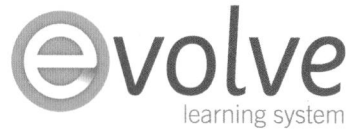
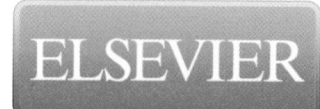
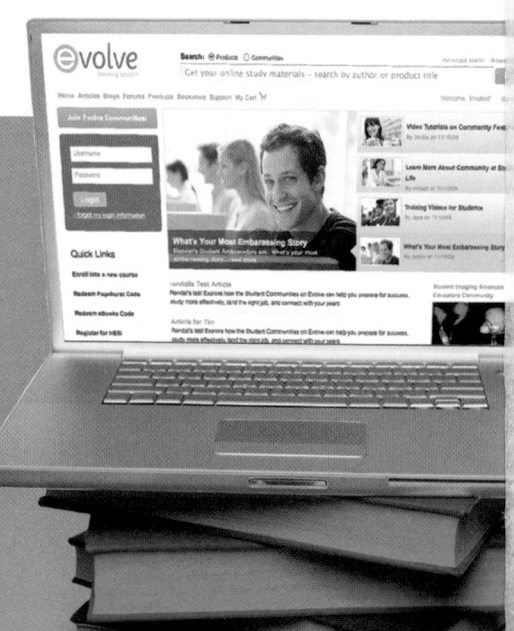

MEDICAL-SURGICAL NURSING IN CANADA

ASSESSMENT AND MANAGEMENT OF CLINICAL PROBLEMS

Third Canadian Edition

MEDICAL-SURGICAL NURSING IN CANADA
ASSESSMENT AND MANAGEMENT OF CLINICAL PROBLEMS

Third Canadian Edition

SHARON L. LEWIS, RN, PhD, FAAN

Research Professor
Castella Distinguished Professor
School of Nursing
University of Texas Health Science Center at San Antonio
San Antonio, Texas

MARGARET McLEAN HEITKEMPER, RN, PhD, FAAN

Professor and Chairperson,
Biobehavioral Nursing and Health Systems
Elizabeth Sterling Soule Endowed Chair in Nursing
School of Nursing;
Adjunct Professor, Division of Gastroenterology
School of Medicine
University of Washington
Seattle, Washington

SHANNON RUFF DIRKSEN, RN, PhD, FAAN

Associate Professor
College of Nursing and Health Innovation
Arizona State University
Phoenix, Arizona

LINDA BUCHER, RN, PhD, CEN, CNE

Mentor/Consultant, Thomas Edison State College
Trenton, New Jersey;
Staff Nurse, Emergency Department
Virtua Memorial Hospital
Mt. Holly, New Jersey;
Professor (Retired), School of Nursing
University of Delaware
Newark, Delaware

IAN M. CAMERA, RN, MSN, ND

Professor
Holyoke Community College
Holyoke, Massachusetts

Canadian Editors

Maureen A. Barry, RN, MScN

Senior Lecturer
Lawrence S. Bloomberg Faculty of Nursing
University of Toronto
Toronto, Ontario

Donna Goodridge, RN, PhD

Professor
College of Nursing
University of Saskatchewan
Saskatoon, Saskatchewan

Sandra Goldsworthy, RN, MSc, CNCC(C), CMSN(C), PhD(c)

Nursing Professor
York University/Georgian/Seneca Collaborative BScN Program
Georgian College
Barrie, Ontario

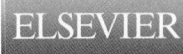

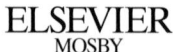

ELSEVIER
MOSBY

Copyright © 2014 Elsevier Canada, a division of Reed Elsevier Canada, Ltd.

Adapted from *Medical-Surgical Nursing: Assessment and Management of Clinical Problems*, 8th edition, by Sharon L. Lewis, Shannon Ruff Dirksen, Margaret McLean Heitkemper, Linda Bucher, and Ian M. Camera.

Copyright © 2011, 2007, 2004, 2000, 1996, 1992, 1987, 1983 by Mosby, Inc., an affiliate of Elsevier Inc.

This adaptation of *Medical-Surgical Nursing*, 8e, by Sharon L. Lewis, RN, PhD, FAAN, Shannon Ruff Dirksen, RN, PhD, Margaret M. Heitkemper, RN, PhD, FAAN, Linda Bucher, RN, PhD, CEN, and Ian M. Camera, RN, MSN, ND is published by arrangement with Elsevier Inc.

Notice

Knowledge and best practice in this field are constantly changing. As new research and expertise broaden our knowledge, changes in practice, treatment, and drug therapy may become necessary.

Practitioners and researchers must always rely on their own experience and knowledge in evaluating and using any information, methods, compounds, or experiments described herein. In using such information or methods they should be mindful of their own safety and the safety of others, including parties for whom they have a professional responsibility.

With respect to any drug or pharmaceutical products identified, readers are advised to check the most current information provided (i) on procedures featured or (ii) by the manufacturer of each product to be administered, to verify the recommended dose or formula, the method and duration of administration, and contraindications. It is the responsibility of practitioners, relying on their own experience and knowledge of their patients, to make diagnoses, to determine dosages and the best treatment for each individual patient, and to take all appropriate safety precautions.

To the fullest extent of the law, neither the Publisher nor the authors, contributors, or editors, assume any liability for any injury and/or damage to persons or property as a matter of products liability, negligence or otherwise, or from any use or operation of any methods, products, instructions, or ideas contained in the material herein.

Library and Archives Canada Cataloguing in Publication

Medical-surgical nursing in Canada : assessment and management of clinical problems / [American editors:] Sharon L. Lewis ... [et al.] ; Canadian editors: Maureen A. Barry, Sandra Goldsworthy, Donna Goodridge. – 3rd Canadian ed.

ISBN 978-1-926648-70-5

1. Nursing–Textbooks. 2. Surgical nursing–Textbooks. I. Lewis, Sharon Mantik II. Barry, Maureen, 1951- III. Goldsworthy, Sandra, 1961- IV. Goodridge, Donna, 1960-

RT41.L49 2013   610.73   C2012-906686-9

ISBN: 978-1-926648-70-5
Ebook ISBN: 978-1-926648-95-8

Vice President, Publishing: Ann Millar
Developmental Editor: Dawn Slawecki
Managing Developmental Editor: Martina van de Velde
Publishing Services Manager: Jeff Patterson
Senior Project Manager: Mary G. Stueck
Copy Editors: Anne Ostroff/Margret Ann McGinnis
Cover Design: Brian Salisbury
Interior Design: Brian Salisbury/Monica Kompter
Typesetting and Assembly: Toppan Best-set Premedia Limited
Printing and Binding: CTPS

Elsevier Canada
905 King Street West, 4th Floor, Toronto, ON, Canada M6K 3G9
Phone: 1-866-896-3331
Fax: 1-866-359-9534

2 3 4 5   18 17 16 15 14

Contents

SECTION 2
Pathophysiological Mechanisms of Disease, *247*

SECTION 5
Problems of Oxygenation: Ventilation, *607*

SECTION 8
Problems of Ingestion, Digestion, Absorption, and Elimination, *1039*

SECTION 9
Problems of Urinary Function, *1265*

SECTION 12
Nursing Care in Specialized Settings, *1921*

About the Authors

Sharon L. Lewis, RN, PhD, FAAN

Sharon Lewis is a Research Professor, School of Nursing and Castella Distinguished Professor at the University of Texas Health Science Center at San Antonio. She received her Bachelor of Science in nursing from the University of Wisconsin–Madison, Master of Science in nursing with a minor in biological sciences from the University of Colorado–Denver, and PhD in immunology from the Department of Pathology at the University of New Mexico School of Medicine. She had a 2-year postdoctoral fellowship from the National Kidney Foundation. Her more than 40 years of teaching experience include inservice education and teaching in associate degree, baccalaureate, master's degree, and doctoral programs in Maryland, Illinois, Wisconsin, New Mexico, and Texas. Favourite teaching areas are pathophysiology, immunology, and family caregiving. She has been actively involved in clinical research for the past 30 years, investigating altered immune responses in various disorders. At this time she is doing research to disseminate her Stress-Busting for Family Caregivers Program. Her free time is spent playing tennis, landscaping, gardening, and being a grandmother.

Shannon Ruff Dirksen, RN, PhD

Shannon Dirksen is Associate Professor at the College of Nursing and Health Innovation, Arizona State University. She received her Bachelor of Science in nursing from Arizona State University, Master of Science in nursing from the University of Arizona, and doctorate in clinical nursing research with a minor in psychology from the University of Arizona. She has over 23 years of undergraduate and graduate teaching experience at the University of Arizona, Edith Cowan University (Western Australia), Intercollegiate College of Nursing–Washington State University, and University of New Mexico. She has been on the faculty at Arizona State University since 1996. She currently teaches nursing theory and research, including evidence-based practice. Her research focuses on individuals diagnosed with cancer. Currently she is investigating symptom clusters in men undergoing treatment for prostate cancer.

Margaret McLean Heitkemper, RN, PhD, FAAN

Margaret Heitkemper is Professor and Chairperson, Department of Biobehavioral Nursing and Health Systems at the School of Nursing, and Adjunct Professor, Division of Gastroenterology at the School of Medicine at the University of Washington. She is also Director of the National Institutes of Health-National Institute for Nursing Research–funded Center for Research on Management of Sleep Disturbances at the University of Washington. In the fall of 2006, Dr. Heitkemper was appointed the Elizabeth Sterling Soule Endowed Chair in Nursing. Dr. Heitkemper received her Bachelor of Science in nursing from Seattle University, a Master of Nursing in gerontologic nursing from the University of Washington, and a doctorate in Physiology and Biophysics from the University of Illinois–Chicago. She has been on faculty at the University of Washington since 1981 and has been the recipient of three School of Nursing Excellence in Teaching awards and the University of Washington Distinguished Teaching Award. In addition, in 2002 she received the Distinguished Nutrition Support Nurse Award from the American Society for Parenteral and Enteral Nutrition (ASPEN), in 2003 the American Gastroenterological Association and Janssen Award for Clinical Research in Gastroenterology, and in 2005 she was the first recipient of the Pfizer and Friends of the National Institutes for Nursing Research Award for Research in Women's Health. She is currently chairperson of the Council for Advancement of Nursing Science (CANS).

Linda Bucher, RN, PhD, CEN

Linda Bucher is currently a Professor at the University of Delaware in Newark, Delaware, and held a joint appointment as a Nursing Research Facilitator at Christiana Care Health System from 2002 to 2010. She received her Bachelor of Science in nursing from Thomas Jefferson University in Philadelphia, her Master of Science in adult health and illness from the University of Pennsylvania in Philadelphia, and her doctorate in nursing from Widener University in Chester, Pennsylvania. Her 34 years of nursing experience has spanned staff and patient education, and teaching in associate, baccalaureate, and graduate nursing programs in New Jersey, Pennsylvania, and Delaware. Her preferred teaching areas include cardiac and emergency nursing and research. She maintains her clinical practice by working per diem as an emergency nurse, is an active member of the American Association of Critical Care Nurses, and enjoys working as a volunteer nurse for Operation Smile. In her free time she enjoys traveling and skiing with her family.

Ian M. Camera, RN, MSN, ND

Ian M. Camera is Professor of Nursing at Holyoke Community College in Holyoke, Massachusetts. He earned his Bachelor of Arts in psychology from Connecticut College, and his Master of Science in Nursing and his Nursing Doctor from the Frances Payne Bolton School of Nursing at Case Western Reserve University, where his research involved applying the human ecology theory of isomorphism to the changing population of homecare agencies in Ohio. He has served as the interim Dean of Health and the Chair of the Associate's Degree in Nursing and Practical Nursing Certificate programs at Holyoke Community College. When not teaching or writing, he enjoys paddling canoes and peddling bicycles with his wife and sons.

Maureen A. Barry, RN, MScN

Maureen A. Barry is a Senior Lecturer and Year 2 Coordinator for the undergraduate program at the Lawrence S. Bloomberg Faculty of Nursing at the University of Toronto. She received her Master of Science in nursing from the University of Toronto. She has been involved in nursing education for over twenty years and has taught in Nova Scotia, Quebec, and Ontario. Her clinical background is adult medicine and surgery and critical care. She has extensive experience in global health, having worked for 5 years in clinics in rural Kenya and Ethiopia and taught medical English in China. More recently, she has done volunteer work during sabbatical time in Zimbabwe and South Africa. She currently teaches medical–surgical nursing and persistent illness and is simulation lead for the Faculty of Nursing undergraduate program. She has won the Teaching Innovation award from the Council of Ontario University Programs in Nursing (COUPN) as well as multiple teaching awards from the University of Toronto. Her primary areas of interest and expertise are clinical teaching, simulation, Web-based learning and technology in nursing education, test theory and development, and global health issues.

Sandra Goldsworthy, RN, MSc, CNCC(C), CMSN(C), PhD(c)

Sandra Goldsworthy is a recognized critical care expert, having worked in this field for more than 20 years. As nursing professor in the Georgian College/York University BScN program, she is also an accomplished practitioner, researcher and author. She received her Bachelor of Science in Nursing at Lakehead University and her Master of Science in Nursing from Queen's University. She is currently pursuing her doctorate in Nursing at the University of British Columbia. She holds a national CNA credential in Critical Care as well as Medical Surgical Nursing. Her research focus is retention of Critical Care nurses. Sandra has conducted and published research involving the use of simulation and PDAs in nursing education. She is currently involved in the delivery of critical care simulation and the mentoring of other educators in this technology. Her recent publications and national and international presentations have concentrated on critical care and technology in nursing. Sandra also sits on the national exam committee for the new CNA Medical/Surgical Nursing Certification exam and is the co-editor of all three editions of *Medical-Surgical Nursing in Canada*. She recently co-authored *Simulation Simplified: A Practical Guide for Nurse Educators* and *Simulation Simplified: Student Laboratory Manual for Critical Care Nursing*.

Donna Goodridge, RN, PhD

Donna Goodridge is a Professor at the College of Nursing at the University of Saskatchewan. She received her Bachelor of Nursing and Master of Nursing from the University of Manitoba, and PhD in interdisciplinary studies from the University of Manitoba. She has over 25 years of clinical experience in various health care settings, including palliative care, home health care, and intensive care. Her research focuses on supportive, community-based care for patients with complex needs, care transitions and health services utilization. Donna is actively involved with several societies affiliated with the Canadian Lung Association and is a director of the Saskatchewan Hospice and Palliative Care Association. She was recently awarded a Queen's Diamond Jubilee Medal by the Governor General for significant achievement in respiratory health. Her border collie ensures her ongoing commitment to running. She and her husband steward an acreage outside of Saskatoon.

Canadian Contributors

Karen Baguley, RN, MScN
Project Manager
Mount Sinai Hospital
Toronto, Ontario

Maureen A. Barry, RN, MScN
Senior Lecturer
Lawrence S. Bloomberg Faculty of Nursing
University of Toronto
Toronto, Ontario

Sandy Bell, RN, BN, MN
Program Director Family Medicine, Rehab/Geriatrics,
    Palliative Care
St. Boniface Hospital
Winnipeg, Manitoba

Veronique M. Boscart, RN, MScN, MEd, PhD
CIHR and Schlegel Chair in Enhancing Care of Seniors
Conestoga College and Schlegel Research Institute of Aging
Kitchener, Ontario

Linda Byrnes, RN, BScN, MA, CIEHP
Faculty, BSN Program
Vancouver Island University
Nanaimo, British Columbia

Rosemary Cashman, MA, MSc(A), NP(A)
Nurse Practitioner, BC Cancer Agency;
Adjunct Professor
University of British Columbia
Faculty of Nursing
Vancouver, British Columbia

Erica Cambly, RN, MN
Lecturer
Lawrence S. Bloomberg Faculty of Nursing
University of Toronto
Toronto, Ontario

Renée Chauvin, RN, BA, BScN, MEd, CNCC
Nurse Manager, ICU
Queensway Carleton Hospital
Ottawa, Ontario

Susan Chernenko, RN(EC), MN, NP
Practice Leader/Program Development
Toronto Lung Transplant Program;
Adjunct Lecturer
Lawrence S. Bloomberg Faculty of Nursing
University of Toronto
Toronto, Ontario

Beth Clarke, RN, MSc(A), MBA, CWOCN
Advanced Practice Nurse (Wound Management)
Bridgepoint Health
Toronto, Ontario

Renee Clarke, RN, BSN, MN
Clinical Instructor/Faculty Resource Person
College of Nursing
University of Saskatchewan
Saskatoon, Saskatchewan

Debra Clendinneng, RN, BScN, MEd, PhD, CPN(C)
Professor of Nursing
Coordinator, Postgraduate Nursing Programs
Algonquin College
Ottawa, Ontario

Shelley L. Cobbett, RN, BN, GnT, MN, EdD
Adjunct Assistant Professor
School of Nursing (Yarmouth Campus)
Dalhousie University
Halifax, Nova Scotia

Daphne Connolly, RN, MN
Clinical Associate
School of Nursing
Saint Francis Xavier University
Antigonish, Nova Scotia

Mary Ann Fegan, RN, BNSc, MN
Senior Lecturer
Lawrence S. Bloomberg Faculty of Nursing
University of Toronto
Toronto, Ontario

Julie H. Fraser, RN, BScN, IIWCC, MN
Clinical Nurse Specialist, Home Health
Fraser Health
Surrey, British Columbia

Sandra Goldsworthy, RN, MSc, CNCC(C), CMSN(C), PhD(c)
Nursing Professor
York University/Georgian/Seneca Collaborative BScN Program
Georgian College
Barrie, Ontario

Donna Goodridge, RN, PhD
Professor
College of Nursing
University of Saskatchewan
Saskatoon, Saskatchewan

Leslie Graham, RN, MN, CNCC
Professor, Nursing
Critical Care eLearning
BScN Collaborative Nursing Program
Durham College
Oshawa, Ontario

Jackie Hartigan-Rogers, RN, MN
Adjunct Assistant Professor
School of Nursing (Yarmouth campus)
Dalhousie University
Halifax, Nova Scotia

Shelly W. Hutchinson, RN, BSN, MN, CRE
COPD Nurse Clinician
LiveWell COPD Program
Saskatoon Health Region
Saskatoon, Saskatchewan

Lynn Jansen, RN, PhD
Acting Associate Dean College of Nursing
Southern Saskatchewan Campus and International Student
    Affairs
University of Saskatchewan
Regina, Saskatchewan

Sarah L. Johnston, RN, MN
Lecturer
Lawrence S. Bloomberg Faculty of Nursing
University of Toronto
Toronto, Ontario

Annemarie F. Kaan, RN, MCN, CCN(C)
Clinical Nurse Specialist—Acute and Chronic Heart Failure
Adjunct Professor
University of British Columbia School of Nursing
St Paul's Hospital
Vancouver, British Columbia

Bridgette Lord, RN, MN, NP–Adult
Clinical Lead, Gattuso Rapid Diagnostic Centre
Princess Margaret Cancer Centre
Toronto, Ontario

J. Jacque E. Lovely, RN, MScN
Program Manager
Ambulatory Care
Alberta Health Services
Edmonton, Alberta

Marian Luctkar-Flude, RN, BScN, MScN
Lecturer
School of Nursing
Queen's University
Kingston, Ontario

Jennifer Macauley, RN, MN
Lecturer—Innovation in Nursing Education
Lawrence S. Bloomberg Faculty of Nursing
University of Toronto
Toronto, Ontario

Joyce Mammel, RN, MN
Content Coordinator
www.MyHealth.Alberta.ca
Calgary, Alberta

Jane McCall, MSN, RN
Nurse Educator, HIV Program
St. Paul's Hospital, Providence Health Care
Vancouver, British Columbia

Christine McCleary, RD, CDE
Registered Dietitian
Lakeridge Health Diabetes Program
Whitby, Ontario

Lynn McCleary, RN, PhD
Associate Professor
Department of Nursing, Faculty of Applied Health Sciences
Brock University
St. Catharines, Ontario

Michael McGillion, RN, PhD
Assistant Professor
Lawrence S. Bloomberg Faculty of Nursing
University of Toronto
Toronto, Ontario

Kelly A. Metcalfe, RN, PhD
Associate Professor
Lawrence S. Bloomberg Faculty of Nursing
University of Toronto
Toronto, Ontario

Barbara L. Mildon, RN, PhD, CHE, CCHN(C)
VP, Professional Practice and Research, and Chief Nurse
    Executive
Ontario Shores Centre for Mental Health Sciences
Whitby, Ontario

Andrea Miller, MHSc, RD
Registered Dietitian
Faculty of Health Sciences
University of Ontario Institute of Technology
Oshawa, Ontario

Tess Montada-Atin, RN(EC), MN, CDE, CNeph(C)
Nurse Practitioner–Adult Diabetes Comprehensive Program
St. Michaels Hospital;
Adjunct Lecturer
Lawrence S. Bloomberg Faculty of Nursing
University of Toronto
Toronto, Ontario

Katarzyna (Kat) Moyer, RN, MSN CMSN(C)
Faculty, Nursing Division
Nursing Education Program of Saskatchewan (NEPS);
Adjunct Professor, University of Regina
Saskatchewan Collaborative Bachelor of Science in Nursing
    Program
Regina, Saskatchewan

Sheila O'Keefe-McCarthy, RN, BScN, MN, CCCN(C), PhD(c)
Lecturer
Lawrence S. Bloomberg Faculty of Nursing
University of Toronto
Toronto, Ontario

Verna C. Pangman, RN, MEd, MN
Senior Instructor
Faculty of Nursing
University of Manitoba
Winnipeg, Manitoba

Janet A. Piper, RN, MScN
Simulation Lab Specialist
School of Health, Wellness and Continuing Education
Sault College of Applied Arts and Technology
Sault Ste. Marie, Ontario

Debbie Rickeard, RN, BA, BScN, MSN, CCRN, CCN(C)
Experiential Learning Specialist
Faculty of Nursing
University of Windsor
Windsor, Ontario

Sheila Rizza, RN(EC), MN NP-Adult, CNCC(C), CCN(C)
Nurse Practitioner, Stroke Prevention Clinic
Humber River Hospital
Toronto, Ontario

Cheryl A. Sams, RN, MSN
Professor, School of Health Sciences
Seneca College of Applied Arts and Technology
Toronto, Ontario

Otto Sanchez, MD, MSc, PhD
Professor
Faculty of Health Sciences
University of Ontario Institute of Technology
Oshawa, Ontario

Angela Sarro, RN(EC), MN, CNN(c)
Nurse Practitioner-Adult
Spine Program
Krembil Neuroscience Centre
Toronto Western Hospital
Toronto, Ontario

Rani H. Srivastava, RN, PhD
Chief of Nursing and Professional Practice
Centre for Addiction and Mental Health;
Assistant Professor
Lawrence Bloomberg Faculty of Nursing
Associate Member, School of Graduate Studies
University of Toronto;
Adjunct Professor
York University School of Nursing
Toronto, Ontario

Beth Swart, RN, MES
Professor
Daphne Cockwell School of Nursing
Ryerson University
Toronto, Ontario

Holly Symonds-Brown, RN, MSN, CPMHN
Faculty Instructor
Faculty of Health and Community Studies, BN Program
Grant MacEwan University
Edmonton, Alberta

Lynne Thibeault, NP-PHC, MEd, DNP
BScN and NP Professor
Confederation College/Lakehead University Emergency Nurse
Thunder Bay Regional Hospital NP-PHC—Norwest Community
    Health Centres
Thunder Bay, Ontario

Christina Vaillancourt, MHSc, RD, CDE
Patient Care Specialist Diabetes and Nephrology
Lakeridge Health
Oshawa, Ontario

Françoise Verville, RN, MN
Adjunct Professor
Saskatchewan Collaborative BScN
Faculty of Nursing
University of Regina SIAST Wascana Campus
Regina, Saskatchewan

Ellen Vogel, PhD, RD, FDC
Dean and Associate Professor
Faculty of Health Sciences
University of Ontario Institute of Technology
Oshawa, Ontario

Judy Watt-Watson, RN, MSc, PhD
Professor Emerita
Lawrence S. Bloomberg Faculty of Nursing
University of Toronto
Toronto, Ontario

Marsha Wood, BN, RN, MN, CNeph(C)
Nurse Practitioner Nephrology
Capital District Health Authority
Halifax, Nova Scotia

Colina Yim, RN(EC), MN
Nurse Practitioner, Hepatology
Toronto Western Hospital Liver Centre
Toronto, Ontario

Rosanra Yoon, NP, MN, CPMHN(C)
Advanced Practice Nurse
Addiction Program
Centre for Addiction and Mental Health;
Adjunct Lecturer
Lawrence S. Bloomberg Faculty of Nursing
University of Toronto
Toronto, Ontario

Patricia G. Yuzik, RN(NP), MN, CON(C)
Lecturer, University of Saskatchewan
Primary Care Nurse Practitioner, Saskatoon Health Region
Saskatoon, Saskatchewan

Contributors to the U.S. 8th Edition

Richard B. Arbour, RN, MSN, CCRN, CNRN, CCNS, FAAN
Critical Care Clinical Nurse Specialist
Albert Einstein Medical Center
Philadelphia, Pennsylvania

Margaret Wooding Baker, RN, PhD, CNL
Associate Professor
University of Washington School of Nursing
Seattle, Washington

Barbara Bartz, RN, MN, CCRN
Nursing Instructor
Yakima Valley Community College
Yakima, Washington

Audrey J. Bopp, RN, MSN, CNS
Assistant Director, School of Nursing
University of Northern Colorado
Greeley, Colorado

Lynne Dantino Bouffard, RN, DNP, FNP, MSN
Director of Cardiovascular Programs
Humana Healthcare
Louisville, Kentucky

Elisabeth G. Bradley, RN, MS, ACNS-BC, CCRN, CCNS
Clinical Leader Cardiovascular Prevention Program
Christiana Care Health System
Newark, Delaware

Lucy Bradley-Springer, RN, PhD, ACRN, FAAN
Associate Professor
University of Colorado School of Medicine
Mountain Plains AIDS Education and Training Center
Denver, Colorado

Linda Bucher, RN, PhD, CEN, CNE
Professor, School of Nursing
College of Health Sciences
University of Delaware
Newark, Delaware;
Staff Nurse, Emergency Department
Virtua Memorial Hospital
Mt. Holly, New Jersey

Jormain Cady, DNP, ARNP, AOCN
Nurse Practitioner
Virginia Mason Medical Center
Department of Radiation Oncology
Seattle, Washington

Ian M. Camera, RN, MSN, ND
Professor
Holyoke Community College
Holyoke, Massachusetts

Deborah Castellucci, RN, MPA, CCRN-CMC
Clinical Nurse Specialist
Thomas Jefferson University Hospital
Philadelphia, Pennsylvania

Olivia Catolico, RN, PhD
Associate Professor, Department of Nursing
Dominican University of California
San Rafael, California

Anne Croghan, MN, ARNP
Nurse Practitioner
Seattle Gastroenterology Associates
Seattle, Washington

Judi Daniels, PhD, ARNP
Course Coordinator
Frontier School of Midwifery and Family Nursing
Richmond, Kentucky

Rose Ann DiMaria-Ghalili, RN, PhD
Associate Professor
College of Nursing and Health Professions
Drexel University
Philadelphia, Pennsylvania

Shannon Ruff Dirksen, RN, PhD, FAAN
Associate Professor
College of Nursing and Health Innovation
Arizona State University
Phoenix, Arizona

Angela J. DiSabatino, RN, MS
Manager, Cardiovascular Clinical Trials
Christiana Care Health System
Newark, Delaware

Laura Dulski, MSN, CNE, RNC-HROB
Assistant Professor
West Suburban College of Nursing
Oak Park, Illinois

Mary Ersek, RN, PhD, FAAN
Associate Professor
University of Pennsylvania
Philadelphia, Pennsylvania

JoAnn Grove, RN, EIS
RN EIS Case Manager
Pueblo Community Health Center
Pueblo, Colorado

Peggi Guenter, RN, PhD, CNSN
Managing Editor for Special Projects
American Society for Parenteral and Enteral Nutrition
Silver Spring, Maryland

Debra Hagler, RN, PhD, ACNS-BC, CNE, ANEF
Clinical Professor
College of Nursing and Health Innovation
Arizona State University
Phoenix, Arizona

Deborah Hamolsky, RN, MS, AOCNS
Nurse Clinician, Educator
Helen Diller Family Cancer Center
Carol Franc Buck Breast Care Center
University of California–San Francisco
San Francisco, California

Carol M. Headley, RN, DNSc, CNN
Dialysis Case Manager
Veterans Affairs Medical Center
Memphis, Tennessee

Margaret McLean Heitkemper, RN, PhD, FAAN
Professor and Chairperson, Biobehavioral Nursing and
    Health Systems
Elizabeth Sterling Soule Endowed Chair in Nursing
School of Nursing;
Adjunct Professor, Division of Gastroenterology
School of Medicine
University of Washington
Seattle, Washington

Teresa E. Hills, RN, MSN, ACNP-BC, CNRN
Neurosurgery/Neurotrauma Critical Care Nurse Practitioner
Christiana Care Health System
Newark, Delaware

Christine R. Hoch, RN, MSN
Nursing Instructor
Delaware Technical and Community College
Newark, Delaware

Joyce A. Jackowski, RN, MS, FNP-BC, AOCNP
Nurse Practitioner
Fairfax Northern Virginia Hematology and Oncology
Arlington, Virginia

Vicki Y. Johnson, RN, PhD, CUCNS
Assistant Professor
University of Alabama School of Nursing at Birmingham
Birmingham, Alabama

Jane Steinman Kaufman, RN, MS, ANP-BC
Clinical Associate Professor
University of North Carolina–Chapel Hill
School of Nursing
Chapel Hill, North Carolina

Judy A. Knighton, RegN, MScN
Clinical Nurse Specialist–Burns
Ross Tilley Burn Centre
Sunnybrook Health Sciences Centre
Toronto, Ontario, Canada

Catherine N. Kotecki, RN, PhD, APN
Associate Dean
Thomas Edison State College
Trenton, New Jersey

Nancy Kupper, RN, MSN
Associate Professor
Tarrant County College
Fort Worth, Texas

Jeffrey Kwong, RN, DNP, MPH, ANP-BC, ACRN
Instructor
University of Colorado School of Medicine
Division of Infectious Diseases
Clinical Education Coordinator
Mountain Plains AIDS Education and Training Center
Denver, Colorado

Carol A. Landis, RN, DNSc, FAAN
Professor and Vice Chair for Research
Department of Biobehavioral Nursing and Health Systems
University of Washington
Seattle, Washington

Cheryl A. Lehman, RN, PhD, CRRN-A, RN-BC, CNS
Associate Professor, Clinical Acute Nursing Department
University of Texas Health Science Center at San Antonio
San Antonio, Texas

Janet Lenart, RN, MN, MPH
Senior Lecturer
School of Nursing, University of Washington
Seattle, Washington

Sharon L. Lewis, RN, PhD, FAAN
Research Professor
Castella Distinguished Professor
School of Nursing
University of Texas Health Science Center at San Antonio
San Antonio, Texas

Kathleen Lucke, RN, PhD
Associate Dean for Academic Affairs
Research Associate Professor
School of Nursing
University at Buffalo
Buffalo, New York

Nancy J. MacMullen, PhD, RNC-HROB, APN/CNS, CNE
Interim Chairperson
Governors State University
University Park, Illinois

Margaret (Peggy) J. Malone, RN, MN, CCRN
Clinical Nurse Specialist, Critical Care
St. John Medical Center
Longview, Washington

Brenda Michel, RN, EdD, CDE
Professor of Nursing
Lincoln Land Community College
Diabetes Educator
Southern Illinois University School of Medicine
Springfield, Illinois

De Ann Fisher Mitchell, RN, PhD
Professor of Nursing
Tarrant County College
Fort Worth, Texas

Teri A. Murray, RN, PhD
Robert Wood Johnson Executive Nurse Fellow
Dean, School of Nursing
Saint Louis University
St. Louis, Missouri

Sherry Neely, RN, MSN, CRNP
Associate Professor
Butler County Community College
Butler, Pennsylvania

Janice A. Neil, RN, PhD
Associate Professor
East Carolina University
College of Nursing
Greenville, North Carolina

Casey Norris, RN, MSN, APRN-BC
Pulmonary Clinical Nurse Specialist
East Tennessee Children's Hospital
Knoxville, Tennessee

Patricia Graber O'Brien, RN, MA, MSN
Former Instructor, College of Nursing
University of New Mexico;
Clinical Research Coordinator
Lovelace Scientific Resources
Albuquerque, New Mexico

DaiWai M. Olson, RN, PhD, CCRN
Assistant Professor of Medicine/Neurology
Duke University Medical Center
Durham, North Carolina

Rosemary C. Polomano, RN, PhD, FAAN
Associate Professor of Pain Practice–Clinician Educator
University of Pennsylvania
School of Nursing
Philadelphia, Pennsylvania

Cory Shaw Retherford, MOM, LAc
Traditional Chinese Medicine Practitioner
Private Practice;
Research Assistant
School of Nursing
University of Texas Health Science Center at San Antonio
San Antonio, Texas

Kathleen Rich, RN, PhD, CCNS, CCRN-CSC, CNN
Cardiovascular Clinical Specialist
La Porte Regional Health System
La Porte, Indiana

Dottie Roberts, RN, EdD(C), MSN, MACI, CMSRN, ONSC-C
Nursing Instructor
South University
Columbia, South Carolina

Sandra Irene Rome, RN, MN, AOCN
Hematology/Oncology Clinical Nurse Specialist
Cedars-Sinai Medical Center
Los Angeles, California

Kathleen Rourke, RN, BSN, ANP, ONP-C
Orthopedic Nurse Practitioner
Harvard Vanguard Medical Associates
West Roxbury, Massachusetts

Marilee Schmelzer, RN, PhD
Associate Professor
The University of Texas at Arlington College of Nursing
Arlington, Texas

Maureen A. Seckel, RN, APN, MSN, ACNS, BC, CCNS, CCRN
Clinical Nurse Specialist Medical Pulmonary Critical Care
Christiana Care Health System
Newark, Delaware

Virginia (Jennie) Shaw, RN, MSN
Associate Professor
University of Texas Health Science Center School of Nursing
San Antonio, Texas

Maura M. Sheridan, RN, BSN, CRNA
Clinical Site Coordinator
Roxanna Canon Arsht Ambulatory Surgery
Christiana Care Health Services
Wilmington, Delaware

Anita Shoup, RN, MSN, CNOR
Clinical Nurse Specialist
Swedish Medical Center
Seattle, Washington

Barbara Sinni-McKeehen, MSN, ARNP, DNC
Dermatology Nurse Practitioner
Bay Pines VA Health Care Center
Bay Pines, Florida

Sarah C. Smith, RN, MA, CRNO, COA
Nurse Manager
University of Iowa Health Care
Department of Nursing, Eye Clinic
Iowa City, Iowa

Colleen R. Walsh, RN, MSN, ONC, CS, ACNP-BC
Faculty, Graduate Nursing
University of Southern Indiana
College of Nursing and Health Professions
Evansville, Indiana

Deirdre D. Wipke-Tevis, RN, PhD
Associate Professor, Coordinator of CNS Area of Study
Sinclair School of Nursing
University of Missouri
Columbia, Missouri

Juvann M. Wolff, RN, ARNP, MN, FNP
Senior Lecturer, Clinical Faculty
University of Washington
School of Nursing
Lake Forest Park, Washington

Russell G. Zaiontz, RN, MSN
Assistant Professor of Nursing
San Antonio College, Department of Nursing Education
San Antonio, Texas

Meg Zomorodi, RN, PhD
Clinical Assistant Professor
University of North Carolina–Chapel Hill
School of Nursing
Chapel Hill, North Carolina

Canadian Reviewers

Connie Barbour, RN, BHScN, MHScN
Professor
Collaborative BScN Program
George Brown College
Toronto, Ontario

Susan Bedrossian, RN, BScN
Nursing Instructor
Faculty of Nursing
John Abbott College
Montreal, Quebec

Ute Beffert, RN, BScN, MEd
Instructor
Nursing Department
John Abbott College
Montreal, Quebec

Debbie Brennick, RN, BScN, MN
Assistant Professor
Department of Nursing
Cape Breton University
Sydney, Nova Scotia

Natasha Bursey, RN, BN
Health Programs Instructor
Aurora College/University of Victoria BSN Program
Inuvik, Northwest Territories

Sharon Carroll, RN, BN, MN
Instructor of Nursing
Medicine Hat College
Medicine Hat, Alberta

Julie Duff Cloutier, RN, BScN, MSc
Assistant Professor
School of Nursing
Laurentian University
Sudbury, Ontario

Corinne Crockett, RN, BScN, MHSc(N)
Instructor
School of Nursing
UBC Okanagan
Kelowna, British Columbia

Dianne Dal Bello, RN, BScN, MScN, ACNP
Professor
BScN Program, McMaster-Mohawk-Conestoga Collaborative
Conestoga College
Kitchener, Ontario

Sheila Epp, RN, BSN, MN
Associate Director
Senior Instructor
School of Nursing
Faculty of Health and Social Development
UBC Okanagan
Kelowna, British Columbia

Barb Fenwick, RN, BScN, MN
Nurse Educator
BSN Program
College of the Rockies
Cranbrook, British Columbia

Pasquale Fiore, RN, BScN, MSc Health Adm, Cert. Ed.
Instructor
Camosun College
Victoria, British Columbia

Laurie Freeman-Gibb, MSN, PhD(c), ANP-BC
Lecturer
Faculty of Nursing
University of Windsor
Windsor, Ontario

Kate Hardie, RN, BScN, MScN, EdD
Senior Lecturer
Lawrence S. Bloomberg Faculty of Nursing
University of Toronto
Toronto, Ontario

Heather G. Hepworth, BSc, RN, MSN/Ed
BSN Program Coordinator, Nurse Educator
College of the Rockies
Cranbrook, British Columbia

Cathryn Jackson, MSN, RN
Instructor
School of Nursing
University of British Columbia
Vancouver, British Columbia

Elsa Jensen, RN, MN
Associate Professor
Saint Francis Xavier University
School of Nursing
Antigonish, Nova Scotia

Sarah L. Johnston, RN, MN
Lecturer
Lawrence S. Bloomberg Faculty of Nursing
University of Toronto
Toronto, Ontario

Joanne Jones, RN, BSN, MSN
Senior Lecturer
School of Nursing
Thompson Rivers University
Kamloops, British Columbia

Michelle Lalonde, RN, MN, PhD(c)
Lecturer
Undergraduate Clinical Coordinator
Lawrence S. Bloomberg Faculty of Nursing
University of Toronto
Toronto, Ontario

Brenda Lane, RN, BScN, DipAdEd, MN, CMSN(c)
University-College Professor
Faculty of Health and Human Services
Vancouver Island University
Nanaimo, British Columbia

Marian Luctkar-Flude, RN, BScN, MScN
Lecturer
School of Nursing
Queen's University
Kingston, Ontario

Jennifer Macauley, RN, MN
Lecturer—Innovation in Nursing Education
Lawrence S. Bloomberg Faculty of Nursing
University of Toronto
Toronto, Ontario

Andrea Miller, RN, BScN, MA
Professor
McMaster-Mohawk-Conestoga BScN Program
Conestoga College
Kitchener, Ontario

Eva Peisachovich, RN, MScN
Sessional Lecturer
School of Nursing
York University
Toronto, Ontario

Lisa Peldjak, RN, BScN
Nursing Faculty
CEGEP Heritage College
Gatineau, Quebec

Jackie Santiago, RN, MEd
Nursing Instructor
Red River College
Winnipeg, Manitoba

Karen Silvester, RN, BSN, MN
Nursing Faculty
North Island College
Vancouver Island, British Columbia

Beth Swart, RN, MES
Professor
Daphne Cockwell School of Nursing
Ryerson University
Toronto, Ontario

Ruth Swart, BSc, BN, RB, MHS
Instructor
Faculty of Nursing
University of Calgary
Calgary, Alberta

Rosemary Wilson, RN(EC), HBScN, MN/NP, PhD
Assistant Professor
School of Nursing
Queen's University
Kingston, Ontario

Jim Wohlgemuth, RN, MN, TCN-B
Instructor
Department of Health Studies and Nursing Education
Grande Prairie Regional College
Grande Prairie, Alberta

Karla Wolsky, RN, BN, MN
NESA BN Programs Chair
School of Health Sciences
Lethbridge College
Lethbridge, Alberta

Pat Woods, MSN, RN
International Coordinator
Langara College School of Nursing
Vancouver, British Columbia

To the Profession of Nursing and to the Important People in Our Lives

My husband Peter, our sons and their families,
Marc and Heidi, Aaron and Roberta, Michael, and Jeremy and Monica,
and our grandchildren Malia, Halle, Aidan, Cian, and Layla
—*Sharon L. Lewis*

My husband John, our children Marshall and Meaghan, my mother Marilyn,
and my siblings Michael, Barbara, and Brian
—*Shannon Ruff Dirksen*

My husband David, our daughters Elizabeth and Ellen,
and our grandson Jaxon James
—*Margaret McLean Heitkemper*

My mother Charlotte, my siblings Millie, Janet, Barb, Rich, and Joanne, and
my very good friend and colleague Catherine
—*Linda Bucher*

My wife Sam, my children Jonas and Julian, and my parents, who have all
taken such good care of each other while I have been writing
—*Ian M. Camera*

My students past, present, and future
—*Maureen A. Barry*

To my husband and three sons for their constant support—I couldn't do it without you!
And, to all of the BScN students (future nurses) and Critical Care RNs I have had the privilege
of teaching and mentoring over the years
—*Sandra Goldsworthy*

To my husband Jim, for always being there and making me laugh
—*Donna Goodridge*

Preface

The Third Edition of *Medical-Surgical Nursing in Canada: Assessment and Management of Clinical Problems* has been thoroughly revised for the Canadian student and incorporates the most current medical–surgical nursing information presented in an attractive, easy-to-use format. More than just a textbook, this is a comprehensive resource set in the Canadian context, containing essential information that nursing students need to prepare for lectures, classroom activities, examinations, clinical assignments, and comprehensive care of patients. In addition to the readable writing style and full-colour illustrations, the text includes many special features to help students learn the medical–surgical nursing content, such as sections that highlight the determinants of health, patient and caregiver teaching, age-related considerations, collaborative care, nutrition, home care, evidence-informed practice, nursing research, patient safety, and much more.

Many aspects of the U.S. Eighth Edition have been incorporated into this edition. Several new features have been added to address some of the rapid changes in practice. Many chapters include new or improved diagrams and photos. Relevant new content from the U.S. Eighth Edition has also been incorporated, ensuring a continuous thread of evidence-informed practice throughout the text. The content has been updated using the most recent important research and newest practice guidelines by Canadian contributors selected for their acknowledged excellence in specific content areas. Specialists in the subject area have reviewed each chapter to ensure accuracy, and the editors have undertaken final rewriting and editing to achieve internal consistency. In other words, all efforts have been made to build on the strengths of the previous Canadian editions and the U.S. Eighth Edition to create an even more effective new Canadian text.

Organization

The content of this book is organized in two major divisions. The first division, Section 1 (Chapters 1 through 13), discusses significant concepts related to adult patients. The second division, Sections 2 through 12 (Chapters 14 through 72), presents nursing assessment and nursing management of medical–surgical problems.

The various body systems are grouped in such a way as to reflect their interrelated functions. Each section is organized around two central themes: assessment and management. Each chapter that deals with the assessment of a body system includes a discussion of the following:

1. A brief review of anatomy and physiology, focusing on background that informs the rationale underlying nursing care
2. Health history and noninvasive physical assessment skills to expand the evidence base on which decisions are made
3. Common diagnostic studies, expected results, and related nursing responsibilities to provide easily accessible information

Chapters on management focus on the pathophysiology, clinical manifestations, laboratory and diagnostic study results, collaborative care, and nursing management of various diseases and disorders. Within each management chapter, the material is organized into assessment, nursing diagnoses, planning, imple-

mentation, and evaluation sections. To emphasize the importance of patient care in various clinical settings, nursing implementation of all major health problems is organized by the following levels of care:

1. Health promotion
2. Acute intervention
3. Ambulatory and home care

Classic Features

- **Canadian context.** Once again, we are pleased to offer you a book that reflects the wide range of expertise of nurses from across Canada. In an effort to better reflect the nursing environments across the country, all chapters have been revised with enhanced Canadian research and statistics. SI units and metric measurements are used throughout the text, and the updated APA format, including digital object identifiers (DOIs), is used for the references.
- **Patient and caregiver teaching** is an ongoing theme throughout the text and is covered by a separate chapter (Chapter 4), as well as 83 **Patient & Caregiver Teaching Guide boxes** throughout the text and 8 more on the Evolve Web site.
- **Community-based nursing and home care** are also emphasized in this edition. Chapter 6 contains the primary discussion, as well as the special Ambulatory and Home Care sections in Nursing Implementation.
- **Collaborative care** is highlighted in special Collaborative Care sections in each of the management chapters and in 89 Collaborative Care tables throughout the text.
- **Culturally Competent Care** is discussed in selected Nursing Management sections highlighting expanded cultural and ethnic content as it relates to specific diseases and disorders.
- **Older Adults** are covered in detail in Chapter 7, and are discussed throughout the text under the headings "Age-Related Considerations" and also in **Age-Related Differences in Assessment tables**.
- **Nutrition** is highlighted throughout the book. Chapter 42 presents **Nutritional Problems,** and **Nutritional Therapy tables** throughout summarize nutritional interventions and promote healthy lifestyles for patients with various health problems.
- **Nursing management** is presented in a consistent and comprehensive format, which includes Health Promotion, Acute Intervention, and Ambulatory and Home Care. In addition, 62 **Nursing Care Plans** appear in the management chapters and on the Evolve Web site.
- **Complementary and alternative therapies** (CATs) are discussed in a separate chapter (Chapter 12) that addresses timely issues in today's health care settings related to these therapies. **Complementary and Alternative Therapies boxes** located in the chapters on disorders expand on the information presented in Chapter 12 and summarize what nurses need to know about such therapies as herbal remedies, acupuncture, and biofeedback.
- **Health research** encourages application of new knowledge into clinical practice. **Nursing Research** and **Interdisciplinary**

Research boxes appear throughout the text, highlighting current research carried out by nurses or by interdisciplinary teams led by or including nurses.

- **Genetics in Clinical Practice boxes** highlight genetic screening and testing, as well as the clinical implications of key genetic disorders that affect adults, as rapid advances in the field of genetics continue to change the way nurses practise.
- **Ethical Dilemmas boxes** promote critical thinking with regard to timely and sensitive issues that nursing students deal with in clinical practice—such as informed consent, treatment decision making, advance directives, and confidentiality.
- **Emergency Management tables** outline the emergency treatment of health problems that are most likely to require rapid intervention.
- **Common Assessment Abnormalities tables** in the assessment chapters alert the nursing student to abnormalities frequently encountered in practice, as well as their possible etiologies.
- **Nursing Assessment tables** summarize the key subjective and objective data related to common diseases.
- **Health History tables** in assessment chapters present key questions related to a specific disease or disorder that will be asked in patient interviews.
- **Nursing Assessment tables** summarize key subjective and objective data related to common diseases, with a sharper focus on issues most relevant to the body system under review. This focus provides for more rapid identification of salient assessment parameters and more effective use of student time.
- **Evidence-Informed Practice boxes** have been enhanced to include updated material that provides synthesis of evidence for application to clinical practice. Many of the studies chosen are systematic reviews of randomized controlled trials from the Cochrane Database. All clinical questions are presented in the PICO format (described in Chapter 1).
- **Determinants of Health boxes** focus on the determinants of health as outlined by Health Canada and the Public Health Agency of Canada as they affect a particular disorder. The determinants are introduced and discussed in detail in Chapter 2 and carried throughout the text in Determinants of Health boxes.
- **Student-friendly pedagogy:**
  - The **Learning Objectives** at the beginning of each chapter help students identify the key content for a specific body system or disorder.
  - The **Key Terms** glossary provides a list of the chapter's most important terms and their definitions. The glossary is also included on the Evolve Web site.
  - The **Electronic Resources** section of the chapter opener draws the students' attention to the supplemental content and exercises provided on the Evolve Web site, making it easier than ever for students to integrate the textbook content with media supplements such as animations, video and audio clips, interactive case studies, and much more.
  - The **Clinical Decision-Making Exercises** appearing at the end of the management chapters include **Case Studies** with discussion questions related to clinical application. The case studies feature photos that "bring patients to life."
  - The **Review Questions** are matched to the learning objectives and thus help students learn the important points in the chapter. Answers are provided on the same page, making the Review Questions a convenient self-study tool.
  - The **Resources** at the end of each chapter contain Weblinks to nursing and health care organizations and tools that provide patient teaching and information on diseases and disorders.

New Features

In addition to the classic strengths of this text, there are several new exciting features:

- *New* chapter—**Chapter 9: Sleep and Sleep Disorders** expands on this key topic that impacts multiple disorders and body systems as well as nearly every aspect of daily functioning.
- *New* Focused Assessment Boxes in all assessment chapters provide brief checklists that help students do a more practical "assessment on the run" or bedside approach to assessment.
- *New* Safety Alert boxes highlight important safety issues.
- *New* Pathophysiology Maps outline complex concepts related to diseases in flowchart format, making them easier to understand.
- *New* Assessment Case Studies available on the Evolve Web site for every assessment chapter help students integrate assessment findings.
- **Patient and caregiver teaching is emphasized as a theme throughout the text.** Chapter 4, Patient and Caregiver Teaching, now emphasizes the increasing importance and prevalence of patient management of chronic illness and conditions, and the role of the caregiver in patient care. Chapter 6, Community-Based Nursing and Home Care, contains a special section on family caregivers. The former Patient and Family Teaching Guides have been renamed Patient & Caregiver Teaching Guides to include non-family caregivers as well.
- **Clinical Decision-Making Exercises** with a Case Study at the end of each management chapter now include a focus on prioritization of patient care, and incorporate multiple disorders so that students learn how to prioritize care and manage patients in the clinical setting.
- *Revised* **Chapter 1: Introduction to Medical-Surgical Nursing Practice in Canada** situates nursing practice within the unique societal contexts that continue to shape the profession of nursing in Canada. Patient-centred care, interprofessional practice and information-communication technologies are forces that have an impact on and are affected by nurses.
- *Revised* **Chapter 2: Cultural Competence and Health Equity in Nursing Care** clearly distinguishes the related concepts of cultural awareness, sensitivity, and competence to provide a strong foundation to practise within the ever-growing cultural diversity that characterizes Canada. Culture is examined as a determinant of health. Health equity is explored in-depth as a concept. New in this edition is a discussion of the relationships between cultural competence, patient safety, and patient- and family-centred care.
- **Chapter 3, Health History and Physical Examination**, has been revised with an emphasis on three types of assessment: emergency, comprehensive, and focused.
- *Revised* **Chapter 5: Chronic Illness.** Nurses are increasingly called on to be active and engaged partners in assisting patients with chronic conditions to live well, which has become Canada's most pressing health care challenge. With a focus on illness as a human experience of symptoms and suffering, this chapter places chronic illness within the larger context of Canadian society. Chapter 5 highlights the determinants of health in relation to chronic illness and includes a discussion of the epidemiology of chronic illness, the physical and psychosocial burden of living with chronic illness, and shared decision-making. "Best buys" for preventing chronic illness as outlined by the World Health Organization are described. The Chronic Care Model, widely used across Canada, forms the cornerstone of this chapter.

- *Revised* **Chapter 46: Nursing Management: Liver, Pancreas, and Biliary Tract Problems.** The revised chapter now includes a new focus on prevention, updated classifications of jaundice, a new section comparing characteristics of hepatitis viruses, a grading scale for hepatic encephalopathy, and tables to assist with interpretation of serological profiles, as well as the most current diagnostic techniques and treatments for liver, pancreas, and biliary tract problems used in Canada. Autoimmune and genetic hepatitis are described in detail.
- *Revised* **Chapter 60: Stroke.** The stroke chapter has been extensively revised and collaborative care, drug therapy, and surgical therapy are now discussed separately for both hemorrhagic and ischemic strokes.
- The content of the **Evolve Web site** that accompanies this text has been significantly enhanced to include the following learning tools:
  - More than 50 in-depth **case studies** include state-of-the-art animations and a variety of interactive learning activities, which provide students with immediate feedback to optimize learning and retention.
  - A dynamic collection of **Multimedia Supplements** includes animations, video clips, and audio clips.
  - A bank of more than **350 multiple-choice Examination Review Questions** aids in test preparation.
  - A **Glossary** provides definitions for key terms in the book and is available as a comprehensive glossary and also one organized by chapter.

A Word on Terminology

In adapting for Canada a text written for the U.S. market, we faced a number of unique challenges, one of which was changing the cultural, ethnic, and racial terminology used in the United States to that used in Canada. In Canada, the term "Black" is more prevalent than "African-Canadian," and hence we have used that term in this text wherever possible. However, it is important to note that much of the research on the race-related aspects of many disorders and diseases has been conducted in the United States in African-American populations. We have, therefore, been careful not to assume that what is true for African-Americans as a cultural and racial entity is necessarily true for all Black people or even all Black people in Canada. Accordingly, where we cite specific research done among *African-Americans,* we have retained that term that refers particularly to Blacks in the United States.

Similarly, there is a difference of opinion as to whether persons of European descent should be called White or Caucasian. Historically, the anthropological term *Caucasian* has included peoples of northern Africa, Western Asia, and India as well as those of Europe and would therefore be inappropriate for our purpose. In any case, the term is no longer in scientific use. We have therefore chosen to refer to white-skinned people simply as "White."

A Word on Laboratory Values

SI units are used for the laboratory values cited throughout the textbook. **Appendix B: Laboratory Values** lists SI units first, followed by U.S. conventional units in parentheses in all relevant instances. It is important to note that reference ranges for laboratory values may vary among laboratories, depending on the

testing techniques used. If discrepancies should exist between the body of the text and Appendix B, the appendix should be considered the final authority.

Learning Supplements for the Student

- The handy **Clinical Companion** presents approximately 200 common medical–surgical conditions and procedures in a concise, alphabetical format for quick clinical reference. Designed for portability, this popular reference includes the essential, need-to-know information for medical–surgical nursing practice. An attractive and functional two-colour design highlights key information for quick, easy reference. This edition features a strong focus on treatments and procedures in which the nurse plays a major role.
- **Evolve Student Resources** are available online at *http://evolve. elsevier.com/Canada/Lewis/medsurg* and include the following valuable learning aids that are organized by chapter:
  - **Over 50 Interactive Case Studies** with state-of-the-art animations and a variety of learning activities that provide students with immediate feedback. Ten of the case studies have been enhanced with photos and narration of the clinical scenarios.
  - MP3-downloadable Audio Key Points for each chapter
  - Printable Key Points summaries for each chapter
  - Content Updates
  - Answer guidelines to the case studies in the textbook
  - Audio Lectures for selected key content areas
  - Customizable Nursing Care Plans
  - 40 Patient and Caregiver Teaching Guide handouts that can be printed and distributed to patients
  - Physical Examination Videos
  - Fluids and Electrolytes Tutorial
  - Electronic Calculators
  - A glossary of key terms, available as a comprehensive alphabetical glossary and organized by chapter
  - Additional resources, including tables, figures, and clinical references
- **Virtual Clinical Excursions (VCE)** is an exciting learning tool that brings learning to life in a "virtual" hospital setting. VCE simulates a realistic, yet safe, nursing environment where the routine and rigours of the average clinical rotation abound. Students can conduct a complete assessment of a patient and set priorities for care, collect data, analyze and interpret data, prepare and administer medications, and reach conclusions about complex problems. Each lesson has a textbook reading assignment and online activities based on "visiting" patients in the hospital. Instructors receive an Implementation Manual with directions for using VCE as a teaching tool.

Teaching Supplements for Instructors

- The **Evolve Instructor Resources** (available online at *http:// evolve.elsevier.com/Canada/Lewis/medsurg*) remain the most comprehensive set of instructor's materials available, containing the following:
  - **Lesson Plans** tie together all chapter resources you need for the most effective class presentations, with sections dedicated to objectives, teaching focus, instructor chapter resources, student chapter resources, answers to chapter questions, and answers to in-class case study discussion.

Teaching strategies include content highlights, student activities, online activities, and large-group activities.

- The **Test Bank** features over 1700 examination test questions with text page references and answers coded for nursing process and cognitive level. The ExamView software allows instructors to create new tests; edit, add, and delete test questions; sort questions by category, cognitive level, difficulty, and question type; and administer and grade online tests.
- The **Image Collection** contains more than 800 full-colour images from the text for use in lectures.
- An extensive collection of **PowerPoint Presentations** includes over 4000 customizable slides for use in lectures. The presentations include illustrations from the image collection and links to applicable animations.
  - A collection of additional "faculty-only" state-of-the-art animations
  - Course management system
  - Access to all student resources listed above
- The **Simulation Learning System** provides a comprehensive package of resources that allow for the integration of simulation within a nursing curriculum. Designed to correspond with the content in the textbook, this innovative product reinforces students' classroom knowledge base and offers the remediation component critical to debriefing—the point of the simulation experience where safe, effective clinical application of knowledge is discovered. Included for each of the scenarios are various resources designed for student and instructor use before, during, and after each simulation.

Acknowledgements

The editors are grateful to the entire editorial team at Elsevier for their leadership and dedication in the preparation of this very comprehensive, but much needed, Canadian medical-surgical textbook. In particular, we wish to thank Ann Millar for recognizing the need for a third edition of the Canadian edition and supporting us during this journey; Dawn Slawecki for her professionalism, sense of humour, patience, and graciousness despite pressing deadlines and for her commitment to the Canadian Lewis project from first to third edition; and Martina van de Velde and Daniela Freitas for their invaluable assistance.

We would like to recognize the commitment and expertise of all the authors, representing diverse areas of practice as well as regions of Canada. It has been a genuine pleasure to work with both the first-time and returning authors on this project. We are also very grateful to the many reviewers for their valuable feedback on earlier versions of this textbook. It takes a large and coordinated team to create a textbook such as this, and we thank everyone for their individual contributions. We are proud to be able to provide a medical–surgical nursing textbook written from a Canadian perspective that provides current and accurate information to enrich the learning of our nursing students.

Concepts in Nursing Practice

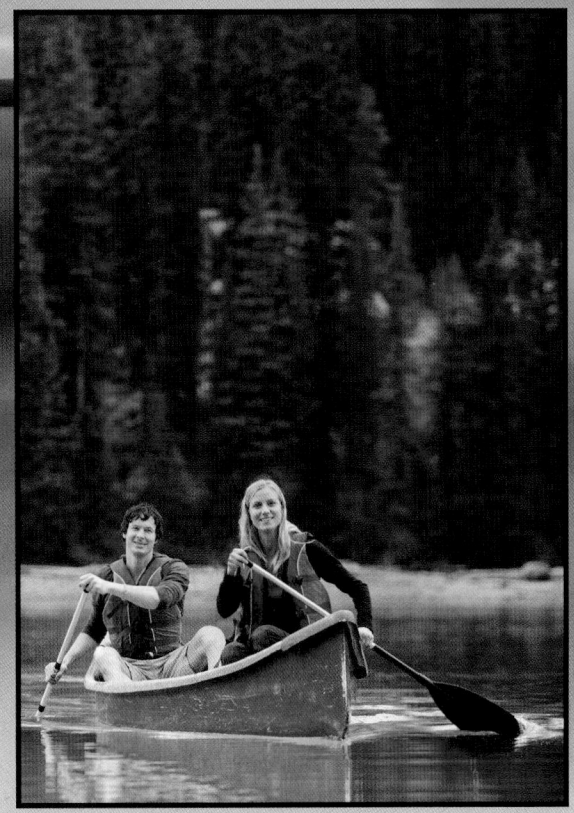

© Leaf/Dreamstime.com

Introduction to Medical-Surgical Nursing Practice in Canada

Written by Donna Goodridge

Based on the original chapter by Patricia Graber O'Brien

LEARNING OBJECTIVES

1. Describe key challenges facing the current Canadian health care system.
2. Situate the practice of professional nursing as a key player on the health care team.
3. Explain the contribution of interprofessional collaboration to high-quality patient outcomes.
4. Describe key attributes of the practice of medical-surgical nursing.
5. Describe the characteristics of evidence-informed practice.
6. Describe the key elements of providing nursing care.
7. Describe the process of preparing and selecting patient outcome statements.
8. Identify the criteria for selecting nursing interventions.
9. Identify the role of evaluation in nursing practice.
10. Describe the importance of documentation to nursing practice and improving patient care.

KEY TERMS

advanced nursing practice An advanced level of clinical nursing practice that maximizes the application of graduate-level education, in-depth nursing knowledge, and expertise in meeting needs of individuals, families, groups, communities, and populations, p. 9

adverse event An event that results in unintended harm to the patient and is related to the care and/or services provided to the patient rather than to the patient's underlying medical condition, p. 4

assessment The collection of subjective and objective information about the patient, p. 10

clinical expertise Ability to use clinical skills and past experience to identify the health states of patients or populations, their risks, their preferences and actions, and the potential benefits of intervention, p. 7

clinical judgement The ways in which nurses come to understand the problems, issues, or concerns of patients; to attend to salient knowledge; and to respond in concerned and involved ways, p. 7

clinical (critical) pathway Includes a nursing care plan, specific interventions for each day of hospitalization, and a documentation tool, p. 15

collaborative problems Potential or actual complications of disease or of treatment that nurses manage together with other health care professionals, p. 13

continuing competence The ongoing ability to integrate and apply the knowledge, skills, judgement, and personal attributes required to practise safely and ethically in a designated role and setting, p. 5

critical thinking The art of analyzing and evaluating thinking with a view to improving it, p. 6

eHealth The use of communication and information technologies in order to support the delivery and integration of clinical care within and across settings, p. 10

evaluation Process of determining if identified outcomes have been met, p. 10

evidence-informed nursing A continuous interactive process involving the explicit, conscientious, and judicious consideration of the best available evidence to provide care, p. 6

expected patient outcomes Goals that articulate what is desired or expected as a result of care, p. 13

implementation The use of nursing interventions to carry out the nursing care plan, p. 10

information and communication technologies (ICT) The tools and applications that support the management of clinical data, information, and knowledge, p. 10

medical-surgical nursing A type of nursing that involves caring for acutely ill adults experiencing complex variations in health, p. 6

Nurse One A Web-based information portal for nurses, p. 9

nursing diagnosis The process of the nurse's identifying and labelling human responses to actual or potential health problems; also, the product of this process as articulated in standard terminology, p. 11

nursing informatics The integration in nursing practice of nursing science, computer science, and information technology to manage and communicate data, information, and knowledge, p. 10

nursing intervention Any treatment, based on clinical judgement and knowledge, that a nurse performs to enhance patient outcomes, p. 13

nursing leadership An attitude and approach that values lifelong learning and a commitment to excellence in practice, p. 17

nursing process An assertive, problem-solving approach to the identification and treatment of patient health problems, p. 10

patient-centred approach An approach that emphasizes patient involvement in care and the individualization of care based on needs, p. 3

planning Setting goals and expected outcomes with the patient and, when feasible, the patient's family and determining strategies for accomplishing the goals, p. 10

regulated health care professionals Paid workers who meet certain requirements that allow them to legally use a specific title and to undertake a specific type of work, p. 4

standard of practice An authoritative statement that sets out the legal and professional basis for nursing practice and describes desirable and achievable level of performance in practice, p. 5

unregulated health workers Paid employees who are not licensed or registered by a regulatory body and may not have mandatory education of practice standards, p. 4

ELECTRONIC RESOURCES

Supplemental content related to Chapter 1 can be found ...

Evolve Web Site   ⊖volve

http://evolve.elsevier.com/Canada/Lewis/medsurg
- Clinical Reference: Laboratory Values
- Content Updates

- Electronic Calculators
- Examination Review Questions
- Glossary
- Key Points (Printable and MP3 Download)

The Canadian Health Care Context

Health care is a subject of keen interest to the public. It was recently ranked as the most important public policy issue for Canadians in a public opinion poll (Canadian Association for Retired Persons, 2011). In Canada, everyone has access to health care through a government-funded universal program, the costs of which are shared by the federal and the provincial or territorial governments. *The Canada Health Act* mandates that all provinces and territories provide coverage for medically necessary procedures. These include most services provided in hospitals and by family doctors. The level of health care funding from the federal government to the provinces and territories depends on the economic health of the country.

In 2003, the first ministers agreed to a 10-year Accord on Health Care Renewal. The Accord committed federal and provincial governments to work toward targeted reforms to improve access, quality, and long-term sustainability of the Canadian health care system (Health Canada, 2011). In 2014, the governments will renegotiate the accord (Canadian Health Coalition, 2011), with many changes expected to result in the way health care is delivered in Canada. There is widespread agreement that our health care system has not kept pace with the changing needs of Canadians. In May 2011, the Canadian Nurses Association (CNA) launched a National Expert Commission entitled "The Health of Our Nation—The Future of Our Health System" (Canadian Nurses Association, 2011a). This commission will

make recommendations to put the patient and family first in health care, with a renewed focus on quality care in both community and institutional settings. The findings of this commission, as well as other initiatives designed to re-engineer our health care system, will have a lasting impact on how nurses practise within the Canadian context.

The Canadian health care system continues to deal with major challenges, including concerns about patient safety, service delivery, fiscal constraints, aging demographics, and the high cost of new technology and drugs.

Romanow (Commission on the Future of Health Care in Canada, 2002), Kirby (Standing Committee on Social Affairs, Science and Technology, 2002), Mazankowski (Premier's Advisory Council on Health for Alberta, 2002), Fyke (Commission on Medicare, 2001), and Dagnone (Patient First Review Commissioner, 2009) have all emphasized the need to accelerate changes within the health care system to ensure sustainability of the system and promote the patient-centred approach desired by the public (Lewis, 2009). A **patient-centred approach** is characterized by: (a) patient involvement in care and (b) individualization of care (Robinson, Callister, Berry, & Dearing, 2008).

Together with the Canadian Medical Association, the CNA has defined a set of key principles designed to guide health care transformation in Canada. These principles are listed in Table 1-1 and are important considerations for all nurses because they will shape the re-engineered health care system of the future.

Table 1-1 Principles to Guide Health Care Transformation in Canada

- *Patient-centred:* Patients must be at the centre of health care, with seamless access to the continuum of care based on their needs.
- *Quality:* Canadians deserve quality services that are appropriate for patient needs, respect individual choice, and are delivered in a manner that is timely, safe, effective, and according to the most currently available scientific knowledge.
- *Health promotion and illness prevention:* The health system must support Canadians in the prevention of illness and the enhancement of their well-being, with attention paid to broader social determinants of health.
- *Equitable:* The health care system has a duty to Canadians to provide and advocate for equitable access to quality care and commonly adopted policies to address the social determinants of health.
- *Sustainable:* Sustainable health care requires universal access to quality health services that are adequately resourced and delivered across the board in a timely and cost-effective manner.
- *Accountable:* The public, patients, families, providers, and funders all have a responsibility for ensuring the system is effective and accountable.

Source: Canadian Nurses Association. (2011). *Nursing and the political agenda.* Retrieved from *http://www.cna-nurses.ca/CNA/issues/matters/ default_e.aspx* © Canadian Nurses Association. Reprinted with permission. Further reproduction prohibited.

Patient Safety

Patient safety is a cornerstone of nursing practice. Entry-to-practice competencies for Registered Nursing recognize the important of the nurse's ability to assess and manage situations that may compromise patient safety (College and Association of Registered Nurses of Alberta, 2006). In spite of the fact that patients turn to the health care system for help with their health conditions, overwhelming evidence has established that significant numbers of patients are harmed as a result of the health care they receive, resulting in permanent injury, increased lengths of stay and even death (World Health Organization, 2011). An **adverse event** is an event that results in unintended harm to the patient and is related to the care and/or services provided to the patient rather than to the patient's underlying medical condition (Canadian Patient Safety Institute, 2008). The 2004 "Canadian Adverse Events Study" confirmed that adverse events are a significant problem in Canadian hospitals (Baker et al., 2004). Table 1-2 describes performance requirements noted by the World Health Organization that facilitate safe practice by health care professionals.

The Profession of Nursing in Canada

Health care in Canada is typically delivered by teams of workers with different responsibilities and scopes of practice. The term **regulated health care professionals** refers to paid workers who meet certain requirements that allow them to legally use a specific title and to undertake a specific type of work (Canadian Institute of Health Information, 2001). Registered Nurses, Registered Psychiatric Nurses, and Licensed Vocational Nurses (LVNs) are examples of regulated providers. In contrast, **unregulated health workers** are paid employees who are not licensed or registered by a regulatory body and may not have mandatory education of

Table 1-2 Requirements for Safe Clinical Practice

GOAL	ACTIONS
Apply patient safety thinking in all clinical activities	Numerous opportunities are available to incorporate patient safety knowledge into practice.
Develop relationships with patients	Relate and communicate with each individual patient as a unique human being who has her or his own experience of her or his illness. Applying clinical skills alone will not necessarily achieve the best outcomes for patients.
Understand that multiple factors are involved in adverse events	Usually, many factors contribute to the occurrence of an adverse event. Using the five "Ws" (who, what, when, where, and why) can keep the discussion focused on the system rather than the individuals involved.
Avoid blaming when an error occurs	Health care providers should support one another when an adverse event occurs. Disclosure of an error when it occurs is an important part of professionalism.
Practise evidence-informed care	Be aware of the nature and use of policies, procedures, clinical guidelines, and protocols used in the agency.
Maintain continuity of care for patients	The health system is made up of many parts that interrelate to produce a continuum of care for patients and families. Important information that is missed or incurred can lead to inadequate care or errors.
Act ethically at all times	Practise according to the Canadian Nurses Association *Code of Ethics* (2009). This document provides guidance about the responsibilities and accountabilities needed to practise nursing safely.

Source: Adapted from the World Health Organization. (2011). *What is patient safety?* Retrieved from *http://www.who.int/patientsafety/education/ curriculum/PSP_MPC_topic-01.pdf*

practice standards (Pan-Canadian Committee on Unregulated Health Workers, 2009). Examples of unregulated health care professionals include "health care aides" and "personal support workers."

Within Canada, nurses are granted the legal authority to use the designation "Registered Nurse" (RN) in accordance with provincial and territorial legislation and regulation. The provincial regulatory bodies set the standards for practice for RNs to protect the public in their province or territory (Canadian Nurses Association, 2011b). RN practice is defined by the Canadian Nurses Association (2007, p. 5) in the following way:

> Registered nurses are self-regulated health-care professionals who work autonomously and in collaboration with others. RNs enable individuals, families, groups, communities and populations to achieve their optimal level of health. RNs coordinate health care, deliver direct services and support patients in their self-care decisions and actions in situations of health, illness, injury and disability in all stages of life.

RNs contribute to the health-care system through their work in direct practice, education, administration, research and policy in a wide array of settings.

Because RNs work with other regulated providers as well as with unregulated workers, the nurse must be aware of both his or her own and other providers' scopes of practice. This is essential to safely enacting key nursing roles such as delegation and prioritization and meeting the standards of practice.

Standards of Practice

A **standard of practice** is an authoritative statement that sets out the legal and professional basis for nursing practice and describes desirable and achievable level of performance (College of Registered Nurses of Nova Scotia, 2004). Standards are intended to promote, guide, direct, and regulate professional nursing practice. Standards of practice demonstrate to the public, government, and other stakeholders that a profession is dedicated to maintaining public trust and upholding the criteria of its professional practice (Canadian Nurses Association, 2011b). Standards of practice are based on the values of the profession and articulated in the *Code of Ethics for Registered Nurses*. Provincial and territorial regulatory bodies for nursing are legally required to set standards for practice for RNs in order to protect the public (Canadian Nurses Association, 2011b). These standards, together with the *Code of Ethics*, form the foundation for nursing practice in Canada.

Given the rapid changes in resources, expectations, and technologies that characterize health care in Canada, the practice of nursing requires a commitment to lifelong learning in order to promote the highest quality of patient outcomes. **Continuing competence** refers to "the ongoing ability of a nurse to integrate and apply the knowledge, skills, judgement and personal attributes required to practise safely and ethically in a designated role and setting" (Joint Statement of the Canadian Nurses Association and the Canadian Association of Schools of Nursing, 2004).

RNs are initially prepared at the baccalaureate level and can go on to pursue further studies at the graduate level. Many nurses also seek recognition of their clinical expertise through certification in 1 of 19 specialty areas of practise through the CNA. Medical-surgical nursing is one of the newest specialties to be recognized through the certification program.

Interprofessional Collaboration. The increasing acuity of patients in the health care system, as well as the growing complexity of interventions designed to promote, restore, and maintain health, means that no one health discipline can work in isolation. In order to help patients achieve optimal health, nurses work in collaboration with a wide range of professionals from many disciplines, including medicine, rehabilitation therapies, social work, diagnostic services, and many others. The CNA recognized the growing importance of interprofessional collaboration in their Position Statement on Interprofessional Collaboration (2011c), described in Table 1-3. Successful collaboration with other health professionals has become a cornerstone of nursing practice.

Nurses function in independent, dependent, and collaborative roles. Each province and territory has a *Nurses' Act* that determines the scope of practice for that region. These acts allow nurses to take on delegated medical responsibilities and have a wider scope of practice when working as nurse practitioners. It is important for nurses to understand how the primary goals of

Table 1-3 Key Principles Facilitating Collaboration Between Health Professionals

1. Focus on the Patient/Client

The needs of individual patients and clients must be the focus of health services. Health professionals work together to optimize the health and wellness of each individual and involve the individual in decision-making about his or her health. Individuals and their families are actively engaged in the prevention, promotion, and management of health problems. Health professionals respect that personal health information must be kept confidential.

2. Population Health Approach

Using assessments of the demographics and health status of a community will ensure the relevance of health services, including the identification of appropriate health professions. Trends in the health of the population are tracked to assess the impact of the services offered.

3. Best Possible Care and Services

Health professionals work together to identify and assess research evidence as a basis for identifying treatment and management of health problems. Health outcomes are continuously evaluated to track the effectiveness and appropriateness of services.

4. Access

The right service is provided at the right time, in the right place, and by the right care provider. Geographical barriers are minimized. Service delivery is respectful of age, gender, culture, language, religion, and lifestyle of patients/clients.

5. Trust and Respect

Each profession brings its own set of knowledge and skills—the result of education, training, and experience—to collaborative health services. Each professional contributes to an individual's health. Shared decision-making, creativity, and innovation allow providers to learn from one another and enhance the effectiveness of their collaborative efforts.

6. Effective Communication

Active listening and effective communication skills facilitate both information sharing and decision making.

The range and complexity of factors that influence health and well-being, as well as disease and illness, require health professionals from diverse health professions to work together in a comprehensive manner. For example, individuals need health information, diagnosis of health problems, support for behavioural change, immunization, screening for disease prevention, and monitoring of management plans for chronic health problems. Working together, the combined knowledge and skills of health professionals become a powerful mechanism to enhance the health of the population served.

Conclusion

Working together can take various forms. At the simplest level, health professionals consult their patients/clients and, when appropriate, one another about the services needed by their patients/clients. In more complex situations, health professionals work more closely, identifying (together with patients/clients) what services are needed, who will provide them, and what adjustments need to be made to the health management plan. The number and type of service health professionals depend on the nature of the health issue and the availability of resources. This is a dynamic process that responds to changing needs.

Source: Enhancing Interdisciplinary Collaboration Project. (2006). *The principles and framework for interdisciplinary collaboration in primary health care.* Ottawa: Author. Retrieved from *http://www.caslpa.ca/PDF/EICP_Principles_and_Framework_final.pdf*

Table 1-4 Comparison of Primary Goals for Nursing and Medicine	
NURSING	**MEDICINE**
Determines responses to health problems, level of wellness, and need for assistance	Determines etiology of illness or injury
Provides physical care, emotional care, teaching, guidance, and counselling	Prescribes medical treatments; performs surgery
Interventions aimed at promoting health, preventing illness/complications, and assisting patients to meet their own needs	Interventions aimed at preventing and curing injury or illness

Source: Lewis, S. L., Dirksen, S. R., Heitkemper, M. M., Bucher, L., & Camera, I. M. (2011). *Medical-surgical nursing: Assessment and management of clinical problems* (8th ed., p. 10). St. Louis: Mosby.

nursing and medicine differ (Table 1-4) to function effectively in these different roles.

What Is Medical-Surgical Nursing?

Medical-surgical nursing is a challenging and dynamic type of nursing that involves caring for acutely ill adults experiencing complex variations in health (Canadian Association of Medical and Surgical Nurses, 2012). Because the scope of medical-surgical nursing is very broad, the nurse practising in this area is expected to develop and maintain a great deal of knowledge and skill. This book provides the beginning nurse with much of the knowledge required to become a safe and competent practitioner.

The medical-surgical nurse is considered a leader and a key member of the interdisciplinary team (Canadian Nurses Association, 2009). Primary responsibilities of the medical-surgical nurse include: prioritization, accountability, advocacy, organization, and coordination of evidence-informed care for multiple patients. Medical-surgical patients and their caregivers come from diverse backgrounds and often possess multiple, complex illnesses, a situation requiring medical-surgical nurses to be well prepared. Given the rapidly changing and complex health concerns that may affect multiple body systems of medical-surgical patients, safe and effective use of technology is an increasingly important competency required by medical-surgical nurses. The effective medical-surgical nurse demonstrates adaptability and a strong commitment to ensuring the best possible patient outcomes.

Medical-surgical nurses practise in diverse environments, ranging from outpatient and primary care environments through the continuum of care to tertiary care hospitals (Canadian Nurses Association, 2009). As the largest single group of nursing professionals in Canada (Canadian Association of Medical and Surgical Nurses, 2012), medical-surgical nurses utilize a broad range of evidence-informed knowledge and clinical skills to address the needs of acutely ill adults and their families. The Canadian Association of Medical and Surgical Nurses is a national organization that promotes excellence through best practice standards to provide high-quality, sage, and ethical care to patients across the continuum of care. Registered nurses may choose to seek recognition of their expertise in this specialty through postlicensure certification offered by the CNA.

Table 1-5 Characteristics of the Well-Cultivated Critical Thinker
A well-cultivated critical thinker:
• Raises vital questions and problems, formulating them clearly and precisely;
• Gathers and assesses relevant information, [and] using abstract ideas to interpret it effectively comes to well-reasoned conclusions and solutions, testing them against relevant criteria and standards;
• Thinks open-mindedly within alternative systems of thought, recognizing and assessing, as need be, their assumptions, implications, and practical consequences; and
• Communicates effectively with others in figuring out solutions to complex problems.

Source: Paul, R., & Elder, L. (2006). *The miniature guide to critical thinking: Concepts and tools* (4th ed., p. 4) Dillon Beach, CA: Foundation for Critical Thinking.

Critical Thinking in Nursing

To provide high-quality care in clinical environments of increasing complexity and greater accountability, nurses need to develop higher-level thinking and reasoning skills.

The ability to engage in critical thinking is widely regarded as a fundamental skill in nursing education and practice. According to the Foundation for Critical Thinking, **critical thinking** is the art of analyzing and evaluating thinking with a view to improving it (Paul & Elder, 2006). Alfaro-LeFevre's (2009) work suggests that critical thinking can be described as "good problem solving" and involves a "commitment to look for the best way, based on the most current research and practice findings." Table 1-5 describes the characteristics of a well-cultivated critical thinker.

According to the CNA (2002), critical thinking is a "complex, active, and purposeful process encompassing the essential skills of interpretation and evaluation and requiring the RN to go beyond the role of performance of skills and interventions." Critical thinking "compels the RN to identify and challenge assumptions, use an organized approach to assessment, check for accuracy and reliability of information, distinguish relevant from irrelevant, normal from abnormal, and recognize inconsistencies, cluster related information, identify patterns and missing information and draw valid conclusions based on evidence, identify different concurrent conclusions and underlying causes, set priorities, and evaluate and correct thinking."

Evidence-Informed Practice

Evidence-informed nursing is a continuous interactive process involving the explicit, conscientious, and judicious consideration of the best available evidence to provide care (Canadian Nurses Association, 2010). Basing health care decisions upon evidence is essential for quality care in all domains of nursing practice. According to the CNA (2010, p. 1), evidence-informed decision-making:

...is essential to optimize outcomes for individual clients, promote healthy communities and populations, improve clinical practice, achieve cost-effective nursing care and ensure accountability and transparency in decision-making within the health-care system.

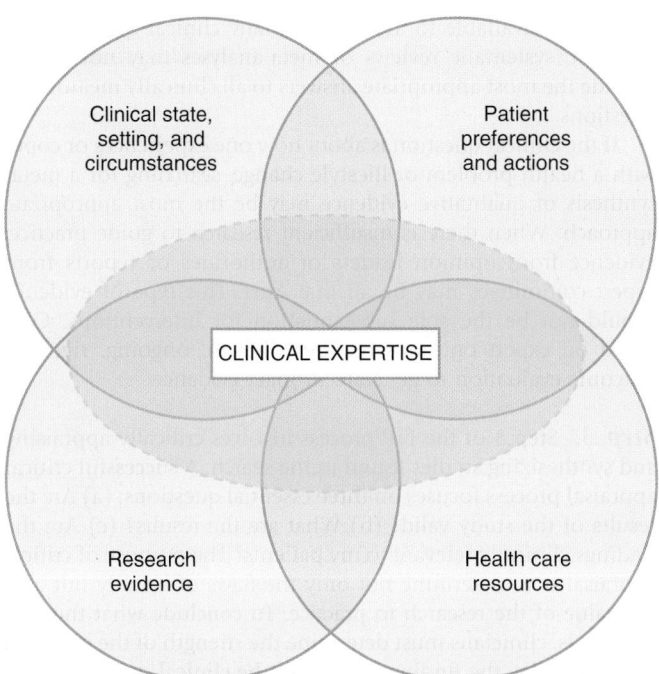

Figure 1-1 A model for evidence-informed clinical decisions.

Source: Adapted by DiCenso, A., Guyatt, G., & Ciliska, D. (2005). In Haynes, R. B., Devereaux, P. J., & Guyatt, G. (2002). Clinical expertise in the area of evidence-based medicine and patient choice. *Evidence-Based Medicine, 7*(2), 36–38. doi:10.1136/ebm.7.2.36

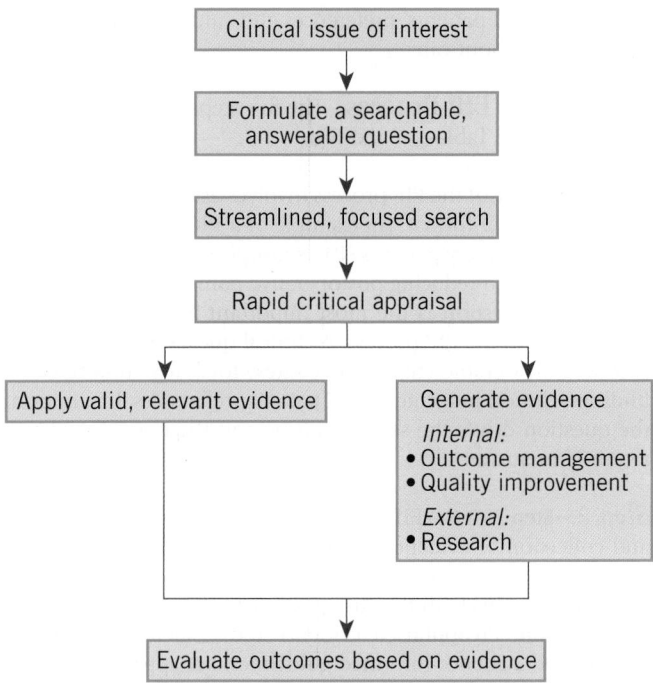

Figure 1-2 Process of evidence-informed practice.

Four primary elements contribute to the practice of evidence-informed nursing (DiCenso, Guyatt, & Ciliska, 2005): (a) clinical state, setting, and circumstances; (b) patient preferences and actions; (c) best research evidence, and (d) health care resources (Figure 1-1). **Clinical expertise,** which integrates these other four components, refers to the nurse's "ability to use clinical skills and past experience to identify the health state of patients or populations, their risks, their preferences and actions, and the potential benefits of intervention; to communicate information to patients and their families; and to provide them with an environment they find comforting and supporting" (DiCenso et al., 2005, p. 5). **Clinical judgement** is defined by Benner, Tanner, and Chesla (2009) as the ways in which nurses come to understand the problems, issues, or concerns of patients; to attend to salient knowledge; and to respond in concerned and involved ways.

Evidence-informed practice (EIP) produces better outcomes in the most effective and efficient way. Application of EIP results in more accurate diagnoses, the most effective and efficient interventions, and the most favourable patient outcomes. The most distinguishing feature of EIP is that the new scientific base for practice is built through a summary of studies on a topic. These summaries are called evidence syntheses, systematic reviews, or integrative reviews, depending on the organization that produces them. The evidence synthesis summarizes all research results into a single conclusion about the state of the science. From this point, the clinician translates the knowledge into a clinical practice guideline, implements it through individual and organizational practice changes, and evaluates it in terms of the effectiveness and efficiency of producing intended health care outcomes (Figure 1-2). Clinical practice guidelines can take the form of protocols, clinical pathways, practice guidelines, policy statements, computer-based protocols, or algorithms.

Best-practice guidelines (BPGs) are increasingly used to guide clinical practice in health care. BPGs are "systematically

Table 1-6 Five Steps of the Evidence-Informed Practice (EIP) Process

1. Ask clinical questions using the **PICO** format:

   P Patient population of interest

   I Intervention or area of interest

   C Comparison of interest or comparison group

   O Outcome(s) of interest

2. Collect the most relevant and best evidence.

3. Critically appraise and synthesize the evidence.

4. Integrate all evidence with one's clinical expertise and patient preferences and values in making a practice decision or change.

5. Evaluate the practice decision or change.

developed statements based on best available evidence to assist practitioners' and patients' decisions about appropriate health care" (Registered Nurses' Association of Ontario, 2006). Examples of the current BPGs include *Adult Asthma Care Guidelines for Nurses: Promoting Control of Asthma; The Assessment and Management of Pain;* and *Client-Centred Care, Nursing Leadership, and Cultural Diversity.*

Throughout this book, evidence-informed clinical practice guidelines are available for selected topics. The EIP boxes provide answers to specific clinical questions. The boxes contain the PICO (*p*atient population of interest, *i*ntervention or area of interest, *c*omparison of interest or comparative group, *o*utcome[s] of interest) question (Table 1-6), critical appraisal of the syntheses of evidence or primary studies, implications for nursing practice, and the source of the evidence. Evidence can support current practice and increase confidence that nursing care will continue to produce the desired outcome, or evidence may require a change in practice. In either case, it is important for nurses to be aware of the role of scientific evidence, their expertise and judgement, and patients' preferences and values in making clinical decisions about care.

Steps in the EIP Process. The five steps of the EIP process are provided in Table 1-5 and Figure 1-2.

Step 1. Step 1 of the EIP process involves asking a clinical question in the PICO format. An example of a PICO question is: "In adult cardiac surgery patients (P), is morphine (I) or fentanyl (C) more effective in reducing postoperative pain (O)?" Formulating the clinical question is the most important and the most challenging step in the EIP process. A clinical question that is searchable and answerable creates the context for integrating research findings, clinical judgement, and patient preferences. In addition, the question drives the search strategy and the type of evidence required to answer it.

Step 2. Step 2 of the EIP process involves an efficient search for and collection of evidence based on the question. The question directs the clinician to the databases that are most appropriate. The search begins with the strongest external evidence to answer the question. Preappraised evidence tools, such as systematic reviews and evidence-informed guidelines, are appropriate time-saving resources in the EIP process (Table 1-7). Systematic reviews of randomized controlled trials (RCTs) are considered the strongest level of evidence to answer questions about interventions (i.e., cause and effect). However, a limited number of systematic

reviews are available to answer the many clinical questions. In addition, systematic reviews or meta-analyses may not always provide the most appropriate answers to all clinically meaningful questions.

If the clinical question is about how one experiences or copes with a health problem or lifestyle change, searching for a meta-synthesis of qualitative evidence may be the most appropriate approach. When there is insufficient research to guide practice, evidence from opinion leaders or authorities or reports from expert committees may be all that exist. This type of evidence should not be the sole substantiation for interventions. Care based on expert opinions requires diligent, ongoing, rigorous outcome evaluation to generate stronger evidence.

Step 3. Step 3 of the EIP process involves critically appraising and synthesizing studies found in the search. A successful critical appraisal process focuses on three essential questions: (a) Are the results of the study valid? (b) What are the results? (c) Are the findings clinically relevant to my patients? The purpose of critical appraisal is to determine not only the flaws of a study but also the value of the research to practice. To conclude what the best practice is, clinicians must determine the strength of the evidence and synthesize the findings related to the clinical question.

Step 4. Step 4 of the EIP process may differ depending on the strength and breadth of the evidence to answer the question. Recommendations from sufficient, strong evidence (e.g., inter-

Table 1-7 Examples of Clinical Questions and Types of Evidence and Where to Find It

QUESTIONS	TYPES OF EVIDENCE TO ANSWER QUESTION	DATABASES WITH EVIDENCE
Therapy: In men with human immunodeficiency virus (HIV) infection, what is the effect of cognitive coping, compared with emotional coping, on mood, distress, and anxiety caused by worsening HIV symptoms?	Evidence-informed guidelines Systematic review of randomized controlled trials (RCTs) Single RCT or group of RCTs	Cochrane Database of Systematic Reviews (CDSR) *(www.cochrane.org)* Database of Abstracts of Reviews of Effects (DARE) *(www.york.ac.uk/inst/crd/darehp.htm)* National Guideline Clearinghouse *(www.guideline.gov)*
Etiology: Are 30- to 50-year-old men with high blood pressure at increased risk for stroke compared with men with normal blood pressure?	Cohort study	MEDLINE CINAHL
Diagnosis or diagnostic test: Is computed tomography (CT) scanning more accurate than ultrasonography in diagnosing appendicitis?	RCT Cohort study	Cochrane Database of Systematic Reviews (CDSR) Database of Abstracts of Reviews of Effects (DARE) National Guideline Clearinghouse MEDLINE CINAHL
Prevention: Over a period of 5 years, is active involvement in an exercise support group better in reducing the risk of cardiovascular disease in obese women, in comparison with the effect of educational programs on lifestyle changes?	Prospective study RCT	MEDLINE CINAHL National Guideline Clearinghouse
Prognosis: Does dietary fat intake influence healthy weight maintenance (body mass index [BMI] <25 kg/m²) in those who have a family history of obesity (BMI >30 kg/m²)?	Cohort study Case-control studies	MEDLINE CINAHL
Meaning: How do young women with rheumatoid arthritis perceive alterations in their daily functioning?	Qualitative study	MEDLINE CINAHL PsycINFO

Additional resources for evidence: Virginia Henderson Library *(www.nursinglibrary.org)*; Joanna Briggs Institute *(www.joannabriggs.edu)*; AHRQ Evidence-Based Practice Centers *(www.ahrq.gov)*; Registered Nurses' Association of Ontario *(www.rnao.org)*.

ventions with systematic reviews of well-designed RCTs) can be implemented in practice in combination with clinicians' expertise and patient preferences. Clinical judgement will influence how patient preferences and values are assessed, integrated, and entered into the decision-making process. For example, although evidence may support the effectiveness of morphine as an analgesic, its use in a patient with renal failure may not be appropriate. In another example, patients may have concerns about the perceived addictive effect of morphine, although evidence may not support these concerns, and prefer fentanyl for pain management. These types of decisions must be based on knowledge of the best available evidence, clinicians' judgement, and patients' perspectives and values.

When there is insufficient evidence, the fourth step could be used to generate data that can be gathered either through outcome management initiatives (i.e., internal evidence) or through the conduct of rigorous research (i.e., external evidence). Clinicians need to partner with research experts to achieve success in these endeavours.

Step 5. Step 5 of the EIP process involves evaluation of identified outcomes in the clinical setting (see Figure 1-1). Outcomes must match the clinical project that has been implemented. For example, when comparing the effectiveness of morphine and fentanyl for pain control, evaluating the cost of each medication will not provide the required data about clinical effectiveness. Outcomes must reflect all aspects of implementation and capture the interdisciplinary contributions elicited by the EIP process.

Implementation of EIP. To implement EIP, nurses continuously seek scientific evidence that supports the care that they provide. The incorporation of evidence should be balanced with clinical expertise and should take into account each patient's unique circumstances and preferences. EIP closes the gap between research and practice, providing more reliable and predictable care than that which is based on tradition, opinion, and a trial-and-error method. EIP provides nurses with a mechanism to manage the explosion of new literature, introduction of new technologies, concern about health care costs, and increasing emphasis on quality care and patient outcomes.

In collaboration with the First Nations and Inuit Health Branch of Health Canada, the CNA launched a Web-based portal for nurses, called *Nurse One* (see the Resources section at the end of this chapter). The portal provides opportunities for accessing libraries and information related to evidence-informed practice and clinical practice issues through a dedicated Web portal. In the future, it will enable nurses to connect with colleagues and health care experts in real time, no matter where they live in Canada.

Advanced Nursing Practice

As the health care system in Canada undergoes changes, advanced nursing practice (ANP) roles are also evolving to optimize patient care within the system. According to the CNA (2008), "advanced nursing practice builds nursing knowledge, advances the profession and contributes to a sustainable and effective health-care system." **Advanced nursing practice** roles focus on health assessment, diagnosis, and treatment of conditions previously considered to be the physician's domain (Figure 1-3). According to the CNA (2008), ANP is "an umbrella term describing an advanced level of clinical nursing practice that maximizes use of graduate educational preparation, in-depth nursing knowledge and exper-

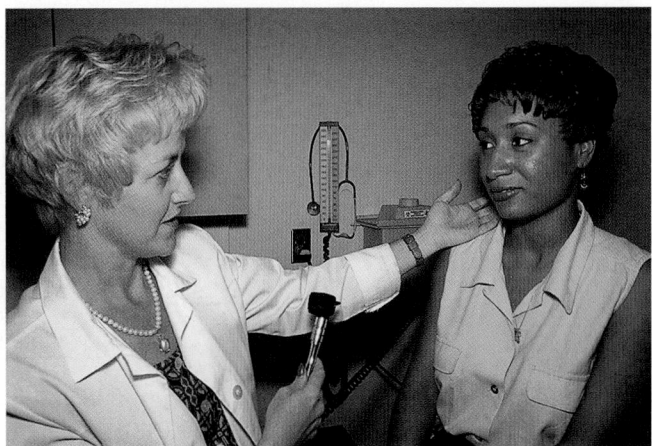

Figure 1-3 Advanced nursing practice (ANP) nurses play an important role in primary care delivery.

Source: Potter, P. A., & Perry, A. G. (1997). *Fundamentals of nursing: Concepts, process and practice* (4th ed.). St. Louis: Mosby.

tise in meeting needs of individuals, families, groups, communities and populations. … ANP extends the boundaries of nursing's scope of practice and contributes to nursing knowledge and the development and advancement of the profession" (Canadian Nurses Association, 2008). Examples of roles within ANP include the clinical nurse specialist (CNS), the nurse practitioner (NP), and the nurse midwife.

In addition to managing and delivering direct patient care, ANP nurses have significant roles in health promotion, case management, administration, and research. There is substantial variation among the provinces and territories in the framework for and specific roles of nurses working in ANP. Practice settings in which an ANP nurse may be employed include primary care, ambulatory care, long-term care, hospital care, community care, as well as in psychiatric and mental health care centres, physicians' offices, family health clinics, and community health facilities (Canadian Nurses Association, 2008). In the ANP role, the nurse's focus may be, for example, on the management of primary care and health promotion for a wide variety of health problems in various specialties; roles include physical examination, diagnosis, treatment of health problems, patient and family education, and counselling. In the management of complex patient care in various clinical specialty areas, the roles of ANP nurses may include direct care, consultation, research, education, case management, and administration.

In 2004, a federal program called the Canadian Nurse Practitioner Initiative (CNPI) was undertaken to facilitate integration and standardization of the ANP role in Canada. This national framework helps the public understand the advanced nurse practitioner's scope of practice and defines qualifications for ANP. The CNA has also asserted that such a framework would allow for a national, coordinated approach to the role of the ANP nurse, while continuing to allow for differences among the provinces and territories in various elements of the framework and enabling focused roles to be created (Canadian Nurses Association, 2008).

Expanding Knowledge and Technology

Rapidly changing technologies and dramatically expanding knowledge in the fields of arts and science affect all areas of health care. Telemedicine, telehealth, and telenursing use virtual

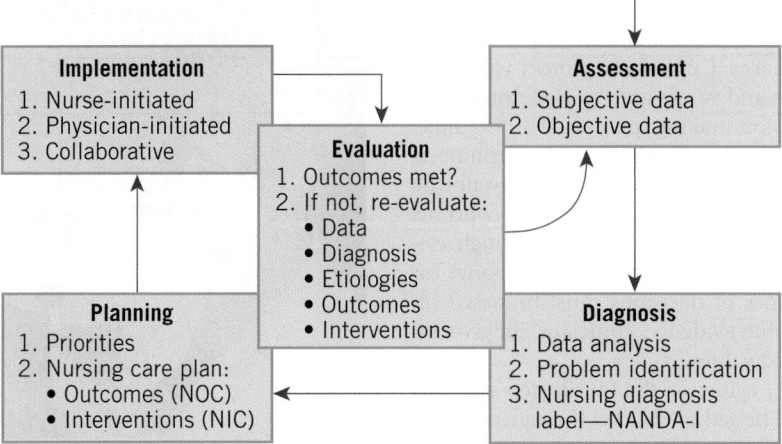

Figure 1-4 The nursing process.

technologies to provide professional education, consultation, and delivery of patient services. **eHealth** refers to the use of communication and information technologies in order to support the delivery and integration of clinical care within and across settings, while **information and communication technologies (ICT)** are tools and applications that support the management of clinical data, information, and knowledge (Registered Nurses' Association of Ontario, 2012). These services are particularly helpful to those working or living in rural and remote parts of Canada. Technology is also increasingly used in nursing education (Bassendowski, 2011).

Nursing informatics is a rapidly growing specialty in nursing. Nursing informatics refers to the integration of nursing science, computer science, and information technology to manage and communicate data, information, and knowledge in nursing practice (Registered Nurses' Association of Ontario, 2012). Nursing informatics facilitates the integration of data, information, and knowledge to support patients, nurses, and other providers in their decision making in all roles and settings.

As the knowledge explosion continues, nurses will be challenged to keep current with new developments in a broad range of areas. Given the growing diversity of Canada's population, nurses must have a good grasp of transcultural nursing and global health issues. Awareness of new developments in the understanding of pathophysiology, psychopathology, and pharmacology and in related areas such as genetics will enable nurses to participate fully in interdisciplinary teamwork. Nurses must also keep abreast of emerging trends in areas such as social determinants of health, environmental health, and food security.

The Nursing Process

The nursing process is one strategy to assist nursing students in understanding the steps involved in providing effective nursing care. The **nursing process** is an assertive, problem-solving approach to the identification and treatment of patient health problems. It provides a framework to organize the knowledge, judgements, and actions that nurses bring to patient care (Wilkinson, 2006). Using the nursing process, the nurse can focus on the unique responses of patients to actual or potential health problems.

Phases of the Nursing Process

The nursing process consists of five phases: assessment, diagnosis, planning, implementation, and evaluation (Figure 1-4). It should be noted that numerous other terms or phrases are also used to describe the steps of the nursing process. **Assessment** involves collecting subjective and objective information about the patient. The nursing diagnosis phase involves analyzing the assessment data, drawing conclusions from the information, and labelling the human response. **Planning** consists of setting goals and expected outcomes with the patient and, when feasible, the patient's family and determining strategies for accomplishing the goals. **Implementation** involves the use of nursing interventions to activate the plan. The nurse also promotes self-care and family involvement, where appropriate. **Evaluation** is an extremely important part of the nursing process that is too often not addressed sufficiently. In the evaluation phase, the nurse first determines whether the identified outcomes have been met. Then the overall accuracy of the assessment, diagnosis, and implementation phases is evaluated. If the outcomes have not been met, new approaches are considered and implemented as the process repeats itself.

Interrelatedness of Phases

The five phases of the nursing process do not occur in isolation from one another. For example, nurses may gather data about the wound condition (assessment) as they change the soiled dressing (implementation). There is, however, a basic order to the nursing process, which begins with assessment. Assessment provides the data on which planning is based. An evaluation of the nature of the assessment data usually follows immediately, resulting in the formulation of a diagnosis. A plan based on the nursing diagnosis then directs the implementation of nursing interventions. Evaluation continues throughout the cycle and provides feedback on the effectiveness of the plan or the need for revision. Revision may be needed in the data collection method, the diagnosis, the expected outcomes or goals, the plan, or the intervention method. Once initiated, the nursing process is not only continuous but also cyclical in nature. There is no limit to the number of times the cycle can be restarted. Application of the nursing process requires sound knowledge of the physical and behavioural

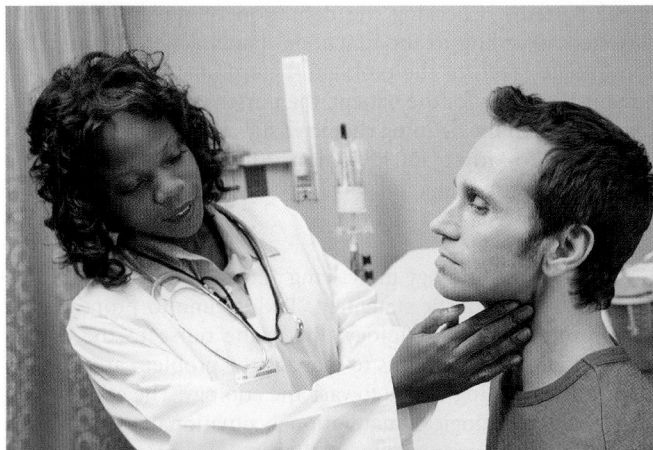

Figure 1-5 Collection of data is a prerequisite to diagnosis, planning, and intervention.

Source: © 2011 JupiterImages Corporation.

sciences and a repertoire of intellectual, interpersonal, and technical skills.

Assessment Phase

Data Collection

Sound data form the foundation for the entire nursing process. Collection of data is a prerequisite to diagnosis, planning, and intervention (Figure 1-5). Humans have needs and problems in biophysical, psychological, sociocultural, spiritual, and environmental domains. A nursing diagnosis made without supporting data pertaining to all of these dimensions can lead to incorrect conclusions and depersonalized care. For example, a hospitalized patient who does not sleep all night may be mistakenly diagnosed as having a disturbed sleep pattern, whereas, in fact, the patient may have worked nights her entire adult life, and it is normal for her to be awake at night. Information concerning her sleeping habits is necessary to provide individualized care to her by ensuring that sleep medication is not routinely administered to her at 2200 hours. The importance of person-centred assessment in the process of clinical decision making cannot be overemphasized. The use of a nursing database (discussed in Chapter 3) is recommended to facilitate data collection.

Because nursing interventions are only as sound as the data on which they are based, the database must be accurate and complete. When possible, collateral information gained from sources such as the patient's record, other health care workers, the patient's family, and the nurse's observations should be validated with the patient. If the patient's statements seem questionable, they should be validated by a knowledgeable person.

Diagnosis Phase

Data Analysis and Problem Identification

The diagnosis phase begins with clustering of information and, after analysis of the assessment data, ends with an evaluative judgement about a patient's health status. Analysis involves sorting through and organizing the information and determining unmet needs as well as the strengths of the patient. The findings are then compared with documented norms to determine whether anything is interfering or could interfere with the patient's needs or ability to maintain his or her usual health pattern.

After a thorough analysis of all available information, one of two possible conclusions is reached: (a) there are no health problems that necessitate nursing intervention or (b) the patient needs nursing assistance to solve a potential or actual health problem. The statements of final conclusions about the health problems are the nursing diagnoses.

Nursing Diagnosis

The term *nursing diagnosis* has many different meanings. To some, it merely connotes the identification of a health problem. More commonly, a nursing diagnosis is viewed as the conclusion about an identified cluster of signs and symptoms. The diagnosis is generally expressed as concisely as possible according to specific guidelines.

Nursing diagnosis is the act of identifying and labelling human responses to actual or potential health problems. Throughout this book, the term *nursing diagnosis* will mean (a) the process of identifying actual and potential health problems and (b) the label or concise statement that describes "a clinical judgement about an individual, family, or community response to actual or potential health problems/life processes. A nursing diagnosis provides the basis for the selection of nursing interventions to achieve outcomes for which the nurse is accountable" (North American Nursing Diagnosis Association International, 2011, p. 515). The human responses that are identified frequently result from a disease process. For example, a patient may have the medical diagnosis of chronic obstructive pulmonary disease (COPD). In this case, the nursing diagnosis would focus on how the COPD affects daily functioning. Examples of patient responses to COPD might be anxiety, activity intolerance, or an inability to maintain a household. Appendix A contains a comprehensive list of nursing diagnoses relevant to care of the medical-surgical patient.

A number of other terms or situations are *not* nursing diagnoses but are often mislabelled as such (NANDA International, 2011). These include the following:
- Medically defined pathological conditions (coronary artery disease)
- Diagnostic tests or studies (upper gastrointestinal series)
- Equipment (nasogastric tube)
- Signs (restlessness)
- Surgical procedures (hysterectomy)
- Treatments (pressure ulcer care)
- Therapeutic goals (performing oral self-care)
- Nursing problems (difficulty in turning patient)
- Therapeutic needs (patient's need for more rest)
- Staff problems (patient being too demanding)

Diagnostic Process

The diagnostic process involves analysis and synthesis of the data collected during assessment of the patient. Data that indicate dysfunctional or risk patterns are clustered, and a judgement about the data is made. It is important to remember that not all conclusions resulting from data analysis lead to nursing diagnoses. Nursing diagnoses describe health states that nurses can legally diagnose and treat. Data may also point to health problems that nurses treat collaboratively with other health care professionals. During this phase of the nursing process, the nurse identifies nursing diagnoses as well as treatments that necessitate collaborative nursing intervention.

Nursing diagnostic statements are considered acceptable when written as two- or three-part statements. When written in three parts, the statement uses the problem–etiology–signs and symptoms (PES) format (Carpenito-Moyet, 2009; Gordon, 2010). A two-part statement is deemed acceptable if the signs and symptoms data are easily available to other nurses caring for the patient through the nursing history or progress notes. "Risk" nursing diagnoses are also two-part statements because signs and symptoms are not relevant. Use of a three-part statement is recommended during the learning process.

Problem (P): a brief statement of the patient's potential or actual health problem (e.g., pain)

Etiology (E): a brief description of the probable cause of the problem; contributing or related factors (e.g., related to surgical incision, localized pressure, edema)

Signs and symptoms (S): a list of the objective and subjective data cluster that leads the nurse to pinpoint the problem; critical, major, or minor defining characteristics (e.g., as manifested by verbalization of pain, isolation, withdrawal)

It is important to remember that gathering the "S" comes first in the diagnostic process, even though it is placed last in the PES format.

Identifying the Problem. The North American Classification of Nursing Diagnoses (NANDA-I, 2011) is one framework that is useful for formulating actual and at-risk nursing diagnoses. Clinically relevant cues are clustered into functional health patterns. (Gordon's [2010] 11 functional health patterns are discussed in Chapter 3.) The process of making a nursing diagnosis from clustered cues begins with the recognition of dysfunc-

tional patterns. Checking the definition of nursing diagnoses classified according to the functional pattern helps identify the appropriate label for the problem. Before final selection of any nursing diagnosis for the patient, the nurse verifies the diagnostic statement with the defining characteristics listed with the diagnosis (Carpenito-Moyet, 2009; Gordon, 2010; NANDA-I, 2011). The most accurate nursing diagnosis is based on the individual patient's data.

Etiology. The etiology underlying a nursing diagnosis is identified in the diagnostic statement. Taking time to properly link the problem with its etiology directs the nurse to the correct interventions. Interventions to manage the problem are planned by directing nursing efforts toward the etiology. The etiology can be a pathophysiological, maturational, situational, or treatment-related factor (Carpenito-Moyet, 2009). The etiology is written after the diagnostic label. These two components are separated by the phrase "related to." For example, in Nursing Care Plan (NCP) 1-1, the nursing diagnosis is "Activity intolerance *related to* fatigue secondary to cardiac insufficiency and pulmonary congestion." The etiology directs the nurse to select the appropriate interventions to modify the factor of fatigue. When the etiology is not included in the diagnosis, the nurse is not able to plan the correct intervention to treat the specific cause of the problem. When possible, the etiology should be validated with the patient. When the etiology is unknown, the statement reads "related to unknown etiology." When identifying risk-for nursing diagnoses, the specific risk factors present in the patient's situation are identified as the etiology.

Multiple etiologies become more common as expertise in the use of nursing diagnoses increases. There is often no single cause of a problem. Many nursing diagnoses presented in the nursing care plans of this book contain multiple etiologies. They can be

NURSING CARE PLAN

Heart Failure*	
NURSING DIAGNOSIS	***Activity intolerance*** *related to* fatigue secondary to cardiac insufficiency and pulmonary congestion *as evidenced by* dyspnea, shortness of breath, weakness, increase in heart rate on exertion, and patient's statement, "I feel too weak to do anything."

Expected Patient Outcomes	**Nursing Interventions and *Rationales***
• Achieves a realistic program of activity that balances physical activity with energy-conserving activities • Vital signs, O₂ saturation, and colour are within normal limits in response to activity	**Energy management** • Encourage alternate rest and activity periods *to reduce cardiac workload.* • Provide calming diversionary activities to promote relaxation *to reduce O₂ consumption and to relieve dyspnea and fatigue.* • Monitor patient's oxygen response (e.g., pulse rate, cardiac rhythm, colour, O₂ saturation, and respiratory rate) to self-care or nursing activities *to determine level of activity that can be performed.* • Teach patient and significant other techniques of self-care *to minimize oxygen consumption (e.g., self-monitoring and pacing techniques for performance of ADLs).* **Activity therapy** • Assist to choose activities consistent with physical, psychological, and social capabilities *to determine level of activity that can be performed.* • Collaborate with occupational, physical, and/or recreational therapists *to plan and monitor activity and exercise program.* • Determine patient's commitment to increasing frequency and/or range of activities *to provide patient with obtainable goals.*

ADLs, activities of daily living; *O₂,* oxygen.

*The complete nursing care plan for heart failure is provided in NCP 37-1 on pp. 943-944.

used as a checklist of possible related factors to be considered when determining the nursing diagnosis specific to an individual patient.

Signs and Symptoms. Signs and symptoms are the clinical cues that, in a cluster, point to the nursing diagnosis (NANDA-I, 2011). The signs and symptoms are often included in the diagnostic statement using the phrase "as evidenced by." The complete nursing diagnostic statement in NCP 1-1 is, "Activity intolerance *related to* fatigue secondary to cardiac insufficiency and pulmonary congestion *as evidenced by* dyspnea, shortness of breath, weakness, increase in heart rate on exertion, and patient's statement, 'I feel too weak to do anything.'"

Collaborative Problems

Collaborative problems are potential or actual complications of disease or of treatment that nurses manage together with other health care professionals (Carpenito-Moyet, 2009). A look at the primary goals of nursing helps in differentiating between nursing and medical diagnoses (see Table 1-3). During the diagnosis phase of the nursing process, the nurse identifies the risks for these physiological complications in addition to nursing diagnoses. Identification of collaborative problems requires knowledge of pathophysiology and possible complications of medical treatment. For example, collaborative problems for the patient with congestive heart failure in NCP 1-1 could include pulmonary edema, hypoxemia, dysrhythmias, and/or cardiogenic shock (Carpenito-Moyet, 2009). In the interdependent role, nurses use both physician-prescribed and nursing-prescribed interventions to prevent, detect, and manage collaborative problems.

Collaborative problem statements are usually written as "potential complication: _____" (e.g., potential complication: pulmonary edema) without a "related to" statement. When potential complications are used in this textbook, "related to" statements have been added to increase understanding and link the potential complication to possible causes.

Planning Phase

Priority Setting

After the nursing diagnoses and collaborative problems are identified, the nurse must determine the urgency of the identified problems. Diagnoses of the highest priority necessitate immediate intervention. Those of lower priority can be addressed at a later time. When setting priorities, the nurse should first intervene for life-threatening problems involving airway, breathing, or circulation issues.

Maslow's hierarchy of needs also acts as a useful guide in determining priorities. These needs include the physical, safety, love and belonging, esteem, and self-actualization (Maslow, 1954). Lower-level needs must be satisfied before a higher level can be attained.

Another guideline in setting priorities is to determine the patient's perception of what is important. When the patient's priorities are not congruent with the actual situation, the nurse may have to give explanations or do some teaching to help the patient understand the need to do one thing before another. Often it is more efficient to meet the patient's priority need before moving on to other priorities.

Identified priorities change as a patient's level of wellness fluctuates. For example, the patient's highest priority in the morning may be a need for information about diabetes mellitus because she is going home and must care for herself. During the teaching session, the patient shows signs of a hypoglycemic reaction. The nurse would interrupt the teaching session to provide a glass of orange juice to avoid a progression of the hypoglycemia to a dangerous level. In this instance, problems relating to risk may have a higher priority than existing (actual) problems.

Identifying Outcomes

After priorities are established, expected outcomes or goals for the patient are identified. *Outcomes* are simply the results of care. **Expected patient outcomes** are *goals* that articulate what is *desired or expected* as a result of care. The terms *goals* and *expected outcomes* are often used interchangeably: both terms describe the degree to which the patient's response, as identified in the nursing diagnosis, should be prevented or changed as a result of nursing care. Expected outcomes should be set with the patient, if feasible, just as priorities of interventions are considered with the patient when possible. Although the ultimate goal for the patient is to maintain or attain a state of dynamic equilibrium at the highest possible level of wellness, the setting of more specific expected outcomes, both short- and long-term, is necessary for systematic evaluation of the patient's progress. Expected patient outcomes identified in the planning stage specify the criteria to be used in the evaluation phase of the nursing process.

The nurse identifies both *long-term* and *short-term* goals by writing specific expected patient outcomes in terms of desired, realistic, measurable patient behaviours to be accomplished by a specific date. For example, a short-term expected outcome for the patient in NCP 1-1 might be, "The patient will maintain normal vital signs in response to activity in 2 days," whereas a long-term expected outcome might be, "The patient will identify a realistic activity level to achieve or maintain by discharge." These outcomes would be evaluated in 2 days and at discharge, and the care plan revised as necessary if the outcomes were not met. However, these statements are less than optimal because they provide no criteria by which to evaluate the patient's degree of progress from admission to discharge. Goals or expected outcomes vary in their degree of specificity; in addition, if the goal is not met, the nurse has no way of knowing how close or how far the patient was from achieving the goal.

Determining Interventions

After patient outcomes are identified, nursing interventions to accomplish the desired status of the patient should be planned. A **nursing intervention** is any treatment, based on clinical judgement and knowledge, that a nurse performs to enhance patient outcomes (Dochterman & Bulechek, 2008). Nursing interventions include both direct and indirect care; nurse-initiated treatments resulting from nursing diagnoses; physician-initiated treatments resulting from medical diagnoses; and daily, essential activities that the patient cannot perform independently (Table 1-8). When choosing an intervention, the nurse considers the following (Dochterman & Bulechek, 2008):
1. Desired patient outcomes
2. Characteristics of the nursing diagnosis
3. Research base associated with the intervention
4. Feasibility of successfully implementing the intervention
5. Acceptability to the patient
6. Capability of the nurse

Table 1-8 Examples of Nursing Activities to Treat Health Care Problems

INTERVENTION	NURSING ACTIVITIES
Nurse-initiated treatments	Encourage patient to cough and deep breathe
Physician-initiated treatments	Administer medications
Essential activity patient cannot perform independently	Provide range of motion exercise

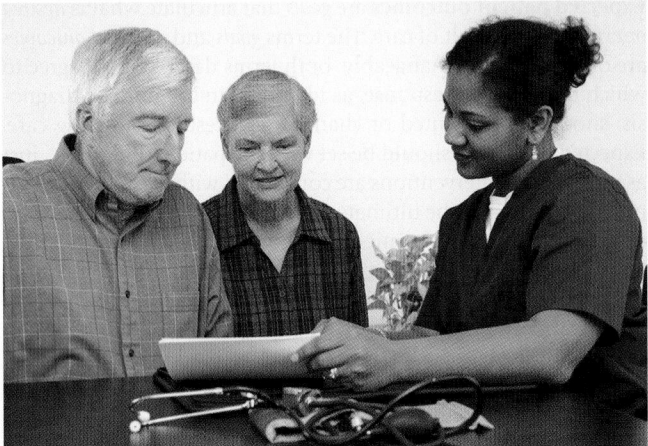

Figure 1-6 Cooperation between the patient and the nurse is necessary in setting goals.

Source: © 2011 JupiterImages Corporation.

Sound knowledge, good judgement, and decision-making ability are necessary to effectively choose the interventions that the nurse will use (Figure 1-6). Although many variables may influence outcomes, nursing interventions should always be chosen in light of their influence on the outcomes of care. In addition, the interventions that are selected should be directed toward altering the etiological factors of the nursing diagnoses. The nurse should foster the use of a research-based approach to interventions. Clinical nursing research that establishes a basis for EIP and that identifies the effectiveness of nursing interventions is being conducted and reported at an increasing rate. In the absence of a nursing research base, scientific principles from the behavioural and biological sciences should guide the selection of interventions.

In addition, the nurse must use ingenuity, intuition, creativity, and past experience when tailoring a plan to meet a patient's needs. Factors such as the availability of help, equipment, time, money, and other resources must also be considered. The nurse must also have the knowledge and skill to be able to carry out the interventions selected. In all cases, the wishes of the patient and the family must be given high priority. This can be challenging in cases in which the patient does not wish to pursue aggressive treatment and health care professionals believe this would be in the patient's best interest. The final selection of interventions remains the choice of the patient as long as the patient is mentally competent (discussed in Chapter 13). Furthermore, the patient or the patient's family often has a wealth of information about measures that were successful or unsuccessful in the past. Significant time and effort can be saved by asking the patient what has been tried and discarded as ineffective.

Implementation Phase

Carrying out the specific, individualized plan constitutes the implementation phase of the nursing process. The nurse performs the activities of interventions or may designate and supervise others who are qualified to intervene. Throughout the implementation phase, the nurse must evaluate the effectiveness of the method chosen to implement the plan. For example, the nurse may determine that the nursing assistant caring for a patient with a mastectomy should not continue to be the person who implements the patient's exercise plan. Perhaps the patient is more depressed than anticipated and would benefit from contact with a nurse who is knowledgeable about changes in body image and sensitive to patient cues that may indicate body image disturbance. The exercise plan might essentially remain the same, but the person implementing the plan would be different and would use different skills to carry out the plan. Referrals to other professionals may also be made when the nurse anticipates that expertise in specialized areas is required to help the patient.

Evaluation Phase

All phases of the nursing process must be evaluated (see Figure 1-4). Evaluation occurs after implementation of the plan but also continuously throughout the process. If evaluation is not carried out, we can have failed or ineffective interventions that are not changed appropriately to achieve desired outcomes.

The nurse evaluates whether sufficient assessment data have been obtained to allow a nursing diagnosis to be made. The diagnosis is, in turn, evaluated for accuracy. For example, was the pain actually related to the wound itself or to pressure from a constricting dressing?

Next the nurse evaluates, with the patient when possible, whether the expected patient outcomes and interventions are realistic and achievable. If not, a new plan should be formulated. This may involve revision of expected patient outcomes and interventions. Consideration must be given to whether the plan should be maintained, modified, totally revised, or discontinued in light of the patient's status.

The effectiveness of each intervention and its contribution to progress toward the expected patient outcome are also evaluated. In addition, the nurse considers whether a different method of implementation of the same plan will provide better results.

Nursing Care Plans

When the nurse has determined the nursing diagnoses, the outcomes, and the interventions for a patient, the plan must be recorded to ensure continuity of care by other nurses and health professionals. The plan should contain specific directions for carrying out the planned interventions, including how, when, for how long, how often, where, by whom, and with what resources the activities should be performed. For example, in NCP 1-1, the nurse may want to specify how the activity of "encourage alternate rest and activity periods" should be implemented—that the patient should rest for 30 minutes following bathing, eating, ambulating to the bathroom, or having visitors. The nurse may also want to specify who should monitor the patient's cardiorespiratory response to activity, what signs should be monitored, and when they should be monitored.

Various methods and formats are used to record the nursing care plan. One of the important factors influencing a choice of care plan format has to do with the frameworks used in a particular agency. Care plans are usually written on a specific form adopted by an institution, but they may also be entered electronically to organize nursing data. Such a computer program enables all nurses caring for the patient to easily print and update the plan as necessary. Every nurse who cares for the patient must be able to have access to the plan, whether handwritten or computer generated, to provide the planned care. The care plan is part of the patient's medical record and may be used in legal proceedings. The nurse must document the patient's nursing care requirements, changes that are made as the plan is implemented, and the outcomes of the nursing interventions. Not every activity that the nurse implements with the patient will be recorded on the care plan. Routine procedures, such as drug and intravenous fluid administration, assessment of vital signs, and other activities prescribed by institutional policies or protocols, may be documented on a variety of other forms.

Standardized care plans are sometimes used as guides for routine nursing care and as a basis for developing individualized care plans. When standardized care plans are used, they should be personalized and specific to the unique needs and problems of each patient.

Beginning in 2009, all nurses practicing in Quebec were required to develop and update "Therapeutic Nursing Plans (TNPs)." The TNP will be a compulsory and permanent part of the client's record.

Concept Maps

A concept map is an alternative method of recording a nursing care plan. In a concept map care plan, the nursing process is recorded in a visual diagram of patient problems and interventions that illustrates the relationships among clinical data. It is used primarily in nursing education to teach nursing process and care planning.

Various formats are used for concept maps, and a variety of shapes, colours, and connecting arrows are used to identify concepts and relationships. In one example, assessment data are used to identify the patient's primary reason for seeking health care. That health state (often a medical diagnosis) is positioned centrally on the map. Positioned around the reason for health care are nursing diagnoses that represent patient responses to the health state. Listed with each nursing diagnosis are the assessment data that support the nursing diagnosis. Diagnostic testing data, treatments, medications, and nursing interventions may be listed with the nursing diagnoses or may be identified in separate areas and connected to the nursing diagnoses with arrows. Figure 1-7 includes a simplified version of a concept map for the patient with heart failure to compare with the care plan format in NCP 1-1.

Clinical (Critical) Pathways

Care related to common health problems experienced by many patients is delineated using clinical (critical) pathways. A **clinical** (critical) **pathway** directs the entire health care team in the daily care goals for select health care problems. It includes a nursing care plan, specific interventions for each day of hospitalization, and a documentation tool.

The clinical pathway organizes and sequences the caregiving process at the patient level to better achieve desired quality and cost outcomes. It is a cyclical process organized for specific case types by all related health care departments. The case types selected for clinical pathways are usually those that occur in high volume and are highly predictable, such as myocardial infarction, stroke, and angina.

The clinical pathway describes the patient care required at specific times in the treatment. A multidisciplinary approach moves the patient toward desired outcomes within an estimated length of stay. The exact content and format of clinical pathways vary among institutions.

Documentation

It is critical that the patient's progress be documented in a systematic way. Proper documentation enables safe and effective patient care. Patient records are also frequently used as evidence when there are legal issues related to negligence and competency. Nurses in Canada should be aware of the Canadian Nurses Protective Society (CNPS). This is the agency that provides liability coverage and is a source of information and education on issues such as documentation and charting.

Many documentation methods and formats are used, depending on personal preference, agency policy, and regulatory standards. Many provinces are now moving to implement electronic health records. Funding and support is available through organizations such as the Canada Health Infoway. Patient progress may be documented by nurses with the use of flow sheets, narrative notes, subjective–objective–assessment–plan (SOAP) charting (described below), clinical pathways, and computer-based charting. Every method or combination of methods is designed to document the assessment of patient status, the implementation of interventions, and the outcome of interventions.

Problem Lists

A multidisciplinary problem list is often developed for each patient. Nurses, physicians, social workers, dietitians, and other health care professionals are encouraged to contribute to the list. Nurses can easily use the problem list as a basis for identifying nursing diagnoses. For example, if one of the identified problems on the list for a patient with a stroke is hemiparesis, appropriate nursing diagnoses for the nurse to consider may be risk for impaired skin integrity and impaired physical mobility.

The problem list is an inherent component of the problem-oriented record, a multidisciplinary patient documentation method. A prescribed method of charting, called SOAP charting, is used with this record.

SOAP Charting

There are several methods of documentation that address the nursing process. The SOAP method is a common way of evaluating and recording patient progress. Some institutions add an I and E and R (i.e., SOAPIER). The "I" stands for *intervention*, the "E" for *evaluation*, and the "R" for *revision* of plan. A SOAP or SOAPIER progress note is problem specific and incorporates the

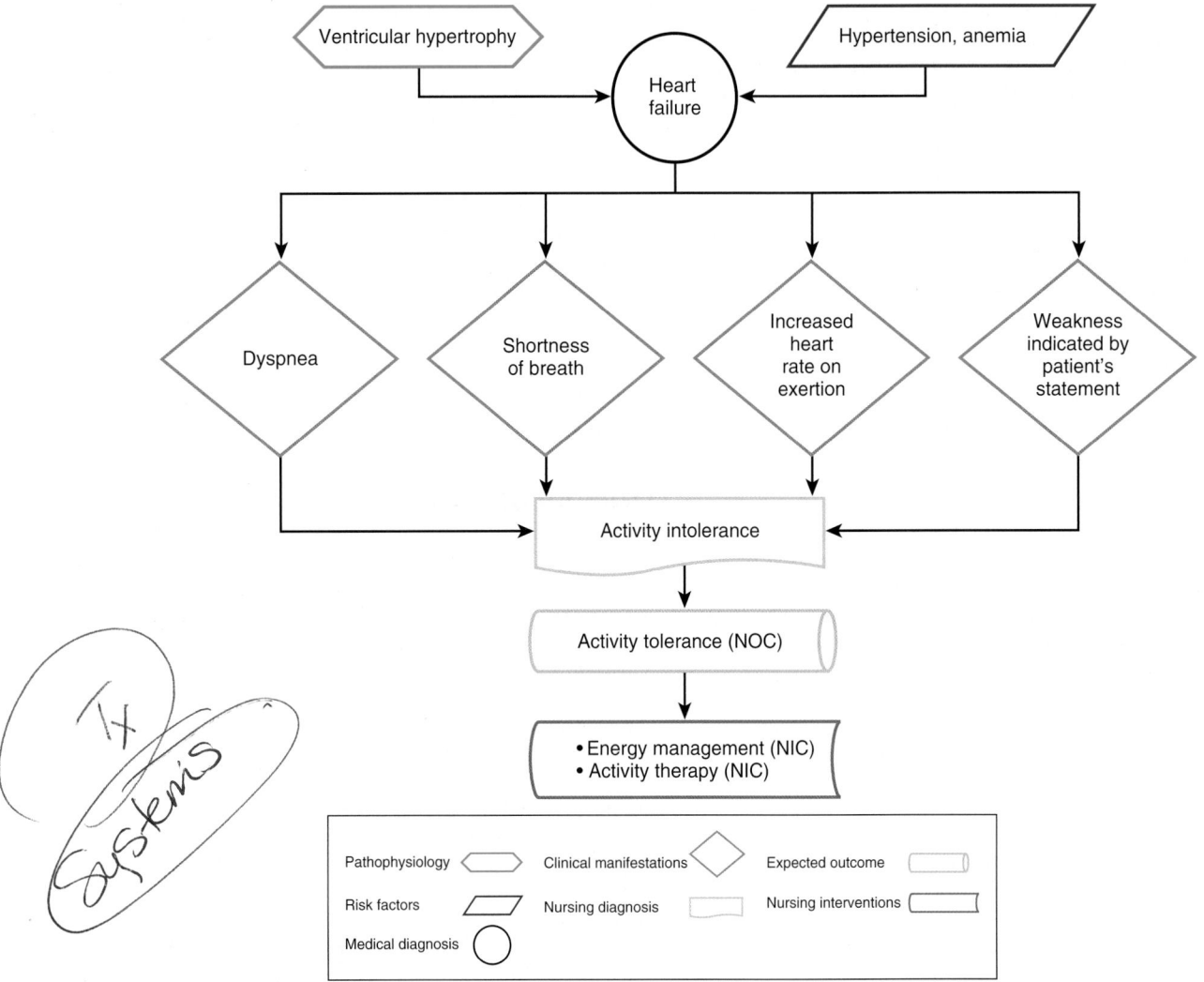

Figure 1-7 Concept map.

elements in Table 1-9. Because the problem list and the record are multidisciplinary, data associated with any identified problem may be recorded by any health care professional. In some institutions, however, nurses write SOAP notes in reference to a list of nursing diagnoses. The following is the process of SOAP documentation:

1. Additional subjective and objective data are gathered related to the area of concern.
2. Based on old and new data, an assessment of the patient's progress toward the expected patient outcome and the effectiveness of each intervention is made.
3. Based on the reassessment of the situation, the initial plan is maintained, revised, or discontinued.

The following is an example of SOAP charting for the nursing diagnosis "risk for infection *related to* traumatized tissue secondary to surgery":

S: Wound is more painful today
O: Temperature of 39.4°C, facial grimacing in response to movement, dressing saturated with purulent drainage
A: Risk for wound infection
P: Notify surgeon, take temperature q2h, reinforce dressing.

Table 1-9 Components of a SOAP Progress Note	
SOAP	**EXPLANATION**
Subjective (S)	Information supplied by patient or knowledgeable other
Objective (O)	Information obtained by nurse directly by observation or measurement, from patient records, or through diagnostic studies
Assessment (A)	Nursing diagnosis or problem based on subjective and objective data
Plan (P)	Specific interventions related to a diagnostic or problem considering diagnostic, therapeutic, and patient education needs

A second method of documentation is the PIE method, which is similar to SOAP charting and is also problem oriented. It does not include assessment data because those are recorded on flow sheets. PIE stands for P—problem, I—intervention, and E—evaluation.

A third documentation format is called DAR progress notes, and this format includes D—data (both subjective and objective), A—action or nursing intervention, and R—response of the patient. It is also called focus charting, and it addresses patient concerns, not just problems.

Charting by exception (CBE) is another method of documentation that focuses on documenting deviations from predefined normal findings. Assessments are standardized on flow sheets, and nurses make a narrative note only when there are exceptions to the standardized statements.

Electronic Health Records (EHR)

Many agencies have adopted electronic documentation. Electronic health records (EHRs) and the Canadian Health Outcomes for Better Information and Care (C-HOBIC) project are examples of electronic collection of health care data, and they are in the process of being implemented across different parts of Canada. An EHR is a complete health record under the custodianship of a health care professional that holds all relevant health information about a person over her or his lifetime (Hodge, 2011). The EHR integrates the output of a number of information systems. Several projects are under way across Canada to develop systems that form the essential building blocks of an EHR, such as digital imaging, summaries of drug prescriptions, and laboratory test results. Provinces and territories across Canada are working together with Canada Health Infoway to accelerate the development of these systems. C-HOBIC is working to develop a strategy for the collection of standardized patient outcome data related to nursing care in EHRs in Saskatchewan and Manitoba (C-HOBIC, 2010). This project introduces a systematic, structured language for admission and discharge assessment of patients receiving acute care, complex continuing care, long-term care, or home care. Data on the following outcomes will be collected: functional status, therapeutic self-care (readiness for discharge), symptom management (e.g., pain, nausea, fatigue, dyspnea), safety (falls, pressure ulcers), and patient satisfaction with nursing care (C-HOBIC, 2010). C-HOBIC will provide real-time information to nurses about how patients are benefitting from care, as well as collecting nursing-related outcomes that provide valuable information about preparing patients for discharge.

Future Challenges of Nursing

Nursing roles continually evolve as our society changes and we learn to integrate new knowledge and technology into current practices. Although nursing is defined in different ways, past and current definitions of nursing have commonalities of health, illness, and caring. It is important that these concepts are addressed in nursing education as greater demands are placed on the profession. Future nursing practice will continue to call for the use of reasoning, analytic thinking skills, and synthesis of rapidly expanding knowledge to assist others to maintain or attain optimal health.

An increasing emphasis on leadership, accountability, courage and persistence, innovation and risk taking, and decision making is essential if nursing is to "get somewhere else." **Nursing leadership** does not refer to only those holding certain positions but also to an attitude and approach that values lifelong learning and a commitment to excellence in practice. In its attempt to keep pace, nursing would do well to remember what the Queen in *Through the Looking Glass* said to Alice: "Now here, you see, it takes all the running you can do to keep in the same place. If you want to get somewhere else, you must run at least twice as fast as that" (Carroll, 1973). This appears to be the future of nursing. Nursing leaders must ask some fundamental questions about what the contribution of nurses must be for the twenty-first century. We must increasingly challenge the status quo by relying on research and the wisdom that comes from asking difficult questions. Nurse–leaders must have an attitude of open-mindedness while remaining grounded in values that overcome the tendency to promote self-interest.

REVIEW QUESTIONS

The number of the question corresponds to the same-numbered objective at the beginning of the chapter.

1. Which of the following is an example of a nursing activity that reflects the Canadian Nurses Association's definition of nursing?
   a. Establishing that the patient with jaundice has hepatitis
   b. Determining the cause of hemorrhage in a postoperative patient based on vital signs
   c. Identifying and treating dysrhythmias that occur in a patient in the coronary care unit
   d. Diagnosing that a patient with pneumonia cannot effectively cough up pulmonary secretions
2. Paid workers who meet certain requirements that allow them to use a specific title and to undertake a specific type of work are referred to as which of the following?
   a. Allied health professionals
   b. Regulated health professionals
   c. Personal support workers
   d. Unregulated health care professionals

3. When a nurse makes an error in practice, what is it important to understand?
   a. She will be blamed for the mistake.
   b. System factors usually contribute to the error.
   c. Her knowledge of evidence-informed practice is inadequate.
   d. She has violated standards of practice.
4. Ensuring the right service is provided at the right time, in the right place, and by the right care provider is known as which of the following?
   a. Patient-centred care
   b. Interprofessional collaboration
   c. Access
   d. A population health approach
5. Medical-surgical nurses do which of the following?
   a. Provide care in acute care hospital settings only
   b. Are required to be certified by the Canadian Nurses Association in this specialty
   c. Address the needs of acutely ill adults and their families
   d. Primarily care for perioperative patients

6. Which of the following is most appropriate to demonstrate the nurse's implementation of evidence-informed practice?
   a. The nurse requires the use of clinical practice guidelines developed by national health agencies.
   b. The nurse uses only findings from randomized clinical trials to plan care for all patient problems.
   c. The nurse uses clinical decision making and judgement to determine what evidence is appropriate for a specific clinical situation.
   d. The nurse statistically analyzes the relationship of nursing interventions to patient outcomes to establish evidence that interventions are appropriate for the patient.

7. "In adults older than age 60 with chronic obstructive pulmonary disease, is structured pulmonary rehabilitation more effective than classroom instruction in reducing the incidence of exacerbation?" In this question, what is the outcome of interest?
   a. Adults older than age 60
   b. Adults with chronic obstructive pulmonary disease
   c. Structured pulmonary rehabilitation
   d. Reduced incidence of exacerbation

8. When the nurse determines that the patient's anxiety must be relieved before effective teaching can be implemented, which phase of the nursing process is being used?
   a. Assessment
   b. Diagnosis
   c. Planning
   d. Evaluation

9. Which of the following is an example of an independent nursing intervention?
   a. Administering blood infusion
   b. Starting an intravenous fluid
   c. Teaching a patient about the effects of prescribed drugs
   d. Administering emergency drugs according to institutional protocols

10. The nurse identifies the nursing diagnosis of *constipation related to laxative misuse* for a patient. What is the most appropriate expected patient outcome related to this nursing diagnosis?
    a. The patient will stop the use of laxatives.
    b. The patient ingests adequate fluid and fibre.
    c. The patient passes normal stools without aids.
    d. The patient's stool is free of blood and mucus.

ANSWERS: 1. d; 2. b; 3. b; 4. c; 5. c; 6. c; 7. d; 8. c; 9. c; 10. c.

REFERENCES

Alfaro-LeFevre, R. (2009). *Critical thinking and clinical judgment* (4th ed.). St. Louis: Saunders.

Baker, G. R., Norton, P. G., Flintoft, V., Blais, R., Brown, A., Cox, J., ..., Tamblyn, R. (2004). The Canadian Adverse Events Study: The incidence of adverse events among hospital patients in Canada. *CMAJ, 170*(11), 1678–1686. doi:10.1503/cmaj.1040498

Bassendowski, S. (Spring 2011). What is your favourite nursing app? *Canadian Journal of Nursing Informatics 6*(2), Technology in Education Column.

Benner, P. E., Tanner, C. A. & Chesla, C. A. (2009). *Expertise in nursing in nursing practice: caring, clinical judgment and ethics.* New York: Springer.

Canadian Association for Retired Persons. (2011). *The most important policy issue.* Retrieved from http://www.carp.ca/2011/09/08/the-most-important-policy-issue-a-k-a-welcome-to-the-twilight-zone/

Canadian Association of Medical and Surgical Nurses. (2012). *About CAMSN.* Retrieved from http://www.medsurgnurse.ca/

Canadian Health Coalition. (2011). *Health accord.* Retrieved from http://healthcoalition.ca/main/issues/health-accord/

Canadian Health Outcomes for Better Information and Care (C-HOBIC). (2010). *About C-HOBIC.* Retrieved from http://www.cna-aiic.ca/c-hobic/about/default_e.aspx

Canadian Institute of Health Information. (2001). *Canada's health care providers.* Retrieved from http://secure.cihi.ca/cihiweb/products/hctenglish.pdf

Canadian Nurses Association. (2002). *Discussion guide for the unique contribution of the registered nurse.* Ottawa: Author. Retrieved from http://www2.cna-aiic.ca/CNA/documents/pdf/publications/unique_role_rn_e.pdf

Canadian Nurses Association (CNA). (2007). *Framework for the practice of registered nurses in Canada.* Retrieved from www2.cna-aiic.ca/CNA/documents/pdf/publications/RN_Framework_Practice_2007_e.pdf

Canadian Nurses Association. (2008). *Advanced nursing practice: A national framework.* Retrieved from http://www2.cna-aiic.ca/CNA/.../pdf/.../ANP_National_Framework_e.pdf

Canadian Nurses Association. (2009). *Medical-surgical nursing certification: Exam blueprint and specialty competencies.* Retrieved from http://www.cna-nurses.ca/CNA/nursing/certification/specialties/default_e.aspx

Canadian Nurses Association (CNA). (2010). *Position statement: Evidence-informed decision-making and nursing practice.* Retrieved from http://www2.cna-aiic.ca/CNA/documents/pdf/publications/PS113_Evidence_informed_2010_e.pdf

Canadian Nurses Association. (2011a). *National expert commission.* Retrieved from http://www.cna-nurses.ca/CNA/about/nec/why/default_e.aspx

Canadian Nurses Association. (2011b). *Standards and best practices.* Retrieved from http://www.cna-aiic.ca/CNA/practice/standards/default_e.aspx

Canadian Nurses Association. (2011c). *Position statement: Interprofessional collaboration.* Retrieved from http://www2.cna-aiic.ca/CNA/documents/pdf/publications/PS117_Interprofessional_Collaboration_2011_e.pdf

Canadian Nurses Association & Canadian Association of Schools of Nursing. (2004). *Joint position statement: Promoting continuing competence for registered nurses.* Retrieved from http://www2.cna-aiic.ca/CNA/documents/pdf/publications/PS77_promoting_competence_e.pdf

Canadian Patient Safety Institute. (2008). *Canadian disclosure guidelines.* Retrieved from http://www.patientsafetyinstitute.ca/English/toolsResources/disclosure/Documents/CPSI%20Canadian%20Disclosure%20Guidelines.pdf

Carpenito-Moyet, L. J. (2009). *Handbook of nursing diagnosis* (13th ed.). Philadelphia: Lippincott.

Carroll, L. (1973). *Alice's adventures in wonderland and through the looking glass.* New York: Collier.

College and Association of Registered Nurses of Alberta (CARNA). (2006). *Entry to practice competencies for the registered nurses profession.* Retrieved from http://www.nurses.ab.ca/carna.../Entry-to-Practice%20Competencies.pdf

College of Registered Nurses of Nova Scotia. (2004). *Standards for nursing practice.* Retrieved from http://www.crnns.ca/documents/standards2004.pdf

Commission on the Future of Health Care in Canada. (2002). *Romanow report proposes sweeping changes to Medicare.* Retrieved from *http://catalogue.iugm.qc.ca/GEIDEFile/Hcc_News_Release.PDF?Archive=191030291921&File=HCC_News_Release_PDF*

Dagnone, T. (2009). *For patient's sake: Commissioner's recommendations.* Retrieved from *http://www.health.gov.sk.ca/patient-first-review*

DiCenso, A., Guyatt, G., & Ciliska, D. (2005). *Evidence-based nursing: A guide to clinical practice.* St. Louis: Mosby.

Dochterman, J., & Bulechek, G. (2008). *Nursing interventions classification (NIC)* (5th ed.). St. Louis: Mosby.

Fyke, K. (2001). *Medicare: Commission on Medicare final report.* Retrieved from *http://www.publications.gov.sk.ca/details.cfm?p=12038*

Gordon, M. (2010). *Manual of nursing diagnosis* (12th ed.). Boston: Jones & Bartlett.

Health Canada. (2011). *Canada's health care system.* Retrieved from *http://www.hc-sc.gc.ca/hcs-sss/pubs/system-regime/2011-hcs-sss/index-eng.php*

Hodge, R. (2011). *EMR, EHR, and PHR—Why all the confusion?* Retrieved from *http://infowayconnects.infoway-inforoute.ca/blog/electronic-health-records/374-emr-ehr-and-phr-%E2%80%93-why-all-the-confusion/*

Lewis, S. (2009). *Patient-centred care: An introduction to what it is and how to achieve it.* Retrieved from *http://www.changefoundation.ca/docs/patient-centred-care-intro.pdf*

Maslow, A. (1954). *Motivation and personality.* New York: Harper & Row.

NANDA International. (2011). *NANDA nursing diagnoses: Definitions and classification 2012–2014.* Philadelphia: Author.

Pan-Canadian Committee on Unregulated Health Workers. (2009). *Valuing unregulated health workers: Highlights of the 2009 Pan-Canadian Symposium.* Retrieved from *http://www.cna-aiic.ca/cna/documents/pdf/publications/UHW_Final_Report_e.pdf*

Paul, R., & Elder, L. (2006). *The miniature guide to critical thinking: Concepts and tools* (4th ed.). Dillon Beach, CA: Foundation for Critical Thinking.

Premier's Advisory Council on Health for Alberta. (2002). *A framework for reform. Government of Alberta.* Retrieved from *http://www.health.alberta.ca/documents/Mazankowski-Report-2001.pdf*

Registered Nurses' Association of Ontario (RNAO). (2006). *Healthy work environments: Best practice guidelines: Developing and sustaining nursing leadership.* Toronto: Author. Retrieved from *http://www.rnao.org/Storage/16/1067_BPG_Sustain_Leadership.pdf*

Registered Nurses' Association of Ontario (RNAO). (2012). *Faculty eHealth resource.* Retrieved from *http://rnao.ca/ehealth/facultyresource*

Robinson, J. H., Callister, L. C., Berry, J. A., & Dearing, K. A. (2008). *Patient-centred care and adherence: Definitions and applications to improve outcomes. Journal of the American Academy of Nurse Practitioners 20,* 600–607. doi:10.1111/j.1745-7599.2008.00360.x

Standing Committee on Social Affairs, Science and Technology. (2002). *The health of Canadians—The federal role. Final Report. Volume 6.* Retrieved from *http://www.parl.gc.ca/Content/SEN/Committee/372/soci/rep/repoct02vol6-e.htm*

Wilkinson, J. (2006). *Nursing process and critical thinking* (4th ed.). Upper Saddle River, NJ: Prentice Hall.

World Health Organization. (2011). *What is patient safety?* Retrieved from *http://www.who.int/patientsafety/education/curriculum/PSP_MPC_topic-01.pdf*

CANADIAN RESOURCES

Canadian Association of Schools of Nursing (CASN)
http://www.casn.ca

Canada Health Infoway
https://www.infoway-inforoute.ca/

Canadian Health Outcomes for Better Information and Care (C-HOBIC) Project
http://www.cna-aiic.ca/c-hobic/about/default_e.aspx

Canadian Nurses Association (CNA)
http://www.cna-nurses.ca

Canadian Nurses Protective Society
http://www.cnps.ca/

Canadian Nursing Informatics Association
http://cnia.ca/

Canadian Patient Safety Institute
http://patientsafetyinstitute.ca

Registered Nurses' Association of Ontario (RNAO)
http://www.rnao.org/bestpractices

Nurse One
http://www.nurseone.ca

RELATED RESOURCES

North American Nursing Diagnosis Association International (NANDA-I)
http://www.nanda.org/

Sigma Theta Tau International (STT)
http://www.nursingsociety.org

ⓔvolve *For additional Internet resources, see the Web site for this book at* **http://evolve.elsevier.com/Canada/Lewis/medsurg**

Cultural Competence and Health Equity in Nursing Care

Written by Rani H. Srivastava

LEARNING OBJECTIVES

1. Define the terms *culture, cultural competence, cultural safety, ethnocentrism, cultural imposition, world view, health literacy,* and *health equity.*
2. Identify the determinants of health and health inequities for Aboriginal populations.
3. Describe the factors that lead to health inequities in culturally diverse populations.
4. Explain the links between cultural competence, patient safety, and patient-/family-centred care.
5. Describe strategies for successfully communicating with a person with limited English proficiency.
6. Examine ways that a nurse's own cultural background may influence how that nurse delivers nursing care.
7. Describe strategies for demonstrating cultural competence and promoting health equity in care encounters.
8. Identify the benefits and challenges associated with a diverse workforce.

KEY TERMS

acculturation Modification of one culture as a result of contact with another culture, p. 24

assimilation Generally a one-way process in which people lose their own cultural identity as they gradually adopt and incorporate characteristics of the dominant cultural group, p. 25

cultural competence The application of knowledge, attitudes, and skills that enhance cross-cultural communication and foster meaningful, respectful interactions with others, p. 25

cultural imposition Imposition of one person's own cultural beliefs and practices, intentionally or unintentionally, on another person or group of people, p. 24

cultural safety Cultural safety analyzes power imbalances, institutional discrimination, colonization, and colonial relationships as they apply to health care and health education, p. 23

culture A way of life characterized by dimensions such as ethnicity, language, religion, sex, socioeconomic class, professional status, age, sexual orientation, group history, and life experiences, p. 24

determinants of health Factors that influence the health of individuals and groups, p. 22

diversity Presence of persons with differences from the majority or dominant group that is assumed to be the norm, p. 25

ethnicity The common social, cultural, linguistic, or religious heritage of a group of people, p. 25

ethnocentrism A tendency of individuals to believe that their way of viewing and responding to the world is the most correct, natural, and superior one, p. 24

explanatory model Set of beliefs regarding what causes the disease or illness and the potential methods that would best treat the condition, p. 26

health disparity The differential burden of diseases, death, and morbidity in ethnic and racial minority groups in comparison with that in nonminority groups, p. 22

health equity The belief that all people—regardless of age, gender, ethnic, or socioeconomic status—have an equal opportunity to develop and maintain health through fair and just access to resources for health, p. 22

health inequity The presence of systematic disparities in health between social groups who have different levels of underlying social advantage or disadvantage that lead to differences in health that are unnecessary, avoidable, unfair, and unjust, p. 22

health literacy Ability to access, understand, and act on information for health, p. 22

race A group characterized by specific biological traits, including skin colour and skeletal hallmarks, p. 25

racialization Social processes that lead to designation of certain groups as different from the dominant groups, on which basis members of the "different" groups are subjected to differential treatment, including unequal access to opportunities, marginalization, and exclusion from services, p. 25

stereotyping The assumption that members of a specific culture, race, or ethnic group automatically have certain characteristics, without further exploration of what they are actually like, p. 25

values The sets of rules by which individuals, families, groups, and communities live, p. 24

world view The way in which people perceive, interpret, and relate to the world around us, p. 24

ELECTRONIC RESOURCES

Supplemental content related to Chapter 2 can be found ...

Evolve Web Site ⊝volve

http://evolve.elsevier.com/Canada/Lewis/medsurg
- Answer Guidelines for Case Study on p. 34
- Clinical Reference: Laboratory Values

- Content Updates
- Electronic Calculators
- Examination Review Questions
- Glossary
- Key Points (Printable and MP3 Download)

The Need for Cultural Competence

By virtue of its First Nations and immigration heritage, Canadian society has been described as a kaleidoscope of cultures, languages, and nationalities. In today's increasingly multicultural environment, nurses come in contact with individuals from many different cultures, as patients and as colleagues, during their professional careers. This diversity can be enriching and can lead to challenges in providing quality care. The changing demographic and cultural composition of Canada and other countries requires that all health care providers understand the influence of culture on health beliefs, practices, and outcomes. This is particularly true for nurses, given the commitment to holistic, patient-centred, and family-centred care. Culture influences individual beliefs about health, illness, care, cure, and even expectations of health care professionals. Understanding these differences is crucial for providing care that is safe, meaningful, and effective for the patient.

Canadian society is generally regarded as an ethnocultural mosaic. Immigration has been and continues to be a significant factor in shaping the social landscape. However, since the 1950s, the immigration patterns have shifted dramatically. Before 1961, 90% of the immigrants to Canada came from Europe and only 3% were Asian-born. By 2006, immigrants born in Asia (including the Middle East) made up 58% of all newcomers to Canada (Statistics Canada, 2008a), and nearly 20% of the Canadian population, or one per five persons, was "foreign-born" (a Statistics Canada term). Since Statistics Canada's definition of foreign-born population does not include nonpermanent residents such as students, individuals with work permits, or refugee claimants, the actual proportion of newcomers to Canadian society is probably higher. According to estimates of Statistics Canada (2011), the proportion of newcomers would reach at least 25% by 2013. Because of the high proportion of newcomers who are also members of visible minorities, this demographic statistic has also increased significantly and continues to grow at a rate that is five times higher than that of the general population growth. The largest visible minority groups in 2006 were South Asian, Chinese,

and Black populations. There is also considerable diversity within the groups. For example, of the Black population, although the majority (52%) are from the Caribbean, the origins of other Black Canadians include various countries in Africa, the British Isles, Canada, and France (Statistics Canada, 2007, 2008a).

Increasing variation in immigrants' countries of origin is also increasing linguistic diversity; 70% of Canadian immigrants report a first language other than English or French (Statistics Canada, 2008a). Of the nearly 150 languages reported as first language, the most frequent was Chinese, followed by Italian, Punjabi, Spanish, German, Tagalog, and Arabic (Statistics Canada, 2008a). These changing demographics lead to new challenges and opportunities in providing health care to a multiethnic population. However, newcomer status is only one marker of cultural diversity. Many visible minority communities have been in Canada for several generations, but they continue to experience racism and health inequities. It must be noted that the term *visible minority* is used by Statistics Canada to refer to people who are nonwhite in race and nonwhite in colour. Many groups may not be visibly distinct but experience discrimination and marginalization on the basis of other identities such as socioeconomic status, sexual orientation, language ability, and physical abilities. Understanding these groups as racialized, regardless of their skin colour, underscores the importance of race and racism as social constructs that expose individuals and groups to inequities. Aboriginal people are the indigenous inhabitants of Canada, but they are not part of the dominant Canadian cultural group; instead, they are considered a minority group and experience many of the challenges faced by newcomers with regard to language and cultural beliefs in accessing health care.*

---

*Use of the term *multiculturalism* is not an acknowledgement of the historical realities of colonization and discrimination that led to social, psychological, and cultural crises in the Aboriginal population and the government's responsibility for it. The need for cultural competence cuts across Aboriginal and non-Aboriginal populations; however, including Aboriginal culture in the wider cultural mix of Canadian society marginalizes the historical legacy of power and repression and the specific self-determination claims of Aboriginal people (Brascoupé & Waters, 2009).

In 2006, the number of people who identified themselves as Aboriginal persons (First Nations people, Métis, and Inuit) surpassed one million and represented 5.4% of the country's total population (Statistics Canada, 2008a; 2008b). Although most Aboriginal people lived in Ontario and the western provinces, this population is increasing across the country and is becoming increasingly urban.

As a result of continuously changing demographics, cultural competence is now recognized as an entry to practice level competency for registered nurses in Canada (Canadian Nurses Association, 2010). However, the dominant ethnocultural heritage in Canadian society is European ancestry, and the dominant language continues to be English, with French predominating only in selected parts of the country. This perspective frames and influences the cultural values of Canadian social systems, including health care, and is the context in which nurses apply their cultural competency skills to ensure high-quality, equitable care for all patients.

Culture as a Determinant of Health

The **determinants of health** are the factors that influence the health of individuals and groups (see Figure 2-1). The primary factors that shape the health of Canadians are not medical treatments or lifestyle choices but rather the living conditions (the economic, social, and political) that they experience (Mikkonen & Raphael, 2010, p. 7; Provincial Health Services Authority, 2011).

These determinants can either improve a person's health status or heighten an individual's risk for disease, injury, and illness. The challenges or advantage may be specific to the individual, or they may be structural and include factors such as income and social status; social support networks; education and literacy; employment/working conditions; social environments; physical environments; personal health practices and coping skills; healthy child development; biology and genetic endowment; gender; and culture and health services, including access,

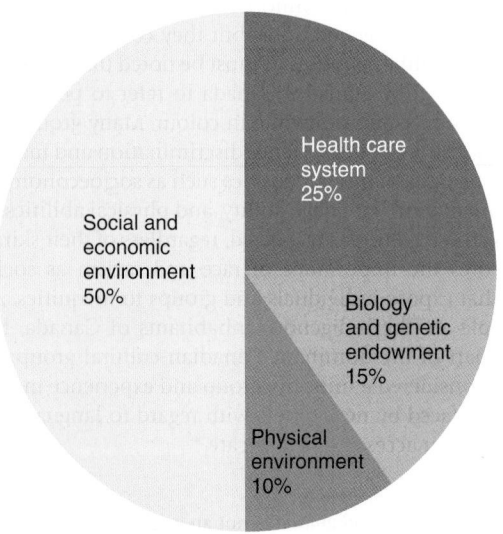

Figure 2-1 Estimated effect of determinants of health on the health status of the population.

Source: Kirby, M. J. L. [2002]. Healthy public policy: Health beyond health care. In *The health of Canadians—The federal role: Final report*, Vol. 6: *Recommendations for reform* [Chapter 13]. Retrieved from *http://www.parl.gc.ca/Content/SEN/Committee/372/SOCI/rep/repoct02vol6part5-e.htm#CHAPTER THIRTEEN*. Reprinted with permission.

focus, and health professional bias (Public Health Agency of Canada, 2003). Because these factors interact with each other, the overall effect can be one of multiple exclusions that are beyond individual control and that lead to compounded adverse effects on health and well-being (Health Nexus and Ontario Chronic Disease Prevention Alliance, 2008).

A **health disparity** is a difference in health status among groups. The term is often used interchangeably with **health inequity.** Health disparities can exist in health outcomes and in health care quality. Disparities in health care outcomes refer to the differential burden of diseases, death, and morbidity in ethnic and racial minority groups in comparison with that of the dominant cultural group. Disparities in health care quality refer to the perceptions of lower-quality care provided to nondominant populations, as a result of factors such as bias and discrimination (Srivastava, 2007b).

Health equity can be defined as "the absence of unfair and avoidable or remediable differences in health among populations or groups defined socially, economically, demographically or geographically" (Solar & Irvin, 2007, p. 7). Health equity is concerned with creating equal opportunities for good health for everyone by decreasing the effect of the social determinants of health and by improving services to enhance access and reduce exclusion. Inequities in health systematically put groups of people who are already socially disadvantaged (because of socioeconomic status, sex, or membership in a minority racial, ethnic, or religious group) at further disadvantage with regard to health. Table 2-1 provides some examples of social and health inequities experienced by marginalized populations, identified through a variety of studies.

The growing evidence of health inequities across a variety of groups is challenging previous assumptions about how to provide quality health care for all in the context of a diverse society. Without cultural competence, patients, families, and communities are at risk for a lack of care or for receiving care that is ineffective or unsafe. Thus cultural competence and health equity are increasingly being seen as fundamental issues of patient safety and quality care, not just as a means to support particular groups within society. Figure 2-2 presents a framework for conceptualizing equity in health care.

As noted in Figure 2-2, equity in health care comprises three dimensions: availability of services, accessibility of services, and acceptability of services. Health literacy and cultural competency are regarded as key components underlying the availability, accessibility, and acceptability of the health system (Provincial Health Services Authority, 2011). **Health literacy** is the extent to which individuals are able to access, understand, and use health information and services. Evidence suggests that nearly 60% of Canadians lack skills to adequately manage their own health (Canadian Council on Learning, 2008). This figure is likely to be higher in the three most vulnerable populations: older adults, immigrants, and unemployed persons. Poor health literacy has been associated with increased prevalence of diabetes, high blood pressure, and poor self-reported health status (Canadian Council on Learning, 2008). The concept also applies to health care systems. Organizations that offer health services share the responsibility for promoting health literacy. Nurses and other health care providers can enhance health literacy by providing services that are accessible and free from discrimination and prejudice and by communicating in ways that facilitate understanding and empower individuals and communities to make informed choices that are relevant and effective. (Health literacy is discussed further in Chapter 4).

Table 2-1 Examples of Health Inequities Experienced by Marginalized Populations

- Aboriginal adults are more than twice as likely to smoke cigarettes as are other adults in Canada. The implications of such high levels of smoking for lung and other kinds of cancers, and for breathing problems, are serious. (Loppie & Wien, 2009)

- Aboriginal Canadians, Canadians of nondominant races, recent immigrants, women, and people with disabilities are especially likely to experience social exclusion. Marginalization and exclusion of individuals and communities from mainstream society constitute a primary factor leading to adult-onset diabetes and a range of other chronic diseases such as respiratory and cardiovascular disease. (Mikkonen & Raphael, 2010)

- The overall suicide rate among First Nation communities is about twice that of the total Canadian population; the rate among Inuit is still higher: 6 to 11 times higher than that among the general population. (Kirmayer, Brass, Holton, Paul, Simpson, & Tait, 2007)

- Aboriginal youth on reserves are five to six times more likely to die of suicide than are their peers in the general population. (Kirmayer et al., 2007)

- Canadians with below-average incomes are three times less likely to fill a prescription because of cost and are 60% less able to obtain a needed test or treatment than are Canadians with above-average incomes. (Bierman et al., 2009)

- Individuals from lower-income neighbourhoods undergo screening for breast, cervical, and colorectal cancer at consistently lower rates than do individuals living in higher income neighbourhoods. (Bierman et al., 2009)

- Disparities faced by the lesbian, gay, bisexual, and transgendered (LGBT) community include less access to insurance and health care services, such as preventive care (e.g., cancer screenings); poorer overall health status; higher rates of smoking, alcohol, and substance abuse; higher risk for mental illnesses such as anxiety and depression; higher rates of sexually transmitted infections, including human immunodeficiency virus (HIV) infection and increased incidence of some cancers (The Joint Commission & The California Endowment, 2011)

- Recent immigrants (less than 5 years in Canada) are less likely to have a primary care physician than are immigrants who have been in the country for 10 or more years and Canadian-born respondents. (Bierman et al., 2009)

Sources: Bierman, A. S., Ahmad, F., Angus, J., Glazier, R. H., Vahabi, M., Damba, C., ... Manuel, D. (2009). Burden of illness. In A. S. Bierman (Ed.), *Project for an Ontario women's health evidence-based report: Vol. 1.* Retrieved from *http://www.powerstudy.ca/the-power-report/the-power-report-volume-1/burden-of-illness*; Joint Commission & The California Endowment. (2011). *Advancing effective communication, cultural competence, and patient- and family-centered care for the lesbian, gay, bisexual, and transgender (LGBT) community.* Retrieved from *http://www.jointcommission.org/lgbt/*; Kirmayer, L., Brass, G. M., Holton, T., Paul, K., Simpson, C., & Tait, C. (2007). *Suicide among Aboriginal people in Canada.* Ottawa: Aboriginal Healing Foundation. Retrieved from *http://www.ahf.ca/downloads/suicide.pdf*; Loppie, C. & Wien, F. (2009). *Health inequalities and social determinants of Aboriginal peoples' health.* Retrieved from *http://www.nccahccnsa.ca/docs/social%20determinates/NCCAH-Loppie-Wien_Report.pdf*; Mikkonen, J., & Raphael, D. (2010). *Social determinants of health: The Canadian facts.* Toronto: York University School of Health Policy and Management. Retrieved from *http://www.thecanadianfacts.org/*

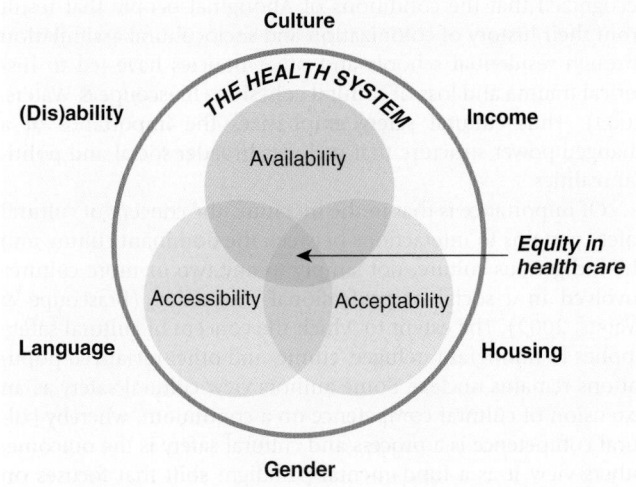

Figure 2-2 A framework for conceptualizing equity in health care.

Source: Provincial Health Services Authority. (2011). *Towards reducing health inequities: A health system approach to chronic disease prevention. A discussion paper* (p. 24). Vancouver, BC: Population & Public Health, Provincial Health Services Authority. Retrieved from *http://www.phsa.ca/NR/rdonlyres/0F19BDB8-2153-49D1-A214-E7D0D0B9DA3B/52162/TowardsReducingHealthInequitiesFinalDiscussionPape.pdf*

The influence of culture on health is significant and multifaceted. The resettlement process for immigrants and refugees presents inherent challenges as individuals experience difficulties in employment, housing, and access to social support. In addition, individuals may face health risks from a social environment, which is largely determined by dominant cultural values that contribute to the perpetuation of conditions such as marginalization, stigmatization, loss or devaluation of language and culture, and lack of access to culturally appropriate diet, activity, and health care services. Culture can also have a direct effect. Culture influences how illness is perceived and experienced, what symptoms are reported, what remedies are sought, and who is consulted in the process. Recognizing the effect of cultural patterns and ways of being is critical in understanding a situation and determining appropriate strategies for engagement.

Exploring the Concepts: Definitions and Meanings

One of the greatest difficulties associated with developing cultural competence in health care has been a lack of clarity regarding the meaning of terms such as *culture* and *cultural competence*, as well as related terms such as *diversity, ethnicity, race,* and *minority*. Terminology related to cultural diversity is often vague, controversial, and subject to multiple interpretations, and it continues to evolve over time. *Cultural competence* is not universally accepted as the term or the framework within which to understand issues of diversity and equity. Increasingly, and particularly in the Canadian context, the concept of **cultural safety** may be more meaningful. This concept was developed in New Zealand to draw attention to the effect of colonization on the health of the indigenous Maori people. In the Canadian context, the term is used largely to draw attention to the historical, social, and political factors that must be considered in the care of the Aboriginal people. The concept is an approach to health care in which it is recognized that the conditions of Aboriginal people that result from their history of colonization and sociocultural assimilation through residential schools and other policies have led to historical trauma and loss of cultural cohesion (Brascoupé & Waters, 2009). Thus cultural safety emphasizes the importance of a changed power structure that includes broader social and political realities.

Of importance is that in the literature, the concept of cultural safety pertains to interactions between the dominant culture and the indigenous culture, not simply to any two or more cultures involved in a social or professional interaction (Brascoupé & Waters, 2009). The extent to which the concept of cultural safety applies to immigrant, refugee, ethnic, and other racialized populations remains unclear. Some authors view cultural safety as an extension of cultural competence on a continuum, whereby cultural competence is a process and cultural safety is the outcome; others view it as a fundamental paradigm shift that focuses on social and political power and redefines the professional–patient relationship with emphasis on self-determination (Brascoupé & Waters, 2009). In this chapter, the term *cultural competence* is used largely because the notion of competence implies acquisition and use of specific knowledge and skills that increase the health care professional's abilities to provide care to a wide range of diverse populations. Three fundamental tenets underlie culturally competent care: (a) the need to uncover one's own assumptions about people and situations; (b) the importance of purposefully seeking out similarities and differences between individuals and groups in order to be responsive to people's varying needs; and (c) the importance of addressing the dynamics of difference that lead to unequal social power and social exclusion at both the individual and the broader systems levels. These tenets form the basis of the relational approach to cultural care (Srivastava, 2008).

The term **culture** is difficult to define. The definitions range from a narrow perspective, whereby culture is associated with race, ethnicity, or religion, to a wide perspective, whereby culture is seen as a broad phenomenon that extends beyond these characteristics to refer to any group with shared values, beliefs, and experiences (Srivastava, 2008). Under this broad definition, culture can include many dimensions, including ethnicity, language, religion, sex, socioeconomic class, professional status, age, sexual orientation, group history, and life experiences (Registered Nurses' Association of Ontario [RNAO], 2007; Srivastava, 2007a). Culture affects ways of perceiving, behaving, and evaluating the world, and it serves as a guide for people's values, beliefs, and practices, including those related to health and illness. Culture is not a static concept and not something that belongs to particular individuals; everyone has a culture. Culture exists at the level of the individual, group, and larger society, and with regard to achieving health equity, the culture of health care providers and the health care system matters as much as the culture of the patient (Srivastava, 2008).

Values are the sets of rules by which individuals, families, groups, and communities live. They are the principles and standards that serve as the basis for beliefs, attitudes, and behaviours. Although all cultures have values, the types and expressions of those values differ from one culture to another. Cultural values develop over time, guide decision making and actions, and affect a person's identity or sense of self. Cultural values are often unconsciously developed and are responsible for many inherent biases, including perceptions of acceptable and unacceptable behaviour. Cultural understanding is learned over time and with exposure and experience. This cultural understanding is often

referred to as the **world view.** A world view is the way in which people perceive, interpret, and relate to the world around them (Srivastava, 2007a) and reflects their beliefs about cosmology, relationships with nature, moral reasoning, and social relationships (Purnell & Paulanka, 2008). Culture is not a static concept; rather, cultural values and understanding evolve over time on the basis of life events and experiences.

Culture has a number of distinguishing features. Table 2-2 highlights six key characteristics. Although individuals within a cultural group have many similarities through their shared values, beliefs, and practices, there is also much diversity within groups. The values, beliefs, and traditions are shared in varying degrees. Individual differences continue to exist, and each person is culturally unique. Although many people equate culture with ethnicity, race, country of origin, or religion, this is an erroneous oversimplification. Factors such as age, gender, class, sexual orientation, and socioeconomic status contribute to an individual's culture and how it influences need, access, and responses to health care (Srivastava, 2008).

Ethnocentrism is a tendency of individuals to believe that their way of viewing and responding to the world is the most correct, natural, and superior one. To some extent, this is a universal tendency, inasmuch each person has the greatest familiarity with and a preference for his or her own way of doing things. However, the conscious or unconscious belief that a particular way is the only way or the best way for everyone is problematic and can lead to categorizing others' beliefs as unusual, inferior, bizarre, and therefore inappropriate. Ethnocentrism can prevent people from considering alternative perspectives and from respecting others' world views. **Cultural imposition,** a closely related concept, is the situation in which one's own cultural beliefs and practices are, intentionally or unintentionally, imposed on another person or group of people. In health care, it can result in disregarding or trivializing a patient's health care beliefs or practices and in planning and providing care without taking into account the cultural beliefs of the patient. Ethnocentrism and risk of cultural imposition can be avoided through self-awareness and awareness of one's own culture, actively learning about other cultures, and developing respect for and recognizing the strengths of other perspectives (RNAO, 2007; Srivastava, 2007a).

Cultural practices change over time through active or passive processes, including acculturation and assimilation. **Acculturation** is the modification of one's own culture as a result of contact

Table 2-2 Key Characteristics of Culture

Culture is ...

- *Learned* through the processes of language acquisition and socialization
- *Shared* by all members of the same cultural group
- *Adapted* to specific conditions such as environmental factors
- *Dynamic* and ever-changing
- *Invisible* and often sensed but not seen
- *Selective* and distinguishes members of one group from another, differentiating between groups

Source: Adapted from Srivastava, R. (2007). Culture care framework I: Overview and cultural sensitivity. In R. Srivastava (Ed.), *The healthcare professional's guide to clinical cultural competence* (pp. 53-74). Toronto: Elsevier Canada.

with another culture (Purnell & Paulanka, 2008). This process may be a gradual change that results in increased numbers of similarities between the two cultures. **Assimilation** is generally a one-way process in which people lose their own cultural identity as they gradually adopt and incorporate characteristics of the dominant cultural group (Purnell & Paulanka, 2008).

Ethnicity refers to characteristics of a group whose members share a common social, cultural, linguistic, or religious heritage (Purnell & Paulanka, 2008). This heritage is passed on through the generations and involves identification with that group. Although shared ethnicity may reflect shared culture, the terms *ethnicity* and *culture* are not interchangeable. **Race** is controversial in that it is both a biological and social construct. The term *race* is sometimes used to highlight biological differences and physical characteristics such as skin colour, bone structure, or blood group. However, the biological basis of race is frequently challenged. Children of mixed-race couples can have varying degrees of skin pigmentation and physical characteristics, and yet they share similar genetic makeup and social culture. As a social construct, race has been used to denote superiority and inferiority, whereby the assigned status limits or increases opportunities and leads to assumptions about individuals and groups; thus the social meaning of race is often more important than the biological meaning (Hyman, 2009). Such categorization or differentiation according to race is described as a process of *racialization*. **Racialization** is closely linked to discrimination, in which members of a particular cultural group are treated unfairly. The term *racialized groups* is used to highlight the fact that race is not an objective biological fact and that health inequities are not a result of static biological differences but rather a product of dynamic race relations in a social context that potentially exposes individuals to racism (Hyman, 2009).

There is a large and growing body of research linking racism to poor health (Bierman et al., 2009; Hyman, 2009; Mikkonen & Raphael, 2010). Racism can take multiple forms. *Institutionalized racism* is experienced through the structures and systems in society that result in exclusion; overt racism is expressed as prejudice and discrimination and experienced as a lack of respect, mistrust, devaluation, scapegoating, dehumanization, and verbal or physical abuse. *Internalized racism* is the situation in which the negative messages are accepted and internalized by the people experiencing the racism; such internalization leads to feelings of low self-worth, resignation, helplessness, and lack of hope (Mikkonen & Raphael, 2010). The effect of racism is also multifaceted. Individuals experiencing racism may resort to high-risk behaviours, such as substance abuse, self-harm, and delays in seeking health care. Racism can influence physical health by causing chronic, negative emotional states such as anxiety, depression, and diminished self-esteem/identity, which, in turn, can have direct effects on biological processes such as the cardiovascular and immune systems and can increase vulnerability to infections, diabetes, high blood pressure, heart attack, stroke, depression, and aggression (Hyman, 2009). Racism also influences health indirectly through differential exposures and opportunities related to other determinants of health such as education and employment (Hyman, 2009).

In **stereotyping**, members of a specific culture, race, or ethnic group are automatically assumed to have characteristics associated with that group, without further exploration of what the individuals—or, for that matter, what the cultural group itself—are actually like. This oversimplified approach does not take into account the individual differences that exist within a culture. Stereotyping can occur with patients or health care professionals.

In health care (as well as most other) settings, being a member of a particular ethnic group does not make the person an expert on other members of that same group. Such stereotyping can lead to false assumptions and negative attitudes that adversely affect a patient's care.

Diversity is another term that is related to culture. For some people, the term simply refers to differences or variations across individuals and social groups, whereas for others, it represents a sum of differences, usually with regard to unequal access to power, privilege, and resources. In general, in the health care context, diversity implies difference from the majority or dominant group that is assumed to be the norm (Canadian Nurses Association, 2010). Diverse groups and communities, in this context, have marginalized status in society, and diversity initiatives often become synonymous with asserting human rights, freedom from discrimination, social justice, and, more recently, health equity.

Cultural Competence

Cultural competence is a complex concept that has evolved from older terms such as *cultural sensitivity* and *cultural awareness*. Whereas cultural sensitivity and awareness refer to an appreciation of and respect for cultural differences, competence takes the concept one step further and refers to the ability to actually apply knowledge and skill appropriately in interactions with patients. It is a process that involves the application of knowledge, attitudes, and skills that enhance cross-cultural communication; foster meaningful, respectful interactions with others; and, in so doing, address issues of exclusion that can affect health outcomes. Cultural competence includes valuing diversity, knowing about cultural norms and traditions of the populations being served, and being sensitive to these differences when providing care (RNAO, 2007). The International Council of Nurses (2007) noted that nurses demonstrate cultural competence by developing self-awareness without letting it have undue influence on their treatment of patients from other backgrounds, by having knowledge and understanding of a patient's culture, by accepting and respecting cultural differences, and by adapting care to be congruent with patient's culture.

Each of the many frameworks and models of cultural competence highlight a different aspect of culture and attributes of cultural competence. However, three key domains are evident across these frameworks: (a) an *affective* domain, which reflects an awareness of and sensitivity to cultural values, needs, and biases; (b) a *behavioural* domain, which reflects skills necessary to be effective in cross-cultural encounters; and (c) a *cognitive* domain, which involves cultural knowledge, as well as theory, research, and cross-cultural approaches to care. Together, these domains can be considered the *ABCs* of cultural competence (Srivastava, 2008). To fully understand the complexities of cultural competence and its relationship to health equity, however, two other domains, *D* and *E*, must also be present: (d) the *dynamics* of difference and (e) the context of care and the supports that are or are not available in the practice *environment*, as well as the goal of *equity* (Srivastava, 2008). Figure 2-3 shows the ABC(DE) framework for cultural competence.

Table 2-3 presents key attributes of the ABC domains of cultural competence. The influence of the dynamics of difference and the environment is evident throughout the affective, behavioural, and cognitive domains and is thus not highlighted separately.

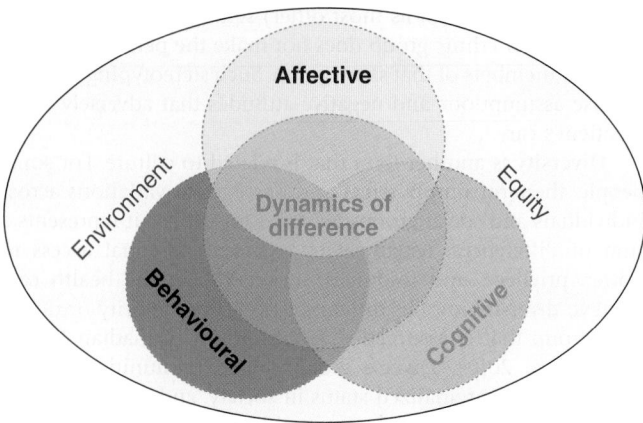

Figure 2-3 The ABC(DE)s of cultural competence.

Source: Adapted from Srivastava, R. (2008). The ABC (and DE) of cultural competence in clinical care. *Ethnicity and Inequalities in Health and Social Care, 8*(1), 25-31 (p. 31)

Affective Domain

The affective domain of cultural competence is concerned with both attitude and awareness. This domain is often seen as the first step toward achieving cultural competence. Openness, a desire to learn, valuing differences, respect for others, and developing humility are characteristic of this domain (Camphina-Bacote, 2009; Cuellar, Brennan, Vito, & de Leon Siantz, 2008; RNAO, 2007; Srivastava, 2008). This domain is characterized by accepting the notion of multiple world views and norms and recognizing that no one way is universally beneficial. *Cultural awareness* is a conscious learning process in which individuals become appreciative of and sensitive to their own culture, as well as the cultures of other people (Camphina-Bacote, 2009). Awareness can be subcategorized into three components: self-awareness, awareness of others, and awareness of the dynamics of difference (Srivastava, 2007a, 2008). Every person is a cultural being; therefore, any nurse–patient interaction is affected by the cultures of both the nurse and the patient. The nurse is influenced not only by his or her cultural background but also by the culture of the nursing profession and the culture of the health care setting in which the interaction occurs. One of the first steps in developing cultural awareness is for the nurse to examine his or her own cultural biases toward people from different cultures and to identify how these views may influence the care encounter (Srivastava, 2008). This is crucial for recognizing ethnocentrism and avoiding cultural imposition. Development of self-awareness requires the nurse to engage in ongoing critical self-reflection and being amenable to feedback from other people.

Awareness of other people as cultural beings is based on recognition of multiple world views and norms. Cultural differences are not issues of right or wrong; they are simply about being different. Cultural awareness also includes an appreciation for the dynamics of difference that exist within the clinician–patient relationship, as well as within the patient's social location in society. Social location refers to one's position in the social hierarchy. Understanding of the effect of social determinants of health and recognition of the historical effect of racism, discrimination, and culturally destructive processes such as the residential schools for the Aboriginal communities are important insights that shape awareness of how differences matter and which differences matter more than in others in particular contexts (Cuellar et al, 2008; Loppie & Wien, 2009; Srivastava, 2007a; 2008).

Behavioural Domain

The behavioural domain concerns the actual application of knowledge and awareness and is also described as cultural skill. Through the intentional use of these skills, the health care provider can perform a comprehensive assessment of not only patients' complaints and symptoms but also their values, beliefs, and practices to determine the most appropriate goals and interventions (Camphina-Bacote, 2009; Srivastava, 2008). Different cultural groups have different beliefs about the causes of illness and the appropriateness of various treatments. It is important for the nurse to try to determine the patient's **explanatory model** (set of beliefs regarding what causes the disease or illness and the methods that would potentially treat the condition best). It is also important to determine how patients' different experiences and beliefs might affect their health and health care. Table 2-4 lists key questions that can be used to learn about the patient's explanatory model of illness and care. These questions do not have to be asked in the order they are listed, and they can be adapted to the situation. Through these questions, the nurse can identify cultural values and beliefs that are important to the patient in that situation.

The behavioural or skills domain is complex and requires competency in awareness, knowledge, and application of the generalized awareness of cultural issues to specific clinical situations. It is also important to develop resources at the individual and organizational levels for ongoing learning, consultation, and referral (Srivastava, 2007b).

Communication. A key area for cultural skill is communication, inasmuch as it is foundational for every aspect of the clinical encounter. Cultural differences are often cited as a barrier to effective communication, leading to poor adherence, dissatisfaction with care, and adverse health outcomes (Teal & Street, 2009). Communication is critical for establishing trust, informed consent, decision making, ability to partner in care, and self-management of chronic illnesses (Surbone, 2008; Teal & Street, 2009). Patient-centred communication is "characterized by communication that elicits and understands the patient's perspective and social context, reaches a shared understanding of the problem and its treatment, and involves patients in choices to the extent they desire" (Teal & Street, 2009, p. 533). From this definition, it is clear that true patient-centred communication involves understanding and integrating a patient's cultural identity and needs. Although patient-centred care and cultural competence have many similarities, the latter requires an explicit understanding of and attention to the dynamics of difference, as well as cultural similarities and differences between the patient's culture and that of the health care provider.

It is not sufficient for nurses to simply learn about cross-cultural communication issues; they must also develop and adapt their communication skills to connect with different cultural groups (RNAO, 2007). Although members of some groups may respond effectively to direct questions, members of others respond more comfortably in interactions that are less direct, in which information is asked for and presented in the third person and more silence and reflection is allowed for. For example, instead of telling a person what to do, a nurse may phrase the teaching in a less directive way: "Many people who experience this illness find it helpful to do …" Nurses must also understand that when a patient says, "Yes," it can have multiple interpretations, including "Go on," "I hear you," "I understand," or "I agree." Thus understanding and agreement must be validated

Table 2-3 The ABCs of Cultural Competence

COMPONENT	DESCRIPTION
Affective (Awareness) Domain	
Attitude	• Humility and a recognition of the need for ongoing learning • Genuine curiosity, desire to learn, and valuing differences • Nonjudgemental stance in encountering situations and perspectives that are different from those of self or the norm • Commitment to the goal of inclusivity and equity • Awareness of own views of differences among people
Awareness of self, others, and dynamics of difference	• Self-awareness of values, beliefs, and biases • Awareness of own social location and privilege • Awareness of challenges with cross-cultural communication • Awareness of cultural influences on information seeking, conflict, and decision making • Recognition of the historical effects of racism and discrimination in society and health care
Behavioural (Skills) Domain	
Assessment	• Ask the correct questions in the correct way (knowing what and knowing how) • Establish trust and health care provider credibility • Elicit patient's explanatory model of illness
Cross-cultural communication	• Determine patient values, strengths, and goals • Adapt own communication style to address cultural nuances and differences in information processing and decision making
Collaborative decision making Empowering and promoting patient choice Advocacy across differences	• Recognize the need for and use of interpreters for language support • Accommodate values and preferences and negotiate approaches to obtain mutually agreed-upon goals • Review cultural conflicts as opportunities to learn from differences • Reframe situations to mitigate biases that exist within the health care provider or the patient • Promote health literacy • Support informed patient choices
Develop resources (personal and organizational) to support practice	• Identify own privilege and use it appropriately to further goals of equity • Recognize and address the dynamics of difference at patient–clinician level and at patient–health care system level • Connect patients with resources within their community to promote greater autonomy and self-management • Explore opportunities to partner with and learn from colleagues, patients, and communities that are culturally different from self or own • Seek out information on different cultural groups through the Internet, media, movies, and visits to cultural and community centres • Seek out the insider cultural perspectives and meanings of events and traditions
Cognitive (Knowledge) Domain	
Generic cultural knowledge	• Understand the effect of culture on health • Understand difference between individualistic and collectivist cultures • Recognize dimensions of care that are likely to be influenced by culture • Identify biophysiological determinants of health and illness in minority groups • Identify social determinants of health: effects of race, culture, health status, employment, and so forth • Understand health disparities and health equity issues • Understand the effect of diversity on team functioning
Specific cultural knowledge	• Learn about commonly held world views and healing traditions • Identify the effect of life events such as migration, settlement, and racism • Develop in-depth knowledge of particular communities served, including religious and cultural beliefs and traditions; cultural strengths and resources; and health inequities particular to the group or groups, such as issues of access to health care, congruence of health care with the culture, and incidence and prevalence of major illnesses • Review care process for own clinical specialty and identify processes and treatments that are particularly susceptible to cultural differences • Not make assumptions on the basis of cultural background; instead, use knowledge as a beginning point for further assessment and inquiry

Source: Adapted from Srivastava, R. (2008). The ABC (and DE) of cultural competence in clinical care. *Ethnicity and Inequalities in Health and Social Care, 8*(1), 25-31; and from Cuellar, N. G., Brennan, A. M., Vito, K., & de Leon Siantz, M. L. (2008). Cultural competence in the undergraduate nursing curriculum. *Journal of Professional Nursing, 24*(3), 143-149. doi:10.1016/j.profnurs.2008.01.004

Table 2-4 Questions for Determining the Patient's Explanatory Model of Illness and Care

1. "What do you call the problem?"
2. "What do you think has caused the problem?"
3. "Why do you think it started when it did?"
4. "What do you think the sickness or illness does to you? How does it work?"
5. "How severe is the sickness? Will it have a long or short course?"
6. "What are the major problems or difficulties this sickness has caused in your life?"
7. "What have you done for this problem up to now?"
8. "What kind of treatment do you think you should receive?"
9. "What are the most important results you hope to achieve from the treatment?"
10. "What do you fear most about the sickness?"
11. "What do you fear most about the treatment?"
12. "Who else should be consulted or involved in your care?"

Source: From Srivastava, R. (2007). Culture care framework I: Overview and cultural sensitivity. In R. Srivastava (Ed.), *The healthcare professional's guide to clinical cultural competence* (p. 89). Toronto: Elsevier Canada. Adapted from Kleinman, A., Eisenberg, L., & Goode, B. (1978). Culture, illness, and care: Clinical lessons from anthropologic and cross cultural research. *Annals of Internal Medicine, 88*, 251-258.

through other means. Negotiation skills are also important in cultural competence because nurses are often required to negotiate interventions and goals that range along the gamut of mainstream and traditional ways of healing. Specific information is presented throughout this book to assist with developing an awareness of cultural differences and learning assessment skills for different cultural groups.

Cultural influences on communication are evident in both verbal and nonverbal communication. Verbal communication includes not only the language or dialect but also the voice tone, volume, timing, and a person's willingness to share thoughts and feelings. Nonverbal communication includes eye contact, use of touch, body language, style of greeting, and the spatial arrangement taken up by the participants. Culture influences the ways that feelings are expressed, as well as which verbal and nonverbal expressions are appropriate in given situations. Culturally competent health care providers are vigilant for miscommunication that can occur in any interaction but is more likely in cross-cultural interactions (Srivastava, 2007c; Teal & Street, 2009).

Meaning of and comfort with silence can vary across cultures. Many Aboriginal people are comfortable with silence and interpret silence as essential for thinking and carefully considering a response. In these interactions, silence shows respect for the other person and demonstrates the importance of the remarks. In traditional Japanese and Chinese cultures, the speaker may stop talking and leave a period of silence for the listener to think about what has been said before continuing. In other cultures (e.g., French, Spanish, and Russian), silence may be interpreted as meaning agreement.

Eye contact varies greatly among cultures. Although nurses are often taught to maintain direct eye contact, patients who are Asian, Arab, or Aboriginal may avoid direct eye contact and consider direct eye contact disrespectful or aggressive. Other variables to consider include the role of sex, age, status, or position on what

is considered to be appropriate eye contact. For example, Muslim-Arab women avoid eye contact with men other than their husbands and when in public situations in order to exhibit modesty.

Touch is another form of communication. Physical contact with patients conveys various meanings, depending on the culture. To perform a comprehensive assessment, touching a patient is necessary. In some cultures, such as the Arab culture, male health care professionals may be prohibited from touching a female patient. Many Asians believe that touching a person's head is a sign of disrespect, especially because the head is believed to be the source of a person's strength. Observing how a patient interacts with others and asking permission to touch before touching are appropriate ways of respecting the patient's cultural values (Srivastava, 2007c).

Another area of importance in communication is the ability to provide effective language support through the use of language aids, including interpreters (College of Nurses of Ontario [CNO], 2009a). Table 2-5 lists strategies for working effectively with interpreters, and Table 2-6 lists strategies for communicating with patients with limited proficiency in English.

Cognitive Domain

Cultural knowledge is a crucial element of cultural competence, but the nature of required knowledge is not always clear. Cultural knowledge can be divided into two categories: generic cultural knowledge and specific cultural knowledge (Lo & Pottinger, 2007; Srivastava, 2007a). Generic cultural knowledge is foundational knowledge that applies across a variety of cultural groups. Specific cultural knowledge focuses on particular cultural populations. Examples of generic cultural knowledge include understanding the relationship between individuals and families across cultures or the effect of life events such as immigration, settlement, and experiencing racism. Generic knowledge also includes familiarity with broad cultural factors that affect health and health care, such as variations in world views and explanatory models of illness, beliefs about care, cure, and caregivers; family roles and expectations; communication styles; the process of migration and settlement; norms about time and personal space; and religiosity and spirituality. Examples of specific cultural knowledge could involve focusing on specific cultural groups, such as the Aboriginal population or the Chinese community, or on the health issues faced by particular populations, such as immigrant women (Srivastava, 2007b).

In addition to determining the kind of generic and specific knowledge that is needed, nurses must critically appraise how knowledge is developed and used. Culture is concerned with shared patterns, not universal truths. Therefore, cultural knowledge should not be used to obscure individual differences, and individualized assessments are important to determine the extent to which the patient shares the beliefs and practices ascribed to the culture. Familiarity with cultural norms is helpful, but caution is warranted in imposing that familiarity on others, which results in stereotyping. It is important for nurses to reflect on how they acquired the knowledge and the extent to which the knowledge is unique to the individual, reflective of the broader cultural group, or reflective of cultural processes in general.

Generic Cultural Knowledge
Communication. Cross-cultural communication was discussed extensively in the previous section. It is important to emphasize that communication challenges extend beyond language and the spoken word. English-speaking patients, too, can

Table 2-5 Working Effectively with Interpreters

General Considerations

- If possible, the interpreter should meet with the patient ahead of time to establish rapport before the interpreting begins.
- Allow extra time for the session.
- Use trained bilingual–bicultural interpreters instead of the patient's family or children.
- Consider personal attributes of the interpreter such as age, gender, ethnicity, and dialect that may influence communication; use an agency interpreter if possible.
- Be aware of common issues such as the following:
  - Words that cannot be translated
  - Being too rushed
  - The interpreter's answering for the patient
  - Conflict between the interpreter and the patient (if this occurs, stop the session immediately!)
- Verify translations to avoid misunderstandings, mistakes, and distortions.

Before the Interpretation Session

- Get to know the interpreter.
- Provide an overview of the situation (patient, goals, and procedures).
- Ask for concerns or issues from the interpreter's perspective.
- Remind interpreter to interpret *everything*.
- Ask the interpreter to share his or her cultural insights with you but to differentiate these from the interpretation itself.
- Reinforce confidentiality.

During the Interpretation Session

- Face the patient directly.
- Speak in the first person.
- Introduce yourself, allowing the interpreter to interpret.
- Describe the role of the interpreter, the interpreter service's mandate, and the purpose of the session.
- Ask the interpreter to introduce himself or herself and his or her role in both languages.
- Address questions to the patient, not to the interpreter.
- Use simple language, and avoid jargon and technical terminology.
- Speak in one- to two-sentence bursts to allow for easier translation.
- Ensure that the interpreter understands what is to be translated.
- Allow the interpreter to ask open-ended questions if necessary to clarify what the patient says.
- Observe the patient for off-target reactions (signalling mistakes in interpretation).
- Observe and evaluate what is going on before you interrupt the interpreter.

After the Interpretation Session and Follow-up Strategies

- Consider providing written instructions as appropriate.
- Ask the patient whether he or she has anything to ask or convey.
- Provide information on how the patient may request an interpreter's services in the future.
- Discuss the process and outcomes of the session with the interpreter.

Table 2-6 Communicating with Patients with Limited English Proficiency

1. Be polite and formal.
2. Gesture to yourself and say your name, offering a handshake, nod, smile, or other greeting. If possible, greet patient in the patient's preferred language. This indicates that you are aware of and respect the patient's culture.
3. Proceed in an unhurried manner. Pay attention to any effort by the patient or family to communicate.
4. Speak in a low, moderate voice. Avoid talking loudly. Remember that there is a tendency to raise the volume and pitch of your voice when the listener appears not to understand. The listener may perceive that you are shouting or angry, or both.
5. Use simple words, such as "pain" instead of "discomfort." Avoid medical jargon, idioms, and slang. Avoid using contractions (e.g., "don't," "can't," "won't"). Use nouns repeatedly instead of pronouns. For example:
   - Do not say: "He has been taking his medicine, hasn't he?"
   - Do say: "Does Janani take medicine?"
6. Pantomime words and simple actions while you verbalize them.
7. Organize what you say, giving information and instructions in the proper sequence. For example:
   - Do not say: "Before you rinse the bottle, sterilize it."
   - Do say: "First, wash the bottle. Second, rinse the bottle."
8. Discuss one topic at a time. Avoid using conjunctions. For example:
   - Do not say: "Are you cold and in pain?"
   - Do say: "Are you cold [while pantomiming]? [Wait for patient's response.] Are you in pain?"
9. Validate understanding by having the patient repeat instructions, demonstrate the procedure, or act out the meaning.
10. Do not ask questions that can be answered with only "yes" or "no."
11. Summarize often, including your understanding of what the person is saying and checking whether your understanding is correct.

Source: Data from Jarvis, C. (2008). *Physical examination and health assessment* (5th ed.). Philadelphia: W. B. Saunders; and from Srivastava, R. (2007). Culture care framework I: Overview and cultural sensitivity. In R. Srivastava (Ed.), *The healthcare professional's guide to clinical cultural competence* (pp. 53-74). Toronto: Elsevier Canada.

experience miscommunication because some words and phrases have meanings and interpretations that are culturally nuanced. Nurses and other health care providers must be vigilant for such variations and potential miscommunication. They must also be knowledgeable about issues in interpretation and translation and be aware of how beliefs about family, authority, and differences in communication styles influence trust, understanding, acceptance, questions and decision making. (See the Clinical Decision-Making Exercise at the end of this chapter.)

Care, Cure, Caregivers, and Healing Systems. Cultural norms have a significant influence on how illness is understood, what remedies are deemed appropriate and desirable, and who provides the care. Whereas in some cultures patients seek professional help, patients in others rely more on family, friends, or spiritual and religious leaders. It is important to ascertain a patient's beliefs about the cause of illness, as well as perceptions of severity, expected treatment, prognosis, and effects (see Table 2-4).

Canadian health care systems and health professions such as nursing also have a cultural basis in the dominant white, Euro-centric culture. The biomedical approach to health care, although regarded as the conventional treatment in North America, is one of several philosophical and scientifically based systems of healing. Other such systems include homeopathy, traditional Chinese medicine, Aboriginal medicine, and Ayurvedic medicine (a form of traditional Hindu medicine). Although it is not possible for a health care provider to have expertise in all the healing systems, familiarity with the major systems and with their basic principles can be helpful (Srivastava, 2007b). Individuals often use multiple healing systems, and a critical part of patient assessment is knowledge of what conventional treatments, as well as other folk or herbal treatments, are being used. Nurses need to understand their role in supporting and providing complementary and alternative therapy (CNO, 2009b).

The Canadian approach to health care delivery is often team based; different members of the team have different roles, and boundaries with regard to who does what are often very clear. In many cultures, people are used to having a single authoritative healer and may regard others as helpers (Srivastava, Srivastava, & Srivastava, 2012). For example, patients may view nurses only as the physicians' handmaidens, or social workers may be viewed as representatives of the state. Lack of familiarity with and misunderstanding of the roles can lead to confusion and risks to patient safety, inasmuch as information may not be disclosed or shared appropriately with the health care team.

Patient values regarding time orientation and personal space can also affect the care delivery process. A frequent source of frustration for many health care providers in hospitals and clinics is that many patients do not seem to value the providers' time and frequently show up late for appointments. This may result from many factors, including issues of transportation, ability to navigate the system, and time orientation. In different cultures, people tend to regard the value of clock time and punctuality in different ways. For some cultures, it is more important to attend to a social role than to arrive on time for an appointment with a health care professional. Hence, the lack of adherence to the appointment time can be attributed to competing demands and a lack of appreciation for the need for punctuality and should not be viewed as blatant disregard or disrespect for the health care providers or the system. The amount of personal space that people are comfortable with and what is considered private also varies across cultures. Many health care processes require close physical contact, discussions of an intimate nature, or both; thus personal boundaries can be particularly significant with regard to patient disclosure and cooperation with activities. Issues concerning personal space and gender often surface during activities involving physical assessment and personal care. Health care professionals must use sensitivity in talking with patients to find approaches that best fit the patients' health care needs and personal preferences. Asking permission before touching, observing and responding to the patients' level of comfort, and asking whether the patient prefers an alternative to how care might be provided are some strategies to ensure that patients' personal space is respected.

Help-seeking is also influenced by system factors, some of which are presented in Table 2-7.

Biology, Physiology, Pharmacology. The racial and ethnic influences on biological and physiological processes are often viewed as controversial because these influences are considered more to be social categories than scientific categories. Although

Table 2-7 Cultural and System Factors Affecting Help Seeking

Economic Factors

- Patients may not obtain health care because they cannot pay the costs associated with travel for health care, medications, or treatments.
- Refugee or illegal immigrant status may deter some patients from using the health care system.
- Patients may lack health insurance.

Health Care System

- Patients may not make or keep appointments because of the time lag between the onset of an illness and an available appointment.
- Hours of operation of health care facilities may not accommodate patients' need to work or use public transportation.
- Patients may be relying on friends and family for transportation, language support, or navigation within the system.
- Patients in rural areas may not have access to particular services.
- Lack of ethnic-specific health care programs and shortages of health care professionals from specific ethnic groups may deter some people from seeking health care.
- Patients may not have a relationship with a primary health care professional and may use emergency departments or urgent care centres for health care.
- Patients may lack knowledge about the availability of existing health care resources and may not know how to navigate the health care system.
- Facility policies may not be culturally sensitive (e.g., hospital policy may limit the number of visitors, which is problematic for people whose cultures value having many family members present).

Beliefs and Practices

- Care provided in established health care programs may not be perceived as culturally relevant.
- Religious beliefs, motivation, or practices may affect a person's decision to seek (or not seek) health care.
- Patients may delay seeking care because of fear or because of a preference for folk medicine and herbal remedies.
- Dietary preferences may affect overall nutritional status, as well as present challenges regarding adherence to specific therapeutic diets.
- Patients may stop treatment or discontinue visits for health care because the symptoms are no longer present and they thus perceive that further care is not required.
- Patients may associate hospitals and extended-care facilities with death.
- Patients may have prior negative experience with culturally insensitive health care professionals or discriminatory practices.
- Patients may mistrust the dominant population and institutions.

it is acknowledged that race is only an approximate biological classification, the clinical realities should not be ignored (Camphina-Bacote, 2007). Gender differences have been increasingly recognized in the prevalence of illness, expression of illness, and response to pharmacological agents. Differences in the occurrence of diseases in different racial and ethnic populations also exist. However, it is important to note that when an illness is prevalent in a culture, neither the individual nor the cultural background is the cause of illness; rather, the broader determinants of health must be assessed to understand and address disparities. Genetic predisposition also varies across racial and ethnic lines. For example, sickle cell disease is a common genetic disorder among people of African descent. Being aware of such illness incidences enables health care providers to perform a focused and thorough assessment and to avoid stereotypical assumptions such as that an Aboriginal patient is a "drunken Indian" when the real issue is diabetic ketoacidosis, or that a young Black man is a drug addict, when really he is experiencing pain from sickle cell disease. Having knowledge of increased vulnerability can enhance clinical decision making and prevent misdiagnosis or unnecessary delays that lead to poor care.

Variations in skin pigmentation, bone density, skin disorders, and pathophysiological features of some illnesses also exist across cultures (Srivastava, 2007d). Nurses need to develop confidence and competence in assessing for conditions such as cyanosis, inflammation, jaundice, and petechiae in patients who are dark skinned because visual inspection alone may not be accurate. Assessment of inflammation can be augmented by palpating the skin for warmth, edema, tightness, or indurations. Cyanosis can be assessed through observations of the sclerae, oral mucosa, nail beds, palms and soles of feet, but jaundice is better assessed through examination of the sclerae of the eyes (Purnell & Paulanka, 2008). Health care providers can establish a baseline by asking the patient and family how the skin looks in comparison with when the patient is feeling "healthy"; observing areas with the least amount of pigment; palpating where possible and appropriate; and comparing skin in corresponding areas (Camphina-Bacote, 2009; Purnell & Paulanka, 2008).

There is increasing evidence that ethnicity influences responses to certain medications. These variations are a result of many factors such as genetics, including body weight, body mass, and differences in metabolism; lifestyle, including diet, nutritional status, smoking, and alcohol use; and simultaneous use of herbal remedies (Camphina-Bacote, 2007; Huang & Temple, 2008; Warren, 2008). Some newly arrived refugees may be particularly vulnerable to malnutrition. Genetic differences in how the body processes particular drugs and its overall effect influence the need for lower or higher therapeutic dose ranges. Ethnic differences have also been found in type of medications ordered, side effects, and treatment response to antidepressants, antipsychotics, and other psychotropic drugs (Chaudhry, Neelam, Duddu, & Hussain, 2008). Dosages of angiotensin II antagonists, angiotensin-converting enzyme (ACE) inhibitors, warfarin, and some drugs such as rosuvastatin (Crestor) may also require adjustments on the basis of ethnicity and genetics (Huang & Temple, 2008). Generic substitution of a trade-name drug can also be problematic for certain ethnic groups because of the particular filler that may be used (Camphina-Bacote, 2007). It is therefore important that nurses are aware of the need for individual variations in dosage and alert to assessment of side effects and suboptimal therapeutic benefit. For nurses working in particular specialty areas, it is important to learn about the ethnocultural variations in response to the particular classification of medications commonly taken by their clinical population.

Family Roles and Relationships. Family roles differ from one culture to another (Figure 2-4). For this reason, it is important for the nurse to determine who should be involved in communication and decision making that are related to health care. For example, individualistic cultures emphasize individual rights, goals, and needs.

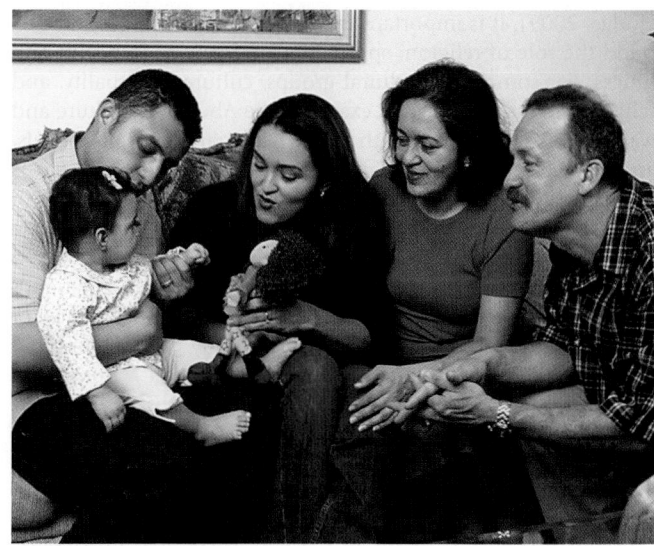

Figure 2-4 Family roles and relationships differ from one culture to another.

Source: © Rick Brady, Riva, MD.

In contrast, collectivist cultures assign greater priority to the needs of the group (family or community), and there is an emphasis on interdependence rather than independence (Debs-Ivall, 2007). In countries such as Canada and the United States, people hold strong beliefs related to autonomy, and each adult individual is expected to make decisions and sign consent forms when receiving health care, whereas in some cultural groups, the head of the household or the eldest son is expected to make health care decisions. In some cultures, affiliation is valued over confrontation, and cooperation is preferred to competition. When the nurse encounters a family that values collectivity over individualism, conflicts may arise in how decisions are made. There may be a delay in treatment while the patient waits for significant family members to arrive before giving consent for a procedure or treatment. In other instances, the patient may make a decision that is best for the family but may have negative or adverse consequences for the patient. Being aware of such values will better prepare the nurse to advocate for and support the patient.

Expectations regarding care giving also vary across cultures. In some cultures, family members are expected to provide care even in the hospital. Some patients may expect health care professionals to provide all care. This expectation is the opposite of the predominant Western expectation of working toward and assuming self-care and independence as quickly as possible.

Spirituality and Religion. Spirituality and religion are aspects of culture that may affect a person's beliefs and decisions about health and illness. *Spirituality* commonly refers to a person's efforts to find purpose, meaning, and a sense of belonging (Camp, 2011; Pesut, Fowler, Taylor, Reimer-Kirkham, & Sawatzky, 2008). *Religion* is a more formal and organized system of beliefs, including belief in or worship of God or gods and involves prayer and one or more rituals. Religion is based on beliefs about life, death, good and evil, and pain and suffering. Religious and spiritual beliefs have been shown to positively influence health outcomes, particularly in the care of patients with mental health and addiction issues (Camp, 2011), and spiritual assessments are often viewed as a required element of quality care (Limb &

Hodge, 2009). It is important for health care providers to understand the role of religion, spirituality, and culture in health and illness. For some ethnocultural groups, culture, spirituality, and religion are inseparable. For example, the Aboriginal culture and way of life are entwined with the religious and spiritual beliefs, and these extend to health and wellness. Similarly, Hinduism is as much a way of life as it is a religion and is also associated with a healing system that may influence perceptions of care and cure (Srivastava et al., 2012).

The nurse can use many interventions to meet a patient's spiritual and religious needs. These interventions include use of prayer, scriptures, listening, and referral. Many patients find that rituals, in the form of prayer, meditation, or other actions, help them during times of illness. Attention to spirituality is an important aspect of holistic care; however, it is important for nurses to be aware of their own assumptions about spirituality and religion and how they may differ from their patients. Not all religions have the same end goals and may, in fact, vary greatly in their central theological questions and objectives (Fowler, 2012). Concepts such as "sin" and "heaven" may be central to Christian theological understanding but are not central concerns in religions such as Buddhism and Hinduism. Even the relationship between the mind, body, and spirit varies among religions (Srivastava et al., 2012). It is therefore important to ascertain what religion and spirituality means to particular individuals and groups, how it may affect health and wellness, and the nurses' role in offering support.

Migration and Settlement. Understanding the influence of migration and resettlement processes on health is another area of generic cultural knowledge. Research indicates that new immigrants tend to be in better overall health than the general resident population. This finding, known as the *healthy immigrant effect,* is not surprising inasmuch as immigrants are screened before being granted admittance to Canada. However, this advantage does not last and, in fact, some groups face higher-than-average risks for illness (Pottie et al., 2011). The deterioration in health is more likely to be reported by recent immigrants of non-European origin. Recent immigrants of colour are also at increased risk for experiencing mental health problems, have higher incidences of housing and food insecurity, and are 50% more likely to visit a physician; however, the adequacy of care is uncertain (Bierman et. al., 2009; Health Nexus and Ontario Chronic Disease Prevention Alliance, 2008; Mikkonen & Raphael, 2010).

Recent immigrants may be at risk for health problems for many reasons. The settlement process is associated with many losses and can cause physical stress and mental distress. New immigrants often experience challenges in areas of the social determinants such as employment, housing, social support, and access to services. Older immigrants are especially affected by changes in role and social position and may be more depressed (Andrews & Boyle, 2008). Factors such as fatigue, stress, and racism—and, for refugees, premigratory circumstances—can result in serious physical and psychological trauma. After migration, factors such employment, housing, and social supports may also play a role in health. Newcomers often face difficulties in accessing the health care system because of a lack of familiarity with the system, limited language proficiency, transportation difficulties, or inability to take time away from other responsibilities related to work and family (Bierman et. al., 2009; Schellenberg & Maheux, 2007). New immigrants are also at risk for social exclusion through underemployment, workplace stress, and unemployment. Workplace stress can be attributed to factors such as poor support from colleagues or supervisors, job insecurity,

and demanding work. Recent immigrants and Canadians of non-dominant races are overrepresented in low-income sector employment and underrepresented in high-income sectors and occupations (Mikkonen & Raphael, 2010). Immigrant women tend to fare even worse than their male counterparts (Health Nexus and Ontario Chronic Disease Prevention Alliance, 2008).

NURSING MANAGEMENT: CULTURAL COMPETENCE IN CARE

Nurse's Self-Assessment

Developing an understanding of one's own culture through reflection and self-assessment is a crucial first step toward cultural competence in clinical care. Evidence indicates that health professionals' attitudes, whether they are conscious of them or not, have a significant influence on their interactions with other people (CNO, 2009a; RNAO, 2007; Srivastava, 2007b). Self-awareness includes being aware of one's motivation and the value that one places on cultural competence (RNAO, 2007). Does it serve merely to avoid problems for the health care professional, or is it a part of learning from differences and achieving equity in health for everyone? In the interest of striving for the latter, nurses must recognize not only their personal culture but also the culture of the nursing profession, as well as that of the health care system. Many tools are available to assist in this process (RNAO, 2007). The need for cultural competence is a fundamental issue of health care quality and patient safety, and achieving it requires a commitment to principles of inclusiveness and equity. Developing cultural competence (see Table 2-3) is a journey in which nurses can begin with generic knowledge and, with time and experience, acquire additional knowledge specific to populations and aspects of care. It is important for the nurse to combine the use of this information and knowledge with critical thinking, however, to ensure that care is provided through a lens of cultural competence without imposition of either the nurse's own values and beliefs or stereotypical views of other people. This approach adds both depth and breadth to the nurse's clinical competence and ability to provide patient-centred care.

Patient Assessment

A cultural assessment should be a fundamental part of all assessments. In some institutions, this assessment may be performed with a structured tool; more often, however, conducting a cultural assessment means asking key questions with regard to language, diet, religion, and acculturation and eliciting the patient's explanatory model of health and illness. This is achieved not only through the questions that are asked (see Table 2-4) but also through the use of cultural knowledge and skill to determine when and how to explore particular issues and, of most importance, being amenable to learning about and working with patient values and beliefs. Table 2-8 lists important components of a holistic assessment.

Nursing Implementation

The first step in any clinical encounter is that of establishing a trusting therapeutic relationship and developing common goals.

Table 2-8 Cultural Assessment

A cultural assessment should include the following:

- Brief history of the cultural group with which the patient identifies (it is important to be aware of significant historical milestones in the country of origin, as well the history of the group in Canada)
- Values orientation
- Cultural sanctions and restrictions
- Communication patterns and style
- Health-related beliefs and practices
- Diet and nutrition
- Education background
- Socioeconomic considerations
- Sources of cultural support (family, friends, organizations)
- Religious and spiritual beliefs

Source: Adapted from Jarvis, C., Browne, A., MacDonald-Jenkins, J., & Luctkar-Flude, M. (2009). *Physical examination and health assessment* (First Canadian ed., Chapter 3). Toronto: Elsevier Canada.

Table 2-9 Nursing Actions to Promote Cultural Competence and Health Equity

- Become aware of your own values, beliefs, and biases.
- Develop humility and a critical awareness that your own expertise is probably ethnocentric.
- Know that racism, heterosexism, classism, sexism, genderism, ageism, ableism, and so forth, are taught, not innate, and that the unlearning process is ongoing.
- Perceive patients/consumers as experts of their own realities.
- Communicate with and about patients in ways that are respectful and accessible.
- Use open-ended questions to understand patients' priorities and perceptions.
- Take responsibility for educating yourself and increase your knowledge and competence to work with people from different backgrounds.
- Advocate with/for patients, and learn how to be an ally across diversity and oppression.
- Challenge discrimination, marginalization, and oppression.
- Assist patients in becoming informed, knowledgeable, and empowered.
- Recognize and address factors at the levels of the individual, organization, and heath care system.
- Embrace learning as an ongoing process.

This can be challenging when care is provided across different languages, priorities, and fundamental beliefs of what is desired and what is acceptable. Consideration of the dynamics of difference is critical. Table 2-9 summarizes nursing actions that are crucial for promoting cultural competence and health equity.

Bridging Cultural Distances

Key characteristics of cultural competence are the ability to effectively apply the ABCDEs of cultural competence—cultural awareness, knowledge, and skills in clinical situations—and the ability to keep in mind the dynamics of difference, supports available through the practice environment, and the goal of equity. Throughout this chapter, strategies that can be used to bridge gaps and differences

Table 2-10 LEARN Model for Cross-Cultural Care

- **L**isten with sympathy and understanding to the patient's perception of the problem.
- **E**xplain your perception of the problem.
- **A**cknowledge and discuss the differences and similarities.
- **R**ecommend treatment.
- **N**egotiate agreement.

Source: Berlin, E. A., & Fowkes, W. C., Jr. (1983). A teaching framework for cross-cultural health care—Application in family practice in cross-cultural medicine. *The Western Journal of Medicine, 12*(139), 93-98.

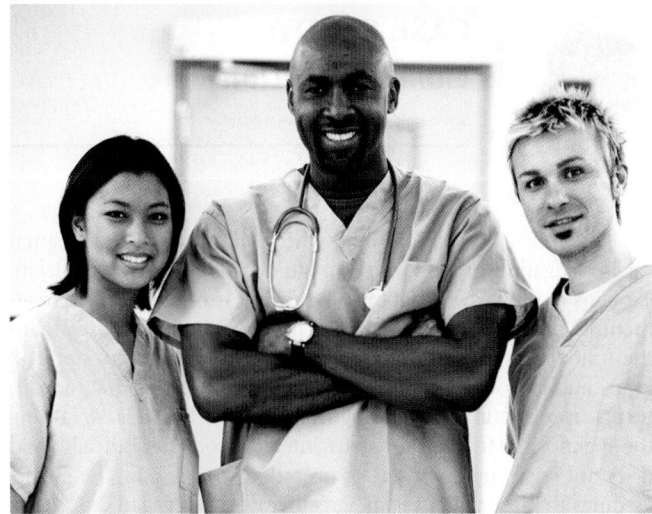

Figure 2-5 Nurses working together in a multicultural health environment.

Source: © JupiterImages Corporation, 2007.

across cultures have been discussed. One model useful for summarizing this discussion is the LEARN model (Table 2-10). First introduced by Berlin and Fowkes (1983), this approach offers simple but comprehensive guidelines for cross-cultural health care. The LEARN model enables the nurse to reveal and acknowledge patients' values and perspectives and practice in a professional manner by sharing his or her expertise. By listening first, the nurse is less likely to give the impression of being hurried or too busy and will be able to tailor explanations in ways that are relevant for the patient.

Working in Diverse Teams

Interactions between patients and health care professionals are not the only situations in which issues of cultural diversity in health care arise. The increasing diversity in society also affects the makeup of the health care team (Figure 2-5). In general, workforce diversity is viewed as a positive attribute and a valuable resource to support the development of cultural competence and the provision of culturally relevant care. A diverse working team creates opportunities for cultural encounters and interactions that can result in greater cultural understanding and better delivery of care (RNAO, 2007). However, diversity in the workforce has challenges. Even though there is a strong belief that culturally competent care necessitates a diverse workforce, workforce diversity does not necessarily result in cultural competence. Research indicates that although culturally diverse groups have a greater potential to generate a greater variety of ideas and other resources than do culturally homogeneous groups, racially and ethnically mixed groups actually experience more conflict and miscommunication than do homogeneous groups (Bassett-Jones, Cornelius, & Brown, 2007). When health care professionals from different cultures and countries work together as members of the health care team, opportunities for miscommunication and conflict naturally arise. The cultural origins of miscommunication and conflict in the workplace are often interconnected with cultural beliefs, values, and etiquette. Examples of such origins are the meaning, purpose, and value of work; family obligations; time orientation; gender roles and sexual orientation; and historical rivalries among groups. Cultural misunderstandings can lead to tensions within the working team, miscommunication, and wrongful assumptions, all of which result in work stress and poor outcomes for patients. These challenges can be minimized through the same principles of respect, empathy, and learning from difference that apply to nurse–patient interactions.

CLINICAL DECISION-MAKING EXERCISE

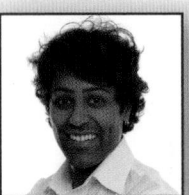

CASE STUDY:
Communication

Source: alberto gagna/iStockphoto.com

Patient Profile

Mr. Jaiswal is a 40-year-old man who is admitted to the hospital for investigation of a tumour. Dr. Stuart, the attending physician, explains to Mr. Jaiswal that the prognosis is excellent and the treatment involves radiation. She plans to schedule the first treatment the following week. Mr. Jaiswal has been in Canada for about 2 years, and although he speaks with an accent, he has had no difficulty in communicating in English. While Dr. Stuart is explaining the diagnosis, Mr. Jaiswal listens intently, nods periodically, and does not raise any questions or objections to the plan. Dr. Stuart assumes that the patient is in agreement with her plan.

Discussion Questions*

1. Would you agree with this assessment?
2. What factors may be influencing Mr. Jaiswal's silence?
3. What actions could be taken by the doctor or you, as the nurse who was present for this discussion, that reflect cultural considerations?

_____

*Based on Teal, C. R., & Street, R. L. (2009). Critical elements of culturally competent communication in the medical encounter: A review and model. *Social Science & Medicine, 68,* 533-543. doi:10.1016/j.socscimed.2008.10.015

ⓔvolve *Answers are available at* **http://evolve.elsevier.com/Canada/Lewis/medsurg**

REVIEW QUESTIONS

The number of the question corresponds to the same-numbered objective at the beginning of the chapter.

1. Which of the following is indicative of forcing one's own cultural beliefs and practices on another person?
   a. Stereotyping
   b. Ethnocentrism
   c. Cultural relativity
   d. Cultural imposition
2. Which of the following is true about inequities between Aboriginal health and the health of the general population?
   a. They result from lifestyle choices.
   b. They result from differences in living conditions, such as housing and education.
   c. They result from conflict between systems of Aboriginal medicine and western health care concepts.
   d. They are decreasing as the Aboriginal population is becoming increasingly urban.
3. Which of the following is true about health inequity?
   a. Health inequities are largely caused by cultural factors compounded by social disadvantage.
   b. Health inequities are largely caused by different beliefs, practices, and lifestyles associated with the cultural communities.
   c. Health inequities can be reduced by improving services to enhance access and reduce exclusion.
   d. In a country in which there is universal access to health care, health inequities are largely an issue of health care quality.
4. Which of the following most accurately describes cultural factors that may affect health?
   a. Diabetes and cancer rates differ by cultural and ethnic groups.
   b. Most patients find that religious rituals help them during times of illness.
   c. There is limited ethnic variation in physiological responses to medications.
   d. Silence during a nurse–patient interaction usually means that the patient understands the instructions.
5. In communications with a patient who speaks a language different from the nurse's, which of the following interventions is important?
   a. Have a family member translate.
   b. Use a trained medical interpreter.
   c. Use specific medical terminology so that there will be no mistakes in the information communicated.
   d. Focus on the translation rather than the nonverbal communication.
6. Why is it important for the nurse to develop cultural self-awareness?
   a. This enables the nurse to clearly articulate the nurse's own values to the patient.
   b. This enables the nurse to prevent ethnocentrism.
   c. This enables the nurse to prevent cultural imposition.
   d. This enables the nurse the opportunity for further personal and professional growth.

7. Which of the following strategies is the most appropriate for demonstrating cultural competence in clinical care?
   a. Explaining to the patient and family how the Canadian health care system works
   b. Connecting the patient with a religious person from the patient's own community
   c. Pairing the patient with a professional from the patient's own cultural community
   d. Exploring the patient's explanatory model of illness

8. How does a diverse workforce influence a nurse's ability to provide care?
   a. It facilitates matching patients with health care professionals of the same ethnicity.
   b. It exposes the nurse to different values, beliefs, and world views.
   c. It leads to greater creativity and innovation and to the development of appropriate interventions for diverse patients.
   d. It meets mandated objectives of the federal and provincial governments.

ANSWERS: 1. d; 2. c; 3. c; 4. a; 5. b; 6. c; 7. d; 8. b.

REFERENCES

Andrews, M., & Boyle, J. (2008). *Transcultural concepts in nursing care* (5th ed.). Philadelphia: Lippincott, Williams & Wilkins.

Bassett-Jones, N., Cornelius, N., & Brown, R. (2007). Delivering diversity management through workplace equality. *Systems Research and Behavioural Science, 24*(1), 59-67. doi:10.1002/sres.762

Berlin, E. A., & Fowkes, W. C., Jr. (1983). A teaching framework for cross-cultural health care—Application in family practice in cross-cultural medicine. *The Western Journal of Medicine, 12*(139), 93-98.

Bierman, A. S., Ahmad, F., Angus, J., Glazier, R. H., Vahabi, M., Damba, C., …, Manuel, D. (2009). Burden of illness. In A. S. Bierman (Ed.), *Project for an Ontario women's health evidence-based report: Volume 1*. Retrieved from *http://www.powerstudy.ca/the-power-report/the-power-report-volume-1/burden-of-illness*

Brascoupé, S., & Waters, C. (2009, November). Cultural safety: Exploring the applicability of the concept of cultural safety to aboriginal health and community wellness. *Journal of Aboriginal Health* 6-41.

Camp, M. (2011). Religion and spirituality in psychiatric practice. *Current Opinion in Psychiatry, 24,* 507-513. doi:10.1097/YCO.0b013e32834bb8f4

Camphina-Bacote, J. (2007). Becoming culturally competent in ethnic pharmacology. *Journal of Psychosocial Nursing, 45*(9), 27-33.

Camphina-Bacote, J. (2009). A culturally competent model of care for African Americans. *Urologic Nursing, 29*(1), 49-54.

Canadian Council on Learning. (2008). *Fact sheet: Health literacy in Canada.* Retrieved from *http://www.ccl-cca.ca/pdfs/HealthLiteracy/HealthLiteracyFactSheetFeb2008E.pdf*

Canadian Nurses Association. (2010). *Promoting cultural competence in nursing.* Ottawa: Author.

Chaudhry, I. B., Neelam, K., Duddu, V., & Hussain, N. (2008). Ethnicity and psychopharmacology. *Journal of Psychopharmacology, 22*(6), 673-680. doi:10.1177/0269881107082105

College of Nurses of Ontario. (2009a). *Culturally sensitive care.* Toronto: Author.

College of Nurses of Ontario. (2009b). *Complementary therapies.* Toronto: Author.

Cuellar, N. G., Brennan, A. M., Vito, K., & de Leon Siantz, M. L. (2008). Cultural competence in the undergraduate nursing curriculum. *Journal of Professional Nursing, 24*(3), 143-149. doi:10.1016/j.profnurs.2008.01.004

Debs-Ivall, S. (2007). Caring for diverse families. In R. H. Srivastava (Ed.), *The healthcare professional's guide to clinical cultural competence* (pp. 144-171). Toronto: Elsevier Canada.

Fowler, M. (2012). Religion in nursing. In M. Fowler, S. Reimer-Kirkham, R. Sawatzky, & E. Johnston Taylor (Eds.), *Religion, religious ethics, and nursing* (pp. 1-26). New York: Springer.

Health Nexus and Ontario Chronic Disease Prevention Alliance. (2008). *Primer to action: Social determinants of health.* Toronto: Author. Retrieved from *www.healthnexus.ca/projects/primer.pdf*

Hyman, I. (2009). *Racism as a determinant of immigrant health.* Retrieved from *http://canada.metropolis.net/pdfs/racism_policy_brief_e.pdf*

Huang, S. M., & Temple, R. (2008). Is this drug or dose for you? Impact and consideration of ethnic factors in global drug development, regulatory review, and clinical practice. *Clinical Pharmacology & Therapeutics, 84*(3), 287-294. doi:10.1038/clpt.2008.144

International Council of Nurses (ICN). (2007). *Cultural and linguistic competence.* Retrieved from *http://www.icn.ch/images/stories/documents/publications/position_statements/B03_Cultural_Linguistic_Competence.pdf*

Limb, G. E., & Hodge, D. R. (2009). Helping child welfare workers improve cultural competence by utilizing spiritual genograms with Native American families and children. *Children and Youth Services Review, 32,* 239-245. doi:10.1016/j.childyouth.2009.08.021

Lo, H. T., & Pottinger, A. (2007). Mental health practice. In R. H. Srivastava (Ed.), *The healthcare professional's guide to clinical cultural competence* (pp. 247-263). Toronto: Elsevier Canada.

Loppie Reading, C. & Wien, F. (2009). *Health inequalities and social determinants of Aboriginal peoples' health.* Retrieved from *http://www.nccah-ccnsa.ca/docs/social%20determinates/NCCAH-loppie-Wien_report.pdf*

Mikkonen, J., & Raphael, D. (2010). *Social determinants of health: The Canadian facts.* Toronto: York University School of Health Policy and Management. Retrieved from *http://www.thecanadianfacts.org/*

Pesut, B., Fowler, M., Taylor, E., Reimer-Kirkham, S., & Sawatzky, R. (2008). Conceptualising spirituality and religion for healthcare. *Journal of Clinical Nursing, 17,* 2803-2810. doi:10.1111/j.1365-2702.2008.02344.x

Pottie, K., Greenway, C., Feightne, J., Welch, V., Swinkels, H., Rashid, M., …, Tugwell, P. (2011). Evidence based clinical guidelines for immigrants and refugees. *Canadian Medical Association Journal, 183*(12), E824-E925. doi:10.1503/cmaj.090313

Provincial Health Services Authority. (2011). *Towards reducing health inequities: A health system approach to chronic disease prevention. A discussion paper.* Vancouver, BC: Population & Public Health, Provincial Health Services Authority. Retrieved from *http://www.phsa.ca/NR/rdonlyres/0F19BDB8-2153-49D1-A214-E7D0D0B9DA3B/52162/TowardsReducingHealthInequitiesFinalDiscussionPape.pdf*

Public Health Agency of Canada. (2003). *What makes Canadians healthy or unhealthy?* Retrieved from *http://www.phac-aspc.gc.ca/ph-sp/determinants/determinants-eng.php#personalhealth*

Purnell, L., & Paulanka, B. (2008). *Transcultural health care: A culturally competent approach* (3rd ed.). Philadelphia: F. A. Davis.

Registered Nurses' Association of Ontario (RNAO). (2007). *Embracing diversity: Developing cultural competence.* Toronto: Author. Retrieved from *www.rnao.org/Page.asp?PageID=122&ContentID=1200*

Schellenberg, G., & Maheux, H. (2007). *Immigrant perspectives on their first four years in Canada. Canadian Social Trends, special edition.* Ottawa: Statistics Canada.

Solar, O., & Irvin, A. (2007). *A conceptual framework for action on the social determinants of health.* Geneva: Commission on Social Determinants of Health, World Health Organization. Retrieved from *http://www.who.int/social_determinants/resources/ csdh_framework_action_05_07.pdf*

Srivastava, R. (2007a). Culture care framework I: Overview and cultural sensitivity. In R. Srivastava (Ed.), *The healthcare professional's guide to clinical cultural competence* (pp. 53-74). Toronto: Elsevier Canada.

Srivastava, R. (Ed.). (2007b). *The healthcare professional's guide to clinical cultural competence.* Toronto: Elsevier Canada.

Srivastava, R. (2007c). Cross cultural communication. In R. Srivastava (Ed.), *The healthcare professional's guide to clinical cultural competence* (pp. 101-124). Toronto: Elsevier Canada.

Srivastava, R. (2007d). Culture care framework II: Culture knowledge, resources, and bridging the gap. In R. Srivastava (Ed.), *The healthcare professional's guide to clinical cultural competence* (pp. 75-100). Toronto: Elsevier Canada.

Srivastava, R. (2008). The ABC (and DE) of cultural competence in clinical care. *Ethnicity and Inequalities in Health and Social Care, 8*(1), 25-31.

Srivastava, R., Srivastava, B. & Srivastava, R. (2012). Hinduism and nursing. In M. Fowler, S. Reimer-Kirkham, R. Sawatzky & E. Johnston Taylor (Eds.), *Religion, religious ethics, and nursing* (pp. 173-196). New York: Springer.

Statistics Canada. (2007). *Immigration in Canada: A portrait of the foreign-born population, 2006 Census* (Catalogue no. 97-557-XIE). Ottawa: Ministry of Industry.

Statistics Canada. (2008a). *Canada's ethnocultural mosaic: 2006 census* (Catalogue no. 97-562-X). Ottawa: Ministry of Industry.

Statistics Canada. (2008b). *Aboriginal Peoples in Canada in 2006: Inuit, Métis and First Nations, 2006 Census* (Catalogue no. 97-558-XIE). Ottawa: Ministry of Industry.

Statistics Canada. (2011). *Insights into the healthy immigrant effect: Mortality by period of immigration and birthplace* (Catalogue no. 82-622-X -No. 008). Ottawa: Ministry of Industry.

Surbone, A. (2008). Cultural aspects of communication in cancer care. *Support Care Cancer, 16,* 235-240. doi:10.1007/s00520-007-0366-0

Teal, C. R., & Street, R. L. (2009). Critical elements of culturally competent communication in the medical encounter: A review and model. *Social Science & Medicine, 68,* 533-543. doi:10.1016/j.socscimed.2008.10.015

Warren, B. J. (2008). Ethnopharmacology: The effect on patients, health care professionals, and systems. *Urologic Nursing, 28*(4), 292-295.

CANADIAN RESOURCES

Aboriginal Nurses Association of Canada
http://www.anac.on.ca
BC Settlement and Multiculturalism
http://www.welcomebc.ca/wbc/immigration/enjoy/leisure/ multiculturalism.page

Canadian Collaboration for Immigrant and Refugee Health (CCIRH)
http://www.ccirh.uottawa.ca/eng/index.html
Canadian Cultural Profiles Project
http://www.cp-pc.ca/
Canadian Ethnocultural Council (CEC)
http://www.ethnocultural.ca/
Citizenship and Immigration Canada
http://www.cic.gc.ca/english/multiculturalism/index.asp
Cultures Canadiennes
http://culturescanada.ca
Cultural Profiles Project
http://www.settlement.org/sys/library_detail.asp?doc_id=1002234
Ethnicity Online
http://www.ethnicityonline.net/
Joint Centre of Excellence for Research on Immigration and Settlement
http://ccrweb.ca/en/org/joint-centre-excellence-research-immigration-and-settlement-toronto-ceris
McMaster University: Cultural Competence
http://www.mcmaster.ca/hres/cultural_competence.html
National Aboriginal Health Organization
http://www.naho.ca/
Ontario Ministry of Children and Youth Services
http://www.children.gov.on.ca/htdocs/English/topics/specialneeds/ achieving_cultural_competence.aspx
Ontario Multicultural Health Applied Research Network
http://www.ryerson.ca/omh/index.html
SickKids Cultural Competence E-Learning Modules Series
http://www.sickkids.ca/culturalcompetence/elearning-modules/ eLearning-modules.html

RELATED RESOURCES

National Standards on Culturally and Linguistically Appropriate Services (Office of Minority Health)
http://minorityhealth.hhs.gov/templates/browse.aspx?lvl=2&lvlID=15
Disparities Solutions Center at Massachusetts General Hospital
http://www2.massgeneral.org/disparitiessolutions/
DiversityRx
http://www.diversityrx.org
Ethnomed
http://ethnomed.org/
National Center for Cultural Competence (Georgetown University, Center for Child and Human Development)
http://www11.georgetown.edu/research/gucchd/nccc/index.html
National Institutes of Health (U.S. Department of Health and Human Services)
http://health.nih.gov/category/MinorityHealth
Think Cultural Health
http://thinkculturalhealth.org/
Transcultural Nursing Society
http://www.tcns.org/

evolve *For additional Internet resources, see the Web site for this book at* **http://evolve.elsevier.com/Canada/Lewis/medsurg**

Health History and Physical Examination

Written by Ian M. Camera

Adapted by Mary Ann Fegan

LEARNING OBJECTIVES

1. Explain the purpose and components of and the techniques related to a patient's health history and physical examination.
2. Obtain a nursing history using a functional health pattern format.
3. Describe the appropriate use and techniques of inspection, palpation, percussion, and auscultation.
4. Differentiate among comprehensive, focused, and emergency types of assessment in terms of indications, purposes, and components.

KEY TERMS

auscultation The act of listening for sounds within the body to evaluate the condition of the heart, the blood vessels, the lungs, the pleura, the intestines, or other organs, p. 45

database Represents all the health information about a patient; it includes the nursing history and physical examination findings, the physician's history and physical examination findings, results of laboratory and diagnostic tests, and information contributed by other health professionals, p. 38

functional health patterns A format designed by Marjorie Gordon to promote systematic data collection to determine the presence of problems amenable to nursing diagnosis and treatment, p. 40

general survey statement Statement of the professional's general impression of a patient, including behavioural observations, p. 44

inspection The visual examination of a part or region of the body to assess normal conditions or deviations from normal, p. 44

medical history A standard format designed to collect data to be used primarily by the physician to determine risk for disease and to diagnose a medical condition, p. 38

negative finding The absence of a sign or symptom usually associated with a problem, p. 44

nursing history The collection and interpretation of a patient's functional health status used primarily by the nurse to support the identification of nursing diagnoses, p. 38

objective data Data relating to the patient's condition that can be observed and measured; also called signs, p. 39

palpation Technique used in physical examination in which the examiner feels the texture, the size, the consistency, and the location of certain body parts with the hands, p. 44

percussion Technique in physical examination of tapping the body directly or indirectly with the fingertips or fist, p. 44

physical examination The systematic assessment of the physical and mental status of a patient, p. 44

positive finding An indication that the patient has or had a sign or symptom associated with the particular problem in question, p. 44

subjective data What the person says about himself or herself either as spontaneously offered information or as a response to direct questioning; also called symptoms, p. 38

ELECTRONIC RESOURCES

Supplemental content related to Chapter 3 can be found …

Evolve Web Site ⊖volve

http://evolve.elsevier.com/Canada/Lewis/medsurg
- Clinical Reference: Laboratory Values
- Content Updates
- Electronic Calculators
- eTables:
  - eTable 3-1: Example of How to Record Findings of Physical Assessment

- eTable 3-2: Head to Toe Assessment
- eTable 3-3: Focused Assessments
- Examination Review Questions
- Glossary
- Key Points (Printable and MP3 Download)
- Physical Examination Video: General Inspection and Measurements

Obtaining a patient's health history and performing a physical examination are activities completed by the nurse during the assessment phase of the nursing process. The information obtained during this phase contributes to a database that identifies the patient's current and past health status and provides a baseline against which future changes can be evaluated. The purpose of the nursing assessment is to enable the nurse to make a judgement or diagnosis about the patient's health status (Jarvis, Browne, MacDonald-Jenkins, & Luctkar-Flude, 2009). Although assessment is identified as the first step of the nursing process, it is performed continuously throughout the nursing process to validate diagnoses, evaluate the patient's response to nursing interventions, and determine the extent to which patient outcomes and goals have been met.

Data Collection

Collection of data about the patient is not solely the nurse's responsibility. The **database** comprises all the health information about a patient. It includes the nursing history and physical examination findings, the physician's history and physical examination findings, results of laboratory and diagnostic tests, and information contributed by other health professionals. Numerous approaches and formats exist for gathering information about the patient in various health care settings. The purpose for which the information is to be used determines the methods of data collection. The nurse and physician both perform a patient history and physical examination, but they use different formats and analyze the data differently because of each discipline's focus.

Medical Focus

A **medical history** is a standard format designed to collect data to be used primarily by the physician to determine risk for disease and to diagnose a medical condition (Table 3-1). The medical history is usually collected by a member of the medical team (physician, resident, or medical student) or an advanced practice nurse (registered nurse [RN], extended class [EC], or RN[EC] or nurse practitioner). The physician's physical examination and the laboratory and diagnostic tests the physician orders assist in establishing a medical diagnosis and evaluating specific medical therapy. The information collected and reported by the physician

is also used by nurses and other health care professionals, but within the focus of their care. For example, the abnormal results of a neurological examination by a physician may assist in the diagnosis of a brain lesion, but the nurse may use those same results to identify a nursing diagnosis of *risk for falls*. The physiotherapist may also use the results to plan therapy involving exercise, splints, or ambulatory aids.

Nursing Focus

The focus of nursing care is the diagnosis and treatment of human responses to actual or potential health problems. The information obtained from the **nursing history** and physical examination is used to determine what responses the patient is exhibiting or could potentially exhibit as a result of a health problem. The nurse is interested in the functional capabilities of the patient. In the patient with a medical diagnosis of diabetes mellitus, for example, one of the patient's responses may be anxiety or a lack of knowledge regarding self-management for the condition. The patient may also experience the physical response of fluid volume deficit because of the abnormal fluid loss caused by hyperglycemia. These human responses to the condition of diabetes can be diagnosed and treated by nurses. During the nursing history interview and physical examination, the nurse obtains the necessary data to support the identification of nursing diagnoses (Figure 3-1).

Types of Data

The database includes both subjective and objective data. **Subjective data** are collected by interviewing the patient during the

Table 3-1 Medical History Format
- Demographic data
- Chief complaint
- History of present illness
- Past health history
- Family health history
- Review of systems

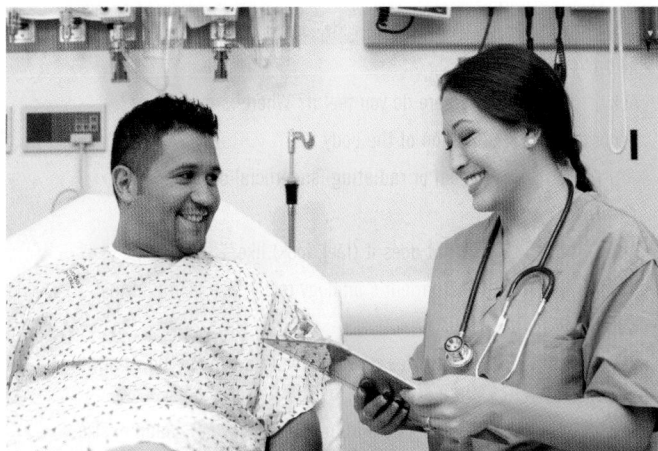

Figure 3-1 Obtaining a nursing history is an important role of the nurse.

Source: © 2011 Jupiterimages Corporation.

nursing history. This body of data includes information that can only be described or verified by the patient. It is what the person tells the nurse about herself or himself either as spontaneously offered information or as a response to direct questioning. Subjective data may also be referred to as *symptoms*. Knowledgeable others, such as family members and caregivers, can also contribute subjective data about the patient.

Objective data are data that can be observed and measured. These types of data are obtained using inspection, palpation, percussion, and auscultation during the physical examination. Objective data are also provided by other health care professionals and diagnostic testing. Objective data are also called *signs*. Although subjective data are usually obtained by interview and objective data are obtained by physical examination, it is common for the patient to provide subjective data while the nurse is performing the physical examination, and it is also common for the nurse to observe objective signs while interviewing the patient during the history.

Interviewing Considerations

The purpose of the patient interview is to obtain a complete health history—subjective data about the patient's past and present health status. Collection of data assists the nurse and the patient in identifying health problems as well as patient strengths and resources. The nurse can use the data to identify areas where the patient may be unable to meet personal needs and therefore requires nursing assistance. The patient perceives this encounter as an indication of how the health care system will provide assistance.

Effective communication is a key factor in the interview process. Creating a climate of trust and respect is critical to establishing a therapeutic relationship, as is the nurse's ability to engage in reflective practice. This concept includes the required capacities of: self-awareness, self-knowledge, empathy, and awareness of boundaries and limits of the professional role (Registered Nurses' Association of Ontario [RNAO], 2006). The nurse must communicate acceptance of the patient as an individual by using an open, responsive, nonjudgemental approach. Individuals communicate not only through language but also in their manner of dress, gestures, and body language. Modes of communication

are learned through one's culture, which influences not only the words, gestures, and posture one uses but also the nature of information that is shared with others. (See Chapter 2 for details on communicating effectively with patients.) In addition to understanding the principles of effective communication, each nurse must develop a personal style of relating to patients. Although no single style fits all people, wording specific questions in certain ways will increase the probability of eliciting the needed information. Ease with asking questions, particularly those related to sensitive areas such as sexual functioning and economic status, comes with experience. The amount of time needed to complete a nursing history may vary with the format used and the experience of the nurse. It may be completed in one or several sessions, depending on the setting and the patient. In the case of an older adult patient with a low energy level, several short sessions may have to be scheduled. Allowing time for the patient to volunteer information about particular areas of concern enables the nurse to work with the patient to identify existing and potential health problems. When a patient is unable to provide the necessary data (e.g., is unconscious or aphasic), the nurse should ask the person who has assumed responsibility for the patient's welfare to provide as much information as possible.

Before beginning the nursing history, the nurse should explain to the patient that the purpose of a detailed history is to collect information that will provide a health profile for comprehensive health care, including health promotion. This detailed information is collected during entry into the health care system, and subsequently, only updates are needed. The nurse should explain that personal and social data are needed to individualize the plan of care. This explanation is necessary because the patient may not be accustomed to sharing personal information and may need to know the purpose of such questioning. The nurse should assure the patient that all information will be kept confidential. The Canadian Nurses Association (CNA) requires that nurses protect the confidentiality of all information gained in the context of the professional relationship and practice within the bounds of relevant laws governing privacy and confidentiality of personal health information. The CNA *Code of Ethics for Registered Nurses* provides helpful guidelines for ensuring confidentiality in nursing practice (Canadian Nurses Association, 2008). To obtain factual, easily categorized information, a direct interview technique can be used. Closed questions such as, "Have you had surgery before?" that require brief, specific responses are used. When asking sensitive personal and social questions, the nurse can communicate the acceptance or normalcy of behaviours by prefacing questions with phrases such as "most people" or "frequently." For example, stating, "Many people taking antihypertensive drugs have concerns about sexual functioning; do you have any you would like to discuss?" shows the patient that a particular situation may not be unique to that patient. Another method of putting the patient at ease is to word the question so that an affirmative answer appears expected. An example of this technique is to ask, "What do you like to drink at a party?" instead of, "Do you drink?" "How often do you drink alcohol?" is another way of obtaining information related to alcohol intake. These questions are open ended, encouraging the patient to discuss the issue in the patient's own words and at his or her own pace (Wilson & Giddens, 2009).

The nurse must judge the reliability of the patient as a historian. An older adult may give a false impression about her or his mental status because of a prolonged response time or visual and hearing impairment. The complexity and long duration of health problems may also make it difficult for an older adult to be an accurate, orderly historian.

It is important that the nurse determine the patient's priority concerns and what the patient expects from the present encounter. Often there is a lack of congruency between the priorities of the patient and those of the nurse. For example, the nurse's priority may be to obtain needed information and complete necessary documentation, whereas the patient is interested only in getting relief from symptoms. Until the patient's priority need is met, the nurse will probably be unsuccessful in obtaining complete data.

The nurse must make a judgement about the amount of information that should be collected on initial contact with the patient. In interviews with older adult patients, patients with long-term chronic disease, patients with pain, and patients in emergency situations, the nurse may choose to ask only those questions that are pertinent to a specific problem and to defer the complete history interview until a more appropriate time.

Symptom Investigation

At any time during assessment, the patient may report a symptom such as pain, fatigue, or weakness. Because symptoms are directly experienced by the patient and not observable to the nurse, the symptom must be investigated. Table 3-2 lists eight areas that should be investigated if a symptom is present. The information that is obtained may help determine the cause of the symptom. For example, if a patient states that he has "pain in his leg at times," the nurse would obtain and record the following information:

> Has right midcalf pain *(location)*, described as "like being stabbed with a knife" *(quality)*. Pain is so severe that it is not possible for the patient to continue walking *(quantity)*. Onset is abrupt, lasting for 1 to 2 minutes; it occurs once or twice daily, and it last occurred on 5/5/12 *(chronology)*. Generally occurs at work when climbing stairs after lunch, but last occurred when cutting lawn *(setting)*. Pain is alleviated by rest for 2 to 3 minutes. The patient has been salting his food "more heavily" than he used to, but "it doesn't help" *(alleviating factor)*. Leg pain is at times accompanied by chest pain that causes some nausea *(associated manifestations)*. The patient has not altered his lifestyle because of the intermittent pain. He thinks it is caused by "muscle cramps from lack of salt" *(personal meaning)*.

Nursing History: Subjective Data

The format used in this chapter for obtaining a nursing history includes an initial collection of important health information followed by assessment of the patient's **functional health patterns** (Table 3-3). Gordon has described an assessment format in which subjective data are collected during assessment of specific functional areas (Gordon, 2010). The format is designed to promote systematic data collection to determine the presence of problems amenable to nursing diagnosis and treatment. Analysis of the data collected with assessment of each functional health pattern facilitates the nursing diagnosis process. It is also important for the nurse to consider the social determinants of health to ensure a complete and relevant health history assessment. The primary factors that shape the health of Canadians are the living conditions that patients experience (Mikkonen & Raphael, 2009).

Table 3-2 Investigation of a Symptom

Location	
Ask	"Where do you feel it? Where is it located?"
Record	Region of the body
	Local or radiating, superficial or deep
Quality	
Ask	"What does it (feel, look) like?"
Record	The patient's analogy (e.g., "like being burned")
Quantity	
Ask	"How often do you have this feeling? How bad is it? On a scale of 0 to 10, rate your pain"
Record	Frequency (mild, moderate, severe), volume, size, extent, pain rating number
Chronology	
Ask	"When was the first time it occurred? Any particular time of day, week, month, or year?"
Record	Time of onset, duration, periodicity and frequency, course of symptoms
Setting	
Ask	"Where are you when this occurs? What are you doing?"
Record	Where patient is when symptom occurs, what patient is doing, if symptom is related to anything
Aggravating or Alleviating Factors	
Ask	"What makes it better? Worse? Is there any activity that seems to cause it? What have you done for it? Did it help? Was there some reason you didn't do anything about it?"
Record	Influence of physical and emotional activities, patient's attempts to alleviate (or treat) the symptom
Associated Manifestations	
Ask	"What other things do you see or feel when it occurs? Has it affected your appetite? Elimination? Sleeping?"
Record	Other symptoms
Meaning of the Symptom to the Patient	
Ask	"How has it affected your life? Why have you sought care now? What do you think may be the cause?"
Record	Patient's statements about the effect of the symptom and the cause of the symptom

Important Health Information

Important health information provides an overview of past and present medical conditions and treatments. Past health history, medications, and surgery or other treatments are included in this part of the history.

Past Health History. The past health history provides information about the patient's prior health status. The patient is specifically asked about major childhood and adult illnesses, injuries, hospitalizations, operations, therapeutic regimens, travel, habits, and the use of supportive devices. Specific questioning is more effective than simply asking if the patient has had any illness or health problems in the past.

Table 3-3 Nursing History: Functional Health Pattern Format

Demographic Data

- Name, address, age, occupation
- Culture and ethnicity

Important Health Information

- Past health history
- Medications/supplements
- Surgery or other treatments

Functional Health Patterns

Health Perception–Health Management Pattern

1. Reason for visit?
2. General state of health?
3. Number of colds in past year?
4. Most important things done to keep healthy? Breast self-examination? Testicular self-examination? Colorectal cancer, hypertension, and cardiac disease risk screening? Papanicolaou (Pap) test? Immunizations such as tetanus, pneumonia, hepatitis, and flu vaccines?
5. Health compliance problems?
6. Cause of illness? Action taken? Results?
7. Things important to you while here?
8. Family health history (e.g., cardiovascular disease, hypertension, cancer, diabetes mellitus, psychiatric illness, genetic disorders)?
9. Illness and injury risk factors: sexual/domestic abuse, violence, use of cigarettes and/or alcohol, substance abuse?
10. Allergies? Immunizations?

Nutritional–Metabolic Pattern

1. Typical daily food intake (describe)? Supplements?
2. Typical daily fluid intake (describe)?
3. Weight loss or gain (amount, time span)?
4. Desired weight?
5. Appetite?
6. Food or eating: Discomfort? Diet restrictions?
7. Change in appetite with anxiety?
8. Heal well or poorly?
9. Skin problems: Lesions? Dryness?
10. Dental problems?
11. Food preferences?
12. Food allergies?

Elimination Pattern

1. Bowel elimination pattern (describe): Frequency? Character? Discomfort? Laxatives? Enemas?
2. Urinary elimination pattern (describe): Frequency? Problem in control? Diuretics?
3. Any external devices?
4. Excess perspiration? Odour problems? Itching?

Activity–Exercise Pattern

1. Sufficient energy for desired or required activities?
2. Exercise pattern? Type? Regularity?
3. Spare time (leisure) activities?
4. Dyspnea? Chest pain? Palpitations? Stiffness? Aching? Weakness?
5. Perceived ability for (code for level):

Feeding _____	Cooking _____	Grooming _____
Bed mobility _____	Bathing _____	Dressing _____
Toileting _____	Shopping _____	General mobility _____

Functional Levels Code

Level 0: Full self-care

Level I: Requires use of equipment or device

Level II: Requires assistance or supervision from another person

Level III: Is dependent and does not participate

Sleep–Rest Pattern

1. Generally rested and ready for daily activities after sleep?
2. Sleep onset problems? Aids? Dreams (nightmares)? Early awakening?
3. Usual sleep rituals?
4. Usual sleep pattern?

Cognitive–Perceptual Pattern

1. Hearing difficulty? Hearing aids?
2. Vision? Wear glasses? Last checked?
3. Any change in taste? Any change in smell?
4. Any recent change in memory?
5. Easiest way to learn things?
6. Any discomfort? Pain (rating on scale 0-10)? How managed?
7. Ability to communicate?
8. Understanding of illness?
9. Understanding of treatments?

Self-Perception–Self-Concept Pattern

1. Self-description? Self-perception?
2. Effect of illness on self-image?
3. Relieving factors?

Role–Relationship Pattern

1. Live alone? Family? Family structure diagram?
2. Difficult family problems?
3. Family problem solving?
4. Family dependence on you for things? How managing?
5. Family's and others' feelings about illness/hospitalization?*
6. Problems with children? Difficulty handling?*
7. Belong to social groups? Have close friends? Feel lonely (frequency)?
8. Work satisfaction (school)? Income sufficient for needs?*
9. Feel part of or isolated from neighbourhood where living?

Continued

Table 3-3 Nursing History: Functional Health Pattern Format—cont'd	
Sexuality–Reproductive Pattern	3. Recent life changes?
1. Any changes or problems in sexual relations?*	4. Problem-solving techniques? Effective?
2. Effect of illness?	**Value–Belief Pattern**
3. Use of contraceptives? Problems?	1. Satisfied with life?
4. When menstruation started? Last menstrual period? Menstrual problems? Gravida? Para?†	2. Religion important in your life?
	3. Conflict between treatment and beliefs?
5. Effect of present condition or treatment on sexuality?	**Other**
6. Sexually transmitted infections?	1. Other important issues?
Coping–Stress Tolerance Pattern	2. Questions?
1. Tense a lot of the time? What helps? Use any medicines, drugs, alcohol?	
2. Have someone to confide in? Available to you now?	

*If appropriate.
†For women.
Source: Adapted from Gordon, M. (2010). *Manual of nursing diagnosis* (12th ed.). Boston: Jones & Bartlett.

Medications. Specific details related to past or present medications are obtained. This includes the use of prescription drugs, over-the-counter drugs, vitamins, herbal products, and dietary supplements. Patients frequently do not consider herbal products and dietary supplements as drugs, and for this reason, or because they fear health care professionals will disapprove, they may not tell health care professionals that they are using these products. Patients at high risk for drug–herb interactions include those taking anticoagulant, antihypertensive, or immune-regulating therapy and patients receiving anaesthesia for surgery, so it is important to specifically ask about their use in an accepting and nonjudgemental manner (see Chapter 12, Table 12-8). Examples of specific prescription and over-the-counter medications to ask about include corticosteroids, birth control pills, antibiotics, diuretics, aspirin, antacids, and laxatives. Older adult patients, in particular, should be questioned about medication routines. Changes in absorption, distribution, metabolism, and excretion of and reaction to drugs, as well as surgery, concurrent disease, and the prevalence of polypharmacy, make drug-related concerns a serious potential problem for older adults (Touhy, Jett, Boscart, & McCleary, 2011).

Surgery or Other Treatments. All injuries, hospitalizations, and surgeries are recorded along with the date of the event, the treatment, and the outcome. The outcome includes whether the problem was completely resolved or if there are residual effects. Blood transfusions received by the patient are also documented.

Functional Health Patterns

The nurse assesses the patient's functional health patterns to identify patient strengths in function and to determine whether dysfunctional health patterns and/or potential dysfunctional patterns exist. Dysfunctional health patterns result in nursing diagnoses, and potential dysfunctional patterns identify risk conditions for problems. Use of the functional health pattern framework for assessment assists the nurse in differentiating between areas for independent nursing intervention and areas requiring collaboration or referral. In addition, the nurse may identify patients with effective function who express a desire for

a higher level of wellness. Table 3–3 provides examples of specific questions appropriate to ask the patient related to the functional health patterns.

Health Perception–Health Management Pattern.

Assessment of the health perception–health management functional health pattern focuses on the patient's perceived level of health and well-being and on personal practices for maintaining health. This includes preventive screening activities, such as breast and testicular examinations; colorectal cancer, hypertension, and cardiac risk factor screening; Papanicolaou (Pap) test; and immunizations such as tetanus, pneumonia, and flu vaccines. The nurse should ask about the type of health care professional that the patient uses. Culture may play a role in who the patient's primary health care professional is. For example, if the patient is Aboriginal Canadian, a traditional healer may be considered as the primary health care professional. If the patient is of Chinese origin, a Chinese healer who practices traditional Chinese medicine may be the primary health care professional.

The questions for this pattern also are aimed at identifying risk factors by obtaining a family history, history of health habits (e.g., smoking, alcohol, drug use), and exposure to environmental hazards. (See Chapter 12 for details on how to assess patients' use of complementary and alternative therapies).

There are several ways to identify the patient's perceived level of health and well-being. First, when questioning the patient, the nurse determines the patient's feelings of effectiveness at staying healthy by asking what helps and what hinders. Next, the patient is asked to describe personal health and any concerns about it. This information should be recorded in the patient's own words. It is often useful to determine whether the patient considers his or her health to be excellent, good, fair, or poor.

In addition, the patient is asked about a family history of major problems, such as cardiovascular disease, hypertension, cancer, diabetes mellitus, psychiatric illness, and genetic disorders. Information about sexual abuse, violence, and drug and alcohol use or abuse should also be obtained. One of the objectives in this pattern is to identify any preventive measures used by the patient to promote personal health.

If the patient is hospitalized, expectations of this hospitalization should be determined. A description of the patient's understanding of the current health problem, including a description of its onset, course, and treatment, should be obtained. Determining what the patient does when ill is important. These questions elicit information about a patient's knowledge of the health problem, awareness of what should be done, and ability to use appropriate resources to manage the problem.

Nutritional–Metabolic Pattern. The processes of ingestion, digestion, absorption, and metabolism are assessed in this pattern. A 24-hour dietary recall should be obtained from the patient. From this information, the nurse can evaluate the quantity and quality of foods and fluids consumed. If a problem is identified, the nurse may request that the patient keep a 3-day food diary for a more careful analysis of dietary intake. Food-frequency questionnaires based on weekly intake are also available to obtain information from the person. Metabolism is evaluated by questioning the patient regarding weight gain, weight loss, energy level, and skin lesions or dryness. (See Chapter 42 for details on assessing nutritional intake.)

The impact on nutrition of psychological factors such as depression, anxiety, and self-concept is assessed. For example, "How is your appetite affected by anxiety?" is an appropriate question. Sociocultural factors such as food budget, who prepares the meals, and food preferences are also assessed.

Determining how the patient's present condition has interfered with eating and appetite is important. If the patient's present condition has produced symptoms such as nausea, gas, or pain, the effect of these symptoms on appetite should be determined. Food allergies and the need for a special or restricted diet should be noted. Additional information about the person's nutritional status can be determined by asking specific questions such as the following:

"How many fruits and vegetables do you eat a day?"
"Give me an example of your usual intake of meat."
"How well do you heal from a wound?"

Elimination Pattern. The nurse assesses bowel, bladder, and skin function in this pattern. The nurse asks about the frequency of bowel and bladder activity. A description of consistency, amount, colour, and unusual odour should be elicited. The patient should be asked if loss of control or pain is associated with defecating or urinating. If laxatives or enemas are used, the frequency, type, and results should be noted. If any collecting devices are used, such as catheter or colostomy equipment, the nurse asks about their use and care.

The skin is assessed again in the elimination pattern in terms of its excretory function. The patient should be asked about the condition of her or his skin and whether edema, pruritus, or excessive perspiration is problematic.

Activity–Exercise Pattern. The patient's usual pattern of exercise, activity, leisure, and recreation is assessed by the nurse. The patient should be questioned about his or her ability to perform activities of daily living. Table 3-3 includes the grading scale for self-care abilities under the activity–exercise pattern. If the patient is unable to perform activities of daily living, such as toileting, eating, and moving independently, the specific problems that limit an activity should be noted. Chest pain, dyspnea, dizziness, intermittent claudication (leg pain when walking short distances), musculoskeletal pain, fatigue, and weakness are problems that commonly result in some degree of self-care deficit.

Sleep–Rest Pattern. This pattern describes the patient's pattern of sleep, rest, and relaxation in a 24-hour period. The individual's perception of the effectiveness of sleep and relaxation is pertinent. This information can be elicited by asking, "Do you feel rested when you wake up?" Most people take sleep for granted unless they have a problem with sleeping.

The patient's usual activities related to bedtime and the usual sleep pattern should be determined. Particular routines, position, medications, and environmental factors used to foster sleep should also be elicited.

Cognitive–Perceptual Pattern. Assessment of this pattern involves a description of all senses (vision, hearing, taste, touch, and smell) and the cognitive functions such as communication, memory, and decision making. In addition, pain is assessed in this pattern. (See Chapter 10 for details on pain assessment.) The patient should be asked about any sensory deficits that affect the ability to perform activities of daily living. Routine eye care, including the date of the last examination, should be elicited. Ways in which the patient compensates for any sensory–perceptual problems should be discussed and noted. Patients should be asked how they communicate best and about their understanding of their illness and treatment. This information is used by the nurse in planning patient teaching.

Self-Perception–Self-Concept Pattern. This pattern describes the patient's self-concept, which is critical in determining the way the person interacts with others. Included are attitudes about self, perception of personal abilities, body image, and general sense of worth.

The nurse should ask the patient for a self-description and how the health condition affects self-attitude. Expressions of helplessness or loss of control frequently reflect an inability to care for oneself.

Role–Relationship Pattern. This pattern describes the roles and relationships of the patient, including major responsibilities. It also examines the patient's self-evaluation of her or his performance of the expected behaviours related to these roles.

The patient should be asked to describe family, social, and work relationships. The nurse should determine whether patterns in these relationships are satisfactory or whether strain is evident. The nurse should note the patient's feelings about his or her role in these relationships and the effect the present condition has on his or her role and relationship.

Sexuality–Reproductive Pattern. This pattern describes satisfaction or dissatisfaction with personal sexuality and describes the reproductive pattern. Assessing this pattern is important because many illnesses, surgical procedures, and medications affect sexual function. A patient's sexual and reproductive concerns may be expressed, teaching needs and treatable problems may be identified, and normal growth and development may be monitored through information obtained in this pattern.

The interview should be appropriate to the sex, age, and developmental stage of the patient. For example, a 40-year-old widowed female patient might be asked if she has any problems related to her genital area, such as vaginal discharge. She also should be asked whether she is sexually active and, if so, whether she practices safer sex. A 25-year-old male patient might be asked about his knowledge and use of condoms.

Specifically, the nurse should determine whether there is a lack of knowledge in relation to sexuality and reproduction.

Whether the patient perceives a problem in the area of sexuality should also be determined. The effect of the patient's present condition or treatment on personal sexuality should be noted.

Obtaining information related to sexuality is often difficult for the nurse. However, it is important to take a health history and screen for sexual function and dysfunction. Based on the complexity of the problem, the nurse may be able to provide limited information or refer the patient to a more experienced professional.

Coping–Stress Tolerance Pattern.

This pattern describes the general coping pattern and the effectiveness of the coping mechanisms. Assessment of this pattern involves analyzing the specific stressors or problems that the patient is confronting, the patient's perception of the stressor, and the patient's response to the stressor.

The major losses or changes experienced by the patient in the previous year are important to document. Current major stressors the patient is confronting are also important. The strategies used by the patient to deal with stressors and relieve tension should be noted. Individuals and groups who make up the patient's social support networks should be recorded.

Value–Belief Pattern.

This pattern describes the values, goals, and beliefs (including spiritual) that guide health-related choices (Gordon, 2010). The patient's ethnic background and the effects of culture and beliefs about health and illness on health practices should be documented. The patient's wishes about continuation of religious practices and the use of religious articles should be noted and honoured. The possibility of a conflict in values or beliefs can be determined by asking a question such as, "Does your plan of care cause any conflict in your value or belief system?"

Physical Examination: Objective Data

General Survey

Following the nursing history, a **general survey statement** is made. The general survey is a statement of the professional's general impression of a patient, including behavioural observations. This initial survey is considered a scanning procedure and begins with the professional's first encounter with the patient and continues during the health history interview.

Although the professional may include other data that seem pertinent, the major areas usually included in the general survey statement are (a) body features, (b) state of consciousness and arousal, (c) speech, (d) body movements, (e) obvious physical signs, (f) nutritional status, and (g) behaviour. Vital signs, height, and weight are often included in the general survey statement. Observations of these areas provide the data for the general survey statement. The following is a sample of a general survey statement:

> Mrs. H. is a 34-year-old Italian woman, BP 130/84, P 88, R 18. No distinguishing body features. Alert but anxious. Speech rapid with trailing thoughts. Wringing hands and shuffling feet during interview. Skin flushed, hands clammy. Overweight relative to height. Sits with eyes downcast and shoulders slumped and avoids eye contact.

Physical Examination

The **physical examination** is the systematic assessment of the physical and mental status of a patient, and findings are considered objective data. Throughout the physical examination, any positive findings are explored using the same criteria as the investigation of a symptom during the nursing history (see Table 3-2). A **positive finding** indicates that the patient has or had the particular problem or sign under discussion. For example, if the patient with jaundice has an enlarged liver, it is a positive finding. Relevant information about this problem should then be gathered.

Negative findings may also be significant. A **negative finding** is the absence of a sign or symptom usually associated with a problem. For example, peripheral edema is common with advanced liver disease. If edema is not present in a patient with advanced liver disease, this should be specifically documented as "no peripheral edema."

Techniques.

Four major techniques are used in performing the physical examination: inspection, palpation, percussion, and auscultation. The physical assessment techniques are usually performed in the sequence of inspection, palpation, percussion, and auscultation. The only exception to this sequence is for the abdominal examination. In this instance, the sequence is inspection, auscultation, percussion, and palpation. Palpation and percussion of the abdomen before auscultation can alter bowel sounds and produce false findings. Not every assessment area requires the use of all four assessment techniques. For example, assessment of the musculoskeletal system requires only inspection and palpation.

Inspection. **Inspection** is the visual examination of a part or region of the body to assess normal conditions or deviations from normal. Inspection is more than just looking. This technique is deliberate, systematic, and focused. The nurse must compare what is seen with the known, generally visible characteristics of the body part being inspected. For example, most 30-year-old men have hair on their legs. Absence of hair may indicate a vascular problem and signals the need for further investigation, or it may be normal for a patient of a particular ethnicity. For example, Aboriginal Canadian men have very little body hair.

Palpation. **Palpation** is the examination of the body through the use of touch. The use of light, moderate, and deep palpation can yield information related to masses, pulsations, organ enlargement, tenderness or pain, swelling, muscular spasm or rigidity, elasticity, vibration of voice sounds, crepitus, moisture, and differences in texture (Weber & Kelley, 2009). The nurse will learn that different parts of the hand are more sensitive and thus suited to certain assessments. For example, the tips of the fingers are used to palpate lymph nodes, the dorsa of hands and fingers are used to assess temperatures, and the palmar surface is best suited for feeling vibrations (Figure 3-2).

Percussion. **Percussion** is an assessment technique involving the production of sound to obtain information about the underlying area. The percussion sound may be produced directly or indirectly. Direct percussion is performed by directly tapping the body with one or two fingers to elicit a sound. Indirect, or mediated, percussion is the more common percussion technique. The middle finger (pleximeter) of the nondominant hand is placed

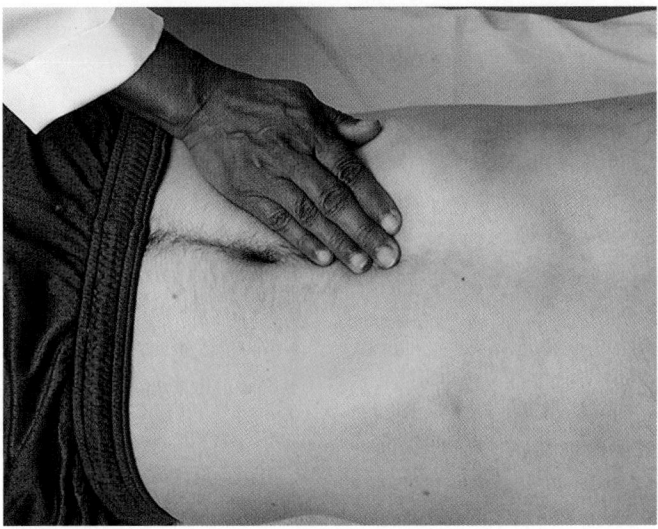

Figure 3-2 Palpation is the examination of the body through the use of touch.

Source: Wilson, S. F., & Giddens, J. F. (2009). *Health assessment for nursing practice* (4th ed., p. 293, Figure 14-8). St. Louis: Mosby.

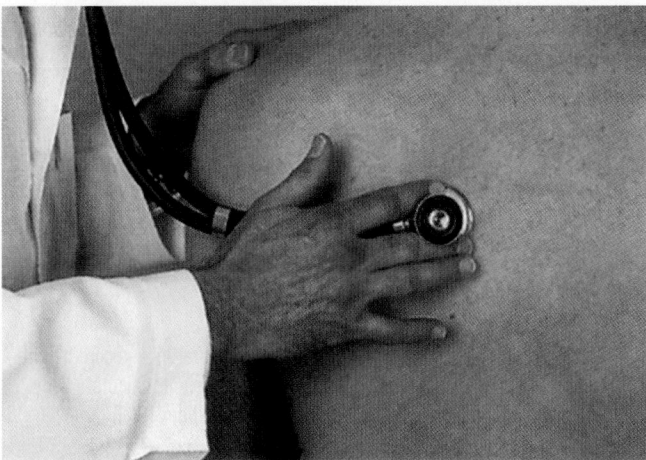

Figure 3-4 Auscultation is listening to sounds produced by the body to assess normal conditions and deviations from normal.

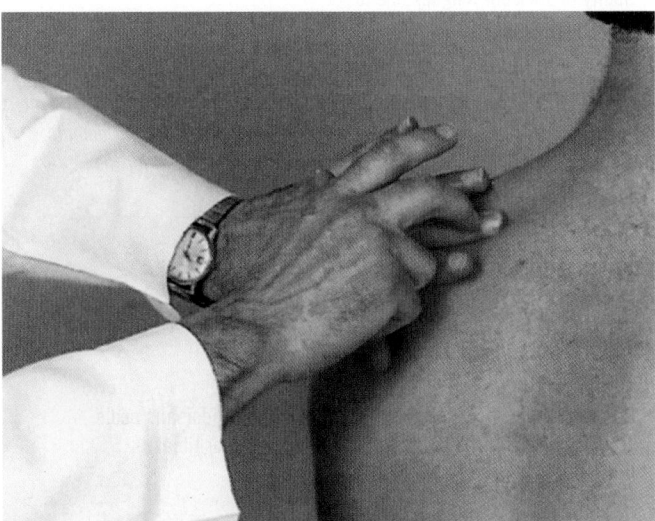

Figure 3-3 Percussion technique: tapping the interphalangeal joint. Only the middle finger of the nondominant hand should be in contact with the skin surface.

Table 3-4 Equipment for Physical Examination	
• Stethoscope (with bell and diaphragm, tubing 38-46 cm)	• Tongue blades
	• Cotton balls
• Wristwatch (with second hand or digitalized)	• Percussion hammer
	• Tuning fork
• Blood pressure cuff	• Alcohol swabs
• Ophthalmoscope–otoscope set	• Patient gown
• Eye chart (wall chart or Snellen pocket eye card)	• Paper cup with water
• Pocket flashlight	• Examining table or bed

firmly against the body surface. The tip of the middle finger of the dominant hand (plexor) strikes the distal phalanx or the distal interphalangeal joint of the pleximeter finger (Figure 3-3). A relaxed wrist and rapid strike produce the best sounds. The sounds and the vibrations produced relative to the underlying structures are evaluated. Deviation from an expected sound may indicate a problem. For example, the usual percussion sound in the right lower quadrant of the abdomen is tympany. Dullness in this area may indicate a problem that should be investigated. (Specific percussion sounds of various body parts and regions are discussed in the appropriate assessment chapters.)

Auscultation. **Auscultation** is listening to sounds produced by the body to assess normal conditions and deviations from

normal. Auscultation is usually indirect and done with a stethoscope to clarify sounds by blocking out extraneous sounds (Figure 3-4). The bell of the stethoscope is more sensitive to low-pitched sounds. The diaphragm of the stethoscope is more sensitive to high-pitched sounds. Auscultation is particularly useful in evaluating sounds from the heart, the lungs, the abdomen, and the vascular system. (Specific auscultatory sounds and techniques are discussed in the appropriate assessment chapters.)

Equipment. The equipment needed for the physical examination should be easily accessible during the examination (Table 3-4). Organizing equipment before the examination saves the time and energy of the patient and the nurse. Lack of organization can discourage the patient and lead to lack of trust and confidence in the nurse. (The uses of specific pieces of equipment are discussed in the appropriate assessment chapters.)

Organization of the Examination. The physical examination should be performed systematically and efficiently. Explanations should be given to the patient as the examination proceeds. The factors to be considered are the nurse's efficiency and the patient's comfort, safety, and privacy. An examiner who is confident and self-assured, as well as considerate and unhurried, will help to reduce any anxiety the patient may be feeling about the exam (Jarvis et al., 2009). The examiner is less likely to forget a procedure, a step in the sequence, or a portion of the body if the same sequence is followed every time. Table 3-5

Table 3-5 Outline for Physical Examination

1. General Survey

Observe general state of health (patient is seated):

- Body features
- State of consciousness and arousal
- Speech
- Body movements
- Physical appearance
- Nutritional status
- Stature

2. Vital Signs

Record vital signs:

- Blood pressure—both arms for comparison
- Apical/radial pulse
- Respiration
- Temperature—record height and weight; calculate body mass index (BMI)

3. Integument

Inspect and palpate skin for the following:

- Colour
- Lesions, breakdown, lacerations
- Scars, tattoos, piercing
- Bruises, rash
- Edema
- Moisture
- Texture
- Temperature
- Turgor
- Vascularity
- Hair pattern
- Capillary refill time

Inspect and palpate nails for the following:

- Colour
- Lesions
- Size
- Flexibility
- Shape
- Angle

4. Head and Neck

Inspect and palpate head for the following:

- Shape and symmetry of skull
- Masses
- Tenderness
- Hair
- Scalp
- Skin
- Temporal arteries
- Temporomandibular joint
- Sensory (CN V, light touch, pain)
- Motor (CN VII, shows teeth, purses lips, raises eyebrows)
- Looks up, wrinkles forehead (CN VII)
- Raises shoulders against resistance (CN XI)

Inspect and palpate (occasionally auscultate) neck for the following:

- Skin (vascularity and visible pulsations)
- Symmetry
- Postural alignment
- Range of motion
- Pulses and bruits (carotid)
- Midline structure (trachea, thyroid gland, cartilage)
- Lymph nodes (preauricular, postauricular, occipital, mandibular, tonsillar, submental, anterior and posterior cervical, infraclavicular, supraclavicular)

Inspect and palpate eyes for the following:

- Visual acuity
- Eyebrows
- Position and movement of eyelids (CN VII)
- Visual fields
- Extraocular movements (CN III, IV, VI)
- Cornea, sclera, conjunctiva
- Pupillary response (CN III)
- Red reflex
- Fundi
- Eyeball tension

Inspect and palpate nose and sinuses for the following:

- External nose—shape; blockage
- Internal nose—patency of nasal passages; shape; turbinates or polyps; discharge
- Frontal and maxillary sinuses

Inspect and palpate ears for the following:

- Placement
- Pinna
- Auditory acuity (Weber's or Rinne test, whispered voice, ticking watch) (CN VIII)
- Mastoid process
- Auditory canal
- Tympanic membrane
- Cone of light and landmarks

Inspect and palpate mouth for the following:

- Lips (symmetry, lesions, colour)
- Buccal mucosa (Stensen's and Wharton's ducts)
- Teeth (absence, state of repair, colour)
- Gums (colour, receding from teeth)
- Tongue for strength (asymmetry, ability to stick out tongue, side to side, fasciculations) (CN XII)
- Palates
- Tonsils and pillars
- Uvular elevation (CN IX)
- Posterior pharynx
- Gag reflex (CN IX and X)
- Jaw strength (CN V)
- Moisture
- Colour
- Floor of mouth

5. Extremities

Observe size and shape, symmetry and deformity, involuntary movements. Inspect and palpate arms, fingers, wrists, elbows, shoulders for the following:

- Strength
- Range of motion
- Crepitus
- Joint pain
- Swelling
- Fluid
- Pulses (radial, brachial)

Inspect and palpate legs for the following:

- Strength of hips
- Edema
- Hair distribution
- Pulses (dorsalis pedis, posterior tibialis)

Test reflexes:

- Biceps
- Triceps
- Brachioradialis
- Patellar
- Achilles
- Plantar

6. Posterior Thorax

Inspect for muscular development, respiratory movement, approximation of AP diameter:

- Palpate for symmetry of respiratory movement, tenderness of CVA, spinous processes, tumours or swelling, tactile fremitus
- Percuss for pulmonary resonance
- Auscultate for breath sounds
- Auscultate for egophony, bronchophony, and whispered pectoriloquy

7. Anterior Thorax

- Assess breasts for configuration, symmetry, dimpling of skin
- Assess nipples for rash, direction, inversion, retraction
- Initiate teaching of or review breast self-examination
- Inspect for apical impulse, other precordial pulsations

Table 3-5 Outline for Physical Examination—cont'd

- Palpate for thrills, lifts, heaves, tenderness over precordium
- Inspect neck for venous distension, pulsations, waves
- Palpate axillae
- Palpate breasts
- Auscultate for rate and rhythm, character of S1 and S2 in the aortic, pulmonic, Erb's point, tricuspid, mitral areas; bruits at carotid, epigastrium; breath sounds

8. Abdomen

- Inspect for scars, shape, symmetry, bulging, muscular position and condition of umbilicus, movements (respiratory, pulsations, presence of peristaltic waves)
- Auscultate for peristalsis, bruits
- Percuss border of liver, four abdominal quadrants
- Palpate to confirm positive findings; check liver (size, surface contour, tenderness); spleen; kidney (size, contour, consistency, tenderness); urinary bladder (distension); femoral pulses; inguinofemoral nodes

9. Completion of Examinations of Extremities

Observe the following:

- Range of motion of hips, knees, ankles, feet
- Crepitus
- Joint pain
- Swelling
- Fluid

- Muscle development
- Coordination (heel to shin)
- Homans' sign
- Proprioception (position sense of great toe)

10. Neurological

Motor status observations	Coordination
• Gait	• Finger to nose
• Toe walk	• Romberg's sign
• Heel walk	• Heel to opposite shin
• Drift	• Spine (scoliosis)

11. Genitalia*

Male External Genitalia

- Inspect penis, noting hair distribution, prepuce, glans, urethral meatus, scars, ulcers, eruptions, structural alterations
- Inspect epidermis of perineum, anus
- Inspect skin of scrotum; palpate for descended testes, masses, pain

Female External Genitalia

- Inspect hair distribution; mons pubis, labia (minora and majora); urethral meatus; Bartholin's, urethral, Skene's glands (may also be palpated, if indicated); introitus; any discharge
- Assess for presence of cystocele, prolapse
- Inspect perineum, anus

AP, anteroposterior; *CN,* cranial nerve; *CVA,* costovertebral angle; *S1* and *S2,* heart sounds.
*If the nurse has the appropriate training, the speculum and bimanual examination of women and the prostate gland examination of men should be performed after this inspection.

---

presents an outline for the physical examination that is organized, logical, and complete. Adaptations of the physical examination often are useful for the older adult patient, who may have age-related problems such as decreased mobility, limited energy, and perceptual changes.

The examination environment, whether in a hospital room, clinic, or patient's home, should be warm and comfortable, quiet, private, and safe. The examiner should always maintain privacy by closing the examination room door, using curtains around the bedside, and having the patient wear a gown during the examination. To help maintain a safe environment and decrease the risk of transmitting infections between patients or between the patient and the examiner, equipment should be kept clean and the examiner should practise good hand hygiene and routine practices.

Recording the Screening Physical Examination.

Only abnormal findings should be recorded during the actual examination. This prevents needless interruptions in the examination to write lengthy normal findings. At the conclusion of the examination, the nurse should combine the normal and abnormal findings in a carefully recorded physical examination. An example of how to record the findings of a physical examination on a healthy adult can be found on the Evolve Web site for this chapter. See Chapter 7, Table 7-2, and the age-related assessment findings in each assessment chapter for helpful references in recording age-related assessment differences.

Types of Assessment

Various types of assessment are used to obtain information about a patient. These approaches can be divided into three types: comprehensive, focused, and emergency (Table 3-6).

The nurse must decide what type of assessment is required for an individual patient based on the clinical situation (e.g., admission history and physical examination, start of shift, throughout shift, acute change in health status, time of discharge). Sometimes the health care agency provides guidelines, and at other times it is a nursing judgement.

Comprehensive Assessment

A *comprehensive assessment* includes a detailed health history and physical examination of one body system or many body systems (see Table 3–6). It is typically done on admission to the hospital or onset of care in a primary care setting.

Focused Assessment

A *focused assessment* is a more abbreviated assessment used to evaluate the status of previously identified problems and monitor for signs of new problems. It can be done when a specific problem (e.g., pneumonia) is identified. The patient's clinical manifestations should alert the nurse to the appropriate focused

Table 3-6 Types of Assessment

DESCRIPTION	WHEN AND WHERE PERFORMED	WHERE FOUND IN BOOK
Comprehensive		
• Detailed assessment of one body or many body systems, including those not directly involved in presenting problem or admission diagnosis. • Used for head-to-toe assessment.	• Onset of care in primary or ambulatory care setting. • On admission to hospital or long-term care setting. • On initial home care visit.	• Assessment chapters for each body system • Outline for physical examination (see Table 3-5) • Head-to-toe or whole-body assessment and checklist available on the Evolve Web site for this book
Focused		
• Abbreviated assessment that focuses on one or more body systems that are the focus of care. • Includes an assessment related to a specific problem (e.g., pneumonia, specific abnormal laboratory findings in a patient). • Used to monitor for signs of new problems.	• Throughout hospital admission—at beginning of a shift and as needed throughout shift. • Revisits in ambulatory care setting or home care setting.	• Focused assessment boxes in each assessment chapter • Tables on nursing assessment of specific diseases throughout book
Emergency		
• Limited to assessing life-threatening conditions (e.g., inhalation injuries, anaphylaxis, myocardial infarction, shock, stroke). • Conducted to ensure survival. Assessment focuses on airway, breathing, circulation and disability. • After life-saving interventions are initiated, a brief systematic assessment is performed to identify any/all other injuries/problems.	• Performed in any setting when signs or symptoms of a life-threatening condition appear (e.g., emergency department, critical care unit, surgical setting, ambulatory care setting, home setting).	• Chapter 71, Tables 71-3 and 71-5 • Emergency management tables throughout the book and listed in Table 71-1

assessment. For example, abdominal pain indicates the need to do a focused examination of the abdomen. Some problems necessitate a focused assessment of more than one body system. A complaint of headache may indicate the need to do musculoskeletal, neurological, and head and neck examinations. Assessment chapters throughout the text will include Focused Assessment Boxes (see eTable 3-3), which are checklists for a more practical "assessment on the run" or bedside approach, and can be used to evaluate the status of previously identified health problems and monitor for signs of new problems.

Emergency Assessment

In an emergency or critical care situation, an *emergency assessment* may be done by rapid, specific questioning of a patient while assessing and maintaining vital functions.

Using Assessment Approaches

Assessment in a hospital inpatient setting, particularly in acute care, is markedly different from assessment in other settings. Focused assessment of the hospitalized patient is frequent and performed by many different people. Such a team approach demands a high degree of consistency among different health care professionals.

While providing ongoing care for a patient, the nurse will be constantly refining her or his mental image of the patient. With experience, the nurse will derive a mental image of the status of a patient from a few very basic details, such as "85-year-old woman admitted for COPD in exacerbation." The nurse's picture

of her becomes clearer as a more complete verbal report is received, such as length of stay, recent laboratory results, physical findings, and vital signs. Next, the nurse performs her or his own assessment using a focused approach. During this assessment, the nurse will confirm or revise the findings that were read in the medical record and received from other health care professionals.

Keep in mind that the process does not end once the nurse has completed her or his first assessment on a patient during rounds. The nurse will have to continue to gather information about her or his patients throughout the shift. Everything that the nurse learned previously about the patient is considered in the light of new information. For example, when the nurse is doing a respiratory assessment on a patient with chronic obstructive pulmonary disease (COPD), crackles are heard in the lungs. This finding should lead the nurse to do a cardiovascular assessment because cardiac problems (e.g., heart failure) can also cause crackles.

Adding to the challenge is the reality that nurses are required to perform such assessments on many patients at once. As the nurse gains experience, the importance of new findings will be more obvious. Assessment case studies are on the Evolve Web site for this text. These assessment cases will help to develop one's assessment skills and knowledge.

Learning Assessment

Once the nurse has gained experience, he or she will stop thinking about what type of assessment is needed. The nurse will not be thinking, "I'd better do a focused assessment now, including the following techniques …" Rather, the nurse will simply know

Table 3-7 Clinical Application of Various Types of Assessment	
The following is an example of how various types of assessment would be used for a patient progressing from the emergency department to an inpatient unit of a hospital.	
TIMELINE	**TYPE OF ASSESSMENT**
Emergency Department	
Patient arrives in acute respiratory distress	Perform emergency assessment (see Table 71-3).
Problem is identified, critical interventions are performed, patient stabilizes	Conduct a focused assessment of the respiratory and related body systems (e.g., cardiovascular). May begin comprehensive assessment of all body systems.
Inpatient Unit	
Patient admitted to a monitored inpatient unit	Complete comprehensive assessment of all body systems.
New nurse arrives at change of shift or midshift reassessment	Perform focused assessment of respiratory system and other related body systems (to determine whether new problems have arisen).

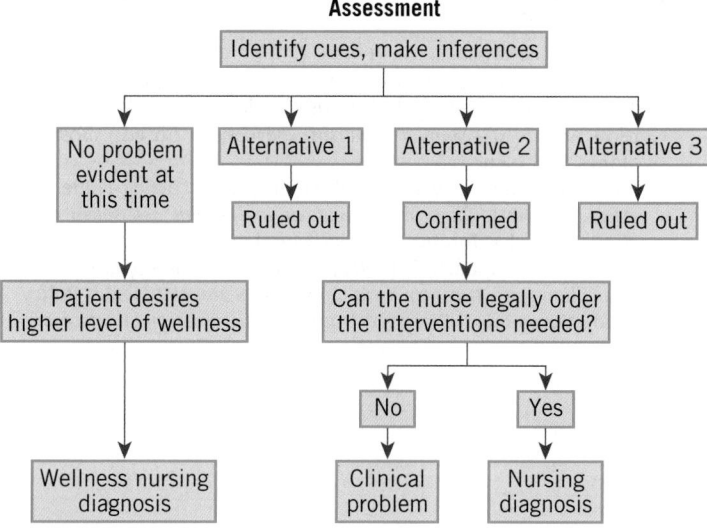

Figure 3-5 Problem identification phase of the nursing process.

the respiratory and related body systems. Then the nurse can obtain a comprehensive assessment of all body systems, whether or not they are involved in the current clinical problem.

Problem Identification and Nursing Diagnoses

After completing the history and physical examination, the nurse clusters and analyzes the data to develop a list of nursing diagnoses and collaborative problems. Figure 3-5 illustrates the problem identification phase of the nursing process. Nursing diagnoses are health-related problems that are managed primarily by nursing care. (Chapter 1 explains the process of establishing nursing diagnoses.)

which pieces of information are most important. The nurse will combine all the necessary techniques to capture those data. However, in the beginning it is helpful to learn about the different types of assessment.

Table 3-7 shows how the nurse can perform different types of assessments based on a patient's progress through a given hospitalization. When a patient arrives at the emergency department (ED) in acute distress, the nurse will perform an emergency assessment based on the principles of airway, breathing, circulation, disability (ABCDs) (see Chapter 71, Table 71-3). Once the patient is stabilized, the nurse can begin a focused assessment of

REVIEW QUESTIONS

The number of the question corresponds to the same-numbered objective at the beginning of the chapter.

1. What is the primary purpose of collecting a nursing history?
   a. To diagnose a medical problem
   b. To investigate the patient's symptoms
   c. To classify subjective and objective data
   d. To support the identification of nursing diagnoses
2. The nurse would place information that the patient revealed about his concern that his illness is threatening his job security in which of the following functional health patterns?
   a. Role–relationship
   b. Cognitive–perceptual
   c. Coping–stress tolerance
   d. Health perception–health management

3. Which of the following techniques would the nurse primarily use to examine the skin of a patient who is complaining of an itchy rash?
   a. Inspection
   b. Palpation
   c. Percussion
   d. Auscultation
4. When would it be most appropriate to perform a focused assessment?
   a. When the patient denies a health problem
   b. When a baseline health maintenance examination is required
   c. When a priority problem or previously identified problem needs to be reassessed
   d. When a specific problem is identified during physical examination

REFERENCES

Canadian Nurses Association (CNA). (2008). *Code of ethics for registered nurses.* Retrieved from *http://www.cna-aiic.ca/cna/documents/pdf/publications/Code_of_Ethics_2008_e.pdf*

Gordon, M. (2010). *Manual of nursing diagnosis* (12th ed.). Boston: Jones & Bartlett.

Jarvis, C., Browne, A., MacDonald-Jenkins, J., & Luctkar-Flude, M. (Eds.). (2009). *Physical examination and health assessment* (1st Canadian ed.). Toronto: Elsevier/Saunders.

Mikkonen, J., & Raphael, D. (2009). *Social determinants of health: The Canadian facts.* Toronto: York University School of Health Policy and Management. Retrieved from *http://www.thecanadianfacts.org*

Registered Nurses' Association of Ontario (RNAO). (2006). *Establishing therapeutic relationships.* Retrieved from *http://www.rnao.org/Storage/15/943_BPG_TR_Supplement.pdf*

Touhy, T. A., Jett, K. F., Boscart, V., & McCleary, L. (2011). *Ebersole and Hess' gerontological nursing and healthy aging* (1st Canadian ed.). Toronto: Mosby.

Weber, J., & Kelley, J. (2009). *Health assessment in nursing* (4th ed.). Philadelphia: Lippincott.

Wilson, S., & Giddens, J. (2009). *Health assessment for nursing practice* (4th ed.). St. Louis: Mosby.

evolve   *For additional Internet resources, see the Web site for this book at* **http://evolve.elsevier.com/Canada/Lewis/medsurg**

Patient and Caregiver Teaching

Written by Linda Bucher and Catherine N. Kotecki
Adapted by Verna C. Pangman

LEARNING OBJECTIVES

1. Identify four specific goals of patient and caregiver teaching.
2. Describe teaching implications of adult learning principles.
3. Describe specific skills that enhance the nurse's effectiveness as a teacher.
4. Identify strategies to manage the barriers to the nurse's teaching effectiveness.
5. Discuss the role of the family in patient teaching.
6. Explain the basic steps in the teaching–learning process.
7. Identify physical, psychological, and sociocultural characteristics of the patient that affect the teaching–learning process.
8. Describe the components of a correctly written learning objective.
9. Identify advantages, disadvantages, and uses of various teaching strategies.
10. Describe common methods of short- and long-term evaluation.

KEY TERMS

androgogy The theoretical basis of adult learning, p. 53

empathy The quality that allows one person to enter into the world of another so as not to judge, sympathize, or correct, but with the goal of establishing mutual understanding, p. 55

facilitator Someone who helps a group of people understand their common objectives and achieve them, without taking a particular position in the discussion, p. 62

family conference A meeting that involves patient, caregiver, and members of the interdisciplinary health care team to discuss treatment and plans for a patient's discharge. p. 52

health literacy The degree to which individuals have the capacity to obtain, process, and understand basic health information and services needed to make appropriate health decisions, p. 57

learning Internal mental change associated with new mastery of content, characterized by rearrangement of neural pathways and behavioural change, p. 52

learning needs The new knowledge and skills that an individual must acquire to be able to meet an objective or a goal, p. 58

learning objectives Written statements that set forth exactly how patients will demonstrate their mastery of the content, p. 60

learning style The way an individual understands and responds to a learning situation; may be visual, auditory, or physical, p. 60

peer teaching Teaching that is conducted within the setting of a peer group such as a self-help or support group, p. 62

self-efficacy A person's belief in his or her ability to cope successfully with and manage a situation, p. 57

stages of behavioural change The six stages of change identified by Prochaska and Velicer (1997) in their article "The Transtheoretical Model of Health Behaviour Change": precontemplation, contemplation, preparation, action, maintenance, and termination, p. 53

teaching A process of deliberately arranging external conditions to promote the mastery of content and the consequent internal change that results in a change in behaviour, p. 52

teaching plan A plan that includes assessment of the patient's ability, need, and readiness to learn; it identifies problems that can be resolved through teaching, p. 52

teaching process The implementation of a plan that includes assessment, diagnosis, the setting of patient outcomes or objectives, intervention, and evaluation, p. 56

Role of Patient and Caregiver Teaching

Teaching patients and caregivers (any family member or significant other) is a dynamic and interactive process. It is one of the most major and challenging roles that nurses face in the current health care system. Constraints on staff time and resources, coupled with the shortened average length of inpatient hospitalizations, can affect the nurse's ability to engage in patient education. Inadequate patient teaching frequently results in devastating consequences for the patient and caregiver. Conversely, teaching patients about promoting, maintaining, and restoring their health is a required nursing skill that most often results in a positive outcome, enhancing the patient's quality of life.

Nurses engage in patient education to help patients and their caregivers focus on optimizing their health and to enable them to cope with acute and chronic health problems. Specifically, teaching goals include maintenance of health, health promotion and prevention of disease, management of illness, and appropriate selection and use of treatment and resources. Furthermore, these goals facilitate maintaining a high level of wellness that is meaningful and relevant for the patient throughout the lifespan. Effective teaching can assist people to make informed decisions about their lifestyle, health practices, and treatment choices. For patients who have acute health problems, quality teaching can prevent complications and promote recovery. For patients with chronic illnesses, increased knowledge can promote self-care and independence.

Patient education can occur wherever nurses practice. Teaching situations include the community, schools, industry, ambulatory care centres, hospitals, long-term care facilities, and homes.

Family conferences are held mainly in hospitals and long-term care settings. These conferences provide opportunities for patients and their caregivers, along with members of the interdisciplinary health care team, to identify needs for information and assistance with health care matters (Fineberg, Kawashima, & Asch, 2011). In fact, the involvement of the caregiver is considered one of the key variables influencing patient outcomes (Bastable, Gramet, Jacobs & Sopczyk, 2011). In family conferences, the nurse uses knowledge and skills to teach the patient and caregiver the availability of resources and strategies to promote health, as well as to assess additional care needs.

The teaching episodes expected from nursing are not complex. For example, teaching a patient to cough effectively and to breathe deeply after surgery can help the patient prevent atelectasis. However, when a patient has specific learning needs concerning management of a health problem or the strategies of health promotion, a teaching plan should be developed and implemented with the patient.

A **teaching plan** is a blueprint for action to achieve the goals and objectives agreed upon by the patient and nurse. For the collaborative plan to be effective, the following elements need to be included: purpose of the plan, goals and objectives, related health content, instructional methods, and time allotment for each objective (Bastable et al., 2011). The nurse then evaluates the effectiveness of the plan. This chapter describes the steps involved in providing patient and caregiver education and discusses factors that contribute to successful educational experiences.

Teaching–Learning Process

Teaching is more than simply imparting information. Learning is more than listening to instruction. According to Kozier and colleagues (2010), **learning** is a cognitive activity that is reflected by a change in behaviour. One critical component of learning is the individual's desire to learn and to act on that learning. This process is known as *compliance* (Kozier et al., 2010). The term *adherence* is often used first to reflect the patient's willingness to follow through on the plan of care. A patient's compliance and adherence together are known as the patient's *ability to follow health-promoting regimens* and are assessed to a large degree by health care providers such as nurses (Bastable, 2008).

Teaching is a process of deliberately arranging external conditions to promote the internal change that results in a change in behaviour. Teaching can be a planned or incidental experience, and it can be conducted with a combination of methods such as instruction, simulation, and assistive technology (computers and communication devices) to influence the patient's knowledge and behaviour (Bastable et al., 2011). The teacher is the one who plans and manages the external conditions to promote learning (Redman, 2007). The challenge for the nurse is to identify and use strategies that are effective in helping patients change behaviours. In patient education, the teaching–learning process involves the patient, the nurse, and the caregiver or social support system. The interdisciplinary team may also partake and can demonstrate accountability and responsibility for patient education on the basis of solid principles of teaching and learning.

Adult Learners

Adult Learning Principles. Through educational research and theoretical development pertaining specifically to adults, investigators have identified specific principles and characteristics that differentiate learning by adults from learning by children. These concepts provide a foundation for the effective teaching of adults. Many of the theories of adult learning have arisen from the work of Knowles (1990), who identified seven principles of **andragogy** (adult learning) that are deemed essential for the nurse to consider when teaching adults. These principles and their implications for patient teaching are presented in Table 4-1.

Table 4-1 Principles of Adult Education Applied to Patient Teaching

PRINCIPLE	TEACHING IMPLICATIONS FOR THE NURSE
Adults are independent learners.	• The teacher is a facilitator who directs the patient to resources but is not the source of all information. • Patients expect to make decisions about their own lives and learning experiences and to take responsibility for those decisions. • Respect for the patient's independence can be reflected in statements such as "What do you think you need to learn about this topic?"
Readiness to learn arises from life's changes.	• Patients see life processes as problems to be solved. • Readiness and motivation to learn are high when new tasks are faced. • Crises in health are "teachable moments."
Past experiences are resources for learning.	• Patients have had many life experiences and have engaged in informal learning for years. • Motivation is increased when patients believe that they already know something about the subject from past experiences. • Identifying past knowledge and experiences can familiarize patients with a new situation and increase their confidence.
Adults learn best when the topic is of immediate value.	• Patients need to apply learning immediately. • Long-term goals may have little appeal. • Short-term, realistic goals should be encouraged. • Education should be focused on information that the patient views as being needed right now.
Adults approach learning as problem solving.	• Patients seek out various resources for specific learning to help them deal with a problem. • Information that is not relevant to the problem is not readily learned. • When relevancy is not recognized by the patient, explanations of the need to learn something should be offered. • Teaching should target the specific problem or circumstance.
Adults see themselves as doers.	• Patients learn better by doing. • Demonstrations, computer activities, and practice of skills should be offered when appropriate.
Adults resist learning when conditions are incongruent with their self-concepts.	• Patients do not learn when they are treated as children and told what they must do. • Patients need control and self-direction to maintain their sense of self-worth.

Determinants of Learning. Because of the combined effects of health care trends and population demographics, the nurse must carefully assess all of the determinants of learning for the patient for whom the nurse has teaching responsibility. The three determinants of learning that require learning assessments are identified in Table 4-2 (Bastable, 2008).

Motivation of Adult Learners. One important factor that is strongly associated with motivation is *emotional readiness* (Bastable, 2008). When a nurse is teaching an adult, it is important to identify what is valued by the adult so that motivation can be enhanced. If the adult perceives a need for information to enhance health or avoid illness, or if the adult has a belief that a behaviour change has health value, motivation to learn is increased. Humans seek out stimulating experiences that increase their desire and effort to learn. Therefore, learning activities must be stimulating to maintain a desire to reach a goal.

When a change in health-related behaviours is recommended, patients and their families may progress through a series of steps before they are willing, or able, to accept the need for and make the change. Six stages of change have been identified in the transtheoretical model of health behaviour change developed by Prochaska and Velicer (1997). The **stages of behavioural change** and their implications for patient teaching are described in Table 4-3. It is important to note that individuals progress through these stages at their own pace and that progression through the stages is often nonlinear and cyclic. Therefore, it is reasonable to expect the patient to experience periods of relapse, whereby the process must be restarted—sometimes repeatedly. Accurate assessment of the patient's stage of change helps the nurse guide the patient through one stage and on to the next.

Nurse as Teacher

Required Skills
Knowledge of Subject Matter. The scope of nursing practice is extensive, and its settings are diverse. Although it is impossible to be expert in all areas, the nurse can develop confidence as a teacher by acquiring knowledge of the matter that is to be taught. For example, if a nurse is teaching a patient about the management of hypertension, the nurse must be able to explain what hypertension is, why it is important to treat the disease, and what the patient needs to know about exercise, diet, and the effects of medication, both expected and untoward. The nurse should be able to teach the patient to use blood pressure equipment to monitor the blood pressure and to identify situations that should be reported to health care professionals. In

Table 4-2 Determinants of Learning

• The needs of the learner. Assist learner to identify, clarify, and prioritize their needs and interests.

• The state of readiness to learn. Seize the moment when the learner demonstrates an interest in learning the material necessary to maintain optimal health.

• The preferred learning style for processing knowledge and information. Assess the various teaching techniques and the teaching learning conditions under which these learners are most likely to perceive, process, store, and recall health-related material.

Source: From Bastable, S. B. (2008). *Essentials of patient education.* Sudbury, MA: Jones & Bartlett.

| | | NURSING |
STAGE	PATIENT BEHAVIOUR	IMPLICATIONS
1. Precontemplation	Is not considering a change; is not ready to learn	Provide support and increase awareness of condition; describe benefits of change and risks of not changing
2. Contemplation	Thinks about a change; may verbalize recognition of need to change; says, "I know I should" but identifies barriers	Introduce what is involved in changing the behaviour; reinforce the stated need to change
3. Preparation	Starts planning the change, gathers information, sets a date to initiate change, shares decision to change with others	Reinforce the positive outcomes of change, provide information and encouragement, develop a plan, help set priorities, and identify sources of support
4. Action	Begins to change behaviour through practice; is tentative and may experience relapses	Reinforce behaviour with reward, encourage self-reward, discuss choices to help minimize relapses and regain focus, and help patient plan how to deal with potential relapses
5. Maintenance	Practises the behaviour regularly; able to sustain the change	Continue to reinforce behaviour; provide additional education on the need to maintain change
6. Termination	Change has become part of lifestyle; behaviour is no longer considered a change	Evaluate effectiveness of the new behaviour; no further intervention is needed

Table 4-3 Stages of Change in the Transtheoretical Model

Source: Adapted from Prochaska, J., & Velicer, W. (1997). The transtheoretical model of health behaviour change. *American Journal of Health Promotion, 12*(1), 38-48. doi:http://dx.doi.org/10.4278/0890-1171-12.1.38

addition, the nurse should provide the patient with sources of additional information such as brochures, appropriate Web sites, and support organizations (e.g., Canadian Heart and Stroke Foundation).

It is not unusual for the patient to ask questions that the nurse may not be able to answer. If the nurse is not sure of the response, the patient should be informed this, the nurse should follow through by seeking additional information to answer the question, and then the nurse should return to the patient to provide the response.

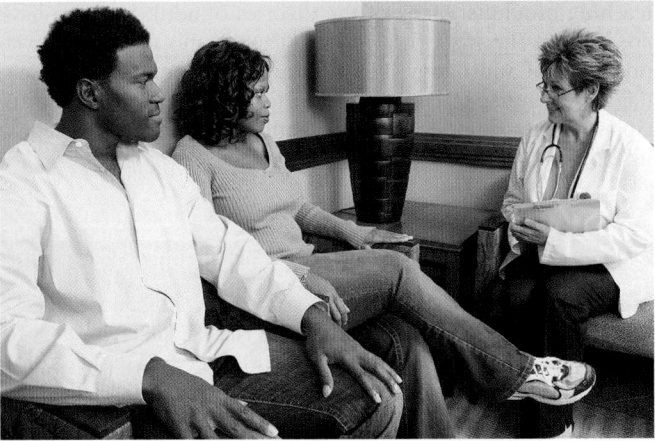

Figure 4-1 Open, relaxed positioning of the patient and nurse at the same eye level promotes communication in teaching and learning.

Source: © 2011 JupiterImages Corporation.

Communication Skills. Patient education is an interactive and dynamic process (Potter, Perry, Ross-Kerr, & Wood, 2010). Through effective communication skills, a nurse can establish a valuable partnership among the nurse himself or herself, the patient, and the caregiver. In such a partnership, a nurse can provide highly supportive environment conducive to the empowerment of the patient and caregivers (Laschinger, Gilbert, Smith & Leslie, 2010).

Empowerment has become increasingly important in the education of patients and caregivers. Empowerment has been found to influence patients' self-efficacy, as well as their participation in decision making and expression of quality of life (Virtanen, Leino-Kilpi, & Salantera, 2007). Specifically, nurses can help patients identify their own internal strengths and self-care abilities, both of which can be called upon to address health care issues. Nurses can facilitate the need for caregivers to support the rights of patients and to ensure that patients have access to the resources necessary to achieve optimal health.

During the teaching process, the nurse should use basic therapeutic communication skills and strategies to support, educate, and empower patients to cope effectively with health-related issues (Arnold & Boggs, 2011). These basic communication skills encompass both verbal and nonverbal components, and they are described in Chapter 3 in the section on the patient interview. The value of effective communication skills is to promote safe and emphatic ways for patients to explore their illness experience. Terms that convey respect for culture, spiritual beliefs, and the educational level of the patient and also that of their caregiver are essential. In communication, the use of medical jargon is unnecessary and can be omitted (Arnold & Boggs, 2011). To provide positive nonverbal messages, it is important for the nurse to sit in an open, relaxed position facing the patient, with his or her eyes level with those of the patient (Figure 4-1).

It is important for the nurse to develop the art of active listening. This means paying attention to what is said, as well as observing the patient's nonverbal cues. The nurse concentrates on the patient as a communicator of vital information and does not interrupt the patient. Nodding in response to the patient's statements and rephrasing and verbally reflecting what the patient is saying help clarify communication. Allowing time for listening without appearing hurried requires thoughtful organization and planning on the part of the nurse. Attentive listening and red-flagging issues allows the nurse to obtain important information needed for the assessment phase of the teaching process.

Empathy. **Empathy** can be defined as having the courage to enter into the world of another so as not to judge, sympathize, or correct but to establish mutual understanding. Empathy means putting aside one's own concerns for a moment and adopting the patient's viewpoint. With regard to patient teaching, empathy means assessing the patient's needs before implementing teaching. For example, the nurse who is working in a rural outpatient clinic is asked to teach a patient with newly diagnosed diabetes the symptoms of hypoglycemia. The nurse enters the room and finds the patient sitting very still, with gaze fixed and mouth slightly ajar. The empathic approach to this situation may include sitting down in a chair next to the patient and discussing the feelings that the patient may be experiencing, before starting the discussion on complications of diabetes.

Barriers to Nurse–Teacher Effectiveness. The perceived lack of time is a major barrier that detracts from the effectiveness of the teaching effort. When time is limited, the nurse should inform the patient at the beginning of the interaction how much time can be devoted to the session. To make the most of limited time, it is critical that the nurse and patient set priorities for the patient's learning so that important teaching can be accomplished during any contact with the patient or caregiver.

Disagreement between the nurse and patient with regard to the expectations of teaching may also be a barrier. The nurse must accept the fact that some patients or caregivers may not be willing to discuss the health problem or its implications. The patient or caregiver may be in denial or hold ideas and values that are in conflict with those of conventional health care. Although the nurse may face hostility or resentment, he or she must respect the patient's response to the health problem.

Another important barrier for the nurse who is attempting to provide patient education is the current health care system. Decreased length of hospitalizations has resulted in the discharge of patients into the community with only the basic elements of educational plans established. At the same time, health care is offering increasingly complex treatment options. This situation results in greater educational needs of the patient and caregiver. Furthermore, patients and caregivers face greater difficulty using resources as the complexity of the health care system increases. Strategies that can be used to address these barriers are presented in Table 4-4.

Caregiver and Social Support

Support provided by the caregiver is important to a patient's sense of physical, psychological, and spiritual well-being. It is important that nurses focus on the caregiver dynamics and interactional patterns (Wright & Leahey, 2009). For example, caregivers who live with chronic disease develop expertise in managing symptoms and adjust their lifestyles and environments. When they meet with nurses, caregivers often bring a wealth of information and personal experience to the encounter. The nurse can initiate conversations about the care and support of the patient and discover that caregivers provide diagnosis, advice, remedies, and support to their family members in both sickness and health. One particularly important nursing strategy is that of

Table 4-4 Suggested Approaches to Overcoming Barriers to Nurse-Teacher Effectiveness

BARRIER	APPROACHES
Lack of time	Preplan. Set realistic goals. Use time with patient efficiently, and use all possible opportunities for teaching, such as when bathing the patient or changing a dressing. Break teaching and practice sessions into small blocks of time. Advocate for time for patient teaching. Carefully document what was taught and the time spent teaching in order to emphasize that it is a primary role of nursing and that it takes time.
Lack of knowledge	Broaden knowledge base. Read, study, and ask questions. Screen teaching materials, participate in other teaching sessions, observe more experienced nurse-teachers, and attend classes.
Disagreement with patient	Establish agreed-upon, written goals. Develop a plan, and discuss it with the patient before teaching begins. Introduce a role model to help illustrate therapeutic expectations. Enlist the aid of family and significant others. Revise expectations; learn to be satisfied with small achievements.
Powerlessness, frustration	Recognize personal reaction to stress. Develop a support system. Rely on friends and family for positive encouragement. Network with other nurses, health professionals, and community leaders to change the situation. Become proactive in legislative processes affecting health care delivery.

commending the caregiver for being supportive to the patient (Wright & Leahey, 2009).

It becomes important for nurses to identify patients who have minimal support and to work collaboratively with other health care professionals to develop networks for these patients. Such a strategy may improve the patients' long-term outcomes.

In many instances, the patient and the caregiver may have differing or conflicting views of the illness, of treatment options and health promotion strategies. Health problems frequently have effects on caregivers' roles and functions. To develop a successful teaching plan, the nurse must view the patient's needs within the context of the caregiver's needs. For example, the nurse may teach a patient with right-sided paresis (weakness) self-feeding techniques with the use of special implements, but at a home visit, the nurse finds the patient being fed by the spouse. On questioning, the spouse reveals that it is too difficult to watch the patient struggle with feeding and that it is easier to feed the patient. This is an example of a situation in which both the patient and the spouse need additional teaching about the goals of self-care. Such situations represent opportunities for home care and community health nurses to partner with acute care nurses by evaluating the teaching that is performed in the hospital and providing ongoing patient teaching in the community.

Process of Patient Education

Patient education is a distinct and definable activity that includes those strategies by which patients and caregivers make informed decisions about the patient's health. These decisions can facilitate proper care for their illnesses and the implementation of health-promotion interventions to facilitate recovery (Schwartz et al., 2010). In fact, participation in patient education helps patients and caregivers obtain the information and education they want and need (Canadian Partnership Against Cancer, 2012).

Many different approaches are used in the process of patient education. However, the approach used most frequently by nurses is actually a parallel of the nursing process. Both the **teaching process** and the nursing process involve development of a plan that includes assessment, diagnosis, setting patient outcomes or objectives, intervention, and evaluation. The teaching process, like the nursing process, may not always flow in sequential order, but the steps serve as checkpoints to ensure that the relevant variables that affect the teaching–learning activity have been considered (Redman, 2007).

Assessment

During the general nursing assessment, the nurse gathers data that determine whether the patient has learning needs that teaching can meet. For example, what does the patient know about the health problem, and how does he or she perceive the current problem? If a learning need is identified, a more refined assessment of need is made, and that problem is addressed with an appropriate teaching process (Billings & Hallstead, 2009). The general nursing assessment also identifies many variables that affect the teaching–learning process, such as the patient's physical and mental state of health and sociocultural characteristics. Caregivers may be included in the assessment, and that information can be used to determine their abilities to care for the patient at home. The assessment that is performed for the purpose of developing a teaching plan includes particularly the physical, psychological, spiritual, and sociocultural characteristics that affect learning, as well as the patient's characteristics that influence the teaching–learning process. Key questions addressing each of these areas are included in Table 4-5.

Physical Characteristics. The age of the patient is an important factor to consider in the teaching plan. The patient's experiences, rate of learning, and ability to retain information are affected by age. Barriers to effective learning, such as sensory impairments (e.g., hearing or vision loss), decrease sensory input and can alter learning. For the patient with impaired vision, magnifying glasses and bright lighting may help with reading teaching materials. Hearing loss can be compensated for with hearing aids or teaching techniques that involve more visual stimuli. Central nervous system function may be affected by disorders of the nervous system, such as stroke and head trauma, but also by other diseases, such as renal disease, hepatic impairment, and cardiovascular failure. Patients with alterations in central nervous system function have difficulty learning and may require that information be presented in small amounts and with frequent repetitions. Manual dexterity is needed to perform procedures such as self-administered injections or blood pressure monitoring. Problems performing manual procedures might be resolved with the use of adaptive equipment.

Table 4-5 Assessment of Characteristics That Affect Patient Teaching: Characteristics and Key Questions

Physical

- What is the patient's age and sex?
- Is the patient acutely ill?
- Is the patient fatigued? In pain?
- What is the primary diagnosis?
- Are there other medical problems?
- What is the patient's current mental status?
- What is the patient's hearing ability? Visual ability? Motor ability?
- What drugs does the patient take? Do they affect learning?
- What is the physical environment in which the teaching will take place: the hospital classroom? The patient's room?

Psychological

- Does the patient appear anxious, afraid, depressed, or defensive?
- Is the patient in a state of denial?
- What is the patient's level of self-efficacy?
- Is the "timing to teach" appropriate?

Sociocultural

- Is the patient employed?
- What is the patient's current or past occupation?
- How does the patient describe his or her financial status?
- What is the patient's educational experience and reading ability?
- What is the patient's living arrangement?
- Does the patient have family or close friends?
- What are the patient's beliefs regarding his or her illness or treatment?
- What is the patient's cultural–ethnic identity?
- Is proposed teaching consistent with the patient's cultural values?
- Has the primary language been assessment for teaching purposes?

Educational

- What does the patient already know?
- What does the patient think is most important to learn first?
- What prior learning experiences establish a frame of reference for current learning needs?
- What is the patient's level of motivation?
- What has the patient's health care provider told the patient about the health problem?
- Is the patient ready to change behaviour or learn?
- Can the patient identify behaviours and habits that would make the problem better or worse?
- How does the patient learn best: through reading? Listening? Physical activities?
- In what kind of environment does the patient learn best: in a formal classroom? In an informal setting, such as home or office? Alone or among peers?
- In what way should the family be involved in patient education?

Pain, fatigue, and certain medications influence the patient's ability to learn. Nobody can learn effectively when in severe pain. When the patient is experiencing pain, the nurse should provide only brief explanations and follow up with more detailed instruction when the pain has been managed. A fatigued and weakened patient cannot learn effectively because of the inability to concentrate. Such inability can be caused by sleep disruption, which is common during hospitalization, and patients are frequently exhausted at the time of discharge. Also, many chemotherapeutic agents cause nausea, vomiting, and headaches that affect the patient's ability to assimilate new information. The nurse must adjust the teaching plan to accommodate these factors by setting high-priority goals that are based on needs and are realistic. Teaching methods should also be adjusted to accommodate for limitations that may arise at any given time in the patient's ability to learn. Moreover, the patient may need follow-up teaching and referral to a health professional who can answer questions that arise after discharge.

Psychological Characteristics.

Psychological factors have a major influence on the patient's ability to learn. Anxiety and depression are common reactions to illness. Although mild anxiety increases the learner's perceptual and learning abilities, moderate and severe anxiety limit learning. For example, the patient with newly diagnosed diabetes who is depressed about the diagnosis may not listen or respond to instructions about blood glucose testing. Engaging with the patient in a discussion about these concerns or referring the patient to an appropriate support group may enable the patient to learn that management of diabetes is possible.

Patients also respond to the stress of illness with a variety of defense mechanisms, such as denial, rationalization, and even humour. A patient who denies having cancer is not receptive to information related to treatment options. A patient using rationalization may imagine any number of reasons for avoiding change or for rejecting instruction; for example, a patient with cardiovascular disease who does not want to change dietary habits may relate stories of persons who have eaten bacon and eggs every morning for years and lived to be 100 years of age. Humour is also used by some patients to filter reality or decrease anxiety. Laughter may be used as an escape from the experience of a threatening situation. A common example of the use of humour is seen when patients assign a name and personality characteristics to an intestinal stoma or even a drainage device. Humour in the teaching process is important and useful, but the nurse must determine when humour is used excessively to avoid facing reality.

One important psychological determinant of successful adoption of new behaviours is the patient's sense of self-efficacy. **Self-efficacy** is a person's belief in his or her ability to cope successfully with, and manage, a situation (see Chapter 5). An individual's belief in his or her capability to produce and regulate events in life affects motivation, thought patterns, behaviour, and emotions (Redman, 2007). Self-efficacy is strongly related to outcomes of illness management (Redman, 2007). Self-efficacy increases when a person gains new skills in managing a threatening situation, but it decreases when the person experiences repeated failure, especially early in the course of events. These findings have significant implications for patient and family teaching. The nurse should plan easily attainable objectives early in the course of teaching, proceeding from simple to more complex content, to establish a positive experience of success. The use of both role play, to rehearse new behaviours, and of peer learning are teaching strategies that can increase feelings of self-efficacy in patients, caregivers, and family members.

Sociocultural Characteristics.

Sociocultural characteristics influence a patient's perception of health, illness, health care, life, and death. Social elements include the patient's lifestyle, status within a family, occupation, income, education, housing arrangement, and living location. Cultural elements include dietary and sleep patterns, exercise, sexuality, language, values, and beliefs. The patient and family may value the presence of an interpreter who can decrease their embarrassment of miscommunication.

Occupation and Income. Knowing the patient's current or past occupation may assist the nurse in determining what vocabulary to use during teaching. For example, an auto mechanic might understand the volume overload associated with heart failure through the metaphor of an engine flooding. An engineer may bring the principles of physics associated with gravity and pressures to bear when discussing vascular problems. This technique of teaching requires creativity but can promote a patient's understanding of pathophysiological processes.

The patient's occupation also gives the nurse an idea about the patient's financial status. Management of chronic health problems is very expensive, and the cost of care should be addressed with the patient or caregiver. The nurse may need to use different teaching resources or improvise materials according to the patient's and caregivers' ability to afford supplies and equipment.

Literacy and Health Literacy. **Health literacy** refers to the ability of people to access and use health information to make appropriate health care decisions and maintain basic health (Canadian Council on Learning, 2007). As the health care environment has become more complex, individuals with limited literacy have been shown to experience greater difficulty in understanding and acting on health information. The result is limited health literacy. Even patients with high general literacy can exhibit low health literacy in the presence of complicated health information.

Knowing whether a patient has poor health literacy skills is critical. Such knowledge enables the nurse to match verbal instructions used and the readability level of materials to the health literacy skills of the patient (Cornett, 2009). Printed educational materials are used extensively for the purpose of teaching patients and caregivers. Depending on the patient's health literacy, nonprint teaching materials, such as videotapes, audiotapes, demonstrations, models, pictograms, and other visual aids, may enable clients to obtain information concerning diagnosis, prognosis, treatment, and health promotion strategies in terms that are understandable. The use of health informatics strategies, such as telehealth, can improve access to health teaching for patients and caregivers in rural or underserviced areas (Hannah, 2007). Virtual education forums are being used extensively as they allow individuals across Canada online access to professionally led educational presentations about how to live well with an illness such as osteoporosis (Osteoporosis Canada, 2011).

Nurses must structure their approach to health care education so that expectancies are consistent with the needs of patients. The nurse must be a facilitator of learning by assisting patients and caregivers to access, use, and evaluate the wide range of available information. The nurse must learn how and when to use technology and remain up to date with new technology-based tools. Doing so enables the nurse to optimize each learning experience (Bastable, 2008). Nurses can empower their patients through the creative use of information technology. For instance, e-mail consultations and clinical information available on the Internet can be provided to patients (Virtanen et al., 2007). By using technology and the information available, patients can become empowered and enlightened to assume more active roles in their own health care. Patients and caregivers are more prepared today than traditionally to engage in a dialogue with the interdisciplinary team about their health care needs.

In the 2003 International Adult Literacy and Skills survey (Organization for Economic Cooperation and Development, 2008), the literacy of participants was categorized into five levels. People with level 1 literacy had very poor skills; for example, they were unable to determine the correct dose of medication from information on the package. People with level 2 literacy required material to be simple and clearly laid out, and only tasks that were not too complex could be included in the material. People at this level could read but had poor test results. They may have had everyday literacy-related coping skills but were unable to meet new demands, such as learning new job skills. People with level 3 literacy had the minimum skills necessary for everyday life in a complex society, such as graduation from high school and acceptance to a postsecondary institution. People at this level were able to integrate several sources of information and solve more complex problems. People with levels 4 and 5 literacy had higher order skills in information processing (Organization for Economic Cooperation and Development, 2008, p. 1).

Another survey revealed that 60% of Canadians lacked the capacity to obtain appropriate health information and act on it to make health-related decisions (Canadian Council on Learning, 2007). Canadian adults with less than a high school education performed much more poorly than did adults with higher levels of education, which indicates that the link between literacy and health promotion and maintenance is very strong. The survey further revealed that higher health literacy resulted in a greater emphasis on healthy behaviours and an enhanced ability to understand and make choices related to health care needs (Canadian Council on Learning, 2007). Figure 4-2 shows the percentage of Canadians whose health literacy skills are considered to be at level 2 and below.

The two most commonly used health literacy tools in health care setting are the Rapid Estimate of Adult Literacy in Medicine (REALM) and the Test of Functional Health Literacy in Adults (TOFHLA; Osborn et al., 2007). The REALM is a test of an individual's ability to recognize and pronounce words, whereas the TOFHLA is a measure of the ability to read, comprehend text, and perform computations involving health-related tasks. The two tests were modelled after general functional literacy measures and provide estimates of literacy ability when applied to health care contexts.

A newer health literacy tool for health care providers is the Newest Vital Sign (Weiss et al., 2005). As a screening tool, it identifies patients at risk for low health literacy. The test result provides information about the patient that allows health care providers to adapt their communication practices in an effort to achieve better health outcomes.

Housing Arrangement and Living Location. The patient should be asked about living arrangements that can affect the teaching–learning process. Whether the patient lives alone, with friends, or with caregivers is a determinant of who else is included in the teaching process. If the patient lives in another city or a rural area, at a distance from the site of teaching, the nurse might be expected to make arrangements for continued teaching in those areas. Modifications of instructions may have to be made if the patient does not have access to electricity, phones, or a computer.

Cultural Considerations. Learning is closely related to the wider culture and the subculture to which a patient belongs. Health practices, beliefs, and behaviour vary by religious, ethnic, and family group. To prevent stereotyping patients according to their appearance, it is important to determine whether the patient identifies with a particular cultural group or practice. Patients could be asked to describe their beliefs regarding health and illness.

A conflict between the patient's cultural beliefs and values and the behaviours promoted by teaching can affect the teaching–learning process. For example, a patient may view being overweight a sign of financial success and sexuality. This patient may have more difficulty accepting the need for diet and exercise unless the importance of blood pressure control is understood.

The nurse must assess the patient's use of cultural remedies and traditional healers. For teaching to be effective, cultural health practices must be incorporated into the teaching plan. In addition, it is important to know who has authority in the patient's culture. Whether this is a community leader, a spiritual leader, or a traditional healer, the patient may defer to the authority's decision making. In this case, the nurse could, if feasible, attempt to work with the decision makers in the patient's cultural group.

Educational Characteristics. Finally, the nurse should assess patient characteristics that are directly related to the development of the teaching plan. These factors include the patient's learning needs, readiness to learn, and learning style.

Learning Needs. **Learning needs** are the new knowledge and skills that an individual must acquire to be able to meet an objective or a goal. The assessment of learning needs should first be used to determine what the patient already knows, whether the patient has misinformation, and whether the patient has any history of experiences with health problems. The learning needs of patients with chronic illnesses are different from those of patients with newly diagnosed health problems. The nurse then identifies the information, the behaviours, or the skills known to improve patient outcomes that should be included in the teaching plan.

What a patient should learn about managing an illness or what behaviours should be changed to promote health may seem obvious to the nurse. However, there is often a significant difference between what health care providers think is important for patients to learn and what patients want to know.

To individualize learning needs for a particular patient, the nurse may give the patient a list of the recommended topics and ask the patient to number the topics in order of importance. Another method includes writing each topic in question format on a single card and asking the patient to sort the cards in priority. For example, some of the questions on the cards for a patient with Parkinson's disease might include, "When is the most important time to take my medications?" and "What can I do to help with the freezing when I walk?" By allowing a patient to

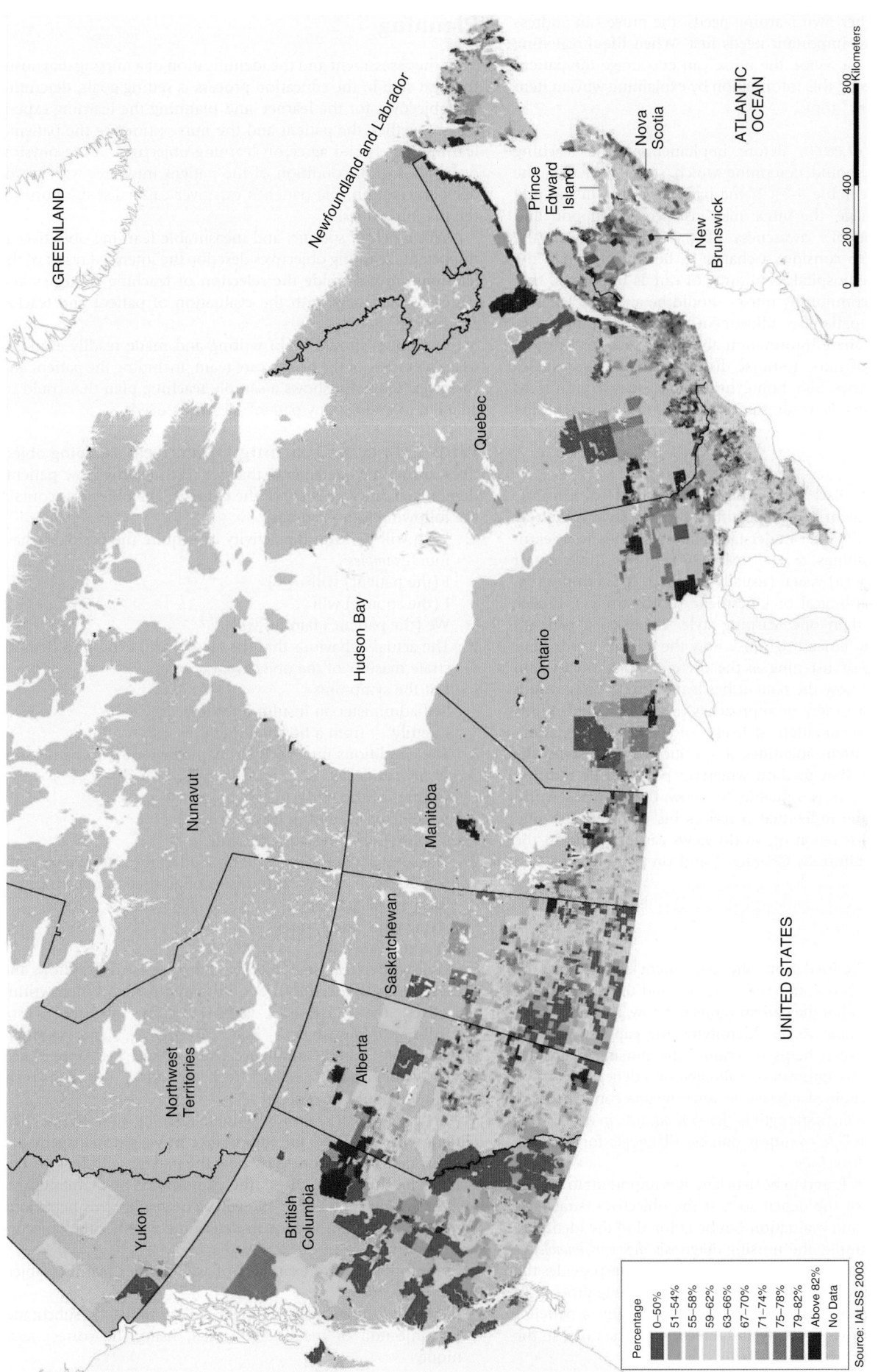

Figure 4-2 The distribution of health literacy in Canada. The analysis and mapping of the health literacy results were conducted by J. Douglas Willms, Canada Research Chair in Human Development at the University of New Brunswick (UNB), with the assistance of Teresa Tang, Geographic Information System (GIS) Programmer at the Canadian Research Institute for Social Policy at UNB.

Source: Canadian Council on Learning. (2007). *Health literacy in Canada: Initial results from the International Adult Literary and Skills Survey*. Retrieved from *http://www.ccl-cca.ca/pdfs/HealthLiteracy/HealthLiteracyinCanada.pdf*

Percentage
- 0–50%
- 51–54%
- 55–58%
- 59–62%
- 63–66%
- 67–70%
- 71–74%
- 75–78%
- 79–82%
- Above 82%
- No Data

Source: IALSS 2003

prioritize his or her own learning needs, the nurse can address the patient's most important needs first. When life-threatening complications are a factor, the nurse can encourage the patient to prioritize learning this information by explaining why an item is a "need-to-know" topic.

Readiness to Learn. Before implementing the teaching plan, the nurse should determine which stage of change the patient is in (see Table 4-3). If the patient is only in the precontemplation stage, the nurse may just provide support and increase the patient's awareness of the problem until the patient is ready to consider a change in behaviour. When the patient leaves the hospital, continuity of care is important; that is, hospital and community nurses should be aware of a transition phase for a patient as adjustment to the community continues. They can share information about the patient's learning stage by means of nurse-to-nurse discharge summaries. Nurses in different agencies and home health care may continue to evaluate the patient's readiness to learn and implement the teaching plan as the patient progresses through the stages of change.

Learning Style. Each person has a distinct style of learning, as individual as his or her personality. **Learning style** is the way in which each individual understands and responds to a learning situation (Billings & Hallstead, 2009). The three major learning styles are (a) visual (usually reading), (b) auditory (listening), and (c) physical or kinesthetic (doing things). People often use more than one learning style. To assess a patient's learning style, the nurse might ask how the patient learns best, whether reading or listening is the preferred method to gain information, and how the patient has learned in the past. Adult learners require a variety of approaches to learning, and nurses must be creative in their delivery of health information. However, if a patient identifies a specific learning style, the nurse should use that method whenever possible. In addition to learning styles, it is valuable to know the patient's world views and how the individual perceives his or her health and illness. Further discussion on world views can be found in the discussions on culture in Chapter 2 and on chronic illness in Chapter 5.

Diagnosis

Information is obtained from the assessment about what the patient knows, believes, and is able to do, and this information is compared with what the patient wants to know, needs to know, and needs to be able to do. Identifying the gap between the known and unknown helps determine the nursing diagnosis. With teaching, a strength can be validated or a deficiency can be corrected. An example of a desirable outcome that could facilitate validation of a patient's strength is "knowledgeable in developing a dietary regimen." A common nursing diagnosis for learning needs is *deficient knowledge.*

If knowledge is found to be deficient, it is important to specify the exact nature of the deficit so that the objectives, strategies, implementation, and evaluation can be tailored to the identified problem. For example, the nursing diagnosis *deficient knowledge related to inability to recognize symptoms of drug toxicity* provides the nurse with a clear direction for the teaching–learning process. In addition to being a nursing diagnosis that validates a patient's strength, it also provides clarity and direction for the nurse in the teaching–learning process.

Planning

After the assessment and the identification of a nursing diagnosis, the next step in the education process is setting goals, determining objectives for the learner, and planning the learning experience. Together, the patient and the nurse prioritize the patient's learning needs and agree on learning objectives. If the physical or psychological condition of the patient interferes with his or her participation, the patient's caregiver can assist the nurse in the planning phase.

Writing clear, specific, and measurable learning objectives is important. Learning objectives describe the intended result of the learning process, guide the selection of teaching strategies and materials, and help with the evaluation of patient and teacher progress.

Objectives should be in writing and made readily available to all members of the health care team, including the patient and caregiver. Table 4-6 shows a sample teaching plan that could be adapted to address any patient's learning needs.

Writing Specific Learning Objectives. **Learning objectives** are written statements that set forth exactly how patients demonstrate their mastery of the content. The objectives contain the following four elements:
1. Who will perform the activity or acquire the desired behaviour; *examples:*
   I (the patient) will …
   I (the spouse) will …
   We (the patient's family) will …
2. The actual behaviour that the learner will exhibit to demonstrate mastery of the objective; *examples:*
   List the symptoms
   Self-administer an insulin injection
   Identify … from a hospital menu
3. The conditions under which the behaviour is to be demonstrated; *examples:*
   In front of the nurse
   Select from a random list
   Choose from a restaurant menu
4. The specific criteria that will be used to measure the patient's success, such as time and degree of accuracy; *examples:*
   With 100% accuracy
   Using correct technique
   Within 3 minutes
   Well-written learning objectives have precise descriptions and include terms that cannot be loosely interpreted. When writing objectives, the nurse uses verbs such as "identify," "list," "describe," "demonstrate," "state," "recognize," and "compare and contrast." Vague, ambiguous terms, such as "appreciate," "learn," "understand," "enjoy," "feel," or "value," cannot be measured and should be avoided.

An example of a poorly written learning objective is "The patient will appreciate the importance of weight management." In this objective, it is not clear how the patient will demonstrate that he or she "appreciates" the importance of maintaining a healthy weight, how he or she will demonstrate this behaviour, or what criteria will be used to determine whether the objective has been met.

The following are examples of well-written learning objectives:
- In front of the nurse, the patient will administer a subcutaneous injection of insulin to herself, using the correct technique.

Table 4-6 Sample Teaching Plan

Purpose: To provide patient with information necessary to correctly change a colostomy appliance

Goal: The patient will be able to affix accurately and independently a colostomy appliance to a stoma

OBJECTIVES	CONTENT OUTLINE	METHOD OF INSTRUCTION	TIME ALLOTTED	RESOURCES	METHOD OF EVALUATION
After a 25-min teaching session, the patient will be able to do the following:					
1. Describe, in order, the steps required to prepare and affix correctly the colostomy appliance (cognitive)	List of the steps Description of the various items required	1:1 instruction	4 min	Description of equipment	Post-testing • Verbal • Written • Other
2. In the presence of the nurse, accurately measure and affix the colostomy appliance to the stoma (psychomotor)	Technique as per hospital policy and procedure Procedure for measuring stoma and affixing the appliance	Demonstration and return demonstration	13 min	All equipment required; e.g., colostomy appliance, measuring grid, adhesive paste (Stomahesive) Stoma model	Observation of return demonstration
3. Express to the nurse any feelings of discomfort regarding the ostomy and its care (affective)	Discuss common concerns Explore patient's feelings	Discussion	8 min	Video of patient vignettes Handouts	Question and answer

Source: Adapted from Bastable, S. B. (2008). *Essentials of patient education.* Sudbury, MA: Jones & Bartlett. Reprinted with permission.

• Given a list of symptoms of heart failure, the patient will identify before discharge from the hospital the early symptoms of heart failure, with 80% accuracy.

When learning objectives are clear and specific, and when they are written down and available in the patient record, all members of the health care team can work together to accomplish the same objectives. Once the objectives of the learning process are clearly stated, the nurse, the patient, and the patient's caregivers should choose the strategy or strategies that are most appropriate for meeting the objectives.

Selecting Teaching Strategies. Selection of a particular strategy is determined by at least three factors: (a) patient characteristics (e.g., age, educational background, degree of illness, culture, learning style); (b) subject matter; and (c) available resources. Some teaching strategies that can be employed to achieve learning objectives are discussed as follows. Each has advantages and disadvantages that render it more or less suitable to a particular patient and learning situation (Figure 4-3).

Lecture. The lecture format is an efficient, versatile, and economical teaching strategy that can be used when the amount of time is limited or when a group of patients and family members can benefit from acquiring a core of basic information. The nurse presents a series of related ideas or facts to one person or to a group. It is important to remember that the average adult learner can remember five to seven points at a time. Disadvantages of the lecture format are that it often has negative "school learning" connotations and that the extent of individual learning is difficult to evaluate.

Lecture–Discussion. The lecture–discussion can overcome some of the disadvantages of the lecture alone. With this strategy, the nurse presents specific information by using the lecture technique and follows up with a discussion, during which patients and their caregivers ask questions and exchange points of view

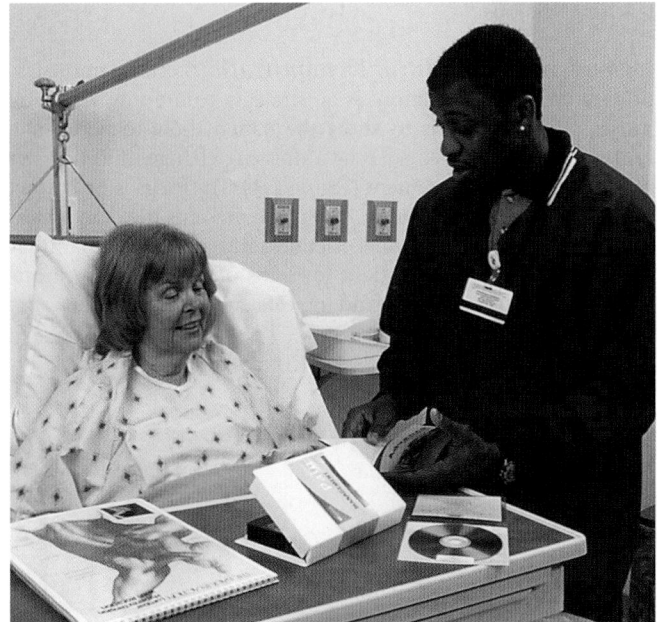

Figure 4-3 Effective teaching with a variety of materials.

with the nurse. This strategy assists the patient in becoming an active participant in the learning process and creates a more informal give-and-take learning environment. Some patients may be reluctant to actively engage in discussions.

Discussion. The purpose of discussion may be to exchange points of view concerning a topic or to arrive at a decision or conclusion. The nurse can discuss content with an individual or with a group, keeping the specific learning objectives in mind and clarifying information as needed. Participants' questions help the nurse identify and correct inaccurate information. This strategy is a good choice when the patient or patients have previous experience with a subject and have information to share, such as smoking cessation or convalescence after coronary artery bypass surgery. The discussion allows the patient or caregivers to participate actively and to apply their own experiences and observations to the learning process.

Group Teaching.   There are two main types of group teaching. In the first, the nurse acts as a **facilitator,** helping the group to share insights about a common problem. As facilitator, the nurse participates by keeping information moving among all group members. The nurse may introduce the patient to an existing group or may recruit a group of patients with similar problems, such as women who have multiple sclerosis.

A second kind of group teaching involves peer teaching. **Peer teaching** is teaching that is conducted within the setting of groups of peers, such as a self-help or support group. In a peer teaching setting, the participants learn from one another without the additional input of an instructor. A support group is a self-help organization that can provide continuing information, shared experiences, acceptance, understanding, and useful suggestions about a problem or concern. Patients with health issues such as cancer, alcoholism, Parkinson's disease, compulsive overeating, diabetes, or heart disease frequently find benefit from peer teaching situations. The nurse should actively look for opportunities to refer a patient or caregiver to a support group. This action should be taken in addition to, not instead of, the nurse's planned teaching sessions.

Demonstration–Return Demonstration.   The demonstration–return demonstration is a strategy commonly used by nurses. The purpose is to show the patient how to perform a motor skill–based task, such as a dressing change, injection, or blood pressure measurement (Figure 4-4). The focus is on correct procedure and its application. The nurse presents the demonstration in an informal manner, defines and explains unfamiliar terms, and watches the patient for signs of confusion or uncertainty. The nurse clarifies and repeats as necessary. Then the patient returns the demonstration with the nurse as observer. The entire process should require no more than 15 to 20 minutes. Achieving motor skills requires practice, and the procedure needs to be practised by the patient between teaching sessions.

Role Play.   Role play is another strategy that the nurse might employ, depending on teaching objectives. This format is most often used when patients need to examine their attitudes and behaviours, when patients need to understand the viewpoints and attitudes of others, or when they need to practise carrying out thoughts, ideas, or decisions. The nurse provides information and clear instructions to role players and observers and provides time for feedback and evaluation. Role playing requires maturity, confidence, and flexibility on the part of the participants. It is important to remember that patients sometimes may feel uncomfortable and inhibited with this method, and it is expected that initial discomfort can be overcome with patience and support. Role playing takes time, and time must be factored into the teaching plan. An example of the use of role playing is that of a wife who needs to rehearse how to talk with her husband about his need to quit smoking. In this case, practising the discussion with the nurse ahead of time is often a helpful strategy.

Use of Audiovisual Materials.   Audiovisual materials, including DVDs, computer-based programs, charts, podcasts, or simple transparencies are commonly used to supplement other teaching strategies. This strategy can enhance the presentation of information because it promotes learning through both visual and auditory stimulation. To use this strategy effectively, the nurse must preview and evaluate the teaching materials for accuracy, completeness, and appropriateness to the learning objectives before showing them to the patient and family. CDs are relatively easy to use and are usually inexpensive. The use of audiovisual materials can be extremely beneficial, particularly when content that is largely visual, such as the steps and processes of procedures (dressing changes, injections, hemodialysis) are taught. Computer-based programs designed for interactive learning of specific health information are widely available.

Use of the Internet.   The use of the Internet, particularly the World Wide Web, for self-education by patients is increasing dramatically. Many patients use their own computers, or those available at public libraries, to access health information on the Internet. The Internet also offers established educational programs designed for specific learners. However, the use of the Internet as a source of information is problematic. It offers a large number of high-quality health resources and poses seemingly unlimited opportunities to inform, teach, and connect health professionals and patients alike; at the same time, much Internet-borne information is incomplete, misleading, or inaccurate.

The nurse is challenged by several factors when using the Internet as a teaching tool. The nurse must have adequate computer competency to review and evaluate information and programs available on the Internet. Personal computer competency is especially necessary to teach patients and caregivers who are unfamiliar with computers, especially older adults, how to access information. All patients who use the Internet must be taught how to identify reliable and accurate information. The nurse should encourage patients to use sites established by the government, universities, or reputable medical or health-related associations (e.g., the Canadian Medical Association, Canadian Diabetes Association, Canadian Heart and Stroke Foundation, and Public Health Agency of Canada). The list of resources at the

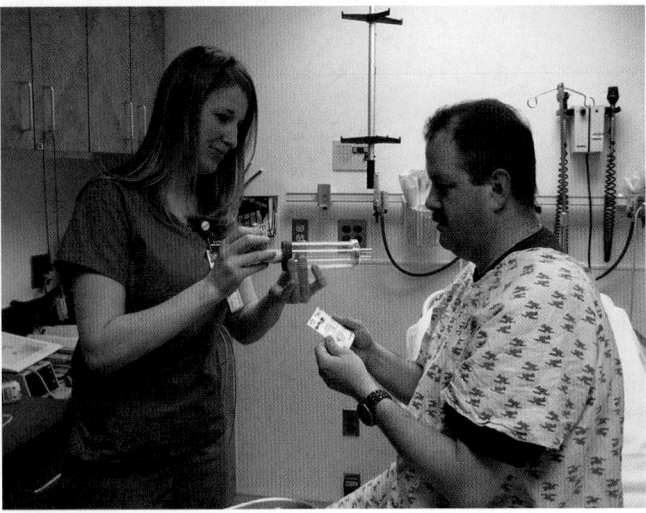

Figure 4-4 Careful teaching using demonstration–return demonstration has been shown to increase the probability of successful learning by the patient.

end of this chapter includes selected reliable patient–education Web sites for the nurse to review and use for patient referral.

Use of Printed Materials. Printed materials are most often used in combination with other teaching strategies presented in this section. For instance, after a lecture on the physiological effects of smoking, the nurse might distribute a pamphlet from the Canadian Cancer Society that reviews and reinforces the topic. Alternatively, the nurse might select a book or magazine article written by a woman who has had a mastectomy and suggest that the patient read this material to prepare for future teaching sessions. Written materials are always recommended for patients whose preferred learning style is reading.

Written material must be appropriate for the reading level of the patient. Before written materials are used with patients, the nurse should evaluate the readability level if it is not indicated on the materials. Because of the extent of health illiteracy, it is recommended that all patient–education materials be written at the fifth- to sixth-grade reading level (Canadian Council on Learning, 2007). At least 40 formulas have been developed to assess the readability of written materials. One easy to use formula that has been used for many years is the Simple Measure of Gobbledygook (SMOG) Readability Formula, developed by G. Harry McLaughlin in 1969. The SMOG formula estimates the years of education a person needs to understand a piece of writing.

If patients are to understand and benefit from all patient education materials, then information must be selected, revised, or redesigned so that even those at the lowest literacy level can comprehend it. To develop low-literacy education materials that can motivate patients to adopt healthier behaviours, the following six steps are recommended:
1. Develop a working team and solicit stakeholder input early.
2. List key concepts to be communicated.
3. Map concepts to a behavioural theory, such as a social cognitive theory. Construct a description of brief interventions to support the use of the written materials.
4. Design the required materials in accordance with low-literacy principles.
5. Refine the materials as necessary by using input from the target populations
6. Assess the success of efforts by using the materials with the target audience. Learn from failures (Seligman, 2007).

Major resources for acquiring relevant printed material include the hospital or care facility library, the pharmacy, the public library, government agencies, universities, voluntary organizations, Web sites, and research centres. Written materials, including computer-based programs, should be reviewed by the nurse before being used. In addition to reading level, the following criteria for review are suggested: (a) accuracy, (b) completeness, (c) whether the material meets specific learning goals, (d) whether pictures and diagrams are used to stimulate interest, (e) whether one main idea or concept is used per pamphlet or program, (f) whether the material contains information the patient would like to know, and (g) whether the material is culture and gender sensitive and appropriate (Redman, 2007).

Implementation

During the implementation phase, the nurse uses the planned strategies to present information and demonstrations. Verbal and nonverbal communication skills, active listening, and empathy are incorporated into the process.

In implementing the teaching plan, the nurse should remember the principles of adult learning and the determinants of learning. Reinforcement and reward are important. Techniques to enhance the teaching process with adults are presented in Table 4-7.

Evaluation

Evaluation is the final step in the learning process. It is a measure of the degree to which the patient has mastered the learning objectives. The nurse monitors the performance level of the patient so that changes can be made as needed. The nurse might find that the patient has already achieved the goals. However, if certain goals are not reached, the nurse should reassess the patient and alter the teaching plan. If the patient has developed new needs, the nurse then plans new goals, content, and strategies accordingly.

For example, an older man with diabetes mellitus entered the hospital with a blood glucose level of 30.5 mmol/L. When the student nurse began to prepare his insulin injection, the nurse asked, "Are you going to observe his technique as he gives himself insulin?" "Oh, no," replied the student nurse, "he has had diabetes for 20 years!" The assumption was that a patient with diabetes would know how to perform this task correctly. The two nurses returned to the patient's room and asked him to prepare an insulin injection. The patient filled the syringe with 20 units of insulin and 20 units of air, instead of 40 units of insulin. After correcting the dosage and questioning the patient more fully, the nurses concluded that the patient could not accurately see the markings on the syringe and that the patient may have been administering insufficient insulin to himself for a long time. The patient's vision was not as good as it had been 20 years earlier, and special equipment and new teaching on how to use it was now necessary for him to administer the insulin safely and accurately.

Evaluation techniques may be short-term or long-term. Short-term evaluation techniques are used to evaluate quickly the

Table 4-7 Techniques to Enhance Patient Learning

- Keep the physical environment relaxed and nonthreatening.
- Maintain a respectful, warm, and enthusiastic attitude.
- Let the patient's expressed needs direct what information is provided.
- Focus on "must-know" information; "nice-to-know" information can be added if time allows.
- Involve the patient and family in the process; emphasize active participation.
- Be aware of and take into consideration the patient's previous experiences.
- Emphasize the relevancy of the information to the patient's lifestyle, and suggest how it may provide an immediate solution to a problem.
- Individualize the teaching plan, even if standardized plans are used.
- Emphasize helping the patient to learn, rather than simply transmitting subject matter.
- Review written materials with the patient.
- Ask frequently for feedback information
- Affirm progress with rewards valued by the patient to reinforce desired behaviours.

patient's mastery of a concept, skill, or behaviour change, and short-term evaluation can be accomplished in the following ways:

1. *Observe the patient directly.* "Let me see how you administer your injection." Through observation, the nurse determines whether the patient has mastered the task, whether further instruction is needed, or whether the patient is ready for new or additional content.

2. *Observe verbal and nonverbal cues.* If the patient asks the nurse to repeat instructions, asks questions, shakes his or her head, loses eye contact, or otherwise expresses doubt about understanding, the patient may be indicating that further instruction is needed or that an alternative approach should be taken.

3. *Ask direct questions.* "What are the major food groups?" "How often must you change your dressing?" "What should you do if you develop chest pain after returning home?" Open-ended questions almost always provide more information about the patient's understanding than do questions that call for only a "yes" or "no" answer.

4. *Use a written measurement tool, graded for accuracy.* Paper-and-pencil tests can actually increase anxiety in patients. Many adults "freeze" when given a test or "go blank" when asked to write something that will be graded. Assess the patient's comfort and learning style before using a written method of evaluation.

5. *Talk with a member of the patient's family or support system.* "Is he eating regularly?" "How is he handling the walker?" "When is she taking her medications?" Because the nurse cannot observe the patient 24 hours a day, the nurse should receive information from other people who have contact with the patient.

6. *Seek the patient's self-evaluation of progress.* By seeking out a patient's opinion, the nurse is allowing the patient to provide input into the evaluation process. Long-term evaluation necessitates follow-up by the nurse, outpatient clinic, or outside agency. The nurse should set up a schedule of visits for the patient before the patient leaves the hospital or clinic

or refer the patient to the proper agencies. The nurse keeps written documentation of follow-up telephone calls or by e-mails to urge the patient to maintain the follow-up schedule. The patient's caregivers should be familiar with the follow-up plan, so that everyone is involved in the patient's long-term progress.

Continuity of Educational Care

The nurse is responsible for communicating with other health professionals involved in the patient's long-term follow-up. The nurse should telephone, visit, or e-mail these health professionals and supply them with the relevant education plan. The data are charted in the patient's medical records for further use.

Documentation of the Educational Process

Documentation is an essential component of the entire teaching–learning transaction. The nurse records everything, from the assessment through short- and long-term plans for evaluation. As mentioned, copies of the documentation should be forwarded to the agency or health care provider providing long-term follow-up. The teaching objectives, the content, the strategies, and the evaluation results should be written clearly and completely because many members of the health care team will use these records in different places and for various reasons.

The Standardized Teaching Plan

Standardized teaching plans are often included in care maps and clinical pathways, and they have become an accepted method of developing a teaching plan. Standardized teaching plans contain widely accepted knowledge and skills that a patient and caregivers need to know with regard to a specific health problem or procedure. However, the nurse should always individualize these plans to meet the patient's specific needs.

CLINICAL DECISION-MAKING EXERCISE

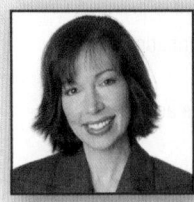

CASE STUDY:
Example of the Teaching Process

Source: © iStockphoto.com/Diane Diederich.

Mrs. Blahavi is admitted to the hospital for preliminary testing and preparation for a hysterectomy. The nurse is aware that a patient undergoing a hysterectomy is often deeply concerned about her self-concept as a woman. The nurse also knows that such patients need to express their feelings in an atmosphere of support and understanding. Therefore, the nurse has sought to listen attentively and ask questions carefully in order to assess the patient's feelings about, and knowledge of, the surgical procedure she is about to undergo. The nurse has asked open-ended questions, such as, "How do you feel about having the surgery?" and "What concerns do you have about undergoing a hysterectomy?"

By establishing both a climate of trust and a counselling relationship, the nurse has completed the assessment that follows.

Biophysical Dimension

Age 44, White female, high-school English teacher and coach of girls' high school basketball team; good general health. Height and weight proportional and average for age. Patient reports that she jogs five evenings a week. No sensory impairment; vision, hearing, and reaction time seem normal.

Psychological Dimension

Patient appears mildly anxious about surgery and seems worried about her husband's acceptance of her sexuality. She is also worried about missing work and leaving her classes to a substitute teacher. She states that she does not "let physical problems get me down," and that she dislikes "pills and hospitals." She states that she is used to "teaching" and not "being taught," and she tries to dominate any conversation or input from the nurse.

Sociocultural Dimension

Married with one child (son), age 23. Mother had a mastectomy at age 51; father healthy. Two younger sisters; both experienced difficult pregnancies but are otherwise healthy. Patient describes caregiver communication as very good. She describes her lifestyle as work oriented and says that her friends are primarily teaching colleagues. She places a high priority on work and family.

Learning Style

Responds well to formal lectures. Enjoys reading and group discussions.

Determining Objectives

After a brief period of rest and adjustment to the unfamiliar hospital environment, Mrs. Blahavi states that she would like to learn more about the details of the upcoming planned surgical procedure. Together, Mrs. Blahavi and the nurse identify the following objectives:

After the teaching session, I (Mrs. Blahavi) will be able to do the following:

1. Describe the surgical procedure to the nurse (hysterectomy).
2. Express to the nurse and my husband my feelings about maintaining an active and fulfilling sex life.

3. Complete arrangements with my family and school principal for convalescence and return to normal activities.
4. List the general recovery experiences that are expected, and state circumstances under which to seek medical advice.
5. Discuss "old wives' tales" regarding hysterectomy and verbalize concerns regarding undergoing the hysterectomy.
6. Identify ways to avoid constipation, weight gain, and potential periods of depression during the recovery period.
7. Identify ways to return comfortably to baseline sexual activities.

Discussion Questions

1. What factors might impede Mrs. Blahavi from learning?
2. What teaching strategies might be the most effective for each learning objective?
3. What observations will inform the nurse that Mrs. Blahavi has met each learning objective (consider verbal and nonverbal behaviours)?
4. How can the learning be reinforced?

evolve *Answers may be found at* **http://evolve.elsevier.com/ Canada/Lewis/medsurg**

REVIEW QUESTIONS

The number of the question corresponds to the same-numbered objective at the beginning of the chapter.

1. The nurse is teaching a middle-aged Italian woman in a clinic about methods to relieve the patient's symptoms of menopause. What is the goal of this teaching episode?
   a. To prevent disease
   b. To maintain health
   c. To alter the patient's cultural belief regarding the use of herbs
   d. To provide information for selection and use of treatment options
2. What should the nurse do when planning experiences with consideration of adult learning principles?
   a. Present material in an efficient lecture format
   b. Recognize that adults enjoy learning regardless of the relevance to their personal lives
   c. Provide opportunities for the patient to learn from other adults with similar experiences
   d. Postpone practice of new skills until the patient can independently practise the skill at home
3. Which of the following skills is necessary for the nurse in the role of teacher?
   a. Determining when patients are too distressed physically or psychologically to learn
   b. Assuring the patient that the nurse understands what is necessary for the patient to learn
   c. Developing standardized teaching plans for use with all patients to save time and overcome time constraints
   d. Presenting information in medical language to increase the patient's vocabulary and understanding of pathophysiology

4. When the nurse is feeling stressed about the limited time available for patient teaching, which of the following strategies would be most beneficial?
   a. Setting realistic goals that have high priority for the patient
   b. Referring the patient to a nurse-educator in private practice for teaching
   c. Observing more experienced nurse-teachers to learn how to teach faster and more efficiently
   d. Providing reading materials for the patient instead of discussing information the patient needs to learn
5. What is the reason for including family members in patient teaching?
   a. They provide most of the care for patients.
   b. Patients have been shown to have better outcomes when caregivers are involved.
   c. The patient may be too ill, or too stressed, by the situation to understand teaching.
   d. They might feel rejected and unimportant if they are not included in the teaching.
6. Which step of the teaching process is involved when the nurse, the patient, and the patient's family decide together what strategies would be best to meet the learning objectives?
   a. Planning
   b. Evaluation
   c. Assessment
   d. Implementation
7. A nurse is spending time with a patient who is undergoing a diagnostic procedure. Which of the following comments by the patient best indicates a teachable moment?
   a. "I have to e-mail a friend in a few moments."
   b. "How long will this procedure take?"
   c. "I have had this procedure before."
   d. "I'm trying not think about it."

8. Which of the following is an example of a correctly written learning objective?
   a. The patient will lose 11.5 kg in 6 weeks.
   b. The patient should understand the implications of the condition.
   c. The patient will read two pamphlets on the subject of breast self-examination.
   d. The patient's spouse will demonstrate to the nurse how to correctly change a colostomy bag before discharge.

9. A patient tells the nurse that she enjoys talking with others and sharing experiences but easily falls asleep when reading. Which of the following teaching strategies would help this patient to learn best?
   a. Role play
   b. Peer teaching
   c. Lecture–discussion
   d. Discussion supplemented with computer programs

10. Which of these approaches would best provide short-term evaluation of teaching effectiveness?
    a. Observing the patient and asking direct questions.
    b. Monitoring the patient for 3 to 6 months after the teaching.
    c. Monitoring for the behaviour change for up to 6 weeks after discharge.
    d. Asking the patient what he or she found helpful about the teaching experience.

ANSWERS: 1. d; 2. c; 3. a; 4. a; 5. b; 6. a; 7. b; 8. d; 9. b; 10. a

REFERENCES

Arnold, E., & Boggs, K. (2011). *Interpersonal relationships: Professional communication skills for nurses* (6th ed.). St. Louis: Elsevier.

Bastable, S. B. (2008). *Essentials of patient education.* Sudbury, MA: Jones & Bartlett.

Bastable, S. B., Gramet, P., Jacobs, K., & Sopczyk, D. (2011). *Health professional as educator.* Sudbury, MA: Jones & Bartlett.

Billings, D., & Hallstead, J. (2009). *Teaching in nursing: A guide for faculty* (3rd ed.). St. Louis: Elsevier.

Canadian Council on Learning. (2007). *Health literacy in Canada: Initial results from the International Adult Literary and Skills Survey.* Retrieved from *www.ccl-cca.ca/pdfs/Healthliteracy/HealthliteracyinCanada.pdf*

Canadian Partnership Against Cancer. (2012). Sustaining action toward a shared vision. Retrieved from *http://www.partnershipagainstcancer.ca/wp-content/uploads/Sustaining-Action-Toward-a-Shared-Vision-Full-Document.pdf*

Cornett, S. (2009). Assessing and addressing health literacy. *Online Journal of Issues in Nursing, 14*(3), 1-21. doi:10.3912/OJIN.Vol-14No03Man02

Fineberg, I., Kawashima, M., & Asch, S. (2011). Communication with families facing life-threatening illness: A research-based model for family conferences. *Journal of Palliative Medicine, 14*(4), 421-427. doi:10.1089/jpm.2010.0436

Hannah, K. (2007). The state of nursing informatics in Canada. *Canadian Nurse, 103*(5), 18-22. Retrieved from *ProQuest.*

Knowles, M. (1990). *The adult learner: A neglected species* (4th ed.). Houston: Gulf Publishing.

Kozier, B., Erb, G., Berman, A., Burke, K., Bouchal, S., & Hirst, S., …, Buck, M. (2010). *Fundamentals of Canadian nursing: Concepts, process, and practice* (2nd Canadian ed.). Toronto: Pearson Canada.

Laschinger, H., Gilbert, S., Smith, L., & Leslie, K. (2010). Towards a comprehensive theory of nurse/patient empowerment: Applying Kanter's empowerment theory to patient care. *Journal of Nursing Management, 18,* 4-13. doi:10.1111/j.1365-2834.2009.01046.x

Organization for Economic Cooperation and Development. (2008). *Adult literacy.* Retrieved from *www.oecd.org/document/2/0,3343,en_2649_39263294_2670850_1_1_1_1,00.html*

Osborn, C., Weiss, B., Davis, T., Skripkauskas, S., Rodrigue, C., Bass, P., & Wolf, M. (2007). Measuring adult health literacy in health care: Performance of the newest vital sign. *American Journal Health Behavior, 31*(Suppl 1), S36-S46. doi:10.5555/ajhb.2007.31.supp.S36

Osteoporosis Canada. (2011). *Virtual education forum.* Retrieved from *http://www.osteoporosis.ca/index.php/ci_id/9166/la_id/1.htm*

Potter, P. A., Perry, A. G., Ross-Kerr, J., & Wood, M. (2010). *Canadian fundamentals of nursing* (4th ed.). Toronto: Elsevier Canada.

Prochaska, J. O., & Velicer, W. F. (1997). The transtheoretical model of health behaviour change. *American Journal of Health Promotion, 12*(1), 38. doi:*http://dx.doi.org/10.4278/0890-1171-12.1.38*

Redman, B. K. (2007). *The practice of patient education: A case study approach* (10th ed.). St. Louis: Mosby.

Seligman, H., Wallace, A., DeWalt, D., Schillinger, D., Arnold, C., Shilliday, B., …, Davis, T. (2007). Facilitating behavior change with low-literacy patient education materials. *American Journal of Health Behavior, 31*(Supp1), S69-S78. doi:10.5555/ajhb.2007.31.supp.S69

Schwartz, F., Hutchings, T., Friedman, A., Quartey, N., Urowitz, S., Wiljer, D., & Smith, R. (2010). Moving towards an organized approach to patient education in Canadian hospitals. *Healthcare Quarterly, 13*(4), 84-88. Retrieved from *http://www.longwoods.com/content/22004*

Virtanen, H., Leino-Kilpi, H., & Salantera, S. (2007). Empowering discourse in patient education. *Patient Education and Counselling, 66,* 140-146. doi:10.1016/j.pec.2006.12.010

Weiss, B., Mays, M., Martz, W., Castro, K., DeWalt, D., Pignone, M., …, Hale, F. (2005). Quick assessment of literacy in primary care: The newest vital sign. *Annals of Family Medicine, 3*(6), 514-522. doi:10.1370/afm.405

Wright, L., & Leahey, M. (2009). *Nurses and families* (5th ed.). Philadelphia: F. A. Davis.

CANADIAN RESOURCES

Canada Public Health Agency, National Literacy and Health
     Program
     http://www.cpha.ca/en/portals/h-l/h-l5.aspx
Canadian Association for the Study of Adult Education (CASAE)
     http://www.casae-aceea.ca/
Health Canada
     http://www.hc-sc.gc.ca/index-eng.php
LD Online (Learning Disabilities and Attention Deficit/
     Hyperactivity Disorder [ADHD])
     http://www.ldonline.org/finding_help/canada.html
Learning Disabilities Association of Canada
     http://www.ldac-acta.ca/
Learning Disabilities Resource Community
     http://www.ldrc.ca/

RELATED RESOURCES

Healthfinder
     Office of Disease Prevention and Health Promotion
     U.S. Department of Health and Human Resources
     http://www.healthfinder.gov
MedicineNet.com
     http://www.medicinenet.com
Medline Plus Health Information
     http://www.nlm.nih.gov/medlineplus

evolve *For additional Internet resources, see the Web site for this book
at* **http://evolve.elsevier.com/Canada/Lewis/medsurg**

LEARNING OBJECTIVES

1. Describe the impact of chronic illness in Canada.
2. Define and describe acute and chronic illness and the relationships between these concepts.
3. Identify key factors contributing to the development of chronic illness.
4. Differentiate between chronic illness and disability.
5. Discuss the psychosocial implications of living with a chronic illness.
6. Describe the ways in which chronic illness may affect family members or significant others.
7. Discuss key conceptual models of chronic illness.
8. Describe the role of self-management in chronic illness.
9. Identify emerging models of providing care to individuals with chronic illness.

KEY TERMS

acute illness Typically characterized by a sudden onset, with signs and symptoms related to the disease process itself, p. 70

best buys Actions that should be undertaken immediately to produce accelerated results in terms of lives saved, diseases prevented, and heavy costs avoided, p. 72

caregiver burden The overall physical, emotional, and financial costs of caregiving, p. 78

chronic illness Health problems that persist over extended periods and that are often (but not always) associated with participation and activity limitations (disability), p. 69

co-morbidity The existence of two or more chronic illness in a person at the same time that are not directly related to each other, p. 71

determinants of health Complex interactions between social and economic factors, the physical environment, and individual behaviours that determine health, p. 70

disability A difficulty in functioning at the body, the personal, or the societal level, in one or more life domains, as experienced by an individual with a health condition in interaction with contextual factors, p. 73

disease A condition that a practitioner views from a pathophysiological model, p. 70

fatigue A subjective, unpleasant symptom that incorporates total body feelings ranging from tiredness to exhaustion, creating an unrelenting overall condition that interferes with individuals' ability to function to their normal capacity, p. 76

health A state of complete physical, mental, and social well-being and not merely the absence of disease or infirmity, p. 70

health-related hardiness (HRH) A personality resource characterized by a sense of control, commitment, and challenge, p. 76

health-related quality of life (HRQL) The subjective experience of the impact of health status on quality of life, p. 77

illness The human experience of symptoms and suffering. This term refers to how the disease is perceived, lived with, and responded to by individuals and their families, p. 70

illness behaviour The varying ways individuals respond to physical symptoms: how they monitor internal states, define and interpret symptoms, make attributions, take remedial actions, and use various sources of informal and formal care, p. 74

illness trajectory A pathway along which the person with an illness progresses, p. 78

informal caregiver A person who provides care without pay and who usually has personal ties to the care recipient, p. 78

lifestyle The choices made by individuals that are influenced by social, economic, and environmental factors, p. 72

modifiable risk factors Factors such as behaviour that can be changed to reduce the risk of developing an illness, p. 72

morbidity Rates of disease, p. 69

mortality Rates of death, p. 69

multimorbidity The simultaneous occurrence of several chronic medical conditions in the same person, p. 71

nonmodifiable risk factors Factors such as age and sex that contribute to the development of an illness but cannot be changed, p. 72

quality of life The degree to which a person enjoys the important possibilities of her or his life, p. 77

self-efficacy The belief that one can successfully execute the behaviour required to produce the desired outcome, p. 75

self-management The daily activities that individuals undertake to keep illness under control, minimize its impact on physical health status and functioning, and cope with the psychosocial sequelae of the illness, p. 80

shared decision making A decision-making process jointly shared by patients and their health care provider, in which the provider is the clinical expert and the patient is the expert in her own life, value, and circumstances (Legare et al., 2009; Godolphin, 2009), p. 75

signs Objective manifestations of a condition, p. 70

stigmatization Being regarded by others as unworthy or disgraceful, p. 77

symptoms The subjective reports of the patient, p. 70

ELECTRONIC RESOURCES

Supplemental content related to Chapter 5 can be found …

Evolve Web Site ⊖volve

http://evolve.elsevier.com/Canada/Lewis/medsurg
- Clinical Reference: Laboratory Values
- Content Updates

- Electronic Calculators
- Examination Review Questions
- Glossary
- Key Points (Printable and MP3 Download)

Few pandemics have resulted in as much suffering and premature death as the current global epidemic of chronic illness (Nolte & McKee, 2008). **Chronic illness** refers to health problems that persist over extended periods and that are often (but not always) associated with participation and activity limitations (disability). Chronic illnesses demand a complex response from patients and families over an extended time period. This response also involves coordinated inputs from a wide range of health professionals, as well as access to essential treatments (Nolte & McKee, 2008). Care for people with chronic illness is ideally embedded within a health care system that promotes patient empowerment.

Unfortunately, the Canadian health care is still largely built around an acute, episodic model of care that is unable to address the needs of those with chronic health problems. The current mismatch between the episodic care orientation of the existing health care system and the needs of people living in the community with chronic illnesses has led to a host of well-documented failures in care provision. These failures include: high rates of hospital readmissions; medical errors; underdiagnosis of conditions; inconsistent monitoring of chronic conditions; lack of patient-centredness; insufficient health education; duplication of resources; inappropriate omission of resources; and preventable injuries (Bodenheimer & Berry-Millett, 2009; Boyd et al., 2007). Innovative models of providing care for people with chronic illness, such as virtual wards, are currently being evaluated in Canada and hold promise for improving care in the future (Canadian Agency for Drugs and Technology, 2012).

Because we need to organize the vast amount of knowledge about the medical–surgical nursing care of people within a cohesive framework, most textbooks are organized along the lines of body systems and common medical diagnoses. It is critical to recognize, however, that medical diagnosis alone does not predict service needs, length of hospitalization, level of care, or functional outcomes and tells us nothing about the person experiencing the condition or how this person will respond to nursing care. The presence of a disease or disorder is not an accurate predictor of outcomes such as receipt of disability benefits, work performance, potential return to work, or likelihood of social integration (Nolte & McKee, 2008). In providing truly holistic and comprehensive care, nurses assume a perspective that includes behavioural, psychosocial, and environmental factors. This chapter seeks to situate the information contained in the remainder of this textbook within such a framework.

The Epidemiology of Chronic Diseases

Chronic heart disease, lung diseases, cancer, and diabetes accounted for well over half (63%) of the 57 million deaths worldwide in 2008 (World Health Organization [WHO], 2011). Cardiovascular diseases (48%) were responsible for the highest proportion of global deaths in 2008 (WHO, 2011). Figure 5-1 illustrates the main causes of global deaths from noncommunicable chronic diseases.

In Canada, chronic illnesses also make a substantial contribution to morbidity and mortality. Canada's aging population, along with the rising rates of some risk factors for chronic diseases, is driving the chronic disease challenge. About two thirds of deaths in Canada each year result from chronic diseases. Table 5-1 illustrates how chronic illnesses affect Canadians.

Morbidity refers to the rates of disease in a population, whereas **mortality** refers to the rates of deaths. Although musculoskeletal conditions such as arthritis and osteoporosis are the most prevalent and costly chronic conditions in Canada, heart disease and stroke were the underlying causes of death for one

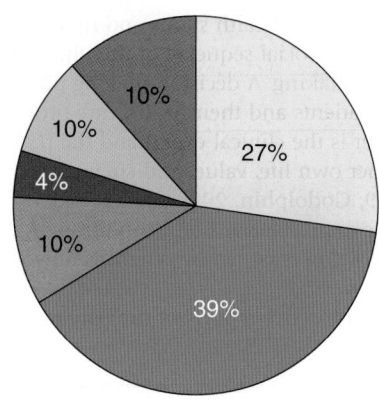

☐ Cancers   ■ Diabetes

■ Cardiovascular diseases   ☐ Digestive diseases

■ Chronic respiratory diseases   ■ Other noncommunicable diseases

Figure 5-1 Main causes of global deaths younger than age 70 years for 2008.

Source: World Health Organization (WHO). (2011). *Global status report on noncommunicable diseases 2010* (p. 11). Geneva: Author. Retrieved from *http://www.who.int/nmh/publications/ncd_report_full_en.pdf*

Table 5-1 Chronic Illness in Canada

Cancer

- About 1 in 3 Canadians will develop cancer in their lifetime
- 177,800 people are diagnosed with cancer each year
- 75,000 Canadians die each year due to cancer

Diabetes

- About 1 in 16 Canadians (6.2%) are living with diabetes and an additional 0.9% of the population (nearly 300,000) is estimated to be undiagnosed
- The prevalence of diabetes increased by 21% from 2002 to 2007
- Among adults 20 years and older, mortality rates for those with diabetes (deaths usually due to a complication of diabetes, like cardiovascular disease) were twice as high as those without diabetes

Cardiovascular Diseases

- 1.6 million Canadians have heart disease or are living with the effects of a stroke
- In 2007, cardiovascular diseases were responsible for about 70,000 deaths
- Death rates have decreased since the late 1960s, probably due to lower smoking rates and improved treatment

Chronic Respiratory Diseases

- Over 3 million Canadians live with a chronic respiratory disease
- Tobacco remains the most important preventable risk factor for chronic respiratory diseases

Source: Public Health Agency of Canada. (2011). *Chronic diseases in Canada*. Reproduced with permission from the Minister of Health, 2012. Retrieved from *http://www.phac-aspc.gc.ca/media/nr-rp/2011/2011_0919-bg-di-eng.php*

---

in three Canadians (Statistics Canada, 2011). Premature death resulting from cardiovascular disease costs the Canadian economy $9.2 billion each year, and cerebrovascular accidents account for $3.2 billion due to direct health care costs (Patra, Popova, Bondy, Flint, & Giescrecht, 2007). An estimated 177,800 new cases of cancer (excluding about 74,100 nonmelanoma skin cancers) and 75,000 deaths will occur in Canada in 2011 (Canadian Cancer Society, 2011). In 2007, cancer surpassed cardiovascular disease (heart and cerebrovascular) as the leading cause of death in Canada (Canadian Cancer Society, 2011). Lung, prostate, breast, and colorectal cancer are the four most common cancer types in Canada and account for over 50% of all new cancer cases (Canadian Cancer Society, 2011). Lung cancer is responsible for more than one quarter of all cancer deaths each year.

Health, Acute Illness, and Chronic Illness

Health and illness may be viewed along a continuum upon which individuals journey throughout life. **Health,** according to the WHO (2011) definition, is a state of complete physical, mental, and social well-being and not merely the absence of disease or infirmity. The state of health is dependent upon complex interactions between multiple social and economic factors, the physical environment, and individual behaviour. These factors are referred to as **determinants of health.** Table 5-2 displays the determinants of health recognized by the Public Health Agency of Canada (PHAC) (2011b).

Disease is a condition that a practitioner views from a pathophysiological model (Lubkin & Larsen, 2009). **Illness,** conversely, is the human experience of symptoms and suffering. This term refers to how the disease is perceived, lived with, and responded to by individuals and their families (Lubkin & Larsen, 2009). Nursing practice must be informed by both knowledge of disease and understanding of the illness experience.

Table 5-3 compares the characteristics of acute and chronic illness. **Acute illness** is typically characterized by a sudden onset, with signs and symptoms related to the disease process itself. **Signs** are typically objective manifestations of a condition, whereas **symptoms** refer to the subjective reports of the patient. Acute illness ends in a relatively short time, sometimes in recovery and sometimes in death (Lubkin & Larsen, 2009). Chronic illness often continues indefinitely. Strauss et al. (1984) viewed chronic illness as an experience of problems that may change but do not go away. The onset of a chronic illness may be sudden, or it may develop insidiously over a long period. Some chronic illnesses are characterized by exacerbations and remissions, whereas other chronic illnesses cause persistent symptoms throughout their course.

Chronic (or noncommunicable) illnesses are typically characterized as having an uncertain etiology, multiple risk factors, long latency, prolonged duration, and a noninfectious origin and can be associated with impairments or functional disability. Cardiovascular disease, diabetes, arthritis and other musculoskeletal diseases, cancers, chronic lung diseases, and chronic neurological disorders (including depression) are conditions recognized by the Centers for Disease Control and Prevention (2011a) as chronic illnesses.

Acute and chronic illnesses can occur in an individual simultaneously. The acute illness may have a profound impact on the person with a pre-existing chronic illness. For example, a person

Table 5-2 Public Health Agency of Canada: Key Determinants of Health

DETERMINANT OF HEALTH	UNDERLYING PREMISE
Income and social status	Health status improves at each step up the income and social hierarchy. High income determines living conditions such as safe housing and ability to buy sufficient good food. The healthiest populations are those societies that are prosperous and have an equitable distribution of wealth.
Social support networks	Support from families, friends, and communities is associated with better health. Such social support networks could be very important in helping people solve problems and deal with adversity as well as in maintaining a sense of mastery and control over life circumstances. The caring and respect that occurs in social relationships, and the resulting sense of satisfaction and wellbeing, seem to act as a buffer against health problems.
Education and literacy	Health status improves with level of education, which is, in turn, tied to socioeconomic status. Education contributes to health and prosperity by equipping people with knowledge and skills for problem solving and helps provide a sense of control and mastery over life circumstances. It increases opportunities for job and income security and job satisfaction. Education also improves people's ability to access and understand information to help keep them healthy.
Employment–working conditions	Unemployment, underemployment, and stressful or unsafe work are associated with poorer health. People who have more control over their work circumstances and fewer stress-related demands of the job are healthier and often live longer than those who have more stressful or riskier types of work and activities.
Social environments	The array of values and norms of a society influences in varying ways the health and well-being of individuals and populations. In addition, social stability, recognition of diversity, safety, good working relationships, and cohesive communities provide a supportive society that reduces or avoids many potential risks to good health. Social or community responses can add resources to an individual's repertoire of strategies to cope with changes and foster health.
Physical environments	The physical environment is an important determinant of health. At certain levels of exposure, contaminants in our air, water, food, and soil can cause a variety of adverse health effects, including cancer, birth defects, respiratory illness, and gastrointestinal ailments. In the built environment, factors related to housing, indoor air quality, and the design of communities and transportation systems can significantly influence our physical and psychological well-being.
Personal health practices and coping skills	These refer to those actions by which individuals can prevent diseases and promote self-care, cope with challenges, develop self-reliance, solve problems, and make choices that enhance health. These influence lifestyle choice through at least five domains: personal life skills, stress, culture, social relationships and belonging, and a sense of control.
Healthy child development	New evidence on the effects of early experiences on brain development, school readiness, and health in later life has sparked a growing consensus about early child development as a powerful determinant of health in its own right. All of the other determinants of health, in turn, affect the physical, social, mental, emotional, and spiritual development of children and youth.
Biology and genetic endowment	The basic biology and organic makeup of the human body are a fundamental determinant of health. Genetic endowment provides an inherited predisposition to a wide range of individual responses that affect health status. Socioeconomic and environmental factors are important determinants of overall health, but in some circumstances, genetic endowment appears to predispose certain individuals to particular diseases or health problems.
Health services	Health services, particularly those designed to maintain and promote health, to prevent disease, and to restore health and function, contribute to the health of the overall population. The health services continuum of care includes treatment and secondary prevention.
Gender	Gender refers to the array of society-determined roles, personality traits, attitudes, behaviours, values, and relative power and influence that society ascribes to the two sexes on a differential basis. "Gendered" norms influence the health system's practices and priorities. Many health issues are a function of gender-based social status or roles.
Culture	Some persons or groups may face additional health risks due to a socioeconomic environment, which is largely determined by dominant cultural values that contribute to the perpetuation of conditions such as marginalization, stigmatization, loss or devaluation of language and culture, and lack of access to culturally appropriate health care and services.

Source: Public Health Agency of Canada. (2011). *What determines health?* Reproduced with permission from the Minister of Health, 2012. Retrieved from *www.phac-aspc.gc.ca/ph-sp/determinants/index.html#determinants*

with longstanding, well-controlled diabetes may experience an acute infection that drastically changes blood glucose and insulin requirements. Similarly, chronic illness may affect the manner in which an acute illness is managed. A person with chronic kidney disease who undergoes surgery will likely require a modified postoperative fluid regimen. The complexity of caring for patients with multiple illnesses, whether acute or chronic, demands a high standard of nursing knowledge and skill. When two or more

chronic illness are found in a person at the same time and are not directly related to each other, this is called **co-morbidity** (Nardi et al., 2007). An example of co-morbidity would be when a patient has heart disease, arthritis, and cancer at the same. **Multimorbidity** is the simultaneous occurrence of several chronic medical conditions, which may or may not be related to each other, in the same person (Campbell-Scherer, 2010). Achieving optimal health for the persons with multimorbidity is

Table 5-3 Characteristics of Acute and Chronic Illness	
ACUTE ILLNESS	**CHRONIC ILLNESS**
Abrupt onset	Gradual onset is common
Limited duration	Unfolds over time; undulating course
Usually single cause	Multivariate causation, changing over time
Diagnosis and prognosis commonly accurate	Diagnosis may be uncertain; prognosis obscure
Self-limited, or specific therapy available	Treatments achieve no definitive results, and therapies have associated adversities
Technological intervention usually effective (laboratory testing, imaging, medication, surgery)	Technological intervention may or may not be helpful
Cure likely with return to normal health	No cure; management over time necessary
Minimal uncertainty	Uncertainty pervasive
Providers knowledgeable; patient inexperienced	Provider and patient partially and reciprocally knowledgeable

Source: Adapted from Holman, H., & Lorig, K. (2004). Patient self-management: a key to effectiveness and efficiency in care of chronic disease. *Public Health Reports, 119*, 239-243. Retrieved from *http://www.ncbi.nlm.nih.gov/pmc/articles/PMC1497631/pdf/15158102.pdf*

challenging because a treatment targeting one condition may make a coexisting condition worse. For example, a patient who is receiving nonsteroidal anti-inflammatory medications to relieve pain from arthritis finds that the medication worsens hypertension and renal disease.

Having multiple chronic medical conditions is associated with many negative outcomes: patients have decreased quality of life, psychological distress, longer hospital stays, more postoperative complications, a higher cost of care, and higher mortality (Fortin, 2007). In addition, multimorbidity affects the care process and may result in complex self-care needs; challenging organizational problems (accessibility, coordination, consultation time); polypharmacy; increased use of emergency facilities; difficulty in applying guidelines; and fragmented, costly, and ineffective care (Fortin, 2007).

Factors Contributing to Chronic Illness

The key determinants of health (see Table 5-2) are also critical considerations in the development of chronic illness. Although some chronic conditions have a specific and unique etiology, there are common factors identified by large, longitudinal studies that play an important role in the development of many types of chronic illness. **Lifestyle** factors such as substance use and misuse and high-risk activities can be harmful to a person's long-term health. The term *lifestyle* not only includes choices made by individuals but also recognizes the influence of social, economic, and environmental factors on the decisions people make about their health.

There is a growing recognition that personal life "choices" are heavily influenced by the socioeconomic environments in which the person lives. A healthy lifestyle can be thought of as a broad description of people's behaviour in three interrelated dimensions: between individuals; individuals within their social environments (e.g., family, peers, community, workplace); and the relationship between individuals and their social environment (PHAC, 2011a). Studies such as the Framingham Heart Study and the Nurses' Health Study have demonstrated clear associations between chronic illness and tobacco use, alcohol misuse, high blood pressure, physical inactivity, obesity, and unhealthy diet (Centers for Disease Control and Prevention, 2011a). Poverty and socioeconomic disadvantage are recognized to have a major impact on the development of chronic illness (Lubkin & Larsen, 2009). Income significantly affects the life expectancy, the ability to obtain and provide nutritious food and good housing, and access to health care (PHAC, 2008). It is estimated that the rate of premature death among all Canadians could be reduced by 20% if all Canadians were as healthy as the richest 20% of Canadians (PHAC, 2008).

Risk Factors for Chronic Illness

Both individuals and communities may possess risk factors for the development of chronic illness (PHAC, 2010). The recognition of these common risk factors and conditions is the conceptual basis for an integrated approach to chronic disease.

Individual risk factors can be classified as background, behavioural, or intermediate. Sex, age, level of education, and genetic characteristics are examples of individual risk factors. Smoking, unhealthy diet, and physical inactivity would fall into the category of behavioural risk factors. Intermediate risk factors include conditions such as diabetes, hypertension, and obesity/overweight. Besides risks that occur at the individual level, community-level factors can also make a significant contribution to the development of chronic illnesses. Examples of community-level risk factors include social and economic conditions, such as poverty, employment, family composition; environmental conditions, such as climate, air pollution; cultural conditions, such as practices, norms, and values; and urbanization, which influences housing, access to products and services (PHAC, 2010).

Figure 5-2 illustrates the conceptual model used by the Centre for Chronic Disease Prevention and Control (2010) at the PHAC to examine risk factors for chronic illness. Although some risk factors, such as age, sex, and genetic makeup, cannot be changed (**nonmodifiable risk factors),** many behavioural risk factors are considered **modifiable** (Centre for Chronic Disease Prevention and Control, 2010). Cultural and environmental risk factors, such as air pollution, may play a significant role in the development of chronic illness and may be modifiable in some cases.

Prevention of Chronic Illness

Prevention of chronic illness is the best way to deal with the chronic disease epidemic. Although not all chronic illnesses are preventable, four behavioural risk factors are considered key contributors to many of these conditions: tobacco use; unhealthy diet; insufficient physical activity, and the harmful use of alcohol (WHO, 2011). Decades of research have determined the most effective means, or "best buys," of preventing chronic illness. **"Best buys,"** according to the WHO (2011), are actions that should be undertaken immediately to produce accelerated results

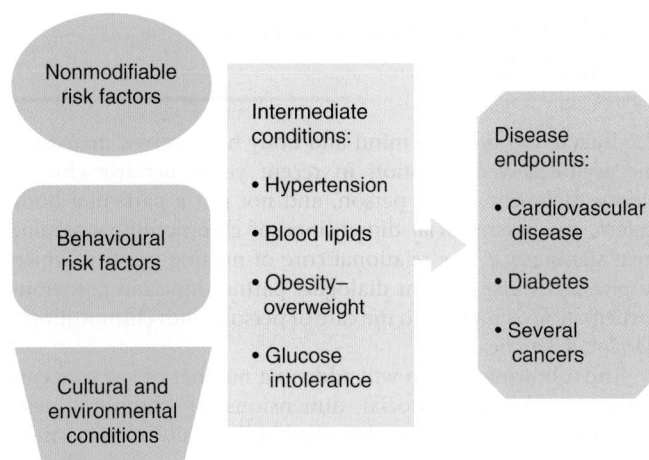

Figure 5-2 Chronic diseases share common risk factors and conditions.

Source: Public Health Agency of Canada: Centre for Chronic Disease Prevention and Control. (2010). *Chronic disease risk factors.* Ottawa: Author. Reproduced with permission from the Minister of Health, 2012. Retrieved from *www.phac-aspc.gc.ca/cd-mc/risk_factors-facteurs_risque-eng.php*

Table 5-4 "Best Buys" for Chronic Illness Prevention

- Protecting people from tobacco smoke and banning smoking in public places
- Warning about the dangers of tobacco use
- Enforcing bans on tobacco advertising, promotion, and sponsorship
- Raising taxes on tobacco
- Restricting access to retailed alcohol
- Enforcing bans on alcohol advertising
- Raising taxes on alcohol
- Reduce salt intake and salt content of food
- Replacing *trans*-fat in food with polyunsaturated fat
- Promoting public awareness about diet and physical activity, including through mass media

Source: World Health Organization (WHO). (2011). *Global status report on preventing noncommunicable diseases 2010.* Geneva: Author. Retrieved from *http://www.who.int/nmh/publications/ncd_report_full_en.pdf*

in terms of lives saved, diseases prevented, and heavy costs avoided. Table 5-4 identifies these "best buys."

The Role of Genetics

Genetics, or the study of how a specific characteristic is passed from one generation to another, has long been recognized to play important roles in the development of certain chronic illnesses. Cystic fibrosis and Huntington's disease are two chronic illnesses for which genetic testing has long been available. Genetic testing can also show an inherited predisposition to several different types of cancer, including breast and ovarian cancer, melanoma, and colon cancer. Research continues to explore the development of screening methods for many other chronic illnesses, such as Alzheimer's disease.

With the completion of human genome sequencing, however, the role of genetic factors will assume increasing importance in prevention, detection, and treatment of many chronic illnesses. The student is referred to Chapter 15 for an in-depth discussion of genetics in nursing practice.

The Role of Aging

Chronic illnesses are on the increase as populations age and individuals live with one or more chronic conditions for decades. The profile of diseases contributing most heavily to death, illness, and disability among Canadians has changed dramatically over the last century. Whereas infectious diseases commonly posed the greatest threat to health in the past, improved sanitation, vaccination, and public health surveillance and the advent of antibiotics have been key factors in prolonging life expectancy rates (Nolte & McKee, 2008). At the time of confederation, in 1867, the average life expectancy in Canada was 42 years, and by 1921, life expectancy had increased to 60 years (Roberts, Clifton, Ferguson, Kampen, & Langlois, 2004). Although life expectancy for Canadians in 2005 was 78.0 years for males and 82.7 years for females, Statistics Canada (2010) projects that males born in 2031 will have an average life expectancy of 81.9 years, and females, 86.0 years.

Aging is associated with the development of many chronic illnesses. As people age, they are more likely to have at least one chronic condition, and the oldest adults (age ≥85 years) are more likely than those age 65-74 years to have at least three chronic conditions (36% versus 20%) (Canadian Institute for Health Information [CIHI], 2011). Cognitive decline becomes much more prevalent in individuals over the age of 85 (Kirkevold, 2010). The most frequently reported chronic conditions among persons aged 65 and older are hypertension (47%, ~2 million seniors) followed by arthritis (27%, ~1.2 million seniors) (CIHI, 2011). The most common combinations of chronic conditions among seniors are: hypertension and arthritis (14%) and hypertension and heart disease (12%) (CIHI, 2011).

Disability in Chronic Illness

Chronic illness is often associated with disability, although many people are not disabled by their chronic illness. **Disability** is a term whose definition continues to be refined after significant global debate. Leonardi, Bickenbach, Ustun, Kostanjsek, and Chatterji (2006) have suggested that disability refers to a difficulty in functioning at the body, the personal, or the societal level, in one or more life domains, as experienced by an individual with a health condition in interaction with contextual factors.

Two different conceptual models of disability have shaped the manner in which we think about disability (WHO, 2002): the medical model and the social model. The medical model views disability as directly caused by disease, trauma, or another health condition. Disability, from the medical model perspective, necessitates medical care provided in the form of individual treatment by providers to "correct" the problem with the individual. The social model of disability, conversely, sees disability as a socially created problem and not an inherent attribute of an individual (Oliver & Barnes, 2010). The social model perspective calls for a political response, because the problem is created by an unaccommodating physical environment brought about by attitudes and other features of the social environment.

The WHO has taken the position that neither the medical nor the social model is fully adequate to define disability, although both models make a significant contribution to the discussion. Disability, according to the WHO (2002), is a complex phenomenon at the levels of both the body and society. Disability always comprises an interaction between features of the person and features of the overall context in which the person lives. In other words, both medical and social responses are appropriate and necessary to the problems associated with disability, but a model of disability that synthesizes both approaches is required. The integration of the medical and social approaches is contained in the bio–psycho–social model, upon which the International Classification of Functioning, Disability and Health, known as the ICF (WHO, 2002), is based. Parallel to the determinants of health (see Table 5-2), disability and functioning are viewed by the ICF as the outcomes of interactions between health conditions (diseases, disorders, and injuries) and contextual factors. Contextual factors are composed of external environmental factors (e.g., social attitudes, architectural characteristics, and legal and social structures, as well as climate, terrain, and so forth) as well as internal personal factors (e.g., gender, age, coping styles, social background, education, profession, past and current experience, overall behaviour pattern, character, and other factors that influence how disability is experienced by the individual).

Figure 5-3 identifies the three levels of human functioning classified by ICF: functioning at the level of body or body part, of the whole person, and of the whole person in a social context. Disability involves dysfunction at one or more of these same levels: impairments, activity limitations, and participation restrictions.

The ICF acknowledges that every human being can experience a decrement in health and thereby experience some degree of disability. Disability is a universal experience at some point in life and is not something that happens only to a minority of individuals. As Susan Sontag (1988, p. 3) notes, "Everyone who is born holds dual citizenship, in the kingdom of the well and the kingdom of the sick."

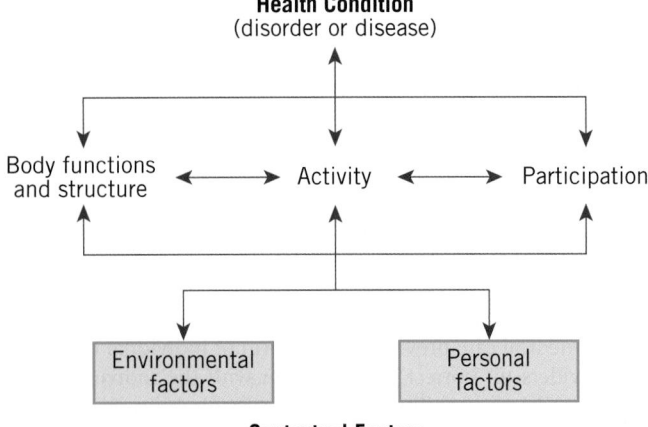

Figure 5-3 The International Classification of Functioning, Disability and Health (ICF) Bio–Psycho–Social Model.

Source: World Health Organization. (2002). *Towards a common language for functioning, disability and health* (p. 9). Geneva: Author. Retrieved from *www.who.int/classifications/icf/en/*

Psychosocial Dimensions of Chronic Illness

The interaction between mind and body has received increasing and well-deserved attention in recent years. Because chronic illness affects the whole person, and not just a particular body system, the psychosocial dimensions of chronic illness assume great significance. The relational core of nursing practice, which emphasizes nurse–patient dialogue, partnership, and conscious participation, is integral to the care of persons with chronic illness (Doane & Varcoe, 2005).

The following section will address a number of key concepts related to the psychosocial dimensions of chronic illness. Although these concepts are described individually in this section, the student should remember that a holistic perspective embraces the many facets of patients as unique individuals, and it is the interplay between these dimensions that shapes the overall experience of chronic illness.

Illness Behaviour

Illness behaviour refers to the varying ways individuals respond to physical symptoms, how they monitor internal states, define and interpret symptoms, make attributions, take remedial actions, and use various sources of informal and formal care (Mechanic, 1995). The "sick role" was first described in 1951 by Talcott Parsons. Sickness was seen by Parsons as a form of deviant behaviour that permitted the avoidance of social responsibilities (Lubkin & Larsen, 2009). A form of learned behaviour, the sick role was achieved through failure to keep well. Table 5-5 describes the characteristics of the sick role.

Parsons' sick-role model, although useful for acute illnesses, has been criticized on many fronts because it does not address important issues related to the chronic illness experience. It fails

Table 5-5 Characteristics of the Sick Role	
COMPONENT OF THE ROLE	**ASSOCIATED BEHAVIOURS AND EXPECTATIONS**
Sick person is exempt from normal social roles.	Dependent on the nature and severity of illness. More severe illness allows patients to be exempt from more roles. Requires legitimization (validation) by a physician.
Sick person is not responsible for his or her condition.	Not responsible for becoming sick, the individual therefore has a right to be cared for. Physical dependency and the right to emotional support are therefore acceptable. Will need a curative process apart from personal willpower or motivation to get well.
Obligation to want to become well.	Being ill is seen as undesirable. Because privileges and exemptions of the sick role can become secondary gains, the motivation to recover assumes primary importance.
Obligation to seek and cooperate with technically competent help.	The patient needs technical expertise that the physician and other health providers have. Cooperation with these providers for the common goal of getting well is mandatory.

Source: Cockerham, W. C. (2001). *Medical sociology* (8th ed., p. 160), Upper Saddle River, NJ: Prentice Hall. © 2001. Electronically reproduced by permission of Pearson Education Inc., Upper Saddle River, New Jersey.

to consider characteristics of chronic illness, the long-term nature of the illness, the reality that an expectation of full recovery is often not reasonable, the management role expected of the patient and family, and the adjustment to permanent change (Lubkin & Larsen, 2009). In the sick-role model, patients are seen as victims of their illness and are subordinate to physicians. This perspective differs significantly from the paradigm of the "expert patient" in which the patient knows his or her condition and its management far better than his or her health care providers (National Health Service, 2011). Unfortunately, many health care providers apply the sick-role model to patients with chronic illnesses in acute care settings (Lubkin & Larsen, 2009). The frequent readmissions often required by patients with chronic illness may create frustration for staff, who are bored by what they see as repetitive, tiresome care (Lubkin & Larsen, 2009). Patients with chronic illness who have experience with the health care system may use their knowledge to gain what they want or need from the system, demanding certain treatments, a specific schedule, or particular routines (Lubkin & Larsen, 2009). These patients may be perceived as "disruptive" to the normal routine of a hospital unit. Lack of sensitivity on the part of health care providers may lay the foundation for energy-draining power struggles with the patient (Thorne, 2006). Findings from an early study by Thorne (1990) documented that chronically ill patients and their families often found that most health care providers could not be trusted to understand the requirements of managing a chronic health condition. Relationships between patients and health care providers were most productive when providers were able to recognize limitations in their own expertise and to respect the expertise of patients and their families. Patients with chronic illness were found to move from "naïve trust" to "disenchantment" and on to a stage of "guarded alliance" in their relationship with health care providers. Nurses must recognize the need to establish credibility and trust with chronically ill patients.

More recent work by Thorne (2006) and Thorne, Oglov, Armstrong, and Hislop (2007) noted the critical importance of communication between patients with chronic illness and health care providers. Communications from health care providers that were helpful included those that provided information in a timely, appropriate, and compassionate manner. Effective communication in health care involves courtesy, respect, and engagement (Thorne, Harris, Mahoney, Con, & McGuinness, 2004). Table 5-6 provides a comparison of effective and problematic communication.

Clarity, a straightforward approach, receptiveness, and responsiveness to questions and written information to complement what was said were helpful characteristics of good communication. Unhelpful communications included those in which there was a mismatch between what patients felt their information needs were at a particular time and the manner in which health care providers supplied this information. It is useful for nurses to reflect on the question: "Am I treating this patient the way I would want to be treated?"

Given their own expertise and experience with health care, many individuals with chronic illness are demanding a new model of care in which they are truly equal partners.

Shared decision making is a decision-making process jointly shared by patients and their health care provider (Legare et al., 2009). It is a central tenet of the patient-centred approach (Godolphin, 2009) described in Chapter 1. Described as a reconciliation of the respect for autonomy and the monopoly and power of the health care system, shared decision making may be considered a "meeting of experts," in which the provider is the clinical expert and the patient is the expert in her or his own life,

Table 5-6 Comparison of Effective and Problematic Patterns of Health Care Communication

DOMAIN	EFFECTIVE COMMUNICATION	PROBLEMATIC ATTITUDES AND BEHAVIOURS
Courtesy (consideration of others)	Politeness Acknowledgement Sincerity	Rudeness Disinterest Being patronizing
Respect (the expression of regard for a specific individual)	Listening Recognition of patient expertise Awareness of social context Empathy Offering information	Discounting patient and caregiver opinions Uncritical acceptance of scientific evidence Withholding information
Engagement (the sense of commitment to the encounter between patient and nurse)	Coaching Teamwork Shared decision-making	Distancing Dismissing Blocking access

Source: Adapted from Thorne, S., Harris, S., Mahoney, A., Con, A., & McGuinness, L. (2004). The context of communication in chronic illness. *Patient Education and Counseling 54*(3), 229-306. doi:10.1016/j.pec.2003.11.009, p. 301.

value, and circumstances (Godolphin, 2009). The partnership between provider and patient works to ensure that the patient's preferences for information and involvement in decision making are respected and that the patient is provided with evidence that will assist her or him to make choices about her or his health care (Godolphin, 2009).

Self-Efficacy

The development and maintenance of self-efficacy is critical to effective self-management of chronic illness. Self-management programs based on self-efficacy principles have been demonstrated to be highly effective in reducing symptoms and facilitating behaviour change (Lubkin & Larsen, 2009). **Self-efficacy** may be considered a type of self-confidence; it is the belief of an individual that he or she can successfully execute the behaviour required to produce the desired outcomes (Bandura, 1977). People's beliefs about their personal efficacy constitute a major aspect of their self-knowledge, according to Bandura's social cognitive theory. Judgements about personal self-efficacy can determine which behaviours will be attempted, how much effort will be devoted to the behaviour, and how long a person will persist in continuing that behaviour. Weight loss, for example, is often recommended as a means of promoting health. The patient's self-efficacy beliefs will influence the strategies the person might use to attempt to lose weight (perhaps calorie reduction or a combined program of calorie reduction and exercise), how much effort they might direct toward this process (a daily walking program or a once per week walking program), and how long they continue their intended program (for a few weeks or several years).

Both outcome expectancies and efficacy expectancies have to be considered in light of self-efficacy. An *outcome expectancy* is the individual's belief that a specific behaviour will lead to certain outcomes. For example, the patient who tells the nurse that exercising helps people to lose weight is voicing an outcome expectancy. An *efficacy expectancy* is the individual's belief that she or he is able to achieve the outcome. The patient who tells the nurse that she or he is not able to exercise is voicing an efficacy expectancy. It is helpful if both outcome and efficacy expectancies are positive. A patient who believes that exercise helps other people lose weight, but it will not help her or him lose weight, might benefit from some of the following influences.

Four primary influences shape an individual's self-efficacy beliefs: mastery; vicarious experience; verbal persuasion and other social influences; and physiological and affective states that help us judge our capability and our vulnerability to dysfunction (Lubkin & Larsen, 2009). Mastery reflects a belief about whether or not "we have what it takes to succeed" and is considered the most influential source of self-efficacy. Many chronic illnesses necessitate the mastery of certain skills, for example, monitoring heart rate and exertion level during exercise, to achieve a sense of self-efficacy. Vicarious experience is the observation of others' performances, from which we learn through modelling and against which we measure our own performance. These experiences inform our self-efficacy beliefs. In our weight loss example, the patient may be encouraged by the example of fellow participants in a walking program who have achieved weight loss through exercise. When people are verbally persuaded that they are capable of performing a certain task, their self-efficacy beliefs may be enhanced. Nurses are in a key position to provide the verbal support the patient may need to undertake the exercise program. Finally, physiological and affective states such as stress impact on our self-efficacy beliefs. The patient may not have the energy to begin a walking program if she or he has just lost her or his job and is experiencing significant financial stress.

Health-Related Hardiness

Health-related hardiness (HRH), a concept first described by Kobasa (1979) and expanded by Pollock, Christian, and Sands (1990) to apply to people with chronic illness, is a personality resource that buffers stress and allows people to experience a high degree of stress without falling ill. Hardy people are considered to possess three general characteristics: control, commitment, and challenge. Control refers to the belief that the individual can influence the events in his or her experience, whereas commitment refers to an ability to feel deeply committed to the activities of life. Challenge is the anticipation of change. The person with HRH, when confronted with a health stressor, possesses sufficient self-mastery and confidence to appraise and modify responses appropriately (control) and cognitively reappraises the health stressor so it is viewed as stimulating and beneficial or an opportunity for growth (challenge). Motivation and competence thus develop to enhance the patient's health status and to facilitate coping with the health stressor (Pollock & Duffy, 1990). There is a substantial evidence base documenting that individuals who have higher levels of hardiness show better psychosocial adaptation to chronic illness. For patients who may be low in hardiness, nurses can make use of interventions that foster a sense of control, commitment, or challenge (Brooks, 2008). These interventions are discussed in the subsequent nursing management chapters.

Mood Disorders

Along with assessments of self-efficacy and health-related hardiness, assessment of the presence of mood disorders such as depression and anxiety is a key element in the nursing assessment of patients with chronic illness. There is a high burden of mood disorders among persons with chronic physical illness. An individual with a chronic physical condition is twice as likely as a person without a chronic physical condition to have a mood disorder (Gadalla, 2008). The likelihood of depression increases with the number of chronic conditions affecting a patient (Gunn et al., 2010). Depressive disorders often accompany chronic illnesses such as heart disease, Parkinson's disease, stroke, human immunodeficiency virus–acquired immune deficiency syndrome (HIV/AIDS) and cancer (Gunn et al., 2010). Prevalence rates of depression for patients with cardiac disease range from 10 to 27%, and 10 to 26% of persons with cancer and between 9 and 26% of persons with diabetes experience depression (Evans et al., 2005; Gadalla, 2008). The burden imposed by mood disorders on persons with chronic illness, their families, and Canadian society is significant. Occupational impairment, disruption in interpersonal relationships, poor health, and suicide may result from mood disorders (Gadalla, 2008). Persons with chronic illness often experience depression or anxiety, potentially affecting their response to treatment of the physical condition. Major depression may adversely affect the course of chronic illness and amplify disability (Evans et al., 2005). The presence of a mood disorder in a person with a chronic physical illness has been found to be associated with short-term disability, the need for help with instrumental activities of daily living, and suicidal ideation (Gadalla, 2008).

It is important to remember that many mood disorders may themselves be considered chronic illnesses. Individuals with mood disorders are also more likely to develop physical conditions. Health care costs for treating a patient with both depression and a chronic physical illness were 50% higher than the costs for treating a person with a physical chronic illness alone (Katon, 2003).

In spite of the evidence that mood disorders are common in persons with chronic physical illness, conditions such as depression remain both underrecognized and undertreated in this population (Gadalla, 2008). The nurse must be alert for the presence or the development of depressive symptoms when caring for patients with chronic illness.

Fatigue

Fatigue is often associated with chronic illness (Whitehead, 2009) and has been described as one of the most distressing symptoms people with chronic illness experience. Fatigue may be both a symptom of an underlying condition and an outcome of that condition. It interferes with normal, customary, and desired activities and pervades every aspect of life (Olson & Morse, 2005). The invisibility of fatigue is one of the most frustrating aspects of the experience, and leads to lack of understanding and misunderstanding by others (Kralik, Telford, Price, & Koch, 2005). The impact of fatigue on functioning is substantial and underrecognized.

Although there is no universally accepted definition of fatigue, it is generally recognized to be a complex, multidimensional experience (Piper, 2003). A classic nursing definition of fatigue was developed by Ream and Richardson (1996, p. 527), who stated that fatigue is "a subjective, unpleasant symptom which incorporates total body feelings ranging from tiredness to exhaustion, creating an unrelenting overall condition which interferes with individuals' ability to function to their normal capacity."

There are many reasons why fatigue is common in people with chronic illness. Pain, mood disorders, sleep problems, physical deconditioning, metabolic abnormalities, infection, dietary problems, hypoxia, and medications can lead to profound fatigue. The experience of fatigue in chronic illness may provoke both psychological and physiological reactions that maintain or exacerbate fatigue in a chronic cycle (Oldervoll, Kaasa, Knobel, & Loge, 2002).

EVIDENCE-INFORMED PRACTICE

Self-Management Education for Patients with Chronic Obstructive Pulmonary Disease

Clinical Question

In people with chronic obstructive pulmonary disease (COPD) (P), what were the settings, methods, and efficacy of COPD self-management education programs (I) on health outcomes and use of health care services (O)?

No comparison group (C) was included.

Best Available Evidence

A systematic review of randomized controlled trials (RCTs).

Critical Appraisal and Synthesis of Evidence

The reviewers assessed a broad range of interventions and health outcomes with different follow-up times. The studies showed a significant reduction in the probability of at least one hospital admission among patients receiving self-management education compared with those receiving usual care (odds ratio [OR] 0.64; 95% confidence interval [CI]; 0.47-0.89). A small but significant reduction was detected in feelings of breathlessness. No significant effects were found in either number of exacerbations, emergency department visits, lung function, exercise capacity, or days lost from work. Inconclusive results were observed in doctor and nurse visits, in symptoms other than dyspnoea, in the use of courses of oral corticosteroids and antibiotics, and in the use of rescue medication.

Conclusions

Self-management education is associated with a reduction in hospital admissions. The data, however, are still insufficient to formulate clear recommendations regarding the form and contents of self-management education programs in COPD. There is an evident need for more large RCTs with a long-term follow-up before more conclusions can be drawn.

Implications for Nursing

Patients with COPD likely experience benefits from self-management education, although the nature and duration of the most effective programs are not clear.

Reference for Evidence

Source: Effing, T., Monninkhof, E. N., van der Valk, P. D. L., Walters, E. H., van de Palen J. J. & Zwernk, M. (2009). *Self-management education for patients with chronic obstructive pulmonary disease.* Cochrane Library. doi:10.1002/14651858. CD002990.pub2

Stigma

People with chronic illness often experience **stigmatization,** which means being regarded by others as unworthy or disgraceful (Kralik, Paterson, & Coates, 2010). Such stigma can have a significant impact on their quality of life. They may be set apart and labelled by others according to the disease they have and the treatments they use. Lubkin and Larsen (2009) note that the elderly and the chronically ill carry a "yoke of undesirability" in health care settings, where caring for these groups is seen as less rewarding in terms of recovery, treatment, and economics than caring for other types of patients. Stigma is an important concept in nursing because it may influence the manner in which care is provided as well as the patient's willingness to disclose information. Individuals who are concerned about being stigmatized if they disclose certain facts may feel threatened and be less likely to share this information (Wellard & Beddoes, 2005). For instance, the person with substance abuse problems may not share information with the nurse about the nature and frequency of her or his drug usage. Lacking this vital information, care decisions may be made that adversely affect patient outcomes.

There are several types of stigma. The stigma of physical deformity relates to situations in which there is a difference between the expected and the valued norm of perfect physical condition and the actual physical condition of the person (Lubkin & Larsen, 2009). The changes or deformities in physical appearance that may occur in chronic illness set the individual apart from others who are not like the individual. The person with multiple sclerosis, for example, may have difficulty walking or require the use of a mobility aid, which can create stigmatization. Character blemishes are another type of stigma (Goffman, 1963). Moral judgements are made about the unworthy character of the individual. Character blemishes are often associated with undesirable traits such as dishonesty, addiction, lack of control, or mental illness (Lubkin & Larsen, 2009). For example, the stigma of character blemish may be experienced by a man with chronic obstructive pulmonary disease (COPD) when others pass judgement about him being responsible for his illness because of a smoking habit he was unable to control. This leads to the scenario of "blaming the victim" and is not uncommon among health care providers.

Quality of Life

Given the many physical and psychosocial challenges inherent in the experience of living with a chronic illness, **quality of life** is a primary outcome measure in evaluating treatment for many health conditions. Quality of life, in its broadest definition, refers to subjective evaluations of both the positive and the negative aspects of life (Centers for Disease Control and Prevention, 2011b). Quality of life is influenced by a host of factors, including financial status, employment, housing, spirituality, social support network, and health. The term **health-related quality of life (HRQL)** has often been used as a way to focus on the ways health affects and is affected by overall quality of life. At an individual level, HRQL usually includes perceptions of physical and mental health status and the key variables that are associated with health status, such as health conditions, functional ability, social support, and socioeconomic status (Centers for Disease Control and Prevention, 2011a). At a community level, HRQL includes resources, conditions, policies, and practices that influence a population's health perceptions and functional status. The concept of HRQL enables health agencies to examine broader areas of healthy public policy around a common theme (Centers for Disease Control and Prevention, 2011a). Although there are many ways to assess health-related quality of life, the Centers for Disease Control 14-item Health Days Measure is widely used in public health as well as clinical research (Moriarty, Zack, & Kobau, 2003).

Living With Chronic Illness

Reduced quality of life, depression, fatigue, and stigma, together with physical symptoms, may make living with a chronic illness a daily challenge for many individuals and their families. Loss of self, "a crumbling away of former self-images without simultaneous development of equally valued new ones" (Charmaz, 1983), is a primary source of suffering for people with chronic illness. Over time, the losses a person sustains as a result of living with a chronic illness cause a decrease in self-esteem. Social isolation, living a restricted life, and being a burden to others all contribute to the loss of self (Charmaz, 1983).

People with chronic conditions use various strategies to try to maintain a "normal life" (Wellard & Beddoes, 2005). Normalization, according to Strauss and colleagues (1984), is a key strategy in living with chronic illness. When individuals fail to exhibit an expected norm, they become viewed as abnormal, having failed to demonstrate what society had expected of them (Wellard & Beddoes, 2005). The person with chronic illness often attempts to achieve what is considered "normal."

Individuals with chronic illness may hide and conceal their disease from others and attempt to pass themselves off as normal, which is an idealized notion of being the same as the rest of the presumably normal population (Wellard & Beddoes, 2005). Although the objective of this behaviour is to fit in with the normal group, this strategy may serve as a constant stress because of the danger of being discovered (Thorne, 1990). "Covering" a visible chronic illness is a strategy employed by some individuals. Covering involves acknowledging the condition while attempting to decrease the anxiety and stress experienced by those who do not have the same condition (Joachim & Acorn, 2000). An example of covering may be making jokes about the condition in an effort to downplay the illness. The nurse must be sensitive to the strategies used by patients with chronic illness and explore with the person whether these strategies are adaptive and helpful or whether they are maladaptive.

Chronic Illness and Caregiving

Living with a chronic illness affects not only the individual affected with the condition but also those in the patient's immediate social network. Nursing assessment of a person with a chronic illness is incomplete without considering the way in which significant others are affected. Families are often called on to provide the often complex and long-term care necessitated by some chronic illnesses. In some cases, care is provided by friends and neighbours. More than 2 million Canadians provide care to people with long-term health problems (CIHI, 2010). The term **informal caregiver** is defined as anyone who provides care without pay and who usually has personal ties to the care recipient (Lubkin & Larsen, 2009).

Family caregivers in Canada are predominantly female and are most likely to be providing care to a spouse or partner or a parent (CIHI, 2010). Even though we often think of older adults as the ones requiring care, it is important to know that older Canadians are often key care providers to spouses, children, grandchildren, friends, and neighbours (CIHI, 2010). One quarter of Canadian caregivers are older than 65 years of age, suggesting that many caregivers themselves may be vulnerable to age-related health problems and high levels of burden (Hollander, Lui, & Chappell, 2009). The overall physical, emotional, and financial cost of caregiving is known as **caregiver burden**. The vast majority of people with chronic conditions live in the community. Only 7% of persons aged 65 and older reside in long-term care facilities (PHAC, 2010). The shift away from institutionalization has meant most of caregiving is now left to families and friends (PHAC, 2010).

The economic value of the informal care provided outside of the health care system is estimated to be in excess of $25 billion dollars annually (CIHI, 2010). The overall health of caregivers, however, has also been demonstrated to be adversely affected by the caregiving experience. Issues arise such as the physical demands of the caregiving role; lack of time to engage in adequate self-care and health promotion activities; the physiological sequelae of psychological distress, predisposing the individual to changes in immune function; and increased risk of hypertension and cardiovascular disease (Pinquart & Sorenson, 2007). Nearly 20,000 informal caregivers (16%) of seniors receiving home care reported distress related to their role. The rates of distress were significantly higher among those providing more than 21 hours of care per week or caring for seniors with symptoms of depression (CIHI, 2010).

The nurse plays a critical role in assessing the level of caregiver distress present, if any, and taking appropriate action to attempt to reduce or eliminate the factors that contribute to the sense of distress.

Conceptual Models of Chronic Illness

Conceptual models are useful in understanding the chronic illness experience, particularly because caring for a patient with a chronic illness requires a different framework for practice than may be useful in caring for a patient with an acute illness. The following section highlights several of the key models of chronic illness.

Illness Trajectory

The concept of an **illness trajectory** was first advanced in 1967 by Glaser and Strauss as a way of understanding the complex, dynamic path of chronic illness. An illness trajectory can be defined as an experiential pathway along which the person with an illness progresses. Some illnesses have more predictable trajectories than others, but all trajectories are subject to individual variation. There have been a number of conceptualizations of illness trajectories. Rolland (1987) identified three critical time phases within the illness trajectory:

- *Crisis phase:* The period before and immediately after diagnosis, when learning to live with symptoms and illness-related demands takes place.
- *Chronic phase:* The time span between initial diagnosis and the final time phase, when the key task is continuing to live as normal a life as possible in the face of the abnormality of having a chronic illness whose outcomes are uncertain.
- *Terminal phase:* This phase is marked by issues surrounding grief and death. Depending on the illness, some patients will enter this phase only after many years.

Further important work in the area of illness trajectories was conducted by Corbin (1998). The authors defined a trajectory

PHASE	DEFINITION	GOAL OF MANAGEMENT
Pretrajectory	Genetic factors or lifestyle behaviours that place an individual or community at risk for the development of a chronic condition.	Prevent onset of chronic illness
Trajectory onset	Appearance of noticeable symptoms; includes period of diagnostic workup as person begins to discover and cope with implications of diagnosis.	Form appropriate trajectory projection and scheme
Stable	Illness course and symptoms are under control. Biography and everyday life activities are being managed within limitations of illness. Illness management centres in the home.	Maintain stability of illness, biography and everyday activities
Unstable	Period of instability to keep symptoms under control or reactivation of illness. Biographical disruption and difficulty in carrying out everyday life activities. Adjustment being made in regimen; care usually taking place at home.	Return to stable
Acute	Severe and unrelieved symptoms or the development of illness complications necessitating hospitalization or bed rest to bring illness course under control. Biographical and everyday life activities temporarily placed on hold or drastically cut back.	Bring illness under control and resume normal biographical and everyday life activities
Crisis	Critical or life-threatening situation necessitating emergency treatment or care. Biography and everyday life activities suspended until crisis passes.	Remove life threat.
Comeback	A gradual return to an acceptable way of life within limits imposed by disability or illness.	Set in motion and continue the trajectory projection and scheme
Downward	Illness course characterized by rapid or gradual physical decline accompanied by increasing disability or difficulty in controlling symptoms.	Adapt to increasing disability with each major downward turn
Dying	Final days or weeks before death. Characterized by gradual or rapid shutting down of body processes, biographical disengagement, and closure and relinquishment of everyday interest and activities	Bring closure, let go, and die peacefully.

Table 5-7 Illness Trajectory Phases and Goals of Management

Source: Corbin, J. (2002). Introduction and overview: Chronic illness and nursing. In R. Hyman & J. Corbin (Eds.), *Chronic illness: Research and theory for nursing practice* (pp. 4-5). New York: Springer.

of the course of an illness over time, identifying nine phases: (a) pretrajectory; (b) trajectory onset; (c) stable; (d) unstable; (e) acute; (f) crisis; (g) comeback; (h) downward; and (i) dying. Table 5-7 describes the phases and the associated goals of management. Although the illness trajectory is set in motion by pathophysiology and changes in health status, there are strategies that can be used by patients, families, and health care providers to shape the course of the trajectory. Shaping means that the illness trajectory can be altered by actions that stabilize the disease course, minimize exacerbations, and better control symptoms (Corbin & Strauss, 1992). This model recognizes that each person's illness trajectory is unique.

These models provide a useful starting point from which to consider the concept of trajectories of chronic illness, although they have been criticized for not fully recognizing individual variation. Wellard and Beddoes (2005), for example, note that the journey of living with chronic illness requires the acquisition of knowledge about the politics of being an ill person in a world of health-centred individuals. For many people with chronic illness, the actual diagnosis that they have a particular condition provides a "feeling of relief" by naming and legitimizing the symptoms they have been experiencing. This feeling of relief may be followed, however, by a process of grieving for the loss of their health and lifestyle. Persons with chronic illness frequently become preoccupied with self, centring on the illness's impact on their lives as a whole (Wellard & Beddoes, 2005).

Shifting Perspectives Model of Chronic Illness

Models that describe living with a chronic illness as a phased process have also been criticized because they imply that an end goal exists and this goal can be reached only if the person has lived long enough to progress through previous stages (Paterson, 2001). The Shifting Perspectives Model of Chronic Illness (Figure 5-4) described by Paterson shows living with a chronic illness as an ongoing, continually shifting process. This perspective of chronic illness contains elements of both illness and wellness. As the reality of the illness experience and its context change, the person's perspective shifts in the degree to which illness or wellness is in the foreground or background of their world (Paterson, 2001). Perspectives of chronic illness are not seen as right or wrong, but as reflections of people's needs and situations.

When illness is in the foreground, individuals are focused on the sickness, suffering, loss, and burden associated with living with a chronic illness. This perspective is marked by self-absorption and difficulty attending to the needs of others (Paterson, 2001). This perspective often occurs in people who are newly diagnosed or overwhelmed by their illness. When wellness is in the foreground, the person attempts to create consonance between self-identity and the identity shaped by the disease and between the construction of the illness by others and by life events

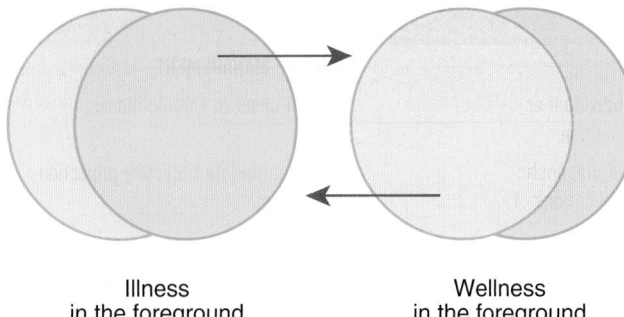

Illness
in the foreground

Wellness
in the foreground

Figure 5-4 The Shifting Perspectives Model of chronic illness.

Source: Paterson, B. (2001). The shifting perspectives model of chronic illness. *Journal of Nursing Scholarship, 33*(1), 21-26 (Figure 1).

(Paterson, 2001). The body is objectified and placed at a distance; it is not allowed to control the person. This perspective can be gained by learning as much as possible about the disease, creating supportive environments, developing skills such as negotiating, identifying the body's unique patterns of response, and sharing knowledge about living with the illness with others. This distance provides for a focus on social, emotional, and spiritual aspects of life, rather than a focus on the diseased body.

The perspective that is in the foreground shifts depending upon circumstances. Perceived threats to control may cause a shift in the foreground from wellness to illness, as may self-help groups that focus on sickness (Paterson, 2001). Returning to having wellness in the foreground may result from changes or interventions that resolve or accommodate the situation that has resulted in the illness focus.

Self-Management

Self-management is the foundation for optimizing health outcomes for people living with chronic illness. A large body of empirical literature demonstrates that successful self-management is related to better overall physical and psychological health outcomes (Battersby, Lawn, & Pols, 2010) **Self-management** refers to the decisions and actions patients undertake that affect their health (Improving Chronic Illness Care, 2011). Every day, patients decide what they are going to eat, whether they will exercise, and to what extent they will take their prescribed medications. These activities, although usually undertaken in cooperation with a health care provider, go beyond merely adhering to a prescribed behavioural regimen. As Glasgow and Anderson (1999, p. 2090) noted:

> Patients are in control. No matter what we as health professionals do or say, patients are in control of these important self-management decisions. When patients leave the clinic or office, they can and do veto recommendations a health professional makes.

The actions people take to manage their conditions are often based on the advice given by health providers. Sometimes, however, they choose not to accept this advice, resulting in less than optimal outcomes (Battersby, Lawn, & Pols, 2010).

Compliance, adherence, and self-care make up the three levels of patient response to health care recommendations on a continuum of self-care. Compliance reflects coercion of the

patient to engage in particular recommendations, whereas adherence implies conformity of the patient with the recommendations. Self-care connotes a therapeutic alliance between the patient and the provider. Adherence is now the term most widely accepted because it incorporates the notion of the patient agreeing with the treatment plan presented by the health care provider.

Partnership between the nurse and the patient, which focuses on an open, caring, mutually responsive, and nondirective dialogue, is a key aspect of relational nursing practice (Jonsdottir, Litchfield, & Pharris, 2004) and is essential in the promotion of self-management. Self-management involves empowering the patient, ensuring some autonomy with respect to adjusting the regimen as necessary. Three sets of tasks must be mastered in order to achieve successful self-management: (a) making informed decisions about care; (b) performing activities aimed at management of the condition; and (c) applying the skills necessary to maintaining adequate psychosocial functioning (Clark, Becker, Janz, Lorig, Rakowski, & Anderson, 1991).

The nurse must be alert to potential barriers to successful self-management. People of low socioeconomic status and those who are marginalized are more difficult to attract and retain in self-management programs (Paterson & Hopwood, 2010). Patients who have limited health literacy may be seriously compromised in their ability to successfully self-manage their conditions. In addition to health literacy, the nurse must be sensitive to the presence of other barriers to self-management, including poorer health, financial constraints, and persistent depressive symptoms (Bayliss, Ellis, & Steiner, 2007). The principles of self-management have been the foundation of numerous chronic illness management programs. Evidence-informed self-management (see, for example, the Evidence-Informed Practice Box on p. 77) starts with the premise that there is a partnership between patients and health providers. New paradigms of self-management examine the beliefs and the problems of people with chronic illness, connecting this information with health providers' views of what knowledge patients must have and what behaviours must change to manage their condition.

The Emerging Paradigm of Chronic Care

Our present health care system is organized around an acute, episodic model of care that fails to meet the needs of many patients, including those with chronic illnesses. Patients, families, caregivers, health care providers, and decision makers must recognize that a new model of care must be enacted that better addresses the needs of those with chronic illness. The shortcomings of the current health care system are well known to the dissatisfied patients, the frustrated families, and the weary staff who have struggled to deal with complexities of chronic illness. There is increasing evidence that patient-centred care, a concept described in Chapter 1, produces better outcomes for patients than traditional approaches (Battersby, Lawn, & Pols, 2010). Table 5-8 describes what patients with chronic illness want from the health care system and what they believe has been missing. These reasonable expectations are embedded within the chronic care model.

Building on the notion of self-management and the need for an integrated, patient-centred system of care, the chronic care model was first advanced by Bodenheimer, Wagner, and Grumbach in 2002. This model predicted that improvements in six interrelated components would improve care for persons with chronic illness. These components are self-management support, clinical information systems, delivery system redesign, decision support, health care organization, and community resources. The original model was expanded to include a greater focus on

prevention and health promotion by Barr et al. in 2003. The Expanded Chronic Care Model (ECCM) appears in Figure 5-5.

The ECCM supports the important role that the social determinants of health play in influencing individual, community, and population health. Support of self-management and the development of personal skills for health and wellness in the ECCM may be accomplished by providing information and enhancing life skills. For example, smoking cessation programs are a cost-effective means of positively affecting health.

Delivery system redesign and reorientation of health services encourage providers to move beyond the provision of cure-focused services to an expanded mandate that promotes a holistic perspective. Decision support encompasses the gathering of evidence not only on disease and treatment but also on staying healthy. Information systems can be used to evaluate established systems and support new ways of providing care. Healthy public policy involves working toward organizational and governmental legislation and policy that foster greater equity in society and leads to safer and healthier goods, services, and environments. The ECCM notes the significant impact of social supports on overall health and quality of life. It promotes the creation of supportive environments that are safe, stimulating, satisfying, and enjoyable. The creation of safe, affordable housing is one example in this area. Finally, strengthening community action involves working together with community groups to set priorities and achieve goals that enhance the health of the community.

Nurses have a vital role to play within the vision of the ECCM and can serve as leaders in the challenge to improve the care of Canadians living with chronic illness.

Table 5-8 What Patients With Chronic Illness Want From the Health Care System

- Access to information concerning:
- Diagnosis and its implications
- Available treatments and their consequences
- Potential impact on the patient's future
- Continuity of care and ready access to it
- Coordination of care, particularly with specialists
- Infrastructure improvements (scheduling, wait times, prompt care)
- Ways to cope with symptoms such as pain, fatigue, disability, and loss of independence
- Ways to adjust to disease consequences such as uncertainty, fear and depression, anger, loneliness, sleep disorders, memory loss, exercise needs, nocturia, sexual dysfunction, and stress

Source: Holman, H., & Lorig, K. (2004). Patient self-management: A key to effectiveness and efficiency in care of chronic disease. *Public Health Reports, 119,* 239-243. Retrieved from *http://www.publichealthreports.org/userfiles/119_3/119239.pdf*

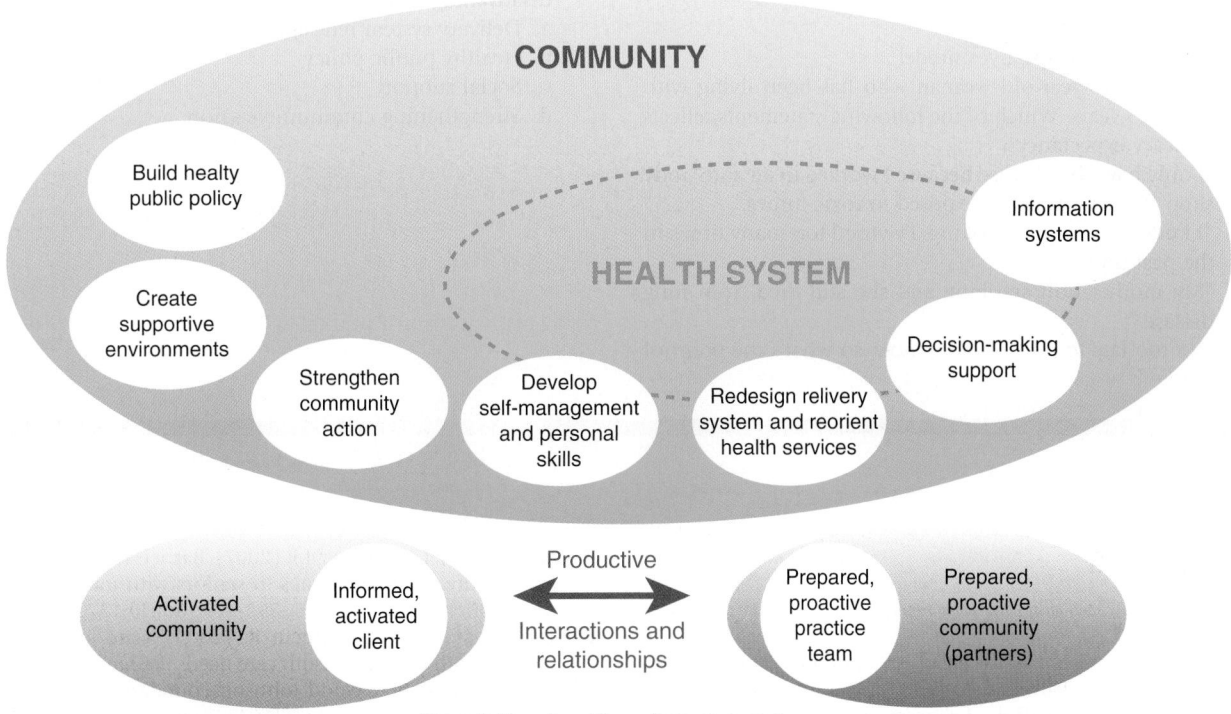

Population health outcomes and functional and clinical outcomes

Figure 5-5 The Expanded Chronic Care Model.

Source: Barr, V., Robinson, S., Marin-Link, B., Underhill, L., Dotts, A., Ravensdale, D., & Salivaras, S. (2003). The Expanded Chronic Care Model: an integration of concepts and strategies from population health promotion and the chronic care model. *Healthcare Quarterly, 7*(1), 73-82.

REVIEW QUESTIONS

The number of the question corresponds to the same-numbered objective at the beginning of the chapter.

1. What is the most common cause of death in Canada?
   a. Cancer
   b. Cardiovascular disease
   c. Respiratory disease
   d. Community-acquired pneumonia

2. The nurse is working with Brian, a 35-year-old with recently diagnosed type 2 diabetes. Which of the following statements by Brian would suggest to the nurse that he understands the nature of chronic illness?
   a. "It's too bad I ate so many sweets as a kid. I wouldn't have diabetes now if I didn't have a sweet tooth."
   b. "Once I start my medication, I won't have to worry about my diabetes."
   c. "I guess that I won't be able to live the same way I used to."
   d. "I know if I take care of myself, I won't run into any complications from diabetes when I'm older."

3. Which of the following are modifiable risk factors for developing chronic illness?
   a. Activity level and sex
   b. Age and genetic background
   c. Air pollution and occupation
   d. Smoking and weight

4. According to the World Health Organization, which of the following best accounts for disability?
   a. The bio–psycho–social model
   b. The medical model
   c. The social model
   d. The shifting perspectives model

5. Marilee is a 47-year-old woman who has been living with COPD for 5 years. Which of the following statements reflects her efficacy expectancy?
   a. "I only have this disease because I worked in an auto body shop for years and was exposed to toxic fumes."
   b. "I know I can't quit smoking. I've tried too many times in the past 5 years."
   c. "My mother quit smoking and she still died from lung disease."
   d. "It's too late to quit smoking now, so what's the point of trying?"

6. In which of the following situations might caregiver burden be most likely to occur?
   a. A husband who must administer medications to his cognitively impaired wife
   b. A daughter who must empty her mother's drains following a mastectomy
   c. A wife with heart failure who must assist her husband to the toilet following a cerebrovascular accident
   d. A neighbour who prepares meals for a patient recently discharged from hospital following cataract surgery

7. Heather has had multiple sclerosis for the last 2 years and is admitted to hospital to manage symptoms of an exacerbation. According to the illness trajectory model, which phase of chronic illness would she be in?
   a. Trajectory onset
   b. Unstable
   c. Acute
   d. Crisis

8. Genevieve, a 53-year-old woman with fibromyalgia, happily reports to the nurse that she has followed her prescribed exercise program for the past month. What would this behaviour be an example of?
   a. Compliance
   b. Adherence
   c. Self-management
   d. Chronic care

9. Within the ECCM, in which domain would the work of a nurse with a citizen group initiative to start a food bank for disadvantaged people fall?
   a. Delivery system redesign
   b. Healthy public policy
   c. Social support
   d. Strengthening community action

ANSWERS: 1. a; 2. c; 3. d; 4. a; 5. b; 6. c; 7. c; 8. b; 9. d

REFERENCES

Bandura, A. (1977). *Social learning theory.* Orrville, OH: Prentice-Hall.

Barr, V. J., Robinson, S., Marin-Link, B., Underhill, L., Dotts, A., Ravensdale, D., & Salivaras, S. (2003). The Expanded Chronic Care Model: An integration of concepts and strategies from population health promotion and the chronic care model. *Hospital Quarterly, 7*(1), 73-82.

Battersby, M., Lawn, S. & Pols, R. (2010). Conceptualization of self-management. In D. Kralik, B. Paterson, & V. Coates (Eds.). *Translating chronic illness research into practice* (pp. 85-110). Chennai, India: Wiley Blackwell.

Bayliss, E., Ellis, J. L., & Steiner, J.F. (2007). Barriers to self-management and quality of life outcomes in seniors with multi-morbidities. *Annals of Family Medicine, 5,* 395-402. doi:10.1370/afm.722

Bodenheimer, T., & Berry-Millett, R. (2009). Care management of patients with complex health care needs. *Research Synthesis Report No. 19.* The Robert Wood Johnson Foundation. Retrieved from *http://www.rwjf.org/files/research/52372caremgt.rpt.revised.pdf*

Bodenheimer, T., Wagner, E. H., & Grumbach, K. (2002). Improving primary care for patients with chronic illness. *JAMA, 288,* 1775-1779. doi:10.1001/jama.288.14.1775

Boyd, C., Boult, C., Shadmi, E., Leff, B., Brager, R., Dunbar, L., & Wegener, S. (2007). Guided care for multi-morbid older adults. *The Gerontologist, 47,* 697-704. doi:10.1093/geront/47.5.697

Brooks, M. V. (2008). Health-related hardiness in individuals with chronic illness. *Clinical Nursing Research, 17*(2), 98-117. doi:10.1177/1054773808316736

Campbell-Scherer, D. (2010). Multimorbidity: A challenge for evidence-based medicine. *Evidence-Based Medicine 15*, 165-166. doi:10.1136/ebm1154

Canadian Agency for Drugs and Technology. (2012). *The use of virtual wards to reduce hospital readmissions in Canada.* Retrieved from *http://www.cadth.ca/en/products/environmental-scanning/environmental-scans/environmental-scan-27*

Canadian Cancer Society. (2011). General cancer statistics at a glance. Retrieved from *http://www.cancer.ca/Canada-wide/About%20cancer/Cancer%20statistics/Stats%20at%20a%20glance/General%20cancer%20stats.aspx?sc_lang=en*

Canadian Institute for Health Information (CIHI). (2010). *Supporting informal caregivers: The heart of home care.* Retrieved from *http://secure.cihi.ca/cihiweb/products/Caregiver_Distress_AIB_2010_EN.pdf*

Canadian Institute for Health Information (CIHI). (2011a). *Seniors and the health care system: What is the impact of multiple chronic conditions?* Retrieved from *http://secure.cihi.ca/cihiweb/products/air-chronic_disease_aib_en.pdf*

Centers for Disease Control and Prevention. (2011b). *Health-related quality of life.* Retrieved from *http://www.cdc.gov/hrqol/concept.htm*

Centers for Disease Control and Prevention. (2011). *Chronic disease prevention and health promotion.* Retrieved from *www.cdc.gov/nccdphp/*

Centre for Chronic Disease Prevention and Control. (2010). *Chronic disease risk factors.* Retrieved from *www.phac-aspc.gc.ca/cd-mc/risk_factors-facteurs_risque-eng.php*

Charmaz, K. (1983). Loss of self: A fundamental form of suffering in the chronically ill. *Sociology of Health and Illness, 5*, 168-195. doi:10.1111/1467-9566.ep10491512

Clark, N. M., Becker, M. N., Janz, N. K., Lorig, K., Rakowski, W., & Anderson, L. (1991). Self-management of chronic disease by older adults. *Journal of Aging and Health, 3*(1), 3-27. doi:10.1177/089826439100300101

Corbin, J. (1998). The Corbin and Strauss chronic illness trajectory model: An update. *Scholarly Inquiry for Nursing Practice, 12*(1), 33-41.

Corbin, J. & Strauss, A. (1992). A nursing model for chronic illness management based upon the trajectory framework. In P. Woong (Ed.), *The chronic illness trajectory framework.* New York: Springer.

Doane, G. H., & Varcoe, C. (2005). *Family nursing as relational inquiry.* Philadelphia: Lippincott Williams & Wilkins.

Evans, D. L., Charney, D. S., Lewis, L., Golden, R. N., Gorman, J. M., Krishnan, K. R., Valvo, W. J. (2005). Mood disorders in the medically ill: scientific review and recommendations. *Biological Psychiatry, 58*(3):175-189.

Fortin, M. (2007). Multimorbidity's many challenges. *BMJ, 334*, 1016-1017. doi:10.1136/bmj.39201.463819.2C

Gadalla, T. (2008). Association of comorbid mood disorders and chronic illness with disability and quality of life in Ontario, Canada. *Chronic Diseases in Canada, 28*, 148-154. Retrieved from *http://www.phac-aspc.gc.ca/publicat/cdic-mcbc/28-4/pdf/cdic28-4-4eng.pdf*

Glaser, B., Strauss, A. (1967). *The discovery of grounded theory: strategies for qualitative research.* New York: Aldine Transaction.

Glasgow, R. E., & Anderson, R. M. (1999). In diabetes care, moving from compliance to adherence is not enough. *Diabetes Care, 22*, 2090-2092. doi:10.2337/diacare.22.12.2092b

Godolphin, W. (2009). Shared decision-making. *Healthcare Quarterly, 12*(Sp), e186-e190. Retrieved from *http://www.longwoods.com/content/20947*

Goffman, E. (1963). *Stigma: Notes on the management of spoiled identity.* Englewood Cliffs, NJ: Prentice Hall.

Gunn, J. M., Ayton, D. R., Densley, K., Pallant, J. F., Chondros, P., Herrman, H. E., & Dowrick, C. (2010). The association between chronic illness, multimorbidity and depressive symptoms in an Australian primary care cohort. *Social Psychiatry and Epidemiology, 47*(2), 175-184. doi:10.1007/s00127-010-0330-z

Hollander, M. J., Liu, G., & Chappell, N. L. (2009). Who cares and how much? The imputed economic contribution to the Canadian healthcare system of middle-aged and older unpaid caregivers providing care to the elderly. *Healthcare Quarterly, 12*(2), 42-49.

Joachim, G., & Acorn, S. (2000). Living with chronic illness: The interface between stigma and normalization. *Canadian Journal of Nursing Research, 32*(3), 37-47.

Jonsdottir, H., Litchfield, M., & Pharris, M. D. (2004). The relational core of nursing practice as partnership. *Journal of Advanced Nursing, 47*, 241-250. doi:10.1111/j.1365-2648.2004.03088_1.x

Katon, W. J. (2003). Clinical and health services relationships between major depression, depressive symptoms and general medical illness. *Biological Psychiatry, 54*, 216-226. doi:10.1016/S0006-3223(03)00273-7

Kirkevold, M. (2010). Translating chronic illness research across the lifespan. In D. Kralik, B. Paterson, & V. Coates (Eds.). *Translating chronic illness research into practice* (pp. 37-56). Chennai, India: Wiley-Blackwell.

Kobasa, S. C. (1979). Stressful events, personality and health: An inquiry into hardiness. *Journal of Personality and Social Psychology, 37*(1), 1-11.

Kralik, D., Paterson, B., & Coates, V. (2010). *Translating chronic illness research into practice.* Chennai, India: Wiley-Blackwell.

Kralik, D., Telford, K., Price, K., & Koch, T. (2005). Women's experiences of fatigue in chronic illness. *Journal of Advanced Nursing, 52*, 372-380. doi:10.1111/j.1365-2648.2005.03602.x

Legare, F., Elwyn, G., Fishbein, M., Fremont, P., Froesch, D., Gagnon, M.-P., …, van der Weijden. (2009). Translating shared decision-making into health care clinical practices: Proof of concepts. *Implementation Science 3*, 2. doi:10.1186/1748-5908-3-2

Leonardi, M., Bickenbach, J., Ustun, T. B., Kostanjsek, N., & Chatterji, S., on behalf of EU MHADIE Consortium. (2006). The definition of disability: What is in a name? *Lancet, 368*, 1219-1221. doi:10.1016/S0140-6736(06)69498-1

Lubkin, I. M., & Larsen, P. D. (2009). *Chronic illness: Impact and interventions* (7th ed.). Toronto: Jones & Bartlett.

Mechanic, D. (1995). The concept of illness behaviour. *Journal of Chronic Diseases, 15*(2), 189-194. doi:10.1016/0021-9681(62)90068-1

Moriarity, D. G., Zack, M. M., & Kobau, R. (2003). The Centers for Disease Control and Prevention's Healthy Days Measures—population tracking of perceived physical and mental health over time. *Health and Quality of Life Outcomes, 1*,37.

Nardi, R., Scanelli, G., Corrao, S., Iori, I., Mathieu, G., & Amatrian, R. (2007). Co-morbidity does not reflect complexity in internal medicine patients. *European Journal of Internal Medicine 18*(5), 359-368.

National Health Service. (2011). *The Expert Patients Programme—What is an expert patient?* London: NHS. Retrieved from *http://www.nhs.uk/Conditions/Expert-patients-programme-/Pages/Whatisanexpertpatient.aspx*

Nolte, E., & McKee, M. (Eds.) (2008). *Caring for people with chronic conditions: A health system perspective.* European Observatory on Health Systems and Health Policies Series, Maidenhead, UK: McGraw Hill. Retrieved from *www.euro.who.int/__data/assets/pdf_file/0006/96468/E91878.pdf*

Oldervoll, L. M., Kaasa, S., Knobel, J., & Loge, J. H. (2002). Exercise reduces fatigue in chronic fatigued Hodgkin's disease survivors—Results from a pilot study. *European Journal of Cancer, 39*(1), 57-63.

Oliver, M., & Barnes, C. (2010). Disability studies, disabled people and the struggle for inclusion. *Journal of Sociology of Education, 31*(5), 547-560. doi:10.1080/0145692.2010.500088

Olson, K., & Morse, J. M. (2005). Delineating the concept of fatigue using a pragmatic utility approach. In J. R. Cutcliffe & H. P. McKenna (Eds.), *The essential concepts of nursing* (pp. 141-159). Toronto: Elsevier Churchill Livingstone.

Parsons, T. (1951). *The social system*. London: The Free Press/ Macmillan.

Paterson, B. (2001). The shifting perspectives model of chronic illness. *Journal of Nursing Scholarship, 33*(1), 21-26. doi:10.1111/j.1547-5069.2001.00021.x

Paterson, B., & Hopwood, M. (2010). The relevance of self-management programmes for people with chronic disease at risk for disease-related complications. In D. Kralik, B. Paterson, & V. Coates (Eds.). *Translating chronic illness research into practice.* (pp. 111-142). Chennai, India: Wiley-Blackwell.

Patra, J., Popova, S., Bondy, J., Flint, R., & Giescrecht, N. (2007). *Economic cost of chronic disease in Canada: 1995-2003.* Ontario Chronic Disease Prevention Alliance and the Ontario Public Health Association. Retrieved from *http://www.cdpac.ca/media.php?mid=260*

Pinquart, M., & Sorensen, S. (2007). Correlates of physical health of informal caregivers: A meta-analysis. *Journal of Gerontology: Psychological Sciences, 62*(2), 126-137.

Piper, B. F. (2003). Fatigue. In V. Carrieri-Kohlman, A. M. Lindsey, & C. M. West (Eds.), *Pathophysiological phenomena in nursing* (3rd ed., pp. 209-234). St. Louis: Saunders.

Pollock, S. E., Christian, B. J., & Sands, D. (1990). Responses to chronic illness: Analysis of psychologic and physiological adaptation. *Nursing Research, 39*(5), 300-304.

Pollock, S. E., & Duffy, M. E. (1990). The Health-Related Hardiness Scale: Development and psychometric analysis. *Nursing Research, 39*, 218-222.

Public Health Agency of Canada. (2008). *Report on the state of public health in Canada*. Retrieved from *http://www.phac-aspc.gc.ca/cphorsphc-respcacsp/2008/pdf/report-eng.pdf*

Public Health Agency of Canada (PHAC). (2010). *The Chief Public Health Officer's Report on the State of Public Health in Canada 2010.* Retrieved from *http://www.phac-aspc.gc.ca/cphorsphc-respcacsp/2010/fr-rc/cphorsphc-respcacsp-06-eng.php*

Public Health Agency of Canada (PHAC). (2011a). *Chronic diseases in Canada.* Retrieved from *http://www.phac-aspc.gc.ca/media/nr-rp/2011/2011_0919-bg-di-eng.php*

Public Health Agency of Canada (PHAC). (2011b). *What determines health?* Retrieved from *www.phac-aspc.gc.ca/ph-sp/determinants/index.html#determinants*

Ream, E., & Richardson, A. (1996). Fatigue: A concept analysis. *International Journal of Nursing Studies, 33*(5), 519-529. doi:10.1016/0020-7489(96)00004-1

Roberts, L. W., Clifton, R. A., Ferguson, B., Kampen, K., & Langlois, S. (2004). *Recent social trends in Canada 1960-2000*. Montreal: McGill-Queen's University Press.

Rolland, J. S. (1987). Chronic illness and the life cycle: A conceptual framework. *Family Process, 26*(2), 203-211. doi:10.1111/j.1545-5300.1987.00203.x

Sontag, S. (1988). *Illness as metaphor*. Toronto: Collins.

Statistics Canada. (2010). *Demographic change*. Retrieved from *http://www.statcan.gc.ca/pub/82-229-x/2009001/demo/int1-eng.htm*

Statistics Canada. (2011). *Mortality, summary list of causes 2008*. Ottawa: Author. Retrieved from *http://www.statcan.gc.ca/bsolc/olc-cel/olc-cel?catno=84F0209X&CHROPG=1&lang=eng*

Strauss, A. L., Corbin, J., Fagerhaugh, S., Glaser, B. G., Maines, D., Suczek, B. & Wiener, C. L. (1984). *Chronic illness and the quality of life*. St. Louis: Mosby.

Thorne, S. (2006). Patient-provider communication in chronic illness: A health promotion window of opportunity. *Family and Community Health, 29*(Suppl. 1S), 4S-11S.

Thorne, S., Harris, S., Mahoney, A., Con, A., & McGuinness, L. (2004). The context of communication in health care. *Patient Education and Counseling 54*(3), 229-306. doi:10.1016/jpec2003.11.009

Thorne, S., Oglov, V., Armstrong, E., & Hislop, T.G. (2007). Prognosticating futures and the human experience of hope. *Palliative and Supportive Care, 5*, 227-239. doi:10.1017/S1478951507000399

Thorne, S. E. (1990). Constructive non-compliance in chronic illness. *Holistic Nursing Practice, 5*(1), 62-69.

Wellard, S. & Beddoes, L. (2005). Constructions of chronic illness. (pp. 113-145). In C. Rogers-Clark, A. McCarthy, & K. Martin-MacDonald (Eds.), *Living with illness: Psychosocial challenges for nursing*. Marrickville, NSW, Australia: Elsevier Australia.

Whitehead, L. (2009). The measurement of fatigue in chronic illness. *Journal of Pain and Symptom Management, 37*(1), 107-128. doi:10.1016/j.jpainsymman.2007.08.019

World Health Organization (WHO). (2002). *Towards a common language for functioning, disability and health. ICF: The International Classification of Functioning, Disability and Health*. Retrieved from *http://www.who.int/classifications/icf/training/icfbeginnersguide.pdf*

World Health Organization (WHO). (2011). *Global status report on noncommunicable diseases 2010* (p. 11). Geneva: Author. Retrieved from *http://www.who.int/nmh/publications/ncd_report_full_en.pdf*

RESOURCES

Canadian Caregiver Coalition
http://www.ccc-ccan.ca/

Canadian Lung Association
http://www.lung.ca

Centre for Chronic Disease Prevention and Control
www.phac-aspc.gc.ca/ccdpc-cpcmc/topics/z_ebic_e.html

Dietitians of Canada Resource Centre
http://www.dietitians.ca/Nutrition-Resources-A-Z/Fact-Sheet-Pages(HTML)/Miscellaneous/Are-organic-foods-better-for-my-health.aspx

Fibromyalgia/Chronic Fatigue Syndrome Canada
http://www.fm-cfs.ca/

Health Council of Canada: Health Care Renewal and Chronic Illness
http://www.healthcouncilcanada.ca/rpt_det.php?id=143

Heart and Stroke Foundation of Canada
http://www.heartandstroke.ca/

Improving Chronic Illness Care (Robert Wood Johnson Foundation)
http://www.improvingchroniccare.org/

"My Tool Box" Chronic Disease Self-Management Program
http://mytoolbox.mcgill.ca/index.php?ref=toolboxworkshopsdetails.html

Public Health Agency of Canada: *Determinants of Health*
http://www.phac-aspc.gc.ca/ph-sp/determinants/index-eng.php

Siteman Cancer Center: "Your Disease Risk" interactive questionnaire
http://www.yourdiseaserisk.wustl.edu

evolve *For additional Internet resources, see the Web site for this book at* **http://evolve.elsevier.com/Canada/Lewis/medsurg**

Community-Based Nursing and Home Care

Written by Barbara L. Mildon and Julie H. Fraser

LEARNING OBJECTIVES

1. Understand the history of community nursing.
2. Define primary health care and explain its importance to the health care system and community health nursing practice.
3. Describe the trends that are threatening the sustainability of Canada's health care system.
4. Describe the role that home care plays in promoting the sustainability of Canada's health care system.
5. Understand how home care in Canada is organized and funded.
6. Describe the practice of the home health nurse, including key clinical competencies.

KEY TERMS

chronic disease management The management of chronic disease through health system elements (information systems, decision support tools, self-management promotion, and realignment of health services) and community elements (supportive environment, health policy, and strengthened community action) (Canadian Public Health Association, 2008), p. 88

family-centred care An approach to nursing care that involves "bringing the perspectives of patients and families directly into the planning, delivery, and evaluation of health care, and thereby improving its quality and safety" (Institute for Patient- and Family-Centered Care [IPFCC], 2011, p. 3), and the core concepts of which include dignity and respect, information sharing, participation, and collaboration (IPFCC, 2011), p. 91

home health nursing A specialized area of nursing practice with roots in community health nursing in which nursing care is delivered in the residence of the patient, or where the patient works or attends school (adapted from the American Nurses Association, 2008, p. 90), p. 86

hospice palliative care Care aimed at "relieving suffering and improving quality of living and dying ... for any patient and/or family living with, or at risk of developing, a life-threatening illness as a result of any diagnosis, with any prognosis, regardless of age, and at the time they have unmet expectations and/or needs, and are prepared to accept care (Canadian Hospice Palliative Care Association, 2002, p. 17), p. 92

nurse practitioners (NPs) "Registered nurses with additional educational preparation and experience who possess and demonstrate the competencies to autonomously diagnose [in some jurisdictions], order and interpret diagnostic tests, prescribe pharmaceuticals, and perform specific procedures within their legislated scope of practice" (Canadian Nurses Association [CNA], 2006, p. 19), emphasizing holism, health promotion, and partnership with individuals, families, and communities (CNA, 2009a, p. 1), p. 87

nursing-sensitive outcomes Outcomes that are "relevant, based on nurses' scope and domain of practice, and for which there is empirical evidence linking nursing inputs and interventions to the outcome" (Doran, 2003, pp. vii-ix), p. 94

primary care The element within primary health care that focuses on the delivery of health care services, including health promotion, illness and injury prevention, and the diagnosis and treatment of illness and injury (Health Canada, 2012), p. 88

primary health care Essential health care based on practical, scientifically sound, and socially acceptable methods and technology made universally accessible to individuals and families in the community through their full participation and at a cost that the community and country can afford (World Health Organization, 1978), p. 88

public health nursing A specialized area of nursing practice, practised in increasingly diverse settings, combining knowledge from public health science, primary health care, nursing science, and the social sciences, and focusing on promoting, protecting and preserving the health of populations with the understanding that a community's health is closely linked to the health of its members and is often reflected first in individual and family health experiences (adapted from Canadian Public Health Association [2010], p. 8), p. 86

ELECTRONIC RESOURCES

Supplemental content related to Chapter 6 can be found...

Evolve Web Site ⊖volve

http://evolve.elsevier.com/Canada/Lewis/medsurg
- Answer Guidelines for Case Study on p. 95
- Clinical Reference: Laboratory Values

- Content Updates
- Electronic Calculators
- Examination Review Questions
- Glossary
- Key Points (Printable and MP3 Download)

The community offers a diversity of exciting and professionally fulfilling roles in which community health nurses (CHNs) make a meaningful difference to the health of individuals, families, communities, and populations. Home and community care has increasingly been recognized as an essential component of the health care system (Canadian Healthcare Association, 2009; Health Council of Canada, 2008a; Nagle, 2008; Ontario Home Care Association, 2011). This chapter is a discussion of community-based nursing, including its history, roles, and practice, with an emphasis on home health care.

In its report of the 2009 nursing workforce, the Canadian Institute for Health Information (CIHI; 2010) reported that 14.2% of registered nurses and 7.8% of licensed practical nurses worked in the community health sector, which includes community health centres, home care nursing agencies or employers, nursing stations (outpost or clinic), and public health departments or units. The percentage of registered psychiatric nurses (found only in western provinces) who worked in the community sector ranged from 20.5 to 25.4%.

The History of Home Health Nursing

Home health nursing (also known as *visiting nursing, district nursing,* and *home care nursing*) is a specialized area of nursing practice with its roots firmly placed in community health nursing. Nursing care is delivered in the residence of the patient, or where the patient works or attends school (American Nurses Association, 2008. p. 90.)

The history of home health nursing in Canada can be traced back through the centuries. Voluntary, charitable organizations were the first to address the health needs of citizens in the community. For example, the Grey Nuns, founded in Montreal in 1738, established hospitals and refuges and travelled to the homes of ill persons to provide care (Allemang, 2000). Thus the philosophy of attending to the well-being of the individual, as well as the health of the community at large, came to uniquely characterize community health nursing (Chalmers & Kristjanson, 1992). In 1897, the Victorian Order of Nurses was established in Canada, followed in 1908 by the Saint Elizabeth Visiting Nurses Association. It has been speculated that this association of volunteerism and charity with community nursing has contributed to the struggle for recognition of the formal education required by CHNs and for appropriate compensation that is still evident today (Chalmers & Kristjanson, 1992).

As this history demonstrates, home health nursing was already well established when public health nursing emerged. Public health nursing came into existence as a result of scientific breakthroughs, including vaccinations, pasteurization, the germ theory of disease, and antisepsis, which provided the basis for preventing infection. The movement of people from rural areas to cities fostered ideal conditions for disease transmission, necessitating new attention to sanitation (Allemang, 2000). In view of these changes, public health nursing focused on health promotion and disease prevention, and home health nurses attended to the needs of people already ill, while also incorporating health promotion and disease prevention into their care. The links between public health and home care nursing were eloquently captured by Emory (1953, p. 29):

> It was from the field of visiting nursing that public health nursing emerged....Public health nursing ... must include health teaching; it may include bedside nursing. Visiting nursing is the giving of bedside care in the homes of the community on a visiting basis; it must include bedside nursing; it should include health teaching; if so it is a branch of public health nursing.

Public health nursing is defined today as a specialized area of nursing practice in which the nurse combines knowledge from public health science, primary health care (including the determinants of health), nursing science, and the social sciences; and focuses on promoting, protecting and preserving the health of populations. Public health nursing recognizes that a community's health is closely linked to the health of its members and is often reflected first in individual and family health experiences. It recognizes that healthy communities and systems that support health contribute to opportunities for health for individuals, families, groups and populations; and practices in increasingly diverse settings such as community health centres, schools, street clinics, youth centres and nursing outposts and with diverse partners to meet the health needs of specific populations (adapted from Canadian Public Health Association, [2010], p. 8.)

The shared history of visiting and public health nursing continues to unify the two groups of CHNs, who are now joined by nurses in many other community-based roles.

Community Health Nursing Roles

CHNs "promote, protect and preserve the health of individuals, families, groups, communities and populations in the settings where they live, work, learn, worship and play in an ongoing and episodic process" (Community Health Nurses of Canada [CHNC], 2011, p. 4). A variety of titles exist for nurses who work in community-based settings. These titles include *public health nurse, home health nurse, prevention nurse, faith community nurse* (also called *parish nurse*), *family practice nurse, outpost* or *rural–remote nurse, case manager, community health centre* or *outreach nurse, occupational health nurse,* and *school nurse.* Additional community health nursing roles have been introduced, including those of the forensic nurse, the sexual assault nurse examiner, the nurse entrepreneur, and the nurse practitioner (also known as a *family* or *adult nurse practitioner*).

Nurse practitioners (NPs) are RNs "with additional educational preparation and experience who possess and demonstrate the competencies to autonomously diagnose [in some jurisdictions], order and interpret diagnostic tests, prescribe pharmaceuticals, and perform specific procedures within their legislated scope of practice" (CNA, 2006, p. 19). NPs blend "clinical diagnostic and therapeutic knowledge, skills and abilities within a nursing framework that emphasizes holism, health promotion and partnership with individuals and families, as well as communities" (CNA, 2009a, p. 1). Their education and experience allows them to function both independently and collaboratively in a range of settings (CNA, 2009a).

The Canadian Public Health Association (2010) published a comprehensive description of the practice of public health/community health nurses whose roles are focused on "health promotion, health protection, disease and injury prevention, health surveillance, population health assessment, as well as emergency preparedness and response" (p. 7). To further delineate the practice of public health nurses, public health nursing discipline-specific competencies were developed and published by the CHNC (2009).

Although the community is the context of care for community-based nurses, they possess an understanding of the entire health system continuum. For example, a person may be hospitalized in a burn unit after suffering burns in a fire at home. When the patient's condition is no longer critically ill, he or she may be transferred to a general medical-surgical unit and then to a rehabilitation facility. Once the patient is back home, a home health nurse may visit to care for unhealed burn injuries, to provide care for other health needs, or both. When the individual is ready to return to work, an occupational health nurse may be involved to facilitate the reintegration to the workplace.

The continuum of care does not always include hospitalization. Health problems may be identified in a variety of outpatient settings, including physicians' offices, workplace health units, health care clinics, or community health centres. For example, a patient may be screened for diabetes mellitus at work. Screening results may prompt a referral to a family physician or nurse practitioner who makes the diagnosis of diabetes. Instead of hospitalization, the patient may be monitored by a chronic disease management nurse or certified diabetes educator in the family practice office or community health centre, who will collaborate with the patient to design a care plan. The care plan may include monitoring and education at a variety of settings, as well as follow-up by a home health nurse to initiate, teach, and monitor the prescribed insulin therapy. In turn, the home health nurse communicates with the appropriate members of the health care team to promote comprehensive, timely, and appropriate patient care.

A Health Care System Under Pressure

Several trends are putting pressure on Canada's health care system and influencing its evolution. The significance of selected trends for CHNs is highlighted in the sections below.

Changing Demographics

The average age of Canadians is increasing (older adults are discussed further in Chapter 7). In 2011, individuals 65 years and older made up 14.4% of the population of Canada, and the median age in Canada was 39.9 years (Statistics Canada, 2011). It has been reported that persons aged 65 and older accounted for 50% of hospital expenditures by provincial/territorial governments in 2009 (CIHI, 2011a). In addition, community-based services for older persons, such as home nursing and personal care support, day care programs, and foot care programs are playing important roles. Canadians 65 years of age and older use more home care services than do younger Canadians (Health Council of Canada, 2008a).

Health Human Resources.   Nurses are the largest group of health care providers in Canada (CIHI, 2010). Concerns about a nursing shortage continue to be raised in Canada (Canadian Nurses Association, 2009b) and globally (World Health Organization, 2010). According to CIHI (2010), nurses aged 40 to 59 represented 57.1% of registered nurses, 54% of licensed practical nurses, and 62% of registered practical nurses. Not only are nurses aging, but also they may also retire before the traditional retirement age of 65 (CIHI, 2010). The health of nurses is also causing concern. A national survey reported that 61% of nurses had taken time off in the previous year for health reasons and that the average number of days absent from work among all nurse respondents was 14.5 per nurse. More nurses than non-nurse health care providers reported musculoskeletal problems, and nurses were more likely to have experienced depression in the previous year than were non-nurse health care providers (Statistics Canada, 2006).

Concern about a shortage of nurses and other health care providers in home care has also been documented (Canadian Home Care Association [CHCA], 2008; Canadian Healthcare Association, 2009; Carter, 2009). Shortages are of concern because they lengthen waiting lists for services, impose a burden on family members who pick up the care of loved ones, and may undermine quality of care if providers feel rushed because of high numbers of patients (CHCA, 2008). Factors contributing to satisfaction and mobility in the home care workforce were explored in two additional studies: one in Ontario (Caplan, 2005) and one in Ontario and Nova Scotia (Shamian, Mildon, Goodwin, Norton, & Talosi, 2006). In both studies, the investigators concluded that employment practices and the lack of security in home care jobs were leading causes of dissatisfaction among home care nurses and other team members. In addition, the CHCA (2008) pointed out that whereas some home care employees view the home setting as maximizing independence, autonomy, and challenge in their work, others find it stressful because of its less structured and less predictable environment.

Patient Safety. Since the release of a report entitled *To Err is Human: Building a Safer Health System* (Institute of Medicine, 1999), the health care system has focused increasingly on enhancing patient safety. Factors influencing safety for home care patients include the fact that a patient's home environment cannot be controlled, the lack of uniformity of procedures in private homes in comparison with hospital units, and a reliance on unpaid or untrained caregivers (Lang, 2010; Lang, Edwards, & Fleiszer, 2008), as well as challenges in coordinating services from hospital to the home, the cost of equipment and supplies, and continuity of care within the home care team. Safety for home care providers is also receiving attention (Stevenson, McRae, & Mughal, 2008). Adverse events in the home include adverse drug events, infections resulting from such interventions as urinary catheterization or venous access, falls, wounds, and accidents related to technology (Masotti, McColl, & Green, 2010).

Sustainability of the Health Care System

Health care costs consume between 30.4% (Quebec) and 47.2% (Nova Scotia) of provincial/territorial budgets in Canada (CIHI, 2011b). These costs have raised an alarm regarding the ability to sustain Canada's health care system and have prompted calls for health system reform or renewal. Policies and programs that address the determinants of health, access to a consistent primary care professional, and a national strategy on chronic disease prevention and management (Morgan, Zamora, & Hindmarsh, 2007) have been identified as elements of health system renewal or reform. These elements are reflected in the philosophy and principles of primary health care.

Primary Health Care. Community health nursing practice is informed and guided by nursing theory and knowledge, social sciences, public health science, and the philosophy and principles of primary health care (CHNC, 2011). According to the Declaration of Alma Ata (World Health Organization, 1978),

> **Primary health care** is essential health care based on practical, scientifically sound, and socially acceptable methods and technology made universally accessible to individuals and families in the community through their full participation and at a cost that the community and country can afford…

There are six key principles of primary health care:

1. Universal access to health care services on the basis of need
2. Focus on the determinants of health as part of a commitment to health equity and social justice
3. Active participation on the parts of individuals and communities in decisions that affect their health and lives
4. Partnership with other disciplines, communities, and sectors for health (intersectoral approach)
5. Appropriate use of knowledge, skills, strategies, technology, and resources
6. Focus on health promotion–illness prevention throughout the life experience from birth to death

Although the terms *primary care* and *primary health care* are often used interchangeably, there is an important difference between them. The focus of **primary care** is disease, and the key participants are health professionals. In contrast, primary health care is both a philosophy and an approach to the delivery of health care. Its focus is system wide, and key participants are intersectoral

partners in the fields of health, social services, housing, and the environment. Primary health care is inclusive of a range of activities from health care of individuals to action on the determinants of health (Smith, Jacobson, & Yiu, 2008). Confusion often arises between the terms *primary care* and *primary health care* because the health professional whom an individual visits for health care is often known as the individual's primary care professional. Moreover, having access to a consistent primary care professional (e.g., a family physician or nurse practitioner) is an essential component of primary health care. Lack of access to a consistent primary care professional may result in more visits to an emergency department or more hospitalizations (Health Council of Canada, 2008b). It may also result in a delay in seeking care, fragmented care, and less effective chronic disease management.

Primary health care is increasingly being embraced as a strategy to shift the health system's emphasis from diagnosis and treatment of illness and injury to health promotion and disease prevention. This shift is also known as *reforming the system*. Decreasing the prevalence and severity of illness through effective chronic disease management has been identified as a key strategy to promote the well-being of Canadians and the sustainability of the health care system (Health Council of Canada, 2008b; Morgan, Zamora, & Hindmarsh, 2007). **Chronic disease management** is the management of chronic disease through health system elements, e.g., information systems, decision support tools, self-management promotion, and realignment of health services, and community elements such as a supportive environment, health policy, and strengthened community action (Canadian Public Health Association, 2008). Primary health care encompasses values and principles that are central to the practice of nurses: promoting health, preventing disease, and working with other members of the multidisciplinary team. Thus it is imperative that all nurses be aware of primary health care philosophy and principles and incorporate them into their practice.

Home Care

Definition and Importance of Home Care

Home care in Canada is defined as "an array of services for people of all ages, provided in the home and community setting, that encompasses health promotion and teaching, curative intervention, end-of-life care, rehabilitation, support and maintenance, social adaptation, and integration and support for the informal (family) caregiver" (CHCA, 2008, p. viii). Home care is *not* one of the insured services covered by the *Canada Health Act*, the legislation that created and protects Canada's universal, publicly funded health care system. Therefore, provinces and territories have no legal obligation to ensure that their citizens have access to home care services. Nonetheless, every province and territory now has a home care program.

Home Care Services

The CHCA (2008) reported that "in general, home care programs in Canada provide a comprehensive range of coordinated health care services for individuals of all ages for the purpose of promoting, maintaining, or restoring health within the context of their daily lives" (p. x). Individuals who are frail or disabled or who have an acute or chronic medical condition are served by home care. They may require intermittent services or full-time assistance 24 hours a day. Family members may also receive home care services such as respite care to support them in their caregiving efforts. Equipment for the home such as electrical beds, wheel-chairs, pressure-relief mattresses, commodes, walkers, raised toilet seats, and other assistive devices may also be provided.

Home care services may be categorized as acute, chronic, palliative, or rehabilitative. In addition, coordination and management of admission to a facility may be provided when it is no longer possible for the individual to remain at home (CHCA, 2008). Services may be provided in the home (e.g., private home or residential facility) or in adult day centres, workplaces, schools, or clinics. Community clinics staffed by home care nurses have been shown to be cost effective and are attractive to patients who are well enough to leave their homes because they can choose their own appointment time and not have to wait in their homes for the nurse's arrival (VanDeVelde-Coke, 2004). However, it is important to note that skilled nursing observation and assessment of the patient's home environment, social supports, caregiver stress, and risk for falls cannot be achieved in the clinic, and thus serious health problems may be overlooked (Pastor, 2006).

Quality and Accountability in Home Care

As a demonstration of quality and accountability, many home care provider organizations voluntarily apply for accreditation from Accreditation Canada. Accreditation is mandatory only in Quebec, where it is obtained through the Quebec Council of Accreditation (CHCA, 2007b).

Standardized home care data has been collected. For example, CIHI has developed the Home Care Reporting System (HCRS), which is a standardized data set to support comparison of specific indicators for home care. At present, British Columbia, the Yukon, Manitoba, Ontario, British Columbia, and Nova Scotia are submitting data generated by their use of the Resident-Assessment Instrument–Home Care (RAI-HC) to the HCRS (CIHI, 2011c). Nurses are involved in collecting such data, which is then used for several purposes. For example, data from the RAI-HC system are now being used to gain a more comprehensive understanding of the health status and demographics of specific groups of home care patients such as those with heart failure (Foebel, Hirdes, Heckman, Tyas, & Tjam, 2011). The data also support quality monitoring and comparison among health care provider organizations (Hutchinson, Draper, & Sales, 2009) and the identification of patient outcomes (Doran et al., 2009).

Funding and Utilization of Home Care Services

The majority of home care is funded by provincial and territorial governments through health budgets that are administered by regional health authorities, departments of health and social services, or local health integration networks and community care access centres (Ontario). The federal government also funds home care services through departments such as the First Nations and Inuit Branch of Health Canada and Veterans Affairs Canada (Table 6-1).

The use of home care services in Canada has grown considerably since the 1990s. In the period 1994 to 1995, the government spent $1.6 billion on home care. By the period 2003 to 2004, home care spending had risen to $3.4 billion and represented 4.2% of total government health spending (Canadian Healthcare Association, 2009). Between 1994 and 2004, the rise in per capita government spending on home care (adjusted for inflation) averaged 6% annually, whereas total government health spending increased by only 5.7% per year. This difference means that efforts to increase the availability of home care services have been effective. However, the average annual increase in the number of

Table 6-1 Funding Mechanisms for Home Care
1. Publicly funded, provincial–territorial health care plan
2. Private insurance (e.g., employment benefit plans)
3. Veterans Affairs Canada
4. First Nations and Inuit Branch of Health Canada
5. Indian and Northern Affairs Canada
6. Workers' Compensation Boards
7. Private payment (also known as *self-payment* or *out-of-pocket payment*)
8. Associations and foundations (e.g., Canadian Red Cross)

patients who received government-subsidized home care between the periods 1994 to 1995 and 2003 to 2004 was only 1%. The fact that spending on home care increased more quickly than the number of patients suggests that home care patients are needing more resources (e.g., nursing visits) to remain in their homes instead of the hospital or other facility (Canadian Healthcare Association, 2009). In turn, the increased need for resources suggests that the acuity of illness in home care patients is rising and the situations of home care patients are more complex. There is also evidence that the volume of nursing and other professional services is increasing in comparison with that of support services such as homemaking and personal support (Wilkins, 2006).

Sometimes the frequency or duration of the government-funded home care services (e.g., the number of nursing visits, the number of hours of supportive care services such as homemaking, and length of time on the program) is not deemed sufficient by the patient or the family. In those instances, they may choose to purchase additional services through either insurance or their own financial resources. The Canadian Healthcare Association (2009) reported that between 2 and 5% of Canadians purchase home care services not funded by government.

Home Health Care Team

Nursing Roles. The home health care team is composed of the *home health nurse* and a variety of team members who work in close collaboration with the patient, the family, and medical practitioners (Table 6-2). Nurses who work on the home health team include registered nurses and licensed practical nurses, as well as nurse practitioners and clinical nurse specialists. Home health nurses are *registered nurses* and *licensed practical nurses* who provide a variety of nursing assessments, planning and implementing of interventions, and teaching to assist individuals in optimizing their health in their home setting. *Nurse practitioners* use their in-depth nursing knowledge and the scope of practice to diagnosis and treat acute and chronic diseases. Nurse practitioners often provide care for homebound patients who do not have access to a primary physician (Canadian Nurses Association, 2008). *Clinical nurse specialists* promote the use of evidence and system changes by providing expert consultation and leadership in guideline and policy development in the community setting (Canadian Nurses Association, 2008). *Unregulated care providers* make an essential contribution to quality of life for the patient by supporting the patient's activities of daily living, including bathing, preparing meals, and performing household chores and personal errands (Canadian Research Network for Care in the Community, 2010). They are an important social connection with patients and are often the team members who spend the most time with them. These individuals also may provide delegated or

Table 6-2 Members of the Home Health Care Team	
MEMBER	**DESCRIPTION**
Community health nurse (CHN)	A registered nurse whose practice specialty promotes the health of individuals, families, communities, and populations and an environment that supports health. A CHN practices in diverse settings such as homes, schools, shelters, churches, community health centres, and on the street (Community Health Nurses of Canada [CHNC], 2011).
Home care or home health nurse	A CHN who uses knowledge from primary health care (including the determinants of health), nursing science, and social sciences to focus on disease prevention, health restoration, and maintenance or palliation for patients, their caregivers, and families (CHNC, 2011) and who generally travels to the patient to provide care.
Case manager	The health care team member who leads the process of case management: "a collaborative patient-driven strategy undertaken by health care professionals and patients to maximize the patient's ability and autonomy through advocacy, communication, education, identification of and access to requisite resources, and service coordination" (Canadian Home Care Association [CHCA], 2007a, p. 2).
Community health worker or home support worker	An unlicensed care provider who assists individuals with activities of daily living (ADLs) such as bathing, dressing, and meal preparation, as well as instrumental ADLs such as housekeeping, shopping, and social recreational activities (Canadian Research Network for Care in the Community, 2010).
Nurse practitioner	"An advance practice nurse who provides direct care focusing on health promotion and the treatment and management of health conditions. [Nurse practitioners] are registered nurses with additional education preparation and experience who possess and demonstrate the competencies to autonomously diagnosis, order, and interpret tests, prescribe pharmaceuticals, and perform specific procedures in their legislated scope of practice" (Canadian Nurses Association, 2008, p. 16).
Clinical nurse specialist	"An advance practice nurse who provides expertise for specialized populations. [Clinical nurse specialists] play a leading role in the development of clinical guidelines and protocols, promote the use of evidence, provide expert support and consultation, and facilitate system change" (Canadian Nurses Association, 2008, p. 16).

assigned nursing care for patients with long-term frequent and predictable health needs (e.g., daily routine medication). Rehabilitation specialists—including physiotherapists, occupational therapists, and speech language pathologists—are crucial members of the home care team, as are social workers, pharmacists, dietitians, and respiratory therapists. The role of the *case manager* is to coordinate the comprehensive care plan and services for the patient, including arranging for and funding services. All members of the home health care team work collaboratively to evaluate the patient's progress, make changes to the care plan, and develop the discharge plan and indicators. The home health care team members actively include the patient's family members in all aspects of care.

Home Health Care Patients

Although home health nurses may care for newborns, young children, teenagers, and adults of all ages, in the period 2009 to 2010, 82% of individuals who received home care services were 65 years of age or older (CIHI, 2011d)—a statistic that reflects Canada's aging population. The most common health conditions assessed in home care patients are cardiovascular disease, musculoskeletal diseases, and other common chronic diseases (e.g., cancer, chronic obstructive pulmonary disease, diabetes). CHNs in all roles play an important part in the prevention and management of chronic illness by (a) promoting regular health screening, (b) incorporating health promotion and disease prevention strategies into their practice, and (c) assisting individuals and families in managing chronic illness in the home.

In addition to the physical and cognitive decline associated with many chronic conditions, many of these individuals live alone. Nearly 40% of home care patients (CIHI, 2011d) receive home support services to assist with both their activities of daily living and instrumental activities of daily living, and close to one third receive nursing services (CIHI, 2011d). The majority of patients who receive home care services require long-term supportive care or acute short-term focused services (e.g., postoperative care); smaller percentages receive end-of-life and rehabilitative

care (CIHI, 2011d). These patient characteristics have implications for home care nurses' role, competencies, and standards.

Home Health Nursing Practice

Overview. Home health nursing is a unique and diverse practice that requires specific clinical competencies. Home health nurses navigate the full spectrum of traffic and weather conditions and cope with unexpected situations ranging from power failures to uncooperative family pets. They work in isolation and use strategies to protect patient privacy and confidentiality within neighbourhoods. Home health nurses need to be extremely organized and be able to work with a high level of autonomy. They require knowledge of community resources and proficiency in time management, case management, communication, and physical, psychosocial, and environmental assessment, as well as in care planning and evaluation. They must understand and work within funding models, service limits, productivity expectations, referral processes, and employer and funder reporting requirements. Many of these competencies differ from those of nurses in other care settings and sectors. Accordingly, the CHNC (2011) developed standards of practice for community health nurses. The following seven interrelated standards of practice form the core expectations for community health nursing:
1. Health promotion
2. Prevention and health protection
3. Health maintenance, restoration, and palliation
4. Professional relationships
5. Capacity building
6. Access and equity
7. Professional responsibility and accountability

On the basis of the standards, detailed practice competencies were developed by CHNC in 2010, and these are described later in this chapter.

Home Health Nursing and Family-Centred Care.
Nursing in the home occurs in a very different context than nursing in the hospital. In the hospital, the health care team has

the dominant role and the environment is controlled. In the home, the patient, caregiver, or family (or a combination of these) plays the dominant role; the nurse is a guest in the house and must adapt to the home environment. Consequently, it is especially important that the home health nurse demonstrates a holistic, nonjudgemental, and family-centred philosophy and negotiates the care with the patient and family.

Family-centred care is "bringing the perspectives of patients and families directly into the planning, delivery, and evaluation of health care, and thereby improving its quality and safety …" (Institute for Patient- and Family-Centered Care [IPFCC], 2011, p. 3). The core concepts of FCC include dignity and respect, information sharing, participation, and collaboration (IPFCC, 2011). According to MacKay (2009), "… [d]ignity and respect directs health care practitioners to listen to their patient and family's choices and perspectives regarding their healthcare and to act on them accordingly. Also, the patient and his/her family's knowledge, beliefs, values, and cultural backgrounds are integrated into the planning and delivery of care. Information sharing requires health care practitioners to communicate and share unbiased and complete information with patients and families. Such information is provided in a timely, thorough and accurate manner so that patients and families are able to actively engage in care and decision-making. Participation includes encouraging patients and families to participate in care and decision-making to the extent in which they choose. Collaboration involves health care leaders consulting with patients and their families to develop policies and programs, implementation and evaluation of care, and professional education." (pp. 6-7).

Family-centred care involves the recognition that an illness experienced by one family member will affect the entire family (Saint Elizabeth Health Care, 2011). Families often provide care for ill members and assist in decision making about all aspects of the care provided. Visits by home care professionals are usually episodic, leaving the family with the burden of care. Home health nursing visits may be as frequent as several times a day or as infrequent as once a month. Visits may be lengthy, such as the initial visit, when the extensive admission assessment is completed; or they may be fairly short, such as visits to assess health status, including wound healing, pain control, or symptom management. Nursing care during a visit may be administered according to a predetermined routine such as one specified in a care pathway, or it may be directed toward newly arising symptoms or health concerns.

In some situations, an older patient may be cared for by a spouse of similar age with chronic illnesses. In other situations, an older parent needing care may live with a busy middle-aged family with dependent children, or a person may be caring for a dying spouse at home. In these situations, it is not uncommon for caregivers to become physically, emotionally, and economically overwhelmed with the responsibilities and demands of caring for a family member (Saint Elizabeth Health Care, 2010; Victorian Order of Nurses, 2009). The home health nurse is a lifeline for the family, helping them understand their loved one's health condition and needs, cope with changing roles and responsibilities, and make decisions about ongoing care arrangements. The focus of care is on empowering the patient and family to meet the identified health care needs and feel in control of their lives. Therefore, decision making and priority setting are shared among patient, family, and nurse, and the goals of care may be short or long term in nature. Referral to various support groups in the community or other resources is one way the nurse can help family members cope. The nurse can also work with the case manager to advocate for additional home care services to reduce the burden of care, such as a personal support worker, more frequent nursing visits, short-term respite placement, or support from a social worker.

Cultural Competence in Home Health Nursing Practice. Home health care is delivered within the context of the family's and the patient's cultural values and beliefs. Strategies to overcome language barriers may be needed, and the home health nurse is more likely than other nurses to encounter the patient's use of healing practices arising from cultural beliefs and the use of home remedies and complementary and alternative therapies. The ability to apply culturally relevant care is included in the competencies expected of home health nurses (CHNC, 2010). The home health nurse demonstrates culturally sensitive care by having a general understanding of how culture can affect beliefs and behaviours (College of Nurses of Ontario, 2009). Building on that understanding, exploring and recognizing the patient's cultural practices, values, and needs and integrating them into the plan of care, or working with the patient and family to resolve concerns about a possible adverse health effect of a cultural practice or complementary therapy are integral to home health nursing (Edmunds & Kinnaird-Iler, 2008). (Culture is discussed in Chapter 2, and complementary and alternative therapies are discussed in Chapter 12.)

Home Health Nursing Practice Knowledge and Skills. It is generally acknowledged that the acuity of home health nursing has been rising steadily and is now very high (Lang & Edwards, 2006). As Lang and Edwards observed,

> Unlike working on a specialized unit in a hospital, home care providers must maintain a *breadth* of general and specific knowledge. This poses a significant safety challenge because of the diversity and varied frequency of health conditions and treatments. It is not unusual to come across particular conditions or treatments only once every few months, making it difficult to maintain competence. This is heightened by the trend for earlier discharge from hospitals and the corresponding increase in the acuity of patients receiving home care services; the lack of resources for continuing education and proficiencies; and the isolated nature of the practice of home care (p. 23).

Specific competencies for home care nurses have been established in Canada (CHNC, 2011) and in the United States (American Nurses Association, 2008). These competencies reflect the knowledge, skills, judgement, and attitudes associated with home care nurse practice. The CHNC (2011) listed three categories of competencies: (1) elements of home health nursing, (2) foundations of home health nursing, and (3) quality and professional responsibility (Table 6-3). Competencies associated with the elements of home health nursing are focused on the nursing activities, functions, goals, and outcomes that are central to home care nursing practice (CHNC, 2011). Competencies associated with the foundations of home care nursing are related to the philosophy of primary health care and the core knowledge related to home care nursing practice (CHNC, 2011). Competencies associated with the quality and professional responsibility are focused on the strategies and activities that demonstrate professionalism and promote quality care (CHNC, 2011). Because many of the standards and competencies related to community health nursing are unique, community health nursing is recognized as a specialty practice by the Canadian Nurses Association. Today, any nurse whose practice is community based may choose to earn a national credential—CCHN(C) (Certified in Community Health Nursing–Canada)—to indicate her or his expertise.

Table 6-3 Specific Competencies for Canadian Home Care Nurses	
Elements of Home Health Nursing	**Foundations of Home Health Nursing**
• Assessment, monitoring, and clinical decision making	• Health promotion
• Care planning and care coordination	• Illness prevention and Health promotion
• Health maintenance, restoration, and palliation	**Quality and Professional Responsibility**
• Teaching and education	• Quality care
• Communication	• Professional responsibility
• Relationships	
• Access and equity	
• Building capacity	

Source: Community Health Nurses of Canada. (2010). *Home health nursing competencies* (version 1.0). Toronto: Author. Retrieved from *http://login.greatbignews.com/UserFiles/289/documents/ HomeHealthNursingCompetenciesVersion1March2010.pdf*

In addition to specific skills, home health nurses require general knowledge of the range of health care equipment or assistive devices used to promote independence. They must also be familiar with the wide variety of medical supplies and devices such as chest and wound drainage tubes, intravenous therapy supplies, urinary catheters, enterostomy supplies, wound care products, enteral feeding equipment (Figure 6-1), central vascular access devices (Figure 6-2), and a variety of infusion pumps. Understanding rehabilitation techniques and terminology is helpful in collaborating with therapists, supporting the patient's progress, and evaluating the plan of care. Home care nurses also use self-management strategies to assist individuals in managing chronic disease; the ideal result is to delay their placement in a residential home or admission to hospital. Clinical documentation skills are also important for reflecting legal and professional accountability and substantiating recommendations made about the patient's needs, the care provided, and the patient's response.

Establishing and maintaining a therapeutic nurse–patient relationship is fundamental for effective home care nursing practice. Therefore, effective communication strategies and techniques are crucial. Teaching must involve the patient and the family. Family members are encouraged to learn how to administer treatments and manage equipment. Such care may seem overwhelming to them initially, and the home health nurse assesses the readiness of the caregiver to assume the care, teaches in a way that is most helpful for the learner, and evaluates the outcomes of care, including the coping of the caregiver.

Hospice palliative care is another important component of home health nursing practice. **Hospice palliative care** is "whole-person health care that aims to relieve suffering and improve the quality of living and dying" (Canadian Hospice Palliative Care Association, 2009, p. 8). Hospice palliative care is not limited to those with cancer diagnoses; it "is appropriate for any patient and/ or family living with, or at risk of developing, a life-threatening illness due to any diagnosis, with any prognosis, regardless of age, and at any time they have unmet expectations and/or needs, and are prepared to accept care" (Canadian Hospice Palliative Care Association, 2009, p. 8). The home health nurse is often the linchpin in achieving the highest possible quality of life for the patient and family throughout the palliative and bereavement experience.

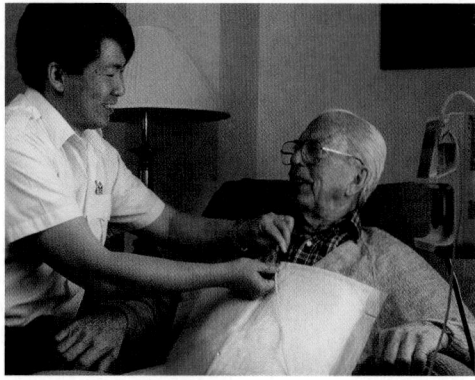

Figure 6-1 Nurse providing skilled care in the home.

Source: Victorian Order of Nurses Canada.

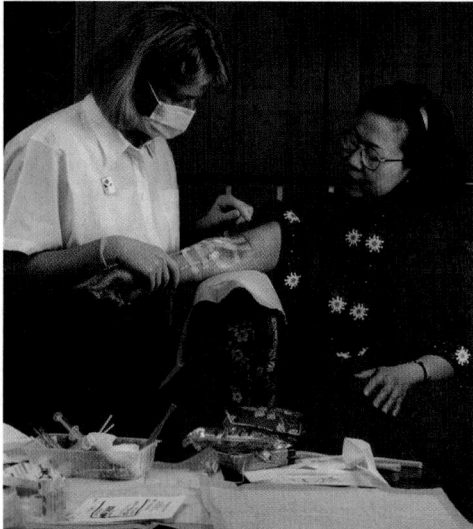

Figure 6-2 Nurse providing peripherally inserted central catheter (PICC) care in the home.

Source: Victorian Order of Nurses Canada.

Trends in Home Health Nursing

New Nursing Graduates and Licensed Practical Nurses in Home Health Nursing. Because of the breadth and depth of knowledge and skills required by the home health nurse, it was widely believed for many years that nurses required a minimum of 2 years of acute care hospital experience before being hired as a home health nurse. Furthermore, registered nurses generally received hiring preference over licensed practical nurses because it was believed that registered nurse preparation provided the best foundation for home care nursing. However, partly because the growing nursing shortage, enhancements to the scope of practice and educational programs for licensed practical nurses, and the need to provide long-term interventions to a growing population with complex and unpredictable care needs, many home health employers now hire both registered nurses and licensed practical nurses right after graduation. To support these new graduates and new home health nurses, a variety of intensive orientation programs and tools have been developed to complement student placement and employment experiences (Meadows, 2009). Figure 6-3 depicts a sample orientation tool.

Competency Assessment Planning and Evaluation Tool (CAPE Tool)
Home Care Nurse, Fraser Health, Surrey, BC

EXCERPT

Date of first assessment	Date of second assessment	Preceptee	Preceptor	Facilitator

CRNBC Standards (College of RNs of BC)			Home Care Nurse Standards	
CRNBC	HCNs		HCNs	
1	5	Responsibility and accountability	1	Promoting health: • Health promotion • Prevention and health protection • Health maintenance restoration and palliation
2	1, 2, 3	Specialized body of knowledge	2	Building individual and community capacity
3	1, 2, 3	Competent application of knowledge	3	Building relationships
4	3, 4	Code of ethics	4	Facilitating access and equity
5	1, 4	Provision of service to the public	5	Demonstrating professional responsibility and accountability
6	5	Self-regulation		

	CRNBC Standards (College of RNs of BC)	Initial Self-Assessment	2.5-Month Self-Assessment	1-Year Self-Assessment	Learning Activities/ Resources	• Reviewed with Mentor/ Preceptor Clinical Educator/CRN Manager Peer • Planned Learning Activities	KEY: 1. Needs education and practice 2. Knowledgeable but needs practice 3. Competent: Independent practice 4. Proficient practice 5. Expert practice Achievement and Validation of Competency (include examples from clinical practice and learning plan) Date and Signature
CRNBC STD.	*COMPETENCY STATEMENTS*						
	1. RESPONSIBILITY/ACCOUNTABILITY/SELF-REGULATION						
1, 6	1. Recognizes own limitations in professional practice and seeks help from appropriate resoures when needed.						
1, 6	2. At all times practices in a safe manner, is accountable, and takes responsibility for own practice.						
	3. Maintains own mental, physical, emotional well being.						
	4. Practices safety and ethically according to: • FH standards, protocols, policies • CRNBC standards of practice/HCN community standards and phibsophy						
	5. Responsible and accountable for regular and prompt attendance at work.						

Figure 6-3 A sample orientation tool.

Source: Fraser Health, Surrey, BC.

Technology in Home Health Nursing Practice. Surgical innovations, such as microscopic surgical techniques that have transformed many operations into day-surgery procedures, and medical interventions, such as advances in life support of premature infants, have allowed individuals to live longer, shifting both acute and long-term care to community-based settings. An array of mechanical devices—including ventilators, infusion pumps, and peritoneal dialysis night cyclers—have been redesigned and miniaturized for portability and ease of use, making it possible for patients to remain at home while receiving intravenous antibiotics, chemotherapy, or total parenteral nutrition. Internet-based education and information programs are now common, and telemonitoring systems are enabling nurses and other health care providers to assess a patient's physical status from a remote location (Figure 6-4).

Digital cameras are now being used to take pictures of complex wounds; the pictures are then transferred via computer to a wound specialist for expert assessment and treatment recommendations (Figure 6-5).

Home care nurses are accessing clinical information and best practice evidence at the point of care by using devices such as smartphones; such devices are also used to document patient health data that in turn is used to monitor and track clinical outcomes (Ontario Ministry of Health and Long-Term Care, 2008). Several of the nursing best practice guidelines published by the Registered Nurses' Association of Ontario are now available as applications for hand-held devices, including the iPhone and Blackberry. Indeed, today's home health nurses are as likely to arrive at the patient's home holding a digital device, a digital camera, or a tablet computer as they would a stethoscope. Computerized clinical documentation systems (Figure 6-6) and electronic health records are now being used by a growing number of home health nurses. The home health nurse is able to review the patient's history and plan of care and update the electronic health record as care is given. The accessibility of electronic health records promotes continuity of care and reduces documentation time.

Measurement of Nursing-Sensitive Outcomes

Nursing-sensitive outcomes are "those that are relevant, based on nurses' scope and domain of practice, and for which there is empirical evidence linking nursing inputs and interventions to the outcomes" (Doran, 2003, pp. vii-ix). Nurses need to know the outcomes associated with their care in order to assess the effectiveness of the patient's care plan and make revisions as indicated. They may also use outcomes data to evaluate their own practice or that of their team or program. Decision makers and funders require outcomes data to support budget needs, program design and delivery, and the development of accountability mechanisms such as balanced scorecards. Research has demonstrated that it is feasible for nurses to collect electronic or

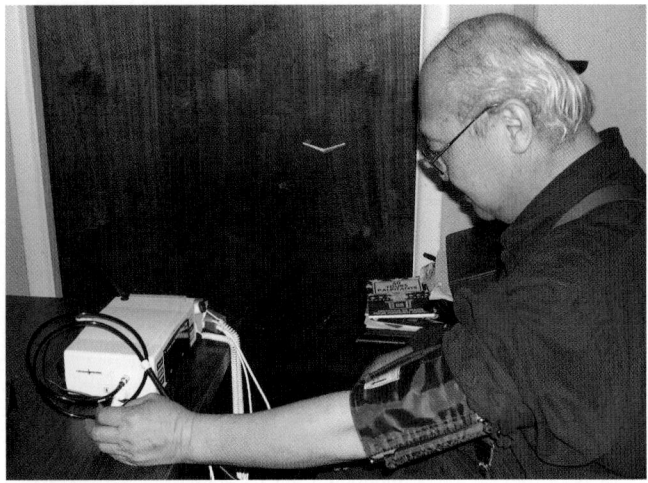

Figure 6-4 Patient at a telemonitoring station in his home.

Source: Saint Elizabeth Health Care, Markham, ON.

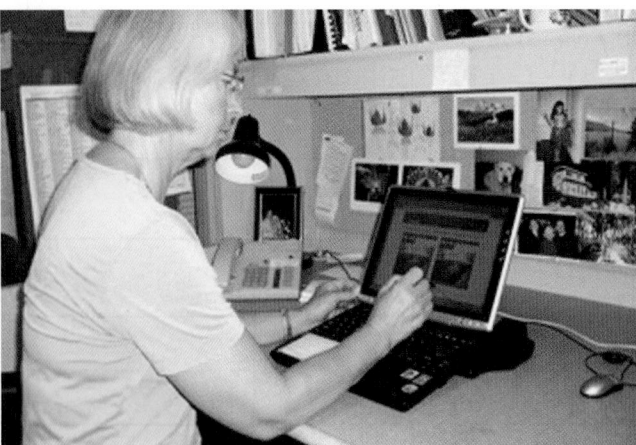

Figure 6-5 Home health nurse examining digital photos of a wound, using the electronic program Pixalere.

Source: Fraser Health, Surrey, BC.

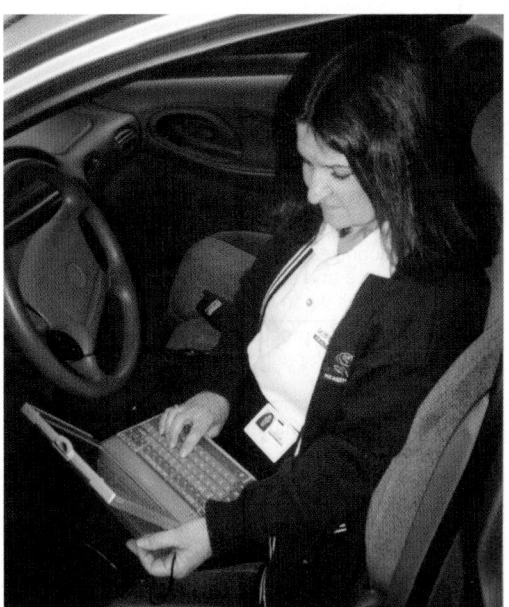

Figure 6-6 Home health nurse using a laptop computer in her car.

Source: Saint Elizabeth Health Care, Markham, ON.

manual data on nursing-sensitive outcomes in home health, acute care hospitals, and long-term care settings (Doran et al., 2004). On the basis of those results, the Canadian Health Outcomes for Better Information and Care (C-HOBIC, 2007) project was launched to test the collection of patient outcome information related to nursing care in the electronic health records of Ontario, Prince Edward Island, and Saskatchewan.

Summary

Nursing in the community represents a dynamic and fulfilling practice specialty for nurses. Community-based nursing is an essential component of the health care system and offers the opportunity to positively influence the health and outcomes of individuals, communities, and populations.

CLINICAL DECISION-MAKING EXERCISE

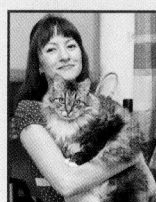

CASE STUDY:
Home Health Care for Patient With Infected Leg Ulcer

Source: © Darkbird77/Dreamstime.com

Patient Profile

Melody Tennant, 43 years old, has been referred to home care for care of her infected leg wound and intravenous antibiotics. She lives alone in an apartment with her cat in an area of town identified as having a high number of calls to the police. Melody worked as a food server but is currently out of work. She is candid with the nurse completing her admission and shares the fact that she has been trying to stop her intravenous drug use for years. Her right lower leg ulcer is the result of injection drugs 6 months ago. The injection site became a "sore" and "just never healed." Melody went to the walk-in clinic when she could no longer stand the pain and her boyfriend noticed her leg was pink and warm to touch. The walk-in clinic physician sent her to the emergency department, where a methicillin-resistant *Staphylococcus aureus* (MRSA)–infected leg wound was diagnosed.

Subjective Data

- Has a history of being hepatitis B positive (3 years)
- Has varicose veins in both legs; worries that the home care nurses will want her to wear support stockings for her varicose veins, and she finds them "ugly."
- Complains of pain in her right lower leg and asks for "something to take the edge off."

Objective Data
Physical Examination
- Peripheral intravenous site (saline lock) in left hand
- Dressing to right lower leg: 10- × 10-cm foam dressing with adhesive edges

- Right lower leg ulcer: 10% pink base, 90% yellow base, irregular flat edges. Wound size is 0.5 cm deep, 7 cm long, 4.4 cm wide. Periwound skin is deep pink, and the diameter of the right lower leg calf is greater than that of the left.

Collaborative Care
- Methadone, 50 mg PO once daily
- Vancomycin, 500 mg intravenously BID
- Multivitamin, 1 tablet PO daily
- High-protein diet

Discussion Questions

1. *Priority decision:* What are the initial priorities for the home health nurse?
2. What other members of the team should be involved in the care of Melody? What are their roles and responsibilities?
3. *Priority decision:* What type of patient education program should be implemented? What are the priority teaching goals to promote self-management?
4. What should the nurse consider in the nutrition assessment? How will the nurse address the economic considerations related to Melody's diet?
5. How can the nurse address Melody's coping skills and use community resources to intervene with her substance use?
6. What types of supplies will Melody need? What diagnostics, teaching, and community resources should accompany the use of these supplies?
7. What types of patient-centred strategies can the nurse use to promote safety for both Melody and the nurse?
8. What are the expected long-term outcomes for Melody?

Ⓔvolve *Answers are available at* **http://evolve.elsevier.com/Canada/Lewis/medsurg**

REVIEW QUESTIONS

The number of the question corresponds to the same-numbered objective at the beginning of the chapter.

1. Which of the following statements is correct about public health nursing?
   a. It predates home health nursing.
   b. It focuses on health promotion and disease prevention.
   c. It does not include health teaching.
   d. It takes place predominantly in private homes.

2. Which of the following statements best describes nurses working in community health settings?
   a. They function autonomously in meeting patient needs.
   b. They focus only on patient needs specific to the setting.
   c. They use the same skills as in acute care settings.
   d. They use case management skills along the continuum of care.

3. Which of the following trends is affecting home care and threatening the sustainability of Canada's health care system?
   a. The long wait times for surgery
   b. The increased number of people hospitalized with acute illness
   c. The shortage of health care providers
   d. The high rate of health care–associated infections

4. Which of the following best describes primary health care?
   a. The first health care professional seen by a patient
   b. Public health nursing
   c. A philosophy that emphasizes health promotion, disease prevention, and patient participation in care
   d. A theoretical model

5. Which of the following statements best reflects the reality of home care services in Canada?
   a. The use of home health services is increasing.
   b. The use of home health services is decreasing.
   c. Home health services are not yet available in all provinces and territories.
   d. Home health services are used more by families than by single patients.

6. Which of the following is a home care nurse competency?
   a. Appreciate and understand the roles and responsibilities and the contributions of other regulated and unregulated health workers involved in the patient's care plan.
   b. Assist patients and their families in recognizing their limited capacity for managing their own health needs according to available resources.
   c. Limit participation in collaborative, interdisciplinary, and intersectoral partnerships to enhance the health of patients and families.
   d. Keep knowledge current to ensure optimal case management is kept to a minimum.

ANSWERS: 1. b; 2. d; 3. c; 4. c; 5. a; 6. a.

REFERENCES

Allemang, M. (2000). *Community nursing: Promoting Canadians' health.* Toronto: W. B. Saunders Canada.

American Nurses Association. (2008). *Home health nursing: Scope and standards of practice.* Silver Spring, MD: Author.

Canadian Healthcare Association. (2009). *Home care in Canada: From the margins to the mainstream.* Ottawa: Author. Retrieved from *http://www.cha.ca/documents/Home_Care_in_Canada_From_the_Margins_to_the_Mainstream_web.pdf*

Canadian Health Outcomes for Better Information and Care (C-HOBIC). (2007). *About C-HOBIC.* Retrieved from *http://www2.cna-aiic.ca/c-hobic/about/default_e.aspx*

Canadian Home Care Association. (2007a). *Implementing case management as a strategy for systems integration: Experiences from the CHCA national partnership project.* Ottawa: Author. Retrieved from *http://www.cdnhomecare.ca/media.php?mid=1557*

Canadian Home Care Association. (2007b). Home care facts: Quality and accountability. Retrieved from *http://www.cdnhomecare.ca/content.php?doc=81*

Canadian Home Care Association. (2008). *Portraits of home care in Canada.* Ottawa: Author.

Canadian Hospice Palliative Care Association. (2002). *A model to guide hospice palliative care: Based on national principles and norms of practice.* Ottawa: Author.

Canadian Hospice Palliative Care Association. (2009). *Canadian hospice palliative care nursing standards of practice.* Ottawa: Canadian Hospice Palliative Care Association Nursing Standards Committee. Retrieved from *http://www.chpca.net/media/7505/Canadian_Hospice_Palliative_Care_Nursing_Standards_2009.pdf*

Canadian Institute for Health Information (2010). Regulated nurses: *Canadian trends, 2005 to 2009.* Ottawa: Author. Retrieved from *http://publications.gc.ca/collections/collection_2011/icis-cihi/H115-48-2009-eng.pdf*

Canadian Institute for Health Information. (2011a). *National health expenditure trends, 1975 to 2011.* Ottawa: Author. Retrieved from *https://secure.cihi.ca/free_products/nhex_trends_report_2011_en.pdf*

Canadian Institute for Health Information. (2011b). *Health spending to reach $200 billion in 2011.* Retrieved from *http://www.cihi.ca/cihi-ext-portal/internet/en/document/spending+and+health+workforce/spending/release_03nov11*

Canadian Institute for Health Information. (2011c). *Home and continuing care news.* Ottawa: Author. Retrieved from *http://www.cihi.ca/CIHI-ext-portal/pdf/internet/HCC_UPDATE_WINTER_11_EN*

Canadian Institute for Health Information. (2011d). Health Care in Canada, 2011. A focus on Seniors and Aging. Retrieved from *https://secure.cihi.ca/free_products/HCIC_2011_seniors_report_en.pdf*

Canadian Nurses Association. (2006). *Practice framework for nurse practitioners in Canada.* Ottawa: Author. Retrieved from *http://www2.cna-aiic.ca/CNA/documents/pdf/publications/cnpi/tech-report/section3/04_Practice%20Framework.pdf*

Canadian Nurses Association. (2008). Advanced nursing practice: A national framework. Retrieved from *http://www2.cna-aiic.ca/CNA/documents/pdf/publications/ANP_National_Framework_e.pdf*

Canadian Nurses Association. (2009a). *Position statement: The Nurse Practitioner.* Ottawa: CNA. Retrieved from *http://www2.cna-aiic.ca/CNA/documents/pdf/publications/PS_Nurse_Practitioner_e.pdf*

Canadian Nurses Association. (2009b). *Tested solutions for eliminating Canada's registered nurse shortage.* Ottawa: Author. Retrieved from *http://www2.cna-aiic.ca/cna/documents/pdf/publications/RN_Highlights_e.pdf*

Canadian Public Health Association. (2008). A tool for strengthening chronic disease prevention and management. Retrieved from *http://www.cpha.ca/en/portals/cd.aspx*

Canadian Public Health Association. (2010). *Public health—Community health nursing practice in Canada: Roles and activities* (4th ed.). Ottawa: Author. Retrieved from *http://www.cpha.ca/uploads/pubs/3-1bk04214.pdf*

Canadian Research Network for Care in the Community. (2010). Home support workers in the continuum of care for older people. Retrieved from *http://www.oanhss.org/AM/Template.cfm?Section=External_Reports&Template=/CM/ContentDisplay.cfm&ContentID=7198*

Caplan, E. (2005). Realizing the potential of home care: Competing for excellence by rewarding results. Retrieved from *http://*

www.homecareontario.ca/public/docs/publications/other-home-care/realizing-potential-of-home-care.pdf

Carter, A. (2009). Nursing shortage predicted to be hardest on home healthcare. *Home Healthcare Nurse, 27*(3), 198.

Chalmers, K. I., & Kristjanson, L. J. (1992). Community health nursing practice. In A. J. Baumgart & J. Larsen (Eds.), *Canadian nursing faces the future* (2nd ed., pp. 153-179). St. Louis: Mosby.

College of Nurses of Ontario. (2009). Practice guideline: Culturally sensitive care. Retrieved from *http://www.cno.org/docs/prac/41040_CulturallySens.pdf*

Community Health Nurses of Canada. (2009). *Public health nursing discipline specific competencies* (version 1.0). Ottawa: Author. Retrieved from *http://www.chnc.ca/documents/CHNC-PublicHealthNursingDisciplineSpecificCompetencies/index.html#/15/zoomed*

Community Health Nurses of Canada. (2010). *Home health nursing competencies* (version 1.0). Toronto: Author. Retrieved from *http://login.greatbignews.com/UserFiles/289/documents/HomeHealthNursingCompetenciesVersion1March2010.pdf*

Community Health Nurses of Canada. (2011). Canadian community health nursing: Professional practice model and standards of practice. Revised March, 2011. Toronto: Author. Retrieved from *http://www.chnc.ca/documents/CHNC-ProfessionalPracticeModel-EN/index.html#/1/*

Doran, D. M. (Ed.). (2003). *Nursing sensitive outcomes: State of the science.* Sudbury, MA: Jones and Bartlett.

Doran, D., Harrison, M. B., Laschinger, H., Hirdes, J., Rukholm, E., Sidani, S.,..., White, P. (2004). Collecting data on nursing-sensitive outcomes in different care settings: Can it be done? What are the benefits? Report of the Nursing and Health Outcomes Feasibility Study. Retrieved from *http://www.ontla.on.ca/library/repository/mon/15000/264600.pdf*

Doran, D. M., Hirdes, J., Poss, J., Jantzi, M., Blais, R., Baker, G. R. & Pickard, J. (2009). Identification of safety outcomes for Canadian home care clients: Evidence from the resident assessment instrument—Home care reporting system concerning emergency room visits. *Healthcare Quarterly, 12, Special Issue,* 40-48.

Edmunds, K., & Kinnaird-Iler, E. (2008). Multicultural clients. In L. L. Stamler & L. Yiu (Eds.), *Community health nursing: A Canadian perspective* (2nd ed., pp. 311-319). Toronto: Pearson Canada.

Emory, F. (1953). *Public health nursing in Canada: Principles and practice* (Rev. ed.). Toronto: Macmillan.

Foebel, A. D., Hirdes, J. P., Heckman, G. A., Tyas, S. L. & Tjam, E. Y. (2011). A profile of older community-dwelling home care clients with heart failure in Ontario. *Chronic Diseases in Canada, 31*(2), 49-57.

Health Canada. (2012). Health system: About primary health care. Retrieved from *http://www.hc-sc.gc.ca/hcs-sss/prim/about-apropos-eng.php*

Health Council of Canada. (2008a). *Fixing the foundation: An update on primary health care and home care renewal in Canada.* Toronto: Author. Retrieved from *http://healthcouncilcanada.ca/tree/2.26-HCC_PHC_Main_web_E.pdf*

Health Council of Canada. (2008b). *Rekindling reform: Health care renewal in Canada, 2003-2008. Summary.* Retrieved from *http://www.homecareontario.ca/public/docs/news/2008/June/rekindling-reform-health-care-renewal-in-canada-03-08-summary-june-08.pdf*

Hutchinson, A. M., Draper, K., & Sales, A. E. (2009). Public reporting of nursing home quality of care: Lessons from the United States experience for Canadian policy discussion. *Healthcare Policy, 5*(2), 87-105.

Institute for Patient- and Family-Centered Care. (2011). Advancing the practice of patient- and family-centered care in hospitals: How to get started. Retrieved from *http://www.ipfcc.org/pdf/getting_started.pdf*

Institute of Medicine. (1999). *To err is human: Building a safer health system.* Washington, DC: Author.

Lang, A. (2010). There's no place like home: Research, practice and policy perspectives regarding safety in home care. *International Journal for Quality in Health Care, 22*(2), 75-76. doi:10.1093/intqhc/mzq007

Lang, A., & Edwards, N. (2006). Safety in home care: Broadening the patient safety agenda to include home care services. Retrieved from *http://www.patientsafetyinstitute.ca/English/research/commissionedResearch/SafetyinHomeCare/Documents/Safety%20in%20Home%20Care.pdf*

Lang, A., Edwards, N., & Fleiszer, A. (2008). Safety in home care: A broadened perspective of patient safety. *International Journal for Quality in Health Care, 20*(2), 130-135. doi:10.1093/intqhc/mzm068

MacKay, L. (2009). Exploring family-centred care among pediatric oncology nurses: A master's thesis, p. 10). Retrieved from *https://www.uleth.ca/dspace/bitstream/handle/10133/2483/mackay,%20lyndsay.pdf?sequence=1*

Masotti, P., McColl, M. A., & Green, M. (2010). Adverse events experienced by homecare patients: A scoping review of the literature. *International Journal for Quality in Health Care, 22*(2), 115-125. doi:10.1093/intqhc/mzq003.

Meadows, C. (2009). Integrating new graduate nurses in home health care. *Home Healthcare Nurse, 27*(9), 561-568. doi:10.1097/01.NHH.0000361929.52668.10

Morgan, M. W., Zamora, N. E., & Hindmarsh, M. F. (2007). An inconvenient truth: A sustainable healthcare system requires chronic disease prevention and management transformation. *Healthcare Papers, 7*(4), 39-42. Retrieved from *http://www.nwlhin.on.ca/uploadedFiles/Home_Page/Integrated_Health_Service_Plan/An%20Inconvenient%20Truth.pdf*

Nagle, L. M. (2008). Show me the way to stay home. *Canadian Journal of Nursing Leadership, 12*(4), 29-32.

Ontario Home Care Association. (2011). *Home care nursing in Ontario.* Hamilton: Author. Retrieved from *http://www.homecareontario.ca/public/docs/news/2011/march/ohca-home-care-nursing-in-ontario.pdf*

Ontario Ministry of Health and Long-Term Care. (2008). *Backgrounder: PDA initiative for Ontario nurses.* Retrieved from *http://www.health.gov.on.ca/en/news/release/2008/may/pda_bg_01_20080512.pdf*

Pastor, D. K. (2006). Home sweet home: A concept analysis of home visiting. *Home Healthcare Nurse, 24*(6), 389-394.

Saint Elizabeth Health Care. (2010). The caregiver compass. Retrieved from *http://www.caretoknow.org/flash/compass/*

Saint Elizabeth Health Care. (2011). What is client-centred care? Client-centred care in the Canadian home and community sector: A review of key concepts. Retrieved from *http://clientcentredcare.caretoknow.org/pdfs/full_report.php#fp_aa*

Shamian, J., Mildon, B., Goodwin, S., Norton, R., & Talosi, R. (2006). Of systems and side effects: Mobility in home care personnel. Retrieved from *http://www.von.ca/doc/Mobility_%20Study.doc*

Smith, D., Jacobson, L., & Yiu, L. (2008). Primary health care. In L. L. Stamler & L. Yiu (Eds.), *Community health nursing: A Canadian perspective* (2nd ed.). Toronto: Pearson.

Statistics Canada. (2006). *Findings from the 2005 National Survey of the Work and Health of Nurses (Cat. No. 83-003-XPE).* Ottawa: Author. Retrieved from *http://www.hc-sc.gc.ca/hcs-sss/alt_formats/hpb-dgps/pdf/pubs/2005-nurse-infirm/2005-nurse-infirm-eng.pdf*

Statistics Canada. (2011). *Canada's population estimates: Age and sex.* Ottawa: Author. Retrieved from *http://www.statcan.gc.ca/daily-quotidien/110928/dq110928a-eng.htm*

Stevenson, R. L., McRae, C., & Mughal, W. A. (2008). Moving to a culture of safety in community home health care. *Journal of Health Services Research and Policy, 13*(Suppl 1), 20-24. doi:10.1258/jhsrp.2007.007016

VanDeVelde-Coke, S. A. (2004). *The effectiveness and efficiency of providing home care visits in nursing clinics versus the traditional home setting.* Ottawa: Canadian Health Services Research Foundation. Retrieved from *http://74.81.206.232/Migrated/PDF/ResearchReports/OGC/coke_final.pdf*

Victorian Order of Nurses. (2009). Caregiving guide. Retrieved from *http://www.von.ca/en/caregiver-guide/healthinfo-family_caregiver.aspx?guide=1*

Wilkins, K. (2006). Government-subsidized home care. *Health Reports, 17*(4), 39-42. Retrieved from *http://publications.gc.ca/Collection-R/Statcan/82-003-XIE/82-003-XIE2005004.pdf*

World Health Organization. (1978). *Primary health care: Report of the International Conference on Primary Health Care, Alma-Ata, USSR, September 6-12, 1978.* Retrieved from *http://whqlibdoc.who.int/publications/9241800011.pdf*

World Health Organization. (2010). A global survey monitoring progress in nursing and midwifery. Geneva: Author. Retrieved from *http://whqlibdoc.who.int/hq/2010/WHO_HRH_HPN_10.4_eng.pdf*

CANADIAN RESOURCES

Canadian Gerontological Nurses Association
http://www.cgna.net
Canadian Home Care Association
http://www.cdnhomecare.ca/
Canadian Institute for Health Information (CIHI)
http://www.cihi.ca
Canadian Nurses Association
http://www.cna-aiic.ca/
Canadian Patient Safety Institute
http://www.patientsafetyinstitute.ca/English/Pages/default.aspx
Canadian Research Network for Care in the Community
http://www.crncc.ca/

Chronic Disease Prevention Alliance of Canada (CDPAC)
http://www.cdpac.ca/
Community Health Nurses of Canada (CHNC)
http://www.chnc.ca
Community Health Nurses Initiatives Group (CHNIG) of the Registered Nurses' Association of Ontario
http://www.chnig.org
Ontario Association of Community Care Access Centres
http://www.oaccac.on.ca
Saint Elizabeth Health Care
http://www.saintelizabeth.com
Victorian Order of Nurses (VON) Canada
http://www.von.ca

RELATED RESOURCES

Home Healthcare Nurses Association
http://www.hhna.org
Institute for Healthcare Improvement
http://www.ihi.org/ihi
National Association for Home Care and Hospice
http://www.nahc.org
National Gerontological Nursing Association
http://www.ngna.org

evolve *For additional Internet resources, see the Web site for this book at* **http://evolve.elsevier.com/Canada/Lewis/medsurg**

CHAPTER

7

Older Adults

Written by Margaret Wooding Baker and Margaret McLean Heitkemper

Adapted by Veronique M. Boscart

LEARNING OBJECTIVES

1. Describe the effects of ageism on the care of older adults.
2. List the major biological theories of aging.
3. Describe the needs of special populations of older adults.
4. Describe nursing interventions to assist chronically ill older adults.
5. Describe common problems of older adults related to acute illness and the role of the nurse in assisting them.
6. Describe challenges and concerns related to the caregiving role.
7. Identify care alternatives to meet specific needs of older adults.
8. Identify the legal and ethical issues related to older adults.
9. Identify the role of the nurse in health screening and promotion and disease prevention for older adults.

KEY TERMS

ageism Negative attitude toward an older adult based on age, p. 100

elder abuse A single, or repeated, act or lack of appropriate action, occurring within any relationship in which there is an expectation of trust, which causes harm or distress to an older person, p. 109

elder mistreatment (EM) An act of commission that harms or threatens to harm an older adult's health or welfare, p. 109

elder neglect An act of omission that harms or threatens to harm an older adult's health or welfare, p. 109

ethnogeriatrics A specialty area of providing culturally competent care to older adults who are identified with a particular ethnic group, p. 108

frail older adults Vulnerable older adults who have declining physical health and resources, p. 107

gerontological nursing The nursing care of older adults, p. 100

long-term care (LTC) facilities A place to live for the older adult who can no longer live alone, needs continuous supervision, has a cognitive and/or physical disability, or is frail, p. 112

nonstochastic theory Hypothesis that aging is programmed by genes, p. 100

polypharmacy Use of multiple medications by an individual, p. 115

stochastic theory Hypothesis that aging is due to chance, p. 100

ELECTRONIC RESOURCES

Supplemental content related to Chapter 7 can be found...

Evolve Web Site ⓔvolve

http://evolve.elsevier.com/Canada/Lewis/medsurg
- Clinical Reference: Laboratory Values
- Content Updates

- Electronic Calculators
- Examination Review Questions
- Glossary
- Key Points (Printable and MP3 Download)

Gerontological nursing is a nursing specialty that revolves around the care of older adults. The nurse delivers care from a person-centred perspective, valuing what is important to the person. This chapter presents specific information about older adults that will assist nurses in providing medical-surgical care to older adults in a variety of settings, such as inpatient care units, clinics, ambulatory care units, community and home health care, long-term and chronic care, nursing homes, and emergency care departments and centres. Gerontological care presents opportunities and challenges that call for highly skilled assessment and creative adaptations of interventions.

Demographics of Aging

Older adults are one of the fastest-growing populations in Canada. Since 1980, the older population has grown about twice as fast as the overall population. As a result, 13.7% of the population were age 65 and older in 2006 (Statistics Canada, 2007a). This rapid growth is expected to continue well into the future. It has been projected that by 2021 there will be almost 7 million older adults, who will represent 19% of the total population; by 2041, there will be over 9 million older adults, who will make up an estimated 25% of the population (Public Health Agency of Canada [PHAC], 2009).

Generally, Canada has a younger population than most Western industrialized countries, yet a large proportion of older adults are immigrants. By 2031, at least one in four Canadians will be an immigrant and about one in three will belong to a visible minority (Statistics Canada, 2011). The number of Aboriginal older adults is predicted to double by 2017 (Turcotte & Schellenberg, 2007). Furthermore, there are significant age-related differences between Canada's provinces and territories; with the largest share of older population in Saskatchewan (14.8%) and Nova Scotia (14.2%), and the smallest in Alberta (10.5%) and Ontario (12.8%) (Statistics Canada, 2007b).

The most rapidly increasing age group is composed of those persons 85 years of age and older. Since the 1960s, this group has increased 250%. The terms *young–old adult* (age 55-75 years) and *old–old adult* (older than 75 years) are used to represent chronological ranges that often present different characteristics and needs.

Gender can have a significant effect on various aspects of aging. Women usually live longer than men. Female Canadians born today have a life expectancy of 83 years and males have a life expectancy of 78.3 years (Statistics Canada, 2010).

Although the majority of adults older than age 65 (83% of men and 75% of women) remain in their home, 17% of men and 25 % of women reside in facility-based care (Cranswick & Dosman, 2008).

Because the needs and expectations of the population are changing rapidly, nurses need to acquire and demonstrate the required knowledge levels, clinical expertise, leadership skills, and a strong understanding of health organizations and policy to deliver the best care possible to older adults.

Attitudes Toward Aging

Today's health care system promotes the concept of aging from a holistic perspective, in which health and wellness are defined as a balance between one's internal and external environment and one's emotional, spiritual, social, cultural, and physical processes.

From this framework, aging is seen as influenced by many factors, including emotional and physical health, developmental stage, socioeconomic status, culture, and ethnicity.

As people age, they are exposed to more and different life experiences. The accumulation of these differences creates a great diversity in the group of older adults. Nurses need to acknowledge and incorporate this diversity and older adults' perceptions of aging in their assessments because it will determine and guide their interventions. Research has indicated that older adults with poor health report a higher perceived age and a lower sense of psychological well-being compared with healthy older adults (Levasseur, St-Cyr Tribble, & Desrosier, 2009). Age is important, but it may not be the most relevant for determining the appropriate care of an individual older adult patient. In approaching aging from a viewpoint of health and well-being, a person's strengths, resilience, resources, and capabilities are emphasized, rather than her or his existing pathological conditions.

Unfortunately, myths and stereotypes about aging are found throughout society and are often supported by media (Rozanova, Northcott, & McDaniel, 2006). These stereotypes provide the basis of commonly held misconceptions that lead to errors in nursing assessments and limitations to interventions. For example, if nurses perceive that most older people are confused or disoriented, necessary assessment for delirium will be neglected, resulting in serious morbidity and mortality for older adults (Capezuti, Zwicker, Mezey, et al., 2007).

This negative attitude based on age is defined as **ageism**. Ageism leads to discrimination and disparities in the care given to the older adult. Research has indicated that nurses who demonstrate an ageist attitude provide lower quality of care towards their patients (Lookinland & Anson, 2008). In today's aging society, it is essential for nurses to demonstrate expertise, knowledge, and practice to care for older adults.

Biological Theories of Aging

Several theories aim at describing the process of aging. From a biological view, aging is defined as the progressive loss of function. The exact etiology or cause of biological aging remains to be determined, yet aging is clearly a multifactorial process involving genetics, oxidative stress, diet, and environment (Desai et al., 2010). Nurses' knowledge of biological changes is important because it allows for differentiation between the normal aging process and health problems that require specific interventions.

Research efforts in the area of biological aging are directed at studying the changes over the lifespan of an organism to increase the average lifespan and the quality of life. The development of new antiaging therapies aims at slowing down or reversing age-related changes. There has long been an interest in slowing down or reversing the effects of aging. However, much more research is needed before it can be determined whether any of these substances delay aging or enhance the functional ability of older adults.

Several theories regarding biological aging are currently proposed and fall into two main categories: stochastic and nonstochastic theories. **Stochastic theories** propose that aging is the result of chance and error, and **nonstochastic theories** propose that aging is *not* related to chance, but is based on predetermined or programmed processes. An overview of biological theories of aging is presented in Table 7-1.

Table 7-1 Summary of Biological Theories of Aging

THEORY	DYNAMICS
Stochastic Theories	
Error	Faulty synthesis of DNA, RNA, or both.
Somatic	Alteration in RNA, DNA, or both; protein or enzyme synthesis causes defective structure or function.
Transcription	Failure of transcription or translation between cells; malfunctions of RNA or related enzymes.
Free radical	Oxidation of fats, proteins, and carbohydrates creates free electrons that attach to other molecules, altering cellular function.
Cross-link	Lipids, proteins, carbohydrates, and nucleic acid react with chemicals or radiation to form bonds that cause an increase in cell rigidity and instability.
Nonstochastic Theories	
Programmed	Biological clock triggers specific cell behaviour at a specific time. Organism is capable of a specific number of cell divisions and has a specific lifespan.
Neuroendocrine	Control mechanisms (pituitary and hypothalamus) regulate interplay between various organs and tissues; efficiency of signals between mechanisms is altered or lost.
Immunological-autoimmunological	Alteration of B and T cells leads to loss of capacity for self-regulation; normal cells or cells with age-related changes are recognized as foreign matter; system reacts by forming antibodies to destroy these cells.
Telomere-telomerase hypothesis	With aging, there is a loss of telomeres (repeated sequences at the ends of DNA). This loss limits the number of times cells can divide.

Stochastic Theories

Stochastic theories explain aging as the result of an accumulation of errors in the synthesis of cellular DNA and RNA, the basic building blocks of the cell (Vijg, 2007, p. 25). Visible signs of aging, such as grey hair, are thought to be the result of the accumulation of these cellular errors. Three of the most common theories of error are somatic, free radical, and cross-link.

Somatic Theory. The somatic mutation theory postulates that aging is a result of lifelong genetic damage (Kennedy, Loeb, & Herr, 2012). This damage may include the progressive accumulation of errors in information-containing molecules. According to *somatic mutation theory*, body cells develop spontaneous mutations in the same way germ cells do. Subsequent cell divisions perpetuate the mutations until organs become inefficient and ultimately fail (Kennedy et al., 2012). Although

this theory is attractive, little evidence exists to support or refute this theory.

Free Radical Theory. The *free radical theory* was initially proposed in 1956 by Harman but, in recent years, has become the focus of new research. A free radical is a highly reactive atom or molecule that carries an unpaired electron and, thus, is prone to combine with another molecule, causing an oxidative process. This process, also called *oxidative stress*, can ultimately disrupt cell membranes and alter DNA and protein synthesis. Common diseases such as atherosclerosis and cancer are associated with oxidative stress (Rak, Klement, & Yu, 2006). Free radicals are natural by-products of many normal cellular processes and are also created under the influence of such environmental factors as smog, tobacco smoke, and radiation. Numerous natural protective mechanisms are in place to prevent oxidative damage. Recent research has focused on the roles of various antioxidants, including vitamins C and E, in slowing down the oxidative process and, ultimately, the aging process. These substances are being investigated for their usefulness in preventing diseases related to aging, such as oral, esophageal, and reproductive cancers, coronary artery disease, and cataracts.

Cross-Link Theory. The *cross-link theory* postulates that, over time and as a result of exposure to chemicals and radiation in the environment, cross-links form between lipids, proteins, and carbohydrates, as well as nucleic acids (Marin-Garcia, 2008). These cross-links result in decreased flexibility and elasticity, and this increases rigidity in tissues (e.g., blood vessels). Such changes in cell structure may explain the observable changes associated with aging, such as wrinkles and a decreased distensibility of arterial blood vessels. However, it is unlikely that such changes account for all of the detrimental physical events associated with aging.

Nonstochastic Theories

Nonstochastic theories describe a *theory of programmed cell death*, proposing that there is an impairment in the ability of the cell to continue dividing (Hayflick, 1973). The neuroendocrine and immunological theory and the telomere-telomerase hypothesis all present nonstochastic perspectives on aging.

Neuroendocrine Theory. The *neuroendocrine theory* proposes that aging occurs because of functional decrements in neurons and associated hormones. It suggests that neural and endocrine changes may be pacemakers for many cellular and physiological aspects of aging. This approach relates the organism's aging to the loss of responsiveness of its neuroendocrine tissue to various signals. An important focus of this theory is the functional changes of the hypothalamic–pituitary system. These changes are accompanied by a decline in functional capacity in other endocrine organs, such as the adrenal and thyroid glands, the ovaries, and the testes (Chahal & Drake, 2007).

Immunological Theory. The *immunological theory* proposes declining functional capacity of the immune system as the basis for the aging process (Fuente & Miquel, 2009). It suggests that aging is not a passive wearing-out of systems but an active self-destruction mediated by the immune system. This theory is based on observing an age-associated decline in T-cell functioning, accompanied by a decrease in resistance and an increase in autoimmune diseases with aging. Whether the immunological changes are determined genetically, regulated by environment, or influenced by endocrine factors remains to be ascertained. The result is an autoimmune phenomenon in which normal body cells are mistaken as foreign and are attacked by the individual's own immune system.

Telomere-Telomerase Hypothesis. The *telomere-telomerase hypothesis* (Shay & Wright, 2005) attributes the process of aging to telomeres. Telomeres are specialized repeated sequences that are present at the ends of DNA strands. Telomerase is the enzyme that synthesizes these repeat sequences. With aging, there is a loss of these strands and a decrease in telomerase activity, both of which affect the number of times a cell can divide. It has also been hypothesized that shortening of the DNA strands is associated with cancer development in older adults (Shay et al., 2005).

Despite the many different theoretical views, the exact cause of aging is unknown. Nurses need to be aware that each older person will present with an individual aging process, which will required a unique approach.

Age-Related Physiological Changes

Age-related changes affect every body system and are part of healthy aging. However, the age at which specific changes become evident differs from person to person and within the same individual. For instance, a person may have greying hair at age 45 but relatively unwrinkled skin at age 80. Nurses need to recognize and assess age-related changes because they form the basis to differentiate from non–age-related changes. Table 7-2 presents an overview of assessments based on age-related physiological changes and associated clinical manifestations.

Older Populations at High Risk

Some subgroups within the older population, such as women, adults with cognitive challenges, and individuals from minority groups, are at a higher risk for developing certain conditions or being misdiagnosed. Some people might belong to several of these subgroups and their care requires skilled expertise in nursing assessment, interventions, and evaluations.

Older Women

Some aging women are confronted with several factors that directly affect the aging process. Issues such as reduced financial resources, a high number of chronic health conditions, and/or informal caregiving responsibilities can all have a significant impact on the health of the older woman. As a result, older women often experience disparities, including unequal access to quality health care (Chapter 2). Nurses should act as advocates for women's equity in the health care system. Advocacy organizations such as the Canadian Women's Health Network can be helpful in this undertaking.

In addition to unequal access to health care, older women are more likely to be victims of family violence than older men, in part because they usually live longer (Hightower, Smith, & Hightower, 2006). The abuse or neglect is often from the older woman's spouse, partner, or adult children; whereas, for an older man, the abuse or neglect is most likely from his adult children

or close friends. Older women have some additional risk factors that can lead to abusive or neglectful situations. Older women are more likely than older men to have experienced a history of emotional, physical, or sexual abuse and are more likely to have disabling conditions, be widowed, or live alone. Because an older woman may have fewer resources, she may be reluctant to leave an abusive relationship (Hightower et al., 2006; Statistics Canada, 2011).

Several resources, organizations, and programs are in place to raise awareness, prevent, diagnose, and address the abuse of older people in Canada. The Registered Nurses Association of Ontario (RNAO) has partnered with the Canadian Nurses Association (CNA) for the Promoting Awareness of Elder Abuse in Long-Term Care Homes (PEACE) pan-Canadian initiative. Resources are listed at the end of the chapter, and nurses should familiarize themselves with this information to address this important health, social, and legal issue.

Older Adults with Cognitive Impairments

The majority of older adults will not have any noticeable decline in mental abilities. There will be some normal age changes, such as a memory lapse or benign forgetfulness, which are significantly different from cognitive impairment. These normal age changes are often referred to as *age-associated memory impairment* (See Table 7-3 on p. 107).

An older adult who is forgetful can benefit from using memory aids, attempting recall in a calm and quiet environment, and actively engaging in memory improvement techniques. Memory aids include clocks, calendars, notes, marked pillboxes, safety alarms on stoves, and identity necklaces or bracelets. Memory improvement techniques include word association, mental imaging, and mnemonics.

Declining physical health is an important factor in cognitive impairment. Older people who experience sensory losses or cerebrovascular disease may show a decline in cognitive functioning. An appropriate cognitive assessment includes functional ability, memory recall, orientation, use of judgement, and appropriateness of emotional state. Standard mental status examinations and behavioural descriptions provide data for determining cognitive status. Cognitive impairment is further discussed in Chapter 62.

Older Adults Living in Rural Settings

Approximately 23% of older Canadians live in rural areas (Turcotte & Schellenberg, 2007) and some face barriers to remain at home, stay active, and stay engaged in their communities. Such barriers include a lack of or limited support available to enable older people to remain independent, as well as very limited housing and transportation options. In addition, older adults in rural and remote areas are frequently required to travel out of their communities for health services, which creates challenges for them and their families (PHAC, 2007). Some research has indicated that older adults living in rural areas present with more symptoms of ill health compared with older adults living in urban areas (Xiaowei, MacKnight, Latta, Mitnitski, & Rockwood, 2007). Furthermore, rural communities offer fewer health-promoting activities, such as structured exercise programs (PHAC, 2007), and are often underserved by health care providers.

Nurses working with older adults in rural communities must clearly recognize the lifestyle values and practices of rural life

Text continued on p. 107

Table 7-2 Age-Related Changes and Associated Clinical Manifestations

SYSTEM	NORMAL AGE CHANGES	CLINICAL MANIFESTATIONS
Cardiovascular		
Cardiac output	• Force of contraction decreased • Fat and collagen increased • Heart muscle decreased • Ventricular wall thickened	• Myocardial oxygen demand increased • Stroke volume and CO decreased • Fatigue, shortness of breath, tachycardia occur • Blood flow to vital organs and periphery decreased
Cardiac rate and rhythm	• Dependence of atrial contraction increased • Loss of fibres from His bundle • Mitral valve stretching • Ventricles slow to relax • Sinus node pacemaker cells decreased	• HR slow to increase with stress • Maximum HR decreased (e.g., 80-year-old person, 120 bpm; 20-year-old person, 200 bpm) • Possible AV block • Recovery time from tachycardia prolonged • Premature beats increased
Structural changes	• Aortic valves sclerotic and calcified • Baroreceptor sensitivity decreased • Mild fibrosis and calcification of valves	• Diastolic murmur present in 50% of older patients • Heart-position landmarks change
Arterial circulation	• Elastin and smooth muscle reduced • Vessel rigidity increased • Vascular resistance increased • Aorta becomes dilated	• Systolic BP modestly increased • Rigid arteries contribute to coronary artery disease and peripheral vascular disease
Venous circulation	• Tortuosity increased	• Inflamed, painful, or cordlike varicosities
Peripheral pulses	• Arteries rigid	• Pulses weaker but equal • Circulation to periphery slowed • Cold feet and hands
Respiratory		
Structures	• Cartilage degeneration • Vertebrae rigid • Strength of muscles decreased • Respiratory muscles atrophy • Rigidity of thoracic wall increased • Ciliary action decreased	• Kyphosis • Anterior-posterior diameter increased • Use of accessory muscles decreased • Chest rigid and barrel-shaped • Respiratory excursion decreased • Cough and deep breathing ability diminished
Change in ventilation and perfusion	• Pulmonary vascular bed decreased • Alveoli decreased • Alveolar walls thickened • Elastic recoil decreased	• Lung compliance decreased • Total lung volume unchanged • Vital capacity decreased • Residual lung volume increased • Mucus thickens • PaO_2 and O_2 saturation decreased • Hyperresonance
Ventilation control	• Response to hypoxia and hypercarbia decreased	• Ability to maintain acid-base balance decreased • Respiratory rate 12-24/min
Integumentary		
Skin	• Collagen and subcutaneous fat decreased • Sweat glands decreased • Epidermal cell turnover slowed • Skin tissue fluid decreased • Capillary fragility increased • Pigment cells decreased • Sebaceous gland activity decreased • Sensory receptors decreased • Thresholds for touch, vibration, heat, and pain increased	• Skin elasticity decreased • Wrinkles and folds increased • Extremity fat lost; fat on trunk increased • Skin heals slowly • Skin dry • Skin tears and bruises easily • Skin colour uneven • Normal skin lesions increased • Ability to respond to heat and cold decreased • Ability to feel light touch decreased • Cutaneous pain sensitivity declines

AV, atrioventricular; *BP*, blood pressure; *bpm*, beats per minute; *CO*, cardiac output; *HR*, heart rate.

Continued

AGE-RELATED DIFFERENCES IN ASSESSMENT

Table 7-2 Age-Related Changes and Associated Clinical Manifestations—cont'd		
SYSTEM	**NORMAL AGE CHANGES**	**CLINICAL MANIFESTATIONS**
Integumentary—cont'd		
Hair	• Melanin decreased • Germ centre and hair follicle decreased in size and number	• Grey or white hair • Hair quantity decreased and thinner • Scalp, pubic, and axillary hair decreased • Facial hair on men decreased • Facial hair on women increased
Nails	• Blood supply to nail bed decreased • Longitudinal striations increased	• Growth slowed • Nails thickened and brittle • Nails easily split • Potential for fungal infection increased
Urinary		
Kidney	• Renal mass decreased • Number of functioning nephrons decreased • Glomerular filtration rate decreased • Renal plasma flow decreased	• Protein in urine increased • Potential for dehydration increased • Creatinine clearance decreased • Serum creatinine and BUN increased • Excretion of toxins and drugs decreased • Nocturia increased
Bladder	• Bladder smooth muscle and elastic tissue decreased	• Capacity decreased • Less control; stress incontinence
Micturition	• Sphincter control decreased	• Frequency, urgency, and nocturia increased
Reproductive		
Male structures	• Prostatic enlargement • Testicular volume decreased • Sperm count decreased • Seminal vesicles atrophy • Serum testosterone constant • Estrogen level increased	• Sexual response less intense • Takes longer to achieve erection • Erection maintained without ejaculation • Force of ejaculation decreased
Female structures	• Estradiol, prolactin, and progesterone diminished • Size of ovaries, uterus, cervix, fallopian tubes, and labia decreased • Associated glands and epithelium atrophied • Elasticity in the pelvic area decreased • Breast tissue decreased • Vaginal pH becomes alkaline	• Responses to changing hormone levels altered • Cervical and vaginal secretions decreased • Intensity of sexual response gradually decreased • Potential for vaginal infections increased • Potential for vaginal and uterine prolapse increased
Gastrointestinal		
Oral cavity	• Dentine decreased • Gingival retraction • Bone density lost • Papillae of tongue decreased • Taste threshold for salt and sugar increased • Salivary secretions decreased	• Taste perception changes • Potential loss of teeth • Gingivitis • Bleeding gums and dry mouth • Oral mucosa dry
Esophagus	• Pressure of lower esophageal sphincter decreased • Motility decreased	• Epigastric distress • Dysphagia • Potential for hiatal hernia and aspiration

BUN, blood urea nitrogen.

AGE-RELATED DIFFERENCES IN ASSESSMENT

Table 7-2 Age-Related Changes and Associated Clinical Manifestations—cont'd		
SYSTEM	**NORMAL AGE CHANGES**	**CLINICAL MANIFESTATIONS**
Gastrointestinal—cont'd		
Stomach	• Gastric mucosa atrophy • Blood flow decreased	• Gastric emptying decreased
Small intestine	• Intestinal villae decreased • Enzyme secretions decreased • Motility decreased	• Intestinal transit slowed • Absorption of fat-soluble vitamins delayed
Large intestine	• Blood flow decreased • Motility decreased • Sensation of defecation urge decreased	• Potential for constipation and fecal impaction
Pancreas	• Pancreatic ducts distended • Lipase production decreased • Pancreatic reserve impaired	• Fat absorption impaired • Glucose tolerance decreased
Liver	• Number and size of cells decreased • Hepatic protein synthesis impaired • Ability to regenerate decreased	• Lower border extends past costal margin • Drug metabolism decreased
Musculoskeletal		
Skeleton	• Intervertebral disc narrowed Cartilage of nose and ears increased	• Height diminished 2.5-10 cm (1-4 in) • Nose and ears lengthen • Kyphosis • Pelvis widens
Bone	• Cortical and trabecular bone decreased	• Bone resorption exceeds bone formation • Potential for osteoporotic fractures
Muscles	• Number of muscle fibres decreased • Muscle fibres atrophy • Muscle regeneration slowed • Contraction time and latency period prolonged • Flexion of joints increased • Ligaments stiffen • Tendons become sclerotic • Tendon flexor reflexes decreased	• Strength decreased • Agility decreased • Rigidity in neck, shoulders, hips, and knees increased • Potential for restless legs syndrome
Joints	• Cartilage erosion • Calcium deposits increased • Water in cartilage decreased	• Mobility decreased • ROM limited • Osteoarthritis
Nervous		
Structure	• Loss of neurons in brain and spinal cord • Brain size decreased • Dendrites atrophy • Major neurotransmitters decreased • Size of ventricles increased	• Conduction of nerve impulses slowed • Peripheral nerve function lost • Reaction time decreased • Response time slowed • Potential for altered balance, vertigo, and syncope • Postural hypotension increased • Proprioception diminished • Sensory input decreased • EEG alpha waves decreased

EEG, electroencephalogram; *ROM*, range of motion.

Continued

AGE-RELATED DIFFERENCES IN ASSESSMENT

Table 7-2 Age-Related Changes and Associated Clinical Manifestations—cont'd

SYSTEM	NORMAL AGE CHANGES	CLINICAL MANIFESTATIONS
Nervous—cont'd		
Sleep	• Deep sleep decreased • REM sleep decreased in old-old adults	• Difficulty falling asleep • Period of wakefulness increased • Sleep time averages 6 hr
Visual		
Eye structure	• Orbital fat lost • Eyebrows and eyelashes grey • Elasticity of eyelid muscles decreased • Tear production decreased	• Eyes sunken • Eyes dry • Potential for ectropion and entropion • Potential for conjunctivitis
Cornea	• Corneal sensitivity decreased • Corneal reflex decreased • Arcus senilis	• Potential for corneal abrasion
Ciliary	• Aqueous humor secretion decreased • Ciliary muscle atrophies	• Ability of lens to accommodate declines • Presbyopia • Peripheral vision decreased
Lens	• Less elastic, more dense	• Lens yellow and opaque • Ability to adapt to light and dark lessened • Tolerance to glare decreased • Incidence of cataracts increased • Night vision impaired
Iris and pupil	• Pigment lost • Pupil size decreased • Vitreous gel debris increased	• Visual acuity decreased • Pupils appear constricted • Floaters
Auditory		
Structure	• Hairs in external auditory canals of men increased • Ceruminal glands decreased	• Potential for conductive hearing loss • Cerumen drier • Sound conduction decreased
Middle ear	• Middle-ear bone joints degenerate • Eardrum thickens	
Inner ear	• Vestibular structures decline • Hair cells lost • Cochlea atrophies • Organ of Corti atrophies	• Sensitivity to high tones and perception of "s," "t," "f," "g" decreased • Understanding of speech decreased • Discrimination of background voice decreased • Equilibrium–balance deficits • Potential for tinnitus
Immune System		
	• Secretory immunoglobulin A (IgA) declines • Thymus gland involuted • Lymphoid tissue decreased • Antibody production impaired • Proliferative response of T and B cells decreased • Autoantibodies increased	• Potential increase for infection on mucosal surfaces • Cell-mediated immune response impaired • Malignancy incidence increased • Response to acute infection reduced • Potential recurrence of latent herpes zoster and tuberculosis • Autoimmune disease increased

REM, rapid eye movement.

AGE-RELATED DIFFERENCES IN ASSESSMENT

Table 7-3 Effects of Aging on Cognitive Functioning

FUNCTION	MANIFESTATIONS OF HEALTHY AGING
Fluid intelligence	Declines during middle age
Crystallized intelligence	Improves
Vocabulary and verbal reasoning	Improves
Spatial perception	Remains constant or improves
Synthesis of new information	Declines during middle age
Mental performance speed	Declines during middle age
Short-term recall memory	Declines during old age
Long-term recall memory	Remains constant

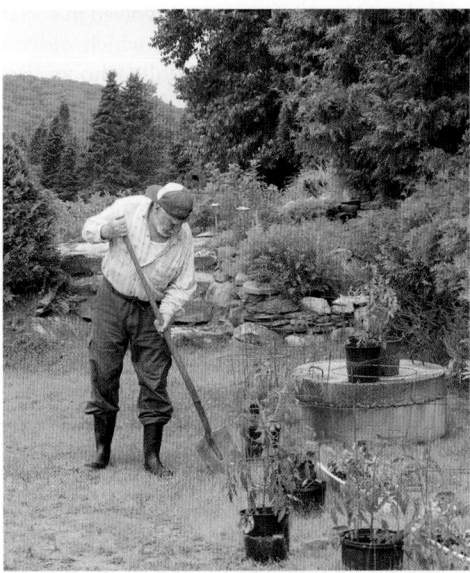

Figure 7-1 Transportation is a possible barrier to providing service to older adults in rural areas.

Source: © 2011 JupiterImages Corporation.

(Figure 7-1) and acknowledge that transportation is a possible barrier to providing service. Alternative service approaches such as computer-based Internet sources and chat rooms, videos, radio, community centres, and church social events should be used to promote healthful practices or to conduct health screening. The development of telehealth devices for monitoring patients in their home environments has enhanced the ability to provide care to isolated individuals.

Older Adults Who Are Homeless

The 2001 Canadian census estimated that approximately 10% of homeless shelter users were 65 years old or older (National Advisory Council on Aging, 2006). Key factors associated with homelessness include (1) a low income, (2) reduced cognitive capacity, and (3) living alone. According to Statistics Canada, 3.6% of males and 7.6% of females 65 years of age are living below the low-income cut-off (LICO). The LICO is the point at which a family is spending 70% or more of their income on necessities (food, clothing, and shelter) (Statistics Canada, 2010). Among older Canadians, single or widowed women are at higher risk for

Table 7-4 Nutritional Assessment of Older Adults

The acronym **SCALES** can remind the nurse to assess important nutritional indicators:

Sadness, or mood change

Cholesterol, high

Albumin, low

Loss or gain of weight

Eating problems

Shopping and food preparation problems

living in poverty. These low-income older people may become homeless because of a lack of affordable housing.

When homeless, the older individual may have increased new health problems or experience an exacerbation of existing problems because most services provided to the homeless population are not designed to reach out to older adults. Long-term care (LTC) placement is often an alternative to homelessness, especially when the individual is cognitively impaired and alone. As a result, a distinct fear of institutionalization may explain why older homeless people do not use shelter- and meal-site services. Homelessness among the elderly requires more research related to risk factors as well as solutions.

Frail Older Adults

Frail older adults is a term used to identify those older adults who, because of declining physical health and resources, are most vulnerable. *Frailty* has been defined as the presence of three or more of the following: unplanned weight loss (≥10 lb in the last year), weakness, poor endurance and energy, slowness, and low activity (Touhy, Jett, Boscart, & McCleary, 2011). Risk factors include disability, multiple chronic illnesses, and the presence of geriatric syndromes. Frailty is not directly related to age per se, although age is a risk factor. Hardiness or psychological strength may be a significant factor in preventing frailty among the elderly.

Most frail older adults have difficulty coping with declining functional abilities and decreasing daily energy. When stressful life events (e.g., the death of a loved one) and daily strain (e.g., caring for an ill spouse) occur, the frail individual may have difficulties with the effects of stress and may become ill. Common health problems of the frail older adult include mobility and strength limitations, sensory impairment, cognitive decline, and falls.

The frail older adult is at particular risk for malnutrition and problems with hydration (Health Canada, 2010). Malnutrition and dehydration are related to sociopsychological factors such as living alone, depression, and/or a low income. Physical factors such as declining cognitive status, inadequate dental care, sensory decreases, physical fatigue, and limited mobility also add to the risks of malnutrition and dehydration. Because many frail older adults have therapeutic diets and multiple drug regimens, their nutritional state may be altered. It is important for the nurse to monitor the frail older adult for adequate calorie, protein, iron, calcium, vitamin D, and fluid intake.

Assessment tools that include a focus on physical, social, and environmental risk factors (Table 7-4) have been developed to monitor the older patient for poor nutritional status. In addition, it is important to review the medications the older adult takes because many medications affect appetite and, therefore, can affect nutritional status. Once the older adult's nutritional needs are identified, interventions can include home-delivered meals, dietary supplements, food stamps, dental referrals, congregate dining sites, home visits with registered dietitians, and vitamin supplements.

Older Adults With Chronic Illness

Daily living with chronic or persistent illness is a reality for many older adults. Although persons of all ages have chronic health problems, illness is most common in the older adult. It is estimated that 81% of Canadian older adults in the community live with at least one chronic condition and 33% of them live with three or more (Gilmour & Park, 2006). The most common conditions for older Canadians are high blood pressure (47%), arthritis (27%), and heart disease (19%) (Canadian Institute for Health Information, 2011). Other chronic persistent conditions such as diabetes, vision problems, and dementia also have a significant impact on health-related quality of life for older adults.

Chronic illness is composed of multiple health problems that have a protracted, unpredictable course. Diagnosis and the acute phase of a chronic persistent illness are often managed in an acute care setting, and all other phases of an illness are usually managed at home. The management of a chronic illness can profoundly affect the lives and the self-concepts of the patient and the family caregiver. Although health status refers to acute and chronic illness, it also includes an individual's level of daily functioning. Functional health includes activities of daily living (ADLs), such as bathing, dressing, eating, toileting, and transfer. Instrumental activities of daily living (IADLs), such as using a telephone, shopping, preparing food, housekeeping, doing laundry, arranging transportation, taking medications, and handling finances, are also included in a functional health assessment.

As age increases, a pattern of declining functional health and increasing disability is seen. Nurses caring for the older adult need to advocate for appropriate, comprehensive assessment in which health and disease states are diagnosed accurately as well as for the utilization of health promotion strategies.

Treatment for chronic conditions can often cause new problems. As one disease is treated, another may be affected. For example, the use of a drug with anticholinergic properties, such as a tricyclic antidepressant, may cause urinary retention (e.g., amitriptyline [Elavil]). In the older adult, disease symptoms are atypical and sometimes silent, that is, asymptomatic. For example, the only symptom of cardiac disease may be fatigue. Pathologies with similar symptoms are often confused. Negative consequences of chronic illness include physical suffering, loss, worry, grief, depression, functional impairment, and increased dependence (Lundman & Jansson, 2007). Daily living with chronic illness can be very difficult for the older adult. The nurse must involve the patient in any decision making related to interventions, goals planning, and quality of life and well-being (Table 7-5).

Table 7-5 Supportive Interventions for Older Adults With Chronic Illness

- Prevent social isolation.
- Control symptoms of the chronic illness.
- Adjust to changes in the course of the disease.
- Prevent and manage episodes of acute illness.
- Carry out prescribed therapies for the chronic illness.
- Use technology to enhance function, independence, and safety.

Socially Isolated Older Adults

As people age and social networks contract, they may become increasingly isolated and lonely. Although social isolation and loneliness are related factors, they are distinctly different concepts. Social isolation is defined as being separated from one's environment to the point of having few satisfying and rewarding relationships. Loneliness, conversely, is one's feeling of dissatisfaction with social contacts in terms of quantity or quality, or both (Cloutier-Fisher & Kobayashi, 2009). Thus, the feeling of loneliness can be present even if the older person is living with someone—with family or in an institution. It is the quality of the social contacts that is critical to the maintenance of well-being and hardiness.

Both social isolation and loneliness have consistently been found to be associated with poorer physical and psychological health (Cloutier-Fisher & Kobayashi, 2009). Although many social, personal, and health factors are involved in social isolation and loneliness, it is difficult to predict which older adults are most at risk for poor health. Older adults who are isolated and lonely should be closely monitored. Keeping these vulnerable older adults engaged in meaningful social relationships and activities is a significant health-promoting intervention, and nurses have an important role to play.

Culturally Competent Care for Older Adults. The term **ethnogeriatrics** is used to describe the specialty area of providing culturally competent care to older people who are identified with a particular ethnic group (Touhy et al., 2011) (Figure 7-2). Canada is officially a multicultural society, and cultural diverse care is an absolute must in order to provide for the needs of a very diverse group of older adults. Vast differences or heterogeneity are found among and within various ethnic groups related to health beliefs and practices, access and utilization of health care, health risks, family dynamics and caregiving, decision-making process and priorities, and responses to interventions and changes in health care policies (McBride & Lewis, 2004). Nurses

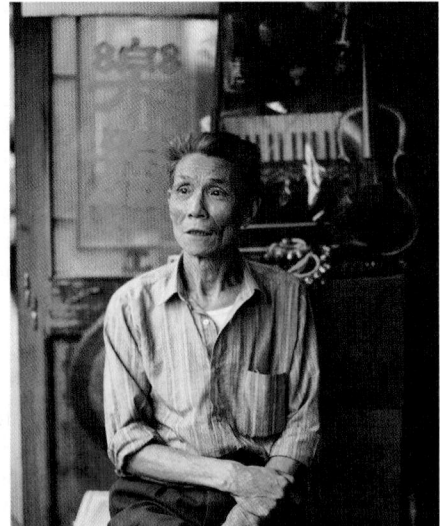

Figure 7-2 Culture and heritage can be important facets of many older adults' lives.

Source: © 2011 JupiterImages Corporation.

are challenged to provide culturally competent care in all types of settings and communities: home care settings, institutionalized settings, day programs, and acute and chronic health care facilities. Whereas it is unrealistic to expect a health provider to be proficient in working with every category and subgroups of minority older persons, it is possible to develop levels of awareness, skills, and sensitivity that can be applied to interactions with ethnic minority older persons and their families. Effective nurses develop cultural competence through knowledge about **ethnicity,** culture, language, and health belief systems and develop the skills needed to optimize intercultural communication (College of Nurses of Ontario [CNO], 2009). The nurse must assess each older adult's ethnic orientation. Several tools or instruments can assist nurses in eliciting health care beliefs and help identify one's perceptions of alternative beliefs (Touhy et al., 2011). Culturally competent care is discussed in Chapter 2.

Social Support and the Older Adult

Social support is essential for all older adults to maintain their level of well-being. Social support occurs at three levels. Family and kinship relations are most often the first level of providers of social support. Second, a semiformal level of support is found in clubs, places of worship, neighbourhoods, and senior citizen centres. Third, the older adult may be linked to a formal system of social welfare agencies, health facilities, and government support. Generally, the nurse is part of the formal support system.

Caregivers

A caregiver is someone who provides supervision and direct care and coordinates services. In 2007, 2.7 million Canadians provided unpaid care to an older adult. About 70% of care is provided to a close family member (Cranswick & Dosman, 2008). Caregiving includes many tasks but focuses mostly on assisting the older person with ADLs and IADLs, providing emotional and social support, and managing health care.

Caregivers often experience their caregiving as rewarding, yet it can also be a physically and emotionally demanding task, even leading to increased medical illnesses and a greater risk of mortality for the caregiver (Zarit, 2006) (Table 7-6).

Some caregivers may develop a sense of being overwhelmed and have feelings of inadequacy, powerlessness, and depression (Kim, Chang, Rose, & Kim, 2011). The stress of caregiving may result in emotional problems such as depression, anger, and resentment. The burden of caregiving separates the individual from others who provide social, emotional, and interactional

Table 7-6 Caregiver Challenges

- Lack of respite or relief from caregiving
- Conflict in the family unit related to decisions about caregiving
- Lack of understanding of the time and energy needed for caregiving
- Inability to meet personal self-care needs, such as socialization and rest
- Inadequate information about specific tasks of caregiving, such as bathing or drug administration
- Financial depletion of resources as a result of a caregiver's inability to work and the increased cost of care

involvement. Time commitments, fatigue, and at times, socially inappropriate behaviours of the dependent older adult contribute to social isolation. The socially isolated caregiver must be identified, and plans should be designed to meet his or her needs for social support and interaction.

Many family members involved in direct caregiving activities also identify rewards associated with this role. Positive aspects of caregiving include knowing that a loved one is receiving good care (often in a home environment), learning and mastering new tasks, and finding opportunities for intimacy. At the same time, the tasks involved in caregiving often provide opportunities for family members to gain greater insights into one another and strengthen their relationships.

The nurse should consider the caregiver as a patient and plan interventions to reduce caregiver strain if necessary. The nurse should communicate a sense of empathy to the caregiver while allowing discussion about the burdens and joys of caregiving. The caregiver can be taught about age-related changes and diseases and specific caregiving techniques. The nurse can also assist the caregiver in seeking help from the formal social support system regarding matters such as respite care, housing, health coverage, and finances. Finally, the nurse should monitor the caregiver for indications of declining health, emotional distress, and caregiver role strain.

Elder Mistreatment and Abuse

Elder abuse can be defined as "any action by someone in a relationship of trust that results in harm or distress to an older person. Neglect is a lack of action by that person in a relationship of trust with the same result" (Seniors Canada, 2009, p. 2). The term **elder mistreatment (EM)** is used to describe acts of commission (elder abuse) or omission (**elder neglect**) that harm or threaten to harm an older adult's health or welfare. An older person may experience more than one form of abuse (Table 7-7). Elder abuse may occur in private homes, when the older person lives alone or with other persons, or in assisted living and any type of health care facilities. Institutional abuse refers to abuse of persons living in LTC homes and residential care facilities.

Overall, EM is an underreported problem and has been difficult to quantify. Estimates of abuse range from 4 to 10% of older Canadians (National Seniors Council, 2007). In a recent Canadian survey, 22% of respondents said they knew an older person who may be experiencing abuse (Environics Research Group, 2008). In the same study, 5% of older respondents said they had experienced abuse. Lack of reporting by victims often stems from the older adult's isolation; impaired cognitive or physical function; feelings of shame, embarrassment, guilt, or self-blame; fear of reprisal; pressure from family members; fear of losing the home and independence; and cultural norms. Lack of reporting by health care providers may be because of lack of confidence in identifying or reporting victims of EM; perceived inability to successfully intervene; and a desire to avoid responsibility for further action. The majority of victims of EM are mentally able women and most abuse is committed by family members (Wahl, 2008). The most common forms of elder abuse are financial abuse and emotional abuse (Centre for Addiction and Mental Health [CAMH], 2008).

The primary risk factors for EM are the characteristics of the abuser. Abusers tend to be adult children who are dependent on the parent for housing and financial means; have a history of violence or antisocial behaviour; are unemployed; and are disabled because of substance abuse or mental illness, or both

Table 7-7 Types of Elder Mistreatment

TYPES	CHARACTERISTICS	MANIFESTATIONS
Physical abuse	Slapping, striking; restraining; incorrect positioning; oversedation with medications	Bruises, bilateral injuries (ankles, wrists), repeated injuries in various stages of healing, oversedation; use of several emergency departments
Physical neglect	Withholding of food, water, medications, clothing, hygiene; failure to provide physical aids such as dentures, eyeglasses, hearing aid; failure to ensure safety	Pressure ulcers on sacral area, heels; loss of body weight; laboratory values showing dehydration (e.g., HCT; serum sodium), malnutrition (serum protein); poor personal hygiene
Psychological or emotional abuse	Berating verbally; harassment; intimidation, threats of punishment or deprivation; treating patient like a child; isolation	Depression, withdrawn behaviour; agitation; ambivalent attitude toward caregiver or family member
Psychological or emotional neglect	Failing to provide social stimulation; leaving alone for long periods; failing to provide companionship	Depression, withdrawn behaviour; agitation; ambivalent attitude toward caregiver or family member
Sexual abuse	Touching inappropriately; forcing sexual contact	Unexplained vaginal or anal bleeding; bruised breasts; unexplained STIs or genital infections
Financial abuse	Denying access to personal resources; stealing money or possessions; coercing to sign contracts or durable power of attorney; making changes in will or trust	Living situation is below level of personal resources; sudden change in personal finances; sudden transfer of assets
Violation of personal rights	Denying right to privacy or right to make decisions regarding health care or living environment; forcible eviction	Sudden inexplicable changes in living situation; confusion

HCT, hematocrit; *STIs,* sexually transmitted infections.

(Department of Justice Canada [DJC], 2009). Victim characteristics, such as frailty, also add to the risk of mistreatment. Frailty increases the likelihood that an older person is unable to seek help or defend herself or himself.

When managing elder abuse, the nurse must be familiar with both federal and provincial laws governing reporting procedures and patient privacy. Information on mandatory reporting can be found on the Canadian Network for Prevention of Elder Abuse Web site.

Institutional EM occurs in LTC facilities as well as other housing situations where older adults receive care. Although the prevalence of institutional EM is difficult to estimate, the problem clearly does exist (Cooper, Selwood, & Livingston, 2007). The types of EM that can occur in institutions do not differ from community types, yet failure to follow the care plan is also considered a form of abuse. In addition, unauthorized use of restraints or use of medication or isolation as punishment is considered abuse. Individual risk factors for mistreatment of residents include frailty, dementia, immobility, and social isolation. Unfortunately, issues arising from the current issues in the health care system contribute to the risk faced by institutionalized older adults, such as insufficient resources and staffing and supervision problems.

The nursing approach to a suspected victim of EM should begin with a carefully taken history and examination for mistreatment. Nurses should assess the individual for the presence of dehydration, malnutrition, pressure ulcers, poor personal hygiene, and lack of compliance with the medical regimen. Key assessment findings include explanations for findings (e.g., injuries) that are not consistent with objective data or contradictory explanations between the patient and the caregiver. The nurse should follow the facility or agency intervention protocol for EM. A screening tool for abuse by a caregiver is available as a pocket tool from the National Initiative for the Care of the Elderly (NICE) (see the Resources at the end of this chapter).

Table 7-8 Nursing Management of Elder Mistreatment

- Mandatory report to the appropriate provincial or territorial body on the suspicion of abuse or neglect.
- Thorough assessment with precise documentation (including photographic documentation).
- Collection and preservation of any physical evidence (e.g., soiled or bloody clothing, bandages, sheets).
- Social services consultation.
- Implementing a safety plan (e.g., hospital admission) if the older person is in immediate danger.

Nursing assessment of the institutionalized older person is similar to that of a community-dwelling older person. In institutionalized settings, nurses should be alert to patterns of recurrent infections, poor hygiene, lack of interest in activities or eating, behavioural changes, new incontinence, sleep problems, and complaints about staff. Risk of mistreatment increases during the evening and night shifts when supervision is limited. Specific nursing interventions to reduce the risk of EM include close management of the patient's plan of care and regular review of the use of restraints and psychotropic medications in addition to the interventions listed in Table 7-8.

Universal Health Care

The older population requires specific consideration within Canada's health care system. With the growth in the older population and the associated increase in chronic health conditions, the health care needs of this population sector are greater than in other population segments.

The Canadian health care system is based on the *Canada Health Act* (1984) and is publicly funded. Health care is administered and delivered by the provinces and territories. The system is referred to by Canadians as "Medicare" and provides for universal comprehensive coverage for "medically necessary" services, including primary health care, care in hospitals, and surgical–dental services. Each province and territory determines which services are publicly funded, so there is significant variation among areas for "not urgent" services such as the provision of home care, LTC, medications outside of hospital, physiotherapy, optometry services, and other services. With the recent focus on Canada's health care reform, there has been increased advocacy for more realistic provision of health care for older adults, including an emphasis on health promotion and expanded community care (Health Canada, 2011; Hollander, Chappell, Prince, & Shapiro, 2007).

Care Alternatives for Older Adults

Most older adults prefer to age at home, but they may have to move to a more restrictive environment at a time of crisis. Several living arrangements and care options for older people are described.

Independent Living Options

Many older adults stay in their place of residence and do not move to a different home or geographic location as they age. The community becomes important to the older adult as an environment that is safe and that supports social contacts. The older adult needs privacy and companionship as well as a sense of belonging. The community should be accessible. The older adult may need housing assistance in the form of property tax relief and assistance with home repair and the cost of utilities (Figure 7-3). A variety of subsidized, low-income housing arrangements are available for older adults in many areas.

For the older adult who chooses to remain in the home as functional abilities decline, some home adaptations and modifications can be made to accommodate for some functional decline, including walker and wheelchair accessibility, increased lighting, and safety devices in bathrooms and kitchens. The *Safe Living Guide—A Guide to Home Safety for Seniors* (see the Resources at the end of this chapter) includes strategies for home adaptations that improve safety and accessibility.

Adult lifestyle communities or retirement communities may be an option for some older adults. These communities are age-segregated, self-contained developments and provide social activities, security, and recreational facilities. Some retirement communities offer expanded health care and social support services. An entrance fee and monthly fees for continuing care are charged. Chapter 6 discusses community-based care settings.

Assisted-living facilities (ALFs) are designed to provide housing and personalized health care. Because over half of community-based older adults require assistance with ADLs or IADLs, this is the most rapidly developing area of care. According to a Canadian Mortgage and Housing Corporation survey, up to 8.4% of Canadians age 75 years and older lived in 2,502 ALFs in 2010. Services vary per facility. Nurses working in this area are challenged by questions related to regulations, use of unregulated care providers, assessment to ensure safe "fit of resident to facility," and shared resident decision making. The Canadian Accreditation Council is developing standards for use in accreditation of ALFs (see the Resources at the end of this chapter).

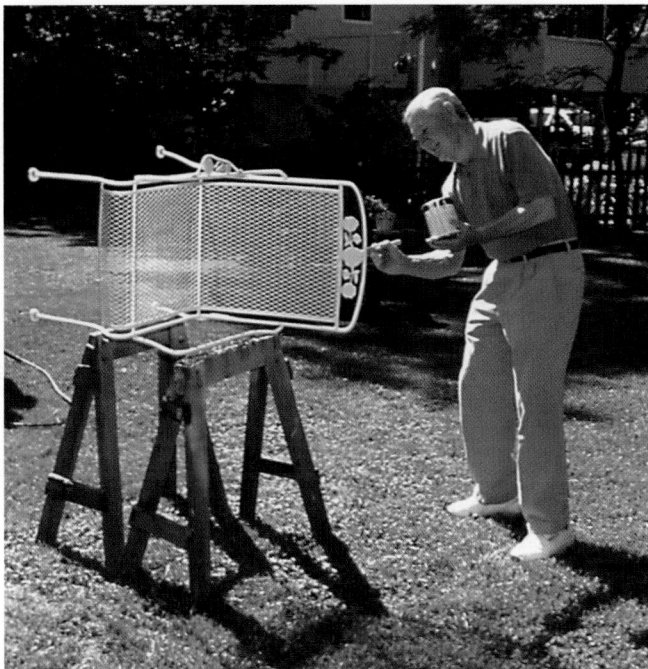

Figure 7-3 Home maintenance is part of an older adult's independent lifestyle.

Source: Rick Brady, Riva, MD.

Community-Based Care for Older Adults

Older adults with special care needs can often be served by services in the community, such as adult day care programs or home health care.

Adult Day Care Programs. *Adult day care (ADC) programs* provide daily supervision, social activities, and ADLs assistance for older adults who are cognitively impaired and/or for persons who have problems with ADLs. The services offered in the ADC programs are based on patient needs. Restorative programs offer health monitoring, therapeutic activities, one-on-one ADLs training, individualized care planning, and personal care services. Programs designed for people with cognitive impairments offer therapeutic recreation, support for family, family counselling, and social involvement. ADC programs provide relief to the caregiver, allow continued employment for the caregiver, and delay institutionalization for the patient. Centres are regulated and standards are set by the province. Costs are not covered by health insurance but are tax deductible as dependent care. The nurse's role consists of knowing the available ADC services and assessing the needs of the patient. The nurse can then help the patient and family in making a good decision.

Home Health Care. Home health care can be a cost-effective care alternative for the older patient who is homebound, yet has health needs that are intermittent or acute. Approximately 900,000 Canadians receive home care services at any given time; most of them are older than age 65 (Canadian Home Care Association [CHCA], 2008). Home health care services offer skilled nursing care and care by other regulated health providers, non-regulated workers, volunteers, friends, and family members, all to support the older adult to remain in the community. Chapter 6 discusses home health care in more detail.

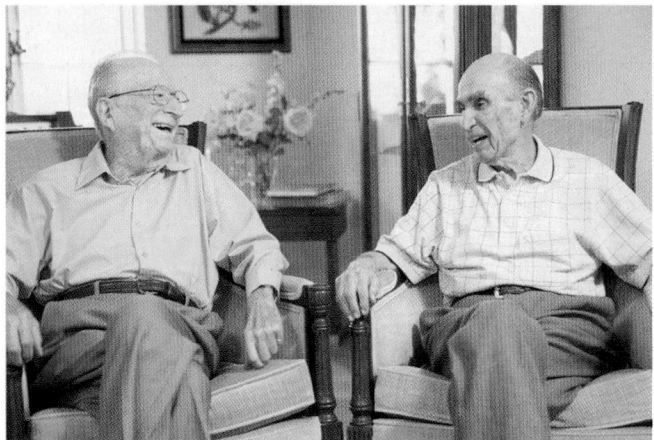

Figure 7-4 Social interaction and acceptance are important for older adults.

Source: © 2011 JupiterImages Corporation.

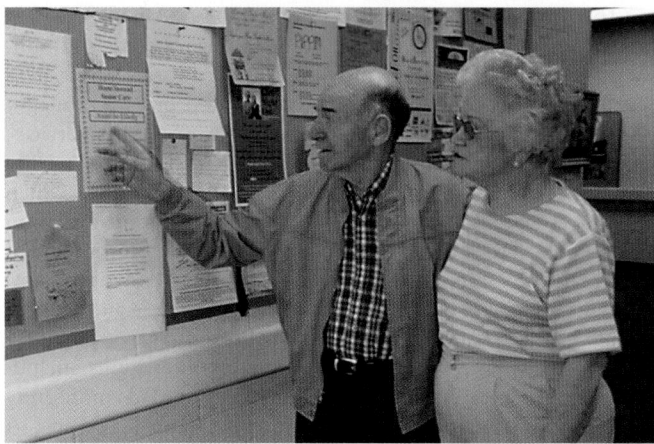

Figure 7-5 Some residential facilities for older adults post notices announcing when free legal help is available.

Source: Rick Brady, Riva, MD.

Long-Term Care Facilities

Long-term care (LTC) facilities are a placement alternative for the older adult who can no longer live alone, who needs continuous supervision, who has three or more ADLs disabilities, or who is frail. Three main factors precipitate placement in an LTC facility: (1) rapid patient deterioration, (2) caregiver inability to continue care, and (3) an alteration in or loss of family support system. Changes in orientation (e.g., increased confusion), incontinence, or a major health event (e.g., stroke) can accelerate placement.

Families and patients often experience guilt and anxiety when an LTC admission seems necessary. LTC homes have made important strides in implementing appropriate interventions to reduce the effects of this relocation, including involving the older adult in the decision to move, adequate visits and preparation before the move, welcoming and orientations when arriving in the new location, and a carefully developed care plan to address the patient's needs. Many LTC homes provide an environment that truly represents the best of caring and quality of life and an extraordinary commitment and dedication of staff. Several initiatives are under way to shift from an institutional model to LTC homes as places that nurture quality of life and well-being for older people (Figure 7-4).

Legal and Ethical Issues

Legal assistance is an issue for many older adults concerned about advance directives, estate planning, taxation issues, and appeals for denied services. In Canada, legal aid is available for all citizens (Figure 7-5). There is some variation between provinces and territories about legal matters affecting capacity, advanced directives, and consent.

Mental capacity is a person's ability to make decisions. It is a legal construct, not a clinical condition (Touhy et al., 2011). To be deemed capable of making a decision, the person must *understand* information that is relevant to making a decision, *evaluate* data, and *appreciate* the consequences of the decision or of not making a decision (Wahl, 2008). People are presumed to have capacity unless there is clear evidence to the contrary and the

person has been legally deemed incapable. Capacity can improve, decrease, or fluctuate (British Columbia Adult Abuse/Neglect Prevention Collaborative [BCAANPC], 2009; Wahl, 2008).

A *power of attorney* (POA) is a legal document and legal device in which one person designates another person (e.g., family member, friend) to act on his or her behalf.

There are primarily two types of advance directives: instruction directives and those that name a substitute decision maker or proxy (Canadian Nurses Association, 1998). An instruction directive (or *living will*) specifies what kinds of interventions are desirable for different health situations. In a proxy directive, the older adult specifies who is to make health care decisions if the person becomes unable to make his or her wishes known. Often, these two terms are used interchangeably; however, they serve different purposes (CNA, 1998). (Advance directives are discussed in Chapter 13.)

The nurse who works with the older adult will encounter areas of ethical concern that influence practice and care. Issues may include the need to evaluate the patient's ability to make decisions, resuscitation, treatment of infections, issues of nutrition and hydration, and transfer to more intensive treatment units.

These situations are often complex and emotionally charged. The nurse can assist the patient, the family, and other health care providers by acknowledging when an ethical dilemma is present, by keeping current on the ethical implications of biotechnology, and by advocating for an institutional ethics committee to help in the decision-making process. For more information, see the Resources section at the end of the chapter.

NURSING MANAGEMENT: OLDER ADULTS

Nursing Assessment

The assessment of the older adult provides the database for the rest of the nursing process; yet it is a complex undertaking. First, it is important to remember that older people may face any health problem with fear or anxiety and that the problem may present in an atypical manner. In addition, health care workers may be perceived as helpful, but institutions may be perceived as negative, potentially harmful places. The nurse beginning an assessment needs to establish a nurse–patient relationship by communicating a sense of concern and care by use of direct and honest statements, appropriate eye contact, and direct touch when appropriate. When beginning the assessment process, the nurse should attend to primary needs first, for example, ensuring that the patient is free of pain, adequately hydrated, and does not need to go to the bathroom. All assistive devices such as glasses and hearing aids should be in place. The interview should be short so the patient does not become fatigued. The nurse should allow adequate time to give information as well as to respond to any questions. The medical history may be lengthy and the nurse must determine what normal age changes are and which information is relevant. If possible, medical records and any current medications should be reviewed.

To truly assess an older adult, a comprehensive geriatric assessment is required. The focus of a comprehensive geriatric assessment is to determine appropriate interventions to maintain and enhance the functional and cognitive abilities of the older adult. This assessment is interdisciplinary and, at a minimum, includes the medical history, the physical examination, a functional abilities assessment, a cognitive assessment, and an assessment of social and financial resources. The interdisciplinary team may include many disciplines, but the minimum components include the nurse, the physician, and the social worker. After the assessment is complete, the interdisciplinary team meets with the patient and family to present the team's findings and recommendations.

Nursing assessment is a key component of the comprehensive geriatric assessment. Elements in a comprehensive nursing assessment include a history using a functional health pattern format (Chapter 3), physical assessment, cognitive assessment, assessment of ADLs and IADLs, and a social–environmental assessment. Evaluation of cognitive status is particularly important for the older adult because results of this evaluation often determine the patient's potential for independent living. Evaluation of the results of a comprehensive nursing assessment helps determine the services needed. A good match between needs and services should be the goal of the assessment. The nurse also collects data regarding community resources that are needed to assist the older person and her or his family to maintain maximal functioning.

The comprehensive nursing assessment should be based on instruments that are reliable, valid, and specific to the older adult. Several standardized assessment tools for gerontology are available and can be used depending on the purpose of the assessment and the status of the older person. Yet, often difficulties arise in the interpretation of the results of findings because of age-related changes and parameters that are not well defined for the older person. The nurse is in an important position to recognize and correct inaccurate interpretation of laboratory tests.

Nursing Diagnoses

With few exceptions, the same nursing diagnoses apply to the older adult as to a younger individual. However, the etiology and defining characteristics are related to age and are unique to the older adult. Table 7-9 lists nursing diagnoses that are seen in older adults as a result of age-related changes. The identification

Table 7-9 Nursing Diagnoses Associated With Age-Related Changes	
Cardiovascular System	**Nervous System**
• Activity intolerance	• Disturbed thought processes
• Decreased cardiac output	• Disturbed sensory perception
• Fatigue	• Hyperthermia
Reproductive System	• Hypothermia
• Disturbed body image	**Urinary System**
• Ineffective sexuality patterns	• Deficient fluid volume
• Sexual dysfunction	• Impaired urinary elimination
Respiratory System	**Senses**
• Impaired gas exchange	• Disturbed body image
• Ineffective airway clearance	• Impaired verbal communication
• Ineffective breathing pattern	• Social isolation
• Risk for aspiration	**Musculoskeletal System**
• Risk for infection	• Impaired physical mobility
Gastrointestinal System	• Chronic pain
• Constipation	• Risk for injury
• Imbalanced nutrition	• Self-care deficit
• Impaired oral mucous membrane	• Sedentary lifestyle
• Integumentary System	**Immune System**
• Impaired skin integrity	• Risk of infection

and management of nursing diagnoses result in higher-quality care and improved patient function.

Planning

When setting goals with the older adult, the nurse must identify the patient's strengths and abilities. Caregivers, if appropriate, should be included in goal development. Personal characteristics such as hardiness, persistence, and the ability to learn contribute to the setting of individualized goals. Priority goals for the older adult may be focused on well-being, such as gaining a sense of control, feeling safe, and reducing stress.

Nursing Implementation

When carrying out a plan of action, the nurse may have to modify the approach and techniques used according to the physical and cognitive status of the older patient. Sensory changes, such as auditory and visionary deficits may interfere with communication. Small body size, common in the frail older adult, may necessitate the use of pediatric equipment (e.g., blood pressure cuff). Bone and joint changes often necessitate assistance with transfers, altered positioning, and use of gait belts and lift devices. The older adult with declining energy reserves may require additional time to complete tasks. A slower pace of interaction, more limited scheduling of interventions and activities, and the use of a bedside commode or other adaptive equipment may be necessary.

Cognitive impairment, if present, calls for careful explanations and a calm approach to avoid producing anxiety in the patient. Depression can result in apathy, malnutrition, and a decline in mobility. Several guidelines and interventions are available to enhance nursing care for people with cognitive impairment (Capezuti, Zwicker, Mezey, et al., 2007; Touhy et al., 2011).

Health Promotion

Health promotion and prevention of health problems in the older adult is one of the most important areas for nurses and is mainly geared toward three areas: reduction in diseases, increased participation in health promotion activities, and targeted services that reduce health hazards. The Division of Aging and Seniors of the PHAC provides federal leadership on health issues affecting older adults, including fall prevention, emergency preparedness, and services in remote communities (PHAC, 2011).

Within gerontology, nurses need to place a high value on health promotion and positive health behaviours. Several programs have been successfully developed for chronic health condition screening, smoking cessation, geriatric foot care, vision and hearing screening, stress reduction, exercise programs, drug usage, crime prevention, elder mistreatment, delirium prevention and treatment and home hazards assessment (RNAO, 2011). The nurse can carry out and teach the older adults about the need for specific preventive services. The nurse interested in older adult health promotion can reference Health Canada's "Healthy Living" Web page (see the Resources at the end of this chapter).

Health promotion and prevention can be included in nursing interventions at any location where nurses and older adult interact and at any level of care delivery. The nurse can use health promotion activities to strengthen self-care, increase personal responsibility for health, and increase independent functioning that will enhance the older adult's well being (Figure 7-6).

Teaching Older Adults.
Throughout the continuum of care, nurses are involved in instructing and teaching the older adult specific self-care practices to enhance health and well-being and modify disease processes (Table 7-10). Individual patient teaching is discussed in Chapter 4.

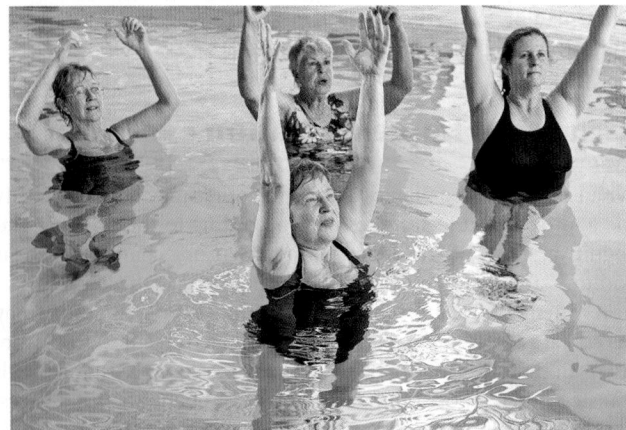

Figure 7-6 Water aerobics is an example of a health promotion activity for older adults.

Source: © 2001 JupiterImages Corporation.

Acute Care Settings

When an emergency arises, and the person cannot be cared for at home or in the ALF, admittance to an acute care hospital might be necessary. Some conditions that might require hospitalization include exacerbations of chronic conditions, stroke, fluid and electrolyte imbalances, pneumonia, and trauma caused by falls. Unfortunately, the complexity of the acute situation often results in the loss of the whole-person perspective and focuses the care only on the diseased part. Nurses' integrated approach and emphasis on individualized care are primordial to restoring an older adult's health and well being within this setting.

Care of the older adult requires an interdisciplinary approach including very succinct nursing components (Table 7-11). Involvement of the patient and the family is essential is supporting the individualized perspective and creating a social support network for when the older adult is discharged.

Geriatric Rehabilitation.
Geriatric rehabilitation interventions are focused on adapting to a new situation or recovering from trauma. Collaborative and interdisciplinary teams focus on building up functional reserve and emotional wellness, using appropriate assistive equipment and supportive personal care, and creating a supportive network in which the older adult can live as independently as possible. The older adult can receive

PATIENT & CAREGIVER TEACHING GUIDE

Table 7-10 Older Adults

CHALLENGES WITH OLDER ADULTS	SPECIFIC STRATEGIES
• Time needed to learn is increased.	• Present material at a slower rate.
• New learning must relate to the patient's actual experience.	• Use visual aids when possible.
• Anxiety and distractions decrease learning.	• Use peer educators when appropriate.
• Lack of willingness to take risks and cautiousness decrease motivation to learn.	• Encourage participation of a spouse or family member.
• Sensory–perceptual deficits and cognitive decline make modified teaching techniques necessary	• Use simple phrases or sentences and provide for repetition.
	• Support the belief that change in behaviour is worth the effort.
	• Emphasize that a person is never too old to learn new things.

Source: Adapted from Rankin, S. H., Stallings, K. D., & London, F. (2004). *Patient education: Principles and practice* (5th ed.). Philadelphia: Lippincott.

Table 7-11 Care of the Hospitalized Older Adult

- Identify those patients at risk for iatrogenic effects of hospitalization.
- Plan and communicate discharge goals and assess needs as soon as a person is admitted.
- Involve interdisciplinary teams and providers who focus on the special needs of older adults.
- Conduct a comprehensive geriatric assessment and be aware of the complexity and interplay of several conditions.
- Involve appropriate community-based services (Chapter 6).

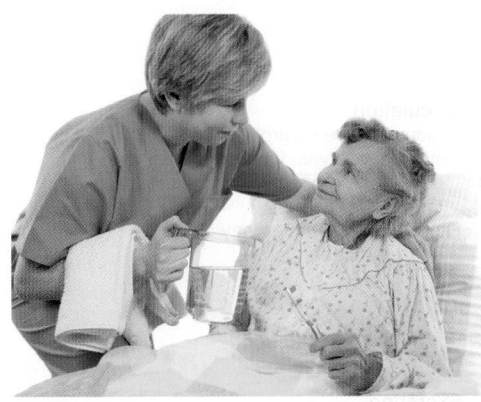

Figure 7-7 The nurse assists a patient in a geriatric rehabilitation facility.

Source: © 2011 JupiterImages Corporation

rehabilitative assistance through inpatient rehabilitation (limited days are covered), day programs, or home care programs (Figure 7-7).

Rehabilitation of the older adult is influenced by several factors. First, the older patient will show greater initial variability in functional capacity than an adult at any other age. Preexisting factors associated with reaction time, visual acuity, fine motor ability, physical strength, cognitive function, and motivation affect the rehabilitation potential of the older adult.

Within the interdisciplinary team, nurses assess and develop interventions for existing chronic illnesses, fears, and anxieties specific to falling; fatigue; sensory–perceptual deficits, malnutrition, and social and financial challenges. The older adult often loses functional ability in the acute care setting because of inactivity and immobility. This deconditioning can occur as a result of unstable acute medical conditions or environmental barriers that limit mobility. The older adult can improve flexibility, strength, and aerobic capacity even into very old age. The interdisciplinary team will develop passive and active range of motion exercises to prevent deconditioning and subsequent functional decline.

Last, the goal of geriatric rehabilitation is to strive for maximal function and physical and cognitive capabilities considering the individual's current health status. For example, a woman with a history of osteoporosis will receive a falls-risk appraisal and specific exercises to build stability and balance. The older adult patient with diabetes will receive a geriatric foot assessment and appropriate follow-up care.

Assistive Devices.

Using appropriate assistive devices such as dentures, glasses, hearing aids, walkers, wheelchairs, adaptive utensils, elevated toilet seats, and skin protective devices can greatly improve independency for the older adult. The need for and use of these devices will be assessed by the interdisciplinary team and findings will be included in the patient's care plan. Electronic monitoring equipment can be used to monitor heart rhythms, blood pressure, potential falls, as well as to locate the wandering patient in the home or LTC facility. Computerized assistive devices can be used to help patients with speech difficulties following stroke, and pocket-sized devices can serve as memory aids.

Safety.

Environmental safety is crucial in the health and independence maintenance of the older adult. With normal sensory age changes, slowed reaction time, decreased thermal and pain sensitivity, changes in gait and balance, and medication effects, the older adult is prone to accidents. Most accidents, such as trips and falls, occur in or around the home. The older adult's impaired thermoregulating system can cause hypothermia and heat prostration (hyperthermia).

The nurse and the care team can provide valuable counsel regarding environmental safety and changes. Measures such as enhanced lighting, coloured step strips, tub and toilet grab bars, and stairway handrails can be effective in "safety-proofing" the living quarters of the older adult. The nurse can also advocate for home fire and security alarms. Uncluttered floor space, railings, increased lighting and night lights, and clearly marked stair edges are some of the easiest and most practical adaptations.

In addition, the older adult who moves to a different location needs a thorough orientation to the environment. The nurse should repeatedly reassure the patient that he or she is safe and attempt to answer all questions. The unit should foster patient orientation by displaying large-print clocks, avoiding complex or visually confusing wall designs, clearly designating doors, and using simple bed and nurse-call systems. Beds should be close to the floor to prevent serious injury from falls. Lighting should be adequate while avoiding glare. Environments that provide consistent caregivers and an established daily routine assist the older patient.

Medication Use.

Medication use in the older adult requires thorough and regular assessment and care planning. The typical older adult fills an average of 35 prescriptions and over-the-counter medications and takes 14 different medications (Ramage-Morin, 2009). The frequency of adverse drug reactions increases as the number of prescribed drugs increases, and as a result, hospital admissions of older adults are often because of drug reactions.

Age-related changes alter the pharmacodynamics and pharmacokinetics of drugs. Drug–drug, drug–food, and drug–disease interactions all influence the absorption, distribution, metabolism, and excretion of drugs. Figure 7-8 illustrates the effects of aging on drug metabolism. The most dramatic changes with aging are related to drug metabolism and clearance. Overall, by age 75 to 80, there is a 50% decline in the renal clearance of drugs. Hepatic blood flow decreases markedly with aging, and the enzymes largely responsible for drug metabolism are decreased as well. Thus the drug half-life is increased in the older patient as compared with one who is younger (Gulick & Jett, 2008).

In addition to changes in the metabolism of drugs, the older adult may have medication-related difficulty resulting from malnutrition and dehydration, cognitive decline, altered sensory perceptions, limited hand mobility, and the high cost of many prescriptions. Common reasons for drug errors made by the older adult are listed in Table 7-12. **Polypharmacy** (the use of multiple medications by a patient who has more than one health problem), overdosage, or forgetting to take medications are recognized as major risk factors for adverse effects in the older adult (Ramage-Morin, 2009).

To accurately assess drug use and knowledge, many nurses ask their older adult patients to bring all medications to the health care appointment (including over-the-counter medications, prescriptions, herbal remedies, and nutritional preparations) that they take regularly or occasionally. The nurse and pharmacist can then accurately assess all medications the older adult is taking, including drugs that the patient may have overlooked or thought unimportant to include. Additional nursing

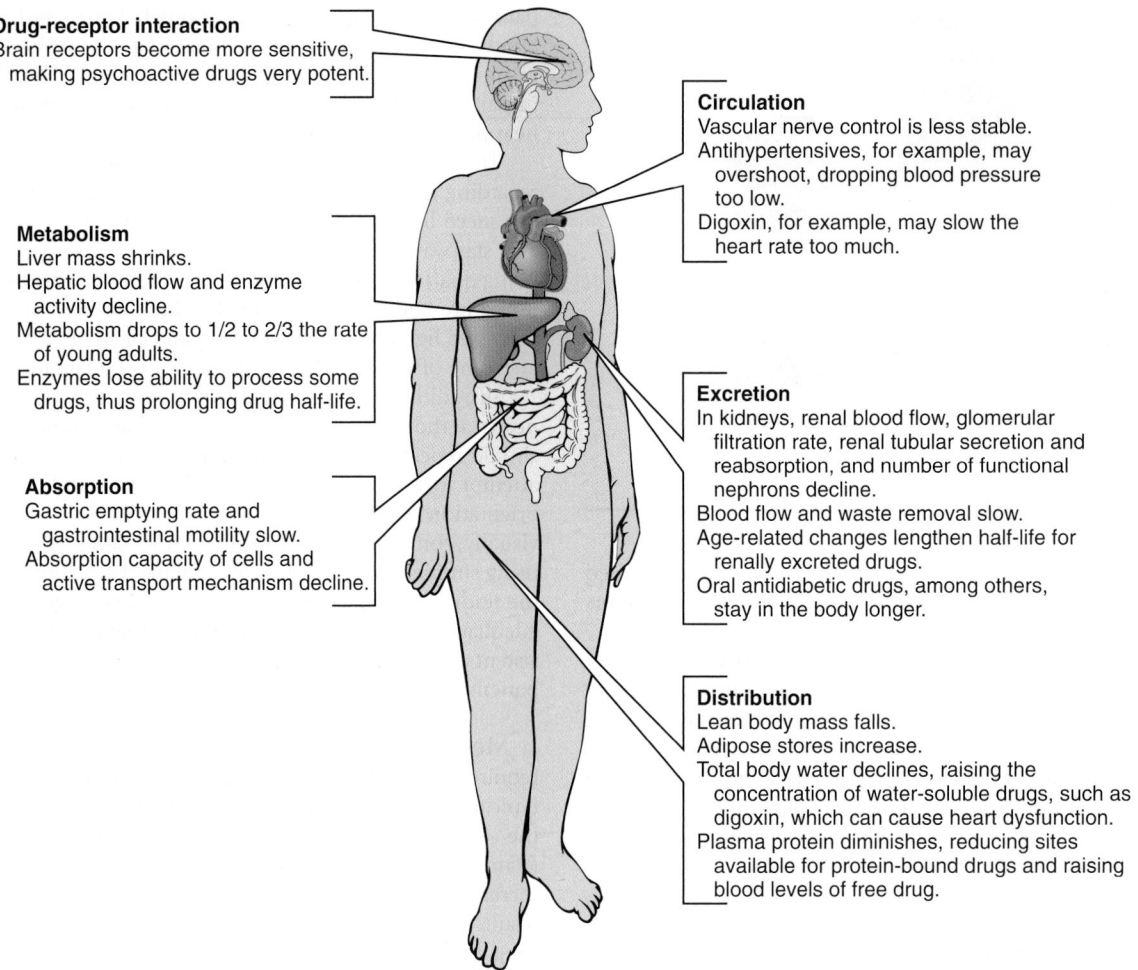

Drug-receptor interaction
Brain receptors become more sensitive, making psychoactive drugs very potent.

Circulation
Vascular nerve control is less stable.
Antihypertensives, for example, may overshoot, dropping blood pressure too low.
Digoxin, for example, may slow the heart rate too much.

Metabolism
Liver mass shrinks.
Hepatic blood flow and enzyme activity decline.
Metabolism drops to 1/2 to 2/3 the rate of young adults.
Enzymes lose ability to process some drugs, thus prolonging drug half-life.

Excretion
In kidneys, renal blood flow, glomerular filtration rate, renal tubular secretion and reabsorption, and number of functional nephrons decline.
Blood flow and waste removal slow.
Age-related changes lengthen half-life for renally excreted drugs.
Oral antidiabetic drugs, among others, stay in the body longer.

Absorption
Gastric emptying rate and gastrointestinal motility slow.
Absorption capacity of cells and active transport mechanism decline.

Distribution
Lean body mass falls.
Adipose stores increase.
Total body water declines, raising the concentration of water-soluble drugs, such as digoxin, which can cause heart dysfunction.
Plasma protein diminishes, reducing sites available for protein-bound drugs and raising blood levels of free drug.

Figure 7-8 The effects of aging on drug metabolism.

Table 7-12 Common Causes of Medication Errors by Older Adults

- Poor eyesight
- Forgetting to take drugs
- Use of nonprescription (over-the-counter) drugs
- Use of medications prescribed for someone else
- Failure to understand instructions or the importance of drug treatment
- Refusal to take medication because of undesirable adverse effects

DRUG THERAPY

Table 7-13 Medication Use by Older Adults

1. Conduct a medication reconciliation review with the physician and the pharmacist.
2. Emphasize medications that are essential.
3. Discuss medication use that is not essential or counterproductive.
4. Screen medication use using a standard assessment tool—including over-the-counter drugs, herbaceuticals, eyedrops and eardrops, antihistamines, and cough syrups.
5. Assess medication interactions.
6. Assess alcohol use.
7. Encourage the use of written or other medication-reminder systems.
8. Monitor drug dosage; normally the dosage should be less than that for the younger person.
9. Encourage the use of one pharmacy.
10. Work with health care providers and pharmacists to establish routine drug profiles on all older adult patients.
11. Advocate (with drug companies) for low-income prescription support services and generic substitutions.
12. Assess financial status and discuss which medications are essential to buy for the older person.

interventions to assist the older adult in following a safe medication routine are listed in Table 7-13.

Several medications are considered inappropriate or dangerous for older adults and are identified on the Beers (1997) list. This list has been recommended as a "best practice" by several Canadian regulating and professional organizations (see the Resources at the end of this chapter for the web link.)

■ **Depression.** Older people have often experienced multiple, simultaneous stressors, such as loss of loved ones, dealing with chronic illness, financial stress, social isolation, and many other stressors. For some older adults, the accumulation of these stressors can result in a mental health issue. The prevalence of mental illness is the same in older adults as in the general population (3-10%), except for a higher prevalence of dementia and delirium (Martens et al., 2007). Rates of depressive symptoms in institutionalized older adults are higher than in the community (Anstey, von Sanden, Sargent-Cox, & Luszcz, 2007). Unfortunately, depression is an underrecognized problem for many older adults.

Depression can exacerbate medical conditions by affecting nutritional intake, mobility, or drug regimens. The older adult who is at high risk for and/or exhibits depressive symptoms should be encouraged to seek treatment. Because a patient often feels unworthy and may withdraw and become isolated, the nurse may have to enlist the support of the family in helping the older adult seek treatment. Nursing assessment consist of observation of appearance and behaviour and examination of cognitive function, functional abilities, anxiety, adjustment reactions, depression, substance abuse, and suicidal risk. A comprehensive guide to assessment and treatment of depression in older adults is available at *http://ConsultGeriRN.org*

Specific interventions include nonpharmacological approaches and, if needed, pharmacological treatment. Depression is often reversible with prompt and appropriate treatment, and 60 to 80% of older people will improve with appropriate medication, psychotherapy and psychosocial interventions, or a combination of these (Kurlowicz & Harvath, 2007).

▧ **Sleep.** Adequacy of sleep is often a concern for the older adult because of altered sleep patterns. Older people experience a marked decrease in deep sleep and are easily aroused. In individuals older than 75, the percentage of sleep time spent in the rapid eye movement (REM) stage decreases. In addition, older adults have difficulty maintaining prolonged sleep. Although the demand for sleep decreases with age, older adults may be disturbed by insomnia and complain that they spend more time in bed but still feel tired. Older people often prefer to spread sleep periods throughout 24 hours with short naps that combined provide adequate rest. Other factors that contribute to sleep difficulties include medical problems, such as sleep apnea and restless legs syndrome, as well as effects of medications (e.g., furosemide [Lasix]). Many times, a later bedtime will promote a better night's sleep and a feeling of being refreshed on awakening.

▧ **Behavioural Management.** Patients with cognitive impairment often are confused and anxious during specific care situations (e.g., while showering) or when left alone. These people might respond with certain behaviours, such as wandering, trying to resist care, or pushing away the care provider. In addressing these responsive behaviours, it is important for the nurses to understand that the person with cognitive impairment is responding to a "perceived threat." Ignoring this behaviour and continuing the care task will only lead to the person becoming more anxious or scared and result in an exacerbation of this responsive behaviour. In caring for people with these behaviours, nurses need to understand *why* the patient is responding in such a way and intervene with competent and compassionate person-centred care.

The nurse should check for changes in vital signs and urinary and bowel patterns that could account for behavioural problems. It is important to use a relational approach with a focus on empathy and nurturing (RNAO, 2011) and to keep care assignments consistent. When the patient is agitated by the

Table 7-14 Evaluating Nursing Care for Older Adults
Evaluation questions may include the following:
1. Has there been an identifiable change in ADLs, IADLs, cognitive status, or disease signs and symptoms?
2. Does the patient consider his or her health and well-being state to be improved?
3. Does the patient think the treatment is helpful?
4. Do the patient and the caregiver think the care is worth the time and cost?
5. Can the nurse document positive changes that support interventions?

ADLs, activities of daily living; *IADLs,* instrumental activities of daily living.

environment, either the patient or the stimulus should be moved. Most responsive behaviours can be redirected by encouraging participation in activities such as holding a towel during the bath or exercising or walking when starting to wander. Reality orientation can be used to recall the patient to time, place, and person. A calming family member can be asked to stay with the patient until the person becomes calmer. The patient should be monitored frequently, and all interventions should be documented. An interdisciplinary approach is important in identifying the best redirective strategies. The use of evidence-informed nursing interventions significantly reduces the use of physical and chemical (drug therapy) restraints (Capezuti, Zwicker, Mezey, et al., 2007; RNAO, 2012).

▧ **Use of Restraints.** Restraints are physical, environmental, or chemical measures used to limit the activity or control the behaviour of a person or a portion of his or her body (RNAO, 2012). Devices such as seat belts, "geri-chairs," or side rails that cannot be removed by the patient are considered physical restraints, and it has been proven that these actually increase a person's risks for falls and injury (Capezuti, Wagner, Brush, et al., 2007). Chemical restraints are any form of psychoactive medication used not to treat illness but to intentionally inhibit a patient's particular behaviour or movement. Several researchers have indicated that antipsychotic medications have limited effectiveness and significant risks for older person with cognitive impairment (Capezuti, Zwicker, Mezey, et al., 2007; RNAO, 2012). Despite abundant research findings, chemical and physical restraints continue to be used in the care of people with responsive behaviours. Several Best Practice Guidelines outline alternatives for care (RNAO, 2011, 2012).

▧ **Evaluation**

The evaluation phase of the nursing process is similar for all patients. Evaluation is ongoing throughout the nursing process. The results of the evaluation direct the nurse to continue the plan of care or revise it as indicated.

When evaluating nursing care with the older adult, the nurse should focus on improving or maintaining the functional and cognitive status and the quality of life and well-being rather than on a cure. Useful questions to consider when evaluating the plan of care for an older adult are included in Table 7-14.

REVIEW QUESTIONS

The number of the question corresponds to the same-numbered objective at the beginning of the chapter.

1. What is the characteristic of ageism?
   a. Denial of negative stereotypes regarding aging
   b. Positive attitudes toward the older adult based on age
   c. Negative attitudes toward the older adult based on age
   d. Negative attitudes toward the older adult based on physical disability

2. Autoimmune diseases increase with aging. Which theory of aging accounts for this phenomenon?
   a. Immune theory of aging
   b. Programmed theory of aging
   c. Neuroendocrine theory of aging
   d. Intrinsic mutation theory of aging

3. Which of the following nursing interventions would promote a sense of self-worth for an ethnic older adult?
   a. Informing the patient about ethnic support services
   b. Allowing the patient to rely on ethnic health beliefs and practices
   c. Using an interpreter to provide explanations and teaching
   d. Emphasizing that a therapeutic diet does not allow ethnic foods

4. Which of the following nursing actions would be helpful to a chronically ill older adult?
   a. Avoid discussing future lifestyle changes.
   b. Inform the patient that the condition is stable.
   c. Treat the patient as a competent manager of the disease.
   d. Encourage the patient to "fight" the disease as long as possible.

5. When older adults become ill, which of the following are they more likely to do than younger adults?
   a. Complain about the symptoms of their problems.
   b. Refuse to carry out lifestyle changes to promote recovery.
   c. Seek medical attention because of limitations on their lifestyle.
   d. Alter their daily living activities to accommodate new symptoms.

6. What should the nurse know about caregivers?
   a. They may need the nurse to assist them in reducing caregiver strain.
   b. They are usually trained health care workers who do not live with the patient.
   c. They are generally strong and healthy but need teaching to carry out care activities.
   d. They are often reluctant to share the burden of caregiving with other family members.

7. For an older adult requiring constant assistance and living with an employed daughter, what is an appropriate care choice?
   a. Adult day care
   b. Nursing home care
   c. A retirement centre
   d. An assisted-living home

8. What is a characteristic of a living will?
   a. Legally binding
   b. Encourages the use of artificial means to prolong life
   c. Allows a person to direct her or his health care in the event of terminal illness
   d. Designates who can act for the patient when the patient is unable to do so for themselves

9. In promoting health for older adults, what is the primary focus of nursing interventions?
   a. Disease management
   b. Controlling symptoms of illness
   c. Teaching positive health behaviours
   d. Teaching the role of nutrition in enhancing longevity

ANSWERS: 1. c; 2. a; 3. a; 4. c; 5. d; 6. a; 7. a; 8. c; 9. c.

REFERENCES

Anstey, K., von Sanden, C., Sargent-Cox, K., & Luszcz, M. (2007). Prevalence and risk factors for depression in a longitudinal, population-based study including individuals in the community and residential care. *American Journal of Geriatric Psychiatry, 15,* 497-505. doi:10.1097/JGP.0b013e31802e21d8

Beers, M. H. (1997). Explicit criteria for determining potentially inappropriate medication use by the elderly: An update. *Archives of Internal Medicine, 157,* 1531-1536.

British Columbia Adult Abuse/Neglect Prevention Collaborative [BCAANPC]. (2009). *Vulnerable adults and capability issues in BC: A provincial strategy document.* Vancouver, BC: Canadian Centre for Elder Law. Retrieved from *http://www.bcli.org/ccel/publications/provincial-strategy-document-vulnerable-adults-and-capability-issues-bc*

Canadian Home Care Association (CHCA). (2008). *Portraits of home care in Canada.* Mississauga, ON: Author. Retrieved from *http://www.cdnhomecare.ca/media.php?mid=1877*

Canadian Institute for Health Information (2011). Seniors and the health care system: What is the impact of multiple chronic conditions? Retrieved from *http://secure.cihi.ca/cihiweb/products/air-chronic_disease_aib_en.pdf*

Canadian Mortgage and Housing Corporation. (2010). Housing market information: Statistics and data. Seniors' housing report and supplementary tables report (2010). Retrieved from *https://www03.cmhc-schl.gc.ca/catalog/productList.cfm?cat=160&lang=en&fr=1336920952910*

Canadian Nurses' Association. (1998). Advance directives; The nurses' role. ISSN 1480-9990. Retrieved at *http://www2.cna-aiic.ca/cna/documents/pdf/publications/Ethics_Pract_Advance_Directives_May_1998_e.pdf*

Capezuti, E., Wagner, L. M., Brush, B. L., Boltz, M., Renz, S., & Talerico, K. A. (2007). Consequences of an intervention to reduce restrictive side rail use in nursing homes. *JAGS, 55*, 334-341. doi:10.1111/j.1532-5415.2007.01082.x

Capezuti, E., Zwicker, D., Mezey, M., Fulmer, T. T., Kluger, M., & Gray-Miceli, D. (2007). *Evidence-based geriatric nursing protocols for best practice.* New York: Springer.

Centre for Addiction and Mental Health (CAMH). (2008). *Improving our response to older adults with substance use, mental health and gambling problems: A guide for supervisors, managers and clinical staff.* Toronto: Author.

Chahal, H. S., & Drake, W. M. (2007). The endocrine system and ageing. *Journal of Pathology, 211*, 173-180. doi:10.1002/path.2110

Cloutier-Fisher, D., & Kobayashi, K. (2009). Examining social isolation by gender and geography: Conceptual and operational challenges using population health data in Canada. *Gender, Place and Culture, 16*, 181-199.

College of Nurses of Ontario (CNO). (2009). Culturally sensitive care. Retrieved from *http://www.cno.org/Global/docs/prac/41040_CulturallySens.pdf*

Cooper, C., Selwood, A., & Livingston, G. (2007). The prevalence of elder abuse and neglect: A systematic review. *Age and Ageing, 37*, 151-160.

Cranswick, K., & Dosman, D. (2008). *Eldercare: What we know today. Canadian Social Trends, 86 (Catalogue 11-008)*, 48-56. Ottawa: Statistics Canada.

Department of Justice Canada (DJC). (2009). *Abuse of older adults: Department of Justice Canada overview paper.* Ottawa: Author. Retrieved from *http://www.justice.gc.ca/eng/pi/fv-vf/facts-info/old-age/pdf/OlderAdultsOverviewPaper.pdf*

Desai, K. M., Chang, T., Wang, H., Banigesh, A., Dhar, A., Liu, J.,…, Wu, L. (2010). Oxidative stress and aging: Is methylglyoxal the hidden enemy? *Canadian Journal of Physiology & Pharmacology, 88*, 273-284. doi:10.1139/Y10-001

Environics Research Group. (2008). *Awareness and perceptions of Canadians toward elder abuse.* Toronto: Author. Retrieved from *http://epe.lac-bac.gc.ca/100/200/301/pwgsc-tpsgc/por-ef/human_resources_social_development_canada/2008/001-08-e/report.pdf*

Fuente, M. D., & Miquel, J. (2009). An update of the oxidation-inflammation theory of aging: The involvement of the immune system in Oxi-Inflamm-Aging. *Current Pharmaceutical Design, 15*, 3003-3026. doi.org/10.2174/138161209789058110

Gilmour, H., & Park, J. (2006). Dependency, chronic conditions and pain in seniors (Catalogue no. 82-003). Supplement to Health Reports, Volume 16. Retrieved from *http://www.statcan.gc.ca/pub/82-003-s/2005000/pdf/9087-eng.pdf*

Gulick, G., & Jett, K. (2008). Geropharmacology. In P. Ebersole, P. Hess, & A. Luggen (Eds.), *Toward healthy aging: human needs and nursing response* (7th ed.). St. Louis: Mosby.

Harman, D. (1956). Aging: A theory based on free radical and radiation chemistry. *Journal of Gerontology, 11*(3):298-300. doi:10.1093/geronj/11.3.298

Hayflick, L. (1973). The biology of human aging. *American Journal of the Medical Sciences, 265*, 432-445.

Health Canada. (2010). *Canada's health and nutrition index: Health indicators.* Ottawa: Author. Retrieved from *http://www.hc-sc.gc.ca/fn-an/surveill/atlas/map-carte/index-eng.php*

Health Canada. (2011). *Canada's health care system (Medicare).* Ottawa: Author. Retrieved from *http://www.hc-sc.gc.ca/hcs-sss/pubs/system-regime/2011-hcs-sss/index-eng.php*

Hightower, J., Smith, M. J., & Hightower, H. C. (2006). Hearing the voices of abused older women. *Journal of Gerontological Social Work, 46*, 205-227. doi:10.1300/J083v46n03_12

Hollander, M. J., Chappell, N. L., Prince, M. J., & Shapiro, E. (2007). Providing care and support for an aging population: Briefing notes on key policy issues. *Healthcare Quarterly, 10*(3), 34-45.

Kennedy, S. R., Loeb, L. A., Herr, A. J. (2012). Somatic mutations in aging, cancer and neurodegeneration. *Mechanisms of Ageing and Development 113*(4), 118-126. doi:10.1016/j.mad.2011.10.009

Kim, H., Chang, M., Rose, K., & Kim, S. (2011). Predictors of caregiver burden in caregivers of individuals with dementia. *Journal of Advanced Nursing, 68*, 846-855. doi:10.1111/j.1365-2648.2011.05787.x

Kurlowicz, L., & Harvath, T. (2007). Depression. In E. Capezuti, D. Swicker, M. Mezey, T. Fulmer, D. Gray-Miceli, & M. Kluger (Eds.), *Evidence-based geriatric nursing protocols for best practice* (3rd ed.). New York: Springer.

Levasseur, M., St-Cyr Tribble, D., & Desrosier, J. (2009). Meaning of quality of life for older adults: Importance of human functioning components. *Archives of Gerontology and Geriatrics, 49*, e91-e100. doi:10.1016/j.archger.2008.08.013

Lookinland, S., & Anson, K. (2008). Perpetuation of ageist attitudes among present and future health care personnel: Implications for elder care. *Journal of Advanced Nursing, 21*, 47-56. doi:10.1046/j.1365-2648.1995.21010047.x

Lundman, B., & Jansson, L. (2007). The meaning of living with a long-term disease: To revalue and be revalued. *Journal of Nursing & Chronic Illness in association with Journal of Clinical Nursing, 16*, 109-115. doi:10.1111/j.1365-2702.2007.01802.x

Marin-Garcia, J. (2008). *Aging and the heart: A post genomic view.* New York: Springer.

Martens, P. J., Fransoo, R., The Need to Know Team, et al. (2007). Prevalence of mental illness and its impact on the use of home care and nursing homes: A population-based study of older adults in Manitoba. *Canadian Journal of Psychiatry, 52*, 581-590.

McBride, M. R., & Lewis, I. D. (2004). African American and Asian American elders: An ethnogeriatric perspective. In J. J. Fitzpatrick, A. M. Villaruel, & C. P. Porter (Eds.), *Annual review of nursing research*, (22nd ed.; pp. 161-214). New York: Springer.

National Advisory Council on Aging. (2006) Seniors in Canada: Report care. Retrieved from *http://www.intraspec.ca/rc2006_e.pdf*

National Seniors' Council. (2007). *Report of the National Seniors Council on elder abuse.* Ottawa: Government of Canada. Retrieved from *http://www.seniorscouncil.gc.ca/eng/research_publications/elder_abuse/2007/hs4_38/page00.shtml*

Public Health Agency of Canada (PHAC). (2007). *Age-friendly rural and remote communities: A guide.* Ottawa: Author. Retrieved from *http://www.phac-aspc.gc.ca/seniors-aines/alt-formats/pdf/publications/public/healthy-sante/age_friendly_rural/AFRRC_en.pdf*

Public Health Agency of Canada (PHAC). (2009). Who are Canadian seniors? Retrieved from *www.phac-aspc.gc.ca/seniorsaines/publications/public/variousvaries/papier-fed-paper/fedreport1-eng.php*

Public Health Agency of Canada (PHAC). (2011). *Aging and seniors.* Ottawa: Author. Retrieved from *http://www.phac-aspc.gc.ca/seniors-aines/index-eng.php*

Rak, J., Klement, P., & Yu, J. (2006). Genetic determinants of cancer coagulopathy. Angiogenesis and disease progression. *Vnitr Lek, 52*, 135-138.

Ramage-Morin, P. L. (2009). *Medication use among senior Canadians. Statistics Canada, Health Reports, 20(1) (Catalogue no. 82-003-X).* Ottawa: Minister of Industry.

Registered Nurses Association of Ontario (RNAO). (2011). *Nursing best practice guidelines.* Toronto: Author. Retrieved from *www.rnao.org/Page.asp?PageID=861&SiteNodeID=133*

Registered Nurses Association of Ontario (RNAO). (2012). *Nursing Best Practice Guidelines. Promoting safety: Alternative approaches to the use of restraints.* Toronto: Author. Retrieved from *http://rnao.ca/bpg/guidelines/promoting-safety-alternative-approaches-use-restraints*

Rozanova, J., Northcott, H. C., & McDaniel, S. A. (2006). Seniors and portrayals of intra-generational and inter-generational inequality in the *Globe and Mail. Canadian Journal on Aging, 25*, 373-386. doi:10.1353/cja.2007.0024

Seniors Canada. (2009). Elder abuse: It's time to face reality. Retrieved from *http://www.seniors.gc.ca/c.4nt.2nt@.jsp?cid=154#f*

Shay, J. W., & Wright, W. E. (2005). Senescence and immortalization: Role of telomeres and telomerase. *Carcinogenesis, 26*, 867-874. doi:10.1093/carcin/bgh296

Statistics Canada. (2007a). *Portrait of the Canadian Population in 2006, by Age and Sex, 2006 Census*. Retrieved from *http://www12.statcan.ca/census-recensement/2006/as-sa/97-551/pdf/97-551-XIE2006001.pdf*

Statistics Canada. (2007b). *A Portrait of Canada's Seniors: 2006.* Retrieved from *http://www.statcan.gc.ca/pub/89-519-x/89-519-x2006001-eng.pdf*

Statistics Canada. (2010). *Life expectancy at birth and at age 65 by sex and by geography*. Ottawa: Ministry of Industry. Retrieved from *http://www.statcan.gc.ca/tables-tableaux/sum-som/l01/cst01/health72a-eng.htm*

Statistics Canada. (2011). Ethnic Diversity and Immigration. Retrieved from *http://www.statcan.gc.ca/pub/11-402-x/2011000/chap/imm/imm-eng.htm*

Touhy, T., Jett, K., Boscart, V. M., & McCleary, L. (2011). *Gerontological nursing and healthy aging (1st Canadian ed.)*. Toronto: Elsevier Canada.

Turcotte, M., & Schellenberg, G. (2007). *A portrait of seniors in Canada*. Ottawa: Minister of Industry.

Vijg, J. (2007). *Aging of the genome. The dual role of DNA in life and death*. Novato, CA: Buck Institute for Aging Research. Retrieved from *http://www.ticklenotes.com/files/Neva0SmalleyGeriatricsLibrary/OxfordUniversityPressAgingoftheGenomeThDualRoleofDNAinLifeandDeath.pdf*

Wahl, J. (2008). *Who assesses capacity under what circumstances?* Toronto: Advocacy Centre for the Elderly. Retrieved from *http://www.advocacycentreelderly.org/appimages/file/Who%20Assesses%20Capacity%20-%20November%202008.pdf*

Xiaowei, S., MacKnight, C., Latta, R., Mitnitski, A. B., & Rockwood, K. (2007). Frailty and survival of rural and urban seniors: Results from the Canadian Study of Health and Aging. *Aging Clinical and Experimental Research, 19*, 145-153.

Zarit, S. H. (2006). Assessment of family caregivers: A research perspective. In *Family Caregiver Alliance, Caregiver assessment: Voices and views from the field, Report from a National Consensus Development Conference (vol. II)*. San Francisco: The Alliance.

CANADIAN RESOURCES

Canadian Accreditation Council
http://www.cacohs.com/
Canadian Association on Gerontology (CAG)
http://www.cagacg.ca
Canadian Centre for Elder Law
http://www.bcli.org/ccel
Canadian Coalition for Seniors' Mental Health: Guideline on the assessment and treatment of depression, delirium, dementia, and suicide risk in older adults
http://www.ccsmh.ca
Canadian Gerontological Nursing Association
http://www.cgna.net
Canadian Meals on Wheels and Senior Meals Programmes
http://www.mealcall.org/canada/index.htm
Canadian Network for the Prevention of Elder Abuse
http://www.cnpea.ca
Canadian Network for the Prevention of Elder Abuse Web site.
http://www.cnpea.ca/mandatory_reporting_table.htm
Canadian Patient Safety Institute: Several guidelines and strategies for medication safety
http://www.patientsafetyinstitute.ca/mobile/english/Home.aspx

Canadian Women's Health Network
http://www.cwhn.ca/indexeng.html
Elder abuse
http://www.seniors.gc.ca/c.4nt.2nt3col@.jsp?geo=&cid=161
Government of Canada—Seniors Canada On-line
http://www.seniors.gc.ca/index.jsp
Health Canada: Healthy Living
http://www.hc-sc.gc.ca/hl-vs/seniors-aines/index_e.html
Health Canada: Just for You—Seniors
http://www.hc-sc.gc.ca/hl-vs/jfy-spv/seniors-aines_e.html
National Clearinghouse on Family Violence—Abuse of Older Adults
http://www.phac-aspc.gc.ca/ncfv-cnivf/familyviolence/age_e.html
National Initiative for the Care of the Elderly
http://www.nicenet.ca
Oaknet Legal Resources by Province and Territory
http://www.oaknet.ca/node/112
Guide to Health and Social Services for Aboriginal People in Manitoba
http://www.wrha.mb.ca/aboriginalhealth/services/files/AHSGuide.pdf
Public Health Agency of Canada—Division of Aging and Seniors
http://www.phac-aspc.gc.ca/seniors-aines/index_pages/aboutis_e.htm
Promoting Awareness of Elder Abuse in Long-Term Care Homes (PEACE) pan-Canadian initiative
http://www.cnpea.ca/iaBPG%20Newsletter%20-%20EA%20final.pdf
Provincial and Territorial Resources on Elder Abuse
http://www.seniors.gc.ca/c.4nt.2nt@.jsp?cid=160
Public Health Agency of Canada: Medication matters: How you can help seniors use medication safely
http://www.phac-aspc.gc.ca/seniors-aines/publications/public/medication/med/index-eng.php
Public Health Agency of Canada: Reaching out: A guide to communicating with Aboriginal seniors
http://www.phac-aspc.gc.ca/seniors-aines/publications/public/various-varies/communicating_aboriginal/index-eng.php
Public Health Agency of Canada: The Safe Living Guide—A Guide to Home Safety for Seniors
http://www.phac-aspc.gc.ca/seniors-aines/publications/public/injury-blessure/safelive-securite/index-eng.php
University of Victoria: Cultural safety learning modules
http://web2.uvcs.uvic.ca/courses/csafety/mod1/index.htm
http://web2.uvcs.uvic.ca/courses/csafety/mod2/notes4.htm
http://web2.uvcs.uvic.ca/courses/csafety/mod3/
VON Canada Caregiver Connect
http://www.caregiver-connect.ca/en-us/caregiverconnectguide/CaregiverHealthInformation/Pages/Whatdoesitmeantobeafamilycaregiver.aspx

RELATED RESOURCES

Hartford Institute for Geriatric Nursing—see the excellent review of Beers Criteria for Potentially Inappropriate Medication Use in the Elderly in their "Try This" section
http://consultgerirn.org/resources

ⓔvolve *For additional Internet resources, see the Web site for this book at* **http://evolve.elsevier.com/Canada/Lewis/medsurg**

Stress and Stress Management

Written by **Sharon L. Lewis** and **Cory Shaw Retherford**
Adapted by **Patricia G. Yuzik**

LEARNING OBJECTIVES

1. Define the terms *stressor, stress, demands, coping, adaptation,* and *allostasis.*
2. Describe the three stages of Hans Selye's general adaptation syndrome.
3. Explain the role of coping in managing stress.
4. Describe the role of the nervous and endocrine systems in the stress process.
5. Describe the effects of stress on the immune system.
6. Describe the effects of stress on health and illness.
7. Describe coping strategies that can be used by persons experiencing stress.
8. List variables that may influence an individual's response to stress.
9. Describe the nursing assessment and management of a patient experiencing stress.

KEY TERMS

alarm reaction First stage of general adaptation syndrome, in which the individual perceives a stressor physically or mentally and the fight-or-flight response is initiated, p. 123

allostasis The means by which the body reestablishes homeostasis when faced with a challenge, p. 123

coping A person's cognitive and behavioural efforts to manage specific external or internal stressors, p. 128

coping resources Internal or external assets, characteristics, or actions that a person uses to manage stress, p. 128

emotion-focused coping A coping strategy that concentrates on methods of managing the emotional response to a problem, p. 128

eustress Stress associated with positive events such as winning an athletic competition, p. 122

general adaptation syndrome The three stages of physical response pattern to stress proposed by Hans Selye, p. 123

problem-focused coping A coping strategy that focuses on managing internal demands, external demands, or obstacles that create the demands, p. 128

psychoneuroimmunology Interdisciplinary science in which investigators seek to understand the interactions among psychological, neurological, and immune responses, p. 126

resilience Being resourceful and flexible and having an available source of coping and problem-solving strategies, p. 124

sense of coherence How a person views the world and his or her existence in it, p. 124

stage of exhaustion Final stage of general adaptation syndrome, which occurs when all the energy for adaptation has been expended, p. 123

stage of resistance Second stage of general adaptation syndrome, in which physiological reserves are mobilized to increase the resistance to stress, p. 123

stress A nonspecific response of the body to any demand made on it, occurring when individuals perceive that they cannot cope adequately with demands being made on them or their well-being is threatened, p. 122

stressors Stress-inducing demands, p. 122

ELECTRONIC RESOURCES

Supplemental content related to Chapter 8 can be found...

Evolve Web Site ⊝volve

http://evolve.elsevier.com/Canada/Lewis/medsurg
- Answer Guidelines for Case Study on p. 133
- Audio Lecture: Stress

- Clinical Reference: Laboratory Values
- Content Updates
- Electronic Calculators
- Examination Review Questions
- Glossary
- Key Points (Printable and MP3 Download)

Stress is a fact of daily living. It can have a positive or negative effect on the mind and body. Stress, especially if it is intense or chronic, is linked to numerous psychological and physiological disorders. Nurses play a very important role in helping patients manage stressful events. Anticipating potentially stressful situations, identifying stress, and implementing appropriate measures to minimize its effect is paramount in health promotion and disease prevention throughout life. Understanding the relationship of stress to physical and emotional health and how people cope with stress is the primary focus of this chapter.

Definition of Stress

Stress is a nonspecific response of the body to any demand made on it (Selye, 1983). Like pain or grief, it is a subjective condition: It is what the affected person says it is. Stress occurs when individuals perceive that they cannot adequately cope with demands being made on them or when their well-being is threatened (Lazarus & Folkman, 1984). These stress-inducing demands are known as **stressors** (Selye, 1983). What is perceived as stressful and the response to the stressor vary greatly among individuals and is influenced by a multitude of factors such as genetic makeup, life experience, family influences, and culture. This is demonstrated in the following examples:
- A woman becomes depressed and refuses to participate in normal self-care activities after a laparoscopic hysterectomy. In this situation, the removal of her uterus is a great stressor because the woman perceives it as a loss of her womanhood and femininity.
- A patient who is told she has type 2 diabetes reacts with a smile. However, the patient is relieved because for weeks she has been worrying that her symptoms were related to terminal cancer.

Many different events, factors, or stimuli can be thought of as stressors. They can be physiological or emotional–psychological (Table 8-1) and positive or negative. The key aspect of stressors is that they require an individual to adapt to a situation (Lazarus & Folkman, 1984). There are differences in the behavioural and physiological adaptive responses to a stressor that are based on the duration of the stressor (acute or chronic) and intensity of the stressor (mild, moderate, or severe). For example, an individual dealing with the chronic stress of caring for a loved one may also be exposed to a multitude of acute episodic stressors (e.g., car accident, influenza).

Daily hassles are experiences and conditions of daily living that are viewed as irritating, frustrating, and distressing. The frequency and intensity of daily hassles have a stronger relationship

Table 8-1 Examples of Stressors	
Physiological	**Emotional/Psychological**
• Burns	• Diagnosis of cancer
• Chronic pain	• Marital problems
• Birth of a baby	• Failing an examination
• Infectious diseases	• Inadequate financial resources
• Excessive noise	• Grieving
• Inadequate nutrition	• Prolonged period of caregiving
• Running a marathon	

with somatic illness than do major life events (Lazarus & Folkman, 1984). Examples of daily hassles are traffic, waiting, misplacing or losing things, deadlines, and planning meals. In contrast to hassles, *uplifts* are defined as positive experiences or temporary joys that are also likely to occur in everyday life (Lazarus & Folkman, 1984). Selye (1983) coined the term **eustress** to refer to stress associated with positive events such as the birth of a baby, going for a run, falling in love, or attending a much-anticipated event. Uplifts may modify the negative effects of daily hassles. Although studies of the effects of negative experiences (hassles or life events) are more plentiful, it is generally accepted that emotions such as laughter and humour are associated with healthy physiological and psychological functioning (Moore, 2008).

Work-Related Stress

Work-related stressors are common. Some demands are intrinsic to the job, such as poor working conditions, work overload, and time pressures. Other demands stem from the individual's role in the organization (e.g., role conflict), career development (e.g., underpromotion), relationships at work (e.g., difficulties in delegating responsibilities), and the organizational climate (e.g., restrictions on behaviour). The extensive research on these factors and their effects validates inclusion of occupation and work experience as essential factors in patient assessment. According to the 2003 Canadian Community Health Survey (Wilkins, 2007), 45% of Canadian health care professionals report significant job-related stress, in comparison to 31% of the general working population. Nurses and student nurses have been studied extensively as groups experiencing high levels of stress and burnout. Decreasing resources for managing increasing workload has been shown to be one of the most significant factors contributing to emotional exhaustion and burnout in Canadian nurses (Jourdain & Chenevert, 2010).

Theories of Stress

Three different but complementary stress theories have influenced most contemporary approaches to the study of stress. The current understanding of stress began with Hans Selye, who performed his research at McGill University in Montreal about 70 years ago. He conceptualized stress as a response to a demand or stressor that elicits a series of physiological changes to which the person must adapt. This process is known as *general adaptation syndrome* and is discussed in the next section.

According to a second stress theory, stress is a stimulus that causes a response. This theory originated with Holmes and Masuda (1966) and Miller and Rahe (1997), who developed a tool, the Social Readjustment Rating Scale, to assess the effects of life changes on health. The major assumption of this theory is that frequent life changes make people more vulnerable to illness. Life changes can range from minor violations of the law to the death of a loved one.

A third stress theory focuses on person–environment interactions and is referred to as the *transaction* or *interaction theory*. Proponents of this theory were Lazarus and Folkman (1984), who emphasized the role of *cognitive appraisal* (Figure 8-1) in assessing stressful situations and selecting coping options. They conceptualized cognitive appraisal as a judgement or evaluative process whereby the individual recognizes the degree of stress and its effect on well-being; this appraisal leads to the use of coping resources that respond to the demand placed upon them.

PATHOPHYSIOLOGY MAP

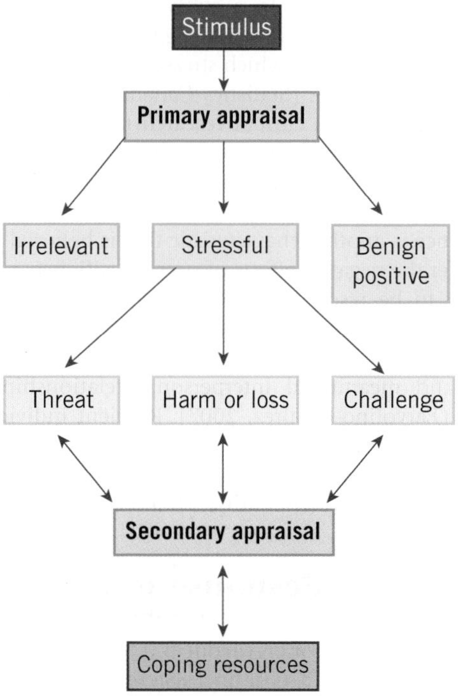

Figure 8-1 Cognitive appraisal process.

General Adaptation Syndrome

Selye's early research showed that stressors from different sources produced a similar physical response. He termed this physical response to stress *general adaptation syndrome.* **General adaptation syndrome** is composed of three stages: alarm reaction, stage of resistance, and stage of exhaustion. Once the environmental event or stressor stimulates the central nervous system, multiple responses occur because of activation of the hypothalamic-pituitary-adrenal axis and the autonomic nervous system.

The first stage of the stress response is the **alarm reaction** of general adaptation syndrome, in which the individual perceives a stressor physically or mentally and the fight-or-flight response is initiated (Figure 8-2). When the stressor is of sufficient intensity to threaten the steady state or homeostasis of the individual, it leads to a series of physiological changes that promote adaptation. This temporarily decreases the individual's resistance and may even result in disease or death if the stress is prolonged and severe.

Ideally, the individual quickly moves from the alarm reaction to the **stage of resistance,** in which physiological reserves are mobilized to increase the resistance to stress. At this time, adaptation may occur. The amount of resistance to the stressor varies among individuals, depending on the level of physical functioning, coping abilities, and total number and intensity of stressors experienced. For example, a person who has been exercising regularly and is physically fit has a greater ability to adapt to the stress of emergency surgery than does a person who is deconditioned and leads a sedentary lifestyle.

Although few overt physical signs and symptoms occur in the resistance stage in comparison with the alarm stage, the person is expending energy in an attempt to adapt. **Allostasis** is the process of achieving homeostasis in the presence of a challenge (Woods, Hall, Campbell, & Angott, 2008). When internal and external resources are adequate, the individual may successfully recover from a stressor and return to his or her baseline state. If homeostasis is not achieved, and if these allostatic responses do not terminate, adaptation does not occur, and the person may move to the final phase of the general adaptation syndrome.

The **stage of exhaustion** is that final stage. It occurs when all of the energy for adaptation has been expended. Physical symptoms of the alarm reaction may briefly reappear in a final effort by the body to survive. A terminally ill person who becomes alert and has stronger vital signs shortly before death exemplifies this. The individual in the stage of exhaustion usually becomes ill and may die if assistance from outside sources is not available. This stage can often be reversed by external sources of adaptive energy, such as medication or psychotherapy. Selye's research indicated that there is a predictable, uniform pattern in the physiological response to various stressors. This finding is attributable in part to the fact that Selye used animal models; such subjects were not capable of representing the complex psychological processing of a stressor.

Factors Affecting Response to Stress

Why do people respond differently to stress, and why do some cope better with stress than do others? Interestingly, some individuals experience significant adverse life events but do not succumb to the effects of stress. Factors that affect an individual's

PATHOPHYSIOLOGY MAP

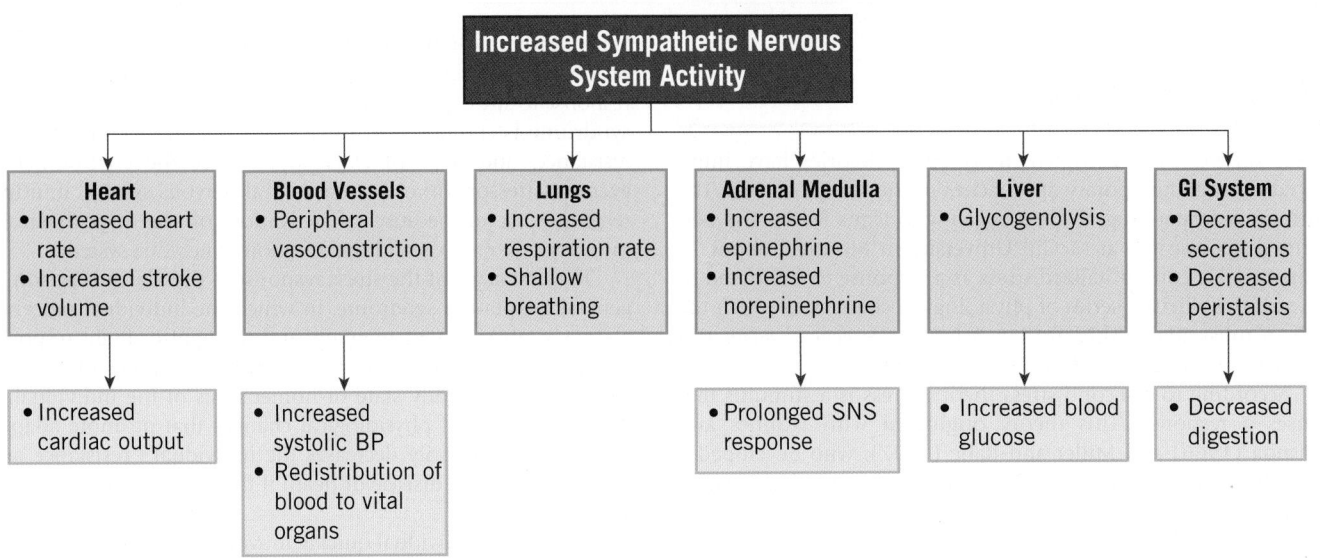

Figure 8-2 "Fight-or-flight" reaction. Alarm reaction responses resulting from increased sympathetic nervous system activity. *BP*, blood pressure; *GI*, gastrointestinal; *SNS*, sympathetic nervous system.

response to stress include internal and external influences, which underscores the importance of using a holistic approach in assessing the effect of stress on an individual.

In attempts to understand why some individuals do not experience negative consequences from stress, researchers have identified key personal characteristics, such as hardiness, sense of coherence, resilience, and attitude as possible factors that buffer the effect of stress. Psychologist Suzanne Kobasa first introduced the concept of *hardiness* in 1979 as a mediating factor in the relationship between stress and illness. She found that hardy people demonstrate commitment, challenge, and control by (a) possessing a clear sense of and commitment to personal values and goals, (b) viewing change as a challenge and opportunity for growth, and (c) believing in an internal rather than external locus of control (as cited in Mathews & Servaty-Seib, 2007). An *internal*

locus of control is the perception that the person's life is self-determined, as opposed to being directed by outside or external events, luck, or chance (an *external locus of control*). Hardiness is discussed in more detail in Chapter 5.

Sense of coherence, first described by Antonovsky (1987), is a concept closely related to hardiness and is thought to be a key determinant of health. Sense of coherence is reflected in an optimistic view of the world and perceived ability to function optimally in that world. An individual with a strong sense of coherence has an enduring tendency to see his or her life as ordered, manageable, and meaningful. In a study of older Canadians, the probability of healthy aging was significantly improved by a strong sense of coherence, which stresses the benefit of a positive attitude throughout life (Statistics Canada, 2004). This finding has been duplicated in current research that supports focusing health care efforts on factors to promote well-being, such as coping with stress, as opposed to focusing on the disease process (Wiesmann & Hannich, 2010).

Resilience is another characteristic that is believed to moderate or buffer the negative effects of stress. **Resilience** is defined as the ability to be resourceful, be flexible, and to recover from stressful situations and return to prior levels of functioning. A higher sense of purpose in life, self-determination, positive social support, and meaningful interpersonal relationships support resiliency (Earvolino-Ramirez, 2007). Resilient individuals tend to employ more effective coping and problem-solving strategies, possess higher self-esteem, and are less likely to perceive an event as stressful or taxing (Steinhardt & Dolbier, 2008).

Physiological Response to Stress

The following discussion is divided into descriptions of the nervous, endocrine, and immune systems. These systems, and thus the physiological stress responses, are interrelated (Figure 8-3). Stress activation of these systems also affects other systems,

PATHOPHYSIOLOGY MAP

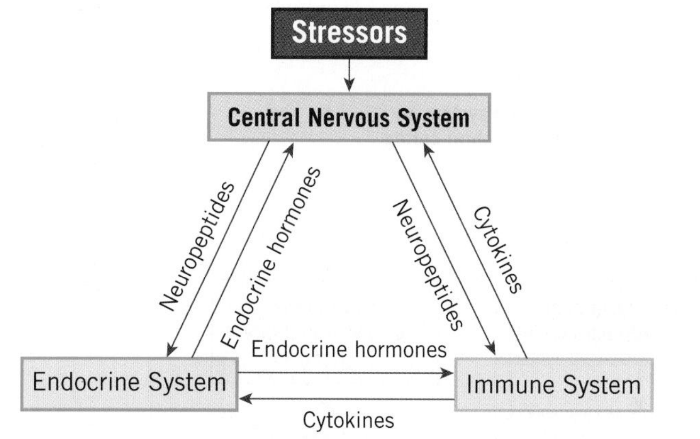

Figure 8-3 Neurochemical links among the nervous, endocrine, and immune systems. The communication among these three systems is bidirectional.

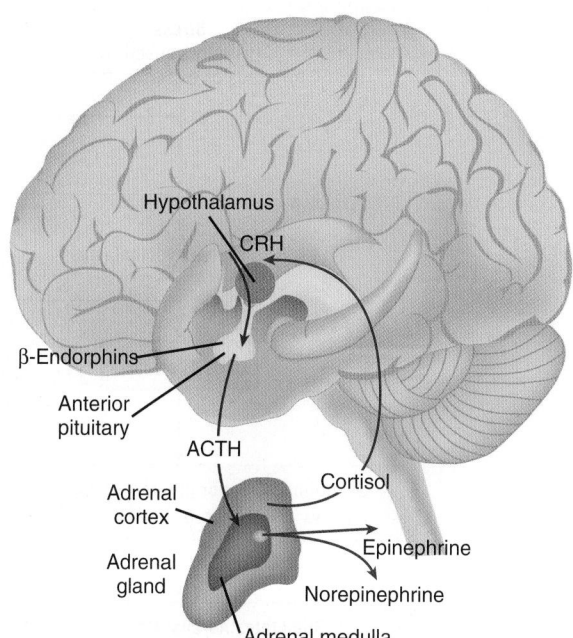

Figure 8-4 Hypothalamic-pituitary-adrenal axis. *ACTH,* adrenocorticotropic hormone; *CRH,* corticotropin-releasing hormone.

such as the cardiovascular, respiratory, gastrointestinal, renal, and reproductive systems.

The complex process by which an event is perceived as a stressor and the body responds is not fully understood. A person's response to a stressor determines the effect it will have on the body. In addition, the body responds physiologically to both actual (physiological) and perceived (emotional/psychological) stressors.

Nervous System

Cerebral Cortex. The cerebral cortex evaluates the emotional–psychological event (stressor) with reference to past experiences and future consequences and plans a course of action. These functions are involved in the perception of a stressor.

Limbic System. The limbic system lies in the inner midportion of the brain near the base of the brain. The limbic system is an important mediator of emotions and behaviour. When the limbic system is stimulated, emotions, feelings, and behaviours that ensure survival and self-preservation may occur.

Reticular Formation. The reticular formation is located between the lower end of the brainstem and the thalamus. It contains the reticular activating system (RAS), which is crucial to the state of wakefulness. When stimulated, the RAS sends impulses to the limbic system and the cerebral cortex, which produce arousal and emotional responses to the stressor. Chronic stimulation of the RAS can lead to sleep disturbances (McCance & Huether, 2010).

Hypothalamus. The hypothalamus, which lies at the base of the brain just above the pituitary gland, has many functions that assist in adaptation to stress. It is the central connection between the nervous and endocrine systems in the stress response. Emotional/psychological (perceived) stressors activate the limbic system, which in turn stimulates the hypothalamus. The hypothalamus sends signals via nerve fibres to stimulate the sympathetic nervous system. It also releases hormones that regulate the secretion of adrenocorticotropic hormone (ACTH) by the

anterior pituitary gland (Figure 8-4). Physiological (actual) stressors may originate in the limbic system or in portions of the brain that receive sensory information, which in turn then stimulate the hypothalamus (see Chapter 50).

Endocrine System

Once the hypothalamus is activated in response to stress, the endocrine system becomes involved. The sympathetic nervous system stimulates the adrenal medulla to release epinephrine and norepinephrine (catecholamines), which initiates a protective reflex called the *fight-or-flight response* (see Figure 8-2). This, along with the actual response of the body to the catecholamines, is referred to as the *sympathoadrenal response.* Stress activates the hypothalamic-pituitary-adrenal axis (see Figure 8-4). In response to stress, the hypothalamus releases corticotropin-releasing hormone, which stimulates the anterior pituitary to release pro-opiomelanocortin (POMC). Both ACTH (a hormone) and β-endorphin (a neuropeptide) are derived from POMC. Endorphins have analgesic-like effects and blunt pain perception during stress situations involving pain stimuli. ACTH, in turn, stimulates the adrenal cortex to synthesize and secrete corticosteroids (e.g., cortisol) and, to a lesser degree, aldosterone. The posterior pituitary increases production of antidiuretic hormone, which leads to water retention and a decrease in urine output (Figure 8-5).

Corticosteroids are essential for the stress response. Cortisol, a primary corticosteroid, produces a number of physiological effects that potentiate or blunt aspects of the stress response, such as increasing blood glucose levels, potentiating the action of catecholamines (epinephrine, norepinephrine) on blood vessels, and inhibiting the inflammatory response. The resulting increases in cardiac output, blood glucose levels, oxygen consumption, and metabolic rate enable the flight-or-fight response (see Figure 8-2). Dilation of blood vessels supplying skeletal muscle increases blood supply to the large muscles, which provides for quick

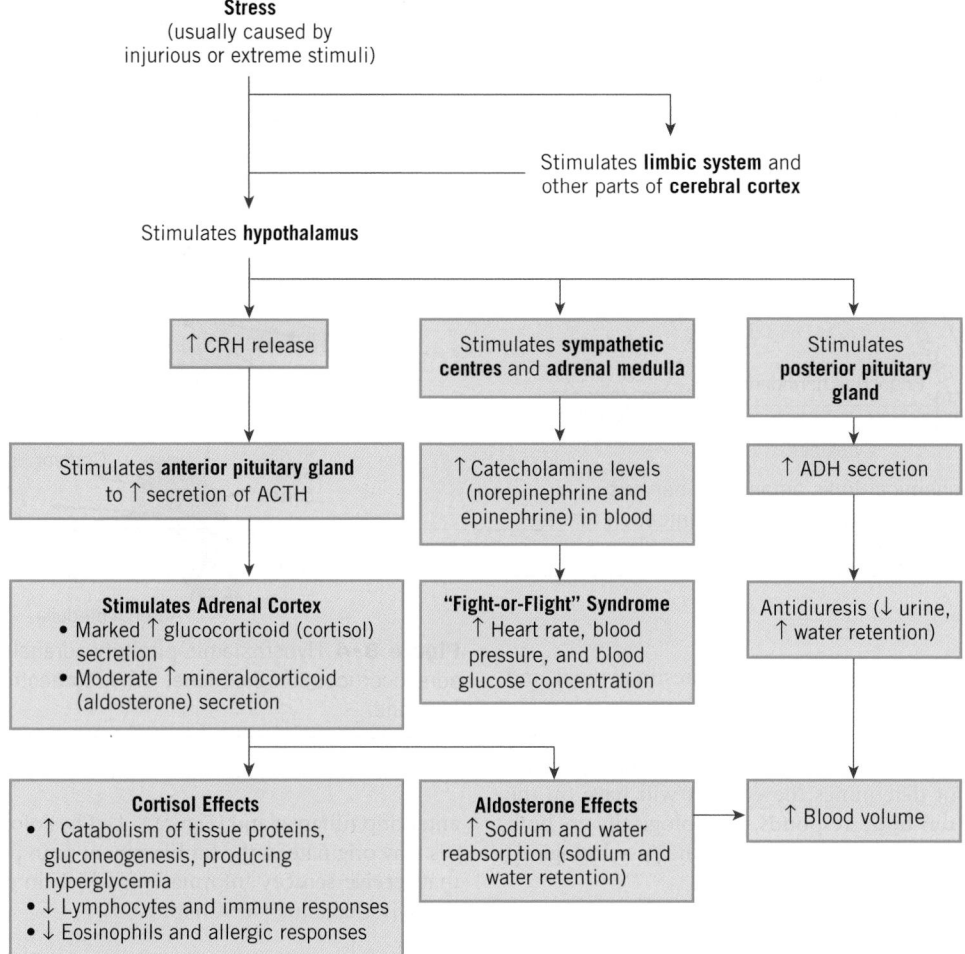

Stress
(usually caused by injurious or extreme stimuli)

Stimulates **limbic system** and other parts of **cerebral cortex**

Stimulates **hypothalamus**

↑ CRH release	Stimulates **sympathetic centres** and **adrenal medulla**	Stimulates **posterior pituitary gland**

Stimulates **anterior pituitary gland** to ↑ secretion of ACTH	↑ Catecholamine levels (norepinephrine and epinephrine) in blood	↑ ADH secretion

Stimulates Adrenal Cortex • Marked ↑ glucocorticoid (cortisol) secretion • Moderate ↑ mineralocorticoid (aldosterone) secretion	"Fight-or-Flight" Syndrome ↑ Heart rate, blood pressure, and blood glucose concentration	Antidiuresis (↓ urine, ↑ water retention)

Cortisol Effects • ↑ Catabolism of tissue proteins, gluconeogenesis, producing hyperglycemia • ↓ Lymphocytes and immune responses • ↓ Eosinophils and allergic responses	Aldosterone Effects ↑ Sodium and water reabsorption (sodium and water retention)	↑ Blood volume

Figure 8-5 Current concepts of the stress syndrome. *ACTH*, adrenocorticotropic hormone; *ADH*, antidiuretic hormone; *CRH*, corticotropin-releasing hormone.

movement, and increased cerebral blood flow heightens mental alertness. The increase in blood volume (which results from increases in extracellular fluid and shunting of blood away from the gastrointestinal system) helps maintain adequate circulation to vital organs in case of traumatic blood loss.

By mediating the inflammatory response, cortisol plays an important role in "turning off" aspects of the stress response, which if uncontrolled can become self-destructive. This is best exemplified by the suppression of proinflammatory mediators, such as the cytokines tumour necrosis factor and interleukin-1. The persistent release of such mediators is believed to initiate organ dysfunction in conditions such as sepsis. Thus corticosteroids act not only to support the adaptive response of the body to a stressor but also act to suppress an overzealous and potentially self-destructive response (McCance & Huether, 2010).

Summary of Neuroendocrine System Stress Response

In summary, the fight-or-flight response is a very important mechanism of the body for adapting to acute stress. This response is triggered by stressors, regardless of whether they are physiological or emotional–psychological. The acute stress response is a state of physiological and psychological arousal characterized by increased sympathetic nervous system activity that leads to increased heart and respiratory rate, increased blood pressure, increased muscle tension, increased brain activity, and decreased skin temperature.

Immune System

Psychoneuroimmunology is an interdisciplinary science in which investigators seek to understand the interactions among psychological, neurological, and immune responses (Segerstrom, 2010). It is now known that the brain is connected to the immune system by neuroanatomical and neuroendocrine pathways; thus stressors have the potential to lead to alterations in immune function (Figure 8-6). The network that links the brain and immune system is bidirectional, allowing for back-and-forth communication among these systems; therefore, not only do emotions modify the immune response but also the products of immune cells send signals back to the brain and alter its activity (see Figure 8-3). Much of the communication from the immune system to the brain is mediated by cytokines, which are crucial in the coordination of the immune response. For example, interleukin-1 (a cytokine made by monocytes) acts on the temperature regulatory centre of the hypothalamus and initiates the febrile response to infectious pathogens (see Figure 14-3).

Nerve fibres extend from the nervous system and reach synapses on cells and tissues (i.e., spleen, lymph nodes) of the

PATHOPHYSIOLOGY MAP

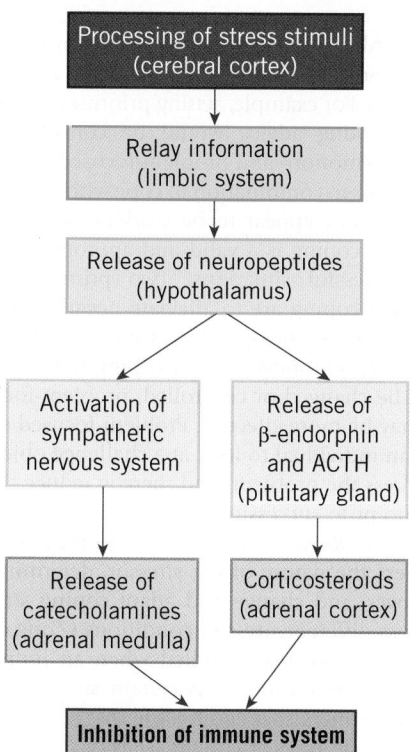

Figure 8-6 The psychological and neuroendocrine response to stress alters immune function. *ACTH*, adrenocorticotropic hormone.

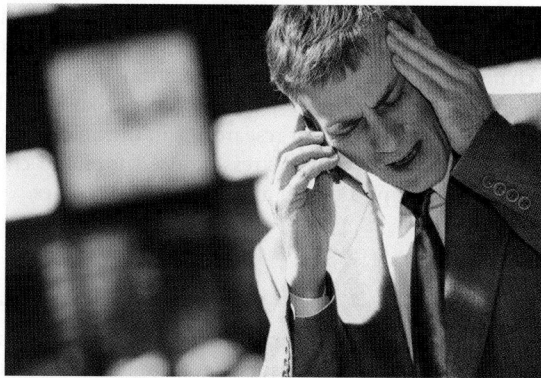

Figure 8-7 Chronic stress can take a toll on the body, resulting in poor concentration and memory problems.

Source: © 2011 JupiterImages Corporation.

Table 8-2 Examples of Conditions Associated With Maladaptation to Stress	
• Angina	• Insomnia
• Asthma	• Irritable bowel syndrome
• Depression	• Low back pain
• Dyspepsia	• Peptic ulcer disease
• Eating disorders	• Sexual dysfunction
• Headaches	

immune system. In turn, the cells of the immune system have receptors for many neuropeptides and hormones, which enable them to respond to nervous and neuroendocrine signals. As a result, the mediation of stress by the central nervous system leads to corresponding changes in immune cell activity.

Both acute and chronic stress can affect immune function. Acute stress stimulates increased proliferation of cellular immune components such as neutrophils and natural killer cells, which are the body's first line of defence against infection (Segerstrom, 2010). The stress response is designed to be beneficial, however, only for acute short-term stress. Chronic stress appears to have a negative effect on both the cellular and humoral (antibody) immune systems (Segerstrom, 2010). Immune responses may be either suboptimal and thus ineffective when needed or hypervigilant, producing chronic inflammatory states that exacerbate chronic stress and predispose affected persons to cardiovascular diseases (Chida & Hamer, 2008).

Effects of Stress on Health

Acute stress leads to physiological changes that are important to human adaptation and survival. However, if stress is excessive or prolonged, these physiological responses can be maladaptive and lead to harm and disease. When a person sustains chronic, unrelieved stress, the body's defences can no longer keep up with the demands. Over time, stress takes a toll (Figure 8-7) and plays a role in the development or progression of conditions related to maladaptation (Table 8-2).

Chronic and intense stress may have profound effects on brain structure and function, especially the hippocampus. The hippocampus plays an important role in long-term memory and other cognitive functions such as spatial learning. Chronic release of corticosteroids in response to stress appears to act in concert with certain neurotransmitters to produce hippocampal damage (Weiss, 2007). Studies in people who have endured traumatic events (e.g., domestic violence, childhood neglect, war) reveal decreased hippocampal volume, activation, and activity (Weiss, 2007). This is thought to explain the memory impairment/fragmentation and dissociation with the traumatic event that are common in posttraumatic stress disorder (Weiss, 2007).

Stress can affect cognitive function, causing deterioration in concentration, memory problems, sleep disturbances, and impairment in decision making. In addition, stress can cause a wide variety of changes in behaviour. Such changes include withdrawing from others or becoming unusually talkative, eating disorders, substance abuse, or becoming irritable (Larzelere & Jones, 2008). Stress can induce fatigue, with the resulting exhaustion limiting a person's ability to cope. Fatigue is discussed in more detail in Chapter 5.

Although hypertension in acute stress is thought to be transient, studies demonstrate a strong association between chronic, maladaptive stress and sustained hypertension, which is a major risk factor for cardiovascular disease (Sparrenberger et al., 2009). Other conditions that may be either precipitated or aggravated by stress include obesity, migraine headaches, irritable bowel syndrome, and peptic ulcers (Larzelere & Jones, 2008). Not only can stress induce immunosuppression, making a person more vulnerable to infectious diseases, but also it may exacerbate or increase the risk of progression of immune-based diseases such as multiple sclerosis, asthma, rheumatoid arthritis, and cancer (Bauer, 2008; Schmidt, Sterlemann, & Müller, 2008). Many questions about stress and the immune response remain unanswered. For example, it is not known how much stress is needed to cause these changes or how much of an alteration in the immune system is necessary before a person becomes susceptible to disease. A current challenge for researchers in the field of psychoneuroimmunology is to study stress-induced immune changes and their relationship to health and to illness outcomes.

Coping

Coping is a person's cognitive and behavioural efforts to manage specific external or internal stressors that seem to exceed available resources (Lazarus & Folkman, 1984). Coping can be either positive or negative. Positive coping includes activities such as exercise and use of social support. Negative coping may include substance abuse and denial. Availability of coping resources affects an individual's ability to cope with stressful situations. **Coping resources** are internal or external assets, characteristics, or actions that a person draws upon to manage stress (Table 8-3).

Coping strategies function broadly in two ways: as problem-focused or emotion-focused efforts (Table 8-4). **Emotion-focused**

Table 8-3 Examples of Coping Resources

INTERNAL COPING RESOURCES

HEALTH, ENERGY, MORALE	PROBLEM-SOLVING SKILLS
Robust health	Collection of information
High energy level	Identification of problem
High morale	Generation of alternatives
Positive beliefs	Social skills
Self-efficacy	Communication skills
Spirituality	Compatibility

EXTERNAL COPING RESOURCES

SOCIAL NETWORKS	UTILITARIAN RESOURCES
Family members	Finances
Co-workers	Self-help books
Social contacts	Social agencies

Table 8-4 Examples of Problem- and Emotion-Focused Coping

STRESSOR	PROBLEM-FOCUSED COPING	EMOTION-FOCUSED COPING
Receiving a diagnosis of terminal cancer	Preparing advanced health care directives	Seeking spiritual guidance from one's place of worship
Exacerbation of chronic obstructive pulmonary disease (COPD)	Quitting smoking	Joining a support group
Renal failure that necessitates frequent travel for dialysis	Arranging for a volunteer driver	Enjoying relaxing music and reading during travel time
Extended hospital stay for stem cell transplantation	Arranging for child/family care before hospital admission	Communicate on Skype with family/friends regularly while in hospital

coping involves managing the emotions that an individual feels when a stressful event occurs. Examples of emotion-focused coping include discussion of feelings with a friend or relaxing in a hot bath. **Problem-focused coping** is a cognitive approach in which the person attempts to find solutions to the problems causing the stress. For example, setting priorities, collecting information, and seeking advice would be considered problem-focused coping. Emotion- and problem-focused strategies can be employed alone or in combination to cope with the same stressor. Although it may not appear to be working toward a solution, emotion-focused coping is a valid and appropriate way to deal with various stressful situations. Two primary purposes of emotion-focused coping are to alleviate negative emotions and to create a sense of well-being. When a situation is unchangeable or uncontrollable, emotion-focused coping may dominate. If a problem can be changed or controlled, problem-focused cognitive coping may be more effective. Problem-focused coping strategies enable an individual to look at a challenge objectively, take action to address the problem, and thereby reduce the stress.

A key concept to successful coping is the use of coping flexibility. *Coping flexibility* is a cognitive process involving the ability to assess the nature of the stressor, determine what one has control over, and change and adapt coping strategies over time and across different stressful conditions (Zong et al., 2010). Stressful situations are best handled when an individual practises flexible coping, inasmuch as certain strategies work more effectively than others, depending on the circumstances, and overreliance on one type of coping strategy can be incapacitating. Regular exercise, especially aerobic movement, results in improved circulation, increased release of endorphins, and an enhanced sense of well-being. Exercise related specifically to stress is well researched and supported. Yang and colleagues (2010) studied 861 young Finnish adults over a 9-year period; those who engaged regularly in moderate to vigorous physical activity once or twice a week reported less job-related strain than did their inactive counterparts. Spirituality addresses a person's ability to remain connected to the world around him or her and creates meaning in that connection. In a study of 117 palliative care nurses in Quebec, spirituality—whether through religious beliefs or the ability to reinterpret experiences and assign positive meaning to them—was shown to mediate bereavement-related stress (Desbiens & Fillion, 2007). Numerous strategies have been shown to prevent or mitigate the effects of stress and are discussed in subsequent sections of this chapter.

Relaxation Strategies

Benson (1975) first described *relaxation response* as a state of physiological and psychological deep rest—the opposite of the stress response. It is characterized by decreased central nervous system and sympathetic nervous system activity, which leads to decreases in heart and respiratory rates, blood pressure, muscle tension, and brain activity and an increase in skin temperature. Benson found that individuals who regularly engage in relaxation strategies are better able to deal with their stressors, increase their sense of control over stressors, and reduce their tension. A systematic review of 14 studies supported Benson's work by demonstrating improved short- and long-term outcomes among patients in critical care units in response to psychosocial support, imagery, and relaxation techniques (Papathanassoglou, 2010). In addition to common strategies discussed in the following section, the relaxation response can be

Table 8-5 Examples of Stress Management Techniques

TECHNIQUE	DESCRIPTION
Thought stopping	A self-directed behavioural approach is used to gain control of self-defeating thoughts. When these thoughts occur, the individual stops the thought process and focuses on conscious relaxation.
Humour	Humour in the form of laughter, cartoons, funny movies, riddles, CDs, comic books, and joke books can be used for both the nurse and the patient.
Assertive behaviour	This behaviour entails open, honest sharing of feelings, desires, and opinions in a controlled way. The individual who has control over his or her life is less subject to stress.
Social support	This may take the form of organized support and self-help groups, relationships with family and friends, professional help, or some combination.
Journal keeping	The individual expresses self in written form, such as personal events, thoughts, feelings, memories, and perceptions. This may allow the individual to increase self-awareness and coping.
Biofeedback	The individual learns to monitor and control physiological responses to stressful or challenging events; these responses include skin temperature, muscle tension, heart rate, brain waves, and skin conductance (see Chapter 12).

CD, compact disc.

elicited through methods listed in Table 8-5. Using a low, steady voice, a nurse can talk a patient through the various relaxation strategies discussed in this chapter.

Relaxation Breathing

The way a person breathes affects every aspect of his or her life. When a person is stressed, muscles tense and breathing becomes shallow and rapid. Therefore, one of the simplest and most effective ways to stop the stress response is to breathe deeply and slowly. It is difficult to maintain tension when breathing in a slow, deep, and relaxed pattern. *Relaxation breathing* forms the basis for most relaxation strategies and can be performed while a person is sitting, standing, or lying down. It is especially useful in reducing stress during a stressful or anxious experience. Techniques for relaxation breathing are presented in Table 8-6.

Before a person practises relaxation breathing, it is important to assess his or her normal breathing pattern. To do this, the person begins by placing one hand gently on the abdomen below the waistline and the other hand on the centre of the chest. Without changing the normal breathing pattern, the person takes several breaths. During inhalation, the person takes notice of which hand rises the most. When relaxation breathing is performed properly, the hand on the abdomen should rise more than the hand on the chest. Chest breathing, which involves the upper chest and shoulders, is associated with inefficient breathing, and often occurs during anxiety and distress. Relaxation

Table 8-6 Relaxation Strategies

Rhythmic Breathing

1. Find a quiet, peaceful environment.
2. Assume a comfortable position, whether sitting or lying down, ensuring that arms and the legs are not crossed.
3. Close your eyes, and breathe in and out slowly, saying, "Breathe in, 2, 3, 4; breathe out, 2, 3, 4." The key is a "signal breath" involving deep inhalation through the nose and forceful exhalation through the mouth. The signal breath precedes and follows each repetition of the exercise.
4. Continue to breathe in an out slowly, using abdominal breathing, feeling more relaxed with each breath. As with any breathing exercise, if a light-headed feeling arises, discontinue exercise for 30 seconds and then start again. Initially, relaxation breathing may feel unusual. With practice it becomes easier, and the relaxing benefits are soon obvious.
5. When you are ready to end a breathing relaxation exercise, count silently from 1 to 3; on 1, move your lower body; on 2, move your upper body; on 3, breathe in deeply, open your eyes, and while breathing out slowly, say silently, "I am relaxed and alert." Stretch as if just waking up.

Progressive Relaxation

See the later section on progressive muscle relaxation, as well as Table 8-7, for more detail.

1. Follow steps 1, 2, 3, and 4 of rhythmic breathing.
2. Once breathing slowly and comfortably, tighten and relax specific muscle groups in ordered succession, concentrating on the feeling of relaxing the muscle. Starting with the feet and moving upward, ending with the face, is an effective technique.
3. Lie still for a few minutes, experiencing the relaxed muscles. Continue to breathe slowly and deeply, feeling tension flow out and relaxation get deeper and deeper with each breath.
4. When you are ready to get up, count backward from 4 to 1 and slowly rise.

Relaxation by Sensory Pacing

1. Follow steps 1 and 2 of rhythmic breathing.
2. Slowly repeat and finish each of the following sentences:

   "Now I am aware of seeing …"
   "Now I am aware of feeling …"
   "Now I am aware of hearing …"
   Repeat and complete each sentence four times, then three times, then twice, and finally once.
3. Allow the eyes to close when they feel heavy.

Modified Autogenic Relaxation

1. Follow steps 1, 2, 3, and 4 of rhythmic breathing.
2. Repeat each of the following phrases to yourself four times, saying the first part of the phrase while breathing in for 2 to 3 seconds, holding the breath for 2 to 3 seconds, and then saying the last part of the phrase while breathing out for 2 to 3 seconds:

BREATHING IN	BREATHING OUT
I am	relaxed.
My arms and legs	are heavy and warm.
My heartbeat	is calm and regular.
My breathing	is free and easy.
My abdomen	is loose and warm.
My forehead	is cool.
My mind	is quiet and still.

breathing, which involves the diaphragm, is natural for newborns and sleeping adults and is associated with efficient breathing.

COMPLEMENTARY & ALTERNATIVE THERAPIES
Stress

In addition to cognitive and behavioural coping strategies, a number of complementary and alternative therapies have been shown to help people to cope with their stress. See Chapter 12 for a discussion of the role of St. John's wort, and kava, in coping with stress. It is important that you read the section on Natural Products to ensure patient safety when considering herbal preparations in managing any disorders. Chapter 12 also discusses other complementary and alternative therapies that may be used when managing stress such as: yoga, therapeutic and healing touch, massage, and prayer.

Meditation

Meditation is an ancient strategy used to relax, as well as to promote mindfulness. Mindfulness cultivates sustained and focused concentration and awareness. Many people practise meditation in response to a deep human need for something transcendental or beyond everyday experiences. However, meditation can also be used as a way to reduce stress and promote well-being. In people who meditate regularly, the brain is reoriented from a stressful fight-or-flight mode to one of acceptance and contentment (Wu & Lo, 2008). Studies have demonstrated possible links between meditation and such health benefits as reversal of coronary artery disease, decreased levels of cortisol and cholesterol levels, increased airflow to the lungs, and improved immunity (Carmody & Baer, 2008; Creswell, Myers, Cole, & Irwin, 2009). In the beginning, individuals typically start with just 5 to 10 minutes of meditation at a time and increase the time as the practice becomes more comfortable. Table 8-7 is a guide to meditation. It is important to note that meditation takes practice, and people are often not successful at first, so beginners should not feel discouraged.

Imagery

Imagery is the use of the mind to generate images that have a calming effect on the body (Table 8-8; Figure 8-8). It involves the use of mental focus and incorporates all the senses to create physiological and emotional changes. It is a simple relaxation technique that requires no equipment other than an active imagination. Guided imagery is a variation of imagery in which images are suggested by another person (either live or a recording).

Imagery can be used in many clinical settings for stress reduction and pain relief. Benefits of imagery include reduction in anxiety, decrease in muscle tension, improvement in comfort during medical procedures, enhancement of immune function, decrease in recovery time after surgery, and improvement in sleep (Eremin et al., 2009; Freeman, et al., 2008; Menzies & Kim, 2008; Trakhtenberg, 2008). A health care professional may use imagery in his or her own life or use guided imagery with his or her patients. Imagery is used to create a safe and special place for mental retreat.

Imagery can also be used to specifically target a disease, problem, or stressor. For example, patients with cancer may imagine sharks gobbling up their cancer cells or radiation and

Table 8-7 Basic Guide to Meditation

- Find a quiet place, with no distractions.
- Sit in a comfortable position, and close your eyes.
- "Shut out the world" so that your brain can stop processing information coming from your senses.
- Pick a word or phrase that means something to you, whose sound or rhythm is soothing when repeated (e.g., "one," "peace," "shalom," "The Lord is my shepherd").
- Breathe slowly, and practise relaxation breathing.
- Say the word or phrase again and again, or try saying it silently to yourself with every exhalation.
- The monotony will help you focus.
- Do not be concerned when other thoughts come to mind; just acknowledge them and return calmly to your word or phrase.
- Continue for 10 to 20 minutes, but even 5 minutes can leave you feeling calm and refreshed. Rise slowly.
- Practise once or twice daily.

Table 8-8 Imagery: Creating a "Special Place"

- Begin by finding a comfortable position, closing your eyes, and taking several slow, deep breaths.
- Imagine a place where you feel completely comfortable and peaceful. It may be a real place or one you imagine; it may one from your past or some place you have always wanted to go.
- Allow this image to take form, slowly. As it takes form in your imagination, look around, to your left, to your right. Enjoy the scenery: the colours, the texture, and the shapes. Engage all senses: sight, hearing, touch, smell.
- Listen carefully to the sounds of your place. What do you hear?
- Is there a gentle breeze or sunshine warming your face? Imagine picking up or touching some favourite objects from this special place. Take in a deep breath through your nose, and notice the rich smells around you. Perhaps your favourite flower is in bloom, or you smell the scents of the ocean.
- Take another deep breath and relax. Enjoy the peace, comfort, and safety of this special place.
- This is your special place. You relax and feel thankful that you are here, in your special place.
- You can return to this place any time that you wish.

chemotherapy entering the body like healing rays of light that destroy cancer cells. Special images can be created to alleviate symptoms (such as pain) or to treat disorders (such as depression); for example, a person may imagine troubles attached to helium balloons and visualize releasing them into the sky. *Relaxation by colour exchange* is a technique that combines rhythmic breathing and imagery. Patients are instructed to focus on an area of pain or tension and assign a colour to it. While breathing in, they can imagine a warm white light coming into their body and surrounding this area. They then imagine the colour of discomfort leaving their body through their breath as they exhale. Imagery can also be used to enhance performance or to process stressful or difficult tasks by allowing one an opportunity to mentally rehearse the difficult or challenging situation. For example, it can be used to help a fearful nurse start an intravenous

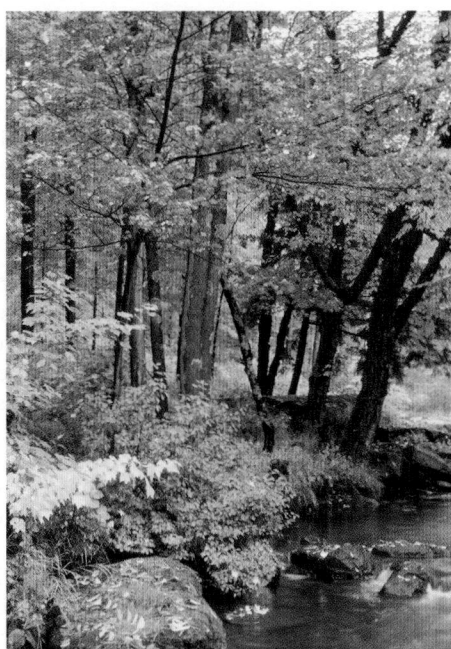

Figure 8-8 Imagery. Creating a "special place" should involve all the senses, such as a place where rustling leaves can be heard, flowers are smelled, wind is felt, and a colourful landscape is seen.

Source: © 2011 JupiterImages Corporation.

infusion or assist a patient who is afraid of undergoing a stressful procedure (e.g., radiation therapy). It should be noted that relaxation by colour exchange is a very new stress reduction technique that does not yet have an evidence base to support its efficacy.

Music for Relaxation

Music can help achieve relaxation and bring about healthy changes in emotional or physical states. Listening to relaxing music may act as a diversion from a stressful situation. In addition, healing vibrations from music can return the mind and body to better balance.

Music has been used in many clinical settings. In general, music appears to affect functions such as such as heart rate, arterial pressure, gastric and bowel secretions, muscle tone, sweat glands, and temperature regulation (Garcia, 2008). It has been shown to decrease anxiety and pain and to evoke the relaxation response (Holm & Fitzmaurice, 2008). Music with low-pitch tones, without words, and that has approximately 60 to 80 beats per minute is considered to be soothing. Mozart's compositions are the most popular form of music used for relaxation. In contrast, fast-tempo music can stimulate and uplift a person.

Music can be incorporated into clinical practice. It is noninvasive, safe, inexpensive, and easy to use. First, it is important to establish the purpose and benefit of using music with the patients in a given clinical setting and to assess each individual patient's interest and preference in music. The patient should be in a comfortable position, and the possibility of interruptions should be minimized: for example, by the use of headphones or earphones. For optimal benefit, music should be played for at least 20 to 30 minutes per day at least twice a day. The patients' response to the music should be evaluated through questions about how it sounds and how it makes them feel.

Another way to use music for relaxation is to simply create one's own music. Singing a song, humming a tune, or playing a musical instrument can be an uplifting experience during stressful times. Music can also be played in the background to help induce relaxation as a person performs housework or office work.

Muscle Relaxation

Muscle tension is a universal reaction to stress. As the stress response sets in, muscles of the entire body tend to tighten. Muscle relaxation is therefore a common method of eliciting the relaxation response. There are two types of muscle relaxation: progressive and passive. *Progressive muscle relaxation* (PMR) involves the tensing and the relaxing of muscles. This method is intended to help differentiate between when a muscle is tensed and when it is relaxed. This recognition enables an individual to reduce muscle tension when it occurs during stress. PMR is based on the principle that when the muscles are relaxed, the mind relaxes. In a session of PMR, relaxation typically begins at the extremities and gradually moves across the whole body. An example of PMR can be found in Table 8-6. Patients with muscle or connective tissue damage or those with low back pain should not use PMR. In addition, PMR should not be used by patients with increased intracranial pressure, uncontrolled hypertension, or severe coronary artery disease.

In *passive muscle relaxation*, on the other hand, the mind focuses only on relaxation of the muscles. It is performed similarly to PMR, moving from one extremity to the rest of the body, with the exception that the muscles are never tightened. In passive muscle relaxation, the focus is simply on relaxing each muscle group separately. This form of muscle relaxation may be used more frequently by individuals who have chronic pain that may be exacerbated by the tension involved during PMR.

NURSING MANAGEMENT: STRESS

Nursing Assessment

Patients face an array of potential stressors, or demands that can have health consequences. Nurses are well positioned to assess patients and their significant others, assist them in identifying periods in which they are at high risk for stress, and implement stress management strategies. Three major areas are important in assessment of stress: demands, human responses to stress, and coping. Stress assessment tools that may be downloaded from the Internet have demonstrated usefulness in the clinical setting. The Perceived Stress Scale is a measure of how stressful a person perceives his or her life at that time (Roberti, Harrington & Storch, 2006). Although further research is needed to connect the identification of stressors with managing them, the Distress Thermometer identifies areas of particular concern to patients (Snowden, White, Christie, Murray, McGowan, & Scott, 2011). Caregiver stress is a well-identified phenomenon that may occur in a variety of situations, such as caring for a spouse with Alzheimer's disease, an older parent, or a child with cancer, and thus should also be considered in a stress assessment. Communication support, adequate education and resources, and a positive approach from nursing staff are shown to improve the quality of life of caregivers (Tamayo, Broxson, Munsell, & Cohen, 2010).

■ Demands

Stressors, or demands, on the patient may include major life changes, events or situations such as disfiguring or debilitating surgery, or daily hassles. Demands may be categorized as external (e.g., job-related situations, extended hospitalization,) or internal (e.g., perception of goals or commitments, physical effects of disease or injury). It is important to keep in mind the many potential stressors that predispose people to stress and take a proactive approach to address them before patients present with stress-related symptoms. The number of simultaneous demands, the duration of these demands, primary appraisal or perception of the demands (see Figure 8-1), previous experience with similar demands, and the patient's family and loved ones' responses to the demands should be considered in the health assessment. Demands may also be categorized as representing harm or loss, threat, or challenge. Eliciting the patient's personal meaning attached to the demand provides useful insight for planning interventions and self-management strategies with patients. Distinct groups such as immigrants and Aboriginal people may have specific stressors such as language barriers and limited understanding of Western medical practices and available resources that may predispose them to stress, and these stressors should be considered when a nursing assessment is performed.

■ Human Responses to Stress

Physiological effects of demands that are appraised as stressful are mediated primarily via the sympathetic nervous system and the hypothalamic-pituitary-adrenal system. Responses such as increased heart rate, increased blood pressure, loss of appetite, hyperventilation, sweating, and dilated pupils are included. Symptomatic experiences may include headache, musculoskeletal pain, gastrointestinal upset, skin disorders, insomnia, and chronic fatigue. In addition, the patient may exhibit some of the stress-related illnesses or diseases of adaptation (see Table 8-2).

Behavioural manifestations may include accident proneness, anxiety, crying, frustration, and shouting. Behaviour in other aspects of life may include absenteeism or tardiness at work, avoiding conversations, or procrastination. Observable cognitive responses include self-reports of excessive demand, inability to make decisions, impaired speech, and forgetfulness or inability to concentrate. Some of these responses may also be apparent in stressed caregivers.

■ Coping

Secondary appraisal by the patient, or the patient's evaluation of coping resources and options, is important to assess (see Figure 8-1). Resources such as supportive family members, adequate finances, and the ability to solve problems are examples of positive resources (see Table 8-3). Knowledge of the patient's resources assists the nurse in supporting existing resources and developing strategies to expand the patient's sources of support to include family, friends, and community resources. Positive social support and possessing a large social network (relatives, friends, spiritual groups, support groups) have been shown to exert powerful effects on the negative distress associated with illness. Conversely, aversive support (punishing, demanding, distancing relationships) may add to life stress and intensify illness-associated pain and distress.

Coping strategies include cognitive and behavioural efforts to meet demands. The use and effectiveness of problem-focused and emotion-focused coping efforts should be addressed (see Table

8-4). These efforts may be categorized as direct action, avoidance of action, seeking information, defence mechanisms, and seeking the assistance of other people. The probability that a certain coping strategy will bring about the desired result is another important aspect to be assessed. Effective coping skills can be taught, and nurses are in a prime position to teach these skills.

■ Nursing Implementation

The first step in managing stress is to become aware of its presence. The role of the nurse is to facilitate and enhance the processes of coping and adaptation that include identifying and expressing stressful feelings. Nursing interventions depend on the severity of the stress experience or demand. The person with multiple traumas expends energy in an attempt to physically survive. The nurse's efforts are directed to life-supporting interventions and to the inclusion of approaches aimed at the reduction of additional stressors to the patient. The individual who has endured significant trauma is much less likely to adapt or recover if faced with additional stressors such as sleep deprivation or an infection.

The importance of cognitive appraisal in the stress experience should prompt the nurse to assess whether changes in the way a person perceives and labels particular events or situations (cognitive reappraisal) are possible. Some experts also propose that the nurse consider the positive effects that result from successfully meeting stressful demands. Greater emphasis should also be placed on the part that cultural values and beliefs can play to enhance or constrain various coping options.

Because dealing with physical, social, and psychological demands is an integral part of daily experiences, the coping behaviours that are used should be adaptive and should not be a source of additional stress to the individual. Generalizing about which coping strategies are the most adaptive is not yet possible. However, in evaluating coping behaviours, the nurse should examine the short-term outcomes (i.e., the effect of the strategy on the reduction or mastery of the demands and the regulation of the emotional response) and the long-term outcomes that relate to health, morale, and social and psychological functioning. Nursing students often experience high levels of stress because of the demands of their educational programs; Table 8-9 provides some useful suggestions for coping.

Various factors affect an individual's response to stressors (see the box on p. 124). Resistance to stress can be increased with a lifestyle that supports optimal health regardless of sex, age, and economic status. Healthy behaviours are also cumulative; that is, the greater the number of these behaviours habitually practised by the individual, the better that person's health is. These behaviours include the following:

1. Sleeping regularly 7 to 8 hours per night
2. Eating breakfast
3. Eating regular, well-balanced meals with minimal, healthy snacking
4. Eating moderately to maintain an ideal weight
5. Exercising moderately
6. Enjoying recreational and relaxing activities with friends
7. Drinking alcohol in moderation or not at all
8. Not smoking (best outcome if the person has never smoked)
9. Learning to successfully handle life's stressors and hassles

Good mental health practices are important for good health as well. These practices result primarily in a realistic, positive self-concept and the ability to solve problems. Teaching problem-solving skills can equip individuals to better handle present and future encounters with stressful circumstances.

Table 8-9 Coping Strategies for the Nursing Student
• Be realistic: do not try to be superhuman.
• Learn to "let go" of things that are outside your control.
• Learn to adapt, and to be flexible.
• Learn acceptance of yourself.
• Share your feelings.
• Keep a sense of humour; laugh often.
• Learn and use relaxation breathing, imagery, meditation, or prayer.
• Live a healthy lifestyle (exercise, nutrition, adequate sleep, not smoking, moderate use of alcohol).
• Develop hobbies.
• Take time to relax every day.
• If it is needed, obtain professional counselling.

Table 8-10 Implementing Stress Management in Clinical Practice
• Learn relaxation–coping techniques by practising them on your own; then practise teaching them to peers before teaching them to patients. Attend seminars and workshops on stress management to learn more.
• Be aware of potential stressors that your patients face.
• Assess your patients for the demands placed on them, their response to these demands, and coping resources being used or available to them.
• Choose the language you use carefully, and be aware of your nonverbal communication. Words or gestures that express overt alarm or ambiguity may increase the stress experience for the patient.
• Pick coping strategies and stress management strategies that are appropriate for your clinical area.
• Take advantage of opportunities to teach coping and relaxation strategies to patients.
• Anticipate setbacks. They provide feedback about what you are doing wrong. Do *not* quit practising!

Stress-reducing activities can be incorporated into nursing practice (Table 8-10). The activities provide mechanisms whereby an individual is able to develop a sense of control of the situation. As stress-reducing practices are incorporated into daily activities, the individual is able to increase his or her confidence and self-reliance and limit the emotional response to the stressful circumstances. Possessing a sense of control over one's life, believing that one is able to overcome adversity, and being committed to that end are important characteristics that can avert the harmful effects inherent in the stress response.

The nurse can assume a primary role in planning stress-reducing interventions. Specific relaxation strategies are presented in Table 8-6. Specific stress-reducing activities within the scope of nursing practice (some of which may require additional training) include relaxation training, guided imagery, cognitive reappraisal,

music therapy, exercise, time management, decisional control, assertiveness training, massage, meditation, and humour (see Table 8-5). There is ample evidence for the effectiveness of stress management interventions in a variety of ill populations. Nurses are in an ideal situation to take the lead in integrating stress management into their practice. Nurses are also well equipped to develop and test the effectiveness of new approaches to manage stress and promote positive health outcomes. However, it is important for the nurse to recognize when the patient, family, or caregivers need to be referred to a professional with advanced training in counselling.

CLINICAL DECISION-MAKING EXERCISE

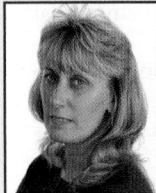

CASE STUDY:
Stress Associated With Cancer Diagnosis and Treatment
Source: © iStockphoto.com/Lisa F. Young

Patient Profile

Mrs. Zyskowski, a Polish immigrant, received a diagnosis of stage II breast cancer at age 44. Her treatment plan included lumpectomy followed by a regimen of chemotherapy and then radiation therapy. She attributed her breast cancer to her depression, which developed while she cared for her mother, who suffered from Alzheimer's disease. Her mother passed away 6 months before the breast cancer diagnosis.

After completion of her lengthy breast cancer therapy, Mrs. Zyskowski's depression worsened. She no longer had her frequent visits to the breast cancer centre, and she missed the interaction with the nurses and other patients. In addition, Mrs. Zyskowski feared that her cancer would recur, and she worried that she would "pass it on" to her two teenage daughters. She would not discuss her fears with her husband or daughters because she did not want to burden them. She began to lose weight and constantly felt fatigued. She felt "alone" with her cancer and lost interest in other aspects of her life. She thought about joining a cancer support group but was embarrassed by her Polish accent.

Discussion Questions

1. Consider Mrs. Zyskowski's situation, and describe the physiological and psychological stressors that she is dealing with. Describe the possible effects of these stressors on her health status.
2. What are some other potential stressors that Mrs. Zyskowski may be experiencing that the nurse should anticipate and assess further for?
3. What specific nursing interventions can be included in Mrs. Zyskowski's management that will enhance her adaptability?
4. On the basis of Mrs. Zyskowski's profile, what resources are available to Mrs. Zyskowski to help her cope with her cancer diagnosis and treatment?
5. Should Mrs. Zyskowski join a cancer support group? If so, how might this benefit her?
6. *Priority decision:* On the basis of the assessment data provided, what are the priority nursing diagnoses? Are there any collaborative problems?

evolve *Answers are available at* **http://evolve.elsevier.com/ Canada/Lewis/medsurg**

REVIEW QUESTIONS

The number of the question corresponds to the same-numbered objective at the beginning of the chapter.

1. How does Selye define stress?
   a. Any stimulus that causes a response in an individual
   b. A response of an individual to environmental demands
   c. A physical or psychological adaptation to internal or external demands
   d. The result of a relationship between an individual and the environment that exceeds the individual's resources

2. A patient who has undergone extensive surgery for multiple injuries has a period of increasing blood pressure, heart rate, and alertness. Which stage of general adaptation syndrome are these symptoms most characteristic of?
   a. The resistance state of general adaptation syndrome
   b. The alarm reaction of the general adaptation syndrome
   c. The stage of exhaustion of general adaptation syndrome
   d. An individual response stereotype

3. Which of the following actions best demonstrates that a patient is using an emotion-focused coping process?
   a. Joining a support group for women with breast cancer
   b. Considering the advantages and disadvantages of the various treatment options
   c. Delaying treatment until her family can take a weekend trip together
   d. Telling the nurse that she has a good prognosis because the tumour is small

4. The nurse would expect which of the following findings in a patient as a result of the physiological effect of stress on the limbic system?
   a. An episode of diarrhea while awaiting painful dressing changes
   b. Refusing to communicate with nurses while awaiting a cardiac catheterization
   c. Inability to sleep the night before beginning to self-administer insulin injections
   d. Increased blood pressure, decreased urine output, and hyperglycemia after a car accident

5. Which of the following best demonstrates that the nurse is applying knowledge of the effects of stress on the immune system?
   a. Encouraging patients to sleep for 10 to 12 hours per day
   b. Encouraging patients to receive regular immunizations when they are stressed
   c. Encouraging patients to use emotion-focused rather than problem-focused coping strategies
   d. Encouraging patients to avoid exposure to upper respiratory infections when physically stressed

6. Chronic stress or daily hassles may place a person at higher risk of developing which of the following conditions?
   a. Osteoporosis
   b. Colds and flu
   c. Low blood pressure
   d. High serum cholesterol

7. During a stressful circumstance that is uncontrollable, which type of coping strategy is the most effective?
   a. Avoidance
   b. Coping flexibility
   c. Emotion-focused coping
   d. Problem-focused coping

8. Which of the following patients is least likely to respond to stress effectively?
   a. One who feels that the situation is directing his or her life
   b. One who sees the situation as a challenge to be addressed
   c. One who has a clear understanding of his or her values and goals
   d. One who uses more problem-focused than emotion-focused coping strategies

9. Which of the following is an appropriate nursing intervention for a patient who has a nursing diagnosis of ineffective coping *related to* inadequate resources?
   a. Controlling the environment to prevent sensory overload and promote sleep
   b. Encouraging the patient's family to offer emotional support by frequent visiting
   c. Arranging for the patient to phone family and friends to maintain emotional bonds
   d. Asking the patient to describe previous stressful situations and how she managed to resolve them

ANSWERS: 1. d; 2. b; 3. c; 4. a; 5. d; 6. b; 7. c; 8. a; 9. d.

REFERENCES

Antonovsky, A. A. (1987). *Unraveling the mystery of health: How people manage stress and stay well*. San Francisco, CA: Jossey-Bass.

Bauer, M. (2008). Chronic stress and immunosenescence: A review. *Neuroimmunomodulation, 15*(4-6), 241-250. doi:10.1159/000156467

Benson, H. (1975). *The relaxation response*. New York: Avon.

Carmody, J., & Baer, R. (2008). Relationships between mindfulness practice and levels of mindfulness, medical and psychological symptoms and well-being in a mindfulness-based stress reduction program. *Journal of Behavioral Medicine, 31*(1), 23-33. doi:10.1007/s10865-007-9130-7

Chida, Y., & Hamer, M. (2008). Chronic psychosocial factors and acute physiological responses to laboratory-induced stress in healthy populations: A quantitative review of 30 years of investigations. *Psychological Bulletin, 134*(6), 829-885. doi:10.1037/a0013342

Creswell, J. D., Myers, H. F., Cole, S. W., & Irwin, M. I. (2009). Mindfulness, meditation training effects on CD4+ T lymphocytes in HIV-1 infected adults: A small randomized controlled trial. *Brain, Behavior and Immunity, 23*, 184-188. doi:10.1016/j.bbi.2008.07.004

Desbiens, J., & Fillion, L. (2007). Coping strategies, emotional outcomes and spiritual quality of life in palliative care nurses. *International Journal of Palliative Nursing, 13*(6), 291-300. Retrieved from *http://www.internurse.com/cgi-bin/go.pl/library/contents.html?uid=1727;journal_uid=14*

Earvolino-Ramirez, M. (2007). Resilience: A concept analysis. *Nursing Forum, 42*(2), 73-82. doi:10.1111/j.1744-6198.2007.00070.x

Eremin, O., Walker, M. B., Simpson, E., Heys, S. D., Ah-See, A. K., Hutcheon, A. W., ... Walker, L. G. (2009). Immuno-modulatory effects of relaxation training and guided imagery in women with locally advanced breast cancer undergoing multimodality therapy: A randomised controlled trial. *The Breast, 18*(1), 17-25. doi:10.1016/j.breast.2008.09.002

Freeman, L., Cohen, L., Stewart, M., White, R., Link, J., Palmer, J., ..., Hild, C. (2008). The experience of imagery as a post-treatment intervention in patients with breast cancer: Program, process, and patient recommendations. *Oncology Nursing Forum, 35*(6), E116-21. doi:10.1188/08.ONF.E116-E121

Garcia, J. E. (2008). Music therapy in oncology. *Clinical and Translational Oncology, 10*(12), 774-776. doi:10.1007/s12094-008-0289-3

Holm, L., & Fitzmaurice, L. (2008). Emergency department waiting room stress: Can music or aromatherapy improve anxiety scores? *Pediatric Emergency Care, 84*(12), 836-838. doi:10.1097/PEC.0b013e31818ea04c

Holmes, T., & Masuda, M. (1966). Magnitude estimations of social readjustments. *Journal of Psychosomatic Research, 11*(2), 219-225.

Jourdain, G., & Chenevert, D. (2010). Job demands—Resources, burnout and intention to leave the nursing profession: A questionnaire survey. *International Journal of Nursing Studies, 47*(6), 709-722. doi:10.1016/j.ijnurstu.2009.11.007

Larzelere, M., & Jones, G. (2008). Stress and health. *Primary Care, 35*(4), 839-856. doi:10.1016/j.pop.2008.07.011

Lazarus, R., & Folkman, S. (1984). *Stress, appraisal, and coping.* New York: Springer.

Mathews, L. L., & Servaty-Seib, H. L. (2007). Hardiness and grief in a sample of bereaved college students. *Death Studies, 31*(3), 183-204.

McCance, K. L., & Huether, S. E. (2010). *Pathophysiology: The biologic basis for disease in adults and children* (6th ed.). St. Louis: Elsevier Mosby.

Menzies, V., & Kim, S. (2008). Relaxation and guided imagery in Hispanic persons diagnosed with fibromyalgia: A pilot study. *Family & Community Health, 31*(3), 204-212. doi:10.1097/01.FCH.0000324477.48083.08

Miller, M. A., & Rahe, R. H. (1997). Life changes scaling for the 1990s. *Journal of Psychosomatic Research, 43*(3), 279-292.

Moore, K. (2008). Is laughter the best medicine? Research into the therapeutic use of laughter and humor in nursing practice. *Whitireia Nursing Journal, 15,* 33-38. http://web.ebscohost.com/ehost/pdfviewer/pdfviewer?sid=26cb10ef-0931-40d0-b814-0cb87da36ba0%40sessionmgr115&vid=6&hid=119

Papathanassoglou, E. (2010). Psychological support and outcomes of ICU patients. *Nursing in Critical Care, 15*(3), 118-128. doi:10.1111/j.1478-5153.2009.00383.x

Roberti, J. W., Harrington, L. N., & Storch, E. A. (2006). Further psychometric support for the 10-item version of the Performance Stress Scale. *Journal of College Counseling, 9*(2), 135-147. Retrieved from http://onlinelibrary.wiley.com/doi/10.1002/j.2161-1882.2006.tb00100.x/abstract

Schmidt, M. V., Sterlemann, V., & Müller, M. B. (2008). Chronic stress and individual vulnerability. *Annals of the New York Academy of Sciences, 1148,* 174-183. doi:10.1196/annals.1410.017

Segerstrom, S. (2010). Resources, stress, and immunity: An ecological perspective on human psychoneuroimmunology. *Annals of Behavioral Medicine, 40*(1), 114-125. doi:10.1007/s12160-010-9195-3

Selye, H. (1983). The stress concept: Past, present, and future. In C. L. Cooper (Ed.), *Stress research: Issues for the eighties.* New York: Wiley.

Snowden, A., White, C. A., Christie, Z., Murray, E., McGowan, C., & Scott, R. (2011). The clinical utility of the distress thermometer: A review. *British Journal of Nursing, 20*(4), 220-227. Retrieved from http://www.internurse.com/cgi-bin/go.pl/library/contents.html?uid=3952;journal_uid=9

Sparrenberger, F., Cichelero, F., Ascoli, A., Fonseca, F., Weiss, G., Berwanger, O., & Fuchs, F. (2009). Does psychosocial stress cause hypertension? A systematic review of observational studies. *Journal of Human Hypertension, 23*(1), 12-19. Retrieved from http://www.nature.com/jhh/journal/v23/n1/full/jhh200874a.html

Statistics Canada. (2004). *Healthy today, healthy tomorrow? Findings from the National Population Health Survey: Healthy aging* (Catalogue no. 82-618-MWE2005004). Ottawa: Health Analysis and Measurement Group.

Steinhardt, M., & Dolbier, C. (2008). Evaluation of a resilience intervention to enhance coping strategies and protective factors and decrease symptomatology. *Journal of American College Health, 56,* 453. doi:10.3200/JACH.56.44.445-454

Tamayo, G. J., Broxson, A., Munsell, M., & Cohen, M. Z. (2010). Caring for the caregiver. *Oncology Nursing Forum, 37*(1):E50-7.

Trakhtenberg, E. C. (2008). The effects of guided imagery on the immune system: A critical review. *International Journal of Neuroscience, 118*(6), 839-855. doi:10.1080/00207450701792705

Weiss, S. (2007). Neurobiological alterations associated with traumatic stress. *Perspectives in Psychiatric Care, 43*(3), 114-122. doi:10.1111/j.1744-6163.2007.00120.x

Wiesmann, U., & Hannich, H. (2010). A salutogenic analysis of healthy aging in active elderly persons. *Research on Aging, 32*(3), 349-371. doi:10.1177/0164027509356954

Wilkins, K. (2007). Work stress among health care providers. *Health Reports, 18*(4), 33-36. Retrieved from http://www.statcan.gc.ca/pub/82-003-x/2006011/article/10367-eng.pdf

Woods, S. J., Hall, R. J., Campbell, J. C., & Angott, D. M. (2008). Physical health and posttraumatic stress disorder symptoms in women experiencing intimate partner violence. *Journal of Midwifery and Women's Health, 53*(6), 538-546. Retrieved from http://www.medscape.com/viewarticle/583188

Wu, S. D., & Lo, P. C. (2008). Inward-attention meditation increases parasympathetic activity: A study based on heart rate variability. *Biomedical Research, 29*(5), 245-250. Retrieved from https://www.jstage.jst.go.jp/article/biomedres/29/5/29_5_245/_article

Yang, X., Telama, R., Hirvensalo, M., Hintsanen, M., Hintsa, T., Pulkki-Ra, L., & Viikari, J. S. A. (2010). The benefits of sustained leisure-time physical activity on job strain. *Occupational Medicine, 60,* 369-375. doi:10.1093/occmed/kqq019

Zong, J., Cao, X., Cao, Y., Shi, Y., Wang, Y., Yan, C., ..., Chan, R. (2010). Coping flexibility in college students with depressive symptoms. *Health & Quality of Life Outcomes, 8,* 66. doi:10.1186/1477-7525-8-66

RESOURCES

Addiction Assessment: Centre for Addiction and Mental Health
http://www.camh.net
Canadian Centre for Occupational Health and Safety
http://www.ccohs.ca/
Canadian Institute of Stress
http://www.stresscanada.org
Canadian Mental Health Association Branches
http://www.addcoach4u.com/support/canadianmentalhealthbr.html
Centre for the Neurobiology of Stress
http://www.utsc.utoronto.ca/~cnstress
Heart and Stroke Foundation of Canada
http://www.heartandstroke.ca
NurseONE
http://www.nurseone.ca
Public Health Agency of Canada
http://www.phac-aspc.gc.ca/chn-rcs/index-eng.php

evolve *For additional Internet resources, see the Web site for this book at* **http://evolve.elsevier.com/Canada/Lewis/medsurg**

Sleep and Sleep Disorders

Written by Carol A. Landis and Margaret McLean Heitkemper

Adapted by Holly Symonds-Brown

LEARNING OBJECTIVES

1. Define *sleep*.
2. Describe physiological sleep mechanisms and stages of sleep.
3. Explain the relationship of various diseases/disorders and sleep disorders.
4. Describe the etiology, clinical manifestations, and collaborative and nursing management of insomnia.
5. Describe the etiology, clinical manifestations, and collaborative and nursing management of narcolepsy.
6. Describe the etiology, clinical manifestations, collaborative care, and nursing management of obstructive sleep apnea.
7. Describe parasomnias, including sleepwalking, sleep terrors, and nightmares.
8. Select appropriate strategies for managing sleep problems associated with shift work.

KEY TERMS

cataplexy A brief and sudden loss of skeletal muscle tone or muscle weakness. Manifestations can range from a brief episode of muscle weakness to complete postural collapse and falling to the ground, p. 144

circadian rhythms The biological rhythms of behaviour and physiology that fluctuate within a 24-hour period of time, p. 138

insomnia Difficulty falling asleep, difficulty staying asleep, waking up too early, or poor quality of sleep, p. 139

narcolepsy A chronic neurological disorder caused by the brain's inability to regulate sleep–wake cycles normally, p. 144

obstructive sleep apnea (OSA) Partial or complete upper airway obstruction during sleep, p. 146

parasomnias Unusual and often undesirable behaviours that occur with sleep or during arousal from sleep, p. 149

sleep disorder One of possibly 70 conditions that result in poor sleep quality, p. 137

sleep-disordered breathing (SDB) Abnormal respiratory patterns associated with sleep. These include snoring, apnea, and hypopnea with increased respiratory effort leading to frequent arousals, p. 145

sleep disturbance Conditions that result in poor sleep quality, p. 137

sleep hygiene A variety of different practices that are important for normal, quality nighttime sleep and daytime alertness, p. 141

sleep terrors A sudden awakening from sleep along with a loud cry and signs of panic. Includes an intense autonomic response including increased heart rate, increased respiration, and diaphoresis, p. 149

wake behaviour Behaviour associated with an activated cortical brain-wave pattern, p. 138

ELECTRONIC RESOURCES

Supplemental content related to Chapter 9 can be found …

Evolve Web Site ⓔvolve

http://evolve.elsevier.com/Canada/Lewis/medsurg
- Clinical Reference: Laboratory Values
- Content Updates

- eTables:
  - eTable 9-1: Pittsburgh Sleep Quality Index
- Examination Review Questions
- Glossary
- Key Points (Printable and MP3 Download)

Sleep

Sleep is a state during which an individual lacks conscious awareness of environmental surroundings and from which one can be easily aroused. Sleep is distinct from unconscious states such as coma, in which the individual cannot be aroused. Sleep is a basic, dynamic, highly organized, and complex behaviour that is essential for normal functioning and survival. Over a lifespan of 70 years, an average individual will spend approximately 20 to 25 years asleep (Buysse et al., 2008). Both behavioural and physiological functions are influenced by sleep. Some of these include memory, mood, cognitive function, hormone secretion, glucose metabolism, immune function, body temperature, and renal function.

Most adults require at least 7 hours of sleep within a 24-hour period. *Insufficient sleep* refers to obtaining less sleep than one requires to be fully awake and alert during the day. The term *fragmented sleep* refers to frequent arousals or actual awakenings that interrupt sleep continuity.

Sleep disorder and **sleep disturbance** are terms used to indicate those conditions that result in poor sleep quality. The classification of sleep disorders is complex, with 70 different types having been identified. Table 9-1 lists the most common sleep disorders based on the American Academy of Sleep Medicine's International Classification of Sleep Disorders (2001).

Over 3 million Canadians have a sleep disorder, and many are unaware that they have a problem (Morin et al., 2011; Public Health Agency of Canada [PHAC], 2009) (Figure 9-1). On average, Canadians sleep approximately 6.5 hours on work days and 7.5 hours on nonwork days. In a recent survey, 40.2% of Canadians reported at least one symptom of insomnia for a minimum of 3 nights a week in the previous month and close to a fifth of the survey respondents reported being dissatisfied with the quality of their sleep (Morin et al., 2011). In another population survey, 58% of Canadians report feeling tired most of the time (Leger Marketing, 2010). Those with chronic health problems or physical disability are at greatest risk for sleep disorders (Tjepkema, 2005).

Many sleep disorders go untreated because health care providers often do not ask and patients often do not talk about sleep problems. Untreated sleep disorders pose considerable health and economic consequences. Sleepiness while driving has become a national epidemic. In 2004, 17.8% of all fatal car collisions and 25.5% of injury-related collisions were associated with driver sleepiness (Elzohairy, 2008). Some work-related accidents have been linked to sleep problems (Kling, McLeod, & Koehoorn, 2010). Each year, sleep disorders, sleep loss, and excessive daytime sleepiness add billions of dollars to the cost of health care and

Table 9-1 Selected Sleep Disorders	
Dyssomnias	• Sleep-disordered breathing
• Inadequate sleep hygiene	• Obstructive sleep apnea
• Insomnia	• Periodic limb movement disorder
• Acute	
• Chronic	• Restless legs syndrome
• Primary	***Parasomnias***
• Secondary (co-morbid)	• Sleepwalking
• Hospital-acquired sleep disorders	• Sleep terrors
• Narcolepsy	• Nightmares
• Circadian rhythm disorders (e.g., jet lag)	

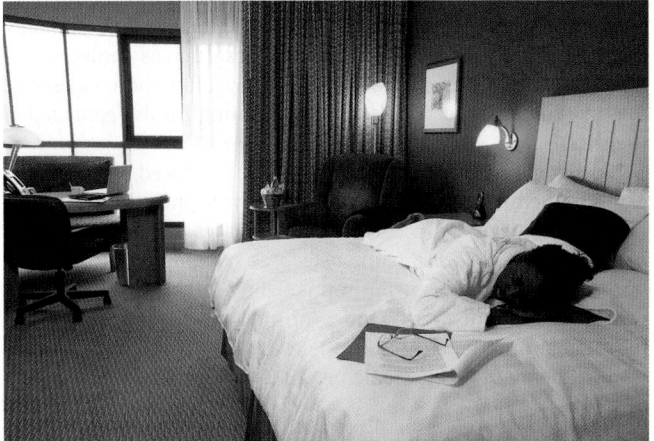

Figure 9-1 Sleep disorders are common in our society.

Source: © 2011 JupiterImages Corporation.

the economic impact of work-related accidents and lost productivity (Kling et al., 2010).

Physiological Sleep Mechanisms

Sleep–Wake Cycle

The nervous system controls the cyclical changes between waking and sleep. No single neuronal structure regulates sleep and waking; rather, a complex arrangement of structures controls these behaviours. Key nuclei in the brainstem, hypothalamus, and thalamus are involved in the regulation of sleep and wake behaviours.

Wake Behaviour. **Wake behaviour** is associated with an activated cortical brain-wave pattern (electroencephalogram [EEG]). The reticular activating system (RAS) in the middle of the brainstem is associated with generalized EEG activation and behavioural arousal. Various neurotransmitters (glutamate, acetylcholine, norepinephrine, dopamine, histamine, serotonin) are involved in wake behaviour. In Alzheimer's disease, there is loss of cholinergic neurons in the basal forebrain, and people with the disease have sleep disturbances. In Parkinson's disease, there is degeneration of dopamine neurons in the substantia nigra, and people with the disease experience excessive daytime sleepiness. Histamine neurons in the hypothalamus stimulate cortical activation and wake behaviour. The sedating properties of many over-the-counter (OTC) medications result from inhibiting one of these arousal systems (especially acetylcholine and histamine).

Neuropeptides also influence wake behaviour. *Orexin* (also called hypocretin) is found in the lateral hypothalamus. Orexin stimulates wake behaviour through activating the RAS. Decreased levels of orexin or its receptors lead to difficulties staying awake and the syndrome called narcolepsy (Nishino et al., 2010). (Narcolepsy is discussed later in this chapter.)

Sleep Behaviour. *Sleep behaviour* is regulated by a variety of neurological structures. Sleep-promoting neurotransmitters and peptides include melatonin, adenosine, somatostatin, growth hormone–releasing hormone, delta-sleep–inducing peptide, prostaglandins, and proinflammatory cytokines (interleukin-1, tumour necrosis factor–alpha, interleukin-6). Proinflammatory cytokines are important in mediating sleepiness and lethargy associated with infectious illness. Peptides, such as cholecystokinin, released by the gastrointestinal tract after food ingestion, may mediate the sleepiness following eating meals (*postprandial sleepiness*).

Melatonin is an endogenous hormone produced by the pineal gland in the brain from the amino acid tryptophan. In the central nervous system (CNS), melatonin decreases sleep latency and increases *sleep efficiency* (time asleep as compared with time in bed). The secretion of melatonin is tightly linked to the environmental light–dark cycle. Under normal day–night conditions, more melatonin is released in the evening as it gets dark (American Academy of Sleep Medicine, 2008).

Circadian Rhythms

Many biological rhythms of behaviour and physiology fluctuate within a 24-hour period of time. These **circadian** (*circa dian*, about a day) **rhythms** persist when people are placed in isolated environments free of external time cues because the rhythms are controlled by internal (endogenous) clock mechanisms. The suprachiasmatic nucleus (SCN) in the hypothalamus is the master clock of the body. The 24-hour cycle is synchronized to the environmental light and dark periods through specific light detectors in the retina. Pathways from the SCN innervate sleep-promoting cells in the anterior hypothalamus and wake-promoting cells of the lateral hypothalamus and brainstem.

Light is the strongest time cue for the sleep–wake rhythm. Because of this, light can be used as a therapy to shift the timing of the sleep–wake rhythm. For example, bright light used early in the morning will cause the sleep–wake rhythm to move to an earlier time; bright light used in the evening will cause the sleep–wake rhythm to move to a later time.

Sleep Architecture

Although there is variability in sleep characteristics and quality, the optimal amount of sleep for most adults is 7 to 8 hours a day in one period of time (Al Lawati, Patel, & Ayaz, 2009). Most adults transition from wake to sleep (*sleep onset latency*) in approximately 10 to 20 minutes.

Once asleep, a person goes through sleep cycles. A typical sleep cycle lasts 90 minutes and is repeated throughout the duration of the person's total sleep time. Based on electrical recordings of brain activity with polysomnography (PSG), sleep can be divided into two major states: *rapid eye movement (REM)* and *non–rapid eye movement (NREM)*.

NREM Sleep. In healthy adults, the largest percentage of sleep time, approximately 75 to 80%, is spent in NREM sleep. NREM sleep is subdivided into three stages (Iber, Ancoli-Israel, Chesson, & Quan, 2007).

Stage 1 occurs in the beginning of sleep, with slow eye movements, and is a transition phase from wakefulness to sleep. It is short in duration, lasting 1 to 7 minutes. The person can be easily awakened.

Stage 2 is a period of sound sleep. The heart rate slows down and the body temperature drops. This stage lasts 10 to 25 minutes.

Stage 3, previously divided into stages 3 and 4, is deep sleep or slow-wave sleep. It is the deepest stage of sleep. This stage lasts 20 to 40 minutes. Dreaming is more common in this stage than in other stages of NREM sleep, although not as common as in REM sleep.

REM Sleep. REM sleep accounts for 20 to 25% of sleep. REM sleep follows NREM sleep. In a healthy adult, REM sleep occurs four to five times during a period of 7 to 8 hours of sleep. This stage is considered paradoxical because the brain waves resemble wakefulness. REM sleep is thought to be important for memory consolidation and is the period when the most vivid dreaming occurs.

Sleep Disorders

Sleep deprivation and poor quality of sleep are associated with changes in body function (Figure 9-2) and health problems (Table 9-2). In patients with chronic illnesses, especially cardiovascular disease and stroke, sleep disorders are directly associated with increased mortality and morbidity (Anic, Titus-Ernstoff, Newcomb, Trentham-Dietz, & Egan, 2010; Bloom et al., 2009). Sleep loss is associated with decreases in immune function and body temperature and endocrine changes, including a decrease in growth hormone levels. Impaired cognitive function and impaired performance on simple behavioural tasks occur within 24 hours of sleep loss. The effects of sleep loss are cumulative. Chronic loss of sleep places the individual at risk for a decrease in cognitive function, depression, impaired daytime functioning, social isolation, and overall reduction in quality of life (Bloom et al., 2009).

An insufficient amount of nighttime sleep has a harmful impact on carbohydrate metabolism and endocrine function. Individuals who report less than 6 hours of sleep a night have a higher body mass index (BMI) and are more likely to be obese.

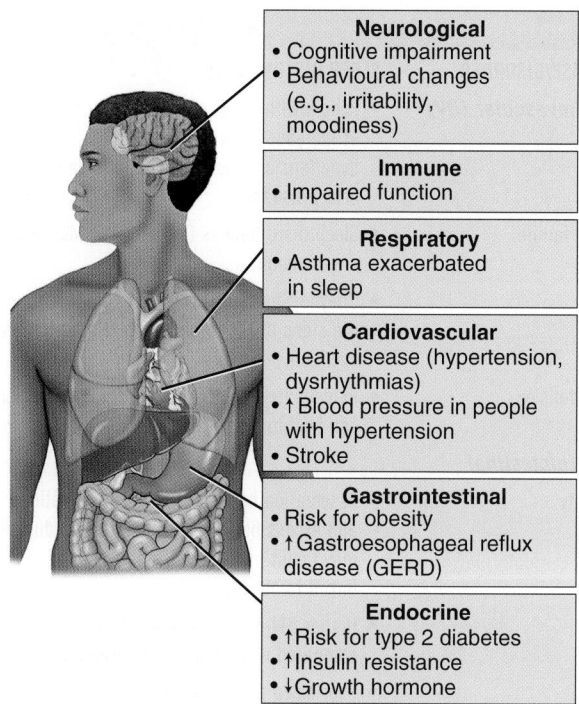

Neurological
- Cognitive impairment
- Behavioural changes (e.g., irritability, moodiness)

Immune
- Impaired function

Respiratory
- Asthma exacerbated in sleep

Cardiovascular
- Heart disease (hypertension, dysrhythmias)
- ↑ Blood pressure in people with hypertension
- Stroke

Gastrointestinal
- Risk for obesity
- ↑ Gastroesophageal reflux disease (GERD)

Endocrine
- ↑ Risk for type 2 diabetes
- ↑ Insulin resistance
- ↓ Growth hormone

Figure 9-2 Effects of sleep deprivation and sleep disorders on the body.

The risk for developing diabetes and glucose intolerance is increased in those individuals with a history of insufficient or poor quality of sleep (Chaput, Després, Bouchard, & Tremblay, 2007; Cappuccio, D'Elia, Strazzullo, & Miller, 2010).

Insomnia

The most common sleep disorder is insomnia. **Insomnia** is defined as difficulty falling asleep, difficulty staying asleep, waking up too early, or poor quality of sleep. Insomnia is a common problem, with approximately one in three adults experiencing it.

Acute insomnia refers to difficulties falling asleep or remaining asleep for at least 3 nights per week over a 2-week period. *Chronic insomnia* is defined by the same symptoms and a daytime complaint (e.g., fatigue, poor concentration, interference with social or family activities) that persist for 1 month or longer. Chronic insomnia occurs in 10 to 15% of Canadians and is more common in women than in men (Morin et al., 2011). Chronic insomnia increases in people older than 45 years of age and is higher in divorced, widowed, and separated individuals as well as in individuals with low socioeconomic status and lower amounts of education (Morin et al., 2011).

Etiology and Pathophysiology

Behaviours, lifestyle, diet, and medications contribute to insomnia. *Inadequate sleep hygiene* refers to those practices or behaviours that are inconsistent with quality sleep. Consumption of stimulants (e.g., caffeine, nicotine, methamphetamine, other drugs of abuse), especially before bedtime, results in insomnia. Insomnia is a common side effect of many medications (e.g., antidepressants, antihypertensives, corticosteroids, psychostimulants, analgesics). Insomnia can be exacerbated or perpetuated by drinking

alcohol to help induce sleep, smoking close to bedtime, taking long naps in the afternoon, sleeping in until late in the morning, nightmares, exercise near bedtime, and jet lag.

Chronic insomnia is classified as either primary or secondary. *Primary* or *idiopathic insomnia* is a lifelong difficulty in initiating and maintaining sleep, resulting in poor daytime functioning. The diagnosis of primary insomnia occurs after medical, neurological, and psychiatric causes have been excluded (Towards Optimized Practice, 2010). The etiology of primary insomnia is not known. Certain individuals may be predisposed or have built-in psychological traits that make them vulnerable to develop insomnia. Individuals with chronic insomnia often report that the onset of disturbed sleep occurred after a stressful life event (e.g., loss of loved one).

Secondary (co-morbid) insomnia is caused by psychiatric illness, medical conditions (see Table 9-2), medications, or substance abuse. The etiology of the co-morbid insomnia may be related to the pathophysiology of the medical condition.

Once chronic insomnia is manifested, symptoms are likely to persist over time. Individuals may engage in behaviours that perpetuate disturbed sleep by keeping irregular sleep–wake schedules, using OTC medications or alcohol as sleep aids, and spending more time in bed trying to sleep. Increased attention to one's environment, worry or fear about not obtaining sufficient sleep, and poor sleep habits can lead to a conditioned arousal.

Clinical Manifestations

Manifestations of insomnia include (1) difficulty falling asleep *(long sleep latency)*, (2) frequent awakenings *(fragmented sleep)*, (3) prolonged nighttime awakenings or awakening too early and not being able to fall back to sleep, and (4) feeling unrefreshed on awakening, called *nonrestorative sleep*. Daytime consequences of insomnia may manifest as feeling tired, having trouble concentrating at work or school, altered mood, and falling asleep during the day. Behavioural manifestations of poor sleep include irritability, forgetfulness, confusion, difficulty staying awake during the day, and anxiety.

Diagnostic Studies

Self-Report. The diagnosis of insomnia is made on the basis of subjective complaints and on an evaluation of a 1- or 2-week sleep diary completed by the patient. In ambulatory care settings, the evaluation of insomnia requires a comprehensive sleep history to establish the type of insomnia and to screen for possible psychiatric, medical, or sleep disorder co-morbidities that would require specific treatment. Questionnaires such as eTable 9-1, Pittsburgh Sleep Quality Index; and eTable 9-2, Epworth Sleepiness Scale, available on the Evolve Web site for this chapter, are examples of questionnaires commonly used to assess sleep quality (Buysse, Reynolds, Monk, Berman, & Kupfer, 1989; Johns, 1991).

Actigraphy. Actigraphy is a relatively noninvasive method of monitoring rest and activity cycles. A small actigraph watch can be worn on the wrist to measure gross motor activity (Figure 9-3). The unit continually records the movements. After the data are collected, they are downloaded to a computer, and algorithms are used to analyze the data.

Polysomnography. A clinical PSG study is not required to establish a diagnosis of insomnia. A PSG study is done only if

Table 9-2 Relationship of Sleep Disturbances to Selected Diseases and Disorders

DISEASE/DISORDER	SLEEP DISTURBANCE	DISEASE/DISORDER	SLEEP DISTURBANCE
Respiratory		**Cardiovascular (CV)**	• People with sleep apnea/sleep disorders are at increased risk for CV disorders including hypertension, dysrhythmias, and coronary artery disease.
Asthma	• Exacerbated during sleep. • Report more insomnia.	Heart failure	• Sleep disturbances (insomnia, PLMD, SDB) are common. • Cheyne-Stokes breathing and central apnea are signs of HF exacerbation related to fluid overload.
Chronic obstructive pulmonary disease (COPD)	• Associated with poor sleep quality, nocturnal O_2 desaturation, and coexisting sleep apnea.		
Obstructive sleep apnea	• Link with heart disease (hypertension, stroke, coronary artery disease, dysrhythmias). • Develop impaired glucose control similar to that which occurs in type 2 diabetes. • Associated with cancer.	Hypertension	• Inadequate sleep in people with hypertension can lead to further elevations in BP.
Renal		**Gastrointestinal**	
End-stage renal disease	• Disrupted nocturnal sleep with excessive daytime sleepiness. • Patients on dialysis have high incidence of SDB, PLMD, and RLS, which is a significant predictor of mortality in these patients.	Obesity	• Association between short sleep duration and excess body weight. Short sleep duration may result in metabolic changes that are linked to obesity. • Higher BMI in people who sleep <6 hr compared with people who sleep >8 hr. • Poor sleep associated with low levels of leptin and high levels of ghrelin.
Immune Disorders		Gastroesophageal reflux disease (GERD)	• Reflux of gastric contents into the esophagus occurs during sleep due to incompetent lower esophageal sphincter.
Human immunodeficiency virus (HIV)	• Sleep disturbances and fatigue are highly prevalent and are associated with survival.	Chronic liver disease	• Associated with excessive sleepiness, nocturnal arousal, and incidence of RLS.
Endocrine		Bowel disorders	• Associated with increased insomnia.
Diabetes	• Insufficient sleep linked to increased risk for type 2 diabetes. • Sleep deprivation in healthy people increases insulin resistance. • Sleep duration and quality are predictors of Hb A1C levels, an important marker of blood glucose control.	**Neurological**	
		Parkinson's disease	• Associated with difficulty initiating or maintaining sleep, parasomnias, and excessive daytime sleepiness.
		Alzheimer's disease	• Many have SDB (frequently sleep apnea). • Circadian rhythm alterations with nocturnal wandering, daytime sleepiness, and sleep disruption and awakening.
Musculoskeletal		Pain (acute and chronic)	• Decreased quantity and quality of sleep. Poor sleep can intensify pain.
Arthritis	• Increased rates of RLS and SDB. Disease activity linked to sleep complaints.	**Cancer**	• Report higher rates of insomnia. • Chemotherapy for cancer treatment associated with fragmented sleep.
Fibromyalgia	• Dysfunctional sleep regulation related to altered circadian rhythms and lower concentrations of sleep-dependent hormones (growth hormone, prolactin).		
Chronic fatigue syndrome	• Sleep disturbances including decreases in total sleep time are reported.		

BMI, Body mass index; *Hb,* hemoglobin; *HF,* heart failure; *PLMD,* periodic limb movement disorder; *RLS,* restless legs syndrome; *SDB,* sleep-disordered breathing.

Sources: US Department of Health and Human Services, National Institutes of Health, & National Heart, Lung and Blood Institute, National Center on Sleep Disorders Research, Trans-NIH Sleep Research Coordinating Committee. (2003). Section 4—Sleep and Health. *2003 National Sleep Disorders Research Plan.* Retrieved from *http://www.nhlbi.nih.gov/health/prof/sleep/res_plan/section4/section4e.html;* Centers for Disease Control and Prevention. (2011). *Sleep and chronic disease.* Retrieved from *http://www.cdc.gov/sleep/about_sleep/chronic_disease.htm;* Tjepkema, M. (2005). Insomnia. *Health Reports, 17,* 9-16.

there are symptoms or signs of a sleep disorder, such as sleep-disordered breathing (discussed later). In a PSG study, electrodes simultaneously record physiological measures that define the main stages of sleep and wakefulness. These measures include (1) muscle tone recorded using an electromyogram (EMG), (2) eye movements recorded with an electro-oculogram (EOG), and (3) brain activity recorded through an EEG. To determine additional characteristics of specific sleep disorders, other measures are made during PSG. These include airflow at the nose and mouth, respiratory effort around the chest and abdomen, heart rate, non-invasive oxygen saturation, and EMG of the anterior tibialis muscles (used to detect periodic leg movements). Finally, a patient's gross body movements are monitored continuously by audiovisual means.

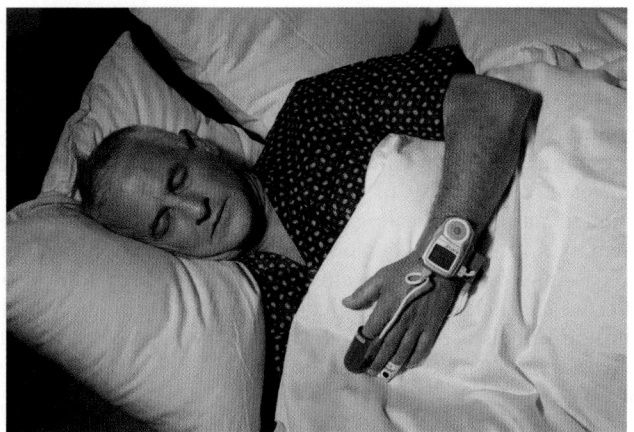

Figure 9-3 Actigraph watch worn while the patient is sleeping.

Source: Courtesy of Itamar Medical, Inc.

COLLABORATIVE CARE
Table 9-3 Insomnia

Diagnostic
- History
  - Self-report sleep log or diary
  - Sleep assessment (see Table 9-6)
  - Pittsburgh Sleep Quality Index*
  - Epworth Sleepiness Scale†
- Physical assessment
- Polysomnography

Collaborative Therapy
- Nondrug
  - Sleep hygiene (see Table 9-4)
- Cognitive behavioural therapy

- Drugs (see Table 9-5)
  - Benzodiazepines
  - Benzodiazepine-receptor–like agents
  - Antidepressants
  - Antihistamines
- Complementary and alternative therapies
  - Melatonin
  - Acupressure
- Acupuncture
- Tai Chi

*See eTable 9-1, available on the Evolve Web site for this chapter.
†See eTable 9-2, available on the Evolve Web site for this chapter.

Collaborative Care

Treatments are oriented toward symptom management (Table 9-3). A key to management is to change behaviours that perpetuate insomnia. This often includes cognitive behavioural strategies and education about sleep, including sleep hygiene. **Sleep hygiene** is a variety of different practices that are important for normal, quality nighttime sleep and daytime alertness (Table 9-4).

Cognitive-Behavioural Therapies.
Cognitive-behavioural therapies (CBTs) are effective in the management of insomnia and should be the first line of therapy (Dirksen & Epstein, 2008; Irwin, Cole, & Nicassio, 2006). CBTs for insomnia include relaxation training, guided imagery, cognitive strategies to address dysfunctional ideas about sleep, and behavioural strategies that target an individual's poor sleep habits. Behavioural therapies for insomnia also include education about good sleep hygiene practices (see Table 9-4). Regular exercise (performed several hours

Table 9-4 Sleep Hygiene

You should include the following instructions when teaching a patient who has sleep disturbances/disorders:
- Do not go to bed unless you are sleepy.
- If you are not asleep after 20 minutes, get out of bed.
- Adopt a regular pattern in terms of bedtime and awakening.
- Begin rituals (e.g., warm bath, light snack, reading) that help you relax each night before bed.
- Get a full night's sleep on a regular basis.
- Keep a regular schedule.
- Do not read, write, eat, watch TV, talk on the phone, or play cards in bed.
- Do not have beer, wine, or any other alcohol within 6 hours of your bedtime.
- Do not have a cigarette or any other source of nicotine before bedtime.
- Do not go to bed hungry, but do not eat a big meal near bedtime either.
- Avoid any strenuous exercise within 6 hours of your bedtime.
- Avoid sleeping pills, or use them cautiously.
- Try to get rid of or deal with things that make you worry.
- Make your bedroom quiet, dark, and a little bit cool.
- Avoid caffeine, nicotine, and alcohol at least 4 to 6 hours before bedtime.

Source: Adapted from American Academy of Sleep Medicine. (2010). *Sleep hygiene: The healthy habits of good sleep.* Retrieved from *http://yoursleep.aasmnet.org/Hygiene.aspx*

before bedtime) may enhance sleep quality. CBTs require individuals to change behaviour. Supporting a patient's behaviour changes requires evaluation of his or her motivation and ability prior to initiating treatments (Towards Optimized Practice, 2010).

Individuals with insomnia are encouraged to not watch television, play video games, or read in bed. Time in bed is limited to the actual time that the individual can sleep. Naps and consumption of large meals, alcohol, and stimulants need to be avoided. Naps are less likely to affect nighttime sleep if they are limited to 20 to 30 minutes.

Drug Therapy.
Hypnotic and anxiolytic medications are effective for the short-term management of insomnia. However, the use of hypnotics in the management of chronic insomnia, particularly in the elderly, is controversial (Passarella & Duong, 2008). Many individuals with insomnia become used to taking OTC or prescription medications to treat insomnia and risk becoming dependent on them, both psychologically and physically (Chapter 11 has more information on substance dependence). *Rebound insomnia* is common with abrupt withdrawal of hypnotic medications. The resulting daytime fatigue can negatively influence the patient's efforts to use nondrug approaches. Classes of medications used to treat insomnia include benzodiazepines, benzodiazepine-receptor–like agents, and antidepressant and antihistamine medications (Table 9-5).

Benzodiazepines. Benzodiazepines such as diazepam (Valium) work by activating the γ-aminobutyric acid (GABA) receptors to promote sleep. The prolonged half-life of some of these

DRUG THERAPY

Table 9-5 Insomnia

Benzodiazepines	Antidepressants
• Nitrazepam (Mogadon)	• Trazodone
• Flurazepam (Dalmane)	**Antihistamines**
• Temazepam (Restoril)	• Diphenhydramine (Benadryl, Nytol, Unisom)
• Triazolam	
Benzodiazepine-Receptor–like Agents	
• Zopiclone (Rhovane, Imovane)	

Source: Health Canada. (2009). *Authorized sleep-aid medications in Canada*. Retrieved from *http://www.hc-sc.gc.ca/ahc-asc/media/advisories-avis/_2009/2009_161-list-eng.php*

agents (e.g., flurazepam [Dalmane]) can result in daytime sleepiness, amnesia, dizziness, and rebound insomnia (Passarella & Duong, 2008). Tolerance to these agents develops slowly, but there is some risk for dependence. It is recommended that the use of benzodiazepines be limited to 2 to 3 weeks. All benzodiazepines have the potential for abuse (see Chapter 11 for more information on benzodiazepine abuse). In addition, benzodiazepines interact with alcohol and other CNS depressants. These agents are no longer recommended as first-line therapy for insomnia.

Benzodiazepine-Receptor–like Agents. Zopiclone (Imovane, Rhovane) is the drug of first choice for insomnia. Because it is a benzodiazepine-receptor agonist, it works similarly to benzodiazepines (Conn & Madan, 2006). Because of the potential delay of activity, it should not be taken with food. This agent has a short half-life, making its duration of action short (Calamaro, 2008).

Antidepressants. Trazodone is an atypical antidepressant that has sedative properties. Trazodone is one of the most common agents prescribed in Canada to treat insomnia. However, the administration of this drug to older adults is controversial.

Antihistamines. Many individuals with insomnia self-medicate with OTC sleep aids. Most OTC agents include diphenhydramine (Benadryl, Nytol, Unisom). These agents are less effective than benzodiazepines and tolerance develops quickly. In addition, there are side effects including daytime sedation, impaired cognitive function, blurred vision, urinary retention, constipation, and risk of increased intraocular pressure. Agents that contain diphenhydramine are not intended for long-term use and should not be used by older adults.

Complementary and Alternative Therapies.

Many types of complementary therapies and herbal products are used as sleep aids. As noted earlier in the chapter, melatonin is a hormone produced by the pineal gland (Ferguson, Rajaratnam, & Dawson, 2010) (see Complementary & Alternative Therapies box). Valerian is an herb that has been used for many years as a sleep aid and to relieve anxiety. However, the research evidence to support the use of valerian to treat insomnia is lacking (Taibi et al., 2008). Acupuncture and acupressure have both been found in several research trials to improve sleep quality (Cao, Pan, Li, & Liu, 2009; Sun, Sung, Huang, Cheng, & Lin, 2010). Acupuncture is an invasive technique that requires a trained provider, and acupressure is a massage technique that can be administered by nursing staff, families, and caregivers (Reza et al., 2010). This area of Chinese medicine has been showing promising results, but continued research is required to help define the specific acupressure points, duration, and longevity of effect (Reza et al., 2010; Sun et al., 2010). Tai Chi is a meditative gentle exercise from Chinese martial and healing arts (Yeh et al., 2008) (see Complementary & Alternative Therapies box). Tai Chi is a nonstrenuous exercise and has relaxation effects that have been found to be effective for increasing sleep quality in older adults and people with cardiac disease (Hosseini, Esfirizi, Marandi, & Rezaei, 2011; Yeh et al., 2008) (see Complementary & Alternative Therapies box below).

COMPLEMENTARY & ALTERNATIVE THERAPIES

Melatonin

Scientific Evidence

Overall, the scientific evidence suggests benefits of melatonin in people who take it for jet lag. The majority of scientific evidence suggests that it decreases the time it takes to fall asleep (sleep latency) and may increase the duration of sleep.

Nursing Implications

- Regarded as safe in recommended doses for short-term use.
- Avoid in patients using warfarin (Coumadin).
- May cause drops in blood pressure. Caution is advised in patients taking drugs that may also lower blood pressure.

Source: Sarris, J., & Byrne, G. J. (2010). A systematic review of insomnia and complementary medicine. *Sleep Medicine Reviews 15*(20), 99–106. doi:10.1016/j.smrv.2010.04.001

COMPLEMENTARY & ALTERNATIVE THERAPIES

Tai Chi Exercise

Scientific Evidence

Several studies including randomized control trials have demonstrated the effectiveness of Tai Chi in improving sleep quality and duration. Because Tai Chi involves relaxation, rhythmic breathing, and exercise, the exact mechanism of action is unclear.

Nursing Implications

- Tai Chi is a well-tolerated accessible nonpharmacological intervention.
- Particularly suited for people with decreased exercise tolerance such as elderly people and those with cardiac conditions.
- Further research using Tai Chi may help specify who can benefit the most from the intervention.

Sources: Irwin, M. R., Olmstead, R., & Motivala, S. J. (2008). Improving sleep quality in older adults with moderate sleep complaints: A randomized controlled trail of Tai Chi Chih. *Sleep, 31*, 1001–1008; Yeh, G., Mietus, J. E., Peng, C. K., Phillips, R., Davis, R. B., Wayne, P. M., ..., Thomas, R. J. (2008). Enhancement of sleep stability with Tai Chi exercise in chronic heart failure: Preliminary findings using an ECG-based spectrogram method. *Sleep Medicine, 9*, 527–536. doi:10.1016/j.sleep.2007.06.003

NURSING MANAGEMENT: INSOMNIA

▪ Nursing Assessment

As a nurse, you are in a key position to assess sleep problems in patients and their family caregivers. Sleep assessment is important in helping patients to identify environmental factors that may contribute to poor sleep. Family caregivers may experience sleep disruptions owing to the necessity of providing care to patients in the home. These sleep disruptions can increase the burden of caregiving.

Both subjective and objective ways are used to assess sleep duration and quality. Report of poor sleep is similar to pain in that it is a subjective complaint. Many patients may not tell their health care provider about their sleep problems. Therefore, the best way to detect sleep problems is to ask about sleep on a regular basis. A sleep history should involve characteristics of sleep, such as the duration and pattern of sleep, and daytime alertness. Before using any questionnaire, the patient's cognitive function, reading level (if a paper form is used), and language are assessed.

Examples of questions to assess sleep are presented in Table 9-6. Also assess the diet. Question the patient about the intake of caffeine and other food stimulants. In addition to asking about how much alcohol is consumed each week, find out whether alcohol is used as a sleep aid. However, some patients may not recall their use of alcohol to promote sleep and others may not volunteer this information.

NURSING ASSESSMENT

Table 9-6 Sleep
The following questions can serve as an initial assessment regarding sleep:
1. What time do you normally go to bed at night? What time do you normally wake up in the morning?
2. Do you often have trouble falling asleep at night?
3. About how many times do you wake up at night?
4. If you do wake up during the night, do you usually have trouble falling back asleep?
5. Does your bed partner say or are you aware that you frequently snore, gasp for air, or stop breathing?
6. Does your bed partner say or are you aware that you kick or thrash about while asleep?
7. Are you aware that you ever walk, eat, punch, kick, or scream during sleep?
8. Are you sleepy or tired during much of the day?
9. Do you usually take one or more naps during the day?
10. Do you usually doze off without planning to during the day?
11. How much sleep do you need to feel alert and function well?
12. Are you currently taking any type of medication or other preparation to help you sleep?

Source: Bloom, H. G., Ahmed, I., Alessi, C. A., Ancoli-Israel, S., Buysse, D. J., Kryger, M. H., ..., Zee, P. C. (2009). Evidence-based recommendations for the assessment and management of sleep disorders in older persons. *Journal of the American Geriatric Society, 57*, 761.

Ask the patient about sleep aids. This includes both OTC and prescription medications. It is important to note the drug dose and frequency of use, as well as any side effects (e.g., daytime drowsiness, dry mouth). Many individuals also consume herbal or dietary supplements to improve sleep, including valerian, melatonin, hops, lavender, passion flower, and skullcap. The exact components and concentrations of herbs and supplements often are unknown, and patients may experience adverse effects. Additional sleep aids include white noise devices or relaxation strategies.

You can encourage individuals to keep a sleep diary for 2 weeks. In the diary, have them record when they go to sleep, when they wake up, and how long they were awake during the night. The number and duration of naps are also recorded. Standardized questionnaires such as the Epworth Sleepiness Scale may be used to assess daytime sleepiness (Johns, 1991).

The patient's medical history can also provide important information about factors that contribute to poor sleep. For example, men with benign prostatic hyperplasia often report frequent awakenings during the night for voiding. Psychiatric problems including depression, anxiety, post-traumatic stress disorder (PTSD), and drug abuse are associated with sleep disturbances. Sleep disturbances often develop as a consequence or complication of a chronic or terminal condition (e.g., heart disease, dementia, cancer, renal failure).

Ask the patient about work schedules as well as cross-country and international travel. Shift work can contribute to reduced or poor-quality sleep. Work-related behaviours resulting from poor sleep may include poor performance, decreased productivity, and job absenteeism.

▪ Nursing Diagnoses

Specific nursing diagnoses related to sleep include insomnia, sleep deprivation, disturbed sleep pattern, and readiness for enhanced sleep.

▪ Nursing Implementation

Nursing interventions depend on the severity and duration of the sleep problem as well as the characteristics of the individual. Optimally, healthy adults should have 7 to 8 hours of sleep a night. Individuals with longer (>9 hours) and shorter (<6 hours) sleep durations may have increased morbidity and mortality risks. Those with short sleep duration have increased risk for weight gain, impaired glucose tolerance and diabetes, hypertension, cardiovascular disease, and stroke. Occasional difficulty getting to sleep or awakening during the night is not unusual. However, prolonged sleep disruptions become problematic.

You can assume a primary role in teaching sleep hygiene (see Table 9-4). Although education about sleep hygiene practices is beneficial, individuals with chronic insomnia will require more in-depth training in cognitive-behavioural strategies. An important component of sleep hygiene is reducing dietary intake of substances containing caffeine. Reducing caffeine intake requires awareness of the caffeine content of certain foods and beverages and the understanding that caffeine and related stimulants such as guarana and yerba mate are not always listed on ingredient labels (Health Canada, 2010). Table 9-7 provides examples of the caffeine content of beverages and foods. Health Canada (2010)

Table 9-7 Caffeine Content of Selected Foods and Beverages

FOOD/BEVERAGE	CAFFEINE (mg)
Coffee, brewed (237 mL)	95-200
Coffee, instant (237 mL)	27-173
Coffee, decaffeinated	5
Tea, leaf or bag (237 mL)	50
Celestial Seasoning herbal tea, all varieties	0
Diet Coke (355 mL)	47
Coca-Cola (355 mL)	45
Dr. Pepper (237 mL)	41
Pepsi-Cola (355 mL)	37
7-Up or Diet 7-Up (355 mL)	0
Root Beer (355 mL)	0
Energy drinks (Red Bull, Monster, Rock Star) (237 mL)	80
Chocolate cake (1 piece)	36
Milk chocolate bar (28 g piece)	7
Dark chocolate bar (28 g piece)	19
Hot chocolate (237 mL)	5

Source: Based on Health Canada. (2010). *It's your health: Caffeine.* Retrieved from *http://www.hc-sc.gc.ca/hl-vs/iyh-vsv/food-aliment/caffeine-eng.php*

recommends no more than 400 mg of caffeine per day for the general adult population and lower amounts for children and women of child-bearing age.

You are also in an ideal position to take the lead in suggesting and implementing change in the home and institutional environment to enhance sleep. Reducing light and noise levels can enhance sleep. Awareness of time passing and watching the clock add to anxieties about not falling asleep or returning to sleep.

Patients require teaching about sleeping medications. With the benzodiazepines and zopiclone (Imovane), the patient is taught to take the drug right before bedtime, be prepared to get a full night's sleep of at least 6 to 8 hours, and not plan activities the next morning that require highly skilled psychomotor coordination. With these agents, the patient should avoid high-fat foods that can alter drug absorption. These medications should not be taken with alcohol or other CNS depressants to avoid oversedation.

Patient follow-up regarding medications is important. Ask the patient about daytime sleepiness, nightmares, and any difficulties in activities of daily living. For patients who have been taking sleeping medications for a period of time, withdrawal of the drug should be tapered.

Sleep Disturbances in the Hospital

Hospitalization, especially in the critical care unit (CCU), is associated with decreases in total sleep time, sleep efficiency, and REM sleep. Pre-existing sleep disorders may be aggravated or triggered in the hospital. Environmental sleep-disruptive factors, psychoactive medications, and acute and critical illness all contribute to poor sleep. Patient symptoms including pain, dyspnea, and nausea can also contribute to sleep loss in the acutely ill patient.

Medications commonly used in acutely and critically ill patients can further contribute to sleep loss. Hospitalized patients are at risk for poor sleep owing in part to circadian rhythm disruptions. The hospital or long-term care facility represents a new environment, and thus, normal cues linked to sleep may be absent.

The hospital and ICU environmental noise (e.g., staff paging system, respirator alarms, bedside monitors, infusion alarms, staff conversations near patients) during both the day and the night can result in sleep difficulties. Bright lights during the night can also disrupt sleep. In addition, patient care activities (e.g., dressing changes, blood draws, vital sign monitoring) will disrupt sleep. Sleep-disordered breathing is a major concern in the ICU. Mechanically ventilated patients have abnormal sleep architecture with a short REM stage and increased fragmentation (Brown & Arora, 2008; Cabello et al., 2008). Poor sleep can last past the patient's ICU admission and can affect the long-term recovery and health (Weinhouse & Schwab, 2006).

Decreased sleep duration influences pain perception. Psychological factors, such as anxiety and depression, will also modify the sleep–pain relationship. Adequate pain management improves the duration and quality of sleep, but medications commonly used to relieve pain, especially opioids, also alter sleep and place the individual at risk for sleep-disordered breathing. Withdrawal of opioids is associated with rebound effects on sleep architecture.

As a nurse, you have a critical role in creating an environment conducive to sleep. This includes the scheduling of medications and procedures. Considering typical sleep architecture when planning interventions and care can be helpful. Scheduling any necessary care episodes to 90 minutes (or a multiple of that) after a patient has fallen asleep has been found to be effective in decreasing sleep disruption. Reducing light and noise levels or use of ear plugs can promote opportunities for sleep. Because, often, patients are having to catch up with sleep during daytime hours, scheduling of care and environmental noise control are needed in the daytime to allow for naps (Weinhouse & Schwab, 2006).

Narcolepsy

Narcolepsy is a chronic neurological disorder caused by the brain's inability to regulate sleep–wake cycles normally. At various times throughout the day, people with narcolepsy experience fleeting urges to sleep. If the urge becomes overwhelming, individuals will fall asleep for periods lasting from a few seconds to several minutes (Nishino et al., 2010).

Narcolepsy affects both men and women. The onset of narcolepsy typically occurs in adolescence or early in the third decade. There are two categories of narcolepsy: narcolepsy with cataplexy and narcolepsy without cataplexy. **Cataplexy** is a brief and sudden loss of skeletal muscle tone or muscle weakness. It can manifest as a brief episode of muscle weakness to complete postural collapse and falling to the ground. Laughter, anger, or surprise often triggers episodes. Approximately 30 to 50% of patients with narcolepsy experience cataplexy (Nishino et al., 2010). Patients with narcolepsy, particularly those with cataplexy, have decreased quality of life because of excessive daytime sleepiness.

Etiology and Pathophysiology

The cause of narcolepsy remains unknown. A deficiency of orexin (hypocretin), a neuropeptide linked to waking, is associated with narcolepsy. The reason for this deficiency is not well understood (Nishino et al., 2010).

Clinical Manifestations and Diagnostic Studies

Symptoms in some patients include brief episodes of sleep paralysis, hallucinations, cataplexy, and fragmented nighttime sleep. *Sleep paralysis* is a temporary (few seconds to minutes) paralysis of skeletal muscles (except respiratory and extraocular muscles) that occurs in the transition from REM sleep to waking. The loss of muscle tone, often triggered by strong emotions, usually lasts less than 2 minutes. During the period of muscle tone loss, the individual remains conscious.

Unwanted episodes of REM sleep occur throughout the day in patients with narcolepsy. These naps are usually of short duration, but they can last for more than 1 hour, and patients feel refreshed afterward. Patients may complain of feeling drowsy and being unable to remain awake while watching a movie, sitting in a classroom, reading, or performing other sedentary activities. As a result, they often show poor performance at work, have reduced quality of life, and are disabled with poor interpersonal relationships.

Narcolepsy is diagnosed based on a history of sleepiness, PSG, and daytime *multiple sleep latency tests* (MSLTs). Short sleep latencies and onset of REM sleep in more than two MSLTs are diagnostic signs of narcolepsy.

Collaborative Care

Drug Therapy. Narcolepsy cannot be cured. But excessive daytime sleepiness and cataplexy, the most disabling symptoms of the disorder, can be controlled in most patients with drug treatment. Drug management of narcolepsy includes amphetamine-like stimulants to relieve excessive daytime sleepiness and antidepressant drug therapy to control cataplexy (Ohayon & Okun, 2006; Bhat & El Solh, 2008) (Table 9-8). CNS stimulant drugs such as dextroamphetamine (Dexedrine) and methylphenidate are used to manage daytime sleepiness. A non-amphetamine wake-promotion drug, modafinil (Alertec) is considered a first-line drug therapy.

A selective norepinephrine reuptake inhibitor atomoxetine (Strattera) and the tricyclic desipramine are effective in the management of cataplexy. High doses of selective serotonin reuptake inhibitors (SSRIs) such as fluoxetine (Prozac) and venlafaxine (Effexor) may be prescribed for management of cataplexy. Sodium oxybate or γ-hydroxybutyrate (Xyrem), a metabolite of GABA, is used in the treatment of cataplexy.

Behavioural Therapy. None of the current drug therapies cure narcolepsy or allow patients to consistently maintain a full, normal state of alertness. As a result, drug therapy is combined with various behavioural strategies. The behavioural therapies for insomnia (discussed earlier in this chapter) are also used for patients with narcolepsy.

Safety precautions, especially when driving, are critically important for patients with narcolepsy. Excessive daytime sleepiness and cataplexy can result in serious injury or death if not treated. Individuals with untreated narcolepsy symptoms are involved in automobile accidents roughly 10 times more frequently than the general population. Among those receiving appropriate treatment, the accident rate is normal (Bhat & El Solh, 2008). You can play a key role in ensuring patient safety and maintaining compliance with prescribed medications.

Patient support groups are also useful for many patients with narcolepsy and their family members. Social isolation can occur because of symptoms. Patients with narcolepsy can be stigmatized as being lazy and unproductive because of lack of understanding about this disorder.

Circadian Rhythm Disorders

Circadian rhythm disorders can occur when the circadian time-keeping system loses synchrony with the environment. Lack of synchrony between the circadian time-keeping system and the environment will disrupt the sleep–wake cycle and affect the patient's ability to have quality sleep. The two common symptoms are insomnia and excessive sleepiness.

Jet lag disorder occurs when an individual's travel results in the crossing of multiple time zones and the person's body time is not synchronized with environmental time. Most individuals crossing at least three time zones will experience jet lag. The number of time zones crossed affects the severity of symptoms and the time it takes to recover. Resynchronization of the body's clock occurs at a rate of about 1 hour per day when travelling eastward and 1.5 hours per day when travelling westward. Melatonin is effective as a sleep aid to help synchronize the body's rhythm. Daytime exposure to daylight assists synchronization of the body clock to environment time.

Several strategies may help to reduce the risk of developing jet lag. Before travel, the individual can start to get in harmony with the time schedule of the destination. When time at destination is brief (i.e., ≤2 days), keeping home-based sleep hours rather than adopting destination sleep hours may reduce sleepiness and jet lag symptoms.

Sleep-Disordered Breathing

The term **sleep-disordered breathing (SDB)** indicates abnormal respiratory patterns associated with sleep. These include snoring, apnea, and hypopnea with increased respiratory effort leading to frequent arousals. Sleep-disordered breathing results in frequent sleep disruptions and alterations in sleep architecture. Obstructive sleep apnea (OSA) is the most commonly diagnosed sleep-disordered breathing problem.

DRUG THERAPY

Table 9-8 Narcolepsy

Wakefulness-Promoting	Antidepressants
• Dextroamphetamine (Dexedrine)	• Tricyclic
• Methamphetamine	• Desipramine
• Methylphenidate (Concerta)	• Selective serotonin reuptake inhibitors (SSRIs)
• Modafinil (Alertec)	• Fluoxetine (Prozac)
Gabaminergic	• Venlafaxine (Effexor)
• Sodium oxybate/γ-hydroxybutyrate (Xyrem)	• Selective norepinephrine reuptake inhibitor (SNRI)
	• Atomoxetine (Strattera)

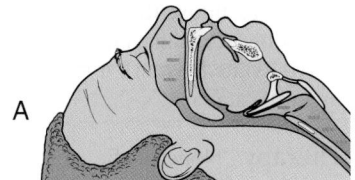

Patient predisposed to OSA

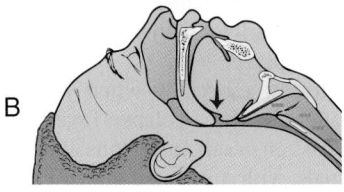

Apneic episode

Nasal CPAP

Figure 9-4 How sleep apnea occurs. **A,** The patient predisposed to obstructive sleep apnea (OSA) has a small pharyngeal airway. **B,** During sleep, the pharyngeal muscles relax, allowing the airway to close. Lack of airflow results in repeated apneic episodes. **C,** With continuous positive airway pressure (CPAP), the airway is splinted open, preventing airflow obstruction.

Source: Courtesy Robert Margulies, Miami, FL. From Smolley, L. A. (1990). How to help patients with obstructive sleep apnea, *Journal of Respiratory Diseases, 11,* 723-732.

Obstructive Sleep Apnea

Obstructive sleep apnea (OSA), also called *obstructive sleep apnea–hypopnea syndrome* (OSAHS), is characterized by partial or complete upper airway obstruction during sleep. *Apnea* is the cessation of spontaneous respirations lasting longer than 10 seconds. *Hypopnea* is a condition characterized by shallow (30–50% reduction in airflow) respirations. Airflow obstruction occurs because of narrowing of the air passages with relaxation of muscle tone during sleep, leading to apnea and hypopnea, or when the tongue and the soft palate fall backward and partially or completely obstruct the pharynx (Figure 9-4).

Each obstruction may last from 10 to 90 seconds. During the apneic period, the patient can experience *hypoxemia* (decreased PaO_2 or SpO_2) and *hypercapnia* (increased $PaCO_2$). These changes are ventilatory stimulants and cause brief arousals, but the patient may not fully awaken. The patient has a generalized startle response, snorts, and gasps, which causes the tongue and soft palate to move forward and the airway to open. Apnea and arousal cycles occur repeatedly, as many as 200 to 400 times during 6 to 8 hours of sleep.

Sleep apnea occurs in at least 3% of the population but is considered to be underreported (PHAC, 2009). The risk increases with obesity (BMI >35 kg/m^2), age older than 50 years, neck circumference greater than 43 cm (17 in), craniofacial abnormalities that affect the upper airway, and acromegaly (Bhat & El

Table 9-9 STOP-BANG		
STOP		
S (Snore): Have you ever been told that you snore?	Yes	No
T (Tired): Are you often tired during the day?	Yes	No
O (Obstruction): Do you know if you stop breathing or has anyone witnessed you stop breathing while you are asleep?	Yes	No
P (Pressure): Do you have high blood pressure or are you on medication to control high blood pressure?	Yes	No
If the person answers "Yes" to two or more of the STOP questions, she or he is at risk for OSA and should contact her or his primary care provider. The second component of this questionnaire (BANG) provides risk assessment of moderate to severe risk of OSA.		
BANG		
B (BMI): Is your body mass index greater than 28?	Yes	No
A (Age): Are you 50 years or older?	Yes	No
N (Neck): Are you a male with a neck circumference greater than 43 cm or a female with a neck circumference greater than 41 cm?	Yes	No
G (Gender): Are you a male?	Yes	No

Source: Chung, F., Yegneswaran, B., Liao, P., Chung, S. A., Vairavanathan, S., Islam, S., ..., Shapiro, C. M. (2008). STOP questionnaire: A tool to screen patients for obstructive sleep apnea. *Anesthesiology, 108,* 812-821. doi:10.1097/ALN.0b013e31816d83e4.

Solh, 2008; PHAC, 2009). Smokers are more likely to have OSA. OSA is twice as common in men as in women. Women with OSA have higher mortality rates. Hypoxemia associated with OSA is greater in those patients with chronic obstructive pulmonary disease (COPD) (Hiestand & Phillips, 2008).

The STOP-BANG questionnaire summarizes the key risk factors and is increasingly used as a screening tool for OSA (Chung et al., 2012) (Table 9-9). The more questions you answer YES to on the BANG portion, the greater your risk of having moderate to severe OSA.

Clinical Manifestations and Diagnostic Studies

Clinical manifestations of sleep apnea include frequent arousals during sleep, insomnia, excessive daytime sleepiness, and witnessed apneic episodes. The patient's bed partner may complain about the patient's loud snoring. The snoring may be so disruptive that both people cannot sleep in the same room. Other symptoms include morning headaches (from hypercapnia or increased blood pressure that causes vasodilation of cerebral blood vessels), personality changes, and irritability.

Complications that can result from untreated sleep apnea include hypertension, right-sided heart failure from pulmonary hypertension caused by chronic nocturnal hypoxemia, and cardiac dysrhythmias. Symptoms of sleep apnea alter many aspects of the patient's lifestyle. Chronic sleep loss predisposes to diminished ability to concentrate, impaired memory, failure to accomplish daily tasks, and interpersonal difficulties. The male patient may experience impotence. Driving accidents are more common in habitually sleepy people. Family life and the patient's ability to maintain employment are often compromised. As a result, the patient may experience severe depression. If problems are identified, appropriate referrals need to be made. Cessation of breathing reported by the bed partner is usually a source of great anxiety because of the fear that breathing may not resume.

Assessment of the patient with OSA includes a thorough sleep and medical history. Symptoms of OSA, including daytime sleepiness, snoring, and witnessed apnea, are obvious characteristics of the disorder. Less obvious symptoms may include cardiovascular symptoms, muscle pain, and mood changes. Patients with OSA frequently have co-morbidities including a history of stroke and cardiovascular disease.

A diagnosis of sleep apnea is made on the basis of PSG. The patient's chest and abdominal movement, oral airflow, nasal airflow, SpO_2, ocular movement, and heart rate and rhythm are monitored. Progression through each sleep stage is determined by monitoring brain waves using EEG. A diagnosis of sleep apnea requires documentation of apneic events (no airflow with respiratory effort) or hypopnea (airflow diminished 30 to 50% with respiratory effort) of at least 10 seconds' duration. OSA is defined as more than five apnea/hypopnea events per hour accompanied by a 3 to 4% decrease in oxygen saturation. Severe apnea can be associated with apneic events of more than 30 to 50 per hour of sleep. Typically, PSG is performed in a sleep laboratory with technicians monitoring the patient. In some instances, portable sleep studies are conducted in the home setting. Overnight pulse oximetry assessment may be an alternative to determine if nocturnal O_2 supplementation is indicated.

NURSING AND COLLABORATIVE MANAGEMENT: SLEEP APNEA

Mild sleep apnea (5 to 10 apnea/hypopnea events per hour) may respond to simple measures. Conservative treatment at home begins with simply sleeping on one's side rather than on the back. Elevating the head of the bed may eliminate OSA in some patients. Instruct the patient to avoid sedatives and consuming alcoholic beverages for 3 to 4 hours before sleep. Sleep medications often make OSA worse. OSA is a potentially life-threatening disorder. Because excessive weight worsens and weight loss reduces sleep apnea, referral to a weight loss program may be indicated. Bariatric surgery reduces OSA (Greenburg, Lettieri, & Eliasson, 2009). Instruct the patient on the dangers of driving or using heavy equipment.

Symptoms may resolve in up to half of patients with OSA who use a special mouth guard, also called an oral appliance, during sleep to prevent airflow obstruction. Oral appliances bring the mandible and tongue forward to enlarge the airway space, thereby preventing airway occlusion. Some individuals find a support group beneficial where concerns and feelings can be expressed and strategies for resolving problems can be discussed.

In patients with more severe symptoms (>15 apnea/hypopnea events per hour), continuous positive airway pressure (CPAP) by mask is the treatment of choice (see Evidence-Informed Practice box). With CPAP, the patient applies a nasal mask that is attached to a high-flow blower. The blower is adjusted to maintain sufficient positive pressure (5 to 25 cm H_2O) in the airway during inspiration and expiration to prevent airway collapse. Some patients cannot adjust to wearing a mask over the nose or mouth or to exhaling against the high pressure. A technologically more sophisticated therapy, bi-level positive airway pressure (BiPAP), can deliver a higher inspiration pressure and a lower pressure during expiration. With BiPAP, the apnea can be relieved with a lower mean pressure and may be better tolerated.

EVIDENCE-INFORMED PRACTICE

Does Continuous Positive Airway Pressure Therapy Relieve Obstructive Sleep Apnea?

Clinical Question
For adults with obstructive sleep apnea (OSA) (P), is continuous positive airway pressure (CPAP) (I) versus no treatment (C) helpful in relieving daytime sleepiness (O)?

Best Available Evidence
- Clinical practice guidelines based on systematic review of randomized controlled trials (RCTs).

Critical Appraisal and Synthesis of Evidence
- 48 RCTs of patients with OSA who received at least 1 week of CPAP.
- Subjective and objective sleepiness, blood pressure, quality of life, and driving performance were assessed.
- CPAP use at night decreased daytime sleepiness for patients with varying OSA severity.

Conclusion
- CPAP helps patients with moderate to severe OSA and in mild OSA if symptoms affect quality of life and daily activities.

Implications for Nursing Practice
- Discuss referral for sleep assessment with patient and primary care provider.
- Teach patient to manage the fit of CPAP mask or nasal device to reduce irritation and discomfort (e.g., nasal dryness, throat irritation).

Reference for Evidence
National Institute for Health and Clinical Excellence (NICE). (2008). Continuous positive airway pressure devices for the treatment of obstructive sleep apnoea-hypopnoea syndrome: A systematic review and economic analysis. London: NICE. Retrieved from *http://www.hta.ac.uk/fullmono/mon1304.pdf*

P, Patient population of interest; *I*, intervention or area of interest; *C*, comparison of interest or comparison group; *O*, outcome(s) of interest (see p. 7).

Although CPAP is highly effective in reducing apnea and hypopnea, compliance is poor. Approximately two thirds of patients using CPAP report side effects such as nasal stuffiness. Adherence to CPAP use is challenging for some patients. First, assess the patient's knowledge about OSA and CPAP and involve the bed partner in education. Evaluate the patient for nasal resistance. Patient-centred selection of mask and device and exposure to CPAP before initiation of therapy have been shown to be important elements associated with successful adherence to CPAP treatment (Weaver & Grunstein, 2008). Interventions such as guided troubleshooting with the equipment and problem solving are helpful strategies to reduce anxiety and enhance adherence to CPAP treatment.

Nasal expiratory positive airway pressure (EPAP) is a relatively new therapy that shows promise for ameliorating OSA (Berry, Kryger, & Massie, 2011). Nasal EPAP uses the patient's own breathing to create positive airway pressure through relatively

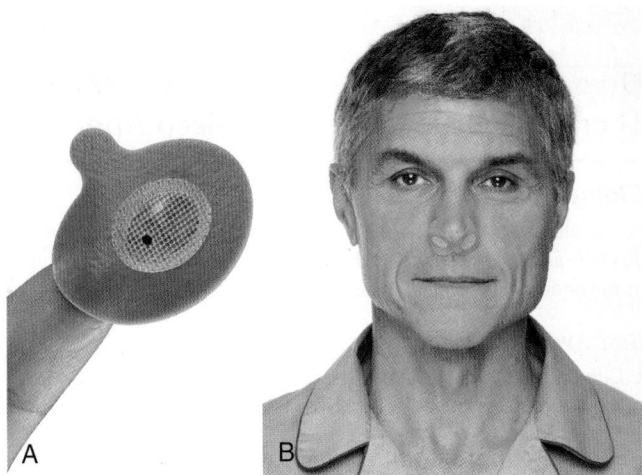

Figure 9-5 A and **B,** Nasal expiratory positive airway pressure (EPAP) device (Provent).

Source: Courtesy of Ventus Medical, Inc.

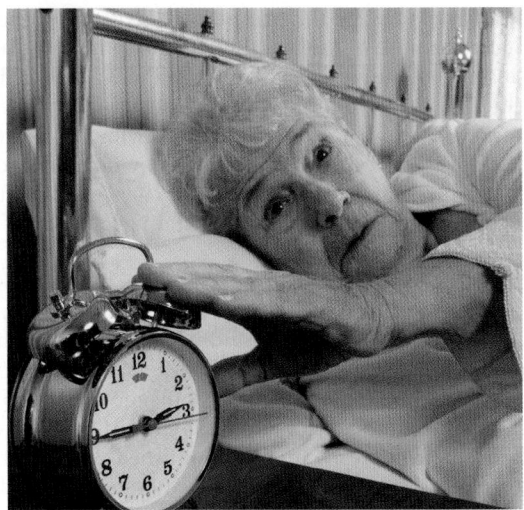

Figure 9-6 Many older people have sleep problems.

Source: © 2011 JupiterImages Corporation.

unobtrusive small valves affixed to each nostril with hypoallergenic adhesive (Figure 9-5). This therapy appears to have a higher degree of patient acceptability and adherence than traditional therapies such as CPAP (Berry et al., 2011).

When patients with a history of OSA are hospitalized, be aware that the administration of opioid analgesics and sedating medications (benzodiazepines, barbiturates, hypnotics) may worsen OSA symptoms by depressing respiration. This will necessitate that the patient wear the CPAP or BiPAP when resting or sleeping (Ross, 2008). If patients have their own CPAP equipment, hospital policy should be checked to determine whether it can be used.

If other measures fail, sleep apnea can be managed surgically. The two most common procedures are uvulopalatopharyngoplasty (UPPP or UP3) and genioglossal advancement and hyoid myotomy (GAHM). UPPP involves excision of the tonsillar pillars, uvula, and posterior soft palate with the goal of removing the obstructing tissue. GAHM involves advancing the attachment of the muscular part of the tongue on the mandible. When GAHM is performed, UPPP is generally performed as well. Depending on the site of the obstruction, symptoms are relieved in up to 80% of patients. Radiofrequency ablation (RFA) alone or in combination with other surgical techniques is also used. RFA is the least invasive of the surgical interventions for OSA.

Complications of airway obstruction or hemorrhage occur most often in the immediate postoperative period. Patients can usually be discharged to home within 1 day following the procedure. Before going home, the patient is taught what to expect during the postoperative recovery period. Patients are told that their throat will be sore. There may be a foul breath odour that may be reduced by rinsing with diluted mouthwash and then salt water after several days. Snoring may persist until the inflammation has subsided. Follow-up of patients after surgery is important. A repeat PSG is performed 3 to 4 months after surgery.

Periodic Limb Movement Disorder

Periodic limb movement disorder (PLMD) is characterized by involuntary, continual movement of the legs and/or arms that affects people only during sleep. Sometimes abdominal, oral, and nasal movement accompanies PLMD. Movements typically occur for 0.5 to 10 seconds, in intervals separated by 5 to 90 seconds. PLMD causes poor-quality sleep, which may lead to sleep maintenance insomnia and/or excessive daytime sleepiness. PLMD and restless legs syndrome (RLS) often occur simultaneously, but they are distinct disorders. (RLS is discussed in Chapter 61.)

PLMD is diagnosed using a detailed history from the patient and/or bed partner and doing a PSG. PLMD is treated by medications aimed at reducing or eliminating the limb movements or the arousals. Dopaminergic drugs (pramipexole [Mirapex] and ropinirole [Requip]) are preferred.

AGE-RELATED CONSIDERATIONS

Sleep

With aging, the most notable change is the decrease in the amount of deep sleep. Older adults report greater problems getting to and maintaining sleep compared with younger adults (Figure 9-6). Older age is associated with overall shorter total sleep time, decreased sleep efficiency, and more awakenings (Bloom et al., 2009; Bombois, Derambure, Pasquier, & Monaca, 2010). Time spent in slow-wave sleep is reduced and fragmentation of sleep is increased by age 50.

Even healthy older adults who do not complain of sleep disturbance have evidence of fragmented sleep, nocturnal wakefulness, and reduced sleep efficiency when studied with PSG. Older adults may attribute their disturbed sleep to normal aging. As a result, they may fail to report symptoms of sleep disorders to their health care providers (Misra & Malow, 2008).

A common misconception is that older people need less sleep than younger people. In fact, the amount of sleep needed as a person ages remains relatively constant. The key issue is that multiple factors impair the ability of older adults to obtain quality sleep.

Insomnia symptoms in the elderly frequently occur with depression, heart disease, body pain, and cognitive problems.

Daily stress and low social support has also been linked with insomnia in older adults (Béland et al., 2010). Insomnia may have detrimental effects on cognitive function in healthy older adults. Older women report more trouble falling asleep and, especially, staying asleep (Bombois et al., 2010). Other sleep disorders (e.g., sleep-disordered breathing) also increase with age and may manifest with insomnia symptoms.

Awakening and getting out of bed during the night to use the bathroom increases the risk for falls. Older adults may use OTC medications or alcohol as a sleep aid (see Chapter 11). This practice can further increase the risk of falls at night. Chronic disturbed sleep in the older adult can result in disorientation, delirium, impaired intellect, disturbed cognition, and/or increased risk of accidents and injury (Garcia, 2008; Halmov, Hanuka, & Horowitz, 2008) (see precipitating factors for delirium in Chapter 62).

Chronic conditions including COPD, diabetes, dementia, chronic pain, and cancer that are more common in older adults can affect sleep quality and increase the prevalence of insomnia (Halmov et al., 2008). Medications used to treat these conditions can contribute to sleep problems. OTC medications also can lead to sleep disturbance. Cough and cold medications, especially those containing pseudoephedrine, caffeine-containing drugs (e.g., combinations of acetaminophen), and drugs containing nicotine (e.g., nicotine gum and transdermal patches) are stimulants. Diphenhydramine, alone or in combination with other drugs, is sedating with anticholinergic effects. Any OTC medication labelled "PM" likely has diphenhydramine and should be used with caution by older adults.

Because many older adults may not tell their health care providers about their sleep problems, a sleeping assessment (see Table 9-6) can be used to detect sleep disturbances. Noise and light levels in the acute care setting may contribute to greater sleep disruption in the older adult (Missildine, 2008).

Drug therapies are more challenging for older adults. Whenever possible, long-acting benzodiazepines should be avoided. Older adults receiving benzodiazepines are at increased risk of daytime sedation, falls, and cognitive and psychomotor impairment (see Table 62-1). Hypnotics should be used for as brief a period as possible, in most cases not exceeding 2 to 3 weeks of treatment (Conn & Madan, 2006).

Metabolism of most hypnotic drugs decreases with aging. The elderly have increased sensitivity to hypnotic and sedative medications. For this reason, drug therapies for sleep disturbances are started at lower doses and monitored carefully.

▪ Parasomnias

Parasomnias are defined as unusual and often undesirable behaviours that occur with sleep or during arousal from sleep. Parasomnias that occur during REM sleep include enuresis (bedwetting), hallucinations, and eating. They are due to CNS activation and often involve complex behaviours. The parasomnia is generally goal-directed, although the person is not aware or conscious of the act. Parasomnias may result in fragmented sleep and fatigue.

Sleepwalking and sleep terrors are arousal parasomnias that occur during NREM sleep. *Sleepwalking* behaviours can range from sitting up in bed, moving objects, and walking around the room to driving a car. During a sleepwalking event, the individual does not speak and may have limited or no awareness of the event. On awakening, the individual does not remember the event. In the ICU, a parasomnia may be misinterpreted as ICU psychosis. In addition, sedated ICU patients can exhibit manifestations of a parasomnia.

Sleep terrors (night terrors) are characterized by a sudden awakening from sleep along with a loud cry and signs of panic. There is an intense autonomic response including increased heart rate, increased respiration, and diaphoresis. Factors in the ICU such as sleep disruption and deprivation, fever, stress (physical or emotional), and exposure to noise and light can contribute to sleep terrors.

Nightmares are a parasomnia characterized by recurrent awakening with recall of the frightful or disturbing dream. These normally occur during the final third of sleep and in association with REM sleep. Nightmares are commonly reported by patients in the ICU and are probably side effects of medication because REM sleep is often absent in critically ill patients. The longer the stay in the ICU, the more likely the patient is to have nightmares. Drug classes most likely to cause nightmares are sedative–hypnotics, beta-adrenergic antagonists, dopamine agonists, and amphetamines.

Special Sleep Needs of Nurses

Nursing is one of several professions that necessitate night shift and rotating shift schedules. In many acute care and long-term care settings, nurses are asked to or volunteer to work a variety of day and night shifts, often alternating and rotating them (Winwood, Winefield, & Lushington, 2006). Unfortunately, nurses who do shift work often report less job satisfaction and more job-related stress (Samaha, Lal, Samaha, & Wyndham, 2007).

Nurses on permanent night or rapidly rotating shifts are at increased risk of experiencing circadian rhythm shift work disorder characterized by insomnia, sleepiness, and fatigue. Nurses on rotating shifts get the least amount of sleep. With repeated periods of inadequate sleep, the sleep debt grows. Poor sleep is the strongest predictor of chronic fatigue in nurses doing shift work. As a result, rotating and night shift schedules pose specific challenges for the individual nurse's health and patient safety.

Shift work alters the synchrony between circadian rhythms and the environment, leading to sleep disruption. Nurses working the night shift are often too sleepy to be fully alert at work and too alert to sleep soundly the next day. Sustained alterations in circadian rhythms such as that imposed by rotating shift work have been linked to negative health outcomes including increased morbidity and mortality risks associated with cardiovascular problems. In addition, mood disorders such as anxiety are higher in nurses who work rotating shifts. Gastrointestinal disturbances are also more common in nurses who do shift work as compared with those who do not.

From a patient safety perspective, disturbed sleep and subsequent fatigue can make for a workplace hazard (errors and accidents) for nurses as well as for their patients. Fatigue can result in diminished or distorted perceptual skills, judgement, and decision-making capabilities. Lack of sleep affects the ability to cope and handle stress. Subsequently, the reduced ability to handle stress may result in physical, mental, and emotional exhaustion (Kling et al., 2010; Samaha et al., 2007).

The problem of sleep disruption is one that is critically important to nursing. Workplace policy and nursing education programs have a significant role to play in helping nurses access strategies to ensure adequate sleep. Several strategies may help reduce the distress associated with rotating shift work. These include brief scheduled periods of on-site napping especially during night shift to help with the chronobiological regulation of sleep (Silva-Costa, Rotenberg, Griep, & Fischer, 2011). Napping during shift has been found to improve recovery time from night shift and enhance safety on the job of shift workers (Takeyama, Kubo, & Itani, 2005). On-site napping may be beneficial only if the amount of domestic work performed in the daytime hours after night shift is limited (Silva-Costa et al., 2011). Maintaining a consistent sleep–wake schedule even on days off is optimum but perhaps unrealistic. For night shift work, scheduling the sleep period just before going to work increases alertness and vigilance, improves reaction times, and decreases accidents during night shift work. Nurses who have control over their work schedules appear to experience less sleep disruption than those whose schedule is imposed (Kilpatrick & Lavoie-Tremblay, 2006). It is important that nurses self-manage the effect of sleep disruption through the use of sleep hygiene practice. Sleep hygiene skills and self-care practices could be considered as required learning for nursing students because sleep quality has been found to decrease as nurses transition from school to workplace (Hasson & Gustavsson, 2010).

CLINICAL DECISION-MAKING EXERCISE

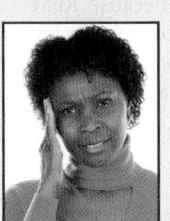

CASE STUDY:
Insomnia

© 2011 Jupiterimages Corporation.

Patient Profile

Donna Parsons, a 49-year-old Black woman, is seen in the primary care clinic for complaints of chronic fatigue. She is postmenopausal based on self-report. In the past year since the end of her periods, she has experienced daily hot flashes and sleep problems. She denies any other health problems. On a usual workday, she drinks two cups of hot tea and one can of diet cola. Currently, she is taking OTC diphenhydramine for sleep. Her partner, who has accompanied her to the clinic, states that her snoring has gotten worse and it is interfering with his sleep.

Subjective Data

- Complains of hot flashes and nighttime sweating
- Complains of daytime tiredness and fatigue
- States she has trouble getting to sleep and staying asleep

Objective Data

Physical Examination
- Laboratory evaluations within normal limits
- Overweight (20% over ideal body weight for height)
- BP 155/92 mm Hg

Diagnostic Studies
- Nighttime polysomnography study reveals episodes of obstructive sleep apnea

Collaborative Care
- CPAP nightly
- Referred for weight reduction counselling

Discussion Questions

1. What are Ms. Parsons' risk factors for sleep apnea?
2. What specific sleep hygiene practices could Ms. Parsons use to improve the quality of her sleep?
3. How does CPAP work?
4. What are the potential health risks associated with sleep apnea?
5. *Priority Decision:* What are the priority nursing interventions for Ms. Parsons?
6. *Priority Decision:* Based on the assessment data provided, what are the priority nursing diagnoses? Are there any collaborative problems?

℮volve　*Answers are available at* **http://evolve.elsevier.com/ Canada/Lewis/medsurg**

REVIEW QUESTIONS

The number of the question corresponds to the same-numbered outcome at the beginning of the chapter.

1. Which of the following definitions best describes sleep?
   a. Loosely organized state similar to coma
   b. State in which pain sensitivity decreases
   c. Quiet state in which there is little brain activity
   d. State in which an individual lacks conscious awareness of the environment

2. Which of the following is true regarding rapid eye movement (REM) sleep?
   a. The EEG pattern is quiescent.
   b. It occurs only once in the night.
   c. It is separated by distinct physiological stages.
   d. The most vivid dreaming occurs during this phase.

3. Sleep loss is associated with which of the following symptoms?
   a. Decreased body mass index
   b. Increased insulin resistance
   c. Enhanced cognitive functioning
   d. Increased immune responsiveness

4. Which of the following points should the nurse emphasize when teaching the patient with primary insomnia?
   a. The importance of daytime naps
   b. The need to exercise before bedtime
   c. The need for long-term use of hypnotics
   d. Avoidance of caffeine-containing beverages before bedtime

5. A nurse is establishing a care plan for a patient who has recently been diagnosed with narcolepsy. Which of the following areas would the nurse want to address as a priority?
   a. Risk for injury
   b. Ineffective coping
   c. Risk for dehydration
   d. Ineffective family coping
6. A patient with sleep apnea would like to avoid using a nasal CPAP device if possible. Which of the following suggestions should the nurse make to help him reach his goal?
   a. Lose excess weight.
   b. Take a nap during the day.
   c. Eat a high-protein snack at bedtime.
   d. Use mild sedatives or alcohol at bedtime.

7. A patient on the surgical unit has a history of parasomnia (sleepwalking). Which of the following is true regarding parasomnia?
   a. Hypnotic medications reduce the risk of sleepwalking.
   b. The patient is often unaware of the activity on awakening.
   c. The patient should be restrained at night to prevent personal harm.
   d. The potential for sleepwalking is reduced by exercise before sleep.
8. Which of the following strategies would reduce sleepiness during nighttime work?
   a. Exercising before work
   b. Sleeping for at least 2 hours before work time
   c. Taking melatonin before working the night shift
   d. Walking for 10 minutes every 4 hours during the night shift

ANSWERS: 1. d; 2. d; 3. b; 4. d; 5. a; 6. a; 7. b; 8. b.

REFERENCES

Al Lawati, N., Patel, S., & Ayas, N. (2009). Epidemiology, risk factors, and consequences of obstructive sleep apnea and short sleep duration. *Progress in Cardiovascular Diseases, 51,* 285-293. doi:10.1016/j.pcad.2008.08.001

American Academy of Sleep Medicine. (2001). *The International Classification of Sleep Disorders, Revised, Diagnostic and coding manual.* Retrieved from *http://www.esst.org/adds/ICSD.pdf*

American Academy of Sleep Medicine. (2008). *Over the counter: Will melatonin cure your sleep problems?* Retrieved from *http://yoursleep.aasmnet.org/article.aspx?id=794*

Anic, G. M., Titus-Ernstoff, L., Newcomb, P. A., Trentham-Dietz, A., & Egan, K. M. (2010). Sleep duration and obesity in a population study. *Sleep Medicine, 11*(5), 447-451. doi:10.1016/j.sleep.2009.11.013

Béland, S. G., Préville, M., Dubois, M., Lorrain, D., Grenier, S., Voyer, P., …, Moride, Y. (2010). Benzodiazepine use and quality of sleep in the community-dwelling elderly population. *Aging & Mental Health, 14,* 843-850. doi:10.1080/13607861003781833

Berry, R. B., Kryger, M. H., & Massie, C. A. (2011). A novel expiratory positive airway pressure (EPAP) device for the treatment of obstructive sleep apnea: A randomized controlled trial. *Sleep, 34,* 479-485.

Bhat, A., & El Solh, A. A. (2008). Management of narcolepsy. *Expert Opinion in Pharmacotherapy, 9,* 1721-1733. doi:10.1517/14656566.9.10.1721

Bloom, H. G., Ahmed, I., Alessi, C. A., Ancoli-Israel, S., Buysse, D. J., Kryger, M. H., …, Zee, P. C. (2009). Evidence-based recommendations for the assessment and management of sleep disorders in older persons. *Journal of the American Geriatric Society, 57,* 761-789. doi:10.1111/j.1532-5415.2009.02220.x

Bombois, S., Derambure, P., Pasquier, F., & Monaca, C. (2010). Sleep disorders in aging and dementia. *Journal of Nutrition, Health, & Aging, 14,* 212-217. doi:10.1007/s12603-010-0052-7

Brown, L. K. & Arora, M. (2008). Nonrespiratory sleep disorders found in ICU patients. *Critical Care Clinics, 24,* 589-611. doi:10.1016/j.ccc.2008.02.001

Buysse, D. J., Angst, J., Gamma, A., Ajdacic, V., Eich, D., & Rössler, W. (2008). Prevalence, course, and comorbidity of insomnia and depression in young adults. *Sleep, 31,* 473-480.

Buysse, D. J., Reynolds, C. F., III, Monk, T. H., Berman, S. R., & Kupfer, D. J. (1989). The Pittsburgh Sleep Quality Index: A new instrument for psychiatric practice and research. *Psychiatry Research, 28,* 193-213.

Cabello, B., Thille, A. W., Drouot, X., Galia, F., Mancebo, J., d'Ortho, M. P., …, Brochard, L. (2008). Sleep quality in mechanically ventilated patients: Comparison of three ventilatory modes. *Critical Care Medicine, 36,* 1749-1755. doi:10.1097/CCM.0b013e3181743f41

Calamaro, C. (2008). Sleeping through the night: Are extended-release formulations the answer? *Journal of the American Academy of Nurse Practitioners, 20*(2), 69-75.

Cao, H., Pan, X., Li, H., & Liu, J. (2009). Acupuncture for treatment of insomnia: A systematic review of randomized controlled trials. *Journal of Alternative and Complementary Medicine, 15*(11), 1171-86.

Cappuccio, F. P., D'Elia, L., Strazzullo, P., & Miller, M. A. (2010). Quantity and quality of sleep and incidence of type 2 diabetes: A systematic review and meta-analysis. *Diabetes Care, 33,* 414-420. doi:10.23337/dc09-1124

Chaput, J. P., Després, J. P., Bouchard, C., & Tremblay, A. (2007). Association of sleep duration with type 2 diabetes and impaired glucose tolerance. *Diabetologia, 50,* 2298-2304. doi:10.1007/s00125-007-0786-x

Chung, F., Subramanyan, R., Liao, P., Sasaki, E., Shapiro, C., & Sun, Y. (2012). High STOP-BANG score indicates a high probability of obstructive sleep apnea. *British Journal of Anesthesia 108,* 768-775.

Conn, D. K., & Madan, R. (2006). Use of sleep-promoting medications in nursing home residents: Risks versus benefits. *Drugs & Aging, 23,* 271-287. doi:1170-229X/06/0004-0271

Dirksen, S. R., & Epstein, D. R. (2008). Efficacy of an insomnia intervention on fatigue, mood, and quality of life in breast cancer survivors. *Journal of Advanced Nursing, 61,* 664-675. doi:10.1111/j.1365-2648.2007.04560.x

Elzohairy, Y. (2008). Fatal and injury fatigue-related crashes on Ontario's roads: A 5-year review. *Highway Safety Roundtable: Working together to understand driver fatigue: Report on symposium proceedings.* Retrieved from *http://www.ibc.ca/en/Car_Insurance/documents/driver_fatigue/Understanding_Driver_Fatigue_HSR-Feb2008.pdf*

Ferguson, S. A., Rajaratnam, S. M., & Dawson, D. (2010). Melatonin agonists and insomnia. *Expert Review of Neurotherapeutics, 10,* 305-318. doi:10.1586/ern.10.1

Garcia, A. D. (2008). The effect of chronic disorders on sleep in the elderly. *Clinics in Geriatric Medicine, 24,* 27-38. doi:10.1016/j.cger.2007.08.008

Greenburg, D. L., Lettieri, C. J., & Eliasson, A. H. (2009). Effects of surgical weight loss on measures of obstructive sleep apnea: A meta-analysis. *American Journal of Medicine, 122,* 535-542. doi:10.1016/j.amjmed.2008.10.037

Halmov, I., Hanuka, E., & Horowitz, Y. (2008). Chronic insomnia and cognitive functioning among older adults. *Behavioral Sleep Medicine, 6,* 32-54. doi:10.1080/15402000701796080

Hasson, D., & Gustavsson, P. (2010). Declining sleep quality among nurses: A population-based four year longitudinal study on the transition from nursing education to working life. *PLoS ONE, 5*(12), 1-6 e14265. doi:10.1371/journal.pone.0014265

Health Canada (2010). It's your health: Caffeine. Retrieved from *http://www.hc-sc.gc.ca/hl-vs/iyh-vsv/food-aliment/caffeine-eng.php*

Hiestand, D., & Phillips, B. (2008). The overlap syndrome: Chronic obstructive pulmonary disease and obstructive sleep apnea. *Critical Care Clinics, 24,* 551-563. doi:10.1016/j.ccc.2008.02.005

Hosseini, H., Esfirizi, M. F., Marandi, S. M., & Rezaei, A. (2011). The effect of Ti Chi exercise on the sleep quality of the elderly residents in Isfahan, Sadeghieh elderly home. *Iranian Journal of Nursing and Midwifery Research, 16,* 1, 55-60. Retrieved from *http://www.ncbi.nlm.nih.gov/pubmed/22039380*

Iber, C., Ancoli-Israel, S., Chesson, A., & Quan, S. F., for the American Academy of Sleep Medicine. (2007). *The AASM manual for the scoring of sleep and associated events: Rules, terminology and technical specifications.* Westchester, IL: American Academy of Sleep Medicine.

Irwin, M. R., Cole, J. C., & Nicassio, P. M. (2006). Comparative meta-analysis of behavioral interventions for insomnia and their efficacy in middle-aged adults and in older adults 55+ years of age. *Health Psychology, 25,* 3-14. doi:10.1037/0278-6133.25.1.3

Johns, M. W. (1991). A new method for measuring daytime sleepiness: The Epworth Sleepiness Scale. *Sleep, 14,* 540-545. Retrieved from *http://www.journalsleep.org/ViewAbstract.aspx?pid=24884*

Kilpatrick, K., & Lavoie-Tremblay, M. (2006). Shiftwork: What health care managers need to know. *Health Care Manager, 25,* 160-166.

Kling, R. N., McLeod, C. B., & Koehoorn, M. (2010). Sleep problems and workplace injuries in Canada. *Sleep, 33,* 611-618. Retrieved from *http://www.journalsleep.org/ViewAbstract.aspx?pid=27783*

Leger Marketing. (2010). *Canadian Broadcasting Corporation: The health of Canadians.* Retrieved from *http://www.cbc.ca/news/pdf/CBCFinalReport.pdf*

Misra, S., & Malow, B. A. (2008). Evaluation of sleep disturbances in older adults. *Clinics in Geriatric Medicine, 24,* 15-26. doi:10.1016/j.cger.2007.08.011

Missildine, K. (2008). Sleep and the sleep environment of older adults in acute care settings. *Journal of Gerontologic Nursing, 34*(6), 15-21.

Morin, C. M., LeBlanc, M., Belanger, L., Ivers, H., Merette, C., & Savard, J. (2011). Prevalence of insomnia and its treatment in Canada. *Canadian Journal of Psychiatry, 56,* 540-548. Retrieved from *http://publications.cpa-apc.org/media.php?mid=1212*

Nishino, S., Okuro, M., Kotorii, N., Anegawa, E., Ishimaru, Y., Matsumara, M., & Kanbayashi, T. (2010). Hypocretin/orexin and narcolepsy: New basic and clinical insights. *Actos Physiologica, 198,* 209-222. doi:10.1111/j.1748-1716.2009.02012.x

Ohayon, M. M., & Okun, M. L. (2006). Occurrence of sleep disorders in the families of narcoleptic patients. *Neurology, 67,* 703-705. doi:10.1212/01.wnl.0000229930.68094.48

Passarella, S., & Duong, M. T. (2008). Diagnosis and treatment of insomnia. *American Journal of Health-System Pharmacy, 65,* 927-934. doi:10.2146/ajhp060640

Public Health Agency of Canada (PHAC). (2009). *What's the impact of sleep apnea on Canadians? Fast facts from the Canadian community health survey—Sleep apnea rapid response.* Retrieved from *http://www.phac-aspc.gc.ca/cd-mc/sleepapnea-apneesommeil/pdf/sleep-apnea.pdf*

Reza, H., Kian, N., Pouresmail, Z., Masood, K., Seyed Bagher, M. S., & Cheraghi, M. A. (2010). The effect of acupressure on quality of sleep in Iranian elderly nursing home residents. *Complementary Therapies in Clinical Practice, 16,* 81-85. doi:10.1016/j.ctcp.2009.07.003

Ross, J. (2008). Obstructive sleep apnea: Knowledge to improve patient outcomes. *Journal of Perianesthesia Nursing, 23,* 273-275. doi:10.1016/j.jopan.2008.05.003

Samaha, E., Lal, S., Samaha, N., & Wyndham, J. (2007). Psychological, lifestyle and coping contributors to chronic fatigue in shift-worker nurses. *Journal of Advanced Nursing, 59,* 221-232. doi:10.1111/j.1365-2648.2007.04338.x

Silva-Costa, A., Rotenberg, L., Griep, R. H., & Fischer, F. M. (2011). Relationship between sleeping on the night shift and recovery from work among nursing workers—The influence of domestic work. *Journal of Advanced Nursing, 67,* 972-981. doi:10.1111/j.1365-2648.2010.05552.x

Sun, J. L., Sung, M. S., Huang, M. Y., Cheng, G. C., & Lin, C. C. (2010). Effectiveness of acupressure for residents of long-term care facilities with insomnia: A randomized controlled trial. *International Journal of Nursing Studies, 47,* 798-805. doi:10.1016/j.inurstu.2009.12.003

Taibi, D. M., Vitiello, M. V., Barsness, S., Elmer, G. W., Anderson, G. D., & Landis, C. A. (2008). A randomized clinical trial of valerian fails to improve self-reported, polysomnographic, and actigraphic sleep in older women with insomnia. *Sleep Medicine, 10,* 319-328. doi:10.1016/j.sleep.2008.02.001

Takeyama, H., Kubo, T., & Itani, T. (2005). The nighttime nap strategies for improving night shift work in the workplace. *Industrial Health, 43,* 24-29.

Tjepkema, M. (2005). Insomnia. *Health Reports, 17*(5), 9-25.

Towards Optimized Practice. (2010). *Clinical practice guidelines: Adult primary insomnia from diagnosis to management.* Retrieved from *http://www.topalbertadoctors.org/cpgs.php?sid=18&cpg_cats=79*

Weaver, T. E., & Grunstein, R. R. (2008). Adherence to continuous positive airway pressure therapy: The challenge to effective treatment. *Proceedings of the American Thoracic Society, 15,* 173-178. doi:10.1513/pats.200708-119MG

Weinhouse, G. L., & Schwab, R. J. (2006). Sleep in the critically ill patient. *Sleep, 29,* 707-716.

Winwood, P. C., Winefield, A. H., & Lushington, K. (2006). Work-related fatigue and recovery: The contribution of age, domestic responsibilities and shiftwork. *Journal of Advanced Nursing, 56,* 438-449. doi:10.1111/j.1365-2648.2006.04011.x

Yeh, G., Mietus, J. E., Peng, C. K., Phillips, R., Davis, R. B., Wayne, P. M., …, Thomas, R. J. (2008). Enhancement of sleep stability with Tai Chi exercise in chronic heart failure: Preliminary findings using an ECG-based spectrogram method. *Sleep Medicine, 9,* 527-536. doi:10.1016/j.sleep.2007.06.003

RESOURCES

American Academy of Sleep Medicine
http://www.aasmnet.org
Better Sleep Council
http://www.bettersleep.org
Canadian Lung Association, Sleep Apnea Resource
http://www.lung.ca/diseases-maladies/apnea-apnee_e.php
Canadian Sleep Society
http://www.canadiansleepsociety.com
Narcolepsy Network
http://www.narcolepsynetwork.org
National Sleep Foundation
http://www.sleepfoundation.org

evolve *For additional Internet resources, see the Web site for this book at* **http://evolve.elsevier.com/Canada/Lewis/medsurg**

CHAPTER 10

Pain

Written by Mary Ersek and Rosemary C. Polomano
Adapted by Michael McGillion, Sheila O'Keefe-McCarthy, and Judy Watt-Watson

LEARNING OBJECTIVES

1. Define pain.
2. Describe the neural mechanisms of pain and pain modulation.
3. Differentiate between nociceptive, neuropathic, somatic, and visceral types of pain.
4. Explain the physical and psychological effects of unrelieved pain.
5. Describe the components of a comprehensive pain assessment.
6. Describe effective pain management techniques used across many professional disciplines.
7. Describe pharmacological and nonpharmacological methods of pain relief.
8. Explain the nurse's role and responsibility in pain management.
9. Discuss ethical issues related to pain and pain management.
10. Evaluate the influence of one's own knowledge, beliefs, and attitudes about pain assessment and management.

KEY TERMS

analgesic ceiling A dosage at which no additional analgesia is produced regardless of further dosage increases, p. 169

breakthrough pain Moderate to severe pain that occurs despite treatment, p. 162

ceiling effect A phenomenon in which increasing dosage of a given medication produces progressively smaller effects, p. 166

dermatomes Areas on the skin that are innervated primarily by a single spinal cord segment, p. 157

equianalgesic dose A dose of one analgesic whose pain-relieving effect is equivalent to that of another analgesic, p. 165

imagery A structured technique in which the patient uses his or her own imagination to develop sensory images that divert focus away from the pain sensation and emphasize other sensory experiences and pleasant memories, p. 175

modulation The activation of descending pathways that exert inhibitory or facilitatory effects on the transmission of pain, p. 159

neuropathic pain Pain caused by damage to nerve cells or changes in spinal cord processing, p. 161

nociception The activation of the primary afferent nociceptors with peripheral terminals (free nerve endings) that respond differently to noxious (tissue-damaging) stimuli, p. 156

nociceptive pain Pain caused by damage to somatic or visceral tissue, p. 160

pain As defined by the International Association for the Study of Pain (IASP): An unpleasant sensory and emotional experience associated with actual or potential tissue damage, or the experience described in terms of such damage, p. 155

pain perception Recognition, definition, and response to pain by the individual experiencing the pain, p. 159

patient-controlled analgesia A system to induce analgesia in which the patient uses a pump to self-administer a dose of opioid when needed, p. 173

physical dependence An expected physiological response to ongoing exposure to pharmacological agents, "a state of adaptation that is manifested by a drug class–specific withdrawal syndrome and can be produced by abrupt cessation, rapid dose reduction, decreasing blood level of the drug, or administration of an antagonist" (American Academy of Pain Medicine, American Pain Society, & American Society of Addiction Medicine, 2001, p. 2), p. 177

suffering The state of severe distress associated with events that threaten the integrity of the person, p. 156

titration Dosage adjustment based on comparison of the adequacy of analgesic effect with the adverse effects produced, p. 166

transduction The conversion of a mechanical, thermal, or chemical stimulus to a neuronal action potential, p. 156

transmission The movement of pain impulses from the site of transduction to the brain, p. 156

trigger point A circumscribed hypersensitive area within a tight band of muscle that is caused by acute or chronic muscle strain, p. 174

windup Part of a constellation of changes in dorsal horn excitability that results in central sensitization. Peripheral tissue damage or nerve injury can cause central sensitization, and continued nociceptive input from the periphery is necessary to maintain it. With ongoing stimulation of slowly conducting unmyelinated C-fibre nociceptors, firing of specialized dorsal horn neurons gradually increases, p. 158

ELECTRONIC RESOURCES

Supplemental content related to Chapter 10 can be found...

Evolve Web Site ⊝volve

http://evolve.elsevier.com/Canada/Lewis/medsurg

Pain

Pain is a complex experience with sensory–discriminative, motivational–affective, and cognitive–evaluative dimensions. For many people, it is a major problem that causes suffering and reduces quality of life. Pain is one of the major reasons that people seek health care, and effective pain relief is a basic human right (Canadian Pain Society, 2010). A thorough understanding of the multiple dimensions of pain is important for effective assessment and management of patients with pain. Many health care providers are involved in the management of a patient's pain. Pain management is practised in all clinical settings and among many different groups of patients. Nurses have a central role in pain assessment and management. Components of the nursing role include (a) assessing pain and documenting and communicating this information to other health care providers, (b) ensuring delivery of effective pain relief measures, (c) evaluating the effectiveness of these interventions, and (d) monitoring ongoing effectiveness of pain management strategies. This chapter presents current knowledge about pain and pain management to enable the nurse to assess and manage pain successfully in collaboration with other health care providers.

Magnitude of the Pain Problem

According to the most recent Canadian Community Health Survey data (2007–2008), more than 1.5 million Canadians 12 to 44 years of age suffer chronic pain, which for 60% interferes with daily activities (Ramage-Morin & Gilmour, 2010). Unrelieved, persistent pain is an epidemic in Canada and the United States. For example, more than 50 million people are affected with musculoskeletal pain such as back pain and arthritis that goes unrelieved for 5 years or more (American Academy of Pain Management, n.d.). In Canada, pain is the most common cause of disability among working-age adults; up to 60% eventually lose their jobs or incur substantial loss of income (Lynch, 2011). Those with chronic pain now gainfully employed are expected to lose up to 28.5 productive working days per year (Boulanger et al., 2007; Lynch, 2011). Unfortunately, cumulative evidence indicates that people across the lifespan, in a variety of settings, continue to experience considerable acute and persistent pain in spite of effective treatment options being available (Hadjistavropoulos & Fine, 2006; Hadjistavropoulos, Hunter, & Fitzgerald, 2009; Lynch, 2011; McGillion et al., 2000; McGillion, Watt-Watson, LeFort, & Stevens, 2007; Watt-Watson et al., 2004). Despite management standards and directives from nongovernmental organizations such as the World Health Organization, the Committee for Research and Ethical Issues of the International Association for the Study of Pain (Zimmerman, 1982), the Joint Commission on Accreditation of Healthcare Organizations (JCAHO) (Wong, 2008), and the Canadian Pain Society (2010), more than four decades of evidence documents inadequate pain management practices as the norm across health care settings and patient populations (Breivik, Collett, Ventafridda, Cohen, & Gallacher, 2006; Tripp, VanDenKerkhof, & McAlister, 2006). For example, chronic pain is estimated to affect at least 50% of older people living in the community and up to 80% of residents of long-term care facilities (Charlton, 2005). People living with cancer—whether the disease is newly diagnosed, being actively treated, or in a more advanced stage—also consistently receive inadequate pain treatment (Lynch, 2011). Consequences of untreated pain include unnecessary suffering, physical dysfunction, psychosocial distress (which manifests in such forms as anxiety or depression), impairment in recovery from acute illness and surgery, immunosuppression, and sleep disturbances (American Geriatrics Society, 2002; Lynch, 2011; Page & Eliyahu, 1997; Pasero, Paice, & McCaffery, 1999). In the acutely ill patient, unrelieved pain can result in increased morbidity as a result of respi-

Table 10-1 Consequences of Unrelieved Pain

SYSTEM	RESPONSES
Endocrine	↑ Adrenocorticotropic hormone (ACTH), ↑ cortisol, ↑ antidiuretic hormone (ADH), ↑ epinephrine, ↑ norepinephrine, ↑ growth hormone, ↑ renin, ↑ aldosterone levels; ↓ insulin, ↓ testosterone levels
Metabolic	Gluconeogenesis, glycogenolysis, hyperglycemia, glucose intolerance, insulin resistance, muscle protein catabolism, ↑ lipolysis
Cardiovascular	↑ Heart rate, ↑ cardiac output, ↑ peripheral vascular resistance, hypertension, ↑ myocardial oxygen consumption, ↑ coagulation
Respiratory	↓ Tidal volume, atelectasis, shunting, hypoxemia, ↓ cough, sputum retention, infection
Genitourinary	↓ Urinary output, urinary retention
Gastrointestinal	↓ Gastric and bowel motility
Musculoskeletal	Muscle spasm, impaired muscle function, fatigue, immobility
Neurological	↓ Cognitive function; mental confusion
Immunological	↓ Immune response

Source: Adapted from McCaffery, M., & Pasero, C. (1999). *Pain: A clinical manual for nursing practice* (2nd ed.). St. Louis: Mosby.

ratory dysfunction, increased heart rate and cardiac workload, increased muscular contraction and spasm, decreased gastrointestinal (GI) motility and transit, and increased catabolism (Cousins & Power, 1999; Table 10-1).

When left untreated, acute pain can also progress to persistent pain problems. For example, multiple reviews of common surgical procedures such as amputation (Behr et al., 2009), hysterectomy (Brandsborg, Nikolajsen, Hansen, Kehlet, & Jensen, 2007), inguinal hernia repair (Aasvang & Kehlet, 2010) and hip arthroplasty (Nikolajsen, Brandsborg, Lucht, Jensen, & Kehlet, 2006) have revealed that 5 to 50% of patients experience persistent pain after surgery, and for some (2 to 10%), this pain is moderate to severe.

The reasons for the undertreatment of pain are varied. Among health care providers, frequently cited reasons include a lack of knowledge and skills to adequately assess and treat pain; misconceptions about pain; and inaccurate and inadequate information regarding addiction, tolerance, respiratory depression, and other adverse effects of opioids (McMillan, Tittle, Hagan, & Laughlin, 2000). Nurses tend to routinely administer the lowest prescribed analgesic dose when a range of doses is prescribed (Erkes, Parker, Carr, & Mayo, 2001). Such practices do little to provide relief from unremitting pain and are not consistent with current pain management guidelines (Moulin et al., 2007; Registered Nurses' Association of Ontario [RNAO], 2002; Watt-Watson, Garfinkel, Gallop, Stevens, & Streiner, 2000). The need to improve pre-licensure pain education for health care providers in Canada is dire. One national study revealed that professionals in only one third of health sciences programs (i.e., dentistry, medicine, nursing, pharmacy, rehabilitation sciences, and veterinary medicine) could identify designated, mandatory curricular content dedicated to pain (Watt-Watson et al., 2009).

Among patients, misconceptions about pain and opioids also play a major role in the under-reporting and undertreatment of pain (Ersek, Kraybill, & Du Pen, 1999; McCaffery & Pasero, 1999). Examples include the belief that pain is inevitable and a result of worsening disease and the desire to be a "good" patient who does not complain (McGillion et al., 2007; Watt-Watson, 1992).

Unfortunately, wait times for expert pain-related care in Canada currently exceed 1 year at more than one third of publicly funded pain clinics (Lynch, 2011), and many regions have no access to appropriate care (Peng et al., 2007).

Definitions of Pain

McCaffery and Pasero's 1979 definition that pain is "whatever and whenever the person says it is" has changed practice by focusing health care providers' attention on the subjectivity of pain (McCaffery & Pasero, 1999). Patients' self-reports about their pain are the key to effective management. This definition at the simplest level may cause problems because patients do not always admit to pain or use the word *pain*. The International Association for the Study of Pain (IASP, 2011) defined **pain** as "An unpleasant sensory and emotional experience associated with actual or potential tissue damage, or described in terms of such damage." The IASP (2011) also stated the following:

> The inability to communicate verbally does not negate the possibility that an individual is experiencing pain and is in need of appropriate pain-relieving treatment. Pain is always subjective. Each individual learns the application of the word through experiences related to injury in early life. Biologists recognize that those stimuli which cause pain are liable to damage tissue. Accordingly, pain is that experience we associate with actual or potential tissue damage. It is unquestionably a sensation in a part or parts of the body, but it is also always unpleasant and therefore also an emotional experience. Experiences which resemble pain but are not unpleasant, e.g., pricking, should not be called pain. Unpleasant abnormal experiences (dysesthesias) may also be pain but are not necessarily so because, subjectively, they may not have the usual sensory qualities of pain. Many people report pain in the absence of tissue damage or any likely pathophysiological cause; usually this happens for psychological reasons. There is usually no way to distinguish their experience from that due to tissue damage if we take the subjective report. If they regard their experience as pain, and if they report it in the same ways as pain caused by tissue damage, it should be accepted as pain. This definition avoids tying pain to the stimulus. Activity induced in the nociceptor and nociceptive pathways by a noxious stimulus is not pain, which is always a psychological state, even though we may well appreciate that pain most often has a proximate physical cause.

Pain therefore is multidimensional and subjective. The IASP definition emphasizes the subjective nature of pain, in which the patient's self-report is the most valid means of assessment. For patients who are nonverbal or cognitively unable to rate pain, nonverbal information is critical for pain assessment.

The IASP (2011) definition underlines the fact that pain can be experienced in the absence of identifiable tissue damage. It is important to differentiate pain that involves perception of a noxious stimulus from pain involving nociception, which may not be perceived as painful. **Nociception** is the activation of the primary afferent nociceptors (PANs) with peripheral terminals (free nerve endings) that respond differently to noxious (tissue-damaging) stimuli. *Nociceptors* function primarily to sense and transmit pain signals. If nociceptive stimuli are blocked, pain is not perceived.

Pain is not synonymous with suffering, although pain can cause substantial suffering. **Suffering** has been defined as the state of severe distress associated with events that threaten the intactness (biopsychosocial integrity) of the person (Cassell, 1982). Suffering can occur in the presence or absence of pain. Pain can also occur with or without suffering. For example, the woman awaiting breast biopsy may suffer emotionally because of anticipated loss of her breast. After the biopsy, she may have pain without suffering if the biopsy result is negative, or she may have pain with suffering if the biopsy result is positive for malignancy. Interventions aimed at relieving pain and suffering may have some commonalities. However, some interventions for suffering are inadequate for pain, just as some interventions for pain are inadequate for suffering.

Dimensions of Pain and the Pain Process

Pain is a complex experience involving several dimensions: *physiological, sensory-discriminative* (i.e., the perception of pain by the individual that addresses the pain location, intensity, pattern, and quality), *motivational-affective,* and *cognitive-evaluative* (Figure 10-1). In 1965, Melzack and Wall built on prior understanding of pain mechanisms in order to develop their gate control theory of pain (Melzack & Wall, 1987). Although the gate control theory is limited to providing a basic understanding of acute pain mechanisms, it is seminal work that remains critical to the understanding of the pain process, including transduction, transmission, perception, and modulation of pain. Pain experience and response result from complex interactions among these dimensions. In the following discussion, each dimension and

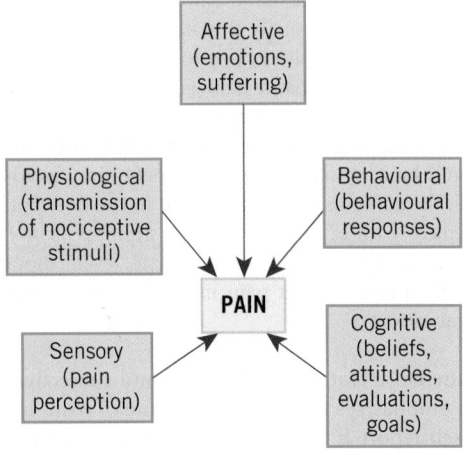

Figure 10-1 Multidimensional nature of pain.

the ways in which different dimensions influence pain are described.

Physiological Dimension of Pain

Understanding the physiological dimension of pain requires knowledge of neural anatomy and physiology. The neural mechanism by which pain is perceived consists of four major steps: transduction, transmission, perception, and modulation (Fields, 1987). Figure 10-2 outlines these four steps.

Transduction. **Transduction** is the conversion of a mechanical, thermal, or chemical stimulus to a neuronal action potential. Transduction occurs at the level of the peripheral nerves, particularly the free nerve endings, or nociceptors. Noxious (tissue-damaging) stimuli can include thermal damage (e.g., sunburn), mechanical damage (e.g., surgical incision, pressure from swelling), or chemical damage (toxic substances). These stimuli cause the release of numerous chemicals into the peripheral microenvironment of the PAN. Some of these chemicals—such as histamines, bradykinin, prostaglandins, nerve growth factor, and acids—activate or sensitize the PAN to excitation (Basbaum & Bushnell, 2002; Basbaum & Jessell, 2000; Basbaum & Julius, 2006; Julius & Basbaum, 2001). If the PAN is activated or excited, it fires an action potential to the spinal cord.

An action potential is necessary to convert the noxious stimulus to an impulse and move the impulse from the periphery to the spinal cord. A pain action potential can result from two sources: (a) a release of the sensitizing and activating chemicals (nociceptive pain) and (b) abnormal processing of stimuli by the nervous system (neuropathic pain); both of these sources produce a change in the charge along the neuronal membrane (Basbaum & Jessell, 2000; Basbaum & Julius, 2006). In other words, when the PAN terminal is transduced, the PAN membrane becomes depolarized: Sodium enters the cell, and potassium exits the cell, thereby generating an action potential. The action potential is then transmitted along the entire length of the neuron to cells in the spinal cord.

Inflammation and the subsequent release of the chemical mediators just listed lower the excitation threshold of PANs and increase the likelihood of transduction. This increased susceptibility is called *sensitization*. Several chemicals, such as leukotrienes, prostaglandins, and substance P, are probably involved in this process of sensitization. It is known that the release of substance P, a chemical stored in the distal terminals of the PAN, sensitizes the PAN and dilates nearby blood vessels, with subsequent development of edema and release of histamine from mast cells (Basbaum & Jessell, 2000).

Therapies directed at altering either the PAN environment or the sensitivity of the PAN are used to prevent the transduction and initiation of an action potential. Decreasing the effects of chemicals released at the periphery is the basis of several pharmacological approaches to pain relief. For example, nonsteroidal anti-inflammatory drugs (NSAIDs) such as ibuprofen (Advil, Motrin) and naproxen (Naprosyn, Aleve), and corticosteroids, such as dexamethasone, exert their analgesic effects by blocking pain-producing chemicals. NSAIDs block the action of cyclo-oxygenase, and corticosteroids block the action of phospholipase, thereby interfering with the production of prostaglandins.

Transmission. **Transmission** is the movement of pain impulses from the site of transduction to the brain (see Figure

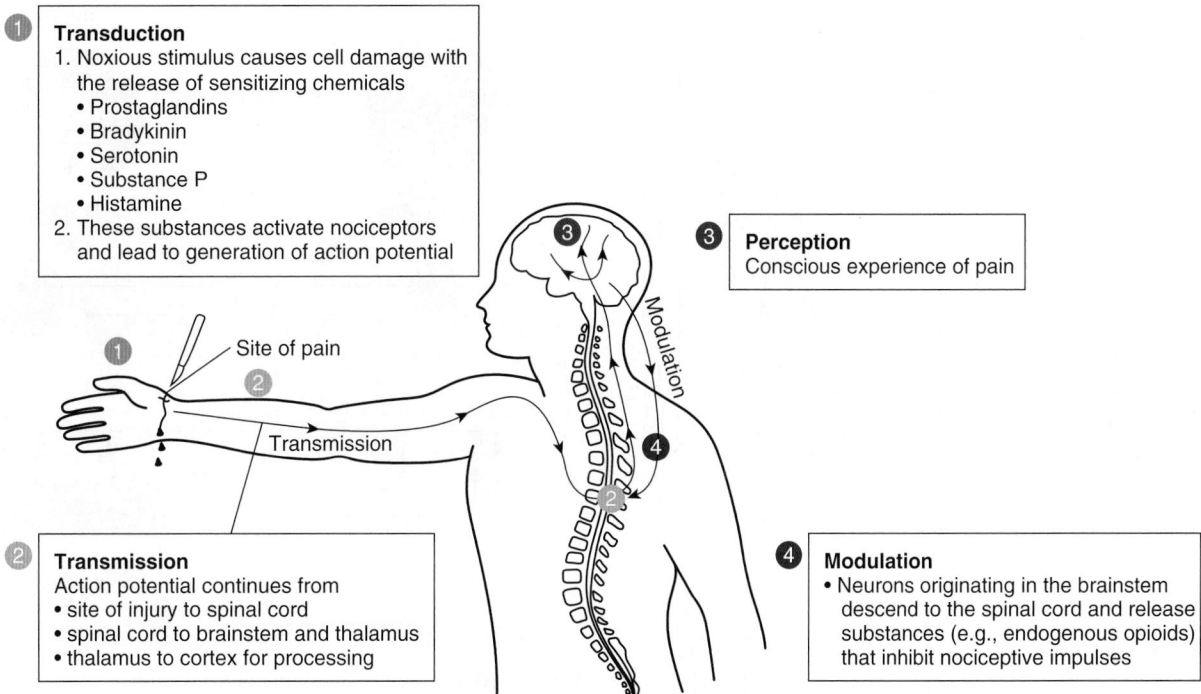

Figure 10-2 Nociceptive pain originates when the tissue is injured. Transduction *(1)* occurs when there is release of chemical mediators. Transmission *(2)* involves the conduct of the action potential from the periphery (injury site) to the spinal cord and then to the brainstem, thalamus, and cerebral cortex. Perception *(3)* is the conscious awareness of pain. Modulation *(4)* involves signals from the brain going back down the spinal cord to modify incoming impulses.

10-2; Fields, 1987). Three segments are involved in nociceptive signal transmission: (a) transmission along the nociceptor fibres to the level of the spinal cord, (b) dorsal horn processing, and (c) transmission to the thalamus and the cortex. Each step in the transmission process is important in pain perception.

Transmission to the Spinal Cord. One nerve cell extends the entire distance from the periphery to the dorsal horn of the spinal cord with no synapses. For example, an afferent fibre from the great toe travels from the toe through the fifth lumbar nerve root into the spinal cord; it is one cell. Once generated, an action potential travels all the way to the spinal cord unless it is blocked by a sodium channel inhibitor or disrupted by a lesion at the central terminal of the fibre (e.g., by a dorsal root entry zone lesion; Fields, 1987).

Two types of peripheral nerve fibres are responsible for the transmission of pain impulses from the site of transduction to the level of the spinal cord: the A fibres (A-alpha, A-beta, and A-delta) and the C fibres. Neurons that project from the periphery to the spinal cord are also referred to as *first-order neurons*. Each type of fibre has different characteristics that determine its conduction rate (Table 10-2). A-alpha and A-beta fibres are large fibres enclosed within myelin sheaths that allow them to conduct impulses at a rapid rate. A-delta fibres are smaller with thinly myelinated sheaths. Because of their smaller size, however, they conduct at a slower rate than the larger A-alpha and A-beta fibres. C fibres are the smallest fibres and are unmyelinated. They conduct at the slowest rate. The conduction rates have important implications for the modulation of noxious information from A-delta and C fibres (Fields, 1987).

Stimulation of different fibres results in different sensations. Stimulation of A-delta fibres results in pain described as pricking,

Table 10-2 Characteristics of Peripheral Nerve Fibres

TYPE OF FIBRE	SIZE	MYELINIZATION	CONDUCTION VELOCITY*
A-alpha	Large	Myelinated	Rapid
A-beta	Large	Myelinated	Rapid
A-delta	Small	Myelinated	Medium
C	Smallest	Not myelinated	Slow

*The conduction rates are important because information carried to the spinal cord by the more rapidly conducting nerve fibres reaches dorsal horn cells sooner than does information carried by the fibres that conduct more slowly.

sharp, well localized, and short in duration. C fibre activation pain is described as a dull, aching, burning sensation and is characterized by its diffuse nature, slow onset, and relatively long duration. The A-alpha (sensory muscle) and A-beta (sensory skin) fibres typically transmit nonpainful sensations such as light pressure to deep muscles, soft touch to skin, and vibration. All of these fibres extend from the peripheral tissues through the dorsal root ganglia to the dorsal horn of the spinal cord. The manner in which nerve fibres enter the spinal cord is central to the notion of spinal dermatomes. **Dermatomes** are areas on the skin that are innervated primarily by a single spinal cord segment. Figure 10-3 illustrates different dermatomes and their innervations.

Drugs that stabilize the neuron membrane and inactivate sodium channels disrupt the transmission of the action potential along the PAN axon. Some drugs, such as local anaesthetics (e.g., bupivacaine [Sensorcaine]) and antiseizure drugs (e.g.,

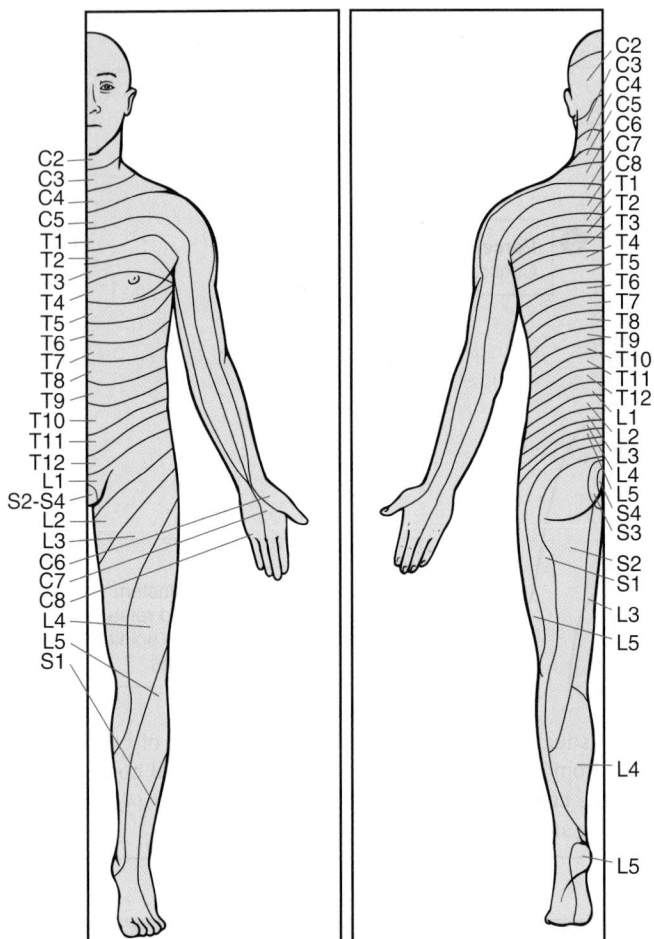

Figure 10-3 Spinal dermatomes representing organized sensory input carried via specific spinal nerve roots. *C*, cervical; *L*, lumbar; *S*, sacral; *T*, thoracic.

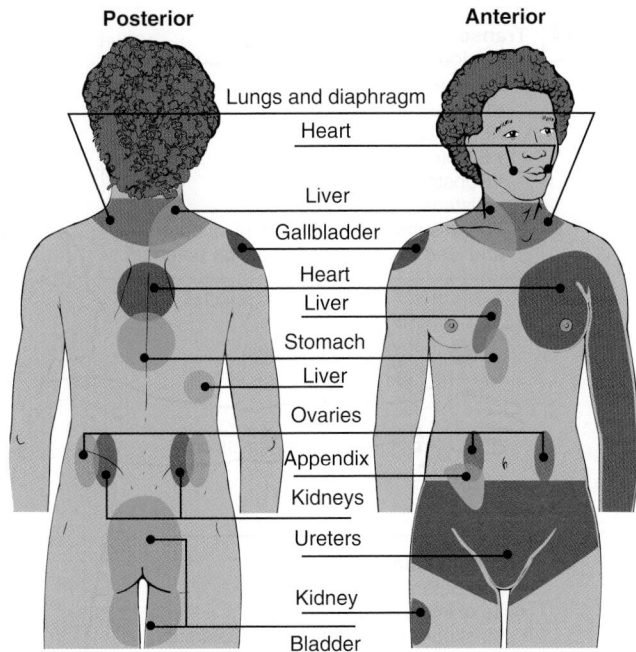

Figure 10-4 Typical areas of referred pain.

carbamazepine [Tegretol], gabapentin [Neurontin]), prevent transmission via this type of mechanism. In diluted concentrations, local anaesthetics are effective in blocking small-fibre transmission without affecting nonpainful sensation (pressure) or motor function. Larger concentrations of local anaesthetics are required to block larger fibres.

Dorsal Horn Processing. Once the nociceptive signal arrives in the central nervous system (CNS), it is processed within the dorsal horn of the spinal cord. This processing includes the release of neurotransmitters from the afferent fibre into the synaptic cleft. These neurotransmitters bind to receptors on nearby cell bodies and dendrites of cells that may be located elsewhere in the dorsal horn. Some of these neurotransmitters (e.g., aspartate, glutamate, substance P) produce activation of nearby cells, whereas others (e.g., γ-aminobutyric acid, serotonin, norepinephrine) inhibit such activation. In turn, these nearby cells release other neurotransmitters. The effects of the complex neurochemistry can facilitate or modulate (i.e., inhibit) transmission of noxious stimuli. In this area, exogenous and endogenous opioids also play an important role by binding to opioid receptors and blocking the release of neurotransmitters, particularly substance P. Endogenous opioids, which include enkephalins and β-endorphins, are chemicals that are synthesized and secreted by

the body. They are capable of producing effects that are similar to those of exogenous opioids such as morphine.

The dorsal horn of the spinal cord contains specialized cells called *wide dynamic range neurons*. These neurons receive input from noxious stimuli primarily carried by A-delta and C fibre afferent pathways (especially from viscera), non-noxious stimuli from A-beta fibres, and indirect input from dendritic projections (Basbaum & Jessell, 2000). Wide dynamic range neurons receive input from both noxious and innocuous stimuli from distant areas; this discovery provides a neural explanation for referred pain. Inputs from both nociceptive fibres and A-beta fibres converge on the wide dynamic range neuron, and when the message is transmitted to the brain, the originating area of the body is poorly localized. The concept of referred pain must be considered when a person with injury to or disease involving visceral organs reports pain in a certain location. The location of a tumour may be distant from the pain location reported by the patient (Figure 10-4). For example, pain from liver disease is located in the right upper abdominal quadrant, but it frequently is referred to the anterior and posterior neck region and to a posterior flank area. If referred pain is not considered in the evaluation of a pain location report, diagnostic tests and therapy could be misdirected.

Sensitization, or enhanced excitability, can also occur at the level of the spinal neurons; this is known as *central sensitization* (Basbaum & Jessell, 2000). Peripheral tissue damage or nerve injury can cause central sensitization, and continued nociceptive input from the periphery is necessary to maintain it (Basbaum & Jessell, 2000). With ongoing stimulation of the slowly conducting unmyelinated C-fibre nociceptors, firing of specialized dorsal horn neurons gradually increases. This process is known as **windup** and is dependent on the activation of *N*-methyl-D-aspartate (NMDA) receptors. NMDA receptors produce alterations in neural processing of afferent stimuli that can persist for long periods. For this reason, an important goal of therapy is to prevent persistent pain by avoiding central sensitization. The NMDA antagonist most commonly used currently is the anaesthetic agent ketamine (Ketalar). Unfortunately, intolerable adverse effects, such as hallucinations, limit its usefulness. Development of newer NMDA-antagonist drugs is ongoing and shows promise for potentially blocking central sensitization with fewer adverse effects.

Transmission to the Thalamus and the Cortex. From the dorsal horn, nociceptive stimuli are communicated to the *third-order neurons*, primarily in the thalamus, and several other areas of the brain. Fibres of dorsal horn projection cells enter the brain through several pathways, including the spinothalamic tract and spinoreticular tract. Distinct thalamic nuclei receive nociceptive input from the spinal cord and have projections to several regions in the cerebral cortex, where the perception of pain is believed to occur.

Perception. **Pain perception** is the recognition, definition, and response to pain by the individual experiencing it. In the brain, nociceptive input is perceived as pain. There is no single, precise location where pain perception occurs. Instead, pain perception involves several brain structures. For example, it is believed that the reticular activating system is responsible for the autonomic response of warning the individual to attend to the pain stimulus; the somatosensory system is responsible for localization and characterization of pain; and the limbic system is responsible for the emotional and behavioural responses to pain. Cortical structures are also thought to be crucial to constructing the meaning of the pain. Therefore, behavioural strategies such as distraction, relaxation, and imagery are effective pain-reducing therapies for many people. By directing attention away from the pain sensation, patients can reduce the sensory and affective components of pain. For example, blood flow to the anterior central gyrus, an area intimately involved with the perception of the unpleasantness of pain, can be altered by hypnosis (Barber, 2001). Prudent nursing practice involves treatment of any noxious stimulus as potentially painful, even in cognitively impaired or comatose patients, who may not respond behaviourally to noxious stimuli. It is important to note that lack of a behavioural response does not necessarily indicate that the person lacks pain perception.

Modulation. **Modulation** involves the activation of descending pathways that exert inhibitory or facilitatory effects on the transmission of pain. Depending on the type and degree of modulation, the nociceptive stimuli may or may not be perceived as pain. Modulation of pain signals can occur at the level of the periphery, the spinal cord, the brainstem, and the cerebral cortex. Centrally, modulation of nociceptive impulses occurs via descending fibres that influence dorsal horn neuronal activity. Complex neurochemistry involving excitatory and inhibitory neurotransmitters such as enkephalin, γ-aminobutyric acid, serotonin, and norepinephrine is involved in this nociceptive modulation; as a result, pain transmission is inhibited (Basbaum & Jessell, 2000). A number of pain management drugs exert their effects through the modulatory systems. For example, tricyclic antidepressants, such as amitriptyline (Elavil), are used in the management of persistent noncancer pain and cancer pain. These agents interfere with the reuptake of serotonin and norepinephrine, thereby increasing their availability to inhibit noxious stimuli and produce analgesia. Baclofen (Lioresal), an analogue of the inhibitory neurotransmitter γ-aminobutyric acid, can interfere with the transmission of nociceptive impulses and thus produce analgesia for many chronic conditions, particularly those accompanied by

DRUG THERAPY

Table 10-3 Interrupting the Pain Pathway

PAIN MECHANISM	MECHANISM OF ACTION
Transduction	
NSAIDs	Block prostaglandin production
Local anaesthetics	Block action potential initiation
Antiseizure agents (e.g., gabapentin [Neurontin])	Block action potential initiation
Corticosteroids	Block action potential initiation
Transmission	
Opioids	Block release of substance P
Perception	
Opioids	Decrease conscious experience of pain
NSAIDs	Inhibit cyclo-oxygenase action
Adjuvants (e.g., antidepressants)	Dependent on specific adjuvant
Modulation	
Tricyclic antidepressants (e.g., amitriptyline [Elavil])	Interfere with reuptake of serotonin and norepinephrine

NSAIDs, nonsteroidal anti-inflammatory drugs.

muscle spasms. Table 10-3 briefly summarizes how pain-relieving drugs can affect pain transduction, transmission, perception, and modulation.

Sensory–Discriminative, Motivational–Affective, Behavioural, Cognitive–Evaluative, and Sociocultural Dimensions of Pain

Pain is subjective and varies from person to person with regard to the experience of the pain and related responses. Because of the complex neural mechanisms of nociceptive processing, pain is a multidimensional sensory and affective experience that has cognitive, behavioural, and sociocultural aspects.

The *sensory-discriminative* component of pain is the recognition of the sensation as painful. Elements of sensory pain include pattern, area, intensity, and nature (PAIN). Information about these elements and knowledge about the pain process are indispensable to clinical decision making and appropriate pain therapy.

The *motivational-affective* component of pain encompasses the emotional responses to the pain experience. These affective responses include anger, fear, depression, and anxiety. Negative emotions impair the patient's quality of life. They become part of a vicious cycle in which pain leads to negative emotions such as depression, which in turn intensifies pain perception, leading to more depression and impairment of function. It is important for nurses to recognize this cycle and intervene quickly and effectively to stop it.

The *behavioural* component of pain comprises the observable actions used to express or control the pain. For example, facial expressions such as grimacing may reflect pain or discomfort. Posturing may be used to decrease pain associated with specific movements. A person often adjusts his or her daily physical and social activities in response to the pain. In this way, pain, especially persistent pain, has profound effects on functioning (Craig, 2006; Flor & Turk, 2006; McGillion et al., 2007).

The *cognitive-evaluative* component of pain consists of beliefs, attitudes, memories, and the meaning of the pain for the individual. The meaning of the pain stimulus can contribute to the pain experience (Arntz & Claassens, 2004). For example, a woman in labour may experience severe pain, but for her it is associated with a joyful event; moreover, she may feel control over her pain because of training she received in prenatal classes and the knowledge that the pain is self-limited. In contrast, a woman with persistent, nonspecific musculoskeletal pain may be plagued by thoughts that the pain is "not real" (Johansson, Hamburg, Westward, & Lindgren, 1999). Similar to this woman, many people with persistent pain may also experience challenges from health care providers and others as to whether their pain is a legitimate experience (Craig, 2005).

Such anxieties, fears, and stressors have been identified as potential intensifiers of perceived pain intensity and related burden (Arntz & de Jong, 1993). The meaning of pain and related responses are critical aspects of nursing pain assessment. The *cognitive* dimension also includes pain-related beliefs and the cognitive coping strategies that people use. For example, some people cope with pain by distracting themselves, whereas others struggle with feelings that the pain is untreatable and overwhelming. Cognitions about the pain contribute to patients' goals for and expectations of pain relief and treatment outcomes. Moreover, factors that affect cognition—such as sedation, dementia, delirium, and mental disability—alter the pain experience and responses to pain.

The *sociocultural* dimension of pain encompasses factors such as demographic features (e.g., age, sex, education, socioeconomic status), support systems, social roles, past pain experiences, and cultural aspects that contribute to the pain experience (Keefe et al., 2000; Watkins, Shifren, Park, & Morell, 1999). Sex, for example, has been found to influence nociceptive processes and the acceptability and usage of and response to analgesics such as NSAIDs and opioids (Gagliese & Melzack, 2006; Holdcroft & Berkley, 2006; Vallerand & Polomano, 2000). Families and caregivers also influence the patient's response to pain through their own beliefs and behaviours. For example, families may discourage the patient from taking opioids because of certain pain-related misconceptions, such as the fear that appropriate treatment with opioids will cause the patient to become addicted. For patients who are unable to care for themselves, family or professional caregivers may also act as "gatekeepers" and administer inadequate doses of analgesics (Ferrell, 2001; Watt-Watson et al., 2000). Culture also affects the experience of pain: specifically, pain expression, drug use, and pain-related beliefs and coping. Thus the sociocultural determinants of pain are also an integral part of a comprehensive pain assessment.

Causes and Types of Pain

Pain is generally classified as nociceptive, neuropathic, or both, according to the underlying pathological process. Nociceptive pain and neuropathic pain have different characteristics (Table 10-4). Because of its temporal nature, pain may be acute or persistent; some people may experience both, depending on the problem (Table 10-5).

Nociceptive Pain

Nociceptive pain is caused by damage to somatic or visceral tissue. *Somatic pain*, characterized as aching or throbbing that is well localized, arises from bone, joint, muscle, skin, or connective tissue. *Visceral pain*, which may result from stimuli such as tumour involvement or obstruction, arises from internal organs such as the intestines and the bladder. Examples of nociceptive pain

Table 10-4 Comparison of Nociceptive and Neuropathic Pain	
NOCICEPTIVE PAIN	**NEUROPATHIC PAIN**
Definition	
Processing of noxious stimuli by an intact nervous system; usually responsive to analgesics (e.g., opioids, NSAIDs) or physical modalities	Abnormal processing of sensory input as a result of injury of the peripheral or central nervous system; treatment includes a variety of analgesics (e.g., antidepressants, opioids, antiseizure drugs)
Types	
Somatic pain: Arises from bone, joint, muscle, skin, or connective tissue; usually aching or throbbing in quality and well localized	*Centrally generated pain:*
	• Deafferentation pain, caused by injury to either the peripheral or central nervous system (e.g., phantom pain may reflect injury to peripheral nerve)
Visceral pain: Arises from organs, such as the gastrointestinal tract and bladder. Can be further subdivided as follows:	• Sympathetically maintained pain, associated with dysregulation of the autonomic nervous system (e.g., reflex sympathetic dystrophy)
	Peripherally generated pain:
• Tumour involvement of the organ capsule that causes aching and fairly well-localized pain	• Painful polyneuropathies, in which pain is felt along the distribution of many peripheral nerves (e.g., diabetic neuropathy, alcohol-nutritional neuropathy, Guillain-Barré syndrome)
• Obstruction of hollow organ that causes intermittent cramping and poorly localized pain	• Painful mononeuropathies, usually associated with a known peripheral nerve injury and in which pain is felt at least partly along the distribution of the damaged nerve (e.g., nerve root compression, trigeminal neuralgia)

Source: Adapted from McCaffery, M., & Pasero, C. (1999). *Pain: A clinical manual for nursing practice* (2nd ed.). St. Louis: Mosby. *NSAIDs,* nonsteroidal anti-inflammatory drugs.

Table 10-5 Differences Between Acute and Persistent Pain

CHARACTERISTIC	ACUTE PAIN	PERSISTENT PAIN
Onset	Sudden	Gradual or sudden
Duration	Usually within the normal time for healing	May start as acute injury but continues past the normal time for healing to occur
Severity	Mild to severe	Mild to severe
Cause of pain	In general, a precipitating illness or event (e.g., surgery) can be identified	May not be known; original cause of pain may differ from mechanisms that maintain the pain
Course of pain	↓ Over time and goes away as recovery occurs	Typically, pain persists and may be ongoing, episodic, or both
Typical physical and behavioural manifestations	Manifestations reflect sympathetic nervous system activation: • ↑ Heart rate • ↑ Respiratory rate • ↑ Blood pressure • Diaphoresis, pallor • Anxiety, agitation, confusion NOTE: Responses normalize quickly owing to adaptation	Predominantly behavioural manifestations: • Changes in affect • ↓ Physical movement and activity • Fatigue • Withdrawal from other people and social interaction
Usual goals of treatment	Pain control with eventual elimination	Minimizing pain to the extent possible; focusing on enhancing function and quality of life

include pain from a surgical incision or a broken bone, arthritis, or cardiac ischemia. Nociceptive pain is usually responsive to nonopioid drugs, as well as to opioids.

Neuropathic Pain

Neuropathic pain is caused by damage to nerve cells or changes in spinal cord processing. Typically described as burning, shooting, stabbing, or electrical in nature, neuropathic pain can be sudden, intense, short-lived, or lingering. Neuropathic pain is difficult to treat, and management includes opioids, antiseizure drugs, and antidepressants. Neuropathic pain can be either central or peripheral in origin. *Deafferentation pain* (injury to either the peripheral or the central nervous system) and *sympathetically maintained pain* (associated with dysregulation of the autonomic nervous system) are considered centrally generated pain. Painful peripheral neuropathies (pain felt along the distribution of multiple peripheral nerves) and painful mononeuropathies (pain felt at least partly along the distribution of the damaged nerve) are considered peripherally generated pain. Examples of neuropathic pain include postherpetic neuralgia, phantom limb pain, diabetic neuropathies, and trigeminal neuralgia.

Table 10-5 lists the classification of pain as acute or persistent. Acute pain and persistent pain have different causes, courses, manifestations, and treatment. Examples of acute pain include postoperative pain, labour pain, pain from trauma (e.g., lacerations, fractures, sprains) and infection (e.g., dysuria), and angina. For acute pain, treatment includes analgesics for symptom control and treatment of the underlying cause (e.g., splinting for a fracture, antibiotic therapy for an infection). Normally, acute pain diminishes over time as healing occurs. Persistent pain continues beyond the normal time expected for healing. Persistent pain is often disabling and accompanied by anxiety and depression (Ramage-Morin & Gilmour, 2010). Sometimes, persistent pain is

further classified as cancer and noncancer pain. Persistent cancer-related pain arises from many causes, including disease progression, diagnostic procedures, anticancer therapies, and infection (Mantyh, 2006). Cancer pain often is considered separately because its cause can be determined, its course differs from that of nonmalignant pain (cancer pain often worsens with documented disease progression), and the use of opioids in treating cancer pain is more widely accepted than for the treatment of noncancer pain (Hoskin, 2006; Mantyh, 2006).

Pain Assessment

The goals of a nursing pain assessment are (a) to describe the patient's sensory, affective, behavioural, cognitive, and sociocultural pain experience for the purpose of implementing pain management techniques and (b) to identify the patient's goal for therapy and resources and strategies for effective self-management. The nurse is responsible for gathering and documenting assessment data and for making collaborative decisions with the patient and other health care providers about pain management. The following sections describe key components in pain assessment.

Sensory–Discriminative Component

Every pain assessment should include evaluation of the sensory-discriminative component: pattern, area, intensity, and nature (PAIN) of the pain. Information about these elements is essential in identifying appropriate therapy for the type and severity of the pain.

Before beginning any assessment, the nurse must recognize that patients may use words other than *pain*. For example, older adults may deny that they have pain but respond positively when asked if they have discomfort, soreness, or aching (Herr &

Garrand, 2001; McGillion et al., 2007). The words that the patient uses in describing pain must be documented, and when the patient is asked about pain, those words should be used consistently.

Pattern of Pain. Pain onset (when it starts) and duration (how long it lasts) are components of the pain pattern. Acute pain typically increases during wound care, ambulation, coughing, and deep breathing. Acute pain associated with surgery or injury tends to diminish over time, with recovery as tissues heal. In contrast, persistent pain may be ongoing, episodic, or both. For example, a person with persistent osteoarthritis pain may experience increased stiffness and pain on arising in the morning. As the joint is gently mobilized, the pain often decreases.

A patient may have constant, around-the-clock pain or discrete periods of intermittent pain. **Breakthrough pain** is moderate to severe pain that occurs despite treatment. Many patients with cancer experience breakthrough pain. It is usually rapid in onset and brief in duration, with highly variable intensity and frequency of occurrence. Episodic, procedural, or incident pain is a transient increase in pain that is caused by a specific activity or event that precipitates the pain. Examples of such events include dressing changes, movement, eating, position changes, and certain procedures such as catheterization.

Figure 10-5 shows one method for the patient to document the pain pattern. This method allows the patient to report how the intensity of the pain changes with time. A similar method could be used to document the changes in the area or nature of the pain.

Area of Pain. The area or location of pain assists in identifying possible causes of the pain and in determining treatment. Some patients may be able to specify one or more precise locations of their pain, whereas others may describe very general areas or comment that they "hurt all over." The location of the pain may also be *referred* from its origin to another site (see Figure 10-4), as described earlier in the chapter. Pain may also *radiate* from its origin to another site. For example, angina pectoris is known to radiate from the chest to the jaw, to the shoulders, or down the left arm. Sciatica is pain that originates from compression or damage to the sciatic nerve or its roots within the spinal cord. The pain is projected along the course of the peripheral nerve, causing painful shooting sensations down the back of the thigh and the inside of the leg.

Typically, information about the location of pain is elicited by asking the patient to (a) describe the site or sites of pain, (b) point to painful areas on the body, or (c) mark painful areas on a body diagram (Figure 10-6). Because many patients have more than one site of pain, it is important to make certain that the patient describes every location and identifies which one is most problematic.

Intensity of Pain. Assessing the severity, or intensity, of pain provides a reliable measurement that is used in determining the type of treatment, as well as evaluating the effectiveness of therapy. Pain scales are useful in helping the patient communicate the intensity of pain and in guiding treatment. Scales must be adjusted to age and level of cognitive development. Numerical scales (e.g., 0 = "no pain" and 10 = "the worst pain"), verbal descriptor scales (e.g., none, a little [1-3], moderate [4-6], and severe [7-10]), or visual analogue scales (a 10-cm line with one end labelled "no pain" and the other end labelled "worst possible pain") can be used by most adults to rate the intensity of their pain (Figure 10-7). For patients who are unable to respond to other pain intensity scales, a series of faces ranging from "smiling" to "crying" can be used. These scales have been investigated for use in a variety of patient populations, including young children and older adults. Results indicate that they provide valid and reliable assessment data (Craig, Prkachin, & Grunau, 2011).

Nature of Pain. The *nature* of pain refers to the quality or characteristics of the pain. Many commonly used words to describe the nature of pain are included in the McGill Pain Questionnaire (MPQ; see the Resources at the end of this chapter). The MPQ is a widely used measure of subjective pain experience with well-established reliability, validity, sensitivity, and discriminative capacity in divergent acute and chronic pain populations (Katz & Melzack, 2011). The MPQ is also a consistently used instrument that provides a description of pain beyond the single dimension of pain intensity (Katz & Melzack, 2011). This measure comprises 20 subclasses of qualitatively and quantitatively ordered verbal descriptors, categorized into four subscales, that describe the sensory, affective, evaluative, and miscellaneous aspects of pain. Sixteen subclasses of descriptors concern the three major dimensions of the pain experience: sensory-discriminative, motivational-affective, and cognitive-evaluative (Katz & Melzack, 2011). The four remaining subclasses of descriptors are classified as "miscellaneous" and are used in the calculation of a total MPQ Pain Rating Index score. The rank value for each descriptor in a given subclass is based on its position in the word set. Rank values are obtained for each aspect of pain and are summed to obtain an overall Pain Rating Index score, which ranges from 0 to 78 (Katz & Melzack, 2011). Two major strengths of the MPQ are that it provides a comprehensive assessment of the nature of pain problems in a short time frame (5 to 10 minutes), and it includes subsets of verbal pain descriptors associated with both nociceptive and neuropathic pain (Katz & Melzack, 2011).

For example, patients may describe neuropathic pain as burning, cold, shooting, stabbing, or itchy. Nociceptive pain may be described as sharp, aching, throbbing, and cramping.

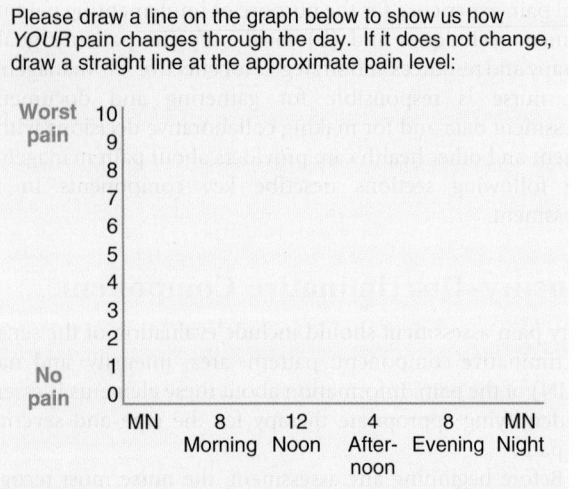

Please draw a line on the graph below to show us how *YOUR* pain changes through the day. If it does not change, draw a straight line at the approximate pain level:

Figure 10-5 A method of tracking pain over time.

Initial Pain Assessment Tool

Date _____

Client's Name _____ Age _____ Room _____

Diagnosis _____ Physician _____

Nurse _____

1. LOCATION: Patient or nurse marks drawing.

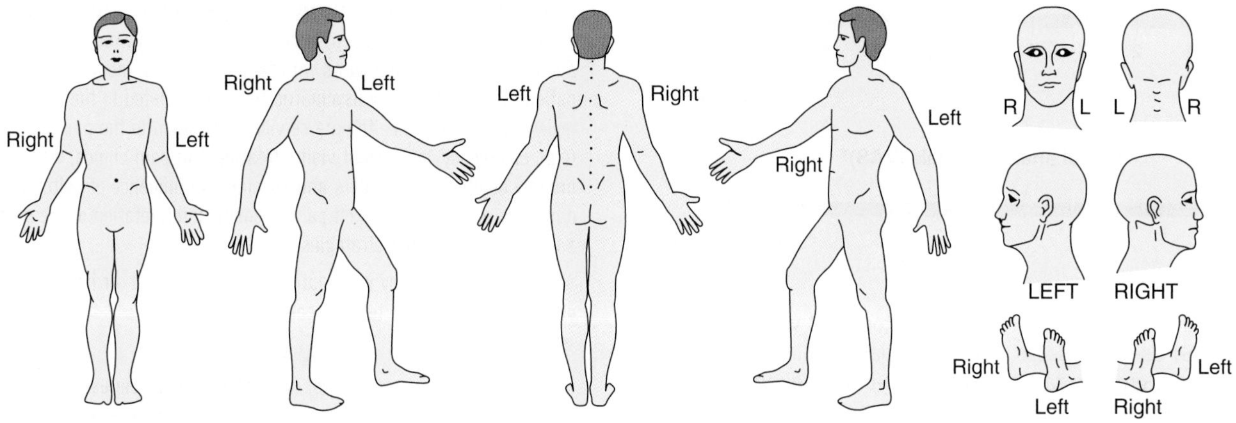

2. INTENSITY: Client rates the pain. Scale used: _____

   Present: _____

   Worst pain gets: _____

   Best pain gets: _____

   Acceptable level of pain: _____

3. QUALITY: (Use client's own words, e.g., prick, ache, burn, throb, pull, sharp) _____

4. ONSET, DURATION, VARIATIONS, RHYTHMS: _____

5. MANNER OF EXPRESSING PAIN: _____

6. WHAT RELIEVES THE PAIN? _____

7. WHAT CAUSES OR INCREASES THE PAIN? _____

8. EFFECTS OF PAIN: (Note decreased function, decreased quality of life.)

   Accompanying symptoms (e.g., nausea) _____

   Sleep _____

   Appetite _____

   Physical activity _____

   Relationship with others (e.g., irritability) _____

   Emotions (e.g., anger, suicidal thoughts and behaviours, crying) _____

   Concentration _____

   Other _____

9. OTHER COMMENTS: _____

10. PLAN: _____

May be duplicated for use in clinical practice. From McCaffery M, Pasero C: Pain: Clinical manual, p. 60. Copyright © 1999, Mosby Inc.

Figure 10-6 Initial pain assessment tool. (May be duplicated for use in clinical practice.)

Source: From McCaffery, M., & Pasero, C. (1999). *Pain: Clinical manual for nursing practice* (2nd ed., p. 60). St. Louis: Mosby.

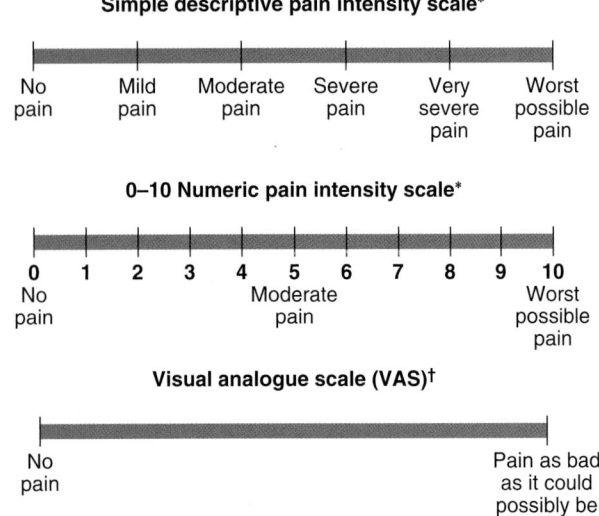

Figure 10-7 Simple descriptive word tool and visual analogue scale (VAS) used to assess a patient's pain.
*If used as a graphic rating scale, a 10-cm baseline is recommended.
†A 10-cm baseline is recommended for VAS scales.

Source: McCormack, H. M., Horne, D. J. & Sheather, S. (1988). Clinical applications of visual analogue scales: a critical review. *Psychological Medicine, 18*(4), 1007-1019.

Motivational–Affective, Behavioural, Cognitive–Evaluative, and Sociocultural Components

Comprehensive pain assessment includes evaluation of all pain dimensions and should be completed upon a patient's admission to a facility or service and repeated at regular intervals in order to evaluate response to treatment. In an acute care setting, time limitations may dictate an abbreviated assessment of the affective, behavioural, cognitive, and sociocultural dimensions of pain. At a bare minimum, patients' expression of pain and the effect of pain on sleep, daily activities, relationships, physical activity, and emotional well-being should be assessed. Strategies that the patient has used or tried to control the pain (effective or not) should also be documented.

When possible and relevant, assessment should also include examination of the psychological and social factors associated with patients' subjective experience of pain and, in particular, the meaning of the pain experience; pain meaning may often feature prominently in patients' treatment progress (DeGood & Cook, 2011). Data related to meaning may be particularly useful in care planning for patients who exhibit high levels of pain-related behaviour or functional impairment or substantial pain-related distress (DeGood & Cook, 2011). Such responses, for example, may be found in patients suffering moderate to severe persistent neuropathic pain after surgery (Herlitz et al., 2008).

Measurement of beliefs related to the meaning of pain is complex. Although a number of standard and reliable measures exist (e.g., Survey of Pain Attitudes [Jensen, Karoly, & Huger, 1987] and Pain Beliefs and Perception Inventory [Williams & Thorn, 1989]), normative data are limited for interpreting individual response profiles for use in the clinical setting (DeGood & Cook, 2011). For clinical assessment purposes, key areas of inquiry with patients about the meaning of pain and related

NURSING ASSESSMENT

Table 10-6 Pain Data

Subjective Data

Important Health Information

Past health history: Includes onset, location, intensity, quality, patterns, and expression of pain; coping strategies; past pain experiences (e.g., in childhood, in family members, other pain problems, pain relief measures used in the past and their effectiveness); pain triggers; effect of pain on emotions, relationships, sleep, work and school, family routines, leisure, and other activities; interviews with family members; meaning of pain to patient; records from any psychiatric treatment related to the pain; review of the use of health care services in relation to the pain problem (e.g., emergency department visits, treatment at pain clinics, visits to primary health care providers and specialists); influence of cultural, ethnic, or religious factors on pain intensity, interpretation of the pain, and pain management strategies

Medications: Use of any prescription, over-the-counter, or herbal products or other drugs for pain relief; alcohol use

Symptoms

Fatigue; limitations in activities; pain related to muscle use; decreased libido; constipation related to opioid or tricyclic drug use (or both); depression; anxiety; mood or self-image problems

Objective Data

- *Complete physical examination*, including evaluation of functional limitations
- *Psychosocial evaluation*

beliefs should include effective pain control in relation to current intervention strategies, pain-related disability, value placed on comfort and solace from other people, and the effect of emotions on the experience of pain.

Comprehensive assessment information is usually necessary to ensure effective treatment, as shown in Table 10-6. Comprehensive pain assessment and intervention ideally involve the entire interdisciplinary pain team, including nurses, physicians and physician assistants, psychologists, physiotherapists, occupational therapists, pharmacists, and social workers.

Pain Treatment

Basic Principles

All pain treatment is guided by the same underlying principles. Although treatment regimens range from short-term management to multimodal, long-term therapy required for many persistent pain problems, all treatment should follow the same basic standards, as stated by the Canadian Pain Society (2010):

- Routine assessment is essential for effective management. Pain is a subjective experience involving multiple characteristics including biological and psychosocial factors, all of which must be considered for comprehensive assessment and management.
- Unrelieved acute pain complicates recovery. Unrelieved pain after surgery or injury results in more complications, longer hospital stays, greater disability, and potentially long-term pain.

- Patients' self-report of pain should be used whenever possible. For patients unable to report pain, a nonverbal assessment method must be used.
- Health professionals have a responsibility to assess pain routinely, to accept patients' pain reports and document them, and to intervene in order to manage pain.
- The best approach to pain management involves patients, families, and health professionals. Patients and families must be informed that they have a right to the best pain care possible and encouraged to communicate the severity of their pain.

Unfortunately, many patients—in particular, vulnerable populations, including infants, children, and adolescents (Ruskin, Amaria, Warnock, & McGrath, 2011); older people (Gauthier & Gagliese, 2011; Holdcroft & Berkley, 2006), adults and children with limited ability to communicate (Hadjistavropoulos, Breau, & Craig, 2011); and patients with past or current substance abuse problems (Jovey, 2010)—are at high risk for suboptimal or inappropriate pain management. For example, approximately 40 to 80% of community-dwelling older patients and 16 to 27% of institutionalized older patients do not receive any treatment for their pain, regardless of pain intensity (Gagliese & Melzack, 2006). Health care providers must understand that adequate pain relief is a basic human right, must be aware of their own biases and misinformation, and must ensure that all patients are treated respectfully.

Treatment must be based on the patient's goals. The patient's and the family's goals for pain treatment should be discussed at the initial pain assessment. Sometimes these goals can be described in terms of pain intensity (e.g., the desire for average pain to decrease from an "8/10" to a "3/10"). Other patients may describe a functional goal (e.g., a person may want the pain to be relieved to an extent that allows him or her to perform daily activities). Over the course of prolonged therapy, these goals should be reassessed, and progress toward meeting them should be documented. If the patient has unrealistic goals for therapy, such as wanting to be completely rid of all persistent arthritis pain, the nurse should work with the patient to establish a more workable goal.

Fourth, treatment plans should involve a combination of drug and nondrug therapies. Although medications are often considered the mainstay of therapy, particularly for moderate to severe pain, nonpharmacological strategies should be incorporated to increase the overall effectiveness of therapy and to allow for the reduction of drug dosages to minimize adverse drug effects. Examples of therapies are discussed later in the chapter.

Fifth, a multidimensional and interdisciplinary approach is necessary for optimal pain management. Pain management clinics generally incorporate the expertise of many health care providers. However, even in situations that do not involve a specialized pain team, multiple perspectives and knowledge should be used.

Sixth, all therapies must be evaluated to ensure that they are meeting the patient's goals. Therapy must be individualized for each patient, and often achievement of an effective treatment plan requires trial and error. Drugs, dosages, and routes are commonly adjusted to achieve maximal benefit while minimizing adverse effects. This trial-and-error process can become frustrating for the patient and family. They need to be reassured that pain relief is possible and that the health care team will continue to work with them to achieve adequate pain relief.

DRUG THERAPY

Table 10-7 Examples of Ways to Manage Adverse Effects of Opioids

- Ensuring a schedule for the dosing regimen to maintain blood levels
- Using stool softeners and stimulant laxatives to prevent constipation
- Using an antiemetic to prevent nausea
- Changing to a different medication in the same class
- Using an administration route that minimizes drug concentrations at the site of the adverse effect (e.g., intraspinal administration of opioids is sometimes used to minimize high drug levels that produce sedation, nausea, and vomiting)

Seventh, adverse drug effects must be prevented or managed. Adverse effects are a major reason for treatment failure and nonadherence despite the fact that most patients can be effectively managed (RNAO, 2002). Adverse effects are managed in one of several ways described in Table 10-7. The nurse plays a key role in monitoring for and treating adverse effects, as well as teaching the patient and family how to minimize adverse effects.

Finally, patient and caregiver teaching should be a cornerstone to the treatment plan. Content should include information about the cause or causes of the pain, pain assessment methods, treatment goals and options, expectations for pain management, instruction regarding the proper use of drugs, management of adverse effects, and nondrug and self-help measures for pain relief (RNAO, 2002). Teaching should be documented, and the patient's and caregiver's comprehension of the teaching should be evaluated.

Drug Therapy for Pain

Although a physician or nurse practitioner prescribes the drugs, it is the nurse's responsibility to evaluate the effectiveness and adverse effects of prescribed drugs. It is also a nursing responsibility to document and communicate the outcomes of analgesic therapy and to suggest changes when appropriate, using knowledge and skills related to several pharmacological and pain management concepts. These include calculating equianalgesic doses, scheduling analgesic doses, titrating opioids, and selecting from the prescribed analgesic drugs.

Equianalgesic Dose. The term **equianalgesic dose** refers to a dose of one analgesic that produces pain-relieving effects equivalent to those of another analgesic. The concept of equivalence is important when substituting one analgesic for another in the event that a particular drug is ineffective or causes intolerable adverse effects and when the administration route of opioids is changed (e.g., from parenteral to oral). In general, opioids are administered in equianalgesic doses, and this is important because no upper dosage limit has been established for many of these drugs. Equianalgesic charts and conversion programs are widely available in textbooks, in clinical guidelines, in health care facility pain protocols, and on the Internet. Table 10-8 provides an example of common equianalgesic dosages compared with 10 mg of parenteral morphine, which is the standard basis for comparison (Brunton, Lazo, & Parker, 2006). Although equianalgesic charts are useful tools, health care providers must understand their limitations. Equianalgesic dosages are approximate, and individual patient response must be routinely assessed. In

Table 10-8 Examples of Common Equianalgesic Doses

DRUG	APPROXIMATE EQUIANALGESIC PARENTERAL DOSAGE	APPROXIMATE EQUIANALGESIC ORAL DOSAGE
Morphine	10 mg q3-4h (presume 24-hr around-the-clock dosing)	30 mg q3-4h
Morphine-like opioid agonists		
Hydromorphone (Dilaudid)	1.5 mg q3-4h	7.5 mg q3-4h
Oxycodone	Not available	20 mg q3-4h
Codeine	120 mg q3-4h	200 mg q3-4h
Methadone*	—	—
Meperidine (Demerol)	75 mg q3h	300 mg q2-3h

*Methadone conversion morphine dose equivalents have not been reliably established. Methadone conversion requires licensed expert assessment that is based on the patient's history of opioid consumption.
Source: Adapted from Brunton, L. L., Lazo, J., & Parker, K. (Eds.). (2006). *Goodman & Gilman's the pharmacological basis of therapeutics* (11th ed.). New York: McGraw-Hill; Hurley, R. W., Cohen, S. P. & Wu, C. L. (2010). Acute pain in adults. In S. M. Fishman, J. C. Ballantyne, & J. P. Rathmell (Eds.), *Bonica's management of pain* (4th ed., pp. 699-723). Baltimore: Lippincott Williams & Wilkins.

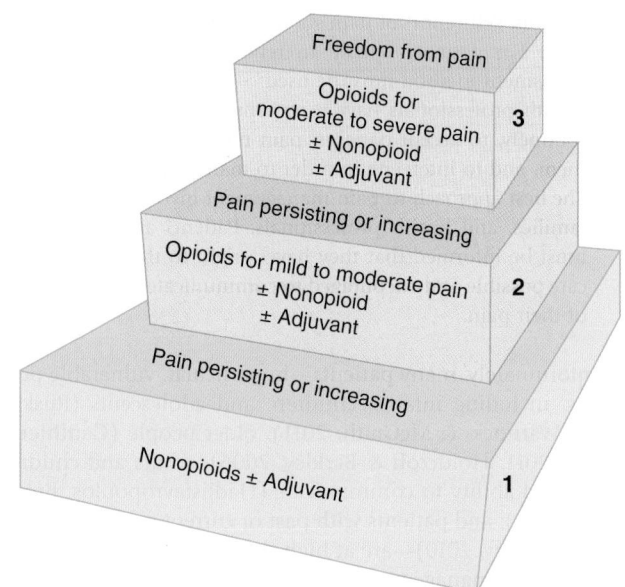

Figure 10-8 The analgesic ladder proposed by the World Health Organization.

Source: World Health Organization. (2008). *WHO's pain ladder.* Retrieved from *http://www.who.int/cancer/palliative/painladder/en/*

addition, discrepancies exist among different published equianalgesic charts (Pereira, Lawlor, Vigano, Dorgan, & Bruera, 2001). All changes in opioid therapy must be carefully monitored and adjusted for the individual patient. When possible, health care providers should use equianalgesic conversions that have been approved for their facility or clinic and should consult a pharmacist before making changes.

Scheduling Analgesics.

Appropriate analgesic scheduling should focus on prevention or ongoing control of pain rather than providing analgesics only after the patient's pain has become moderate to severe. A patient should receive medication before painful procedures and activities that are expected to produce pain. Similarly, a patient with constant pain should receive analgesics around the clock rather than on an as-needed basis. These strategies control pain before it starts and usually result in lower analgesic requirements. Fast-acting drugs should be used for incident or breakthrough pain, whereas long-acting analgesics are more effective for constant pain. Examples of fast-acting and sustained-release analgesics are described later in this section.

Titration.

Analgesic **titration** is dosage adjustment that is based on assessment of the adequacy of analgesic effect versus the adverse effects produced. The amount of analgesic needed to manage pain varies widely, and titration is an important strategy in addressing this variability. An analgesic dosage can be titrated upward or downward, depending on the situation. For example, in a postoperative patient, the dosage of analgesic generally decreases over time as the acute pain resolves. On the other hand, opioids for persistent, severe chronic noncancer pain may be titrated upward over the course of therapy to maintain adequate

pain control; this requires expert specialty care according to Canadian guidelines for chronic opioid therapy (National Opioid Use Guideline Group [NOUGG], 2010). The goal of titration is to use the lowest dosage of opioid that provides effective pain control with the fewest adverse effects (Brunton et al., 2006).

Analgesic Ladder.

Several national and international groups have published practice guidelines recommending a systematic plan for using analgesic drugs. One widely used system is the analgesic ladder proposed by the World Health Organization (WHO; Figure 10-8). The WHO treatment plan emphasizes that different drugs are administered, depending on the severity of pain, by means of a three-step ladder approach. Step 1 drugs are used for mild pain, step 2 for mild to moderate pain, and step 3 for moderate to severe pain. If pain persists or increases, drugs from the next higher step are used to control the pain. The steps are not meant to be sequential if someone has moderate to severe pain: for this person, the analgesics given would be the stronger analgesics listed in steps 2 and 3.

Drug Therapy for Mild Pain.

When pain is mild (1-3 on a scale of 0 to 10), nonopioid analgesics (aspirin and other salicylates, other NSAIDs, and acetaminophen) may be used (Table 10-9). These agents are characterized by the following: (a) their analgesic properties have a **ceiling effect:** that is, increasing the dose beyond an upper limit provides no greater analgesia; (b) they do not produce tolerance or physical dependence; and (c) many are available without a prescription. It is important to monitor over-the-counter analgesic use to avoid serious problems related to drug interactions, adverse effects, and overdosage.

A number of nonopioid analgesics such as acetylsalicylic acid (ASA, aspirin) and NSAIDs inhibit the chemicals that activate the PAN (Figure 10-9). Thus when these agents are used, the PAN is transduced less often or a larger stimulus is needed to produce transduction.

DRUG THERAPY

Table 10-9	Comparison of Selected Nonopioid Analgesics	
DRUG	**ANALGESIC EFFICACY IN COMPARISON TO STANDARDS**	**NURSING CONSIDERATIONS**
Acetaminophen (Tylenol)	Comparable with aspirin	Rectal suppository available; sustained-release preparations available; maximum daily dosage of 4 g
Salicylates		
Acetylsalicylic acid (aspirin)	Standard for comparison	Rectal suppository available; sustained-release preparations available Possibility of upper GI bleeding
Nonsteroidal anti-inflammatory drugs (NSAIDs)		
Ibuprofen (Motrin, Advil)	Superior at 200-650 mg of aspirin	Usually well tolerated despite the potential for upper GI bleeding
Indomethacin	25 mg comparable with 650 mg of aspirin	Not routinely used because of high incidence of adverse effects; rectal, intravenous, and sustained-release oral forms available
Ketorolac (Toradol)	30-60 mg equivalent to 6-12 mg of morphine	Treatment should be limited to maximum of 7 days; may precipitate renal failure in dehydrated patients
Diclofenac (Voltaren)	25-50 mg BID to TID; has a longer duration than 650 mg of aspirin	Available in oral, ophthalmic, and topical preparations
Cyclo-oxygenase-2 (COX-2) inhibitors		
Meloxicam (Mobicox)	Similar to other NSAIDs	May cause fewer GI adverse effects, including bleeding, than do other NSAIDs, but risk is still present; is more costly than other NSAIDs

BID, twice per day; *GI,* gastrointestinal; *TID,* three times per day.

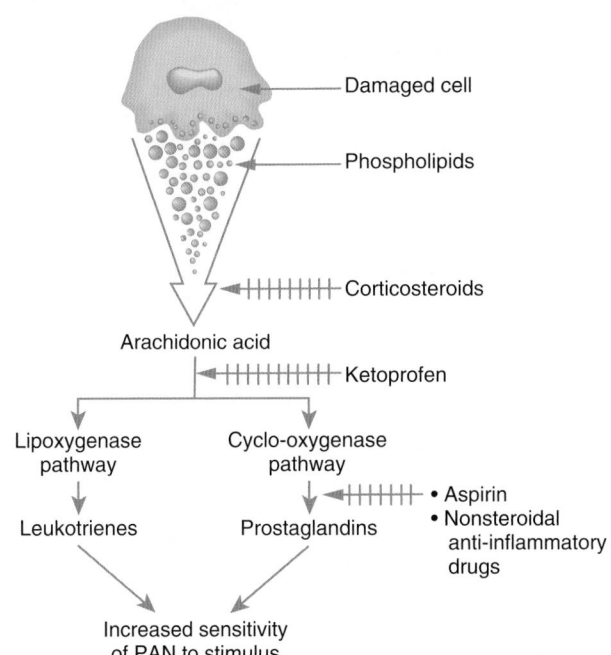

Figure 10-9 Schematic representation of two pathways that lead to the production of chemicals that cause the primary afferent nociceptor *(PAN)* to be more easily excited. Drugs that block the synthesis of these chemicals are also shown.

Aspirin is effective for mild pain, but its use is limited by its common adverse effects, including gastric upset and bleeding. Other salicylates such as choline magnesium trisalicylate cause fewer GI disturbances and bleeding abnormalities. Similarly to aspirin, acetaminophen (Tylenol) has analgesic and antipyretic effects, but it has no antiplatelet or anti-inflammatory effects. Acetaminophen is well tolerated; however, dosages higher than 4000 mg per day, acute overdosage, or use by patients with alcoholism or liver disease can result in severe hepatotoxicity.

The NSAIDs represent a broad class of drugs with varying efficacy and adverse effects. Some NSAIDs possess analgesic efficacy equal to that of aspirin, whereas others have somewhat higher efficacy (Brunton et al., 2006). Patients vary greatly in their responses to a specific NSAID, so when one NSAID does not provide relief, another should be tried. NSAIDs inhibit the cyclo-oxygenase-1 (COX-1) and -2 (COX-2) enzymes, which produce prostaglandins involved in inflammation. Because prostaglandins also play a key role in protecting the lining of the stomach from acids, adverse effects of NSAIDs can be serious and include bleeding tendencies secondary to decreased platelet aggregation, GI problems ranging from dyspepsia to ulceration and hemorrhage, renal insufficiency, and, on occasion, CNS dysfunction. For certain chronic conditions, such as rheumatoid arthritis and osteoarthritis, NSAIDs that more selectively inhibit cyclo-oxygenase-2 (COX-2) only are used (Brunton et al., 2006). The COX-2 enzyme does not play a role in protecting the stomach or intestinal tract, and therefore its selective inhibition is not associated with the same risk of injury to these organs as the inhibition of COX-1. A common example of a COX-2 inhibitor is meloxicam (Mobicox).

Drug Therapy for Mild to Moderate Pain. When pain is moderate in intensity (4 to 6 on a scale of 0 to 10) or mild but persistent despite nonopioid therapy, step 2 drugs are indicated. Drugs commonly used for mild to moderate pain are listed in Table 10-10.

One class of step 2 drugs is opioids. Opioids include many drugs (Table 10-11; also see Table 10-10) that produce their effects by binding to receptors. Opioid receptors are found in the central nervous system, on the terminals of sensory nerves, and on the

DRUG THERAPY

Table 10-10 Opioid Analgesics Commonly Used for Mild to Moderate Pain

DRUG	COMMENTS	NURSING CONSIDERATIONS
Morphine-Like Agonists		
Codeine	Weak opioid: Many preparations include combination with nonopioid analgesics; codeine is a prodrug and metabolized to morphine; 1-30% of people metabolize too efficiently and 10-20% are unable to metabolize it	For mild to moderate pain, preparations of codeine and other opioids are limited by the dosage of nonopioid analgesic (e.g., the maximum dosage of acetaminophen is 4 g/day)
Oxycodone (slow-release formulation is OxyContin)	May be given alone or combined with acetaminophen; immediate- and slow-release preparations are available	For moderate to severe pain; usually well tolerated
Tramadol (Ultram)	Maximum dosage is 400 mg/day	May cause seizures, although this is rare
Mixed Agonist–Antagonists		
Pentazocine (Talwin)	*Not recommended*	Can precipitate withdrawal in people taking opioids on a regular basis; frequently causes psychotomimetic effects
Butorphanol	Not available orally; not scheduled under *Controlled Substance Act*; butorphanol nasal spray is used to treat migraine headaches	May precipitate withdrawal in people taking opioids on a regular basis; may cause psychotomimetic effects

Source: Adapted from Lynch, M., & Watson, C. P. N. (2006). The pharmacotherapy of chronic pain: A review. *Pain Research and Management, 11*(1), 11-38.

DRUG THERAPY

Table 10-11 Opioids Commonly Used for Severe Pain

DRUG	COMMENTS	NURSING CONSIDERATIONS
Morphine	Standard comparison for opioid analgesics; sustained-release preparation (MS Contin) available	For all opioids: use with caution in people with impaired ventilation, bronchial asthma, increased intracranial pressure, liver failure; in some people the metabolite M6G may cause excessive vomiting and hallucinations, necessitating a change of opioid
Morphine-Like Agonists		
Hydromorphone (Dilaudid)	—	Well tolerated
Methadone	Good oral potency; 24- to 36-hr half-life, which necessitates careful monitoring	Licence required to prescribe; accumulates with repeated doses; on days 2-5, dosage size and frequency must be reduced
Fentanyl (Duragesic)	Available as sublingual tablet, as injection, or, for persistent pain, as transdermal preparation (Duragesic)	Immediate onset after administration by intravenous route; within 7-8 min after intramuscular route; onset after transdermal route may take several hours
Meperidine (Demerol)	Not recommended Short duration of action (2-3 hr)	Not well absorbed through oral route and should not be used; normeperidine (toxic metabolite with half-life of 14-21 hr) accumulates with repetitive dosing, causing central nervous system excitation and seizures; naloxone potentiates excitation and must not be used; avoid in patients taking monoamine oxidase inhibitors (e.g., selegiline)
Mixed Agonist–Antagonists		
Butorphanol	Not available orally; not scheduled under *Controlled Substance Act*	May precipitate withdrawal in opioid-dependent patients

Source: Adapted from Inturrisi, C., & Lipman, A. (2010). Opioid analgesics. In S. M. Fishman, J. C. Ballantyne, & J. P. Rathmell (Eds.), *Bonica's management of pain* (4th ed., pp. 1174-1175). London: Wolters-Kluwer/Lippincott Williams & Wilkins.

surface of immune cells (Brunton et al., 2006). There are three major opioid receptors, traditionally referred to as mu, kappa, and delta. The receptors have been reclassified as OP1 (delta), OP2 (kappa), and OP3 (mu) (Brunton et al., 2006). Most clinically useful opioids bind to the mu receptors. Mu agonists include morphine, oxycodone, hydromorphone (Dilaudid), and methadone. Opioid *agonists* (e.g., morphine) bind to the receptors and cause analgesia. *Antagonists* (e.g., naloxone) bind to the receptors but do not produce analgesia; they also block other effects of opioid receptor activation, such as sedation and respiratory depression. Mixed *agonist–antagonists*, such as pentazocine (Talwin) and butorphanol, should not be used because they bind

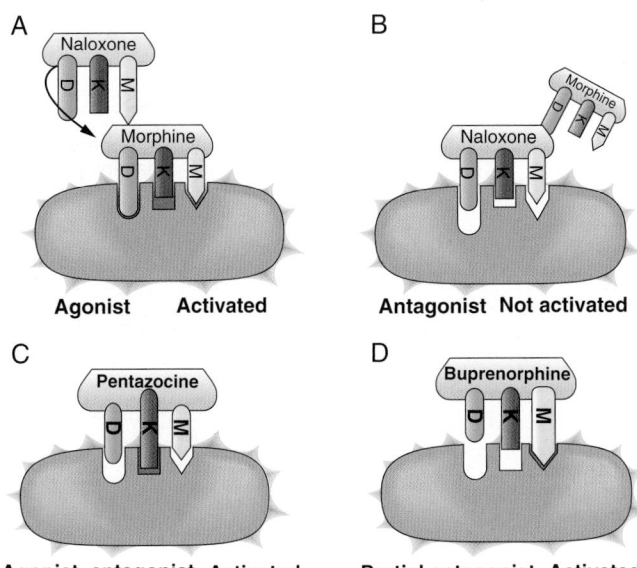

Figure 10-10 Opioid receptor subtypes. **A,** Agonist action. **B,** Antagonist action. **C,** Agonist–antagonist action. **D,** Partial antagonist action. *M,* mu receptor; *K,* kappa receptor; *D,* delta receptor.

as agonists on the kappa receptor and as weak antagonists or partial agonists on the mu receptor (Figure 10-10). When a mixed agonist–antagonist is given to someone taking an agonist (e.g., morphine), it will act like an agonist–antagonist, such as naloxone, and reverse any analgesic effect. These opioid agonist–antagonists also cause more dysphoria and agitation. In addition, they have an **analgesic ceiling** (a dosage at which no additional analgesia is produced regardless of further dosage increases) and can precipitate withdrawal if used in a client who is physically dependent on agonist drugs.

At step 2, prescriptions for commonly used opioids are often for products combining an opioid with a nonopioid analgesic (e.g., oxycodone or codeine plus acetaminophen [Tylenol No. 3]), which may limit the opioid dose that can be given. Oxycodone is now administered for severe pain as well. Although propoxyphene (Darvon) is classified as a step 2 drug, it is not recommended in analgesia guidelines because its effectiveness is limited and its toxic metabolite can cause seizures. Propoxyphene is not approved for use in Canada. A third type of medication available for mild to moderate pain is tramadol (Ultram). Tramadol is a weak mu-receptor agonist and is thought to inhibit the reuptake of norepinephrine and serotonin. It has approximately the same efficacy as Tylenol No. 3. The most common adverse effects, which are similar to those of other opioids, include nausea, constipation, dizziness, and sedation.

Drug Therapy for Moderate to Severe Pain. Step 3 drugs are recommended for moderate to severe pain (4 to 10 on a scale of 0 to 10) or when step 2 drugs do not produce effective pain relief. Most commonly used step 3 analgesics are mu-receptor agonists, although these drugs also bind with the other receptors. These drugs are effective for moderate to severe pain because they are potent, have no analgesic ceiling, and can be delivered via many routes of administration. Step 3 drugs are listed in Table 10-11.

Morphine is the standard of comparison for all other opioid analgesics. Equianalgesic charts generally list dosages in equivalent morphine dosages. Morphine is one of the opioids most commonly prescribed for moderate to severe pain, although fentanyl (Duragesic), hydromorphone (Dilaudid), methadone (Metadol), and oxycodone also are used extensively. A long-acting morphine formulation (MS Contin) is available to treat moderate to severe persistent pain in patients who require continuous, around-the-clock therapy for an extended period. Meperidine (Demerol), a mu-receptor agonist, is no longer recommended for acute or persistent pain because of the high incidence of neurotoxicity (e.g., seizures) associated with the accumulation of its neurotoxic metabolite, normeperidine. Moreover, any adverse effect cannot be reversed by naloxone, which potentiates the effect of normeperidine. In addition, a hyperpyrexic syndrome with delirium, which can cause death, can occur if meperidine is given to patients taking monoamine oxidase inhibitors (Brunton et al., 2006). Although step 3 opioids have no analgesic ceiling, people can experience dose-limiting adverse effects. In opioid-naïve patients, adverse effects include constipation, nausea and vomiting, sedation, respiratory depression, and pruritus. With continued use, most adverse effects diminish; the exception is constipation. Less common adverse effects include urinary retention, myoclonus, dizziness, confusion, and hallucinations.

Constipation is the most common opioid adverse effect. Because tolerance to opioid-induced constipation does not occur, a bowel regimen should be instituted at the beginning of opioid therapy and should continue for as long as the person takes opioids. Although dietary roughage, fluids, and exercise should be encouraged to the extent possible, these measures rarely are sufficient by themselves. Thus most affected patients should immediately begin taking a gentle stimulant laxative (e.g., senna [Senokot]) plus a stool softener (e.g., docusate sodium [Colace]). Other agents (e.g., milk of magnesia, bisacodyl [Dulcolax], lactulose) can be added if necessary. Left untreated, constipation can lead to fecal impaction and paralytic ileus that can be difficult to differentiate from obstruction.

Nausea often is a problem in opioid-naïve patients. The use of antiemetics such as metoclopramide, hydroxyzine, or a phenothiazine (e.g., prochlorperazine) can prevent or minimize opioid-related nausea and vomiting until tolerance develops, which usually occurs within 1 week. Metoclopramide is particularly effective when a patient complains of gastric fullness. Opioids delay gastric emptying, and this effect can be reversed by metoclopramide. If nausea and vomiting are severe and persistent, as with morphine because of the metabolite M6G, changing to a different opioid such as oxycodone or hydromorphone may be necessary.

Concerns about sedation and respiratory depression are two of the most common fears associated with opioids. Sedation may occur initially in opioid-naïve patients, although patients may be sleep deprived if they have been handling unrelieved pain at home before admission. Respiratory depression is rare in opioid-tolerant patients when opioids are titrated to analgesic effect. Individuals at risk for respiratory depression include opioid-naïve patients, older patients, and patients with underlying lung disease. If respiratory depression occurs and stimulating the patient (calling and shaking patient) does not reverse the somnolence or increase the respiratory rate and depth, naloxone (0.4 mg in 10 mL saline), an opioid antagonist, can be administered intravenously or subcutaneously in 0.5-mL increments every 2 minutes. However, if the patient has been taking opioids regularly for more than a few days, naloxone should be used judiciously and titrated carefully because its use can precipitate severe, agonizing pain, profound withdrawal symptoms, and seizures. Because the half-life (60 to 90 min) of naloxone is shorter than that of most opioids, nurses should monitor the patient's respiratory rate because it can drop again 1 to 2 hours after naloxone administration.

Itching may occur with opioids, most frequently when they are administered via intraspinal routes. An antihistamine such as diphenhydramine (Benadryl) often is effective. If other measures are ineffective, a low-dose opioid antagonist (e.g., naloxone) or a mixed agonist–antagonist can be used, but the patient must be carefully assessed for reversal of analgesia and withdrawal.

SAFETY ALERT

- The most appropriate opioid depends on the patient's clinical profile and the nature of the pain problem (e.g., mild to moderate, severe).

- Patients should be advised that opioids could cause cognitive effects, impairing their ability to drive.

- For postoperative patients who are breastfeeding, it is important to recognize that some women rapidly metabolize codeine to morphine. This places the infant at risk for fatal opioid toxicity. If codeine is prescribed to breastfeeding mothers, consultation with the physician and other health care team members is crucial to ensure careful monitoring (NOUGG, 2010). The patient should be advised to monitor the infant for signs of CNS depression, including poor feeding and limpness. The health care provider should be contacted immediately if any infant signs of CNS depression are noted.

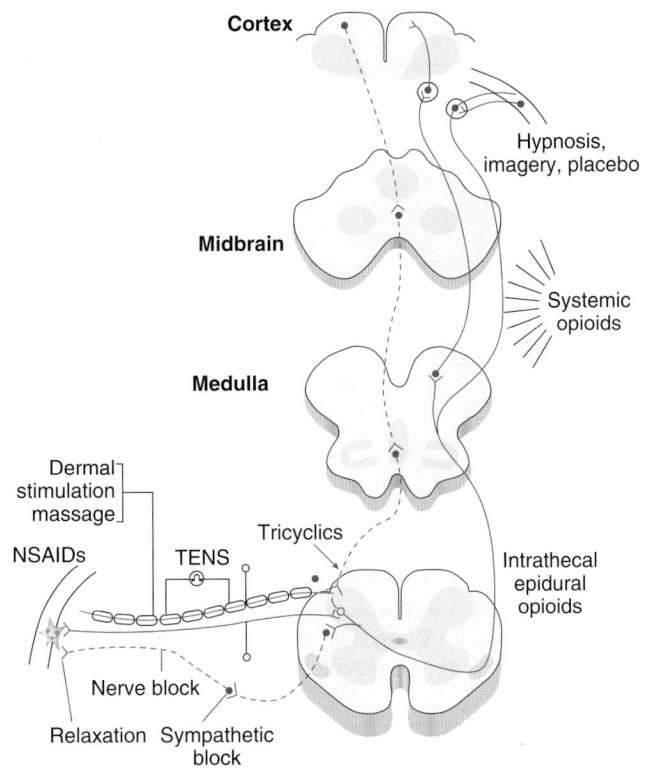

Figure 10-11 The sites of commonly used pharmacological and nonpharmacological analgesic therapies. *NSAIDs,* nonsteroidal anti-inflammatory drugs; *TENS,* transcutaneous electrical nerve stimulation.

Adjuvant Analgesic Therapy. Adjuvant analgesic therapies are drugs used in conjunction with opioid and nonopioid analgesics. Adjuvants are sometimes referred to as *coanalgesics.* They include drugs that enhance pain therapy through one of three mechanisms: (a) enhancing the effects of opioids and nonopioids, (b) possessing analgesic properties of their own, or (c) counteracting the adverse effects of other analgesics. Commonly used analgesic adjuvants are listed in Table 10-12. Figure 10-11 shows the sites of actions of pharmacological and nonpharmacological therapies for pain. Adjuvant drugs are used at every step in the WHO ladder.

Antidepressants. Tricyclic antidepressants have analgesic properties at dosages lower than those effective for depression. They enhance the descending inhibitory system by preventing synaptic reuptake of serotonin and norepinephrine. Higher levels of serotonin and norepinephrine in the synaptic cleft inhibit the transmission of nociceptive signals in the CNS. Tricyclic antidepressants have been shown to be effective for a variety of pain syndromes, especially those involving neuropathic pain. Anticholinergic effects such as dry mouth, urinary retention, sedation, and orthostatic hypotension may lessen patients' acceptance of the drug and adherence to the regimen. Selective serotonin reuptake inhibitors (e.g., paroxetine [Paxil], sertraline [Zoloft], and fluoxetine [Prozac]) have not been as effective in treating pain (Brunton et al., 2006).

Antiseizure Agents. Antiseizure drugs such as gabapentin (Neurontin), carbamazepine (Tegretol), and clonazepam (Rivotril) stabilize the membrane of the neuron and prevent transmission. These agents are effective for some neuropathic pain and prophylactic treatment of headaches (Brunton et al., 2006).

Corticosteroids. Corticosteroid medications, which include dexamethasone and methylprednisolone (Medrol), are used to treat several types of pain, including acute and persistent cancer pain, pain secondary to spinal cord or brain compression, and some neuropathic pain syndromes. Mechanisms of action are unknown but may involve the ability of corticosteroids to decrease edema and inflammation and, in some cases, to shrink tumours. Corticosteroids have many adverse effects, especially when used chronically in high dosages. Adverse effects include hyperglycemia, fluid retention, dyspepsia and GI bleeding, impairment in healing, muscle wasting, osteoporosis, and susceptibility to infection.

Local Anaesthetics. Oral, parenteral, and topical applications of local anaesthetics are used to interrupt transmission of pain signals to the brain. Local anaesthetics are given for acute pain resulting from surgery or trauma. Persistent neuropathic pain also may be controlled with local anaesthetics. Adverse effects can include dizziness, paraesthesias, and seizures (at high dosages). Incidence and severity of adverse effects depend on dosage and route of administration. These agents also affect cardiac conductivity and may cause dysrhythmias and myocardial depression (Brunton et al., 2006).

Administration Routes. Opioids and other analgesic agents can be delivered via many routes. This flexibility allows the health care provider to (a) target a particular anatomical source of the pain, (b) achieve therapeutic blood levels rapidly when necessary, (c) avoid certain adverse effects through localized administration,

DRUG THERAPY

Table 10-12 Adjuvant Drugs Used for Pain Management

DRUG	SPECIFIC INDICATION	NURSING CONSIDERATIONS
Corticosteroids	Inflammation	Avoid high dosage for long-term use
Antidepressants		
Amitriptyline (Elavil)	Neuropathic pain	Monitor for anticholinergic adverse effects
Bupropion		
Desipramine		
Doxepin (Sinequan)		
Imipramine		
Maprotiline		
Nortriptyline (Aventyl)		
Venlafaxine		
Antiseizure Agents		
Carbamazepine (Tegretol)	Neuropathic pain	Start with low dosages, increase slowly to appropriate level for effect
Clonazepam (Rivotril)		Clonazepam and carbamazepine: Check liver function, renal function, electrolytes, and blood cell counts at baseline, at 2 wk, and at 6 wk
Gabapentin (Neurontin)		
Pregabalin (Lyrica)		
Oxcarbazepine (Trileptal)		Gabapentin: Monitor for idiosyncratic adverse effects (e.g., ankle swelling, ataxia)
Topiramate (Topamax)		
Valproic acid (Epival, Depakene)		
Muscle Relaxant		
Baclofen (Lioresal)	Neuropathic pain (e.g., trigeminal neuralgia, muscle spasms)	Monitor for weakness, urinary dysfunction; avoid abrupt discontinuation because of CNS irritability
Anaesthaetics: Systemic or Oral		
Mexiletine	Diabetic neuropathy; neuropathic pain	Monitor for adverse effects, including dizziness, perioral numbness, paresthesias, tremor; can cause seizures, dysrhythmias, and myocardial depression at high dosages; avoid in patients with pre-existing cardiac disease
Anaesthaetics: Local		
Topical EMLA (eutectic mixture of local anaesthetics): lidocaine 2.5% + prilocaine 2.5%	Local skin analgesic before venipuncture, incision; possibly effective for postherpetic neuralgia	Must be applied under an occlusive dressing (e.g., Tegaderm, DuoDERM) or on an anaesthetic disc; absorption from the genital mucosa is more rapid and onset time is shorter (5-10 min) than after application to intact skin; common adverse effects include mild erythema, edema, skin blanching
Capsaicin	Pain associated with arthritis, postherpetic neuralgia, diabetic neuropathy	Apply sparingly, rub well into affected area; wash hands with soap and water after application; adverse effects include skin irritation (burning, stinging) at the application site and cough
Psychostimulants		
Dextroamphetamine (Dexedrine)	Managing opioid-induced sedation	Adverse effect is insomnia; avoid administering late in the day; usually well tolerated at low dosages
Methylphenidate (Ritalin)		

and (d) provide analgesia when patients are unable to swallow. The following discussion highlights the uses and nursing considerations for analgesics delivered through a variety of routes.

Oral. In general, oral administration is the route of choice for the patient with a functioning GI system. Oral drugs are usually less expensive than those delivered by other routes. Many opioids are available in oral preparations, such as liquid and tablet formulations. To obtain analgesia equivalent to that pro-vided by doses administered intramuscularly or intravenously, oral doses must be higher. For example, 10 mg of parenteral morphine is equivalent to approximately 30 mg of oral mor-phine (see Table 10-8). Higher dosages are required for opioid-naïve patients because of the first-pass effect of hepatic metabolism. This means that oral opioids initially are absorbed from the GI tract into the portal circulation and shunted to the liver (Brunton et al., 2006). Partial metabolism in the liver occurs before the drug enters systemic circulation and becomes available to peripheral receptors or can cross the blood–brain barrier and access CNS opioid receptors, which is necessary to produce analgesia. Oral opioids are as effective as parenteral opioids if the dose administered is large enough to compensate for the first-pass metabolism.

Oral preparations also are available in immediate-release and sustained-release preparations. For example, morphine is available in immediate-release solutions or tablets. These products are effective in providing rapid, short-term pain relief; concentration in the blood typically peaks within 30 to 60 minutes. Sustained-release oral morphine tablets are administered every 8 to 12 hours; the most common preparation is morphine ER (MS Contin). As with other sustained-release preparations, this product should not be crushed, broken, or chewed. Oxycodone also comes in a sustained-release capsule (OxyContin). Other opioids with sustained-release formulations include hydromorphone and tramadol. The time to maximum blood plasma dose concentration typically ranges from 30 to 60 minutes and from 2 to 4 hours for immediate-release and sustained-release formulations, respectively (Kalso, 2010).

Sublingual and Buccal. Opioids administered under the tongue or held in the mouth and absorbed into systemic circulation are exempt from the first-pass effect. Although morphine is commonly administered to patients with cancer pain via the sublingual route, little of the drug is absorbed from the sublingual tissue. Instead, much of the drug is dissolved in saliva and swallowed, and thus its metabolism is similar to that of oral morphine.

Intranasal. Intranasal administration allows delivery of medication to highly vascular mucosa and avoids the first-pass effect. Butorphanol is one of the few intranasal analgesics available. This drug is most commonly indicated for migraine headaches. Several intranasal opioid agents are being investigated.

Rectal. The rectal route is often overlooked but is particularly useful when the patient cannot take an analgesic by mouth. Rectal suppositories that are effective for pain relief include hydromorphone (Dilaudid) and morphine.

Transdermal. Fentanyl (Duragesic) is available as a transdermal patch system for application to nonhairy skin. This delivery system is useful for the patient who cannot tolerate oral analgesic drugs. Absorption from the patch is slow. Therefore, transdermal fentanyl is not suitable for rapid dosage titration but can be effective if the patient's pain is stable and the dosage required to control it is known. Patches may have to be changed every 48 hours rather than the recommended 72 hours, depending on individual patient responses.

Currently, creams and lotions containing 10% trolamine salicylate (e.g., Aspercreme, Myoflex cream) are available. These agents have been recommended by the manufacturers for joint and muscle pain. This aspirin-like substance is absorbed locally. The topical route of administration precludes gastric irritation, but the other adverse effects of high-dosage salicylate are not necessarily prevented.

Ointments, lotions, gels, liniments, and balms (most of which are over-the-counter products) are sometimes applied to the skin to achieve pain relief. Common ingredients include methyl salicylate combined with camphor, menthol, or both. On application, these agents usually produce a strong hot or cold sensation and should not be used after massage or a heat treatment, when blood vessels are already dilated. Skin testing is advisable when the patient has not used the particular agent before because the strengths of the agents vary and different intensities of sensation are produced. These products are indicated for arthralgia, bursitis, myalgia, and tendinitis.

Other topical analgesic agents, such as capsaicin (e.g., Icy Hot) and prilocaine plus lidocaine (eutectic mixture of local anaesthetics [EMLA]), also provide analgesia. Derived from red chili pepper, capsaicin depletes and prevents reaccumulation of substance P in the peripheral sensory neurons. It can control pain associated with postherpetic neuralgia, diabetic neuropathy, and arthritis. EMLA is useful for control of pain associated with venipunctures, ulcer debridement, and possibly postherpetic neuralgia. The area to which EMLA is applied should be covered with a plastic wrap for 30 to 60 minutes before a painful procedure begins.

Parenteral Routes. The parenteral route includes subcutaneous and intravenous administration. The only opioid that must be injected intramuscularly is meperidine, and this drug is not recommended because its toxic metabolite, normeperidine, can accumulate with repeated administration, causing CNS excitation (Brunton et al., 2006). Single-dose administration (subcutaneous or intravenous) is possible via parenteral routes. The intramuscular route, although frequently used, is not recommended because these injections cause significant pain, result in unreliable absorption, and with chronic use can result in abscesses and fibrosis. Onset of analgesia after subcutaneous administration is slow, and thus the subcutaneous route is rarely used for acute pain management. However, continuous subcutaneous infusions are effective for persistent cancer pain. This route is especially helpful for people with abnormal GI function and limited venous access. Intravenous administration is the best option when immediate analgesia and rapid titration are necessary. Continuous intravenous infusions provide excellent steady-state analgesia through stable blood levels.

Intraspinal Delivery. Intraspinal (epidural or intrathecal) opioid therapy involves inserting a catheter into the subarachnoid space (for intrathecal delivery) or the epidural space (for epidural delivery) and injecting an analgesic, either by intermittent bolus doses or continuous infusion (see e-Figure 10-1 on the Evolve Web site). Percutaneously placed temporary catheters are used for short-term therapy (2-4 days), and surgically implanted catheters are used for long-term therapy. Although the lumbar region is the most common site of placement, epidural catheters may be placed at any point along the neuroaxis (cervical, thoracic, lumbar, or caudal). Intraspinally administered analgesics are highly potent because they are delivered close to the receptors in the dorsal horn of the spinal cord. Thus much lower doses of analgesics are needed for intraspinal delivery in comparison with other routes, including intravenous. Drugs that are delivered intraspinally include morphine, fentanyl, and hydromorphone. Nausea, itching, and urinary retention are common adverse effects of intraspinal opioids.

Complications of intraspinal analgesia include catheter displacement and migration, neurotoxicity (especially of certain agents when infused intraspinally), and infection. Clinical manifestations of catheter displacement or migration depend on catheter location. Movement of a catheter out of the intrathecal or epidural space causes a decrease in pain relief with no improvement even when additional analgesic is administered. Correct placement of an intrathecal catheter can be checked by aspirating cerebrospinal fluid. Migration of a catheter into a blood vessel causes an increase in drug adverse effects because of systemic drug distribution. A number of drugs and chemicals are highly neurotoxic when administered intraspinally. These include many substances such as preservatives (e.g., alcohol and phenol), antibiotics, potassium, and total parenteral nutrition supplements. To avoid inadvertent injection of intravenous drugs into an intraspinal catheter, the catheter should be clearly marked as an intraspinal access device, and only preservative-free drugs should be injected.

Infection rarely occurs with intraspinal analgesia. However, it is a serious complication that can be difficult to detect. The skin around the exit site should be carefully assessed for inflammation, drainage, or pain. Signs and symptoms of an intraspinal infection include diffuse back pain, pain or paresthesias during bolus injection, and unexplained sensory or motor deficits. Fever may or may not be present. Acute bacterial infection (meningitis) is manifested by fever, headache, and altered mental status. Infection is avoided with regular, meticulous wound care and with the use of sterile technique in caring for the catheter and injecting drugs.

Patient-Controlled Analgesia. A specific type of subcutaneous, intravenous, or intraspinal delivery system is **patient-controlled analgesia** (PCA), or *demand analgesia.* PCA is an infusion system that allows the patient to self-administer a dose of opioid through a pump when needed: The patient pushes a button to receive a bolus infusion of an analgesic. PCA is used widely for the management of acute pain, including postoperative pain and cancer pain. Often, the patient also receives an additional continuous, basal infusion (known as *PCA plus basal*) at a preset dose and rate. The addition of a continuous basal infusion to a PCA regimen improves nighttime pain relief and promotes better sleep postoperatively. Common opioids used in the PCA administration method include morphine and hydromorphone (Dilaudid).

Use of PCA begins with patient teaching. The patient needs to understand the benefits and principles of PCA therapy, the mechanics of obtaining a drug dose (i.e., the operation of the pump and button), and how to titrate the drug to achieve good pain relief. The patient should be encouraged to use the PCA pump prophylactically by self-administering the analgesic before ambulation, physiotherapy, and dressing changes. The patient also needs to be reminded that apart from the involved health care providers, he or she is the only person who should press the button. The patient should also be assured that he or she cannot "overdose" because the pump is programmed to deliver a maximum number of doses per hour; pressing the button after the maximum dose is administered will not result in additional analgesic. If the maximum doses are inadequate to relieve pain, the pump can be reprogrammed to increase the amount or frequency of administration (this requires an order from the physician or nurse practitioner). In addition, bolus doses can be given by the nurse if they are included in the physician's orders. The patient should also be encouraged to report possible adverse effects such as nausea and vomiting or pruritus so that they can be managed effectively. To make a smooth transition from infusion PCA to oral therapy, the dosage of oral drug should be increased (as ordered) as the PCA analgesic is tapered.

Surgical Therapy for Pain

Nerve Blocks. Nerve blocks are used to reduce pain by temporarily or permanently interrupting transmission of nociceptive input. This is achieved with local anaesthetics or neurolytic agents (e.g., alcohol, phenol). Neural blockade with local anaesthetics is sometimes used for perioperative pain. For intractable persistent pain, nerve blocks are used when more conservative therapies fail. Nerve blocks have been a successful pain management technique for more localized persistent pain states, such as peripheral vascular disease, trigeminal neuralgia, causalgia, and some cancer pain. A nerve block may be considered advantageous in managing localized pain caused by malignancy and in debilitated patients who could not otherwise withstand a surgical procedure for pain relief.

Interventional Therapy

Therapeutic Nerve Blocks. Nerve blocks generally involve one-time or continuous infusion of local anaesthetics into a particular area to produce pain relief. Such relief is also referred to as *regional anaesthesia.* Nerve blocks interrupt all afferent and efferent transmission to the area and thus are not specific to nociceptive pathways. They include local infiltration of anaesthetics into a surgical area (e.g., for excision of a breast lump, inguinal hernia surgery, intra-articular infiltration after joint surgery) and injection of anaesthetics into a specific nerve (e.g., occipital or pudendal nerve) or nerve plexus (e.g., brachial or celiac plexus; Curatolo & Bogduk, 2010). Nerve blocks often are used during and after surgery to manage pain. For longer-term relief of chronic pain syndromes, local anaesthetics can be administered via a continuous infusion (Ilfeld, 2010).

For intractable chronic pain, neuroablative nerve blocks (see next section) with phenol or alcohol may be used. For example, a neurolytic celiac plexus block may be induced for pain caused by pancreatic cancer, or an intercostal neurolytic block may be induced for post-thoracotomy pain. Heat and microwaves, used in many neurolytic procedures, produce nerve tissue destruction (Curatolo & Bogduk, 2010).

Neuroablative Techniques. *Neuroablative interventions* are performed for severe pain that is unresponsive to all other therapies. Neuroablative techniques destroy nerves, thereby interrupting pain transmission. Destruction is accomplished by surgical resection or thermocoagulation, including radiofrequency coagulation. Neuroablative interventions that destroy the sensory division of a peripheral or spinal nerve are classified as neurectomies, rhizotomies, and sympathectomies. Neurosurgical procedures that ablate the lateral spinothalamic tract are classified as cordotomies if the tract is interrupted in the spinal cord or as tractotomies if the interruption is in the medulla or the midbrain of the brainstem. Figure 10-12 depicts the sites of neurosurgical procedures for pain relief. Both cordotomy and tractotomy can be performed with the aid of local anaesthesia by a percutaneous technique.

Neuroaugmentation. Neuroaugmentation involves electrical stimulation of the brain and the spinal cord. Spinal cord stimulation is performed much more often than deep brain stimulation. Technological advances have enabled the use of multiple leads and multiple electrode terminals so as to stimulate large areas. In Canada and the United States, common uses of spinal cord stimulation are for chronic back pain secondary to nerve damage that is unresponsive to other therapies (Simpson, Meyerson, & Linderoth, 2006) and chronic refractory angina (Ekre, Eliasson, Norrsell, Wahrborg, & Mannheimer, 2002).

Potential complications include those related to the surgery (bleeding and infection), migration of the generator (which usually is implanted in the subcutaneous tissues of the upper gluteal or pectoralis area), and nerve damage. Stimulation of deep brain structures (e.g., thalamus) was performed in the 1970s and 1980s to achieve pain control but is rarely performed today.

Nonpharmacological Therapy for Pain

Nonpharmacological pain management strategies can reduce the dose of an analgesic required to control pain and thereby minimize adverse effects of drug therapy. Some strategies are believed to alter ascending nociceptive input or stimulate descending pain modulation mechanisms. Nonpharmacological pain relief methods can be categorized as physical or cognitive strategies (Table 10-13).

Physical Pain Relief Strategies

Massage. Massage is a common therapy for pain, and many massage techniques exist. Examples include moving the hands or fingers over the skin slowly or briskly with long strokes or in circles (superficial massage) or applying firm pressure to the skin to maintain contact while massaging the underlying tissues

(deep massage). Specific massage techniques include acupressure and trigger-point massage. A **trigger point** is a circumscribed hypersensitive area within a tight band of muscle that is the result of acute or chronic muscle strain. Several common trigger points have been identified on the neck, back, and arms. Trigger-point massage is performed either by application of strong, sustained digital pressure, deep massage, or gentler massage with ice followed by muscle heating. (Massage is discussed further in Chapter 12).

Therapeutic Exercise. Therapeutic exercise is a critical part of the treatment plan for patients with chronic pain, particularly those with musculoskeletal pain. Research findings support the effectiveness of many types of exercise for a variety of painful conditions (McLean et al., 2010; Watson, Main, & Smeets, 2010). Many patients become physically deconditioned as a result of their pain, which in turn can exacerbate pain. Exercise acts through many mechanisms to relieve pain: It enhances circulation and cardiovascular fitness, reduces edema, increases muscle strength and flexibility, and enhances physical and psychosocial functioning. A safe exercise program should be tailored to the physical needs and lifestyle of the patient and should include mild to moderate aerobic exercise, stretching, and strengthening exercises. The program also should be supervised by trained personnel (e.g., psychologist, physiatrist, registered nurse with specialty training, exercise physiologist, physiotherapist). Examples of exercise programs include yoga, Tai Chi, walking regimens, and water aerobics.

Transcutaneous Electrical Nerve Stimulation. Transcutaneous electrical nerve stimulation (TENS) involves the delivery of an electric current through electrodes applied to the skin surface over the painful region, at trigger points, or over a peripheral nerve. A TENS system consists of two or more electrodes connected by lead wires to a small, battery-operated stimulator (Figure 10-13). Usually, a physiotherapist is responsible for

Table 10-13 Nonpharmacological Therapies for Pain	
Physical Therapies	**Cognitive Therapies**
• Acupuncture	• Distraction
• Application of heat and cold	• Hypnosis
• Exercise	• Imagery
• Massage	• Relaxation strategies
• Percutaneous electrical nerve stimulation (PENS)	• Self-management
• Transcutaneous electrical nerve stimulation (TENS)	

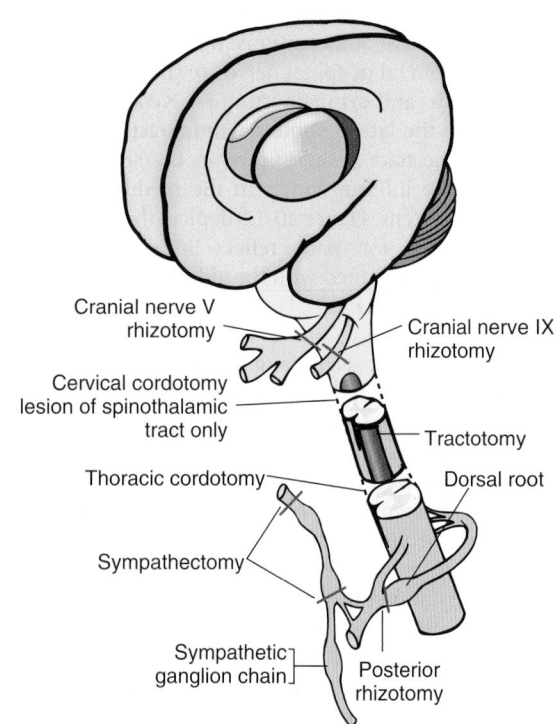

Figure 10-12 Sites of neurosurgical procedures for pain relief.

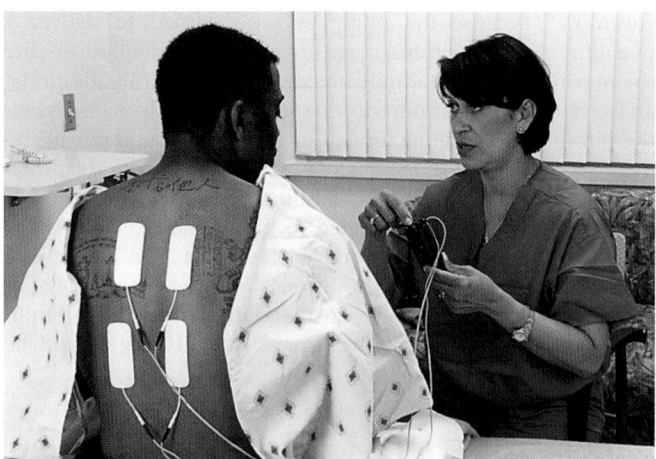

Figure 10-13 Initial transcutaneous electrical nerve stimulation (TENS) treatment being given by a physiotherapist to assess effectiveness in pain relief.

Source: Rick Brady, Riva, MD.

administering TENS therapy, although nurses also can be trained in the technique.

TENS has been enthusiastically embraced by some pain health care providers, although there is little scientific evidence from well-designed clinical trials to support its effectiveness (Barlas & Lundeberg, 2006). Strong evidence in favour of TENS was obtained in studies of patients with dysmenorrhea or angina pectoris and in some groups of patients with neuropathic pain (Barlas & Lundeberg, 2006).

Application of Heat. Heat therapy is the application of either moist or dry heat to the skin. Heat therapy can be either superficial or deep. Superficial heat can be applied through an electric heating pad (dry or moist), a hot pack, hot moist compresses, or a hot water bottle. For exposure to large areas of the body, patients can immerse themselves in a hot bath, shower, or whirlpool. Physical therapy departments provide deep-heat therapy through such techniques as short-wave diathermy, microwave diathermy, and ultrasound therapy. Patient teaching regarding heat therapy is described in Table 10-14.

Application of Cold. Cold therapy involves the application of either moist or dry cold to the skin. Dry cold can be applied by means of an ice bag and moist cold by means of towels soaked in ice water, cold hydrocollator packs, or immersion in a bath or under running cold water. Icing with ice cubes or blocks of ice made to resemble Popsicles is another technique used for pain relief. Cold therapy is believed to be more effective than heat for a variety of painful conditions, including acute pain from trauma or surgery, acute flares of arthritis, muscle spasms, and headache. Patient teaching regarding cold therapy is described in Table 10-14.

Cognitive Techniques. Techniques to alter the affective, cognitive, and behavioural components of pain include a variety of cognitive strategies and behavioural approaches. Some of these techniques require little training and often are adopted independently by the patient. For others, a trained therapist must administer therapy.

Distraction and Imagery. Distraction involves redirection of attention on something and away from the pain. It is a simple but powerful strategy to relieve pain. Distraction can be achieved by engaging the patient in any activity that can hold his or her attention (e.g., watching TV, conversing, listening to music, playing a game). It is important to match the activity with the patient's energy level and ability to concentrate. **Imagery** is a structured technique in which the patient's own imagination is used to develop sensory images that divert focus away from the pain. (See Chapter 8 for additional information.)

Hypnosis. Research supports the effectiveness of self-hypnosis training for many types of chronic pain, particularly those aggravated by tension and stress (Elkins et al., 2007). Despite these promising results, there is a lack of consensus on a standardized approach to hypnotic interventions across clinical trials. Moreover, the current evidence has been obtained from small studies and lacks long-term follow up (Elkins et al., 2007). Hypnosis training should be administered and monitored only by specially trained clinicians. (See Chapter 12 for additional information.)

Relaxation Strategies. The goal of the various relaxation strategies is to achieve a state that is free from anxiety and muscle tension. Relaxation reduces stress, decreases acute anxiety, distracts from pain, alleviates muscle tension, combats fatigue, facilitates sleep, and enhances the effectiveness of other pain relief measures (Flor & Turk, 2006). Elicitation of the relaxation response requires a quiet environment, a comfortable position, and a mental device as a focus of concentration (e.g., a word, a sound, or the person's breathing). Relaxation strategies include relaxation breathing, music, imagery, meditation, and progressive muscle relaxation. (See Chapter 8 for additional information.)

Self-Management. Self-management training is gaining momentum in Canada as an effective, adjunctive strategy for managing the effect of persistent pain on day-to-day functioning and quality of life (LeFort, Gray-Donald, Rowat, & Jeans, 1998; McGillion et al., 2008; Stinson et al., 2008). Self-management training programs are typically conducted in groups with a focus on helping participants increase their daily pain management skills and decrease the negative consequences of persistent pain, such as social isolation. By structured rehearsal of various cognitive and behavioural self-management techniques (e.g., energy conservation, pacing, sleep promotion, relaxation, communication skills, and safe exercise), patients and family members learn to set realistic weekly goals that are directed at increasing overall functional capacity and emotional well-being. Strong evidence (see the Nursing Research box) supports the effectiveness of self-management training for (a) improving participants' perceived self-efficacy or ability to achieve selected goals, (b) reducing pain, and (c) improving perceived quality of life (LeFort et al., 1998; McGillion et al., 2008; Stinson et al., 2008). Nurses who facilitate self-management intervention programs require specialized training in self-efficacy–enhancing mechanisms, managing groups, and assessing patients' readiness to engage in pain self-management.

PATIENT & CAREGIVER TEACHING GUIDE

Table 10-14 Application of Heat and Cold

When patients use superficial heating techniques, they should be taught the following:

- Do not use heat on an area that is being treated with radiation therapy, is bleeding, has decreased sensation, or has been injured in the past 24 hours.
- Do not use any menthol-containing products (e.g., Vicks VapoRub) with heat applications because this may cause burns.
- Cover the heat source with a towel or cloth to prevent burns.

When patients use superficial cold techniques, they should be taught the following:

- Cover the cold source with a cloth or towel.
- Do not apply cold to areas that are being treated with radiation therapy, have open wounds, or have poor circulation.
- If it is not possible to apply the cold directly to the painful site, try applying it directly above or below the painful site or on the opposite side of the body on the corresponding site (e.g., left elbow if the right elbow hurts).

NURSING RESEARCH

Pain Self-Management

Citation

McGillion, M., Watt-Watson, J., Stevens, B., LeFort, S., Coyte, P., & Graham, A. (2008). Randomized controlled trial of a psychoeducation program for the self-management of chronic cardiac pain. *Journal of Pain and Symptom Management, 26,* 126-140.

Purpose

Chronic stable angina is a major form of chronic pain in Canada with major negative effects on health-related quality of life (HRQL), including pain, poor general health status, and inability to self-manage pain. This randomized clinical trial evaluated the effect of a low-cost 6-week angina psychoeducation program, titled the Chronic Angina Self-Management Program (CASMP), on HRQL, self-efficacy, and resourcefulness to self-manage anginal pain.

Methods

One hundred thirty participants were randomly assigned to the CASMP (a standardized, 6-week self-management program) or to 3-month waiting list usual care; 117 completed the study. The mean age of participants was 68; 80% were male. General HRQL, angina pain, self-efficacy, and resourcefulness were measured at baseline and 3 months after the test.

Results and Conclusions

Significant improvements in physical functioning, general health, angina pain, and self-efficacy to manage pain were found for CASMP participants at 3 months, in comparison with those who received usual care.

Implications for Nursing Practice

These data indicate that the nurse-facilitated CASMP was effective for improving angina pain and related aspects of physical functioning and general health. Further research is needed to examine the ability of the CASMP to improve patients' angina pain over the long term.

NURSING MANAGEMENT: PAIN

The nurse is an important member of the multidisciplinary pain management team. The nurse acts as planner, educator, patient advocate, interpreter, and supporter of the patient in pain and the patient's family or caregivers. Because any patient in a wide variety of care settings (e.g., home, hospital, clinic) can be in pain, the nurse must be knowledgeable about current therapies and flexible in trying new approaches to pain management. The extent of the nurse's involvement depends on the unique factors associated with the patient, the setting, and the cause of the pain. Many nursing roles were described earlier in this chapter: conducting pain assessments, administering therapies, monitoring for adverse effects, and teaching patients and caregivers. However, the success of these actions depends on the nurse's ability to establish a trusting relationship with the patient and caregivers

and to address the concerns that they have regarding pain and its treatment.

Effective Communication

Patients need to feel confident that their reporting of pain will be believed and will not be perceived as "complaining." The patient and the family also need to know that the nurse considers the pain significant and understands that pain may disrupt a person's life. The nurse must communicate concern about the patient and assure the patient that he or she is committed to helping the patient obtain pain relief and cope with any unrelieved pain. Pharmacological and nonpharmacological interventions should be incorporated into the treatment plan, and the patient should be supported through the period of trial and error that may be necessary to implement an effective therapeutic plan. It also is important to clarify responsibilities of pain relief. The nurse should help the patient understand the roles of the health care team members, as well as the roles and expectations of the patient.

In addition to addressing specific aspects of pain assessment and treatment, the nurse evaluates the total effect that the pain may have on the lives of the patient and family. Thus, other possible nursing diagnoses must also be considered. Table 10-15 lists possible nursing diagnoses that may be appropriate for assessing and managing pain. Table 10-16 addresses teaching needs of patients and caregivers in relation to pain management.

NURSING ASSESSMENT

Table 10-15 Pain-Related Nursing Diagnoses

• Activity intolerance	• Hopelessness
• Acute pain	• Ineffective coping
• Anxiety	• Ineffective role performance
• Chronic pain	• Interrupted family processes
• Constipation	• Powerlessness
• Disturbed sleep pattern	• Risk for self-mutilation
• Fatigue	• Social isolation
• Fear	• Thought processes, disturbed

PATIENT & CAREGIVER TEACHING GUIDE

Table 10-16 Pain Management: Teaching Needs

The goals of teaching related to pain management include the expectation that the patient and the caregivers understand the following:

- Need to maintain a record of pain level and effectiveness of treatment
- No need to wait until pain becomes severe to take drugs or use nondrug therapies for pain relief
- The possibility that the dosage of medication may have to be adjusted over time to maximize long-term effectiveness
- Potential adverse effects and complications that are associated with opioid therapy or therapies; common adverse effects can include nausea and vomiting, constipation, sedation and drowsiness, itching, urinary retention, sweating
- Need to report when pain is not relieved to tolerable levels

Barriers to Effective Pain Management

Pain is a complex, multidimensional, and subjective experience, and its management is influenced greatly by psychosocial, socio-cultural, and legal and ethical factors. These factors include emotions, behaviours, misconceptions, and attitudes of patients and family members about pain and use of pain therapies. Achieving effective pain management requires careful consideration of these factors.

Concerns regarding tolerance, dependence, and addiction are common barriers to effective pain management, inasmuch as these phenomena are often misunderstood. Patients, family members, and health care providers often share these concerns. It is important for the nurse to understand and to be able to explain the differences among these various concepts (Jovey, 2010).

Tolerance

Tolerance is "a state of adaptation in which exposure to a drug induces changes that result in a diminution of one or more of the drug's effects over time" (NOUGG, 2010, p. 126). In the case of opioids, steady-state dosing can lead to tolerance of unwanted opioid adverse effects (Jovey, 2010). However, development of tolerance to an opioid itself is characterized by the need for increasing or more frequent doses of the opioid to maintain the same degree of analgesic effect. Although tolerance is not as common as once thought, it is essential to assess for increased analgesic needs in patients receiving chronic opioid therapy (Jovey, 2010). The first sign of tolerance may be that the patient begins to experience regular end-of-dose failure. If manifestations of possible tolerance appear, appropriate evaluations should be made to rule out other causes of increased analgesic needs, such as disease progression or infection. Approaches to managing tolerance are (a) to increase the dosage of the analgesic, (b) to substitute another drug in the same class (e.g., changing from morphine to oxycodone), or (c) to add a drug from a different drug class that will augment pain relief without increasing adverse effects. It is important to note that there is no ceiling effect for opioid-agonist drugs and to recognize that "The occurrence of tolerance to opioids, in and of itself, does not imply addiction" (Jovey, 2010, p. 320).

Physical Dependence

Like tolerance, **physical dependence** is an expected physiological response to ongoing exposure to pharmacological agents: Physical dependence is "a state of adaptation manifested by a drug class–specific withdrawal syndrome that can be produced by abrupt cessation, rapid dose reduction, decreasing blood level of the drug, and/or administration of an antagonist" (NOUGG, 2010, p. 124). Symptoms of opioid withdrawal are listed in Table 10-17. When opioids are no longer needed to provide pain relief, a tapering schedule should be used in conjunction with careful monitoring. A typical tapering schedule begins with calculating the 24-hour dose used by the patient and dividing by 2. Of this decreased amount, 25% is given every 6 hours. After 2 days, the daily dose is reduced by an additional 25% every 2 days until the 24-hour oral dose is 30 mg (morphine equivalent) per day. After

Table 10-17 Manifestations of Withdrawal From Opioids	
Type	**Response**
• Mood	• Anxiety, agitation
• Physical and behavioural	• Restlessness
	• Diaphoresis
	• Fever
	• Flu-like symptoms (i.e., nausea, muscle aches)
	• Tremor
	• Tachycardia

2 days on this minimum dosage, the opioid is then discontinued. Despite this slow weaning schedule, the nurse should assess carefully for signs and symptoms of opioid withdrawal. In addition to assessing and preventing opioid withdrawal, it is also important to recognize that other commonly prescribed drugs for pain also can induce physical dependence and therefore must be slowly tapered. These include benzodiazepines and muscle relaxants.

Addiction

Addiction is defined as "a primary, chronic, neurobiological disease, with genetic, psychosocial, and environmental factors influencing its development and manifestations. It is characterized by behaviours that include one or more of the following: impaired control over drug use, compulsive use, continued use despite harm, and craving" (NOUGG, 2010, p. 124). Tolerance and physical dependence are not indicators of addiction. Rather, they are normal physiological responses to chronic exposure to certain drugs, including opioids.

Substance use disorders, including illicit drug use and misuse of prescription opioids, affect about 10% of the general population (Jovey, 2010). The available data are of limited quality and suggest that in patients being treated for chronic pain, the risk of concurrent substance abuse or addiction is generally the same or higher than in patients without those disorders (Jovey, 2010). For patients without a history of substance use disorder, the risk is thought to be significantly lower. For example, a 2010 Cochrane Review revealed that signs of addiction were present in 0.3% of patients without a documented history of substance use disorder who were being treated with opioids for chronic noncancer pain (Noble et al., 2010). People with a history of addiction can be managed successfully on opioids for their pain with careful monitoring. In these populations, the risk of addiction may be higher. Expectations of the health care team and the patient must be discussed openly and documented. Signs and symptoms of possible addiction must be monitored and interventions promptly initiated.

In addition to fears about addiction, physical dependence, and tolerance, other barriers hinder effective pain management. These include concern about adverse effects, difficulties with remembering to take drugs, desire to handle pain stoically, and not wanting to distract the health care provider from treating the disease. Table 10-18 lists examples of patient-related barriers to effective pain management, and includes strategies to address the barriers.

PATIENT & CAREGIVER TEACHING GUIDE

Table 10-18 Reducing Patient-Related Barriers to Pain Management

BARRIER	NURSING CONSIDERATIONS	BARRIER	NURSING CONSIDERATIONS
Fear of addiction	• Provide accurate definition of addiction. • Explain that addiction is uncommon in patients taking opioids for pain relief.	Desire to be stoic	• Explain that although stoicism is a valued behaviour in many cultures, failure to report pain can result in undertreatment and severe, unrelieved pain.
Fear of tolerance	• Provide accurate definition of tolerance. • Teach that tolerance is a normal physiological response to chronic opioid therapy. If tolerance does develop, the drug may have to be changed (e.g., morphine in place of oxycodone). • Teach that there is no upper limit to pure opioid agonists (e.g., morphine). Dosages can be increased indefinitely, and the patient should not save drugs for when the pain is worse. • Teach that tolerance to analgesic effects of opioids develops more slowly than do many adverse effects (e.g., sedation, respiratory depression). Tolerance does not ameliorate constipation; thus a regular bowel program should be started early.	Forgetting to take analgesic	• Provide and teach use of pill containers. • Provide methods of record keeping for drug use. • Recruit family members as appropriate to assist with the analgesic regimen.
		Fear of distracting the health care provider from treating the disease	• Explain that reporting pain is important for treating both the disease and its symptoms.
Concern about adverse effects	• Teach methods to prevent and to treat common adverse effects. • Emphasize that adverse effects such as sedation and nausea decrease with time. • Explain that different drugs have unique adverse effects and that other pain drugs can be tried to reduce the specific adverse effect. • Teach nondrug therapies to minimize the dosage of drug needed to control pain.	Concern that pain signifies disease progression	• Explain that increased pain or analgesic needs may reflect tolerance. • Emphasize that new pain may come from a non–life-threatening source (e.g., muscle spasm, urinary tract infection). • Institute pharmacological and nonpharmacological strategies to reduce anxiety. • Ensure that the patient and family members have current, accurate, comprehensive information about the disease and the prognosis. • Provide psychological support.
Fear of injections	• Explain that oral medicines are preferred. • Emphasize that even if the oral route becomes unusable, transdermal or indwelling parenteral routes can be used rather than injections.	Sense of fatalism	• Explain that research has shown that pain can be managed in most patients. • Explain that with most therapies, a period of trial and error is necessary. • Emphasize that adverse effects can be managed.
Desire to be a "good" patient	• Explain that patients are partners in their care and that the partnership requires open communication on the parts of both patient and nurse. • Emphasize to patients that they have a responsibility to keep the nurse informed about their pain.	Ineffective medication	• Teach that there are multiple options within each category of medication (e.g., opioids, NSAIDs) and that another medication from the same category may provide better relief. • Emphasize that finding the best treatment regimen often requires trial and error. • Incorporate nondrug approaches in treatment plan.

NSAIDs, nonsteroidal anti-inflammatory drugs.

Source: Adapted from Ersek, M. (1999). Enhancing effective pain management by addressing patient barriers to analgesic use. *Journal of Hospice & Palliative Nursing, 1,* 87-96.

Institutionalizing Pain Education and Management

Besides patient and family barriers, other major barriers to effective pain management arise in connection with the health care provider: inadequate education, misconceptions about pain, and lack of organizational support. Traditionally, medical and nursing school curricula have included little time teaching future physicians and nurses about pain and effective pain management, although this is changing. This lack of emphasis was partially responsible for the insufficiency of health care providers' knowledge of and skills to treat pain adequately. Moreover, pain assessment and treatment were not priorities in clinical practice. Health care providers have misconceptions about pain. Similar to patients, many clinicians confuse physical dependence, tolerance, and addiction and are more likely to assess pain by observing behaviours rather than believing or eliciting a patient's report (Jovey, 2010).

Over the past few decades, some improvements have been made in overcoming these barriers. Some prelicensure, undergraduate health care programs are now devoting more time to addressing pain (Hunter et al., 2008; Watt-Watson et al., 2004), and there is growing interest in inter-professional educational intervention trials for practising health care providers that target common pain-related misconceptions (McGillion et al., 2011; see the following Nursing Research Box).

The International Association of the Study of Pain has published a core curriculum on pain that was developed for the learning needs of a range of health care provider groups. Provincial organizations such as the RNAO have also developed evidence-informed practice guidelines on pain that are readily accessible (see the Resources section at the end of this chapter for the Weblinks).

Health care institutions are also directing more, much needed attention to their support of pain management. Researchers and health care providers have documented the central role of institutional commitment and practices in changing clinical practice; without institutional support, pain outcomes are unlikely to change. The pain management standards from the Canadian Pain Society's (2010) *Position Statement on Pain Relief* (see the Resources section at the end of this chapter) emphasize that patients have a right to the best pain relief possible and that measures to prevent or reduce acute pain are a priority.

Ethical Issues in Pain Management

Fear of Hastening Death by Administering Analgesics

It is common for the health care provider, patient, and family members to be concerned that providing sufficient drug to relieve pain will precipitate the death of a terminally ill person (Beauchamp & Childress, 2008). The ethical justification for administering analgesics despite the possibility of hastening death follows the bioethical principle of the *rule of double effect*: that if an unwanted consequence (i.e., hastened death) occurs as a result of an action taken to achieve a moral good (i.e., pain relief), the action is justified according to ethical theory because the nurse's intent is to relieve pain and not to hasten death (Beauchamp & Childress, 2008). Unrelieved pain is associated with higher suicide rates and a sense of hopelessness (Lynch, 2011).

Use of Placebos in Pain Assessment and Treatment

Placebos have been used inappropriately in the past to determine whether patients' pain was "real." Use of medication placebos for pain, such as giving saline injections instead of an opioid, or giving oral dosages of inappropriate drugs, such as meperidine, 50 mg by mouth, is unethical.

NURSING RESEARCH

Pain-Related Misconceptions and Pain Assessment Skills for Health Care Providers

Citation

McGillion, M., Dubrowski, A., Stremler, R., Watt-Watson, J., Campbell, F., McCartney, C., ... Silver, I. (2011). The Postoperative Pain Assessment Skills pilot trial. *Pain Research and Management, 16,* 433-439.

Purpose

Pain-related misconceptions among health care providers are common and contribute to the ineffectiveness of postoperative pain assessment. Although so-called standardized patients (SPs) (healthy people trained to portray the history, symptoms, characteristics, and concerns of actual patients), have been effectively used to improve health care providers' assessment skills, not all centres have SP programs. This pilot equivalence randomized controlled trial was an examination of the efficacy of an alternative simulation method—deteriorating patient-based simulation—versus SPs for improving interprofessional pain knowledge and assessment skills.

Methods

Seventy-two health care providers were randomly assigned to receive a 3-hour standardized patient or patient-based simulation intervention. Measures were taken at baseline, immediately after intervention, and 2 months after intervention. The primary outcome was health care providers' pain assessment performance, as measured by the Post-operative Pain Assessment Skills Tool (PAST). Secondary outcomes included health care providers' knowledge of pain-related misconceptions and perceived satisfaction and quality of the simulation. These outcomes were measured with the Pain Beliefs Scale (PBS), the Satisfaction with Simulated Learning Scale (SSLS), and the Simulation Design Scale (SDS), respectively. Participants' *t*-tests were used to test for overall group differences in postintervention PAST, SSLS, and SDS scores. One-way analysis of covariance was conducted to test for overall group differences in PBS scores.

Results and Conclusions

Patient-based simulation and SP groups did not differ on post-test PAST, SSLS, or SDS scores. Knowledge of pain-related misconceptions (Pain Beliefs Scale) was also similar between groups.

Implications for Nursing Research and Practice

These pilot data indicated that patient-based simulation is an effective simulation alternative for nurses' and other health care providers' education on postoperative pain assessment, with improvements in performance and knowledge comparable to those after standardized patient-based simulation. A larger equivalence trial is warranted to examine the effectiveness of deteriorating patient-based simulation versus standardized patients.

AGE-RELATED CONSIDERATIONS: PAIN

Persistent noncancer pain is a common problem in older adults and is often associated with significant physical disability and psychosocial problems. Estimates of the prevalence of persistent pain problems among community-dwelling older adults are reported to be at least 50% (Charlton, 2005). Among institutionalized older adults, 80% report at least one unresolved pain problem (Charlton, 2005). The most common sources of pain among older adults are musculoskeletal conditions, such as osteoarthritis and low back pain, and previous fracture sites. Persistent pain often results in depression, sleep disturbance, decreased mobility, increased use of health care services, and physical and social role dysfunction. Despite its high prevalence, pain in older adults often is inadequately assessed and treated (Gagliese & Melzack, 2006). There are several barriers to pain assessment in the older patient. In general, the barriers discussed earlier in the chapter are more prevalent among this population. For example, many older patients believe that pain is a normal, inevitable part of aging. They may also believe that nothing can be done to relieve the pain. Older adults may not report pain for fear of being a "burden" or a "bad" patient. They may have greater fears of taking opioids than do patients in other age-groups (Gagliese & Melzack, 2006). Also, older patients are more likely to use words such as "aching," "soreness," or "discomfort" rather than "pain." Despite their reluctance to report pain, current research indicates that pain tolerance actually decreases with age (Gagliese & Melzack, 2006). For all these reasons, nurses must be vigilant in asking older people about their pain and its effect.

Another barrier to pain assessment in older adults is the relatively high prevalence of cognitive, sensory–perceptual, and motor problems that interfere with a person's ability to process information and to communicate. Examples of these problems include dementia and delirium, poststroke aphasia and paraplegia, and language barriers. Also, hearing and vision deficits may complicate assessment. Therefore, pain assessment tools may have to be adapted for older adults. For example, it may be necessary to use a large-print pain intensity scale. Although there is some concern that older adults have difficulty using pain scales, it has been documented that many older adults, even those with mild to moderate cognitive impairment, can use quantitative scales accurately and reliably. There is some evidence that older adults have difficulty using visual analogue scales and that numerical rating scales and verbal descriptor scales are preferable (Gagliese & Melzack, 2006) (see Figure 10-7).

As for other patients with persistent pain, a thorough physical examination should be performed and the history thoroughly documented to identify causes of pain, possible therapies, and potential problems. Because depression and functional impairments are common among older adults with pain, the possibility of these also must be assessed.

Although recommendations for older people with pain are similar to those for other age groups, treatment of pain in older adults is complicated by several factors. First, older adults metabolize drugs more slowly than do younger patients and thus are at greater risk for higher blood levels and adverse effects. For this reason, the adage "start low and go slow" is applied to analgesic therapy in this age group. Second, the use of NSAIDs in older adults is associated with a high frequency of serious GI bleeding. For this reason, acetaminophen should be used whenever possible. Third, many older people take multiple drugs for one or more chronic conditions. The addition of analgesics can result in dangerous drug interactions and more adverse effects. Fourth, cognitive impairment and ataxia can be exacerbated when analgesics such as opioids, antidepressants, and anticonvulsant drugs are used, which again necessitates that health care providers titrate drugs slowly and monitor carefully for adverse effects.

Treatment regimens for older adults must incorporate nondrug modalities. Exercise and patient teaching are particularly important nonpharmacological interventions for older adults with persistent pain. The roles of family and paid caregivers also should be included in the treatment plan.

Special Populations

Cognitively Impaired Individuals

Although patient self-report is the "gold standard" of pain assessment in most circumstances, severe cognitive impairment often prevents patients from communicating clearly about their pain. For these individuals, behavioural and physiological changes may be the only indicators that they are in pain. Therefore, the nurse must be astute at recognizing behavioural symptoms of pain.

Several scales have been developed to assess pain in cognitively impaired older patients (Hadjistavropoulos et al., 2009). Typically, these scales help assess pain according to common behavioural indicators such as the following:

- Vocalization: moaning, grunting, crying, sighing
- Facial expressions: grimacing, wincing, frowning, clenching teeth
- Breathing: noisy, laboured
- Body movements: restlessness, rocking, pacing
- Body tension: clenching fist, resisting movement
- Consolability: inability to be consoled or distracted

Because it is not possible to validate the meaning of the behaviours, nurses should rely on their own knowledge of the patient's usual behaviour. If the nurse does not know the patient's baseline behaviours, she or he should obtain this information from other caregivers, including family members. When pain behaviours are present, pain therapy should be instituted on an empirical basis, and patients should be carefully reassessed to evaluate treatment effectiveness.

Patients With Substance Abuse Problems

Individuals with a past or current substance abuse disorder have the right to receive effective pain management. A comprehensive pain assessment is imperative, including a detailed history, physical examination, psychosocial assessment, and diagnostic workup to determine the cause of the pain. The use of screening tools to determine the possible risk of addiction has been described (Jovey, 2010). The goal of the pain assessment is to facilitate the establishment of a treatment plan that will relieve the individual's pain effectively, as well as prevent or minimize withdrawal symptoms.

Opioids may be used effectively and safely in patients with substance dependence when indicated for pain control. Opioid agonist–antagonist agents (e.g., pentazocine [Talwin], butorphanol) should not be used in this population because they may precipitate withdrawal. The use of "potentiators" and psychoactive drugs that do not have analgesic properties should also be avoided. In individuals who are tolerant to CNS depressants, larger doses of opioids or increased frequency of drug administration is necessary to achieve pain relief.

Pain management for people with addiction is challenging and requires expert leadership and consultation for assessment and facilitation of a planned, multidisciplinary team approach according to current Canadian guidelines (NOUGG, 2010). Team members must be aware of their own attitudes and misconceptions about people with substance abuse problems, which may result in undertreatment of pain.

CLINICAL DECISION-MAKING EXERCISE

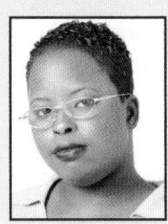

CASE STUDY:
Pain

Source: © 2007 JupiterImages Corporation.

Patient Profile

Mrs. Cato is a 112-kg, 43-year-old Caribbean woman admitted for an incision and drainage of a right renal abscess. Her renal function is not impaired.

Subjective Data

- Lives alone.
- Desires 0 pain during therapy but will accept 1 to 2 on a scale of 0 to 10.
- Reports incision-area pain as a 2 or 3 between dressing changes and as a 10 during dressing changes.
- States sharp, throbbing pain persists 1 to 2 hours after dressing change.
- Reports pain between dressing changes controlled by two oxycodone (Percocet) tablets.
- Reports that morphine, 2 mg intravenously, barely affects pain during dressing changes.

Objective Data

- Requires twice-a-day dry-to-dry dressing changes for 1 week.
- Morphine, 2 to 15 mg intravenously, for every dressing change.
- Percocet, 1 to 2 tablets, for breakthrough pain between dressing changes.

Discussion Questions

1. Initially, what dosage of intravenous morphine should be given?
2. Describe the assessment data that supports the dosage selected in Question 1.
3. How long should the nurse wait after the intravenous morphine dose to begin the dressing change?
4. If an initial dose of 6 mg intravenous morphine reduces the pain to a 6 during the dressing change, what nursing action is indicated for the next dressing?
5. What nursing action is indicated if Mrs. Cato has pain 5 hours after her dressing change?
6. When Mrs. Cato is discharged needing dressing changes for 3 days at home, how would the home care nurse organize her care? The nurse knows that Mrs. Cato has obtained adequate pain relief with 8 mg intravenous morphine.

evolve   Answers are available at **http://evolve.elsevier.com/Canada/Lewis/medsurg**

REVIEW QUESTIONS

The number of the question corresponds to the same-numbered objective at the beginning of the chapter.

1. How is pain best described?
   a. A creation of a person's imagination
   b. An unpleasant, subjective experience
   c. A maladaptive response to a stimulus
   d. A neurological event resulting from activation of nociceptors
2. Which of the following inhibiting neurotransmitters is known for its involvement in pain modulation?
   a. Dopamine
   b. Acetylcholine
   c. Prostaglandin
   d. Norepinephrine
3. Which of the following words is most likely to be used to describe neuropathic pain?
   a. Dull
   b. Mild
   c. Aching
   d. Burning
4. Which of the following is true of unrelieved pain?
   a. It is to be expected after major surgery.
   b. It is to be expected in a person with cancer.
   c. It is dangerous and can lead to many physical and psychological complications.
   d. It is an annoying sensation, but it is not as important as other physical care needs.

5. Which of the following is a critical step in the pain assessment process?
   a. Assessment of critical sensory components
   b. Teaching the patient about pain therapies
   c. Conducting a comprehensive pain assessment
   d. Provision of appropriate treatment and evaluation of its effect
6. Which of the following is an example of distraction to provide pain relief?
   a. TENS
   b. Music
   c. Exercise
   d. Biofeedback
7. Which of the following is an appropriate nonopioid analgesic for mild pain?
   a. Oxycodone (Percocet)
   b. Ibuprofen (Advil)
   c. Lorazepam (Ativan)
   d. Cyclobenzaprine
8. Which of the following is an important nursing responsibility related to pain?
   a. Encourage the patient to stay in bed.
   b. Help the patient appear to not be in pain.
   c. Believe what the patient says about the pain.
   d. Assume responsibility for eliminating the patient's pain.

9. A nurse is administering a prescribed dose of an intravenous opioid titrated for a person with severe pain related to a terminal illness. Which of the following actions is reflective of this practice?
   a. Euthanasia
   b. Assisted suicide
   c. Enabling the patient's addiction
   d. Palliative pain management

10. A nurse believes that patients with the same type of tissue injury should have the same amount of pain. Which of the following statements best describes this belief?
    a. It will contribute to appropriate pain management.
    b. It is an accurate statement about pain mechanisms and an expected goal of pain therapy.
    c. The nurse's belief will have no effect on the type of care provided to people in pain.
    d. It is a common misconception about pain and a major contributor to ineffective pain management.

ANSWERS: 1. b; 2. d; 3. d; 4. c; 5. c; 6. b; 7. b; 8. c; 9. d; 10. d.

REFERENCES

Aasvang, E. K., & Kehlet, H. (2010). Persistent sensory dysfunction in pain-free herniotomy. *Acta Anaesthesiologica Scandinavica, 54*, 291-298. doi:10.1111/j.1399-6576.2009.02137.x

American Academy of Pain Management. (n.d.). *Pain issues: Pain is an epidemic.* Sonora, CA: Author. Retrieved from *http://www.aapainmanage.org/literature/Articles/PainAnEpidemic.pdf*

American Academy of Pain Medicine, American Pain Society, & American Society of Addiction Medicine. (2001). *Consensus statement: Definitions related to the use of opioids for the treatment of pain.* Retrieved from *http://www.asam.org/advocacy/find-a-policy-statement/view-policy-statement/public-policy-statements/2011/12/15/definitions-related-to-the-use-of-opioids-for-the-treatment-of-pain-consensus-statement*

American Geriatrics Society. (2002). The management of persistent pain in older persons. *Journal of the American Geriatric Society, 50*(Suppl. 6), 1-20. doi:10.1046/j.1532-5415.50.6s.1.x

Arntz, A., & Claassens, L. (2004). The meaning of pain influences its experienced intensity. *Pain, 109*, 20-25. doi:10.1016/j.pain.2003.12.030

Arntz, A., & de Jong, P. (1993). Anxiety, attention and pain. *Journal of Psychosomatic Research, 37*, 423-432. doi:0022.3999/93 36.00.00

Barber, J. (2001). Hypnosis. In J. D. Loeser, S. M. Butler, C. R. Chapman, & D. C. Turk (Eds.), *Bonica's management of pain* (3rd ed., pp. 1768-1778). Baltimore: Lippincott Williams & Wilkins.

Barlas, P., & Lundeberg, T. (2006). Transcutaneous electrical nerve stimulation and acupuncture. In S. B. McMahaon & M. Koltzenburg (eds.). *Melzack and Wall's Textbook of Pain*, pp. 583-590. Philadelphia: Elsevier Churchill Livingstone.

Basbaum, A., & Bushnell, M. C. (2002). Pain: Basic mechanisms. In M. A. Giamberardino (Ed.), *Pain 2002—An updated review: Refresher course syllabus* (pp. 3-14). Seattle: IASP Press.

Basbaum, A., & Jessell, T. (2000). The perception of pain. In E. Kandel, J. Schwartz, & T. Jessell (Eds.), *Principles of neural science* (4th ed., pp. 472-490). New York: McGraw-Hill.

Basbaum, A., & Julius, D. (2006). Toward better pain control. *Scientific American, 294*(6), 60-67. doi:10.1038/scientificamerican 0606-60

Beauchamp, T. L., & Childress, J. F. (2008). *Principles of biomedical ethics* (6th ed.). New York: Oxford University Press.

Behr, J., Friedly, J., Molton, I., Morgenroth, D., Jensen, M. P., & Smith, D. G. (2009). Pain and pain-related interference in adults with lower-limb amputation: Comparison of knee-disarticulation, transtibial, and transfemoral surgical sites. *Journal of Rehabilitation Research and Development, 46*, 963-972. doi:10.1682/JRRD.2008.07.0085

Boulanger, A., Clark, A. J., Squire, P., Cui, E., & Horbay, G. L. A. (2007). Chronic pain in Canada: Have we improved manage-ment of chronic non-cancer pain? *Pain Research and Management, 12*, 39-47.

Brandsborg, B., Nikolajsen, L., Hansen, C. T., Kehlet, H., & Jensen, T. S. (2007). Risk factors for chronic pain after hysterectomy: A nationwide questionnaire and database study. *Anesthesiology, 106*, 1003-1012. doi:10.1097/01.anes.0000265161.39932.e8

Breivik, H., Collett, B., Ventafridda, V., Cohen, R., & Gallacher, D. (2006). Survey of chronic pain in Europe: Prevalence, impact on daily life and treatment. *European Journal of Pain, 10*, 287-333. doi:10.1016/j.ejpain.2005.06.009

Brunton, L. L., Lazo, J., & Parker, K. (Eds.). (2006). *Goodman & Gilman's The pharmacological basis of therapeutics* (11th ed.). New York: McGraw-Hill.

Canadian Pain Society. (2010). *Position statement on pain treatment as a human right.* Retrieved from *http://www.canadianpainsociety.ca/en/about_policy.html*

Cassell, E. J. (1982). The nature of suffering and the goals of medicine. *New England Journal of Medicine, 306*, 639. doi:10.1056/NEJM198203183061104

Charlton, J. E. (2005). *Core curriculum for professional education in pain* (3rd ed.). Seattle, WA: IASP Press.

Cousins, M., & Power, I. (1999). Acute and postoperative pain. In P. D. Wall & R. Melzack (Eds.), *Textbook of pain* (4th ed., pp. 447-492). Edinburgh: Churchill Livingstone.

Craig, K. (2006). Emotions and psychobiology. In S. B. McMahon & M. Koltzenburg (Eds.), *Melzack and Wall's textbook of pain* (5th ed., pp. 231-240). Philadelphia: Elsevier.

Craig, K. D. (2005). Assessment of credibility. In R. F. Schmidt & W. D. Willis (Eds.), *Encyclopedic reference of pain* (pp. 491-493). New York: Springer.

Craig, K. D., Prkachin, K. M., & Grunau, R. E. (2011). The facial expression of pain. In D. C. Turk & R. Melzack (Eds.), *Handbook of pain assessment* (3rd ed., pp. 117-134). New York: Guilford.

Curatolo, M., & Bogduk, N. (2010). Diagnostic and therapeutic nerve blocks. In S. M. Fishman, J. C. Ballantyne, & J. P. Rathmell (Eds.), *Bonica's management of pain* (4th ed., pp. 1401-1423). Baltimore: Lippincott Williams & Wilkins.

DeGood, D. E., & Cook, A. J. (2011). Psychosocial assessment, comprehensive measures, and measures specific to pain beliefs and coping. In D. C. Turk & R. Melzack (Eds.), *Handbook of pain assessment* (3rd ed., pp. 67-97). New York: Guilford.

Ekre, O., Eliasson, T., Norrsell, H., Wahrborg, P., & Mannheimer, C. (2002). Long-term effects of spinal cord stimulation and coronary artery bypass grafting on quality of life and survival in the ESBY study. *European Heart Journal, 23*, 1938-1945. doi:10.1053/euhj.2002.3194

Elkins, G., Jensen, M. P., & Patterson, D. R. (2007). Hypnotherapy for the management of chronic pain. *The International Journal of Clinical and Experimental Hypnosis, 55*(3), 275-287. doi:10.1080/00207140701338621.

Erkes, E. B., Parker, V. G., Carr, R. L., & Mayo, R. M. (2001). An examination of critical care nurses' knowledge and attitudes regarding pain management in hospitalized patients. *Pain Management Nursing, 2,* 47-53. doi:10.1053/jpmn.2001.23177

Ersek, M., Kraybill, B. M., & Du Pen, A. R. (1999). Factors hindering patients' use of medication for cancer pain. *Cancer Practice, 7,* 226-232. doi:10.1016/j.pain.2007.10.02

Ferrell, B. R. (2001). Pain observed: The experience of pain from the family caregiver's perspective. *Clinics in Geriatric Medicine, 17,* 595-609. doi:10.1016/S0749-0690(05)70099-9

Fields, H. (1987). *Pain.* Toronto: McGraw-Hill.

Flor, H., & Turk, D. C. (2006). Cognitive and learning aspects. In S. B. McMahon & M. Koltzenburg (Eds.), *Melzack and Wall's textbook of pain* (5th ed., pp. 241-258). Philadelphia: Elsevier.

Gagliese, L., & Melzack, R. (2006). Pain in the elderly. In S. B. McMahon & M. Koltzenburg (Eds.), *Melzack and Wall's textbook of pain* (5th ed., pp. 1169-1179). Philadelphia: Elsevier.

Gauthier, L. R., & Gagliese, L. (2011). Assessment of pain in older persons. In D. C. Turk & R. Melzack (Eds.), *Handbook of pain assessment* (3rd ed., pp. 242-259). New York: Guilford.

Hadjistavropoulos, T., Breau, L. M., & Craig, K. D. (2011). Assessment of pain in adults and children with limited ability to communicate. In D. C. Turk & R. Melzack (Eds.), *Handbook of pain assessment* (3rd ed., pp. 260-280). New York: Guilford.

Hadjistavropoulos, T., & Fine, P. G. (2006). Chronic pain in older persons: Prevalence, assessment and management. *Reviews in Clinical Gerontology, 16,* 231-241. doi:10.1017-S0959259807002201.

Hadjistavropoulos, T., Hunter, P., & Fitzgerald, T. D. (2009). Pain assessment and management in older adults: Conceptual issues and clinical challenges. *Canadian Psychology, 50*(4), 241-254. doi:10.1037-a0015341

Herlitz, J., Brandup-Wognsen, G., Caidahl, K., Haglid, M., Heartford, M., Karlson, B. W., ..., Sjöland, H. (2008). Symptoms of chest pain and dyspnea and factors associated with chest pain and dyspnea 10 years after coronary artery bypass grafting. *American Heart Journal, 156*(3), 580-587. doi:10.1016/j.ahj.2008.04.017

Herr, K., & Garrand, L. (2001). Assessment and measurement of pain in older adults. *Clinics in Geriatric Medicine, 17,* 457. doi:10.1016/S0749-0690(05)70080-X

Holdcroft, A., & Berkley, K. J. (2006). Sex and gender differences in pain and its relief. In S. B. McMahon & M. Koltzenburg (Eds.), *Melzack and Wall's textbook of pain* (5th ed., pp. 1181-1197). Philadelphia: Elsevier.

Hoskin, P. (2006). Cancer pain: Treatment overview. In S. B. McMahon & M. Koltzenburg (Eds.), *Melzack and Wall's textbook of pain* (5th ed., pp. 1141-1157). Philadelphia: Elsevier.

Hunter, J., Watt-Watson, J., McGillion, M., Raman-Wilms, L., Cockburn, L., Lax, L., ..., Salter, M. (2008). An interfaculty pain curriculum: Lessons learned from six years experience. *Pain, 140,* 74-86. doi:10.1016/j.pain.2008.07.010

Ilfeld, B. (2010). Continuous peripheral nerve blocks for treating acute pain in the hospital and the ambulatory environment. In J. Mogil (Ed.), *Pain 2010—An updated review: Refresher course syllabus* (pp. 303-312). Seattle: IASP Press.

International Association for the Study of Pain. (2011). *IASP taxonomy: Changes in the 2011 list.* [Online taxonomy update from Merskey, H., & Bogduk, N. (Eds.). (1994). Part III: Pain terms, a current list with definitions and notes on usage. In *Classification of chronic pain* (2nd edition, pp. 209-214), Seattle: IASP Press, IASP Task Force on Taxonomy.] Retrieved from *http://www.iasp-pain.org/AM/Template.cfm?Section=Pain_Defi...isplay.cfm&ContentID=1728*

Jensen, M. P., Karoly, P., & Huger, R. (1987). The development and preliminary validation of an instrument to assess patients' attitudes toward pain. *Journal of Psychosomatic Research, 31,* 393-400. doi:10.1016/0022-3999(87)90060-2

Johansson, E. E., Hamburg, K., Westward, G., & Lindgren, G. (1999). The meanings of pain: An exploration of women's descriptions of symptoms. *Social Science & Medicine, 48,* 1791-1802. doi:10.1016/S0277-9536(99)00080-5

Jovey, R. D. (2010). Pain and addiction: Prevalence, neurobiology, definitions. In J. Mogil (Ed.), *Pain 2010—An updated review: Refresher course syllabus* (pp. 315-321). Seattle: IASP Press.

Julius, D., & Basbaum, A. (2001). Molecular mechanisms of nociception. *Nature, 413,* 203-210. doi:10.1038/35093019

Kalso, E. (2010). Clinical pharmacology of opioids in the treatment of pain. In J. Mogil (Ed.), *Pain 2010—An updated review: Refresher course syllabus* (pp. 207-215). Seattle: IASP Press.

Katz, J., & Melzack, R. (2011). The McGill Pain Questionnaire: Development, psychometric properties, and usefulness of the long form short form, and short form–2. In D. C. Turk & R. Melzack (Eds.), *Handbook of pain assessment* (3rd ed., pp. 45-66). New York: Guilford.

Keefe, F. J., Lefebvre, J. C., Egert, J. R., Affleck, G., Sullivan, M. J., & Caldwell, D. S. (2000). The relationship of gender to pain, pain behaviour, and disability in osteoarthritis patients: The role of catastrophizing. *Pain, 87,* 325-334.

LeFort, S., Gray-Donald, K., Rowat, K. M., & Jeans, M. E. (1998). Randomized controlled trial of a community-based psychoeducation program for the self-management of chronic pain. *Pain, 74,* 297-306. doi:10.1016/S0304-3959(97)00190-5

Lynch, M. E. (2011). The need for a Canadian pain strategy. *Pain Research and Management, 16*(2), 77-80.

Mantyh, P. W. (2006). Cancer pain: Causes, consequences and therapeutic opportunities. In S. B. McMahon & M. Koltzenburg (Eds.), *Melzack and Wall's textbook of pain* (5th ed., pp. 1087-1098). Philadelphia: Elsevier.

McCaffery, M., & Pasero, C. (1999). *Pain: A clinical manual for nursing practice* (2nd ed.). St. Louis: Mosby.

McGillion, M., Dubrowski, A., Stremler, R., Watt-Watson, J., Campbell, F., McCartney, C., ..., Silver, I. (2011). The Postoperative Pain Assessment Skills pilot trial. *Pain Research and Management, 16,* 433-439.

McGillion, M., Watt-Watson, J., LeFort, S., & Stevens, B. (2007). Positive shifts in the perceived meaning of cardiac pain following a psychoeducation program for chronic stable angina. *Canadian Journal of Nursing Research, 39*(2), 48-65. doi:10.1016/j.jpainsymman.2007.09.015

McGillion, M., Watt-Watson, J., Stevens, B., LeFort, S., Coyte, P., & Graham, A. (2008). Randomized controlled trial of a psychoeducation program for the self-management of chronic cardiac pain. *Journal of Pain and Symptom Management, 26,* 126-140. doi:10.1016/j.jpainsymman.2007.09.015

McLean, J. P., Chimes, G. P., Press, J. M., Hearndon, M. L., Willick, S. E., & Herring, S. A. (2010). Basic concepts in biomechanics and musculoskeletal rehabilitation. In S. M. Fishman, J. C. Ballantyne, & J. P. Rathmell (Eds.), *Bonica's management of pain* (4th ed., pp. 1294-1312). Baltimore: Lippincott Williams & Wilkins.

McMillan, S. C., Tittle, M., Hagan, S., & Laughlin, J. (2000). Management of pain and pain-related symptoms in hospitalized veterans with cancer. *Cancer Nursing, 23,* 327-336. doi:10.1097/00002820-200010000-00001

Melzack, R., & Wall, P. D. (1987). *The challenge of pain.* New York: Penguin Books.

Moulin, D. E., Clark, A. J., Gilron, I., Ware, M. A., Watson, C. P., Sessle, B. J., ..., Canadian Pain Society. (2007). Pharmacological management of chronic neuropathic pain—Consensus statement and guidelines from the Canadian Pain Society. *Pain Research & Management, 12*(1), 13-21.

National Opioid Use Guideline Group [NOUGG]. (2010). *Canadian guideline for safe and effective use of opioids for chronic non-cancer pain.* Retrieved from *http://nationalpaincentre.mcmaster.ca/opioid/*

Nikolajsen, L., Brandsborg, B., Lucht, U., Jensen, T. S., & Kehlet, H. (2006). Chronic pain following total hip arthroplasty: A nationwide questionnaire study. *Acta Anaesthesiologica Scandinavica, 50,* 495-500. doi:10.1111/j.1399-6576.2006.00976.x

Noble, M., Treadwell, J. R., Tregear, S. J., Coates, V. H., Wiffen, P. J., Akafomo, C., & Scholles, K. M. (2010). Long-term opioid management for chronic non-cancer pain. *Cochrane Database of Systematic Reviews, No. 1,* CD006605. doi:10.1002/14651858. CD006605.pub2

Page, G. G., & Eliyahu, S. (1997). The immune-suppressive nature of pain. *Seminars in Oncology Nursing, 13*(1), 10-15. doi:10.1016/ S0749-2081(97)80044-7

Pasero, C., Paice, J. A., & McCaffery, M. (1999). Basic mechanisms underlying the causes and effects of pain. In M. McCaffery & C. Pasero (Eds.), *Pain: Clinical manual* (2nd ed.). St. Louis: Mosby.

Peng, P., Choiniere, M., Dion, D., Intrater, H., Lefort, S., Lynch, M., ..., STOPPAIN Investigators Group. (2007). Challenges in accessing multidisciplinary pain treatment facilities in Canada. *Canadian Journal of Anaesthesiology, 54,* 977-984. doi:10.1007/ BF03016631

Pereira, J., Lawlor, P., Vigano, A., Dorgan, M., & Bruera, E. (2001). Equianalgesic dose ratios for opioids. A critical review and proposals for long-term dosing. *Journal of Pain Symptom Management, 22,* 672-687. doi:10.1016/S0885-3924(01)00294-9

Ramage-Morin, L., & Gilmour, H. (2010). Chronic pain at ages 12 to 44 (Statistics Canada Catalogue no. 82-003-XPE). *Health Reports, 21*(4). Retrieved from *http://www.statcan.gc.ca/pub/82-003-x/2010004/article/11389-eng.pdf*

Registered Nurses' Association of Ontario (RNAO). (2002). *Assessment and management of pain.* Toronto, ON: Author. Retrieved from *http://www.rnao.org/Page.asp?PageID=924&ContentID=720*

Ruskin, D. A., Amaria, K. A., Warnock, F., & McGrath, P. A. (2011). Assessment of pain in infants, children, and adolescents. In D. C. Turk & R. Melzack (Eds.), *Handbook of pain assessment* (3rd ed., pp. 213-241). New York: Guilford.

Simpson, B. A., Meyerson, B. A., & Linderoth, B. (2006). Spinal cord and brain stimulation. In S. B. McMahon & M. Koltzenburg (Eds.), *Melzack and Wall's textbook of pain* (5th ed., pp. 563-582). Philadelphia: Elsevier.

Stinson, J., Toomey, P. C., Stevens, B. J., Kagan, S., Duffy, C. M., Huber, A., ..., Feldman, B. M. (2008). Asking the experts: Exploring the self-management needs of adolescents with arthritis. *Arthritis and Rheumatism, 59*(1), 65-72. doi:10.1002/art.23244/full

Tripp, D. A., VanDenKerkhof, E. G., & McAlister, M. (2006). Prevalence and determinants of pain and pain-related disability in urban and rural settings in southeastern Ontario. *Pain Research and Management, 11,* 225-233.

Vallerand, A. H., & Polomano, R. C. (2000). The relationship of gender to pain. *Pain Management Nursing, 1*(Suppl. 3), 8-15. doi:10.1053/jpmn.2000.9759

Watkins, K. W., Shifren, K., Park, D. C., & Morell, R. W. (1999). Age, pain and coping with rheumatoid arthritis. *Pain, 82,* 217-228. doi:10.1016/S0304-3959(99)00047-0

Watson, P. J., Main, C. J., & Smeets, R. J. E. M. (2010). Basics: Management and treatment of low back pain. In J. Mogil (Ed.), *Pain 2010—An updated review: Refresher course syllabus* (pp. 361-380). Seattle: IASP Press.

Watt-Watson, J. (1992). Misbeliefs about pain. In J. Watt-Watson & M. Donovan (Eds.), *Pain management: Nursing perspective* (pp. 36-58). St. Louis: Mosby.

Watt-Watson, J., Garfinkel, P., Gallop, R., Stevens, B., & Streiner, D. (2000). The impact of nurses' empathic responses on patients' pain management in acute care. *Nursing Research, 4,* 191-200. doi:10.1097/00006199-200007000-00002

Watt-Watson, J., McGillion, M., Hunter, J., Choiniere, M., Clark, A. J., Dewar, A., ..., Webber, K. (2009). A survey of prelicensure pain curricula in health science faculties in Canadian Universities. *Pain Research and Management, 14,* 439-444.

Watt-Watson, J., Stevens, B., Katz, J., Costello, J., Reid, D., & David, T. (2004). Impact of preoperative education on pain outcomes after coronary artery bypass graft surgery. *Pain, 109,* 73-85. doi:10.1016/j.pain.2004.01.012

Williams, D. A., & Thorn, B. E. (1989). An empirical assessment of pain beliefs. *Pain, 36,* 351-358. doi:10.1016/0304-3959(89) 90095-X

Wong, D. (2008). *Joint Commission on Accreditation of Healthcare Organizations (JCAHO). Pain standards: Implications for clinical practice.* Retrieved from *http://www.ncbi.nlm.nih.gov/pubmed/11706454*

Zimmerman, M., for the Committee for Research and Ethical Issues of the International Association for the Study of Pain. (1982). *Ethical guidelines for pain research in humans.* Retrieved from *http://www.iasp-pain.org/AM/Template.cfm?Section=General_ Resource_Links&Template=/CM/HTMLDisplay.cfm&ContentID= 3052#humans*

CANADIAN RESOURCES

Canadian Pain Coalition
http://www.canadianpaincoalition.ca
Canadian Pain Society position statement on pain relief
http://www.pulsus.com/journals/pdf_frameset.jsp?jnlKy=7&atlKy=610 4&isArt=t&jnlAdvert=Pain&adverifHCTp=_NP&sTitle=Canadia nPainSocietypositionstatementonpainrelief, Pulsus Group Inc&HCtype=Consumer
Canadian Guideline for Safe and Effective Use of Opioids for Non-Cancer Pain (NOUGG)
http://nationalpaincentre.mcmaster.ca/opioid/
McGill Pain Questionnaire
http://www.chcr.brown.edu/pcoc/MCGILLPAINQUEST.PDF
Registered Nurses' Association of Ontario Best Practice Guidelines: Assessment and Management of Pain
http://rnao.ca/bpg/guidelines/assessment-and-management-pain

RELATED RESOURCES

Agency for Healthcare Research and Quality
http://www.ahcpr.gov
American Pain Society
http://www.ampainsoc.org
City of Hope Pain & Palliative Care Resource Center
http://prc.coh.org/eol.asp
Core Curriculum for Professional Education in Pain
http://issuu.com/iasp/docs/core-corecurriculum?mode=embed&layout= http%3A%2F%2Fskin.issuu.com%2Fv%2Fdarkicons%2Flayout. xml&showFlipBtn=true
International Association for the Study of Pain
http://www.iasp-pain.org

evolve *For additional Internet resources, see the Web site for this book at* **http://evolve.elsevier.com/Canada/Lewis/medsurg**

Written by Patricia Graber O'Brien

Adapted by Rosanra Yoon

LEARNING OBJECTIVES

1. Gain a broad understanding of the prevalence of substance use in Canada.
2. Situate substance use within the continuum of use perspective.
3. Discuss the core aspects of a collaborative nursing therapeutic relationship in working with people experiencing substance use–related problems.
4. Describe the harm-reduction model.
5. Discuss screening and assessment of people experiencing substance use–related problems.
6. Identify common substances of abuse, their effects, and associated health consequences.
7. Discuss nursing interventions for smoking cessation, alcohol dependence, and opioid dependency.
8. Describe the nursing management of patients who experience intoxication, overdose, or withdrawal from stimulants, depressants, or hallucinogens.
9. Describe nursing management of the surgical patient with substance use.
10. Discuss the nursing management of pain in the patient who is substance dependent.
11. Describe the use of motivational interviewing to initiate behaviour change in patients with addictions.
12. Discuss substance use problems specific to the older adult.

KEY TERMS

addiction Problematic use of a substance resulting in negative personal and social consequences marked by increasing loss of control over use and compulsive use of the substance despite harms associated with use, p. 193

brain reward system A system involving the mesolimbic and mesocortical pathways; responsible for creating the sensation of pleasure for certain behaviours that reinforces behaviours associated with pleasure. p. 187

craving An intense desire for a particular substance, p. 188

cross-tolerance The development of resistance to one or more effects of a drug as a result of tolerance developed to a similar drug, p. 202

cue-induced craving Craving that occurs in the presence of people, places, or things previously associated with drug taking, p. 188

Korsakoff's syndrome A neurological condition that is caused by thiamine deficiency related to chronic consumption and/or malnutrition that is nonreversible and affects memory and cognition, p. 202

lapses Very short periods of substance use followed by quick return to maintaining nonuse, p. 210

motivational interviewing A collaborative person-centred, counselling approach that elicits behaviour change by working with the person to explore and resolve ambivalence, p. 210

opiates Natural and semisynthetic substances that have been derived from the opium poppy, such as opium, morphine, and codeine. p. 206

opioids Umbrella term that includes the opiates as well as many synthetic narcotic agents, p. 206

physical dependence Physiological adaptation to ongoing exposure to pharmacological agents such that use and cessation of use cause an expected physiological response, p. 211

psychological dependence Emotional and psychological reliance on a substance because of the pleasurable and reinforcing effects of the substance, p. 188

potentiation A drug interaction causing an accumulative response greater than the sum of the individual responses to each drug, p. 202

relapse Problematic substance use after a period of nonuse, p. 188

substance dependence A pattern of problematic substance use marked by an increase in frequency of use and compulsive use despite significant personal and social harms as well as the development of tolerance and withdrawal symptoms associated with the substance, p. 187

substance use Problematic use or misuse of substance(s) despite the associated negative personal and social consequences as a result of the substance(s), p. 186

tolerance The development of requiring increasing amounts of a substance to achieve the same effect, p. 188

transtheoretical model of change A framework of behaviour change that provides a contextual approach for clinicians working with people demonstrating differing stages of change that include precontemplation, contemplation, preparation, action, maintenance, lapse, and relapse, p. 210

Wernicke's encephalopathy An inflammatory, hemorrhagic, degenerative condition of the brain associated with long-term alcohol abuse, p. 202

withdrawal Constellation of physiological and psychological responses that occur when there is abrupt cessation or reduced intake of a substance on which an individual is dependent, p. 191

withdrawal management Interventions and processes aimed at addressing the physiological and psychological symptoms that occur in response to stopping a substance on which physiological and psychological dependence has developed, p. 202

ELECTRONIC RESOURCES

Supplemental content related to Chapter 11 can be found …

Evolve Web Site ⊖volve

http://evolve.elsevier.com/Canada/Lewis/medsurg
- Answer Guideline for Case Study on p. 212
- Clinical Reference: Laboratory Values
- Content Updates
- Customizable Nursing Care Plan: Alcohol Withdrawal
- Electronic Calculators

- eTables:
  - eTable 11-1: RNAO Practice Recommendations for Smoking Cessation Interventions: The "Ask, Advise, Assist, Arrange" Protocol
  - eTable 11-2: Patient & Caregiver Teaching Guide: Smoking and Tobacco Use Cessation
- Examination Review Questions
- Glossary
- Key Points (Printable and MP3 Download)

Substance Use in Canada

Substance use and abuse affect a broad spectrum of Canadians, regardless of age, gender, socioeconomic class, educational levels, cultural backgrounds, or geographic region. As such, it is important for nurses to routinely assess for substance use with every individual in all practice settings and to determine whether the pattern of use is problematic. **Substance use** may be defined as the problematic use or misuse of substance(s) despite the associated negative personal and social consequences.

According to the Canadian Alcohol and Drug Use Monitoring Survey in 2010 (Health Canada, 2011a), 77% of Canadians age 15 years and older reported past-year consumption of alcohol; 10.7% reported cannabis use; 11% reported use of either cocaine, cannabis, speed, Ecstasy, or hallucinogens; and 26% reported having taken a psychoactive pharmaceutical medication (Table 11-1). The results of the 2010 Canadian Tobacco Use Monitoring Survey (CTUMS) (Health Canada, 2011b) indicate 4.7 million Canadians aged 15 years and older are current smokers, of which 13% reported smoking an average of 15.1 cigarettes per day. Nurses have a key role in screening, assessing, and promoting healthy choices regarding the use of substances as well as screening and assessing for problematic use.

Furthermore, the costs related to substance use–related problems in Canada across sectors, including health care, corrections, and law enforcement, in addition to lost productivity, was estimated to exceed $39.8 billion annually (Rehm et al., 2006). However, the economic costs associated with substance use are overshadowed by the significant personal and social costs to Canadians and their families experiencing substance use that are manifested as poor physical and mental health, stress, relationship strain, and increased morbidity and mortality related to substance use.

Substance Use From a Continuum of Use Perspective

People with substance use problems have often been categorized, especially among health care providers, into those whose use is classified as substance use and those whose use is classified as substance dependence. Increasingly, it has become apparent that situating substance use on a continuum of use allows for a broader understanding of a wider range of substance use across populations (Figure 11-1) (Herie & Skinner, 2010). This perspective captures substance use across a spectrum of use that ranges from nonuse to substance dependence. This allows for health risks and associated harms related to differing levels of use to be routinely screened and assessed, regardless of where along the spectrum a person is situated. A good example is the case of the person who has had a one-time high-risk use of heroin resulting in a near overdose. A one-time accidental overdose does not necessarily warrant a classification of substance dependence.

Table 11-1 Highlights From the Canadian Alcohol and Drug Use Monitoring Survey (CADUMS) 2010

Alcohol

- 77% of Canadians reported drinking alcohol in the past year.
- 80.2% of men and 73.9% of women reported alcohol use in the past year.
- Heavy frequent drinking among youth age 15-24 years of age was approximately three times higher (9.4%) than for adults (3.3%).
- Average age of first alcohol consumption was 15.9 years.
- 14.6% of Canadians reported experiencing at least one harm in the course of their life as result of alcohol consumption.

Cannabis

- The prevalence of past-year use of cannabis reported by youth was 25.1%, three times higher than the rate reported by adults (7.9%).
- The rate of cannabis use among males (14.6%) was double that of cannabis use among women (7.1%).
- The average age of initiation of cannabis use among youth was 15.7 years.

Other Drug Use

- Among Canadians 15 years and older, the prevalence of past-year cocaine or crack use decreased from 1.9% in 2004 to 1.2% in 2010, whereas past-year use of hallucinogens (0.9%), Ecstasy (0.7%), and speed (0.5%) is comparable with the rates of use reported in 2004.
- Among youth aged 15 to 24 years, past-year use of at least one of five illicit drugs (cocaine or crack, speed, hallucinogens, Ecstasy, and heroin) decreased from 11.3% in 2004 to 7.0% in 2010.
- The rate of drug use by youth 15-24 years of age remains much higher than that reported by adults 25 years and older: nine times higher for past-year use of any drug excluding cannabis (7.9% vs. 0.8%).
- The rates of psychoactive pharmaceutical use and abuse remain comparable with the rates reported in 2009: 26.0% of respondents age 15 years and older indicated that they had used an opioid pain reliever, a stimulant, or a sedative or tranquilizer in the past year and 0.3% reported that they used any of these drugs to get high in the past year.

Source: Health Canada. (2011a). *Canadian Alcohol and Drug Use Monitoring Survey: Summary of results for 2010.* Retrieved from *http://www.hc-sc.gc.ca/hc-ps/drugs-drogues/stat/_2010/summary-sommaire-eng.php*

Important assessment parameters include pattern, frequency of use, adverse personal and social outcomes, and continued compulsive use despite harms (Gitlow, 2007; Kahan & Wilson, 2002). Skill and knowledge regarding the intervention and management of overdoses, intoxication, and withdrawal from substances of abuse are vital aspects of nursing practice.

Neurophysiology of Substances of Abuse

Substances of abuse are psychoactive in nature, meaning they affect key areas of the brain involved in pleasure and reinforcement. Caffeine is one example of a substance of abuse. Caffeine is a stimulant with reinforcing psychoactive qualities that result in mental alertness and enhanced mood. If taken regularly over a period of time, abrupt cessation of caffeine can lead to mild withdrawal symptoms. Substances with a higher index of abuse engage the reward pleasure system of the brain more intensely and quickly. These include substances such as cocaine or nicotine that require very little time to engage the brain reward pathways. Substances with higher risk for dependency are those that possess fast onset and intense psychoactive characteristics (Reiss, Fiellin, Miller, & Scutz, 2009).

Substances of abuse increase the availability of dopamine in the "pleasure" area of the mesolimbic system of the brain. This mechanism has been identified as the **brain reward system,** creating the sensation of pleasure for certain behaviours that include necessary behaviours required for survival of the human species, such as eating and sex (Shuckit, 2006).

Normally, dopamine is released at a slow rate by neurons in the mesolimbic system, producing normal affect or mood. Both endogenous and exogenous opiates have been found to increase the firing rate of dopaminergic neurons. Cocaine has been shown to decrease the reuptake of dopamine at the synapse, thereby decreasing its breakdown and increasing the amount of available dopamine. Nicotine, alcohol, marijuana, amphetamines, and caffeine also increase dopaminergic neuron activity at the synapse. The resulting increase in mesolimbic dopamine produces mood elevation and euphoria, factors that provide strong motivation to repeat the experience. Substances of abuse also increase the availability of other neurotransmitters, such as serotonin and γ-aminobutyric acid (GABA), but dopamine's effect on the reward system appears to be pivotal to the process of substance use and dependency.

Substance dependence results from the prolonged effects of psychoactive substances on the brain. Repeated use of substances of abuse changes the neural circuitry involving the dopamine neurotransmitter system and reduces the responsiveness of

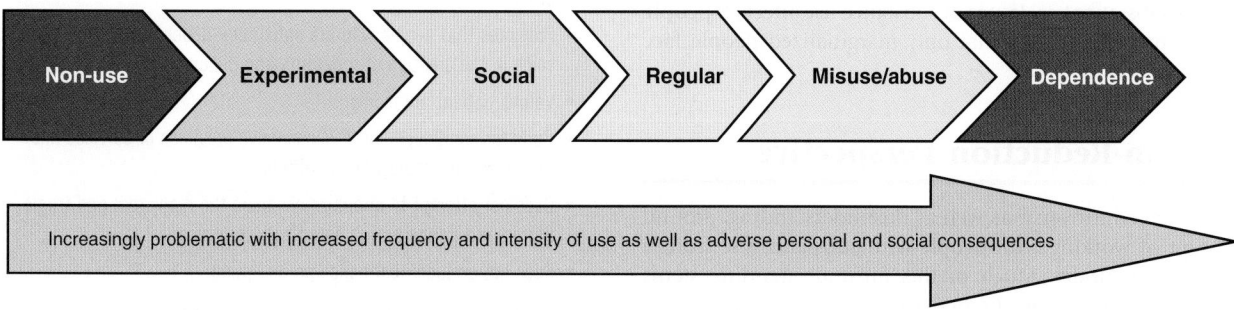

Figure 11-1 Continuum of use for substance use.

Source: Herie, M., & Skinner, W. (2010). *Substance abuse in Canada* (p. 20: Figure 1-2, Risk continuum and continuum of substance use). Toronto: Oxford University Press.

dopamine receptors. This decreased responsiveness leads to **tolerance,** the need for a larger dose of a drug to obtain the original euphoria, and also reduces the sense of pleasure from experiences that previously resulted in positive feelings. Without the substance, the individual experiences depression, anxiety, and irritability. To feel even normal, the individual must take the substance.

Furthermore, a key aspect of substances of abuse is the formation of the memory of the pleasurable experience of the substance that is long-lasting even in periods of nonuse. Drug **craving,** the intense desire for a substance, usually experienced after decreased use or abstinence, is the result of the memory aspect related to the brain reward pathway. An important type of craving experienced by people who have experienced problematic substance use or dependency is the experience of **cue-induced craving** that occurs in the presence of people, places, or things that they have previously associated with taking the substance. Cue-induced craving may occur after long periods of abstinence and is a common cause of **relapse,** or returning to substance use after a period of abstinence.

Stigma, Prejudice, and Attitudes Toward People Experiencing Substance-Related Problems

People with substance use–related problems face significant stigma and prejudice largely perpetuated by pejorative images of substance use in media and society at large. Misinformation and misunderstanding regarding the biopsychosocial aspects of substance use and associated health complications are key factors contributing to the generally accepted perspective that substance use and dependency are a matter of personal choice. Substance use is, however, intimately linked to the effects of substances on the neurophysiology of the brain reward system. Substance use is a complex condition that involves the whole person. Underlying mental health needs and physiological and **psychological dependence** with serious health complications are factors that require supportive intervention.

Positive engagement with health care providers that is nonjudgemental, collaborative, and transparent in nature is fundamental in engaging people to talk about the role and impact of substance use on their life and health. A positive interaction and dialogue about substance use with a health care provider significantly improve health outcomes and increase the likelihood that the person will engage in reducing the harms associated with substance use. Nurses are essential in engaging people in a collaborative and nonjudgemental manner about substance use. This requires nurses to reflect upon their own views and understanding of substance use. Issues of substance use affect all people despite the prevailing myth that only marginalized people face problems of substance use.

The Harm-Reduction Perspective

There is much controversy, as well as misunderstanding, around the concept of working with people with substance use from a harm-reduction model. Much of this misunderstanding stems from the focus of discussions being based on the question of "allowing the person to use the substance" versus abstinence, which misses the point of harm reduction all together. Harm reduction focuses on reducing the harms associated with use across the continuum of use, which includes high-risk use to abstinence. The harms targeted for reduction include the very real personal, social, and physical harms related to use of a substance from a public health perspective (Canadian Nurses Association [CNA], 2011). Examples of harm reduction across the continuum of use include interventions such as laws against drinking and driving and nonsmoking bylaws that protect people from the associated harms related to alcohol and smoking that are inclusive of all people, as well as evidence-informed interventions such as needle exchange programs and safer sex education that reduce the harms associated with high-risk substance use without demanding that the person stop use.

Harm reduction is based on a collaborative approach in working with people with substance use whereby patients have autonomy and choice in accessing treatment and services that promote wellness and recovery. Foundational to harm reduction is respect for patient autonomy, a nonjudgemental empathetic approach that honours the patient's inherent dignity and ability to make informed decisions (Bierness, Jesseman, Notarandrea, & Perron, 2008). Table 11-2 lists the principles of harm reduction. Nurses have a key responsibility to provide accurate and timely health information to support patient autonomy in making healthy choices and avoiding risks associated with substance use.

Health Complications of Substance Use

Health complications and harms related to substances of abuse are related to three general factors: the substance, the route, and related high-risk behaviours. First, the inherent properties of the substance itself will have specific physiological harms associated with its use such as liver damage related to alcohol use and emphysema related to smoking. Second, the route by which the substance is taken will pose specific harms. Harms associated with oral consumption are different in nature from those associated with inhalation or intravenous use. Third, high-risk sexual behaviours, exposure to violence and trauma, and placing one's personal safety at risk may occur during substance use (Table 11-3).

Table 11-2 Principles of Harm Reduction
Harm Reduction
• Is a public health alternative to the moral/criminal and disease models of drug use
• Accepts that at any given time some people are not ready to choose abstinence
• Promotes low-threshold access to services as an alternative to traditional, high-threshold approaches
• Accepts that substance use occurs and works to minimize its harmful effects
• Promotes that people who are substance-dependent should have a voice in the creation of programs and policies designed to serve them
• Values patient autonomy
• Calls for nonjudgemental, noncoercive provision of services and resources for people who use drugs
• Does not attempt to minimize or ignore the many real and tragic harms and dangers associated with drug use
• Does not exclude abstinence as an option

Source: Adapted from Harm Reduction Coalition. (n.d.). *Principles of harm reduction.* Retrieved from *http://harmreduction.org/about-us/principles-of-harm-reduction/*; and Marlatt, G. A. (1996). Harm reduction: Come as you are. *Addictive Behaviours, 21,* 779-788. doi:10.1016/0306-4603(96)00042-1

Table 11-3 Common Health Problems Related to Substance Use

SUBSTANCE	HEALTH PROBLEMS*	SUBSTANCE	HEALTH PROBLEMS*
Nicotine and smoking	COPD	Opioids	Sexual dysfunction
	Cancers of lung, mouth, larynx, esophagus, stomach, pancreas, bladder, prostate, cervix		Gastric ulcers
			Glomerulonephritis
	Coronary artery disease, peripheral artery disease		Opioid-induced constipation
	Peptic ulcer disease, GERD	Cannabis	Bronchitis, chronic sinusitis
Cocaine	Nasal sores, septal necrosis or perforation		Memory impairment
	Chronic sinusitis		Impaired immune function
	"Crack lung" pneumonia		Reproductive dysfunction
	Cardiac dysrhythmias, myocardial ischemia and infarction		Psychosis
	Stroke	**High-Risk Behaviours**	**Health Problems**
	Psychosis	Intravenous Use	Blood clots, phlebitis, skin infections
Amphetamines	Cardiac dysrhythmias, myocardial ischemia and infarction		Hepatitis B and C
			HIV/AIDS
	Death of brain cells		Other infections: endocarditis, tuberculosis, pneumonia, meningitis, tetanus, bone and joint infections, lung abscesses
	Syndrome of uncontrollable tremors		
Caffeine	Gastrointestinal irritation, peptic ulcer disease, GERD		
	Anxiety, sleep disruption	Snorting drugs	Nasal sores, septal necrosis or perforation
	Elevated blood pressure		Chronic sinusitis
Alcohol	Gastritis, peptic ulcer disease	Risky sexual behaviour	HIV/AIDS
	Esophageal varices		Hepatitis B and C
	Cirrhosis of the liver, pancreatitis		Other sexually transmitted infections
	Cancers of esophagus, stomach, head and neck, lung	Personal	Malnutrition, impaired immunity
	Dementias		Accidental injuries and soft tissue trauma
	Decreased bone density		Head injuries
	Hypertension		Falls
	Thiamine deficiency		Victims of violence
Sedative– hypnotics	Memory impairment		Driving or operating heavy machinery under the influence of substances
	Respiratory depression		
	Risk for falls and fractures		

COPD, chronic obstructive pulmonary disease; GERD, gastroesophageal reflux disease; HIV/AIDS, human immunodeficiency virus–acquired immunodeficiency syndrome.

*Throughout the text, the health problems related to substance use are discussed in the appropriate chapters where substance use–related behaviours are identified as risk factors for these problems.

Sources: Dodgen, C. E., & Shea, W. M. (2000). *Substance abuse disorders: Assessment and treatment.* San Diego: Academic; and Shuckit, M. A. (2006). *Drug and alcohol abuse: A clinical guide to diagnosis and treatment* (6th ed.). New York: Springer Science and Business Media.

NURSING MANAGEMENT: ACUTE INTERVENTION FOR ADDICTIVE BEHAVIOURS

Nursing Implementation

Acute Intervention

Acute care situations precipitated by substance use involve acute intoxication, overdose, or withdrawal (Table 11-4). Intoxication responses usually last less than 24 hours and are directly related to the ingestion of psychoactive drugs. Intoxication effects are generally dose related, and symptoms often include the desired effects of using the drug. Overdose leads to toxic reactions that may include respiratory and circulatory arrest and other life-threatening complications. Overdose occurs with the ingestion of an excessive dose of one drug or when a combination of similarly acting drugs is used. The nurse should be aware that intoxication and overdose may occur in a hospitalized patient dependent on substances if visitors provide substances. Table 11-5 provides a timeline of commonly abused substances and routes to assist in anticipating intoxication, overdose, and withdrawal manifestations.

Overdose. A drug overdose is an emergency situation, and management is based on the type of substance involved. Drug overdose can be accidental or intentional. If multiple substances have been ingested, a complex and potentially confusing clinical picture can result. The first priority of care in overdose is always the patient's ABCs (airway, breathing, and circulation). Continuous monitoring of neurological status, including level of consciousness and respiratory and cardiovascular function, is critical until the patient is stable. Vital signs and intake and output should

Table 11-4 Effects of Frequently Used Substances

SUBSTANCE	PHYSIOLOGICAL AND PSYCHOLOGICAL EFFECTS	EFFECTS OF OVERDOSE	WITHDRAWAL SYMPTOMS
Stimulants			
Nicotine	Increased arousal and alertness; performance enhancement; increased heart rate, cardiac output, and blood pressure; cutaneous vasoconstriction; fine tremor, decreased appetite; antidiuretic effect; increased gastric motility	Rare: Nausea, abdominal pain, diarrhea, vomiting, dizziness, weakness, confusion, decreased respirations, seizures, death from respiratory failure	Craving, restlessness, depression, hyperirritability, headache, insomnia, decreased blood pressure and heart rate, increased appetite
Cocaine Amphetamines: amphetamine, dextroamphetamine (Dexedrine), methamphetamine, crystal methamphetamine (crystal meth), methylenedioxy-methamphetamine (MDMA, Ecstasy), methylphenidate (Ritalin), phenmetrazine (Preludin)	Euphoria, grandiosity, mood swings, hyperactivity, hyperalertness, restlessness, anorexia, insomnia, hypertension, tachycardia, marked vasoconstriction, tremor, dysrhythmias, seizures, dilated pupils, diaphoresis	Agitation; increased temperature, heart rate, respiratory rate, blood pressure; cardiac dysrhythmias, myocardial infarction, hallucinations, seizures, possible death	Severe craving, severely depressed mood, exhaustion, prolonged sleep, apathy, irritability, disorientation
Caffeine	Mood elevation, increased alertness, nervousness, jitteriness, irritability, insomnia; increased respirations, heart rate, and force of myocardial contraction; relaxation of smooth muscle, diuresis	Rare: Hyperstimulation, nervousness, confusion, psychomotor agitation, anxiety, dizziness, tinnitus, muscle twitching, elevated blood pressure, tachycardia, extrasystoles, increased respiratory rate	Headache, irritability, drowsiness, fatigue
Depressants			
Alcohol Sedative–hypnotics • Barbiturates: phenobarbital (Phenobarb), pentobarbital amobarbital (Amytal) • Benzodiazepines: diazepam (Valium), chlordiazepoxide (Librax), alprazolam (Xanax) • Nonbarbiturates–nonbenzodiazepines: methaqualone (Quaalude), chloral hydrate (Noctec)	Initial relaxation, emotional lability, decreased inhibitions, drowsiness, lack of coordination, impaired judgement, slurred speech, hypotension, bradycardia, bradypnea	Shallow respirations; cold, clammy skin; weak, rapid pulse; hyporeflexia, coma, possible death	Anxiety, agitation, insomnia, diaphoresis, tremors, delirium, seizures, possible death
Opioids			
Heroin Morphine Opium Codeine Fentanyl (Duragesic) Meperidine (Demerol) Hydromorphone (Dilaudid) Pentazocine (Talwin) Oxycodone hydrochloride (OxyNEO) Oxycodone (Percocet) Methadone	Analgesia, euphoria, drowsiness, detachment from environment, relaxation, constricted pupils, constipation, nausea, decreased respiratory rate, slurred speech, impaired judgement, decreased sexual and aggressive drives	Slow, shallow respirations; clammy skin; constricted pupils; coma; possible death	Watery eyes, dilated pupils, runny nose, yawning, tremors, pain, chills, fever, diaphoresis, nausea, vomiting, diarrhea, abdominal cramps

Table 11-4 Effects of Frequently Used Substances—cont'd

SUBSTANCE	PHYSIOLOGICAL AND PSYCHOLOGICAL EFFECTS	EFFECTS OF OVERDOSE	WITHDRAWAL SYMPTOMS
Cannabis			
Marijuana Hashish	Relaxation, euphoria, lack of motivation, slowed time sensation, abrupt mood changes, impaired memory and attention, impaired judgement, reddened eyes, dry mouth, lack of coordination, decreased reflexes, tachycardia, increased appetite	Fatigue, paranoia, panic reactions, hallucinogen-like psychotic states	None except for rare insomnia, hyperactivity
Hallucinogens			
Lysergic acid diethylamide (LSD) Psilocybin (mushrooms) Dimethyltryptamine (DMT) Diethyltryptamine (DET) 3,4 Methylenedioxyamphetamine (MDA) Methylenedioxymethamphetamine (MDMA, Ecstasy) Mescaline (peyote) Phencyclidine (PCP)	Perceptual distortions, hallucinations, delusions (PCP), depersonalization, heightened sensory perception, euphoria, mood swings, suspiciousness, panic, impaired judgement, increased body temperature, hypertension, flushed face, tremor, dilated pupils, constricted pupils (PCP), nystagmus (PCP), violence (PCP)	Prolonged effects and episodes, anxiety, panic, confusion, blurred vision, increases in blood pressure and temperature. Seizures, coma, death (PCP), skeletal muscle contraction, dehydration, paranoia, psychosis	None
Inhalants			
Aerosol propellants Fluorinated hydrocarbons Nitrous oxide (in deodorants, hair spray, pesticide, whipped cream spray, spray paint, cookware coating products) Solvents (gasoline, kerosene, nail polish remover, typewriter correction fluid, cleaning solutions, lighter fluid, paint, paint thinner, glue) Anaesthetic agents (nitrous oxide, chloroform) Nitrites (amyl nitrite, butyl nitrite)	Euphoria, decreased inhibitions, giddiness, slurred speech, illusions, drowsiness, clouded sensorium, tinnitis, nystagmus, dysrhythmias, cough, nausea, vomiting, diarrhea; irritation to eyes, nose, mouth	Anxiety, respiratory depression, cardiac dysrhythmias, loss of consciousness, sudden death, suicide	None

be monitored. Emergency management of overdose and toxicity of central nervous system (CNS) stimulants and CNS depressants is presented later in the chapter in Tables 11-7 and 11-11.

Pharmacological agents are administered as ordered to counteract toxic effects of drugs. Naloxone and flumazenil may be administered when a depressant effect is present but the ingested drug is unknown. Naloxone rapidly reverses the effects of opioids, and flumazenil reverses the effects of benzodiazepine overdose. The effects of these antagonists necessitate frequent monitoring because these drugs have a short half-life and may need to be readministered after the initial reversal of toxic effects. Specific antagonists are not available for other drugs of abuse, but a variety of other medications may be used to control symptoms.

The patient who has overdosed on sedative–hypnotics other than benzodiazepines must be treated aggressively and may require dialysis to decrease the drug level and to prevent irreversible CNS-depressant effects and death. Gastric lavage and administration of activated charcoal may be instituted if the drug was taken orally within 4 to 6 hours. CNS stimulants are not used in the treatment of depressant-drug overdose.

As soon as the patient is stable, a thorough history and physical examination must be completed. When the patient is unwilling or unable to give a history, a collateral history should be obtained from the patient's significant others. Recent drug and alcohol use, including the type, amount, and time of use, and the presence of any chronic illnesses, are important in the continuing treatment of the patient. A patient who intentionally overdosed should not be allowed to return home until seen by a psychiatric professional.

Withdrawal. In general, **withdrawal** signs and symptoms are opposite in nature from the direct effects of the drug (see Table 11-4). Because abused substances are psychoactive, changes are consistently noted in the neurological system. These changes often manifest as acute anxiety and protracted depression. Withdrawal from CNS depressants, including alcohol, benzodiazepines, and barbiturates, can be dangerous and may be life threatening. The nurse must be alert to the possibility of withdrawal in any patient who has a history of substance use. The nurse should also suspect substance dependence in patients who

Table 11-5 Onset, Peak, Duration, and Withdrawal Onset of Abused Substances

SUBSTANCE AND ROUTE	ONSET	PEAK	DURATION	ONSET OF WITHDRAWAL SYMPTOMS
Inhaled				
Nicotine	Immediate	5 min	5-15 min	3-4 hr
Marijuana	5-20 min	30-60 min	3-7 hr	—
Cocaine	Immediate	5-30 min	60 min	9 hr
Inhalants	Immediate	10-15 min	20-45 min	—
Intravenous				
Cocaine	Immediate	10-20 min	20-30 min	2 hr
Opioids	Immediate	60-90 min	2-4 hr	8-10 hr
Amphetamines	Immediate	10-20 min	20-30 min	2 hr
Oral				
Alcohol	15-20 min	60-90 min	12-14 hr	6-12 hr
Amphetamines	10-30 min	60-90 min	2-4 hr	8-10 hr
Sedative–hypnotics	15-30 min	2-4 hr	4-12 hr	12-16 hr
Caffeine	10-20 min	30 min	3-7 hr	12-24 hr
Opioids	30 min	2 hr	4-8 hr	8-10 hr
Intranasal				
Cocaine	3-5 min	5-30 min	2-4 hr	4 hr
Amphetamines	3-5 min	5-20 min	45 min	2 hr
Buccal				
Nicotine	10-15 min	20-30 min	30-60 min	1-2 hr

discharge themselves against medical advice. This may occur when patients are not being treated appropriately and need the substance to prevent withdrawal symptoms. In withdrawal from all abused substances, nursing management includes monitoring physiological function, ensuring safety and comfort, preventing the progression of symptoms, providing reassurance and orientation, and motivating the patient to engage in long-term treatment (Department of Health, England, 2007).

◼ **Perioperative Care.** An individual who abuses substances is more likely to have accidents and injuries that necessitate surgery. All trauma victims must be carefully assessed for signs and symptoms of substance overdose and withdrawal that could lead to adverse drug interactions with analgesics or anaesthetics. During elective surgery in both inpatient and outpatient surgical settings, the patient dependent on substances is at high risk for postoperative complications and death. Preoperative assessment must include a thorough health history and assessment of substance use, including questions related to nicotine and caffeine use. Respiratory changes in smokers make introduction of endotracheal and suction tubes more difficult and increase the risk for postoperative respiratory problems. Postoperative headaches may be caused by caffeine withdrawal in heavy users. During the patient's surgical recovery period, the nurse should be alert for signs and symptoms of drug interactions with pain medications or anaesthesia or for signs of withdrawal. Special nursing considerations for the substance-abusing patient undergoing surgery are presented in Table 11-6.

Special precautions must be taken for the patient who is intoxicated or alcohol dependent and requires surgery. Alcohol use may be overlooked in an accident victim if there are injuries

Table 11-6 Considerations for Patients With Problematic Substance Use Who Are Undergoing Surgery

- Standard amounts of anaesthetic and analgesic drugs may not be sufficient if patient is cross-tolerant.
- Increased doses of pain medications may be required if patient is cross-tolerant.
- Anaesthetic agents may have a prolonged sedative effect if the patient has liver dysfunction. This situation necessitates an extended observation period.
- Patients have an increased susceptibility to cardiac and respiratory depression.
- Patients have an increased risk for bleeding, postoperative complications, and infection.
- Withdrawal symptoms from substances may be delayed for up to 5 days because of effects of anaesthetics and pain medications.
- Dosage of pain medications must be reduced gradually.

that cause CNS depression, and many people are undiagnosed as alcoholics at the time of admission for elective surgery. Optimally, health problems such as malnutrition, dehydration, and infection should be treated before surgery is performed. The patient who is alcohol dependent but is not currently drinking usually requires an increased level of anaesthesia because of cross-tolerance. The intoxicated individual needs a decreased level of anaesthesia because of the synergistic effect of the alcohol.

Whenever possible, surgery is postponed in intoxicated individuals until the blood alcohol content (BAC) is less than

43 mmol/L (0.2 mg %). Synergistic effects occur with anaesthesia when the BAC is over 33 mmol/L (0.15 mg %), and a patient with a BAC over 54 mmol/L (0.25 mg %) has a significantly increased surgical risk and risk of death. Acute withdrawal and delirium tremens (DTs) may be triggered by surgery and the cessation of alcohol consumption. Surgery should be delayed for at least 48 to 72 hours, if possible, or intravenous (IV) alcohol may be given to prevent withdrawal if immediate surgery is required. Alcohol interferes with pulmonary function, decreased liver function affects metabolism of many drugs, and the medical problems associated with alcohol use may affect the outcome of surgery. Vital signs, including body temperature, must be closely monitored to identify signs of withdrawal, possible infections, and respiratory or cardiac problems. Anaesthetics and pain medications used in the acute period can delay withdrawal symptoms for up to 5 days postoperatively (Carroll, Angst, & Clark, 2004).

■ **Acute Pain Management Considerations.** Care providers may demonstrate reluctance to treat acute pain with opioid medications in people with substance use problems. However, it must be noted that the effective treatment of acute pain is a key priority for all people, and the use of opioid analgesia for acute pain for people with substance use issues is appropriate.

If the patient acknowledges opioid use, it is important to determine the types and the amounts of drugs used. It is best to avoid exposing the patient to the drug of abuse, and effective equianalgesic doses of other opioids may be determined if daily drug doses are known. Withdrawal symptoms can exacerbate pain and lead to medication-seeking behaviour. Toxicology screens may be helpful in determining recently used substances. Discussing these findings with the patient is essential.

Severe pain should be treated with opioids, and at much higher doses than those used with drug-naive patients. The use of one opioid is preferred. A mixed opioid agonist–antagonist such as butorphanol or a partial agonist such as buprenorphine should be avoided because these may precipitate withdrawal symptoms. Nonopioid and adjuvant analgesics and nonpharmacological pain relief measures may also be used as appropriate. To maintain opioid blood levels and prevent withdrawal symptoms, analgesics should be provided around the clock. Supplemental doses should be used to treat breakthrough pain. Although controversial for treating people with substance use problems, patient-controlled analgesia (PCA) may improve pain and provide more effective control (Alford, Compton, & Samet, 2006).

A written agreement or treatment plan that describes the pain management should be developed with the patient. The plan should ensure that pain will be treated based on the patient's perception and report of pain, but also clearly outline the gradual tapering of the analgesic dose, eventual substitution of parenteral analgesics with long-acting oral preparations, and possibly cessation of opioids by the time of discharge (Alford et al., 2006).

Stimulants and Stimulant Withdrawal

Substances in this category of agents stimulate the CNS and generally cause increased alertness, increased heart rate, and a sense of euphoria.

Withdrawal from cocaine and amphetamines does not usually cause obvious physical symptoms, but physical and behavioural manifestations do occur. Craving for the drug is intense during the first hours to days of drug cessation and may continue for weeks. It is unusual for an individual dependent on stimulants to be hospitalized for management of withdrawal symptoms. However, the nurse may identify withdrawal symptoms in a patient dependent on cocaine or amphetamines who is hospitalized for management of other health problems. Nursing management of withdrawal symptoms is supportive and includes measures to decrease agitation and restlessness in the early phase and allowing the patient to sleep and eat as needed in later phases. Mild symptoms of stimulant withdrawal can also be experienced by the patient dependent on caffeine when meals and fluids are withheld before diagnostic testing or during a surgical experience. Withdrawal symptoms are also experienced by patients dependent on nicotine when smoking restrictions are applied. A nicotine replacement system should be provided for tobacco users to control symptoms of withdrawal when they are hospitalized.

Nicotine

Characteristics

Tobacco use is the leading cause of preventable premature death, disease, and disability in Canada and is responsible for the loss of one third of potential years of life because of tobacco-related cancer, one quarter of years of potential life lost to cardiovascular disease, and one half of potential years of life lost to respiratory diseases (Registered Nurses' Association of Ontario [RNAO], 2007). Nicotine is a psychoactive substance present in the tobacco plant and is the alkaloid that causes dependence. Its rapid onset of action makes it one of the most rapidly addicting of substances of abuse. It is estimated that 4.7 million Canadians aged 15 years and older are current smokers (Health Canada, 2010b). Considering the magnitude and severity of the risks associated with nicotine dependence, it is crucial that nurses screen and provide interventions for nicotine dependence.

Physiological Effects of Use

Nicotine is primarily responsible for a person's **addiction** to tobacco products, including cigarettes. During smoking, nicotine is absorbed quickly into the bloodstream and travels to the brain in a matter of seconds. Nicotine causes addiction to cigarettes and other tobacco products that is similar to the addiction produced by using heroin and cocaine (Health Canada, 2009).

When nicotine is absorbed, it produces a wide range of effects in the peripheral nervous system and CNS through action at nicotinic receptors. Responses include increased blood pressure, heart rate, cardiac output, coronary blood flow, and cutaneous vasoconstriction. These effects result in stimulation of the cardiovascular system and increased myocardial oxygen consumption. In the brain, the action of nicotine on nicotinic receptors causes general CNS stimulation with increased alertness and arousal. In the gastrointestinal (GI) tract, stimulation of nicotinic receptors increases GI motility and secretion. Through both peripheral nervous system and CNS effects, nicotine also causes changes in the endocrine system, including release of prolactin, growth hormone, vasopressin, endorphins, and adrenocorticotropic hormone with a subsequent increase in cortisol (Shuckit, 2006).

Although people with nicotine dependence report that nicotine use causes a depressant effect with relaxation and relief of anxiety, it is thought that these effects actually occur when periodic nicotine withdrawal is relieved by further nicotine. The effects of nicotine are listed in Table 11-4.

The strong psychological dependence associated with nicotine use is supported by the fact that it rapidly acts on the pleasure-producing mesolimbic area of the brain. Physiological dependence occurs with regular heavy use and is evidenced by increased tolerance and withdrawal symptoms following attempts to stop smoking. Withdrawal symptoms may occur within the first few hours after stopping, peak in 24 to 48 hours, and last from a few weeks to several months. Symptoms include craving, restlessness, and hyperirritability (O'Hara & Patel, 2006). Additional symptoms of withdrawal are presented in Table 11-6. After withdrawal subsides, cue-induced craving may cause smoking relapse.

Health Complications

The complications of nicotine abuse are related to the dose and the method of ingestion. Cigarette smoking is the single most preventable cause of death. Cigarette smoking also causes chronic lung disease, cardiovascular disease, stroke, and cataracts. Smoking during pregnancy can cause stillbirth, low birth weight, sudden infant death syndrome (SIDS), and other serious pregnancy complications (Health Canada, 2007a). Cigarette smoke contains more than 4000 chemical agents, including over 60 carcinogens (Canadian Lung Association, 2012). In addition, many of these substances, such as carbon monoxide, tar, arsenic, and lead, are poisonous and toxic to the human body.

The chronic respiratory irritation caused by cigarette smoke is the most important risk factor in the development of lung cancer and chronic obstructive pulmonary disease (COPD). The toxic gases inhaled in cigarette smoke constrict the bronchi, paralyze the cilia, thicken the mucus-secreting membranes, dilate the distal airways, and destroy the alveolar walls. Tar in cigarette smoke contains several hundred chemicals, most of which are carcinogenic.

Chronic irritation from smoking also is a factor in the increased incidence of cancer of the mouth, larynx, and esophagus in those who smoke tobacco in any form. Carcinogens absorbed into the blood from tobacco smoke may be responsible for the increased incidence in smokers of cancers of the bladder, prostate, and pancreas.

Together with the increased myocardial oxygen consumption that nicotine causes, carbon monoxide significantly decreases the oxygen available to the myocardium. The result is an even greater increase in heart rate and myocardial oxygen consumption that may lead to myocardial ischemia.

Passive, or involuntary, smoking occurs when nonsmokers are exposed to cigarette smoke, often in the presence of poor ventilation. Smoking in public places is increasingly being banned across Canada. Children whose parents smoke have a higher prevalence of respiratory symptoms and respiratory disease. Provinces such as British Columbia, Nova Scotia, and Ontario have passed legislation banning adults from smoking in closed environments such as cars when children are present, with other provinces soon to follow suit (Canadian Lung Association, 2008b). In adults, involuntary, or second-hand, smoking is associated with decreased pulmonary function, increased risk for lung cancer, and increased mortality rates from coronary artery disease (Shuckit, 2006).

Women are at greater risk than men for smoking-related diseases (Canadian Lung Association, 2008a). Women who smoke have almost double the risk of myocardial infarction than men and may also have nearly double the risk of lung cancer as men. Smoking in women is associated with greater menstrual bleeding and duration of dysmenorrhea as well as greater variability in menstrual cycle length. In addition, there is strong evidence that breast and cervical cancer risks are increased among women who smoke (World Health Organization [WHO], 2008).

Although those who use smokeless tobacco (snuff, plug, and leaf) have less risk of lung disease than smokers, the use of smokeless tobacco is not without complications. Holding tobacco in the mouth increases the risk of cancer of the mouth, cheek, tongue, and gingiva nearly fifty-fold (WHO, 2008). Smokeless tobacco users also experience the wide systemic effects of nicotine.

All users of nicotine in any form may develop complications that are directly related to the effects of nicotine itself. Such complications may include an increased risk for peripheral arterial disease, delayed wound healing, reproductive disorders, peptic ulcer disease, and gastroesophageal reflux disease (GERD) (Canadian Lung Association, 2008a). Common health problems associated with tobacco use are presented in Table 11-3.

Collaborative Care: Nursing Interventions for Nicotine Dependence

A combination of medications, behavioural approaches, and support is believed to be most effective in addressing nicotine dependence and long-term tobacco cessation. Nurses have a pivotal role in engaging patients about smoking.

Prevention of Tobacco Use. Prevention of tobacco use in children and adolescents is the emphasis of primary and secondary prevention of substance use. Most current Canadian adult smokers began daily smoking by age 15. According to Health Canada (2007b), the proportion of youth who smoke is approximately 20%. Young adults (age 20–24 years) have the highest reported prevalence of smoking at 27%. Because nicotine abuse is highly correlated with illicit drug and alcohol use, especially in adolescents, if tobacco use is not started and maintained during childhood and adolescence, there is a much better chance that other drugs will not be abused as this population ages. Programs developed to help children explore the external influences (e.g., peer pressure) that may cause one to start smoking and that help them identify alternative behaviours make it less likely for children to start smoking. An emphasis on the health hazards of tobacco use, as well as on those of other addictive behaviours, should be part of the total curriculum beginning in elementary schools.

Tobacco Use Cessation. Because tobacco use is the leading cause of preventable illness and death in Canada, nurses have a crucial role in screening, assessing, and providing interventions to support people with smoking cessation. The RNAO's "Ask, advise, assist, arrange" algorithm (2007) is an effective approach in working collaboratively with people with nicotine dependence. These guidelines identify minimal and intensive clinical interventions that should be used at each patient encounter, depending on the time available (see eTable 11-1, available on the Evolve Web site for this chapter). These interventions are designed to identify tobacco users, encourage them to quit, determine their willingness to quit, assist them in quitting, and arrange for follow-up to prevent relapse. In fact, 80% of smokers who are screened and advised to stop smoking reported that they in fact wanted help to stop smoking (RNAO, 2007). Simply screening for and assessing for smoking has significant impact as an intervention to help people quit smoking. Smoking cessation is the single most effective intervention to increase quality of life and decrease the morbidity and mortality directly caused by smoking (see eTable 11-2, Patient & Caregiver Teaching Guide: Smoking and Tobacco Use Cessation, available on the Evolve Web site for this chapter.)

Nicotine Replacement Therapy and Pharmcotherapeutic Interventions for Nicotine Dependence. A variety of nicotine replacement systems, available in the form of gum (nicotine polacrilex [Nicorette]), transdermal patches (Habitrol, Nicoderm), nasal spray, and nicotine inhalers, can be used to reduce the craving and withdrawal symptoms associated with tobacco cessation. These agents enable a smoker to replace nicotine consumption previously obtained from smoking cigarettes with a system that provides slower delivery of the drug and elimination of the carcinogens and gases associated with tobacco smoke. Nicotine replacement therapy is not generally recommended for pregnant women and people who have recently experienced an acute myocardial infarction, have unstable angina, or have life-threatening dysrhythmias.

Participation in tobacco cessation programs is recommended in conjunction with nicotine replacement therapy to help people who use tobacco obtain important behavioural skills while they receive some relief from nicotine withdrawal symptoms. Behavioural approaches help patients to obtain skills in relapse prevention and to avoid high-risk situations for smoking relapse, such as those that promote cue-induced craving. Tobacco cessation programs also promote development of other coping skills, such as cigarette refusal skills, assertiveness, alternative activities to cope with stress, and use of peer support systems (Canadian Lung Association, 2008a).

Pharmacotherapeutic options for nicotine dependence are also available to assist with smoking cessation. Bupropion (Zyban) is an antidepressant approved as an aid to quit smoking. It is a relatively weak inhibitor of neuronal uptake of norepinephrine, serotonin, and dopamine. It reduces the urge to smoke, reduces some symptoms of withdrawal, and helps prevent weight gain associated with smoking cessation. Varenicline (Champix) is a relatively new drug used to aid smoking cessation (Health Canada, 2007c). Varenicline is unique in that it has both agonist and blocking actions at nicotinic receptors. Its agonist activity at one subtype of nicotinic receptors provides some replacement nicotine effects. By blocking another subtype of nicotinic receptors, it also blocks the action of nicotine and prevents stimulation of the mesolimbic dopamine system. Thus, it both eases the withdrawal symptoms and at the same time precludes enjoyment from cigarettes should a person resume smoking.

Helping individuals to stop smoking or using tobacco is one area in which every nurse has a professional role. It has been reported that 80% of smokers said they would like to quit, but only half of those were encouraged to do so by health care providers (Bialous & Sarna, 2004). Because fewer than 5% of smokers are successful on their first attempt at quitting and the average smoker requires multiple attempts before being successful, some health care providers have become cynical with regard to counselling their patients to abstain from tobacco use. However, smoking a few cigarettes during a cessation attempt (a slip) is much different from resuming the full smoking habit (a relapse).

The advice and motivation provided by health care providers can be a powerful force in smoking cessation. Several excellent resources the nurse can use to help patients quit smoking are available at the RNAO website, *www.rnao.org*. See the *Best Practice Guidelines on Smoking Cessation*, Appendix D, "The Benefits of Quitting Smoking"; from *Integrating Smoking Cessation into Daily Nursing Practice*, see Appendix H, "Ask, Advise, Assist, Arrange Protocol"; and Appendix L, "Quit Smoking: First-Line Medications Compared." Links to these documents may be found in the Resources at the end of this chapter.

Cocaine

Characteristics

The Canadian Addiction Survey in 2004 (Canadian Centre on Substance Abuse, 2011) disclosed that 10.3% of those older than age 15 had reported using cocaine in their lifetime, a significantly higher proportion than the 3.8% reported 10 years earlier. Cocaine and "crack" (a freebase form of cocaine whereby cocaine is mixed with other substances such as baking soda to increase supply) are powerful, short-acting CNS stimulants (Figure 11-2). Powder cocaine, because of its fine texture and purity, can be easily snorted intranasally or injected; however, crack has a chalk-like consistency and, therefore, cannot be snorted easily. It must be manipulated either by placing it in a pipe to smoke it or by melting it down with a heat source and then adding liquid for the purpose of intravenous use.

Effects of Use

All stimulants work in part by increasing the amount of dopamine in the brain, producing euphoria and increasing energy and alertness. This action on the brain reward system magnifies pleasure and leads to rapid dependence. In addition to stimulation of the CNS, cocaine and other stimulants also affect the peripheral nervous system and the cardiovascular system. Effects include adrenaline-like actions that lead to increased heart rate, blood pressure, and body temperature; dysrhythmias; marked vasoconstriction; tremors of the hands; nausea or vomiting; and diminished appetite. Additional physical and psychological effects are presented in Table 11-7. Chronic use may lead to impairment of concentration and memory, irritability, mood swings, paranoia, and depression (Shuckit, 2006).

The most common method of administration of cocaine is intranasal (snorting), but it may be smoked as "crack" cocaine or in "freebase" form, injected intravenously, taken orally, or absorbed through mucous membranes. Smoking and IV methods result in the fastest absorption and the highest "rush." Peak blood levels develop within 5 to 30 minutes with most methods of administration, and the longest-lasting effects occur following intranasal ingestion (Dodgen & Shea, 2000). However, it must be noted that effects of cocaine use are short, which is the main reason why people who use cocaine are compelled to seek out and purchase more and more cocaine throughout the day to sustain the euphoric effects and why a great deal of money can be spent on cocaine over a short period of use. During periods of use, the person may not be sleeping, eating, or taking care of himself or herself. Because of its highly stimulating effect on the CNS, cocaine intoxication poses significant medical concerns.

Cocaine withdrawal is usually accompanied by an intense psychological response of dysphoria, fatigue, and irritability. In

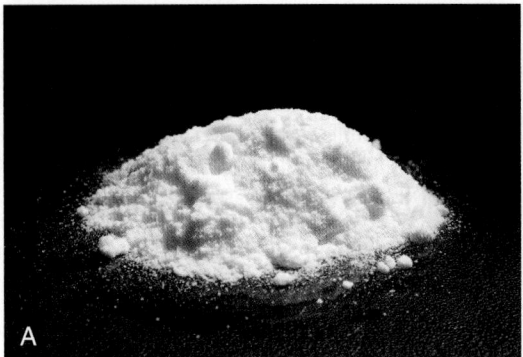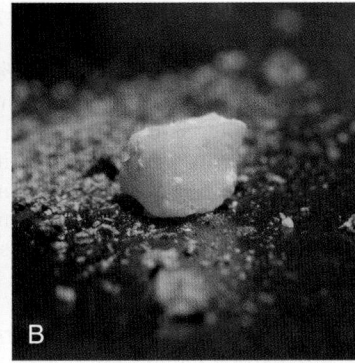

Figure 11-2 A, Powder cocaine, which can be easily snorted or injected. **B,** Crack cocaine, a chalklike derivative of cocaine whereby cocaine is mixed with other substances such as baking soda.

Source: **A,** © Fet/Dreamstime.com; **B,** © Mark Harvey/Alamy.

Table 11-7 Effects of Cocaine and Amphetamine Use

	EARLY EFFECTS	LONG-TERM EFFECTS
Central nervous system	Excitation, euphoria, restlessness, talkativeness	Depression, hallucinations, tremors, visual disturbances, seizures, headache, insomnia, stroke
Cardiovascular system	Tachycardia, hypertension, angina, dysrhythmias, palpitations	Dysrhythmias, hypotension, congestive heart failure, myocardial infarction, cardiomyopathy
Respiratory system	Increased respiratory rate, dyspnea, chest pain, epistaxis	Chronic cough, inflamed throat, congestion of lungs, brown or black sputum production, pneumonia, respiratory distress and/or arrest, pulmonary edema, rhinorrhea, rhinitis, erosion and perforation of the nasal septum
Reproductive system	Heightened sexual desire, delayed orgasm and ejaculation; women may have difficulty achieving orgasm	Difficulty in maintaining erection and ejaculation; loss of interest in sexual activity; women may develop aberrant sexual behaviour
Gastrointestinal system	Decreased appetite	Dehydration, weight loss, nausea; intestinal ischemia may cause gangrenous bowel
Psychological	Behaviour changes or mood swings	Depression or suicidal thoughts

the first 9 hours to 14 days, withdrawal is characterized by intense craving and cocaine-seeking behaviour. There is marked agitation, feelings of depression, exhaustion, and a need to sleep. Table 11-7 describes the effects of cocaine and amphetamine use. Eventually mood is stabilized, but a desire to return to the drug, especially prompted by cue-induced craving, remains for a long period of time (Shuckit, 2006).

Complications

Complications are directly related to the route of administration, type of cocaine, dose, and individual vulnerabilities (see Table 11-3). Of particular concern is the purity of crack cocaine. The other substances added to the cocaine to make crack are widely variable, usually unknown, and questionable. Levamisole, a toxic chemotherapy medication no longer allowed for human use (but available for use for deworming of pigs), has been found in crack taken by people who presented to emergency departments with near-fatal presentations of low white blood counts.

Routes of administration have important health complications. Intravenous administration may result in collapse and scar-

ring of the veins at the injection site, cellulitis, wound abscess, endocarditis, hepatitis B virus (HBV) and hepatitis C virus (HCV) infection, and human immunodeficiency virus (HIV) infection. With intranasal use, the nasal septum and mucosa may be damaged, and frequent sniffing and rhinitis are common signs of chronic intranasal use. Pulmonary damage from smoking crack may be apparent as evidenced by black or dark brown sputum and a form of pneumonia known as "crack lung." Bilateral loss of eyebrow and eyelash hair may occur during "freebasing." Dental caries and loose or broken teeth are also frequently seen as a consequence of using cocaine by any route.

A *stimulant psychosis* may occur with the chronic use of any stimulant. A cocaine psychosis usually progresses from paranoid delusions to visual hallucinations of "snow lights" (coloured lights perceived when cocaine is administered) and tactile hallucinations of bugs crawling under the skin. Skin excoriations from scratching; needle marks; and elevated blood pressure, heart rate, and temperature are findings that help differentiate a stimulant psychosis from schizophrenia (Shuckit, 2006).

Acute cocaine toxicity may be manifested by cardiac palpitations, tachycardia, increased respiratory rate, and fever. At high levels of overdose, seizures, hypertension, and dysrhythmias or myocardial ischemia can occur. The patient experiences restlessness, paranoia, agitated delirium, confusion, and stereotypical repetitive behaviours. Death is often related to stroke, fatal dysrhythmias, or myocardial infarction (Shuckit, 2006).

Collaborative Care

Emergency management of cocaine intoxication will depend on the findings regarding the patient at the time of treatment and may be complicated by the possibility that the patient has combined the use of cocaine with heroin, alcohol, or phencyclidine hydrochloride (PCP). Emergency management of cocaine toxicity is presented in Table 11-8.

Amphetamines

The different types of amphetamines and related drugs such as methylphenidate are stimulant drugs that speed up the CNS. These drugs act like adrenaline, a hormone that is one of the body's natural stimulants. Other drugs with similar effects include cocaine, Ecstasy, ephedrine, caffeine, and many others.

The Centre for Addiction and Mental Health (CAMH) (2006) reported an increase in methamphetamine use among specific populations in Canada, including participants in the club scene and homeless youth. The prevalence of methamphetamine use among Toronto street youth was approximately 37% (CAMH, 2006), making this a serious problem.

Characteristics

Amphetamine is a synthetic drug and, with its derivatives and similar stimulants, is strictly regulated. Specific drugs classified as amphetamines are identified in Table 11-4. Amphetamines may be prescribed for treatment of narcolepsy, attention deficit disorders, and weight control. However, methamphetamine and smokable methamphetamine crystals ("crystal meth," "ice") are in great demand on the street. The methamphetamine that is produced for recreational use is made in illicit laboratories with fairly inexpensive and often toxic or flammable ingredients. The chemicals and processes used vary from laboratory to laboratory, affecting the strength, purity, and effect of the final product (CAMH, 2006).

Effects of Use

Amphetamines are similar to cocaine and stimulate the CNS and peripheral nervous system and the cardiovascular system to produce euphoria, hyperactivity, and increased heart rate and blood pressure. Initial use results in increased alertness, improved performance, relief of fatigue, and anorexia. As with cocaine use, amphetamines used over time may lead to irritability, anxiety, paranoia, and hostile and violent behaviours (see Table 11-7).

Amphetamines are usually taken orally. Rapid effects are obtained by smoking, snorting, or IV injection. Amphetamines have a longer half-life than cocaine and, because they are more

EMERGENCY MANAGEMENT

Table 11-8 Cocaine and Amphetamine Toxicity

ETIOLOGY	ASSESSMENT FINDINGS	INTERVENTIONS
Intranasal, inhalation, parenteral, oral, vaginal, rectal, or sublingual administration of cocaine; oral or parenteral administration of amphetamines	*Cardiovascular* • Palpitations • Tachycardia • Hypertension • Dysrhythmias • Myocardial ischemia or infarction *Central Nervous System* • Feeling of impending doom • Euphoria • Agitation • Combativeness • Seizures • Hallucinations • Confusion • Paranoia • Fever *Other* • Track marks • Consumption of bags of cocaine	*Initial* • Ensure patent airway • Anticipate need for intubation if respiratory distress evident • Establish IV access and initiate fluid replacement as appropriate • Obtain a 12-lead ECG • Treat ventricular dysrhythmias as appropriate with lidocaine, bretylium, or procainamide • Administer IV haloperidol for psychosis • Administer IV diazepam (Valium) or lorazepam (Ativan) for seizures • Naloxone IV should be given if CNS depression is present and concurrent opiate use is suspected • Anticipate the need for propranolol (Inderal) or labetalol for hypertension and tachycardia *Ongoing* • Monitor vital signs, level of consciousness, cardiac rhythm • Use restraints only if needed to protect the patient and staff

CNS, central nervous system; *ECG,* electrocardiogram; *IV,* intravenous.

often taken orally, have a longer effect. Withdrawal symptoms of amphetamines are similar to those of cocaine use and are presented in Table 11-4.

Complications

Toxic reactions to amphetamines are similar to those of cocaine. Increased levels of stimulation, sometimes described as "over-ramping," may result in amphetamine psychosis, paranoia, seizures, and death (see Tables 11-4 and 11-8). Without medical intervention, death may occur as a result of dysrhythmias, myocardial infarction, hyperthermia, or cerebral hemorrhage. Withdrawal symptoms are characterized by intense dysphoria and craving and, as such, place the person at risk for self-harm and impulsivity.

Collaborative Care

Patients often seek treatment for complications of amphetamine abuse such as panic reactions or temporary psychosis related to intoxication, overdose, or withdrawal. Emergency management of amphetamine toxicity is the same as that for cocaine and is presented in Table 11-8.

Caffeine

Characteristics

Caffeine is the most widely used psychoactive substance in the world, and its use to promote alertness and alleviate fatigue is safe in most people. Although weaker than other stimulant drugs, caffeine shares characteristics of intoxication, tolerance, and withdrawal symptoms with regular and consistent patterns. One cup of coffee contains approximately 90 to 150 mg of caffeine, with drip preparation yielding the highest amount of caffeine. A cup of tea averages 30 to 100 mg of caffeine, depending on the brewing method. Traditional cola soft drinks average 25 to 50 mg of caffeine (Shuckit, 2006), although "energy drinks" may contain up to 80 mg or more. The consumption of energy drinks high in caffeine content among children and youth is a growing health concern. In addition to being a component of many beverages, caffeine is found in numerous prescription and over-the-counter (OTC) analgesics, stimulants, appetite suppressants, and cold and flu preparations.

Effects of Use

Caffeine is a relatively weak CNS stimulant. It is a diuretic and a myocardial stimulant. It relaxes smooth muscles, promotes vasodilation, constricts cerebral arteries, increases gastric acid secretion, and enhances contraction of skeletal muscles. Oral doses of 200 mg (two cups of coffee) can elevate mood, produce insomnia, increase irritability, cause anxiety, and offset fatigue. Chronic or heavy intake of 500 mg or more per day is known to cause intoxication manifested by nervousness, insomnia, gastric hyperacidity, muscle twitching, confusion, tachycardia or cardiac dysrhythmias, and psychomotor agitation. The effects of caffeine are presented in Table 11-4.

Physical and psychological dependence on caffeine has been found with chronic use of more than 500 mg/day. However, dependence may occur in some individuals at lower doses, especially in children and youth who have smaller body mass. The

most commonly reported withdrawal symptoms are headache, irritability, drowsiness, and fatigue that occur within 12 to 24 hours following abstinence (see Table 11-4). Caffeine withdrawal may be responsible for some cases of headache that occur after general anaesthesia.

Complications

Chronic and heavy use of caffeine may cause GI upset, including abdominal pain, diarrhea, and heartburn. Habitual users are reported to have slightly higher blood pressure, heart rates, and basal metabolic rates (see Table 11-4). Because symptoms of chronic use develop gradually, most people with caffeine dependence do not link sleep disruption, anxiety, and other symptoms with caffeine intake. Women with high consumption of caffeine are at particular risk for loss of bone mineral density, a risk in the development of osteoporosis later in life. In toxic doses, caffeine influences behaviour patterns and may precipitate panic states.

Collaborative Care

Management of the patient with symptoms of caffeine dependence includes assisting the patient to gradually reduce or stop the intake of caffeine. A list of caffeinated products itemizing their caffeine content may be helpful to the patient who quits coffee only to unknowingly substitute other foods and beverages containing caffeine. Substituting decaffeinated beverages may also help. Decaffeinated coffee and tea contain 2 to 4 mg of caffeine per cup. Toxic reactions to caffeine and lethal doses of caffeine are managed symptomatically, with attention to maintaining respirations and controlling hypertension, dysrhythmias, and seizures.

Depressants

Substances classified as depressants have common physiological effects and include alcohol, sedatives, hypnotics, and opioid narcotics. Depressants are also widely recognized for their abuse potential, which leads to rapid development of tolerance, dependence, and medical emergencies involving overdose and withdrawal.

Alcohol

Characteristics

Alcohol is the most widely consumed substance of abuse in North America. In Canada, 77% of the population age 15 or older drink alcohol (Health Canada, 2011a). The use of alcohol, whether by occasional drinkers or by those who are alcohol dependent, is linked to negative consequences, including automobile accidents, arrests, violence, poor job performance, trauma, and associated injuries requiring emergency intervention.

Alcohol dependence is currently viewed as a chronic, progressive, potentially fatal condition if left untreated. Numerous factors appear to be interrelated in the development of alcohol dependence and may include genetic and biological factors, psychosocial factors, and cultural–environmental background. Alcohol dependence generally occurs over a period of years and may be preceded by heavy social drinking.

Health teaching about the risks associated with consuming more than the recommended low-risk drinking guidelines (Table 11-9) is essential. Although there is evidence of the health benefits of consuming wine, it must be noted that the health benefits are associated with low consumption of 1 standard drink (142 mL [5 oz.] glass of 12% alcohol wine), and in fact, consumption of more than this amount is associated with adverse health risks such as increased risk for hypertension and cardiovascular disease.

Effects of Use

Alcohol affects almost all cells of the body and has complex effects on the neurons in the CNS. Alcohol depresses all areas and functions of the CNS, leading to slowed respirations and heart rate and also affects memory, judgement, and coordination (Herie & Skinner, 2010). Alcohol is absorbed rapidly and widely distributed to body organs; it is mostly metabolized by the enzyme alcohol dehydrogenase by the liver and is metabolized at a constant rate of 10 g of alcohol per hour (Kahan, 2000). Absorption is slower in the presence of water or food, especially proteins and fats. Faster absorption occurs when alcohol is mixed with carbonated liquids. Owing to having a smaller volume of distribution, women have significantly lower rates of metabolism and will have higher blood alcohol levels than men after the same amount of alcohol intake (CAMH, 2006). As such, Canada's low-risk drinking guidelines recommend that women limit consumption to 10 standard drinks per week, with no more than 2 drinks per day most days, and that men limit consumption to no more than 15 standard drinks per week with no more than 3 drinks per day most days.

The effects of alcohol are related to the concentration of alcohol and individual susceptibility. The concentration of alcohol in the body can be determined by assessing the BAC. Alcohol may be measured in the blood within 15 to 20 minutes of ingestion, peaks in 60 to 90 minutes, and is excreted in 12 to 24 hours. BAC is affected by the amount consumed, the drinking rate, body size and composition, drink concentration, and hormones (Table 11-10). As such, children and youth who have lower body mass are more susceptible to the effects of alcohol. The relationship between BAC and behaviour is different in a person who has developed tolerance to alcohol and its effects. This individual is commonly able to drink large amounts without obvious impairment and perform complex tasks without problems at BAC levels several times higher than levels that would produce obvious impairment in a person who has less tolerance. Comparatively, in most people who have not developed tolerance, a BAC of 160 mg % (34 mmol/L) will cause obvious signs of intoxication, whereas, in individuals with developed tolerance, a BAC of up to 280 to 320 mg % (60 or 70 mmol/L) will present as within normal functioning. Coma can develop in most people at BAC levels between 400 and 560 mg % (90 and 120 mmol/L) (Kahan, 2000). Also, people who have developed high tolerance to the effects of alcohol have greater risk for complicated withdrawal from alcohol that can lead to seizures and death. Table 11-11 compares problematic drinking with alcohol dependence.

Alcohol Intoxication

Intoxication is evidenced with increasing BAC and results in behavioural and physical changes (see Table 11-10). Behavioural effects may include relaxation, sedation, disinhibition, aggres-

Table 11-9 Canada's Low-Risk Drinking Guidelines

Drinking is a personal choice. If you choose to drink, these guidelines can help you decide when, where, why, and how.

Guideline 1

Reduce your long-term health risks by drinking no more than:

- 10 drinks per week for women, with no more than 2 drinks per day most days
- 15 drinks per week for men, with no more than 3 drinks per day most days

Plan nondrinking days every week, to avoid developing a habit.

Guideline 2

Reduce your risk of injury and harm by drinking no more than 3 drinks (for women) and 4 drinks (for men) on any single occasion.

Plan to drink in a safe environment. Stay within the weekly limits outlined in Guideline 1.

Guideline 3

Do not drink when you are:

- Driving a vehicle or using machinery and tools
- Taking medicine or other drugs that interact with alcohol
- Doing any kind of dangerous physical activity
- Living with mental or physical health problems
- Living with alcohol dependence
- Pregnant or planning to be pregnant
- Responsible for the safety of others
- Making important decisions

Guideline 4

If you are pregnant, planning to become pregnant, or before breastfeeding, the safest choice is to drink no alcohol at all.

Guideline 5

If you are a child or youth, you should delay drinking until your late teens. Talk with your parents about drinking. Alcohol can harm the way your brain and body develop.

If you are drinking, plan ahead, follow local alcohol laws, and stay within the limits outlined in Guideline 1.

For These Guidelines, "a Drink" Means

- 341 mL (12 oz.) bottle of 5% alcohol beer, cider, or cooler
- 142 mL (5 oz.) glass of 12% alcohol wine
- 43 mL (1.5 oz.) serving of 40% distilled alcohol (e.g., rye, rum, gin)

  Low-risk drinking helps to promote a culture of moderation. Low-risk drinking supports healthy lifestyles.

Tips

- Set limits for yourself and abide by them.
- Drink slowly. Have no more than 2 drinks in any 3 hours.
- For every drink of alcohol, have 1 nonalcoholic drink.
- Eat before and while you are drinking.
- Always consider your age, body weight, and health problems that might suggest lower limits.
- Although drinking may provide health benefits for certain groups of people, do not start to drink, or increase your drinking, for health benefits.

Source: National Alcohol Strategy Advisory Committee. (2012). Canada's Low-Risk Alcohol Drinking Guidelines. Ottawa: Canadian Centre on Substance Abuse. Retrieved from: *http://www.ccsa.ca/eng/priorities/alcohol/canada-low-risk-alcohol-drinking-guidelines/Pages/default.aspx#guide*

Table 11-10 Blood Alcohol Concentration and Related Effects

BAC* mg/dL (mg%)	PSYCHOPHYSIOLOGICAL EFFECT
20 (0.02)	Light and moderate drinkers begin to feel some effects. Approximate BAC is reached after 1 drink.†
40 (0.04)	Most people begin to feel relaxed.
60 (0.06)	Judgement is mildly impaired. People are less able to make rational decisions about their capabilities (e.g., driving skills).
80 (0.08)	Definite impairment of muscle coordination and driving skills occurs. Person is legally intoxicated according to Canada's Criminal Code.‡
100 (0.1)	Clear deterioration of reaction time and control is observed. Person is legally intoxicated in most provinces and territories. Some provinces permit slightly higher levels than those permitted by the federal government.
120 (0.12)	Vomiting occurs unless this level is reached slowly.
150 (0.15)	Balance and movement are impaired. Equivalent of one-half pint of whiskey is circulating in the bloodstream.
300 (0.3)	Many people lose consciousness.
400 (0.4)	Most people lose consciousness, and some die. For 50% of adult humans, 0.4 mg % is the accepted lethal dose.§
450 (0.45)	Breathing stops; person eventually dies.

BAC, blood alcohol concentration.
*BAC is generally recorded in milligrams percent (mg %) or milligrams of alcohol per decilitre (mg/dL) of blood. Percentage is used for legal definitions of intoxication. BAC is dependent on how much alcohol is consumed, how fast it is consumed, and the person's weight.
†One drink is 360 mL beer, 150 mL wine, or 30 mL distilled spirits, all of which provide the same amount of alcohol.
‡Canada Safety Council. (2009). *Canada's blood alcohol laws among the strictest in the Western world.* Retrieved from *http://canadasafetycouncil.org/news/canada-s-blood-alcohol-laws-among-strictest-western-world*; provincial blood alcohol limits for drivers vary.
§Brick, J. (2005). *Online fact—Driving while impaired.* Center for Alcohol Studies, Rutgers University. Retrieved from *http://alcoholstudies.rutgers.edu/onlinefacts/dwi.html*

Table 11-11 Problematic Drinking versus Alcohol Dependence

OBJECTIVE MEASURES	PROBLEMATIC DRINKING	ALCOHOL DEPENDENCE
Number of drinks/wk	Male: >15 Female: >10	>40-60/wk
Drinks moderately (<4/day)	Often	Rarely
Tolerance	Mild	Marked
Withdrawal symptoms	No	Often
Neglect of major responsibilities	No	Yes
Socially stable	Usually	Not often

Source: Adapted from Kahan, M., & Wilson, L (Eds.). (2002). *Managing alcohol, tobacco and other drug problems: A pocket guide for physicians and nurses* (Chapter 7, p. 32). Toronto: Centre for Addiction and Mental Health.

doses of this drug. It is important to obtain as accurate a history as possible, using collateral information as necessary, and assess for injuries, trauma, diseases, and hypoglycemia. The basic principles of the ABCs must be implemented. Vital signs and level of consciousness should be monitored. Generally, the heart rate is normal in uncomplicated intoxication but elevated in withdrawal.

Complications Associated With Chronic Alcoholism

Patients with chronic consumption may experience Wernicke's encephalopathy. These patients should be assessed for ocular abnormalities, including nystagmus and paralysis of the lateral rectus muscles, as well as ataxia and a global confusion state. Untreated or progressive Wernicke's encephalopathy may lead to Korsakoff's psychosis. Because symptoms of encephalopathy may be difficult to distinguish from intoxication or withdrawal and because Wernicke's encephalopathy is potentially reversible, IV thiamine is often administered to intoxicated patients. Patients with alcohol intoxication may also be hypoglycemic from a lack of food intake. Glucose solutions may precipitate Wernicke's encephalopathy in a previously unaffected patient, so thiamine should be started before treatment with IV glucose solution in all patients with alcoholism and continued until the patient resumes a normal diet.

The nurse should remain with the patient as much as possible, orienting to reality as necessary. Agitation and anxiety are common, and the patient should be assessed for increasing belligerence and a potential for violence. The patient is also at high risk for injury because of lack of coordination and impaired judgement, and protective measures should be used. It is critical to continue assessment and interventions until the BAC has decreased to at least 0.1 mg % and until any associated disorders or injuries have been ruled out. A BAC of 0.1 mg % is usually reached within 6 to 10 hours (Canada Safety Council, 2009).

Alcohol Withdrawal

After excessive drinking, individuals may experience hangovers manifested by malaise, nausea, headache, thirst, and a general feeling of fatigue. In people with alcohol dependence, sudden

sion, impaired judgement, irritability, euphoria, depression, and emotional lability. Physical signs include slurred speech, lack of motor coordination, nystagmus, and flushing resulting from dilation of peripheral blood vessels. Disturbances in memory and blackouts may occur in dependent drinkers. People are at higher risk for self-injurious behaviours while intoxicated, as a result of impaired judgement and impulsivity. In addition, nurses should ask people about histories of having blackouts while intoxicated. People are also at risk of significant mood disregulation and depression in the context of intoxication, and risk for suicide is an important consideration. Fatalities caused by drinking and driving, head injuries, physical trauma, and violence are closely linked to alcohol intoxication.

Acute Alcohol Intoxication. Acute alcohol intoxication may manifest as an emergency primarily because of the narrow range between the intoxicating, the anaesthetic, and the lethal

NURSING CARE PLAN 11-1

Alcohol Withdrawal

NURSING DIAGNOSIS	*Risk for injury related to* sensorimotor deficits, seizure activity, and confusion
Expected Patient Outcomes	**Nursing Interventions and *Rationales***
• Reports no falls or injuries • Experiences decrease in tremors and psychomotor activity • Reports no seizures • Verbalizes risk for injury associated with alcohol use before discharge	• Assess for risk factors such as impaired mobility (e.g., unsteady gait), sensory deficits, tremors, impaired judgement, confusion, seizure activity *to plan appropriate preventive measures.* • Assess for signs of injury such as lacerations, bruises, or burns *to treat appropriately.* • Monitor vital signs frequently, especially heart rate, *because prompt recognition of extreme autonomic nervous system response is necessary for early intervention to prevent progression of symptoms.* • Administer benzodiazepines as ordered to control hyperactivity, thiamine *to reduce neurological complications (e.g., Wernicke's encephalopathy),* and antiseizure medications as ordered *to prevent seizures.* • Use seizure precautions *to prevent injury.*
NURSING DIAGNOSIS	*Disturbed sensory perception (auditory and/or visual) related to* sensory overload *as evidenced by* impaired interpretation of environmental stimuli, disorientation, and hallucinations
Expected Patient Outcomes	**Nursing Interventions and *Rationales***
• Reports no hallucinations • Remains oriented to person, place, and time	• Assess patient's orientation and cognition *to determine appropriate interventions.* • Provide quiet and nonstimulating environment *to reduce external stimuli and calm overactive CNS.* • Orient to nurse and environment with each contact; use calm, approach; provide consistent staff; explain procedures and what is expected *to assist in orientation and decrease anxiety.* • Administer benzodiazepines as ordered *to reduce CNS stimulation.* • Administer antipsychotic medication (e.g., haloperidol [Haldol]) if ordered *to decrease severity of hallucinations.* (Be aware that Haldol lowers the seizure threshold.
NURSING DIAGNOSIS	*Ineffective breathing pattern as evidenced by* rapid respirations, dyspnea, and use of accessory muscles
Expected Patient Outcomes	**Nursing Interventions and *Rationales***
• Maintains effective breathing • Reports no indications of hypoxia	• Monitor respiratory rate, depth, and pattern *so appropriate interventions may be taken.* • Position patient on side and in semi-Fowler's position *to reduce possibility of aspiration and to enhance lung expansion by lowering diaphragm.* • Monitor effects of medications given for withdrawal *to detect respiratory depression.* • Encourage coughing and deep breathing *to prevent complications of hypoventilation.* • Administer supplemental oxygen *to treat hypoxia.*

CNS, central nervous system.

cessation of consumption, "going cold turkey," may have life-threatening effects owing to medical complications caused by alcohol withdrawal.

A patient with alcohol dependence who is hospitalized for other illnesses, health conditions, or trauma often develops alcohol withdrawal when the ingestion of alcohol is abruptly stopped. The signs and symptoms of alcohol withdrawal generally begin 6 to 12 hours after the patient's last drink and may last for 3 to 5 days (see Table 11-5). The most common severe manifestations are hallucinations and seizures. The progression of early symptoms to DTs can be prevented by administration of benzodiazepines, such as lorazepam (Ativan). Thiamine and multiple vitamins are important to prevent development of Wernicke's encephalopathy and Korsakoff's psychosis. A quiet, calm environment is important to prevent exacerbation of symptoms. The use of restraints and IV lines should be avoided whenever

possible. Supportive care is needed to ensure adequate rest and nutrition. The nursing care plan for the patient in alcohol withdrawal is presented in Nursing Care Plan 11-1.

Characteristic symptoms include tremulousness, anxiety, increased heart rate, increased blood pressure, sweating, nausea, hyperreflexia, and insomnia (see Table 11-4). Seizures are most likely to occur 12 to 72 hours after the last drink in untreated alcohol withdrawal (Table 11-12). Alcohol-withdrawal delirium, or DTs, is a medically serious complication that may occur from 30 to 120 hours after the last drink of untreated alcohol withdrawal that can result in death. People at highest risk for developing DTs are individuals who are elderly with a history of regular alcohol consumption with few or no periods of abstinence, or history of complicated alcohol withdrawal, and/or undergoing physiological stress such as surgery or medical intervention. Delirium components include disorientation, visual or

Table 11-12 Stages of Alcohol Withdrawal

MINOR	INTERMEDIATE	MAJOR
Autonomic hyperactivity: • Nausea/vomiting • Coarse tremor • Sweating • Tachycardia • Hypertension	Autonomic hyperactivity: • Seizures • Dysrhythmias (atrial fibrillation, supraventricular/ventricular tachycardia) • Hallucinations (auditory/visual)	Delirium tremens: • Severe agitation • Gross tremulousness • Global confusion • Disorientation • Auditory, tactile, visual hallucinations • Psychomotor and autonomic hyperactivity (e.g., hypertension, fever)
Symptoms tend to appear within 6-12 hr of last drink	Withdrawal seizures usually occur between 12-72 hr after drinking has stopped	Typically occur 5-6 days after severe, untreated withdrawal
Symptoms usually resolve within 48-72 hr	Seizure protocol: 20 mg Valium qhr × 3 doses min	Sudden death can occur

Source: Kahan, M., & Wilson, L. (Eds.). (2002). *Managing alcohol, tobacco and other drug problems: A pocket guide for physicians and nurses* (pp. 38-47). Toronto: Centre for Addiction and Mental Health.

auditory hallucinations, and increased hyperactivity. Death may be caused by hyperthermia, peripheral vascular collapse, or cardiac failure. Key nursing intervention and management of alcohol withdrawal is based on early and accurate assessment in order to prevent complications of untreated withdrawal that can lead to seizures and complications. Nurses should assess for tachycardia, dehydration, fever, diaphoresis, dysrhythmias, and liver impairment, in addition to cognition and level of consciousness. Treatment of intermediate withdrawal usually involves the administration of diazepam in order to prevent withdrawal-related seizure. For those with poor liver function or who are elderly, lorazepam is preferred. The Clinical Institute Withdrawal Assessment for Alcohol (Table 11-13) is a standardized assessment tool that can be used to assess and monitor for withdrawal symptoms caused by alcohol withdrawal; it provides a symptom-triggered approach to management and intervention using benzodiazepine medications such as diazepam and lorazepam to prevent complicated withdrawal.

If there is any indication of alcohol or other CNS-depressant use when a patient is hospitalized, the nurse should always question when the patient last used the substance. This information will help the nurse anticipate drug interactions or the time of possible onset of withdrawal symptoms.

Complications

Acute alcohol toxicity may occur with binge drinking or the use of alcohol with other CNS depressants. Alcohol-induced CNS depression leads to respiratory and circulatory failure manifested by depressed respirations, hypotension, hypothermia, and a decreased level of consciousness (see Table 11-4).

Individuals who abuse alcohol are subject to many health problems. Physical complications of chronic alcohol abuse are outlined in Table 11-14 and are frequently the reasons that alcohol-dependent individuals seek health care.

Complications may also arise from the interaction of alcohol with commonly prescribed or OTC drugs. Drugs that interact with alcohol in an additive manner include antihypertensives, antihistamines, antianginals, and salicylates (aspirin). Alcohol taken with aspirin may cause or exacerbate GI bleeding. Alcohol taken with acetaminophen may increase the risk of liver damage. Potentiation and cross-tolerance with other CNS depressants also

may occur. **Potentiation,** a drug interaction causing a response greater than the sum of the individual responses to each drug, occurs when an additional CNS depressant is taken with alcohol, increasing the effect. Heavy drinkers may be tolerant (require an increased dose for effect) to other depressant drugs such as benzodiazepines or opioids, even if they have never used these drugs. This is called **cross-tolerance** and refers to resistance to one or more of the effects of one drug because of tolerance developed to a similar drug (Shuckit, 2006).

One complication of chronic alcohol abuse is **Wernicke's encephalopathy,** an inflammatory, hemorrhagic, degenerative condition of the brain. Wernicke's encephalopathy is caused by a thiamine deficiency resulting from poor diet and alcohol-induced suppression of thiamine absorption. This syndrome is readily reversible with administration of thiamine. Untreated or progressive Wernicke's encephalopathy may lead to **Korsakoff's psychosis,** an irreversible form of amnesia characterized by loss of short-term memory and an inability to learn (Johnson, 2004).

Collaborative Care

Initial treatment of alcohol dependency is aimed at **withdrawal management** (interventions and processes aimed at addressing the physiological and psychological symptoms that occur in response to stopping a substance on which physiological and psychological dependence has developed) as necessary and stabilization of the patient's condition. In toxic reactions, naloxone, an opiate antagonist, may be given if opioids have been used with alcohol. Supportive measures are used to promote ventilation and circulation until the alcohol is metabolized. The patient who is intoxicated and has rising BAC should not be given other depressants because of their additive effects.

Management of alcohol withdrawal frequently includes the use of medications to decrease symptoms, increase the level of comfort, and decrease the risk of seizures and DTs. Table 11-15 presents the clinical manifestations of alcohol withdrawal and suggested drug treatment.

Although cessation of drinking is the short-term goal that is accomplished through withdrawal management, rehabilitation and sustained abstinence are the primary long-term goals. Patients should be referred to inpatient or intensive outpatient programs

Table 11-13 Clinical Institute Withdrawal Assessment for Alcohol (CIWA)

Patient Name:_____ (Last Name, First Name)

Time:_____ Total Score (max score = 67)_____ Temp: _____ BP:_____/_____ Apex rate:_____ Resps:_____ Initials:____

Time:_____ Total Score (max score = 67)_____ Temp: _____ BP:_____/_____ Apex rate:_____ Resps:_____ Initials:____

_____ _____ (print name and credentials) (signature)

(dd/mm/yyyy):_____ F0136-20100721 Chart Tab: Assessments/Plans Patient ID Label

NAUSEA & VOMITING: Ask "Do you feel sick to your stomach? Have you vomited?" Observation.

0 No nausea/vomiting

1

2

3

4 Intermittent nausea with dry heaves

5

6

7 Constant nausea, frequent dry heaves & vomiting

TREMOR: Arms extended and fingers spread apart. Observation.

0 No tremor

1 Not visible, but can be felt fingertip to fingertip

2

3

4 Moderate, with patient's arms extended

5

6

7 Severe, even with arms not extended

PAROXYSMAL SWEATS: Observation.

0 No sweat visible

1 Barely perceptible sweating, palms moist

2

3

4 Beads of sweat obvious on forehead

5

6

7 Drenching sweats

ANXIETY: Ask "Do you feel nervous?" Observation.

0 No anxiety, at ease

1 Mildly anxious

2

3

4 Moderately anxious, or guarded, so anxiety is inferred

5

6

7 Acute panic as seen in severe delirium or acute schizophrenic reactions

TACTILE DISTURBANCES: Ask: "Have you any itching, pins and needles sensations, any burning, any numbness or do you feel bugs crawling on or under your skin?" Observation.

0 None

1 Very mild itching, pins and needles, burning or numbness

2 Mild itching, pins and needles, burning or numbness

3 Moderate itching, pins and needles, burning or numbness

4 Moderately severe hallucinations

5 Severe hallucinations

6 Extremely severe hallucinations

7 Continuous hallucinations

AUDITORY DISTURBANCES: Ask: "Are you more aware of sounds around you? Are they harsh? Do they frighten you? Are you hearing anything that is disturbing to you? Are you hearing things you know are not there?" Observation.

0 Not present

1 Very mild harshness or ability to frighten

2 Mild harshness or ability to frighten

3 Moderate harshness or ability to frighten

4 Moderately severe hallucinations

5 Severe hallucinations

6 Extremely severe hallucinations

7 Continuous hallucinations

VISUAL DISTURBANCES: Ask: "Does the light appear to be too bright? Is its colour different? Does it hurt your eyes? Are you seeing anything that is disturbing to you? Are you seeing things you know are not there?" Observation.

0 Not present

1 Very mild sensitivity

2 Mild sensitivity

3 Moderate sensitivity

4 Moderately severe hallucinations

5 Severe hallucinations

6 Extremely severe hallucinations

7 Continuous hallucinations

HEADACHE, FULLNESS IN HEAD: Ask: "Does your head feel different? Does it feel like there is a band around your head?" Do not rate for dizziness or lightheadedness. Otherwise, rate severity.

0 Not present

1 Very mild

2 Mild

3 Moderate

4 Moderately severe

5 Severe

6 Very severe

7 Extremely severe

Continued

Table 11-13 Clinical Institute Withdrawal Assessment for Alcohol (CIWA)—cont'd

AGITATION: Observation.	**ORIENTATION & CLOUDING OF SENSORIUM:** Ask: "What day is this? Where are you? Who am I?"
0 Normal activity	0 Oriented and can do serial additions
1 Somewhat more than normal activity	1 Cannot do serial additions or is uncertain about date
2	2 Disoriented for date by no more than 2 calendar days
3	3 Disoriented for date by more than 2 calendar days
4 Moderately fidgety and restless	4 Disoriented for place and/or person
5	
6	
7 Paces back and forth during most interview, or constantly thrashes about	

Source: Brands, B., Kahan, M., Selby, P., & Wilson, L. (Eds.). (2000). *Management of alcohol, tobacco and other drug problems: A physician's manual* (p. 77). Toronto: Centre for Addiction and Mental Health.

Table 11-14 Effects of Chronic Alcohol Abuse

BODY SYSTEM	SYSTEM EFFECTS
Central nervous system	Alcoholic dementia; Wernicke's syndrome (confusion, nystagmus, paralysis of ocular muscles, ataxia); Korsakoff's syndrome (confabulation, amnesic disorder); impairment of cognitive function, psychomotor skills, abstract thinking, and memory; depression, attention deficit, labile moods, seizures, sleep disturbances
Peripheral nervous system	Peripheral neuropathy including pain, paresthesias, weakness
Immune system	Increased risk for tuberculosis and viral infections, especially pneumonia; increased risk for cancer of oral cavity, pharynx, esophagus, liver, colon, rectum, and possibly breast
Hematological system	Bone marrow depression, anemia, leukopenia, thrombocytopenia, blood clotting abnormalities
Musculoskeletal system	Painful or tender swelling of large muscle groups; painless progressive muscle weakness and wasting; osteoporosis
Cardiovascular system	Elevated pulse and blood pressure; decreased exercise tolerance; cardiomyopathy (irreversible); increased risk for hemorrhagic stroke, coronary artery disease, hypertension, sudden cardiac death
Hepatic system	Steatosis (reversible)—nausea, vomiting, hepatomegaly Alcoholic hepatitis (reversible)—anorexia, nausea, vomiting, fever, chills, abdominal pain, cirrhosis; cancer
Gastrointestinal system	Gastritis, peptic ulcer, esophagitis, esophageal varices, enteritis, colitis, Mallory-Weiss tear, pancreatitis
Digestive system	Decreased appetite, indigestion, malabsorption, vitamin deficiencies
Urinary system	Diuretic effect from inhibition of antidiuretic hormone
Endocrine and reproductive system	Altered gonadal function, testicular atrophy, decreased beard growth, decreased libido, diminished sperm count, gynecomastia, glucose intolerance, early menopause, fetal alcohol spectrum disorder (FASD)
Integumentary system	Palmar erythema, spider angiomas, rosacea, rhinophyma

for continued support and treatment. Treatment includes behavioural therapy and may also include drugs that block the desired effects of alcohol, such as naltrexone (ReVia), or agents that prevent drinking by causing aversive consequences when alcohol is consumed, such as disulfiram (Antabuse) and citrated calcium carbimide (Temposil).

Sedative–Hypnotics

Characteristics

Commonly abused sedative–hypnotic agents include barbiturates, benzodiazepines, and barbiturate-like drugs. Benzodiazepine-class medications are effective and important in the treatment of panic attacks and severe anxiety. However, in practice, benzodiazepine medications are widely prescribed for generalized anxiety

and at times for sleep disturbance for long periods of time, which can contribute to the development of tolerance and risk for misuse.

Subsequently, the person may become tolerant to the effects and increase the dose and frequency of use without medical advice or indication. The second and more common pattern involves illegal sources, often begins with intermittent use by teenagers or young adults at parties and the potential for misuse or dependency.

Effects of Use

Sedative–hypnotic drugs act primarily on the CNS, causing sedation at low doses and sleep at high doses. Excessive amounts produce an initial euphoria and an intoxication that includes impaired judgement, slurred speech, and loss of inhibitions and motor coordination. Although benzodiazepines are believed to

Table 11-15 Clinical Manifestations of Alcohol Withdrawal and Suggested Drug Treatment

Clinical Manifestations	Drug Treatment

• Gross tremors
• Seizures
• Hallucinations
• Delirium tremens (DTs)
• Minor withdrawal syndrome
  • Tremulousness, anxiety
  • Increased heart rate
  • Increased blood pressure
  • Sweating
  • Nausea
  • Hyper-reflexia
  • Insomnia
• Major withdrawal (DTs)
  • Altered level of consciousness
  • Visual–auditory hallucinations
  • Increased hyperactivity without seizures
	• Benzodiazepines (e.g., chlordiazepoxide [Librax])
	• Thiamine (prevents Wernicke's encephalopathy)
	• Multivitamins (folic acid, B vitamins)
	• Phenytoin (Dilantin) for seizures or past history of seizures
	• Magnesium sulphate (if serum magnesium is low)
	• Temazepam (Restoril) for sedation
	• Haloperidol for hallucinations

NOTE: For DTs, provide intravenous fluids (do not overhydrate), cooling blanket, well-lit quiet room, consistent staff, and frequent checks of vital signs; check for hypoglycemia; assess any other health problems.

have a wide margin of safety, they are not without adverse reactions, including rebound anxiety and insomnia with short-acting drugs, and confusion and memory loss with long-acting drugs. The drugs are usually taken orally, but barbiturates may be injected intravenously (Shuckit, 2006). The effects of sedative–hypnotics are presented in Table 11-4.

Tolerance to the sedative effects develops rapidly, necessitating higher doses to achieve euphoria. Tolerance may not develop to the brainstem-depressant effects, so an increased dose may trigger hypotension and respiratory depression, resulting in death.

Withdrawal from sedative–hypnotics can be very serious. The patient may develop anxiety, tremors, weakness, nausea with or without vomiting, muscle cramps, and increased reflexes. After 24 hours, the patient is craving the drug and may experience delirium, seizures, and respiratory and cardiac arrest (see Table 11-4). Symptoms of withdrawal peak on the second or third day for short-acting drugs (e.g., alprazolam [Xanax], pentobarbital) and on the seventh or eighth day for long-acting drugs (e.g., diazepam [Valium], chlordiazepoxide [Librax], phenobarbital [Phenobarb]) (Kosten & O'Connor, 2003).

Complications

An overdose of a sedative–hypnotic may cause death as a result of respiratory depression. Symptoms of overdose are listed in Table 11-16. Complications associated with IV use of the drugs (e.g., blood-borne infections) can also occur.

EMERGENCY MANAGEMENT

Table 11-16 Overdose of Depressant Drugs

ETIOLOGY	ASSESSMENT FINDINGS	INTERVENTIONS
Ingestion, inhalation, or injection of CNS depressants—accidental or intentional	• Aggressive behaviour • Agitation • Confusion • Lethargy • Stupor • Hallucinations • Depression • Slurred speech • Pinpoint pupils • Nystagmus • Seizures • Needle tracks • Cold, clammy skin • Rapid, weak pulse • Slow or rapid shallow respirations • Decreased O$_2$ saturation • Hypotension • Dysrhythmia • ECG changes • Cardiac or respiratory arrest	**Initial** • Ensure patent airway • Anticipate intubation if respiratory distress evident • Establish IV access • Obtain temperature • Obtain 12-lead ECG • Obtain information about substance (name, route, when taken, amount) • Obtain specific drug levels or comprehensive toxicology screen • Obtain a health history including drug use and allergies • Administer antidotes as appropriate • Perform gastric lavage if necessary • Administer activated charcoal and cathartics as appropriate **Ongoing** • Monitor vital signs, temperature, level of consciousness, O$_2$ saturation, cardiac rhythm

CNS, central nervous system; ECG, electrocardiogram; IV, intravenous.

Withdrawal from Sedative–Hypnotics. Withdrawal from sedative–hypnotics can be highly variable, and the severity and the onset of symptoms depend on many factors, including the drug, the pattern of use, the dose and duration of use, and the presence of concurrent alcohol use. Symptoms may begin 12 hours after cessation of a short-acting drug and more than 100 hours after cessation of a long-acting drug. Withdrawal from high doses is potentially life-threatening and necessitates close monitoring in an inpatient setting. Management of withdrawal from sedative–hypnotic agents is symptomatic and includes a gradual reduction in drug dosage. Long-acting agents such as diazepam (Valium), chlordiazepoxide (Librax), clonazepam, or phenobarbital may be substituted for the drug and tapered after stabilization. Mild to moderate symptoms can persist for 2 to 3 weeks after a 3- to 5-day period of acute symptoms.

Collaborative Care

Overdoses of benzodiazepines may be treated with flumazenil, a specific benzodiazepine antagonist. There are no known antagonists to counteract the effects of other sedative–hypnotic drugs. Emergency life support measures must be taken in cases of overdose. Table 11-16 presents emergency management of CNS depressants. Treatment of an individual dependent on a sedative–hypnotic calls for gradual withdrawal of the drug. Hospitalization is recommended during drug withdrawal for individuals who have been abusing large amounts of the drugs in order to safely manage their symptoms.

Abrupt cessation of the drug is not recommended because of the risk of seizures and complicated withdrawal. Medically supervised tapering off over an extended period of time is recommended for withdrawal management of people with benzodiazepine dependency.

Opioids

Characteristics

Opiates are substances, such as morphine and codeine, that are directly derived from the opium poppy. **Opioids** is an umbrella term that includes the opiates in addition to the many semisynthetic and synthetic narcotic agents used as analgesics. Commonly abused opioids are identified in Table 11-4. Narcotic antagonists include naloxone.

Heroin and fentanyl are commonly used street drugs, but recently, the IV use of controlled-release oxycodone has become epidemic. Although the rates of opioid dependency are lower than for other illegal drugs, their use is associated with high levels of crime, violence, HIV infection, and death from overdose.

Heroin use is considered an increasingly marginal form of drug use among illicit opioid users in Canada, particularly outside of Vancouver and Montreal (port cities that are major heroin import points). Instead, the use of prescription opioids in varying forms has become the predominant form of illicit opioid use (Fischer, Rehm, Patra, & Cruz, 2006).

The vast majority of people who are prescribed opioid medications for analgesia do not develop problematic or aberrant use patterns. Opioid medications are important in the treatment of acute and chronic pain. However, certain risk factors will increase the risk of developing dependency and include factors such as a past or current personal history of substance use, history of sexual trauma, concurrent mental health conditions such as depression or anxiety, and a family history of substance use (Kahan, Srivastava, Wilson, Gourlay, & Midmer, 2006).

Effects of Use

By acting on opiate receptors and neurotransmitter systems in the CNS, opioids cause CNS depression and a major effect on the brain reward system. As drugs of abuse, they are taken orally, sniffed, smoked, or taken intravenously.

The primary effects include analgesia, drowsiness, slurred speech, detachment from the environment, hunger, decreased respiratory rate, GI peristalsis, and decreased pupil size. Tolerance to the analgesic effects of opioids develops slowly, whereas tolerance to the euphoric psychological effects develops much more quickly; therefore, for people who are misusing opioids for the sense of euphoria will require increasingly high amounts to achieve the same effect. Hand in hand, physiological tolerance develops quickly as well. Of note is that physiological tolerance to opioids is lost very quickly as well, in as short a time as a few days of abstinence, which can lead to fatal overdoses should people resume taking the same amount they had been accustomed to taking after a period of abstinence.

Opioid Overdose

Signs of overdose of opioids include pinpoint pupils, clammy skin, depressed respiration, sedation, and decreased level of consciousness that can lead to coma and death if the overdose is not treated. Opioid overdose is a medical emergency and should be treated in an acute medical setting. Treatment includes administration of a naloxone infusion and maintaining airways. Giving naloxone 0.4 mg to 2.0 mg intravenously puts the person into withdrawal temporarily, and as such, repeat doses may be required. Unintentional overdose frequently occurs with recreational use of the drugs because of the unpredictability in potency and purity as well as in cases of resuming use of the same amount after a period of abstinence owing to loss of tolerance. Signs of overdose are presented in Table 11-4.

Opioid Withdrawal

Withdrawal from opioids occurs with decreased amounts or cessation of the drug after a period of moderate to heavy use. Symptoms may include craving, abdominal cramps, diarrhea, nausea, and vomiting and is extremely uncomfortable and similar to a bout of stomach flu (Table 11-17). Additional symptoms are presented in Table 11-6. Opioid withdrawal usually peaks 2 to 3 days after the last use and resolves by days 5 to 7. Interventions to support withdrawal include comfort measures such as heat packs for myalgias and medications for symptomatic relief that include antidiarrheal agents, antiemetics, nonsteroidal anti-inflammatory agents, and clonidine.

Complications

A key consideration in people with regular chronic use of opioids is opioid-induced constipation, which can lead to bowel obstruction. A key point of health teaching for patients is to advise them to avoid bulk-forming laxatives, which in fact will make the constipation worse. What is recommended are osmotic agents that will aid in the relief of opioid-induced constipation. But of key concern is the risk of death caused by unintentional overdose

Table 11-17 Symptoms of Opioid Withdrawal versus Opioid Intoxication

OPIOID OVERDOSE	OPIOID WITHDRAWAL
Early Signs	• Dysphoric mood
• Nodding off/drowsiness	• Nausea or vomiting
• Slurred speech	• Abdominal cramps
• Emotional lability	• Myalgia (muscle pain)
• Myosis	• Lacrimation (teary eyes)
Late Signs	• Rhinorrhea (runny nose)
• Respiratory depression	• Mydriasis, piloerection
• Prolonged QT interval	• Sweating
• Ventricular arrhythmias	• Diarrhea
• Coma	• Yawning
(Centre for Addiction and Mental Health, 2007)	• Fever
	• Insomnia
	• Anxiety
	• Agitation
	• Fatigue
	• Tachycardia
	(CPSO, 2005)

Source: Registered Nurses' Association of Ontario. (2009). *Supporting clients on methadone maintenance treatment: Clinical Best Practice Guidelines* (p. 107, Appendix H). Toronto: Author. Retrieved from *http://rnao.ca/sites/rnao-ca/files/Supporting_Clients_on_Methadone_Maintenance_Treatment.pdf*

resulting from loss of tolerance. Health problems associated with opioid use are presented in Table 11-2.

Collaborative Care

Best outcomes are achieved with psychosocial interventions plus pharmacotherapy. Opioid dependency is a chronic and relapsing condition, and thus, a long-term treatment approach is taken (Sherbaum & Specka, 2008). Engagement in treatment affords the person the opportunity to have the time and mental and emotional resources to look at improving health, and coping.

Goals include:
• Reducing or stopping use
• Reducing current and future harms associated with use
• Improvement in quality of life and well-being of the person (WHO, 2009)

Substitution Therapy/Maintenance.
Pharmacological treatment using methadone or buprenorphine in combination with psychosocial intervention has been found to be very effective, with only 20 to 30% of people experiencing relapse or treatment failure (National Institute for Health and Clinical Evidence [NICE], 2007; Maremmani & Gerra, 2010).

Methadone. Methadone has very good outcomes for people who are opioid dependent as evidenced by treatment retention and improvements to psychosocial well-being and quality of life (Mattick, Breen, Kimber, & Davoli, 2003). Methadone is a very long-acting agonist opioid that, at the right dose, allows the

person who takes it to feel comfortable and withdrawal symptom-free for 24 hours. This is in contrast to opioids of abuse such as heroin and nonmedical prescription opioids that have a very short period of action, leading to the quick onset of withdrawal and subsequent reseeking behaviour. Numerous episodes of withdrawal throughout the day lead to the development of tolerance and a pattern of dependence (Kahan & Marsh, 2000).

People can access treatment for methadone maintenance therapy by connecting with a methadone provider/clinic. Methadone is dispensed as a liquid mixed with juice that is taken daily. Until a period of stability is achieved as evidenced by improved psychosocial functioning and abstinence from substance use, the person is dosed daily at a pharmacy. With stability, take-home doses of methadone are provided. Methadone is a potent long-acting medication that requires the person to take on responsibilities to ensure safe storage and handling of take-home doses. In the surgical setting, it is important to review the routine and medication history of the person who is taking methadone to ensure that there have been no missed doses; it is also essential to confirm when the person last took the dose, to avoid double dosing and overdosage. Upon discharge, close coordination must be undertaken to ensure that the person can resume dosing in the community to avoid any missed doses.

Methadone can be sedating; thus, people on methadone maintenance therapy should be advised to avoid sedating substances such as alcohol and benzodiazepines.

Buprenorphine. Buprenorphine has properties of being both a partial opioid agonist and an antagonist and is less sedating than methadone. It is available as a sublingual oral tablet for substitution therapy. It is taken once daily and, like methadone, allows the person to be withdrawal symptom–free at the right dose for 24 hours. Buprenorphine has a better safety profile than methadone, in that the risk of overdose is much lower, because buprenorphine binds to more receptors. Therefore, if additional other opioids are used, they have fewer receptors to bind to, thereby reducing the risk of overdosage (Handford et al., 2011).

Hallucinogens

Hallucinogens are a variety of psychoactive substances that act to produce a change in level of consciousness, alter mood, and induce hallucinations. Table 11-4 identifies common hallucinogens and their effects.

Cannabis

Characteristics

Cannabis, or marijuana, is generally the first illegal drug used by young people, and its use is more common in adolescents and young adults. Patterns of use are similar to those for alcohol in that there is occasional use, misuse resulting in temporary problems, and abuse or dependence associated with a high potential for future problems.

In Canada, cannabis is usually sold as marijuana. The key active ingredient in cannabis responsible for most of the psychoactive effects is tetrahydrocannabinol (THC). Although a number of potential benefits of THC have been reported, the only approved THC preparation is dronabinol (Marinol). Dronabinol is available by prescription to control nausea and vomiting resulting from cancer chemotherapy and to stimulate the appetite in patients with acquired immunodeficiency syndrome (AIDS) (Health Canada, 2008).

Effects of Use

At low to moderate doses, THC produces fewer physiological and psychological alterations than do other classes of psychoactive drugs, including alcohol. Although its mechanism of action is uncertain, THC affects dopamine and other neurotransmitter activity and a variety of receptors in the brain. When marijuana is smoked, effects usually occur in about 20 to 30 minutes and may last up to 7 hours. Because it is stored in body fat, it is eliminated slowly, resulting in a half-life of 2 to 7 days (Health Canada, 2008).

Marijuana produces three principal effects: euphoria, sedation, and hallucinations. The most commonly affected organs are the brain and the cardiovascular and respiratory systems. Decreased sperm production and a decrease in reproductive hormones in both men and women may occur. Signs of intoxication are presented in Table 11-4. Problems of chronic use include impaired short-term memory, decreased motor coordination, tremors, and increased heart and respiratory rates. A condition known as *amotivational syndrome* characterized by apathy, dullness, and disinterest may also occur.

Complications

Complications of marijuana use are generally mild and transient. Heavy use may cause health problems identified in Table 11-4. It may precipitate seizures in people with epilepsy, psychotic episodes in people with schizophrenia, and ketoacidosis in people with diabetes mellitus. Marijuana may also complicate pre-existing conditions in people with heart disease.

Cannabis Intoxication. In acute marijuana intoxication, the nurse should perform a physical examination, a toxicology screen, and a thorough history. The approach is basically the same for treating panic, flashbacks, and toxic reactions related to the use of marijuana or other hallucinogens. An individual with cannabis intoxication or other acute problems related to cannabis use is seldom hospitalized. The main interventions are to provide a quiet environment and to support and reassure the patient by explaining what is happening. The patient should understand that the level of intoxication may fluctuate over several days as metabolites are released.

Collaborative Care

Acute reactions, including intoxication and withdrawal, are usually mild and time limited. An individual may be treated for toxic reactions to a combination of drugs that includes marijuana or may seek treatment for panic reactions. Treatment is directed toward relief of symptoms, and the administration of drugs is avoided if possible.

Inhalants

Inhalation is the major route of ingestion for a number of common household and industrial volatile substances. Forms of use include sniffing, huffing, bagging, and spraying. Because inhalants are readily accessible, are inexpensive, and produce a rapid high, their use among preadolescents and adolescents is high.

There are four main classes of inhalants: volatile solvents, aerosols, anaesthetic agents, and nitrites. They act as CNS depressants but are also extremely damaging to the cardiovascular and respiratory systems. Common agents and their effects are presented in Table 11-4. Sudden death may result from direct toxic effects, aspiration of gastric contents, trauma, and suffocation (Dodgen & Shea, 2000).

NURSING MANAGEMENT: ADDICTIVE BEHAVIOURS

Nursing Assessment and Screening

Early recognition and identification of a patient with substance dependence is crucial to successful treatment outcomes for any health problem. Because the nurse may fail to recognize signs and symptoms of abuse in a patient who does not fit the stereotype of an "addict," and because most patients will under-report problems associated with substance use, an assessment of drug and alcohol use should be performed for all patients. The history should include questioning about the use of all substances, including prescribed medications, OTC drugs, herbal and homeopathic products, caffeine, tobacco, alcohol, and recreational drugs, noting pattern, amount, frequency of use, reasons for use, and reasons for nonuse.

Although a variety of screening tools are available, a tool that is easily used by nurses to identify alcohol dependence is the Alcohol Use Disorders Identification Test (AUDIT) (Table 11-18). A person with a score of 8 points or less is considered to not have problematic use, whereas 9 points or above suggests problematic use and warrants further assessment. Another instrument frequently used is the CAGE (cut down, annoy, guilt, eye-opener drinks) questionnaire (Table 11-19). In addition, if the patient provides information concerning drug use that is inconsistent with assessment findings, the nurse should question the patient further. It must be emphasized that screening is not diagnostic or equivalent to a comprehensive assessment because it serves only to trigger the screener to need to assess further for a potential problematic pattern.

Physical assessment also reveals clues about substance use. The nurse must be alert to signs and symptoms of the many health problems associated with substance use that may be apparent during the physical examination. Assessment of the patient's general appearance and nutritional status, and examination of the abdomen, the skin, and the cardiovascular, respiratory, and neurological systems, often reflect problems associated with substance use.

Nursing Diagnoses

Nursing diagnoses for the patient in alcohol withdrawal may include, but are not limited to, those presented in Nursing Care Plan 11-1. In addition, other nursing diagnoses for an individual with substance use may include, but are not limited to, the following:

- Impaired coping related to negative consequences of substance use.

Table 11-18 Alcohol Use Disorders Identification Test (AUDIT)

PLEASE ANSWER EACH QUESTION BY CHECKING ONE OF THE CIRCLES IN THE SECOND COLUMN.		SCORE	PLEASE ANSWER EACH QUESTION BY CHECKING ONE OF THE CIRCLES IN THE SECOND COLUMN.		SCORE
1. How often do you have a drink containing alcohol?	○ Never	(0)	6. How often during the last year have you needed a first drink in the morning to get yourself going after a heavy drinking session?	○ Never	(0)
	○ Monthly or less	(1)		○ Less than monthly	(1)
	○ 2-4 times/mo	(2)		○ Monthly	(2)
	○ 2-4 times/wk	(3)		○ Weekly	(3)
	○ 4+ times/wk	(4)		○ Daily or almost daily	(4)
2. How many drinks containing alcohol do you have on a typical day when you are drinking?	○ 1 or 2	(0)	7. How often during the last year have you had a feeling of guilt or remorse about drinking?	○ Never	(0)
	○ 3 or 4	(1)		○ Less than monthly	(1)
	○ 5 or 6	(2)		○ Monthly	(2)
	○ 7 to 9	(3)		○ Weekly	(3)
	○ 10 or more	(4)		○ Daily or almost daily	(4)
3. How often do you have six or more drinks on one occasion?	○ Never	(0)	8. How often during the last year have you been unable to remember what happened the night before because you had been drinking?	○ Never	(0)
	○ Less than monthly	(1)		○ Less than monthly	(1)
	○ Monthly	(2)		○ Monthly	(2)
	○ Weekly	(3)		○ Weekly	(3)
	○ Daily or almost daily	(4)		○ Daily or almost daily	(4)
4. How often during the last year have you found that you were not able to stop drinking once you had started?	○ Never	(0)	9. Have you or someone else been injured as a result of your drinking?	○ No	(0)
	○ Less than monthly	(1)		○ Yes, but not in the last year	(2)
	○ Monthly	(2)			(4)
	○ Weekly	(3)		○ Yes, during the last year	
	○ Daily or almost daily	(4)			
5. How often in the last year have you failed to do what was normally expected of you because you were drinking?	○ Never	(0)	10. Has a relative, friend, doctor, or other health worker been concerned about your drinking or suggested that you cut down?	○ No	(0)
	○ Less than monthly	(1)		○ Yes, but not in the last year	(2)
	○ Monthly	(2)			(4)
	○ Weekly	(3)		○ Yes, during the last year	
	○ Daily or almost daily	(4)			

Scoring for AUDIT: Questions 1 through 8 are scored 0, 1, 2, 3, or 4. Questions 9 and 10 are scored 0, 2, or 4 only. The minimum score (nondrinkers) is 0, and the maximum possible score is 40. A score of 9 or more indicates hazardous or harmful alcohol consumption.
Source: Saunders, J. B., Aasland, O., Babor, T. F., de la Fuente, J., & Grant, M. (1993). Development of the Alcohol Use Disorders Screening Test (AUDIT), WHO collaborative project on early detection of persons with harmful alcohol consumption. II. *Addiction, 88,* 791. doi:10.1111/j.1360-0443.1993.tb02093.x

- Impaired thought processes related to drug or alcohol consumption.
- Risk for infection related to IV drug use or high-risk behaviours in the context of active substance use.
- Impaired nutrition: less than body requirements related to lack of nutritional intake.
- Ineffective health maintenance related to progression of substance use.
- Family strain and relationship difficulty related to substance use by significant member.

▮ Planning

Essential to the nursing care of people with whom substance use is routine, early screening and assessment of substance use is a

standard of practice across all practice settings with all patients, because the risk of overlooking or not screening for substance use is a critical aspect that can increase unforeseen adverse outcomes to the health intervention at hand. In addition, nurses need to have the capacity to be able to effectively assess for, manage, and evaluate patients experiencing intoxication, overdose, and withdrawal syndromes because these clinical situations will arise in all settings, from the emergency department to a surgical environment. But most importantly, the positive nonjudgemental and supportive engagement and therapeutic dialogue that take place as nurses provide assessment, intervention, and management of substance use–related health sequelae are fundamental in increasing health outcomes for the person experiencing substance use–related health problems. Involving and including family members in the planning of the patient's care that is directed by the patient's choice is very important in supporting best outcomes for the patient.

Table 11-19 CAGE Questionnaire Adapted to Include Drugs (CAGE AID)

Have you felt you ought to cut down on your drinking *(or drug use)*?

_____Yes _____No

Have people annoyed you by criticizing your drinking *(or drug use)*?

_____Yes _____No

Have you felt bad or guilty about your drinking *(or drug use)*?

_____Yes _____No

Have you ever had a drink (or used drugs) first thing in the morning to steady your nerves or get rid of a hangover *(or to get the day started)*?

_____Yes _____No

Note: In the general population, two or more positive answers indicates a need for a more in-depth assessment.
Source: Fleming, M. F., & Barry, K. L. (1992). *Addictive disorders.* St. Louis: Mosby; and Ewing, J. A. (1984). Detecting alcoholism: The CAGE questionnaire. *Journal of the American Medical Association, 252,* 1905-1907. doi:10.1001/jama.1984.03350140051025

Table 11-20 Key Aspects of Successful Motivational Interviewing

- Express empathy.
- Provide positive reinforcement and encouragement for gains made by the patient.
- Listen rather than tell.
- Gently persuade, with the understanding that change is up to the patient.
- Develop discrepancy between patient's goals or values and current behaviour, helping the patient recognize the discrepancies between where he or she is and where he or she hopes to be.
- Avoid argument and direct confrontation, which can cause defensiveness and a power struggle.
- Adjust to, rather than oppose, patient resistance.
- Focus on the patient's strengths to support the hope and optimism needed to make changes.

Nursing Implementation

Health Promotion

Prevention of substance use problems and addictive behaviours includes primary, secondary, and tertiary prevention. Primary prevention targets primarily adolescents and young adults with education about effects, negative outcomes, and effects of continued use of addictive substances. Secondary prevention focuses on early detection of substance use, interventions through peer or employee assistance programs, and continuing education about substance-free alternatives and stress management techniques. Tertiary prevention occurs when individuals have established dependence and includes motivating individuals to enter addiction treatment and referral to treatment and relapse prevention programs.

Motivational Interviewing: Engaging in a Supportive Dialogue With People With Problematic Substance Use

The nurse is in a unique position to motivate and facilitate behaviour change while caring for patients in primary and acute care settings. When patients seek care for health problems related to substance use or when hospitalization interferes with the patient's normal use of substances, the patient's awareness of problems associated with addictive behaviours is increased. Intervention by nurses at this time can be a crucial factor in promoting behaviour change.

Motivational interviewing is a directive, patient-centred counselling style for eliciting behaviour change by helping patients to explore and resolve ambivalence (Rollnick & Miller, 1995) that can be effectively used by nurses. Motivational interviewing uses nonconfrontational interpersonal communication techniques to motivate patients to change behaviour by eliciting the patient to talk about her or his substance use. As such, the key aspect is that the patient is able to hear herself or himself speak and gain awareness of her or his views and values of her or his substance use. The role of the nurse is to listen and reflect back to the person what she or he is saying, bring to light positive change talk, and recognize that ambivalence is normal and expected when anyone is confronted with having to make a change.

The stages of change identified in the **transtheoretical model of change** include precontemplation, contemplation, preparation, action, maintenance, and termination (Prochaska & Velicer, 1997), as described in Chapter 4. The stages are not viewed as linear but, rather, as a cycle through which patients move back and forth. During the process of change, relapse and small **lapses** are part of the journey and are a normal aspect of behaviour change. Patients who do not change behaviours or who return to substance use after a period of cessation are often labelled "noncompliant" and "unmotivated." However, this development may reflect a normal relapse or may indicate that the interventions used do not consider the patient's stage of change. Therefore, it is important for the nurse to identify the patient's current stage of readiness for change and the stage to which the patient is moving. Patients who are in the early stages of change need and use different kinds of motivational support from those of patients at later stages of change.

Motivational interviewing includes the use of any intervention that enhances the patient's motivation for change. The interventions are those that respect the patient's autonomy and establish a nonjudgemental, collaborative relationship (Canadian Network of Substance Abuse and Allied Professionals, 2007). The key aspects of successful motivational interviewing are presented in Table 11-20.

In the precontemplation stage, patients are not concerned about their substance use and are not considering changing their behaviour. For example, when asked whether smoking contributes to his or her shortness of breath, the patient denies any connection because "I never had it before and I've smoked for years." During this stage, it is most important for the nurse to help the patient increase awareness of risks and problems related to the current behaviour and to create doubt about the use of substances (Canadian Network of Substance Abuse and Allied Professionals, 2007). Asking what the patient thinks could happen if the behaviour is continued, providing evidence of the problem such as abnormal laboratory values, and offering factual information about the risks of substance use are important strategies. Although patients may not be ready to change behaviour while experiencing an acute health problem, the seeds of doubt can be sown. In other cases, such as when a patient experiences a life-threatening condition, there may be an immediate awareness of the problem and motivation to change.

A patient in the contemplation stage of change often experiences ambivalence. The patient understands that the behaviour is a problem and that change is necessary, yet feels that change is too difficult or that the pleasures of continuing the behaviour are worth the risks. This can be seen in the patient who says, "I know that I have to stop drinking. This car accident almost killed me. And one more traffic ticket while I'm intoxicated means I'll lose my licence. But all my friends drink, and it is the only way I can relax. I don't think I can do it." During this stage of change, the nurse should help the patient thoughtfully consider the positive and the negative aspects of the substance use, gently trying to tip the balance in favour of beneficial behaviour. Helping the patient discover internal motivators in addition to those external motivators (e.g., accidents, traffic tickets, legal and health problems, costs) that push the patient toward change can move the patient from contemplating change to preparation and action. Summarizing the patient's concerns and affirming the patient's ambivalence are useful techniques. Throughout this process, the patient's personal choices and responsibilities for change should be emphasized (Canadian Network of Substance Abuse and Allied Professionals, 2007).

As the patient moves from contemplation to preparation, a commitment to change can be strengthened by helping the patient develop self-efficacy. Self-efficacy in this case is the patient's optimism that substance use behaviours can be changed, and the nurse should support even the smallest effort to change. Movement through action and maintenance stages of change requires continued support to increase the patient's involvement and participation in treatment.

The resolution of acute health problems or discharge from the hospital often occurs before the patient moves to the preparation and action stages of change. It is critical that, as the patient develops readiness to change in the contemplative stage of change, the continuation of the change process be supported by referral to appropriate community and outpatient resources.

◼ Ambulatory and Home Care

Before treatment and rehabilitation for addiction are considered, acute health problems must be resolved. Many of the patients with substance use problems who the nurse encounters in hospitals and primary care centres seek care because of health problems associated with substance use, not to receive care for the addiction. It is the nurse's responsibility, in collaboration with physicians, social workers, and addiction specialists, to address the patient's substance problem and motivate the patient to change behaviours and seek treatment for the addiction. Although the nurse working in the medical–surgical setting is not usually involved in long-term treatment of patients with addictive behaviours, it is the nurse's responsibility to identify the problem, increase the patient's awareness of the problem, and to refer the patient to inpatient and outpatient programs in the community that provide treatment and rehabilitation. Failure to confront the patient's addiction, thus enabling the patient's addictive behaviour, is a breach of professional responsibility.

ETHICAL DILEMMAS
Duty to Report

Situation

A patient who has been treated for severe alcohol withdrawal complications discloses to you that he is a long-distance truck driver and has been working for the past 10 years. As part of your substance use assessment, it appears that he has developed high tolerance to alcohol with daily consumption with short periods of abstinence since his divorce last year. He had no previous substance use history or problematic substance use before last year.

Important Points for Consideration

- Nurses have an ethical obligation to prevent harm to patients and the public.
- Nurses are responsible to communicate concerns regarding harms to the patient as well as communicating them to the patient's team of health care providers.
- Being knowledgeable about the legal reporting obligations regarding driver licensing for each province is key.

Clinical Decision-Making Questions

1. How should the nurses handle this situation?
2. What are the provisions of your province's legal reporting obligations regarding impaired driving?

AGE-RELATED CONSIDERATIONS

Substance misuse and substance use in older adults are much less likely to be recognized by nurses and other health care providers than in younger adults. Older adults do not fit the image that people in today's society have of those who abuse substances. In addition, patterns of substance use in older adults are considerably different from those in younger and middle-aged adults. Because alcohol and substance use among older adults is often mistaken for other conditions (e.g., neuropathy, anemia, mental status changes) associated with the aging process, the problem is often undiagnosed and untreated.

Although illicit drug use is minimal in older adults, older adults have the highest use of OTC and prescription drugs (Ramage-Morin, 2009). The prescription drugs used by older adults are primarily psychoactive in nature, including sedative, hypnotic, anxiolytic, and opioid agents. Older women are more likely than men to become dependent on prescription drugs, especially benzodiazepines (Voyer, Cohen, Lauzon, & Collin, 2004). Simultaneous use of OTC drugs, prescription drugs, and alcohol occurs in many older adults. This presents a pattern of drug misuse and abuse that is not commonly seen in younger populations.

The effects of alcohol and other psychoactive substances increase with aging. Age-related decreases in circulation, metabolism, and excretion slow the body's detoxification of drugs, potentiate tolerance, and accelerate **physical dependence** (physiological adaptation to ongoing exposure such that use and cessation cause an expected physiological response). Physiological changes that accompany aging may lead to intoxication at levels of intake that may not have been a problem earlier in life.

The adverse effects of interaction of alcohol and other drugs also increase with aging. When taken with alcohol, sedative–hypnotic drugs, minor tranquilizers, and CNS depressants have additive and synergistic effects. Misuse and abuse of psychoactive agents, either alone or in combination, by older adults may cause confusion, disorientation, delirium, memory loss, and neuromuscular impairment. The effects of alcohol and drug use can also be mistaken for medical or psychiatric conditions common among older adults, such as insomnia, depression, poor nutrition, heart failure, and frequent falls. Withdrawal symptoms also occur in the older adult when alcohol, opioids, or sedative–hypnotics are abruptly stopped and may be more severe than in younger individuals. Because of the possibility of alcohol use in older adults, the nurse should always consider that behaviour changes in the older patient may be caused by alcohol use or withdrawal.

Identification of substance misuse, abuse, and dependence in the older patient presents a challenge. Family members who are concerned about a patient's possible problem are important sources of information. Evidence of addictive disorders is not always obvious in the older adult, and manifestations may be similar to those caused by common health problems of the elderly. As with all patients, it is important for the nurse to discuss all drug and alcohol use with older patients, including OTC, herbal, and homeopathic drug use. The patient's knowledge of medications that are currently being taken should be assessed.

Questionnaires customarily used to screen for alcoholism such as the AUDIT have been found to be not as accurate in screening for problematic use in older adults (Alto, Alho, Halme, & Seppa, 2011). Screening tools such as the Short Michigan Alcohol Screening Test—Geriatric Version (MAST-G) have been shown to fare better in screening for alcohol-related health consequences in the older adult population (Naegle, 2008).

It is important to screen for warning signs such as unexplained falls, neglect of personal hygiene, and complaints of mood, sleep, or memory problems.

Smoking and other tobacco use is also an issue in older adults. Older adults who have been chronic smokers for decades can feel unable to stop or may feel that there is no benefit to stopping at an advanced age. However, smoking contributes to and exacerbates many chronic illnesses found in the older population, and smoking cessation at any age is beneficial. In fact, many older adults want to quit smoking.

Patient education for the older adult includes teaching about the desired effects, possible adverse effects, and appropriate use of prescribed and OTC drugs. The nurse should recommend that the patient use only one pharmacy because many pharmacies maintain a drug profile on each individual that may prevent problems with drug interactions. Patients should be advised not to drink alcohol when using prescribed and OTC drugs. Where there is no medical condition or possible drug interaction that would preclude the use of alcohol, older patients should be advised to limit their alcohol intake to one drink per day.

Developmental, physical, and psychosocial changes that occur with aging contribute to the late-onset abuse of alcohol and other drugs by older adults. The older adult may have difficulty coping with losses that occur with increasing age, such as retirement, death of family and friends, relocation, social isolation, and poor health.

Knowing that older people may respond to the stresses of age with alcohol or drug use, the nurse should monitor people who are experiencing losses and identify those who are having difficulty coping. When risks are noted, these individuals can be taught coping skills and introduced to support services. Home visits by a nurse provide a good source of assessment of the problems and also provide valuable support. When the nurse suspects an alcohol or substance dependence in the older patient, the nurse should refer the patient for treatment. It is a mistaken belief that older people have little to gain from alcohol and drug dependence treatment. The rewards of treatment can lead to greater quality and quantity of life for older adults.

CLINICAL DECISION-MAKING EXERCISE

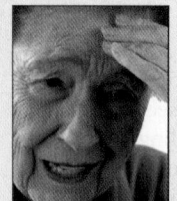

CASE STUDY:
Substance Misuse and Abuse

Source: © iStockphoto.com/Lisa Kyle Young.

Patient Profile

Mrs. Carla Muller, a 78-year-old woman, is admitted to the emergency department after falling and injuring her right shoulder and arm. She has been widowed for 4 years and lives alone. Recently, her best friend died. Her only family is a daughter who lives out of town. When the nurse contacts the daughter by phone, she tells the nurse that her mother has appeared to become more disoriented and confused over the past year when she has talked to her on the phone.

Subjective Data

- Is complaining of severe pain in her right shoulder and upper arm.
- Admits she had some wine in the late afternoon to stimulate her appetite.
- Has experienced several falls in the past 2 months.
- Reports that she fell after taking her sleeping pill, prescribed by her physician because she does not sleep well.
- Speech is hesitant and slurred.
- Says she smokes about half a pack of cigarettes a day.

Objective Data

Physical Examination

- Oriented to person and place, but not time.
- Blood pressure 162/94, pulse 92, respirations 24.
- Bruising and edema of right upper arm.
- Tremors of hands.

Diagnostic Tests

- Radiographic examination reveals comminuted fracture of the proximal humerus necessitating surgical repair.
- Blood alcohol concentration (BAC) 26 mmol/L (0.12 mg %).
- Complete blood count: hemoglobin 106 g/L hematocrit 0.38 (38%).

Discussion Questions

1. What other information is needed to assess Mrs. Muller's condition?
2. How should questions regarding these areas be addressed?
3. What factors may contribute to Mrs. Muller's use of psychoactive substances?
4. *Priority Decision:* What priority nursing interventions are appropriate during Mrs. Muller's preoperative period?
5. What possible complications and other health problems may become apparent during Mrs. Muller's postoperative recovery?
6. What nursing interventions are appropriate following Mrs. Muller's surgery?
7. *Priority Decision:* Based on the assessment data presented, what are the priority nursing diagnoses for Mrs. Muller? Are there any collaborative problems?

evolve *Answers are available at* **http://evolve.elsevier.com/ Canada/Lewis/medsurg**

REVIEW QUESTIONS

The number of the question corresponds to the same-numbered objective at the beginning of the chapter.

1. Which of these statements is true?
   a. Only a small percentage of Canadians are affected by substance use issues.
   b. Tobacco is the leading cause of preventable morbidity and mortality.
   c. The highest incidence of substance use is among youth.
   d. Substance use is more prevalent in urban areas.

2. What term best describes a pattern of compulsive, continued use of a substance despite significant personal harms and withdrawal syndromes?
   a. Abuse
   b. Substance dependence
   c. Tolerance
   d. Addictive behaviour

3. When engaging a patient experiencing substance use or dependency, which of the following is the nursing intervention based on?
   a. A comprehensive and thorough screening and assessment of substance use.
   b. A holistic biopsychosocial approach to care.
   c. Nonjudgemental, collaborative therapeutic relationship that honours patient autonomy and choice.
   d. Assessment of safety concerns and stabilization of acute illness.

4. When using a harm-reduction approach with patients experiencing substance use problems, what is the key aim of the nurse?
   a. To provide harm-reduction supplies and health teaching.
   b. Not to coerce or force the individual to quit his or her substance use.
   c. To ensure that patients have access to health care services.
   d. To reduce the harms associated with substance use.

5. When screening and assessing for substance use, which of the following are some key aspects to cover?
   a. Use of substances, pattern of use, route, frequency of use, and date and time of last use.
   b. Medical history and psychiatric history.
   c. Social supports.
   d. Legal history.

6. What is a long-term effect of addictive substances on the brain?
   a. Increased availability of dopamine
   b. Destruction of the mesolimbic system
   c. Loss of pleasure from experiences that previously resulted in enjoyment
   d. Potentiation of effects of similar drugs taken when the individual is drug free

7. Which of the following is the most appropriate nursing intervention for a patient who is seen at the clinic for increasing shortness of breath but who is not interested in quitting smoking?
   a. Accept the patient's decision and do not intervene until the patient expresses a desire to quit.
   b. Realize that some smokers will never quit and that trying to assist them only increases the patient's and the nurse's frustration.
   c. Increase the patient's motivation to quit by explaining that continued smoking will only increase the breathing problems.
   d. Ask the patient at every clinic visit to identify the relevance, the risks, and the benefits of quitting and what barriers to quitting are present.

8. Which of the following would suggest to the nurse that a patient is experiencing a cocaine overdose?
   a. Craving, restlessness, and irritability
   b. Agitation, cardiac dysrhythmia, and seizures
   c. Diarrhea, nausea and vomiting, and confusion
   d. Slow, shallow respirations, hyporeflexia, and blurred vision

9. A patient who is dependent on IV barbiturates is scheduled for surgery following an automobile accident. What is important for the nurse to recognize in this case?
   a. The patient may need less pain medication during the postoperative period.
   b. The patient should be provided with tapering doses of barbiturates following surgery.
   c. The patient may have an immediate onset of withdrawal symptoms when given anaesthetic and analgesic agents.
   d. The patient has a low risk for physical withdrawal symptoms but is likely to experience craving and drug-seeking behaviour during the postoperative period.

10. Which of the following is important in pain management of patients dependent on opioids or other CNS depressants?
    a. Realize the goal is to treat acute pain.
    b. Avoid treating the pain.
    c. Understand that opioid analgesia may worsen an addictive disease.
    d. Addiction treatment remains a priority while the patient is in pain.

11. In which of the following behaviours should the nurse engage during motivational interviewing with a patient?
    a. Insist that the patient maintain abstinence while undergoing therapy.
    b. Relate motivational techniques to the patient's stage of behaviour change.
    c. Use any method of communication that will make the patient change behaviour.
    d. Ask a prescribed set of questions to increase the patient's awareness of addiction behaviours.

12. To which factors are substance use problems in older adults most commonly related?
    a. Use of drugs and alcohol as a social activity
    b. Misuse of prescribed and OTC drugs and alcohol
    c. Continued use of illegal drugs initiated during middle age
    d. A pattern of binge drinking for weeks or months with periods of sobriety

ANSWERS: 1. b; 2. b; 3. c; 4. d; 5. a; 6. c; 7. d; 8. b; 9. b; 10. a; 11. b; 12. b.

REFERENCES

Alford, D. P., Compton, P., & Samet, J. H. (2006). Acute pain management for patients receiving maintenance methadone or buprenorphine therapy. *Annals of Internal Medicine, 144*, 127-134.

Alto, M., Alho, H., Halme, J. T., & Seppa, K. (2011). The Alcohol Use Disorders Identification Test (AUDIT) and its derivatives in screening for heavy drinking among the elderly. *International Journal of Geriatric Psychiatry, 26*, 881-885. doi:10.1002/gps.2498.

Bialous, S. A., & Sarna, L. (2004). Sparing a few minutes for tobacco cessation. *American Journal of Nursing, 104*(12), 61-62.

Bierness, D. J., Jesseman, R., Notarandrea, R., & Perron, M. (2008). *Harm reduction: What's in a name?* Ottawa: Canadian Centre on Substance Abuse. Retrieved from *http://www.ccsa.ca/2008%20 CCSA%20Documents2/ccsa0115302008e.pdf*

Canada Safety Council. (2009). Canada's blood alcohol laws—An international perspective. Retrieved from *http://canadasafety council.org/sites/default/files/PDF_en/bac_study-2009-final.pdf*

Canadian Centre on Substance Abuse. (2011). Canadian Addiction Survey (CAS). Retrieved from *http://www.ccsa.ca/eng/priorities/ research/canadianaddiction/pages/default.aspx*

Canadian Lung Association. (2008a). Facts about smoking. Retrieved from *http://www.lung.ca/protect-protegez/tobacco-tabagisme/facts-faits/index_e.php#truth*

Canadian Lung Association. (2008b). Our kids deserve it: Lung Association launches national push for smoke-free cars. Retrieved from *http://www.newswire.ca/en/releases/archive/January 2008/23/c3135.html*

Canadian Lung Association. (2012). What's in cigarettes? Retrieved from *http://www.lung.ca/protect-protegez/tobacco-tabagisme/facts-faits/what-que_e.php*

Canadian Network of Substance Abuse and Allied Professionals. (2007). Motivational interviewing. Retrieved from *http://www. cnsaap.ca/cnsaap/ProfessionalToolkits/Motivational+Interviewing ?Language=EN*

Canadian Nurses Association (CNA). (2011). *Harm reduction & criminally illegal drugs: Implications for nursing policy, practice, education and research.* Ottawa: Author.

Carroll, I. R., Angst, M. S., & Clark, J. D. (2004). Management of perioperative pain in patients chronically consuming opioids. *Regional Anesthesia and Pain Medicine, 29*, 576-591. doi:10.1016/j. rapm.2004.06.009

Centre for Addiction and Mental Health (CAMH). (2006). Information about crystal meth. Retrieved from *http://www.camh.net/ About_Addiction_Mental_Health/Drug_and_Addiction_Information/ crystal_meth_information.html*

Centre for Addiction and Mental Health. (2007). *ED management of methadone overdose.* Toronto: Centre for Addiction and Mental Health.

College of Physicians and Surgeons of Ontario. (2005). *Methadone Maintenance Guidelines.* Toronto: College of Physicians and Surgeons of Ontario. Retrieved from *http://www.cpso.on.ca/publica-tions/MethadoneGuideNov05.pdf*

Department of Health (England) and the Devolved Administrations. (2007). *Drug misuse and dependence: UK guidelines on clinical management.* London: Department of Health (England), the Scottish Government, Welsh Assembly Government, and Northern Ireland Executive. Retrieved from *http://www.nta.nhs.uk/ publications/documents/clinical_guidelines_2007.pdf*

Dodgen, C. E., & Shea, W. M. (2000). *Substance use disorders: Assessment and treatment.* San Diego, CA: Academic.

Fischer, B., Rehm, J., Patra, J., & Cruz, M. F. (2006). Changes in illicit opioid use across Canada. *Canadian Medical Association Journal, 175*, 1351. doi:10.1503/cmaj.060729

Gitlow, S. (2007). *Substance use disorders: A practical guide* (2nd ed.). Philadelphia: Lippincott Williams & Wilkins.

Handford, C., Kahan, M., Srivastava, A., Cirone, S., Sanghera, S., Palda, V., ... Selby, P. (2011). *Buprenorphine/naloxone for opioid dependence: Clinical practice guideline.* Toronto: Centre for Addiction and Mental Health.

Health Canada. (2007a). *Smoking and your body—Pregnancy.* Ottawa: Author. Retrieved from *http://www.hc-sc.gc.ca/hc-ps/tobac-tabac/ body-corps/preg-gros-eng.php*

Health Canada. (2007b). *Smoking in Canada: An overview.* Ottawa: Author. Retrieved from *http://www.hc-sc.gc.ca/hl-vs/ tobactabac/research-recherche/stat/_ctums-esutc_fs-if/2003-smokfum-eng.php*

Health Canada. (2007c). *Notice of decision for Champix.* Ottawa: Author. Retrieved from *http://www.hc-sc.gc.ca/dhp-mps/prodpharma/ sbd-smd/phase1-decision/drug-med/nd_ad_2007_champix_104007-eng.php*

Health Canada. (2008). *Medical use of marihuana: Information for health care professionals.* Ottawa: Author. Retrieved from *http:// www.hc-sc.gc.ca/dhp-mps/marihuana/how-comment/medpract/ infoprof/clinical-clinique-eng.php*

Health Canada. (2009). *Health concerns: Smoking and your body: Addiction.* Ottawa: Author. Retrieved from *http://www.hc-sc.gc.ca/hc-ps/ tobac-tabac/body-corps/addiction-dependance-eng.php*

Health Canada. (2011a). Canadian Alcohol and Drug Use Monitoring Survey: Summary of Results for 2010. Retrieved from *http:// www.hc-sc.gc.ca/hc-ps/drugs-drogues/stat/_2010/summary-sommaire-eng.php*

Health Canada. (2011b). *Canadian Tobacco Use Monitoring Survey (CTUMS): Summary of annual results for 2010*. Ottawa: Author. Retrieved from *http://www.hc-sc.gc.ca/hc-ps/tobac-tabac/research-recherche/stat/_ctums-esutc_2010/ann_summary-sommaire-eng.php*

Herie, M., & Skinner, W. (2010). *Substance abuse in Canada*. Toronto: Oxford University Press.

Johnson, B. A. (2004). The biologic basis of alcohol dependence. *Advanced Studies in Medicine, 2*, 48-53.

Kahan, M. (2000). Alcohol: Metabolism and acute effects. In B. Brands, M. Kahan, P. Selby, & L. Wilson (Eds.), *Management of alcohol, tobacco and other drug problems: A physician's manual* (pp. 71-75). Toronto: Centre for Addiction and Mental Health.

Kahan, M., & Marsh, D. (2000). Intoxication, overdose and withdrawal. In B. Brands, M. Kahan, P. Selby, & L. Wilson (Eds.), *Management of alcohol, tobacco and other drug problems: A physician's manual* (pp. 225-233). Toronto: Centre for Addiction and Mental Health.

Kahan, M., & Wilson, L. (2002). *Managing alcohol, tobacco and other drug problems: A pocket guide for physicians and nurses*. Toronto: Centre for Addiction and Mental Health.

Kahan, M., Srivastava, A., Wilson, L., Gourlay, D., Midmer, D. (2006). Misuse of and dependence on opioids: Study of chronic pain patients. *Canadian Family Physician, 52*, 1081-1087.

Kosten, T. R., & O'Connor, P. G. (2003). Management of drug and alcohol withdrawal. *New England Journal of Medicine, 348*, 1786-1795. doi:10.1056/NEJMra020617

Maremmani, I., & Gerra, G. (2010). Buprenorphine-based regimens and methadone for the medical management of opioid dependence: Selecting the appropriate drug for treatment. *American Journal on Addictions, 19*, 557-68.

Mattick, R. P., Breen, C., Kimber, J., & Davoli, M. (2003[Rev. 2009]). Methadone maintenance therapy versus no opioid replacement therapy for opioid dependence. *Cochrane Database Syst Rev, 2*, CD002209; Cochrane Database of Systematic Reviews.

Naegle, M. (2008). Screening for alcohol use and misuse in older adults: Using the short Michigan alcoholism screening test—Geriatric version. *American Journal of Nursing, 108*(11), 50-58. doi:10.1097/01.NAJ.0000339100.32362.d9

National Institute for Health and Clinical Evidence (NICE). (2007). Methadone and buprenorphine for the management of opioid dependence. Retrieved from *http://www.nice.org.uk/nicemedia/live/11606/33833/33833.pdf*

O'Hara, J., & Patel, J. (2006). Smoking cessation. In V. P. Arcangelo & A. M. Peterson (Eds.), *Pharmacotherapeutics for advanced practice: A practical approach*. Philadelphia: Lippincott Williams & Wilkins.

Prochaska, J. O., & Velicer, W. F. (1997). The transtheoretical model of health behaviour change. *American Journal of Health Promotion, 12*, 38-48. doi:10.4278/0890-1171-12.1.38

Ramage-Morin, P. L. (2009). *Medication use among senior Canadians (Cat. no. 82-003-X)*. Ottawa: Statistics Canada. Retrieved from *http://www.statcan.gc.ca/pub/82-003-x/2009001/article/10801-eng.pdf*

Registered Nurses Association of Ontario (RNAO). (2007). *Integrating smoking cessation into daily nursing practice: Nursing Best Practices Guideline*. Toronto: RNAO.

Rehm, J., Baliunas, D., Brochu, S., Fischer, B., Gnam, W., Patra, J., et al. (2006). *The costs of substance abuse in Canada 2002*. Ottawa: Canadian Centre on Substance Abuse. Retrieved from *http://www.ccsa.ca/2006%20CCSA%20Documents/ccsa-011332-2006.pdf*

Reiss, R., Fiellin, D. A., Miller, S. C., & Scutz, R. (2009). (Eds). *Principles of addiction medicine* (4th ed.). Philadelphia: Wolters Kluwer/Lippincott Williams & Wilkins.

Rollnick, S., & Miller, W. R. (1995). What is motivational interviewing? *Behavioural and Cognitive Psychotherapy, 23*, 325-334. doi:10.1017/S135246580001643X

Sherbaum, N., & Specka, M. (2008). Factors influencing the course of opiate addiction. *International Journal of Methods in Psychiatric Research, 17*(Suppl), S39-S44.

Shuckit, M. A. (2006). *Drug and alcohol abuse: A clinical guide to diagnosis and treatment* (6th ed.). New York: Springer Science and Business Media.

Voyer, P., Cohen, D., Lauzon, S., & Collin, J. (2004). Factors associated with psychotropic drug use among community-dwelling older persons: A review of empirical studies. *BMC Nursing, 3*, 3. doi:10.1186/1472-6955-3-3

World Health Organization (WHO). (2008). *Tobacco-free initiative: Cancer*. Geneva: Author. Retrieved from *http://www.who.int/tobacco/research/cancer/en/index.html*

World Health Organization (WHO). (2009). Guidelines for the psychosocially assisted pharmacological treatment of opioid dependence. Geneva: Author. Retrieved from *http://www.who.int/substance_abuse/publications/opioid_dependence_guidelines.pdf*

CANADIAN RESOURCES

Canadian Cancer Society
http://www.cancer.ca/?sc_lang=en
Canadian Centre on Substance Abuse (CCSA)
http://www.ccsa.ca
Canadian Foundation for Drug Policy
http://www.cfdp.ca
Canadian Institute for Health Information
http://www.cihi.ca
Canadian Network of Substance Abuse and Allied Professionals
http://www.cnsaap.ca
Centre for Addiction and Mental Health
http://www.camh.net
Program Training and Consultation Centre
http://www.ptcc-cfc.on.ca
Project Create
http://www.addictionmedicine.ca
Public Health Agency of Canada: Substance Use/Addictions
http://www.phac-aspc.gc.ca/chn-rcs/saa-toxicomanie-eng.php
Registered Nurses' Association of Ontario (RNAO) Best Practice Guideline: Integrating Smoking Cessation into Daily Nursing Practice
http://rnao.ca/sites/rnao-ca/files/Integrating_Smoking_Cessation_into_Daily_Nursing_Practice.pdf
Appendix D: The Benefits of Quitting Smoking
Appendix H: Ask, Advise, Assist, Arrange Protocol
Appendix L: Quit Smoking First-Line Medications Compared
The Lung Association
http://www.lung.ca

RELATED RESOURCES

Alcoholics Anonymous
http://www.alcoholics-anonymous.org
Division of Public Health and Primary Health Care
http://www.dphpc.ox.ac.uk
International Nurses Society on Addictions
http://www.intnsa.org
Narcotics Anonymous
http://www.na.org
WHO Department of Mental Health and Substance Dependence
http://www.who.int/mental_health

evolve *For additional Internet resources, see the Web site for this book at* **http://evolve.elsevier.com/Canada/Lewis/medsurg**

12

Complementary and Alternative Therapies

Written by Virginia (Jennie) Shaw

Adapted by Linda Byrnes

LEARNING OBJECTIVES

1. Describe commonly used complementary and alternative therapies.
2. List indications for the use of traditional Chinese medicine (TCM).
3. Describe the general types of herbal therapy and indications for their use.
4. List concepts to be included in patient teaching with regard to herbal supplements.

5. Describe the practice of holistic nursing.
6. Describe the process of assessing patients' use of complementary and alternative therapies.
7. Describe the roles of the nurse in integrating complementary and alternative therapies into nursing practice.

KEY TERMS

acupuncture A family of procedures involving stimulation of anatomical points on the body by a variety of techniques, including the penetration of the skin with thin, solid, metallic needles that are manipulated by the hands or by electrical stimulation, p. 218

alternative therapies Therapies used as the primary treatment instead of traditional Western health practices, p. 217

complementary therapies Therapies used alongside traditional Western health practices recommended by a person's health care provider, p. 217

healing touch A biofield therapy that encompasses a group of noninvasive techniques that utilize the hands to clear, energize, and balance the human and environmental energy fields, p. 224

herbal therapy The use of individual herbs or combinations of herbs for therapeutic benefit to treat, prevent, or cure disease, p. 220

holistic nursing Nursing practice that incorporates mind–body–spirit principles into the development of a caring/healing relationship with patients, p. 226

massage therapy Therapy involving the manipulation of soft tissues and joints of the body to improve health and promote healing, p. 221

prayer A form of communication or fellowship with a divine entity or the sacred, p. 225

therapeutic touch A method of detecting and balancing human energy, p. 224

traditional Chinese medicine A treatment modality based on restoring and maintaining the balance of vital energy (Qi); interventions include acupressure, acupuncture, Chinese herbology, cupping, moxibustion, nutrition, meditation, Tai Chi, and Qi gong, p. 217

ELECTRONIC RESOURCES

Supplemental content related to Chapter 12 can be found...

Evolve Web Site ⊖volve

http://evolve.elsevier.com/Canada/Lewis/medsurg
• Answer Guidelines for Case Study on p. 227
• Audio Lecture: Traditional Chinese Medicine

• Clinical Reference: Laboratory Values
• Content Updates
• Electronic Calculators
• Examination Review Questions
• Glossary
• Key Points (Printable and MP3 Download)

The general health of Canadians is steadily improving, as evidenced by lower mortality rates and increased life expectancy. Biomedical and technological advances have contributed to these improvements. However, conventional therapy has been less helpful in alleviating symptoms of chronic illnesses. Chronic health challenges are at an epidemic high. Furthermore, conventional (Western, mainstream) approaches to health care tend to be depersonalized and often fail to account for all aspects of an individual, including not only body but also mind and spirit. Increasing access to global perspectives has resulted in greater exposure to healing philosophies from many cultures, suggesting many new ideas about health and healing to consumers and health care providers (Fontaine, 2011).

A variety of terms have been used to describe health-related approaches that are considered outside the mainstream of the system of health care dominant in Canada. The terms currently used in Western cultures to describe such approaches include *alternative, complementary, integrative, nontraditional, unconventional, holistic, natural,* and *unorthodox.* Currently, the term most frequently used to refer to such modalities and practices is *complementary and alternative therapies.* According to Health Canada (2009, 2011), **complementary therapies** are therapies that accompany traditional North American health practices, whereas **alternative therapies** are used instead of traditional health practices. Of note is that most of these therapies were developed outside the mainstream of conventional biomedical approaches and are generally available without medical authorization. Furthermore, many of these modalities are similar to autonomous nursing interventions such as touch, massage, stress management, and activities to facilitate wellness and enrich health.

Complementary and alternative therapies are harmonious with many of the values of nursing (Canadian Nurses Association, 1999, 2008). These values include a view of humans as holistic beings, an emphasis on healing, recognition that the professional–patient relationship should be a partnership, and a focus on health promotion and illness prevention. Nursing's interest in complementary and alternative perspectives is reflected in the formation of specialty nursing groups. For example, the Canadian Holistic Nurses Association (CHNA) (CHNA, 2011a) was established to recognize holistic nursing as a specialty and to further the development of holistic nursing practice in order to ensure that professional holistic practices are made available to the people of Canada for health promotion and health maintenance.

Health care providers have raised important questions about the effectiveness and safety of complementary and alternative approaches in view of their increased use by consumers. In response to this need in Canada, the Canadian Interdisciplinary Network for Complementary and Alternative Medicine Research (IN-CAM) was established to foster excellence in complementary and alternative medicine (CAM) research (Andrews & Boon, 2005). The objectives are to build a sustainable network that facilitates and supports research, promoting knowledge transfer among researchers and thus avoiding the duplication of research efforts (see the Resources at the end of this chapter). It is difficult to classify the enormous array of complementary and alternative health practices. For analytical purposes, the National Center for Complementary and Alternative Medicine (NCCAM) (NCCAM, 2010) classified these therapies into specific groups: natural products, mind–body medicine, manipulative and body-based practices, and other CAM practices. Table 12-1 includes descriptions of major categories. Tables 12-2, 12-3, 12-4, and 12-5 include descriptions of selected therapies within each category. The list

Table 12-1 NCCAM Categories of Complementary and Alternative Therapies

CATEGORY	DESCRIPTION
Mind–body medicine	Therapy focused on the effects of mind–body practices on the brain, mind, body, and behaviours. Science of psychoneuroimmunology demonstrates the strength of this mind–body connection (see Table 12-2).
Natural products	Substances found in nature that are used for their effect on health and wellness (see Table 12-3).
Manipulative and body-based practices	Therapies that manipulate and focus on systems of the body (see Table 12-4).
Other CAM practices	Therapies not included in the other categories of CAM therapies (see Table 12-5).

CAM, complementary and alternative medicine.
Source: National Center for Complementary and Alternative Medicine (NCCAM) (NCCAM, 2010). Retrieved from *http://nccam.nih.gov/health/whatiscam*

continually changes as practices proven safe and effective become accepted as "mainstream" health care practices.

Alternative Medical Systems

Alternative medical systems involve complete methods of health-related theory and practice that have been developed outside of the Western biomedical model. Many are traditional systems that are practised by individuals in different cultures throughout the world. Traditional Chinese medicine is one of the subcategories that NCCAM has identified.

Traditional Chinese Medicine

Traditional Chinese medicine (TCM) is one of the world's oldest and most comprehensive medical systems. Over several thousand years, it has evolved with cultural and philosophical developments, as well as extensive clinical observation and testing. Several major concepts constitute Chinese medicine. The principle of *yin and yang* is a core tenet of Chinese art, philosophy, and science, as well as TCM. Various states are associated with yin energies (feminine energy, cold, heavy, moist, negative) and yang energies (masculine energy, hot, dry, light, positive). Yin and yang are viewed as dynamic, interacting, and interdependent energies, neither of which can exist without the other, each containing some part of the other within it (Figure 12-1). These energies are a part of everything in nature and must be maintained in a harmonious state of balance to achieve optimal health. Imbalance is associated with illness. TCM modalities are used to restore balance between yin and yang energies.

Strengths of TCM include its individualized system of diagnosis and treatment, as well as its focus on prevention. Assessment tools include a comprehensive health history, tongue examination, and pulse examination. TCM includes an array of modalities, the most common choices being acupuncture and Chinese herbal medicine. These modalities are used together to replenish and soothe the flow of Qi throughout the body. When

Table 12-2 Mind–Body Medicine

EXAMPLES	DESCRIPTION
Relaxation breathing	Slow diaphragmatic breathing and exercises, used to elicit the relaxation response. See Chapter 8 for further information.
Meditation	State of being with increased concentration and awareness. Focuses one's attention and increases self-awareness. Two branches exist: (a) inclusive/mindfulness and (b) exclusive/concentrative. Mindfulness meditation focuses on "living in the moment" without judgement. Concentrative meditation involves "moving inward," often initiated by concentrating on the breath, a mantra, or an object. Outcomes may include relaxation, spiritual growth, and personal healing.
Biofeedback	Method of learned control of physiological responses of the body (Fontaine, 2011). Information about one or more physiological functions is received, interventions are used, and a feedback loop allows for voluntary control of certain functions.
Yoga	Activity that includes mental and physical exercises, ethical principles, and guidelines for healthy living. Part of the Ayurvedic medical system. Canadians use yoga more for its physical benefits and for stress reduction.
Imagery	Use of the mind to generate images that have a calming effect on the body. Involves use of vision, sound, smell, and taste, as well as the senses of movement, position, and touch. Outcomes may include reduction of anxiety, relaxation, enhanced immunity, and changes in hormonal responses.
Hypnosis/ hypnotherapy	Attainment of a state of attentive, focused concentration with suspension of some peripheral awareness. May be effective in promoting healing, decreasing pain, managing chronic illness, and preparing for surgery and other procedures (Fontaine, 2011).
Music therapy	Includes listening to music and creating music. Type of music used is individually determined. Outcomes may include relaxation, decreased anxiety, and decreased pain.
Art therapy	Involves creative expression through a variety of artistic mediums. May be used to facilitate expression of emotions, memories, and conscious and unconscious concerns. Outcomes may include decreased stress, as well as facilitation of healing from past distress or trauma.
Journalling	Involves writing down one's feelings, thoughts, perceptions, personal events, or memories. Outcomes may include stress reduction, as well as personal development through self-reflection.
Animal-assisted therapy (AAT)	Use of specifically trained animals to assist in attainment of health care goals. An example is hippotherapy (use of horseback riding) to meet physiotherapy and rehabilitation goals. Animal-assisted activities (AAAs) include use of trained animals for motivational, educational, and recreational objectives. An example is placement of animals in assisted-living facilities.

Table 12-3 Natural Products

EXAMPLES	DESCRIPTION
Herbal therapy	Use of unrefined plant-based products to treat, prevent, or cure disease. Effects are slow and less dramatic than effects of pharmaceutical drugs.
Nutraceuticals	Vitamin and mineral supplements. Best source of vitamins and minerals is a well-balanced diet. Nonetheless, many Canadians take supplements regularly.
Nutritional therapy	Special diets for health promotion. Such diets must be studied for potential benefit.
Aromatherapy	Use of plants' essential oils for their beneficial effect. Canadians seek out this therapy primarily for stress reduction and use these oils via inhalation or topically. In other cultures, essential oils are used more comprehensively in health care.
Homeopathy	Therapy based on the adage "like cures like." Remedies are specially prepared from the same substance that causes the symptom or problem. Extremely small amounts of the substance are used for the remedy. The remedies are generally safe and free from interactions with other medications. Remedies are believed to work through an energy transfer.
Naturopathy	Therapy based on promotion of health rather than symptom management. Focus is on enhancing the body's natural healing response through a variety of individualized interventions such as nutrition, herbology, homeopathy, physical therapies, and counselling. Naturopathic physicians are graduates of accredited naturopathic medical schools, and licensing varies by province.
Probiotic therapy	Use of live microorganisms that are similar to those found in the human digestive tract and that assist in and aid with digestion.

yin and yang are in balance, Qi (pronounced "chee"), or the fundamental life force, flows evenly through the body, leading to good health. *Qi* is a form of energy found in all life; when it is disrupted, illness and pain can occur. **Acupuncture** involves the insertion of fine needles into the circulation of Qi underneath the skin's surface (Figure 12-2). Specific points are selected on the basis of the diagnosis and the nature of the complaint. With proper point selection and manipulation, acupuncture corrects disruptions in the flow of Qi.

Chinese herbs are used to supplement the effects of an acupuncture treatment. Taken regularly over time, Chinese herbal formulas strengthen the body's ability to correct its own imbalance so that regular treatments are no longer necessary. Herbs are selected on the basis of specific assessment findings and complaint history; formulas are individually created to match the patient's needs. Other TCM interventions include acupressure, moxibustion, cupping, Chinese massage, meditative physical exercise (e.g., Tai Chi and Qi gong), and nutrition counselling.

Table 12-4 Manipulative and Body-Based Methods

EXAMPLES	DESCRIPTION
Manipulative and Body-Based Methods	
Chiropractic therapy	Therapy that restores and maintains health by proper alignment of the spine through a variety of adjustment and manipulation techniques. Correct spinal alignment facilitates self-healing and improves health and well-being.
Pressure point therapy	Application of finger and hand pressure to specific areas of body (acupressure points defined by charts of energy meridians) to improve energy flow, relieve pain, and stimulate the body's innate healing abilities.
Massage therapy	Manipulation of soft tissues to improve health and promote healing. Outcomes include relaxation, reduced tension, improved immune function, increased flexibility, and pain relief.
Energy Therapies	
Hand-mediated biofield energies	Therapeutic touch involves the use of the practitioner's hands to assess and balance the patient's energy field. Healing intent is incorporated. This technique is based on the belief that healing is facilitated when the human energy field is in balance.
Healing touch	A technique that includes therapeutic touch as well as other energy healing modalities. Primarily used by nurses.
Reiki	A Japanese therapy that involves use of the hands to affect the human energy field, with the intent to heal.

Table 12-5 Other CAM Practices

EXAMPLES	DESCRIPTION
Manipulation of energy fields: Bioelectromagnetics	Magnet therapy: Based on the principle that every animal, plant, and mineral has an electromagnetic field that allows other objects to interact with it as part of one unified energy system (Fontaine, 2011); magnets are frequently used to reduce pain, relieve swelling and inflammation, and promote healing of soft tissue and bone.
Whole Medical Systems	
Ayurvedic	Based on the balance of mind, body, and spirit; developed in India. Disease is viewed as an imbalance between a person's life force (*prana*) and basic metabolic condition (*dosha*). Interventions include breathing exercises, nutrition, detoxification, herbs, meditation, and yoga.
Traditional Chinese medicine (TCM)	Based on restoring and maintaining the balance of vital energy (*Qi*). Interventions include acupressure, acupuncture, Chinese herbology, cupping, moxibustion, nutrition, meditation, Tai Chi, and Qi gong. One of the world's oldest, most holistic medical systems.
Spiritual Therapies	
Aboriginal health care	Based on a spiritual domain whereby all things have "spirit." Community is valued and plays a role in the healing process. Gratitude to and harmony with nature are central themes. Medicine men and women use herbs and natural medicines, spiritual rituals, and ceremony. It is imperative that nurses recognize the importance of incorporating Aboriginal healing traditions in the care of Aboriginal patients (Beaulieu, 2012; Hunter, Logan, Barton, & Goulet, 2004; Phillips, 2010)
Prayer	Involves communication with a deity or the sacred. Found in all cultures. A frequently used therapy. Nurses may incorporate prayer into their practice.

CAM, complementary and alternative medicine.

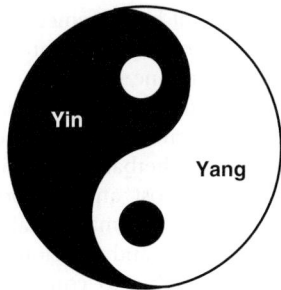

Figure 12-1 Symbol of yin and yang. The circle representing the whole is divided into yin (black) and yang (white). The small circles of opposite colour within those regions illustrate that within the yin, there is yang, and within the yang, there is yin. The dynamic curve dividing them indicates that yin and yang are continuously shifting in balance. Thus yin and yang create each other, control each other, and transform into each other. When yin and yang are in balance, Qi (pronounced "chee"), or the fundamental life force, flows evenly through the body, leading to good health.

Tai Chi and Qi gong are slow movement exercises in which breathing must be focused.

Clinical Applications of Acupuncture.

Acupuncture is the primary treatment modality used by TCM practitioners. In 1983, the Chinese Medicine and Acupuncture Association of Canada was federally incorporated in order to unite practitioners of TCM and acupuncture in Canada.

Clinical studies have indicated that acupuncture is effective in reducing pain, fighting inflammation, accelerating wound healing, and promoting nerve regeneration. It is also effective in treating many causes of nausea and vomiting (Berman, et al., 2004; Birch, Hesselink, Jonkman, & Hecker, 2004; Fontaine, 2011; Shirato, 2005). Table 12-6 has a more complete listing of the uses of acupuncture.

Acupuncture is considered a safe therapy when the practitioner has been appropriately trained and uses disposable needles. Patients should review the credentials of their practitioners.

Acupressure.

Acupressure is a natural, hands-on healing therapy based on the same principles as acupuncture. Finger

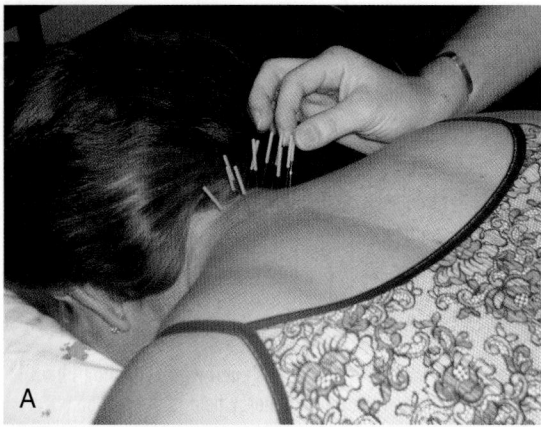

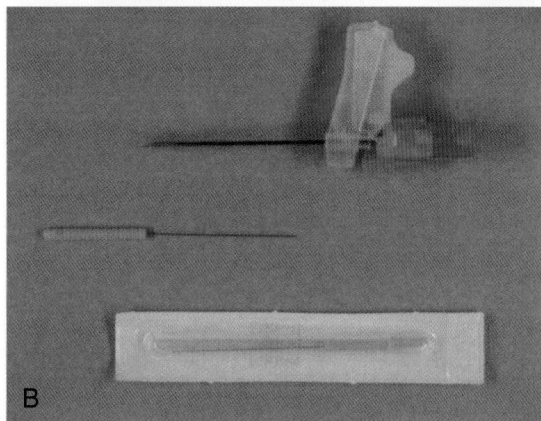

Figure 12-2 Acupuncture. **A,** TCM practitioner placing acupuncture needles. The needles are placed along the meridians to balance the flow of Qi. **B,** Comparison of injection needles and acupuncture needles. Injection needles are larger and hollow in the centre. Acupuncture needles are very thin and solid. They are so flexible that a guide tube is used during insertion.

Source: Courtesy Cory Shaw, San Antonio, TX

Table 12-6 Conditions for Which Acupuncture May Be Beneficial	
Pain Management	**Gynecological and Obstetric Conditions**
• Low back pain	• Induction of labour
• Headache pain	• Infertility
• Osteoarthritis	• Menopausal symptom
• Cervical neck pain	Dysmenorrhea
• Musculoskeletal and myofascial pain	
• Fibromyalgia	**Asthma**
Surgical Analgesia	**Gastrointestinal Conditions**
• Procedural analgesia	
• Postoperative pain	• Irritable bowel syndrome
• Postoperative nausea and vomiting	• Chronic constipation
Chemotherapy-Induced Nausea	**Substance Abuse**
Neurological Disorders	• Smoking cessation
• Acute stroke	• Opioid dependence
• Stroke rehabilitation	

pressure is applied along the body's energy meridians. Acupressure works by accessing and releasing blocked or congested energy in the body. Acupressure can be used for many conditions, including postoperative nausea, chemotherapy-induced nausea, and headaches. Jo Shin Do and reflexology are also forms of pressure-point therapies that stimulate certain areas within the body to help balance the body's energies (Fontaine, 2011).

Mind–Body Medicines

Mind–body interventions include a variety of techniques designed to facilitate the mind's capacity to affect bodily function. These include behavioural, psychological, social, and spiritual approaches to health. Specific examples of therapies and approaches are included in Table 12-2. NCCAM considers behavioural approaches such as psychotherapy, certain uses of hypnosis, biofeedback, patient education, and support groups as "mainstream" within the category of mind–body methods. Nurses frequently use many of these biobehavioural approaches.

Natural Products

Biologically based therapies include herbal therapies (phytotherapy), special diet therapies, and orthomolecular medicine (see Table 12-3).

Herbal Therapies

Herbal therapy is the use of individual herbs or combinations of herbs for therapeutic benefit. An herb is a plant or plant part (bark, roots, leaves, seeds, flowers, or fruit) that produces and contains chemical substances that act on the body. It is estimated that approximately 25,000 plant species are used medicinally throughout the world, and approximately 30% of modern prescription drugs are derived from plants. Botanical medicine is the oldest known form of medicine; archaeological evidence suggests that Neanderthals used plant-based remedies 60,000 years ago. Today, about 80% of the world's population relies extensively on plant-derived remedies (Fontaine, 2011).

Since the early 1980s, interest in herbal therapies has increased in countries whose health care practices are dominated by the biomedical model. Interest in herbal products is related to several factors, including the high cost and the potential for severe adverse effects associated with pharmaceutical drugs. Herbal remedies are considered "natural" and therefore may be viewed as safer. They are directly available to consumers and appeal to consumers, which allows individuals to assume more autonomy with regard to their health care.

More than 73% of Canadians now consume natural health products in the form of traditional herbal products, vitamins and mineral supplements, and homeopathic preparations. To ensure that these products are safe, Health Canada established the Office of Natural Health Products in 2008. In January 2004, the Natural Health Products regulations were implemented to ensure the safety of over-the-counter (OTC) products. In contrast, in the United States, herbal products used for medicinal value are classified as dietary supplements. As such, they lie outside the jurisdiction of many of the safety and regulatory rules covering foods and drugs.

Clinical Applications of Herbal Therapy.
Medicinal plants work in much the same way as drugs; both are absorbed and trigger biological effects that can be therapeutic. Many have more than one physiological effect and thus can be used for more than one condition. A number of herbs have been determined to be safe and effective for a variety of conditions. Boxes with descriptions of herbs related to specific diseases are found throughout this book (see the accompanying Complementary & Alternative Therapies box).

COMPLEMENTARY & ALTERNATIVE THERAPIES

Complementary & Alternative Therapies Throughout This Text

Information related to the following complementary and alternative therapies can be found throughout this text.

- Acupuncture
- Bilberry
- Biofeedback
- Echinacea
- Garlic
- Ginger
- Ginkgo biloba
- Ginseng
- Glucosamine
- Goldenseal
- Guided imagery
- Herbs and supplements that affect blood clotting
- Herbs and supplements that affect blood glucose levels
- Herbs and supplements used for menopause
- Herbs and surgical patients
- Herbs that affect healing
- Lipid-lowering agents
- Milk thistle
- Music therapy
- Saw palmetto
- Valerian
- Zinc

Although most herbal therapies can safely be used without professional assistance, adverse effects and interactions with prescription drugs have been described. Adverse effects resulting from the use of herbal remedies may be under-reported, which thus promotes the impression that herbal remedies are completely safe to use. Because consumers tend not to discuss their use of herbal therapies with their primary health care provider, herb–drug interactions may also be under-reported. For example, patients who are scheduled for surgery should be advised to stop taking herbal remedies 2 to 3 weeks before surgery. Patients who are being treated with conventional drug therapy should be advised to discontinue herbal remedies that produce similar pharmacological effects because the combination may lead to an excessive reaction or to unknown interaction effects. General patient teaching guidelines related to herbal therapy use are presented in Table 12-7.

Patients should be advised that if they take herbal therapies, they should adhere to the suggested dosage. If herbal preparations are taken in high doses, they can be toxic. The potency of a particular herbal remedy can vary widely because of factors such as where and how it was grown, as well as harvesting and processing methods. Herbal medicines should be purchased only from reputable manufacturers. Health Canada (2011) advises Canadians to use only herbal products that have been approved for sale

PATIENT & CAREGIVER TEACHING GUIDE

Table 12-7   Herbal Therapies

- Ask the patient about use of herbal therapies. Document a complete history of herbal use, including amounts, brand names, and frequency of use. Ask the patient about allergies.
- Investigate whether herbs are used instead of or in addition to traditional medical treatments. Find out whether herbal therapies are used to prevent disease or to treat an existing problem.
- Instruct the patient to inform the health care provider of any intention to take herbal treatments before doing so.
- Make the patient aware of the risks and benefits associated with herbal use, including drug reactions when herbs are taken in combination with other drugs.
- Advise the patient using herbal therapies to be aware of any adverse effects while taking herbal treatments and to immediately report them to the health care provider.
- Make the patient aware that moisture, sunlight, and heat may alter the components of herbal treatments.
- Inform the patient of the need to be aware of the reputation of the manufacturers of herbal products and the safety of the product before buying herbal treatments.
- Encourage the patient to read labels of herbal therapies carefully. Advise the patient not to take more of an herb than is recommended.
- Inform the patient that most herbal therapies should be discontinued at least 2 to 3 weeks before surgery.
- Inform the patient that the employees of health food stores may not have any educational background in the actions, interactions, and efficacies of the herbal therapies sold in the store they are working in. It is the responsibility of the patient to ensure that the information received comes from someone who has the appropriate background and education to be providing that information.

under the Natural Health Products regulations. If the product has been assessed, it will have a Drug Identification Number (DIN) or Natural Products Number (NPN) on its label. This certifies that the product has passed a review of formulation, labelling, and instructions for use. Because of the potential for adverse effects, pregnant women, nursing mothers, and older adults with liver or cardiovascular disease should use caution in consuming herbal products. Commonly used herbs are listed in Table 12-8. Some common herbs are shown in Figure 12-3. Commonly used dietary supplements are found in Table 12-9.

Manipulative and Body-Based Practices

Manipulative and body-based practices include interventions and approaches to health care that are based on manipulation or movement of the body. Examples include chiropractic therapy, pressure point therapies, massage, and hand-mediated biofield therapies. Massage therapy is one of the body-based practices used commonly by nurses.

Massage Therapy

Massage therapy includes a range of techniques with which the practitioner manipulates the soft tissues and joints of the body. Involving touch and movement, massage is typically delivered with the hands, although elbows, forearms, or feet

Table 12-8 Commonly Used Herbs*

NAME	USES INFORMED BY SCIENTIFIC EVIDENCE	COMMENTS
Aloe	Constipation	• Should be used no longer than 7 days for constipation • May cause electrolyte imbalances • May lower blood glucose level
Black cohosh	Menopausal symptoms	• Generally safe when used for up to 6 months by healthy, nonpregnant women • May lower blood pressure
Echinacea	Treatment of upper respiratory tract infections	• Should be used with caution by patients with conditions affecting the immune system • May lead to liver inflammation • Short-term use is recommended
Evening primrose	Eczema, skin irritation	• Contraindicated in individuals with seizure disorders
Feverfew	Migraine headache prevention	• May increase risk of bleeding • Stopping long-term use may lead to withdrawal symptoms
Garlic	High cholesterol level	• May increase risk of bleeding • May lower blood glucose level
Ginger	Nausea and vomiting of pregnancy	• May increase risk of bleeding • Use during pregnancy should not exceed 1 g/day • Supervision by health care provider is recommended for pregnant women considering use of ginger
Ginkgo biloba	Intermittent claudication	• Generally well tolerated in recommended dosages for up to 6 months • May increase risk of bleeding • May affect blood glucose levels
Ginseng (*Panax* species, including Asian and American ginseng)	Improvement of mental performance Lower blood glucose level in type 2 diabetes mellitus	• May lower blood glucose levels • May reduce effectiveness of warfarin • Should be avoided by patients with hormone-sensitive conditions, such as breast cancer
Hawthorn	Mild to moderate heart failure	• May add to the effects of cardiac glycosides, antihypertensives, and cholesterol-lowering drugs
Kava	Anxiety	• Should be used only under the supervision of a health care provider • Should be avoided by patients with liver problems and by patients taking medications that affect the liver • May increase sedation caused by some herbs or supplements • Should be used with caution with herbs or supplements that are metabolized by the kidneys
Milk thistle	Hepatitis caused by viruses or alcohol; cirrhosis	• May lower blood glucose levels • May interfere with the liver's cytochrome P450 enzyme system
St. John's wort	Short-term treatment of mild to moderate depression	• May lead to serious interactions with herbs, supplements, OTC drugs, or prescription drugs • Interferes with metabolism of drugs that act through the cytochrome P450 enzyme system • May lead to increased adverse effects when taken with other antidepressants • Advise patients to consult a health care provider before self-medicating with St. John's wort

OTC, over-the-counter.

*Advise patients who are pregnant or lactating to consult a health care practitioner before they use any herbs. Scientific evidence for the use of most herbs during pregnancy or lactation is limited.

Source: Natural Standard (*http://www.naturalstandard.com*).

may be used. Massage techniques are used in body work, sports training, physiotherapy, nursing, chiropractic therapy, osteopathy, and naturopathy. Benefits of massage relate to its effects on the musculoskeletal, circulatory, lymphatic, and nervous systems. Massage also positively affects mental and emotional states. Massage therapy continues to grow in popularity; most people who use massage therapy do so as a means of reducing stress.

Clinical Applications of Massage Therapy. Until the 1970s, nurses were taught to perform "P.M. care," which consisted of a back rub and other measures to promote relaxation and

Table 12-9 Commonly Used Dietary Supplements*

NAME	USES INFORMED BY SCIENTIFIC EVIDENCE	COMMENTS
Chondroitin sulfate	Osteoarthritis	Should be used with caution in patients with bleeding disorders or taking anticoagulants
Coenzyme Q_{10}	Hypertension	May decrease blood glucose levels
Fish oil/omega-3 fatty acids	Hypertension	Taking large doses may increase risk of bleeding
	Hypertriglyceridemia	May increase blood glucose levels in patients with diabetes
	Cardiovascular disease prevention	May increase low-density lipoprotein (LDL) level
Glucosamine	Osteoarthritis	May decrease effectiveness of insulin or other drugs used to control blood glucose levels
		May increase risk of bleeding
Melatonin	Jet lag	Should be avoided by patients taking warfarin
	Sleep enhancement	Should be used with caution by patients taking anticoagulants or antihypertensive drugs
		Should be used with caution by patients with diabetes or hypoglycemia
		Should be used with caution by patients with seizure disorder
		May increase cholesterol levels
Probiotics (live bacteria or yeast)	Re-establishing gut flora, especially after prolonged antibiotic therapy	—

Source: http://www.naturalstandard.com

*Advise patients who are pregnant or lactating to consult a health care provider before they use any supplements. Scientific evidence for use during pregnancy or lactation is limited.

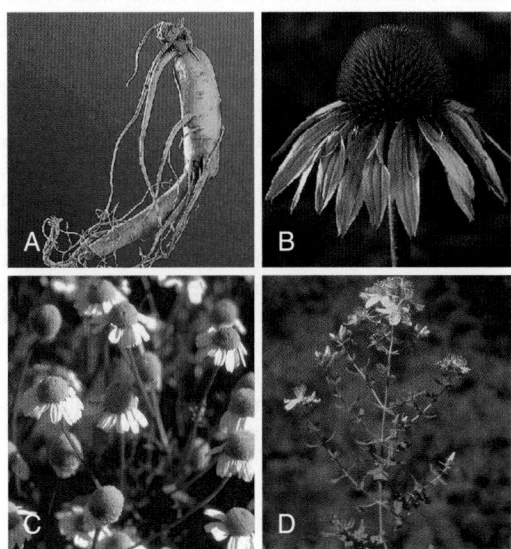

Figure 12-3 Herbs. **A,** Ginseng. **B,** Echinacea. **C,** Chamomile. **D,** St. John's wort.

Source: Blake, S. (1999). *Alternative remedies* (CD-ROM). St. Louis: Mosby.

sleep. After that time, P.M. care and back rubs became the exception rather than the rule. Yet today, with the increased focus on providing holistic care, nurses are again recognizing the benefits of massage. Massage is a form of touch and also a form of caring, communication, and comfort (Fontaine, 2011). The role of the nurse in massage differs from that of the registered massage therapist. Whereas massage therapists can provide more comprehensive massage therapies, nurses can use specific massage techniques as part of nursing care, when indicated by findings in

patient assessment. For example, a back massage can be used to help promote sleep. For a bedridden patient, gentle massage can stimulate circulation. When a nurse determines that massage may be indicated in meeting a patient goal, the nurse must first assess the patient's preference regarding touch and massage. The nurse should consider cultural and social beliefs and discuss potential benefits with the patient. The indicated plan of care (e.g., hand massage, back massage) can then be implemented, and reassessment can be performed after the massage.

Massage Techniques. Nursing use of massage typically begins with *effleurage,* or gliding strokes, to promote relaxation. Stroking is done from distal to proximal, along the long axis of the muscle (Figure 12-4, *A*). After relaxing the muscles with effleurage, *pétrissage,* or a kneading stroke, may be used to gently lift and knead the muscle (see Figure 12-4, *B*). Gently scented lotions or diluted essential oils may be included in the massage. Forms of massage are often used for pregnant women. Essential oils should not be used for massage on a pregnant patient because they can be harmful to the fetus (Fontaine, 2011).

A simple hand massage (Figure 12-5) can be used for a calming and relaxing effect, especially for patients who are anxious or agitated. When a patient is frustrated or agitated, a hand massage can act as a distraction and return the person to a calm state.

Family members can be taught to perform massage on their loved one, providing a way for family members to participate in patient care. This can be therapeutic for both the patient and the family, even when the loved one is mentally ill or unresponsive. Massage is beneficial during all aspects of the life continuum. During the end-of-life process, hospice nurses may incorporate massage into their nursing care, inasmuch as the massaging touch can lessen pain and restlessness. Massage is contraindicated in patients who have had recent injuries, trauma, or, recent surgery;

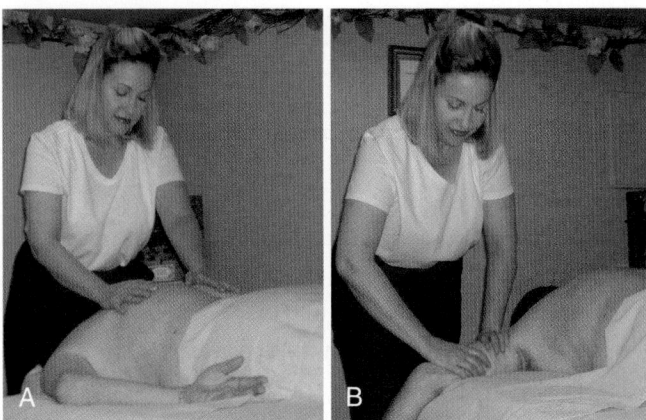

Figure 12-4 Massage. **A,** With the use of effleurage to relax the back. **B,** With the use of pétrissage to relax arm muscles.

Source: Lori Karhu, RMT, RN, San Antonio, TX.

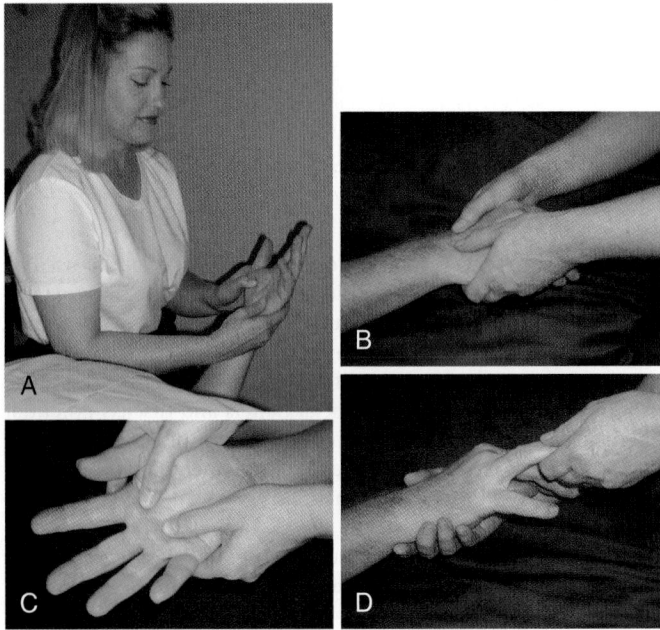

Figure 12-5 A, Hand massage. **B,** Technique of hand massage: Bend the wrist backward and forward to relax the wrist, then massage the wrist and top of the hand, using circular movements. **C,** Massage the palm of the hand with the cushions of the thumbs, using circular movements. **D,** Massage each finger from the base to the tip.

Source: Lori Karhu, RMT, RN, San Antonio, TX.

and in patients with open wounds, deep venous thrombosis, inflammation or infections, bleeding, edema, or decreased sensation. Massage therapy is also contraindicated when a patient has used alcohol or recreational drugs.

Hand-Mediated Biofield Energies

Energy therapies are those that involve the manipulation of energy fields. They focus on energy fields originating within the body (biofields or human energy fields) (Brennan, 1987) or those from other sources (electromagnetic fields). Examples of

biofield (human energy field) therapies include therapeutic touch, healing touch, and Reiki. Biofield (human energy field) healing therapies (see Table 12-4) are based on the theory that energy systems in the body need to be balanced and repatterned to enhance healing. Some forms of energy therapy manipulate biofields (human energy fields) by applying pressure or manipulating the body by placing the hands in, or through, these fields. To obtain specialty certification with regard to the CHNA (CHNA, 2011b), the nurse must have completed a prerequisite of Level I Therapeutic Touch or Level I Healing Touch.

Therapeutic Touch. **Therapeutic touch** is a method of detecting, balancing, and repatterning the human energy field. It is a contemporary interpretation of several ancient healing practices. It involves the conscious use of the hands to direct or modulate human energy fields. Therapeutic touch was developed in the 1970s by a nurse, Dolores Krieger, and a traditional healer, Doris Kunz. According to Krieger (1997), therapeutic touch is based on the assumptions that a human being is an open energy system, a balanced flow of energy underlies good health, and illness is a reflection of an imbalance in an individual's energy field.

Clinical Applications of Therapeutic Touch. During the actual treatment, nurses use their hands to assess the patient's energy field. Hands are positioned 5 to 15 cm from the body. The energy field is assessed for bilateral similarities or differences in the flow of energy. The next step is clearing and balancing the energy field. Nurses then work with the energy field of the patient involving the intentionality (the conscious effort to bring about healing or to be healed) of the patient and the intentionality of the nurse. The session ends with a smoothing of the energy. Therapeutic touch is not a diagnostic tool but is used as a form of treatment in conjunction with a biomedical treatment plan. Research has been conducted on the effectiveness of therapeutic touch for a wide range of conditions, including wound healing; sleep promotion; enhancement of immune function; and the reduction of anxiety, agitation, postoperative pain, tension headache, and stress. The research findings have been inconclusive, which indicates the need for further research. Specialized instruction is needed to perform therapeutic touch. Some individuals are able to "feel" the energy field more readily than others. However, with patience, determination, and a desire to help others, anyone (including family members) can learn to use therapeutic touch.

Healing Touch. **Healing touch** is a nurse-based program founded in the 1980s by a nurse, Janet Mentgen. It is a biofield therapy that encompasses a group of non-invasive techniques that utilize the hands to clear, energize, and balance the human and environmental energy fields. Healing touch employs the gentle placement of the nurse's hands on or near the patient's clothed body. In accordance with established guidelines, the nurse assesses the patient's energy field, realigns energy flow, eliminates energy blockages, reactivates the mind–body–spirit connection, and then evaluates the process (Healing Touch Canada, 1998). It is an organized system designed to assist the patient to self-heal. The patient, not the nurse, determines the effectiveness (Maville, Bowen, & Benham, 2008).

Clinical Applications of Healing Touch. Research on energy therapies is in the early stage of development. However, research does indicate that healing touch may be effective in (a) reducing anxiety, (b) improving muscle relaxation, (c) reducing stress, (d) promoting wound healing, and (e) reducing pain (Maville et al., 2008). Education on healing touch is a multilevel program leading to certification in healing touch. Information on classes, resources, and practice is available at the Healing Touch International Web site (see the Resources at the end of this chapter).

Other Complementary and Alternative Medicine Practices

Spiritual Therapies

Prayer. **Prayer** (described in Table 12-5) is one of the mind–body interventions used most commonly by all cultures, and yet it is difficult to define. Viewed globally, prayer can be described as connecting with the sacred. An ancient healing practice, prayer has been acknowledged in health care literature. Terms such as *distant healing, mental healing,* and *spiritual healing* are used, as researchers attempt to study the outcomes of prayer. The term *theosomatic medicine* has been developed to describe the study of health as related to an apparent connection between a deity and the human body. In exploring this connection, religious involvement has been found to be generally associated with lower levels of illness and higher levels of wellness. Prayer has been linked to the prevention of illness and to healing from disease (Fontaine, 2011).

Forms of Prayer. Forms of prayer include meditative prayer, ritualistic prayer, colloquial prayer, and intercessory (or petitionary) prayer. Meditative prayer involves openness to the divine and does not require words or thoughts. Ritualistic prayer involves repeated words and phrases and is commonly associated with formal liturgy. Colloquial prayer involves spontaneous thought and conversation with the divine. Intercessory prayer involves making a request for specific needs to be met (Fontaine, 2011).

Clinical Applications of Prayer. Nurses are committed to spiritual care as part of their holistic practice. Spiritual assessments can guide nurses in identifying patients' needs. Different formats or tools may be used. Patients often under-report or do not report their use of alternative and complementary modalities to their health care provider because they are afraid of being judged or of not having their health care needs met. It is important that the nurse be nonjudgemental and amenable to the patient's needs.

Nurses need knowledge about prayer practices, awareness of what patients want, cross-cultural wisdom about how people pray, and rigorous research to examine the effects of prayer. Nursing literature indicates that prayer is an intervention valued by many patients (Fontaine, 2011). Patients may request intercessory prayer: that is, for someone to pray with them or for them. Self-reflection is important in this situation. Knowing his or her own beliefs and values, the nurse can decide to meet the patient's request directly. However, many nurses feel uncomfortable praying with their patients. Barriers to praying with patients include lack of time, personal discomfort, lack of experience, and lack of private space (Fontaine, 2011). For whatever reason, if the nurse feels uncomfortable or is unable to address the patient's request directly, the nurse may consult with a spiritual director or religious leader. In most hospitals, chaplains of various faiths and denominations are available to meet with patients. Because many patients find prayer comforting, especially during times of illness, nurses must ensure that spiritual needs are met. Nurses also report using prayer in more personal ways (Fontaine, 2011; Helming, 2011). Nurses who are hesitant to pray with their patients often say that they do pray for their patients. They also describe using prayer before their shift or as they start their day, seeking inner guidance for effective nursing care. Nurses may use prayer for emotional support, motivation, spiritual awareness, or enhanced professional performance.

AGE-RELATED CONSIDERATIONS: COMPLEMENTARY AND ALTERNATIVE THERAPIES

Older adults with non–life-threatening, chronic conditions are most likely to use complementary and alternative therapies. For older adults, safety concerns involve herb–drug interactions/ toxicity from polypharmacy and age-related changes in pharmacokinetics (Scholz, Holmes, & Marcus, 2008). Decreased renal and liver function may slow metabolism and excretion of herbs and dietary supplements. Because older patients are a more vulnerable population, the nurse must discuss the risks and benefits of using herbal products, while encouraging patients to inform their health provider of any herbal product or dietary supplement that they are taking.

NURSING MANAGEMENT: COMPLEMENTARY AND ALTERNATIVE THERAPIES

The role of the nurse with regard to complementary and alternative therapies is evolving. Roles of the nurse may include (a) assessing patients' use of complementary and alternative therapies and their risk for complications or adverse interactions with conventional therapies; (b) serving as a resource about complementary or alternative therapies, including teaching patients about complementary and alternative options, providing information about evidence concerning effectiveness, and making referrals to qualified practitioners; (c) serving as a provider of therapies for which the nurse obtains training and certification, such as therapeutic touch or acupuncture; and (d) conducting research about complementary and alternative approaches. The nurse must be able to perform these roles nonjudgementally. If patients believe they are being judged because of their use of complementary or alternative therapies, they will stop communicating and will withhold this information from their health care providers.

A resource for nurses and patients in Canada with regard to complementary and alternative therapies and practitioners is the Natural Health Practitioners of Canada (NHPC). "The NHPC is dedicated to promoting the art and science of natural health practices, to serving the needs and maintaining the professional standards of natural health practitioners in Canada, and to improving health care in Canada" (NHPC, 2011).

▪ Assessment

Collection of data on patients' use of complementary and alternative therapies is part of a thorough nursing assessment. It is especially important because most patients do not voluntarily tell their health care provider about their use of these therapies. However, they usually share this information with a nurse when asked. Nurses must ask general open-ended questions, while remaining nonjudgemental and respectful of the patient's response.

Examples of assessment questions to ask include the following:

1. What are you doing to maintain or improve your health and well-being?
2. How involved are you in planning and carrying out your health-related care?
3. What is your view of the ideal relationship between yourself and your primary health care provider?
4. Do you have any conditions that have not responded to conventional medicine? If so, have you tried any other approaches?
5. Are you using any vitamin, mineral, dietary, herbal supplements, or energy-based therapies?
6. Are you interested in obtaining information about alternative or complementary approaches?

Along with assessing use, the nurse needs to document the effectiveness of interventions that are used.

▪ Serving as a Resource and Promoting Safety

According to the Canadian Nurses Association's *Code of Ethics,* nurses must respect and promote people's autonomy and help them both express their health needs and obtain desired information in order to make informed decisions. A wide variety of therapies fall within the category of complementary and alternative therapies, and some of these therapies may be ineffective or even harmful. However, patients self-select these therapies, generally without consulting a health care provider. Safety concerns encompass the reliability of information, the safety and effectiveness of therapies, and the regulation of practitioners. Regarding sources of information, patients most commonly get their information from health food stores, informal word of mouth, books, magazines, and the Internet. Patients need to be encouraged to seek professional assistance with these decisions. If a patient questions the nurse on how to find a registered practitioner of natural health practices in Canada, the nurse can refer the patient to the Natural Health Care Practitioners of Canada (NHCPC) Web site (see the Resources at the end of this chapter). This organization maintains a directory of registered natural health practitioners in Canada. Serving as a patient advocate, the nurse provides information on both conventional therapies and complementary and alternative therapies. Patients should be advised that complementary therapies do not replace conventional therapies but can often be used in combination with conventional therapies. By providing information for the patient, the nurse fosters informed decision making.

To serve as a resource for patients, nurses must first develop their own knowledge base. Even if specific information about complementary and alternative therapies is not provided in basic nursing programs, nurses are educated to be critical thinkers and problem solvers. Thus nurses are prepared to seek ongoing education regarding complementary and alternative therapies and to continue to read and critique research on these therapies.

As ethical practitioners, nurses need to be aware of their biases and judgements with regard to complementary and alternative therapies. Biased and judgemental attitudes do not allow the nurse to provide the best care possible for the patient.

▪ Providing Holistic Self-Care and Holistic Nursing Practice

Some individuals choose to become nurses because they want to care for others—to be a caregiver for their patients. This is a compelling reason to choose nursing. Yet many nurses fail to recognize that "caring for others" can occur only when their values and practices include "care for self" (Fontaine, 2011). Self-care (caring for one's own general level of health and well-being) is essential on both a personal and professional level. On a personal level, self-care involves commitment to maintaining one's own level of wellness. Keeping one's mind, body, and spirit healthy is required so that one has the strength to care for others. On a professional level, self-care is important because nurses are role models. They are role models for family, friends, patients, health care providers, and the community. By demonstrating self-care practices, nurses motivate other people to achieve greater health and wellness. Learning about complementary and alternative therapies can be one pathway to self-care. Initially, nurses are eager to learn about complementary and alternative therapies so that they can provide better patient care and be holistic in their approach. However, nurses often find that these therapies can also be used personally to enhance their own level of health and wellness. Because many different therapies are included as part of complementary and alternative therapies, each individual nurse should be able to find ways to promote personal well-being. Examples of therapies commonly used by nurses for personal well-being include relaxation breathing, meditation, prayer, yoga, massage, and music.

It is essential that the "caregiver" first care for himself or herself. Professional nursing from its onset included care of the whole person, which is the concept of mind–body–spirit. However, the Western biomedical model, with its focus on the physical body, caused nursing practice to transform into a more "medical" model. The increase in the use of complementary and alternative therapies provides an opportunity for nursing to return to its origin and a focus on holistic nursing practice. **Holistic nursing** incorporates mind–body–spirit principles into the development of a caring–healing relationship with patients. Core concepts of holistic nursing include the following: (a) The nurse accepts patients as they are, without judgement and with compassion; (b) the nurse's care is based on holism and integrates mind–body–spirit principles; (c) the nurse serves as a facilitator, recognizing the patient's capacity for self-healing; (d) the nurse incorporates self-care and self-responsibility, recognizing the greater interconnectedness of all individuals; and (e) the nurse's practice is guided by holistic education and research (Dossey, Keegan, & Guzzetta, 2005).

Nursing interventions include therapeutic listening and empathy. The nurse also promotes a therapeutic environment and honours cultural diversity. The holistic nurse may also choose to integrate complementary and alternative therapies as part of nursing practice, recognizing the value of both conventional and complementary and alternative therapies.

▪ Serving as a Provider

Nursing has a long history of providing therapies that have been considered complementary and alternative. These include massage, relaxation therapy, music therapy, and therapeutic touch, as well as other strategies to promote comfort, reduce stress, improve coping, and promote symptom relief. The practice of nursing is defined in legislation throughout Canada and commonly includes promoting, maintaining, and restoring health and assessing and providing care through supportive, preventative, therapeutic, rehabilitative, and palliative means. Nurses also "facilitate and respect the patient's informed choice to use alternative and complementary therapies" (Canadian Nurses Association, 2011). The requirements for use of a specific complementary or alternative therapy are not different from those for other nursing interventions. The nurse should have specific training in the use of the therapy and should be aware of the evidence base that addresses the conditions for which the therapy is indicated, the effectiveness of the therapy, and the potential for adverse outcomes or synergistic effects. Nurses are responsible for ensuring that the patient has given consent for a given therapy. The patient must be aware of the proposed benefit and any potential risks involved. The nurse must document the effectiveness of the interventions. A mechanism must be in place to evaluate the care outcomes.

Participating in Research

Nurses are responsible for critiquing and applying relevant research findings to their practice, as well as participating in the identification of researchable problems. Using summaries of research evidence on complementary and alternative therapies is one strategy for developing evidence-informed approaches. Participating on teams whose focus is to develop evidence-informed protocols that address appropriate use of complementary and alternative therapies is another effective approach. Practising with a questioning mind can facilitate identification of research questions that can be investigated with research-trained health care providers. Types of research considerations that can be addressed through questions include describing the extent of patients' use of specific therapies, exploring patients' experiences of using various complementary and alternative therapies, and documenting the effectiveness of therapies commonly used by nurses.

Patient interest and participation in complementary and alternative therapies is increasing. Therefore, nurses must be knowledgeable about the multiple therapies available and must develop effective strategies to document the use of these therapies. It is also important for nurses to keep abreast of the current research in this area to provide accurate information to both patients and other health care providers. Nurses are well positioned to become the link between conventional therapy and complementary and alternative therapies.

CLINICAL DECISION-MAKING EXERCISE

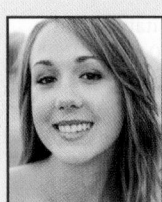

CASE STUDY:
University Student With Abdominal Distress

Source: Corbis/Jim Craigmyle.

Patient Profile

Jane Craigo, a 21-year-old university student, was seen in the student health centre for increasing episodes of abdominal fullness and discomfort with alternating diarrhea and constipation.

Subjective Data

- Reports that irritable bowel syndrome was diagnosed several years ago.
- Was told to eat more fibre, but nothing has seemed to be effective in reducing her abdominal distress.
- Is taking a heavy course load this semester.

- Has to work 20 hours each week for her work-study contract.
- Eats mainly fast foods and drinks several colas daily.

Discussion Questions

1. Assess what Ms. Craigo is currently doing to help alleviate the symptoms.
2. Explain the psychological stressors that may be contributing to Ms. Craigo's abdominal discomfort.
3. Describe how her current diet may be affecting her, both physiologically and psychologically.
4. What complementary or alternative therapy (or therapies) would be appropriate for Ms. Craigo?
5. How would you recommend complementary therapies to her physician? What arguments could you use to support their use?

evolve   Answers are available at **http://evolve.elsevier.com/ Canada/Lewis/medsurg**

REVIEW QUESTIONS

The number of the question corresponds to the same-numbered objective at the beginning of the chapter.

1. Which of the following statements best describes complementary and alternative therapies?
   a. They are used as a primary form of treatment.
   b. They contradict the values of nursing.
   c. They are based on extensive scientific research.
   d. They were developed outside the Western biomedical model.

2. Which of the following patients is most likely to benefit from treatment by a traditional Chinese medicine practitioner?
   a. A patient with pneumonia
   b. A patient with mental illness
   c. A patient with chronic back pain
   d. A postoperative patient with low blood pressure

3. Which of the following is a common complication of the use of garlic, ginkgo biloba, and ginger?
   a. Allergic reactions
   b. Clotting alterations
   c. Skin photosensitivity
   d. Increased blood pressure

4. Which of the following concepts should be included in patient teaching with regard to use of herbal products?
   a. All herbal products are safe to use.
   b. Herbal products are effective immediately.
   c. Herbal products' labels give all essential information.
   d. Use of herbal products must be reported to the patient's health care provider.

5. Which of the following statements describes holistic nursing?
   a. Holistic nursing focuses on physical health.
   b. Holistic nursing is practised only by experienced nurses.
   c. Holistic nursing promotes self-care and self-responsibility.
   d. Holistic nursing is based on the biomedical model of health care.

6. In assessing a patient's use of complementary and alternative therapies, which of the following actions is a priority to include?
   a. Assess the patient's compliance with all treatment modalities.
   b. Determine the patient's knowledge of the therapies that he or she is using.
   c. Use the term "alternative therapies" when assessing the patient's use of these therapies.
   d. Reinforce the benefits of traditional Western medicine.

7. Which of the following best describes the role of the nurse involved with complementary and alternative therapies?
   a. Caring for patients rather than caring for self.
   b. Prescribing the appropriate herbal therapies for a patient.
   c. Serving as a resource to guide patients in the safe use of therapies.
   d. Advocating for use of complementary and alternative therapies instead of conventional health care.

ANSWERS: 1. d; 2. c; 3 b.; 4. d; 5. c; 6. b.; 7. c.

REFERENCES

Andrews, G. J., & Boon, H. (2005). CAM in Canada: Places, practices, research. *Complementary Therapies in Clinical Practice, 11*(1), 21-27.

Beaulieu, T. (2012). *Exploring indigenous and western therapeutic integration: Perspectives and experiences of indigenous elders (dissertation)*. Toronto: University of Toronto.

Berman, B., Lao, L., Langenberg, P., Lee, W., Gilpin, A., & Hochberg, M. (2004). Effectiveness of acupuncture as adjunctive therapy in osteoarthritis of the knee. *Annals of Internal Medicine, 141*(12), 901-910.

Birch, S., Hesselink, J. K., Jonkman, F. A., & Hecker, T. (2004). Clinical research on acupuncture (part 1). *Journal of Alternative and Complementary Medicine, 10*(3), 468-480.

Brennan, B. (1987). *Hands of light: A guide to healing through the human energy field*. Toronto: Bantam Books.

Canadian Holistic Nurses Association. (2011a). *About us*. Retrieved from http://www.chna.ca/Default.aspx?pageId=812652

Canadian Holistic Nurses Association. (2011b). *Specialization program in holistic nursing*. Retrieved from http://www.chna.ca/specialization.

Canadian Nurses Association (CNA). (1999, July). Complementary therapies—Finding the right balance. *Nursing Now: Issues and Trends in Canadian Nursing*. Retrieved from http://www2.cna-aiic.ca/CNA/documents/pdf/publications/ComplimentaryTherapies_July1999_e.pdf

Canadian Nurses Association (CNA). (2008). *Code of ethics for registered nurses*. Ottawa: Author. Retrieved from http://www2.cna-aiic.ca/CNA/documents/pdf/publications/Code_of_Ethics_2008_e.pdf

Canadian Nurses Association (CNA). (2011). *Registered Nurses Examination: Competencies June 2010–May 2015*. Ottawa: Author. Retrieved from http://www2.cna-aiic.ca/CNA/nursing/rnexam/competencies/default_e.aspx

Dossey, B., Keegan, L., & Guzzetta, C. (2005). *Holistic nursing: A handbook for practice*. Sudbury, MA: Jones & Bartlett.

Fontaine, K. L. (2011). *Complementary and alternative therapies for nursing* (3rd ed.). Upper Saddle River, NJ: Pearson Education.

Healing Touch Canada. (1998). *What is healing touch?* Retrieved from http://www.healingtouchcanada.net/htc/newwhat.html

Health Canada. (2009). *Health promotion approach: Natural health products and complementary and alternative health care*. Ottawa: Author. Retrieved from http://www.hc-sc.gc.ca/dhp-mps/pubs/complement/index-eng.php

Health Canada. (2011). *Natural health products*. Ottawa: Author. Retrieved from http://www.hc-sc.gc.ca/dhp-mps/prodnatur/index-eng.php

Helming, M. B. (2011). Healing through prayer: A qualitative study. *Holistic Nursing Practice, 25*(1), 33-44. doi:10.1097/HNP.0b013e3181fe2697

Hunter, L., Logan, J., Barton, S., & Goulet, J. (2004). Linking Aboriginal healing traditions to holistic nursing practice. *Journal of Holistic Practice, 22*(3), 267-284. doi:10.1177/0898010104266750

Krieger, D. (1997). *Therapeutic touch inner workbook: Ventures in transpersonal healing*. Santa Fe, NM: Bear.

Maville, J. A., Bowen, J. E., & Benham, G. (2008). Effect of healing touch on stress perception and biological correlates. *Holistic Nursing Practice, 22*(2), 103-110. doi:10.1097/01.HNP.0000312659.21513.f9

National Center for Complementary and Alternative Medicine. (2010). *What is complementary and alternative medicine?* Retrieved from http://nccam.nih.gov/health/whatiscam

Natural Health Practitioners of Canada (NHPC). (2011). *About us*. Retrieved from http://www.nhpcanada.org/about-us/

Phillips, M. (2010). *Understanding resilience through revitalizing traditional ways of healing in a Kanien'keha:ka community (master's thesis)*. Montreal: Concordia University. Retrieved from http://spectrum.library.concordia.ca/7071/

Scholz, B. A., Holmes, H. M., Marcus, D. M. (2008). Use of herbal medications in elderly patients. *Annals of Long-Term Care, 16*(12): 24-28.

Shirato, S. (2005). How CAM helps systemic lupus erythematosus. *Holistic Nursing Practice, 19*(1), 36-39.

CANADIAN RESOURCES

Acupuncture Canada
http://www.acupuncture.ca

Acupuncture Foundation of Canada Institute (AFCI)
http://www.afcinstitute.com

Canadian Association for Parish Nursing Ministry
http://www.capnm.ca

Canadian Association of Naturopathic Doctors (CAND)
http://www.naturopathicassoc.ca

Canadian Chiropractic Association
http://www.ccachiro.org
Canadian Holistic Nurses Association
http://www.chna.ca/
Canadian Interdisciplinary Network for Complementary and
Alternative Medicine Research (IN-CAM)
http://www.incamresearch.ca
Massage Therapy Alliance of Canada (MTAC)
http://massage.ca/professional_development.html
College of Traditional Chinese Medicine & Pharmacology
Canada
http://www.ctcmpc.com/
Health Canada: Health Promotion Approach: Natural Health
Products and Complementary and Alternative Health Care
http://www.hc-sc.gc.ca/dhp-mps/pubs/complement/index_e.html
Healing Touch Canada
http://www.healingtouchcanada.net/

Natural Health Care Practitioners of Canada
http://www.nhpcanada.org
Registered Nurses' Association of Ontario (RNAO)
Complementary Therapies Nurses' Interest Group (CTNIG)
http://www.rnao-ctnig.org/

RELATED RESOURCES

National Center for Complementary and Alternative Medicine
(NCCAM)
http://nccam.nih.gov

ⓔvolve *For additional Internet resources, see the Web site for this book
at* **http://evolve.elsevier.com/Canada/Lewis/medsurg**

Palliative Care
at the End of Life

Written by Margaret McLean Heitkemper
Adapted by Donna Goodridge

LEARNING OBJECTIVES

1. Describe nursing management of common physical manifestations at the end of life.
2. Describe nursing management of common psychosocial manifestations at the end of life.
3. Explain the process of grief and bereavement.
4. Discuss some of the variables that affect end-of-life care.

5. Discuss key ethical and legal issues related to palliative care.
6. Explore the special needs of family caregivers of a dying patient.
7. Discuss the special needs of the nurse who cares for dying patients and their families.

KEY TERMS

advance care planning An ongoing process of discussion among a patient, the family, and health providers, aimed at improving care decisions at the end of life, p. 235

advance directives Documents that specify the care the patient wishes to receive in the event that he or she becomes unable to participate in treatment decision making, p. 235

bereavement A sense of deprivation or loss generated by the death of a valued other, p. 233

brain death The final clinical expression of complete and irreversible neurological failure, p. 232

Cheyne-Stokes respiration Abnormal pattern of respiration characterized by alternating periods of apnea and deep, rapid breathing, p. 231

certification of death The legally required completion of a death certificate stating the cause of death, p. 240

death The irreversible cessation of circulatory and respiratory function or the irreversible cessation of all functions of the entire brain, including the brainstem, p. 231

end-of-life care Care provided in the last days or weeks of life, p. 231

grief The emotional and behavioural response to loss, p. 233

hospice A concept of care that provides compassion, concern, and support for the dying; may also refer to a facility where inpatient care is provided to the dying, p. 236

mourning The social customs and cultural practices that are carried out following a death, p. 233

palliative care Care designed to prevent and relieve suffering at any stage of illness, p. 231

pronouncement of death Determination that life has ceased based on a physical assessment, p. 240

ELECTRONIC RESOURCES

Supplemental content related to Chapter 13 can be found . . .

Evolve Web Site ⊝volve

http://evolve.elsevier.com/Canada/Lewis/medsurg
- Clinical Reference: Laboratory Values
- Content Updates

- Electronic Calculators
- Examination Review Questions
- Glossary
- Interactive Case Study: Chronic Myelogenous Leukemia Including End-of-Life Care
- Key Points (Printable and MP3 Download)

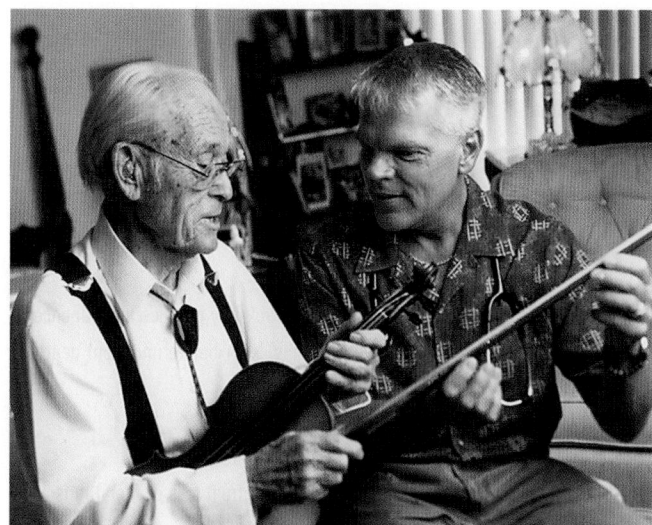

Figure 13-1 One goal of end-of-life care is to improve the quality of the patient's remaining life.

Source: Kathleen A. Pollard, RN, MSN, CHPN, Phoenix, AZ.

The fundamental processes of life and death have intrigued humankind for millennia. Artists, writers, philosophers, scientists, religious leaders, and many others have pondered the meaning of life and death. In Western society, however, mortality and the death experience are often difficult and awkward topics to discuss and accept. Still, death is as real a part of life as birth.

The concepts of death and dying were rarely discussed or studied in the West before the 1960s. Many times, patients who were not expected to survive were placed in isolated hospital areas, were given less than quality care, and died without appropriate medical care. Family members, faith communities, or both were usually the care providers.

Today, with the reality of an aging Canadian population and the increasing number of persons with chronic diseases, terminal illness and dying are not viewed as the taboo topics that they once were. The special needs of the dying and the terminally ill are now acknowledged and integrated into care. Death and dying are researched by scientists, health care providers, theologians, and laypersons. Information concerning death and dying can be found in both popular and professional literature.

End-of-life care (EOL care) is the term often used to describe care provided in the last days or weeks of life (Subcommittee of the Standing Senate Committee on Social Affairs, Science and Technology, 2000), whereas **palliative care** is an approach that improves the quality of life of patients and their families facing problems associated with life-threatening illness (World Health Organization [WHO], 2011). The time from diagnosis of a terminal illness to death varies considerably, depending on the patient's diagnosis and the extent of disease. EOL care focuses on physical and psychosocial needs at the end of life for the patient and the patient's family. The goals for EOL care are to (1) provide comfort and supportive care during the dying process, (2) improve the quality of the remaining life (Figure 13-1), and (3) help ensure a dignified death. The Senate of Canada Report entitled *Quality End-of-Life Care: The Right of Every Canadian* stated that EOL care must be an unshakable core value of Canada's health care system. Each person has the right to skilled, compassionate, and respectful care at the end of life. However, it is estimated that only 5% of Canadians receive integrated and interdisciplinary EOL care (Quality End of Life Care Coalition, 2010). The Canadian Hospice Palliative Care Association strategy to improve EOL care includes service delivery by interdisciplinary teams; patient access and availability to services; professionals' skill in pain and symptom management; and the provision of support for caregivers and family members.

Physical Manifestations at End of Life

Death occurs when all vital organs and systems cease to function. **Death** is the irreversible cessation of circulatory and respiratory function or the irreversible cessation of all functions of the entire brain, including the brainstem. Trauma and disease processes can affect physical manifestations at the end of life. As death approaches, metabolism is reduced and the body gradually slows down until all function ends. Generally, respirations become increasingly erratic and gradually stop. Then the heart stops beating within a few minutes. Physical manifestations of approaching death are listed in Table 13-1.

Sensory Changes

With decreased oxygenation and circulation to the brain, there are alterations in the interpretation of sensory input. Sensory changes can include blurred vision, decreased sense of taste and smell, and decreased pain and touch perception. The blink reflex is eventually lost, and the patient appears to stare. The sense of touch decreases first in the lower extremities because of circulatory alterations. Hearing is commonly believed to be the last sense to remain intact at the end of life.

Circulatory and Respiratory Changes

With decreased oxygenation and altered circulation causing metabolic changes, the heart rate slows and weakens, and the blood pressure falls progressively. Respirations may be rapid or slow, shallow, and irregular. Breath sounds may become wet and noisy, both audibly and on auscultation. Noisy, wet-sounding respirations are caused by mouth breathing and accumulation of secretions in the upper airways. **Cheyne-Stokes respiration** is a pattern of breathing characterized by alternating periods of apnea and deep, rapid breathing. This type of breathing is often seen as a person nears death.

There is decreased circulation, especially noticeable on the skin. The extremities become pale, mottled, and cyanotic. The skin feels cool to the touch, first in the feet and legs, then progressing to the hands and arms, and finally to the torso. The skin may feel warm because of an elevated body temperature that is related to an underlying disease process and changes in hypothalamic function.

Loss of Muscle Tone

As death becomes imminent, metabolic changes cause the muscular system to gradually weaken, leading to rapidly declining functional abilities. Facial muscles lose tone, causing the jaw to sag. Decreased muscle coordination leads to difficulty in speaking. Swallowing becomes increasingly difficult, and the gag reflex is eventually lost. Gastrointestinal motility and peristalsis diminish, leading to constipation, gas accumulation, distension, and

Table 13-1 Physical Manifestations of Approaching Death

SYSTEM	MANIFESTATIONS	SYSTEM	MANIFESTATIONS
Sensory system		Gastrointestinal system	• Loss of appetite and thirst sensations
Hearing	• Usually last sense to disappear		• Slowing of digestive tract and possible cessation of function (may be exacerbated by pain-relieving drugs)
Touch	• Decreased sensation		
	• Decreased perception of pain and touch		• Accumulation of gas
Taste and smell	• Decreased with disease progression		• Distension
Sight	• Blurring of vision		• Loss of sphincter control may produce incontinence
	• Sinking and glazing of eyes		• Bowel movement may occur before imminent death or at time of death
	• Blink reflex absent	Musculoskeletal system	• Increasing weakness
	• Eyelids may remain half open		• Gradual loss of ability to move
Integumentary system	• Mottling on hands, feet, arms, and legs		• Sagging of jaw resulting from loss of facial muscle tone
	• Cold, clammy skin		
	• Cyanosis of nose, nail beds, and knees		• Difficulty speaking
	• "Waxlike" skin when very near death		• Swallowing can become more difficult
Respiratory system	• Increased respiratory rate		• Difficulty maintaining body posture and alignment
	• Cheyne-Stokes respiration (abnormal pattern of respiration characterized by alternating periods of apnea and deep, rapid breathing)		• Loss of gag reflex
			• Jerking seen in patients receiving large amounts of opioids (myoclonus)
	• Inability to cough or clear secretions, resulting in grunting, gurgling, or noisy congested breathing (death rattle)	Cardiovascular system	• Increased heart rate; later slowing and weakening of pulse
			• Irregular rhythm
	• Irregular breathing, gradually slowing down to terminal gasps (may be described as "guppy breathing")		• Decrease in blood pressure
			• Delayed absorption of drugs administered intramuscularly or subcutaneously
Urinary system	• Gradual decrease in urinary output		
	• Patient may be incontinent of urine		
	• Patient may be unable to urinate (urinary retention)		

possible nausea. Pain-relieving drugs may exacerbate these gastrointestinal manifestations. The ability of the urinary system to function and produce urine decreases. Loss of sphincter control can lead to fecal and urinary incontinence.

Brain Death

Brain death is best understood as brain arrest, or the final clinical expression of complete and irreversible neurological failure (Shemie et al., 2006). Neurological death is the irreversible loss of the capacity for consciousness with the irreversible loss of all brainstem functions, including the capacity to breathe.

Severe brain injury is a prerequisite for neurological determination of death (NDD); NDD is a prerequisite for cadaveric organ donation. NDD is diagnosed by rigorous tests at the bedside to demonstrate deep, unresponsive coma; absent respiratory effort; absent gag and cough reflexes; and the bilateral absence of other reflexes as listed in Table 13-2 (Shemie et al., 2006). Potentially reversible causes of neurological injury, such as unresuscitated shock, hypothermia, severe metabolic disorders and abnormalities, peripheral nerve or muscle dysfunction, and clinically significant drug intoxications, are considered confounding factors that must be ruled out before the diagnosis of NDD is made. Currently, legal and medical standards in Canada require that two physicians determine the presence of NDD.

Table 13-2 Canadian Minimum Clinical Criteria for Neurological Determination of Death in Adults

• Established etiology capable of causing neurological death in the absence of reversible conditions capable of mimicking neurological death

• Deep unresponsive coma with bilateral absence of motor responses, excluding spinal reflexes

• Absent brainstem reflexes as defined by absent gag and cough reflexes and the bilateral absence of
  • Corneal responses
  • Pupillary responses to light, with pupils at midsize or greater
  • Vestibulo-ocular responses
• Absent respiratory effort
• Absent confounding factors

Source: Shemie, S., Doig, C., Dickens, B., Byrne, P., Wheelock, B., Rocker, G., …, Teitelbaum, J. (2006). Brain arrest: The neurological determination of death and organ donor management in Canada. *Canadian Medical Association Journal, 174*(Suppl), S1-S30. Reprinted by permission of the publisher. © 2006 Canadian Medical Association.

Table 13-3 Psychosocial Manifestations of Approaching Death

- Altered decision making
- Anxiety about unfinished business (including asking for forgiveness and forgiving others)
- Decreased socialization
- Fear of loneliness
- Fear of meaninglessness
- Fear of pain
- Helplessness
- Life review
- Peacefulness
- Restlessness
- Saying goodbyes
- Unusual communication
- Vision-like experiences, often involving communication with deceased relatives
- Withdrawal

Table 13-4 Comparison of Stages of Grieving

KÜBLER-ROSS (1969)	MARTOCCHIO (1985)	RANDO (1993)
Denial	Shock and disbelief	Avoidance
Anger and bargaining	Yearning and protest	Confrontation
Depression	Anguish, disorganization, and despair	
Acceptance	Reorganization and restoration	Accommodation

Psychosocial Manifestations at End of Life

Just as people live in different ways, they also experience the process of dying differently. A wide range of feelings and emotions may affect the dying patient and family at different times in the dying trajectory at the end of life. Specific psychosocial manifestations are listed in Table 13-3. Most patients and families struggle with a terminal diagnosis and the realization that there is no cure. Time may be needed to process the impending death and to formulate emotional responses. The patient and the family may feel overwhelmed, fearful, powerless, and fatigued. The patient's needs and wishes must be respected. Patients need time to ponder their thoughts and express their feelings. Response time to questions may be sluggish because of fatigue, weakness, and confusion.

> The dying process has been compared to the birthing process, and the analogy is useful. Both birthing and dying are natural parts of life that involve physical, psychological, and spiritual dimensions. There's nothing clean or easy about either one. And these natural processes have been going on as long as life has existed; medicalization is but a recent trend (Sanderson, 2007; pp. 280-281).

Bereavement, Grief, and Mourning

Although these terms are often used interchangeably, they refer to different processes. **Bereavement** is a sense of deprivation or loss generated by the death of a valued other. In conjunction with grief, it is through bereavement that significant others who survive respond to the loss of the loved one. It is important to note that bereavement for the family and significant others may begin before the death occurs. Working through the bereavement process helps the dying person and significant others adapt to the loss.

Grief is the emotional and behavioural response to loss. It is an emotional reaction that is necessary to maintain both emotional and physical well-being. The grieving process is an individual experience associated with thoughts, feelings, and behaviours. Grieving related to loss from death is a complex and intense emotional experience. **Mourning** refers to the social customs and cultural practices that are carried out following a

death; it is a process of incorporating the experience of loss into the lives of the bereaved.

Grief is manifested in a variety of ways. Every loss is as different as each person is unique. There are no guidelines to predict grief reactions, although the first year of bereavement is often most intense. Individuals experience different aspects of the grieving process at different times. Cultural beliefs, religious influences or spiritual beliefs, and the individual's value system influence grief reactions. The intensity of grief is driven by an individual's personality, the strength of the relationship with the dying person, concurrent life crises, coping resources, and the availability of support systems. Health care providers such as nurses can also experience grief when the patients they care for die, especially when those patients have been under their care for a long period of time (Heidrich, 2007).

Many different theories explaining grief and the grieving process have been articulated over the years. Kübler-Ross (1969), Martocchio (1985), and Rando (1993) have each identified stages of grief. Table 13-4 compares these theories. Kübler-Ross identified denial, anger, bargaining, depression, and acceptance as the five stages of grieving. Martocchio presented five clusters of grief to include (1) shock and disbelief; (2) yearning and protest; (3) anguish, disorganization, and despair; (4) identification of bereavement; and (5) reorganization and resolution. Rando defined three phases of responses to grieving: avoidance, confrontation, and accommodation.

Grief is a complex process, and individuals may neither progress through the stages in a linear fashion nor experience all stages. Martin and Elder (1993) view grief as a continuous process wherein the individual tries to make sense of the loss. The authors describe a figure-eight pattern with an inward path of protest, despair, and detachment and an outward path of exploration, hope, and investment. Individuals may begin at any phase and may pass through a phase many times. A key aspect of this model is the "circle of influence," which refers to the people in the griever's life who influence the grief process.

Grief that is helpful or that assists the person in accepting the reality of death is called *adaptive grief*. Adaptive grief is a healthy response. It may be associated with grieving before a death actually occurs or when the reality that death is inevitable is realized. The process of resolution in normal grief, or *uncomplicated grief* may take months to years. *Anticipatory grief* occurs in anticipation of the death event and may allow for emotional and practical adjustments to be made that facilitate coping. *Prolonged grief disorder* can manifest as chronic grief when the intensity does not wane after the first year. The bereaved person becomes "bogged down" in the grieving process and may experience intensive intrusive thoughts, severe pangs of emotion, unusual sleep disturbances, and maladaptive loss of interest in personal activities. It is estimated that one in five bereaved individuals experiences prolonged grief disorder (Kersting & Kroker, 2010). Failure to accomplish the essential tasks involved in grieving may result in *unresolved grief* that can last a lifetime.

The grief that occurs when an individual experiences a loss that cannot be publicly acknowledged or supported is referred to as *disenfranchised grief* and may also be known as "grieving in secret" (Doka, 1995). This type of grief can occur when individuals are in relationships outside of the socially accepted norm. For example, a mistress involved with a married man may not receive adequate social support if her lover dies. Similarly, grief that arises from losses as a result of miscarriage, abortion, or infertility is not always viewed as "legitimate" grief by some societies. The grief process takes time, energy, and work. Goals for the grieving process include resolving emotions, reflecting on the dying person, expressing feelings of loss and sadness, and valuing what has been shared.

Variables Affecting End-of-Life Care

People experiencing the inevitability of death are in need of caregivers who are knowledgeable about personal issues and attitudes that affect the end of life experience. The attitudes of the dying person, the family and significant others, and nurses affect the death experience.

Health care providers must be aware of religious and cultural differences, which are often intertwined, as they care for patients and families. Just as religion and culture affect the preferences and expectations of patients and families at the end of life, these variables also affect the attitudes and responses of health care providers involved (Frost, Cook, Heyland, & Fowler, 2011). An adequate understanding of cultural, religious, and familial influences is beneficial when focusing on the dying person's and the family's needs, wants, and fears. Although there may be influences from culture, religion, and family, the uniqueness of each person will create a very individual set of circumstances at the end of life. It is critical for the nurse to check out her or his assumptions about the preferences for end of life with the patient and family for whom she or he is caring.

As a multicultural society that continues to grow in diversity, Canada is now home to an ever-growing range of ethnic groups from all over the globe. Culture and religious beliefs affect a person's understanding of and reaction to pain and other symptoms, impending death, and loss. Health care providers must be aware of the impact that cultural differences and religious beliefs have on the care of the terminally ill. It is important to keep in mind that there is great variation within any given group and not assume that all persons from a culture will adhere to specific norms. For example, some Aboriginal patients follow traditional cultural teachings that need to be respected during EOL care, whereas others may adhere to Western religious beliefs.

Some cultures believe that death and dying are private matters to be shared only with significant others. Often, feelings are repressed or internalized. People who believe in "toughing it out" or "being strong" may not express themselves when they are experiencing a tragic loss. In caring for dying patients and their families, the nurse should assess cultural factors such as language barriers, nutritional issues, communication patterns, social customs, decision making, and death rituals. (Culturally competent care is discussed in Chapter 2.)

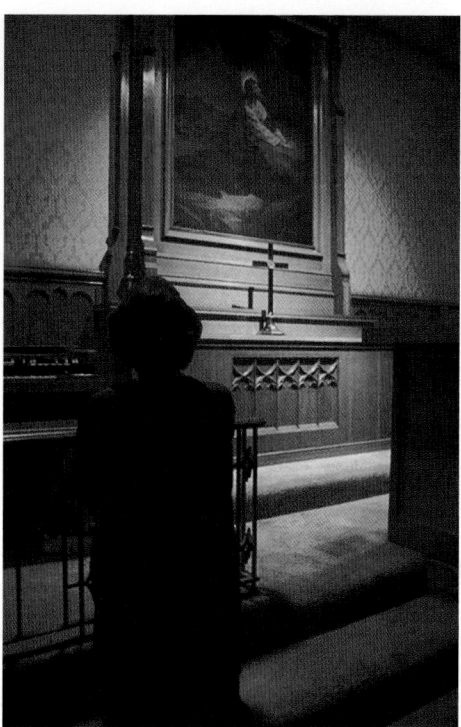

Figure 13-2 Spiritual needs are a critical consideration in end-of-life care.

Source: Potter, P. A., Perry, A. G., Ross-Kerr, J., & Sirotnik, M. (1997). *Canadian fundamentals of nursing* (p. 447, Figure 25-5). St. Louis: Mosby–Year Book.

Assessment of spiritual needs in EOL care is a key consideration as patients and families search for meaning (Figure 13-2). Spirituality is not the same as religion. A person may be of no particular faith, but have a deep spirituality. At the end of life, patients often question their beliefs about a higher power, their own journey through life, religion, and an afterlife. Some patients may choose to pursue a spiritual path. Some may not. Their individual choice has to be respected.

Deep-seated spiritual tensions may surface for some patients when they deal with their terminal diagnosis and related issues. Spiritual distress may occur along with a challenge to and a questioning of beliefs and values surrounding the past, present, and future.

Some dying patients are secure in their faith about the future. It is common to observe patients relinquishing material values of life and focusing on values they believe will lead them on to another place.

Differences among cultural, religious, and spiritual beliefs and values are innumerable. Nursing assessments of beliefs and preferences should be completed on an individual basis to avoid stereotyping individuals with particular behaviours and belief systems. (Culture is discussed in Chapter 2.)

Legal and Ethical Issues Affecting End-of-Life Care

Patients and families struggle with many decisions during the experience of terminal illness and dying. The decisions may involve the choices about treatments, such as cardiopulmonary resuscitation or admission to intensive care units, as well as more common health care decisions, such as the use of antibiotics during the final days of life.

Legal Documents Used in End-of-Life Care

In Canada, it is recognized that mentally competent adults have the right to make decisions regarding their health care, including the right to request or refuse life-sustaining treatment. Although health care providers have a duty to uphold the patient's right to self-determination, the central role of the family in decision making is increasingly being recognized.

Advance care planning (ACP) is an ongoing process of discussion among a patient, the family, and health providers aimed at improving care decisions at the end of life. **Advance directives,** or "living wills," are one type of ACP (Health Canada, 2009), written documents prepared by competent persons outlining their treatment wishes in the event that they become incapacitated. They have been widely advocated as a means of ensuring that treatment preferences are respected.

There are two major types of advance directives: instructional and proxy directives. Instructional directives include living wills or treatment directives. Proxy directives are also referred to as power of attorney for personal care. Most Canadian provinces have legislation allowing people to appoint substitute decision makers in the event that they become incompetent. The power of attorney for personal care specifies who is to make decisions for the patient when the patient is no longer able to make the decisions for himself or herself. Table 13-5 identifies common legal and ethical documents used in EOL care.

Copies of generic advance directive forms can be obtained from local medical associations, law offices, the Internet, and the Office of the Public Guardian and Trustee. However, a person may write her or his wishes without special forms. Verbal directives may be given to physicians with specific instructions. In the event that the person is not capable of communicating her or his wishes, the family and the physician can agree on what measures will or will not be taken. The physician should record the family's decision.

Since the early 1980s, cardiopulmonary resuscitation (CPR) has become common practice in health care. Patients who suffered respiratory or cardiac arrest have often been administered CPR unless a *do-not-resuscitate (DNR) order* was provided by the physician. Many times, patients and families have had no choice as to whether CPR was used. In recent years, much has been written concerning the right to die and the right to choose. Many people believe that the patient or the patient's family has the right to decide whether CPR will be used. It is no longer the sole decision of the physician.

A physician's order should be written to include the information concerning the patient's or family's wishes for the use of CPR. A DNR order means that CPR will not be attempted but does not preclude the use of other forms of treatment or care. Several different types of CPR decisions can be made. All-encompassing heroic measures, which may include CPR, drugs, and mechanical ventilation, can be referred to as a *full code*.

Another term sometimes used to replace "no code" or DNR is the term *allow natural death* (AND). This term more accurately conveys what actually happens. All comfort measures associated with pain control and symptom management are carried out. However, the natural physiological progression to death is not delayed or interrupted.

Withholding or withdrawing treatments can be included in an advance directive. This could include a list of medical treatments that a patient would or would not want to receive in various circumstances. This may include interventions such as CPR, admission to an intensive care unit, tube feeding, and blood transfusions.

The nurse must be aware of legal issues and the wishes of the patient. Advance care plans and organ donor information should be kept in the medical record and their location and content noted on the patient's record, the nursing care plan, or both. All caregivers responsible for the patient need to know the patient's wishes. In addition, the nurse is responsible for becoming familiar with provincial, local, and agency procedures for end-of-life documentation.

Persons who are legally competent may choose organ donation. Any body part or the entire body may be donated. The decision to donate organs or to provide anatomical gifts may be made by a person before death. The decision to donate organs may be made by immediate family members following death. Neurological death has to be established for organ donation to

Table 13-5 Common Documents Used in End-of-Life Care

DOCUMENT	DESCRIPTION	SPECIAL CONSIDERATIONS
Advance directive	A general term used to describe documents that give instructions about future medical care and treatments	• Specific measures to be used or withheld may be specified.
Do not resuscitate (DNR) Do not attempt resuscitation (DNAR)	A written physician's order instructing health care providers not to attempt cardiopulmonary resuscitation (CPR)	• Any specific measures to be used or withheld must be specified. DNR does NOT mean "do not treat." Symptom management is a key component of end-of-life care.
Living will	A lay term used frequently to describe any number of documents that give instructions about future medical care and treatments or the wish to be allowed to die without heroic or extraordinary measures should the patient be unable to communicate for self	• Living wills may be prepared by the individual or by the individual in consultation with a lawyer.
Power of attorney for personal care	A term used to describe a document that names the person or persons authorized to make decisions regarding personal care (e.g., housing, food, hygiene, health care) when the ill person is unable to do so for self	• The person appointed may be called a substitute decision maker, agent, or proxy.

take place. In addition, cardiac function must be maintained by artificial means during the removal of some organs. In reality, few people at end of life meet the criteria for organ donation to take place, other than in the case of severe trauma without serious pre-existing illness. Contraindications to donation often include sepsis, cancer, and various infectious diseases.

Canadians can make their wishes known by filling out their provincial organ donor card. Both organ and tissue donations follow specific legal guidelines. Legal requirements and facility policies for organ or tissue donation must be followed.

ETHICAL DILEMMAS
End-of-Life Care

Situation

Jane is a terminally ill 50-year-old woman with metastatic breast cancer. She has developed severe bone pain that is not adequately controlled by her current dosage of intravenous (IV) morphine. She moans at rest and verbalizes severe pain from any movement to reposition her. Even though she appears to sleep at intervals, she requests pain medicine frequently, and her family is demanding additional pain medicine for her. At the team conference, the nurses have discussed the need for more effective pain control but are concerned that additional pain medicine could hasten her death.

Important Points for Consideration

- Adequate pain relief is an important outcome for all patients, but in particular for patients who are terminally ill. The *principle of beneficence* imposes the obligation to provide the necessary care to benefit the patient.
- One goal of treatment of the terminally ill is to provide adequate pain control to alleviate suffering. This goal is based on the *principle of nonmaleficence*: preventing or reducing harm to the patient. The secondary effect of hastening the patient's death is ethically justified. This is referred to as the principle of *double effect*.
- *Euthanasia*, the deliberate act of hastening death, is not legal in Canada at present.
- Adequate pain relief at the end of life continues to be a major concern of health care professionals and consumers.

Clinical Decision-Making Questions

1. In the above situation, what type of discussion needs to occur among members of the health care team, the patient, and the family as this phase of the care of the terminally ill is approached?
2. Distinguish between assisted suicide and euthanasia and between promotion of comfort and relief of pain in dying patients.

Palliative Care and Hospice

In Canada, *palliative care* and *hospice* are often used interchangeably, although in some areas, *hospice* refers to those organizations with a residential facility. The term *hospice palliative care* refers to the convergence of hospice and palliative care into one movement with the same principles and norms of practice. The Canadian Hospice Palliative Care Association (2011b) defines

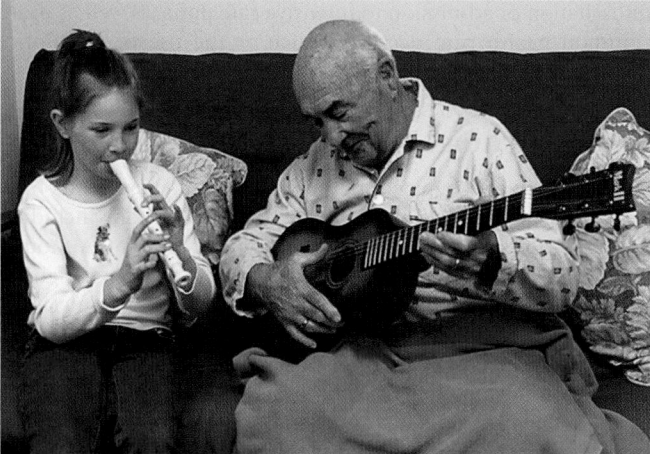

Figure 13-3 Hospice care is designed to provide compassion, concern, and support for the dying.

Source: Rick Brady, Riva, MD.

palliative care as "care aimed at relief of suffering and improving the quality of life for persons who are living with or dying from advanced illness or are bereaved. . . . The goal of palliative care is comfort and dignity for the person living with the illness as well as the best quality of life for both this person and his or her family."

Hospice is a concept of care that provides compassion, concern, and support for the dying (Figure 13-3). Hospice exists to provide support and care for persons in the last phases of incurable diseases so they might live as fully and as comfortably as possible at home or in a homelike setting. Hospice care ensures that patient and family needs are the focus of any intervention.

> You matter because you are you and you matter to the last moment of your life. We will do all we can not only to help you die peacefully, but to live until you die (Clark, 2002).

There are over 600 hospice palliative care programs and services in Canada (G. Adams, personal communication to Canadian Hospice Palliative Care Association, June 23, 2008). The Canadian Hospice Palliative Care Association is a charitable non-profit association whose mission is to provide leadership in hospice palliative care in Canada (Canadian Hospice Palliative Care Association, 2011a). The association strives to achieve this mission by supporting research, promoting education and training, improving public awareness of hospice palliative care, and advocating for increased programs and services.

Hospice care is often provided in the home, with inpatient care reserved for acute pain management or respite care for families or caregivers in need of a break. Every province and territory in Canada has a home care program that provides EOL care or palliative care services. This may include nursing services, personal support, physiotherapy, occupational therapy, social work, medical supplies, equipment, assistive devices, and respite care for family caregivers. Basic palliative care costs are usually covered under the *Canada Health Act*. Other costs may be covered by private insurance plans. The home care program works in collaboration with community services and hospice organizations. Inpatient hospice settings have been deinstitutionalized to make the atmosphere as relaxed and homelike as possible (Figure 13-4). Staff and volunteers are available to the patient and family.

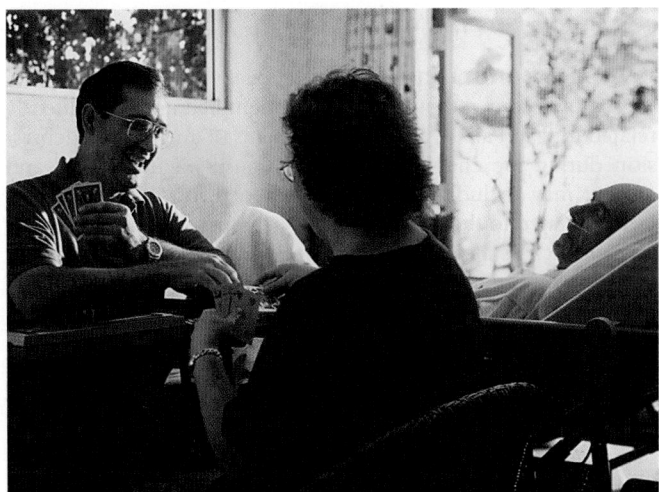

Figure 13-4 Inpatient hospice settings have been deinstitutionalized to make the atmosphere as relaxed and homelike as possible.

Source: Kathleen A. Pollard, RN, MSN, CHPN, Phoenix, AZ.

A multidisciplinary team approach often provides holistic health care.

A medically supervised interdisciplinary team of professionals and volunteers provides EOL care whether in a free-standing hospice or in a palliative care unit. The palliative care nurse is an integral part of and plays a pivotal role in coordination of the team. Nurses work collaboratively with palliative care physicians, pharmacists, dietitians, physiotherapists, social workers, personal support workers, spiritual care providers, and volunteers to provide care and support to the patient and family members. Palliative care nurses are educated in pain control and symptom management. As with home health care, hospice nursing calls for excellent teaching skills, compassion, flexibility, and adaptability to patient needs.

For several reasons, the decision to begin hospice palliative care can be difficult. Patients, families, and physicians may lack information about this type of care. Some patients or family members wrongly believe that palliative care excludes active treatment. Physicians may be reluctant to refer to palliative care services because they sometimes view a patient's decline as their personal failure.

Bereavement counselling is an important aspect of hospice and palliative care programs. The objective of a bereavement program is to provide support to and assist survivors in the transition to a life without the deceased person. Grief support is incorporated into the plan of care for family members and significant others during the patient's illness, as well as after the death.

NURSING MANAGEMENT: END OF LIFE

Nursing care of terminally ill and dying patients is holistic and encompasses all aspects of psychosocial and physical needs. Nursing care focuses on psychosocial manifestations and the grieving process, as well as the physical changes that are associated with dying. The patient and the family need to be the focus of nursing care. Respect, dignity, and comfort are important for

the patient and for the family. In addition, nurses and other care providers must recognize their own needs when dealing with grief and dying.

Nursing Assessment

Assessment of the terminally ill or dying patient varies with the patient's condition and the proximity of approaching death. In general, the assessment is limited to essential data. The nurse documents the specific event or change that brought the patient into the health care facility. The patient's medical diagnoses, medication profile, and allergies are recorded. If the patient is alert, a brief review of the body systems to detect important signs and symptoms should be completed. Discomfort, fatigue, pain, nausea, constipation, and dyspnea are carefully assessed so prompt interventions can be implemented.

The functional assessment of activities of daily living elicits information about the patient's abilities, food and fluid intake, patterns of sleep and rest, and response to the stress of terminal illness. Coping abilities of the patient and the family should also be assessed.

The physical assessment is abbreviated and focuses on changes that accompany terminal illness and the specific disease process. The frequency of assessment depends on the patient's stability but is done at least every 8 hours. As changes occur, assessment and documentation must be done more frequently.

As death approaches, neurological assessment is especially important and includes level of consciousness, presence of reflexes, and pupil responses. Evaluation of vital signs, skin colour, and temperature helps identify changes in circulation. Respiratory status, character and pattern of respirations, and characteristics of breath sounds are monitored and described. Monitoring nutritional and fluid intake, urinary output, and bowel function provides data for assessment of renal and gastrointestinal functioning. Skin condition must be assessed on an ongoing basis because skin becomes fragile and may easily break down.

It is important to be sensitive and not to burden the dying patient with repetitive, unnecessary assessments. Health history data that are available in the chart should be used when available rather than tiring the patient with an interview. However, it is important to assess the patient's status frequently. A variety of assessment tools are available, including the Palliative Performance Scale, the McGill Quality of Life Questionnaire, the Brief Fatigue Inventory, the Edmonton Symptom Assessment System, the Karnofsky Performance Scale, and the Brief Pain Inventory. These instruments can be easily accessed at the End of Life Toolkit Web page (see the Resources at the end of this chapter).

Nursing Diagnoses

Several nursing diagnoses deal with psychosocial manifestations (Table 13-6) and physical manifestations (Table 13-7) associated with EOL care.

Planning

Planning for EOL care entails a holistic approach. Care must be coordinated, focusing on both the patient's needs and the needs of the family members and significant others. Education, counselling, advocacy, and support for the patient and the family are

Table 13-6 Nursing Diagnoses: Psychosocial Manifestations at the End of Life

- Adjustment, impaired
- Anxiety, death
- Confusion, acute
- Confusion, chronic
- Coping, ineffective
- Denial, ineffective
- Family processes, interrupted
- Fear
- Grieving, anticipatory
- Grieving, dysfunctional
- Hopelessness
- Loneliness, risk for
- Sleep pattern, disturbed
- Social interaction, impaired
- Social isolation
- Sorrow, chronic
- Spiritual distress
- Spiritual well-being, readiness for enhanced
- Thought processes, disturbed
- Verbal communication, impaired

Table 13-7 Nursing Diagnoses: Physical Care at the End of Life

- Airway clearance, ineffective
- Aspiration, risk for
- Bed mobility, impaired
- Bowel incontinence
- Breathing pattern, ineffective
- Cardiac output, decreased
- Constipation
- Diarrhea
- Fatigue
- Gas exchange, impaired
- Infection, risk for
- Injury, risk for
- Nausea
- Nutrition, imbalanced: less than body requirements
- Oral mucous membrane, impaired
- Pain, acute
- Pain, chronic
- Physical mobility, impaired
- Self-care deficit
- Skin integrity, impaired
- Swallowing, impaired
- Thermoregulation, ineffective
- Tissue integrity, impaired
- Tissue perfusion, ineffective
- Urinary elimination, impaired
- Urinary incontinence, total

priorities. Psychosocially, nursing goals centre on the patient's abilities to express and share feelings with others. Nursing care goals during the last stages of life involve comfort measures and physical maintenance care.

Education of both the patient and the family is an important part of the nurse's planning in EOL care. Families need ongoing information on the disease, the dying process, and any care that will be provided. They need support to cope with many issues during this period of their lives. Denial and grieving may be barriers to learning and understanding at the end of life for both the patient and the family members. Nurses must take the time to develop a comprehensive plan to support, educate, and evaluate patients and families in EOL care issues.

Nursing Implementation

Nursing interventions for the dying patient focus on comfort and improving the quality of life. Psychosocial care and physical care are interrelated for both the dying patient and the family members or significant others.

Psychosocial Care

Anxiety and Depression. Anxiety is an uneasy feeling caused by a source that is not easily identified and is frequently related to fear. Patients often exhibit signs of anxiety and depression during the end of life period. Causes of depression and anxiety may include pain that is out of control, psychosocial factors related to the disease process or impending death, altered physiological states, and some medications. Encouragement, support, and education decrease some of the anxiety. Management of anxiety may include both pharmacological and nonpharmacological interventions.

Anger. Anger is a normal and common response to fear, grief, powerlessness, or hopelessness. The grieving person cannot be compelled to accept the many losses that occur at the end of life. Surviving family members may feel anger at the person who is leaving them. There is a need to acknowledge and encourage the expression of emotions. Nurses are sometimes a target of anger and must understand what is happening. It is usually not helpful to react personally when confronted with an angry patient or family member.

Fear. Fear is a common feeling associated with dying. The nurse frequently assists the dying person to cope with fears. Specific fears associated with dying may be fear of the unknown, fear of pain, fear of loneliness and abandonment, and fear of meaninglessness.

Fear of Pain. There is a tendency to associate death with pain. Common sayings such as "on pain of death" or "a violent death" have influenced the way that death is perceived. A dying person who has lost a loved one to a painful death may expect the same type of experience. Subsequently, many people assume that pain always accompanies death. Physiologically, there is no reason to assume that death itself is painful. Psychologically, pain may occur based on the anxieties and separations related to dying. Terminally ill patients who do experience physical pain should have pain-relieving drugs available. The patient and the family need assurance that drugs will be given promptly when needed, and that adverse effects of drugs can and will be managed.

Patients can participate in their own pain relief by discussing pain-relief measures and their effects. Most patients want their pain relieved while minimizing the adverse effects of grogginess or sleepiness. The nurse must work with the patient to achieve a balance between pain relief and drowsiness that is most acceptable to the patient.

Fear of Shortness of Breath. Respiratory diseases and shortness of breath may occur for some patients at the end of life and are very distressing for the patient and his or her family. Current therapies include opioids, bronchodilators, and oxygen. Anxiety-reducing medications may be helpful in relieving shortness of breath.

Fear of Loneliness and Abandonment. Most terminally ill and dying people do not want to be alone and fear loneliness. Many dying patients are afraid that loved ones who are unable to cope with the patient's imminent death will abandon them. Dying patients typically want someone whom they know and trust to stay with them (Figure 13-5). This may be a loved one or a caregiver. A simple, caring presence provides support and

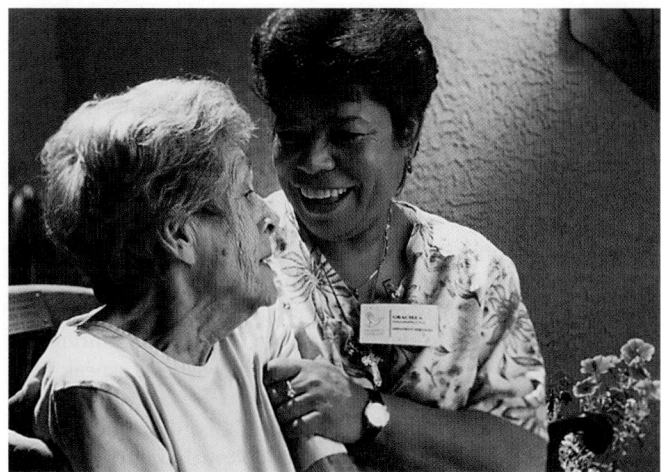

Figure 13-5 Dying patients typically want someone whom they know and trust to stay with them.

Source: Kathleen A. Pollard, RN, MSN, CHPN, Phoenix, AZ.

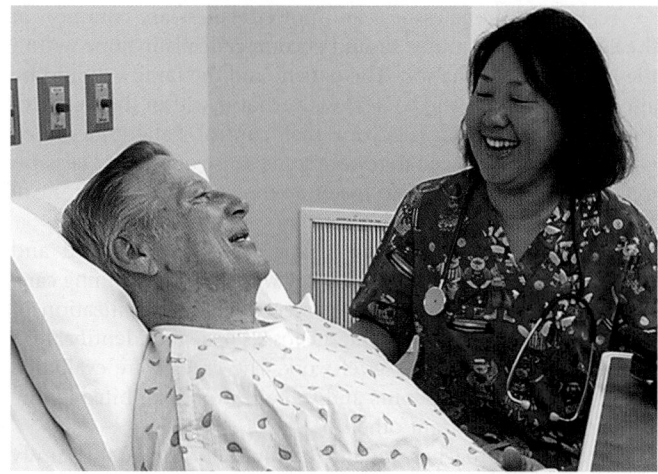

Figure 13-6 Therapeutic communication is an important aspect of end-of-life nursing care.

Source: Kathleen A. Pollard, RN, MSN, CHPN, Phoenix, AZ.

comfort. Neither words nor actions are necessary unless the patient requires something. Holding hands, touching, and listening are considered to be high-quality nursing responses. Simply providing companionship allows the dying person a sense of security.

Fear of Meaninglessness. Fear of meaninglessness leads most people to review their lives. They review their intentions during life, examining actions and expressing regrets about what might have been. Life review helps patients recognize the value that their lives have held. Nurses and family members can help patients review their lives. The worth of the dying person must be expressed. The nurse can assist patients and their families in identifying the positive qualities of the patient's life. The sharing of thoughts and feelings may provide comfort for the patient. The nurse must respect and accept the practices and rituals associated with the patient's life review while remaining nonjudgemental.

Communication. Therapeutic communication is an important nursing intervention used to assist the dying patient and the family (Figure 13-6). Empathy and active listening are essential communication components in EOL care. *Empathy* is the identification with and understanding of another's situation, feelings, and motives, or some combination of the three. *Listening* is an active process required in the development of empathy toward another's feelings.

There may be silence as patients and families process the many changes they are experiencing. Words may be difficult to find or no longer needed. Respecting the need for silence conveys the nurse's acceptance and empathy.

Patients and families need to be allowed time to express their feelings and thoughts. Making time to listen and interact in a sensitive way enhances the relationship among the nurse, the patient, and the family. Listening is essential. There may be silence. Frequently, silence is related to the overwhelming feelings experienced at the end of life. Silence can also allow time to gather thoughts. Listening to the silence sends a message of acceptance and comfort.

Unusual communication by the patient may take place at the end of life. Frequently, near the end of life, the patient's com-munication may become confused, disoriented, or garbled. Patients may speak to or about family members or others who have predeceased them, give instructions to those who will survive them, or speak of projects yet to be completed (Ufema, 2007). Active, careful listening allows for the identification of specific patterns in the dying person's communication and decreases the risk for inappropriate labelling of behaviours.

Grief. Resolution of grief is the primary focus for anticipatory and dysfunctional grieving. Interventions are similar for these two types of grieving, and therefore, they are addressed together. Specific interventions are planned for the specific stage of the grief process or the specific feelings expressed by the patient or family. Goals for grief resolution include patient expression of feelings related to grief, acknowledgement of the impending loss, and demonstrations of behaviours that reflect progress in grief resolution.

Priority interventions for grief must focus on providing an environment that allows the patient to express feelings. Open discussion of feelings helps both the patient and the family work toward resolution of the grief process. The patient should be free to express feelings of anger, fear, or guilt without judgement on the part of the nurse. The patient and the family need to know that the grief reaction is normal. Respect for the patient's privacy and need or desire to talk (or not to talk) is important. Honesty in answering questions and giving information is essential. Families and patients need encouragement to continue their usual activities as much as possible. They need to discuss their activities and maintain some control over their lives. At times, it helps to discuss what can and cannot change. Assistance with planning for the future or for the funeral may be needed according to the patient's or the family's coping abilities.

Anger is a common and normal response to grief. It is important to understand that the grieving person cannot be forced to accept the loss. The surviving family members may be angry at the dying loved one who is leaving them. There is a need to acknowledge and encourage the expression of feelings but at the same time realize how difficult it is to come to terms with grief. Nurses are sometimes the target of the anger and must understand what is happening and not react on a personal level.

Feelings of hopelessness and powerlessness are common at the end of life. The nurse should encourage realistic hope within the limits of the situation. The patient and the family should be allowed to identify and to deal with what is within their control and to recognize what is beyond their control. Patient-identified goals can be encouraged to restore some sense of power. Decision making about care can also foster a sense of power and control for the patient.

Evaluation of the specific coping skills demonstrated and expressed by the patient or the family will assist in planning care. Outcome criteria for goal achievement include verbalization of specific feelings, expression that the loss is real, and identification of specific progress in the grief work. The criteria are evaluated based on specific behaviours and verbalizations exhibited by the patient or the significant others.

As death approaches, the nurse should encourage the family to respond appropriately to the psychosocial manifestations at the end of life. Table 13-8 discusses management of psychosocial manifestations near death.

Physical Care

Nursing management related to physical care at the end of life deals with symptom management and caring, rather than treatments for curing a particular disease or disorder. Meeting the patient's physiological and safety needs is the priority. Physical care focuses on the needs for oxygen, nutrition, pain relief, mobility, elimination, and skin care. People who are dying deserve and require the same physical care as people who are expected to recover. Nursing management at the end of life focuses on symptom management. Table 13-9 delineates the physical care at the end of life.

Pronouncement of Death

In many jurisdictions and agencies, registered nurses are legally able to pronounce that death has occurred. Pronouncement of death differs from certification of death (Registered Nurses Association of British Columbia, 2011). **Pronouncement of death** is defined as determination that life has ceased based on a physical assessment. **Certification of death** is defined as the legally required completion of a death certificate stating the cause of death. Certification of death can be undertaken only by a physician or a coroner. The employing agency is responsible for setting the policy regarding nurse pronouncement of death within the agency.

When pronouncing an individual dead, it is helpful to first acknowledge the family, using statements such as "I'm sorry for your loss . . ."; or "This must be very difficult for you . . ". The family can be invited to stay in the room for the pronouncement. It is appropriate to ask whether the family wishes to speak with a chaplain if one is not already present.

To make the pronouncement of death, confirm the identity of the patient by checking the armband. Note the general appearance of the body, and ascertain that the patient does not rouse to verbal or tactile stimuli. Check for the absence of heart sounds and the carotid pulse. Look and listen for the absence of spontaneous respirations and the absence of the pupillary light reflex (College and Association of the Registered Nurses of Alberta [CARNA] 2011). In the health record, document the time, the date, and the findings of the assessment and whether the family has been notified or an autopsy is required. The agency policy should be checked to determine whether it is necessary to notify the provincial coroner.

Last Offices

After the patient is pronounced dead, the nurse respectfully prepares or delegates preparation of the body for immediate viewing by the family with consideration for cultural customs and in accord with agency policies and procedures. In general, the nurse closes the patient's eyes, replaces dentures, and washes the body as needed (placing pads under the perineum to absorb urine and feces) and may remove tubes and dressings, depending on the setting. The body should be straightened, leaving the pillow to support the head and prevent pooling of blood and

Table 13-8 Nursing Management: Psychosocial Care at the End of Life

CHARACTERISTIC	NURSING MANAGEMENT
Withdrawal	
Patient near death may withdraw from others and from the physical environment.	• Families may be distressed by the patient's withdrawal. Reinforce that this is a normal part of the dying process and support the family. Converse as if the patient is alert, using a soft voice and gentle touch.
Unusual Communication	
Patient may become restless and agitated or perform repetitive tasks. Unusual communication may indicate that an unresolved issue is preventing the dying person from letting go.	• Encourage the family to tell the dying person, "It's okay to go."
Vision-Like Experiences	
Patient may talk to persons who are not there or see places and objects not visible. Vision-like experiences assist the dying person in coming to terms with meaning assigned to life and transitioning from it.	• Affirm the dying person's experience as a part of transition from this life.
Saying Goodbyes	
It is important for the patient and family members to acknowledge their sadness, mutually forgive one another, and say goodbye.	• Encourage the dying person and the family members to verbalize their feelings of sadness, loss, and forgiveness; to touch, hug, and cry. • Allow the patient and family privacy to express their feelings and comfort one another.

Table 13-9 Nursing Management: Physical Care at the End of Life

CHARACTERISTIC	NURSING MANAGEMENT
Pain	
• Pain may be a major symptom associated with terminal illness and the one most feared. • Pain can be acute or chronic. • Physical and emotional irritations can aggravate pain.	• Assess pain thoroughly and regularly to determine the quality, intensity, location, and pattern, as well as contributing and relieving factors. • Minimize possible skin irritations such as those caused by wetness, heat or cold, and pressure. • Administer medications around the clock in a timely manner and on a regular basis to provide constant relief rather than waiting until the pain is unbearable and then trying to relieve it. • Provide complementary and alternative therapies such as guided imagery, massage, acupressure, heat and cold, therapeutic touch, distraction, and relaxation techniques as needed. • Evaluate the effectiveness of pain relief measures frequently to ensure that the patient is on an appropriate and adequate drug regimen. • Do not delay or deny pain relief measures to a terminally ill patient.
Delirium	
• A state characterized by confusion, disorientation, restlessness, clouding of consciousness, incoherence, fear, anxiety, excitement, and often, hallucinations. • May be misidentified as depression, psychosis, anger, or anxiety. • Use of opioids or corticosteroids (and many other medications) in end-of-life care may cause delirium. • Underlying disease process may contribute to delirium. • Generally considered a reversible process.	• Perform a thorough assessment for reversible causes of delirium, including pain, constipation, and urinary retention. • Provide a room that is quiet, well lighted, and familiar to reduce the effects of delirium. • Reorient the dying person to person, place, and time with each encounter. • Adjustments in narcotic type and dosage may be required to counteract opioid toxicity. • Some providers find that hydration using hypodermoclysis may improve delirium. • Administer ordered benzodiazepines, sedatives, and antipsychotics as needed. • Stay physically close to frightened patient. Reassure in a calm, soft voice with touch and slow strokes of the skin. • Provide family members with emotional support and encouragement in their efforts to cope with the behaviours associated with delirium. • Encourage the family to participate in the care for the patient.
Restlessness	
• May occur as death approaches and cerebral metabolism slows.	• Assess for spiritual distress as a cause for restlessness and agitation. • Do not restrain. • Create a soothing environment. • Limit the number of persons at the bedside. • Limit other stimuli and activity.
Dysphagia	
• May occur because of extreme weakness and changes in level of consciousness.	• Identify the least invasive alternative routes of administration for drugs needed for symptom management. • Administer frequent oral care.
Dehydration	
• May occur during the last days of life. • Hunger and thirst are rare in the last days of life. • As the end of life approaches, patients tend to take in less food and fluid.	• Assess condition of mucous membranes frequently to prevent excessive dryness, which can lead to discomfort. • Maintain complete, regular oral care to provide for comfort and hydration of mucous membranes. • Do not force the patient to eat or drink. • Encourage consumption of ice chips and sips of fluids, or use moist cloths to provide moisture to the mouth. • Use moist cloths and swabs for unconscious patients to prevent aspiration. • Apply lubricant to the lips and oral mucous membranes as needed. • Reassure family that cessation of food and fluid intake is a natural part of the process of dying.

Continued

Table 13-9 Nursing Management: Physical Care at the End of Life—cont'd

CHARACTERISTIC	NURSING MANAGEMENT
Dyspnea • Subjective symptom. • Accompanied by fear of suffocation and anxiety. • Underlying disease process can exacerbate dyspnea.	• Assess respiratory status regularly. • Elevate the head or position patient on side to improve chest expansion. • Use a fan or air conditioner to facilitate movement of cool air. • Administer supplemental oxygen as ordered. • Administer drugs (depending on underlying cause of dyspnea) such as opioids, sedatives, diuretics, antibiotics, corticosteroids, and bronchodilators as ordered to relieve congestion and coughing and to decrease apprehension.
Pooling of Secretions • Coughing and expectorating secretions become difficult.	• Position patient on side supported with pillows with head down, or if secretions are excessive, in semiprone position. • Use anticholinergic medications (scopolamine or glycopyrrolate [Robinul]) as ordered.
Weakness and Fatigue • Expected at the end of life. • Metabolic demands related to disease process contribute to weakness and fatigue.	• Assess the patient's tolerance for activities. • Time nursing interventions to conserve energy. • Assist the patient to identify and complete valued or desired activities. • Provide support as needed to maintain positions in bed or chair. • Provide frequent rest periods. • Monitor for risk of falls.
Myoclonus • Mild to severe jerking or twitching sometimes associated with high use of opioids. • Patient may complain of involuntary twitching of upper and lower extremities.	• Assess for the initial onset and the duration and any discomfort or distress experienced by patient. • If myoclonus is distressing or becoming more severe, discuss possible drug therapy modifications with the physician. • Changes in opioid medication may alleviate or decrease myoclonus.
Skin Breakdown • Skin integrity is difficult to maintain at the end of life. • Immobility, urinary and bowel incontinence, dry skin, nutritional deficits, anemia, friction, and shearing forces lead to a high risk for skin breakdown. • Disease and other processes may impair skin integrity. • As death approaches, circulation to the extremities decreases and they become cool, mottled, and cyanotic.	• Assess the skin for signs of breakdown. • Implement protocols to prevent skin breakdown by controlling drainage and odour and keeping the skin and any wound areas clean. • Perform wound assessments as needed. • Follow appropriate nursing management protocol for dressing wounds. • Consider use of special pressure-relieving air mattresses. • Follow appropriate nursing management protocol for a patient who is immobile, but consider what outcomes of skin integrity are realistic and in keeping with maintaining comfort. • Follow appropriate nursing management to prevent skin irritations and breakdown from urinary and bowel incontinence. • Use blankets to cover for warmth; never apply heat. • Prevent the effects of shearing forces.
Bowel Patterns • Constipation can be caused by immobility, use of opioid medications, lack of fibre in the diet, and dehydration. • Diarrhea may occur as muscles relax or from a fecal impaction related to the use of opioids and immobility.	• Assess bowel function. • Assess for and remove fecal impactions. • Encourage movement and physical activities as tolerated. • Encourage fibre in the diet if appropriate. • Encourage fluids if appropriate. • Use suppositories, laxatives, or enemas if ordered.

Table 13-9 Nursing Management: Physical Care at End of the Life—cont'd	
CHARACTERISTIC	**NURSING MANAGEMENT**
Urinary Incontinence	
• May result from disease progression or changes in the level of consciousness. • As death becomes imminent, the perineal muscles relax.	• Assess urinary function. • Use absorbent pads for urinary incontinence. • Follow the appropriate nursing protocol for the consideration and use of indwelling or external catheters. • Follow appropriate nursing management to prevent skin irritations and breakdown from urinary incontinence.
Anorexia, Nausea, and Vomiting	
• Anorexia is normal at the end of life. • May be caused by complications of disease process. • Drugs contribute to nausea. • Constipation, impaction, and bowel obstruction can cause anorexia, nausea, and vomiting.	• Ketosis caused by anorexia causes the release of endorphins, which are thought to provide some natural analgesia. • Assess the patient for complaints of nausea, vomiting, or both. • Assess possible contributing causes of nausea or vomiting. • Have family members provide the patient's favourite foods. • Educate the family about the normal lessening of appetite as death draws near. • Discuss modifications to the drug regimen with the health care provider. • Provide antiemetics before meals if ordered. • Offer and provide frequent meals with small portions of favourite foods. • Offer culturally appropriate foods. • Provide frequent mouth care, especially after vomiting.

discolouration of the face. The family should then be allowed privacy and as much time as they need with the deceased person. In the case of an unexpected or unanticipated death, preparation of the body for viewing or release to a funeral home depends on provincial law and agency policies and procedures.

The loss of a loved person is one of the most intensely painful experiences any human being can suffer (Bowlby, 2000).

Special Needs of Caregivers in End-of-Life Care

Special Needs of Family Caregivers

The dying process can be a long and arduous journey for everyone involved. Being present throughout a family member's dying process can be highly stressful for family members. The role of the nurse includes working and communicating with the patient, supporting the patient's concerns, helping the patient resolve any unfinished business, working with other family members and friends, and dealing with the caregiver's own needs and feelings. An understanding of the grieving process as it affects both the patient and the family caregivers is of great importance. Assistance from spiritual care providers can be invaluable to both the patient and the family.

Recognizing signs and behaviours among family members who may be at risk for abnormal grief reactions is an important nursing intervention. These may include dependency and negative feelings about the dying person, inability to express feelings, concurrent life crises, a history of depression, difficult reactions to previous losses, perceived lack of social or family support, low self-esteem, multiple previous bereavements, alcoholism and substance use, or some combination.

Family caregivers and other family members often need encouragement to care for themselves. They need to prioritize their own activities and maintain some control over their lives. At times, it helps to discuss what can and cannot change.

Grieving relatives, friends, and significant others can provide emotional support for one another. Nurses must be sensitive to the importance of significant others who are not necessarily relatives. Resources such as community counselling and local support may assist some people in working through their grief. Generally, simply allowing the involved people to express their feelings helps to resolve the grief. Family members should be encouraged to facilitate the building of a support system of extended family, friends, faith community, and clergy. The family members should have access to people whom they can call on at any time to express any feelings that they are experiencing. Caregivers and family members should also be provided time to be alone.

Family members need to be encouraged to take care of themselves in ways that address their unique needs (e.g., keeping a journal can help the caregiver express feelings that may be difficult to express verbally). Eating a balanced diet at regular times will provide for the caregiver's well-being. Nourishing the spirit as well as the body is important for the family member to consider. Humour is important, and its sensitive use from time to time can provide distraction and relieve stress-filled situations.

Special Needs of Nurses

Many nurses who care for dying patients do so because they are passionate about providing quality EOL care. Most nurses care for dying patients at some point in their careers. However, caring for dying patients is intense and emotionally charged. A bond or connection often develops among the patient, the family, and the nurse. Nurses need to carefully reflect upon how grief affects them personally. The nurse who is responsible for the care of terminally ill or dying patients is not immune to feelings of loss. It is common for nurses to feel helpless and powerless when dealing with death. Feelings of sorrow, guilt, and frustration can be highlighted by sharing with colleagues, who often have similar feelings.

The nurse must come to recognize and acknowledge what can and cannot be controlled. Recognizing personal feelings allows openness in exchanging feelings with the patient and the family. Realizing that it is acceptable to cry with the patient or the family during the grief process is essential to the nurse's well-being.

Self-care is a key aspect of alleviating stress for the nurse. Involvement in hobbies or other interests, scheduling time for oneself, maintaining a peer support system, and developing a support system beyond the workplace are usually helpful. Crises and grief result in varying forms of stress for nurses. Many agencies provide care for their team members through professionally assisted groups, informal discussion sessions, and flexible time schedules.

Terminal illness and dying are extremely intimate and intense journeys that affect the patient, the family, and the health care team. Caring for patients and their families at the end of life is both a challenging and a rewarding experience. EOL care offers an opportunity to apply the skills and personal commitments that nurses bring to their profession.

REVIEW QUESTIONS

The number of the question corresponds to the same-numbered objective at the beginning of the chapter.

1. Mr. Riesling is in the terminal stages of lung cancer. On assessment, it is noted that he has alternating periods of apnea and deep, rapid breathing. Which of the following is the correct terminology to use in documenting this assessment data?
   a. Tachypnea
   b. Stertorous respirations
   c. Dyspnea
   d. Cheyne-Stokes respirations

2. Mrs. MacLeod has inoperable pancreatic cancer. Until recently, she has been very active with her book club, but she no longer wants to attend. Which common end of life psychological manifestation is she demonstrating?
   a. Decreased socialization
   b. Decreased disease progression
   c. Decreased sense of helplessness
   d. Decreased perception of pain and touch

3. Mohammed's father died 2 years ago. He has repeatedly asked his mother to donate his deceased father's belongings to charity, but his mother has refused. She often sits in the bedroom, crying and talking to her long-dead husband. What type of grief is Mohammed's mother experiencing?
   a. Adaptive grief
   b. Disruptive grief
   c. Anticipatory grief
   d. Prolonged grief

4. Mrs. Rana is in the terminal stages of her disease and experiences choking when she is given food or fluids. The family is concerned that she is starving. What is the most helpful response from the nurse?
   a. "If you give her food, she will choke to death."
   b. "I can order you a tray and you can try to feed her if you like."
   c. "People who are dying usually don't experience discomfort from hunger or thirst the way they did in the past."
   d. "I will see if tube feeding could be started for her."

5. Mr. Makoni did not have an advance directive when he suffered a serious stroke. Who is responsible for identifying end of life measures to be instituted when the patient cannot communicate his or her specific wishes?
   a. Adult children
   b. Notary and attorney
   c. Physician and family
   d. Physician and nursing staff

6. When Mr. Naidu was diagnosed with renal failure, his new wife asked his children from a previous marriage to help with their father's care. Each of the children refused to help. Mrs. Naidu cared for her husband without help until his death. Which behaviours of the children indicate that they may be at risk for abnormal grief reactions? (Check all that apply.)
   a. Dependency and negative feelings about the deceased person
   b. Lack of experience with other deaths in the family
   c. Difficulties with substance misuse
   d. Strong social cohesion between the children

7. Mei Lee has been working full time as a nurse with terminally ill patients for 3 years. She has been experiencing irritability and mixed emotions when expressing sadness since four of her patients died on the same day. What should she change to optimize the quality of her nursing care?
   a. Full-time work schedule
   b. Past feelings toward death
   c. Patterns for dealing with grief
   d. Demands for involvement in care

ANSWERS: 1. d; 2. a; 3. d; 4. c; 5. c; 6. a; 7. c.

REFERENCES

Bowlby, J. (2000). *Notes on symptom control in hospice and palliative care* (rev. ed.). Essex, UK: Hospice Education Institute.

Canadian Hospice Palliative Care Association. (2011a). About us. Retrieved from *http://www.chpca.net/mission-vision*

Canadian Hospice Palliative Care Association. (2011b). Frequently asked questions. Retrieved from *http://www.chpca.net/FAQs#1*

Clark, D. (2002). *Cicely Saunders, founder of the modern-day hospice movement.* New York: Oxford University Press.

College and Association of the Registered Nurses of Alberta. (2011). Pronouncement of death. Retrieved from *http://www.nurses.ab.ca/ Carna-Admin/Uploads/Pronouncement%20of%20Death_1.pdf*

Doka, K. J. (1995). Disenfranchised grief. In L. A. De Spelderg & A. L. Strickland (Eds.), *The path ahead.* Mountain View, CA: Mayfield.

Frost, R., Cook, D., Heyland, D., & Fowler, R. (2011). Patient health-care professional decision-making influencing end-of-life decision-making during critical illness: A systematic review. *Critical Care Medicine 39*(5), 1174-1189. doi:10.1097/CCM. 0b013e31820eacf2

Health Canada. (2009). *Implementation guide to advance care planning in Canada: A case study of two health authorities.* Ottawa: Author. Retrieved from *http://www.hc-sc.gc.ca/hcs-sss/pubs/palliat/2008-acp-guide-pps/index-eng.php*

Heidrich, D. A. (2007). The dying process. In K. K. Kuebler, D. E. Heidrich, & P. Esper (Eds.), *Palliative and end-of-life care: Clinical practice guidelines* (pp. 33-45). St. Louis: Saunders/Elsevier.

Kersting, A., & Kroker, K. (2010). Prolonged grief as a distinct disorder, specifically affecting female health. *Archives of Women's Mental Health, 13*(1), 27-28. doi:10.1007/s00737-009-0112-3

Kübler-Ross, E. (1969). *On death and dying.* New York: Macmillan.

Martin, K., & Elder, S. (1993). Pathways through grief: A model of the process. In J. Morgan (Ed.). *Personal care in an impersonal world: A multidimensional look at bereavement.* New York: Baywood.

Martocchio, B. C. (1985). Grief and bereavement healing through hurt. *Nursing Clinics of North America, 20,* 327.

Quality End of Life Care Coalition. (2010). Blueprint for Action 2010 to 2020. Retrieved from *http://www.qelccc.ca/uploads/files/ information_and_resources/Blueprint_for_Action_2010_to_2020_ April_2010.pdf*

Rando, T. A. (1993). *Treatment of complicated mourning.* Champaign, IL: Research Press.

Registered Nurses Association of British Columbia. (2011). Pronouncement of death. Pub. 456. Retrieved from *https:// www.crnbc.ca/Standards/LegalIssues/Pages/Default.aspx*

Sanderson, C. A. (2007). *End of life: A nurses' guide to compassionate care.* Ambler, PA: Lippincott Williams & Wilkins.

Shemie, S., Doig, C., Dickens, B., Byrne, P., Wheelock, B., Rocker, G., ..., Teitelbaum, J. (2006). Brain arrest: The neurological determination of death and organ donor management in Canada. *Canadian Medical Association Journal, 174*(Suppl), S1-S30.

Subcommittee of the Standing Senate Committee on Social Affairs, Science and Technology. (2000). *Quality end-of-life care: The right of every Canadian.* Ottawa: Senate of Canada. Retrieved from *http://www.parl.gc.ca/Content/SEN/Committee/362/upda/rep/ repfinjun00-e.htm*

Ufema, J. (2007) *Insights on death and dying.* Philadelphia: Lippincott Williams & Wilkins.

World Health Organization (WHO). (2011). WHO definition of palliative care. Retrieved from *http://www.who.int/cancer/palliative/ definition/en/*

CANADIAN RESOURCES

Advance Care Planning
http://www.advancecareplanning.ca

Canadian Cancer Society
http://www.cancer.ca

Canadian Home Care Association
http://www.cdnhomecare.ca/

Canadian Hospice Palliative Care Association
http://www.chpca.net

Canadian Virtual Hospice
http://www.virtualhospice.ca

Casey House Hospice
http://www.caseyhouse.com

Hospice Association of Ontario
http://www.hospice.on.ca

Palliative Care Association of Alberta
http://www.albertapalliative.net

Temmy Letner Centre for Palliative Care
http://www.tlcpc.org/

Toronto Palliative Care Network
http://www.tpcn.ca/

Trillium Gift of Life Network
http://www.giftoflife.on.ca

Victoria Hospice Society
http://www.victoriahospice.org

RELATED RESOURCES

Browns University End of Life Toolkit
http://www.chcr.brown.edu/pcoc/toolkit.htm

evolve   *For additional Internet resources, see the Web site for this book at* **http://evolve.elsevier.com/Canada/Lewis/medsurg**

Pathophysiological Mechanisms of Disease

SECTION OUTLINE

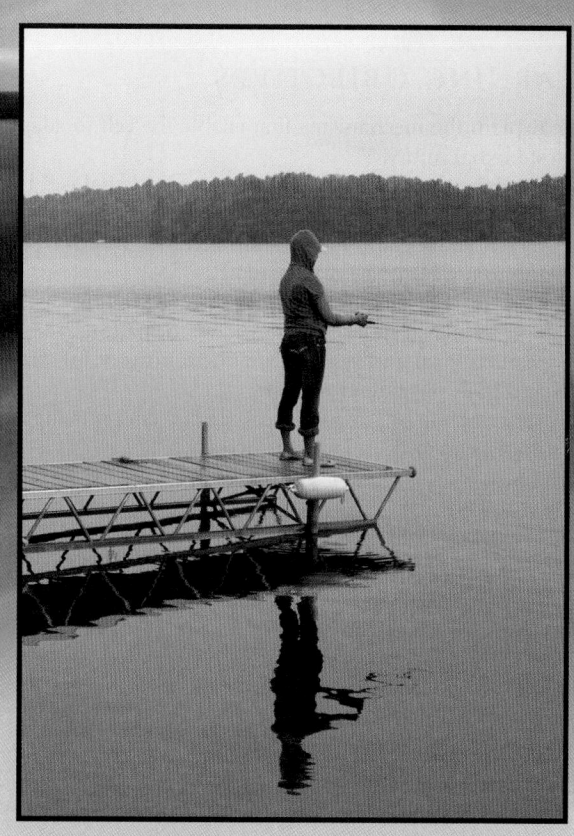

Source: Leobruce/Dreamstime.com

Inflammation and Wound Healing

Written by Russell G. Zaiontz and Sharon L. Lewis
Adapted by Beth Clarke

LEARNING OBJECTIVES

1. Explain the mechanisms that enable the cell to adapt to sublethal injury.
2. Describe the causes and mechanisms of lethal cell injury.
3. Differentiate among types of cell necrosis.
4. Describe the components and functions of the mononuclear phagocyte system.
5. Describe the inflammatory response, including vascular and cellular responses and exudate formation.
6. Explain local and systemic manifestations of inflammation and their physiological bases.
7. Describe the pharmacological, dietary, and nursing management of inflammation.
8. Differentiate among healing by primary, secondary, and tertiary intention.
9. Describe the factors that delay wound healing and common complications of wound healing.
10. Describe the risk assessment process for pressure ulcers.
11. Discuss measures to prevent the development of pressure ulcers.
12. Explain the causes and clinical manifestations of pressure ulcers.
13. Discuss collaborative and nursing management of a patient with pressure ulcers.

KEY TERMS

adhesions Bands of scar tissue between or around organs, p. 259

anaplasia Cell differentiation to a more immature or embryonic form, p. 250

apoptosis Programmed, normally occurring cell death, p. 250

atrophy Decrease in the size of a tissue or organ caused by a reduction in the number or size of the individual cells, p. 249

dehiscence Separation and disruption of previously joined wound edges, p. 259

dry gangrene Ischemic necrosis without superimposed bacterial action, p. 250

dysplasia Abnormal differentiation of dividing cells that results in changes in the size, shape, and appearance of the cells, p. 250

evisceration Protrusion of intestines through a wound when wound edges separate to a certain extent, p. 259

fibroblasts Immature connective tissue cells that migrate into the healing site and secrete collagen, p. 256

fistula an abnormal passage between organs or a hollow organ and the skin, p. 259

hyperplasia An increase in the number of cells as a result of increased cellular division, p. 249

hypertrophic scar Inappropriately large, red, raised, and hard scar that remains confined to the wound edges and regresses in time, p. 260

hypertrophy An increase in the size of cells that results in increased tissue mass without cell division, p. 249

inflammatory response A sequential reaction to cell injury that neutralizes and dilutes the inflammatory agent, removes necrotic materials, and establishes an environment suitable for healing and repair, p. 251

integrins Cell receptors that mediate attachment between endothelial cells and surrounding tissues, involved in leukocyte extravasation during the immune response, p. 252

keloid Permanent protrusion of scar tissue that extends beyond the wound edges and may form tumour-like masses, p. 260

lethal injury Irreversible injury that causes cell death, p. 249

metaplasia Reversible transformation of one cell type into another, p. 250

necrosis Death of a tissue (cell death on a large scale) or part of a tissue with cellular reaction to the dead cells, p. 250

pressure ulcer A localized injury to the skin, underlying tissue, or both, usually over a bony prominence, as a result of pressure or pressure in combination with shear or friction, p. 265

regeneration Replacement of lost cells and tissues with cells of the same type, p. 255

repair Healing that results from replacement of lost cells by connective tissue, p. 255

selectins Cell surface carbohydrate-binding proteins that mediate cell adhesion, involved in leukocyte extravasation during the immune response, p. 252

shearing force Pressure exerted on the skin when it adheres to the bed and the underlying skin layers slide in the direction of body movement, p. 265

sublethal injury Alteration of function without causing cell death, p. 249

wet gangrene Ischemic necrosis with superimposed bacterial action, p. 250

ELECTRONIC RESOURCES

Supplemental content related to Chapter 14 can be found...

Evolve Web Site ⊝volve

http://evolve.elsevier.com/Canada/Lewis/medsurg
- Answer Guidelines for Case Study on p. 272
- Content Updates
- Customizable Nursing Care Plans
  - Fever
  - Pressure Ulcer
- Electronic Calculators
- eFigures:
  - eFigure 14-1: Margination, Diapedesis, and Chemotaxis of White Blood Cells

- eFigure 14-2: Sequential Activation and Biological Effects of the Complement System
- eTables:
  - eTable 14-1: Wound Classification by Etiology
  - eTable 14-2: Wound Classification by Systems
- Examination Review Questions
- Glossary
- Interactive Case Study: Pressure Ulcers
- Key Points (Printable and MP3 Download)

Cell Injury

Cell injury can be sublethal or lethal. **Sublethal injury** alters function without causing cell death. The changes caused by this type of injury are potentially reversible if the injurious stimulus is removed. **Lethal injury** is an irreversible process that causes cell death.

Cell Adaptation to Sublethal Injury

Cell adaptations to sublethal injuries are common and are part of many normal physiological processes, but they may also result from pathological changes. For example, prolonged exposure to sunlight stimulates melanin production, which provides protection of deeper skin layers; increased melanin production causes tanning of the skin. Lack of muscular activity can lead to atrophy and decreased muscle tone. Adaptive processes of the cell include hypertrophy, hyperplasia, atrophy, and metaplasia. Other responses, which are considered maladaptive, are dysplasia and anaplasia.

Hypertrophy. **Hypertrophy** is an increase in the size of cells, which results in increased tissue mass without cell division. It is usually caused by the response of an organ or a select area of tissue to an increased demand for work. An example of physiological hypertrophy is that in the skeletal muscles, known as *muscle hypertrophy*. Muscle hypertrophy results from an increase in the size of muscle fibres in response to an increase in cellular protein, which occurs during weight training. Other examples of physiological hypertrophy include uterus enlargement during

pregnancy from hormonal stimulation and enlargement of the sex organs during puberty. An example of pathological hyperplasia is enlargement of the heart in a person with severe hypertension to compensate for the increased resistance to its pumping action. Removal of one kidney results in an increase in the size of the remaining kidney because of the increased work demand.

Hyperplasia. **Hyperplasia** is an increase in the number of cells as a result of increased cellular division. This process is reversible when the stimulus for cellular division is removed. Compensatory hyperplasia is an adaptive process whereby cells of certain organs regenerate. For example, if portions of the liver are removed, the remaining cells undergo increased mitosis to compensate for the cells removed. Hormonal hyperplasia occurs primarily in structures responsive to estrogen, such as the breasts and the uterus. For example, the uterus undergoes hyperplasia during pregnancy, and the female breast undergoes hyperplasia during lactation. An example of pathological hyperplasia is endometrial hyperplasia, caused by excessive hormone stimulation. In this condition, high amounts of estrogen or an imbalance between estrogen and progesterone leads to excessive growth of the endometrium.

Atrophy. **Atrophy** is a decrease in the size of a tissue or organ caused by a reduction in the number or the size of the individual cells. It frequently occurs as a result of disease (e.g., musculoskeletal disease), lack of blood supply (e.g., thrombus formation), the natural aging process (e.g., atrophy of ovaries after menopause), inactivity (e.g., decreased muscle size), and nutritional deficiency.

Metaplasia. Metaplasia is the reversible transformation of one cell type into another. An example of physiological metaplasia is the change of circulating monocytes to macrophages as they migrate into inflamed tissues. An example of pathophysiological metaplasia is the change of normal pseudostratified columnar epithelium of the bronchi to squamous epithelium in response to chronic cigarette smoking. If the irritating stimulus (the cigarette smoke) is removed, the bronchial metaplasia may be reversible.

Dysplasia. Dysplasia is an abnormal differentiation of dividing cells that results in changes in the size, shape, and appearance of these cells. Minor dysplasia is found in some areas of inflammation. Dysplasia is potentially reversible if the stimulus for the change is removed. Dysplasia is frequently a precursor of malignancy, as in cervical dysplasia.

Anaplasia. Anaplasia is cell differentiation to a more immature or embryonic form. Malignant tumours are often characterized by anaplastic cell growth.

Causes of Lethal Cell Injury

Many different agents and factors can cause lethal cell injury (Table 14-1). The mechanisms of actual cell death may include deterioration of the nucleus, such as pyknosis (nuclear condensation and shrinking), karyolysis (dissolution of nucleus and contents), disruption of cell metabolism, and rupture of the cell membrane.

Microbial invasion often results in cell injury and death. Infection occurs when pathogens (microorganisms capable of producing disease) invade and multiply in body tissue.

Cell Apoptosis and Necrosis

Apoptosis and necrosis are the two fundamental types of cell death. Individual cell death is a normal event in some regenerating tissues, such as skin and gut epithelium, and during embryogenesis. Programmed cell death is termed **apoptosis.** Human health is dependent on this process (Saltsman, 2011). However, cell death is *not* a normal event in developed tissues such as those of the brain and becomes a serious occurrence when many cells are involved in such organs as the liver, when it is considered necrosis.

Necrosis is death of a tissue (cell death on a large scale) or part of a tissue with cellular reaction to the dead cells (Saltsman, 2011). Different types of tissue necrosis tend to occur in different organs or tissues (Table 14-2, Figure 14-1). **Dry gangrene** refers to the dry, shrivelled, darkened area (see Figure 14-1), and **wet gangrene** refers to liquefied necrotic tissue.

Table 14-1 Causes of Lethal Cell Injury

CAUSE	EFFECT ON CELL
Hypoxia or ischemic injury	Compromised cell metabolism, acute or gradual cell death
Physical agents	
Heat	Denaturation of protein, acceleration of metabolic reactions
Cold	Decreased blood flow from vasoconstriction, slowed metabolic reactions, thrombosis of blood vessels, freezing of cell contents that forms crystals and can cause cell to burst
Radiation	Alteration of cell structure and activity, alteration of enzyme systems, mutations
Electrothermal injury	Interruption of neural conduction, fibrillation of cardiac muscle, coagulative necrosis of skin and skeletal muscle
Mechanical trauma	Transfer of excess kinetic energy to cells, causing rupture of cells, blood vessels, tissue; examples include the following: *Abrasion:* scraping of skin or mucous membrane *Laceration:* severing of vessels and tissue *Contusion (bruise):* crushing of tissue cells causing hemorrhage into skin *Puncture:* piercing of body structure or organ *Incision:* surgical cutting
Chemical injury	Alteration of cell metabolism, interference with normal enzymatic action within cells
Microbial injury	
Viruses	Taking over of cell metabolism and synthesis of new particles that may cause cell rupture; cumulative effect may produce clinical disease
Bacteria	Destruction of cell membrane or cell nucleus, production of lethal toxins
Immunological*	
Antigen–antibody response	
Autoimmune	Release of substances (histamine, complement) that can injure and damage cells Activation of complement, which destroys normal cells and produces inflammation
Neoplastic growth	Cell destruction from abnormal and uncontrolled cell growth
Normal substances (e.g., digestive enzymes, uric acid)	Release into abdomen, causing peritonitis and crystallization of excess accumulation in joints and renal tissue

*See Chapter 16 for a more detailed discussion.

Table 14-2 Types of Necrosis

TYPE	DESCRIPTION
Coagulative necrosis	Caused by ischemia. Ischemia results in decreased adenosine triphosphate (ATP), increased cytosolic Ca^{2+}, and free radical formation, each of which eventually causes membrane damage. A myocardial infarct is an example of a localized area of coagulative necrosis.
Liquefactive necrosis	Usually caused by focal bacterial infections because they can attract polymorphonuclear leukocytes (PMNs). The enzymes in the PMNs are released to fight the bacteria but also dissolve the tissues nearby, causing an accumulation of pus and effectively liquefying the tissue. An abscess is an example of a liquefactive necrotic process.
Caseous necrosis	A distinct form of coagulative necrosis that occurs in mycobacterial infections (e.g., tuberculosis) or in tumour necrosis, in which the coagulated tissue no longer resembles the cells but is in chunks of unrecognizable debris.
Gangrene	Necrosis of an appendage (usually the limbs). The term may also be used to describe necrosis of an appendix or gallbladder. This form of necrosis applies to ischemic necrosis, usually with superimposed bacterial action (wet gangrene) but sometimes in toes without bacterial effects (dry gangrene or mummification).

Source: Adapted from Krafts, K.(2012). A quick summary of six types of necrosis. Retrieved from *http://www.pathologystudent.com/?p=5770*

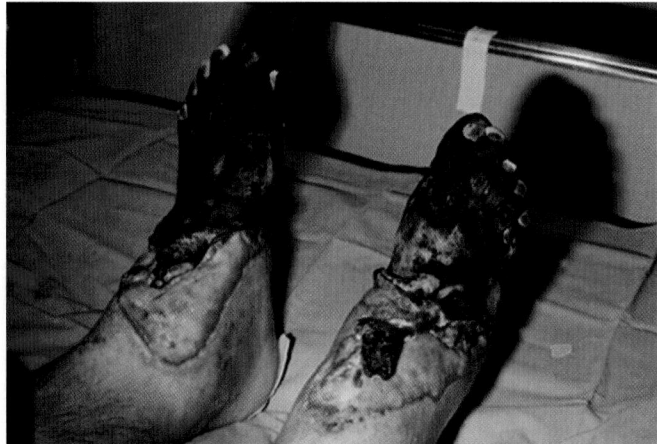

Figure 14-1 Gangrene of the toes. Gangrenous necrosis 6 weeks after frostbite injury.

Source: Courtesy Cameron Bangs, MD. From Auerbach, P. S. (2007). *Wilderness medicine* (5th ed., p. 201, Figure 8-3, *A*). St. Louis: Mosby.

Table 14-3 Locations and Names of Macrophages*

LOCATION	NAME
Connective tissue	Histiocytes
Liver	Kupffer cells
Lung	Alveolar macrophages
Spleen	Free and fixed macrophages
Bone marrow	Fixed macrophages
Lymph nodes	Free and fixed macrophages
Bone tissue	Osteoclasts
Central nervous system	Microglial cells
Peritoneal cavity	Peritoneal macrophages
Pleural cavity	Pleural macrophages
Skin	Histiocytes, Langerhans cells
Synovium	Type A cells

*In addition, monocytes become macrophages once they leave the blood and enter the tissues.

Defence Against Injury

To protect against injury and infection, the body has various defence mechanisms: (a) the skin and mucous membranes (see Chapter 25); (b) the mononuclear phagocyte system; (c) the inflammatory response; and (d) the immune system (see Chapter 16).

Mononuclear Phagocyte System

The *mononuclear phagocyte system* consists of monocytes and macrophages and their precursor cells. In the past, the mononuclear phagocyte system was called the *reticuloendothelial system*. However, it is not a body system with distinctly defined tissues and organs. Rather, it consists of phagocytic cells located in various tissues and organs (Table 14-3). The phagocytic cells are either fixed or free (mobile). The macrophages of the liver, spleen, bone marrow, lungs, lymph nodes, and nervous system (microglial cells) are fixed phagocytes. The monocytes (in blood) and the macrophages found in connective tissue (histiocytes) are mobile, or wandering, phagocytes.

Monocytes and macrophages originate in the bone marrow. Monocytes spend a few days in the blood and then enter tissues and change into macrophages. Tissue macrophages are larger and more phagocytic than monocytes.

The functions of the macrophage system include recognition and phagocytosis of foreign material such as microorganisms, removal of old or damaged cells from circulation, and participation in the immune response (see Chapter 16).

Inflammatory Response

The **inflammatory response** is a complex, nonlinear process and is a key aspect of many disease processes. It is a biological response to cell injury by pathogens, irritants, or chronic health conditions. It neutralizes and dilutes the inflammatory agent, removes necrotic materials, and establishes an environment suitable for healing and repair. The term *inflammation* should not be confused with *infection*. Infections almost always cause inflammation, but not all inflammations are caused by infections. Furthermore, neutropenic individuals may not mount an inflammatory response to infection. An infection involves invasion of tissues or cells by microorganisms such as bacteria, fungi, and viruses. Inflammation can also be caused by nonliving agents such as heat, radiation, trauma, and allergens (see Table 14-1). Under these conditions, the presence of an infection represents a superimposed invasion of microorganisms.

The mechanism of inflammation is basically the same regardless of the injuring agent. The intensity of the response depends on the extent and the severity of injury and on the reactive capacity of the injured person. The inflammatory response can be divided into a vascular response, a cellular response, formation of exudate, and healing. Figure 14-2 illustrates the vascular and cellular responses to injury.

Vascular Response. After cell injury, arterioles in the area briefly undergo transient vasoconstriction, which is stimulated by the sympathetic nervous system. Platelets adhere to vessels and aggregate to seal the injured area, forming a fibrin-platelet clot, and release proinflammatory mediators such as histamine, which cause vasodilation. This results in *hyperemia* (increased blood flow in the area) in which filtration pressure increases, causing endothelial cell retraction and increase in capillary permeability. Movement of fluid from capillaries into tissue spaces is thus facilitated. Initially composed of serous fluid, this inflammatory exudate later contains plasma proteins, primarily albumin, which exerts oncotic pressure that further draws fluid from blood vessels, and the tissue become edematous.

As the plasma protein fibrinogen leaves the blood, it is activated by the products of the injured cells to become fibrin. Fibrin strengthens the blood clot formed by platelets. In tissue, the clot functions to trap bacteria, to prevent their spread, and to serve as a framework for the healing process.

Cellular Response. Phagocytes produce nitric oxide, whose role in the inflammatory response is to inhibit vascular smooth muscle contraction and growth, platelet aggregation, and leukocyte adhesion to endothelium. Cytokines are released by macrophages, which causes endothelial cells to express cellular adhesion molecules (**selectins** and **integrins**). The blood flow through capillaries in the area slows as fluid is lost and viscosity increases. Neutrophils and monocytes move to the inner surface of the capillaries (margination) and then, in ameboid manner, through the capillary wall (*diapedesis*) to the site of injury.

Chemotaxis is the directional migration of white blood cells (WBCs) along a concentration gradient of chemotactic factors, which are substances that attract WBCs to the site of inflammation. Chemotaxis is the mechanism for ensuring accumulation of neutrophils and monocytes at the focus of injury. (eFigure 14-1, which shows chemotaxis, is available on the Evolve Web site for this chapter.)

Neutrophils. Neutrophils are the first leukocytes to arrive at the site of inflammation (usually within 6 to 12 hours). They

PATHOPHYSIOLOGY MAP

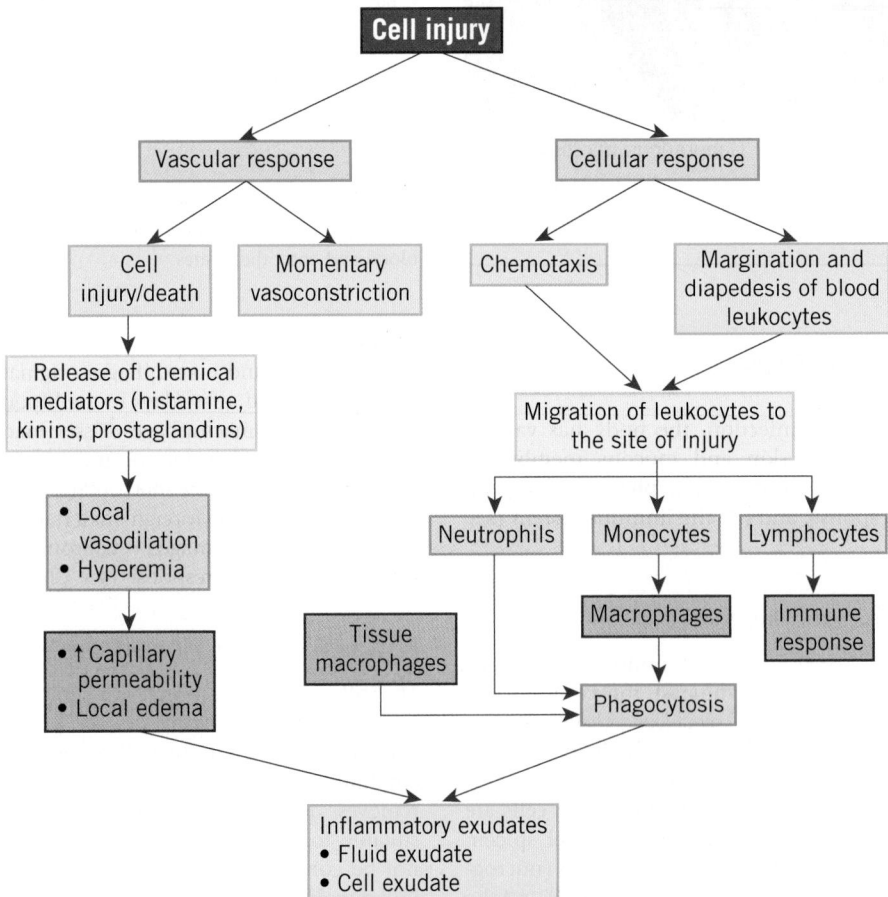

Figure 14-2 Vascular and cellular responses in inflammation.

phagocytize (engulf) bacteria, other foreign material, and damaged cells. Because of their short lifespan (24 to 48 hours), dead neutrophils soon accumulate. In time, a mixture of dead neutrophils, digested bacteria, and other cell debris accumulates as a creamy substance *(pus)*.

To keep up with the demand for neutrophils, the bone marrow releases more neutrophils into circulation. This results in elevation of the WBC count, especially the neutrophil count. Sometimes the demand for neutrophils increases to the extent that the bone marrow releases immature forms of neutrophils (bands) into circulation. (Mature neutrophils are called *segmented neutrophils*.) The finding of increased numbers of band neutrophils in circulation is called *a shift to the left* and is commonly observed in patients with acute bacterial infections. (See Chapter 32 for a discussion of neutrophils.)

Monocytes. Monocytes are the second type of phagocytic cells that migrate from circulating blood. They are attracted by chemotactic factors and usually arrive at the site within 3 to 7 days after the onset of inflammation. On entering the tissue spaces, monocytes transform into macrophages. Together with the tissue macrophages, they assist in phagocytosis of the inflammatory debris. The macrophage role is important in cleaning the area before healing can occur. Macrophages have a long lifespan; they can multiply and may stay in the damaged tissues for weeks and are important in orchestrating the healing process.

In some cases, macrophages perform tasks other than phagocytosis. They may accumulate and fuse to form a *multinucleated giant cell.* The giant cell attempts to phagocytize particles too large for macrophages and is then encapsulated by collagen, which leads to the formation of a granuloma. A classic example of this process occurs with the tubercle bacillus in the lung. Although the bacillus is walled off, a chronic state of inflammation exists. The granuloma formed is a cavity of necrotic tissue.

Lymphocytes. Lymphocytes arrive later at the site of injury. Their primary role is related to humoral and cell-mediated immunity (see Chapter 16).

Eosinophils and Basophils. Eosinophils and basophils have a more selective role in inflammation. Eosinophils are released in large quantities during an allergic reaction. They release chemicals that act to control the effects of histamine and serotonin. They are also involved in phagocytosis of the allergen-antibody complex. Eosinophils contain highly caustic chemicals that are capable of destroying a parasite's cell surfaces. The histamine and heparin that basophils carry in their granules are released during inflammation.

Chemical Mediators. Mediators of the inflammatory response are presented in Table 14-4.

Complement System. The complement system is a major mediator of the inflammatory response. Major functions of the complement system are enhanced phagocytosis, increased vascular permeability, chemotaxis, and cellular lysis. All of these activities are important in the inflammatory response.

When the complement system is activated, the components are generated in the sequential order of C1, C4, C2, C3, C5, C6, C7, C8, and C9 (eFigure 14-2, which shows the complement cascade, is available on the Evolve Web site for this chapter). The numbering reflects the order of their discovery. Some components have subparts designated by lowercase letters, such as C3a, C3b, and C5a. The primary pathway for activation of the complement system is through fixation of component C1 to an antigen-antibody complex. Immunoglobulins G and M are responsible for fixing complement. Each activated complex can act on the next component, which creates a cascade effect.

An alternative pathway exists in which C3 is activated without prior antigen-antibody fixation. Bacterial products, lipopolysaccharides, and neutrophil proteases can stimulate the complement sequence at the C3 level with activation of C5 through C9.

Complement activation increases phagocytosis through opsonization and chemotaxis. *Opsonization* occurs when the antigen, in combination with complement factor C3b and immunoglobulin, sticks to the surface of phagocytic cells. This leads to

Table 14-4 Mediators of Inflammation

MEDIATOR	SOURCE	MECHANISMS OF ACTION
Histamine	Stored in granules of basophils, mast cells, platelets	Causes vasodilation and increased vascular permeability by stimulating contraction of endothelial cells and creating widened gaps between cells
Serotonin	Stored in platelets, mast cells, enterochromaffin cells of GI tract	Causes vasodilation and increased vascular permeability by stimulating contraction of endothelial cells and creating widened gaps between cells; stimulates smooth muscle contraction
Kinins (e.g., bradykinin)	Produced from precursor factor kininogen as a result of activation of Hageman factor (XII) of clotting system	Cause contraction of smooth muscle and dilation of blood vessels; result in stimulation of pain
Complement components (C3a, C4a, C5a)	Anaphylatoxic agents generated from complement pathway activation	Stimulate histamine release; stimulate chemotaxis
Fibrinopeptides	Produced from activation of the clotting system	Increase vascular permeability; stimulate chemotaxis for neutrophils and monocytes
Prostaglandins and leukotrienes	Produced from arachidonic acid	Prostaglandins E_1 and E_2 cause vasodilation; leukotriene B_4 stimulates chemotaxis
Cytokines	For information on cytokines, see Table 16-3	

GI, gastrointestinal.

Table 14-5 Types of Inflammatory Exudate

TYPE	DESCRIPTION	EXAMPLES
Serous	Results from fluid that has low cell and protein content; seen in early stages of inflammation or when injury is mild	Skin blisters, pleural effusion
Catarrhal	Found in tissues in which cells produce mucus; mucus production is accelerated by inflammatory response	Runny nose in association with upper respiratory tract infection
Fibrinous	Occurs with increasing vascular permeability and fibrinogen leakage into interstitial spaces; excessive amounts of fibrin coating of tissue surfaces may cause tissues to adhere	Adhesions
Purulent (pus)	Consists of WBCs, microorganisms (dead and alive), liquefied dead cells, and other debris	Furuncle (boil), abscess, cellulitis (diffuse inflammation in connective tissue)
Hemorrhagic	Results from rupture or necrosis of blood vessel walls; consists of RBCs that escape into tissue	Hematoma

RBCs, red blood cells; *WBCs,* white blood cells.

more rapid phagocytosis. In addition, complement component C5a promotes chemotaxis.

The components C3a, C5a, and C4a are termed *anaphylatoxins* and bind to receptors on mast cells and basophils, thus triggering histamine release. Histamine causes smooth muscle contraction, vasodilation, and an increase in vascular permeability.

The entire complement sequence of C1 to C9 must be activated for cell lysis to occur. The final components (C8, C9) act on the cell surface, causing rupture of the cell membrane and lysis. Bacteria, red blood cells, and nucleated cells are susceptible to the lysis.

Prostaglandins and Leukotrienes. Prostaglandins are substances that can be synthesized from the phospholipids of cell membranes of most body tissues, including blood cells. On stimulation by chemotactic factors or phagocytosis or after cell injury, phospholipids can be converted to arachidonic acid, which is then oxidized by two different pathways.

The *cyclooxygenase metabolic pathway* leads to the production of prostaglandins of the D, E, F, and I series and thromboxanes (formed on activation of platelets). Prostaglandins of the E and I series are potent vasodilators and inhibit platelet and neutrophil aggregation. Prostaglandin E_2 (PGE_2) can also sensitize pain receptors to arousal by stimuli that would normally be painless. PGE_2 is also a potent pyrogen, acting on the temperature-regulating area of the hypothalamus. Thromboxane A_2 is a potent vasoconstrictor and platelet-aggregating agent. Prostaglandins are generally considered proinflammatory, contributing to increased blood flow, edema, and pain. Metabolism of arachidonic acid by the lipoxygenase pathway leads to the production of leukotrienes. Leukotriene B_4 is a potent chemotactic factor. Leukotrienes C_4, D_4, and E_4 form the slow-reacting substance of anaphylaxis (SRS-A), which constricts smooth muscles of bronchi and increases capillary permeability.

Drugs that inhibit prostaglandin synthesis are useful clinically. Nonsteroidal anti-inflammatory drugs (NSAIDs), one type of these drugs, are a prototype drug treatment for many acute and chronic inflammatory conditions. Acetylsalicylic acid blocks platelet aggregation; it also has anti-inflammatory action. Prostacyclin (prostaglandin I_2) has been used to prevent platelet deposition in extracorporeal systems, such as hemodialysis and heart-lung bypass oxygenators.

Table 14-6 Local Manifestations of Inflammation

MANIFESTATIONS	CAUSE
Redness	Hyperemia from vasodilation
Heat	Increased metabolism at inflammatory site
Pain	Change in pH; change in local ionic concentration; nerve stimulation by chemicals (e.g., histamine, prostaglandins); pressure from fluid exudates
Swelling	Fluid shift to interstitial spaces; fluid exudates accumulation
Loss of function	Swelling and pain

Another group of drugs that inhibit prostaglandins are corticosteroids. They are valuable in the treatment of asthma because they inhibit leukotriene production and thus prevent bronchoconstriction. (Other mediators of the inflammatory response are described in Table 14-4.)

Exudate Formation. Exudate consists of fluid and leukocytes that move from the circulation to the site of injury. The nature and quantity of exudate depend on the type and the severity of the injury and the tissues involved (Table 14-5).

Clinical Manifestations. The local response to inflammation includes the manifestations of redness, heat and swelling (caused by increased blood flow), pain (caused by release of chemical mediators that stimulate nerve endings), and loss of function (Table 14-6). Systemic manifestations of inflammation include leukocytosis with a shift to the left, malaise, nausea and anorexia, increased pulse and respiratory rate, and fever.

Leukocytosis results from the increased release of leukocytes from the bone marrow. The circulating number of one or more types of leukocytes may be increased. Inflammatory reactions are accompanied by the vaguely defined constitutional symptoms of malaise, nausea, anorexia, and fatigue. The causes of these systemic changes are poorly understood but are probably complement activation and the release of cytokines (soluble factors secreted by WBCs that act as intercellular messengers) from stimulated WBCs. Three of these cytokines—interleukin-1,

PATHOPHYSIOLOGY MAP

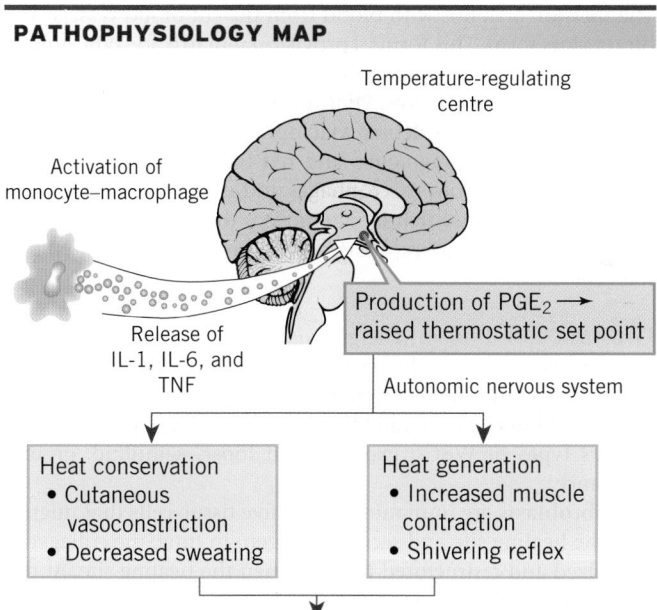

FEVER

Figure 14-3 Production of fever. When monocytes or macrophages are activated, they secrete cytokines such as interleukin-1 (IL-1), interleukin-6 (IL-6), and tumour necrosis factor (TNF), which reach the hypothalamic temperature-regulating centre. These cytokines promote the synthesis and secretion of prostaglandin E_2 (PGE_2) in the anterior hypothalamus. PGE_2 increases the thermostatic set point, and the autonomic nervous system is stimulated, resulting in shivering, muscle contraction, and peripheral vasoconstriction.

Table 14-7 Stages of the Febrile Response	
STAGE	**CHARACTERISTICS**
Prodromal	Nonspecific complaints such as mild headache, fatigue, general malaise, muscle aches
Chill	Cutaneous vasoconstriction, "goose pimples," pale skin; feeling of being cold; generalized, shaking chill; shivering causing body to reach new temperature set by control centre in hypothalamus
Flush	Sensation of warmth throughout body; cutaneous vasodilation; warming and flushing of skin
Defervescence	Sweating; decrease in body temperature

interleukin-6, and tumour necrosis factor—are important in causing the generalized symptoms of inflammation, such as malaise, as well as inducing fever. An increase in pulse and respiration follows the rise in metabolism as a result of an increase in body temperature. (Cytokines are discussed in Chapter 16.)

Fever. The onset of fever is triggered by the release of cytokines. The most potent of these cytokines are interleukin-1, interleukin-6, and tumour necrosis factor (released from mononuclear phagocyte cells). α-Interferon (α-IFN), β-interferon (β-IFN), and γ-interferon (γ-IFN) are also cytokines that can stimulate the responses to cause a fever (Dinarello & Porat, 2011). These pyrogenic cytokines cause fever by their ability to initiate metabolic changes in the temperature-regulating centre (Figure 14-3). The synthesis of PGE_2 is the most critical metabolic change. PGE_2 acts directly to increase the thermostatic set point. The hypothalamus then activates the sympathetic branch of the autonomic nervous system to stimulate increases in muscle tone and shivering and decreases in perspiration and blood flow to the periphery. Epinephrine released from the adrenal medulla increases the metabolic rate. The net result is fever.

With the physiological thermostat fixed at a higher-than-normal temperature, the rate of heat production is increased until the body temperature reaches the new set point. As the set point is raised, the hypothalamus signals an increase in heat production and conservation to raise the body temperature to the new level. At this point, the affected individual feels chilled and shivers. The shivering response is the body's method of raising

the body's temperature until the new set point is attained. The body is hot, and yet an individual paradoxically piles on blankets and may go to bed to get warm. When the circulating body temperature reaches the set point of the core body temperature, the chills and warmth-seeking behaviour cease (Dinarello & Porat, 2011). The febrile response is classified into four stages, described in Table 14-7.

The released cytokines and the fever they trigger activate the body's defence mechanisms. Beneficial aspects of fever include increased killing of microorganisms, increased phagocytosis by neutrophils, and increased proliferation of T cells. Higher body temperatures may also enhance the activity of interferon, the body's natural virus-fighting substance (see Chapter 16).

Types of Inflammation. The basic types of inflammation are acute, subacute, and chronic. In *acute inflammation*, the healing occurs in 2 to 3 weeks and usually leaves no residual damage. Neutrophils are the predominant cell type at the site of inflammation. A *subacute inflammation* has the features of the acute process but lasts longer. For example, infective endocarditis is a smouldering infection with acute inflammation, but it persists throughout weeks or months (see Chapter 39).

Chronic inflammation lasts for weeks, months, or even years. The injurious agent persists or repeatedly injures tissue. The predominant cell types present at the site of inflammation are lymphocytes and macrophages. Examples of chronic inflammation include rheumatoid arthritis and tuberculosis. Tuberculosis is a type of chronic granulomatous inflammation. A chronic inflammatory process is debilitating and can be devastating. The prolongation and chronicity of any inflammation may be the result of an alteration in the immune response. C-reactive protein is an acute-phase protein whose plasma concentration increases in response to inflammation, and thus it is a useful inflammatory marker.

Healing Process

The final phase of the inflammatory response is healing. Healing includes the two major components of regeneration and repair. **Regeneration** is the replacement of lost cells and tissues with cells of the same type. **Repair** is healing as a result of lost cells being replaced by connective tissue. Repair is the more common type of healing and usually results in scar formation.

Table 14-8 Regenerative Ability of Different Types of Tissues

TISSUE TYPE	REGENERATIVE ABILITY
Epithelial	
Skin, linings of blood vessels, mucous membranes	Cells readily divide and regenerate
Connective Tissue	
Bone	Active tissue heals rapidly
Cartilage	Regeneration possible but slow
Tendons and ligaments	Regeneration possible but slow
Blood	Cells actively regenerate
Muscle	
Smooth	Regeneration usually possible (particularly in GI tract)
Cardiac	Damaged muscle replaced by connective tissue
Skeletal	Connective tissue replaces severely damaged muscle; some regeneration in moderately damaged muscle occurs
Nerve	
Neurons	Generally nonmitotic; do not replicate and replace themselves if irreversibly damaged
Glial	Cells regenerate; scar tissue often forms when neurons are damaged

GI, gastrointestinal.

Regeneration

The ability of cells to regenerate depends on the cell type (Table 14-8). Labile cells—such as cells of the skin, lymphoid organs, bone marrow, and mucous membranes of the gastrointestinal, urinary, and reproductive tracts—divide constantly. Injury to these organs is followed by rapid regeneration.

Stable cells retain their ability to regenerate but do so only if the organ is injured. Examples of stable cells are liver, pancreas, kidney, and bone cells.

Permanent cells do not regenerate. Examples of these cells are neurons of the central nervous system and cardiac muscle cells. Damage to neurons of the central nervous system or to heart muscle can lead to permanent loss. Healing occurs by repair with scar tissue.

Repair

Repair is a more complex process than regeneration. Most injuries heal by connective tissue repair. Repair healing occurs by primary, secondary, or tertiary intention (Figure 14-4).

Primary Intention. *Primary intention* healing takes place when wound margins are neatly approximated, as in a surgical incision or a paper cut. A continuum of processes is associated with primary healing (Table 14-9). These processes include three phases:

Initial Phase. The initial phase lasts for 3 to 5 days. The edges of the incision are first aligned and sutured (or stapled) in place.

The incision area fills with blood from the cut blood vessels, and blood clots form. This forms a provisional matrix for WBC migration. An acute inflammatory reaction occurs. The area of injury is composed of fibrin clots, erythrocytes, neutrophils (both dead and dying), and other debris. Macrophages ingest and digest cellular debris, fibrin fragments, and red blood cells. Extracellular enzymes derived from macrophages and neutrophils help digest fibrin. As the wound debris is removed, the fibrin clot serves as a meshwork for future capillary growth and migration of epithelial cells.

Granulation Phase. The *granulation (fibroblastic, proliferative, reconstructive)* phase is the second step and lasts from 5 days to 3 weeks. The components of granulation tissue include proliferating fibroblasts; proliferating capillary sprouts (angioblasts); various types of WBCs; exudate; and loose, semifluid, ground substance.

Fibroblasts are immature connective tissue cells that migrate into the healing site and secrete collagen. In time, the collagen is organized and restructured to strengthen the healing site. At this stage, it is termed *fibrous* or *scar tissue.*

During the granulation phase, the wound is pink and vascular. Numerous red granules (young budding capillaries) are present. At this point, the wound is friable, at risk for dehiscence, and resistant to infection.

Surface epithelium at the wound edges begins to regenerate. In a few days, a thin layer of epithelium migrates across the wound surface. The epithelium thickens and begins to mature, and the wound now closely resembles the adjacent skin. In a superficial wound, re-epithelialization may take 3 to 5 days.

Maturation Phase and Scar Contraction. The maturation phase, in which scar contraction occurs, overlaps with the granulation phase. It may begin 7 days after the injury and continue for several months or years. Collagen fibres are further organized, and the remodelling process occurs. Fibroblasts disappear as the scar becomes stronger. The active movement of the myofibroblasts causes contraction of the healing area, helping to close the defect and bring the skin edges closer together. A mature scar is then formed. In contrast to granulation tissue, a mature scar is virtually avascular and pale, and the site may be more painful at this phase than in the granulation phase.

Secondary Intention. Wounds that occur from trauma, ulceration, and infection and have large amounts of exudate and wide, irregular wound margins, with extensive tissue loss, may not have edges that can be approximated. The inflammatory reaction may be greater than in primary healing. This results in more debris, cells, and exudate. The debris may have to be cleaned away (debrided) before healing can take place.

In some instances, a primary incision may become infected, which creates additional inflammation. The wound may reopen, and healing by secondary intention takes place.

The process of healing by secondary intention is essentially the same as by primary healing. The major differences are the larger defect and the gaping wound edges. Healing and granulation take place from the edges inward and from the bottom of the wound upward until the defect is filled. There is more granulation tissue, and the result is a much larger scar.

Tertiary Intention. *Tertiary intention* (delayed primary intention) healing occurs with delayed suturing of a wound in which two layers of granulation tissue are sutured together. This occurs

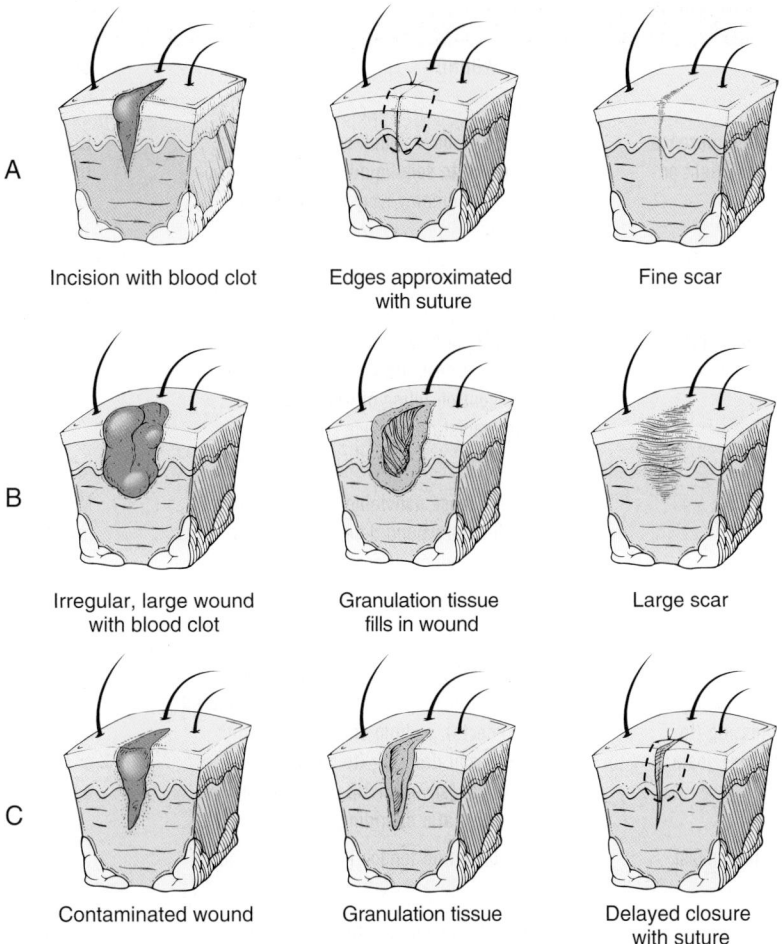

Figure 14-4 Types of wound healing. **A,** Primary intention. **B,** Secondary intention. **C,** Tertiary intention.

Table 14-9 Phases in Primary Intention Healing	
PHASE	**ACTIVITY**
Initial (3 to 5 days)	Approximation of incision edges; migration of epithelial cells; clot serving as meshwork for starting capillary growth
Granulation (5 days to 4 weeks)	Migration of fibroblasts; secretion of collagen; abundance of capillary buds; fragility of wound
Scar contracture (7 days to several months)	Remodelling of collagen; strengthening of scar

when a contaminated wound is left open and sutured closed after the infection is controlled. It also occurs when a primary wound becomes infected, is opened, is allowed to granulate, and is then sutured. Tertiary intention usually results in a larger and deeper scar than does primary or secondary intention.

Wound Classification

Identifying the cause of a wound is essential for classifying the wound properly. Wounds can be classified by cause (surgical or nonsurgical; acute or chronic), level of contamination, or depth of tissue affected (superficial, partial thickness, or full thickness) (Wound, Ostomy and Continence Nurses Society, 2011). A superficial wound involves only the epidermis. Partial-thickness wounds extend into the dermis. Full-thickness wounds have the deepest layer of tissue destruction because they involve the subcutaneous tissue and sometimes even extend into the fascia and underlying structures such as muscle, tendon, or bone (see Figure 27-3 on p. 584).

Another system that is sometimes used clinically to classify open wounds is based on the colour of the wound (red, yellow, black) rather than on the depth of tissue destruction (Table 14-10, Figure 14-5). It can be applied to any wound allowed to heal by secondary intention, including surgical wounds left to heal without skin closure because of a risk for infection. A wound may have two or three colours at the same time. In this situation, the wound is classified according to the least desirable colour present.

Delay of Healing

In a healthy person, wounds heal at a normal, predictable rate. Little can be done to accelerate this process. However, some factors delay wound healing. These are summarized in Table 14-11.

Table 14-10 Red-Yellow-Black Concept of Wound Care

RED WOUND	YELLOW WOUND	BLACK WOUND
Characteristics		
Traumatic or surgical wound, possible presence of serosanguineous drainage, pink to bright or dark red healing or chronic wounds with granulating tissue	Presence of yellow slough or soft necrotic tissue; liquid to semiliquid slough with exudate ranging from creamy ivory to yellow-green	Black, grey, or brown adherent necrotic tissue; possible presence of pus
Purpose of Treatment		
Healing		
Protection and gentle, atraumatic cleansing; filling of wound defects; control of bacteria; maintenance of moisture	Wound cleansing to remove nonviable tissue and absorb excess drainage; debridement; bacteria control; filling of wound defects; providing moisture balance	Debridement of eschar and nonviable tissue; control of odour; control of bacteria
Nonhealing		
—	Removal of loose nonviable tissue; control of odour; filling of wound defects; control of bacteria; promotion of comfort	Maintenance of wound; no debridement of intact eschar; control of odour; control of bacteria; promotion of comfort
Dressings and Therapy		
Healing		
Transparent film, clear acrylic dressing, hydrogel (if additional moisture is required), calcium alginate, or hydrophilic dressing (to absorb exudate and fill wound defects), foam	Hydrocolloid, hydrogel, calcium alginate, or hydrophilic dressing (to absorb exudate and fill wound defects), sodium chloride dressing, foam, charcoal dressing (to control odour), antimicrobial (silver, PHMB, or cadexomer iodine), enzymatic debriding agent	Hydrocolloid, hydrogel, sodium chloride dressing, foam, charcoal dressing (to control odour), antimicrobial (silver, PHMB, or cadexomer iodine), enzymatic debriding agent
Exposed bone and tendon must remain moist	Exposed bone and tendon must remain moist	
Nonhealing		
—	Povidone-iodine, cover with dry dressing	Povidone-iodine, cover with dry dressing

PHMB, polyhexamethylene biguinide.

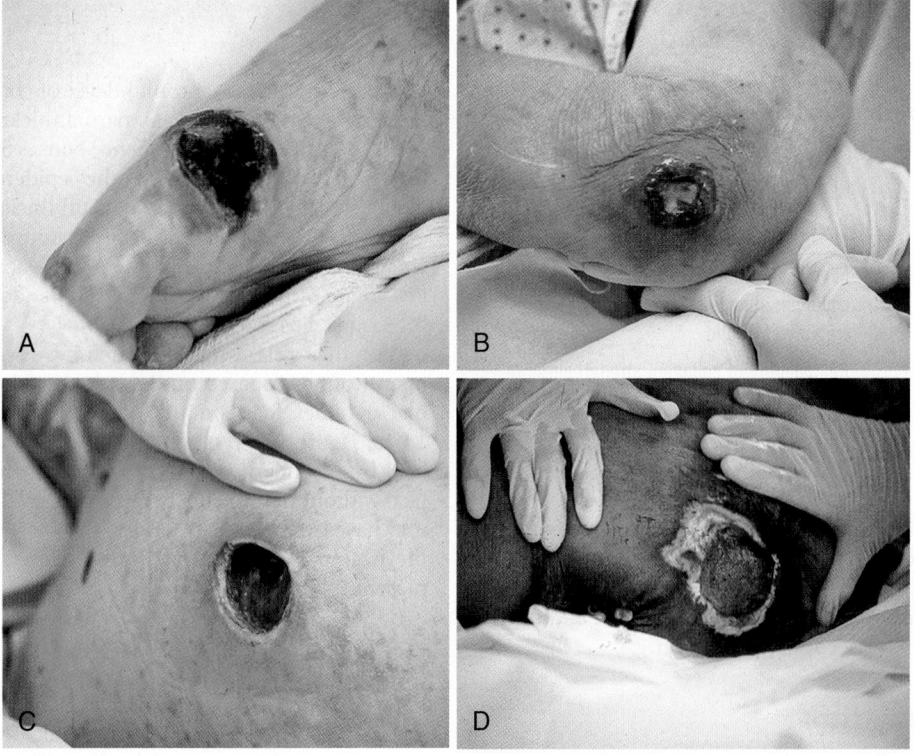

Figure 14-5 Wounds classified by colour assessment. **A,** Black wound. **B,** Yellow wound. **C,** Red wound. **D,** Mixed-colour wound.

Source: Courtesy Molnlyche Health Care, Eddystone, PA. In Potter, P. A., & Perry, A. G. (2009). *Fundamentals of nursing* (7th ed., p. 1285, Figure 48-7). St. Louis: Mosby.

Table 14-11 Factors Delaying Wound Healing

FACTOR	EFFECT ON WOUND HEALING
Nutrition	
Vitamin C deficiency	Delays formation of collagen fibres and capillary development
Protein deficiency	Decreases supply of amino acids for tissue repair
Zinc deficiency	Impairs epithelialization
Inadequate blood supply	Decreases supply of nutrients to injured area, decreases removal of exudative debris, inhibits inflammatory response
Smoking	Nicotine is a potent vasoconstrictor and impedes blood flow to healing areas, which results in tissue ischemia and impairs wound healing
Corticosteroid drugs	Impair phagocytosis by WBCs, inhibit fibroblast proliferation and function, depress formation of granulation tissue, inhibit wound contraction
Infection	Increases inflammatory response and tissue destruction
Anemia	Causes less oxygen to be supplied at tissue level
Advanced age	Slows collagen synthesis by fibroblasts, impairs circulation, imposes need for longer time for epithelialization of skin, alters phagocytic and immune responses
Obesity	Decreases blood supply in fatty tissue
Diabetes mellitus	Decreases collagen synthesis, retards early capillary growth, impairs phagocytosis (result of hyperglycemia), reduces supply of O_2 and nutrients secondary to vascular disease
Poor general health	Causes generalized absence of factors necessary to promote wound healing
Mechanical friction on wound	Destroys granulation tissue, prevents apposition of wound edges
Cold temperature	Decreases cellular activity and fibroblast proliferation
Excessive moisture	Promotes formation of hypergranulation tissue, which prevents the migration of epithelial cells

WBCs, white blood cells.

Complications of Healing

Complications of wound healing may include adhesions, contractures, dehiscence and evisceration, excess granulation tissue, fistula formation, infection, hemorrhage, and formation of hypertrophic scars and keloids.

Adhesions. **Adhesions** are bands of scar tissue between or around organs. Adhesions may occur in the abdominal cavity or between the lungs and pleura. Adhesions in the abdomen may cause an intestinal obstruction. Adhesions between the lungs and the pleura necessitate decortication, or stripping of pleura, to enable normal ventilation.

Contractures. Wound contraction is necessary for healing. This process may become abnormal when contraction is excessive and results in deformity or *contracture.* A shortening of muscle or scar tissue results from excessive fibrous formation, especially if the wound is near a joint. Contractures frequently occur in burn injuries, in which extensive skin and subcutaneous tissue are lost (see Chapter 27).

Dehiscence. **Dehiscence** is the separation and disruption of previously joined wound edges. It usually occurs when a primary healing site bursts open (Figure 14-6). There are three possible contributing causes of dehiscence. First, an infection may cause an inflammatory process. Second, the granulation tissue may not be strong enough to withstand the forces imposed on the wound; for example, during the granulation phase of wound healing, the patient is at risk for wound dehiscence. Third, obese individuals are at a high risk for dehiscence because adipose tissue interferes with healing. **Evisceration** occurs when wound edges separate to the extent that intestines protrude through the wound.

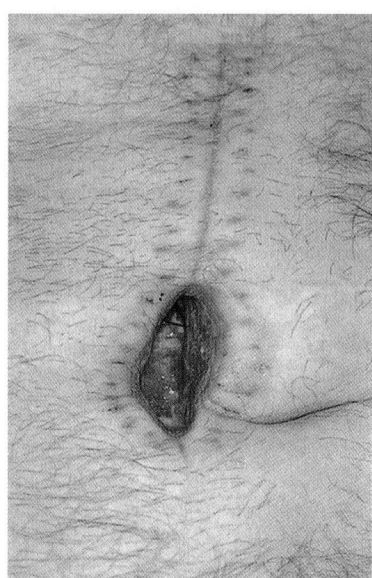

Figure 14-6 Dehiscence after a cholecystectomy.

Source: From Bale, S., & Jones, V. (2006). *Wound care nursing: A patient-centered approach* (2nd ed., p. 20, Figure 1.11). St. Louis: Mosby.

Excess Granulation Tissue. *Excess granulation tissue* or hypergranulation tissue ("proud flesh") may protrude above the surface of the healing wound. If the granulation tissue is cauterized or cut off, healing continues in a normal manner.

Fistula Formation. A **fistula** is an abnormal passage between organs or a hollow organ and the skin.

Infection. The patient is at an increased risk of *infection* when the wound contains necrotic tissue, blood supply is decreased, immune function is depressed, the patient is malnourished, the patient has multiple stressors present, or the patient is diabetic.

Hemorrhage. Bleeding is normal immediately after tissue injury and ceases with clot formation. *Hemorrhage* occurs as abnormal internal or external blood loss caused by suture failure, clotting abnormalities, dislodged clot, infection, or erosion of a blood vessel by a foreign object (tubing, drains) or infection process.

Formation of Hypertrophic Scars and Keloids.

Hypertrophic scars and keloid form when the body produces excess collagen tissue. A **hypertrophic scar** is inappropriately large, red, raised, and hard (Figure 14-7). However, it remains confined to the wound edges and regresses in time. In contrast, a **keloid** is an even greater protrusion of scar tissue that extends beyond the wound edges and may form tumour-like masses (Figure 14-8). Keloids are permanent, without any tendency to subside. The patient with keloids often complains of tenderness, pain, and hyperesthesia, particularly in the early stages of development.

A predisposition to keloid formation is thought to be hereditary and occurs more often in dark-skinned people, particularly Black persons. Neither complication is life-threatening, but both can have serious cosmetic implications.

Collaborative Care

Collaborative care related to inflammation and infection is highly variable. It depends on the causative agent, the degree of injury, and the patient's condition. Superficial skin injuries may need only cleansing. Adhesive strips may be used instead of sutures. The treatment plan can include covering these wounds with a film dressing to ensure that the healing environment is moist and to provide protection from trauma. Deeper skin wounds can be closed by suturing the edges together. If the wound is contaminated, it must be converted into a clean wound before healing can occur nor-

mally. Debridement of a wound that has multiple fragments or devitalized tissue may be necessary. If the source of inflammation is a nonvital internal organ (e.g., appendix, ruptured spleen), surgical removal of the organ is the treatment of choice.

Drug Therapy. Drugs are used to decrease the inflammatory response (Table 14-12). Antihistamine drugs may also be used to inhibit the action of histamine. (Antihistamines are discussed in Chapters 16 and 29.)

Nutritional Therapy. Special nutritional measures facilitate wound healing. A high fluid intake is needed to replace fluid loss from perspiration and exudate formation. An increased metabolic rate intensifies water loss. For every 1°C increase in temperature above 37.8°C, metabolism increases by 13%.

A diet high in protein, carbohydrate, and vitamins with moderate fat intake is necessary to promote healing. Protein is needed to correct the negative nitrogen balance that results from the increased metabolic rate. Protein is also necessary for synthesis of immune factors, leukocytes, fibroblasts, and collagen. Carbohydrate is needed for the increased metabolic energy required for inflammation and healing. If carbohydrate intake is deficient, the body breaks down protein for the needed energy. Fats are also a necessary component in the diet to help in the synthesis of fatty acids and triglycerides, which are part of the cellular membrane. Vitamin C is needed for capillary synthesis, capillary formation, and resistance to infection. The B-complex vitamins are necessary as coenzymes for many metabolic reactions. If a vitamin B deficiency develops, metabolism of protein, fat, and carbohydrate is disrupted. Vitamin A is also needed in healing because it aids in the process of epithelialization. It increases collagen synthesis and tensile strength of the healing wound. Patients are sometimes given vitamin A to counteract the effects of steroids on wound healing.

If the patient is unable to eat, enteral feedings and supplements should be the first choice if the gastrointestinal tract is functional. Parenteral nutrition is indicated when enteral feedings are contraindicated or not tolerated. (Enteral and parenteral nutrition are discussed in Chapter 42.)

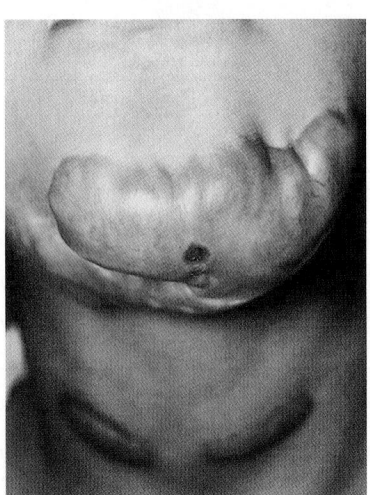

Figure 14-7 Hypertrophic scarring.

Source: Courtesy Dr. C. Lawrence, Wound Healing Research Unit, Cardiff, Wales, UK. In Bale, S., & Jones, V. (2006). *Wound care nursing: A patient-centered approach* (2nd ed., p. 16, Figure 1.9). St. Louis: Mosby.

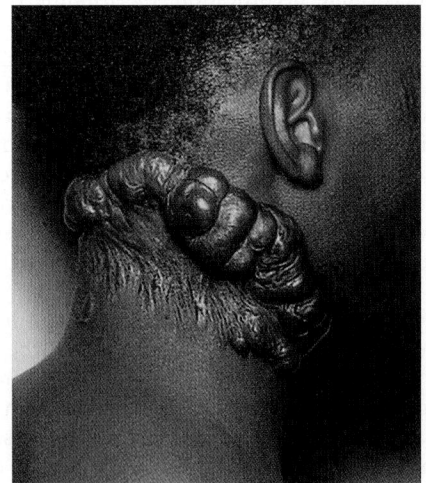

Figure 14-8 Keloid scarring.

Source: Courtesy Dr. C. Lawrence, Wound Healing Research Unit, Cardiff, Wales, UK. In Bale, S., & Jones, V. (2006). *Wound care nursing: A patient-centered approach* (2nd ed., p. 17, Figure 1.10). St. Louis: Mosby.

DRUG THERAPY
Table 14-12 Inflammation and Healing

DRUG	MECHANISMS OF ACTION
Antipyretic Drugs	
Salicylates (aspirin)	Lower temperature by action on heat-regulating centre in hypothalamus, resulting in peripheral dilation and heat loss; interfere with formation and release of prostaglandins; selectively depress CNS
Acetaminophen (Tylenol)	Lowers temperature by action on heat-regulating centre in hypothalamus
NSAIDs (e.g., ibuprofen [Motrin, Advil])	Inhibit synthesis of prostaglandins
Anti-inflammatory Drugs	
Salicylates	Inhibit synthesis of prostaglandins, reduce capillary permeability
Corticosteroids	Interfere with tissue granulation, induce immunosuppressive effects (decreased synthesis of lymphocytes), prevent liberation of lysosomes
NSAIDs (e.g., ibuprofen [Motrin], naproxen [Naprosyn], celecoxib [Celebrex])	Inhibit synthesis of prostaglandins
Vitamins	
Vitamin A	Accelerates epithelialization
Vitamin B complex	Acts as coenzymes
Vitamin C	Assists in synthesis of collagen and new capillaries
Vitamin D	Facilitates calcium absorption

CNS, central nervous system; *NSAIDs,* nonsteroidal anti-inflammatory drugs.

NURSING MANAGEMENT: INFLAMMATION AND HEALING
Nursing Implementation
Health Promotion

The best management of inflammation is the prevention of infection, trauma, surgery, and contact with potentially harmful agents. This is not always possible; for example, a simple mosquito bite causes an inflammatory response. Because occasional injury is inevitable, concerted efforts to minimize inflammation and infection are needed.

Adequate nutrition is essential so that the body has the necessary factors to promote healing when injury occurs. Individuals at risk for wound-healing problems are those with malabsorption problems (e.g., Crohn's disease, gastrointestinal surgery, liver disease), deficient intake or high energy demands (e.g., malignancy, major trauma or surgery, sepsis, fever), or diabetes. An individual should always be considered at risk for wound-healing problems if the following have occurred: (a) loss of 20% or more of total body weight in the preceding 6 months or (b) 10% loss of total body weight in the preceding 2 months.

The manifestations of inflammation and infection must be recognized early so that appropriate treatment can begin. Treatment may be rest, drug therapy, or specific care of the injured site. Immediate treatment may prevent the extension and complications of inflammation.

Acute Intervention
Observation and Vital Signs. The ability to recognize the clinical manifestations of inflammation is important. In the individual who is immunosuppressed (e.g., taking corticosteroids or receiving chemotherapy), the classic manifestations of inflammation may be masked. In this individual, early symptoms of inflammation may be malaise or "just not feeling well."

Observation and recording of wound characteristics are essential. The consistency, colour, and odour of any drainage should be recorded and reported if abnormal for the situation. *Staphylococcus* and *Pseudomonas* organisms commonly cause purulent drainage. Exudate from wounds colonized with *Pseudomonas* often has a distinctive bright "highlighter" yellow or green appearance.

Vital signs are important to note with any inflammation, especially when an infectious process is present. When infection is present, temperature may rise, and pulse and respiration rates may increase. If a wound infection develops in a postoperative patient, vital signs change within 3 to 5 days after surgery.

Fever. The most important aspect of fever management should be determining its cause. Although fever is usually regarded as harmful, an increase in body temperature is an important host defence mechanism. Steps are frequently taken to lower body temperature to relieve the anxiety of the patient and medical personnel. Because mild to moderate fever usually does little harm, imposes no great discomfort, and may benefit host defence mechanisms, antipyretic drugs are rarely essential for patient welfare. Moderate fevers (up to 39.5°C) usually produce few problems in most patients. However, if the patient is very young or very old, is extremely uncomfortable, or has a significant medical problem (e.g., severe cardiopulmonary disease, brain injury), the use of antipyretics should be considered. Fever in an immunosuppressed patient should be treated rapidly and antibiotic therapy begun because infections can rapidly progress to septicemia.

Fever (especially if the temperature exceeds 40°C) can be damaging to body cells, and delirium and seizures can occur. At

NURSING CARE PLAN 14-1

Fever	
NURSING DIAGNOSIS	*Hyperthermia related to* infection *as evidenced by* increased body temperature and increased heart and respiratory rate
Expected Patient Outcomes	**Nursing Interventions and *Rationales***
• Maintains temperature below 37.8°C	• Assess for rapid respirations and pulse; damp skin, clothing, and bed clothes; unwillingness or inability to ingest fluids; signs of dehydration such as dry lips and tongue, poor skin turgor, sunken eyes *to determine risk for or presence of fluid volume deficit.* • Encourage fluid intake of 3 to 4 L/day if tolerated *to replace fluid lost as a result of fever and diaphoresis.* • Monitor vital signs q2-4h *because increasing pulse, rapid respirations, and decreasing blood pressure can indicate hypovolemia.* • Administer intravenous fluids if necessary *to replace fluid loss if oral intake is inadequate.* • Monitor intake and output accurately, and carefully estimate insensible losses *to evaluate need for replacement.*
NURSING DIAGNOSIS	*Risk for deficient fluid volume related to* increased metabolic rate, diaphoresis, and decreased oral intake
Expected Patient Outcomes	**Nursing Interventions and *Rationales***
• Experiences no signs of dehydration	• Assess patient's temperature q2-4h *to monitor temperature.* • Administer antipyretic drugs q3-4h if ordered. • Keep environmental temperature at 21.1°C. • Avoid heavy layers of clothing or bed covers *to aid in lowering body temperature.* • Change linen frequently if patient is diaphoretic *to prevent shivering and subsequent rise in body temperature from muscular activity.*

temperatures higher than 41°C, regulation by the hypothalamic temperature control centre becomes impaired, and damage can occur to many cells, including those in the brain.

Older adults have a blunted febrile response to infection (Dinarello & Porat, 2011). The body temperature may not rise to the level expected for a younger adult, or the onset of fever may be delayed. The blunted response can delay diagnosis and treatment. By the time fever (as defined for younger adults) is present, the illness may be severe.

Several drugs are commonly used to lower the body temperature set point in the hypothalamus. Aspirin specifically blocks prostaglandin synthesis in the hypothalamus and elsewhere in the body. Acetaminophen acts on the heat-regulating centre in the hypothalamus. Some NSAIDs (e.g., ibuprofen [Motrin, Advil]) have antipyretic effects. Corticosteroids are antipyretic through the dual mechanisms of inhibiting interleukin-1 production and preventing prostaglandin synthesis. The action of these drugs results in dilation of superficial blood vessels, increased skin temperature, and sweating.

Antipyretics should be given around the clock to prevent acute swings in temperature. Chills may be evoked or perpetuated by the intermittent administration of antipyretics. These agents cause a sharp decrease in temperature. When the antipyretic wears off, the body may initiate a compensatory involuntary muscular contraction (i.e., chill) to raise the body temperature back up to its previous level. This unpleasant adverse effect of antipyretic drugs can be prevented by administering these agents regularly and frequently at 2- to 4-hour intervals. Although sponge baths increase evaporative heat loss, there is no evidence that they decrease the body temperature unless antipyretic drugs have been given to lower the set point; otherwise, the body will initiate

compensatory mechanisms (e.g., shivering) to restore body heat. The same principle applies to the use of cooling blankets; they are most effective in lowering body temperature when the set point has also been lowered. The nursing care of the patient with a fever is presented in Nursing Care Plan 14-1.

Rest and Immobilization. Rest and immobilization of the inflamed area promote healing by decreasing the inflammatory process, assisting in the repair process, and decreasing metabolic needs. Immobilization with a cast, splint, or bandage lessens wound debris and the possibility of hemorrhage. The repair process is facilitated by allowing fibrin and collagen to form across the wound edges with little disruption. Rest helps the body better use its nutrients and oxygen for the healing process.

Elevation. Elevation of an injured extremity reduces the edema at the inflammatory site and increases venous return. Elevation helps reduce pain and improve the circulation of blood, which provides the oxygen and nutrients needed for healing.

Oxygenation. Adequate oxygenation of the inflamed area is essential because oxygen promotes the differentiation of fibroblasts and collagen synthesis. Oxygen is also essential for cell growth and division. A patient with arterial disease, hypovolemia, or hypotension is at great risk for infection and may benefit from oxygen administration.

Heat and Cold. Applications of heat and cold are somewhat controversial interventions. At the time of initial trauma, cold application is usually appropriate because it causes vasoconstriction and decreases swelling, pain, and congestion from increased metabolism in the area of inflammation. Heat may be used later (e.g., after 24 to 48 hours) and when swelling has subsided to promote healing by increasing the circulation to the inflamed site and subsequent removal of debris. Heat is also used to localize the inflammatory agents. Warm, moist heat may help debride the wound site if necrotic material is present.

Wound Management. The type of wound management and dressings required depend on the type, the extent, and the characteristics of the wound (Registered Nurses' Association of Ontario [RNAO], 2007). The purposes of wound management include (a) cleaning a wound to remove any dirt and debris from the wound bed, (b) treating infection to prepare the wound for healing, and (c) protecting a clean wound from trauma so that it can heal normally. Treatment of pressure ulcers is discussed in more detail later in this chapter.

For wounds that heal by primary intention, it is common to cover the incision with a dry, sterile dressing that is removed as soon as the drainage stops or in 2 to 3 days. Protective sprays or wipes that form a transparent film on the skin may be used for dressings on a clean incision or injury. Sometimes a surgeon leaves a surgical wound uncovered.

Wound healing management by secondary intention depends on the cause of the wound and the type of tissue in the wound. In this type of management, the red-yellow-black concept of wound care (see Table 14-10 and Figure 14-5), transparent film dressings or other dressings are commonly used. Examples of wound dressing types are presented in Table 14-13.

Red Wound. A *red wound* can be a superficial or deep wound if it is clean and red or pink in appearance. Examples include skin tears, pressure ulcers, partial-thickness or second-degree burns, and wounds created surgically that are allowed to heal by secondary intention. The goal of treatment is gentle cleansing and protection of the wound. Clean wounds that are granulating and re-epithelializing should be kept slightly moist and protected from further trauma until they heal naturally. A dressing that keeps the wound surface clean and slightly moist is optimal in promoting epithelialization. Transparent films or clear acrylic dressings are semiocclusive and can be permeated by oxygen. Systemic antibiotics may be given, or antimicrobials such as bacitracin, neomycin, and povidone-iodine can be used if the wound is infected; the wound is then covered with a sterile dressing. Unnecessary manipulation during dressing changes may destroy new granulation tissue and break down fibrin formation.

Yellow Wound. A *yellow wound* has nonviable necrotic tissue, which creates an ideal environment for bacterial growth. The goal of treatment is removal of nonviable tissue and absorption of excessive drainage. This can be facilitated by the use of hydrogel or absorptive dressings (e.g., calcium alginate, hydrofibre, hypertonic gauze) with a secondary dressing. This approach facilitates autolytic debridement, a selective process in which the body's own enzymes are used to selectively rehydrate, soften and liquefy slough. Hydrocolloids are also used to treat yellow wounds. The inner component of these dressings interacts with the exudate, forming a hydrated gel over the wound. When the dressing is removed, the gel separates and stays over the wound. The wound must be cleansed gently to prevent damage to newly formed tissue. These dressings are

designed to be left in place for up to 7 days or until leakage occurs around the dressing.

Enzymatic debriding agents may also be used to eliminate nonviable necrotic tissue from the wound (*enzymatic debridement*).

Black Wound. A *black wound* is covered with thick, dry, necrotic tissue called *eschar* that is black, brown, or grey. Examples of black wounds include full-thickness or third-degree burns and gangrenous ulcers. The risk of wound infection increases in proportion to the amount of necrotic tissue present. The immediate treatment is debridement of the nonviable eschar. The debridement method used depends on the amount of debris and the condition of the wound tissue. There are several approaches to debridement:

1. *Surgical debridement.* This quickest method of debridement is indicated when large amounts of tissue are nonviable and the patient has sepsis. Sharp surgical debridement is selective and can be performed in the operating room or at the patient's bedside, depending on the extent of necrotic material.

2. *Mechanical debridement.* This method is used when debris is minimal. A common form of mechanical debridement is wet-to-dry dressings in which open-mesh gauze is moistened with normal saline, packed into the wound surface, and allowed to dry. Wound debris adheres to the dressing. When the dressing is removed, the debris is trapped in the gauze and is mechanically separated from the wound bed. One disadvantage to this method is that it is nonselective and destroys some healthy tissue. Mechanical debridement can be painful, and the patient should receive appropriate pain management before the removal of a wet-to-dry dressing.

   Topical antimicrobials and bactericidals (e.g., povidone-iodine, sodium hypochlorite [Dakin's solution], hydrogen peroxide, and chlorhexidine) should be used with caution in wound care because they can damage the new epithelium of healing tissue. They should never be used to treat clean granulating wounds.

   Another method of mechanical debridement is pressurized wound irrigation, in which water is delivered at high or low pressure to remove bacteria, foreign matter, and necrotic tissue from the wound. It is important to ensure that the pressure is not too high, as this could drive bacteria and debris deeper into the wound and damage granulation tissue. Whirlpool is another method of mechanical debridement that can be effective at loosening and removing surface wound debris, but it should be used with caution because it can cause tissue maceration and bacterial cross-contamination. Mechanical debridement should not be used for clean granulating wounds.

3. *Autolytic debridement.* Hydrogels, semiocclusive dressings, or occlusive dressings (see Table 14-13) may be used to promote softening of dry eschar by autolysis. This is a slow but selective and painless process that enables the body's own endogenous enzymes to break down necrotic tissue. These types of dressings are used in noninfected wounds with necrotic tissue and adequate circulation. The use of a skin protectant around the wound helps prevent maceration.

4. *Enzymatic debridement.* In this method, a topical ointment containing proteolytic enzymes is applied to the necrotic tissue in the wound and then covered with a moist dressing such as saline-moistened gauze and changed daily. Santyl

Table 14-13 Types of Wound Dressings

TYPE	DESCRIPTION	EXAMPLES
Gauze	Provides absorption of exudate. Supports debridement if applied and kept moist. Can be used to maintain moistness of wound surface. Can be used as filler dressings in sinus tracts.	NuGauze (numerous products available)
Nonadherent dressing	Woven or nonwoven dressings may be impregnated with petrolatum or antimicrobials. Minimally absorbent. Used on minor wounds or skin tears.	Adaptic, Jelonet, Bactigras, Inadine
Transparent film	Semipermeable membrane that permits gaseous exchange between wound bed and environment. Minimally absorbent so that environment is kept moist in presence of exudate. Bacteria do not penetrate membrane. Used for dry, noninfected wounds, wounds with minimal drainage, or stage 1 pressure ulcers to help prevent friction and shear.	Bioclusive, OpSite, Tegaderm, Mefilm
Acrylic clear	Used for superficial and partial-thickness wounds with light drainage.	Tegaderm Absorbent
Hydrocolloid dressing	Occlusive dressing does not allow O_2 to diffuse from atmosphere to wound bed. Occlusion does not interfere with wound healing and supports debridement. Used for superficial and partial-thickness wounds with light to moderate drainage.	Comfeel, DuoDERM, Restore, Tegasorb
Foam	Product comes in many shapes and sizes. Absorbs moderate to heavy amount of exudate. Used for partial- or full-thickness wounds or infected wounds.	Allevyn, Hydrasorb, Lyofoam, Mepilex, Biatain, Tegaderm Foam
Alginate, calcium alginate, and hydrofibre dressings	Large volume of exudate can be absorbed. Dressing forms a gel-like substance that supports autolytic debridement and maintains moistness of wound surface. Fills wound cavities and obliterates dead space. Available in rope or sheet form. For partial- or full-thickness wounds or infected wounds with heavy drainage. Should not be used for lightly draining or dry wounds because they can desiccate the wound bed. Require a secondary dressing.	Aquacel, Kaltostat, Tegagen, Seasorb, Fibracol, Algisite, Algisite M, Melgisorb
Hypertonic dressing	Sheet, ribbon, or gel impregnated with sodium chloride concentrate. Should not be used on dry wounds (which should be treated with a hydrogel). May be painful on sensitive tissue.	Mesalt, Hypergel
Hydrogel	Gently eliminates necrotic tissue by autolytic debridement. Maintains moistness of wound surface. Provides limited absorption of exudate. Available as sheet, gel, and impregnated gauze. Requires a secondary dressing. Used for partial- or full-thickness wounds with minimal drainage, and necrotic wounds. Has a cooling effect on the wound and thus is effective in managing pain.	IntraSite Gel, DuoDERM Gel, Normlgel, Nu-Gel, Tegagel, Tegaderm Hydrogel wound filler
Charcoal dressing	Dressing that contains odour-absorbent charcoal layered within the product. Some products contain silver to enhance antimicrobial capability.	Actisorb, Carbonet, CarboFLEX
Antimicrobial dressing	Broad spectrum against bacteria. Silver, PHMB, cadexomer iodine with vehicle for delivery: sheets, foams, alginates, ribbons, gels, or paste. Products are not to be used on patients with known hypersensitivity to any product components.	Acticoat, AMD Antimicrobial Foam, Iodosorb, Allevyn Ag, Mepilex Ag, Aquacel Ag, Contreet, Silvercel, Silvasorb, Tegaderm Ag Mesh
Biological dressing	Living human fibroblasts provided in sheets at ambient or frozen temperatures. Extracellular matrix. Collagen-containing preparations. Hyaluronic acid. Never to be used on wounds with infections or sinus tracts, on wounds with excessive exudate, or on patients with hypersensitivity to any of the product components.	Apilgraf, Oasis Wound Matrix, Biostep, Promogran, Tegaderm Matrix

Source: Information on antimicrobials and biological dressings adapted from Sibbald, G., Orsted, H., Coutts, P., & Keast, D. (2006). Best practice recommendations for preparing the wound bed: Update. *Wound Care Canada, 4*(1), 309-405.
PHMB, polyhexamethylene biguinide.

collagenase is the only product in this category currently available in Canada. The wound pH must be between 6 and 8 for optimal enzyme activity; therefore, cleansing products containing detergents or heavy metals such as mercury or silver should not be used.

■ **Negative-Pressure Wound Therapy.** This therapy involves the application of negative pressure (suction) to the wound bed. The type and application of dressing vary by manufacturer. Wound types suitable for this therapy include chronic, acute, traumatic, and dehisced wounds; partial-thickness burns; ulcers (e.g., diabetic, pressure); flaps; and grafts. For further information on negative-pressure wound therapy, refer to the Ontario Ministry of Long-Term Care document *Negative Pressure Wound Therapy* in the Resources at the end of this chapter.

■ **Hyperbaric Oxygen Therapy.** Hyperbaric oxygen therapy is the systemic delivery of oxygen at increased atmospheric pressures. The patient is placed in an enclosed chamber in which 100% oxygen is administered at 1.5 to 3.0 times the normal atmospheric pressure. This form of therapy accelerates granulation tissue formation and wound closure by increasing blood and tissue oxygen content in hypoxic tissues, which stimulates fibroblast proliferation and collagen synthesis.

■ **Psychological Implications.** The patient may be distressed at the thought or sight of an incision or wound because of fear of scarring or disfigurement. Drainage from a wound may also cause alarm. The patient needs to understand the healing process and the normal changes that occur as the wound heals. When a nurse is changing a dressing, inappropriate facial expressions on the nurse's face can alert the patient to problems with the wound or the nurse's ability to care for it. Wrinkling of the nose by the nurse may convey disgust to the patient. A nurse should also be careful not to focus on the wound to the extent that the patient is not treated as a total person.

■ **Ambulatory and Home Care**

Because patients are currently being discharged earlier after surgery and many undergo surgery as outpatients, it is important that the patient, the family, or both know how to care for surgical wounds and perform dressing changes. Wound healing may not be complete for 4 to 6 weeks or longer. Adequate rest and good nutrition should be continued throughout this time. Physical and emotional stress should be minimized. Observing the wound for complications such as contractures, adhesions, and infection is important. The patient should be able to recognize the signs and symptoms of infection and note changes in wound colour and the amount of drainage. The health care professional should be notified of any signs of abnormal wound healing.

Medications often are taken for a period after recovery from an acute infection. Drug-specific adverse effects should be reviewed with the patient; the patient should be instructed to contact the health care provider if any of these effects occur. Awareness of the necessity to continue the drugs for the specified time is an important point to teach the patient. For example, a patient who is instructed to take an antibiotic for 10 days may stop taking the drug after 5 days because symptoms disappear. However, the organism may not be entirely eliminated, and it may also become resistant to the antibiotic if the drug is not continued.

Pressure Ulcers

Causes and Pathophysiological Features

A **pressure ulcer** is a localized injury to the skin or underlying tissue, usually over a bony prominence as a result of pressure or pressure in combination with shear, friction, or both.

According to the most recent information available, the prevalence of pressure ulcers in Canada is 25% in acute care, 30% in nonacute care, 22% in mixed health care settings, and 15% in community care (Woodbury & Houghton, 2004). Cole and Nesbitt (2004) found the incidence of pressure ulcers in an Ontario community hospital to be 18%. A number of contributing or confounding factors are also associated with pressure ulcers; the significance of these factors is yet to be elucidated (National Pressure Ulcer Advisory Panel [NPUAP], 2009). The most common site for pressure ulcers is the sacrum; heels are the second most common site. Factors that influence the development of pressure ulcers include the amount of pressure (intensity), the length of time the pressure is exerted on the skin (duration), and the ability of the patient's tissue to tolerate the externally applied pressure. It has yet to be determined whether pressure ulcers are formed by tissue destruction occurring from

Table 14-14 Risk Factors for Pressure Ulcers	
• Advanced age	• Mental deterioration
• Anemia	• Neurological disorders
• Contractures	• Nutritional deficiencies
• Diabetes mellitus	• Obesity
• Elevated body temperature	• Pain
• Immobility	• Prolonged surgery
• Impaired circulation	• Prolonged use of steroids
• Incontinence	• Vascular disease
• Low diastolic blood pressure (<60 mm Hg)	

the bone outward to the skin or from the epidermis inward toward the deeper tissue layers surrounding the bony prominence (Bryant, 2010). Besides pressure, **shearing force** (pressure exerted on the skin when it adheres to the bed and the underlying skin layers slide in the direction of body movement), *friction* (two surfaces rubbing against each other), and *excessive moisture* (incontinence or perspiration) contribute to pressure ulcer formation (RNAO, 2007). Factors that increase a patient's risk for the development of pressure ulcers are presented in Table 14-14.

Clinical Manifestations

The clinical manifestations of pressure ulcers depend on the extent of the tissue that is involved. Pressure ulcers are staged according to their deepest level of tissue damage. Table 14-15 illustrates the pressure ulcer stages according to the NPUAP (2009) guidelines. When slough or necrotic eschar is present, it is not possible to stage the ulcer until the devitalized tissue is removed by debridement. Clinicians may describe such pressure ulcers as *unstageable* (RNAO, 2007).

If a pressure ulcer becomes infected, the patient may display signs of infection, such as leukocytosis and fever. In addition, the pressure ulcer may increase in size, odour, and drainage; have necrotic tissue; and be indurated, warm, and painful. The most common complication of a pressure ulcer is recurrence. Therefore, it is important to note the location of previously healed pressure ulcers in an initial admission assessment of a patient.

Research has revealed that as deeper ulcers heal, fat, muscle, and dermis are replaced with granulation tissue, and so the original integrity of the tissue is lost. Reverse staging—that is, stating that a stage III ulcer has healed into a stage II ulcer—is thus not appropriate. Rather, the ulcer would be known as a "healing stage III ulcer."

NURSING AND COLLABORATIVE MANAGEMENT: PRESSURE ULCERS

Care of a patient with a pressure ulcer encompasses local care of the wound and support measures of the whole person, such as adequate nutrition, pain management, control of other medical conditions, and pressure relief. Evidence-informed practice is to keep a pressure ulcer slightly moist, rather than dry, to enhance re-epithelialization. In addition to the nurse, other members of

Table 14-15 Staging of Pressure Ulcers

DEFINITION AND DESCRIPTION	DIAGRAM	CLINICAL PRESENTATION
(Suspected) Deep Tissue Injury Purple or maroon localized area of discoloured intact skin or blood-filled blister resulting from the damage to underlying soft tissue from pressure, shear, or both. This tissue may be painful, firm, mushy, boggy, and warmer or cooler than adjacent tissue. Deep tissue injury may be difficult to detect in individuals with dark skin tones. Evolution of the wound may include a thin blister over a dark wound bed. The wound may further evolve and become covered by thin eschar. Evolution may be rapid and expose additional layers of tissue even with optimal treatment.	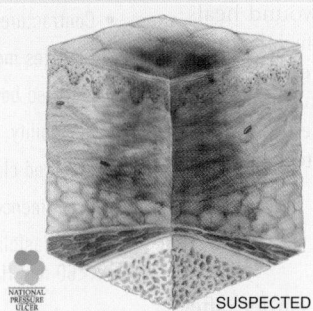 SUSPECTED DEEP TISSUE INJURY®	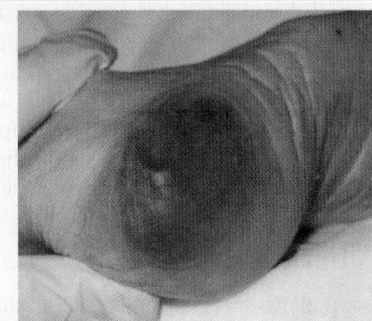
Stage I A stage I pressure ulcer is described as intact skin with nonblanchable redness of a localized area, usually over a bony prominence. A wound in darkly pigmented skin may not have visible blanching; its colour may differ from that of the surrounding area. The area may be painful, firm, soft, and warmer or cooler than adjacent tissue. Stage I ulcers may be difficult to detect in individuals with dark skin tones. Stage I ulcers may indicate that affected persons are "at risk" (a heralding sign of risk) for skin breakdown.	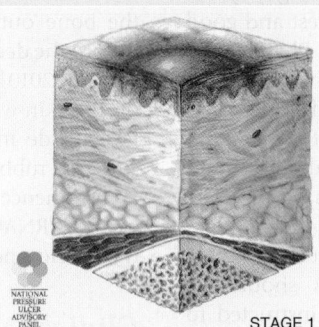 STAGE 1	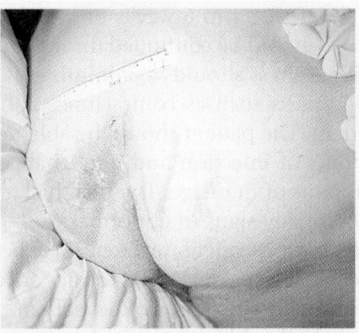
Stage II Partial-thickness loss of dermis, seen as a shallow open ulcer with a red-pink wound bed, without slough. May also appear as an intact or open (ruptured) serum-filled blister. Manifests as a shiny or dry shallow ulcer without slough or bruising. This stage should not be used to describe skin tears, tape burns, perineal dermatitis, maceration, or excoriation. Bruising indicates possible deep tissue injury.	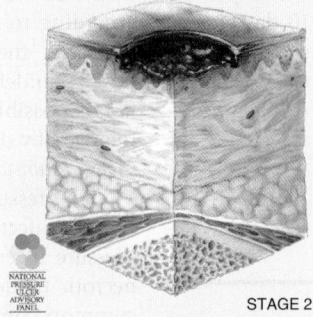 STAGE 2	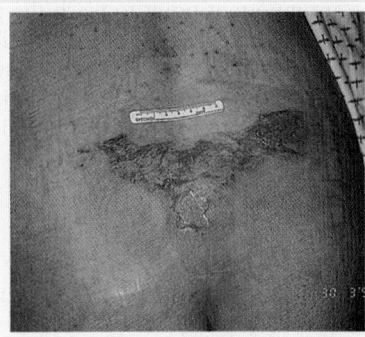
Stage III Full-thickness tissue loss. Subcutaneous fat may be visible, but bone, tendon, or muscle is not exposed. Slough may be present but does not obscure the depth of tissue loss. May include undermining and tunneling. The depth of a stage III ulcer varies by anatomical location. The bridge of the nose, the ear, the occiput, and the malleolus do not have subcutaneous tissue, and stage III pressure ulcers in these locations can be shallow. In contrast, areas of significant adiposity can develop extremely deep stage III pressure ulcers. Bone and tendon are not visible or directly palpable.	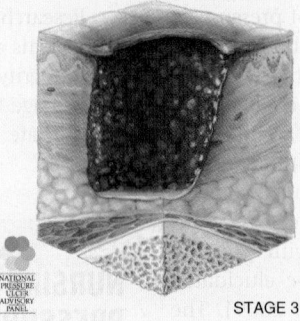 STAGE 3	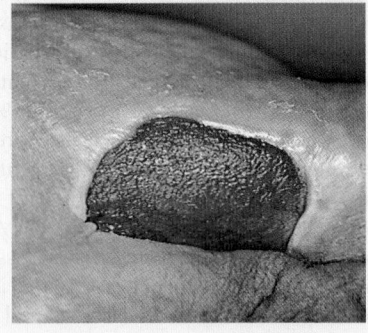

Table 14-15 Staging of Pressure Ulcers—cont'd

DEFINITION AND DESCRIPTION	DIAGRAM	CLINICAL PRESENTATION
Stage IV Full-thickness tissue loss in which bone, tendon, or muscle is exposed. Slough or eschar may be present on some parts of the wound bed. These often include undermining and tunnelling. The depth of a stage IV pressure ulcer varies by anatomical location. The bridge of the nose, the ear, the occiput, and the malleolus do not have subcutaneous tissue, and these ulcers can be shallow. Stage IV ulcers can extend into muscle and supporting structures (e.g., fascia, tendon, or joint capsule), making osteomyelitis possible. Exposed bone or tendon is visible or directly palpable.	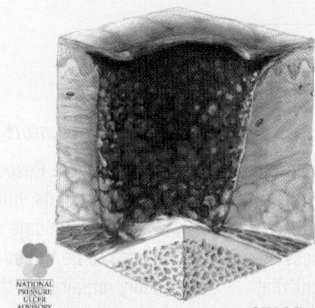 STAGE 4	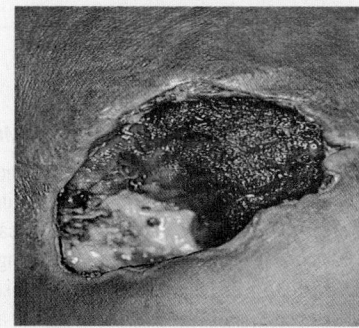
Unstageable Full-thickness tissue loss in which the base of the ulcer is covered by slough (yellow, tan, gray, green, or brown) or eschar (tan, brown, or black), or both, in the wound bed. Until enough slough or eschar is removed to expose the base of the wound, the true depth, and therefore the wound stage, cannot be determined. Stable (dry, adherent, intact without erythema or fluctuance) eschar on the heels serves as "the body's natural cover" and should not be removed.	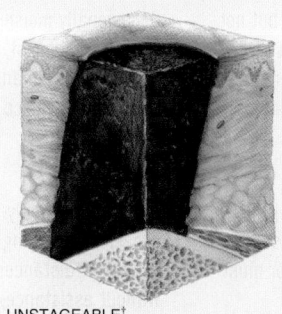 UNSTAGEABLE†	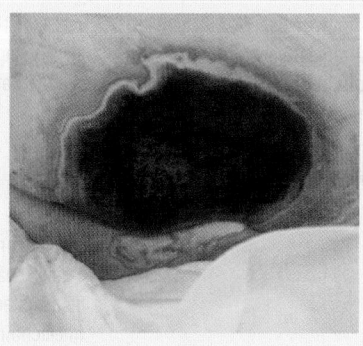

NOTE: For additional information regarding the staging of pressure ulcers, refer to the Registered Nurses' Association of Ontario (RNAO). (2007). *Assessment and management of stage I to IV pressure ulcers (Revised): Best practice guideline,* available at *http://www.rnao.org/Storage/29/2371_BPG_Pressure_Ulcers_I_to_IV.pdf*

*From Fleck, C. A. (2007). Deep tissue injury: What, why, and when? *Wound Care Canada, 5*(2), 10-53.
†Courtesy of Alison Anger, RN(EC), PHC-NP, BScN, MSc, ET.
Source: From National Pressure Ulcer Advisory Panel (NPUAP). (2009). NPUAP pressure ulcer prevention: Quick reference guide, and Pressure ulcer treatment: Quick reference guide, October 2009. Retrieved from *http://www.epuap.org/guidelines/Final_Quick_Treatment.pdf*

the health care team, such as the plastic surgeon, the dietitian, the physiotherapist, and the occupational therapist, can provide valuable input into the complex treatment necessary to prevent and manage pressure ulcers. Both conservative and surgical strategies are used in the treatment of pressure ulcers, depending on the stage and the condition of the ulcer. Therapeutic and nursing management are discussed together because the activities are interrelated.

Nursing Assessment

Patients should be assessed for pressure ulcer risk initially on admission to the hospital and at periodic intervals thereafter on the basis of the patient's condition and the care setting (RNAO, 2007).

SAFETY ALERT
- In acute care, reassess the patient every 24 hours.
- In long-term care, reassess a resident weekly for the first 4 weeks and after admission at least monthly or every 3 months.
- In home care, reassess the patient at each nurse visit.

For example, in acute care, a patient should be reassessed every 24 hours; in long-term care, a resident should be reassessed weekly for the first 4 weeks after admission and then at least monthly or every 3 months; in home care, a person should be reassessed during every nurse visit.

Risk assessment should be performed with a validated assessment tool such as the Braden scale (Table 14-16). To obtain a patient's pressure ulcer risk assessment score on the Braden scale, the nurse adds the numerical scores for the factors in each of the six subscales (sensory perception, moisture, activity, mobility, nutrition, and friction and shear). Scores can range from 6 to 23. The lower the numerical score on the Braden scale, the higher is the patient's predicted risk of developing a pressure ulcer. Incremental changes in the score indicate the level of risk: no risk (19 to 23), at risk (15 to 18), moderate risk (13 to 14), high risk (10 to 12), and very high risk (≤9). Knowing the level of risk can determine how aggressive the preventive measures should be. The Braden scale has also been modified (Braden Q scale) for use with the pediatric population (Noonan, Quigley, & Curley, 2011).

Identification of stage I pressure ulcers may be difficult in patients with dark skin. Table 14-17 presents techniques to help assess darker skin. Subjective and objective data that should be obtained from a person with a pressure ulcer are presented in Table 14-18.

Table 14-16 Braden Scale for Predicting Pressure Sore Risk

Patient's Name _____

Evaluator's Name _____

Date of Assessment _____

		POINT VALUE		
1	**2**	**3**	**4**	**SCORE**
Sensory Perception: Ability to Respond Meaningfully to Pressure-Related Discomfort				
Completely limited: Unresponsive (does not moan, flinch, or grasp) to painful stimuli, due to diminished level of consciousness or sedation or limited ability to feel pain over most of body	Very limited: Responds only to painful stimuli; cannot communicate discomfort except by moaning or restlessness or has a sensory impairment that limits the ability to feel pain or discomfort over half of body	Slightly limited: Responds to verbal commands, but cannot always communicate discomfort or the need to be turned or has some sensory impairment that limits ability to feel pain or discomfort in one or two extremities	No impairment: Responds to verbal commands; has no sensory deficit that would limit ability to feel or to voice pain or discomfort	
Moisture: Degree to Which Skin Is Exposed to Moisture				
Constantly moist: Skin is kept moist almost constantly by perspiration, urine, and so on; dampness is detected every time patient is moved or turned	Very moist: Skin is often, but not always, moist; linen must be changed at least once per shift	Occasionally moist: Skin is occasionally moist, necessitating an extra linen change approximately once per day	Rarely moist: Skin is usually dry; linen… requires changing [only] at routine intervals	
Activity: Degree of Physical Activity				
Bedfast: Confined to bed	Chairfast: Ability to walk [is] severely limited or nonexistent; cannot bear own weight or must be assisted into chair or wheelchair	Walks occasionally: Walks occasionally during day, but for very short distances, with or without assistance; spends most of each shift in bed or chair	Walks frequently: Walks outside room at least twice per day and inside room at least once every 2 hours during waking hours	
Mobility: Ability to Change and Control Body Position				
Completely immobile: Does not make even slight changes in body or extremity position without assistance	Very limited: Makes occasional slight changes in body or extremity position but unable to make frequent or significant changes independently	Slightly limited: Makes frequent though slight changes in body or extremity position independently	No limitation: Makes major and frequent changes in position without assistance	
Nutrition: Usual Food Intake Pattern				
Very poor: Never eats a complete meal; rarely eats more than half of any food offered; eats two servings or less of protein (meat or dairy products) per day; takes fluids poorly; does not take a liquid dietary supplement or is NPO and/or maintained on clear liquids or IVs for more than 5 days	Probably inadequate: Rarely eats a complete meal and generally eats only about half of any food offered; protein intake includes only three servings of meat or dairy products per day; occasionally will take a dietary supplement or receives less than optimum amount of liquid diet or tube feeding	Adequate: Eats over half of most meals; eats four servings of protein (meat or dairy products) per day; occasionally will refuse a meal, but will usually take a supplement when offered or is on a tube feeding or total parenteral nutrition regimen that probably meets most of nutritional needs	Excellent: eats most of every meal; never refuses a meal; eats four or more servings of protein (meat or dairy products); occasionally eats between meals; does not require supplementation	
Friction and Shear				
Problem: Requires moderate to maximum assistance in moving; complete lifting without sliding against sheets is impossible; frequently slides down in bed or chair, necessitating frequent repositioning with maximum assistance; spasticity, contractures, or agitation leads to almost constant friction	Potential problem: Moves feebly or requires minimum assistance; during a move, skin probably slides to some extent against sheets, chair, restraints, or other devices; maintains relatively good position in chair or bed most of the time but occasionally slides down	No apparent problem: Moves in bed and in chair independently and has sufficient muscle strength to lift up completely during move; maintains good position in bed or chair		

Source: From Braden, B., & Bergstrom, N. (1994). Predictive validity of the Braden scale for pressure sore risk in a nursing home population. *Research in Nursing & Health, 17,* 459. Copyright © Barbara Braden and Nancy Bergstrom. All rights reserved.

IVs, intravenous nutrition; *NPO,* nothing by mouth (status).

Nursing Diagnoses

Nursing diagnoses for the patient with a pressure ulcer may include, but are not limited to, those presented in Nursing Care Plan 14-2.

Planning

The overall goals are that the patient with a pressure ulcer will (a) have no deterioration of the ulcer stage, (b) reduce or eliminate the factors that lead to pressure ulcers, (c) have improved nutritional status, (d) have increased mobility, (e) not develop an infection in the pressure ulcer, (f) have healing of pressure ulcers, and (g) have no recurrence.

Nursing Implementation

Health Promotion

A primary nursing responsibility is the identification of patients at risk for the development of pressure ulcers (see Tables 14-14 and 14-16) and implementing strategies to prevent pressure ulcers for those identified as being at risk. Prevention remains the best treatment for pressure ulcers. Devices such as support surfaces, special transfer equipment, and heel boots are useful in reducing pressure and shearing force. However, they are not adequate substitutes for frequent repositioning. Once a patient has been identified as being at risk for pressure ulcer development, prevention strategies should be implemented (Table 14-19).

Table 14-17 Assessing Patients With Dark Skin

- Look for changes in skin colour, such as skin that is darker (purplish, brownish, bluish) than surrounding skin.
- Use natural light or a halogen light source to accurately assess the skin colour. Fluorescent light casts blue light, which can make skin assessment difficult.
- Assess the skin temperature of the area by using your hand. The area may initially feel warm, then cooler.
- Touch the skin to feel its consistency. Boggy or edematous feel may indicate a stage I pressure ulcer.
- Ask the patient if he or she has any pain or itchy sensation.

SAFETY ALERT

- Reposition the patient frequently to prevent pressure ulcers.
- Use devices to reduce pressure and shearing force (e.g., alternating pressure mattresses, foam mattresses, wheelchair cushions, padded commode seats, boots [foam, air], lift sheets) as appropriate.
- These devices are not adequate substitutes for frequent repositioning.

NURSING ASSESSMENT
Table 14-18 Pressure Ulcers

Subjective Data

Important Health Information

Past health history: Stroke, spinal cord injury; prolonged bed rest or immobility; circulatory impairment; poor nutrition; altered level of consciousness; history of previous pressure ulcer; immunological abnormalities; advanced age; diabetes; anemia; trauma

Medications: Use of narcotics, hypnotics, systemic corticosteroids, nicotine

Surgery or other treatments: Recent surgery

Symptoms

Incontinence of urine, feces, or both; weakness, debilitation, inability to turn and position body; pain or altered cutaneous sensation in pressure ulcer area; decreased awareness of pressure on body areas; decreased fluid, calorie, or protein intake; vitamin or mineral deficiencies

Objective Data

General

Obesity; emaciation; clinically significant malnutrition as indicated by low serum albumin level, decreased total lymphocyte count, and decreased body weight (15% less than ideal body weight); contractures

Integumentary

Diaphoresis, edema, and discoloration, especially over bony areas such as sacrum, hips, elbows, heels, knees, ankles, shoulders, and ear rims, progressing to increased tissue damage characteristic of ulcer stages*

Possible Findings

Leukocytosis if infection present, positive cultures for microorganisms from pressure ulcer

*See Table 14-15.

PATIENT & CAREGIVER TEACHING GUIDE
Table 14-19 Pressure Ulcer

1. Identify and explain risk factors and causes of pressure ulcers to the patient and family.

2. Assess the patient for risk at time of first hospital or home visit, whenever the patient's condition changes, and thereafter at regular intervals on the basis of care setting (every 24 hours for acute care or every visit in home care).

3. Teach caregivers the care techniques for incontinence. When incontinence occurs, cleanse the patient's skin immediately with incontinence cleanser, and use moisture barrier and absorbent pads or briefs.

4. Demonstrate correct positioning to decrease risk of skin breakdown. Instruct caregivers to reposition bed-bound patient at least every 2 hours and chair-bound patient every hour. *Never* position the patient directly on the pressure ulcer.

5. Assess resources of patients requiring pressure ulcer care at home (i.e., adequacy of caregiver availability and skill, finances, and equipment). When dressings are selected, consider cost, ability of wound to heal, and caregiver time.

6. Teach patient and/or caregiver to use "no touch" clean technique when changing dressings. Instruct caregivers on disposal of contaminated dressings.

7. Teach patient and caregivers to inspect skin daily. Assess and document pressure ulcer status at least weekly; doing so may necessitate help from patient and caregivers.

8. Evaluate effectiveness of the plan of care.

NURSING CARE PLAN 14-2

Pressure Ulcer

NURSING DIAGNOSIS	*Impaired skin integrity* related to pressure and inadequate circulation *as evidenced by* pressure ulcer.
Expected Patient Outcomes	**Nursing Interventions and *Rationales***
• Maintains intact skin • Experiences healing of wound without complications	• Use an established risk assessment tool to identify causative factors such as activity, mobility, presence or absence of sensory deficits, nutrition and hydration status, circulation and oxygenation, and skin moisture status *to assist in the formulation of a care plan to reduce factors that can contribute to the development or progression of the pressure ulcer.* • Document wound stage and characteristics on a regular basis in relation to location, length, width, and depth of wound; amount of granulation tissue visible or epithelialization; necrotic tissue; local or systemic infection; and description of exudate, including volume, colour, consistency, and odour *to provide baseline and ongoing data for monitoring pressure ulcer.* • Use support surfaces for the patient's bed and chair that fit with the plan of care and goals of treatment *to provide pressure reduction and increase circulation to the relevant site or sites.* • Institute and document position change schedule q2h *to prevent prolonged pressure in one area.* • Keep patient's heels off bed. Suspend patient's heels with devices as needed (heel boots). Keep head of bed at or below 30-degree angle and bed flat when not contraindicated *to avoid sacral, buttock, and heel pressure.* • Use assistive devices (e.g., trapeze, turning sheets, lifts) *to aid patient movement and reduce potential for shear.* • Protect patient's skin from excess moisture (perspiration, wound drainage, incontinence) *to prevent maceration.* • Institute intake of 2000 to 3000 calories per day (more if metabolic demands are increased), vitamin/mineral supplements (if there are deficiencies), and 2000 mL per day of fluid *to provide calories, protein, and fluids necessary for tissue repair.* • Initiate prescribed treatment based on pressure ulcer characteristics in accordance with RNAO Best Practice Guidelines* *to provide the optimal environment for wound healing.* • Assess the psychosocial impact of pressure ulcer on the patient and caregivers, and provide support or make referrals to other health care professionals as indicated *to provide holistic patient care.* • Teach patient and family about cause, prevention, and treatment of pressure ulcer *to prevent recurrence* (see Table 14-19).

*Registered Nurses Association of Ontario (RNAO). (2007). *Assessment and management of stage I to IV pressure ulcers* (*Revised*): *Best Practice Guideline.* Retrieved from *http://rnao.ca/bpg/guidelines/assessment-and-management-stage-i-iv-pressure-ulcers*

■ **Acute Intervention.** Once a pressure ulcer has developed, the nurse should initiate interventions that are based on the ulcer characteristics (e.g., stage, size, location, amount of exudate, type of wound, presence of infection or pain) and the patient's general status (e.g., nutritional state, level of mobility).

■ *Measuring the wound.* The size of the pressure ulcer should be carefully documented. A wound-measuring tape can be used to note the ulcer's maximum length and width in centimetres (Figure 14-9). To find the depth of the ulcer, gently place a sterile cotton-tipped applicator into the deepest part of the ulcer. The length of the portion of the applicator that probed the ulcer can then be measured.

■ *Documentation.* Healing of the wound can be documented with several available pressure ulcer healing tools such as the NPUAP Pressure Ulcer Scale of Healing (PUSH) tool. Some agencies require that pictures of the pressure ulcer be taken initially and at regular intervals during the course of treatment.

Local care of the pressure ulcer may involve debridement, wound cleaning, application of a dressing, and relief of pressure. It is important to select the appropriate support surface for both bed and chair or wheelchair to relieve pressure and keep the patient off of the pressure ulcer.

■ *Debridement.* When a pressure ulcer that has necrotic tissue or eschar (except for dry, stable, necrotic heels), the tissue must be removed by surgical, mechanical, enzymatic, or autolytic debridement methods (RNAO, 2007). Once the pressure ulcer has been successfully debrided and has a clean, granulating base, the goal is to provide an appropriate wound environment that supports moistness for wound healing and prevents disruption of the newly formed granulation tissue. Reconstruction of the pressure ulcer site by operative repair, including skin grafting, skin flaps, musculocutaneous flaps, or free flaps, may be necessary.

■ *Wound Irrigation.* Pressure ulcers should be cleaned with noncytotoxic solutions that do not kill or damage cells, especially fibroblasts. Solutions such as sodium hypochlorite, acetic acid, povidone-iodine, and hydrogen peroxide are cytotoxic and therefore should not be used to clean pressure ulcers (RNAO, 2007). It is also important to use enough irrigation pressure (4 to 15 psi) to clean the pressure ulcer adequately without causing trauma or damage to the wound (RNAO, 2007).

■ *Local Wound Care.* After the pressure ulcer has been cleansed, it should be covered with an appropriate dressing. Some factors to consider in selecting a dressing are maintenance of a moist environment, prevention of wound desiccation (drying out), ability to absorb the wound drainage, location of the wound, amount of caregiver time, cost of the dressing, presence of infection, and setting of care delivery (RNAO, 2007). A wet-to-dry dressing should never be used on a clean, granulating pres-

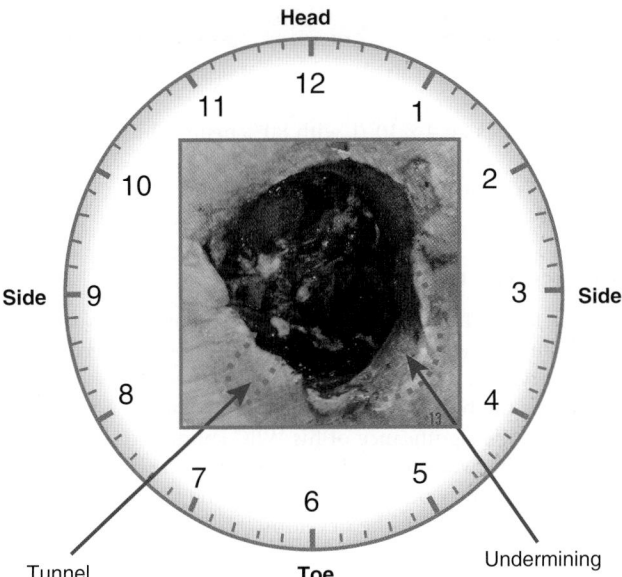

Figure 14-9 Wound measurements are made in centimetres. The first measurement is oriented from head to toe, the second is from side to side, and the third is the depth (if any). Any tunnelling (when a cotton-tipped applicator is placed in the wound, the applicator moves) or undermining (when a cotton-tipped applicator is placed in wound, there is a "lip" around the wound) is charted like a clock, the 12 o'clock position being toward the patient's head. This wound would be charted as a full-thickness, red wound, 7 cm × 5 cm × 3 cm, with a 3-cm tunnel at the 7 o'clock position and 2 cm undermining from the 3 o'clock to 5 o'clock positions.

Source: Courtesy Robert B. Babiak, RN, BSN, CWOCN, San Antonio, TX.

INTERDISCIPLINARY RESEARCH

Wound Pain

Citation

Woo, K., Sibbald, G., Fogh, K., Glynn, C., Krasner, D., Leaper, D. ..., Teot, L. (2008). Assessment and management of persistent (chronic) and total wound. *International Wound Journal, 5*(2), 205-215.

Purpose

To improve the health care professional's awareness and management of chronic wound pain.

Methods

Medline, CINAHL and PubMed databases were used to identify articles, guidelines, and studies addressing chronic wound pain that were then reviewed and summarized. The authors drafted 10 proposal statements, which were reviewed by an interprofessional panel and health care leaders.

Results and Conclusions

The panel concluded that chronic wounds should be assumed to be painful unless patients indicate otherwise and highlighted benefits of optimal pain management for patient ADLs and well-being. Wound pain should be assessed on a regular basis and a search for treatable causes explored when increased pain is identified. Procedural wound pain merits special attention. Building on a therapeutic relationship between the patient and team, both pharmacological and nonpharmacological management strategies were recommended, as was engagement of patients and caregivers in assessment and planning, and communication of the pain management plan to patient, caregivers, and interdisciplinary team members.

Implications for Nursing Practice

Controlling wound pain can play a major role in improving patient quality of life. Nurses must ensure that the assessment of wound pain is incorporated into their everyday practice.

sure ulcer; this type of dressing should be used only for mechanical debridement of the wound. For further information on preparing the wound bed and localized wound care, refer to the Canadian Association of Wound Care Web site (see the Resources at the end of this chapter). (Dressings are discussed in Table 14-13.)

Stage II through stage IV pressure ulcers are considered to be contaminated or colonized with bacteria. It is important to remember that for patients with chronic wounds or who are immunocompromised, the clinical signs of infection (purulent exudate, odour, erythema, induration, warmth, tenderness, edema, pain, fever, and elevated WBC count) may not be present even though the pressure ulcer is infected.

The maintenance of adequate nutrition is an important nursing responsibility for the patient with a pressure ulcer (RNAO, 2007). Often, the patient is debilitated and has a poor appetite secondary to inactivity. Clinically significant malnutrition is defined as a serum albumin level lower than 30 g/L, total lymphocyte count lower than 1.8×10^9/L, or body weight decrease of more than 5% over a 6- to 12-month period (Bryant, 2010). Oral feedings must be adequate in calories, proteins, fluids, vitamins, and minerals to meet the patient's nutritional requirements. The intake needed to correct and maintain a nutritional balance may be 30 to 35 calories per kilogram per day and 1.25 to 1.50 g of protein per kilogram per day. Nasogastric feedings can be used to supplement the oral feedings. If necessary, parenteral nutrition consisting of amino acid and glucose solutions is used when oral

and nasogastric feedings are inadequate. (Parenteral and enteral nutrition are discussed in Chapter 42.) Nursing Care Plan 14-2 outlines the care for the patient with a pressure ulcer.

Ambulatory and Home Care. Pressure ulcers affect the quality of life of patients and their caregivers. Because the recurrence of pressure ulcers is common, the education of both the patient and the care provider in prevention techniques is extremely important (see Table 14-19). The care provider needs to know the causes of pressure ulcers, prevention techniques, early signs, nutritional support, and care techniques for actual pressure ulcers. Because many patients with a pressure ulcer require extensive care for other health problems, it is important that the nurse support the caregiver in confronting the added responsibility of pressure ulcer treatment.

Evaluation

Expected outcomes for the patient with a pressure ulcer are presented in Nursing Care Plan 14-2.

CLINICAL DECISION-MAKING EXERCISE

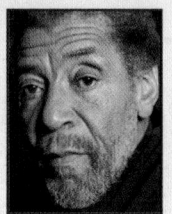

CASE STUDY:
Inflammation and Infection

Source: © iStockphoto.com/Gisele Gaze.

Patient Profile

Mr. Roger, a 58-year-old man, is admitted to the hospital emergency department with partial-thickness burns that involved his face, neck, and upper trunk. He also has a lacerated right leg. His injuries occurred about 24 hours earlier, when he fell out of a tree onto his gas grill (which was lit) while he was trying to get his cat.

Subjective Data

- Complains of slightly hoarse voice and irritated throat
- States that he tried to treat himself because he does not regularly see the same primary care health professional
- Has been coughing up sooty sputum
- Complains of severe pain in left hip

Objective Data

Physical Examination
- Leg wound is gaping and looks infected; temperature is 38.4°C
- Radiographs reveal a fractured right tibia and fractured left hip

Laboratory Studies
- WBC count is 26.4×10^9/L with 80% neutrophils (10% bands)

Collaborative Care
- Surgery is performed to repair the left hip

Discussion Questions

1. What clinical manifestations of inflammation did Mr. Roger exhibit, and what are their pathophysiological mechanisms?
2. What type of exudate formation developed?
3. What is the basis for the elevated temperature?
4. What is the significance of his WBC count and differential?
5. Because his wound was deep, primary tissue healing was not possible. How would you expect healing to take place? What complications could he develop?
6. What are Mr. Roger's risk factors for developing a pressure ulcer?
7. *Priority Decision:* On the basis of the assessment data provided, what are the priority nursing diagnoses? Are there any collaborative problems?

ⓔvolve *Answers are available at* **http://evolve.elsevier.com/ Canada/Lewis/medsurg**

REVIEW QUESTIONS

The number of the question corresponds to the same-numbered objective at the beginning of the chapter.

1. In which context is physiological hyperplasia commonly found?
   a. A distended urinary bladder
   b. The female breast during lactation
   c. The bronchi of a chronic cigarette smoker
   d. An enlarged myocardium in heart failure
2. When radiation therapy is used in the treatment of cancer, how does it achieve the desired effect, which is death of cancer cells?
   a. Altering cellular metabolism and activity
   b. Producing mutations that interfere only with cancer cell function
   c. Accelerating metabolic reactions to reduce the normal life span of cells
   d. Stimulating synthesis of new particles that cause cell rupture and death
3. What is a common cause of coagulation necrosis?
   a. Autophagocytosis
   b. Pulmonary embolus
   c. Malignant brain tumour
   d. Peripheral vascular disease
4. Which of the following will be experienced by a patient with an impaired mononuclear phagocyte system?
   a. Increased circulation of histamine
   b. Decreased susceptibility to infection
   c. Decreased vascular response to cell injury
   d. Decreased surveillance for damaged or mutated cells
5. Which response of the inflammatory process is affected by the complement system during opsonization?
   a. Healing
   b. Cellular
   c. Vascular
   d. Formation of exudate
6. Which of the following is the most likely cause of fever that accompanies inflammation?
   a. Activation of the complement system
   b. Release of interleukin-1, interleukin-6, and tumour necrosis factor from monocytes
   c. Increased production and activity of neutrophils
   d. Massive vasodilation during the vascular response
7. A patient has an open, infected surgical wound that is treated with irrigations and moist gauze dressings. Which of the following should the nurse expect of this wound?
   a. It is classified as a black wound.
   b. It must heal by tertiary intention.
   c. It heals by regeneration of epithelial cells.
   d. It heals by the same processes as an uninfected deep wound.
8. Why do contractures frequently occur after burn healing?
   a. Secondary infection
   b. Lack of adequate blood supply
   c. Weakness of connective tissue
   d. Excess fibrous tissue formation
9. Why are rest and immobilization important measures of acute care for wound healing?
   a. They decrease the inflammatory response.
   b. They increase the circulation to the affected area.
   c. They increase the body's production of corticosteroids.
   d. They are mechanisms known to increase cytokine production.

10. An 85-year-old patient is assessed to have a score of 15 on the Braden scale. What does this score suggest?
    a. The patient has an existing stage I pressure ulcer.
    b. The patient is at risk for developing a pressure ulcer.
    c. The patient is in need of a daily pressure ulcer risk assessment.
    d. The patient is not at risk for developing a pressure ulcer at this time.

11. A 65-year-old patient who had a stroke and is confined to bed is assessed to be at risk for the development of a pressure ulcer. On the basis of this information, which of the following should the nurse implement?
    a. Begin a schedule of turning every 2 hours.
    b. Have the patient maintain a high-fat diet.
    c. Keep head of bed elevated to 90 degrees at all times.
    d. Vigorously massage reddened bony prominences daily.

12. An 82-year-old man who is being cared for at home by his family has a pressure ulcer that is 1 cm wide by 2 cm long. The wound is shallow, measuring 0.5 cm in depth, and pink tissue is completely visible on the wound bed. What stage is this pressure ulcer?
    a. Stage I
    b. Stage II
    c. Stage III
    d. Stage IV

13. Which one of the following orders should a nurse question as part of the plan of care for a patient with a stage III pressure ulcer?
    a. Cover the ulcer with foam dressing.
    b. Turn and position the patient every 2 hours.
    c. Clean the ulcer every shift with Dakin's solution.
    d. Assess for pain and medicate before dressing change.

ANSWERS: 1. b; 2. a; 3. b; 4. d; 5. b; 6. b; 7. d; 8. d; 9. a; 10. b; 11. a; 12. b; 13. c.

REFERENCES

Bryant, R. A. (2010). *Acute and chronic wounds—Nursing management* (4th ed.). St. Louis: Mosby.

Cole, L., & Nesbitt, C. (2004). A three-year multiphase pressure ulcer prevalence/incidence study in a regional referral hospital. *Ostomy/ Wound Management, 50*(11), 32-40. Retrieved from *http:// www.o-wm.com/article/3259*

Dinarello, C. A., & Porat, R. (2011). Fever and hyperthermia. In D. Longo, A. Fauci, D. Kasper, S. Hauser, J. Jameson, & J. Loscalzo (Eds.), *Harrison's principles of internal medicine* (18th ed.). Toronto: McGraw-Hill.

National Pressure Ulcer Advisory Panel (NPUAP). (2009). NPUAP clinical practice guidelines, October 2009. Retrieved from *http:// www.npuap.org/wp-content/uploads/2012/02/Final_Quick_ Prevention_for_web_2010.pdf*

Noonan, C., Quigley, S., & Curley, M. (2011). Using the Braden Q Scale to predict pressure ulcer risk in pediatric patients. *Journal of Pediatric Nursing, 26*(6), 566-575. doi:10.1016/j.pedn.2010. 07.006

Registered Nurses' Association of Ontario (RNAO). (2007). Assessment and management of stage I to IV pressure ulcers (Revised). Retrieved from *http://rnao.ca/bpg/guidelines/assessment- and-management-stage-i-iv-pressure-ulcers*

Saltsman, K. (2011). *The last chapter: Cell aging and death.* Bethesda, MD: National Institute of General Medical Sciences. Retrieved from *http://publications.nigms.nih.gov/insidethecell/chapter5.html*

Woodbury, M. G., & Houghton, P. E. (2004). Prevalence of pressure ulcers in Canadian health-care settings. *Ostomy/Wound Manage- ment, 50*(10), 22-28.

Wound, Ostomy and Continence Nurses Society. (2011). WOCN Society position statement: Pressure ulcer staging. Retrieved from *http://www.wocn.org/resource/resmgr/Docs/pressure_ulcer_staging. pdf*

CANADIAN RESOURCES

Canadian Association for Enterostomal Therapists
http://www.caet.ca
Canadian Association of Wound Care
http://www.cawc.net
Community and Hospital Infection Control Association (CHICA)—Canada
http://www.chica.org

Ontario Ministry of Health and Long-Term Care
http://www.health.gov.on.ca/en/
Public Health Agency of Canada
http://www.phac-aspc.gc.ca
Registered Nurses' Association of Ontario (RNAO)—Best Practice Guidelines
http://rnao.ca/bpg
Toronto Medical Laboratories and Mount Sinai Hospital Department of Microbiology, MicroWeb
http://www.microbiology.mtsinai.on.ca

RELATED RESOURCES

Agency for Health Care Policy
http://www.ahrq.gov/
Centers for Disease Control and Prevention
http://www.cdc.gov
European Pressure Ulcer Advisory Panel (EPUAP)
http://www.epuap.org
European Wound Management Association
http://www.ewma.org
International Federation of Infection Control
http://www.theific.org/
National Pressure Ulcer Advisory Panel
http://www.npuap.org
Ostomy Wound Management
http://www.o-wm.com/
Ontario Medical Advisory Secretariat and Ministry of Long-Term Care. (2006). *Negative Pressure Wound Therapy*
http://www.health.gov.on.ca/english/providers/program/mas/tech/ reviews/pdf/rev_npwt_070106.pdf.
World Council of Enterostomal Therapists
http://www.wcetn.org
World Health Organization
http://www.who.int/en
World Wide Wounds
http://www.worldwidewounds.com
Wound, Ostomy and Continence Nurses Society
http://www.wocn.org

evolve *For additional Internet resources, see the Web site for this book* at **http://evolve.elsevier.com/Canada/Lewis/medsurg**

15

Genetics

Written by Kelly A. Metcalfe

LEARNING OBJECTIVES

1. Define common terms related to genetics and genetic disorders: autosome, carrier, heterozygous, homozygous, mutation, recessive, and sex-linked.
2. Describe the basic principles of genetics.
3. Compare and contrast the most common categories of genetic disorders.
4. Describe taking a family history or pedigree using the common nomenclature.
5. Identify the common types of genetic testing.
6. Outline the role of the nurse in working with patients and families with possible or actual genetic conditions.
7. Identify ethical, legal, and psychosocial issues related to genetics and genetic testing.

KEY TERMS

allele One of two or more alternative forms of a gene that can occupy a particular chromosomal locus; Table 15-1, p. 276

amniocentesis Transabdominal puncture of the amniotic sac under ultrasound guidance using a needle and syringe in order to remove amniotic fluid to detect genetic and biochemical disorders, p. 281

autosome Any chromosome that is not a sex chromosome; Table 15-1, p. 276

carrier An individual who carries a copy of a mutated gene for a recessive disorder; Table 15-1, p. 276

chorionic villus sampling (CVS) Aspiration of fetal trophoblastic tissue (chorionic villi) by either transcervical or transabdominal approach for prenatal evaluation of the chromosomal, enzymatic, and DNA status of the fetus, p. 281

deoxyribonucleic acid (DNA) A nucleic acid that forms the chromosomes in human cells, p. 275

gene therapy An experimental technique that is used to replace or functionally repair defective or missing genes with normal genes, p. 282

genetics The study of inheritance, p. 275

genotype An individual's genetic makeup, p. 275

heterozygous Having two different alleles for one given gene; Table 15-1, p. 276

homozygous Having two identical alleles for one given gene; Table 15-1, p. 276

mutation A change in the DNA sequence of a gene affecting the original expression of the gene, p. 277

recessive allele An allele that has no noticeable effect on the phenotype in a heterozygous individual; Table 15-1, p. 276

ribonucleic acid (RNA) A single-stranded nucleic acid that translates DNA genetic information into protein, p. 276

sex-linked gene A gene located on a sex chromosome; Table 15-1, p. 276

transcription The process through which RNA is synthesized from the DNA template, p. 276

translation The process through which the codon sequence is converted into amino acids, p. 277

ELECTRONIC RESOURCES

Supplemental content related to Chapter 15 can be found ...

Evolve Web Site ⊖volve

http://evolve.elsevier.com/Canada/Lewis/medsurg
- Clinical Reference: Laboratory Values

- Content Updates
- Electronic Calculators
- Examination Review Questions
- Glossary
- Key Points (Printable and MP3 Download)

Genomics is a central science for all nursing practice because essentially all diseases and conditions have a genetic or genomic component. Health care for all persons will increasingly include genetic and genomic information along the pathways of prevention, screening, diagnostics, prognostics, selection of treatment, and monitoring of treatment effectiveness.

Consensus Panel on Genetic/Genomic Nursing Competencies (2009, p. 1).

Genetics has a great impact on health and disease. The study of genetics has become increasingly important for health care providers. More than 10,000 identified genetic disorders known to be inherited in predictable patterns in families have been identified and classified (Online Mendelian Inheritance in Man [OMIM], n.d.). Common disorders such as heart disease and most cancers arise from a complex interplay among multiple genes and between genes and factors in the environment (Berry & Hern, 2004; Lashley, 2005).

The identification of a genetic basis for many diseases has affected the study of genetics and its relevance to nurses. This has directly influenced the care of patients at risk for or diagnosed with a disease that has a genetic basis. Nurses need to know the basic principles of genetics, be familiar with the impact that genetics has on health and disease, and be prepared to assist the patient and family in dealing with genetics issues (Calzone et al., 2010). In addition, nurses must become knowledgeable regarding the application of genetic discoveries to clinical care and assume leadership in preparing to meet consumers' needs for the future (Lea, 2009). Nurses are at the interface of translating new human genome research discoveries into clinical practice and will increasingly care for individuals and families who have a genetic condition or a genetic component to their health.

Human Genome Project

The Human Genome Project (HGP) is one of the most significant health-related advances of modern times. The HGP began in 1990 as an international effort to analyze the structure of human DNA and determine the location on chromosomes of all human genes. The human genome was completely sequenced by 2003. The project mapped all 30,000 to 40,000 human genes (the human genome) and determined the complete sequence of more than 3 billion DNA bases. It involved more than 2000 scientists from 20 institutions in six countries. The legal, social, and ethical issues that may arise from the project are also being addressed.

The HGP will help improve the diagnosis of disease, allow for earlier detection of genetic predisposition to disease, and play a critical role in determining risk assessment for genetic-related diseases. A comprehensive Web site covering the topic of the HGP can be found at Human Genome Project Information (see the Resources at the end of this chapter.)

Basic Principles of Genetics

Genetics is the study of inheritance. Table 15-1 presents a glossary of terms commonly used in the study of genetics.

Chromosomes, Genes, and DNA

Humans have approximately 30,000 *genes* in their genetic makeup, or *genome*. A person's genetic makeup is called the **genotype,** and how these genes express themselves is called the *phenotype*. Genes are contained in *chromosomes*, and chromosomes are located within the cell nucleus (Figure 15-1). There are 46 chromosomes, and these occur in pairs in all human cells of the body with the exception of reproductive cells (oocytes and sperm), which contain 23 chromosomes. Genes on each of the chromosome pairs are *homologous* to each other, meaning that they have the same position and order. One copy is inherited from the mother, and one copy is inherited from the father during conception. Twenty-two pairs of chromosomes, called *autosomes*, are the same in both men and women. The twenty-third pair is referred to as the sex chromosomes. A male has an X and a Y chromosome, and a female has two X chromosomes (Figure 15-2).

The composition of each gene in the human genome is specified in the **deoxyribonucleic acid (DNA)** of the 46 chromosomes. Each individual gene is made up of a piece of DNA. DNA is a chemical that contains genetic instructions for making proteins that are necessary for proper bodily functioning. Genes are responsible for making proteins and control the rate at which they are made.

The DNA carries the chemical information that allows the precise transmission of genetic information from one cell to its daughter cell and from one generation to the next. The specific structure of DNA is a double helix in which two strands (polynucleotide chains) run in opposite directions (Figure 15-3). The two strands are held together by hydrogen bonds between pairs of bases: adenine (A), thymine (T), guanine (G), and cytosine (C). DNA is composed of a sugar (deoxyribose), a phosphate group, and one of the four nitrogenous bases. One unit, a sugar group combined with a phosphate group and one of the four bases, is called a *nucleotide*. The bases on each strand of DNA are paired in a specific manner. Adenine always pairs with thymine, and guanine pairs with cytosine. The specific nature of the genetic information encoded in the human genome lies in the sequence of As, Ts, Gs, and Cs on the two strands of the double helix along each of the chromosomes.

Table 15-1 Glossary of Genetic Terms	
TERM	**DEFINITION**
Allele	One of two or more alternative forms of a gene that can occupy a particular chromosomal locus
Autosome	Any chromosome that is not a sex chromosome
Carrier	Individual who carries a copy of a mutated gene for a recessive disorder
Chromosome	Gene-carrying structure in the nucleus of all human cells consisting of DNA and protein
Codominance	Two dominant versions of a trait that are both expressed in the same individual
Congenital	Condition present at birth
Dominant allele	Gene that is expressed in the phenotype of a heterozygous individual
Gene	Unit of hereditary information located on a specific part of a chromosome
Genome	Total genetic information of an organism
Hereditary	A disease or condition being transmitted from parent to offspring
Heterozygous	Having two different alleles for one given gene
Homozygous	Having two identical alleles for one given gene
Locus	Position of a gene on a chromosome
Mutation	Change in the DNA sequence of a gene affecting the expression of the gene (changing the original manner of expression)
Oncogene	Gene that is able to initiate and contribute to the conversion of normal cells to cancer cells
Pedigree	Family tree that contains the genetic characteristics and disorders of that particular family
Phenotype	Clinically expressed traits of an individual
Proto-oncogenes	Normal cellular genes that are important regulators of normal cellular processes; mutations can activate them to become oncogenes
Recessive allele	Allele that has no noticeable effect on the phenotype in a heterozygous individual
Sex-linked gene	Gene located on a sex chromosome
Trait	Physical characteristic that one inherits, such as hair and eye colour

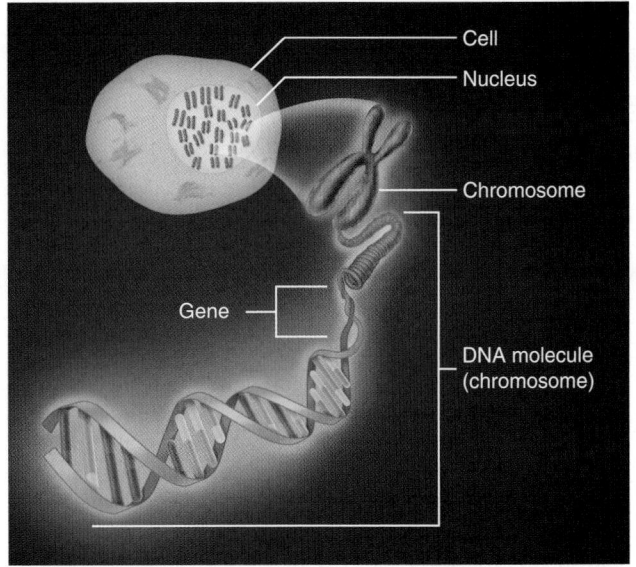

Figure 15-1 Human DNA.

Source: Redrawn from National Cancer Institute. (2005). *Gene testing: DNA.* Retrieved from *http://www.cancer.gov/cancertopics/understandingcancer/genetesting/page2*

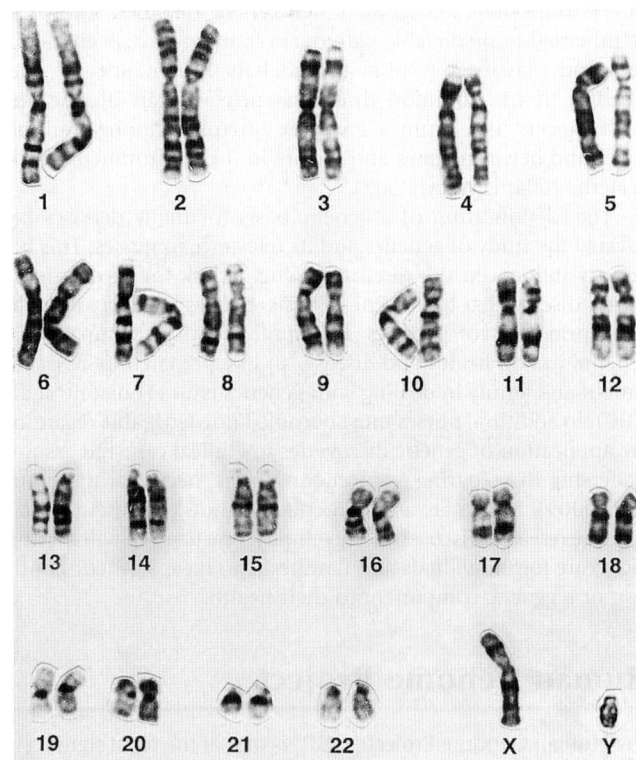

Figure 15-2 Human chromosomes.

Source: Turnpenny, P. D. (2007). *Emery's elements of medical genetics* (13th ed., p. 34, Figure 3-5). Edinburgh/Philadelphia: Churchill Livingstone/Elsevier.

How Proteins Are Made

DNA must undergo replication, transcription, and translation before a functional protein is made. A new DNA strand must be synthesized before cell division. In order to do this, the two DNA strands separate and unwind and become templates for new strands. DNA is formed and replicated in the cell nucleus, whereas protein synthesis takes place in the cytoplasm of the cell. Two processes take place when the genetic code is transported from the cell nucleus to the cytoplasm: transcription and translation, the latter following the former (Figure 15-4). **Ribonucleic acid (RNA)** is the nucleic acid that is involved in these processes. RNA is similar to DNA; however, it is composed of only one strand (as opposed to two strands in DNA), and the nitrogenous base thymine (T) is replaced with uracil (U). **Transcription** takes place

when RNA is synthesized from the DNA template. Genes are made up of coding (exons) and noncoding (introns) regions. In transcription, the noncoding regions (introns) are removed. As a result, a messenger RNA (mRNA) is created and can move across the nuclear membrane into the cytoplasm. This is where, based on the sequence of the mRNA, the protein is manufactured.

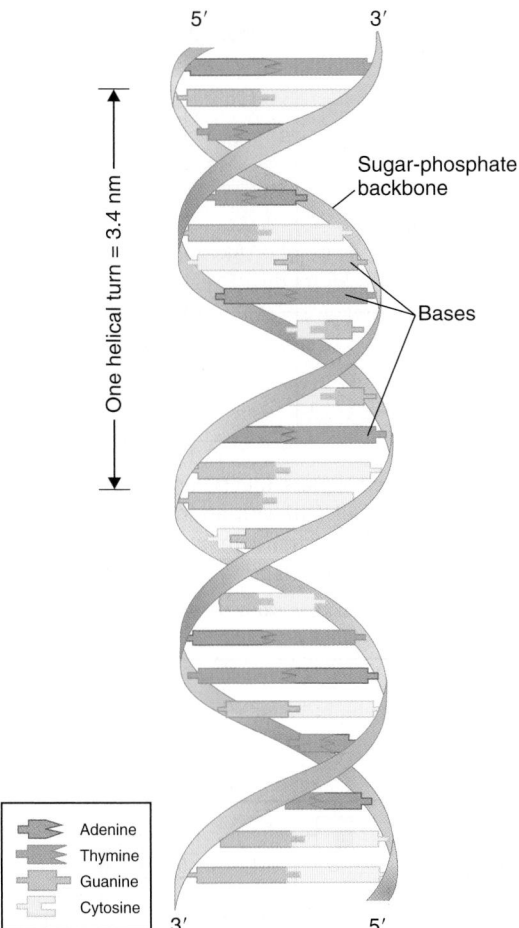

Figure 15-3 The DNA double helix, with sugar-phosphate backbone and nitrogenous bases.

Source: Jorde, L., Cary, J., & Bamshad, M. (2010). *Medical genetics* (4th ed., p. 7, Figure 2-3). St. Louis, MO: Mosby.

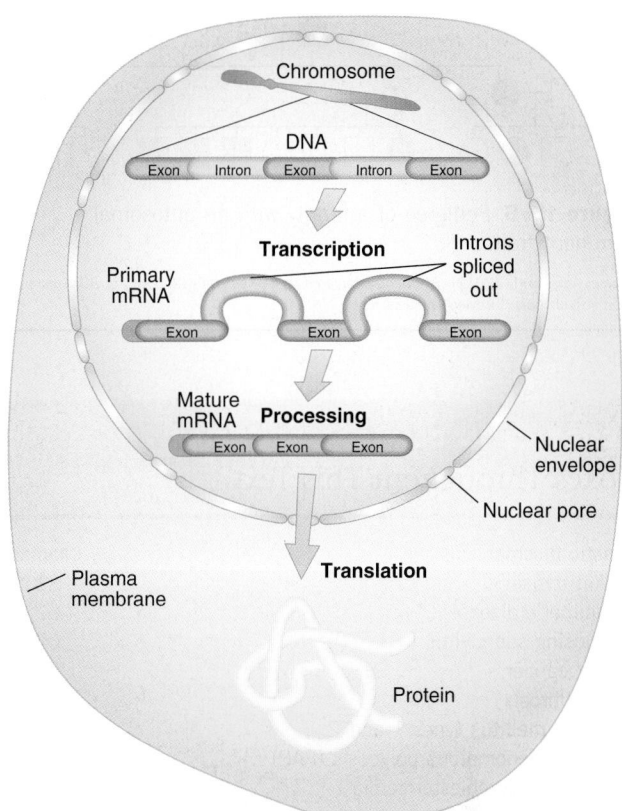

Figure 15-4 A summary of the steps leading from DNA to protein creation. Replication and transcription occur in the cell nucleus. The mRNA is then transported to the cytoplasm, where translation of the mRNA into amino acid sequences composing a protein occurs.

Source: Jorde, L., Cary, J., & Bamshad, M. (2010). *Medical genetics* (4th ed., p. 10, Figure 2-7). St. Louis: Mosby.

After transcription is complete, **translation** occurs. This is the process through which the codon sequence is converted into amino acids. Codons are made up of three nucleotides (e.g., CCG) and specify the production of one amino acid. Proteins are made up of many amino acids. Translation is accomplished by a cytoplasmic particle called the *ribosome.*

Genes are generally stable and are passed from one generation to the next. However, sometimes a change in the gene occurs, and this is referred to as a **mutation.** Mutations can occur in the germline (sperm and eggs) or in the somatic (body) cells after fertilization. Germline mutations are those that are passed from one generation to the next and account for familial syndromes. Approximately 2% of the DNA is composed of sequences that code for specific proteins, and the other 98% is made up of noncoding regions. It is when there is a change in the sequence of the coding sequence of a structural gene that the protein may not be formed correctly.

Primary Categories of Genetic Conditions

Within each human, alterations in genes or in combinations of them can cause genetic disorders. These disorders can be classified into three categories: (1) single gene disorders; (2) chromosomal disorders; and (3) multifactorial disorders.

Single Gene Disorders

These disorders are caused by individual genes. The mutation may be present on only one chromosome of a pair (matched with a normal allele on the homologous chromosome) or on both chromosomes of the pair. These disorders usually exhibit obvious and characteristic inheritance patterns in families and are also referred to as *mendelian.* Examples of single gene disorders include cystic fibrosis, Marfan syndrome, and sickle cell anemia. There are three primary single gene or mendelian inheritance patterns: (1) autosomal dominant; (2) autosomal recessive; and (3) X-linked recessive. If the mutant gene is located on an autosome, the genetic disorder is called *autosomal.* If the mutant gene is on the X chromosome, the genetic disorder is called *X linked.*

Autosomal Dominant. An autosomal dominant trait is one that manifests in the heterozygous state, that is, in a person who has both an abnormal (mutated) and a normal gene. The mutated gene dominates the other normal gene. Families with conditions that suggest autosomal dominant inheritance exhibit several characteristics:

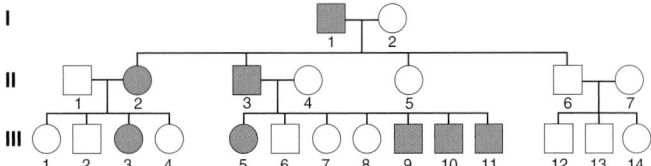

Figure 15-5 Pedigree of a family with an autosomal dominant trait.

Source: Adkison, L. (2012). *Elsevier's integrated review: genetics* (2nd ed., p. 30, Figure 3-2). Philadelphia: Elsevier/Saunders.

GENETICS IN CLINICAL PRACTICE
Boxes Throughout This Text

Genetic Disorder	Chapter
α₁-Antitrypsin	31
Alzheimer's disease	62
Ankylosing spondylitis	67
Breast cancer	54
Cystic fibrosis	31
Diabetes mellitus types 1 and 2	52
Familial adenomatous polyposis (FAP)	45
Familial hypercholesterolemia	36
Hemachromatosis	33
Hemophilia A and B	33
Hereditary nonpolyposis colorectal cancer (HNPCC)	45
Huntington's disease	61
Ovarian cancer	56
Polycystic kidney disease	48
Sickle cell disease	33

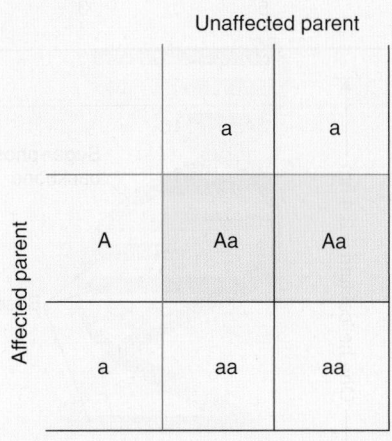

Figure 15-6 Punnett square illustrates the mating of an unaffected individual *(aa)* with an individual who is heterozygous for an autosomal dominant disease gene *(Aa)*. The genotypes of affected offspring are shaded.

Source: Jorde, L., Cary, J., & Bamshad, M. (2010). *Medical genetics* (4th ed., p. 60, Figure 4-2). St. Louis, MO: Mosby.

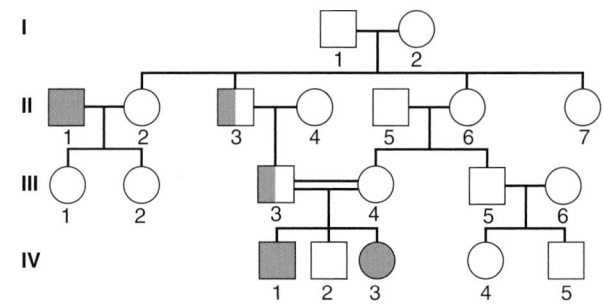

Figure 15-7 Pedigree of a family with an autosomal recessive trait.

Source: Adapted from Adkison, L. (2012). *Elsevier's integrated review: genetics* (2nd ed., p. 31, Figure 3-3). Philadelphia: Elsevier/Saunders.

1. The affected offspring has one affected parent (with each pregnancy in an affected parent, there is a 50% chance that the characteristic will be passed to the child).
2. Unaffected persons do not transmit the trait to their children.
3. Males and females are equally likely to inherit the trait.
4. The trait does not skip generations.

Some examples of autosomal dominant disorders are achondroplasia, Marfan syndrome, neurofibromatosis type 1, and brachydactyly. See Figure 15-5 for an example of a pedigree of a family with an autosomal dominant trait. (Conventional symbols used in pedigrees are defined in Figure 15-11, on p. 280.)

Punnett squares can be used to determine inheritance possibilities. The Punnett square in Figure 15-6 illustrates the mating of an affected parent with the autosomal dominant trait and an unaffected parent. The probability that the affected parent will pass on the mutated gene to a child is 0.5. Therefore, on average, 50% of the offspring will inherit the trait.

Autosomal Recessive. In the majority of recessive conditions, an affected offspring results from a mating between two unaffected carriers of the mutated gene. The offspring inherits two copies of the mutated gene, one from each parent, which results in the offspring exhibiting the disorder. The parents of these offspring do not exhibit the trait associated with having the mutation because they each carry only one copy of the mutated gene (they are heterozygous carriers). Families with conditions that suggest autosomal recessive inheritance exhibit several characteristics:

1. Most affected individuals have parents that have normal phenotypes (do not exhibit the trait).
2. On average, 1 in 4 children is affected.
3. Males and females are equally likely to be affected.
4. Affected persons who mate with normal persons tend to have phenotypically normal children.

Some examples of autosomal recessive disorders are albinism, cystic fibrosis, and phenylketonuria. See Figure 15-7 for an example of a pedigree of a family with an autosomal recessive trait. The Punnett square illustrating the mating of two heterozygous parents of an autosomal recessive gene is shown in Figure 15-8.

X-Linked Recessive. An X-linked recessive trait is one determined by a gene carried on the X chromosome, and it usually manifests only in males. In males, there is only one X chromosome (the other is a Y chromosome), whereas females have two X chromosomes. A male with a mutation in a gene on the X chromosome will exhibit the disorder, because he has no corre-

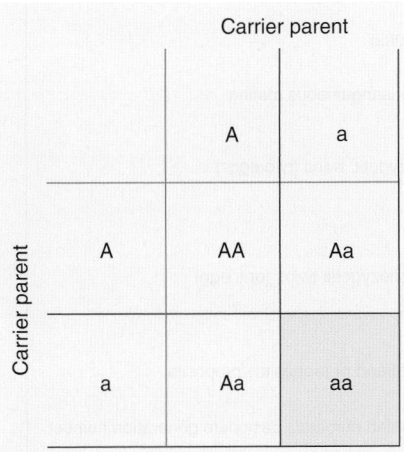

Figure 15-8 Punnett square illustrates the mating of two heterozygous carriers of an autosomal recessive gene. The genotype of the affected offspring is *shaded*.

Source: Jorde, L., Cary, J., & Bamshad, M. (2010). *Medical genetics* (4th ed., p. 61, Figure 4-5). St. Louis: Mosby.

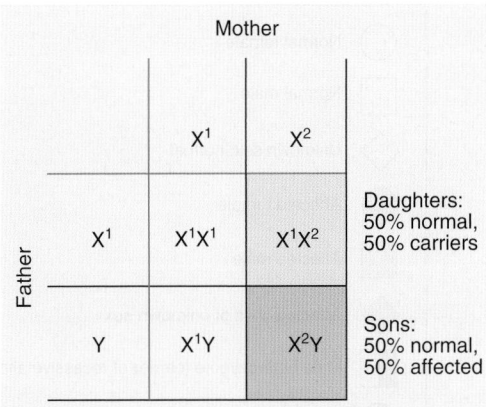

Figure 15-10 Punnett square representation of the mating of a heterozygous female who carries an X-linked recessive disease gene with a normal male. X^1, Chromosome with normal allele; X^2, chromosome with disease allele.

Source: Jorde, L., Cary, J., & Bamshad, M. (2010). *Medical genetics* (4th ed., p. 85, Figure 5-4). St. Louis: Mosby.

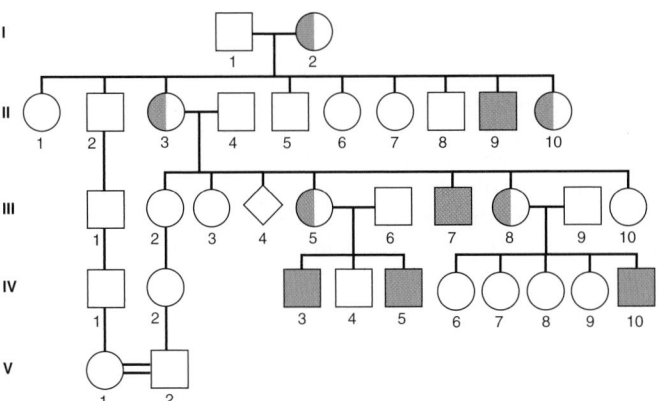

Figure 15-9 X-linked inheritance of hemophilia A among descendants of Queen Victoria (I-2) of England. Roman numerals, generation number; arabic numbers, individuals within generations

Source: Adkison, L. (2012). *Elsevier's integrated review: genetics* (2nd ed., p. 33, Figure 3-4). Philadelphia: Elsevier/Saunders.

sponding normal gene to mask the mutated gene's effects. Diseases inherited in an X-linked manner are transmitted by healthy heterozygous female carriers to males, who are thus affected, as well as by affected males to their carrier daughters, with a future risk to male grandchildren. Families with conditions that suggest X-linked recessive inheritance exhibit several characteristics:

1. Unaffected males do not transmit the disorder.
2. All daughters of an affected male are heterozygous carriers.
3. Heterozygous women transmit the mutant allele to 50% of the sons (who are affected) and to 50% of the daughters (who are heterozygous carriers).

Some examples of X-linked recessive disorders are hemophilia A and Duchenne muscular dystrophy (DMD). See Figure 15-9 for an example of a pedigree of a family with an autosomal recessive trait. The Punnett square in Figure 15-10 illustrates the mating of a female carrier of an X-linked recessive disorder and a normal male.

Chromosomal Disorders

Abnormalities of chromosomes may be either numerical or structural and may involve one or more autosomes, sex chromosomes, or both together. The most common type of clinically significant chromosomal abnormality involves the number of chromosomes *(aneuploidy)*. In this situation, there are either extra or missing chromosomes. Aneuploidy results from an error during meiotic cell division, creating a sperm or an egg with too many or too few chromosomes, which is passed on to the offspring during conception. Most aneuploid offspring have either trisomy (three chromosomes) or monosomy (only one chromosome)—instead of the normal pair of chromosomes. The most common trisomy is trisomy 21 (Down syndrome). In these offspring, there are three copies of chromosome 21. Other examples of aneuploidy are trisomy 13 and trisomy 18. Monosomy for an entire chromosome is almost always lethal, with the exception of monosomy for the X chromosome, as seen in Turner's syndrome.

Chromosomal disorders can also be the result of abnormalities of chromosome structure. Structural rearrangements result from chromosome breakage and subsequent reconstitution in an abnormal combination. These new configurations can be either balanced or unbalanced. In balanced rearrangements, the chromosome is complete, with no loss or gain of genetic material. These rearrangements are generally harmless except in rare cases where one of the breakpoints damages an important functional gene. When a chromosome rearrangement is unbalanced, the chromosomal complement contains an incorrect amount of chromosome material, and the clinical effects are usually serious.

Multifactorial Inheritance

Disorders that are caused by multifactorial inheritance occur as a result of an interaction between one or more genes (polygenic) or between one or more genes and environmental influences. Multifactorial inheritance is thought to be the basis for most common diseases, including cancer, heart disease, and multiple sclerosis. A primary characteristic of this type of inheritance is familial aggregation of diseases. Multifactorial conditions tend to run in families, but the pattern of inheritance is not as predictable

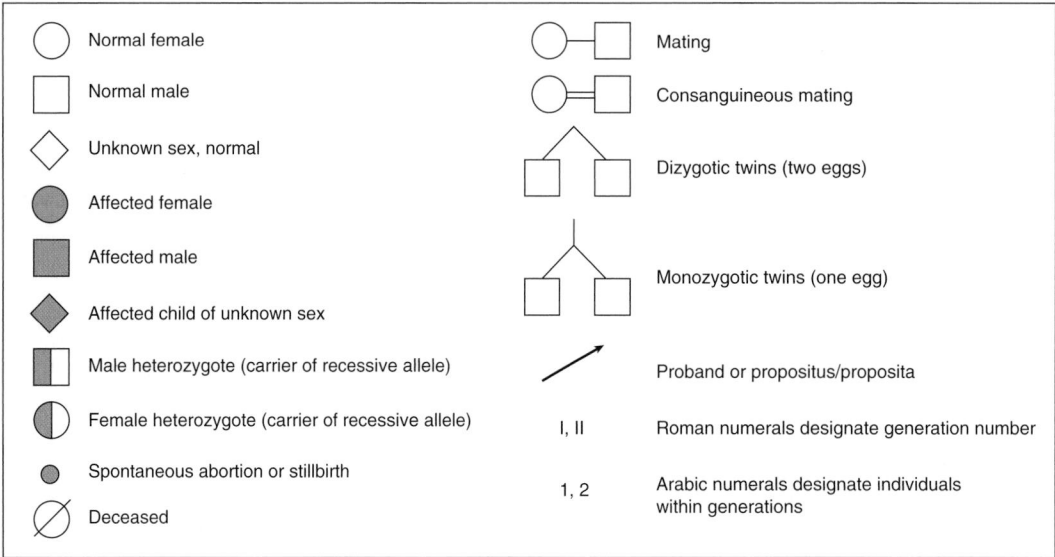

Figure 15-11 Conventional symbols used in pedigrees.

Source: Adkison, L. (2012). *Elsevier's integrated review: genetics* (2nd ed., p. 30, Figure 3-1). Philadelphia: Elsevier/Saunders.

as with single gene disorders. The chance of recurrence is also less than the risk for single gene disorders. The degree of risk of a multifactorial disorder occurring in relatives is related to the number of genes they share in common with the affected individual. The closer the degree of relationship, the more genes they have in common. The degree of risk also increases with the severity of the disorder. Although multifactorial conditions run in families, the risk is generally less than the 25 or 50% seen in mendelian conditions. Identical twins, exactly alike genetically, may not always have the same condition when inheritance is multifactorial. This indicates that there are nongenetic factors that also play a role in the expression of multifactorial traits. For instance, the risk of coronary heart disease increases with smoking or obesity, and the risk of emphysema in individuals with α_1-antitrypsin deficiency increases greatly with smoking.

Characteristics of multifactorial inheritance include the following:

1. There is a similar risk for first-degree relatives (offspring, siblings, or parents).
2. Identical twins are not 100% concordant, indicating that there are nongenetic factors involved.
3. The greater the number of affected relatives, the higher the recurrence risk.
4. The severity of the disorder and occasionally the sex of the affected individual may modify the risk.

Genetics in Clinical Practice

Taking a Family History

A detailed three-generation family history, or pedigree, offers great insight into possible genetic conditions within a family. A pedigree is a symbolic representation of family members indicating specific details about each individual. General family history screening should be obtained for each family member, with details for at least three generations. Information (including age, disease status, and vital status) should be collected on the patient, his or her children, and the patient's siblings, parents, aunts,

uncles, and grandparents. Standard nomenclature should be used when constructing a pedigree (Figure 15-11). This initial pedigree can highlight certain areas, such as those pertinent to a specific condition (e.g., cancer), for further questioning. A pedigree targeting the possibility of a hereditary cancer syndrome will gather even more details about the incidence of cancer, the types of cancer, ages at diagnosis, and outcomes. Information about paternal and maternal ethnicity should also be gathered because some genetic mutations are found more commonly in certain ethnic groups.

Genetic Testing

Genetic testing is the analysis of DNA, chromosomes, proteins, or metabolites, or some combination. Testing can be done on blood or other bodily samples and involves looking for a genetic mutation that indicates the presence or absence of a genetic condition or predisposition to a genetic condition. Genetic testing can be used in a multitude of ways. A genetic screening test may be useful in determining the potential risk for development of a disease in one's lifetime. Such tests may be done in a variety of settings and at any point during the lifespan, including prenatally, at birth, or throughout childhood and adulthood. Some tests screen for the possibility of a disease and are predictive of expression of disease. Other tests are done to determine whether an individual is a carrier of a mutated gene, which may be passed on to an offspring.

Prenatal Diagnosis and Screening. The main objective of prenatal diagnosis is to give parents information so they can make informed decisions during pregnancy. The potential benefits of prenatal testing include the following: (1) decreasing the anxiety of at-risk parents (when test results return as normal); (2) providing risk information to parents before conception so an informed choice can be made regarding future pregnancies; (3) allowing parents to prepare psychologically for the birth of an affected child; and (4) providing risk information to parents when pregnancy termination is an option. Prenatal diagnostic tests can be either invasive (e.g., amniocentesis, chorionic villus

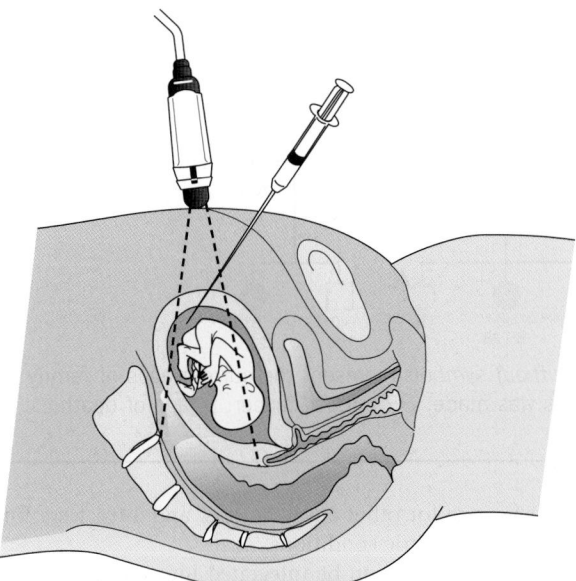

Figure 15-12 A schematic illustration of an amniocentesis, in which 20 to 30 mL of amniotic fluid is withdrawn trans-abdominally (with ultrasound guidance), usually at 15 to 17 weeks' gestation.

Source: Jorde, L., Cary, J., & Bamshad, M. (2010). *Medical genetics* (4th ed., p. 268, Figure 13-4). St. Louis: Mosby.

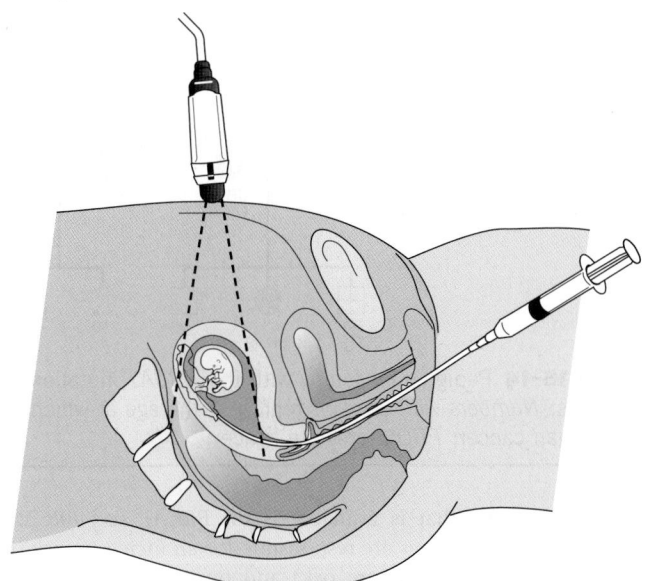

Figure 15-13 A schematic illustration of a transcervical chorionic villus sampling procedure. With ultrasound guidance, a catheter is inserted, and several milligrams of villus tissue is aspirated.

Source: Jorde, L., Cary, J., & Bamshad, M. (2010). *Medical genetics* (4th ed., p. 269, Figure 13-5). St. Louis: Mosby.

sampling) or noninvasive (e.g., maternal serum screening, ultra-sonography).

Amniocentesis. **Amniocentesis** is traditionally performed 15 to 17 weeks after a pregnant woman's last menstrual period. It can be used to diagnose neural tube defects, chromosome abnormalities, metabolic disorders, and molecular defects. A needle is inserted through the abdominal wall into the amniotic sac while the fetus is being monitored using ultrasound (Figure 15-12). Between 20 and 30 mL of amniotic fluid, which contains living cells (amniocytes) shed by the fetus, is removed. Cytogenetic studies are done after culture of the amniocytes. Common indications for amniocentesis are (1) maternal age older than 35 years; (2) previous child with chromosome abnormality; (3) history of structural chromosome abnormality in one parent; (4) family history of genetic defect that is diagnosable by biochemical or DNA analysis; and (5) risk of neural tube defect. There is approximately a risk of 0.5% to 1% of miscarriage associated with this procedure (Mujezinovic & Alfirevic, 2007).

Chorionic Villus Sampling. **Chorionic villus sampling** (CVS) is done in the first trimester, usually between 11 and 12 weeks' gestation. It is performed by aspirating fetal trophoblastic tissue (chorionic villi) by either the transcervical or the transabdominal approach for prenatal evaluation of the chromosomal, enzymatic, and DNA status of the fetus (Figure 15-13).

Compared with amniocentesis, CVS has the advantage of providing a diagnosis much earlier in a pregnancy than amniocentesis for couples who may consider termination as an option. CVS is associated with a slightly higher risk of miscarriage (1 to 1.5%) (Mujezinovic & Alfirevic, 2007).

Screening for Carriers of Genetic Disease. This type of genetic screening is done on healthy individuals (i.e., those

unaffected with a genetic condition) to determine whether they carry a mutation that could be passed to offspring and cause genetic diseases. Typically, this test is done for autosomal recessive and X-linked disorders. Individuals may opt for this type of genetic screening if there is a family history of a genetic disease or if they are in an ethnic group that has a greater risk of carrying a certain genetic mutation. Examples of disorders for which testing is available are Tay-Sachs disease, cystic fibrosis, and fragile X syndrome.

Presymptomatic and Predisposition Testing. Predictive testing includes both presymptomatic and predisposition testing. In presymptomatic testing, an individual has genetic testing to determine whether she or he carries a genetic mutation for a genetic disorder. Typically, individuals electing this testing are members of a family that exhibits a genetic disorder. An example of this would be genetic testing for Huntington's disease. This is an adult-onset condition and involves progressive neurological degeneration. The gene responsible for Huntington's disease is 100% penetrant, that is, everyone who inherits this mutation will exhibit the disease. There is no cure for this disorder, so everyone who inherits the mutation will die of the disease. For members of families in which Huntington's disease is present, the decision to undergo predictive testing may be difficult. In Canada, the uptake rate for predictive testing is approximately 18% of the estimated Canadian population at risk for the disease (Creighton et al., 2003).

Genetic testing is also available to determine an individual's predisposition for developing a genetic condition and is now used in prenatal, pediatric, and adult populations. Many genes that, when mutated, cause an individual to be predisposed to a disease (i.e., the individual has an increased risk of developing the disease) have been identified. However, not all individuals who have the genetic mutation will get the disease. An example

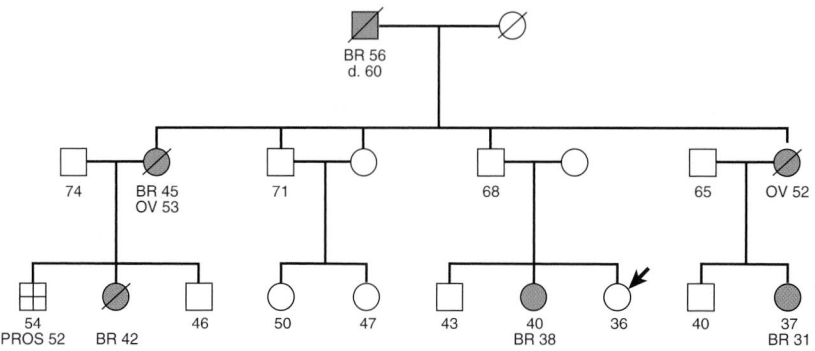

Figure 15-14 Pedigree for family with the *BRCA1* mutation. *Numbers without symbols* represent the current ages of family members. *Numbers with symbols* represent the age at which the diagnosis was made. *BR*, breast cancer; *d*, age of death; *OV*, ovarian cancer; *PROS*, prostate cancer.

of genetic testing that is available is for *BRCA1* and *BRCA2*. Mutations in these genes are responsible for an increased risk of breast cancer (≤80% lifetime risk) and ovarian cancer (≤60% lifetime risk) (Chen & Parmigiani, 2007). Typically, families that carry mutations in these genes have numerous members who have been diagnosed with breast or ovarian cancers (Figure 15-14). Other characteristics that suggest a possible *BRCA1* or *BRCA2* mutation in a family are onset of breast cancer at young age (<50 years), male breast cancer, and bilateral breast cancer (cancer in both breasts). The advantage of testing for mutations in *BRCA1* and *BRCA2* is that women at high risk for developing breast and ovarian cancers can be identified before the development of cancer. These women can then begin vigilant breast and ovarian cancer screening at an earlier age, or they can elect for preventive options. Included in preventive options are prophylactic surgery (both bilateral mastectomy and bilateral oophorectomy) or chemopreventive drugs (e.g., tamoxifen). Each option offers varying cancer risk reduction, and there are both medical and psychological adverse effects that may result. In a recent Canadian publication, uptake of preventive options by women with a *BRCA1* or *BRCA2* mutation was reported. Twenty-one percent of women had a prophylactic mastectomy, 54% of women had a bilateral oophorectomy (preventive removal of the ovaries), and 6% took tamoxifen (Metcalfe et al., 2007).

Genetic Counselling

Genetic counselling is the process of helping people understand and adapt to the medical, psychological, and familial implications of genetic contributions to disease (National Society of Genetic Counselors [NSGC], 2008). This process integrates the following:

• Interpretation of family and medical histories to assess the chance of disease occurrence or recurrence.
• Education about inheritance, testing, management, prevention, resources, and research.
• Counselling to promote informed choices and adaptation to the risk or condition.

Andermann and Narod (2002) reported on current practices of genetic counsellors in Ontario who serve a population of over 11 million people. The cost of most genetic counselling was covered by the provincial health plan. There were no private genetic services, and there were no patient copayments. The report found that 45% of genetic consultations were for preconception or prenatal diagnosis, 22% were for breast and ovarian

cancer, 5% were for other adult cancers, and 14% were for the evaluation of pediatric conditions.

Although genetics can be integrated into most nurses' practices, some nurses specialize in genetics. Genetic nurses have specialized education and training in genetics in addition to generic training in health care practice and seek to care for people's genetic and genomic health (International Society of Nurses in Genetics [ISONG], 2010). Genetic nurses help people at risk for or affected by diseases with a genetic component to achieve and maintain health. They perform risk assessments, analyze the genetic contribution to disease risk, and discuss the impact of risk on health care management for individuals and families. They also provide genetic education, provide nursing care to patients and families, and conduct research in genetics. The ISONG is an organization of nurses around the world who work in genetics (see the Resources at the end of this chapter.).

Genetic counsellors are health professionals with specialized graduate degrees and experience in the areas of medical genetics and counselling. They provide information and support to families who have members with birth defects or genetic disorders and to families who may be at risk for a variety of inherited conditions. They identify families at risk, investigate the problem that the family has, interpret information about the disorder, analyze inheritance patterns and risks of recurrence, and review available options with the family. Genetic counsellors also provide supportive counselling to families, serve as patient advocates, and refer individuals and families to community or provincial and territorial support services (NSGC, 2008).

Gene Therapy

Gene therapy is an experimental technique that is used to replace or functionally repair defective or missing genes with normal genes. A normal gene can be inserted into a human chromosome to counteract the effects of a missing or abnormal gene. Although gene therapy is a promising treatment option for a number of diseases (including inherited disorders, some types of cancer, and certain viral infections), the technique remains risky and is still under study to make sure that it will be safe and effective. Gene therapy is currently being tested only for the treatment of diseases that have no other cures (National Library of Medicine, 2008b).

The first approved gene therapy trials involved children with severe combined immunodeficiency disease caused by adenosine deaminase deficiency. T lymphocytes from these children were obtained, and the missing gene was inserted into these T cells (Figure 15-15). The new T cells were then reinjected into the

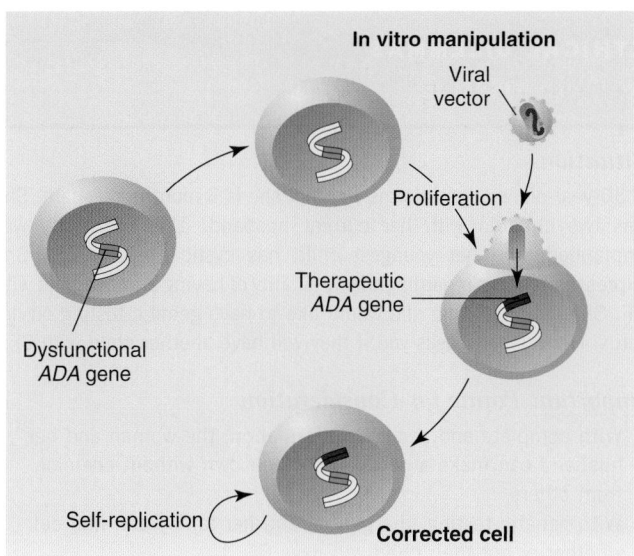

In vitro manipulation

Viral vector

Proliferation

Therapeutic *ADA* gene

Dysfunctional *ADA* gene

Self-replication

Corrected cell

Figure 15-15 Gene therapy for adenosine deaminase (ADA) deficiency attempts to correct this immunodeficiency state. The viral vector containing the therapeutic *ADA* gene is inserted into the patient's lymphocytes. These cells can then make the ADA enzyme.

children's bloodstreams. The gene signalled the cells to produce the missing enzyme, and these children were capable of developing a functioning immune system.

Gene therapy has promise for treating a wide array of problems that do not respond to conventional methods of intervention. Although no gene therapy is used in clinical practice, the treatment strategies closest to being incorporated into mainstream therapies include those that address immunodeficiency disease, hemophilia, and ischemic vascular disease. Before gene therapy can become a practical approach to treating disease, scientists must find improved methods of delivering the genes to directly target the affected cells and must ensure that the new genes can be controlled by the body (National Library of Medicine, 2008a).

Methods of Gene Delivery. One of the major hurdles in gene therapy is finding a way to insert the gene into the body. Genes that are inserted directly into a cell usually do not function. Instead, a carrier, called a *vector,* is used to deliver the gene. The most common vectors are attenuated or modified versions of viruses. The viruses are modified so they cannot cause disease when used in humans (National Library of Medicine, 2008b).

Some types of viruses, such as retroviruses, integrate their genetic material (including the new gene) into a chromosome in the human cell. Other viruses, such as adenoviruses, introduce their DNA into the nucleus of the cell, but the DNA is not integrated into a chromosome.

The vector can be injected or given by the intravenous (IV) route directly into a specific tissue in the body, where it is taken up by the individual cells. Alternatively, a sample of the patient's cells can be removed and exposed to the vector in a laboratory setting. The cells containing the vector are returned to the patient. If the treatment is successful, the new gene delivered by the vector will make a functioning protein.

Examples of Gene Therapy for Cancer. One of the first gene therapy protocols used in treating cancer patients involved

the addition of a gene for tumour necrosis factor (TNF). The vector with the gene for TNF was inserted into lymphocytes aimed at sites of malignant melanoma. This approach allows a high dose of TNF to be delivered to the tumour only and avoids systemic adverse effects.

The purpose of the multidrug resistance (MDR) clinical gene therapy trials is to modify the effects of high-dose chemotherapy in bone marrow cells by inserting the MDR gene. Bone marrow stem cells are separated and cultured with a virus carrying the genetic material for the MDR gene. The virus transfers the MDR gene into the patient's stem cells. These stem cells and their offspring become resistant to the toxic effects of chemotherapy by acquiring the ability to pump the chemotherapeutic drugs out of the cells before the drugs are able to kill the cells.

NURSING MANAGEMENT: GENETICS

Nurses must be knowledgeable about the fundamentals of genetics. By understanding the influence that genetics has on health and disease, the nurse can assist the patient and family in making critical decisions related to genetic issues, such as genetic testing. The nurse also should collaborate with the team or physician to involve a genetics counsellor. The nurse should be able to give patients and their families accurate information pertaining to genetics, genetic diseases, and probabilities of genetic disorders. Inheritance patterns can be assessed by the nurse and explained to the patient and family through the use of Punnett squares (see Figures 15-6, 15-8, and 15-10) or family pedigrees (see Figures 15-5, 15-7, and 15-9). Maintaining patient confidentiality and respecting the patient's values and beliefs are critical because the information from the counsellor may have major implications for many persons who are involved. Examples of applications of genetics in nursing practice include (Consensus Panel, 2009):

- Recognizing a newborn infant that is at risk for morbidity and mortality because of genetic metabolism errors
- Identifying an asymptomatic adolescent who is at high risk for hereditary colorectal cancer based on his or her family history
- Identifying a couple who is at risk for having a child with a genetic condition
- Assisting with the selection of a drug or dose of a drug, based on genetic markers, in the treatment of an adult with cancer
- Helping an individual or family with questions related to genetic information or services to find reliable information

Genetic testing may raise many psychological issues. Knowledge of a carrier status of a genetic disorder may influence a person's career plans and decisions for marriage and childbearing. It may also affect significant others when grappling with serious life and health care issues. Furthermore, there are ethical concerns: Who should know the result of a genetic test? How should society or the government protect the privacy of individuals' test results and protect individuals from discrimination? Genetic information should not be misused to stigmatize individuals or particular ethnic groups. Attention must be paid to better understand psychosocial needs of individuals and societal responses and health care policy related to genetic testing.

There are many ethical issues that may arise when dealing with genetic testing. Genetic results offer individuals insight into conditions that may already exist or that may develop in the future. This type of information may cause ethical dilemmas. Prenatal genetic testing may raise ethics issues for parents. For example, if parents are informed prenatally that their baby has a genetic condition, decisions about the future of the pregnancy must be considered. If a baby is identified as having trisomy 21 (Down syndrome), it is unclear how severe the condition might be. There will be physical and developmental abnormalities; however, it is difficult to predict the extent of these abnormalities. This may make it difficult for parents to decide if termination of the pregnancy is an option for them. In addition, for some individuals, cultural and religious beliefs may factor into this decision making.

Genetic testing for adult-onset conditions also may raise ethical dilemmas. With testing for adult-onset conditions (e.g., breast cancer), issues related to "duty to warn" may surface. If a woman is told that she has a *BRCA1* mutation, there are significant implications for her blood relatives. Once a *BRCA1* mutation is identified in a family, all blood relatives are eligible to receive genetic testing for the specific mutation. However, if an individual does not share her genetic test results with her family, the family members may be unaware of their chance of having the *BRCA1* mutation and their significantly increased risk of developing breast cancer. This may result in a family member not having the opportunity to elect for a cancer prevention option and developing breast cancer as a result.

Ethical issues must be considered carefully when working with families undergoing genetic testing. These issues are often dealt with in genetic counselling that is offered by genetic counsellors or genetic nurses. The Committee on Assessing Genetic Risks, Division of Health Sciences Policy, Institute of Medicine, emphasizes autonomy, confidentiality, privacy, and equity as essential to analysis of questions related to genetic testing (Andrews, Fullarton, Holtzman, & Motulsky, 1994). Nurses must be aware of these ethical principles when providing care to individuals and families.

ETHICAL DILEMMAS
Genetic Testing

Situation

A 30-year-old woman informs you that she is 3 months pregnant. She has two children with her current husband. This pregnancy was unplanned, and her youngest child has cystic fibrosis (CF). She expresses concern regarding the possibility of having another child with CF. She mentions that she would like to have genetic testing on her fetus. Her husband asks you if they will have another child with CF.

Important Points for Consideration

- With complete and accurate information, the woman and her husband can make a decision on their own without coercion from others.
- With genetic testing, the patient and her family can find out whether or not their child will have CF.
- Genetic counselling is recommended before and after obtaining genetic testing because of the complexity of the information and the emotional issues involved.
- The nurse, knowing that CF is an autosomal recessive condition, can use Punnett squares (see Figures 15-6, 15-8, and 15-10) to show the woman and her husband the probability of having another child with CF.

Clinical Decision-Making Questions

1. What information would you give the patient regarding genetic testing in order for her and her husband to make a decision?
2. What options are available for this couple?
3. How would you assist this couple in making a decision about possibly terminating the pregnancy if the results of the genetic testing show that the fetus tested positive for the CF gene?

REVIEW QUESTIONS

The number of the question corresponds to the same-numbered objective at the beginning of the chapter.

1. If a person is heterozygous for a given gene, what does it mean?
   a. The person is a carrier for a genetic disorder.
   b. The person is affected by the genetic disorder.
   c. The person has two identical alleles for the gene.
   d. The person has two different alleles for the gene.
2. Which of the following statements best describes genomics?
   a. The study of genetic disorders in families
   b. The study of inheritance
   c. The study of the interaction between genes and the environment
   d. The comprehensive study of the genetic information of an organism

3. Which of the following statements is correct about a father who has an X-linked recessive disorder and a wife with a normal genotype?
   a. The father will pass the carrier state to his male children.
   b. The father will pass the carrier state to all of his children.
   c. The father will pass the carrier state to his female children.
   d. The father will not pass on the genetic mutation to any of his children.
4. What is a family pedigree?
   a. The family ancestry traced through the father
   b. The family line of descent through the mother
   c. The depiction of an autosome recessive gene disorder
   d. A family tree drawn in the form of a diagram
5. Which of the following would be a reason for a patient or potential parents to undergo genetic testing?
   a. To determine the sex of an unborn child through amniocentesis
   b. To predict the potential for developing diabetes
   c. To help couples at risk of genetic disorders to make an informed choice before conception
   d. To screen for the possibility of undiagnosed breast cancer

6. Which of the following is the best response for the nurse who is asked by a pregnant woman about the risk associated with invasive prenatal testing?
   a. Amniocentesis is associated with a 1 to 5% risk of miscarriage.
   b. Chorionic villus sampling (CVS) is associated with a much lower risk of miscarriage than amniocentesis because it is less invasive.
   c. Both amniocentesis and CVS are associated with a low risk of miscarriage (<1.5%).
   d. CVS is the preferred method of prenatal testing because it can be done as late as 18 weeks' gestation.

7. Why might prenatal genetic testing cause ethical dilemmas for parents?
   a. The sex of the child would be known.
   b. Decisions about the future of the pregnancy (including termination) would be left to the parents.
   c. Health care providers would know about the genetic conditions of the unborn child.
   d. Family members might question the couple's decision to undergo genetic testing.

ANSWERS: 1. d; 2. d; 3. c; 4. d; 5. c; 6. c; 7. b.

REFERENCES

Andermann, A., & Narod, S. A. (2002). Genetic counselling for familial breast and ovarian cancer in Ontario. *Journal of Medical Genetics, 39,* 695-696. doi:10.1136/jmg.39.9.695

Andrews, L., Fullarton, J., Holtzman, N., & Motulsky, A. (Eds). (1994). *Assessing genetic risks: Implications for health and social policy.* Ch. 8: Social, Legal, and Ethical Implications of Genetic Testing, pp. 247-289.Washington, DC: National Academy Press.

Berry, T. A., & Hern, M. J. (2004). Genetic practice, education, and research: An overview for advanced practice nurses. *Clinical Nurse Specialist, 18,* 126-132. doi:10.1097/00002800-200405000-00012

Calzone, K. A., Cashion, A., Feetham, S., Jenkins, J., Prows, C. A., Williams, J. K., & Wung, S. F. (2010). Nurses transforming health care using genetics and genomics. *Nursing Outlook, 58,* 26-35. doi:10.10106/j.outlook.2009.05.001.

Chen, S., & Parmigiani, G. (2007). Meta-analysis of BRCA1 and BRCA2 penetrance. *Journal of Clinical Oncology, 25,* 1329-1333. doi:10.1200/JCO.2006.09.1066

Consensus Panel on Genetic/Genomic Nursing Competencies (2009). *Essentials of genetic and genomic nursing: Competencies, curricula guidelines, and outcome indicators* (2nd ed.). Silver Spring, MD: American Nurses Association. Retrieved from *http://www.genome.gov/Pages/Careers/HealthProfessionalEducation/geneticscompetency.pdf*

Creighton, S., Almqvist, E. W., MacGregor, D., Fernandez, B., Hogg, H., Beis, J., ..., Hayden, M. R. (2003). Predictive, pre-natal and diagnostic genetic testing for Huntington's disease: The experience in Canada from 1987 to 2000. *Clinical Genetics, 63,* 462-475. doi:10.1034/j.1399-0004.2003.00093.x

International Society of Nurses in Genetics (ISONG). (2010). Provision of quality genetic services and care: Building a multidisciplinary, collaborative approach among genetic nurses and genetic counselors. Retrieved from *http://www.isong.org/*

Lashley, F. R. (2005). *Clinical genetics in nursing practice.* New York: Springer.

Lea, D. H. (2009). Basic genetics and genomics: A primer for nurses. *OJIN: Online Journal of Issues in Nursing, 14*(2) (Feb. 17). Retrieved from *http://www.nursingworld.org/MainMenuCategories/ANAMarketplace/ANAPeriodicals/OJIN/TableofContents/Vol142009/No2May09/Articles-Previous-Topics/Basic-Genetics-and-Genomics.html*

Metcalfe, K., Ghadirian, P., Rosen, B., Foulkes, W., Kim-Sing, C., Eisen, A, ..., Narod, S. (2007). Variation in rates of uptake of preventive options in BRCA1 and BRCA2 mutation carriers across Canada. *Open Medicine, 1,* E92-E98. Retrieved from *http://www.openmedicine.ca/article/view/12/50*

Mujezinovic, F., & Alfirevic, Z. (2007). Procedure-related complications of amniocentesis and chorionic villous sampling: A systematic review. *Obstetrics & Gynecology, 110,* 687-694. doi:10.1097/01.AOG.0000278820.54029.e3

National Library of Medicine. (2008a). Genetics home reference: Your guide to understanding genetic conditions. Retrieved from *http://ghr.nlm.nih.gov/*

National Library of Medicine. (2008b). Handbook: Gene therapy—Experimental techniques, safety, ethics, and availability. Retrieved from *http://ghr.nlm.nih.gov/handbook/therapy?show=all*

National Society of Genetic Counselors (NSGC). (2008). FAQs about genetic counselors and the NSGC. Retrieved from *www.nsgc.org/consumer/faq_consumers.cfm*

Online mendelian inheritance in man (OMIM®). (n.d.). McKusick-Nathans Institute of Genetic Medicine, Johns Hopkins University (Baltimore, MD) and National Center for Biotechnology Information, National Library of Medicine (Bethesda, MD). Retrieved from *www.ncbi.nlm.nih.gov/omim/*

CANADIAN RESOURCES

Canadian Directory of Genetic Support Groups
http://www.lhsc.on.ca/programs/medgenet/
Genetic Resources Ontario
http://www.geneticresourcesontario.ca/
Genome Program
http://www.genomecanada.ca
Inherited Metabolic Disorders Clinic
http://www.medicalgenetics.ca/inherited.html
Public Health Agency of Canada
http://www.hc-sc.gc.ca/hbp/lcdc

RELATED RESOURCES

American College of Medical Genetics and Genomics
http://www.acmg.net
Centers for Disease Control and Prevention, Public Health Genomics
http://www.cdc.gov/genomics
Gene Clinics, Testing & Support Groups
http://www.geneclinics.org
Gene Tests
http://www.genetests.org
Genetic Alliance
http:// www.geneticalliance.org
Genetics Program for Nursing Faculty
http:// www.cincinnatichildrens.org/ed/clinical/gpnf/default.htm
International Society of Nurses in Genetics (ISONG)
http:// www.isong.org/
National Human Genome Research Institute
http://www.nhgri.nih.gov
Online Mendelian Inheritance in Man
http://www.ncbi.nlm.nih.gov/omim/
Understanding Gene Testing
http://www.accessexcellence.org/AE/AEPC/NIH

evolve   *For additional Internet resources, see the Web site for this book at* **http://evolve.elsevier.com/Canada/Lewis/medsurg**

CHAPTER

16

Altered Immune Response and Transplantation

Written by Sharon L. Lewis

Adapted by Susan Chernenko

LEARNING OBJECTIVES

1. Describe the functions and components of the immune system.
2. Compare and contrast humoral and cell-mediated immunity regarding lymphocytes involved, types of reactions, and effects on antigens.
3. Identify the five types of immunoglobulins and their characteristics.
4. Differentiate among the four types of hypersensitivity reactions in terms of immunological mechanisms and resulting alterations.
5. Identify the clinical manifestations and emergency management of a systemic anaphylactic reaction.
6. Describe the assessment and collaborative care of a patient with chronic allergies.
7. Describe the causes, the clinical manifestations, and the treatment modalities of autoimmune diseases.

8. Explain the relationship between the human leukocyte antigen system and certain diseases.
9. Describe the causes and categories of immunodeficiency disorders.
10. Describe the various kinds of organ transplantation and the types of rejection that may be experienced after transplantation.
11. Identify the types and adverse effects of immunosuppressive therapy.
12. Describe alternative strategies that have been explored to address organ donor shortages.
13. Describe new technologies in immunology, including hybridoma technology, recombinant DNA technology, and gene therapy.

KEY TERMS

anergy Immunodeficient condition characterized by lack of or diminished reaction to an antigen or a group of antigens, p. 293

antigen A substance that elicits an immune response, p. 287

apheresis The use of a procedure that separates components of the blood followed by the removal of one or more of those components, p. 303

autoimmunity An immune reaction to self-proteins; the immune system no longer differentiates self from nonself, p. 302

cell-mediated immunity Immune responses that are initiated through specific antigen recognition by T cells, p. 292

cytokines Soluble factors secreted by white blood cells and a variety of other cells in the body, p. 289

human leukocyte antigen (HLA) system A series of linked genes that occur together on the sixth chromosome in humans that plays an important part in the body's immune response to foreign substances, p. 303

humoral immunity Antibody-mediated immunity, p. 290

hypersensitivity reaction An overreactive immune response against foreign antigens or failure to maintain self-tolerance that may result in tissue damage, p. 293

immunocompetence The ability of the body's immune system to identify and inactivate or destroy foreign substances, p. 293

immunodeficiency The inability of the immune system to protect the body adequately, p. 304

immunosuppressive therapy Therapy with the goal of adequately suppressing the immune response enough to prevent rejection of the transplanted organ but not to prevent overwhelming infection, p. 307

monoclonal antibodies Homogeneous populations of identical antibody molecules produced by specialized tissue cell culture lines, p. 310

organ transplantation The transfer of a whole or partial organ from one individual to another for the purpose of replacing the recipient's damaged or failing organ with a working one from the donor, p. 305

ELECTRONIC RESOURCES

Supplemental content related to Chapter 16 can be found...

Evolve Web Site ⊖volve

http://evolve.elsevier.com/Canada/Lewis/medsurg
- Animations:
  - Activation and Function of B Cells
  - Function of T Cytotoxic Memory Cells and T Cytotoxic Cells

- Clinical Reference: Laboratory Values
- Content Updates
- Electronic Calculators
- Examination Review Questions
- Glossary
- Key Points (Printable and MP3 Download)

Normal Immune Response

Immunity is a state of responsiveness to foreign substances such as microorganisms and tumour proteins. Immune responses serve three functions (Coico & Sunshine, 2009):
1. *Defence.* The body protects against invasions by microorganisms and prevents the development of infection by attacking foreign antigens and pathogens.
2. *Homeostasis.* Damaged cellular substances are digested and removed. Through this mechanism, the body's different cell types remain uniform and unchanged.
3. *Surveillance.* Mutations continually arise in the body but are normally recognized as foreign cells and destroyed.

Types of Immunity

Immunity is classified as innate (natural) or acquired. *Innate immunity* exists in a person without prior contact with an antigen. This type of immunity involves a nonspecific response; neutrophils and monocytes are the white blood cells (WBCs) primarily involved. One type of innate immunity that is not antigen specific is the type that is present at birth (Coico & Sunshine, 2009). Humans are naturally immune to some of the infectious agents that cause illnesses in other species. *Acquired immunity* is the development of immunity, either actively or passively (Table 16-1).

Active Acquired Immunity.
Active acquired immunity results from the invasion of the body by foreign substances such as microorganisms, which leads to the development of antibodies and sensitized lymphocytes. With each reinvasion of the microorganisms, the body responds more rapidly and vigorously to fight off the invader. Active acquired immunity may result naturally from a disease or artificially through inoculation of a less virulent antigen (e.g., immunization). Because antibodies are synthesized, immunity takes time to develop but is long-lasting.

Passive Acquired Immunity.
In *passive acquired immunity,* the host receives, rather than synthesizes, antibodies to an antigen. This may take place naturally through the transfer of immunoglobulins across the placental membrane from mother to fetus. Artificial passive acquired immunity occurs through injection with γ-globulin (serum antibodies). The benefit of this immunity is its immediate effect. Unfortunately, passive immunity is short-lived because the host does not synthesize the antibodies and consequently does not retain memory cells for the antigen.

Table 16-1 Types of Acquired Specific Immunity

Active
Natural
Natural contact with antigen through clinical infection (e.g., disease and recovery from chicken pox, measles, and mumps)
Artificial
Immunization with antigen (e.g., immunization with live or killed vaccines)
Passive
Natural
Transplacental and colostrum-mediated transfer from mother to infant (e.g., maternal immunoglobulins in neonate)
Artificial
Injection of serum from immune human (e.g., injection of human γ-globulin)

Antigens

An **antigen** is a substance that elicits an immune response. Most antigens are composed of proteins. However, other substances such as large-size polysaccharides, lipoproteins, and nucleic acids can act as antigens. All the body's cells have antigens on their surface that are unique to that person and enable the body to recognize self-substances. The immune system becomes "tolerant" to the body's own molecules and therefore is nonresponsive to self-substances.

Lymphoid Organs

The lymphoid system is composed of central (or primary) and peripheral lymphoid organs. The *central lymphoid organs* are the thymus gland and bone marrow. The *peripheral lymphoid organs* are the tonsils; gut-, genital-, bronchial-, and skin-associated lymphoid tissues; lymph nodes; and spleen (Figure 16-1).

Lymphocytes are produced in the bone marrow and eventually migrate to the peripheral organs. The thymus is important in the differentiation and maturation of T lymphocytes and is therefore essential for a cell-mediated immune response. During childhood, the thymus gland is large; however, it shrinks with age, thus becoming a collection of reticular fibres, lymphocytes, and connective tissue in older persons.

Lymphoid tissue is found in the submucosa of the respiratory (bronchus-associated), genitourinary (genital-associated), and gastrointestinal (gut-associated) tracts. This tissue protects the

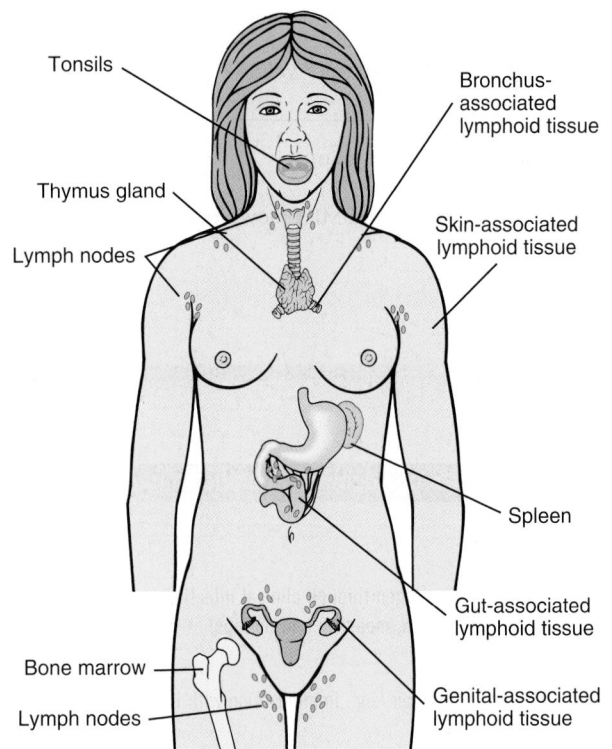

Tonsils

Bronchus-associated lymphoid tissue

Thymus gland

Lymph nodes

Skin-associated lymphoid tissue

Spleen

Gut-associated lymphoid tissue

Bone marrow

Lymph nodes

Genital-associated lymphoid tissue

Figure 16-1 Organs of the immune system.

body surface from external microorganisms. The tonsils are a typical example of lymphoid tissue.

The skin-associated lymph tissue primarily consists of lymphocytes and Langerhans cells (a type of resident macrophage) found in the epidermis of skin. When Langerhans cells are depleted, the skin can neither initiate an immune response nor support a skin-localized delayed hypersensitivity response.

When antigens are introduced into the body, they may be carried by the bloodstream or lymph channels to regional lymph nodes. The antigens interact with B and T lymphocytes and macrophages in the lymph node. The two important functions of lymph nodes are (a) filtration of foreign material brought to the site and (b) circulation of lymphocytes.

The spleen is important as the primary site for filtering foreign substances from the blood. It consists of two kinds of tissue: white pulp containing B and T lymphocytes and red pulp containing erythrocytes. Macrophages line the pulp and the sinuses of the spleen. The spleen is the major site of immune responses to bloodborne antigens. If the spleen is removed in childhood, the individual may be predisposed to life-threatening septicemia.

Cells Involved in Immune Response

Mononuclear Phagocytes. The *mononuclear phagocyte system* includes monocytes in the blood and macrophages found throughout the body. (See Chapter 14 for a more complete description of macrophages.) Mononuclear phagocytes have a critical role in the immune system. They are responsible for capturing, processing, and presenting the antigen to the lymphocytes, which stimulates a humoral or cell-mediated immune response. Capturing is accomplished through phagocytosis. The macrophage-bound antigen, which is highly immunogenic, is presented to circulating T or B lymphocytes and thus triggers an immune response (Figure 16-2).

Lymphocytes. Lymphocytes are produced in the bone marrow (Figure 16-3). Lymphocytes differentiate into B and T lymphocytes.

B Lymphocytes. In birds, *B lymphocytes* (bursa-equivalent lymphocytes) mature under the influence of the bursa of Fabricius. However, this lymphoid organ does not exist in humans. The bursa-equivalent tissue in humans is the bone marrow. B cells differentiate into *plasma cells* when activated and produce antibodies (immunoglobulins) (Table 16-2).

T Lymphocytes. Cells that migrate from the bone marrow to the thymus differentiate into *T lymphocytes* (thymus-dependent cells). The thymus secretes hormones, including thymosin, that stimulate the maturation and differentiation of T lymphocytes. T cells make up 70% to 80% of the circulating lymphocytes and are responsible primarily for immunity to intracellular viruses, tumour cells, and fungi. T cells live from a few months to an individual's lifespan and account for long-term immunity.

T lymphocytes can be categorized into T cytotoxic, T helper, and T suppressor cells. Antigenic characteristics of WBCs have been classified through the use of monoclonal antibodies. These antigens are classified as *clusters of differentiation,* or *CD, antigens.* Many types of WBCs, especially lymphocytes, are referred to by their CD designations. All mature T cells have the CD3 antigen (Chaplin, 2006).

T Cytotoxic Cells. T cytotoxic cells are involved in attacking antigens on the cell membrane of foreign pathogens and releasing cytolytic substances that destroy the pathogen. These cells have antigen specificity and are sensitized by exposure to the antigen (Chaplin, 2006). Like B lymphocytes, some sensitized T cells do not attack the antigen but remain as memory T cells. As in the humoral immune response, a second exposure to the antigen results in a more intense and rapid cell-mediated immune response.

T Helper and T Suppressor Cells. T helper (CD4) cells and T suppressor (CD8) cells are involved in the regulation of cell-mediated immunity and the humoral antibody response. These two cell types are often referred to as *immunoregulatory cells.* In many autoimmune diseases, the number of T suppressor cells decreases in proportion to the number of T helper cells, which results in an overaggressive immune response. The human immunodeficiency virus (HIV) invades T helper cells, thus decreasing their number and function. Therefore, individuals with HIV infection do not mount an aggressive immune response and are at an increased risk for opportunistic infections and malignancies.

Natural Killer Cells. Natural killer (NK) cells are also involved in cell-mediated immunity. These cells are not T or B cells but are large lymphocytes with numerous granules in the cytoplasm. Prior sensitization is not required for the generation of NK cells. These cells are involved in recognition and killing of virus-infected cells, tumour cells, and transplanted grafts; however, the mechanism of recognition is not fully understood. NK cells have a significant role in immune surveillance for malignant cell changes.

Dendritic Cells. Dendritic cells are a system of cells that play a significant role in cell-mediated immune response. They are found in the skin (those are called *Langerhans cells*), the lining of the nose, the lungs, the stomach, and the intestines, and when in

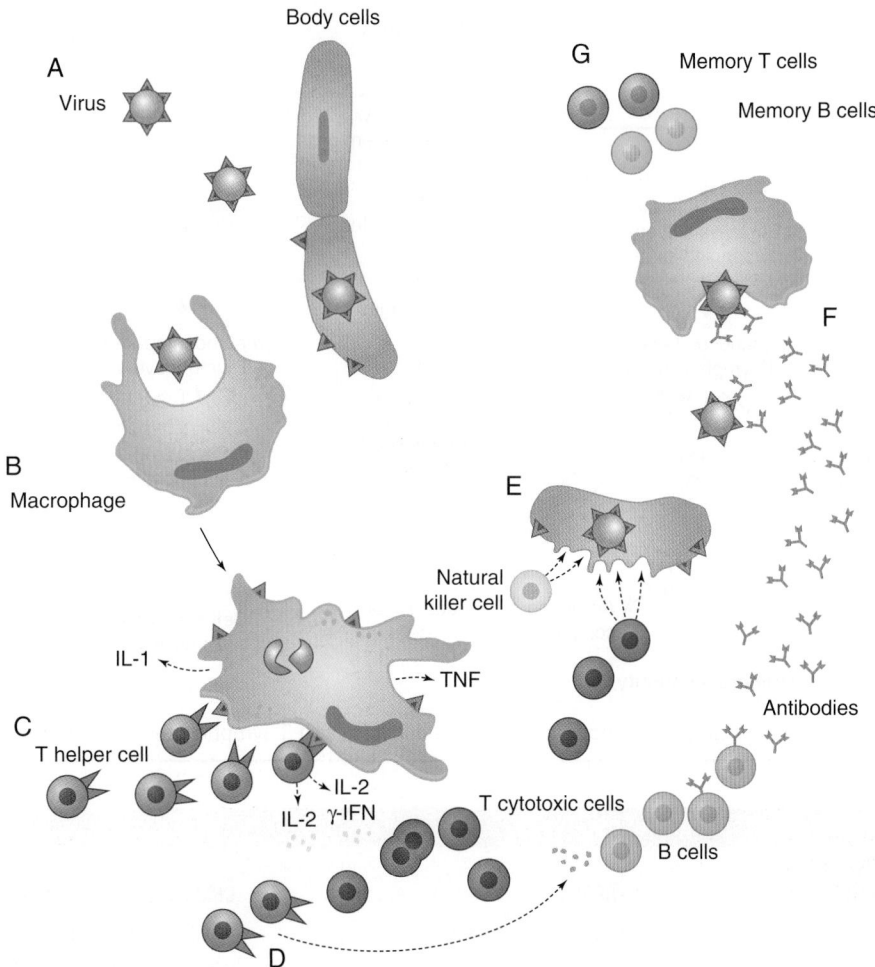

Figure 16-2 The immune response to a virus. **A,** A virus invades the body through a break in the skin or another portal of entry. The virus must make its way inside a cell in order to replicate itself. **B,** A macrophage recognizes the antigens on the surface of the virus. The macrophage digests the virus and displays pieces of the virus (antigens) on its surface. **C,** T helper cells recognize the antigen displayed and bind to the macrophage. This binding stimulates the production of cytokines (interleukin-1 [IL-1] and tumour necrosis factor [TNF]) by the macrophage and interleukin-2 (IL-2) and γ-interferon (γ-IFN) by the T helper cells. These cytokines are intercellular messengers that provide communication among the cells. **D,** IL-2 instructs other T helper cells and T cytotoxic cells to proliferate (multiply). T helper cells release cytokines, causing B cells to multiply and produce antibodies. **E,** T cytotoxic cells and natural killer cells destroy infected body cells. **F,** The antibodies bind to the virus and mark it for macrophage destruction. **G,** Once the virus is gone, activated T and B cells are turned off by suppressor T cells. Memory B and T cells remain behind to respond quickly if the same virus attacks again.

an immature state, they can be found in the blood. Their primary function is to capture antigens at sites of contact with the external environment (e.g., skin, mucous membranes) and then transport this antigen until it encounters a T cell with specificity for the antigen. Dendritic cells, in this role, have an important function in activating the immune response.

Cytokines

The immune response involves complex interactions of T cells, B cells, monocytes, and neutrophils. These interactions depend on **cytokines** (soluble factors secreted by WBCs and a variety of other cells in the body) that act as messengers between the cell types. Cytokines instruct cells to alter their proliferation, differentiation, secretion, or activity. At least 100 different cytokines are currently known, and they can be classified into distinct categories (Chaplin, 2010). Some of these cytokines are listed in Table 16-3. In general,

the interleukins act as immunomodulatory factors, colony-stimulating factors act as growth-regulating factors for hematopoietic cells, and interferons are antiviral and immunomodulatory.

Cytokines serve a beneficial role in immune function but can also have detrimental effects such as those observed in chronic inflammation, autoimmune diseases, and sepsis. Cytokines such as colony-stimulating factors (see Chapters 18 and 33), interferons (see Chapter 18), and interleukin-2 (see Chapter 18) are used clinically to (a) stimulate the bone marrow to make WBCs and (b) treat various malignancies. In addition, inhibitors of cytokines such as soluble tumour necrosis factor (TNF) receptor–antagonist and interleukin-1 are being used in clinical trials as anti-inflammatory agents. (Clinical uses of cytokines are listed in Table 16-4.)

Interferon helps the body's natural defences attack tumours and viruses. Three types of interferon have been identified (see Table 16-3). In addition to their direct antiviral properties, inter-

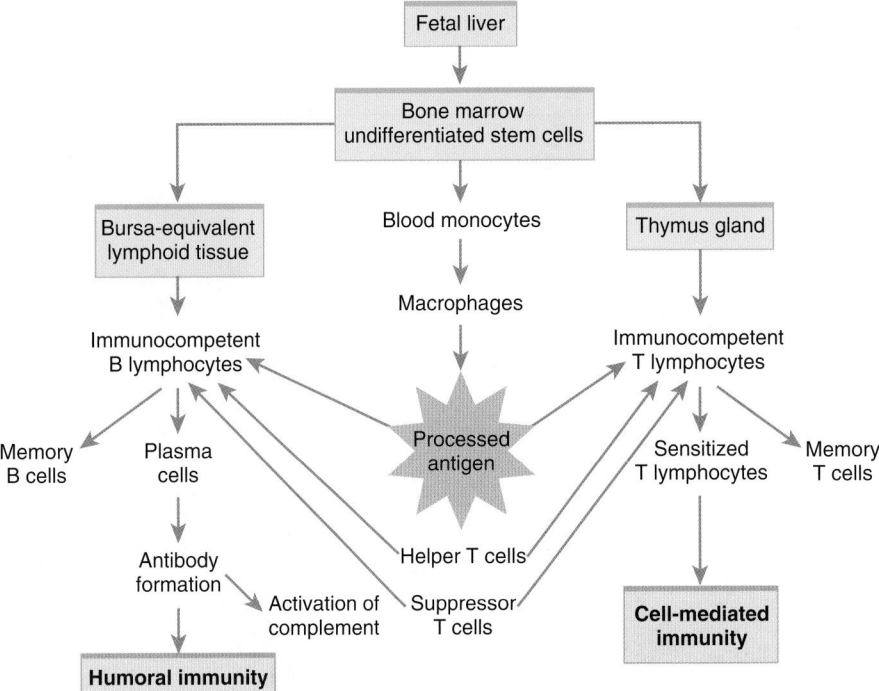

Figure 16-3 Relationships and functions of macrophages, B lymphocytes, and T lymphocytes in an immune response.

Table 16-2 Characteristics of Immunoglobulins			
CLASS	**RELATIVE SERUM CONCENTRATION (%)**	**LOCATION**	**CHARACTERISTICS**
IgG	76	Plasma, interstitial fluid	Is only immunoglobulin that crosses placenta
			Is responsible for secondary immune response
IgA	15	Body secretions, including tears, saliva, breast milk, colostrum	Lines mucous membranes and protects body surfaces
IgM	8	Plasma	Is responsible for primary immune response
			Forms antibodies to ABO blood antigens
IgD	1	Plasma	Is present on lymphocyte surface
			Assists in the differentiation of B lymphocytes
IgE	0.002	Plasma, interstitial fluids	Causes symptoms of allergic reactions
			Fixes to mast cells and basophils
			Assists in defence against parasitic infections

Ig, immunoglobulin.

ferons have immunoregulatory functions, which include enhancement of NK cell production and activation and inhibition of tumour cell growth. Interferon is not directly antiviral but produces an antiviral effect in cells by reacting with them and inducing the formation of a second protein termed *antiviral protein* (Figure 16-4). This protein mediates the antiviral action of interferon by altering the cell's protein synthesis and prevents the virus from replicating.

Comparison of Humoral and Cell-Mediated Immunity

Humans need both humoral and cell-mediated immunity to remain healthy. Each type of immunity has unique properties and different modes of action. Table 16-5 is a comparison of humoral and cell-mediated immunity.

Humoral Immunity. **Humoral immunity** is antibody-mediated immunity. The term *humoral* comes from the Greek word *humor*, which means "body fluid." Antibodies are produced by plasma cells (differentiated B cells) and are found in plasma; therefore, the term *humoral immunity* is used. Production of antibodies is an essential component in a humoral immune response. Each of the five classes of immunoglobulins— immunoglobulins G, A, M, D, and E (IgG, IgA, IgM, IgD, and IgE)—has specific characteristics (see Table 16-2).

When a pathogen (especially a bacterium) enters the body, it may encounter a B lymphocyte specific for antigens located on that bacterial cell wall. In addition, a monocyte or macrophage may phagocytize the bacteria and present its antigens to a B lymphocyte. The B lymphocyte recognizes the antigen because it has receptors on its cell surface specific for that antigen. When the antigen comes in contact with the cell surface receptor, the B cell

Table 16-3 Types and Functions of Cytokines

TYPE	PRIMARY FUNCTIONS	TYPE	PRIMARY FUNCTIONS
Interleukins		IL-14	Stimulates proliferation of activated B cells
Interleukin (IL)–1	Augments the immune response; inflammatory mediator; promotes maturation and clonal expansion of B cells; enhances activity of NK cells; activates T cells, activates macrophages	IL-15	Mimics IL-2 effects; stimulates proliferation of T cells and NK cells
		IL-16	Proinflammatory cytokine; chemoattractant of T cells, eosinophils, and monocytes
IL-2	Induces proliferation and differentiation of T cells; plays role in activation of T cells, NK cells, and macrophages; stimulates release of other cytokines (α-IFN, TNF, IL-1, IL-6)	IL-17	Promotes release of IL-6, IL-8, G-CSF; enhances expression of adhesion molecules
		IL-18	Induces α-IFN, IL-2, and GM-CSF production; important role in development of T helper cells; enhances NK activity; inhibits production of IL-10
IL-3 (multicolony-stimulating factor)	Hematopoietic growth factor for hematopoietic precursor cells	IL-19	Similar to IL-10
		IL-20	Similar to IL-10
IL-4	B cell growth factor; stimulates proliferation and differentiation of B cells; induces proliferation of T cells; stimulates growth of mast cells	IL-21	Similar to IL-2, IL-4, and IL-5
		IL-22	Similar to IL-10
IL-5	Promotes B cell growth and differentiation; promotes growth and differentiation of eosinophils	IL-23	Similar functions to IL-12; promotes memory T cell proliferation
IL-6	Enhances the inflammatory response; plays role in B cell stimulation; promotes differentiation of B cells into plasma cells; stimulates antibody secretion; induces fever; has synergistic effects with IL-1 and TNF	IL-24	Similar to IL-10
		Interferons	
		α-Interferon (α-IFN)	Inhibits viral replication; activates NK cells and macrophages; has antiproliferative effects on tumour cells
IL-7	Promotes growth of T and B cells; increases expression of IL-2 and its receptor	β-Interferon (β-IFN)	Inhibits viral replication; inhibits certain white blood cells; used in the treatment of multiple sclerosis
IL-8	Involved in chemotaxis of neutrophils and T cells; stimulates superoxide and granule release	γ-Interferon (γ-IFN)	Activates macrophages, neutrophils, and NK cells; promotes B cell differentiation; inhibits viral replication
IL-9	Acts as mitogen, supporting proliferation in absence of antigen; enhances T cell survival; plays role in mast cell activation	**Tumour Necrosis Factor**	
		Tumour necrosis factor (TNF)	Activates macrophages and granulocytes; promotes the immune and inflammatory responses; kills tumour cells; is responsible for extensive weight loss associated with chronic inflammation and cancer
IL-10	Inhibits cytokine production by T and NK cells; promotes B cell proliferation and antibody responses; is potent suppressor of macrophage function		
IL-11	Is a multifunctional regulator of hematopoiesis and lymphopoiesis; plays role in osteoclast formation; elevates platelet count; inhibits proinflammatory cytokine production	**Colony-Stimulating Factors**	
		G-CSF	Stimulates proliferation and differentiation of neutrophils; enhances functional activity of mature PMNs
IL-12	Promotes α-IFN production; plays role in induction of T helper cells; activates NK cells; stimulates proliferation of activated T and NK cells	GM-CSF	Stimulates proliferation and differentiation of PMNs and monocytes
IL-13	Promotes B cell growth and differentiation; inhibits proinflammatory cytokine production	M-CSF	Promotes the proliferation, differentiation, and activation of monocytes and macrophages

G-CSF, granulocyte colony–stimulating factor; *GM-CSF,* granulocyte-macrophage colony–stimulating factor; *M-CSF,* macrophage colony–stimulating factor; *NK,* natural killer; *PMN,* polymorphonuclear neutrophil.

becomes activated, and most B cells differentiate into plasma cells (see Figure 16-3). The mature plasma cell secretes immunoglobulins. Some stimulated B lymphocytes remain as memory cells.

The primary immune response is evident 4 to 8 days after the initial exposure to the antigen (Figure 16-5). IgM is the first type of antibody formed. Because of the large size of the IgM molecule, this immunoglobulin is confined to the intravascular space. As the immune response progresses, IgG is produced and can move from intravascular to extravascular spaces.

When the individual is exposed to the antigen the second time, a secondary antibody response occurs. This response occurs faster (1 to 3 days), is stronger, and lasts for a longer time than a primary response. Memory cells account for the memory of the first exposure to the antigen and the more rapid production of antibodies. IgG is the primary antibody found in a secondary immune response.

IgG crosses the placental membrane and provides the newborn with passive acquired immunity for at least 3 months. Infants may also get some passive immunity from IgA in breast milk and colostrum.

Cell-Mediated Immunity. Immune responses that are initiated through specific antigen recognition by T cells provide

Table 16-4 Clinical Uses of Cytokines

CYTOKINE	CLINICAL USES
α-Interferon	
(Intron A)	Hepatitis B and C
	Kaposi's sarcoma
	Hairy cell leukemia
	Lymphomas
	Leukemias
	Melanoma
	Renal cell carcinoma
	Multiple myeloma
β-Interferon	
β-Interferon-1b (Betaseron)	Multiple sclerosis
β-Interferon-1a (Avonex, Rebif)	
Colony-Stimulating Factors: G-CSF, GM-CSF	
Filgrastim (Neupogen)	Neutropenia
Soluble Tumour Necrosis Factor Receptor	
Etanercept (Enbrel)	Rheumatoid arthritis
Interleukin-2	
Aldesleukin (Proleukin)	Renal cell carcinoma
	Malignant melanoma
	Lymphoma
	Acute myelocytic leukemia
Erythropoietin	
(Aranesp, Eprex)	Anemia
Interleukin-1 Receptor Antagonist	
Anakinra (Kineret)	Rheumatoid arthritis

G-CSF, granulocyte colony–stimulating factor; *GM-CSF,* granulocyte-macrophage colony–stimulating factor.

Table 16-5 Comparison of Humoral Immunity and Cell-Mediated Immunity

CHARACTERISTICS	HUMORAL IMMUNITY	CELL-MEDIATED IMMUNITY
Cells involved	B lymphocytes	T lymphocytes, macrophages
Products	Antibodies	Sensitized T cells, lymphokines
Memory cells	Present	Present
Protection	Bacteria	Fungus
	Viruses (extracellular)	Viruses (intracellular)
	Respiratory and gastrointestinal pathogens	Chronic infectious agents
		Tumour cells
Examples	Anaphylactic shock	Tuberculosis
	Atopic diseases	Fungal infections
	Transfusion reaction	Contact dermatitis
	Bacterial infections	Graft rejection
		Destruction of cancer cells

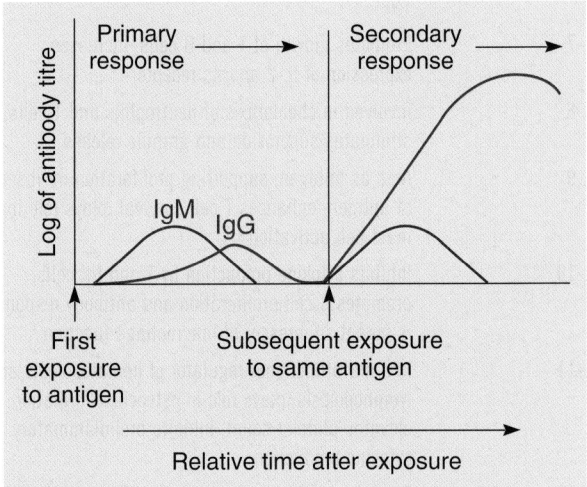

Figure 16-5 Primary and secondary immune responses. The introduction of antigen induces a response dominated by two classes of immunoglobulins: immunoglobulin M (IgM) and immunoglobulin G (IgG). IgM predominates in the primary response; some amount of IgG appears later. After the host's immune system is primed, another challenge with the same antigen induces the secondary response, in which some IgM and large amounts of IgG are produced.

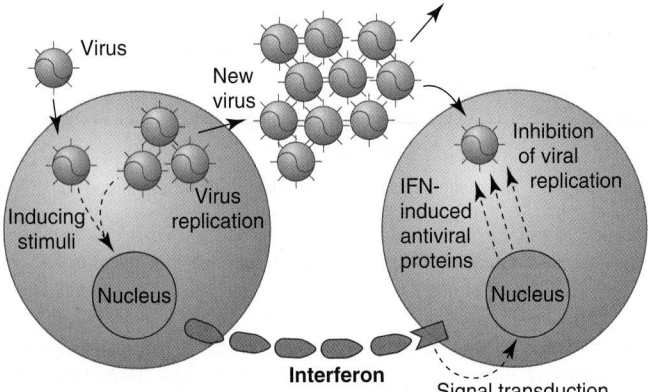

Figure 16-4 Mechanism of action of interferon. The virus attacks a cell. The cell begins to synthesize viral DNA and interferon. Interferon serves as an intercellular messenger. Interferon induces the production of antiviral proteins. The virus is not able to replicate in the cell.

cell-mediated immunity. Although these reactions were initially considered to be solely mediated by T cells, several cell types and factors are now known to be involved in cell-mediated immunity. The cell types involved include T lymphocytes, macrophages, and NK cells. Cell-mediated immunity is of primary importance in (a) immunity against pathogens that survive inside of cells, including viruses and some bacteria (e.g., *Mycobacterium* species); (b) fungal infections; (c) rejection of transplanted tissues; (d) contact hypersensitivity reactions; and (e) tumour immunity.

Table 16-6 Effects of Aging on the Immune System

- Thymic involution
- ↓ Cell-mediated immunity
- ↓ Delayed hypersensitivity response
- ↓ IL-1 and IL-2 synthesis
- ↓ Expression of IL-2 receptors
- ↓ Proliferative response of T and B cells
- ↓ Primary and secondary antibody responses
- ↓ Autoantibodies

IL-1, interleukin-1; *IL-2*, interleukin-2.

AGE-RELATED CONSIDERATIONS: EFFECTS OF AGING ON THE IMMUNE SYSTEM

With advancing age, the effectiveness of the immune system declines (Weiskopf, Weinberger, & Grubeck-Loebenstein, 2009; Table 16-6). The primary clinical evidence for this immunosenescence is the high incidence of tumours in older adults. Older persons become increasingly susceptible to infections (e.g., influenza, pneumonia) from pathogens against which the immune system had fought off successfully earlier in life.

Aging does not affect all aspects of the immune system. The bone marrow is relatively unaffected by increasing age. However, aging has a pronounced effect on the thymus, which decreases in size and activity. These changes in the thymus are probably a primary cause of immunosenescence. Both T and B cells show deficiencies in activation, transit time through the cell cycle, and subsequent differentiation. However, the most significant alterations involve T cells. As thymic output of T cells diminishes, the differentiation of T cells increases. Consequently, memory cells accumulate, rather than new precursor cells responsive to previously unencountered antigens.

Delayed hypersensitivity response, as determined by skin testing with injected antigens, is frequently decreased or absent in older adults. This altered response reflects **anergy** (an immunodeficient condition characterized by lack of or diminished reaction to an antigen or a group of antigens). The clinical consequences of a decline in cell-mediated immunity are evident.

Altered Immune Response

Immunocompetence is the state in which the body's immune system can identify and inactivate or destroy foreign substances. When the immune system is incompetent or underresponsive, severe infections, immunodeficiency diseases, and malignancies may occur. When the immune system overreacts, hypersensitivity disorders such as allergies and autoimmune diseases may occur.

Hypersensitivity Reactions

An overreactive immune response against foreign antigens or failure to maintain self-tolerance can result in tissue damage. This is termed a **hypersensitivity reaction.** A type of hypersensitivity response is the failure of the body to recognize self-proteins, which causes the body to react against its own protein. The dis-

eases that occur as a result of immune responses against self-antigens are termed *autoimmune diseases.*

Hypersensitivity reactions may be classified according to the source of the antigen, the time sequence (immediate or delayed), or the basic immunological mechanisms causing the injury. Four types of hypersensitivity reactions exist. Types I, II, and III are immediate and are examples of humoral immunity. Type IV is a delayed hypersensitivity reaction and is related to cell-mediated immunity. Table 16-7 summarizes the four types of hypersensitivity reactions.

Type I: Anaphylactic Reactions. *Anaphylactic reactions* are type I reactions that occur only in susceptible persons who are highly sensitized to specific allergens. IgE antibodies, produced in response to the allergen, have a characteristic property of attaching to mast cells and basophils (Figure 16-6; see Chapter 31, Figure 31-2). Within these cells are granules containing potent chemical mediators (histamine, serotonin, slow-reacting substance of anaphylaxis [SRS-A], eosinophil chemotactic factor of anaphylaxis, kinins, and bradykinin). (Leukotriene components of SRS-A are discussed in Chapters 14 and 31 and Figure 14-7.) On the first exposure to the allergen, IgE antibodies are produced and bind to mast cells and basophils. On any subsequent exposures, the allergen links with the IgE bound to mast cells or basophils and triggers degranulation of the cells and the release of chemical mediators from the granules. These chemical mediators attack target organs, causing clinical symptoms of allergy (Khan & Kemp, 2011). These effects include smooth muscle contraction, increased vascular permeability, vasodilation, hypotension, increased secretion of mucus, and itching. Fortunately, the mediators are short acting, and their effects are reversible. The mediators and their effects are summarized in Table 16-8.

A genetic predisposition to the development of allergic diseases exists. The capacity to become sensitized to an allergen, rather than the specific allergic disorder, appears to be an inherited trait. For example, a father with asthma may have a son who has allergic rhinitis.

The clinical manifestations of an anaphylactic reaction depend on whether the mediators remain local or become systemic and whether they affect particular organs. When the mediators remain localized, a cutaneous response termed the *wheal-and-flare reaction* occurs. This reaction is characterized by a pale wheal (pink, raised, edematous, pruritic areas) containing edematous fluid, surrounded by a red flare from the hyperemia. The reaction occurs in minutes or hours and is usually not dangerous. A classical example of a wheal-and-flare reaction is the mosquito bite. The wheal-and-flare reaction serves a diagnostic purpose as a means of demonstrating allergic reactions to specific allergens during skin tests.

Common allergic reactions include anaphylaxis and atopic reactions.

Anaphylaxis. Anaphylaxis is an example of an extreme secondary immune response that occurs when mediators are released systemically (e.g., after injection of a drug, after an insect sting). The reaction occurs within minutes and can be life threatening as a result of bronchial constriction and subsequent airway obstruction and vascular collapse. The target organs affected are depicted in Figure 16-7. Initial symptoms include edema and itching at the site of the exposure to the allergen. Shock can occur rapidly and is manifested by rapid, weak pulse; hypotension; dilated pupils; dyspnea; and possibly cyanosis. This is compounded by bronchial edema and angioedema. Death occurs if

Table 16-7 Types of Hypersensitivity Reactions

TYPE I: ANAPHYLACTIC REACTIONS	TYPE II: CYTOTOXIC REACTIONS	TYPE III: IMMUNE-COMPLEX REACTIONS	TYPE IV: DELAYED HYPERSENSITIVITY REACTIONS
Antigen			
Exogenous pollen, food, drugs, dust	Cell surface of RBCs Basement membrane	Extracellular fungal, viral, bacterial	Intracellular or extracellular
Antibody Involved			
IgE	IgG IgM	IgG IgM	None
Complement Involved			
No	Yes	Yes	No
Mediators of Injury			
Histamine SRS-A	Complement lysis Neutrophils	Neutrophils Complement lysis	Cytokines T cytotoxic cells Monocytes, macrophages Lysosomal enzymes
Examples			
Allergic rhinitis Asthma	Transfusion reaction Goodpasture's syndrome	Serum sickness Systemic lupus erythematosus Rheumatoid arthritis	Contact dermatitis Tumour rejection Transplant rejection
Skin Test			
Wheal and flare	None	Erythema and edema in 3 to 8 hours	Erythema and edema in 24 to 48 hours (e.g., tuberculin test)

IgE, immunoglobulin E; *IgM,* immunoglobulin M; *RBC,* red blood cell; *SRS-A,* slow-reacting substance of anaphylaxis.

emergency treatment is not initiated. Treatment can range from epinephrine administered subcutaneously for mild symptoms to full circulatory support with oxygen and vasopressor therapy (Peavy & Metcalfe, 2008). Some of the important allergens leading to anaphylactic shock in hypersensitive persons are listed in Table 16-9.

Atopic Reactions. An estimated 20% of the population are *atopic,* which means they have an inherited tendency to become sensitive to environmental allergens. The atopic diseases that can result are allergic rhinitis, asthma, atopic dermatitis, urticaria, and angioedema.

Allergic rhinitis, or hay fever, is the most common type I hypersensitivity reaction. It may occur year round (perennial allergic rhinitis), or it may be seasonal (seasonal allergic rhinitis). Airborne substances such as pollens, dust, or moulds are the primary cause of allergic rhinitis. Perennial allergic rhinitis may be caused by dust, moulds, and animal dander. Seasonal allergic rhinitis is commonly caused by pollens from trees, weeds, or grasses. The target areas affected are the conjunctivae of the eyes and the mucosa of the upper respiratory tract. Symptoms include nasal discharge, sneezing, lacrimation, mucosal swelling with airway obstruction, and pruritus around the eyes, nose, throat, and mouth. (Treatment of allergic rhinitis is discussed in Chapter 29.)

Many cases of *asthma* have an allergic component. Many affected patients have a history of atopic disorders (e.g., infantile eczema, allergic rhinitis, food intolerances). In asthma, SRS-A and histamine are responsible primarily for action on the bronchioles (see Chapter 31, Figure 31-2). These mediators produce bronchial smooth muscle constriction, excessive secretion of viscous mucus, edema of the mucous membranes of the bronchi, and decreased lung compliance. Because of these physiological alterations, affected patients manifest dyspnea, wheezing, coughing, sensation of tightness in the chest, and thick sputum. (Pathophysiology and management of asthma are discussed in Chapter 31.)

Atopic dermatitis is a chronic, inherited skin disorder characterized by exacerbations and remissions. It is caused by several environmental allergens that are difficult to identify. Although patients with atopic dermatitis have elevated IgE levels and positive results on skin tests, the histopathological features do not represent the typical, localized wheal-and-flare type I reactions. The skin lesions are more generalized and involve vasodilation of blood vessels, which results in interstitial edema with vesicle formation (Figure 16-8). (Dermatitis is discussed in Chapter 26.)

Urticaria (hives) is a cutaneous reaction against systemic allergens that occurs in atopic persons. It is characterized by transient wheals that vary in size and shape and may occur throughout the body. Urticaria develops rapidly after exposure to an allergen and may last minutes or hours. Histamine causes localized vasodilation (erythema), transudation of fluid (wheal), and flaring. Flaring is caused by dilation of blood vessels on the edge of the wheal in response to a reaction augmented by the sympathetic nervous system. Histamine is responsible for the pruritus associated with the lesions. (Urticaria is discussed further in Chapter 26.)

Angioedema is a localized cutaneous lesion similar to urticaria but involving deeper layers of the skin and the submucosa. The principal areas of involvement include the eyelids, the lips, the tongue, the larynx, the hands, the feet, the gastrointestinal tract,

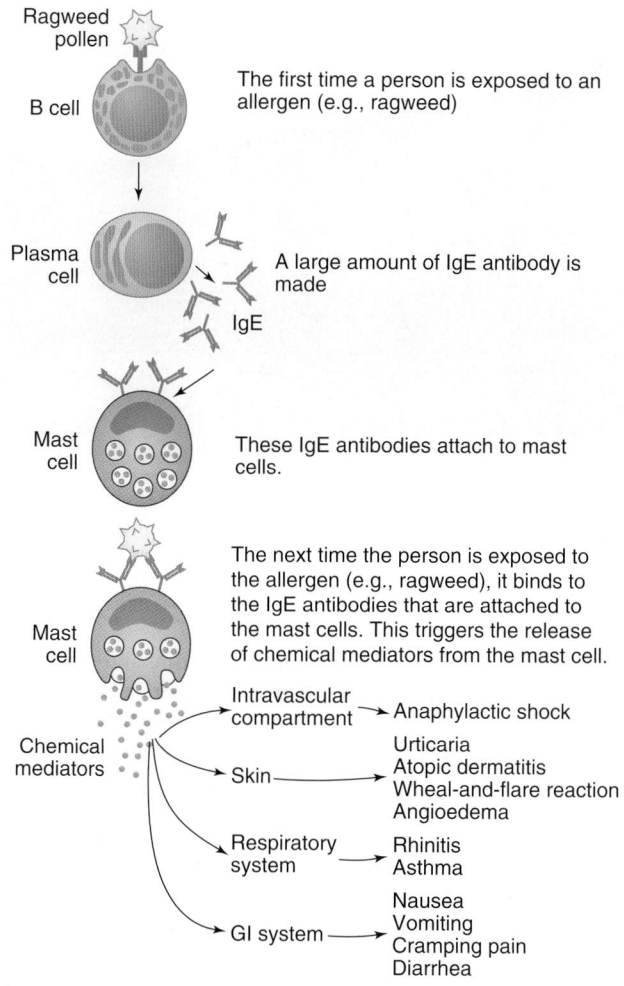

Figure 16-6 Steps in a type I allergic reaction. *GI*, gastrointestinal; *IgE*, immunoglobulin E.

Table 16-8 Mediators of Allergic Response		
TYPE AND SOURCE	**BIOLOGICAL ACTIVITY**	**CLINICAL OUTCOMES**
Histamine		
Mast cell and basophil granules	Increases vascular permeability; constricts smooth muscle; stimulates irritant receptors	Edema of airways and larynx; bronchial constriction; urticaria, angioedema, pruritus; nausea, vomiting, diarrhea; shock
Leukotrienes		
Metabolites of arachidonic acid by lipoxygenase pathway	Constrict bronchial smooth muscle; increase vascular permeability	Bronchial constriction; enhanced effect of histamine on smooth muscle
Prostaglandins		
Metabolites of arachidonic acid by cyclooxygenase pathway	Stimulate vasodilation; constrict smooth muscle	Wheal-and-flare reaction on skin; hypotension; bronchospasm
Platelet-Activating Factor		
Mast cell	Aggregates platelets; stimulates vasodilation	Increase in pulmonary artery pressure; systemic hypotension
Kinins		
Kininogen	Stimulates slow, sustained smooth muscle contraction; increases vascular permeability; stimulates secretion of mucus; stimulates pain receptors	Angioedema with painful swelling; bronchial constriction
Serotonin		
Platelets	Increase vascular permeability; stimulate smooth muscle contraction	Mucosal edema; bronchial constriction
Anaphylatoxins		
C3a, C4a, C5a from complement activation	Stimulate histamine release	Edema of airways and larynx; bronchial constriction; urticaria, angioedema, pruritus; nausea, vomiting, diarrhea; shock

and the genitalia. Swelling usually begins in the face and then progresses to the airways and other parts of the body. Dilation and engorgement of the capillaries secondary to release of histamine cause the diffuse swelling. Welts are not apparent as in urticaria; the outer skin appears normal or has a reddish hue. The lesions may burn, sting, or itch and, if in the gastrointestinal tract, can cause acute abdominal pain. The swelling may occur suddenly or over several hours and usually lasts for 24 hours.

Type II: Cytotoxic and Cytolytic Reactions. Cytotoxic and cytolytic reactions are type II hypersensitivity reactions involving the direct binding of IgG or IgM antibodies to an antigen on the cell surface. Antigen–antibody complexes activate the complement system, which mediates the reaction. Cellular tissue is destroyed in one of two ways: (a) activation of the complement cascade resulting in cytolysis or (b) enhanced phagocytosis.

Target cells frequently destroyed in type II reactions are erythrocytes, platelets, and leukocytes. Some of the antigens involved are the ABO blood group, Rh factor, and drugs. Pathophysiological disorders characteristic of type II reactions include ABO incompatibility transfusion reaction, Rh incompatibility transfusion reaction, autoimmune and drug-related hemolytic anemias, leukopenia, thrombocytopenia, erythroblastosis fetalis (hemolytic disease of the newborn), and Goodpasture's syndrome. Tissue damage usually occurs rapidly.

Hemolytic Transfusion Reactions. A classic type II reaction occurs when a recipient receives ABO-incompatible blood from a donor. Naturally acquired antibodies to antigens of the ABO blood group are in the recipient's serum but are not present on the erythrocyte membranes (see Chapter 32, Table 32-10). For example, a person with type A blood has anti-B antibodies, a person with type B blood has anti-A antibodies, a person with type AB blood has no antibodies, and a person with type O blood has both anti-A and anti-B antibodies.

If the recipient receives a transfusion with incompatible blood, antibodies immediately coat the foreign erythrocytes,

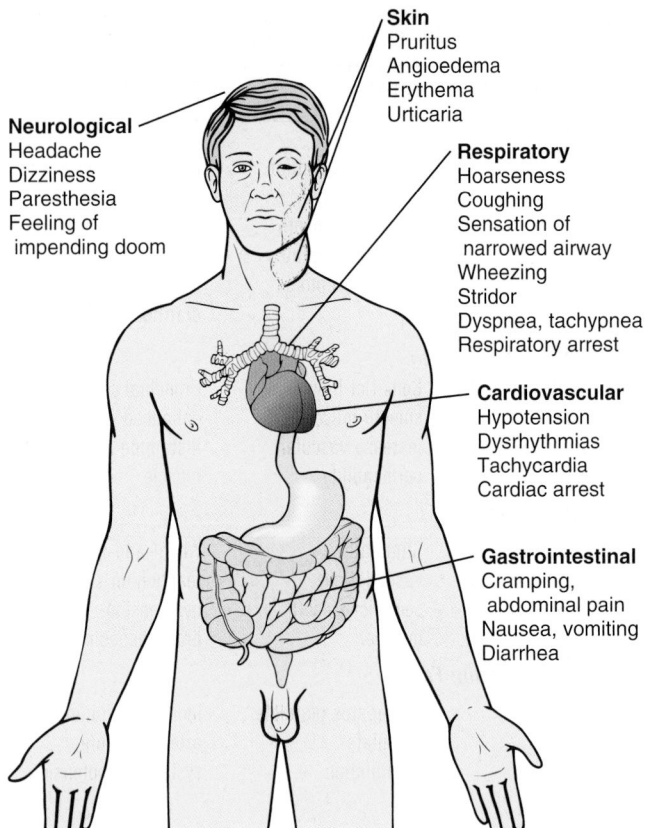

Neurological
Headache
Dizziness
Paresthesia
Feeling of
 impending doom

Skin
Pruritus
Angioedema
Erythema
Urticaria

Respiratory
Hoarseness
Coughing
Sensation of
 narrowed airway
Wheezing
Stridor
Dyspnea, tachypnea
Respiratory arrest

Cardiovascular
Hypotension
Dysrhythmias
Tachycardia
Cardiac arrest

Gastrointestinal
Cramping,
 abdominal pain
Nausea, vomiting
Diarrhea

Figure 16-7 Clinical manifestations of a systemic anaphylactic reaction.

Table 16-9 Allergens That Cause Anaphylactic Shock	
Drugs	Milk
Penicillins	Peanuts
Insulins	Fish
Tetracycline	Strawberries
Chemotherapeutic agents	**Animal Sera**
Nonsteroidal anti-inflammatory drugs	Tetanus antitoxin
Sulfonamides	Diphtheria antitoxin
Aspirin	Rabies antitoxin
Local anaesthetics	Snake venom antitoxin
Cephalosporins	**Treatment Measures**
Insect Venoms	Blood products (whole blood and components)
Hymenoptera*	Allergenic extracts in hyposensitization therapy
Foods	
Eggs	Iodine-contrast media for intravenous pyelography or angiography
Nuts	
Shellfish	
Chocolate	

*Wasps, hornets, yellow jackets, bumblebees, and ants.

causing agglutination (clumping). The clumping of cells blocks small blood vessels in the body, using and thus depleting existing clotting factors, which leads to bleeding. Within hours, neutrophils and macrophages phagocytize the agglutinated cells. As complement is fixed to the antigen, cytolysis occurs. Cellular lysis

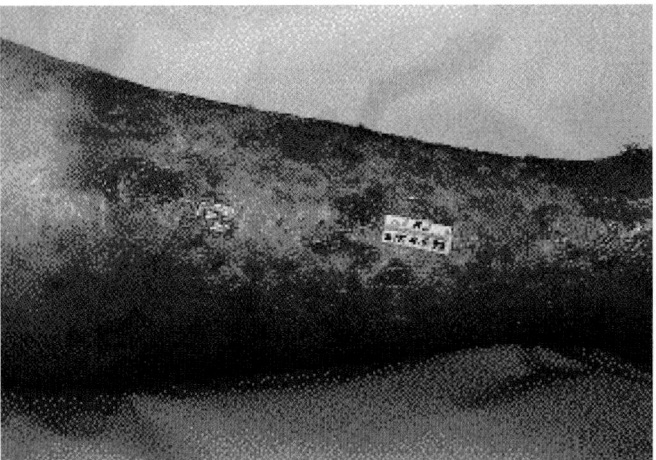

Figure 16-8 Eczema of the lower leg.

Source: From Morison, M. J., Moffatt, C., Bridel-Nixon, J., & Bale, S. [1997]. *A colour guide to the nursing management of chronic wounds* [2nd ed.]. Edinburgh: Mosby.

causes the release of hemoglobin into the urine and plasma. In addition, a cytotoxic reaction causes vascular spasms in the kidney that further block the renal tubules. Acute renal failure can result from hemoglobinuria. (Blood transfusions are discussed in Chapter 33.)

Goodpasture's Syndrome. *Goodpasture's syndrome* is a rare disorder involving the lungs and the kidneys. An antibody-mediated autoimmune reaction occurs involving the glomerular and alveolar basement membranes. The circulating antibodies combine with tissue antigen to activate complement, which causes deposits of IgG to form along the basement membranes of the lungs or the kidneys. This reaction may result in pulmonary hemorrhage and glomerulonephritis. Corticosteroids, immunosuppressive drugs (e.g., cyclophosphamide [Procytox]), and plasmapheresis have been effective in slowing the rapid progression of the disease. (Goodpasture's syndrome is discussed further in Chapter 48.)

Type II: Immune-Complex Reactions. Tissue damage in immune-complex reactions, which are type III reactions, occurs secondary to antigen–antibody complexes. Soluble antigens combine with immunoglobulins of the IgG and IgM classes to form complexes that are too small to be effectively removed by the mononuclear phagocyte system. Therefore, the complexes are deposited in tissue or small blood vessels. They cause the fixation of complement and the release of chemotactic factors that lead to inflammation and destruction of the involved tissue.

Type III reactions may be either local or systemic and either immediate or delayed. The clinical manifestations depend on the number of complexes and their location in the body. Common sites for deposit are the kidneys, the skin, the joints, blood vessels, and the lungs. Severe type III reactions are associated with autoimmune disorders such as systemic lupus erythematosus (SLE), acute glomerulonephritis, and rheumatoid arthritis. (SLE and rheumatoid arthritis are discussed further in Chapter 67, and acute glomerulonephritis is discussed further in Chapter 48.)

Type IV: Delayed Hypersensitivity Reactions. A *delayed hypersensitivity reaction*—a type IV reaction—is also a cell-

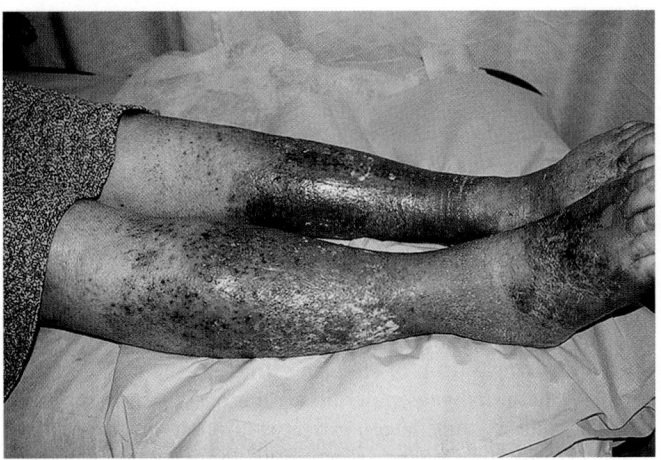

Figure 16-9 Contact dermatitis in reaction to rubber.

Source: From Morison, M. J., Moffatt, C., Bridel-Nixon, J., & Bale, S. [1997]. *A colour guide to the nursing management of chronic wounds* [2nd ed.]. Edinburgh: Mosby.

mediated immune response. Although cell-mediated immune responses are usually protective mechanisms, tissue damage occurs in delayed hypersensitivity reactions.

The tissue damage in a type IV reaction does not occur in the presence of antibodies or complement. Rather, sensitized T lymphocytes attack antigens or release cytokines, some of which attract macrophages into the area. These macrophages and enzymes are responsible for most of the tissue destruction. A delayed hypersensitivity reaction takes 24 to 48 hours to occur.

Clinical examples of a delayed hypersensitivity reaction include contact dermatitis (Figure 16-9); hypersensitivity reactions to bacterial, fungal, and viral infections; and transplant rejection. Some types of drug sensitivity reactions also fit this category.

Contact Dermatitis. Allergic contact dermatitis is an example of a delayed hypersensitivity reaction involving the skin. The reaction occurs when the skin is exposed to substances that easily penetrate the skin to combine with epidermal proteins. The substance then becomes antigenic, and over a period of 7 to 14 days, memory cells for the antigen form. On subsequent exposure to the substance, a sensitized person develops eczematous skin lesions within 48 hours. The most common potentially antigenic substances encountered are metal compounds (e.g., nickel, mercury); rubber compounds; catechols present in poison ivy, poison oak, and poison sumac; cosmetics; and some dyes.

In acute contact dermatitis, the skin lesions appear erythematous and edematous and are covered with papules, vesicles, and bullae. The involved area is very pruritic but may also burn or sting. When contact dermatitis becomes chronic, the lesions resemble atopic dermatitis because they are thickened, scaly, and lichenified. The main difference between contact dermatitis and atopic dermatitis is that contact dermatitis is localized and restricted to the area exposed to the allergens, whereas atopic dermatitis is usually widespread.

Microbial Hypersensitivity Reactions. The classic example of a microbial cell-mediated immune reaction is the body's defence against the tubercle bacillus. Tuberculosis results from invasion of lung tissue by the highly resistant tubercle bacillus. The organism itself does not directly damage the lung tissue.

However, antigenic material released from the tubercle bacilli reacts with T lymphocytes, initiating a cell-mediated immune response. The resulting response causes extensive caseous necrosis of the lung.

After the initial cell-mediated immune reaction, memory cells remain; therefore, subsequent contact with the tubercle bacillus or an extract of purified protein from the organism causes a delayed hypersensitivity reaction. This is the basis for the purified protein derivative (PPD) tuberculosis skin test, which yields results 48 to 72 hours after the injection. (Tuberculosis is discussed in Chapter 30.)

Allergic Disorders

Although an alteration of the immune system may be manifested in many ways, allergies or type I hypersensitivity reactions are most frequent.

Assessment

For a thorough assessment of a patient with allergies, a complete health history must be documented, and a physical examination, diagnostic workup, and skin testing for allergens must be performed.

Health History. A comprehensive history that covers family allergies, past and current allergies, and social and environmental factors is essential. The information may be obtained from the patient or the patient's caregiver.

Family history, including information about atopic reactions in relatives, is especially important in identifying at-risk patients. The specific disorder, clinical manifestations, and treatments prescribed should be assessed.

Identifying past and current allergens that may have triggered a reaction is essential for controlling or preventing allergic reactions. The patient's use of any over-the-counter or prescription medications used to treat the allergies should be documented.

In addition to identification of the allergen, information about the clinical manifestations and the course of allergic reaction should be obtained. In female patients, assessment of symptoms during pregnancy, menstruation, or menopause may have significance. Social factors (patient's lifestyle and stressors), environmental factors, and physical environment should be reviewed in connection with the appearance of allergic symptoms. Questions about pets, trees, plants, air pollutants, floor coverings, and cooling and heating systems in the home or workplace can provide valuable information about potential allergens. In addition, a daily or weekly food diary may be helpful. Of particular importance is a screening for any reaction to medications.

Physical Examination. A comprehensive head-to-toe physical examination should be given to a patient with allergies, with particular attention focused on the site of the allergic manifestations. A comprehensive assessment that includes subjective and objective data should be obtained from the patient (Table 16-10).

Diagnostic Studies

Many specialized immunological techniques can be performed to detect abnormalities of lymphocytes, eosinophils, and immunoglobulins. A complete blood cell count (CBC) and serological tests are commonly performed.

NURSING ASSESSMENT

Table 16-10 Allergies

Subjective Data

Important Health Information

Past health history: Recurrent respiratory problems; seasonal exacerbations; unusual reactions to insect bites or stings; past and present allergies; altered home and work environment, presence of pets; family history of allergies

Medications: Unusual reactions to any medications; use of over-the-counter drugs; use of medications for allergies

Symptoms

Food intolerances; vomiting; abdominal cramps, diarrhea; fatigue; hoarseness, cough, dyspnea; itching, burning, stinging of eyes, nose, throat, or skin; chest tightness; malaise

Objective Data

Integumentary

Rashes, including urticaria, wheal-and-flare, papules, vesicles, bullae; dryness, scaliness, scratches, irritation

Eyes, Ears, Nose, and Throat

Eyes: Conjunctivitis; lacrimation; rubbing or excessive blinking; dark circles under the eyes ("allergic shiner")

Ears: Diminished hearing; immobile or scarred tympanic membranes; recurrent ear infections

Nose: Nasal polyps; nasal voice; nose twitching; itchy nose; rhinitis; pale, boggy mucous membranes; sniffling; repeated sneezing; swollen nasal passages; recurrent, unexplained nosebleeds; crease across the bridge of nose ("allergic salute")

Throat: Continual throat clearing; swollen lips or tongue; red throat; palpable neck lymph nodes

Respiratory

Wheezing, stridor; thick sputum

Possible Findings

Eosinophilia of serum, sputum, or nasal and bronchial secretions; ↑ serum IgE levels; positive skin tests; abnormal chest and sinus radiographs

Ig, immunoglobulin.

A CBC with WBC differential is required, with an absolute lymphocyte count and eosinophil count. Cellular immunodeficiency is diagnosed if the lymphocyte count is lower than 1.2×10^9/L. T cell and B cell quantification is used to diagnose specific immunodeficiency syndromes. The eosinophil count is elevated with type I hypersensitivity reactions involving IgE. The serum IgE level is also generally elevated in type I hypersensitivity reactions and serves as a diagnostic indicator of atopic diseases.

The radioallergosorbent test (RAST) is an in vitro diagnostic test for IgE antibodies to specific allergens. The RAST is helpful in confirming reactivity to various foods or drugs in individuals with a history of severe anaphylactic reactions.

Sputum and nasal and bronchial secretions also may be tested for the presence of eosinophils. If asthma is suspected, pulmonary function tests for vital capacity, forced expiratory volume, and maximum midexpiratory flow rates may yield helpful findings.

Skin Tests. Skin testing is generally used to confirm specific sensitivity in patients with atopic disease after the history has suggested possible allergens for testing.

Procedure. Skin testing may be performed by one of two methods: (a) a cutaneous scratch or prick or (b) an intracutaneous injection. The areas of the body usually used in testing are the arms and the back. Allergen extracts are applied to the skin in rows with a corresponding control site opposite the test site. Saline or another diluent is applied to the control site. In the scratch test, the epidermal skin layer is scratched with a lancet, and the allergen extract is applied at the site. The prick test involves placing a drop of allergen extract on the skin and then piercing the underlying epidermis with a needle. In the intracutaneous method, the allergen extract is injected intradermally in rows. Because the allergic reaction is more severe with this method, the test is used only for persons who did not react to cutaneous methods.

Results. If a person is hypersensitive to an allergen, a positive reaction typically occurs within minutes after insertion in the skin and may last for 8 to 12 hours. A positive reaction is manifested by a local wheal-and-flare response. The size of the positive reaction is not always correlated with the severity of allergy symptoms. False-positive and false-negative results may occur. Negative results from skin testing do not necessarily mean the person does not have an allergic disorder, and positive results do not necessarily mean that the allergen was causing the clinical manifestations. Positive results imply that the person is sensitized to that allergen. Therefore, correlating skin test results with the patient's history is important.

Precautions. A highly sensitive person is always at risk for developing an anaphylactic reaction to skin tests. Therefore, a patient should never be left alone during the testing period. Sometimes, skin testing is completely contraindicated, and the RAST is used. If a severe reaction does occur with a cutaneous test, the extract is immediately removed, and anti-inflammatory topical cream is applied to the site. For intracutaneous testing, the arm is used so that a tourniquet can be applied during a severe reaction. A subcutaneous injection of epinephrine may also be necessary.

Collaborative Care

After an allergic disorder is diagnosed, the therapeutic treatment is aimed at reducing exposure to the offending allergen, treating the symptoms, and, if necessary, desensitizing the person through immunotherapy. All health care workers must be prepared for the rare but life-threatening anaphylactic reaction, which necessitates immediate medical and nursing interventions. It is extremely important that all of a patient's allergies be listed on the chart, the nursing care plan, and the medication record.

Anaphylaxis. Anaphylactic reactions occur suddenly in hypersensitive patients after exposure to the offending allergen. They may occur after parenteral injection of drugs (especially antibiotics), blood products, and insect stings. The cardinal principle in therapeutic management is speed: (a) in recognizing signs and symptoms of an anaphylactic reaction, (b) in establishing and maintaining a patent airway, (c) in preventing spread of the allergen with the use of a tourniquet, (d) in administering drugs, and (e) in performing treatment for shock (Peavy & Metcalfe, 2008).

Table 16-11 summarizes the emergency treatment of anaphylactic shock.

Mild symptoms such as pruritus and urticaria can be controlled by administration of 0.2 to 0.5 mL of epinephrine, diluted 1:1000, given subcutaneously every 20 minutes according to the health care provider's orders or a hospital emergency drug protocol. An intravenous infusion should be initiated to provide a route for administration of 0.5 mL of epinephrine, diluted 1:10,000, at 5- to 10-minute intervals; volume expanders; and vasopressor agents such as dopamine (Intropin) if intractable hypotension occurs.

Oxygen should be delivered through a nonrebreather mask. If progressive hypoxia develops, endotracheal intubation or a tracheostomy is required for oxygen delivery. Other agents can also be used, including an antihistamine such as diphenhydramine (Benadryl) intravenously or intramuscularly for urticaria and angioedema.

In more severe cases of anaphylaxis, hypovolemic shock may occur because of the loss of intravascular fluid into interstitial spaces that is secondary to increased capillary permeability. Peripheral vasoconstriction and stimulation of the sympathetic nervous system occur to compensate for the fluid shift. However, unless shock is treated early, the body will no longer be able to compensate, and irreversible tissue damage will occur, leading to death. (Hypovolemic shock is further discussed in Chapter 69.)

Chronic Allergies.
Most allergic reactions are chronic and are characterized by remissions and exacerbations of symptoms. Treatment focuses on identification and control of allergens, relief of symptoms through drug therapy, and hyposensitization of a patient to an offending allergen.

Allergen Recognition and Control. The nurse plays an important role in helping the patient make lifestyle adjustments to minimize exposure to the offending allergens and offers preventive measures that will help control the allergic symptoms. The nurse must reinforce that the patient will never be desensitized or completely symptom free, even with drug therapy and immunotherapy.

Of primary importance is the need to identify the offending allergen, at times performed through skin testing. In the case of food allergies, an elimination diet is sometimes helpful. If an allergic reaction occurs, all food previously eaten should be avoided at first and then gradually reintroduced sequentially until the offending food is identified.

Many allergic reactions, especially asthma and urticaria, may be aggravated by fatigue and emotional stress. The nurse can initiate a stress management program with the patient through relaxation techniques when the patient comes for repeated immunotherapy treatments.

Sometimes, control of allergic symptoms necessitates environmental control, including changing an occupation, moving to a different climate, or giving up a favourite pet. In the case of airborne allergens, sleeping in an air-conditioned room, damp-dusting daily, covering mattresses and pillows with hypoallergenic covers, and wearing a mask outdoors may be helpful.

With an identified drug allergy, the patient should be instructed not only to avoid the drug but also to notify all health care providers of drug intolerance. The patient should wear a medical alert bracelet listing the particular drug allergy and have the offending drug listed on all medical and dental records.

For a patient allergic to insect stings, commercial bee-sting kits containing preinjectable epinephrine and a tourniquet are

EMERGENCY MANAGEMENT
Table 16-11 Anaphylactic Shock

CAUSE	ASSESSMENT FINDINGS	INTERVENTIONS
• Injection of, inhalation of, ingestion of, or topical exposure to substance that produces profound allergic response • See Table 16-9 for more complete listing.	See Figure 16-7.	**Initial** • Ensure patent airway. • Remove insect stinger if it is present. • Administer epinephrine 1:1000, 0.2 to 0.5 mL SC for mild symptoms; repeat at 20-minute intervals. • Epinephrine 1:10,000, 0.5 mL IV at 5- to 10-minute intervals for severe reaction. • Administer high-flow oxygen via nonrebreather mask. • Place patient in recumbent position, and elevate his or her legs. • Keep patient warm. • Administer diphenhydramine (Benadryl) IM or IV. • Administer histamine H_2 blockers such as cimetidine. • Maintain patient's blood pressure with fluids, volume expanders, vasopressors (e.g., dopamine, norepinephrine bitartrate [Levophed]). **Ongoing Monitoring** • Monitor vital signs, respiratory effort, oxygen saturation, level of consciousness, and cardiac rhythm. • Anticipate intubation in cases of severe respiratory distress. • Anticipate cricothyrotomy or tracheostomy in cases of severe laryngeal edema.

IM, intramuscularly; *IV,* intravenously; *SC,* subcutaneously.

available. The nurse should instruct the patient on the technique of applying the tourniquet and self-injecting the subcutaneous epinephrine. Such patients also should wear a medical alert bracelet and carry a bee-sting kit whenever they go outdoors.

Drug Therapy. The major categories of drugs used for symptomatic relief of chronic allergic disorders include antihistamines, sympathomimetic or decongestant drugs, corticosteroids, antipruritic drugs, and mast cell–stabilizing drugs. Many of these drugs may be obtained over the counter.

Antihistamines. Antihistamines are the best drugs for treatment of allergic rhinitis and urticaria; however, they are less effective for severe allergic reactions (see Chapter 29, Table 29-2). They act by competing with histamine for H_1-receptor sites and thus blocking the effect of histamine. Best results are achieved if they are taken as soon as allergy signs and symptoms appear. Antihistamines can be used effectively to treat edema and pruritus but are relatively ineffective in preventing bronchoconstriction. With seasonal rhinitis, antihistamines should be taken during peak pollen seasons. (Antihistamines are discussed further in Chapter 29.)

Sympathomimetic or Decongestant Drugs. The major sympathomimetic drug is epinephrine (Adrenalin), which is the drug of choice to treat an anaphylactic reaction. Epinephrine is a hormone produced by the adrenal medulla that stimulates α- and β-adrenergic receptors. Stimulation of the α-adrenergic receptors causes vasoconstriction of peripheral blood vessels. Stimulation of β-adrenergic receptors causes relaxation of the bronchial smooth muscles. Epinephrine also acts directly on mast cells to stabilize them against further degranulation. The action of epinephrine lasts only a few minutes. For the treatment of anaphylaxis, the drug must be given parenterally (usually subcutaneously).

Several specific, minor sympathomimetic drugs differ from epinephrine because they can be taken orally or nasally and last for several hours. Included in this category are phenylephrine (Neo-Synephrine) and pseudoephedrine (Sudafed). The minor sympathomimetic drugs are used primarily to treat allergic rhinitis.

Corticosteroids. Nasal corticosteroid sprays are very effective in relieving the symptoms of allergic rhinitis (see Chapter 29, Table 29-2). Occasional patients may experience such severe manifestations of allergies that a brief course of oral corticosteroids is required.

Antipruritic Drugs. Topically applied antipruritic drugs protect the skin and provide relief from itching. They are most effective when the skin is not broken. Common over-the-counter drugs include calamine lotion, coal tar solutions, and camphor. Menthol and phenol may be added to other lotions to produce an antipruritic effect. Some more potent drugs for which a prescription is needed include trimeprazine; however, they should be used with great caution because of the associated risk of agranulocytosis.

Mast Cell–Stabilizing Drugs. Nedocromil (Alocril) is a mast cell-stabilizing agent that inhibits the release of histamines, leukotrienes, and other agents from the mast cell after antigen–IgE interaction. They are available as an inhalant nebulizer solution, a nasal spray, or an oral pill. They are used in the management of asthma (see Chapter 31) and allergic rhinitis (see Chapter 29) and have only minor adverse effects.

Leukotriene Receptor Antagonists. Leukotriene-receptor antagonists block leukotriene, one of the major mediators of the allergic inflammatory process. They may be used in the treatment of allergic rhinitis and asthma. These medications can be taken orally. For more information, refer to Chapters 29 and 31.

Immunotherapy. Immunotherapy is the recommended treatment for control of allergic symptoms when the allergen cannot be avoided and drug therapy is not effective. Relatively few patients with allergies have symptoms so intolerable that they require allergy immunotherapy. Immunotherapy is absolutely indicated only in individuals with anaphylactic reactions to insect venom. It involves administration of small titres of an allergen extract in increasing strengths until hyposensitivity to the specific allergen is achieved. For best results, the patient should continue to avoid the offending allergen whenever possible because complete desensitization is impossible.

Mechanism of Action. The IgE level is elevated in atopic individuals. When IgE combines with an allergen in a hypersensitive person, a reaction occurs in which histamine is released in various body tissues. Allergens more readily combine with IgG than with other immunoglobulins. Therefore, immunotherapy involves injecting allergen extracts that will stimulate increases in IgG levels. The binding of IgG to allergen-reactive sites interferes with allergen binding to mast cell–bound IgE, preventing mast cell degranulation and thus reducing the number of reactions that cause tissue damage. The goal of long-term immunotherapy is to maintain high levels of "blocking" IgG. In addition, allergen-specific T suppressor cells develop in individuals receiving immunotherapy.

Method of Administration. The allergens included in immunotherapy are chosen on the basis of the results of skin testing with a panel of allergens found in the local geographic area. Immunotherapy involves the subcutaneous injection of titrated amounts of allergen extracts biweekly or weekly. The dose is small at first and is increased slowly until a maintenance dosage is reached. In general, it takes 1 to 2 years of immunotherapy to reach the maximal therapeutic effect. Therapy may be continued for about 5 years. After that, discontinuing therapy is considered. In many patients, a decrease in symptoms is sustained after the treatment is discontinued. For patients with severe allergies or sensitivity to insect stings, maintenance therapy is continued indefinitely. Best results are achieved when immunotherapy is administered throughout the year.

NURSING MANAGEMENT: IMMUNOTHERAPY

The nurse is often the professional primarily responsible for administering immunotherapy. Adverse reactions should always be anticipated, especially when a new strength of the dose is used, after a previous reaction, or after a dose is missed. Early signs and symptoms indicative of a systemic reaction include pruritus, urticaria, sneezing, laryngeal edema, and hypotension. Emergency measures for anaphylactic shock should be initiated immediately. A local reaction should be described according to the degree of redness and swelling at the injection site. If the area is greater than the size of a quarter in an adult, the reaction should be reported to the health care provider so that the allergen dosage may be decreased.

Immunotherapy always carries the risk of a severe anaphylactic reaction. Therefore, when injections are given, a health care provider, emergency equipment, and essential drugs should be available.

Accurate record keeping is invaluable because it can prevent an adverse reaction to the allergen extract. Before giving the injection, the nurse should check the patient's name with the name on the vial, check the vial strength, the amount of the previous dose, the date of the previous dose, and any reaction information previously identified.

The nurse should always administer the allergen extract in an extremity away from a joint so that a tourniquet can be applied in the event of a severe reaction. The site should be rotated for each injection. Before giving an injection, the nurse must aspirate for blood to ensure the allergen extract is not injected into a blood vessel. An injection directly into the bloodstream can potentiate an anaphylactic reaction. After the injection is given, the patient should be carefully observed for 20 minutes because systemic reactions typically occur immediately. However, the patient should be warned that a delayed reaction can occur as long as 24 hours later.

Latex Allergies

Allergies to latex products have become a problem of increasing proportion, affecting both patients and health care providers. The increase in allergic reactions has coincided with the sharp increase in glove use related to the introduction of universal precautions against infectious diseases in 1987. It is estimated that 8% to 17% of health care providers regularly exposed to latex are sensitized. The more frequent and prolonged the exposure to latex, the greater the likelihood of developing a latex allergy (Peavy & Metcalfe, 2008).

In addition to gloves, many products used in health care contain latex: for example, blood pressure cuffs, stethoscopes, tourniquets, intravenous tubing, syringes, electrode pads, oxygen masks, tracheal tubes, colostomy and ileostomy pouches, urinary catheters, anaesthetic masks, and adhesive tape. Latex proteins can become aerosolized through powder on gloves and can result in serious reactions when inhaled by sensitized individuals.

Types of Latex Allergies.
Two types of latex allergies that can occur are type IV allergic contact dermatitis and type I allergic reactions. Type IV contact dermatitis is caused by the chemicals used in the manufacturing process of latex gloves. It is a delayed reaction that occurs within 6 to 48 hours. Typically, the person first has dryness, pruritus, fissuring, and cracking of the skin, followed by redness, swelling, and crusting at 24 to 48 hours. The dermatitis may extend beyond the area of physical contact with the allergen. Chronic exposure can lead to lichenification, scaling, and hyperpigmentation.

A type I allergic reaction is a response to the natural rubber latex proteins and occurs within minutes of contact with the proteins. These types of allergic reactions can manifest as various reactions ranging from skin redness, urticaria, rhinitis, conjunctivitis, or asthma to full-blown anaphylactic shock. Systemic reactions to latex may result from exposure to latex protein via various routes, including the skin, mucous membranes, lungs, or blood.

NURSING AND COLLABORATIVE MANAGEMENT: LATEX ALLERGIES

The identification of patients and health care providers who are sensitive to latex is crucial in the prevention of adverse reactions. A thorough health history and history of any allergies should be documented, especially for patients with any complaints of latex contact symptoms. Not all latex-sensitive individuals can be identified, even with a carefully documented and thorough history. Risk factors include long-term multiple exposures to latex products (e.g., health care personnel, individuals who have undergone multiple surgical procedures, rubber industry workers). People with latex allergies may also have a history of hay fever, asthma, and allergies to certain foods (latex-food syndrome) such as avocados, guava, kiwi, bananas, water chestnuts, hazelnuts, tomatoes, potatoes, peaches, grapes, and apricots.

The U.S. National Institute for Occupational Safety and Health (NIOSH) and the Canadian Centre for Occupational Health and Safety (CCOHS) have published recommendations for preventing allergic reactions to latex in the workplace (CCOHS, 2009; NIOSH, n.d.). In summary, they include the following points:
1. Use nonlatex gloves for activities that are not likely to involve contact with infectious materials (e.g., food preparation, housekeeping).
2. Use powder-free gloves with reduced protein content.
3. Do not use oil-based hand creams or lotions when wearing gloves.
4. After removing gloves, wash hands with mild soap, and dry thoroughly.
5. Frequently clean work areas that are contaminated with latex-containing dust.
6. Know the symptoms of latex allergy, including skin rash; hives; flushing; itching; nasal, eye, or sinus symptoms; asthma; and shock.
7. If symptoms of latex allergy develop, avoid direct contact with latex gloves and products.
8. Wear a medical alert bracelet, and carry an epinephrine pen.

Latex precaution protocols should be used for patients identified as having either a positive reaction to a latex allergy test or a history of signs and symptoms related to latex exposure. Many health care facilities have created latex-free product carts that can be used for patients with latex allergies.

Multiple Chemical Sensitivities

Multiple chemical sensitivities—also known as *idiopathic environmental intolerances*—is the term for an acquired disorder in which certain people who are exposed to various chemicals and food in the environment have many symptoms related to multiple body systems. These symptoms are usually subjective and are not found during physical examination. The patient experiences wide-ranging symptoms, but evidence of pathological processes or physiological dysfunction is lacking.

This disorder occurs primarily in women. Symptoms include fatigue, headache, nausea, pain, dizziness, mouth irritation, disorientation, and cough. Almost any chemical can initiate the symptoms. Food additives, drugs, and naturally occurring food, including drinking water, often cause sensitivity. However, odour appears to be the principal trigger. Gas exhaust, perfumes, cigarette smoke, plastics, pesticides, and industrial solvents are some of the most common odours associated with multiple chemical sensitivities. The uniqueness of this disorder is that symptoms occur at levels below the established guidelines of toxic levels and concentrations.

The causes of multiple chemical sensitivities are thought to be immunological, psychological, toxicological, and sociological. Diagnosis is usually made based on a patient's health history as there is no established test to diagnose multiple chemical sensitivities. Diagnostic tests that are used include provocation-neutralization and immunological testing (e.g., CBC, lymphocyte subsets, antibody titres). Immunological testing, however, has not been widely accepted as a diagnostic test. In the provocation-neutralization test, the patient is exposed to certain environmental substances to produce symptoms and then at higher and lower dosages to initiate the disappearance of symptoms.

Treatment includes minimizing exposure to known irritants, elimination of foods causing sensitivity, and regular exercise. Complementary and alternative therapies such as physiotherapy and complementary and alternative therapies such as massage, prayer, and meditation are also recommended.

Autoimmunity

Autoimmunity is an immune reaction to self-proteins: the immune system no longer differentiates self from nonself. For unknown reasons, immune cells that are normally unresponsive (tolerant of self-antigens) are activated. Both T cells and B cells have the ability to tolerate self-antigens. Therefore, an alteration in T cells alone or in both B cells and T cells can produce autoantibodies and autosensitized T cells to cause pathophysiological tissue damage. The particular autoimmune disease manifested depends on which self-antigen is involved (Chaplin, 2010).

Autoimmune diseases tend to occur in clusters, so that one individual may have more than one autoimmune disease (e.g., rheumatoid arthritis and Addison's disease), or the same or related autoimmune diseases may be found in other members of the same family. This observation has led to the concept of genetic predisposition to autoimmune disease.

Theories of Causation

The cause of autoimmune diseases remains largely unknown; however, a combination of etiological factors are believe to contribute to its development. Age is thought to play a role because the number of circulating autoantibodies increases in persons older than 50 (Coico & Sunshine, 2009).

Genetic Susceptibility. Most autoimmune diseases have a genetic basis. Most of the research work in this area correlates certain human leukocyte antigen (HLA) types with an autoimmune condition. (HLA and disease association are discussed later in this chapter.)

Initiation of Autoreactivity. Even in a genetically predisposed person, some triggering event is necessary for the initiation of autoreactivity. This event may include infection with agents such as a virus (Coico & Sunshine, 2009). Viral infections can alter cells or tissues that make them antigenic. There is some

Table 16-12 Examples of Autoimmune Diseases*	
Systemic Diseases	**Endocrine System**
Systemic lupus erythematosus (SLE)	Addison's disease
	Thyroiditis
Rheumatoid arthritis	Hypothyroidism
Progressive systemic sclerosis (scleroderma)	Type 1 diabetes mellitus
Mixed connective tissue disease	**Gastrointestinal System**
Organ-Specific Diseases	Pernicious anemia
Blood	Ulcerative colitis
Autoimmune hemolytic anemia	**Kidney**
Immune thrombocytopenic purpura	Goodpasture's syndrome
	Glomerulonephritis
Central Nervous System	**Liver**
Multiple sclerosis	Primary biliary cirrhosis
Guillain-Barré syndrome	Autoimmune hepatitis
Muscle	**Eye**
Myasthenia gravis	Uveitis
Heart	
Rheumatic fever	

*These diseases are discussed in various chapters throughout the book.

evidence that viruses may be involved in the development of multiple sclerosis and type 1 diabetes mellitus. Rheumatic fever and rheumatic heart disease are autoimmune responses triggered by streptococcal infection and mediated by antibodies against group A β-hemolytic streptococci that cross-react with heart muscles, heart valves, and synovial membranes.

Drugs can also be precipitating factors in autoimmune diseases. Hemolytic anemia can result from administration. Procainamide can induce the formation of antinuclear antibodies and cause a lupus-like syndrome.

Hormones also have a role in autoimmune diseases, and more women than men are affected. During pregnancy, symptoms of many autoimmune diseases improve; however, after delivery, the disease frequently worsens.

Autoimmune Diseases

In general, autoimmune diseases are grouped according to organ-specific and systemic diseases. (Table 16-12 lists examples of autoimmune diseases.) SLE is a classic example of a systemic autoimmune disease characterized by damage to multiple organs. It occurs most frequently in women, with onset at 20 to 40 years of age. The cause is unknown, but there appears to be a loss of self-tolerance for the body's own DNA antigens.

In SLE, tissue injury appears to be the result of the formation of antinuclear antibodies. For an unknown reason (possibly a viral infection), the cell membrane is damaged and DNA is released into the systemic circulation, where it is viewed as nonself material. This DNA is normally sequestered inside the nucleus of cells. On release into circulation, the DNA antigen reacts with an antibody. Some antibodies are involved in immune-complex formation, and others may cause damage directly. Once the complexes are deposited, complement is activated and further damages the tissue, especially the renal glomerulus. (SLE is discussed further in Chapter 67.)

Apheresis

Apheresis has been effectively used to treat autoimmune diseases and other diseases and disorders. **Apheresis** is the use of a procedure in which components of the blood are separated and then one or more of those components is removed. Prefixes are often used to describe any particular apheresis procedure, depending on the blood components being collected. *Cytapheresis* is a general term for cell separation and removal. *Plateletpheresis* is the removal of platelets, usually for collection from normal individuals to infuse into patients with low platelet counts (e.g., patients taking chemotherapy who develop thrombocytopenia). *Leukocytapheresis* is a general term indicating the removal of WBCs, a technique used in chronic myelogenous leukemia to remove high numbers of leukemic cells. *Lymphocytapheresis* is used to decrease high lymphocyte counts, as in individuals with chronic lymphocytic leukemia.

Plasmapheresis. *Plasmapheresis* is the removal of plasma-containing components that cause or are thought to cause disease. When plasma is removed, it is replaced by substitution fluids such as saline or albumin. Therefore, the term *plasma exchange* more accurately describes this procedure.

Plasmapheresis has been used to treat autoimmune diseases such as SLE, glomerulonephritis, Goodpasture's syndrome, myasthenia gravis, thrombocytopenic purpura, rheumatoid arthritis, and Guillain-Barré syndrome. Apheresis procedures are also performed on healthy donors to obtain plasma and selected blood components to administer to other patients receiving replacement therapy.

The rationale for performing therapeutic plasmapheresis in autoimmune disorders is to remove pathological substances present in plasma. Many disorders for which plasmapheresis is being used are characterized by circulating autoantibodies (usually of the IgG class) and antigen–antibody complexes. Immunosuppressive therapy has been used to prevent recovery of IgG production, and plasmapheresis has been used to prevent antibody rebound.

In addition to removing antibodies and antigen–antibody complexes, plasmapheresis may also remove inflammatory mediators (e.g., complement) that are responsible for tissue damage. In the treatment of SLE, plasmapheresis is usually reserved for patients in an acute attack who are unresponsive to conventional therapy.

Plasmapheresis involves the removal of whole blood through a needle inserted in one arm and circulation of the blood through a cell separator. Inside the separator, the blood is divided into plasma and its cellular components by centrifugation or membrane filtration. A needle is inserted into the opposite arm for return of the blood to the patient. Plasma, platelets, WBCs, or erythrocytes can be separated selectively. The undesirable component is removed, and the remainder is returned to the patient. The plasma is generally replaced with normal saline, lactated Ringer's solution, fresh-frozen plasma, plasma protein fractions, or albumin. When blood is manually removed, only 500 mL may be taken at one time. However, with the use of apheresis procedures, more than 4 L of plasma can be removed in 2 to 3 hours.

As with administration of other blood products, nurses must be aware of adverse effects associated with plasmapheresis. The most common complications are hypotension and citrate toxicity. Hypotension is usually the result of vasovagal reaction or transient volume changes. Citrate is used as an anticoagulant and may cause hypocalcemia, which may manifest as headache, paresthesias, and dizziness.

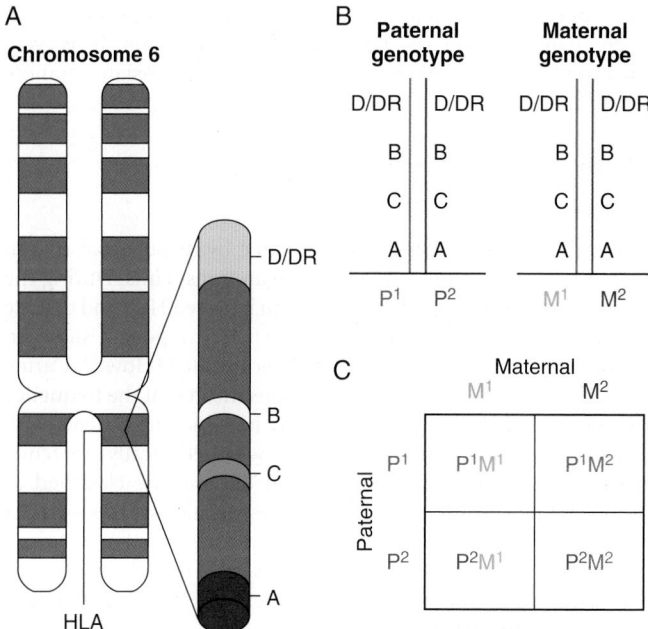

Figure 16-10 Patterns of human leukocyte antigen (HLA) inheritance. **A,** HLA genes are located on chromosome 6. **B,** The two haplotypes of the father are labelled P^1 and P^2, and the haplotypes of the mother are labelled M^1 and M^2. Each child inherits two haplotypes, one from each parent. **C,** Therefore, only four combinations—P^1M^1, P^1M^2, P^2M^1, P^2M^2—are possible, and the offspring have a 25% chance of having identical HLA haplotypes.

Histocompatibility

Human Leukocyte Antigen System

The **human leukocyte antigen (HLA) system** consists of a series of linked genes that occur together on the sixth chromosome and plays an important part in the body's immune response to foreign substances (Coico & Sunshine, 2009). The products of these genes include the cell membrane antigens of the HLA series. Because of its importance in the study of tissue matching, the chromosomal region incorporating the HLA genes is termed the *major histocompatibility complex*. The genes determining the products recognized as the HLA-A, HLA-B, HLA-C, HLA-D, and HLA-DR antigens are clustered together (Figure 16-10). HLA antigens are present on all nucleated cells and platelets.

An important characteristic of HLA genes is that they are highly polymorphic. Each HLA locus can have many different possible alleles. The specific allele is identified by a number. With many alleles possible at each HLA locus, many combinations exist. For example, a person could have the alleles A6, B7, C8, D1, and DR7. Each person has two antigens for each locus, one inherited from each parent. Both antigens of a locus are expressed independently (i.e., they are codominant). The entire set of A, B, C, D, and DR antigens located on one chromosome is termed a *haplotype*. A complete set of antigens located on a chromosome is inherited as a unit (haplotype). One haplotype is inherited from each parent (see Figure 16-10).

Because of the polymorphic nature of the HLA system, it is an ideal marker for genetic studies and is therefore a useful tool in settling paternity disputes. The frequencies of HLAs vary considerably among different races. For example, HLA-B8 is relatively common among European Americans, but it is very uncommon in First Nations people and South Asian Japanese persons.

Human Leukocyte Antigen and Disease Associations

The early interest in HLA was stimulated by its potential role in matching donors and recipients of organ transplants. During the last few years, interest in the association between HLA and disease has grown. Strong associations between HLA type and susceptibility to certain diseases have been demonstrated (Howell, Carter, & Clark, 2010). HLA-disease associations mean that the frequency of a defined HLA allele is significantly increased in patients with a certain disease when compared with ethnically matched controls. Most of the HLA-associated diseases are classified as autoimmune disorders. Examples of associations between HLA types and diseases include (a) the presence of HLA-B27 with ankylosing spondylitis, (b) the presence of HLA-DR2 and HLA-DR3 with SLE, and (c) the presence of HLA-DR3 and HLA-DR4 with diabetes mellitus.

The discovery of HLA associations with certain diseases is a major breakthrough in understanding the genetic bases of these diseases. It is now known that at least part of the genetic basis of HLA-associated diseases lies in the HLA region, but the actual mechanism or mechanisms involved in these associations are still unknown. However, most individuals who inherit an HLA type associated with a disease never actually develop the disease.

The association between HLA and certain diseases is at present of little practical clinical importance. Nevertheless, there is promise for the development of clinical applications in the future. For example, in families with certain autoimmune diseases, it may be possible to identify the members who are at greatest risk for developing the same or a related autoimmune disease. These persons would need close medical supervision, implementation of preventive measures (if possible), and early diagnosis and treatment to prevent chronic complications.

Histocompatibility Studies

The purpose of histocompatibility testing is to identify the HLAs for both donors and potential recipients. A serological test is used to type for the antigens at all five loci (A, B, C, D, and DR). Lymphocytes are isolated from peripheral blood and then combined with serum that contains antibodies to HLAs. Currently, only the A, B, and DR antigens are thought to be clinically significant for transplantation. Because there are two antigens at each locus, a total of six antigens are identified. In certain cadaveric solid organ transplantations, an attempt is made to match as many antigens as possible between the HLA-A, HLA-B, and HLA-DR loci. Antigen matches of five and six antigens and certain four-antigen matches have been found to have better clinical outcomes (i.e., the patient is less likely to reject the transplanted organ), especially with kidney and bone marrow transplants.

Another test called a *crossmatch* is performed at the time a living donor is being evaluated and just before organ removal from cadaveric donors. In a crossmatch, serum from the recipient is mixed with donor lymphocytes to test for any preformed cytotoxic (anti-HLA) antibodies to the potential donor organ. A positive crossmatch indicates that the recipient has cytotoxic antibodies to the donor, which is an absolute contraindication to transplantation. The potential recipient may have been exposed to antigens similar to those of the donor by means of previous blood transfusions, pregnancy, or a previous organ transplant. If transplanted, the organ would undergo hyperacute rejection. A negative crossmatch indicates that no preformed antibodies are present and it is safe to proceed with transplantation.

Crossmatching is also performed to detect preformed cytotoxic antibodies in the recipient serum to HLAs on lymphocytes from random donors. In this situation, the recipient serum is mixed with a randomly selected panel of donor lymphocytes, rather than with specific donor lymphocytes, to determine reactivity. This is called the *panel of reactive antibodies* (PRA) and indicates the recipient's sensitivity to various HLAs. The results are calculated in percentages. A high PRA percentage indicates that the person has a large number of cytotoxic antibodies, which means that the chance of finding a crossmatch-negative donor is poor. In patients awaiting transplantation, a PRA panel is usually performed on a regular basis.

Immunodeficiency Disorders

The condition in which the immune system does not adequately protect the body is **immunodeficiency.** Immunodeficiency disorders involve an impairment of one or more immune mechanisms, which include (a) phagocytosis, (b) humoral response, (c) cell-mediated immune response, (d) complement, and (e) a combined humoral and cell-mediated deficiency. Immunodeficiency disorders are primary if the immune cells are improperly developed or absent and secondary if the deficiency is caused by illnesses or treatment. Primary immunodeficiency disorders are rare and often serious, whereas secondary disorders are more common and less severe.

Primary Immunodeficiency Disorders

The basic categories of primary immunodeficiency disorders are (a) phagocytic defects, (b) B cell deficiency, (c) T cell deficiency, and (d) a combined B cell and T cell deficiency (Arason, Jorgensen, & Ludviksson, 2010; Table 16-13).

Secondary Immunodeficiency Disorders

Some important factors that may cause secondary immunodeficiency disorders are listed in Table 16-14. Drug-induced immunosuppression is the most common. Immunosuppressive therapy is prescribed for patients to treat autoimmune disorders and to prevent transplant rejection. In addition, immunosuppression is a serious adverse effect of drugs used in cancer chemotherapy. Generalized leukopenia often results, leading to a decreased humoral and cell-mediated immune response. Therefore, secondary infections are common in immunosuppressed patients.

Stress may alter the immune response. This response involves interrelationships among the nervous, endocrine, and immune systems (see Chapter 8).

The immune system is in a hypofunctional state in young children and older adults. Laboratory studies have demonstrated that immunoglobulin levels decrease with age and therefore lead to a suppressed humoral immune response in older adults. Thymic involution occurs with aging, along with decreases in the numbers of T cells. The incidence of malignancies and autoimmune diseases increases with aging and may be related to immunological alterations.

Table 16-13 Primary Immunodeficiency Disorders		
DISORDER	**AFFECTED CELLS**	**GENETIC BASIS**
Chronic granulomatous disease	PMNs, monocytes	Sex-linked
Job syndrome	PMNs, monocytes	—
Bruton's (X-linked) hypogammaglobulinemia	B	Sex-linked
Common variable hypogammaglobulinemia	B	—
Selective IgA, IgM, or IgG deficiency	B	Some sex-linked
DiGeorge's syndrome (thymic hypoplasia)	T	—
Severe combined immunodeficiency disease	Stem, B, T	Sex-linked or autosomal recessive
Ataxia telangiectasia	B, T	Autosomal recessive
Wiskott-Aldrich syndrome	B, T	Sex-linked
Graft-versus-host disease	B, T	—

IgA, immunoglobulin A; *IgG*, immunoglobulin G; *IgM*, immunoglobulin M; *PMN*, polymorphonuclear neutrophil.

Table 16-14 Causes of Secondary Immunodeficiency	
• Drug-induced immunodeficiency	• Anaesthesia
• Chemotherapy drugs	• Trauma
• Corticosteroids	• Burns
• Stress	• Predisposing factors
• Age	• Acquired immunodeficiency syndrome (AIDS)
• Infants	• Alcoholic cirrhosis
• Older adults	• Chronic renal disease
• Malnutrition	• Diabetes mellitus
• Dietary deficiency	• Malignancies
• Cirrhosis	• Systemic lupus erythematosus
• Cachexia	
• Radiation	
• Surgery	

Malnutrition alters cell-mediated immune responses. When protein is deficient over a prolonged period, atrophy of the thymus gland occurs and lymphoid tissue decreases. In addition, the susceptibility to infections always increases.

Radiation destroys lymphocytes either directly or through depletion of stem cells. As the radiation dose is increased, more bone marrow atrophies, which leads to severe pancytopenia and suppression of immune function.

Surgical removal of lymph nodes, thymus, or spleen can suppress the immune response. Splenectomy in children is especially dangerous and may lead to septicemia from simple respiratory infections.

Hodgkin's disease greatly impairs the cell-mediated immune response, and patients may die from severe viral or fungal infec-

tions. (Hodgkin's disease is discussed further in Chapter 33.) Viruses, especially rubella, may cause immunodeficiency by direct cytotoxic damage to lymphoid cells. Systemic infections can place such a demand on the immune system that resistance to a secondary or subsequent infection is impaired.

Graft-Versus-Host Disease

Graft-versus-host (GVH) disease occurs when an immunoincompetent (immunodeficient) patient receives a transfusion or transplant with immunocompetent cells. A GVH response may result from the infusion of any blood product containing viable lymphocytes, as in therapeutic blood transfusions, and from the transplantation of fetal thymus, fetal liver, or stem cells. In most transplantation situations, the biggest concern is the host's rejection of the graft. However, in GVH disease, the graft rejects the host or recipient tissue.

The GVH response may begin 7 to 30 days after transplantation. Once the reaction is started, little can be done to modify its course. The exact mechanism involved in this reaction is not completely understood. However, it involves donor T cells attacking and destroying vulnerable host cells.

The target organs for the GVH phenomenon are the skin, the gastrointestinal tract, and the liver. The skin disease may be a maculopapular rash, which may be pruritic or painful. It initially involves the palms and the soles of the feet but can progress to a generalized erythema with bullous formation and desquamation. The liver disease may manifest as mild jaundice with elevated levels of liver enzymes and progress to hepatic coma. The intestinal disease may be manifested by mild to severe diarrhea, severe abdominal pain, gastrointestinal bleeding, and malabsorption. The biggest problem with GVH disease is differing types of infection at different time periods. Bacterial and fungal infections predominate immediately after transplantation, when granulocytopenia is occurring. Later, the development of interstitial pneumonitis is the predominant problem.

Once GVH disease is established, no treatment is adequate. Although corticosteroids are often used, the susceptibility to infection then increases. The use of immunosuppressive agents (e.g., methotrexate, cyclosporine) has been most effective as preventive rather than a treatment measure. Irradiated blood products before administration is another measure to prevent T cell replication.

Organ Transplantation

During the 1960s, organ and tissue transplantation was considered an experimental procedure reserved for patients with critical end-stage medical disease. However, as a result of advances in medical technology and surgical procedures and improved immunosuppressive regimens, organ transplantation has resulted in improved survival and quality of life. **Organ transplantation** is the transfer of a whole or partial organ from one individual to another for the purpose of replacing the recipient's damaged or failing organ with a working one from the donor. Commonly transplanted organs and tissues include the heart, lungs, liver, kidneys, pancreas, corneas, skin, bone marrow, heart valves, bone, and connective tissues (Figure 16-11). Corneas are transplanted to prevent or correct blindness, and skin grafts are used to assist in managing burns. Bone marrow or stem cells are transplanted to help patients with leukemias and other hematological malignancies.

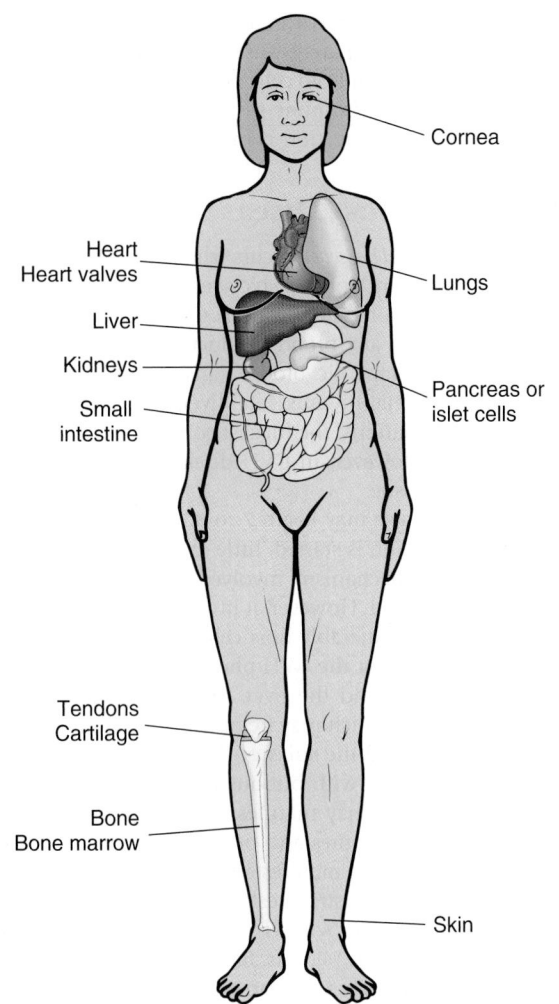

Figure 16-11 Tissues and organs that can be transplanted.

Organs can be successfully transplanted together; for example, a patient may receive both a pancreas transplant for pancreatic insufficiency and a kidney transplant for renal failure.

Some organs may be transplanted in segments rather than in their entirety. Liver and lung lobes may be transplanted, or an intestine may be used in segments, thus allowing one person's organ donation to benefit multiple recipients. This technique not only enables living donors to donate part of an organ while maintaining their functioning organ but also addresses the high rate of mortality among patients on the waiting list that results from poor organ donation rates. Organ donations can be taken from two sources: deceased (cadaveric) and living donors. Patients are matched to available donors through ABO blood and HLA typing, medical urgency, time on the waiting list, and body size. Most organs currently used originate from deceased donors. The majority of living donors are relatives of the recipient, although a number are also nonrelated living donors.

In order to become an organ or tissue donor, an individual either signs an organ and tissue donor card or registers his or her consent through the provincial registry. However, despite registering as an organ or tissue donor, the individual is encouraged to discuss the decision with loved ones because doctors will not proceed with donation without the consent of family members. (Organ donation is discussed further in Chapter 71.)

Nurses caring for a patient in the critical care unit or emergency department who has a diagnosis of brain death should discuss with the health care team the option of organ donation for the patient's family. The local organ procurement organization should then be contacted to speak with the family.

Transplant Rejection

Rejection is one of the major contributing factors for organ loss after solid organ transplantation. Organ rejection occurs if the HLA profile of the donor organ does not identically match that of the recipient. Rejection can be prevented through close matching of ABO and Rh status and HLA profiles of the donor and recipient. Unfortunately, because many differing HLA profiles have been found in humans, a perfect match is impossible, with the exception of tissue matching of identical twins. Three forms of rejection can develop: hyperacute, acute, or chronic. Prevention, early diagnosis, and treatment of rejection are essential for long-term graft function.

Hyperacute Rejection. *Hyperacute rejection* (also called *antibody-mediated* or *humoral rejection*) occurs minutes to hours after transplantation. Hyperacute rejection may result from antibody development through a number of mechanisms, some of which are not clearly understood. Recipients who have received prior blood transfusions may have antibodies to major histocompatibility complex antigens from the transfused blood that may match those in the graft (donated organ), which results in hyperacute rejection. Furthermore, multiple prior pregnancies may have exposed the woman to paternal antigens of the fetus, resulting in the development of antibodies. In the absence of these factors, antibody-mediated rejection may occur nonetheless, and the cause often remains unknown.

Acute Rejection. Acute rejection most commonly occurs days to months after transplantation. This type of rejection is mediated by the recipient's T cytotoxic lymphocytes, which attack the foreign organ (Figure 16-12). Many transplant recipients experience at least one rejection episode after transplantation. These episodes are usually reversible with alteration in or additional immunosuppressive therapy that may include increased corticosteroid doses or polyclonal or monoclonal antibody treatment. Unfortunately, increased doses of immunosuppressants increase the risk for infection.

Chronic Rejection. Chronic rejection is a process that occurs over months to years and is considered irreversible. The transplanted organ is infiltrated with large numbers of T and B cells, which is characteristic of an ongoing, low-grade, immune-mediated injury. Chronic rejection is more common in some organ transplants than others. For example, chronic lung rejection or bronchiolitis obliterans syndrome results from inflammation and fibrosis of the small airways (Banner, Polak, & Yacoub, 2007). Chronic liver rejection is rare and typically is a result of repeated episodes of acute rejection (Movahedi, Holt, & Saab, 2010).

No definitive therapy is yet available for chronic rejection. Switching immunosuppressive therapy to tacrolimus (Prograf) or mycophenolate mofetil (CellCept) has yielded some improvement for patients; however, treatment has largely been supportive. Ultimately, the prognosis for patients with chronic rejection remains poor, and if possible, such patients should be offered the option of retransplantation.

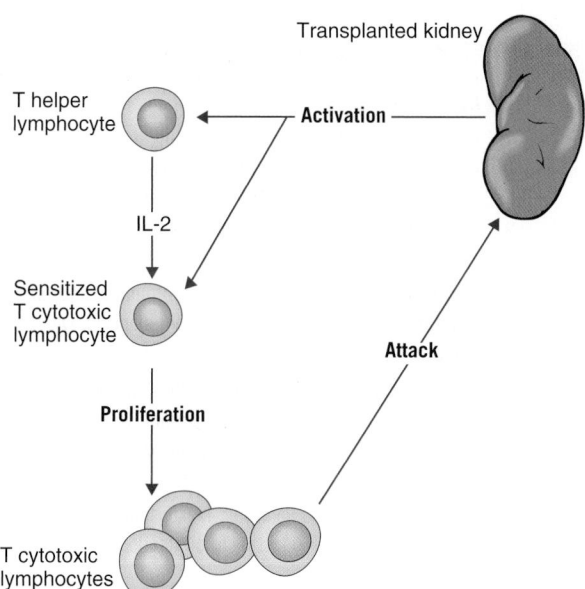

Figure 16-12 Mechanism of action of T cytotoxic lymphocyte activation and attack of transplanted tissue. The transplanted organ (e.g., kidney) is recognized as foreign, and the immune system is activated. T helper cells are activated to produce interleukin-2 (IL-2), and T cytotoxic lymphocytes are sensitized. After the T cytotoxic cells proliferate, they attack the transplanted organ.

Immunosuppressive Therapy

The goal of **immunosuppressive therapy** is to adequately suppress the immune response to prevent rejection of the transplanted organ and yet maintain sufficient immunity to prevent overwhelming infection. Many of the medications used to achieve immunosuppression have adverse effects. In a combination of medications that work in different phases of the immune response, lower doses of each drug produce effective immunosuppression and minimize adverse effects (Pellegrino & Mancini, 2011). Immunosuppressive protocols are highly variable among transplant centres, and different combinations of medications are used. Most patients are initially on triple therapy, which includes a calcineurin inhibitor, a corticosteroid, and either mycophenolate mofetil or azathioprine (Imuran). The major immunosuppressive agents are (a) calcineurin inhibitors, including cyclosporine (Sandimmune, Neoral) and tacrolimus; (b) corticosteroids (prednisone, methylprednisolone [Solu-Medrol] by intravenous route); (c) mycophenolate mofetil; and (d) sirolimus (Rapamune). Azathioprine (Imuran) and cyclophosphamide (Procytox) were used in the past but are now being replaced with safer, newer-generation drugs. Antithymocyte globulin, antilymphocyte globulin, and muromonab-CD3 are medications administered intravenously for short periods to prevent early rejection (induction therapy) or to reverse acute rejection. The most common drugs, routes of administration, mechanisms of action, and adverse effects are listed in Table 16-15.

Calcineurin Inhibitors

This group of drugs includes tacrolimus and cyclosporine. The mechanism of action of these drugs is to prevent the production and release of interleukin (IL)–2, IL-4, and γ-interferon by interfering with calcineurin binding. These cytokines are needed to promote T cell proliferation and activation. Therefore, these drugs prevent a cell-mediated attack against the transplanted organ (Figure 16-13; also see Chapter 49). These drugs do not cause bone marrow suppression or alterations of the normal inflammatory response. They are typically used in combination with corticosteroids and mycophenolate mofetil. Adverse effects of calcineurin inhibitors are dose related and involve nephrotoxicity; therefore, drug levels are closely monitored. Neoral, a microemulsion of cyclosporine, has replaced Sandimmune because of its improved absorption (Pellegrino & Mancini, 2011). Neoral and Sandimmune are not biocompatible and should never be interchanged for one another.

Tacrolimus is 100 times more potent than cyclosporine, allowing for smaller doses to be administered. It does not cause hirsutism or gingival hyperplasia, which are common adverse effects of cyclosporine. Its most significant adverse effects include neurotoxic manifestations, such as tremor and altered mental status, and diabetes.

Sirolimus

Sirolimus is a newer immunosuppressive agent with structural similarities to tacrolimus but a different mechanism of action. Sirolimus suppresses lymphocyte proliferation and inhibits B cells from synthesizing antibodies. At relatively low doses, it has a synergistic effect with cyclosporine, tacrolimus, and corticosteroids. Everolimus (Certican) is similar to sirolimus. It is approved for use in kidney transplantation; however, it remains in the clinical trials phase for heart and liver transplantation.

Mycophenolate Mofetil

Mycophenolate mofetil (CellCept) is a lymphocyte-specific inhibitor of purine synthesis with suppressive effects on both T and B lymphocytes. This drug appears to be most effective when used in combination with tacrolimus or cyclosporine. Its effects are additive because it acts later in the lymphocyte activation pathway by a different mechanism. It is used in place of azathioprine at many transplantation centres because of its lymphocyte-specific effects. It has also been shown to decrease the incidence of late graft loss. The major limitation of this drug is its gastrointestinal toxic effects, including nausea, vomiting, and diarrhea. In many cases, the adverse effects can be diminished by reduction in the dose or administration of smaller doses more frequently. Myfortic is an enteric-coated form of mycophenolate mofetil that has a similar adverse effect profile (Khurana & Brennan, 2011).

Polyclonal Antibodies (Antithymocyte Globulin and Antilymphocyte Globulin)

Antilymphocyte globulin and antithymocyte globulin are used as induction therapy or to treat acute rejection. The purpose of induction therapy is to provide significant immunosuppression to an individual immediately after transplantation to prevent early rejection. These agents are prepared by immunizing horses or rabbits with human lymphoid material (thymocytes, lymph nodes, or spleen cells). The antibody made against the human lymphocytes is then purified and administered intravenously. The actual mechanism of action of antithymocyte globulin and antilymphocyte globulin remains unclear, but they induce lymphopenia and decrease the proliferative response of T

DRUG THERAPY

Table 16-15 Immunosuppressive Therapy

AGENT	ROUTE	MECHANISM OF ACTION	ADVERSE EFFECTS
Corticosteroids: prednisone, methylprednisolone (Solu-Medrol)	PO, IV	Suppress inflammatory response; inhibit cytokine production and T cell activation	Peptic ulcers, hypertension, GI bleeding, osteoporosis, aseptic necrosis, Na$^+$ and H$_2$O retention, acne, muscle weakness, easy bruising, delayed healing, hyperglycemia, ↑ appetite, mood alterations, leukopenia, cataracts, dyslipidemia, ↓ resistance to infection
Tacrolimus (Prograf)	PO, IV	Calcineurin inhibitor; prevents production and release of IL-2, IL-4, and α-interferon; inhibits production of T cytotoxic lymphocytes	Nephrotoxicity, neurotoxicity, seizures, tremors, nausea and vomiting, hyperglycemia, hypertension, alopecia, lymphoma, ↓ resistance to infection
Cyclosporine (Sandimmune, Neoral*)	PO, IV PO	Calcineurin inhibitor; prevents production and release of IL-2, IL-4, and α-interferon; inhibits production of T cytotoxic lymphocytes	Nephrotoxicity, neurotoxicity, headaches, seizures, tremors, hyperglycemia, hypertension, nausea and vomiting, dyslipidemia, gingival hyperplasia, hirsutism, hepatotoxicity, lymphoma, ↓ resistance to infection
Mycophenolate mofetil (CellCept)	PO, IV	Antimetabolite that inhibits purine synthesis; suppresses proliferation of T and B cells	Diarrhea, nausea and vomiting, leukopenia, thrombocytopenia, ↓ resistance to infection, ↑ incidence of malignancies
Sirolimus (Rapamune)	PO	Suppresses lymphocyte proliferation; inhibits B cells from synthesizing antibodies	Diarrhea, dyslipidemia, hypercholesterolemia, arthralgias, delayed wound healing, thrombocytopenia, ↓ resistance to infection, ↑ incidence of malignancies
Muromonab-CD3 (OKT3)	IV push	Monoclonal antibody that binds to CD3 receptors on lymphocytes, causing cell lysis; inhibits function of cytotoxic T cells	Fever, chills, tachycardia, pulmonary edema, muscle and joint pain, diarrhea, hypertension or hypotension, aseptic meningitis, ↓ resistance to infection, ↑ incidence of malignancies
Basiliximab (Simulect)	IV	Monoclonal antibody that acts as IL-2 receptor antagonist by inhibiting the binding of IL-2; inhibits T cell activation and proliferation	Generally no adverse effects
Polyclonal antibody serums: ATG, ALG (Thymoglobulin, ATGAM)	IV	Polyclonal antibodies directed against lymphocytes; particularly deplete T cells	Serum sickness (fever, chills, muscle and joint pain), tachycardia, back pain, shortness of breath, hypotension, anaphylaxis, leukopenia, thrombocytopenia, rash, ↓ resistance to infection, ↑ incidence of malignancies

ALG, antilymphocyte globulin; *ATG*, antithymocyte globulin; *GI*, gastrointestinal; *IL-2*, interleukin-2; *IL-4*, interleukin-4; *IV*, intravenous (route); *PO*, by mouth.
*Neoral is a microemulsion with better absorption than Sandimmune.

lymphocytes, possibly as a result of the generation of T suppressor lymphocytes.

Allergic reactions to the foreign proteins from the host animal, manifested by fever, arthralgias, and tachycardia, are common but usually not severe enough to preclude use. These adverse effects can be attenuated by administering the preparation slowly, over 4 to 6 hours, and administering premedication such as acetaminophen (Tylenol), diphenhydramine (Benadryl), and methylprednisolone (Solu-Medrol). The main toxic effects of polyclonal antibodies are lymphopenia and thrombocytopenia, caused by antibody contaminants that are not completely removed during preparation of the antibodies.

Monoclonal Antibodies

Monoclonal antibodies are used for preventing and treating acute rejection episodes. (Monoclonal antibodies are discussed later in this chapter.) Muromonab-CD3 was the first monoclonal antibody to be used in clinical transplantation. It is a mouse monoclonal antibody that binds with the CD3 antigen found on the surface of human thymocytes and mature T cells. It is an anti–antigen receptor antibody that interferes with the function of the T lymphocyte, the pivotal cell in the response to graft rejection. It is administered via intravenous push daily for 7 to 14 days. All T cells are affected, rather than just the subset active in graft rejection. Within minutes after the initial infusion of muromonab-CD3, the number of circulating T cells decreases significantly.

A flu-like syndrome occurs during the first few days of treatment, as a result of cytokine release. Adverse effects include fever, rigors, headache, myalgias, and various gastrointestinal disturbances. To reduce the expected adverse effects of muromonab-CD3, patients should receive acetaminophen, diphenhydramine, and intravenous corticosteroids before the dose is administered.

A newer generation monoclonal antibody, basiliximab (Simulect; Khurana & Brennan, 2011), is also a hybrid of mouse and human antibodies, but it has fewer adverse effects than muromonab-CD3 because large parts of the molecule have been replaced with human IgG.

New Immunosuppressive Therapy

The search continues for immunosuppressants that specifically target the cells responsible for rejection, are easy to administer, and limit drug toxicity. Two categories of novel immunosuppressants are small molecules and biological agents. The develop-

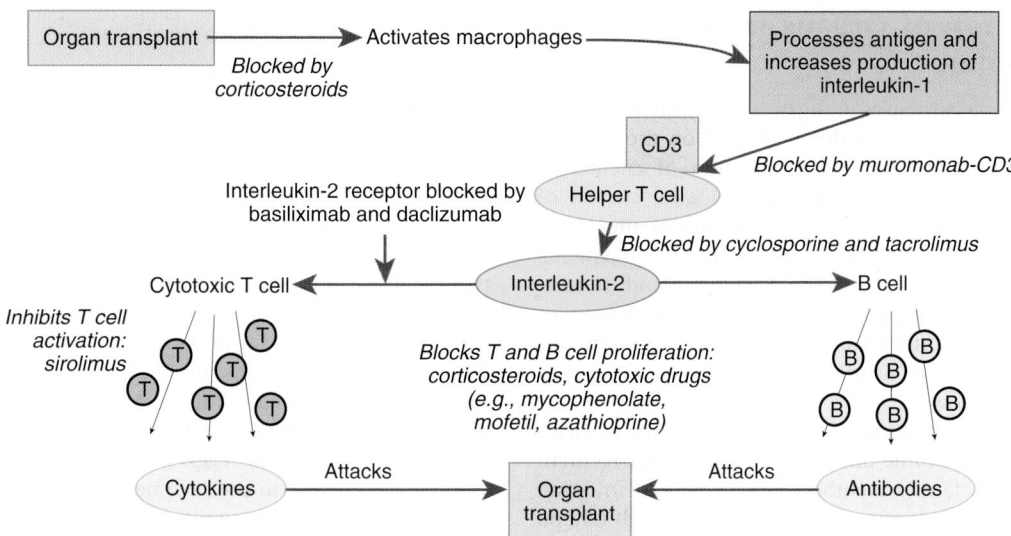

Figure 16-13 Sites of action for immunosuppressive agents.

Source: From McKenry, L., Tessier, E., & Hogan, M. [2006]. *Mosby's pharmacology in nursing* [22nd ed., p. 1161, Figure 63-1]. St. Louis: Mosby.

ment of a new generation of "small molecules" endowed with immunosuppressive properties and potentially without the many adverse effects of the older immunosuppressants is under way. Many drugs currently available that suppress the activation of the immune system lack specificity in terms of their molecular targets; therefore, they potentially generate many adverse effects. Examples of small molecule agents are Janus kinase (JAK) inhibitors and aEB071, a protein-kinase inhibitor. A biological agent still in clinical trials is belatacept.

Antibody-mediated rejection has increasingly been recognized as a major problem. New strategies to address this concern have been with the use of rituxan, an anti-CD20 agent used for B cell malignancies. Two newer agents under investigation are the complement inhibitor eculizumab and the proteasome inhibitor bortezomib. Bortezomib shows promise for primary or refractory antibody-mediated rejection and may also have a role in anti-HLA desensitization. It is currently being tested in trials with other desensitization strategies, such as rituxan, plasmapheresis, and intravenous immunoglobulin (Malek, 2011).

Alternative Strategies

In the past decade, there has been a rapid rise in solid organ transplantation worldwide because of the increased incidence of organ failure and greater improvements in post-transplantation outcomes. However, cadaveric organ donation rates have not met the demands needed; thus waiting lists are long, and increasing numbers of patients die waiting for a suitable organ (Abouna, 2008; Shemie, 2006). The number of patients waiting for an organ transplant in Canada in 2010 was 4,529, but only 423 cadaveric organs were recovered. Approximately 247 people die annually waiting for an organ transplant in Canada; that means 21 people die each month awaiting transplantation, mostly of a liver or kidney (Canadian Institute for Health Information, 2010). Various strategies worldwide have been implemented to offset the critical organ shortage, some with modest success, others remaining under scientific investigation and ethical debate (see the "Ethical Dilemmas" box).

ETHICAL DILEMMAS
Transplantation

Situation
A 24-year-old female patient is admitted to hospital with evidence of acute organ rejection. The patient informs the nurse in confidence that she does not take her antirejection medications regularly because she is very busy with work and school. The patient also states that she usually feels so well that she does not think she needs to take them every day. She asks the nurse not to inform the health care team that she has been missing some of her antirejection medications.

Important Points for Consideration
- Building a trusting relationship with patients is key in the health care environment; however, the larger implications for the patient's health supersede the issue of confidentiality. There are some limits to confidentiality, including potential or real harm to self or others.
- The nurse is a member of the treatment team.
- Organ rejection can cause reduced organ function and potential loss of the graft and subsequent death for the patient. With complete information, the patient can understand the importance of adherence to the medication regimen.

Critical Thinking Questions
1. How would you respond to this patient's request for confidentiality? Would you inform the treatment team? If so, would you tell the patient you are informing them?
2. What information would you give the patient regarding the importance of taking her anti-rejection medications?
3. How could you work with the patient who has a busy schedule and forgets to take her medications?

Transplantation of Organs from Deceased Donor

One of the most rapid increases in organ recovery rates has been from deceased persons who are declared dead on the basis of cardiopulmonary criteria (irreversible cessation of circulatory and respiratory function) rather than neurological criteria of "brain death" (irreversible loss of all functions of the entire brain, including the brainstem; Steinbrook, 2007). Such patients typically are on a ventilator because of devastating and irreversible brain injury (not complete brain death) from trauma or intracranial bleeding. Furthermore, in some of these patients, complete cessation of the heartbeat with subsequent cardiac resuscitation was followed by irreversible brain injury as the result of a long period of anoxia (lack of oxygen). Further treatment has been deemed futile and end-of-life care management implemented. Often, family members express interest in organ donation. The potential donor must meet cardiac death criteria at onset of asystole or absence of a heartbeat. In order to avoid conflict of interest, those involved in end-of-life care or declaration of death of the potential donor are not involved in the care of the transplant recipient. Organs most commonly recovered for donation include the kidneys, the liver, the pancreas, and the lungs (Steinbrook, 2007). In 2010 in Canada, 45 organs were recovered after deceased cardiac death and successfully transplanted into recipients (Canadian Institute for Health Information, 2010).

Xenotransplantation

Xenotransplantation is the replacement of a patient's diseased and malfunctioning organ with an organ harvested from another species. Animals considered as a possible source of organs for human use include primates (because of their genetic similarities to humans) and pigs (because of their large availability). Organs from primates have been largely dismissed because of logistical difficulties. The pig is believed to be the most appropriate candidate because of comparable organ size, large litters, and rapid gestation. Difficulties in successful organ transplantation from one species to another, as in from pig to human, include multiple biological barriers. First, the significant degree of antigen disparity means that there is more for the human immune system to recognize and reject. Second, the possibility of diseases "jumping" the species barrier and infecting humans, such as porcine endogenous retroviruses, is one of the main reasons why people remain skeptical and concerned regarding xenotransplantation. This possibility has decreased enthusiasm for xenotransplantation as an alternative to allogeneic organ transplantation (Cozzi, Bosio, Seveso, Vadori, & Ancona, 2006). However, despite strong skepticism, much scientific research and advancement in this area continues.

Ex Vivo Transplantation

A novel strategy to help overcome donor lung shortages has been through the development of normothermic ex vivo lung perfusion (EVLP). The injured donor lungs are reassessed and conditioned through the EVLP system by mimicking the lung's natural physiological environment and by providing oxygen and other substrates necessary for active metabolism. Through the use of EVLP, therapeutic interventions can be performed in the donor lungs that reduce the degree or negative influence of pulmonary edema, pulmonary emboli, gastric aspiration, pneumonia, and lung inflammation (Cypel, Yeung, & Keshavjee, 2011).

Stem Cell Transplantation

Stem cells are the subject of much discussion. It is believed that the use of stem cells may allow for the regeneration of lost tissue and restoration of function in many chronic diseases such as Parkinson's disease, Alzheimer's disease, heart disease, diabetes mellitus, and spinal cord injuries.

Stem cells are cells in the body that have the ability to differentiate into other cells. Stem cells can be divided into two types: embryonic and adult. *Embryonic stem cells* have the ability to become any one of the hundreds of types of cells in the human body. They are derived from human embryo cells that are 4 to 5 days old. These stem cells are pluripotent and can differentiate into any cell type that they are stimulated to become. Because of their versatility, embryonic stem cells are preferred for use in medical research. Donor eggs, like stem cells, can be used with existing adult tissue to produce new tissue. In a process known as *nuclear transfer* or *therapeutic cloning*, the nucleus is removed from the egg and replaced with the nucleus of the desired tissue. Then, as the egg divides, a 200-cell blastocyst of the desired tissue is created. *Adult stem cells* are undifferentiated cells that are found in small numbers in most adult tissues; they have been discovered in the skin, the gastrointestinal tract, and bone marrow. They are also found in newborns and can be extracted from umbilical cord blood. The primary roles of adult stem cells in the body are to maintain and repair tissues in which they are found. They are usually thought of as multipotent cells, giving rise to a closely related family of cells within the tissue. For example, hematopoietic stem cells form all the various cells in blood, whereas skin stem cells produce new skin cells. Scientists hope that adult stem cells can be coaxed into providing tissue for unrelated organs.

Stem cells found within the bone marrow are the body's site of hematopoiesis. The cells are prolific by design and are already being donated in the treatment of certain diseases, such as leukemia. Cells similar to the stem cells found in bone marrow can be found in the umbilical cord and blood from the placenta. These cells are used in situations similar to those of bone marrow. Studies are being conducted to find future uses that will allow the cells to become other tissues in the body (National Institutes of Health, 2011). With increasing waiting lists for organ transplantation, embryonic stem cell research may be the key to solving the problem of organ shortages through organ regeneration. However, conflicts exist regarding creating embryonic stem cells for therapeutic purposes such as organ development, with much debate over the definition of human life at the earliest stages versus a potentially life-saving therapy. Much discussion continues in this area internationally.

New Technologies in Immunology

Hybridoma Technology: Monoclonal Antibodies

Monoclonal antibodies are homogeneous populations of identical antibody molecules produced by specialized tissue cell culture lines. They are manufactured through cell fusion techniques and standard in vitro tissue culture systems (Figure 16-14). The two essential biological components are immunized mice or rats and myeloma tumour cell lines, which are of lymphoid origin. Single antibody-forming cells (lymphocytes) from rodents previously immunized with antigen are fused with myeloma cells to create hybrid cells with properties of both parent cell types. Like the myeloma parent cell, the hybrids have an unlimited capacity to

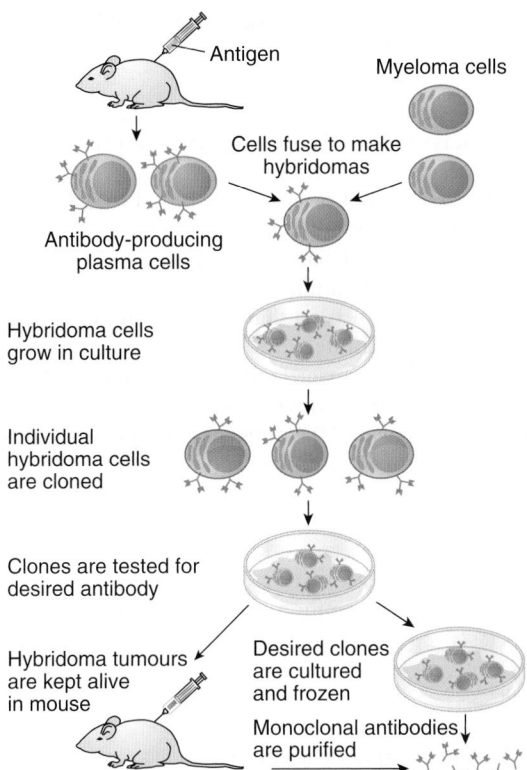

Figure 16-14 Monoclonal antibodies are identical antibodies made by clones of a single antibody-producing cell. The target antigen is injected into a mouse. Plasma cells are harvested from the spleen of the mouse and fused with myeloma cells. The fused cells, or hybridomas, are then cloned. A clone can secrete monoclonal antibodies over a long period.

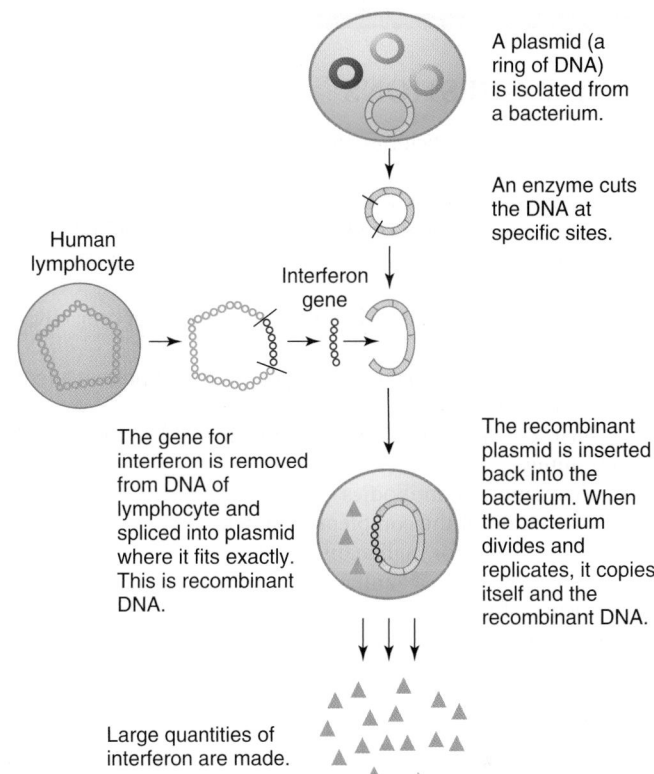

Figure 16-15 Mass production of interferon by recombinant gene technology.

reproduce. The hybrids produce the single type of antibody molecule that they inherited from the normal, antibody-forming parent cell. Hybrid cells derived in this way can produce unlimited quantities of specific antibodies. With appropriate selection techniques, producing monoclonal antibodies to virtually any antigen is possible. Because the monoclonal antibodies are a completely homogeneous population, their use incurs fewer problems than does that of conventional polyclonal antisera.

Monoclonal antibodies are used widely in many areas of medicine and biological science. Thousands of monoclonal antibodies have been made against many different types of antigens. Monoclonal antibodies have begun to replace conventional antibodies in blood banking and are used in the identification of organisms in bacteriology laboratories. Monoclonal antibodies have also been extensively used in radioimmunoassays to measure serum levels of various substances (e.g., parathyroid hormone). They have been useful in quantifying types of WBCs and subtypes of lymphocytes and in the diagnosis of leukemia. More recently, monoclonal antibodies have been used in the treatment of malignancies (see Chapter 18). They have been used to treat transplant rejection episodes, to purge bone marrow of tumour cells in bone marrow transplants, and to remove mature T cells that cause GVH disease in bone marrow transplant recipients.

A major limitation of monoclonal antibody use for humans is that they are mouse antibodies and therefore can elicit an antibody response by the host against the foreign agent. Human hybridomas have been produced through the use of human myelomas. These hybrids synthesize human monoclonal antibodies and are therefore advantageous for in vivo use in diagnosis and therapy.

Recombinant DNA Technology

Recombinant DNA technology, a form of genetic engineering, involves taking segments of DNA from one type of organism and combining them with genes from a second organism (Figure 16-15). When the cell divides, the DNA is transcribed, and a specific protein coded by the DNA is made. In this way, relatively simple organisms such as *Escherichia coli*, yeast, or mammalian tissue culture cells can be used to make large quantities of human proteins. This process is used to make human insulin and cytokines (e.g., α-interferon, interleukin-2), as well as many other substances.

Polymerase Chain Reaction

When rapid genetic diagnosis is necessary, polymerase chain reaction (PCR) can provide a way to make many copies of a DNA or RNA sequence in only a few hours. PCR involves the artificial replication of a DNA or RNA sequence. The DNA or RNA strands can be separated to form new templates that are used for replication. PCR requires only small amounts of sample (e.g., blood, buccal swabs, secretions), in contrast to other laboratory assays. PCR is used extensively in forensic medicine to identify DNA of criminal suspects by using samples from blood, hair, and semen. PCR can also be used as a confirmatory test in HIV testing. This is especially important when an infant of a mother who is seropositive for HIV antibodies is also HIV-seropositive. In this situation, it is not known whether the antibodies in the infant's blood are from the infant or the mother. PCR techniques can be used on the infant's lymphocytes to determine whether the infant is infected with HIV.

REVIEW QUESTIONS

The number of the question corresponds to the same-numbered objective at the beginning of the chapter.

1. What is the function of monocytes in immunity?
   a. They stimulate the production of T and B lymphocytes.
   b. They produce antibodies on exposure to foreign substances.
   c. They bind antigens and stimulate natural killer cell activation.
   d. They capture antigens by phagocytosis and present them to lymphocytes.

2. Which of the following is a function of cell-mediated immunity?
   a. Formation of antibodies
   b. Activation of the complement system
   c. Surveillance for malignant cell changes
   d. Opsonization of antigens to allow phagocytosis by neutrophils

3. Which immunoglobulin from maternal transmission protects newborns in the first 6 months of life from bacterial infections?
   a. IgG
   b. IgA
   c. IgM
   d. IgE

4. Which primary immunological disorder typically occurs in a type I hypersensitivity reaction?
   a. Binding of IgG to an antigen on a cell surface
   b. Deposit of antigen–antibody complexes in small vessels
   c. Release of lymphokines to interact with specific antigens
   d. Release of chemical mediators from IgE-bound mast cells and basophils

5. Which response may alert the nurse that a possible anaphylactic shock reaction may be occurring immediately after a patient has received an intramuscular penicillin injection?
   a. Edema and itching at the injection site
   b. Sneezing and itching of the nose and eyes
   c. A wheal-and-flare reaction at the injection site
   d. Chest tightness and production of thick sputum

6. Which is the most appropriate response when a person requests a friend who is a nurse to administer his allergy shot?
   a. It is illegal for nurses to administer injections outside of a medical setting.
   b. He or she is qualified to do it if the friend has epinephrine in an injectable syringe provided with his extract.
   c. Avoiding the allergens is a more effective way of controlling allergies, and allergy shots are not usually effective.
   d. Immunotherapy should only be administered in a setting where emergency equipment and drugs are available.

7. A patient is undergoing plasmapheresis for treatment of SLE. What does plasmapheresis do?
   a. Removes T lymphocytes in her blood that are producing antinuclear antibodies
   b. Removes normal particles in her blood that are being damaged by autoantibodies
   c. Exchanges her plasma that contains antinuclear antibodies with a substitute fluid
   d. Replaces viral-damaged cellular components of her blood with replacement whole blood

8. Association between HLA antigens and diseases is most commonly found in what disease conditions?
   a. Malignancies
   b. Infectious diseases
   c. Neurological diseases
   d. Autoimmune disorders

9. What is the most common cause of secondary immunodeficiencies?
   a. Drugs
   b. Stress
   c. Malnutrition
   d. Human immunodeficiency virus

10. Which of the following accurately describes rejection after transplantation?
    a. Hyperacute rejection can be treated with mycophenolate mofetil (CellCept).
    b. Acute rejection can be treated with sirolimus or tacrolimus.
    c. Chronic rejection can be treated with tacrolimus or cyclosporine.
    d. Hyperacute rejection can usually be avoided in kidney transplantation if crossmatching is done before the transplantation.

11. If a person is experiencing an acute rejection of a transplanted organ, which of the following drugs would most likely be used?
    a. Tacrolimus
    b. Cyclosporine
    c. Muromonab-CD3
    d. Mycophenolate mofetil

12. Which of the following statements best describes cardiac death in a deceased donor?
    a. Severe brain damage; coma has progressed to a state of wakefulness without detectable awareness
    b. Irreversible loss of all functions of the entire brain, including the brainstem
    c. Devastating and irreversible brain injuries (not complete brain death) from trauma or intracranial bleeding; complete cessation of the heartbeat may have occurred, and after subsequent cardiac resuscitation, irreversible brain injury results from a long period of lack of oxygen
    d. Inability to be awakened; fails to respond normally to pain or light, does not have sleep–wake cycles, and does not take voluntary actions

REFERENCES

Abouna, G. M. (2008). Organ shortage crisis: Problems and possible solutions. *Transplantation Proceedings, 40*(1), 34-38. doi:10.1016/j.transproceed.2007.11.067

Arason, G. J., Jorgensen, G. H., & Ludviksson, B. R. (2010). Primary immunodeficiency and autoimmunity: Lessons from human diseases. *Scandinavian Journal of Immunology, 71*(5), 317-328. doi:10.1111/j.1365-3083.2010.02386.x

Banner, R. B., Polak, M., & Yacoub, M. H. (2007). *Lung transplantation* (1st ed.). Cambridge, UK: Cambridge University Press.

Canadian Centre for Occupational Health and Safety. (2009). Latex allergy. Retrieved from *http://www.ccohs.ca/oshanswers/diseases/latex.html*

Canadian Institute for Health Information. (2010). *2010 Summary statistics, January 1 to December 31st, 2010*. Ottawa: Author. Retrieved from *http://www.cihi.ca/CIHI-ext-portal/pdf/internet/REPORT_STATS2010_PDF_EN*

Chaplin, D. D. (2006). Overview of the immune response. *Journal of Allergy and Clinical Immunology, 117*(2, Suppl. Mini-Primer), S430-S435. doi:10.1016/j.jaci.2005.09.034

Chaplin, D. D. (2010). Overview of the immune response [Review]. *Journal of Allergy and Clinical Immunology, 125*(2, Suppl. 2), S3-S23. doi:10.1016/j.jaci.2009.12.980

Coico, R., & Sunshine, G. (2009). *Immunology: A short course* (6th ed.). Hoboken, NJ: Wiley.

Cozzi, E., Bosio, E., Seveso, M., Vadori, M., & Ancona, E. (2006). Xenotransplantation—Current status and future perspectives. *British Medical Bulletin, 75-76*, 99-114. doi:10.1093/bmb/ldh061

Cypel, M., Yeung, J. C., & Keshavjee, S. (2011). Novel approaches to expanding the lung donor pool: Donation after cardiac death and ex vivo conditioning [Review]. *Clinics in Chest Medicine, 32*(2), 233-244. doi:10.1016/j.ccm.2011.02.003

Howell, W. M., Carter, V., & Clark, B. (2010). The HLA system: Immunobiology, HLA typing, antibody screening and crossmatching techniques. *Journal of Clinical Pathology, 63*(5), 387-390. doi:10.1136/jcp.2009.072371

Khan, B. Q., & Kemp, S. F. (2011). Pathophysiology of anaphylaxis. *Current Opinion on Allergy and Clinical Immunology, 11*(4), 319-325. doi:10.1097/ACI.0b013e3283481ab6

Khurana, A., & Brennan, D. C. (2011). Current concepts of immunosuppression and side effects. In H. Liapis & H. L. Wang (eds.), *Pathology of solid organ transplantation* (pp. 11-30). Berlin: Springer-Verlag. doi:10.1007/978-3-540-79343-4_2

Malek, S. K. (2011). Marching toward new, non-nephrotoxic immunosuppressive agents [Editorial]. *Nephrology Times, 4*(4), 2-3. doi:10.1097/01.NEP.0000398057.65793.df

Movahedi, Z., Holt, C. D., & Saab, S. (2010). Liver transplant: A primer [Review]. *Experimental and Clinical Transplantation, 8*(2), 83-90.

National Institute for Occupational Safety and Health. (n.d.). *NIOSH alert: Preventing allergic reactions to natural rubber latex in the workplace* (DHHS [NIOSH] Publication No. 97-135). Retrieved from *http://www.cdc.gov/niosh/pdfs/97-135sum.pdf*

National Institutes of Health. (2011). *Stem cell basics* [home page]. Retrieved from *http://stemcells.nih.gov/info/basics/basics6.asp*

Peavy, R. D., & Metcalfe, D. D. (2008). Understanding the mechanisms of anaphylaxis. *Current Opinion in Allergy and Clinical Immunology, 8*(4), 310-315. doi:10.1097/ACI.0b013e3283036a90

Pellegrino, B., & Mancini, M. (2011). Immunosuppression. Retrieved from *http://emedicine.medscape.com/article/432316-overview*

Shemie, S. D. (2006). Brain arrest to neurological determination of death to organ utilization: The evolution of hospital-based organ donation strategies in Canada. *Canadian Journal of Anesthesia, 53*(8), 747-752. doi:10.1007/BF03022789

Steinbrook, R. (2007). Organ donation after cardiac death. *New England Journal of Medicine, 357*(3), 209-213. doi:10.1056/NEJMp078066

Weiskopf, D., Weinberger, B., & Grubeck-Loebenstein, B. (2009). The aging of the immune system. *Transplant International, 22*(11), 1041-1050. doi:10.1111/j.1432-2277.2009.00927.x

CANADIAN RESOURCES

Asthma Society of Canada
http://www.asthma.ca

Canadian Association for Clinical Microbiology and Infectious Diseases
http://www.cacmid.ca/

Canadian Centre for Occupational Health and Safety (CCOHS)
http://www.ccohs.ca

Canadian Society of Allergy and Clinical Immunology (CSACI)
http://www.csaci.ca/

Genome Program
http://www.genomecanada.ca/

Trillium Gift of Life Network website
http://www.giftoflife.on.ca

RELATED RESOURCES

Centers for Disease Control and Prevention, Office of Genomics and Disease Prevention
http://www.cdc.gov/genomics

National Human Genome Research Institute, National Institutes of Health
http://www.nhgri.nih.gov

National Institute of Nursing Research (NINR), Division of Intramural Research
http://www.ninr.nih.gov/ResearchAndFunding/DivisionofIntramuralResearch/default.htm

Understanding Gene Testing
http://www.accessexcellence.org/AE/AEPC/NIH

ⓔvolve   *For additional Internet resources, see the Web site for this book at* **http://evolve.elsevier.com/Canada/Lewis/medsurg**

Infection and Human Immunodeficiency Virus Infection

Written by Jeffrey Kwong and Lucy Bradley-Springer
Adapted by Jane McCall

LEARNING OBJECTIVES

1. Discuss the impact of emerging and re-emerging infections on health care.
2. Review infection prevention and control strategies.
3. List the modes and variables involved in the transmission of the human immunodeficiency virus (HIV).
4. Describe the pathophysiology of HIV infection.
5. Outline HIV disease progression against the spectrum of untreated HIV infection.
6. List the diagnostic criteria for acquired immune deficiency syndrome (AIDS).
7. Explain the methods of testing for HIV infection.
8. Discuss the collaborative management of HIV infection.
9. Discuss the long-term consequences of HIV infection and treatment of HIV infection.
10. Explain the characteristics of opportunistic diseases associated with AIDS.
11. Describe the nursing management of HIV-infected patients and those at risk for HIV infection.
12. Compare and contrast the methods of HIV prevention that eliminate risk and those that decrease risk.

KEY TERMS

acquired immunodeficiency syndrome (AIDS) End stage of chronic HIV infection; a syndrome involving a defect in cell-mediated immunity that has a long incubation period and is manifested by various opportunistic infections and cancers, p. 326

acute retroviral syndrome Symptoms accompanying the development of HIV-specific antibodies (seroconversion), including a flulike syndrome of fever, swollen lymph glands, sore throat, headache, malaise, nausea, muscle and joint pain, diarrhea, or a diffuse rash, or some combination, p. 325

bacteria One-celled microorganisms that are found virtually everywhere on earth and are involved in fermentation, putrefaction, infectious diseases, and nitrogen fixation, p. 315

emerging infectious disease A disease of infectious origin that newly appears in a population, or whose incidence in humans has increased within the recent past or threatens to increase in the near future, including those infections that appear in new geographic areas or increase abruptly (WHO, 2005, p. 1), p. 315

fungi Organisms similar to plants, but lacking in chlorophyll; pathogenic fungi cause infections that are usually localized, but may become disseminated in an immunocompromised individual, p. 315

human immunodeficiency virus (HIV) Retrovirus that causes HIV infection and AIDS, p. 324

opportunistic diseases Infections and cancers that occur in immunosuppressed patients that can lead to disability, disease, and death, p. 325

oral hairy leukoplakia An Epstein-Barr virus infection that causes painless, white, raised lesions on the lateral aspect of the tongue, p. 326

protozoa Single-cell, animal-like microorganisms that normally live in soil and bodies of water, but can cause infection when introduced into the human body, p. 315

retroviruses Viruses that replicate in a "backward" manner, going from RNA to DNA, p. 324

reverse transcriptase An enzyme made by HIV and other retroviruses that helps the virus replicate back from RNA to DNA, p. 324

viral load The number of HIV particles in the blood, p. 322

viremia Large amounts of virus in the blood, p. 325

viruses Infectious agents consisting of either RNA or DNA and a protein envelope; can reproduce only in the cells of a living organism, p. 315

window period Time period of 2 months after infection during which an infected individual will not test positive for HIV antibodies, p. 327

ELECTRONIC RESOURCES

Supplemental content related to Chapter 17 can be found ...

Evolve Web Site ⊝volve

http://evolve.elsevier.com/Canada/Lewis/medsurg
- Answer Guideline for Case Study on p. 341
- Clinical Reference: Laboratory Values
- Content Updates
- eFigures:
  - eFigure 17-1: Proper Placement of the Male Condom
  - eFigure 17-2: Proper Placement of the Female Condom
- Electronic Calculators
- Examination Review Questions

- Glossary
- Interactive Case Study: Human Immunodeficiency Virus (HIV) Infection and Acquired Immunodeficiency Syndrome (AIDS)
- Key Points (Printable and MP3 Download)
- Patient & Caregiver Teaching Guides:
  - The Proper Use of Drug-Using Equipment
  - Signs and Symptoms that HIV-Infected Clients Need to Report
  - Use of Antiretroviral Drugs
  - The Right Way to Use Antibiotics

Infections

An infection is an invasion of the body by a *pathogen* (any microorganism that causes disease) and the resulting signs and symptoms that develop in response to the invasion. Infections can be divided into two categories: localized and systemic. A localized infection is limited to a small area. Systemic infections are widespread throughout the body and are often spread via the blood.

Causes of Infections

A number of microorganisms can cause infections. The most common are bacteria, viruses, fungi, and protozoa. **Bacteria** are one-celled microorganisms that are found virtually everywhere on earth and are involved in fermentation, putrefaction, infectious diseases, and nitrogen fixation. They were first observed by Anton Van Leeuwenhoek, who named them "animalcules." A number of bacteria are considered to be normal flora. Under normal circumstances, they live harmoniously in or on the human body without causing disease. These normal flora act protectively and prevent the overgrowth of other microorganisms. *Escherichia coli,* for example, are bacteria that are normal flora in the large intestine (Huether & McCance, 2012).

Bacteria cause disease in two ways. They can enter the body and grow inside human cells (e.g., tuberculosis [TB]), or they can secrete toxins that damage cells. Bacteria are divided into categories based on the shape of their cells. Cocci, including streptococci and staphylococci, are round cells. Bacilli are rod shaped and include tetanus and TB. Curved rods include *Vibrio* bacteria, one of which causes cholera. Table 17-1 lists common pathogenic bacteria and the diseases that they cause (Huether & McCance, 2012; Pommerville, 2009).

Viruses can also cause infections. The word *virus* comes from the Latin term meaning poison. Unlike bacteria, viruses are not cells. They consist of either RNA or DNA and a protein envelope. Viruses can reproduce only in the cells of a living organism and are, therefore, obligate parasites. Examples of diseases caused by viruses are presented in Table 17-2 (Huether & McCance, 2012).

Fungi are organisms similar to plants, but they lack chlorophyll. Mycosis is any disease caused by a fungus. Pathogenic fungi cause infections that are usually localized to a small area but can become disseminated in an immunocompromised person. Athlete's foot and ringworm are two common mycotic infections. Some fungi are normal flora in various places in the body, but when overgrowth occurs, disease can result. Overgrowth of *Candida albicans,* for example, causes oral candidiasis (thrush), esophageal candidiasis, intestinal symptoms, and vaginitis, depending on the affected site (Huether & McCance, 2012). Other fungi and their respective mycotic infections are listed in Table 17-3. Fungal infections of the lungs are presented in Chapter 30, Table 30-13, and fungal infections of the skin in Chapter 26, Table 26-7.

Protozoa are single-cell, animal-like microorganisms. Protozoa can be divided into four categories: amebas, ciliates, flagellates, and sporozoa. Protozoa normally live in soil and bodies of water. When introduced into the human body, infection can result. Amebic dysentery and giardiasis are caused by protozoan parasites. Malaria is caused by a sporozoa called *Plasmodium malariae* (Huether & McCance, 2012; Pommerville, 2009).

Emerging Infections

An **emerging infectious disease** is a disease of infectious origin that newly appears in a population, or whose incidence in humans has increased within the recent past or threatens to increase in the near future, including those infections that appear in new geographic areas or increase abruptly (WHO, 2005, p. 1). Examples of emerging infections are described in Table 17-4. Emerging infectious diseases can originate from unknown sources, contact with animals, changes in known diseases, natural disasters, or even biological warfare. For example, severe acute respiratory syndrome (SARS) and the West Nile virus come from animal sources, whereas others, such as *Staphylococcus aureus,* have emerged as a result of a previously treatable organism developing resistance to antibiotics. Climate change has resulted in increased vegetation in some regions that leads to increases in rodent numbers and hantavirus. Climate change is also associated with an expanded range of insect populations including

Table 17-1 Common Disease-Causing Bacteria

TYPE	DISEASES CAUSED
Clostridium organisms	
C. botulinum	Food poisoning with progressive muscle paralysis
C. tetani	Tetanus (lockjaw)
Corynebacterium diphtheriae	Diphtheria
Escherichia coli	Urinary tract infections, peritonitis
Haemophilus organisms	
H. influenzae	Nasopharyngitis, meningitis, pneumonia
H. pertussis	Whooping cough
Helicobacter pylori	Peptic ulcers, gastritis
Klebsiella and Enterobacter organisms	Urinary tract infections, peritonitis, pneumonia
Legionella pneumophila	Pneumonia (legionnaires' disease)
Mycobacterium organisms	
M. leprae	Hansen's disease (leprosy)
M. tuberculosis	Tuberculosis
Neisseria organisms	
N. gonorrhoeae	Gonorrhea, pelvic inflammatory disease
N. meningitidis	Meningococcemia, meningitis
Proteus organisms	Urinary tract infections, peritonitis
Pseudomonas aeruginosa	Urinary tract infections, meningitis
Salmonella organisms	
S. typhi	Typhoid fever
Other Salmonella organisms	Food poisoning, gastroenteritis
Shigella organisms	Shigellosis, diarrhea with abdominal pain and fever (dysentery)
Staphylococcus aureus	Skin infections, pneumonia, urinary tract infections, acute osteomyelitis, toxic shock syndrome
Streptococcus organisms	
S. faecalis	Genitourinary infection, infection of surgical wounds
S. pneumoniae	Pneumococcal pneumonia
S. pyogenes (group A β-hemolytic streptococci)	Pharyngitis, scarlet fever, rheumatic fever, acute glomerulonephritis, erysipelas, pneumonia
S. pyogenes (group B β-hemolytic streptococci)	Urinary tract infections
S. viridans	Bacterial endocarditis
Treponema pallidum	Syphilis

Table 17-2 Common Disease-Causing Viruses

TYPE	DISEASES CAUSED
Adenoviruses	Upper respiratory tract infection, pneumonia
Arbovirus	Syndrome of fever, malaise, headache, myalgia; aseptic meningitis; encephalitis
Coronavirus	Upper respiratory tract infection
Coxsackieviruses A and B	Upper respiratory tract infection, gastroenteritis, acute myocarditis, aseptic meningitis
Echoviruses	Upper respiratory tract infection, gastroenteritis, aseptic meningitis
Hepatitis	
A	Viral hepatitis
B	Viral hepatitis
C	Viral hepatitis
D	Viral hepatitis
E	Viral hepatitis
Herpesviruses	
Cytomegalovirus (CMV)	Gastroenteritis; pneumonia and retinal damage in immunosuppressed individuals, infectious mononucleosis–like syndrome
Epstein-Barr	Mononucleosis, Burkitt's lymphoma (possibly)
Herpes simplex, type 1	Herpes labialis ("fever blisters"), genital herpes infection
Herpes simplex, type 2	Genital herpes infection
Varicella-zoster	Chickenpox; shingles
HIV	HIV infection, AIDS
Influenza A and B	Upper respiratory tract infection
Mumps	Parotitis, orchitis in postpubertal males
Papovavirus	Warts
Parainfluenza types 1-4	Upper respiratory tract infection
Parvovirus	Gastroenteritis
Poliovirus	Poliomyelitis
Pox viruses	Smallpox
Reoviruses 1, 2, 3	Upper respiratory tract infection
Respiratory syncytial virus	Gastroenteritis, respiratory tract infection
Rhabdovirus	Rabies
Rhinovirus	Upper respiratory tract infection, pneumonia
Rotaviruses	Gastroenteritis
Rubella	German measles
Rubeola	Measles
West Nile virus	Flulike symptoms, meningitis, encephalitis

AIDS, acquired immune deficiency syndrome; *CMV*, cytomegalovirus; *HIV*, human immunodeficiency virus.

Table 17-3 Common Disease-Causing Fungi

ORGANISM	DISEASES CAUSED	ORGANS AFFECTED
Aspergillus fumigatus	Aspergillosis	Lungs*
	Otomycosis	Ears
Blastomyces dermatitidis	Blastomycosis	Lungs, various organs
Candida albicans	Candidiasis	Intestines
	Vaginitis	Vagina
	Thrush	Skin,† mouth
Coccidioides immitis	Coccidioidomycosis	Lungs*
Pneumocystis jiroveci	*Pneumocystis* pneumonia	Lungs*
Sporothrix schenckii	Sporotrichosis	Skin, lymph vessels
Trichophyton spp.	Tinea pedis	Skin†
Microsporum spp.	Tinea capitis	
Epidermophyton spp.	Tinea corporis	

*See Table 30-13: Fungal Infections of the Lung.
†See Table 26-7: Common Fungal Infections of the Skin and Mucous Membranes.

Table 17-4 Examples of Emerging Infections

MICROBE	RELATED DISEASE
Bacteria	
Borrelia burgdorferi	Lyme disease
Campylobacter jejuni	Diarrhea
Escherichia coli O157:H7	Hemorrhagic colitis, hemolytic uremic syndrome
Helicobacter pylori	Peptic ulcer disease
Legionella pneumophila	Legionnaires' disease
Vibrio cholerae O139	New strain associated with epidemic cholera
Virus	
Ebola virus	Ebola hemorrhagic fever
Hantavirus	Hemorrhagic fever associated with severe pulmonary syndrome
Hepatitis C	Parenterally transmitted hepatitis
Hepatitis D	Parenterally transmitted hepatitis
Hepatitis E	Enterically transmitted hepatitis
HIV	HIV disease and AIDS
HHV-6	Roseola subitum
HHV-8	Associated with Kaposi's sarcoma and Castleman's disease in immunosuppressed patients, patients with AIDS
West Nile virus	West Nile fever
Avian influenza A (H5N1) virus	Avian flu
Parasite	
Cryptosporidium parvum	Acute and chronic diarrhea

AIDS, acquired immunodeficiency syndrome; *HHV,* human herpesvirus; *HIV,* human immunodeficiency virus.

disease-carrying mosquitoes (Lashley & Durham, 2007). Earthquakes, such as the recent large one in Haiti, are associated with the spread of water-borne diseases such as cholera. The battle against infectious disease is an age-old problem. However, modern technologies have changed the rules of the game. Global travel, population density, encroachment into new environments, and misused antibiotics have all increased the risk for widespread new or untreatable infectious diseases (Canadian Communicable Disease Report, 2007).

It is interesting that, only a generation ago, many believed that science had conquered infectious disease. Unfortunately, infections remain the leading cause of death worldwide. More than 30 newly recognized infectious diseases have emerged in the last 3 decades, including human immunodeficiency virus (HIV) infection, Lyme disease, hepatitis C, SARS, avian flu, and Ebola virus. In addition, some diseases once thought to be under control, including TB and drug-resistant strains of other bacteria, have re-emerged (Canadian Communicable Disease Report, 2007; Madoff & Kasper, 2008).

Studies in zoonosis (the science of transmission of diseases from animals to humans) indicate that many known infectious diseases come from animals and insects (vectors). The SARS outbreak in China in 2003, for instance, was linked to the civet cat, a small carnivorous mammal found throughout much of Asia and Africa. (SARS is discussed in Chapters 30, 70, and 72.) Animalborne infections are difficult to predict and prevent.

West Nile virus is transmitted by a virus carried by mosquitoes. Mosquitoes acquire the virus as they draw blood from infected birds (Rossi, Ross, & Evans, 2010). The virus does not cause illness in the mosquito but can be transferred to uninfected animals and humans as the mosquito continues to feed. Bird deaths are an indicator of the spread of the West Nile virus and can serve as an early warning sign of an outbreak that can spread quickly if action is not taken in a timely manner (Canadian Communicable Disease Report, 2007; Madoff & Kaspar, 2008). (West Nile virus is discussed in Chapter 59.) Another serious disease transmitted by animals is Lyme disease, which is caused by the bite of a black-legged tick. Lyme disease is most common in northeastern and north central United States, as well as the west coast, including British Columbia.

Sometimes, an organism alters its normal path of transmission. In the past, influenza A viruses were typically spread from birds to pigs to humans. Recently, in cases such as the avian flu outbreak, the virus has been spread directly from chickens to humans. This was first demonstrated in Hong Kong in 1997 and also in the Netherlands in 2003. Infected people generally suffer from conjunctivitis or mild influenza-like symptoms. However, 130 deaths related to avian flu have occurred (Public Health Agency of Canada [PHAC], 2006). Upon discovery of an outbreak, all chickens in the area are typically slaughtered to remove the source of the infection.

The Ebola virus is an emerging disease that has presented an ongoing challenge to public health since it was first seen in 1976. Ebola virus causes a severe hemorrhagic fever and is usually lethal. Therapeutic and preventive measures are extremely limited. The natural reservoir and path of transmission of the virus are unknown, which makes it impossible to effectively combat the disease.

Re-Emerging Infections

Vaccines and proper medications have led to the near eradication of some infections. However, infective agents can always re-emerge if conditions are right. Table 17-5 illustrates some diseases that have re-emerged in recent decades.

For example, the incidence of TB was steadily decreasing beginning in the mid-1950s. However, in the 1990s, the declining trend stabilized and incidence levelled out to 7 cases/100,000 people in Canada (Ontario Agency for Health Protection and Promotion, 2009). There has since been a scaled-up, and there was a steady decline in TB rates between 1999 and 2010 (PHAC, 2011; PHAC, 2012) with the rate currently sitting at 5 cases/100,000 people (PHAC, 2010c). One factor that led to the increase in TB cases was the increase in people with HIV, whose depressed immune systems allow pathogens such as TB bacilli to cause disease. There has been an increase in drug-resistant TB, although, in Canada, the rates remain relatively low (PHAC, 2010a). International travel creates a new dilemma for the local eradication of diseases. Measles, for instance, is no longer considered endemic in Canada, but it remains a leading cause of morbidity in developing countries. Some measles cases in Canada have been found in people with recent travel to these measles-endemic countries (PHAC, 2005).

Table 17-5 Examples of Re-Emerging Infections

MICROBE	DESCRIPTION
Bacteria	
Diphtheria	Localized infection of mucous membranes or skin
Escherichia coli 0157:H7	Acute infection causing abdominal cramping, inflammatory colitis, profuse diarrhea, and hemolytic uremic syndrome
Pertussis	Acute, highly contagious respiratory disease that is characterized by loud whooping inspiration; also known as whooping cough
Tuberculosis	Chronic infection caused by *Mycobacterium tuberculosis*; transmitted by inhalation of infected droplets (see Chapter 30)
Virus	
Dengue fever	Acute infection transmitted by mosquitoes and occurring mainly in tropical and subtropical regions
Parasite	
Giardiasis	Diarrheal illness that usually originates in fecal-contaminated water; also known as traveller's diarrhea

Resistant Organisms

Antibiotic-resistant organisms (AROs), also called multidrug-resistant organisms (MDROs) or "superbugs," are bacteria whose growth and reproduction are unaffected by particular antibiotics. Microorganisms can become resistant to classic antibiotics (e.g., penicillin) as well as newer antibiotic and antiviral agents.

Methicillin-resistant *Staphylococcus aureus* (MRSA), vancomycin-resistant enterococci (VREs), and penicillin-resistant *Streptococcus pneumoniae* are three of the most troublesome resistant bacteria currently causing problems in North America. Table 17-6 describes the most common antibiotic-resistant bacteria.

Bacteria are highly adaptable organisms that have evolved genetic and biochemical means of resisting antimicrobial actions. Genetic mechanisms include mutation and acquisition of new DNA. Biochemically, bacteria resist antibiotics by producing enzymes that destroy or inactivate the drugs. Drug target sites are then altered so that the antibiotic cannot bind to or enter the bacteria. If the drug cannot enter the cell, it cannot kill the bacteria (Centers for Disease Control and Prevention [CDC], 2008a). MRSA can be acquired in a hospital setting as well as in the community. Health care workers exposed to MRSA can become infected and spread the infection to other health care workers and patients. The organism can remain viable for days on environmental surfaces and clothing. Hospital patients most at risk include those who are immunosuppressed (e.g., receiving chemotherapy), have invasive devices (e.g., indwelling catheters), or have breaks in the skin barrier (e.g., surgical wound). VREs are hardier than MRSA and can remain viable on environmental surfaces for weeks. An antiseptic soap such as chlorhexidine is needed to kill these bacteria (DeBaun, 2008). Health Canada (1999) and the Canadian Communicable Disease Report (2007) recommend that infection control for AROs consist of routine practices or standard precautions (see Tables 17-8 and 17-9 later in the chapter), which should be used for all patient care. Certain gram-negative bacteria have developed the ability to produce β-lactamase, an enzyme that makes them resistant to third-generation cephalosporins (e.g., ceftriaxone, cefixime [Suprax]). Infections caused by these bacteria appear with signs and symptoms similar to those of nonresistant strains but require different antibiotics to be effectively treated. Culture specimens should be tested to determine whether the bacteria is β-lactamase producing and that the organism is sensitive to the antibiotic selected for treatment (Chopra et al., 2008).

Drug resistance is a particularly difficult problem when dealing with infectious diseases. Health care providers can contribute to the development of drug-resistant organisms. They can do this by (1) administering antibiotics for viral infections,

Table 17-6 Common Antibiotic-Resistant Organisms and Treatment

BACTERIA	RESISTANT TO	PREFERRED TREATMENT
Staphylococcus aureus	Methicillin	Vancomycin
Staphylococcus epidermidis	Methicillin	Vancomycin
Enterococcus faecalis	Vancomycin (Vancocin), streptomycin, gentamicin (Garamycin)	Penicillin G or ampicillin
Enterococcus faecium	Vancomycin, streptomycin, gentamicin	Penicillin G or ampicillin
Streptococcus pneumoniae	Penicillin G	Ceftriaxone, cefotaxime (Claforan)
Klebsiella pneumoniae	Third-generation cephalosporins (e.g., ceftazidime [Fortaz])	Imipenem/cilastatin (Primaxin), meropenem (Merrem IV)

Table 17-7   Decreasing Risk for Antibiotic-Resistant Infection

1. **Do Not Take Antibiotics to Prevent Illness.** Doing this increases your risk for developing resistant infection.

   Exceptions include taking antibiotics before certain surgeries and taking antibiotics before dental work if you have a heart valve disorder.

2. **Wash Your Hands Frequently.** Handwashing is the single most important thing you can do to prevent an infection.

3. **Follow Directions.** Not taking your antibiotic as prescribed or skipping doses can encourage the development of antibiotic-resistant bacteria.

4. **Finish Your Antibiotic.** Do not stop taking your antibiotic when you feel better. If you stop taking your antibiotic early, the hardiest bacteria survive and multiply. Eventually you could develop an infection resistant to many antibiotics. You should never have leftover antibiotics.

5. **Do Not Request an Antibiotic for Flu or Colds.** If your health care provider says that you do not need an antibiotic, chances are you do not. Antibiotics are effective against bacterial infections but not viruses, which cause colds and flus.

6. **Do Not Take Leftover Antibiotics.** People often save unfinished antibiotics for later use or borrow leftover drugs from family or friends. This is dangerous because (1) the leftover antibiotic may not be appropriate for you, (2) your illness may not be a bacterial infection, (3) old antibiotics can lose their effectiveness and in some cases can even be fatal, and (4) there will not be enough doses in a leftover bottle to allow for a full treatment.

(2) succumbing to pressures from patients to prescribe unnecessary antibiotic therapy, (3) using inadequate drug regimens to treat infections, or (4) using broad-spectrum or combination agents for infections that should be treated with first-line medications. Patients who miss doses or do not take antibiotics for the full duration of the prescribed therapy also contribute to the development of resistance. In addition, limited resources or access to medications makes it difficult for some patients to get adequate treatment for infections. Patients and their families should be taught that the proper use of antibiotics (Table 17-7) is crucial to treatment success and prevention of drug-resistant pathogens.

Health Care–Associated Infections

Health care–associated infections (HAIs) (formerly called *nosocomial infections*) are infections that are acquired as a result of exposure to a microorganism in any setting where health care is delivered (e.g., acute or long-term care, ambulatory clinic, home) and are related to receiving health care (Siegel, Rhinehart, Jackson, & Chiarello, 2006). An estimated 8000 people die in Canadian hospitals each year as a result of infections acquired during their hospitalization (Zoutman et al., 2003). According to a 2002 prevalence study of HAIs by the Canadian Nosocomial Infection Surveillance Program (CNISP), the prevalence of HAIs in adults was 10.5% (PHAC, 2007a). Surgical patients are at greater risk. In addition, some bacteria that are not normally pathological can cause infections in patients who are immunocompromised as a result of illness or treatment of illness. HAIs can be caused by any

organism, but certain bacteria, including *E. coli, S. aureus, Enterobacter aerogenes, Clostridium difficile,* and various types of streptococci, are the more common culprits. At least 30% of HAIs can be prevented by following infection prevention strategies (Ontario Ministry of Health and Long-Term Care, 2007). HAIs are often transmitted from patient to patient through direct contact by health care providers. Hand hygiene (handwashing or use of alcohol-based hand rub) between patient visits and procedures as well as appropriate use of personal protective equipment (PPE) such as gloves remain the first lines of defence in preventing the spread of HAIs. It is important to remember that *C. difficile* is not killed by alcohol-based hand rub. Handwashing with soap and water must be followed in this instance. Isolated infections can be caused when bacteria that are normally present in one area of the body are introduced into another area. Therefore, care must be taken to change gloves and use hand hygiene when moving from one task to another, even when working with one patient (CDC, 2007a).

AGE-RELATED CONSIDERATIONS: INFECTION IN OLDER ADULTS

For older adult patients, the rate of HAI is two to three times higher than for younger patients. Individuals in long-term care facilities have a greater incidence of illness and are at special risk. Age-related changes of decreased immunocompetence, the presence of co-morbidities, and an increase in disability all contribute to higher infection rates (High et al., 2009). Infections common in older adults include pneumonia, urinary tract infections, skin infections, and TB (High et al., 2009). Urinary tract infections are the most common HAIs in older adults residing in long-term care facilities. They are often found in patients who have indwelling catheters. Infections in older adults often have atypical presentations, and cognitive and behavioural changes appear before alterations occur in laboratory values (High et al., 2009). Suspicion of disease should typically begin when changes in ability to perform daily activities or in cognitive function occur. Fever should not be relied on to indicate infection in older adults because many have lower core body temperatures and decreased immune responses. In addition, underlying diseases, increased frequency of drug reactions, and institutionalization can all complicate the management of the older adult with infection.

Infection Prevention and Control

Infection Precautions

If a patient develops an infection that is considered a risk to others, infection precautions may be needed. The purpose of these precautions is to prevent the transmission of organisms from patients to health care providers, from health care providers to patients, and from one patient to another. The CDC issue isolation precaution guidelines that are used in many health care institutions in Canada and around the world. Health Canada has issued similar recommendations (Health Canada, 1999).

Both sets of guidelines contain two levels of precautions (Table 17-8): *routine practices or standard precautions,* which are designed for the care of all patients in hospitals and health care facilities regardless of their diagnosis or presumed infection

Table 17-8 Summary of Routine Practices and Additional Precautions for Preventing the Transmission of Infection in Health Care

ROUTINE PRACTICES OR STANDARD PRECAUTIONS	ADDITIONAL OR TRANSMISSION-BASED PRECAUTIONS: AIRBORNE*	ADDITIONAL OR TRANSMISSION-BASED PRECAUTIONS: DROPLET*	ADDITIONAL OR TRANSMISSION-BASED PRECAUTIONS: CONTACT
When to Use			
All patients	Use in addition to routine practices or standard precautions for patients known to be or suspected of being infected with microorganisms transmitted by airborne droplet (e.g., measles, varicella, tuberculosis). Requires negative-pressure room.	Use in addition to routine practices or standard precautions for patients known to be or suspected of being infected with microorganisms transmitted by droplets (e.g., *Haemophilus influenzae, Neisseria meningitidis, Streptococcus pneumoniae, Mycoplasma pneumoniae,* febrile respiratory illness).	Use in addition to routine practices or standard precautions for specified patients known to be or suspected of being infected with epidemiologically important microorganisms that can be transmitted by direct contact with patient or environmental surfaces (e.g., enteric pathogens, multidrug-resistant bacteria, *Clostridium difficile,* herpes simplex).
Hand Hygiene			
Perform hand hygiene (the removal or killing of microorganisms on the hands). This is done either by handwashing or by using alcohol-based hand rubs. Using alcohol-based hand rubs is more effective than washing hands (even with antibacterial soap) when hands are not visibly soiled. Hand hygiene should be performed (1) before initial patient contact or contact with the patient's environment, (2) before aseptic procedures, (3) after body fluid exposure risk, and (4) after contact with a patient or the patient's environment.	Same as routine practices or standard precautions.	Same as routine practices or standard precautions.	Same as routine practices or standard precautions.
Gloves			
Wear nonsterile gloves when touching blood, body fluids, secretions, excretions, and contaminated items; put on clean gloves just before touching mucous membranes and nonintact skin; remove gloves promptly after use, before touching noncontaminated items, environmental surfaces, or going to another patient.	Same as routine practices or standard precautions.	Same as routine practices or standard precautions.	In addition to glove use as described in routine practices or standard precautions, wear gloves when entering the room and whenever providing direct patient care or having hand contact with potentially contaminated surfaces or items in patient's environment.
Mask, Eye Protection, Face Shield			
Wear mask and eye protection or face shield to protect mucous membranes of eyes, nose, and mouth during procedures and patient care activities likely to generate splashes or sprays of blood, body fluids, secretions, and excretions. Wear within 1 m of coughing patient.	In addition to routine practices or standard precautions, wear respiratory protection when entering room of patient known to have or suspected of having tuberculosis. NOTE: check the facility's policy for use of respirator.	In addition to routine practices or standard precautions, wear a mask.	Same as routine practices or standard precautions.

Table 17-8 Summary of Routine Practices and Additional Precautions for Preventing the Transmission of Infection in Health Care—cont'd

ROUTINE PRACTICES OR STANDARD PRECAUTIONS	ADDITIONAL OR TRANSMISSION-BASED PRECAUTIONS: AIRBORNE*	ADDITIONAL OR TRANSMISSION-BASED PRECAUTIONS: DROPLET*	ADDITIONAL OR TRANSMISSION-BASED PRECAUTIONS: CONTACT
Gown			
Wear clean, nonsterile gown to protect skin and prevent soiling of clothing during procedures and patient care activities likely to generate splashes or sprays of blood, body fluids, secretions, or excretions or likely to cause soiling of clothing; remove gown promptly when tasks are completed; wash hands.	Same as routine practices or standard precautions.	Same as routine practices or standard precautions.	Wear clean, nonsterile gown if substantial contact is anticipated with patient, surfaces, or items in environment; wear gown if patient is incontinent or has diarrhea, an ileostomy, a colostomy, or uncontained wound drainage; remove gown carefully when tasks are completed; wash hands.
Linen			
Handle, transport, and process used linen in manner that prevents skin and mucous membrane exposure, contamination of clothing, and environmental soiling.	Same as routine practices or standard precautions.	Same as routine practices or standard precautions.	Same as routine practices or standard precautions.
Patient Transport			
	Limit movement and transport of patient from room to instances of essential purposes only; if transport or movement is necessary, minimize patient dispersal of droplet nuclei by placing surgical mask on patient, if possible.	Limit movement and transport of patient from room to instances of essential purposes only; if transport or movement is necessary, minimize patient dispersal of droplet nuclei by masking patient, if possible.	Limit movement and transport of patient from room to instances of essential purposes only; if transport is necessary, ensure that precautions are maintained to minimize contamination of environmental surfaces or equipment.

*In the case of certain infections (e.g., chickenpox and disseminated zoster), a combination of airborne and contact transmission precautions may be required. For certain other infections (e.g., influenza and invasive group A streptococcus), a combination of droplet and contact precautions is required.
Source: Provincial Infectious Diseases Advisory Committee (PIDAC). (2008 [revised 2010]). Best practices for hand hygiene in all health care settings. Retrieved from *http://www.ontla.on.ca/library/repository/mon/25009/312519.pdf*; and Health Canada. (1999). Routine practices and additional precautions for preventing the transmission of infection in health care. Canadian Communicable Disease Report, 25, S4. Retrieved from *http:// www.opseu.org/hands/cdr25s4e.pdf*

status, and *additional precautions or transmission-based precautions,* which are used for patients known to be or suspected of being infected with epidemiologically important pathogens that can be transmitted by airborne or droplet transmission or by contact with dry skin or contaminated surfaces.

The routine practices or standard precautions system applies to (1) blood; (2) all body fluids, secretions, and excretions regardless of whether they contain visible blood; (3) nonintact skin; and (4) mucous membranes. Routine practices or standard precautions are designed to reduce the risk of transmission of microorganisms from both recognized and unrecognized sources of infection in hospitals. Routine practices or standard precautions should be applied to all patients regardless of diagnosis or infection status.

Additional or transmission-based precautions are designed for patients suspected or documented of being infected with highly transmissible or epidemiologically important pathogens for which additional precautions beyond routine practices or standard precautions are needed to interrupt transmission in

hospitals. The three types of additional or transmission-based precautions are *airborne precautions, droplet precautions,* and *contact precautions.* They may be used in combination for diseases that have multiple routes of transmission. When used either by themselves or in combination, these precautions are used in addition to routine practices or standard precautions.

Preventing Occupational Infections in Health Care Workers

In 2002, Health Canada issued updated standards for preventing and controlling occupational infections in health care workers. These standards mandated that any employer whose employees are potentially exposed to blood from needles and other sharps must implement sharps safety devices wherever feasible. Many provinces have implemented mandatory use of safety-engineered needles and needle-free infusion devices. In addition, employees at risk need to be provided with appropriate PPE. Health care workers must minimize or eliminate exposure to infectious mate-

Table 17-9 Health Canada Recommendations for the Use of Personal Protective Equipment for Health Care Workers

EQUIPMENT	INDICATIONS FOR USE
Medical gloves	Should be worn for all procedures that might involve direct skin or mucous membrane contact with blood or fluid capable of transmitting bloodborne pathogens. May also be indicated for other activities (e.g., procedures involving other infectious agents, toxins, or contaminated equipment).
Masks and protective eyewear (e.g., goggles, safety glasses) or face shields	Should be worn to protect mucous membranes, nonintact skin, and conjunctiva during procedures that are likely to generate splashes of blood or fluids capable of transmitting bloodborne pathogens.
Gowns or aprons	Should be worn during procedures that are likely to generate splashes of blood or fluid capable of transmitting bloodborne pathogens. Assessment of the specific risk will determine the type of gown required (e.g., fluid-resistant).

Source: Based on Health Canada. (1997). Preventing the transmission of blood-borne pathogens in health care and public service settings. Full recommendations available at *http://www.collectionscanada.gc.ca/webarchives/20071124030210/http://www.phac-aspc.gc.ca/publicat/ccdr-rmtc/97vol23/23s3/index.html*

rial. When that is not possible, appropriate PPE must be selected. These include gloves, clothing, and facial protection (Table 17-9). Appropriate PPE will vary depending on the situation (Health Canada, 2002).

In the event that a health care worker is exposed to blood or body fluids, as a result of either a needle stick or a mucous membrane splash, the worker should seek immediate medical attention to assess the level of risk for acquiring a bloodborne virus from the incident. If the risk is deemed serious enough to put the person at risk for acquiring HIV, postexposure prophylaxis (PEP) will be initiated. There is no PEP for hepatitis C virus. Statistics have been compiled since the early 1990s about the rates of HIV seroconversion in health care workers as a result of an accidental exposure, and in fact, the rates are extremely low, but there have been documented cases, so it is important for nurses to use routine practices or standard precautions with every patient with whom they come into contact (Department of Health, 2008; McCall, McMillan, & Pielak, 2005).

Human Immunodeficiency Virus Infection

The history of the human immunodeficiency virus (HIV) epidemic in Canada and the United States has unfolded over the last 3 decades. HIV had been circulating in sub-Saharan Africa since the early 1920s (Pepin, 2011), but it was not until 1981 that public health officials documented the presence of a new disease that would become known as the *acquired immunodeficiency syndrome* (AIDS). By 1985, the causative agent, HIV, had been identified, and AIDS was determined to be the end stage

of chronic HIV infection. In addition, an antibody test was developed and routes of transmission were determined. Drug therapy to treat the infection became available in 1987 with the release of zidovudine (ZDV, azidothymidine [AZT], Retrovir) and has since expanded. Since 1994, several important advances have been made, including the development of laboratory tests to assess the number of HIV particles in the blood **(viral load)**, the production of new drugs, combination drug therapy, the ability to test for antiretroviral drug resistance, treatment to decrease the risk of transmission from mother to baby (McCall, Vicol, & Tsang, 2009; Stek, 2008), and the use of treatment as prevention (Montaner, 2011). In developed countries around the world, these advances have led to decreases in the number of HIV-related deaths, improved quality of life, and decreases in the number of children born with HIV (PHAC, 2010c). Unfortunately, these advances are not effective or available for all those who need them. Although great progress has been made, the HIV epidemic is not over, there are signs that it is levelling off, with fewer new infections each year, but it continues to take its toll with approximately 7000 people being newly infected every day (United Nations AIDS [UNAIDS], 2010). Nursing care for patients with HIV infection continues to be a critical need that must change as new findings and treatment advances emerge.

Significance of the Problem

Almost 1.5 million people were living with HIV in North America at the end of 2008, with an estimated 70,000 new infections and 26,000 HIV-related deaths that year (UNAIDS, 2009). Of those living with the infection, 260,000 (25%) were adolescent and adult women and 11,000 were children younger than age 15. At the end of 2008, Health Canada estimated there were approximately 65,000 people in Canada living with HIV (including those living with AIDS) and that approximately 17,000, or 30%, were not aware that they were infected (PHAC, 2010b). In addition, treatment has provided major advances in the ability to keep HIV-infected people healthy for longer periods, and the death rate has fallen dramatically (Centre for Infectious Disease Prevention and Control, 2007). Globally, HIV has been devastating. Since the beginning of the pandemic, more than 60 million people have been infected, and more than 30 million of those have died (UNAIDS, 2011). At the end of 2009, an estimated 33.3 million people—including 2.2 million children younger than age 15—were living with HIV. During that year, 2.6 million people were newly infected with HIV and over 1.8 million died of HIV-related causes (UNAIDS, 2010). The number of new HIV infections in Canada in 2009 did not decrease and may have increased slightly compared with 2005 (Health Canada, 2010b). The burden of HIV is not evenly distributed. Since the beginning of the epidemic, sub-Saharan Africa has been the most devastated, but Asia, Russia, Central America, and South America also have rampant epidemics. In developing countries, the major mode of transmission is through heterosexual sex, and women and children bear a large part of the burden of illness. Industrialized countries have fared better but have not been able to eliminate the infection or provide appropriate care to all HIV-infected individuals (World Health Organization [WHO], 2007). For the most part, HIV remains a disease of marginalized individuals: those who are disenfranchised by virtue of sex, race, sexual orientation, poverty, drug use, or lack of access to health care (PHAC, 2007b).

Transmission of HIV

HIV is a fragile virus. It can be transmitted only under specific conditions that allow contact with infected body fluids, including blood, semen, vaginal secretions, and breast milk. Transmission of HIV occurs through sexual intercourse with an infected partner, exposure to HIV-infected blood or blood products, as a result of either contaminated transfusion or needle sharing, and perinatal transmission during pregnancy at the time of delivery or through breastfeeding (Health Canada, 2010a).

HIV-infected individuals can transmit HIV to others within a few days after becoming infected. After that, the ability to transmit HIV is lifelong. Transmission of HIV is subject to the same requirements as other microorganisms: a large enough amount of the virus must enter the body of a susceptible host. Duration and frequency of contact, volume of fluid, virulence and concentration of the organism, and host immune status all affect whether infection actually occurs after an exposure. The viral load in the blood, the semen, the vaginal secretions, or the breast milk of the "donor" is an important variable. In HIV infection, large amounts of virus can be found in the blood during the first 2 to 6 months after infection and again during the late stages of the disease (Figure 17-1). Unprotected sexual or blood exposure to an infected individual is more risky during these periods, although HIV can be transmitted during all phases of the disease (CDC, 2012).

HIV is not spread casually. The virus cannot be transmitted through hugging, dry kissing, shaking hands, sharing eating utensils, using toilet seats, or attending school or working with an HIV-infected person. It is not transmitted through tears, saliva, urine, emesis, sputum, feces, or sweat. Repeated studies have failed to demonstrate transmission of the virus by respiratory droplets, enteric routes, or casual encounters in any setting. Health care workers have a very low risk of acquiring HIV at work, even after a needle-stick injury (McCall et al., 2005; CDC, 2010). Should a health care worker become exposed, she or he should follow the hospital policy for reporting needle-stick incidents.

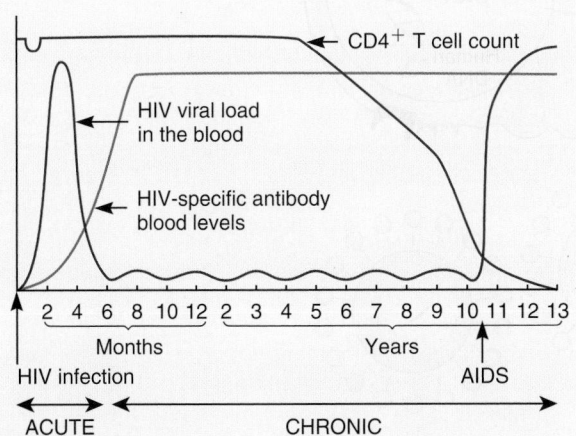

Figure 17-1 Viral load in the blood and CD4+ T cell counts across the spectrum of untreated human immunodeficiency virus (HIV) infection. *AIDS*, acquired immune deficiency syndrome.

Sexual Transmission

Sexual contact with an HIV-infected partner is the most common mode of transmission. Sexual activity provides an opportunity for contact with semen, vaginal secretions, and blood, all of which have lymphocytes that contain HIV.

Although men who have sex with men (MSM) still account for most cases of HIV in Canada and the United States, heterosexual transmission is becoming more prevalent and is now the most common method of infection for women. The most risky form of sexual intercourse is unprotected anal intercourse (Sanchez et al., 2006). During any form of sexual intercourse (anal, vaginal, or oral), the risk of infection is greater for the partner who receives the semen, although infection can also be transmitted to an inserting partner. This increased risk occurs because the receiver has prolonged contact with the semen. This helps explain why women are more easily infected than men during heterosexual intercourse. Sexual activities that involve blood, such as during menstruation or as a result of trauma to tissues, also increase the risk of transmission. In addition, the presence of genital lesions caused by other sexually transmitted infections (STIs) (e.g., herpes, syphilis) increases the likelihood of infection (Toblan & Quinn, 2009).

Contact With Blood and Blood Products

HIV is transmitted by exposure to contaminated blood through the accidental or intended sharing of injection equipment. Sharing equipment to inject illegal drugs is a major means of transmission in many large metropolitan areas and is becoming more common in smaller cities and rural areas. Once used, equipment used to inject any drug, whether prescribed or not, is contaminated, potentially with HIV, other bloodborne organisms, or both, and sharing that equipment can result in disease transmission (AIDS InfoNet, 2009a; CDC, 2010).

In Canada, an estimated 1150 individuals were infected with HIV through blood transfusions between 1978 and 1985. In 1985, the practices of routine screening of blood donors to identify at-risk individuals and testing donated blood for the presence of HIV were implemented, thereby improving the safety of the blood supply. HIV infection as a result of blood transfusions is now unlikely. In 2001, a new, highly sensitive nucleic acid amplification test (NAAT) was implemented by the Canadian Blood Services to detect HIV genetic material in blood of potential donors. The NAAT has a much shorter window period than antibody testing and is now the standard test for donated blood in Canada.

Puncture wounds are the most common means of work-related transmission. The risk of infection after a needle-stick exposure to HIV-infected blood is 0.3 to 0.4% (or 3-4 out of 1000). The risk is higher if the exposure involves blood from a patient with a high viral load, a deep puncture wound, a needle with a hollow bore and visible blood, a device used for venous or arterial access, or a patient who dies within 60 days. Splash exposures of blood on skin with an open lesion present some risk, but it is much lower than from a puncture wound (McCall et al., 2005; Hamlyn & Easterbrook, 2007).

Perinatal Transmission

Perinatal transmission is the most common route of infection for children. Transmission from an HIV-infected mother to her infant can occur during pregnancy, at the time of delivery, or after

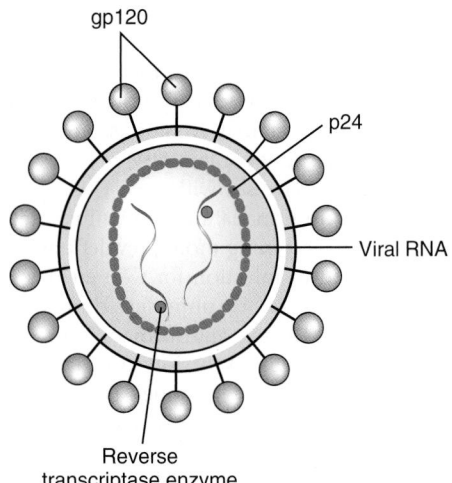

gp120

p24

Viral RNA

Reverse
transcriptase enzyme

Figure 17-2 HIV is surrounded by an envelope made up of proteins (including gp120) and contains a core of viral RNA and proteins (including p24).

birth through breastfeeding (CDC, 2007b). On average, 25% of infants born to untreated HIV-infected women will be born with HIV. Fortunately, with the use of antiretroviral therapy (ART), transmission has been reduced to less than 2% (CDC, 2009d). Risk of transmission from breastfeeding is between 7 and 22% (Dunn, Newell, Ades, & Peckham, 1992).

Pathophysiology

Human immunodeficiency virus (HIV) is an RNA virus that was discovered in 1983. RNA viruses are called **retroviruses** because they replicate in a "backward" manner (going from RNA to DNA). Like all viruses, HIV cannot replicate unless it is inside a living cell. HIV can enter a cell when the gp120 "knobs" (Figure 17-2) on the viral envelope bind to specific CD4 receptor sites and CCR5 and CXCR4 co-receptor sites on the cell's surface (Figure 17-3). Once bound, viral genetic material enters the cell. In the cell, viral RNA is transcribed into a double strand of viral DNA with the assistance of **reverse transcriptase,** an enzyme made by HIV and other retroviruses. At this point, viral

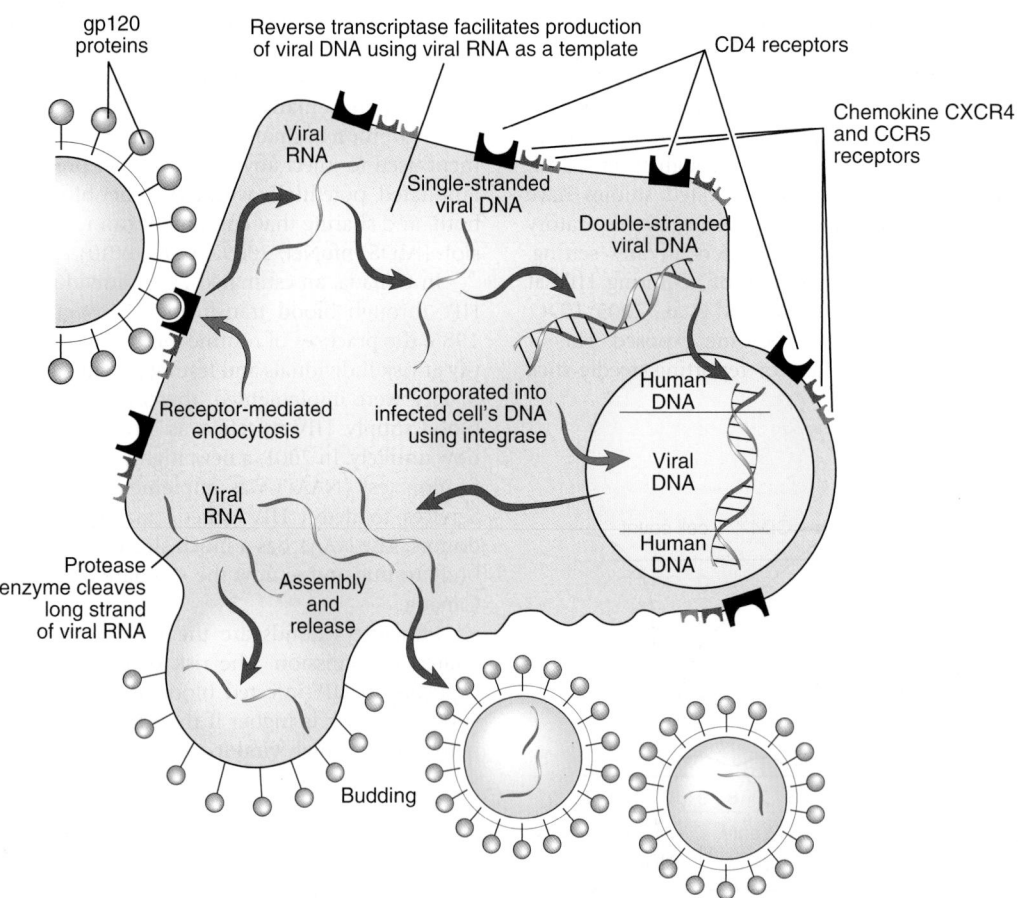

Figure 17-3 HIV has gp120 glycoproteins that attach to CD4 and chemokine CXCR4 and CCR5 receptors on the surface of CD4⁺ T cells. Viral RNA then enters the cell, produces viral DNA in the presence of reverse transcriptase, and incorporates itself into the cellular genome in the presence of integrase, causing permanent cellular infection and the production of new virions. New viral RNA develops initially in long strands that are cut in the presence of protease and leave the cell through a budding process that ultimately contributes to cellular destruction.

DNA can enter the cell's nucleus and, using an enzyme called integrase, splice itself into the genome, becoming a permanent part of the cell's genetic structure. There are two consequences of this action: (1) because all genetic material is replicated during cellular division, all daughter cells from the infected cell will also be infected; and (2) because the genome now contains viral DNA, the cell's genetic codes can direct the cell to make HIV. Production of HIV within the cell is a complicated process that results in long strands of HIV RNA. These are cut into appropriate lengths with the assistance of the enzyme protease during the budding sequence (AIDS InfoNet, 2009b; Ortiz & Silvestri, 2009).

Initial infection with HIV results in **viremia** (large amounts of virus in the blood). This is followed within a few weeks by a prolonged period during which HIV levels in the blood remain low even without treatment (see Figure 17-1). During this time, which may last for 10 to 12 years, there are few clinical symptoms. It was initially thought that this phase represented a latency period during which very little viral activity occurred. It is now known that HIV replication occurs at rapid and constant rates in the blood and lymph tissues from early in the infection. A steady-state viral load can be maintained in the body of infected individuals for many years. To do this, 108 to 109 new viruses are produced each day. A major consequence of rapid replication is that copy errors are made, causing mutations that contribute to difficulties in treatment and vaccine development (AIDS InfoNet, 2009b; Ortiz & Silvestri, 2009).

In a normal immune response, foreign antigens interact with B cells and T cells. In the initial stages of HIV infection, these cells respond and function normally. B cells make HIV-specific antibodies that are effective in reducing viral loads in the blood, and activated T cells mount a cellular immune response to viruses trapped in the lymph nodes (O'Bryne & MacPherson, 2008; Ortiz & Silvestri, 2009).

HIV infects human cells that have CD4 receptors on their surfaces. These include lymphocytes, monocytes and macrophages, astrocytes, and oligodendrocytes. Immune dysfunction in HIV disease is caused predominantly by damage to and destruction of CD4$^+$ T cells (also known as T helper cells or CD4$^+$ T lymphocytes). These cells are targeted because they have more CD4 receptors on their surfaces than other CD4 receptor–bearing cells. This is unfortunate because CD4$^+$ T cells play a key role in the ability of the immune system to recognize and defend against pathogens. Adults normally have approximately 800 to 1200 CD4$^+$ T cells per microlitre (μL) of blood (normal ranges may vary). The normal lifespan of a CD4$^+$ T cell is about 100 days, but HIV-infected CD4$^+$ T cells will die after an average lifespan of only 2 days (O'Byrne & MacPherson, 2008; Ortiz & Silvestri, 2009). The compromise of the immune system is also caused by the chronic state of immune activation that is a result of HIV infection. This activation leads to elevated inflammatory markers and destruction of T helper cells (Wasserman, Segal-Maurer, Wehbeh, & Rubin, 2011).

Viral activity destroys about 1 billion CD4$^+$ T cells every day. Fortunately, the bone marrow and the thymus are able to produce enough CD4$^+$ T cells to replace the destroyed cells for many years. Eventually, however, the ability of HIV to destroy CD4$^+$ T cells exceeds the body's ability to replace the cells. The result is a decline in the CD4$^+$ T-cell count and a decrease in immune capability. Generally, the immune system will remain healthy with more than 500 CD4$^+$ T cells per microlitre. Immune problems start to occur when the count drops to 200 to 499 CD4$^+$ T cells per microlitre. Severe problems develop

with less than 200 CD4$^+$ T cells per microlitre and a CD4 fraction of less than 15%. In HIV infection, a point is eventually reached where so many CD4$^+$ T cells are destroyed that not enough remain to regulate immune responses (see Figure 17-1). The major concern related to immune suppression is the development of **opportunistic diseases** (infections and cancers that occur in immunosuppressed patients that can lead to disability, disease, and death) (CDC, 2009b; O'Byrne & MacPherson, 2008).

Clinical Manifestations and Complications

The typical course of untreated HIV infection follows the pattern shown in Figure 17-4. However, it is important to remember that HIV is highly individualized. The information depicted in Figure 17-4 represents data from large groups of people and should not be used to predict an individual's lifespan after HIV infection.

Acute Infection

Development of HIV-specific antibodies *(seroconversion)* is frequently accompanied by a flulike syndrome of fever, swollen lymph glands, sore throat, headache, malaise, nausea, muscle and joint pain, diarrhea, and/or a diffuse rash. These symptoms, called **acute retroviral syndrome,** generally occur 1 to 3 weeks after the initial infection and last for 1 to 2 weeks, although some of the symptoms may continue for several months. During this time, a high level of HIV in the blood is noted and CD4$^+$ T-cell counts fall temporarily but quickly return to baseline (see Figure. 17-1). In most people, acute retroviral symptoms are moderate and may be mistaken for a cold or flu. In some people, neurological complications, such as aseptic meningitis, peripheral

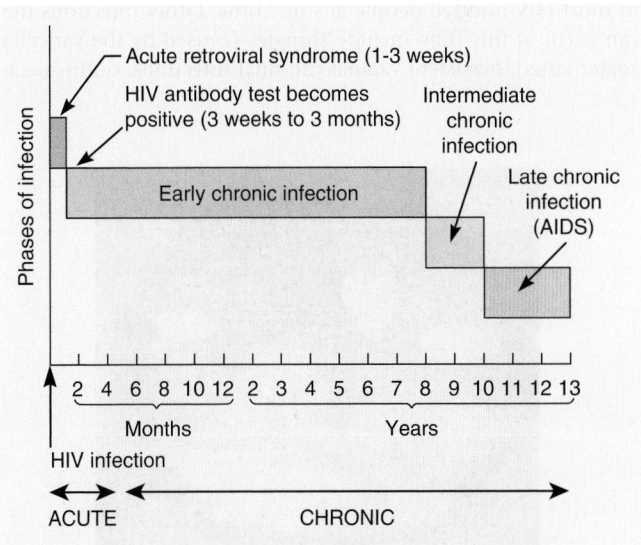

Figure 17-4 Timeline for the spectrum of untreated human immunodeficiency virus (HIV) infection. The timeline represents the course of the illness from the time of infection to the clinical manifestations of disease. *AIDS,* acquired immune deficiency syndrome.

neuropathy, facial palsy, or Guillain-Barré syndrome, have developed (Valenti, 2008).

Chronic HIV Infection

Early Chronic Infection. The median interval between untreated HIV infection and a diagnosis of AIDS is about 10 years. During this time, CD4$^+$ T-lymphocyte counts remain above 500 cells per microlitre (normal or slightly decreased), and the viral load in the blood will be low. This phase has been referred to as asymptomatic disease, but fatigue, headache, low-grade fever, night sweats, persistent generalized lymphadenopathy (PGL), and other symptoms often occur (CDC, 2008b).

Because most of the symptoms during early infection are vague and nonspecific for HIV, people may not be aware that they are infected. The PHAC (2010d) estimates that approximately 30% of individuals infected with HIV are unaware of their status. During this time, infected people continue activities that may include high-risk sexual and drug-using behaviours, creating a public health problem because infected people can transmit HIV to others even if they have no symptoms. Personal health is also affected because people who do not know they are infected have no motivation to seek treatment or to make changes in health habits that could beneficially alter the quality and quantity of their lives.

Intermediate Chronic Infection. When the CD4$^+$ T-cell count drops to 200 to 500 cells per microlitre, the viral load rises and HIV advances to a more active stage. Symptoms seen in earlier phases tend to become worse, causing persistent fever, frequent drenching night sweats, chronic diarrhea, recurrent headaches, and fatigue severe enough to interrupt normal routines. Other problems that may occur at this time include localized infections, lymphadenopathy, and nervous system manifestations (CDC, 2008b).

The most common infection associated with this phase of HIV disease is oropharyngeal candidiasis, or thrush (Figure 17-5). *Candida* rarely causes problems in healthy adults, but it will occur in most HIV-infected people at some time. Other infections that can occur at this time include shingles (caused by the varicella-zoster virus), persistent vaginal candidal infections, outbreaks of oral or genital herpes, bacterial infections, and Kaposi's sarcoma (KS) (Figure 17-6). **Oral hairy leukoplakia,** an Epstein-Barr virus infection that causes painless, white, raised lesions on the lateral aspect of the tongue, can also occur (Figure 17-7). Oral lesions may provide the earliest indication of HIV infection.

Late Chronic Infection or AIDS. A diagnosis of **acquired immune deficiency syndrome (AIDS)** cannot be made until the HIV-infected patient meets the criteria established by the WHO (2007).

These criteria (Table 17-10) are more likely to occur when the immune system becomes severely compromised. As the viral load increases, decreases in the absolute number of lymphocytes, as well as the percentage of lymphocytes, may also occur, and the risk of developing one or more of the opportunistic diseases that contribute to disability and death increases (AIDS InfoNet, 2009b; Ortiz & Silvestri, 2009).

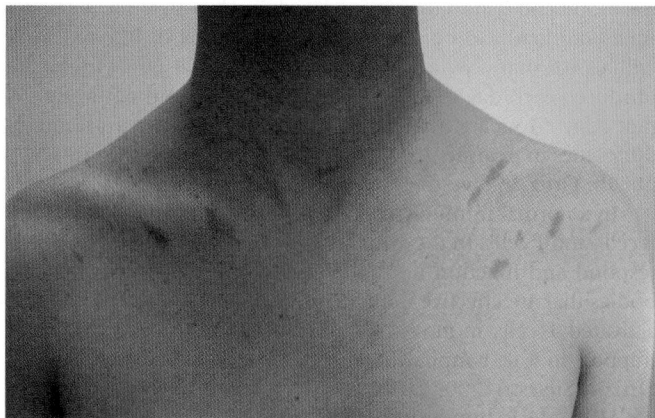

Figure 17-6 Kaposi's sarcoma (KS). Malignant vascular lesion on the torso. KS lesions can appear anywhere on the skin surface or on internal organs. Lesions vary in size from pinpoint to very large and may appear in a variety of shades.

Source: Courtesy Jeffrey Kwong.

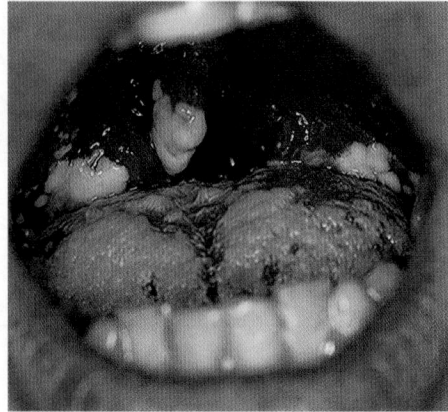

Figure 17-5 Oral thrush involving the hard and soft palate surfaces.

Source: Emond, R., Welsby, P., & Rowland, H. (2003). *Colour atlas of infectious diseases* (4th ed.). Edinburgh: Mosby.

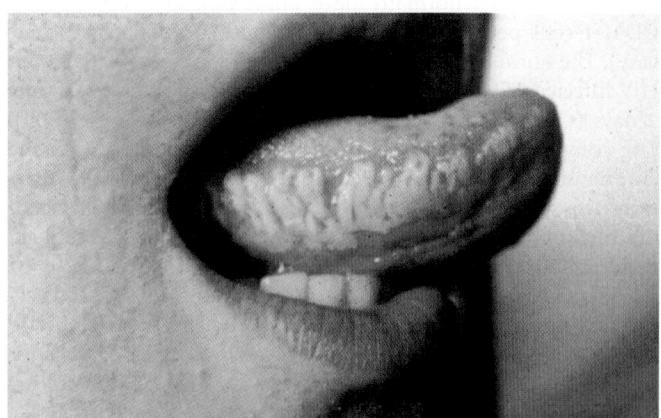

Figure 17-7 Oral hairy leukoplakia on the lateral aspect of the tongue.

Source: Set of slides published in 1992 by Jon Fuller, MD, and Howard Libman, MD, at Boston University School of Medicine, Boston.

Table 17-10 Diagnostic Criteria for AIDS

AIDS is diagnosed when an individual with HIV develops at least one of these conditions:

- HIV wasting syndrome (*wasting* is defined as a loss of 10% or more of ideal body mass)
- *Pneumocystis* pneumonia
- Recurrent bacterial pneumonia
- Chronic herpes simplex virus infection
- Esophageal candidiasis
- Extrapulmonary tuberculosis
- Kaposi's sarcoma
- Cytomegalovirus disease (other than liver, spleen, or lymph nodes)
- Central nervous system toxoplasmosis
- HIV encephalopathy
- Extrapulmonary cryptococcosis (including meningitis)
- Disseminated nontuberculous mycobacteria infection
- Progressive multifocal leukoencephalopathy (PML)
- Chronic cryptosporidiosis
- Chronic isosporiasis
- Disseminated mycosis (coccidiomycosis or histoplasmosis)
- Recurrent nontyphoid *Salmonella* bacteremia
- Lymphoma (cerebral or B-cell non-Hodgkin's)
- Invasive cervical carcinoma
- Atypical disseminated leishmaniasis
- Symptomatic HIV-associated nephropathy
- Symptomatic HIV-associated cardiomyopathy

AIDS, acquired immune deficiency syndrome; *HIV*, human immunodeficiency virus.
Source: World Health Organization (WHO). (2007). WHO Case definitions of HIV for surveillance and revised clinical staging and immunological classification of HIV-related disease in adults and children. Geneva: World Health Organization. Retrieved from *http://www.who.int/hiv/pub/guidelines/HIVstaging150307.pdf*

Opportunistic diseases, often a reactivation of a prior infection, generally do not occur in the presence of a functioning immune system. Numerous infections, a variety of malignancies, wasting, and dementia can result from HIV-related immune impairment (Table 17-11). Organisms that do not usually cause disease in people with functioning immune systems can cause severe, debilitating, disseminated, and life-threatening infections during this stage. Several opportunistic diseases are likely to occur at the same time, further compounding the difficulties of diagnosis and treatment. Advances in HIV treatment have led to significant decreases in opportunistic diseases because successful treatment helps maintain a functioning immune system (CDC, 2009b).

Diagnostic Studies

Diagnosis of HIV Infection

The most useful screening tests for HIV are those that detect HIV-specific antibodies. The major problem with these tests is that there is a median delay of 2 months after infection before antibodies can be detected (see Figure 17-1). This creates a **window period** during which an infected individual will not test positive for HIV antibodies. HIV-antibody screening is generally done in the sequence shown in Table 17-12. This process produces highly accurate results. New "rapid" HIV-antibody tests provide results in 20 minutes and are strongly recommended by the CDC (2006). Rapid testing is highly reliable and provides immediate feedback to patients who can then be counselled about treatment and prevention. Positive rapid tests must be confirmed as described in Table 17-12, but results can be given to the patient as soon as they are available (Armington, 2005). This is an important advantage because many people do not return to get their test results, which is necessary when other tests are used.

Laboratory Studies in HIV Infection

The progression of HIV infection is monitored by two tests: $CD4^+$ T-cell counts and CD4 fraction. As the disease progresses, there is usually a decrease in the number of $CD4^+$ T cells, a marker for decreased immune function (see Figure 17-1). However, $CD4^+$ T-cell counts, although extremely important, reveal only part of the clinical picture because, even in uninfected people, CD4 counts vary greatly from day to day, making accurate assessment of immune status difficult. In contrast, CD4 fraction is a stable number for most people with a normal range of 27 to 60%. A CD4 fraction of less than 15% is associated with immune compromise. Laboratory tests that measure viral activity also allow a better assessment of clinical status and disease progression. Viral load (also referred to as viral burden) counts the number of viral particles in a sample of blood. Viral loads can be determined with HIV RNA polymerase chain reaction (PCR) or branched-chain DNA (bDNA) tests. Viral load is reported as less than 40 copies per millilitre, a definitive number between 40 and 10 million, or greater than 10 million. These tests provide information that helps determine when to initiate therapy, the efficacy of therapy, and whether clinical goals are being met (CDC, 2008b).

A variety of abnormal laboratory tests of the blood are common in untreated HIV infection and may be caused by HIV, opportunistic diseases, or complications of drug or radiation therapy. A decreased white blood cell (WBC) count is often seen, especially low neutrophil counts (neutropenia); low platelet counts (thrombocytopenia) may be caused by antiplatelet antibodies or drug therapy; and anemia is associated with the chronic disease process as well as with common adverse effects of some of the antiretroviral agents. Altered liver function tests are common. These may be caused by disease processes or drug therapy and may be more common with newer drug therapy. Early identification of co-infection with hepatitis B virus (HBV) and/or hepatitis C virus is important because these infections may have a more serious course in the patient with HIV infection and may ultimately limit options for ART (Anema, Wood, & Montaner, 2008).

It is now possible to test for resistance to antiretroviral drugs in people being treated for HIV infection. Two types of assays are used: genotype and phenotype. The genotype assay detects drug-resistant viral mutations that are present in the reverse transcriptase and protease genes. The phenotype assay measures the growth of the virus in various concentrations of antiretroviral drugs (much like bacteria–antibiotic sensitivity tests). These assays are especially useful in making decisions about new drug combinations in patients who are not responding to their current therapies (CDC, 2008b). Genotyping is usually done before the

DRUG THERAPY

Table 17-11 Manifestations and Treatment of Common Opportunistic Diseases Associated With HIV Infection

ORGANISM AND DISEASE	CLINICAL MANIFESTATIONS	PROPHYLAXIS* AND TREATMENT†
Candida albicans	Thrush, esophagitis, vaginitis; whitish yellow patches in mouth, esophagus, GI tract, vagina	Treatment: fluconazole (Diflucan), clotrimazole, nystatin, itraconazole (Sporanox); if fluconazole refractory: amphotericin B (Fungizone)
		Secondary prophylaxis (only if subsequent episodes are frequent or severe recurrences): fluconazole (Diflucan), itraconazole (Sporanox)
Castleman's disease (caused by HHV-8)	Generalized malaise, night sweats, rigors, fever, anorexia, weight loss	Treatment: antivirals such as IV ganciclovir or oral valganciclovir
	Will have lymphadenopathy, hepatosplenomegaly, ascites, edema, pulmonary and pericardial effusions	Chemotherapy, either mono or combined: the CHOP protocol is most recommended
Cervical cancer	Cancerous lesions in the cervix	Surgical excision of the cancerous lesion
	Vaginal bleeding, pain during intercourse	Chemotherapy
		Radiotherapy
Coccidioides immitis	Pneumonia: fever, weight loss, cough	Treatment: amphotericin B (Fungizone), fluconazole (Diflucan), itraconazole (Sporanox)
		Secondary prophylaxis (to prevent recurrence of documented disease): fluconazole (Diflucan), amphotericin B (Fungizone), itraconazole (Sporanox)
CNS lymphoma	Cognitive dysfunction, motor impairment, aphasia, seizures, personality changes, headache	Treatment: radiation, chemotherapy
Cryptococcus neoformans	Meningitis, cognitive impairment, motor dysfunction, fever, seizures, headache	Treatment: amphotericin B (Fungizone), fluconazole (Diflucan), itraconazole (Sporanox)
		Secondary prophylaxis (to prevent recurrence of documented disease): fluconazole (Diflucan), amphotericin B (Fungizone), itraconazole (Sporanox)
		Therapeutic lumbar punctures to reduce intracranial pressure
Cryptosporidium muris	Gastroenteritis, watery diarrhea, abdominal pain, weight loss	Treatment: antidiarrheals, nitazoxanide (Alinia), paromomycin (Humatin)
CMV	Retinitis: retinal lesions, blurred vision, loss of vision	Treatment: ganciclovir (Cytovene), foscarnet (Foscavir), cidofovir (Vistide), valganciclovir (Valcyte)
	Esophagitis, stomatitis: difficulty swallowing; colitis, gastritis: bloody diarrhea, pain, weight loss	Secondary prophylaxis (to prevent recurrence of documented disease): ganciclovir (Cytovene), foscarnet (Foscavir), cidofovir (Vistide), valganciclovir (Valcyte)
	Pneumonitis: respiratory symptoms	
	Neurological disease: CNS manifestations	
HBV	Jaundice, fatigue, abdominal pain, loss of appetite, nausea, vomiting, joint pain; 30% may have no signs or symptoms	Primary prevention: HBV vaccine series; screen and vaccinate those with no evidence of previous HBV infection; encourage for IDU, sexually active MSM, sexual partners or household contacts of HBV-infected individuals, and those with HCVs; HAV vaccine series should be given to prevent additive effects and advanced liver damage; screen and vaccinate those without evidence of previous HAV infection
		Treatment: adefovir dipivoxil (Hepsera), α-interferon, lamivudine, entecavir (Baraclude)
HCV	Jaundice, fatigue, abdominal pain, loss of appetite, nausea, vomiting, dark urine; 80% may have no signs or symptoms	Prophylaxis: none for HCV; HAV and HBV vaccines series should be given to prevent additive effects and advanced liver damage; screen and vaccinate those without evidence of previous HAV or HBV infection
		Treatment: α-interferon, ribavirin (Virazole), boceprevir
HSV	HSV1 (Type 1): orolabial and mucocutaneous vesicular and ulcerative lesions; keratitis: visual disturbances; encephalitis: CNS manifestations	Treatment: acyclovir (Zovirax), famciclovir (Famvir), valacyclovir (Valtrex), foscarnet (Foscavir), cidofovir (Vistide)
	HSV2 (Type 2): genital and perianal vesicular and ulcerative lesions	Secondary prophylaxis (only if subsequent episodes are frequent or severe): acyclovir (Zovirax), famciclovir (Famvir), valacyclovir (Valtrex)

Table 17-11 Manifestations and Treatment of Common Opportunistic Diseases Associated With HIV Infection—cont'd

ORGANISM AND DISEASE	CLINICAL MANIFESTATIONS	PROPHYLAXIS* AND TREATMENT†
Histoplasma capsulatum	Pneumonia: fever, cough, weight loss Meningitis: CNS manifestations; disseminated disease	Treatment: amphotericin B (Fungizone), itraconazole (Sporanox), fluconazole (Diflucan) Secondary prophylaxis (to prevent recurrence of documented disease): itraconazole (Sporanox), amphotericin B (Fungizone)
Influenza virus	Fever (usually high), headache, extreme tiredness, dry cough, sore throat, runny or stuffy nose, muscle aches; nausea, vomiting, and diarrhea can occur	Primary prevention: inactivated trivalent influenza virus vaccine; provide annually, before influenza virus season; revaccinate if initial vaccine was given when CD4+ T cell count was <200 per microlitre Treatment: supportive therapy
JC papovavirus	PML, CNS manifestations, mental and motor declines	Treatment: supportive therapy
KS (caused by HHV-8)	Vascular lesions on the skin, mucous membranes, and viscera, with wide range of presentation: firm, flat, raised, or nodular; pinpoint to several centimetres in size; hyperpigmented, multicentric; can cause lymphedema and disfigurement, particularly when confluent; not usually serious unless it occurs in the respiratory or GI systems	Treatment (dependent on severity of lesions): cancer chemotherapy, α-interferon, local radiation; cryotherapy for skin lesions
MAC	Gastroenteritis, watery diarrhea, weight loss	Primary prophylaxis (initiate when CD4+ T cells <50 per microlitre): clarithromycin (Biaxin) or azithromycin (Zithromax), rifabutin (Mycobutin). Prophylaxis may be stopped when CD4+ T cell count of >100 per microlitre is documented for 6-12 mo; restart if CD4+ T cell count falls to <50 per microlitre. Rule out disseminated disease or TB. Treatment: clarithromycin (Biaxin), ethambutol, rifabutin (Mycobutin), azithromycin (Zithromax), ciprofloxacin (Cipro), levofloxacin (Levaquin), amikacin
Mycobacterium tuberculosis	Respiratory and disseminated disease; productive cough, fever, night sweats, weight loss	Primary prophylaxis (initiate if TB testing is ≥0.5-mm reactive, after high-risk exposure, or if prior positive TB testing without treatment): INH + pyridoxine for 9 mo; consider directly observed therapy. Rule out active disease, extrapulmonary disease, or drug-resistant strain, all of which require multidrug therapy. Treatment: INH, rifampin (Rifadin), rifabutin (Mycobutin), pyrazinamide, ethambutol
PJP	Pneumonia, nonproductive cough, hypoxemia, progressive shortness of breath, fever, night sweats, fatigue	Primary prophylaxis: initiate when CD4+ T cells <200 per microlitre: TMP/SMX (Septra), dapsone, dapsone with pyrimethamine, folinic acid, aerosolized pentamidine, atovaquone. Adverse effects of TMP/SMX and dapsone (especially rash, fever, and anemia) are common and may limit use. Treatment: TMP/SMX, pentamidine, dapsone, trimethoprim, clindamycin, primaquine, atovaquone (Mepron); with hypoxia, use corticosteroids
Toxoplasma gondii	Encephalitis, cognitive dysfunction, motor impairment, fever, altered mental status, headache, seizures, sensory abnormalities	Primary prophylaxis: initiate with positive toxoplasmosis IgG titre when CD4+ T cells <100 per microlitre: TMP/SMX or dapsone with pyrimethamine + folinic acid or atovaquone ± pyrimethamine + folinic acid Treatment: pyrimethamine + folinic acid + sulfadiazine, clindamycin, azithromycin (Zithromax), atovaquone (Mepron)
VZV	Shingles: erythematous maculopapular rash along dermatomal planes, pain, pruritus Ocular: progressive outer retinal necrosis	Primary prophylaxis: VZIG administered only after significant exposure to chickenpox or shingles for patients with no history of disease or negative VZV antibody test Treatment: acyclovir (Zovirax), famciclovir (Famvir), valacyclovir (Valtrex)

CHOP, cyclophosphamide, hydroxydaunomycin, Oncovin, prednisone; *CMV*, cytomegalovirus; *CNS*, central nervous system; *GI*, gastrointestinal; *HAV*, hepatitis A virus; *HBV*, hepatitis B virus; *HCV*, hepatitis C virus; *HHV*, human herpesvirus; *HIV*, human immunodeficiency virus; *HSV*, herpes simplex virus; *IDU*, injection drug use; *IgG*, immunoglobulin G; *INH*, isoniazid; IV, intravenous; JC, "John Cunningham" virus; *KS*, Kaposi's sarcoma; *MAC*, *Mycobacterium avium* complex; *MSM*, men who have sex with men; *PJP*, *Pneumocystis jiroveci* pneumonia; *PML*, progressive multifocal leukoencephalopathy; *TB*, tuberculosis; *TMP/SMX*, trimethoprim-sulfamethoxazole; *VZIG*, varicella-zoster immune globulin; *VZV*, varicella-zoster virus.

*If available. In most cases, effective antiretroviral therapy is the best prevention for all opportunistic diseases.

†In most cases, adequate antiretroviral therapy is the best treatment for all opportunistic diseases.

Source: B.C. Centre for Excellence in HIV/AIDS (BCCFE). (2007). Therapeutic guidelines for opportunistic infections. Vancouver: Author. Retrieved from *http://www.cfenet.ubc.ca/our-work/initiatives/therapeutic-guidelines/opportunistic-infection-therapeutic-guidelines*

Table 17-12 HIV Antibody Test Screening Process

All HIV testing should be accompanied by pretest and post-test counselling. The following additional steps are used in the process of testing blood for antibodies to HIV:

1. A highly sensitive EIA is done to detect serum antibodies that bind to HIV antigens on test plates. Blood samples with negative findings on this test are reported as negative. The EIA test can be done either with a conventional blood sample or with a rapid point of care test.
   - Post-test counselling should include an assessment of risk behaviours and especially seek to identify recent risks.
   - If recent risks are found, encourage retesting at 3 weeks, 6 weeks, and 3 months.
2. If the EIA of the blood shows positive findings, the test is repeated.
3. If the findings of the EIA of the blood are repeatedly positive, a more specific confirming test, such as the WB or IFA, is done.
   - WB testing uses gel electrophoresis on purified HIV antigens. These are incubated with serum samples. If antibody in the serum is present, it can be detected.
   - IFA is used to identify HIV in infected cells. Blood is treated with a fluorescent antibody against p17 or p24 antigen and then examined using a fluorescent microscope.
4. Blood that is reactive in all of the first three steps is reported as positive for HIV antibodies.
5. If the results are inconclusive, the following steps are taken:
   - If in-depth risk assessment reveals that the individual does not have a history of high-risk activities, reassure the patient that he or she is extremely unlikely to be infected with HIV, and suggest retesting in 3 months.
   - If in-depth risk assessment reveals that the individual does have a history of high-risk activities, repeat antibody test at 1, 2, and 6 months; discuss harm reduction measures to protect partners from infection; consider tests for HIV-antigen detection such as an NAAT.

EIA, enzyme immunoassay; *HIV,* human immunodeficiency virus; *IFA,* immunofluorescence assay; *NAAT,* nucleic antigen amplification test; *WB,* Western blot.

patient starts his or her first treatment regimen because it is possible to acquire resistant virus. The PHAC (2010a) estimates that approximately 9% of individuals have resistant virus at the time of infection.

Another test that is frequently done before putting patients on ART is a human leukocyte antigen (HLA) B5701 antigen test. If this test is positive, the patient will most likely have a hypersensitivity to abacavir, one of the nucleoside reverse transcriptase inhibitors.

A test that may be performed is therapeutic drug monitoring (TDM). TDM is indicated for patients who continue to have replicating virus in the presence of ART without evidence of nonadherence. It will determine whether the patient is effectively metabolizing her or his ART regimen and has a therapeutic level of drug in her or his system.

Collaborative Care

Collaborative management of the HIV-infected patient focuses on monitoring HIV disease progression and immune function, initiating and monitoring ART, preventing the development of opportunistic diseases, detecting and treating opportunistic diseases, managing symptoms, and preventing or decreasing the complications of treatment. Ongoing assessment and health care professional–patient interactions are required to accomplish these objectives (CDC, 2009a; Kwong, 2009).

The initial visit provides an opportunity to gather baseline data and to establish rapport. A complete history and physical examination, including an immunization history and psychosocial and dietary evaluations, should be conducted. Findings from the history, assessment, and laboratory tests help determine the patient's needs. This is a good time to initiate patient education related to the spectrum of HIV disease, treatment, preventing transmission to others, improving health, and family planning. Patient input should be used to develop a plan of care, and necessary referrals can be made. It is important to remember that a newly diagnosed patient may be in a state of shock or denial and be unable to understand or retain information. The nurse should be prepared to repeat and clarify information over the course of several months. If case reports are required by the public health department, they should be completed at this time (Canadian Nurses Association, 2006; Kwong, 2009).

Drug Therapy for HIV Infection

The goals of drug therapy in HIV infection are to (1) decrease the viral load, (2) maintain or raise CD4+ T-cell counts, (3) delay the development of HIV-related symptoms and opportunistic diseases and 4) prevent transmission. Guidelines on the use of antiretroviral agents are updated regularly (Thompson et al., 2010). HIV treatment guidelines incorporate the use of the following principles:

1. Treatment decisions should be individualized by risk for disease progression indicated by higher viral loads and lower CD4+ T-cell counts and by a patient's desires for therapy.
2. Combination ART suppresses HIV replication and limits the potential for antiretroviral resistance, which is the major factor limiting treatment effect. The most effective means to suppress HIV replication is simultaneous initiation of at least three effective antiretroviral drugs from at least two different drug classes used in optimum schedules and full dosages. In general, patients are started on two nucleoside (or nucleotide) reverse transcriptase inhibitors (NRTIs) and a nonnucleoside reverse transcriptase inhibitor (NNRTI) or a protease inhibitor (PI) that is boosted with ritonavir. The nucleosides and nucleotides are considered the backbone of ART.
3. Women should receive optimal ART regardless of pregnancy status.
4. HIV-infected persons, even those with viral loads below detectable limits and those on effective ART, should be considered infectious and should avoid behaviours associated with transmission of HIV and other infectious pathogens (CDC, 2008b; O'Byrne & MacPherson, 2008). There is evidence, however, that the risk of HIV transmission decreases with lower viral loads. There is an increasing acceptance of the need to start ART at a higher CD4 because it has become clear that a suppressed viral load leads to significantly lower infectivity (Montaner, 2011).

Recommendations for starting therapy in the chronically infected patient are summarized in Table 17-13.

Currently approved drugs include four groups that inhibit the ability of HIV to make a DNA copy early in replication, one group that inhibits the ability of the virus to reproduce in the late stages of replication, and one group that prevents entry of HIV into the

Table 17-13 Recommendations for Initiating Antiretroviral Therapy in Treatment-Naïve Adults with Established HIV-1 Infection*

MEASURE	RECOMMENDATION (RATING)
Symptomatic HIV disease	Antiretroviral therapy recommended
Asymptomatic HIV disease	
CD4⁺ cell count <500 microlitres	Antiretroviral therapy recommended
CD4⁺ cell count ≥500 microlitres†	Antiretroviral therapy should be considered unless patient is an elite controller or has stable CD4 count and low level viremia in the absence of ART
Pregnant women	Treatment recommended
HIV RNA >100,000 copies/mL	Treatment recommended
Rapid decline in CD4 count >100 microlitres/yr	Treatment recommended
Active hepatitis B or C co-infection	Treatment recommended
Active or high risk for cardiovascular disease	Treatment recommended
HIV associated nephropathy	Treatment recommended
Symptomatic primary HIV infection	Treatment recommended
Risk for secondary transmission is high (e.g., serodiscordant couples)	Treatment recommended

ART, antiretroviral therapy; *HIV*, human immunodeficiency virus.
*In nonpregnant adults only. For all individuals, regardless of whether they are receiving treatment, intensive counselling to prevent secondary transmission is recommended.
†Considerations include high viral load (>100,000 HIV RNA copies/mL), rapid decline in CD4 cell count (>100/microlitre/yr), high risk of cardiovascular disease, active hepatitis B or C co-infections, or presence of HIV-associated nephropathy.
Source: Thompson, M. A., Aberg, J. A., Cahn, P., Montaner, J. S. G., Rizzardini, G., ..., Schooley, R. T. (2010). Antiretroviral treatment of adult HIV infection: 2010 recommendations of the International AIDS Society—USA panel. *Journal of the American Medical Association, 304*(3), 321-333.

cell (Table 17-14). *Nucleoside reverse transcriptase inhibitors* (NRTIs), *nonnucleoside reverse transcriptase inhibitors* (NNRTIs), and *nucleotide reverse transcriptase inhibitors* (NtRTIs) work by inhibiting the activity of reverse transcriptase, *protease inhibitors* (PIs) work by interfering with the activity of the enzyme protease, and integrase inhibitors work by interfering with the enzyme integrase. Fusion inhibitors (entry inhibitors) work by inhibiting the binding of HIV to cells. A major problem with most drugs used in ART is that resistance develops rapidly when they are used alone or taken in inadequate doses. For that reason, combinations of three or more antiretroviral drugs, prescribed at full strength, should be used. PIs and NNRTIs also have a number of dangerous and potentially lethal interactions with other commonly used drugs, including over-the-counter drugs and herbal therapies (CDC, 2008b; Davis et al., 2009). For example, St. John's wort can interfere with ART (AIDS InfoNet, 2011). Some herbs (e.g., echinacea, astragalus) should not be used because they can enhance the replication of HIV.

Table 17-14 Mechanisms of Action of Drugs Used to Treat HIV Infection

DRUG CLASSIFICATION	MECHANISM OF ACTION
Nonnucleoside reverse transcriptase inhibitors (NNRTIs)	Combine with reverse transcriptase enzyme to block the process needed to convert HIV RNA into HIV DNA
Nucleoside reverse transcriptase inhibitors (NRTIs)	Insert a bit of protein (a nucleoside) into the developing HIV DNA chain, blocking further development of the chain and leaving the production of the new strand of HIV DNA incomplete
Nucleotide reverse transcriptase inhibitors (NtRTIs)	Inhibit the action of reverse transcriptase
Protease inhibitors (PIs)	Prevent the protease enzyme from cutting HIV proteins into the proper lengths needed to allow viable virions to assemble and bud out from the cell membrane
Integrase inhibitors	Prevents viral DNA integration into the CD4⁺ cell chromosome
Fusion inhibitors (entry inhibitors)	Prevent binding of HIV to cells, thus preventing entry of HIV into healthy cells

HIV, human immunodeficiency virus; *RNA*, ribonucleic acid.

Treatment protocols can reduce viral loads by 90 to 99% in most cases, but adverse effects and other problems are common (Thompson et al., 2010). Antiretroviral agents used in HIV infection and their adverse effects are detailed in Table 17-15. Some patients will not be able to use combination therapies because of the expense, adverse effects, or inability to adhere to required schedules. Combination ART is more cost effective than the cost of advancing disease (Long, Brandeau, & Owens, 2010), but the drugs are not readily available in less developed countries.

Drug Therapy for Opportunistic Diseases

Management of HIV is complicated by the many opportunistic diseases that can develop as the immune system deteriorates. A preferred approach to opportunistic diseases is to prevent their occurrence. A number of opportunistic diseases associated with HIV can be delayed or prevented through the use of adequate ART, vaccines (including hepatitis B, influenza, and pneumococcal), and disease-specific prevention measures. Prophylaxis, used according to established criteria, contributes significantly to preventing morbidity and mortality. Although it is usually not possible to eradicate opportunistic diseases once they occur, treatments are available that can control them. Advances in the prevention, diagnosis, and treatment of opportunistic diseases have contributed significantly to increased life expectancy (CDC, 2009b). Table 17-11 lists prophylaxis and treatments for some common HIV-related opportunistic diseases.

Vaccination

Despite considerable research, a vaccine for HIV still eludes scientists. The problems that impede HIV vaccine development are

DRUG THERAPY

Table 17-15 Antiretroviral Agents Used in Treatment of HIV Infection*†

DRUG	ADVERSE EFFECTS	DRUG	ADVERSE EFFECTS
Nucleoside reverse transcriptase inhibitors (NRTIs)	Adverse effects common to NRTIs: Lactic acidosis with hepatic steatosis is a rare but potentially life-threatening problem; lipodystrophy, especially fat atrophy and mitochondrial toxicity.	Efavirenz (Sustiva)	Dizziness, trouble concentrating, unusual dreams, confusion, anxiety, depression, diarrhea, encephalopathy; false-positive cannabinoid test
Zidovudine (azidothymidine [AZT], ZDV, Retrovir)	Nausea, vomiting, anemia, leukopenia, fatigue, headache, insomnia, pancreatitis	Rilpivirine	Depression, insomnia, headache
Didanosine (dideoxyinosine [ddI], Videx, Videx-EC [time-release])	Nausea, diarrhea, peripheral neuropathy (dosage related and reversible), pancreatitis	Atripla (tenofovir, emtricitabine and efavirenz combination)	See above
Stavudine (d4T, Zerit)	Peripheral neuropathy, nausea, pancreatitis	Protease Inhibitors (PIs)	Adverse effects common to PIs: dysglycemia, hyperlipidemia, lipodystrophy
Lamivudine (3TC)	Minimal toxicities, nausea, nasal congestion	Saquinavir (Invirase)	Diarrhea, nausea, headache
Abacavir (Ziagen)	Nausea; hypersensitivity reaction, including fever, nausea, vomiting, diarrhea, lethargy, malaise, sore throat, shortness of breath, cough, rash; may produce life-threatening event if hypersensitivity is rechallenged	Indinavir (Crixivan)	Nausea, diarrhea, asymptomatic hyperbilirubinemia, interstitial nephritis, kidney stones (patient should drink 2-4 L of fluid a day)
Emtricitabine (FTC, Emtriva)	Headache, diarrhea, nausea, rash, skin discoloration	Ritonavir (Norvir)—most often used in low doses with other PIs to boost effect	Nausea, diarrhea, vomiting, taste perversion, circumoral and perioral paresthesia, hepatitis
Combivir (lamivudine and zidovudine combination)	Combines adverse effects of lamivudine and zidovudine	Nelfinavir (Viracept)	Diarrhea, flatulence, nausea, rash
Trizivir (lamivudine, zidovudine, and abacavir combination)	Combines adverse effects of lamivudine, zidovudine, and abacavir	Kaletra (lopinavir and ritonavir combination)	Nausea, diarrhea, taste perversion, perioral and circumoral paresthesia, hepatitis
Kivexa (abacavir and lamivudine)	Combines adverse effects of lamivudine and abacavir	Atazanavir (Reyataz)	Nausea, diarrhea, hyperbilirubinemia
Nucleotide reverse transcriptase inhibitor (NtRTI)		Fosamprenavir (Lexiva)	Diarrhea, nausea, vomiting, headache
Tenofovir DF (Viread)	Nausea, vomiting, diarrhea	Tipranavir (Aptivus)	Nausea, diarrhea, headache, clinical hepatitis, increased serum transaminases, hepatic decompensation, symptoms of sulpha allergy, rash, or photosensitivity
Truvada (tenofovir and emtricitabine combination)	Combines adverse effects of tenofovir and emtricitabine	Darunavir (Prezista)	Diarrhea, nausea, headache
Atripla (tenofovir, emtricitabine and efavirenz combination)	Nausea and vomiting, cough, increased pigmentation on soles of feet and palms of hands, diarrhea, drowsiness, indigestion, headache, strange dreams, fatigue	Integrase Inhibitor	
		Raltegravir	Diarrhea, nausea, headache, fever
		Entry Inhibitor	
Nonnucleoside Reverse Transcriptase Inhibitors (NNRTIs)	Adverse effects common to NNRTIs: rash, erythema multiforme, increased liver enzymes, hepatotoxicity	Enfuvirtide (Fuzeon)	ISRs, fatigue, nausea, diarrhea, insomnia, peripheral neuropathy, hypersensitivity reaction, pneumonia
Nevirapine (Viramune)	GI upset, headache, generalized rash	Maraviroc	Persistent cough, URT infections, and GI upset
Delavirdine (Rescriptor)	Headache, fatigue, GI upset, neutropenia, pruritus	Combination Therapy	
		Atripla: tenofovir (NtRTI) + emtricitabine (NRTI) + efavirenz (NNRTI)	Combined adverse effects of tenovir, emtricitabine, and efavirenz

GI, gastrointestinal; *ISRs*, injection site reactions; *URT*, upper respiratory tract.
*Current recommendations for therapy mandate combinations of three or more of these drugs. Treatment with only one drug is rarely acceptable.
†Many of these drugs cause serious and potentially fatal interactions when used in combination with other commonly used drugs, some of which are available over the counter.

Source: British Columbia Centre for Excellence in HIV/AIDS. (2011). Therapeutic guidelines: Antiretroviral treatment of adult HIV infection. Vancouver: Author. Retrieved from *http://www.cfenet.ubc.ca/our-work/initiatives/therapeutic-guidelines/adult-therapeutic-guidelines*; Montessori, V., Press, N., Harris, M., Akagi, L., & Montaner, J. S. G. (2004). Adverse effects of antiretroviral therapy for HIV infection. Canadian Medical Association Journal, 170(2), 229-238.

numerous. HIV lives inside cells, where it can "hide" from circulating immune factors. HIV also mutates rapidly, so that infected individuals develop HIV variants that may not all respond to a simple vaccine (Greenwood, Salisbury, & Hill, 2011). In addition, two strains of HIV (HIV-1 and HIV-2) cause AIDS, and at least nine *clades* (subtypes) of HIV-1 exist around the world. Development of an effective vaccine for clade B (the predominant group in the Americas and Western Europe) may not be effective in developing countries, where the need is even greater (Watkins, 2009; Ramachandran & Shanmughavle, 2009; Buchbinder, 2009).

There are also social, ethical, and economic issues related to vaccination. Vaccine efficacy will eventually have to be established in human testing: How will volunteers be recruited? How will true protection be determined? Will volunteers be exposed to HIV after immunization to test immunity? Because HIV is a global problem, with developing countries bearing the brunt of the epidemic, there is also concern about developing a vaccine that can be widely distributed in a short amount of time at an acceptable cost. Will vaccines, once developed, be accepted? Despite the overwhelming nature of these issues, considerable research is in progress. Vaccines in various stages of development are being tested. The development of a successful vaccine would be extremely helpful in controlling the epidemic but would not replace current prevention methods because no vaccine is likely to be 100% effective (Buchbinder, 2009).

NURSING MANAGEMENT: HIV INFECTION

Nursing Assessment

Nursing assessment for individuals not known to be infected with HIV should focus on behaviours that could put the person at risk for HIV infection and other sexually transmitted and bloodborne diseases. Nurses can help individuals assess risks by asking four basic questions: (1) Have you ever had a blood transfusion or used clotting factors? If so, was it before 1985? (2) Have you ever shared needles, syringes, or other injecting equipment with another person? (3) Have you ever had a sexual experience in which your penis, vagina, rectum, or mouth came into contact with another person's penis, vagina, rectum, or mouth? and (4) Have you ever had an STI? These questions provide the minimum data needed to initiate a risk assessment. A positive response to any of these questions requires an in-depth exploration of the issues specific to the identified risk (CDC, 2009c; Mountain Plains AIDS Education and Training Center, n.d.).

Further assessment is needed when an individual has been diagnosed with HIV infection. Subjective and objective data that should be obtained are presented in Table 17-16. Ongoing nursing assessments are essential because early recognition and treatment of problems can decrease the progression of HIV infection. A complete history and thorough systems review can help the nurse identify problems in a timely manner.

Nursing Diagnoses

Nursing diagnoses related to HIV infection are dictated by several variables: the stage (e.g., is prevention of HIV infection the issue? Are there concerns related to ongoing infection? Is the patient in terminal phases of the disease?), presence of specific etiological

problems (e.g., respiratory distress, depression, wasting), and social factors (e.g., issues related to self-esteem, sexuality, family interactions, finances). Because HIV infection is a complex and individually experienced disease, a broad spectrum of nursing diagnoses may include, but not be limited to, those presented in Table 17-17.

Planning

Prevention of HIV infection presents a number of challenges for the patient, many of which are related to the difficulties of behaviour change. Nurses can be instrumental in this process. Nursing interventions to prevent disease transmission depend on assessment of the patient's individual risk behaviours, knowledge, and skill deficits. Nursing orders based on these assessments will encourage the patient to learn safer, healthier, and less risky behaviours. Infection with HIV affects the entire range of a person's life, from physical health to social, emotional, economic, and spiritual well-being. Once a person is infected, treatment cannot eliminate HIV from the body. The overriding goals of therapy, therefore, are to keep the viral load as low as possible for as long as possible; to maintain or restore a functioning immune system; to improve the patient's quality of life; to reduce the potential for transmission of the virus, and to reduce HIV-related disease, disability, and death and prevent reinfection. Nursing interventions can assist the patient to (1) adhere to drug regimens; (2) promote a healthy lifestyle; (3) prevent opportunistic disease; (4) protect others from HIV; (5) maintain or develop healthy, supportive relationships; (6) maintain activities and productivity; (7) come to terms with issues related to disease, death, and spirituality; and (8) cope with the frequent symptoms caused by HIV and its treatments (Swanson, 2010; Canadian Nurses Association, 2006). Goals are individualized and change as new treatment protocols develop or as HIV disease progresses.

Nursing Implementation

The complexity of HIV disease is related to its chronic nature. As with most chronic and infectious diseases, primary prevention and health promotion are the most effective health care strategies. When prevention fails, however, disease results. HIV has no cure and continues for life. If the patient does not access ART, it causes increasing physical disability, contributes to impaired health, and ultimately causes death.

Nursing interventions at every stage of HIV disease can be instrumental in improving the quality and quantity of the patient's life. Nurses who emphasize a holistic and individualized approach to care are well suited to and capable of providing optimal care to these patients. Table 17-18 presents a synopsis of nursing goals, assessments, and interventions at each stage of HIV infection.

Health Promotion

A major goal of health promotion is to prevent disease. Even with recent successes in the treatment of HIV, prevention is crucial for control of the epidemic. Another goal of health promotion is to detect disease early so that, if primary prevention has failed, early intervention can be implemented (CDC, 2006, 2009a).

Prevention of HIV Infection. HIV infection is preventable. At this time, education and behaviour change are the most

NURSING ASSESSMENT

Table 17-16 HIV-Infected Patient

Subjective Data	**Eyes**
Important Health Information	Presence of exudate; retinal lesions or hemorrhage; papilledema
Past health history: Route of infection; hepatitis; other STIs; tuberculosis; foreign travel; frequent viral, fungal, or bacterial infections; alcohol and drug use	**Respiratory**
	Tachypnea, dyspnea, intercostal retractions; crackles, wheezing, productive of nonproductive cough
Medications: Use of immunosuppressive drugs	**Cardiovascular**
Symptoms	Pericardial friction rub, murmur, bradycardia, tachycardia
Malaise, chronic fatigue, weight loss, anorexia, nausea, vomiting; lesions, bleeding, or ulcerations of lips, mouth, gums, tongue, or throat; sensitivity to acidic, salty, or spicy foods; difficulty swallowing; abdominal cramping	**Gastrointestinal**
	Mouth lesions, including blisters (HSV), white-grey patches (*Candida*), painless white lesions on lateral aspect of the tongue (hairy leukoplakia), discolorations (KS); gingivitis, tooth decay or loosening; redness or white patchy lesions of throat; vomiting, diarrhea, incontinence; rectal lesions; hyperactive bowel sounds, abdominal masses, hepatosplenomegaly
Skin rashes, lesions, or colour changes; pruritus; nonhealing wounds	
Persistent diarrhea, change in character of stools; painful urination	
Cough, shortness of breath	**Musculoskeletal**
Insomnia; night sweats	Muscle wasting
Headaches, stiff neck, chest pain, rectal pain, retrosternal pain	**Neurological**
Blurred vision, photophobia, diplopia, loss of vision; hearing impairment; confusion, forgetfulness, attention deficit, changes in mental status, memory loss, personality changes, muscle weakness, difficulty walking; paresthesias, hypersensitivity in feet	Ataxia, tremors, lack of coordination; sensory loss; slurred speech, aphasia; memory loss, apathy, agitation, depression, inappropriate behaviour; decreasing levels of consciousness, seizures, paralysis, coma
	Reproductive
Lesions on genitalia (internal or external), pruritus or burning in vagina, painful sexual intercourse, changes in menstruation, vaginal or penile discharge	Genital lesions or discharge, abdominal tenderness secondary to PID
	Possible Findings
Objective Data	Positive HIV antibody assay (EIA or ELISA, confirmed by WB or IFA); detectable viral load levels by bDNA or PCR, ↓ CD4+ lymphocytes, reversal of CD4:CD8 ratio; ↓ WBC count, lymphopenia, anemia, thrombocytopenia; electrolyte imbalances; abnormal liver function tests; ↑ cholesterol, triglycerides, and blood glucose
General	
Lethargy, persistent fever, lymphadenopathy, peripheral wasting, fat deposits in truncal areas and upper back; social withdrawal	
Integumentary	
Decreased skin turgor, dry skin, or diaphoresis; pallor, cyanosis; lesions, eruptions, discolorations, or bruises of skin and mucous membranes; vaginal or perianal excoriation; alopecia, delayed wound healing	

bDNA, branched-chain deoxyribonucleic acid; *EIA,* enzyme immunoassay; *ELISA,* enzyme-linked immunosorbent assay; *HIV,* human immunodeficiency virus; *HSV,* herpes simplex virus; *IFA,* immunofluorescence assay; *KS,* Kaposi's sarcoma; *PCR,* polymerase chain reaction; *STIs,* sexually transmitted infections; *WB,* Western blot; *WBC,* white blood cell.

Table 17-17 Nursing Diagnoses: Human Immunodeficiency Virus Infection

Anxiety	Nutrition, *imbalanced*: less than body requirements
Body image, *disturbed*	
Caregiver role strain	Oral mucous membrane, *impaired*
Coping, *ineffective*	Pain, acute or chronic
Confusion	Powerlessness
Decisional conflict	Relocation stress syndrome
Denial, *ineffective*	Self-care deficit
Diarrhea	Self-esteem, *chronic low*
Disuse syndrome, *risk for*	Self-esteem, *situational low*
Fatigue	Shortness of breath
Family processes, *interrupted*	Sleep pattern, *disturbed*
Fear	Social isolation
Grieving	Spiritual distress
Headache	Therapeutic regimen management, *ineffective*
Hyperthermia	
Noncompliance or nonadherence	Thought processes, *disturbed*

effective prevention tools. Educational messages should be specific to the patient's need, culturally sensitive, language appropriate, and age specific. Nurses are excellent resources for this type of education, but nurses must be comfortable with and know how to talk about sensitive topics such as sexuality and drug use (Magnan & Reynolds, 2006).

Prevention behaviours have been known and recommended since the mid-1980s. It is important to remember that a range of activities can reduce the risk of HIV infection and that individuals will choose different techniques. The goal is for the person to develop safer, healthier, and less risky behaviours than are currently being used. These techniques can be divided into *safe activities* (those that eliminate risk) and *risk-reducing activities* (those that decrease risk but do not eliminate it). The more consistently and correctly prevention methods are used, the more effective they are in preventing HIV infection.

Research shows that the majority of new HIV infections were transmitted by individuals who were not aware that they were infected. An estimated 25% to 30% of HIV-infected people in Canada do not know that they are infected (PHAC, 2010b). These facts helped the CDC develop four strategies in the *Advancing HIV Prevention* (AHP) initiative: (1) HIV testing should be a part of

Table 17-18 Nursing Interventions in Human Immunodeficiency Virus Disease

LEVELS OF CARE; GOALS	ASSESS	INTERVENTIONS
Health Promotion		
1. Prevent HIV infection 2. Detect HIV infection early	*Risk factors:* What behaviours or social, physical, emotional, pathological, and immune factors place the patient at risk? Does the patient need to be tested for HIV?	Education, including knowledge, attitudes, and behaviours, with an emphasis on risk reduction, to accomplish the following: • General population: cover general information • Pregnant women: general information and information specific to HIV infection and pregnancy. Offer prenatal HIV testing in the first trimester. Individual patient: specific to assessed need Empower patients to take control of prevention measures. Provide HIV-antibody testing with pretest and post-test counselling.
Acute Intervention		
1. Promote health and limit disability 2. Manage problems caused by HIV infection	*Physical health:* Is patient experiencing problems? *Mental health status:* How is the patient coping? *Resources:* Does the patient have family and social support? Is the patient accessing community services? Is money or insurance a problem? Does the patient have access to spiritual support?	Provide case management. Educate regarding HIV, the spectrum of infection, options for care, signs and symptoms to watch for, treatment options, immune enhancement, harm reduction, and ways to adhere to treatment regimens. Refer to needed resources. Establish long-term, trusting relationship with patient, family, and significant others. Provide emotional and spiritual support. Provide care during acute exacerbations: recognition of life-threatening developments, life support, rapid intervention with treatments and drugs, patient and family emotional support during crisis, comfort, and hygiene needs. Develop resources for legal needs: discrimination prevention, wills and powers of attorney, child care wishes. Empower patient to identify needs, direct care, and seek services.
Ambulatory and Home Care		
1. Maximize quality of life 2. Resolve life and death issues	*Physical health:* Are new symptoms developing? Is the patient experiencing drug adverse effects or interactions? *Mental health:* How is the patient coping? What adjustments have been made? *Finances:* Can the patient maintain health care and basic standards of living? *Family, social, and community supports:* Are these available? Is the patient using supports in an effective manner? Do family or significant others need education, encouragement, or stress relief? *Spirituality issues:* Does the patient desire support from a religious organization? Are spirituality issues private and personal? What assistance does the patient need?	Continue case management. Educate about changing treatment options and continued adherence. Empower patient to continue to direct care and to make desires known to family members and significant others. Continue physical care for chronic disease process: treatments, drugs, comfort, and hygiene needs. Support patient and family and significant others in a trusting relationship. Refer to resources that will assist in meeting identified needs. Promote health maintenance measures. Assist with end-of-life issues: resuscitation orders, comfort measures, funeral plans, and the like. Refer to palliative care.

HIV, human immunodeficiency virus.

routine health care based on risk assessment and clinical need, (2) rapid HIV testing should also be used to diagnose HIV outside of traditional care settings (e.g., in community-based organizations and at health fairs), (3) providers should work with HIV-infected patients and their partners to change risky behaviours and decrease the risks of HIV transmission, and (4) perinatal transmission should be further reduced by universally offering HIV tests to pregnant women and appropriate treatment to those found to be infected (CDC, 2006).

■ *Decreasing Risks Related to Sexual Intercourse.* Safe sexual activities significantly decrease the risk of exposure to HIV in semen and vaginal secretions. Abstaining from all sexual activity is the most effective way to accomplish this goal, but there are safe options for those who cannot or do not wish to abstain. *Outercourse* (limiting sexual behaviour to activities in which the mouth, penis, vagina, or rectum does not come into contact with a partner's mouth, penis, vagina, or rectum) is safe because there is no contact with blood, semen, or vaginal secretions. Outer-

Table 17-19 Proper Use of the Male Condom

- Use only condoms (rubbers) that are made out of latex or polyurethane. "Natural skin" condoms have pores that are large enough for HIV to penetrate.
- Store condoms in a cool, dry place and protect them from trauma. The friction caused by carrying them in a back pocket, for instance, can wear down the latex.
- Do not use a condom if the expiration date has passed or if the package looks worn or punctured.
- Lubricants used in conjunction with condoms must be water soluble. Oil-based lubricants can weaken latex and increase the risk of tearing or breaking.
- Nonlubricated, flavoured, or unflavoured condoms can provide protection during oral intercourse.
- The condom must be placed on the erect penis before any contact is made with the partner's mouth, vagina, or rectum to prevent exposure to pre-ejaculatory secretions that may contain HIV.
- See eFigure 17-1 for proper steps in male condom placement.
- Remove the penis and condom from the partner's vagina or rectum immediately after ejaculation and before the erection is lost. Hold the condom at the base of the penis and remove both penis and condom at the same time. This keeps semen from leaking around the condom as the penis becomes flaccid.
- Remove the condom after use, wrap in tissue, and discard. Do not flush down the toilet because this can cause plumbing problems.
- Condoms are not reusable! A new condom must be used for every act of intercourse.

HIV, human immunodeficiency virus.

Table 17-20 Proper Use of the Female Condom

- Female condoms consist of a polyurethane sheath with two spring-form rings.
  The smaller ring is inserted into the vagina and holds the condom in place internally. This ring can be removed if the condom is to be used for anal intercourse. It should not be removed if the condom is to be used for vaginal intercourse.
  The larger ring surrounds the opening to the condom. It functions to keep the condom in place while protecting the external genitalia.
- Use only water-soluble lubricants with female condoms.
  Female condoms come prelubricated and with a tube of additional lubricant.
  Lubrication is needed to protect the condom from tearing during sexual intercourse and can also decrease the noise that results from friction of the penis against the condom.
- Some men have reported that the female condom feels better than the male condom. Other men like male condoms better. The only way to find out which type of condom works best is to try them both.
- Practise inserting the female condom. The steps for proper insertion are shown in Figure 17-8. Lubrication makes the condom slippery, but do not get discouraged—just keep trying.
- During sexual intercourse, ensure that the penis is inserted into the female condom through the outer ring. It is possible for the penis to miss the opening, thus making contact with the vagina and defeating the purpose of the condom.
- Do not use a male condom at the same time as a female condom.
- After intercourse, remove the condom before standing up.
  Twist the outer ring to keep the semen inside, gently pull the condom out of the vagina, and discard.
- Do not flush down the toilet because this can cause plumbing problems.
- Do not reuse a female condom.

course includes massage, masturbation, mutual masturbation ("hand job"), telephone sex, and other activities that meet the "no contact" requirements. *Insertive sex* between partners who are not infected with HIV or not at risk of becoming infected with HIV is considered to be safe.

Reducing the risk of sexual activities through the use of barriers decreases the risk of contact with HIV. Barriers should be used when engaging in insertive sexual activity (oral, vaginal, or anal) with a partner who is known to be HIV infected or with a partner whose HIV status is not known. The most commonly used barrier is the male condom. Male condoms have been shown to be almost 100% effective in preventing the transmission of HIV when used correctly and consistently. (The proper use and placement of the male condom are presented in eFigure 17-1 on the Evolve Website for this chapter.) Major points for the correct use of male condoms are discussed in Table 17-19. Female condoms are also available. Use can be complicated, so careful instruction and practice are necessary (Table 17-20) (The proper use and placement of the female condom are presented in eFigure 17-2 on the Evolve Website for this chapter.). In addition, squares of latex (known as dental dams) or plastic food wrap can be used to cover the external female genitalia during oral sexual activity.

Decreasing Risks Related to Substance Use. Substance use, including alcohol and tobacco, is harmful. It can cause immune suppression and malnutrition as well as a host of psychosocial problems. However, substance use in and of itself does not cause HIV infection. The major risk for HIV infection is related to sharing injecting equipment or having unsafe sexual experiences while under the influence of substances. The basic rules are as follows: (1) Do not inject illicit drugs; (2) If you do inject illicit drugs, do not share equipment; and (3) Do not have sexual intercourse when under the influence of any drug (including alcohol) that impairs decision-making ability (AIDS InfoNet, 2009a).

The safest mechanism is to abstain from substances. Although this is the best option for those who do not currently use substances, it may not be a viable alternative for users who are not prepared to quit or for those who have no access to treatment services. The risk of HIV for individuals who use drugs can be eliminated if they use alternatives to injecting, such as smoking, snorting, or ingesting the drug. Risk for HIV can also be eliminated if users do not share injecting equipment. Injecting equipment ("works") includes needles, syringes, cookers (spoons or bottle caps used to mix the drug), cotton, and rinse water. None of this equipment should be shared. Another safe tactic is for the user to have access to sterile equipment. This can be accomplished through community needle and syringe exchange programs (NSEPs) and supervised injection sites that provide sterile equipment to users in exchange for used equipment. Opposition to these programs is supported by the fear that ready access to

PATIENT & CAREGIVER TEACHING GUIDE

Table 17-21 Proper Use of Injection Equipment

- When injecting drugs, it is always preferable to use new, sterile syringes, needles, cookers, and cotton (works).
- Find out if there is a needle and syringe exchange program in your community. If there is, take used equipment in and you will be provided with new works.
- Swab skin with an alcohol preparation before injecting.
- Use a tourniquet to assist in locating veins.
- Always inject with the bevel facing up on the needle.
- If you must share your equipment, it is very important to clean the works thoroughly with bleach before use.
- First, rinse the used needle and syringe twice with tap water.
- Then, fill the syringe with full-strength household bleach, shake for 30 seconds, and squirt the bleach out.
- Repeat the bleaching process a second time, being sure to shake the bleach-filled syringe for 30 seconds.
- Finally, rinse equipment twice with tap water.
- Do not share your bleach or rinse water.
- Do not share your cooker. If you must share your cooker, clean it with bleach and water before using it again.
- Supervised injection sites are another viable alternative for preventing the spread of infection and there is political will to open sites in various parts of the country.

injecting supplies will increase drug use. However, studies have shown that in communities where exchange programs have been established, drug use does not increase, rates of HIV infection are controlled, and an overall cost benefit results (Des Jarlais, McKnight, Goldblatt, & Purchase, 2009).

Cleaning equipment before use is a risk-reducing activity. It decreases the risk for those who share equipment (Table 17-21). This process takes time and may be difficult for a person in drug withdrawal.

Decreasing Risks of Perinatal Transmission. The best way to prevent HIV infection in infants is to prevent HIV infection in women. Women who are already infected with HIV should be asked about their reproductive desires. Women who choose not to have children need to have birth control methods discussed in detail. Should they become pregnant, abortion may be desired and should be discussed in conjunction with other options.

If HIV-infected pregnant women are appropriately treated during pregnancy, the rate of perinatal transmission can be decreased from 25% to less than 2%. The current standard of care is that all women who are pregnant or contemplating pregnancy should be counselled about HIV infection, informed of their choices, routinely offered access to voluntary HIV-antibody testing, and, if infected, offered optimal ART (CDC, 2007b).

Decreasing Risks at Work. The risk of infection from occupational exposure to HIV is small but real. The Canadian Centre for Occupational Health and Safety (CCOHS) requires employers to protect workers from exposure to blood and other potentially infectious materials. Precautions and safety devices decrease the risk of direct contact with blood and body fluids. Precautions for the prevention of occupational exposure to bloodborne diseases are discussed earlier in this chapter. Should

significant exposure to HIV-infected fluids occur, PEP with combination ART based on the type of exposure, the volume of the exposure, and the status of the source patient has been shown to significantly decrease the risk of infection. The possibility of treatment makes reporting of all blood exposures even more critical (Department of Health, 2008).

HIV Testing and Counselling. Testing is the only sure way to determine whether a person has HIV infection. Any individual who is at risk for HIV infection should be encouraged to be tested. When findings are negative, testing can relieve anxieties about past behaviours and provide opportunities for prevention education. When findings are positive, testing provides the needed impetus to seek treatment and to protect sexual and drug-using partners. All testing for HIV should be accompanied by pretest and post-test counselling (Table 17-22) as mandated by the Minister of Public Works and Government Services Canada in 2007.

Acute Intervention

Early Intervention. Early intervention after detection of HIV infection can promote health and limit or delay disability. Because the course of HIV is variable, assessment is very important. Nursing interventions are based on and tailored to patient needs noted during assessment. The nursing assessment in HIV disease should focus on early detection of symptoms, opportunistic diseases, and psychosocial problems (see Table 17-8).

Initial Response to a Diagnosis of HIV. Reactions to a positive HIV-antibody test are similar to the reactions of people who are diagnosed with any life-threatening, debilitating, or chronic illness. They include anxiety, panic, fear, depression, denial, hopelessness, thoughts of suicide, anger, and guilt (CDC, 2006). Many of these reactions are also seen in the patient's family members, friends, and caregivers. As time passes, patients and their loved ones must confront common issues associated with a life-threatening illness. These include difficult treatment decisions; feelings of loss, anger, powerlessness, depression, and grief; social isolation imposed by self or others; altered concepts of the physical, social, emotional, and creative self; thoughts of suicide; and the possibility of death (Bogart et al., 2008). The nurse can help the patient gain control. Empowerment is particularly important because the individual with HIV infection often experiences multiple losses, including an overwhelming feeling of loss of control. Empowerment is facilitated by education and honest discussions about the patient's health status and treatment options.

Antiretroviral Therapy. Multidrug-therapy protocols have been shown to significantly reduce viral loads and reverse clinical progression of HIV (Thompson et al., 2010). However, nurses must be aware that the protocols are complex, the drugs have adverse effects and interactions, and they do not work for everyone. All of these factors contribute to problems with adherence to treatment, a dangerous situation because of the risk of developing drug resistance. It is important for patients to maintain a minimum of 95% adherence to their ART protocol in order to avoid resistance (Bangsberg & Machtinger, 2009). Frequently, nurses are the health care providers who work most closely with patients who are trying to cope with these issues. Nurses can support patients to be adherent to their regimen. Some interventions to support adherence include education about (1) the

Table 17-22 Pretest and Post-Test Counselling Associated With HIV-Antibody Testing

General Guidelines

1. People who are being tested for HIV are frequently fearful about the test results.
   - Establish rapport with the patient.
   - Assess the patient's ability to understand HIV counselling.
   - Determine the patient's ability to access support systems.
2. Explain the benefits of testing.
   - Testing provides an opportunity for education that can decrease the risk of new infections.
   - Infected individuals can be referred for early intervention and support programs.
3. Discuss negative aspects of testing.
   - Confidentiality issues: breaches of confidentiality have led to discrimination.
   - A positive test affects all aspects of the patient's life (e.g., personal, social, economic) and can raise difficult emotions (anger, anxiety, guilt, and thoughts of suicide).

Pretest Counselling

1. Determine the patient's risk factors and when the last risk occurred. Counselling should be individualized according to these parameters.
2. Provide education to decrease future risk of exposure.
3. Provide education that will help the patient protect sexual and drug-sharing partners.
4. Discuss problems related to the delay between infection and an accurate test. Testing will have to be repeated at intervals for up to 6 months after each possible exposure. Discuss the need to use measures to decrease the risks to the patient and the patient's partners during that interval.
5. Discuss the possibility of false-negative tests, which are most likely to occur during the window period.
6. Assess support systems. Provide telephone numbers and resources as needed.

7. Discuss the responses the patient anticipates having to the test results (positive and negative).
8. Outline assistance that will be offered if the test is positive.

Post-Test Counselling

1. If the test is negative, reinforce pretest counselling and prevention education. Remind the patient that the test must be repeated at intervals for up to 6 months after the most recent exposure risk.
2. If the test is positive, understand that the patient may be in shock and not hear much of what the nurse says.
3. Provide resources for medical and emotional support, and help the patient get immediate assistance.
   - Evaluate suicide risk and follow-up as needed.
   - Determine need to test others who have had risky contact with the patient.
   - Discuss retesting to verify results. This tactic supports hope for the patient, but more importantly, it keeps the patient in the system. While waiting for the second test result, the patient has time to think about and adjust to the possibility of being HIV infected.
   - Encourage optimism.
4. Remind the patient that effective treatments are available; HIV is not a death sentence.
5. Review health habits that can improve the immune system.
6. Arrange for the patient to speak to HIV-infected people who are willing to share with and assist newly diagnosed patients during the transition period.
7. Reinforce that a positive HIV test means that the patient is infected but does not necessarily mean that the patient has progressed to AIDS.
8. Educate to prevent new infections. HIV-infected people should be instructed to avoid donating blood, organs, or semen; to avoid sharing razors, toothbrushes, or other household items that may contain blood or other body fluids; and to protect sexual and needle-sharing partners from blood, semen, and vaginal secretions.

AIDS, acquired immune deficiency syndrome; *HIV,* human immunodeficiency virus.

---

advantages and disadvantages of new treatments, (2) the dangers of nonadherence to therapeutic regimens, (3) how and when to take each drug, (4) drug interactions to prevent, (5) monitoring the patient for depression, (6) managing addiction, and (7) adverse effects that must be reported to the primary care provider (Swanson, 2010). Table 17-23 provides guidance for patient teaching in these areas.

■ *When to Start Antiretroviral Therapy.* ART has been in a state of continuous change since the first antiretroviral drug was released in 1987. When new drugs were developed, health care providers had the ability to combine and substitute drugs. However, as new treatments improve the quality and quantity of patients' lives, problems emerge. For a while, the preferred treatment strategy was known as "hit it early, hit it hard." This was thought to be appropriate because decreasing the viral load provides for better health outcomes. However, adverse effects and lack of adherence caused many patients to question their ability to sustain ART for long periods of time. For this reason, new guidelines suggest that treatment can be delayed until the CD4 count drops below 500 (Thompson et al., 2010).

Given patient readiness, without which lack of adherence may be a problem, treatment should be initiated at a CD4 count

of 500 because suppressing viral loads is helpful in reducing transmission rates (Montaner, 2011) and because it has become apparent that a CD4 count of less than 500 is associated with non–AIDS-related issues such as cardiovascular disease, renal disease, and some cancers (Thompson et al., 2010). Nurses can provide in-depth education and counselling for patients as they struggle to make this decision.

■ *Adherence.* Adherence to drug regimens is a critical component of drug therapy for people with HIV infection and an area in which nurses are uniquely well prepared to provide assistance. Taking drugs as ordered (right dose and time) every day is important for all drug therapy. The difference with HIV is that missing a dose can lead to viral mutations that allow HIV to become resistant to the drug (CDC, 2008b; Roberson, 2009). The difficulty of adhering consistently is clear to anyone who has tried to take a 10-day course of antibiotics. Patients with HIV infection have to take anywhere from 3 to 20 pills a day, at precise times during the day. This process must be repeated every day for the rest of their lives even though they often suffer uncomfortable adverse effects. Nurses have learned that helping people adhere to difficult treatment regimens requires a number of things. The most important is to remember that each patient is a unique

Table 17-23 Use of Antiretroviral Drugs

Resistance to antiretroviral drugs is a major problem in treating HIV infection. To decrease the risk of developing resistance:

1. Take at least three different antiretroviral drugs at a time; discuss other options with your health care provider.

2. Know what medications you are taking and how to take them (some have to be taken with food, some must be taken on an empty stomach, some cannot be taken together). If you do not understand, ask. Get your nurse to write the instructions clearly for you.

3. Take the full dose prescribed, and take it on schedule. If you cannot take the drug because of adverse effects or other problems, report it to your health care provider.

4. Take all of the drugs prescribed. It is important that you take them more than 95% of the time. Do not quit taking one drug while continuing the others. If you cannot tolerate one of your drugs, your health care provider will recommend a completely new set of drugs.

5. Many of the antiretroviral drugs interact with other drugs, including a number of common drugs you can buy without a prescription. Be sure your health care provider and pharmacist know all of the drugs that you are taking, and do not take any new drugs without checking for possible interactions.

6. The goal of antiretroviral therapy is to decrease the amount of virus in your blood. This is called your viral load. Viral load can be determined by tests such as the PCR or bDNA. The results are reported in absolute numbers. The goal is to get your viral load to an undetectable level. Most health care providers will check this number on a regular basis whether you are taking antiretroviral agents or not.

7. In 2 to 4 weeks after you start on drug therapy (or change your therapy), your health care provider will test your viral load to find out if the drugs are working. These results are reported in absolute numbers or in logs (a mathematical concept). All you have to know is that you want to see the viral load drop. If reports are in logs, you want to see a drop of at least 1 log, which means that 90% of your viral load has been eliminated. If your viral load drops by 2 logs, your viral load will have been 95% eliminated. If your viral load drops by 3 logs, your viral load will have been 99% eliminated.

8. An undetectable viral load means that the amount of virus is extremely low and viruses cannot be found in the blood using the current technology. It does not mean that the virus is gone, because much of the virus will be in lymph nodes and organs where the tests cannot detect it. It also does not mean that you are no longer able to transmit HIV to others; you will need to continue protecting all of your sexual and drug-using partners.

AIDS, acquired immune deficiency syndrome; *bDNA,* branched-chain DNA; *HIV,* human immunodeficiency virus; *PCR,* polymerase chain reaction.

Table 17-24 Signs and Symptoms That HIV Patients Need to Report

Report the Following Signs and Symptoms Immediately to a Health Care Provider

- Any change in level of consciousness: lethargy, hard to arouse, unable to arouse, unresponsive, unconscious
- Headache accompanied by nausea and vomiting, changes in vision, changes in ability to perform coordinated activities, or after any head trauma
- Vision changes: blurry or black areas in vision field, new floaters
- Persistent shortness of breath related to activity and not relieved by a short rest period
- Nausea and vomiting accompanied by abdominal pain
- Dehydration: unable to eat or drink because of nausea, diarrhea, or mouth lesions; severe diarrhea or vomiting; dizziness when standing
- Yellow discoloration of the skin
- Any bleeding from the rectum that is not related to hemorrhoids
- Pain in the flank with fever and unable to urinate for more than 6 hours
- New onset of weakness in any part of the body, new onset of numbness that is not obviously related to pressure, new onset of difficulty speaking
- Chest pain not obviously related to cough
- Seizures
- New rash accompanied by fever
- New oral lesions accompanied by fever
- Severe depression, anxiety, hallucinations, delusions, or possible danger to self or others

Report the Following Signs and Symptoms Within 24 Hours

- New or different headache; constant headache not relieved by aspirin or acetaminophen
- Headache accompanied by fever, nasal congestion, or cough
- Burning, itching, or discharge from the eyes
- New or productive cough
- Vomiting two or three times a day
- Vomiting accompanied by fever
- New, significant, or watery diarrhea (>6 times a day)
- Painful urination, bloody urine, urethral discharge
- New, significant rash (widespread, painful, itchy, or following a path down the leg or arm, around the chest, or on the face)
- Difficulty eating because of mouth lesions
- Vaginal discharge, pain, or itching

individual who will have different ways of coping and of learning. Patients can be helped with technologies such as blister packs, electronic reminders, beepers, or timers on pillboxes. Group support and individual counselling can also help, but the best assistance may be learning about the patient's life and assisting with problem solving within the constraints of that life (CDC, 2008b; Knobel et al., 2009; Roberson, 2009).

■ *Health Promotion.* HIV disease progression may also be delayed by promoting a healthy immune system, whether the patient chooses to use ART or not. Useful interventions for HIV-infected patients include (1) nutritional support to maintain lean body mass and ensure appropriate levels of vitamins and micro-nutrients; (2) moderation or elimination of alcohol intake, smoking, and drug use; (3) adequate rest and exercise; (4) stress reduction; (5) avoidance of exposure to new infectious agents; (6) mental health counselling; and (7) involvement in support groups and community activities. In the absence of ART, however, disease progression can be delayed only for a finite amount of time.

Patients should be taught to recognize symptoms that may indicate disease progression or drug adverse effects so that prompt medical care can be initiated. Table 17-24 provides an overview of symptoms that patients should report. In general, patients should have as much information as needed to make informed decisions about health care. These decisions then dictate the appropriate interventions.

■ **Acute Exacerbations.** Chronic diseases are characterized by acute exacerbations of recurring problems. This is especially true in HIV disease, where infections, cancers, debility, and psychosocial and economic issues may interact to overwhelm the patient's ability to cope. Nursing care becomes more complex if the patient's immune system deteriorates and new problems arise to compound existing difficulties. When opportunistic diseases or difficult adverse effects of treatment develop, symptom management, education, and emotional support are necessary (Portillo, Holzemer, & Chou, 2007).

Nursing care assumes primary importance in helping patients prevent the many opportunistic diseases associated with HIV infection. The best prevention of opportunistic disease is adequate treatment of the underlying HIV infection.

■ **Ongoing Care.** HIV-infected patients share problems experienced by all individuals with chronic diseases, but these problems are exacerbated by social constructs surrounding HIV. Chronic diseases are characterized by negative social attitudes that label the patient as weak willed or immoral for being sick. In HIV, this stigma is compounded by several factors. HIV-infected people may be seen as lacking control over urges to have sex or use drugs. It is then easy to jump to the conclusion that they brought the disease on themselves and, therefore, somehow deserve to be sick. Behaviours associated with HIV infection may be viewed as immoral (e.g., homosexuality, having many sexual partners) and are sometimes illegal (e.g., injecting heroin, sex work). The fact that infected individuals can transmit the virus to others furthers the negative, stigmatizing social concept of HIV. Social stigmatization supports discrimination in all facets of life. According to the Canadian Human Rights Commission (1986) policy on HIV/AIDS, all Canadians have the right to equality and dignity without discrimination, regardless of HIV/AIDS status.

The chronic nature of HIV infection can cause family stress, social isolation, dependence, frustration, lowered self-image, loss of control, and economic pressures. An interesting observation is that all of these variables may have contributed to the patient's infection in the first place. Low self-esteem, searching for social contact, frustration, and economic difficulties all contribute to drug use and risky sexual behaviours.

■ **Disease and Drug Adverse Effects.** Physical problems related to HIV disease or the treatment of HIV can interrupt the patient's ability to maintain a desired lifestyle. HIV-infected patients frequently experience anxiety, fear, diarrhea, depression, peripheral neuropathy, pain, nausea and vomiting, and fatigue. These are symptoms that nurses deal with routinely, and the interventions for them do not change significantly based on the primary diagnosis. Individual considerations will, of course, influence the way that the nurse approaches the patient. Nursing management of diarrhea, for instance, still includes helping patients collect specimens, recommending dietary changes, encouraging fluid and electrolyte replacement, instructing the patient about skin care, and managing skin breakdown around the perianal area. Nursing approaches for fatigue in HIV include teaching patients to assess fatigue patterns, determine contributing factors, set activity priorities, conserve energy, schedule rest periods, exercise, and avoid substances such as caffeine, nicotine, alcohol, and other drugs that may disturb sleep (Swanson, 2010).

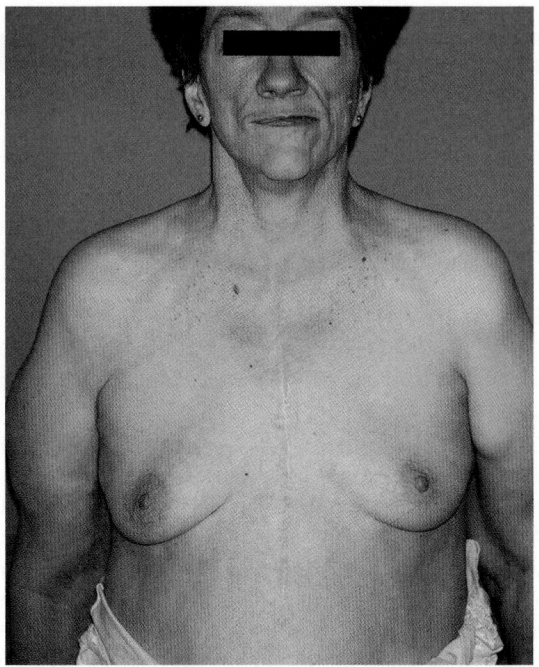

Figure 17-8 Lipodystrophy manifestations.

Source: James, W. D., Berger, T., & Elston, D. (2006). *Andrews' diseases of the skin: Clinical dermatology* (10th ed.) St. Louis: Saunders.

Over the past several years, a new set of metabolic disorders has emerged among HIV-infected patients, especially those who have been infected for a long time and who have been on ART. These disorders include changes in body shape (fat deposits in the abdomen, the upper back, and the breasts, along with fat loss in the arms, the legs, and the face) caused by lipodystrophy (Figure 17-8), dyslipidemia (elevated triglycerides and decreases in high-density lipoproteins), insulin resistance and hyperglycemia, bone disease (osteoporosis, osteopenia, avascular necrosis), lactic acidosis, and cardiovascular disease. It is still not clear why these disorders develop, but it is probably a combination of factors such as long-term infection with HIV, adverse effects of ART, genetic predisposition, and chronic stress (Leung & Glesby, 2011).

Management of metabolic disorders currently focuses on detecting problems early, dealing with the symptoms, and helping the patient cope with new problems and additional drugs. It is important to recognize and treat these problems early, especially because cardiovascular disease and lactic acidosis are potentially fatal complications. A frequent first intervention is to change ART, because some drugs are more often associated with these problems (see Table 17-15). Lipid abnormalities are generally treated with lipid-lowering drugs, dietary changes, and exercise. Insulin resistance is treated with hypoglycemic drugs and weight loss. Bone disease may be improved with exercise, dietary changes, and calcium and vitamin D supplements (Bradley-Springer, 2005; Barbaro & Iacobellis, 2009; Martinez, Larrousse, & Gatelli, 2009).

Body changes that combine fat accumulation and wasting are major problems for patients with this syndrome. Human growth hormone, testosterone, and anabolic steroids have been used to help resolve these changes, but the results are inconclusive. Some patients may undergo plastic surgery procedures such as liposuction or facial implants to deal with the body changes associated with fat redistribution. There is little evidence that exercise or dietary changes make any difference. Nursing interventions must focus on helping the patient make treatment decisions and on dealing with negative changes in body image (Portillo et al., 2007).

▌ **Terminal Care.** Despite exciting new developments in the treatment of HIV infection, many patients will experience disease progression, disability, and death. Sometimes, these occur because treatments do not work for the patient. Some patients will never access treatment. Research has shown that patients who are poor, female, or Aboriginal are less likely to access treatment (Joy et al., 2008). This can be devastating because of the media hype related to "miracle" recoveries among those for whom the drugs work. In other cases, patients may make a calculated decision to forego further treatment, allowing the disease to progress toward death. This may be especially difficult for family members and loved ones to accept. Nursing care during the terminal phase of any disease must focus on keeping the patient comfortable, facilitating emotional and spiritual acceptance of the finite nature of life, and helping the patient's significant others deal with grief and loss. Nurses become pivotal care providers during the terminal phase of illness, especially in HIV disease, where patients and families often choose terminal care at home. (End-of-life care is discussed in Chapter 13.)

▌ Evaluation

The expected outcomes are that the patient at risk for HIV infection will do the following:

- Analyze personal risk factors
- Develop and implement a personal plan to decrease risks
- Get tested for HIV

The expected outcomes are that the patient with HIV infection will:

- Describe basic aspects of the effects of HIV on the immune system
- Compare and contrast various treatment options for HIV disease
- Work with a team of health care providers to achieve optimal health
- Prevent transmission of HIV to others

ETHICAL DILEMMAS
Duty to Treat

Situation

A nurse in a community clinic has just discovered that Ms. M., a patient with respiratory problems, has human immunodeficiency virus (HIV) infection. The nurse is concerned about contact with Ms. M. and her body fluids. She requests that she not be assigned to Ms. M.'s care. The nurse believes that she has the right to refuse to care for Ms. M. because she has her own family to support and protect.

Important Points for Consideration

- According to the Canadian Nurses Association (CNA) *Code of Ethics*, the nurse must not discriminate in the provision of nursing care based on cultural or socioeconomic background or health status.
- Health care providers have contact with patients every day who may have infectious blood or other body fluids.
- Infection precautions are instituted to protect health care workers from potentially infectious blood or other body fluids.
- There are two situations in which nurses can refuse to care for patients if employers are notified in advance: (1) when caring for a patient would conflict with a nurse's deeply held religious belief or (2) when there might be greater potential harm to the nurse than benefit to the patient (e.g., if the nurse were immunocompromised).
- The Canadian Human Rights Commission Policy (1986) on HIV/AIDS (acquired immune deficiency syndrome) prohibits discrimination based on HIV/AIDS status.
- If a nurse's primary concern is personal safety, the nurse needs to re-examine her or his commitment to the nursing profession.

Clinical Decision-Making Questions

1. How should the nurse address this issue if the other nurse was a colleague?
2. If nurses could select which patients they would care for, how would that affect their ability to care for patients in general?

CLINICAL DECISION-MAKING EXERCISE

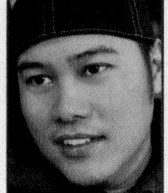

CASE STUDY:
At Risk for HIV Disease
Source: © iStockphoto.com/Mike Manzano.

Patient Profile

Mr. Emilio Chavez, a 20-year-old university student, comes to the student health centre with pain on urination.

Subjective Data

- Describes pain as, "Just like it felt when I had the clap last year"
- Provides a history of sexual activity since age 15; reports lifetime sexual partners as six women and two men
- Denies injected-drug use, tobacco use, or corticosteroid therapy
- Uses alcohol (mainly beer) at weekend parties and has smoked marijuana, but not recently
- Recent sexual activity has been on weekends during or after beer parties

Objective Data

Physical Examination
- 180 cm (5 ft, 11 in) tall, 76 kg (168 lb), temperature 38° C, purulent urethral discharge noted

Laboratory Studies
- Urine test for *Neisseria gonorrhoeae* is positive

Collaborative Care

- Intramuscular (IM) injection with 250 mg ceftriaxone
- Doxycycline 100 mg orally twice daily for 7 days

Discussion Questions

1. Why should Mr. Chavez be encouraged to be tested for human immunodeficiency virus (HIV)?
2. How will the nurse counsel Mr. Chavez about the testing process? How can the nurse help him prepare for the test and the test results?
3. What further questions will the nurse need to ask Mr. Chavez before the nurse can determine his educational needs?
4. Ask a classmate to be "Mr. Chavez" and role-play HIV risk assessment, risk-reduction counselling, and pretest and post-test counselling.
5. *Priority Decision:* What are the main considerations to cover when teaching about barrier methods of protection? Are there cultural components that may affect the nurse's approach to teaching about condoms?
6. How will the nurse discuss the issue of partner notification with Mr. Chavez?
7. *Priority Decision:* If Mr. Chavez's HIV test is positive, what are the priority nursing diagnoses most likely to apply? If his HIV test is negative, what priority nursing diagnoses most likely apply?

ⓔvolve *Answers are available at* **http://evolve.elsevier.com/ Canada/Lewis/medsurg**

REVIEW QUESTIONS

The number of the question corresponds to the same-numbered objective at the beginning of the chapter.

1. Which three items in the following list are a source of emerging infections?
   a. Plants
   b. Animals
   c. Biological warfare
   d. Antibiotic resistance

2. Which of the following antibiotic-resistant organisms are resistant to normal hand soap?
   a. Vancomycin-resistant enterococci
   b. Methicillin-resistant *Staphylococcus aureus*
   c. Penicillin-resistant *Streptococcus pneumoniae*
   d. β-Lactamase–producing *Klebsiella pneumoniae*

3. How does the transmission of human immunodeficiency virus (HIV) occur?
   a. Most commonly as a result of sexual contact
   b. In all infants born to women with HIV infection
   c. Only when there is a large viral load in the blood
   d. Frequently in health care workers with needle-stick exposures

4. Which is the common physiological change after HIV infection?
   a. The virus replicates mainly in B lymphocytes before spreading to CD4+ T cells in lymph nodes.
   b. The immune system is impaired predominantly by infection and destruction of CD4+ T cells.
   c. Infection of monocytes may occur, but these cells are destroyed by antibodies produced by oligodendrocytes.
   d. A long period develops during which the virus is not found in the blood and there is little viral replication.

5. Which of the following statements is false?
   a. Infection with HIV results in a chronic disease with acute exacerbations.
   b. Untreated HIV infection can remain in the early chronic stage for a decade or more.
   c. Late-stage infection is often called acquired immune deficiency syndrome (AIDS).
   d. Opportunistic diseases occur more often when the CD4+ T-cell count is high and the viral load is low.

6. When is a diagnosis of AIDS made?
   a. When an HIV-infected patient develops an AIDS-defining illness
   b. When an HIV-infected patient has an increasing amount of HIV in the blood
   c. When an HIV-infected patient has a reversal of the CD4:CD8 ratio less than 2 : 1
   d. When an HIV-infected patient has oral hairy leukoplakia, an infection caused by Epstein-Barr virus

7. What does screening for HIV infection generally involve?
   a. Laboratory analysis of blood to detect HIV antigen
   b. Electrophoretic analysis of HIV antigen in plasma
   c. Laboratory analysis of blood to detect HIV antibodies
   d. Analysis of lymph tissues for the presence of HIV RNA

8. What is the indication for use of antiretroviral drugs?
   a. Cure acute HIV infection
   b. Treat opportunistic diseases
   c. Decrease viral RNA levels
   d. Supplement radiation and surgery

9. Which of the follow statements about opportunistic diseases in HIV infection is correct?
   a. Usually occur one at a time
   b. Generally slow to develop and progress
   c. Occur in the presence of immunosuppression
   d. Curable with appropriate pharmacological intervention

10. Which of the following statements about metabolic adverse effects of antiretroviral therapy (ART) is false?
    a. These are an annoying set of symptoms that are ultimately harmless.
    b. Changes in body shape and size are often difficult for HIV-infected patients to accept.
    c. Lipid abnormalities include increases of triglycerides and decreases in high-density cholesterol.
    d. Insulin resistance and dyslipidemia can be treated with drugs to control blood glucose and decrease cholesterol.

11. Which of the following eliminates the risk of transmission of HIV?
    a. Using sterile equipment to inject drugs
    b. Cleaning equipment used to inject drugs
    c. Taking zidovudine (azidothymidine [AZT], ZDV, Retrovir) during pregnancy
    d. Using latex barriers to cover genitals during sexual contact

12. Of the following, which is the most appropriate nursing intervention to help an HIV-infected patient adhere to the treatment regimen?
    a. Give the patient a DVD and a brochure to view and read at home.
    b. Volunteer to "set up" a drug pillbox for a week at a time.
    c. Inform the patient that the adverse effects of the drugs are bad but that they go away after a while.
    d. Assess the patient's lifestyle and find adherence cues that fit into the patient's lifestyle.

ANSWERS: 1. b; 2. a; 3. a; 4. b; 5. d; 6. a; 7. c; 8. c; 9. c; 10. a; 11. a; 12. d.

REFERENCES

AIDS InfoNet. (2009a). Drug use and HIV: Fact Sheet 154. Retrieved from *http://www.aidsinfonet.org/fact_sheets/view/154*

AIDS InfoNet. (2009b). The HIV lifecycle: Fact sheet 400. Retrieved from *http://www.aidsinfonet.org/fact_sheets/view/400*

AIDS InfoNet. (2011). Fact sheet 729: St. Johns wort (hypericin). Retrieved from *http://www.aidsinfonet.org/fact_sheets/view/729*

Anema, A., Wood, E., & Montaner, J. (2008). The use of highly active retroviral therapy to reduce HIV incidence at the population level. *Canadian Medical Association Journal, 179*(1), 13-14. doi:10.1503/cmaj.071809

Armington, K. (2005). Integrating rapid HIV testing into fast-paced private practice settings. *PRN Notebook, 10*, 7.

Bangsberg, D. R., & Machtinger, E. L. (2009). *Adherence to HIV antiretroviral therapy. HIV Insite Knowledge Base Chapter*. San Francisco, CA: University of California San Francisco. Retrieved from *http://www.hivinsite.ucsf.edu/InSite?page=kb-03-02-09*

Barbaro, G., & Iacobellis, G. (2009). Metabolic syndrome associated with HIV and highly active antiretroviral therapy. *Current Diabetes Report, 9*(1), 37-42. doi:10.1007/sl11892-009-008-7

Bogart, L. M., Cargill, B. O., Kennedy, D., Ryan, G., Murphy, D. A., Elijah, J., & Schuster, M. A. (2008). HIV related stigma among people with HIV and their families: A qualitative analysis. *AIDS and Behavior, 12*(3), 244-254. doi:10.1007/s10461-007-9231-x

Bradley-Springer, L. (Ed.). (2005). *HIV symptom management*. Akron, OH: Association of Nurses in AIDS Care (ANAC).

Buchbinder, S. (2009). The epidemiology of new HIV infections and interventions to limit HIV transmission. *Topics in HIV Medicine, 17*(2), 37-43.

Canadian Communicable Disease Report. (2007). Canadian Communicable Disease Report. Retrieved from *http://www.phac-aspc.gc.ca/publicat/ccdrrmtc/07vol33/index-eng.php*

Canadian Human Rights Commission. (1986). Policy on HIV/AIDS. Retrieved from *http://www.chrc-ccdp.ca/legislation_policies/aids-en.asp*

Canadian Nurses Association. (2006). Position statement: Bloodborne pathogens: Registered nurses and their ethical obligations. Retrieved from *http://www.cna-aiic.ca/CNA/documents/pdf/publications/PS86_Blood_Borne_Pathogen_e.pdf*

Centers for Disease Control and Prevention (CDC). (2006). Revised recommendations for HIV testing of adults, adolescents and pregnant women in health care settings. Retrieved from *http://www.cdc.gov/mmwr/preview/mmwrhtml/rr5514a1.htm*

Centers for Disease Control and Prevention (CDC). (2007a). Guidelines for isolation precautions: Preventing transmission of infectious agents in hospital settings. Retrieved from *http://www.cdc.gov/hicpac/2007IP/2007isolationprecautions.html*

Centers for Disease Control and Prevention (CDC). (2007b). HIV and its transmission. Retrieved from *http://www.cdc.gov/hiv/pubs/facts/transmission.htm*

Centers for Disease Control and Prevention (CDC). (2007b). Mother to child (perinatal) HIV transmission and prevention. Retrieved from *http://www.cdc.gov/hiv/topics/perinatal/resources/factsheets/perinatal.htm*

Centers for Disease Control and Prevention (CDC). (2008a). Guidelines for the use of antiretroviral agents in HIV-1 infected adults and adolescents. Retrieved from *http://www.aidsinfo.nih.gov*

Centers for Disease Control and Prevention (CDC). (2008b). Trends in tuberculosis—United States. *Morbidity and Mortality Weekly Report, 58*(10).

Centers for Disease Control and Prevention (CDC). (2009a). Advancing HIV prevention: New strategies for a changing epidemic. Retrieved from *http://www.cdc.gov/mmwr/preview/mmwrhtml/mm5215a1.htm*

Centers for Disease Control and Prevention (CDC). (2009b). Guidelines for the prevention and treatment of opportunistic infections in HIV-infected adults and adolescents: Recommendations from CDC, the National Institutes of Health, and the HIV Medicine Association of the Infectious Diseases Society of America. Retrieved from *http://www.aidsinfo.nih.gov*

Centers for Disease Control and Prevention (CDC). (2009c). Incorporating HIV prevention into medical care settings. Retrieved from *http://www.cdc.gov/hiv/topics/prev-prog/AHP/resources/factsheets/PICS.htm*

Centers for Disease Control and Prevention (CDC). (2009d). Public Health Service Task Force recommendations for use of antiretroviral drugs in pregnant HIV-1-infected women for maternal health and interventions to reduce perinatal HIV-1 transmission in the United States. Retrieved from *http://aidsinfo.nih.gov*

Centers for Disease Control and Prevention (CDC). (2010). How is HIV passed from one person to another? Retrieved from *http://www.cdc.gov/hiv/resources/qa/transmission.htm*

Centers for Disease Control and Prevention. (2012). HIV and the law: HIV transmission risk. Retrieved from *http://www.cdc.gov/hiv/law/transmission.htm*

Centre for Infectious Disease Prevention and Control. (2007). *HIV/AIDS Epi Updates*. Ottawa, ON: Public Health Agency of Canada.

Chopra, I., Schofield, C., Everett, M., O'Neill, A., Miller, K., Wilcox, M., …, Corvallin, P. (2008). Treatment of health-care associated infections caused by gram-negative bacteria: A consensus statement. *Lancet, 8*(2), 133-139. doi:10.1016/S1473-3099(08)70018-5

Davis, A., Johnson, S. C., Kiser, J., Hindman, J. (2009). *A pharmacist's guide to antiretroviral medications for HIV-infected adults and adolescents*. Denver, CO: Mountain Plains Education and Training. Retrieved from *http://www.mpaetc.org*

DeBaun, B. (2008). Evaluation of the antimicrobial properties of an alcohol free 2% chlorhexidine gluconate solution. *AORN Journal, 87*(5), 925-933. doi:10.1016/j.aorn.2008.02.001

Department of Health. (2008). *HIV post-exposure prophylaxis: Guidance from the United Kingdom chief medical officers' expert advisory group on AIDS*. Department of Health: London. Retrieved from *http://www.dh.gov.uk/prod_consum_dh/groups/dh_digitalassets/@dh/@en/documents/digitalasset/dh_089997.pdf*

Des Jarlais, D. C., McKnight, C., Goldblatt, C., & Purchase, D. (2009). Doing harm reduction better: Syringe exchange in the United States. *Addiction, 104*(9), 1441-1446. doi:10.1111/j.1360.0443.2008.02465.x

Dunn, D. T., Newell, M. L., Ades, A., & Peckham, E. (1992). Risk of human immunodeficiency virus type 1 transmission through breastfeeding. *Lancet, 340*(8819), 585-588. doi:10.1016/0140-6736(92)92115-v

Greenwood, B., Salisbury, D., & Hill, A. V. S. (2011). Vaccines and global health. *Philosophical Transactions of the Royal Society, 366*(1579), 2733-2742. doi:10.1098/rstb.2011.0076

Hamlyn, E., & Easterbrook, P. (2007). Occupational exposure to HIV and the use of post-exposure prophylaxis. *Occupational Medicine, 57*(5), 329-336. doi:10.1093/occmed/kqm046

Health Canada. (1999). Routine practices and additional precautions for preventing the transmission of infection in health care. *Canada Communicable Disease Report, 25*, S4.

Health Canada. (2002). Preventing the transmission of blood-borne pathogens in health care and public service settings. 23S3, May 1997. Update. In Prevention and Control of Occupational Infections in Health Care. *Canadian Communicable Disease Report, 28*, SI, 1-264.

Health Canada. (2010a). HIV/AIDS. Retrieved from *http://www.hc-sc.gc.ca/hl-vs/iyh-vsv/diseases-maladies/hiv-vih-eng.php*

Health Canada. (2010b). HIV/AIDS Epi Update, July 2010. Retrieved from *http://www.phac-aspc.gc.ca/aids-sida/publication/epi/2010/1-eng.php*

High, K. P., Bradley, S. F., Gravenstein, S., Mehr, D. R., Quagliarello, V. J., Richards, C., …, Yoshikawa, T. T. (2009). Clinical practice guideline for management of fever and infection in older residents of long-term care facilities: 2008 update by the Infectious Diseases Society of America. *Journal of the American Geriatric Society, 57*(3), 375-394. doi:10.1111/j.1532-5415.2009.02175x

Huether, S. E., & McCance, K. L. (2012). *Understanding pathophysiology*, 5th ed. St. Louis: Elsevier/Mosby.

Joy, R., Druyts, E. F., Brandson, E. K., Lima, V. D., Rustand, C. A., Zhang, W., …, Hogg, R. S. (2008). Impact of neighbourhood level socioeconomic status on HIV disease progression in a universal health care setting. *Journal of Acquired Immunodeficiency Syndrome, 47*(4), 500-505. doi:10.1097/QA1.0b013e3181648dfd

Knobel, H., Urbine, O., Conzalez, A., Sorli, M. L., Montero, M., Carmona, A., …, Guelar, A. (2009). Impact of different patterns of non-adherence on the outcome of highly active antiretroviral therapy in patients with long term followup. *HIV Medicine, 10*(6), 364-369. doi:10.1111/j.1468-1293.2009.00696.x

Kwong, J. (2009). *First visit basics: Initiating care for the HIV-infected patient*. Denver, CO: Mountain Plains Education and Training. Retrieved from *http://www.mpaetc.org*

Lashley, F., Durham, J. (ed.) (2007). *Emerging infectious diseases*, 2nd ed. New York: Jones and Bartlett.

Leung, V. L., & Glesby, M. J. (2011). Pathogenesis and treatment of HIV lipohypertrophy. *Current Opinions in Infectious Diseases, 24*(1), 43-49. doi:10.1097/QCO.06013e3283420eef

Long, E. F., Brandeau, M. L., & Owens, D. K. (2010). The cost-effectiveness and population outcomes of expanded HIV screening and antiretroviral treatment in the United States. *Annals of Internal Medicine, 153*(12), 778-789.

Madoff, L. C., & Kasper, D. L. (2008). Introduction to infectious disease: Host-pathogen interaction. In A. S. Fauci, E. Braunwald, D. L. Kaspar, S. L. Hauser, D. L. Longo, J. L. Jameson, & J. Loscalzo (Eds.), *Harrison's principles of internal medicine*. New York: McGraw-Hill.

Magnan, M. A., & Reynolds, K. (2006). Barriers to addressing patient sexuality concerns across five areas of specialization. *Clinical Nurse Specialist, 20*(6), 285-292.

Martinez, E., Larrousse, M., & Gatell, J. M. (2009). Cardiovascular disease and HIV infection: Host, virus or drugs? *Current Opinion in Infectious Diseases, 22*(1), 28-34. doi:10.1097/QCO.06013e328320a849

McCall, J., McMillan, N., & Pielak, K. (2005). Accidental exposure guidelines: What you should know. *Nursing BC, 37*(5), 16-20.

McCall, J., Vicol, L., & Tsang, G. (2009). Healthy mothers, healthy babies: Preventing vertical transmission of HIV/AIDS. *Nursing BC, 41*(2), 26-30.

Montaner, J. S. (2011). Treatment as prevention: A double hat trick. *Lancet, 378*(9787), 208-209. doi:10.1016/50140-6736(11)60821-0

Mountain Plains AIDS Education and Training Center. (n.d.). STD/HIV Risk assessment: A quick reference guide. Retrieved from *http://www.mpaetc.org*

O'Bryne, P., & MacPherson, P. (2008). Understanding HIV viral load: Implications for counselling. *Canadian Journal of Public Health, 99*(3), 189-191.

Ontario Agency for Health Protection and Promotion. (2009). Slide Presentation: Tuberculosis: Out with the Old, in with the New: Diagnostic Challenges and Possibilities. Retrieved from *http://www.oahpp.ca/resources/documents/presentations/2009oct8/TB_Diagnostic%20laboratory%20in%20Ontario_Fran_Oct%202009.pdf*

Ontario Ministry of Health and Long-Term Care. (2007). Infection prevention and control: Core competency education. Retrieved from *http://www.health.gov.on.ca/english/providers/program/infectious/infect_prevent/ipccce_mn.html*

Ortiz, A. M., & Silvestri, G. (2009). Immunopathogenesis of AIDS. *Current Infectious Disease Report, 11*(3), 239-245. doi:10.1007/s11908-009-0035-1

Pepin, J. (2011). *The origin of AIDS*. Cambridge, UK: Cambridge University Press.

Pommerville, J. C. (2009). *Alcamo's fundamentals of microbiology* (2nd ed). Boston: Jones & Bartlett.

Portillo, C. J., Holzemer, W. L., & Chou, F. (2007). HIV symptoms. *Annual Review of Nursing Research, 25*, 259-291.

Public Health Agency of Canada (PHAC). (2005). *Canada's report on HIV/AIDS 2005*. Ottawa: PHAC. Retrieved from *http://www.phac-aspc.gc.ca/aids-sida/publication/reports/report05/2-eng.php*

Public Health Agency of Canada (PHAC). (2006). *Avian influenza*. Ottawa: PHAC. Retrieved from *http://www.phac-aspc.gc.ca/influenza/avian-eng.php*

Public Health Agency of Canada (PHAC). (2007a). *The Canadian Nosocomial Infection Surveillance Program: Point prevalence study*. Ottawa: Author. Retrieved from *http://www.phac-aspc.gc.ca/nois-sinp/projects/pps-eng.php*

Public Health Agency of Canada (PHAC). (2007b). *Populations at risk*. Ottawa: Author. Retrieved from *http://www.phac-aspc.gc.ca/aids-sida/populations-eng.php*

Public Health Agency of Canada (PHAC). (2010a). *Drug resistance in Canada*. Ottawa: Author. Retrieved from *http://www.phac-aspc.gc.ca/tbpc-latb/pubs/tbdrc10/index-eng.php*

Public Health Agency of Canada (PHAC). (2010b). *HIV/AIDS epi updates—July 2010*. Ottawa: Author. Retrieved from *http://www.phac-aspc.gc.ca/aids-sida/publication/index-eng.php#er*

Public Health Agency of Canada (PHAC). (2010c). *International tuberculosis incidence rates*. Ottawa: Author. Retrieved from *http://www.phac-aspc.gc.ca/tbpc-latb/itir-eng.php*

Public Health Agency of Canada. (2010d). *At a glance—HIV and AIDS in Canada: Surveillance report to December 31, 2010*. Health Canada: Ottawa. Retrieved from *http://www.phac-aspc.gc.ca/aids-sida/publication/servreport/2010/dec/index-eng.php*

Public Health Agency of Canada (PHAC). (2011). *Tuberculosis in Canada, 2009 – Pre-Release*. Retrieved from *http://www.phac-aspc.gc.ca/tbpc-latb/pubs/tbcan09pre/index-eng.php*

Public Health Agency of Canada (PHAC). (2012). Tuberculosis in Canada 2010 – Pre-Release. Retrieved from *http://www.phac-aspc.gc.ca/tbpc-latb/pubs/tbcan10pre/index-eng.php*

Ramachandran, R., & Shanmughavle, P. (2009). Role of microbicides in the prevention of HIV and sexually transmitted diseases—

A review. *Current HIV Research, 7*(3), 279-286. doi:10.2174/157016209788347921

Roberson, D. (2009). Factors influencing adherence to antiretroviral therapy for HIV-infected female inmates. *Journal of the Association of Nurses in AIDS Care, 20*(1), 50-61, doi:10.1016/j.jana.2008.05.008

Rossi, S. L., Ross, T. M., & Evans, J. D.(2010). West Nile virus. *Clinics in Laboratory Medicine, 30*(1), 47-65. doi:10.1016/j.cll.2009.10.006

Sanchez, T., Finlayson, T., Drake, A., Behel, S., Cribbin, M., DiNenno, E., ..., Lamsky, A. (2006). Human immunodeficiency virus (HIV) risk, prevention and testing behaviors—United States National HIV Behavioral Surveillance System: Men who have sex with men, November 2003—April 2005. *Morbidity and Mortality Weekly Report, 55*(SS-6), 1-16.

Siegel, J. D., Rhinehart, E., Jackson, M., & Chiarello, L. (2006). Management of multidrug-resistant organisms in healthcare settings. Centers for Disease Control and Prevention. Retrieved from *http://www.cdc.gov/hicpac/pdf/MDRO/MDROGuideline2006.pdf*

Stek, A. M. (2008). Antiretroviral treatment in pregnancy. *Current Opinion in HIV/AIDS, 3*(2), 155-160. doi:10.1097/COH.0b013e3282f50bfe

Swanson, B. (Ed.) (2010). *ANAC's core curriculum for HIV/AIDS nursing* (3rd ed.). Sudbury, MA: Jones and Bartlett.

Thompson, M. A., Aberg, J. A., Cahn, P., Montaner, J. S. G., Rizzardini, G., Telenti, A., ..., Schooley, R. T. (2010). Antiretroviral treatment of adult HIV infection: 2010 recommendations of the International AIDS Society—USA panel. *Journal of the American Medical Association, 304*(3), 321-333. doi:10.1001/jama.2010.1004

Toblan, A. A., & Quinn, T. C. (2009). Herpes simplex type 2 and syphilis infection with HIV: An evolving synergy in transmission and prevention. *Current Opinion in HIV/AIDS, 4*(4), 294-299. doi:10.1097/COH.0b013e32832c1881

United Nations AIDS (UNAIDS). (2009). 2009 Epidemic Update. Retrieved from *http://www.unaids.org/en/dataanalysis/epidemiology/2009aidsepidemicupdate*

United Nations AIDS (UNAIDS). (2010). *Global Report: UNAIDS Report on the Global AIDS Epidemic.* Geneva: Author. Retrieved from *http://www.unaids.org/globalreport/Global_report.htm*

United Nations AIDS (UNAIDS). (2011). Global AIDS response continues to show results as a record number of people access treatment and rates of new HIV infection fall by nearly 25%. Retrieved from *http://www.unaids.org/en/resources/presscentre/pressreleaseandstatementarchive/2011/June/20110603praids30/#d.en.60161*

Valenti, W. M. (2008). *Acute retroviral syndrome: A challenge for primary care.* AIDS Reader, 18, 294.

Wasserman, P., Segal-Maurer, S., Wehbeh, W., & Rubin, D. S. (2011). Wasting disease, chronic immune activation and inflammation in HIV infected patients. *Topics in Clinical Nutrition, 26*(1), 14-28. doi:10.1097/TIN.0b013e318209e3a0

Watkins, D. (2009). HIV vaccine development. *Topics in HIV Medicine, 17*(2), 35-36.

World Health Organization. (2005). *Combating Emerging Infectious Diseases in the South-East Asia Region.* Retrieved from *http://203.90.70.117/PDS_DOCS/B0005.pdf*

World Health Organization (WHO). (2007). *WHO case definitions of HIV for surveillance and revised clinical staging and immunological classification of HIV-related disease in adults and children.* Geneva: World Health Organization. Retrieved from *http://www.who.int/hiv/pub/guidelines/HIVstaging150307.pdf*

Zoutman, D. E., Ford, B. D., Bryce, E., Gourdeau, M., Hebert, G., Henderson, E., ..., Paton, S. (2003). The state of infection surveillance and control in Canadian acute care hospitals. *American Journal of Infection Control, 31*(5), 266-273. doi:10.1067/mic.2003.139

CANADIAN RESOURCES

BC Centre for Excellence in HIV/AIDS
http://www.cfenet.ubc.ca
Canadian Aboriginal AIDS Network
http://www.caan.ca
Canadian AIDS Society
http://www.cdnaids.ca
Canadian AIDS Treatment Information Exchange (CATIE)
http://www.catie.ca
Canadian Association of Nurses in AIDS Care
http://www.canac.org
Canadian Blood Services
http://www.bloodservices.ca
Canadian Centre for Occupational Health and Safety
http://www.ccohs.ca
Canadian Nurses Association Code of Ethics for Registered Nurses
http://www.cna-aiic.ca/CNA/documents/pdf/publications/Code_of_Ethics_2008_e.pdf
http://www.cna-aiic.ca/cna/documents/pdf/publications/CodeofEthics2002_e.pdf
Canadian Public Health Association
http://www.cpha.ca
Canadian Treatment Action Council
http://www.ctac.ca
Canadian Working Group on HIV and Rehabilitation
http://www.hivandrehab.ca
Community and Hospital Infection Control Association Canada
http://www.chica.org/
Health Canada—HIV and AIDS
http://www.hc-sc.gc.ca/hc-ps/dc-ma/aids-sida-eng.php
Canadian: *http://www.hc-sc.gc.ca/english/diseases/aids.html*
HIV/AIDS Epi Update
http://www.phac-aspc.gc.ca/publicat/epiu-aepi/index.html#HIV
HIV/AIDS Legal Network
http://www.aidslaw.ca
HIV Anti-Discrimination Campaign
http://www.doyou.cpha.ca
Positive Living Society of BC
http://www.positivelivingbc.org
Positive Women's Network
http:// www.pwn.bc.ca
Proceedings of the Consensus Conference on Infected Health Care Workers: Risk for Transmission of Blood-borne Pathogens
http://www.phac-aspc.gc.ca/publicat/info/infbbp-eng.php
http://www.phac-aspc.gc.ca/publicat/ccdr-rmtc/98vol24/24s4/index.html
Public Health Agency of Canada
http://www.phac-aspc.gc.ca
Public Health Agency of Canada—Surveillance and Risk Assessment Division (SRAD)
http://www.phac-aspc.gc.ca/aids-sida/about/surv-eng.phphast-vsmt/index.html

RELATED RESOURCES

AIDS Education Global Information System (AEGIS)
http://www.aegis.com
HIV/AIDS Clinical Treatment Information Service (ATIS)
http://www.hivatis.org
Joint United Nations Programme on HIV/AIDS (UNAIDS)
http://www.unaids.org

evolve *For additional Internet resources, see the Web site for this book at* **http://evolve.elsevier.com/Canada/Lewis/medsurg**

Written by Jormain Cady and Joyce A. Jackowski

Adapted by Rosemary Cashman

LEARNING OBJECTIVES

1. Describe the prevalence, the incidence, and the death rates of cancer in Canada.
2. Describe the biological processes involved in cancer.
3. Differentiate the three phases of cancer development.
4. Describe the role of the immune system in relation to cancer.
5. Describe the use of the classification systems for cancer.
6. Explain the role of the nurse in the prevention and detection of cancer.
7. Explain the use of surgery, radiation therapy, chemotherapy, and biological therapy in the treatment of cancer.
8. Differentiate between external beam radiation and brachytherapy.
9. Identify the classifications of chemotherapeutic agents and methods of administration.
10. Describe the effects of radiation therapy and chemotherapy on normal tissues.
11. Identify the types and effects of biological therapy agents.
12. Describe the nursing management of patients receiving radiation therapy, chemotherapy, and biological therapy.
13. Describe the nutritional therapy for patients with cancer.
14. Describe the complications that can occur in advanced cancer.
15. Describe the appropriate psychosocial support of the patient with cancer and the patient's family.

KEY TERMS

benign neoplasm A localized tumour that has a fibrous capsule, limited potential for growth and metastasis, a regular shape, and cells that are well differentiated, p. 350

biological therapy Treatment involving the use of biological agents such as interferons, interleukins, monoclonal antibodies, and growth factors to modify the relationship between the host and the tumour, p. 372

bone marrow transplantation The transplantation of bone marrow from healthy donors (allogeneic transplantation) or from marrow that has been purged of disease and reinfused back to the donor (autologous transplantation) to stimulate production of normal blood cells, p. 376

brachytherapy "Closed" radiation delivery system in which radioactive materials are implanted or inserted directly into the tumour or close to the tumour, p. 365

cancer A group of more than 200 diseases characterized by uncontrolled and unregulated growth of cells, p. 347

carcinogens Agents that cause cancer, p. 350

carcinoma in situ A lesion with all the histological features of cancer except invasion of surrounding areas, p. 355

carcinomas Malignant tumours that originate from embryonal ectoderm and endoderm, p. 354

histological grading A pathology-based system for grading tumours according to appearance and other features of cells that are predictive of growth rate and invasiveness; tumour grade helps determine treatment and prognosis, p. 355

immunological surveillance The response of the immune system to antigens of the malignant cells, p. 353

malignant neoplasms Tumours that tend to grow, invade, and metastasize; usually have an irregular shape and are composed of poorly differentiated cells, p. 350

metastasis Spread of cancer from the initial or primary site to a distant site, p. 351

nadir The lowest level of the peripheral blood cell counts that occurs secondary to destruction of circulating and proliferating progenitor blood cells by chemotherapy, p. 363

oncogenes Excessively or inappropriately active genes that encode proteins whose actions promote cellular proliferation and have the potential to induce cancer, p. 349

proto-oncogenes Normal genes that regulate cellular processes and proliferation but may undergo mutations that lead to the development of cancer cells, p. 349

radiation The emission and distribution of energy through space or a material medium, p. 364

sarcomas Malignant tumours that originate from embryonal mesoderm, which normally becomes connective tissue, muscle, bone, and fat, p. 355

staging Classifying the extent and spread of disease, p. 355

tumour angiogenesis The process of the formation of blood vessels within the tumour itself, p. 352

tumour-associated antigens Antigens on tumour cell surfaces, not present on normal cells, that may be targeted by antineoplastic therapies, p. 352

tumour suppressor genes Normal genes that regulate cellular processes and proliferation and normally suppress the development of cancer cells, p. 349

vesicants Agents, including some chemotherapeutic drugs, that are capable of causing tissue blistering, p. 360

ELECTRONIC RESOURCES

Supplemental content related to Chapter 18 can be found…

Evolve Web Site ⊖volve

http://evolve.elsevier.com/Canada/Lewis/medsurg
- Clinical Reference: Laboratory Values
- Content Updates
- Electronic Calculators
- eTables:
  - eTable 18-1: Karnofsky Functional Performance Scale
  - eTable 18-2: Screening Guidelines for Early Detection of Cancer in Asymptomatic People
- eTable 18-3: Four *R*s of Radiology
- eTable 18-4: Nutritional Therapy: Protein Foods With High Biological Value
- eTable 18-5: Nutritional Therapy: High-Calorie Foods
- Examination Review Questions
- Glossary
- Key Points (Printable and MP3 Download)

Definition and Incidence

Cancer is a group of more than 200 diseases characterized by uncontrolled and unregulated growth of cells. It can occur in persons of all ages and all ethnicities and is a major health problem. In 2011, it was estimated that 177,800 new cancer cases (excluding 74,100 nonmelanoma skin cancers) would be diagnosed and that 75,000 people would die from cancer in Canada (Canadian Cancer Society's Steering Committee on Cancer Statistics, 2011). As the population ages, the incidence of cancer rises. Among persons with cancer, 42% of new cases and 59% of deaths caused by cancer occur in those who are at least 70 years of age. Cancer is more common among boys and men younger than 20 and older than 60 than in girls and women of the same ages, but more cancer cases and deaths occur among women between the ages of 20 and 59. Approximately 43% of Canadians will develop cancer during their lifetimes, and 27% of those will die from the disease; the mortality rate is slightly greater for men than women. Of new cancer cases, about 50,000 (30%) affect those between ages 20 and 59, and 13,000 (18%) die of cancer-related causes, with significant repercussions on Canadian families and the economy (Canadian Cancer Society's Steering Committee on Cancer Statistics, 2011). Estimated cancer incidence and mortality by site (type) and sex are presented in Tables 18-1 and 18-2.

Prevalence is the total number of people who are living with a diagnosis of cancer. Advances in research in the areas of early detection, treatment, and supportive therapies have resulted in more people surviving cancer, especially in the pediatric population. Prevalence is, therefore, more often and more usefully defined as those still alive 10 years after the initial diagnosis with cancer. One per 44 Canadians (2.3% of the population) received a cancer diagnosis in the previous 10 years (Canadian Cancer

Table 18-1 New Cases for Cancer by Site (Type) and Sex, Canada, 2011

MALE		FEMALE	
TYPE	NEW CASE ESTIMATE	TYPE	NEW CASE ESTIMATE
Prostate	25,500	Breast	23,400
Lung	13,200	Lung	12,200
Colorectal	12,500	Colorectal	9,700
Non-Hodgkin's lymphoma	4,200	Non-Hodgkin's lymphoma	3,400
Bladder, kidney	5,400	Uterus	4,700
Melanoma (skin)	3,100	Melanoma	2,500

Source: Canadian Cancer Society's Steering Committee on Cancer Statistics. (2011). *Canadian Cancer Statistics 2011*. Toronto: Canadian Cancer Society.

Table 18-2 Estimated Deaths for Cancer by Site and Sex, Canada, 2011

MALE		FEMALE	
TYPE	DEATHS	TYPE	DEATHS
Lung	11,300	Lung	9,300
Prostate	4,100	Breast	5,100
Colorectal	5,000	Colorectal	3,900
Pancreas	1,900	Pancreas	1,950
Non-Hodgkin's lymphoma	1,700	Ovary	1,750

Source: Canadian Cancer Society's Steering Committee on Cancer Statistics (2011). *Canadian Cancer Statistics 2011*. Toronto: Canadian Cancer Society.

Society's Steering Committee on Cancer Statistics, 2011). Since 2008, cancer has been the leading cause of death in every Canadian province, accounting for 30% of all deaths, with heart disease in second place (21% of deaths) (Statistics Canada, 2011). Lung cancer remains the leading cause of premature death from cancer (Canadian Cancer Society's Steering Committee on Cancer Statistics, 2011), and tobacco use has long been recognized as a significant risk for the development of this and other types of cancer. Smoking prevalence and amount have declined in the Canadian population overall; however, smoking rates among Aboriginal peoples are more than twice as high as those in the general population, with particularly high rates (54-65%) among Aboriginal youth (Canadian Cancer Society, 2005). Cancer incidence and mortality are tracked by province through cancer registries. There are variations between eastern and western regions; for example, both incidence and death rates are higher in the eastern regions of Canada. Statistics document the incidence and prevalence of cancer but cannot reveal the physiological and psychosocial effect of cancer on individuals, families, and society. Nurses play a critical role in shaping attitudes and promoting behaviours that prevent the development of cancer or facilitate adjustment to living with cancer.

Progress Made in Cancer Prevention: Modifiable Risk Factors

Many well-known and common cancer risk factors are preventable. For example, in addition to tobacco use, known risk factors include excessive body weight, lack of physical activity, unhealthy eating habits, and excessive exposure to the sun. Several of these factors are related to other chronic diseases such as diabetes, kidney failure, chronic obstructive lung disease, and cardiovascular disease. The Canadian Cancer Society reports that 60% of Canadians do not eat recommended amounts of fruits and vegetables, about half (54% of women and 44% of men) are physically inactive, 15% are obese, and 56% of men and 39% of women are at an unhealthy weight (Canadian Cancer Society, 2005). All of these risk factors are within the control of each individual to modify. If these lifestyle factors were modified, the rates of cancers and other chronic diseases would be reduced (Table 18-3). Concerted efforts in health promotion and disease prevention strategies are required in every province to alert and educate the public about what they can do to achieve improvements in health and longevity.

Table 18-3 Potentially Preventable Cancer Cases and Deaths According to Selected Modifiable Risk Factors, Canada, 2005

RISK FACTOR	ESTIMATED NO. CASES	ESTIMATED NO. CANCER DEATHS
Tobacco use	44,700	20,850
Unhealthy diet, physical inactivity, excess body weight	44,700	20,850
Sun	65,840	725
Alcohol	4,470	2,085

Source: Adapted from Canadian Cancer Society. (2005). Canadian cancer statistics 2005, p. 81. Retrieved from *http://www.cancer.ca/ canada-wide/about%20cancer/cancer%20statistics/~/media/CCS/Canada%20 wide/Files%20List/English%20files%20heading/pdf%20not%20in%20 publications%20section/Canadian%20Cancer%20Statistics%20-%20 2005%20-%20EN%20-%20PDF_401594768.ashx*

Biological Processes of Cancer

The term *cancer* encompasses many diseases of multiple causes that can arise in any cell of the body capable of evading regulatory controls over proliferation and differentiation. Two major dysfunctions present in the process of cancer are defective cellular *proliferation* (growth) and defective cellular *differentiation*.

Defects in Cellular Proliferation

Normally, most tissues of the human adult contain a population of predetermined, undifferentiated cells known as *stem cells*. *Predetermined* means that the stem cells of a particular tissue will ultimately differentiate and become mature, functioning cells of that tissue and only that tissue.

Cell proliferation originates in the stem cell and begins when the stem cell enters the cell cycle (Figure 18-1). The time from when a cell enters the cell cycle to the time the cell divides into two identical cells is called the *generation time of the cell*. A mature cell continues to function until it degenerates and dies.

All cells of a tissue are controlled by an intracellular mechanism that determines when cellular proliferation is necessary. Under normal conditions, a state of dynamic equilibrium is constantly maintained (i.e., cellular proliferation equals cellular degeneration). Normally, the process of cellular division and proliferation is activated only in the event of cellular degeneration or death. Cellular proliferation also occurs if the body has a physiological need for more cells. For example, a normal increase in white blood cell (WBC) count occurs in the presence of infection.

Another explanation for the phenomenon of proliferation control in normal cells is *contact inhibition*. Normal cells "respect" the boundaries and territory of the cells surrounding them; they do not invade a territory that is not their own. The neighbouring cells are thought to inhibit cellular growth through the physical contact of the surrounding cell membranes. Cancer cells grown in tissue culture are characterized by loss of contact inhibition. These cells have no regard for cellular boundaries and will grow on top of one another and also on top of or between normal cells.

The rate of normal cellular proliferation differs in each body tissue. In some tissues, such as bone marrow, hair follicles, and epithelial lining of the gastrointestinal (GI) tract, the rate of cellular proliferation is rapid. In other tissues, such as myocardium, neurons, and cartilage, cellular proliferation is slow or does not occur at all.

Cancer cells usually proliferate in the manner and at the same rate as the normal cells of the tissue from which they arise. However, cancer cells respond differently than normal cells to the intracellular signals that regulate the state of dynamic equilibrium. Cell division in cancer is dysregulated and haphazard.

According to the stem cell theory, the loss of intracellular control of proliferation results from a mutation of the stem cells (Tannock, Hill, Bristow, & Harrington, 2005). The stem cells are viewed as the target or the origin of cancer development. The DNA of the stem cell is substituted or permanently rearranged. When this happens, the stem cell is mutated. Once the cell has mutated, one of three things can occur: (a) the cell can die, either from the damage resulting from the mutation or from initiation of a programmed cellular suicide called *apoptosis*; (b) the cell can recognize the damage and repair itself; or (c) the mutated cell can survive and pass along the damage to its daughter cells. Mutated

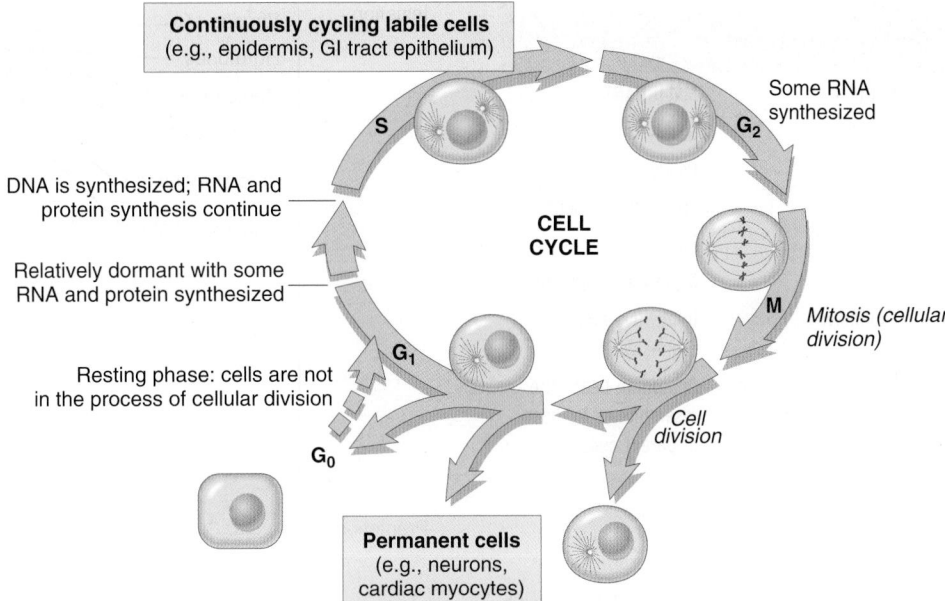

Figure 18-1 Cell life cycle and metabolic activity. Generation time is the period from one M (mitosis) phase to the next. Cells not in the cycle but capable of division are in the resting phase (G_0). *DNA*, deoxyribonucleic acid; *RNA*, ribonucleic acid.

Source: Adapted from Kumar, V., Abbas, A. K., Fausto, N., & Aster, J. C. (2010). *Robbins and Cotran pathologic basis of disease* (8th ed., p. 86, Fig 3-7). Philadelphia: W. B. Saunders.

cells that survive have the potential to become malignant (i.e., cells with invasive and metastatic potential), especially if the progeny cells acquire additional mutations.

A common misconception regarding the characteristics of cancer cells is that the mitotic rate is more rapid than that of any normal body cell. In most situations, cancer cells proliferate at the same rate as the normal cells of the tissue from which they originate. Whereas normal cell proliferation is regulated according to the body's needs, however, proliferation of the cancer cells is indiscriminate and continuous. In this way, with each cell division creating two or more offspring cells, the tumour mass continuously doubles in size: 1 cell → 2 cells → 4 cells → 8 cells → 16 cells and so on. This is termed the *pyramid effect*. The time required for a tumour mass to double in size is known as its *doubling time*.

Proliferating cells rely on a genetic blueprint for tissues and organs, which is found on chromosomes within the nucleus of the cell. Structures called *telomeres,* consisting of a repeated DNA code, are found at the end of chromosomes and serve to protect the genetic data within the chromosomes and facilitate normal cell division. Each time a cell divides, the telomere becomes shorter, and a small sequence of genetic material is not copied. Ultimately, the cell is unable to undergo further division, becomes inactive (senescent), and dies. Cancer cells produce an enzyme called *telomerase* that prevents telomere shortening and allows the cells to escape senescence and death. Telomerase thus promotes the immortalization of cells and has a role in the development of cancer, as well as the process of aging.

Defects in Cellular Differentiation

Cellular differentiation is normally an orderly process in which the cell progresses from a state of immaturity to a state of maturity. Because all body cells are derived from fertilized ova, all cells have the potential to perform all body functions. As cells differentiate,

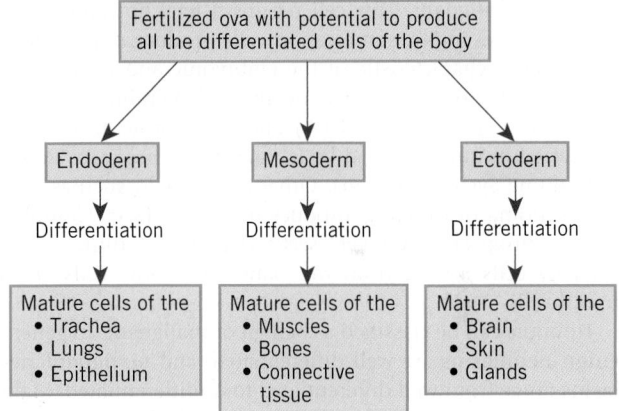

Figure 18-2 Normal cellular differentiation.

this potential is repressed, and the mature cell is capable of performing only specific functions (Figure 18-2).

In cellular differentiation, the phasing out of cellular potential is stable and orderly. Under normal conditions, the differentiated cell is stable and does not *dedifferentiate* (i.e., revert to a previous undifferentiated state).

The exact mechanism that controls cellular differentiation and proliferation is not completely understood. Two types of normal genes are important regulators of normal cellular processes: **proto-oncogenes** promote growth, whereas **tumour suppressor genes,** such as tumour protein 53, suppress growth. Both can be affected by mutations. Those that alter the expression of proto-oncogenes can activate them to function as **oncogenes** (tumour-inducing genes). Mutations that alter tumour suppressor genes render them inactive, which results in a loss of their tumour suppressor actions (Ewart-Toland & Balmain, 2004).

Table 18-4 Comparison of Benign and Malignant Neoplasms		
CHARACTERISTIC	**BENIGN**	**MALIGNANT**
Encapsulated	Usually	Rarely
Differentiated	Normally	Poorly
Metastasis	Absent	Frequently present
Recurrence	Rare	Possible
Vascularity	Slight	Moderate to marked
Mode of growth	Expansive	Infiltrative and expansive
Cell characteristics	Fairly normal; similar to those of parent cells	Abnormal; bear little resemblance to those of parent cells

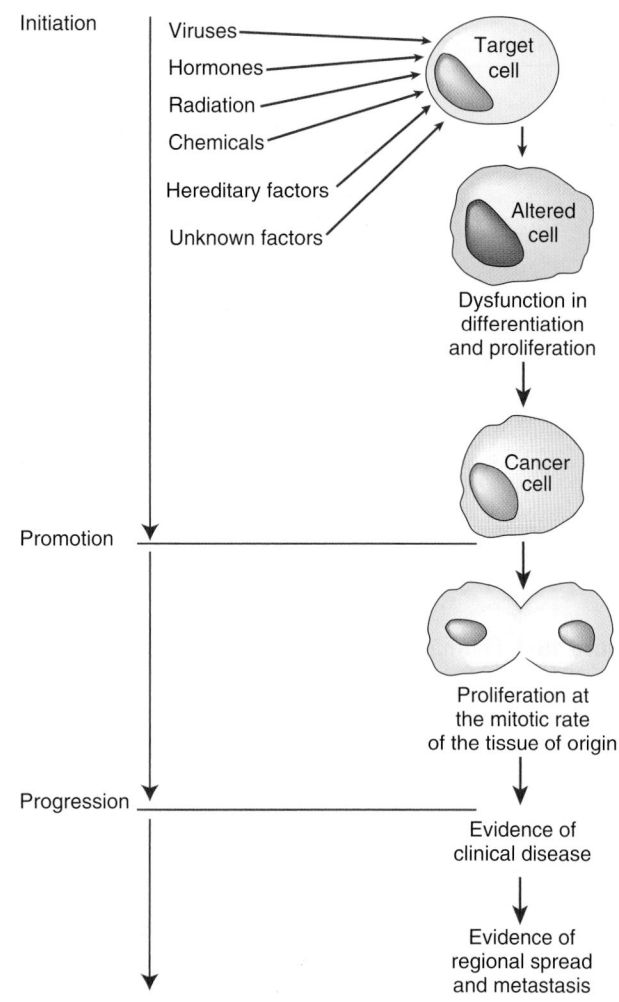

Figure 18-3 Process of cancer development.

The proto-oncogene has been described as the genetic lock that keeps the cell in its mature functioning state. When this lock is "unlocked," as may occur through exposure to **carcinogens** (cancer-causing agents capable of producing cellular alterations) or oncogenic viruses, genetic alterations and mutations occur. The abilities and properties that the cell had during fetal development are again expressed. Oncogenes interfere with normal cell expression under some conditions, causing the cell to become malignant. This cell regains a fetal appearance and function. For example, some cancer cells produce new proteins, such as those characteristic of the embryonic and fetal periods of life. These proteins, located on the cell membrane, include carcinoembryonic antigen (CEA) and α-fetoprotein. They can be detected in human blood by laboratory studies (see "Role of the Immune System" section). Other cancer cells, such as small cell carcinoma of the lung, produce hormones (see "Complications Resulting From Cancer" section) that are ordinarily produced by cells arising from the same embryonic cells as the tumour cells.

Tumours can be classified as benign or malignant. In general, **benign neoplasms** are well differentiated, and **malignant neoplasms** range from well differentiated to undifferentiated. Malignant tumour cells have the ability to invade and metastasize, unlike benign neoplasms. Other differences between benign and malignant neoplasms are listed in Table 18-4.

Development of Cancer

In this section, a theoretical model of the development of cancer is described. The cause and development of each type of cancer are likely to be multifactorial. It is not known how many tumours have a chemical, environmental, genetic, immunological, or viral origin. Cancers may arise spontaneously from causes that are thus far unclear.

It is a common belief that the development of cancer is a rapid, haphazard event. However, the natural history of cancer is an orderly process comprising several stages and occurring over a period of time. These stages are *initiation, promotion,* and *progression* (Figure 18-3).

Initiation. The first stage, *initiation,* is a mutation in the cell's genetic structure resulting from an inherited mutation, an error that occurs during DNA replication or after exposure to a carcinogen. This altered cell has the potential for developing into a *clone* (progeny of a single cell) of neoplastic cells.

Many carcinogens are detoxified by protective enzymes and harmlessly excreted. If this protective mechanism fails, carcinogens can enter a cell's nucleus and alter DNA. The cell may die or repair itself. However, if cell death or repair does not occur before cell division, the cell replicates into daughter cells, each with the same genetic alteration. Carcinogens may be chemical, radioactive, or viral in nature. In addition, some genetic anomalies increase the susceptibility of individuals to certain cancers. Common characteristics of carcinogens are that their effects in the stage of initiation are usually irreversible and additive.

Chemical Carcinogens. Chemicals were identified as cancer-causing agents in the latter part of the eighteenth century, when Percival Pott noted that chimney sweeps had a higher incidence of cancer of the scrotum in association with exposure to soot residues in chimneys. Over time, more chemical agents were identified as actual and potential carcinogens. Evidence indicated that individuals undergoing sustained exposure to certain chemicals had a greater incidence of certain cancers than others. Because of the long latency period from the time of exposure to the development of cancer, identifying cancer-causing chemicals is difficult. Chemicals that cause cancer in animals may or may not cause the same specific cancer in humans. Some chemicals are cancer causative in their environmental form, but others must first undergo specific changes to become carcinogenic.

Certain drugs have also been identified as carcinogens. Drugs that are capable of interacting with DNA (e.g., alkylating agents) and immunosuppressive agents have the potential to cause neoplasms in humans. The use of alkylating agents (e.g., cyclophosphamide and nitrogen mustards), either alone or in combination with radiation therapy, has been associated with an increased incidence of acute myelogenous leukemia in persons treated for Hodgkin's disease, non-Hodgkin's lymphomas, and multiple myeloma. These secondary leukemias are relatively refractory to treatment. Secondary leukemia has also been observed in persons who have undergone transplantation surgery and taken immunosuppressive drugs.

Radiation. Early in the twentieth century, ionizing radiation was found to cause cancer in almost any human body tissue. The safe threshold for exposure to radiation is not known, and there is considerable debate surrounding the effect of exposure to low-dose radiation over time. Radiation damages cellular DNA. Certain malignancies have been linked to radiation:

1. Leukemia, lymphoma, thyroid cancer, and other cancers increased in incidence in the general population of Hiroshima and Nagasaki after the atomic bomb explosions.
2. A higher incidence of bone cancer occurs in persons exposed to radiation in certain occupations, such as radiologists, radiation chemists, and uranium miners.
3. Thyroid cancer has a higher incidence among persons who have received radiation to the head and neck area for treatment of a variety of disorders, such as acne, tonsillitis, sore throat, or enlarged thyroid gland.
4. The incidence of childhood cancer is higher among children exposed to radiation during fetal life.

Ultraviolet (UV) radiation has long been associated with melanoma, squamous cell carcinoma, and basal cell carcinoma of the skin. Skin cancer is by far the most common type of cancer in North America. Melanoma is a particularly aggressive skin cancer that responds poorly to treatment. Although the cause of melanoma is probably multifactorial, mounting evidence suggests that UV radiation secondary to sunlight exposure is linked to the development of melanoma.

Viral and Bacterial Carcinogens. Certain DNA and RNA viruses, termed *oncogenic viruses,* can transform the cells they infect and induce malignant transformation. Viruses have been identified as causative agents of cancer in animals and humans. For example, cells from patients with Burkett's lymphoma have consistently shown evidence of the presence of the Epstein-Barr virus (EBV) in vitro. This virus also causes infectious mononucleosis; the precise process through which an infectious disease versus a lymphoma develops is unclear. Persons with acquired immunodeficiency syndrome (AIDS), which is caused by a retrovirus, have a higher incidence of Kaposi's sarcoma (see Chapter 17). Other viruses that have been linked to the development of cancer include hepatitis B and C viruses, associated with hepatocellular carcinoma, and human papillomavirus, associated with squamous cell carcinomas such as cervical cancers. *Helicobacter pylori* is a bacterium found in the stomach of two thirds of the world's population and is implicated in the development of gastric and duodenal ulcers, as well as of some gastric cancers.

Genetic Susceptibility. Cancer-related genes have been identified that increase an individual's susceptibility to the development of certain cancers. For example, a woman with mutations in the gene *BRCA1* or *BRCA2* has a 40 to 85% risk of developing breast cancer in her lifetime. However, 95% of women who develop breast cancer do not possess these genetic mutations. On the basis of current knowledge, it is believed that only 5 to 10% of cancers have a strong genetic link (Loud & Hutson, 2011).

Promotion. A single alteration of the genetic structure of the cell is not sufficient to result in cancer. However, the odds of cancer development are increased with the presence of promoting agents. *Promotion,* the second stage in the development of cancer, is characterized by the reversible proliferation of the altered cells. Consequently, with an increase in the altered cell population, the likelihood of sustained mutagenesis is increased.

An important distinction between initiation and promotion is that the activity of promoters is reversible. This is a key concept in cancer prevention. Promoting factors include dietary fat, obesity, cigarette smoking, and alcohol consumption. The withdrawal or reduction of these factors can reduce the risk of cancer development.

Several promoting factors exert activity against specific types of body tissues or organs, and these agents tend to promote specific kinds of cancer. For example, cigarette smoke is a promoting agent in bronchogenic carcinoma and, in conjunction with alcohol intake, promotes esophageal and bladder cancers. Some carcinogens (*complete carcinogens*) are capable of both initiating and promoting the development of cancer. Tobacco is an example of a complete carcinogen, capable of initiating and promoting cancer.

A period of time, ranging from 1 to 40 years, elapses between the initial genetic alteration and the actual clinical evidence of cancer. This period, called the *latency period,* is now theorized to comprise both the initiation and the promotion stages in the natural history of cancer (DeVita, Lawrence, & Rosenberg, 2011). The variation in the length of time that elapses before the cancer becomes clinically evident is associated with the mitotic rate of the tissue of origin and environmental factors. For most cancers, the process of developing takes years or even decades.

For the disease process to become clinically evident, the cells must reach a critical mass. A 1-cm tumour (the size usually detectable on palpation) contains 1 billion cancer cells. A 0.5-cm tumour is the smallest that can be detected by current diagnostic measures, such as magnetic resonance imaging (MRI).

Progression. *Progression* is the final stage in the natural history of a cancer. This stage is characterized by increased growth rate of the tumour, as well as by increased invasiveness and spread of the cancer to a distant site **(metastasis).** Certain biochemical and morphological alterations take place during this stage, enabling the tumour to survive and thrive in its primary environment and throughout the process of metastasis.

Some cancers metastasize early in the process of development (e.g., premenopausal breast cancer), whereas others spread regionally and rarely metastasize (e.g., glioblastoma multiforme, basal cell carcinoma of the skin). Certain cancers seem to have an affinity for a particular tissue or organ as a site of metastasis (e.g., colon cancer spreads to the liver); other cancers are unpredictable in their pattern of metastasis (e.g., melanoma). Frequent sites of metastasis are the lungs, the brain, the bone, the liver, and the adrenal glands (Figure 18-4). Metastasis is a multistep process

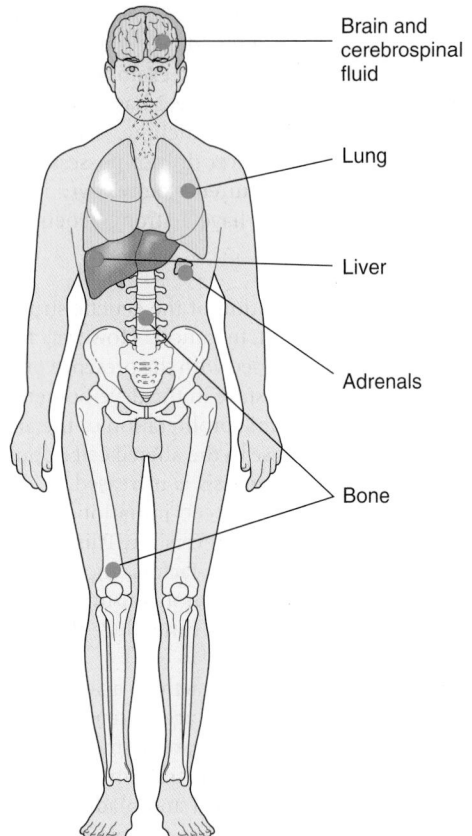

Figure 18-4 Main sites of bloodborne metastasis.

Source: Stevens, A., & Lowe, J. (2000). *Pathology: Illustrated review in color* (2nd ed.). London: Mosby.

beginning with the rapid growth of the primary tumour (Figure 18-5). As the tumour increases in size, development of its own blood supply is crucial for its survival and growth. The process of the formation of blood vessels within the tumour itself is termed **tumour angiogenesis** and is facilitated by tumour angiogenesis factors produced by the cancer cells. As the tumour grows, it can begin to mechanically invade surrounding tissues, growing into areas of the least resistance.

Certain subpopulations of tumour cells are able to detach from the primary tumour, invade the tissue surrounding the tumour, and penetrate the walls of lymph or vascular vessels for metastasis to a distant site. Unique capabilities of some tumour cells facilitate this process. First, rapid proliferation of malignant cells causes mechanical pressure that lead to penetration of surrounding tissues. Second, certain cells have decreased cell-to-cell adhesion in comparison with normal cells. This property allows these cancer cells to physically detach from their site of origin and invade vascular and organ structures. In addition, motility factors are produced by both tumour and normal cells, and changes in the tumour's cytoskeleton further facilitates movement of tumour cells. Some cancer cells produce matrix metalloproteases (MMPs), a family of lytic enzymes that can erode the basement membrane (a tough barrier surrounding tissues and blood vessels) of the tumour itself, as well as lymph and blood vessels, muscles, nerves, and most epithelial boundaries, allowing for the spread of the tumour. Once free from the primary tumour, metastatic tumour cells frequently travel to distant organ sites via

lymphatic and hematogenous routes. Because these two routes are interconnected, it is theorized that tumour cells metastasize via both routes.

Hematogenous metastasis involves several steps, beginning with the penetration of blood vessels by primary tumour cells via the release of MMPs, as described previously. The tumour cells then enter the circulation, adhere to small blood vessels of distant organs, and penetrate these vessels, again with the assistance of MMPs. Most tumour cells do not survive this process and are destroyed by mechanical mechanisms (e.g., turbulence of blood flow) and cells of the immune system. However, the formation of a combination of tumour cells, platelets, and fibrin deposits may protect some tumour cells from destruction in blood vessels.

In the lymphatic system, tumour cells may be "trapped" in the first lymph node confronted, or they may bypass regional lymph nodes and travel to more distant lymph nodes, This phenomenon, termed *skip metastasis,* is exhibited in malignancies such as esophageal cancers and is the basis for questions about the effectiveness of dissection of regional lymph nodes for the prevention of some distant metastases (Abeloff, Armitage, Niederhuber, Kastan, & McKenna, 2008). Tumour cells that do survive the process of metastasis must create and maintain an environment in the distant organ site that is favourable to their growth and development. This is facilitated by the ability of tumour cells to evade cells of the immune system and to produce a vascular supply within the metastatic site similar to that developed in the primary tumour site. Vascularization is critical for the supply of nutrients to the metastatic tumour and for the removal of waste products. MMPs contribute to vascularization through release of angiogenesis promoters such as vascular endothelial growth factor (VEGF).

Cells of the primary tumour and metastatic site may develop from a single cell or may be a *clone* (a cell or cells derived from a single cell of origin). However, as the primary and metastatic sites develop, the cells quickly become more heterogeneous as they repeatedly undergo spontaneous genetic mutations. The heterogeneous nature of the cells in primary and metastatic tumours makes them difficult to treat, inasmuch as they are more likely to become resistant to chemotherapy and radiation therapy. Surgical removal may be effective for some small, circumscribed tumours.

Role of the Immune System

This section is limited to a discussion of the role of the immune system in the recognition and destruction of tumour cells. (For a detailed discussion of immune system function, see Chapter 16.)

The immune system has the potential to distinguish normal (self) from abnormal (nonself) cells. For example, cells of transplanted organs can be recognized by the immune system as nonself entities and thus elicit an immune response. This response can ultimately result in the rejection of the organ. Similarly, cancer cells can be perceived as nonself entities and elicit an immune response that results in their rejection and destruction. However, unlike transplanted cells, cancer cells arise from normal "self" cells, and although mutated and thus different, the immune response that is mounted against cancer cells may be inadequate to reject and destroy the cancer cells.

Some cancer cells have changes on their cell surface antigens as a result of malignant transformation. These antigens are termed **tumour-associated antigens** (Figure 18-6). It is believed that one of the functions of the immune system is to respond to tumour-associated antigens. The response of the immune system to anti-

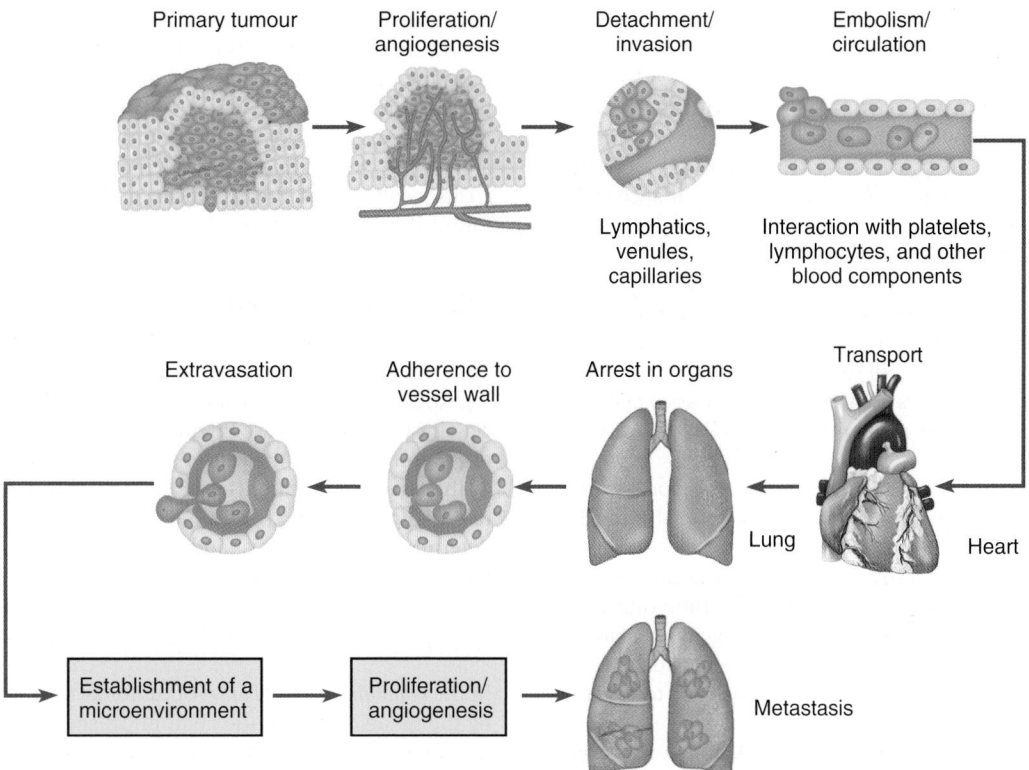

Figure 18-5 The pathogenesis of cancer metastasis. To produce metastases, tumour cells must detach from the primary tumour and enter the circulation, survive in circulation, adhere to capillary basement membrane, gain entrance into the organ parenchyma, respond to growth factors, proliferate and induce angiogenesis, and evade host defences.

Source: Fidler, I. T. (2003). The pathogenesis of cancer metastasis: The "seed and soil" hypothesis revisited, *Nature Reviews Canada, 3,* 453-458. doi:10.1038/nrc1098

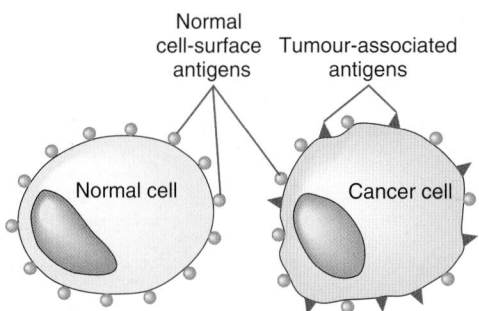

Figure 18-6 Tumour-associated antigens appear on the cell surface of malignant cells.

gens of the malignant cells is termed ***immunological surveillance.*** Lymphocytes continually check cell surface antigens and detect and destroy cells with abnormal or altered antigenic determinants. It has been proposed that malignant transformation occurs continuously and that the malignant cells are destroyed by the immune response. Under most circumstances, immunological surveillance prevents these transformed cells from developing into clinically detectable tumours.

Virtually every cell type involved in normal immune responses and every function used to inactivate or remove antigens has been demonstrated in immune responses to tumours. These immune responses involve cytotoxic T cells, natural killer (NK) cells, macrophages, and B lymphocytes.

Cytotoxic T cells are thought to play a dominant role in resisting tumour growth. These cells are capable of killing tumour cells. T cells are also important in the production of cytokines (e.g., interleukin-2 [IL-2] and γ-interferon [γ-IFN], which stimulate T cells), NK cells, B cells, and macrophages.

NK cells are able to directly lyse tumour cells spontaneously without any prior sensitization. These cells are stimulated by γ-IFN and IL-2 (released from T cells), which results in increased cytotoxic activity.

Monocytes and macrophages have several important roles in tumour immunity. Macrophages can be activated by γ-IFN (produced by T cells) to become nonspecifically lytic for tumour cells. Macrophages also secrete cytokines, including interleukin-1 (IL-1), tumour necrosis factor (TNF), and colony-stimulating factors. The release of IL-1, coupled with the presentation of the processed antigen, stimulates T lymphocyte activation and production. α-Interferon augments the killing ability of NK cells. TNF causes hemorrhagic necrosis of tumours and exerts cytocidal or cytostatic actions against tumour cells. Colony-stimulating factors regulate the production of various blood cells in the bone marrow and stimulate the function of various WBCs.

B lymphocytes produce specific antibodies that bind to tumour cells and destroy these cells by complement fixation and lysis. These antibodies are often detectable in the serum and the saliva of an affected patient. In some persons, antibodies that are specific for both the person's own tumour and a similar tumour in other persons have been found (Kobayashi, Miaskowski, Wallhagen, & Smith-McCune, 2000).

Escape Mechanisms From Immunological Surveillance.

The process by which cancer cells evade the immune system is termed *immunological escape*. Theorized mechanisms by which cancer cells can escape immunological surveillance include (a) suppression of factors that stimulate T cells to react to cancer cells, (b) weak surface antigens that allow cancer cells to "sneak through" immunological surveillance, (c) the development of tolerance of the immune system to some tumour antigens, (d) suppression of the immune response by products secreted by cancer cells, (e) the induction of suppressor T cells by the tumour, and (f) blocking antibodies that bind tumour-associated antigens, thus preventing their recognition by T cells (Figure 18-7).

Oncofetal Antigens.

Oncofetal antigens are a type of tumour antigen. They are found on both the surface and the inside of cancer cells, as well as fetal cells. These antigens are an expression of the shift of cancerous cells to a more immature metabolic pathway, an expression usually associated with embryonic or fetal periods of life. The reappearance of fetal antigens in malignant disease is not well understood, but it is believed to occur as a result of the cell's regaining its embryonic capability to differentiate into many different cell types.

Examples of oncofetal antigens are CEA and α-fetoprotein. CEA is found on the surface of cancer cells derived from the GI tract and from normal cells from the fetal gut, liver, and pancreas. Normally, it disappears during the last 3 months of gestation. CEA was originally isolated from colon cancer cells. However, elevated CEA levels have also been found in nonmalignant conditions (e.g., cirrhosis of the liver, ulcerative colitis, and heavy smoking). At present, the major value of CEA is its use as an indicator of the success of cancer treatment. For example, the persistence of elevated preoperative CEA titres after surgery indicates that the tumour is not completely removed. A rise in CEA levels after chemotherapy or radiation therapy may indicate recurrence or spread of the cancer.

α-Fetoprotein is produced by malignant liver cells, as well as fetal liver cells. α-Fetoprotein levels have also been found to be elevated in some cases of testicular carcinoma, viral hepatitis, and nonmalignant liver disorders. α-Fetoprotein has diagnostic value in primary cancer of the liver (hepatoma), but it is also produced in metastases to the liver. The detection of α-fetoprotein is of value in tumour detection and determination of tumour progression.

Other examples of oncofetal antigens currently being studied are CA-125, found in ovarian carcinoma; CA-19-9, found in pancreatic, colon, and breast cancer; and prostate-specific antigen, found in prostate cancer.

Classification of Cancer

Tumours can be classified according to anatomical site, histological analysis (grading), and extent of disease (staging). Tumour classification systems are intended to provide a standardized way to (a) communicate the cancer status of a patient to the members of the health care team, (b) assist in determining the most effective treatment plan, (c) evaluate the treatment plan, (d) help determine the prognosis, and (e) compare patients with similar conditions for statistical purposes.

Anatomical Site Classification

In the *anatomical classification* of tumours, the tumour is identified by the tissue of origin, the anatomical site, and the behaviour of the tumour (i.e., benign or malignant; Table 18-5). **Carcinomas** originate from embryonal *ectoderm* (skin and glands) and *endoderm* (mucous membrane linings of the respiratory, GI, and gen-

Table 18-5 Anatomical Classification of Tumours		
SITE	**BENIGN**	**MALIGNANT**
Epithelial Tissue Tumours*	Suffix: *-oma*	Suffix: *-carcinoma*
Surface epithelium	Papilloma	Carcinoma
Glandular epithelium	Adenoma	Adenocarcinoma
Connective Tissue Tumours†	Suffix: *-oma*	Suffix: *-sarcoma*
Fibrous tissue	Fibroma	Fibrosarcoma
Cartilage	Chondroma	Chondrosarcoma
Striated muscle	Rhabdomyoma	Rhabdomyosarcoma
Bone	Osteoma	Osteosarcoma
Nervous Tissue Tumours	Suffix: *-oma*	Suffix: *-oma*
Pineal region	Pineocytoma	Pineoblastoma
Nerve cells	Ganglioneuroma	Neuroblastoma
Hematopoietic Tissue Tumours		
Lymphoid tissue	—	Hodgkin's disease, non-Hodgkin's lymphoma
Plasma cells	—	Multiple myeloma
Bone marrow	—	Lymphocytic and myelogenous leukemia

*Body surfaces, lining of body cavities, and glandular structures.
†Supporting tissue, fibrotic tissue, and blood vessels.

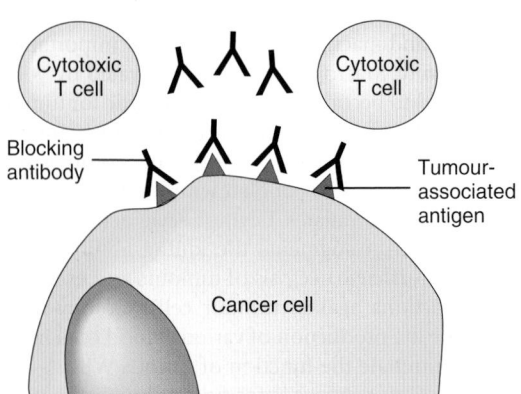

Figure 18-7 Blocking antibodies prevent T cells from interacting with tumour-associated antigens and from destroying the malignant cell.

itourinary tracts). **Sarcomas** originate from embryonal mesoderm (connective tissue, muscle, bone, and fat). Lymphomas and leukemias originate from the hematopoietic system.

Histological Analysis Classification

In **histological grading** of tumours, the appearance of cells and the degree of differentiation are evaluated. For many tumour cells, four grades are used:

Grade I: Cells differ slightly from normal cells (mild dysplasia) and are well differentiated.

Grade II: Cells are more abnormal (moderate dysplasia) and moderately differentiated.

Grade III: Cells are very abnormal (severe dysplasia) and poorly differentiated.

Grade IV: Cells are immature and primitive (anaplasia) and undifferentiated; cell of origin is difficult to determine.

Classifying Extent of Disease

Classifying the extent and spread of disease is termed **staging**. This classification system is based on a description of the extent of the disease rather than on cell appearance. The extent to which the disease has spread has important ramifications for prognosis. Although there are similarities in the staging of cancers, there are many differences based on a thorough knowledge of the natural history of each specific type of cancer.

Clinical Staging.
The clinical staging classification system determines the extent of the disease process of cancer within the body by stages:

Stage 0: cancer in situ

Stage I: tumour limited to the tissue of origin; localized tumour growth

Stage II: limited local spread

Stage III: extensive local and regional spread

Stage IV: metastasis

This classification system has been used as a basis for staging in cancer of the cervix (see Chapter 56, Table 56-11) and Hodgkin's disease (see Chapter 33, Figure 33-16).

TNM Classification System.
The *TNM classification system* represents the standardization of the clinical staging of cancer by the Geneva-based International Union Against Cancer. This classification system (Table 18-6) is used to determine the extent of the disease process of cancer according to three parameters: tumour size (T), degree of regional spread to the lymph nodes (N), and metastasis (M).

Staging of the disease may be performed initially and at repeated intervals. Clinical diagnostic staging is performed at the time of diagnosis to determine the most effective treatment plan. Examples of diagnostic studies that may be performed to assess for spread of disease include bone and liver scans, ultrasonography, computed tomography, and MRI.

Surgical staging is used to describe the extent of the disease process after biopsy or surgical exploration. For example, a laparotomy and a splenectomy may be performed in the staging of Hodgkin's disease. During staging laparotomy, lymph node biopsy samples are obtained, and margins of any masses are marked with metal clips. These clips are used as markers when radiotherapy is used as a treatment modality.

After the extent of the disease is determined, the stage classification is not changed. The original description of the extent of the tumour remains part of the original record. If additional treatment is needed, or if treatment fails, treatment restaging is performed to determine the extent of the disease process at the time of retreatment.

Carcinoma in situ is a commonly used term in classification of cancer. It is defined as a lesion with all the histological features of cancer except invasion. If left untreated, carcinoma in situ eventually becomes invasive.

In addition to tumour classification systems, there are also classification systems that can be used to describe the functional status of the patient with cancer. The Karnofsky Performance Status scale is an example of a functional assessment scale. (This scale is presented in eTable 18-1, available on the Evolve Web site for this chapter.)

Prevention and Detection of Cancer

The nurse has a prominent role in the prevention and detection of cancer. Early detection and prompt treatment are directly responsible for increased survival rates among patients with cancer. Public education should include the following recommendations:

1. Reduce or eliminate exposure to carcinogens and cancer promoters, such as cigarette smoke and sun exposure.
2. Eat a balanced diet that includes fresh fruits, vegetables, omega-3 fatty acids, and fibre, and reduce intake of cholesterol and saturated fats. Following *Eating Well With Canada's Food Guide* helps to ensure a healthy diet (Health Canada, 2011) (see Chapter 42, Figure 42-1).
3. Participate regularly (a minimum of 30 minutes, 5 times per week) in mild to moderate physical activity such as biking, walking, or running.
4. Maintain a healthy weight for your body type.
5. Limit alcohol use to one or two drinks per day.
6. Get to know your body. Learn and practise self-examination (e.g., breast self-examination, testicular self-examination). Report any changes to your doctor or dentist.
7. Follow cancer screening guidelines (see eTable 18-2, *Summary of Canadian Cancer Society Recommendations for Early Detection of Cancer in Asymptomatic People*, available on the Evolve Web site for this chapter). Early detection of cancer has a positive effect on prognosis.
8. Know the seven warning signs of cancer (Table 18-7).

Table 18-6 TNM Classification System	
Primary Tumour Size (T)	
T_0	No evidence of primary tumour
T_{is}	Carcinoma in situ
T_1-T_4	Ascending degrees of increase in tumour size and involvement
Involvement of Regional Lymph Nodes (N)	
N_0	No evidence of disease in lymph nodes
N_1-N_3	Ascending degrees of nodal involvement
N_x	Regional lymph nodes unable to be assessed clinically
Distant Metastases (M)	
M_0	No distant metastases
M_1	Distant metastases

Table 18-7 Seven Warning Signs of Cancer	
C	**C**hange in bowel or bladder habits
A	**A** sore that does not heal
U	**U**nusual bleeding or discharge from any body orifice
T	**T**hickening or a lump in the breast or elsewhere
I	**I**ndigestion or difficulty in swallowing
O	**O**bvious change in a wart or mole
N	**N**agging cough or hoarseness

When the public is educated about cancer, care should be taken to minimize the fear that surrounds the diagnosis. Teaching strategies that address the specific needs of the target audience (e.g., the needs of older adults in comparison with those of high school students and of new immigrants to Canada) are most effective. Although the general public requires information that supports healthy behaviours, those at an increased risk of cancer are the target population for effective cancer control. These individuals must be motivated to learn to change negative health behaviours in order to achieve and maintain an optimal state of health. Nurses can have a definite effect in convincing people that change in lifestyle patterns will have a positive influence on health. To be successful, nurses must identify potential challenges and barriers and develop appropriate strategies to facilitate uptake of information about effective cancer control.

Diagnosis of Cancer

The threat of a cancer diagnosis creates tremendous anxiety for an individual and his or her family. Patients typically undergo several days to weeks of diagnostic studies. During this time, fear of the unknown may be more stressful than the actual diagnosis of cancer.

While the patient is waiting for the results of the diagnostic studies, the nurse should be available to actively listen to the patient's concerns. Communication plays a pivotal role in the provision of optimal patient care. Essential elements of the establishment of a therapeutic relationship with the patient are the ability to listen, ask questions sensitively, and avoid false reassurances. During this time of high anxiety, the patient needs repetition and reinforcement of information, the opportunity to ask questions, and clarification of the diagnostic workup. Explanations should be clear and tailored to meet the specific needs of patients and families. Content that is particularly threatening or detailed may overwhelm patients and should thus be provided with sensitivity to the individual's ability to absorb the information. Written information at the level of the patient's literacy level is helpful for reinforcement of verbal information.

A diagnostic plan for the person in whom cancer is suspected includes health history, potential or actual risk factors, physical examination, and specific diagnostic studies. (The specifics of the health history and the screening physical examination are presented in Chapter 3.)

The health history includes particular emphasis on risk factors, such as family history of cancer, exposure to or ingestion of known carcinogens (e.g., cigarette smoking, exposure to occupational pollutants or chemicals), diseases characterized by chronic inflammation (e.g., ulcerative colitis), and drug ingestion (e.g., hormone therapy). Other important information is related to dietary habits, ingestion of alcohol, lifestyle, and patterns and degree of coping with perceived stressors.

The physical examination should be thorough, with particular attention to the respiratory system, the GI system (including the colon, rectum, and liver), the lymphatic system (including the spleen), the breasts, the skin, the reproductive system (testes and prostate gland in men; cervix, uterus, and ovaries in women), and the musculoskeletal and neurological systems.

The choice of diagnostic studies depends on the suspected primary or metastatic site or sites of the cancer. (Specific procedures related to each body system are discussed in the respective assessment chapters.) Studies that may be conducted in the process of diagnosing cancer include the following:

1. Cytology studies (e.g., Papanicolaou [Pap] test)
2. Hematology and chemistry studies (e.g., complete blood cell count [CBC], liver and renal function tests)
3. Sigmoidoscopic or colonoscopic examination (including fecal occult blood test)
4. Radiological studies (e.g., chest radiography, mammography, computed tomography, MRI)
5. Radioisotope scans (e.g., bone, lung, liver, brain)
6. Assays for the presence of oncofetal antigens, such as CEA and α-fetoprotein, or of genetic markers, such as *BRCA1* and *BRCA2*
7. Bone marrow examination (if a hematolymphoid malignancy is suspected)
8. Biopsy

Biopsy. The *biopsy* procedure is the definitive means of diagnosing cancer, and the results guide treatment decisions. In a biopsy, a piece of tissue is surgically removed from the suspect area for histological examination by a pathologist. This examination helps determine whether the tissue is benign or malignant, the anatomical tissue from which the tumour arises, and the degree of cellular differentiation (i.e., how closely the specimen cells resemble the normal cells of the tissue).

The procedure may be a needle biopsy, an incisional biopsy, or an excisional biopsy. In a *needle biopsy*, cells and tissue fragments are obtained through a large-bore needle guided into the tissue of investigation (e.g., bone marrow, prostate gland, breast, liver, or kidney tissues).

Incisional biopsy performed with a scalpel or dermal punch is a common technique for obtaining a tissue sample: for example, from a skin lesion. The premise that incisional biopsy may contribute to the spread of cancer has not been proven.

Excisional biopsy involves removal of the entire tumour. It is usually used for small tumours (<2 cm in diameter), skin lesions, intestinal polyps, and breast masses. This procedure can be therapeutic in addition to diagnostic. When a tumour is not easily accessible, a major surgical procedure (laparotomy, thoracotomy, craniotomy) is necessary to obtain the tumour tissue. Biopsy specimens of the GI tract, respiratory tract, and genitourinary system can usually be obtained by endoscopic procedures, such as flexible sigmoidoscopy.

Collaborative Care

Goals and Modalities

The goal of cancer treatment is cure, control, or palliation (Figure 18-8). Factors determining the therapeutic approach include the cell type of the cancer, the location and size of the tumour, and

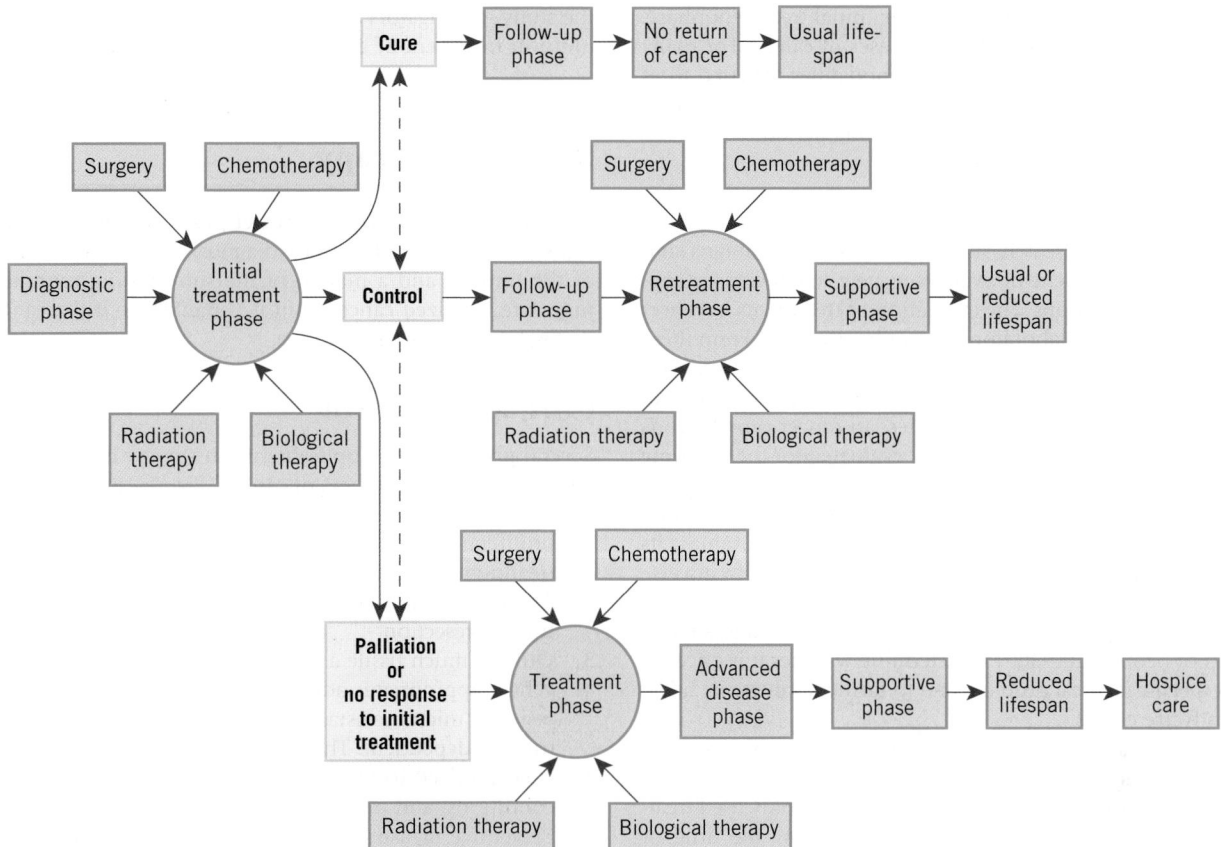

Figure 18-8 Goals of cancer treatment.

Source: Adapted from Krakoff, I. H. (1996). Systemic treatment of cancer. *CA: A Cancer Journal for Clinicians, 46*, 134.

the extent of the disease. The patient's physiological and psychological status and personal desires are also important elements in determining the treatment plan. All factors influence the goals of care, the modalities chosen for treatment, and the length of time the treatment is administered. Evidence-informed treatment guidelines have been developed in a number of provinces to guide treatment decisions. Examples include provincial guidelines in British Columbia and Ontario (see the Resources at the end of this chapter).

When caring for the patient with cancer, the nurse should know the goals of the treatment plan to communicate with and support the patient. When cure is the goal, treatment that has the greatest likelihood of eradicating the disease is offered. With many kinds of cancer, therapy has the potential for inducing permanent remission; therapy may be an initial course of treatment or treatment that extends for several weeks, months, or years. Basal cell carcinoma of the skin is usually cured by surgical removal of the lesion or by several weeks of radiation therapy. Acute lymphocytic leukemia in children has the potential for cure. The treatment plan for this type of cancer includes the administration of several chemotherapeutic drugs on a scheduled basis over a span of 6 months to several years. Head and neck cancers may be cured with combination therapy that includes surgery and radiation, with or without chemotherapy. The risk of disease recurrence differs according to the tumour type. In general, the risk for recurrent disease is greatest after completion of treatment and gradually decreases with the passage of time. Tumours

with a rapid mitotic rate (e.g., testicular cancer) are considered to be in remission if cancer is not detected in a 2-year time span after treatment. For tumours that have a slower mitotic rate (e.g., postmenopausal breast cancer), the patient must be free of disease 20 years or longer before he or she can be considered cured of cancer.

Control is the goal of the treatment plan for many cancers that cannot be completely eradicated but are responsive to cancer therapies. The patient undergoes the initial course of therapy and is continued on maintenance therapy for a time or monitored closely so that early signs and symptoms of disease recurrence or progression can be detected. These cancers usually are not cured but are controlled by therapy for variably extended periods in a manner similar to other chronic illnesses, such as diabetes mellitus, chronic lung disease, and congestive heart failure. An example of this type of cancer is chronic lymphocytic leukemia (see Chapter 33).

Palliation may also be a goal of the treatment plan. With palliation, relief or control of symptoms and the optimization of quality of life are the primary objectives, rather than cure or control of the disease process. Radiation therapy to relieve the pain of bone metastasis is an example of a palliative cancer treatment. Palliative care may be undertaken for days, weeks, months, or years.

The goals of cure, control, and palliation are achieved through the use of four treatment modalities: surgery, radiation therapy, chemotherapy, and biological therapy. These modalities can be used alone or in any combination in the initial treatment phase, as well as in the repeated treatment phases of cancer. For many cancers, two or more of the treatment modalities (referred to as *concurrent, combined-modality,* or *multimodality therapy*) are used to achieve the goal of cure or control for a long period.

Clinical Trials

A *clinical trial* is a research study conducted on humans and designed with the intent of evaluating new treatments or supportive care interventions. The evaluation of treatments in cancer research begins in the laboratory with animal studies. From these studies, the treatments determined to be most effective, with reasonable levels of toxicity, are further evaluated in a series of studies on patients with cancer. Progress in cancer care depends on research. New drugs or treatments, evaluated for the first time in human beings, are studied in three phases:

- In *phase I trials,* researchers test a new drug or treatment in a small group of people (20-80) for the first time to evaluate its safety, determine a safe dosage range, and identify adverse effects.
- In *phase II trials,* the study drug or treatment is given to a larger group of people (100-300) to determine whether it is effective for a specific medical problem and to further evaluate its safety and adverse effects.
- In *phase III trials,* the study drug or treatment is given to large groups of people (1000-3000) to confirm its effectiveness, monitor adverse effects, compare it with commonly used treatments, and collect information that will allow the drug or treatment to be used safely.

Institutional review boards in each agency that conducts research closely guard the rights of the patients participating in clinical trials. These boards not only review clinical trials at their inception but also continue to review and monitor each study until its completion. Informed consent is a process in which the clinical trial physician and nurse give the patient full information regarding the nature of the treatment being evaluated and the potential risks and benefits of entering the clinical trial. The patient must understand that he or she may decide to leave a clinical trial at any time or refuse to participate in the trial without threat of compromised care or treatment.

The guidelines for the administration of a research protocol are included in the study's protocol and are monitored closely by the study investigators and clinical trial nurses to ensure safe and uniform treatment of patients.

Surgical Therapy

Surgery is the oldest form of cancer treatment and was for many years the only method of cancer diagnosis and treatment. Removal of the tumour and a margin of the surrounding normal tissue may cure localized cancers, but it is ineffective if the cancer has metastasized to other locations.

Cure and Control

Several principles are applicable when surgery is used to cure or control the disease process of cancer (Figure 18-9):

1. Cancer that arises from a tissue with a slow rate of cellular proliferation or replication is the most amenable to surgical treatment.
2. A margin of normal tissue must surround the tumour at the time of resection.
3. Only as much tissue as necessary is removed.
4. When appropriate, adjuvant therapy is used to eliminate residual micrometastases. The risk for metastatic disease is tumour dependent. The decision regarding adjuvant therapy is customized to the patient's tumour type, stage, comorbid conditions, and preferences.
5. Preventive measures are used to reduce the surgical seeding of cancer cells.
6. The usual sites of regional spread may be surgically removed for diagnostic or therapeutic purposes.

Examples of surgical procedures used for cure or control of cancer include radical neck dissection, lumpectomy, mastectomy, pneumonectomy, orchiectomy, thyroidectomy, and bowel resection.

A *debulking* or *cytoreductive* procedure may be used if the tumour cannot be completely removed (e.g., is attached to a vital organ). When this occurs, as much tumour as possible is removed, and the patient may be given chemotherapy or radiation therapy. This type of surgical procedure may increase the effectiveness of chemotherapy or radiation therapy because the target disease is reduced.

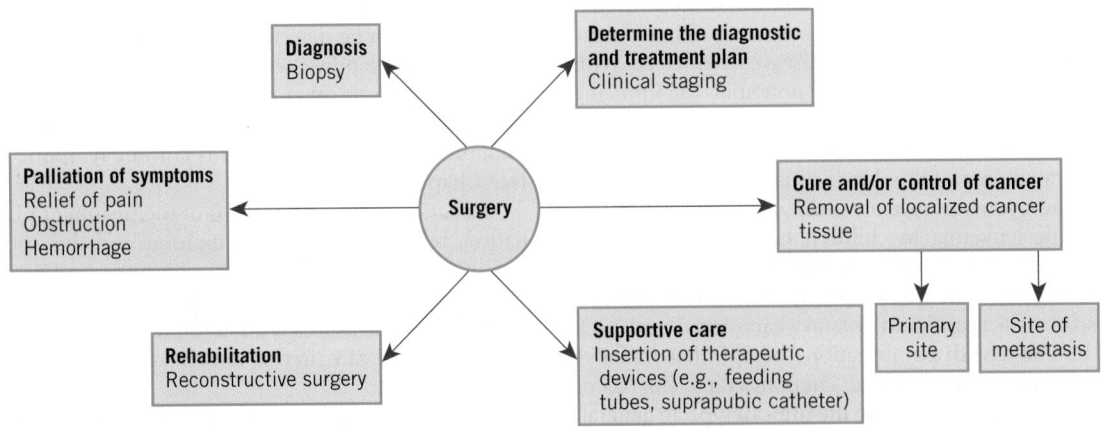

Figure 18-9 Role of surgery in the treatment of cancer.

Supportive and Palliative Surgical Procedures

Surgical procedures can also be used to provide supportive care and palliate symptoms throughout the disease process of cancer. Examples of supportive surgical procedures include the following:

1. Insertion of feeding tubes in the stomach for patients with head and neck cancers or cancer of the esophagus.
2. Creation of a colostomy to allow healing of rectal abscess.
3. Suprapubic cystostomy in cases of advanced prostatic cancer.

When cure or control of cancer is no longer possible, relief from distressing symptoms may be achieved through surgical procedures, including the following:

1. Debulking of tumour to relieve pain or pressure.
2. Colostomy for the relief of a bowel obstruction (see Chapter 45).
3. Laminectomy for the relief of a spinal cord compression (see Chapter 63).

Rehabilitative Management

Cancer surgery may cause a change in a person's body image or function. It may be difficult for the patient to cope with these changes, on top of the distress of a diagnosis of cancer, while he or she attempts to maintain usual lifestyle patterns. As the treatment for certain cancers becomes more effective, the length of time that a patient must live with an alteration created by treatment will be increased. If quality of life is to be maintained, the body image must be one that the patient is able to accept and cope with on a daily basis. The rehabilitative role of surgery in cancer care has grown in prominence to improve patients' quality of life. Breast reconstruction after a mastectomy is an example of a rehabilitative surgical procedure. The use of prostheses, such as artificial eyes or limbs, and the care of ostomies are other major contributions to rehabilitative management.

Chemotherapy

The use of chemicals as a systemic therapy for cancer has been evolving. In the 1940s, chemotherapy was in its infancy. Nitrogen mustard, a chemical warfare agent used in World Wars I and II, was used in the treatment of lymphoma and acute leukemia, and a folic acid antimetabolite (5-fluorouracil) was found to have antitumour activity. In the 1970s, chemotherapy was established as an effective treatment modality for cancer. Chemotherapy is now used in the treatment of many solid tumours and is the primary therapy for hematological malignancies, including leukemia and lymphoma. Chemotherapy has evolved significantly to become a therapeutic option that can cure some cancers, control others, or palliate symptoms when cure or control is no longer achievable (Figure 18-10). Although practice standards in different provinces vary, nurses administering chemotherapy must be specifically trained in the protocols, administration, and possible adverse effects (Canadian Association of Nurses in Oncology, 2006).

Effect on Cells

The effect of chemotherapy is at the cellular level. All cells, whether malignant or normal, enter the cell cycle for replication and proliferation (see Figure 18-1). The effects of the chemo-

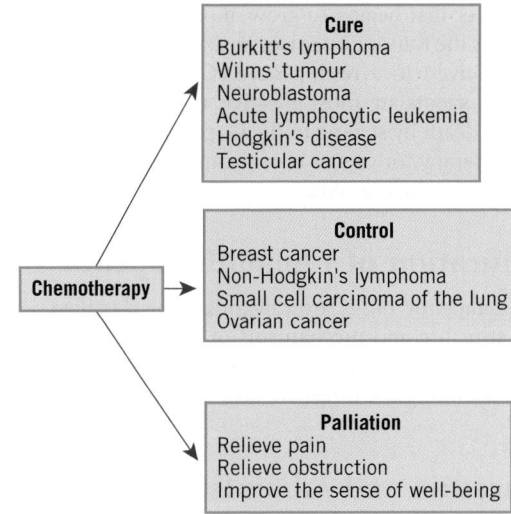

Figure 18-10 Goals of chemotherapy.

therapeutic agents are described in relationship to the cell cycle. The two major categories of chemotherapeutic drugs are cell cycle phase–nonspecific and cell cycle phase–specific drugs.

Cell cycle phase–nonspecific chemotherapeutic drugs have their effect on the cells that are in the process of cellular replication and proliferation, as well as those in the resting phase (G_0).

Cell cycle phase–specific chemotherapeutic drugs have their effect on cells that are in the process of cellular replication or proliferation (G_1, S_1, G_2, or M). These drugs exert their most significant effect during specific phases of the cell cycle. Cell cycle phase–specific and cell cycle phase–nonspecific agents are often administered in combination with one another. The aim of this approach is to promote a better response through the use of agents that function by differing mechanisms and at different points in the cell cycle.

The goal of chemotherapy is to reduce the number of cancer cells present in the primary tumour site and metastatic tumour site or sites (Otto, 2004). Several factors determine the response of cancer cells to chemotherapy:

1. *Mitotic rate of the tissue from which the tumour arises.* The more rapid the mitotic rate, the greater the response to chemotherapy. Chemotherapy is the treatment of choice for acute leukemia, Wilms' tumour (in conjunction with surgery), and neuroblastoma. These cancer cells have a rapid rate of cellular proliferation.
2. *Size of the tumour.* The lower the tumour burden (i.e., the fewer cancer cells), the greater the response to chemotherapy.
3. *Age of the tumour.* The younger the tumour, the greater the response to chemotherapy. Developing tumours have a higher percentage of proliferating cells.
4. *Location of the tumour.* Certain anatomical sites provide a protected environment, or "sanctuary," from the effects of chemotherapy. For example, only a few drugs (such as nitrosoureas and temozolomide) cross the blood–brain barrier.
5. *Presence of resistant tumour cells.* Mutation of cancer cells within the tumour mass can result in variant cells that are resistant to chemotherapy. Resistance can also occur because of the biochemical inability of some cancer cells to convert the drug to its active form. This resistance is passed on to new daughter cells.

As cancer first begins to grow, most of the cells are actively dividing. As the tumour increases in size, more cells become inactive and convert to a resting state (G_0). Because most chemotherapeutic agents are most effective against dividing cells, cells can escape death by staying in the G_0 phase. The major challenge of chemotherapy for cancer is overcoming the drug resistance of resting and noncycling cells.

Classification of Chemotherapeutic Drugs

Chemotherapeutic drugs are categorized or classified according to their structure and mechanisms of action (Table 18-8). Each drug in a particular classification has many similarities, but major differences among the drugs are also evident.

Preparation and Administration of Chemotherapeutic Agents

It is very important to know the specific guidelines for administration of chemotherapeutic drugs. These drugs may also pose occupational hazards for health care professionals. A health care provider preparing or administering chemotherapeutic agents may absorb the drug through inhalation of particles and through skin contact when reconstituting a powder in an open ampule. There may also be some risk in handling the body fluids and excreta of patients receiving chemotherapy. Guidelines for the safe handling of chemotherapeutic agents have been developed by the National Institute for Occupational Safety and Health (NIOSH) and the Oncology Nursing Society (see the Resources at the end of this chapter).

Methods of Administration

Several routes are used to administer chemotherapeutic agents (Table 18-9). The oral and intravenous routes are the most commonly used. The major concerns associated with the intravenous administration of antineoplastic drugs are the potential for irritation or damage to the vessels; problems with the venous access device or catheter, including infection; and *extravasation* (infiltration of drugs into tissues surrounding the infusion site), which causes local tissue damage. Many chemotherapeutic drugs are irritants or **vesicants,** agents that cause severe local tissue breakdown and necrosis when accidentally infiltrated into the skin (Figure 18-11).

Pain is the cardinal symptom of extravasation, although extravasation has been known to occur without causing pain. Swelling, redness, and the presence of vesicles on the skin are other signs of extravasation. After a few days, the tissue may begin to ulcerate and necrose, and closure with skin grafts is often required.

In order to minimize these risks and to avoid physical discomfort, chemotherapeutic agents may be administered by means of a central venous access device. Cancer care increasingly involves combination therapies that entail venous access; therefore, the use of these devices has increased. Central venous access devices are placed in large blood vessels and enable frequent, continuous, or intermittent administration of chemotherapeutic agents, biological therapeutic agents, and other products. They are indicated in instances of limited venous access, intensive chemotherapy, continuous infusion of vesicant agents, and projected long-term need for venous access. (Central venous access devices are discussed further in Chapter 19 on pp. 412-416.)

The advantages of venous access devices are that they provide for rapid dilution of chemotherapeutic agents, decreased incidence of extravasation, and reduced need for venipuncture. In addition to their usefulness in administration of chemotherapeutic agents, venous access devices can be used to administer additional fluids such as blood products, parenteral nutrition, or other drugs, as well as for venous blood sampling. The disadvantages are that central catheters can be a source of systemic infection, particularly if the patient becomes immunosuppressed during therapy. Three major types of venous access devices used in oncology care are tunnelled catheters, peripherally inserted central catheters, and implanted infusion ports. (See Chapter 19 for a detailed discussion of these venous access devices.)

Infusion Pumps. Infusion pumps are used primarily for the continuous infusion of chemotherapeutic agents by intravenous, subcutaneous, intra-arterial, and epidural routes. Infusion pumps can be worn externally or implanted surgically. The various types of external infusion pumps have different mechanisms of action, components, and capabilities.

Implanted infusion pumps are used primarily for intra-arterial administration of chemotherapeutic agents (Figure 18-12). This approach enables continuous infusion of the chemotherapeutic agent directly to the area of the tumour while sparing the patient the systemic effects of the drug. Some implanted pumps have two silicone septa. The second septum can be used for bolus medication administration. The most common use of this method of chemotherapeutic administration has been hepatic artery infusion in the treatment of liver metastasis, usually from primary colon cancer.

Implanted pumps also consist of a catheter that is threaded into the designated artery. The catheter is attached to a pump apparatus that consists of two chambers: an inner chamber that serves as the drug reservoir and an outer chamber that contains vapour pressure, which provides a source of power for the pump. The pump is implanted surgically in a subcutaneous pocket. Access to the pump is via a silicone septum with a Huber-point needle. Flow rate of the pump can be affected by drug concentration, the length and diameter of the Silastic catheter, and the patient's body temperature. Thus dose alterations may be required if the patient experiences a change in temperature or travels to higher altitudes. Complications that have been associated with implanted infusion pumps include infection, thrombosis, clotting of the catheter, and pump malfunction.

Other access devices used in the treatment of the person with cancer include the Tenckhoff catheter used in the administration of intraperitoneal chemotherapeutic agents and the Ommaya reservoir, which delivers agents directly to the central nervous system (CNS).

Regional Administration of Chemotherapeutic Agents

Regional treatment with chemotherapy involves the delivery of the drug directly to the tumour site. The advantage of administering chemotherapy by this method is that higher concentrations of the drug can be delivered to the tumour with reduced systemic toxicity. Several regional delivery methods have been developed, including intra-arterial, intraperitoneal, intrathecal or intraventricular, and intravesical bladder chemotherapy.

Intra-Arterial Chemotherapy. In intra-arterial chemotherapy, the drug is delivered to the tumour via the arterial vessel

DRUG THERAPY

Table 18-8 Classification of Chemotherapeutic Drugs

MECHANISMS OF ACTION	EXAMPLES
Alkylating Agents	
Cell Cycle Phase–Nonspecific Agents	
Damage DNA by causing breaks in the double-strand helix (similar to the effect of radiation therapy); if repair does not occur, cells die immediately (cytocidal) or when they attempt to divide (cytostatic)	Mechlorethamine (nitrogen mustard), cyclophosphamide (Procytox), chlorambucil (Leukeran), melphalan (Alkeran), busulfan (Myleran), dacarbazine (DTIC), lomustine (CCNU, CEENU), oxaliplatin (Eloxatin), streptozocin (Zanosar), cisplatin, carboplatin
Antimetabolites	
Cell Cycle Phase–Specific Agents (Primarily S Phase)	
Interfere with enzyme function and synthesis of DNA by mimicking naturally occurring metabolites required by the cell for synthesis of DNA and RNA (cytocidal)	Methotrexate, cytarabine (Cytosar), fluorouracil (5-FU), mercaptopurine (6-MP), thioguanine (6-TG), fludarabine (Fludara), hydroxyurea (Hydrea), gemcitabine (Gemzar), cladribine (Leustatin)
Antitumour Antibiotics	
Cell Cycle Phase–Nonspecific Agents	
Modify function of DNA and interfere with transcription of RNA (cytocidal or cytostatic)	Doxorubicin (Adriamycin), bleomycin (Blenoxane), mitomycin, daunorubicin (Daunomycin), dactinomycin (Cosmegen), idarubicin (Idamycin), epirubicin (Ellence), mitoxantrone
Plant Alkaloids (Mitotic Inhibitors)	
Cell Cycle Phase–Specific Agents (G_2 and M Phases)	
Interrupt cellular replication in mitosis at metaphase (cytocidal)	Vinblastine, vincristine, etoposide (VePesid), paclitaxel (Taxol), docetaxel (Taxotere), teniposide (Vumon)
Nitrosoureas	
Cell Cycle Phase–Nonspecific Agents	
Similar to alkylating agents; break DNA helix and interfere with DNA replication (cytocidal or cytostatic)	Carmustine (BCNU), lomustine (CCNU, CEENU)
Corticosteroids	
Cell Cycle Phase–Nonspecific Agents	
Disrupt the cell membrane and inhibit synthesis of protein; decrease circulating lymphocytes; inhibit mitosis; depress immune system; increase feeling of well-being	Cortisone, hydrocortisone (Cortef), methylprednisolone (Medrol), prednisone, dexamethasone
Hormone Therapy	
Cell Cycle Phase–Nonspecific Agents	
Interfere with hormone receptors and proteins, inhibiting tumour growth	Androgens (testosterone), estrogens, progestins
Aromatase Inhibitors	
Inhibit the enzyme aromatase, a cytochrome P450 enzyme involved in estrogen synthesis	Anastrozole (Arimidex), letrozole (Femara), exemestane (Aromasin)
Selective Estrogen Receptor Modulator (SERM)	
Selectively modulates estrogen receptors, thus acting as an estrogen antagonist	Raloxifene (Evista)
Miscellaneous	
Destroys exogenous supply of L-asparagine, which is needed for cellular proliferation; L-asparagine can be synthesized by normal cells, but not cancer cells	L-Asparaginase (Elspar)
Antiestrogens used in breast cancer	Tamoxifen (Nolvadex), fulvestrant (Faslodex)
Suppresses mitosis at interphase, appears to alter preformed DNA, RNA, and protein	Procarbazine (Matulane)

DNA, deoxyribonucleic acid; *RNA,* ribonucleic acid.
NOTE: Each cancer agency in Canada has a formulary of protocols and practice guidelines; strict adherence to these guidelines is critical in the clinical setting. With new clinical trial research, drug protocols change; thus, the list above may not remain current.

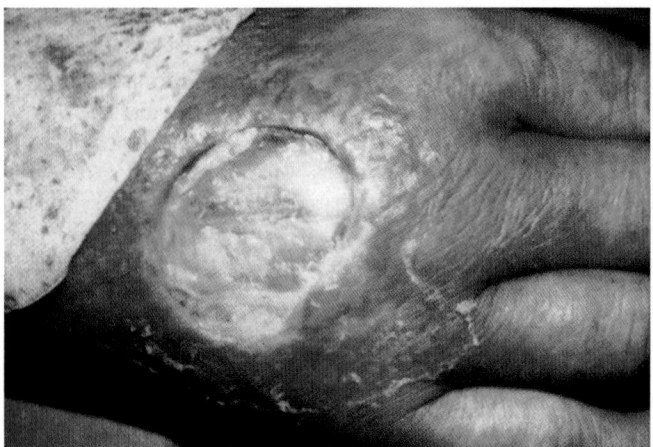

Figure 18-11 Extravasation injury from infiltration of chemotherapeutic drug.

Source: Sauerland, C., Engelking, C., Wickham, R., & Corbi, D. (2006). Vesciant extravasation part I: Mechanisms, pathogenesis, and nursing care to reduce risk. *Oncology Nursing Forum, 33*(6), 1134-1141.

DRUG THERAPY

Table 18-9 Methods of Administration of Chemotherapeutic Drugs

METHOD	EXAMPLES
Oral	Cyclophosphamide
Intramuscular	Bleomycin
Intravenous	Doxorubicin, vincristine
Intracavitary (pleural, peritoneal)	Radioisotopes, alkylating agents, methotrexate
Intrathecal	Methotrexate, cytarabine
Intra-arterial	Dacarbazine (DTIC), 5-fluorouracil (5-FU), methotrexate, floxuridine
Perfusion	Alkylating agents
Continuous infusion	5-FU, methotrexate, cytarabine
Subcutaneous	Cytarabine

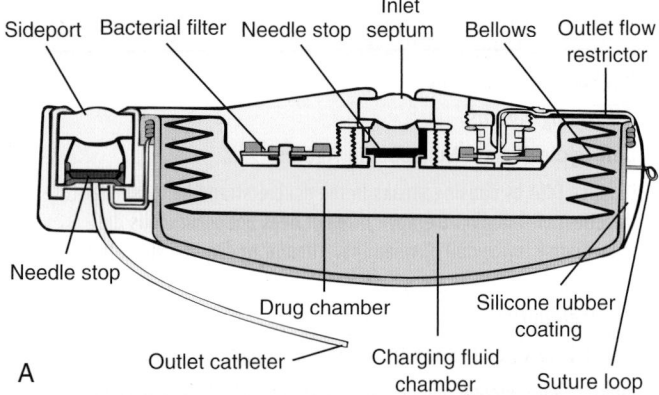

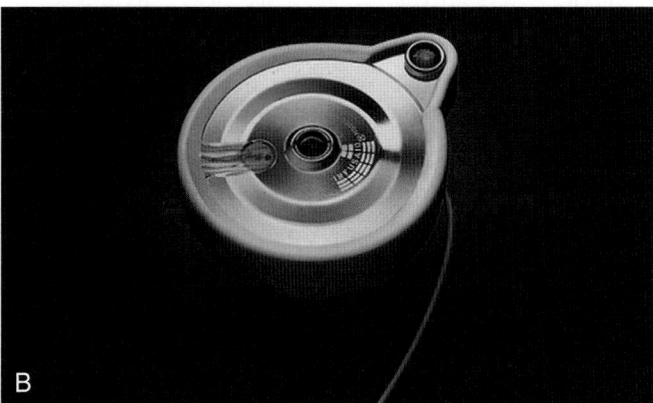

Figure 18-12 A, Cross-section of the implantable pump displaying its two chambers: the drug chamber (inner) and the charging fluid chamber (outer). As the drug chamber is filled, the bellows expand, compressing the charging fluid in the outer chamber. The resulting increased pressure in the outer chamber forces the drug through a membrane filter and preset flow restrictor, thus ensuring a nearly constant flow. **B,** Infusaid pump.

Source: Courtesy Strato/Infusaid, Inc., Norwood, MA.

supplying the tumour. This method has been used for the treatment of osteogenic sarcoma; cancers of the head and neck, the bladder, the brain, and the cervix; melanoma; primary liver cancer; and metastatic liver disease. One method of intra-arterial drug delivery involves the surgical placement of a catheter that is subsequently connected to an external infusion pump or an implanted infusion pump for infusion of the chemotherapeutic agent. In general, intra-arterial chemotherapy results in reduced systemic toxicity. The type of toxicity experienced by the patient depends on the site of the tumour being treated.

Intraperitoneal Chemotherapy. Intraperitoneal chemotherapy involves the delivery of chemotherapeutic agents to the peritoneal cavity for treatment of peritoneal metastases from primary colorectal and ovarian cancers and malignant ascites. Temporary Silastic catheters (Tenckhoff, Hickman, and Groshong) are percutaneously or surgically placed into the peritoneal cavity for short-term administration of chemotherapeutic agents. Alternatively, an implanted port can be used to administer che-

motherapeutic agents intraperitoneally. Complications of peritoneal chemotherapy include abdominal pain; catheter occlusion, dislodgement, and migration; and infection (Langhorne, Fulton, & Otto, 2007).

Intrathecal or Intraventricular Chemotherapy. Cancers that metastasize to the CNS—most commonly breast, lung, and GI cancers; leukemia; and lymphoma—are difficult to treat because the blood–brain barrier often prevents distribution of chemotherapeutic agents to this area. One method used to treat metastasis to the CNS is intrathecal chemotherapy. This method involves a lumbar puncture and injection of chemotherapeutic drugs into the subarachnoid space. However, this method has resulted in incomplete distribution of the drug in the CNS, particularly to the cisternal and ventricular areas.

To ensure more uniform distribution of chemotherapeutic drugs to the cisternal and ventricular areas, an Ommaya reservoir is often inserted. An Ommaya reservoir is a Silastic, dome-shaped disc with an extension catheter that is surgically implanted through the cranium into a lateral ventricle. In addition to providing more consistent drug distribution, the Ommaya reservoir averts the need for repeated painful lumbar punctures.

Complications of intrathecal or intraventricular chemotherapy include headache, nausea, vomiting, fever, and nuchal rigidity (Aiello-Laws & Rutledge, 2008).

Intravesical Bladder Chemotherapy.

Many patients with superficial transitional cell cancer of the bladder have recurrent disease after traditional surgical therapy. Instillation of chemotherapeutic agents into the bladder promotes destruction of cancer cells and reduces the incidence of recurrent disease. Additional benefits of this therapy include reduced urinary and sexual dysfunction. The chemotherapeutic agent is instilled into the bladder via a urinary catheter and retained for 1 to 3 hours. Complications of this therapy include dysuria, urinary frequency, hematuria, and bladder spasms.

Effects of Chemotherapy on Normal Tissues

Chemotherapeutic agents cannot selectively distinguish between normal cells and cancer cells. The experience of adverse effects and toxic effects results from the destruction of normal cells, especially those that proliferate rapidly, such as the cells of the bone marrow, the GI lining, and the integumentary system (Table 18-10). The body's response to the products of cellular destruction in the circulation may cause fatigue, anorexia, and taste alterations.

The adverse effects of these drugs can be classified as acute, delayed, or chronic. Acute toxic effects include vomiting, allergic reactions, and dysrhythmias. Delayed effects include mucositis, alopecia, and bone marrow suppression. Mucositis can result in mouth sores, gastritis, and diarrhea. Chronic toxicity involves damage to organs such as the heart, the liver, the kidneys, and the lungs.

Treatment Plan

When chemotherapy is used in the treatment of cancer, several drugs may be given in combination. Multidrug regimens have proved to be particularly effective in the treatment of many types of cancer. The drugs given are carefully selected to kill the cancer cells most effectively and yet allow the normal cells to repair themselves and proliferate. The dose of each drug is carefully calculated according to the body weight or the body surface area (i.e., body weight and height) of the patient being treated. The principles of combination chemotherapy include the following:

1. The drugs used in the treatment plan are effective against the cancer being treated.
2. When drugs are given in combination, a synergistic effect occurs.
3. The combination includes cell cycle phase–specific drugs, cell cycle phase–nonspecific drugs, and drugs that have different mechanisms of action.
4. The combination includes drugs that have different toxic adverse effects.
5. The combination includes drugs that cause nadirs at different time intervals. The **nadir** is the lowest level of the peripheral blood cell counts (particularly WBC) that occurs secondary to bone marrow depression. The nadir after administration of most chemotherapeutic drugs occurs in 7 to 28 days.

An example of a treatment regimen is the FOLFOX regimen (folinic acid, fluorouracil, and oxaliplatin; Table 18-11). The agents in this drug protocol differ in mechanisms of action, toxic adverse effects, and nadir, but the combination is synergistic in nature, and the dosage schedule includes a time of drug administration and a time of rest from drug administration. The rest period is necessary to allow the normal cells to proliferate and repair the damaged tissue. The patient is evaluated before the administration of each course of chemotherapy to determine how well he or she is tolerating the treatment and whether the normal cells have recovered sufficiently for the next dose to occur.

Radiation Therapy

Radiation therapy is a local treatment modality for cancer. It is one of the oldest methods of cancer treatment. Historically,

Table 18-10 Cells With Rapid Rate of Proliferation

CELLS AND GENERATION TIME	EFFECT OF CELL DESTRUCTION
Bone marrow stem cell: 6-24 hr	Myelosuppression; infection, bleeding, anemia
Neutrophils: 12 hr	Leukopenia, infection
Epithelial cells lining the gastrointestinal tract: 12-24 hr	Anorexia, stomatitis, esophagitis, nausea and vomiting, diarrhea
Ova or testes: 24-36 hr	Reproductive dysfunction
Cells of the hair follicle: 24 hr	Alopecia

DRUG THERAPY

Table 18-11 FOLFOX Chemotherapeutic Drug Schedule

Schedule: FOLFOX + bevacizumab (Avastin) is given to treat advanced colon cancer. FOLFOX* includes 5-fluorouracil ("FOL") administered as a continuous intravenous infusion over 46 hours on days 1 and 2; leucovorin (folinic acid; "F") administered intravenously over 2 hours on days 1 and 2; and oxaliplatin (Eloxatin; "OX") administered intravenously over 2 hours on day 1. Bevacizumab is administered intravenously over 2 hours on day 1. This schedule is repeated every 2 weeks. The number of cycles depends on a patient's situation.

| | WEEK 1 | | | WEEK 3 | | | WEEK 5 | | | WEEK 7 | | |
DRUG	DAY 1	DAY 2	DAY 3	DAY 1	DAY 2	DAY 3	DAY 1	DAY 2	DAY 3	DAY 1	DAY 2	DAY 3
5-Fluorouracil	↔	↔		↔	↔		↔	↔		↔	↔	
Leucovorin (folinic acid)	↔	↔		↔	↔		↔	↔		↔	↔	
Oxaliplatin (Eloxatin)	↔			↔			↔			↔		
Bevacizumab (Avastin)	↔			↔			↔			↔		

*There are slightly different versions of the FOLFOX regimen.

Table 18-12 Tumour Radiosensitivity			
HIGH RADIOSENSITIVITY	**MODERATE RADIOSENSITIVITY**	**MILD RADIOSENSITIVITY**	**POOR RADIOSENSITIVITY**
Ovarian dysgerminoma	Skin carcinoma	Soft tissue sarcomas (e.g., chondrosarcoma)	Osteosarcoma
Testicular seminoma	Oropharyngeal carcinoma	Gastric adenocarcinoma	Malignant melanoma
Hodgkin's disease	Esophageal carcinoma	Renal adenocarcinoma	Malignant gliomas
Non-Hodgkin's lymphoma	Breast adenocarcinoma	Colon adenocarcinoma	Testicular nonseminoma
Wilms' tumour	Uterine and cervical carcinoma		
Neuroblastoma	Prostate carcinoma		
	Bladder carcinoma		

workers exposed to radiation had a higher incidence of skin desquamation and developed carcinomas of the fingers. Both Marie Curie and her daughter Irène Joliot-Curie developed leukemia as a result of radiation exposure (Kaplan, 1979).

The observation that radiation exposure caused tissue damage led scientists to explore the use of radiation to treat tumours. The hypothesized association was that if radiation resulted in the destruction of the highly mitotic skin cells of workers, it could be used in a controlled way to prevent the continued growth of highly mitotic cancer cells. It was not until the 1960s that sophisticated equipment and treatment planning facilitated the delivery of adequate radiation doses to tumours and tolerable doses to normal tissues. Today, radiotherapy has a central role in the treatment of cancer.

Effects of Radiation

Radiation is the emission and distribution of energy through space or a material medium. The energy produced by radiation, when absorbed into tissue, produces ionization and excitation. This local energy and the resultant generation of free radicals breaks chemical bonds in DNA, which may lead to lethal or sublethal damage. Lethal damage causes sufficient chromosomal disruption that the cell is unable to replicate. Sublethal DNA damage may be repaired between radiation doses or, alternatively, may accumulate with repetitive doses, leading to cell death. Cancer cells are especially vulnerable to the effects of cumulative radiation doses, because they are less capable of repairing sublethal damage than normal cells. When repetitive, *fractionated* (or divided) doses of radiation are delivered to a tumour, damage to malignant cells is maximized, and normal cells are more likely to recover. The principles of radiotherapy dosing and fractionation are guided by cellular response to radiation, known as the *four Rs* of radiobiology: repair of cellular damage, redistribution of cells in the cell cycle, repopulation, and reoxygenation of hypoxic tumour areas (see eTable 18-3 on the Evolve Web site for this chapter).

Cellular Death and Tissue Reactions. *Cellular death* related to radiation is defined as an irreversible loss of proliferative capacity. Cells may undergo several mitoses and then die. A cell that retains its proliferative capacity is a clonogenic cell because it is able to produce new clones or colonies of similar cells. After radiation, cancer is considered controlled if the cells that remain are nonclonogenic.

Cellular sensitivity to radiation varies throughout the cell cycle; cells are most sensitive in the M and G_2 phases and least sensitive during the S or synthesis phase (see Figure 18-1). Cells treated during the M and G_2 phases of the cell cycle are more likely to suffer lethal damage. The damage to DNA in cells that are not in the M phase will be expressed when division occurs.

The amount of time that is required for the manifestations of radiation damage is determined by the mitotic rate of the tissue. Sufficient cells within the tissue must be killed to establish a noticeable effect. This is true in both normal and cancer cells. Rapidly dividing cells in the GI tract, oral mucosa, and bone marrow will die fast or exhibit other early acute responses to radiation. Tissues with slowly proliferating cells—such as those of cartilage, bone, and kidneys—manifest late responses to radiation.

This differential rate of cellular death explains the timing of clinical manifestations related to radiation therapy. Normal cells within the radiation field are also affected by treatment. For each normal cell type, there is a maximally tolerated radiation dose. Administration of radiation above the maximally tolerated doses results in limited ability of normal cells to recover from damage and in potentially irreversible adverse effects. Treatment planning and computerized dosimetry ensure that normal tissue tolerance is not exceeded (Behrend, 2011).

Table 18-12 describes the relative radiosensitivity of a variety of tumours. In responsive tumours, even a large tumour burden is affected by therapy. In less responsive tumours, a large tumour burden may result in a slower and perhaps incomplete response.

Simulation and Treatment

Simulation is a part of radiation treatment planning used to determine the optimal treatment method. The patient lies on a table in the treatment position. Under fluoroscopy, the critical normal structures to be included in the treatment field or portal are identified. An image is taken to verify the field, and marks are placed on the skin so that the field can be reproduced on a daily basis. Immobilization devices (e.g., casts, bite blocks, thermoplastic face masks) are typically used to help the patient maintain a stable position (Figure 18-13). Computerized dosimetry, accomplished with computed tomographic scanning, is used to produce a treatment plan for delivering the maximum amount of radiation to the tumour within the acceptable dosage limits for normal tissue.

External Radiation. Teletherapy *(external beam irradiation)* is the most common form of radiation treatment delivery. With this technique, the patient is exposed to radiation from a megavoltage treatment machine. The radiation source may include cobalt-60, which emits gamma rays from a radioactive source. Therapy may be delivered by a cyclotron, which produces

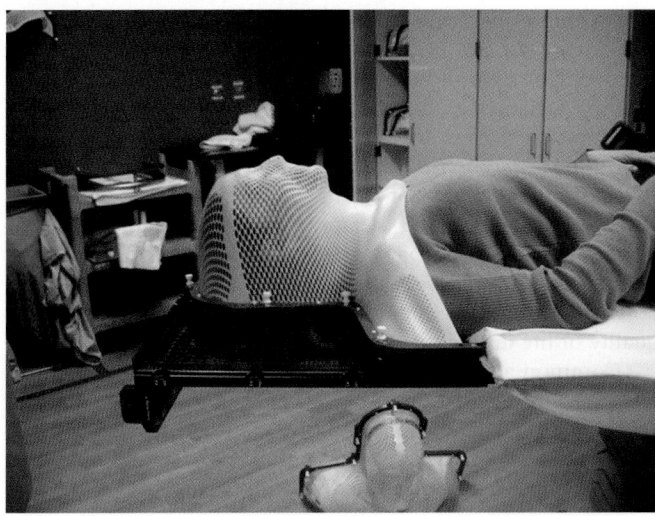

Figure 18-13 Immobilization device. Use of a head holder and immobilization mask may be used to ensure accurate positioning for daily treatment of head and neck cancer.

Source: Courtesy Jormain Cady, Virginia Mason Medical Center, Seattle, WA.

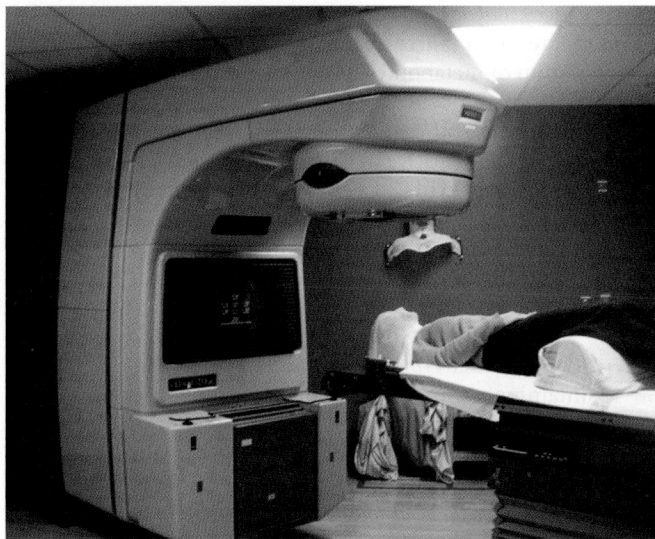

Figure 18-14 Linear accelerator. Varian Clinac EX linear accelerator with multiple photon and electron energies available for use according to the treatment plan. Patient is positioned on radiation treatment table for treatment of head and neck cancer.

Source: Courtesy Jormain Cady, Virginia Mason Medical Center, Seattle, WA.

neutrons or protons, or by a linear accelerator, which generates ionizing radiation from electricity and can have multiple energies (Figure 18-14).

Internal Radiation. Another radiation delivery system is **brachytherapy** ("close" treatment). In this method, radioactive materials are implanted or inserted directly into the tumour or close to the tumour. An implant may be temporary; the source is placed into a catheter or tube inserted into the tumour area and left in place for several days. This method is commonly used for

Table 18-13 Measurement of Radiation	
UNIT	**DEFINITION**
Curie (Ci)	A measure of the number of atoms of a particular radioisotope that disintegrate in 1 second
Roentgen (R)	A measure of the radiation required to produce a standard number of ions in air; a unit of exposure to radiation
Rad	Measurement of radiation dosage absorbed by the tissues
Rem	Measurement of the biological effectiveness of various forms of radiation on the human cell (1 rem = 1 rad)
Gray (Gy)	100 rads = 1 Gy
Centigray (cGy)	1 Gy = 100 cGy

tumours of the head and neck and for prostate and gynecological malignancies. Implants may also be permanent, whereby radioactive seeds are inserted into tumours: for example, in the prostate. Brachytherapy is clinically appropriate when the radiation dose necessary to eradicate the tumour exceeds the dose tolerance of nearby normal tissues. The sources used in brachytherapy are not as energetic or penetrating as those used in the external beam machines and thus deliver most of the dose locally. External beam radiation and brachytherapy may be used in combination.

Caring for the person with a radiation implant requires that the nurse be aware that the patient is radioactive. Patients with temporary implants are radioactive during the time the source is in place. If the patient has a permanent implant, the radioactive exposure to the outside and to other people is low, and the patient may be discharged with precautions. The principles of time, distance, and shielding are used when caring for the person with an implant. Nursing care should be organized so that time spent in direct contact with the patient is kept to a minimum. The patient should be informed of these restrictions before the implantation procedure. The radiation safety officer determines how much time at a specific distance can be spent with the patient, according to the dose delivered by the implant. Because the source is nonpenetrating, small differences in distance are critical. Only care that must be delivered near the source, such as checking placement of the implant, is performed in close proximity. Shielding, if available, should be used, and the health care provider should not deliver care without wearing a film badge. This badge indicates any radiation exposure. The film badge should not be shared, should not be worn anywhere other than at work, and should be returned according to the agency's protocol.

Measurement of Radiation

Several different units are used to measure radiation (Table 18-13). Grays (Gy) and centigrays (cGy) are the units currently used in clinical practice.

Goals of Radiation Therapy

The goals of radiation therapy are cure, control, and palliation. To accomplish these treatment goals, radiation therapy can be used alone or as an adjuvant treatment modality with surgery, chemotherapy, biological therapy, or some combination of these.

Cure is the goal when radiation therapy is used alone for treating patients with basal cell carcinoma of the skin, tumours confined to the vocal cords, and stage I or IIA Hodgkin's disease. Radiation therapy can be combined with surgery and chemotherapy to cure certain cancers; for example, (a) stages IIB, IIIA, and IIIB Hodgkin's disease (in combination with chemotherapy); (b) Ewing's sarcoma (in combination with chemotherapy); (c) head and neck cancer (in combination with surgery and chemotherapy); and (d) stages I and II breast cancer (in combination with surgery).

Control of the disease process for a time may be a reasonable goal in some situations. Initial treatment is offered at the time of diagnosis, and additional treatment may be instituted if symptoms of disease recur. Most patients enjoy a satisfactory quality of life during the symptom-free period. Radiation therapy can be combined with surgery to further enhance the local control of cancer. It can be given preoperatively to reduce the size of the tumour so that it can be more easily resected, or it can be given postoperatively to destroy any remaining tumour cells. Intraoperative radiation therapy is now available at some research centres. In this procedure, radiation is administered directly to the site of the tumour during surgery.

Inoperable tumours can be treated with radiation therapy. These tumours are large and have extended regionally. An example of an inoperable cancer treated for control with radiation therapy is small (oat) cell cancer of the lung.

Palliation is often the goal of radiation therapy, with the aim of controlling symptoms resulting from the disease process. Tumours can be reduced in size to relieve symptoms such as pain and obstruction. Examples of the use of radiation therapy for palliation include relief from the following:

1. Pain associated with bone metastasis
2. Pain and neurological symptoms associated with brain metastasis
3. Spinal cord compression
4. Intestinal obstruction
5. Superior vena cava obstruction
6. Bronchial or tracheal obstruction
7. Bleeding (e.g., bladder and intrabronchial)

NURSING MANAGEMENT: RADIATION THERAPY AND CHEMOTHERAPY

The nurse has an important role in educating patients about their treatment regimens and the management of adverse effects and disease symptoms. Teaching should be tailored to the needs and abilities of patients and their families. Nurses can also assist patients to cope with the psychosocial issues associated with a cancer diagnosis. Anxiety and fear may pervade a patient's day-to-day experience and become a barrier to his or her ability to navigate through treatment. The nurse can mobilize a collaborative team of health care providers, community resources, and the patient's family to provide and reinforce information, facilitate transportation to the cancer centre, and ensure adequate physical, emotional, and spiritual support. One of the most important responsibilities of the nurse is that of differentiating between toxic effects of treatments and progression of the malignant process. The nurse must also distinguish tolerable adverse effects from acute toxic effects of chemotherapeutic agents. For example,

nausea and vomiting are expected and controllable adverse effects of many drugs. However, if paraesthesia occurs with the use of vincristine or signs of heart failure appear with the use of doxorubicin (Adriamycin), these serious reactions must be reported to the physician so that drug dosages can be modified or the drug discontinued. Some toxic effects associated with chemotherapy may not be reversible. For example, ototoxicity may be an irreversible effect of cisplatin therapy, especially at high doses. Periodic testing of hearing may be necessary to monitor for this toxic effect. A nurse also advises patients about the availability of supportive therapies (e.g., antiemetics, antidiarrheals) to optimize quality of life during treatment.

Common adverse effects and specific nursing considerations related to problems caused by cancer therapy are presented in Table 18-14. Fatigue, anorexia, bone marrow suppression, skin reactions, mucosal reactions, and pulmonary, GI, and reproductive effects are discussed in the following sections.

Nursing Implementation

Fatigue

Fatigue is a commonly reported adverse effect of cancer therapy, affecting 70% to 100% of patients with cancer (Prue, Rankin, Allen, Gracey, & Cramp, 2006). The pathophysiological mechanisms that result in cancer treatment–induced fatigue are unclear. Accumulation of metabolites from the destruction of cells during treatment is one probable cause. The metabolites include lactate, hydrogen ions, and other end products of cellular destruction and result in decreased muscle strength. Alterations in energy production in the patient with cancer may also result from cachexia, anorexia, fever, and infection. Fatigue associated with radiotherapy generally begins during the third to fourth week of treatment, persists after treatment ends, and then gradually subsides. Chemotherapy-related fatigue may become chronic after therapy. Factors such as weight loss, anemia, depression, nausea, and other symptoms exacerbate the sensation of fatigue.

Maintaining good nutrition and adequate hydration, alternating periods of rest and activity, relying on family members for assistance with responsibilities, and managing pain and anxiety may help reduce fatigue. The nurse can prepare patients for the expected adverse effect of fatigue, so that they do not assume that it is a sign of treatment failure. A patient may report more energy on some days than on others. Encouraging the patient to identify days or times during the day when he or she feels better may assist in understanding his or her body's responses and maximizing energy reserves. Ignoring the fatigue or overstressing the body when fatigue is tolerable may lead to an increase in symptoms. Mild physical activity programs are usually within the abilities of patients and have been found to ameliorate symptoms of fatigue, lessen anxiety, and facilitate sleep in patients with cancer (Fillion et al., 2008). Family caregivers of patients with cancer are also prone to fatigue and poor energy levels (Passik & Kirsh, 2005). Remaining as active as the patient is able has been shown to improve mood and avoid the debilitating cycle of fatigue-depression-fatigue that can occur.

Anorexia

Anorexia may develop as a general reaction to treatment. The mechanisms underlying the development of anorexia are unclear, but several theories exist. Macrophages release TNF and IL-1 in

Table 18-14 Nursing Management of Problems Caused by Radiation Therapy and Chemotherapy

PROBLEM	CAUSE	NURSING MANAGEMENT
Gastrointestinal System		
Stomatitis, mucositis, esophagitis	Destruction of cells in radiation treatment field. Destruction of epithelial cells by chemotherapy Inflammation and ulceration, which result from rapid cell destruction	• Be aware that eating, swallowing, and talking may be difficult and necessitate changes in diet and fluid intake. • Encourage patient to use artificial saliva. • Assess oral mucosa daily. Teach the patient to do this, and encourage the patient to practise good oral hygiene. • Use evidence-informed guidelines and protocols to minimize the occurrence or reduce the severity of oral mucositis. • Discourage use of irritants such as tobacco and alcohol, spicy foods, and drinks. • Apply topical anaesthetics, such as Xylocaine Viscous or oxethazaine.
Nausea and vomiting	Cellular breakdown, which stimulates vomiting centre in brain Drugs, which also stimulate vomiting centre Destruction of GI lining by radiation and chemotherapy	• Counsel the patient to eat and drink when not nauseated. • Administer antiemetics, and teach the patient and family caregiver when to use antiemetic therapy to maximize symptom control.
Anorexia	Release of TNF and IL-1 from macrophages, which has appetite-suppressant effect General reaction to therapy	• Use diversional activities (if appropriate). • Monitor the patient's weight. • Encourage the patient to eat small, frequent meals of high-protein, high-calorie foods (e.g., Ensure or other supplements). • Reassure family caregivers, and teach them to provide gentle encouragement to the patient.
Diarrhea	Denuding of epithelial lining of intestines	• Suggest low-fibre, low-residue diet. • Increase fluids. • Provide antidiarrheal agents as needed.
Constipation	Autonomic nervous system dysfunction Neurotoxic effects of plant alkaloids (vincristine, vinblastine) Use of opioids	• Encourage the patient to use a diary to monitor bowel movements and report to the health care team as needed. • Provide stool softeners and laxatives as needed. • Encourage intake of high-fibre foods.
Hepatotoxicity	Toxic effects from chemotherapeutic drugs	• Monitor liver function values.
Hematological System		
Anemia	Bone marrow depressed secondary to therapy Malignant infiltration of bone marrow by cancer	• Monitor hemoglobin and hematocrit levels. • Encourage intake of foods that promote RBC production (see Chapter 33, Table 33-5).
Leukopenia	Depression of bone marrow secondary to chemotherapy or radiation therapy Febrile neutropenia Infection resulting from immunosuppression (most frequent cause of morbidity and death in patients with cancer) Infection in respiratory and genitourinary systems (usual sites of infection)	• Monitor WBC count, especially neutrophils. • Educate and counsel patients and family caregivers to do the following: Monitor changes in temperature, and report any elevation immediately to the health care team. Advise the patient to maintain good personal hygiene, including frequent handwashing. Recommend that the patient report any signs of infection (swelling, unusual cough, vomiting, severe headache, redness) immediately at the nearest hospital. Advise the patient to avoid large crowds and people with infections.
Thrombocytopenia	Bone marrow depression secondary to chemotherapy Malignant infiltration of bone marrow Spontaneous bleeding, which can occur with platelet counts at or below 20×10^9/L	• Observe for signs of bleeding (e.g., petechiae, ecchymosis). • Monitor hemoglobin, hematocrit, and platelet counts. • Counsel use of a soft-bristle toothbrush and electric razor.

GI, gastrointestinal; *IL-1*, interleukin 1; *RBC*, red blood cell; *TNF*, tumour necrosis factor; *WBC*, white blood cell.

Continued

Table 18-14 Nursing Management of Problems Caused by Radiation Therapy and Chemotherapy—cont'd

PROBLEM	CAUSE	NURSING MANAGEMENT
Integumentary System		
Alopecia (usually temporary with chemotherapy and usually permanent in response to radiation)	Destruction of hair follicles by chemotherapy or radiation to scalp	• Suggest ways to cope with hair loss (e.g., hairpieces, scarves, wigs). • Discuss effect of hair loss on self-image. • Recommend cutting long hair before therapy. • Advise the patient to avoid excessive shampooing, brushing, and combing of hair. • Recommend avoiding use of electric hair dryers, curlers, and curling irons.
Skin reactions	Extravasation of vesicant chemotherapeutic drugs Radiation therapy damage to skin	• Protect the patient from extravasation through careful attention to delivery of chemotherapeutic drugs and assessment of venous access. • Recommend lubricating dry skin with nonirritating creams. • Recommend avoiding the use of harsh soaps. • Advise the patient to wear loose clothing and cotton underwear; avoid tight garments. • Inform the patient that photosensitivity may occur.
Genitourinary System		
Cystitis	Destruction of cells lining the bladder by chemotherapy Adverse effect of radiation when located in treatment field	• Monitor manifestations such as urgency, frequency, and hematuria. • Discuss these changes with the patient.
Reproductive dysfunction	Damage of cells of testes or ova by therapy	• Provide information about effects on fertility and referral to fertility resources (e.g., sperm banking) before radiation to the pelvis, high-dose chemotherapy, or bone marrow transplantation.
Nephrotoxicity	Accumulation of drugs in the kidney and tumour lysis, which cause necrosis of proximal renal tubules	• Monitor BUN and serum creatinine levels.
Nervous System		
Increased intracranial pressure	Radiation-related edema in central nervous system	• Administer steroids and pain medication. • Monitor neurological status.
Peripheral neuropathy	Paraesthesias, areflexia, skeletal muscle weakness, and smooth muscle dysfunction, which can occur as adverse effects of plant alkaloids and cisplatin	• Monitor for such manifestations in patients receiving these drugs.
Respiratory System		
Pneumonitis (develops 2-3 mo after start of treatment) Fibrosis (develops after 6-12 mo and is evident on radiographs)	Radiation Adverse effects of some chemotherapeutic drugs	• Monitor for dry, hacking cough; fever; and exertional dyspnea.
Cardiovascular System		
Pericarditis and myocarditis (complication when chest wall is radiated; may occur up to 1 yr after treatment)	Inflammation secondary to radiation injury Adverse effect of some chemotherapeutic drugs	• Monitor for clinical manifestations of these disorders. • Monitor heart function with ECG studies and cardiac ejection fractions.
Cardiotoxicity	Some chemotherapeutic drugs (e.g., doxorubicin, daunorubicin) can cause ECG changes and rapidly progressive heart failure	• Drug therapy may have to be modified.

Table 18-14 Nursing Management of Problems Caused by Radiation Therapy and Chemotherapy—cont'd

PROBLEM	CAUSE	NURSING MANAGEMENT
Biochemical		
Hyperuricemia, secondary gout, and obstructive uropathy	Cell destruction by chemotherapy	• Monitor uric acid levels. • Allopurinol (Zyloprim) may be given as a prophylactic measure. • Encourage high fluid intake.
Multidimensional Effects		
Fatigue	Increased metabolic rate Anabolic processes that result in accumulation of metabolites from cell breakdown	• Counsel the patient that fatigue is an expected adverse effect of therapy but that there are ways to manage fatigue, such as sleep hygiene, moderate exercise, and pacing activities. • Encourage the patient to rest when fatigued, to maintain usual lifestyle patterns as closely as possible, and to pace activities in accordance with energy level.
Pain	Compression or infiltration of tumour involving nerves Inflammation, ulceration, or necrosis of tissues	• Use an analgesic ladder to provide basis for pain medication administration. • Teach use of imagery, relaxation therapy, and other alternative measures (see Chapters 8 and 12).

BUN, blood urea nitrogen (serum urea [nitrogen]); *ECG*, electrocardiographic; *GI*, gastrointestinal; *IL-1*, interleukin 1; *RBC*, red blood cell; *TNF*, tumour necrosis factor; *WBC*, white blood cell.

an attempt to fight the cancer. Both TNF and IL-1 have an appetite-suppressing (anorexic) effect. It is hypothesized that as tumours are destroyed by therapy, increased levels of these factors are released into the system and cross the blood–brain barrier, affecting the satiety centre. Large tumours produce more of these factors, thus resulting in the cachexia observed in patients with advanced cancer. In addition, radiation treatments to the head and neck and the GI system exacerbate eating difficulties. Anorexia peaks at about 4 weeks of treatment and seems to resolve more quickly than fatigue when treatment ends.

The patient with anorexia needs to be monitored carefully during treatment to ensure that weight loss does not become excessive. Body weight should be measured at least twice weekly. Small, frequent meals of high-protein, high-calorie foods are better tolerated than large meals (see eTables 18-4 and 18-5 on the Evolve Web site for this chapter). Nutritional supplements may be required.

■ Bone Marrow Suppression

Myelosuppression is a common and significant effect of many chemotherapeutic modalities and may also occur with radiotherapy. Chemotherapy is a systemic treatment with the ability to affect every vulnerable cell in the body, whereas radiotherapy is delivered locally, so that only the cells within the treatment field are affected. Concurrent chemoradiation generally increases the risk of bone marrow toxicity. The onset of bone marrow suppression is related to the lifespan of the blood cell type. WBCs are affected within 1 week, platelets in 2 to 3 weeks, and red blood cells (RBCs) in 2 to 3 months. The severity of myelosuppression is related to the type and the dose of chemotherapeutic drug or the specific radiation field and to the extent of bone marrow reserves. In the adult, about 40% of active marrow is in the pelvis, and 25% is in the thoracic and lumbar vertebrae.

Blood cell counts (including WBCs, neutrophils, RBCs, and platelets) must be closely monitored. Neutropenia is most common in patients receiving chemotherapy and puts them at risk for serious infections or sepsis. WBC growth factors may be used to stimulate regeneration of adequate numbers of leuko-cytes and prevent treatment delays. Thrombocytopenia may cause spontaneous bleeding or hemorrhage and may necessitate a platelet transfusion if counts fall below 20×10^9/L. If anemia occurs and the hemoglobin level drops below 6 mmol/L, the patient may require blood transfusions. Radiation therapy is more effective against well-oxygenated cells. Therefore, there is a concern that a hemoglobin level below 130 g/L may not provide for adequate oxygenation of cells in the treatment field (Prosnitz, Yao, Farrell, & Brizel, 2005).

■ Skin Reactions

Like the bone marrow, the skin cells are rapidly proliferating and are therefore vulnerable to the effects of radiation and chemotherapy. Both acute and chronic changes can occur in the skin within the radiation field. The skin-sparing property of modern radiation equipment limits the severity of these reactions. Although the skin reaction begins as early as the first treatment, it is initially transitory. Erythema may develop 1 to 24 hours after a single treatment. Erythema is an acute response followed by dry desquamation (Figure 18-15). If the rate of cellular sloughing is faster than the ability of the new epidermal cells to replace dead cells, a wet desquamation occurs, with exposure of the dermis and oozing of serum (Figure 18-16). Skin reactions are particularly evident in areas subjected to pressure, such as behind the ear and in gluteal folds, the perineum, the breast, the collar line, and bony prominences.

Although skin care protocols vary among institutions, they are founded on basic skin care principles (D'Haese et al., 2005). Dry reactions are uncomfortable and result in pruritus. Wet reactions result in discomfort and drainage. Dry skin should be lubricated with a nonirritating lotion or solution that contains no metal, alcohol, perfume, or additives that irritate the skin. Wet reactions must be kept clean and protected from further damage. Prevention of infection and facilitation of wound healing are the therapeutic goals.

Irradiated skin should be protected from extremes of temperature to prevent trauma. Heating pads, ice packs, and hot water bottles cannot be used in the treatment field. Constricting

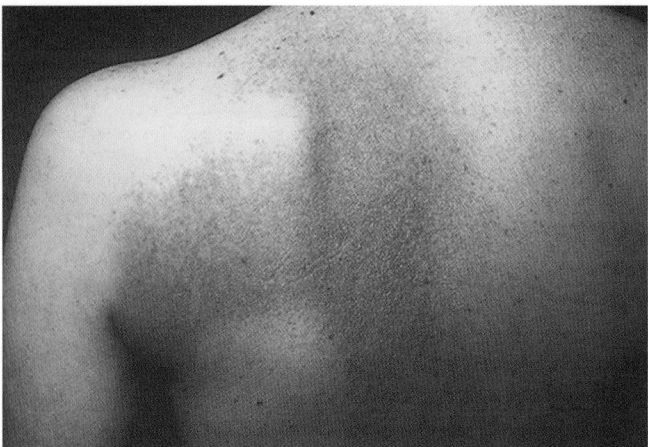

Figure 18-15 Dry desquamation.

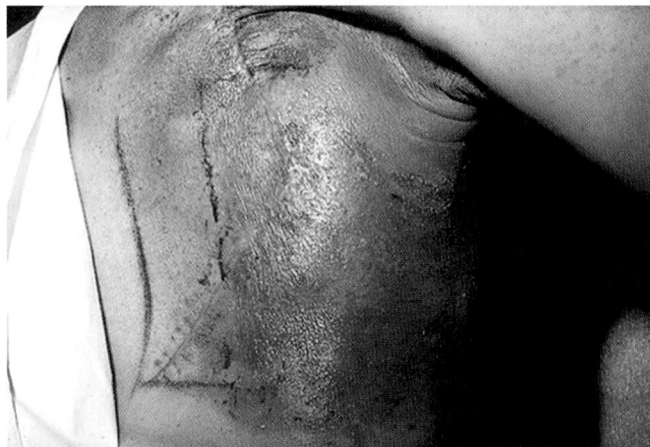

Figure 18-16 Wet desquamation.

garments, rubbing, harsh chemicals, and deodorants may also traumatize the skin and should be avoided. The use of corticosteroids and hydrogen peroxide is controversial because of their interference with wound healing. The guidelines presented in Table 18-15 are not intended to replace protocols or guidelines developed by the cancer agency or hospital program.

Alopecia (hair loss) is restricted to the radiation field when caused by radiotherapy but affects all body hair (including eyelashes and eyebrows) when caused by chemotherapeutic agents. For some patients, hair loss causes profound distress. Chemotherapy-induced alopecia is temporary; hair regrowth begins 3 to 4 weeks after therapy is terminated. Radiotherapy-induced hair loss may be temporary or permanent, depending on the dose administered. Patients may be directed to the Canadian Cancer Society's "Look Good, Feel Better" program for support and advice about wigs and head coverings.

▪ Oral, Oropharyngeal, and Esophageal Reactions

The mucosal lining of the GI tract is sensitive to the effects of radiation therapy and to certain antineoplastics, especially 5-fluorouracil. As a result, nutritional status may be compromised by treatment. Salivary flow often decreases, with resultant

PATIENT & CAREGIVER TEACHING GUIDE
Table 18-15 Radiation Skin Reactions

1. Gently cleanse the skin in the treatment field with a mild soap (Ivory, Dove), tepid water, a soft cloth, and a gentle patting motion. Rinse thoroughly and pat dry.

2. Apply nonmedicated, nonperfumed, moisturizing lotion or creams, such as baby lotion, oil, aloe gel, or cream to alleviate dry skin. This substance must be gently cleansed from the treatment field before each treatment and reapplied after. (Note: Care differs from institution to institution.) Dusting with cornstarch may reduce itching.

3. Rinse the area with saline solution. Expose the area to air as often as possible. If copious drainage is present, nonadhesive absorbent dressings are warranted, and they must be changed as soon as they become wet. Observe the area daily for signs of infection.

4. Avoid wearing tight-fitting clothing such as brassieres, girdles, and belts over the treatment field.

5. Avoid wearing harsh fabrics, such as wool and corduroy. A lightweight cotton garment is best. If possible, expose the treatment field to air.

6. Use gentle detergents such as Ivory Snow to wash clothing that will come in contact with the treatment field.

7. Avoid direct exposure to the sun. If the treatment field is in an area that is exposed to the sun, wear protective clothing such as a wide-brimmed hat during exposure to the sun. (Note: In general, people should avoid sun exposure regardless of whether they are in treatment or not; use of protective clothing and sunscreen on exposed areas should be recommended.)

8. Prevent application of heat from all sources (hot water bottles, heating pads, and sun lamps) on the treatment field.

9. Avoid exposing the treatment area to cold temperatures (ice bags or cold weather).

10. Avoid swimming in salt water or in chlorinated pools during the time of treatment.

11. Avoid the use of all medication, deodorants, perfumes, powders, or cosmetics on the skin in the treatment field. Tape, dressings, and adhesive bandages should also be avoided unless permitted by the radiation therapist. Avoid shaving the hair in the treatment field.

12. Continue to protect sensitive skin after the treatment is completed by doing the following:
    a. Avoid direct exposure to the sun. A sunscreen agent and protective clothing must be worn if there is potential for exposure to the sun.
    b. If shaving is necessary in the treatment field, use an electric razor.

xerostomia (dry mouth), during radiotherapy to the head and neck. Food must be dissolved in saliva to be tasted. Taste loss is progressive during therapy, and by the end of treatment, patients often report that all food has lost its flavour. Thick saliva is less able to perform the functions of cleansing teeth and moistening food. Difficulty swallowing, which characterizes esophageal reactions, further impedes eating. Patients report feeling that they have a "lump" as they swallow and that "foods get stuck."

Meticulous oral assessment and prompt intervention are essential to prevent infection and facilitate nutritional intake (McGuire, Correa, Johnson, & Wienandts, 2006). Oral care includes pretreatment evaluation by a dentist to perform all necessary dental work before the initiation of treatment. The patient must be taught to examine the mouth and gums daily. Mucous membranes, characteristics of saliva, and ability to swallow must be assessed regularly. The patient should also be taught how to perform oral care at least before and after each meal and at bedtime. A saline solution of 1 teaspoon of salt in 1 L of water is an effective cleansing agent. One teaspoon of sodium bicarbonate may be added to the oral care solution to decrease odour, alleviate pain, and dissolve mucin. Tooth brushing and flossing are critical unless contraindicated by decreased platelet counts. Compliance with this protocol significantly reduces the risk of radiation caries, which develops as a result of loss of saliva. Saliva substitutes are available and may be offered to patients, although many patients find that drinking small amounts of water frequently has an equivalent effect.

Antacids, diphenhydramine (Benadryl), and viscous lidocaine (Xylocaine) have been mixed in equal proportions to use as a component of oral care. The solutions may be swallowed to alleviate esophagitis. Any coating solution must be cleansed and not allowed to build up on the mucosa, where it could serve as a medium for infection. Infection, particularly with *Candida albicans*, can occur in individuals receiving head and neck radiation, and its incidence increases dramatically in protocols involving concomitant chemotherapy. Antifungal agents may be prescribed to treat the infection. Alleviation of mucositis may be achieved through the use of coating and analgesic compounds. Palifermin (Kepivance) has been shown to be effective in reducing the severity and duration of oral mucositis in patients receiving stem cell transplants and cryotherapy involving ice chips helps to prevent mucositis associated with 5-fluorouracil and melphalan therapy. The use of sucralfate, chlorhexidine, antimicrobial lozenges, and colony-stimulating factor mouthwash is not recommended (Keefe et al., 2007).

Feedings of soft, nonirritating high-protein and high-calorie foods should be offered frequently throughout the day. Extremes of temperature, as well as tobacco and alcohol, should be avoided. Nutritional supplements (e.g., Ensure) as an adjunct to meals and fluid intake may be encouraged. The patient should be weighed at least twice each week to monitor weight loss. Families are an integral part of the health care team. As taste loss increases, the family's role in assisting the patient to eat becomes increasingly critical. If family members are not available, alternative support such as volunteers and home aides are indicated.

Pulmonary Effects

Pulmonary effects of cancer therapies may be irreversible and progressive. The effects of radiation on the lung include both acute and late reactions. Radiation doses in the lung are magnified because the dose cannot be reduced through tissue. Pneumonitis can be an acute inflammatory reaction related to radiation. This reaction is often asymptomatic, although cough, fever, and night sweats may increase. Treatment with bronchodilators, expectorants, bed rest, and oxygen is preferable to treatment with corticosteroids.

The most common pulmonary toxic effects associated with chemotherapy include pulmonary edema, interstitial fibrosis, and pneumonitis. The chemotherapeutic agents most strongly associated with these complications include bleomycin, busulfan, carmustine, cyclophosphamide, and some targeted agents (e.g., gefitinib [Iressa]). The pulmonary effects of treatments may be difficult to distinguish from those related to the disease and

are frightening to the patient because they may involve an exacerbation of the symptoms that precipitated the cancer diagnosis. Cough and dyspnea may increase. The cough becomes more productive because alveoli that had been blocked are opened as the tumour responds to treatment. As treatment continues, the cough can become dry as the mucosa begins to be altered by the radiation. Cough suppressants may be indicated for use at night.

Oxygen, if prescribed for symptomatic pneumonitis, must be used judiciously if the patient has chronic obstructive pulmonary disease (see Chapter 31). Oxygen therapy in these patients can cause carbon dioxide retention and respiratory acidosis and may be lethal. If the patient experiences dyspnea, anxiety may be pronounced. Lying flat on the radiation treatment table and being alone in the room may potentiate anxiety.

Gastrointestinal Effects

The mucosa of the GI tract is highly proliferative: Surface cells are replaced every 2 to 6 days, and thus they are highly vulnerable to cancer therapies. The intestinal mucosa is one of the most radiosensitive tissues. Radiation alters gastric secretion by direct injury to cells. The secretion of mucus, hydrochloric acid, and pepsin decreases with further treatment. Nausea, vomiting, and diarrhea are early responses to irradiation of the GI tissue and may occur immediately after the first treatment. The occurrence of these symptoms in response to cancer therapies may be related to the release of serotonin from the GI tract, which then stimulates the chemoreceptor trigger zone and the vomiting centre in the brain. Further GI irritation is related to direct injury to epithelial cells.

Several antiemetic drugs are available (see Chapter 44 and Table 44-1). Metoclopramide, ondansetron (Zofran), granisetron (Kytril), aprepitant (Emend), and dexamethasone have been used to decrease nausea and vomiting caused by chemotherapy. The introduction of antiemetic clinical practice guidelines and effective implementation of the guidelines into the oncology settings are essential methods for managing this treatment adverse effect (Herrstedt, 2008). Administration of antiemetics before treatment alleviates the patient's experience of nausea and vomiting. The patient may find that eating a light meal of nonirritating food before treatment is also helpful. *Anticipatory nausea and vomiting* may develop in the patient receiving radiation or chemotherapy when these symptoms are poorly controlled. This conditioned response results in the experience of nausea and vomiting when the patient encounters cues associated with the treatment: for example, walking through the doors of the cancer centre or merely seeing the oncologist, even outside of the treatment centre. In some individuals, this response persists after treatment ends. Aggressive emesis control, including the use of prophylactic antiemetics and antianxiety agents, is recommended.

The patient experiencing nausea and vomiting must be assessed for signs and symptoms of dehydration and alkalosis. Fluid intake is recorded to ensure that the volume consumed and retained is adequate. Diarrhea may be a reaction of the bowel mucosa to radiation. The small bowel is extremely sensitive and does not tolerate significant radiation doses. Administering treatments when the patient has a full bladder may serve to move the small bowel out of the treatment field. Nonirritating diets and low-residue diets, as well as antidiarrheal and antispasmodic drugs, are recommended. Lukewarm sitz baths may alleviate discomfort and cleanse the rectal area. The rectal area must be kept scrupulously clean and dry to maintain mucosal integrity. The nurse should inspect the perianal area. Number, volume, consistency, and character of stools per day should be recorded by patients, as should any potentially aggravating or alleviating factors related to bowel movements. Adequate food and fluid intake promote healing and mucosal integrity. Systemic analgesia is warranted for the painful skin irritations that may develop.

Reproductive Effects

The effects of radiation and chemotherapy on the ovary and testes are determined by the dose delivered and the type of chemotherapy used. The testes are highly sensitive to radiation, and protection of the testicles is achieved whenever possible. Doses of 15 to 30 cGy temporarily decrease the sperm count; aspermia results at 35 to 230 cGy. In some cases, 200 cGy may result in permanent aspermia. In the patient receiving 300 to 600 cGy, the sperm count either recovers in 2 to 5 years or does not recover at all. Pretreatment status may be a significant factor because a low sperm count and loss of motility are seen in individuals with testicular cancer and Hodgkin's disease before any therapy. Combined modality treatment or prior chemotherapy with alkylating agents enhances and prolongs the effects of radiation on the testes. When radiation is used alone with conventional doses and appropriate shielding, testicular recovery often occurs. Compromised reproductive function in men may also result from erectile dysfunction after pelvic radiation and its related vascular and neurological effects.

The radiation dose necessary to induce ovarian failure changes with age. Permanent cessation of menses occurs at 500 to 1000 cGy in 95% of women younger than 40 years, and at 375 cGy the percentage increases to a greater level in women older than 40 years. Unlike the testes, the ovaries have no avenue for repair; therefore, the ovaries are shielded whenever possible. Other factors that influence reproductive or sexual functioning in women include reactions in the cervix and endometrium. These tissues withstand a high radiation dose with minimal sequelae, which accounts for the ability to treat endometrial and cervical cancer with high external and brachytherapeutic doses. Acute reactions such as tenderness, irritation, and loss of lubrication compromise sexual activity. Late effects of combined internal and external therapy include loss of elasticity, loss of lubrication, and vaginal shortening related to fibrosis. Supportive nursing care during brachytherapy for gynecological cancer is critical to the well-being and psychological functioning of women experiencing this treatment (Stilos, Doyle, & Daines, 2008).

The patient and the patient's partner require information about the expected effects of treatment in relation to reproductive and sexual issues. Potential infertility can be a significant consequence for the individual, and counselling is indicated. Pretreatment harvesting of sperm or ova may be considered. Specific suggestions to manage adverse effects that have an effect on sexual functioning include use of a water-soluble vaginal lubricant and a vaginal dilator after pelvic irradiation. The nurse must be competent in discussing issues related to sexuality, offering specific suggestions, and making referrals for ongoing counselling when indicated (Katz, 2007).

Late Effects of Radiation and Chemotherapy

Cancer survivors are achieving higher rates of long-term remission and survival because of advancements in treatment modali-

ties. However, these forms of therapy (especially radiation and chemotherapy) may produce long-term sequelae termed *physiological late effects* that occur months to years after cessation of therapy. Every body system can be affected to some extent by chemotherapy and radiation therapy. The effects of radiation on the body's tissues are caused by cellular hypoplasia of stem cells and alterations in the fine vasculature and fibroconnective tissues. In addition to the acute toxic effects, chemotherapy can have long-term effects related to the loss of cells' proliferative reserve capacity. The additive effects of multiagent chemotherapy before, during, or after a course of radiotherapy can significantly increase the resulting physiological late effects.

The cancer survivor may also be at risk for leukemias and other secondary malignancies resulting from therapy for the primary cancer. However, the potential risk for developing a second malignancy does not contraindicate the use of cancer treatment. The overall risk of developing neoplastic complications is low, and the latency period may be long.

The cancer treatments most frequently implicated in causing secondary malignancy are the alkylating chemotherapeutic agents and high-dose radiation, which can induce cancers at the exposure site. The exact mechanism of oncogenesis secondary to radiation and chemotherapy remains unclear. It could be related to interactions between immunosuppressive factors, direct cellular damage, and carcinogenic effects, along with other environmental carcinogens.

Acute leukemias occurring as secondary malignancies have been most widely reported after treatment for Hodgkin's disease, but they also occur in survivors of ovarian, lung, and breast cancers. Secondary malignancies other than leukemias include multiple myeloma after radiation therapy for breast cancer; non-Hodgkin's lymphoma after treatment for Hodgkin's disease; and cancers of the bladder, the kidney, and the ureters after the use of cyclophosphamide. Radiation therapy for breast, lung, ovarian, uterine, and thyroid cancers, non-Hodgkin's lymphoma, and Hodgkin's disease has been linked to secondary osteosarcoma of the rib, scapula, clavicle, humerus, sternum, ilium, and pelvis. Fibrosarcomas have been reported several years after radiation therapy for astrocytoma, glioblastoma, and pituitary adenoma. Unfortunately, secondary malignancies are usually resistant to therapy, but supportive care and palliative care are options for the patient.

Biological and Targeted Therapy

Biological therapy is treatment involving the use of biological agents such as interferons, interleukins, monoclonal antibodies, and growth factors to modify the relationship between the host and the tumour. Biological agents are assuming a larger role in cancer treatment, either alone or in combination with surgery, radiation therapy, and chemotherapy. An understanding of the principles of cellular interaction underlies the development of agents that modify the relationship between the host and the tumour by altering the biological response of the host to the tumour cells. Biological agents may affect host–tumour response in three ways: (a) They have direct antitumour effects; (b) they restore, augment, or modulate host immune system mechanisms; and (c) they have other biological effects, such as interfering with the cancer cells' ability to metastasize or differentiate (Table 18-16, Figure 18-17).

Tumour cells express tumour antigens on their surfaces that can be recognized and destroyed by the body's immune cells.

DRUG THERAPY

Table 18-16 Biological and Targeted Therapy

DRUG	MECHANISM OF ACTION	INDICATIONS	ADVERSE EFFECTS
Cytokines and Immunomodulators			
α-Interferon (Intron A)	Inhibits DNA and protein synthesis. Suppresses cell proliferation. Increases cytotoxic effects of NK cells	Hairy cell leukemia, chronic myelogenous leukemia, malignant melanoma, renal cell carcinoma, non-Hodgkin's lymphoma, ovarian cancer, multiple myeloma, Kaposi's sarcoma, pancreatic carcinoma	Flu-like syndrome (fever, chills, myalgia, headache), cognitive changes, fatigue, nausea, vomiting, anorexia, weight loss
Interleukin-2 (aldesleukin [Proleukin])	Stimulates proliferation of T and B cells. Activates NK cells	Metastatic renal cell cancer, metastatic melanoma	Same as those of α-interferon; capillary leak syndrome, resulting in hypotension; bone marrow suppression
Levamisole	Potentiates monocytes and macrophage function	Duke's stage C colon cancer (given in combination with 5-fluorouracil)	Diarrhea, metallic taste, nausea, fever, chills, mouth sores, headache
Bacillus Calmette-Guérin vaccine	Induces an immune response that prevents angiogenesis of tumour	In situ bladder cancer	Flu-like syndrome, nausea, vomiting, rash, cough
Tyrosine Kinase Inhibitors			
Cetuximab (Erbitux)	Inhibits epidermal growth factor receptor, which is coupled with tyrosine kinase	Colorectal cancer, in combination with radiotherapy for head and neck carcinoma	Rash, dry skin, infusion reactions, interstitial lung disease, fatigue, fever
Erlotinib (Tarceva) and gefitinib (Iressa)	Same as for cetuximab	Non–small cell lung cancer	Rash, diarrhea, interstitial lung disease
Imatinib (Gleevec)	Inhibits *bcr-abl* tyrosine kinase	Chronic myeloid leukemia	Nausea, diarrhea, myalgia, fluid retention
Sorafenib (Nexavar)	Inhibits several tyrosine kinases, some of which are involved in angiogenesis	Advanced renal cell carcinoma	Rash, diarrhea, hypertension; redness, pain, swelling, or blisters on hands and feet
Monoclonal Antibody to CD20			
Rituximab (Rituxan)	Binds CD20 antigen, causing cytotoxicity	Non-Hodgkin's lymphoma (B cell)	Fever, chills, nausea, headache, angioedema
Ibritumomab tiuxetan–yttrium-90 (Zevalin)	Binds CD20 antigen, causing cytotoxicity and radiation injury	Non-Hodgkin's lymphoma (B cell)	Bone marrow suppression, fatigue, nausea, chills
Tositumomab, tositumomab–iodine-131 (Bexxar)	Binds CD20 antigen, causing immune attack and radiation injury	Non-Hodgkin's lymphoma (B cell)	Bone marrow suppression, fever, chills, nausea, headache
Angiogenesis Inhibitor			
Bevacizumab (Avastin)	Binds vascular endothelial growth factor, thereby inhibiting angiogenesis	Colorectal cancer	Hypertension, colon bleeding and perforation, impaired wound healing, thromboembolism, diarrhea
Proteosome Inhibitor			
Bortezomib (Velcade)	Inhibits proteasome activity, which functions to regulate cell growth	Multiple myeloma	Bone marrow suppression, nausea, vomiting, diarrhea, peripheral neuropathy, fatigue
Monoclonal Antibodies			
Gemtuzumab ozogamicin (Mylotarg)	Binds CD33 antigen (expressed on leukemic cells) to deliver cytotoxic drug into the DNA	Acute myeloid leukemia	Bone marrow suppression, fever, chills, nausea
Alemtuzumab (Campath)	Binds CD52 antigen (found on T and B cells, monocytes, NK cells, neutrophils)	Chronic lymphocytic leukemia (B cell)	Bone marrow suppression, chills, fever, vomiting, diarrhea, fatigue
Trastuzumab (Herceptin)	Binds HER-2	Breast cancer (HER-2 positive)	Cardiotoxicity

HER-2, human epidermal growth factor receptor 2; *NK*, natural killer.

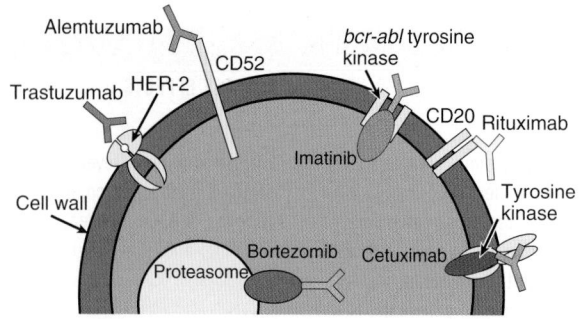

Figure 18-17 Sites of action of targeted therapy. *HER-2*, Human epidermal growth factor receptor 2.

Cytokines are glycoprotein products of immune cells, such as lymphocytes and macrophages, and are capable of defence functions. Cytokines include interferons, interleukins, colony-stimulating factors, and tumour necrosis factor. Interferons were the first type of cytokine to be studied as a cancer therapy. Interferons protect cells infected by viruses from attack by other viruses and inhibit replication of viral DNA. The antiproliferative effects of interferons are not completely understood. However, they have been shown to inhibit DNA and protein synthesis in some tumour cells and to stimulate the expression of tumour antigens on tumour cell surfaces. Because the interferons have antiviral and antitumour effects, they are used to treat a number of medical conditions, including hepatitis C and Kaposi's sarcoma. The severity of adverse effects of interferons depends on the dose and the route of administration. One of the most common adverse effects is flu-like syndrome, which includes fever, chills, myalgia, and headache. Targeted therapy interferes with cancer growth by targeting specific cellular receptors and pathways that are important for tumour growth. The targeted therapies are more selective for specific molecular targets than cancer drugs and are thus able to kill cancer cells without damaging normal cells. Targeted therapies include tyrosine kinase inhibitors, monoclonal antibodies, antiangiogenic agents such as VEGF receptor inhibitors, and interleukins.

Tyrosine kinases are important enzymes that activate the signaling pathways regulating cell proliferation and survival. For example, epidermal growth factor receptor (EGFR) is expressed in cells of epithelial origin, which rely on these receptors for repair and maintenance. EGFR is overexpressed in a wide variety of tumours, including non–small cell lung cancer, head and neck cancers, and pancreatic tumours and gliomas. Overexpression of EGFR is correlated with poor prognosis, increased recurrence rates, and resistance to chemotherapy. As such, it is an appealing target for cancer therapy. Erlotinib (Tarceva) and gefitinib (Iressa) are examples of EGFR tyrosine kinase inhibitors used in the treatment of non–small cell lung cancer.

Produced by B lymphocytes, monoclonal antibodies are antibodies (immunoglobulins) that are capable of binding to specific target cells, including tumour cells. Monoclonal antibodies can be unconjugated or conjugated. Unconjugated monoclonal antibodies are used alone to attack tumour cells directly. Conjugated monoclonal antibodies are attached to agents such as radioisotopes, toxins, chemotherapeutic agents, and other biological agents. The goal of this approach is to deliver the monoclonal antibody complex directly to the targeted cancer cells for their ultimate destruction. The antibodies also may stimulate an immune response in patients (Viele, 2005). Hybridoma technology for the production of monoclonal antibodies is described in Chapter 16.

The first monoclonal antibody approved for use in oncological treatment was rituximab (Rituxan), an unconjugated monoclonal antibody directed against the CD20 antigen found on the surface of B lymphocytes. Human epidermal growth factor receptor 2 (HER-2) is overexpressed in certain cancers (especially breast cancer) and is associated with more aggressive disease and decreased rates of survival. Trastuzumab (Herceptin) is an unconjugated monoclonal antibody that binds to HER-2 and inhibits the growth of breast cancer cells that express the HER-2 protein.

The most common type of conjugated monoclonal antibody is an immunotoxin, a molecule formed when a monoclonal antibody is conjugated to a plant or bacterial cell toxin. The most frequently used bacterial toxins to date have been *Pseudomonas* exotoxin and diphtheria toxin. Unfortunately, immunotoxins have shown poor clinical efficacy thus far and are associated with significant toxic effects.

Administration of monoclonal antibodies is by the infusion method. Patients may experience infusion-related symptoms, which can include fever, chills, urticaria, mucosal congestion, nausea, diarrhea, and myalgias. There is also a risk, although rare, of anaphylaxis associated with the administration of monoclonal antibodies. This potential exists because most monoclonal antibodies are produced by mouse lymphocytes and thus represent a foreign protein to the human body. Onset of anaphylaxis can occur within 5 minutes of administration and can be a life-threatening event. (See Chapter 16 for a discussion of nursing management of anaphylaxis.) Other toxic effects of monoclonal antibodies may include hepatotoxicity, bone marrow depression, and CNS effects. Patients who receive trastuzumab may also experience cardiac dysfunction, especially when it is administered in higher doses or in combination with anthracycline antibiotics such as doxorubicin (Adriamycin).

Angiogenesis inhibitors work by preventing the mechanisms and pathways necessary for the vascularization of tumours. Bevacizumab (Avastin), a recombinant human monoclonal antibody, is active against the VEGF molecule, a crucial regulator of normal and pathological angiogenesis. Undesirable adverse effects of bevacizumab include hypertension, hemorrhage, and thromboembolic events. Its use is indicated in the treatment of colorectal cancer, and trials are being conducted to treat a number of other cancers.

Interleukins are a family of cytokines that act primarily between lymphocytes to induce activation of the immune system or alteration in the functional capacity of tumour cells. To date, 29 interleukins have been discovered, and each is designated by number, but only IL-2 has been approved as an anticancer agent. Aldesleukin (Proleukin) is a recombinant form of IL-2 used in the treatment of metastatic renal cell carcinoma, acute myelogenous leukemia, and lymphoma.

A major toxic effect of IL-2 therapy is capillary leak syndrome, which occurs as a result of changes in capillary permeability and vascular tone. As a consequence of the increase in capillary permeability, fluids shift from intravascular to extravascular compartments. This causes intravascular fluid depletion. Manifestations of capillary leak syndrome include hypotension, peripheral edema, ascites, interstitial pulmonary infiltrates, weight gain, and decreased systemic vascular resistance. Additional toxic effects of IL-2 therapy include renal, cardiovascular, pulmonary, GI, and integumentary toxic effects; bone marrow suppression; and changes in cognitive function. (NOTE: Provincial care programs and drug benefits programs may vary; the nurse should consult the agency's protocols and formulary.)

Hematopoietic Growth Factors

Colony-Stimulating Factors. Colony-stimulating factors are a family of glycoproteins produced by various cells. These glycoproteins stimulate production, maturation, regulation, and activation of cells of the hematological system. After release, colony-stimulating factors attach to receptors on the cell surface of peripheral blood cells and hematopoietic precursors (precursors of mature blood cells). They then stimulate production, maturation, release from the bone marrow, and functional ability of blood cells. The name of the colony-stimulating factor is based on the specific cell line it affects: granulocyte colony–stimulating factor (G-CSF), granulocyte-macrophage colony–stimulating factor (GM-CSF), macrophage colony–stimulating factor (M-CSF or CSF-1), and multicolony-stimulating factor (interleukin-3 [IL-3]).

Colony-stimulating factors have a number of potential clinical uses. They may hasten recovery from bone marrow depression after standard and high-dose chemotherapy and bone marrow transplantation or decrease bone marrow suppression associated with administration of chemotherapeutic agents. Colony-stimulating factors may also re-establish bone marrow function in aplastic anemia, myelodysplastic syndrome, and leukemia and may be effective in the management of sepsis.

G-CSF is available as filgrastim (Neupogen) for the treatment of neutropenia. Pegfilgrastim (Neulasta) is a longer-acting form of filgrastim. G-CSF stimulates the production and function of neutrophils. It can be administered subcutaneously or by intravenous infusion. The most commonly reported adverse effect of G-CSF therapy is medullary bone pain, which occurs most often in the lower back, the pelvis, and the sternum. This pain generally develops at the time the neutrophil count begins to recover and lasts for about 24 hours. The pain associated with G-CSF therapy is usually relieved with nonnarcotic analgesics.

GM-CSF is available as sargramostim (Leukine, Prokine) for the treatment of (a) neutropenia associated with bone marrow transplantation, (b) bone marrow transplant failure or delay in bone marrow engraftment, and (c) acute myelogenous leukemia after chemotherapy. GM-CSF stimulates the production and function of neutrophils, eosinophils, and monocytes. In addition, GM-CSF stimulates these cells to produce cytokines. GM-CSF can be administered either subcutaneously or by intravenous infusion. The most common adverse effects associated with GM-CSF administration include medullary bone pain (similar to the bone pain associated with G-CSF administration), leukocytosis, and eosinophilia.

IL-3 is a multipotential stimulator of hematopoietic stem cells. IL-3 has been shown to stimulate the growth of neutrophils, monocytes, eosinophils, basophils, and platelet cell lines. IL-3 is being investigated for the treatment of bone marrow failure and for its ability to enhance myeloid recovery after chemotherapy, radiotherapy, and bone marrow transplantation. M-CSF is also undergoing investigation for its potential role in cancer treatment.

Erythropoietin. Erythropoietin is a colony-stimulating factor responsible for stimulating growth of the erythroid precursor cells that ultimately mature into RBCs. Erythropoietin is produced naturally by the kidneys. Erythropoietin was initially approved for the management of chronic anemia associated with end-stage renal disease. Subsequently, approval was expanded to include the use of erythropoietin (Eprex) for the management of chemotherapy-related anemia. Darbepoetin alfa (Aranesp), a long-acting form of erythropoietin, is now available.

Toxic and Adverse Effects of Biological Agents

The administration of one biological agent usually induces the endogenous release of others. The release and action of these biological agents result in systemic immune and inflammatory responses. The toxic effects and adverse effects of biological agents are related to dose and schedule. Common adverse effects, especially with interferons, include constitutional flu-like symptoms such as headache, fever, chills, myalgias, fatigue, malaise, weakness, photosensitivity, anorexia, and nausea. The severity of the flu-like symptoms associated with interferon therapy generally decreases over time. Acetaminophen administered every 4 hours, as prescribed, often reduces the severity of the flu-like syndrome. The patient is commonly premedicated with acetaminophen in an attempt to prevent or decrease the intensity of these symptoms. In addition, large amounts of fluids help decrease the intensity of symptoms.

Tachycardia and orthostatic hypotension are also commonly reported. IL-2 and monoclonal antibodies can cause capillary leak syndrome, with resulting pulmonary edema. Other toxic and adverse effects may involve the CNS and the renal, hepatic, and cardiovascular systems. These effects are found particularly with interferons and IL-2.

NURSING MANAGEMENT: BIOLOGICAL THERAPY

Problems experienced by the patient receiving biological therapy may differ in type or severity from those observed with more traditional forms of cancer therapy. For example, capillary leak syndrome and pulmonary edema are problems that necessitate critical care nursing expertise. Bone marrow depression occurring with biological agent administration is generally more transient and mild than that observed with chemotherapy, but fatigue associated with biological therapy can be so severe that it may constitute a dose-limiting toxic effect.

Nursing interventions for flu-like syndrome include the administration of acetaminophen before treatment and every 4 hours after treatment. Intravenous meperidine (Demerol) has been used to control the severe chills associated with some biological agents. Other nursing measures include monitoring of vital signs and temperature, planning for periods of rest for the patient, and assisting with activities of daily living.

With interferon and IL-2 therapy, numerous neurological deficits have been observed. The nature and extent of these problems have not been completely elucidated. However, these problems are frightening to the patient and the family, who must be taught to observe for neurological problems (e.g., confusion, memory loss, difficulty making decisions, insomnia), report their occurrence, and institute appropriate safety and support measures. (NOTE: Provincial care programs and drug benefits programs may vary: the nurse should consult the agency's protocols and formulary.)

Bone Marrow and Stem Cell Transplantation

Bone marrow transplantation (BMT) is an effective, lifesaving procedure for a number of malignant and nonmalignant diseases (Table 18-17). BMT allows for the safe use of very high doses of chemotherapeutic agents or radiation to patients whose tumours are resistant or unresponsive to standard doses of chemotherapeutic agents and radiation. BMT offers hope to many patients whose disease is responsive to increased doses of systemic therapy. In recent years, the numbers of BMT and transplantation programs in Canada have increased dramatically.

Whether the diagnosis is a malignant or nonmalignant disease, the goal of BMT is cure. Cure rates are still low but are steadily increasing. Even if there is no cure, most transplantation procedures result in a period of remission. BMT is an intensive procedure with many risks, and some patients die from complications of BMT or from relapse of the original disease. Because it is a highly toxic therapy, the patient must weigh the significant risks of treatment-related death or treatment failure (relapse) against the hope of cure.

Types of Bone Marrow Transplants

Bone marrow transplants can be allogeneic, autologous, or syngeneic. In *allogeneic marrow transplantation*, the infused bone marrow is acquired from a donor who has been determined to be matched to the recipient in terms of human leukocyte antigen (HLA) tissue typing. HLA typing involves testing WBCs to identify genetically inherited antigens common to both donor and recipient that are important in compatibility of transplanted tissue. (HLA tissue typing is discussed in Chapter 16.) The donor is often a family member, but an unrelated donor may be found through a bone marrow registry. The goal is to administer large doses of systemic therapy and then "rescue" the bone marrow through the engraftment and subsequent normal proliferation and differentiation of the donated marrow in the recipient. The most common indication for allogeneic transplantation is leukemia.

In *autologous marrow transplantation*, patients receive their own bone marrow. The aim of this approach is to enable patients to receive intensive chemotherapy or radiation while supporting them with their own bone marrow. In this type of BMT, the patient's own marrow is removed, treated, stored, and reinfused. *Syngeneic marrow transplantation* involves obtaining stem cells from one identical twin and infusing them into the other. Identical twins have identical HLA types and are a perfect match.

Procedures

Harvest Procedures. Bone marrow can be "harvested" through a procedure conducted in the operating room with the patient under general or spinal anaesthesia in which multiple bone marrow aspirations are carried out, usually from the iliac crest, but also from the sternum. The entire harvesting procedure usually takes 1 to 2 hours, and the patient can be discharged after recovery. After the procedure, the donor may experience pain at the collection site, which can be treated with mild analgesics. The donor's body replaces the bone marrow in a few weeks.

After harvesting, autologous bone marrow may be treated *(purged)* to remove cancer cells. Many different pharmacological, immunological, physical, and chemical agents have been used for this purpose. The bone marrow is then frozen *(cryopreserved)* and stored until it is used for transplantation. In allogeneic transplantation, the marrow can be harvested, processed, and infused into the recipient within a few hours of donation.

Preparative Regimens. In malignant diseases, the goal of BMT is to rescue the marrow after the patient has received high doses of chemotherapeutic agents, with or without radiation, aimed at treating the underlying disease. After harvesting of the marrow, the patient is given high-dose chemotherapy with or without radiation therapy. Total body irradiation can be used for immunosuppression or to treat the disease.

After the therapy, the marrow that was removed is thawed and administered to the patient intravenously to replace the destroyed marrow. The stem cells reconstitute, or "rescue," the recipient's hematopoietic system. Usually 2 to 4 weeks are required for the transplanted marrow to start producing hematopoietic blood cells. During this pancytopenic period, it is critical for the patient to be in a protective isolation environment and receive supportive care. RBC and platelet transfusions are usually necessary to maintain the necessary quantity of circulating RBCs and platelets.

Complications. Bacterial, viral, and fungal infections are common after BMT. Prophylactic antibiotic therapy may reduce their incidence. A potentially serious complication of allogeneic transplant is graft-versus-host disease. This occurs when the T lymphocytes from the donated marrow (graft) recognize the recipient (host) as foreign and begin to attack certain organs such as the skin, the liver, and the intestines. Graft-versus-host disease is discussed in Chapter 16. Another major adverse event is inadequate oral intake, which results in dehydration and malnutrition and thereby necessitates intensive nutritional support through a variety of interventions, such as oral supplementation and enteral feeding (McDiarmid, 2002).

Peripheral Stem Cell Transplantation

An alternative to the harvest procedure is *peripheral stem cell transplantation* (PSCT). Peripheral or circulating stem cells are capable of repopulating the bone marrow. PSCT is a type of transplantation that differs from BMT primarily in the method of stem cell

Table 18-17 Uses for Bone Marrow Transplantation	
MALIGNANT DISEASES	**NONMALIGNANT DISEASES**
• Acute and chronic myelogenous leukemia	• Sickle cell disease
• Acute lymphocytic leukemia	• Thalassemia
• Hodgkin's lymphoma	• Aplastic anemia
• Non-Hodgkin's lymphoma	• Immunodeficiency diseases
• Myelodysplastic syndrome	• Severe autoimmune diseases
• Multiple myeloma	
• Neuroblastoma	
• Sarcoma	
• Testicular cancer	
• Ovarian cancer	

collection. Because the blood contains fewer stem cells than does the bone marrow, stem cells from the bone marrow can be mobilized into the peripheral blood through chemotherapy or hematopoietic growth factors. Common growth factors that are used are GM-CSF and G-CSF. The donor's blood is collected, the peripheral stem cells are separated by means of a cell separator machine, and then the blood is returned through a venous line to the patient. This procedure is called *leukapheresis* and usually takes 2 to 4 hours to complete. In autologous transplantation, the stem cells are purged to kill any cancer cells and then frozen and stored until used for transplantation. Although many of the same steps (harvesting, intensive chemotherapy, reinfusion) of BMT are used in PSCT, the hematological recovery period in PSCT is shorter and has fewer, less severe complications (McAdams & Burgunder, 2004).

Cord Blood Stem Cells

Umbilical cord blood is rich in hematopoietic stem cells, and successful allogeneic transplantation has been performed with the use of this source. Cord blood can be HLA typed and cryopreserved. A disadvantage of cord blood is the possibly insufficient numbers of stem cells for transplantation into adults.

Gene Therapy

Gene therapy involves the transfer of exogenous genes (transgenes) into the cells of patients in an effort to correct the defective gene. The effect of gene therapy for cancer can be a temporary gene transfer with the additional goal of instigating an immune response to the transgene. The use of this new therapeutic approach for cancer is currently investigational. Several clinical trials are under way to evaluate the safety, tolerability, and efficacy of gene therapy for malignancies such as melanoma, brain tumours, and mesothelioma. (Gene therapy is discussed in Chapter 16.)

Complications Resulting From Cancer

The patient may develop complications related to the continual growth of the malignancy or the adverse effects of treatment.

Nutritional Problems

Malnutrition. The patient with cancer often experiences protein and calorie malnutrition, characterized by depletion of fat and muscle. (Assessment of the degree of malnutrition is discussed in Chapter 42.) Foods suggested for increasing the protein intake to facilitate repair and regeneration of cells are presented in eTable 18-4, available on the Evolve Web site for this chapter. High-caloric foods that provide energy and minimize weight loss are presented in eTable 18-5 on the Evolve Web site. A sample high-calorie, high-protein diet is presented in eTable 42-5.

The nurse should suggest a referral to a dietitian as soon as a 5% weight loss is noted or if the patient has the potential for protein and caloric malnutrition. Albumin and prealbumin levels should be monitored. Once a 4.5-kg weight loss occurs, it is difficult to maintain the nutritional status. The patient can be taught to use nutritional supplements in place of milk when cooking or baking. Foods to which nutritional supplements can

be easily added include scrambled eggs, pudding, custard, mashed potatoes, cereal, and cream sauces. Packages of instant breakfast can be used as indicated or sprinkled on cereals, desserts, and casseroles.

If the malnutrition cannot be treated with dietary intake, it may be necessary to use enteral or parenteral supplementation as an adjunct nutritional measure. (Enteral and parenteral nutrition are discussed in Chapter 42.)

Altered Taste Sensation. It is theorized that cancer cells release substances that resemble amino acids and stimulate the bitter taste buds. The patient may also experience an alteration in the sweet taste sensation and in the sour and the salty taste sensations. Meat may taste bitter to the patient. The physiological basis of these taste alterations is unclear. It is important to help the patient (a) understand the changes that will be experienced and (b) find foods that are appealing. Many Canadians are from different cultural and ethnic groups, and the nurse must be aware of possible differences in the meal preparation and selection that are amenable to the patient. Frequently, the patient may feel compelled to eat certain foods because those foods are believed to be beneficial. The patient can be encouraged to experiment with spices and other seasoning agents to taste in an attempt to mask the taste alterations.

Infection

Infection can cause death in a patient whose immune system is suppressed as a result of cancer treatment. The usual sites of infection include lungs, genitourinary system, mouth, rectum, peritoneal cavity, and blood (septicemia). Infection occurs as a result of the ulceration and necrosis caused by the tumour, compression of vital organs by the tumour, and neutropenia caused by the disease process or the treatment of cancer. A critical aspect of nursing care is teaching about infection risk associated with neutropenia. A patient with a body temperature of 38°C (100.5°F) or higher should come to be seen at the hospital or cancer centre as soon as possible. Assessment most often includes signs and symptoms of fever, determination of possible cause, and complete blood cell count.

Many patients are neutropenic when an infection develops. In such individuals, infection causes significant morbidity and may be rapidly fatal if not treated promptly. The classical manifestations of infection are often not present in a patient with neutropenia and a depressed immune system. (Neutropenia is discussed in Chapter 33.) (See the Evidence-Informed Practice box on nursing interventions and infection.)

Oncological Emergencies

Oncological emergencies are life-threatening events that can occur as a result of cancer or cancer treatment. These emergencies can be obstructive, metabolic, or infiltrative.

Obstructive Emergencies. Obstructive emergencies are caused primarily by tumour obstruction of an organ or a blood vessel. Obstructive emergencies include superior vena cava syndrome, spinal cord compression syndrome, third space syndrome, and intestinal obstruction.

Superior Vena Cava Syndrome. Superior vena cava syndrome results from obstruction of the superior vena cava by a tumour. The clinical manifestations include facial edema, periorbital

Do Nursing Interventions Prevent or Reduce Infection in Patients With Cancer?

Clinical Question

In patients with cancer (P), do nursing interventions (I) prevent or reduce infection (O) in patients who received the intervention (C)?

Best Available Evidence

Systematic review

Critical Appraisal and Synthesis of Evidence

One hundred two research articles, systematic reviews, and meta-analyses from 1995 to 2005 that focused on nursing interventions aimed at preventing infection were reviewed. Three criteria determined the assessment of the level of evidence for the interventions: quality of evidence, magnitude of the outcome, and concurrence of the evidence.

Conclusion

Pharmacological and nonpharmacological nursing interventions play a critical role in the prevention of infection in patients with cancer.

Implications for Nursing Practice

There is strong evidence to support the use of the following practices for the prevention of infection in patients with cancer:

- Hand hygiene with soap and water or an antiseptic hand rub
- Colony-stimulating factors for patients undergoing chemotherapy with more than a 20% risk of febrile neutropenia
- Influenza vaccine annually
- Trimethoprim-sulfamethoxazole to prevent *Pneumocystis jiroveci* pneumonia for patients at risk
- Antifungal, antibacterial, and antiviral prophylaxis for selected patients at risk
- Restrictions on visitors with respiratory infections
- Protective gowns if soiling with respiratory secretions is anticipated
- Environmental interventions (keep windows closed; use of anterooms or high-efficiency particulate air filters and negative-pressure rooms)

Reference for Evidence

Zitella, L. J., Friese, C. R., Hauser, J., Gobel, B. H., Woolery, M., O'Leary, C., & Andrews, F. A. (2006). Putting evidence into practice: Prevention of infection. *Clinical Journal of Oncology Nursing, 10*(6), 739-750.

edema, distension of veins of the neck and chest, headache, and seizures. A mediastinal mass is often visible on chest radiographs. The most common causes are Hodgkin's disease, non-Hodgkin's lymphoma, and lung cancer. Superior vena cava syndrome is considered a serious medical problem, and management usually involves radiation therapy to the site of obstruction and treatment of the primary tumour. Chemotherapeutic agents may be administered concurrently with the radiation therapy (Moore, 2005).

Spinal Cord Compression. *Spinal cord compression* is a neurological emergency caused by the presence of a malignant tumour in the epidural space of the spinal cord. The most common primary tumours that produce this problem are those of the breast, lung, prostate, GI system, and kidneys and melanoma (Held-Warmkessel, 2005). Lymphomas also pose a risk if diseased lymph tissue invades the epidural space. The manifestations are back pain that is intense, localized, and persistent, accompanied by vertebral tenderness and aggravated by the Valsalva manoeuvre; motor weakness and dysfunction; sensory paraesthesia and loss; and autonomic dysfunction. One of the clinical symptoms that reflect autonomic dysfunction is a change in bowel or bladder function. The nurse should carefully assess for potential signs or symptoms related to cord compression. Radiation therapy is used for the patient with slowly progressive neurological deficits and radiosensitive tumours. Surgery is usually recommended for the patient with rapidly progressive neurological signs, especially if the tumours are relatively radiologically resistant.

Third Space Syndrome. *Third space syndrome* involves a shifting of fluid from the vascular space to the interstitial space that is primarily secondary to extensive surgical procedures, biological therapy, or septic shock. Initially, affected patients exhibit signs of hypovolemia, including hypotension, tachycardia, low central venous pressure, and decreased urine output. Treatment includes fluid, electrolyte, and plasma protein replacement. During recovery, hypervolemia can occur, resulting in hypertension, elevated central venous pressure, weight gain, and shortness of breath. Treatment generally involves reduction in fluid administration and fluid balance monitoring.

Intestinal Obstruction. Chapter 45 contains a complete discussion of intestinal obstruction.

Metabolic Emergencies. Metabolic emergencies are caused by the production of ectopic hormones directly from the tumour or are secondary to cancer treatment. Ectopic hormones can arise in tumours because their cells are less differentiated than normal cells, enabling re-expression of genes that are suppressed in normal development. Metabolic emergencies include syndrome of inappropriate antidiuretic hormone (SIADH), hypercalcemia, tumour lysis syndrome (TLS), septic shock, and disseminated intravascular coagulation.

Syndrome of Inappropriate Antidiuretic Hormone. SIADH results from abnormal or sustained production of antidiuretic hormone (ADH; see Chapter 51). SIADH occurs most frequently with carcinoma of the lung but can also occur with cancers of the pancreas, duodenum, brain, esophagus, colon, ovary, prostate, bronchus, and nasopharynx and with leukemia, mesothelioma, reticulum cell sarcoma, Hodgkin's disease, thymoma, and lymphosarcoma. Cancer cells in these tumours are actually able to manufacture, store, and release ADH. The chemotherapeutic agents vincristine and cyclophosphamide (Procytox) also stimulate the release of ADH from the pituitary or tumour cells. Symptoms of SIADH include weight gain, weakness, anorexia, nausea, vomiting, personality changes, seizures, and coma. Treatment of SIADH includes fluid restriction and, in severe cases, intravenous administration of 3% sodium chloride solution.

Hypercalcemia. Hypercalcemia can occur in the presence of cancer that involves the bone, as in metastatic disease of the bone or multiple myeloma, or when a parathyroid hormone–like substance is secreted by cancer cells in the absence of bone metastasis (Shuey & Brant, 2004). Hypercalcemia resulting from malignancies that have metastasized occurs most frequently in patients with lung, breast, kidney, colon, ovarian, or thyroid cancer. Hypercalcemia resulting from secretion of parathyroid hormone–like substance occurs most frequently in patients with hypernephromas; squamous cell carcinoma of the lung; head and neck, cervical, and esophageal cancer; lymphomas; and leukemia. Immobility and dehydration can contribute to or exacerbate hypercalcemia.

The primary manifestations of hypercalcemia include apathy, depression, fatigue, muscle weakness, electrocardiographic changes, polyuria and nocturia, anorexia, nausea, and vomiting. Serum levels of calcium in excess of 3 mmol/L can be life-threatening. Chronic hypercalcemia can result in nephrocalcinosis and irreversible renal failure. The long-term treatment of hypercalcemia is aimed at the primary disease. Acute hypercalcemia is treated by hydration (3 L/day), diuretic administration (particularly loop diuretics), and a bisphosphonate, a drug that inhibits the action of osteoclasts. Infusion of a bisphosphonate is the treatment of choice.

Tumour Lysis Syndrome. Acute TLS is a metabolic complication that occurs in some patients with cancer and is frequently triggered by chemotherapy. It results from the rapid destruction of a large number of tumour cells, which can cause fatal biochemical changes. TLS is often associated with tumours that have high growth rates and are sensitive to the effects of chemotherapy. If not identified and treated quickly, TLS can result in acute renal failure.

The four hallmark signs of TLS are hyperuricemia, hyperphosphatemia, hyperkalemia, and hypocalcemia. TLS usually occurs within the first 24 to 48 hours after the initiation of chemotherapy and may persist for approximately 5 to 7 days. The primary goal of TLS management is preventing renal failure and severe electrolyte imbalances. The primary treatment includes increasing urine production through hydration therapy and decreasing uric acid concentrations through administration of allopurinol (Del Toro, Morris, & Cairo, 2005).

Septic Shock and Disseminated Intravascular Coagulation. Septic shock is discussed in Chapter 69, and disseminated intravascular coagulation is discussed in Chapter 33.

Infiltrative Emergencies. Infiltrative emergencies occur when malignant tumours infiltrate major organs secondary to cancer therapy. The most common infiltrative emergencies are cardiac tamponade and carotid artery rupture.

Cardiac Tamponade. Cardiac tamponade results from fluid accumulation in the pericardial sac, constriction of the pericardium by tumour, or pericarditis secondary to radiation therapy for the chest. Manifestations include a heavy feeling over the chest, shortness of breath, tachycardia, cough, dysphagia, hiccups, hoarseness, nausea, vomiting, excessive perspiration, decreased level of consciousness, pulsus paradoxus, distant or muted heart sounds, and extreme anxiety. Emergency management is aimed at reduction of fluid around the heart and includes surgical establishment of a pericardial window or an indwelling pericardial catheter. Supportive therapy includes administration of oxygen therapy, intravenous hydration, and vasopressor therapy.

Carotid Artery Rupture. Rupture of the carotid artery occurs most frequently in patients with cancer of the head and neck

secondary to invasion of the arterial wall by tumour or erosion after surgery or radiation therapy. Bleeding can manifest as minor oozing or, in the case of a bursting of the artery, spurting of blood. In the presence of bursting, pressure should be applied to the site with a finger. Intravenous fluid and blood products are administered in an attempt to stabilize the patient for surgery. Surgical management involves ligation of the carotid artery above and below the rupture site and reduction of local tumour.

Management of Cancer Pain

Moderate to severe pain occurs in approximately 50% of patients receiving active treatment for cancer and in 80% of those with advanced cancer. Despite progress made in cancer therapies, the incidence of cancer-related pain has not changed in decades. Undertreatment of cancer pain is common and has serious outcomes on patients' quality of life and ability to function, and it increases the burden on family caregivers (Ferrell & Virani, 2008).

Inadequate pain assessment is the greatest barrier to effective pain management (Miaskowski et al., 2005). Data such as vital signs and patient behaviours are not reliable indicators of pain, especially long-standing, chronic pain. Therefore, it is essential that every patient with cancer be assessed for pain by the question "Do you have pain?" If the patient's self-report is affirmative, further data are obtained and documented initially and at regular intervals regarding the onset, the location, and the intensity of the pain, what it feels like, and how it is relieved. Patterns of change also should be assessed. The patient's pain report must be accepted as the primary source of assessment data. Drug therapy includes nonsteroidal anti-inflammatory medications, opioids, and adjuvant pain medications. Analgesic medications should be administered on a regular schedule, around the clock, with additional doses as needed for breakthrough pain. Oral administration of the medication is preferred. It is important to remember that with opioid drugs, such as morphine, the appropriate dose is whatever is necessary to control the pain with the least intrusive adverse effects. Principles of patient-controlled analgesia should also be followed. Fear of addiction is not warranted but must be addressed as part of patient teaching relevant to pain control because for both the patient and the nurse, it represents a significant barrier to appropriate pain management.

Nonpharmacological interventions, including relaxation therapy and imagery, can be effectively used to manage pain (see Chapter 12). (Additional strategies to relieve pain are discussed in Chapter 10.) For more information on cancer pain management, refer to cancer agency clinical practice guidelines, such as those on the BC Cancer Agency Web site (see the Resources at the end of this chapter).

Psychosocial Care

Psychosocial care is an important aspect of cancer care. Supportive care includes services and strategies to help cancer patients and their families cope with the cancer experience. Because of the effectiveness of cancer treatment, cancer is cured in many patients, or the disease is controlled for long periods. In view of this trend in survival, an optimal quality of life must be maintained after the diagnosis of cancer. By understanding the effect of cancer on the person and the family and by promoting services that can provide financial, social, and psychological counselling, the nurse can be more effective in assisting patients and families throughout their cancer experience.

A diagnosis of cancer may precipitate a crisis in the lives of the patient and his or her family, and repercussions may affect all aspects of their lives. Common fears experienced by the patient with cancer include disfigurement, dependency, unrelieved pain, financial depletion, abandonment, and death.

To cope with these fears, the patient with cancer may use and experience different behavioural patterns: shock, anger, denial, bargaining, depression, helplessness, hopelessness, rationalization, acceptance, and intellectualization. These behavioural patterns may occur at any time during the process of cancer. However, some patterns appear to occur more frequently or at a greater intensity at certain specific stages of the disease process. The following factors may determine how a patient will cope with the diagnosis of cancer:

1. *Ability to cope with stressful events in the past* (e.g., loss of job, major disappointment): By simply asking how the patient has coped with stressful events, the nurse can gain an understanding of the patient's coping patterns, the effectiveness of the usual coping patterns, and the usual coping time framework.

2. *Availability of significant others:* Patients who have effective support systems tend to cope more effectively than do patients who do not have a meaningful, available support system.

3. *Ability to express feelings and concerns:* Patients who are able to express feelings and needs and who seek and ask for help appear to cope more effectively than do patients who internalize feelings and needs.

4. *Age at the time of diagnosis:* Age determines the coping strategies to a great degree. For example, a young mother with cancer may have concerns that differ from those of a 70-year-old woman with cancer.

5. *Extent of disease:* Cure or control of the disease process is usually easier to cope with than the reality of terminal illness.

6. *Disruption of body image:* Such disruption (e.g., by radical neck dissection, alopecia, mastectomy) may intensify the psychological effect of cancer.

7. *Presence of symptoms:* Symptoms such as fatigue, nausea, diarrhea, and pain may intensify the psychological effect of cancer.

8. *Past experience with cancer:* If past experiences with cancer have been negative, the patient will probably view his or her current status as negative.

9. *Attitude associated with the cancer:* A patient who feels in control and has a positive attitude about cancer and cancer treatment is better able to cope with the diagnosis and treatment of cancer than is a patient who feels hopeless, helpless, and out of control.

To facilitate the development of a hopeful attitude about cancer and to support the patient and the family during the various stages of the process of cancer, the nurse should act on the following suggestions:

1. Be available and continue to be available for discussion with the patient and family, especially during difficult times.

2. Actively assess the patient's needs for counselling and refer him or her to appropriate services when necessary.

3. Listen actively to fears and concerns.

4. Offer strategies to enhance coping behaviours.

5. Provide essential information as the patient asks for it, and be sensitive to information overload.

6. Establish a therapeutic relationship based on trust and confidence; be open, honest, and caring in the approach.

7. Be "present" with the patient to offer comfort and assurance that you care about him or her.

8. Understand and collaborate with the patient to set realistic, reachable short- and long-term goals.

9. Encourage the patient to maintain usual lifestyle patterns.

10. Maintain hope. Hope varies, depending on the status of the patient: hope that the symptoms are not serious, hope that the treatment is curative, hope for independence, hope for relief of pain, hope for a longer life, or hope for a peaceful death. Hope provides control over what is occurring and is the basis of a positive attitude toward cancer and cancer care.

11. Consider the spiritual aspects of care; support patients in exploring their belief systems and in finding meaning that transcends cultural and religious boundaries (Skalla & McCoy, 2006). Nurses can assist patients in identifying their strengths and developing skills to cope with the emotional aspects of having cancer.

12. Encourage and facilitate patients' participation in their care. This may include considering their interest in the use of integrative therapies such as support groups, mind–body

ETHICAL DILEMMAS
Medical Futility

Situation

A 65-year-old woman has breast cancer with metastasis to the liver and bone. The family asks the nurse why their mother is not receiving chemotherapy. In addition, they want to make certain that she will be resuscitated should her heart stop. They are aware of her diagnosis and that she may have less than 1 month to live. The nurse was told in morning rounds that the woman does not want any treatment that would prolong her life.

Important Points for Consideration

- If the patient is competent, the patient is legally and ethically the decision maker regarding his or her own care in consultation with the patient's family and the health care team as desired.
- Members of the health care team have no obligation to provide care that is medically futile. Care that is futile may be inappropriate, prolong dying, or provide little or no benefit to the patient.
- Palliative care is health care that would provide comfort, control pain, reduce symptoms, or improve the quality of her remaining life, as defined by the patient.
- Patients or families do not have a right to demand treatment that offers no clear benefit to the patient.
- The nurse should work in collaboration with other members of the health care team to have discussions with the family members, ease the acceptance of their mother's diagnosis, incorporate their mother's goals into the plan of care, discuss a do-not-resuscitate (DNR) order and a referral to hospice, and plan for her eventual death.

Clinical Decision-Making Questions

1. How can the nurse help the patient communicate her wishes to her family?
2. How can the nurse and the health care team help the family plan end-of-life care that incorporates the wishes of their mother?

modalities, nutritional supplements, and herbal therapies. The "unofficial" use of complementary and alternative medicines in oncology is widespread and has the potential to help (e.g., by relieving symptoms) or to harm (e.g., through associated toxic effects or by preventing or diminishing the effects of proven therapies). Patients may need support in understanding the difference between complementary and alternative therapies and the risks and benefits associated with complementary and alternative medicine (Deng et al., 2009).

Organizations and journals available as resources for the nurse are listed in the Resources section at the end of this chapter The Ethical Dilemmas box considers nurse-family interactions when treatment is considered medically futile.

AGE-RELATED CONSIDERATIONS: CANCER

Cancer is usually a disease of aging. Most cancers occur in people older than 65 years. Cancer is the leading cause of death in people 65 to 74 years of age. Clinical manifestations of cancer in an older adult may be mistakenly attributed to age-related changes and ignored by the person (Coleman, Hutchins, & Goodwin, 2005).

Older adults are particularly vulnerable to the complications of both cancer and cancer therapy. This is because of their decline in physiological functioning, social and emotional resources, and cognitive function. The functional status of an older adult should be taken into consideration when a treatment plan is selected (Extermann & Hurria, 2007). Age alone is not a good predictor of tolerance or response to treatment.

Because of advances in the treatment of cancer, cancer therapies benefit an increasing number of older adults, including patients with suboptimal health. Some important questions to consider when cancer is diagnosed in an older person include the following: Will the treatment provide more benefit than harm? Will the patient be able to tolerate the treatment safely? What is the patient's choice of therapy?

REVIEW QUESTIONS

The number of the question corresponds to the same-numbered objective at the beginning of the chapter.

1. Which of the following is consistent with recent trends in the incidence and death rates of cancer?
   a. Lung cancer is the most common type of cancer in men.
   b. Breast cancer is the leading cause of cancer deaths in women.
   c. A higher percentage of women than men have lung cancer.
   d. The incidence of cancer increases as the population ages.

2. Which feature is characteristic of cancer?
   a. An increasing differentiation of cells
   b. The production of toxins that alter cells
   c. The rapid, explosive proliferation of cells
   d. Cell growth that escapes normal control

3. Which is a characteristic feature of the stage of progression in the development of cancer?
   a. Oncogenic viral transformation of target cells
   b. A reversible steady growth facilitated by carcinogens
   c. A period of latency before clinical detection of cancer
   d. The proliferation of cancer cells in spite of host control mechanisms

4. What is the primary protective role of the immune system in relation to malignant cells?
   a. Surveillance for cells with tumour-associated antigens
   b. The binding with free antigen released by malignant cells
   c. The production of blocking factors that immobilize cancer cells
   d. The response to a new set of antigenic determinants on cancer cells

5. What is the primary difference between benign and malignant neoplasms?
   a. The rate of cell proliferation
   b. The site of malignant tumour
   c. The requirements for cellular nutrients
   d. The characteristic of tissue invasiveness

6. Which nursing roles are important for the prevention and detection of cancer?
   a. Health promotion in relation to eating low-fibre, refined-carbohydrate diets
   b. Teaching about cancer risk factors
   c. Encouraging the public to participate in regular screening tests for all detectable cancer sites
   d. Using people's natural fear of cancer to motivate changes in unhealthy lifestyles

7. Which principle underpins a therapeutic approach to cancer?
   a. Surgery is the single most effective treatment for cancer.
   b. Initial treatment is always directed toward cure of the cancer.
   c. A combination of treatment modalities is effective for controlling many cancers.
   d. None of the above.

8. Which points would be part of nursing teaching for a patient undergoing brachytherapy of the cervix?
   a. The patient will learn that she must undergo simulation to locate the treatment area.
   b. The patient will be taught about the treatment and need for staff time limitations in relation to her care.
   c. The patient will be taught that she may experience desquamation of the skin on the abdomen and upper legs.
   d. The patient will require shielding of the ovaries during treatment to prevent ovarian damage.

9. Which is the most effective method of administering a chemotherapeutic agent that is a vesicant?
   a. Give it orally.
   b. Give it intra-arterially.
   c. Use an Ommaya reservoir.
   d. Use a central venous access device.

10. Why does stomatitis, a common adverse effect of chemotherapeutic agents, occur?
    a. The site of the malignancy is near the oral cavity.
    b. The general health of the patient with cancer is poor.
    c. Chemotherapeutic drugs have a local and irritating effect on epithelial cells.
    d. Rapidly dividing cells of the mucous membranes of the mouth are being destroyed.

11. In teaching the patient about IL-2, which information will the nurse include?
    a. It stimulates the immune system.
    b. It inhibits DNA and protein synthesis in tumour cells.
    c. It decreases the antigenic expression of antigens on tumour cell surfaces.
    d. It prevents bone marrow suppression associated with chemotherapy.

12. Which information will the nurse provide to a patient receiving radiation therapy or chemotherapy?
    a. Effective birth control methods should be used for the rest of the patient's life.
    b. Notify the health care team if nausea and vomiting are experienced during treatment so that these can be managed.
    c. After successful treatment, a return to the person's previous functional level occurs.
    d. The cycle of fatigue-depression-fatigue that may occur during treatment can be reduced by restricting activity.

13. Which is an inappropriate nursing intervention to promote nutrition in the patient with cancer?
    a. Providing bland, pureed food because the person's taste sensation is altered
    b. Providing increased protein for normal cell recovery and immune system function
    c. Encouraging the patient to eat a high-calorie, high-protein snack every few hours to prevent weight loss
    d. Alerting the physician that nutritional supplements may be needed when the patient has a 4-kg weight loss

14. What is the primary cause of syndrome of SIADH in cancer?
    a. Autoimmune reaction
    b. Gram-negative septicemia
    c. Invasiveness of cancer cells
    d. Ectopic hormonal production

15. A patient has recently received a diagnosis of early-stage breast cancer. Which of the following is most appropriate for the nurse to focus on?
    a. Maintaining the patient's hope
    b. Preparing a will and advance directives
    c. Discussing replacement child care for patient's children
    d. Discussing the patient's past experiences with her grandmother's cancer

ANSWERS: 1. d; 2. d; 3. d; 4. a; 5. d; 6. b; 7. c; 8. b; 9. d; 10. d; 11. a; 12. b; 13. a; 14. d; 15. a

REFERENCES

Abeloff, M. D., Armitage, J. D., Niederhuber, J. E., Kastan, M. B., & McKenna, W. G. (2008). *Abeloff's clinical oncology* (4th ed.). New York: Churchill Livingstone.

Aiello-Laws, L. & Rutledge, D. N. (2008). Management of adult patients receiving intraventricular chemotherapy for the treatment of leptomeningeal metastases. *Clinical Journal of Oncology Nursing, 12*(3), 429-435. doi:10.1188/08.CJON.429-435

Behrend, S. W. (2011). Radiation treatment planning. In C. H. Yarbro, D. Wujcik, & B. H. Gobel (Eds.), *Cancer nursing: Principles and practice* (7th ed.). Sudbury, MA: Jones & Bartlett.

Canadian Association of Nurses in Oncology. (2006). *Standards of care, roles, and competencies*. Ottawa: Author.

Canadian Cancer Society. (2005). Progress in cancer prevention: Modifiable risk factors. In *Canadian cancer statistics 2005*. Toronto: Canadian Cancer Society.

Canadian Cancer Society's Steering Committee on Cancer Statistics. (2011). *Canadian Cancer Statistics 2011*. Toronto, ON: Canadian Cancer Society.

Coleman, E., Hutchins, L., & Goodwin, J. (2005). An overview of cancer in the older adult. *Medsurg Nursing, 13*(75), 2.

Del Toro, G., Morris, E., & Cairo, M. S. (2005). Tumor lysis syndrome: Pathophysiology, definition, and alternative treatment approaches. *Clinical Advances in Hematology & Oncology, 3*(1), 54.

Deng, G. E., Prenkel, M., Cohen, L., Cassilth, B. R., Abrams, D. I., Capodice, J. L., …, Sagar, S. (2009). Evidence-based clinical practice guidelines for integrative oncology: Complementary therapies and botanicals. *Journal of the Society for Integrative Oncology, 7*(3), 85-120. doi:10.2310/7200.2009.0019

DeVita, V. T., Lawrence, T. S., & Rosenberg, S. A. (Eds.). (2011). *DeVita, Hellman, and Rosenberg's cancer: Principles and practice of oncology*, 9th ed., Philadelphia: Lippincott, Williams & Wilkins.

D'Haese, S., Bate, T., Claes, S., Boone, A., Vanvoorden, V., & Efficace, F. (2005). Management of skin reactions during radiotherapy: A study of nursing practice. *European Journal of Cancer Care, 14*, 28. doi:10.1016/j.ejon.2009.10.006

Ewart-Toland, A., & Balmain, A. (2004). The genetics of cancer susceptibility: From mouse to man. *Toxicologic Pathology, 32*(Suppl. 1), 26. doi:10.1080/01926230490424716

Extermann, M., & Hurria, A. (2007). Comprehensive geriatric assessment for older patients with cancer. *Journal of Clinical Oncology, 25* (14), 1824-1831. doi:10.1200/JCO.2007.10.6559

Ferrell, B. R., & Virani, R. (2008). National guidelines for palliative care: A roadmap for oncology nurses. *Oncology, 22*(2, Suppl.; Nurse Ed.), 28-34.

Fillion, L., Gagnon, P., LeBlond, F., Gélinas, C., Savard, J., Dupuis, R., …, Larochelle, M. (2008). A brief intervention for fatigue management in breast cancer survivors. *Cancer Nursing, 31*(2), 145-159.

Health Canada. (2011). Eating well with Canada's Food Guide. Retrieved from *http://www.hc-sc.gc.ca/fn-an/food-guide-aliment/order-commander/index-eng.php#a1*

Held-Warmkessel, J. (2005). Managing critical cancer. *Nursing, 35*, 58.

Herrstedt, J. (2008). Antiemetics: An update and the MASCC guidelines applied in clinical practice. *Nature Clinical Practice Oncology, 5*(1), 32-43. doi:10.1038/ncponc1021

Kaplan, H. (1979). Historic milestones in radiobiology and radiation therapy. *Seminars in Oncology, 4*, 479.

Katz, A. (2007). *Breaking the silence on cancer and sexuality: A handbook for healthcare providers*. Pittsburgh: Oncology Nursing Society.

Keefe, D. M., Schubert, M. M., Elting, L. S., Sonis, S. T., Epstein, J. B., Raber-Durlacher, J. E., …, Peterson, D. E. (2007). Updated clinical practice guidelines for the prevention and treatment of mucositis. *Cancer, 109*(5), 820-831. doi:10.1002/cncr.22484

Kobayashi, A., Miaskowski, C., Wallhagen, M., & Smith-McCune, K. (2000). Recent developments in understanding the immune response to human papilloma virus infection and cervical neoplasia. *Oncology Nursing Forum, 27,* 643.

Langhorne, M. E., Fulton, J., & Otto, S. E. (2007). *Oncology nursing: Clinical reference.* St. Louis: Mosby.

Loud, J. T., & Hutson, S. P. (2011). Genetic risk and hereditary cancer syndromes. In C. H. Yarbro, D. Wujcik, & B. H. Gobel (Eds.), *Cancer nursing: Principles and practice* (7th ed.). Sudbury, MA: Jones & Bartlett.

McAdams, F. W., & Burgunder, M. R. (2004). Transplant course. In S. Ezzone (Ed.), *Hematopoietic stem cell transplantation: A manual for nursing practice.* Pittsburgh: Oncology Nursing Society.

McDiarmid, S. (2002). Nutritional support of the patient receiving high-dose therapy with hematopoietic stem cell support. *Canadian Oncology Nursing Journal, 12*(2), 102-115.

McGuire, D. B., Correa, M. E., Johnson, J., & Wienandts, P. (2006). The role of basic oral care and good clinical practice principles in the management of oral mucositis. *Supportive Care in Cancer, 14*(6), 541-547. doi:10.1007/s00520-006-0051-8

Miaskowski, C., Clearly, J., Burney, R., Coyne, P., Finley, R., Foster, R., …, Zahrbock, C. (2005). *Guideline for the management of cancer pain in adults and children (APS Clinical Practice Guidelines Series, No 3).* Glenview, IL: American Pain Society.

Moore, S. (2005). Superior vena cava syndrome. In C. H. Yarbro, M. H. Frogge, & M. Goodman (Eds.), *Cancer nursing: Principles and practice* (6th ed.). Sudbury, MA: Jones & Bartlett.

Otto, S. (2004). *Oncology nursing: clinical reference.* St. Louis: Mosby.

Passik, S. D., & Kirsh, K. L. (2005). A pilot examination of the impact of cancer patients' fatigue on their spousal caregivers. *Palliative & Supportive Care, 3*(4), 273-279. doi:10.1017/S1478951505050431

Prosnitz, R. G., Yao, B., Farrell, C. L., & Brizel, D. M. (2005). Pretreatment anemia is correlated with the reduced effectiveness of radiation and concurrent chemotherapy in advanced head and neck cancer. *International Journal of Radiation Oncology Biology Physics, 61*(4), 1087-95. doi.org/10.1016/j.ijrobp.2004.07.710

Prue, G., Rankin, J., Allen, J., Gracey, J., & Cramp, F. (2006). Cancer-related fatigue: A critical appraisal. *European Journal of Cancer, 42,* 846-63. doi:10.1016/j.ejca.2005.11.026

Shuey, K. M., & Brant, J. M. (2004). Hypercalcemia of malignancy: Part II. *Clinical Journal of Oncology Nursing, 8*(3), 321-323. doi:10.1188/04.CJON.321-323

Skalla, K. A., & McCoy, J. P. (2006). Spiritual assessment of patients with cancer: The moral authority, vocational, aesthetic, social, and transcendent model. *Oncology Nursing Forum, 33*(4), 745-751. doi:10.1188/06.ONF.745-751

Statistics Canada. (2011). Leading Causes of Death in Canada, 2008. Cat no. 84-215-X. Retrieved from *http://www.statcan.gc.ca/pub/84-215-x/2011001/hl-fs-eng.htm*

Stilos, K., Doyle, C., & Daines, P. (2008). Addressing the sexual health needs in patients with gynecological cancers. *Clinical Journal of Oncology Nursing, 12*(3), 457-463. doi:10.1188/08.CJON.457-463

Tannock, I. F., Hill, R. P., Bristow, R. G., & Harrington, L. (Eds.). (2005). *The basic science of oncology* (4th ed.). New York: McGraw-Hill.

Viele, C. (2005). Keys to unlock cancer: Targeted therapy. *Oncology Nursing Forum, 32*(5), 935-940. doi:10.1188/05.ONF.935-940

CANADIAN RESOURCES

BC Cancer Agency
Cancer Management Guidelines
  http://www.bccancer.bc.ca/HPI/CancerManagementGuidelines/default.htm
Pain & Symptom Management
  http://www.bccancer.bc.ca/HPI/CancerManagementGuidelines/SupportiveCare/PainSymptomManagement
Canadian Association of Nurses in Oncology (CANO)
  http://www.cano-acio.ca

Canadian Association of Provincial Cancer Agencies (CAPCA)
  http://www.capca.ca
Canadian Association of Psychosocial Oncology (CAPO)
  http://www.capo.ca
Canadian Breast Cancer Research Alliance (CBCRA)
  http://www.breast.cancer.ca
Canadian Cancer Society
  http://www.cancer.ca
Our Cancer Information Service
  http://www.cancer.ca/canada-wide/support%20services/cancer%20information%20service.aspx
Canadian Hospice Palliative Care Association
  http://www.chpca.net
Canadian Institute of Health Information (CIHI)
Canadian Oncology Nursing Journal (CONJ)
  http://cano.malachite-mgmt.com/?page=CONJOnline
Cancer Care Ontario
Program in Evidence-Based Care: Practice Guidelines
  https://www.cancercare.on.ca/cms/One.aspx?portalId=1377&pageId=10144
Cancer News on the Net
  http://www.cancernews.com
Cancer Research Society
  http://www.cancer-research-society.ca
Canadian Strategy for Cancer Control: A Cancer Plan for Canada
  http://www.partnershipagainstcancer.ca/wp-content/uploads/CSCC_CancerPlan_20061.pdf
Cancer Symptoms
  http://www.cancersymptoms.org
Colorectal Cancer Association of Canada
  http://www.colorectal-cancer.ca/
Evidence-informed Treatment Guidelines in British Columbia
  http://www.bccancer.bc.ca
Evidence-informed Treatment Guidelines in Ontario
  https://www.cancercare.on.ca
Institute for Clinical Evaluative Studies (ICES)
  http://www.ices.on.ca
National Cancer Institute, Canada
  http://oicr.on.ca/institution/national-cancer-institute-canada
Psychosocial Oncology Research Training (PORT)
  http://www.port.mcgill.ca
Prostate Cancer Canada Network (CPCN)
  http://prostatecancer.ca/

RELATED RESOURCES

American Association for Cancer Education (AACE)
  http://www.aaceonline.com
International Society of Nurses in Cancer Care
  http://www.isncc.org
National Coalition for Cancer Survivorship (NCS)
  http://www.canceradvocacy.org
National Institute for Occupational Safety and Health (NIOSH)
Preventing Occupational Exposures to Antineoplastic and Other Hazardous Drugs in Health Care Settings
  http://www.cdc.gov/niosh/docs/2004-165/pdfs/2004-165.pdf
OncoLink (cancer information site)
  http://www.oncolink.upenn.edu
Oncology Nursing Society
(Including guidelines for the safe handling of chemotherapeutic agents)
  http://www.ons.org
Union for International Cancer Control
  http://www.uicc.ch

evolve *For additional Internet resources, see the Web site for this book at* **http://evolve.elsevier.com/Canada/Lewis/medsurg**

Fluid, Electrolyte, and Acid–Base Imbalances

Written by Audrey J. Bopp
Adapted by Otto Sanchez

LEARNING OBJECTIVES

1. Describe the composition of the major body fluid compartments.
2. Define the following processes involved in the regulation of the movement of water and electrolytes between the body fluid compartments: diffusion, osmosis, filtration, hydrostatic pressure, oncotic pressure, and osmotic pressure.
3. Describe the etiology, laboratory diagnostic findings, clinical manifestations, and nursing and collaborative management of the following disorders:
   a. Water excess and deficit
   b. Sodium and volume imbalances: hypernatremia and hyponatremia
   c. Potassium imbalance: hyperkalemia and hypokalemia
   d. Magnesium imbalance: hypermagnesemia and hypomagnesemia
   e. Calcium imbalance: hypercalcemia and hypocalcemia
   f. Phosphate imbalance: hyperphosphatemia and hypophosphatemia
4. Identify the processes of acid–base regulation.
5. Discuss the etiology, laboratory diagnostic findings, clinical manifestations, and nursing and collaborative management of the following acid–base imbalances: metabolic acidosis, metabolic alkalosis, respiratory acidosis, and respiratory alkalosis.
6. Describe the composition and indications for use of common intravenous fluid solutions.
7. Discuss types and nursing management of commonly used central venous access devices.

KEY TERMS

acidosis An abnormal increase in blood acidity; a pH less than 7.35, p. 405

active transport A process requiring energy in which molecules move through a membrane against the concentration gradient, p. 388

alkalosis An abnormal decrease in blood acidity; a pH greater than 7.45, p. 405

anions Negatively charged ions, p. 386

buffers A solution or system that maintains a stable pH, p. 405

cations Positively charged ions, p. 386

diffusion The movement of molecules from an area of high concentration to one of low concentration, p. 387

electrolytes Substances whose molecules dissociate or split into ions when placed in solution, p. 386

facilitated diffusion The movement of molecules from an area of high concentration to one of low concentration, assisted by a membrane carrier molecule, p. 387

fluid spacing A term describing the distribution of body water in different body compartments, p. 390

homeostasis The state of equilibrium in the internal environment of the body, naturally maintained by adaptive responses, p. 385

hydrostatic pressure The force within a fluid compartment, exerted by water pressure, p. 389

hypertonic Solutions in which solutes are more concentrated than they are in the intracellular compartment, p. 389

hypotonic Solutions in which solutes are less concentrated than they are in the intracellular compartment, p. 389

ions Electrically charged particles, p. 386

isotonic Solutions in which the concentration of solutes equals that of the intracellular compartment, p. 389

oncotic pressure Osmotic pressure exerted by colloids in solution, p. 389

osmolality A measure of the total solute concentration per kilogram of solvent, p. 388

osmolarity A measure of the total solute concentration per litre of solution, p. 388

osmosis The movement of water between two compartments separated by a membrane permeable to water but not to a solute, p. 388

osmotic pressure The amount of pressure required to stop the osmotic flow of water, p. 388

pH The negative logarithm of hydrogen ion concentration, p. 404

tetany Increased nerve excitability and sustained muscle contraction, p. 402

valence The electrical charge of an ion, p. 386

ELECTRONIC RESOURCES

Supplemental content related to Chapter 19 can be found …

Evolve Web Site ⊖volve

http://evolve.elsevier.com/Canada/Lewis/medsurg
- Answer Guideline for Case Study on p. 416
- Clinical Reference: Laboratory Values
- Content Updates

- Electronic Calculators
- Examination Review Questions
- Fluid and Electrolyte Tutorial
- Glossary
- Interactive Case Study: Hyponatremia/Fluid Volume Imbalance
- Key Points (Printable and MP3 Download)

Homeostasis

Body fluids and electrolytes play an important role in homeostasis. **Homeostasis** is the state of equilibrium in the internal environment of the body, naturally maintained by adaptive responses that promote healthy survival (Mosby, 2009). Maintenance of the composition and volume of body fluids within narrow normal limits is necessary to maintain homeostasis (McCance & Huether, 2010). During normal metabolism, the body produces many acids. These acids alter the internal environment of the body, including fluid and electrolyte balances, and must also be regulated to maintain homeostasis. Many diseases and their treatments have the ability to affect fluid and electrolyte balance. For example, a patient with metastatic breast cancer may develop hypercalcemia. Chemotherapy prescribed to treat the cancer may result in nausea and vomiting and, subsequently, dehydration and acid–base imbalances. Correction of the dehydration with intravenous (IV) fluids must be monitored closely to prevent fluid overload.

It is important for the nurse to anticipate the potential for alterations in fluid and electrolyte balance associated with certain disorders and medical therapies, to recognize the signs and symptoms of imbalances, and to intervene with the appropriate action. This chapter describes the normal control of fluids, electrolytes, and acid–base balance; etiologies that disrupt homeostasis and resultant manifestations; and actions that the health care provider can take to prevent or restore fluid, electrolyte, and acid–base balance.

Water Content of the Body

Water is the primary component of the body, accounting for approximately 60% of adult body weight. Water is the solvent in which body salts, nutrients, and wastes are dissolved and transported. Water content varies with sex, body mass, and age (Figure 19-1). In men, the percentage of body weight that is composed of water is generally greater than in women because men tend to

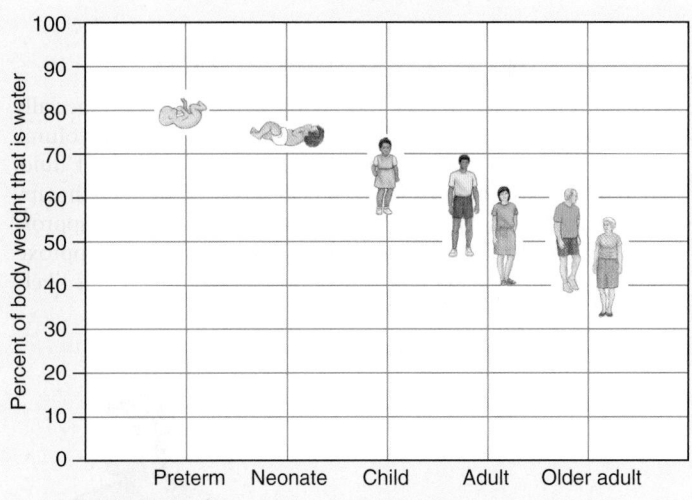

Figure 19-1 Changes in body water content with age.

Source: Copstead-Kirkhorn, L. C., & Banasik, J. L. (2010). *Pathophysiology* (4th ed., p. 594, Figure 24-2). St. Louis: Mosby.

have more lean body mass. Fat cells contain less water than an equivalent volume of lean tissue (Kee, Paulanka, & Polek, 2009). In older adults, body water content averages 45 to 55% of body weight. In infants, water content is 70 to 80% of the body weight. Thus, infants and the elderly are at a higher risk for fluid-related problems.

Body Fluid Compartments

The two major fluid compartments in the body are intracellular and extracellular (Figure 19-2). Approximately two thirds of body water is located within cells and is termed *intracellular fluid* (ICF); the ICF constitutes approximately 42% of body weight. The body of a 70-kg man would contain approximately 42 L of water, of which 30 L would be intracellular. *Extracellular fluid* (ECF) consists of fluid spaces between cells (interstitial fluid and lymph) and the plasma space. The ECF consists of one third of the body water, or about 17% of the total weight; this would amount to about 11 L in a 70-kg man. About one third of the ECF is in the plasma space (3 L in a 70-kg man), and two thirds is in the interstitial space (8 L in a 70-kg man).

A third, small, but important fluid compartment is the *transcellular space*, accounting for approximately 1 L. It includes fluid in the cerebrospinal space, the gastrointestinal (GI) tract, and the pleural, synovial, and peritoneal spaces. If the transcellular fluid is not resorbed, its loss (e.g., by vomiting) can produce serious fluid and electrolyte imbalances. A "third space" syndrome can develop when an increase in transcellular fluid occurs at the expense of fluid in other compartments, for instance, after intestinal paralysis or in postcirrhotic ascites, hydrocephaly, or pleural and pericardial effusions.

Functions of Body Water

Body fluids are in constant motion transporting nutrients, electrolytes, and oxygen to cells and carrying waste products away from cells. Water is necessary in the regulation of body temperature. In addition, it lubricates joints and membranes and is a medium for food digestion (Kee et al., 2009).

Calculation of Fluid Gain or Loss

One litre of water weighs 1 kg. Body weight change, especially sudden change, is an excellent indicator of overall fluid volume loss or gain. For example, if a patient drinks 240 mL of fluid, weight gain will be 0.24 kg. A patient receiving diuretic therapy who loses 2 kg in 24 hours has experienced a fluid loss of approximately 2 L. An adult patient who is fasting might lose approximately 0.5 to 1 kg per day. A weight loss exceeding this is likely caused by loss of body fluid.

Electrolytes

Electrolytes are substances whose molecules dissociate or split into ions when placed in solution. **Ions** are electrically charged particles. **Cations** are positively charged ions. Examples include sodium (Na^+), potassium (K^+), calcium (Ca^{2+}), and magnesium (Mg^{2+}) ions. **Anions** are negatively charged ions. Examples include bicarbonate (HCO_3^-), chloride (Cl^-), and phosphate (PO_4^{3-}) ions. Most proteins bear a negative charge and are thus anions. The electrical charge of an ion is termed its **valence.** Cations and anions combine according to their valences. (Terminology related to body fluid chemistry is presented in Table 19-1.)

Table 19-1 Terminology Related to Body Fluid Chemistry	
Anion	Ion that carries a negative charge
Cation	Ion that carries a positive charge
Electrolyte	Substance that dissociates in solution into ions (charged particles); a molecule of sodium chloride (NaCl) in solution becomes Na^+ and Cl^-
Nonelectrolyte	Substance that does not dissociate into ions in solution; examples include glucose and urea
Osmolality	A measure of the total solute concentration per kilogram of solvent
Osmolarity	A measure of the total solute concentration per litre of solution
Solute	Substance that is dissolved in a solvent
Solution	Homogeneous mixture of solutes dissolved in a solvent
Solvent	Substance that is capable of dissolving a solute (liquid or gas)
Valence	The degree of combining power of an ion

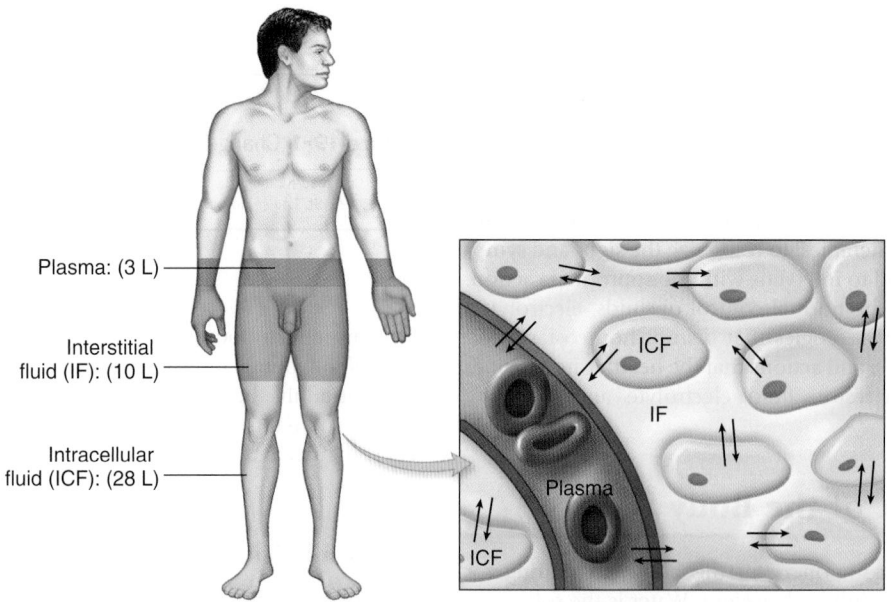

Figure 19-2 Relative volumes of three body fluids. Values represent fluid distribution in a young male adult. *ICF,* intercellular fluid; *IF,* interstitial fluid.

Source: Thibodeau, G. A., & Patton, K. T. (2010). *The human body in health and disease* (5th ed., p. 570, Figure 20-1). St. Louis: Mosby.

Measurement of Electrolytes

The measurement of electrolytes is important to the nurse in evaluating electrolyte balance as well as in determining the composition of electrolyte preparations. The concentration of electrolytes can be expressed in milligrams per decilitre (mg/dL), millimoles per litre (mmol/L), or milliequivalents per litre (mEq/L). The international standard for measuring electrolytes is mmol/L. One mole (mol) of a substance is the molecular (or atomic) weight of that substance expressed in grams; hence, a millimole (mmol) of a substance is the atomic weight in milligrams. Sodium's atomic weight is 23 mg; therefore, 23 mg of sodium is 1 mmol of sodium. Sodium and chloride are monovalent elements that carry one electron and will match one to one: 1 mmol of sodium combines with 1 mmol of chloride.

An element with two electrons, such as calcium, will require two monovalent partners. To avoid keeping track of how to match millimoles, the milliequivalent is the favoured unit of measure for electrolytes. The following formula is used to convert millimoles to milliequivalents:

$$mEq = mmol/L \times valence$$

Electrolytes in body fluids are active chemicals that unite in varying combinations. Thus, it is more practical to express their concentration as a measure of chemical activity (or milliequivalents) rather than as a measure of weight. Ions combine milliequivalent for milliequivalent: they match 1 to 1. For example, 1 mEq (1 mmol) of sodium combines with 1 mEq (1 mmol) of chloride, and 1 mEq (0.5 mmol) of calcium combines with 1 mEq (1 mmol) of chloride. This combining power of electrolytes is important to maintaining the balance of positively charged (cation) and negatively charged (anion) ions within body fluids.

Electrolyte Composition of Fluid Compartments

Electrolyte composition varies between the ECF and the ICF. The overall concentration of the electrolytes is approximately the same in the two compartments. However, concentrations of specific ions differ greatly (Figure 19-3). In the ICF, the most prevalent cation is potassium, with small amounts of magnesium and sodium. The prevalent anion is phosphate, with some protein and a small amount of bicarbonate. In the ECF, the main cation is sodium, with small amounts of potassium, calcium, and magnesium. The primary ECF anion is chloride, with small amounts of bicarbonate, sulphate, and phosphate anions. The plasma has substantial amounts of protein. However, the amount of protein in the plasma is less than in the ICF. There is a small amount of protein in the interstitium.

Mechanisms Controlling Fluid and Electrolyte Movement

Different processes are involved in the movement of electrolytes and water between the ICF and the ECF. Electrolytes move according to their concentration and electrical gradients toward the areas of lower concentration and toward areas with the opposite charge. Some of the processes include simple diffusion, facilitated diffusion, and active transport. Water movement is driven by two forces: hydrostatic pressure and osmotic pressure.

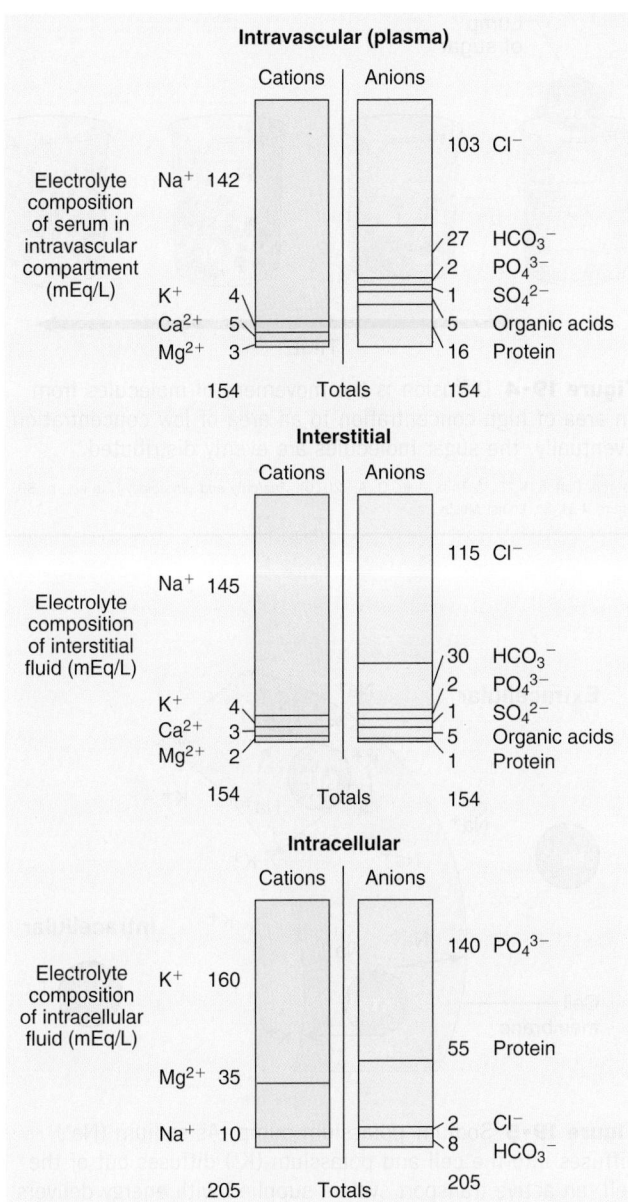

Figure 19-3 Electrolyte content of fluid compartments.

Diffusion

Diffusion is the movement of molecules from an area of high concentration to one of low concentration (Figure 19-4) in liquids, gases, and solids. Net movement of molecules stops when the concentrations are equal in both areas. The membrane separating the two areas must be permeable to the diffusing substance for the process to occur. Simple diffusion requires no external energy. Gases (e.g., oxygen, nitrogen, carbon dioxide) and substances (e.g., urea) can permeate cell membranes and are distributed throughout the body.

Facilitated Diffusion

Because of the composition of cellular membranes, some molecules diffuse slowly into the cell. However, when they are combined with a specific carrier molecule, the rate of diffusion accelerates. Like simple diffusion, **facilitated diffusion** moves

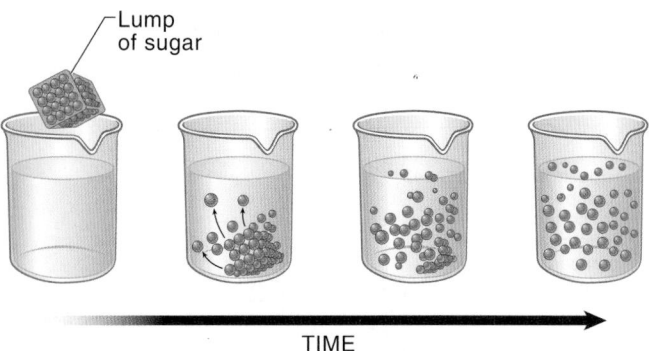

Figure 19-4 Diffusion is the movement of molecules from an area of high concentration to an area of low concentration. Eventually, the sugar molecules are evenly distributed.

Source: Patton, K. T., & Thibodeau, G. A. (2010). *Anatomy and physiology* (7th ed., p. 89, Figure 4-1). St. Louis: Mosby.

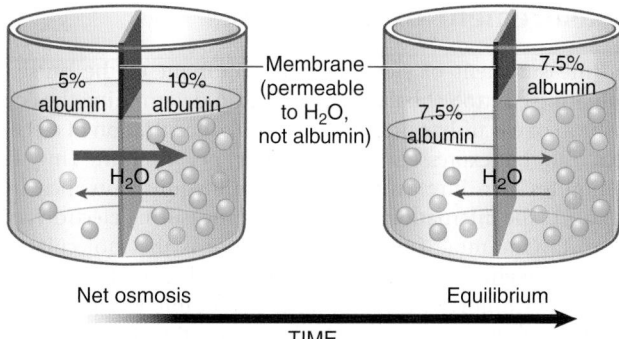

Figure 19-6 Osmosis is the process of water movement through a semipermeable membrane from an area of low solute concentration to an area of high solute concentration.

Source: Patton, K. T., & Thibodeau, G. A. (2010). *Anatomy and physiology* (7th ed., p. 92, Figure 4-3). St. Louis: Mosby.

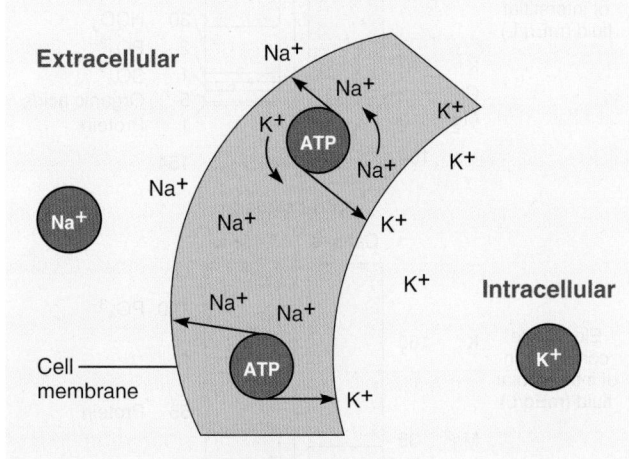

Figure 19-5 Sodium–potassium pump. As sodium (Na⁺) diffuses into the cell and potassium (K⁺) diffuses out of the cell, an active transport system supplied with energy delivers Na⁺ back to the extracellular compartment and K⁺ to the intracellular compartment. *ATP*, adenosine triphosphate.

molecules from an area of high concentration to one of low concentration, is passive, and requires no energy other than that of the concentration gradient. Unlike simple diffusion, there must be a membrane carrier molecule to facilitate the rate of diffusion. Glucose transport into cells is a clinically important example as it occurs through GLUT4, a transport protein activated by binding of insulin to its receptor.

Active Transport

Active transport is a process requiring energy in which molecules move against the concentration gradient. The concentrations of sodium and potassium differ greatly intracellularly and extracellularly (see Figure 19-3). By active transport, sodium moves out of the cell and potassium moves into the cell to maintain this concentration difference (Figure 19-5). The energy source for the sodium–potassium pump is adenosine triphosphate (ATP), which is produced in the mitochondria.

Osmosis

Osmosis is the movement of water between two compartments separated by a membrane permeable to water but not to a solute. Water moves through the membrane from an area of low solute concentration to an area of high solute concentration (Figure 19-6); that is, water moves from the more dilute compartment (has more water) to the side that is more concentrated (has less water). The semipermeable membrane prevents movement of solute particles. Osmosis requires no outside energy sources and stops when the concentration differences disappear or when hydrostatic pressure builds and is sufficient to oppose any further movement of water. Diffusion and osmosis are important in maintaining the fluid volume of body cells and the concentration of the solute.

Osmotic pressure is the amount of pressure required to stop the osmotic flow of water. Osmotic pressure can be understood by imagining a chamber in which two compartments are separated by a semipermeable membrane (see Figure 19-6). Water will move to the more concentrated side of the vessel until the pressure generated by the height of the higher column of water will oppose further movement.

Osmotic pressure is determined by the concentration of solutes in solution. It is measured in milliosmoles and may be expressed as either fluid osmolarity or fluid osmolality. **Osmolality** measures the osmotic force of solute per unit of weight of solvent (mOsm/kg or mmol/kg). **Osmolarity** measures the total milliosmoles of solute per unit of total volume of solution (mOsm/L). Although osmolality and osmolarity are often used interchangeably, osmolality is properly used to describe fluids inside the body, and osmolarity pertains to fluids outside the body (Porth, 2010). Osmolality is the criterion typically tested to evaluate the concentration of plasma and urine.

Measurement of Osmolality. Osmolality is approximately the same in the various body fluid spaces. Determining osmolality is important because it indicates the water balance of the body. To assess the state of the body water balance, one can measure or estimate plasma osmolality. Normal plasma osmolality is between 285 and 295 mmol/kg. A value greater than 295 mOsm/kg indicates that the concentration of particles is too great or that the water content is too little. This condition is termed *water deficit*. A value less than 285 mmol/kg indicates too little solute for the amount of water or too much water for the amount of solute. This condition is termed *water excess*. Both conditions are clinically significant.

Plasma and urine osmolality can be measured in most clinical laboratories. Because the major determinants of the plasma osmolality are sodium, glucose, and urea, one can calculate the effective plasma osmolality based on the concentrations of those compounds by using the following equation:

$$\text{Effective osmolality} = 2 \times (Na^-)p + (\text{glucose})/18$$

where $(Na^-)p$ and (glucose) are the plasma concentrations of sodium and glucose in mEq/L and mg/dL, respectively. The sodium concentration is multiplied by 2 to account for the presence of an equivalent number of anions. Glucose concentration is divided by one tenth of its molecular weight to calculate the number of osmotically active particles per litre.

It is sometimes recommended that the blood urea nitrogen (BUN)* be included in the calculation of plasma osmolality. This is done by adding a third term to the effective osmolality equation (+ BUN/2.8), with the BUN expressed in mg/dL. However, the urea moves freely between body fluid compartments; it has no lasting effect on water movement across cell boundaries and is sometimes dubbed an "ineffective osmole." One can estimate the actual osmolality more accurately by including the BUN. However, the measure of the effective plasma osmolality without consideration of the BUN term is the more physiologically meaningful estimate. Osmolality of urine can range from 100 to 1300 mOsm/kg, depending on the amount of antidiuretic hormone (ADH) and the renal response to it.

Osmotic Movement of Fluids.

Cells are affected by the osmolality of the fluid that surrounds them. Fluids with the same osmolality as the cell interior are termed **isotonic**. Solutions in which the solutes are less concentrated than they are in cells are termed **hypotonic** (hypo-osmolar). Those with solutes more concentrated than they are in cells are termed **hypertonic** (hyperosmolar).

Normally, the ECF and the ICF are isotonic to one another; hence, no net movement of water occurs. In the metabolically active cell, there is a constant exchange of substances between the compartments, but no net gain or loss of water occurs.

If a cell is surrounded by hypotonic fluid, water moves into the cell, causing it to swell and possibly to burst. If a cell is surrounded by hypertonic fluid, water leaves the cell to dilute the ECF; the cell shrinks and may eventually die (Figure 19-7).

Hydrostatic Pressure

Hydrostatic pressure is the force within a fluid compartment. In the blood vessels, hydrostatic pressure is the blood pressure generated by the contraction of the heart. Hydrostatic pressure in the vascular system gradually decreases as the blood moves through the arteries until it is about 40 mm Hg at the arterial end of a capillary. Because of the size of the capillary bed and fluid movement into the interstitium, the pressure decreases to about 10 mm Hg at the venous end of the capillary. Hydrostatic pressure is the major force that pushes water out of the vascular system at the capillary level.

_____
*Serum urea (nitrogen).

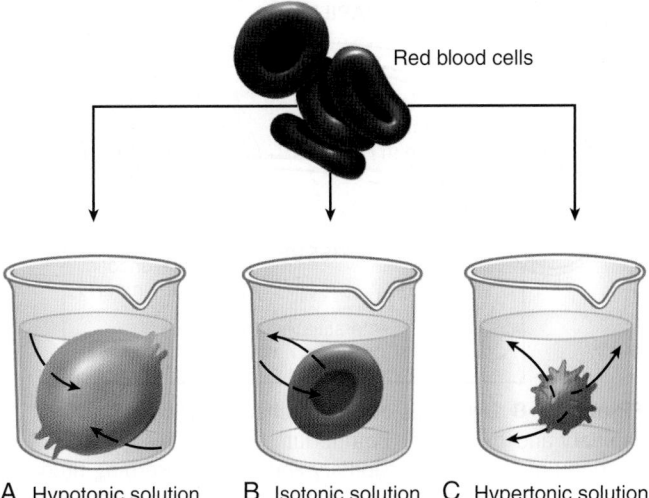

Red blood cells

A Hypotonic solution   B Isotonic solution   C Hypertonic solution

Figure 19-7 Effects of water status on red blood cells. *A,* Hypotonic solution (H_2O excess) results in cellular swelling. *B,* Isotonic solution (normal H_2O balance) results in no change. *C,* Hypertonic solution (H_2O deficit) results in cellular shrinking.

Source: Adapted from Patton, K. T., & Thibodeau, G. A. (2010). *Anatomy and physiology* (7th ed., p. 93, Figure 4-5). St. Louis: Mosby.

Oncotic Pressure

Oncotic pressure (colloidal osmotic pressure) is osmotic pressure exerted by colloids in solution. The major colloid in the vascular system contributing to the total osmotic pressure is protein. Protein molecules attract water, pulling fluid from the tissue space to the vascular space (Porth, 2010). Unlike electrolytes, the large molecular size prevents proteins from leaving the vascular space through pores in capillary walls. Plasma oncotic pressure is approximately 25 mm Hg. Some proteins are found in the interstitial space; they exert an oncotic pressure of approximately 1 mm Hg.

Fluid Movement in Capillaries

There is normal movement of fluid between the capillary and the interstitium. The amount and direction of movement are determined by the interaction of (1) capillary hydrostatic pressure, (2) plasma oncotic pressure, (3) interstitial hydrostatic pressure, and (4) interstitial oncotic pressure.

Capillary hydrostatic pressure and interstitial oncotic pressure cause the movement of water out of the capillaries. Plasma oncotic pressure and interstitial hydrostatic pressure cause the movement of fluid into the capillary. At the arterial end of the capillary (Figure 19-8), capillary hydrostatic pressure exceeds plasma oncotic pressure, and fluid is moved into the interstitium. At the venous end of the capillary, the capillary hydrostatic pressure is lower than plasma oncotic pressure, and fluid is drawn back into the capillary by the oncotic pressure created by plasma proteins.

Fluid Shifts

If capillary or interstitial pressures are altered, fluid may abnormally shift from one compartment to another, resulting in edema or dehydration.

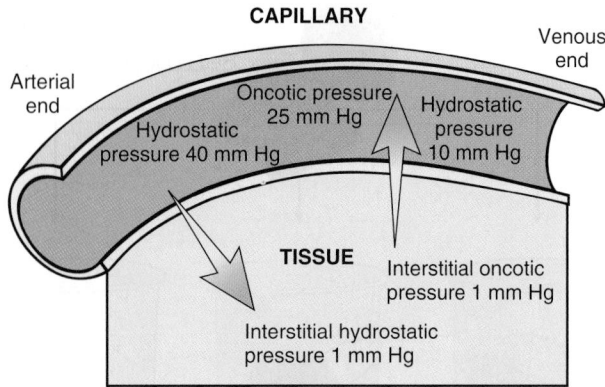

Figure 19-8 Dynamics of fluid exchange between the capillary and the tissue. Equilibrium exists between forces filtering fluid out of the capillary and forces absorbing fluid back into the capillary. Note that the hydrostatic pressure is greater at the arterial end of the capillary than at the venous end. The net effect of pressures at the arterial end of the capillary causes a movement of fluid into the tissue. At the venous end of the capillary, there is net movement of fluid back into the capillary.

Shifts of Plasma to Interstitial Fluid. Accumulation of fluid in the interstitium (edema) occurs if venous hydrostatic pressure rises, plasma oncotic pressure decreases, or interstitial oncotic pressure rises. Edema may also develop if there is an obstruction of lymphatic outflow that causes decreased removal of interstitial fluid.

Elevation of Venous Hydrostatic Pressure. Increasing the pressure at the venous end of the capillary inhibits fluid movement back into the capillary. Causes of increased venous pressure include fluid overload, congestive heart failure, liver failure, obstruction of venous return to the heart (e.g., tourniquets, restrictive clothing, venous thrombosis), and venous insufficiency (e.g., varicose veins).

Decrease in Plasma Oncotic Pressure. Fluid remains in the interstitium if the plasma oncotic pressure is too low to draw fluid back into the capillary. Decreased oncotic pressure is seen when the plasma protein content is low. This can result from excessive protein loss (renal disorders), deficient protein synthesis (liver disease), and deficient protein intake (malnutrition).

Elevation of Interstitial Oncotic Pressure. Trauma, burns, and inflammation can damage capillary walls and allow plasma proteins to accumulate in the interstitium. The resultant increased interstitial oncotic pressure draws fluid into the interstitium and holds it there.

Shifts of Interstitial Fluid to Plasma. Fluid is drawn into the plasma space whenever there is an increase in the plasma osmotic or oncotic pressure. This could happen with administration of colloids, dextran, mannitol, or hypertonic solutions. Fluid is drawn from the interstitium. In turn, water is drawn from cells via osmosis, equilibrating the osmolality between the ICF and the ECF.

Increasing the tissue hydrostatic pressure is another way of causing a shift of fluid into plasma. The wearing of elastic compression gradient stockings or hose to decrease peripheral edema is a therapeutic application of this effect.

Fluid Movement Between Extracellular Fluid and Intracellular Fluid

Changes in the osmolality of the ECF alter the volume of cells. Increased ECF osmolality (water deficit) pulls water out of cells until the two compartments have a similar osmolality. Water deficit is associated with symptoms that result from cell shrinkage as water is pulled into the vascular system. For example, neurological symptoms are caused by altered central nervous system (CNS) function as brain cells shrink. Decreased ECF osmolality (water excess) develops as the result of gain or retention of excess water. In this case, cells swell. Again, the primary symptoms are neurological as a result of brain cell swelling as water shifts into the cells.

Fluid Spacing

Fluid spacing is a term sometimes used to describe the distribution of body water. *First spacing* describes the normal distribution of fluid in the ICF and ECF compartments. *Second spacing* refers to an abnormal accumulation of interstitial fluid (i.e., edema). *Third spacing* occurs when fluid accumulates in a portion of the body from which it is not easily exchanged with the rest of the ECF. Third-spaced fluid is trapped and essentially unavailable for functional use. Examples of third spacing are ascites, sequestration of fluid in the abdominal cavity with peritonitis, and edema associated with burns.

Regulation of Water Balance

Hypothalamic Regulation

Water balance is maintained by a balance of intake and excretion. A body fluid deficit or increase in plasma osmolality is sensed by hypothalamic osmoreceptors, which in turn stimulate thirst and ADH release. Thirst causes the patient to drink water. Hypothalamic ADH, which is stored in the posterior pituitary, induces water reabsorption in the renal distal and collecting tubules. Together, these factors result in increased free water in the body and decreased plasma osmolality. Once plasma osmolality is normalized, secretion of ADH is suppressed, thus restoring urinary excretion.

An intact thirst mechanism is critical because it is the primary protection against the development of hyperosmolality. The patient who cannot recognize or act on the sensation of thirst is at risk for fluid deficit and hyperosmolality. The sensitivity of the thirst mechanism decreases in older adults.

The desire to consume fluids is also affected by social and psychological factors not related to fluid balance. A dry mouth will cause the patient to drink, even when there is no measurable body water deficit. This will be normally compensated by equivalent water excretion. A psychiatric patient may display psychogenic polydipsia that may lead to water intoxication.

Pituitary Regulation

Under hypothalamic control, the posterior pituitary releases ADH, which causes the distal tubules and collecting ducts in the kidneys to regulate water retention by becoming more permeable to water. Water is reabsorbed from the tubular filtrate into the blood and not excreted in urine. Factors that stimulate ADH release include increased plasma osmolality, stress, nausea, nicotine, and morphine. For instance, it is common for the postoperative patient to have a lower serum osmolality after surgery, possibly because of the stress of surgery and narcotic analgesia.

A pathological condition seen occasionally is *syndrome of inappropriate antidiuretic hormone* (SIADH) (see Chapter 51). Causes of SIADH include abnormal ADH production in CNS disorders (e.g., brain tumours, brain injury) and certain malignancies (e.g., small cell lung cancer). The inappropriate ADH secretion causes water retention, which produces a decrease in plasma osmolality below the normal value and a relative increase in urine osmolality with a decrease in urine volume.

Reduction in the release or action of ADH produces diabetes insipidus (see Chapter 51). A copious amount of dilute urine is excreted because the renal tubules and collecting ducts do not appropriately reabsorb water. The patient with diabetes insipidus exhibits extreme polyuria and, if alert, polydipsia (excessive thirst). Symptoms of dehydration and hypernatremia develop if the water losses are not adequately replaced.

Adrenal Cortical Regulation

ECF volume is maintained by a combination of hormonal influences. ADH affects only water reabsorption. Hormones released by the adrenal cortex help regulate both water and electrolytes. Two groups of hormones secreted by the adrenal cortex are glucocorticoids and mineralocorticoids. The glucocorticoids (e.g., cortisol) primarily have an anti-inflammatory effect and increase serum glucose levels, whereas the mineralocorticoids (e.g., aldosterone) enhance sodium retention and potassium excretion (Figure 19-9). When sodium is reabsorbed, water follows as a result of osmotic changes.

Cortisol is the most common example of a naturally occurring glucocorticoid. In large doses, cortisol has both glucocorticoid (glucose-elevating and anti-inflammatory) and mineralocorticoid (sodium-retention) properties. The adrenocortical

hormone cortisol is secreted normally and whenever stress levels are increased. Many body systems, including fluid and electrolyte balance, are affected by stress (Figure 19-10).

Aldosterone is a naturally occurring mineralocorticoid with potent sodium-retaining and potassium-excreting capability. The secretion of aldosterone may be stimulated by decreased renal perfusion or decreased sodium delivery to the distal portion of the renal tubule. The kidneys respond by secreting renin into the plasma. Angiotensinogen produced in the liver and normally found in blood is acted on by the renin to form angiotensin I, which converts to angiotensin II, which stimulates the adrenal cortex to secrete aldosterone. In addition to the renin–angiotensin mechanism, increased plasma potassium, decreased plasma sodium, and increased release of adrenocorticotropic hormone (ACTH) from the anterior pituitary all act directly on the adrenal cortex to stimulate the secretion of aldosterone (see Figure 19-9).

Renal Regulation

The primary organs for regulating fluid and electrolyte balance are the kidneys (see Chapter 47). The kidneys regulate water balance through adjustments in urine volume. Similarly, urinary excretion of most electrolytes is adjusted so that a balance is maintained between overall intake and output. The total plasma volume is filtered by the kidneys many times each day. In the average adult, the kidney reabsorbs 99% of this filtrate, producing approximately 1.5 L of urine per day. As the filtrate moves through the renal tubules, selective reabsorption of water and

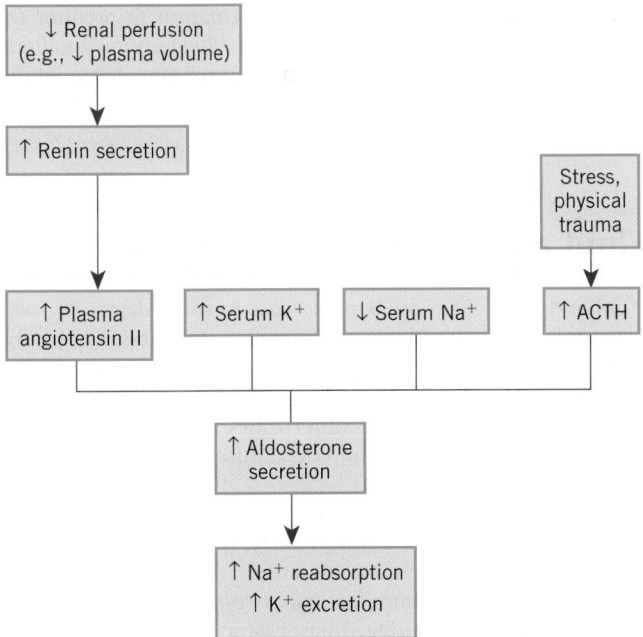

Figure 19-9 Factors affecting aldosterone secretion. *ACTH*, adrenocorticotropic hormone.

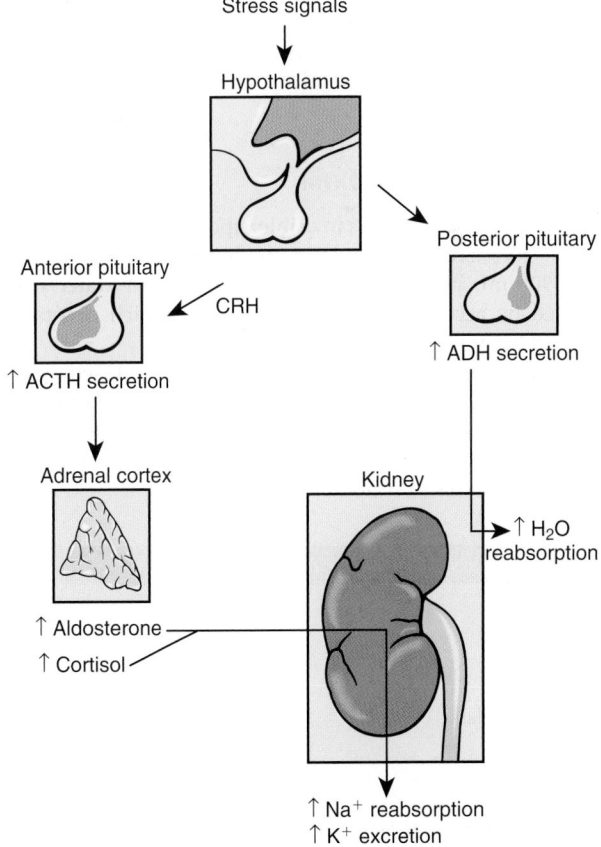

Figure 19-10 Effects of stress on fluid and electrolyte balance. *ACTH*, adrenocorticotropic hormone; *ADH*, antidiuretic hormone; *CRH*, corticotropin-releasing hormone.

electrolytes and secretion of electrolytes result in the production of urine that is greatly different in composition and concentration than the plasma. This process helps maintain normal plasma osmolality, electrolyte balance, blood volume, and acid–base balance. The renal tubules are the site for the actions of ADH and aldosterone.

With severely impaired renal function, the kidneys cannot maintain fluid and electrolyte balance. This condition results in edema, potassium and phosphorus retention, acidosis, and other electrolyte imbalances (see Chapter 49). Renal function is typically decreased in the older adult, placing the patient at increased risk for fluid and electrolyte imbalances. In particular, the ability to concentrate urine may be reduced in the older adult.

Cardiac Regulation

Atrial natriuretic factor (ANF) is a hormone released by the cardiac atria in response to increased atrial pressure (increased volume). The primary actions of ANF are vasodilation and increased urinary excretion of sodium and water, which decreases blood volume (McCance & Huether, 2010).

Gastrointestinal Regulation

Daily water intake and output are between 2000 and 3000 mL (Table 19-2). The GI tract accounts for most of the water intake. Water intake includes fluids, water from food metabolism, and water present in solid foods. Lean meat is approximately 70% water, whereas the water content of many fruits and vegetables approaches 100%.

Most of the body's water is excreted by the kidneys. A small amount of water is normally eliminated by the GI tract in feces, but diarrhea and vomiting can lead to significant fluid and electrolyte loss.

Insensible Water Loss

Insensible water loss, which is invisible vaporization from the lungs and the skin, assists in regulating body temperature. Normally, about 900 mL per day is lost. The amount of water loss is increased by accelerated body metabolism, which occurs with increased body temperature and exercise.

Water loss through the skin should not be confused with the vaporization of water excreted by sweat glands. Only water is lost by insensible perspiration. Excessive sweating *(sensible perspiration)* caused by fever or high environmental temperatures may lead to large losses of water and electrolytes.

Table 19-2 Normal Fluid Balance in the Adult

Intake	
Fluids	1200 mL
Solid food	1000 mL
Water from oxidation	300 mL
Total	**2500 mL**
Output	
Insensible loss (skin and lungs)	900 mL
Urine	1500 mL
In feces	100 mL
Total	**2500 mL**

AGE-RELATED CONSIDERATIONS: FLUID AND ELECTROLYTES

The older adult experiences normal physiologic changes that increase susceptibility to fluid and electrolyte imbalances. Structural changes to the kidney and a decrease in the renal blood flow lead to a decrease in the glomerular filtration rate, decreased creatinine clearance, the loss of the ability to concentrate urine and conserve water, and narrowed limits for the excretion of water, sodium, potassium, and hydrogen ions. Hormonal changes include a decrease in renin and aldosterone and an increase in ADH and atrial natriuretic peptides (ANP) (Ebersole, Hess, Touhy, Jett, & Luggen, 2008). Loss of subcutaneous tissue and thinning of the dermis lead to increased loss of moisture through the skin and an inability to respond to heat or cold quickly. Older adults experience a decrease in the thirst mechanism resulting in decreased fluid intake despite increases in osmolality and serum sodium level. The frail elderly, especially if ill, are at increased risk of free-water loss and subsequent development of hypernatremia secondary to impairment of the thirst mechanism and barriers to accessible fluids (Amella, 2004).

Healthy older adults usually consume adequate fluids to remain well hydrated. However, functional changes may occur that affect the individual's ability to independently obtain fluids. Musculoskeletal changes, such as stiffness of the hands and fingers, can lead to a decreased ability to hold a glass or cup. Mental status changes, such as confusion or disorientation, or changes in ambulation status may lead to a decreased ability to obtain fluids. As a result of incontinent episodes, the older adult may intentionally restrict fluid intake (Amella, 2004).

To help the older adult patient, the health care provider must understand the homeostatic changes that occur in the elderly. It is important to avoid the pitfalls of ageism, wherein elderly patients' fluid and electrolyte problems may be inappropriately attributed to the natural processes of aging. The nurse needs to adapt assessment and nursing implementation to account for these physiologic and functional changes. Suggestions for alterations in nursing care for the older adult are presented throughout this chapter and in Chapter 7.

Fluid and Electrolyte Imbalances

Fluid and electrolyte imbalances occur to some degree in most patients with a major illness or injury because illness disrupts the normal homeostatic mechanism. Some fluid and electrolyte imbalances are directly caused by illness or disease (e.g., burns, congestive heart failure). At other times, therapeutic measures (e.g., IV fluid replacement, diuretics) cause or contribute to fluid and electrolyte imbalances.

The imbalances are commonly classified as *deficits* or *excesses.* Each imbalance is discussed separately. (For normal values, see Table 19-3.) In actual clinical situations, more than one imbalance occurring in the same patient is common. For example, a patient undergoing prolonged nasogastric suction will lose Na^+, K^+, H^+, and Cl^-. These imbalances may result in a deficiency of both Na^+ and K^+ as well as metabolic alkalosis and fluid volume deficit.

Sodium and Volume Imbalances

Sodium plays a major role in maintaining the concentration and the volume of the ECF. Sodium is the main cation of the ECF and the primary determinant of ECF osmolality. Sodium imbalances are typically associated with parallel changes in osmolality. Because of its impact on osmolality, sodium affects the water distribution between the ECF and the ICF. Sodium is also important in the generation and transmission of nerve impulses and the regulation of acid–base balance. Serum sodium is measured in milliequivalents per litre or millimoles per litre.

The GI tract absorbs sodium from foods. Typically, daily intake of sodium far exceeds the body's daily requirements. Sodium leaves the body through urine, sweat, and feces. The kidneys are the primary regulator of sodium balance. The kidneys regulate the ECF concentration of sodium by excreting or retaining water under the influence of ADH. Aldosterone also plays a part in sodium regulation by promoting sodium reabsorption from the renal tubules. The serum sodium level reflects the ratio of sodium to water, not necessarily the loss or gain of sodium. Thus, changes in the serum sodium level may reflect either a primary water imbalance, a primary sodium imbalance, or a combination of the two. Sodium imbalances are typically associated with imbalances in ECF volume (Figures 19-11 and 19-12).

Hypernatremia

Common causes of hypernatremia are listed in Table 19-4. An elevated serum sodium may occur with water loss or sodium gain. Because sodium is the major determinant of the ECF osmolality, hypernatremia causes hyperosmolality. In turn, hyperosmolality causes a shift of water out of the cells, which leads to cellular dehydration.

As discussed earlier, the primary protection against the development of hyperosmolality is thirst. As the plasma osmolality increases, the thirst centre in the hypothalamus is stimulated, and the individual seeks fluids.

Hypernatremia is not a problem in an alert person who has access to water, can sense thirst, and is able to swallow. Hypernatremia secondary to water deficiency is often the result of an impaired level of consciousness or an inability to obtain fluids. The unconscious patient and the cognitively impaired are at risk because of an inability to express thirst and act on it.

Several clinical states can produce water loss and hypernatremia. A deficiency in the synthesis of ADH or its release from the posterior pituitary gland (central diabetes insipidus) or a decrease in kidney responsiveness to ADH (nephrogenic diabetes insipidus) can result in profound diuresis, causing a water deficit and hypernatremia. Hyperosmolality can result from administration of concentrated hyperosmolar tube feedings and osmotic diuretics (mannitol) as well as hyperglycemia associated with uncontrolled diabetes mellitus. These situations result in osmotic diuresis. Dilute urine is lost, leaving behind a high solute load. Other causes of hypernatremia include excessive sweating and increased sensible losses from high fever.

Sodium intake in excess of water intake can also lead to hypernatremia. Examples of sodium gain include IV administration of hypertonic saline or sodium bicarbonate, use of sodium-containing drugs, excessive oral intake of sodium (ingestion of seawater), and primary aldosteronism (hypersecretion of aldosterone) caused by a tumour of the adrenal glands.

The clinical manifestations of hypernatremia are listed in Table 19-4. Symptoms are primarily the result of changes in the

Table 19-3 Normal Serum Electrolyte Values	
ELECTROLYTE	**NORMAL VALUE**
Anions	
Bicarbonate (HCO_3^-)	21-28 mmol/L
Chloride (Cl^-)	98-106 mmol/L
Phosphate (PO_4^{3-})	0.97-1.45 mmol/L
Protein	64-83 g/L
Cations	
Potassium (K^+)	3.5-5.0 mmol/L
Magnesium (Mg^{2+})	0.65-1.05 mmol/L
Sodium (Na^+)	135-145 mmol/L
Calcium (Ca^{2+}) (total)	2.25-2.75 mmol/L
Calcium (ionized)	1.05-1.30 mmol/L

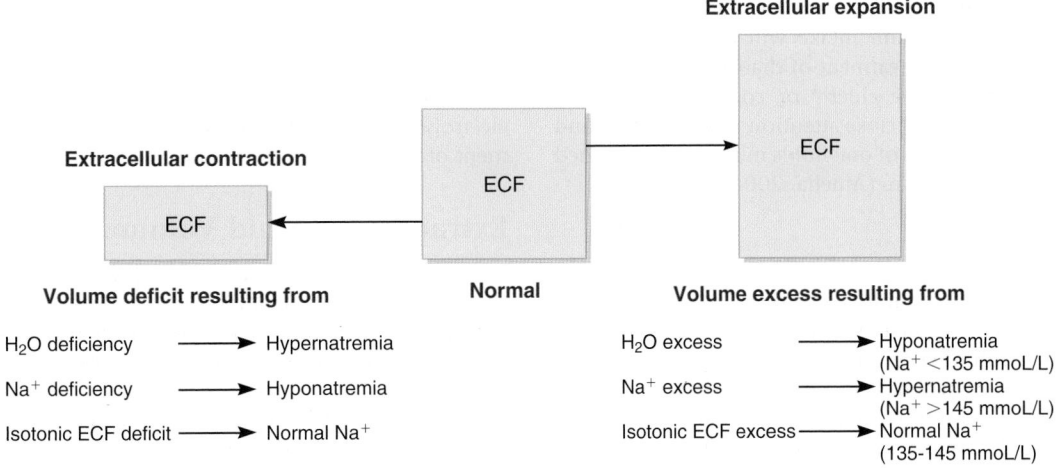

Figure 19-11 Differential assessment of extracellular fluid (ECF) volume.

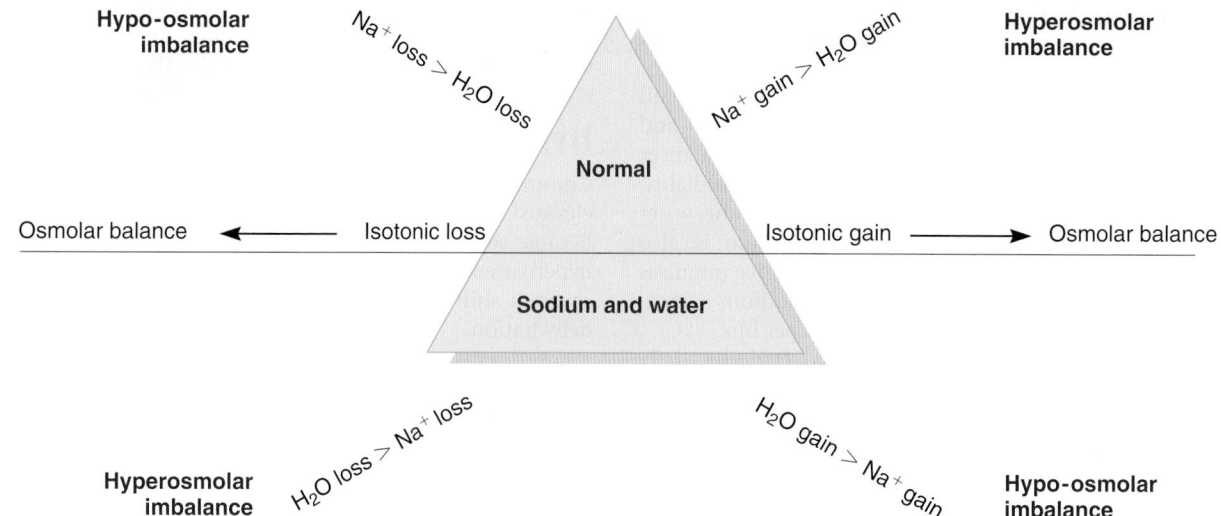

Figure 19-12 Isotonic gains and losses affect mainly the extracellular fluid (ECF) compartment, with little or no water movement into the cells. Hypertonic imbalances cause water to move from inside the cell into the ECF to dilute the concentrated sodium, causing cell shrinkage. Hypotonic imbalances cause water to move into the cell, causing cell swelling.

plasma osmolality that lead to changes in the volume of cellular water. Dehydration of neurons leads to neurological manifestations such as intense thirst, lethargy, agitation, seizures, and even coma. Sodium excess also has a direct effect on the irritability and conduction of neurons, causing them to be more easily excited. Patients with hypernatremia will also exhibit the symptoms of any accompanying volume imbalance.

Collaborative Care. The goal of treatment in hypernatremia that is caused by either water loss or sodium gain is to treat the underlying cause. In primary water deficit, the continued water loss must be prevented, and water replacement must be provided. If oral fluids cannot be ingested, IV solutions of 5% dextrose in water or hypotonic saline may be given initially. Serum sodium levels must be reduced gradually to prevent too rapid a shift of water back into the cells. Overly rapid correction of hypernatremia can result in cerebral edema. The risk is greatest in the patient who has developed hypernatremia over several days or longer.

The goal of treatment for sodium excess is to dilute the sodium concentration with salt-free IV fluids, such as 5% dextrose in water, and to promote excretion of the excess sodium by administering diuretics. Sodium intake will also be restricted. (See Chapter 51 for specific treatment of diabetes insipidus.) To prevent hypernatremia in the elderly or cognitively impaired patient, it is important to pay close attention to fluid intake and losses. Regular administration of oral fluids must be incorporated into these patients' plan of care (Amella, 2004).

Hyponatremia

Hyponatremia may result from loss of sodium-containing fluids or from water excess. Hyponatremia causes extracellular hypo-osmolality with a shift of water into the cells.

Common causes of hyponatremia caused by water excess are inappropriate use of sodium-free or hypotonic IV fluids. This may occur in patients after surgery or major trauma, during administration of fluids in patients with renal failure, or in patients with psychiatric disorders associated with excessive water intake. SIADH will result in dilutional hyponatremia caused by abnor-

mal retention of water. (See Chapter 51 for a discussion of the causes of SIADH.)

Losses of sodium-rich body fluids from the GI tract, the kidney, or the skin indirectly result in hyponatremia. Because these fluids are either isotonic or hypotonic, sodium is lost with an equal or greater proportion of water. However, hyponatremia develops as the body responds to the fluid volume deficit with activation of the thirst mechanism and by releasing ADH. The resultant retention of water lowers the sodium concentration (Kee et al., 2009).

Symptoms of hyponatremia are related to cellular swelling and are first manifested in the CNS (Kee et al., 2009). The excess water lowers plasma osmolality, shifting fluid into brain cells. The clinical manifestations of hyponatremia are listed in Table 19-4.

Collaborative Care. In hyponatremia that is caused by water excess, fluid restriction is often all that is needed to treat the problem. If severe symptoms (seizures) develop, small amounts of IV hypertonic saline solution (3% sodium chloride [NaCl]) are given to restore the serum sodium level while the body is returning to a normal water balance. Treatment of hyponatremia associated with abnormal fluid loss includes fluid replacement with sodium-containing solutions. Replacing losses with commercially available oral rehydration fluids containing electrolytes instead of pure water may help prevent the development of hyponatremia in the home setting.

Extracellular Fluid Volume Imbalances

ECF volume deficit (hypovolemia) and ECF volume excess (hypervolemia) are commonly occurring clinical conditions (Table 19-5). ECF volume imbalances are typically accompanied by one or more electrolyte imbalances. As previously discussed, volume imbalances are often associated with changes in the serum sodium level. Fluid volume deficit can occur with abnormal loss of body fluids (e.g., diarrhea, fistula drainage, hemorrhage, polyuria), decreased intake, or a plasma–to–interstitial fluid shift. Fluid volume excess may result from excessive intake of fluids, abnormal retention of fluids (e.g., congestive heart

Table 19-4 Water and Sodium Imbalances: Causes and Clinical Manifestations

WATER EXCESS: HYPONATREMIA (Na⁺ <135 mmol/L)	WATER DEFICIT: HYPERNATREMIA (Na⁺ >145 mmol/L)
Causes	
Sodium Loss	**Water Loss (Sodium Concentration)**
• GI losses: diarrhea, vomiting, fistulas, NG suction	• ↑ Insensible water loss or perspiration (high fever, heatstroke)
• Renal losses: diuretics, adrenal insufficiency, Na⁺ wasting renal disease	• Diabetes insipidus
• Skin losses: burns, wound drainage	• Osmotic diuresis
Water Gain (Sodium Dilution)	**Sodium Gain**
• SIADH	• IV hypertonic NaCl
• Congestive heart failure	• IV sodium bicarbonate
• Excessive hypotonic IV fluids	• IV excessive isotonic NaCl
• Primary polydipsia	• Primary hyperaldosteronism
	• Saltwater near-drowning
Clinical Manifestations	
Decreased ECF Volume (Sodium Loss)	**Decreased ECF Volume (Water Loss)**
• Irritability, apprehension, confusion	• Intense thirst; dry, swollen tongue
• Postural hypotension	• Restlessness, agitation, twitching
• Tachycardia	• Seizures, coma
• Rapid, thready pulse	• Weakness
• ↓ CVP	• Postural hypotension, ↓ CVP
• ↓ Jugular venous filling	• Weight loss
• Nausea, vomiting	
• Dry mucous membranes	
• Weight loss	
• Tremors, seizures, coma	
Normal or Increased ECF Volume (Water Gain)	**Normal or Increased ECF Volume (Sodium Gain)**
• Headache, lassitude, apathy	• Intense thirst
• Weakness, confusion	• Restlessness, agitation, twitching
• Nausea, vomiting	• Seizures, coma
• Weight gain	• Flushed skin
• ↑ BP, ↑ CVP	• Weight gain
• Muscle spasms, seizures, coma	• Peripheral and pulmonary edema
	• ↑ BP, ↑ CVP

BP, blood pressure; *CVP*, central venous pressure; *ECF*, extracellular fluid; *GI*, gastrointestinal; *IV*, intravenous; *NG*, nasogastric; *SIADH*, syndrome of inappropriate antidiuretic hormone.

Table 19-5 Causes of ECF Volume Imbalances

ECF VOLUME DEFICIT	ECF VOLUME EXCESS
Increased Loss	**Increased Retention**
• Vomiting	• Congestive heart failure
• Diarrhea	• Cushing's syndrome
• Fistula drainage	• Chronic liver disease with portal hypertension
• GI tract suction	• Long-term use of corticosteroids
• Excessive sweating	• Renal failure
• Third space fluid shifts (e.g., burns, intestinal obstruction)	
• Overuse of diuretics	
• Hemorrhage	
Decreased Intake	**Increased Intake**
• Nausea	• Rare with adequate renal function
• Anorexia	• Excessive IV administration of fluids
• Inability to drink	
• Inability to obtain water	

ECF, extracellular fluid; *GI*, gastrointestinal; *IV*, intravenous.

failure, renal failure), or interstitial–to–plasma fluid shift. Although shifts in fluid between the plasma and the interstitium do not alter the overall volume of the ECF, these shifts do result in changes in the clinically important intravascular volume.

Collaborative Care. The goal of treatment for fluid volume deficit is to correct the underlying cause and to replace both water and electrolytes. Balanced IV solutions, such as lactated Ringer's solution, are usually given. Isotonic NaCl is used when rapid volume replacement is indicated. Blood is administered when volume loss is caused by blood loss.

The goal of treatment for fluid volume excess is removal of sodium and water without producing abnormal changes in the electrolyte composition or osmolality of ECF. The primary cause must be identified and treated. IV therapy is usually not indicated for this type of fluid imbalance. Diuretics and fluid restriction are the primary forms of therapy. Restriction of sodium intake may also be indicated. If the fluid excess leads to ascites or pleural effusion, an abdominal paracentesis or thoracentesis may be necessary.

NURSING MANAGEMENT: SODIUM AND VOLUME IMBALANCES

■ Nursing Diagnoses

Nursing diagnoses and collaborative problems for the patient with various fluid and sodium imbalances include, but are not limited to, the following:
ECF volume excess:

- Excess fluid volume *related to* increased sodium and water retention.
- Ineffective airway clearance *related to* sodium and water retention.

- Risk for impaired skin integrity *related to* edema.
- Disturbed body image *related to* altered body appearance secondary to edema.
- Potential complications: pulmonary edema, ascites.

ECF volume deficit:

- Deficient fluid volume *related to* excessive ECF losses or decreased fluid intake.
- Decreased cardiac output *related to* excessive ECF losses or decreased fluid intake.
- Potential complication: hypovolemic shock.

Hypernatremia:

- Risk for injury *related to* altered sensorium and seizures secondary to abnormal CNS function.

Hyponatremia:

- Risk for injury *related to* altered sensorium and decreased level of consciousness secondary to abnormal CNS function.

Nursing Implementation

Intake and Output

The use of 24-hour intake and output records gives valuable information regarding fluid and electrolyte problems. Sources of excessive intake or fluid losses can be identified on a properly recorded intake-and-output flow sheet. Intake should include oral, IV, and tube feedings and retained irrigants. Output includes urine, excess perspiration, wound or tube drainage, vomitus, and diarrhea. Fluid loss from wounds and perspiration should be estimated. Urine specific gravity measurements can be done. Readings of greater than 1.030 indicate a concentrated urine, whereas those of less than 1.005 indicate a dilute urine.

Cardiovascular Changes

Monitoring the patient for cardiovascular changes is necessary to prevent or detect complications from sodium and volume imbalances. Signs and symptoms of ECF volume excess and deficit are reflected in changes in blood pressure, pulse force, and jugular venous visibility. In fluid volume excess, the pulse is full and bounding. Because of the expanded intravascular volume, the pulse is not easily obliterated. Increased volume causes distended neck veins (jugular venous distension) and increased blood pressure.

In mild to moderate fluid volume deficit, compensatory mechanisms include sympathetic nervous system stimulation of the heart and peripheral vasoconstriction. Stimulation of the heart increases heart rate and, combined with vasoconstriction, maintains blood pressure within normal limits. A change in position from lying to sitting or standing may elicit a further increase in heart rate or a decrease in blood pressure (orthostatic hypotension). If vasoconstriction and tachycardia provide inadequate compensation, hypotension occurs when the patient is recumbent. Severe fluid volume deficit can cause a weak, thready pulse that is easily obliterated and flattened neck veins. Severe, untreated fluid deficit will result in shock.

Respiratory Changes

Both fluid excess and fluid deficit affect respiratory status. Fluid excess results in pulmonary congestion and pulmonary edema as increased hydrostatic pressure in the pulmonary vessels forces fluid into the alveoli. The patient will experience shortness of breath, irritative cough, and moist crackles on auscultation (Kee et al., 2009). The patient with fluid deficit will demonstrate an increased respiratory rate because of decreased tissue perfusion and resultant hypoxia.

Neurological Changes

Changes in neurological function may occur with sodium and water imbalances. With increased water volume and hyponatremia, water moves by osmosis into the brain cells. Alternatively, decreased water volume and hypernatremia cause water to shift out of the brain cells, with resultant shrinkage. In addition, profound volume depletion may cause an alteration in sensorium secondary to reduced cerebral tissue perfusion.

Assessment of neurological function includes evaluation of (1) the level of consciousness, which includes responses to verbal and painful stimuli and the determination of a person's orientation to time, place, and person; (2) pupillary response to light and equality of pupil size; and (3) voluntary movement of the extremities, degree of muscle strength, and reflexes. Nursing care focuses on maintaining patient safety.

Daily Weights

Accurate daily weight measurements provide the easiest measurement of volume status. An increase of 1 kg is equal to 1000 mL (1 L) fluid retention (provided the person has maintained usual dietary intake or has not been on nothing-by-mouth [NPO] status). However, weight changes can be relied on only if obtained under standardized conditions. Obtaining an accurate weight depends on the patient being weighed at the same time every day, wearing the same garments, and on the same carefully calibrated scale. Excess bedding should be removed, and all drainage bags should be emptied before the weighing. If bulky dressings or tubes are present, which may not necessarily be used every day, a notation regarding these variables should be recorded on the flow sheet or nursing notes.

Skin Assessment and Care

Clues to fluid volume deficit and excess can be detected by inspection of the skin. Skin should be examined for turgor and mobility. Normally, a fold of skin, when pinched, will readily move and, on release, will rapidly return to its former position. Skin areas over the sternum, the abdomen, and the anterior forearm are the usual sites for evaluation of tissue turgor (Figure 19-13). The preferred areas to assess for tissue turgor in the older person are areas where decreases in skin elasticity are less significant, such as the forehead or over the sternum (Larson, 2003).

Decreased skin turgor is less predictive of fluid deficit in older persons because of the loss of tissue elasticity (Ebersole et al., 2008). In ECF volume deficit, skin turgor is diminished; there is a lag in the pinched skinfold's return to its original state (referred to as *tenting*). The skin may be cool and moist if there is vasoconstriction to compensate for the decreased fluid volume.

Mild hypovolemia usually does not stimulate this compensatory response; consequently, the skin will be warm and dry. Volume deficit may also cause the skin to appear dry and wrinkled. These signs may be difficult to evaluate in the older adult because the patient's skin may be normally dry, wrinkled, and nonelastic. Oral mucous membranes will be dry, the tongue may be furrowed, and the individual often complains of thirst. Routine

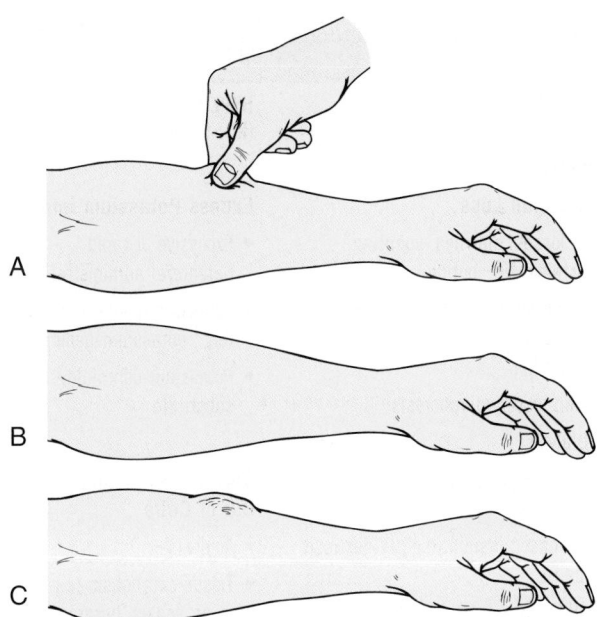

Figure 19-13 Assessment of skin turgor. **A** and **B,** When normal skin is pinched, it resumes shape in seconds. **C,** If the skin remains wrinkled for 20 to 30 seconds, the patient has poor skin turgor.

oral care is critical to the comfort of the dehydrated patient and the patient who is on fluid restrictions for management of fluid volume excess.

Skin that is edematous may feel cool because of fluid accumulation and a decrease in blood flow secondary to the pressure of the fluid. The fluid can also stretch the skin, causing it to feel taut and hard. Edema is assessed by pressing with a thumb or forefinger over the edematous area. A grading scale is used to standardize the description if an indentation (ranging from 1+ [slight, 2-mm indentation] to 4+ [pitting, 8-mm indentation]) remains when pressure is released. The areas to be evaluated for edema are those where soft tissues overlie a bone. Skin areas over the tibia, the fibula, and the sacrum are the preferred sites.

Good skin care for the person with fluid volume excess or deficit is important. Edematous tissues must be protected from extremes of heat and cold, prolonged pressure, and trauma. Frequent skin care and changes in position will protect the patient from skin breakdown. Elevation of edematous extremities helps promote venous return and fluid reabsorption. Dehydrated skin needs frequent care without the use of soap. The application of moisturizing creams or oils will increase moisture retention and stimulate circulation.

◼ Other Nursing Measures

The rates of infusion of IV fluid solutions should be carefully monitored. Attempts to "catch up" should be approached with extreme caution, particularly when large volumes of fluid or certain electrolytes are involved. This is especially true in patients with cardiac, renal, or neurological problems. Patients receiving tube feedings need supplementary water added to their enteral formula. The amount of water will depend on the osmolarity of the feeding and the patient's condition.

The patient with nasogastric suction should not be allowed to drink water because it will increase the loss of electrolytes. Occasionally, the patient may be given small amounts of ice chips to suck. A nasogastric tube should always be irrigated with isotonic saline solution and not with water. Water causes diffusion of electrolytes into the gastric lumen from mucosal cells; the electrolytes are then suctioned away.

Nurses in hospital and community settings should encourage and often assist the older or debilitated patient to maintain an adequate oral intake. This may be accomplished by giving patients a drink as part of the morning care, encouraging extra sips of fluid with drugs, and including a drink of fluids as part of one-on-one conversations.

Potassium Imbalances

Potassium is the major ICF cation, with 98% of the body potassium being intracellular. For example, potassium concentration within muscle cells is approximately 140 mmol; potassium concentration in the ECF is 3.5 to 5.0 mmol. The sodium–potassium pump in cell membranes maintains this concentration difference by pumping potassium into the cell and sodium out, a process fuelled by the breakdown of ATP. The ratio of ECF potassium to ICF potassium is the major factor in the resting neuron's membrane potential. Many of the symptoms related to potassium imbalance are caused by changes in the ratio of ECF to ICF potassium (increased or decreased ECF potassium) (McCance & Huether, 2010).

Potassium is critical for many cellular and metabolic functions. It is necessary for the transmission and conduction of nerve impulses, maintenance of normal cardiac rhythms, and skeletal and smooth muscle contraction. As the major intracellular cation, potassium regulates intracellular osmolality and promotes cellular growth. Potassium moves into cells during the formation of new tissues and leaves the cell during tissue breakdown (McCance & Huether, 2010). Potassium also plays a role in acid–base balance, which is discussed in acid–base regulation later in this chapter.

Diet is the source of potassium. The typical Western diet contains approximately 50 to 100 mEq of potassium daily, mainly from fruits, dried fruits, and vegetables. Many salt substitutes contain substantial potassium. Patients may receive potassium from parenteral sources, including IV fluids, stored transfused blood, and potassium–penicillin.

The kidneys are the primary route for potassium loss. About 90% of the daily potassium intake is eliminated by the kidneys; the remainder is lost in the stool and sweat. If kidney function is significantly impaired, toxic levels of potassium may be retained. There is an inverse relationship between sodium and potassium reabsorption in the kidneys. Factors that cause sodium retention (e.g., low blood volume, increased aldosterone level) cause potassium loss in the urine. Large urine volumes can be associated with excess loss of potassium in the urine. The ability of the kidneys to conserve potassium is weak even when body stores are depleted (McCance & Huether, 2010).

Disruptions in the dynamic equilibrium between ICF and ECF potassium often cause clinical problems. Among the factors causing potassium to move from the ECF to the ICF are the following:
• Insulin
• Alkalosis

- β-Adrenergic stimulation (catecholamine release in stress, coronary ischemia, delirium tremens, or administration of β-adrenergic agonist drugs)
- Rapid cell building (administration of folic acid or cobalamin [vitamin B$_{12}$] to patients with megaloblastic anemia, resulting in marked production of red blood cells [RBCs])

Factors that cause potassium to move from the ICF to the ECF include acidosis, trauma to cells (as in massive soft tissue damage or in tumour lysis), and exercise. Both digoxin-like drugs and β-adrenergic blocking drugs (e.g., propanolol [Inderal]) can impair entry of potassium into cells, resulting in the higher ECF potassium concentration. Causes of potassium imbalance are summarized in Table 19-6.

Hyperkalemia

Hyperkalemia (high serum potassium) may be caused by a massive intake of potassium, impaired renal excretion, shift of potassium from the ICF to the ECF, or a combination of these factors. The most common cause of hyperkalemia is renal failure. Hyperkalemia is also common in patients with massive cell destruction (e.g., burn or crush injury, tumour lysis), rapid transfusion of aged blood, and catabolic state (e.g., severe infections). Metabolic acidosis, particularly when the chloride is normal, is associated with a shift of potassium ions from the ICF to the ECF as hydrogen ions move into the cell. Adrenal insufficiency leads to retention of potassium ions in the serum because of aldosterone deficiency. Certain drugs, such as potassium-sparing diuretics (e.g., spironolactone [Aldactone], triamterene) and angiotensin-converting enzyme (ACE) inhibitors (e.g., enalapril [Vasotec], lisinopril [Prinivil]), may contribute to the development of hyperkalemia. Both of these types of drugs reduce the kidneys' ability to secrete and therefore excrete excess potassium (see Table 19-6).

Clinical Manifestations. Hyperkalemia causes membrane depolarization, altering cell excitability. Skeletal muscles become weak or paralyzed. The patient may experience cramping leg pain. Leg muscles are affected initially; respiratory muscles are spared. Disturbances in cardiac conduction occur as the potassium level rises (Kee et al., 2009). Ventricular fibrillation or cardiac standstill may occur. Cardiac depolarization is impaired, leading to flattening of the P wave and widening of the QRS wave. Repolarization occurs more rapidly, resulting in shortening of the Q–T interval and causing the T wave to be narrower and more peaked. Figure 19-14 illustrates the electrocardiographic (ECG) effects of hypokalemia and hyperkalemia. Abdominal cramping and diarrhea occur from hyperactivity of smooth muscles. Other clinical manifestations are listed in Table 19-6.

NURSING AND COLLABORATIVE MANAGEMENT: HYPERKALEMIA

▪ Nursing Diagnoses

Nursing diagnoses and collaborative problems for the patient with hyperkalemia include, but are not limited to, the following:
- Risk for injury *related to* lower extremity muscle weakness and seizures.
- Potential complication: dysrhythmias.

Table 19-6 Potassium Imbalances: Causes and Clinical Manifestations

HYPOKALEMIA (K$^+$ <3.5 mmol/L)	HYPERKALEMIA (K$^+$ >5.5 mmol/L)
Causes	
Potassium Loss	**Excess Potassium Intake**
• GI losses: diarrhea, vomiting, fistulas, NG suction	• Excessive or rapid parenteral administration
• Renal losses: diuretics, hyperaldosteronism, magnesium depletion	• Potassium-containing drugs (e.g., potassium-penicillin)
• Skin losses: diaphoresis	• Potassium-containing salt substitute
• Dialysis	
Shift of Potassium Into Cells	**Shift of Potassium Out of Cells**
• Increased insulin (e.g., IV dextrose load)	• Acidosis
• Alkalosis	• Tissue catabolism (e.g., fever, sepsis, burns)
• Tissue repair	• Crush injury
• ↑ Epinephrine (e.g., stress)	• Tumour lysis syndrome
Lack of Potassium Intake	**Failure to Eliminate Potassium**
• Starvation	• Renal disease
• Diet low in potassium	• Potassium-sparing diuretics
• Failure to include potassium in parenteral fluids if NPO	• Adrenal insufficiency
	• ACE inhibitors
Clinical Manifestations	
• Fatigue	• Irritability
• Muscle weakness	• Anxiety
• Leg cramps	• Abdominal cramping, diarrhea
• Nausea, vomiting, ileus	• Weakness of lower extremities
• Soft, flabby muscles	• Paresthesias
• Paresthesias, decreased reflexes	• Irregular pulse
• Weak, irregular pulse	• Cardiac standstill if hyperkalemia sudden or severe
• Polyuria	
• Hyperglycemia	
Electrocardiogram Changes	
• ST segment depression	• Tall, peaked T wave
• Flattened T wave	• Prolonged P–R interval
• Presence of U wave	• ST depression
• Ventricular dysrhythmias (e.g., PVCs)	• Loss of P wave
• Bradycardia	• Widening QRS
• Enhanced digitalis effect	• Ventricular fibrillation
	• Ventricular standstill

ACE, angiotensin-converting enzyme; *GI,* gastrointestinal; *IV,* intravenous; *NG,* nasogastric; *NPO,* nothing by mouth; *PVC,* premature ventricular contraction.

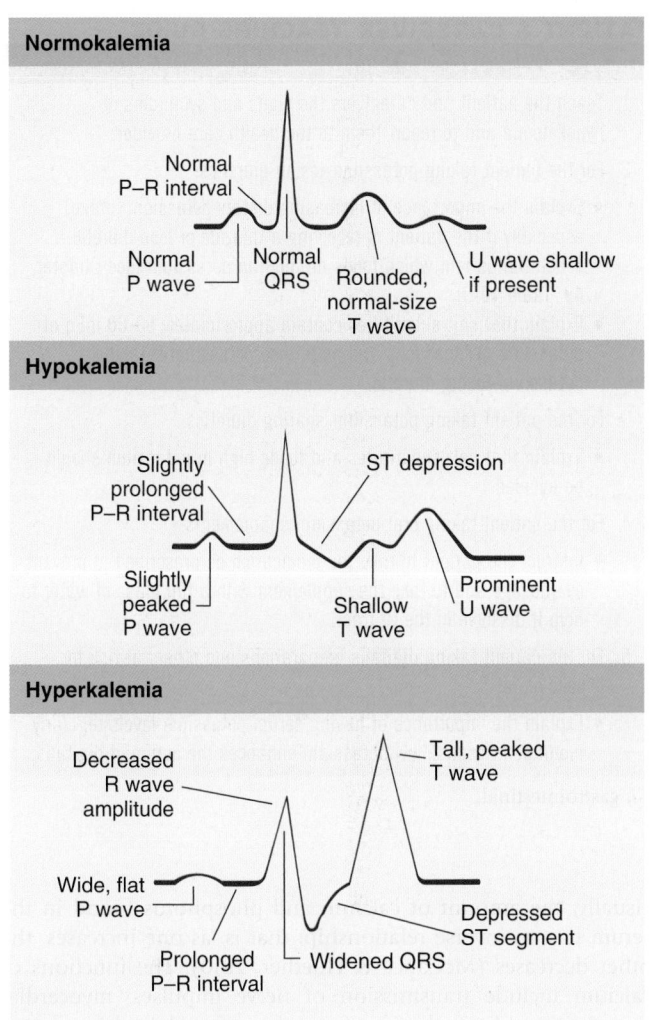

Normokalemia

Normal
P–R interval

Normal
P wave

Normal
QRS

Rounded,
normal-size
T wave

U wave shallow
if present

Hypokalemia

Slightly
prolonged
P–R interval

ST depression

Slightly
peaked
P wave

Shallow
T wave

Prominent
U wave

Hyperkalemia

Decreased
R wave
amplitude

Tall, peaked
T wave

Wide, flat
P wave

Prolonged
P–R interval

Widened QRS

Depressed
ST segment

Figure 19-14 Electrocardiographic changes associated with alterations in potassium status.

Source: Redrawn from McCance, K. L., & Huether, S. E. (2010). *Pathophysiology: The biologic basis for disease in adults and children* (6th ed., p. 1104, Figure 29-13). St. Louis: Mosby.

■ Nursing Implementation

Treatment of hyperkalemia consists of the following (see Chapter 49, Table 49-4):

1. Eliminate oral and parenteral potassium intake.
2. Increase elimination of potassium. This is accomplished via diuretics, dialysis, and use of ion-exchange resins such as sodium polystyrene sulphonate (Kayexalate). Increased fluid intake can enhance renal potassium elimination.
3. Force potassium from the ECF to the ICF. This is accomplished by administration of IV insulin (along with glucose so the patient does not become hypoglycemic) or via administration of IV sodium bicarbonate in the correction of acidosis. Rarely, a β-adrenergic agonist (e.g., epinephrine) is administered.
4. Reverse the membrane effects of the elevated ECF potassium by administering calcium gluconate intravenously. Calcium ion can immediately reverse the effect of the depolarization on cell excitability.

In cases in which the elevation of potassium is mild and the kidneys are functioning, it may be sufficient to withhold potas-

sium from the diet and IV sources and increase renal elimination by administering fluids and possibly diuretics. Kayexalate, which is administered via the GI tract, binds potassium in exchange for sodium, and the resin is excreted in feces (see Chapter 49). All patients with clinically significant hyperkalemia should be monitored electrocardiographically to detect dysrhythmias and to monitor the effects of therapy. Patients with moderate hyperkalemia should additionally receive one of the treatments to force potassium into cells, usually IV insulin and glucose. The patient experiencing dangerous cardiac dysrhythmias should receive IV calcium gluconate immediately; this serves to protect the patient while the potassium is being eliminated and forced into cells. Hemodialysis is an effective means of removing potassium from the body in the patient with renal failure.

Hypokalemia

Hypokalemia (low serum potassium) can result from abnormal losses of potassium from a shift of potassium from ECF to ICF or, rarely, from deficient dietary potassium intake. The most common causes of hypokalemia are abnormal losses, via either the kidneys or the GI tract. Abnormal losses occur when the patient is diuresing, particularly in the patient with an elevated aldosterone level. Aldosterone is released when the circulating blood volume is low; it causes sodium retention in the kidneys but loss of potassium in the urine. Magnesium deficiency may contribute to the development of potassium depletion. Low plasma magnesium stimulates renin release and subsequently increases aldosterone levels, which results in potassium excretion. GI tract losses of potassium secondary to diarrhea, laxative abuse, vomiting, and ileostomy drainage can cause hypokalemia.

Metabolic alkalosis can cause a shift of potassium into cells in exchange for hydrogen, thus lowering the potassium in the ECF and causing symptomatic hypokalemia. Hypokalemia is sometimes associated with the treatment of diabetic ketoacidosis because of a combination of factors, including an increased urinary potassium loss and a shift of potassium into cells with the administration of insulin and correction of acidosis. A less common cause of hypokalemia is the sudden initiation of cell formation; for example, the formation of RBCs as in treatment of anemia with cobalamin, folic acid, or erythropoietin.

Clinical Manifestations. Hypokalemia alters resting membrane potential. It most commonly is associated with hyperpolarization, or increased negative charge within the cell. This causes excitability problems in many types of tissue. The most serious clinical problems are cardiac. The incidence of potentially lethal ventricular dysrhythmias is increased in hypokalemia. Patients should be monitored with ECG for signs of hypokalemia. These changes include impaired repolarization, resulting in a flattening of the T wave and eventually in emergence of a U wave. The P wave amplitude may increase and may become peaked (see Figure 19-14). Patients taking digoxin experience increased digoxin toxicity if their serum potassium is low. Skeletal muscle weakness and paralysis may occur with hypokalemia. As with hyperkalemia, symptoms are most often observed in the legs. Respiratory muscles and those innervated by cranial nerves are not involved. Muscle cramping and muscle cell breakdown (known as rhabdomyolysis) can be caused by hypokalemia. This can lead to myoglobin in the plasma and the urine, which can, in turn, lead to renal failure.

Smooth muscle function is altered by hypokalemia. The patient may experience decreased GI motility (e.g., paralytic ileus), altered airway responsiveness, and impaired regulation of arteriolar blood flow, possibly contributing to muscle cell breakdown. Finally, hypokalemia can impair function in nonmuscle tissue. With prolonged hypokalemia, the kidneys are unable to concentrate urine, and diuresis occurs. Release of insulin is impaired, often causing hyperglycemia. Clinical manifestations of hypokalemia are presented in Table 19-6.

NURSING AND COLLABORATIVE MANAGEMENT: HYPOKALEMIA

▪ Nursing Diagnoses

Nursing diagnoses and collaborative problems for the patient with hypokalemia include, but are not limited to, the following:
• Risk for injury *related to* muscle weakness and hyporeflexia.
• Potential complication: dysrhythmias.

▪ Nursing Implementation

Hypokalemia is treated by giving potassium chloride (KCl) supplements and increasing dietary intake of potassium. KCl supplements can be given orally or intravenously. Except in severe deficiencies, KCl is never given unless there is urine output of at least 0.5 mL/kg of body weight per hour. KCl supplements added to IV solutions should never exceed 60 mmol (mEq/L). The preferred level is 40 mmol. The rate of IV administration of KCl should not exceed 10 to 20 mEq/hr to prevent hyperkalemia and cardiac arrest. When given intravenously, potassium may cause pain in the area of the vein where it is entering. Central IV lines should be used when rapid correction of hypokalemia is necessary. Potassium may also be replaced with potassium phosphate. Patients should be taught methods to prevent hypokalemia, depending on their individual situations. Patients at risk should obtain regular serum potassium levels to monitor for hypokalemia (Table 19-7).

SAFETY ALERT
• KCl given intravenously must always be diluted.
• Never give KCl via IV push or in concentrated amounts.
• IV bags containing KCl should be inverted several times to ensure even distribution in the bag.
• Never add KCl to a hanging IV bag to prevent giving a bolus dose.

Calcium Imbalances

Calcium is obtained from ingested foods. However, only about 30% is absorbed in the GI tract. More than 99% of the body's calcium is combined with phosphorus and concentrated in the skeletal system. Bones serve as a readily available store of calcium. Thus, wide variations in serum calcium levels are avoided by regulating the movement of calcium into or out of the bone.

PATIENT & CAREGIVER TEACHING GUIDE
Table 19-7 Prevention of Hypokalemia

1. Teach the patient and caregivers the signs and symptoms of hypokalemia and to report them to the health care provider.

2. For the patient taking potassium-losing diuretics:
   • Explain the importance of increasing dietary potassium intake, especially if the patient is receiving a thiazide or loop diuretic.
   • Teach the patient which foods are high in potassium (see Chapter 49, Table 49-9).
   • Explain that salt substitutes contain approximately 50-60 mEq of potassium per teaspoon and help raise potassium if taking a potassium-losing diuretic.

3. For the patient taking potassium-sparing diuretics:
   • Explain that salt substitutes and foods high in potassium should be avoided.

4. For the patient taking oral potassium supplements:
   • Instruct the patient to take the medication as prescribed to prevent overdosage and to take the supplement with a full glass of water to help it dissolve in the GI tract.

5. For the patient taking digitalis preparations and others at risk for hypokalemia:
   • Explain the importance of having serum potassium levels regularly monitored because low potassium enhances the action of digitalis.

GI, gastrointestinal.

Usually, the amount of calcium and phosphorus found in the serum has an inverse relationship; that is, as one increases, the other decreases (McCance & Huether, 2010). The functions of calcium include transmission of nerve impulses, myocardial contractions, blood clotting, formation of teeth and bone, and muscle contractions.

Calcium is present in the serum in three forms: free or ionized; bound to protein (primarily albumin); and complexed with phosphate, citrate, or carbonate. The ionized form is the biologically active form. Approximately one half of the total serum calcium is ionized.

Calcium is typically measured in milligrams per decilitre (mg/dL). As usually reported, serum calcium levels reflect the total calcium level (all three forms), although ionized calcium levels may be reported separately. The levels listed in Table 19-8 reflect total calcium levels. Changes in serum pH will alter the level of ionized calcium without altering the total calcium level. Acidosis decreases calcium binding to albumin, leading to more ionized calcium, and alkalosis increases calcium binding, leading to decreased ionized calcium. Alterations in serum albumin levels affect interpretation of total calcium levels. Low albumin levels result in a drop in the total calcium level, although the level of ionized calcium does not change as much.

Calcium balance is controlled by parathyroid hormone (PTH), calcitonin, and vitamin D (McCance & Huether, 2010). PTH is produced by the parathyroid gland. Its production and release are stimulated by low serum calcium levels. PTH increases bone resorption (movement of calcium out of bones), increases GI absorption of calcium, and increases renal tubule reabsorption of calcium.

Calcitonin is produced by the thyroid gland and is stimulated by high serum calcium levels. It opposes the action of PTH and, thus, lowers the serum calcium level by decreasing GI absorption,

Table 19-8 Calcium Imbalances: Causes and Clinical Manifestations

HYPOCALCEMIA (Ca²⁺ <2.25 mmol/L)	HYPERCALCEMIA (Ca²⁺ >2.74 mmol/L)
Causes	
Decreased Total Calcium	**Increased Total Calcium**
• Chronic renal failure	• Multiple myeloma
• Elevated phosphorus	• Other malignancy
• Primary hypoparathyroidism	• Prolonged immobilization
• Vitamin D deficiency	• Hyperparathyroidism
• Magnesium deficiency	• Vitamin D overdose
• Acute pancreatitis	• Thiazide diuretics
• Loop diuretics	• Milk–alkali syndrome
• Chronic alcoholism	
• Diarrhea	
• ↓ Serum albumin (patient is usually asymptomatic because of normal ionized calcium level)	
Decreased Ionized Calcium	**Increased Ionized Calcium**
• Alkalosis	• Acidosis
• Excess administration of citrated blood	
Clinical Manifestations	
• Easy fatigability	• Lethargy, weakness
• Depression, anxiety, confusion	• Depressed reflexes
• Numbness and tingling in extremities and region around mouth	• Decreased memory
• Hyperreflexia, muscle cramps	• Confusion, personality changes, psychosis
• Chvostek's sign	• Anorexia, nausea, vomiting
• Trousseau's sign	• Bone pain, fractures
• Laryngeal spasm	• Polyuria, dehydration
• Tetany, seizures	• Nephrolithiasis
	• Stupor, coma
Electrocardiogram Changes	
• Elongation of ST segment	• Shortened ST segment
• Prolonged Q–T interval	• Shortened Q–T interval
• Ventricular tachycardia	• Ventricular dysrhythmias
	• Increased digitalis effect

tumour secretion of a parathyroid-related protein, which stimulates calcium release from bones. Hypercalcemia is also associated with vitamin D overdose. Prolonged immobilization results in bone mineral loss and increased calcium concentration. Hypercalcemia rarely occurs from increased calcium intake (e.g., ingestion of antacids containing calcium, excessive administration during cardiac arrest).

Excess calcium blocks the effect of sodium in skeletal muscles, which leads to reduced excitability of both muscles and nerves (McCance & Huether, 2010). Manifestations of hypercalcemia include decreased memory, confusion, disorientation, fatigue, muscle weakness, constipation, cardiac dysrhythmias, and renal calculi (see Table 19-8).

NURSING AND COLLABORATIVE MANAGEMENT: HYPERCALCEMIA

▪ Nursing Diagnoses

Nursing diagnoses and collaborative problems for the patient with hypercalcemia include, but are not limited to, the following:
• Risk for injury *related to* neuromuscular and sensorium changes.
• Potential complication: dysrhythmias.

▪ Nursing Implementation

The basic treatment of hypercalcemia is promotion of excretion of calcium in urine by administration of a loop diuretic (e.g., furosemide [Lasix], ethacrynic acid [Edecrin]) and hydration of the patient with isotonic saline infusions. In hypercalcemia, the patient must drink 3000 to 4000 mL of fluid daily to promote the renal excretion of calcium and to decrease the possibility of renal calculi formation.

Synthetic calcitonin can also be administered to lower serum calcium levels. A diet low in calcium may be prescribed. Mobilization with weight-bearing activity is encouraged to enhance bone mineralization. In hypercalcemia associated with malignancy, the drug of choice is pamidronate (Aredia), which inhibits the activity of osteoclasts. Pamidronate is preferred because it does not have cytotoxic adverse effects and it inhibits bone resorption without inhibiting bone formation and mineralization.

increasing calcium deposition into bone, and promoting renal excretion.

Vitamin D is formed through the action of ultraviolet rays on a precursor found in the skin or is ingested in the diet. Vitamin D is important for absorption of calcium from the GI tract. Causes of calcium imbalances are listed in Table 19-8.

Hypercalcemia

About two thirds of hypercalcemia cases are caused by hyperparathyroidism, and one third are caused by malignancy, especially from breast cancer, lung cancer, and multiple myeloma (Wilson, Shannon, & Stang, 2011). Malignancies lead to hypercalcemia through bone destruction from tumour invasion or through

Hypocalcemia

Any condition that causes a decrease in the production of PTH may result in the development of hypocalcemia. This may occur with surgical removal of a portion of or injury to the parathyroid glands during thyroid or neck surgery. Acute pancreatitis is another potential cause of hypocalcemia. Lipolysis, a consequence of pancreatitis, produces fatty acids that combine with calcium ions, decreasing serum calcium levels. The patient who receives multiple blood transfusions can become hypocalcemic because the citrate used to anticoagulate the blood binds with the calcium. Sudden alkalosis may also result in symptomatic hypocalcemia despite a normal total serum calcium level. The high pH increases calcium binding to protein, decreasing the amount of ionized calcium. Hypocalcemia can occur if the diet is low in calcium or if there is increased loss of calcium with

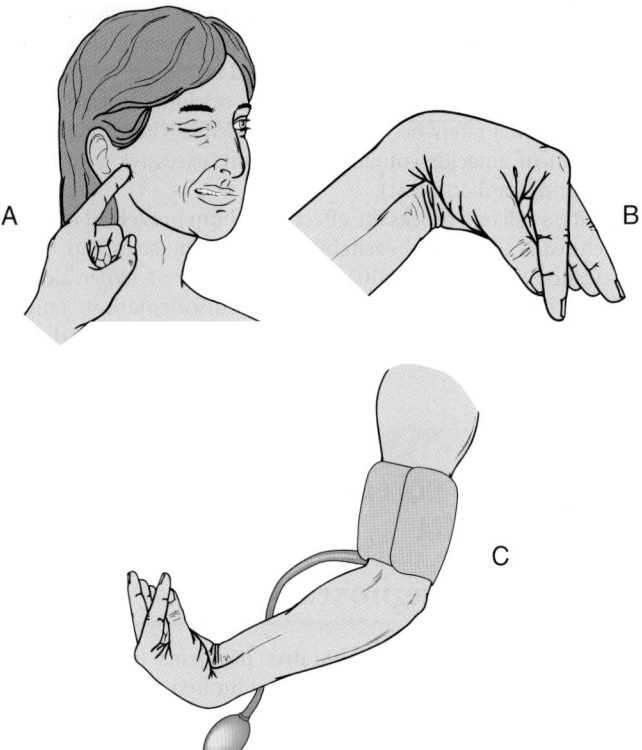

Figure 19-15 Tests for hypocalcemia. **A,** Chvostek's sign is contraction of facial muscles in response to a light tap over the facial nerve in front of the ear. **B,** Trousseau's sign is a carpal spasm induced by **C,** inflating a blood pressure cuff above the systolic pressure for a few minutes.

laxative abuse and malabsorption syndromes. (See Table 19-8 for the clinical manifestations and etiologies of hypocalcemia.)

Low calcium levels allow sodium to move into excitable cells, increasing depolarization. This results in increased nerve excitability and sustained muscle contraction that is referred to as **tetany.** Clinical signs of tetany include Trousseau's and Chvostek's signs. *Trousseau's sign* refers to carpal spasms induced by inflating a blood pressure cuff on the arm (Figure 19-15). The blood pressure cuff is inflated above the systolic pressure. Carpal spasms become evident within 3 minutes if hypocalcemia is present. *Chvostek's sign* is contraction of facial muscles in response to a tap over the facial nerve in front of the ear (see Figure 19-15), and it also indicates hypocalcemia with latent tetany. Other manifestations of tetany are laryngeal stridor, dysphagia, and numbness and tingling around the mouth or in the extremities.

Because calcium is necessary for cardiac contractions, hypocalcemia results in decreased cardiac contractility and ECG change. Clinical manifestations of hypocalcemia are listed in Table 19-8.

NURSING AND COLLABORATIVE MANAGEMENT: HYPOCALCEMIA

Nursing Diagnoses

Nursing diagnoses and collaborative problems for the patient with hypocalcemia include, but are not limited to, the following:

- Risk for injury *related to* tetany and seizures.
- Potential complications: fracture, respiratory arrest.

Nursing Implementation

Treatment of hypocalcemia is primarily aimed at correcting the cause. Hypocalcemia can be treated with oral or IV calcium supplements. Calcium is not given by the intramuscular route because it will precipitate in the muscle. IV preparations of calcium, such as calcium gluconate, are administered when severe symptoms of hypocalcemia are impending or present. A diet high in calcium-rich foods is usually ordered along with vitamin D supplements for the patient with hypocalcemia. Oral calcium supplements, such as calcium carbonate, may be used when patients are unable to consume enough calcium in the diet, such as those who do not tolerate dairy products. Pain and anxiety must be adequately treated in the patient with suspected hypocalcemia because hyperventilation-induced respiratory alkalosis can precipitate hypocalcemic symptoms. Any patient who has had thyroid or neck surgery must be observed closely in the immediate postoperative period for manifestations of hypocalcemia because of the proximity of the surgery to the parathyroid glands.

Phosphate Imbalances

Phosphorus is a primary anion in the ICF and is essential to the function of muscle, RBCs, and the nervous system. It is deposited with calcium for bone and tooth structure. It is also involved in the acid–base buffering system, in the mitochondrial energy production of ATP, in cellular uptake and use of glucose, and as an intermediary in the metabolism of carbohydrates, proteins, and fats.

Maintenance of normal phosphate balance requires adequate renal functioning because the kidneys are the major route of phosphate excretion. A small amount is lost in the feces. A reciprocal relationship exists between phosphorus and calcium in that a high serum phosphate level tends to cause a low calcium concentration in the serum.

Hyperphosphatemia

The major condition that can lead to hyperphosphatemia is acute or chronic renal failure that results in an altered ability of the kidneys to excrete phosphate. Other causes include chemotherapy for certain malignancies (lymphomas), excessive ingestion of milk or phosphate-containing laxatives, and large intakes of vitamin D that increase GI absorption of phosphorus (Table 19-9).

Clinical manifestations of hyperphosphatemia (presented in Table 19-9) primarily relate to metastatic calcium–phosphate precipitates. Ordinarily, calcium and phosphate are deposited only in bone. However, an increased serum phosphate concentration along with calcium precipitates readily, and calcified deposits can occur in soft tissue such as joints, arteries, skin, kidneys, and corneas (see Chapter 49). Other manifestations of hyperphosphatemia are neuromuscular irritability and tetany, which are related to the low serum calcium levels often associated with high serum phosphate levels.

Table 19-9 Phosphate Imbalances: Causes and Clinical Manifestations	
HYPOPHOSPHATEMIA (PO_4^{3-} <0.97 mmol/L)	**HYPERPHOSPHATEMIA** (PO_4^{3-} >1.45 mmol/L)
Causes	
• Malabsorption syndrome	• Renal failure
• Nutritional recovery syndrome	• Chemotherapeutic agents
• Glucose administration	• Enemas containing phosphorus (e.g., Fleet Enema)
• Total parenteral nutrition	• Excessive ingestion (e.g., milk, phosphate-containing laxatives)
• Alcohol withdrawal	
• Phosphate-binding antacids	
• Recovery from diabetic ketoacidosis	• Large vitamin D intake
• Respiratory alkalosis	• Hypoparathyroidism
Clinical Manifestations	
• Central nervous system dysfunction (confusion, coma)	• Hypocalcemia
• Rhabdomyolysis	• Muscle problems; tetany
• Renal tubular wasting of Mg^{2+}, Ca^{2+}, HCO_3^-	• Deposition of calcium–phosphate precipitates in skin, soft tissue, cornea, viscera, blood vessels
• Cardiac problems (dysrhythmias, decreased stroke volume)	
• Muscle weakness, including respiratory muscle weakness	
• Osteomalacia	

Table 19-10 Causes of Magnesium Imbalances	
HYPOMAGNESEMIA	**HYPERMAGNESEMIA**
• Diarrhea	• Renal failure (especially if patient is given magnesium products)
• Vomiting	
• Chronic alcoholism	
• Impaired GI absorption	• Excessive administration of magnesium for treatment of eclampsia
• Malabsorption syndrome	
• Prolonged malnutrition	• Adrenal insufficiency
• Large urine output	
• NG suction	
• Poorly controlled diabetes mellitus	
• Hyperaldosteronism	

GI, gastrointestinal; *NG*, nasogastric.

Management of hyperphosphatemia is aimed at identifying and treating the underlying cause. Ingestion of foods and fluids high in phosphorus (e.g., dairy products) should be restricted. Adequate hydration and correction of hypocalcemic conditions can enhance the renal excretion of phosphate. For the patient with renal failure, measures to reduce serum phosphate levels include calcium supplements, phosphate-binding agents or gels, and dietary phosphate restrictions (see Chapter 49).

Hypophosphatemia

Hypophosphatemia (low serum phosphate) is seen in the patient who is malnourished or has malabsorption syndromes. Other causes include alcohol withdrawal and use of phosphate-binding antacids. Hypophosphatemia may also occur during parenteral nutrition with inadequate phosphorus replacement. Table 19-9 lists causes of phosphorus imbalances.

Most of the clinical manifestations of hypophosphatemia (presented in Table 19-9) relate to a deficiency of ATP or 2,3-diphosphoglycerate (2,3-DPG), an enzyme in RBCs. Both conditions result in impaired cellular energy resources and oxygen delivery to tissues. Hemolytic anemia may occur because of the fragility of the RBCs. Acute manifestations include CNS depression, confusion, and other mental changes. Other manifestations include muscle weakness and pain, dysrhythmias, and cardiomyopathy.

Management of a mild phosphorus deficiency may involve oral supplementation and ingestion of foods high in phosphorus (e.g., dairy products). Severe hypophosphatemia can be serious

and may require IV administration of sodium phosphate or potassium phosphate. Frequent monitoring of serum phosphate levels is necessary to guide IV therapy. Sudden symptomatic hypocalcemia, secondary to increased calcium phosphorus binding, is a potential complication of IV phosphorus administration.

Magnesium Imbalances

Magnesium is the second most abundant intracellular cation. Approximately 50 to 60% of the body's magnesium is contained in bone. Magnesium functions as a coenzyme in the metabolism of carbohydrates and protein. It is also involved in metabolism of cellular nucleic acids and proteins. Magnesium concentration is regulated by GI absorption and renal excretion. The kidneys are able to conserve magnesium in times of need and excrete excesses. Factors that regulate calcium balance (e.g., PTH) appear to influence magnesium balance. Manifestations of magnesium balance are often mistaken for calcium imbalances. Because magnesium balance is related to calcium and potassium balance, all three cations should be assessed together (Kee et al., 2009). Causes of magnesium imbalances are listed in Table 19-10. Magnesium acts directly on the myoneural junction, and neuromuscular excitability is profoundly affected by alterations in serum magnesium.

Hypomagnesemia (low serum magnesium level) produces neuromuscular and CNS hyperirritability. A high serum magnesium level *(hypermagnesemia)* depresses neuromuscular and CNS functions. Magnesium is important for normal cardiac function. There is an association between hypomagnesemia and cardiac dysrhythmias, such as premature ventricular contractions and ventricular fibrillation (Kee et al., 2009). However, it is not clear how hypomagnesemia and insulin resistance are related.

Hypermagnesemia

Hypermagnesemia usually occurs only with an increase in magnesium intake accompanied by renal insufficiency or failure. A patient with chronic renal failure who ingests products containing magnesium (e.g., Maalox, milk of magnesia) will have a problem with excess magnesium. Magnesium excess could develop in the pregnant woman who receives magnesium sulphate for the management of eclampsia.

Initial clinical manifestations of a mildly elevated serum magnesium concentration include lethargy, drowsiness, and nausea and vomiting. As the levels of serum magnesium increase, deep tendon reflexes are lost; somnolence follows, and then respiratory and, ultimately, cardiac arrest can occur.

Management of hypermagnesemia should focus on prevention. Persons with renal failure should not take magnesium-containing drugs and must be cautioned to review all over-the-counter drug labels for magnesium content. The emergency treatment of hypermagnesemia is IV administration of calcium chloride or calcium gluconate to physiologically oppose the effects of the magnesium on cardiac muscle. Promoting urinary excretion with fluid will decrease serum magnesium levels. The patient with impaired renal function will require dialysis because the kidneys are the major route of excretion for magnesium.

Hypomagnesemia

A major cause of magnesium deficiency is prolonged fasting or starvation. Chronic alcoholism commonly causes hypomagnesemia as a result of insufficient food intake. Fluid loss from the GI tract interferes with magnesium absorption. Another potential cause of hypomagnesemia is prolonged parenteral nutrition without magnesium supplementation. Many diuretics increase the risk of magnesium loss through renal excretion (Kee et al., 2009). In addition, osmotic diuresis caused by high glucose levels in uncontrolled diabetes mellitus increases renal excretion of magnesium. The significant clinical manifestations include confusion, hyperactive deep tendon reflexes, tremors, and seizures. Magnesium deficiency also predisposes to cardiac dysrhythmias. Clinically, hypomagnesemia resembles hypocalcemia and may contribute to the development of hypocalcemia as a result of the decreased action of PTH. Hypomagnesemia may also be associated with hypokalemia that does not respond well to potassium replacement. This occurs because intracellular magnesium is critical to normal function of the sodium–potassium pump.

Mild magnesium deficiencies can be treated with oral supplements and increased dietary intake of foods high in magnesium (e.g., green vegetables, nuts, bananas, oranges, peanut butter, chocolate). If the condition is severe, parenteral IV or IM magnesium (e.g., magnesium sulfate) should be administered. Too rapid administration of magnesium can lead to cardiac or respiratory arrest.

Protein Imbalances

Plasma proteins, particularly albumin, are a significant determinant of plasma volume. Because of their large molecular size, they remain in the vascular space and contribute to the colloidal oncotic pressure. Causes of protein imbalances are listed in Table 19-11. Hypoproteinemia can occur over time. Causes related to intake are anorexia, malnutrition, starvation, fad dieting, and poorly balanced vegetarian diets. Poor absorption of protein can occur in certain GI malabsorptive diseases, such as pancreatic insufficiency and inflammatory bowel disease. Protein can shift out of the intravascular space with inflammation. Increased breakdown of proteins occurs with elevated basal metabolic rates and catabolic states, such as fever, infection, and certain malignancies. Increased use of protein occurs with cell growth and repair after surgical wounds or burns. Hemorrhage with loss of RBCs can be a cause of protein deficit. Impaired synthesis of

Table 19-11 Causes of Protein Imbalances	
HYPOPROTEINEMIA	**HYPERPROTEINEMIA**
• Decreased food intake	• Dehydration
• Starvation	• Hemoconcentration
• Diseased liver	
• Massive burns	
• Loss of albumin in renal disease	
• Major infection	

albumin occurs in liver failure. The kidneys can lose large amounts of protein, especially albumin, in nephrotic syndrome (see Chapter 48).

Clinical manifestations of protein deficit include edema (from decreased oncotic pressure), slow healing, anorexia, fatigue, anemia, and muscle loss that results from the breakdown of body tissue to meet the body's need for protein. Intravascular fluid readily accumulates in the peritoneal cavity, producing ascites, when the vascular oncotic pressure is decreased in hypoproteinemia.

Management of protein deficit includes providing a high-carbohydrate, high-protein diet and dietary protein supplements. If the patient cannot meet the needs for protein orally, enteral nutrition or total parenteral nutrition may be used. (Protein-calorie malnutrition is discussed in Chapter 42.)

Hyperproteinemia is rare, but it can occur with dehydration-induced hemoconcentration.

Acid–Base Imbalances

The body normally maintains a steady balance between acids produced during metabolism and bases that neutralize and promote the excretion of the acids. Many health problems may lead to acid–base imbalances in addition to fluid and electrolyte imbalances. Patients with diabetes mellitus, chronic obstructive pulmonary disease, and kidney disease frequently develop acid–base imbalances. Vomiting and diarrhea may cause loss of acids and bases in addition to fluids and electrolytes. The kidneys are an essential buffer system for acids, and in the older adult, the kidneys are less able to compensate for an acid load. The older adult also has decreased respiratory function, leading to impaired compensation for acid–base imbalances. In addition, tissue hypoxia from any cause may alter acid–base balance. The nurse must always consider the possibility of acid–base imbalance in patients with serious illnesses.

pH and Hydrogen Ion Concentration

The acidity or alkalinity of a solution depends on its hydrogen ion (H^+) concentration. An increase in H^+ concentration leads to acidity; a decrease leads to alkalinity. (Definitions related to acid–base balance are presented in Table 19-12.)

Despite the fact that acids are produced by the body daily, the H^+ concentration of body fluids is small (0.0004 mEq/L). This tiny amount is maintained within a narrow range to ensure optimal cellular function. H^+ concentration is usually expressed as a negative logarithm (symbolized as **pH**) rather than in milliequivalents. The use of the negative logarithm means that the lower the pH, the higher the H^+ concentration. In contrast

Table 19-12 Terms in Acid–Base Physiology

Acid	Donor of hydrogen ion (H⁺); separation of an acid into H⁺ and its accompanying anion in solution
Acidemia	Signifying an arterial blood pH <7.35
Acidosis	Process that adds acid or eliminates base from body fluids
Alkalemia	Signifying an arterial blood pH >7.45
Alkalosis	Process that adds base or eliminates acid from body fluids
Anion gap	Calculation approximating normally unmeasured anions in the plasma; helpful in differential diagnosis of acidosis
Base	Acceptor of hydrogen ions; chemical combining of acid and base when hydrogen ions are added to a solution containing a base; bicarbonate (HCO_3^-) is most abundant base in body fluids
Buffer	Substance that reacts with an acid or base to prevent a large change in pH
pH	Negative logarithm of the H⁺ concentration

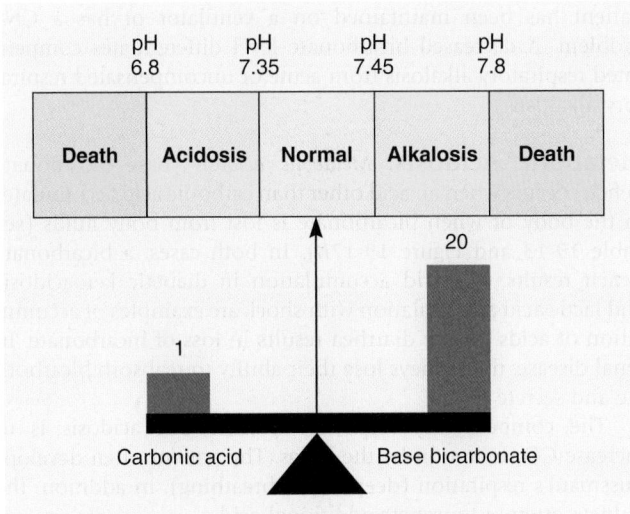

Figure 19-16 The normal range of plasma pH is 7.35 to 7.45. A normal pH is maintained by a ratio of 1 part carbonic acid to 20 parts bicarbonate.

to a pH of 7, a pH of 8 represents a ten-fold decrease in H⁺ concentration.

The pH of a chemical solution may range from 1 to 14. A solution with a pH of 7 is considered neutral. An acid solution has a pH less than 7, and an alkaline solution has a pH greater than 7. Blood is slightly alkaline (pH 7.35-7.45); if its pH drops below 7.35, the person has **acidosis,** even though the blood may never become truly acidic. If the blood pH is greater than 7.45, the person has **alkalosis** (Figure 19-16).

Acid–Base Regulation

The body's metabolic processes constantly produce acids. These acids must be neutralized and excreted to maintain acid–base balance. Normally, the body has three mechanisms by which it regulates acid–base balance to maintain the arterial pH between 7.35 and 7.45. These mechanisms are the buffer systems, the respiratory system, and the renal system.

The regulatory mechanisms react at different speeds. Buffers react immediately; the respiratory system responds in minutes and reaches maximum effectiveness in hours; and the renal response takes 2 to 3 days to respond maximally, but the kidneys can maintain balance for a long period.

Buffer System. The buffer system is the fastest-acting system and the primary regulator of acid–base balance. **Buffers** act chemically to change strong acids into weaker acids or to bind acids to neutralize their effect. The buffers in the body include carbonic acid–bicarbonate, monohydrogen–dihydrogen phosphate, intracellular and plasma protein, and hemoglobin buffers.

A buffer consists of a weakly ionized acid or a base and its salt. Buffers function to minimize the effect of acids on blood pH until they can be excreted from the body. The carbonic acid (H_2CO_3)–bicarbonate (HCO_3^-) buffer system neutralizes hydrochloric acid (HCl) in the following manner:

$$\underset{\text{(strong acid)}}{HCl} + \underset{\text{(strong base)}}{NaH_2CO_3} \rightarrow \underset{\text{(salt)}}{NaCl} + \underset{\text{(weak acid)}}{H_2CO_3}$$

In this way, HCl is prevented from making a large change in the solution's pH, and more H_2CO_3 is formed. The carbonic acid, in turn, is broken down to H_2O and CO_2. The CO_2 is excreted by the lungs. In this process, the buffer system maintains the 20:1 ratio between bicarbonate and carbonic acid and the normal pH.

The phosphate buffer system is composed of sodium and other cations in combination with HPO_4^{2-} and $H_2PO_4^-$. This buffer system acts in the same manner as the bicarbonate system. Strong acids are neutralized to form a weak acid of sodium biphosphate, which can be excreted in the urine, and NaCl:

$$Na_2HPO_4 + HCl \rightarrow NaCl + NaH_2PO_4$$

When a strong base is added to the system, it is neutralized to form a weak base and H_2O:

$$NaOH + NaH_2PO_4 \rightarrow Na_2HPO_4 + H_2O$$

Intracellular and extracellular proteins are an effective buffering system throughout the body. The protein buffering system acts like the bicarbonate system. Some of the amino acids of proteins contain free acid radicals such as —COOH, which can dissociate into CO_2 and H⁺. Other amino acids have basic radicals such as —NH₃OH, which can dissociate into NH³⁺ and OH⁻; the OH⁻ can combine with an H⁺ to form H_2O.

Using the "chloride shift" mechanism, hemoglobin regulates pH by shifting chloride in and out of RBCs in exchange for bicarbonate. This shift is regulated by the level of oxygen in blood.

The cell can also act as a buffer by shifting hydrogen in and out of the cell. With an accumulation of H⁺ in the ECF, the intracellular compartment can accept hydrogen in exchange for another cation (e.g., Na⁺).

The body buffers an acid load better than it neutralizes base excess. Buffers cannot maintain pH without the adequate functioning of the respiratory and renal systems.

Respiratory System. The lungs help maintain a normal pH by excreting CO_2 and water, which are by-products of cellular metabolism. When released into circulation, CO_2 enters

RBCs and combines with H_2O to form H_2CO_3. The carbonic acid dissociates into hydrogen ions and bicarbonate. The free hydrogen is buffered by hemoglobin molecules, and the bicarbonate diffuses into the plasma. In the pulmonary capillaries, this process is reversed, and CO_2 is formed and excreted by the lungs. The overall reversible reaction is expressed as the following:

$$CO_2 + H_2O \leftrightarrow H_2CO_3 \leftrightarrow H^+ + HCO_3^-$$

The amount of CO_2 in the blood directly relates to carbonic acid concentration and subsequently to H^+ concentration. With increased respirations, less CO_2 remains in the blood. This leads to less carbonic acid and fewer H^+. With decreased respirations, more CO_2 remains in the blood. This leads to increased carbonic acid and more H^+.

The rate of excretion of CO_2 is controlled by the respiratory centre in the medulla in the brainstem. If increased amounts of CO_2 or H^+ are present, the respiratory centre stimulates an increased rate and depth of breathing. Respirations are inhibited if the centre senses low H^+ or CO_2 levels.

As a compensatory mechanism, the respiratory system acts on the $CO_2 + H_2O$ side of the reaction by altering the rate and depth of breathing to "blow off" (through hyperventilation) or "retain" (through hypoventilation) CO_2. If a respiratory problem is the cause of an acid–base imbalance (e.g., respiratory failure), the respiratory system cannot play its usual role to correct a pH alteration.

Renal System. Under normal conditions, the kidneys reabsorb and conserve all of the bicarbonate they filter. The kidneys can generate additional bicarbonate and eliminate excess H^+ as compensation for acidosis. The three mechanisms of acid elimination include (1) secretion of small amounts of free hydrogen into the renal tubule, (2) combination of H^+ with ammonia (NH_3) to form ammonium (NH_4^-), and (3) excretion of weak acids.

The body depends on the kidneys to excrete a portion of the acid produced by cellular metabolism. Thus, the kidneys normally excrete an acidic urine (average pH = 6). As a compensatory mechanism, the pH of the urine can decrease to 4 and increase to 8. If the renal system is the cause of an acid–base imbalance (e.g., renal failure), it loses its ability to correct a pH alteration.

Alterations in Acid–Base Balance

An acid–base imbalance is produced when the ratio of 1:20 between acid and base content is altered (Table 19-13). A primary disease or process may alter one side of the ratio (e.g., CO_2 retention in pulmonary disease). The compensatory process attempts to maintain the other side of the ratio (e.g., increased renal bicarbonate reabsorption). When the compensatory mechanism fails, an acid–base imbalance results. The compensatory process may be inadequate because either the pathophysiological process is overwhelming or there is insufficient time for the compensatory process to function.

Acid–base imbalances are classified as respiratory or metabolic. *Respiratory imbalances* affect carbonic acid concentrations; *metabolic imbalances* affect the base bicarbonate. Therefore, acidosis can be caused by an increase in carbonic acid (respiratory acidosis) or a decrease in bicarbonate (metabolic acidosis). Alkalosis can be caused by a decrease in carbonic acid (respiratory alkalosis) or an increase in bicarbonate (metabolic alkalosis). Imbalances may be further classified as acute or chronic. Chronic imbalances allow greater time for compensatory changes.

Respiratory Acidosis. *Respiratory acidosis* (carbonic acid excess) occurs whenever there is hypoventilation (see Table 19-13). Hypoventilation results in a buildup of CO_2; subsequently, carbonic acid accumulates in the blood. Carbonic acid dissociates, liberating H^-, and there is a decrease in pH. If CO_2 is not eliminated from the blood, acidosis results from the accumulation of carbonic acid (Figure 19-17A).

To compensate, the kidneys conserve bicarbonate and secrete increased concentrations of H^+ into the urine. In acute respiratory acidosis, the renal compensatory mechanisms begin to operate within 24 hours. Therefore, even in anticipation of the kidneys' compensating for the imbalance, a normal serum bicarbonate level usually can be found.

Respiratory Alkalosis. *Respiratory alkalosis* (carbonic acid deficit) occurs with hyperventilation (see Table 19-13). Anxiety, CNS disorders, sepsis, and mechanical overventilation all increase ventilation and decrease the partial pressure of carbon dioxide (PCO_2; the amount of CO_2 gas dissolved in the blood). This leads to decreased carbonic acid and alkalosis (see Figure 19-17A).

Compensated respiratory alkalosis is uncommon unless the patient has been maintained on a ventilator or has a CNS problem. A decreased bicarbonate level differentiates compensated respiratory alkalosis from acute or uncompensated respiratory alkalosis.

Metabolic Acidosis. *Metabolic acidosis* (base bicarbonate deficit) occurs when an acid other than carbonic acid accumulates in the body or when bicarbonate is lost from body fluids (see Table 19-13 and Figure 19-17B). In both cases, a bicarbonate deficit results. Ketoacid accumulation in diabetic ketoacidosis and lactic acid accumulation with shock are examples of accumulation of acids. Severe diarrhea results in loss of bicarbonate. In renal disease, the kidneys lose their ability to reabsorb bicarbonate and secrete H^+.

The compensatory response to metabolic acidosis is to increase CO_2 excretion by the lungs. The patient often develops Kussmaul's respiration (deep, rapid breathing). In addition, the kidneys attempt to excrete additional acid.

Metabolic Alkalosis. *Metabolic alkalosis* (base bicarbonate excess) occurs when a loss of acid (prolonged vomiting or gastric suction) or a gain in bicarbonate (ingestion of baking soda) occurs (see Table 19-13 and Figure 19-17B). The compensatory mechanism is a decreased respiratory rate to increase plasma CO_2. Renal excretion of bicarbonate also occurs.

Mixed Acid–Base Disorders. A mixed acid–base disorder occurs when two or more simple disorders are present at the same time. The pH will depend on type, severity, and acuity of each of the simple disorders involved. Respiratory acidosis combined with metabolic alkalosis (e.g., chronic obstructive pulmonary disease treated with diuretic therapy) may result in a near-normal pH, whereas respiratory acidosis combined with metabolic acidosis will cause a greater decrease in pH than either disorder alone. An example of a mixed acidosis appears in a patient in cardiopulmonary arrest. Hypoventilation elevates the CO_2 level, and anaerobic metabolism produces lactic acid. An example of a mixed alkalosis is the case of a patient who is hyperventilating

Table 19-13 Acid–Base Imbalances

COMMON CAUSES	PATHOPHYSIOLOGY	LABORATORY FINDINGS
Respiratory Acidosis		
• Chronic obstructive pulmonary disease	• CO_2 retention from hypoventilation	• ↓ Plasma pH
• Barbiturate or sedative overdose		• ↑ PCO_2
• Chest wall abnormality (e.g., obesity)	• Compensatory response to HCO_3^- retention by kidney	• HCO_3^- normal (uncompensated)
• Severe pneumonia		• ↑ HCO_3^- (compensated)
• Atelectasis		• Urine pH >6 (compensated)
• Respiratory muscle weakness (e.g., Guillain-Barré syndrome)		
• Mechanical hypoventilation		
Respiratory Alkalosis		
• Hyperventilation (caused by hypoxia, pulmonary emboli, anxiety, fear, pain, exercise, fever)	• Increased CO_2 excretion from hyperventilation	• ↑Plasma pH
		• ↓ PCO_2
• Stimulated respiratory centre caused by septicemia, encephalitis, brain injury, salicylate poisoning	• Compensatory response of HCO_3^- excretion by kidney	• HCO_3^- normal (uncompensated)
		• ↓ HCO_3^- (compensated)
• Mechanical hyperventilation		• Urine pH >6 (compensated)
Metabolic Acidosis		
• Diabetic ketoacidosis	• Gain of fixed acid, inability to excrete acid or loss of base	• ↓ Plasma pH
• Lactic acidosis		• PCO_2 normal (uncompensated)
• Starvation	• Compensatory response of CO_2 excretion by lungs	• ↓ PCO_2 (compensated)
• Severe diarrhea		• ↓ HCO_3^-
• Renal tubular acidosis		• Urine pH >6 (compensated)
• Renal failure		
• Gastrointestinal fistulas		
• Shock		
Metabolic Alkalosis		
• Severe vomiting	• Loss of strong acid or gain of base	• ↑ Plasma pH
• Excess gastric suctioning		• PCO_2 normal (uncompensated)
• Diuretic therapy*	• Compensatory response of CO_2 retention by lungs	• ↑ PCO_2 (compensated)
• Potassium deficit		• ↑ HCO_3^-
• Excess $NaHCO_3$ intake		• Urine pH >6 (compensated)
• Excessive mineralocorticoids		

PCO_2, partial pressure of CO_2.
*Commonly used diuretics such as thiazides and furosemide are known to produce mild alkalosis by affecting tubular excretion of electrolytes and bicarbonate.

because of postoperative pain and is also losing acid secondary to nasogastric suctioning.

Clinical Manifestations

Clinical manifestations of acidosis and alkalosis are summarized in Tables 19-14 and 19-15. Because a normal pH is vital to all cellular reactions, the clinical manifestations of acid–base imbalances are generalized and nonspecific. The actual compensatory mechanisms also produce some clinical manifestations. For example, the deep, rapid respirations of a patient with metabolic acidosis are an example of respiratory compensation. In alkalosis, hypocalcemia may concurrently be found and accounts for many of the clinical manifestations.

Blood Gas Values. Arterial blood gas (ABG) values provide valuable information about a patient's acid–base status,

the origin of the imbalance, an idea of the body's ability to regulate pH, and a reflection of the patient's overall oxygen status. Diagnosis of acid–base disturbances and identification of compensatory processes are done by performing the following five steps:

1. Determine whether the pH is acidotic or alkalotic. Use 7.4 as the starting point. Label values less than 7.4 as acidotic and values greater than 7.4 as alkalotic.
2. Analyze the PCO_2 to determine whether the patient has respiratory acidosis or alkalosis. CO_2 is controlled by the lungs and is thus considered the respiratory component of the ABG. Because CO_2 forms carbonic acid when dissolved in blood, high CO_2 levels indicate acidosis and low CO_2 levels indicate alkalosis.
3. Analyze the HCO_3^- to determine whether the patient has metabolic acidosis or alkalosis. HCO_3^-, the metabolic component of the ABG, is controlled primarily by the kidneys.

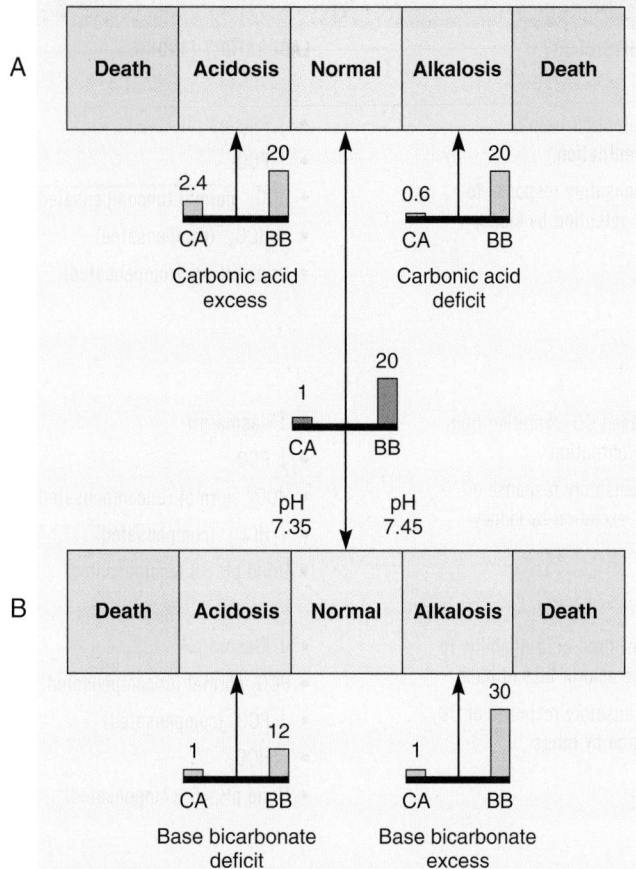

Figure 19-17 Kinds of acid–base imbalances. **A,** Respiratory imbalances caused by carbonic acid (CA) excess and CA deficit. BB, base bicarbonate. **B,** Metabolic imbalances caused by BB deficit and BB excess.

Table 19-14 Clinical Manifestations of Acidosis	
RESPIRATORY (↑ PCO₂)	**METABOLIC (↓ HCO₃⁻)**
Neurological	
• Drowsiness	• Drowsiness
• Disorientation	• Confusion
• Dizziness	• Headache
• Headache	• Coma
• Coma	
Cardiovascular	
• ↓ Blood pressure	• ↓ Blood pressure
• Ventricular fibrillation (related to hyperkalemia from compensation)	• Dysrhythmias (related to hyperkalemia from compensation)
• Warm, flushed skin (related to peripheral vasodilation)	• Warm, flushed skin (related to peripheral vasodilation)
Gastrointestinal	
• No significant findings	• Nausea, vomiting, diarrhea, abdominal pain
Neuromuscular	
• Seizures	• No significant findings
Respiratory	
• Hypoventilation with hypoxia (lungs are unable to compensate when there is a respiratory problem)	• Deep, rapid respirations (compensatory action by the lungs)

PCO_2, partial pressure of CO_2.

Because HCO_3^- is a base, high levels of HCO_3^- result in alkalosis and low levels result in acidosis.

4. Determine whether the CO_2 or the HCO_3^- matches the acid or base alteration of the pH. For example, if the pH is acidotic and the CO_2 is high (respiratory acidosis) but the HCO_3^- is high (metabolic alkalosis), the CO_2 is the parameter that matches the pH derangement. The patient's acid–base imbalance would be diagnosed as respiratory acidosis.

5. Decide whether the body is attempting to compensate for the pH change. If the parameter that does not match the pH is moving in the opposite direction, the body is attempting to compensate. In step 4, the HCO_3^- is alkalotic; this is in the opposite direction of respiratory acidosis and considered compensation. If compensatory mechanisms are functioning, the pH will return toward 7.4. When the pH is back to normal, the patient has *full compensation*. The body will not overcompensate for pH changes.

Table 19-16 lists normal blood gas values, and Table 19-17 provides a sample ABG with interpretation. (Refer to the laboratory findings column of Table 19-13 for the ABG findings of the four major acid–base disturbances.) Table 19-18 shows how the ROME (respiratory, opposite, metabolic, equivalent) mnemonic can be used for understanding acid–base imbalances.

Knowledge of the patient's clinical situation and the physiological extent of renal and respiratory compensation enables the clinician to identify mixed acid–base disorders.

Blood gas analysis will also show the PCO_2 and oxygen saturation. These values are used to identify hypoxemia. ABGs are usually obtained. The values of blood gases differ slightly between arterial and venous samples (see Table 19-16). (Blood gases are discussed further in Chapter 28.)

Assessment of Fluid, Electrolyte, and Acid–Base Imbalances

Subjective Data

Important Health Information

Past Health History. The patient should be questioned about any past health history of problems involving the kidneys, the heart, the GI system, or the lungs that could affect the present fluid, electrolyte, and acid–base balance. Information about specific diseases such as diabetes mellitus, diabetes insipidus, chronic obstructive pulmonary disease, ulcerative colitis, and Crohn's disease should be obtained from the patient. The patient should also be questioned about the incidence of a prior fluid, electrolyte, or acid–base disorder.

Medications. An assessment of the patient's current and past use of medications is important. The ingredients in many drugs,

Table 19-15 Clinical Manifestations of Alkalosis

RESPIRATORY ($\downarrow$ PCO$_2$)	METABOLIC ($\uparrow$ HCO$_3^-$)
Neurological	
• Lethargy	• Dizziness
• Lightheadedness	• Irritability
• Confusion	• Nervousness
	• Confusion
Cardiovascular	
• Tachycardia	• Tachycardia
• Dysrhythmias (related to hypokalemia from compensation)	• Dysrhythmias (related to hypokalemia from compensation)
Gastrointestinal	
• Nausea	• Anorexia
• Vomiting	• Nausea
• Epigastric pain	• Vomiting
Neuromuscular*	
• Tetany	• Tremors
• Numbness	• Hypertonic muscles
• Tingling of extremities	• Muscle cramps
• Hyperreflexia	• Tetany
• Seizures	• Tingling of fingers and toes
Respiratory	
• Hyperventilation (lungs are unable to compensate when there is a respiratory problem)	• Hypoventilation (compensatory action by the lungs)

PCO$_2$, Partial pressure of CO$_2$.
*Alkalosis decreases calcium binding to protein.

Table 19-16 Normal Arterial and Venous Blood Gas Values

PARAMETER	ARTERIAL	VENOUS
pH	7.35-7.45	7.31-7.41
PCO$_2$	35-45 mm Hg	SvO$_2$ is a better indicator of change in acid–base balance
Bicarbonate (HCO$_3^-$)	21-28 mmol/L	21-28 mmol/L
PO$_2$*	80-100 mm Hg	40-50 mm Hg
SvO$_2$	$\geq$95%	60-80%
Base excess	$\pm$2.0 mEq/L	$\pm$2.0 mEq/L

PCO$_2$, partial pressure of carbon dioxide; *PO$_2$*, partial pressure of oxygen; *SvO$_2$*, venous oxygen saturation.
*Decreases above sea level and with increasing age.

especially over-the-counter drugs, are often overlooked as sources of sodium, potassium, calcium, magnesium, and other electrolytes. Many prescription drugs, including diuretics, corticosteroids, and electrolyte supplements, can cause fluid and electrolyte problems.

Surgery or Other Treatments. The patient should be asked about past or present renal dialysis, kidney surgery, or bowel

Table 19-17 Arterial Blood Gas (ABG) Analysis

ABG VALUES	ANALYSIS
pH 7.30 PCO$_2$ 25 mm Hg HCO$_3^-$ 16 mEq/L	1. pH <7.4 indicates acidosis. 2. PCO$_2$ is low, indicating respiratory alkalosis. 3. HCO$_3^-$ is low, indicating metabolic acidosis. 4. Metabolic acidosis matches the pH. 5. The CO$_2$ does not match but is moving in the opposite direction, which indicates the lungs are attempting to compensate for the metabolic acidosis.

Interpretation

This ABG is interpreted as metabolic acidosis with partial compensation. If the pH returns to the normal range, the patient is said to have full compensation.

ABG, arterial blood gas; *HCO$_3^-$*, bicarbonate; *PCO$_2$*, partial pressure of CO$_2$.

Table 19-18 ROME: Memory Device for Acid–Base Imbalances

For acid–base imbalances, the mnemonic Rome can be used.
In **Respiratory** conditions, the pH and the PaCO$_2$ go in **Opposite** directions.
- In respiratory alkalosis, the pH is $\uparrow$ and the PaCO$_2$ is $\downarrow$.
- In respiratory acidosis, the pH is $\downarrow$ and the PaCO$_2$ is $\uparrow$.

In **Metabolic** conditions, the pH and the HCO$_3^-$ go in the same direction (equal or **Equivalent**). The PaCO$_2$ may also go in the same direction.
- In metabolic alkalosis, pH and HCO$_3^-$ are $\uparrow$ and the PaCO$_2$ is $\uparrow$ or normal.
- In metabolic acidosis, pH and HCO$_3^-$ are $\downarrow$ and the PaCO$_2$ is $\downarrow$ or normal.

Respiratory		pH	PaCO$_2$
Opposite	Acidosis	$\downarrow$	$\uparrow$
	Alkalosis	$\uparrow$	$\downarrow$
Metabolic		**pH**	**HCO$_3^-$**
Equivalent	Acidosis	$\downarrow$	$\downarrow$
	Alkalosis	$\uparrow$	$\uparrow$

HCO$_3^-$, bicarbonate; *PaCO$_2$*, arterial partial pressure of carbon dioxide.

surgery resulting in a temporary or permanent external collecting system such as a colostomy or nephrostomy.

Other Subjective Data. If the patient is currently experiencing a problem related to fluid, electrolyte, and acid–base balance, a careful description of the illness, including onset, course, and treatment, should be obtained.

The patient should be questioned regarding diet, especially whether she or he has been on a special diet such as a weight-reducing, low-sodium, or fad diet. If the patient is on a special diet, such as low sodium or high potassium, her or his ability to comply with the dietary prescription should be determined.

Note should be made of the patient's usual bowel and bladder habits. Any deviations from the expected elimination pattern, such as diarrhea, nocturia, or polyuria, should be carefully documented.

The patient's exercise pattern is important to determine because excessive perspiration secondary to exercise could result in a fluid and electrolyte problem. Also, the patient's exposure to extremely high temperatures as a result of leisure or work activity should be determined. The patient should be asked what practices are followed to replace fluid and electrolytes lost through excessive perspiration.

The patient should be queried about any changes in sensations, such as numbness, tingling, *fasciculations* (uncoordinated twitching of a single muscle group), or muscle weakness, that could indicate a fluid and electrolyte problem. In addition, both the patient and the caregivers should be asked whether any changes in mentation or alertness have been noted, such as confusion, memory impairment, or lethargy.

Objective Data

Physical Examination.
There is no specific physical examination to assess fluid, electrolyte, and acid–base balance. Common abnormal assessment findings of major body systems offer clues to possible imbalances (Table 19-19).

Laboratory Values.
Assessment of serum electrolyte values is a good starting point for identifying fluid and electrolyte imbalance (see Table 19-3). However, serum electrolyte values often provide only cursory information. They reflect the concentration of that electrolyte in the ECF but do not necessarily provide information concerning the concentration of the electrolyte in the ICF. For example, the majority of the potassium in the body is found intracellularly. Changes in serum potassium values may be the result of a true deficit or excess of potassium or may reflect the movement of potassium into or out of the cell over the course of acid–base imbalances.

An abnormal serum sodium level may reflect a sodium problem or, more likely, a water problem. A reduced hematocrit value could indicate anemia, or it could be caused by fluid volume excess. Other laboratory tests that are helpful in evaluating the presence of or risk for fluid, electrolyte, and acid–base imbalances include serum and urine osmolality, serum glucose, BUN (serum urea [nitrogen]), serum creatinine, urine specific gravity, and urine electrolytes.

In addition to arterial and venous blood gases, serum electrolytes can provide important information concerning a patient's acid–base balance. Changes in the serum bicarbonate (often reported as total CO_2 or CO_2 content on an electrolyte panel) will indicate the presence of metabolic acidosis (low bicarbonate level) or alkalosis (high bicarbonate level). Calculation of the *anion gap* (serum sodium level minus chloride and bicarbonate levels) can help determine the source of metabolic acidosis. The anion gap is increased in metabolic acidosis associated with acid gain (e.g., lactic acidosis, diabetic ketoacidosis) but remains normal (10-14 mmol/L) in metabolic acidosis caused by bicarbonate loss (e.g., diarrhea).

COMMON ASSESSMENT ABNORMALITIES
Table 19-19 Fluid and Electrolyte Imbalances

FINDING	POSSIBLE CAUSE
Skin	
Poor skin turgor	Fluid volume deficit
Cold, clammy skin	Na^+ deficit, shift of plasma to interstitial fluid
Pitting edema	Fluid volume excess
Flushed, dry skin	Na^+ excess
Pulse	
Bounding pulse	Fluid volume excess, shift of interstitial fluid to plasma
Rapid, weak, thready pulse	Shift of plasma to interstitial fluid, Na^+ deficit, fluid volume deficit
Weak, irregular, rapid pulse	Severe K^+ deficit
Weak, irregular, slow pulse	Severe K^+ excess
Blood Pressure	
Hypotension	Fluid volume deficit, shift of plasma to interstitial fluid, Na^+ deficit
Hypertension	Fluid volume excess, shift of interstitial fluid to plasma
Respirations	
Deep, rapid breathing	Compensation for metabolic acidosis
Shallow, slow, irregular breathing	Compensation for metabolic alkalosis
Shortness of breath	Fluid volume excess
Moist crackles	Fluid volume excess, shift of interstitial fluid to plasma
Skeletal Muscles	
Cramping of exercised muscle	Ca^{2+} deficit, Mg^{2+} deficit, alkalosis
Carpal spasm (Trousseau's sign)	Ca^{2+} deficit, Mg^{2+} deficit, alkalosis
Flabby muscles	K^+ deficit
Positive Chvostek's sign	Ca^{2+} deficit, Mg^{2+} deficit, alkalosis
Behaviour or Mental State	
Picking at bedclothes	K^+ deficit, Mg^{2+} deficit
Indifference	Fluid volume deficit, Na^+ deficit
Apprehension	Shift of plasma to interstitial fluid
Extreme restlessness	K^+ excess, fluid volume deficit
Confusion and irritability	K^+ deficit, fluid volume excess, Ca^{2+} excess, Mg^{2+} excess, H_2O excess
Decreased level of consciousness	H_2O excess

Oral Fluid and Electrolyte Replacement

In all cases of fluid, electrolyte, and acid–base imbalances, the treatment is directed toward correction of the underlying cause. The specific diseases or disorders that cause these imbalances are discussed in various chapters throughout this text. Mild fluid and electrolyte deficits can be corrected using oral rehydration solutions containing water, electrolytes, and glucose. Glucose not only provides calories but also promotes sodium absorption in the small intestine. Commercial oral rehydration solutions are now available in markets and pharmacies for home use.

Intravenous Fluid and Electrolyte Replacement

IV fluid and electrolyte therapy are commonly used to treat many different fluid and electrolyte imbalances. Many patients need maintenance IV fluid therapy only while they cannot take oral fluids (e.g., during and after surgery). Other patients need corrective or replacement therapy for losses that have already occurred. The amount and the type of solution are determined by the normal daily maintenance requirements and by imbalances identified by laboratory results. Table 19-20 provides a list of commonly prescribed IV solutions. The available selections have remained fairly constant over the years. With IV fluid

Table 19-20 Composition and Use of Commonly Prescribed Crystalloid Solutions

SOLUTION	TONICITY	mOsm/kg	GLUCOSE (g/L)	INDICATIONS AND CONSIDERATIONS
Dextrose in Water				
5%	Isotonic, but physiologically hypotonic	278	50	• Provides free water necessary for renal excretion of solutes • Used to replace water losses and treat hypernatremia • Provides 170 cal/L • Does not provide any electrolytes
10%	Hypertonic	556	100	• Provides free water only, no electrolytes • Provides 340 cal/L
Saline (NaCl)				
0.45%	Hypotonic	154	0	• Provides free water in addition to Na^+ and Cl^- • Used to replace hypotonic fluid losses • Used as maintenance solution, although it does not replace daily losses of other electrolytes • Provides no calories
0.9%	Isotonic	308	0	• Used to expand intravascular volume and replace extracellular fluid losses • Only solution that may be administered with blood products • Contains Na^+ and Cl^- in excess of plasma levels • Does not provide free water, calories, other electrolytes • May cause intravascular overload or hyperchloremic acidosis
3.0%	Hypertonic	1026	0	• Used to treat symptomatic hyponatremia • Must be administered slowly and with extreme caution because it may cause dangerous intravascular volume overload and pulmonary edema
Dextrose in Saline				
5% in 0.225%	Isotonic	355	50	• Provides Na^+, Cl^-, and free water • Used to replace hypotonic losses and treat hypernatremia • Provides 170 cal/L
5% in 0.45%	Hypertonic	432	50	• Same as 0.45% NaCl except provides 170 cal/L
5% in 0.9%	Hypertonic	586	50	• Same as 0.9% NaCl except provides 170 cal/L
Multiple Electrolyte Solutions				
Ringer's solution	Isotonic	309	0	• Similar in composition to plasma except that it has excess Cl^-, no Mg^{2+}, and no HCO_3^- • Does not provide free water or calories • Used to expand the intravascular volume and replace extracellular fluid losses
Lactated Ringer's (Hartmann's) solution	Isotonic	274	0	• Similar in composition to normal plasma except does not contain Mg^{2+} • Used to treat losses from burns and lower GI tract • May be used to treat mild metabolic acidosis but should not be used to treat lactic acidosis • Does not provide free water or calories

GI, gastrointestinal.
Source: Adapted from Heitz, U. E., & Horne, M. M. (2005). *Pocket guide to fluid, electrolyte, and acid-base balance* (5th ed., p. 70, Table 6-3). St. Louis: Mosby.

replacement therapy, local complications may occur, including phlebitis, ecchymosis, extravascular fluid infiltration, infection, thrombosis, and venous spasm. Systemic complications may also occur, such as bacteremia and sepsis, air embolism, and pulmonary edema.

Solutions

Hypotonic. A hypotonic solution provides more water than electrolytes, diluting the ECF. Osmosis then produces a movement of water from the ECF to the ICF. After osmotic equilibrium has been achieved, the ICF and the ECF have the same osmolality, and both compartments have been expanded. Examples of hypotonic fluids are given in Table 19-20. Maintenance fluids are usually hypotonic solutions (e.g., 0.45% NaCl [saline]) because normal daily losses are hypotonic. Additional electrolytes (e.g., KCl) may be added to maintain normal levels. Hypotonic solutions have the potential to cause cellular swelling, and patients should be monitored for changes in mentation that may indicate cerebral edema (Porth, 2010).

Although 5% dextrose in water is considered an isotonic solution, the dextrose is quickly metabolized, and the net result is the administration of free water (hypotonic) with proportionately equal expansion of the ECF and ICF. One litre of a 5% dextrose solution provides 50 g of dextrose, or 170 calories. Although this amount of dextrose is not enough to meet caloric requirements, it helps prevent ketosis associated with starvation. Pure water must not be administered intravenously because it would cause hemolysis of RBCs.

Isotonic. Administration of an isotonic solution expands only the ECF. There is no net loss or gain from the ICF. An isotonic solution is the ideal fluid replacement for a patient with an ECF volume deficit. Examples of isotonic solutions include lactated Ringer's solution and 0.9% NaCl. Lactated Ringer's solution contains sodium, potassium, chloride, calcium, and lactate (the precursor of bicarbonate) in about the same concentrations as those of the ECF. It is contraindicated for use in the presence of lactic acidosis because of the body's decreased ability to convert lactate to bicarbonate.

Isotonic saline (0.9% NaCl) has a sodium concentration (154 mmol/L) somewhat higher than plasma (135-145 mmol/L) and a chloride concentration (154 mmol/L) significantly higher than the plasma chloride level (98-106 mmol/L or mEq/L). Thus, excessive administration of isotonic NaCl can result in elevated sodium and chloride levels. Isotonic saline may be used when a patient has experienced both fluid and sodium losses or as vascular fluid replacement in hypovolemic shock.

Hypertonic. A hypertonic solution initially raises the osmolality of ECF and expands it. It is useful in treatment of hypovolemia and hyponatremia. Examples are listed in Table 19-20. In addition, the higher osmotic pressure draws water out of the cells into the ECF. Hypertonic solutions (e.g., 3% NaCl) necessitate frequent monitoring of blood pressure, lung sounds, and serum sodium levels and should be used with caution because of the risk for intravascular fluid volume excess as well as intracellular dehydration (Porth, 2010).

Although concentrated dextrose and water solutions (≥10% dextrose) are hypertonic solutions, once the dextrose is metabolized, the net result is the administration of water. The free water provided by these solutions will ultimately expand both the ECF and the ICF. The primary use of these solutions is in the provi-

sion of calories. Concentrated dextrose solutions may be combined with amino acid solutions, electrolytes, vitamins, and trace elements to provide total parenteral nutrition (see Chapter 42). Solutions containing 10% dextrose or less may be administered through a peripheral IV line. Solutions with greater concentrations of dextrose must be administered through a central line so that there is adequate dilution to prevent shrinkage of RBCs.

Intravenous Additives. In addition to the basic solutions that provide water and a minimum amount of calories and electrolytes, there are additives to replace specific losses. These additives were mentioned previously during the discussion of the particular electrolyte deficiencies. KCl, CaCl, $MgSO_4$, and HCO_3^- are common additives to the basic IV solutions.

Recommendations for giving potassium vary, but in general, no more than 10 to 20 mEq per hour is considered safe for routine administration. Potassium can be safely diluted as 40 mEq/L of solution, with a maximum of 60 mEq/L. It must never be administered undiluted or by IV push because it can cause fatal cardiac reactions.

Plasma Expanders. Plasma expanders stay in the vascular space and increase the osmotic pressure. Plasma expanders include colloids, dextran, and hetastarch. Colloids are protein solutions such as plasma, albumin, and commercial plasmas. Albumin is available in 5% and 25% solutions. The 5% solution has an albumin concentration similar to that of plasma and will expand the intravascular fluid millilitre for millilitre. In contrast, the 25% albumin solution is hypertonic and will draw additional fluid from the interstitium. Dextran is a complex synthetic sugar. Because dextran is metabolized slowly, it remains in the vascular system for a prolonged period but not as long as the colloids. It pulls additional fluid into the intravascular space. (Indications for plasma volume expanders are discussed in Chapter 69.)

If the patient has lost blood, whole blood or packed RBCs are necessary. Packed RBCs have the advantage of giving the patient primarily RBCs; the blood bank can use the plasma for blood components. Whole blood, with its additional fluid volume, may cause circulatory overload. Although packed cells have a decreased plasma volume, they will increase the oncotic pressure and pull fluid into the intravascular space. Loop diuretics may be administered with blood to prevent symptoms of fluid volume excess in anemic patients who are not volume depleted. (Administration of blood is discussed in Chapter 33.)

Central Venous Access Devices

Central venous access devices (CVADs) are catheters that are placed in large blood vessels (e.g., subclavian vein, jugular vein) of people who require frequent access to the vascular system. In contrast to CVADs, the basic IV catheter is inserted into a peripheral vein in the hand, inside of the arm, or antecubital fossa and is used for short-term IV access. Central venous access can be achieved by three different methods: centrally inserted catheters, peripherally inserted central catheters (PICCs), or implanted ports. Centrally inserted catheters and implanted ports must be placed by a physician whereas PICCs can be inserted by a nurse with specialized training.

CVADs permit frequent, continuous, rapid, or intermittent administration of fluids and medications. They allow for the

Do Heparin Flushes of Central Venous Catheters Decrease Occlusions?

Clinical Question

For patients with intermittently used central venous catheters (P), do heparin solution flushes (I) versus normal saline flushes (C) decrease catheter occlusions (O)?

Best Available Evidence

Systematic review of 2 previous systematic reviews, 6 clinical practice guidelines, and 22 research articles

Critical Appraisal and Synthesis of Evidence

- Adult patients with a central venous catheter or peripherally inserted central catheter. Excluded patients with implanted ports.
- Outcomes were catheter patency, catheter-related bloodstream infections (CRBSIs), and heparin-induced thrombocytopenia (HIT) rates.
- Weak evidence that heparin flushing reduces catheter occlusions.
- No evidence that heparin flushing reduces bloodstream infections.

Conclusions

- Insufficient evidence exists on effectiveness of flushing catheters with heparin.
- More trials are needed on central venous access maintenance procedures to guide evidence-informed practice.

Implications for Nursing Practice

- Maintenance of catheter patency is critical.
- Flushing devices with saline solution may be a safe and effective alternative to heparin flushes for catheter maintenance.

Reference for Evidence

Mitchell, M. M., Anderson, B. J., Williams, K., & Umscheid, C. A. (2009). Heparin flushing and other interventions to maintain patency of central venous catheters: A systematic review. *Journal of Advanced Nursing*, *65*(10), 2007-2021. doi:10.1111/j.1365-2648.2009.05103.x

P, patient population of interest; *I*, intervention or area of interest; *C*, comparison of interest or comparison group; *O*, outcome(s) of interest (see p. 6).

Table 19-21 Indications for Central Venous Access Device*

MEDICAL CONDITION	INDICATIONS FOR USE
Medication administration	
Cancer	Chemotherapy, infuse irritating or vesicant medications
Infection	Long-term administration of antibiotics
Pain	Long-term administration of pain medication
Drugs at risk to cause phlebitis	Epoprostenol (Flolan), calcium chloride, potassium chloride, amiodarone (Cordarone)
Nutritional replacement	Infusion of PN
	Able to infuse higher dextrose solutions through CVAD than peripheral line
Blood samples	Multiple blood draws for diagnostic tests over a period of time
Blood transfusions	Infusion of blood or blood products acutely, as well as over a period of time
Renal failure	Perform hemodialysis (especially on an acute basis) or continuous renal replacement therapy
Shock, burns	Infusion of high volumes of fluid and electrolyte replacement
Hemodynamic monitoring	Used to measure CVP to assess fluid balance
Heart failure	Perform ultrafiltration
Autoimmune disorders	Perform plasmapheresis

CVAD, central venous access device; *CVP*, central venous pressure; *PN*, parenteral nutrition.
*This list is not all-inclusive, and these are examples only.

of or damage to the device being used. The major disadvantages of CVADs are an increased risk of systemic infection and the invasiveness of the procedure.

Centrally Inserted Catheters

Centrally inserted catheters (also called central venous catheters [CVCs]) are inserted into a vein in the neck or chest (subclavian or jugular) or groin (femoral) with the tip resting in the distal end of the superior vena cava (Figure 19-18). These catheters are single-, double-, triple-, or quadruple-lumen catheters, and they are inserted with the aid of local or general anaesthesia. The other end of the catheter is either nontunnelled or tunnelled through subcutaneous tissue and exits through a separate incision on the chest or abdominal wall. A Dacron cuff on the catheter serves to stabilize the catheter and may decrease the incidence of infection by impeding bacteria migration along the catheter beyond the cuff. Accurate placement must be verified by chest radiograph before the catheter can be used. Care requirements include injection cap change, cleansing, flushing, and dressing change. The exact frequency and procedures for these requirements vary and are outlined in the institution's policy.

administration of drugs that are potential vesicants, blood and blood products, and parenteral nutrition. They may also be used for hemodynamic monitoring and venous blood sampling. These devices are indicated for patients who have limited peripheral vascular access or who have a projected need for long-term vascular access. Table 19-21 provides examples of medical conditions in which CVADs are used. The Infusion Nurses Society recommends considering a long-term CVAD if the patient will need therapy for more than 1 year (Ludeman, 2007).

Advantages of CVADs include a reduced need for multiple venipunctures, decreased risk of extravasation injury, and immediate access to the central venous system. Although the incidence is decreased, extravasation can still occur if there is displacement

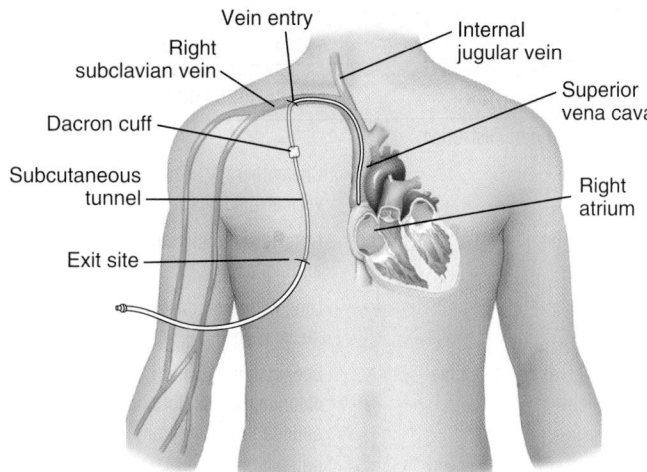

Figure 19-18 Tunnelled central venous catheter. Note tip of the catheter in the superior vena cava.

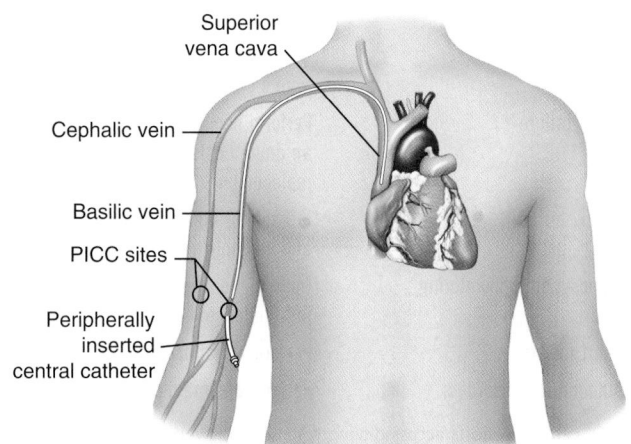

Figure 19-19 Peripherally inserted central catheter (PICC) can be inserted using the basilic or cephalic vein.

Specific types of long-term central catheters are Hickman catheters, which require clamps to make sure the valve is closed, and Groshong catheters, which have a valve that opens as fluid is withdrawn or infused and remains closed when not in use.

Peripherally Inserted Central Catheters

PICCs are CVCs inserted into a vein in the arm rather than a vein in the neck or chest. They are single- or multiple-lumen, nontunnelled catheters that are up to 60 cm in length with gauges ranging from 24 to 16. PICC lines are inserted at or just above the antecubital fossa (usually cephalic or basilic vein) and advanced to a position with the tip ending in the distal one third of the superior vena cava (Figure 19-19). They are intended for patients who need vascular access for 1 week to 6 months though they can be in place for longer periods of time.

The technique for placement of a PICC line involves insertion of the catheter through a needle with the use of a guidewire or forceps to advance the line. Advantages of the PICC over a CVC are lower infection rate, fewer insertion-related complications, decreased cost, and insertion at the bedside or outpatient area.

Complications of PICC lines include catheter occlusion and phlebitis (Table 19-22). If phlebitis occurs, it usually appears within 7 to 10 days following insertion. The arm in which a PICC is in place should not be used for blood pressure readings or blood drawing (Hadaway, 2008).

Implanted Infusion Ports

Implanted infusion ports consist of a CVC connected to an implanted, single or double subcutaneous injection port (Figure 19-20, *A*). The catheter is placed into the desired vein and the other end is connected to a port that is surgically implanted in a subcutaneous pocket on the chest wall. The port consists of a metal sheath with a self-sealing silicone septum. Drugs are injected through the skin into the port. After being filled, the reservoir slowly releases the medicine into the bloodstream.

The port is accessed via the septum by means of a special Huber-point needle that has a deflected tip, which prevents damage to the septum that could make the port useless (Figure 19-20, *B*) (Ludeman, 2007). Huber-point needles are also available with the tip at a 90-degree angle for longer infusions. Implanted ports are good for long-term therapy and have a low risk of infection. Because the port is hidden, it offers cosmetic advantages.

Implanted ports have been developed that are safe for injections of radiopaque contrast media at high pressures and controlled rates. For patients who already have poor peripheral venous access, the ability to use the port to inject contrast media decreases discomfort from venipuncture and helps lower the risk for extravasation of vesicant contrast media (Smith, 2008). Care requirements include regular flushing. Formation of "sludge" (accumulation of clotted blood and drug precipitate) may also occur within the port septum.

Complications

The potential for complications associated with CVADs is always present. Astute monitoring and assessment may assist in early identification of potential complications. Table 19-22 lists common possible complications, potential causes, clinical manifestations, and interventions.

NURSING MANAGEMENT: CENTRAL VENOUS ACCESS DEVICES

Nursing management of CVADs includes assessment, dressing change and cleansing, injection cap changes, and flushing. Although different types of CVADs may have specific institution policies and procedures, there are some general guidelines to be followed.

Catheter and insertion site assessment includes inspection of the site for redness, edema, warmth, drainage, and tenderness or pain. Observation of the catheter for misplacement or slippage is important. A comprehensive pain assessment should be performed, particularly noting any complaints of chest or neck discomfort, arm pain, or pain at the insertion site (Hadaway, 2008).

Dressing change and cleansing of the catheter insertion site should be performed according to institution policies and procedures using strict sterile technique. Transparent semipermeable dressings or gauze and tape can be used. If the site is bleeding, a gauze dressing may be preferable; otherwise, transparent dressings have some advantages over gauze and tape. They allow

Table 19-22 Potential Complications of Central Venous Access Devices

POSSIBLE CAUSE	CLINICAL MANIFESTATIONS	NURSING AND COLLABORATIVE MANAGEMENT
Catheter Occlusion		
• Clamped or kinked catheter • Tip against wall of vessel • Thrombosis • Precipitate buildup in lumen	• Sluggish infusion or aspiration • Unable to infuse and/or aspirate	• Instruct patient to change position, raise arm, and cough • Assess for and alleviate clamping or kinking • Flush with normal saline using a 10-mL syringe; do not force flush • Fluoroscopy to determine cause and site • Anticoagulant or thrombolytic agents
Embolism		
• Catheter breaking • Dislodgement of thrombus • Entry of air into circulation	• Chest pain • Respiratory distress (dyspnea, tachypnea, hypoxia, cyanosis) • Hypotension • Tachycardia	• Administer oxygen • Clamp catheter • Place patient on left side with head down (air emboli) • Notify physician
Catheter-Related Infection (Local or Systemic)		
• Contamination during insertion or use • Migration of organisms along catheter • Immunosuppressed patient	• Local: redness, tenderness, purulent drainage, warmth, edema • Systemic: fever, chills, malaise	**Local** • Culture of drainage from site • Warm, moist compresses • Catheter removal if indicated **Systemic** • Blood cultures • Antibiotic therapy • Antipyretic therapy • Catheter removal if indicated
Pneumothorax		
• Perforation of visceral pleura during insertion	• Decreased or absent breath sounds • Respiratory distress (cyanosis, dyspnea, tachypnea) • Chest pain • Distended unilateral chest	• Administer oxygen • Position in semi-Fowler's position • Prepare for chest tube insertion
Catheter Migration		
• Improper suturing • Insertion site trauma • Changes in intrathoracic pressure • Forceful catheter flushing • Spontaneous	• Sluggish infusion or aspiration • Edema of chest or neck during infusion • Patient complaint of gurgling sound in ear • Dysrhythmias • Increased external catheter length	• Fluoroscopy to verify position • Assist with removal and new CVAD placement

CVAD, central venous access device.

observation of the site without dressing removal and may be left in place for up to 1 week if clean, dry, and intact. Change any dressing immediately if it becomes damp, loose, or visibly soiled (Hadaway, 2008).

Cleanse the skin around the catheter insertion site according to institution policy. Usually, a chlorhexidine-based preparation, povidone-iodine, or isopropyl alcohol is used. Chlorhexidine persists longer than either povidone-iodine or isopropyl alcohol, offering improved residual kill of bacteria. When using chlorhexidine, cleanse the skin using a back-and-forth scrub rather than a circular motion, because it is the recommended technique. Generating friction during skin preparation is a key to infection prevention (Rosenthal, 2007; Weinstein, 2007). The area should

be allowed to air dry completely before the new dressing is applied. Chlorhexidine preparations dry quickly; povidone-iodine requires a drying time of at least 2 minutes (Hadaway, 2008). Secure the lumen ports to the skin above the dressing site. Document the date and time of the dressing change and the nurse's initials, per institution procedure.

Injection caps must be changed at regular intervals using strict sterile technique according to institution policy or when they are damaged from excessive punctures. Teach the patient to turn the head to the opposite side of the CVAD insertion site during cap change. If the catheter cannot be clamped, instruct the patient to lie flat in bed and perform the Valsalva manoeuvre whenever the catheter is open to air to prevent an air embolism.

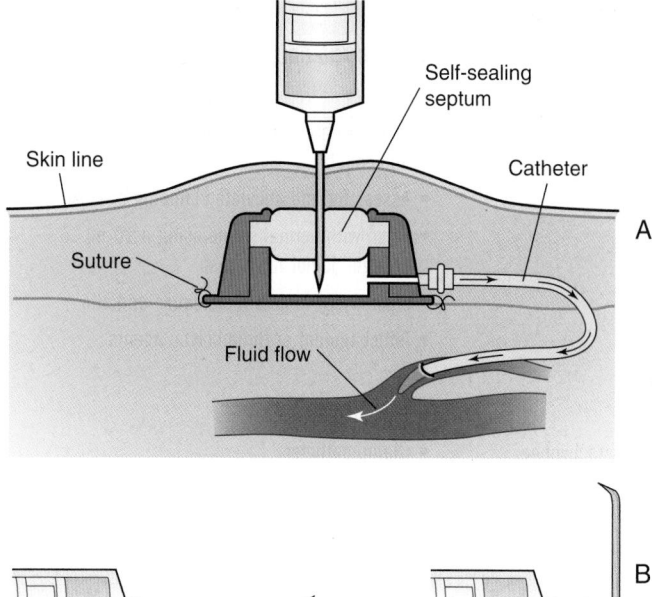

Figure 19-20 A, Cross-section of implantable port displaying access of the port with the Huber-point needle. Note the deflected point of the Huber-point needle, which prevents coring of the port's septum. **B,** Two Huber-point needles used to enter the implanted port. The 90-degree needle is used for top-entry ports for continuous infusion.

Source: **A,** Courtesy Pharmaceia Deltec, Inc., St. Paul, MN.

Flushing is one of the most effective ways to maintain lumen patency and to prevent occlusion of the CVAD. It also keeps incompatible drugs or fluids from mixing. Use a normal saline solution in a syringe that has a barrel capacity of 10 mL or more to avoid excess pressure on the catheter. If resistance is felt, force should not be applied. This could result in a ruptured catheter or create an embolism if a thrombus is present. Because of the risk of contamination and infection, prefilled syringes or single-dose vials are preferred over multiple-dose vials. When flushing, the push–pause method is preferred over a continual even push of saline into the catheter. The push–pause technique creates turbulence within the catheter lumen, promoting the removal of debris that adheres to the catheter lumen. This technique involves injecting the saline with a rapid alternating push–pause motion, instilling 1 to 2 mL with each push on the syringe plunger.

Removal of Central Venous Access Devices

Removal of CVADs should be done according to institution policy and the nurse's scope of practice. In many agencies, nurses with demonstrated competency can remove PICCs and nontunnelled CVCs. The procedure involves removing the sutures, if present, gently withdrawing the catheter while instructing the patient to perform the Valsalva manoeuvre as the last 5 to 10 cm of the catheter is withdrawn (Ludeman, 2007). Pressure should be immediately applied to the site with sterile gauze to prevent air from entering and to control bleeding. The catheter tip should be inspected to determine that it is intact. After hemostasis is achieved, an antiseptic ointment and sterile dressing should be applied to the site.

CLINICAL DECISION-MAKING EXERCISE

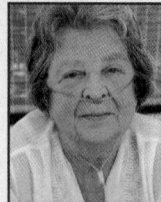

CASE STUDY:
Fluid and Electrolyte Imbalance

Source: ©iStockphoto.com/Jessica Jones Photography.

Patient Profile

Sarah Spiegel, a 73-year-old woman with lung cancer, has been receiving chemotherapy on an outpatient basis. She completed her third treatment 5 days ago and has been experiencing nausea and vomiting for 2 days even though she has been taking prochlorperazine as directed. Ms. Spiegel's daughter brings her to the hospital, where she is admitted to the medical unit. The admitting nurse performs a thorough assessment.

Subjective Data

- Complains of lethargy, weakness, and a dry mouth
- States she has been too nauseous to eat or drink anything for 2 days

Objective Data

- Heart rate 110, pulse thready
- Blood pressure 100/65 mm Hg

- Weight loss of 2.2 kg since she received her chemotherapy treatment 5 days ago
- Dry oral mucous membranes

Discussion Questions

1. Based on her clinical manifestations, what fluid imbalance does Ms. Spiegel have?
2. What additional assessment data should the nurse obtain?
3. What are the patient's risk factors for fluid and electrolyte imbalances?
4. The nurse draws blood for a serum chemistry evaluation. What electrolyte imbalances are likely to be found and why?
5. The physician orders dextrose 5% in 0.45% saline to infuse at 100 mL/hr. What type of solution is this, and how will it help Ms. Spiegel's fluid imbalance?
6. *Priority Decision:* What are the priority nursing interventions for Ms. Spiegel?
7. *Priority Decision:* Based on the assessment data presented, what are the priority nursing diagnoses? Are there any collaborative problems?

⊘volve *Answers are available at* **http://evolve.elsevier.com/ Canada/Lewis/medsurg**

REVIEW QUESTIONS

The number of the question corresponds to the same-numbered objective at the beginning of the chapter.

1. In which of the following fluid compartments is the majority of the body's water contained?
   a. Interstitial
   b. Intracellular
   c. Extracellular
   d. Intravascular

2. Which mechanism is involved with equalizing the fluid concentration when the blood plasma has a higher osmolality than the intracellular fluid in blood cells?
   a. Osmosis
   b. Diffusion
   c. Active transport
   d. Facilitated diffusion

3a. Which of the following is a clinical indication of dehydration?
   a. Weight loss
   b. Full, bounding pulse
   c. Engorged neck veins
   d. Kussmaul's respiration

3b. Which of the following nursing actions is required in hyponatremia?
   a. Fluid restriction
   b. Administration of hypotonic intravenous fluids
   c. Administration of a cation exchange resin
   d. Increased water intake for patients on nasogastric suction

3c. Which of the following should the nurse monitor for when a patient is receiving a loop diuretic?
   a. Restlessness and agitation
   b. Paresthesias and irritability
   c. Weak, irregular pulse and poor muscle tone
   d. Increased blood pressure and muscle spasms

3d. Which of the following patients would be at greatest risk for the potential development of hypermagnesemia?
   a. An 83-year-old man with lung cancer and hypertension
   b. A 65-year-old woman with hypertension taking β-adrenergic blockers
   c. A 42-year-old woman with systemic lupus erythematosus and renal failure
   d. A 50-year-old man with benign prostatic hyperplasia and a urinary tract infection

3e. For which of the following is it especially important for the nurse to assess in a patient who has just undergone a total thyroidectomy?
   a. Weight gain
   b. Depressed reflexes
   c. Positive Chvostek's sign
   d. Confusion and personality changes

3f. Care of the patient experiencing hyperphosphatemia secondary to renal failure includes which of the following?
   a. Calcium supplements
   b. Potassium supplements
   c. Magnesium supplements
   d. Fluid replacement therapy

4. How do the lungs act as an acid-base buffer?
   a. By increasing respiratory rate and depth when CO_2 levels in the blood are high, reducing acid load
   b. By increasing respiratory rate and depth when CO_2 levels in the blood are low, reducing base load
   c. By decreasing respiratory rate and depth when CO_2 levels in the blood are high, reducing acid load
   d. By decreasing respiratory rate and depth when CO_2 levels in the blood are low, increasing acid load

5. A patient has the following arterial blood gas results: pH 7.52; $PaCO_2$ (partial pressure of carbon dioxide in the arterial blood) 30 mm Hg; HCO_3^- 24 mmol/L. The presence of which acid-base disturbance do these results indicate?
   a. Metabolic acidosis
   b. Metabolic alkalosis
   c. Respiratory acidosis
   d. Respiratory alkalosis

6. What is the typical fluid replacement for the patient with a fluid volume deficit?
   a. Dextran
   b. 0.45% Saline
   c. Lactated Ringer's
   d. 5% dextrose in 0.45% saline

7. The nurse is unable to flush a central venous access device and suspects occlusion. Which of the following would be the best nursing intervention?
   a. Apply warm moist compresses to the insertion site.
   b. Attempt to force 10 mL of normal saline into the device.
   c. Place the patient on the left side with head-down position.
   d. Instruct the patient to change positions, raise arm, and cough.

ANSWERS: 1. b; 2. a; 3a. a; 3b. a; 3c. c; 3d. c; 3e. c; 3f. d; 4. a; 5. d; 6. c; 7. d.

REFERENCES

Amella, E. J. (2004). Feeding and hydration issues for older adults with dementia. *Nursing Clinics of North America, 39*(3), 607. doi:10.1016/j.cnur.2004.02.014

Ebersole, P., Hess, P., Touhy, T. A., Jett, K., & Luggen, A. S. (2008). *Toward healthy aging* (7th ed.). St. Louis: Mosby.

Hadaway, L. C. (2008). Central venous access devices. *Nursing, 3*(5), 26-33.

Kee, J. L., Paulanka, B. J., & Polek, C. (2009). *Handbook of fluids, electrolytes and acid-base imbalances* (3rd ed.). Clifton Park, NJ: Delmar.

Larson, K. (2003). Fluid balance in the elderly. *Geriatric Nursing, 24*(5), 306. doi:10.1016/S0197-4572(03)00247-7

Ludeman, K. (2007). Choosing the right vascular access device. *Nursing, 37*(9), 38-41.

McCance, K. L., & Huether, S. E. (2010). *Pathophysiology: The biologic basis for disease in adults and children* (6th ed.). St. Louis: Mosby.

Mosby. (2009). *Mosby's dictionary of medicine, nursing, and health professions* (8th ed.). St Louis: Mosby.

Porth, C. M. (2010). *Pathophysiology: Concepts of altered health states* (8th ed.). Philadelphia: Lippincott.

Rosenthal, K. (2007). Peak technique: CVAD site prep with pep. *Nursing Made Incredibly Easy, 5*(6), 23-25.

Smith, L. H. (2008). Implanted ports, computed tomography, power injectors, and catheter rupture. *Clinical Journal of Oncology Nursing, 12*(5), 809-812. doi:10.1188/08.CJON.809-812

Weinstein, S. M. (2007). *Plumer's principles and practice of intravenous therapy* (8th ed.). Philadelphia: Lippincott Williams & Wilkins.

Wilson, B. A., Shannon, M. A., & Stang, C. L. (2011). *Pearson intravenous drug guide 2011-2012* (2nd ed.). Prentice Hall.

RESOURCES

Acid-Base Physiology @ The Anaesthesia Education Web site
http://www.anaesthesiamcq.com/AcidBaseBook/ABindex.php

Acid-Base Tutorial
http://www.acid-base.com/

Body Fluid Volumes Calculator
http://www.globalrph.com/body_fluid_volumes.htm

L. Ibsen, Oregon Health & Science University, Doernbecher Children's Hospital
http://www.ohsu.edu/xd/health/services/providers/ ibsenl.cfm?searchResult=yes

The Virtual Anesthesia Textbook
http://www.virtual-anaesthesia-textbook.com/vat/acidbase.html

ⓔvolve   *For additional Internet resources, see the Web site for this book at* **http://evolve.elsevier.com/Canada/Lewis/medsurg**

Perioperative Care

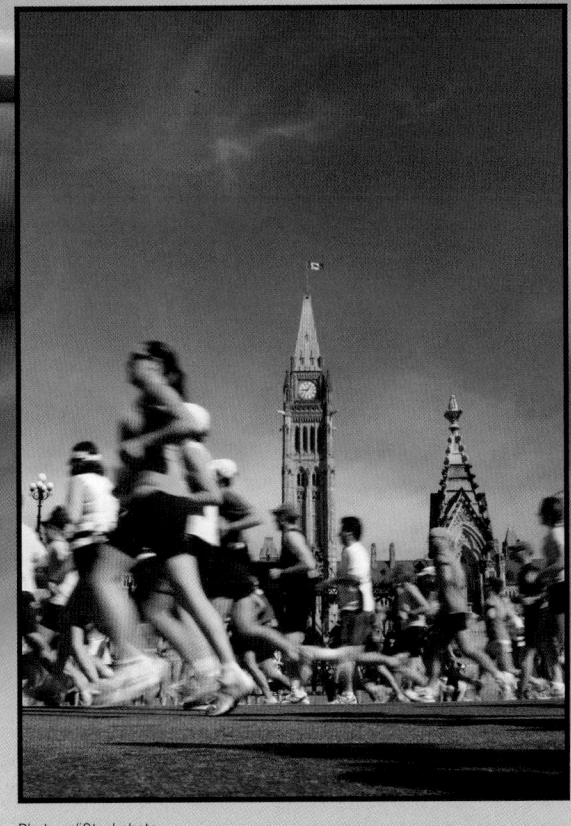

Photawa/iStockphoto

Nursing Management: Preoperative Care

Written by Janice A. Neil

Adapted by Debra Clendinneng

LEARNING OBJECTIVES

1. Identify the common purposes and settings of surgery.
2. Describe the purpose and components of a preoperative nursing assessment.
3. Interpret the significance of data related to the health status and operative risk of the patient about to undergo surgery.
4. Explain the components and purpose of informed consent for surgery.
5. Describe the nursing role in the physical, psychological, and educational preparation of the patient undergoing surgery.

6. Discuss the day-of-surgery preparation for the patient undergoing surgery.
7. Identify the purposes and types of preoperative medications.
8. Identify the special considerations of preoperative preparation for the older adult patient undergoing surgery.

KEY TERMS

ambulatory surgery Also called *same-day surgery*; refers to surgery performed so that the patient can be discharged on the same day, p. 421
elective surgery Surgery that is planned, p. 421
emergency surgery Surgery that is unexpected and urgent, p. 421
informed consent An active, shared decision-making process between the provider and the recipient of health care; this

process protects the patient, the surgeon, and the hospital and its employees, p. 431
same-day admission Admission to hospital on the same day that the surgery will take place, p. 421
surgery The art and science of treating diseases, injuries, and deformities by operation and instrumentation, p. 421

ELECTRONIC RESOURCES

Supplemental content related to Chapter 20 can be found …

Evolve Web Site ⊖volve

http://evolve.elsevier.com/Canada/Lewis/medsurg
• Answer Guideline for Case Study on p. 435
• Clinical Reference: Laboratory Values

• Content Updates
• Electronic Calculators
• Examination Review Questions
• Glossary
• Key Points (Printable and MP3 Download)

The Canadian health care system focuses on wellness, disease prevention, health maintenance, and health promotion (D'Amico, Barbarito, Twomey, & Harder, 2012, p. 3). There is still the need, however, to care for patients with diseases or conditions that require surgical interventions. **Surgery** can be defined as the art and science of treating diseases, injuries, and deformities by operation and instrumentation. The surgical procedure involves the interaction of the patient with the entire surgical team. Surgery may be performed for any of the following purposes:

1. *Diagnosis:* determination of the presence or extent of pathological abnormality (e.g., lymph node biopsy or bronchoscopy).
2. *Cure or repair:* elimination or repair of a pathological condition (e.g., removal of a ruptured appendix or benign ovarian cyst) or repair of anatomy (e.g., fracture repair).
3. *Palliation:* alleviation of symptoms without cure (e.g., cutting a nerve root [rhizotomy] to remove symptoms of pain or creating a colostomy to bypass an inoperable bowel obstruction).
4. *Prevention:* removal of a premalignant or partial colectomy in a patient with familial adenomatous polyposis to prevent cancer.
5. *Exploration:* surgical examination to determine the nature or extent of a disease (e.g., laparotomy).
6. *Cosmetic improvement:* repairing a burn scar or changing breast shape.

Specific suffixes are commonly used in combination with identifying a body part or organ in naming surgical procedures (Table 20-1).

Surgical Settings

Surgery may arise with unexpected urgency (**emergency surgery**) or be a carefully planned event (**elective surgery**). Although Canadian provinces had initiatives to reduce wait times for elective surgery, in 2011, on average, Canadians experienced a total waiting time of 19.0 weeks from the referral from a general practitioner to their elective surgical treatment (Barua, Rovere, & Skinner, 2011).

Elective Inpatient Surgery

Patients requiring one or more overnight stays are now *usually* admitted the day of their surgery (**same-day admission**). This is because of changes in fiscal conditions, surgical techniques, and technology.

Ambulatory surgery is also called *same-day surgery*. In Canada, the majority of surgeries are performed so that the patient can be discharged on the same day. Ambulatory surgery can be conducted in emergency departments, endoscopy clinics, doctors' offices, and outpatient surgery units in hospitals. These procedures can be performed with the use of a general, regional, or local anaesthetic; usually take less than 2 hours; necessitate less than a 3- to 4-hour stay in the postanaesthesia care unit (PACU) or postanaesthetic recovery room (PARR); and do not necessitate an overnight hospital stay. In some cases, the patient will stay in the hospital overnight after surgery, especially if the patient is having difficulty with pain control, nausea, or vomiting.

Regardless of where the surgery is performed, the nurse is vital in preparing the patient for surgery, caring for the patient during surgery, and facilitating the patient's recovery following surgery. To perform these functions effectively, the nurse must have certain basic information. First, the nurse must have knowledge of the nature of the disorder necessitating surgery and any coexisting disease processes. Second, the nurse must identify the individual patient's response to the stress of surgery. Third, the nurse must assess the results of appropriate preoperative diagnostic tests. Finally, the nurse must consider the bodily alterations and potential risks and complications associated with the surgical procedure and any coexisting medical problems. The nurse caring for the patient before surgery is likely to be different from the nurse in the operating room (OR), PACU, intensive care unit (ICU), or surgical unit. Thus, communication and documentation of important preoperative assessment findings are essential.

The preoperative nursing measures included in this chapter are those that are applicable to the preparation of any patient undergoing surgery. Specific measures in preparation for specific surgical procedures (e.g., abdominal, thoracic, or orthopedic surgery) are covered in appropriate chapters of this text.

Patient Interview

The patient may be seen multiple times by many members of the health care team before surgery. To save the patient from having to repeat the same information over and over, the nurse should check the documentation for information before asking common questions. Regardless of the source of information, one of the most important nursing actions is the preoperative interview. In Canada, the patient is most often seen in the preoperative admission clinic (PAC), or the hospital preoperative area. The site of the interview and the time remaining before surgery will dictate the depth and completeness of the interview. Important findings must be documented and communicated to others so that continuity of care will be maintained.

The nursing preoperative interview will likely occur on the day of surgery. The primary purposes of the interview with the patient about to undergo surgery are to (1) obtain patient health information, (2) determine the patient's expectations about

Table 20-1 Suffixes Describing Common Surgical Procedures				
SUFFIX	**MEANING**	**GENERAL SURGERY**	**ORTHOPEDIC SURGERY**	**UROLOGICAL SURGERY**
-ectomy	Excision/removal	Appendectomy	Discectomy	Nephrectomy
-oscopy	Looking into	Gastroscopy	Knee arthroscopy	Cystoscopy
-ostomy	Creation of opening into	Colostomy		Ureterostomy
-otomy	Cutting into/incision	Tracheotomy	Arthrotomy	Cystotomy
-plasty	Repair/reconstruction	Mammoplasty	Total hip arthroplasty	Ureteroplasty

surgery and anaesthesia, (3) provide and clarify information about the surgical experience, (4) assess the patient's emotional state and readiness for surgery, and (5) provide discharge planning and postoperative teaching for the patient (see Chapter 22). The interview also provides an opportunity for the patient and the caregivers to ask questions about surgery, anaesthesia, and postoperative care. Patients commonly ask about taking routine medications before surgery such as insulin, heart or blood pressure medication, or bowel preparations. Patients need to know when they can return to normal activities. The nurse who is aware of a patient's and caregivers' needs and perception of stressors can provide or arrange for the support needed during the perioperative period.

Nursing Assessment of the Patient Before Surgery

All patients coming to the OR must have a comprehensive physical assessment completed by a physician and recorded on their chart. Before surgery, the nurse is required to do a focused preoperative assessment and each hospital or facility will have a concise preoperative checklist for the nurse to complete. This helps identify risk factors and plan care to ensure patient safety throughout the surgical experience. Goals of the assessment are the following:

1. Determine the psychological status of the patient and reinforce coping strategies.
2. Determine physiological factors related and unrelated to the surgical procedure that may contribute to operative risk factors.
3. Establish baseline data for comparison in the intraoperative and postoperative periods.
4. Identify prescription medications, over-the-counter drugs, and herbal medications taken by the patient that may affect the surgical outcome.
5. Ensure that the results of all preoperative laboratory and diagnostic tests are documented and communicated to appropriate personnel.
6. Identify cultural and ethnic factors that may affect the surgical experience.
7. Determine whether the patient has received adequate information from the surgeon to make an informed decision to have surgery, and ensure that the consent form is signed by the patient and physician.
8. Identify any psychosocial needs of the patient, and assess the patient's ability to cope with stressors and change to lifestyle. Ensure that the patient has supports in place for the postoperative period.
9. Confirm that appropriate preoperative consultations with members of the health care team such as cardiologists, internal medicine, physiotherapists and occupational therapists, or wound care nurses have been done.

Subjective Data

Psychosocial Assessment.
Surgery, whether minor or major, can be a frightening event. The psychological and physiological reactions to the surgery elicit the body's stress response, a desirable mechanism that enables the body to cope, adapt, and heal in the postoperative period. If stressors or the response to the stressors is excessive, the stress response can increase anaes-

thetic risk, postoperative pain, and wound healing (Bailey, 2010). Many factors influence the patient's susceptibility to stress, including age, past experiences, current health, and socioeconomic status. The nurse must assess and plan interventions in order to provide information support and interventions during the perioperative period so the patient can manage stress (Bailey, 2010). (See Chapter 8 for a discussion of stress.)

Emotional reactions to impending surgery intensify at both extremes of the age spectrum. For older adults, hospitalization for surgery may represent physical decline or loss of mobility and independence. They may fear being placed in a long-term care facility, which can be viewed as a place to die. The nurse is instrumental in alleviating anxieties and restoring the self-esteem of these surgical patients (see "Age-Related Considerations" at the end of the chapter).

Children and their caregivers experience anxiety related to pediatric surgery despite increased knowledge of perioperative events (Tourigny, Clendinneng, Chartrand, & Gaboury, 2011). Nurses help reassure anxious parents and reduce children's emotional distress by correcting erroneous ideas and providing timely information in the perioperative period.

The nurse must use common language and avoid medical jargon when speaking to the patient and his or her caregivers during the perioperative period. If the patient and caregivers do not speak English, it would be ideal to have an interpreter to help with the dissemination of information. Not all hospitals have the ability to provide an interpreter, so families will often bring an English-speaking representative with them to the preoperative interview. (The use of interpreters is discussed in Chapter 2.)

The nurse should use words and language that are familiar to the patient to increase the patient's understanding of surgical consent and the surgical process, and to help decrease anxiety. To psychologically assess a patient for surgery, a nurse must consider stressors that can negatively affect the patient (Table 20-2). It is important for the nurse to be able to identify these stressors within a short period. The most common psychological factors experienced by a patient about to undergo surgery include anxiety, fear, and loss of hope.

Anxiety. Patients may be anxious when facing surgery because of the unknown. Anxiety can arise from lack of knowledge, which may range from not knowing what to expect during the surgical experience to uncertainty about the outcome of surgery and the potential findings, when the surgery is for diagnostic purposes. The patient may have totally unrealistic expectations of the surgery itself or the outcome of the surgery. Although not all patients want the same depth of information, preoperative education that includes information about the intraoperative, postoperative and recovery periods may help decrease anxiety (Bailey, 2010). Preoperative education that includes information about the intraoperative, postoperative and recovery periods helps decrease their anxiety (Bailey, 2010). The surgeon should be informed whether the patient requires any additional information or if anxiety seems excessive.

The patient may experience anxiety when surgical or anaesthetic interventions, for example, blood transfusions, are in conflict with her or his religious and cultural beliefs. The requesting physician should discuss the need for blood replacement with the patient and obtain an informed consent noting patient consent or refusal for transfusion on the patient's chart (*Transfusion Medicine,* 2011). Patients may also experience preoperative anxiety because of waiting lists or fear of possible cancellations of surgery.

Table 20-2 Psychosocial Assessment of the Patient Before Surgery

Situational Changes

- Determine support systems, including family, other caregivers, significant others, group and institutional structure, and religious and spiritual orientation.
- Define current degree of personal control, decision making, and independence.
- Consider the impact of surgery and hospitalization on family and dependents and financial impacts related to recovery time and medical expenses.
- Identify the presence of hope and anticipation of positive results.

Concerns With the Unknown

- Identify specific areas and depth of anxiety and fears.
- Identify expectations of surgery, changes in current health status, and effects on daily living.

Concerns With Body Image

- Identify current roles or relationships and view of self.
- Determine perceived or potential changes in role or relationships and their impact on body image.

Past Experiences

- Review previous surgical experiences, hospitalizations, and treatments.
- Determine responses to those experiences (positive and negative).
- Identify current perceptions of surgical procedure in relation to the above and information from others (e.g., a neighbour's view of a personal surgical experience).

Knowledge Deficit

- Identify what amount and type of preoperative information this specific patient wants to receive.
- Assess understanding of the surgical procedure, including preparation, care, interventions, preoperative activities, restrictions, and expected outcomes.
- Identify the accuracy of information the patient has received from others, including the health care team, family, friends, and the media.

Common Fears. There are many reasons patients may fear surgery. The most prevalent is the potential for death or permanent disability resulting from surgery. Sometimes, the fear arises after hearing or reading about the risks during the informed consent process. Other fears can be pain, change in body image, or results of a diagnostic procedure.

Fear of death can be extremely stressful for the patient. If the nurse identifies that a patient has a fear of death, this concern must be communicated to the physician immediately. It may be important that the surgeon talks with the patient to understand where the fear of death is coming from. An increase in fear and anxiety may affect a patient's postoperative recovery.

Fear of pain and discomfort during and after surgery is very common. If the fear appears extreme, the nurse should notify the anaesthesiologist so that appropriate preoperative medication (such as an antianxiety medication) can be ordered. The patient should be reassured that medications are available to minimize or eliminate pain during and after surgery. Drugs can be given that provide an amnesic effect so that the patient will not remember what occurs during the surgical episode. These medications can cause temporary cognitive deficits following surgery, and the patient should be told before surgery that this is common. The nurse should stress that the patient should ask for medications following surgery if pain is present and that taking these medications will not contribute to an addiction. It is important to remember that not all medications may completely eliminate a patient's pain or anxiety. (Pain is discussed in Chapter 10.)

Fear of mutilation or alteration in body image can occur whether the surgery is minor, such as a bunion repair, or radical, such as amputation. Even the presence of just a small scar on the body can be bothersome to some patients. The nurse must listen to and assess the patient's concern about this aspect of surgery with an open, nonjudgemental attitude.

Fear of anaesthesia may arise from the unknown, from tales of others' bad experiences, or from personal past experience. Some patients are concerned about information provided about hazards or complications (e.g., brain damage, paralysis, family history of malignant hypothermia). Other patients have a fear of losing control while under the influence of anaesthesia. If these fears or questions are identified, the nurse should inform the anaesthesiologist immediately so that he or she can talk further with the patient. The patient should also be reassured that a nurse and the anaesthesiologist will be present at all times during surgery.

Fear of disruption of life functioning or patterns may be present in varying degrees. It can range from fear of permanent disability or loss of life to concerns about physical limitations after surgery. Concerns about separation from family and about how the spouse or children are managing are common. Financial concerns may be related to an anticipated loss of income because of missed work. If the nurse identifies any of these fears, consultation with a social worker, a spiritual or cultural advisor, a psychologist, or family members may prove valuable in providing assistance to the patient.

Hope. Most psychological factors related to surgery seem to be negative, but hope stands out as a positive attribute (Arman & Rehnsfeldt, 2007). Hope may be the patient's strongest method of coping, and to deny or minimize hope may negate the positive mental attitude necessary for a quick and full recovery. There are many routine surgeries that will have a positive outcome. These can be the surgeries that repair (e.g., plastic surgery for burn scars), rebuild (e.g., total joint replacement to minimize pain and improve function), or save and extend life (e.g., repair of aneurysm, coronary artery bypass surgery). The nurse should assess and support the presence of hope and the patient's anticipation of positive results.

Past Health History.

The nurse should ask about diagnosed medical conditions in the patient's past as well as current health problems. Hospital guidelines for preoperative review of the patient's past health history and other subjective data will be available to assist in asking the patient about specific problems. An organized approach elicits better information than just asking whether the patient has had any medical problems. Initially, the nurse should determine whether the patient understands the reason for surgery. For example, the patient scheduled for a total knee replacement may indicate that the reason for the surgery is increasing problems with pain and mobility. Detailed information on past hospitalizations should be documented. Any previous surgeries and dates of the surgeries should also be documented. Any problems with previous surgeries or reactions to previous anaesthetics should be identified. For example, the patient may have experienced a bad wound infection or a reaction to an analgesic following a prior surgery.

Women should be asked about their menstrual and obstetrical history. An obstetrical history should include the date of the patient's last menstrual period and the number of pregnancies and deliveries the patient has had. If the patient states that she might be pregnant, information should be immediately given to the surgeon to avoid maternal and subsequent fetal exposure to anaesthetics during the first trimester. Questioning regarding reproductive functioning may be embarrassing for a teenager in the presence of parents or guardians. The nurse may elect to ask these questions with parents or guardians out of the room.

Possible inherited conditions may be identified by asking about the patient's family health history. A family history of cardiac and endocrine disease should be recorded. For example, if a patient reports a mother or father with hypertension, sudden cardiac death, myocardial infarction, or coronary artery disease, the nurse should be alerted to the possibility that the patient may also have a similar predisposition or condition. A family history of diabetes should also be investigated because of the familial predisposition to both type 1 and type 2 diabetes mellitus. Tendencies toward these conditions may be exacerbated during surgery and affect physiological function during and after surgery. Inherited traits, such as sickle cell trait, may contribute to the choice of anaesthesia and surgical outcome and must be considered in the family histories (Drain & Odom-Forren, 2009, p. 694). Anaesthesia care providers also obtain information about the patient's family history, especially adverse reactions to or problems with anaesthesia such as malignant hyperthermia, a rare metabolic disease characterized by hyperthermia with rigidity of skeletal muscles that can result in death The genetic predisposition for malignant hyperthermia is now well documented, and plans of care include minimizing complications associated with this condition (Rothrock, 2011). (Malignant hyperthermia is discussed in Chapter 21.)

Medications. Current medication use, including the use of over-the-counter drugs and herbal products, should be documented. In many settings, patients are asked to bring their bottles of medications with them when attending the PAC. This will enable the nurse to more accurately chart the names and dosage of drugs because patients frequently cannot remember specific details if they use a large number of drugs. For example, it is important to investigate whether the patient is taking the drug as ordered or has stopped taking the drug because of cost, adverse effects, or the feeling that ongoing therapy is no longer needed.

Drugs and herbal products may interact with anaesthetics, often increasing or decreasing potency and effectiveness, or they may be needed during surgery to maintain physiological function. It is especially important to consider the effects of drugs used for heart disease, hypertension, immunosuppression, seizure control, anticoagulation, and endocrine replacement. Insulin or oral hypoglycemic agents may require dosage or agent adjustments during the perioperative period because of increased body metabolism, decreased caloric intake, stress, and anaesthesia. Use of acetylsalicylic acid is common in many people, but it inhibits platelet aggregation and may contribute to postoperative bleeding complications. Surgeons often require that patients not take any aspirin for at least 2 weeks before surgery. It is also important to stress that stopping some medications abruptly can cause complications. The preoperative nurse should check with an anaesthesiologist to ensure which medications should be stopped and which should be taken the day of surgery.

The use of herbal therapy and dietary supplements is prevalent today. Many patients do not disclose to health care providers that they take these supplements unless specifically asked (Shorofi & Arbon, 2010). Therefore, it is essential to specifically ask about the use of vitamins, herbal supplements, and other alternative substances (see Chapter 12, Table 12-8). These products may interfere with anaesthesia and potentially cause complications during surgery (American Society of Anesthesiologists, 2010). Complications from herbal products can include effects on blood pressure, increased sedation, cardiac effects, electrolyte alterations, and inhibition of platelet aggregation. In patients taking anticoagulants or platelet aggregation inhibitors, the use of specific herbal products can cause excessive postoperative bleeding that may necessitate a return to the OR. These types of supplements must be discontinued before surgery as ordered by the physician (Drain & Odom-Forren, 2009, p. 279). Some effects of specific herbs that can be of concern during the perioperative period are identified in the Complementary & Alternative Therapies box.

COMPLEMENTARY & ALTERNATIVE THERAPIES

Effects of Herbs and Supplements During the Perioperative Period

Herb	Perioperative Considerations
Echinacea	May cause inflammation of the liver if used with certain medications
Feverfew	May inhibit platelet activity and increase bleeding
Garlic	May increase bleeding, especially in patients taking anticoagulants
Ginger	May increase bleeding, especially in patients taking anticoagulants
Ginkgo biloba	May increase bleeding, especially in patients taking anticoagulants
Ginseng	May increase bleeding, especially in patients taking anticoagulants; may cause increased heart rate or elevated BP
Goldenseal	May cause increased BP; may increase swelling
Kava	May prolong the effects of certain anaesthetics or antiseizure medications; may cause liver injury
Licorice	Certain preparations may cause elevated BP, swelling, or electrolyte imbalance
Saw palmetto	May have additive effects with other hormone therapies
St. John's wort	May prolong the effects of anaesthetic agents
Valerian	May prolong the effects of certain anaesthetics or antiseizure medications; may cause liver injury
Vitamin E	May increase bleeding, especially in patients taking anticoagulants; may affect thyroid gland function; in high doses, may cause increased BP in patients who already have high BP

BP, blood pressure.

Source: Excerpted from *What you should know about herbal and dietary supplement use and anesthesia* of the American Society of Anesthesiologists. (2003). A copy of the text can be obtained from American Society of Anesthesiologists, 520 N. Northwest Highway, Park Ridge, Illinois, 60068-2573.

The nurse must also ask the patient about possible recreational drug use, abuse, and addiction. The substances most likely to be abused include tobacco, alcohol, opioids, marijuana, and cocaine. Questions should be asked matter-of-factly, and the nurse should stress that recreational drug use may affect the type and amount of anaesthesia that will be needed. When patients become aware of the potential interactions of these drugs with anaesthetics, most patients will respond honestly about their drug use. Chronic alcohol use will place the patient undergoing surgery at risk because of lung, gastrointestinal, or liver damage. When liver function is decreased, metabolism of anaesthetic agents is prolonged, nutritional status is altered, and the potential for postoperative complications is increased. Alcohol withdrawal can also occur during lengthy surgery or in the postoperative period. This can be a life-threatening event, but it can be avoided with appropriate planning and management (see Chapter 11).

When assessing medication use, drug intolerance and drug allergies should be considered. Drug intolerance usually results in adverse effects that are uncomfortable or unpleasant for the patient but are not life threatening. These effects can include nausea, constipation, diarrhea, or *idiosyncratic* (opposite from expected) reactions. A true drug allergy produces hives, an anaphylactic reaction, or both; this causes cardiopulmonary compromise, including hypotension, tachycardia, bronchospasm, and possibly pulmonary edema. By being aware of drug intolerance and drug allergies, it will be possible to maintain patient comfort, safety, and stability. For example, some anaesthetic agents contain sulphur, so the anaesthesiologist should be notified if a history of allergy to sulphur is given. If a drug intolerance or drug allergy is noted, it must be documented, and an allergy wristband should be put on the patient on the day of surgery.

All findings of the medication history should be documented and communicated to the intraoperative and postoperative personnel. Although the anaesthesiologist will determine the appropriate schedule and dose of the patient's routine medications before and after surgery based on the medication history, the nurse must ensure that all of the patient's medications are identified, administer the medications as ordered, and monitor the patient for potential interactions and complications.

Allergies. The nurse should inquire about nondrug allergies, including allergies to foods, chemicals, tape, and pollen. The patient with a history of any allergic responsiveness has a greater potential for demonstrating hypersensitivity reactions to drugs administered during anaesthesia.

Patients should also be screened for possible latex allergies (Operating Room Nurses Association of Canada [ORNAC], 2011, p. 299) (see Chapters 16 and 21). The Canadian Society of Allergy and Clinical Immunology (CSACI) recommends that patients be questioned in the following five areas:
1. Risk factors
2. Contact dermatitis
3. Contact urticaria (hives)
4. Aerosol reactions
5. History of reactions that suggest an allergy to latex

High-risk groups include health care personnel and patients with spina bifida or genitourinary tract anomalies. Additional risk factors include food allergies to papain (meat tenderizer), avocados, kiwi, bananas, papayas, chestnuts, potatoes, tomatoes, celery, peaches, and other fruit with stones. Latex allergies can produce local or systemic reactions including anaphylaxis (ORNAC, 2011, p. 298).

Review of Systems. A thorough body systems review is performed and documented before surgery by members of the perioperative team. This review of systems is described in detail in Chapter 3. The following are specific to the day of surgery. The surgeon does a preoperative physical examination (PE) and patient history and orders appropriate preoperative laboratory tests and consultations.

In the immediate preoperative period, there is seldom time for the nurse to do a full physical assessment, so nurses rely on the chart documentation. The following are important points for the nurse to assess immediately before surgery to ensure a seamless, safe experience for the patient.

Nervous System. Preoperative evaluation of neurological functioning includes assessing the patient's ability to respond to questions, follow commands, and maintain orderly thought patterns. Alterations in the patient's hearing (aids) and vision (glasses, glaucoma) may affect responses and ability to follow directions. The ability to pay attention, concentrate, and respond appropriately must be documented to use as the baseline for postoperative comparison.

Impaired cognitive function may affect the patient's ability to prepare for surgery, and the nurse must determine whether all preoperative procedures were carried out—for example, bowel preparations. If confusion is noted and persistent, it is important to determine whether there are appropriate resources and support to assist the patient after surgery.

Cognitive function is an area of major importance in the assessment of older adult patients. The older adult may have intact mental abilities before surgery, but the stress of surgery, dehydration, hypothermia, and drugs may contribute to the development of postoperative delirium. Nonverbal elder patients and those with chronic conditions such as Alzheimer's disease must be assessed for their interpretation of pain before surgery so that postoperative pain scales can be used effectively (Rothrock, 2011, p. 1167). These preoperative findings are extremely important for postoperative comparison.

Cardiovascular System. The purpose of evaluating cardiovascular function is to determine the presence of pre-existing disease or existing problems so that the patient can be efficiently monitored during the surgical and recovery periods. If there is a history of cardiac problems, including hypertension, angina, dysrhythmias, congestive heart failure, myocardial infarction, or use of pacemakers or implanted cardiac devices, the patient may need a cardiology and anaesthesia consult before surgery.

If pertinent, clotting and bleeding times and other relevant laboratory results must be on the chart before surgery. For example, the patient who receives digitalis therapy will have serum potassium levels drawn before surgery, and results must be available. If the patient has a history of congenital, rheumatic, or valvular heart disease, antibiotic prophylaxis before surgery may be given to decrease the risk of bacterial endocarditis (see Chapter 37).

Respiratory System. The patient should be asked about any recent or chronic upper respiratory infections. The presence of an upper airway infection may result in the cancellation or postponement of elective surgery because the patient has an increased anaesthetic risk. If the patient has a respiratory history, he or she will have an anaesthetic consult before surgery and an appropriate workup.

If a patient has asthma, the nurse should inquire about the patient's recent use of inhaled or oral corticosteroids and bronchodilators. The patient with a severe active airway infection, chronic obstructive pulmonary disease, or asthma is at risk for pulmonary complications, including bronchospasm, laryngospasm, hypoxemia, and atelectasis.

The patient who smokes should be encouraged to stop at least 6 weeks before surgery to decrease the risk of intraoperative and postoperative respiratory complications, but may find this difficult during such a stressful time (Lauerman, 2008) (see the Registered Nurses' Association of Ontario [RNAO], 2011 e-learning course *Helping People Quit Smoking*). The greater the patient's pack-years of smoking, the greater the patient's risk for pulmonary complications.

Obesity; spinal, chest, or airway deformities; and sleep apnea can compromise respiratory function. Depending on the patient's history and PE findings, baseline pulmonary function tests and arterial blood gases may be ordered before surgery.

Urinary System. Before surgery, the present urinary system status should be noted and documented. Results of any renal function tests, such as serum creatinine and blood urea nitrogen (serum urea [nitrogen]), ordered before surgery should be available on the chart before surgery.

Male patients who have problems voiding may have an enlarged prostate, which would hinder the insertion of a urinary catheter during surgery and also impair voiding in the postoperative period. This information is documented for the perioperative team. The nurse should inform patients if they are going to have a catheter after surgery.

Integumentary System. Any skin rashes, boils, ulcers, or other dermatological conditions should be noted. A history of pressure ulcers may necessitate extra padding during surgery, and skin problems may affect postoperative healing.

Musculoskeletal System. Mobility problems should also be noted in all affected joints. Mobility restrictions may influence intraoperative and postoperative positioning and affect ambulation. Spinal anaesthesia may be difficult if the patient cannot flex her or his lumbar spine adequately to allow easy needle insertion. If the neck is affected, intubation and airway management may be difficult.

Endocrine System. Diabetes mellitus is a risk factor for both anaesthesia and surgery. The patient with diabetes is at risk for the development of hypoglycemia, hyperglycemia, ketosis, cardiovascular alterations, delayed wound healing, and infection. Preoperative capillary blood glucose tests should be done to determine baseline levels. It is important to clarify with the patient's surgeon or anaesthesiologist whether the patient should take the usual dose of insulin on the day of surgery. Some practitioners prefer that the patient take only half of the usual dose; others ask that the patient take either the usual dose or no insulin at all. Regardless of the preoperative insulin orders, the patient's capillary blood glucose will be determined periodically and managed, if necessary, with regular (short-acting, rapid-onset) insulin.

It should also be determined whether the patient has a history of thyroid dysfunction. Either hyperthyroidism or hypothyroidism can place the patient at surgical risk because of alterations in metabolic rate. If the patient takes a thyroid replacement

drug, the nurse should check with the anaesthesiologist about administration of the drug the day of surgery. If the patient has a history of thyroid dysfunction, laboratory tests may be ordered to determine current levels of thyroid function.

Immune System. Following Routine Practices in the OR protects patients and personnel from unknown, undiagnosed infectious diseases (ORNAC, 2011, p. 89). Patients with active chronic infections, such as hepatitis, acquired immune deficiency syndrome, and tuberculosis may have surgery; however, if the patient has a history of a compromised immune system or takes immunosuppressive drugs, it must be documented. Impairment of the immune system can lead to delayed wound healing and postoperative infections. If the patient has an acute infection (e.g., active skin rash, acute sinusitis, flu), elective surgery is frequently cancelled. (Infection control guidelines are discussed in Chapter 17.)

Fluid and Electrolyte Status. The patient should be questioned about vomiting, diarrhea, or difficulty swallowing. Drugs that the patient takes that alter fluid and electrolyte status, such as diuretics, should also be identified because serum electrolyte levels may need to be evaluated before surgery. Most patients have restricted fluids because of nothing-by-mouth (NPO) status before surgery, and it is the responsibility of the anaesthesiologist to administer intravenous (IV) fluids and electrolyte therapy to maintain proper hydration.

Nutritional Status. Nutritional extremes require consideration in the perioperative period. For example, with extreme obesity, notification a day before surgery allows the perioperative nurse time to prepare the necessary equipment and instrumentation. Obesity stresses the cardiac and pulmonary systems and may make access to the surgical site and anaesthesia administration more difficult. It predisposes the patient to delayed emersion from anaesthesia and wound healing and increases the likelihood of thromboembolic complications after surgery (Phillips, 2012).

Malnutrition is a result of inadequate intake of protein or calories. It can cause poor tolerance of anaesthetic agents, altered wound healing, and susceptibility to infections and has an increased risk of morbidity and mortality (Phillips, 2012). The older adult is often at risk for malnutrition and fluid volume deficits. If the patient is very thin, the perioperative team should be notified in order to have adequate pressure-reducing positioning devices (pressure points on all patients are protected routinely) on the operating bed. Pressure reduction helps prevent pressure ulcers, especially during lengthy procedures. Nutritional deficiencies impair the ability to recover from surgery, so if the nutritional problem is severe, surgery may be postponed until the patient's weight and nutritional deficiencies are corrected.

Dietary habits may affect postoperative recovery and should be identified if the patient will remain in the hospital after surgery. Patients who consume large quantities of coffee or soft drinks containing high caffeine levels should be identified. Acute caffeine abstinence increases brain blood flow, an effect that may account for withdrawal headaches, fatigue, and decreased alertness after surgery (University of Vermont, 2009).

Nursing Assessment: Patient About to Undergo Surgery. The review of the patient's health provides valuable data about the patient's physical and psychological status as well

HEALTH HISTORY

Table 20-3 Patient About to Undergo Surgery

Subjective Data

Past Health History

- Have you had surgeries in the past?* Which ones?* Did you have any complications?*
- Have you or any family members ever experienced any problems with anaesthesia?*
- Do you have any past hospitalizations?*
- Do you have any chronic health conditions?*
- Do you have a history of high blood pressure or cardiac disease?*
- Do you have any history of dyspnea, coughing, hemoptysis, COPD, or asthma?*

Current Health History

- What is your usual or present height and weight? Have you had a recent weight gain or loss?*
- Do you at present have an upper respiratory infection?*
- Do you wear glasses, contact lenses, or a hearing aid?*
- Do you smoke?* If yes, how many packs daily? For how many years?
- What is your usual use of alcohol?
- Do you have any problems healing?*
- Do you have any musculoskeletal problems that might affect positioning during surgery or activity level after surgery?*
- Do you have any limitation in mobility of your neck?* (might affect intubation for surgery)
- Do you require any special equipment for ambulation?*
- How would you describe your pain tolerance? What methods have you found effective for pain relief?
- Do you have anxiety related to the surgery?
- Will you have the support you feel you need following discharge?

Medications

- Are you currently taking any prescribed medications, over-the-counter medications, or herbal or vitamin supplements?*
- Do you have any allergies or sensitivities to any foods or medications?*

COPD, chronic obstructive pulmonary disease.
*If yes, describe.

Table 20-4 Preoperative Rating of Patient's Physical Status

RATING	EXAMPLES
I. Healthy patient with no systemic disease	Patient with no significant past or present health problems
II. Mild systemic disease without functional limitations	Patient with a history of asthma controlled with β-adrenergic agonist inhaler
III. Severe systemic disease associated with definite functional limitations	Patient with history of chronic asthma controlled with β-adrenergic agonist inhaler and inhaled corticosteroids; not wheezing
IV. Severe systemic disease that is an ongoing threat to life	Patient with history of asthma, poorly controlled with β-adrenergic agonists and corticosteroids; PaO$_2$ of 50 mm Hg; wheezing; changes on chest radiograph
V. Patient unlikely to survive for more than 24 hours with or without surgery	Patient in status asthmaticus, intubated and on ventilator, receiving corticosteroids and aminophylline intravenously

PaO$_2$, arterial partial pressure of oxygen.

as cultural values and beliefs related to his or her health care. Questions to ask a patient about to undergo surgery are listed in Table 20-3.

Objective Data

Physical Examination. In Canada, each province or territory and health authority may have its own policies on preoperative health assessments, but it is important to have a PE documented on the chart in case surgical complications arise. This examination may be done in advance of surgery or on the day of surgery.

Findings from the patient's history and PE will enable the anaesthesiologist to assign the patient a physical status rating for anaesthesia administration reference (Table 20-4). This rating is an indicator of the patient's fitness for anaesthesia and surgery (Pudner, 2010, p. 5).

Many physiological stressors may put the patient at risk for surgical complications, whether the surgery is an elective or an emergency procedure. A physiological assessment of the patient who is about to undergo surgery is presented in Table 20-5. If the PE is done immediately before surgery, it will be a more focused assessment because of the impending procedures that must be completed before surgery. The nurse should review the documentation already present on the patient's chart, including the review of systems and the physician's PE report. All findings must be documented, with any relevant findings immediately communicated to members of the perioperative team.

Laboratory and Diagnostic Testing. The need for preoperative laboratory and electrocardiogram testing is determined based on the patient's history, and the risk of the surgical procedure (Hepner, 2009). For example, if the patient is taking an anticoagulant (including aspirin), a coagulation profile may be done; a patient on diuretic or digoxin therapy may need to have a potassium level obtained; a patient taking medications for dysrhythmias will have a preoperative electrocardiogram. Blood glucose monitoring should be done for patients with diabetes. Findings may necessitate dosage or agent adjustments during the perioperative period because of increased body metabolism, decreased caloric intake, stress, and anaesthesia. Regulation of the stability of the blood glucose levels during surgery will promote a more positive outcome. Commonly ordered preoperative laboratory tests can be found in Table 20-6.

Offices and PACs may do the preoperative tests days before surgery. Thus, the nurse must ensure that all laboratory reports are on the chart. Lack of these reports may result in a delay or cancellation of the surgery.

Table 20-5 Physiological Assessment of the Patient Before Surgery*

Neurological System

- Determine orientation to time, place, and person.
- Identify presence of confusion, disorderly thinking, or inability to follow commands.
- Identify past history of strokes, transient ischemic attacks, or diseases of the central nervous system such as Parkinson's disease or multiple sclerosis.
- Identify history of headaches or issues with vision or hearing.

Cardiovascular System

- Identify acute or chronic problems; focus on the presence of angina, hypertension, heart failure, and recent history of myocardial infarction.
- Palpate baseline radial pulse for rate and characteristics.
- Inspect for edema, noting location and severity.
- Take baseline blood pressure.
- Identify any drug or herbal product that may affect coagulation (e.g., aspirin, ginkgo biloba, ginger).
- Review laboratory and diagnostic tests for cardiovascular function when indicated.

Respiratory System

- Identify acute or chronic problems; note the presence of infection or chronic obstructive pulmonary disease (COPD).
- Assess history of smoking and encourage the patient to stop prior to surgery by educating him or her on the increased risk of complications.†
- Determine baseline respiratory rate and rhythm, regularity of pattern, and pulse oximetry.
- Observe for cough, dyspnea, use of accessory muscles of respiration, and cyanosis.

Urinary System

- Identify any pre-existing disease and ability of the patient to void. Prostate enlargement may affect catheterization during surgery and ability to void after surgery.
- Review laboratory and diagnostic tests for renal function when indicated.

Hepatic System

- Review past history of substance abuse, especially alcohol and intravenous drug use.
- Review laboratory and diagnostic tests for liver when indicated.

Endocrine and Hematological Systems

- Identify pre-existing problems with bleeding or hematological and endocrine disorders.

Integumentary System

- Assess mucous membranes for dryness and intactness.
- Determine skin status; note drying, bruising, or breaks in integrity of surface.
- Inspect skin for rashes, boils, or infection, especially around the planned surgical site.
- Assess skin moisture and temperature.
- Inspect the mucous membranes and skin turgor for presence of dehydration.
- Identify any history of problems with wound healing.

Musculoskeletal System

- Examine skin–bone pressure points and pressure ulcers.
- Assess for limitations in joint pain, range of motion, and muscle weakness.
- Assess mobility, gait, and balance.

Gastrointestinal–Nutritional System

- Identify history of gastrointestinal disorders or problems with elimination.
- Determine food and fluid intake patterns and any recent weight loss.
- Weigh patient.
- Assess for the presence of dentures and bridges (loose dentures or teeth may be dislodged during intubation).

*See related body system chapters for more specific assessments and related laboratory studies.
†Ontario Anesthesiologists. (2012). *Why stop smoking for safer surgery*. Retrieved from *http://www.ontarioanesthesiologists.ca/stop-smoking-safe-surgery/why-stop-smoking-for-safer-surgery/*

NURSING MANAGEMENT: PATIENT ABOUT TO UNDERGO SURGERY

Preoperative nursing interventions are derived from the nursing assessment and must reflect each individual patient's specific needs. Physical preparations will be determined by the pending surgery and the routines of the surgery setting. Psychological preparations should be tailored to each patient's needs. Preoperative teaching may be minimal or extensive. General information for surgery should be given.

▪ Preoperative Teaching

The patient has a right to know what to expect and how to participate effectively during the surgical experience. Preoperative

teaching increases patient satisfaction and may reduce fear, anxiety, stress (the duration of hospitalization), and recovery time following discharge. Barriers to effective teaching may be because of language, culture, the time available and the patient's anxiety level, and motivation—the patient must find the information valuable in order to retain it (Pudner, 2010, p. 9). Further, the nurse's teaching ability adds to the patient's retention of information (Drain & Odom-Forren, 2009, pp. 391-392).

In most surgical settings, patients often attend the PAC within a month of their scheduled surgery. However, there are always cases in which surgery is unplanned. Even in such situations, there is still time for the nurse to present information to the patient and her or his family about the surgery and the postoperative period. The only time patients may not receive any information about their surgery is in an emergency situation where time does not present itself for teaching. Generally, in the PAC, information is presented to the patient in written, verbal, and

Table 20-6 Common Preoperative Laboratory Tests

TEST	AREA ASSESSED
Urinalysis	Renal status, hydration, urinary tract infection and disease
Chest radiograph	Pulmonary disorders, cardiac enlargement
Blood studies: RBC, Hgb, Hct, platelets, WBC, WBC differential	Anemia, immune status, infection
Electrolytes	Metabolic status, renal function, diuretic adverse effects
ABGs, oximetry	Pulmonary and metabolic function
Prothrombin (INR) or partial thromboplastin time	Bleeding tendencies
Blood glucose	Metabolic status, diabetes mellitus
Creatinine	Renal function
Blood urea nitrogen*	Renal function
Electrocardiogram	Cardiac disease, electrolyte abnormalities
Pulmonary function studies	Pulmonary status
Liver function tests	Liver function
Type, screen, and crossmatch	Blood availability for replacement (elective surgery patients may have own blood available—autologous)
Pregnancy	Reproductive status

ABGs, arterial blood gases; *Hct,* hematocrit; *Hgb,* hemoglobin; *INR,* international normalized ratio; *RBC,* red blood cell; *WBC,* white blood cell.

*Serum urea (nitrogen).

video forms. Written materials are provided for patients and caregivers to use for review and reinforcement.

In preparing the patient for surgery, the nurse identifies the patient's educational needs by determining his or her knowledge level, perceptions of surgery and ability to understand the information provided. Patients who receive basic information about the sequence of events, the surgical procedure, and postoperative recovery have reduced anxiety (Bailey, 2010).

Generally, preoperative teaching concerns three types of information: sensory, process, and procedural. Different patients, with varying cultures, backgrounds, and experience, may want different types of information. With *sensory information,* patients want to know what they will see, hear, smell, and feel during the surgery. The nurse may tell them that the OR will be cold, but they can ask the perioperative nurse for a warm blanket; the lights in the OR are very bright; or there will be lots of sounds that are unfamiliar and there may be specific smells present. Patients wanting *process information* may not want specific details but desire the general flow of what is going to happen. Patients can be advised that a nurse and anaesthesiologist will speak with them in the preoperative unit then they will go to the OR and, when they wake up, they will be in the PACU. After this, they will be transferred back to their postoperative room or home. With *procedural information,* desired details are more specific; for example, an IV line will be started while patients are in the holding area, and in the OR, patients will be asked to move

onto the narrow bed and a safety strap will be put over their thighs.

Preoperative patient teaching must be communicated to the postoperative care nurses so learning can be reinforced. Because nurses have limited time for teaching, the team approach is usually used. Nurses in the PAC initiate the teaching, the perioperative nurses continue it, and the postoperative and discharge nurses reinforce and supplement it. Community nurses must be aware if the patient has continuing learning needs because they may be the ones who visit the patient at home, in the community, or in extended care facilities after surgery. All teaching should be documented in the patient's medical record. A patient and caregiver teaching guide for preoperative preparation is presented in Table 20-7. Additional information related to patient teaching may be found in Chapter 4.

General Surgery Information

Preoperative teaching includes essential information that the patient desires and needs to know during the surgical experience (Bailey, 2010). This information must be tailored to each individual patient and reflect the specific surgery. The nurse should determine what will best serve the particular patient rather than routinely giving information that may or may not be relevant (Table 20-8). All patients should receive instruction about deep breathing, incentive spirometry, coughing, and moving after surgery. This is essential because patients may not want to do these activities after surgery unless they are taught the rationale for them and practise them before surgery. Patients and caregivers should be told whether there will be tubes, drains, monitoring devices, or special equipment after surgery and that these devices enable the nurse to safely care for the patient.

Examples of individualized teaching may include how to use incentive spirometers or postoperative, patient-controlled analgesia pumps. The patient could also receive surgery-specific information, such as a patient with a total joint replacement having an immobilizer, a patient getting an epidural catheter for postoperative pain control, or a patient requiring extensive surgery being told about waking up in the ICU.

Ambulatory Surgery Information

The ambulatory surgery patient or the patient admitted to hospital the day of surgery will need to receive information before admission. The teaching is generally done in the surgeon's office or PAC and reinforced on the day of surgery. Some ambulatory surgical centres have the staff telephone the patient the evening before surgery to answer last-minute questions and to reinforce teaching.

Information for the patient includes the time to arrive at the surgical centre and the time of surgery. Arrival time is usually a minimum of 2 hours before the scheduled time of surgery to allow for the completion of the preoperative assessment and paperwork preparation. Information can also include the day-of-surgery events such as patient registration, parking, what to wear, what to bring, and the need to have a responsible adult present for transportation home after surgery.

Preoperative preadmission information can include the need for a preoperative shower, an enema, and food and fluid restrictions. The Canadian Anaesthesiologists' Society has published fluid restriction guidelines that take into consideration age and pre-existing medical conditions as well as safe anaesthesia delivery (Merchant et al., 2010) (Table 20-9). Providing the patient

PATIENT & CAREGIVER TEACHING GUIDE
Table 20-7 Preoperative Preparation

Sensory Information

- Holding area is often noisy.
- Drugs and cleaning solutions may be smelled.
- Operating room can be cold; warm blankets are available.
- Talking may be heard in the OR but will be distorted because of masks. Questions should be asked if something is not understood.
- OR bed will be narrow. A safety strap will be applied over the knees.
- Lights in the OR can be very bright.
- Machines (ticking and pinging noises) may be heard when awake. Their purpose is to monitor and ensure safety.

Procedural Information

- What to bring and what type of clothing to wear to the ambulatory surgery centre
- Any changes in time of surgery
- Fluid and food restrictions
- Physical preparation required (e.g., bowel or skin preparation)
- Purpose of frequent vital signs assessment
- Pain control and other comfort measures (this includes any pain scales that a specific hospital might use to assess pain)
- Why turning, coughing, and deep breathing using incentive spirometry after surgery is important; practice sessions must be done before surgery. (Some hospitals use incentive spirometry to assist patients with deep breathing and coughing. It is also important to show patients how to use a pillow to assist them with splinting after surgery.)
- Insertion of intravenous lines
- Procedure for anaesthesia administration
- Importance of mobility, transferring, and postoperative exercises should be introduced.

Process Information

Information About General Flow of Surgery

- Admission area
- Preoperative holding area, OR, and recovery area
- Families can usually stay in holding area until surgery.
- Families may be able to enter recovery area as soon as patient is awake.
- Identification of any technology that may be present on awakening, such as monitors and central lines

Where Families Can Wait During Surgery

- Patient and family members need to be encouraged to verbalize concerns.
- OR staff will notify family when surgery is completed.
- Surgeon will usually talk with family following surgery.

OR, operating room.

Table 20-8 Summary of Preoperative Teaching

TOPIC	WHAT TO TEACH THE PATIENT
Nutrition	• Most surgeries require NPO after midnight
	• Increase diet slowly
	• Nausea is common—there are medications to help with this
Ambulation	• Ambulate early
	• May have immobilizers, have to use assistive devices
	• Leg exercises
	• May have to wear antiembolism stockings after surgery
Breathing	• Perform deep breathing and coughing exercises
	• Splinting
	• Use of incentive spirometer
Grooming	• Take a bath or shower morning of surgery
	• Remove nail polish, artificial fingernails, hair clips, and jewellery before surgery
	• Dentures and eyeglasses will be removed and stored during surgery
	• Remove prosthetics
	• No contact lenses permitted
Medications	• Take preoperative medication as ordered
	• Stop taking prescribed medications, OTC medications, and herbal remedies as suggested by the physician, anaesthesiologist, or surgeon
Pain control	• Ask for pain medication as needed
	• Types of pain control (epidural, PCA)
Drains, dressings, and tubings	• Tell patient about any drains (e.g., Jackson Pratt, hemovac)
	• Dressings (staples, sutures) to be expected
	• Tubing: IV, NG, or epidural tubing
Safety	• Call for assistance to get out of bed
	• Use call bell
	• Do not climb over the side rails
Preoperative information	• Parking
	• Time to be at hospital and time of surgery
	• Waiting areas for family
	• Length of expected stay

IV, intravenous; *NG,* nasogastric; *NPO,* nothing-by-mouth status; *OTC,* over-the-counter; *PCA,* patient-controlled analgesia.

with the rationale for adhering to NPO orders can significantly increase the patient's perception of their importance (Baril & Portman, 2007). Protocols may vary if the patient is having local anaesthesia or the surgery is scheduled for late in the day. Varying NPO protocols exist; the NPO protocol of each surgical facility should be followed. Restriction of fluids and food is designed to minimize the potential risk of aspiration and to decrease the risk

of postoperative nausea and vomiting. The patient who has not followed this instruction may have surgery delayed or cancelled, so it is vital that the patient undergoing surgery understands and adheres to these restrictions (see the Evidence-Informed Practice box "How Long Should Patients Fast before Elective Surgery?").

Legal Preparation for Surgery

Legal preparation for surgery consists of checking that all required forms have been correctly signed and are present in the chart and

Table 20-9 Preoperative Fasting Recommendations of the Canadian Anesthesiologists' Society	
LIQUID AND FOOD INTAKE	**MINIMUM FASTING PERIOD (HR)**
Clear liquids (e.g., water, clear tea, black coffee, carbonated beverages, and fruit juice without pulp)	2
Breast milk	4
Nonhuman milk, including infant formula	6
Light meal (e.g., toast and clear liquids)	6
Regular or heavy meal (may include fried or fatty food)	8

Source: Merchant, R., Chartrand, D., Dain, S., Dobson, J., Kurrek, M., LeDez, K., …, Shukla, R. (2012). *Canadian Anesthesiologists' Society Guidelines to the practice of anaesthesia* (rev. ed., 2012). *Canadian Journal of Anaesthesia, 59*(1), 63-102. doi:10.1007/s12630-011-9609-0

that the patient and family clearly understand what is going to happen. The most important of these forms is the signed consent form for the surgical procedure on the correct side (right or left), with no abbreviations, and for blood transfusion. Other forms can include those that have been completed for advance directives, living wills, and power of attorney (see Chapter 13).

Consent for Surgery

Before nonemergency surgery can be legally performed, the patient must voluntarily sign an informed consent in the presence of a witness. **Informed consent** is an active, shared decision-making process between the provider and the recipient of care. This process protects the patient, the surgeon, and the hospital and its employees. Every surgical facility has its own required informed consent form, and the nurse should become familiar with both the form and the process of obtaining consent in that institution.

Conditions that must exist for consent to be valid include the following (Burkhardt, Nathaniel, & Walton, 2010, p. 150):
- It must relate to the treatment.
- It must be informed.
- It must be voluntary.
- It cannot be obtained through misrepresentation or fraud.

There must be adequate disclosure of the diagnosis; the purpose of the proposed treatment; the risks and consequences of the proposed treatment; the probability of a successful outcome; the availability, benefits, and risks of alternative treatments (see the Ethical Dilemmas box); and the prognosis if treatment is not instituted. The patient must have the capacity to comprehend the information being provided. Preoperative drugs may interfere with patient comprehension, so the operative consent must be voluntarily signed before any preoperative medication is given. Consent can be withdrawn at any time by the patient so preoperative verification by the nurse is an integral part of the assessment (Pudner, 2010). Although the physician is ultimately responsible for obtaining the consent, in most institutions, the nurse may witness the patient's signature on the consent form. At this time, the nurse can be a patient advocate, verifying that the patient (or a family member) understands the consent form and its implications and that consent for surgery is truly voluntary. The nurse will contact the surgeon and explain the

EVIDENCE-INFORMED PRACTICE

How Long Should Patients Fast Before Elective Surgery?

Clinical Question
Should patients (P) be NPO (I) after midnight or for a shortened period (C) before elective surgery (O)?

Best Available Evidence
Systematic review of "randomized controlled trials" to evaluate the effect on surgical patient well-being that included thirst and hunger, anxiety and pain, and nausea and vomiting. Further, the review looked at fasting effects on different adult populations regarding perioperative complications such as aspiration and regurgitation.

Critical Appraisal and Synthesis of Evidence
- 22 trials (with 38 randomized controlled comparisons)
- Healthy adults not at risk for regurgitation or aspiration
- No evidence showed that a shortened fast period increased patients' risk for aspiration or complication intraoperatively compared with risk for those patients who were NPO after midnight.
- Patients who were able to have water to drink before surgery also had a significantly lower gastric volume.

Conclusion
Based on extensive evidence, the CAS and ASA revised practice guidelines for preoperative fasting in healthy patients undergoing elective procedures (see Table 20-9).

Implications for Nursing Practice
More collaboration between nurses and surgeons is needed to ensure that fasting instructions conform to CAS and ASA guidelines and that patients understand them.

References for Evidence
Brady, M. C., Kinn, S., Stuart, P., & Ness, V. (2010). Preoperative fasting for adults to prevent perioperative complications. *Cochrane Database of Systematic Reviews*, 2003, Issue 4. Art. No.: CD004423. DOI:10.1002/14651858 CD004423 Retrieved from *http://summaries.cochrane.org/ CD004423/preoperative-fasting-for-adults-to-prevent-perioperative-complications*

ASA, American Society of Anesthesiologists; *CAS*, Canadian Anaesthesiologists Society; *NPO*, nothing by mouth; *PICO: P*, patient population of interest; *I*, interventions or area of interest; *C*, comparison of interest or comparison group; *O*, outcome(s) of interest.

need for additional information if the patient is unclear about operative plans. The patient needs to be informed that permission may be withdrawn at any time, including after the permit has been signed.

In Canada, if the patient is a minor, is unconscious, or has diminished capacity to sign the consent, the written permission may be given by a legally appointed representative or responsible family member. Hospital policies should be consulted for further clarification.

In Canada, a true medical emergency may override the need to obtain consent. Exceptions for obtaining consent in an emer-

Informed Consent

Situation

The nurse discusses a patient's impending surgery in the preoperative holding area. It becomes obvious that this competent adult patient was not fully informed of the alternatives to this surgery. She has signed the consent form but clearly was not fully informed about her treatment options.

Important Points for Consideration

- Informed consent requires that patients have complete information about the proposed treatment and its possible consequences as well as alternative treatments and possible consequences.
- Risks and benefits of each treatment option must also be explained in order for patients to weigh treatment options.
- An opportunity to have questions answered about the various treatment options and their possible outcomes is also an important element of informed consent.
- Health care providers must ensure that they provide complete information for patients to make fully informed decisions and must not decide what is best for patients.

Clinical Decision-Making Questions

1. What should the nurse do?
2. What is the nurse's role as patient advocate in the informed consent process?

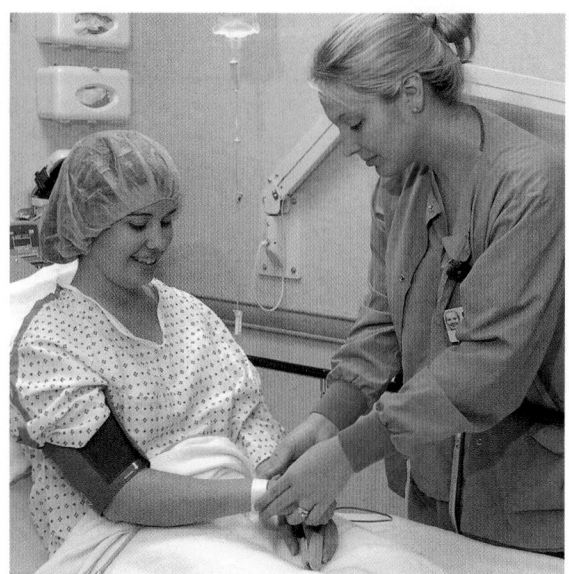

Figure 20-1 The nurse performs a safety check by verifying that the patient has an identification band (wristband) as part of the preoperative preparations before she goes to surgery.

Source: Courtesy Susan R. Volk, MSN, RN, CCRN, CPAN, Staff Development Specialist, Christiana Care Health System, Newark, DE.

gency situation include when the patient exhibits a life- or limb-threatening episode, when the patient is unable to consent for the procedure because of circumstances beyond her or his control.

A *mature minor* is a child or adolescent with an advanced level of understanding who is deemed by the physician obtaining the consent to have the intelligence, education, and experience to give informed consent for a procedure. Children and adolescents should be assessed for capability to consent on an individual basis (Burkhardt et al., 2010, p. 153). Each province or territory has its own legislation for obtaining consent; this may also vary according to institution.

▪ Day-of-Surgery Preparation

▪ Nursing Role

Day-of-surgery preparation will vary a great deal depending on whether the patient is an inpatient or an outpatient. The nursing responsibility immediately before surgery includes final preoperative teaching, assessment, and communication of pertinent findings and ensuring that all preoperative preparation orders have been completed and that records and reports are present and complete to accompany the patient to the OR. It is especially important to verify the presence of a signed operative consent, laboratory data, a history and PE report, a record of any consultations, baseline vital signs, and nurses' notes.

If the patient is an inpatient, it will be the responsibility of the nurse to ensure that the patient is ready and appropriately prepared for surgery. If the patient is an outpatient, the patient or the family member will share the responsibility for preoperative preparation.

Most institutions require that a patient has showered or bathed before surgery and that a patient is dressed in a hospital gown with no underclothes. Some surgery centres allow the patient to wear underwear, depending on the surgical procedure to be performed. The patient should wear no cosmetics because observation of skin colour will be important. Nail polish should be removed because the pulse oximeter, used to monitor oxygenation, will be placed on the patient's fingertip and cannot distinguish blood oxygen through coloured nail polish. An identification band is put on the patient and, if applicable, so is an allergy band (Figure 20-1). It is also very important to ensure that, if the patient has been typed and screened for possible blood transfusion, a blood band be applied to the patient's wrist. All patient valuables are returned to a family member or locked up according to institutional protocol. If the patient prefers not to remove a wedding ring, the ring can be taped securely to the finger to prevent loss. All other jewellery (including all body piercings) and prostheses, including dentures, contact lenses, and glasses, are generally removed to prevent loss or damage. Hearing aids are usually left in place to allow the patient to better follow instructions. Glasses and hearing aids, if removed, must be returned to the patient as soon as possible following surgery.

The patient must void shortly before surgery, and this should be documented. Urination before surgery prevents involuntary elimination under anaesthesia and reduces the possibility of urinary retention during early postoperative recovery. This should be done before the administration of any preoperative medication. Many preoperative medications can interfere with balance and could lead to a fall when the patient is in the bathroom. The nurse should determine that all preoperative preparations have been completed and that the signed consent for surgery is present before giving any preoperative medications.

Preoperative requirements	Initials	Day of surgery	Initials
Height _____ Weight _____		Surgical site marked Y N NA	
Isolation? _____ Type _____		ID band on patient	
Allergies noted on chart		Allergy band on patient Y NA	
Vital signs (Initial) T_____ P_____ R_____ BP_____		Vital signs Time _____ T_____ P_____ R_____ BP_____	
Chart Review		**Procedures**	
H&P on chart		NPO since _____	
H&P within 30 days? Y N		Capillary blood glucose Y N	
Signed and witthessed informed consent form on chart		Preoperative skin prep Y N Shower Scrub Shave	
Signed consent for blood administration Y NA		Makeup, nail polish, false fingernails, and false eyelashes removed Y NA	
Blood type and crossmatch Y NA		Hospital gown applied Y NA	
Name plate on chart		**Valuables Y N**	
Old chart requested and sent Y NA		Dentures _____	
Diagnostic Results		Wig or hairpiece _____	
Hb/Hct _____ / _____ NA		Eyeglasses _____	
PT/INR/PTT _____ / _____ / _____ NA		Contact lenses _____	
CXR _____ NA		Hearing aid _____	
ECG _____ NA		Prosthesis _____	
Other labs		Jewellery _____	
		Clothing _____	
Final chart review: New forms added		Disposition of valuables Family Rings taped Safe	
Signed off		Voided/catheter Time _____	
		Preooperative medications given Time _____ NA	
Time to OR _____ Date _____ Transported to OR by _____ Final check by _____ RN		Preoperative antibiotics given Time _____ NA	

Figure 20-2 Preoperative checklist. *BP*, blood pressure; *CXR*, chest x-ray scan; *ECG*, electrocardiogram; *H&P*, history and physical examination; *Hb*, hemoglobin; *Hct*, hematocrit; *ID*, identification; *INR*, international normalized ratio; *N*, no; *NA*, not applicable; *NPO*, nothing by mouth; *OR*, operating room; *P*, pulse; *PT*, prothrombin time; *PTT*, partial thromboplastin time; *R*, respiration; *T*, temperature; *Y*, yes.

SAFETY ALERT

Use a preoperative checklist (Figure 20-2) to ensure that all preoperative preparations have been completed before the patient is given any sedating medications.

▪ Preoperative Medications

Preoperative medications are used for a variety of reasons (Table 20-10). A patient may receive a single drug or a combination of drugs (Table 20-11). Benzodiazepines and barbiturates are used for their sedative and amnestic properties. Anticholinergics may be given to reduce secretions. Narcotics may be given to decrease intraoperative anaesthetic requirements and to decrease pain. Antiemetics may be given to decrease nausea and vomiting after surgery.

DRUG THERAPY

Table 20-10 Purposes of Preoperative Medications

- Provide analgesia
- Prevent nausea and vomiting
- Promote sedation and amnesia
- Decrease anaesthetic requirements
- Facilitate induction of anaesthesia
- Relieve apprehension and anxiety
- Prevent autonomic reflex response
- Decrease respiratory and gastrointestinal secretions

DRUG THERAPY

Table 20-11 Frequently Used Preoperative Medications

CLASS	DRUG	PURPOSE AND EFFECTS
Benzodiazepines	Midazolam	Reduce anxiety
	Diazepam (Valium)	Induce sedation
	Lorazepam (Ativan)	Induce amnesia
Narcotics	Morphine	Relieve discomfort during preoperative procedures
	Meperidine (Demerol)	
	Fentanyl	
Histamine H$_2$-receptor antagonists	Cimetidine	Increase gastric pH
	Famotidine (Pepcid)	Decrease gastric volume
	Ranitidine (Zantac)	
Antacids	Sodium citrate	Increase gastric pH
Antiemetics	Metoclopramide	Increase gastric emptying
Anticholinergics	Atropine	Decrease oral and respiratory secretions
	Glycopyrrolate	

Other medications that may be administered before surgery include antibiotics, eye drops, and routine prescription drugs. Antibiotics may be administered throughout the perioperative period for a patient with a history of congenital or valvular heart disease to prevent the development of infective endocarditis, for patients in whom wound contamination is either a potential risk or in whom wound infection could have serious postoperative consequences (e.g., cardiac and joint replacement surgery). Antibiotics are most commonly administered by IV route and may be started either before surgery or in the OR with optimal initiation 30 minutes before the incision time. Provincial reporting of prophylactic antibiotic use rates for specific surgical interventions to monitor Surgical Site Infections are required by some provinces (Baker, 2009).

Eye drops are commonly ordered and administered before surgery for the patient undergoing cataract and other eye surgery. Many times, the patient will require multiple sets of eye drops administered at 5-minute intervals. It is important to administer these drugs as ordered and on time to adequately prepare the eye for surgery.

A standard protocol for what routine medications are always given on the day of surgery and those that are never given on the day of surgery does not exist. In order to facilitate patient teaching and eliminate confusion about the medications, it is very important to carefully check written preoperative orders and to clarify which medications should and should not be taken on the day of surgery. If there is any question, the nurse should clarify the orders with the anaesthesiologist. Most patients will be advised to take routine cardiac, antihypertensive, and asthma medications on the day of surgery. In the case of insulin, it is important to clarify the time and amount of the last dose before surgery.

Premedications may be administered by oral, IV, subcutaneous, or intramuscular routes. Oral medications should be given 60 to 90 minutes before the patient goes to the OR. Because patients are fluid restricted before surgery, the patient should swallow these medications with a minimal amount of water. Intramuscular and subcutaneous injections should be given 30 to 60 minutes before arrival at the OR (minimally 20 minutes). IV medications are usually administered to the patient after arrival in the preoperative holding area or OR. The drug administration must be charted immediately. The patient should be told the effects of the medications, such as relaxation, drowsiness, and dryness of the mouth.

■ Transportation to the Operating Room

If the patient is an inpatient, in most institutions, the OR staff sends transport personnel to the patient's room with a stretcher to transport the patient to surgery. The nurse assists the patient in transferring from the hospital bed to the OR stretcher, and the side rails of the stretcher are raised and secured. Some hospitals allow patients to be transported to the OR in their hospital beds, especially in instances in which the patient may have difficulty transferring from a stretcher to a bed after surgery (i.e., total joint replacement, Caesarean section). The nurse should ensure that the completed chart goes with the patient.

If the patient is an outpatient, the patient may be transported to the OR by stretcher or wheelchair or, in the absence of premedication, may even walk, accompanied, to the OR. In all cases, it is important for the nurse to ensure patient safety during transport. The method of transportation and who transported the patient should be documented by the nurse responsible for the transfer.

The family or caregivers should be instructed where to wait for the patient during surgery. Many hospitals have a surgical waiting room where OR personnel communicate the status of the patient to the family. It is in this waiting room that the surgeon can locate the family after surgery and where families can be notified that the surgery is complete. Some hospitals provide pagers to waiting family members so that they may eat or do errands during the surgery.

While the patient is in surgery, the inpatient nurse can prepare the patient's room in consideration of the patient's needs after surgery. There must be equipment for vital signs assessment, which will be the first priority of the receiving nurse. The bed is remade and raised to stretcher height, and if necessary, disposable pads are placed for any anticipated drainage. The nurse should also ensure that there is a basin, soap, towels, and clean gown available in the patient's room. Any additional necessary equipment, including IV poles, oxygen, suction, kidney basin, and additional pillows for positioning, should also be placed in the room. The room should be organized to facilitate entry of the stretcher or hospital bed. By having these items readily available and the room ready, patient transfer from the PACU or PARR will be smooth.

CULTURALLY COMPETENT CARE: PATIENT ABOUT TO UNDERGO SURGERY

The nurse should include cultural and ethnic considerations when assessing and implementing care for the preoperative needs of a patient. For example, culture, not necessarily related to ethnicity, might determine one's expression of pain, coping strategies, family expectations, and ability to verbally express needs for an optimal level of quality of life (Walter et al., 2007). Canadians may belong to any number of diverse groups that have many cultural variations. Decisions made because of cultural variations must be respected and valued. (Culturally competent care is discussed in Chapter 2.)

AGE-RELATED CONSIDERATIONS: OLDER ADULT PATIENT ABOUT TO UNDERGO SURGERY

Many surgical procedures are performed on patients older than 65 years of age, and surgery can be safely performed even on those in their 90s. Frequently performed procedures in the older adult are cataract extraction, coronary and vascular procedures, prostate surgery, herniorrhaphy, cholecystectomy, total knee and hip replacements, and repair of fractured hips.

The nurse must be particularly alert when assessing and caring for the older adult patient undergoing surgery. An event that has little effect on a younger patient may be overwhelming to the older patient. The risks associated with anaesthesia and surgery increase in the older patient (Rothrock, 2011, p. 1161). It is important to assess the physiological reserve of the geriatric patient, because frailty is predictive of postoperative outcomes (Makary et al., 2010). As a whole, the older the patient, the greater the risk of complications after surgery. The geriatric population has specific assessments and considerations. For instance, it is important to consider the physiological status or condition of the patient in planning care and not simply the chronological age. The patient's biological age rather than the chronological age is important to consider in planning surgery and assessing risks. A 75-year-old woman may be biologically healthy and be more like a 60 year old in physiological responses. Conversely, a 55 year old with multiple chronic health problems may biologically be more like a 75 year old. The surgical risk in the older adult relates to normal physiological aging and changes that compromise organ function, reduce reserve capacity, and limit the body's ability to adapt to stress. This decreased ability to cope with stress, frequently compounded by the additional burden of one or more chronic illnesses, and the surgery itself increase the risk of complications.

When preparing the older adult for surgery, it is important to obtain a detailed history and complete PE. Preoperative laboratory tests, an electrocardiogram, laboratory results, and a chest radiograph can be important in planning the choice and technique of anaesthesia. When caring for a geriatric patient, more than one physician may be involved. It is important for the nurse to help coordinate the care and the physicians' orders for the patient.

Consideration of family support is important with the older adult. With the increase in same-day surgical procedures and shorter postoperative hospitalization, family support is an important consideration in the continuity of care for the older patient.

The nurse must remember that many older adults have sensory deficits. Vision and hearing may be diminished, and bright lights may bother those with eye problems. Thought processes and cognitive abilities may be slowed or impaired. This does not mean that every elderly person has cognitive deficits. Sensory function and cognition must be assessed and documented (Clayton, 2008). Physical reactions are often slowed as a result of mobility and balance problems. All of these changes may necessitate that more time be allowed for the older adult to complete preoperative testing and understand preoperative instructions.

Some older adults live in long-term care facilities. Transportation from these agencies must be coordinated so that timely arrival allows for surgery preparation. If a long-term care patient is cognitively impaired, a falls-risk assessment should be completed. A legal representative of the patient must be present to provide consent for surgery if the patient cannot sign for himself or herself.

Adding to the stress of the surgical procedure, even a minimally invasive one, the perceived situational change and loss may be overwhelming to the older adult. The threat to independence, lifestyle, and self-esteem may result in ineffective coping. The nurse must be particularly supportive and help the older adult cope with the surgical experience.

CLINICAL DECISION-MAKING EXERCISE

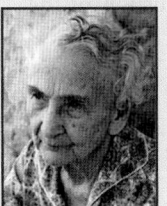

CASE STUDY
Patient About to Undergo Surgery

Source: © iStockphoto.com/bbear

Patient Profile

Mrs. Mary Goodswimmer, an 82-year-old First Nations retired librarian, is admitted to the hospital with compromised circulation of the right lower leg and a necrotic right foot. She was diagnosed with diabetes 40 years ago and takes insulin to maintain appropriate blood glucose levels. She is scheduled for surgery today for a below-knee amputation under spinal anaesthesia. She had a light breakfast at 0600 hours and a glass of apple juice at 1000 hours but has not had anything since. It is now 1300 hours of the day of surgery.

Subjective Data

- History of type 2 diabetes mellitus for 40 years
- History of renal problems
- History of vision problems
- Surgical history that includes a Caesarean section at age 30 and a cholecystectomy at age 65; did not heal well following the last surgery
- Blood glucose has not been well controlled
- Pension cheques barely cover the cost of living and medications
- Lives alone but has family that wants her to move in with them following surgery
- Uses herbs to control diabetes and frequently refuses to take insulin

Objective Data

Physical Examination

- Alert, cognitively intact, anxious, elderly woman with complaints of numbness and lack of feeling in right leg
- Weight, 65 kg; height, 160 cm
- Wears glasses
- Has macular degeneration in her right eye

Diagnostic Studies

- Admission laboratory blood glucose level was 29.8 mmol/L
- Morning finger-stick blood glucose level was 5.39 mmol/L
- Doppler pulses for lower right leg very weak; absent in right foot
- Doppler pulses in left leg present, weak in left foot
- Serum creatinine 221 mmol/L

Collaborative Care

- Scheduled for a below-the-knee amputation of the right leg as the last case of the day

Discussion Questions

1. What factors may influence Mrs. Goodswimmer's response to hospitalization and surgery?
2. *Priority Decision:* Given Mrs. Goodswimmer's history, what priority preoperative nursing assessments would you want to complete and why?
3. *Priority Decision:* What priority topics would you include in Mrs. Goodswimmer's preoperative teaching plan?
4. *Priority Decision:* Based on the assessment data presented, identify the priority nursing diagnoses and related interventions. Are there any collaborative problems?

🅔volve *Answers are available at* **http://evolve.elsevier.com/ Canada/Lewis/medsurg**

REVIEW QUESTIONS

The number of the question corresponds to the same-numbered objective at the beginning of the chapter.

1. Which of the following surgical procedures involves removal of a body organ?
   a. Colostomy
   b. Laparotomy
   c. Mammoplasty
   d. Cholecystectomy
2. Which of the following is one of the most important goals of the preoperative assessment by the nurse?
   a. Determine whether the patient's psychological stress is too high to undergo surgery.
   b. Identify what information the patient needs to understand before surgery.
   c. Establish baseline data for comparison of the patient's status in the intraoperative and postoperative periods.
   d. Determine whether the patient's surgery should be done on an inpatient, an outpatient, or a same-day admission basis.
3. A patient who is scheduled for a hysterectomy reports using ginkgo biloba to improve her memory. Which of the following questions is the most important for the perioperative nurse to ask the patient?
   a. "How long have you used ginkgo biloba?"
   b. "How have you been able to tell if this herb is effective?"
   c. "Have you been taking this herb during the last several weeks?"
   d. "Have you experienced any adverse effects of taking this herbal product?"
4. What is the nurse's role when assisting a patient with informed consent before an operative procedure?
   a. Obtains the consent when a surgeon cannot
   b. Asks the patient to explain what surgical procedure she or he is having and ensures that the patient understands the operation to be performed
   c. Explains all the risks of the surgical procedure
   d. Ensures that the patient signs the consent form before preoperative sedation is given

5. What is a **priority** nursing intervention that will assist a patient about to undergo surgery in coping with fear of pain?
   a. Describe the degree of pain expected.
   b. Explain the availability of pain medication.
   c. Divert the patient when talking about pain.
   d. Inform the patient of the frequency of pain medication.
6. What is the last nursing intervention that should be performed before a patient is transported to the operating room?
   a. Ask the patient to void in the bathroom.
   b. Check chart for signed consent form.
   c. Administer preanaesthetic medications.
   d. Lock up the patient's jewellery and money.
7. What should the nurse administering preoperative medications recognize before administering the medication?
   a. Preoperative medications are used only to decrease patient anxiety.
   b. Intravenous medications can be administered only by an anaesthesiologist on the day of surgery.
   c. A preoperative diazepam (Valium) tablet should be administered within 15 minutes of scheduled surgery.
   d. Preoperative narcotics given to decrease pain may help reduce intraoperative anaesthetic requirements.
8. What is a primary consideration in the instruction of the older patient about to undergo surgery?
   a. Using large-print material
   b. Teaching early in the morning
   c. Standing very close to aid communication
   d. Recognizing that cognitive function may be decreased

REFERENCES

American Society of Anesthesiologists. (2010). *Herbal supplements and anesthesia*. Park Ridge, IL: Author.

Arman, M., & Rehnsfeldt, A. (2007). The "little extra" that alleviates suffering. *Nursing Ethics, 14*(3), 372-386. doi:10.1177/0969733007075877

Bailey, L. (2010). Strategies for decreasing patient anxiety in the perioperative setting. *American Operating Room Nursing Journal, 92*(4), 445-460. doi:10.1016/j.aorn.2010.04.017

Baker, M. (2009). Public reporting of CLI, VAP and SSI (prophylactic antibiotic use) rates. Retrieved from *http://www.health.gov.on.ca/patient_safety/pro/ssi/pro_resource/pres_baker_ssi_20090404.pdf*

Baril, P., & Portman, H. (2007). Preoperative fasting: Knowledge and perceptions. *AORN Journal, 86*(4), 609-617. doi:10.1016/j.aorn.2007.09.003

Barua, B., Rovere, M., & Skinner, B. (2011). Waiting your turn: Wait times for health care in Canada. 2011 report. Studies in Health Policy. Fraser Institute. Retrieved from *http://www.fraserinstitute.org/uploadedFiles/fraser-ca/Content/research-news/research/publications/waiting-your-turn-2011.pdf*

Burkhardt, M., Nathaniel, A., & Walton, N. (2010). *Ethics and issues in contemporary nursing*. Toronto: Nelson.

Clayton, J. L. (2008). Special needs of older adults undergoing surgery. *AORN Journal, 87*(3), 557-570. doi:10.1016/j.aorn.2008.02.006

D'Amico, D., Barbarito, C., Twomey, C., & Harder, N. (2012). *Health and physical assessment in nursing*. Toronto: Pearson Canada.

Drain, C., & Odom-Forren, J. (2009) *Perianesthesia nursing*. St. Louis: Saunders Elsevier.

Hepner, D. (2009). The role of testing in the preoperative evaluation. *Cleveland Clinic Journal of Medicine, 76*(4), S22-S27. doi:10.3949/ccjm.76.s4.04

Lauerman, C. J. (2008). Surgical patient education related to smoking. *AORN Journal, 87*(3), 599-609. doi:10.1016/j.aorn.2007.09.015

Makary, M., Segev, D., Pronovost, P., Syin, D., Bandeen-Roche, K., Patel, P., ..., Fried, L. (2010). Frailty as a predictor of surgical outcomes in older patients. *Journal of American College of Surgeons, 210*(6), 901-908. doi:10.1016/j.jamcollsurg.2010.01.028

Merchant, R., Bosenberg, C., Brown, K., Chartrand, D., Dain, S., Dobson, J., ..., Shukla, R. (2010). Guidelines to the practice of anesthesia: Revised ed. 2010. *Canadian Journal of Anesthesia, 57*(1), 58-87. doi:10.1007/s12630-009-9209-4

Ontario Anesthesiologists. (2012). Why stop smoking for safer surgery. Retrieved from *http://www.ontarioanesthesiologists.ca/stop-smoking-safe-surgery/why-stop-smoking-for-safer-surgery/*

Operating Room Nurses Association of Canada (ORNAC). (2011). *Standards, guidelines, and position statements for perioperative registered nursing practice* (10th ed.). Halifax, NS: ORNAC.

Phillips, N. (2012). Principles of asepsis and sterile techniques. In N. Phillips (Ed.). *Operating room technique* (12th ed.). St. Louis: Mosby.

Pudner, R. (2010). *Nursing the surgical patient*. St. Louis: Elsevier.

Registered Nurses' Association of Ontario (RNAO). (2011). *Helping people quit smoking*. Toronto: Author. Retrieved from *http://elearning.rnao.ca/*

Rothrock, J. (2011). *Alexander's care of the patient in surgery* (14th ed.). St. Louis: Elsevier Mosby.

Shorofi, S., & Arbon, P. A., (2010). Complementary and alternative medicine (CAM) among hospitalised patients: An Australian study. *Complementary Therapies in Clinical Practice, 16*(2), 86-91. doi:10.1016/j.ctcp.2009.09.009

Tourigny, J., Clendinneng, D., Chartrand, J., & Gaboury, I. (2011). Evaluation of a virtual tour for children undergoing same-day surgery and their parents. *Pediatric Nursing 37*(4), 117-183.

Transfusion Medicine. (2011). *Informed consent for transfusion*. Toronto: Canadian Blood Services. Retrieved from *http://www.transfusionmedicine.ca/*

University of Vermont. (2009, May 1). Caffeine withdrawal headache explained: Your brain on—and off—caffeine. *Science Daily*. Retrieved from *http://www.sciencedaily.com/releases/2009/05/090501162805.htm*

Walter, M. H., Woronuk, J. I., Tan, H. K., Lenz, U., Koch, R., Boening, K. W., & Pinchbeck, Y. J. (2007). Determinants of oral health-related quality of life in a cross-cultural German-Canadian sample. *Journal of Public Health, 15*, 43-50. doi:10.1007/s10389-006-0077-x

RESOURCES

Resources for this chapter are listed in Chapter 22 on page 478.

evolve   *For additional Internet resources, see the Web site for this book at* **http://evolve.elsevier.com/Canada/Lewis/medsurg**

Nursing Management: Intraoperative Care

Written by Anita Shoup and Maura M. Sheridan*
Adapted by Debra Clendinneng

LEARNING OBJECTIVES

1. Describe the roles of the perioperative nurse, nurse anaesthesiologist, and registered nurse first assistant.
2. Name three different areas of the surgical suite and the proper attire for each area.
3. Describe the physical environment of the operating room and the holding area.
4. Describe the functions of the members of the surgical team.
5. Identify needs experienced by the patient undergoing surgical procedures.
6. Describe basic principles of aseptic technique used in the operating room.
7. Discuss the importance of safety in the positioning of patients.
8. Differentiate between general and regional or local anaesthesia, including advantages, disadvantages, and rationale for choice of the anaesthetic technique.
9. Identify the basic techniques used to induce and maintain general anaesthesia.
10. Discuss techniques for administering local and regional anaesthesia.

KEY TERMS

anaesthesiologist A specialist physician who administers the anaesthetic, p. 442

circulating nurse A perioperative nurse who is not scrubbed, gowned, or gloved and remains in an unsterile field, p. 441

epidural block Injection of a local anaesthetic into the epidural (extradural) space via either a thoracic or a lumbar approach, p. 451

general anaesthesia The loss of sensation with loss of consciousness, skeletal muscle relaxation, analgesia, and elimination of the somatic, autonomic, and endocrine responses, including coughing, gagging, vomiting, and sympathetic nervous system responsiveness, p. 448

holding area Also called the preoperative holding area; a special waiting area inside or adjacent to the surgical suite, p. 440

local anaesthesia The loss of sensation without loss of consciousness, p. 448

malignant hyperthermia A rare metabolic disease characterized by hyperthermia with rigidity of skeletal muscles that can result in death, p. 453

operating room (OR) A unique acute care setting specially designed for surgery, with strict geographical,

environmental, and bacteriological control and restricted flow of personnel; the traditional setting for surgery. Can be located within hospitals or in separate clinical or physicians' surgery offices, p. 440

perioperative nurse A nurse who practises in a variety of settings (OR, ambulatory care, clinics, physicians' offices, and communities) who focuses on identifying and meeting the individual needs throughout the perioperative period of the patient undergoing surgery, p. 439

procedural sedation Moderately depressed level of consciousness used for managing patient pain and anxiety but which maintains the patient's protective airway reflexes. Patient may be monitored by a nurse with appropriate rescue training, p. 448

regional anaesthesia The loss of sensation to a region of the body without loss of consciousness when a specific nerve or group of nerves is blocked with the administration of a local anaesthetic, p. 448

scrub nurse A perioperative nurse who is gowned and gloved in sterile attire, follows the designated scrub procedure, and remains in the sterile field, p. 441

---

*Contributed anaesthesia content.

spinal anaesthesia The injection of a local anaesthetic into the cerebrospinal fluid found in the subarachnoid space, usually below the level of L2, p. 451

surgeon The physician who performs the surgical procedure, p. 441

surgical suite A controlled environment designed to minimize the spread of infectious organisms and allow a smooth flow of patients, personnel, and instruments and equipment needed to provide safe patient care; divided into the unrestricted, the semirestricted, and the restricted areas, p. 439

ELECTRONIC RESOURCES

Supplemental content related to Chapter 21 can be found . . .

Evolve Web Site ⊝volve

http://evolve.elsevier.com/Canada/Lewis/medsurg
- Clinical Reference: Laboratory Values
- Content Updates

- Electronic Calculators
- Examination Review Questions
- Glossary
- Key Points (Printable and MP3 Download)

The **perioperative nurse** provides individualized nursing to patients throughout the surgical continuum. In order to address the patient's complex physiological, psychological, sociocultural, and spiritual responses to the surgical event, perioperative nurses require basic and expanded knowledge, skills, and abilities. The Operating Room Nurses Association of Canada (ORNAC) *Standards of Practice* present the evidence-informed rationale for the structure and resources required in the perioperative environment that promotes safe, effective patient care (ORNAC, 2011, p. 17). Since 1995, perioperative nurses have been able to attain national certification through the Canadian Nurses Association (2008) and the designation Certified Perioperative Nurse (Canada). This certification reinforces ORNAC's mission to promote and advance excellence in perioperative patient care (ORNAC, 2011, p. 21). Expanded roles of the perioperative nurse include registered nurse first assistant (RNFA) and nurse anaesthesiologist.

The advent of advanced surgical technologies, improvements in the administration of anaesthesia, and changes in the Canadian health care system have altered where and how surgery is delivered. Depending on the acuity of the surgical procedure, it can be performed in diverse environments like hospital operating rooms, ambulatory care settings, and clinics. Today, the majority of surgery is minimally invasive and done on an outpatient basis. This eliminates the need for hospital admission, decreasing postoperative pain, and recuperation and allows for an earlier return to the patient's normal lifestyle (Rothrock, 2011, p. 205). The impact for the surgical team is shorter procedures requiring quicker turnovers and less time available for perioperative teaching of the patient and caregivers. The perioperative nurse knows that all surgical procedures have a potential for complications. These nurses refer to research and national patient safety standards and embed safe practice into the perioperative environment (Canadian Patient Safety Institute, 2009). This is accomplished through establishing and maintaining an aseptic environment, keeping current on new technologies, and continuing to advocate for safe patient care, for instance, in the implementation of the Safe Surgery Checklist—an interprofessional time out before the surgical incision to verify patient information

(Canadian Patient Safety Institute, 2009). In a 2009 global research project involving over 3000 surgical patients, the postoperative death rate before the implementation of the checklist was 1.5%; after implementation, it was reduced to 0.8%. Postoperative complications for inpatients went from 11% to 7%. The implementation of the checklist was associated with marked improvement in patient safety (Haynes et al., 2009). (See the Resources at the end of this chapter for the Canadian adaptation of the Surgical Safety Checklist.)

Physical Environment

Department Layout

The **surgical suite** is a controlled environment designed to minimize the spread of infectious organisms and allow a smooth flow of patients, personnel, and the instruments and equipment needed to provide safe patient care. The suite is divided into three distinct areas: the unrestricted, the semirestricted, and the restricted. The *unrestricted* area is where personnel in street clothes can interact with those in scrub uniforms. These areas typically include the holding area, a point of entry for patients, staff locker rooms, and the communication centre or nursing station. The *semirestricted* area includes the peripheral support areas and corridors. Authorized personnel can access semirestricted areas but must wear surgical attire and cover all head and facial hair. In the *restricted* area, including the ORs, the scrub sink areas, and the clean core, personnel wear masks to supplement their surgical attire (ORNAC, 2011, p. 110). This physical layout is designed to reduce cross-contamination. Clean and sterile supplies and equipment should be separated from waste and supplies contaminated by patient contact by space, time, and traffic patterns. An example is the movement of sterile surgical supplies from the medical device reprocessing department (MDRD) through the clean core and into the OR for surgery. Supplies contaminated after surgery are transported through the peripheral areas back to the decontamination area of the MDRD (ORNAC, 2011, p. 111).

Holding Area

The **holding area,** frequently called the *preoperative holding area,* is a special waiting area inside or adjacent to the surgical suite. The size varies according to hospital design and can range from a centralized area to accommodate numerous patients to a small designated area immediately outside the actual room scheduled for the surgical procedure. In the holding area, the perioperative nurse makes the final identification and assessment before the patient is transferred into the OR for surgery. Many minor procedures can also be performed in the holding area, such as catheter insertions for intravenous (IV) and invasive monitoring (central venous pressure and arterial line), peripheral and spinal nerve blocks, epidural catheter insertion, and preoperative drug administration. Depending on the location of the holding unit, some institutions permit the family or a friend to wait with the patient until it is time to be transferred to the OR because this helps relieve patient anxiety.

Operating Room

The **operating room (OR)** is a unique acute care setting (Figure 21-1), that is usually adjacent to the *postanaesthesia care unit* (PACU) and the surgical intensive care unit (ICU). This allows for quick postoperative transportation of the surgical patient. Close proximity to anaesthesia and surgical personnel promotes collaboration during postanaesthesia recovery and intensive care follow-up, especially if complications arise.

ORs are designed using infection control principles. Transmission of dust and microorganisms is controlled by HEPA (high-efficiency particulate air) filters in the ventilating systems, and controlled airflow and proper air exchange provides physical comfort and helps remove toxic fumes and anaesthetic gas fumes (ORNAC, 2011). Positive air pressure in the rooms and keeping the doors closed prevents air from back-flowing from the halls and corridors to the OR (Rothrock, 2011, p. 89). Materials that are easily disinfected are used. Physical safety and comfort are aided by the use of OR furniture that is adjustable and easily cleaned and moved. All equipment is checked frequently to ensure proper functioning and electrical safety. The lighting is designed to provide a low- to high-intensity range for a precise view of the surgical site. A communication system provides a means for the delivery of routine and emergency messages (ORNAC, 2011).

The temperature is controlled to remain between 20°C and 24°C, and the humidity is regulated at 30% to 60% to facilitate patient comfort under the surgical drapes, team comfort during the procedure, and an environment that inhibits bacterial incubation and growth (ORNAC, 2011, p. 250). The privacy of the patient is achieved by restricting access to the OR by unnecessary hospital personnel and visitors (Figure 21-2).

Surgical Team

Registered Nurse

ORNAC describes the scope of perioperative registered nursing practice as a continuum of nursing activities that focuses on identifying and meeting the patient's individual needs throughout the perioperative experience (ORNAC, 2011). Competencies include: practising professionally, providing physical and supportive care, promoting a safe environment, responding to urgent situations, and managing resources (ORNAC, 2011, p. 53).The perioperative nurse orchestrates the preparation of the OR with other members of the surgical team. When the patient arrives in the surgical suite, the nurse is usually the first member of the surgical team to greet her or him. The nurse is the patient's advocate throughout the intraoperative experience. For instance, the patient's individual plan of care may include ensuring comfortable positioning, placement of a warming blanket, and negotiating with the anaesthesiologist to preserve the patient's autonomy by leaving her or his hearing aids in until the patient

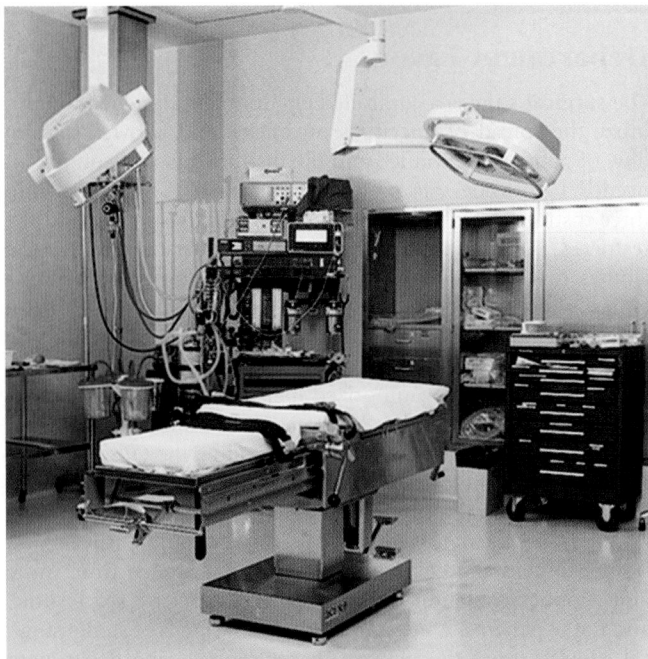

Figure 21-1 Traditional operating room.

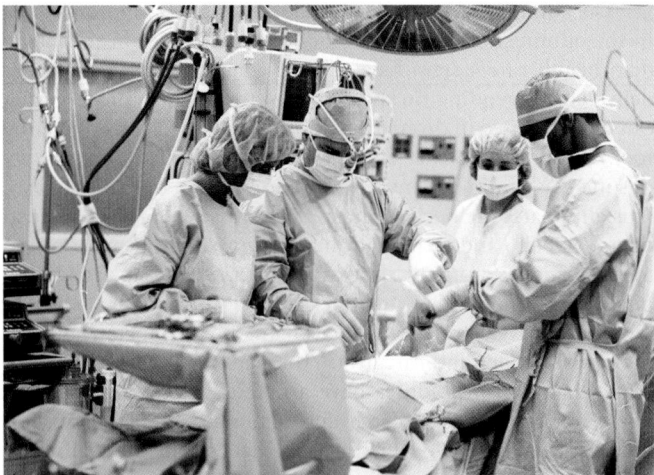

Figure 21-2 The complexity of the operative procedure does not permit the presence of extra personnel or visitors.

is anaesthetized. As well as communicating about the upcoming experience, the nurse helps reduce the patient's anxiety through proximity and touch (Phillips, 2013a).

Different roles may be assumed by the perioperative nurse that involve either sterile or nonsterile activities. If the nurse is not scrubbed, gowned, and gloved and remains in the unsterile field, the function of *circulating* is implemented and the nurse is referred to as the **circulating nurse**. Some specific intraoperative activities of the circulating nurse are outlined in Table 21-1. The nurse who follows the designated scrub procedure is gowned and gloved in sterile attire and remains in the sterile field implements the function of *scrubbing* and is termed the **scrub nurse**. The scrub nurse's duties include setting priorities and ensuring an efficient aseptic set-up for the surgical procedure, monitoring aseptic technique throughout the procedure, performing the surgical count concurrently with the circulating nurse, and acting as the patient's advocate during the surgical procedure (ORNAC, 2011).

Perioperative nurses use critical thinking in ongoing patient assessment and when responding to changing patient conditions. Examples of nursing activities that characterize each phase surrounding the surgical experience are presented in Table 21-2.

The nurse in the circulating role documents nursing and medical activities throughout the perioperative period. Intraoperative documentation includes, but is not limited to (ORNAC, 2011, pp. 196-200):

- Naming all personnel involved in patient care in the OR.
- Recording event times, additional interventions such as radiographic scanning or fluoroscopy, and the surgical procedure performed.
- Documenting the patient's positioning, surgical skin preparation, and placement of dispersive pad.
- Documenting patient monitoring devices and type of anaesthesia.
- Recording all equipment used on the patient including settings, serial numbers, and the like.
- Noting information for prosthetic implants and other devices left in the patient such as catheters and drains.
- Logging of specimens and documenting blood loss and the surgical count.
- Making a note of any untoward events.

Practical Nurse

In many Canadian institutions, a trained practical nurse performs the scrubbing function. The scrubbed person assists the surgeon by passing instruments and implementing other technical functions during the surgical procedure. This role is supervised and can also be assumed by a registered nurse (RN).

Surgeon and Assistant

The **surgeon** is the physician who performs the surgical procedure. The surgeon may be the patient's primary physician or one who was selected by the patient's physician or the patient. The surgeon is primarily responsible for the following:

1. Preoperative medical history and physical assessment, including need for surgical intervention, choice of surgical procedure, and management of preoperative workup.
2. Obtaining informed consent and explaining all the risks and complications associated with surgery and alternate treatment options.

Table 21-1 Activities of the Circulating Nurse
Circulating Role
The perioperative Registered Nurse shall practice in a manner that:
2.1 Assesses the physical status of the patient
2.2 Develops, modifies and documents the individualized plan of care, or a clinical pathway to meet the specific needs of the patient
2.3 Provides resources for the health care team to function efficiently
2.4 Provides physical comfort measures specific to each surgical patient
2.5 Provides appropriate care during the admission, pre-induction, induction, intraoperative, and emergence phases
2.6 Performs the surgical count procedure concurrently with the scrub nurse and documents accurately
2.7 Uses a surgical conscience to maintain and monitor the integrity of the sterile field
2.8 Reduces risk by providing continuous, astute, and vigilant observation of the surgical team throughout the surgical phase meeting the health care team and patient's needs
2.9 Acts as the patient's advocate throughout the perioperative period
2.10 Responds appropriately to complications and unexpected events during the perioperative period
2.11 Organizes and coordinates appropriate resources in a timely manner in preparation for the subsequent patient
2.12 Provides and assists with procedures/devices required to complete patient care following the surgical procedure
2.13 Assists in the patient transfer and postoperative positioning
2.14 Accurately and appropriately documents nursing, surgical, and other health care team activities during the perioperative period
2.15 Promotes appropriate communication techniques to keep noise levels at a minimum
2.16 Assists with patient transport to a receiving unit and communicates pertinent patient information
2.17 Organizes and coordinates appropriate resources to ensure an efficient theatre turnover

Source: Operating Room Nurses Association of Canada (ORNAC). (2011). *Standards, guidelines, and position statements for perioperative registered nursing practice* (10th ed., p. 55). Halifax, NS: Author.

3. Patient safety and surgical management in the OR.
4. Postoperative management of the patient.

The surgeon's assistant can be a physician who functions in an assisting role during the surgical procedure. The assistant usually holds retractors to expose surgical areas and assists with hemostasis and suturing. In some instances, especially in educational settings, the assistant may perform some portions of the operative procedure under the direct supervision of the surgeon. In some institutions, the surgeon's assistant is an RNFA, an advanced practice nurse who functions in the role of assistant under the direct supervision of the physician.

Registered Nurse First Assistant

The RNFA is an RN with advanced education, skills, and knowledge of surgery who facilitates and supports the health needs of

Table 21-2 Examples of Nursing Activities Surrounding the Surgical Experience

Before Assessment	Monitoring of Physical Status
Home, Clinic, Holding Area	• Monitors and reports changes in patient's vital signs
• Initiates preoperative assessment	• Monitors blood loss
• Plans teaching methods appropriate to patient's needs	• Monitors urine output as applicable
• Involves family and other caregivers in interview and education	**Monitoring of Psychological Status**
Surgical Unit	• Provides emotional support to patient
• Completes preoperative assessment	• Stands near or touches patient during procedures and induction
• Coordinates patient teaching with other nursing staff	• Ensures patient's right to privacy is maintained
• Develops a plan of care	• Communicates patient's emotional status to other appropriate members of health care team
Surgical Suite	**After Evaluation**
• Identifies patient	**Postanaesthesia, Discharge Area**
• Verifies surgical site	• Determines patient's immediate response to surgical intervention
• Assesses patient's level of consciousness, skin integrity, mobility, emotional status, and functional limitations	• Monitors vital signs
• Reviews chart	• Safely administers appropriate medications
Planning	**Surgical Unit**
• Determines a plan of care that incorporates and respects patient's value system, lifestyle, ethnicity, and culture	• Evaluates effectiveness of nursing care in OR using patient outcome criteria
• Ensures all supplies and equipment needed for surgery are available, functioning properly, and sterile if appropriate	• Determines patient's level of satisfaction with care given during perioperative period
During Implementation	• Evaluates products used in care of patient in OR
Maintenance of Safety	• Determines patient's psychological status
• Ensures integrity of sterile field	• Assists with discharge planning
• Ensures that sponge, needle, and instrument counts are correct	**Home, Clinic**
• Positions patient to ensure correct alignment, exposure of surgical site, and prevention of injury	• Seeks patient's perception of surgery in terms of effects of anaesthetic agents, impact on body image, immobilization
• Prevents chemical injury from preparation solutions, pharmaceuticals, and the like	• Determines family's perceptions of surgery and ability to cope and function during recuperation phase of the surgery
• Ensures safe use of electrical equipment, lasers, and radiation	
• Safely labels and administers appropriate medications	
• Handles, labels, documents and establishes chain of custody for specimens	

OR, operating room.

the perioperative patient. The scope of practice of the RNFA allows him or her to collaborate with the surgeon in planning preoperative, intraoperative, and postoperative patient care. RNFAs assist in surgery under the direct supervision of the surgeon (ORNAC, 2011, p. 43).

Anaesthesiologist

According to the Canadian Anesthesiologists' Society (CAS) (2011), an **anaesthesiologist** is a physician who is responsible for a patient's medical care before, during, and shortly after surgery. Anaesthesiologists are vital members of the surgical team. They have expert knowledge of the extremely potent drugs used in surgery and are responsible for preoperative anaesthetic assessments; delivery, maintenance, and reversal of the anaesthesia; and care of a patient's recovery until discharged from the PACU. In larger ORs and teaching hospitals, there may be respiratory ther-

apists who get advanced training and work with the anaesthesia team as anaesthesia assistants.

Advanced Nursing Practice Roles

Registered Nurse Anaesthesia Assistant. A registered nurse anaesthesia assistant (RNAA) is an RN with advanced education, knowledge, and skills in the anaesthesia specialty who works in collaboration with and under supervision from an anaesthesiologist throughout the perioperative period (ORNAC, 2011, p. 17).

An additional category of anaesthesia provider is the nurse practitioner with a diploma in anaesthesia care. These nurse practitioners with specialist education in anaesthesia care complement and collaboratively provide a range of anaesthesia care and related services in preoperative, perioperative, postoperative, and ambulatory care settings.

The scope and responsibilities state that graduates will be able to:

1. Use anaesthetic drugs properly and monitor and regulate the replacement of fluids and blood
2. Interpret data from patient monitoring
3. Recognize and correct complications
4. Provide patient resuscitation when indicated
5. Manage patient pain
6. Participate in anaesthetic research, education, and administrative functions (University of Toronto, 2009).

The OR is a complex, unpredictable environment. All members of the perioperative team must be proficient in their practice and be constantly striving to improve their competence. Perioperative teams can work efficiently together in all specialty areas to ensure patient safety (Phillips, 2013b, p. 56). Effective teams demonstrate exceptional communication skills, trust, interprofessional collaboration, and shared leadership.

NURSING MANAGEMENT: PATIENT BEFORE SURGERY

The preoperative assessment of the patient about to undergo surgery establishes baseline data for intraoperative and postanaesthesia care. Assessment data that are provided by the patient and family in the holding area and data from the inpatient nursing units are verified and are important to ensure that a plan of care can be developed (Rothrock, 2011).

Psychosocial Assessment

The perioperative nurse who cares for the patient in the OR must be knowledgeable about the patient's surgical experience and have the ability to prioritize patient care. This knowledge allows for informative and reassuring explanations, especially to the anxious patient. General questions regarding surgery or anaesthesia can usually be answered by the perioperative nurse. Examples of these questions include, "When will I go to sleep?" "Who will be in the room?" "How much of my body will be exposed and to whom?" "When will I wake up?" Specific questions relating to details of the surgical procedure and anaesthesia may be referred to the surgeon or anaesthesiologist (Phillips, 2013a).

Physical Assessment

A thorough physical assessment should be made during the preoperative preparation of the patient (see Chapter 20). *Vital signs* are important as baseline data to evaluate the effects of intraoperative medications and body positioning. *Height* and *weight* of the patient guide the nurse regarding the width and length of the operating bed. It is also necessary to have an accurate weight because the dosage of many medications in the OR is ordered per kilogram. The need for extra warmth is indicated by the patient's age, metabolic problems, and planned surgical procedures. Some *allergic reactions* may be avoided with such simple measures as effective preoperative screening. The *condition* of the skin will alert the team to the potential for infection as a result of open or closed skin lesions. Knowledge of *skeletal and muscle impairments* helps

prevent injury during positioning. Perceptual difficulty, such as a *vision or hearing impairment,* will guide the nurse in adapting communication techniques to individual needs. An *altered level of consciousness* necessitates the practice of increased safety. Communicating identified sources of *pain* to other health team members prevents subjecting the patient to unnecessary discomfort.

Chart Review

Required chart data vary with hospital policy, patient condition, and specific surgical procedures. Because ambulatory surgery facilities tend to have a healthier population, fewer tests may be required. Minimum requirements for the health record include (ORNAC, 2011, p. 163):

• Documentation of consent
• Preoperative checklist
• History and physical examination

Admitting the Patient

Hospital policy designates the protocol to be followed when admitting the patient to the holding area and OR suite. The perioperative nurse is responsible for identifying herself or himself to the patient using name and job title. The nurse should communicate a caring attitude that makes the patient feel comfortable. The identification process includes asking the patient to state his or her name, the surgeon's name, and the operative procedure and site of surgery. This active communication process reduces the risk of error. The nurse compares hospital identification numbers with the patient's own identification band and chart (ORNAC, 2011, p. 163). The admitting procedure is continued with verification of the preoperative checklist, care for personal belongings, checking for informed consent, and validating that the correct preoperative medication was administered (ORNAC, 2011, p. 164). There must be time allowed for replying to any last-minute questions. The nurse completes the review of the chart and documents any abnormalities or changes. Comfort measures are instituted to keep the patient warm and relaxed. The patient may be seen and assessed by the surgeon or anaesthesiologist, or both, before anaesthesia induction.

NURSING MANAGEMENT: PATIENT DURING SURGERY

Room Preparation

Before transferring the patient into the scheduled OR, the nurse spends significant time preparing the room to ensure privacy, safety, and prevention of infection. Surgical attire (pants and shirts, masks, protective eyewear, and caps or hoods) is worn by all persons entering the OR suite (Figure 21-3). All electrical and mechanical equipment is checked for proper functioning. Each

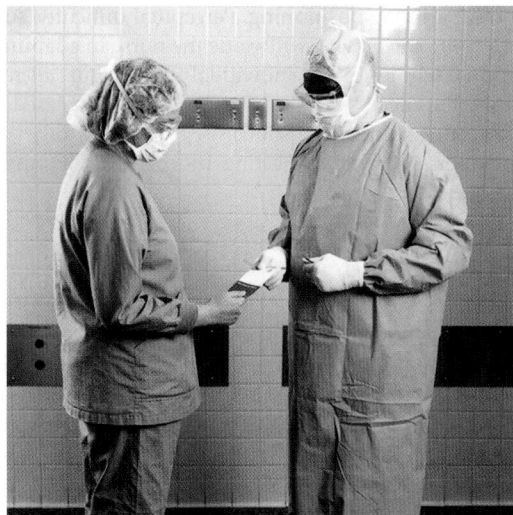

Figure 21-3 Surgical attire is worn by all persons entering the operating room suite.

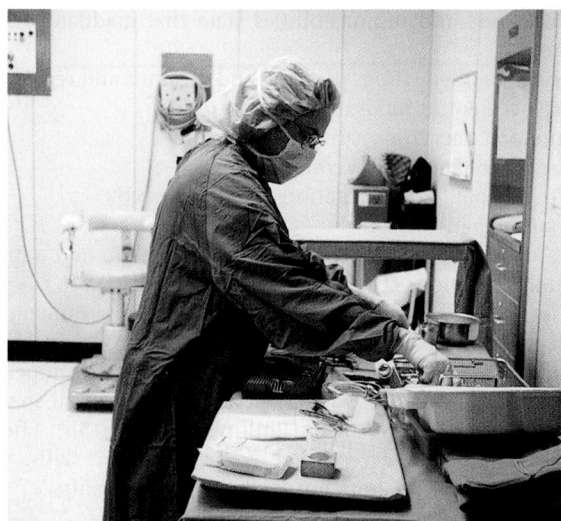

Figure 21-4 A sterile field is created before surgery.

Source: Courtesy of The Methodist Hospital, Houston, TX. Photograph by Donna Dahms, RN, CNOR.

sterile, surgical item is opened in a specific manner for the scrub nurse to handle and place systematically on the instrument table (Phillips, 2013a). The perioperative nurse determines the type of surgical count, full or partial, which depends on the surgery being done. Counts are conducted and documented in accordance with ORNAC guidelines and hospital policy (ORNAC, 2011, p. 167).

During the procedure, the functions of the team members are well delineated. The scrub person will scrub hands and arms, put on *sterile* gown and gloves, and touch only those items in the *sterile* field. The circulating nurse remains in the *unsterile* field and implements those activities that involve touching all *unsterile* items and the patient. Every person on the surgical team shares the responsibility for monitoring aseptic practice and initiating corrective action when a sterile field is compromised (Phillips, 2013a).

Transferring the Patient

Once the patient has been properly identified and the OR has been adequately prepared, the patient is transported into the room for the surgery. Each time a patient is transferred from one bed to another, the wheels of the stretcher should be locked, and a sufficient number of personnel should be available to lift, guide, and prevent accidental falling. Once the patient is on the operating bed, a safety strap should be placed across the patient's thighs. At this time, the electrocardiogram monitor leads, oxygen saturation monitor, and blood pressure cuff are usually applied, and an IV catheter is inserted if it was not started before surgery.

Scrubbing, Gowning, and Gloving

Before entering the sterile field, all sterile members of the surgical team (surgical assistant, surgeon, and nurse) are required to cleanse their hands and arms by using a surgical hand antiseptic or scrub agent. The surgical hand antiseptic/scrub is a broad-spectrum agent that kills microorganisms on contact and also supplies persistent protection because it reduces the regrowth of microorganisms. There are different procedures for water-based

and waterless hand preparation, and personnel must follow the manufacturer's written instructions and hospital policy (ORNAC, 2011, p. 116).

Once the scrub procedure is completed, the team members enter the room to put on surgical gowns and gloves. Because the gowns and gloves are sterile, it is permissible for the scrubbed individuals to manipulate and organize all sterile items for use during the procedure.

Basic Aseptic Technique

To prevent infections, aseptic technique is practised in the OR. This is implemented through the creation and maintenance of a sterile field (Figure 21-4). The centre of the sterile field is the site of the surgical incision. Items in the sterile field include instruments, supplies, and equipment that have been sterilized by appropriate sterilization methods.

There are specific principles that the team members should understand to practise aseptic technique correctly. Unless these principles are followed, the safety of the patient is compromised, and the potential for postoperative infection is increased. These include principles for dispensing sterile supplies (ORNAC, 2011), and for maintaining a sterile field in the OR (Table 21-3). In addition to following the principles of aseptic technique, the surgical team is responsible for following the guidelines established by ORNAC to protect the patient and the team from exposure to blood-borne pathogens. Routine practice (formally known as standard precautions) should be used when caring for all patients. Additional protocols (e.g., airborne, droplet, or contact) should be used to manage infections spread by those specific methods of transmission (ORNAC, 2011, pp. 91-93). These guidelines emphasize standard and transmission-based precautions (see Table 17-8), engineering and work practice controls, and the use of personal protective equipment such as gloves, gowns, aprons, caps, face shields, masks, and protective eyewear (see Table 17-9 and Figure 21-3). This is especially important in the OR environment because of the high potential for exposure to bloodborne pathogens.

Table 21-3 Maintaining a Sterile Field in the Operating Room

Practice

7.4.1 Opened sterile supplies/set-up shall not be left unattended. They shall be continuously monitored for possible contamination.

7.4.2 Unsterile persons shall not reach over the sterile field.

7.4.3 Sterile persons shall not reach over unsterile areas.

7.4.4 Sterile persons shall stay within the sterile field. Sterile persons shall not walk around or go outside the theatre.

7.4.5 The scrub team should remain close to, and face the sterile field. Movement shall be between sterile areas only. If position changes are necessary, scrubbed personnel shall pass face to face or back to back. When changing positions, the scrub personnel should avoid changing levels; they either sit or stand. Hands shall be kept above waist level.

7.4.6 Talking should be kept to a minimum.

7.4.7 Unsterile health care team members shall remain at least 30 cm (1 ft.) from the sterile field. Movement is from unsterile to unsterile areas. They should not pass between sterile fields.

7.4.8 The sterile set-up shall not be covered.

7.4.9 Cover unsterile equipment with sterile barriers before placing them over or in the sterile field.

7.4.10 Breaks in aseptic technique shall be monitored, documented and corrective action taken as soon as safely possible.

Source: Operating Room Nurses Association of Canada (ORNAC). (2011). *Standards, guidelines, and position statements for perioperative registered nursing practice* (10th ed., pp. 123–124). Halifax, NS: Author.

Assisting the Anaesthesiologist

The perioperative circulating nurse often works with the anaesthesiologist to prepare the patient for the administration of the anaesthetic. The nurse must understand the types of anaesthetic modalities, for example, general, spinal, epidural, and blocks, and the pharmacological effects of the agents. Nurses must respond collaboratively to unexpected complications and emergency situations, so they must know the location of all emergency drugs and equipment in the OR area (ORNAC, 2011, p. 278).

The circulating nurse may be involved in helping establish monitoring of the surgical patient such as:
- Temperature, pulse, and respiration
- Blood pressure
- Electrocardiogram
- Oxygen saturation
- Arterial, central venous pressure, and pulmonary artery lines
- Input and output (urine, blood loss)

If the patient is to have a general anaesthetic, the nurse remains at the patient's side to ensure safety and to assist the anaesthesiologist. The nurse's responsibilities may include ensuring all necessary equipment is available and functional (i.e., suction is on and laryngoscope is fully lighted, initiating monitoring, and assisting in securing the patient's airway). This is commonly done by inserting a laryngeal mask airway (LMA) or endotracheal tube (ET) (Figure 21-5). After IV drug-induced loss of consciousness, the anaesthesiologist can place an LMA or administer a neuromuscular blocking drug intravenously that leads to skeletal muscle relaxation. This enables the anaesthesiologist to perform a direct laryngoscopy followed by tracheal intubation. Under direct supervision of the anaesthesiology provider, the circulating nurse may assist by applying cricoid pressure, supporting head positioning, administering oxygen, and inflating the ET tube (ORNAC, 2011, p. 276).

For insertion of epidural catheters or administration of spinal anaesthetic or blocks, the circulating nurse assists the anaesthesiologist by ensuring appropriate supplies are accessible and by positioning the patient for the anaesthetic intervention (ORNAC, 2011, p. 277).

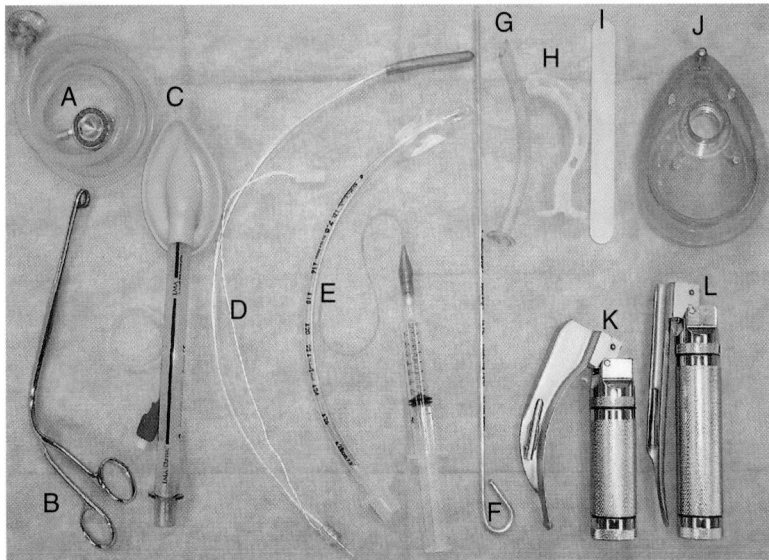

Figure 21-5 Commonly used anaesthesia equipment. *A,* Precordial stethoscope. *B,* McGill forceps. *C,* Laryngeal mask airway. *D,* Esophageal stethoscope with esophageal temperature monitor. *E,* Endotracheal tube. *F,* Intubating stylet for endotracheal tube. *G,* Nasal airway. *H,* Oral airway. *I,* Tongue blade. *J,* Mask. *K,* "Stubby" laryngoscope handle with MacIntosh (curved) fibreoptic laryngoscope blade. *L,* Miller (straight) fibreoptic laryngoscope blade and handle.

Source: Rothrock, J. C. (2011). *Alexander's care of the patient in surgery* (14th ed., p. 129, Figure 4-2). St. Louis: Mosby.

▪ Positioning the Patient

Positioning the patient is a critical part of every procedure. The entire perioperative team must have in-depth knowledge about the surgical procedure, patient time on the OR bed, what position the patient will be in, and any patient limitations such as arthritis or joint replacements that require special care (Fawcett, 2011, p. 167). The main goal is to optimize surgical exposure; however, positions necessary for surgery may result in undesirable effects such as hypotension, oxygen desaturation, and peripheral nerve injuries. Proper positioning is a team effort that follows administration of the anaesthetic. The anaesthesiologist indicates when to begin the positioning and assists the surgeon, nurses, and auxiliary staff to comply with recommended positioning practices that ensure safety (Fawcett, 2011, p. 167).

The position of the patient should allow for accessibility to the operative site, administration and monitoring of anaesthetic agents, and maintenance of the patient's airway. When positioning for the surgical procedure, care must be used to (1) provide correct skeletal alignment; (2) prevent undue pressure on nerves, skin over bony prominences, and eyes; (3) provide for adequate thoracic excursion; (4) prevent occlusion of arteries and veins; (5) provide modesty in exposure; and (6) recognize and respect individual needs such as previously assessed aches, pains, or deformities.

It is a nursing responsibility to secure the extremities, provide adequate padding and support, and obtain sufficient physical or mechanical help to avoid unnecessary straining of self or patient (ORNAC, 2011, p. 178).

Various positions in which the patient may be placed include supine, prone, Trendelenburg, lateral decubitus, and lithotomy (Figure 21-6). The supine is the most common position used. It is suited for surgery involving the abdomen, the heart, and the breast. A variation of the supine position is the Trendelenburg position. This position can be used in lower abdominal or pelvic surgery, where it is necessary to visualize the pelvic organs. The prone position allows easy access for back surgeries

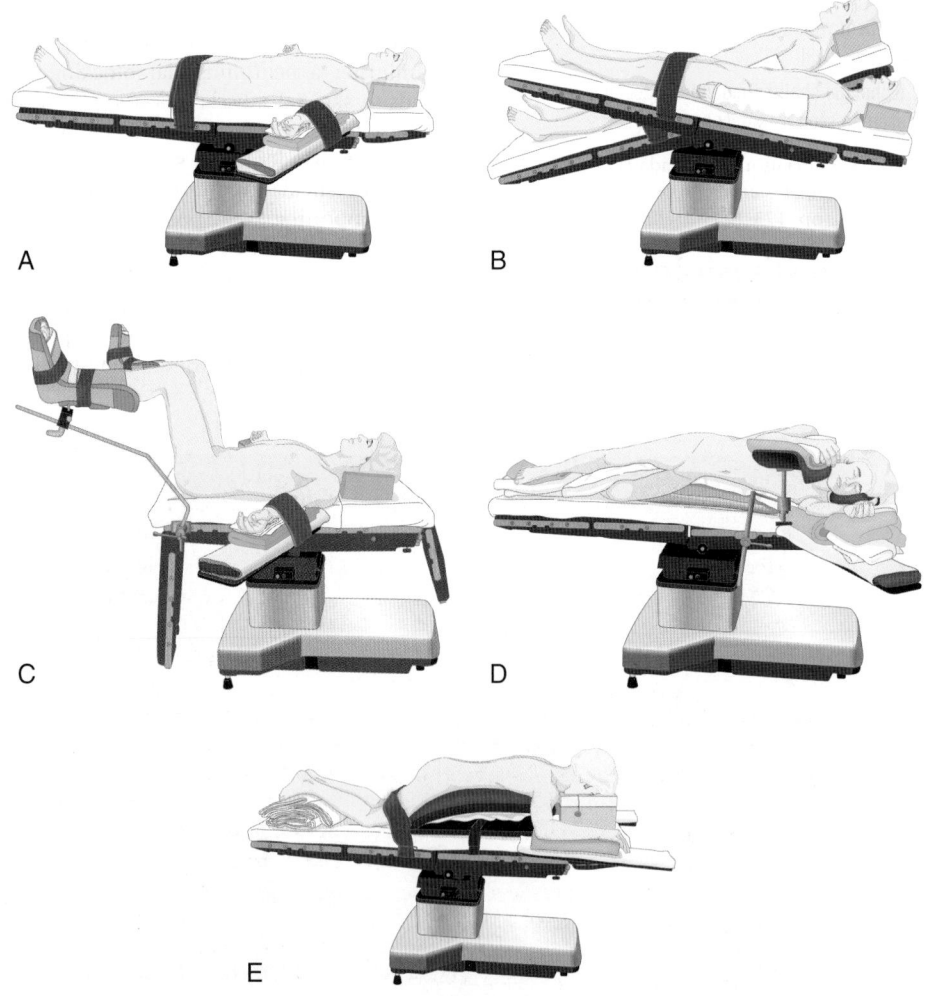

Figure 21-6 Common intraoperative patient positioning. **A,** Supine position: abdominal surgery. **B,** Trendelenburg position: pelvic surgery. **C,** Lithotomy position: abdominal perineal resection. **D,** Lateral decubitus position: thoracic surgery. **E,** Prone position with a Wilson frame: spinal surgery.

Source: Miller, R.D. (Ed.). (2010). *Miller's anesthesia* (7th ed., pp. 1153, Figure 36-1; p. 1155, Figure 36-5; p. 1157, Figure 36-6; p. 1158, Figure 36-10; p. 1160, Figure 36-14). Philadelphia: Churchill-Livingstone.

(e.g., laminectomies). The lithotomy position is used for some types of pelvic organ surgery (e.g., vaginal hysterectomy).

Whatever position is required for the procedure, great care is taken to prevent injury to the patient. Because anaesthesia has blocked the nerve impulses, the patient will not feel pain or discomfort or stress being placed on nerves, muscles, bones, or skin. Improper positioning could potentially result in muscle strain, joint damage, pressure ulcers, nerve damage, and other untoward effects (Phillips, 2013a).

General anaesthesia causes peripheral vessels to dilate. Position changes affect where the pooling of blood occurs. If the head of the OR bed is raised, the lower torso will have increased blood volume and the upper torso may become compromised. Hypovolemia and cardiovascular disease can further compromise the patient's status. Consequently, the perioperative nurse, working with the entire surgical team, carefully plans and implements the patient's positioning and then closely monitors the patient throughout the surgical procedure.

Once the patient is positioned, the circulating nurse applies an adhesive, flexible, gel pad called a dispersive electrode so the electrosurgical unit (ESU) or electrocautery unit can be used by the surgeon to cauterize blood vessels and cut tissue. The dispersive electrode is a safety device that prevents electrical burns. It acts as a ground allowing the electrical current used to cauterize to return from the patient back to the ESU. The electrode is placed by the circulating nurse on a well-muscled, dry, clean area as close to the operative site as possible. Places to avoid are bony areas, over any implanted prosthesis, and scar tissue. If the current from the ESU does not return through the dispersive electrode, burning can occur (ORNAC, 2011, pp. 229-230; Phillips, 2013a). An alternative method for grounding the patient is to use a specifically designed gel mattress on the OR bed that connects to the ESU. Patient contact with the mattress provides adequate protection against electrical burns.

Preparing the Surgical Site

The purpose of skin preparation, or "prepping," is to reduce the number of organisms available to migrate to the surgical wound. The task of preparing is usually the responsibility of the circulating nurse.

Before surgical skin preparation, all gross debris, excess hair, and piercing body jewellery are removed. The shave preparation is a controversial topic with several studies showing mixed results (Tanner, Woodings, & Moncaster, 2008), so surgical units must form their own policy and procedures. Evidence-informed recommendations state the following:

- If ordered, the shave preparation is performed as close to the time of surgery as possible to reduce the risk for microbial growth in breaks in the skin.
- To protect the patient's privacy, shaving should be performed in the preoperative holding area. If it is done in the OR, nurses must follow hospital policy and remove all loose hair from the operative site.
- Electric clippers are recommended and should be used on wetted skin and hair.
- Reusable electric clippers should be cleaned and disinfected after use; single-use shaving heads are disposed of in sharps containers.
- Patients should not perform a self-shave or use a depilatory before surgery.

- An alternative for keeping the hair out of the surgical wound, especially for cranial incisions, is to apply a nonflammable gel to the hair (ORNAC 2011; Phillips, 2013a).

The skin preparation starts when the nurse verifies the incision preparation area, which should be marked with indelible ink. An inspection is done by the perioperative nurse who notes and documents any lesions, irritation, or abrasions on or near the incision site (Phillips, 2013a, p. 511). The incision site is cleansed using an agent having fast-acting, broad-spectrum, persistent antimicrobial action and that is nontoxic and nonallergenic to the patient (Phillips, 2013a, p. 514). The area is scrubbed in a circular motion from the clean area (site of the incision) to the dirty area (periphery) with the exception of the umbilicus. If there is an incision in proximity to the umbilicus, the umbilical area is prepared first, then the preparation is continued in a circular fashion, to the periphery (ORNAC, 2011; Phillips, 2013a). Preparation technique varies with the type of surgery being done, the preparation supplies available, and hospital policy (ORNAC, 2011, pp. 146-147). After preparation of the skin, the sterile members of the surgical team drape the area. Only the site to be incised is left exposed.

Safety Considerations

All surgical procedures, regardless of where they take place, can put the patient at risk for injury. These injuries can be infections, physical injury from positioning or equipment used, or from the surgery itself. Lasers and ESUs can cause injury to the patient and the surgical staff. The perioperative nurse must be familiar with fire safety issues to protect the patient and staff against burns. Airborne contaminants produced during laser procedures may contain trace hydrocarbons, including acetone, isopropanol, toluene, formaldehyde, and cyanide. Smoke can cause respiratory irritation and has mutagenic and carcinogenic potential. Smoke evacuators are used in the OR.

SAFETY ALERT

The risk of wrong patient/wrong site surgery has catastrophic implications. The Canadian Patient Safety Institute (2009) developed a Safe Surgery Checklist that is being successfully implemented in Canadian hospitals. The OR staff gather for a briefing before anaesthesia induction, and a *surgical time out* or *pause* just before the incision is done by the surgeon, anaesthesiologist, and nurse who all verbally confirm:

- Patient identity
- Site, side, and level of surgery
- Procedure being performed
- Antibiotic prophylaxis: was initial dose given and repeat dose necessary?
- Final surgical positioning of patient
- Whether anyone has any other questions or concerns before proceeding

The postoperative debriefing is a review of intraoperative patient care and identification of any concerns for patient recovery. These data become part of the hand-off information to the PACU/ICU nursing staff as part of the transfer of accountability (Canadian Patient Safety Institute, 2009).

Classification of Anaesthesia

Anaesthesia is classified according to the effect that it has on the patient's sensorium (central nervous system) and pain perception. **General anaesthesia** is the loss of sensation with loss of consciousness, skeletal muscle relaxation, analgesia, and elimination of the somatic, autonomic, and endocrine responses, including coughing, gagging, vomiting, and sympathetic nervous system responsiveness. **Local anaesthesia** is the loss of sensation without loss of consciousness. Local anaesthesia may be induced topically or via infiltration intracutaneously or subcutaneously. **Regional anaesthesia** is the loss of sensation to a region of the body without loss of consciousness when a specific nerve or group of nerves is blocked with the administration of a local anaesthetic (e.g., spinal, epidural, or peripheral nerve block).

Procedural sedation (formerly *conscious sedation*) refers to the technique of administering IV sedatives or procedural agents with or without analgesics. Procedural sedation with analgesia results in depressed levels of consciousness but patients do maintain independent control of their airway and, subsequently, oxygenation. In this manner, patients can tolerate unpleasant procedures while maintaining their protective airway reflexes (Odom-Forren, 2011, p. 82).

General Anaesthesia

General anaesthesia is usually the technique of choice for patients who (1) are having surgical procedures that require significant skeletal muscle relaxation, last for long periods of time, require awkward positions because of the location of the incision site, or require control of respiration; (2) are extremely anxious; (3) refuse or have contraindications for local or regional anaesthetic techniques; and (4) are uncooperative because of their emotional status, lack of maturity, intoxication, head injury, or pathophysiological processes that do not permit them to remain immobile for any length of time.

General anaesthesia may be administered intravenously, by inhalation, or rectally. A *balanced technique* (use of drugs from different classes) is the most common method used for general anaesthesia. Table 21-4 presents common anaesthetic drugs with advantages and disadvantages of and nursing interventions that are indicated for patients receiving the agents.

Intravenous Induction Agents. Virtually all routine general anaesthetic protocols for use with adults begin with an IV induction agent, such as midazolam or propofol (Diprivan). These agents induce a pleasant sleep, with a rapid onset of action that patients find desirable. A single dose lasts only a few minutes, which is long enough for an ET to be placed and an inhalation agent to be started.

Inhalation Agents. Inhalation agents are the foundation of general anaesthesia. The inhalation agents used for general anaesthesia may be volatile liquids (liquid at room temperature) or gases (gas at room temperature). Volatile liquids are administered through a specially designed vaporizer after being mixed with oxygen as a carrier gas.

Inhalation agents enter the body through the alveoli in the lungs. They may be administered through a mask, an ET, an LMA, or a tracheostomy. Ease of administration and rapid excretion by ventilation make them desirable agents. One undesirable characteristic is the irritating effect of inhalation agents on the respiratory tract. Complications that may arise are coughing, *laryngospasm* (muscular constriction of the larynx), bronchospasm, increased secretions, and respiratory depression (Thompson, 2007). Inhalation agents are most commonly administered via an ET placed into the trachea once the patient has been induced with an IV agent. The ET permits control of ventilation and airway protection, both for patency and to prevent aspiration. Complications of endotracheal intubation include those primarily associated with its insertion and removal. These include damage to teeth and lips, laryngospasm, laryngeal edema, postoperative sore throat, and hoarseness caused by injury or irritation of the vocal cords or surrounding tissues.

Adjuncts to General Anaesthesia. The administration of general anaesthesia is rarely limited to one agent. Drugs added to an inhalation anaesthetic (other than an IV induction agent) are termed *adjuncts*. Adjunctive drugs are usually given for analgesia and amnesia. Sometimes, these drugs are given to counteract adverse effects of anaesthesia before surgery, intraoperatively, and after surgery. These agents are added to the anaesthetic regimen specifically to achieve unconsciousness, analgesia, amnesia, muscle relaxation, or autonomic nervous system control (Phillips, 2013a). (See Table 21-5 for adjuncts to general anaesthesia.) Adjuncts include opioids (narcotics), benzodiazepines, neuromuscular blocking agents (muscle relaxants), and antiemetics. In some cases, PACU nurses may observe that patients have a deeper level of sedation than would be expected when any single neurological blocking agent is given alone. See Table 21-4 for neuromuscular blocking agents.

DRUG THERAPY

Table 21-4 General Anaesthesia

DRUG	ADVANTAGE	DISADVANTAGE	NURSING IMPLICATIONS
Preoperative Agents			
Lorazepam (Ativan)	Excellent for patients with anxiety	Must be administered cautiously to patients with hepatic or renal disease, and pediatric and geriatric patients	Ensure patients have signed consent before administering any premedication Ensure siderails on stretchers or beds are up
Midazolam	Short acting; excellent for inducing amnesia	Has a slower induction than thiopental	Can be used for a premedication as well as an agent for induction and maintenance of anaesthesia; no pain on injection; often used in conjunction with regional anaesthetic

DRUG THERAPY

Table 21-4 General Anaesthesia—cont'd

DRUG	ADVANTAGE	DISADVANTAGE	NURSING IMPLICATIONS
Induction Agents			
Propofol (Diprivan)	Ideal for short outpatient procedures because of rapid onset of action and elimination; may be used for maintenance of anaesthesia as well as induction	May cause bradycardia and other dysrhythmias, hypotension, apnea, phlebitis, nausea and vomiting, hiccups	Short action leads to minimal postoperative effects; monitor injection site for phlebitis; cardiac monitoring if patient condition is unstable
Ketamine (Ketalar)	Can be administered by IV or IM route; potent analgesic and amnestic	May cause hallucinations and nightmares, increased intracranial and intraocular pressure, increased heart rate, hypertension	—
Inhalation Gases			
Volatile Liquids			
Isoflurane (Forane) Desflurane (Suprane) Sevoflurane	All volatile liquids: muscle relaxation, low incidence of nausea and vomiting *Isoflurane:* less cardiac depression, devoid of toxicity to body organs *Desflurane:* rapid induction and emergence, most widely used volatile agent *Sevoflurane:* predictable effects on cardiovascular and respiratory systems, rapid acting, nonirritating to respiratory system	All volatile liquids: myocardial depression, early onset of postoperative pain because of rapid elimination	Assess and treat pain during early anaesthesia recovery; assess for adverse reactions such as cardiopulmonary depression with hypotension and prolonged respiratory depression, confusion, and nausea and vomiting
Gaseous Agents			
Nitrous oxide (N_2O)	Potentiates volatile agents, allowing a reduction in both their dosage and their adverse effects, and increases the rate of induction	Weak anaesthetic, rarely used alone; must be administered with oxygen to prevent hypoxemia	Produces little or no toxicity; monitor for effects of volatile liquids when N_2O used as an adjunct
Induction: Depolarizing Muscle Relaxant			
Succinylcholine	Used with intubation or short cases; rapid onset	Can trigger MH crisis	Requires refrigeration; may cause fasciculations
Induction: Nondepolarizing Muscle Relaxants			
Intermediate Onset and Duration			
Atracurium	Used with intubation, maintenance of relaxation	May have slight histamine release	Requires refrigeration
Rocuronium (Zemuron)	Rapid onset, maintenance of relaxation	Can increase heart rate (vagolytic)	Eliminated by the kidney and the liver
Longer Onset and Duration			
Pancuronium	Onset 1-3 min Maintenance of relaxation	May increase heart rate and blood pressure	Eliminated via the kidneys
Reversal: Cholinergic Agent			
Neostigmine bromide (Prostigmin)	Reverses nondepolarizing neuromuscular blocker in 3-15 min	Cardiac arrhythmias	Given with atropine sulphate or glycopyrrolate; prevents breakdown of acetylcholine
Anticholinergics			
Atropine sulphate (Atropine)	Blocks effect of acetylcholine; can decrease vagal tone; increases heart rate, suppresses salivary, gastric, and bronchial secretions	May cause dry mouth, CNS symptoms (dizziness)	Used in the treatment of bradycardia
Glycopyrrolate	Blocks effect of acetylcholine; can decrease vagal tone; increases heart rate; suppresses salivary, gastric, and bronchial secretions	Can have prolonged duration of effects	Does not cross blood–brain barrier; has lower incidence of dysrhythmias than atropine sulphate
Edrophonium (Tensilon)	Rapid onset, well matched to atropine sulphate	Bradycardia may occur in some patients; increases respiratory tract secretions	Ensure patient is monitored by ECG when drug is used; have suctioning equipment available

CNS, central nervous system; *ECG,* electrocardiogram; *IM,* intramuscular; *IV,* intravenous; *MH,* malignant hyperthermia.

DRUG THERAPY

Table 21-5 Adjuncts to General Anaesthesia

AGENTS	USES DURING ANAESTHESIA	ADVERSE EFFECTS	NURSING INTERVENTIONS
Opioids			
Fentanyl Morphine sulphate Sufentanil (Sufenta) Alfentanil (Alfenta)	Induce and maintain anaesthesia, reduce stimuli from sensory nerve endings, provide analgesia during surgery and anaesthetic recovery	Respiratory depression, stimulation of vomiting centre, possible bradycardia and peripheral vasodilation (when combined with anaesthetics), high incidence of pruritus with both regional and IV administration	Assess respiratory status, monitor pulse oximetry findings, protect airway in anticipation of vomiting, use standing orders for antipruritics such as diphenhydramine
Benzodiazepines			
Midazolam Diazepam (Valium) Lorazepam (Ativan)	Induce and maintain anaesthesia	Potentiation of the effects of opioids, increasing the potential for respiratory depression; hypotension and tachycardia	Monitor cardiopulmonary status, level of consciousness
Antiemetics			
Ondansetron (Zofran) Metoclopramide Dimenhydrinate (Gravol) Promethazine Droperidol	Prevention of vomiting with aspiration during surgery, counteract the emetic effects of inhalation agents and opioids; droperidol often used during surgery; others more often used after surgery	*Droperidol:* dysrhythmias, laryngospasm, bronchospasm, tachycardia, hypotension, central nervous system alterations, extrapyramidal reactions; contraindicated for use in patients with Parkinson disease or hypomagnesemia *Other antiemetics:* headache, dizziness, sedation, malaise, fatigue, musculoskeletal pain, shivers, diarrhea, acute dystonic reactions, cardiovascular alterations; contraindicated for use with patients with hypomagnesemia	Monitor cardiopulmonary status, level of consciousness, and ability to move limbs *Droperidol:* administer with caution in patients with heart disease

IV, intravenous.

Opioids. Opioids are used before surgery for sedation and analgesia, intraoperatively for induction and maintenance of anaesthesia, and after surgery for pain management. Opioids alter the perception of pain and the response to painful stimuli. When administered before the end of a surgical procedure, the residual analgesia often carries over into the PACU, allowing the patient to awaken relatively pain free.

All opioids produce dose-related respiratory depression. Respiratory depression may be difficult to detect in the OR and, therefore, necessitates close observation and pulse oximetry monitoring. Respiratory depression can be reversed with naloxone. However, its use is often associated with a reversal of the analgesic effects of the narcotics as well.

Benzodiazepines. Sedative–hypnotic benzodiazepines are widely used as premedication before surgery for their amnestic effects, as agents for the induction and maintenance of anaesthesia, for procedural sedation, as supplemental IV sedation during local and regional anaesthesia, and for postoperative anxiety and agitation. Because of its excellent amnestic property, shorter duration of action, and absence of pain on injection, midazolam is at present the most frequently used benzodiazepine. The other agents are limited in their usefulness because of their long duration of action. In both ambulatory surgery settings and procedural sedation, midazolam is the most common anaesthesia adjunct used. It is commonly administered by IV or intramuscular route. Flumazenil is a specific benzodiazepine antagonist that may be used to reverse marked benzodiazepine-induced respiratory depression.

Neuromuscular Blocking Agents. Neuromuscular blocking agents (muscle relaxants) are used as adjuncts to general anaesthesia to facilitate endotracheal intubation and to optimize surgical working conditions by providing relaxation (paralysis) of skeletal muscles. Neuromuscular blocking agents interrupt the transmission of nerve impulses at the neuromuscular junction. Based on their mechanisms of action, neuromuscular blocking agents are classified as either depolarizing or nondepolarizing muscle relaxants. The effects of nondepolarizing muscle relaxants are frequently reversed toward the end of the surgery by the administration of anticholinesterase agents (e.g., neostigmine [Prostigmin], pyridostigmine [Mestinon], edrophonium [Tensilon]).

Disadvantages of the use of muscle relaxants are of special concern to the anaesthesiologist and postanaesthesia nurse. The duration of their action may be longer than the surgical procedure, and reversal agents may not be effective in completely eliminating the residual effects. The patient should be carefully observed for airway patency and adequacy of respiratory muscle movement. Lack of movement or poor return of reflexes and strength may indicate the need for an artificial airway and ventilator. If the patient is intubated, the ET should not be removed without careful assessment of return of muscular strength, level of consciousness, and the minute volume (respiratory rate times tidal volume [amount of air inhaled and exhaled during a normal ventilation]).

Antiemetics. Antiemetics are used before surgery, intraoperatively, and after surgery to prevent and treat nausea and vomiting associated with the administration of anaesthesia. Antiemetics listed in Table 21-5 are most frequently used before and after surgery.

Local Anaesthesia

Local anaesthetics block the initiation and transmission of electrical impulses along nerve fibres. With progressive increases in local anaesthetic concentration, the transmission of autonomic, then somatic sensory, and finally somatic motor impulses is blocked. This produces autonomic nervous system blockade, anaesthesia, and skeletal muscle paralysis in the area of the affected nerve.

Local anaesthesia allows an operative procedure to be performed on a particular part of the body without loss of consciousness or sedation. Because there is little systemic absorption of the drug, recovery is rapid with little residual drug "hangover." The duration of action of the local anaesthetic frequently carries over into the postoperative period, providing continued analgesia. In addition, the use of a local anaesthetic in a regional technique provides an alternative to a general anaesthetic in a physiologically compromised patient.

The disadvantages of local anaesthetics include the technical difficulty and discomfort that may be associated with injections, inadvertent IV administration producing hypotension and potential seizures, and the inability to precisely match the duration of action of the agents administered to the duration of the surgical procedure.

Methods of Administration. There are a variety of methods for administering local anaesthetics (Table 21-6). *Topical application* is application of the agent directly to the skin, mucous membranes, or open surface. Eutectic mixture of local anaesthetics (lidocaine and prilocaine) in a skin cream form can be applied to the skin to produce localized dermal anaesthesia (see Chapter 10). Anaesthetic cream should be applied to the site 30 to 60 minutes before painful procedures. *Local infiltration* is the injection of the agent into the tissues through which the surgical incision will pass.

Regional (peripheral) nerve block is achieved by the injection of a local anaesthetic into or around a specific nerve or group of nerves. Nerve blocks may be used to provide intraoperative anaesthesia and postoperative analgesia and for the diagnosis and treatment of chronic pain. Examples of common regional nerve blocks include brachial plexus, intercostal, and retrobulbar blocks. IV regional nerve block (Bier block) is the IV injection of

a local anaesthetic into an extremity following mechanical exsanguination using a compression bandage and a tourniquet. This type of block provides not only analgesia but also the ability to work in a bloodless field.

Spinal and Epidural Anaesthesia. Spinal and epidural anaesthesia are also types of regional anaesthesia. **Spinal anaesthesia** involves the injection of a local anaesthetic into the cerebrospinal fluid found in the subarachnoid space, usually below the level of L2. The local anaesthetic mixes with cerebrospinal fluid, and depending on the extent of its spread, various levels of anaesthesia are achieved. Because the local anaesthetic is administered directly into the cerebrospinal fluid, a spinal anaesthetic produces an autonomic, sensory, and motor blockade. Patients experience vasodilation and may become hypotensive as a result of the autonomic block, feel no pain as a result of the sensory block, and are unable to move as a result of the motor block. The duration of action of the spinal anaesthetic depends on the agent selected and the dose administered. A spinal anaesthetic may be used for procedures involving the lower abdomen, the groin, the perineum, or a lower extremity.

An **epidural block** involves injection of a local anaesthetic into the epidural (extradural) space via either a thoracic or a lumbar approach. The anaesthetic agent does not enter the cerebrospinal fluid but works by binding to nerve roots as they enter and exit the spinal cord. By using a low concentration of local anaesthetic, sensory pathways are blocked, but motor fibres remain intact. In higher doses, both sensory and motor fibres are blocked (Figure 21-7). Epidural anaesthesia may be used as the sole anaesthetic for a surgical procedure, or a catheter may be placed to allow for intraoperative use with continued use into the postoperative period for analgesia, using lower doses of epidurally administered local anaesthetic, usually in combination with an opioid. Epidural anaesthesia is commonly used for vascular

Table 21-6 Methods for Administering Local Anaesthesia
• Topical application
• Local infiltration
• Regional injection
• Peripheral nerve block
• Intravenous regional block (Bier block)
• Spinal anaesthesia (block)
• Epidural anaesthesia (block)

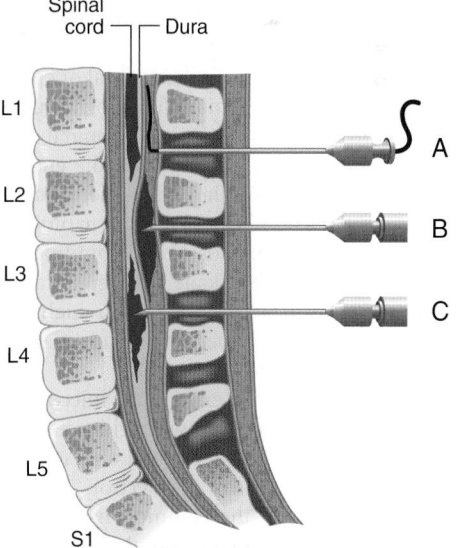

Figure 21-7 Location of needle point and injected anaesthetic relative to dura. *A,* Epidural catheter. *B,* Single-injection epidural. *C,* Spinal anaesthesia. (Interspaces most commonly used are L4-5, L3-4, and L2-3.)

Source: Rothrock, J. C. (2011). *Alexander's care of the patient in surgery* (14th ed., p. 134, Figure 4-7). St. Louis: Mosby.

Table 21-7 Differences Between Epidural and Spinal Anaesthetics

DRUGS	INJECTION SPACE	POTENTIAL COMPLICATIONS	POSTOPERATIVE MONITORING
Spinal Anaesthetic (Local)			
Bupivacaine (Marcaine) Lidocaine Tetracaine	Most commonly used interspaces: L4-5, L3-4, and L2-3	Hypotension, total spinal anaesthesia, post–dural puncture headache	Vital signs Motor and sensory block Urinary output and bladder distension Assess for headache
Spinal Anaesthetic (Analgesia)			
Fentanyl Morphine sulphate (preservative free)	Most commonly used interspaces: L4-5, L3-4, and L2-3	Hypotension; pruritus; urinary retention; nausea, vomiting; infection; epidural hematoma; oversedation *Contraindications:* Septicemia, ↑ ICP, hypovolemia, neurological disease, anticoagulation therapy, spinal fracture	Vital signs Motor and sensory block Urinary output and bladder distension Assess for headache
Epidural Anaesthetic (Local)			
Ropivacaine Lidocaine Bupivacaine	Between the ligamentum flavum and the dura	Bupivacaine can be associated with cardiac toxicity if injected intravascularly	Respiratory assessment Vital signs Sedation score
Epidural Anaesthetic (Analgesia)			
Morphine sulphate (preservative free) Fentanyl Sufentanil (Sufenta)	The dura	Hypotension; pruritus; urinary retention; nausea, vomiting; infection; epidural hematoma; oversedation *Contraindications:* Septicemia, ↑ ICP, hypovolemia, neurological disease, anticoagulation therapy, spinal fracture	Urinary output and bladder distension Assess for pruritus, nausea, or vomiting Pain assessment Assess for catheter migration (numbness or tingling) Assess dressing and insertion site Headaches

ICP, intracranial pressure.

procedures involving the lower extremity and hip and knee replacement surgeries. (Table 21-7 lists some differences between epidural and spinal anaesthetics.)

During the surgical procedure when spinal or epidural anaesthesia is used, the patient can remain fully conscious or sedation can be achieved intravenously. The onset of spinal anaesthesia is faster than that seen with an epidural, but the end results with either approach are usually similar. The patient must be closely observed for signs of autonomic nervous system blockade, including hypotension, bradycardia, nausea, and vomiting. There is less autonomic nervous system blockade with epidural anaesthesia than with spinal anaesthesia. Should "too high" a block be achieved, the patient may experience inadequate respiratory excursion and apnea (ORNAC, 2011, p. 291).

One advantage of epidural (extradural) injection over spinal (subarachnoid) injection is a decreased incidence of headache. A headache may be experienced after spinal anaesthesia following leakage of spinal fluid at the site of injection. The incidence of headache is decreasing with the common use of smaller-gauge spinal needles (25- to 27-gauge) and the use of noncutting, "pencil-point" spinal needles. A headache following an epidural may occur when a 17- to 18-gauge needle is advanced too far and the dura is punctured, resulting in the leakage of cerebrospinal fluid (ORNAC, 2011).

Procedural Sedation

The primary goals of procedural sedation are to reduce the patient's anxiety, discomfort, and pain and to facilitate coopera-

tion because the patient is able to respond appropriately to verbal commands. Procedural sedation is frequently used not only for minor surgical procedures but also for diagnostic procedures such as endoscopy and wound debridement, central line and chest tube placement, and reduction of fractures and dislocations. Nurses may monitor these patients if they have the expanded knowledge, skills, and judgement to do so within their scope of practice. If the patient requires deeper sedation during the procedure, there is a potential for loss of airway control, so an anaesthesia care provider must be present (Odom-Forren, 2011, p. 83; ORNAC, 2011, pp. 283-287). Table 21-8 lists risk factors for complications with procedural sedation.

Patient After Surgery

Through constant observation of the surgical progress, the anaesthesiologist anticipates the end of the surgical procedure and uses appropriate types and doses of anaesthetic agents so that their effects will be minimal at the end of the surgical procedure. This also allows greater physiological control of the patient during the transfer to the PACU or designated recovery area.

The anaesthesiologist and the perioperative nurse or another member of the surgical team accompany the patient to the PACU. A report of the patient's status and the procedure is communicated. The OR nurse evaluates the patient's response to nursing care based on outcome criteria established when the plan of care was developed and transfers the accountability of nursing care to the health care providers using a written and verbal report. The verbal report of nursing care provides continuity of care from one

Table 21-8 Risk Factors for Complications With Procedural Sedation

PATIENT RISK FACTOR	INTERVENTION
Airway abnormalities	Evaluate airway and presence of sleep apnea prior to sedation.
ASA classification III or greater	Assess Class III patients individually and arrange anaesthesia consult for Classes IV and V.
Chronic obstructive pulmonary disease	Bronchodilators given prior to procedure. Make sure to titrate sedatives in small increments.
Chronic renal failure	Do not use long-lasting opioids and administer small incremental doses of sedatives.
Coronary artery disease	Allow patient to take routine cardiac medications on day of procedure. Do not over- or undersedate. Give supplemental oxygen during procedure.
Drug addiction	Administer short-acting sedatives in incremental doses. Do not use reversal agents.
Extremes of age: pediatric to older adults	Administer individual and incremental doses.
Obesity	Give oral histamine H_2 antagonist and titrate sedatives in small increments.

Source: Adapted from Odom-Forren, J. (2011). Perioperative patient safety and procedural sedation. In D. Watson (Ed.), *Perioperative safety* (p. 85). St. Louis: Mosby Elsevier.
ASA, American Society of Anesthesiologists.

health care provider to another and decreases risk of error. The report should include the following (ORNAC, 2011, p. 280):
• Name and age of patient
• Preoperative diagnosis and co-morbid medical problems
• Preoperative medications
• Time of next antibiotic dose
• Operative procedure performed
• Intake/output, vital signs
• Allergies
• Drains, catheters, dressing/packing
• Intraoperative positioning and postoperative skin assessment
• Physical issues such as loose teeth, deafness, blindness, arthritis
• Psychological disorders and language barriers
• Existence of advance directives

AGE-RELATED CONSIDERATIONS: PATIENT DURING SURGERY

Although anaesthetic agents have become safer and more predictable, older adults often demonstrate varying and unique responses to medications. Because of this, anaesthetic drugs should be carefully titrated when given to older adults. Physiological changes in aging, and comorbidities, may alter the patient's response not only to the anaesthetic but to blood and fluid loss and replacement, hypothermia, pain, and the tolerance of the surgical procedure and positioning (Westhead, 2007). The older adult's response to all anaesthetic agents must be carefully monitored

and the postoperative recovery assessed before the patient is left without close supervision (e.g., transferred from the PACU to a surgical unit).

Many older adults experience a decrease in their ability to communicate and follow directions as a result of alterations in vision or hearing. These factors pose a special need for clear and concise communication in the OR, especially when preoperative sedation is superimposed on the existing sensory deficit. Skin elasticity in the older adult is decreased because of loss of collagen. As a result, the skin is sensitive to injury from tape, electrodes, warming and cooling blankets, and certain types of dressings. In addition, the older adult often has osteoporosis and osteoarthritis. These factors reinforce the need for careful transferring, lifting, and positioning techniques.

Emergency Events in the Operating Room

Unanticipated intraoperative events occasionally occur. Although some are more predictable than others (e.g., cardiac arrest in an unstable patient, massive blood loss during trauma surgery), all demand immediate intervention by all members of the OR team. Such events include anaphylactic reactions, malignant hyperthermia (MH), major blood loss, and intraoperative death (ORNAC, 2011, pp. 296-298; 302-305).

Anaphylactic Reactions

Anaphylaxis is the most severe form of an allergic reaction, manifesting with life-threatening pulmonary and circulatory complications. Initial clinical manifestations of anaphylaxis may be masked by anaesthesia. Anaesthesiologists administer an array of drugs to patients, such as anaesthetics, antibiotics, blood products, and plasma expanders, and because any parenterally administered material can theoretically produce an allergic response, vigilance and rapid intervention are essential. An anaphylactic reaction causes hypotension, tachycardia, bronchospasm, and possibly, pulmonary edema. Antibiotics and latex are responsible for many perioperative allergic reactions. (Anaphylaxis is discussed in Chapter 16.)

Latex allergy remains a concern in the perioperative setting, despite the move for surgical products to be produced from materials other than natural rubber latex. Reactions to natural rubber latex range from urticaria to anaphylaxis, with symptoms appearing immediately or at some time during the surgical procedure.

Policies and procedures must be available so the health care team can provide a latex-safe environment for patients with potential or actual latex allergy (ORNAC, 2011, p. 298). (Latex allergies are discussed in Chapter 16.)

Malignant Hyperthermia

Malignant hyperthermia (MH) is a rare metabolic disease characterized by hyperthermia with rigidity of skeletal muscles that can result in death. It occurs in affected people exposed to certain anaesthetic agents. Succinylcholine (Anectine), especially in conjunction with volatile inhalation agents, appears to be the primary trigger of the disorder, although other factors, such as stress, trauma, and heat, have been implicated. It usually occurs during general anaesthesia, but it may manifest in the recovery period as well. It is autosomal dominant in inheritance but is variable in its genetic penetrance, so predictions based on family history are important but inconsistent. (Autosomal dominant disorders are discussed in Chapter 15.) The fundamental defect is hypermetabolism of skeletal muscle resulting from altered control of intracellular calcium, leading to muscle contracture, hyperthermia, hypoxemia, lactic acidosis, and hemodynamic and cardiac alterations.

Tachycardia, tachypnea, hypercarbia, and ventricular dysrhythmias are generally seen but are nonspecific to MH. MH is generally diagnosed after all other causes of the hypermetabolism are ruled out. The rise in body temperature is a delayed sign of MH.

Unless there is a prompt initiation of appropriate intervention, MH can result in cardiac arrest and death. The definitive treatment of MH is prompt administration of dantrolene (Dantrium), which slows metabolism and provides symptomatic support to correct hemodynamic instability, acidosis, hypoxemia, and elevated temperature. A treatment protocol in the form of an interactive MH-emergency iPhone application or a hardcopy poster is available from the Malignant Hyperthermia Association of the United States (see the Resources section at the end of this chapter).

To prevent MH, it is important for the nurse to obtain a careful family history and be alert to susceptibility perioperatively. The patient known or suspected to be at risk for MH can be anaesthetized with minimal risk if appropriate precautions are taken. Patients with MH should be informed of the condition so that family members may be genetically tested (ORNAC, 2011).

Major Blood Loss

Surgery always poses a risk for blood loss. If major blood loss occurs during surgery, it is the circulating nurse's responsibility to assist the anaesthesiologist with replacement of the loss. Blood transfusions and fluid volume expanders (Pentaspan) are the most common ways to replace major blood loss in the OR. The circulating nurse should monitor and record all fluid accumulation in the suction container. It is also extremely important to note how much irrigation is used because both blood and irrigation solution can accumulate together. In cases of major blood loss, it might be important to weigh surgical sponges to account for blood that has accumulated in the operative site. Anaesthesiologists may monitor a patient's laboratory values (hemoglobin, blood gases) intraoperatively to help determine whether intraoperative blood transfusions are needed.

New and Future Considerations

Changes in technology and new developments in science and research data lead to better treatment for the patient undergoing surgery. One example is the revision of fasting guidelines for healthy patients undergoing elective surgery (Rothrock, 2011, p. 118). (Chapter 20 details preoperative fasting guidelines used by the Canadian Anesthesiologists' Society.)

Another example is "bloodless surgery," which is becoming more of a reality (Crum & Valenti, 2007). Various techniques can minimize blood loss during and after surgery, and others allow the surgical team to manage blood loss without the need for a blood transfusion. These include drug therapy and techniques for managing low hematocrit, hemostatic agents to enhance clotting and control bleeding, surgical devices and techniques to locate and stop internal bleeding, and surgical and anaesthetic techniques to limit blood loss. In cases of extreme blood loss, an autologous blood salvage unit can be used to suction the patient's blood from the sterile field and filter and process it for infusion back to the patient. This equipment is complex and should be used by specially trained individuals (Rothrock, 2011, p. 1197). There are also new alternatives to blood transfusions, such as erythropoietin, deliberate hypotension, and normovolemic hemodilution. Research is also continuing on the development of a synthetic, oxygen-carrying blood alternative.

A third example is robotic devices, which are being used in some ORs to assist in laparoscopic surgery. Surgical intervention using robotics, combined with advances in computer technology and communication systems, has made telepresence surgery a reality. This allows surgeons at a distance to perform laparoscopic surgery using remote-controlled robots (Rothrock, 2011, p. 223).

REVIEW QUESTIONS

The number of the question corresponds to the same-numbered objective at the beginning of the chapter.

1. What is the perioperative nurse's primary responsibility for the care of the patient undergoing surgery?
   a. Developing an individualized plan of nursing care for the patient
   b. Carrying out specific tasks related to surgical policies and procedures
   c. Ensuring that the patient has been assessed for safe administration of anaesthesia
   d. Performing a preoperative history and physical assessment to identify patient needs

2. What is the proper attire for the semirestricted area of the surgery department?
   a. Street clothing
   b. Surgical attire and head cover
   c. Surgical attire, head cover, and mask
   d. Street clothing with the addition of shoe covers

3. What is one characteristic of the operating room (OR) environment that facilitates the prevention of infection in the surgical patient?
   a. Adjustable lighting
   b. Conductive furniture
   c. Filters in the ventilating system
   d. Explosion-proof electrical plugs

4. What is one perioperative team activity that is carried out in the OR before the incision is made?
   a. Check electrical equipment.
   b. Count instruments and supplies.
   c. Conduct a time out or pause and review the Surgical Safety Check List.
   d. Ensure the patient has been typed and screened for blood transfusion.

5. What is the most important intervention to perform when a patient arrives to the OR with musculoskeletal impairments?
   a. Ensure proper preparation of the skin.
   b. Ensure the anaesthesiologist uses muscle relaxants.
   c. Ensure positioning on the OR bed to prevent injury.
   d. Provide detailed explanations about the surgical activities.

6. Which of the following is not acceptable when putting items on the sterile field?
   a. Opening the sterile package and handing the sterile item to the scrub nurse
   b. Placing sterile items carefully on the sterile back table while avoiding reaching over the field
   c. Opening sterile packages onto a clean, dry surface, providing the wrapper fully covers the surface
   d. Flipping the item from a paper peel pack onto the sterile field

7. Which of the following is not a consideration when positioning the surgical patient?
   a. Provision of modesty for the patient
   b. Avoiding compression of nerve tissue
   c. Provision of correct skeletal alignment
   d. Ensuring that students in the room can see the operative site

8. Mrs. Jones is scheduled for an abdominal hysterectomy. She is extremely anxious and has a tendency to hyperventilate when upset. What is the most appropriate type of anaesthetic for Mrs. Jones?
   a. A spinal block
   b. An epidural block
   c. A general anaesthetic
   d. A local anaesthetic

9. Why is intravenous induction for general anaesthesia the method of choice for most patients?
   a. The patient is not intubated.
   b. The agents are nonexplosive.
   c. Induction is rapid and pleasant.
   d. The odour of the agent is not offensive.

10. What is the name for the injection of the local anaesthetic into the tissues through the surgical incision?
    a. Nerve block
    b. Local infiltration
    c. Topical application
    d. Regional application

ANSWERS: 1. a; 2. b; 3. c; 4. c; 5. c; 6. d; 7. d; 8. c; 9. c; 10. b.

REFERENCES

Canadian Anesthesiologists' Society. (2011). Guidelines to the practice of anesthesia. *Supplement to the Canadian Journal of Anesthesia, 58*, 74-107. doi:10.1007/s12630-010-9416

Canadian Nurses Association. (2008). Perioperative nursing certification exam development guidelines. Retrieved from *http://www2.cna-aiic.ca/cna/documents/pdf/publications/CERT_Perioperative_e.pdf*

Canadian Patient Safety Institute. (2009). Surgical safety checklist and scorecard. Retrieved from *http://signup.patientsafetyinstitute.ca/English/toolsResources/sssl/Pages/SSSLDocuments.aspx?File=3*

Crum, E., & Valenti, J. (2007). Can a bloodless surgery program work in the trauma setting? *Nursing, 37*(7), 54-56.

Fawcett, D. (2011). Prevention of positioning injuries. In D. Watson (Ed.), *Perioperative safety* (pp. 167-178). St. Louis: Mosby Elsevier.

Haynes, A., Weiser, T., Berry, W., Lipsitz, S., Breizat, A., Dellinger, E., …, Gawande, A. A. (2009). A surgical safety checklist to reduce morbidity and mortality in a global population. *New England Journal of Medicine, 360*, 491-499.

Odom-Forren, J. (2011). Perioperative patient safety and procedural sedation. In D. Watson (Ed.), *Perioperative safety*. St. Louis: Mosby Elsevier.

Operating Room Nurses Association of Canada (ORNAC). (2011). *Standards, guidelines, and position statements for perioperative registered nursing practice* (10th ed.). Halifax, NS: Author.

Phillips, N. (2013a). Principles of asepsis and sterile techniques. In N. Phillips (Ed.), *Berry & Kohn's operating room technique* (12th ed.). St. Louis: Mosby.

Phillips, N. (2013b). The perioperative patient care team and professional credentialing. In N. Phillips (Ed.), *Berry & Kohn's operating room technique* (12th ed.). St. Louis: Mosby.

Rothrock, J. (2011). *Alexander's care of the patient in surgery* (14th ed.). St. Louis: Elsevier/Mosby.

Tanner, J., Woodings, D., & Moncaster, K. (2008). Preoperative hair removal to reduce surgical site infection. *Cochrane Database of Systematic Reviews, 2*. Art. No. CD004122. doi:10.1002?14651858. CD004122.pub3

Thompson, C. A. (2007). Prevention of respiratory depression becomes safety foundation's new goal. *American Journal of Health System Pharmacy, 64*, 798-799. doi:10.2146/news070035

University of Toronto. (2009). Proposal for Master of Nursing (Nurse Practitioner Field) Concurrent Diploma in Anesthesia Care. Retrieved from *http://portal.sgs.utoronto.ca/gws/ProposalView.aspx?id=1925*

Westhead, C. (2007). Perioperative nursing management of the elderly patient. *Canadian Operating Room Nursing Journal, 25*(3), 34-40.

CANADIAN RESOURCES

Canadian Anesthesiologists' Society
http://www.cas.ca

Malignant Hyperthermia Unit – Ottawa Hospital
http://www.ottawahospital.on.ca/wps/portal/Base/TheHospital/ClinicalServices/DeptPgrmCS/Departments/Anesthesiology/MalignantHyperthermiaUnit

National Association of PeriAnesthesia Nurses of Canada
http://www.napanc.org/

Ontario PeriAnesthesia Nurses Association
http://www.opana.org

Operating Room Nursing Association of Canada
http://www.ornac.ca

Surgical Safety Checklist—Canadian Version
http://www.saferhealthcarenow.ca/EN/Interventions/SafeSurgery/Pages/SurgicalSafetyChecklist.aspx

RELATED RESOURCES

Malignant Hyperthermia Association of the United States
http://www.mhaus.org/

evolve *For additional Internet resources, see the Web site for this book at* **http://evolve.elsevier.com/Canada/Lewis/medsurg**

Nursing Management: Postoperative Care

Written by Christine R. Hoch

Adapted by Debra Clendinneng

LEARNING OBJECTIVES

1. Identify the components of an initial postanaesthesia assessment.
2. Identify the nursing responsibilities in admitting patients to the postanaesthesia care unit (PACU).
3. Explain the etiology and nursing assessment and management of potential problems of patients in the PACU.
4. Describe the initial nursing assessment and management after transfer from the PACU to the general care unit.
5. Explain the etiology and nursing assessment and management of potential problems during the postoperative period.
6. Identify the information needed after surgery by the patient in preparation for discharge.

KEY TERMS

airway obstruction A blockage of the patient's airway, most commonly caused by the patient's tongue, p. 459

atelectasis An abnormal condition characterized by the collapse of alveoli, p. 461

bronchospasm The result of an increase in bronchial smooth muscle tone with resultant closure of small airways, p. 462

delayed awakening Longer-than-expected duration of postoperative unconsciousness, usually caused by prolonged drug action and, rarely, by neurological injury, p. 465

emergence delirium A neurological alteration that occurs in some patients awakening from anaesthesia after surgery; can include behaviours such as restlessness, agitation, disorientation, thrashing, and shouting; also called violent emergence, p. 465

epidural analgesia The infusion of pain-relieving medications through a catheter placed into the epidural space surrounding the spinal cord, p. 467

hiccups Intermittent spasms of the diaphragm caused by irritation of the phrenic nerve, which innervates the diaphragm, p. 469

hypothermia A core temperature of less than 36°C; occurs when heat loss exceeds heat production, p. 467

hypoventilation Deficient ventilation of the lungs, characterized by a decreased respiratory rate or effort, hypoxemia, and an increasing arterial partial pressure of carbon dioxide ($PaCO_2$), p. 462

hypoxemia Low oxygen tension in the blood (PaO_2 <60 mm Hg), characterized by a variety of nonspecific clinical signs and symptoms, p. 461

paralytic ileus A small-bowel obstruction that results when peristalsis stops, p. 469

patient-controlled analgesia (PCA) Self-administration of predetermined doses of analgesia by the patient, with the goals of providing immediate analgesia and maintaining a constant blood level of the analgesic agent, p. 467

syncope Fainting that may occur with decreased cardiac output, fluid deficits, or defects in cerebral perfusion, p. 464

wound dehiscence Separation and disruption of previously joined wound edges, p. 471

wound evisceration Protrusion of the visceral organs though a wound opening, p. 471

ELECTRONIC RESOURCES

Supplemental content related to Chapter 22 can be found…

Evolve Web Site ⊖volve

http://evolve.elsevier.com/Canada/Lewis/medsurg
- Answer Guidelines for Case Study on p. 476
- Clinical Reference: Laboratory Values
- Content Updates

- Customizable Nursing Care Plan: Postoperative Patient
- Electronic Calculators
- Examination Review Questions
- Glossary
- Interactive Case Study: Surgery
- Key Points (Printable and MP3 Download)

The postoperative period begins immediately after surgery and continues until the patient is discharged from medical care. This chapter focuses on the common features of postoperative nursing care for the patient undergoing surgery. After surgery, the primary focus is on protecting the patient, who has been put in physiological risk during surgery, and preventing complications while the body heals. The problems and nursing care related to specific surgical procedures are discussed in the appropriate chapters of this text.

Postoperative Care in the Postanaesthesia Care Unit

The patient's immediate recovery period occurs in a *postanaesthesia care unit* (PACU). It is located adjacent to the operating room (OR) to minimize transportation of the patient immediately after surgery and to provide ready access to anaesthesia and surgical personnel. Three phases of postanaesthesia care provide different levels of care, depending on the patient's surgical procedure, anaesthesia, and individualized needs (Table 22-1).

Postanaesthesia Care Unit Admission

The initial admission of the patient to the PACU is a transfer of care from the anaesthesiologist and perioperative nurse to the PACU nurse. This collaboration fosters a smooth transfer of care to the PACU and plays a role in deciding the phase to which the patient is assigned.

Postanaesthesia Care Unit Progression. Patients move through the phases of care in the PACU depending on their condition. A patient who is stable and recovering well is admitted to Phase I care and may rapidly be discharged to either Phase II care or an inpatient unit. This *rapid postanaesthesia care unit progression* (RPP) can occur with inpatients or outpatients. Another accelerated system of care, *fast-tracking*, involves admitting ambulatory surgery patients who have received general, regional, or local anaesthesia directly to Phase II care. Patients' safety must be the primary consideration when determining what level of postoperative care is provided.

Initial Assessment. On patient admission to the PACU, the anaesthesiologist and perioperative nurse give a verbal report to the admitting PACU nurse. Table 22-2 summarizes the components of a complete anaesthesia report. While the patient is in the PACU, priority care includes monitoring and management of respiratory and circulatory function, pain, temperature, and surgical site and assessing the patient's response to the reversal of anaesthetic, such as sedation score and level of spinal block.

Table 22-1 Phases of Postanaesthesia Care

Phase I
- Care during the immediate postanaesthesia period
- ECG and more intense monitoring
- Goal: Prepare patient for transfer to Phase II or inpatient unit

Phase II
- Ambulatory surgery patients
- Goal: Prepare patient for transfer to extended observation, home, or extended care facility

Extended Observation
- Extended care/observation unit
- Goal: Prepare patient for self-care

ECG, electrocardiogram.
Source: American Society of PeriAnesthesia Nurses. (2008). *2008-2010 standards of perianesthesia nursing practice.* Cherry Hill, NJ: ASPAN.

Table 22-2 Postanaesthesia Admission Report

General Information	Intraoperative Management
• Patient name	• Anaesthetic medications received
• Age	• Other medications received before surgery or intraoperatively
• Anaesthesiologist name	
• Surgeon name	
• Surgical procedure	• Blood loss
Patient History	• Fluid replacement totals, including blood transfusions
• Indication for surgery	
• Medical history, medications, allergies	• Urine output
	Intraoperative Course
	• Unexpected anaesthetic events or reactions
	• Unexpected surgical events
	• Vital signs and monitoring trends
	• Results of intraoperative laboratory tests

Table 22-3 Initial Postanaesthesia Care Unit Assessment

Airway	Neurological
• Patency	• Level of consciousness
• Oral or nasal airway	• Orientation
• Endotracheal tube	• Sensory and motor status
Breathing	**Gastrointestinal–Genitourinary**
• Respiratory rate and quality	• Intake (fluids, irrigations)
• Auscultated breath sounds	• Output (emesis, urine, drains)
• Pulse oximetry	**Surgical Site**
• Supplemental oxygen	• Dressings and drainage
Circulation	**Pain**
• ECG monitoring—rate and rhythm	• Incision
	• Other
• Blood pressure	
• Temperature and colour of skin	
• Peripheral pulses	

ECG, electrocardiogram.

Table 22-4 Clinical Manifestations of Inadequate Oxygenation

Central Nervous System	Integumentary System
• Restlessness	• Cyanosis
• Agitation	• Prolonged capillary refill
• Muscle twitching	• Flushed and moist skin
• Seizures	• Observe for colour, sensation, and movement (CSM)
• Coma	
Cardiovascular System	**Respiratory System**
• Hypertension	• Alterations ranging from increased to absent respiratory effort
• Hypotension	• Use of accessory muscles
• Tachycardia	• Abnormal breath sounds
• Bradycardia	• Abnormal arterial blood gases
• Dysrhythmias	**Renal System**
	• Urine output 30 mL/hr

Assessment should begin with an evaluation of the airway, breathing, and circulation (ABC) status of the patient (Table 22-3). The first priority is to establish a patent airway. The patient may need stimulation to take deep breaths, be repositioned to the right side, or require a chin tilt. If these measures do not work, an oral or nasal airway may be used.

Evidence of respiratory compromise requires prompt intervention so pulse oximetry monitoring is initiated on admission because it provides a noninvasive means of assessing the adequacy of oxygenation.

Oxygen therapy will be used if the patient has had general anaesthesia or if the anaesthesiologist orders it. Oxygen therapy is given via nasal cannula or face mask. Oxygen aids in eliminating anaesthetic gases and meets the increased demand for oxygen needed owing to decreased blood volume or increased cellular metabolism. If the patient requires postoperative ventilation, a ventilator is provided. During the initial assessment, signs of inadequate oxygenation and ventilation should be identified (Table 22-4).

Electrocardiographic (ECG) monitoring may be initiated to determine cardiac rate and rhythm. Deviations from preoperative findings should be noted and evaluated. Blood pressure (BP) should be measured and compared with baseline readings. Invasive monitoring (e.g., arterial BP monitoring) that was initiated in the OR will be monitored in the PACU. *Body temperature, skin colour* and condition, and capillary refill should also be assessed. Any evidence of inadequate circulatory status requires prompt intervention. The *initial neurological assessment* focuses on level of consciousness; orientation; sensory and motor status; and size, equality, and reactivity of the pupils. Hearing is the first sense to return in the unconscious patient, so the nurse should explain all activities to the patient from the moment of admission to the PACU including that the surgery is completed, the patient is in the recovery room, and that the family or significant other has been notified.

Occasionally, patients may wake up agitated in what is referred to as *emergence delirium* (Figure 22-1), a condition in which patients may be disoriented to place, time, and person and exhibit bizarre behaviour after anaesthesia (Rothrock, 2011, p. 1167). According to Radtke and colleagues (2010), 5% of the

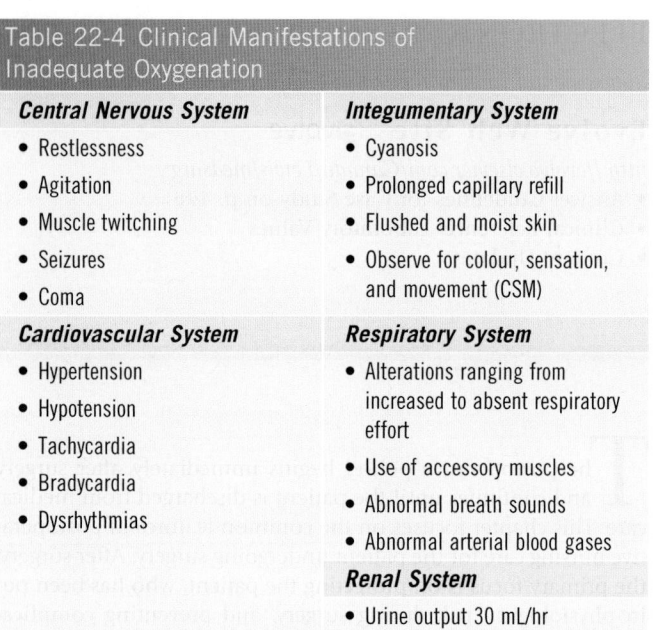
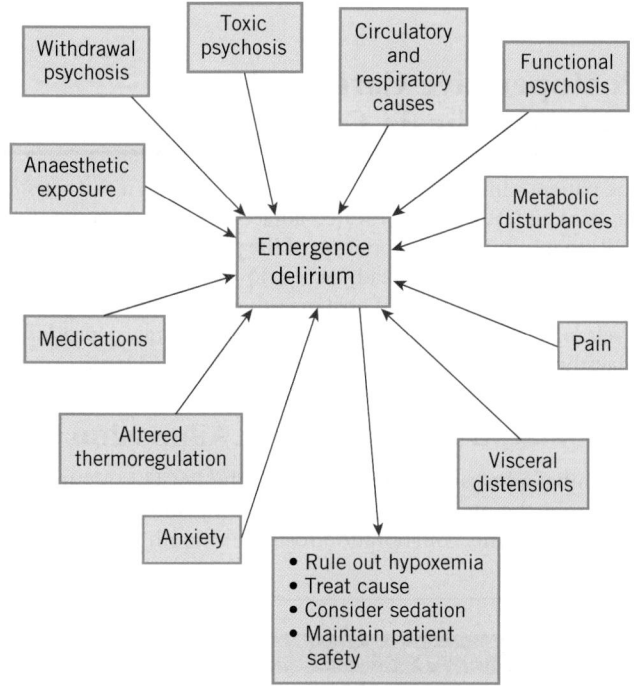

Figure 22-1 Emergence delirium in the postanaesthesia care unit: contributing factors and treatment.

Source: Redrawn from Rothrock, J. C. (2011). *Alexander's care of the patient in surgery* (14th ed., p. 277, Figure 9-7). St. Louis: Mosby.

population experiences emergence delirium and it affects primarily pediatric and older adult patients. Other contributing factors include inadequate pain control while emerging from anaesthesia and in the PACU, large intraoperative blood loss, and the use of sevoflurane, isoflurane, or analgesics. This delirium is usually noted about half an hour after surgery but may manifest in up to 24 hours in the elderly. It is a reversible state and most cases resolve spontaneously with only supportive nursing care (Hudek, 2009).

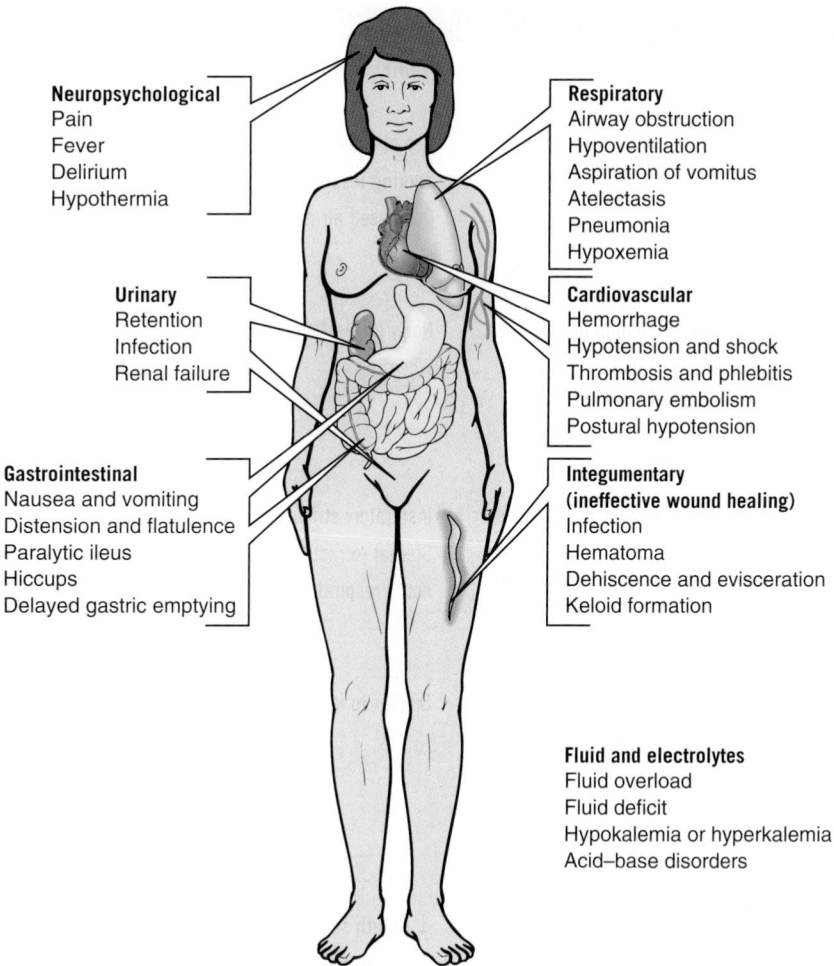

Neuropsychological
Pain
Fever
Delirium
Hypothermia

Respiratory
Airway obstruction
Hypoventilation
Aspiration of vomitus
Atelectasis
Pneumonia
Hypoxemia

Urinary
Retention
Infection
Renal failure

Cardiovascular
Hemorrhage
Hypotension and shock
Thrombosis and phlebitis
Pulmonary embolism
Postural hypotension

Gastrointestinal
Nausea and vomiting
Distension and flatulence
Paralytic ileus
Hiccups
Delayed gastric emptying

Integumentary
(ineffective wound healing)
Infection
Hematoma
Dehiscence and evisceration
Keloid formation

Fluid and electrolytes
Fluid overload
Fluid deficit
Hypokalemia or hyperkalemia
Acid–base disorders

Figure 22-2 Potential problems in the postoperative period.

If the patient had a regional anaesthetic (e.g., spinal or epidural), sensory and motor blockade may still be present, and the patient should be assessed for sensation and movement.

The assessment of the *urinary system* focuses on intake and output and fluid balance. Intraoperative fluid totals are communicated as part of the anaesthesia report. The PACU nurse should note the presence of all intravenous (IV) lines, irrigation solutions and infusions, and output devices such as catheters. IV infusions are regulated according to postoperative orders. If the patient is nauseous or vomiting, the nurse should administer antiemetic medications as ordered. The colour and amount of emesis should be charted.

The *surgical site* is assessed by the PACU nurse. The condition of any dressings and the colour and amount of any drainage from the incision site or wound drains should be charted. All data obtained in the admission assessment are documented on a PACU record, a form specific to postanaesthesia and postsurgical care.

After the initial assessment is completed, the PACU nurse continues to apply the skills of ongoing assessment, diagnosis, and intervention and notes the patient's response to intervention. The goal of PACU care is to identify actual and potential patient problems that may occur as a result of anaesthetic administration and surgical intervention and to intervene appropriately. Common postoperative problems the nurse should anticipate include airway compromise (obstruction), respiratory insuffi-

ciency (hypoxemia and hypercarbia), cardiac compromise (hypotension, hypertension, and dysrhythmias), neurological compromise (emergence delirium and delayed awakening), hypothermia, pain, and nausea and vomiting (Figure 22-2). Each of these problems and appropriate nursing interventions are discussed in this chapter.

Potential Alterations in Respiratory Function

Etiology

Postanaesthesia Care Unit. In the immediate postanaesthetic period, the most common causes of airway compromise include obstruction, hypoxemia, and hypoventilation (Table 22-5). Patients at particular risk include those who have had general anaesthesia; are older; have a smoking history or lung disease; are obese; or have undergone airway, thoracic, or abdominal surgery. However, respiratory complications may occur with any patient who has been anaesthetized.

Airway obstruction is most commonly caused by blockage of the airway by the patient's tongue (Figure 22-3). The base of the tongue falls backward against the soft palate and occludes the pharynx. It is most pronounced in the supine position and in the patient who is extremely sleepy after surgery. Less common causes

Table 22-5 Common Immediate Postoperative Respiratory Complications

COMPLICATIONS AND CAUSES	MECHANISMS	MANIFESTATIONS	INTERVENTIONS
Airway Obstruction			
Tongue falling back	Muscular flaccidity associated with decreased consciousness and muscle relaxants	Use of accessory muscles Snoring respirations Decreased air movement	Patient stimulation Jaw thrust Chin lift Artificial airway Position patient on side
Retained thick secretions	Secretion stimulation by anaesthetic agents Dehydration of secretions	Noisy respirations Wheezing	Suctioning Deep breathing and coughing IV hydration IPPB with mucolytic agent Chest physical therapy
Laryngospasm	Irritation from endotracheal tube or anaesthetic gases Most likely to occur after removal of endotracheal tube	Inspiratory stridor (crowing respiration) Sternal retraction Acute respiratory distress	O_2 therapy Positive pressure ventilation IV muscle relaxant Lidocaine Corticosteroids
Laryngeal edema	Allergic drug reaction Mechanical irritation from intubation Fluid overload	Similar to laryngospasm	O_2 therapy Antihistamines Corticosteroids Sedatives Possible intubation
Hypoxemia			
Atelectasis	Bronchial obstruction caused by secretions or decreased lung volumes	↓ Breath sounds ↓ O_2 saturation	O_2 therapy Deep breathing Incentive spirometry Early mobilization
Pulmonary edema	↑ Hydrostatic pressure ↓ Interstitial pressure ↑ Capillary permeability	Crackles Infiltrates seen on chest radiograph Fluid overload ↓ O_2 saturation Productive cough with clear to pink sputum	O_2 therapy Diuretics Fluid restriction
Pulmonary embolism	Thrombus dislodged from peripheral venous system; lodged in pulmonary arterial system	Acute tachypnea Dyspnea Tachycardia Hypotension ↓ O_2 saturation	O_2 therapy Cardiopulmonary support Anticoagulant therapy
Aspiration	Inhalation of gastric contents	Bronchospasm Atelectasis Crackles Respiratory distress ↓ O_2 saturation	O_2 therapy Cardiac support Antibiotics
Bronchospasm	Increased smooth muscle tone with closure of small airways	Wheezing Dyspnea Tachypnea ↓ O_2 saturation	O_2 therapy Bronchodilators

Table 22-5 Common Immediate Postoperative Respiratory Complications—cont'd

COMPLICATIONS AND CAUSES	MECHANISMS	MANIFESTATIONS	INTERVENTIONS
Hypoventilation			
Depression of central respiratory drive	Medullary depression from anaesthetics, narcotics, or sedatives	Shallow respirations ↓ Respiratory rate, apnea ↓ PaO_2 ↑ $PaCO_2$	Stimulation Reversal of narcotics or benzodiazepines Mechanical ventilation Deep breathing
Poor respiratory muscle tone	Neuromuscular blockade Neuromuscular disease	As above	Reversal of paralysis Mechanical ventilation
Mechanical restriction	Tight casts, dressings, positioning, and obesity prevent lung expansion	As above	Elevate head of bed Repositioning Loosen dressings
Pain	Shallow breathing to prevent incisional pain	As above Complaints of pain Guarding behaviour	Narcotic analgesic therapy in reduced dosage

IPPB, intermittent positive pressure breathing; *IV*, intravenous; *PaCO₂*, arterial partial pressure of carbon dioxide; *PaO₂*, arterial partial pressure of oxygen.

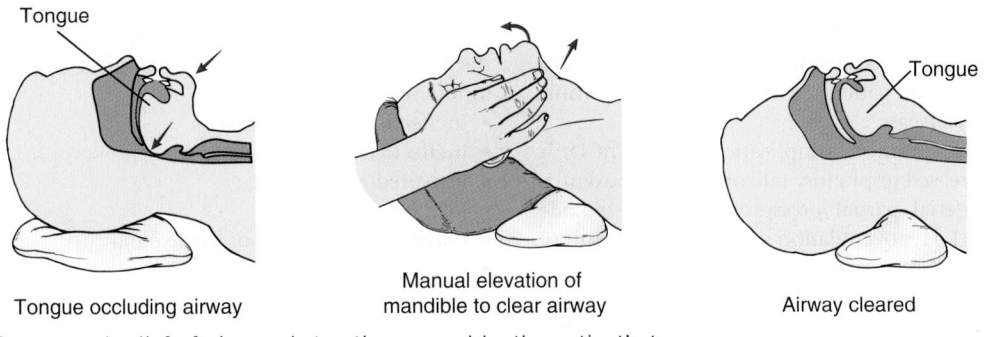

Figure 22-3 Causes and relief of airway obstruction caused by the patient's tongue.

Tongue occluding airway / Manual elevation of mandible to clear airway / Airway cleared

of airway obstruction include laryngospasm, retained secretions, and laryngeal edema.

Hypoxemia, an arterial partial pressure of oxygen (PaO_2) of less than 60 mm Hg, is characterized by a variety of non-specific clinical signs and symptoms, ranging from agitation to somnolence, hypertension to hypotension, and tachycardia to bradycardia. Pulse oximetry will indicate a low oxygen saturation (<90-92%). Arterial blood gas analysis can confirm hypoxemia if the pulse oximetry indicates low O_2 saturation. Low oxygen saturation may be corrected by encouraging deep breathing and coughing or by increasing the amount of oxygen delivered.

The most common cause of postoperative hypoxemia is atelectasis. **Atelectasis** (alveolar collapse) may be the result of bronchial obstruction caused by retained secretions or decreased respiratory excursion. Atelectasis occurs when mucus blocks bronchioles or when the amount of alveolar surfactant (the substance that holds the alveoli open) is reduced (Figure 22-4). As air becomes trapped beyond the plug and is eventually absorbed, the alveoli collapse. Atelectasis may affect a portion or an entire lobe of the lungs.

Other causes of hypoxemia that may occur in the PACU include pulmonary edema, pulmonary embolism, aspiration, and bronchospasm.

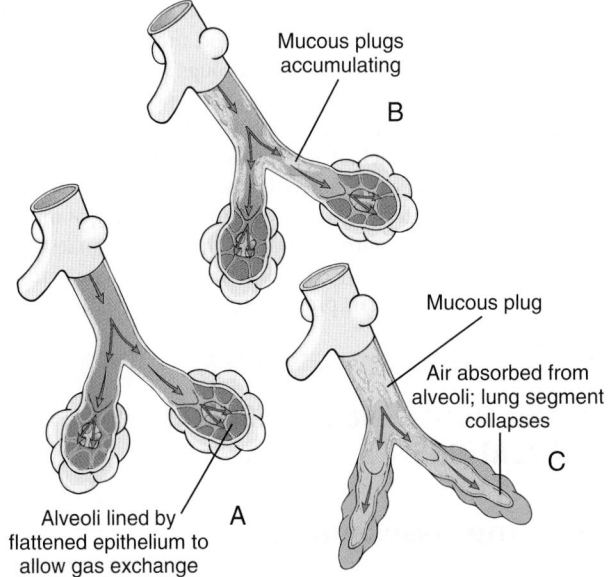

Mucous plugs accumulating

B

Mucous plug

Air absorbed from alveoli; lung segment collapses

C

Alveoli lined by flattened epithelium to allow gas exchange

A

Figure 22-4 Postoperative atelectasis. **A,** Normal bronchiole and alveoli. **B,** Mucous plugs in bronchioles. **C,** Collapse of alveoli caused by atelectasis following absorption of air.

Pulmonary edema is caused by an accumulation of fluid in the alveoli and may be the result of fluid overload; left ventricular failure; or prolonged airway obstruction, sepsis, or aspiration. Pulmonary edema is characterized by hypoxemia, crackles on auscultation, decreased pulmonary compliance, and the presence of infiltrates seen on chest radiograph.

Aspiration of gastric contents into the lungs is a potentially serious airway emergency with symptoms of bronchospasm, hypoxemia, atelectasis, interstitial edema, alveolar hemorrhage, and respiratory failure. Gastric aspiration may result in laryngospasm, infection, and pulmonary edema. Because of the serious consequences of gastric aspiration, prevention, as opposed to treatment, is the goal. Patients identified as being at risk (obese, pregnant, history of hiatal hernia, gastroesophageal reflux disease, peptic ulcer, or trauma) may be premedicated with a histamine H_2-receptor antagonist (e.g., famotidine [Pepcid]) before induction of anaesthesia. The anaesthesiologist will take special precautions to protect the airway during induction of and emergence from anaesthesia.

Bronchospasm is the result of an increase in bronchial smooth muscle tone with resultant closure of small airways. Airway edema develops, causing secretions to build up in the airway. The patient will have wheezing, dyspnea, use of accessory muscles, hypoxemia, and tachypnea. Bronchospasm may be caused by aspiration, endotracheal intubation, suctioning, or chemical mediator release as a result of an allergic response. (Allergic responses are discussed in Chapter 16.) Bronchospasm is seen more frequently in patients with asthma and chronic obstructive pulmonary disease.

Hypoventilation, a common complication in the PACU, is characterized by a decreased respiratory rate or effort, hypoxemia, and an increasing arterial partial pressure of carbon dioxide ($PaCO_2$) (hypercapnia). Hypoventilation may occur as a result of depression of the central respiratory drive (secondary to anaesthesia or pain medication), poor respiratory muscle tone (secondary to neuromuscular blockade or disease), or a combination of both.

Clinical Unit. Common causes of respiratory problems for postoperative patients in the clinical unit are atelectasis and pneumonia especially after abdominal and thoracic surgery. The postoperative development of mucous plugs and decreased surfactant production are directly related to hypoventilation, constant recumbent position, ineffective coughing, and history of smoking. Increased bronchial secretions occur when the respiratory passages have been irritated by heavy smoking, acute or chronic pulmonary infection or disease, and the drying of mucous membranes that occurs with intubation, inhalation anaesthesia, and dehydration. Without intervention, microorganisms grow in the stagnant mucus and can progress to pneumonia.

NURSING MANAGEMENT: RESPIRATORY COMPLICATIONS

Nursing Assessment

For an adequate respiratory assessment, the nurse in both the PACU and the clinical unit settings must evaluate airway patency; chest symmetry; and the depth, rate, and character of respirations. The chest wall should be observed for symmetry of movement with a hand placed lightly over the xiphoid process. Impaired ventilation may initially be detected by the observation of slowed breathing or diminished chest and abdominal movement during the respiratory cycle. It should also be determined whether abdominal or accessory muscles are being used for breathing. Observable use of these muscles may indicate respiratory distress. Breath sounds should be auscultated anteriorly, laterally, and posteriorly. Decreased or absent breath sounds will be detected when airflow is diminished or obstructed. The presence of crackles or wheezes necessitates notification of physician.

Regular monitoring of vital signs and use of pulse oximetry in conjunction with thorough respiratory assessment permit the nurse to recognize early signs of respiratory complications. The presence of hypoxemia from any cause may be reflected by rapid breathing, gasping, apprehension, restlessness, and a rapid or thready pulse.

The characteristics of sputum or mucus should be noted and recorded. Mucus from the trachea and throat is colourless and thin in consistency. Sputum from the lungs and bronchi can be thick with a slight yellow or pink tinge.

Nursing Diagnoses

Nursing diagnoses and collaborative problems related to potential postoperative respiratory complications for the patient in the PACU and clinical unit include, but are not limited to, the following:

- Ineffective airway clearance
- Ineffective breathing pattern
- Impaired gas exchange
- Risk for aspiration
- Potential complication: hypoxemia
- Potential complication: pneumonia
- Potential complication: atelectasis

Nursing Implementation

Postanaesthesia Care Unit

Nursing interventions are designed to both prevent and treat respiratory problems. Proper positioning of the patient to facilitate respirations and protect the airway is essential. Unless contraindicated by the surgical procedure, the unconscious patient is positioned in a lateral "recovery" position (Figure 22-5). This recovery position keeps the airway open and reduces the risk of aspiration if vomiting occurs. Once conscious, the patient is usually returned to a supine position with the head of the bed elevated. This position maximizes expansion of the thorax by decreasing the pressure of the abdominal contents on the diaphragm.

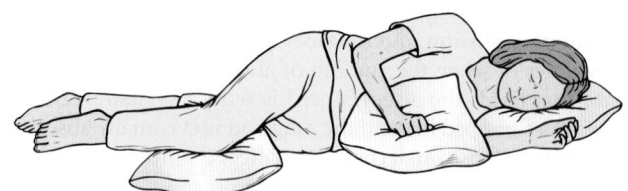

Figure 22-5 Position of patient during recovery from general anaesthesia.

◼ Clinical Unit

Deep breathing is encouraged to facilitate gas exchange and promote the return to consciousness. The patient should be taught to take in slow, deep breaths, ideally through the nose, to hold the breath, and to then slowly exhale. This type of breathing is also useful as a relaxation strategy when the patient is anxious or in pain. Other nursing interventions appropriate for specific respiratory complications are detailed in Table 22-5.

Deep breathing and coughing techniques in the postoperative phase help the patient prevent alveolar collapse and move respiratory secretions to larger airway passages for expectoration. The patient should be assisted to breathe deeply 10 times every hour while awake. The use of an incentive spirometer is helpful in providing visual feedback of respiratory effort (Harton, Grap, Savage, & Elswick, 2007). The nurse should teach the patient to use an incentive spirometer, which involves the following: inhale into the mechanism, hold the ball for about 3 seconds, and then exhale. This procedure should be done 10 to 15 times, and then the nurse should encourage the patient to cough. It is recommended that an incentive spirometer should be used every 2 hours while awake (University of Pittsburgh Medical Center, 2011). Diaphragmatic or abdominal breathing is accomplished by inhaling slowly and deeply through the nose, holding the breath for a few seconds, and then exhaling slowly and completely through the mouth. The patient's hands should be placed lightly over the lower ribs and upper abdomen. This allows the patient to feel the abdomen rise during inspiration and fall during expiration.

Effective coughing is essential in mobilizing secretions (see Chapter 30). If secretions are present in the respiratory passages, deep breathing often will move them up to stimulate the cough reflex without any voluntary effort by the patient, and then they can be expectorated. Splinting an abdominal incision with a pillow or a rolled blanket provides support to the incision and aids in coughing and expectoration of secretions (Figure 22-6).

The patient's position should be changed every 1 to 2 hours to allow full chest expansion and increase perfusion of both lungs. Ambulation, not just sitting in a chair, should be aggressively carried out unless contraindicated by the surgical procedure performed or other concurrent diagnoses. Adequate and regular analgesic medication should be provided because incisional pain often is the greatest deterrent to patient participation in effective ventilation and ambulation. The patient should also be reassured that these activities will not cause the incision to separate. Adequate hydration, either parenteral or oral, is essential to maintain the integrity of mucous membranes and to keep secretions thin and loose for easy expectoration.

Potential Alterations in Cardiovascular Function

Etiology

Postanaesthesia Care Unit. In the immediate postanaesthetic period, the most common cardiovascular complications include hypotension, hypertension, and dysrhythmias. Patients at greatest risk for alterations in cardiovascular function include those with altered respiratory function or a cardiac history, older adults, and debilitated or critically ill patients.

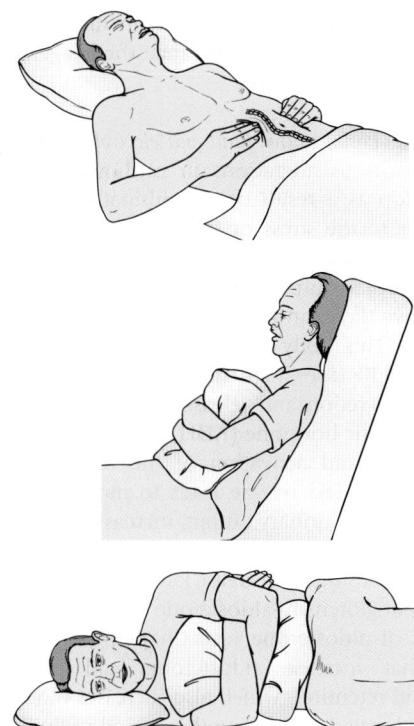

Figure 22-6 Techniques for splinting wound when coughing.

Hypotension is evidenced by signs of hypoperfusion to the vital organs, especially the brain, the heart, and the kidneys. Clinical signs of disorientation, loss of consciousness, chest pain, oliguria, and anuria reflect hypoxemia and the loss of physiological compensation. Intervention must be timely to prevent the devastating complications of cardiac ischemia or infarction, cerebral ischemia, renal ischemia, and bowel infarction.

The most common cause of hypotension in the PACU is unreplaced fluid and blood loss, which may lead to hypovolemic shock. Hemorrhage is always a risk of surgery and can occur internally, requiring assessment for changes in level of consciousness and vital signs. If changes are detected, treatment is directed toward restoring circulating volume. If there is no response to fluid administration, cardiac dysfunction should be presumed to be the cause of hypotension.

Primary cardiac dysfunction, as may occur in the case of myocardial infarction, cardiac tamponade, or pulmonary embolism, results in an acute fall in cardiac output. Secondary myocardial dysfunction occurs as a result of the negative chronotropic (rate-derived) and negative inotropic (force-derived) effects of drugs, such as β-adrenergic blockers, digoxin, or narcotics. Other causes of hypotension include decreased or low systemic vascular resistance and dysrhythmias; measurement errors that may occur if a BP cuff is incorrectly sized may lead to an erroneous finding of hypotension.

Hypertension, a common finding in the PACU, is most frequently the result of sympathetic nervous stimulation that may be the result of pain, anxiety, bladder distension, or respiratory compromise. Hypertension may also be the result of hypothermia or pre-existing hypertension. It may be seen after vascular and cardiac surgery as a result of revascularization.

Dysrhythmias are often the result of an identifiable cause other than myocardial injury. The leading causes include hypokalemia, hypoxemia, hypercarbia, alterations in acid–base status, circulatory instability, and pre-existing heart disease. Hypothermia, pain, surgical stress, and many anaesthetic agents are also capable of causing dysrhythmias.

Clinical Unit.
Postoperative fluid and electrolyte imbalances are contributing factors to alterations in cardiovascular function. They may develop as a result of a combination of the body's normal response to the stress of surgery, excessive fluid losses, and improper IV fluid replacement. The body's fluid status directly affects cardiac output. Fluid retention during the first 2 to 5 postoperative days can be the result of the stress response (see Chapter 8). This body response serves to maintain both blood volume and BP (see Chapter 8, Figure 8-6). Fluid retention results from the secretion and release of two hormones by the pituitary—antidiuretic hormone (ADH) and adrenocorticotropic hormone (ACTH)—and activation of the renin–angiotensin–aldosterone system. ADH release leads to increased H_2O reabsorption and decreased urinary output, increasing blood volume. ACTH stimulates the adrenal cortex to secrete aldosterone. Fluid losses resulting from surgery decrease kidney perfusion, stimulating the renin–angiotensin–aldosterone system and causing marked release of aldosterone (see Chapter 19). Both of the mechanisms that increase aldosterone lead to significant sodium and fluid retention, which also increases blood volume.

Fluid overload may occur during this period of fluid retention when IV fluids are administered too rapidly, when chronic (e.g., cardiac or renal) disease exists, or when the patient is an older adult. Conversely, fluid deficit may be related to slow or inadequate fluid replacement, which leads to decreases in cardiac output and tissue perfusion. Untreated preoperative dehydration or intraoperative or postoperative losses from vomiting, bleeding, wound drainage, or suctioning may be contributing factors to fluid deficits.

Hypokalemia can be a consequence of urinary and gastrointestinal tract losses, and it results when potassium is not replaced in IV fluids. Low serum potassium levels directly affect the contractility of the heart and, thus, may also contribute to decreased cardiac output and overall body tissue perfusion. Adequate replacement of potassium usually entails administration of 40 mEq/d. However, it should not be given until adequate renal function has been established. A urine output of at least 30 mL/hr is generally considered indicative of adequate renal function.

Cardiovascular status is also affected by the state of tissue perfusion or blood flow. The stress response contributes to an increase in clotting tendencies in the postoperative patient by increasing platelet production. *Deep venous thrombosis* (DVT) may form in leg veins as a result of inactivity, body position, and pressure, all of which lead to venous stasis and decreased perfusion. DVT, especially common in older adults and obese or immobilized individuals, is a potentially life-threatening complication because it may lead to pulmonary embolism. Patients with a history of DVT have a greater risk for pulmonary embolism. Pulmonary embolism should be suspected in any patient complaining of tachypnea, dyspnea, and tachycardia, particularly when the patient is already receiving oxygen therapy. Manifestations may include chest pain, hypotension, hemoptysis, dysrhythmias, or heart failure. Definitive diagnosis requires pulmonary angiography. Superficial thrombophlebitis is an uncomfortable but less ominous complication that may develop in a leg vein as a result of venous stasis or in the arm veins as a result of irritation from IV catheters or solutions. If a piece of a clot becomes dislodged and travels to the lung, it can cause a pulmonary infarction of a size proportionate to the vessel in which it lodges.

Syncope (fainting) is another factor that reflects the cardiovascular status. It may indicate decreased cardiac output, fluid deficits, or defects in cerebral perfusion. Syncope frequently occurs as a result of orthostatic hypotension, a fall in BP when the patient sits or stands. It results from peripheral dilation in which blood leaves the central body organs, most notably the brain, and moves to the periphery, causing the person to feel faint. Assess for orthostatic hypotension by following these steps (Kozier et al., 2010, p. 688):

- Place the patient in the supine position for 5 minutes to allow BP and pulse to stabilize.
- Record the patient's pulse and BP.
- Assist the patient to sit or stand and support him or her in case of faintness.
- After 1 to 3 minutes in the upright position, recheck the pulse and BP.
- Record the results—if the pulse rate increases by 20 beats per minute (bpm) or there is a decrease in systolic or diastolic BP of over 10 mm Hg, it is indicative of orthostatic hypotension.

NURSING MANAGEMENT: CARDIOVASCULAR PROBLEMS

Nursing Assessment

The most important aspect of the cardiovascular assessment is frequent monitoring of vital signs. They are usually monitored every 15 minutes or more often until they stabilize, and then at less frequent intervals. Postoperative vital signs should be compared with preoperative and intraoperative readings to determine when the signs are stabilizing at a normal level for the patient's condition. The anaesthesiologist or surgeon should be notified if the following occur:

1. Systolic BP is less than 90 mm Hg or greater than 160 mm Hg.
2. Pulse rate is less than 60 bpm or greater than 120 bpm.
3. Pulse pressure (difference between systolic and diastolic pressures) narrows.
4. BP gradually decreases during several consecutive readings.
5. An irregular cardiac rhythm develops.
6. There is a significant variation from preoperative readings.

Cardiac monitoring is recommended for patients who have a history of cardiac disease and for all older adult patients who have undergone major surgery, regardless of whether they have cardiac problems. The apical–radial pulse should be assessed carefully, and any irregularities should be reported.

Assessment of skin colour, temperature, and moisture provides valuable information for detecting cardiovascular problems. Hypotension accompanied by a normal pulse and warm, dry, pink skin usually represents the residual vasodilating effects of anaesthesia and suggests only a need for continued observation. Hypotension accompanied by a rapid pulse and cold, clammy, pale skin may be caused by impending hypovolemic shock and necessitates immediate treatment.

Specific assessment of cardiovascular function includes the regular monitoring of the patient's BP, heart rate, pulse, and skin temperature and colour. Peripheral circulation, dressing, and drains should also be assessed. Results should be compared with the preoperative status and the immediate postoperative and intraoperative findings.

Nursing Diagnoses

Nursing diagnoses and collaborative problems related to potential cardiovascular complications for the patient in the PACU and the clinical unit include, but are not limited to, the following:

- Decreased cardiac output
- Deficient fluid volume
- Excess fluid volume
- Ineffective peripheral tissue perfusion
- Activity intolerance
- Potential complication: hypovolemic shock
- Potential complication: venous thromboembolism

Nursing Implementation

Postanaesthesia Care Unit

Nursing interventions in the PACU are designed to prevent and treat cardiovascular complications. Treatment of hypotension should always begin with oxygen therapy to promote oxygenation of hypoperfused organs. Volume status should be assessed as described, and errors of BP measurement should be ruled out. Because the most common cause of hypotension is fluid loss, IV fluid boluses will be given to normalize BP. Primary cardiac dysfunction may necessitate drug intervention. Peripheral vasodilation and hypotension may necessitate administration of vasoconstrictive agents to normalize systemic vascular resistance.

Treatment of hypertension will centre on addressing the cause of sympathetic nervous system stimulation and eliminating the precipitating cause. Treatment may include the use of analgesics, assistance in voiding, and correction of respiratory problems. Rewarming will correct hypothermia-induced hypertension. If the patient has pre-existing hypertension or has undergone cardiac or vascular surgery, drug therapy designed to reduce BP will usually be required.

Because the majority of dysrhythmias seen in the PACU have identifiable causes, treatment is directed toward eliminating the cause. Correction of these physiological alterations will, in most instances, correct the dysrhythmias. In the event of life-threatening dysrhythmias, protocols of advanced cardiac life support will be applied (see Chapter 38).

Clinical Unit

An accurate intake and output record should be kept during the postoperative period, and laboratory findings (e.g., electrolytes, hematocrit) should be monitored. Nursing responsibilities relating to IV management are critical during this period. In particular, the nurse should be alert for symptoms of too slow or too rapid a rate of fluid replacement. Assessment should also be made of the infusion site for discomfort and the hazards associated with the *IV administration of potassium*, such as *cardiac arrest* and pain in the area of the vein where it is entering (Cornish, Hyland, & Koczmara, 2006). Thirst is one of the most annoying discomforts of postoperative patients. This may be related to the drying effects of anticholinergic drugs, anaesthetic gases, and fluid deficits. Adequate and regular mouth care is helpful while the patient cannot ingest food or drink by mouth.

Patients should alternatively flex and extend all joints 10 to 12 times every 1 to 2 hours while awake. The muscular contraction produced by these exercises and by ambulation facilitates

venous return from the lower extremities. The ambulating patient should pick up the feet rather than shuffling them so that muscular contraction is maximized. When confined to bed, the patient should alternately flex and extend the legs. When the patient is sitting in a chair or lying in bed, there should be no pressure to impede venous flow through the popliteal space. Crossed legs, pillows behind the knees, and extreme elevation of the knee gatch must be avoided.

Some surgeons routinely prescribe use of elastic stockings or mechanical aids such as sequential compressive devices to stimulate and enhance the massaging and milking actions that are transmitted to the veins when leg muscles contract. The nurse must remember that these aids are useless if the legs are not exercised and may actually impair circulation if the legs remain inactive or if the devices are sized or applied improperly. When in use, elastic stockings must be removed and reapplied at least twice daily for skin care and inspection. The skin of the heels and post-tibial areas is particularly susceptible to increased pressure and breakdown (MacLellan & Fletcher, 2007). The use of unfractionated heparin or low–molecular weight heparin is a prophylactic measure for venous thrombosis and pulmonary embolism (Graber, Dachs, & Darby-Stewart, 2008; Rocha, Imberti, & Paschina, 2007). Advantages of low–molecular weight heparin over unfractionated heparin include (1) less major bleeding, (2) decreased incidence of thrombocytopenia, (3) better absorption, (4) longer duration of action, (5) as effective or more effective, and (6) no laboratory monitoring required (Geerts et al., 2008; Janjigian & Muhs, 2008).

Before the patient may ambulate, the nurse can first raise the head of the patient's bed for 1 to 2 minutes and then assist the patient to sit on the side of the bed while monitoring the radial pulse for rate and quality. If no changes or complaints are noted, ambulation can be started. Nurses should use transfer belts or have adequate personnel to assist ambulation if the patient is unsteady or unable to transfer herself or himself. If the patient complains of feeling faint during ambulation, the nurse should provide assistance to ease the patient to a supine position until recovery is evidenced by BP stability. If faintness occurs, it is often frightening for the patient but poses no real physiological danger, although injury can result from a fall.

Potential Alterations in Neurological Function

Etiology

Postanaesthesia Care Unit. After surgery in the PACU, emergence delirium remains the neurological alteration that causes the most concern to the practitioner. **Emergence delirium** can include behaviours such as restlessness, agitation, disorientation, thrashing, and shouting. This condition may be caused by anaesthetic agents, hypoxia, bladder distension, pain, electrolyte abnormalities, presence of an endotracheal tube, or the patient's state of anxiety before surgery. Nurses may be able to affect the patient's recovery by using interventions to decrease anxiety. If delirium occurs, the nurse should first suspect hypoxia.

Delayed awakening may also be a problem after surgery. Fortunately, the most common cause of delayed awakening is prolonged drug action, particularly of narcotics, sedatives, and inhalational anaesthetics, as opposed to neurological injury. Normally, awakening can be predicted by the anaesthesiologist based on the drugs used in surgery.

NURSING MANAGEMENT: NEUROLOGICAL COMPLICATIONS

▪ Nursing Assessment

The patient's level of consciousness, orientation, and ability to follow commands should be assessed. The size, reactivity, and equality of the pupils should be determined. The patient's sensory and motor status should be noted. If the patient had a regional anaesthetic, the level of anaesthetic effect should also be determined by assessing the level of numbness and number of dermatomes blocked. If the neurological status is altered, possible causes should be determined.

▪ Nursing Diagnoses

Nursing diagnoses related to potential neurological complications for the patient in the PACU and the clinical unit include, but are not limited to, the following:
- Disturbed sensory perception
- Risk for injury
- Disturbed thought processes
- Impaired verbal communication

▪ Nursing Implementation

▪ Postanaesthesia Care Unit

The most common cause of postoperative agitation is hypoxemia, so the nurse needs to evaluate respiratory function. Once hypoxemia has been ruled out and all potentially known causes have been addressed, sedation may prove beneficial in controlling the agitation and provide patient and staff safety. Emergence delirium is usually time limited and will resolve before the patient is discharged from the PACU. Delays in awakening usually resolve spontaneously with time. If necessary, benzodiazepines and narcotics may be pharmacologically reversed with antagonists.

Until the patient is awake and able to communicate effectively, it will be the responsibility of the PACU nurse to act as a patient advocate and to maintain patient safety at all times. Measures to accomplish this include having the side rails up, securing IV lines and artificial airways, verifying the presence of identification and allergy bands, and monitoring physiological status.

▪ Clinical Unit

On the postoperative unit, the nurse prevents or manages postoperative delirium by maintaining fluid and electrolyte balance, ensuring adequate nutrition and sleep, providing pain management, ensuring proper bowel and bladder function, and aiding early mobilization. Specific aids, such as clocks, calendars, and photographs, help orient the patient.

Psychological problems in the postoperative period can be limited by providing adequate support for the patient such as listening to and talking with him or her, explaining, reassuring, and encouraging caregiver presence.

Some common alterations in neurological function seen on the clinical unit may be related to medications for pain management, sleep deprivation, or sensory overload. It is important for the nurse to complete a central nervous system assessment for all patients who have undergone surgery. The nurse must ensure that patients who are receiving pain medication are responsive and oriented to person, place, and time; sensation and motor function must also be assessed in any patient who has received a spinal or epidural anaesthetic. An ice pack may be used to check a patient's motor block as the effects of the spinal anaesthetic are resolving.

Pain and Discomfort

Etiology

Postanaesthesia Care Unit. Despite the availability of analgesic drugs and pain-relieving techniques, pain remains a common problem and a significant fear for the patient in the PACU and during the postoperative period. Pain may be the result of surgical manipulation, positioning, or the presence of internal devices such as an endotracheal tube or catheter, or it may occur as the patient begins to mobilize after surgery. Pain is a common reason for a prolonged stay in the PACU (Mackintosh, 2007).

Clinical Unit. On the surgical unit, postoperative pain is caused by the interaction of a number of physiological and psychological factors. Skin and underlying tissues have been traumatized by the incision and retraction during surgery (Hutchison, 2007), and there may be reflex muscle spasms around the incision. Anxiety and fear, sometimes related to the anticipation of pain, create tension and further increase muscle tone and spasm. The effort and movement associated with deep breathing, coughing, and changing position may aggravate pain by creating tension or pull on the incisional area.

When the internal viscera are cut, no pain is felt. However, pressure in the internal viscera elicits pain. Therefore, deep visceral pain may signal the presence of a complication such as intestinal distension, bleeding, or abscess formation.

NURSING MANAGEMENT: PAIN

▪ Nursing Assessment

▪ Postanaesthesia Care Unit

Pain assessment may be difficult in the PACU and in the early postoperative period on the clinical unit. The patient may not be able to verbalize the presence or severity of pain. The nurse should observe for behavioural clues of pain such as a wrinkling face or brow, a clenched fist, moaning, diaphoresis, or an increased pulse rate.

▪ Clinical Unit

Postoperative pain is usually most severe within the first 48 hours and subsides thereafter. Variation is considerable, according to the procedure performed and the patient's individual pain tolerance or perception (Lauzon Clabo, 2008). The patient should be observed for indications of pain (e.g., restlessness) and questioned about the degree and characteristics of the pain. Identifying the location of the pain is important. It is also important that the nurse assess the effectiveness of all pain control (e.g., epidural catheters, patient-controlled analgesia [PCA]). Incisional pain is to be expected, but other causes of pain, such as a full bladder, may also be present. All patients must be assessed for pain using one of the following rating scales: verbal descriptor, numeric rating, or visual analogue (Flaherty, 2008). (See Chapter 10 for a more detailed discussion of pain assessment.)

Nursing Diagnoses

Nursing diagnoses for the patient experiencing pain and discomfort in the PACU and clinical unit include, but are not limited to, the following:

- Acute pain
- Anxiety

Nursing Implementation

Postanaesthesia Care Unit

The most effective interventions for pain include both pharmacological and nonpharmacological approaches (Chaturvedi & Chaturvedi, 2007). IV narcotics provide the most rapid relief. Drugs are administered slowly and titrated to allow for optimal pain management with minimal to no adverse drug effects. More sustained relief may be obtained through the use of epidural catheters, PCA, or regional anaesthetic blockade. Comfort measures, including touch, reuniting the patient and family, and rewarming, also contribute to patient comfort.

Pain management is most likely to be successful if the treatment plan is initiated with involvement of the patient, the anaesthesiologists, and the PACU nurse. The goals should be to determine the most effective therapy, drug, and dose and the best response to therapy. Once the patient is discharged from the PACU to an inpatient unit, the nurse will replace the PACU nurse as a member of the pain management team. (For more information on nursing assessment and management of patients in pain, see Chapter 10.)

Clinical Unit

On the surgical unit, postoperative pain relief is a nursing responsibility because the surgeon's orders for analgesic medication and other comfort measures are usually written on an as-needed basis. During the first 48 hours or longer, narcotic analgesics (e.g., morphine) are required to relieve moderate to severe pain. After that time, non-narcotic analgesics, such as nonsteroidal anti-inflammatory agents, may be sufficient as pain intensity decreases.

Effective pain management will reduce harmful complications and promote optimal healing, prevent complications, and allow patients to participate in necessary activities (Rothrock, 2011). Administration of analgesic medication should be timed to ensure that it is in effect during activities that may be painful for the patient, such as ambulating. Although narcotic analgesics are often essential for the postoperative patient's comfort, there are adverse effects. Constipation, nausea and vomiting, respiratory depression, and hypotension are the most common adverse effects of opioids. Before administering any analgesic, the nurse should first assess the nature of the patient's pain, including location, quality, and intensity. If it is incisional pain, analgesic

administration is appropriate. If it is chest or leg pain, medication may simply mask a complication that must be reported and documented. If it is gas pain, narcotic medication can aggravate it. The nurse should notify the physician and request a change in the order if the analgesic either fails to relieve the pain or makes the patient excessively lethargic or somnolent.

Patient-controlled analgesia (PCA) and epidural analgesia are two alternative approaches for pain control. The goals of PCA are to provide immediate analgesia and to maintain a constant, steady blood level of the analgesic agent. PCA involves self-administration of predetermined doses of analgesia by the patient (Rothrock, 2011; Viscusi, 2008). The route of delivery may be IV, oral, or epidural. (PCA is discussed in Chapter 10.)

Epidural analgesia is the infusion of pain-relieving medications through a catheter placed into the epidural space surrounding the spinal cord. The goal of epidural analgesia is delivery of medication directly to opiate receptors in the spinal cord. The administration may be intermittent or constant and is monitored by the nurse. Epidural analgesia may also be controlled by the patient (Viscusi, 2008). The overall effectiveness and the technique of administration result in a constant circulating level and a total reduced dose of medication.

Potential Alterations in Temperature

Etiology

Postanaesthesia Care Unit. Hypothermia, a core temperature of less than 36°C, occurs when heat loss exceeds heat production (American Society of PeriAnesthesia Nurses [ASPAN], 2009). Hypothermia may be the result of loss of heat from a warm body to a cold OR or loss of heat from exposed body organs to the air.

Although all patients are at risk for hypothermia, those especially vulnerable are the elderly, children younger than 2 years—especially neonates—and burn patients (Rothrock, 2011, p. 276). Long surgical procedures and prolonged general anaesthesia place the patient at an increased risk for hypothermia. Complications from hypothermia may include increased likelihood of surgical site infection, bleeding, and morbid cardiac incidences (Ledrick, Caudell, & Bowman, 2008; Rothrock, 2011; Weirich, 2008).

In the PACU, temperature may be taken orally or via the tympanic membrane or the axilla. The colour and approximate temperature of the skin should also be assessed.

Active rewarming of hypothermic patients involves the application of external warming devices, including warm blankets, heated aerosols, radiant warmers, forced air warmers, and heated water mattresses. When using any external warming device, body temperature should be monitored at 30-minute intervals, and care should be taken to prevent skin injuries. Oxygen therapy via nasal prongs or mask is used to treat the increased demand for oxygen accompanying the increase in body temperature. Shivering is usually quickly suppressed by opioids.

Clinical Unit. Temperature variation in the postoperative period provides valuable information about the patient's status. Fever may occur at any time during the postoperative period (Table 22-6). A mild elevation (≤38°C) during the first 48 hours usually reflects the surgical stress response. A moderate elevation (>38°C) is caused more frequently by respiratory congestion or

Table 22-6 Significance of Postoperative Temperature Changes		
TIME AFTER SURGERY	**TEMPERATURE**	**POSSIBLE CAUSES**
≤12 hr	Hypothermia to 36°C	Effects of anaesthesia
		Body heat loss in surgical exposure
First 24-48 hr	Elevation to 38°C	Inflammatory response to surgical stress
	>38°C	Lung congestion, atelectasis
Third day and later	Elevation above 37.7°C	Wound infection
		Urinary infection
		Respiratory infection
		Phlebitis

Table 22-7 Postoperative Diets
Clear Fluids
Broth, gelatin, water, tea, black coffee
Fluids
Milk, coffee with cream, cream soups
Soft Diet
Fish, cottage cheese, pasta, eggs, mousse, pudding
Full Diet
Regular diets
Patients can also be placed on special diets, such as diabetic or low sodium.

atelectasis and less frequently by dehydration. After the first 48 hours, a moderate to marked elevation (>37.7°C) is usually caused by infection.

NURSING MANAGEMENT: POTENTIAL TEMPERATURE COMPLICATIONS

▪ Nursing Assessment

Frequent assessment of the patient's temperature in the days after surgery is important to detect patterns of hypothermia or fever that may be present in the postoperative period. The nurse should observe the patient for early signs of inflammation and infection so that any complications that arise may be treated in a timely manner. Infections may include:

- Wound
- Respiratory tract
- Urinary tract (secondary to catheterization)
- IV site superficial thrombophlebitis (temperature elevation between 7 and 10 days after surgery)
- Hospital-associated diarrhea caused by *Clostridium difficile*
- Septicemia (microorganisms enter bloodstream during surgery especially in gastrointestinal or genitourinary procedures)

▪ Nursing Diagnoses

Nursing diagnoses related to potential postoperative temperature complications may include, but are not limited to, the following:

- Hypothermia
- Risk for imbalanced body temperature
- Hyperthermia

▪ Nursing Implementation

▪ Postanaesthesia Care Unit

Passive rewarming (i.e., shivering) raises basal heat metabolism. Active rewarming requires the application of external warming devices and may include use of warm blankets, heated aerosols, radiant warmers, forced-air warmers, or heated water mattresses (Cooper, 2006). When using any external warming device, body temperature should be monitored at 15-minute intervals, and care should be taken to prevent skin injuries. The nurse should also pay close attention to the patient with an increase in temperature, especially for symptoms of malignant hyperthermia because symptoms may not be evident until the postoperative phase. (See the discussion of malignant hyperthermia in Chapter 21). In addition, oxygen therapy via nasal prongs or mask is used to treat the increased demand for oxygen accompanying the increase in body temperature. (See Chapter 71 for additional management of hypothermia.)

▪ Clinical Unit

The nurse's role with respect to postoperative fever may be preventive, diagnostic, therapeutic, or some combination. The patient's temperature is usually measured every 4 hours for the first 48 hours after surgery and then less frequently if no problems develop. Meticulous care is maintained with regard to the wound and the IV site, and airway clearance is encouraged. If fever develops, chest radiographs may be done, and depending on the suspected cause, cultures of the wound, urine, or blood are obtained. If infection is the source of the fever, antibiotics are started as soon as cultures have been obtained. If the fever rises above 39.4°C, antipyretic drugs and body-cooling measures may be employed.

Potential Gastrointestinal Problems

Etiology

Postanaesthesia Care Unit. Nausea and vomiting are significant problems in the immediate postoperative period. These problems are responsible for unanticipated hospital admission of day-surgery patients, increased patient discomfort, delays in discharge, and patient dissatisfaction with the surgical experience.

Clinical Unit. Slowed gastrointestinal motility and altered patterns of food intake may lead to the development of several distressing postoperative symptoms that are most pronounced after abdominal surgery. Nausea and vomiting may be caused by the action of anaesthetics or narcotics, delayed gastric emptying, slowed peristalsis resulting from the handling of the bowel during surgery, and resumption of oral intake too soon after surgery (Table 22-7).

NURSING MANAGEMENT: GASTROINTESTINAL PROBLEMS

Nursing Assessment

Nausea and Vomiting

Postoperative nausea and vomiting (PONV) occurs because of stimuli from organs and tissues traumatized during surgery that are carried by afferent neurons of the vagus nerve to the emetic center in the brain. Nurses must be aware that there are patients who are predisposed to this complication:

- Pediatric patients ages 6 to 14 years
- Female patients
- Patients with motion sickness
- Nonsmokers
- Anxious patients

Types of surgical interventions that also predispose patients to PONV include breast, eyes, ears, nose and throat, cranial, gynecological and abdominal scopes, and laparotomy (Mathias, 2008).

Any procedure longer than 45 to 60 minutes duration can also lead to PONV.

Preventive measures include the administration of antiemetics such as ondansetron (Zofran) before emergence of anaesthesia (Macksey, 2010, p. 73). After surgery, the nurse should question the patient about feelings of nausea and administer antiemetics as ordered. If vomiting occurs, it is important to determine and document the quantity and the characteristics (including colour) of the emesis.

Ileus

Postoperative Ileus.
Fifty percent of patients who have bowel surgery experience postoperative ileus (POI), a transient cessation of bowel motility that prevents effective passage of intestinal contents and may affect the patient's tolerance of oral intake. Most cases of POI resolve spontaneously within 2 to 3 days with supportive treatment (Mukherjee et al., 2011). Recent studies suggest that starting a clear-liquid diet for some types of POI and initiating early ambulation and pharmacological interventions such as μ-opioid antagonists before and after surgery and bisacodyl (Dulcolax) suppositories in the early postoperative phase may decrease the duration of the ileus (Zeinali, Stulberg, & Delaney, 2009). Patients who experience vomiting should receive IV therapy. Abdominal distension may require insertion of a nasogastric tube for symptomatic relief; however, this practice is now known to increase the length of time to resolve POI (Zeinali et al., 2009).

Paralytic Ileus.
Ileus that persists for more than 3 days after surgery is called **paralytic ileus**. Peristalsis stops and the patient complains of abdominal pain, distension, nausea, vomiting, and poor appetite. Nursing care on the postoperative unit consists of monitoring for abdominal distension by measuring the patient's abdominal girth. The abdomen should be auscultated in all four quadrants to determine presence, frequency, and characteristics of the bowel sounds. Bowel sounds are frequently absent or diminished, and the abdomen will sound tympanic to percussion. The return of normal bowel sounds and motility is usually accompanied by the passage of flatus. When paralytic ileus does not resolve spontaneously, the patient may require diagnostic tests to rule out mechanical blockage that would require surgical intervention.

Nursing Diagnoses

Nursing diagnoses and collaborative problems related to potential gastrointestinal complications in the PACU and clinical unit may include, but are not limited to, the following:

- Nausea
- Risk for aspiration
- Risk for deficient fluid volume
- Imbalanced nutrition: less than body requirements
- Potential complication: fluid and electrolyte imbalance
- Potential complication: hiccups

Nursing Implementation

Postanaesthesia Care Unit

Intervention for *nausea and vomiting* is primarily the use of antiemetic or prokinetic drugs (see Chapter 44). In the PACU, oral fluids should be given only as indicated and tolerated. IV fluids will provide hydration until the patient is able to tolerate oral fluids. Care should also be taken to prevent aspiration if the patient vomits while still sleepy from anaesthesia. Having suction equipment readily available at the bedside and positioning the patient in the lateral recovery position will help protect the patient from aspiration (see Figure 22-4). Other interventions that may be effective include placing the patient in the upright position; slow, deep breathing; mouth care; distraction; and emotional support.

Clinical Unit

Depending on the nature of the surgery, the patient may resume oral intake as soon as the gag reflex returns. While the patient is on nothing by mouth status, IV infusions are given to maintain fluid and electrolyte balance. When oral intake is allowed, clear liquids are started and the IV infusion is continued, usually at a reduced rate. If oral intake is well tolerated by the patient, the IV is discontinued and the diet is advanced until a regular diet is tolerated.

The nurse should assess the patient regularly to detect the resumption of normal intestinal peristalsis as evidenced by the return of bowel sounds and the passage of flatus. The patient may need to be encouraged to expel flatus and reassured that expulsion is necessary and desirable. Gas pains, which tend to become pronounced on the second or third postoperative day, may be relieved by ambulation and frequent repositioning. Positioning the patient on the right side permits gas to rise along the transverse colon and facilitates its release. Resumption of a normal diet after bowel sounds have returned will also enhance the return of normal peristalsis. If the patient does not improve with conservative measures, she or he will be reassessed and may require additional surgery. **Hiccups** (singultus) are intermittent spasms of the diaphragm caused by irritation of the phrenic nerve, which innervates the diaphragm. Postoperative sources of direct irritation of the phrenic nerve may be gastric distension, intestinal obstruction, intra-abdominal bleeding, or a subphrenic abscess. Indirect irritation of the phrenic nerve may be produced by acid–base or electrolyte imbalances. Reflex irritation may come from drinking hot or cold liquids or from the presence of a nasogastric tube. Hiccups usually last a short time and subside spontaneously; occasionally, they may be persistent but are rarely debilitating.

Potential Alterations in Urinary Function

Etiology

Low Urine Output. *Postoperative oliguria* refers to a decrease in urine output (<500 mL/d) (Kozier et al., 2010) in the first 24 hours after a major operation regardless of fluid intake. This low output is caused by increased aldosterone and antidiuretic hormone secretion resulting from the stress of surgery, fluid restriction before surgery, and loss of fluids during surgery, drainage, and diaphoresis. By the second or third day, after fluid has been mobilized and the immediate stress reaction subsides, the patient will begin to have increasing urinary output that returns to the normal level of 0.5 to 1 mL/kg/hr (~60 mL/hr). Persistent oliguria can indicate inadequate renal perfusion and pending renal failure. Restoring renal blood flow and urine production can prevent renal failure.

Acute urinary retention can occur in the postoperative period for a variety of reasons. Surgery on the urinary tract can cause swelling, and bleeding may result in pink- or red-tinged urine. Anaesthesia depresses the nervous system, allowing the bladder to fill more completely than normal before the urge to void is felt. Spinal anaesthesia can impede voluntary voiding because it decreases the patient's awareness of the need to void. Anticholinergic, antispasmodic, and narcotic drugs are a few examples of medications that may interfere with the ability to initiate voiding or to empty the bladder completely.

Retention is more likely to occur after lower abdominal or pelvic surgery, because spasms or guarding of the abdominal and pelvic muscles interferes with their normal function in micturition. Pain may alter perception and interfere with the patient's awareness of the less intense sensation arising as the bladder fills. Voiding ability is probably impaired to the greatest extent by immobility and the recumbent position in bed. Lack of skeletal muscle activity decreases smooth muscle (bladder detrusor) tone, and the supine position reduces the ability to relax the perineal muscles and the external sphincter.

NURSING MANAGEMENT: POTENTIAL URINARY PROBLEMS

Nursing Assessment

The urine of the patient after surgery should be examined for both quantity and quality. The colour, amount, consistency, and odour of the urine should be noted. Indwelling catheters should be assessed for patency, and urine output should be approximately 60 mL/hr. Most people urinate approximately 200 mL of urine within 6 to 8 hours after surgery. If no voiding occurs, the abdominal contour should be inspected and the bladder palpated and percussed for distension. In some institutions, bladder scanners are used to detect bladder volumes. Urinary testing may

be ordered on the postoperative unit primarily to determine kidney function or infections (Kozier et al., 2010). Nurses may be required to do testing for:

- Specific gravity
- Urinary pH
- Ketones
- Protein
- Occult blood
- Creatinine clearance test
- Urine cultures

Nursing Diagnoses

Nursing diagnoses and collaborative problems related to potential urinary complications for the patient after surgery include, but are not limited to, the following:

- Impaired urinary elimination
- Potential complication: acute urinary retention

Nursing Implementation

The nurse may facilitate voiding by normal positioning of the patient—sitting for women and standing for men. Providing reassurance to the patient regarding the ability to void and the use of techniques such as running water, drinking water, or pouring warm water over the perineum may also be of assistance. Ambulation, preferably to the bathroom, and the use of a bedside commode are additional helpful measures to promote voiding.

The surgeon often leaves an order to catheterize the patient in 8 to 12 hours if voiding has not occurred. The nurse should first try other measures to induce voiding. In assessing the need for catheterization, the nurse should consider fluid intake during and after surgery and determine bladder fullness (e.g., palpable fullness above the symphysis pubis, discomfort when pressure is applied over the bladder, the presence of the urge to void). Urinary tract infections are the most common complication associated with urinary catheterization, so nurses should be sure patients are catheterized only when absolutely necessary, proper aseptic protocol is followed when performing the catheterization, and the catheter is removed as soon as it is no longer required (Kozier et al., 2010).

Potential Alterations in the Integument

Etiology

Surgery generally involves an incision through the skin and underlying tissues. An incision disrupts the protective skin barrier; therefore, wound healing is one of the major concerns during the postoperative period (Mazaris, Varkarakis, & Jarrett, 2007). With information on wound management doubling every 12 to 18 months, nurses must remain current in new trends (Canadian Association of Wound Care and Canadian Association for Enterostomal Therapy, n.d.).

An adequate nutritional state is essential for wound healing. Amino acids are readily available for the healing process because of the catabolic effects of the stress-related hormones (e.g., cortisol). The patient who maintains adequate oxygenation and is well nourished before surgery can tolerate the postoperative delay in nutritional intake for several days. The patient with at least one co-morbidity, such as hypertension, diabetes, cardiovascular disease, and neurological disorders, is more prone to problems of wound healing. Incidence of wound sepsis is higher in patients who are malnourished, immunosuppressed, or older or who have had a prolonged hospital stay or a lengthy surgical procedure lasting more than 3 hours.

Surgical site infections (SSIs) occur within 30 days after surgery or within 1 year of implant surgery. They are characterized by a combination of purulent discharge; the isolation of organisms, most commonly *Staphylococcus aureus* (Roy, Brull, & Eichhorn, 2011); a reopening incision; and physician or radiological diagnosis. SSIs are a common adverse hospital event that increases length of hospital stay, mortality, and readmission rate for treatment (Attrell & Armstrong, 2007).

SSI manifestations include local redness, swelling, and increasing pain and tenderness at the site. Systemic manifestations are fever and leukocytosis. Owing to the fact that evidence of wound infection often becomes apparent after discharge from hospital, frequently community nurses are responsible for wound care in the home. A Canadian study found that surgical wounds accounted for 31% to 38% of all wounds being managed in the community (Hurd, Zuiliani, & Posnett, 2008). Wounds are a significant, costly, and preventable barrier to the successful recovery from routine surgical interventions (Health Service Executive, 2009). Box 22-1 provides guidelines for the prevention of SSIs. Wound healing and complications are discussed in Chapter 14.

NURSING MANAGEMENT: SURGICAL WOUNDS

▪ Nursing Assessment

Nursing assessment of the wound and dressing requires knowledge of the type of wound, drains inserted, and expected drainage related to the specific type of surgery (Rothrock, 2011).

Assessment includes (Kozier et al., 2010, p. 1046):
- *Appearance:* Colour of wound, bruising, redness, approximation of the incision.
- *Size:* Note the general size and shape of the wound and any signs of the wound opening (i.e., dehiscence or evisceration).
- *Drainage:* Check the dressing for colour, odour, and amount of drainage on the dressing.
- *Edema:* Excessive swelling may be indicative of wound complications.
- *Pain:* Moderate incisional pain is expected up to 5 days after surgery, but sudden onset or persistent severe pain may indicate infection or hemorrhage.
- *Drains:* Note the placement and security of the drain or tube. Check the collection device; empty as required and document.

A small amount of serous or drainage is common from any type of wound. Drainage is expected to change from sanguineous (red) to serosanguineous (pink) to serous (clear yellow). Purulent drainage indicates an SSI. The drainage output should decrease over hours or days, depending on the type of surgery. **Wound dehiscence** (separation and disruption of previously joined wound edges) may be preceded by a sudden discharge of brown, pink, or clear drainage. **Wound evisceration** (protrusion of the visceral organs though a wound opening) can also occur after surgery and

is considered a medical emergency. If evisceration occurs, place sterile saline-soaked towels over any extruding tissue, keep the patient on nothing by mouth status, observe the patient for signs and symptoms of shock, and call the surgeon immediately.

▪ Nursing Diagnoses

Nursing diagnoses related to surgical wounds of the patient after surgery include, but are not limited to, the following:
- Risk for infection
- Potential complication: impaired wound healing

▪ Nursing Implementation

When drainage occurs on the dressing, the type, amount, colour, consistency, and odour of drainage should be noted and recorded. Expected drainage from tubes is outlined in Table 22-8. The effect of position changes on drainage should also be assessed. The surgeon should be notified of any excessive or abnormal drainage and significant changes in vital signs.

Immediately after surgery, the incision may be initially covered with a dressing. Surgical wound dressings are left dry and untouched for a minimum of 48 hours after surgery. This permits re-establishment of the protective, natural bacteria-proof barrier. Dressing changes are done by the nurse according to agency policy. Wound healing and care are discussed in Chapter 14.

Potential Alterations in Psychological Function

Etiology

Anxiety and depression may occur in the postoperative patient. These states may be more pronounced in the patient who has had radical surgery (e.g., colostomy) or amputation or whose findings suggest a poor prognosis (e.g., inoperable tumour). A history of a neurotic or psychotic disorder should alert the nurse to the possibility of postoperative anxiety and depression. However, these responses may develop in any patient as part of the grief response to loss of a body organ or disturbance in body image and may be exacerbated by a lowered response to stress. The patient who lives alone or requires rehabilitation after surgery may also develop anxiety and depression when faced with the need for assistance after surgery until strength and independence can be regained. The discharge nurse may refer a patient to home care before discharge if the nurse ascertains that the patient may need assistance after returning home.

In caring for the older adult, nurses in Canada must be cognizant of the increasing incidence in delirium, dementia, and depression in the elder population. Nurses must possess the knowledge and skills to screen and differentiate between these conditions that can have overlapping clinical features (Registered Nurses' Association of Ontario [RNAO], 2010).

After surgery, confusion or delirium may arise from physiological sources including fluid and electrolyte imbalances, hypoxemia, drug effects, sleep deprivation, and sensory alteration, deprivation, or overload.

Delirium tremens may also occur after surgery as a result of alcohol withdrawal. Delirium tremens is a reaction characterized

BOX 22-1 Guidelines for Prevention of Surgical Site Infections

Surgical site infections (SSIs) account for 14 to 16% of all hospital-acquired infections. An understanding of the Centers for Disease Control and Prevention guideline ranking system enables nurses to weigh factors that are viewed as effective in preventing SSIs. Category I rankings (including IA and IB) are applicable to all settings and should be adopted. Subcategories A and B differ only in the strength of supporting research and evidence. Category II rankings are supported by less research and evidence. They may be appropriate for addressing specific situations or patient populations. The Unresolved category offers no recommendation for some practices, either because little research is available to support their effectiveness or because there is no consensus regarding their efficacy. That category is not addressed here.

Rankings

Category	Supporting Research and Evidence
IA	Strongly recommended for implementation and supported by well-designed experimental, clinical, or epidemiological studies
IB	Strongly recommended for implementation and supported by some experimental, clinical, or epidemiological studies and strong theoretic rationale
II	Suggested for implementation and supported by suggestive clinical or epidemiological studies or theoretical rationale

Recommendations

Preoperative—partial and modified

Preparation of the Patient

Category IA

- When possible, identify and treat infections remote to the surgical site before elective operation; postpone surgery until resolved. Do not remove hair from operative site unless necessary to facilitate surgery. If hair is removed, do immediately before surgery, preferably with electric clippers.

Category IB

- Adequately control serum blood glucose in diabetics and particularly avoid hyperglycemia perioperatively.
- Encourage cessation of tobacco use (cigarettes, cigars, pipes, chewing/dipping) 30 days before surgery.
- Do not withhold necessary blood products from surgical patients to prevent SSIs.

- Require patients to shower or bathe the night before operative procedure.
- Wash incision site to remove gross contamination before performing antiseptic skin preparation.

Category II

- Prepare skin in concentric circles from incision site.
- Keep preoperative stay in hospital as short as possible.

Surgical Team Members

Category 1B

- Keep nails short and do not wear artificial nails.
- Perform a preoperative surgical scrub/surgical hand antisepsis (hands and forearms up to the elbows) for at least 2 to 5 minutes using an appropriate antiseptic. After performing the surgical scrub/surgical hand antisepsis, keep the hands up and away from the body. Dry hands with a sterile towel, and don a sterile gown and gloves.
- Educate and encourage surgical personnel who have signs and symptoms of transmissible infections to report conditions promptly to supervisory personnel.
- Develop well-defined policies concerning patient care responsibilities when personnel have potentially transmissible infectious conditions.
- Do not routinely exclude surgical personnel who are colonized with organisms such as *Staphylococcus aureus* or group A streptococcus, unless such personnel have been linked epidemiologically to dissemination of the organism in the health care setting.

Category II

- Clean underneath each fingernail before performing the first surgical scrub of the day.
- Do not wear hand or arm jewellery.

Postoperative Incision Care

Category IB

- Protect with a sterile dressing for 24 to 48 hours after surgery incisions that have been closed primarily.
- Wash hands before and after dressing changes and any contact with the surgical site.

Category II

- When an incision dressing must be changed, use sterile technique.
- Educate the family regarding proper incision care, symptoms of SSI, and the need to report such symptoms.

Source: Reprinted from Rothrock, J. C. (2011). *Alexander's care of the patient in surgery* (14th ed., p. 260). St. Louis: Mosby. Adapted from Mangram, A. J., Horan, T. C., Pearson, M. L., Silver, L.C., Jarvis, W. R., & The Hospital Infection Control Practices Advisory Committee. (1999). *Guideline for prevention of surgical site infection, 1999.* National Center for Infectious Diseases, Hospital Infections Program; Centers for Disease Control and Prevention; Public Health Service, & US Department of Health and Human Services. Retrieved from *http://www.cdc.gov/hicpac/pdf/SSIguidelines.pdf*

Table 22-8 Expected Drainage From Tubes and Catheters

SUBSTANCE	DAILY AMOUNT	COLOUR	ODOUR	CONSISTENCY
Indwelling Catheter				
Urine*	500-700 mL, 1-2 days postoperative; 1500-2500 mL thereafter output 0.5-1 mL/kg/hr)	Clear, yellow	Ammonia	Watery
Nasogastric Tube, Gastrostomy Tube				
Gastric contents	≤1500 mL/day	Pale, yellow–green, brown Bloody following gastrointestinal surgery	Sour	Watery
Hemovac, Jackson-Pratt				
Wound drainage	Variable with procedure	Variable with procedure Usually serosanguineous	Same as wound dressing	Variable
T Tube				
Bile	500 mL	Bright yellow to dark green	Acid	Thick

*See Chapter 47.

by restlessness, insomnia and nightmares, tachycardia, apprehension, confusion and disorientation, irritability, and auditory or visual hallucinations. (Management of delirium tremens is discussed in Chapter 11.)

NURSING MANAGEMENT: PSYCHOLOGICAL FUNCTION

■ Nursing Diagnoses

Nursing diagnoses related to potential postoperative alterations in psychological function include, but are not limited to, the following:
• Anxiety
• Ineffective coping
• Disturbed body image
• Decisional conflict

■ Nursing Implementation

Nurses must observe and evaluate the patient's behaviour and plan appropriate interventions to ensure proper treatment of symptoms, prevent adverse outcomes, and improve patients' quality of life on discharge. Supportive measures include taking time to listen and talk with the patient, offering explanations and reassurance, and working collaboratively with family or significant others for discharge planning.

The nurse should discuss the patient's expectation of activity and what assistance will be needed following discharge. The older patient may be particularly distressed that an immediate return to home is not feasible. The patient must be included in discharge planning and should be provided with the information and support to make informed decisions about continuing care.

The recognition of the alcohol withdrawal syndrome in a patient not previously known to be an alcoholic presents a particular challenge. Any unusual or disturbed behaviour should be reported immediately so that diagnosis and treatment may be instituted.

Table 22-9 Postanaesthesia and Ambulatory Surgery Discharge Criteria

Postanaesthesia Discharge Criteria
• Patient awake (or baseline)
• Vital signs stable
• No excess bleeding or drainage
• No respiratory depression
• Oxygen saturation >90%
• Report given

Ambulatory Surgery Discharge Criteria
• All PACU discharge criteria met
• No IV narcotics for last 30 minutes
• Minimal nausea and vomiting
• Voided (if appropriate to surgical procedure or orders)
• Able to ambulate if age appropriate and not contraindicated
• Responsible adult present to accompany patient
• Written discharge instructions given and understood

PACU, postanaesthesia care unit; IV, intravenous.

Discharge From the Postanaesthesia Care Unit

The patient leaving the PACU may be discharged to an intensive care unit, an inpatient unit, an ambulatory care unit, or home. The choice of discharge site is based on patient acuity, access to follow-up care, and the potential for postoperative complications. The decision to discharge the patient from the PACU is based on written discharge criteria which can take the form of a standardized scoring system used to determine the patient's general condition and readiness for discharge from the PACU. Examples of discharge criteria are provided in Table 22-9.

Care of the Postoperative Patient on the Clinical Unit

Before discharging the patient from the PACU to the clinical unit, the PACU nurse provides a verbal report about the patient to the receiving nurse. The report summarizes the operative and post-anaesthetic period.

The nurse receiving the patient on the clinical unit assists PACU transport personnel in transferring the patient from the PACU stretcher onto the bed. Care must be taken to protect IV lines, wound drains, dressings, and traction devices. The use of a draw sheet or transfer board and sufficient personnel facilitates transfer of the patient.

Vital signs should be obtained, and patient status should be compared with the report provided by the PACU. Documentation of the transfer is then completed, followed by a more in-depth assessment (Table 22-10). Postoperative orders and appropriate nursing care are then initiated.

Although many of the potential problems that may occur in the PACU are time limited to the immediate postoperative period, a number of potential complications may occur during the extended postoperative recovery period on the clinical unit. Nursing assessment and management are based on awareness of the potential complications of surgery in general as well as complications specific to the surgical procedure. A comprehensive nursing care plan for the postoperative patient is available on the Evolve Web site for this chapter).

Planning for Discharge and Follow-Up Care

Ambulatory and Inpatient Surgery Discharge

Ambulatory. Ambulatory surgery accounts for up to 80% of all surgical procedures in Canada and the United States

---

Table 22-10 Nursing Assessment and Care of Patient on Admission to Clinical Unit: General Anaesthetic Versus Spinal or Epidural Anaesthetic

General Anaesthetic	*Spinal or Epidural Anaesthetic*
1. Record time of patient's return to unit.	1. Record time of patient's return to unit.
2. Take baseline vital signs.	2. Take baseline vital signs.
3. Assess airway and breath sounds.	3. Assess airway and breath sounds.
4. Assess neurological status, including level of consciousness and movement of extremities.	4. Assess neurological status, including level of consciousness and movement of extremities.
5. Assess wound, wound closure and dressing, and drainage tubes.	• Assess spinal insertion or epidural insertion site; ensure that there is a continuous epidural infusion in place and that the dressing and catheter are secure.
• Note type and amount of drainage.	• Assess motor and sensory blockade from spinal anaesthetic.
• Note any packing to an open wound.	5. Assess wound, wound closure, dressing, and drainage tubes.
• Connect tubing to gravity or suction drainage.	• Note type and amount of drainage.
6. Assess colour and appearance of skin.	• Note any packing to an open wound.
7. Assess urinary status.	• Connect tubing to gravity or suction drainage.
• Note time of voiding.	6. Assess colour and appearance of skin.
• Note presence of catheter, if any, and total output.	7. Assess urinary status.
• Check for bladder distension or urge to void.	• Note time of voiding.
• Note catheter patency; check integrity of insertion site and size of Foley catheter.	• Note presence of catheter, if any, and total output.
8. Assess pain and discomfort.	• Check for bladder distension or urge to void.
• Note last dose and type of pain control.	• Note catheter patency; check integrity of insertion site and size of Foley catheter.
• Note current pain intensity.	8. Assess pain and discomfort.
9. Position for comfort, safety (bed in low position, side rails up).	• Note last dose and type of pain control.
10. Check IV infusion.	• Note current pain intensity.
• Note type of solution.	9. Position for comfort, safety (bed in low position, side rails up).
• Note amount of fluid remaining.	10. Check IV infusion.
• Note flow rate.	• Note type of solution.
11. Attach call light within patient's reach, and orient patient to use of call light.	• Note amount of fluid remaining.
12. Ensure that emesis basin and tissues are available.	• Note flow rate.
13. Determine emotional condition and support needed.	11. Attach call light within patient's reach, and orient patient to use of call light.
14. Check for presence of family member or significant other.	12. Ensure that emesis basin and tissues are available.
15. Orient patient and family to immediate environment.	13. Determine emotional condition and support.
16. Check and carry out postoperative orders.	14. Check for presence of family member or significant other.
	15. Orient patient and family to immediate environment.
	16. Check and carry out postoperative orders.

IV, intravenous.

(Hughes, 2007) and has many advantages, including patient convenience, lower rates of hospital-acquired infections, and reduced costs.

Because these patients are in the health care setting for such a short amount of time, it is difficult to do all the required teaching. Optimally, the patient and any caregivers should be contacted 1 or more days before surgery to collect assessment data and to provide teaching that will be needed after surgery. The patient's anxiety level is lower at this time and learning may be enhanced.

The patient leaving an ambulatory surgery setting must be mobile and alert to provide a degree of self-care when discharged to home. Postoperative pain must be controlled. Overall, the patient must be stable and near the level of preoperative functioning for discharge from the unit. On discharge, instructions specific to the type of anaesthesia received and the surgery are given to the patient and caregiver verbally and reinforced with written directions. The patient may not drive and must be accompanied by a responsible adult at the time of discharge. A follow-up evaluation of the patient's status is made by telephone, and any specific questions and concerns are addressed.

Although ambulatory surgical procedures are minimally invasive, the nurse must carefully determine not only readiness for discharge but also home care needs of the individual. It is important to determine availability of assistive personnel (e.g., family, friends), access to a pharmacy for prescriptions, access to a phone in the event of an emergency, and access to follow-up care.

Discharge from the Clinical Unit.

Preparation for the patient's discharge should be an ongoing process throughout the surgical experience that begins during the preoperative period. The informed patient is, therefore, prepared as events unfold and gradually assumes greater responsibility for self-care during the postoperative period. As the day of discharge approaches, the nurse should be certain that the patient and any caregivers have the following information:

1. Care requirements of wound site and any dressings, including bathing recommendations.
2. Action and possible adverse effects of any drugs; when and how to take them.
3. Activities allowed and prohibited; when various physical activities can be resumed safely (e.g., driving a car, returning to work, sexual intercourse, leisure activities).
4. Dietary restrictions or modifications.
5. Symptoms to be reported (e.g., development of incisional tenderness or increased drainage, discomfort in other parts of the body).
6. Where and when to return for follow-up care.
7. Answers to any individual questions or concerns.

The nurse should specifically document in the record the discharge instructions provided to the patient and family. For the patient, the postoperative phase of care continues and extends into the recuperative period. Assessment and evaluation of the patient after discharge may be accomplished by a follow-up call or by a visit from a nurse (e.g., home health nurse).

Increasingly, patients are being discharged from hospital with many medical or surgical needs. They may be transferred to transitional care facilities, to long-term care facilities, or directly to their homes (see Chapter 6). When discharged directly to home, it is expected that the patient, with assistance from family, friends, or home health care, will continue self-care in the home. This may include dressing changes, wound care, catheter or drain care, home antibiotics, or continued physical therapy. Working through

the discharge planner for the hospital unit or the case manager, the nurse can facilitate the transition of care from hospital-based to community-based and home care, without jeopardizing the quality of care.

NURSING RESEARCH

Knowledge of Surgical Patients

Clinical Question

In ambulatory surgical patients (P), what are patients' knowledge expectations (I) before admission and their perceptions of received knowledge (C) 2 weeks after discharge (O)?

Best Available Evidence

A descriptive comparison cross-sectional study using pretests and post-tests was used.

Critical Appraisal and Synthesis of Evidence

The population of this study consisted of 120 patients receiving orthopedic care. The *Hospital Patient's Knowledge Expectations Scale and Hospital Patient's Received Knowledge Scale* was developed at an earlier date to collect data on patients before and after surgery. Six subscales were measured: biophysiological, functional, experimental, ethical, social, and functional. All patients participated in a 30-minute education session face-to-face with a nurse. Empirical data were collected twice: before the ambulatory surgery and 2 weeks after surgery. It was found that patients' knowledge expectations varied, especially on the experimental dimensions and the social dimensions.

Conclusion

More generalized knowledge is needed to assist with the development, planning, and implementation of patient education.

Implications for Nursing

It is important to assess patient knowledge and modify education according to patient needs. Patients who are more knowledgeable about their operation can prevent postoperative complications.

Reference for Evidence

Heikkinen, K., Lenio-Kilpi, H., Hiltunen, A., Johansson, K., Kalijonen, A., Rankinen, S., ..., Salantera, S. (2007). Ambulatory orthopedic surgery patients' knowledge expectations and perceptions of received knowledge. *Journal of Advanced Nursing*, *60*(3), 270-278. doi:10.1111/j.1365-2648.2007.04408.x

PICO: P, Patient population of interest; I, interventions or area of interest; C, comparison of interest or comparison group; O, outcome(s) of interest.

AGE-RELATED CONSIDERATIONS: PATIENT AFTER SURGERY

The older patient deserves special consideration after surgery (Clayton, 2008). The older adult has a decrease in respiratory function, including decreased ability to cough, decreased thoracic compliance, and decreased lung tissue. These alterations in pulmonary status lead to an increase in the work of ventilation and a decreased ability to readily eliminate pharmacological agents. Reactions to anaesthetic agents must be carefully monitored and their postoperative elimination assessed before the patient is left without close supervision. Pneumonia is a common postoperative complication in older adults.

Vascular function in the older adult is altered because of atherosclerosis and decreased elasticity in the blood vessels. Cardiac function is often compromised, and compensatory responses to changes in BP and volume are limited. Circulating blood volume is decreased, and hypertension is common. Cardiovascular parameters must be closely monitored throughout surgery and the postoperative period.

Drug toxicity is a potential problem in the older adult. Renal perfusion in the older adult normally decreases, with a reduction in the ability to eliminate drugs that are excreted by the kidney. Decreased liver function in the older adult also leads to decreased drug metabolism and thus increased drug activity. Renal and liver function must be carefully assessed in the postoperative phase of the patient's care to prevent drug overdose and toxicity.

Observing for changes in mental status is an important part of postoperative care in older adults. Postoperative delirium is common in the elderly in the postoperative period (Redelmeier, 2007).

Factors such as age, alcohol abuse, low baseline cognition, severe metabolic derangement, hypoxia, hypotension, and type of surgery appear to contribute to postoperative delirium. Anaesthetics, notably anticholinergic drugs and benzodiazepines,

increase the risk for delirium. One way that the nurse can differentiate delirium from dementia is to observe for alterations in the level of consciousness, which may indicate a diagnosis of delirium rather than dementia (Bodolea et al., 2008; Kojima & Narita, 2006). In patients with an acute change in mental status, a potentially reversible cause should be considered, such as an infection or an adverse effect of analgesic medication. (Dementia and delirium are discussed in Chapter 62.)

Pain is a multidimensional experience, and assessment should include how pain affects function, mood, activities, and quality of life. Older patients may be hesitant to request pain medication. They may believe that pain is an inevitable consequence of surgery and they need to just tolerate it. Nurses may not appropriately assess pain in patients who do not report their pain. Some older patients are hesitant to learn how to use PCA machines. The nurse should know that the surgery will usually result in pain, and if untreated, pain could have a negative effect on recovery. (Pain is discussed in Chapter 10.)

A comprehensive, multidisciplinary approach to caring for the health needs of the older adult patient is recommended by health professionals working with this population. When the older adult must undergo surgery, this approach to care during the perioperative period can improve the outcome and decrease the risk for these patients.

CLINICAL DECISION-MAKING EXERCISES

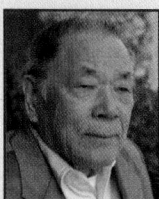

CASE STUDY:
Patient After Surgery
Source: © iStockphoto.com/Nancy Louie.

Patient Profile
Edward Lee, a 74-year-old Chinese Canadian retired university professor, has just undergone surgery for a fractured hip. He fell off of a ladder while painting his house. The surgery, performed while the patient was under general anaesthesia, was uneventful.

Subjective Data
- Was in excellent health before fall
- Played tennis three times each week
- Walked 30 to 50 km/wk
- Always had problems sleeping
- Difficulty hearing, wears hearing aid
- Upset with injury and its impact on activity
- Has no relatives or friends to assist with care

Objective Data
- Admitted to PACU with abduction pillow between his legs, two peripheral IV catheters, a self-suction drain from the hip dressing, and an indwelling urinary catheter

Collaborative Care
- Postoperative orders
- Vital signs per PACU routine

- Dextrose 5% in 0.45 normal saline at 100 mL/hr
- Morphine via patient-controlled analgesia 1 mg q6min (30 mg max in 4 hr) for pain
- Advance diet as tolerated
- Triflow spirometry q1h

Discussion Questions
1. What are the potential postanaesthesia problems that the nurse might expect with Mr. Lee?
2. *Priority Decision:* What priority nursing interventions would be appropriate to prevent these complications from occurring?
3. What factors may predispose Mr. Lee to the following problems: atelectasis, infection, pulmonary embolism, and nausea and vomiting?
4. How should it be determined when Mr. Lee is sufficiently recovered from general anaesthesia to be discharged to the clinical unit?
5. What potential postoperative problems might the nurse on the clinical unit expect?
6. *Priority Decision:* Based on the assessment data presented, identify two priority nursing diagnoses. Are there any collaborative problems?

Answers are available at **http://evolve.elsevier.com/Canada/Lewis/medsurg**

REVIEW QUESTIONS

The number of the question corresponds to the same-numbered objective at the beginning of the chapter.

1. What is the priority assessment by the nurse as soon as the patient enters the postanaesthesia care unit (PACU)?
   a. Urinary output
   b. Electrocardiogram monitoring
   c. Level of consciousness
   d. Airway patency and respiratory status

2. Which of the following nursing interventions is indicated during the patient's recovery from general anaesthesia in the PACU?
   a. Placing the patient in a prone position
   b. Encouraging deep breathing and coughing
   c. Restraining patients during episodes of emergence delirium
   d. Withholding analgesics until the patient is discharged from PACU

3. Which of the following patients is at greatest risk for postoperative nausea and vomiting?
   a. A 14-year-old, 40-kg, boy following an orchiopexy under general anaesthesia
   b. An 81-year-old, 55-kg, woman following a cystoscopy under local anaesthesia
   c. A 45-year-old, 70-kg, man following an arthroscopy under epidural anaesthesia
   d. A 23-year-old, 125-kg, woman following a diagnostic laparoscopy under general anaesthesia

4. Following admission of the patient to the clinical unit after surgery, which of the following pieces of assessment data requires the most immediate attention?
   a. Oxygen saturation of 80%
   b. Respiratory rate of 13/min
   c. Blood pressure of 90/60 mm Hg
   d. Temperature of 34.6°C

5. Which of the following urine outputs would be a concern for a nurse's care for a patient on his first postoperative day?
   a. 1500 mL
   b. 1000 mL
   c. 500 mL
   d. 2000 mL

6. What is the *priority* information the nurse should advise the patient of in preparation for discharge after surgery?
   a. A time frame for when various physical activities can be resumed
   b. The rationale for abstinence from sexual intercourse for 4 to 6 weeks
   c. The need to call hospital clinical unit to report any abnormal signs or symptoms
   d. The necessity of a referral to nutritional centre for management of dietary restrictions

ANSWERS: 1. d; 2. b; 3. d; 4. a; 5. c; 6. c.

REFERENCES

American Society of PeriAnesthesia Nurses (ASPAN). (2009). ASPAN's evidence-based clinical practice guidelines for the promotion of perioperative normothermia. *Journal of Perianesthesia Nursing, 24*, 693-700. doi:10.1016/j.jopan.2009.09.001

Attrell, E., & Armstrong, P. (2007). Surgical site infection: Surveillance in a home-care setting. *Wound Care Canada, 5*(2), 44-48.

Bodolea, C., Hagau, N., Coman, I., Pintea, S., Alina, I. C., Cristea, T., & Negrutiu, S. (2008). Postoperative cognitive dysfunction in elderly patients: An integrated psychological and medical approach. *Journal of Cognitive and Behavioral Psychotherapies, 8*(1), 117-132.

Canadian Association of Wound Care and Canadian Association for Enterostomal Therapy. (n.d.). The wound care instrument: Collaborative appraisal and recommendations for education. Retrieved from *http://www.cawc.net and http://www.caet.ca*

Chaturvedi, S., & Chaturvedi, A. (2007). Postoperative pain and its management. *Indian Journal of Critical Care Medicine, 11*(4), 204-211. doi:10.4103/0972-5229.37716

Clayton, J. L. (2008). Special needs of older adult undergoing surgery. *AORN Journal, 87*(3), 557-570. doi:10.1016/j.aorn.2008.02.006

Cooper, S. (2006). The effects of preoperative warming on patients' postoperative temperatures. *Association of periOperative Registered Nurses Journal, 83*(5), 1074-1084.

Cornish, P., Hyland, S., & Koczmara, C. (2006). Enhancing safety with potassium phosphates injection. *ISMP Canada Safety Bulletin (ISMP Canada, 2006, April 25)*. Retrieved from *http://www.ismp-canada.org/download/caccn/CACCN-Winter07.pdf*

Flaherty, E. (2008). Using pain-rating scales with older adults. *American Journal of Nursing, 108*(6), 40-47. doi:10.1097/01.NAJ.0000324375.02027.9f

Geerts, W., Bergqvist, D., Pineo, G. F., Heit, J. A., Samama, C. M., Lassen, M. R., & Colwell, C. W. (2008). Prevention of venous thromboembolism: American College of Chest Physicians evidence-based clinical practice guidelines (8th ed.). *Chest, 133*(6), 381S. doi:10.1378/chest.08-0656

Graber, M., Dachs, R., & Darby-Stewart, A. (2008). Is unfractionated heparin equivalent to low-molecular-weight heparin for venous thromboembolism? *American Family Physician: Journal Club, 77*(11), 1492-1493. Retrieved from *http://www.aafp.org/afp/2008/0601/p1492.html*

Harton, S., Grap, M. J., Savage, L., & Elswick, R. K. (2007). Frequency and predictors of return to incentive spirometry volume baseline after cardiac surgery. *Progress in Cardiovascular Nursing, 22*(1), 7-12. doi:10.1111/j.0889-7204.2007.05199.x

Health Service Executive. (2009). National best practice and evidence based guidelines for wound management. Retrieved from *http://www.hse.ie/eng/services/Publications/services/Primary/woundguidelines.pdf*

Hudek, K. (2009). Emergence delirium: A nursing perspective. *AORN Journal, 89*(3), 509-520.

Hughes, A. (2007). Day surgery: Trends in practice. *Prospectus 9 topics 9 views*. Retrieved from *http://www.prospectus.ie/documents/83679309_topics_9_views.pdf*

Hurd, T., Zuiliani, N., & Posnett, J. (2008). Evaluation of the impact of restructuring wound management practices in a community care provider in Niagara, Canada. *International Wound Journal*, 5(2), 296-304.

Hutchison, R. (2007). Challenges in acute post-operative pain management. *American Journal Health-System Pharmacy*, 64(4), 2-5. doi:10.2146/ajhp060679

Janjigian, M. P., & Muhs, B. E. (2008). Current treatment of acute lower extremity deep venous thrombosis. *International Journal of Lower Extremity Wounds*, 7(1), 15-20. doi:10.1177/1534734608314566

Kojima, Y., & Narita, M. (2006). Postoperative outcome among elderly patients after general anesthesia. *Acta Anaesthesiological Scandinavica*, 50, 19-25.

Kozier, B., Erb, G., Berman, A., Synder, S., Bouchal, D. S., Hirst, S., ... Buck, M. (2010). *Fundamentals of Canadian nursing: Concepts, process and practice*. Toronto: Pearson.

Lauzon Clabo, L. (2008). An ethnography of pain assessment and the role of social context on two postoperative units. *Journal of Advanced Nursing*, 61(5), 531-539. doi:10.1111/j.1365-2648.2007.04550.x

Ledrick, D., Caudell, M. J., & Bowman, M. J. (2008). Hypothermia and hyperthermia: Treating temperature disruptions. *Practical Summaries in Acute Care*, 3(2), 9-16.

Mackintosh, C. (2007). Assessment and management of patients with post-operative pain. *Nursing Standard*, 22(5), 49-55.

Macksey, L. (2010). *Nurse anesthesia pocket guide* (2nd ed.). Toronto: Jones and Bartlett Publishers.

MacLellan, D. G., & Fletcher, J. P. (2007). Mechanical compression in the prophylaxis of venous thromboembolism. *Australian and New Zealand Journal of Surgery*, 77, 418-423. doi:10.1111/j.1445-2197.2007.04085.x

Mathias, J. M. (2008). Protect your patients from nausea and vomiting. *OR Manager*, 24(4), 27-28.

Mazaris, E., Varkarakis, I., & Jarrett, T. (2007). Abdominal fascial wound and skin closure: Current techniques and materials. *Contemporary Urology*, 19(5), 38-43.

Mukherjee, S., Otah, E., Otah, K., Serrano, O., Walker, J., & Cooperman, A. (2011). Ileus. *Medscape reference drugs, diseases and procedures*. Retrieved from *http://emedicine.medscape.com/article/178948-overview*

Radtke, F. M., Franck, M., Hagemann, L., Seeling, M., Wernecke, K. D., & Spies, C. D. (2010). Risk factors for inadequate emergence after anesthesia: Emergence delirium and hypoactive emergence. *Minerva Anestesiologica*, 76(6), 394-403.

Redelmeier, D. (2007). New thinking about postoperative delirium. *Canadian Medical Association Journal*, 177(4), 424. doi:10.1503/cmaj.070932

Registered Nurses' Association of Ontario (RNAO). (2010). Screening for delirium, dementia and depression in older adults. Retrieved from *http://rnao.ca/sites/rnao-ca/files/Screening_for_Delirium_Dementia_and_Depression_in_the_Older_Adult.pdf*

Rocha, E., Imberti, D., & Paschina, E. (2007). Low-molecular-weight heparins: Before or after surgery? New concepts and evidence. *Clinical Drug Investigations*, 27(5), 357-366. doi:10.2165/00044011-200727050-00007

Rothrock, J. (2011). *Alexander's care of the patient in surgery* (14th ed.). St. Louis: Elsevier.

Roy, R., Brull, S., & Eichhorn, J. (2011). Surgical site infections and the anesthesia professionals' Microbiome: We've all been slimed! Now what are we going to do about it? *Anesthesia & Analgesia*, 112(1), 4-7. doi:10.1213/ANE.0b013e3181fe4942

University of Pittsburgh Medical Center. (2011). Incentive spirometry. Retrieved from *http://www.upmc.com/healthatoz/patienteducation/b/pages/incentive-spirometry.aspx*

Viscusi, E. (2008). Patient-controlled drug delivery for acute postoperative pain management: A review of current and emerging technologies. *Regional Anesthesia and Pain Medicine*, 33(2), 146-158. doi:10.1016/j.rapm.2007.11.005

Weirich, T. L. (2008). Hypothermia/warming protocols: Why are they not widely used in the OR? *AORN Journal*, 87(2), 333-344. doi:10.1016/j.aorn.2007.08.021

Zeinali, F., Stulberg, J., & Delaney, C. (2009). Pharmacological management of postoperative ileus. *Canadian Journal of Surgery*, 52(2) 153-157.

CANADIAN RESOURCES

Allergy and Asthma Information Association
http://www.aaia.ca
Canadian Allergy, Asthma, and Immunology Foundation
http://www.allergyfoundation.ca
Canadian Anesthesiologists' Society
http://www.cas.ca/
Canadian Association of Wound Care
http://cawc.net/index.php
Canadian Pain Society
http://www.canadianpainsociety.ca
National Association of PeriAnesthesia Nurses of Canada
http://www.napanc.org
Operating Room Nurses Association of Canada
http://www.ornac.ca
Registered Nurses' Association of Ontario
http://rnao.ca/

RELATED RESOURCES

American College of Surgeons
http://www.facs.org
American Latex Allergy Association
http://latexallergyresources.org/
American Society of Anesthesiologists
http://www.asahq.org
American Society of PeriAnesthesia Nurses (ASPAN)
http://www.aspan.org
Association of periOperative Registered Nurses (AORN)
http://www.aorn.org

ⓔvolve   *For additional Internet resources, see the Web site for this book at* **http://evolve.elsevier.com/Canada/Lewis/medsurg**

Problems Related to Altered Sensory Input

4

SECTION OUTLINE

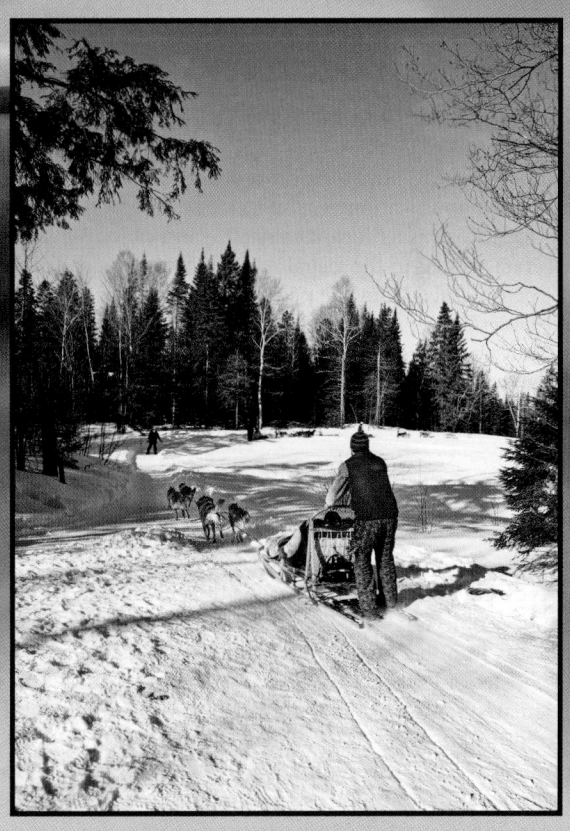

Brand X Pictures/Jupiter Images/Getty Images/Thinkstock

Nursing Assessment: Visual and Auditory Systems

Written by Sarah C. Smith and Sherry Neely

Adapted by Marian Luctkar-Flude

LEARNING OBJECTIVES

1. Describe the structures and functions of the visual and auditory systems.
2. Describe the physiological processes involved in normal vision and hearing.
3. Identify the significant subjective and objective assessment data related to the visual and auditory systems that should be obtained from the patient.
4. Describe the appropriate techniques used in the physical assessment of the visual and auditory systems.
5. Differentiate normal from common abnormal findings of a physical assessment of the visual and auditory systems.
6. Relate age-related changes in the visual and auditory systems to differences in assessment findings.
7. Describe the determinants of health that may be evident in the assessment of the visual and auditory systems.
8. Describe the purpose, the significance of results, and the nursing responsibilities related to diagnostic studies of the visual and auditory systems.

KEY TERMS

accommodation The convergence of the eyes and the constriction of the pupils when the eyes focus from a far to near object, p. 483

aqueous humor A clear, watery fluid that fills the anterior and posterior chambers of the eye, p. 481

astigmatism A refractive error caused by unevenness in the cornea, p. 481

conjunctiva A transparent mucous membrane that covers the inner surfaces of the eyelids and extends over the sclera, p. 483

hyperopia Inability of the eye to focus on nearby objects, p. 481

lens A biconvex, avascular, transparent structure located behind the iris, p. 483

myopia Inability of the eye to focus on objects far away, p. 481

nystagmus An abnormal involuntary repetitive movement of the eyes, p. 494

PERRLA Acronym that stands for "pupils are equal, round, and reactive to light and accommodation," p. 490

presbyopia A hyperopic shift to farsightedness resulting from a loss of elasticity of the lens of the eye, p. 481

retina The innermost layer of the eye that extends and forms the optic nerve, p. 483

sclera An opaque structure composed of collagen fibres that form the "white" of the eye, p. 483

tinnitus The sensation of a ringing sound in the ears, p. 494

vertigo The sensation that a person or objects around the person are moving or spinning; usually stimulated by movement of the head, p. 494

ELECTRONIC RESOURCES

Supplemental content related to Chapter 23 can be found…

Evolve Web Site ⊖volve

http://evolve.elsevier.com/Canada/Lewis/medsurg
- Animation: Weber Test
- Assessment Case Study
- Clinical Reference: Laboratory Values
- Content Updates
- Electronic Calculators
- Examination Review Questions
- Glossary

- Key Points (Printable and MP3 Download)
- Physical Examination Videos:
  - Eyes
  - Ears
- Video Clips:
  - Evaluation: Central Vision and Visual Acuity
  - Evaluation: Pupil Responses, Direct and Consensual
  - Inspection and Palpation: External Eye
  - Inspection and Palpation: External Ear
  - Inspection: Ear Canal

The Visual System

Structures and Functions

The visual system consists of the external tissues and structures surrounding the eye, the external and internal structures of the eye, the refractive media, and the visual pathway. The external structures are the eyebrows, eyelids, eyelashes, lacrimal system, conjunctiva, cornea, sclera, and extraocular muscles. The internal structures are the iris, lens, ciliary body, choroid, and retina. The entire visual system is important for visual function. Light reflected from an object in the field of vision passes through the transparent structures of the eye and, in doing so, is *refracted* (bent) so that a clear image can fall on the retina. From the retina, the visual stimuli travel through the visual pathway to the occipital cortex, where they are perceived as an image.

Structures and Functions of Vision

Eyeball. The eyeball, or globe, is composed of three layers (Figure 23-1). The tough outer layer is composed of the sclera and the transparent cornea. The middle layer consists of the uveal tract (iris, choroid, and ciliary body), and the innermost layer is the retina. The anterior chamber lies between the iris and the posterior surface of the cornea, whereas the posterior chamber lies between the anterior surface of the lens and the posterior surface of the iris. These chambers are filled with aqueous humor secreted by the ciliary body. The anatomic space *(vitreous cavity)* between the posterior lens and the retina is filled with a gel substance *(vitreous humor* or *vitreous).*

Refractive Media. For light to reach the retina, it must pass through a number of structures: the cornea, the aqueous humor, the lens, and the vitreous humor. All of these structures must remain clear for light to reach the retina and stimulate the photoreceptor cells. The cornea, which is normally transparent, is the first structure through which light passes. It is responsible for the majority of light refraction necessary for clear vision (Smith, 2008).

Aqueous humor, produced by the ciliary process, is a clear, watery fluid that fills the anterior and posterior chambers of the anterior cavity of the eye. It drains through the trabecular meshwork located in the angle. This circular canal conveys fluid into scleral veins, which enter the circulation of the body. The aqueous humor bathes and nourishes the lens and the endothelium of the cornea. Normal intraocular pressure is between 10 and 21 mm Hg; excess production or decreased outflow can cause an elevation in this pressure, a condition termed *glaucoma.*

The lens is a biconvex structure located behind the iris and supported in place by the fibres of the ciliary zonules. The primary function of the lens is to bend light rays, which enables them to fall onto the retina. Anything altering the clarity of the lens affects light transmission.

Vitreous humor is located in the vitreous cavity, the large area behind the lens and in front of the retina (see Figure 23-1). Light passing through the vitreous humor may be blocked by any nontransparent substance within, such as the cellular debris (often called *floaters).* The effect on vision varies, depending on the amount, type, and location of the substance blocking the light.

Refractive Errors. Refraction is the ability of the eye to bend light rays so that they fall on the retina. In the normal eye, parallel light rays are focused through the lens into a sharp image on the retina. The state that enables this process is termed *emmetropia,* which means that light is focused exactly on the retina, not in front of it or behind it. The condition in which the light does not focus properly is called a *refractive error.*

The individual with **myopia** can see near objects clearly (nearsightedness), but objects in the distance appear blurred. The individual with **hyperopia** can see distant objects clearly (farsightedness), but close objects appear blurred. **Astigmatism** is caused by an unevenness in the cornea, which results in visual distortion. **Presbyopia** is a form of hyperopia, or farsightedness, that occurs as a normal process of aging, usually beginning around age 40.

Visual Pathways. Once the image travels through the refractive media, it is focused on the retina, inverted, and reversed left to right. For example, if the visualized object is in the upper part

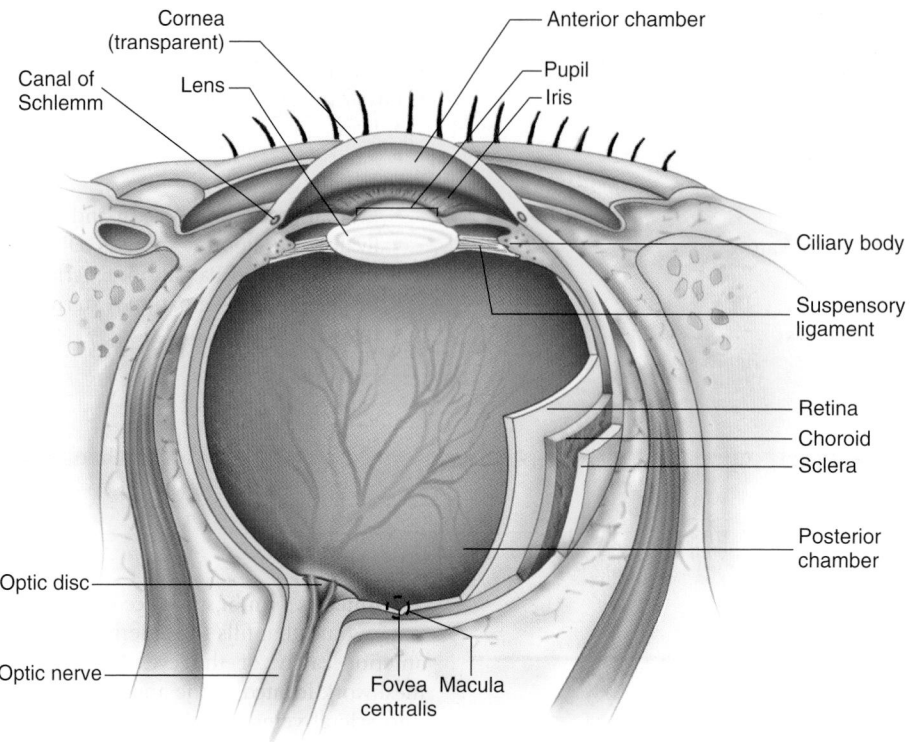

Figure 23-1 The human eye.

Source: Adapted from Patton, K. T., & Thibodeau, G. A. (2010). *Anatomy and physiology* (7th ed., p. 515, Figure 15-21). St. Louis: Mosby.

of the left temporal visual field, it is focused in the lower part of the nasal retina, upside down, and as a mirror image. From the retina, the impulses travel through the optic nerve to the optic chiasm, where the nasal fibres of each eye cross over to the other side. Fibres from the left field of both eyes form the left optic tract and travel to the left occipital cortex. The fibres from the right field of both eyes form the right optic tract and travel to the right occipital cortex. Because of this arrangement of the nerve fibres in the visual pathways, it is possible to determine the anatomic location of abnormalities in those nerve fibres from the specific visual field defect (Figure 23-2).

External Structures and Functions

Eyebrows, Eyelids, and Eyelashes. Eyebrows, eyelids, and eyelashes serve an important role in protecting the eye. They provide a physical barrier to dust and foreign particles (Figure 23-3). The eye is further protected by the surrounding bony orbit and by fat pads located below and behind the *globe,* or eyeball.

The upper and lower eyelids join at the medial and lateral canthi. The upper eyelid blinks spontaneously approximately 15 times a minute. Blinking distributes tears over the anterior surface of the eyeball and helps control the amount of light entering the visual pathway.

The eyelids open and close through the action of muscles innervated by cranial nerve (CN) VII, which is the facial nerve. Muscular action also helps hold the eyelids against the eyeball.

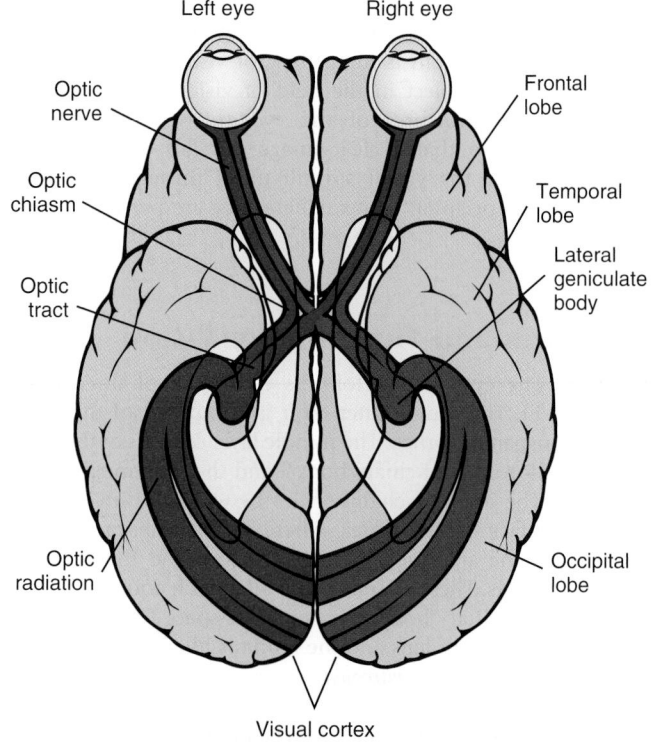

Figure 23-2 The visual pathway. Fibres from the nasal portion of each retina cross over to the opposite side of the optic chiasma, terminating in the lateral geniculate body of the opposite side. The location of a lesion in the visual pathway determines the resulting visual defect.

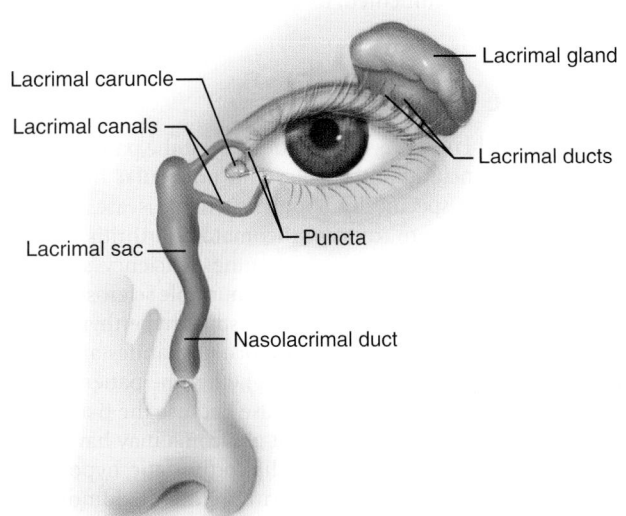

Lacrimal caruncle

Lacrimal canals

Lacrimal sac

Lacrimal gland

Lacrimal ducts

Puncta

Nasolacrimal duct

Figure 23-3 External eye and lacrimal apparatus. Tears produced in the lacrimal gland pass over the surface of the eye and enter the lacrimal canal. From there, the tears are carried through the nasolacrimal duct to the nasal cavity.

Conjunctiva. The **conjunctiva** is a transparent mucous membrane that covers the inner surfaces of the eyelids (the palpebral conjunctiva) and extends over the sclera (the bulbar conjunctiva), forming a "pocket" under each eyelid. Glands in the conjunctiva secrete mucus and tears.

Sclera. The **sclera** is composed of collagen fibres meshed together to form an opaque structure commonly referred to as the "white" of the eye. The sclera forms a tough shell that helps protect the intraocular structures.

Cornea. The transparent and avascular cornea allows light to enter the eye (see Figure 23-1). The curved cornea refracts (bends) incoming light rays to help focus them on the retina. The cornea consists of five layers: the epithelium, Bowman's layer, the stroma, Descemet's membrane, and the endothelium. The epithelium consists of a layer of cells that helps protect the eye. Epithelial cells regenerate when damaged. The stroma consists of collagen fibrils.

Lacrimal Apparatus. The lacrimal system consists of the lacrimal gland and ducts, the lacrimal canals and puncta, the lacrimal sac, and the nasolacrimal duct. In addition to the lacrimal gland, other glands provide secretions to make up the mucous, aqueous, and lipid layers of the tear film. The tear film moistens the eye and provides oxygen to the cornea.

Extraocular Muscles. Each eye is moved by three pairs of extraocular muscles and controlled by three cranial nerves: (a) superior and inferior rectus muscles (CN III), (b) medial (CN III) and lateral rectus muscles (CN VI), and (c) superior (CN IV) and inferior oblique muscles (CN III). Neuromuscular coordination enables simultaneous movement of the eyes in the same direction (*conjugate movement*).

Internal Structures and Functions

Iris. The iris (plural: *irides*) is the colourful part of the eye. This structure has a small, round opening in its centre, the *pupil*, which allows light to enter the eye. The pupil constricts through action of the iris sphincter muscle (innervated by CN III [oculomotor nerve]) and dilates through action of the iris dilator muscle (innervated by CN V [trigeminal nerve]) to control the amount of light that enters the eye.

Lens. The **lens** is a biconvex, avascular, transparent structure located behind the iris. It is supported by small fibres that comprise the *anterior and posterior ciliary zonules*. The primary function of the lens is to bend light rays so that they fall onto the retina. The shape of the lens is modified by action of the ciliary body as part of **accommodation,** the convergence of the eyes and the constriction of the pupils that occurs when the eye refocuses from a far object to a near object. This enables a person to focus on near objects, as in reading a book.

Ciliary Body. The ciliary body consists of the ciliary muscles, which surround the lens and lie parallel to the sclera; the ciliary zonules, which attach to the lens capsule; and the ciliary processes, which constitute the terminal portion of the ciliary body. The ciliary processes lie behind the peripheral part of the iris and secrete aqueous humor.

Choroid. The choroid is a highly vascular structure that serves to nourish the ciliary body, the iris, and the outer portion of the retina. It lies inside and parallel to the sclera and extends from the area where the optic nerve enters the eye to the ciliary body (see Figure 23-1).

Retina. The **retina** is the innermost layer of the eye that extends and gives rise to the optic nerve. Neurons make up the major portion of the retina. Therefore, retinal cells cannot regenerate if destroyed. The retina lines the inside of the eyeball, extending from the area of the optic nerve to the ciliary body (see Figure 23-1). It is responsible for converting images into a form that the brain can understand and process as vision. The retina is composed of two types of photoreceptor cells: rods and cones. Rods are stimulated in dim or darkened environments, and cones are receptive to colours in bright environments. The centre of the retina is the *fovea centralis*, a pinpoint depression composed only of densely packed cones (Thibodeau & Patton, 2012). This area of the retina provides the sharpest visual acuity. Surrounding the fovea is the *macula*, an area smaller than 1 square millimetre, which has a high concentration of cones and is relatively free of blood vessels. With the exception of the macula, the retina is nourished by retinal arterioles and veins. This blood supply enters the eye through the optic disc, located nasally from the macula. The optic disc is the area where the optic nerve (CN II) exits the eyeball. Within the disc is the physiological cup, a depression that can be visualized through the pupil with the ophthalmoscope. The retinal veins and arteries can also be visualized in this way and can provide information about the condition of the vascular system in general.

The visual system may be affected by biological and genetic determinants of health, and by personal health practices (see the Determinants of Health box "Visual System").

DETERMINANTS OF HEALTH
Visual System

Biology and Genetics

- Patients with darker skin tones may also have small brown macules on the sclera (Jarvis, Browne, MacDonald-Jenkins, & Luctkar-Flude, 2009).
- Vision problems are more common in those who are older, have diabetes, are of African descent, or have a strong family history of glaucoma, age-related macular degeneration, or retinopathies (Clinical Practice Guidelines Expert Committee, 2007).
- Vision problems are more common among new immigrants and refugees than in the general Canadian population (Pottie et al., 2011).
- Aboriginal people are three to four times more likely to experience lower case type 2 diabetes than non-Aboriginal Canadians (Health Canada, 2011) and tend to have more advanced diabetic retinopathy changes (Ross, McKenna, Mozejko, & Fick, 2007).
- Women are at greater risk for age-related macular degeneration and glaucoma (National Coalition for Vision Health, 2007).
- Males are more than twice as likely as females to experience eye trauma (National Coalition for Vision Health, 2007).
- Men are more likely than women to have colour blindness (Jarvis et al., 2009).

Personal Health Practices

- Smoking is associated with a greater risk of developing age-related macular degeneration, glaucoma, and cataracts (Muzychka, 2009).
- Exposure to ultraviolet B light (i.e., sunlight) is associated with a greater risk of developing cataracts (National Coalition for Vision Health, 2007).

AGE-RELATED CONSIDERATIONS: THE VISUAL SYSTEM

Every structure of the visual system is subject to changes as the individual ages. Whereas many of these changes are relatively benign, others may compromise visual acuity severely in the older adult. The psychosocial effect of poor vision or blindness can be highly significant. Visual impairment increases with age; vision loss doubles every decade after age 40 and triples after age 75 (Muzychka, 2009, p. 19). Age-related changes in the visual system and differences in assessment findings are presented in Table 23-1.

Assessment

Assessment of the visual system may be as simple as determining a patient's visual acuity or as complex as collecting complete subjective and objective data pertinent to the visual system. To perform an appropriate ophthalmic evaluation, the nurse must determine which parts of the data collection are important for each patient. Table 23-2 lists suggested questions to ask while the health history is documented, to obtain subjective data related to the visual system.

Subjective Data

Past Health History. Information about the patient's health history should include both ocular and nonocular history. The nurse should ask specifically about systemic diseases—such as diabetes, hypertension, cancer, rheumatoid arthritis, sexually transmitted infections, acquired immune deficiency syndrome, muscular dystrophy, myasthenia gravis, multiple sclerosis, inflammatory bowel disease, and hypothyroidism or hyperthyroidism—because many of these diseases have ocular manifestations. It is particularly important to determine whether the patient has any history of cardiac or pulmonary disease because the β-adrenergic blocker eye drops often used to treat glaucoma may have serious adverse effects, including bradycardia, orthostatic hypotension, bronchospasm, and congestive heart failure (Skidmore-Roth, 2012).

The nurse should ask the patient about previous trauma to the head. Also, inquiring about headaches is important because migraines may create visual disturbances.

A history of tests for visual acuity should be obtained, including the date of the most recent examination and change in glasses or contact lens prescriptions, as well as testing for glaucoma and what the results were. The nurse should specifically ask about a history of strabismus, amblyopia, cataracts, retinal detachment, refractive surgery, glaucoma, and any trauma to the eye, its treatment, and sequelae.

Medications. If the patient takes any medications, the nurse should obtain a complete list, including over-the-counter medicines, eye drops, herbal therapies, or dietary supplements. Many patients do not think that over-the-counter drugs, eye drops, or herbal therapies are "real" drugs and may not mention their use unless specifically questioned. However, many of these drugs have ocular effects. For example, many preparations for colds contain a form of epinephrine (e.g., pseudoephedrine) that can dilate the pupil. The nurse should also note the use of any antihistamines or decongestants because these drugs can cause ocular dryness. The nurse should specifically ask whether the patient uses any prescription drugs such as corticosteroids, thyroid medications, oral hypoglycemic agents, or insulin. Long-term use of corticosteroids can contribute to development of glaucoma or cataracts. It is especially important to note whether the patient is taking any β-adrenergic blocker eye drops because they may potentiate the effects of corticosteroids.

The nurse should also ask female patients whether they are taking birth control pills or are pregnant because hormonal changes can affect the wearing of contact lenses. Finally, the nurse should determine whether the patient has allergies to medications or other substances.

Surgery or Other Treatments. Surgical procedures related to the head, eye, or brain should be noted. Brain surgery and subsequent swelling can cause pressure on the optic nerve or tract, resulting in visual alterations. Any laser procedures to the eye should also be documented, as should the effect of any eye surgery or laser treatment on visual acuity.

Nutrition and Elimination. The patient's intake of vitamins and trace minerals can be important to ocular health. Supplementation with vitamins C and E, and the phytochemicals lutein

AGE-RELATED DIFFERENCES IN ASSESSMENT

Table 23-1 Visual System

CHANGES	DIFFERENCES IN ASSESSMENT FINDINGS
Eyebrows and Eyelashes	
Loss of pigment in the hair	Greying of eyebrows, eyelashes
Eyelids	
Loss of orbital fat, decreased muscle tone	Entropion, ectropion, mild ptosis
Tissue atrophy, prolapse of fat into eyelid tissue	Blepharodermachalasis (excessive upper eyelid skin)
Plaques	Xanthelasma
Conjunctiva	
Tissue damage related to chronic exposure to ultraviolet light or to other chronic environmental exposure	Pinguecula (small, yellowish spot seen usually on the medial aspect of the conjunctiva)
Sclera	
Lipid deposition	Yellowish (as opposed to bluish) scleral colour
Cornea	
Cholesterol deposits in peripheral cornea	Arcus senilis (milky or yellow ring encircling periphery of cornea; see Figure 23-3)
Tissue damage related to chronic exposure	Pterygium (thickened, triangular bit of pale tissue that extends from the inner canthus of the eye to the nasal border of the cornea)
Decrease in water content, atrophy of nerve fibres	Decreased corneal sensitivity and corneal reflex
Epithelial changes	Loss of corneal lustre
Accumulation of lipid deposits	Blurring of vision
Lacrimal Apparatus	
Decreased tear secretion	Dryness
Malposition of the eyelid that results in tears overflowing the eyelid margins instead of draining through the puncta	Tearing, irritated eyes
Iris	
Increased rigidity of iris	Decreased pupil size
Dilator muscle atrophy or weakness	Slower recovery of pupil size after light stimulation
Loss of pigment	Change of iris colour
Shrinking and stiffening of ciliary muscle	Decrease in near vision and accommodation
Lens	
Biochemical changes in lens proteins, oxidative damage, chronic exposure to ultraviolet light	Cataracts
Increased rigidity of lens	Presbyopia
Opacities in the lens (may also be related to opacities in the cornea and the vitreous humor)	Complaints of glare, impairment of night vision
Accumulation of yellow substances	Yellow colouring of lens
Retina	
Retinal vascular changes related to atherosclerosis and hypertension	Narrowed, pale, straighter arterioles; acute branching
Decrease in cones	Changes in colour perception, especially blue and violet
Loss of photoreceptor cells, retinal pigment, epithelial cells, and melanin	Decreased visual acuity, appearance of drusen
Age-related macular degeneration as a result of vascular changes	Loss of central vision
Vitreous Humor	
Liquefaction and detachment of the vitreous humor	Increased complaints of "floaters"

HEALTH HISTORY

Table 23-2 Visual System: Questions for Obtaining Subjective Data

Vision Difficulty

- Describe the change in your vision. Describe how this affects your daily life.
- Do you have any visual difficulties or change in your visual acuity?* Did it come on slowly or progress slowly? Does it affect one or both eyes? Is it constant or intermittent? Do you see spots move in front of your eyes?*
- Do you have a blind spot?*
- Do you have any night blindness?*
- For older adults: Are you experiencing any visual difficulties when you climb stairs or drive at night?
- Do you use any visual aids such as glasses or contact lenses?

Eye Pain

- Do you have any eye pain?*

Strabismus or Diplopia

- Have you ever had a history of crossed eyes, or do you have double vision?*

Redness or Swelling

- Do you have redness or swelling in your eyes?*
- Do you have any discharge or watering from your eyes?*

Family History

- Do you have a family history of diseases such as atherosclerosis, diabetes, thyroid disease, hypertension, arthritis, or cancer that might affect your eyes?*
- Do you have a family history of ocular problems such as cataracts, tumours, glaucoma, refractive errors (especially myopia and hyperopia), or retinal degenerative conditions (e.g., macular degeneration, retinal detachment, retinitis pigmentosa)?*

Nutrition and Elimination

- Do you take any nutritional supplements?
- Does your visual problem affect your ability to obtain and prepare food?*
- Do you have to strain to void or defecate?*

Sleep

- Is your vision affected by the amount of sleep you get?*
- Is your sleep affected by your eye problem?*

Reproduction–Sexuality

- Has your eye problem caused a change in your sex life?*
- For women: Are you pregnant? Do you use birth control pills?

Self-Care History

- Do you have regular eye examinations? When was your last test?
- Do you wear glasses or contact lenses? When was the last time your eye prescription was checked? Was it changed?
- Have you ever been tested for colour vision?*
- Do you wear protective eyewear (sunglasses, safety goggles, or hats)?*
- Do you wear contact lenses? If so, how do you take care of them?
- If you use eye drops, how do you instill them?
- Do you spend long periods of time in the sun?* Do you wear sunglasses?
- Do you smoke, or are you regularly exposed to second-hand smoke?
- Have you ever been tested for glaucoma?* Results?

Social and Occupational History

- Do you have any problems at work or home because of your eyes?*
- Does your eye problem affect your ability to read?*
- Have you made any changes in your social activities because of your eyes?*
- Are your activities limited in any way by your eye problem?*
- Are there any environmental conditions at home or work that may have an effect on your eyes (e.g., smoke, dust, chemicals, flying sparks)?* If so, do you use goggles for eye protection?
- Do you participate in any leisure activities that have the potential for eye injury?*
- Do you work for long hours at the computer?*

Coping Abilities

- How does your eye problem make you feel about yourself?
- If you have a vision loss, how do you cope?* Are you able to maintain your same living environment?* Do you use large-print books or Braille?*

*If yes, describe.

Source: Adapted from Jarvis, C., Browne, A. J., MacDonald-Jenkins, J., & Luctkar-Flude, M. (2009). *Physical examination & health assessment* (1st Canadian ed., pp. 304-306). Toronto: Elsevier Canada.

and zeaxanthin may help prevent or delay the progression of eye diseases such as cataracts, glaucoma, and age-related macular degeneration (Rhone & Basu, 2008).

The nurse should assess the patient's usual pattern of elimination and determine the potential for constipation in the patient who has undergone or will undergo ophthalmological surgical procedures. Straining to defecate (the Valsalva manoeuvre) can raise intraocular pressure. Although there is some evidence that elevating the intraocular pressure in the course of normal activities is not detrimental in relation to the surgical incision made during eye surgery, many surgeons do not want such patients to strain.

Self-Care History. The nurse should assess the patient's ocular health care activities. The patient may not recognize the importance of eye safety practices, such as wearing protective eyewear during potentially hazardous activities or while playing sports, or avoiding noxious fumes and other eye irritants. Information about the use of sunglasses in bright light should be obtained. Prolonged exposure to ultraviolet light can affect the retina and has been linked to an increase in cataracts. Nighttime driving habits and any problems encountered should be noted. Today, millions of people wear contact lenses, but many do not care for them properly (Sweeney, Holden, Evans, Ng, & Cho, 2009). The type of contact lenses used and the patient's wearing and care habits may indicate a need for teaching. Today, many individuals work for long hours in front of computers; eye strain can be a common problem. The nurse should ask about the patient's time spent in working on computers or handheld devices. The 20/20 rule can be promoted: Every 20 minutes, patients should look away from their computer screen for 20 seconds (American Optometric Association, 2011).

Regular eye examinations should be discussed. Environmental exposures at home or work can cause trauma or irritation to the eyes; eye protection should be discussed. Patients should be asked whether they smoke or are regularly exposed to second-hand smoke. Smokers are at greater risk for developing age-related macular degeneration. If patients use eye drops, the nurse should ascertain whether they are aware of correct methods for instilling drops to avoid contamination of the container.

Social and Occupational Health History. The patient's ability to maintain necessary or desired roles and responsibilities in home, work, and social environments can be negatively affected by ocular problems. For example, macular degeneration may decrease the patient's visual acuity to a level inadequate for functioning at work. In many occupations, employees work in conditions in which eye injury may occur. For example, factory workers may be at risk from flying debris. Information should be obtained about eye safety practices, such as use of goggles or safety glasses. Workers can also be exposed to eyestrain in the office from video display terminals, poor lighting, and glare. An ergonomic consultation may be beneficial.

The patient with diabetes may not be able to see well enough to self-administer insulin. This patient may resent the dependence on a family member who takes over this function. The patient with *exophthalmos* (marked protrusion of eyeballs) may be embarrassed by his or her appearance and avoid usual social activities. The nurse should sensitively inquire whether the patient's preferred roles and responsibilities have been affected by the ocular problem.

The nurse should also inquire about leisure activities during which the patient may incur an ocular injury. For example, during gardening, woodworking, and other craft activities, foreign bodies can enter the cornea or conjunctiva or even penetrate the globe. Injuries to the globe or the bony orbit can also occur after blows to the head or eye during sports activities such as racquetball, baseball, and tennis. Cross-country skiers may develop corneal fungal ulcers after an abrasion caused by low-hanging tree limbs. Other leisure activities such as needlepoint, fly tying, or bird watching may have high-level visual demands and produce eye strain.

Coping Abilities. Patients with visual loss or visual problems may experience many emotions intensely and have difficulty coping with the resulting changes. A more comprehensive psychosocial assessment should be performed for patients who indicate mood changes or difficulty coping.

Objective Data

Physical Examination. Physical examination of the visual system includes inspecting ocular structures and determining their functional status. Assessment of ocular structures should include examining the ocular adnexa, the external eye, and internal structures. Some structures, such as the retina and blood vessels, must be visualized with the aid of equipment, such as the ophthalmoscope. Physiological functional assessment includes determining the patient's visual acuity and ability to judge closeness and distance, assessing extraocular muscle function, evaluating visual fields, observing pupil function, and measuring intraocular pressure.

Table 23-3 Normal Physical Assessment of the Visual System
• Visual acuity: 20/20 in both eyes; no diplopia
• External eye structures: symmetrical and without lesions or deformities
• Lacrimal apparatus: nontender and without drainage
• Conjunctiva: clear; sclera: white
• Pupils: equal, round, and reactive to light and accommodation (PERRLA)
• Lens: clear
• Extraocular movements: intact
• Disc margins: sharp
• Retinal vessels: normal, with no hemorrhages or spots

Assessment of the visual system may include all of the components described in the following material, or it may be as brief as measuring the patient's visual acuity. The nurse assesses what is appropriate and necessary for the specific patient. All of the following assessments are in the nurse's scope of practice, but some require special training. A normal physical assessment of the visual system is outlined in Table 23-3. Age-related visual changes and differences in assessment findings are listed in Table 23-1. Assessment techniques related to vision are summarized in Table 23-4. Common abnormalities found during assessment are listed in Table 23-5.

Initial Observation. The initial observation of the patient can provide information that will help the nurse focus the assessment. The patient with impaired colour vision may dress in clothing with unusual colour combinations. The patient with diplopia may hold the head in a skewed position in an attempt to see a single image. The patient with a corneal abrasion or photophobia may cover the eyes with the hands or wear dark glasses to try to block out room light. The nurse can make a crude estimate of depth perception by extending a hand for the patient to shake.

During the initial observation, the nurse should also observe overall facial and ophthalmic appearance of the patient. The eyes should be symmetrical and normally positioned on the face. The globes should not have a bulging or sunken appearance.

Assessing Functional Status

Visual Acuity. Before the patient receives any care, the nurse should record the patient's visual acuity for medical and legal reasons.

To assess distance visual acuity, the patient sits or stands 6 metres (20 feet) from the Snellen chart with the usual correction (glasses or contact lenses) left in place unless they are used solely for reading. The nurse asks the patient to cover the left eye with an eye spoon and read through the chart to the smallest line of letters that the patient can possibly discern. The nurse notes the smallest line the patient can read with 50% or fewer errors. The nurse then asks the patient to cover the right eye, and the process is repeated. At the left of most rows of the Snellen chart is a fraction (e.g., "20/30") in which the numerator represents the distance the patient is from the chart and the denominator represents the distance at which a normal eye could see the letters in the row. For example, a patient with a visual acuity of 20/30 sees at 20 feet what the patient with no vision problems would see at

NURSING ASSESSMENT

Table 23-4 Assessment Techniques: Visual System

TECHNIQUE	DESCRIPTION	PURPOSE
Basic Techniques		
Visual acuity testing	Patient reads from Snellen chart at a distance of 6 m (distance vision test) or Jaeger's chart at a distance of 35 cm (near vision test); examiner notes smallest print that patient can read on each chart.	To determine patient's distance and near visual acuity
Confrontation visual field test	Patient faces examiner, covers one eye, fixates on examiner's face, and counts number of fingers that the examiner brings into patient's field of vision.	To determine whether patient has a full field of vision, without obvious scotomas
Pupil function testing	Examiner shines light into patient's pupil and observes pupillary response; each pupil is examined independently; examiner also checks for consensual and accommodative response.	To determine whether patient has normal pupillary response
Extraocular muscle functioning	Patient faces examiner, holds head still, and follows (with eyes only) object that examiner moves through 6 cardinal positions of gaze. Examiner also uses corneal light reflex test.	To determine whether muscles and cranial nerves III, IV, and VI are functioning normally
Colour vision testing	Patient identifies numbers or paths formed by pattern of dots in a series of colour plates.	To determine patient's ability to distinguish colours
Advanced Techniques*		
Tono-Pen tonometry	Covered end of probe gently touches the anaesthetized corneal surface several times; examiner records several readings to obtain a mean intraocular pressure (see Figure 23-6).	To measure intraocular pressure (normal pressure is 10-22 mm Hg)
Ophthalmoscopy	Examiner holds ophthalmoscope close to patient's eye, shining light into back of eye and looking through aperture on ophthalmoscope; examiner adjusts dial to select one of the lenses in ophthalmoscope that produces the desired amount of magnification to inspect ocular fundus.	To provide magnified view of retina and optic nerve head
Keratometry	Examiner aligns the projection and notes the readings of corneal curvature.	To measure the corneal curvature; often performed before fitting of contact lenses, before refractive surgery, or after corneal transplantation

*Performed by qualified health care provider.

COMMON ASSESSMENT ABNORMALITIES

Table 23-5 Visual System

FINDING	DESCRIPTION	POSSIBLE CAUSE AND SIGNIFICANCE
Subjective Data		
Pain	Foreign body sensation	Superficial corneal erosion or abrasion; can result from contact lens wear or trauma or from foreign body in the conjunctiva or cornea
	Severe, deep, throbbing	Anterior uveitis, acute glaucoma, infection; acute glaucoma also associated with nausea, vomiting
Photophobia	Persistent abnormal intolerance to light	Inflammation or infection of cornea or anterior uveal tract (iris and ciliary body), conjunctivitis
Blurred vision	Gradual or sudden inability to see clearly	Refractive errors, corneal opacities, cataracts, migraine aura, retinal changes (detachment, macular degeneration)
Spots, floaters	Patient describes seeing spots, "spider webs," "curtain," or floaters within the field of vision	Most common cause is liquefaction of the vitreous humor (benign phenomenon); other possible causes include hemorrhage into the vitreous humor, retinal holes, or retinal tears
Dryness	Discomfort, sandy or gritty sensation, irritation, or burning	Decreased tear formation or changes in tear composition because of aging or various systemic diseases
Diplopia	Double vision	Abnormalities of extraocular muscle action related to muscle or cranial nerve abnormality
Glare	Headache, ocular discomfort, reduced visual acuity	Related to corneal inflammation or to opacities in cornea, lens, or vitreous humor that scatter the incoming light; can also result from light scatter around edges of an intraocular lens; worse at night, when pupil is dilated

COMMON ASSESSMENT ABNORMALITIES

Table 23-5 Visual System—cont'd

FINDING	DESCRIPTION	POSSIBLE CAUSE AND SIGNIFICANCE
Objective Data		
Eyelids		
Allergic reactions	Redness, excessive tearing, and itching of eyelid margins	Many possible allergens; associated eye trauma can occur from rubbing itchy eyelids
Hordeolum (sty)	Small, superficial white nodule along eyelid margin	Infection of a sebaceous gland of eyelid; causative organism is usually bacterial (most commonly *Staphylococcus aureus*)
Blepharitis	Redness, swelling, and crusting along eyelid margins	Bacterial invasion of eyelid margins; often chronic
Ptosis	Drooping of upper eyelid margin; unilateral or bilateral	Mechanical causes as a result of eyelid tumours or excess skin; myogenic causes such as myasthenia gravis or neurogenic causes
Entropion	Inward turning of upper or lower eyelid margin, unilateral or bilateral	Congenital causes resulting in development abnormalities
Ectropion	Outward turning of lower eyelid margin	Mechanical causes as a result of eyelid tumours, herniated orbital fat, or extravasation of fluid
Conjunctiva		
Conjunctivitis	Redness, swelling of conjunctiva; may be itchy	Bacterial or viral infection; may be allergic response or inflammatory response to chemical exposure
Subconjunctival hemorrhage	Appearance of blood spot on sclera; may be small or can affect entire sclera	Conjunctival blood vessels rupture, leaking blood into the subconjunctival space
Cornea and Sclera		
Corneal abrasion	Localized painful disruption of the epithelial layer of cornea; can be visualized with fluorescein dye	Trauma; overwear or improper fit of contact lenses
Jaundice	Yellow discoloration* of the entire sclera	Related to liver dysfunction or hemolytic disease
Globe		
Exophthalmos	Protrusion of globe beyond its normal position within bony orbit; sclera often visible above iris when eyelids are open	Intraocular or periorbital tumours; hyperthyroidism; Crouzon's syndrome
Pupil		
Anisocoria	Pupils are unequal (constricted)	Central nervous system disorders; in a small percentage of the population, slight difference in pupil size is normal
Abnormal response to light or accommodation	Pupils respond asymmetrically or abnormally to light stimulus or accommodation	Central nervous system disorders, general anaesthesia
Iris		
Heterochromia	Irides are different colours†	Congenital causes (Horner's syndrome); acquired causes (chronic iritis, metastatic carcinoma, diffuse iris nevus or melanoma)
Extraocular Muscles		
Strabismus	Deviation of eye position in one or more directions	Overaction or underaction of one or more extraocular muscles
Lens		
Cataract	Opacification of lens; pupil can appear cloudy or white when opacity is visible behind pupil opening	Aging, trauma, diabetes, long-term systemic corticosteroid therapy
Visual Field Defect		
Peripheral	Partial or complete loss of peripheral vision	Glaucoma; interruption of visual pathway (e.g., tumour); migraine headache
Central	Loss of central vision	Macular disease

*Yellow colour is normal after a diagnostic study necessitating intravenous fluorescein injection.

†Most cases of heterochromia occur by chance and are not associated with any other symptoms or problems.

30 feet. The larger the denominator, the worse the visual acuity. If vision is poorer than 20/30, the patient should be referred to an ophthalmologist or optometrist (Jarvis et al., 2009). *Legal blindness* is defined as the best corrected vision in the better eye of 20/200 or worse. If a patient cannot read letters, the nurse can use an eye chart with pictures, numbers, or symbols, such as the Stycar graded-balls test, the Sheridan-Gardiner letter-matching test, or the Snellen E chart.

To evaluate visual acuity when the patient is unable to see even the largest letters, the nurse holds up a number of fingers in front of the patient at successively closer distances and asks the patient to count them. If the patient cannot count the fingers, the nurse asks the patient to indicate whether he or she can see hand motion or light from a penlight in front of the face.

If the patient has a complaint of near vision problems, and for all patients 40 years of age or older, the nurse tests near visual acuity. The patient is instructed to hold a Jaeger chart 35 cm (14 inches) from the eyes. The nurse covers the patient's left eye with an eye spoon, asks the patient to read successively smaller lines of print from the chart, and records the visual acuity corresponding to the smallest line of print that the patient can read comfortably. The procedure is repeated with the right eye covered. A normal result is 14/14. A result of 14/20 means the person can read at 14 inches what someone with normal vision reads at 20 inches. If a screening card is not available, near vision acuity can be assessed by asking the patient to read from a newspaper.

Extraocular Muscle Functions. The nurse observes the corneal light reflex to evaluate for weakness or imbalance of the extraocular muscles. In a darkened room, the nurse asks the patient to look straight ahead while a penlight is shone directly on the cornea. The light reflection should be located in the centre of both corneas as the patient faces the light source.

To assess eye movement, the nurse should hold a finger or object 25 to 30 cm from the patient's nose. The patient is asked to follow the movement of the object or finger with only his or her eyes through the six cardinal positions of gaze (Figure 23-4). This test can indicate weakness or paralysis in the extraocular muscles or dysfunction in a cranial nerve (oculomotor nerve [CN III], trochlear nerve [CN IV], and abducens nerve [CN VI]). The nurse should pay attention to the ends of each gaze position, inasmuch as weakness appears there first (Williams, 2006).

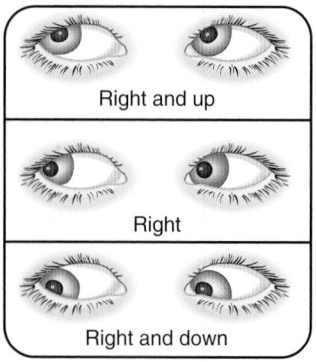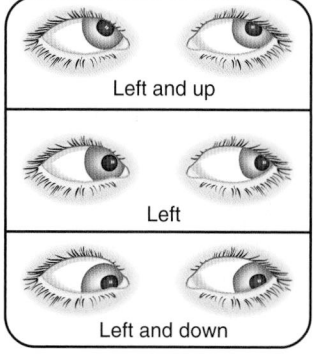

Right and up | Left and up
Right | Left
Right and down | Left and down

Figure 23-4 Six cardinal positions of gaze.

Source: Adapted from Kanski, J. J. (2009). *Clinical ophthalmology: A synopsis* (2nd ed.). New York: Butterworth-Heinemann.

Pupil Function. To determine pupil function, the nurse inspects the pupils and their reactions to light. Pupils should be equal in size and round and should react briskly to light. Pupil size is noted before reaction to light is checked. With age, pupil size decreases (Williams, 2006). In a small percentage of the population, pupils are unequal in size (anisocoria). Pupils should react to light directly (pupil constricts when a light shines into the eye) and consensually (pupil of one eye constricts when a light shines into opposite eye). Accommodation should also be present: When the patient looks at a distant object 0.6 to 0.9 metres away and then is asked to focus on an object 7 to 8 cm from the nose, the nurse should observe convergence of the eyes and constriction of the pupils. Normal pupil function may be documented as **PERRLA** (pupils equal, round, reactive to light and accommodation).

Assessing Structures. The visual system is unique because the nurse can directly inspect not only the external structures but also many of the internal structures by using special equipment such as the ophthalmoscope and the slit-lamp microscope, which enables examination of conjunctiva, sclera, cornea, anterior chamber, iris, lens, vitreous humor, and retina under magnification. The *ophthalmoscope,* a handheld instrument with a light source and magnifying lenses, is held close to the patient's eye to visualize the posterior part of the eye. Little pain or discomfort is associated with these examinations.

Eyebrows, Eyelashes, and Eyelids. All structures should be present, symmetrical, and without deformities, redness, or swelling. Eyelashes extend outward from the eyelid margins. In normal closing, the upper and lower eyelid margins just touch. The lacrimal puncta should be open and positioned properly against the globe. If the sac is inflamed, pressure over the lacrimal sac may cause purulent material to ooze from the puncta.

Conjunctiva and Sclera. The nurse can easily examine the conjunctiva and sclera at the same time, evaluating colour, smoothness, and presence of any lesions or foreign bodies. The conjunctiva covering the sclera is normally clear, with fine blood vessels visible. These blood vessels are more common in the periphery.

The sclera is normally white, but it may take on a yellowish hue in older individuals because of lipid deposition. A pale blue cast caused by scleral thinning can also be normal in older adults and infants (who have naturally thinner sclerae). A slightly yellow cast may also be found in some dark-skinned persons.

Cornea. The cornea should be clear, transparent, and shiny. The iris should appear flat and not bulge toward the cornea. The area between the cornea and iris should be clear, with no blood or purulent material visible in the anterior chamber.

Iris. Both irides should be of similar colour and shape. However, a colour difference between the irides is normal in a small proportion of individuals. Round or notched areas of missing iris tissue are often the result of cataract or glaucoma surgery. A triangular area may indicate an iridectomy scar, whereas a circular one may be a result of laser surgery (Williams, 2006). The nurse should determine the cause of these round, notched, or triangular areas and document the findings.

Retina and Optic Nerve. To assess these structures, the nurse uses an ophthalmoscope to magnify the ocular structures and bring them into crisp focus (Figure 23-5). The ability to directly view arteries, veins, and the optic nerve in this manner is unique. The nurse directs the beam of light from the

Optic disc   Fovea centralis

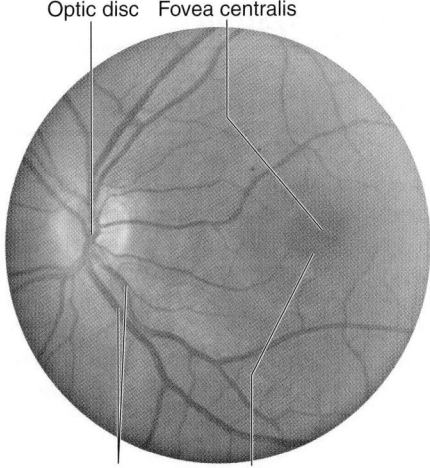

Retinal blood vessels   Macula

Figure 23-5 Illustration of magnified view of retina through the ophthalmoscope.

Source: Newell, F. W. (1992). *Ophthalmology: Principles and concepts* (7th ed.). St. Louis: Mosby.

ophthalmoscope obliquely into the patient's pupils and should note the appearance of a *red reflex*. This reflex is a result of light's reflecting off the retina. Any dense area in the lens or nontransparent material in the vitreous humor decreases the red reflex. The optic nerve or disc is examined for size, colour, and abnormalities. The optic disc is creamy yellow with distinct margins. A slight blurring of the nasal margin is common.

A central depression in the disc, called the *physiologic cup*, is the exit site for the optic nerve. The cup should be less than one half the diameter of the disc. Normally, no hemorrhages or exudates are present in the fundus (retinal background). Careful inspection of the fundus can reveal the presence of retinal holes, tears, detachments, or lesions. Small hemorrhages can be associated with diabetes or hypertension and can appear in various shapes, such as dots or flames. Finally, the nurse examines the macula for shape and appearance. This area of high reflectivity is devoid of any blood vessels.

The nurse can obtain important information about the vascular system and the central nervous system through direct visualization with an ophthalmoscope. Skilled use of this instrument requires practice.

Focused Assessment. A focused assessment (see the Focused Assessment box "Visual System") may be performed by a generalist nurse when a patient is admitted to a medical-surgical unit or outpatient clinic. Inspection of the eyes may be performed routinely as part of the assessment of a hospitalized patient. In addition, the nurse should assess for and document use of glasses or contact lenses. Assessment of PERRLA may be performed routinely as part of neurological assessment of a hospitalized patient (see Chapter 59).

Special Assessment Techniques

Colour Vision. Testing the patient's ability to distinguish colours can be an important part of the overall assessment because some occupations may require accurate colour discrimination. The Ishihara colour test determines the patient's ability to distinguish a pattern of colour in a series of colour plates. Older adults have a loss of colour discrimination at the blue end

of the colour spectrum and loss of sensitivity throughout the entire spectrum, especially when cataracts are present.

Stereopsis. *Stereoscopic vision* allows a patient to see objects in three dimensions. Any event causing a patient to have monocular vision (e.g., enucleation, patching) results in loss of stereoscopic vision, impairing the individual's ability to judge distances. This condition can have serious consequences: for example, if the patient trips over a step when walking or follows too closely behind another vehicle when driving.

Intraocular Pressure. Testing intraocular pressure is important because high intraocular pressure is a major risk factor for glaucoma. Intraocular pressure can be measured by a variety of methods, including the Tono-Pen (Figure 23-6). Use of the Tono-Pen is common because it is simple and the results are very accurate. The surface of the anaesthetized cornea is touched lightly several times with the covered end of the probe. The instrument records several readings and provides a mean measurement on a digital light-emitting diode (LED) screen located on the front surface. Normal intraocular pressure ranges from 10 to 22 mm Hg.

Diagnostic Studies

Diagnostic studies provide important information to the nurse monitoring the patient's condition and planning appropriate interventions. These studies are considered objective data. Table 23-6 presents the most common basic diagnostic studies of the visual system.

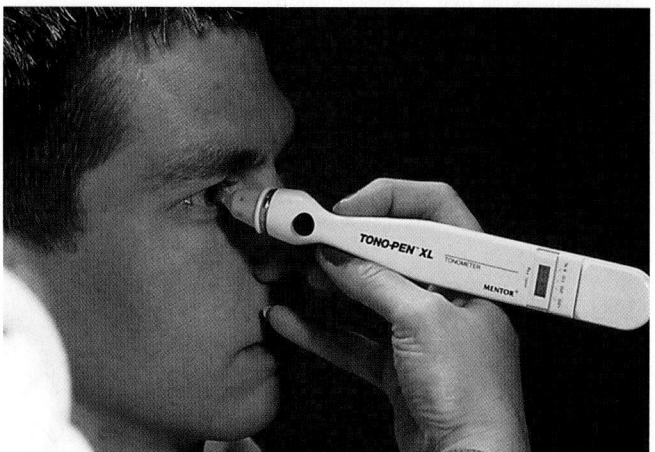

Figure 23-6 Tono-Pen tonometry.

Source: Courtesy Eye Institute, Department of Ophthalmology and Visual Services, University of Iowa Health Care, Iowa City, Iowa.

The Auditory System

Structures and Functions

The auditory system is composed of the peripheral and central auditory systems. The peripheral system includes the structures of the ear itself: external, middle, and inner ear (Figure 23-7). This system is concerned with the reception and perception of sound. The external and middle portions of the ear function to conduct and amplify sound waves from the environment. The inner ear serves functions of hearing and balance. The central system (the brain and its pathways) integrates and assigns meaning to what is heard.

External Ear

The external ear consists of the *auricle* (pinna) and the external auditory canal. The auricle is composed of cartilage and connective tissue covered with epithelium, which also lines the external auditory canal (see Figure 23-7). The external auditory canal is a slightly S-shaped tube about 2.5 cm in length in the adult. The skin that lines the canal contains fine hairs and sebaceous (oil) glands and ceruminous (wax) glands. The oil and wax lubricate the ear canal, keep it free from debris, and kill bacteria (Herlihy & Maebius, 2007).

Hair is present in the outer half of the canal. The inner half of the ear canal is highly sensitive. The function of the external ear and canal is to collect and transmit sound waves to the

DIAGNOSTIC STUDIES

Table 23-6 Visual System

STUDY	DESCRIPTION AND PURPOSE	NURSING RESPONSIBILITY*
Refractometry	Subjective measure of refractive error; multiple lenses are mounted on rotating wheels. While patient sits looking through apertures at Snellen acuity chart, lenses are changed; patient chooses lenses that make acuity sharpest. Cycloplegic drugs are used to paralyze accommodation during refraction process.	Procedure is painless; patient may need help holding the head still. Pupil dilation makes it difficult for the patient to focus on near objects; dilation may last from 3-4 hr.
Ultrasonography	A-scan probe is placed on patient's anaesthetized cornea; used primarily for axial length measurement for calculating power of intraocular lens implanted after cataract extraction. B-scan probe is applied to patient's closed eyelid; used more often than A-scan for diagnosis of ocular disorders such as intraocular foreign bodies or tumours, opacities in the vitreous humor, retinal detachments.	Procedure is painless (cornea is anaesthetized).
Fluorescein angiography	Fluorescein (a nonradioactive, noniodine dye) is intravenously injected into antecubital or other peripheral vein, followed by serial photographs (over 10-min period) of the retina through dilated pupils. Provides diagnostic information about flow of blood through pigment epithelial and retinal vessels; often used in patients with diabetes to accurately locate areas of diabetic retinopathy before laser destruction of neovascularization.	Fluorescein is toxic to tissue if extravasation occurs; systemic allergic reactions are rare, but the nurse should be familiar with emergency equipment and procedures. The patient should be informed that dye can sometimes cause transient nausea or vomiting and transient yellow discoloration of urine and skin.
Amsler grid test	Test is self-administered with a handheld card printed with a grid of lines (similar to graph paper); patient fixates on centre dot and records any abnormalities of the grid lines, such as wavy, missing, or distorted areas. Test is used to monitor macular problems.	Regular testing is necessary to identify any changes in macular function.

*Patient education regarding the purpose and method of testing is a nursing responsibility for all diagnostic procedures.

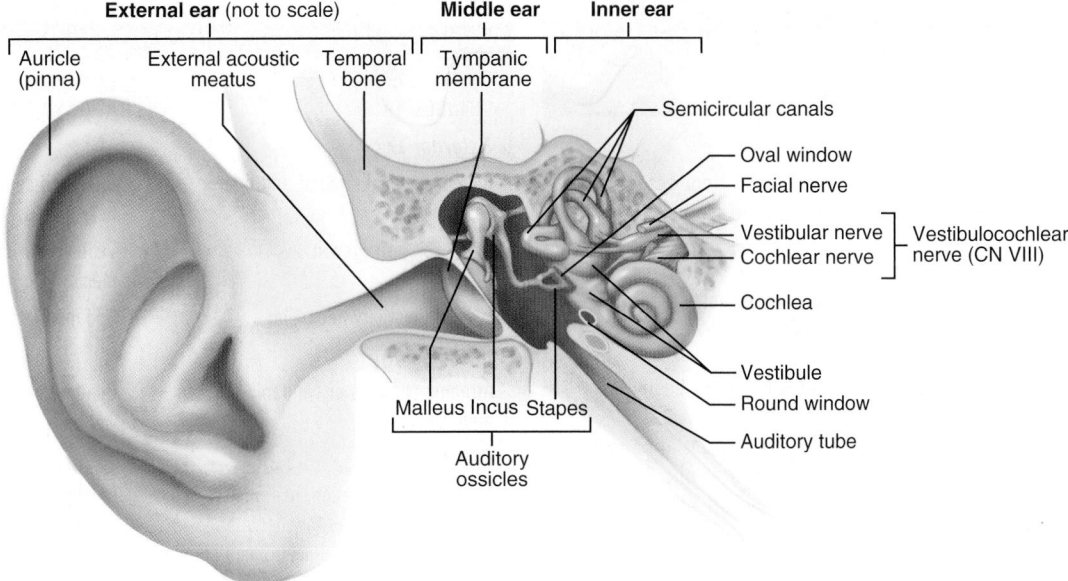

Figure 23-7 External, middle, and inner ear. CN, cranial nerve.

Source: Patton, K. T., & Thibodeau, G. A. (2010). *Anatomy and physiology* (7th ed., p. 506, Figure 15-11). St. Louis: Mosby.

tympanic membrane (eardrum). This shiny, translucent, pearl-grey membrane is composed of epithelial cells, connective tissue, and mucous membrane. It serves as a partition and instrument of sound transmission between the external auditory canal and middle ear.

Middle Ear

The middle ear cavity is an air space located in the temporal bone. Mucosa lines the middle ear and is continuous from the nasal pharynx via the Eustachian (auditory) tube. The Eustachian tube functions to equalize atmospheric air pressure between the middle ear and throat and allows the tympanic membrane to move freely. It opens during yawning and swallowing. Blockage of this tube can occur with allergies, nasopharyngeal infections, or enlarged adenoids. The middle ear contains three tiny bones: *malleus, incus,* and *stapes* (ossicles). Vibrations of the tympanic membrane cause the ossicles to move and transmit sound waves to the oval window. This oval-window vibration causes fluid in the inner ear to move and stimulate hearing receptors. The round window sits below the oval window and is covered with a thin membrane called the *fenestra cochlea;* it also opens into the inner ear and acts as a pressure valve that moves outward as fluid pressure builds in the inner ear. The superior part of the middle ear is called the *epitympanum* (attic). It also communicates with air cells within the mastoid bone. The facial nerve (CN VII) passes above the oval window of the middle ear. The thin, bony covering of the facial nerve can become damaged by chronic ear infection, skull fracture, or trauma during ear surgery. Such damage can cause problems with voluntary facial movements, eyelid closure, and taste discrimination. Permanent damage to the facial nerve can also result.

Inner Ear

The inner ear is composed of a bony labyrinth (maze) surrounding a membrane. This complex contains the functional organs for hearing and balance. The receptor organ for hearing is the *cochlea,* a coiled structure. It contains the *organ of Corti,* whose tiny hair cells respond to stimulation of selected portions of the basilar membrane according to pitch. This stimulus is converted into an electrochemical impulse and then transmitted by the cochlear branch of the vestibulocochlear nerve (CN VIII; formerly called the *acoustic nerve*) to the temporal lobe of the brain to process and interpret the sound.

Three semicircular canals and the vestibule make up the organ of balance. These structures make up the membranous labyrinth, which is housed in the bony labyrinth. The membranous labyrinth is filled with endolymphatic fluid, and the bony labyrinth is filled with perilymphatic fluid. The fluid cushions these two sensitive organs and communicates with the brain and the subarachnoid spaces of the brain. The nervous stimuli are communicated by the vestibular portion of CN VIII. Debris or excessive pressure within the lymphatic fluid can cause disorders such as vertigo.

Transmission of Sound and Implications for Hearing Loss

Sound waves are conducted by air (air conduction) and picked up by the auricles and the auditory canal. The sound waves strike the tympanic membrane, causing it to vibrate. The central area of the tympanic membrane is connected to the malleus, which also starts to vibrate, transmitting the vibration to the incus and then the stapes. As the stapes moves back and forth, it pushes the membrane of the oval window in and out. Movement of the oval window produces waves in the perilymph. Pathological disturbances in the external ear canal or within the middle ear may cause a conductive hearing loss, resulting in an alteration in the patient's perception of or sensitivity to sounds. Older adult patients may exhibit decreased hearing as a result of impacted cerumen in the ear canal.

Once sound has been transmitted to the liquid medium of the inner ear, the vibration is picked up by the tiny sensory hair cells of the cochlea, which initiate nerve impulses. These impulses are carried by nerve fibres to the main branch of the acoustic

DETERMINANTS OF HEALTH
Auditory System

Biology and Genetics

- There is a higher prevalence of corrected and uncorrected hearing impairment among Canadian men than women (Corna, Wade, Streiner, & Cairney, 2009).
- Persons of European or African descent are likely to have wet cerumen that is moist and brown or tan, whereas persons of Asian or Native American descent are likely to have dry cerumen that is flaky and grey (Miller, 2012).
- Cerumen becomes drier, harder, coarser, and more easily impacted as persons age.
- Elderly persons, young children, and the cognitively impaired are at high risk for cerumen impaction (Roland et al., 2008).
- Otitis media is more common and more severe in Aboriginal, Inuit, and Hispanic people (Jarvis et al., 2009).
- Infections such as otitis media are more common in children, whereas otosclerosis is more common in young adults (Jarvis et al., 2009).
- Of Canadians over 75 years old, 50% have developed a hearing loss, and this increases to 80% for those over 85 (Bance, 2007).

AGE-RELATED DIFFERENCES IN ASSESSMENT

Table 23-7 Auditory System

CHANGES	DIFFERENCES IN ASSESSMENT FINDINGS
External Ear	
Increased production of and drier cerumen	Impacted cerumen; potential hearing loss
Increased hair growth	Visible hair, especially in men
Loss of elasticity in cartilage	Collapsed ear canal
Middle Ear	
Atrophic changes of tympanic membrane	Conductive hearing loss
Inner Ear	
Hair cell degeneration, neuron degeneration in auditory nerve and central pathways, reduced blood supply to cochlea, calcification of ossicles	Presbycusis, diminished sensitivity to high-pitched sounds, impairment in speech reception, tinnitus
Less effective vestibular apparatus in semicircular canals	Alterations in balance and body orientation

portion of CN VIII and then to the brain. Disruptions of the inner ear or along the nerve pathway from the inner ear to the brain can result in sensorineural hearing loss. This may result in an alteration of the patient's perception of or sensitivity to specific tones. Impairment within the central auditory system causes *central hearing loss.* This type of hearing loss causes difficulty in understanding the meaning of words that are heard. (Types of hearing loss are discussed further in Chapter 24.) Biological and genetic determinants can also affect hearing quality (see the Determinants of Health box "Auditory System").

The bones of the skull can also transmit sound directly to the inner ear (bone conduction). This can be demonstrated by placing the stem of a vibrating tuning fork on the patient's head, against the skull.

AGE-RELATED CONSIDERATIONS: THE AUDITORY SYSTEM

Age-related changes of the auditory system can result in hearing impairment. *Presbycusis,* or hearing loss caused by aging, can also result from insults from a variety of sources. Noise exposure, vascular or systemic diseases, poor or inadequate nutrition, ototoxic drugs, and pollution during the lifespan can damage delicate hair cells of the organ of Corti or cause atrophy of lymph-producing cells. Sound transmission is diminished by calcification of the ossicles. Dry cerumen in the external canal can also interfere with transmission of sound. **Tinnitus,** or ringing in the ears, may accompany hearing loss that results from the aging process.

Hearing loss, especially in the older adult, can have serious implications for the quality of life, including progressive physical and psychosocial dysfunction (Seidel, Ball, Dains, & Benedict, 2011). As the average lifespan increases, the number of people

with hearing loss will also increase. Early identification of problems will ensure that patients in their seventh and eighth decades are more active and healthy.

Age-related changes in the auditory system and differences in assessment findings are presented in Table 23-7.

Assessment

Assessment of the auditory system includes assessment of the *vestibular* (balance) system because the auditory and vestibular systems are so closely related. It is often difficult to separate symptoms from the two systems. The nurse should, if necessary, help the patient describe symptoms and problems in order to differentiate the source of the problems. Health history questions to ask a patient with an auditory problem are listed in Table 23-8.

Problems with balance may manifest as nystagmus or vertigo. **Nystagmus** is abnormal eye movements that may be observed by other people as twitching of the eyeball or may be described by the patient as a blurring of vision with head or eye movement. **Vertigo** is a sense that the person or objects around the person are moving or spinning and is usually stimulated by movement of the head. Dizziness is a sensation of being off-balance that occurs when the person is standing or walking. It does not occur when the person is lying down.

Initially, the nurse should try to categorize symptoms related to balance and distinguish them from symptoms related to hearing loss or tinnitus. The symptoms can be combined later in the assessment to help make the diagnosis and plan for treatment.

Subjective Data

Important Health History
Current Health of Auditory System. The nurse should inquire about earache or pain in the ear. Such pain may be caused

HEALTH HISTORY

Table 23-8 Auditory System: Questions for Obtaining Subjective Data

Earache

- Do you have earache or another kind of pain in your ear?*
- Where is it located? Can you describe the pain?
- Do you have any symptoms of a cold or a sore throat?*
- What measures have you used to relieve the pain?* Were they effective?

Discharge

- Have you experienced discharge from your ears? How much and what colour?
- Have you had ear infections? How frequent? How were they treated?

Hearing Loss

- Was the hearing loss sudden or gradual?*
- Is it all your hearing or just hearing of certain sounds that has decreased?
- Where do you notice the hearing loss (e.g., conversations in a crowd, telephone conversations, watching television)?
- Have you travelled by airplane recently?
- How does the hearing loss affect your life at home and at work?
- Do you have any allergies that result in ear problems?*
- How does your hearing loss affect your daily life?

Environmental Noise

- Do you have loud noise in your home or work environment?*
- Do you work near loud noises such as heavy machinery or drums in a band?

Tinnitus

- Have you ever experienced ringing, crackling, or buzzing in your ears?*
- Does the noise seem louder at certain times?*
- When does it bother you the most?
- What things have you tried that help?

Vertigo

- Have you felt vertigo—a spinning sensation?*
- Have you felt dizzy, as if you were falling or losing your balance?*
- Do you ever experience lightheadedness or giddiness?*
- Have you ever fallen because of the dizziness?*
- How does your dizziness affect your daily life?*

Nutrition and Elimination

- Do you have any food allergies that affect your ears?*
- Do you notice any differences in symptoms with changes in your diet?*
- Does your ear problem cause nausea that interferes with your food intake?*
- Does chewing or swallowing cause you any ear discomfort?
- Does straining during a bowel movement cause you ear pain?*

Activities of Daily Living and Exercise

- Does your ear problem cause you to change your usual activity or exercise?*
- Do you need help with certain activities (e.g., lifting, bending, climbing stairs, driving, speaking) because of symptoms?*
- Do you have any limitations in activities of daily living because of your symptoms?*
- Is your sleep disturbed by symptoms of pain, tinnitus, or dizziness?*

Self-Care History

- When did you last have your ears checked?
- How do you clean your ears?
- Do you use any devices to improve your hearing (e.g., hearing aid, special volume control, headphones for television or audio devices)?*
- How long have you used a hearing aid? Do you have any problems using or maintaining your hearing aid?*
- Do you use any means to protect your ears such as headphones or earplugs?* When?
- Do you use personal sound systems such as iPods or MP3 players?*

Coping Abilities

- Is your ability to communicate and understand affected by your symptoms?*
- Have changes in your hearing affected your self-esteem or feeling of independence?*
- What effect has your ear problem had on your work, family, or social life?
- Do you feel able to cope with your hearing or balance problem? If no, describe.
- Do you consider your ear problem a stressor?*

*If yes, describe.

Source: Adapted from Jarvis, C., Browne, A. J., MacDonald-Jenkins, J., & Luctkar-Flude, M. (Eds.). (2009). *Physical examination and health assessment* (1st Canadian ed., pp. 346-348). Toronto: Elsevier Canada.

by ear disease such as infection or may be referred pain originating in the teeth or temporomandibular joint. Pain is associated with some ear problems, particularly those involving the middle ear. If pain is present, the patient should be asked to describe the pain and the treatments used for relief. The effect on the pain level when the auricle is moved or the tragus is palpated should be noted.

If the patient has experienced any ear infections or has a history of chronic ear infections, this may contribute to increased hearing loss. Pus or bloody discharge may indicate an ear infection, whereas a clear discharge may consist of cerebrospinal fluid, particularly if the patient has received any head trauma. The nurse should note the time of onset of the hearing loss and whether it

is sudden or gradual. The person who noted the onset should be recorded, whether the patient, a family member, or a significant other. Gradual hearing losses are most often noted by persons who communicate regularly with the patient. Sudden losses and those exacerbated by some other condition are most often reported by the patient. If a hearing loss is identified in an older adult patient, the nurse can use the questions from the Hearing Handicap Inventory for Older Persons (Table 23-9). The higher the score on the inventory, the more severe the hearing handicap. Referral is recommended for individuals scoring 10 or higher on the inventory.

If the patient has experienced any ringing, crackling, or buzzing sensation, the nurse should note time of onset and

Table 23-9 The Hearing Handicap Inventory for Older Persons*

Does a hearing problem cause you

1. (E) To feel embarrassed when meeting new people?
2. (E) To feel frustrated when talking to members of your family?
3. (S) To have difficulty understanding when someone speaks in a whisper?
4. (E) To feel handicapped?
5. (S) To have difficulty when visiting friends, relatives, or neighbours?
6. (S) To attend religious services less often than you would like?
7. (E) To have arguments with family members?
8. (S) To have difficulty when listening to television or radio?
9. (E) To feel that your hearing limits or hampers your personal or social life?
10. (S) To have difficulty when in a restaurant with relatives and friends?

*Overall scoring: *yes* = 4 points; *sometimes* = 2 points; *no* = 0 points. (E), emotional handicap question; (S), social handicap question.
Source: Adapted from Bance, M. (2007). Hearing and aging. *Canadian Medical Association Journal, 176*(7), 925-927. By permission of the publisher. © 1982 Canadian Medical Association.

whether the patient is taking any medications that might cause tinnitus.

Symptoms such as dizziness, tinnitus, and hearing loss are recorded in detail in the patient's own words. This careful description could help differentiate the cause.

Health History. Many problems related to the ear are sequelae of childhood illnesses or result from problems of adjacent organs. Consequently, a careful assessment of past health problems is important.

The patient should be questioned about previous problems regarding the ears, especially problems experienced during childhood. The frequency of acute middle ear infections (otitis media), perforations of the eardrum, drainage, and history of mumps, measles, or scarlet fever should be recorded. Congenital hearing loss can result from infectious diseases (e.g., rubella, influenza, or syphilis), teratogenic medications, or hypoxia in the first trimester of pregnancy. Head injury should be documented because it can result in hearing loss. Information about food and environmental allergies is important because they can cause the Eustachian tube to become edematous and prevent aeration of the middle ear.

Medications. The nurse should obtain information about current or past medications that are *ototoxic* (cause damage to CN VIII) and can produce hearing loss, tinnitus, and vertigo. The amount and frequency of aspirin use is important because tinnitus can result from high aspirin intake. Aminoglycosides, any other antibiotics, salicylates, antimalarial agents, chemotherapeutic drugs, diuretics, and nonsteroidal anti-inflammatory drugs are groups of drugs that are potentially ototoxic (Lehne, 2012). Careful monitoring for hearing and balance problems is essential. Many drugs produce hearing loss that may be reversible if treatment is stopped. The nurse should also inquire about the use of herbal or alternative therapies, including ear candling. Health Canada (2006) does not recommend ear candling

because patients have experienced burns and hearing loss as a result.

Surgery or Other Treatments. The nurse should obtain information regarding previous hospitalizations for ear surgery (e.g., myringotomy, tympanoplasty), as well as for tonsillectomy and adenoidectomy. Use of and satisfaction with a hearing aid should be documented. Problems with impacted cerumen should also be noted.

Family History. Information regarding family members with hearing loss and type of hearing loss is important. Some congenital hearing loss is hereditary. The age at onset of presbycusis also follows a familial pattern.

Nutrition and Elimination. Both alcohol and sodium affect the amount of endolymph in the inner ear system. Patients with Ménière's disease generally notice some improvement in their symptoms with alcohol restriction and a low-sodium diet. Improvements and exacerbations associated with food intake should be noted. The patient should also be questioned about any ear pain or discomfort that occurs with chewing or swallowing, which might decrease nutritional intake. This situation is often associated with a problem in the middle ear.

Assessment of clenching or grinding of the teeth helps differentiate problems of the ear from referred pain of the temporomandibular joint. The nurse should ask about dental problems and dentures.

Elimination patterns and their association with ear problems are mainly of interest in patients with perilymph fistula or patients immediately after surgery. Frequent constipation or straining with bowel or bladder elimination may interfere with healing of a perilymph fistula or its repair. A patient who has just undergone stapedectomy especially needs to prevent the increase in intracranial (and consequent inner ear) pressure associated with straining during bowel movements. Stool softeners may be ordered postoperatively for a patient who reports chronic problems with constipation.

Activities of Daily Living and Exercise. Activity and exercise review is most important in assessing a patient with vestibular problems. If vertigo is a problem, the patient should be questioned about the onset, duration, and frequency of this symptom. Patients who have Ménière's disease demonstrate increasing inability to compensate for environmental input as the day progresses. Symptoms are experienced particularly in the evening. In contrast, patients with chronic vertigo syndrome (benign paroxysmal positional vertigo) note that the symptoms improve throughout the day as adjustment to the visual and positional input from the environment occurs. The nurse and the patient should identify a list of activities and exercises that aggravate and relieve dizziness and vertigo or cause nausea or vomiting. Frequent repetition of an activity that causes symptoms (habituation) may help the body adjust so that the activity is no longer a problem.

A patient with chronic tinnitus should be questioned about sleep problems. Tinnitus can disturb sleep and activities conducted in a quiet environment. Affected patients should be asked whether they have used or tried any masking devices or techniques to drown out the tinnitus. The nurse should also assess for snoring because it can be caused by swelling or hypertrophy of tissue in the nasopharynx. This excessive tissue can impair the functioning of the Eustachian tube and cause the sensation of ear fullness or pain.

Self-Care History. Patients should be questioned about personal practices such as the last ear examination, use of cotton ear swabs, use of earphones for personal listening devices, and practices used to preserve hearing. Patients should be questioned about contact with environments that have excessive noise levels, such as work with jet engines and machinery, firing of firearms, and electronically amplified music. The use of protective ear covers or earplugs is good practice for persons in high-noise environments and is important to document.

If the patient is a swimmer, the frequency and duration of swimming and use of ear protection should be documented. It is also important to note the type of water (pool, lake, or ocean) in which the swimming takes place to help identify contact with contaminated water. Placement of any item in the ear, including hearing aids, that can cause trauma to the skin increases risk of infection.

Coping Abilities. Patients should be questioned about the effect the ear problem has had on family life, work responsibilities, and social relationships. Hearing loss can result in strained family relations and misunderstandings. Failure to acknowledge hearing loss and failure to seek treatment can further hinder family relationships.

Many jobs rely on the ability to hear accurately and respond appropriately. If a hearing loss is present, the nurse should gather detailed information of its effect on the patient's job. The patient should be assisted to realistically evaluate the job situation.

Hearing loss often leaves the patient feeling isolated from valued social relationships. The nurse should historically document social activities such as playing cards, going to movies, and attending religious functions from before and since the hearing loss occurred. Comparison of the frequency and enjoyment of the events can indicate whether a problem is present.

The unpredictability of vertigo attacks can have devastating effects on all aspects of a patient's life. Ordinary activities such as driving, child care, housework, climbing stairs, and cooking all acquire an element of danger. The patient should be asked to describe the effect of the vertigo on the many roles and responsibilities of life. Compensatory practices to avoid the development of dangerous situations should also be noted.

The nurse should determine whether hearing loss or deafness has interfered with the patient's establishment of a satisfactory sex life. Although intimacy does not depend on the ability to hear, it could interfere with establishing or maintaining a relationship.

Objective Data

Physical Examination. During the health history interview, the nurse can collect valuable objective data regarding the patient's ability to hear. Clues such as posturing of the head and appropriateness of responses should be noted. Does the patient ask to have certain words repeated? Does the patient intently watch the examiner but miss comments when not looking at the examiner? Such observations are significant and should be recorded. This is also important because many patients are unaware of hearing loss or do not admit to changes in hearing until moderate losses have occurred. A normal assessment of the ear is described in Table 23-10.

Table 23-10 Normal Physical Assessment of the Auditory System
• Ears: symmetrical in location and shape
• Auricles and tragus: nontender, without lesions
• Canal: clear; tympanic membrane: intact; landmarks and light reflex: intact
• Able to hear low whisper at 30 cm; Rinne's test results: air conduction is better than bone conduction; Weber's test results: no lateralization

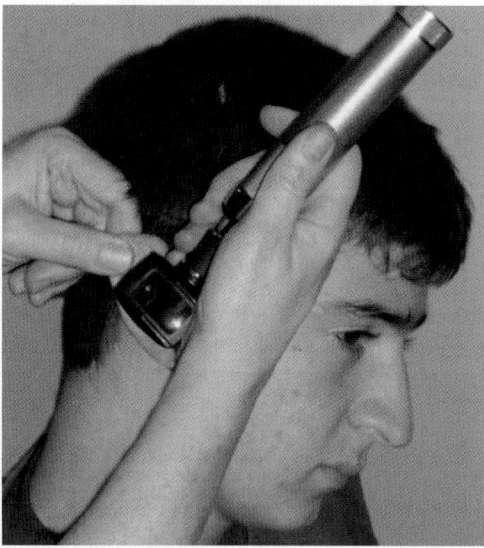

Figure 23-8 Otoscopic examination of the adult ear. Auricle is pulled up and back. The hand holding the otoscope is braced against the face for stabilization.

Source: Courtesy Maureen Barry.

Age-related changes of the auditory system and differences in assessment findings are listed in Table 23-7.

External Ear. The external ear is inspected and palpated before examination of the external canal and tympanum. The auricle, preauricular area, and mastoid area are observed for symmetry of both ears, colour of skin, temperature, nodules, swelling, redness, and lesions. The auricle and mastoid areas are then palpated for tenderness and nodules. Grasping the auricle may elicit a pain response, especially if inflammation of the external ear or canal is present.

External Auditory Canal and Tympanum. Before inserting an otoscope, the nurse should inspect the canal opening for patency, palpate the tragus, and gently move the auricle to check for discomfort. A speculum only slightly smaller than the size of the ear canal is selected. The patient's head is tipped to the opposite shoulder. The top of the auricle is grasped and gently pulled up and backward in adults and slightly down and backward in children to straighten the canal. The otoscope, held in the examiner's hand and stabilized on the patient's head by the examiner's fingers, is inserted slowly (Figure 23-8). A tight seal of the speculum is essential during this step of the examination. The canal is observed for size and shape, and the colour, amount, and type of cerumen. The tympanic membrane separates the external ear from the middle ear. If a large amount of cerumen is present, the tympanic membrane may not be visible. The tympanic membrane is observed for colour, landmarks, contour, and intactness (Figure 23-9). It is pearl-grey, white, or pink; shiny; and translucent. The handle *(manubrium)* of the malleus and the end

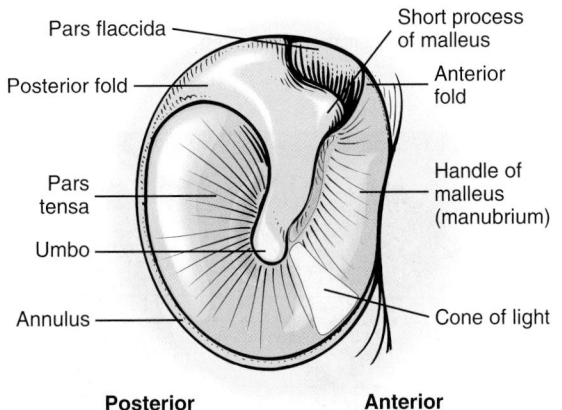

Pars flaccida
Posterior fold
Pars tensa
Umbo
Annulus
Short process of malleus
Anterior fold
Handle of malleus (manubrium)
Cone of light
Posterior   **Anterior**

Figure 23-9 Illustration of normal landmarks of the right tympanic membrane, as seen through an otoscope.

(umbo) are formed from the short process of the malleus and should be visible through the membrane. The somewhat anterior position and concave shape of the tympanic membrane causes the light from the otoscope to reflect back as a cone of light with crisp edges. If the tympanic membrane is bulging or retracted, the edges of the light reflex do not have the cone shape; instead, the reflected light spreads out or moves and has irregular edges (diffuse). The circumference of the tympanum is thickened into a dense, whitish, fibrous ring, or *annulus*, except in the superior area. The tympanum within the annulus *(pars tensa)* is taut. Above the short process of the malleus is the *pars flaccida*, the flaccid part of the tympanum. The malleolar folds are anterior and posterior to the short process of the malleus. The middle and inner ear cannot be examined with the otoscope because of the tympanic membrane. Table 23-11 summarizes common assessment abnormalities of the auditory system.

Focused Assessment. A focused assessment (see the Focused Assessment box "Auditory System") may be performed by a generalist nurse when a patient is admitted to a medical-surgical unit or outpatient clinic. Inspection of the ears may be performed routinely as part of the assessment of a hospitalized patient. In addition the nurse should assess for the presence of a hearing aid and document whether or not the patient has been using it.

COMMON ASSESSMENT ABNORMALITIES

Table 23-11 Auditory System

FINDING	DESCRIPTION	POSSIBLE CAUSE AND SIGNIFICANCE
External Ear and Canal		
Sebaceous cyst behind ear	Usually within skin, possible presence of black dot (opening to sebaceous gland)	Removal or incision and drainage if painful
Tophi	Hard nodules in the helix or antihelix consisting of uric acid crystals	Associated with gout, metabolic disorder; further diagnosis needed
Impacted cerumen	Wax that has not normally been excreted from the ear; no visualization of eardrum	Decreased hearing possible, sensation of fullness in auditory canal; removal necessary before otoscopic examination can be conducted
Discharge in canal	Infection of external ear, usually painful	Swimmer's ear, infection of external ear; possibly caused by ruptured eardrum and otitis media
Swelling of pinna, pain	Infection of glands of skin, hematoma caused by trauma	Aspiration (for hematoma)
Scaling or lesions	Change in usual appearance of skin	Seborrheic dermatitis, squamous cell carcinoma, atrophic dermatitis
Exostosis	Bony growth extending into canal, causing narrowing of canal	Possible interference with visualization of tympanum; usually asymptomatic
Tympanum		
Retracted eardrum	Appearance of shorter, more horizontal malleus; cone of light is absent or bent	Vacuum in middle ear, blockage of Eustachian tube, negative pressure in middle ear
Hairline fluid level, yellow-amber bubbles above fluid level	Caused by transudate of blood and serum; meniscus of fluid produces hairline appearance	Serous otitis media
Bulging red or blue eardrum, lack of landmarks	Middle ear filled with fluid (pus, blood)	Acute otitis media, perforation possible
Perforation of eardrum (central or marginal)	Previous perforations of the eardrum that have failed to heal; thin, transparent layer of epithelium surrounding eardrum	Chronic otitis media, mastoiditis
Recruitment	Disproportionate loudness of sound from malfunction of inner ear	Difficulty in using hearing aid

Auditory System

Use this checklist to make sure the key assessment steps have been performed.

Subjective

Ask the patient about any of the following and note responses

Changes in hearing	Y	N
Ear pain	Y	N
Ear drainage	Y	N

Objective: Physical Examination

Inspect

Alignment and position of ears on head	✓
Size, shape, symmetry, colour, and skin intactness	✓
External auditory meatus for discharge or lesions	✓

Assess

Hearing, according to ability to respond to conversation, respond to a whisper, or hear a ticking watch	✓

Diagnostic Studies

Table 23-12 describes diagnostic studies commonly used to assess the auditory system.

Tests for Hearing Acuity

Tests involving the whispered and the spoken voice can provide gross screening information about the patient's ability to hear. Audiometric testing provides more detailed information that can be used for diagnosis and treatment.

In the *whispered voice test,* the examiner stands 30 to 60 cm to the side of the patient and, after exhaling, speaks in a low whisper. A louder whisper is used if the patient does not respond correctly. Spoken voice, increasing in loudness, is similarly used. The patient is asked to repeat numbers or words or answer questions. Each ear is tested. The ear not being tested is masked by the patient, who occludes the ear, or by the examiner, who moves a finger rapidly, close to the ear canal.

Tuning-Fork Tests. Tuning-fork tests aid in differentiating between conductive and sensorineural hearing loss. Tuning forks of 512 Hz are generally used for this examination. Both skill and experience are required to ensure accurate results. If a problem is suspected, further evaluation by pure-tone audiometry is essential. The most common tuning-fork tests are Rinne's test and Weber's test.

For Rinne's test, the base of an activated tuning fork is held first against the mastoid bone and then 1 to 5 cm in front of the ear canal. The patient reports whether the sound is louder behind the ear (on the mastoid bone) or next to the ear canal. When the sound is no longer perceived behind the ear, the fork is moved next to the ear canal until the patient indicates that the sound is no longer heard. The test result is positive when the patient reports that air conduction is heard longer than bone conduction. This can indicate normal hearing or a sensorineural loss. If the patient hears the tuning fork better by bone conduction, the test result is negative, indicating that a conductive hearing loss is present.

For Weber's test, an activated tuning fork is placed on the midline of the skull, the forehead, or the teeth. The patient is asked to indicate where the sound is heard best. In conditions of normal auditory function, the patient perceives a midline tone best. If a patient has a conductive hearing loss in one ear, sound is heard louder (lateralizes) in that ear. If a sensorineural loss is present, sound is louder (lateralizes) in the unaffected ear.

Results of tuning fork tests are subjective. The patient with inconsistent test results or questionable results should be referred for more objective audiometric evaluation.

Audiometry. *Audiometry* is beneficial as a screening test for hearing acuity and as a diagnostic test for determining the degree and type of hearing loss. The audiometer produces pure tones at varying intensities to which the patient can respond. Sound is characterized by the number of vibrations or cycles that occur each second. *Hertz* (Hz) is the unit of measurement used to classify the frequency of a tone; the higher the frequency, the higher the pitch. Hearing loss can affect certain sound frequencies. The specific pattern produced on the audiogram by these losses can assist in the diagnosis of the type of hearing loss. The intensity or strength of a sound wave is expressed in terms of decibels (dB), ranging from 0 to 110 dB. The intensity of a sound required to make any frequency barely audible to the average normal ear is 0 dB. *Threshold* refers to the signal level at which pure tones are detected (pure tone thresholds) or the signal level at which the patient correctly hears 50% of the signals (speech detection thresholds).

Normal speech is approximately 40 to 65 dB; a soft whisper is 20 dB. Normally, a child and a young adult can hear frequencies from about 16 to 20,000 Hz, but hearing is most sensitive between 500 and 4000 Hz. This range is similar to that of the frequencies contained in speech. A 40- to 45-dB loss in these frequencies causes moderate difficulty in hearing normal speech. A hearing aid may be helpful because it makes sound information louder, although not clearer. A hearing aid may not be helpful to a patient who has problems with discrimination of sounds or sound information because the consonants are still not heard well enough to make speech understandable.

Screening Audiometry. Screening audiometry is the testing of large numbers of persons with a fast, simple test to detect possible hearing problems. A pass–fail criterion is used to screen persons who will or will not be given additional diagnostic testing. Persons who fail the screening should be referred to an audiologist for pure-tone (threshold) audiometry.

Pure-Tone Audiometry. A pure-tone audiometer produces tones at specific frequencies and intensities and is used by an audiologist to determine the hearing range of the patient in terms of decibels and hertz. Tinnitus can cause inconsistent results.

Specialized Tests

Specialized tests of the auditory system are most often performed in an outpatient setting by an audiologist. An audiologist can perform many additional tests with the use of audiometers and computers that record electrical activity from the middle ear, the inner ear, and the brain (see Table 23-11). The test most

DIAGNOSTIC STUDIES

Table 23-12　Auditory System

STUDY	DESCRIPTION AND PURPOSE	NURSING RESPONSIBILITY
Auditory		
Pure tone audiometry	Sounds are presented through earphones in soundproof room. Patient responds nonverbally when sound is heard. Response is recorded on an audiogram. Purpose is to determine patient's hearing range in terms of decibels (dB) and hertz (Hz) for diagnosing conductive and sensorineural hearing loss. Tinnitus can cause inconsistent results.	Nurse does not usually participate in examination.
Bone conduction	Tuning fork is placed on mastoid process, and hearing by bone conduction is recorded. Diagnoses conductive hearing loss.	Nurse may perform test.
One- and two-syllable word lists	Words are presented and recorded at comfortable level of hearing to determine percentage correct and word understanding.	Nurse may perform test.
Auditory evoked potential	Procedure is similar to electroencephalography (see Chapter 58 and Table 58-9). Electrodes are attached to patient in darkened room. Electrodes are placed typically at vertex, mastoid process, or earlobes and forehead. A computer is used to isolate auditory from other electrical activity of the brain.	Nurse should explain procedure to patient. Nurse should not leave patient alone in the darkened room.
Electrocochleography	Test is useful for uncooperative patient or for patient who cannot volunteer useful information. Test records electrical activity in the cochlea and auditory nerve.	Nurse does not usually participate in examination.
Auditory brainstem response	Study measures electrical peaks along auditory pathway of inner ear to brain and provides diagnostic information related to acoustical neuromas, brainstem problems, and stroke.	Nurse does not usually participate in examination.
Tympanometry (impedance audiometry)	Useful in diagnosis of middle ear effusions. A probe is placed snugly in the external ear canal, and positive and negative pressures are then applied. Compliance of the middle ear is then noted in response to the pressures.	Nurse does not usually participate in examination.
Vestibular		
Caloric test stimulus	Endolymph of the semicircular canals is stimulated by irrigation of cold (20°C) or warm (36°C) solution into ear. Patient is seated or in supine position. Observation of type of nystagmus, nausea and vomiting, falling, or vertigo is helpful in diagnosing disease of labyrinth. Decreased response indicates decreased function and thus disease of vestibular system. Other ear is tested similarly, and results are compared.	Nurse instructs patient to eat light meal before test, to prevent nausea. Nurse observes patient for vomiting and assists patient if necessary. Nurse ensures patient safety.
Electronystagmography	Electrodes are placed near patient's eyes, and movement of eyes (nystagmus) is recorded on graph during specific eye movements and when ear is irrigated. Study aids in diagnosing diseases of vestibular system.	Nurse instructs patient to eat light meal before test, to prevent nausea. Nurse observes patient for vomiting and assists patient if necessary. Nurse ensures patient safety.
Posturography	Study is a balance test in which one semicircular canal can be isolated from others to determine site of lesion.	Nurse informs patient that test is time consuming and uncomfortable but that the test can be discontinued any time at patient's request.
Rotary chair testing	The patient is seated in a chair driven by a motor under computer control. Test is an evaluation of peripheral vestibular system.	Nurse instructs patient to eat light meal before test, to prevent nausea. Nurse observes patient for vomiting and assists patient if necessary. Nurse ensures patient safety.

commonly performed by audiologists is pure-tone audiometry. Audiologists can also test air conduction and bone conduction to aid in differentiating sensorineural from conductive hearing losses (Chernecky & Berger, 2008). Nursing responsibilities include (a) explaining the examination in general terms to the patient, (b) informing the patient of any dietary restrictions such as no caffeine or other stimulants, and (c) informing the patient whether sedation will be used.

More sophisticated tests are available to determine the origin of certain hearing losses. These include evoked potential studies (also called *auditory brainstem response*) and electrocochleography. Computed tomography and magnetic resonance imaging are used to diagnose the site of a lesion, such as a tumour of the auditory nerve.

Test for Vestibular Function

Table 23-12 describes diagnostic studies commonly used to assess vestibular function. Results of these tests can be altered by use of caffeine, other stimulants, sedatives, and antivertigo agents.

ⓔvolve   An assessment case study of the visual and auditory systems is available at *http://evolve.elsevier.com/Canada/Lewis/medsurg*

REVIEW QUESTIONS

The number of the question corresponds to the same-numbered objective at the beginning of the chapter.

1. In a patient who has a hemorrhage in the vitreous cavity of the eye, where is the blood accumulating?
   a. In the aqueous humor
   b. Between the lens and the retina
   c. Between the cornea and the lens
   d. In the space between the iris and the lens
2. Why might intraocular pressure increase?
   a. Edema of the corneal stroma
   b. Dilation of the retinal arterioles
   c. Blockage of the lacrimal canals and ducts
   d. Increased production of aqueous humor by the ciliary process
3. Which of the following should the nurse question patients about if they are using eye drops to treat glaucoma?
   a. Use of corrective lenses
   b. Their usual sleep pattern
   c. A history of heart or lung disease
   d. Sensitivity to opioids or depressants
4. For a patient with an ophthalmic problem, the nurse should always assess for which of the following?
   a. Visual acuity
   b. Pupillary reactions
   c. Intraocular pressure
   d. Confrontation visual fields
5. Which of the following normal findings would the nurse expect to find during assessment of the auditory system?
   a. Absence of the cone of light
   b. Pearl-grey tympanic membrane
   c. Lateralization with Weber's test
   d. Bone conduction greater than air conduction
6. What is the cause of arcus senilis?
   a. Tissue atrophy
   b. Decreased pupil size
   c. Opacities in the lens
   d. Cholesterol deposits in the cornea
7. Which of the following determinants of health have an influence on the visual system?
   a. Income, social status, and social support networks
   b. Personal health practices, gender, biology and genetics
   c. Social environment, education, and healthy child development
   d. Health and social services, employment, and working conditions
8. Before fluorescein is injected for angiography, what is of most importance?
   a. Obtaining an emesis basin
   b. Asking whether the patient is fatigued
   c. Administering a topical anaesthetic
   d. Determining whether the patient has a peripheral scotoma

ANSWERS: 1. b; 2. d; 3. c; 4. a; 5. b; 6. d; 7. b; 8. d.

REFERENCES

American Optometric Association. (2011). *Computer vision syndrome.* Retrieved from *http://www.aoa.org/x5253.xml*

Bance, M. (2007). Hearing and aging. *Canadian Medical Association Journal, 176*(7), 925-927. doi:10.1503/cmaj.07007

Brunetti, L., Santell, J. P., & Hicks, R. W. (2007). The impact of abbreviations on patient safety. *The Joint Commission Journal on Quality and Patient Safety, 33*(9), 576-583. Retrieved from *http://psnet.ahrq.gov/public/Brunetti_JCJQPS_2007.pdf*

Chernecky, C., & Berger, B. (2008). *Laboratory tests and diagnostic procedures.* Philadelphia: Elsevier Saunders.

Clinical Practice Guideline Expert Committee. (2007). Canadian Ophthalmological Society evidence-based clinical practice guidelines for the periodic eye examination in adults in Canada. *Canadian Journal of Ophthalmology, 42,* 39-45. doi:10.3129/canjophthalmol.06-126e

Corna, L. M., Wade, T. J., Streiner, D. L., & Cairney, J. (2009). Corrected and uncorrected hearing impairment in older Canadians. *Gerontology, 55,* 468-476. doi:10.1159/000219589

Health Canada. (2006). *Ear candling.* Ottawa: Author. Retrieved from *http://www.hc-sc.gc.ca/iyh-vsv/med/ear-oreille_e.html*

Health Canada. (2011). *First Nations, Inuit and Aboriginal health: Diabetes.* Ottawa: Author. Retrieved from *http://www.hc-sc.gc.ca/fniah-spnia/diseases-maladies/diabete/index-eng.php*

Herlihy, B., & Maebius, N. (2007). *Human body in health and illness* (3rd ed.). St. Louis: Elsevier Saunders.

Jarvis, C., Browne, A. J., MacDonald-Jenkins, J., & Luctkar-Flude, M. (2009). *Physical examination & health assessment* (1st Canadian ed.). Toronto: Saunders Elsevier.

Lehne, R. (2012). *Pharmacology for nursing care.* (8th ed.). Philadelphia: Saunders.

Miller, C. A. (2012). *Nursing for wellness in older adults* (6th ed.). Philadelphia: Lippincott Williams & Wilkins.

Muzychka, M. (2009). *Environmental scan of vision health and vision loss in the provinces and territories of Canada.* Toronto: National Coalition for Vision Health. Retrieved from *http://www.visionhealth.ca/news/NCVHVersionSeptember29F,2009.pdf*

National Coalition for Vision Health. (2007). *Foundations for a Canadian vision health strategy: Towards preventing avoidable blindness and promoting vision health.* Retrieved from *http://www.visionhealth.ca/projects/documents/Foundations-For-A-Canadian-Vision-Health-Strategy.pdf*

Pottie, K., Greenaway, C., Feightner, J., Welch, V., Swinkels, H., Rashid M., ..., Tugwell, P. (2011). Evidence-based clinical guidelines for immigrants and refugees: Vision health, *Canadian Medical Association Journal, 183*(12), E898-E900. doi:10.1503/cmaj.090313

Rhone, M., & Basu, A. (2008). Phytochemicals and age-related eye diseases. *Nutrition Reviews, 66*(8), 465-472. doi:10.1111/j.1753-4887.2008.00078.x

Roland, P. S., Smith, T. L., Schwartz, S. R., Rosenfeld, R. M., Ballachanda, B., Earll, J. M., ..., Wetmore, S., (2008). Clinical practice guideline: Cerumen impaction. *Otolaryngology—Head and Neck Surgery, (139),* S1-S21. doi:10.1016/j.otohns.2008.06.026

Ross, S. A., McKenna, A., Mozejko, S., & Fick, G. H. (2007). Diabetic retinopathy in native and non-native Canadians. *Experimental Diabetes Research,* vol. 2007: Article ID 76271. doi:10.1155/2007/76271

Seidel, H., Ball, J. W., Dains, J. E., & Benedict, G. W. (2011). *Mosby's guide to physical examination* (7th ed.). St. Louis: Mosby.

Skidmore-Roth, L. (2012). *Mosby's 2013 nursing drug reference* (26th ed.). St. Louis: Mosby.

Smith, S. D. (2008). Basic ocular anatomy, *Insight, 33*(3), 19-23.

Sweeney, D., Holden, B., Evans, K., Ng, V., & Cho, P. (2009). Best practice contact lens care: A review of the Asia Pacific Contact Lens Care Summit. *Clinical and Experimental Optometry, 92*(2), 78-89. doi:10.1111/j.1444-0938.2009.00353.x

Thibodeau, G., & Patton, K. (2012). *Structure and function of the body* (14th ed.). St Louis: Mosby.

Williams, M. (2006). Examining the eyes of an older person. *Medscape.* Retrieved from *http://www.medscape.org/viewarticle/547645*

RESOURCES

Resources for this chapter are listed after Chapter 24, on page 539.

ⓔvolve *For additional resources, see the Web site for this book at* **http://evolve.elsevier.com/Canada/Lewis/medsurg**

CHAPTER 24

Nursing Management: Visual and Auditory Problems

Written by Sarah C. Smith and Sherry Neely

Adapted by Sandy Bell

LEARNING OBJECTIVES

1. Describe the types of refractive errors and appropriate corrections.
2. Describe the causes of and collaborative care for extraocular disorders.
3. Explain the pathophysiological processes and clinical manifestations of selected intraocular disorders, and describe nursing management and collaborative care of the patient with selected intraocular disorders.
4. Describe the nursing measures that promote the health of the eyes and ears.
5. Explain the general preoperative and postoperative care of the patient undergoing surgery in the eye or the ear.
6. Summarize the action and uses of drug therapy for treating patients with problems of the eyes and the ears.
7. Explain the pathophysiological processes and clinical manifestations of common ear problems, and describe nursing management and collaborative care of common ear problems.
8. Compare the causes, management, and rehabilitative potential of conductive and sensorineural hearing loss.
9. Explain the use and care of assistive devices for eye and ear problems, and describe the relevant patient teaching.
10. Describe the common causes and assistive measures for uncorrectable visual impairment and deafness.
11. Describe the measures used to assist the patient in adapting psychologically to decreased vision and hearing.

KEY TERMS

age-related macular degeneration (AMD) An eye disease that begins after age 60 that progressively destroys the macula (the central portion of the retina), causing irreversible loss of central vision, p. 519

amblyopia Reduced vision or no vision in an affected eye that may develop in childhood if refractive errors are not corrected, p. 504

astigmatism A condition caused by irregular corneal curvature in which the incoming light rays are bent unequally and do not converge at a single point of focus on the retina, p. 504

blepharitis Inflammation of the eyelid margins, p. 509

cataract An abnormal progressive condition of the lens of the eye, characterized by an opacity within the lens, p. 513

conjunctivitis An infection or inflammation of the conjunctiva, caused by bacterial or viral infection, allergy, or environmental factors, p. 509

enucleation Removal of the eye, p. 525

glaucoma A group of disorders characterized by increased intraocular pressure and the consequences of elevated pressure, optic nerve atrophy, and peripheral visual field loss, p. 520

hordeolum An infection of the sebaceous glands in the eyelid margin, p. 508

hyperopia A condition affecting the accommodation of the lens of the eye in which incoming rays of light reach the retina before they converge into a focused image; this results in defective vision of near objects, p. 504

keratitis An inflammation or infection of the cornea that can be caused by a variety of microorganisms or by other factors, p. 510

Ménière's disease An inner ear disease that causes symptoms of episodic vertigo, tinnitus, fluctuating sensorineural hearing loss, and a sensation of aural fullness, p. 530

myopia A condition affecting the accommodation of the lens of the eye in which the visual images converge into a focus in front of the retina of the eye; this results in defective vision of distant objects, p. 504

otosclerosis A hereditary condition in which irregular ossification occurs on the footplate of the stapes in the oval window, which results in decreased hearing acuity, p. 529

presbycusis Hearing loss associated with normal aging, p. 535

presbyopia A decrease in the accommodative ability of the eye to focus on near objects as a result of normal aging. p. 504

refractive error A condition that prevents light rays from converging into a single focus on the retina, p. 504

retinal detachment A separation of the sensory retina and the underlying pigment epithelium, with fluid accumulation between the two layers, p. 517

retinopathy The process of microvascular damage of the retina; may develop slowly or rapidly, p. 517

ELECTRONIC RESOURCES

Supplemental content related to Chapter 24 can be found...

Evolve Web Site ⊖volve

http://evolve.elsevier.com/Canada/Lewis/medsurg
- Answer Guideline for Case Study on p. 536
- Clinical Reference: Laboratory Values
- Content Updates

- eFigure 24-1: Refractive Errors
- eNCP24-1: Eye Surgery
- Electronic Calculators
- Examination Review Questions
- Glossary
- Interactive Case Study: Cataract Surgery
- Key Points (Printable and MP3 Download)

Visual Problems

Visual problems include correctable and uncorrectable problems involving the outer or inner functioning of the eye or both. Fear of vision loss is second only to fear of cancer (Muzychka, 2009). Loss of some or all vision doubles the difficulties associated with activities of daily living, halves the ease of social functioning, doubles the risk of falls, triples the risk of depression, quadruples the risk of hip fractures, and doubles mortality rates (Muzychka, 2009).

Correctable Refractive Errors

Refractive error is the most common visual problem and the most easily correctable cause of vision loss (Muzychka, 2009). This defect prevents light rays from converging into a single focus on the retina. Defects are a result of irregularities of the corneal curvature, the focusing power of the lens, or the length (i.e., depth) of the eye from the front surface to the rear of the vitreous cavity. The major symptom is blurred vision. In some cases, the patient may also complain of ocular discomfort, eyestrain, or headaches. The principal refractive errors of the eye can be corrected by the use of lenses in the form of eyeglasses or contact lenses, by refractive surgery, or by surgical implantation of an artificial lens. Refractive errors in young children should be corrected because children may develop **amblyopia** (reduced or no vision in the affected eye) if such errors go uncorrected (Canadian Ophthalmological Society, 2007a). Undetected and untreated refractive errors and cataracts in persons older than 65 can lead to falls and unintentional injuries, such as fractures. Falls and fractures are of particular concern because of the effect on the individual's independence and long-term health (Bell, Hawranik, & McCormac, 2011).

> **SAFETY ALERT**
> Upon admission to hospital, older patients should undergo vision screening and, when it is warranted, be referred to an appropriate eye care specialist.

Several refractive errors (myopia, hyperopia, and presbyopia) involve the accommodative ability of the eye. *Accommodation* is the adjustment in the focal length of the lens of the eye, which allows images at different distances to be focused on the retina.

Myopia (nearsightedness) is a condition affecting the accommodation of the lens of the eye in which the visual images come to a focus in front of the retina of the eye; this results in defective vision of distant objects. Myopia is the most common refractive error and is more common among women than among men. (Refractive errors are depicted in eFigure 24-1 available on the Evolve Web site for this chapter.)

Hyperopia (farsightedness) is a condition affecting the accommodation of the lens of the eye in which incoming rays of light reach the retina before they converge into a focused image; this results in defective vision of near objects.

Presbyopia is farsightedness that results from a decrease in the accommodative ability of the eye to see near objects. As a result of aging, the lens becomes larger, firmer, and less elastic. The first sign of presbyopia is often the need to hold reading material farther away.

Other correctable refractive errors include astigmatism and aphakia. **Astigmatism** is caused by an irregular corneal curvature. This irregularity causes the incoming light rays to be bent unequally. Consequently, the light rays do not converge in a single point of focus on the retina. Astigmatism can occur in conjunction with any of the other refractive errors.

Aphakia is the absence of the lens. Without the focusing ability of the lens, images are projected behind the retina. In rare cases, the lens may be absent congenitally, or it may be removed during cataract surgery. A lens that is traumatically injured is removed and replaced with an intraocular lens implant. The lens accounts for approximately 30% of ocular refractive power. The absence of the lens results in a significant refractive error (Smith, 2008).

Nonsurgical Corrections

Corrective Glasses. Myopia, hyperopia, presbyopia, astigmatism, and aphakia can be modified with an appropriate corrective lens. Myopia necessitates a "minus" *(concave)* corrective lens, whereas hyperopia and presbyopia all necessitate a "plus" *(convex)* corrective lens. Glasses for presbyopia are often called *reading glasses* because they are usually worn only for close work. The presbyopic correction may be combined with a correction for another refractive error, such as myopia or astigmatism. If these combined glasses are bifocal or trifocal, the presbyopic correction is in the lower portion of the lens. A newer type of corrective for presbyopia, the progressive lens, is actually a multifocal lens in which the transition from near to far correction is graduated seamlessly over a range in the middle area of the lens. This eliminates the visible lines between the different corrective lenses. The lower lens in multifocal glasses may predispose older people to falls because viewing the environment through their lower lenses impairs the important visual capabilities (contrast sensitivity and depth perception) for detecting environmental hazards, particularly in unfamiliar environments (Haran et al., 2009).

Aphakic glasses are very thick, and so they are heavy and considered unattractive. The high degree of correction also causes images to be magnified about 25%. With the surgical procedures available and common today, patients seldom wear aphakic glasses for correction because of the associated visual problems.

Contact Lenses. Contact lenses are another way to correct refractive errors and are available in rigid and soft types. The rigid types are available in standard and gas-permeable forms. Their care requires separate solutions for cleaning, storing and wetting. The soft types are available in many forms. The most commonly used soft contact lenses are the standard and disposable forms, which are less durable and more expensive than rigid forms. Contact lenses generally provide better vision than do glasses because the patient has more normal peripheral vision without the distortion and obstruction of glasses and their frames. This is especially true with high refractive errors. Contact lenses are made from various plastic and silicone substances, which are very permeable to oxygen, have a high water content, and thus enable longer wearing time with greater comfort. If the oxygen supply to the cornea is decreased, the cornea becomes swollen, visual acuity decreases, and the patient experiences severe discomfort.

Altered or decreased tear formation can make wearing contact lenses difficult. Tear production can be decreased by medications such as antihistamines, decongestants, diuretics, hormone medications such as oral contraceptives, and the hormones produced during pregnancy. Environmental factors such as wind, fans, and dust may also decrease the tear film. Allergic conjunctivitis with itching, tearing, and redness can also affect contact lens wear.

In general, the nurse must know whether the patient wears contact lenses, the pattern of wear (daily versus extended), and care practices. Shining a light obliquely on the eyeball can help the nurse visualize a contact lens. The patient should know the signs and symptoms of contact lens problems that must be managed by the eye care professional. The patient may remember these symptoms better if the nurse uses the mnemonic device *RSVP: redness, sensitivity, vision problems, and pain.*

SAFETY ALERT

Stress the importance of removing contact lenses immediately when the patient experiences RSVP symptoms.

Corneal Moulding. *Corneal moulding*, also called *orthokeratology*, is the use of specially designed, rigid, gas-permeable contact lenses to alter the shape of the cornea. It reduces or corrects myopia and moderate degrees of astigmatism. The cornea is moulded by fitting progressively flatter rigid contact lenses and requires regular wearing of "retainer" contact lenses to maintain corneal shape.

Surgical Therapy

Surgical procedures are designed to eliminate or reduce the need for eyeglasses or contact lenses and correct refractive errors by changing the focus of the eye. Surgical management for refractive errors includes laser surgery, intraocular lens (IOL) implantation, and thermal procedures.

Laser Surgery. *Laser-assisted in situ keratomileusis* (LASIK) may be considered for patients with low to moderately high degrees of myopia, hyperopia, and astigmatism. It has revolutionized refractive surgery, and millions of LASIK procedures have been performed worldwide. The procedure first involves using a laser or surgical blade to create a thin flap in the cornea. Through new "wave-front" technology, the laser is then programmed to use a map of the patient's cornea to sculpt the cornea and correct the refractive error. The flap is then repositioned and adheres on its own without sutures in a few minutes. Glare, halos, starbursts and poor night vision are negative consequences for some patients despite uncomplicated and successful surgery (Sutton & Kim, 2010).

Photorefractive keratectomy is indicated for low to moderate degrees of myopia, hyperopia, and astigmatism and is a good option for a patient with insufficient corneal thickness for a LASIK flap. In photorefractive keratectomy, only the epithelium is removed and the laser sculpts the cornea to correct the refractive error. *Laser-assisted epithelial keratomileusis* (LASEK) is similar to photorefractive keratectomy except that the epithelium is replaced after surgery.

Implantation. *Intracorneal ring segments* are two semicircular pieces of plastic that are implanted between the layers of the cornea to treat mild forms of myopia. They are designed to change the shape of the cornea by adjusting the focusing power. Intracorneal ring segments can be removed, and the cornea usually returns to its original shape within a few weeks.

Refractive intraocular lens (refractive IOL) implantation is an option for patients with severe myopia or hyperopia. Like cataract surgery, it involves the removal of the patient's natural lens and implantation of an IOL, which is a small plastic lens to correct a patient's refractive error. Because this requires entering the eye, the risk of complications is higher. New accommodating IOLs will correct both myopia and presbyopia.

Phakic intraocular lenses (phakic IOLs) are sometimes referred to as *implantable contact lenses*. They are implanted into the eye without removal of the eye's natural lens. They are used for patients with severe myopia and hyperopia. Unlike the refractive IOL, the phakic IOL is placed in front of the eye's natural lens. Leaving the natural lens in the eye preserves the ability of the eye to focus for reading vision. Artisan is one type of phakic IOL used for moderate to severe myopia.

Thermal Procedures. *Laser thermal keratoplasty* and *conductive keratoplasty* are procedures for patients with hyperopia or presbyopia. Through the use of laser or high-frequency radio waves, heat is applied to the peripheral area of the cornea to tighten it like a belt and make the central cornea steeper. Only the less dominant eye is treated, and the desired effect is monovision. Monovision enables one eye to focus at close proximity; the other eye is left untreated or, if needed, is treated to focus at a

Table 24-1 Definition of Blindness in Canada

Legal blindness is defined as follows:

- Central visual acuity for distance of 20/200 or worse in the better eye (with correction).
- Visual field of no greater than 20 degrees in its widest diameter or in the better eye.

distance. A preoperative trial with contact lenses is a useful test to determine whether a patient will adapt to the intended refractive outcome.

Uncorrectable Visual Impairment

In 2006, 836,000 Canadians were identified as having a *seeing disability,* defined as either difficulty seeing ordinary newsprint with corrective lenses if usually worn, or difficulty seeing the face of someone 4 metres across a room with corrective lenses if usually worn (National Coalition for Vision Health, 2011). The partially sighted individual may actually have significant vision. It is important in working with the visually impaired patient to understand that a person classified as blind may have useful vision. Appropriate responses and interventions depend on the nurse's understanding of an individual patient's visual abilities.

Levels of Visual Impairment

Total blindness is defined as no light perception and no usable vision. *Functional blindness* is present when the patient has some light perception but no usable vision. The patient with either total or functional blindness may use vision substitutes such as guide dogs and canes for ambulation. Vision enhancement techniques are not helpful.

There are approximately 108,000 legally blind Canadians (visual acuity less than 20/200) and another 278,000 with visual impairment (visual acuity between 20/50 and 20/200; National Coalition for Vision Health, 2011). Most vision impairment and blindness is caused by conditions such as age-related macular degeneration, glaucoma, diabetic retinopathy, and cataracts. These conditions are preventable, or treatable, or both. The number of blind individuals is expected to double within 10 years (Muzychka, 2009).

The *legally blind individual* meets the criteria developed by the federal government to determine eligibility for government programs and income tax benefits (Table 24-1). A legally blind individual may have some usable vision. The *partially sighted individual* who is not legally blind has a corrected visual acuity greater than 20/200 in the better eye and greater than 20 degrees of visual field, but the visual acuity is 20/50 or worse in the better eye. The patient who is partially sighted but also legally blind can benefit greatly from vision enhancement techniques.

NURSING MANAGEMENT: VISUAL IMPAIRMENT

Nursing Assessment

It is important to determine how long a patient has had a visual impairment because recent loss of vision has particular implica-

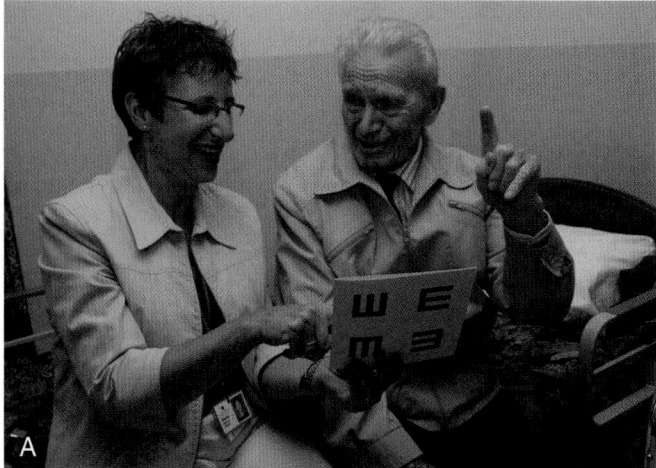

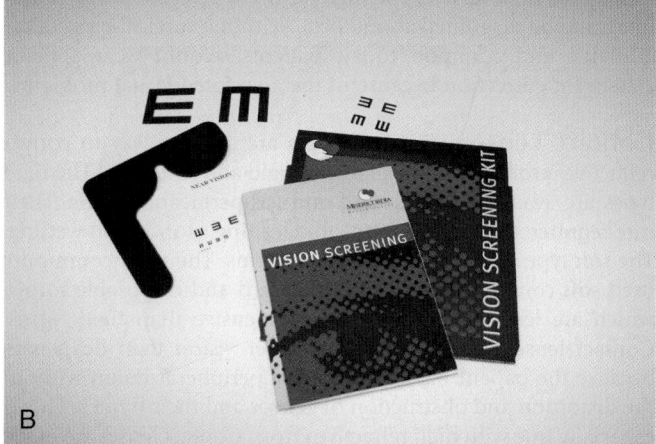

Figure 24-1 A, An older patient undergoing vision screening with the Focus on Falls Prevention Program Vision Screening Tool. **B,** Focus on Falls Prevention Program Vision Screening Tool.

Source: Courtesy Focus on Falls Prevention Vision Screening Program, Winnipeg, Manitoba.

tions for nursing care. To determine how the patient's visual impairment affects normal functioning, the nurse should question the patient about the level of difficulty encountered when he or she performs certain tasks. For example, the nurse may ask how much difficulty the patient has when reading a newspaper, writing a check, moving from one room to the next, or viewing television. Other questions can help the nurse determine the personal meaning that the patient attaches to the visual impairment. The nurse can ask how the vision loss has affected specific aspects of the patient's life, whether the patient has lost a job, or in what activities the patient no longer engages because of the visual impairment. Techniques such as describing where personal items are located, warning the patient when the nurse will be providing direct care, and informing the patient where food items are located on the tray are helpful strategies (Jensen, 2012). In older patients in all health care settings, vision can be assessed with the evidence-informed Focus on Falls Prevention Program Vision Screening Tool (Figure 24-1). This tool was specifically adapted and designed to screen vision in older patients and has proved to be successful in effectively identifying such patients who require a referral to an eye specialist. Improving vision in older patients can prevent falls and associated fractures (Bell et al., 2011).

The patient may attach many negative meanings to the impairment because of societal opinions about blindness. For example, the patient may view the impairment as punishment or view himself or herself as useless and burdensome. It is also important to determine the patient's primary coping strategies, the patient's emotional reactions, and the availability and strength of the patient's support systems.

Nursing Diagnoses

Nursing diagnoses depend on the degree of visual impairment and how long it has been present. Nursing diagnoses for the visually impaired patient include, but are not limited to, the following:

- Disturbed sensory perception *related to* visual deficit
- Risk for injury *related to* visual impairment and inability to see potential dangers
- Self-care deficits *related to* visual impairment
- Fear *related to* inability to see potential danger or accurately interpret environment
- Grieving *related to* loss of functional vision

Planning

The overall goals are that the patient with recently impaired vision or the patient with impaired adjustment to long-standing visual impairment will (a) make a successful adjustment to the impairment, (b) verbalize feelings related to the loss, (c) identify personal strengths and external support systems, and (d) use appropriate coping strategies. If the patient has been functioning at an appropriate or acceptable level, the goal is to maintain the current level of function.

Nursing Implementation

Health Promotion

When a partially sighted patient is at risk for preventable further visual impairment, the nurse should encourage the patient to seek appropriate health care. For example, the patient with vision loss from glaucoma may prevent further visual impairment by complying with prescribed therapies and suggested ophthalmological evaluations.

Acute Intervention

The nurse provides emotional support and direct care to patients with visual impairment of recent onset. Active listening and facilitating are important components of nursing care for such a patient. The nurse should allow the patient to express anger and grief and should help the patient identify fears and successful coping strategies. The family is intimately involved in the experiences that follow vision loss. With the patient's knowledge and permission, the nurse should include family members in discussions and encourage members to express their concerns.

Many people are uncomfortable around a blind or partially sighted individual because they are not sure what behaviours are appropriate. Sensitivity to the person's feelings without being overly solicitous or stifling the person's independence is vital in creating a therapeutic nursing presence.

The nurse should always communicate in a normal conversational tone and manner with the patient and address the patient directly, not the family member or friend who may accompany the patient. Common courtesy dictates introducing oneself and any other persons who approach a blind or partially sighted patient and saying goodbye on leaving. Making eye contact with the partially sighted patient accomplishes several objectives. It ensures that the nurse speaks while facing the patient so that the patient has no difficulty hearing the nurse. The nurse's head position confirms that the nurse is attentive to the patient. Also, establishing eye contact ensures that the nurse can observe the patient's facial expressions and reactions.

Orientation to the environment lessens patients' anxiety or discomfort and facilitates independence. In orienting a partially sighted or blind patient to a new area, the nurse should identify one object as the focal point and describe the location of other objects in relation to it. For example, the nurse may say, "The bed is straight ahead, approximately 10 steps. The chair is to the left of the bed, and the nightstand is to the right, near the head of the bed. The bathroom is to the left of the foot of the bed." The nurse should explain any activities or noises occurring in the patient's immediate surroundings.

The nurse should assist the patient in ambulating to each major object in the area, using the *sighted-guide technique.* When using this technique, the nurse stands slightly in front and to one side of the patient and offers an elbow for the patient to hold. The nurse serves as the sighted guide, walking slightly ahead of the patient with the patient holding the back of the nurse's arm. When using this technique in any situation, the nurse describes the environment to help orient the patient. For example, the nurse may say, "We're going through an open doorway and approaching two steps down. There is an obstacle on the left." To assist the patient to sit, place one of his or her hands on the back of the chair.

The nurse should be familiar with common vision deficits such as cataracts, refractive errors, macular degeneration, glaucoma, and diabetic retinopathy and their associated nursing strategies for care. For example, age-related macular degeneration entails loss of central vision, and the patient is best cared for by being approached from the side. This condition affects a person's ability to see detail required for reading, writing, preparing meals, and recognizing faces. Caring for the patient with glaucoma, which entails loss of peripheral vision, is better when the nurse directly faces the patient. Vision loss from glaucoma primarily affects a person's mobility, especially in a dynamic moving environment (Haslbeck, Anderson, Markowitz, & Feder, 2009).

Ambulatory and Home Care

Rehabilitation after partial or total loss of vision can foster independence, self-esteem, and productivity. The nurse should know what services and devices are available for a partially sighted or blind patient and should be prepared to make appropriate referrals for those services and devices. For legally blind patients and those with low-degree vision, the primary resource for services is the Canadian National Institute for the Blind. A list of agencies that serve the partially sighted or blind patient is available from this institute (see the Canadian Resources at the end of this chapter).

Braille or audio books for reading and a cane or guide dog for ambulation are examples of vision substitution techniques. These are usually most appropriate for patients with no functional vision. For most patients who have some remaining vision, vision enhancement techniques can provide enough help to learn to ambulate, read printed material, and accomplish activities of daily living.

Optical Devices for Vision Enhancement.

Telescopic lenses for near or far vision and magnifiers of various types can often enhance the patient's remaining vision enough to enable him or her to perform many otherwise impossible tasks and activities. Most of these devices require some training and practice for successful use. Closed-circuit television can provide magnification up to 60 times, allowing some patients to read, write, use computers, and do crafts. Although these systems are expensive and their portability is limited, they are available in some public or university libraries.

Nonoptical Methods for Vision Enhancement.

Approach magnification is a simple but sometimes overlooked technique for enhancing the patient's residual vision. The nurse can recommend that the patient sit closer to the television or hold books closer to the eyes, which the patient may be reluctant to do unless encouraged. Contrast enhancement techniques include watching television in black and white, placing dark objects against a light background (e.g., a white plate on a black place mat), using a black felt-tip marker to write, and using contrasting colours (e.g., a red stripe at the edge of steps or curbs). Increased lighting can be provided by halogen lamps, direct sunlight, or gooseneck lamps that can be aimed directly at the reading material or other near objects. Large type is often helpful, especially in conjunction with other optical or nonoptical vision enhancements.

Evaluation

The following are overall expected outcomes for the patient with severe visual impairment:

- The patient's participation in activities of daily living and other activities will be assessed regularly to monitor vision care needs.
- The patient will be able to express adaptive coping strategies.
- The patient will not experience a decrease in self-esteem or social interactions.
- The patient will function safely within her or his own environment.

AGE-RELATED CONSIDERATIONS: VISUAL IMPAIRMENT

Older adult patients are at an increased risk for vision loss because of cataracts, glaucoma, diabetic retinopathy, and macular degeneration. An older patient may have other deficits, such as cognitive impairment or limited mobility, that further affect the ability to function in usual ways. Societal devaluation of older adults may compound the self-esteem or isolation issues associated with the older patient's visual impairment. Financial resources may meet normal needs but can be inadequate in meeting increased demands of vision services or devices.

Older patients may become confused or disoriented when visually compromised. The combination of decreased vision and confusion increases the risk of falls, which have potentially serious consequences for older adults. Decreased vision may compromise an older patient's ability to function, causing con-

cerns about maintaining independence and damaging the patient's self-image. Decreased manual dexterity may make the instillation of prescribed eye drops difficult for some older adults. It is important to provide proper instruction and demonstration. Having the patient demonstrate the technique is an important aspect of nursing education and reassurance for patients. Eye drop assistive devices are available for purchase at pharmacies in Canada, and their use can be suggested.

Eye Trauma

Although the eyes are well protected by the bony orbit and by fat pads, everyday activities can result in ocular trauma. Ocular injuries can involve the ocular adnexa, the superficial structures, or the deeper ocular structures. Eye trauma is one of the leading causes of vision impairment in Canada; according to estimates, the incidence of eye injuries is more than 100,000 per year. The Canadian National Institute for the Blind estimates that each day approximately 200 Canadian workers suffer injuries to their eyes; many of these injuries are serious enough to cause workers to lose work time, and some can lead to permanent eye damage or blindness (Muzychka, 2009). A Canadian online eye injury registry has been developed to gather data about the pattern and types of eye injuries that occur. Table 24-2 outlines emergency management of the patient with an eye injury. Types of ocular trauma include blunt injuries, penetrating injuries, and chemical exposure injuries. Causes of ocular injuries include automobile accidents, falls, sports and leisure activity injuries, assaults, and work-related situations. Trauma is often a preventable cause of visual impairment. Almost 90% of all eye injuries could be prevented by the wearing of protective eyewear during potentially hazardous work, hobbies, or sports activities. The nurse's role in individual and community education is extremely important in reducing the incidence of ocular trauma.

Extraocular Disorders

Inflammation and Infection

One of the most common conditions encountered by the ophthalmologist is inflammation or infection of the external eye. Many external irritants or microorganisms affect the eyelids and conjunctiva and can involve the avascular cornea. The nurse is responsible for teaching the patient appropriate interventions related to the specific disorder.

Hordeolum. An external **hordeolum** (commonly called a *sty*) is an infection of the sebaceous glands in the eyelid margin (Figure 24-2). The most common bacterial infective agent is *Staphylococcus aureus.* The affected area rapidly becomes red, swollen, circumscribed, and acutely tender. The nurse should instruct the patient to apply warm, moist compresses at least four times a day until it improves. This may be the only treatment necessary. If there is a tendency for recurrence, the patient should be taught to perform eyelid scrubs daily. In addition, use of appropriate antibiotic ointments or drops may be indicated.

Chalazion. A *chalazion* is a chronic inflammatory granuloma of the meibomian (sebaceous) glands in the eyelid. A hordeolum may evolve into a chalazion. A chalazion may also occur as a response to the material released into the eyelid when a blocked

EMERGENCY MANAGEMENT

Table 24-2 Eye Injury

CAUSE	INTERVENTIONS
Blunt Injury: Fist; other blunt objects	***Initial***
Penetrating Injury: Fragments such as glass, metal, wood; knife, stick, or other large object	• Determine mechanism of injury.
	• Ensure airway, breathing, and circulation.
Chemical Injury: Alkaline; acid	• Assess for other injuries.
Thermal Injury: Direct burn from curling iron or other hot surface; indirect burn from ultraviolet light (e.g., welding torch, sun lamp)	• Assess for chemical exposure.
	• Begin ocular irrigation immediately in case of chemical exposure; do not stop until emergency personnel arrive to continue irrigation. Sterile, pH-balanced, physiological solution is best; if it is unavailable, use any nontoxic liquid. Use sterile saline or water if saline is unavailable.
Foreign Bodies: Glass; metal; wood; plastic	
Trauma: Blunt; penetrating or perforating	
Burns: Chemical; thermal	• Assess visual acuity.
POSSIBLE ASSESSMENT FINDINGS DEPENDING ON CAUSE	• Do not put pressure on the eye.
• Pain	• Instruct patient not to blow nose.
• Photophobia	• Do not attempt to treat the injury (except as noted previously for chemical exposure).
• Redness: diffuse or localized	
• Swelling	• Stabilize foreign objects.
• Ecchymosis	• Cover the eye or eyes with dry, sterile patches and a protective shield.
• Tearing	• Do not give the patient food or fluids.
• Blood in the anterior chamber	• Elevate head of bed to 45 degrees.
• Absent eye movements	• Do not put medication or solutions in the eye unless ordered by physician.
• Fluid drainage from eye (e.g., blood, CSF, aqueous humor)	• Administer analgesia as appropriate.
• Abnormal or decreased vision	***Ongoing Monitoring***
• Visible foreign body	• Reassure the patient.
• Prolapsed globe	• Monitor pain.
• Abnormal intraocular pressure	• Anticipate surgical repair for penetrating injury, globe rupture, or globe avulsion.
• Visual field defect	

CSF, cerebrospinal fluid; *UV,* ultraviolet.

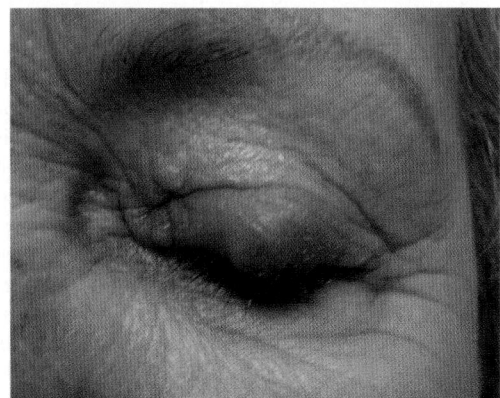

Figure 24-2 External hordeolum (sty) on the upper eyelid caused by staphylococcal infection.

Source: Courtesy Cory J. Bosanko, OD, FAAO, Eye Centers of Tennessee, Crossville, Tennessee.

gland ruptures. The chalazion usually appears on the upper eyelid as a swollen, tender, reddened area that may be painful. Initial treatment is similar to that for a hordeolum. If warm, moist compresses are ineffective in causing spontaneous drainage, the ophthalmologist may surgically remove the lesion (this is nor-mally an office procedure), or the ophthalmologist may inject the lesion with corticosteroids.

Blepharitis. **Blepharitis** is a chronic inflammatory process of the eyelid margin. It is a common eye disorder throughout the world and can affect any age group. The cause is unknown and probably multifactorial. Bacteria have been implicated in playing a significant role. It may be associated with several systemic diseases such as rosacea or seborrhea dermatitis. It is related to other ocular conditions such as dry eye, chalazion, conjunctivitis, and keratitis. Symptoms include a burning sensation, irritation, tearing, photophobia, blurred vision, and redness of the conjunctiva. These symptoms are usually worse in the morning because the inflamed eyelids are in close contact with the ocular surface and tear production is decreased overnight as a result of less blinking. Basic treatment includes a long-term commitment to eyelid hygiene. Warm compresses and washing the eyelid margins with baby shampoo diluted in water and applied gently with a cotton dipped swab are recommended. An antibiotic-corticosteroid ointment can be used for short periods only. A combination of omega-3 fatty acids and flaxseed oil is considered an adjunctive therapy (Bernardes & Bonfioli, 2010).

Conjunctivitis. **Conjunctivitis** is an inflammation of the conjunctiva, the mucous membrane that lines the eyelids and covers the white of the eyeball. The most common cause is a viral infection. Symptoms include redness, discharge, burning, and sometimes itching and light sensitivity. It can occur in one or both eyes and is contagious. Careful hand hygiene and use of individual or disposable towels helps prevent the spread of the condition (Callahan, 2012).

Bacterial Infections. Acute bacterial conjunctivitis (pinkeye) is a common infection. Although it occurs in every age group, epidemics commonly occur among children because of their poor personal hygiene habits. In adults and children, the most common causative microorganism is *S. aureus*. *Streptococcus pneumoniae* and *Haemophilus influenzae* are other common causative agents, but they are seen more often in children than in adults. A patient with bacterial conjunctivitis may complain of irritation, tearing, redness, and a mucopurulent drainage. Although this initially occurs in one eye, it generally spreads within 48 hours to the unaffected eye (Mahmood & Narang, 2008). The infection is usually self-limiting, but treatment with antibiotic drops shortens the course of the disorder.

Viral Infections. Conjunctival infections may be caused by many different viruses. A patient with viral conjunctivitis may complain of tearing, foreign body sensation, redness, and mild photophobia. This condition is usually mild and self-limiting. However, it can be severe, with considerable discomfort and subconjunctival hemorrhaging. Adenovirus conjunctivitis may be contracted in contaminated swimming pools and through direct contact with an infected patient. Treatment is usually palliative. If the patient is severely symptomatic, topical corticosteroids provide temporary relief but will not cure the infection. Antiviral drops are ineffective and therefore not indicated for use.

Chlamydial Infections. Trachoma is a chronic conjunctivitis caused by *Chlamydia trachomatis* (serotypes A through C). It is a major cause of blindness worldwide. It affects approximately 84 million people, and 8 million of these patients suffer from visual impairment (World Health Organization, 2011). This preventable eye disease is transmitted mainly via contact with the hands and by flies. Adult inclusion conjunctivitis (AIC) is caused by *C. trachomatis* (serotypes D through K). Manifestations of both trachoma and AIC are mucopurulent ocular discharge, irritation, redness, and eyelid swelling. For unknown reasons, AIC does not carry the long-term consequences of trachoma. AIC also differs from trachoma in that it is common in economically developed countries, whereas trachoma is most commonly seen in underdeveloped countries. Antibiotic therapy is usually effective for trachoma and AIC.

Although antibiotic treatment may be successful in adults with AIC, these patients have a high risk of concurrent chlamydial genital infection, as well as other sexually transmitted infections. The nurse's teaching plan for this patient should include the implications of AIC for sexual activity and reproductive health.

Allergic Conjunctivitis. Conjunctivitis caused by exposure to some allergen can be mild and transitory, or it can be severe enough to cause significant swelling, sometimes causing the conjunctiva to balloon beyond the eyelids. The defining symptom of allergic conjunctivitis is itching (Mahmood & Narang, 2008). The patient may also complain of burning, redness, and tearing. In the acute stage, the patient may also have white or clear exudate. If the condition is chronic, the exudate is thicker and becomes mucopurulent. The patient may develop allergic conjunctivitis in response to pollens, in addition to animal dander, ocular solutions and medications, or even contact lenses. The nurse should instruct the patient to avoid the allergen if it is known. Artificial tears can be effective in diluting the allergen and washing it from the eye. Effective topical medications include antihistamines and corticosteroids.

Keratitis. Keratitis is an inflammation or infection of the cornea that can be caused by a variety of microorganisms or by other factors. The condition may involve the conjunctiva, the cornea, or both. When it involves both, the disorder is termed *keratoconjunctivitis*.

Bacterial Infections. When the epithelial layer is disrupted, the cornea can become infected by a variety of bacteria. Topical antibiotics are generally effective, but eradicating the infection may require subconjunctival antibiotic injection or, in severe cases, intravenous antibiotics. Risk factors include mechanical or chemical corneal epithelial damage, contact lens wear, debilitation, nutritional deficiencies, immunosuppressed states, and use of contaminated products (e.g., lens care solutions and cases, topical medications, cosmetics).

Viral Infections. Herpes simplex virus (HSV) keratitis is the most frequently occurring infectious cause of corneal blindness in the Western hemisphere. It is a growing problem, especially among immunosuppressed patients. It may be caused by HSV-1 or HSV-2 (genital herpes), although HSV-2 ocular infection is much less common. The resulting corneal ulcer has a characteristic dendritic (tree-branching) appearance (Khare, Symons, & Do, 2008). Pain and photophobia are common. In up to 40% of patients, herpetic keratitis heals spontaneously. The spontaneous healing rate increases to 70% if the cornea is debrided to remove infected cells. Collaborative therapy includes corneal debridement, followed by topical therapy with trifluridine (Viroptic) for 2 to 3 weeks. Topical corticosteroids are usually contraindicated because they contribute to lengthening of the course and possible deeper ulceration of the cornea. Drug therapy may also include oral acyclovir (Zovirax).

The varicella-zoster virus causes both chickenpox and herpes zoster ophthalmicus. Herpes zoster ophthalmicus may occur by reactivation of an endogenous infection that has persisted in latent form after an earlier attack of varicella or by direct or indirect contact with a patient with chickenpox or herpes zoster. It occurs most frequently in older adults and in immunosuppressed patients. Collaborative care of a patient with acute herpes zoster ophthalmicus may include opioid or nonopioid analgesics for the pain, topical corticosteroids to reduce inflammation, antiviral agents such as acyclovir (Zovirax) to reduce viral replication, mydriatic agents to dilate the pupil and relieve pain, and topical antibiotics to combat secondary infection. The patient may apply warm compresses and povidone-iodine gel to the affected skin (gel should not be applied near the eye).

Epidemic keratoconjunctivitis is the most serious ocular adenoviral disease. Epidemic keratoconjunctivitis is spread by direct contact, including sexual activity. In the medical setting, contaminated hands and instruments can be the source of spread. The patient may complain of tearing, redness, photophobia, and sensation of foreign body. In most patients, the disease involves only one eye. Treatment is primarily palliative and includes ice packs and dark glasses. In severe cases, therapy can include mild topical corticosteroids to temporarily relieve symptoms and

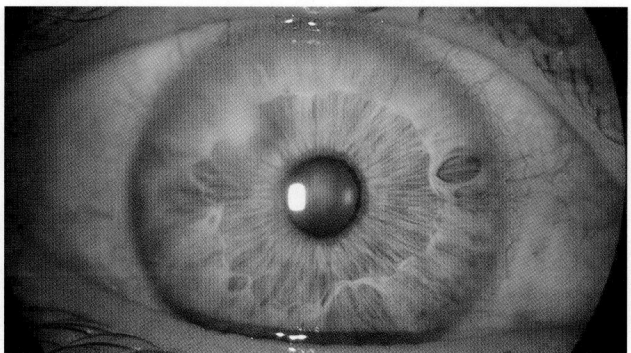

Figure 24-3 Corneal ulcer. Infection associated with poor contact lens care.

Source: Courtesy Cory J. Bosanko, OD, FAAO, Eye Centers of Tennessee, Crossville, Tennessee.

topical antibiotic ointment. The nurse's most important role is to teach the patient and family members the importance of good hygienic practices to avoid spreading the disease.

Other Causes of Keratitis. Keratitis may also be caused by fungi (most commonly *Aspergillus, Candida,* and *Fusarium* species), especially in the case of ocular trauma in an outdoor setting in which fungi are prevalent in the soil and moist organic matter. *Acanthamoeba* keratitis is caused by a parasite that is associated with contact lens wear, probably as a result of using contaminated lens care solutions or cases. Homemade saline solution is particularly susceptible to *Acanthamoeba* contamination. The nurse should instruct all patients who wear contact lenses about good lens care practices. Medical treatment of fungal and *Acanthamoeba* keratitis is difficult. The *Acanthamoeba* organism is resistant to most drugs. If antimicrobial therapy fails, the patient may require corneal transplantation.

Exposure keratitis occurs when the patient cannot adequately close the eyelids. The patient with exophthalmos (protruding eyeball) caused by thyroid eye disease or masses posterior to the globe is susceptible to exposure keratitis.

Corneal Ulcer. Tissue loss caused by infection of the cornea produces a *corneal ulcer* (infectious keratitis) (Figure 24-3). The infection can be caused by bacteria, viruses, or fungi. Corneal ulcers are often very painful, and patients may feel as if a foreign body is in the eye. Other symptoms can include tearing, purulent or watery discharge, redness, and photophobia. Treatment is generally aggressive to prevent permanent loss of vision. Antibiotic, antiviral, or antifungal eye drops may be prescribed as frequently as every hour, night and day, for the first 24 hours. An untreated corneal ulcer can result in corneal scarring and perforation (hole in the cornea). Corneal transplantation may be indicated.

NURSING MANAGEMENT: INFLAMMATION AND INFECTION

Nursing Assessment

The nurse should assess ocular changes—such as edema, redness, decreasing visual acuity, the sensation that a foreign body is

present, or discomfort—and document the findings in the patient's record. In the assessment, the nurse should also consider the psychosocial aspects of the patient's condition, especially when the patient has visual impairment in association with the condition.

Nursing Diagnoses

Nursing diagnoses for the patient with inflammation or infection of the external eye include, but are not limited to, the following:
- Acute pain *related to* irritation or infection of the external eye
- Anxiety *related to* uncertainty of cause of disease and outcome of treatment
- Disturbed sensory perception (visual) *related to* diminished or absent vision

Planning

The overall goals are that the patient with inflammation or infection of the external eye will (a) avoid spread of infection, (b) maintain an acceptable level of comfort and functioning during the course of the specific ocular problem, (c) maintain or improve visual acuity, (d) comply with the prescribed therapy, and (e) engage in appropriate health-seeking behaviours.

Nursing Implementation

Health Promotion

Careful asepsis and frequent, thorough hand hygiene are essential to prevent spreading organisms from one eye to the other, to other patients, to family members, and to the nurse. The patient and family require information about avoiding sources of ocular irritation or infection and responding appropriately if an ocular problem occurs. The patient with infective disorders that may be transmitted sexually or who has an associated sexually transmitted infection needs specific information about those disorders. Inform the patient about the appropriate use and care of lenses and lens care products.

Acute Intervention

Apply warm or cool compresses if indicated for the patient's condition. Darkening the room and providing an appropriate analgesic are other comfort measures. If the patient's visual acuity is decreased, the nurse may need to modify the patient's environment or activities for safety.

The patient may require eye drops as frequently as every hour. If the patient receives two or more different types of drops, the nurse should stagger the eye drop dosing to promote maximum absorption. For example, if two different eye drops are ordered hourly, the nurse should administer one kind of drop on the hour and the other kind of drop on the half-hour unless otherwise prescribed. This staggered schedule promotes maximum absorption. The patient who needs frequent eye drop administration may experience sleep deprivation.

Ambulatory and Home Care

The patient's primary need in the home environment is for information about required care and how to accomplish that care. The patient and family also need information about proper techniques for medication administration. If the patient's vision is compromised, the nurse should provide suggestions for alternative ways to accomplish necessary daily activities and self-care. The patient who wears contact lenses and develops infections should discard all opened or used lens care products and cosmetics to decrease the risk of re-infection from contaminated products (a common problem and a probable source of infection for many patients).

▮ Evaluation

The overall expected outcomes for the patient with inflammation or infection of the external eye are as follows:

- The patient will cooperate with the treatment plan.
- The patient will experience relief of ocular discomfort.
- The patient will effectively cope with functional changes if visual acuity is decreased.
- The patient will obtain specific information to prevent recurrent disease.

Dry Eye Disorders

Keratoconjunctivitis sicca (dry eyes) is a common complaint, particularly of older adults and individuals with certain systemic diseases such as scleroderma and systemic lupus erythematosus. Dry eyes affect the patient's quality of life by causing pain and irritation that typically worsen throughout the day. This condition also affects the person's general health and sense of well-being, his or her perception of visual function, and his or her visual performance, as well as limiting daily activities (Tavares, Fernandes, Bernardes, Bonfioli, & Soares, 2010). This condition is caused by a decrease in the quality or quantity of the tear film, and treatment is directed at the underlying cause. If it is caused by lacrimal duct dysfunction, the condition may respond to hot compresses and eyelid massage. With decreased tear secretion, the patient may use artificial tears or ointments. They should be used sparingly because preservatives in the drops or overuse can cause further ocular irritation. In severe cases, closure of the lacrimal puncta may be necessary. Patients with dry eyes in association with dry mouth may have Sjögren's syndrome (see Chapter 67).

Strabismus

Strabismus is a condition in which the patient cannot consistently focus both eyes simultaneously on the same object (Figure 24-4). One eye may deviate inward *(esotropia)*, outward *(exotropia)*, upward *(hypertropia)*, or downward *(hypotropia)*. Strabismus in adults may be caused by thyroid disease, neuromuscular problems of the eye muscles, entrapment of the extraocular muscles in orbital floor fractures, retinal detachment repair, or cerebral lesions. The primary complaint with strabismus is double vision.

Corneal Disorders

Corneal Scars and Opacities

The cornea is a transparent tissue that allows light rays to enter the eye and focus on the retina, thus producing a visual image.

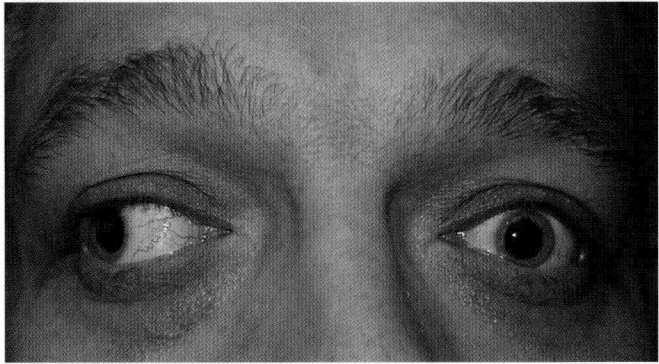

Figure 24-4 Strabismus with right exotropia and fixation of the left eye.

Source: Courtesy Cory J. Bosanko, OD, FAAO, Eye Centers of Tennessee, Crossville, Tennessee.

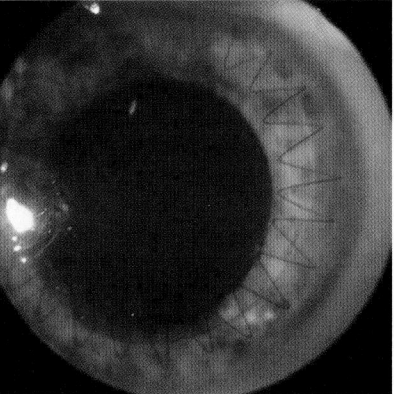

Figure 24-5 Sutures on a donated cornea after penetrating keratoplasty (corneal transplantation).

Source: Courtesy Cory J. Bosanko, OD, FAAO, Eye Centers of Tennessee, Crossville, Tennessee.

Any wound causes the cornea to become abnormally hydrated and decreases the normal transparency. A rigid contact lens can be effective in correcting the irregular astigmatism that results from corneal scars. In other situations, the treatment for corneal scars or opacities is *penetrating keratoplasty* (corneal transplantation). In this surgical procedure, the ophthalmic surgeon removes the full thickness of the patient's cornea and replaces it with a donor cornea that is sutured into place (Figure 24-5). Corneal problems leading to blindness are uncommon, but if they occur, corneal transplantation can preserve vision that otherwise would be lost.

The time between the donor's death and the removal of the tissue should be as short as possible. Most surgeons prefer this interval to be 4 hours or less. The eye banks test donors for human immunodeficiency virus (HIV) and hepatitis B and C viruses. The tissue is preserved in a special nutritive solution, and it can be kept for up to 5 days in the storage medium, if used for transplantation. Improved methods of tissue procurement and preservation, refined surgical techniques, postoperative topical corticosteroids, and careful follow-up have decreased the incidence of graft rejection. Matching the blood type of the donor and the recipient may also improve the success rate (National Eye Institute, n.d.).

Keratoconus

Keratoconus is a noninflammatory, usually bilateral disease that is familial but has no well-defined inheritance pattern. It can be associated with Down syndrome, atopic dermatitis, Marfan's syndrome, aniridia (congenital absence of the iris), and retinitis pigmentosa (hereditary disease characterized by bilateral primary degeneration of the retina beginning in childhood and progressing to blindness by middle age).

The anterior cornea thins and protrudes forward, taking on a cone shape. Keratoconus usually appears during adolescence and slowly progresses between the ages of 20 and 60 years. The only symptom is blurred vision caused by the variable astigmatism associated with the altered corneal shape. The astigmatism may be corrected with glasses or rigid contact lenses. INTACS inserts, for example, are two clear plastic lenses surgically inserted on the cornea's perimeter to reduce astigmatism and myopia. INTACS inserts are generally used to delay the need for corneal transplantation when contact lenses or glasses no longer help a patient achieve adequate vision. The cornea can perforate as central corneal thinning progresses. In advanced cases, a penetrating keratoplasty is indicated before perforation occurs.

Intraocular Disorders

Cataract

A **cataract** is an area of opacity within the lens. The patient may have a cataract in one or both eyes. If cataracts are present in both eyes, one cataract may affect the patient's vision more than the other. Cataracts are one of the leading causes of vision loss in Canada. Nearly 2.5 million Canadians have some form of cataract, and this number is expected to double by 2031 (Buhrmann et al., 2007). Of Canadians aged 65 to 69, 25% have cataracts, and this proportion increases to 70% among those 80 years of age and older (Buhrmann et al., 2007). Cataract removal is the most common surgical procedure for Canadians older than 65 years.

Causes and Pathophysiological Processes. Although most cataracts are age related (*senile cataracts*), they can be associated with other factors. These include blunt or penetrating trauma, congenital factors such as maternal rubella, exposure to radiation or ultraviolet light, certain drugs such as systemic corticosteroids or long-term topical corticosteroids, and ocular inflammation (Kirkwood, 2008). Patients with diabetes mellitus tend to develop cataracts at a younger age than do patients without diabetes.

Cataract development is mediated by a number of factors. In senile cataract formation, it appears that altered metabolic processes within the lens cause an accumulation of water and alterations in the lens fibre structure. These changes affect lens transparency, causing vision changes (Kirkwood, 2008).

Clinical Manifestations. Patients with cataracts may complain of a decrease in vision, abnormal colour perception, and glare. Glare results from light scatter caused by the lens opacities, and it may be significantly worse at night when the pupil dilates. The visual decline is gradual, but the rate of cataract development varies from patient to patient. Secondary glaucoma can also occur if the enlarging lens causes an increase in intraocular pressure (IOP).

COLLABORATIVE CARE

Table 24-3 Cataract

Diagnostic	**Acute Care: Surgical Therapy**
• History and physical examination	**Preoperative**
• Visual acuity measurement	• Mydriatic, cycloplegic agents (see Table 24-4)
• Ophthalmoscopy (direct and indirect)	• Nonsteroidal anti-inflammatory drugs
• Slit-lamp microscopy	• Topical antibiotics
• Glare testing, potential acuity testing in selected patients	• Antianxiety medications
• Keratometry and A-scan ultrasonography (if surgery is planned)	**During Surgery**
	• Removal of lens:
	• Phacoemulsification (see Figure 24-4)
• Other tests (e.g., visual field perimetry) may be indicated to differentiate visual loss of cataract from visual loss of other causes	• Extracapsular extraction
	• Correction of surgical aphakia
	• Intraocular lens implantation (most frequent type of correction)
Collaborative Therapy	• Contact lens
Nonsurgical	**Postoperative**
• Prescription change for glasses	• Topical antibiotic
• Strong reading glasses or magnifiers	• Topical corticosteroid or other anti-inflammatory drug
• Increased lighting	• Mild analgesic agent if necessary
• Lifestyle adjustment	• Eye shield and activity as preferred by patient's surgeon
• Reassurance	

Diagnostic Studies. Diagnosis is based on decreased visual acuity or other complaints of visual dysfunction. The opacity is directly observable by ophthalmoscopic or slit-lamp microscopic examination. A totally opaque lens creates the appearance of a white pupil. Table 24-3 outlines other diagnostic studies that may be helpful in evaluating the visual effect of a cataract.

Collaborative Care. The presence of a cataract does not necessarily indicate a need for surgery. For many patients, the diagnosis is made long before they actually decide to have surgery. Nonsurgical therapy may postpone the need for surgery. Collaborative care for cataracts is described in Table 24-3.

Nonsurgical Therapy. Currently, no treatment to "cure" cataracts other than surgical removal is available. If the cataract is not removed, the patient's vision will continue to deteriorate. However, specific strategies may help the patient. Often, changing the patient's eyewear prescription can improve the level of visual acuity, at least temporarily. Other visual aids, such as strong reading glasses or magnifiers of some type, may help the patient with close vision. Increasing the amount of light to read or accomplish other near-vision tasks is another useful measure. The patient may be willing to adjust his or her lifestyle to accommodate for visual decline. For example, if glare makes it difficult to drive at night, a patient may elect to drive only during daylight hours and to have a family member drive at night. Sometimes, informing and reassuring the patient about the disease process makes the patient comfortable about choosing nonsurgical measures, at least temporarily.

Surgical Therapy. When one or a combination of specific strategies no longer provides an acceptable level of visual function, the patient is an appropriate candidate for surgery. The patient's occupational needs and lifestyle changes are also factors affecting the decision to undergo surgery. In some instances, factors other than the patient's visual needs may influence the need for surgery. Lens-induced problems such as increased IOP may necessitate lens removal. Opacities may prevent the ophthalmologist from obtaining a clear view of the retina in the patient with diabetic retinopathy or other sight-threatening pathological conditions. In those cases, the cataract may be removed to allow visualization of the retina and adequate management of the problem.

Preoperative Phase. The patient's preoperative preparation should include an appropriate documentation of the history and a physical examination. Because almost all patients undergo the procedure under anaesthesia, many physicians and surgical facilities do not require an extensive preoperative physical assessment. However, most patients with cataracts are older adults and may have several medical problems that should be evaluated and controlled before surgery. The surgeon may order preoperative antibiotic eye drops. The patient should not have food or fluids for approximately 6 to 8 hours before surgery. Almost all patients with cataracts are admitted to a surgical facility on an outpatient basis (see the Evidence-Informed Practice box). The patient is normally admitted several hours before surgery to allow adequate time for necessary preoperative procedures.

The instillation of dilating and nonsteroidal anti-inflammatory eye drops helps maintain pupil dilation and reduce inflammation, respectively. One type of drug used for dilation is a *mydriatic*, an α-adrenergic agonist that produces pupillary dilation by causing contraction of the iris dilator muscle. Another type of drug is a *cycloplegic*, an anticholinergic agent that produces paralysis of accommodation (cycloplegia) and thus pupillary dilation (mydriasis) by blocking the effect of acetylcholine on the ciliary body muscles or iris sphincter muscle. Examples of mydriatic and cycloplegic agents are listed in Table 24-4, and nursing considerations are discussed on p. 516. The patient often receives preoperative antianxiety medication before the injection of local anaesthetic.

SAFETY ALERT

- For patients using cycloplegic and mydriatic agents, instruct patient to wear dark glasses to minimize photophobia.
- Monitor for signs of systemic toxicity (e.g., tachycardia, central nervous system effects).

Intraoperative Phase. Cataract extraction is an intraocular procedure. In rare cases, intracapsular extraction is performed, in which the entire lens is removed with the capsule intact (this procedure may be necessary in instances of trauma). More commonly, extracapsular extraction is performed, in which the anterior capsule is opened and the lens nucleus and cortex are removed, leaving the remaining capsular bag intact. In extracapsular extraction, the surgeon can remove the lens nucleus by "scooping" it out with a lens loop or by *phacoemulsification*, in which the nucleus is fragmented by ultrasonic vibration and

EVIDENCE-INFORMED PRACTICE
What Surgical Location Has Better Outcomes for Cataract Surgery?

Clinical (PICO) Question
In adults with cataracts (P), does day surgery (I) or inpatient surgery (C) result in better visual acuity 4 months postoperatively, and which surgical location is safer and more cost effective (O)?

Best Available Evidence
Systematic review of randomized controlled trials (RCTs)

Critical Appraisal and Synthesis of Evidence
- Meta-analysis of two RCTs ($n = 1284$). Only one study with 1034 subjects was methodologically sound, and evidence is based primarily on this study.
- No significant differences in visual acuity were found as measured with the Snellen chart 4 months after surgery.
- Significantly more early complications (e.g., increased intraocular pressure) were reported in the day-surgery patients, with no relevance to vision acuity at 4 months.
- Costs for inpatient surgery were 20% higher than those for day surgery.
- Quality-of-life scores, patient satisfaction, and cataract symptom scores were similar for both patient groups.

Conclusions
- Day surgery is safe and, subjectively, preferred by patients.
- Day surgery provides the same visual outcome as inpatient surgery.

Implications for Nursing Practice
- Provide information that day-surgery outcomes are comparable to those of inpatient surgery and less costly.
- Quality of life may be improved if day surgery allows the patient to begin home recuperation sooner.

Reference for Evidence
Fedorowicz, Z., Lawrence, D., Gutierrez, P., & van Zuuren, E. J. (2011). Day care versus in-patient surgery for age-related cataract. *Cochrane Database of Systematic Reviews*, (7), CD004242. doi:10.1002/14651858.CD004242.pub4

PICO: P, patient population of interest; *I*, intervention or area of interest; *C*, comparison of interest or comparison group; *O*, outcome(s) of interest.

aspirated from inside the capsular bag (Riaz et al., 2006; Figure 24-6). In either case, the remaining cortex is aspirated with an irrigation and aspiration instrument. The choice of placement and type of incision varies among surgeons. Corneoscleral incisions necessitate closure with sutures, whereas scleral tunnel incisions are self-sealing and necessitate no closing suture. The incision required for phacoemulsification is considerably smaller than that required with intracapsular or standard extracapsular surgery.

In almost all cases today, an intraocular lens is implanted at the time of cataract extraction surgery. Because most patients undergo an extracapsular procedure, the lens of choice is a posterior chamber lens that is implanted in the capsular bag behind

DRUG THERAPY

Table 24-4 Topical Medications for Pupil Dilation

EXAMPLES	ONSET	DURATION	COMMENTS
Mydriatic Agents			
Phenylephrine hydrochloric acid (Mydfrin)	45-60 min	4-6 hr	May cause tachycardia and elevated blood pressure, especially in older adult patient; can cause a reflexive decrease in heart rate when blood pressure rises; punctal occlusion should be used to limit systemic absorption
Cycloplegic Agents			
Tropicamide (Mydriacyl)	20-40 min	4-6 hr	1% Solution used in cycloplegic refraction; 0.5% solution used in fundus examination
Cyclopentolate HCl acid (Cyclogyl)	30-75 min	6-24 hr	Has been associated with psychotic reactions and behavioural disturbances; used in cycloplegic refraction, fundus examination, and uveitis
Homatropine hydrobromide (Isopto Homatropine)	30-60 min	1-3 days	Used in cycloplegic refraction, uveitis; may be used for pupil dilation to allow patient to see around a central lens opacity
Atropine (Isopto Atropine)	30-180 min	6-12 days	Used in cycloplegic refraction, uveitis

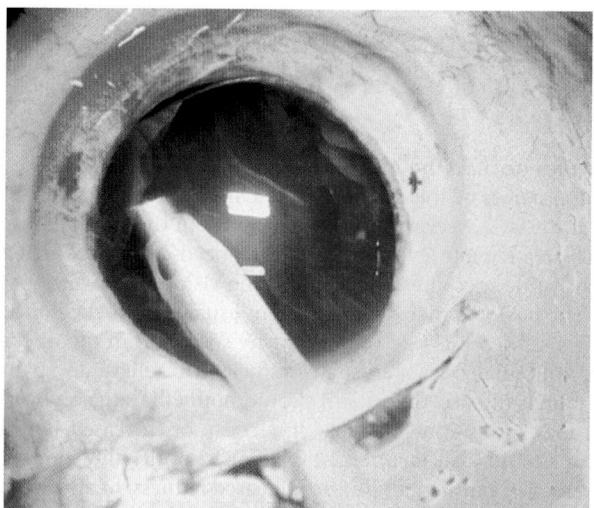

Figure 24-6 Phacoemulsification of a cataractous lens through a self-sealing, scleral-tunnel incision. Note the circular opening in the anterior lens capsule.

the iris. At the end of the procedure, additional medications such as antibiotics and corticosteroids may be administered (DeCroos & Afshari, 2008). Depending on the type of anaesthetic, the patient's eye is covered with a patch or protective shield. If used, a patch or protective shield is usually worn overnight and removed during the first postoperative visit.

Postoperative Phase. Unless complications occur, the patient is usually ready to go home as soon as the effects of sedative agents have worn off. Postoperative medications usually include antibiotic drops to prevent infection and corticosteroid drops to decrease the postoperative inflammatory response. There is some evidence that postoperative activity restrictions and nighttime eye shielding are unnecessary. However, many ophthalmologists still prefer that the patient avoid activities that increase the IOP, such as bending or stooping, coughing, or lifting.

The ophthalmologist usually examines the patient two or three times throughout the 6 to 8 weeks after surgery. During each postoperative examination, the ophthalmologist measures the patient's visual acuity, checks anterior chamber depth, assesses corneal clarity, and measures IOP. A flat anterior chamber may cause adhesions of the iris and cornea. The cornea may become hazy or cloudy from intraoperative trauma to the endothelium. Even on the operative day, the patient's uncorrected visual acuity in the operative eye may be good. However, it is not unusual or indicative of any problem if the patient's visual acuity is reduced immediately after surgery. Administration of the postoperative eye drops is gradually reduced in frequency and finally discontinued when the eye has healed. When the eye is fully recovered, the patient receives a final prescription for glasses. Although the majority of the postoperative refractive error is corrected with the intraocular lens, the patient still needs corrective eyewear for near vision and for any residual refractive error (Leyland & Pringle, 2006). The newest innovation is a multifocal IOL that corrects for both near and distance vision. Regardless of the type of IOL used, patients may still need glasses to achieve their best visual acuity.

NURSING MANAGEMENT: CATARACTS

▪ Nursing Assessment

The nurse should assess the patient's visual acuity for distance and near objects. If the patient is to undergo surgery, the nurse should especially note the visual acuity in the patient's unoperated eye. With this information, the nurse can determine how visually compromised the patient may be while the operative eye is healing. In addition, the nurse should assess the psychosocial effect of the patient's visual disability and the patient's level of knowledge regarding the disease process and therapeutic options. Postoperatively, it is important to assess the patient's level of comfort and ability to follow the postoperative regimen.

▪ Nursing Diagnoses

Nursing diagnoses for the patient with a cataract include, but are not limited to, the following:

- Self-care deficits *related to* visual deficit
- Anxiety *related to* lack of knowledge about the surgical and postoperative experience

■ Planning

Preoperatively, the overall goals are that the patient with a cataract will (a) make informed decisions regarding therapeutic options and (b) experience minimal anxiety. Postoperatively, the overall goals are that the patient with a cataract will (a) understand and comply with postoperative therapy, (b) maintain an acceptable level of physical and emotional comfort, and (c) remain free of infection and other complications.

■ Nursing Implementation

■ Health Promotion

There are no proven measures to prevent cataract development. However, it is wise (and certainly does no harm) to suggest that the patient wear sunglasses, avoid extraneous or unnecessary radiation, and maintain good nutrition and appropriate intake of antioxidant vitamins (e.g., vitamins C and E). Also information about vision enhancement techniques should be provided to the patient who chooses not to undergo surgery.

■ Acute Intervention

Preoperatively, the patient with cataracts needs accurate information about the disease process and the treatment options, especially because cataract surgery is considered an elective procedure. Although cataracts are not a life-threatening condition, the patient needs to know that without surgery, some degree of visual disability will develop. The nurse should be available to give the patient and the family or caregivers information to help them make an informed decision about appropriate treatment.

For the patient who elects to have surgery, the nurse is able to provide information, support, and reassurance about the surgical and postoperative experience that can reduce or alleviate the patient's anxiety.

When administering topical medications for pupil dilation before surgery (see Table 24-4 for examples), note that patients with dark irides may need a larger dose. Photophobia is common; therefore, decreasing the room lighting is helpful. These medications produce transient stinging and burning and are contraindicated for use in patients with narrow-angle glaucoma because angle-closure glaucoma may be produced. Mydriatic agents can produce significant cardiovascular effects.

> **SAFETY ALERT**
>
> Immediately after eye drops are administered, patients should close their eyes and apply gentle pressure with fingers to the inside corner of the eye (punta) for 2 to 3 minutes. This retards drainage of the solution from the intended area and helps prevent rapid systemic reactions (Bartlett, 2010).

Table 24-5 outlines patient and caregiver teaching after eye surgery. Patients with a patch should be informed that they will not have depth perception until the patch is removed (usually within 24 hours). This necessitates special considerations to avoid possible falls or other injuries. The patient with significant visual impairment in the unoperated eye requires more assistance while the operated eye is patched. Once the patch is removed (usually within 24 hours), most patients with visual impairment in the unoperated eye have adequate vision for necessary

PATIENT & CAREGIVER TEACHING GUIDE

Table 24-5   After Eye Surgery

Teach patient or both patient and caregiver the following:

1. Proper hygiene and eye care techniques to ensure that medications, dressings, or surgical wound are not contaminated during necessary eye care

2. Signs and symptoms of infection and when and how to report those to allow early recognition and treatment of possible infection

3. Importance of complying with postoperative restrictions on head positioning, bending, coughing, and Valsalva's manoeuvre to optimize visual outcomes and prevent increased intraocular pressure

4. How to instill eye medications with the use of aseptic techniques and to comply with prescribed eye medication regimen to prevent infection

5. How to monitor pain and take prescribed medication for pain as directed and to report pain not relieved by prescribed medication

6. Importance of continued follow-up as recommended to maximize potential visual outcomes

Source: American Society of Ophthalmic Registered Nurses. (2004). *Core curriculum for ophthalmic nursing* (2nd ed.). Dubuque, IA: Kendall/Hunt.

activities because the implanted IOL provides immediate visual rehabilitation in the operated eye. On occasion, a patient may require 1 or 2 weeks for the visual acuity in the operated eye to reach an adequate level for most visual needs. Such a patient also needs some special assistance until the vision improves.

The postoperative cataract patient usually experiences little or no pain. There may be some scratchy sensation in the operated eye. Mild analgesics are usually sufficient to relieve any pain. If the pain is intense, the patient should notify the surgeon because this may indicate hemorrhage, infection, or increased IOP. The nurse should also instruct the patient to notify the surgeon of increased or purulent drainage, increased redness, or any decrease in visual acuity. (A nursing care plan for the patient after eye surgery is available on the Evolve Web site for this chapter.)

■ Ambulatory and Home Care

For the patient with cataracts who has not undergone surgery, the nurse can suggest ways in which the patient may modify activities or lifestyle to accommodate the visual deficit caused by the cataract. The nurse should also provide the patient with accurate information about appropriate long-term eye care.

Patients with cataracts who undergo surgery remain in the surgical facility for only a few hours. The patient and the family are responsible for almost all postoperative care. It is essential that the nurse give them written and verbal instructions before discharge. These teachings should include information about postoperative eye care, activity restrictions, medications, follow-up visit scheduling, and signs and symptoms of possible complications. The patient's family should be included in the instruction because some patients may have difficulty with self-care activities, especially if the vision in the unoperated eye is poor. The nurse should provide an opportunity for the patient and family to demonstrate any necessary self-care activities. Most patients experience little visual impairment after surgery.

IOL implants provide immediate visual rehabilitation, and many patients achieve a usable level of visual acuity within a few days after surgery. Also, the patient's eye may remain patched for only 24 hours, and many patients have good vision in the unoperated eye. A few patients may experience significant visual impairment postoperatively: those who do not have an IOL implanted at the time of surgery, those who require several weeks to achieve a usable level of visual acuity after surgery, and those with poor vision in the unoperated eye. For such patients, the time between surgery and receiving aphakic glasses or contacts can be a period of significant visual disability. The nurse can suggest ways in which the patient and the family can modify activities and the environment to maintain an adequate level of safe functioning. Suggestions may include getting assistance with going up stairs, removing scatter or area rugs and other potential obstacles, keeping furniture in the same place, preparing meals for freezing before surgery, or obtaining audio books for diversion until visual acuity improves.

Evaluation

The overall expected outcomes for the patient who has cataract surgery are as follows:
- The patient will have improved vision.
- The patient will be better able to take care of himself or herself.
- The patient will have minimal to no pain.
- The patient will be optimistic about expected outcomes.

AGE-RELATED CONSIDERATIONS: CATARACTS

Most patients with cataracts are older adults. When an older patient is visually impaired, even temporarily, the patient may experience a loss of independence, lack of control over her or his life, and a significant change in self-perception. Societal devaluation of older individuals complicates these experiences. Many older patients need emotional support and encouragement, as well as specific suggestions to allow a maximum level of independent function. Assure older patients that cataract surgery can be accomplished safely and comfortably with minimal sedation. A study in which nonagenarians (individuals aged 90 to 99) were compared with octogenarians (aged 80 to 90) revealed that nonagenarians are not at increased risk of ocular complications from cataract surgery (Tseng et al., 2011).The use of outpatient surgery for cataract surgery is particularly beneficial for older patients who may become confused or disoriented during hospitalization.

Retinopathy

Retinopathy is a process of microvascular damage to the retina. It can develop slowly or rapidly and lead to blurred vision and progressive vision loss. In adults, retinopathy is most often associated with diabetes mellitus and hypertension.

Diabetic retinopathy is the leading cause of visual disability and blindness in Canadians with long-standing uncontrolled diabetes (diabetes is discussed in Chapter 52). Because diabetes has been diagnosed in 1.3 million Canadians, the incidence of diabetic retinopathy will continue to increase. In a Canadian study of diabetic retinopathy in native and non-native Canadians, the data indicated that ethnicity does play a significant role in the development and severity of diabetic retinopathy, but potential risk factors are not significantly different (Ross, McKenna, Mozejko, & Fick, 2007). *Nonproliferative retinopathy* is the most common form of diabetic retinopathy and is characterized by capillary microaneurysms, retinal swelling, and hard exudates. Macular edema represents a worsening of the retinopathy as plasma leaks from macular blood vessels. This can lead to a severe loss of central vision. As the disease advances, *proliferative retinopathy* may occur where new blood vessels grow. However, these blood vessels are abnormal, fragile, and predisposed to leak, thus causing severe vision loss. Fluorescein angiography is used to detect diabetic macular edema, which may be treated with laser photocoagulation. An angiogram is a type of photograph of the retinal blood vessels that helps with these diagnoses. In fluorescein angiography, fluorescein dye is used to highlight blood vessels in the photographs, so that the vessels can be identified and evaluated; the examination does not involve X-rays, radioactive materials, or iodine-based dyes, as do other types of angiography. Both the appearance and nonappearance of dye in the photographs are clues to diagnosis and treatment. In laser photocoagulation, the heat from a laser is used to seal or destroy abnormal, leaking blood vessels in the retina for the treatment of macular edema.

Hypertensive retinopathy is caused by blockages in retinal blood vessels that result from hypertension. (Hypertension is discussed in Chapter 35.) These changes may not initially affect a person's vision. On a routine eye examination, retinal hemorrhages and macular swelling can be noted. Sustained, severe hypertension can cause swelling of the optic disc and nerve (*papilledema*), leading to sudden visual loss. Treatment, which may be required on an emergency basis, focuses on lowering the blood pressure. Normal vision is restored in most affected patients with treatment of the underlying cause of the hypertension.

Retinal Detachment

A **retinal detachment** is a separation of the sensory retina and the underlying pigment epithelium, with fluid accumulation between the two layers. The incidence of nontraumatic retinal detachment is approximately 1 per 10,000 individuals each year. This number is higher when aphakic individuals are included because retinal detachment is more likely to occur in aphakic patients. In the patient with no other risk factors who has had a retinal detachment in one eye, the risk of detachment in the second eye is 2% to 25%. Almost all patients with an untreated, symptomatic retinal detachment become blind in the involved eye.

Cause and Pathophysiological Processes

There are many causes of retinal detachment. The most common cause, *retinal break*, is an interruption in the full thickness of the retinal tissue, and it can be classified as a tear or hole. *Retinal holes* are atrophic retinal breaks that occur spontaneously. *Retinal tears* can occur as the vitreous humor shrinks during aging and pulls on the retina. The retina tears when the traction force exceeds the strength of the retina. Once there is a break in the retina, liquid vitreous humor can enter the subretinal space between the sensory layer and the retinal pigment epithelium layer, causing a *rhegmatogenous* retinal detachment. Less frequently, retinal detachment can occur when abnormal membranes mechanically pull on the retina. These are called *tractional* detachments. A third type of retinal detachment is the *secondary*

Table 24-6 Risk Factors for Retinal Detachment

- Increasing age
- Severe myopia
- Eye trauma
- Retinopathy (diabetic)
- Cataract or glaucoma surgery
- Family or personal history

Source: National Eye Institute/National Institutes of Health. (2009). *Facts about retinal detachment.* Retrieved from *http://www.nei.nih.gov/health/retinaldetach/retinaldetach.asp#c*

COLLABORATIVE CARE

Table 24-7 Retinal Detachment

Diagnostic	During Surgery
• History and physical examination	• Laser photocoagulation
• Visual acuity measurement	• Cryoretinopexy
• Ophthalmoscopy (direct and indirect)	• Scleral buckling procedure
• Slit-lamp microscopy	• Draining of subretinal fluid
• Ultrasonography if cornea, lens, or vitreous humor is hazy or opaque	• Vitrectomy
	• Intravitreal bubble
Collaborative Therapy	**Postoperative**
Preoperative	• Topical antibiotic
• Mydriatic, cycloplegic eye drops (Table 24-4)	• Topical corticosteroid
	• Analgesia
• Photocoagulation of retinal break that has not progressed to detachment	• Mydriatics
	• Positioning and activity as preferred by patient's surgeon

or *exudative* detachment, which occurs in conditions that allow fluid to accumulate in the subretinal space (e.g., choroidal tumours, intraocular inflammation). Risk factors for retinal detachment are listed in Table 24-6.

Clinical Manifestations

Patients with a detaching retina describe symptoms that include *photopsia* (light flashes), floaters, and a "cobweb," "hairnet," or ring in the field of vision. Once the retina has detached, the patient describes a painless loss of peripheral or central vision, "like a curtain" coming across the field of vision. The area of visual loss corresponds to the area of detachment. If the detachment is in the superior nasal retina, the visual field loss is in the inferior temporal area. If the detachment is small or develops slowly in the periphery, the patient may not be aware of a visual problem. The effects of a retinal detachment can be viewed online at VisionSimulations.com (see the Related Resources at the end of this chapter).

Diagnostic Studies

Visual acuity measurements should be the first diagnostic procedure with any complaint of vision loss (Table 24-7). The retinal detachment can be directly visualized through direct and indirect ophthalmoscopy or slit-lamp microscopy in conjunction with a special lens to view the far periphery of the retina. Ultrasonography may be useful for identifying a retinal detachment if the retina cannot be directly visualized (e.g., when the cornea, the lens, or the vitreous humor is hazy or opaque).

Collaborative Care

The ophthalmologist carefully evaluates the patient with retinal breaks to determine whether prophylactic laser photocoagulation or cryopexy is necessary to avoid possible retinal detachment. Some retinal breaks are not likely to progress to detachment. The ophthalmologist simply monitors the patient, giving precise information about the warning signs and symptoms of impending detachment and instructing the patient to seek immediate evaluation if any of those signs or symptoms occurs. Most ophthalmologists refer patients with retinal detachments to a retinal specialist. Treatment of retinal detachment has two objectives: to seal any retinal breaks and to relieve inward traction on the retina. Several techniques are used to accomplish these objectives.

Surgical Therapy
Laser Photocoagulation and Cryopexy. These techniques seal retinal breaks by creating an inflammatory reaction that causes a chorioretinal adhesion or scar. *Laser photocoagulation* involves using an intense, precisely focused light beam, such as the argon laser, to create an inflammatory reaction. The light is directed at the area of the retinal break. This produces a scar that seals the edges of the hole or tear and prevents fluid from collecting in the subretinal space and causing a detachment. The retinal specialist may use photocoagulation alone if there is a single small tear with little or no detachment in the periphery and minimal subretinal fluid. For retinal breaks accompanied by significant detachment, the retinal specialist may use photocoagulation intraoperatively in conjunction with scleral buckling. Tears or holes without accompanying retinal detachment may be treated prophylactically with laser photocoagulation if the retinal specialist judges them to be at high risk of progressing to retinal detachment. When used alone, laser therapy is an outpatient procedure that usually necessitates only topical anaesthesia, and the patient usually experiences minimal adverse symptoms during or after the procedure.

An alternative method used to seal retinal breaks is *cryopexy.* This procedure involves using extreme cold to create the inflammatory reaction that produces the sealing scar. The ophthalmologist applies the cryoprobe instrument to the external globe in the area over the tear. This is usually done on an outpatient basis and with the use of a local anaesthetic. As with photocoagulation, cryotherapy may be used alone or during scleral buckling surgery. The patient may experience significant discomfort and eye pain after cryopexy. Encourage the patient to take the prescribed pain medication after the procedure.

Scleral Buckling. *Scleral buckling* is an extraocular surgical procedure that involves compressing the globe so that the pigment epithelium, the choroid, and the sclera move toward the detached retina. The retinal surgeon sutures a silicone implant against the sclera at the site of the retinal tear to push the sclera towards the tear and this causes the sclera to buckle inward. This not only helps seal retinal breaks but also helps relieve inward traction on the retina. The surgeon may place an encircling band over the implant if there are multiple retinal breaks, if the surgeon cannot

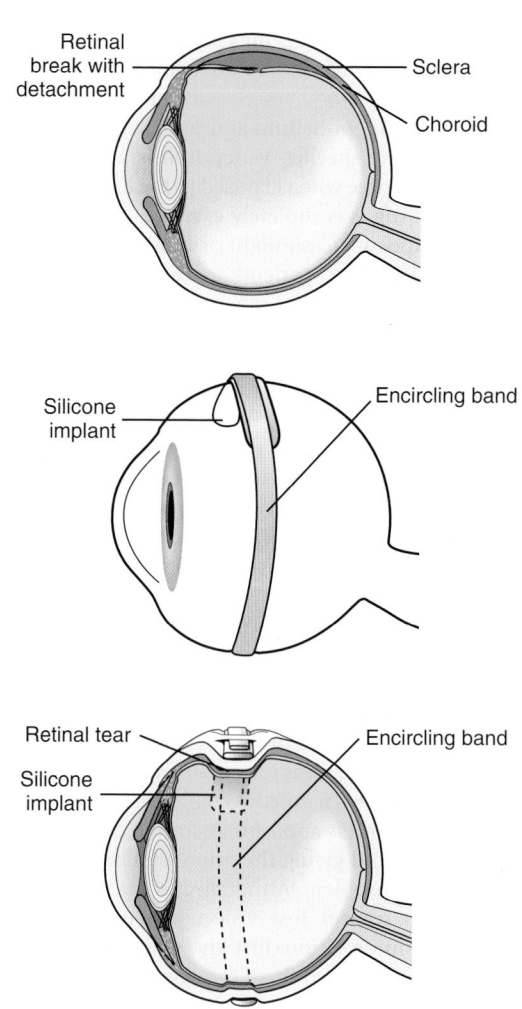

Figure 24-7 Retinal break with detachment *(top)*; surgical repair by scleral buckling technique *(middle and bottom)*.

locate suspected breaks, or if there is widespread inward traction on the retina (Figure 24-7). To drain any subretinal fluid, a small-gauge needle is inserted to facilitate contact between the retina and the buckled sclera. Scleral buckling is usually accomplished with the use of a local anaesthetic, and the patient may be discharged on the first postoperative day. Scleral buckling surgery is often performed as an outpatient procedure.

Intraocular Procedures. In addition to the extraocular procedures described, retinal surgeons may use one or more intraocular procedures in treating some retinal detachments. *Pneumatic retinopexy* is the intravitreal injection of a gas to form a temporary bubble in the vitreous humor that closes retinal breaks and provides apposition of the separated retinal layers. Because the intravitreal bubble is temporary, this technique is combined with laser photocoagulation or cryotherapy. The patient with an intravitreal bubble must position the head so that the bubble is in contact with the retinal break. It may be necessary for the patient to maintain this position as much as possible for up to several weeks.

Vitrectomy (surgical removal of the vitreous humor) may be used to relieve traction on the retina, especially when the traction results from proliferative diabetic retinopathy. Vitrectomy may be combined with scleral buckling to provide a dual effect in relieving traction. In *proliferative vitreoretinopathy,* membranes develop in the vitreous cavity and on the retinal surface, exerting traction that causes folds in the retina. Vitrectomy may be combined with membrane peeling to relieve traction in those cases.

Postoperative Considerations in Scleral Buckling and Intraocular Procedures. Reattachment is successful in 90% of scleral buckling procedures for retinal detachments. Visual prognosis varies, depending on the extent, the length, and the area of detachment. Postoperatively, the patient may be on bed rest and may require special positioning to maintain proper position of an intravitreal bubble. The patient may need multiple topical medications, including antibiotics, anti-inflammatory agents, or dilating agents. Activity recommendations vary according to the physician's preference, the extent of the detachment, and the particular repair procedure.

In most cases, retinal detachment is an urgent situation, and the patient is confronted suddenly with the need for surgery. The patient needs emotional support, especially during the immediate preoperative period when preparations for surgery can lead to additional anxiety. When the patient experiences postoperative pain, the nurse should administer prescribed pain medications and teach the patient to take the medication as necessary after being discharged. The patient may go home within a few hours of surgery or may remain in the hospital for several days, depending on the surgeon and the type of repair.

Discharge planning and teaching are important, and the nurse should begin these processes as early as possible because the patient does not remain hospitalized long. Patient and caregiver teaching after eye surgery is discussed in Table 24-5. The patient is at risk for retinal detachment in the other eye. Therefore, the nurse should teach the patient the signs and symptoms of retinal detachment. The nurse can also promote use of proper protective eyewear to help avoid retinal detachments related to trauma.

The level of activity restriction after surgery for retinal detachment varies greatly. The nurse should verify the prescribed level of activity with each patient's surgeon and help the patient plan for any necessary assistance related to activity restrictions.

Age-Related Macular Degeneration

Age-related macular degeneration (AMD) is an eye disease that begins after age 60 that progressively destroys the macula (the central portion of the retina), causing irreversible central vision loss. It is the most common cause of irreversible central vision loss in persons older than 60 in Canada. More than 250,000 Canadians have the most advanced type (Muzychka, 2009). The number of Canadians with AMD is expected to double in 25 years (Buhrmann et al., 2007). AMD is divided into two forms: dry (nonexudative) and wet (exudative). People with dry AMD, which is the more common form (90% of all cases), may often notice that tasks requiring close vision become more difficult. In this form, the macular cells start to atrophy, leading to a slowly progressive and painless vision loss.

Wet AMD is the more severe form. Untreated, the majority of patients with wet AMD become functionally blind. Wet AMD accounts for 90% of the cases of AMD-related blindness. Wet AMD has a more rapid onset and is noted by the development of abnormal blood vessels in or near the macula. Only 10% to 15% of patients with dry AMD go on to develop the wet form.

Causes and Pathophysiological Processes

AMD is related to retinal aging. Genetic factors also appear to play a major role, and family history is a major risk factor for AMD. A gene responsible for some cases of AMD has been identified. People who currently smoke are twice as likely to develop late AMD as are nonsmokers (Buhrmann et al., 2007). Other risk factors include obesity, race, and sex (women appear to be more at risk; National Eye Institute, 2009). It is believed that antioxidant nutrients are protective against the development or progression, or both, of AMD. New evidence suggests that β-carotene and vitamin E may play a detrimental role, however. Mechanisms of protection are also being discovered among non-antioxidant nutrients such as omega-3 fatty acids and the B vitamins. A proper nutritious diet is thought to be more protective than nutritional supplements. The nutrients with the strongest evidence of a protective effect include zinc, lutein, zeaxanthin, DHA (docosahexaenoic acid) and EPA (eicosapentaenoic acid). Older patients are at higher risk of zinc deficiency, which may increase their risk of vision loss from AMD (Olson, Erie, & Bakri, 2011).

The dry form of AMD starts with the abnormal accumulation of yellowish extracellular deposits called *drusen* in the retinal pigment epithelium. The atrophy and degeneration of macular cells then result. Wet AMD is characterized by the growth of new blood vessels from their normal location in the choroid to an abnormal location in the retinal epithelium. As the new blood vessels leak, scar tissue gradually forms. Acute vision loss may occur in some cases, with bleeding from subretinal neovascular membranes.

Clinical Manifestations

The patient may complain of blurred and darkened vision, the presence of *scotomas* (blind spots in the visual field), and *metamorphopsia* (distortion of vision). Many people may not notice unilateral early changes in their vision if the other eye is not affected.

Diagnostic Studies

In addition to visual acuity measurement, the primary diagnostic procedure is ophthalmoscopy. The examiner looks for drusen and other fundus changes associated with AMD. The Amsler grid test may help define the involved area, and the result provides a baseline for future comparison. Fundus photography and intravenous angiography with fluorescein or indocyanine green dyes, or both, may be helpful in further defining the extent and type of AMD.

Collaborative Care

Vision often does not improve for most people with AMD. Limited treatment options for patients with wet AMD include several medications that are injected directly into the vitreous cavity. Pegaptanib (Macugen), ranibizumab (Lucentis), and bevacizumab (Avastin) are selective inhibitors of endothelial growth factor that helps to slow vision loss in wet AMD. Adverse effects of the drugs include blurred vision, eye irritation, eye pain, and photosensitivity. The injections are given at 4- to 6-week intervals, depending on which drug is being used. Retinal instability is determined by ocular coherence tomography, which allows the physician to identify fluid in the central retinal to determine the need for continued intravitreal injections.

Photodynamic therapy entails the use of verteporfin (Visudyne) intravenously and a "cold" laser to excite the dye. This procedure destroys the abnormal blood vessels without permanent damage to the retinal pigment epithelium and photoreceptor cells. Criteria for its use are very specific. Verteporfin is a photosensitizing drug that becomes active when exposed to the low-level laser light waves. Until the drug is completely excreted by the body, it can be activated by exposure to sunlight or other high-intensity light such as halogen. Therefore, patients are cautioned to avoid direct exposure to sunlight and other intense forms of light for 5 days after treatment. After receiving therapy, patients must be completely covered because any exposure to skin by sunlight could activate the drug in that area, resulting in a thermal burn.

People at risk for developing advanced AMD should (in consultation with their health care provider) consider supplements of vitamins and minerals. The cessation of smoking may also help in halting the progression of dry AMD to a more advanced stage. In current clinical trials aimed at reducing the progression of AMD and slowing the associated vision loss, researchers are examining the effectiveness of corticosteroid preparations injected directly into the vitreous cavity. The slow-release deposit of corticosteroids under the conjunctiva is also under investigation.

Many patients with low-vision assistive devices can continue reading and retain a license to drive during the daytime and at lowered speeds. The permanent loss of central vision has significant psychosocial implications for nursing care. Nursing management of the patient with uncorrectable visual impairment is discussed on p. 516 and is appropriate for the patient with AMD. The nurse should avoid giving the impression that "nothing can be done" about the problem. Although it is true that therapy will not help patients recover lost vision, much can be done to augment the remaining vision. Just knowing that the health care provider has not abandoned them can give these patients a more positive outlook.

Glaucoma

Glaucoma is the name of not one disease but rather a group of disorders characterized by elevated intraocular pressure (IOP) and the consequences of elevated pressure, optic nerve atrophy, and peripheral visual field loss.

IOP is regulated by the formation and reabsorption of aqueous humor. The presence of glaucoma is directly related to the balance or imbalance of this fluid. Glaucoma is the second most common reason for vision loss in Canadians. More than 250,000 Canadians have chronic open-angle glaucoma, the most common form of the disease; however, only 50% of them are aware that they do (Muzychka, 2009). Risk factors for glaucoma include family history, age, nearsightedness, ethnicity (e.g., individuals of African descent are more likely to develop the disease), and diabetes. The incidence of glaucoma increases with age. Blindness from glaucoma is largely preventable with early detection and appropriate treatment.

Causes and Pathophysiological Processes

The cause of glaucoma is related to the consequences of elevated IOP. A proper balance between the rate of aqueous humor production (referred to as *inflow*) and the rate of aqueous humor reabsorption (referred to as *outflow*) is essential to maintain the IOP within normal limits. The place where the outflow occurs is called the "angle" as it is the angle where the iris meets the cornea.

When the rate of inflow is greater than the rate of outflow, IOP can rise above the normal limits. If IOP remains elevated, permanent vision loss may occur.

Primary open-angle glaucoma (POAG) is the most common type of glaucoma. In POAG, the outflow of aqueous humor is decreased through the trabecular meshwork. The drainage channels become clogged, and damage to the optic nerve can then result (Sharts-Hopko & Glynn-Milley, 2009).

Primary angle-closure glaucoma (PACG) is caused by a reduction in the outflow of aqueous humor that results from angle closure. This is usually caused by the bulging forward of the lens as a result of an aging process. Angle closure may also occur as a result of pupil dilation in the patient with anatomically narrow angles. Dilation causes peripheral iris bulging with the same outcome of covering the trabecular meshwork and blocking the outflow channels. An acute attack may be precipitated by situations in which the pupil remains in a partially dilated state long enough to cause an acute and significant rise in the IOP. This may occur because of drug-induced mydriasis, emotional excitement, or darkness. Drug-induced mydriasis may occur not only from topical ophthalmic preparations but also from many systemic medications (both prescription and over-the-counter drugs). The nurse should check drug records and documentation before administering medications to the patient with angle-closure glaucoma and instruct the patient not to take any mydriasis-producing medications.

In *secondary glaucoma*, IOP increases as a result of other ocular or systemic conditions that may block the outflow channels in some way, such as inflammation from trauma or ocular tumours.

Clinical Manifestations

POAG develops slowly and without symptoms. The patient with POAG reports no symptoms of pain or pressure. The patient usually does not notice the gradual visual field loss until peripheral vision has been severely compromised. Eventually, the patient with untreated glaucoma has "tunnel vision" in which only a small centre field can be seen and all peripheral vision is absent.

Acute angle-closure glaucoma causes definite symptoms, including sudden, excruciating pain in or around the eye. This is often accompanied by nausea and vomiting. Visual symptoms include blurred vision, ocular redness, and seeing coloured halos around lights. The acute rise in IOP may also cause corneal edema, which gives the cornea a frosted appearance.

Manifestations of subacute or chronic angle-closure glaucoma appear more gradually. The patient who has had a previous, unrecognized episode of subacute angle-closure glaucoma may report a history of blurred vision, ocular redness, eye or brow pain, or seeing coloured halos around lights. The effects of glaucoma can be viewed online at VisionSimulations.com (see the Related Resources at the end of this chapter).

Diagnostic Studies

IOP is usually elevated in glaucoma. Normal IOP is 10 to 21 mm Hg. In the patient with elevated pressures, the ophthalmologist usually repeats the measurements over time to verify the elevation. In open-angle glaucoma, IOP is usually between 22 and 32 mm Hg. In acute angle-closure glaucoma, IOP may be 50 mm Hg or higher.

In open-angle glaucoma, slit-lamp microscopy reveals a normal angle. In angle-closure glaucoma, the examiner may note a markedly narrow or flat anterior chamber angle, an edematous cornea, a fixed and moderately dilated pupil, and ciliary

injection. Gonioscopy allows better visualization of the anterior chamber angle.

Measures of peripheral and central vision provide other diagnostic information. Whereas central acuity may remain 20/20 even in the presence of severe peripheral visual field loss, visual field perimetry may reveal subtle changes in the peripheral retina early in the disease process, long before actual scotomas develop. In chronic open-angle glaucoma, when visual field defects begin to appear, the initial scotoma is a small, football-shaped defect that gradually progresses to a nasal and superior field defect. In acute angle-closure glaucoma, central visual acuity is reduced if the patient has corneal edema, and the visual fields may be markedly decreased.

As glaucoma progresses, *optic disc cupping* occurs. This is visible with direct or indirect ophthalmoscopy (Figure 24-8). The optic disc becomes wider, deeper, and paler (light grey or white). Optic disc cupping may be one of the first signs of chronic open-angle glaucoma. Optic disc photographs are useful for comparison over time to demonstrate an increase in the cup-to-disc ratio and progressive blanching.

Collaborative Care

The primary focus of glaucoma therapy is to keep the IOP low enough to prevent the patient from developing optic nerve damage. This damage is manifested by increasing visual field loss

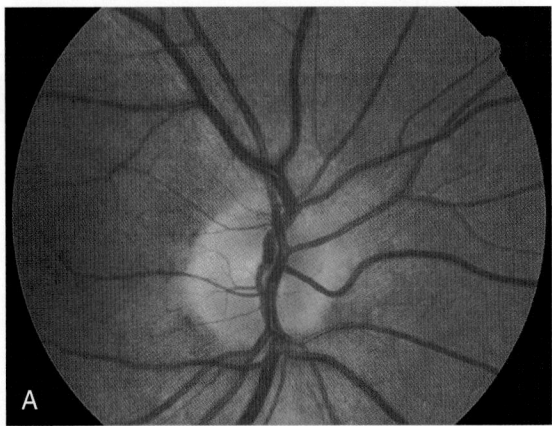
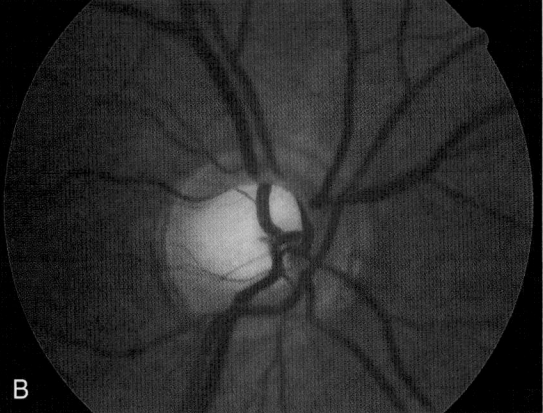

Figure 24-8 The optic disc. **A,** In the normal eye, the optic disc is pink with little cupping. **B,** In glaucoma, the optic disc is bleached, and optic cupping is present. (Note the appearance of the retinal vessels, which travel over the edge of the optic cup and appear to dip into it.)

COLLABORATIVE CARE

Table 24-8 Glaucoma

Diagnostic	Collaborative Therapy
• History and physical examination	**Ambulatory or Home Care for Open-Angle Glaucoma**
• Visual acuity measurement	**Drug Therapy***
• Tonometry	• β-Adrenergic blockers
• Ophthalmoscopy (direct and indirect)	• α-Adrenergic agonists
	• Cholinergic agents (miotics)
• Slit-lamp microscopy	• Carbonic anhydrase inhibitors
• Gonioscopy	**Surgical Therapy**
• Visual field perimetry	• Argon laser trabeculoplasty
• Fundus photography	• Trabeculectomy with or without filtering implant
	Acute Care for Angle-Closure Glaucoma
	• Topical cholinergic agent
	• Hyperosmotic agent
	• Laser peripheral iridotomy
	• Surgical iridectomy

*See Table 24-9.

and progressive optic disc cupping. Specific therapies vary with the type of glaucoma. The diagnostic and collaborative care of glaucoma is summarized in Table 24-8.

Chronic Open-Angle Glaucoma.

Initial treatment in chronic open-angle glaucoma is with drugs (Table 24-9). As with all drug therapy, the patient must understand that continued treatment and supervision are necessary because the drugs control but do not cure the disease.

Argon laser trabeculoplasty (ALT) is a therapeutic option to lower IOP when medications are not successful or when the patient either cannot or will not use the drug therapy as recommended. Argon laser trabeculoplasty is an outpatient procedure that necessitates only topical anaesthesia. The topical drops anaesthetize the cornea before the gonioscopy lens is applied, allowing visualization of the treatment area. Approximately 50 laser "spots" are evenly spaced around the superior or inferior 180 degrees of the trabecular meshwork. The laser stimulates scarring and contraction of the trabecular meshwork, opening the outflow channels. Argon laser trabeculoplasty reduces IOP in approximately 75% of cases. A second 180-degree area may be treated in a subsequent procedure. The patient uses topical corticosteroids for approximately 3 to 5 days after the procedure. The most common complication is an acute postoperative rise in IOP. Because the decrease in pressure is gradual, the patient continues taking the preoperative glaucoma medication. The ophthalmologist examines the patient 1 week after the procedure and again 4 to 6 weeks after surgery.

DRUG THERAPY

Table 24-9 Acute and Chronic Glaucoma

DRUG	ACTION	ADVERSE EFFECTS	NURSING CONSIDERATIONS
β-Adrenergic Blockers			
Betaxolol (Betoptic)	Cardioselective β_1-blocker; probably decreases aqueous humor production	Transient discomfort; systemic reactions rarely reported but include bradycardia, heart block, pulmonary distress, headache, depression	Topical drugs; minimal effect on pulmonary and cardiovascular parameters. Contraindicated for use in patient with bradycardia, cardiogenic shock, or overt cardiac failure. Systemic absorption can have additive effect with systemic β_1-blocking agents.
Levobunolol (Betagan) Timolol maleate (Timoptic)	Noncardioselective β_1- and β_2-blockers; probably decrease aqueous humor production	Transient ocular discomfort, blurred vision, photophobia, blepharoconjunctivitis, bradycardia, decreased BP, bronchospasm, headache, depression	Topical drops; same as betaxolol; these noncardioselective β_2-blockers are also contraindicated for use in patients with asthma or severe COPD.
α-Adrenergic Agonists			
Apraclonidine (Iopidine) Brimonidine (Alphagan, apo-Brimonidine)	α-Adrenergic agonists; probably decrease aqueous humor production	Ocular redness; irregular heart rate	Topical drops; used to control or prevent acute post–laser procedure IOP rise (used before and immediately after ALT and iridotomy, Nd:YAG laser capsulotomy) Teach patient at risk for systemic reactions to occlude puncta.
Latanoprost (Xalatan)	Prostaglandin-F analogue	Increased brown iris pigmentation, ocular discomfort and redness, dryness, itching, and sensation of foreign body	Topical drops Teach patient not to take more than 1 drop per evening and to remove contact lens 15 min before instilling.

DRUG THERAPY

Table 24-9 Acute and Chronic Glaucoma—cont'd

DRUG	ACTION	ADVERSE EFFECTS	NURSING CONSIDERATIONS
Cholinergic Agents (Miotics)			
Carbachol (Isopto Carbachol)	Parasympathomimetic; stimulates iris sphincter contraction, causing miosis and opening of trabecular meshwork, facilitating aqueous outflow; also partially inhibits cholinesterase	Transient ocular discomfort, headache, ache in brow area, blurred vision, decreased adaptation to darkness, syncope, excessive salivation, dysrhythmias, vomiting, diarrhea, hypotension, retinal detachment in susceptible individual (rare)	Topical drops Caution patient about decreased visual acuity caused by miosis, particularly in dim light.
Pilocarpine (Isopto Carpine)	Parasympathomimetic; stimulates iris sphincter contraction, causing miosis and opening of trabecular meshwork, facilitating aqueous humor outflow	Same as those of carbachol	Topical drops Same cautions as for carbachol
Carbonic Anhydrase Inhibitors			
Systemic			
Acetazolamide (Apo-Acetazolamide) Methazolamide (Apo-Methazolamide)	Decreases aqueous humor production	Paraesthesias, especially "tingling" sensation in extremities; hearing dysfunction or tinnitus; loss of appetite; taste alteration; GI disturbances; drowsiness; confusion	Oral nonbacteriostatic sulphonamides Anaphylaxis and other sulpha type of allergic reactions may occur in patient allergic to sulpha. Diuretic effect can lower electrolyte levels. Ask patient about aspirin use; drug should not be given to patient receiving high-dose aspirin therapy.
Topical			
Brinzolamide (Azopt) Dorzolamide (Trusopt)	Decreases aqueous humor production	Transient stinging, blurred vision, redness	Same as for systemic agents
Combination Therapy			
Timolol maleate and dorzolamide (Cosopt)	Combination of two drugs (β-adrenergic blocker and topical carbonic anhydrase inhibitors)	Same as those for timolol maleate and dorzolamide (described previously)	—
Hyperosmolar Agents			
Mannitol solution (Osmitrol)	Increases extracellular osmolarity so intracellular water moves to the extracellular and vascular spaces, reducing IOP	Nausea, vomiting, diarrhea, thrombophlebitis, hypertension, hypotension, tachycardia	Intravenous solution; used in acute glaucoma attacks or preoperatively when decreased IOP is desired Assess patient for susceptibility to pulmonary edema and HF before administering hyperosmolar agents.

ALT, argon laser trabeculoplasty; *BP,* blood pressure; *COPD,* chronic obstructive pulmonary disease; *GI,* gastrointestinal; *HF,* heart failure; *IOP,* intraocular pressure; *Nd:YAG,* neodymium:yttrium–aluminum–garnet (laser).

A filtering procedure, such as *trabeculectomy*, may be indicated if medical management and laser therapy are not successful. In this procedure, the surgeon makes conjunctival and scleral flaps, removes part of the iris and trabecular meshwork, and closes the scleral flap loosely. Aqueous humor may now "percolate" out through the area of missing iris, where it is trapped under the repaired conjunctiva and absorbed into the systemic circulation. The success rate of this filtering surgery is 75% to 85%. The subconjunctival application of mitomycin or 5-fluorouracil may increase the success rate by preventing scarring and subsequent closure of the opening created during surgery.

Implantation of a shunt is another surgical option, usually reserved for patients in whom filtration surgery has failed. It involves surgical placement of a small plastic drainage tube and reservoir to shunt aqueous humor from the anterior chamber and the surrounding tissue absorbs the fluid.

Acute Angle-Closure Glaucoma. Acute angle-closure glaucoma is an ocular emergency that necessitates immediate intervention. Miotics and oral or intravenous hyperosmotic agents are usually successful in immediately lowering the IOP (see Table 24-8). A laser peripheral iridotomy or surgical iridectomy is necessary for long-term treatment and prevention of subsequent episodes. These procedures allow the aqueous humor to flow through a newly created opening in the iris and into normal outflow channels. One of these procedures may also be performed on the other eye as a precaution because many affected patients experience a second acute attack in the other eye.

Secondary Glaucoma. Secondary glaucoma is managed by treatment of the underlying problem and by the use of antiglaucoma drugs. If treatment fails, glaucoma can progress to absolute glaucoma, which causes the eye to become hard, sightless, and usually painful and necessitates enucleation (surgical removal of the eye).

NURSING MANAGEMENT: GLAUCOMA

▪ Nursing Assessment

Because glaucoma is a chronic condition that necessitates long-term management, the nurse must carefully assess the patient's ability to understand the rationale for the prescribed therapy and to comply with the treatment regimen. In addition, the nurse should assess the patient's psychological reaction to the diagnosis of a potentially sight-threatening chronic disorder. The nurse must include the patient's caregiver in the assessment process because the chronic nature of this disorder affects the family in many ways. Some families may become the primary providers of necessary care, such as eye drop administration, if the patient is unwilling or unable to accomplish these self-care activities. The nurse also assesses visual acuity, visual fields, IOP, and fundus changes when appropriate.

▪ Nursing Diagnoses

Nursing diagnoses for the patient with glaucoma include, but are not limited to, the following:
- Risk for injury *related to* visual acuity deficits
- Self-care deficits *related to* visual acuity deficits
- Acute pain *related to* pathophysiological process and surgical correction
- Noncompliance *related to* the inconvenience and adverse effects of glaucoma medications

▪ Planning

The overall goals are that the patient with glaucoma will (a) have no progression of visual impairment, (b) understand the disease process and the rationale for therapy, (c) comply with all aspects of therapy (including medication administration and follow-up care), and (d) have no postoperative complications.

▪ Nursing Implementation

▪ Health Promotion

Loss of vision from glaucoma is a preventable problem. It is important to teach the patient and caregiver about the risk of glaucoma. The nurse should stress the importance of early detection and treatment in preventing visual impairment. This knowledge should encourage the patient to seek appropriate ophthalmic health care. The patient should know that the incidence of glaucoma increases with age and that a comprehensive ophthalmic examination is invaluable in identifying persons with glaucoma or those at risk of developing glaucoma. The Canadian Ophthalmological Society (2007b) recommended an eye examination every 3 to 5 years until the age of 40 and then every 2 to 4 years until the age of 65. Patients with risk factors such as family history of glaucoma and those of African descent should have annual eye examinations. Because so many eye diseases tend to occur in older adults, those older than 65 should have an examination every 2 years (annually if they have any risk factors) (Canadian Ophthalmological Society, 2007b).

▪ Acute Intervention

Acute nursing interventions are directed primarily toward patients with acute angle-closure glaucoma and surgical patients. A patient with acute angle-closure glaucoma requires immediate IOP-lowering medication, which the nurse must administer in a timely and appropriate manner according to the ophthalmologist's prescription. This patient may also be uncomfortable, and appropriate nursing comfort interventions may include darkening the environment, applying cool compresses to the patient's forehead, and providing a quiet and private space for the patient. Most surgical procedures for glaucoma are outpatient procedures. In the acute situation, the patient needs postoperative instructions and may require nursing comfort measures to relieve discomfort related to the procedure. Patient and caregiver teaching after eye surgery is discussed in Table 24-5.

▪ Ambulatory and Home Care

Because of the chronic nature of glaucoma, the patient needs encouragement to follow the therapeutic regimen and follow-up recommendations prescribed by the ophthalmologist. The patient needs accurate information about the disease process and treatment options, including the rationale underlying each option. In addition, the patient needs information about the purpose, the frequency, and the technique for administration of prescribed antiglaucoma agents. In addition to verbal instructions, all patients should receive written instructions that contain the same information. The nurse may encourage the patient to comply by helping the patient identify the most convenient and appropriate times for medication administration or by advocating a change in therapy if the patient reports unacceptable adverse effects.

▪ Evaluation

The overall expected outcomes are the following for the patient with glaucoma:
- The patient will have no further loss of vision.
- The patient will comply with recommended therapy.
- The patient will safely function within his or her own environment.
- The patient will obtain relief from pain associated with the disease and surgery.

AGE-RELATED CONSIDERATIONS: GLAUCOMA

Many older patients with glaucoma have systemic illnesses or take systemic medications that may affect their therapy. In particular, patients who take a β-adrenergic blocking agent for glaucoma may experience an additive effect if they are also taking a systemic β-adrenergic blocking drug. All β-adrenergic blocking glaucoma agents are contraindicated for use in patients with bradycardia, those with greater than first-degree heart block, those in cardiogenic shock, and those with overt cardiac failure. The noncardioselective β-adrenergic blocker glaucoma agents are also contraindicated for use in patients with severe chronic obstructive pulmonary disease or asthma. The hyperosmolar agents may precipitate heart failure or pulmonary edema in susceptible patients. Older patients receiving high-dose aspirin therapy for rheumatoid arthritis should not take carbonic anhydrase inhibitors. The α-adrenergic agonists can cause tachycardia or hypertension, which may have serious consequences in older patients. The nurse must teach older patients to occlude the puncta to limit the systemic absorption of glaucoma medications.

Intraocular Inflammation and Infection

The term *uveitis* is used to describe inflammation of the uveal tract, the retina, the vitreous cavity, or the optic nerve. This inflammation may be caused by bacteria, viruses, fungi, or parasites. *Cytomegalovirus retinitis* (CMV retinitis) is an opportunistic infection that occurs in patients with acquired immune deficiency syndrome (AIDS) and in other immunosuppressed patients. The causes of sterile intraocular inflammation include autoimmune disorders, AIDS, malignancies, and disorders associated with systemic diseases such as juvenile rheumatoid arthritis and inflammatory bowel disease. Pain and photophobia are common symptoms.

Endophthalmitis is an extensive intraocular inflammation of the vitreous cavity. Bacteria, viruses, fungi, or parasites can all induce this serious but rare inflammatory response. The mechanism of infection may be endogenous, in which the infecting agent arrives at the eye through the bloodstream, or exogenous, in which the infecting agent is introduced through a surgical wound or a penetrating injury. In most cases, endophthalmitis is a devastating complication of intraocular surgery or penetrating ocular injury and can lead to irreversible blindness within hours or days. Manifestations include ocular pain, photophobia, decreased visual acuity, headaches, upper eyelid edema, reddened and swollen conjunctiva, and corneal edema.

> **SAFETY ALERT**
>
> Patients discharged after eye surgery are instructed to seek immediate emergency ophthalmological care if any of manifestations of endophthalmitis occur.

When all the layers of the eye (vitreous humor, retina, choroid, and sclera) are involved in the inflammatory response, the patient has *panophthalmitis*. In the final stages of extensive cases, the scleral coat may undergo bacterial or inflammatory dissolution.

Subsequent rupture of the globe spreads the infection into the orbit or eyelids.

Treatment of intraocular inflammation depends on the underlying cause. Intraocular infections must be treated with antimicrobial agents, which may be delivered topically, subconjunctivally, intravitreally, systemically, or in some combination. Sterile inflammatory responses must be treated with anti-inflammatory agents such as corticosteroids. The site and the severity of the sterile inflammatory response determine whether topical, subconjunctival, or systemic corticosteroids are necessary.

The patient with intraocular inflammation is usually uncomfortable and may be noticeably anxious and frightened. The patient may fear sudden and total loss of vision. Provide accurate information and emotional support to the patient and the family. In severe cases, enucleation may be necessary. When patients lose visual function or even the entire eye, they grieve over the loss. The nurse's role includes helping patients through the grieving process.

Enucleation

Enucleation is the removal of the eye. The primary indication for enucleation is blindness and pain in an eye. This may result from absolute glaucoma, infection, or trauma. Enucleation may also be indicated in ocular malignancies, although many malignancies can be managed with cryotherapy, radiation, and chemotherapy. An extremely rare indication is *sympathetic ophthalmia*, in which the nontraumatized eye develops an inflammatory response after the primary eye trauma. In this situation, the traumatized eye is enucleated. The surgical procedure includes severing the extraocular muscles close to their insertion on the globe, inserting an implant to maintain the intraorbital anatomy, and suturing the ends of the extraocular muscles over the implant. The conjunctiva covers the joined muscles, and a clear conformer is placed over the conjunctiva until the permanent prosthesis is fitted. A pressure dressing helps prevent postoperative bleeding.

Postoperatively, the nurse observes the patient for signs of complications, including excessive bleeding or swelling, increased pain, displacement of the implant, or temperature elevation. Patient teaching should include instructions about the instillation of topical ointments or drops and wound cleansing. The nurse should also instruct the patient how to insert the conformer into the socket in case it falls out. The patient is often devastated by the loss of an eye, even when enucleation occurs after a lengthy period of painful blindness. The nurse should recognize and validate the patient's emotional response and provide support to the patient and the family or caregiver.

Approximately 6 weeks after surgery, the wound is sufficiently healed for the permanent prosthesis. The prosthesis is fitted by an ocular specialist and designed to match the remaining eye. The patient should learn how to remove, cleanse, and insert the prosthesis. Special polishing is required periodically to remove dried protein secretions.

Ocular Tumours

Benign and malignant tumours can occur in many areas of the eye, including the conjunctiva, retina, and orbit. Malignancies of the eyelid include basal cell and squamous cell carcinomas (see Chapter 26). Diagnostic testing may include ultrasonography, magnetic resonance imagining (MRI), and fine-needle aspiration biopsy (Fu, Hayden, & Singh, 2008). Treatment is determined by the status of the involved eye.

Ocular Manifestations of Systemic Diseases

Many systemic diseases are accompanied by significant ocular manifestations. Although it is not the purpose of this discussion to provide a full description of these disorders, it is important for the nurse to recognize that many systemic diseases produce ocular symptoms. Conversely, ocular signs and symptoms may be the first finding or complaint in a patient with a systemic disease. One example is the patient with undiagnosed diabetes who seeks ophthalmic care for blurred vision. A thorough history and careful examination of the patient can reveal that the underlying cause of the blurred vision is lens swelling caused by hyperglycemia. Another example is the patient who seeks care for a conjunctival lesion. The ophthalmologist may be the first health care professional to make the diagnosis of AIDS on the basis of the presence of a conjunctival Kaposi's sarcoma. Table 24-10 lists some systemic diseases and disorders and the associated ophthalmic manifestations.

Auditory Problems

External Ear and Canal

Trauma

Trauma to the external ear can cause injury to the subcutaneous tissue that may result in a hematoma. If the hematoma is not aspirated, inflammation of the membranes of the ear cartilage (perichondritis) can result. Antibiotics are administered to prevent infection. Blows to the ear can also cause a conductive hearing loss if there is damage to the ossicles in the middle ear or if a perforation of the tympanic membrane results. Head trauma that injures the temporal lobe of the cerebral cortex can impair the ability to understand the meaning of sounds.

External Otitis

The skin of the external ear and the ear canal is subject to the same problems as skin anywhere on the body. *External otitis* involves inflammation or infection of the epithelium of the auricle and the ear canal. Frequent swimming may alter the flora of the external canal, resulting in an infection often referred to as "swimmer's ear." Trauma caused by picking the ear or the use of sharp objects, such as hairpins, frequently causes the initial break in the skin. Piercing of auricular cartilage carries a greater risk of infection than soft-tissue piercing (Lee & Gold, 2011).

Causes. Infections, dermatitis, or both may cause external otitis. Bacteria or fungi may be the cause. The bacteria most commonly cultured are *Pseudomonas aeruginosa*, *Klebsiella* species, *Proteus* species, *Escherichia coli*, and *S. aureus*. The fungi most commonly involved are *Candida albicans* and *Aspergillus* organisms and thrive in warm, moist climates. The warm, dark environment of the ear canal provides a good medium for the growth of microorganisms. Fungi are often the causative agents of external otitis.

Table 24-10 Ocular Manifestations of Systemic Diseases or Disorders

SYSTEMIC PROBLEM	OCULAR MANIFESTATIONS
AIDS	Herpes zoster ophthalmicus, keratitis (bacterial and viral), CMV retinitis, endophthalmitis (bacterial and fungal), cotton-wool spots and microvasculopathy of the retina, KS of eyelids or conjunctiva
Diabetes mellitus	Fluctuating refractive errors, diabetic retinopathy, macular edema, premature cataract development, increased incidence of glaucoma
Down syndrome	Myopia, cataracts, nystagmus, strabismus, keratoconus, upward and outward slant of palpebral fissures
Hypertension	Cotton-wool spots and hemorrhage of the retina, retinal lipid deposits
Systemic lupus erythematosus	Dry eye, retinal changes, uveitis, scleritis
Rheumatoid arthritis	Dry eye, keratitis, scleritis
Infections	
Botulism	Blurred vision; ptosis; diplopia; fixed, dilated pupil
Endocarditis	Subconjunctival or retinal petechiae
Tuberculosis	Conjunctivitis, keratitis, uveitis
Herpes	Herpes simplex keratitis
CMV infection	CMV retinitis
Measles	Conjunctivitis, keratitis, retinopathy
Histoplasmosis	Chorioretinal lesions, subretinal neovascularization
Toxoplasmosis	Necrotic retinal lesions, vitreal inflammation, retinochoroiditis
Lyme disease	Conjunctivitis, keratitis, episcleritis, panophthalmitis, retinal detachment, diplopia
Syphilis	Conjunctivitis, keratitis, uveitis, retinal detachment, macular edema, lens dislocation, glaucoma (congenital syphilis)
Temporal arteritis	Vision loss; palsies of CN III, IV, and VI; nystagmus; ptosis
Thyroid disease	Eyelid retraction, eyelid lag, exophthalmos, abnormal eye movement, increased IOP
Vitamin deficiencies	
A	Night blindness, corneal ulceration
B	Optic neuropathy, corneal changes, retinal hemorrhage, nystagmus
C	Hemorrhage in anterior chamber, retina, conjunctiva
D	Exophthalmos

AIDS, acquired immunodeficiency syndrome; *CMV*, *cytomegalovirus*; *CN*, cranial nerve; *IOP*, intraocular pressure; *KS*, Kaposi's sarcoma.

Malignant external otitis is an infection caused by *P. aeruginosa*. The infection occurs mainly in older adult patients with diabetes. It can spread from the external ear to the parotid gland and temporal bone (osteomyelitis) and is difficult to treat.

Clinical Manifestations and Complications. Pain *(otalgia)* is one of the first signs of external otitis. Even in mild cases, the patient may experience pain that is disproportionate to the infection. The swelling of the bony ear canal as a result of the inflammatory process causes pain. Pain is especially noted on movement of the auricle or on application of pressure to the tragus (directly in front of the ear). Drainage from the ear may be serosanguineous or purulent. If it is the result of an infection caused by *Pseudomonas* organisms, the drainage is green and has a musty smell. Temperature is elevated when tissue is involved extensively. The swelling of the ear canal can block hearing and cause dizziness. Facial nerve paralysis may occur with malignant external otitis.

NURSING MANAGEMENT: EXTERNAL OTITIS

Diagnosis of external otitis is made by observation with the otoscope light; the examiner uses the largest speculum that the patient's ear will accommodate without causing the patient unnecessary discomfort. The eardrum may be normal if it can be seen. Culture and sensitivity studies of the drainage may be done. Mild analgesics usually control the pain. After the ear canal is cleansed, a wick of cotton is placed in the canal to help deliver the antibiotic eardrops. Cotton wicks should be used with caution in young patients and in confused or psychotic patients, who may push them farther into the ear. Topical antibiotics include polymyxin B, neomycin, and chloramphenicol (Pentamycetin). Nystatin (Nyaderm) is used for fungal infections. Corticosteroids may also be used to decrease inflammation unless the infection is fungal, in which case their use is contraindicated. If the surrounding tissue is involved, systemic antibiotics are prescribed. Warm, moist compresses or heat may be applied. Improvement should occur in 48 hours, but 7 to 14 days are required for complete resolution.

Careful handling and disposal of material saturated with drainage is important. The patient should wash hands before and after administering otic drops (eardrops). The drops should be administered at room temperature. Cold drops can cause dizziness in the patient, as a result of the stimulation of the semicircular canals, and heated drops can burn the tympanum. To prevent contamination of the entire bottle of drops, the tip of the dropper should not touch the ear during administration,. The ear is positioned so that the drops can run down the canal. This position should be maintained for 2 minutes after eardrop administration to allow dispersion of drops. Sometimes drops are ordered to be placed onto a wick of cotton that is placed in the ear canal. In that case, the nurse should instruct the patient not to push the cotton farther into the ear. The nurse should also instruct the patient on methods to reduce the risk of external otitis (Table 24-11).

Cerumen and Foreign Bodies in the External Ear Canal

Impacted cerumen (earwax) can cause discomfort and decrease hearing. As people age, the earwax becomes dense and drier. Hair

PATIENT & CAREGIVER TEACHING GUIDE
Table 24-11 Prevention of External Otitis

The following instructions should be included in teaching the patient or caregiver:

1. Do not put anything in your ear canal unless requested by your health care provider.
2. Report itching if it becomes a problem.
3. Cerumen (earwax) is normal.
   - It lubricates and protects the canal.
   - Report chronic excessive cerumen if it impairs your hearing.
4. Keep your ears as dry as possible.
   - Use earplugs if you are prone to swimmer's ear.
   - Turn your head to each side for 30 sec at a time to help water run out of the ears.
   - Do not dry with cotton-tipped applicators.
   - A hair dryer set to low and held at least 6 in from the ear can speed water evaporation.

Table 24-12 Manifestations of Cerumen Impaction

- Hearing loss
- Otalgia
- Tinnitus
- Vertigo
- Cough
- Cardiac depression (vagal stimulation)

becomes thicker and coarser, entrapping the hard, dry cerumen in the canal. Water that enters the canal during a shower or swimming may cause swelling of the cerumen, which results in complete blockage of the canal. Symptoms of cerumen impaction are outlined in Table 24-12. Management involves irrigation of the canal with body-temperature solutions. Special syringes, varying from the simple bulb syringe to special irrigating equipment used in the health care professional's office or clinic, can be used. The patient is placed in a sitting position with an emesis basin under the ear. The auricle is pulled up and back, and the flow of solution is directed above or below the impaction. It is important that the ear canal not be completely occluded with the syringe tip. If irrigation does not remove the cerumen, mild lubricant drops may be used to soften it. Irrigation may then be effective in removing the impacted cerumen. It may need to be removed by a physician who uses an operating microscope, suction, and microsurgical instruments.

Ear candling is a popular alternative remedy that some members of the public use. In this procedure, one end of a hollow tube of fabric is coated with beeswax and inserted into the ear and the other end is ignited. It is marketed as a way to draw cerumen out of the ear through a "chimney effect" produced by the burning candle. Although no reliable data are available on ear candling, limited research has shown that it is implausible, ineffective, and potentially unsafe (Armstrong, 2009).

The list of foreign objects removed from ears is extensive and includes animate, inanimate, vegetable, and mineral objects. Attempts to remove an object occasionally result in its being pushed further into the canal. An otolaryngologist should remove the object. Vegetable matter tends to swell and may create a secondary inflammation, making removal more difficult.

Animate objects must be immobilized before removal. Mineral oil or lidocaine can be used to drown an insect. The organism can then be removed with microscope guidance. The use of a general anaesthetic or medication to produce conscious sedation may be necessary, depending on the level of patient cooperation. In rare cases, it may be necessary to make a canal incision to remove the foreign body.

The patient should be instructed to keep objects out of the ear. Ears should be cleaned only with a washcloth and finger. Hairpins and cotton-tipped applicators should especially be avoided. Penetration of the middle ear by a cotton-tipped applicator can cause serious injury to the tympanic membrane and ossicles and may result in facial paralysis as a result of nerve damage. The use of cotton-tipped applicators can also pack cerumen against the tympanic membrane and impair hearing.

Malignancy of the External Ear

Malignancies of the external ear (other than skin cancers) and canal are uncommon. Because of long-term sun exposure, the superior border of the auricle is at risk for the development of skin cancer, which can initially appear as rough sandpaper-like lesions. The most common malignant neoplasms of the auricle are basal cell and squamous cell cancers. These skin cancers can be excised surgically and are usually not life-threatening. Cancer of the ear often results in cosmetic deformities that are difficult to reconstruct. An important nursing role is teaching the patient about the danger of sun exposure and the importance of using hats and sunscreen when outdoors.

Middle Ear and Mastoid

Acute Otitis Media

Acute otitis media is an infection of the tympanum, ossicles, and space of the middle ear. Swelling of the auditory tube from colds or allergies can trap bacteria, causing a middle ear infection. Pressure from the inflammation pushes on the tympanic membrane, causing it to become red, bulging, and painful. It is usually a childhood disease because in children the auditory tube that drains fluids and mucus from the middle ear is shorter and narrower, and its position is flatter, than that in adults (Patton & Thibodeau, 2010). Pain, fever, malaise, and reduced hearing are signs and symptoms of infections. Referred pain from the temporomandibular joint, teeth, gums, sinuses, or throat may also cause adult ear pain. Clinical practice guidelines include strategies such as observation, antibiotics and pain control (Thornton, Parrish, & Swords, 2011).

Collaborative care involves the use of antibiotics to eradicate the causative organism. Amoxicillin is the current therapy of choice in North America. Surgical intervention is generally reserved for the patient who does not respond to medical treatment. A *myringotomy* involves an incision in the tympanum to release the increased pressure and exudate from the middle ear. A tympanostomy tube may be placed for short- or long-term drainage. Prompt treatment of an episode of acute otitis media generally prevents spontaneous perforation of the tympanic membrane. In the adult patient for whom allergy may be a causative factor, antihistamines may also be prescribed.

Otitis Media with Effusion

Otitis media with effusion is an inflammation of the middle ear in which a collection of fluid is present in the middle ear space. The fluid may be thin, mucoid, or purulent. This condition is commonly called *serous otitis media,* "glue ear," or *secretory otitis media.* The fluid usually collects because of a malfunction of the eustachian tube, which commonly follows upper respiratory or chronic sinus infections, barotrauma (caused by pressure change), or otitis media. If the eustachian tube does not open and allow equalization of atmospheric pressure, negative pressure within the middle ear causes fluid to seep from the tissues.

Complaints include a feeling of fullness of the ear, a "plugged" feeling or popping sensation, and decreased hearing. The patient does not experience pain, fever, or discharge from the ear. Pneumatic otoscopy is a critical assessment tool in differentiating otitis media with effusion from acute otitis media. It is normal to have otitis media with effusion for weeks to months after an episode of acute otitis media. It usually resolves in 75% to 90% of cases without treatment but may recur.

Chronic Otitis Media and Mastoiditis

Etiology and Pathophysiology. Untreated or repeated attacks of acute otitis media may lead to a chronic condition. Chronic infection of the middle ear is more common in persons who experience episodes of acute otitis media in early childhood. Organisms involved in chronic otitis media include *S. aureus, Proteus mirabilis,* and *P. aeruginosa.* Because the mucous membrane is continuous, both the middle ear and the air cells of the mastoid can be involved in the chronic infectious process.

Clinical Manifestations. *Chronic otitis media* is characterized by a purulent exudate and inflammation that can involve the ossicles, eustachian tube, and mastoid bone. It is often painless. Nausea and episodes of dizziness can occur. The patient may complain of hearing loss that may be a result of destruction of the ossicles, a tympanic membrane perforation, or the accumulation of fluid in the middle ear space. On occasion, a facial palsy or an attack of vertigo may alert the patient to this condition.

Complications. Untreated conditions can result in perforation of the tympanic membrane and the formation of a cholesteatoma (a mass of epithelial cells and cholesterol in the middle ear). Its enlarging tumour-like behaviour may destroy the adjacent bones, including the ossicles. Unless removed surgically, a cholesteatoma can cause extensive damage to the structures of the middle ear, can erode the bony protection of the facial nerve, may create a labyrinthine fistula, or can even invade the dura, threatening the brain.

Diagnostic Studies. Otoscopic examination may reveal colour changes, decreased tympanic membrane mobility, and a marginal or central perforation of the tympanic membrane (Figure 24-9). Culture and sensitivity tests are necessary to identify the organisms involved so that the appropriate antibiotic therapy can be prescribed. Audiography may demonstrate no loss in hearing or a loss as great as 50 to 60 dB if the ossicles have been partially destroyed or separated. Sinus radiographic studies, MRI, or computed tomography of the temporal bone may demonstrate bone destruction, absence of ossicles, or the presence of a mass.

COLLABORATIVE CARE

Table 24-13 Chronic Otitis Media

Diagnostic	Collaborative Therapy

• History and physical examination
• Otoscopic examination
• Culture and sensitivity of middle ear drainage
• Mastoid radiograph
	• Ear irrigations
	• Otic, oral, or parenteral antibiotics
	• Analgesics
	• Antiemetics
	• Surgery
	   • Tympanoplasty*
	   • Mastoidectomy

*See Table 24-14.

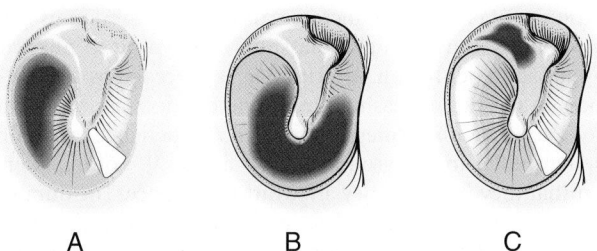

A   B   C

Figure 24-9 Three common tympanic perforations (indicated by shaded area). **A,** Small central perforation (hearing is usually good). **B,** Large central perforation around the handle of the malleus (hearing is usually poor). **C,** Marginal perforation of Shrapnell's membrane (hearing is usually good). Cholesteatomas commonly occur in patients with a marginal perforation that does not heal.

Collaborative Care. The aims of treatment are to clear the middle ear of infection, repair the perforation, and preserve hearing (Table 24-13). Systemic antibiotic therapy is initiated on the basis of the culture and sensitivity results. In addition, the patient may need to undergo frequent evacuation of drainage and debris in an outpatient setting. Otic and oral antibiotics are used to reduce infection. In many cases of chronic otitis media, the causative agent is resistant to antibiotics.

Surgical Therapy. Chronic tympanic membrane perforations often do not heal with conservative treatment, and surgery is necessary. Surgery involving reconstruction of the tympanic membrane or the ossicular chain is called a *tympanoplasty*. A *mastoidectomy* is often performed with a tympanoplasty to remove diseased tissue and the source of infection. Removal of tissue stops at the middle ear structures that appear capable of functioning in the conduction of sound. A *myringoplasty* is surgical reconstruction limited to repair of a tympanic membrane perforation.

NURSING MANAGEMENT: CHRONIC OTITIS MEDIA

▪ After Tympanoplasty

Routine preoperative care is provided before tympanoplasty and includes teaching postoperative expectations (Table 24-14). Post-

PATIENT & CAREGIVER TEACHING GUIDE

Table 24-14 After Ear Surgery

1. Avoid sudden head movements.
2. Do not try to get out of bed without assistance.
3. Take drugs to reduce dizziness if prescribed.
4. Change positions slowly.
5. Avoid getting the head wet (including showering) until directed by surgeon.
6. Report fever, pain, an increase in hearing loss, or drainage from the ear.
7. Do not cough or blow the nose because this causes increased pressure in the eustachian tube and middle ear cavity and disrupts healing.
8. If you need to cough or sneeze, leave the mouth open to help reduce the pressure.
9. Avoid crowds because respiratory infections may be contracted.
10. Avoid situations in which pressure or popping in the ears is normally experienced, such as high elevations or airplane travel.

operative concerns are the avoidance of complications, such as disruption of the repair during the healing phase and facial nerve paralysis.

After surgery, the patient is positioned flat and side-lying with the operative side up. It is normal to have impaired hearing during the postoperative period if there is packing in the ear. A cotton-ball dressing is used for an endaural incision. The patient should be instructed to change the cotton packing and dressing daily. If a postauricular incision is used and a drain is in place, a mastoid dressing is used. A small gauze pad is cut to fit behind the ear, and fluffs are applied over the ear to prevent the outer circular head dressing from placing pressure on the auricle. Monitor the amount and type of drainage postoperatively, as well as the tightness of the dressing, to prevent tissue necrosis.

Otosclerosis

Otosclerosis, a hereditary autosomal dominant disease, is the fixation of the footplate of the stapes in the oval window. Spongy bone develops from the bony labyrinth, causing immobilization of the footplate of the stapes, which reduces the transmission of vibrations to the inner ear fluids. It is a common cause of conductive hearing loss in young adults, especially women, and may accelerate during pregnancy. Otosclerosis is bilateral in about 80% of cases. Although hearing loss is typically bilateral, one ear may show faster hearing loss progression. The patient is often unaware of the problem until the loss becomes so severe that communication is difficult.

Otoscopic examination may reveal a reddish blush of the tympanum (Schwartze's sign) caused by the vascular and bony changes within the middle ear. Tuning-fork tests help identify the conductive component of the hearing loss. On Rinne's test, sound is heard longer when the stem of the tuning fork is touching the mastoid bone (bone conduction) than when placed next to the ear (air conduction). In Weber's test, the sound is heard better through the skull bone in the ear than through air when conductive hearing loss is greater. Audiography demonstrates good hearing by bone conduction, but air conduction demonstrates

COLLABORATIVE CARE

Table 24-15 Otosclerosis

Diagnostic	Collaborative Therapy

• History and physical examination
• Otoscopic examination
• Rinne's test (512-Hz tuning fork)
• Weber's test
• Audiometry
• Tympanometry
	• Hearing aid
	• Surgery (stapedectomy or fenestration)
	• Drug therapy
	  • Sodium fluoride with vitamin D
	  • Calcium carbonate

poor hearing (air–bone gap). Usually, at least a difference of 20 to 25 dB between air and bone conduction levels of hearing is observed in otosclerosis.

Collaborative Care. The hearing loss associated with otosclerosis may be stabilized by the use of sodium fluoride with vitamin D and calcium carbonate to retard bone resorption and encourage calcification of bony lesions. Amplification of sound by a hearing aid can be effective because the inner ear function is normal. Surgical treatment involves partial removal of the stapes *(stapedectomy)* or complete removal with prosthesis insertion *(fenestration)*. Collaborative care of otosclerosis is described in Table 24-15.

Patients usually undergo surgery under local anaesthesia with sedation. The ear with poorer hearing is repaired first, and the other ear may be operated on 6 months to 1 year later. An endaural incision is made under visualization through the operating microscope. Gelfoam is used on the incision flap to limit bleeding. A cotton ball is placed in the ear canal, and a small dressing is used to cover the ear.

During surgery, patients often report an immediate improvement in hearing in the operated ear. Because of the accumulation of blood and fluid in the middle ear, the hearing level decreases postoperatively but improves with healing. After stapedectomy, 90% of patients experience an improvement in hearing, in many instances to near normal.

NURSING MANAGEMENT: OTOSCLEROSIS

Nursing management of patients undergoing stapedectomy or fenestration is similar to that for patients who have undergone tympanoplasty. Postoperatively, patients may experience dizziness, nausea, and vomiting as a result of intraoperative stimulation of the labyrinth. Some patients demonstrate nystagmus because of disturbance of the perilymph fluid. Care should be taken to decrease sudden movements by patients that may induce or exacerbate dizziness. Actions such as coughing, sneezing, lifting, bending, and straining during bowel movements should also be minimized.

Inner Ear Problems

Three symptoms that indicate disease of the inner ear are vertigo, sensorineural hearing loss, and tinnitus. Symptoms of vertigo arise from the vestibular labyrinth, whereas hearing loss and tinnitus arise from the auditory labyrinth. Manifestations of inner ear problems overlap with some manifestations of central nervous system disorders.

Ménière's Disease

Ménière's disease (endolymphatic hydrops) is characterized by symptoms caused by inner ear disease, including episodic vertigo, tinnitus, fluctuating sensorineural hearing loss, and aural fullness. Sudden, severe attacks of vertigo with nausea and vomiting cause significant disability for the patient with Ménière's disease. Symptoms usually begin between the ages of 30 and 60 years.

The cause of the disease is unknown, but it results in an excessive accumulation of endolymph in the membranous labyrinth. The volume of endolymph increases until the membranous labyrinth ruptures, causing high-potassium endolymph to mix with low-potassium perilymph. Attacks may be preceded by a sense of fullness in the ear, increasing tinnitus, and a decrease in hearing acuity. Patients with Ménière's disease may experience the feeling of being pulled to the ground ("drop attacks"). Some patients report that they feel as if they are whirling in space. The duration of attacks may be hours or days, and attacks may occur several times a year. Autonomic symptoms include pallor, sweating, nausea, and vomiting.

The clinical course of the disease is highly variable. Low-pitched tinnitus may be present continuously in the affected ear, or it may be intensified during an attack. It is often described as a "roar" or "like the ocean." Hearing loss fluctuates; when attacks continue, hearing recovery is often less complete with each episode; eventually, patients may suffer permanent hearing loss.

NURSING AND COLLABORATIVE MANAGEMENT: MÉNIÈRE'S DISEASE

Collaborative care of Ménière's disease (Table 24-16) includes diagnostic tests to rule out central nervous system disease. Audiography demonstrates a mild, low-frequency sensorineural hearing loss. Vestibular tests indicate decreased function.

A glycerol test may aid in the diagnosis of Ménière's disease. An oral dose of glycerol is given, followed by serial audiography over 3 hours. Improvement in hearing or speech discrimination supports a diagnosis of Ménière's disease. The improvement is attributed to the osmotic effect of glycerol that pulls fluid from the inner ear. Although a positive test result is diagnostic of Ménière's disease, a negative test result does not rule out the condition.

During the acute attack, antihistamines, anticholinergics, and benzodiazepines can be used to decrease the abnormal sensation and lessen symptoms such as nausea and vomiting. Acute vertigo is treated symptomatically with bed rest, sedation, and antiemetics or antivertigo drugs for motion sickness, administered orally, rectally, or intravenously. The patient requires reassurance and counselling that the condition is not life-threatening. Management between attacks may include diuretics, antihistamines, and a low-sodium diet. Diazepam may be used to reduce the vertigo. Over a period of time, most patients respond to the prescribed medications but must learn to live with the unpredictability of the attacks. The remainder of patients may, in time, require surgical intervention.

COLLABORATIVE CARE

Table 24-16 Ménière's Disease

Diagnostic	Surgical Therapy
• History and physical examination	**Conservative Surgical Intervention**
• Audiometric studies, including speech discrimination, tone decay	• Endolymphatic shunt
	• Vestibular nerve section
• Vestibular tests, including caloric test, positional test	**Destructive Surgical Intervention**
• Electronystagmography	• Labyrinthotomy
• Neurological examination	• Labyrinthectomy
• Glycerol test	**Ambulatory or Home Care**
Collaborative Therapy	• Diuretics
Acute Care	• Antihistamines
Drug Therapy (one or more)	• Calcium channel blockers
• Sedatives	• Sedatives
• Anticholinergics	• Hydrops diet: restriction of sodium, caffeine, nicotine, alcohol, and foods with monosodium glutamate (MSG)
• Vasodilators	
• Antihistamines	

Frequent and incapacitating attacks, reduced quality of life, and a resultant threat of unemployment are indications for surgical intervention. The endolymphatic sac is surgically decompressed to reduce the pressure on the cochlear hair cells and to prevent further damage and hearing loss. If relief is not achieved with endolymphatic shunt surgery and hearing remains good, the vestibular nerve may be resected to alleviate vertigo and preserve hearing (Sajjadi & Paparella, 2008). When involvement is unilateral, surgical ablation of the labyrinth, resulting in loss of the vestibular and hearing cochlear function, is performed. Careful management can decrease the possibility of progressive sensorineural loss in many patients.

Nursing interventions are planned to minimize vertigo and provide for patient safety. During an acute attack, the patient is kept in a quiet, darkened room in a comfortable position. The patient needs to be taught to avoid sudden head movements or position changes. Fluorescent or flickering lights or television may exacerbate symptoms and should be avoided. An emesis basin should be available because vomiting is common. To minimize the patient's risk of falling, the nurse should keep the side rails up and the bed low in position when the patient is in bed. The patient should be instructed to call for assistance when getting out of bed. Medications and fluids are administered parenterally, and intake and output are monitored. When the attack subsides, the patient should be assisted with ambulation because he or she may remain unsteady. Similar nursing care is provided after surgical ablation of the labyrinth. Patients who undergo ablation have severe tinnitus and vertigo, which decrease during a period of days or weeks as the brain adjusts to loss of vestibular input and postural stability is regained.

Therapies have been unable to prevent the progressive cochlear dysfunction of Ménière's disease, although hearing can be restored through hearing rehabilitative strategies and auditory stimulation in affected individuals. Many patients continue to be disabled by the severe tinnitus and chronic imbalance that accompany this disease (Semaan & Megerian, 2011).

Benign Paroxysmal Positional Vertigo

Benign paroxysmal positional vertigo (BPPV) is a common cause of vertigo. In BPPV, free-floating debris in the semicircular canal causes vertigo to occur with specific head movements, such as those involved with getting out of bed, rolling over in bed, and sitting up from lying down (Kerber, 2009). The debris ("ear rocks") is composed of small crystals of calcium carbonate derived from the utricle in the inner ear. The utricle may be injured by head trauma, infection, or degeneration as a result of the aging process. In many patients, however, a cause cannot be found.

Symptoms include dizziness, vertigo, light-headedness, loss of balance, and nausea. There is no hearing loss, and symptoms tend to be intermittent. The symptoms of BPPV may be confused with those of Ménière's disease. Diagnosis is based on the results of auditory and vestibular tests.

Although BPPV is a bothersome problem, it is rarely serious unless a person falls. Epley's manoeuvre (canalith repositioning procedure) is effective in providing symptom relief for many patients. In this manoeuvre, the ear debris is moved to a less sensitive part of the ear. The manoeuvre moves these particles from areas in the inner ear that cause symptoms and repositions them into areas where they do not cause these problems. Epley's manoeuvre does not address the actual presence of particles of debris; rather, it changes their location.

Labyrinthitis

Labyrinthitis is an inflammation of the inner ear affecting the cochlear and vestibular portions of the labyrinth. Infection can enter from the meninges, the middle ear, or the bloodstream. Symptoms include vertigo, tinnitus, and sensorineural hearing loss on the affected side. This condition has been rare since the advent of antibiotics. *Nystagmus*, an abnormal rhythmic, jerking movement of the eyes, accompanies the vertigo.

The most common complication of labyrinthitis is meningitis. It is important for the nurse to assess for changes in level of consciousness, headache, and nuchal rigidity (stiff neck). Affected patients may become very lethargic or easily agitated. It is important for the nurse to document these assessment findings even if they are normal. (Meningitis is discussed in Chapter 59.)

Acoustic Neuroma

An acoustic neuroma (or *vestibular schwannoma*) is a benign tumour that occurs where the acoustic nerve (cranial nerve [CN] VIII) enters the internal auditory canal or the temporal bone from the brain. It is important that the condition be diagnosed early because the tumour can compress the facial nerve and arteries within the internal auditory canal. Once the tumour has expanded and become an intracranial neoplasm, more extensive surgery is necessary, which reduces the chances of preserving hearing and normal facial nerve function. Watchful waiting, or observation, after diagnosis has become a more common treatment strategy as tumours are diagnosed at smaller sizes. Practitioners manage this condition better now than in the past, inasmuch as improved imaging and heightened awareness leads to earlier diagnosis (Quesnel & McKenna, 2011).

Early symptoms are associated with CN VIII compression and destruction. They include unilateral, progressive, sensorineural hearing loss; unilateral tinnitus; and mild, intermittent vertigo. One of the earliest symptoms of an acoustic neuroma is reduced touch sensation in the posterior ear canal. Diagnostic tests include neurological, audiometric, and vestibular tests; computed tomography; and MRI with gadolinium enhancement.

Surgery to remove small tumours is performed through the middle cranial fossa or the retrolabyrinthine approach, which preserves hearing and vestibular function. A translabyrinthine approach is usually used for medium-sized tumours and when hearing is minimal. Although hearing is destroyed by this approach, advantages include good access to the tumour and preservation of the facial nerve. Retrosigmoid (suboccipital) or transotic approaches are used for large tumours (>3 cm). It is almost impossible to preserve hearing when the tumour is larger than 2 cm.

Hearing Loss and Deafness

Hearing loss is the fastest growing and one of the most prevalent, chronic conditions facing Canadians today (Hearing Foundation of Canada, 2010). Hearing loss has many causes; age-related presbycusis and noise-induced hearing loss are two of the most common. Nearly half of the persons who need assistance with hearing disorders are 65 years of age or older. With the aging of the population, hearing loss is increasing. At age 50, one of every eight persons is hearing impaired. A disturbing trend is the number of young adults showing signs of hearing loss. The tiny hair cells located inside the ear pick up sound waves and convert them into electrical signals that the brain can interpret. When loud sounds are listened to constantly, the vibrations destroy the tiny hair cells, which contributes to hearing loss. Unlike other cells in the body, hair cells never grow back once they are damaged. A survey of adolescents aged 12 to 18 indicated that although they were aware of the risks of exposure to loud music from audio devices (such as MP3 players) on their hearing, they expressed low personal vulnerability to music-induced hearing loss (Vogel, Brug, Hosli, van der Ploeg, & Raat, 2008). Earbuds are of particular concern because volumes must be high in order to block out environmental distractions (Portnuff, Fligor, & Arehart, 2011). Causes of hearing loss are listed in Figure 24-10.

Types of Hearing Loss

Conductive Hearing Loss. *Conductive hearing loss* occurs when conditions in the outer or middle ear impair the transmission of sound through air to the inner ear. A common cause is otitis media with effusion (Rajesh & Pallavi, 2007). It is caused by conditions interfering with air conduction, such as impacted cerumen and foreign bodies, middle ear disease, otosclerosis, and stenosis of the external auditory canal.

Audiography demonstrates an air–bone gap of at least 15 decibel (dB). The term *air–bone gap* represents the situation in which hearing sensitivity is better by bone conduction than by air conduction. Affected patients may speak softly because they hear their own voices, which are conducted by bone, as being loud. Such patients hear better in a noisy environment. A hearing aid is helpful for a patient with a loss of 40 to 50 dB or more if the cause cannot be corrected.

Sensorineural Hearing Loss. *Sensorineural hearing loss* is caused by impairment of function of the inner ear or the vestibulocochlear nerve (CN VIII). Congenital and hereditary factors, noise trauma lasting over time, aging (presbycusis), Ménière's disease, and ototoxicity can cause sensorineural hearing loss. Systemic diseases, such as tuberculosis, syphilis, Lyme disease, cytomegalovirus, HIV, and Paget's disease of the bone, can also lead

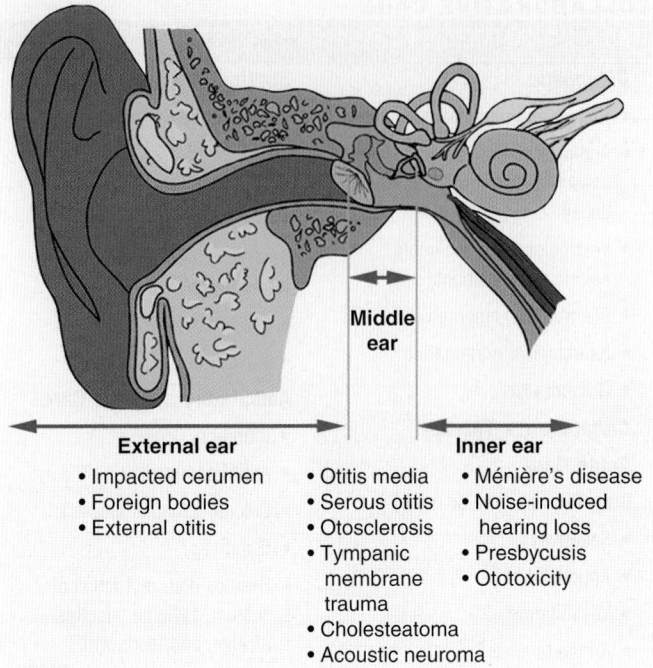

External ear	Middle ear	Inner ear
• Impacted cerumen	• Otitis media	• Ménière's disease
• Foreign bodies	• Serous otitis	• Noise-induced
• External otitis	• Otosclerosis	hearing loss
	• Tympanic	• Presbycusis
	membrane	• Ototoxicity
	trauma	
	• Cholesteatoma	
	• Acoustic neuroma	

Figure 24-10 Causes of hearing loss, by location.

to sensorineural deafness. Immune diseases, diabetes mellitus, bacterial meningitis, and trauma are also causes of this type of hearing loss.

The two main problems associated with sensorineural loss are (a) the inability to understand speech despite the ability to hear sound and (b) the lack of understanding of the problem by other people. The ability to hear high-pitched sounds diminishes with sensorineural hearing loss. Consonants are high-pitched sounds that give intelligibility to speech. Words become difficult to distinguish, and sound becomes muffled. Audiography demonstrates a loss in decibel levels at the 4000-Hz level, which can progress to the 2000-Hz level. A hearing aid may help the patient who has a loss of 30 dB or more by reducing the strain of trying to hear, but the sounds are still muffled.

Mixed Hearing Loss. Mixed hearing loss is caused by a combination of conductive and sensorineural losses. Careful evaluation is needed before corrective surgery for conductive loss is planned because the sensorineural component of the hearing loss will still remain.

Central and Functional Hearing Loss. Central hearing loss is caused by a problem along the pathway from the inner ear to the auditory region of the brain or in the brain itself. Patients with central hearing loss are unable to understand or to put meaning to the incoming sound. Careful documentation of the history is helpful because there is usually a reference to deafness within the family. Referral to qualified hearing and speech services is indicated.

Functional hearing loss may be caused by an emotional or a psychological factor. The patient does not seem to hear or respond to pure tone subjective hearing tests, but no organic cause can be identified. Psychological counselling may help.

Classification of Hearing Loss. Hearing loss can also be classified by the decibel level or loss as recorded on audiography. Normal hearing includes sound at the 0- to 15-dB range. With slight hearing loss, the softest sounds heard are in the 16- to 25-dB range; with mild impairment, the 26- to 40-dB range; with moderate impairment, the 41- to 55-dB range; with moderately severe impairment, the 56- to 70-dB range; with severe impairment, the 71- to 90-dB range; and with profound deafness, more than 91 dB. Many cases of profound deafness are congenital.

Clinical Manifestations. Manifestations that indicate hearing loss include asking other people to speak up, answering questions inappropriately, not responding when not looking at the speaker, straining to hear, cupping the hand around the ear, showing irritability with others who do not speak up, and increasing sensitivity to slight increases in noise level. Often, the patient is unaware of minimal hearing loss or may compensate by using these mannerisms. Family and friends who get tired of repeating or talking loudly are often first to notice hearing loss.

Deafness is often called the "unseen handicap" because it is not until conversation is initiated with a deaf adult that the difficulty in communication is realized. It is important that the health professional be aware of the need for thorough validation of the deaf person's understanding of health teaching. Descriptive visual aids can be helpful.

Interference in communication and interaction with other people can be the source of many problems for the patient and family or caregivers. Many patients refuse to admit to, or may be unaware of, impaired hearing. Irritability is common because of the concentration with which the patient must listen to understand speech. The loss of clarity of speech is most frustrating to a patient with sensorineural hearing loss. The patient may hear someone speaking but not understand it. Withdrawal, suspicion, loss of self-esteem, and insecurity are commonly associated with advancing hearing loss.

Table 24-17 Range of Sounds Audible to the Human Ear	
DECIBELS	**EXAMPLES**
Normal Sounds	
0	Faintest sound heard by human ear
30	Whisper, quiet library
50	Rainfall, refrigerator
60	Normal conversation, sewing machine, typewriter
70	Freeway traffic
Hazardous Sounds	
70–110	Personal stereo (levels at 110 dB or more can cause serious risk)
84–108	Home and car audio
85	Electric razor or busy street
	Continued noise at this level can cause hearing loss if exposure continues for 8 hr or more
89–96	Music in fitness class
90–110	Music in dance bars, subway, power tools
90–122	Rock concert, sandblasting, auto horn, and race cars
	People who frequently attend rock concerts experience some irreversible loss
150	Fireworks, jet engine
	Brief exposure can cause pain and injuries to unprotected ears
170	Shotgun firing

Source: American Academy of Otolaryngology. (2011). *Loudness scale.* Retrieved from *http://www.entnet.org/HealthInformation/loudnessScale.cfm;* and American Academy of Otolaryngology. (2011). *Noise and hearing protection: Sound measurements.* Retrieved from *http://www.entnet.org/HealthInformation/hearingProtection.cfm*

NURSING AND COLLABORATIVE MANAGEMENT: HEARING LOSS AND DEAFNESS

Health Promotion

Environmental Noise Control

Hearing loss can be caused by acute loud noise (acoustic trauma) or by the chronic exposure to loud noise (noise-induced hearing loss). Acoustic trauma causes hearing loss from mechanical destruction of parts of the organ of Corti. Some function may be recovered in the first weeks after injury, but the remaining loss is permanent. Noise-induced hearing loss is probably caused by high-intensity stimulation of the cochlea that results in mechanical damage of the hair cells and basal membrane in the organ of Corti.

Sensorineural hearing loss as a result of increased and prolonged environmental noise, such as amplified sound, is occurring in young adults at an increasing rate. A new disorder, coined "iPod ear," refers to hearing loss from MP3 players because volumes are often turned up to mask background noise. Young adults should be encouraged to keep amplified music at a reasonable level and limit their exposure time. Health teaching must emphasize avoidance of continued exposure to noise levels greater than 85 to 95 dB. Table 24-17 describes the range of sounds audible to humans. A study conducted on music-induced hearing loss reported that nearly half of the respondents admitted experiencing symptoms such as tinnitus or hearing loss after exposure to loud music. Health care providers were the least likely source of awareness of music-induced hearing loss, despite the respondents' favouring provider education for hearing protection through behaviour modification. Most respondents indicated they would wear protective ear wear if made aware of the hearing loss risk, especially if informed by health care professionals (Quintanilla-Dieck, Artunduaga, & Eavey, 2009).

In work environments known to have high noise levels (>85 dB), ear protection should be worn. Canadian Occupational Health and Safety regulations Part VII, Sections 7.1 to 7.8, deal with workplace noise (Department of Justice Canada, 2011). A variety of protectors that are worn over the ears or in the ears to prevent hearing loss are available. Periodic audiometric screening should be part of the health maintenance policies of industry. This provides baseline data on hearing to measure subsequent hearing loss.

Employees should participate in hearing conservation programs in work environments. A hearing conservation program should include noise exposure analysis, provision for control of noise exposure (hearing protectors), measurements of hearing, and employee–employer notification and education. Often, a multidisciplinary team including an industrial hygienist, an engineer, a nurse, and an audiometric technician is responsible for such a program.

Ear protection should be worn during skeet shooting and other recreational pursuits with high noise levels. Hearing loss caused by noise is not reversible.

Immunizations

Various viruses can cause deafness as a result of fetal damage and malformations affecting the ear. Childhood and adult immunizations—including the immunization for measles, mumps, and rubella—should be promoted. The period of greatest risk for birth defects caused by rubella infection is during the first trimester of gestation. Infection during the first 8 weeks of gestation is associated with an 85% incidence of congenital rubella syndrome, which commonly involves sensorineural deafness. Women of childbearing age should be tested for immunity. A rubella antibody titre of 1 : 8 or higher shows that the individual has immunity to rubella. If the titre is lower, immunization with live vaccine should be given, after which the woman should avoid pregnancy for at least 3 months. Immunization must be delayed if the woman is pregnant. Women who are susceptible to rubella can be vaccinated safely during the postpartum period.

Ototoxic Substances

Ototoxic drugs and chemicals used in industry (e.g., toluene, carbon disulphide, mercury) may damage the inner ear (Hoet & Lison, 2008). Drugs commonly associated with ototoxicity include salicylates, diuretics, antineoplastic drugs, and antibiotics. Patients who are receiving ototoxic drugs or are exposed to ototoxic chemicals should be monitored for signs and symptoms associated with ototoxicity, including tinnitus, sensorineural hearing loss, and vestibular dysfunction. If these symptoms develop, immediate withdrawal of the drug may prevent further damage and may cause the symptoms to disappear.

Assistive Devices and Techniques

Hearing Aids

It is important that a patient with a suspected hearing loss undergo a hearing assessment by a qualified audiologist, including examination and audiometric testing. If use of a hearing aid is indicated, it should be fitted by an audiologist or by a speech and hearing specialist. Many types of hearing aids are available, each with advantages and disadvantages (Figure 24-11). The conventional hearing aid serves as a simple amplifier. An implanted hearing system is available to treat moderate to severe sensorineural hearing loss.

For patients with bilateral hearing impairment, binaural hearing aids provide the best sound lateralization and speech discrimination. The nurse must give careful instruction on its use and maintenance and must assist the patient during the period of adjustment. The goal of hearing aid therapy is improved hearing with consistent use. Patients who are motivated and optimistic about using a hearing aid are more successful users. The nurse should determine the patient's readiness for hearing aid therapy, including whether the patient acknowledges a hearing problem, how the patient feels about wearing a hearing aid, how

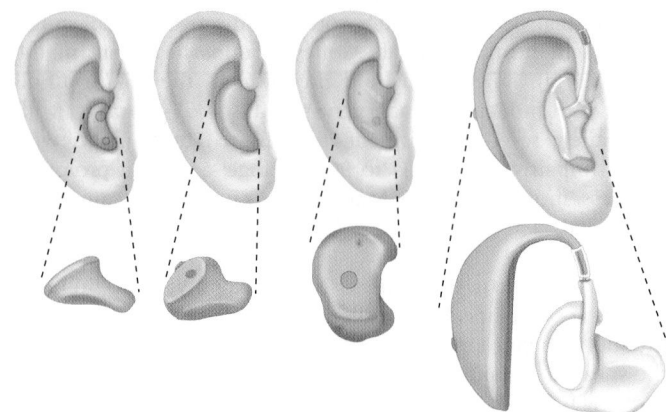

Figure 24-11 Types of hearing aids.

much the hearing loss affects the patient's life, and whether the patient has any difficulty manipulating small objects such as putting a battery in a hearing aid.

Initially, use of the hearing aid should be restricted to quiet situations in the home. The patient must first adjust to voices (including the patient's own) and household sounds. The patient should also experiment by increasing and decreasing the volume, as situations require. When the patient adjusts to the increase in sounds and background noise, he or she is ready to try a different listening environment, such as a small gathering at which several people will be talking simultaneously. Next, the environment can be expanded to the outdoors. After adapting to controlled situations, the patient is ready to encounter environments such as the shopping mall or grocery store. Adjustment to different environments occurs gradually, depending on the individual patient.

When the hearing aid is not being worn, it should be placed in a dry, cool area where it will not be inadvertently damaged or lost. The battery should be disconnected or removed. Battery life averages 1 week, and patients should be advised to purchase only a month's supply at a time. Ear moulds should be cleaned weekly or as needed. Toothpicks or pipe cleaners may be used to clear a clogged ear tip.

Speech Reading

Speech reading, commonly called *lip reading,* can be helpful in increasing communication. It enables patients to achieve approximately 40% understanding of the spoken word. Patients are able to use visual cues associated with speech, such as gestures and facial expression, to help clarify the spoken message. In speech reading, many words look alike (e.g., "rabbit," "woman"). If a patient wears glasses, the glasses should be used to facilitate speech reading. The nurse can help the patient by using and teaching verbal and nonverbal communication techniques as described in Table 24-18. If a hearing aid is used, it should be readily available to the patient.

Sign Language

Sign language is used as a form of communication for deaf people. It is a visual–spatial language that involves gestures and facial features such as eyebrow motion and lip-mouth movements.

Table 24-18 Communication With Patients Who Have Hearing Impairments	
Nonverbal Aids	**Verbal Aids**
• Draw attention with hand movements.	• Speak normally and slowly.
• Have face in good light.	• Do not overexaggerate facial expressions.
• Avoid covering mouth or face with hands.	• Do not overenunciate.
• Avoid chewing, eating, and smoking while talking.	• Use simple sentences.
• Maintain eye contact.	• Rephrase sentence; use different words.
• Avoid distracting environments.	• Write name or difficult words.
• Avoid careless expression that the patient may misinterpret.	• Do not shout.
• Use touch.	• Speak in normal voice directly into better ear.
• Move close to the patient's better ear.	
• Avoid standing in front of light source.	

Sign language is not universal. American Sign Language is used in the United States and the English-speaking parts of Canada.

Cochlear Implant

The *cochlear implant* is used as a hearing device for people with severe to profound deafness who obtain little to no benefit from hearing aids. The implant is an electronic hearing device that stimulates nerves within the inner ear. The system consists of a surgically implanted induction coil beneath the skin behind the ear and an electrode wire placed in the cochlea (Figure 24-12). The implanted parts interface with an externally worn speech processor. The system stimulates auditory nerve fibres with an electric current so that signals reach the brainstem's auditory nuclei and ultimately the auditory cortex. The implant is intended for patients whose sensorineural hearing loss is either congenital or acquired. The ideal candidate is one who has become deaf after acquiring speech and language. The adult who was born deaf or became deaf before learning to speak may be considered a candidate for a cochlear implant if she or he has followed an aural-oral educational approach (Miyamoto & Kirk, 2006).

The implant offers people with profound deafness the ability to hear environmental sounds, including speech, at comfortable loudness levels. Multichannel cochlear implants also serve as aids to speech production. Extensive training and rehabilitation are essential in order to receive maximum benefit from these implants. The positive aspects of a cochlear implant include providing sound to the person who otherwise hears none, improving speech reading ability, monitoring the loudness of the person's own speech, improving the sense of security, and decreasing feelings of isolation. With continued research, the cochlear implant may offer the possibility of aural rehabilitation for individuals with a wide variety of hearing impairments.

The U.S. Food and Drug Administration has created an informational Web site on cochlear implants (see the Related Resources

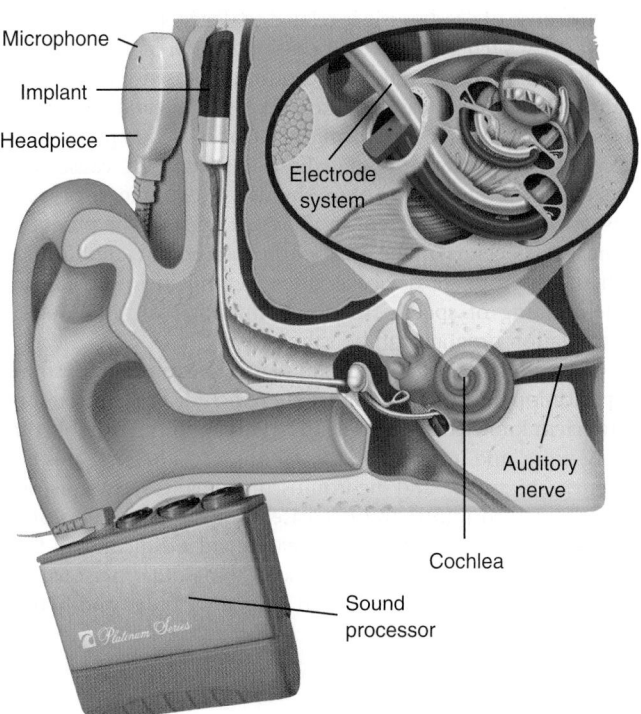

Figure 24-12 Cochlear implant.

Source: Courtesy Advanced Bionics Corp., Valencia, California.

at the end of this chapter). The site includes an animated movie to help visualize the implants and how they work.

Assisted Listening Devices

Numerous devices are now available to assist hearing-impaired persons. The nurse can explore the use of direct amplification devices, amplified telephone receivers, alerting systems that flash when activated by sound, an infrared system for amplifying the sound of the television, and a combination FM receiver and hearing aid according to a patient's needs. Patients with profound deafness may be assisted by text-telephone alerting systems that flash when activated by sound, by closed captioning on television, and by a specially trained dog. The dogs are trained to alert their owners to specific sounds within the environment. This increases safety and independence for the owners.

AGE-RELATED CONSIDERATIONS: HEARING LOSS

Presbycusis, which is hearing loss associated with aging, includes the loss of peripheral auditory sensitivity, a decline in word recognition ability, and associated psychological and communication issues. Because consonants (high-frequency sounds) are the letters by which spoken words are recognized, the ability of an older person with presbycusis to understand the spoken word is greatly affected. Vowels are heard, but some consonants fall into the high-frequency range and cannot be differentiated. This may lead to confusion and embarrassment because of the difference in what was said and what was heard.

The cause of presbycusis is related to degenerative changes in the inner ear such as loss of hair cells, reduction of blood supply, diminution of endolymph production, decreased basilar membrane flexibility, and loss of neurons in the cochlear nuclei. Noise exposure is thought to be a common factor related to presbycusis. Table 24-19 describes the classification of specific causes and associated hearing changes of presbycusis. More than one type of presbycusis are often present in the same person. The prognosis for hearing depends on the cause of the loss. Sound amplification with the appropriate device is often helpful in improving the understanding of speech. In other situations, an audiological rehabilitation program can be valuable.

Older adults are often reluctant to use a hearing aid for sound amplification. Reasons cited most often include cost, appearance, insufficient knowledge about hearing aids, amplification of competing noise, and unrealistic expectations. Most hearing aids and batteries are small, and neuromuscular changes such as stiff fingers, enlarged joints, and decreased sensory perception often make the care and handling of a hearing aid a difficult and frustrating experience for an older person. Some older persons also tend to accept their losses as part of getting older and believe there is no need for treating them.

Table 24-19 Classification of Presbycusis

TYPE	HEARING CHANGE	PROGNOSIS
Sensory		
Atrophy of auditory nerve; loss of sensory hair cells	Loss of high-pitched sounds	Little effect on speech understanding; good response to sound amplification
Neural		
Degenerative changes in cochlea and spinal ganglion	Loss of speech discrimination	Amplification alone not sufficient
Metabolic		
Degenerative changes in cochlea and spinal ganglion	Uniform loss for all frequencies accompanied by recruitment*	Good response to hearing aid
Cochlear		
Stiffening of basilar membrane, which interferes with sound transmission in the cochlea	Hearing loss increases from low to high frequencies; speech discrimination affected with higher frequency losses	Ameliorated by appropriate forms of amplification

*Abnormally rapid increase in loudness as sound intensity increases.

CLINICAL DECISION-MAKING EXERCISE

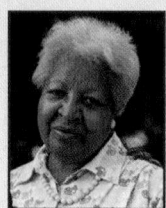

CASE STUDY:
Glaucoma and Diabetic Retinopathy

Source: © 2007 JupiterImages Corporation

Patient Profile

Lena Andrews is a 73-year-old Black woman with rheumatoid arthritis and diabetic retinopathy with a 20-year history of type 2 diabetes mellitus. She returns to the eye clinic for continued evaluation and care of the POAG and re-examination for changes in diabetic retinopathy. Her current medical regimen for POAG includes topical timolol maleate, 0.5% extended (Timoptic XE), once daily in each eye, and latanoprost (Xalatan), 0.005%, in each eye, at bedtime. The examiner noted that she has signs of nonproliferative retinopathy, exhibiting new formations of microaneurysms, hard exudates of the retina, and macular edema.

Subjective Data

- She can no longer read the newspaper and reports that medication labels are difficult to read.
- She states she is not always successful in getting the eye drops instilled because her hands are gnarled and painful from rheumatoid arthritis.

Objective Data

- Distant and near visual acuity are stable at 20/50 in the right eye and 20/70 in the left eye. This is a reduction from 20/40 in both eyes at her visit.

- Intraocular pressures are stable at 20 mm Hg in both eyes.
- There is new microaneurysm formation and hard exudates in both eyes.
- Fluorescein angiography reveals diabetic macular edema in both eyes.

Collaborative Care

- Laser photocoagulation therapy to treat diabetic macular edema
- Continuation of previous glaucoma drop regimen and reassessments
- Follow-up examination for diabetic macular edema in 8 weeks

Discussion Questions

1. What is the cause of Ms. Andrews' new nonproliferative retinopathy?
2. Why might laser photocoagulation be an appropriate therapy for macular edema?
3. What is the purpose of the fluorescein angiography?
4. *Priority decision.* What priority topics should be discussed in discharge teaching?
5. In what way could glaucoma cause vision loss if Ms. Andrews' eye pressures are not properly monitored?
6. *Priority decision.* What are the priority nursing interventions for Ms. Andrews?
7. *Priority decision.* On the basis of the assessment data, what are the priority nursing diagnoses? Are there any collaborative problems?

evolve *Answers are available at* **http://evolve.elsevier.com/ Canada/Lewis/medsurg**

REVIEW QUESTIONS

The number of the question corresponds to the same-numbered objective at the beginning of the chapter.

1. Why does presbyopia occur in older individuals?
   a. The retina degenerates.
   b. The lens becomes inflexible.
   c. The corneal curvature becomes irregular.
   d. It is associated with cataract development.

2. What is the most important nursing intervention for patients with epidemic keratoconjunctivitis?
   a. Applying patches to the affected eyes
   b. Accurately measuring intraocular pressure
   c. Monitoring near visual acuity every 4 hours
   d. Teaching patient and family members good hygiene techniques

3. What should patients with eye inflammation or an eye infection be taught?
   a. Wear dark glasses to prevent irritation from UV light.
   b. Acute conditions commonly lead to chronic problems.
   c. Apply a cold compress with pressure to the inflamed area frequently.
   d. Regular, careful hand hygiene may prevent the infection from spreading.

4. Women of childbearing age should be tested for immunity to rubella before becoming pregnant. When can a rubella infection cause hearing problems for the fetus?
   a. If exposure is after 20 weeks of gestation
   b. If exposure is before 16 weeks of gestation
   c. If the mother had rubella before age 18 years
   d. If the mother is vaccinated during the postpartum period

5. What should the nurse do to prepare patients for retinal detachment surgery?
   a. Explain how to care for an ocular prosthesis.
   b. Assure patients that they can expect 20/20 vision after surgery.
   c. Teach the family how to recognize when the patient is hallucinating.
   d. Assess the patient's level of knowledge about retinal detachment and provide information appropriate to the situation.

6. The nurse is teaching an adult patient how to administer antibiotic eardrops. Which of the following instructions is important to include in the teaching?
   a. Cool the drops so that they decrease swelling in the canal.
   b. Be careful to avoid touching the tip of the dropper bottle to the ear.
   c. Placement of a cotton wick to assist in administering the drops is not recommended.
   d. Keep the head tilted for 5 to 7 minutes after administering the drops to prevent them from running out of the ear canal.

7. In which of the following patients would the nurse suspect otosclerosis from assessment findings of hearing loss?
   a. A 26-year-old woman who has three biological children younger than 5 years of age
   b. A 52-year-old man whose hearing loss is accompanied by vertigo and tinnitus
   c. A 42-year-old Black woman who has a history of serous otitis media
   d. A 63-year-old man who can hear high-pitched sounds more effectively than low-pitched sounds

8. Which of the following statements best describes a patient who has a sensorineural hearing loss?
   a. The patient has difficulty understanding speech.
   b. The patient experiences clearer sounds with the use of a hearing aid.
   c. The patient may have a reversal of damage caused by ototoxic drugs.
   d. The patient hears low-pitched sounds better than high-pitched sounds.

9. Which of the following would the nurse teach the patient with extended-wear contact lenses?
   a. The lenses may be moistened with saliva if necessary.
   b. The lenses may be worn for up to 1 week without removal.
   c. Any saline solution may be used for moistening as long as it is hypertonic.
   d. The person may continue lens wear if he or she experiences only mild to moderate irritation or redness.

10. Which of the following strategies would best assist the nurse in communicating with a patient who has a hearing loss?
    a. Overenunciate speech
    b. Exaggerate facial expression
    c. Raise the voice to a higher pitch
    d. Write out all questions and responses

11. Which of the following statements best describes patients with permanent visual impairment?
    a. They feel most comfortable with other visually impaired persons.
    b. They may feel threatened when others make eye contact during a conversation.
    c. They usually need others to speak louder so they can communicate appropriately.
    d. They may experience the same grieving process that is associated with other losses.

ANSWERS: 1. b; 2. d; 3. d; 4. b; 5. d; 6. b; 7. a; 8. a; 9. b; 10. a; 11. d.

REFERENCES

Armstrong, C. (2009). Diagnosis and management of cerumen impaction. *American Family Physician, 80*(9), 1011-1013. Retrieved from *http://www.aafp.org/afp/2009/1101/p1011.html*

Bartlett, J. D. (2010). *Ophthalmic drug facts* (22nd ed.). Philadelphia: Lippincott Williams & Wilkins.

Bell, S., Hawranik, P. G., & McCormac, K. (2011). Focus on falls prevention: A quality improvement initiative. *AER Journal: Research and Practice in Visual Impairment and Blindness, 4*(3), 133.

Bernardes, T. F., & Bonfioli, A. A. (2010). Blepharitis. *Seminars in Ophthalmology, 25*(3), 79-83. doi:10.3109/08820538.2010.488562

Buhrmann, R., Hodge, W., Beardmore, J., Baker, G., Lowcock, B., Pan, I., & Bovell, A. (2007). *Foundations for a Canadian vision health strategy: Towards preventing avoidable blindness and promoting vision health.* Retrieved from *http://www.visionhealth.ca/projects/documents/Foundations-For-A-Canadian-Vision-Health-Strategy.pdf*

Callahan, D. (2012). Conjunctivitis. *Digital Journal of Ophthalmology.* Retrieved from *http://www.djo.harvard.edu/site.php?url=/patients/pi/410*

Canadian Ophthalmological Society. (2007a). *Amblyopia: Treat "lazy eye" in early childhood.* Retrieved from *http://www.eyesite.ca/english/public-information/eye-conditions/pdfs/Amblyopia_e.pdf*

Canadian Ophthalmological Society. (2007b). Evidence-based clinical practice guidelines for the periodic eye examinations in adults in Canada. *Canadian Journal of Ophthalmology, 42*(1), 39-45. doi:10.3129/can j ophthalmol.06-126e

DeCroos, F. C., & Afshari, N. A. (2008). Perioperative antibiotics and anti-inflammatory agents in cataract surgery. *Current Opinion in Ophthalmology, 19*(1), 22-26. doi:10.1097/ICU.0b013e3282f30577

Department of Justice Canada. (2011). *Canada occupational health and safety regulations.* Retrieved from *http://laws.justice.gc.ca/eng/regulations/SOR-86-304/index.html.*

Fu, E., Hayden, B., & Singh, A. (2008). Intraocular tumors. *Ultrasound Clinic, 3*(2), 229-244. doi:10.1016/j.cult2008.04.002. doi:10.1016/j.cult.2008.04.002.

Haran, M. J., Lord, S. R., Cameron, I. D., Ivers, R. Q., Simpson, J. M., Lee, B. B., ..., Severino, C. (2009). Preventing falls in older multifocal glasses wearers by providing single-lens distance glasses: The protocol for the VISIBLE randomised controlled trial. *BMC Geriatrics, 9*(1), 10. doi:10.1186/1471-2318-9-10

Haslbeck, C., Anderson, L., Markowitz, M., & Feder, K. (2009). Tips and resources for occupational therapists (OTs) working with people with vision loss (Conference notes). *Canadian Association of Occupational Therapists Conference 2009.*

Hearing Foundation of Canada. (2010). *Statistics.* Retrieved from *http://www.thfc.ca/cms/en/KeyStatistics/KeyStatistics.aspx?menuid=87*

Hoet, P., & Lison, D. (2008). Ototoxicity of toluene and styrene: State of current knowledge. *Critical Reviews in Toxicology, 38*(2), 127-170. doi:10.1080/10408440701845443

Jensen, L. (2012). Working with clients with vision loss. *Canadian Nurse, 108*(3), 28-33.

Kerber, K. (2009). Vertigo and dizziness in the emergency department. *Emergency Medicine Clinics of North America, 27*(1), 39-viii. doi:10.1016/j.emc.2008.09.002

Khare, G. D., Symons, R. C., & Do, D. V. (2008). Common ophthalmic emergencies. *International Journal of Clinical Practice, 62*(11), 1776-1784. doi:10.1111/j.1742-1241.2008.01855.x

Kirkwood, B. (2008). Clinical assessment of patients with cataract. *Insight—Journal of the American Society of Ophthalmic Registered Nurses, 33*(3), 10-17.

Lee, T. C., & Gold, W. L. (2011). Necrotizing pseudomonas chondritis after piercing of the upper ear. *Canadian Medical Association Journal, 183*(7), 819-821. doi:10.1503/cmaj.100018

Leyland, M., & Pringle, E. (2006). Multifocal versus monofocal intraocular lenses after cataract extraction. *Cochrane Database of Systematic Reviews (Online), 4*(4), CD003169. doi:10.1002/14651858.CD003169.pub2

Mahmood, A., & Narang, A. (2008). Diagnosis and management of acute red eye. *Emergency Medical Clinics of North America, 26*(1), 35-55. doi:10.1016/j.emc.2007.10.002

Miyamoto, R. T., & Kirk, K. I. (2006). Cochlear implants and other implantable auditory prostheses. In B. J. Bailery, J. T. Johnson, & S. D. Newlands (Eds.), *Head and neck surgery—Otolaryngology.* Philadelphia: Lippincott Williams & Wilkins.

Muzychka, M. (2009). *Environmental scan of vision health and vision loss in the provinces and territories of Canada.* Toronto: National Coalition for Vision Health. Retrieved from *http://www.eyesite.ca/resources/NCVH-environment-scanSept2009.pdf*

National Coalition for Vision Health. (2011). *FAQ.* Retrieved from *http://www.visionhealth.ca/faq.htm*

National Eye Institute. (2009). *Facts About age-related macular degeneration.* Retrieved from *http://www.nei.nih.gov/health/maculardegen/armd_facts.asp*

National Eye Institute. (n.d.). *Facts about the cornea and corneal disease [NEI health information].* Retrieved from *http://www.nei.nih.gov/health/cornealdisease/*

Olson, J. H., Erie, J. C., & Bakri, S. J. (2011). Nutritional supplementation and age-related macular degeneration. *Seminars in Ophthalmology, 26*(3), 131-136. doi:10.3109/08820538.2011.577131

Patton, K. T., & Thibodeau, G. A. (2010). *Anatomy & physiology* (7th ed.). St. Louis: Mosby.

Portnuff, C. D. F., Fligor, B. J., & Arehart, K. H. (2011). Teenage use of portable listening devices: A hazard to hearing? *Journal of American Academy of Audiology, 22*(10), 663-667.

Quesnel, A. M., & McKenna, M. J. (2011). Current strategies in management of intracanalicular vestibular schwannoma. *Current Opinion in Otolaryngology and Head and Neck Surgery, 19*(5), 335-340. doi:10.1097/MOO.0b013e32834a3fa7

Quintanilla-Dieck, M. de L., Artunduaga, M. A., & Eavey, R. D. (2009). Intentional exposure to loud music: The second MTV.com survey reveals an opportunity to educate. *Journal of Pediatrics, 155*(4), 550-555. doi:10.1016/j.jpeds.2009.04.053

Rajesh, M., & Pallavi, M. (2007). Drainage of effusion in otitis media: A historical review. *Internet Journal of Otorhinolaryngology, 6*(2). Retrieved from *http://www.ispub.com/journal/the-internet-journal-of-otorhinolaryngology/volume-6-number-2/drainage-of-effusion-in-otitis-media-a-historical-review.html*

Riaz, Y., Mehta, J. S., Wormald, R., Evans, J. R., Foster, A., Ravilla, T., & Snelligan, T. (2006). Surgical interventions for age-related cataract. *Cochrane Database of Systematic Reviews (Online), 4*(4), CD001323. doi:10.1002/14651858.CD001323.pub2

Ross, S. A., McKenna, A., Mozejko, S., & Fick, G. H. (2007). Diabetic retinopathy in native and nonnative Canadians. *Experimental Diabetes Research, 2007*, 762-71. doi:10.1155/2007/76271

Sajjadi, H., & Paperella, M. (2008). Ménière's disease. *Lancet, 372*(9636), 406-414. doi:10.1016/S0140-6736(08)61161-7

Semaan, M. T., & Megerian, C. A. (2011). Ménière's disease: A challenging and relentless disorder. *Otolaryngologic Clinics of North America, 44*(2), 383-403. doi:10.1016/j.otc.2011.01.010

Sharts-Hopko, N. C., & Glynn-Milley, C. (2009). Primary open-angle glaucoma. *American Journal of Nursing, 109*(2), 40-47. doi:10.1097/01.NAJ.0000345434.37734.ee

Smith, S. (2008). Basic ocular anatomy. *Insight: The Journal of the American Society of Ophthalmic Registered Nurses, Inc. 33*(3), 19-25.

Sutton, G. L., & Kim, P. (2010). Laser in situ keratomileusis in 2010—A review. *Clinical & Experimental Ophthalmology, 38*(2), 192-210. doi:10.1111/j.1442-9071.2010.02227.x

Tavares, F. de P., Fernandes, R. S., Bernardes, T. F., Bonfioli, A. A., & Soares, E. J. (2010). Dry eye disease. *Seminars in Ophthalmology, 25*(3), 84-93. doi:10.3109/08820538.2010.488568

Thornton, K., Parrish, F., & Swords, C. (2011). Topical vs. systemic treatments for acute otitis media. *Pediatric Nursing, 37*(5).

Retrieved from *http://www.pediatricnursing.net/issues/11sepoct/abstr5.html*

Tseng, V. L., Greenberg, P. B., Wu, W.-C., Jiang, L., Li, E., Kang, J. M., …, Friedmann, P. D. (2011). Cataract surgery complications in nonagenarians. *Ophthalmology, 118*(7), 1229-1235. doi:10.1016/j.ophtha.2010.11.023

Vogel, I., Brug, J., Hosli, E. J., van der Ploeg, C. P. B., & Raat, H. (2008). MP3 players and hearing loss: Adolescents' perceptions of loud music and hearing conservation. *Journal of Pediatrics, 152*(3), 400-404.e1. doi:10.1016/j.jpeds.2007.07.009

World Health Organization. (2011). *Prevention of blindness and visual impairment: Trachoma.* Retrieved from *http://www.who.int/blindness/causes/trachoma*

CANADIAN RESOURCES

Alberta Association of the Deaf
http://www.aadnews.ca/

Alliance for Equality of Blind Canadians
http://www.blindcanadians.ca/

AMD Alliance International
http://www.amdalliance.org/

BC and Alberta Guide Dog Services
http://www.bcguidedog.com/

Canadian Association of the Deaf
http://www.cad.ca/

Canadian Association of Optometrists
http://opto.ca/

Canadian Council of the Blind (CCB)
http://www.ccbnational.net/Wuzzy/

The Canadian Deafblind and Rubella Association
http://www.cdbraontario.ca/index_e.php

Canadian Glaucoma Society
http://www.cgs-scg.org/

Canadian Hard of Hearing Association
http://www.chha.ca/chha/

Canadian Hearing Society
http://www.chs.ca/

Canadian Helen Keller Centre
http://www.chkc.org/

Canadian National Institute for the Blind (CNIB)
http://www.cnib.ca/en/

Canadian Ophthalmological Society
http://www.eyesite.ca/english/index.htm

Deafblind Services Society of British Columbia
http://www.deafblindservices.com/

Foundation Fighting Blindness
http://www.blindness.org/

Hearing Foundation of Canada
http://www.thfc.ca/Default.aspx

Misericordia Health Centre: Buhler Eye Care Centre
http://www.misericordia.mb.ca/Programs/EyeCare.html

Misericordia Health Centre: Focus on Falls Prevention Vision Screening Program
http://www.misericordia.mb.ca/AboutUs/VisionScreening.html

Montreal Association for the Blind
http://www.mabmackay.ca/

National Coalition for Vision Health
http://www.visionhealth.ca/

Society of Deaf and Hard of Hearing Nova Scotians
http://sdhhns.org/

University of Ottawa Eye Institute
http://www.ottawahospital.on.ca/wps/portal/Base/TheHospital/ClinicalServices/DeptPgrmCS/Programs/EyeInstitute

RELATED RESOURCES

American Academy of Audiology
http://www.audiology.org/Pages/default.aspx

American Academy of Ophthalmology
http://www.aao.org/

American Society of Cataract and Refractive Surgery
http://ascrs.org/

American Society of Ophthalmic Registered Nurses
http://www.asorn.org/

Glaucoma Research Foundation
http://www.glaucoma.org/

International Hearing Dog, Inc.
http://www.ihdi.org/Home.html

International Hearing Society
http://ihsinfo.org/IhsV2/Home/Index.cfm

The Macula Foundation
http://maculafoundation.org/

National Eye Institute of the National Institutes of Health
http://www.nei.nih.gov/

National Consortium on Deaf-Blindness
http://www.nationaldb.org/

VisionSimulations.com
http://visionsimulations.com/

University of Michigan Kellogg Eye Center
http://www.kellogg.umich.edu/

U.S. Food and Drug Administration
Cochlear Implants
http://www.fda.gov/MedicalDevices/ProductsandMedicalProcedures/ImplantsandProsthetics/CochlearImplants/default.htm

evolve *For additional Internet resources, see the Web site for this book at* **http://evolve.elsevier.com/Canada/Lewis/medsurg**

Nursing Assessment: Integumentary System

Written by Barbara Sinni-McKeehen

Adapted by Cheryl A. Sams

LEARNING OBJECTIVES

1. Describe the structures and the functions of the integumentary system.
2. Describe age-related changes in the integumentary system and differences in assessment findings.
3. Identify the significant subjective and objective data related to the integumentary system that should be obtained from a patient.
4. Describe specific assessments to be made during the physical examination of the skin and the appendages.
5. Compare the critical components for describing primary and secondary lesions.

6. Describe the appropriate techniques used in the physical assessment of the integumentary system.
7. Summarize the structural and assessment differences in light- and dark-skinned individuals.
8. Differentiate normal from common abnormal findings of a physical assessment of the integumentary system.
9. Describe the purpose, significance of results, and nursing responsibilities related to diagnostic studies of the integumentary system.

KEY TERMS

alopecia Partial or complete lack of hair resulting from normal aging, endocrine disorder, drug reaction, anticancer medication, or skin disease, p. 544

apocrine sweat glands Glands with no known function that are located mainly in the axillae, breast areolae, umbilical and anogenital areas, external auditory canals, and eyelids. They secrete a thick milky substance of unknown composition that becomes odoriferous when altered by skin surface bacteria, p. 542

dermis Connective tissue below the epidermis, p. 542

eccrine sweat glands Function to cool the body by evaporation, to excrete waste products through the pores of the skin, and to moisturize surface cells, p. 543

epidermis The thin avascular superficial layer of the skin; made up of an outer dead cornified portion that serves as a protective barrier and a deeper, living portion that folds into the dermis, p. 541

erythema Skin redness from dilation of blood vessels that occurs in patches of variable size and shape and is caused by heat, certain drugs, alcohol, ultraviolet rays, and other problems, Table 25-9, p. 549

hirsutism Male distribution of hair in women occurs and is caused by an abnormality of ovaries or adrenal glands, decrease in estrogen level, or familial trait, Table 25-9, p. 549

intertriginous Describing an area where opposing skin surfaces touch and may rub, such as skin folds of groin, axilla, abdomen, or breast, p. 545

keloid An overgrowth of collagenous scar tissue at the site of a skin injury, particularly a wound or a surgical incision; the new tissue is elevated, rounded, and firm, p. 548

keratinocytes Cells synthesized from epidermal cells in the basal layer; they produce a specialized protein, keratin, that is vital to the protective barrier function of the skin, p. 542

melanocytes Cells contained in the deep, basal layer (stratum germinativum) of the epidermis that contain melanin, a pigment that gives colour to the skin and hair and protects the body from damaging ultraviolet sunlight, p. 541

mole (nevus) Benign overgrowth of melanocytes occurs as a defect of development; excessive numbers and large, irregular moles are often familial, Table 25-9, p. 549

pruritus Itching, p. 544

sebaceous glands Oil-producing glands that produce sebum, which prevents the skin and hair from becoming dry, p. 542

ELECTRONIC RESOURCES

Supplemental content related to Chapter 25 can be found…

Evolve Web Site ⊖volve

http://evolve.elsevier.com/Canada/Lewis/medsurg
- Assessment Case Study
- Clinical Reference: Laboratory Values
- Content Updates
- eFigures:
  - eFigure 25-1: Traction Alopecia
  - eFigure 25-2: Keloid scarring

- Electronic Calculators
- Examination Review Questions
- Glossary
- Key Points (Printable and MP3 Download)
- Physical Examination Videos:
  - Back and Posterior Chest
  - Feet, Legs, and Hips
  - Head and Face

The integumentary system is the largest body organ and comprises skin, hair, nails, and glands. The skin is further divided into three layers—epidermis, dermis, and subcutaneous tissue—and is illustrated in Figure 25-1.

Structures and Functions of the Skin and Appendages

Structures

The epidermis is the outermost layer of the skin. The dermis, the second skin layer, contains collagen bundles and supports the nerve and vascular network. The subcutaneous layer is not part of the skin, lies below the dermis, and is composed primarily of fat and loose connective tissue.

Epidermis. The **epidermis,** the thin avascular superficial layer of the skin, is made up of an outer dead cornified portion that serves as a protective barrier and a deeper, living portion that folds into the dermis. Together these layers measure 0.05 to 0.1 mm in thickness. The epidermis is nourished by blood vessels in the dermis. The epidermis regenerates with new cells every 28 days. The two types of epidermal cells are the melanocytes (5%) and the keratinocytes (95%) (Patton & Thibodeau, 2010).

Melanocytes are contained in the deep, basal layer (stratum germinativum) of the epidermis. They contain melanin, a pigment that gives colour to the skin and hair and protects the body from

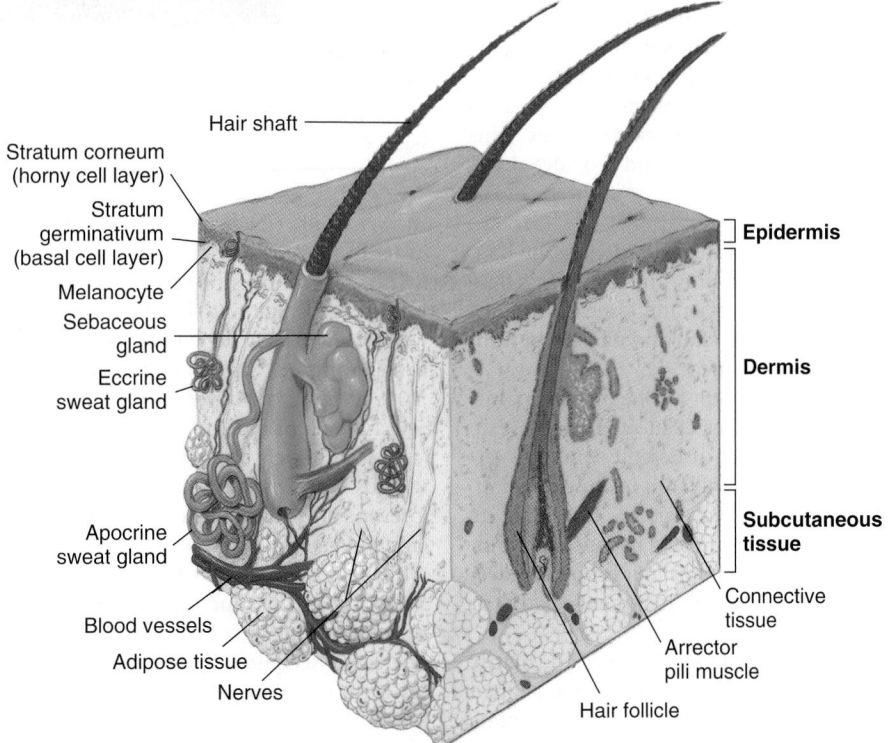

Figure 25-1 Microscopic view of the skin in longitudinal section.

Source: Jarvis, C. (2008). *Physical examination and health assessment* (5th ed., p. 222, Figure 12-1). St. Louis: Saunders.

damaging ultraviolet (UV) sunlight. Sunlight and hormones stimulate melanosomes (within the melanocyte) to produce melanin. The wide range of skin and hair colours is caused by the amount of melanin produced; more melanin results in darker skin colour (Goldsmith et al., 2012).

Keratinocytes are synthesized from epidermal cells in the basal layer. Initially, these cells are undifferentiated. As they mature (keratinize), they move to the surface, where they flatten and die to form the outer skin layer (stratum corneum). Keratinocytes produce a fibrous protein, keratin, which is vital to the protective barrier function of the skin. The upward movement of keratinocytes from the basement membrane to the stratum corneum takes approximately 4 weeks. If dead cells slough off too rapidly, the skin will appear thin and eroded. If new cells form faster than old cells are shed, the skin becomes scaly and thickened. Changes in this cell cycle account for many skin problems, such as psoriasis.

Dermis.
The **dermis** is the connective tissue below the epidermis. Dermal thickness varies from 1 to 4 mm. The dermis is highly vascular and assists in body temperature and blood pressure regulation. The dermis is divided into two layers, an upper thin papillary layer and a deeper, thicker reticular layer. The papillary exposed surface ridges form congenital patterns called fingerprints and footprints. The reticular layer contains collagen, elastic and reticular fibres.

Collagen forms the greatest part of the dermis and is responsible for the mechanical strength of the skin. The primary cell type in the dermis is the *fibroblast*. Fibroblasts produce collagen and elastin and are important in wound healing. Elastin fibres, nerves, lymphatic vessels, hair follicles, and sebaceous and sweat glands are also found in the dermis.

Subcutaneous Tissue.
The subcutaneous tissue is often discussed with the skin because it attaches the skin to underlying tissues such as the muscle and bone. The subcutaneous tissue contains loose connective tissue and fat cells that provide insulation. The anatomic distribution of subcutaneous tissue varies according to gender, heredity, age, and nutritional status. This layer also stores lipids, regulates temperature, and provides shock absorption.

Skin Appendages.
Appendages of the skin include the hair, the nails, and glands (sebaceous, apocrine, and eccrine). These structures develop from the epidermal layer and receive nutrients, electrolytes, and fluids from the dermis. Hair and nails form from specialized keratin that becomes hardened.

Hair grows on most of the body except for the lips, the palms of the hands, and the soles of the feet (Patton & Thibodeau, 2012). The colour of the hair is a result of heredity and is determined by the type and the amount of melanin in the hair shaft. Hair grows approximately 1 cm/mo. On average, 100 hairs are lost each day; the rate of growth is not affected by cutting (Goldsmith et al., 2012). Baldness results when lost hair is not replaced. This absence of hair may be disease- or treatment-related or caused by heredity.

Nails grow from under the matrix of the nail plate. The matrix is commonly called the *lunula*, which is the white crescent-shaped area visible through the nail root (Figure 25-2). The nail plate adheres to and is supported by the nail bed. The cuticle is the part of the skin that extends a small distance on the nail plate before being shed (like the stratum corneum). Fingernails grow at a rate of 0.7 to 0.84 mm/wk, with toenail growth 30% to 50%

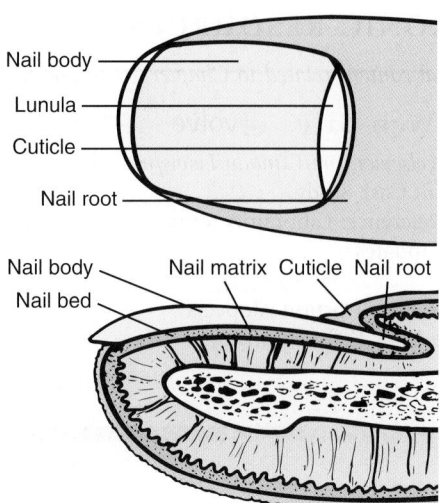

Figure 25-2 Structure of a nail.

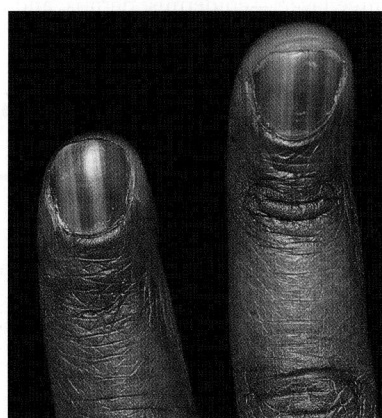

Figure 25-3 Pigmented nail bed normally seen with dark skin colour.

Source: Habif, T. P. (2004). *Clinical dermatology: A color guide to diagnosis and therapy* (4th ed., p. 868, Figure 25-5). St. Louis: Mosby.

slower. Nails can be injured by direct trauma. A lost fingernail usually regenerates in 3 to 6 months, but a lost toenail may require 12 months or more. Nail growth may vary according to the person's age and health. Nail colour ranges from pink to yellow or brown depending on skin colour. Pigmented bands (melanonychea striata) occur in the nail bed in approximately 90% or more of all people with dark skin (Figure 25-3).

Two major types of glands are associated with the skin: sebaceous and sweat (apocrine and eccrine) glands. The **sebaceous glands** secrete *sebum*, which is emptied into the hair follicles to prevent skin and hair dryness. Sebum is somewhat bacteriostatic and fungistatic and consists mainly of lipids. These glands depend on sex hormones, particularly testosterone, to regulate sebum secretion and production. Sebum secretion varies across the lifespan according to sex hormone levels, increased levels generating increased secretion by the sebaceous glands. The development of acne with puberty and sebum secretion demonstrates this positive correlation. Sebaceous glands are present on all areas of the skin except the palms and soles and are most abundant on the face, the scalp, the upper chest, and the back.

The **apocrine sweat glands** are located mainly in the axillae, the breast areolae, the umbilical and anogenital areas, the external auditory canals, and the eyelids. They secrete a thick milky substance whose precise composition is unknown; this becomes odoriferous when altered by skin surface bacteria. These glands enlarge and become active at puberty owing to reproductive hormones.

The **eccrine sweat glands** are widely distributed over the body, except in a few areas, such as the lips. Two square centimetres of skin contains about 1000 of these sweat glands. Sweat is a transparent watery solution composed of salts, ammonia, urea, and other wastes. The main function of these glands is to cool the body by evaporation, excrete waste products through the pores of the skin, and moisturize surface cells.

Functions of the Integumentary System

The primary function of the skin is to protect the underlying tissues of the body by serving as a surface barrier to the external environment. The skin also acts as a barrier against invasion by bacteria and viruses and prevents excessive water loss. The fat of the subcutaneous layer insulates the body and provides protection from trauma.

The skin with its nerve endings and special receptors provides sensory perception for environmental stimuli that supply information to the brain related to pain, heat and cold, touch, pressure, and vibration. The skin controls heat regulation by responding to changes in internal and external temperature with vasoconstriction or vasodilation. Related to heat regulation is the skin's function of excretion. Between 600 and 900 mL of water is lost daily through insensible perspiration that helps maintain homeostasis through fluid and electrolyte balance. In addition, sebum and sweat are secreted by the skin and lubricate the skin surface. Endogenous synthesis of vitamin D, which is critical to calcium and phosphorus balance, occurs in the epidermis. Vitamin D is synthesized by the action of UV light on vitamin D precursors in epidermal cells.

The aesthetic functions of the skin include the mirroring of various emotions, such as anger or embarrassment, as well as displaying the individual identity of a person. The role of absorption at the cutaneous level is well known, and an increasing number of drugs are effectively delivered via patches applied directly to the skin.

AGE-RELATED CONSIDERATIONS: EFFECTS OF AGING ON THE INTEGUMENTARY SYSTEM

In young children, the skin is normally smooth, nonoily, slightly dry, and warm. As the skin ages, many changes will occur. Although many changes are not serious except for their cosmetic value, others are more serious and need careful evaluation. Age-related changes of the integumentary system and differences in assessment findings are listed in Table 25-1.

The rate of age-related skin changes is influenced by heredity and a personal history of sun exposure, hygiene practices, nutrition, and general state of health. Skin changes related to aging include decreased turgor, thinning, dryness, wrinkling, vascular lesions, increased skin fragility, and benign neoplasms.

The junction between the dermis and the epidermis becomes flattened, and the epidermis contains fewer melanocytes. In addition, the dermis loses volume and has fewer blood vessels. Scalp, pubic, and axillary hair becomes depigmented and thinner. A loss of melanin results in grey or white hair. The nail

AGE-RELATED DIFFERENCES IN ASSESSMENT

Table 25-1 Integumentary System

DIFFERENCES IN CHANGES	ASSESSMENT FINDINGS
Skin	
• Decreased subcutaneous fat, muscle laxity, degeneration of elastic fibres, collagen stiffening	Increased wrinkling, sagging breasts and abdomen, redundant flesh around eyes, slowness of skin to flatten when pinched together (tenting)
• Decreased extracellular water, surface lipids, and sebaceous gland activity	Dry, flaking skin with possible signs of excoriation caused by scratching
• Decreased activity of apocrine and sebaceous glands	Dry skin with minimal to no perspiration, skin colour uneven
• Increased capillary fragility and permeability	Evidence of bruising
• Increased focal melanocytes in basal layer with pigment accumulation	Solar lentigines on face and back of hands
• Diminished blood supply	Decrease in rosy appearance of skin and mucous membranes; skin is cool to touch; diminished awareness of pain, touch, temperature, and peripheral vibration
• Decreased proliferative capacity	Diminished rate of wound healing
• Decreased immunocompetence	Increase in neoplasms
Hair	
• Decreased melanin and melanocytes	Grey or white hair
• Decreased oil	Dry, coarse hair; scaly scalp
• Decreased density of hair	Thinning and loss of hair; loss of hair in outer half or outer third of eyebrow and back of legs
• Cumulative androgen effect; decreasing estrogen levels	Facial hirsutism; baldness
Nails	
• Decreased peripheral blood supply	Thick, brittle nails with diminished growth
• Increased keratin	Longitudinal ridging
• Decreased circulation	Prolonged return of blood to nails on blanching

plate thins, and nails become brittle, thicker, and more prone to splitting and yellowing. Nails, especially toenails, may also thicken with age.

Chronic UV exposure is the major contributor to photoaging and wrinkling of the skin (Helfrich, Sachs, & Voorhees, 2008). Photoaging refers to cumulative damage done to the skin from prolonged exposure, over a person's lifetime, to UV radiation (Figure 25-4). The wrinkling of sun-exposed areas such as the face and hands is more marked than in sun-shielded areas such as the buttocks. Poor nutrition contributes to aging of the skin resulting from a decreased intake of protein, calories, and vitamins. With aging, collagen fibres stiffen, elastic fibres degenerate, and the amount of subcutaneous tissue decreases.

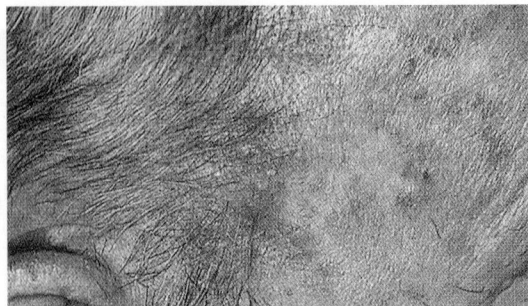

Figure 25-4 Photoaging. Irregular pigmentation and keratoses occur on sun-damaged skin on the forehead.

Source: Gawkrodger, D. (2008). *Dermatology* (4th ed.). Edinburgh: Churchill Livingstone.

These changes, with the added effects of gravity, lead to wrinkling (see Figure 25-4).

Benign neoplasms related to the aging process can occur on the skin. These growths include seborrheic keratoses, vascular lesions such as cherry angiomas, and skin tags. Actinic keratosis, which appears on areas of chronic sun exposure, occurs especially in the person who has a fair complexion and light eyes (blue, green, or hazel). These premalignant cutaneous lesions place an individual at increased risk for squamous cell and basal cell carcinomas. The photoaged person is more susceptible to skin cancers because of decline in the capacity to repair cellular deoxyribonucleic acid (especially DNA) damage caused by UV exposure. Chronic UV exposure from tanning beds causes the same damage as UV from the sun.

Decreased subcutaneous fat leads to an increased risk of traumatic injury, hypothermia, and skin shearing, which may lead to pressure ulcers. With aging, the apocrine and eccrine sweat glands atrophy, causing dry skin and decreased body odour. The growth rate of the hair and nails decreases as a result of atrophy of the involved structures. Hormonal and vitamin deficiencies can cause dry, thin hair and **alopecia** (partial or complete lack of hair).

The visible effects of aging on the skin and hair may have a profound psychological effect on many people. A youthful look may be tied to a person's self-image. Although fine wrinkling of the skin, thinning hair, and brittle nails are normal changes with aging, they may result in an altered self-image (Jarvis, Browne, MacDonald-Jenkins, & Luctkar-Flude, 2009).

Assessment of the Integumentary System

A general assessment of the skin begins at the initial contact with the patient and continues throughout the examination. Specific areas are examined during examination of other body sites unless the reason for seeking care is a dermatological problem. A general statement about the physical condition of the skin should be recorded (Table 25-2), and specific problems should be noted under the appropriate system. Health history questions presented in Table 25-3 should be asked when a skin problem is noted.

Objective Data

Physical Examination. Primary skin lesions develop on previously unaltered skin. The common characteristics of primary

Table 25-2 Normal Physical Assessment of the Integumentary System
Skin: Evenly pigmented; no petechiae, purpura, lesions, or excoriations; warm, good turgor
Nails: Pink, oval, and adhere to nail base with 160-degree angle
Hair: Shiny and full; amount and distribution appropriate for age and gender; no flaking of scalp, forehead, or pinna

skin lesions are shown in Table 25-4. Secondary skin lesions are lesions that change with time or because of a factor such as scratching or infection. Secondary skin lesions are shown in Table 25-5. General principles when conducting an assessment of the skin are as follows:

1. Have a private examination room of moderate temperature with good lighting; a room with exposure to daylight is preferred.
2. Ensure that the patient is comfortable and in a dressing gown that allows easy access to all skin areas.
3. Be systematic and proceed from head to toe.
4. Compare symmetrical parts.
5. Perform a general inspection and then a lesion-specific examination.
6. Use the metric system when taking measurements.
7. Use appropriate terminology and nomenclature when reporting or documenting.
   Photographs are useful when accurate findings are needed.

Inspection. Inspect the skin for general colour and pigmentation, vascularity, bruising, and the presence of lesions or discolorations. The critical factor in assessment of skin colour is change. A skin colour that is normal for a particular patient can be a sign of a pathological condition in another patient. The colour of the skin depends on the amount of melanin (brown), carotene (yellow), oxyhemoglobin (red), and reduced hemoglobin (bluish red) present at a particular time. The most reliable areas in which to assess erythema, cyanosis, pallor, and jaundice are the areas of least pigmentation, such as sclerae, conjunctivae, nail beds, lips, and buccal mucosa. The true skin colour is best observed in photo-protected areas, such as the buttocks. Activity, sun (UV) exposure, emotions, cigarette smoking, and edema, as well as respiratory, renal, cardiovascular, and hepatic disorders, can all directly affect the colour of the skin. The nurse should also ask whether there is any **pruritus** (itching) and inspect the patient's skin for evidence of scratching. Table 25-6 describes assessment variations in light- and dark-skinned individuals.

Examine the skin for possible problems related to vascularity, such as areas of bruising, and vascular and purpuric lesions, such as *angioma* (benign tumour of blood or lymph vessels), *petechiae* (tiny purple spots on skin), or *purpura* (bleeding disorder causing ecchymosis or petechiae). Reaction to direct pressure should be noted. If a lesion blanches on direct pressure and then refills, the redness is caused by dilated blood vessels. If the discoloration remains, it is the result of subcutaneous or intradermal bleeding or the presence of a nonvascular lesion. Note any pattern of bruising, for example, in the shape of the hand or fingers, or bruises at different stages of resolution. These may be indications of other health problems or abuse and should be further investigated.

If lesions are found on the skin, their colour, size, distribution, location, and shape should be recorded. Skin lesions are

HEALTH HISTORY

Table 25-3 Integumentary System: Questions for Obtaining Subjective Data

Past History

- Any history of previous trauma, surgery, or prior disease that involves the skin?*
- Do you have any dermatological manifestations of systemic problems such as jaundice (liver disease), delayed wound healing (diabetes mellitus), cyanosis (respiratory disorder), or pallor (anemia)?*
- Do you have a history of chronic or unprotected exposure to UV light such as use of tanning beds or history of radiation treatments?*
- Have you had any skin-related problems that occurred as a result of taking prescription or OTC medications?*
- Have you ever taken vitamins, hormones, antibiotics, corticosteroids, or antimetabolites?
- Are you taking any complementary or alternative medicine?*
- Are you using any medications to treat hair loss?*
- Have you used prescription or OTC medications to treat a primary skin problem such as acne or a secondary skin problem such as itching? If so, please state the name, length of use, method of application, and effectiveness of the medication.
- Did you ever have any surgery on your skin, including cosmetic surgery?*
- Do you have any body art, piercings, or tattoos?* Did you experience any complications such as skin infections, allergic reactions, dental problems, or MRI burns?
- Have you ever had a skin biopsy?* If so, what were the results?
- Have you had any treatments specific for a skin problem (e.g., phototherapy, radiation therapy, cosmetic "peels")?

Family History

- Do you have any family history of any skin diseases, including congenital and familial diseases (e.g., alopecia and psoriasis) and systemic diseases with dermatological manifestations (e.g., diabetes, thyroid disease, cardiovascular diseases, immune disorders)?
- Any family and personal history of skin cancer, particularly melanoma?

Social, Environment, or Occupational History

- Do you have any pets?
- Do you have any food, pet, or drug allergies?*
- Do you have any unusual skin reactions to insect bites and stings?*

- Are there any environmental skin irritants at your current or previous work place or home?*
- Do your leisure activities involve the use of any chemicals that are potentially toxic to the skin?*

Self-Care History

- Describe your daily hygiene practices.
- What skin products are you currently using?
- Do you do anything to protect yourself from the sun?* How frequently do you use sun protection and what is the SPF number of your sunscreen products?
- Has your birth control method, if used, caused a skin problem?*

Cognitive–Perceptual

- Do you have any unusual sensations of heat, cold, or touch?*
- Do you have any pain associated with your skin condition?*
- Do you have any joint pain?*

Nutritional History

- Are there any changes in the condition of your skin, hair, nails, and mucous membranes that might be related to dietary changes?*
- Do you have food allergies that cause a skin reaction?

General

- Describe any current skin condition, including onset, course, and treatment (if any).
- Describe any changes in the condition of your skin, hair, nails, and mucous membranes.
- Have you noticed any changes in skin pigmentation? Any changes in the size or shape or colour of a mole? Any excessive bruising? Any unusual hair loss? Any change in the strength, colour, or nature of your nails? Any pruritus or itching?
- Have you noticed any changes in the way sores or lesions heal?*
- Have you noticed changes in your skin related to excessive sweating, dryness, or swelling?*
- Does your skin condition keep you awake or awaken you after you have fallen asleep?*

MRI, magnetic resonance imaging; *OTC*, over-the-counter; *SPF*, sun protection factor; *UV*, ultraviolet.
*If yes, describe.
Source: Based on Jarvis, C., Browne, A. J., MacDonald-Jenkins, J., & Luctkar-Flude, M. (Eds.). (2009). *Physical examination and health assessment* (1st Canadian ed., pp. 225–229). Toronto: Elsevier Canada.

usually described in terms related to the lesions' configuration (solitary or pattern in relation to other lesions [Table 25-7]) and distribution (arrangement of lesions over an area of skin [Table 25-8]).

During systematic inspection, it is important to note any unusual odours. Skin sites that contain lesions, such as rashes that are colonized with yeast or bacteria, are often found in **intertriginous** areas where opposing skin surfaces touch and may rub (e.g., axilla, overhanging abdominal folds, groin, breast) and are often associated with distinctive odours (Figure 25-5). Tattoos and needle-track marks should be examined and noted for location and the characteristics of the surrounding skin area.

Inspection of the hair should include an examination of all body hair. Note the distribution, the texture, and the quantity of hair. Changes in the normal distribution of body hair and growth

may indicate an endocrine or vascular disorder. Inspection of the nails should include a careful examination of nail shape, thickness, curvature, and surface. Note any grooves, pitting, or ridges or detachment from the nail bed. Changes in nail smoothness or thickness can occur with anemia, psoriasis, thyroid problems, decreased vascular circulation, and some infectious organisms.

Palpation. Palpate the skin to provide information about temperature, turgor and mobility, moisture, and texture. Temperature of the skin is best assessed by using the back of the hand on the patient's skin. The skin should be warm without being hot. The temperature of the skin increases when blood flow to the dermis is increased. There will be a localized temperature increase with burns and local inflammation. A generalized increase will result from fever. A decreased body temperature

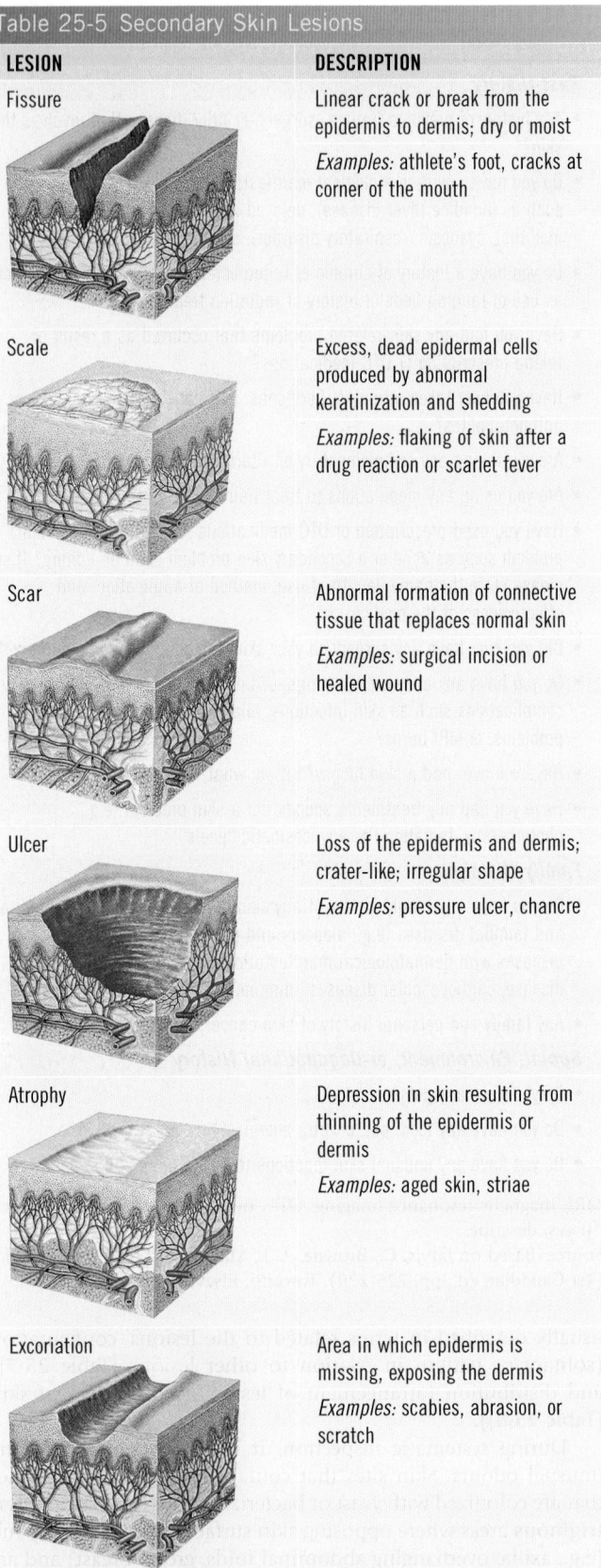

Table 25-4 Primary Skin Lesions

LESION	DESCRIPTION
Macule	Circumscribed, flat area with a change in skin colour; <1 cm in diameter *Examples:* freckles, petechiae, measles, flat mole (nevus)
Papule	Elevated, solid lesion; <1 cm in diameter *Examples:* wart (verruca), elevated moles
Vesicle	Circumscribed, superficial collection of serous fluid; <1 cm in diameter *Examples:* varicella (chicken pox), herpes zoster (shingles), second-degree burn
Plaque	Circumscribed, elevated superficial, solid lesion; >1 cm in diameter *Examples:* psoriasis, seborrheic and active keratoses
Wheal	Firm, edematous, irregularly shaped area; diameter variable *Examples:* insect bite, urticaria
Pustule	Elevated, superficial lesion filled with purulent fluid *Examples:* acne, impetigo

Source: Diagrams of macule, papule, vesicle, plaque, wheal, and pustule from Thibodeau, G. A., & Patton, K. T. (2010). *The human body in health and disease* (5th ed., p. 140, Table 6-1). St. Louis: Mosby.

Table 25-5 Secondary Skin Lesions

LESION	DESCRIPTION
Fissure	Linear crack or break from the epidermis to dermis; dry or moist *Examples:* athlete's foot, cracks at corner of the mouth
Scale	Excess, dead epidermal cells produced by abnormal keratinization and shedding *Examples:* flaking of skin after a drug reaction or scarlet fever
Scar	Abnormal formation of connective tissue that replaces normal skin *Examples:* surgical incision or healed wound
Ulcer	Loss of the epidermis and dermis; crater-like; irregular shape *Examples:* pressure ulcer, chancre
Atrophy	Depression in skin resulting from thinning of the epidermis or dermis *Examples:* aged skin, striae
Excoriation	Area in which epidermis is missing, exposing the dermis *Examples:* scabies, abrasion, or scratch

Source: Diagrams of fissure, ulcer, atrophy, and excoriation from Thibodeau, G. A., & Patton, K. T. (2010). *The human body in health and disease* (5th ed., p. 140, Table 6-1). St. Louis: Mosby; diagrams of scale, scar, and atrophy from Wilson, S. F., & Giddens, J. F. (2009). *Health assessment in nursing practice.* (4th ed., p. 132, Table 10-3). St. Louis: Mosby.

Table 25-6 Assessment Variations in Light- and Dark-Skinned Individuals

CLINICAL SIGN	LIGHT SKIN	DARK SKIN
Cyanosis	Greyish blue tone, especially in nail beds, earlobes, lips, mucous membranes, and palms and soles of feet	Ashen or greyish colour most easily seen in the conjunctiva of the eye, mucous membranes, and nail beds
Ecchymosis	Dark red, purple, yellow, or green colour, depending on age of bruise	Purple to brownish black; difficult to see unless occurring in an area of light pigmentation
Erythema	Reddish tone, possibly accompanied by increased skin temperature secondary to localized inflammation	Deeper brown or purple skin tone with evidence of increased skin temperature secondary to inflammation
Jaundice	Yellowish colour of skin, sclera, fingernails, palms of hands, and oral mucosa	Yellowish green colour most obviously seen in sclera of eye (do not confuse with yellow eye pigmentation, which may be evident in dark-skinned patients), palms of hands, and soles of feet
Pallor	Pale skin colour that may appear white or ashen, also evident on lips, nail beds, and mucous membranes	Underlying red tone in brown or black skin is absent. Light-skinned Black patients may have yellowish brown skin; dark-skinned Black patients may appear ashen or grey
Petechiae	Lesions appear as small, reddish purple pinpoints, best observed on abdomen and buttocks	Difficult to see; may be evident in the buccal mucosa of the mouth or the conjunctiva of the eye
Rash	May be visualized as well as felt with light palpation	Not easily visualized, but may be felt with light palpation
Scar	Generally heals, showing narrow scar line	Higher incidence of keloid development, resulting in a thickened, raised scar (see Figure 14-8, eFigure 25-2)

Table 25-7 Lesion Configuration Terminology

NAME	APPEARANCE
Annular	Ring shaped
Gyrate	Spiral shaped
Iris lesions	Concentric rings or "bull's eyes"
Linear	In a line
Nummular, discoid	Coinlike
Polymorphous	Occurring in several forms
Punctuate	Marked by points or dots
Serpiginous	Snakelike

Table 25-8 Lesion Distribution Terminology

TERM	DESCRIPTION
Asymmetrical	Unilateral distribution
Confluent	Merging together
Diffuse	Wide distribution
Discrete	Separate from other lesions
Generalized	Diffuse distribution
Grouped	Cluster of lesions
Localized	Limited areas of involvement that are clearly defined
Satellite	Single lesion in close proximity to a large grouping
Solitary	A single lesion
Symmetrical	Bilateral distribution
Zosteriform	Bandlike distribution along a dermatome area

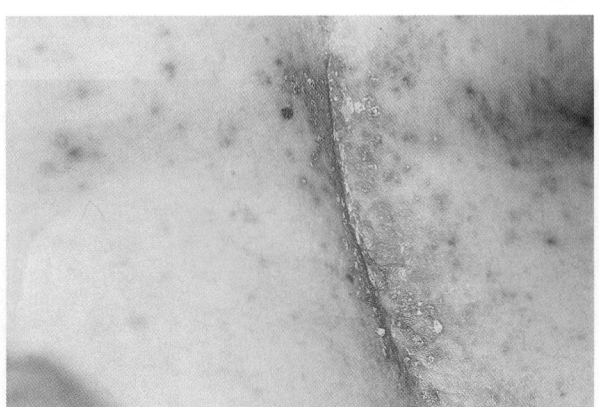

Figure 25-5 Intertrigo. Rash in body folds with *Candida* infection.

Source: Graham-Brown, R., Bourke, J., & Cunliffe, T. (2008). *Dermatology: Fundamentals of practice.* Edinburgh: Mosby.

may occur when shock or other circulatory problems, chilling, or infection is present.

Turgor and mobility refer to the elasticity of the skin. The nurse should assess turgor by gently pinching an area of skin under the clavicle or on the back of the hand. Skin with good turgor should move easily when lifted and should immediately return to its original position when released. There is a loss of turgor with dehydration and aging that often causes tenting (Table 25-9).

Moisture of the skin is the dampness or dryness of the skin. Moisture increases in intertriginous areas and with high humidity. The amount of moisture on the skin varies with environmental temperature, muscular activity, body weight, and body temperature. The skin should be intact with no flaking, scaling, or cracking. Skin generally becomes drier with increasing age.

Texture refers to the fineness or coarseness of the skin. The skin should feel smooth and firm with the surface evenly thin in most areas. Thickened callus areas are normal on the soles and palms and relate to weight bearing. Increased thickness is often work related and a result of excessive pressure. Common assessment abnormalities of the skin are described in Table 25-9.

Risk assessment to predict a patient's pressure ulcer risk should be done using a validated assessment tool such as the Braden Scale. (See Chapter 14, Table 14-16 for the Braden Scale for Predicting Pressure Sore Risk.)

A focused assessment is used to evaluate the status of previously identified integumentary problems and to monitor for signs of new problems (see Table 25-9). A focused assessment of the integumentary system is presented in the box below.

Assessment of Dark Skin Colour

A normal range of differences exists in the physical examination of skin, hair, and nails. Genetic factors determine the skin colour of the individual, which can vary from white to dark brown with overtones of yellow, olive, and red. The darker skin tones result from the reflection of light as it strikes the underlying skin pigment. An increased amount of melanin pigment produced by the melanocytes causes the darker skin colour. This increased melanin forms a natural sunshield for dark skin and results in a decreased incidence of skin cancer in these individuals.

The structures of dark skin are no different than those of lighter skin, but they are often more difficult to assess (see Table 25-6). Assessment of colour is more easily made in areas where the epidermis is thin and pigmentation is not influenced by sun exposure, such as the lips, mucous membranes, nail beds, and protected areas such as the buttocks. Palmar and plantar surfaces are lighter than other skin areas in darker-skinned individuals. Rashes are often difficult to observe and may need to be palpated. Wrinkling resulting from sun exposure is more apparent in light-skinned individuals than in dark-skinned individuals (Wilson & Giddens, 2009).

Individuals with dark skin are predisposed to certain skin and hair conditions. These conditions include *pseudofolliculitis,* an inflammatory response to ingrown hairs with pustules and papules likely caused by ingrown hairs from close shaving; *traction alopecia,* trauma from hair rollers or tight braiding of the hair (see eFigure 25-1, available on the Evolve Web site for this chapter); and **keloid,** an overgrowth of collagenous tissue at site of skin injury (see eFigure 25-2 on the Evolve Web site, and Figure 14-8 on p. 262). Pigment changes to darker skin include *vitiligo,* which is total loss of pigment in the affected area (Figure 25-6); *dermatosis papulosa nigra,* small, pigmented wartlike papules commonly found on the face; *Naevus of Ota* is a slate-grey or blue-grey birthmark located on the forehead and face around the eye area, which may also involve the sclera (Figure 25-7); and *mongolian spots,* benign bluish black macules. Because of the darkness of the skin of some individuals, colour often cannot be used as an indicator of systemic conditions (e.g., skin flushing with fever). Cyanosis may be difficult to determine because a normal bluish hue occurs in dark-skinned persons.

Diagnostic Studies of the Integumentary System

Diagnostic studies provide important information to the nurse in monitoring the patient condition and planning appropriate interventions. These studies are considered to be objective data. Table 25-10 contains diagnostic studies common to the integumentary system.

The main diagnostic techniques related to skin problems are inspection of an individual lesion and a careful history related to the problem. If a definitive diagnosis cannot be made by these techniques, additional tests may be indicated such as dermatoscopy (examination of the skin through a lighted instrument with optical magnification).

Biopsy is one of the most common diagnostic tests used in the evaluation of a skin lesion. A biopsy is indicated in all conditions in which a malignancy is suspected or a specific diagnosis is questionable. Techniques include punch, incisional, excisional, and shave biopsies. The method used is related to factors such as

---

FOCUSED ASSESSMENT
Integumentary System

Use this checklist to make sure the key assessment steps have been done.

Subjective
Ask the patient about any of the following and note responses

Hair loss (unusual or rapid)	Y	N
Changes in the skin (e.g., lesions, bruising)	Y	N
Nail discoloration	Y	N

Objective: Diagnostic
Check for the following for results and critical values

Biopsy results	✓
Albumin	✓

Objective: Physical Examination
Inspect

Skin for colour, integrity, scars, lesions, signs of breakdown	✓
Facial and body hair for distribution, colour, quantity, and hygiene	✓
Nails for shape, contour, colour, thickness, and cleanliness	✓
Dressings if present	✓

Palpate

Skin for temperature, texture, moisture, thickness, turgor, and mobility	✓

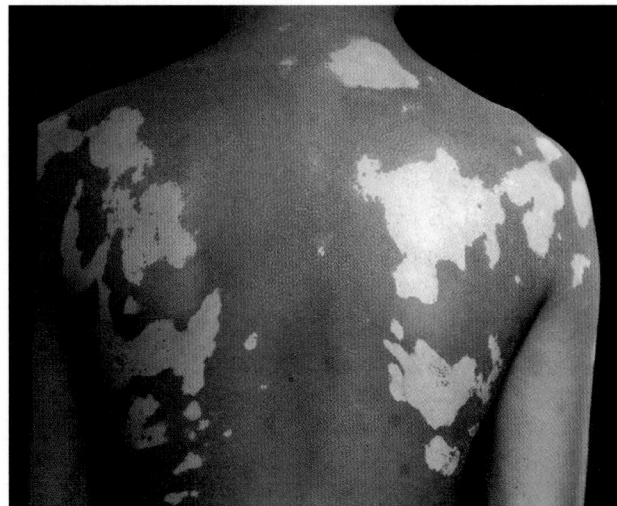

Figure 25-6 Vitiligo. Total loss of pigment in the affected area.

Source: Graham-Brown, R., Bourke, J., & Cunliffe, T. (2008). *Dermatology: Fundamentals of practice.* Edinburgh: Mosby.

the site of the biopsy, the cosmetic result desired, and the type of tissue to be obtained.

Other diagnostic procedures used include stains and cultures for fungal, bacterial, and viral infections. Direct immunofluorescence is a special technique used on biopsy specimens and may be indicated in certain conditions such as bullous diseases and systemic lupus erythematosus; indirect immunofluorescence is performed on a sample of blood. Patch testing (Figure 25-8) and photopatch testing may be used in the evaluation of allergic contact dermatitis and photoallergic reactions (Goldsmith, et al., 2012).

COMMON ASSESSMENT ABNORMALITIES

Table 25-9 Integumentary System

FINDING	DESCRIPTION	POSSIBLE ETIOLOGY AND SIGNIFICANCE
Alopecia	Loss of hair (localized or general; especially the head, but there can be hair loss on other parts of the body as well, from patches to total body hair loss) (see eFigure 25-1)	Heredity, friction, rubbing, traction, trauma, stress, infection, inflammation, chemotherapy, pregnancy, emotional shock, tinea capitis, immunological factors or unknown causation
Angioma	Tumour consisting of blood or lymph vessels	Normal increase with aging, liver disease, pregnancy, varicose veins
Carotenemia (carotenosis)	Yellow discoloration of skin, no yellowing of sclerae, most noticeable on palms and soles	Ingestion of vegetables containing carotene (e.g., carrots, squash), hypothyroidism
Comedo (acne lesion)	Enlarged hair follicle plugged with sebum, bacteria, and skin cells; can be open (blackhead) or closed (whitehead)	Hereditary, certain drugs, hormonal changes with puberty and pregnancy
Cyanosis	Slightly bluish grey or dark purple discoloration of the skin and mucous membranes caused by presence of excessive amounts of reduced hemoglobin in capillaries	Cardiorespiratory problems; vasoconstriction, asphyxiation, anemia, leukemia, and malignancies
Cyst	Sac containing fluid or semisolid material	Obstruction of a duct or gland, parasitic infection
Ecchymosis	Large, bruiselike lesion caused by collection of extravascular blood in dermis and subcutaneous tissue	Trauma, bleeding disorders
Erythema	Redness occurring in patches of variable size and shape	Heat, certain drugs, alcohol, ultraviolet rays, any problem that causes dilation of blood vessels to the skin
Hematoma	Extravasation of blood of sufficient size to cause visible swelling	Trauma, bleeding disorders
Hirsutism	Male-pattern distribution of hair in women	Abnormality of ovaries or adrenal glands, decrease in estrogen level, familial trait
Hypopigmentation	Congenital or acquired loss of melanin resulting in lighter depigmented areas	Genetic, chemical, and pharmacological agents, nutritional factors, burns, inflammation and infection, vitiligo (patchy loss of skin pigment common on hands, face, and genital region (Figure 25-6)
Intertrigo	Dermatitis of overlying surfaces of the skin	Moisture, irritation, obesity; may be complicated by *Candida* infection (see Figure 25-5)
Jaundice	Yellow (in Whites) or yellowish brown (in Blacks) discoloration of the skin, best observed in the sclera secondary to increased bilirubin in the blood	Liver disease, red blood cell hemolysis, pancreatic cancer, common bile duct obstruction
Keloid	Hypertrophied scar beyond margin of incision or trauma (see Figure 14-8 and eFigure 25-2)	Predisposition more common in Blacks
Lichenification	Thickening of the skin with accentuated skin markings	Repeated scratching, rubbing, and irritation usually due to pruritus or neurosis
Mole (nevus)	Benign overgrowth of melanocytes	Defects of development; excessive numbers and large, irregular moles; often familial
Petechiae	Pinpoint, discrete deposit of blood <1-2 mm in the extravascular tissues and visible through the skin or mucous membrane	Inflammation, marked dilation, blood vessel trauma, blood dyscrasia that results in bleeding tendencies (e.g., thrombocytopenia)
Telangiectasia	Visibly dilated, superficial, cutaneous small blood vessels, commonly found on face and thighs	Aging, acne, sun exposure, alcohol, liver failure, corticosteroids, radiation, certain systemic diseases, skin tumours
Tenting	Failure of skin to return immediately to normal position after gentle pinching	Aging, dehydration, cachexia
Varicosity	Increased prominence of superficial veins	Interruption of venous return (e.g., from tumour, incompetent valves, inflammation), commonly found on lower legs with aging
Vitiligo	Complete absence of melanin (pigment) resulting in chalky white patch (see Figure 25-6)	Autoimmune, familial, thyroid disease

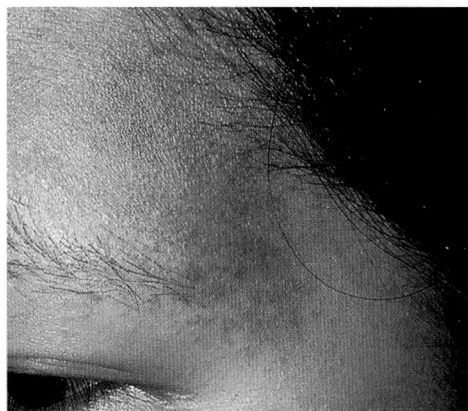

Figure 25-7 Naevus of Ota. Flat grey to blue pigmentation in the upper trigeminal area, which is more common in dark-skinned individuals.

Source: Gawkrodger, D. (2008). *Dermatology* (4th ed.). Edinburgh: Churchill Livingstone.

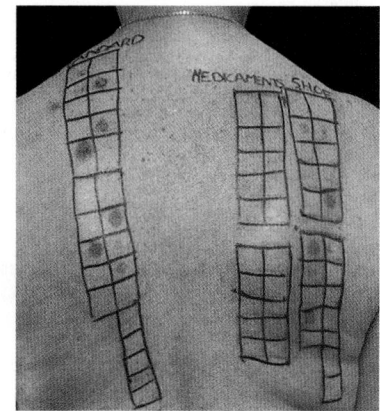

Figure 25-8 Patch test. Results from an application of possible allergens to the skin shows positive reactions in the sites labelled "standard" and "shoe."

Source: Graham-Brown, R., Bourke, J., & Cunliffe, T. (2008). *Dermatology: Fundamentals of practice*. Edinburgh: Mosby.

DIAGNOSTIC STUDIES

Table 25-10 Integumentary System

STUDY	DESCRIPTION AND PURPOSE	NURSING RESPONSIBILITY
Biopsy		
Punch	Special punch biopsy instrument of appropriate size used. Instrument rotated to appropriate level to include dermis and some fat. Suturing may or may not be done. Provides full-thickness skin for diagnostic purposes.	Verify that consent form is signed (if needed). Assist with preparation of site, anaesthesia, procedure, and hemostasis. Apply dressing, and give postprocedure instructions to patient. Properly identify specimen.
Excisional	Useful when good cosmetic results and/or entire removal desired. Skin closed with subcutaneous and skin sutures.	Same as above.
Incisional	Wedge-shaped incision made in lesion too large for excisional biopsy. Useful when larger specimen than shave biopsy is needed.	Same as above.
Shave	Single-edged razor blade used to shave off superficial lesions or small sample of a large lesion. Provides full-thickness specimen of stratum corneum. Provides thin specimen for diagnostic purposes.	Same as above.
Microscopic Tests		
Potassium hydroxide (KOH)	Hair, scales, or nails examined for superficial fungal infection. Specimen is put on a glass slide and potassium hydroxide solution of 10-20% concentration added.	Instruct patient regarding purpose of test. Prepare slide.
Tzanck test (Wright's and Giemsa stains)	Fluid and cells from vesicles examined. Used to diagnose herpes infections. Specimen put on slide, stained, and examined microscopically.	Inform patient of purpose of test. Use sterile technique for collection of fluid.
Culture	The test identifies fungal, bacterial, and viral organisms. For *fungi*, scraping or swab of skin performed. For *bacteria*, material obtained from intact pustules, bullae, or abscesses. For *viruses*, vesicle or bulla scraped and exudate taken from base of lesion.	Instruct patient regarding purpose and procedure. Properly identify specimen. Follow instructions for storage of specimen if not immediately sent to laboratory.
Mineral oil slides	To check for infestations, scrapings placed on slide with mineral oil and viewed microscopically.	Instruct patient about purpose of test. Prepare slide.
Immunofluorescent studies	Some cutaneous diseases have specific, abnormal antibody proteins that can be identified by fluorescent studies. Both skin and serum can be examined.	Inform patient about purpose of test. Assist in obtaining specimen. For punch biopsy of tissue, place specimen in special fixative (e.g., Michel's) and not formalin
Miscellaneous		
Wood's lamp (black light)	Examination of skin with long-wave ultraviolet light causes specific substances to fluoresce (e.g., *Pseudomonas* organisms, fungal infections, vitiligo).	Explain purpose of examination. Inform patient that it is not painful. Room is darkened for examination.
Patch test	Used to determine whether patient is allergic to any testing material. Small amount of potentially allergenic material applied, usually to skin on back.	Explain purpose and procedure to patient. Instruct patient to return in 48-72 hr for removal of allergens and evaluation. Inform patient if re-evaluation is needed at 96 hr (see Figure 25-8).

An assessment case study of the integumentary system is available at *http://evolve.elsevier.com/Canada/Lewis/medsurg*

REVIEW QUESTIONS

The number of the question corresponds to the same-numbered objective at the beginning of the chapter.

1. What is the primary function of the skin?
   a. Insulation
   b. Protection
   c. Sensation
   d. Absorption
2. Which of the following is an age-related change in the skin?
   a. Oily scalp
   b. A loss of collagen
   c. Thinner, flexible nails
   d. Improved blood supply
3. When assessing the sleep and rest routines in relation to the skin, which of the following would the nurse question the patient regarding?
   a. The presence of dry, flaky skin
   b. Occupational exposure to irritants
   c. Self-care habits related to daily hygiene
   d. The presence of dark circles under the eyes
4. During the physical examination of a patient's skin, which of the following would the nurse do?
   a. Use a flashlight if the room is poorly lit.
   b. Note cool, moist skin as a normal finding.
   c. Pinch up a fold of skin to assess for turgor.
   d. Perform a lesion-specific examination first and then a general inspection.
5. Which of the following skin lesions is described as circumscribed, superficial, elevated, solid, and greater than 0.5 cm in diameter?
   a. Plaque
   b. Papule
   c. Pustule
   d. Wheal
6. What is the most appropriate technique to assess the skin for temperature and moisture?
   a. Palpation
   b. Inspection
   c. Percussion
   d. Auscultation
7. Which of the following are individuals with dark skin more likely to develop?
   a. Keloids
   b. Wrinkles
   c. Skin rashes
   d. Skin cancer
8. On inspection of the patient's skin, the nurse notes the complete absence of melanin pigment in patchy areas on the patient's hands. What is this condition called?
   a. Vitiligo
   b. Carotenemia
   c. Telangiectasia
   d. Lichenification
9. When is diagnostic testing recommended for skin lesions?
   a. When a health history cannot be obtained
   b. When a more definitive diagnosis is needed
   c. When percussion reveals an abnormal finding
   d. When treatment with prescribed medication has failed

ANSWERS: 1. b; 2. b; 3. d; 4. c; 5. a; 6. a; 7. a; 8. a; 9. b

REFERENCES

Goldsmith, L., Katz, S., Gilchrest, B., Paller, A., Leffell, D., & Wolff, K. (2012). *Fitzpatrick's dermatology in general medicine* (8th ed.). New York: McGraw-Hill.

Helfrich, Y., Sachs, D., & Voorhees, J. (2008). Overview of skin aging and photoaging. *Dermatology Nursing 20*(3), 177-183. Retrieved from *http://www.dermatologynursing.net/ceonline/2010/article20177183.pdf*

Jarvis, C., Browne, A., MacDonald-Jenkins, J., & Luctkar-Flude, M. (2009). *Physical examination and health assessment* (1st Canadian ed.). Toronto: Elsevier Canada.

Patton, K. T., & Thibodeau, G. A. (2010). *Anatomy and physiology* (7th ed.). St. Louis: Mosby.

Thibodeau, G. A., & Patton, K. T. (2012). *Structure and function of the body* (14th ed.). St. Louis: Mosby.

Wilson, S., & Giddens, J. (2009). *Health assessment for nursing practice* (4th ed.). St. Louis: Mosby.

For additional Internet resources, see the Web site for this book at **http://evolve.elsevier.com/Canada/Lewis/medsurg**

Nursing Management: Integumentary Problems

Written by Barbara Sinni-McKeehen

Adapted by Cheryl A. Sams

LEARNING OBJECTIVES

1. Specify health promotion practices related to the integumentary system.
2. Explain the etiology, clinical manifestations, and nursing and collaborative management of common acute dermatological problems.
3. Describe the psychological and physiological effects of chronic dermatological conditions.
4. Explain the etiology, clinical manifestations, and collaborative management of malignant dermatological disorders.
5. Explain the etiology, clinical manifestations, and collaborative management of bacterial, viral, and fungal infections of the integument.
6. Explain the etiology, clinical manifestations, and collaborative management of infestations and insect bites.
7. Explain the etiology, clinical manifestations, and collaborative management of allergic dermatological disorders.
8. Explain the etiology, clinical manifestations, and collaborative management care related to benign dermatological disorders.
9. Describe the dermatological manifestations of common systemic diseases.
10. Explain the indications and nursing management related to common cosmetic procedures and skin grafts.

KEY TERMS

acne vulgaris An eruption of blackheads, cysts, papules, and pustules on an inflamed base that develops during puberty and adolescence because of androgenic stimulation of sebum secretion with plugging of follicles by keratinization, associated with *Propionibacterium acnes,* p. 565

actinic keratosis A slowly developing, localized thickening and scaling of the outer layers of the skin consisting of hyperkeratotic papules and plaques as a result of chronic, prolonged exposure to the sun; also known as solar keratosis, p. 557

basal cell carcinoma (BCC) A malignant epithelial cell tumour arising from epidermal basal cells that begins as a papule and enlarges peripherally, developing a central crater that erodes, crusts, and bleeds, p. 557

cellulitis An inflammation of subcutaneous, loose connective tissue, Table 26-5, p. 561

cryosurgery The use of subfreezing temperatures to destroy epidermal lesions, p. 572

curettage The removal and scooping away of tissue using an instrument with a circular cutting edge attached to a handle, p. 571

dysplastic nevus syndrome (DNS) A pattern of atypical moles, p. 560

herpes zoster Varicella-zoster virus infection, characterized by an eruption of groups of vesicles on one side of the body along the course of a nerve, caused by inflammation of ganglia and dorsal nerve roots. The condition is self-limited but may be accompanied by or followed by severe postherpetic pain, p. 562

impetigo A condition characterized by pruritus and an eruption of vesiculopustular lesions with a honey-coloured crust surrounded by erythema. Most commonly on the face, caused by Group A β-hemolytic streptococci, staphylococci, or combination of both, Table 26-5, p. 561

lichenification A thickening of skin as a result of the proliferation of keratinocytes, with accentuation of the normal markings of the skin, p. 573

malignant melanoma A tumour arising in melanocytes, p. 557

psoriasis An inherited condition that is common and is characterized by the eruption of reddish, silver-scaled maculopapules, predominantly on the elbows, knees, scalp, and trunk, p. 565

pruritus Itching, p. 573
squamous cell carcinoma (SCC) A malignant neoplasm of keratinizing epidermal cells, p. 557
sun protection factor (SPF) A method of measuring the effectiveness of a sunscreen in filtering and absorbing ultraviolet B light (UVB) radiation, p. 553

urticaria An eruption of wheals that are itchy and usually systemic in origin; it may be caused by hypersensitivity to foods or drugs, foci of infection, physical agents such as exercise, heat, cold, light, friction, or physical stimuli, Table 26-9, p. 565

ELECTRONIC RESOURCES

Supplemental content related to Chapter 26 can be found…

Evolve Web Site ⊖volve

- Answer Guideline for Case Study on p. 577
- Clinical Reference: Laboratory Values
- Content Updates

Health Promotion

Health promotion practices related to the skin often parallel practices appropriate for general good health. The skin reflects both physical and psychological well-being. Specific health promotion activities appropriate to good skin health include avoidance of environmental hazards, adequate rest and exercise, adequate hygiene and nutrition, and use of self-examination and treatment.

Environmental Hazards

Sun Exposure. Years of exposure to the sun are cumulative and damaging. The ultraviolet (UV) rays of the sun cause degenerative changes in the dermis, resulting in premature aging (e.g., loss of elasticity, thinning, wrinkling, drying of the skin). Prolonged and repeated sun exposure is a major factor in precancerous and cancerous lesions (Health Canada, 2008). Actinic keratoses, basal cell carcinoma, squamous cell carcinoma (SCC), and malignant melanoma are dermatological problems associated directly or indirectly with sun exposure. The earth's ozone layer, which protects the world's creatures from excessive exposure to UV radiation, continues to thin because of environmental pollutants, leading to increased risk of sun damage and skin cancer.

It is important for the nurse to emphasize safe sun practices to patients. Specific wavelengths of the sun (Table 26-1) have different effects on the skin. Sunlight is composed of visible light and UV light. Both types can damage the skin and increase the risk of skin cancer. When sun exposure is excessive, the turnover time of the skin is shortened and results in peeling. Fair-skinned persons should be especially cautious about excessive sun exposure because they have less melanin and, thus, less natural protection.

There are two types of topical sunscreens that filter ultraviolet A light (UVA) and ultraviolet B light (UVB) wavelengths—chemical and physical. Chemical sunscreens are light creams, lotions, or sprays that are designed to absorb or filter UV light, resulting in diminished UV light penetration into the epidermis.

Table 26-1 Wavelengths of the Sun and Effects on Skin

WAVELENGTH	EFFECT
Long (UVA) Responsible for tanning due to increased melanin production	Can produce elastic tissue damage and actinic skin damage; contributes to formation of skin cancer
Middle (UVB) Responsible for sunburns	Causes sunburn and cumulative effect of sun damage; major factor in development of skin cancer
Short (UVC)	Does not reach earth; blocked by atmosphere

UVA, ultraviolet A light; *UVB,* ultraviolet B light; *UVC,* ultraviolet C light.

Physical sunscreens are thick, opaque, heavy creams that reflect UV radiation. They block all UVA and UVB radiation as well as all visible light.

Sunscreen products are rated according to their **sun protection factor (SPF)** (Health Canada, 2010a). This is a method of measuring the effectiveness of a sunscreen in filtering and absorbing UVB radiation. There is no similar rating of products to screen UVA. Broad-spectrum products indicate a wide range of absorbance, particularly for UVB wavelengths (Table 26-2).

Consumers need to select the sunscreen most appropriate for their needs (see Table 26-2). Waterproof sunscreens should be used by swimmers and persons who perspire profusely. Specific products have different pre-exposure application directions.

The general recommendation is that everyone should use a sunscreen with a minimum SPF of 15 daily (Health Canada, 2010a). Sunscreens with an SPF of 15 or more filter 92% of the UVB responsible for erythema and make sunburn unlikely in most individuals when applied appropriately. The Canadian Dermatology Association (CDA) recommends a broad-spectrum sunscreen with an SPF of 30 or higher to prevent premature aging

Table 26-2 Sunscreen Ingredients and Ultraviolet Light Protection

SUNSCREEN INGREDIENTS	ULTRAVIOLET LIGHT PROTECTION
Chemical	
Benzophenones	UVA and UVB
PABA and PABA esters	UVB
(Removed from many sunscreen products because of clothing staining, allergic reactions, including contact dermatitis)	
Cinnamates	UVB
Salicylates	UVB
Miscellaneous	
Methyl anthranilate	UVB
Parsol (Avobenzone)	UVA
Physical Sunscreens	
Titanium dioxide	UVA and UVB
Zinc oxide	UVA and UVB

PABA, para-aminobenzoic acid; *UVA,* long wavelength of ultraviolet light; *UVB,* middle wavelength of ultraviolet light.

of the skin (photoaging). The CDA also recommend sunscreens up to 60 SPF for outdoor workers, athletes, and spectators (CDA, 2011a). Sunscreen should be applied 15 to 30 minutes before going outside. It must be reapplied after swimming or profusely sweating to maintain good sun protection even if the product is waterproof. Sunscreens with physical filters such as zinc oxide or titanium dioxide that scatter and reflect both UVA and UVB rays are recommended for prominent parts like the nose, cheeks, shoulders, and ears (Health Canada, 2010a). It is important to follow specific product instructions.

The CDA has developed a cooperative program with sunscreen manufacturers. To obtain CDA approval and to have the CDA logo printed on their products, the companies must meet the following criteria: UVB of at least 15 SPF; broad-spectrum UVA block; noncomedogenic, nonirritating, hypoallergenic; and minimally or nonperfumed. The CDA-approved sunscreens are listed on the CDA Web site.

The nurse plays an important role in educating the public about sun safety. In addition to sunscreen protection, sun exposure can be decreased by staying indoors from 1100 hours until 1600 hours during daylight savings time or between 1000 hours until 1500 hours standard time. Shaded areas and umbrellas for outdoor activities can decrease sunlight contact. Hats with the minimum of 8-cm brims or the legionnaire style of hat with a back flap that protects the head, neck, and ears are important to wear. Tightly woven clothing that covers the body is also helpful. Wet T-shirts and sheer fabrics add little to sun protection.

Eyes also absorb energy and UV rays that can potentially cause retinal damage and may be a contributing factor in cataract development. Sunglasses that are dark enough to be comfortable in the light without reducing or distorting vision, with UVA and UVB protection, are an important choice to protect the fragile eye (Health Canada, 2010b). Wraparound sunglasses provide more protection from sunlight rays, helping prevent unfiltered sun rays from entering the eyes through the side.

Even on overcast days, serious sunburn can occur because up to 80% of UV rays can penetrate the clouds. Other factors that increase sunburn risk include being at high altitudes; being in snow, which reflects 85% of the sun's rays; and being in or near water.

The CDA recommends that Canadians check the daily UV index from Environment Canada, which is broadcast on A.M. radio and television, and on the Environment Canada and the Weather Network Web sites. The UV index indicates the level of intensity of the sun's UV rays. There are five categories: low, moderate, high, very high, and extreme (Health Canada, 2008). The months from late April until August usually have the highest UV index in Canada, although in April, May, and June, it is not as hot and sunscreen is less likely to be applied (CDA, 2008).

Tanning booths and sun lamps are still being commonly used to artificially tan skin. There is increasing concern, which is supported by research that links SCC to UV radiation, which consists mostly of UVA rays. The CDA has launched a public service campaign to increase the awareness of the danger of tanning beds, particularly in the 18-year-old and younger age-groups. UVA exposure through tanning beds can increase a person's risk of developing melanoma by 75% if used before the age of 35 (CDA, 2011b). The CDA (2011c) has identified melanoma as the third most common cancer in young women in the 15- to 29-year-old age-group, representing 11% of new cases. In addition, tanning beds also cause significant photoaging. Individuals who should never use tanning beds: are younger than 18 years of age, have fair or freckled skin, burn easily, have a lot of moles, have had previous skin cancer or a family history of skin cancer, or use medication that increases sensitivity to UV (CDA, 2011b). Canada regulates the tanning salon industry by public health authorities, and treatments are limited to patrons older than age 16, include protective goggles, and limit the maximum dosage to 15 kJ/m^2 annually from the tanning equipment (Health Canada, 2005). The CDA has published a position statement that the application of self-tanning products is safe (CDA, 2000). From a nursing perspective, it is important to teach people that the self-tanning products do not provide sun protection unless sunscreen has been added to the product or is applied separately with sun exposure.

Certain topical and systemic medications potentiate the effect of the sun, even with brief exposure. Categories of drug therapy that may contain common photosensitizing medications are listed in Table 26-3. The nurse should be aware that many drugs are included in these categories, and the photosensitivity of each individual drug should be examined. The chemicals in these medications absorb light and release energy that harms cells and tissues. The clinical manifestations of drug-induced photosensitivity are similar to those of exaggerated sunburn, with swelling; erythema; papular, plaquelike lesions; and vesicles. Skin that is at risk for photosensitivity reactions can be protected by the use of sunscreen products. Nurses have a role in educating patients who are taking these drugs about their photosensitizing effect.

Irritants and Allergens. There are two types of contact dermatitis. *Irritant contact dermatitis* is produced by direct chemical injury to the skin. *Allergic contact dermatitis* is an antigen-specific, Type IV delayed hypersensitivity response. This response requires sensitization and occurs only in individuals who are predisposed to react to a particular antigen (see Chapter 14).

Counsel patients to avoid known irritants (e.g., ammonia, harsh detergents). Skin patch testing (application of allergens)

DRUG THERAPY

Table 26-3 Categories of Drugs That May Cause Photosensitivity

CATEGORIES	EXAMPLES
Anticancer drugs	Methotrexate, vinorelbine
Antidepressants	Amitriptyline, clomipramine (Anafranil), doxepin (Apo-Doxepin)
Antidysrhythmics	Quinidine, amiodarone (Cordarone)
Antihistamines	Diphenhydramine (Benadryl), clemastine (Tavist)
Antimicrobials	Tetracycline, sulphamethoxazole, azithromycin (Zithromax), ciprofloxacin (Cipro)
Antifungals	Ketoconazole (Nizoral)
Antipsychotics	Chlorpromazine, haloperidol (Apo-Haloperidol)
Diuretics	Furosemide (Lasix), hydrochlorothiazide
Hypoglycemics	Tolbutamide (Apo-Tolbutamide), chlorpropamide (Apo-Chlorpropamide)
Nonsteroidal anti-inflammatory drugs	Diclofenac, piroxicam (Apo-Piroxicam), sulindac (Apo-Sulin)

can sometimes be helpful in determining the most likely sensitizing agent. Sometimes the health care provider is the first to detect a contact allergy to various metals, gloves (latex), and adhesives. The nurse must also be aware that prescribed and over-the-counter (OTC) topical and systemic drugs used to treat a variety of conditions may contain fragrances and preservatives that cause dermatological reactions. Health Canada (2010c) provides a Web site that maintains a database of suspected adverse reactions, including dermatological problems, to Canadian-marketed health products.

Radiation. Although most radiology departments are extremely cautious in protecting both themselves and their patients from the effects of excessive radiation, the nurse should help the patient make decisions about radiological procedures. Radiographic studies are invaluable in both diagnosis and therapy, but they can cause serious adverse effects to the skin, including erythema, dry and moist desquamation, edema, and hypopigmentation and hyperpigmentation. In the 1940s and 1950s, cystic acne was treated with radiation. These patients have an increased incidence of carcinoma.

Rest and Sleep

Sleep is restorative to the skin as well as to the rest of the body. Pruritic skin diseases often interfere with sleep. These patients require the nurse's assistance in improving their quality of sleep, which increases their itching tolerance and decreases skin damage from scratching.

Exercise

Exercise increases circulation and dilates the blood vessels. In addition to the healthy glow produced by exercise, the psychological effects can also improve one's appearance and mental outlook. However, caution must be used to avoid or protect from overexposure to heat, cold, and sun during outdoor exercise.

Hygiene

Hygienic practices are influenced by and should match the skin type, the lifestyle, and the culture of the patient. The normal acidity of the skin (pH 4.2 to 5.6) and perspiration protect against bacterial overgrowth. Most soaps are alkaline and cause a neutralization of the skin surface and loss of protection. The use of milder soaps such as Ivory and nonsoap (lipid-free) cleansers, as well as avoiding hot water and vigorous rubbing, can noticeably decrease local irritation and inflammation. Skin piercings where jewellery has been inserted can be cared for with antibacterial soaps that do not contain sulphites.

In general, the skin and hair should be washed often enough to remove excess oil and excretions and to prevent odour. Older persons should avoid the use of harsh soaps and shampoos because of the increasing dryness of their skin and scalp. Moisturizers should be used immediately after bath or shower, while the skin is still damp, to seal in this moisture.

Cleansing and moisturizing are very important to keep the skin in good condition to prevent skin breakdown that provides a portal for infection. In the harsh Canadian climate, cold weather and heating can often create dry and pruritic skin conditions.

DETERMINANTS OF HEALTH
Integumentary Problems

Biology and Genetic Endowment

- Canadians of African descent, Asians, and Aboriginals have a lower incidence of skin cancer than White Canadians.
- Skin assessment may be difficult in individuals with darker skin. The oral mucous membranes and the conjunctiva are areas where pallor, cyanosis, and jaundice are more readily detected. The palms of the hands and the soles of the feet can also be used for assessment of the skin of darker individuals.
- Melanoma can occur in dark-skinned individuals but often goes unrecognized until the advanced stages.
- When darker skin heals following injury or inflammation, it tends to be hypopigmented or hyperpigmented.

Nutrition

A well-balanced diet adequate in all food groups can produce healthy skin, hair, and nails (see *Canada's Food Guide* in Chapter 42). Important elements of nutritional skin support include the following:

1. *Vitamin A:* Essential for maintenance of normal cell structure, specifically epithelial cells. It is necessary for normal wound healing. The absence of vitamin A causes dryness of the conjunctiva and poor wound healing.
2. *Vitamin B complex:* Essential for complex metabolic functions. Deficiencies of niacin and pyridoxine (B_6) manifest as dermatological symptoms such as erythema, bullae, and seborrhoea-like lesions.
3. *Vitamin C (ascorbic acid):* Essential for connective tissue formation and normal wound healing. Absence of vitamin C

causes symptoms of scurvy, including petechiae, bleeding gums, and purpura.

4. *Vitamin D₃ (cholecalciferol):* Essential for bone health. It is produced naturally by cutaneous photosynthesis after UVB exposure. A deficiency interferes with normal prothrombin synthesis in the liver and can lead to bruising.
5. *Vitamin K:* Essential for synthesizing blood clotting factors. A deficiency interferes with normal prothrombin synthesis in the liver and can lead to bruising.
6. *Protein:* Necessary in amounts adequate for cell growth and maintenance. It is also necessary for normal wound healing.
7. *Unsaturated fatty acids:* Necessary to maintain the function and integrity of cellular and subcellular membranes in tissue metabolism, especially linoleic and arachidonic acids.

A deficiency of biotin, a water-soluble B-complex vitamin, may result in rashes and alopecia. The effectiveness of biotin supplements has not been proved. Foods high in biotin include liver, cauliflower, salmon, carrots, bananas, soy flour, cereals, and yeast.

Obesity has an adverse effect on the skin. The increase in subcutaneous fat can lead to stretching and overheating (see Chapter 43). Overheating secondary to the greater insulation provided by fat causes an increase in sweating, which inflames and dries the skin. Obesity also has an influence on the development of type 2 diabetes mellitus, which may cause skin symptoms such as velvety dark skin of neck and body folds (acanthosis nigricans), rash in the intertriginous sites (intertrigo), skin tags (acrochordons), impaired arterial and venous flow, and other skin complications. Obesity is also a risk factor for poor wound healing (see Chapter 43).

Self-Treatment

The nurse must increase the patient's awareness of the dangers of self-diagnosis and treatment. The increasing variety of OTC skin preparations can confuse the consumer.

In the nurse's general instructions to the patient, the nurse should stress the duration of the treatment and the need to follow package directions closely. Skin problems are generally slow to produce symptoms and slow to resolve. If the package insert of an OTC drug says its use should not exceed 7 days, this warning should be heeded. Instruct the patient to always follow package directions for use of OTC drugs. If any systemic signs of inflammation or extension of the skin problem (e.g., an increased number of lesions or increased erythema or swelling) develop, self-care should be stopped and professional help should be sought.

Malignant Skin Neoplasms

Skin cancer is the most common cancer diagnosed in Canada and the world. Skin cancers are either nonmelanoma or melanoma. Skin cancer rates have been steadily increasing since the early 1980s. At the time of writing, it was predicted that more than 74,000 new cases of basal and squamous carcinomas would be diagnosed in Canada in 2012 (Canadian Cancer Society's Steering Committee on Cancer Statistics, 2011). Canadians who were born in the 1990s have a 1 in 6 risk of developing skin cancer during their lifetimes (CDA, 2011d).

The presence of a persistent skin lesion that does not heal is highly suspicious for malignancy and should be examined by a health care provider. Malignant neoplasms of the skin exhibit

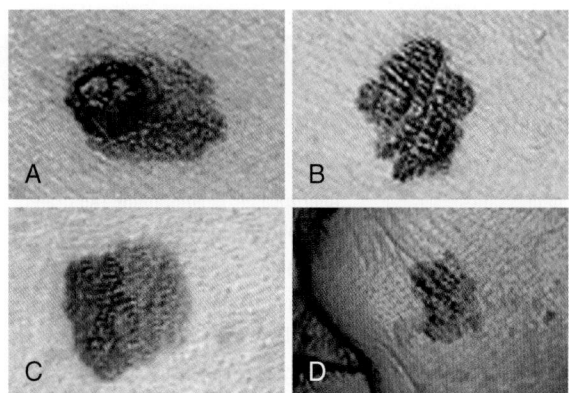

Figure 26-1 The ABCDEs of melanoma. **A,** Asymmetry: one half is unlike the other half. **B,** Border irregularity: edges are ragged, notched, or blurred. **C,** Colour: varied pigmentation; shades of tan, brown, and black. **D,** Diameter: greater than 6 mm (diameter of a pencil eraser). **E,** Evolving; changing appearance (not pictured; change in shape, size, colour, or other characteristic is noted over a length of time).

Source: The Skin Cancer Foundation, New York, NY.

characteristics similar to those of other malignant conditions (see Chapter 18). Although skin malignancies generally grow slowly, persistent lesions that do not heal should be biopsied. Adequate and early treatment can often lead to a highly favourable prognosis. The fact that skin lesions are so visible increases the likelihood of early detection and diagnosis. Teach patients to self-examine their skin at least on a monthly basis. The cornerstone of the skin self-examination is the "ABCDE rule" (Figure 26-1). Examination of skin lesions for *a*symmetry, *b*order irregularity, *c*olour change or variation, *d*iameter of 6 mm or more, and *e*volving in appearance is simple to teach patients and easy to remember. Emphasize to patients that lesions once flat and now raised, or once small and recently growing or changing in appearance, are warning signs.

Risk Factors

Risk factors for skin malignancies include having a fair skin type (blonde or red hair and blue or green eyes), history of chronic sun exposure, family history of skin cancer, and exposure to tar and systemic arsenic compounds. Environmental factors that increase the risk of skin malignancies include living near the equator, outdoor occupations, and frequent outdoor recreational activities. Behavioural factors such as commercial indoor and outdoor tanning and immunosuppression by smoking are controllable risk factors for skin malignancies. Patients treated with photochemotherapy with oral methoxsalen (psoralen) and UVA radiation (PUVA) may be at greater risk of melanoma. Dark-skinned persons are less susceptible to skin cancer because of the naturally occurring increased melanin, an effective sunscreen, but they can develop melanoma, most often on the palms, the soles, and the mucous membranes.

Nonmelanoma Skin Cancers

Nonmelanoma skin cancers, either basal cell carcinoma (BCC) or SCC, are the most common forms of skin cancer (CDA, 2011d).

About 75% of nonmelanoma skin cancers are BCC and 25% are SCC (Canadian Cancer Society, 2012a). Nonmelanoma skin cancers develop from the epidermis and do not develop from melanocytes, the skin cells that make melanin, as melanoma skin cancers do. The most common sites for development of nonmelanoma skin cancer are in sun-exposed areas and include the face, head, neck, back of the hands, and arms.

Although the number of deaths attributable to nonmelanoma skin cancer is relatively small, the tumours have an inherent potential for severe local destruction, permanent disfigurement, and disability. The most common etiological factor is chronic sun exposure. The risk of developing this type of cancer increases with age, particularly after age 50 (CDA, 2011d). There are many psychosocial implications when an individual is diagnosed with skin cancer. The impact of cancer is discussed in Chapter 18. Avoidance of exposure to the midday sun and the use of protective clothing and sunscreens beginning early in life can help prevent the formation of skin malignancies later in life.

Actinic Keratosis

Actinic keratosis, also known as solar keratosis, consists of hyperkeratotic papules and plaques occurring on sun-exposed areas. Actinic keratosis is a premalignant form of SCC that affects nearly all of the older White population. It is the most common precancerous skin lesion. The clinical appearance of actinic keratosis can be highly varied. The typical lesion is an irregularly shaped, flat, slightly erythematous papule with indistinct borders and an overlying hard keratotic scale or horn (Table 26-4). Many forms of treatment are used, including cryosurgery, 5-fluorouracil (5-FU), surgical removal, tretinoin (Retin-A), imiquimod (Aldara), diclofenac, chemical peeling agents, dermabrasion, and laser resurfacing. Any lesion that persists should be evaluated for possible biopsy.

Basal Cell Carcinoma

Basal cell carcinoma (BCC) is a locally invasive malignancy arising from epidermal basal cells. It is the most common type of skin cancer and also the least deadly. BCC usually occurs in middle-aged to older adults. Clinical manifestations are described in Table 26-4 (see also Figure 26-2). The cancerous cells of BCC almost never spread beyond the skin. However, if left untreated, massive tissue destruction may result. Some BCCs are pigmented with curled borders and an opaque appearance and may be misinterpreted as a melanoma. A tissue biopsy is needed to confirm the diagnosis.

Multiple treatment modalities are used depending on the tumour location and histological type, history of recurrence, and patient characteristics. Treatment modalities include electrodesiccation and curettage, surgical excision, cryosurgery, radiation therapy, Mohs' micrographic surgery, topical chemotherapy (5-FU or imiquimod), and photodynamic therapy. (These treatments are discussed later in this chapter.) Electrodesiccation and curettage, cryosurgery, and excision all have a cure rate greater than 90% when used correctly on primary lesions. Location and size are important factors in determining the best treatment.

Squamous Cell Carcinoma

Squamous cell carcinoma (SCC) is a malignant neoplasm of keratinizing epidermal cells (Figure 26-3). It frequently occurs on sun-exposed skin. SCC is less common than BCC. SCC can be

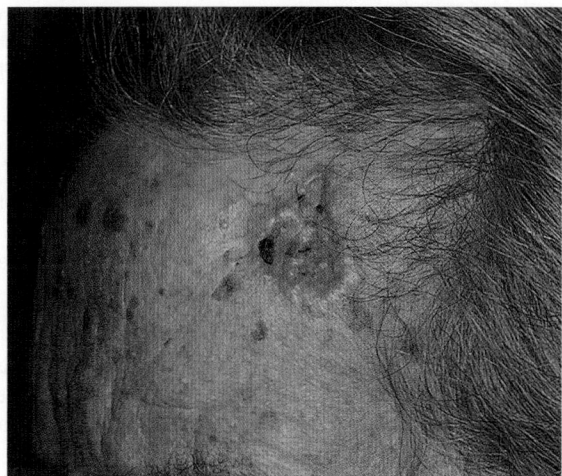

Figure 26-2 Basal cell carcinoma. Note rolled border and central erosion. Pearly papule with slight erythema.

Source: Swartz, M. H. (2010). *Textbook of physical diagnosis: History and examination* (6th ed., p. 159, Figure 8-33). Philadelphia: Saunders.

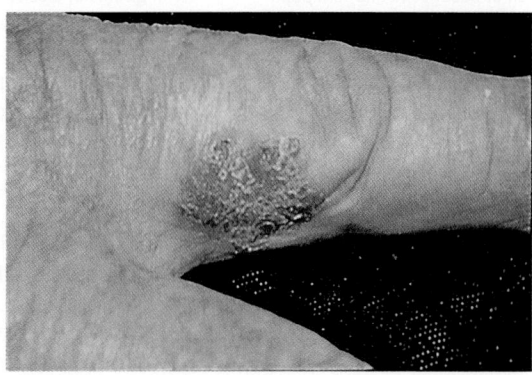

Figure 26-3 Squamous cell carcinoma of the finger.

Source: Goldstein, B. G., & Goldstein, A. O. (1997). *Practical dermatology* (2nd ed.). St. Louis, Mosby. Courtesy Department of Dermatology, Medical College of Georgia, Augusta, GA.

very aggressive, has the potential to metastasize, and may lead to death if not treated early and correctly. Pipe, cigar, and cigarette smoking contributes to the formation of SCC on the mouth and lips.

The clinical manifestations of SCC are described in Table 26-4. A biopsy should always be performed when a lesion is suspected to be SCC. Treatment consists of electrodesiccation and curettage, excision, radiation therapy, intralesional injection of 5-FU or methotrexate, and Mohs' surgery. There is a high cure rate with early detection and treatment.

Malignant Melanoma

Malignant melanoma is a tumour arising in melanocytes, which are the cells producing melanin. Melanoma has the ability to metastasize to any organ, including the brain and the heart. This is the most deadly skin cancer, and its incidence is increasing faster than any other cancer. It was estimated that 5800 Canadians would be diagnosed in 2012 and 970 would die from it (Canadian Cancer Society, 2012b).

Table 26-4 Premalignant and Malignant Conditions of the Skin

ETIOLOGY AND PATHOPHYSIOLOGY	CLINICAL MANIFESTATIONS	TREATMENT AND PROGNOSIS
Actinic Keratoses		
Actinic (sun) damage (precursor of squamous cell carcinoma)	Flat or slightly elevated, dry, hyperkeratotic scaly papule; possibly flat, rough, or verrucous (wartlike); adherent scale, which returns when removed; often multiple; rough scale on red base; often on erythematous sun-exposed areas; increase in number with age	Cryosurgery, chemical caustics, topical application of 5-FU over entire area for 14-21 days or topical application of imiquimod (Aldara) over ≥8 wk; recurrence possible even with adequate treatment
Atypical/Dysplastic Nevi		
Morphologically between common acquired nevi and melanoma; may be precursor of cutaneous malignant melanoma	Often >5 mm; irregular border, possibly notched; variegated colour mixture of tan, brown, black, red, and pink with single mole; presence of at least one flat portion, often at edge of mole; frequently multiple; uncommon before puberty; most common site is the back, but possible in uncommon mole sites such as scalp or buttocks	Marker of increased risk for melanoma; careful monitoring of persons suspected of familial tendency to melanoma or dysplastic nevi; excisional biopsy for suspicious lesions
Basal Cell Carcinoma		
Change in basal cells; no maturation or normal keratinization; continuing division of basal cells and formation of enlarging mass; related to excessive sun exposure, genetic skin type, x-ray radiation, scars, and some types of nevi; basal cells possibly pigmented	*Nodular and ulcerative:* Small, slowly enlarging papule; borders semitranslucent or "pearly," with overlying telangiectasia; erosion, ulceration, and depression of centre; normal skin markings lost (see Figure 26-2)\n*Superficial:* Erythematous, sharply defined, barely elevated multinodular plaques with varying scaling and crusting; similar to eczema but not pruritic	Excisional surgery, chemosurgery, electrosurgery, cryosurgery; 90% cure rate; slow-growing tumour that invades local tissue; metastasis rare; 5-FU and imiquimod (Aldara) for superficial lesions
Squamous Cell Carcinoma		
Frequent occurrence on previously damaged skin (e.g., from sun, radiation, scar); malignant tumour of squamous (prickle) cell of epidermis; invasion of dermis, surrounding skin; metastasis possible	*Superficial:* Thin, scaly, erythematous plaque without invasion into the dermis\n*Early:* Firm nodules with indistinct borders; scaling and ulceration; opaque\n*Late:* Covering of lesion with scale or horn from keratinization; most common on sun-exposed areas such as face and hands (see Figure 26-3)	Surgical removal, cryosurgery, radiation therapy, chemosurgery, Mohs' procedure or microscopically controlled excision, and electrodesiccation and curettage; untreated lesion possibly metastasizes to regional lymph nodes; high cure rate with early detection and treatment
Cutaneous T Cell Lymphoma (Mycosis Fungoides)		
Origination in skin; chronic, slowly progressing disease; possible etiologies of environmental toxins and chemical exposure	Classic presentation involving three stages—patch, plaque, and tumour; history of persistent macular eruption followed by gradual appearance of indurated plaques.	UVB in patch stage, PUVA, topical nitrogen mustard, radiation therapy, systemic chemotherapy, extracorporeal photopheresis; 5-year life expectancy with only skin manifestations and no treatment; greatly decreased survival rate with generalized erythroderma with exfoliation and abnormal cells in bloodstream (Sézary syndrome)
Malignant Melanoma		
Neoplastic growth of melanocytes anywhere on skin, eyes, or mucous membranes; classification according to major histological mode of spread; potential invasion and widespread metastases	Irregular colour, surface, and border; variegation of colour including red, white, blue, black, grey, and brown; flat or elevated, eroded or ulcerated; often <1 cm in size; most common sites in males are back, then chest; in females, most common sites are legs, then back (see Figure 26-1)	Wide surgical excision, down to fascia, and possible sentinel lymph node evaluation depending on the depth; correlation of survival rate with depth of invasion; poor prognosis unless diagnosis and treatment early; spreading by local extension, regional lymphatic vessels, and bloodstream; adjuvant therapy after surgery may be indicated if lesion >1.5 mm in depth

5-FU, 5-fluorouracil; *PUVA,* psoralen plus ultraviolet A light (phototherapy); *UVB,* ultraviolet B light.

The exact cause of melanoma is unknown. Risk factors include chronic UV exposure without protection or overexposure to artificial light such as from a tanning bed. Persons with fair skin and eyes have less melanin and, thus, less protection from UV radiation. Severe and frequent childhood sunburns are another risk factor. Genetic factors such as a prior diagnosis of melanoma and having a first-degree relative diagnosed with melanoma increase a person's risk. A mutated gene has been identified in some families who have a high familial incidence of melanoma. Other factors include hormonal and immunological factors or a recreational lifestyle that leads to greater sun exposure. Multiple and atypical moles, particularly atypical dysplastic nevi, are other factors that puts a person more at risk (Canadian Cancer Society, 2012b).

EVIDENCE-INFORMED PRACTICE

Can Postherpetic Neuralgia Be Prevented With Oral Acyclovir?

Clinical Question

In patients with herpes zoster (P), is oral acyclovir effective (I) versus placebo (C) in preventing PHN (O) at 6 months after initial infection (T)?

Best Available Evidence

Systematic review of RCTs

Critical Appraisal and Synthesis of Evidence

- Five RCTs evaluated oral acyclovir and 1 RCT evaluated oral famciclovir (*n* = 1211).
- Patients had varying degrees of herpes zoster severity. Antiviral agents were given within 72 hours after onset of herpes zoster rash.
- Presence of PHN at site of shingles rash measured for 6 months.
- No significant difference between antiviral (either acyclovir or famciclovir) or placebo in preventing PHN after rash onset.

Conclusions

- Oral acyclovir did not reduce incidence of PHN.

Implications for Nursing

- Assess patient for several years after herpes zoster onset for continuing discomfort.
- PHN treatments may not be effective for many patients.
- Burning, incapacitating pain of acute herpes zoster and continuing PHN may lead to altered mood, fatigue, insomnia, and social isolation.
- Provide supportive counselling and referral for chronic neuralgia pain.

Reference for Evidence

Li, Q., Chen, N., Yang, J., Zhou, M., Zhou, D., Zhang, Q., & He, L. (2009). Antiviral treatment for preventing postherpetic neuralgia. *Cochrane Database of Systematic Reviews*, Issue 2. Art. No.: CD006866. doi:10.1002/14651858.CD006866.pub2

PHN, postherpetic neuralgia; *PICO: P*, patient population of interest; *I*, intervention or area of interest; *C*, comparison of interest or comparison group; *O*, outcome(s) of interest; *T*, time (this element is not always included in the PICO format); *RCTs*, randomized controlled trials.

Types of Melanoma

The four types of cutaneous melanoma are superficial spreading melanoma (SSM), lentigo maligna melanoma (LMM), acral–lentiginous melanoma (ALM), and nodular melanoma (NM).

SSM is the most common type, is the most curable, and often occurs on chronically sun-exposed areas such as the legs and the upper back. It frequently arises from a pre-existing mole. LMM is commonly located on the face and is often found in older adult patients. Precursor lesions are called *lentigines* and appear as flat, brown, irregular patches. These patches increase in size for many years before the development of cancer occurs. ALM appears on soles, palms, mucous membranes, and terminal phalanges. ALM is more common in Asian persons and persons with dark skin. NM occurs more often in men and can be located anywhere on the body. It is believed to be a more aggressive type of melanoma that develops and invades rapidly. ALM is the most frequently misdiagnosed melanoma because it resembles a benign lesion such as a blood blister or polyp or even a BCC.

Clinical Manifestations

About one third of melanomas occur in existing nevi or moles; about 20% occur in dysplastic nevi (see Table 26-4). Melanoma frequently occurs on the lower legs and on the back in women and on the trunk, the head, and the neck in men. Because most melanoma cells continue to produce melanin, melanoma tumours are often dark brown or black. Individuals should consult their health care provider immediately if their moles or lesions show any of the clinical signs (ABCDEs) of melanoma (see Figure 26-1). Any sudden or progressive increase in the size, the colour, or the shape of a mole should be checked. When melanoma begins in the skin, it is called cutaneous melanoma. Melanoma can also occur in the eyes, the meninges, the lymph nodes, the digestive tract, and anywhere else in the body where melanocytes are found.

Collaborative Care

Pigmented lesions suspected to be melanoma should never be shave-biopsied, shave-excised, or electrocauterized. All suspicious lesions should be biopsied using an excisional biopsy technique. The most important prognostic factor is tumour thickness at the time of the diagnosis. Two methods to determine thickness are currently being used. The *Breslow measurement* indicates tumour depth in millimetres, and the *Clark level* indicates the number of skin layers involved (1-5); the higher the number, the deeper the melanoma.

Treatment depends on the site of the original tumour, stage of the cancer, and the patient's age and general health. The initial treatment of malignant melanoma is surgery. Melanoma that has spread to the lymph nodes or nearby sites usually requires additional therapy such as chemotherapy, biological therapy (e.g., α-interferon, interleukin-2), or radiation therapy. Examples of chemotherapy agents that are used include dacarbazine, temozolomide (Temodal), procarbazine (Matulane), carmustine (BiCNU), and lomustine (CeeNU). Gene and vaccine therapies are currently being examined as additional treatment options (see Chapter 15 for discussion of these therapies). Topical immune therapy (imiquimod [Aldara]) is being investigated in the treatment of LMM.

The staging of melanoma (stages 0-4) is based on tumour size, nodal involvement, and presence of metastasis. In stage 0, the melanoma is confined to one place (in situ) in the epidermis. Melanoma is nearly 100% curable by excision if diagnosed at stage 0. The 5-year survival rate (75-95%) in stage 1 can vary depending on the sentinel node biopsy results, which indicate whether metastasis has occurred. If spread to regional lymph nodes has occurred (stage 3), the patient has a 61.7% chance of 5-year survival (Howlader et al., 2011). If metastasis to other organs occurs (stage 4), treatment then is palliative.

Atypical/Dysplastic Nevus

An abnormal nevus pattern called **dysplastic nevus syndrome,** places a person at increased risk of melanoma. Approximately 2 to 8% of the White population has moles classified as dysplastic nevi (DNs). DNs, or atypical moles, are moles that are larger than usual (>5 mm across) with irregular borders and various shades of colour. These nevi may have the same ABCDE characteristics as melanoma, but they are less pronounced. The earliest clinically detectable abnormality associated with DNs is an increase in the number of morphologically normal–looking nevi at around age 2 to 6 years. Another proliferation occurs around adolescence, and new nevi continue to appear throughout the person's life. The average number of normal nevi in adults is about 40; individuals with DNs may have over 100 normal-appearing nevi. The nurse should obtain a detailed family history related to melanoma and DNs. The risk of developing melanoma doubles with the presence of one DN, and having multiple DNs increases the risk up to twelve-fold.

Skin Infections and Infestations

Bacterial Infections

The skin provides an ideal environment for bacterial growth with an abundant supply of nutrients, water, and warm temperature. The skin is covered with numerous microorganisms, especially bacteria. *Staphylococcus aureus* and group A β-hemolytic streptococci are the major types of bacteria responsible for primary and secondary skin infections; Figure 26-4 shows impetigo.

Bacterial infection occurs when the balance between the host and the microorganisms is altered. This can occur as a primary

infection following a break in the skin. It can also occur as a secondary infection in already damaged skin or as a sign of a systemic disease (Table 26-5).

Healthy persons can develop bacterial skin infections. Predisposing factors such as moisture, obesity, atopic dermatitis, systemic corticosteroids and antibiotics, and chronic disease such as diabetes mellitus all increase the likelihood of infection (Figure 26-5). Good hygiene practices and general good health inhibit bacterial infections. If an infection is present, the resulting drainage is infectious. Good skin hygiene and infection control practices are necessary to prevent spread of the infection.

Viral Infections

Viral infections of the skin are as difficult to treat as viral infections anywhere in the body. When a virus infects a cell, a skin lesion may develop (Figure 26-6). Lesions can also result from an inflammatory response to the viral infections. Herpes simplex,

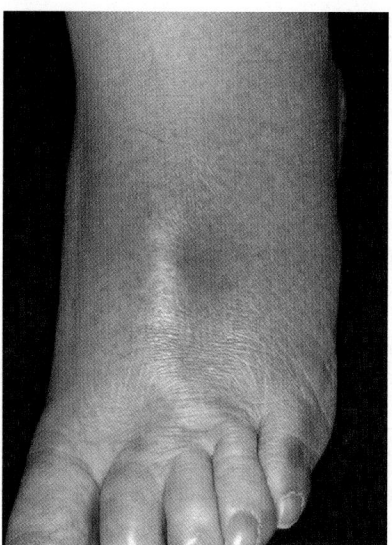

Figure 26-5 Cellulitis with characteristic erythema, tenderness, and edema.

Source: Habif, T. P. (2004). *Clinical dermatology: A color guide to diagnosis and therapy* (4th ed., p. 274, Figure 9-11). St. Louis: Mosby.

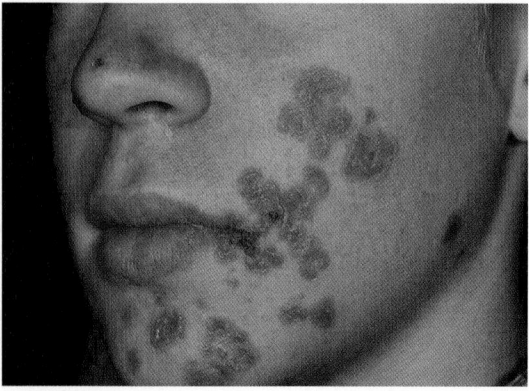

Figure 26-4 Impetigo. Superficial pustules covered by a thick, honey yellow–coloured crust.

Source: Habif, T. P. (2004). *Clinical dermatology: A color guide to diagnosis and therapy* (4th ed., p. 270, Figure 9-6). St. Louis: Mosby.

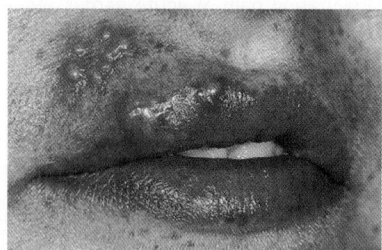

Figure 26-6 Herpes viral infection on the lips. Typical presentation with vesicles on the lips and extending onto the skin.

Source: Habif, T. P. (1996). *Clinical dermatology: A color guide to diagnosis and therapy* (3rd ed.). St. Louis: Mosby.

Table 26-5 Common Bacterial Infections of the Skin

ETIOLOGY AND PATHOPHYSIOLOGY	CLINICAL MANIFESTATIONS	TREATMENT AND PROGNOSIS
Impetigo		
Group A β-hemolytic streptococci, staphylococci, or combination of both; associated with poor hygiene; primary or secondary infection; contagious	Vesiculopustular lesions that develop thick, honey-coloured crust surrounded by erythema; pruritic; most common on face as primary infection (see Figure 26-4)	*Systemic Antibiotics* Oral penicillin, benzathine penicillin G by IM route, erythromycin *Local Treatment* Warm saline or aluminum acetate soaks followed by soap-and-water removal of crusts; topical antibiotic cream or ointment (Bactroban); with no treatment, glomerulonephritis possible when streptococcal strain nephritogenic; meticulous hygiene essential
Folliculitis		
Usually staphylococci; present in areas subjected to friction, moisture, rubbing, or oiliness; increased incidence in patients with diabetes mellitus	Small pustule at hair follicle opening with minimal erythema; development of crusting; most common on scalp, beard, extremities in men; tender to touch	Antistaphylococcal soap (e.g., Hibiclens, Lever 2000, Dial) and water cleansing; topical antibiotics (e.g., Bactroban); warm compresses of water or aluminum acetate solution; healing usually without scarring; if lesions extensive and deep, possible scarring and loss of involved hair follicles, and treatment with systemic antibiotics necessary
Furuncle		
Deep infection with staphylococci around hair follicle, often associated with severe acne or seborrheic dermatitis	Tender erythematous area around hair follicle; draining pus and core of necrotic debris on rupture; most common on face, back of neck, axillae, breasts, buttocks, perineum, thighs; painful	Incision and drainage; packing may be required; antibiotics, meticulous care of involved skin, frequent application of warm, moist compresses
Furunculosis		
Increased incidence in patients who are obese, diabetic, chronically ill, or regularly exposed to moisture or pressure	Lesions as above; malaise, regional adenopathy, elevated body temperature	Warm, moist compresses; systemic antibiotic after culture and sensitivity study of drainage (usually semisynthetic, penicillinase-resistant, oral penicillin such as cloxacillin); measures to reduce surface staphylococci include antimicrobial cream to nares, armpits, and groin and antiseptic to entire skin; often recurrent with scarring; incision and drainage of soft lesions; prevention or correction of predisposing factors; meticulous personal hygiene
Carbuncle		
Multiple, interconnecting furuncles	Many pustules appearing in erythematous area, most common at nape of neck	Treatment same as furuncles; often recurrent despite production of antibodies; healing slow with scar formation
Cellulitis		
Inflammation of subcutaneous tissues; possibly secondary complication or primary infection; often following break in skin; *Staphylococcus aureus* and streptococci usual causative agents; deep inflammation of subcutaneous tissue from enzymes produced by bacteria	Hot, tender, erythematous, and edematous area with diffuse borders; chills, malaise, and fever (see Figure 26-5)	Moist heat, immobilization and elevation, systemic antibiotic therapy, hospitalization if severe; progression to gangrene possible if untreated
Erysipelas		
Superficial cellulitis primarily involving the dermis; group A β-hemolytic streptococci	Red, hot, sharply demarcated plaque that is indurated and painful; bacteremia possible; most common on face and extremities; toxic signs, such as fever, ↑ white blood cell count, headache, malaise	Systemic antibiotics—usually penicillin; hospitalization often required

IM, intramuscular.

herpes zoster (Figure 26-7), and warts are the most common viral infections affecting the skin (Table 26-6).

Fungal Infections

Because of the large number of identified fungi, it is almost impossible to avoid exposure to some pathological varieties. However, some fungi, including candidiasis and tinea unguium (Figures 26-8 and 26-9), can cause infections of the skin, hair, and nails (Snow, 2008). Common fungal infections of the skin are presented in Table 26-7.

Microscopic examination of the scraping of suspicious skin lesions in 10 to 20% potassium hydroxide (KOH) is an easy, inexpensive diagnostic measure to determine the presence of fungus. The appearance of hyphae (threadlike structures) is indicative of a fungal infection.

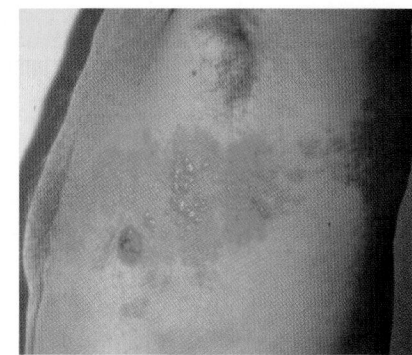

Figure 26-7 Herpes zoster (shingles) on the anterior chest, confined to one dermatome.

Source: Lemmi, F. O., & Lemmi, C. A. E. (2000). *Physical assessment findings*. Philadelphia: Saunders.

Table 26-6 Common Viral Infections of the Skin

ETIOLOGY AND PATHOPHYSIOLOGY	CLINICAL MANIFESTATIONS	TREATMENT AND PROGNOSIS
Herpes Simplex Virus Types 1* and 2		
Generally oral or genital HSV-1 or HSV-2; both are recurrent lifelong viral infections that return to skin and mucous membranes to cause recurrence when exacerbated by sunlight, trauma, menses, stress, and systemic infection; contagious to those not previously infected; transmission by respiratory droplets or virus-containing fluid, such as saliva or cervical secretions; no protection against subsequent infection in other areas with episodes of infection in one area (see Figure 26-6)	*First Episode* Symptoms occurring 3-7 days or more after contact; painful local reaction; single or grouped vesicles on erythematous base; systemic symptoms, such as fever and malaise, possible or asymptomatic presentation possible (see Figure 26-6) *Recurrent* Small; recurrence in similar spot; characteristic grouped vesicles on erythematous base	Symptomatic medication such as antiviral agents (e.g., acyclovir [Zovirax], famciclovir [Famvir], and valacyclovir [Valtrex]); soothing, moist compresses; petrolatum to lesions; scarring not usual result Vaccines not currently available
Herpes Zoster (Shingles)		
Activation of the varicella-zoster virus; incidence increases with age; frequent occurrence in immunosuppressed patients; potentially contagious to anyone who has not had varicella or who is immunosuppressed	Linear distribution along dermatome of grouped vesicles on erythematous base; usually unilateral and on trunk, face, and lumbosacral areas; burning, pain, and neuralgia preceding outbreak; mild to severe pain during outbreak (see Figure 26-7)	Symptomatic; antiviral agents such as acyclovir, famciclovir, and valacyclovir within 72 hr to prevent PHN; wet compresses, Silvadene to ruptured vesicles; analgesia; mild sedation at bedtime; gabapentin (Neurontin) indicated in the treatment of PHN; usual healing without complications, but scarring and PHN possible; vaccine (Zostavax) to prevent shingles is available for adults 60 yr or older who previously had chickenpox
Verruca Vulgaris		
Caused by HPV; spontaneous disappearance in 1-2 yr possible; mildly contagious by autoinoculation; specific response dependent on body part affected; prevalence greater in youth and immunosuppressed	Circumscribed, hypertrophic, flesh-coloured papule limited to epidermis; painful on lateral compression	Multiple treatments, including surgery—blunt dissection with scissors or curette; liquid nitrogen therapy; blistering agents—cantharidin; keratolytic agents—salicylic acid; CO₂ laser destruction; treatment can result in scarring
Plantar Warts		
Caused by HPV	Wart on bottom surface of foot, growing inward because of pressure of walking or standing; painful when pressure applied; interrupted skin markings; cone-shaped with black dots (thrombosed vessels) when wart removed	Topical immunotherapy (imiquimod), cryosurgery, and salicylic acid

HPV, human papillomavirus; *HSV,* herpes simplex virus; *PHN,* postherpetic neuralgia.
*Herpes simplex is also discussed in Chapter 55.

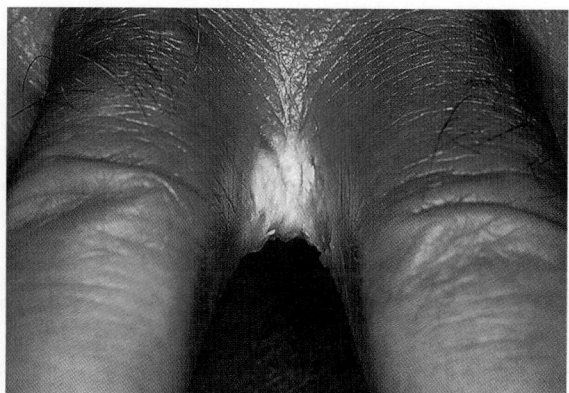

Figure 26-8 Candidiasis in interdigital cleft. Occurs in workers whose constantly wet hands are not dried often.

Source: Gawkrodger, D. (2002). *Dermatology: An illustrated colour text* (3rd ed.). Edinburgh: Churchill Livingstone.

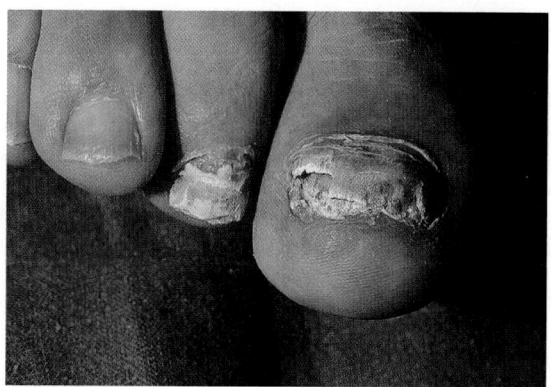

Figure 26-9 Tinea unguium (onychomycosis). Fungal infection of toenails. Crumbly, discoloured, and thickened nails.

Source: Gawkrodger, D. (2002). *Dermatology: An illustrated colour text* (3rd ed.). Edinburgh: Churchill Livingstone.

Table 26-7 Common Fungal Infections of the Skin and the Mucous Membranes

ETIOLOGY AND PATHOPHYSIOLOGY	CLINICAL MANIFESTATIONS	TREATMENT AND PROGNOSIS
Candidiasis		
Caused by *Candida albicans*; also known as moniliasis; 50% of adults symptom-free carriers; presenting in warm, moist areas such as groin area, oral mucosa, and submammary folds; HIV infection, chemotherapy, radiation, and organ transplantation related to depression of cell-mediated immunity that allows yeast to become pathogenic	*Mouth* White, cheesy plaque, resembles milk curds *Vagina* Vaginitis, with red, edematous, painful vaginal wall, white patches; vaginal discharge; pruritus; pain on urination and intercourse *Skin* Diffuse papular erythematous rash with pinpoint satellite lesions around edges of affected area (see Figure 26-8)	Microscopic examination and culture; azole antifungals (e.g., fluconazole, ketoconazole), or other specific medication such as vaginal suppository or oral lozenge; abstinence from intercourse or use of condom; eradication of infection with appropriate medication; skin hygiene to keep area clean and dry; Mycostatin powder effective on nonmucosal skin lesions
Tinea Corporis		
Various dermatophytes, commonly referred to as ringworm	Typical annular (ringlike) scaly appearance, well-defined margins; erythematous	Cool compresses; topical antifungals for isolated patches; creams or solutions of miconazole (Monistat), clotrimazole (Canesten), and ketoconazole
Tinea Cruris		
Various dermatophytes, commonly referred to as jock itch	Well-defined scaly plaques in groin area; does not affect mucous membrane	Topical antifungal cream or solution
Tinea Pedis		
Various dermatophytes, commonly referred to as athlete's foot	Interdigital scaling and maceration; scaly plantar surfaces sometimes with erythema and blistering; may be pruritic; possibly painful	Topical antifungal cream, gel, solution, spray, or powder
Tinea Unguium (Onychomycosis)		
Various dermatophytes; incidence increases with age	Only a few nails on one hand may be affected; toenails more commonly affected; scaliness under distal nail plate; brittle, thickened, broken, or crumbling nails with yellowish discoloration (see Figure 26-9)	Topical antifungal cream or solution if unable to tolerate systemic treatment; oral antifungal (terbinafine [Lamisil], itraconazole [Sporanox]); topical antifungal (minimal effectiveness) if unable to tolerate system drug; thinning of toenails if needed; nail avulsion (removal) is an option

HIV, human immunodeficiency virus.

Infestations and Insect Bites

The possibilities for exposure to infestations (harbouring insects or worms) and insect bites are numerous. In many instances, an allergy to the venom plays a major role in the reaction. In other cases, the clinical manifestations are a reaction to the eggs, the feces, or the body parts of the invading organism (Figure 26-10). Some individuals react with a severe hypersensitivity (anaphylaxis), which can be life threatening. (Anaphylaxis is discussed in Chapter 14.)

Prevention of insect bites by avoidance or by the use of repellents is somewhat effective. Meticulous hygiene related to personal articles, clothing, bedding, and examination and care of pets, as well as careful selection of sexual partners, can reduce the incidence of infestations. Routine inspection is necessary in geographic areas where there is a risk of tick bites and Lyme disease (Table 26-8).

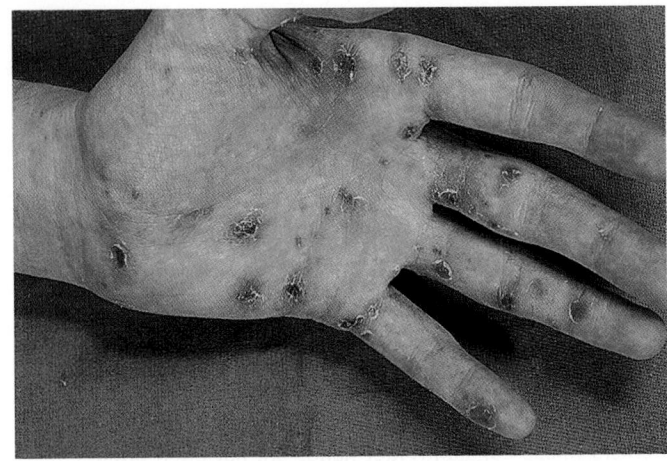

Figure 26-10 Scabies infestation on hand.

Source: Gawkrodger, D. (2002). *Dermatology: An illustrated colour text* (3rd ed.). Edinburgh: Churchill Livingstone.

Table 26-8 Common Infestations and Insect Bites

ETIOLOGY AND PATHOPHYSIOLOGY	CLINICAL MANIFESTATIONS	TREATMENT AND PROGNOSIS
Bees and Wasps		
Hymenoptera	Intense, burning, local pain; swelling and itching; severe hypersensitivity possibly leading to anaphylaxis	Cool compresses; local application of antipruritic lotion; antihistamines if indicated; usually uneventful recovery
Bedbugs		
Cimicidae; feeding periodic, usually at night; present in furniture, walls during day	Wheal surrounded by vivid flare; firm urticaria transforming into persistent lesion; severe pruritus; often grouped in threes appearing on noncovered parts of body	Bedbug controlled by chlorocyclohexane; lesions usually requiring no treatment; severe itching possibly necessitating use of antihistamines or topical corticosteroids
Pediculosis (Head Lice, Body Lice, Pubic Lice)		
Pediculus humanus, var. *capitis*; *Pediculus humanus,* var. *corporis*; *Phthirus pubis*; obligate parasites that suck blood, leave excrement and eggs on skin, live in seams of clothing (if body lice) and in hair as nits; transmission of pubic lice often by sexual contact	Minute, red, noninflammatory; points flush with skin; progression to papular wheal-like lesions; pruritus; secondary excoriation, especially parallel linear excoriations in intrascapular region; firmly attached to hair shaft in head and body lice	γ-Benzene hexachloride or pyrethrins to treat various parts of body; application as directed; screen and treat all possible close contacts: bed partners, playmates, shared head gear
Scabies		
Sarcoptes scabiei; mite penetrates stratum corneum, deposits eggs; allergic reaction resulting from presence of eggs, feces, mite parts; transmission by direct physical contact, only occasionally by shared personal items; rarely seen in dark-skinned people	Severe itching, especially at night, usually not on face; presence of burrows, especially in interdigital webs, flexor surface of wrists, genitals, and anterior axillary folds; erythematous papules (may be crusted), possible vesiculation, interdigital web crusting (see Figure 26-10)	5% permethrin topical lotion, one overnight application with second application 1 wk later, may yield 95% eradication; treat environment with plastic covering for 5 days, launder all clothes and linen with bleach; treat sexual partner; antibiotics if secondary infections present; possible residual pruritus up to 4 wk after treatment; recurrence possible if inadequately treated
Ticks		
Borrelia burgdorferi (spirochete transmitted by ticks in certain areas) causes Lyme disease; endemic in Nova Scotia, southern and eastern Ontario, southeast in Manitoba, and southern British Columbia, with isolated occurrences in the southern part of the provinces bordering the United States; migratory birds can carry the ticks, and it may be present in unidentified regions. Occurrence is on the increase because of global warming and increased animal dispersement (Ogden et al., 2009).	Spreading, ringlike rash 3-4 wk after bite; rash commonly in groin, buttocks, axillae, trunk, and upper arms and legs; warm, itchy, or painful rash; flulike symptoms; cardiac, arthritic, and neurological manifestations possible; unreliable laboratory test; no acquired immunity	Oral antibiotics, such as doxycycline, tetracycline; intravenous antibiotics for arthritic, neurological, and cardiac symptoms; rest and healthy diet; good prognosis with treatment (see discussion of Lyme disease in Chapter 67)

Table 26-9 Common Allergic Conditions of the Skin

ETIOLOGY AND PATHOPHYSIOLOGY	CLINICAL MANIFESTATIONS	TREATMENT AND PROGNOSIS
Allergic Contact Dermatitis		
Manifestation of delayed hypersensitivity, absorbed agent acting as antigen, sensitization after several exposures, appearance of lesions 2-7 days after contact with allergen	Red, hivelike papules and plaques; sharply circumscribed with occasional vesicles; usually pruritic; area of dermatitis frequently takes shape of causative agent (e.g., metal allergy and dermatitis on ring finger)	Topical or systemic corticosteroids if severe, antihistamines; skin lubrication; elimination of contact allergen; avoidance of irritating affected area
Urticaria		
Usually allergic phenomenon; presence of erythema and edema in upper dermis resulting from a local increase in permeability of capillaries (usually from histamine response)	Spontaneously occurring and raised or irregularly shaped wheals; varying size; usually multiple; a single lesion usually resolves in 24 hr; can occur anywhere on the body	Removal of source, if known; antihistamine therapy; cool compresses, possibly systemic corticosteroids
Drug Reaction		
Any drug that acts as antigen and causes hypersensitivity reaction is possible cause; certain drugs more prone to reactions (e.g., penicillin); not all reactions are allergic, some are intolerance (e.g., gastric upset; some reactions may be life threatening requiring immediate and intensive care	Rash of any morphology; often red, macular and papular, semiconfluent, generalized rash with abrupt onset; appearance as late as 14 days after cessation of drug; possibly pruritic; some reactions may be life threatening, require immediate and intensive care	Withdrawal of drug if possible; antihistamines, topical or systemic corticosteroids may be necessary depending on severity of symptoms
Atopic Dermatitis		
Genetically influenced, chronic, relapsing disease associated with immunological irregularity involving inflammatory mediators, exaggerated by a cutaneous response to environmental allergens; associated with allergic rhinitis and asthma; most severe in childhood	Multiple presentations include acute, subacute, and chronic stages; all are pruritic; acute stage with bright erythema, oozing vesicles, with extreme pruritus; subacute phase with scaly, light red to red-brown plaques; chronic stage has thickened skin with accentuation of skin markings (lichenification), possible hypopigmentation or hyperpigmentation; dry skin; common in an antecubital and popliteal space in adults	Lubrication of dry (xerotic) skin; restoration of skin barrier function; topical immunomodulators (pimecrolimus [Elidel], tacrolimus [Protopic]); corticosteroids, phototherapy for severe inflammation and pruritus; reduction of stress reduces flare; antibiotics for secondary infection as needed

Allergic Dermatological Problems

Dermatological problems associated with allergies and hypersensitivity reactions may present a challenge to the clinician (Table 26-9). The pathophysiology related to allergic and contact dermatitis is discussed in Chapter 14. A careful family history and discussion of exposure to possible offending agents provide valuable data. Patch testing involves the application of allergens to the patient's skin (usually on the back) for 48 hours, after which the test sites are examined for erythema, papules, vesicles, or all of these. Patch testing is used to aid in determining possible causative agents. The best treatment of allergic dermatitis is avoidance of the causative agent. The extreme pruritus of contact dermatitis and its potential for chronicity make it a frustrating problem for patient, nurse, and dermatologist, especially if the offending agent cannot be identified.

Benign Dermatological Problems

The list of benign dermatoses is extensive; nonetheless, some of the most commonly seen and distressing problems include psoriasis, acne vulgaris, and seborrheic keratoses. Benign problems are summarized in Table 26-10.

Psoriasis is a common benign disorder that currently affects 1 million people in Canada (CDA, 2011e). The disease usually develops in individuals between 15 and 25 years old. One third of all people with psoriasis report that they have at least one relative with the disease. A majority of people have mild disease that is characterized as affecting at least 3% of the body. Severe disease exists when psoriasis affects over 10% of the body. The chronicity of psoriasis can be severe and disabling as people withdraw from social contacts because of visible lesions (Figure 26-11). Quality of life is also negatively affected. Psoriatic arthritis affects 10 to 30% of all persons with psoriasis (CDA, 2011e). (Psoriatic arthritis is discussed in Chapter 66.)

Diseases with Dermatological Manifestations

Dermatological manifestations of various diseases are listed in Table 26-11. The health care provider should always consider the possibility that a particular dermatosis is a clue to an internal, less obvious problem.

Table 26-10 Common Benign Conditions of the Skin

ETIOLOGY AND PATHOPHYSIOLOGY	CLINICAL MANIFESTATIONS	TREATMENT AND PROGNOSIS
Acne Vulgaris		
Inflammatory disorder of sebaceous glands; more common in teenagers but possible development and persistence in adulthood; flare can occur before menses, with use of corticosteroids and androgen-dominant birth control pills	Noninflammatory lesions, including open comedones (blackheads) and closed comedones (whiteheads) Inflammatory lesions, including papules, pustules, and cysts; most common on face, neck, and upper back Nodular or inflammatory acne produces deeper lesions and can lead to significant scarring (Figure 26-12)	Mechanical removal of multiple lesions with comedo extractor; topical benzoyl peroxide or other antimicrobial; topical retinoids, systemic antibiotics; aim of treatment is to suppress new lesions and minimize scarring; spontaneous remission possible; often improvement with exposure to sun Use of isotretinoin (Accutane) for severe nodulocystic and/or inflammatory, conglobata, and recalcitrant acne to possibly provide lasting remission; contraindicated for use in pregnant women or women intending to become pregnant while on drug or when breastfeeding; should not donate blood for 1 mo following treatment; monitoring of liver function and pregnancy tests, cholesterol, and triglycerides essential; the CDA supports the use of isotretinoin with education for the physician and the patient to ensure safe administration of the drug* Health Canada* issued safety alert about the possible association between Accutane and the occurrence of depression or suicidal ideation in young people; signs of depression must be carefully monitored when the drug is being used; Health Canada† also issued another safety alert about the occurrence of very rare reports of severe skin reactions (e.g. erythema multiforme, Stevens-Johnson syndrome, and toxic epidermal necrolysis) associated with Accutane use.
Nevi (Moles)		
Grouping of normal cells derived from melanocyte-like precursor cells	Hyperpigmented areas that vary in form and colour; flat, slightly elevated, haloid, verrucoid, polypoid, dome-shaped, sessile, or papillomatous; preservation of normal skin markings; hair growth possible	No treatment necessary except for cosmetic reasons; skin biopsy for diagnosis
Psoriasis		
Autoimmune chronic dermatitis, which involves excessively rapid turnover of epidermal cells; family predisposition; usually develops before age 40	Sharply demarcated, silvery, scaling plaques on the scalp, elbows, and knees; palms, soles, and fingernails possibly affected; itching burning pain; localized or general, intermittent or continuous; symptoms vary from mild to severe (see Figure 26-11)	Goal is to reduce inflammation and suppress rapid turnover of epidermal cells; topical treatment may be time consuming; usually topical or systemic corticosteroids, tar, anthralin; intralesional injection of corticosteroids for chronic plaques; sunlight; natural or artificial UVB, PUVA, UVA ultraviolet light, alone or with topical or systematic potentiation (psoralen) and clobetasol propionate 0.05% spray (Clobex); systemic treatments: antimetabolite (methotrexate) Biological therapy adalimumab (Humira), immunosuppressant (cyclosporine), retinoid (acitretin), etanercept (Enbrel), infliximab (Remicade) for moderate to severe plaque form of disease; no cure, but control is possible
Seborrheic Keratoses		
Benign, familial, genetically determined growths; found in increasing number with age; no association with sun exposure; exact etiology unknown	Irregularly round or oval, flat-topped papules or plaques; surface often verrucous (warty); well-defined shape, appearance of being glued on; increase in pigmentation with age of lesion; usually multiple and possibly itchy (Figure 26-13)	Removal by curettage or cryosurgery for cosmetic reasons or to eliminate source of irritation; minimal scarring; biopsy if unable to differentiate from melanoma

*Health Canada. (2009). *Drugs and health products: Important information on Accutane*, Hoffman Laroche Canada. Retrieved from *http://www.hc-sc.gc.ca/ dhp-mps/medeff/advisories-avis/prof/_2001/accutane_hpc-cps-eng.php*

†Health Canada. (2010). *Drugs and health products: Accutane (Isotretinoid) association of severe skin reactions for health professionals.* Retrieved from *http:// www.hc-sc.gc.ca/dhp-mps/medeff/advisories-avis/prof/_2010/accutane_2_hpc-cps-eng.php*

Table 26-10 Common Benign Conditions of the Skin—cont'd

ETIOLOGY AND PATHOPHYSIOLOGY	CLINICAL MANIFESTATIONS	TREATMENT AND PROGNOSIS
Acrochordons (Skin Tags)		
Common after midlife; appearance on neck, axillae, and upper trunk secondary to mechanical friction or redundant skin (associated with obesity)	Small, skin-coloured, irregularly round or oval, often verrucous papules or plaques; well-defined shape, appearance of being stuck on; may become irritated	No treatment medically unless for sites of repeated trauma or cosmetic reasons; surgical removal possible; usually just "clipping off" without anaesthesia
Lipoma		
Benign tumour of adipose tissue, often encapsulated, most common in 40- to 60-yr-old age-group	Rubbery, compressible, round mass of adipose tissue; single or multiple; variable in size, possibly extremely large; most common on trunk, back of neck, and forearms	Usually no treatment, biopsy to differentiate from liposarcoma, excision usual treatment (when indicated)
Vitiligo		
Unknown cause; genetically influenced, often precipitated by an event such as illness or a crisis; most noticeable in dark-skinned persons and those with a tan; complete absence of melanocytes; noncontagious	Focal amelanosis (complete loss of pigment); macular; variation in size and location; usually symmetrical and may be permanent	Topical steroids often successful in small areas; attempts at repigmentation of larger areas with exposure to UVA and psoralens; depigmentation of pigmented skin with extensive disease (>50% of body involved); cosmetics and stains for camouflage and to de-emphasize vitiliginous areas
Lentigo		
Increased number of normal melanocytes in basal layer of epidermis; senile lentigos ("liver" or "age spots") related to aging and sun exposure	Hyperpigmented, brown to black, flat macula or patch; single or multiple; usually on sun-exposed areas; potential for progression to lentigo maligna (melanoma in situ) in advanced years	Evaluate carefully for progression; treatment only for cosmetic purposes is liquid nitrogen; laser resurfacing; possible recurrence in 1-2 yr; biopsy if suspicious of melanoma

CDA, Canadian Dermatology Association; *IM,* intramuscular (route); *IV,* intravenous (route); *PUVA,* psoralen plus ultraviolet A light; *UVA,* ultraviolet A light; *UVB,* ultraviolet B light.

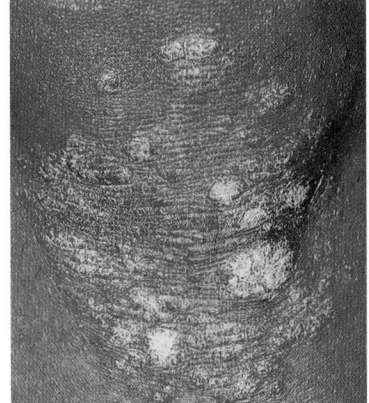

Figure 26-11 Psoriasis. Characteristic inflammation and scaling.

Source: Patton, K. T., & Thibodeau, G. A. (2010). *Anatomy and physiology* (7th ed., p. 185, Figure 6-27). St. Louis: Mosby.

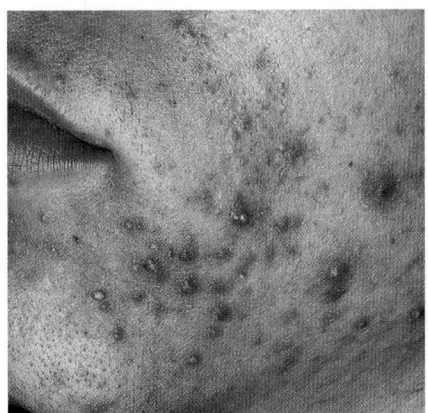

Figure 26-12 Acne vulgaris. Papules and pustules.

Source: James, W. D., Berger, T., & Elston, D. (2006). *Andrews' diseases of the skin: Clinical dermatology* (10th ed.). Philadelphia: Saunders.

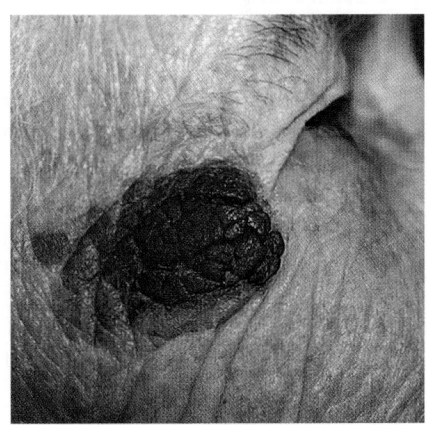

Figure 26-13 Seborrheic keratoses. Deeply pigmented, rough, and warty surface.

Source: Callen, J. P., & Greer, K. E. (1993). *Color atlas of dermatology*. Philadelphia: Saunders.

Table 26-11 Diseases With Dermatological Manifestations*

SYSTEMIC PROBLEM	DERMATOLOGICAL MANIFESTATIONS	SYSTEMIC PROBLEM	DERMATOLOGICAL MANIFESTATIONS
Endocrine		Hypervitaminosis A	Hair loss, dry skin
Hyperthyroidism	Increased sweating; warm skin with persistent flush; thin nails; vitiligo; alopecia; fine, soft hair	Vitamin B₁ (thiamine) deficiency	Edema, redness of soles of feet
Hypothyroidism	Cold, dry, pale to yellow skin; slightly hyperkeratotic epidermis with follicular plugging; generalized nonpitting edema; dry, coarse, brittle hair; brittle, slow-growing nails	Vitamin B₂ (riboflavin) deficiency	Red fissures at corner of mouth, glossitis
		Nicotinic acid (niacin) deficiency	Pellagra; redness of exposed areas of hand or foot, face or neck; infected dermatitis
Glucocorticoid excess (Cushing's syndrome)	Atrophy; striae; epidermal thinning; telangiectasia; acne; decreased subcutaneous fat over extremities; thin, loose dermis; impaired wound healing; increased vascular fragility; mild hirsutism; excessive collection of fat over clavicles, back of neck, abdomen, and face; increased incidence of pyodermas (purulent bacterial dermatitis)	Vitamin C deficiency	Petechiae, purpura, bleeding gums
		Immune	
		HIV infection	Kaposi's sarcoma, eosinophilic folliculitis
		Cancer of breast, stomach, lung, uterus, kidney, ovary, colon, bladder	Metastasis to skin
Addison's disease	Loss of body hair (especially axillary), generalized hyperpigmentation (accentuated in folds)	Hodgkin's disease	Pruritus and nonspecific erythemas
Androgen excess	Enlarged facial pores, male sex characteristics, acne, acceleration of coarse hair growth	Lymphomas	Papules, nodules, plaques, pruritus
		Cardiovascular	
Androgen deficiency—postpuberty	Development of sparse hair; marked reduction in sebum production	Rheumatic heart disease	Petechiae, urticaria, nodules, erythema nodosum and multiforme
		Periarteritis nodosa	Periarteritis nodules
Hypoparathyroidism	Opaque, brittle nails with transverse ridges; coarse, sparse hair with patchy alopecia; eczematous and exfoliative dermatitis; hyperkeratotic and maculopapular eruptions	Thromboangiitis obliterans (Buerger's disease)	Superficial migrating thrombophlebitis, pallor or cyanosis, gangrene, ulceration
		Peripheral arterial disease	Loss of hair on hands and feet; delayed capillary filling; dependent rubour (redness); pain
Hyperpituitarism (acromegaly)	Coarsened skin, deepened lines; increased oiliness and sweating; acne; increased number of nevi, hyperpigmentation; hypertrichosis (excess hair growth)	Venous stasis ulcers	Leathery, brownish skin on lower leg; pruritus, concave lesion with edema; scar tissue with healing
		Respiratory	
Diabetes mellitus	Erythematous plaques of shin spots, delayed wound healing, neuropathy	Inadequate oxygenation secondary to respiratory disease	Cyanosis
Gastrointestinal		**Hematological**	
Ulcerative colitis, Crohn's disease	Mouth ulcers, erythema nodosum	Anemia	Pallor, hyperpigmentation, pale mucous membranes, hair loss, nail dystrophy
Liver disease and biliary tract obstruction	Jaundice, itching, pigmentary abnormalities, alterations in nails and hair, spider angiomas, telangiectasia	Clotting disorders	Purpura, petechiae, ecchymosis
		Renal	
Deficiency of essential fatty acids	Scaly skin	Chronic kidney disease	Dry skin, pruritus, uremic frost, pallor, dry skin, bruises
Malabsorption syndrome	Acquired ichthyosis (dry, scaly skin)	**Reproductive**	
		Primary syphilis	Chancre
Cystic fibrosis	Abnormal sweat gland function resulting in failure to conserve sodium	Secondary syphilis	Generalized skin lesions, alopecia
		Tertiary syphilis	Gummas
Musculoskeletal and Connective Tissue		Paget's disease	Eczematous patch of nipple and areola
Systemic lupus erythematosus	Discoid lesions, maculopapular semiconfluent rash (butterfly rash)	**Neurological**	
Scleroderma	Leathery hardening and stiffness of skin	Chronic sensory polyneuropathies	Trophic changes in skin resulting from sensory denervation, pressure ulcers, anaesthesia, paresthesias
Dermatomyositis	Edema; purplish red upper eyelids; scaly, macular erythema over knuckles	Spinal cord trauma	
Metabolic			
Lipidoses	Xanthomas		
Vitamin A deficiency	Generalized dry hyperkeratoses		

HIV, human immunodeficiency virus.
*Refer to the discussion of the systemic disease for specific information.

Certain life changes are recognized to be associated with dermatoses. At puberty, male- or female-pattern hair growth will be evident as a secondary sex characteristic. Increased apocrine gland activity can lead to body odour. The increased sebaceous gland activity stimulated by androgens can result in seborrhea and acne.

Collaborative Care: Dermatological Problems

Diagnostic Studies

A careful history is of prime importance in the diagnosis of skin problems. The clinician must be skilled at detecting any evidence that could lead to the etiology of the extraordinary number of skin diseases and conditions. After a careful history and physical examination, inspect individual lesions. On the basis of the history, the physical examination, and appropriate diagnostic tests, either medical, surgical, or combination therapy is planned.

Collaborative Care

Many different treatment methods are used in dermatology. Advances in this field have brought relief to sufferers of many previously chronic, untreatable conditions. Many of the specific therapeutic treatments require specialized equipment and are usually reserved for use by the dermatologist. Many clinicians prescribe drug therapy. The effectiveness of topical therapy can often be related to the base (or vehicle) in which the medication is prepared. Table 26-12 summarizes the common agents used as bases for topical preparations and their therapeutic considerations.

Phototherapy. Two types of UV light, or a combination of the two types (UVA, UVB), are used to treat many dermatological conditions. UV wavelengths cause erythema, blistering, desqua-

DRUG THERAPY

Table 26-12 Common Bases for Topical Medications

AGENT	THERAPEUTIC CONSIDERATIONS
Powder	Promotion of dryness, lubricates skinfold areas to prevent irritation; increase in evaporation, absorbing of moisture possible, common base for antifungal preparations; protect patient from inhaling
Lotion	Oil and water emulsions; cooling and drying, with residual powder film after evaporation of water; useful in subacute pruritic eruptions
Cream	Emulsions of oil and water, most common base for topical medications; lubrication, protection
Ointment	Oil with differing amounts of water added in suspension; lubrication and prevention of dehydration; petrolatum most common
Paste	Mixture of powder and ointment, used when drying effect necessary because moisture is absorbed
Gel	Nongreasy combination of propylene glycol and water; may contain alcohol; used for acute exudative inflammation (e.g., contact dermatitis)

mation, and pigmentation and may cause a temporary suppression of basal cell mitosis followed by a rebound increase in cell turnover.

PUVA is a form of phototherapy. The photosensitizing drug psoralen is given to patients 90 minutes before exposure to UVA to enhance the effect of UV light in the UVA spectrum. Usually, a moisturizing agent is applied to the affected area in a thin layer before exposure to UVB. Conditions that are responsive to effective wavelengths with or without drugs include atopic dermatitis, cutaneous T-cell lymphoma, pruritus, psoriasis, and vitiligo (Tope & Bhardwaj, 2008).

UV light in the specific wavelengths can be produced artificially. Therapeutic doses of UVA and UVB can be measured and used to treat spectrum-specific diseases. Frequent skin assessments must be performed on all patients receiving phototherapy. Inappropriate or excessive exposure to UV light can result in BCC or SCC, as well as severe erythema or burn to the skin. Patients should be cautioned about the potential hazards of using photosensitizing chemicals and further exposure to UV rays from sunlight or artificial UV light during the course of phototherapy. Protective eyewear that blocks 100% of UV light is prescribed for patients receiving PUVA because psoralen is absorbed by the lens of the eye. The eyewear is used to prevent cataract formation. Instruct patients to use the eyewear for 24 hours after taking the medication when outdoors or near a bright window because UVA penetrates glass. The immunosuppressive effects related to the use of PUVA require careful ongoing monitoring of these patients.

Phototherapy is a method for treating spectrum-specific diseases. The patient's eyes must be protected during the phototherapy session.

Radiation Therapy. The use of radiation for the treatment of cutaneous malignancies varies greatly according to local practice and availability. Even if radiation therapy is planned, a biopsy must first be performed to obtain a pathological diagnosis. Radiation to malignant cutaneous lesions is a painless treatment. It produces minimal damage to surrounding tissue. It is a particularly effective treatment for the older adult or the debilitated patient who cannot tolerate minor surgical procedures and for such areas as nose, eyelids, and canthal areas, where preservation of the surrounding tissue is of prime consideration. Careful shielding is necessary to prevent ocular lens damage if the irradiated area is around the eyes.

Radiation therapy usually necessitates multiple visits to a radiology department. It is most effective on lesions above the neck. However, it produces permanent hair loss (alopecia) of the irradiated areas. Other adverse effects include telangiectasia, atrophy, hyperpigmentation, depigmentation, ulceration, chronic radiodermatitis, BCC, and SCC. (Radiation therapy is discussed in Chapter 18.)

Total-body skin irradiation (body is bombarded with high-energy electrons) may be the treatment of choice or adjunctive therapy for cutaneous T-cell lymphoma. Treatment follows a lengthy course. Patients experience varying degrees of hair loss and radiation dermatitis with transient loss of sweat gland function. This treatment causes premature aging of the skin.

Laser Technology. Laser treatment is expanding rapidly as an efficient surgical tool for many types of dermatological problems (Table 26-13). Lasers are able to produce measurable, repeatable, consistent zones of tissue damage. They can cut, coagulate, and vaporize tissue to some degree. The wavelength

Table 26-13 Use of Laser Treatments for Skin Conditions	
• Acne scars	• Port-wine stain
• Skin lesions	• Vascular lesions
• Hemangiomas	• Tattoos
• Leg veins	• Resurfacing of skin
• Rosacea	• Psoriasis
• Pigmented nevi	• Wrinkles
• Hair removal	• Epidermal pigment

determines the type of delivery system used and the intensity of the energy delivered.

The surgical use of laser energy requires a focusing device to produce a small, high-density spot of energy that can be carefully focused on the surgical site and controllably directed to the operative site. Written policies and procedures should cover laser safety and be reviewed by all personnel working with laser equipment. Laser light does not accumulate and cannot cause cumulative cellular changes or damage.

Several types of lasers are available in most offices and hospitals. The CO_2 laser is the most common vaporizing and cutting tool for most tissues. The argon laser emits light that is primarily absorbed by hemoglobin and helps in the treatment of vascular and other pigmented lesions. Other, less common lasers include the use of copper and gold vapours, and neodymium : yttrium–aluminum–garnet (Nd : YAG) laser. Laser uses include coagulation of vascular lesions, skin resurfacing, removal of birthmarks, and the treatment of BCCs, condylomas, plantar warts, and keloids.

Laser technology is increasingly being used for cosmetic treatments (see Table 26-13). The effectiveness of the treatment depends on a variety of factors which include: choice of the correct laser equipment, training and skills of the laser operator, beam wavelength, power settings, duration of the energy pulse, and colour of the skin or hair. Teach the patient about risks of laser treatments, which include pain; reddened, bruised, and swollen skin; burns; infection; and permanent scarring and discoloration if the wrong equipment or technique is used (Health Canada, 2004). The CDA (2012) has indicated their growing concern with the largely unregulated laser industry. Health Canada monitors hair removal lasers and Ontario directs the local public health office to check for sanitary conditions. The equipment is used in many settings such as doctors' offices, salons, and spas. The laser operators are often physicians, nurses, and aestheticians who may have limited training and experience. Inform the patient as to how to find a safe laser facility.

Drug Therapy

Antibiotics. Antibiotics are used both topically and systemically to treat dermatological problems, and they are often used in combination. If used, topical antibiotics should be applied in a thin film lightly to clean skin. Common OTC topical antibiotics include polymyxin B sulphate–neomycin sulphate (Neosporin; often causes allergic contact dermatitis), bacitracin, and polymyxin B. Prescription topical antibiotics include mupirocin (used for superficial *Staphylococcus* such as impetigo, gentamicin (used for *Staphylococcus* and most Gram-negative organisms), and erythromycin (used for Gram-positive cocci [staphylococci and streptococci] and Gram-negative cocci and bacilli). Topical

erythromycin and clindamycin are used in the treatment of acne vulgaris. Topical metronidazole is used to treat rosacea and bacterial vaginosis. Many of the more popular systemic antibiotics are not used topically because of the danger of allergic contact dermatitis.

If there are signs of systemic infection, a systemic antibiotic should be used. Systemic antibiotics are useful in the treatment of bacterial infections and acne vulgaris. The most frequently used are synthetic sulphur, penicillin, erythromycin, and tetracycline (or doxycycline). These drugs are particularly useful for erysipelas, cellulitis, carbuncles, and severe, infected eczema. Culture and sensitivity of the lesion can guide the choice of antibiotic. Patients require drug-specific instructions on the proper technique of taking or applying antibiotics.

Corticosteroids. Corticosteroids are particularly effective in treating a wide variety of dermatological conditions and can be used topically, intralesionally, or systemically. Topical corticosteroids are used for their local anti-inflammatory action as well as for their antipruritic effects. Attempts to diagnose a lesion should be made before a corticosteroid preparation is applied because corticosteroids will mask the clinical manifestations. Once a sufficient amount of medication is dispensed, limits should be set on the duration and the frequency of application. The potency of a particular preparation is related to the concentration of active drug in the preparation. With prolonged use, the more potent corticosteroid formulations can cause adrenal suppression, especially if a large surface area is covered and occlusive dressings are used. High-potency corticosteroids may produce adverse effects when their use is prolonged, including atrophy of the skin resulting from impaired cell mitosis and capillary fragility and susceptibility to bruising. In general, dermal and epidermal atrophy does not occur until a corticosteroid has been used for 2 to 3 weeks. If drug use is discontinued at the first sign of atrophy, recovery usually occurs in several weeks. Rosacea eruptions, severe exacerbations of acne vulgaris, and dermatophyte infections may also occur. Rebound dermatitis is not uncommon when therapy is stopped, and this can be reduced by tapering the use of high-potency topical corticosteroids when the patient improves.

Low-potency corticosteroids such as hydrocortisone act more slowly but can be used for a longer period without producing serious adverse effects. Low-potency corticosteroids are safe to use on the face and intertriginous (opposing skin surfaces) areas, such as the axillae. The ointment form represents the most efficient delivery system. Creams and ointments should be applied in thin layers and slowly massaged into the site one to three times a day as prescribed. Accurate and adequate topical therapy is often the key to a successful outcome.

Intralesional corticosteroids are injected directly into or just beneath the lesion. This method provides a reservoir of medication with an effect lasting several weeks to months. Intralesional injection is commonly used in the treatment of psoriasis, alopecia areata (patchy hair loss), cystic acne, hypertrophic scars, and keloids. Triamcinolone acetonide (Kenalog) is the most common drug used for intralesional injection.

Systemic corticosteroids can have remarkable results in the treatment of dermatological conditions. However, they often have undesirable systemic effects (see Chapter 51). Corticosteroids can be administered as short-term therapy for acute conditions such as contact dermatitis caused by poison ivy. Long-term corticosteroid therapy for dermatological conditions is reserved for chronic bullous (blistering) disorders, for severe systemic effects of collagen and immunologic responses, and as a last resort when other therapies have failed.

Antihistamines. Oral antihistamines are used to treat conditions that exhibit urticaria, angioedema, and pruritus. Dermatological problems such as atopic dermatitis, contact dermatitis, and other allergic cutaneous reactions can be mediated with the use of histamine blockers. Antihistamines compete with histamine for the receptor site, thus preventing its effect. Antihistamines may have anticholinergic and/or sedative effects. Several different antihistamines may have to be tried before the satisfactory therapeutic effect is achieved. Sedating antihistamines such as hydroxyzine (Atarax) and diphenhydramine (Benadryl) are often preferred for pruritus because the tranquillizing and sedative effects offer symptomatic relief. The patient should be warned about sedative effects, a particular problem when driving or operating heavy machinery. Antihistamines such as fexofenadine (Allegra), cetirizine (Reactine), and loratadine (Claritin) bind to peripheral histamine receptors, providing antihistamine action without sedation. These nonsedating antihistamines are generally not effective for controlling pruritus. Antihistamines should be used with caution in older adults because of their long half-life and their anticholinergic effects.

Topical Fluorouracil. Fluorouracil (5-FU) is a topical cytotoxic agent with selective toxicity for sun-damaged cells. 5-FU is available in four strengths (0.5%, 1%, 2%, and 5%). It is used for the treatment of premalignant skin disease, especially actinic keratosis, and some malignant skin diseases. Because systemic absorption of the drug is minimal, systemic adverse effects are virtually nonexistent. Patient compliance is a consideration in the use of 5-FU because of erythema and pruritus within 3 to 5 days and painful, eroded areas over the damaged skin within 1 to 3 weeks, depending on skin thickness of site. Treatment must continue with applications one (only in the 0.5% strength) to two times a day for 2 to 6 weeks. Healing may take up to 4 weeks after medication is stopped. Low-potency topical steroids are often prescribed and increase patient compliance with therapy. Because 5-FU is a photosensitizing drug, the patient must be educated to avoid sunlight during treatment. Patients should be educated about the effect of the medication, and should be warned that they will look worse before they look better. Compliance depends on thoroughness of the instruction, and a written handout should always be given. After effective treatment, treated skin is smooth and free of actinic keratoses, although it may recur in treated areas and multiple courses of chemotherapy may be necessary over the years for individuals with severely sun-damaged skin.

Immunomodulators. Topical immunomodulators, such as pimecrolimus (Elidel) and tacrolimus (Protopic), are newer nonsteroidal medications used to treat atopic dermatitis. They work by suppressing an overreactive immune system. The adverse effects are minimal and may include a transient burning or feeling of heat at the application site. An increased risk of skin cancer and precancerous lesions may be associated with these drugs. Another topical immunomodulator, imiquimod (Aldara), acts to stimulate the production of α-interferon and other cytokines to enhance cell-mediated immunity. It boosts the immune response only where applied and is safe for transplant patients. This medication is used for external genital warts, actinic keratoses, and superficial BCC. Most patients using this cream experience skin reactions including redness, swelling, blistering, excoriations, peeling, itching, and burning.

Diagnostic and Surgical Therapy

Skin Scraping. Scraping is done with a scalpel blade to obtain a sample of surface cells (stratum corneum) for microscopic inspection and diagnosis. The most common tests of skin scrapings are potassium hydroxide (KOH) for fungus and mineral oil examination for scabies.

Electrodesiccation and Electrocoagulation. Electrical energy can be converted to heat by the tip of an electrode. This results in tissue being destroyed by burning. The major uses of this type of therapy are point coagulation of bleeding vessels to obtain hemostasis and destruction of small *telangiectasias* (dilation of groups of superficial capillaries and venules). *Electrodesiccation* usually involves more superficial destruction, and a monopolar electrode is used. *Electrocoagulation* has a deeper effect, with better hemostasis and an increased possibility of scarring. A dipolar electrode is used for electrocoagulation.

Curettage. Curettage is the removal and scooping away of tissue using an instrument with a circular cutting edge attached to a handle (Figure 26-14). Although the curette is not usually strong enough to cut normal skin, it is useful for scooping many types of small skin tumours and superficial lesions, such as such as warts, actinic keratoses, and small BCCs and SCCs. The area to be curetted is anaesthetized before the procedure. Hemostasis is obtained by use of one of several methods: electrocoagulation, ferric subsulphate (Monsel's solution), gelatin foam, aluminum chloride, or a gauze pressure dressing. A small scar and hypopigmentation may form. The specimen should be sent for biopsy.

Punch Biopsy. Punch biopsy is a common dermatological procedure used to obtain a tissue sample for histological study or to remove small lesions. Its use is generally reserved for lesions smaller than 0.5 cm. Before local anaesthesia is used, the biopsy area is outlined so that landmarks will not be obscured by the anaesthetizing agent. The biopsy punch instrument cores out a small cylinder of skin when its sharp edge is twirled between the fingers (Figure 26-15). The core of skin is snipped from the subcutaneous fat and appropriately preserved for examination in a fixative solution. Hemostasis is achieved by using methods as with curettage, but sites of 4 mm or larger are often closed with sutures. Other types of biopsies are discussed in Table 26-10.

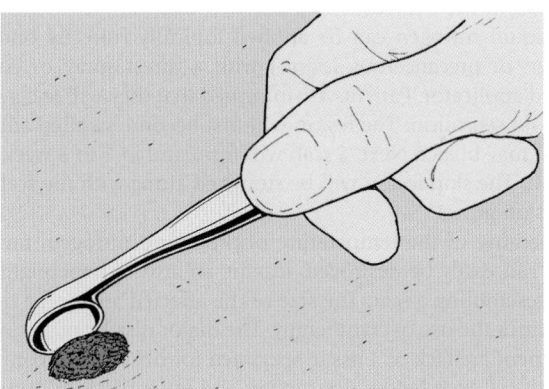

Figure 26-14 Curettage. The superficial growth is removed by a gentle scooping technique.

Source: Gawkrodger, D. (2002). *Dermatology: An illustrated colour text* (3rd ed.). Edinburgh: Churchill Livingstone.

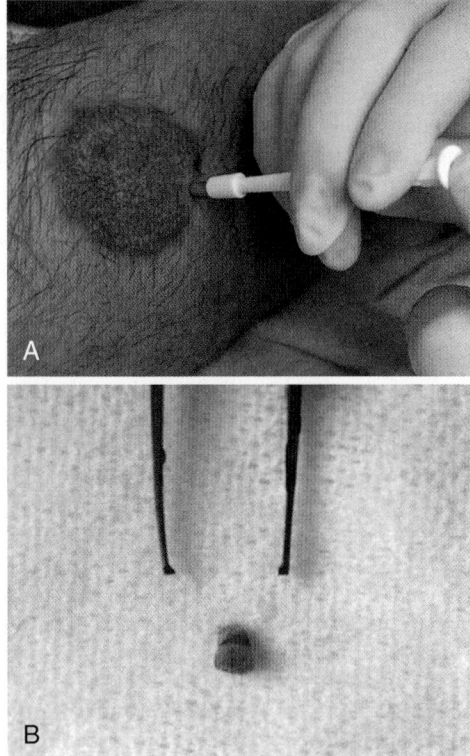

Figure 26-15 Punch biopsy. **A,** Removal of skin for diagnostic purposes. **B,** Specimen obtained.

Source: Graham-Brown, R., Bourke, J., & Cunliffe, T. (2008). *Dermatology: Fundamentals of practice*. Edinburgh: Mosby.

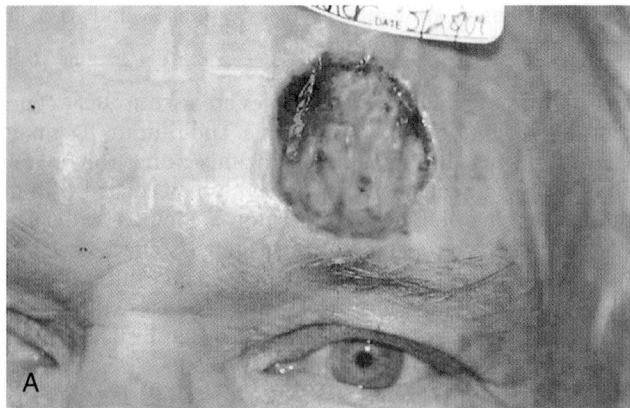

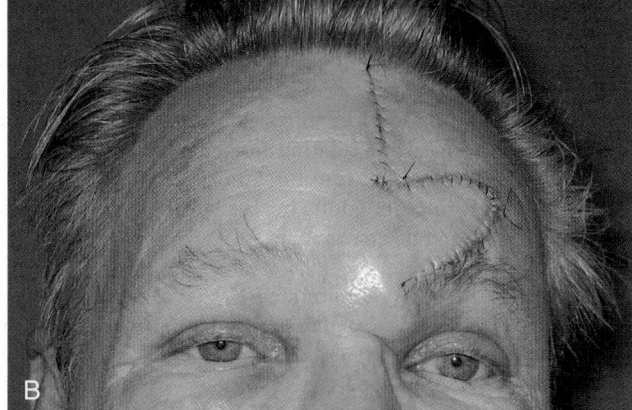

Figure 26-16 A, Removal of melanoma by Mohs' surgery. **B,** Following plastic surgery using a skin flap to repair defect.

Source: Courtesy Peter Bonner.

Cryosurgery. **Cryosurgery** is the use of subfreezing temperatures to destroy epidermal lesions. Cryosurgery is a useful treatment for common benign, precancerous conditions including common and genital warts, cutaneous tags, thin seborrheic keratoses, lentigines, actinic keratoses, and many other less common skin conditions. Topical liquid nitrogen is the agent most commonly used for cryosurgery (Graham-Robin, Bourke & Cunliffe, 2008). The mechanism of injury involves direct cellular freezing as well as vascular stasis (stoppage or slowdown in the flow of blood), which develops after thawing. Intracellular ice formation causes the cell to rupture during thaw, leading to cell death and necrosis of the treated tissue.

Liquid nitrogen can be applied topically (directly onto the benign or precancerous lesion) with a direct spray or cotton-tipped applicator. Patients are informed that they will feel a stinging cold sensation. The lesion will first become swollen and red, and it may blister. Next, a scab will form and in 1 to 3 weeks will fall off. The skin lesion will be sloughed along with the scab and new skin grows.

Because of the temperature of the liquid nitrogen, melanocytes can easily be destroyed, leaving an area of hyperpigmentation resembling a scar. The size of the affected area to be treated may limit the use of cryotherapy. The major disadvantages of this treatment are lack of a tissue specimen for histological confirmation of cell type before destruction and potential for destruction of adjacent healthy tissue.

Excision. Excision should be considered if the lesion involves the dermis. Complete closure of the excised area usually results in a good cosmetic result.

A specific type of excision is the *Mohs' surgery* (Figure 26-16), which is a microscopically controlled removal of a cutaneous malignancy. This procedure sections the surgical specimen horizontally so that 100% of the surgical margin can be examined. Tissue is removed in thin layers, and all margins of the specimen are mapped to determine whether any malignant cells remain. Any residual tumour not removed by the first surgical excision can be removed in serial excisions performed the same day. The benefits are preservation of normal tissue, producing the smallest possible wound, and complete removal of the cancer. Although this can be lengthy procedure, it is performed as an outpatient under local anaesthesia.

NURSING MANAGEMENT: DERMATOLOGICAL PROBLEMS

Ambulatory and Home Care

Dermatological conditions are not common reasons for hospitalization. Many hospitalized patients will exhibit concurrent skin problems that warrant nursing intervention and patient education.

If the patient is in an acute care setting, the nurse will both administer and teach the appropriate treatments. If the patient is in an outpatient setting, the nursing focus is on patient teaching, with opportunities provided for demonstration and repeated demonstration. Subsequent visits provide the opportunity to evaluate patient understanding and treatment effectiveness.

Nursing interventions related to dermatological conditions fall into broad categories. They are applicable to many skin problems in both inpatient and outpatient settings. A nursing care plan for the patient with chronic skin lesions is available on the Evolve Web site for this chapter.

Wet Dressings

Wet dressings are commonly used when there is oozing from the skin, which usually indicates infection and/or inflammation. Salt water or a prescribed solution (i.e., Domeboro powder) is applied to the skin by soaking (a foot or hand) or applying compresses onto a larger area. Wet dressings are also used to relieve itching, suppress inflammation, and debride a wound. In addition, wet dressings increase penetration of topical medications, promote sleep by relieving discomfort, and enhance removal of scales, crusts, and exudate. Such materials as thin sheeting, gauze sponges, thermal underwear, or tube socks can be used for dressings. Ingenuity is sometimes required when odd-shaped parts of the body must be covered.

Place the prescribed dressing into fresh solution, squeezed until it is no longer dripping, and then applied to the affected area, avoiding normal skin tissue. If the desired effect is drying, soaks or compresses are left in place for 20 minutes, three times daily for 2 to 3 days. Care must be taken to prevent overdrying because new problems may result, such as fissuring. Wet dressings for uses other than drying should be left in place 10 to 30 minutes, two to four times a day as ordered. If the skin appears macerated (softened), the dressings should be discontinued for 2 to 3 hours. Protect the patient from discomfort and chilling by using linens and bedclothes with pads or plastic.

Wet dressings do not need to be sterile. Tap water at room temperature is the most common solution in areas in which water quality is adequate. Filtered or sterile water may be indicated in some locations. Wet dressings should be cool when an anti-inflammatory effect is desired and tepid when the purpose is to debride an infected, crusted lesion. These treatments are excellent ways to remove the scabs left by the collection of debris at a wound site.

Baths

Baths are appropriate when large body areas need to be treated. They also have sedative and antipruritic effects. Some medications, such as oilated oatmeal (Aveeno) and sodium bicarbonate, can be added directly to the bath water. One cup of the mixture can be added to 2 cups of water and then added to the bath water. Fill the tub and cover affected areas. Both the bath water and the prescribed solution should be at a lukewarm (tepid) temperature. The patient can soak for 15 to 20 minutes three or four times a day, depending on the severity of the dermatitis and the patient's discomfort. It is important to stress to the patient that the skin must not be rubbed dry with a towel but gently patted to prevent increasing irritation and inflammation. The addition of oils makes the bathtub extremely slippery and should be avoided. If oils are used in the tub, the utmost caution must be used in transferring patient to prevent accidents. To sustain the hydrating effect, cream or emollients (moisturizer) or topical agents should be applied to the skin directly after the bath. This helps retain the moisture in the hydrated cells.

Topical Medications

A thin layer of ointment, cream, lotion or solution, or gel should be applied to clean skin and spread evenly in a downward motion. Thickly applied topicals waste medication and leave the skin greasy. Alternatively, the medication may be applied directly onto the dressings. Pastes are designed to protect the affected area. They should be applied thickly with a tongue blade or a gloved hand. Draining lesions and lesions with greasy medication can be covered with a light dressing to prevent soiling clothes. Patients need specific directions on the proper application technique of prescribed topical medications.

Control of Pruritus

Pruritus (itching) can be caused by almost any physical or chemical stimulus to the skin (such as drugs, insects), dry skin, and any scaling skin disorder. The itch sensation is carried by the same nonmyelinated nerve fibres as pain. If the epidermis is damaged or absent, the sensation will be felt as pain rather than an itch.

The itch–scratch cycle must be broken to prevent excoriation and lichenification. Control of pruritus is also important because it is difficult to diagnose a lesion that is excoriated and inflamed. Certain circumstances make itching worse. Anything that causes vasodilation, such as heat or rubbing, should be avoided. Dryness of the skin lowers the itch threshold and increases the itch sensation.

The nurse can use or teach the patient about the various methods that may be helpful to break the itch–scratch cycle. A cool environment may cause vasoconstriction and decrease itching. Topically applied menthol, camphor, or phenol can be used to numb the itch receptors. Systemic antihistamines can be used if necessary to provide relief while the underlying cause of the pruritus is diagnosed and treated. The principal adverse effect of most antihistamines is sedation. This may be desirable because pruritus is often worse at night and can interfere with sleep.

Wet dressings can be used effectively to relieve pruritus. Thin cotton sheets or thermal underwear is placed in warm water, wrung out, and placed over the pruritic area. After 10 to 15 minutes, the dressing is removed and the skin is patted dry (not rubbed) and a lubricant or medication applied. This procedure can be repeated as necessary for comfort.

Lichenification is a thickening of skin as a result of the proliferation of keratinocytes with accentuation of the normal markings of the skin (Graham-Robin et al., 2008) Lichenification is caused by chronic scratching or rubbing of the skin and is often associated with atopic dermatoses and pruritic conditions. Although any area of the body may be affected, the nape of the neck, shins, hands, and forearms are common sites. Excoriations may be evident in the lichenified skin as a result of the pruritus and scratching.

Prevention of Spread

Although most skin problems are not contagious, infection precautions indicate the need for gloves with open or bleeding wounds. Procedures should be explained to avoid demoralizing an already sensitive patient. The most common contagious lesions that the nurse should be cautious with include impetigo, *Staphylococcus*, pyoderma, primary chancre and secondary syphilis lesions, scabies, and pediculosis. Careful handwashing and safe disposal of soiled dressings are the best means of preventing spread of skin problems.

■ Prevention of Secondary Infections

Open lesions on the skin are susceptible to invasion by other viral, bacterial, or fungal organisms. Meticulous hygiene, handwashing, and dressing changes are important to minimize potential for secondary infections. In addition, the patient should be warned about scratching lesions, which can cause excoriations and create a portal of entry for pathogens. The patient's nails should be trimmed short to minimize trauma from scratching.

■ Specific Skin Care

Nurses are often in a position to advise patients regarding care of the skin following simple dermatological surgical procedures, such as skin biopsy, excision, and cryosurgery. Patient follow-up should be individualized. In general, instructions include dressing changes, use of topical antibiotics, and the signs and symptoms of infection. After a dermatological procedure, any oozing wound should be cleansed twice a day or as ordered by the care provider with a saline solution. Soap and water can be used to clean a non-oozing wound. An antibiotic ointment or plain petrolatum may then be applied with a dressing that is both absorbent and nonadherent.

Wounds that are kept moist and covered heal more rapidly and with less scarring. The initial crust that forms should be left undisturbed as a protective coating for the damaged skin beneath. Healing crusts that have been moisturized and protected will separate naturally from healed epidermis.

A wound that required sutures can be covered with a variety of different dressings. Sutures will generally be removed in 4 to 14 days depending on the site. Sometimes alternating sutures are removed after the third day. Incision lines may require daily cleansing, usually with plain tap water. If necessary, a topical antibiotic is applied, and the wound is either covered with a dry sterile dressing or left open to air. The patient may experience some swelling and discomfort in the first 24 hours during the first phase of wound healing. Ice packs may be applied over the surgical dressing to reduce edema. Mild analgesics such as acetaminophen should control the discomfort. The patient needs to know the manifestations of inflammation, such as redness, fever, or increased pain or swelling, and signs of infection, such as purulent drainage. If these manifestations occur, they should be reported to the health care provider.

■ Psychological Effects of Chronic Dermatological Problems

Emotional stress can occur for persons who suffer from chronic skin problems such as psoriasis, atopic dermatitis, or acne. The sequelae of chronic skin problems can include social and employment problems with subsequent financial implications, a poor self-image, problems with sexuality, and increasing and progressive frustration. The usual lack of overt systemic illness coupled with the visibility of the skin lesions often presents a real problem to the patient.

The nurse must continue to be optimistic and help the patient comply with the prescribed regimen. The patient must be allowed to verbalize the "Why me?" question, even though there is no

ready answer. Reinforcement of the prescribed hygiene and treatment measures is an important part of the teaching plan. Dermatology patient support groups are listed on the CDA Web site. These groups are extremely helpful for patient support and accurate education materials.

Many lesions can be camouflaged with the skillful use of cosmetics. Individual sensitivity to product ingredients must always be considered in the selection of a cosmetic product. Oil-free, hypoallergenic cosmetics are available and can sometimes be beneficial to the allergic patient. Rehabilitative cosmetics are available to help camouflage and de-emphasize such lesions as *vitiligo* (loss of pigmentation), *melasma* (tan to brown patches on the face), or healed postoperative wound sites. These commercially available products are opaque, smudge resistant, and water resistant. In addition to specific skin conditions that tend to chronicity, other factors affecting the outcome of long-term dermatological problems include skin type, history of previous exacerbations, family history, complications, intolerance to therapy, environmental factors, lack of adherence to the prescribed regimen, endocrine factors, and psychological factors. Lesions that follow a chronic pattern often are associated with lichenification and scarring.

■ Physiological Effects of Chronic Dermatological Problems

Scarring and lichenification are the result of chronic dermatological problems. Scars occur when ulceration takes place and reflect the pattern of healing in the area. Scars are pink and vascular at first. With time, they become avascular and white (scars on individuals with darker skin may be hyperpigmented) and increasingly strong. Different regions of the body scar differently, such as the face and neck, which heal fairly well because they are well vascularized. Scar formation is described in Chapter 14.

The location of the scar is the determining factor with respect to its cosmetic implications. Facial scars are the most damaging psychologically because they are so visible. Creative use of cosmetics can do much to mask the scarring of chronic skin conditions. The best treatment is prevention of scarring by control of the problem in the acute phase.

Cosmetic Procedures

The array of cosmetic procedures is vast, indeed, almost limitless. Cosmetic procedures can include chemical peels, toxin injections, collagen fillers, laser surgery, breast augmentation and reduction (see Chapter 54), laser surgery, facelift, eyelid lift, and liposuction. Common cosmetic topical procedures are presented in Table 26-14. Other types of common cosmetic injection procedures include the injection of botulinum toxins (Botox), collagen (Zyplast), and hyaluronic acid fillers (Restylane, Perlane). Transitory adverse effects such as mild redness, pain, swelling, and bruising may occur.

The reasons for undergoing these procedures are as varied as the techniques. The most common reason that people suffer the discomfort and financial expense (most are not covered by insurance) of a cosmetic procedure is to improve their body image. People project their personal image of themselves. If they feel better about themselves after having cosmetic procedures, they

Table 26-14 Common Cosmetic Topical Procedures

TRETINOIN (RETIN-A, RENOVA)	CHEMICAL PEELS	MICRODERMABRASION	ALPHA HYDROXY ACIDS (e.g., GLYCOLIC ACID, LACTIC ACID)
Indications			
Improves appearance of aged and photodamaged skin and the reduction of actinic keratoses	Improves appearance of aged and photodamaged skin, acne scarring, freckles, actinic and seborrheic keratoses	Smoother appearance of photodamaged and wrinkled skin	Similar indications as for microdermabrasion; also called a "minipeel"
Description			
Applied initially every other day, aiming for nightly applications as tolerated; treatment stopped if inflammation is severe; maximum response in 8-12 mo	Solution applied (e.g., solid carbon dioxide, trichloracetic acid) in varying amounts to the skin, causing a controlled burn; loss of melanin occurs	Removal of the epidermis and top dermal layer by application of aluminum oxide or baking soda crystals; re-epithelialization of abraded surface then occurs	Low concentrations (<10%) found in many skin care products that consumers can apply to the skin; higher concentration (50-70%) given only by a health care provider
Adverse Drug Events			
Erythema, swelling, flaking, photosensitivity, hypopigmentation; teratogenic; increases phototoxicity if also taking other photosensitive drugs (see Table 26-3)	Moderate swelling and crusting for 1 wk; redness persisting 6-8 wk; pink tone possible for several months; photosensitivity	Light pink tone that resolves within 24 hr; photosensitivity	Photosensitivity, minimal stinging and redness at lower concentrations; severe redness, oozing, and flaking skin may occur for 1-4 wk at higher concentrations
Patient Teaching			
Apply emollients (e.g., petroleum jelly) and sunscreen (SPF 15 or higher), use sun avoidance measures, avoid use of abrasive or drying facial cleanser if there is severe sensitivity (e.g., excess blistering, peeling); notify health care provider of severe sensitivity	Use sunscreen; avoid sun for 6 mo to prevent hyperpigmentation	Generous application of emollients and sunscreen	Use sunscreen

SPF, sun protection factor.

will often act more confident and self-assured. Often social position and economic considerations are part of the decision. Increased longevity provides a larger population to whom cosmetic procedures are especially appealing.

Regardless of the patient's reasons, the nurse should maintain a supportive, nonjudgemental attitude about these cosmetic procedures. If the patient wishes to change or enhance a body feature perceived as unattractive and has realistic expectations about the outcome, the nurse should support this decision. The reasons for undergoing the surgery are as varied as the techniques.

Body Art and Tattoos

Body art through tattoos and skin piercings is becoming increasingly popular among both genders. A tattoo is a permanent design that is made by injecting dyes into the skin's epidermal layer via a machine that creates tiny skin pricks. There are significant safety risks that are important for the patient to consider before having it done. The risks from unsafe tattooing and piercing include transmission of bloodborne diseases such as human immunodeficiency virus, hepatitis, and skin infections. The following safety guidelines should be followed to decrease the risk of infections: tattoo shop certification by the local public health unit; reputable tattoo artist; good hand hygiene and wearing of gloves; thorough skin disinfection; new disposable razors; new tattooing dye, tattoo and piercing needles; and sterile jewellery.

The patient should be up-to-date with the hepatitis B vaccine. The tattoo dye contains metal and a magnetic resonance imaging scan may not be able to be done over a tattooed site. Educate the patient on how to care for the tattoo and piercing at home in order to minimize infection risk. Important points include: washing hands thoroughly before applying lotions or ointments to the tattooed or pierced area and before rotating jewellery as well as observing for signs of infection (pain, swelling, redness, or high temperature) and allergic reactions. Oral piercings require specific care: careful mouth hygiene (ideal bacterial breeding ground), plastic jewellery because metal chips the teeth, checking for loose pieces that could be a choking risk, and a mouth guard when playing sports (Simcoe Muskoka Health Unit, 2011).

Elective Surgery

Laser Surgery. When a laser beam enters the skin, the light can affect skin structures by scattering, being absorbed, or passing through different layers. The spectrum of clinical application for each laser depends on the depth of the wavelength emitted and the operator technique. Alteration in technique, such as pulse duration and the number of passes over the skin, vary the result (Health Canada, 2004). New handpiece technology with multiple spot size and cooling device additions have also generated new flexibility in laser technology.

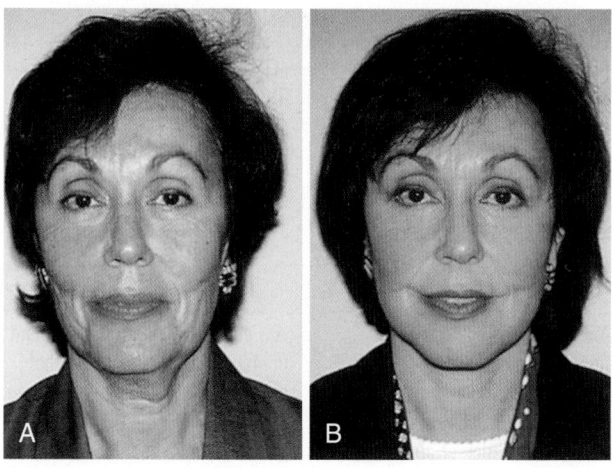

Figure 26-17 Facelift. **A,** Before surgery. **B,** After surgery.

Source: Pastorek, N., & Bustillo, A. (2005). Deep plane face lift. *Facial Plastic Surgery Clinics of North America, 13,* 433-449.

Lasers can reduce fine wrinkles around the lips or eyes and remove facial lesions (see Table 26-13). Swelling, redness, and bruising are common after treatment. The treated areas usually are kept moist with ointment or occlusive dressings (surgical bandages) for the first few days. The treated skin must be protected from the sun.

Facelift. A facelift *(rhytidectomy)* is the lifting and repositioning of the lower two thirds of the face and neck to improve appearance. Indications for this procedure include the following:

1. Redundant soft tissue resulting from disease (e.g., acne scarring).
2. Asymmetrical redundancy of soft tissues (e.g., facial palsy).
3. Redundant soft tissue resulting from trauma.
4. Preauricular lesions.
5. Redundant soft tissues resulting from solar elastosis (sagging of the skin as a result of sun damage), changes in body weight, and the effects of gravity.
6. Restoration of body image.

The surgical approach and the lines of incisions vary according to the nature of the deformity and the position of the hairline. Eyelid lifts *(blepharoplasty)* with similar indications are performed to remove redundant tissue and possibly improve the field of vision. Prevention of hematoma formation is the most important postoperative consideration. Ice packs are usually applied during the first 24 to 48 hours to reduce swelling and decrease the possibility of hematoma formation. Complications can occur if the person smokes or is involved in vigorous exercise. Usually, there is minimal pain. Antibiotics are used at the discretion of the surgeon. Infection is not a common problem (see Figure 26-17).

Liposuction. Liposuction is a technique for removing subcutaneous fat to improve facial and body contours. Although not a substitute for diet and exercise, it can be successful in removing areas of fat from virtually any body area that is resistant to other techniques.

Although relatively free of complications, possible contraindications for the procedure include use of anticoagulants, uncontrolled hypertension, diabetes mellitus, and poor cardiovascular status. Persons younger than 40 years of age with good skin

elasticity are the best candidates. However, patients ranging in age from 16 to 70 years can be treated successfully.

The procedure is usually performed on an outpatient basis with the aid of local anaesthesia. One or more sessions may be necessary, depending on the size of the area to be treated. A blunt-tipped cannula is inserted through a 1.3-cm incision and pushed into the fat to break it loose from the fibrous stroma. Multiple repeated thrusts disrupt the fat and create tunnels. The loosened fat is removed with a powerful suction. The area is taped because firm bandaging helps contour the skin and reduce the chance of postoperative bleeding and fluid accumulation. It may take several months for the final results to be evident.

NURSING MANAGEMENT: COSMETIC SURGERY

Many cosmetic surgical procedures are performed in well-equipped day-surgery units or in office surgery suites. Several nursing interventions are appropriate for the patient who has cosmetic surgery, regardless of where the surgery was done.

Preoperative Management

A major preoperative management consideration relates to informed consent and realistic expectations of what cosmetic surgery can accomplish. Although this information is usually provided by the surgeon, the nurse should reinforce this information and answer questions and concerns. For instance, a facelift has little or no effect on deep wrinkling of the forehead and temples, deep nasolabial grooves, or vertical lip wrinkles. Before- and after-treatment photographs of similar cases are often useful in helping the patient to set realistic expectations.

The nurse's teaching plan should include the time frame for healing. Because the third phase of wound healing does not become complete for 1 year, immediate, complete results should not be anticipated. The oozing, crusting stage of the abrasive procedure must be explained so the patient can plan time off from work if necessary. The final results of the cosmetic procedure are affected by the patient's age, general state of health, extent of procedure, and skin type. If a health problem is present, efforts should be made to correct or control the problem before the procedure is performed.

Postoperative Management

Most of the cosmetic procedures are not extremely painful. Usually, mild analgesics are sufficient to keep the patient comfortable.

Although infection is not a common problem after cosmetic surgery, the nurse should assess the surgical sites for signs of infection. Inform the patient of signs of infection and tell him or her to report any such signs and symptoms immediately so that appropriate antibiotic intervention can be started.

If the surgery involved alteration in the circulation to the skin, such as in a facelift, a careful monitoring of adequate circulation is necessary. Warm, pink skin that blanches on pressure indicates that adequate circulation is present in the surgical area. Supportive, compressed dressings and ice packs may be necessary early in the postoperative period.

Skin Grafts

Uses

Skin grafts may be necessary to provide protection to underlying structures or to reconstruct areas for functional or cosmetic purposes. Ideally, wounds heal by primary intention. However, large surgically created wounds, trauma, and chronic wounds can cause extensive tissue destruction, making primary intention healing impossible. In these cases, skin grafting may be necessary to close the defect. Improved surgical techniques make it possible to graft skin, bone, cartilage, fat, fascia, muscles, and nerves. For cosmetically pleasing results, the colour, thickness, texture, and hair-growing nature of skin used for grafting must be chosen to match the recipient site. (Skin grafting is discussed in Chapter 27.)

Types

The two types of skin grafts are free grafts and skin flaps. Free grafts are further classified according to the method of providing a blood supply to the grafted skin. One method is to transfer the graft (epidermis and part or all of the dermis) to the recipient site from the donor site. If the graft is an *autograft* (from the patient's own body) or an *isograft* (from an identical twin), it will revascularize and become fixed to the new site. Chapter 27 discusses full- and split-thickness skin grafts in detail. Another method of free skin grafting is by *reconstructive microsurgery*. With the use of an operating microscope, circulation is immediately established in the free flap by anastomosis of the blood vessels from the skin flap to the vessels in the recipient site.

Skin flaps involve moving a section of skin and subcutaneous tissue from one part of the body to another without terminating the vascular attachment. The vascular attachment is called a *pedicle*.

Skin flaps are used to cover wounds with a poor vascular bed, when padding is needed, and to cover wounds over cartilage and bone. There may be a need for intermediate flap placement if the recipient site is far removed from the donor site. For instance, a skin flap from the thigh to the head would require an intermediate graft. The flap is advanced to the recipient site when circulation is well established at the intermediate site. The type of flap and the route of transfer are determined according to the needs of the patient and the nature of the defect to be repaired.

Soft tissue expansion is a technique for providing skin for resurfacing a defect, such as a burn scar; for removing a disfiguring mark, such as a tattoo; or as a preliminary step in breast reconstruction. A subcutaneous tissue expander of an appropriate size and shape is placed under the skin, usually as an outpatient procedure. Weekly expansion with saline solution can be done in a health care setting or by the patient at home. This expansion procedure is repeated until the skin reaches the size needed for the repair. This may take from several weeks to 3 to 4 months. Once sufficient skin is available, the old incision is opened, the expander is removed, and the soft tissue is ready to be used as an advancement flap. The tissue expander next to a defect retains the primary tissue characteristics such as colour and texture.

CLINICAL DECISION-MAKING EXERCISE

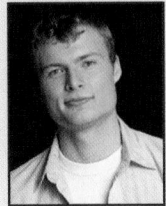

CASE STUDY:
Malignant Melanoma and Dysplastic Nevi

Justin Horrocks/iStockphoto

Patient Profile

Michel Dufault, 37, is a White, fair-skinned, blue-eyed park ranger who enjoys fishing and river rafting. He comes to the clinic for evaluation of a changing mole.

Subjective Data

- History of a mole on his left lower leg from birth that has become scaly, hard, and lumpy over the last 3 months
- Father and older sister treated for malignant melanoma in the last 10 years
- Anxious that the mole might be cancer and necessitate extensive disfiguring surgery

Objective Data

Physical Examination

- Has a 6-mm nevus, blue-black in colour, scalloped with vaguely defined borders
- Has a large number of small nevi (>50) on back, legs, and arms
- Two dysplastic nevi found on back

Diagnostic Studies

- Excisional biopsy confirmed malignant melanoma
- Further diagnostic tests indicate the melanoma is stage 0

Discussion Questions

1. What risk factors for malignant melanoma does this patient have?
2. What manifestations does the patient show that are usually associated with malignant melanoma?
3. What is the prognosis for a patient with this stage of malignant melanoma?
4. What treatment options are there for this patient?
5. How would the nurse address Mr. Dufault regarding his anxiety over the treatment outcomes?
6. *Priority Decision:* What is the priority of care for Mr. Dufault?
7. What would the nurse include in a patient teaching plan to address future sun exposure for this patient?
8. *Priority Decision:* Based on the assessment data presented, what are the priority nursing diagnoses? Are there any collaborative problems?

evolve *Answers are available at* **http://evolve.elsevier.com/ Canada/Lewis/medsurg**

REVIEW QUESTIONS

The number of the question corresponds to the same-numbered objective at the beginning of the chapter.

1. Which of the following should be contained in the sunscreen that the nurse advises a patient with photosensitivity to use?
   a. Cinnamates
   b. Benzophenones
   c. Methyl anthranilate
   d. PABA (para-aminobenzoic acid)

2. What should the nurse teach a patient who is using topical corticosteroids to treat an acute dermatitis?
   a. The cream form is the most efficient system of delivery.
   b. Topical low-potency corticosteroids can cause systemic adverse effects.
   c. Creams and ointments should be applied with a glove in small amounts to prevent further infection.
   d. Abruptly discontinuing the use of topical corticosteroids will cause a reappearance of the dermatitis.

3. A patient with psoriasis tells the nurse that she has quit her job as a receptionist because she feels her appearance is disgusting to customers. Which of the following nursing diagnoses best describes this patient's response?
   a. Ineffective coping related to lack of social support
   b. Impaired skin integrity related to presence of lesions
   c. Anxiety related to lack of knowledge of the disease process
   d. Social isolation related to decreased activities secondary to fear of rejection

4. The nurse is teaching a patient with malignant melanoma about this disorder. What is the prognosis of the patient most dependent on?
   a. The thickness of the lesion
   b. The degree of colour change in the lesion
   c. How much superficial spread the lesion has
   d. The amount of ulceration present in the lesion

5. Which of the following disorders is the patient most at risk of spreading?
   a. Tinea pedis
   b. Impetigo on the face
   c. Candidiasis of the nails
   d. Psoriasis on the palms and soles

6. A mother and her two children have been diagnosed with pediculosis corporis at a health centre. Which of the following is an appropriate measure in treating this condition?
   a. Washing the body with pyrethrins
   b. Topical application of griseofulvin
   c. Moist compresses applied frequently
   d. Administration of systemic antibiotics

7. What is a common site for the lesions associated with atopic dermatitis?
   a. Buttocks
   b. Temporal area
   c. Antecubital space
   d. Palmar surface of the feet

8. During assessment of a patient, the nurse notes an area of red, sharply defined plaques covered with silvery scales that are mildly itchy on the patient's knee and elbow. Which of the following is the correct finding?
   a. Lentigo
   b. Psoriasis
   c. Actinic keratoses
   d. Seborrheic keratoses

9. What would a dermatological manifestation of Cushing's syndrome include?
   a. Telangiectasia
   b. Thickened skin
   c. Increased sweating
   d. Generalized hyperpigmentation

10. Which of the following is an important patient teaching after a chemical peel?
    a. Avoidance of sun exposure
    b. Application of firm bandages
    c. Limitation of vigorous exercise
    d. Use of mild heat to prevent drying

ANSWERS: 1. b; 2. d; 3. d; 4. a; 5. b; 6. a; 7. c; 8. b; 9. a; 10. a.

REFERENCES

Canadian Cancer Society. (2012a). Skin: Nonmelanoma. *Canadian cancer encyclopedia.* Retrieved from *http://info.cancer.ca/E/CCE/cceexplorer.asp?tocid=47*

Canadian Cancer Society. (2012b). Skin: Melanoma. *Canadian cancer encyclopedia.* Retrieved from *http://info.cancer.ca/E/CCE/cceexplorer.asp?tocid=46*

Canadian Cancer Society's Steering Committee on Cancer Statistics. (2011). *Canadian Cancer Statistics 2011.* Toronto, ON: Canadian Cancer Society. Retrieved from *http://www.cancer.ca/Canada-wide/About%20cancer/Cancer%20statistics/~/media/CCS/Canada%20wide/Files%20List/English%20files%20heading/PDF%20-%20Policy%20-%20Canadian%20Cancer%20Statistics%20-%20English/Canadian%20Cancer%20Statistics%202011%20-%20English.ashx*

Canadian Dermatology Association (CDA). (2000). *Position statement on the use of self-tanning creams.* Retrieved from *www.dermatology.ca/english/public-patients/positions_e.html#self*

Canadian Dermatology Association (CDA). (2008). *UV index.* Retrieved from *www.dermatology.ca*

Canadian Dermatology Association (CDA). (2011a). *Sun safety for outdoor workers.* Retrieved from *http://www.dermatology.ca/outdoorworkers.html*

Canadian Dermatology Association (CDA). (2011b). *Indoor tanning is out.* Retrieved from *http://www.dermatology.ca/indoortanning/index.html*

Canadian Dermatology Association (CDA). (2011c). *Canadian Dermatology Association 2011 melanoma fact sheet.* Retrieved from *http://www.dermatology.ca/wp-content/uploads/2012/01/2011-Melanoma-Factsheet-EN.pdf*

Canadian Dermatology Association (CDA). (2011d). *Canadian Dermatology Association 2011 skin cancer fact sheet.* Retrieved from *http://www.dermatology.ca/wp-content/uploads/2012/01/2011-Skin-Cancer-Stats-EN.pdf*

Canadian Dermatology Association (CDA). (2011e). *Psoriasis.* Retrieved from *http://www.dermatology.ca/skin-hair-nails/skin/psoriasis/#!/skin-hair-nails/skin/psoriasis/living-with-psoriasis/*

Canadian Dermatology Association (CDA). (2012). *It doesn't hurt to ask: @CdnDermatology releases new video on laser hair removal.* Retrieved from *http://www.dermatology.ca/wp-content/uploads/2012/06/2012-Laser-video-Media-RELEASE.pdf*

Graham-Robin, R., Bourke, J., & Cunliffe. T. (2008). *Dermatology: Fundamentals of practice.* Edinburgh: Royal College of General Practitioners, Elsevier.

Health Canada. (2004). *It's your health: Laser cosmetic treatments.* Retrieved from: *http://www.hc-sc.gc.ca/hl-vs/iyh-vsv/med/laser-eng.php*

Health Canada. (2005). *Guidelines for tanning salon owners, operators and users.* Retrieved from *www.hc-sc.gc.ca/ewh-semt/pubs/radiation/tan-bronzage/index_e.html*

Health Canada. (2008). *Healthy living: The UV index and your local forecast.* Retrieved from *http://www.hc-sc.gc.ca/hl-vs/sun-sol/protect-protegez/index-uv-indice-eng.php*

Health Canada. (2010a). *It's your health: Sunscreens.* Retrieved from *http://www.hc-sc.gc.ca/hl-vs/iyh-vsv/life-vie/sun_soleil-eng.php*

Health Canada. (2010b). *It's your health: Sunglasses.* Retrieved from *www.hc-sc.gc.ca/hl-vs/iyh-vsv/prod/glasses-lunettes-eng.php*

Health Canada. (2010c). *Med effects Canada. Adverse reaction database.* Retrieved from *www.hc-sc.gc.ca/dhp-mps/medeff/databasdon/instructions-eng.php*

Howlader, N., Noone, A. M., Krapcho, M., Neyman, N., Aminou, R., Waldron, W., …, Edwards, B. K. (Eds.). (2011). *SEER cancer statistics review, 1975-2008.* National Cancer Institute. Retrieved from *http://seer.cancer.gov/csr/1975_2008/*, based on November 2010 SEER data submission, posted to the SEER Web site, 2011.

Ogden, N. H., Robbin, L., Muhammad, M., Sockett, P. N., & Artsob, H. (2009). The emergence of Lyme disease in Canada. *CMAJ, 180(12)*, 1221-1224. doi:10.1503/cmaj.080148

Simcoe Muskoka Heath Unit. (2011). *Tattooing and piercing: Make it safe.* Retrieved from *http://www.simcoemuskokahealth.org/Topics/SexualHealth/NeedlesSharps/TattooingAndPiercing.aspx*

Snow, M. (2008). Fighting fungal infections: Stopping tinea in its tracks. *Nursing, 38(7)*, 62-63. Retrieved from *http://www.nursingcenter.com/pdf.asp?AID=800828*

Tope, W. D., & Bhardwaj, S. S. (2008). Photodynamic therapy. In J. L. Bolognia, J. L. Jorizzo, & R. P. Rapini (Eds.), *Dermatology* (2nd ed., pp. 2071-2080). St. Louis: Mosby Elsevier.

CANADIAN RESOURCES

Canadian Cancer Society
  http://www.cancer.ca
Canadian Dermatology Association
  http://www.dermatology.ca
Canadian Dermatology Foundation
  http://www.cdf.ca
Canadian Dermatology Nurses Association
  http://www.cdernurse.org
Canadian Melanoma Foundation
  http://www.derm.ubc.ca/division/cmf/cmf1.htm
Canadian Skin Patient Alliance
  http://www.skinpatientalliance.ca/skin-conditions-diseases/vitiligo
Canadian Society of Plastic Surgeons
  http://www.plasticsurgery.ca
Canadian Society of Plastic Surgery Nurses
  http://www.cspsn.org/pdfs
Derm Web
University of British Columbia, Division of Dermatology Web site
  http://www.derm.ubc.ca
Eczema Society of Canada
  http://www.eczemahelp.ca
Lupus Canada
  http://www.lupuscanada.org
Melanoma Network
  http://www.melanomanetwork.ca
Psoriasis Society of Canada
  http://www.psoriasissociety.org
Rosacea Awareness Program
  http://www.rosaceainfo.com
Save Your Skin Foundation
  http://www.saveyourskin.ca
Scleroderma Society of Canada
  http://www.scleroderma.ca/

RELATED RESOURCES

AcneNet
  http://www.derm-infonet.com/acnenet/index.html
American Academy of Dermatology
  http://www.aad.org
American Academy of Facial Plastic and Reconstructive Surgery
  http://www.aafprs.org/
American Society of Plastic and Reconstructive Surgical Nurses
  https://www.aspsn.org/
Dermatology Foundation
  http://www.dermfnd.org

evolve   *For additional Internet resources, see the Web site for this book* at **http://evolve.elsevier.com/Canada/Lewis/medsurg**

Written by Judy A. Knighton
Adapted by Jackie Hartigan-Rogers

LEARNING OBJECTIVES

1. Explain the causes of burn injuries and prevention strategies.
2. Differentiate between partial- and full-thickness burns.
3. Apply the parameters used to determine the severity of burns.
4. Compare the pathophysiological processes, clinical manifestations, complications, and collaborative management throughout the three burn phases.
5. Compare the fluid and electrolyte shifts during the emergent and the acute burn phases.
6. Differentiate the nutritional needs of the patient with a burn injury throughout the three burn phases.

7. Compare the various burn wound care techniques and surgical options for partial-thickness versus full-thickness burn wounds.
8. Prioritize nursing interventions in the management of the physiological and psychosocial needs of the patient throughout the three burn phases.
9. Examine the various physiological and psychosocial aspects of burn rehabilitation.
10. Design a plan of care to prepare the burn patient and family for discharge.

KEY TERMS

burn Injury to the tissues of the body caused by heat, chemicals, electric current, or radiation, p. 581

chemical burns Result from tissue injury and destruction from acids, alkalis, and organic compounds, p. 581

contracture An abnormal, usually permanent condition of a joint, characterized by flexion and fixation, p. 602

cultured epithelial autograft Skin grafts grown from biopsy specimens obtained from the patient's own skin, p. 599

debridement Removal of necrotic tissue from a wound to prevent infection and promote healing, p. 593

electrical burns Result from intense heat generated from an electric current, p. 582

escharotomy Incision into necrotic tissue from a severe burn performed when eschar formation compromises circulation, p. 590

excision and grafting Procedure during which eschar is removed down to the subcutaneous tissue or fascia, depending on the degree of injury, and a graft is then placed on clean, viable tissue to achieve good adherence, p. 598

full-thickness burn Destruction of all skin elements and subcutaneous tissues, with possible involvement of muscles, tendons, and bones, p. 584

partial-thickness burn Varying degrees of epidermal and dermal skin injury in which some skin elements remain viable for regeneration, p. 584

smoke and inhalation injuries Damage to the tissues of the respiratory tract as a result of the inhalation of hot air or noxious chemicals, p. 581

thermal burns Burns caused by flame, flash, scald, or contact with hot objects, p. 581

ELECTRONIC RESOURCES

Supplemental content related to Chapter 27 can be found…

Evolve Web Site ⊝volve

- Answer Guidelines for Case Study on p. 604
- Clinical Reference: Laboratory Values
- Content Updates

- Electronic Calculators
- eNCP 27-1: Thermal Burn Injury
- Examination Review Questions
- Glossary
- Interactive Case Study: Burns
- Key Points (Printable and MP3 Download)

A burn is an injury to the tissues of the body caused by heat, chemicals, electrical current, or radiation. The resulting effects are influenced by the temperature of the burning agent, the duration of contact time, and the type of tissue that is injured.

According to data collected from three Canadian burn centres, the majority of patients with burns (85%) who receive specialized burn care suffered injuries as a result of exposure to fire or flames (54%), scalds (25%), and electrical injuries (6%; American Burn Association, 2011). Unfortunately, there is a lack of data on Canadian burn-injured patients (Burton, Sharma, Harrop, & Lindsay, 2009).

Although burn incidence has decreased over the past several decades, burn injuries are still numerous, and most should be viewed as preventable (Taira et al., 2011). Future prevention initiatives need to focus on behaviours that lead to increased risk, such as supervision of young children by older siblings, playing with fire, cooking, and fire-related dangers (Taira et al., 2011). The focus of burn prevention programs has shifted from concentrating on individual blame and changing individual behaviours to include more legislative changes. The aim of these changes is to make improvements in the environment. Coordinated national programs include child-resistant lighters, nonflammable children's clothing, tap water antiscalding devices, stricter building codes, hardwired smoke detectors and alarms, and fire sprinklers. Nurses can advocate for burn risk reduction strategies in the home. Occupational health nurses can also educate workers to reduce the incidence of burn injuries in the work setting (Tables 27-1 and 27-2).

Types of Burn Injury

Thermal Burns

Thermal burns are burns caused by flame, flash fire, scalding, or contact with hot objects. They are the most common type of burn injury (Figure 27-1; see Table 27-2).

Chemical Burns

Chemical burns result from tissue injury and destruction from acids, alkalis, and organic compounds. In addition to skin damage, eyes can be injured if they are splashed with a chemical. Acids are found in many household cleaners and include hydrochloric, oxalic, and hydrofluoric acid. Alkali burns can be more difficult to manage than acid burns because alkaline substances

Table 27-1 Common Locations and Sources of Burn Injury	
Occupational Hazards	**Home**
• Tar	**Kitchen and Bathroom**
• Chemicals	• Microwaved food
• Hot metals	• Hot water heaters set at 60°C or higher
• Steam pipes	
• Combustible fuels	• Steam, hot grease, or liquids from cooking
• Fertilizers and pesticides	**General Household**
• Electricity from power lines	• Fireplaces (gas, wood)
• Sparks from live electric sources	• Open space heaters
	• Frayed or defective wiring
	• Radiators (home, automobile)
	• Outdoor grills (propane, charcoal)
	• Multiple extension cords per outlet
	• Carelessness with cigarettes, matches, candles
	• Flammable liquids (e.g., starter fluid, gasoline, kerosene)

are not neutralized by tissue fluids as readily as are acid substances. Alkalis adhere to tissue, causing protein hydrolysis and liquefaction. Alkalis are found in oven and drain cleaners, fertilizers, and heavy industrial cleaners. Organic compounds, including phenols and petroleum products, produce contact burns and systemic toxicity. Phenols are found in chemical disinfectants; petroleum products include creosote and gasoline.

Smoke and Inhalation Injury

Smoke and inhalation injuries are damage to the tissues of the respiratory tract that result from the inhalation of hot air or noxious chemicals. Fortunately, gases are cooled to body temperature before they reach the lung tissue. Although damage to the respiratory mucosa can occur, it seldom happens because the vocal cords and glottis close as a protective mechanism. Redness and airway swelling (edema) may result when damage occurs. Because smoke inhalation injuries are a major predictor of mortality in burn-injured patients, a rapid assessment is critical (Mlcak, Suman, & Herndon, 2007).

Table 27-2 Types of Burn Injury and Risk Reduction Strategies	
TYPES	**RISK REDUCTION STRATEGIES**
Flame or contact	• Never leave candles unattended or near open windows or curtains. • Encourage use of "child-resistant" lighters. • Encourage use of home fire exit drills. • Never use gasoline or other flammable liquids as accelerants. • Never leave hot oil unattended while cooking. • Never smoke in bed. • Consider a flame-retardant smoking apron for older adults and "at-risk" people. • Exercise caution when microwaving food and beverages.
Inhalation	• Install smoke and carbon monoxide detectors.
Electrical	• Avoid and/or repair frayed wiring. • Ensure electrical power source is shut off before beginning repairs. • Wear protective eyewear and gloves when conducting electrical repairs. • Avoid outdoor activities during electrical (i.e., lightning) storms.
Scald	• Lower hot water temperature to the "lowest point" or 40°C. • Use antiscalding devices with showerhead or faucet fixtures. • Supervise bathing with small children, older adults, or anyone whose physical movement, physical sensation, or judgement is impaired. • After running bath water, check temperature with hand or with bath thermometer.
Chemical	• Store chemicals safely in approved containers, and label clearly. • Ensure safety of workers, students handling chemicals (education, protective eyewear, gloves, masks, clothing).

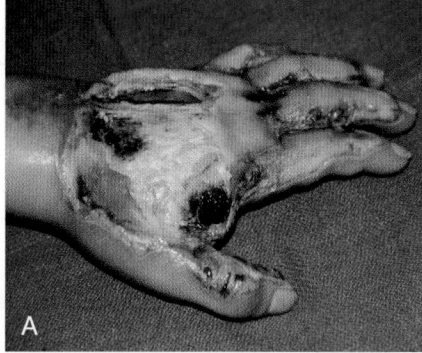
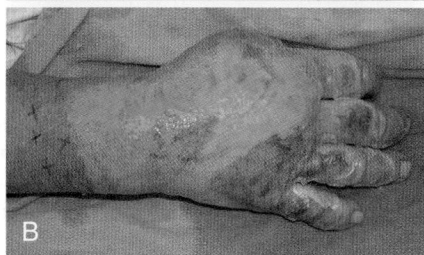
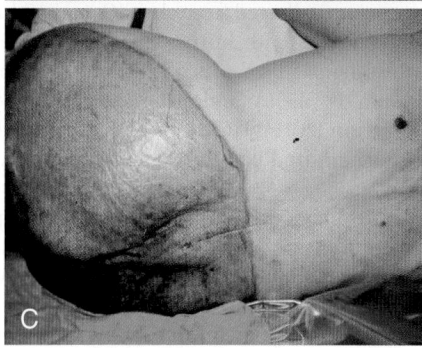

Figure 27-1 Types of burn injury. **A,** Full-thickness thermal burn. **B,** Partial-thickness thermal burn. **C,** Full-thickness scalding burn secondary to immersion in hot water.

Source: Courtesy Judy A. Knighton, RN, MScN, Toronto.

There are three types of smoke and inhalation injuries:

1. *Carbon monoxide poisoning.* Carbon monoxide poisoning and asphyxiation account for the majority of deaths at a fire scene. Carbon monoxide is produced by the incomplete combustion of burning materials. It is subsequently inhaled and displaces oxygen (O_2) on the hemoglobin molecule, causing carboxyhemoglobinemia, hypoxia, and, when the carbon monoxide levels exceed 20%, death. With severe carbon monoxide poisoning, skin colour is often described as "cherry red" in appearance. Carbon monoxide poisoning may occur in the absence of burn injury to the skin (e.g., smoke inhalation during a fire).

2. *Inhalation injury above the glottis.* In general, an inhalation injury above the glottis (*upper airway injury*) is thermally produced and may be caused by the inhalation of hot air, steam, or smoke. Mucosal burns of the oropharynx and larynx are manifested by redness, blistering, and edema. Mechanical obstruction can occur quickly, which represents a true medical emergency. Clues to the occurrence of this injury include the presence of facial burns, singed nasal hair, hoarseness, painful swallowing, darkened oral and nasal membranes, carbonaceous sputum, history of being burned in an enclosed space, and clothing burns around the chest and neck.

3. *Inhalation injury below the glottis.* An inhalation injury below the glottis (*lower airway injury*) is usually chemically produced. Tissue damage is related to the duration of exposure to smoke or toxic fumes. Clinical manifestations such as pulmonary edema may not appear until 12 to 24 hours after the burn, and then they may manifest as acute respiratory distress syndrome (see Chapter 70).

Electrical Burns

Electrical burns are the result of intense heat generated from an electric current (Figure 27-2). Direct damage to nerves and vessels, causing tissue anoxia and tissue death, can also occur. The severity of the electrical injury depends on the amount of voltage, tissue resistance, current pathways, amount of surface area in contact with the current, and length of time that the current

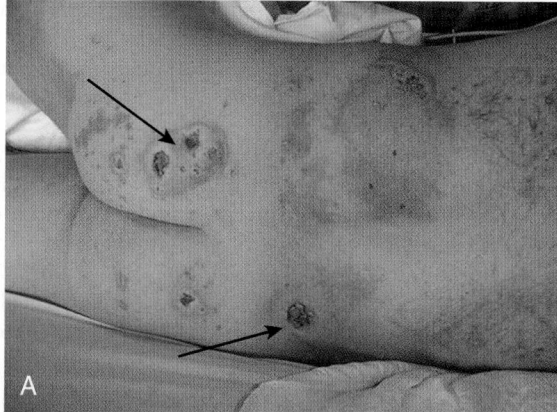

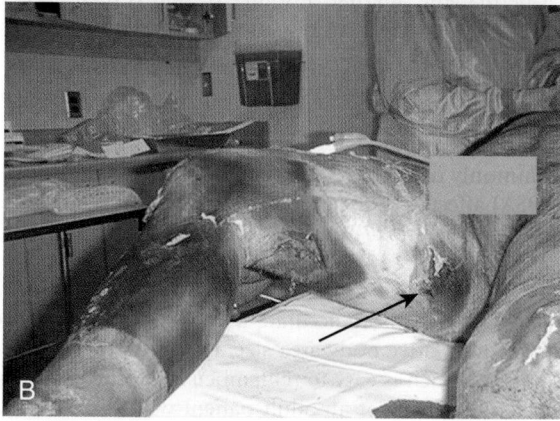

Figure 27-2 Electrical injury produces heat coagulation of blood supply and contact area as electric current passes through the skin. **A,** Electrical injury to the back and buttock. **B,** Electrical injury to the leg.

Source: Courtesy Judy A. Knighton, RN, MScN, Toronto.

---

flow was sustained. Tissue densities offer various amounts of resistance to electric current. For example, fat and bone offer the most resistance, whereas nerves and blood vessels offer the least resistance. Current that passes through vital organs (e.g., brain, heart, kidneys) produces more life-threatening sequelae than does current that passes through other tissues. In addition, electric sparks may ignite the patient's clothing, causing a combination of thermal and electrical injury.

As with inhalation injury, the patient with electrical injury must be assessed rapidly. Transfer to a burn unit is indicated. The severity of an electrical injury can be difficult to determine inasmuch as most of the damage is below the skin (the "iceberg effect"). Determination of electric current contact points and history of the injury may help determine the probable path of the current and potential areas of injury. Contact with electric current can cause muscle contractions strong enough to fracture the long bones and the vertebrae. Another reason to suspect long bone or spinal fractures is a fall resulting from the electrical injury. For this reason, all patients with electrical burns should be considered at risk for a potential cervical spine injury. Cervical spine immobilization must be used during transport and subsequent diagnostic testing to confirm or rule out any injury.

Electrical injury puts the patient at risk for dysrhythmias or cardiac arrest, severe metabolic acidosis, and myoglobinuria, which can lead to acute tubular necrosis. The electric shock event

Table 27-3 Criteria for Transfer of the Patient With Burn Injuries

Patients with the following burn injuries should be referred to a burn unit:

- Combination partial- and full-thickness burns of 10% or more in children <10 years or adults >50 years
- Combination partial- and full-thickness burns >20% in other age-group (>10 and <50 years)
- Full-thickness burns ≥5% of body surface (any age)
- Partial- and full-thickness burns of face, eyes, ears, hands, feet, genitalia, or perineum or over major joints
- Circumferential chest or extremity burns
- Any inhalation injury, high voltage electrical burns, lightning, significant chemical burns
- Any patient requiring social or emotional counselling services
- Presence of pre-existing illness that may complicate recovery (e.g., diabetes mellitus)

Source: *Clinical Practice Guidelines for Nurses in Primary Care.* Health Canada. Reviewed July 2011. Reproduced with permission from the Minister of Health, 2012. Retrieved from *http://www.hc-sc.gc.ca/ fniah-spnia/services/nurs-infirm/clini/adult/skin-peau-eng.php*

can cause immediate cardiac standstill or ventricular fibrillation. Delayed cardiac dysrhythmias or arrest may also occur without warning during the first 24 hours after injury.

Myoglobin from injured muscle tissue and hemoglobin from damaged red blood cells (RBCs) are released into the circulation whenever massive muscle and blood vessel damage occurs. The released myoglobin pigments are then transported to the kidneys, where they can mechanically block the renal tubules because of their large size. This process can result in acute tubular necrosis and eventual acute renal failure if not appropriately treated (see Chapter 49).

Cold Thermal Injury

Cold thermal injury, or frostbite, is discussed in Chapter 71.

Classification of Burn Injury

The treatment of burns is related to the severity of the injury. Severity is determined by (a) depth of burn, (b) extent of burn calculated in percentage of total body surface area, (c) location of burn, and (d) patient risk factors. Health Canada has established referral criteria that recommend which burn injuries should be treated in burn units, in which specialized facilities and personnel are available for handling this type of trauma (Table 27-3). The majority of patients with minor burn injuries that do not necessitate referral can be managed in community hospitals by non–burn unit personnel on an outpatient basis. Goals of care include wound healing, prevention of infection, pain management, prevention of complications, and return to preinjury function.

Depth of Burn

Burn injury involves the destruction of the integumentary system. The skin is divided into three layers: the epidermis, the dermis, and subcutaneous tissue (Figure 27-3). The *epidermis*, or nonvascular outer layer of the skin, is approximately as thick as a sheet of paper. It is composed of many layers of nonliving epithelial cells that provide a protective barrier to the skin, hold in fluids and electrolytes, help regulate body temperature, and keep harmful agents in the external environment from injuring or invading the body. The *dermis*, which lies below the epidermis, is approximately 30 to 45 times thicker than the epidermis. The dermis contains connective tissues with blood vessels and highly specialized structures consisting of hair follicles, nerve endings, sweat glands, and sebaceous glands. Under the

dermis lies the *subcutaneous tissue*, which contains major vascular networks, fat, nerves, and lymphatic vessels. The subcutaneous tissue acts as a heat insulator for underlying structures, which include the muscles, tendons, bones, and internal organs.

Burns have been and continue to be defined by degrees: first-, second-, third-, and fourth-degree burns. The American Burn Association recommends a more precise definition of burns, classifying them according to depth of skin destruction: **partial-thickness burn** and **full-thickness burn** (see Figure 27-3). Skin-reproducing (re-epithelializing) cells are located throughout the dermis and along the shafts of the hair follicles and sebaceous glands. If there is significant damage to the dermis (e.g., a full-thickness burn), not enough skin cells remain to regenerate new skin. A permanent, alternative source of skin is then needed. In Table 27-4, the various burn classifications are compared according to the depth of injury.

Extent of Burn

Two commonly used guides for determining the *total body surface area* (TBSA) affected or the extent of a burn wound are the *Lund-Browder chart* (Figure 27-4, *A*) and the *rule-of-nines chart* (Figure 27-4, *B*). (First-degree burns, equivalent to a sunburn, are not included when TBSA burned is calculated.) The Lund-Browder chart is considered more accurate because the patient's age, in proportion to relative body-area size, is taken into account. The rule of nines, which is easy to remember, is considered adequate for initial assessment of an adult patient with burn injury. For irregular or odd-shaped burns, the patient's hand (including the fingers) is approximately 1% of TBSA.

An additional tool is the *Sage Burn Diagram*, a free, Internet-based tool available for estimating TBSA burned (see the Resources at the end of this chapter). The extent of a burn is often revised after edema has subsided and demarcation of the zones of injury have occurred.

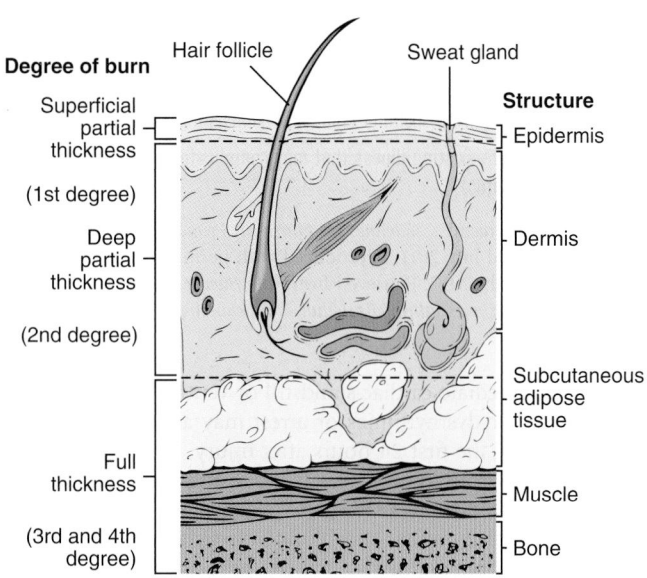

Figure 27-3 Illustration of cross-section of skin, indicating the depth of burn and structures involved.

Table 27-4 Classification of Burn Injury Depth			
CLASSIFICATION	**CLINICAL APPEARANCE**	**POSSIBLE CAUSE**	**STRUCTURES INVOLVED**
Partial-Thickness Skin Destruction			
Superficial: first-degree burn	Erythema, blanching on pressure, pain and mild swelling, no vesicles or blisters (although after 24 hr, skin may blister and peel)	Superficial sunburn Quick heat flash	Superficial epidermal damage with hyperemia; tactile and pain sensation intact
Deep: second-degree burn	Fluid-filled vesicles that are red, shiny, wet (if vesicles have ruptured); severe pain caused by nerve injury; mild to moderate edema	Flame Flash Scalding Contact burns Chemical burns Tar Electric current	Epidermis and dermis involved to varying depth; skin elements, from which epithelial regeneration occurs, remain viable
Full-Thickness Skin Destruction			
Third- and fourth-degree burns	Dry, waxy white, leathery, or hard skin; visible thrombosed vessels; insensitivity to pain because of nerve destruction; possible involvement of muscles, tendons, and bones	Flame Scalding Chemical burns Tar Electric current	All skin elements and local nerve endings destroyed; coagulation necrosis present; surgical intervention for healing

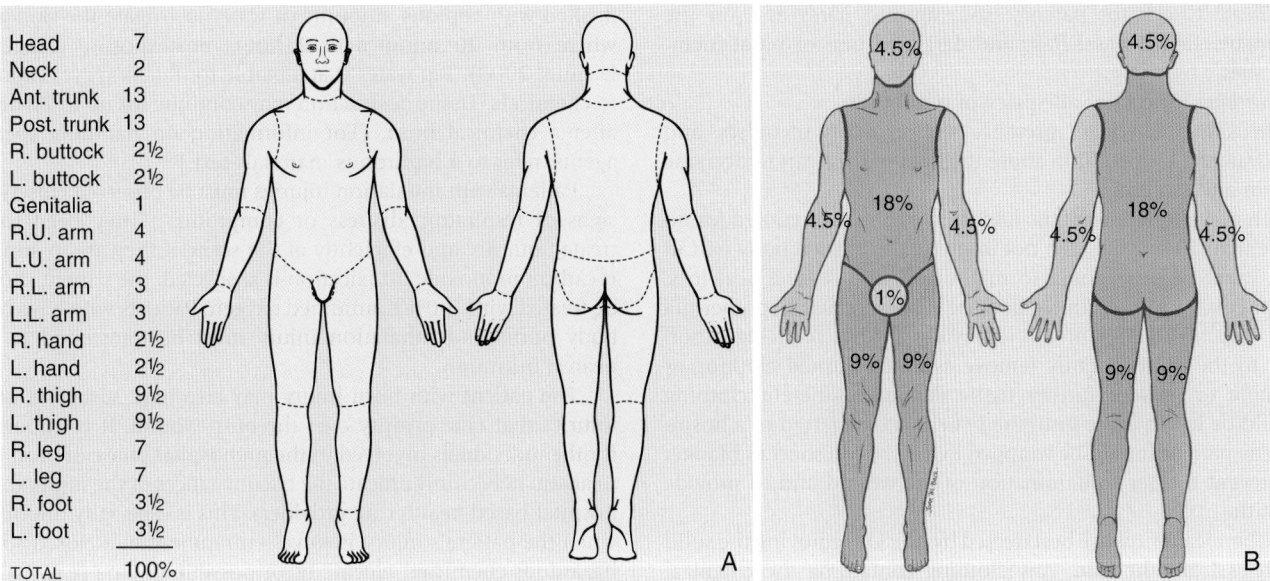

Head	7
Neck	2
Ant. trunk	13
Post. trunk	13
R. buttock	2½
L. buttock	2½
Genitalia	1
R.U. arm	4
L.U. arm	4
R.L. arm	3
L.L. arm	3
R. hand	2½
L. hand	2½
R. thigh	9½
L. thigh	9½
R. leg	7
L. leg	7
R. foot	3½
L. foot	3½
TOTAL	100%

Figure 27-4 A, Lund-Browder chart. By convention, when filling out this chart, the examiner colours areas of partial-thickness injury in blue and areas of full-thickness injury in red. Superficial partial-thickness burns are not calculated. **B,** Rule-of-nines chart. *Ant.,* anterior; *L.,* left; *L.L.,* left lower; *L.U.,* left upper; *Post.,* posterior; *R.,* right; *R.L.,* right lower; *R.U.,* right upper.

Source: Rothrock, J. C. (2007). *Alexander's care of the patient in surgery* (13th ed.). St. Louis: Mosby.

Location of Burn

The severity of the burn injury is related to the location of the burn wound. Burns to the face and neck and circumferential burns to the chest or back can result in mechanical obstruction secondary to edema or leathery, devitalized tissue formation (*eschar*), which may inhibit respiratory function. These injuries may also include possible inhalation injury and respiratory mucosal damage.

Burns of the hands, feet, joints, and eyes are of concern because they make self-care very difficult and may jeopardize future function. Burns of the hands and the feet are challenging to manage because of superficial vascular and nerve supply systems and the need to maintain their function during healing.

Burns to the ears and the nose are susceptible to infection because of poor blood supply to the cartilage. Burns to the buttocks or perineum are highly susceptible to infection. Circumferential burns to the extremities can cause circulatory compromise distal to the burn and, subsequently, neurological impairment of the affected extremity. Patients may also develop compartment syndrome (see Chapter 65) from direct heat damage to the muscles; edema may result, and preburn vascular problems can be exacerbated.

Patient Risk Factors

The older adult heals more slowly and usually experiences more difficulty with rehabilitation than a younger adult. Any patient with pre-existing cardiovascular, respiratory, or renal disease has a poorer prognosis for recovery because of the tremendous demands placed on the body by a burn injury. The patient with diabetes mellitus or peripheral vascular disease is at high risk for poor healing and gangrene, especially with foot and leg burns. General physical debilitation from any chronic disease—including alcoholism, drug abuse, or malnutrition—renders the patient less physiologically able to recover from a burn injury. In addition,

the patient with a burn injury who has concurrently sustained other injuries—fractures, head injuries, or other trauma—has a poorer prognosis for recovery.

Phases of Burn Management

Historically, burn management has been organized chronologically into three phases that correspond to the key priority of each particular phase: emergent (resuscitative), acute (wound healing), and rehabilitative (restorative). The care overlaps from one phase to another. For example, although the emergent phase is seen as beginning in the emergency department, care often begins in the prehospital phase, depending on the skill level of paramedics at the scene. Planning for rehabilitation begins on the day of the burn injury or admission to the burn unit. Formal rehabilitation begins as soon as functional assessment can be performed. Wound care is the primary focus of the acute phase, but it also takes place in both the emergent and rehabilitative phases.

Prehospital Care

At the scene of the injury, priority is given to removing the person from the source of the burn and stopping the burning process. Rescuers must also protect themselves from being injured. In the case of electrical injuries, initial management involves removal of the patient from contact with the electric source.

Small thermal burns (<10% of TBSA) should be covered with a clean, cool, tap water–dampened towel for the patient's comfort and protection until definitive medical care is instituted. Cooling of the injured area (if small) within 1 minute helps minimize the depth of the injury. If the burn area is large (>10% of TBSA) or an electrical or inhalation burn is suspected, attention needs to be focused first on the so-called ABCs:

- *Airway:* Check for patency, soot around nares and on the tongue, singed nasal hair, and darkened oral or nasal membranes.
- *Breathing:* Check for adequacy of ventilation.
- *Circulation:* Check for presence and regularity of pulses, and elevate the burned limb above the level of the heart to decrease pain and swelling.

To prevent hypothermia, large burns should be cooled for no more than 10 minutes. Do not immerse the burned body part in cool water because doing so might lead to extensive heat loss. Never cover a burn with ice because this can cause hypothermia and vasoconstriction of blood vessels, further reducing blood flow to the injury. Gently remove as much burned clothing as possible to prevent further tissue damage. Adherent clothing should be left in place until the patient is transferred to a hospital. The patient should be wrapped in a dry, clean sheet or blanket to prevent further contamination of the wound and to provide warmth.

Chemical burns are best treated by quickly removing the solid particles from the skin. Any clothing containing the chemical must also be removed as the burning process continues while the chemical is in contact with the skin. The affected area should be flushed with copious amounts of water to irrigate the skin anywhere from 20 minutes to 2 hours postexposure (Singer & Dagum, 2008). Tap water is acceptable for flushing eyes exposed to chemicals. Tissue destruction may continue for up to 72 hours after a chemical burn. (For information on handling specific agents, refer to a hazardous materials text.)

Patients with inhalation injuries must be observed closely for signs of respiratory distress or compromise. They need to be treated quickly and efficiently at the scene if they are to survive. If carbon monoxide intoxication is suspected, the patient should be treated with 100% humidified oxygen. Patients who have both body burns and inhalation injury must be transferred to the nearest burn unit.

The patient with burn injury may also have sustained other injuries that take priority over the burn wound. It is important for the individuals involved in the prehospital phase of burn care to adequately communicate the circumstances of the injury to the hospital-based health care providers. This is especially important when the patient's injury involves entrapment in a closed space, hazardous chemicals, electricity, or possible trauma (e.g., fall).

Prehospital management and emergency management are described for chemical burns (Table 27-5), inhalation injury

EMERGENCY MANAGEMENT

Table 27-5 Chemical Burns

CAUSE	ASSESSMENT FINDINGS	INTERVENTIONS
• Acids • Alkalis • Organic compounds	• Burning • Redness, swelling of injured tissue • Degeneration of exposed tissue • Discoloration of injured skin • Localized pain • Edema of surrounding tissue • Tissue destruction may continue up to 72 hr • Respiratory distress if chemical inhaled • Decreased muscle coordination (if organophosphate is involved) • Paralysis	**Initial** • Assess airway, breathing, and circulation before decontamination procedures are done. • Stabilize cervical spine. • Provide supplemental oxygen as needed. • Anticipate intubation with significant inhalation injury, circumferential full-thickness burns to the neck and chest, or large TBSA burn. • Brush dry chemical from skin before irrigation. • Remove nonadherent clothing, shoes, watches, jewellery, and, if face was exposed, glasses or contact lenses. • Flush chemical from wound and surrounding area with copious amounts of saline solution or water. • For chemical burn of the eye, flush from inner to outer corner of eye with water unless lactated Ringer's solution is available. • Cover burned areas with dry dressings or clean sheet. • Establish IV access with two large-bore catheters if burn >15% of TBSA. • Begin fluid replacement. • Insert urinary catheter if adult burn >15% of TBSA. • Elevate burned limb above level of heart to decrease edema. • Administer IV analgesic agents, and assess effectiveness frequently. • Contact poison control centre for assistance. **Ongoing Monitoring** • Monitor airway if patient was exposed to chemicals. • Monitor urine output. • Consider possibility of systemic effect of identified chemical, and monitor and treat accordingly. • Monitor pH of eye if patient was exposed to chemicals.

IV, intravenous; *TBSA,* total body surface area.

EMERGENCY MANAGEMENT

Table 27-6 Inhalation Injury

CAUSE	ASSESSMENT FINDINGS	INTERVENTIONS
• Exposure of respiratory tract to intense heat or flames • Inhalation of noxious chemicals, smoke, or carbon monoxide	• History of being trapped in an enclosed space, of being in an explosion, or of clothing catching fire • Rapid, shallow respirations • Increasing hoarseness • Coughing • Singed nasal or facial hair • Darkened oral or nasal membranes • Smoky breath • Carbonaceous sputum • Productive cough with black, grey, or bloody sputum • Irritation of upper airways or burning pain in throat or chest • Difficulty swallowing • Cherry-red skin colour (carbon monoxide levels >20%) • Restlessness, anxiety • Altered mental status, including confusion, coma • Decreased oxygen saturation • Dysrhythmias	***Initial*** • Assess airway, breathing, and circulation. • Stabilize cervical spine. • Assess for inhalation injury. • Provide 100% humidified oxygen. • Monitor vital signs, level of consciousness, oxygen saturation, and cardiac rhythm. • Remove nonadherent clothing, jewellery, and, if face was exposed, glasses or contact lenses. • Establish IV access with two large-bore catheters if burn >15% of TBSA. • Begin fluid replacement. • Insert urinary catheter if burn >15% of TBSA. • Elevate burned limb above level of heart to decrease edema. • Measure arterial blood gas and carboxyhemoglobin levels, and obtain chest radiograph. • Administer IV analgesic agent, and assess effectiveness frequently. • Identify and treat other associated injuries (e.g., fractures, pneumothorax, head injury). • Cover burned areas with dry dressings or clean sheet. • Anticipate need for fibreoptic bronchoscopy or intubation. ***Ongoing Monitoring*** • Monitor airway. • Monitor urine output. • Monitor vital signs, level of consciousness, respiratory status, oxygen saturation, and cardiac rhythm.

IV, intravenous; *TBSA,* total body surface area.

(Table 27-6), electrical burns (Table 27-7), and thermal burns (Table 27-8).

Emergent Phase

The *emergent (resuscitative) phase* is the period of time required to resolve the immediate, life-threatening problems resulting from the burn injury. This phase usually lasts up to 72 hours from the time of the burn. The primary concerns are the onset of hypovolemic shock and the formation of edema. The phase ends when fluid mobilization and diuresis begin.

Pathophysiological Changes

Fluid and Electrolyte Shifts. The greatest initial threat to a patient with a major burn is hypovolemic shock (Nicol & Huether, 2012). It is caused by a massive shift of fluids out of the blood vessels as a result of increased capillary permeability and can begin as early as 20 minutes after the burn injury. As the capillary walls become more permeable, water, sodium, and, later, plasma proteins (especially albumin) move into interstitial spaces and other surrounding tissue (Figure 27-5). The colloidal osmotic pressure decreases with progressive loss of protein from the vascular space. This results in the shifting of more fluid out of the vascular space into the interstitial spaces (Figure 27-6). (Fluid accumulation in the interstitium is termed *second spacing.*) Fluid also moves to areas that normally have minimal to no fluid, a phenomenon termed *third spacing.* Examples of third spacing in burn injury are exudate and blister formation, as well as edema in nonburned areas.

Other sources of fluid loss during this period are insensible losses by evaporation from large, denuded body surfaces and the respiratory system. The normal insensible loss of 30 to 50 mL per hour is increased in severely burned patients. The net result of the fluid shifts and loses is intravascular volume depletion. Decreased blood pressure, increased heart rate, and other manifestations of hypovolemic shock are clinically detectable signs of intravascular volume depletion (see Chapter 69). If it is not corrected, irreversible shock and death may result. The circulatory status is also impaired because of hemolysis of RBCs. The RBCs are hemolyzed by circulating factors (e.g., oxygen free radicals) released at the time of the burn, as well as by the direct insult of the burn injury. Thrombosis in the capillaries of burned tissue causes an additional loss of circulating RBCs. Elevation of the hematocrit is commonly caused by hemoconcentration, which

EMERGENCY MANAGEMENT

Table 27-7 Electrical Burns

CAUSE	ASSESSMENT FINDINGS	INTERVENTIONS
Alternating Current	• Leathery, white, or charred skin	**Initial**
• Electric wires	• Burn odour	• Remove patient from electric source while protecting rescuer.
• Utility wires	• Loss of consciousness	• Assess airway, breathing, and circulation.
Direct Current	• Impaired touch sensation	• Stabilize cervical spine.
• Lightning	• Minimal or no pain	• Provide supplemental O_2 as needed.
• Defibrillator	• Dysrhythmias	• Monitor vital signs, level of consciousness, respiratory status, oxygen saturation, and cardiac rhythm.
	• Cardiac arrest	• Check pulses distal to burns.
	• Location of contact points	• Remove nonadherent clothing, shoes, watches, jewellery, glasses, or contact lenses if face was exposed.
	• Diminished peripheral circulation in injured extremity	• Cover burned areas with dry dressing or clean sheet.
	• Thermal burns if clothing ignites	• Establish IV access with two large-bore catheters if burn >15% of TBSA.
	• Fractures or dislocations from force of current	• Begin fluid replacement.
	• Head or neck injury if fall occurred	• Measure arterial blood gas to assess acid–base balance.
	• Depth and extent of wound difficult to visualize; injury should be presumed more severe than what is seen	• Insert urinary catheter if burn >15% of TBSA.
		• Elevate burned limb above level of heart to decrease edema.
		• Administer IV analgesic agent, and assess effectiveness frequently.
		• Identify and treat other associated injuries (e.g., fractures, pneumothorax, head injury).
		Ongoing Monitoring
		• Monitor airway.
		• Monitor vital signs, cardiac rhythm, level of consciousness, respiratory status, oxygen saturation, and neurovascular status of injured limbs.
		• Monitor urine output.
		• Monitor urine for development of myoglobinuria secondary to muscle breakdown and hemoglobinuria secondary to RBC breakdown.
		• Anticipate possible administration of $NaHCO_3$ to alkalinize the urine and maintain serum pH >6.0.

IV, intravenous; *NaHCO₃*, sodium bicarbonate; *RBC*, red blood cell; *TBSA*, total body surface area.

results from fluid loss. After fluid balance has been restored, hematocrit levels are lowered as a result of dilution.

Major shifts in sodium and potassium also occur during this phase. Sodium rapidly shifts to the interstitial spaces and remains there until edema formation ceases (Figure 27-7). A potassium shift develops initially because injured cells and hemolyzed RBCs release potassium into the circulation. (Fluid and electrolyte shifts are discussed in Chapter 19.)

Toward the end of the emergent phase, capillary membrane permeability is restored if fluid replacement is adequate. Fluid loss and edema formation cease. Interstitial fluid gradually returns to the vascular space (see Figure 27-7). Clinically, diuresis is noted with low urine specific gravities.

Inflammation and Healing. Burn injury causes coagulation necrosis, in which tissues and vessels are damaged or destroyed. Neutrophils and monocytes accumulate at the site of injury. Fibroblasts and newly formed collagen fibrils appear and

begin wound repair within the first 6 to 12 hours after injury. (The inflammatory response is discussed in Chapter 14.)

Immunological Changes. Burn injury causes widespread impairment of the immune system. The skin barrier to invading organisms is destroyed, bone marrow depression occurs, and circulating levels of immunoglobulins are decreased. The function of white blood cells (WBCs) becomes defective. The inflammatory cytokine cascade triggered by tissue damage impairs the function of lymphocytes, monocytes, and neutrophils, which increases the patient's risk for infection.

Clinical Manifestations

Patients with burns are likely to be in shock from hypovolemia. In many cases, the areas of full-thickness and deep partial-thickness burns are initially anaesthetic because the nerve endings have been destroyed. Superficial to moderate partial-thickness

Table 27-8 Thermal Burns

CAUSE	ASSESSMENT FINDINGS	INTERVENTIONS
• Hot liquids or solids	***Partial-Thickness Burn***	***Initial***
• Flash flame	**Superficial; First-Degree Burn**	• Assess airway, breathing, and circulation.
• Open flame	• Redness	• Stabilize cervical spine.
• Steam	• Pain	• Assess for inhalation injury.
• Hot surface	• Moderate to severe tenderness	• Provide supplemental oxygen as needed.
• Ultraviolet rays	• Minimal edema	• Monitor vital signs, level of consciousness, respiratory status, oxygen saturation, and cardiac rhythm.
	• Blanching with pressure	• Remove nonadherent clothing, shoes, watches, jewellery, glasses or contact lenses, if face was exposed.
	Deep; Second-Degree Burn	• Cover burned areas with dry dressing or clean sheet.
	• Moist blebs, blisters	• Establish IV access with two large-bore catheters if burn >15% of TBSA.
	• Mottled white, pink to cherry red discoloration	• Begin fluid replacement.
	• Hypersensitive to touch or air	• Insert urinary catheter if burn >15% of TBSA.
	• Moderate to severe pain	• Elevate burned limb above level of heart to decrease edema.
	• Blanching with pressure	• Administer IV analgesic agent, and assess effectiveness frequently.
	Full-Thickness; Third- or Fourth-Degree Burn	• Identify and treat other associated injuries (e.g., fractures, pneumothorax, head injury).
	• Dry, leathery eschar	***Ongoing Monitoring***
	• White, waxy, dark brown, or charred appearance	• Monitor airway.
	• Strong burn odour	• Monitor vital signs, cardiac rhythm, level of consciousness, respiratory status and oxygen saturation.
	• Impaired sensation when touched	• Monitor urine output.
	• Absence of pain with severe pain in surrounding tissues	
	• Lack of blanching with pressure	

IV, intravenous; *TBSA,* total body surface area.

PATHOPHYSIOLOGY MAP

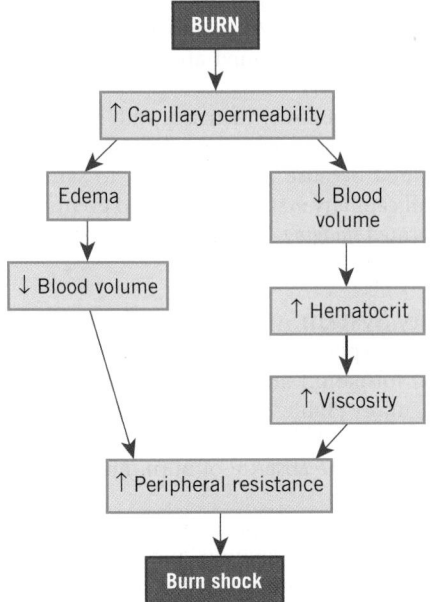

Figure 27-5 At the time of major burn injury, there is increased capillary permeability. All fluid components of the blood begin to leak into the interstitium, causing edema and a decrease in blood volume. Hematocrit increases, and the blood becomes more viscous. The combination of decreased blood volume and increased viscosity produces increased peripheral resistance. Burn shock, a type of hypovolemic shock, rapidly ensues, and if it is not corrected, death can result.

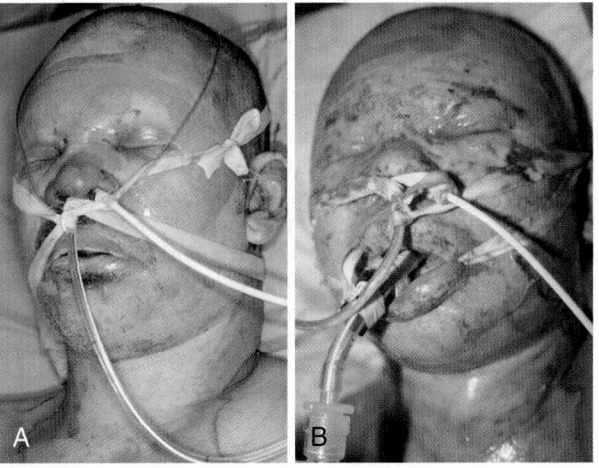

Figure 27-6 A, Facial edema before fluid resuscitation. **B,** Facial edema after 24 hours.

Source: Adapted from AACN. (2009). *Advanced Critical Care Nursing.* (p. 1216, Figure 44-2) St. Louis: Saunders.

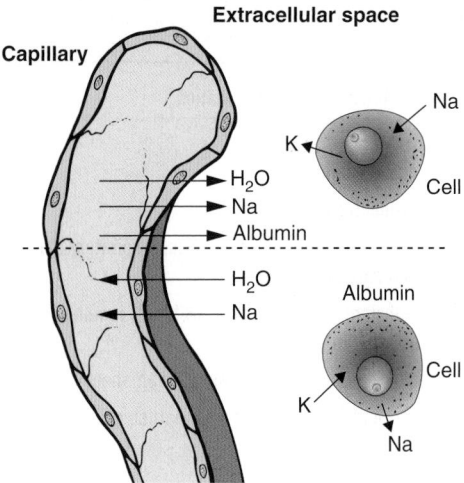

Figure 27-7 The effects of burn shock are shown above the dotted line. As the capillary seal is lost, interstitial edema develops. The cellular integrity is also altered, with sodium (Na) moving into the cell in abnormal amounts and potassium (K) leaving the cell. The shifts after the resolution of burn shock are shown below the dotted line. The water and sodium move back into the circulating volume through the capillary. The albumin remains in the interstitium. Potassium is transported into the cell, and sodium is transported out as the cellular integrity returns.

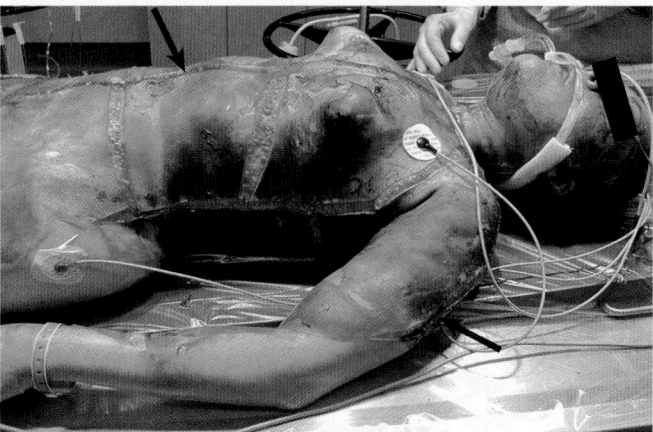

Figure 27-8 Escharotomies of the chest and arm (indicated by *arrows*).

Source: Courtesy Judy A. Knighton, RN, MScN, Toronto.

Table 27-9 Manifestations of Respiratory Injury Associated With Burns
Upper Airway Injury
Edema, hoarseness, difficulty swallowing, copious secretions, stridor, substernal and intercostal retractions, total airway obstruction
Lower Airway Injury
Strongly assumed if patient was trapped in a fire in an enclosed space or clothing caught fire and if patient has facial burns or singed nasal or facial hair; symptoms include dyspnea, carbonaceous sputum, wheezing, hoarseness, altered mental status.

burns are painful. Blisters filled with fluid and protein may develop in partial-thickness burns. Fluid is not actually lost from the body as much as it is sequestered in the interstitial spaces and third spaces. Patients with a larger burn area may have signs of adynamic ileus, such as absent or decreased bowel sounds, as a result of the body's response to massive trauma and potassium shifts. Shivering may occur as a result of chilling that is caused by heat loss, anxiety, or pain. Ongoing nursing assessment of the ABCs, vital signs, cardiac rhythm, oxygenation, and level of consciousness are priorities during the emergent phase of burn care.

Most patients with burn injuries are quite alert and can provide answers to questions shortly after the injury or until they are intubated. They are often frightened and benefit from calm reassurance and simple explanations by all health care providers. Unconsciousness or altered mental status in a patient with burn injury is usually not a result of the burn. The most common reason for unconsciousness or altered mental status is hypoxia associated with smoke inhalation. Other possibilities include head trauma, history of substance abuse, or excessive amounts of sedation or pain medication.

Complications

The three major organ systems most susceptible to complications during the emergent phase of burn injury are the cardiovascular, respiratory, and urinary systems.

Cardiovascular System. Complications of burns in the cardiovascular system include dysrhythmias and hypovolemic shock, which may progress to irreversible shock. Circulation to the extremities can be severely impaired by circumferential burns and subsequent edema formation. These processes occlude the blood supply by acting like a tourniquet. If they are untreated, ischemia, paresthesias, necrosis, and eventually gangrene can occur. To restore circulation to compromised extremities, an **escharotomy** (a scalpel or electrocautery incision through the full-thickness eschar) is frequently performed after the patient's transfer to a burn unit (Figure 27-8).

Initially, blood viscosity increases with burn injuries because of the fluid loss that occurs in the emergent period. Microcirculation is impaired because of the damage to skin structures that contain small capillary systems. These two events result in a phenomenon termed *sludging*. Sludging can be corrected by adequate fluid replacement.

Respiratory System. The respiratory system is especially vulnerable to two types of injury: (a) upper airway burns, which cause edema formation and obstruction of the airway, and (b) lower airway injury (Table 27-9). Upper airway distress may occur with or without smoke inhalation, and airway injury at either level may occur in the absence of burn injury to the skin.

Upper Airway Injury. Upper airway injury results from direct heat injury or edema formation and can lead to mechanical airway obstruction and asphyxia. The edema associated with an upper respiratory tract burn injury can be massive and the onset insidious. Mechanical obstruction of the airway is not limited to patients with flame burns to the upper airway. Swelling that accompanies scalding of the face and neck can be lethal, as can pressure from the accumulated edema that compresses the airway externally. Flame burns to the neck and chest may contribute to respiratory difficulty because the inelastic eschar becomes tight and constricting as a result of the underlying edema.

Lower Airway Injury. *Lower airway* (or inhalation) injury refers to a direct insult at the alveolar level secondary to the inhalation of toxic fumes or smoke. The result is interstitial edema, which prevents the diffusion of oxygen from the alveoli into the circulatory system (Mlcak et al., 2007). Fibreoptic bronchoscopy and carboxyhemoglobin blood levels can be used to confirm a suspected inhalation injury. Another diagnostic indicator may be a history of prolonged exposure to smoke or fumes. Sputum may contain carbon. The nurse must be especially sensitive to signs of impending respiratory distress—such as increased agitation, restlessness, or change in the rate or character of respirations—because the symptoms may not be present immediately. In general, the extent of TBSA burn is not correlated with severity of inhalation injury because inhalation injury is a factor of time exposure, in addition to the type and density of the material inhaled. The initial chest radiograph may appear normal on admission; changes are noted over the next 24 to 48 hours. ABG values may also be within the normal range on admission and then change during hospitalization.

Other Cardiopulmonary Problems. Burn-injured patients with pre-existing heart disease (e.g., myocardial infarction) or lung disease (e.g., chronic obstructive pulmonary disease) are at risk for complications. If fluid replacement is too vigorous, such patients can develop heart failure or pulmonary edema. Invasive measures (e.g., hemodynamic monitoring) may be necessary to monitor fluid resuscitation.

Burn-injured patients with pre-existing respiratory problems are more likely to develop a respiratory infection. Pneumonia is a common complication of major burns and the leading cause of death in patients with an inhalation injury. Debilitation, abundant microbial flora, and relative immobility predispose such patients to the development of pneumonia. Burn-injured patients are at risk for the development of venous thromboembolism. Risk for venous thromboembolism is increased if one or more of the following conditions are present: advanced age, morbid obesity, extensive or lower-extremity burns, concomitant lower-extremity trauma, or prolonged immobility.

Urinary System. The most common complication of the urinary system in the emergent phase is acute tubular necrosis. If the patient becomes hypovolemic, blood flow to the kidneys is decreased, causing renal ischemia. If this continues, acute renal failure may develop.

With full-thickness and electrical burns, myoglobin (from muscle cell breakdown) and hemoglobin (from RBC breakdown) are released into the bloodstream and occlude renal tubules. Adequate fluid replacement and diuretics can counteract myoglobin and hemoglobin obstruction of the tubules.

NURSING AND COLLABORATIVE MANAGEMENT: EMERGENT PHASE

In the emergent phase, patient survival depends on rapid and thorough assessment and intervention (Hackenschmidt, 2007). The nurse, in collaboration with a physician, usually makes the initial assessment of depth and extent of the burn and coordinates the actions of the health care team. In a community hospital, decisions must be made as to whether the patient requires inpatient or outpatient care and, in the case of inpatient care, whether the patient remains in that hospital or is transferred to the closest regional burn unit (see Table 27-3). From the onset of the burn event until the patient is stabilized, nursing and collaborative management consists predominantly of airway management, fluid therapy, and wound care (Table 27-10).

Although the burn management can be chronologically categorized as emergent, acute, and rehabilitative, the overall care requirements are not so easily classified. Depending on the acuity of the patient's condition, the duration of time spent in each phase varies greatly, and conditions improve and worsen unpredictably on an almost daily basis. Care changes accordingly. Whereas physiotherapy and occupational therapy are a focus of the acute and rehabilitative phases, proper positioning and splinting begin at the time of admission. Support and teaching of patients and caregivers begin on admission and intensify in the rehabilitative phase. See the accompanying nursing care plan eNCP 27-1 (Thermal Burn Injury) on the Evolve Web site for this chapter.

■ Airway Management

Airway management frequently involves early endotracheal (preferably orotracheal) intubation. Early intubation eliminates the necessity for emergency tracheostomy after respiratory problems have become apparent. In general, patients with major injuries involving burns to the face and neck require intubation within 1 to 2 hours after burn injury. (Intubation is discussed in Chapter 68.) After intubation, such patients are placed on ventilatory assistance, and the delivered oxygen concentration is determined from an assessment of ABG values. Extubation may be indicated when the edema resolves, usually 3 to 6 days after burn injury, unless severe inhalation injury is involved. Escharotomies of the chest wall may be needed to relieve respiratory distress secondary to circumferential, full-thickness burns of the neck and trunk (see Figure 27-8).

Within 6 to 12 hours after injury in which smoke inhalation is suspected, a fibreoptic bronchoscopy should be performed to assess the lower airway. Significant findings include the appearance of carbonaceous material, mucosal edema, vesicles, erythema, hemorrhage, and ulceration.

When intubation is not performed, treatment of inhalation injury includes administration of 100% humidified oxygen as needed. Patients should be placed in a high Fowler's position unless this is contraindicated (e.g., because of spinal injury), and coughing and deep breathing every hour should be encouraged. Patients should be repositioned every 1 to 2 hours, and chest physiotherapy and suctioning performed as necessary. If respiratory failure develops, intubation and mechanical ventilation are initiated. Positive end-expiratory pressure may be used to prevent collapse of the alveoli and progressive respiratory failure (see Chapter 68). Bronchodilators may be administered to treat severe bronchospasm. Carbon monoxide poisoning is treated by administering 100% oxygen until carboxyhemoglobin levels return to normal. The use of hyperbaric oxygen therapy remains controversial.

■ Fluid Therapy

Establishing IV access is critical for fluid resuscitation and drug administration. At least two large-bore intravenous access routes must be obtained for patients with burns over more than 15% of

COLLABORATIVE CARE

Table 27-10 Patient With Burn Injury

EMERGENT PHASE	ACUTE PHASE	REHABILITATION PHASE
Fluid Therapy		
• Assess fluid needs.* • Begin IV fluid replacement. • Insert urinary catheter. • Monitor intake and output.	• Continue to monitor intake and output. • Continue to replace fluids, depending on patient's clinical response.	• Discuss possible reconstructive surgery. • Prepare for discharge home or transfer to rehabilitation unit or hospital.
Wound Care		
• Start daily shower and wound care. • Debride as necessary. • Assess extent and depth of burns. • Administer tetanus toxoid or tetanus antitoxin.	• Continue daily shower and wound care. • Assess wound daily and adjust dressing protocols as necessary. • Observe for complications (e.g., infection). • Continue debridement (if necessary).	—
Pain and Anxiety		
• Assess and manage pain and anxiety.	• Continue to assess for and treat pain and anxiety.	—
Psychosocial Care		
• Provide support to patient and family during initial crisis phase.	• Continue to provide ongoing support/counselling/education to patient and family about physical and emotional aspects of care and recovery. • Begin to anticipate discharge needs.	• Continue to counsel and teach patient and family. • Continue to encourage and assist patient in resuming self-care.
Respiratory Therapy		
• Assess oxygenation needs. • Provide supplemental oxygen as needed. • Intubate if necessary. • Monitor respiratory status.	• Continue to assess oxygenation needs. • Continue to monitor respiratory status. • Monitor for signs of complications (e.g., pneumonia).	—
Physical and Occupational Therapy		
• Place patient in position that prevents contracture formation and reduces edema. • Assess need for splints or devices such as air beds and gel mattress to decrease tissue ischemia and potential for skin breakdown. • Turn and reposition patient frequently to allow for appropriate circulation to tissues.	• Have patient begin daily therapy program for maintenance of range of motion. • Assess need for splints and anticontracture positioning. • Encourage and assist patient with self-care as possible.	• Continue to prevent or minimize contractures, and assess likelihood for scarring (surgery, physical and occupational therapy, splinting, or pressure garments).
Nutritional Therapy		
• Assess nutritional needs and begin feeding patient by most appropriate route as soon as possible.	• Continue to assess diet to support wound healing.	—
Other Therapy		
	Early Excision and Grafting • Provide temporary homografts. • Provide permanent autografts. • Care for donor sites. **Rehabilitation Phase** • Continue to counsel and teach patient and family. • Continue to encourage and assist patient in resuming self-care. • Continue to prevent or minimize contractures, and assess likelihood for scarring (surgery, physical and occupational therapy, splinting, or pressure garments). • Discuss possible reconstructive surgery. • Prepare for discharge home or transfer to rehabilitation unit or hospital.	• Discuss possible reconstructive surgery. • Prepare for discharge home or transfer to rehabilitation unit or hospital.

IV, intravenous.
*See Tables 27-11 and 27-12.

Table 27-11 Formulas for Estimating Fluid Replacement of an Adult Patient With Burn Injury

FORMULA	FIRST 24 HR CRYSTALLOIDS	SECOND 24 HR COLLOIDS	GLUCOSE IN WATER
Brooke (modified)	Lactated Ringer's solution: 2 mL/kg per percentage of TBSA burned; 50% given during first 8 hr; 50% given during next 16 hr	0.3-0.5 mL/kg per percentage of TBSA burned	Amount to replace estimated evaporative losses
Parkland (Baxter)	Lactated Ringer's solution: 4 mL/kg per percentage of TBSA burned; 50% given during first 8 hr; 25% given during next 8 hr; 25% given during the following 8 hr	0.3-0.5 mL/kg per percentage of TBSA burned	Amount to replace estimated evaporative losses

TBSA, total body surface area.

TBSA. It is critical to establish IV access that can accommodate large volumes of fluid. For patients with burns over more than 30% of TBSA, a central line for fluid and drug administration, as well as a line for blood sampling, should be considered if frequent ABGs or invasive BP monitoring is needed.

A standardized chart is used to assess to the extent of the burn wound (see Figure 27-4). This allows for the accurate estimation of fluid resuscitation requirements.

The type of fluid replacement is determined by size and depth of burn, age of the patient, and individual considerations, such as pre-existing chronic illness. Each burn unit has a preference for a replacement regimen. Fluid replacement is accomplished with crystalloid solutions (usually lactated Ringer's solution), colloids (albumin), or a combination of the two. Paramedics generally administer IV saline until the patient's arrival at the hospital.

The Parkland (Baxter) formula for fluid replacement is the formula most commonly used to estimate fluid replacement; the modified Brooke formula is second most commonly used (Tables 27-11 and 27-12). It is important to remember that all formulas yield estimates, and those estimates must be titrated on the basis of the patient's physiological response. For example, in patients with an electrical injury, fluid requirements may be greater than normal.

Colloidal solutions (e.g., albumin) may be given. However, administration is recommended in the first 12 to 24 hours after the burn injury, when capillary permeability returns to normal or near normal. After this time, the plasma remains in the vascular space and expands the circulating volume. The replacement volume is calculated on the basis of the patient's body weight and TBSA burned (e.g., 0.3 to 0.5 mL/kg per percentage of TBSA burned).

The adequacy of fluid replacement is best assessed according to clinical parameters. Urine output, the most commonly used parameter, and cardiac parameters are defined as follows:
1. *Urine output:* The goal is 0.5 to 1 mL/kg/hour and 75 to 100 mL/hour in patients with electrical burn and evidence of hemoglobinuria or myoglobinuria.
2. *Cardiac factors:* Mean arterial pressure is greater than 65 mm Hg, systolic blood pressure is greater than 90 mm Hg, and heart rate is less than 120 beats/minute. Mean arterial pressure and blood pressure are most appropriately measured by means of an arterial line. Peripheral measurement is often invalid because of vasoconstriction and edema.

Table 27-12 Fluid Resuscitation With the Parkland (Baxter) Formula*

Formula

4 mL of lactated Ringer's solution per kilogram of body weight per percentage of TBSA burned = Total fluid requirements for first 24 hr after burn

Application

50% of total in first 8 hr

25% of total in second 8 hr

25% of total in third 8 hr

Example

For a 70-kg patient with a burn on 50% of TBSA:

4 mL × 70 kg × 50% of TBSA burned	=	14,000 mL or 14 L in 24 hr
50% of total in first 8 hr	=	7000 mL (875 mL/hr)
25% of total in second 8 hr	=	3500 mL (436 mL/hr)
25% of total in third 8 hr	=	3500 mL (436 mL/hr)

*Formulas are guidelines. Fluid is administered at a rate to produce 0.5-1.0 mL/kg/hr of urine output.
TBSA, total body surface area.

Wound Care

Once a patent airway, adequate circulation, and adequate fluid replacement have been established, the priority is care of the burn wound. Full-thickness burn wounds are dry and waxy-white to dark brown or black and have only minor, localized sensation because the nerve endings have been destroyed. Partial-thickness burn wounds appear pink to cherry-red and are wet and shiny with serous exudate. These wounds may or may not have intact blisters and are painful when touched or exposed to air.

Cleansing and gentle debridement, with the use of scissors and forceps, can occur in a cart shower (Figure 27-9), a regular shower, or the patient's bed or stretcher. Extensive, surgical debridement is performed in the operating room (Figure 27-10). During **debridement,** necrotic skin is removed. Releasing escharotomies and fasciotomies can be carried out in the emergent phase, usually in burn units by burn physicians. Care should

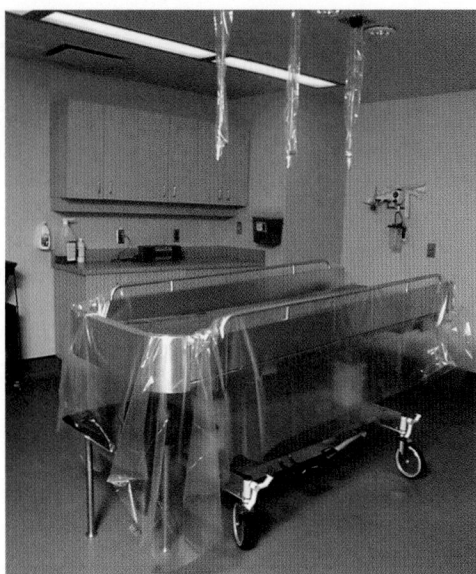

Figure 27-9 Cart shower. Showering presents an opportunity for physical therapy, as well as wound care.

Source: Courtesy Judy A. Knighton, RN, MScN, Toronto.

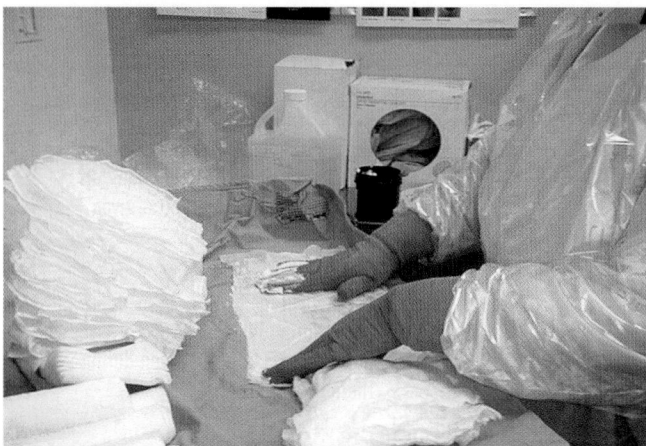

Figure 27-11 Application of silver sulphadiazine cream to saline-moistened gauze.

Source: Courtesy Judy A. Knighton, RN, MScN, Toronto.

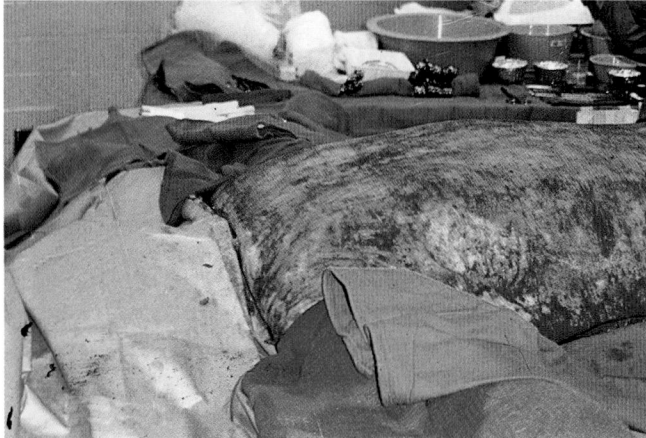

Figure 27-10 Surgical debridement of full-thickness burns is necessary to prepare the wound for grafting.

be taken to accomplish these procedures as quickly and effectively as possible.

Patients find the initial wound care to be both physically and psychologically demanding. Providing emotional support is invaluable and assists in building an important sense of trust in the nurse–patient relationship. Patients are showered with tap water, not exceeding 40°C. A once-daily shower and dressing change in the morning, followed by a dressing change in the patient's room in the evening, is a common routine in many burn units. Some of the newer antimicrobial dressings can be left in place from 3 to 14 days, thereby decreasing the frequency of dressing changes.

Infection is the most serious risk leading to further tissue injury and possible sepsis (Nicol & Huether, 2012). The source of infection in burn wounds is the patient's own flora, predominantly from the skin (burned and unburned), respiratory tract, and gastrointestinal tract. The prevention of cross-contamination between one patient and another is a priority for all members of the health care team.

Two approaches to burn wound treatment are the open method and the use of multiple dressing changes. In the *open method*, the patient's burn is covered with a topical antimicrobial and has no dressing over the wound. In the *multiple-dressing change* or *closed method*, sterile gauze dressings are impregnated with or laid over a topical antimicrobial (Figure 27-11). These dressings are changed at various intervals, from every 12 to 24 hours to once every 14 days, depending on the product. Most burn units support the concept of moist wound healing and use dressings to cover the burned areas, except for the burned face.

When the patient's open burn wounds are exposed, staff must wear personal protective equipment (e.g., disposable hats, masks, gowns, gloves). When removing contaminated dressings and washing the dirty wound, the nurse may use nonsterile, disposable gloves. Sterile gloves are used in applying ointments and sterile dressings. In addition, the room must be kept warm (approximately 29.4°C). The nurse removes all personal protective equipment when he or she is finished treating one patient and dons new personal protective equipment before treating another patient. This is necessary to avoid transmitting organisms from one patient to another, a significant risk especially when more than one patient is in a room. Careful handwashing and the use of alcohol hand gel, both inside and outside each patient room, is also necessary to prevent cross-contamination. After the dressing change is completed, the equipment and immediate environment are thoroughly cleaned and disinfected. The use of plastic liners on equipment is helpful in reducing the potential contamination of the equipment and facilitates cleaning.

Coverage is the primary goal for burn wounds (Atiyeh & Costagliola, 2007). In the major burn wound (>50% of TBSA), there is rarely enough unburned skin for immediate grafting. This necessitates the use of other temporary wound closure methods. *Allograft (homograft) skin* (usually from cadavers) is used, along with newer biosynthetic options, with varying frequency among burn units (Table 27-13).

Table 27-13 Sources of Grafts		
SOURCE	**GRAFT NAME**	**COVERAGE**
Porcine skin	Heterograft or xenograft (different species)	Temporary (3 days to 2 wk)
Cadaveric skin	Homograft or allograft (same species)	Temporary (3 days to 2 wk)
Patient's own skin	Autograft	Permanent
Patient's own skin and cell cultures	Cultured epithelial autograft (CEA)	Permanent
Porcine collagen bonded to silicone membrane	Biobrane	Temporary (10-21 days)
Bovine collagen and glycosaminoglycan bonded to silicone membrane	Integra	Permanent
Acellular dermal matrix derived from donated human skin	AlloDerm	Permanent

Other Care Measures

For certain parts of the body (e.g., face, eyes, hands, arms, ears, perineum), nursing care must be particularly meticulous. The face is highly vascular and subject to a great amount of edema. It is often covered with ointments and gauze but not wrapped, to limit pressure on delicate facial structures. Eye care for corneal burns or edema includes antibiotic ointments (Jang et al., 2006). All patients with facial burns should undergo an ophthalmological examination soon after admission. Periorbital edema can prevent opening of the eyes and be frightening to the patient. The nurse must provide assurance that the swelling is not permanent. Instillation of methylcellulose drops or artificial tears into the eyes for moisture provides additional comfort for patients.

Hands and arms should be extended and elevated on pillows to minimize edema. Splints may need to be applied to burned hands and feet to maintain them in positions of function. Ears should be kept free of pressure because of their poor vascularization and predisposition to infection. A patient with ear burns should not rest the head on pillows because pressure on the cartilage may cause chondritis and the ear may stick to the pillowcase, causing pain and bleeding. The patient's head can be elevated with a rolled towel placed under the shoulders, with care to avoid pressure necrosis. The same holds true for a patient with neck burns. Pillows are removed and a rolled towel is placed under the shoulders to hyperextend the neck and prevent neck wound contracture.

The perineum must be kept as clean and dry as possible. In addition to providing hourly urine outputs, an indwelling catheter prevents urine contamination of the perineal area. Regular, once- to twice-daily perineal and catheter care in the presence or absence of a perineal burn wound is essential.

Routine laboratory tests are performed to monitor fluid and electrolyte balance. ABGs are measured to determine adequacy of ventilation and perfusion in all patients with suspected or confirmed inhalation or electrical injury.

Physiotherapy is begun immediately, sometimes during showering and dressing changes and before new dressings are applied. Early range-of-motion exercises are necessary to facilitate mobilization of the extravasated fluid back into the vascular bed. Exercise of body parts also maintains function, prevents contracture, and reassures the patient that movement is still possible.

Drug Therapy

Analgesics and Sedatives

Analgesics are ordered to promote patient comfort. Early in the postburn period, pain medications should be given intravenously because (a) onset of action is fastest with this route; (b) gastrointestinal function is slowed or impaired as a result of shock or paralytic ileus; and (c) medications injected intramuscularly are not absorbed adequately in burned or edematous areas, and so medications pool in the tissues. When fluid mobilization begins, the interstitial accumulation of previous intramuscular medications could cause inadvertent overdose.

Opioids commonly used for pain control are listed in Table 27-14. The need for analgesia must be re-evaluated frequently because patients' needs may change and tolerance to medications may develop over time. Initially, opioids are the drugs of choice for pain control. When administered appropriately, these drugs should provide adequate pain management. Sedative/hypnotics and antidepressant agents can also be given with analgesics to control the anxiety, insomnia, and/or depression that patients may experience (see Table 27-14). Managing burn pain is a unique and complex challenge, and it is critical that the nurse remember that pain is a subjective experience. Analgesic requirements can vary tremendously from one patient to another. The extent and depth of burn may not be correlated with pain intensity. Hospital pharmacists, psychiatrists, and multidisciplinary pain services are valuable resources for the more complex patient situations. Effective pain control depends on assessment, prompt analgesia with dosages titrated to achieve effect, and regular evaluation (Richardson & Mustard, 2009).

Tetanus Immunization

Tetanus toxoid is given routinely to all patients with burn injuries because of the likelihood of anaerobic contamination of the burn wound. If the patient has not received an active immunization within 10 years before the burn injury, tetanus immunoglobulin should be considered.

Antimicrobial Agents

After the wound is cleansed, topical agents are applied (see Figure 27-11) and covered with a light dressing. Systemic antibiotics are not routinely used to control burn wound flora because there is little or no blood supply to the burn eschar and, consequently, there is little delivery of the antibiotic to the wound. In addition, the routine use of systemic antibiotics increases the chance of developing multidrug-resistant organisms. Some topical burn agents penetrate the eschar, thereby inhibiting bacterial invasion of the wound. Silver-impregnated dressings (e.g., Acticoat, Silverlon, Aquacel Ag) can be left in place anywhere from 3 to 14 days and are used in many burn units. Silver sulphadiazine (Silvadene, Flamazine) and mafenide acetate (Sulfamylon) creams are also used. They are effective against many organisms. Sepsis remains

Table 27-14 Drugs Commonly Used in Burn Treatment

TYPES AND NAMES OF DRUGS	PURPOSE
Nutritional Support	
Vitamins A, C, E, and multivitamins	Promote wound healing
Minerals: zinc, iron (ferrous sulphate)	Promote cell integrity and hemoglobin formation
Analgesia	
Morphine	All promote pain control
Sustained-release morphine (MS Contin)	
Hydromorphone (Dilaudid)	
Fentanyl	
Oxycodone and acetaminophen (Percocet)	
Methadone	
Nonsteroidal anti-inflammatory drugs (e.g., ketorolac [Toradol])	
Adjuvant analgesics (e.g., gabapentin [Neurontin])	
Sedation/Hypnosis	
Haloperidol	Produces antipsychotic and sedative effects
Lorazepam (Ativan)	Diminishes anxiety
Midazolam	Provides short-acting amnestic effects
Antidepressant Therapy	
Sertraline (Zoloft)	Reduce depression, improves mood
Citalopram (Celexa)	
Anticoagulation Therapy	
Enoxaparin (Lovenox)	Prevent venous thromboembolism
Heparin	
Gastrointestinal Support	
Ranitidine (Zantac)	Decrease stomach acid and risk of Curling's ulcer
Esomeprazole (Nexium)	
Mylanta, Maalox	Neutralizes stomach acid

a leading cause of death in patients with major burns because it may lead to multiple organ dysfunction syndrome (see Chapter 69). Systemic antibiotic therapy is initiated when invasive burn wound sepsis is clinically diagnosed or when some other source of infection is identified (e.g., pneumonia).

Fungal infections may develop in the patient's mucous membranes (mouth and genitalia) as a result of systemic antibiotic therapy and low resistance in the host. The offending organism is usually *Candida albicans*. Oral infection is treated with nystatin (Mycostatin) mouthwash. When a normal diet is resumed, yogourt or *Lactobacillus* (Lacidofil) may be given by mouth to reintroduce the normal intestinal flora that have been destroyed by antibiotic therapy.

◼ Venous Thromboembolism Prophylaxis

For burn-injured patients at risk for venous thromboembolism (e.g., those with lower extremity burns, obese patients) and if

there are no contraindications, it is recommended that low-molecular-weight heparin (enoxaparin [Lovenox]) or low-dose unfractionated heparin be started as soon as it is considered safe to do so. For burn-injured patients who are at high risk for bleeding, it is recommended that mechanical prophylaxis against venous thromboembolism with sequential compression devices or graduated compression stockings, or both, be used until the bleeding risk decreases and heparin can be started (Pannucci, Osborne, & Wahl, 2011; see Table 27-14).

◼ Nutritional Therapy

Once fluid replacement needs have been addressed, nutrition takes priority in the initial emergent phase. Early and aggressive nutritional support within several hours of the burn injury can decrease mortality risks and complications, optimize healing of the burn wound, and minimize the negative effects of hypermetabolism and catabolism (Chan & Chan, 2009). Nonintubated patients with a burn over less than 20% of TBSA are generally able to eat enough to meet their nutritional requirements. Intubated patients and those with larger burns require additional support. Enteral feedings (gastric or intestinal) have almost entirely replaced parenteral feeding. Early enteral feeding, usually with smaller bore tubes, preserves gastrointestinal function, increases intestinal blood flow, promotes optimal conditions for wound healing, and prevents complications (e.g., Curling's ulcer). The patient with a large burn (>20% of TBSA) can develop paralytic ileus within a few hours as a result of the body's response to major trauma. If a large nasogastric tube is inserted on admission, gastric residuals should be checked frequently to detect delayed gastric emptying. Bowel sounds should be assessed every 8 hours. In general, feedings can begin slowly at 20 to 40 mL/hour and increased to the goal rate within 24 to 48 hours.

A *hypermetabolic state* proportional to the size of the wound occurs after a major burn injury. Resting metabolic expenditure may be increased by 50% to 100% above normal in patients with major burns. Core temperature is elevated. Catecholamines, which stimulate catabolism and heat production, are increased. Massive catabolism can occur and is characterized by protein breakdown and increased gluconeogenesis. Failure to supply adequate calories and protein leads to malnutrition and delayed healing. Calorie-containing nutritional supplements and milkshakes are often administered because of the great need for calories. Protein powder can also be added to food and liquids. Supplemental vitamins may be given as early as the emergent phase, with iron supplements often started in the acute phase (see Table 27-14).

Acute Phase

The *acute phase* begins with the mobilization of extracellular fluid and subsequent diuresis. This phase is concluded when the burned area is completely covered by skin grafts or when the wounds are healed. This may take weeks or many months.

Pathophysiological Changes

Burn injury involves pathophysiological changes in many body systems. Diuresis from fluid mobilization occurs, and the patient is less edematous. Areas that are full- or partial-thickness burns are more evident than in the emergent phase. Bowel sounds return. The patient may now become aware of the enormity of the situation and benefit from additional psychosocial support. Some healing begins as WBCs surround the burn wound and phagocytosis occurs. Necrotic tissue begins to slough. Fibroblasts lay down matrices of the collagen precursors that eventually form granulation tissue. A partial-thickness burn wound heals from the edges and from the dermal bed below if kept free from infection and *desiccation* (dryness). However, full-thickness burn wounds, unless extremely small, must be covered by skin grafts. In some cases, healing time and length of hospitalization are decreased by early excision and grafting.

Clinical Manifestations

Partial-thickness wounds form eschar, which begins separating fairly soon after injury. Once the eschar is removed, re-epithelialization begins at the wound margins and appears as red or pink scar tissue. Epithelial buds from the dermal bed eventually close in the wound, which then heals spontaneously without surgical intervention, usually within 10 to 21 days.

Margins of full-thickness eschar take longer to separate. As a result, full-thickness wounds necessitate surgical debridement and skin grafting for healing.

Laboratory Values

Because the body is attempting to re-establish fluid and electrolyte homeostasis in the initial acute phase, it is important to monitor serum electrolyte levels closely.

Sodium. *Hyponatremia* can develop from excessive gastrointestinal suction, diarrhea, and excessive water intake. Manifestations of hyponatremia include weakness, dizziness, muscle cramps, fatigue, headache, tachycardia, and confusion. The patient with burn injuries may also develop *water intoxication,* a dilutional form of hyponatremia. To avoid this condition, the patient should drink fluids other than water, such as juice, soft drinks, or nutritional supplements.

Hypernatremia may occur after successful fluid replacement if copious amounts of hypertonic solutions were required. Other causes may be related to tube-feeding therapy or inappropriate fluid administration. Manifestations of hypernatremia include thirst; dry, coated tongue; lethargy; confusion; and possibly seizures.

Potassium. *Hyperkalemia* is noted if the patient has renal failure, adrenocortical insufficiency, or massive deep muscle injury (e.g., electrical burn) with large amounts of potassium released from damaged cells. Cardiac dysrhythmias and ventricular failure can occur with elevated potassium levels. Muscle weakness and electrocardiographic changes are observed clinically (see Chapter 19).

Hypokalemia occurs with vomiting, diarrhea, prolonged gastrointestinal suction, and prolonged intravenous therapy without potassium supplementation. A constant potassium loss occurs through the burn wound.

Manifestations of hypokalemia include fatigue, muscle weakness, leg cramps, paraesthesias, and decreased reflexes (see Chapter 19).

Complications

Infection. The body's first line of defence, the skin, is destroyed by burn injury. Pathogens often proliferate before phagocytosis has adequately begun. The burn wound becomes colonized with organisms. If the bacterial density at the junction of the eschar with underlying viable tissue rises to greater than 10^5/g of tissue, the burn wound is considered infected (Greenhalgh et al., 2007). In the presence of an infection, localized inflammation, induration, and sometimes suppuration can occur at the burn wound margins. Partial-thickness burns can convert to full-thickness wounds when the infecting organisms invade viable, adjacent, unburned tissue. Invasive wound infections may be treated with systemic antibiotics on the basis of culture results.

Burn wound infection may progress to transient bacteremia and sepsis as a result of burn wound manipulation (e.g., after showering and debridement). Manifestations of sepsis include hypothermia or hyperthermia, increased heart and respiratory rates, decreased BP, and decreased urine output. Patients may exhibit mild confusion, chills, malaise, and loss of appetite. The WBC count is usually between 10 and 20×10^9/L.

There are functional defects in the WBCs, and the patient remains immunosuppressed for a time after the burn injury. The causative organisms of sepsis are usually gram-negative bacteria (e.g., *Pseudomonas, Proteus* organisms), which increase the risk for septic shock.

When sepsis is suspected, cultures are immediately obtained from all possible sources, including the burn wound, blood, urine, sputum, oropharynx, perineal regions, and the intravenous site. However, treatment should not be delayed pending results of the culture and sensitivity studies. Therapy begins with antibiotics appropriate for the usual residual flora of the particular burn unit. The topical antibiotic in use may be continued or be changed to another agent. At this stage, the patient's condition is critical, and vital signs must be monitored closely. Collaboration with infectious disease specialists is important to ensure appropriate antibiotic coverage.

Cardiovascular and Respiratory Systems. The same cardiovascular and respiratory system complications present in the emergent phase may continue into the acute phase of care. In addition, new problems might arise, necessitating timely intervention.

Neurological System. Neurologically, the patient usually has no physical symptoms, unless severe hypoxia from respiratory injuries or complications from electrical injuries occur. However, some patients may demonstrate certain behaviours that are not completely understood. A patient can become extremely disoriented, may become withdrawn or combative, and may have hallucinations and frequent nightmare-like episodes. Delirium is more acute at night and occurs more often in older patients. Consultation with psychiatric or geriatric services is helpful in quickly diagnosing and treating delirium or similar behaviours. The nurse can then focus on strategies to orient and reassure a confused or agitated patient. This is a transient state, lasting from a day or two to several weeks. Various causes have been considered, including electrolyte imbalance, stress, cerebral edema, sepsis, sleep disturbances, and the use of analgesics and anti-anxiety drugs.

Musculoskeletal System. The musculoskeletal system is particularly prone to complications during the acute phase. As the burns begin to heal and scar tissue forms, the skin is less supple and pliant. Range of motion may be limited, and contractures can occur. The muscles in the body tend to shorten in a flexed position. The patient should be encouraged to stretch and move the burned body parts as much as possible. Splinting can be beneficial in preventing or reducing contracture formation. Attention to repositioning and the use of devices such as air beds and gel mattresses may also be necessary to decrease the potential for tissue ischemia and skin breakdown.

Gastrointestinal System.

The gastrointestinal system may also exhibit complications during this phase. Paralytic ileus results from sepsis. Diarrhea may be caused by the use of enteral feedings or antibiotics. Constipation can occur as a side effect of opioid analgesics, decreased mobility, and a low-fibre diet. *Curling's ulcer* is a type of gastroduodenal ulcer characterized by diffuse superficial lesions (including mucosal erosion). It is caused by a generalized stress response to decreased blood flow to the gastrointestinal tract during the emergent phase; this response results in decreased production of mucus and increased secretion of gastric acid. The best measure for preventing Curling's ulcer is feeding the patient as soon as possible after the injury. Antacids, H_2-histamine blockers (e.g., ranitidine [Zantac]), and proton pump inhibitors (e.g., esomeprazole [Nexium]) are used prophylactically to neutralize stomach acids and inhibit the secretion of histamine and hydrochloric acid (see Table 27-14). Patients with major burns also have occult blood in their stools during the acute phase.

Endocrine System.

A transient increase in blood glucose levels may occur because of stress-mediated cortisol and catecholamine release, which results in the increased mobilization of glycogen stores, gluconeogenesis, and the subsequent production of glucose. Insulin production and release of insulin is also increased. However, insulin's effectiveness is decreased because of relative insulin insensitivity; consequently, the blood glucose level is elevated. Later, hyperglycemia can be caused by the increased caloric intake necessary to meet some patients' metabolic requirements. When this occurs, the treatment is supplemental intravenous insulin, not decreased feeding. Serum glucose levels are checked frequently, and an appropriate amount of insulin is given if hyperglycemia is present. Glucometers may be used to assess blood glucose at the patient's bedside; serum glucose samples yield more accurate results than does capillary blood analysis by glucometer. As the patient's metabolic demands are met and less stress is placed on the entire system, this stress-induced condition is reversed.

NURSING AND COLLABORATIVE MANAGEMENT: ACUTE PHASE

The predominant therapeutic interventions in the acute phase are (a) wound care, (b) excision and grafting, (c) pain management, (d) physical and occupational therapy, (e) nutritional therapy, and (f) psychosocial care.

Wound Care

The goals of wound care are to (a) prevent infection by cleansing and debriding the area of necrotic tissue that would promote bacterial growth and (b) promote wound re-epithelialization, successful skin grafting, or both.

Wound care consists of daily observation, assessment, cleansing, debridement, and dressing reapplication. Nonsurgical debridement, dressing changes, topical antimicrobial therapy, graft care, and donor site care are performed as often as necessary, depending on the topical cream or dressing ordered. Enzymatic debridement materials made of natural ingredients, such as papain, may be used for the *enzymatic debridement* of burn wounds, which speeds up the removal of necrotic tissue from the healthy wound bed. Wounds are cleansed with soap and water or with normal saline–moistened gauze to gently remove the old antimicrobial agent and any loose necrotic tissue, scabs, or dried blood. During the debridement phase, the wound is covered with topical antimicrobial creams (e.g., silver sulphadiazine, silver-impregnated dressings; see the Evidence-Informed Practice box "Does Silver Sulphadiazine Promote Burn Healing?"). When the partial-thickness burn wounds have been fully debrided, a protective, coarse or fine-meshed, grease-based (paraffin or petroleum) gauze dressing is applied to protect the re-epithelializing cells as they resurface and close the open wound bed. If grafting is necessary, the meshed, split-thickness skin graft may be protected with the same greasy gauze dressings next to the graft, followed by middle and outer dressings. With facial grafts, the unmeshed sheet graft is left open, so it is possible for *blebs* (serosanguineous exudates) to form between the graft and the recipient bed. Blebs prevent the graft from permanently attaching to the wound itself. The evacuation of blebs is best performed by aspiration with a tuberculin syringe and only by professionals who have received instruction in this specialized skill. (Dressings are discussed in Chapter 14 and Table 14-10.)

Excision and Grafting

Current therapeutic management of full-thickness burn wounds involves early removal of the necrotic tissue, followed by application of split-thickness autograft skin (Nicol & Huether, 2012). This therapy has changed the management of burn injuries and decreased the mortality rate among patients. In the past, patients with major burns had low rates of survival because healing and wound coverage took so long that patients usually died of sepsis or malnutrition. Currently, as a result of earlier intervention, mortality and morbidity rates have been greatly reduced. Many patients, especially those with major burns, are taken to the operating room for wound excision on day 1 or 2 (resuscitation phase). The wounds are covered with a biological dressing or allograft for temporary coverage until permanent grafting can be accomplished (see Table 27-13).

During the procedure of **excision and grafting**, devitalized tissue (eschar) is excised down to the subcutaneous tissue or the fascia, depending on the degree of injury. Surgical excision can result in massive blood loss, and blood conservation techniques are used to limit this complication. Topical application of epinephrine or thrombin, application of extremity tourniquets, or application of a fibrin sealant (ARTISS) all work to decrease surgical blood loss (Foster et al., 2008).

Once hemostasis has been achieved, a graft is then placed on clean, viable tissue to achieve good adherence. Whenever possible, the freshly excised wound is covered with *autograft* (the person's own) skin (see Table 27-13). Fibrin sealant has been used to attach skin grafts to the wound bed. Grafts can also be stapled

EVIDENCE-INFORMED PRACTICE

Does Silver Sulphadiazine Promote Burn Healing?

Clinical Question

For patients with superficial and partial-thickness burns (P), does silver sulphadiazine (I) versus biosynthetic dressings (C) reduce healing time (O)?

Best Available Evidence

Systematic review of randomized controlled trials (RCTs)

Critical Appraisal and Synthesis of Evidence

- 26 RCTs
- Outcomes were wound healing time, pain, and number of dressing changes required.
- Biosynthetic dressings were associated with decreased time to heal and reduced pain during dressing changes.
- Using silver sulphadiazine dressings for the full course of treatment needs to be reconsidered as some studies showed delayed wound healing and increased number of dressing changes.

Conclusions

There is a lack of high quality RCTs on dressing treatments for superficial and partial-thickness burns. Most of the 26 RCTs were methodologically lacking. Despite some findings that were promising, the current evidence is of limited usefulness to practitioners who need to choose suitable burn dressings for their patients.

Implications for Nursing

- Silver sulphadiazine, the traditional covering for burns, might not be the best choice for the management of superficial and partial-thickness burns. More comparative studies are needed on the topic.
- Burn dressing choice should be based on promotion of healing, ease of application and removal, dressing change requirements, cost, and patient comfort.

Reference for Evidence

Wasiak, J., Cleland, H., & Campbell, F. (2008). Dressings for superficial and partial thickness burns, *Cochrane Database of Systematic Reviews*, (4), CD002106. doi:10.1002/14651858. CD002106.pub3

P, patient population of interest; *I*, intervention or area of interest; *C*, comparison of interest or comparison group; *O*, outcome(s) of interest (see pp. 7-8).

or sutured into place (Figure 27-12, *A*). A temporary allograft (skin obtained from another human being) can be used to test the suitability of the recipient site to accept a graft. The allograft is then removed several days later in the operating room and an autograft applied.

With early excision, function is restored and scar tissue formation is minimized. Clots between the graft and the wound keep the graft from adhering to the wound. Frequent observation for bleeding and circulation problems and appropriate nursing interventions can help identify and manage complications that would interfere with graft survival. Facial, neck, and hand burns require skilful nursing care to identify and manage clots quickly for the best functional and aesthetic outcomes.

Skin from another area of the patient's own body is taken for grafting by means of a dermatome, which removes a thin (14/1000 to 16/1000) split-thickness layer of skin from an unburned site (see Figure 27-12). This sample of skin can be meshed (usually a ration of 1.5:1) to allow for greater wound coverage, or it may be applied as an unmeshed sheet graft for a better cosmetic result when grafting the face, neck, and hands. The site from which this skin was taken now becomes a new open wound.

The goals of donor site care are to promote rapid, moist wound healing, decrease pain at the site, and prevent infection. The choices of dressings vary among burn centres and include transparent dressings (e.g., Opsite), xenograft, silver sulphadiazene, silver impregnated dressings, calcium alginate, and hydrophilic foam dressings (see Figure 27-12, *C*). Nursing care of the donor site is specific to the dressing selected. Several of the newer dressing materials offer decreased healing time, which facilitates earlier reharvesting of skin at the same site. The average healing time for a donor site is 10 to 14 days (see Figure 27-12, *D*).

Cultured Epithelial Autografts

In the patient with large body surface area burns, only a limited amount of unburned skin may be available as donor sites for grafting, and some of that available skin may be unsuitable for harvesting. **Cultured epithelial autograft** (CEA) is a method of obtaining permanent skin from a person with limited available skin for harvesting. CEA is grown from biopsy specimens obtained from the patient's own unburned skin (Atiyeh & Costagliola, 2007). In some burn units, this procedure is performed on suitable patients as soon as possible after admission. The specimens are sent to a commercial laboratory, where the keratinocytes from the biopsy sample are grown in a culture medium containing epidermal growth factor. After approximately 18 to 25 days, the keratinocytes have expanded up to 10,000 times and form confluent sheets that can be used as skin grafts. The cultured skin is returned to the burn unit, where it is placed on the patient's excised burn wounds. Because CEA tissue is made only of epidermal cells, meticulous care is required to prevent shearing injury or infection. CEA tissue generally form a seamless, smooth replacement skin tissue (Figure 27-13). Problems related to CEA include infection, contracture development, and poor graft take as a result of loss of thin epidermal skin during healing.

Artificial Skin

To be successful, artificial skin must perform all functions of the natural skin and consist of both dermal and epidermal elements. The Integra artificial skin dermal regeneration template is an example of a successful skin replacement system available in burn care today. Its application requires a high degree of skill. As with CEA, it is indicated for use in the treatment of life-threatening full-thickness or deep partial-thickness burn wounds when conventional autograft is not available or advisable, as in older adult patients or patients at high risk from complications of anaesthesia. It has also been successfully used in surgical reconstructive procedures for burns. As with CEA, it needs to be applied within a few days of admission for greatest success.

Integra artificial skin has a bilayer membrane composed of acellular dermis and silicone. The wound is debrided, the bilayer membrane is placed dermal layer down, and the wound is wrapped with dressings in the operating room. The dermal layer

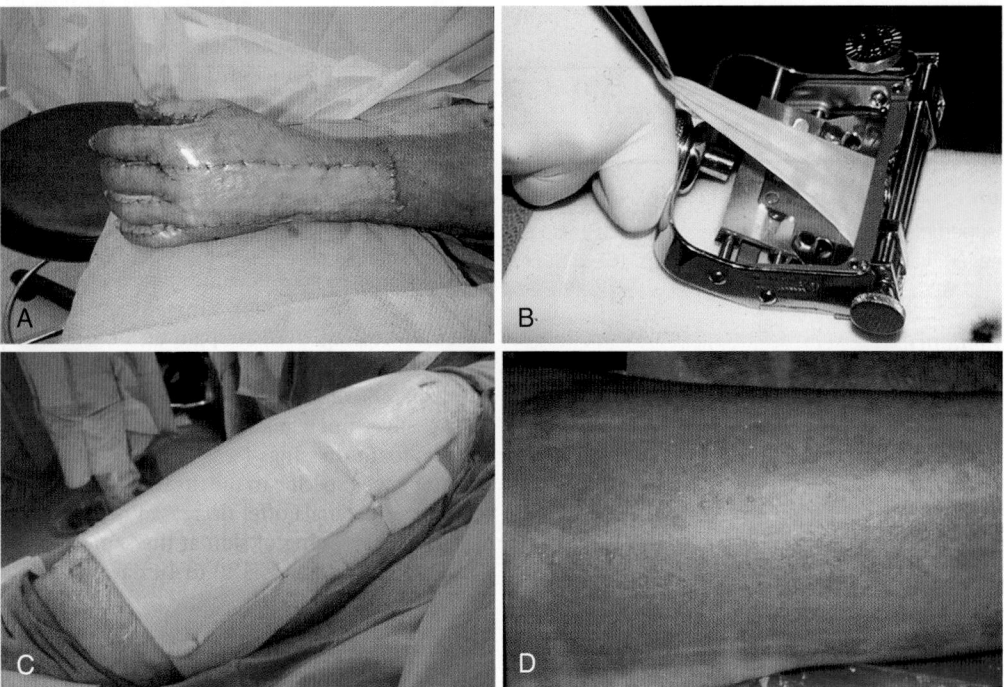

Figure 27-12 Split-thickness skin grafting. **A,** Freshly applied split-thickness sheet skin graft to the hand. **B,** Split-thickness skin graft is harvested from a patient's thigh with a dermatome. **C,** Donor site is covered with a hydrophilic foam dressing. **D,** Healed donor site.

Source: Courtesy Judy A. Knighton, RN, MScN, Toronto.

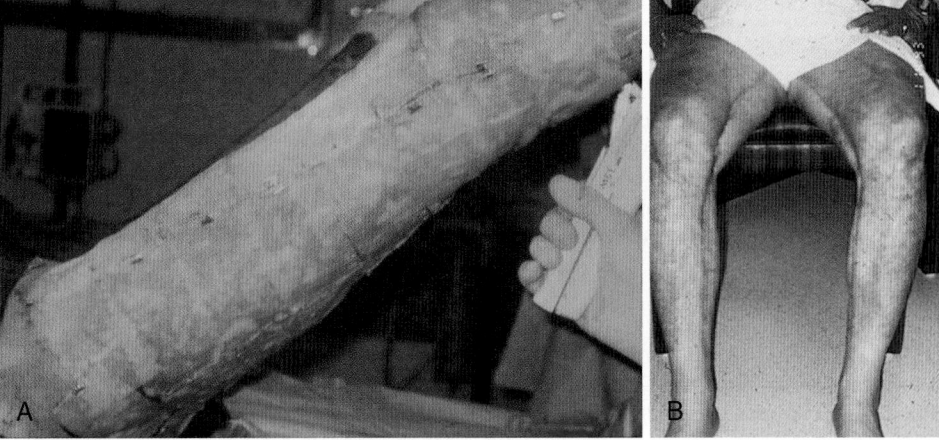

Figure 27-13 Cultured epithelial autograft (CEA). **A,** Intraoperative application of CEA. **B,** Appearance of healed CEA.

functions as a biodegradable template that induces organized regeneration of new dermis by the body. The silicone layer remains intact for 3 weeks as the dermal layer degrades and epidermal autografts become available. At this point, the silicone is removed during a second surgical procedure and replaced by the patient's own epidermal autografts. In some situations, burn units use CEA as the source of epidermis.

Another currently available dermal replacement is AlloDerm, a cryopreserved allogenic dermis (Yim et al., 2010). Human allograft dermis, harvested from cadavers, is decellularized to render it immunogenic, and then it is freeze-dried. Once thawed, AlloDerm is rehydrated with ultrathin epidermal autografts immediately before placement on a newly excised wound.

Pain Management

One of the most critical functions a nurse performs on behalf of a patient with burn injuries is individualized and ongoing pain assessment and management. Many aspects of burn care cause pain. However, patients experience moments of relative comfort if they receive adequate analgesia. A coordinated understanding of both the physiological and psychological aspects of pain is essential if the nurse is to intervene with actions that are beneficial. (General pain management is discussed in Chapter 10.) Patients with burn injuries experience two kinds of pain: (a) continuous, background pain that might be present throughout the day and night and (b) treatment-induced pain associated with dressing changes, ambulation, and rehabilitation activities. Initial treatment is pharmacological (see Table 27-14). With background pain, a continuous intravenous infusion of an opioid allows for a steady, therapeutic level of medication. If an intravenous infusion is not present, slow-release twice-a-day opioid medications (e.g., MS Contin) are indicated. Around-the-clock oral analgesics can also be used. Breakthrough doses of pain medication need to be available regardless of the regimen selected. Anxiolytics, which frequently potentiate analgesics, are also indicated and include lorazepam (Ativan) and midazolam.

For treatment-induced pain, premedication with an analgesic and an anxiolytic via the intravenous or oral route is required. For patients with an intravenous infusion, a potent short-acting analgesic, such as fentanyl, is useful. During treatment or activity, doses should be low but just high enough to keep the patient as comfortable as possible. Elimination of all the pain is difficult to achieve, and most patients indicate satisfaction with "tolerable" levels of discomfort. Pain management is complex and ever-changing throughout the patient's hospital stay and after discharge.

Pain can also be managed through nonpharmacological strategies. Mind–body interventions such as relaxation, hypnosis, guided imagery, biofeedback, and music therapy are considered adjuncts to traditional pharmacological treatment of pain. They are not meant to be used exclusively to control pain but may help some patients cope with the painful aspects of care, both in the hospital and after discharge (see Chapters 8 and 12).

An important point to remember about pain management is that the more control the patient has in managing the pain, the more successful the chosen strategies are. Patient-controlled analgesia is used in selected circumstances in some burn units, with varying degrees of success. (Patient-controlled analgesia is discussed in Chapters 10 and 22.) Active patient participation has also been found to be effective for some patients in anticipating and coping with treatment-induced pain.

▪ Physical and Occupational Therapy

Rigorous physical therapy throughout burn recovery is imperative to maintain muscle strength and optimal joint function. A good time for exercise is during and after wound cleansing, when the skin is softer and bulky dressings are removed. Passive and active range-of-motion exercises should be performed on all joints. The patient with neck burns must sleep without pillows or with the head hanging slightly over the top of the mattress to encourage hyperextension. Custom-fitted splints are designed to keep joints in functional position. These must be re-examined frequently to ensure an optimal fit with no undue pressure that might lead to skin breakdown or nerve damage.

▪ Nutritional Therapy

The goal of nutritional therapy during the acute burn phase is to provide adequate calories and protein to promote healing. The patient with burn injury is in a hypermetabolic and highly catabolic state as a result of the burn injury. Decreasing catecholamine release by minimizing pain, fear, anxiety, and cold can maximize the patient's comfort and conserve energy. Infection also increases the metabolic rate.

Meeting daily caloric requirements is crucial and should begin within the first 1 to 2 days after the burn injury. The daily estimated caloric needs must be regularly calculated by a dietitian and readjusted as the patient's condition changes (e.g., wound healing, sepsis).

If the patient is on a mechanical ventilator or unable to consume adequate calories by mouth, a small-bore feeding tube is placed and enteral feedings are initiated. When the patient is extubated, a swallowing assessment should be performed by a speech-language pathologist before the oral feeding is commenced. The alert patient should be encouraged to eat high-protein, high-carbohydrate foods to meet increased caloric needs. Family members should be encouraged to bring in favourite foods from home. Patients' appetite is usually diminished, and constant encouragement may be necessary to achieve adequate intake. Ideally, weight loss should not be more than 10% of preburn weight. The nurse then records the patient's caloric intake daily on calorie-count sheets, which are monitored by the dietitian. Patients are weighed routinely to evaluate progress.

▪ Psychosocial Care

The patient and family have many needs for psychosocial support during the often lengthy, unpredictable, and complex course of care (Klein et al., 2011). The social worker and nursing staff have important support and counselling roles to play. Pastoral care may also be appropriate for some patients and their families. (Patient and family emotional needs are discussed later in this chapter on p. 605 and in Chapter 6.)

Rehabilitation Phase

The formal *rehabilitation phase* begins when the patient's burn wounds have healed and the patient is able to resume a level of self-care activity. This can occur as early as 2 weeks or as long as 7 to 8 months after the burn injury. Goals for this period are (a) to assist the patient in resuming a functional role in society and (b) rehabilitation after functional and cosmetic reconstructive surgery. Rehabilitation-focused activities that have been taking place during the earlier emergent and acute phases now begin in earnest once the patient's wounds have healed.

Pathophysiological Changes and Clinical Manifestations

Burn wounds heal either by primary intention or by grafting. Layers of epithelialization begin rebuilding the tissue structure destroyed by the burn injury. Collagen fibres, present in the new scar tissue, assist with healing and add strength to weakened areas. The new skin appears flat and pink. In approximately 4 to 6 weeks, the area becomes raised and hyperemic. If adequate range of motion is not instituted, the new tissue shortens, which causes a contracture. Mature healing is reached in about 12 months, by which time suppleness has returned and the pink or red colour has faded to a slightly lighter hue than the surrounding unburned tissue. It takes longer for more heavily pigmented skin to regain its dark colour because many of the melanocytes have been destroyed. In many cases, the skin never regains its original colour. Paramedical cosmetic camouflage—the

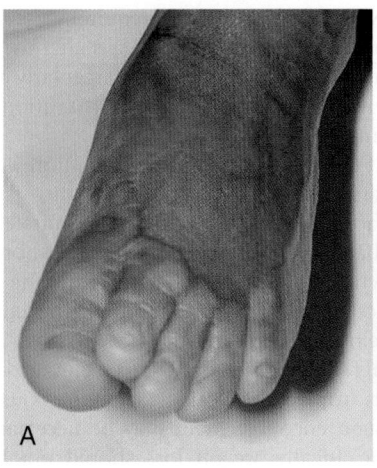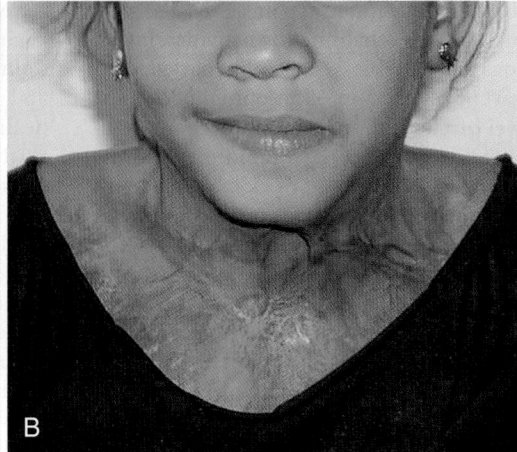

Figure 27-14 Contractures. **A,** Foot. **B,** Neck.

Source: Courtesy Judy A. Knighton, RN, MScN, Toronto, and Linda Bucher, RN, PhD.

implantation of pigment within the skin—can help even out unequal skin tones and improve the patient's overall appearance and self-image.

Scarring has two components: discoloration and contour. The discoloration of scars fades somewhat with time. However, scar tissue tends to develop altered contours; that is, it is no longer flat or slightly raised but becomes elevated and enlarged above the original burned injury area. It is believed that pressure can help keep a scar flat. Gentle pressure can be maintained on the healed burn with custom-fitted pressure garments (e.g., Jobst garments). They should never be worn over unhealed wounds and are removed only for short periods during bathing.

These garments are worn up to 24 hours a day for as long as 12 to 18 months. Patients typically experience discomfort from itching where healing is occurring. Application of water-based moisturizers and use of oral antihistamines (e.g., diphenhydramine [Benadryl]) help reduce the itching. Massage oil, silicone gel sheeting (e.g., Biodermis), gabapentin (Neurontin), and injectable steroids also may be helpful (Brooks, Malic, & Judkins, 2008). As "old" epithelium is replaced by new cells, flaking occurs. The newly formed skin is extremely sensitive to trauma.

Blisters and skin tears are likely to develop from slight pressure or friction. In addition, these newly healed areas can be hypersensitive or hyposensitive to cold, heat, and touch. Grafted areas are more likely to be hyposensitive until peripheral nerve regeneration occurs. Healed burn areas must be protected from direct sunlight for about 3 months to prevent hyperpigmentation and sunburn injury.

Complications

The most common complications during the rehabilitative phase are skin and joint contractures and hypertrophic scarring (Figure 27-14). A **contracture** (an abnormal condition of a joint characterized by flexion and fixation) develops as a result of the shortening of scar tissue in the flexor tissues of a joint (Schneider et al., 2008). Areas that are most susceptible to contracture formation include anterior and lateral neck areas, axillae, antecubital fossae, fingers, groin areas, popliteal fossae, knees, and ankles. These areas encompass major joints. Not only does the skin over these areas develop contractures, but also the underlying tissues, such

as the ligaments and tendons, have a tendency to shorten in the healing process.

Because of pain, patients with burn injuries prefer to assume a flexed position for comfort. This position predisposes wounds to contracture formation. Positioning, splinting, and exercise should be instituted to minimize this complication (Schneider et al., 2008). These procedures should be continued until the skin matures. Therapy is aimed at the extension of body parts because the flexors are stronger than the extensors. Burned legs may be wrapped with elastic (e.g., tensor [ACE]) bandages to assist with circulation to leg graft and donor sites before ambulation. This additional pressure prevents blister formation, promotes venous return, and decreases pain and itchiness. Once the skin is completely healed, less fragile, custom-fitted pressure garments can replace the elastic bandages.

NURSING AND COLLABORATIVE MANAGEMENT: REHABILITATION PHASE

During the rehabilitation phase, both the patient and the family are actively encouraged to participate in care. Because the patient may go home with small, unhealed wounds, education and "hands-on" instruction in dressing changes and wound care are needed. If necessary, home care nursing services should be arranged to assist with care for the first few weeks after discharge. An emollient water-based cream (e.g., Vaseline Intensive Care Extra Strength) that penetrates into the dermis should be used routinely on healed areas to keep the skin supple and well moisturized, which will decrease itching and flaking. Oral antihistamines may be used if itching persists. Reconstructive surgery is frequently required after a major burn. It is important for the patient to understand the need for or possibility of further surgery before leaving the hospital.

The continuous role of exercise and physical/occupational therapy cannot be overemphasized. Constant encouragement and reassurance are necessary to maintain a patient's morale, particularly once the patient realizes that recovery can be slow and rehabilitation may need to be a primary focus for at least the next 6 to 12 months.

Because of the tremendous psychological effect of burn injury, health care providers should be particularly sensitive and attuned to the patient's emotions and concerns. It is essential that patients be encouraged to discuss their fears regarding loss of their lifestyle as they once knew it, loss of function, temporary or permanent deformity and disfigurement, return to work and home life, and financial burdens resulting from a long and potentially costly hospitalization and rehabilitation. Care should also be taken to address individual spiritual and cultural needs because both these facets of a patient's life play a role in recovery. Pastoral care and cultural groups may be helpful resources to the patient, the family, and the health care team. In earlier discussions with family members in the emergent and acute phases, the different meanings of a burn injury in different cultures and, in particular, for the patient's loved one are probably identified. Patients can then be assisted toward a realistic and positive appraisal of their particular situation, emphasizing what they can do instead of what they cannot do.

A person's self-esteem is usually adversely affected by a burn injury (Moi, Vindenes, & Gjengedal, 2008). In some individuals, an overwhelming fear may be the loss of relationships because of perceived or actual physical disfigurement. In a society in which physical beauty is valued, alterations in body image can result in psychological distress. Encouraging appropriate independence, an eventual return to preburn activities, and interactions with other burn survivors will involve the patient in familiar activities that may bring comfort and help restore self-esteem. Counselling, which may have started in the acute phase of care, can be offered after discharge. Patients appreciate reassurance that their emotions during this period of adjustment are normal and that frustration is to be expected as they attempt to resume a normal lifestyle.

AGE-RELATED CONSIDERATIONS: BURNS

Older adult patients with burns present many challenges for the burn team. The normal aging process puts such patients at risk for injury because of the possibility of an unsteady gait, limited eyesight, and diminished hearing. As people age, skin becomes drier, more wrinkled, and looser. The dermal layer thins, there is a loss of elastic fibres, the amount of subcutaneous adipose tissue decreases, and vascularity decreases. As a result, the thinner dermis, with reduced blood flow, sustains deeper burns with poorer rates of healing (Gómez & Cancio, 2007).

Once injured, older adults have more complications in the emergent and acute phases of burn resuscitation because of pre-existing medical conditions. For example, among older patients with diabetes, heart failure, or chronic obstructive pulmonary disease, morbidity and mortality rates exceed those of healthy, younger patients. In older adult patients, pneumonia is a frequent complication, burn wounds and donor sites take longer to heal, and surgical procedures are not as well tolerated. Weaning from a ventilator can be a challenge, and delirium from medication and anaesthesia may be a distressing, although usually self-limiting, outcome. It usually takes longer for older patients to become rehabilitated to the point at which they can safely return home. For some, a return home to independent living may not be possible. As the population ages, developing strategies to prevent burn injuries in this population is a priority (Staats, 2008).

Emotional Needs of the Patient and Caregivers

For the nurse to adequately manage the enormous range of emotional responses that the patient with burn injury may exhibit, it is important to have an understanding of the circumstances of the burn, family relationships, and previous coping experiences with stressful stimuli. At any time, the various emotions of fear, anxiety, anger, guilt, and depression may be experienced (Table 27-15).

A common emotional response is regression. The patient may revert to behaviour that helped in coping with stressful situations in the past. This response can be healthy and is usually short-lived. Major emotional challenges confront patients and families throughout the recovery of the patient with burn injuries and perhaps for years to come. As more and more independence is expected from the patient, new fears must be confronted: "Can I do it?" "Am I a desirable partner or parent?" Open and frequent communication among the patient, family members, close friends, and burn team members is essential.

Burn survivors frequently experience thoughts and feelings that are frightening and disturbing, such as guilt about the burn accident, reliving the experience, fear of death, concern about future therapy and surgery, frustrations with ongoing discomfort and wound breakdown, and, perhaps, hopelessness about the future. Families may share some or all of these feelings. At times, family members may feel helpless to assist their loved one. Continued support from trusted and familiar burn team members is essential. Assisting with aspects of care helps family members reconnect with their loved one and assists with the transition home. Many burn survivors and their families remark on the powerful learning experience of the burn and a renewed appreciation of life, despite the ongoing challenges of a prolonged and challenging recovery. Acknowledgement that their many feelings are real and valid can be therapeutic for patients and their families.

Table 27-15 Emotional Responses of Patients With Burn Injury*	
EMOTION	**POSSIBLE VERBAL EXPRESSION**
Fear	"Will I die?"
	"What will happen next?"
	"Will I be disfigured?"
	"Will my family and friends still love me?"
Anxiety	"I feel out of control."
	"What's going to happen to me?"
	"When will I look normal again?"
Anger	"Why did this happen to me?"
	"The nurses enjoy hurting me."
	"I hope the person who did this to me dies."
Guilt	"If only I'd been more careful."
	"I'm being punished because I did something wrong."
Depression	"It's no use going on like this."
	"I don't care what happens to me."
	"I wish people would leave me alone."

*List is not all-inclusive.

The stress of the burn injury occasionally precipitates a time-limited psychiatric or psychological crisis. Many patients realize that coping with this experience is beyond their ability. Assessment by a psychiatrist who can prescribe appropriate medication, if needed, and begin short-term counselling is frequently helpful. Early psychiatric intervention is essential if the patient has been previously treated for a psychiatric illness or if the injury was a suicide attempt. The diagnosis of post-traumatic stress disorder is made in a number of patients with burn injuries (McKibben, Bresnick, Wiechman Askay, & Fauerbach, 2008). Treatment typically begins in the hospital, but links to community resources must be made before discharge to ensure continuity of psychological care. Once the patient is discharged, referral to a psychiatrist, psychologist, mental health counsellor, social worker, or psychiatric clinical nurse specialist may be helpful if concerns are raised at burn clinic follow-up.

Patients with burn injuries have a significant need to receive information about sexuality and intimacy (Rimmer et al., 2010). Physical appearance is altered in patients who have sustained a major burn. Acceptance of any changes is difficult at first for a patient and the significant other. The nature of skin injury in itself causes modifications in processing sexual stimuli. Touch is an important part of sexuality, and immature scar tissue may make the sensation of touch unpleasant or may dull it. This is usually transient, but the patient and partner need to know that it is normal and must receive anticipatory guidance from the health care team to avoid undue emotional strain.

Patient and family support groups may be beneficial in meeting the patient and family's emotional needs at any phase of the recovery process. Speaking with other people who have experienced burn trauma can be beneficial, both in terms of reaffirming that the feelings of the patient are normal and in allowing for the sharing of helpful advice. The Phoenix Society (see the Resources at the end of this chapter) is an international and highly respected burn survivors' support group that has been offering invaluable support and resources to burn survivors, family members, and burn team personnel for many years.

Special Needs of the Nursing Staff

Warm, trusting, mutually satisfying relationships frequently develop between patients with burn injuries and nursing staff, not only during hospitalization but also during the long-term rehabilitation period. Sometimes the bond can be so strong that the patient has difficulty separating from the hospital and staff. The frequency and intensity of family contact can also be rewarding, as well as draining, to the nurse. Nurses new to burn nursing often find it difficult to cope with not only the deformities caused by burn injury but also the odours, the unpleasant sight of wounds, and the reality of the pain that accompanies the burn and its treatment.

Many nurses come to know that the care they provide makes a critical difference in helping patients not only to survive but also to cope with and triumph over a severe and multifaceted injury. It is this belief that allows and inspires nurses to provide meaningful care to patients with burn injury and their families.

Ongoing support services for the burn nurse or critical incident stress debriefings led by a psychiatrist, psychologist, psychiatric clinical nurse specialist, or social worker may be helpful (Kornhaber & Wilson, 2011). Peer support groups (e.g., American Burn Association, Canadian Association of Burn Nurses, International Society for Burn Injuries) can serve a similar purpose by helping nursing staff cope with difficult feelings they may experience when caring for patients with burn injuries. Burn nursing is physically, psychologically, and intellectually demanding; it has many challenges and inherent rewards. Attention to self-care is important to maintain a positive attitude and healthy work–life balance. Time with family and friends and rest and relaxation at home are essential parts of self-care and living a life with purpose and fulfillment.

CLINICAL DECISION-MAKING EXERCISE

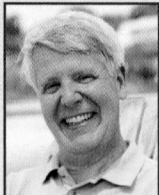

CASE STUDY:
Burn Injury

Source: © 2007 JupiterImages Corporation.

Patient Profile

Elliott Curtis, a 65-year-old married White man, is brought to the emergency department with burns to his face and right arm and hand from a kitchen grease fire. He arrives with an 18-gauge intravenous line with lactated Ringer's solution infusing at 100 mL/hour, and he is receiving 100% humidified oxygen by mask.

Subjective Data

- Complains of impaired vision and swallowing difficulties
- Cannot remember the accident
- Expresses a great deal of fear
- States he has "diabetes and high blood pressure"

Objective Data

Physical Examination

- Patient is awake, alert, and oriented but in obvious distress.
- Eyes are red and irritated.
- Voice is hoarse; nasal hair is singed.
- Face is reddened, with blisters noted on the nose and mouth.
- Right arm and hand have shiny, bright red, wet wounds.
- Patient is shivering.

Discussion Questions

1. *Priority Decision:* What are the priorities of care in the pre-hospital environment? How should Mr. Curtis's airway, breathing, and circulation be managed?
2. *Priority Decision:* What signs and symptoms indicate that Mr. Curtis likely has an inhalation injury? What priority interventions can be anticipated?
3. What pain medications might be considered to relieve his pain?
4. Which of the criteria for admission to the hospital burn unit does Mr. Curtis meet?

5. What metabolic disturbances would be expected soon after Mr. Curtis's admission? Explain the physiological basis for these changes.
6. How might Mr. Curtis's comorbid conditions affect his burn care and rehabilitation?
7. What measures should be taken to support Mr. Curtis's family?

8. *Priority Decision:* On the basis of the assessment data presented, develop three priority nursing diagnoses, and identify any collaborative problems.

evolve *Answers are available at* **http://evolve.elsevier.com/ Canada/Lewis/medsurg**

REVIEW QUESTIONS

The number of the question corresponds to the same-numbered objective at the beginning of the chapter.

1. Which of the following prevention strategies would the nurse focus on when teaching about fire safety?
   a. Use only hardwired smoke detectors.
   b. Set hot water temperature at 60°C.
   c. Encourage regular home fire exit drills.
   d. Never permit older adults to cook unattended.
2. Which of the following injuries is least likely to result in a full-thickness burn?
   a. Sunburn
   b. Scalding injury
   c. Chemical burn
   d. Electrical injury
3. What would the nurse expect to find when assessing a patient with a partial-thickness burn?
   a. Exposed fascia
   b. Dry, waxy appearance
   c. Red, shiny, wet appearance
   d. Absence of blanching with pressure
4. Which of the following describes the assessment of the extent of burns?
   a. Rating the location of burns at specific body sites
   b. Determining the presence of pre-existing risk factors
   c. Estimating the ratio of full-thickness to partial-thickness burns
   d. Using guides to indicate burn location relative to total body surface
5. Which of the following fluid and electrolyte shifts occurs during the early emergent phase?
   a. Adherence of albumin to vascular walls
   b. Movement of potassium into the vascular space
   c. Sequestering of sodium and water in interstitial fluid
   d. Hemolysis of RBCs from large volumes of rapidly administered fluid
6. Which of the following must the patient do in order to maintain a positive nitrogen balance in a major burn?
   a. Eat a high-protein, low-fat, high-carbohydrate diet.
   b. Increase normal adult caloric intake by about three times.
   c. Eat at least 1500 calories per day in small, frequent meals.
   d. Eat rice and whole wheat for the chemical effect on nitrogen balance.

7. A patient has 25% of TBSA burned from a car fire. His wounds have been debrided and covered with a silver sulphadiazine–impregnated dressing. What should the nurse's priority intervention for wound care be?
   a. To reapply a new dressing without disturbing the wound bed
   b. To observe the wound for signs of infection during dressing changes
   c. To apply cool compresses for pain relief in between dressing changes
   d. To wash the wound aggressively with soap and water three times a day
8. Which of the following is most effective in terms of pain management for the patient with burn injuries?
   a. The nurse administers opioids on a set schedule around the clock.
   b. The patient has as much control over the management of the pain as possible.
   c. The nurse has total freedom to administer opioids within a dosage and frequency range.
   d. Painful dressing changes and repositioning are delayed until the patient's pain is totally relieved.
9. Which of the following therapeutic measures is used to prevent hypertrophic scarring during the rehabilitative phase of burn recovery?
   a. Applying pressure garments
   b. Repositioning the patient every 2 hours
   c. Performing active range-of-motion exercises at least every 4 hours
   d. Massaging the new tissue with water-based moisturizers
10. The nurse is providing discharge instructions related to wound care. Which statement indicates that the patient understands the instructions?
    a. "I can expect occasional periods of low-grade fever and can take Tylenol every 4 hours."
    b. "I must wear my elastic garment all day and can only remove it when I am going to bed."
    c. "I will need to take sponge baths at home to avoid exposing the wounds to unsterile bath water."
    d. "If any unhealed areas break open I should cover them with a sterile dressing and then immediately report it."

ANSWERS: 1. c; 2. a; 3. c; 4. d; 5. c; 6. a; 7. b; 8. b; 9. a; 10. d.

REFERENCES

American Burn Association. (2011). 2011 National Burn Repository: Report of Data from 2001-2010. Analysis of Canadian and international records p 109-112. Retrieved from *http://www.ameriburn.org/2012NBRAnnualReport.pdf*

Atiyeh, S. B., & Costagliola, M. (2007). Cultured epithelial autograft (CEA) in burn treatment: Three decades later. *Burns, 33*(4), 405-413. doi:10.1016/j.burns.2006.11.002

Brooks, J. P., Malic, C. C., & Judkins, K. C. (2008). Scratching the surface—Managing the itch associated with burns: A review of current knowledge. *Burns, 34,* 751-760. doi:10.1016/j.burns.2007.11.015

Burton, K. R., Sharma, V. K., Harrop, R., & Lindsay, R. (2009). A population-based study of the epidemiology of acute adult burn injuries in the Calgary health region and factors associated with mortality and hospital length of stay from 1995 to 2004. *Burns, 35*(4), 572-579. doi:10.1016/j.burns.2008.10.003

Chan, M. M., & Chan, G. M. (2009). Nutritional therapy for burns in children and adults. *Nutrition, 25,* 261-269. doi:10.1016/j.nut.2008.10.011

Foster, K., Greenhalgh, D., Gamelli, R. L., Mozingo, D., Gibran, N., Neumeister, M., ..., FS41UVHS/D Clinical Study Group. (2008). Efficacy and safety of a fibrin sealant for adherence of autologous skin grafts to burn wounds: Results of a phase 3 clinical study. *Journal of Burn Care & Research, 29,* 293-303. doi:10.1097/BCR.0b013e31816673f8

Gómez, R., & Cancio, L. C. (2007). Management of burn wounds in the emergency department. *Emergency Medicine Clinics of North America, 25,* 135-146. doi:10.1016/j.emc.2007.01.005

Greenhalgh, D. G., Saffle, J. R., Homes, J. H. IV, Gamelli, D. G., Palmieri, T. L., Horton, J. W., ..., American Burn Association Consensus Conference on Burn Sepsis and Infection Group. (2007). American Burn Association consensus conference to define sepsis and infection in burns. *Journal of Burn Care & Research, 28*(6), 776-790. doi:10.1097/BCR.0b013e3181599bc9

Hackenschmidt, A. (2007). Burn trauma priorities for a patient with 80% total body surface area burns. *Journal of Emergency Nursing, 33*(4), 405-408. doi:10.1016/j.jen.2007.05.007

Jang, Y. C., Kim, Y. J., Lee, J. W., Oh, S. J., Han, K. W., Lee, J. W., & Han, T. H. (2006). Face burns caused by flambé drinks. *Journal of Burn Care & Research, 27*(1), 93-96. doi:10.1097/01.bcr.0000192264.90796.23

Klein, M. B., Lezotte, D. C., Heltshe, S., Fauerbach, J., Holavanahalli, R. K., Rivara, F. P., ..., Engrav, L. (2011). Functional and psychosocial outcomes of older adults after burn injury: Results from a multicenter database of severe burn injury. *Journal of Burn Care & Research, 32*(1), 66-78. doi:10.1097/BCR.0b013e31820336a

Kornhaber, R. A., & Wilson, A. (2011). Building resilience in burns nurses: A descriptive phenomenological inquiry. *Journal of Burn Care & Research, 32*(4):481-488.

McKibben, J. B. A., Bresnick, M. G., Wiechman Askay, S. A., & Fauerbach, J. A. (2008). Acute stress disorder and posttraumatic stress disorder: A prospective study of prevalence, course and predictors in a sample with major burn injuries. *Journal of Burn Care & Research, 29*(1), 22-35. doi:10.1097/BCR.0b013e31815f59c4

Mlcak, R. P., Suman, O. E., & Herndon, D. N. (2007). Respiratory management of inhalation injury. *Burns, 33*(1), 2-13. doi:10.1016/j.burns.2006.07.007

Moi, A. L., Vindenes, H. A., & Gjengedale, E. (2008). The experience of life after burn injury: a new bodily awareness. *Journal of Advanced Nursing, 64*(3), 278-286.

Nicol, N. H., & Huether, S. E. (2012). Structure, function, and disorders of the integument. In S. E. Huether & K. L. McCance (Eds.), *Understanding pathophysiology* (5th ed., pp. 1060-1064). St. Louis: Mosby.

Pannucci, C. J., Osborne, N. H., & Wahl, W. L. (2011). Venous thromboembolism in thermally injured patients: Analysis of the National Burn Repository. *Journal of Burn Care & Research, 32*(1), 6-12. doi:10.1097/BCR.0b013e318204b2ff

Richardson, P., & Mustard, L. (2009). The management of pain in the burns unit. *Burns, 35*(7), 921-936. doi:10.1016/j.burns.2009.03.003

Rimmer, R. B., Rutter, C. E., Lessard, C. R., Pressman, M. S., Jost, J. C., Bosch, J., ..., Caruso, D. M. (2010). Burn care professionals' attitudes and practices regarding discussions of sexuality and intimacy with adult burn survivors. *Journal of Burn Care & Research, 31,* 579-589. doi:10.1097/BCR.0b013e3181e4d66a

Schneider, J. C., Holavanahalli, R., Helm, P., O'Neil, C., Goldstein, R., & Kowalske, K. (2008). Contractures in burn injury part II: Investigating joints of the hand. *Journal of Burn Care & Research, 29*(4), 606-613. doi:10.1097/BCR.0b013e31817db8e1

Singer, A. J., & Dagum, A. B. (2008). Current management of acute cutaneous wounds. *New England Journal of Medicine, 359*(10), 1037-1046. doi:10.1056/NEJMra0707253

Staats, D. O. (2008). Health promotion in older adults: What clinicians can do to prevent accidental injuries. *Geriatrics, 63*(4), 12-17.

Taira, B. R., Cassara, G., Meng, H., Salama, M. N., Chohan, J., Sandoval, S., & Singer, A. J. (2011). Predictors of sustaining burn injury: Does the use of common prevention strategies matter? *Journal of Burn Care & Research, 32*(1), 20-25. doi:10.1097/BCR.0b013e318204b2eb

Yim, H., Cho, Y. S., Seo, C. H., Lee, B. C., Ko, J. H., Kim, D., ..., Kim, J. H. (2010). The use of AlloDerm on major burn patients: AlloDerm prevents post-burn joint contracture. *Burns, 36,* 322-328. doi:10.1016/j.burns.2009.10.018

CANADIAN RESOURCES

Canadian Association of Burn Nurses
http://www.cabn.ca
Canadian Burn Foundation
http://www.canadianburnfoundation.org/whoweare.php

RELATED RESOURCES

American Burn Association
http://www.ameriburn.org
Burn Foundation
http://www.burnfoundation.org
Changing Faces
http://www.changingfaces.org.uk
International Society for Burn Injuries
http://www.worldburn.org
Phoenix Society for Burn Survivors
http://www.phoenix-society.org
SageDiagram
http://www.sagediagram.com

evolve *For additional Internet resources, see the Web site for this book at* **http://evolve.elsevier.com/Canada/Lewis/medsurg**

Problems of Oxygenation: Ventilation

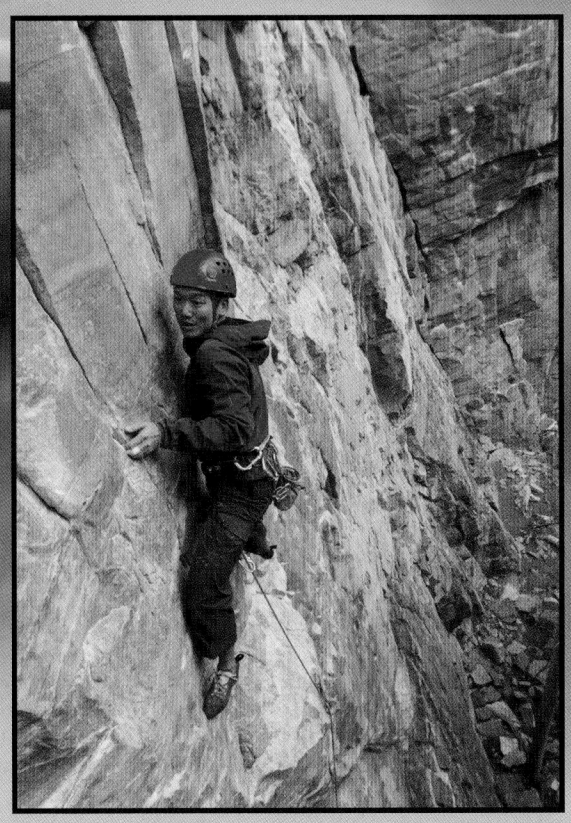

Scott Hailstone/iStockphoto

Nursing Assessment: Respiratory System

Written by Casey Norris

Adapted by Leslie Graham

LEARNING OBJECTIVES

1. Describe the structures and functions of the upper respiratory tract, the lower respiratory tract, and the chest wall.
2. Describe the process that initiates and controls inspiration and expiration.
3. Describe the process of gas diffusion within the lungs.
4. Identify the respiratory defence mechanisms.
5. Describe the significance of arterial blood gas values and the oxygen–hemoglobin dissociation curve in relation to respiratory function.
6. Identify the signs and symptoms of inadequate oxygenation and the implications of these findings.
7. Describe age-related changes in the respiratory system and differences in assessment findings.
8. Identify the significant subjective and objective data related to the respiratory system that should be obtained from a patient.
9. Describe the techniques used in physical assessment of the respiratory system.
10. Differentiate normal from common abnormal findings in a physical assessment of the respiratory system.
11. Describe the purpose, significance of results, and nursing responsibilities related to diagnostic studies of the respiratory system.

KEY TERMS

adventitious sounds Extra breath sounds that are abnormal, p. 622

chemoreceptor A receptor that responds to a change in the chemical composition (partial pressure of arterial carbon dioxide [$PaCO_2$] and pH) of the fluid around it, p. 615

compliance A measure of the elasticity of the lungs and thorax, p. 612

crackles Short, low-pitched sounds caused by passage of air through an airway intermittently occluded by mucus, unstable bronchial wall, or fold of mucosa, p. 622

dyspnea Shortness of breath; difficulty breathing that may be caused by certain heart or lung conditions, strenuous exercise, or anxiety, p. 617

elastic recoil The tendency for the lungs to recoil after being stretched or expanded, p. 612

fremitus Vibration of the chest wall produced by vocalization, p. 620

mechanical receptors Receptors located in the lungs, upper airways, chest wall, and diaphragm; stimulated by a variety of physiological factors, such as irritants, muscle stretching, and alveolar wall distortion. Signals from the stretch receptors aid in the control of respiration. As the lungs inflate, pulmonary stretch receptors activate the inspiratory centre to inhibit further lung expansion, p. 615

pleural friction rub Creaking or grating sound that results when roughened, inflamed surfaces of the pleura rub together; evident during inspiration, expiration, or both; no change with coughing, p. 622

surfactant A lipoprotein that lowers the surface tension in the alveoli, reduces the amount of pressure needed to inflate the alveoli, and decreases the tendency of the alveoli to collapse, p. 610

tidal volume Volume of air exchanged with each breath, p. 610

ventilation Inspiration (movement of air into the lungs) and expiration (movement of air out of the lungs), p. 612

wheezes Continuous high-pitched squeaking sounds caused by rapid vibration of bronchial walls, p. 622

ELECTRONIC RESOURCES

Supplemental content related to Chapter 28 can be found...

Evolve Web Site ⊝volve

- Animations:
  - Patterns of Respiration
  - Percussion Tones Throughout the Chest
  - Pulmonary Circulation
- Assessment Case Study: Respiratory System
- Audio Clips:
  - Bronchial Breath Sounds
  - Bronchovesicular Breath Sounds
  - High-Pitched Crackles
  - High-Pitched Wheeze
  - Low-Pitched Crackles
  - Low-Pitched Wheeze
  - Pleural Friction Rub
  - Stridor
  - Vesicular Breath Sounds

- Content Updates
- Electronic Calculators
- Examination Review Questions
- Glossary
- Key Points (Printable and MP3 Download)
- Physical Examination Videos:
  - Anterior Chest, Lungs, and Heart
  - Lungs
- Video Clips:
  - Inspection and Palpation: Breathing and Chest Expansion, Anterior Chest
  - Inspection and Palpation: Respirations, Chest Expansion, and Tactile Fremitus, Posterior Chest
  - Inspection and Percussion: Diaphragmatic Excursion
  - Inspection: Nose
  - Palpation: Tactile Fremitus, Posterior Chest
  - Percussion: Anterior Thorax

Structures and Functions of the Respiratory System

The primary purpose of the respiratory system is gas exchange, which involves the transfer of oxygen and carbon dioxide from the atmosphere to the blood. The respiratory system is divided into two parts: the upper respiratory tract and the lower respiratory tract (Figure 28-1). The upper respiratory tract includes the nasal cavity, the pharynx, the adenoids, the tonsils, the epiglottis, the larynx, and the trachea. The major structures of the lower respiratory tract are the bronchi, the bronchioles, the alveolar ducts, and the alveoli. With the exception of the right and left main-stem bronchi, all lower airway structures are contained within the lungs. The right lung is divided into three lobes (upper, middle, and lower) and the left lung into two lobes (upper and lower; Figure 28-2). The structures of the chest wall (ribs, pleura, muscles of respiration) are also essential for respiration.

Upper Respiratory Tract

The nose, made of bone and cartilage, is divided into two nares by the nasal septum. The interior of the nose is shaped into rolling projections called *turbinates* that increase the surface area for warming and moistening air. The internal portion of the nose opens directly into the sinuses. The nasal cavity is connected to the pharynx, a tubular passageway that is subdivided into three parts: In descending order, they are the nasopharynx, the oropharynx, and the laryngopharynx.

Breathing through the narrow nasal passages (rather than mouth breathing) provides protection for the lower airway. The nose is lined with mucous membrane and small hairs. Air entering the nose is warmed to near body temperature, humidified to nearly 100% water saturation, and filtered to remove particles larger than 10 micrometres (μm) (e.g., dust, bacteria).

The olfactory nerve endings (receptors for the sense of smell) are located in the roof of the nose. The adenoids and the tonsils, which are small masses of lymphatic tissue, are found in the nasopharynx and the oropharynx, respectively.

The epiglottis is a small flap of tissue at the base of the tongue. During swallowing, the epiglottis covers the larynx, preventing solids and liquids from entering the lungs. A condition such as a stroke that alters swallowing ability may impair the function of the epiglottis, thus predisposing to aspiration.

After passing through the oropharynx, air moves through the laryngopharynx and the larynx, where the vocal cords are located, and then down into the trachea. The trachea is a cylindrical tube about 10 to 12 cm long and 1.5 to 2.5 cm in diameter. The support of U-shaped cartilages keeps the trachea open but allows the adjacent esophagus to expand for swallowing. The trachea bifurcates into the right and left main-stem bronchi at a point called the *carina*. The carina is located at the level of the manubriosternal junction, also called the *angle of Louis*. The carina is highly sensitive, and touching it during suctioning causes vigorous coughing (Thibodeau & Patton, 2010).

Lower Respiratory Tract

Once air passes the carina, it is in the lower respiratory tract. The main-stem bronchi, the pulmonary vessels, and nerves enter the lungs through a slit called the *hilum*. The right main-stem bronchus is shorter, wider, and straighter than the left main-stem bronchus. For this reason, aspiration is more likely to occur in the right lung than in the left lung.

The main-stem bronchi subdivide several times to form the lobar, segmental, and subsegmental bronchi. Further divisions form the bronchioles. The most distant bronchioles are called the *respiratory bronchioles*. Beyond these lie the alveolar ducts and the alveolar sacs (Figure 28-3). The bronchioles are encircled by smooth muscles that constrict and dilate in response to various stimuli. The terms *bronchoconstriction* and *bronchodilation* are

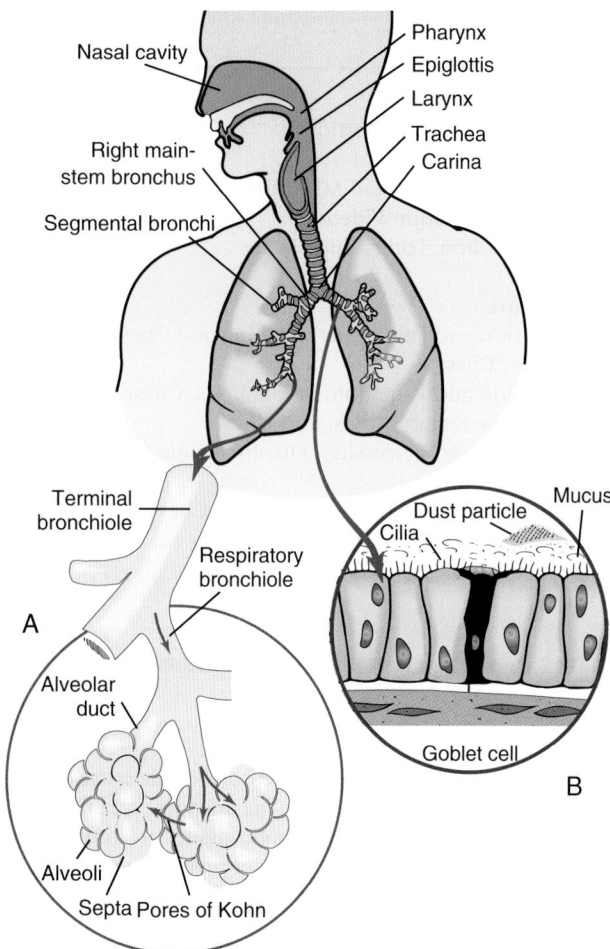

Figure 28-1 Structures of the respiratory tract. **A,** Pulmonary functional unit. **B,** Ciliated mucous membrane.

Source: Redrawn from Price, S. A., & Wilson, L. M. (2003). *Pathophysiology: Clinical concepts of disease processes* (6th ed.). St. Louis: Mosby.

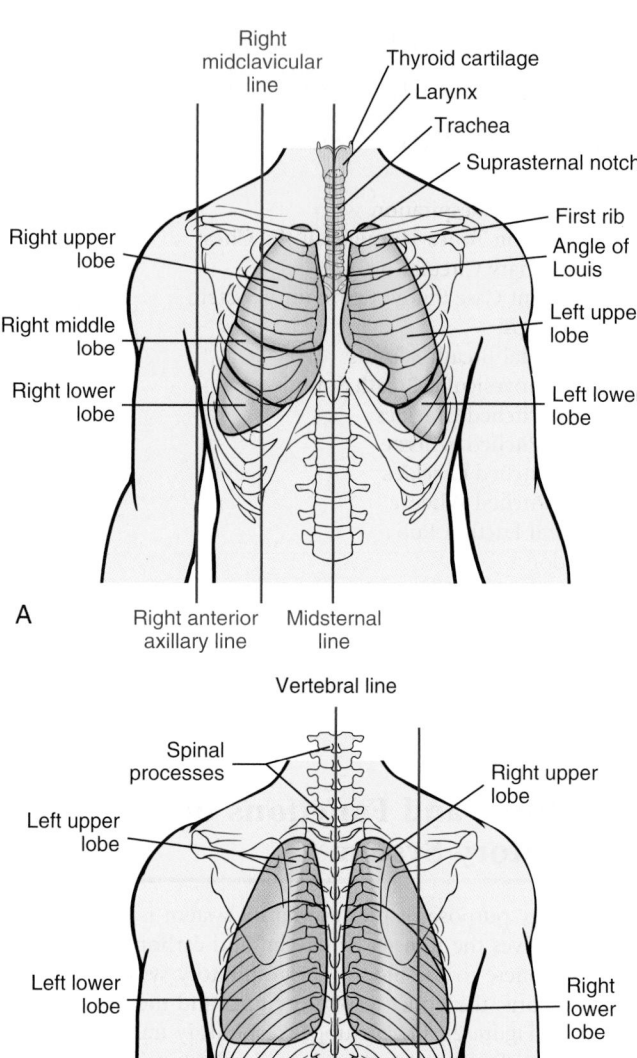

Figure 28-2 Landmarks and structures of the chest wall. **A,** Anterior view. **B,** Posterior view.

Source: Thompson, J. M., McFarland, G., & Tucker, S. (2002). *Mosby's clinical nursing* (5th ed.). St. Louis: Mosby.

used to refer to a decrease or increase in the diameter of the airways that is caused by contraction or relaxation of these muscles.

No exchange of oxygen or carbon dioxide takes place until air enters the respiratory bronchioles. The area of the respiratory tract from the nose to the respiratory bronchioles serves only as a conducting pathway and is therefore termed the *anatomical dead space* (V_D). This space must be filled with every breath, but the air that fills it is not available for gas exchange. In adults, a normal **tidal volume,** or volume of air exchanged with each breath, is about 500 mL. Of each 500 mL inhaled, about 150 mL is V_D.

After moving through the conducting zone, air reaches the respiratory bronchioles and the alveoli (Figure 28-4). *Alveoli* are small sacs that form the functional unit of the lungs. The alveoli are interconnected by pores of Kohn, which allow movement of air from alveolus to alveolus (see Figure 28-1). Bacteria can also move through these pores; as a result, a respiratory infection can extend to previously noninfected areas. The 300 million alveoli in the adult have a total volume of about 2500 mL and a surface area for gas exchange that is about the size of a tennis court. The alveolar–capillary membrane (Figure 28-5) is very thin—less

than 5 µm thick—and is the site of gas exchange. In conditions such as pulmonary edema, excess fluid fills the interstitial space and the alveoli, markedly impairing gas exchange (Thibodeau & Patton, 2010; Wagner, Johnson, & Hardin-Pierce, 2009; Weinberger, 2009).

Surfactant. The lung can be conceptualized as a collection of 300 million bubbles (alveoli), each 0.3 mm in diameter. Such a structure is inherently unstable and, as a consequence, the alveoli have a natural tendency to collapse. The alveolar surface is composed of cells that provide structure and cells that secrete surfactant (see Figure 28-5). **Surfactant,** a lipoprotein that lowers the surface tension in the alveoli, reduces the

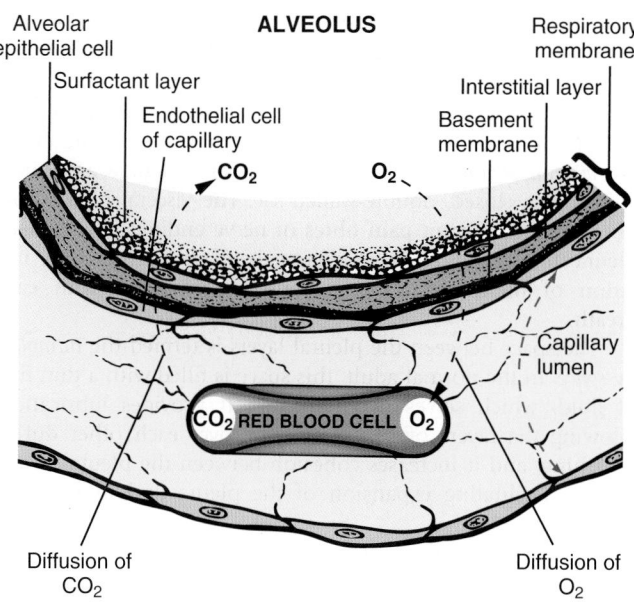

Conducting airways					Respiratory unit
Trachea	Bronchi, segmental bronchi	Sub-segmental bronchi	Bronchioles		Alveolar ducts, alveoli
			Non-respiratory	Respiratory	

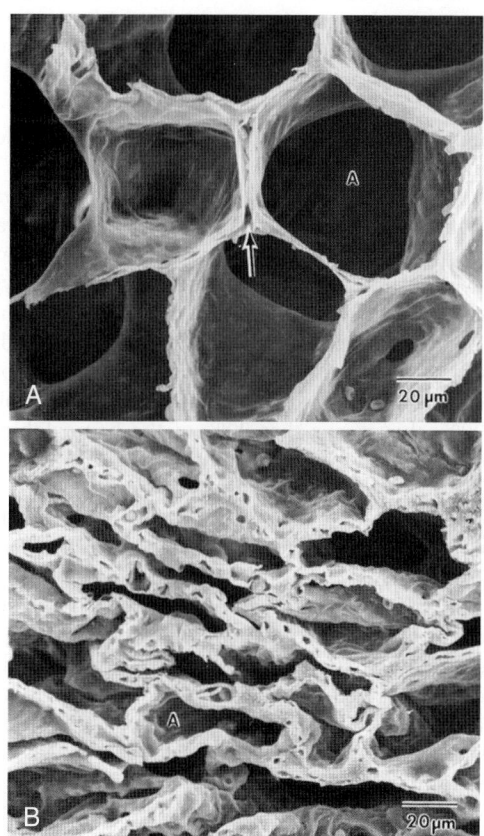

| Generations | 8 | 15 | 21-22 | 24 | 28 |

Figure 28-3 Structures of lower airways.

Source: From Thompson, J. M., McFarland, G., & Tucker, S. (2002). *Mosby's clinical nursing* (5th ed.). St. Louis: Mosby.

Figure 28-5 A small portion of the respiratory membrane, greatly magnified. An extremely thin interstitial layer of tissue separates the endothelial cell and basement membrane on the capillary side from the epithelial cell and surfactant layer on the alveolar side of the respiratory membrane. The total thickness of the respiratory membrane is less than 5 μm.

Figure 28-4 Scanning electron micrograph of lung parenchyma. **A,** Alveoli *(A)* and alveolar capillary *(arrow)*. **B,** Effects of atelectasis. Alveoli *(A)* are partially or totally collapsed.

Source: **A,** From Bone, R. C., Dantzker, D. R., George, R. B., et al. (Eds.), (1993). *Pulmonary and critical care medicine* (Vol. 1). St. Louis: Mosby; **B,** From Albertine, K. H., Williams, M. C., & Hyde, D. M. (2005). Anatomy of the lungs. In Mason, R. J., Broaddus, V. C., Murray, J. F., & Nadel, J. A. (Eds.), *Murray and Nadel's textbook of respiratory medicine* (4th ed.). Philadelphia: W. B. Saunders.)

amount of pressure needed to inflate the alveoli and decreases the tendency of the alveoli to collapse. Normally, each person takes a slightly larger breath, termed a *sigh,* after every five to six breaths. This sigh stretches the alveoli and promotes surfactant secretion.

When insufficient surfactant is present, the alveoli collapse. The term *atelectasis* refers to collapsed, airless alveoli (see Figure 28-4). The patient who has just undergone surgery is at risk for postoperative atelectasis because of the effects of anaesthesia and restricted breathing with pain (see Chapter 22). In acute respiratory distress syndrome, lack of surfactant contributes to widespread atelectasis (Huether & McCance, 2012). (Acute respiratory distress syndrome is discussed further in Chapter 70.)

Blood Supply. The lungs have two different types of circulation: pulmonary and bronchial. The pulmonary circulation provides the lungs with blood for gas exchange. The pulmonary artery receives deoxygenated blood from the right ventricle of the heart and branches so that each pulmonary capillary is directly connected with many alveoli. Oxygen–carbon dioxide exchange occurs at this point. The pulmonary veins return oxygenated blood to the left atrium of the heart.

The bronchial circulation starts with the bronchial arteries, which arise from the thoracic aorta. The bronchial circulation provides oxygen to the bronchi and other pulmonary tissues. Deoxygenated blood returns from the bronchial circulation through the azygos vein into the left atrium.

Chest Wall

The chest wall is shaped, supported, and protected by 24 ribs (12 on each side). The ribs and the sternum protect the lungs and the heart from injury and are collectively sometimes called the *thoracic cage*. The structures of the chest wall include the thoracic cage, the pleura, and the respiratory muscles.

The chest cavity is lined with a membrane called the *parietal pleura*, and the lungs are lined with a membrane called the *visceral pleura*. The parietal and visceral pleurae are joined and form a closed, double-walled sac. The visceral pleura does not have any afferent pain fibres or nerve endings. The parietal pleura, however, does have afferent pain fibres. Therefore, irritation of the parietal pleura causes severe pain with each breath.

The space between the pleural layers is termed the *intrapleural space*. In the normal adult, this space is filled with a thin film of fluid, which serves two purposes: It provides lubrication, allowing the layers of pleura to slide over each other during breathing, and it increases cohesion between the pleural layers, thereby facilitating expansion of the pleura and lung during inspiration.

Normally, the pleural space contains 20 to 25 mL of fluid. Fluid is drained from the pleural space by the lymphatic circulation. Several pathological conditions may cause the accumulation of greater amounts of fluid, termed *pleural effusions*. Pleural fluid may accumulate because malignant cells block lymphatic drainage or because there is an imbalance between intravascular and oncotic fluid pressures, as occurs in congestive heart failure. The presence of purulent pleural fluid with bacterial infection is called *empyema*.

The diaphragm is the major muscle of respiration. During inspiration, the diaphragm contracts, pushing the abdominal contents downward. At the same time, the external intercostal muscles and scalene muscles contract, increasing the lateral and anteroposterior dimension of the chest. This causes the size of the thoracic cavity to increase and intrathoracic pressure to decrease, so that air can enter the lungs.

The diaphragm is made up of two hemidiaphragms, each innervated by the right and left phrenic nerves. The phrenic nerves arise from the spinal cord between C3 and C5, the third and fifth cervical vertebrae. Injury to the phrenic nerve results in hemidiaphragmatic paralysis on the side of the injury. Complete spinal cord injuries above the level of C3 result in total diaphragmatic paralysis, and affected patients are dependent on mechanical ventilation (Herlihy & Maebius, 2010).

Physiology of Respiration

Ventilation. **Ventilation** involves *inspiration* (movement of air into the lungs) and *expiration* (movement of air out of the lungs). Air moves in and out of the lungs because intrathoracic pressure changes in relation to pressure at the airway opening. Contraction of the diaphragm and of the intercostal and scalene muscles increases chest dimensions, thereby decreasing intrathoracic pressure. Gas flows from an area of higher pressure (atmospheric) to one of lower pressure (intrathoracic). When inspiration is difficult, neck and shoulder muscles can assist the effort. Some conditions (e.g., phrenic nerve paralysis, rib fractures, neuromuscular disease) may limit diaphragm or chest wall movement and cause the patient to breathe with smaller tidal volumes. As a result, the lungs do not fully inflate, and gas exchange is impaired.

In contrast to inspiration, expiration is passive. The elastic recoil of the chest wall and lungs allows the chest to passively return to its normal position. Intrathoracic pressure rises, causing air to move out of the lungs. Exacerbations of asthma or emphysema cause expiration to become an active, laboured process (see Chapter 31). Abdominal and intercostal muscles assist in expelling air during laboured breathing.

Elastic Recoil and Compliance. **Elastic recoil** is the tendency for the lungs to recoil after being stretched or expanded. The elasticity of lung tissue is attributable to the elastin fibres that are found in the alveolar walls and that surround the bronchioles and capillaries.

Compliance (distensibility) is a measure of the elasticity of the lungs and the thorax. When compliance is decreased, inflation of the lungs is more difficult. Examples of conditions in which compliance is decreased include those that increase fluid in the lungs (e.g., pulmonary edema, acute respiratory distress syndrome); diseases that make lung tissue less elastic (e.g., pulmonary fibrosis, sarcoidosis); and conditions that restrict lung movement (e.g., pleural effusion). Compliance is decreased as a result of aging and when there is destruction of alveolar walls and loss of tissue elasticity, as in emphysema.

Diffusion. Oxygen and carbon dioxide move back and forth across the alveolar capillary membrane by diffusion. The overall direction of movement is from the area of higher concentration to the area of lower concentration. Thus oxygen moves from alveolar gas (atmospheric air) into the arterial blood, and carbon dioxide from the arterial blood into the alveolar gas. Diffusion continues until equilibrium is reached (see Figure 28-5).

The ability of the lungs to oxygenate arterial blood adequately is determined by examination of the arterial oxygen tension (PaO_2; also referred to as the *partial pressure of oxygen in arterial blood*) and arterial oxygen saturation (SaO_2). Oxygen is carried in the blood in two forms: dissolved oxygen and hemoglobin-bound oxygen. The PaO_2 represents the amount of oxygen dissolved in the plasma and is expressed in millimetres of mercury. The SaO_2 is the amount of oxygen bound to hemoglobin in comparison with the amount of oxygen the hemoglobin can carry. The SaO_2 is expressed as a percentage. For example, if the SaO_2 is 90%, this means that 90% of the hemoglobin attachments for oxygen have oxygen bound to them.

Oxygen–Hemoglobin Dissociation Curve. The affinity of hemoglobin for oxygen is described by the *oxygen–hemoglobin (oxyhemoglobin) dissociation curve* (Figure 28-6). Oxygen delivery to the tissues depends on the amount of oxygen transported to the tissues and the ease with which hemoglobin gives up oxygen once it reaches the tissues. In the upper flat portion of the curve, fairly large changes in the PaO_2 cause small changes in hemoglobin saturation. For this reason, if the PaO_2 drops from 100 to 60 mm Hg, the saturation of hemoglobin changes only 7% (from the normal 97% to 90%). In other words, the hemoglobin remains 90% saturated despite a 40–mm Hg drop in the PaO_2. This portion of the curve also explains why a patient is considered adequately oxygenated when the PaO_2 is higher than 60 mm Hg. Increasing the PaO_2 above this level does little to improve hemoglobin saturation.

The lower portion of the oxyhemoglobin dissociation curve indicates a different type of phenomenon. As hemoglobin is desaturated, larger amounts of oxygen are released for tissue use. This is an important method of maintaining the pressure gradient between the blood and the tissues. It also ensures an adequate oxygen supply to peripheral tissues, even if oxygen delivery is compromised.

Many factors alter the affinity of hemoglobin for oxygen. When the oxygen dissociation curve shifts to the left, blood picks up oxygen more readily in the lungs but delivers oxygen less readily to the tissues. This occurs in alkalosis, in hypothermia, and with a decrease in arterial carbon dioxide tension (PaCO$_2$; also referred to as the *partial pressure of carbon dioxide in the arterial blood*) (see Figure 28-6). A patient with a condition that causes a leftward shift of the curve, such as hypothermia that follows open heart surgery, may be given higher concentrations of oxygen until the body temperature normalizes. This helps compensate for decreased oxygen unloading in the tissues. When the curve shifts to the right, the opposite occurs: Blood picks up oxygen less rapidly in the lungs but delivers oxygen more readily to the tissues. This occurs in acidosis, in hyperthermia, and when the PaCO$_2$ is increased.

Two methods are used to assess the efficiency of gas transfer in the lung: analysis of arterial blood gas (ABG) values and oximetry. These measures are usually adequate if the patient is stable and not critically ill. Many critically ill patients have a condition that impairs tissue oxygen delivery. In such patients, cardiac output, tissue oxygen consumption, mixed venous oxygen tension (PvO$_2$), and venous oxygen saturation (SvO$_2$) may also be assessed (Urden, Stacy, & Lough, 2010; see Chapter 68).

Arterial Blood Gases. ABGs are measured to determine oxygenation status and acid–base balance. ABG analysis includes measurement of the PaO$_2$, PaCO$_2$, pH, and bicarbonate (HCO$_3^-$) in arterial blood. The SaO$_2$ is either calculated or measured during this analysis. Blood for ABG analysis can be obtained by arterial puncture or from an arterial catheter in the radial or the femoral artery. Both techniques are invasive and allow only intermittent analysis. Continuous intra-arterial blood gas monitoring is also possible via a fibreoptic sensor or an oxygen electrode inserted into an arterial catheter. An arterial catheter enables ABG sampling without repeated arterial punctures.

Normal ABG values are given in Table 28-1. The normal PaO$_2$ decreases with advancing age. The normal PaO$_2$ also varies in relation to the distance above sea level. At higher altitudes, the barometric pressure is lower, and thus inspired oxygen pressure and PaO$_2$ are lower (see Table 28-1). Most airplanes are pressurized to approximate an altitude of 2400 m above sea level. A normal person can expect a 16- to 32-mm Hg fall in PaO$_2$ at this altitude (McCance & Huether, 2010). A patient who is already receiving oxygen therapy or a patient whose PaO$_2$ is lower than 72 mm Hg while he or she is breathing room air needs a careful evaluation before air travel. Supplemental oxygen or a change in litre flow may be required during the flight.

Mixed Venous Blood Gases. For patients with normal or near-normal cardiac status, an assessment of PaO$_2$ or SaO$_2$ is usually sufficient to determine adequate oxygenation. Patients with impaired cardiac output or hemodynamic instability may have inadequate tissue oxygen delivery or abnormal oxygen consumption. The amount of oxygen delivered to the tissues or consumed can be calculated.

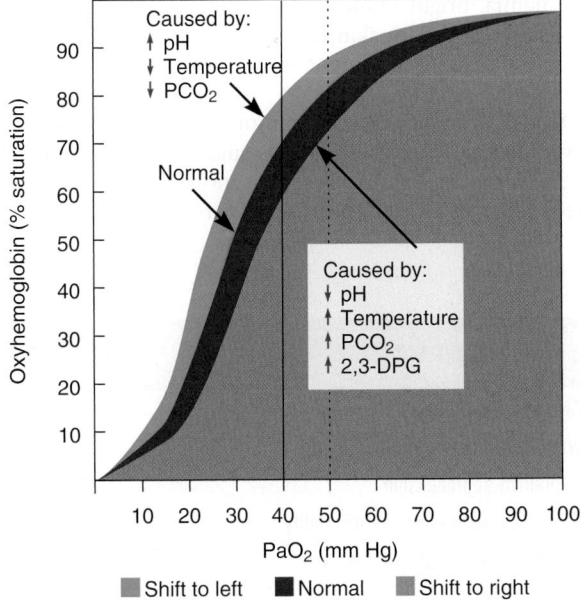

Figure 28-6 Oxygen–hemoglobin dissociation curve. A shift to the left indicates the hemoglobin's increased affinity for oxygen. A shift to the right indicates the hemoglobin's decreased affinity for oxygen. *2,3-DPG*, 2,3-diphosphoglycerate; *PaO$_2$*, partial pressure of oxygen in arterial blood; *PCO$_2$*, partial pressure of carbon dioxide.

Table 28-1 Normal Arterial and Venous Blood Gas Values*			
	ARTERIAL BLOOD GASES		**VENOUS BLOOD GASES**
LABORATORY VALUE	**BP AT SEA LEVEL: 760 mm Hg**	**BP AT 1609 METRES ABOVE SEA LEVEL: 629 mm Hg**	**MIXED VENOUS BLOOD GASES**
pH	7.35-7.45	7.35-7.45	7.31-7.41
Partial pressure of oxygen	80-100 mm Hg	65-75 mm Hg	40-50 mm Hg
Oxygen saturation	≥95%†	≥95%†	60-80%†
Partial pressure of carbon dioxide	35-45 mm Hg	35-45 mm Hg	SvO$_2$ is a better indicator for change in acid–base balance
HCO$_3^-$	21-28 mmol/L	21-28 mmol/L	21-28 mmol/L

BP, barometric pressure; *HCO$_3^-$*, bicarbonate.

*Assumes patient is ≤60 years of age and breathing room air.

†The same normal values apply to both the venous oxygen saturation value (obtained by mixed venous blood gas sampling or oximetry via catheter) and the oxygen saturation value (obtained by pulse oximetry).

A catheter positioned in the pulmonary artery, termed a *pulmonary artery catheter*, is used for mixed venous sampling (see Chapter 68). Blood drawn from a pulmonary artery catheter is termed a *mixed venous blood gas sample* because it consists of venous blood that has returned to the heart from all tissue beds and "mixed" in the right ventricle. Normal mixed venous values are listed in Table 28-1. When tissue oxygen delivery is inadequate or when inadequate oxygen is transported to the tissues by the hemoglobin, the PvO_2 and SvO_2 fall.

Oximetry.

ABG values provide accurate information about oxygenation and acid–base balance. However, they are invasive, necessitate laboratory analysis, and create the risk of bleeding from an arterial puncture. Arterial oxygen saturation can be monitored continuously by means of a *pulse oximetry* probe on a finger, a toe, an ear, the forehead, or the bridge of the nose (Figure 28-7).

A pulse oximeter emits two wavelengths of light, one red and one infrared, which pass from a light-emitting diode (positioned on one side of the probe) to a photodetector (positioned on the opposite side). Well-oxygenated blood absorbs light differently from deoxygenated blood. The oximeter determines the amount of light absorbed by the vascular bed and calculates the saturation. The oxygen saturation value obtained by pulse oximetry (SpO_2) and heart rate are displayed on the monitor as digital readings (see Figure 28-7, *B*). The normal SpO_2 is higher than 95%.

Pulse oximetry is particularly valuable in intensive care and perioperative areas, where sedation or decreased consciousness might mask hypoxia (Table 28-2). SpO_2 is assessed during each routine check of vital signs in many inpatient areas. Changes in SpO_2 can be detected quickly and treated (Table 28-3). Oximetry is also used during exercise testing and when flow rates are adjusted during long-term oxygen therapy. Pulse oximetry alone does not provide information about ventilation status and acid–base balance. Therefore, ABG measurements are also needed periodically.

Values obtained by pulse oximetry are less reliable if the SpO_2 is lower than 70%. At this level, the oximeter tends to underestimate saturation and may display an artificially low value. Pulse oximetry is also inaccurate if hemoglobin variants (e.g., carboxyhemoglobin, methemoglobin) are present. Other factors that can alter the accuracy of pulse oximetry include motion, low perfusion, anemia, bright fluorescent lights, intravascular dyes, thick acrylic nails, and dark skin colour. If there is doubt about the accuracy of the SpO_2 reading, ABGs should be measured to verify accuracy.

Oximetry can also be used to monitor SvO_2 via a pulmonary artery catheter. A decrease in SvO_2 suggests that less oxygen is being delivered to the tissues or that more oxygen is being consumed. Changes in SvO_2 provide an early warning of a change

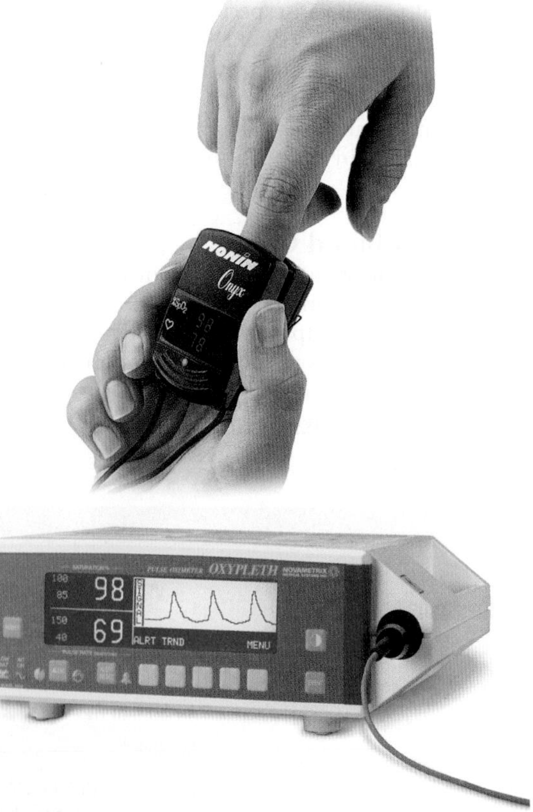

Figure 28-7 A, Portable pulse oximeter displays oxygen saturation (SpO_2) and pulse rate. **B,** A pulse oximeter displays the oxygen saturation and pulse rate as a digital reading.

Sources: **A,** Courtesy Nonin Medical Inc., Plymouth, Minnesota; **B,** Courtesy Respironics, Inc., Murrysville, Pennsylvania.

Table 28-2 Signs and Symptoms of Inadequate Oxygenation	
SIGNS AND SYMPTOMS	**ONSET**
Central Nervous System	
Unexplained apprehension	Early
Unexplained restlessness or irritability	Early
Unexplained confusion or lethargy	Early or late
Combativeness	Late
Coma	Late
Respiratory	
Tachypnea	Early
Dyspnea on exertion	Early
Dyspnea at rest	Late
Use of accessory muscles	Late
Retraction of interspaces on inspiration	Late
Pause for breath between sentences, words	Late
Cardiovascular	
Tachycardia	Early
Mild hypertension	Early
Dysrhythmias (e.g., premature ventricular contractions)	Early or late
Hypotension	Late
Cyanosis	Late
Cool, clammy skin	Late
Other	
Diaphoresis	Early or late
Decreased urinary output	Early or late
Unexplained fatigue	Early or late

PaO₂	SpO₂	CONSIDERATIONS
≥70%	≥95%	Adequate unless patient is hemodynamically unstable or has O₂ unloading problem. With a low cardiac output, dysrhythmias, a leftward shift of the oxyhemoglobin dissociation curve, or carbon monoxide inhalation, higher values may be desirable. Benefits of a higher arterial O₂ level must be balanced against the risk of O₂ toxicity.
60%	90%	Adequate in almost all patients. Values are at steep part of O₂–hemoglobin dissociation curve. Oxygenation is adequate, but margin of error is less than for higher values.
55%	88%	Adequate for patients with chronic hypoxemia if no cardiac problems occur. These values are also used as criteria for prescription of continuous O₂ therapy.
40%	75%	Inadequate but may be acceptable on a short-term basis if the patient also has CO₂ retention. In this situation, respirations may be stimulated by a low PaO₂. Thus, the PaO₂ cannot be raised rapidly. O₂ therapy at a low concentration (24-28%) will gradually increase the PaO₂. Monitoring for dysrhythmias is necessary.
<40%	<75%	Inadequate. Tissue hypoxia and cardiac dysrhythmias can be expected.

Table 28-3 Critical Values for PaO₂ and SpO₂*

PaO₂, partial pressure of oxygen in arterial blood; *SpO₂*, the oxygen saturation value obtained by pulse oximetry.
*The same critical values apply for SpO₂ and arterial oxygen saturation (SaO₂). Values pertain to rest or exertion.

in cardiac output or tissue oxygen delivery. Normal SvO₂ is 60 to 80%.

Oxygen Delivery. Information from ABG values or oximetry is used to assess adequacy of oxygenation. Several questions must be asked to determine whether oxygenation is adequate:
1. What is the patient's SpO₂ or PaO₂ in comparison with expected normal values (see Table 28-1)?
2. What is the degree of hypoxemia, and what is the trend? Has SpO₂ or PaO₂ declined rapidly? A sudden drop in blood oxygen level can be life-threatening. A gradual decline is tolerated with fewer symptoms. Critical values for SpO₂ and PaO₂ are given in Table 28-3.
3. Is the patient exhibiting signs or symptoms of inadequate oxygenation? Changes in central nervous system, respiratory, cardiovascular, and renal function occur when tissue oxygen delivery is inadequate (see Table 28-2). Because the brain is highly sensitive to a decrease in tissue oxygen delivery, the first evidence of hypoxemia may be apprehension, restlessness, or irritability. If these signs or symptoms are observed, a change in the management plan is needed.
4. What is the oxygenation status with activity or exercise? To assess for desaturation with activity, pulse oximetry is used to monitor SpO₂ levels during a standardized 6-minute walk distance test or during activities of daily living. An SpO₂ value of 88% or less during exertion indicates the need for supplemental oxygen (McCance & Huether, 2010).

Control of Respiration

The respiratory centre in the brainstem medulla responds to chemical and mechanical signals from the body. Impulses are sent from the medulla to the respiratory muscles through the spinal cord and phrenic nerves.

Chemoreceptors. A **chemoreceptor** is a receptor that responds to a change in the chemical composition (PaCO₂ and pH) of the fluid around it. Central chemoreceptors are located in the medulla and respond to changes in the hydrogen ion (H⁺) concentration. An increase in the H⁺ concentration (*acidosis*) causes the medulla to increase the respiratory rate and tidal volume. A decrease in H⁺ concentration (*alkalosis*) has the oppo-

site effect. Changes in PaCO₂ regulate ventilation primarily by their effect on the pH of the cerebrospinal fluid. When the PaCO₂ level is increased, more CO₂ is available to combine with H₂O and form carbonic acid (H₂CO₃). This lowers the pH of the cerebrospinal fluid and stimulates an increase in respiratory rate. The opposite process occurs with a decrease in PaCO₂ level.

Peripheral chemoreceptors are located in the carotid bodies at the bifurcation of the common carotid arteries and in the aortic bodies above and below the aortic arch. The peripheral chemoreceptors respond to decreases in PaO₂ and pH and to increases in PaCO₂. These changes also cause stimulation of the respiratory centre.

In a healthy person, an increase in PaCO₂ or a decrease in pH causes an immediate increase in the respiratory rate. The process is extremely precise. The PaCO₂ does not vary more than about 3 mm Hg if lung function is normal. Conditions such as chronic obstructive pulmonary disease (COPD) alter lung function and may result in chronically elevated PaCO₂ levels. In these circumstances, patients are relatively insensitive to further increases in PaCO₂ as a stimulus to breathe and may be maintaining ventilation largely because of a hypoxic drive from the peripheral chemoreceptors (see Chapter 31).

Mechanical Receptors. Mechanical receptors (juxtacapillary and irritant) are located in lungs, upper airways, chest wall, and diaphragm. They are stimulated by a variety of physiological factors, such as irritants, muscle stretching, and alveolar wall distortion. Signals from the stretch receptors aid in the control of respiration. As the lungs inflate, pulmonary stretch receptors activate the inspiratory centre to inhibit further lung expansion. This is termed the *Hering-Breuer reflex* and prevents overdistension of the lungs. Impulses from the mechanical sensors are sent through the vagus nerve to the brain. Juxtacapillary receptors (J receptors) are believed to cause the rapid respiration (tachypnea) observed in patients with pulmonary edema. These receptors are stimulated by the entry of fluid into the pulmonary interstitial space.

Respiratory Defence Mechanisms

Respiratory defence mechanisms are efficient in protecting the lungs from inhaled particles, microorganisms, and toxic gases.

The defence mechanisms include filtration of air, the mucociliary clearance system, the cough reflex, reflex bronchoconstriction, and alveolar macrophages.

Filtration of Air.

Nasal hairs filter the inspired air. In addition, the abrupt changes in direction of airflow that occur as air moves through the nasopharynx and larynx increase air turbulence. This causes particles and bacteria to contact the mucosa lining these structures. Most large particles (>5 μm in diameter) are removed in this manner.

The velocity of airflow slows greatly after it passes the larynx, facilitating the deposition of smaller particles (1-5 μm in size). They settle like sand in a river, a process termed *sedimentation*. Particles less than 1 μm in size are too small to settle in this manner and are deposited in the alveoli. One example of small particles that can build up is coal dust, which can lead to pneumoconiosis (see Chapter 30). Particle size is important. Particles larger than 5 μm are less dangerous because they are removed in the nasopharynx or bronchi and do not reach the alveoli.

Mucociliary Clearance System.

Below the larynx, movement of mucus is accomplished by the mucociliary clearance system, commonly referred to as the *mucociliary escalator*. This term is used to indicate the interrelationship between the secretion of mucus and the ciliary activity. Mucus is continually secreted at a rate of about 100 mL per day by goblet cells and submucosal glands. It forms a mucous blanket that contains the impacted particles and debris from distal lung areas (see Figure 28-1). The small amount of mucus normally secreted is swallowed without being noticed. Secretory immunoglobulin A in the mucus contributes to protection against bacteria and viruses (Tortora & Derrickson, 2010).

Cilia cover the airways from the level of the trachea to the respiratory bronchioles (see Figure 28-1). Each ciliated cell contains approximately 200 cilia, which beat rhythmically about 1000 times per minute in the large airways, moving mucus toward the mouth. The ciliary beat is slower further down the tracheobronchial tree. As a consequence, particles that penetrate more deeply into the airways are removed less rapidly. Ciliary action is impaired by dehydration, smoking, inhalation of high oxygen concentrations, infection, and ingestion of drugs such as atropine, anaesthetics, alcohol, and cocaine. Patients with chronic bronchitis and cystic fibrosis have repeated upper respiratory infections. Cilia are often destroyed during these infections, which results in impaired secretion clearance, a chronic productive cough, and frequent respiratory infections.

Cough Reflex.

The cough is a protective reflex action that clears the airway by a high-pressure, high-velocity flow of air. It is a backup for mucociliary clearance, especially when this clearance mechanism is overwhelmed or ineffective. Coughing is effective in removing secretions only above the subsegmental level (large or main airways). Secretions below this level must be moved upward by the mucociliary mechanism or by interventions such as postural drainage before they can be removed by coughing.

Reflex Bronchoconstriction.

Another defence mechanism is reflex bronchoconstriction. In response to the inhalation of large amounts of irritating substances (e.g., dusts, aerosols), the bronchi constrict in an effort to prevent entry of the irritants. In conditions of hyperreactive airways, such as asthma, bronchoconstriction occurs after inhalation of cold air, perfume, or other strong odours.

Alveolar Macrophages.

Because ciliated cells are not found below the level of the respiratory bronchioles, the primary defence mechanism at the alveolar level is performed by alveolar macrophages. *Alveolar macrophages* rapidly phagocytize inhaled foreign particles such as bacteria. The debris is moved to the level of the bronchioles for removal by the cilia or is removed from the lungs by the lymphatic system. Particles (e.g., coal dust, silica) that cannot be adequately phagocytized tend to remain in the lungs for indefinite periods and can stimulate inflammatory responses (see Chapter 30). Because alveolar macrophage activity is impaired by cigarette smoke, smokers who are employed in an occupation with heavy dust exposure (e.g., mining, foundries) are at an especially high risk for lung disease.

AGE-RELATED CONSIDERATIONS: EFFECTS OF AGING ON THE RESPIRATORY SYSTEM

Age-related changes in the respiratory system can be divided into alterations in structure, defence mechanisms, and respiratory control. Structural alterations include a decrease in elastic recoil of the lung and a decrease in chest wall compliance. Calcification of the costal cartilages inhibits thorax expansion. Many older adults have a barrel-shaped thorax as result of an increased anteroposterior diameter. Older people may develop kyphosis, which is a curvature of the spine. Severe kyphosis may limit both mobility and cardiopulmonary function. Within the lung, the number of functional alveoli decreases. Small airways in the lung bases close earlier in expiration. As a consequence, more inspired air is distributed to the lung apices, and ventilation is less matched to perfusion, which causes a lowering of the PaO_2. The PaO_2 associated with a given age can be calculated by means of the following equation:

$$PaO_2 \text{ (mm Hg)} = 103.5 - (0.42 \times \text{Age in years})$$

For example, the normal PaO_2 for a patient 80 years of age is 70 mm Hg [103.5 − (0.42 × 80)]; in comparison, the normal PaO_2 for a 25-year-old person is 93 mm Hg [103.5 − (0.42 × 25)].

Respiratory defence mechanisms are less effective in older persons because of a decline in cell-mediated immunity and formation of antibodies. The alveolar macrophages are less effective at phagocytosis. Older patients have a less forceful cough and fewer and less functional cilia. Formation of secretory immunoglobulin A, an important mechanism in neutralizing the effect of viruses, is also diminished.

In addition, respiratory control is altered, and thus the response to changes in blood oxygen or carbon dioxide level becomes more gradual. The PaO_2 drops to a lower level, and the $PaCO_2$ rises to a higher level, before the respiratory rate changes.

The extent of these changes varies among persons of the same age. Older patients—who have experienced many years of exposure to smoking, air pollutants, and other environmental toxins—are at risk for a host of other conditions (Hoffman Wold, 2008; Jarvis, Browne, MacDonald-Jenkins, & Luctkar-Flude, 2009). Age-related changes in the respiratory system and differences in assessment findings are listed in Table 28-4.

AGE-RELATED DIFFERENCES IN ASSESSMENT

Table 28-4 Respiratory System

CHANGES	DIFFERENCES IN ASSESSMENT FINDINGS
Structure	
↓ Elastic recoil	Barrel shape of chest
↓ Chest wall compliance	↓ Chest wall movement
↑ Anteroposterior diameter	↓ Respiratory excursion
↓ Functioning alveoli	↓ Vital capacity*
	↑ Functional residual capacity*
	Diminished breath sounds, particularly at lung bases
	↓ PaO_2 and SaO_2; normal pH and $PaCO_2$
Defence Mechanisms	
↓ Cell-mediated immunity	↓ Cough effectiveness
↓ Specific antibodies	↓ Secretion clearance
↓ Cilia function	↑ Risk of upper respiratory infection, influenza, and pneumonia; respiratory infections may be more severe and last longer
↓ Cough force	
↓ Alveolar macrophage function	
Respiratory Control	
↓ Response to hypoxemia	Greater ↓ in PaO_2 and ↑ in $PaCO_2$ before respiratory rate changes
↓ Response to hypercapnia	Significant hypoxemia or hypercapnia may develop from relatively small incidents
	Retained secretions, excessive sedation, or positioning that impairs chest expansion may substantially alter PaO_2 or SpO_2 values

*See Table 28-13 for definitions of terms related to lung volumes and capacities.
PaCO_2, arterial carbon dioxide tension; *PaO_2*, arterial oxygen tension; *SaO_2*, arterial oxygen saturation; *SpO_2*, oxygen saturation value obtained by pulse oximetry.

Assessment of the Respiratory System

Correct diagnosis depends on an accurate health history and a thorough physical examination (Table 28-5). A respiratory assessment can be performed as part of a comprehensive physical examination or as a focused evaluation. Whether all or part of the history and physical examination is completed is based on problems presented by the patient and the degree of respiratory distress. If respiratory distress is severe, only pertinent information should be obtained; a thorough assessment should be deferred until the patient's condition stabilizes. Table 28-6 outlines subjective and objective data that may emerge during the assessment that provide clues to the presence of respiratory problems.

Subjective Data

Important Health Information

Past Health History. The nurse should discuss with the patient the types of respiratory illnesses that the patient experi-enced during childhood (e.g., croup, respiratory syncytial virus, asthma, pneumonia, frequent colds).

The nurse should determine the frequency of upper respiratory problems (e.g., colds, sore throats, sinus problems, allergies) and whether weather changes exacerbate these problems. Patients with allergies should be questioned about possible precipitating factors such as medications, pollen, smoke, or exposure to animal dander. Characteristics of the allergic reaction—such as runny nose, wheezing, scratchy throat, or sensation of tightness in the chest—and the severity of the reaction should be documented. The frequency of asthma exacerbations and cause, if known, should also be determined. Prior use of a peak expiratory flow-meter and personal best values can be helpful information in determining the patient's current asthma status.

A history of lower respiratory tract problems, such as asthma, COPD, pneumonia, and tuberculosis, should also be documented (see the Determinants of Health box on tuberculosis in Canada, Chapter 30, p. 669). Respiratory symptoms are often manifestations of problems that involve other body systems. Therefore, the patient should be asked whether he or she has a history of other health problems in addition to those involving the respiratory system. For example, patients with cardiac dysfunction may experience **dyspnea** (shortness of breath) as a consequence of congestive heart failure. Patients with human immunodeficiency virus (HIV) infection may experience frequent respiratory infections because immune function is compromised.

Medications. Patients should be questioned carefully about prescription and over-the-counter (OTC) drugs used to manage respiratory problems, such as antihistamines, bronchodilators, corticosteroids, cough suppressants, and antibiotics. Information about the reason for taking the medication, its name, the dose and frequency, length of time taken, its effect, and any adverse effects should be obtained.

If a patient is using oxygen to ease a breathing problem, the amount, the method of administration, and effectiveness of the therapy should be documented. Safety practices related to using oxygen should also be assessed.

Patients should be questioned with regard to the OTC and herbal remedies used to treat respiratory illnesses such as the common cold, sore throat, and laryngitis.

Surgery or Other Treatments. The nurse should determine whether a patient has been hospitalized for a respiratory problem. If so, the dates, therapy (including surgery), and current status of the problem should be recorded. The nurse should ask about the use and results of respiratory treatments such as nebulizer, humidifier, and airway clearance modalities, including a flutter valve, high-frequency chest oscillation, postural drainage, and percussion.

Current Health History. If a patient has a cough, the nurse should evaluate the quality of the cough. For example, a loose-sounding cough indicates the presence of secretions; a dry, hacking cough indicates airway irritation or obstruction; a harsh, barking cough is suggestive of upper airway obstruction from inhibited vocal cord movement related to subglottic edema. The nurse should assess whether the cough is weak or strong and whether it is productive or nonproductive of secretions. Determining the onset and chronicity of a cough is helpful in the differential diagnosis process. The pattern of the cough is determined from answers to questions such as the following: What

HEALTH HISTORY

Table 28-5 Respiratory System: Questions for Obtaining Subjective Data

Past Health History

- Do you have frequent colds or very severe colds, or both?*
- Do you have any chronic health conditions?* Allergies?*
- Do you have a history of high blood pressure or heart disease?*
- Do you have any history of shortness of breath, coughing, blood in your phlegm, COPD, bronchitis, emphysema, asthma, or pneumonia?*
- Do you have a family history of allergies, tuberculosis, or asthma?

Medications

- Are you currently taking any prescribed medications, over-the-counter medications, or herbal or vitamin supplements?*
- Are you using home oxygen? If so, what amount and how is it delivered? Is it effective?
- Do you have any allergies or sensitivities to any foods or medications?*

Surgery or Other Treatments

- Have you been hospitalized for a respiratory problem in the past?*

Current Health History

- What is your usual or present height and weight? Have you recently gained or lost weight?*
- Are there any environmental conditions at home or work that may have an effect on your respiratory health (e.g., smoke, dust, chemicals)?*
- Do you currently have an upper respiratory infection?*
- Do you use any equipment to manage respiratory symptoms (e.g., home oxygen therapy equipment, metered-dose inhaler with spacer or nebulizer for medication administration, positive airway pressure device for relief of sleep apnea)?

Self-Care History

- Have you received immunization for influenza (flu) and pneumococcal pneumonia (Pneumovax)? When?
- Do you smoke?* If yes, how many packs daily? For how many years? Do you smoke cigarettes or cigars? Have you ever tried to quit? Are you living with someone who smokes?
- When was your last tuberculosis skin test and chest radiograph?

Symptoms

Cough

- Do you have a cough, and if so, when did it start? How often do you cough? Does it wake you up at night? Does activity affect your cough?* What alleviates your cough?
- Do you cough up sputum? How much do you expectorate? What colour is your sputum? Are you coughing up blood?

Shortness of Breath

- Are you ever short of breath during exercise?* At rest?*
- Do you get too short of breath to do the things you want to do?* (NOTE: To determine the intensity of dyspnea, the Medical Research Council Dyspnea Scale [see Chapter 31, Figure 31-11] or a visual analogue scale may be helpful [Registered Nurses' Association of Ontario, 2010]; see Figure 28-8.)
- Do breathing problems cause you to awaken during the night?*
- Can you lie flat at night? If not, how many pillows do you use? Do you need to sleep upright in a chair?
- What do you do when you get short of breath?
- Are you or your sleep partner aware of any snoring?

Chest Pain With Breathing

- Do you experience chest pain with breathing?* Where exactly is the pain located? What precipitates the pain? What alleviates the pain?
- Do you have a history of lung diseases such as COPD?

Source: Based on Jarvis, C., Browne, A. J., MacDonald-Jenkins, J., & Luctkar-Flude, M. (Eds.). (2009). *Physical examination and health assessment* (1st Canadian ed., pp. 444-446). Toronto: Elsevier Canada.
*If yes, describe.
COPD, chronic obstructive pulmonary disease.

Table 28-6 Clues to Respiratory Problems

MANIFESTATION	DESCRIPTION
Shortness of breath (dyspnea)	Distressing sensation of uncomfortable breathing. Most common complaint of people with respiratory problems. Person may become accustomed to sensation and not recognize its presence. Difficult to evaluate because it is a subjective experience.
Wheezing	May or may not be heard by patient. May be described as "chest tightness."
Pleuritic chest pain	Described on a continuum from discomfort during inspiration to intense, sharp pain at the end of inspiration. Pain is usually aggravated by deep breathing and coughing.
Cough	Characteristics and timing of cough are important diagnostic clues.
Sputum production	Material coughed up from lungs. Contains mucus, cellular debris, or microorganisms and may contain blood or pus. Amount, colour, and constituents of sputum constitute important diagnostic information.
Hemoptysis	Coughing up of blood; sputum may be grossly bloody, frankly bloody, or blood-tinged. Precipitating events should be investigated.
Audible changes	Voice changes such as hoarseness and muffling, stridor (whistling sound during inspiration), or a barking cough may indicate abnormalities of upper airway, vocal cord dysfunction, or gastroesophageal reflux disease.
Fatigue	Sense of overwhelming tiredness, not completely relieved by sleep or rest.

has been the pattern of coughing? Has it been regular or irregular, and related to a time of day or weather, certain activities, talking, or deep breaths? Has the cough changed over time? What efforts have been tried to alleviate the coughing? Were any prescription or OTC drugs tried?

If a patient has a productive cough, the following characteristics of sputum should be evaluated: amount, colour, consistency, and odour. The amount should be quantified in teaspoons, tablespoons, or cups per day. The nurse should note any recent increases or decreases in the amount. The normal colour is clear or slightly whitish. If a patient smokes cigarettes, the sputum is usually clear to grey with occasional specks of brown. Patients with COPD may exhibit clear, whitish, or slightly yellow sputum, especially in the morning on rising. If a patient reports any change in sputum from baseline colour to yellow, pink, red, brown, or green, pulmonary complications should be suspected. Changes in consistency of sputum to thick, thin, or frothy should be noted. These changes may indicate dehydration, postnasal drip or sinus drainage, or possible pulmonary edema. Normally sputum should be odourless. A foul odour is suggestive of an infectious process. The patient should be asked whether the sputum was produced along with a position change (e.g., increased with lying down) or a change in activity.

Patients should be questioned about a family history of respiratory problems that may be genetic or familial tendencies, such as asthma, emphysema resulting from α_1-antitrypsin deficiency, or cystic fibrosis. A history of family exposure to tubercle bacilli should be noted.

The nurse should conduct case finding surveillance in accordance with the *Best Practices in Surveillance and Infection Prevention and Control for Febrile Respiratory Illness* (Ministry of Health and Long Term Care Ontario, 2010). This surveillance includes determining whether a patient has a new or worse cough or shortness of breath and whether the patient is feeling feverish. The nurse would also ask where the patient has lived and travelled, particularly in the past 14 days. Questions regarding travel and febrile illness symptoms would also apply to family or household members who reside in the same residence as the patient or who have close physical contact, or both. Risk factors for tuberculosis include prior residence in Asia, Africa, or Latin America. Risk factors for avian influenza A include recent trips to China, and those for severe acute respiratory syndrome (SARS) include recent travel to China and other parts of Asia. It is important for the nurse to take droplet or airborne precautions with patients being assessed for new respiratory illness (Public Health Ontario, 2011).

The nurse should also ask about current and past smoking habits and quantify exposure in pack-years by multiplying the number of packs smoked per day by the number of years smoked. For example, a person who smoked one pack per day for 15 years has a 15 pack-year history. The risk of lung cancer rises in direct proportion to the number of pack-years smoked. Smoking increases the risk of COPD and exacerbates symptoms of asthma and chronic bronchitis. In addition to asking about cigarette use, it is important to find out the use of any tobacco products, including cigars, pipes, chewing tobacco, and smokeless tobacco products. Information about exposure to second-hand smoke is also important. The nurse should also ask whether efforts have been made to quit the use of these tobacco products, including the use of prescription, OTC, and herbal remedies.

The nurse should ask whether the patient received immunization for influenza (flu) and pneumococcal pneumonia (Pneu-movax). Influenza vaccine should be administered yearly in the fall (Public Health Agency of Canada, 2007). Pneumococcal vaccine is recommended for persons 65 years of age or older and for individuals with chronic cardiovascular disease, chronic pulmonary disease, or diabetes mellitus. The current recommendation is one dose of Pneumovax vaccine for adults aged 65 or older. This vaccine is also recommended in immunocompromised persons (e.g., transplant recipients; Public Health Agency of Canada, 2006).

Patients should be asked whether they use equipment to manage respiratory symptoms, such as home oxygen therapy equipment, metered-dose inhaler (MDI) with spacer or nebulizer for medication administration, and positive airway pressure device for relief of sleep apnea. Patients should be questioned about the type of equipment used, frequency of use, its therapeutic effect, and any adverse effects. Patients who use an MDI should be asked to demonstrate its use. Many patients do not know how to use MDI devices correctly (see Chapter 31).

Objective Data

Physical Examination. Vital signs, including temperature, pulse, respirations, and blood pressure, are important data to collect before examination of the respiratory system.

Nose. The nose is inspected for patency, inflammation, deformities, symmetry, and discharge. Each naris (nostril) is checked for air patency with respiration while the other naris is briefly occluded. The nurse tilts the patient's head backward and pushes the tip of the nose upward gently. With a nasal speculum and a good light, the interior of the nose is inspected. The mucous membrane should be pink and moist, with no evidence of edema (bogginess), exudate, or bleeding. The nasal septum should be observed for deviation, perforations, and bleeding. Some nasal deviation is normal in an adult. The turbinates should be observed for polyps, which are abnormal, fingerlike projections of swollen nasal mucosa. Polyps may result from long-term irritation of the mucosa, as from allergies. Any discharge should be assessed for colour and consistency. The presence of purulent and malodorous discharge could indicate the presence of a foreign body. Watery discharge could be secondary to allergies or could represent cerebrospinal fluid. Bloody discharge could be secondary to trauma. Thick mucosal discharge could indicate the presence of infection.

Mouth and Pharynx. Using a good light source, the nurse inspects the interior of the mouth for colour, lesions, masses, gum retraction, bleeding, and poor dentition. The tongue is inspected for symmetry and presence of lesions. The nurse observes the pharynx by pressing a tongue blade against the middle of the back of the tongue. The pharynx should be smooth and moist, with no evidence of exudate, ulcerations, swelling, or postnasal drip. The colour, symmetry, and any enlargement of the tonsils are noted. The nurse stimulates the gag reflex by placing a tongue blade along the side of the pharynx behind the tonsil. A normal response (gagging) indicates that cranial nerves IX (glossopharyngeal nerve) and X (vagus nerve) are intact and that the airway is protected. Each side of the pharynx should be checked for the gag reflex.

Neck. The nurse inspects the neck for symmetry and presence of tender or swollen areas. The lymph nodes are palpated while the patient is sitting erect with the neck slightly flexed. Palpation progresses from the nodes around the ears to the nodes at the base of the skull and then to those located under the angles of the mandible to the midline. The nodes may be small, mobile, and nontender (shotty nodes), which is not a sign of a pathological condition. Nodes that are tender, hard, or fixed indicate disease. The location and characteristics of any palpable nodes are described.

Thorax and Lungs. Imaginary lines can be pictured on the chest to help in identifying abnormalities (see Figure 28-2). The locations of abnormalities can be described in relation to these lines (e.g., 2 cm from the right midclavicular line).

Chest examination is best performed in a well-lit, warm room, with measures taken to ensure the patient's privacy. Either the anterior or the posterior aspect of the chest may be examined first.

Inspection. The anterior aspect of the chest should be exposed while the patient is sitting upright or with the head of the bed upright. The patient may need to lean forward to support himself or herself on the bedside table in order to facilitate breathing. First, the nurse observes the patient's appearance and notes any evidence of respiratory distress, such as tachypnea or use of accessory muscles. Next, the nurse determines the shape and symmetry of the chest. Chest movement should be equal on both sides, and the anteroposterior diameter should be less than the transverse diameter. Normal anteroposterior diameter is less than the transverse diameter by a ratio of 1:2. An increase in anteroposterior diameter (e.g., barrel-shaped chest) may be a normal age-related change or a result of lung hyperinflation, as seen with emphysema. The nurse observes for abnormalities in the sternum, such as *pectus carinatum* (a prominent protrusion of the sternum) and *pectus excavatum* (an indentation of the lower sternum above the xiphoid process).

Next, the nurse should observe the respiratory rate, depth, and rhythm. The normal rate is 12 to 20 breaths per minute; in older persons, it is 16 to 25 breaths per minute. Inspiration should take half as long as expiration (ratio of inspiration to expiration is 1:2). The nurse should observe for abnormal breathing patterns, such as Kussmaul's (rapid, deep breathing), Cheyne-Stokes (abnormal pattern of respiration characterized by alternating periods of apnea and deep, rapid breathing), or Biot's (irregular breathing with apnea every four to five cycles) respiration (Seidel, Ball, Dains, & Benedict, 2011). Skin colour provides clues to respiratory status. In dark-skinned patients, cyanosis is best observed in the conjunctivae, lips, palms, and soles of the feet. Causes of cyanosis include hypoxemia and decreased cardiac output. The fingers should be inspected for evidence of *clubbing* (an increase in the angle between the base of the nail and the fingernail to 180 degrees or more, usually accompanied by an increase in depth, bulk, and sponginess of the end of the finger). Nail beds should also be inspected for cyanosis.

When the nurse is inspecting the posterior aspect of the chest, the patient should lean forward with arms folded. This position moves the scapula away from the spine, so there is more exposure of the area to be examined. The observations that were made on the anterior part of the chest are made in the same sequence on the posterior part. In addition, any spinal curvature is noted. Spinal curvatures that affect breathing include kyphosis, scoliosis, and kyphoscoliosis.

Palpation. The nurse determines tracheal position by gently placing the index fingers on either side of the patient's trachea

just above the suprasternal notch and gently pressing backward. Normal tracheal position is midline; deviation to the left or right is abnormal. Tracheal deviation occurs away from the side of a tension pneumothorax or a neck mass but toward the side of a pneumonectomy or lobar atelectasis (Wilson & Giddens, 2009). The nurse determines symmetry of chest expansion and extent of movement at the level of the diaphragm. The nurse places the hands over the lower anterior aspect of the patient's chest wall along the costal margin and moves them inward until the thumbs meet at midline. The patient is asked to breathe deeply, and the nurse observes the movement of the thumbs away from each other. Normal expansion is 2.5 cm. On the posterior side of the chest, the nurse places the hands at the level of the patient's tenth rib and moves the thumbs until they meet over the patient's spine (Figure 28-8).

Normal chest movement is symmetrical. Expansion is asymmetrical when air entry is limited by conditions involving the lung (e.g., atelectasis, pneumothorax) or the chest wall (e.g., incisional pain). Expansion is symmetrical but diminished in conditions that produce a hyperinflated or barrel-shaped chest or in neuromuscular conditions (e.g., amyotrophic lateral sclerosis, spinal cord lesions). Movement may be absent or asymmetrical over a pleural effusion, an atelectasis, or a pneumothorax.

Fremitus is an abnormal palpable vibration caused by the passage of air past thick bronchial mucus. The nurse can feel it with the hand on the chest while the patient takes a deep inspiration, and it may change or clear with coughing. It is produced by vocalization. To elicit tactile fremitus, the nurse places the palms of the hands against the patient's chest and asks the patient to repeat a phrase such as "ninety-nine." The nurse moves the hands from side to side and from top to bottom on the patient's chest (Figure 28-9). All areas of the chest should be palpated, and vibrations from an area on one side should be compared with those from the corresponding area on the other side. Tactile fremitus is most intense in the first and second interspaces lateral to the sternum and between the scapulae because these areas are closest to the major bronchi. Fremitus is less intense farther away from these areas.

Increase, decrease, or absence of fremitus should be noted. Fremitus is increased when the lung becomes filled with fluid or

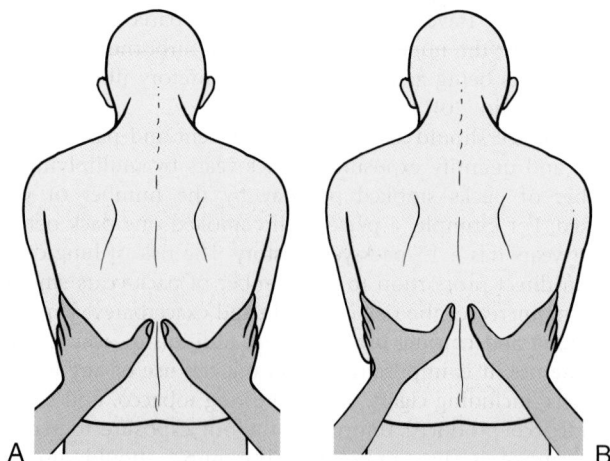

Figure 28-8 Estimation of thoracic expansion. **A,** Exhalation. **B,** Maximal inhalation.

Source: Adapted from Wilkins, R. L., Stoller, J. K., & Scanlan, C. L. (2009). *Egan's fundamentals of respiratory care* (9th ed., p. 333, Fig 15-5). St. Louis: Mosby.

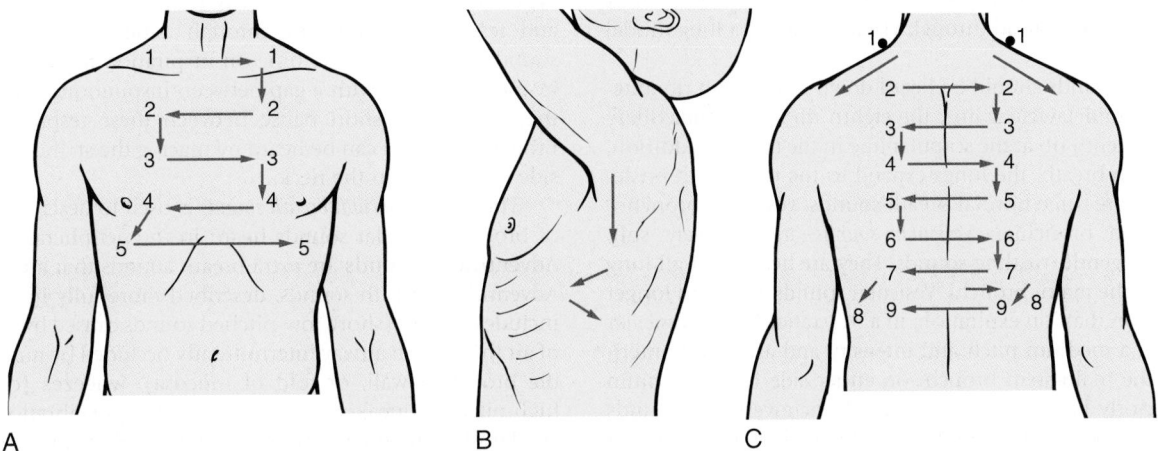

Figure 28-9 Sequence for examination of the chest. **A,** Anterior sequence. **B,** Lateral sequence. **C,** Posterior sequence. For palpation, the nurse places the palms of the hands in the position designated as *1* on the right and left sides of the chest. The nurse compares the intensity of vibrations. Then the nurse repeats for all positions in each sequence. For percussion, the nurse taps the chest at each designated position, moving downward from side to side, while comparing percussion notes. For auscultation, the nurse places the stethoscope at each position and listens to at least one complete inspiratory and expiratory cycle.

Table 28-7 Percussion Sounds	
SOUND	**DESCRIPTION**
Resonance	Low-pitched sound heard over normal lungs
Hyperresonance	Loud, lower-pitched sound than normal resonance heard over hyperinflated lungs, as in chronic obstructive lung disease and acute asthma
Tympany	Drumlike, loud, empty quality heard over gas-filled stomach or intestine or over pneumothorax
Dull	Medium-intensity pitch and duration heard over areas of "mixed" solid and lung tissue, such as over the top area of the liver, partially consolidated lung tissue (pneumonia), or fluid-filled pleural space
Flat	Soft, high-pitched sound of short duration heard over very dense tissue where air is not present

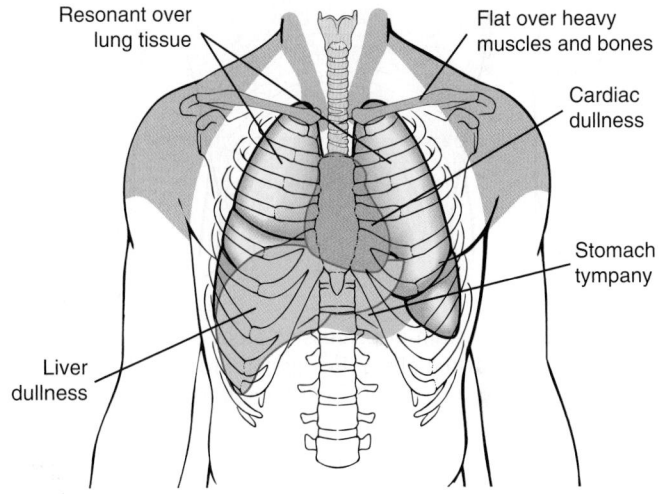

Figure 28-10 Diagram of percussion areas and sounds in the anterior aspect of the chest.

Source: From Thompson, J. M., McFarland, G., & Tucker, S. (2002). *Mosby's clinical nursing* (5th ed.). St. Louis: Mosby.

more dense. This is noted with pneumonia, with lung tumours, and above a pleural effusion (the lung is compressed upward). Fremitus is decreased if the hand is farther from the lung (e.g., pleural effusion) or the lung is hyperinflated (e.g., as in barrel-shaped chest). Absence of fremitus may be noted with pneumothorax or atelectasis. The anterior aspect of the chest is more difficult to palpate for fremitus because of the presence of large muscles and breast tissue.

Percussion. Percussion is performed to assess density or aeration of the lungs. Percussion sounds are described in Table 28-7. (The technique for percussion is described in Chapter 3.)

The anterior aspect of the chest is usually percussed with the patient in a semisitting or supine position. Starting above the clavicles, the nurse percusses downward, interspace by interspace (see Figure 28-9). The area over lung tissue should be resonant, with the exception of the area of cardiac dullness (Figure 28-10). For percussion of the posterior chest, the patient should sit leaning forward with arms folded. The posterior chest should be resonant over lung tissue to the level of the diaphragm (Figure 28-11).

Auscultation. During chest auscultation, the patient is instructed to breathe slowly and deeply in through the nose and out through the mouth. The nurse should proceed by comparing opposite areas of the chest, from the lung apices to the bases (see Figure 28-9). The stethoscope should be placed over lung tissue, not over bony prominences. At each placement of the stethoscope, the nurse should listen to at least one cycle of inspiration and expiration. Note the pitch (e.g., high, low), the duration of sound, and presence of any adventitious or abnormal sounds. The location of normal auscultatory sounds is more easily understood through visualization of a lung model (Figure 28-12).

The lung sounds should be heard down to the sixth rib anteriorly at the midclavicular line, the eighth rib at the midaxillary line, and the tenth rib at the scapular line in the back. In addition, during a deep breath, the lungs expand to the twelfth rib posteriorly. There are three normal breath sounds: vesicular, bronchovesicular, and bronchial. *Vesicular sounds* are relatively soft, low-pitched, gentle, rustling sounds. They are heard over all lung areas except the major bronchi. Vesicular sounds are heard longer on inspiration than on expiration, in a 3 : 1 ratio. *Bronchovesicular sounds* have a medium pitch and intensity and are heard anteriorly over the main-stem bronchi on either side of the sternum and posteriorly between the scapulae. Bronchovesicular sounds are heard for the same length of time on inspiration as on

expiration (1 : 1). *Bronchial sounds* are louder and higher pitched and resemble air blowing through a hollow pipe. Bronchial sounds last for a shorter time on inspiration than on expiration by a ratio of 2 : 3, with a gap between inspiration and expiration that reflects the short pause between these respiratory cycles. Bronchial sounds can be heard by placing the stethoscope alongside the trachea in the neck.

The term *abnormal breath sounds* is used to describe bronchial or bronchovesicular sounds heard in the peripheral lung fields. **Adventitious sounds** are extra breath sounds that are abnormal. Adventitious breath sounds, described more fully in Table 28-9, include **crackles** (short, low-pitched sounds caused by the passage of air through an airway intermittently occluded by mucus, unstable bronchial wall, or fold of mucosa), **wheezes** (continuous high-pitched squeaking sound caused by rapid vibration of bronchial walls), and **pleural friction rub** (a creaking or grating sound that occurs when roughened, inflamed surfaces of the pleura rub together; it is evident during inspiration, expiration, or both; and does not change with coughing).

A record of the normal physical assessment of the respiratory system is shown in Table 28-8. Common assessment abnormalities of the thorax and lungs are listed in Table 28-9. Chest examination findings in common pulmonary problems are listed in Table 28-10. Age-related changes in the respiratory system and assessment findings are listed in Table 28-4.

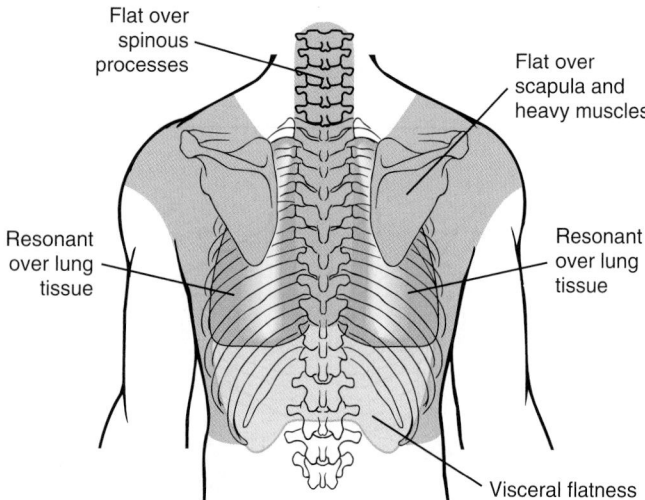

Figure 28-11 Diagram of percussion areas and sounds in the posterior aspect of the chest. Percussion proceeds from the lung apices to the lung bases, and sounds from opposite areas of the chest are compared.

Source: From Thompson, J. M., McFarland, G., & Tucker, S. (2002). *Mosby's clinical nursing* (5th ed.). St. Louis: Mosby.

Table 28-8 Normal Physical Assessment of the Respiratory System
• Nose is symmetrical with no deformities. Nasal mucosa is pink and moist with no edema, exudate, blood, or polyps. Nasal septum is straight, without perforations.
• Oral mucosa is light pink and moist, with no exudate or ulcerations.
• Tonsils are not inflamed or enlarged.
• Pharynx is smooth, moist, and pink.
• Trachea is midline. No nodes are palpable.
• Chest is elliptical in shape, and chest expansion is symmetrical. Respirations are regular and nonlaboured, at the rate of 14/min. Breath sounds noted throughout both lung fields, without crackles or wheezes. No axillary nodes are palpable.

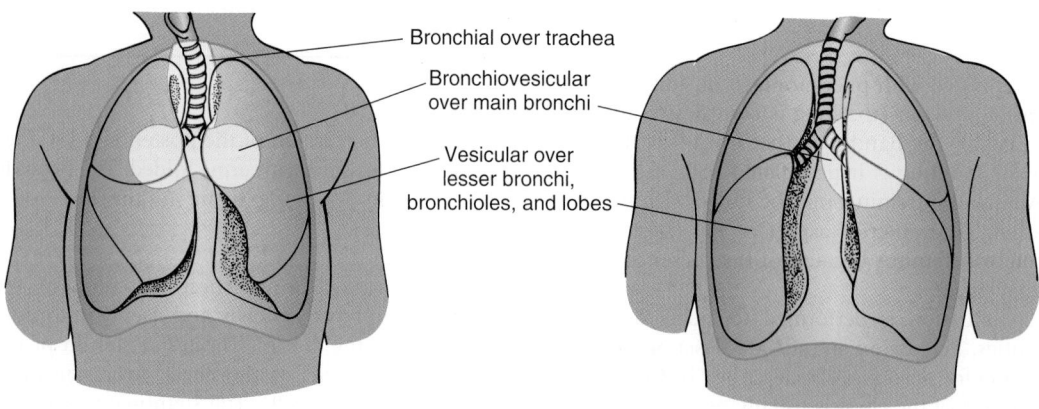

Figure 28-12 Normal auscultatory sounds.

Source: From Beare, P. G., & Myers, J. L. (1998). *Adult health nursing* (3rd ed.). St. Louis: Mosby.

COMMON ASSESSMENT ABNORMALITIES

Table 28-9 Respiratory System

FINDING	DESCRIPTION	POSSIBLE ETIOLOGY AND SIGNIFICANCE*
Inspection		
Pursed-lip breathing	Exhalation through mouth with lips pursed together to slow exhalation	COPD, asthma; suggests ↑ breathlessness; strategy taught to slow expiration, reduce dyspnea
Tripod position; inability to lie flat	Learning forward with arms and elbows supported on overbed table	COPD, asthma in exacerbation, pulmonary edema; indicates moderate to severe respiratory distress
Accessory muscle use; intercostal retractions	Neck and shoulder muscles used to assist breathing; muscles between ribs pull in during inspiration	COPD, asthma in exacerbation, secretion retention; indicates severe respiratory distress, hypoxemia
Splinting	Voluntary ↓ in tidal volume to ↓ pain on chest expansion	Thoracic or abdominal incision; chest trauma, pleurisy
↑ Anteroposterior diameter	Anteroposterior chest diameter equal to transverse diameter; slope of ribs more horizontal (90 degrees) to spine	COPD, asthma, cystic fibrosis; lung hyperinflation; advanced age
Tachypnea	Rate >20 breaths/min; >25 breaths/min in older adults	Fever, anxiety, hypoxemia, restrictive lung disease; ↑ above normal respiratory rate reflects increased work of breathing
Kussmaul's respirations	Regular, rapid, and deep respirations	Metabolic acidosis; ↑ in rate aids body in ↑ CO_2 excretion
Cyanosis	Bluish colour of skin, best seen in earlobes, under the eyelids, or in nail beds	↓ Oxygen transfer in lungs, ↓ cardiac output; nonspecific, unreliable indicator
Clubbing of fingers	↑ Depth, bulk, sponginess of distal digit of finger	Chronic hypoxemia; cystic fibrosis, lung cancer, bronchiectasis
Abdominal paradox	Inward (rather than normal outward) movement of abdomen during inspiration	Inefficient and ineffective breathing pattern; nonspecific indicator of severe respiratory distress
Palpation		
Tracheal deviation	Leftward or rightward movement of trachea from normal midline position	Nonspecific indicator of change in position of mediastinal structures; medical emergency if caused by tension pneumothorax
Altered tactile fremitus	Increase or decrease in vibrations	↑ In pneumonia, pulmonary edema; ↓ in pleural effusion, lung hyperinflation; absent in pneumothorax, atelectasis
Altered chest movement	Diminished movement (can be asymmetrical or symmetrical) of two sides of chest with inspiration	Asymmetrical movement caused by atelectasis, pneumothorax, pleural effusion, splinting; symmetrical but diminished movement caused by barrel shape of chest, restrictive disease, neuromuscular disease
Percussion		
Hyperresonance	Loud, lower-pitched sound over areas that normally produce a resonant sound	Lung hyperinflation (COPD), lung collapse (pneumothorax), air trapping (asthma)
Dullness	Medium-pitched sound over areas that normally produce a resonant sound	↑ Density (pneumonia, large atelectasis), ↑ fluid pleural space (pleural effusion)
Auscultation		
Fine crackles	Series of short, explosive, high-pitched sounds heard just before the end of inspiration; result of rapid equalization of gas pressure when collapsed alveoli or terminal bronchioles suddenly snap open; sound is similar to that heard when rolling hair between fingers just behind ear	Interstitial fibrosis (asbestosis), interstitial edema (early pulmonary edema), alveolar filling (pneumonia), loss of lung volume (atelectasis), early phase of congestive heart failure

Continued

COMMON ASSESSMENT ABNORMALITIES

Table 28-9 Respiratory System—cont'd

FINDING	DESCRIPTION	POSSIBLE ETIOLOGY AND SIGNIFICANCE*
Coarse crackles	Series of short, low-pitched sounds caused by air passing through airway intermittently occluded by mucus, unstable bronchial wall, or fold of mucosa; evident on inspiration and, at times, expiration; similar sound to blowing through straw under water; increase in bubbling quality with more fluid	Congestive heart failure, pulmonary edema, pneumonia with severe congestion, COPD
Wheezes	Continuous high-pitched squeaking sound caused by rapid vibration of bronchial walls; first evident on expiration but possibly evident on inspiration as obstruction of airway increases; possibly audible without stethoscope	Bronchospasm (caused by asthma), airway obstruction (caused by foreign body; tumour; viscous, thick increased secretions), COPD, pneumonia, bronchiectasis
Stridor	Continuous musical sound of constant pitch; result of partial obstruction of larynx or trachea	Croup, epiglottitis, vocal cord edema after extubation, foreign body
Absence of breath sounds	No sound evident over entire lung or area of lung	Pleural effusion, main-stem bronchi obstruction, large atelectasis, pneumonectomy, lobectomy
Pleural friction rub	Creaking or grating sound that occurs when roughened, inflamed surfaces of the pleura rub together; evident during inspiration, expiration, or both; no change with coughing; usually uncomfortable, especially on deep inspiration	Pleurisy, pneumonia, pulmonary infarct

COPD, chronic obstructive pulmonary disease.
*Only common causes are listed. (These conditions are discussed further in Chapters 29 through 31.)

Table 28-10 Chest Examination Findings in Common Pulmonary Problems

PROBLEM	INSPECTION	PALPATION	PERCUSSION	AUSCULTATION
Chronic bronchitis	Barrel shape of chest; cyanosis; possible clubbing of fingers	—	Resonant	Crackles over deflated areas; wheeze may be present
Emphysema	Barrel shape of chest; tripod position; use of accessory muscles	↓ Chest expansion	Hyperresonant or dull if consolidation is present	Crackles diminished if no exacerbation is present
Asthma (during an exacerbation)	Prolonged expiration; tripod position; pursed lips	↓ Chest expansion; ↓ Fremitus if hyperinflation is present	Hyperresonance	Wheezes; ↓ breath sounds are ominous sign if no improvement occurs (represent severely diminished air movement)
Pneumonia	Tachypnea; use of accessory muscles; cyanosis	Unequal movement with lobar involvement; ↑ fremitus over affected area	Dull over affected areas	Early: bronchial sounds Later: crackles; wheezes
Atelectasis	No change unless entire segment or lobe is involved	If small, no change If large, ↓ movement on affected side; ↑ fremitus	Dull over affected areas	Crackles (may disappear with deep breaths); absence of sounds if large
Pulmonary edema	Tachypnea; laboured respirations; cyanosis	↓ Chest expansion or normal movement	Dull or normal, depending on amount of fluid	Fine or coarse crackles
Pleural effusion	Tachypnea; use of accessory muscles	↓ Chest expansion ↑ Fremitus above effusion; absence of fremitus over effusion	Dull	Diminished or absent over effusion; egophony over effusion
Pulmonary fibrosis	Tachypnea	↓ Chest expansion	Normal	Crackles

A focused assessment is performed to evaluate the status of previously identified respiratory problems and to monitor for signs of new problems (see Chapter 3, Table 3-6). A focused assessment of the respiratory system is presented in the Focused Assessment box below.

FOCUSED ASSESSMENT
Respiratory System

Subjective
Ask the patient about any of the following and note responses

Shortness of breath	Y	N
Wheezing	Y	N
Sputum production (colour, quantity)	Y	N
Pain with breathing	Y	N
Cough	Y	N

Objective: Diagnostic
Check the following laboratory results for critical values

Arterial blood gas measurements	✓
Chest radiographic examination	✓
Hct, Hb measurements	✓

Objective: Physical Examination
Observe

Respirations for rate, quality, and pattern	✓

Inspect

Skin and nails for integrity and colour	✓
Neck for position of trachea	✓
Shape, symmetry, and movement of chest wall	✓

Palpate

Chest and back for masses	✓

Auscultate

Lung (breath) sounds	✓

Diagnostic Studies of the Respiratory System

Blood Studies

Common blood studies used to assess the respiratory system are the determinations of hemoglobin (Hb), hematocrit (Hct), and ABGs. Table 28-11 describes nursing responsibilities associated with these tests.

Oximetry

Oximetry is used to noninvasively monitor SpO_2 and SvO_2 (see Tables 28-1 and 28-3). Nursing care associated with oximetry is discussed in Table 28-11.

Sputum Studies

Sputum samples can be obtained by expectoration, tracheal suction, or bronchoscopy, a technique in which a flexible bronchoscope is inserted into the airways. The specimens may be examined for culture and sensitivity to identify an infecting organism (e.g., *Mycobacterium, Pneumocystis jiroveci*) or to confirm a diagnosis (e.g., malignant cells). Nursing responsibilities for specimen collection are described in Table 28-11. Regardless of whether specimen tests are ordered, it is important to observe the sputum for colour, blood, volume, and viscosity.

Skin Tests

Skin tests may be performed to test for allergic reactions or exposure to tubercle bacilli or fungi. Skin tests involve the intradermal injection of an antigen. A positive result indicates that the patient has been exposed to the antigen. It does not indicate that disease is currently present. A negative result indicates that the patient has not been exposed or that cell-mediated immunity is depressed, as occurs in HIV infection.

Nursing responsibilities are similar for all skin tests. First, to prevent a false-negative reaction, the nurse should be certain that the injection is intradermal and not subcutaneous. After the injection, the sites should be circled and the patient instructed not to remove the marks. When charting administration of the antigen, the nurse should draw a diagram of the forearm and hand and label the injection sites. The diagram is especially helpful when more than one test is administered.

When reading test results, the nurse should use a good light. If an induration is present, a marking pen should be brought in from the periphery on all four sides of the induration. As the pen touches the raised area, a mark should be made. The nurse then determines the diameter of the induration in millimetres. Reddened, flat areas are not measured. Reactions that indicate a positive and potential negative tuberculin skin test (TST) are described in Table 28-12. In Canada, 10 mm is the standard measurement that indicates whether tuberculosis is present. Canadian health care settings use tuberculin purified protein (Tubersol) for skin tests. If any patient has had a previous bacille Calmette-Guérin (BCG) vaccination, it will affect results. This is significant especially for people from Quebec, Newfoundland, and Aboriginal populations, who regularly received this vaccine from 1940 through the 1980s.

Radiological Studies

Chest Radiography. Chest radiographic examination is the most common method for assessing the respiratory system. It is also used to assess progression of disease and response to treatment. The views most commonly used are posteroanterior and lateral. (See Table 28-11 for nursing responsibilities related to chest radiographic examinations.)

Computed Tomography. Computed tomography (CT) may be used to examine cross-sections of the entire body. CT is used to evaluate areas that are difficult to assess by conventional radiographic study, such as the mediastinum, the hilum, and the pleura. With enhancement by a contrast medium, high-resolution technique, or newer spiral CT, even pulmonary arteries can be inspected for emboli.

Magnetic Resonance Imaging. While in a strong magnetic field, the alignment of spinning nuclei can be changed with a superimposed radiofrequency, and the rate at which they return to alignment with the field can be measured. In magnetic resonance imaging (MRI), this technique is used to produce images

DIAGNOSTIC STUDIES

Table 28-11 Respiratory System

STUDY	DESCRIPTION AND PURPOSE	NURSING RESPONSIBILITY
Blood Studies		
Hemoglobin measurement	Value reflects amount of hemoglobin available for combination with oxygen. Venous blood is used. Normal level for men is 140-180 g/L; normal level for women is 120-160 g/L.	Explain procedure and its purpose.
Hematocrit measurement	Value reflects ratio of red blood cells to plasma cells. Increased hematocrit (polycythemia) found in chronic hypoxemia. Venous blood is used. Normal for men is 0.42-0.52; normal for women is 0.37-0.47.	Explain procedure and its purpose.
ABG measurements	ABGs are measured to assess acid–base balance, ventilation status, need for oxygen therapy, change in oxygen therapy, or change in ventilator settings.* Arterial blood is obtained through puncture of radial or femoral artery or through arterial catheter. Continuous ABG monitoring is also possible via a sensor or electrode inserted into the arterial catheter.	Indicate whether patient is using O_2 (percentage, amount per minute). Avoid change in oxygen therapy or interventions (e.g., suctioning, position change) for 20 min before obtaining sample. Assist with positioning (e.g., palm up, wrist slightly hyperextended if radial artery is used). Collect blood into heparinized syringe. To ensure accurate results, expel all air bubbles, and place sample on ice, unless it will be analyzed in less than 1 min. Apply pressure to artery for 5 min after specimen is obtained to prevent hematoma at the arterial puncture site.
Oximetry	Test monitors arterial or venous oxygen saturation. Oximetry is used for intermittent or continuous monitoring and exercise testing.†‡ Device attaches to finger, forehead, earlobe, or nose for SpO_2 monitoring or is contained in a pulmonary artery catheter for SvO_2 monitoring.	Apply probe to finger, forehead, earlobe, or bridge of nose. When interpreting SpO_2 and SvO_2 values, first assess patient status and presence of factors that can alter accuracy of pulse oximeter reading. For SpO_2, these include motion, low perfusion, bright lights, use of intravascular dyes, acrylic nails, dark skin colour. For SvO_2, these include change in O_2 delivery or O_2 consumption. For SpO_2, notify health care professional of $\pm 4\%$ change from baseline or $\downarrow$ to <90%. For SvO_2, notify health care professional of $\pm 10\%$ change from baseline or $\downarrow$ to <60%.
Sputum Studies		
Culture and sensitivity	Purpose is to diagnose bacterial infection, select antibiotic, and evaluate treatment. Single sputum specimen is collected in a sterile container.	Instruct patient on how to produce a good specimen (see Gram stain). If patient cannot produce specimen, bronchoscopy may be used (see Figure 28-13).
Gram stain	Staining of sputum enables classification of bacteria into Gram-negative and Gram-positive types. Results guide therapy until culture and sensitivity results are obtained.	Instruct patient to expectorate sputum into the container after coughing deeply. Obtain sputum (mucoid-like), not saliva. Obtain specimen in early morning because secretions accumulate during night. If sputum production is unsuccessful, try increasing oral fluid intake unless fluids are restricted. Collect sputum in sterile container (sputum trap) during suctioning or by aspirating secretions from the trachea. Send specimen to laboratory promptly.
Acid-fast smear and culture	Test is performed to collect sputum for acid-fast bacilli (tuberculosis). A series of three early morning specimens is used.	Instruct patient on how to produce a good specimen (see Gram stain). Cover specimen and send to laboratory for analysis.
Cytology	Purpose is to determine presence of abnormal cells that may indicate malignant condition. Single sputum specimen is collected in special container with fixative solution.	Send specimen to laboratory promptly. Instruct patient on how to produce a satisfactory specimen (see Gram stain). If patient cannot produce specimen, bronchoscopy may be used (see Figure 28-13).

DIAGNOSTIC STUDIES

Table 28-11 Respiratory System—cont'd

STUDY	DESCRIPTION AND PURPOSE	NURSING RESPONSIBILITY
Radiology		
Chest radiograph	Test is used to screen, diagnose, and evaluate change. Most common views are posteroanterior and lateral.	Instruct patient to undress to waist, put on gown, and remove any metal objects (e.g., jewellery, watch) between neck and waist.
Computed tomography (CT)	Test is performed for diagnosis of lesions difficult to assess by conventional radiographic studies, such as those in the hilum, the mediastinum, and the pleura. Images show structures in cross-section.	Same as for chest radiograph.
Magnetic resonance imaging (MRI)	Test is used for diagnosis of lesions difficult to assess by CT (e.g., lung apex near the spine).	Same as for chest radiograph. Instruct the patient to remove all metal objects (e.g., jewellery, watch) before test.
Ventilation–perfusion (V̇/Q̇) scan	Test is used to identify areas of the lung not receiving airflow (ventilation) or blood flow (perfusion). It involves injection of radioisotope and inhalation of small amount of radioactive gas (xenon). A gamma-detecting device records radioactivity. Ventilation without perfusion is suggestive of pulmonary embolus.	Same as for chest radiograph. No precautions needed afterward because the gas and isotope transmit radioactivity for only a brief interval.
Pulmonary angiography	Study is used to visualize pulmonary vasculature and locate obstruction or pathological conditions such as pulmonary embolus. Contrast medium is injected through a catheter into the pulmonary artery or right side of the heart.	Same as for chest radiograph. Know that contrast injection may cause flushing, warm sensation, and coughing. Check pressure dressing site after procedure. Monitor blood pressure, pulse, and circulation distal to injection site. Report and record significant changes.
Positron emission tomography (PET)	Test is used to distinguish benign and malignant lung nodules. It involves IV injection of a radioisotope with short half-life.	Same as for chest radiograph. No precautions needed afterward because isotope transmits radioactivity for only a brief interval.
Endoscopic Examinations		
Bronchoscopy	Flexible fibreoptic scope is used for diagnosis, biopsy, specimen collection, or assessment of changes. It may also be used to suction mucous plugs or to remove foreign objects. Study is typically performed in outpatient procedure room.	Instruct patient to be on NPO status for 6-12 hr. Obtain informed consent. Give sedative if it is ordered. After procedure, keep patient on NPO status until gag reflex returns, and monitor for laryngeal edema; monitor for recovery from sedatives. If biopsy was performed, monitor for hemorrhage and pneumothorax.
Mediastinoscopy	Test is used for inspection and biopsy of lymph nodes in mediastinal area.	Prepare patient for surgical intervention. Obtain informed consent. Afterward, monitor as for bronchoscopy.
Biopsy		
Lung biopsy	Specimens may be obtained by transbronchial or open-lung biopsy. This test is used to obtain specimens for laboratory analysis.	Same as for bronchoscopy if procedure is performed with bronchoscope, and same as for thoracotomy (see Chapter 30) if open-lung biopsy is performed. Obtain informed consent.
Other		
Thoracentesis	Test is used to obtain specimen of pleural fluid for diagnosis, to remove pleural fluid, or to instill medication. The physician inserts a large-bore needle through the chest wall into pleural space. A chest radiograph is always obtained after procedure to check for pneumothorax.	Explain procedure to patient, and obtain informed consent before procedure. Position patient sitting upright with elbows on an overbed table and feet supported. Instruct patient not to talk or cough, and assist during procedure. Observe for signs of hypoxia and verify breath sounds in all fields after procedure. Send labelled specimens to laboratory.
Pulmonary function test	Test is used to evaluate lung function. It involves use of a spirometer to diagram air movement as patient performs prescribed respiratory manoeuvres.†	Avoid scheduling test immediately after mealtime. Avoid administration of inhaled bronchodilator for 6 hr before procedure. Explain procedure to patient. Allow patient to rest after the procedure.

ABG, arterial blood gas; *NPO*, nothing by mouth; *SpO₂*, the oxygen saturation value obtained by pulse oximetry; *SvO₂*, venous oxygen saturation.
*For normal values, see Tables 28-1.
†For normal values, see Table 28-14.
‡For critical values, see Table 28-3.

Table 28-12　The First Dimension of Interpretation of the Tuberculin Skin Test: Size

Positive Reactions

Reaction (Induration) Size	Situation in Which Reaction is Considered Positive
0-4 mm	HIV infection with immune suppression is present *and* the expected likelihood of TB infection is high (e.g., patient is from a population with a high prevalence of TB infection, is a close contact of patient with an active contagious case, or has abnormal radiographic results)
5-9 mm	HIV infection
	Close contact of patient with an active contagious case
	Children suspected of having TB disease
	Chest radiograph shows abnormalities with fibronodular disease
	Other immune suppression: TNF-α inhibitors, chemotherapy
≥10 mm	All others

False-Negative Reactions

Cause	Example
Technical	Poor injection technique
Biological	Immune suppression caused by advanced age; treatment with corticosteroids (at least 15 mg/day of prednisone or equivalent for 1 mo or more); cancer therapy agents; HIV infection, especially if CD4 count <500 × 106/L; and possibly TNF-α inhibitors
	Malnutrition, particularly after recent weight loss
	Severe illness, which can include active TB, major viral illness (mononucleosis, mumps, or measles, but not the common cold)
	Immunization within the previous 4 wk with measles, mumps, rubella, varicella (chickenpox), or yellow fever vaccine
	Very young age (<6 mo); the validity of tuberculin skin test results in infants younger than 6 mo is unknown

HIV, human immunodeficiency virus; *TB,* tuberculosis; *TNF,* tumour necrosis factor.

Source: Adapted from Long, R., & Ellis, E. (Eds.). (2007.) *Canadian tuberculosis standards* (6th ed., pp. 61, 63). Ottawa, ON: Public Health Agency of Canada. Retrieved from *http://www.phac-aspc.gc.ca/tbpc-latb/pubs/pdf/tbstand07_e.pdf.* Reproduced with the permission of the Minister of Public Works and Government Services Canada, 2009.

of body structures. MRI has limited indications. It is most useful when evaluating images near the lung apex or the spine and for distinguishing vascular from nonvascular structures.

Ventilation–Perfusion Scan. A ventilation–perfusion scan is used primarily to check for the presence of a pulmonary embolus. There is no specific preparation or aftercare. A radioisotope is administered intravenously for the perfusion portion of the test; it outlines the pulmonary vasculature, which is then photographed. For the ventilation portion, the patient inhales a radioactive gas, which outlines the alveoli, and another photograph is taken. Normal scans show homogeneous radioactivity. Diminished appearance or absence of radioactivity is suggestive of lack of perfusion or airflow.

Pulmonary Angiography. Pulmonary angiography is used to confirm the diagnosis of an embolus if findings of the lung scan are inconclusive. A series of radiographs is taken after radiopaque dye is injected into the pulmonary artery. This test also detects congenital and acquired lesions of the pulmonary vessels.

Positron Emission Tomography. Positron emission tomography (PET) scans involve the use of radionuclides with short half-lives. PET scans are used to distinguish benign and malignant solitary pulmonary nodules. Because uptake of glucose is increased in malignant lung cells, the PET scan, in which an intravenous glucose preparation is used, can demonstrate the presence of malignant lung cells.

Endoscopic Examinations

Bronchoscopy. *Bronchoscopy* is a procedure in which the bronchi are visualized through a fibreoptic tube. Bronchoscopy may be used to obtain biopsy specimens, assess changes resulting from treatment, and remove mucous plugs or foreign bodies. Small amounts (30 mL) of sterile saline may be injected through the bronchoscope and withdrawn and examined for cells. This technique, termed *bronchoalveolar lavage,* is used to diagnose *Pneumocystis jiroveci* pneumonia (PCP) (Figure 28-13).

Bronchoscopy can be performed in an outpatient procedure room, in a surgical suite, or at the bedside in the critical care unit or on a medical-surgical floor, with the patient lying down or seated. After the nasal pharynx and oral pharynx are anaesthetized with local anaesthetic, the bronchoscope is coated with lidocaine (Xylocaine) and inserted, usually through the nose, and threaded down into the airways. A bronchoscopy can be performed on mechanically ventilated patients through the endotracheal tube. The nursing care for patients undergoing this procedure is described in Table 28-11.

Mediastinoscopy. For mediastinoscopy, an endoscope is inserted through a small incision in the suprasternal notch and advanced into the mediastinum to inspect and biopsy lymph nodes. The test is used to diagnose carcinoma, granulomatous infections, and sarcoidosis. The procedure is performed in the operating room, and the patient is given a general anaesthetic.

Lung Biopsy

Lung biopsy may be performed transbronchially or as an open-lung procedure. The purpose is to obtain tissue, cells, or secretions for evaluation. Transbronchial lung biopsy involves passing a forceps or needle through the bronchoscope for a specimen (Figure 28-14). Specimens can be cultured or examined for malignant cells. A combination of transbronchial lung biopsy and bronchoalveolar lavage is used to differentiate infection and rejection in lung transplant recipients. Nursing care is the same as for fibreoptic bronchoscopy. Open-lung biopsy is used when pulmonary disease cannot be diagnosed by other procedures. The patient receives a general anaesthetic, the chest is opened with

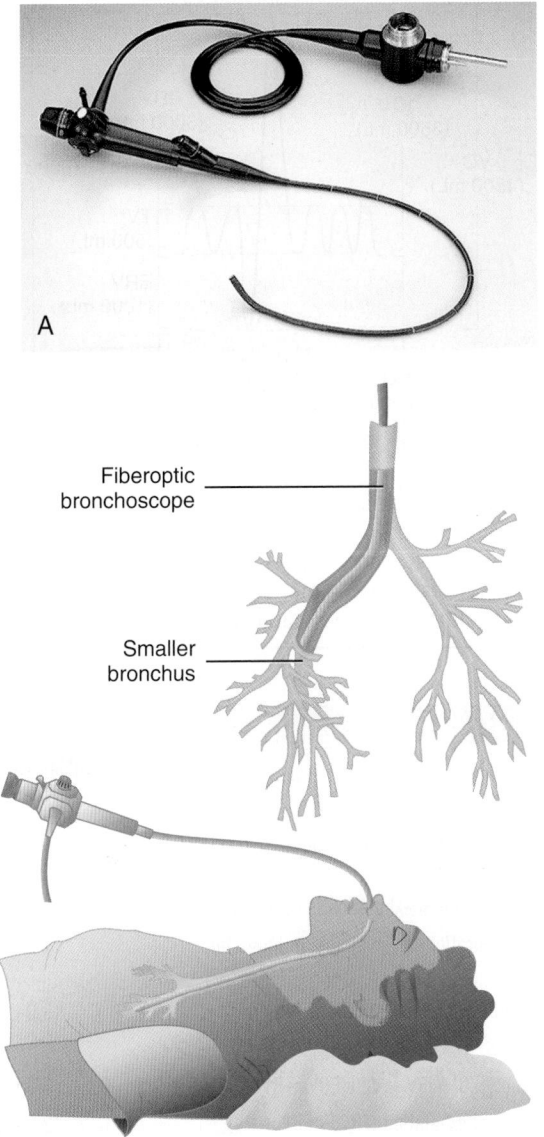

Figure 28-13 Fibreoptic bronchoscopy. **A,** The transbronchoscopic balloon-tipped catheter and the flexible fibreoptic bronchoscope. **B,** Procedure. The catheter is introduced into a small airway, and the balloon inflated with 1.5 to 2 mL air to occlude the airway. To perform bronchoalveolar lavage, 30 mL aliquots of sterile saline solution are injected and withdrawn, with gentle aspiration after each injection. Specimens are sent to the laboratory for analysis.

Sources: **A,** Courtesy Olympus America, Melville, New York; **B,** Beare, P. G., & Myers, J. L. (1998). *Adult health nursing* (3rd ed.) St. Louis: Mosby.

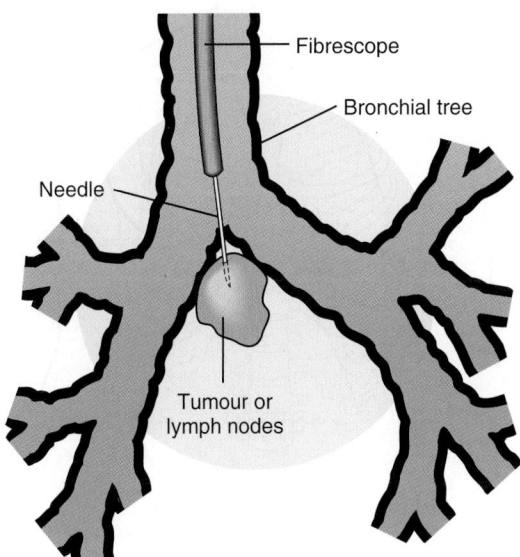

Figure 28-14 Transbronchial needle biopsy. In this diagram, a transbronchial biopsy needle penetrates the bronchial wall and enters a mass of subcarinal lymph nodes or tumour.

Source: Redrawn from Du Bois, R. M., & Clarke, S. W. (1987). *Fiberoptic bronchoscopy in diagnosis and management.* Orlando, FL: Grune & Stratton.

a thoracotomy incision, and a biopsy specimen is obtained. Nursing care for the procedure is the same as after thoracotomy (see Chapter 30).

Thoracentesis

Thoracentesis is the insertion of a needle through the chest wall into the pleural space to obtain specimens for diagnostic evaluation, remove pleural fluid, or instill medication into the pleural space (Figure 28-15). The patient is positioned sitting upright with elbows on an overbed table and feet supported. The skin is cleansed, and a local anaesthetic (lidocaine [Xylocaine]) is instilled subcutaneously. A chest tube may be inserted to enable further drainage of fluid. Nursing care is described in Table 28-11.

Pulmonary Function Tests

Pulmonary function tests (PFTs) are conducted to measure lung volumes and airflow. The results of PFTs are used to diagnose pulmonary disease, monitor disease progression, evaluate disability, and evaluate response to bronchodilators. In PFTs, a spirometer is used. The patient's age, sex, height, and weight are entered into the PFT computer to calculate predicted values. The patient inserts a mouthpiece, takes as deep a breath as possible, and exhales as hard, fast, and long as possible. Verbal coaching is given to ensure that the patient continues blowing out until exhalation is complete. The computer determines the actual value achieved, predicted (normal) value, and percentage of the predicted value for each test. A normal actual value is 80% to 120% of the predicted value. Normal values for PFTs are shown in Tables 28-13 and 28-14 and in Figure 28-16.

Home spirometry may be used to monitor lung function in persons with asthma or cystic fibrosis, as well as before and after lung transplantation. Changes in spirometry values at home can warn of early lung transplant rejection or infection. Feedback from a peak expiratory flowmeter can increase the sense of control achieved when persons with asthma learn to modify activities and medications in response to changes in rates of peak expiratory flow.

Pulmonary function parameters can also be used to determine the need for mechanical ventilation or the readiness to be weaned from ventilatory support. Measurements of vital capacity, maximum inspiratory pressure, and minute ventilation are used to make this determination (see Table 28-13).

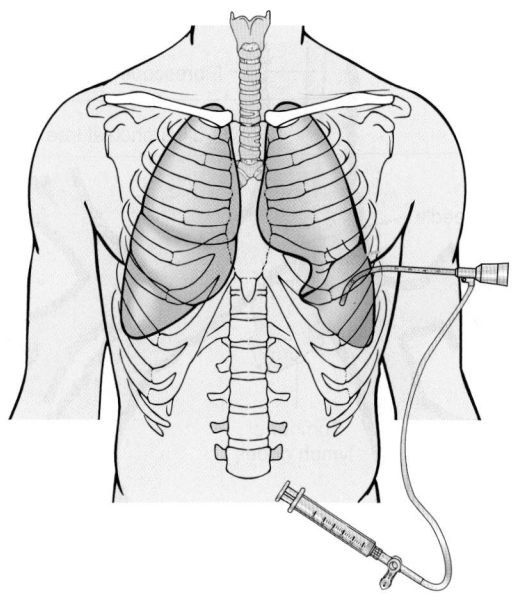

Figure 28-15 Thoracentesis. A catheter is positioned in the pleural space to remove accumulated fluid.

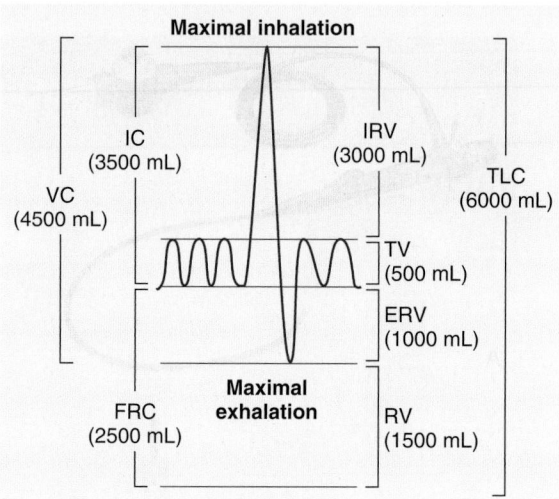

Figure 28-16 Relationship of lung volumes and capacities. *ERV*, expiratory reserve volume; *FRC*, functional residual capacity; *IC*, inspiratory capacity; *IRV*, inspiratory reserve volume; *RV*, residual volume; *TLC*, total lung capacity; *TV*, total volume; *VC*, vital capacity.

Table 28-13 Lung Volumes and Capacities

PARAMETER	DEFINITION	NORMAL VALUE
Volumes		
Tidal volume (V_T)	Volume of air inhaled and exhaled with each breath; only a small proportion of total capacity of lungs	0.5 L
Expiratory reserve volume (ERV)	Additional air that can be forcefully exhaled after normal exhalation is complete	1.0 L
Residual volume (RV)	Amount of air remaining in lungs after forced expiration; air available in lungs for gas exchange between breaths	1.5 L
Inspiratory reserve volume (IRV)	Maximum volume of air that can be inhaled forcefully after normal inhalation	3.0 L
Capacities		
Total lung capacity (TLC)	Maximum volume of air that lungs can contain (TLC = IRV + V_T + ERV + RV)	6.0 L
Functional residual capacity (FRC)	Volume of air remaining in lungs at end of normal exhalation (FRC = ERV + RV); increase or decrease possible with lung disease	2.5 L
Vital capacity (VC)	Maximum volume of air that can be exhaled after maximum inspiration (VC = IRV + V_T + ERV); generally higher in men	4.5 L
Inspiratory capacity (IC)	Maximum volume of air that can be inhaled after normal expiration (IC = V_T + IRV)	3.5 L

Table 28-14 Common Measures of Pulmonary Function

MEASURE	DESCRIPTION	NORMAL VALUE*
Forced vital capacity (FVC)	Amount of air that can be quickly and forcefully exhaled after maximum inspiration	>80% of predicted
Forced expiratory volume in first second of expiration (FEV_1)	Amount of air exhaled in first second of FVC; valuable clue to severity of airway obstruction	>80% of predicted
FEV_1/FVC	Ratio of value for FEV_1 to value for FVC; useful in differentiating obstructive and restrictive pulmonary dysfunction	>80% of predicted
Forced midexpiratory flow rate ($FEF_{25-75\%}$)	Measurement of airflow rate in middle half of forced expiration; early indicator of disease of small airways	>80% of predicted
Maximal voluntary ventilation (MVV)	Deep breathing as rapidly as possible for specified period; test for airflow, muscle strength, coordination, airway resistance; important factor in exercise tolerance	≈170 L/min
Peak expiratory flow rate (PEFR)	Maximum airflow rate during forced expiration; aids in monitoring bronchoconstriction in asthma	≤600 L/min
Maximum inspiratory pressure (MIP) or negative inspiratory force (NIF)	Amount of negative pressure generated on inspiration; indication of ability to breathe deeply and cough	≤80 cm H_2O

*Normal values vary with height, weight, age, and sex of patient.

Exercise Testing

Exercise testing is used in diagnosis, in determining exercise capacity, and for disability evaluation. A complete exercise test involves walking on a treadmill while expired oxygen and carbon dioxide, respiratory rate, heart rate, and rhythm are monitored. A modified test (desaturation test) may also be used. In that case, only SpO_2 is monitored. A desaturation test can also be used to determine the oxygen flow needed to maintain the SpO_2 at a safe level during activity or exercise in patients who use home oxygen therapy.

A timed walk can also be used to measure exercise capacity. The patient is instructed to walk as far as possible during a timed period (6 or 12 minutes), to stop when short of breath, and to continue when able. The distance walked is measured, and the data are used to monitor progression of disease or improvement after rehabilitation.

evolve *An assessment case study of the respiratory system is available at* **http://evolve.elsevier.com/Canada/Lewis/medsurg**

REVIEW QUESTIONS

The number of the question corresponds to the same-numbered objective at the beginning of the chapter.

1. Which of the following is the mechanism that stimulates the release of surfactant?
   a. Fluid accumulation in the alveoli
   b. Alveolar collapse from atelectasis
   c. Alveolar stretch from deep breathing
   d. Air movement through the alveolar pores of Kohn

2. Which of the following causes air to enter the thoracic cavity during inspiration?
   a. Contraction of the accessory abdominal muscles
   b. Increased carbon dioxide and decreased oxygen in the blood
   c. Stimulation of the respiratory muscles by the chemoreceptors
   d. Decreased intrathoracic pressure relative to pressure at the airway

3. Which of the following measures the lungs' ability to adequately oxygenate the arterial blood?
   a. Arterial oxygen tension
   b. Carboxyhemoglobin level
   c. Arterial carbon dioxide tension
   d. Venous carbon dioxide tension

4. Which of the following is the most important respiratory defence mechanism distal to the respiratory bronchioles?
   a. Alveolar macrophage
   b. Impaction of particles
   c. Reflex bronchoconstriction
   d. Mucociliary clearance mechanism

5. Which of the following is caused by a rightward shift of the oxygen–hemoglobin dissociation curve?
   a. Metabolic alkalosis
   b. Postoperative hypothermia
   c. Release of oxygen at the tissue level
   d. Greater affinity of oxygen for hemoglobin

6. Which of the following are very early signs or symptoms of inadequate oxygenation?
   a. Dyspnea and hypotension
   b. Apprehension and restlessness
   c. Cyanosis and cool, clammy skin
   d. Increased urine output and diaphoresis

7. Which of the following would the nurse expect to find during the respiratory assessment of the older adult?
   a. Hypercapnia while at rest
   b. Increased breath sounds in the lung apices
   c. Decreased pH and increased $PaCO_2$ levels
   d. Increased anteroposterior chest diameter

8. Which of the following should the nurse inquire about when assessing activity and exercise related to respiratory health?
   a. Dyspnea during rest or exercise
   b. Recent weight loss or weight gain
   c. Willingness to wear oxygen in public
   d. Ability to sleep through the entire night

9. Which of the following is the best tool to assess for the vibration of tactile fremitus?
   a. Palms
   b. Fingertips
   c. Stethoscope
   d. Index fingers

10. Which of the following is an abnormal assessment finding of the respiratory system?
    a. Presence of fremitus
    b. Inspiratory chest expansion of 2.5 cm
    c. Percussion resonance over the lung bases
    d. Symmetrical chest expansion and contraction

11. Which of the following is performed to remove pleural fluid for analysis?
    a. Thoracentesis
    b. Bronchoscopy
    c. Pulmonary angiography
    d. Sputum culture and sensitivity

ANSWERS: 1. c; 2. d; 3. a; 4. a; 5. c; 6. b; 7. d; 8. a; 9. a; 10. a; 11. a.

REFERENCES

Herlihy, B., & Maebius, N. K. (2010). *The human body in health and illness* (4th ed.). Philadelphia: W. B. Saunders.

Hoffman Wold, G. (2008). *Basic geriatric nursing* (4th ed.). St. Louis: Mosby.

Huether, S. E., & McCance, K. L. (2012). *Understanding pathophysiology* (5th ed.). St. Louis: Mosby.

Jarvis, C., Browne, A., MacDonald-Jenkins, J., & Luctkar-Flude, M. (2009). *Physical examination & health assessment* (1st Canadian ed.). Toronto: Elsevier Canada.

McCance, K. L., & Huether, S. E. (2010). *Pathophysiology: The biologic basis for disease in adults and children* (6th ed.). St. Louis: Mosby.

Ministry of Health and Long Term Care Ontario (2010). *Best Practices in Surveillance and Infection Prevention and Control for Febrile Respiratory Illness*, retrieved from *http://www.oahpp.ca/resources/documents/pidac/RPAP%20Annex%20B%20Prevention%20Transmission%20Acute%20Respiratory%20Infection.pdf*

Public Health Agency of Canada. (2006). *Canadian immunization guide* (7th ed.). Retrieved from *http://www.phac-aspc.gc.ca/publicat/cig-gci/p03-eng.php*

Public Health Agency of Canada. (2007). *Canadian tuberculosis standards* (6th ed.—2007). Retrieved from *http://www.phac-aspc.gc.ca/tbpc-latb/pubs/tbstand07-eng.php*

Public Health Ontario. (2011). *Ontario Influenza and Respiratory Infection Surveillance Program, 2011-2012* [Memorandum]. Retrieved from *http://www.oahpp.ca/resources/documents/flubulletin/2011-12-surveillance-package.pdf*

Registered Nurses' Association of Ontario (RNAO). (2010). Nursing care of dyspnea: The 6th vital sign in individuals with chronic obstructive pulmonary disease. *Nursing Best Practice Guidelines.* Toronto: Author. Retrieved from *http://rnao.ca/sites/rnao-ca/files/Nursing_Care_of_Dyspnea_-The_6th_Vital_Sign_in_Individuals_with_Chronic_Obstructive_Pulmonary_Disease.pdf*

Seidel, H. M., Ball, J., Dains, J., & Benedict, G. W. (2011). *Mosby's guide to physical examination* (7th ed.). St. Louis: Mosby.

Thibodeau, G. A., & Patton, K. T. (2010). *Anatomy and physiology* (7th ed.). St. Louis: Mosby.

Tortora, G., & Derrickson, B. (2010). *Principles of anatomy and physiology* (13th ed.). Hoboken, NJ: Wiley.

Urden, L., Stacy, K., & Lough, M. (2010). *Critical care nursing* (6th ed.). St. Louis: Mosby.

Wagner, K., Johnson, K., & Hardin-Pierce, M. (2009). *High acuity nursing* (5th ed.). Upper Saddle River, NJ: Prentice-Hall.

Weinberger, S. E. (2009). *Principles of pulmonary medicine* (5th ed.). Philadelphia: W. B. Saunders.

Wilson, S. F., & Giddens, J. F. (2009). *Health assessment for nursing practice* (4th ed.). St. Louis: Mosby.

RESOURCES

Resources for this chapter are listed in Chapter 31 on p. 761.

evolve   *For additional Internet resources, see the Web site for this book at* **http://evolve.elsevier.com/Canada/Lewis/medsurg**

Nursing Management: Upper Respiratory Problems

Written by Casey Norris
Adapted by Leslie Graham

LEARNING OBJECTIVES

1. Describe the clinical manifestations and nursing management of problems of the nose.
2. Describe the clinical manifestations and nursing management of problems of the paranasal sinuses.
3. Describe the clinical manifestations and nursing management of problems of the pharynx and the larynx.
4. Discuss the nursing management of the patient who requires a tracheostomy.
5. Identify the steps involved in performing tracheostomy care and suctioning an airway.
6. Describe the risk factors and warning symptoms associated with head and neck cancer.
7. Discuss the nursing management of the patient with a laryngectomy.
8. Describe the methods used in voice restoration for the patient with temporary or permanent loss of speech.

KEY TERMS

allergic rhinitis The reaction of the nasal mucosa to a specific allergen, p. 635

deviated septum A deflection of the normally straight nasal septum, p. 634

epistaxis Nosebleed, p. 634

esophageal speech A method of swallowing air, trapping it in the esophagus, and releasing it to create sound, p. 655

nasal polyps Benign mucous membrane masses that form slowly in response to repeated inflammation of the sinus or the nasal mucosa, p. 641

rhinoplasty Surgical reconstruction of the nose; performed for cosmetic reasons or to improve airway function when trauma or developmental deformities result in nasal obstruction, p. 634

tracheostomy The stoma (opening) that results from the tracheotomy, p. 642

tracheotomy A surgical incision into the trachea for the purpose of establishing an airway, p. 642

ELECTRONIC RESOURCES

Supplemental content related to Chapter 29 can be found…

Evolve Web Site ⊖volve

- Animation: Anatomic Location of Sinuses
- Answer Guidelines for Case Study on p. 656
- Content Updates
- Customizable Nursing Care Plans:
  - Total Laryngectomy and/or Radical Neck Surgery
  - Tracheostomy

- Electronic Calculators
- Examination Review Questions
- Glossary
- Interactive Case Study: Head and Neck Cancer: Laryngectomy With Tracheostomy
- Key Points (Printable and MP3 Download)
- Patient & Caregiver Teaching Guides:
  - Acute or Chronic Sinusitis
  - How to Reduce Symptoms of Allergic Rhinitis

Structural and Traumatic Disorders of the Nose

Deviated Septum

Deviated septum is a deflection of the normally straight nasal septum. It is most commonly caused by trauma to the nose or arises from a congenital disproportion in which the size of the septum is not proportional to the size of the nose. On inspection, the septum is bent to one side, altering the air passage. Symptoms are variable. The patient may experience obstruction to nasal breathing, nasal edema, or dryness of the nasal mucosa with crusting and bleeding (epistaxis). A severely deviated septum may block drainage of mucus from the sinus cavities, resulting in infection (sinusitis) (Thibodeau & Patton, 2010).

Medical management of deviated septum includes nasal allergy control as in allergic rhinitis (see p. 635). For patients with severe symptoms, a nasal septoplasty (surgical realignment of the septum) is performed to reconstruct and properly align the deviated septum.

Nasal Fracture

Nasal fracture is most often caused by trauma of substantial force to the middle of the face. Some cases of facial trauma can be prevented by using protective sports equipment and protecting against falls. Complications of a nasal fracture include airway obstruction, epistaxis, meningeal tears, and cosmetic deformity.

Nasal fractures are classified as unilateral, bilateral, or complex. A *unilateral fracture* typically produces little or no displacement. *Bilateral fractures,* the most common, give the nose a flattened look. Powerful frontal blows cause *complex fractures,* which may also shatter the frontal bones. Diagnosis is based on the health history, direct observation, and radiographic findings.

On inspection, the nurse should assess the patient's ability to breathe through each nostril and note the presence of edema, bleeding, or hematoma (Emergency Nurses Association, 2010). There may be ecchymosis under one or both eyes. Ecchymosis involving both eyes is often termed *raccoon eyes.* The nose is inspected internally for evidence of septal deviation, hemorrhage, or clear drainage, which suggests leakage of cerebrospinal fluid (CSF). If clear drainage is observed, a specimen may be sent to the laboratory to determine if it is CSF. Injury of sufficient force to fracture nasal bones results in considerable swelling of soft tissues. With extensive swelling, it may be difficult to verify the extent of deformity or to repair the fracture until several days later when the edema subsides (Monahan, 2009).

The goals of nursing management are to reduce edema, prevent complications, and provide emotional support. Ice may be applied to the face and nose to reduce edema and bleeding. When a fracture is confirmed, the goal of management is to realign the fracture using closed or open reduction (septoplasty, rhinoplasty). These procedures re-establish cosmetic appearance and proper function of the nose and provide an adequate airway. After the patient undergoes nasal surgery, the patient should be assessed for the ability to mouth breathe. Nasal intubation or nasogastric tube should be avoided in any patient suspected of a nasal fracture (Rothrock, 2011).

Rhinoplasty

Rhinoplasty, the surgical reconstruction of the nose, is performed for cosmetic reasons or to improve airway function when trauma or congenital deformities result in nasal obstruction. Assessment of the patient's expectations is a critical aspect in preparation for a rhinoplasty. Expected results of surgery should be explained frankly and truthfully to prevent disappointment (Rothrock, 2011).

Collaborative Care

Rhinoplasty is performed as an outpatient procedure using regional anaesthesia. Nasal tissue may be added or removed, and the nose may be lengthened or shortened. Plastic implants are sometimes used to reshape the nose. After surgery, nasal packing may be inserted to apply pressure and prevent bleeding or septal hematoma formation. Nasal septal splints (small pieces of plastic or Silastic) may be inserted to help prevent scar tissue formation between the surgical site and the lateral nasal wall. Adhesive-strip skin closures are placed to hold the skin against the septal cartilage. Typically, nasal packing is removed the day after surgery, and the splint is removed in 3 to 5 days. A small dressing under the nostrils is changed as often as every 2 hours during the first 24 hours. The patient is instructed to prevent pressure on surgical site by sneezing through mouth (Sagrillo & Kunz, 2008).

NURSING MANAGEMENT: NASAL SURGERY

Examples of nasal surgery include rhinoplasty, septoplasty, and nasal fracture reductions. Before surgery, the patient should be instructed to not take aspirin-containing drugs or nonsteroidal anti-inflammatory drugs (NSAIDs) for 2 weeks to reduce the risk of bleeding. Nursing interventions during the immediate postoperative period include assessment of respiratory status, pain management, and observation of the surgical site for hemorrhage and edema. Teaching is important because the patient must be able to detect complications at home (Rothrock, 2011). There is an interim period while edema and ecchymosis resolve before the final cosmetic effect can be achieved.

Epistaxis

Epistaxis (nosebleed) occurs in all age groups, especially in children and the elderly. Epistaxis may be caused by trauma, foreign bodies, nasal spray abuse, street drug use, anatomical malformation, allergic rhinitis, or tumours. Any condition that prolongs bleeding time or alters platelet counts will predispose the patient to epistaxis. Bleeding time may also be prolonged if the patient takes aspirin or NSAIDs. Conditions such as hypertension do not increase the risk of epistaxis (Emergency Nurses Association, 2010; Supriya, Shakeel, Veitch, & Wong, 2010). Elevated blood pressure, however, makes bleeding more difficult to control.

Children and young adults have a tendency to develop anterior nasal bleeding, whereas older adults more commonly have posterior nasal bleeding. Anterior bleeding usually stops spontaneously or can be self-treated; posterior bleeding may require medical treatment (Supriya et al., 2010).

NURSING AND COLLABORATIVE MANAGEMENT: EPISTAXIS

Simple first aid measures should be attempted first to control epistaxis. The nurse should (1) keep the patient quiet; (2) place the patient in a sitting position, leaning forward, or if not possible, in a reclining position with head and shoulders elevated; (3) apply direct pressure by pinching the entire soft lower portion of the nose for 10 to 15 minutes; (4) apply ice compresses to the forehead and have the patient suck on ice; (5) apply digital pressure if bleeding continues; and (6) obtain medical assistance if bleeding does not stop (Emergency Nurses Association, 2010).

If first aid is not effective, management involves localization of the bleeding site and application of a vasoconstrictive agent, cauterization, or anterior packing by a health care provider. Anterior packing may consist of ribbon gauze impregnated with antibiotic ointment that is wedged firmly in the desired location and remains in place for 48 to 72 hours. If posterior packing is required, the patient should be hospitalized. Inflatable balloons may be used as a nasal pack, or gauze rolls may be inserted (Figure 29-1). Strings attached to the packing are brought to the outside and taped to the cheek for ease of removal. A nasal sling (a folded 2 × 2–inch gauze pad) should be taped over the nares to absorb drainage (Christensen & Kockrow, 2011).

Posterior packing may alter respiratory status, especially in older adults. Some patients experience *hypoventilation* causing *hypercapnia* (increase in the partial pressure of carbon dioxide in arterial blood [$PaCO_2$]) and *hypoxemia* (decrease in the partial pressure of oxygen in arterial blood [PaO_2]) sufficient to lead to cardiac dysrhythmias or respiratory arrest. The nurse should closely monitor respiratory rate, heart rate and rhythm, oxygen saturation using pulse oximetry (SpO_2), and level of consciousness and observe for signs of aspiration (Aghababian et al., 2011).

Packing is painful because sufficient pressure must be applied to stop the bleeding. Nasal packing predisposes to infection from bacteria (e.g., *Staphylococcus aureus*) present in the nasal cavity. The patient should receive a mild narcotic analgesic for pain (e.g., acetaminophen with codeine) and an antibiotic effective against staphylococci to protect against infection.

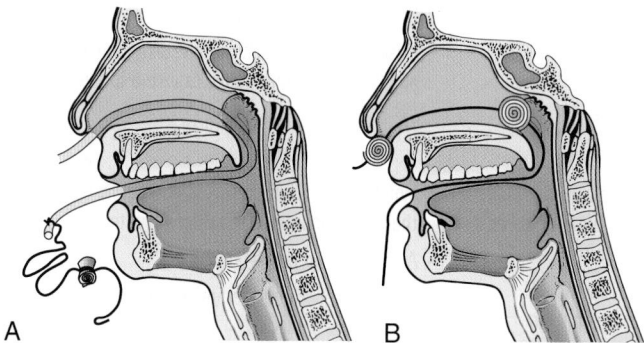

Figure 29-1 Method for placing posterior nasal pack. **A,** Catheter is passed through the bleeding side of the nose and pulled out through the mouth with a hemostat. Strings are tied to the catheter, and the pack is pulled up behind the soft palate and into the nasopharynx. **B,** Nasal pack in position in the posterior nasopharynx. Dental roll at the nose helps maintain correct position.

Posterior packs are left in place for no longer than 48 hours because of the incidence of toxic shock syndrome and are usually removed by the surgeon. Before removal, the patient should be medicated for pain because this procedure is very uncomfortable. After removal, the nares may be gently cleaned and lubricated with petroleum jelly.

Failure of posterior packing to control epistaxis indicates the need for surgery or radiological embolization of the affected artery (Aghababian et al., 2011). The most common surgical procedure of this nature involves ligation of the internal maxillary artery performed through a Caldwell-Luc incision under the upper lip to gain access to the artery.

The patient can be discharged after being taught about home care. The patient should be instructed to avoid vigorous nose blowing, strenuous activity, lifting, and straining for 4 to 6 weeks. The patient should be taught to sneeze with the mouth open and to avoid the use of aspirin-containing products or NSAIDs (Rothrock, 2011).

Inflammation and Infection of the Nose and Paranasal Sinuses

Allergic Rhinitis

Allergic rhinitis is the reaction of the nasal mucosa to a specific allergen. Attacks of seasonal rhinitis usually occur in the spring and fall and are caused by allergy to pollens from trees, flowers, or grasses. The typical attack lasts for several weeks during times when pollen counts are high, then disappears, and recurs at the same time the following year. Perennial rhinitis is present intermittently or constantly. Symptoms are usually caused by specific environmental triggers such as pet dander, dust mites, moulds, or cockroaches (Tickle & Sewell, 2007). Because symptoms of perennial rhinitis resemble the common cold, the patient may believe the condition is a continuous or repeated cold.

Clinical Manifestations

Manifestations of allergic rhinitis are nasal congestion; sneezing; watery, itchy eyes and nose; altered sense of smell; and thin, watery nasal discharge. The nasal turbinates appear pale, boggy, and swollen. With chronic exposure to allergens, the patient's responses include headache, congestion, pressure, postnasal drip, and nasal polyps (Shoup, 2011). The patient may complain of cough, hoarseness, snoring, or the recurrent need to clear the throat.

NURSING AND COLLABORATIVE MANAGEMENT: ALLERGIC RHINITIS

Several steps are used in managing allergic rhinitis. The most important step involves identifying and avoiding triggers of allergic reactions (Table 29-1). The patient should be instructed to keep a diary of times when the allergic reaction occurs and the activities that precipitate the reaction. Steps can then be taken to avoid these triggers.

Drug therapy involves using nasal sprays, leukotriene receptor antagonists (LTRAs) (Tickle & Sewell, 2007), antihistamines, and decongestants to manage symptoms (Table 29-2). Intranasal cor-

Table 29-1 How to Reduce Symptoms of Allergic Rhinitis

1. Avoidance of allergens is the best treatment.

2. Avoid house dust. Use the approach "less is best." Focus on the bedroom. Remove carpeting. Limit furniture. Enclose pillows, mattress, and springs in air-tight, vinyl encasements. Limit clothing in the bedroom to items used frequently. Place clothing in air-tight, zipper-sealed, vinyl clothes bags. Install an air filter. Close the air-conditioning vent into the room.

3. Avoid house dust mites. Wash bedding in hot water 55°C weekly. Wear a mask when vacuuming. Double-bag the vacuum cleaner. Install a filter on the outlet port of the vacuum cleaner. Avoid sleeping or lying on upholstered furniture. Remove carpets that are laid on concrete. If possible, have someone else clean the house.

4. Avoid mould spores. The three *D*s that promote growth of mould spores are *d*arkness, *d*ampness, and *d*rafts. Avoid places where humidity is high (e.g., basements, camps on the lake, clothes hampers, greenhouses, stables, barns). Dehumidifiers may be helpful in humid weather and in damp spaces. Ventilate closed rooms, open doors, and install fans. HEPA (high-efficiency particulate air) filters may be beneficial. Consider adding windows to dark rooms. Consider keeping a small light on in closets. A basement light with a timer that provides light several hours a day may decrease mould growth.

5. Avoid pollens. Stay inside with closed doors and windows during high-pollen season. Avoid the use of fans. Install an air conditioner with a good air filter. Wash filters weekly during high pollen season. Put the car air conditioner on "recirculate" when driving. Get someone else to tend to your yard.

6. Avoid pet allergens. Remove pets from the interior of the home. Clean the living area thoroughly. Do not expect instant relief. Symptoms usually do not improve significantly for 2 months following pet removal.

7. Avoid smoke. The presence of a smoker will sabotage the best of all possible symptom reduction programs.

Source: Adapted from Thompson, E., & Poore, R. (2010). Allergic rhinitis. *BCHealthGuideOnline.* Retrieved from *http://www.healthlinkbc.ca/kb/content/special/hw33436.html#hw33621*

DRUG THERAPY

Table 29-2 Allergic Rhinitis and Sinusitis

PREPARATION	MECHANISM OF ACTION	ADVERSE EFFECTS	NURSING ACTIONS
Corticosteroids			
Nasal Spray			
Beclomethasone (Apo-Beclomethasone) Budesonide (Rhinocort) Flunisolide (Apo-Flunisolide) Fluticasone (Flonase) Triamcinolone (Nasacort) Ciclesonide (Omnaris)	Inhibits inflammatory response. At recommended dosage, systemic adverse effects are unlikely because of low systemic absorption. Systemic effects may occur with greater-than-recommended dosages.	Mild transient nasal burning and stinging; in rare instances, localized fungal infection with *Candida albicans*	• Teach patient correct use. • Instruct patient to use on regular basis and not PRN. • Explain to patient that the spray acts to decrease inflammation over time and does not have an immediate effect. • Discontinue use if nasal infection develops.
Mast Cell Stabilizer			
Nasal Spray			
Cromolyn spray (Apo-Cromolyn)	Inhibits degranulation of sensitized mast cells that occurs after exposure to specific antigens.	Minimal adverse effects; occasional burning or nasal irritation	• Teach patient correct use. • Reinforce that spray prevents symptoms. • Begin 2 wk before pollen season starts and use throughout pollen season. • If isolated allergy, such as cat, use prophylactically (i.e., 10-15 min before exposure to allergen).
Leukotriene Receptor Antagonists (LTRAs)			
Antagonists			
Zafirlukast (Accolate) Montelukast (Singulair)	Antagonize or inhibit leukotriene activity, thereby inhibiting airway edema and bronchoconstriction through decreasing inflammatory process.	Headaches, dizziness, rash, altered liver function tests, abdominal pain *Zafirlukast:* Monitor PT levels and theophylline levels if patient is taking coumadin or theophylline	• Monitor liver function tests periodically while on therapy. Discontinue if values elevate. • Administer on empty stomach. • Do not discontinue therapy without consulting health care provider. • Not to be used for acute attacks.
Anticholinergic			
Nasal Spray			
Ipratropium bromide (Atrovent)	Blocks hypersecretory effects by competing for binding sites on the cell. Reduces rhinorrhea in the common cold, allergic and nonallergic rhinitis.	Dryness of the mouth and nose may occur Does not cause systemic adverse effects	• Teach patient correct use. • Reinforce that spray prevents symptoms, with onset of action within 1 hr of use. • May reduce need for other rhinitis medications.

DRUG THERAPY

Table 29-2 Allergic Rhinitis and Sinusitis—cont'd

PREPARATION	MECHANISM OF ACTION	ADVERSE EFFECTS	NURSING ACTIONS
Antihistamines			
First-Generation Agents			
Ethanolamines Clemastine (Tavist) Diphenhydramine (Benadryl) *Ethylenediamines* Tripelennamine (PBZ; PBZ-SR) *Alkylamines* Brompheniramine (Dimetane) Chlorpheniramine (Chlor-Tripolon)	Bind with H$_1$ receptors on target cells, blocking histamine binding. Relieve acute symptoms of allergic response (itching, sneezing, excessive secretions, mild congestion).	First-generation agents cross blood–brain barrier, bind to H$_1$ receptors in brain, cause sedation (diminished alertness, slow reaction time, somnolence) and stimulation (restless, nervous, insomnia) Some drugs (e.g., ethanolamines) are more likely to cause sedation Patients vary in their sensitivity to these adverse effects. The next most common adverse effects involve the GI system and include loss of appetite, epigastric distress, constipation, or diarrhea May cause palpitations, tachycardia, urinary retention or frequency	• Warn patient that operating machinery and driving may be dangerous because of sedative effect. Drowsiness usually passes after 2 wk of treatment. • Teach patient to report palpitations, change in heart rate, change in bowel, bladder habits. • Instruct patient not to use alcohol with antihistamines because of additive depressant effect. • Rapid onset of action, no drug tolerance with prolonged use. • Limited use with sinusitis.
Second-Generation Agents			
Loratadine (Claritin) Cetirizine (Reactine) Fexofenadine (Allegra) Desloratadine (Aerius)	—	Second-generation agents have limited affinity for brain H$_1$ receptors; cause minimal sedation; few effects on psychomotor activities, bladder function	• Teach patient to expect few, if any, adverse effects. • More expensive than classical antihistamines. • Rapid onset of action, no drug tolerance with prolonged use. *General interactions:* • Do not take with alcohol or any form of tranquilizer or sedative. • Do not take with any monoamine oxidase inhibitor.
Decongestants			
Oral			
Pseudoephedrine (Sudafed)	Stimulate adrenergic receptors on blood vessels, promote vasoconstriction and reduce nasal edema and rhinorrhea.	CNS stimulation, causing insomnia, excitation, headache, irritability, increased blood and ocular pressure, dysuria, palpitations, tachycardia	• Advise patient of adverse reactions. • Advise that use of some preparations is contraindicated for patients with cardiovascular disease, hypertension, diabetes, glaucoma, prostate hyperplasia, hepatic and renal disease. • Teach patient that these drugs should not be used for more than 3 days or more than three or four times a day. • Longer use increases risk of rebound vasodilation, which can increase congestion.
Topical (Nasal Spray)			
Oxymetazoline (Dristan) Phenylephrine (Neo-Synephrine)	Same as above. Blocks action of histamine.	Same as above, plus rhinitis medicamentosa (rebound nasal congestion) Headache, bitter taste, somnolence, nasal irritation	—

CNS, central nervous system; *GI*, gastrointestinal; *H₁*, histamine 1; *PRN*, as needed; *PT*, prothrombin time.

ticosteroid and cromolyn sprays are effective for seasonal and perennial rhinitis. Nasal corticosteroid sprays are used to decrease inflammation locally; there is little absorption in the systemic circulation, and therefore, systemic adverse drug events are rare. Relief may require combining a nasal corticosteroid spray and an antihistamine. The patient using nasal inhalers needs careful instructions about proper use. Nasal decongestant sprays can be used for up to 5 days because they can cause a rebound effect from prolonged use (Tickle & Sewell, 2007).

Immunotherapy ("allergy injections") may be used if drugs are not tolerated, or ineffective, when a specific, unavoidable allergen is identified. Immunotherapy involves controlled exposure to small amounts of a known allergen through frequent (at least weekly) injections with the goal to decrease sensitivity. (The mechanisms involved in the allergic response and immunotherapy are discussed in Chapter 14.)

Acute Viral Rhinitis

Acute viral rhinitis (common cold or acute coryza) is caused by viruses that invade the upper respiratory tract. It is the most prevalent infectious disease and is spread by airborne droplet sprays emitted by the infected person while breathing, talking, sneezing, or coughing or by direct hand contact. Frequency increases in the winter months, when people stay indoors and overcrowding is more common. Other factors, such as chilling, fatigue, physical and emotional stress, and compromised immune status, may increase susceptibility. The patient with acute viral rhinitis typically first experiences tickling, irritation, sneezing, or dryness of the nose or nasopharynx followed by copious nasal secretions, some nasal obstruction, watery eyes, elevated temperature, general malaise, and headache. After the early profuse secretions, the nose becomes more obstructed, and the discharge is thicker. Within a few days, the general symptoms improve, nasal passages reopen, and normal breathing is re-established (Goldman & Ausiello, 2007).

NURSING AND COLLABORATIVE MANAGEMENT: ACUTE VIRAL RHINITIS

Supportive therapy such as rest, fluids, proper diet, antipyretics, and analgesics is the recommended treatment. Complications of acute viral rhinitis include pharyngitis, sinusitis, otitis media, tonsillitis, and lung infections. Antibiotics do not have a role in the treatment of viral rhinitis during the cold season; the patient with a chronic illness or a compromised immune status should be advised to avoid crowded, close situations and other persons who have obvious cold symptoms. Frequent hand hygiene and avoiding hand-to-face contact may help prevent direct spread.

Interventions are directed toward relieving annoying and uncomfortable symptoms. The patient should be encouraged to drink increased amounts of fluids to liquefy secretions. Antihistamine or decongestant therapy reduces postnasal drip and significantly decreases severity of cough, nasal obstruction, and nasal discharge. The patient should also be taught to recognize the symptoms of secondary bacterial infection, such as a temperature higher than 38°C (100.4°F); purulent nasal exudate;

tender, swollen glands; and a sore, red throat. In the patient with pulmonary disease, signs of infection include a change in consistency, colour, or volume of the sputum. Because infection can progress rapidly, the patient with chronic respiratory disease may be taught to begin antibiotics in response to sputum changes (Goldman & Ausiello, 2007).

Influenza

Approximately 10 to 25% of Canadians could get the flu during flu season, which runs from November to April. Although the majority recover completely, an estimated 4000 to 8000, mostly seniors, die every year from flu-related pneumonia. Many others die from other complications of flu. Much of the influenza-related morbidity and mortality could be prevented by vaccination of high-risk groups (Table 29-3). Over 50 million doses of flu vaccine were purchased by the Government of Canada for distribution to all Canadians (Health Canada, 2009).

There are three groups of influenza viruses (A, B, and C; note that influenza C has little pathogenic potential). Influenza viruses have a remarkable ability to change over time. This accounts for widespread disease and the need for annual vaccination against new strains. Fewer cases of influenza result when a minor change in the virus occurs because most persons have partial immunity. Birds are natural carriers of influenza A viruses. Currently, avian influenza H5N1 is circulating in Southeast Asia and parts of Europe, infecting many poultry populations and some humans. This strain is highly pathogenic to birds and has infected a limited number of people. There is no evidence this virus is transmitted from person to person.

The Canadian Pandemic Influenza Plan was updated in 2010 to reflect current infection control practices. It outlines preventive activities as well as ongoing surveillance for a pandemic influenza

Table 29-3 Target Groups for Influenza Immunization

Groups at High Risk

- Adults and children with cardiac or pulmonary disease
- Adults ≥65 yr old
- Healthy children between 6 and 23 mo
- Pregnant females, in the third trimester, if their delivery date is in influenza season
- Residents of nursing homes or long-term care facilities
- People with chronic conditions such as diabetes, anemia, cancer, immunodeficiency, immunosuppression, renal disease, or conditions that compromise management of respiratory secretions
- Children or adolescents on long-term acetylsalicylic acid therapy
- Health care workers, and those who provide essential community services, and other caregivers and household contacts capable of transmitting influenza to the above at-risk groups
- People at high risk of influenza complications
- People who are also travelling to areas where the flu virus is likely to be circulating

Source: Public Health Agency of Canada (PHAC). (2010). *Canadian immunization guide, 2007* (8th ed., Table 6). Retrieved from *http://www.phac-aspc.gc.ca/publicat/cig-gci/p04-inf-eng.php#table6*

outbreak. It is based on the World Health Organization guidelines to mobilize global efforts to manage pandemic influenza (Public Health Agency of Canada [PHAC], 2010).

Clinical Manifestations

The onset of flu is typically abrupt with systemic symptoms of cough, fever, and myalgia often accompanied by a headache and sore throat. Milder symptoms, similar to those of the common cold, may also occur. Physical findings are usually minimal, with normal assessment on chest auscultation. Dyspnea and diffuse crackles are signs of pulmonary complications. In uncomplicated cases, symptoms subside within 7 days. Some patients, particularly older adults, experience weakness or lassitude that persists for weeks. The convalescent phase may be marked by hyperactive airways and a chronic cough. Important diagnostic factors include the patient's health history, clinical findings, and the presence of other cases of influenza in the community.

The most common complication of influenza is pneumonia. The patient who develops secondary bacterial pneumonia experiences gradual improvement of influenza symptoms, then worsening cough and purulent sputum. Treatment with antibiotics is usually effective if started early.

NURSING AND COLLABORATIVE MANAGEMENT: INFLUENZA

The nurse should advocate regular handwashing as an effective strategy to reducing the risk of influenza. The nurse should also advocate influenza vaccination for patients at high risk during routine office visits or, if hospitalized, at the time of discharge (see Table 29-3). The vaccine is 70 to 90% effective in preventing influenza in adults. To be effective, the vaccine must be given in the fall (mid-October) before exposure occurs. Although all healthy people between 2 and 65 years old should be encouraged to receive the vaccination, high priority should also be given to groups that can transmit influenza to high-risk persons, such as health care workers. By being vaccinated, the nurse can decrease the risk of transmitting influenza to those who have less ability to cope with the effects of this illness. Despite obvious benefits, many persons are reluctant to be vaccinated. Current vaccines are highly purified, and reactions are extremely uncommon. Soreness at the injection site is usually the only adverse effect. The only contraindications are for children younger than 6 months, people who have a hypersensitivity to eggs, or those who had a reaction to a previous immunization. People with a previous history of Guillain-Barré syndrome following a vaccination should avoid future vaccinations.

The primary goals in nursing management are supportive measures directed toward relief of symptoms and prevention of secondary infection. The patient should drink plenty of fluids and get plenty of rest. Older adults and those with a chronic illness may require hospitalization. Drug therapy with amantadine, oseltamivir (Tamiflu), or zanamivir (Relenza) may be given to prevent or decrease symptoms of influenza in high-risk patients. Amantadine is effective only against influenza A. These drugs prevent the virus from budding and spreading to other cells. For maximum benefit, they should be initiated as soon as possible and ideally within 2 days of the onset of symptoms. They shorten the duration and severity of influenza and can be used prophylactically for control of outbreaks. Zanamivir is administered using an inhaler. Amantadine and oseltamivir are taken orally (PHAC, 2010).

COMPLEMENTARY & ALTERNATIVE THERAPIES

Goldenseal

Clinical Uses

Common cold, respiratory and gastrointestinal infections, wound healing, cirrhosis of the liver, gallbladder inflammation, peptic ulcers.

Effects

Has a wide variety of effects such as anti-inflammatory properties, antimicrobial, and immunostimulating actions. Goldenseal can stimulate the flow of bile.

Nursing Implications

Because of the anticoagulant effects, goldenseal should not be used for longer than 2 weeks. Large doses may cause gastrointestinal distress (e.g., diarrhea, vomiting) and possible nervous system effects. Commonly combined with echinacea in preparations. May be used in conjunction with antibiotics. Should not be used concurrently with anticoagulants, antihypertensives, β-adrenergic blockers, or calcium channel blockers. Should not be used if person has heart or vascular disease, especially hypertension, heart failure, or dysrhythmias.

Sources: Christensen & Kockrow, 2011; Rothrock, 2011.

Sinusitis

Sinusitis develops when the ostia (exit) from the sinuses is narrowed or blocked by inflammation or hypertrophy (swelling) of the mucosa (Figure 29-2). The secretions that accumulate behind the obstruction provide a rich medium for growth of bacteria, viruses, and fungi, all of which may cause infection. Bacterial sinusitis is most commonly caused by *Streptococcus pneumoniae, Haemophilus influenzae,* or *Moraxella catarrhalis* (Dykewicz & Hamilos, 2010). Viral sinusitis follows an upper respiratory infection in which the virus penetrates the mucous membrane and decreases ciliary transport. Fungal sinusitis is uncommon and is usually found in patients who are debilitated or immunocompromised.

Acute sinusitis usually results from an upper respiratory infection, allergic rhinitis, swimming, or dental manipulation, all of which can cause inflammatory changes and retention of secretions. When acute sinusitis follows viral rhinitis, symptoms worsen after 5 to 7 days and are worse than the original rhinitis. *Chronic sinusitis* is a persistent infection usually associated with allergies and nasal polyps. Chronic sinusitis generally results from repeated episodes of acute sinusitis that result in irreversible loss of the normal ciliated epithelium lining the sinus cavity.

Clinical Manifestations

Acute sinusitis causes significant pain over the affected sinus, purulent nasal drainage, nasal obstruction, congestion, fever, and malaise. The patient looks and feels sick. Assessment involves inspection of the nasal mucosa and palpation of the sinus points for pain. Findings that indicate acute sinusitis include a hyperemic and edematous mucosa, enlarged turbinates, and tenderness over the involved sinuses. The patient may have recurrent headaches that change in intensity with position changes or when secretions drain (Christensen & Kockrow, 2011).

Chronic sinusitis is difficult to diagnose because symptoms may be nonspecific. The patient is rarely febrile. Although there may be facial pain, nasal congestion, and increased drainage, severe pain and purulent drainage are often absent. Symptoms may mimic those seen with allergies. Radiographic studies of the sinuses or a sinus computed tomography (CT) scan may be performed to confirm the diagnosis. CT scans may show the sinuses to be filled with fluid or the mucous membrane to be thickened. Nasal endoscopy with a flexible scope may be used to examine the sinuses, obtain drainage for culture, and restore normal drainage.

Many patients with asthma have sinusitis. The link between these diseases is unclear. Sinusitis may trigger asthma by stimulating reflex bronchospasm. Appropriate treatment of sinusitis often causes a reduction in asthma symptoms (Dykewicz & Hamilos, 2010).

NURSING AND COLLABORATIVE MANAGEMENT: SINUSITIS

If allergies are the precipitating cause of sinusitis, the patient needs to be instructed in ways to reduce sinus inflammation and infection, including environmental control of allergies and appropriate drug therapy (see section on allergic rhinitis earlier in this chapter). Treatment of acute sinusitis includes antibiotics to treat the infection, decongestants to promote drainage, nasal corticosteroids to decrease inflammation, and mucolytics to promote mucous flow (Table 29-4). Classical (first-generation) antihistamines increase the viscosity of mucus and promote continued symptoms, so they should be avoided. Nonsedating (second-generation) antihistamines do not cause this problem. Antibiotic therapy is usually continued for 10 to 14 days for acute sinusitis.

If symptoms do not resolve, the antibiotic should be changed to a broader-spectrum agent. With chronic sinusitis, mixed bacterial flora are often present and infections are difficult to eliminate. Broad-spectrum antibiotics may be used for 4 to 6 weeks.

The patient should be encouraged to increase fluid intake (six to eight glasses daily) and use nasal cleaning techniques. This may include taking a hot shower in the morning and the evening followed by blowing the nose thoroughly. Other interventions to

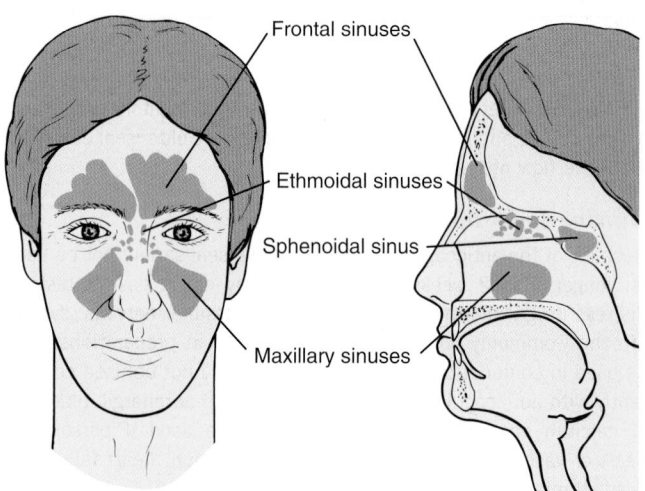

Figure 29-2 Location of the sinuses.

Table 29-4 Acute or Chronic Sinusitis

1. Keep well hydrated by drinking six to eight glasses of water daily to liquefy secretions.

2. Take hot showers twice daily; use a steam inhaler (15-min vaporization of boiled water), bedside humidifier, or nasal saline spray to promote secretion drainage.

3. Report temperature of ≥38°C, which may indicate infection.

4. Follow prescribed medication regimen:
   - Take analgesics to relieve pain.
   - Take decongestants or expectorants, or both, to relieve swelling and to thin mucus.
   - Take antibiotics, as prescribed, for infection. Be sure to take entire prescription and report continued symptoms or a change in symptoms.
   - Administer nasal sprays correctly.

5. Do not smoke, and avoid exposure to smoke. Smoke is an irritant and may worsen symptoms.

6. If allergies predispose to sinusitis, follow instructions regarding environmental control, drug therapy, and immunotherapy to reduce the inflammation and prevent sinus infection.

7. Avoid use of nasogastric tube inserted via the nares.

cleanse the nasal passages and promote drainage include irrigating the nose with salt water—2.5 to 5 mL of salt/L of water (Egan & Hickner, 2009)—or inhaling steam.

The patient with persistent or recurrent sinus complaints not alleviated by medical therapy may require nasal endoscopic surgery to relieve blockage caused by hypertrophy or septal deviation. This is an outpatient procedure usually performed under local anaesthesia (Christensen & Kockrow, 2011).

Obstruction of the Nose and Paranasal Sinuses

Polyps

Nasal polyps are benign mucous membrane masses that form slowly in response to repeated inflammation of the sinus or the nasal mucosa. Polyps, which appear as bluish, glossy projections in the nares (nostril), can exceed the size of a grape. The patient may be anxious, fearing they are malignant. Clinical manifestations include nasal obstruction, nasal discharge (usually clear mucus), and speech distortion. Nasal polyps can be removed with endoscopic or laser surgery, but recurrence is common. Topical or systemic corticosteroids may slow polyp growth (Christensen & Kockrow, 2011).

Foreign Bodies

A variety of foreign bodies may lodge in the upper respiratory tract. Inorganic foreign bodies such as buttons and beads may cause no symptoms, lie undetected, and be accidentally discovered on routine examination. Organic foreign bodies such as wood, cotton, beans, peas, and paper produce a local inflammatory reaction and nasal discharge, which may become purulent and foul smelling. Foreign bodies should be removed from the nose through the route of entry. Sneezing with the opposite nostril closed may be effective in assisting the removal of foreign bodies. Irrigation of the nose or pushing the object backward should not be done because either could cause aspiration and airway obstruction. If sneezing or blowing the nose does not remove the object, the patient should see a health care provider.

Problems Related to the Pharynx

Acute Pharyngitis

Acute pharyngitis is an acute inflammation of the pharyngeal walls. It may include tonsils, palate, and uvula. It can be caused by a viral, bacterial, or fungal infection. Viral pharyngitis accounts for approximately 70% of cases. Acute follicular pharyngitis ("strep throat") results from β-hemolytic streptococcal invasion and accounts for an additional 5 to 15% of episodes (Christensen & Kockrow, 2011). Fungal pharyngitis, especially candidiasis, can develop with prolonged use of antibiotics or inhaled corticosteroids or in immunosuppressed patients, especially those with human immunodeficiency virus (HIV).

Clinical Manifestations

Symptoms of acute pharyngitis range in severity from complaints of a "scratchy throat" to pain so severe that swallowing is difficult. Both viral and strep infections appear as a red and edematous pharynx, with or without patchy yellow exudates. Appearance is not always diagnostic. Cultures or a rapid strep antigen test is done to establish the cause and direct appropriate management. Inadequate treatment of acute streptococcal pharyngitis can result in rheumatic heart disease or glomerulonephritis.

White, irregular patches suggest fungal infection with *Candida albicans*. In diphtheria, a grey-white false membrane, termed a *pseudomembrane*, is seen covering the oropharynx, nasopharynx, and laryngopharynx and sometimes extending to the trachea.

NURSING AND COLLABORATIVE MANAGEMENT: ACUTE PHARYNGITIS

The goals of nursing management are infection control, symptomatic relief, and prevention of secondary complications. The patient with documented strep throat is treated with antibiotics. *Candida* infections are treated with nystatin, an antifungal antibiotic. The preparation should be swished in the mouth as long as possible before it is swallowed, and treatment should continue until symptoms are gone. The patient should be encouraged to increase fluid intake. Cool, bland liquids and gelatin will not irritate the pharynx; avoid citrus juices because they can be irritating to the throat.

Peritonsillar Abscess

Peritonsillar abscess is a complication of acute pharyngitis or acute tonsillitis when bacterial infection invades one or both tonsils. The tonsils may enlarge sufficiently to threaten airway patency. The patient experiences a high fever, leukocytosis, and chills. Intravenous antibiotic therapy is given along with needle aspiration or incision and drainage of the abscess. An emergency tonsillectomy may be performed, or an elective tonsillectomy may be scheduled after the infection has subsided.

Problems Related to the Trachea and Larynx

Airway Obstruction

Airway obstruction may be complete or partial. *Complete airway obstruction* is a medical emergency. *Partial airway obstruction* may occur as a result of aspiration of food or a foreign body. In addition, partial airway obstruction may result from laryngeal edema following extubation, laryngeal or tracheal stenosis, central nervous system (CNS) depression, and allergic reactions. Symptoms include stridor, use of accessory muscles, suprasternal and intercostal retractions, wheezing, restlessness, tachycardia, and cyanosis. Prompt assessment and treatment are essential because partial obstruction may quickly progress to complete obstruction. Interventions to re-establish a patent airway include the obstructed airway (Heimlich) manoeuvre (see Chapter 71), cricothyroidotomy, endotracheal intubation, and tracheostomy. Unexplained or recurrent symptoms indicate the need for additional tests, such as a chest radiography, pulmonary function tests, and bronchoscopy.

Tracheostomy

A **tracheotomy** is a surgical incision into the trachea for the purpose of establishing an airway. A **tracheostomy** is the stoma (opening) that results from the tracheotomy. Indications for a tracheostomy are to (1) bypass an upper airway obstruction, (2) facilitate removal of secretions, (3) permit long-term mechanical ventilation, and (4) permit oral intake and speech in the patient who requires long-term mechanical ventilation. Most patients who require mechanical ventilation are initially managed with an endotracheal tube, which can be quickly inserted in an emergency. (Care of the patient with an endotracheal tube is discussed in Chapter 68.) A tracheostomy requires surgical dissection and is, therefore, not typically an emergency procedure. Percutaneous tracheostomy can be performed emergently at the bedside with decreased risk of complications (Engels, Bayshaw, Meier, Brindley, 2008).

Several advantages make a tracheostomy the better option for long-term nursing management. With a tracheostomy, patient comfort may be increased without a tube in the mouth. The patient is able to eat and talk with a tracheostomy because the tube enters lower in the airway (Figure 29-3). With this type of

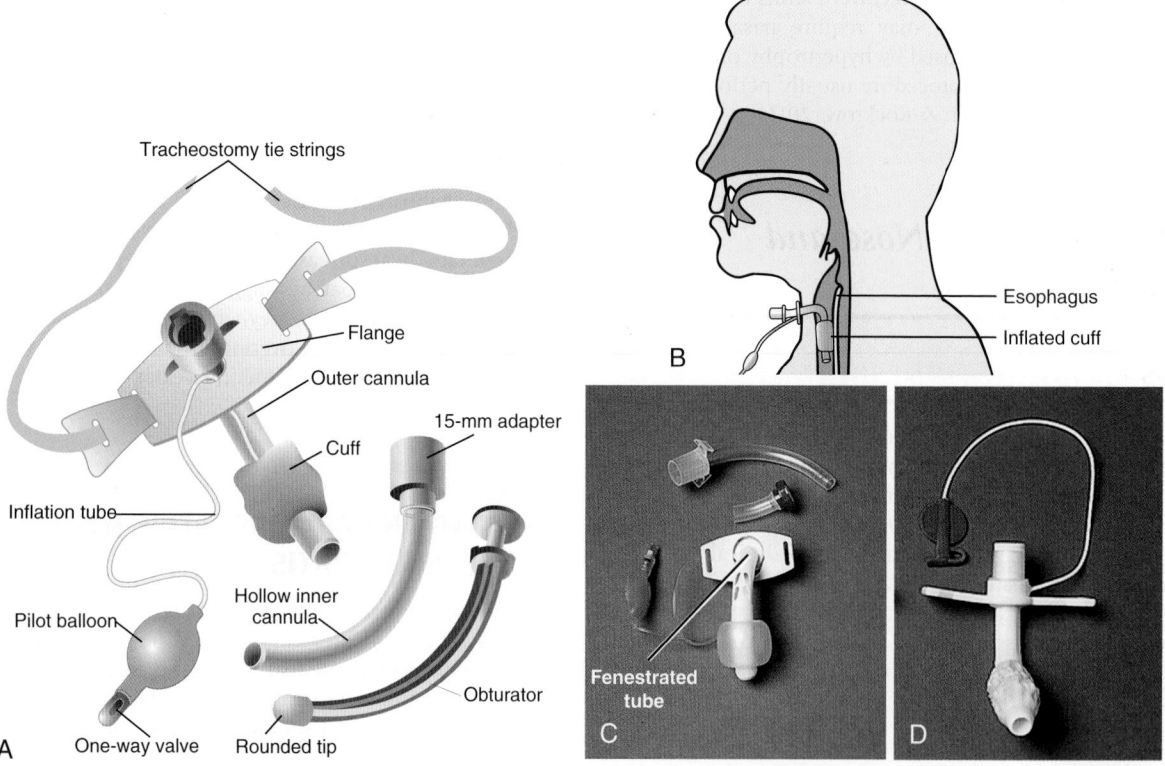

Figure 29-3 Types of tracheostomy tubes. **A,** Parts of a tracheostomy tube. **B,** Tracheostomy tube inserted in the airway with an inflated cuff. **C,** Fenestrated tracheostomy tube with cuff, inner cannula, decannulation plug, and pilot balloon. **D,** Tracheostomy tube with a foam cuff and obturator (one cuff is deflated on tracheostomy tube). (See Table 29-5 and NCP 29-1 for related nursing management.)

insertion airway adjunct, the patient is potentially able to wean from the ventilator. Because the tracheostomy tube is more secure, mobility may be increased (Urden, Stacy, & Lough, 2010).

NURSING MANAGEMENT: TRACHEOSTOMY

■ Providing Tracheostomy Care

Before the tracheotomy procedure, the nurse should explain to the patient and caregivers the purpose of the procedure and inform them that the patient will not be able to speak while an inflated cuff is used. A number of complications can occur with tracheostomies (Table 29-5).

A variety of tubes are available to meet individual patient needs (Table 29-6). All tracheostomy tubes contain a faceplate or flange, which rests on the neck between the clavicle and an outer cannula. In addition, all tubes have an obturator, which is used when inserting the tube (see Figure 29-3, C). A spare tracheostomy set should be kept at the bedside in case of accidental decannulation (Skillings & Curtis, 2011).

Some tracheostomy tubes also have an inner cannula, which can be removed for cleaning (see Figure 29-3, B). The cleaning procedure removes mucus from the inside of the tube. If humidification is adequate, mucus may not accumulate and a tube without an inner cannula can be used. Care of the patient with a tracheostomy involves suctioning the airway to remove secretions (Figure 29-4 and Table 29-7) and cleaning around the stoma. In addition, tracheostomy care includes changing tracheostomy ties (Figure 29-5 and Table 29-8). If an inner cannula is used, whether disposable or nondisposable, tracheostomy care also involves inner cannula care (Lynn-McHale Weigand, 2011) (see Table 29-8).

Both cuffed and uncuffed tracheostomy tubes are available. A tracheostomy tube with an inflated cuff is used if the patient is at risk of aspiration or needs mechanical ventilation. Because an inflated cuff exerts pressure on tracheal mucosa, it is important to inflate the cuff with the minimum volume of air required to obtain an airway seal. Cuff inflation pressure should not exceed 20 mm Hg or 25 cm H_2O because higher pressures may compress tracheal capillaries, limit blood flow, and predispose to tracheal necrosis. An alternative approach, termed the *minimal leak technique* (MLT), involves inflating the cuff with the minimum amount of air to obtain a seal and then withdrawing 0.1 mL of air. A disadvantage of MLT is the risk of aspiration from secretions leaking around the cuff. MLT should not be used if the tracheostomy was placed to bypass an upper airway obstruction, such as with patients who have undergone head and neck surgery (Skillings & Curtis, 2011).

In some patients, cuff deflation is performed to remove secretions that accumulate above the cuff. Before deflation, the patient should cough up secretions, if possible, and the tracheostomy tube and mouth should be suctioned (see Figure 29-4 and Table 29-7). This step is important to prevent secretions from being aspirated during deflation. The cuff is deflated during exhalation because the exhaled gas helps propel secretions into the mouth. The patient should also cough or be suctioned after cuff deflation. The cuff should be reinflated during inspiration. The volume of air required to inflate the cuff should be monitored daily because this volume may increase if there is tracheal dilation from cuff pressure. The nurse should assess the ability of the patient to protect the airway from aspiration and remain with the patient when the cuff is initially deflated unless the patient can protect the airway from aspiration and breathe without respiratory distress.

When the patient can protect the airway from aspiration and does not require mechanical ventilation, a cuffless tracheostomy tube should be used.

Retention sutures are often placed in the tracheal cartilage when the tracheostomy is performed. The free ends should be taped to the skin in a place and manner that leaves them accessible if the tube becomes dislodged. Care should be taken not to dislodge the tracheostomy tube during the first few days when the stoma is not mature (healed). Because tube replacement can be difficult, several precautions are required: (1) a replacement tube of equal or smaller size is kept at the bedside, readily available for emergency reinsertion; (2) tracheostomy tapes are not changed for at least 24 hours after the insertion procedure; and (3) the first tube change is performed by a physician usually no sooner than 7 days after the tracheotomy.

The retention sutures (if present) are grasped and the opening is spread. A hemostat can also be used to spread the opening to facilitate replacing the tube. Another method is to insert a suction catheter to allow passage of air and to serve as a guide

Table 29-5 Complications of Tracheostomies

COMPLICATION	CAUSES	NURSING MANAGEMENT
Abnormal bleeding	Surgical intervention Erosion or rupture of blood vessel, or both	• Monitor bleeding • Notify physician if it continues or is excessive
Tube dislodgement	Excessive manipulation or suctioning	• Ensure ties are secure • Keep obturator, hemostat, and new tracheostomy tube at bedside
Obstructed tube	Dried or excessive secretions	• Assess patient's respiratory status • Suction as necessary • Maintain humidification • Perform tracheostomy care • Ensure adequate hydration
Subcutaneous emphysema	Air escapes from the incision to the subcutaneous tissue	• Monitor subcutaneous emphysema • Reassure patient and family
Tracheoesophageal fistula	Tracheal wall necrosis leading to fistula formation	• Monitor cuff pressure • Monitor patient for coughing and choking while eating or drinking
Tracheal stenosis	Narrowing of tracheal lumen owing to scarring caused by tracheal irritation	• Monitor cuff pressure • Ensure prompt treatment of infections • Ensure ties are secure

Table 29-6 Characteristics and Nursing Management of Tracheostomies

TUBE	CHARACTERISTICS	NURSING MANAGEMENT
Tracheostomy tube with cuff and pilot balloon (see Figure 29-3, *A* and *B*)	When properly inflated, low-pressure, high-volume cuff distributes cuff pressure over large area, minimizing pressure on tracheal wall.	**Procedure for Cuff Inflation** • *Spontaneously breathing patient:* Inflate cuff to minimal occlusion pressure by slowly injecting air into the cuff until no sound is heard after deep breath or during inhalation with manual resuscitation bag. If using MLT, remove 0.1 mL of air while maintaining seal. MLT should not be used if there is risk of aspiration. • *Immediately after cuff inflation:* Verify pressure is within accepted range (≤20 mm Hg or ≤25 cm H$_2$O) with a manometer. Record cuff pressure and volume of air used for cuff inflation in chart. **Care of Patients With an Inflated Cuff** • Monitor and record cuff pressure q8h. Cuff pressure should be ≤20 mm Hg or ≤25 cm H$_2$O to allow adequate tracheal capillary perfusion. If necessary, remove or add air to the pilot tubing using a syringe and stopcock. Afterward, verify cuff pressure is within accepted range with manometer. • Report inability to keep the cuff inflated or need to use progressively larger volumes of air to keep cuff inflated. Potential causes include tracheal dilation at the cuff site or a crack or slow leak in the housing of the one-way inflation valve. If the leak is caused by tracheal dilation, the physician may intubate the patient with a larger tube. Cracks in the inflation valve may be temporarily managed by clamping the small-bore tubing with a hemostat. The tube should be changed within 24 hr.
Fenestrated tracheostomy tube (Shiley, Portex) with cuff, inner cannula, and decannulation plug (see Figures 29-3, *B* and 29-6, *A*)	When inner cannula is removed, cuff deflated, and decannulation plug inserted, air flows around tube, through fenestration in outer cannula, and up over vocal cords. Patient can then speak.	• Signs or symptoms of aspiration need further evaluation by a speech pathologist or radiologist. • *Never* insert decannulation plug in tracheostomy tube until cuff is deflated and inner cannula removed. Prior insertion will prevent patient from breathing (no air inflow). This may precipitate a respiratory arrest. • Assess for signs of respiratory distress when a fenestrated cannula is first used. If this occurs, the cap should be removed, the inner cannula replaced, and the cuff reinflated. • Cuff management as described above.
Speaking tracheostomy tube (Portex, National) with cuff, two external tubings (see Figure 29-6, *B*)	Has two tubings, one leading to cuff and second to opening above the cuff. When port is connected to air source, air flows out of opening and up over the vocal cords, allowing speech with cuff inflated.	• Once tube is inserted, wait 2 days before use so that the stoma can close around the tube and prevent leaks. • When patient desires to speak, connect port to compressed air (or oxygen). Be certain to identify correct tubing. If gas enters the cuff, it will overinflate and rupture, necessitating an emergency tube change. Use lowest flow (typically 4-6 L/min) that results in speech. High flows dehydrate mucosa. • Cover port adaptor. This will cause the air to flow upward. Instruct patient to speak in short sentences because voice becomes a whisper with long sentences. • Disconnect flow when patient does not want to speak to prevent mucosal dehydration. • Cuff management as described above.
Tracheostomy tube (Bivona Fome-Cuf) foam-filled cuff (see Figure 29-3, *C*)	Cuff is filled with plastic foam. Before insertion, cuff is deflated. After insertion, cuff is allowed to fill passively with air. Pilot tubing is not capped, and no cuff pressure monitoring is required.	• Before insertion, withdraw all air from the cuff using a 20-mL syringe. Cap pilot balloon tubing to prevent re-entry of air. After tracheostomy is inserted, remove cap from pilot tubing allowing cuff to passively reinflate. • Do not inject air into tubing or cap pilot balloon tubing while in patient. Air will flow in and out in response to pressure changes (head turning). Place tag on tubing, alerting staff not to cap or inflate cuff. • Deflate cuff daily via pilot balloon to evaluate integrity of cuff. Also assess ability to easily deflate cuff. Difficulty deflating cuff indicates a need for tube change. If aspirate returns with air, the cuff is no longer intact. • Tube can be used for up to 1 mo in patients on home mechanical ventilation. Good choice for patients who require inflated cuff at home because teaching about cuff pressure is simplified.

MLT, minimal leak technique.

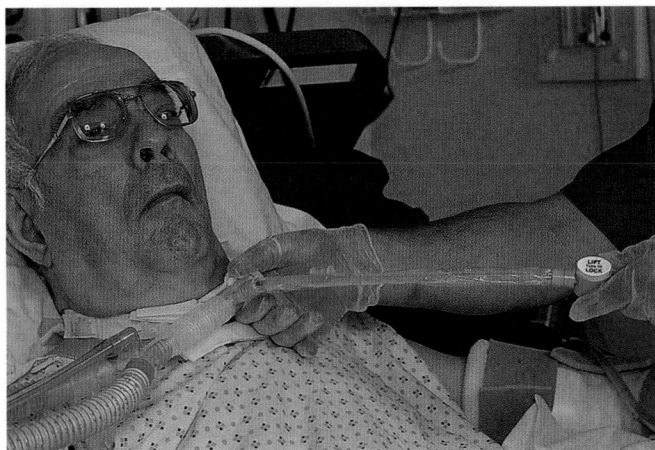

Figure 29-4 Suctioning tracheostomy with closed system suction catheter.

Source: Potter, P. A., Perry, A. G., Stockert, P. A., & Hall, A. (2011). *Basic nursing: Essentials for practice* (7th ed., p. 826, Step 4a). St. Louis: Mosby.

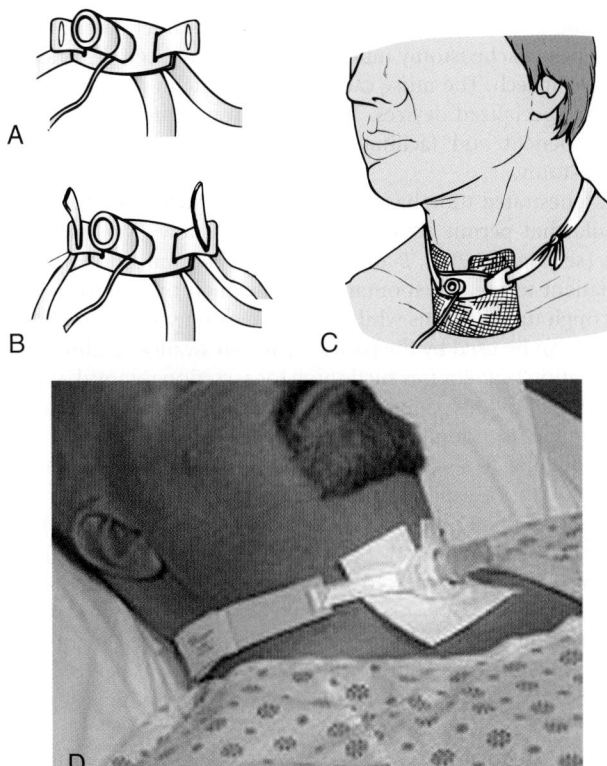

Figure 29-5 Changing tracheostomy ties. **A,** A slit is cut about 2.5 cm (1 in) from the end. The slit end is put into the opening of the faceplate. **B,** A loop is made with the other end of the tape. **C,** The tapes are tied together with a double knot on the side of the neck, avoiding any blood vessels. **D,** A tracheostomy tube holder can be used in place of twill ties to make tracheostomy tube stabilization more secure.

Source: **D,** Dale Medical Products, Inc.

Table 29-7 Procedure for Suctioning a Tracheostomy Tube

1. Assess the need for suctioning q2h. Indications include coarse crackles or wheezes over large airways, moist cough, and restlessness or agitation if accompanied by decrease in SpO_2 or PaO_2. Do not suction routinely or if patient is able to clear secretions with cough.

2. If suctioning is indicated, explain procedure to patient.

3. Collect necessary sterile equipment: suction catheter (no larger than half the lumen of the tracheostomy tube), gloves, water, cup, and drape. If a closed tracheal suction system is used, the catheter is enclosed in a plastic sleeve and reused. No additional equipment is needed.

4. Adjust suction pressure until the dial reads between 100 and 150 mm Hg pressure (for adults) with tubing occluded. For infants and children, the pressure should read between 50 and 100 mm Hg, depending upon the size of the child. (NOTE: The nurse should check the institution or agency's policy and procedure manuals for specific guidelines.)

5. Wash hands. Put on goggles and gloves.

6. Use sterile technique to open package, fill cup with water, put on gloves, and connect catheter to suction. Designate one hand as contaminated for disconnecting, bagging, and operating the suction control. Suction water through the catheter to test the system.

7. Assess SpO_2 and heart rate and rhythm to provide baseline for detecting change during suctioning.

8. Provide preoxygenation by using a reservoir-equipped MRB connected to 100% oxygen; or asking the patient to take three to four deep breaths while administering oxygen. The method chosen will depend on the patient's underlying disease and acuity of illness. The patient who has had a tracheostomy for an extended period and is not acutely ill may be able to tolerate suctioning without use of an MRB.

9. Gently insert catheter *without suction* to minimize the amount of oxygen removed from the lungs. Insert the catheter approximately 13 to 15 cm (5-6 inches). Stop if an obstruction is met.

10. Withdraw the catheter 1 to 2 cm (0.5-0.75 inches) and apply suction intermittently while withdrawing catheter in a rotating manner. If secretion volume is large, apply suction continuously.

11. *Limit suction time to 10 seconds.* Discontinue suctioning if heart rate decreases from baseline by 20 beats per minute, increases from baseline by 40 beats per minute, a dysrhythmia occurs, or SpO_2 decreases to less than 90%.

12. After each suction pass, oxygenate with three to four breaths by MRB, or deep breaths with oxygen.

13. Single-use catheters should not be reintroduced into the tracheostomy tube. (Check the institution's policy and procedure manuals.)

14. Repeat procedure until airway is clear. Limit insertions of suction catheter to as few as needed.

15. Return oxygen concentration to prior setting.

16. Suction the oropharynx or use mouth suction.

17. Dispose of catheter by wrapping it around fingers of gloved hand and pulling glove over catheter. Discard equipment in proper waste container.

18. Auscultate to assess changes in lung sounds. Record time, amount, and character of secretions and response to suctioning.

MRB, manual resuscitation bag.

Table 29-8 Tracheostomy Care

1. Explain procedure to patient.

2. Use tracheostomy care kit or collect necessary sterile equipment (e.g., suction catheter, gloves, water, basin, drape, tracheostomy ties, tube brush or pipe cleaners, 4 × 4s, normal saline or sterile water, and tracheostomy dressing [optional]). NOTE: Clean rather than sterile technique is used at home.

3. Position patient in semi-Fowler's position.

4. Assemble needed materials on bedside table next to patient.

5. Wash hands. Put on goggles and clean gloves.

6. Auscultate chest sounds. If wheezes or coarse crackles are present, suction the patient if unable to cough up secretions (see Table 29-7). Remove soiled dressing and clean gloves.

7. Open sterile equipment, pour sterile normal saline into basins, and put on sterile gloves.

8. Unlock and remove inner cannula, if present. Many tracheostomy tubes do not have inner cannulas. Care for these tubes includes all steps except for inner cannula care.

9. If disposable inner cannula is used, replace with new cannula. If a nondisposable cannula is used, the following applies:

   a. Immerse inner cannula in sterile normal saline, and clean inside and outside of cannula using tube brush or pipe cleaners.
   b. Rinse in normal saline. Shake to dry.
   c. Insert inner cannula into outer cannula with the curved part downward and lock in place.

10. Remove dried secretions from stoma, outer cannula, and neck plate, using 4 × 4 soaked in normal saline. Gently pat area around the stoma dry.

11. Maintain position of tracheal retention sutures, if present, by taping above and below the stoma.

12. Change tracheostomy ties. Secure new ties to flanges before removing the old ones. Tie tracheostomy ties securely with room for one finger between ties and skin (see Figure 29-5). To prevent accidental tube removal, secure the tracheostomy tube by gently applying pressure to the flange of the tube during the tie changes. *Do not change tracheostomy ties for first 72 hours after the tracheotomy procedure.*

13. As an alternative, some patients prefer tracheostomy ties made of Velcro, which are easier to adjust.

14. If drainage is excessive, place dressing around tube (see Figure 29-5). A tracheostomy dressing or unlined gauze should be used. Do not cut the gauze because threads may be inhaled or wrap around the tracheostomy tube. Change the dressing frequently. Wet dressings promote infection and stoma irritation.

15. Repeat care three times a day and as needed.

for insertion. The tracheostomy tube should be threaded over the catheter and the suction catheter removed. If the tube cannot be replaced, assess the level of respiratory distress. Minor dyspnea may be alleviated by use of semi-Fowler's position until assistance arrives. Severe dyspnea may progress to respiratory arrest. If this situation occurs, the stoma should be covered with a sterile dressing, and the patient should be ventilated with bag–mask ventilation until help arrives.

After the first tube change, the tube should be changed approximately once a month. When a tracheostomy has been in place for several months, the healed tract will be well formed.

The patient can then be taught to change the tube using a clean technique at home. Teaching will vary depending on how ill the patient is and what device has been selected.

Swallowing Dysfunction

The patient who cannot protect the airway from aspiration requires an inflated cuff. However, an inflated cuff may promote swallowing dysfunction because the cuff interferes with the normal function of muscles used to swallow. For this reason, it is important to evaluate the risk for aspiration with the cuff deflated. The patient may be able to swallow without aspirating when the cuff is deflated but not when it is inflated. The cuff may then be left deflated or a cuffless tube substituted (Figure 29-6).

Speech with a Tracheostomy Tube

A number of techniques promote speech in the patient with a tracheostomy. The spontaneously breathing patient may be able to talk by deflating the cuff, which allows exhaled air to flow upward over the vocal cords. This can be enhanced by the patient occluding the tube with a finger or plug. Frequently, a small cuffless tube is inserted so exhaled air can pass freely around the tube. These tracheostomy tubes and valves have been designed to facilitate speech. The nurse can be an advocate in promoting use of these specialized devices. Their use can provide great psychological benefit and facilitate self-care for the patient with a tracheostomy.

A fenestrated tube has openings on the surface of the outer cannula that permit air from the lungs to flow over the vocal cords (see Figures 29-3, *B* and 29-6, *A*). A fenestrated tube allows the patient to breathe spontaneously through the larynx, speak, and cough up secretions while the tracheostomy tube remains in place. It can be used by the patient who can swallow without risk of aspiration but requires suctioning for secretion removal. It may also be used by the patient who requires mechanical ventilation for less than 24 hours a day (e.g., during sleep).

Before the fenestrated tube is used, the patient's ability to swallow without aspiration is determined (see Table 29-5 and Nursing Care Plan [NCP] 29-1). If there is no aspiration, (1) the inner cannula is removed, (2) the cuff is deflated, and (3) the decannulation cap is placed in the tube (see Figure. 29-6, *A*). It is important to perform the steps in order because severe respiratory distress may result if the tube is capped before the inner cannula is removed and the cuff deflated. When a fenestrated cannula is first used, the nurse should frequently assess the patient for signs of respiratory distress.

If the patient is not able to tolerate the procedure, the cap should be removed, the inner cannula replaced, and the cuff reinflated. A disadvantage of fenestrated tubes is the potential for development of tracheal polyps from tracheal tissue granulating into the fenestrated openings (Skillings & Curtis, 2011).

A speaking tracheostomy tube has two pigtail tubings. One tubing connects to the cuff and is used for cuff inflation, and the second connects to an opening just above the cuff (see Figure 29-6, *B*). When the second tubing is connected to a low-flow (4-6 L/min) air source, sufficient air moves up over the vocal cords to permit speech. The patient can then speak, although the cuff is inflated.

When a speaking tracheostomy valve is used, a cuffless tube must be in place or the cuff deflated to allow exhalation

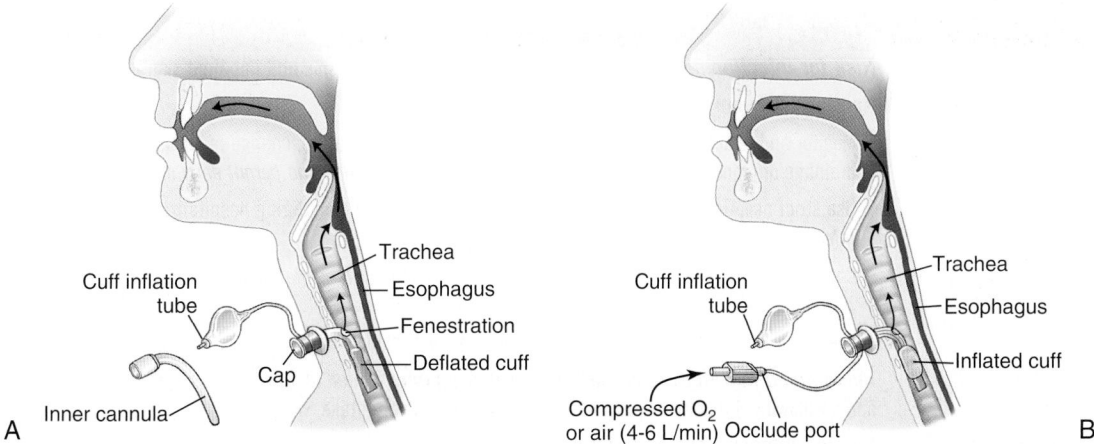

Figure 29-6 Speaking tracheostomy tubes. **A,** Fenestrated tracheostomy tube with cuff deflated, inner cannula removed, and tracheostomy tube capped to allow air to pass over the vocal cords. **B,** Speaking tracheostomy tube. One tube is used for cuff inflation. The second tube is connected to a source of compressed air or oxygen. When the port on the second tube is occluded, air flows up over the vocal cords, allowing speech with an inflated cuff. (See Table 29-5 and NCP 29-1 for related nursing management.)

NURSING CARE PLAN 29-1

Tracheostomy

NURSING DIAGNOSIS	**Ineffective airway clearance** *related to* presence of tracheostomy tube and difficulty expectorating sputum *as evidenced by* adventitious breath sounds, tenacious secretions, increase in restlessness, and ineffective or absent cough
Expected Patient Outcomes	**Nursing Interventions and *Rationales***
• Maintains patent airway • Expectorates secretions without need to suction airway • Has clear lung sounds • Has normal SpO_2	• Assess for respiratory distress (e.g., abnormal breath sounds, dyspnea, SpO_2 <90%) to determine need for interventions. • Clear secretions by encouraging coughing or by suctioning to clear airway. • Keep head of bed elevated 30 to 40 degrees to allow a more forceful cough and to relieve dyspnea. • Provide humidification and hydration to liquefy secretions. • Encourage coughing, deep breathing, and ambulation to assist in mobilizing secretions. • Clean and/or change inner cannula, if present, as per agency policy to minimize buildup of secretions on inside lumen of cannula. • Maintain minimum cuff pressure while obtaining airway seal by measuring with manometer at no more than 25 cm H_2O pressure or with MLT to minimize pressure on trachea. MLT cannot be used if tracheostomy is to bypass upper airway obstruction such as with head and neck surgery. • If cuff is to be deflated, deflate during exhalation and reinflate during inhalation. Clear mouth and trachea before and after deflation by coughing or suctioning to minimize aspiration. • Keep tracheostomy tube tied securely, allowing room for one finger between ties and skin, to secure tube from dislodging. • Secure a second tracheostomy tube (same size) and hemostat to the head of the bed to maintain airway in case of accidental decannulation.
NURSING DIAGNOSIS	**Impaired verbal communication** *related to* use of artificial airway and cuff *as evidenced by* inability to speak and signs of frustration
Expected Patient Outcomes	**Nursing Interventions and *Rationales***
• Communicates needs	• Provide call bell within easy reach and respond immediately, in person, *to allay anxiety.* • Assess patient's ability to read and write; provide with magic slate, pad and pencil, communication board with illustrations of requests, electrolarynx (Cooper-Rand) *as alternative means of communication.* • Reassure patient that speech will return when tube can be removed (if total laryngectomy has not been performed) *to allay fear that situation is permanent.* • Suggest use of speaking tubes (small, cuffless tube, fenestrated tube, speaking valve, speaking tracheostomy tube) *to permit speech.* • Encourage gesturing *to communicate needs and desires.*

Continued

NURSING CARE PLAN 29-1

Tracheostomy—cont'd

NURSING DIAGNOSIS	*Risk for infection* related to bypass of airway defence mechanisms and impaired skin integrity
Expected Patient Outcomes	**Nursing Interventions and *Rationales***
• Maintains normal white blood cell count • Has normal temperature • Has clear mucus • Has no erythema or purulent secretions from stoma site	• Monitor and report elevated white blood cell count and temperature, change in colour of secretions, purulent drainage or redness around the site *to identify signs of infection and permit early medical intervention.* • Use strict aseptic technique for suctioning and tracheostomy care during hospitalization *to reduce occurrence of infection.* • Change oxygen-delivery equipment per agency policy *to prevent contaminated tubing from being a source of infection.* • Keep stoma clean and dry, and perform frequent tracheostomy care *to reduce risk of infection.*
NURSING DIAGNOSIS	*Imbalanced nutrition: less than body requirements* related to decreased oral intake, altered taste sensation, and swallowing difficulty *as evidenced by* inadequate caloric intake, weight loss
Expected Patient Outcomes	**Nursing Interventions and *Rationales***
• Reports usual appetite • Maintains or progresses toward normal body weight	• Provide ongoing assessment of oral intake and caloric count *to assess adequacy of diet.* • Monitor weight *to provide information for evaluation.* • Provide high-calorie, high-protein food and beverages *to maximize nutritional intake.* • Thicken foods and beverages if needed *to ease swallowing and minimize aspiration.* • Assess for swallowing dysfunction *to determine if presence of inflated cuff is predisposing to aspiration.* • Assess oral mucosa, lips, and tongue q4h; perform mouth care q2-4h and PRN *to promote patient comfort and appetite.*
NURSING DIAGNOSIS	*Impaired swallowing* related to tracheostomy tube *as evidenced by* inability to swallow without difficulty and/or without aspiration
Expected Patient Outcomes	**Nursing Interventions and *Rationales***
• Swallows normally • Experiences no aspiration	• Assess swallow and gag reflexes by deflating cuff; note coughing *because it is an indicator of aspiration.* • A formal swallowing evaluation may be done by a speech pathologist or radiologist to assess for aspiration.
NURSING DIAGNOSIS	*Ineffective therapeutic regimen management* related to lack of knowledge about care of tracheostomy at home *as evidenced by* questioning about care (patient or family or both), agitation, and restlessness when planning for discharge
Expected Patient Outcomes	**Nursing Interventions and *Rationales***
• Demonstrates techniques by patient and significant others for tracheostomy care • Verbalizes expected outcomes and when to contact health care providers if problems arise	• Assess ability of patient and significant other to provide care at home, including tracheostomy tube care, stoma care, airway care, and ability to respond appropriately to emergencies, *to determine if home care is feasible.* • Teach good handwashing technique *to minimize risk for infection.* • Teach clean tracheostomy tube care and home preparation of sterile saline solution *so patient can care for self at home.* • Teach clean suctioning, if needed, *so patient can care for self at home.* • Teach patient and significant other the signs and symptoms to report to health care providers such as changes in secretions (yellow, green, or blood-tinged) or elevated temperature (or both) *because these may be early signs of respiratory infection.* • Make referral of patient to home health nurse *to provide ongoing assistance and support.*
NURSING DIAGNOSIS	*Risk for hypoxemia* related to misplaced or improperly functioning tube, accumulated secretions
Nursing Goals	**Nursing Interventions and *Rationales***

• Monitor for signs of hypoxemia
 • Carry out appropriate medical and nursing interventions
	• Assess patient for restlessness, agitation, confusion, tachycardia, bradycardia, dysrhythmias, or SpO₂ less than 90% *to detect presence of hypoxemia.*
	 • Elevate head of bed if tolerated *to maximize lung expansion and effective cough.*
	 • Auscultate chest *to determine need for suctioning.* If coarse crackles or wheezes are present and patient cannot cough and clear secretions, suction airway.
	 • If unable to pass suction catheter, tube is dislodged and emergency measures must be implemented.
	 • Monitor tube and inner cannula placement *to ensure proper positioning.*
	 • If tube is dislodged or misplaced:
	     • Assess the level of respiratory distress to determine whether patient can breathe without tube for a short interval.
	     • Grasp the retention sutures (if present) or hemostat and spread opening.
	     • Notify physician. If distress is severe, ventilate with bag–mask until assistance arrives to ensure adequate ventilation.

MLT, minimal leak technique; *PRN,* as needed.

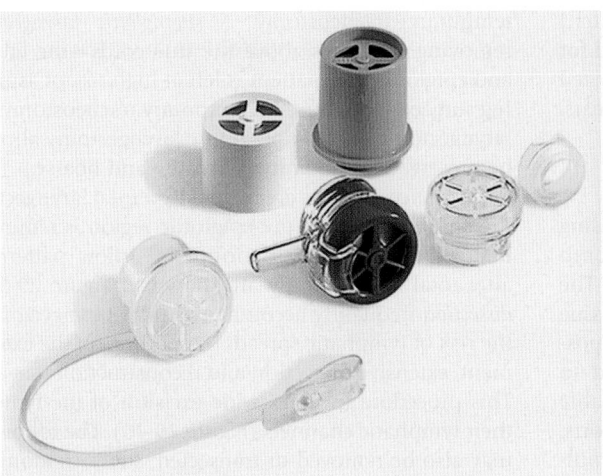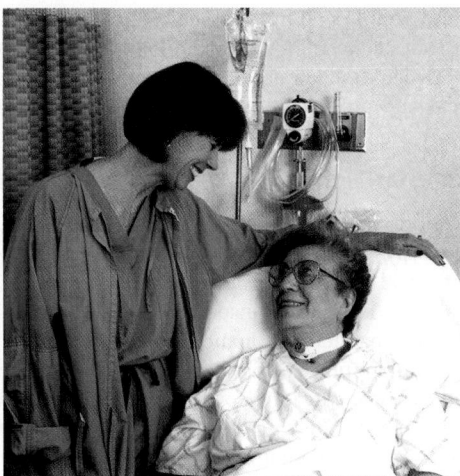

Figure 29-7 Passy-Muir speaking tracheostomy valve. The valve is placed over the hub of the tracheostomy tube after the cuff is deflated. Multiple options are available and can be used for ventilated and nonventilated patients. The valve contains a one-way valve that allows air to enter the lungs during inspiration and redirects air upward over the vocal cords into the mouth during expiration.

Source: Passy-Muir, Inc., Irvine, California.

(Figure 29-7). Ability to tolerate cuff deflation without aspiration or respiratory distress must also be evaluated in patients using this device. If there is no aspiration, the cuff is deflated and the valve is placed over the tracheostomy tube opening. The speaking valve contains a thin plastic diaphragm that opens on inspiration and closes on expiration. During inspiration, air flows in through the valve. During expiration, the diaphragm prevents exhalation and air flows upward over the vocal cords and into the mouth.

If speaking devices are not used, the patient should be provided with a paper and pencil or magic slate. A word (communication) board can usually be obtained from speech therapy, or one can be devised with pictures of common needs and an alphabet for spelling words.

◾ Decannulation

When the patient can adequately exchange air and expectorate secretions, the tracheostomy tube can be removed. The stoma is closed with tape strips and covered with an occlusive dressing. The dressing must be changed if it gets soiled or wet. The patient should be instructed to splint the stoma with the fingers when coughing, swallowing, or speaking. Epithelial tissue begins to form in 24 to 48 hours, and the opening will close in several days. Surgical intervention to close the tracheostomy is not required (Skillings & Curtis, 2011).

Laryngeal Polyps

Laryngeal polyps may develop on the vocal cords from vocal abuse (e.g., excessive talking, singing) or irritation (e.g., intubation, cigarette smoking). The most common symptom is hoarseness. Polyps may be treated conservatively with voice rest. Surgical removal may be indicated for large polyps, which may cause dyspnea and stridor. Polyps are usually benign but may be removed because they may later become malignant.

Head and Neck Cancer

Head and neck cancer arises from mucosal surfaces and is typically squamous cell in origin. This category of tumours includes those of the paranasal sinuses, the oral cavity, and the nasopharynx, oropharynx, and larynx. (Cancer of the oral cavity is discussed in Chapter 44.) It was estimated that there would be 3600 new cases of oral cancer in Canada in 2011, with a steady decline in new cases over the past 20 years attributed to a decline in smoking. It was also estimated that there would be 1150 deaths from oral cancer and 490 from cancer of the larynx. Males tend to be affected two to five times more than females (Canadian Cancer Society Steering Committee on Cancer Statistics, 2011). Although this type of cancer is not common, disability is great because of the potential loss of voice, disfigurement, and social consequences. Most (90%) head and neck cancers occur in individuals 50 years or older after prolonged use of tobacco and alcohol.

Clinical Manifestations

Early signs and symptoms of head and neck cancer vary with the tumour location. Cancer of the oral cavity may first be signalled by a painless growth in the mouth, an ulcer that does not heal, or a change in fit of dentures. Pain is a late symptom that may be aggravated by acidic food. Cancers of the oropharynx, hypopharynx, and supraglottic larynx rarely produce early symptoms and are usually diagnosed in late stages. The patient may complain of persistent unilateral sore throat or otalgia (ear pain). Hoarseness may be a symptom of early laryngeal cancer. If a lump in the neck or hoarseness lasts longer than 2 weeks, a medical evaluation is indicated. Some patients experience what feels like a lump in the throat or a change in voice quality.

Late stages of head and neck cancers have easily detectable signs and symptoms, including pain, dysphagia, decreased mobility of the tongue, airway obstruction, and cranial nerve neuropathies. The nurse should thoroughly examine the oral cavity, including the areas under the tongue and the dentures. The floor of the mouth, the tongue, and the lymph nodes in the neck should be bimanually palpated. There may be thickening of the normally soft and pliable oral mucosa. *Leukoplakia* (white patch) or *erythroplakia* (red patch) may be seen and should be noted for later biopsy. Both leukoplakia and carcinoma in situ (localized to a defined area) may precede invasive carcinoma by many years.

Diagnostic Studies

If lesions are suspected, the upper airways may be examined using indirect laryngoscopy, which involves using a laryngeal mirror to visualize the laryngeal area, or a flexible nasopharyngoscope. The larynx and vocal cords are visually inspected for lesions and tissue mobility. A CT scan, magnetic resonance imaging (MRI), or positron emission tomography (PET) scan may be performed to detect local and regional spread. Neoplastic tissue is identifiable because it contains tissue of greater density or because it distorts, displaces, or destroys normal anatomic structures. Typically, multiple biopsy specimens are obtained to determine the extent of the disease (Goldman & Ausiello, 2007).

Collaborative Care

The stage of the disease will be determined based on tumour size (T), number and location of involved nodes (N), and extent of metastasis (M). TNM staging classifies disease over the range between stage I through stage IV and guides treatment. Choice of treatment is based on medical history, extent of disease, cosmetic considerations, urgency of treatment, and patient choice. Approximately one third of patients with head and neck cancers have highly confined lesions that are stage I or II at diagnosis. Such patients can undergo radiation therapy or surgery with the goal of cure.

Radiation therapy may be effective in curing early vocal cord lesions. This therapy is usually successful in eliminating the tumour while preserving the quality of the voice. If radiation therapy is not successful or the lesion is too advanced for this therapy, surgery may be performed. A *cordectomy* (partial removal of one vocal cord) is used when there is a superficial tumour involving one cord (Figure 29-8). A *hemilaryngectomy* involves removal of one vocal cord or part of a cord and necessitates a temporary tracheostomy. A *supraglottic laryngectomy* involves removing structures above the true cords—the false vocal cords and epiglottis. The patient is left at high risk of aspiration following surgery and requires a temporary tracheostomy. Both a hemilaryngectomy and a supraglottic laryngectomy allow the voice to be preserved, but quality is breathy and hoarse.

Advanced lesions are treated by a total laryngectomy in which the entire larynx and pre-epiglottic region is removed and a permanent tracheostomy performed. Airflow patterns before and after total laryngectomy are shown in Figure 29-9. *Radical neck dissection* frequently accompanies total laryngectomy to decrease the risk of lymphatic spread. Depending on the extent of involvement, extensive dissection and reconstruction may be performed. This procedure involves wide excision of the lymph nodes and their lymphatic channels (Figure 29-10). The following structures may also be removed or transected: sternocleidomastoid muscle and other closely associated muscles, internal jugular vein, mandible, submaxillary gland, part of the thyroid and parathyroid glands, and the spinal accessory nerve.

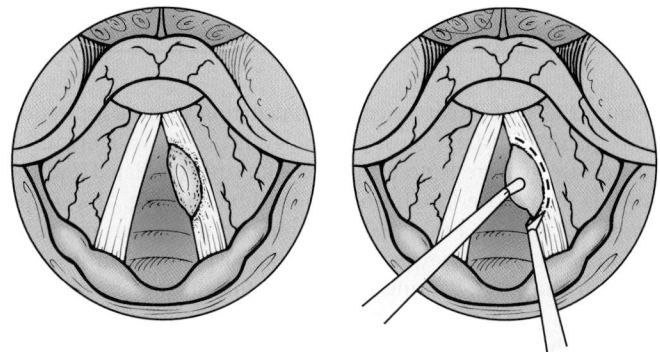

Figure 29-8 Excision of laryngeal cancer. This cancer of the right vocal cord meets criteria for resection by transoral cordectomy. The cord is fully mobile and the lesion can be fully exposed. It does not approach or cross the anterior commissure.

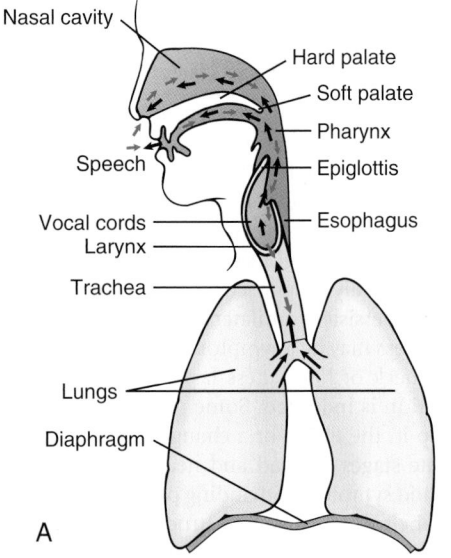

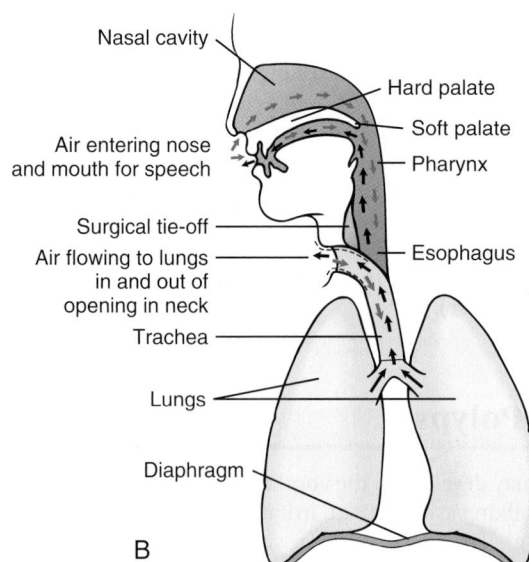

Figure 29-9 A, Normal airflow in and out of the lungs. **B,** Airflow in and out of the lungs after total laryngectomy. Patients using esophageal speech trap air in the esophagus and release it to create sound.

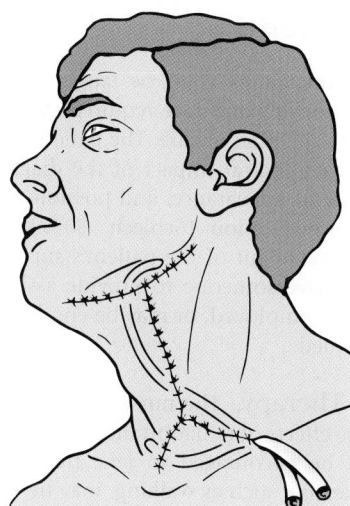

Figure 29-10 Radical neck incision with drains in place.

Table 29-9 Steps for Performing the Supraglottic Swallow

1. Take a deep breath to aerate lungs.
2. Perform Valsalva's manoeuvre to approximate cords.
3. Place food in mouth and swallow. Some food will enter airway and remain on top of closed vocal cords.
4. Cough to remove food from top of vocal cords.
5. Swallow so food is moved from top of vocal cords.
6. Breathe after cough–swallow sequence to prevent aspiration of food collected on top of vocal cords.

A *modified neck dissection* is performed whenever possible as an alternative to a radical neck dissection. The dissection is modified by sparing as many structures as possible to limit disfigurement and functional loss. A modified neck dissection usually involves dissection of the major cervical lymphatic vessels and lateral cervical space with preservation of nerves and vessels, including the sympathetic and vagus nerves, spinal accessory nerves, and internal jugular vein. Neck dissection with vocal cord cancer usually involves one side of the neck. However, if the lesion is midline, a bilateral neck dissection may be performed. When a bilateral neck dissection is performed, it is always modified on at least one side to minimize structural and functional deficits (Rothrock, 2011).

The patient may refuse surgical intervention for advanced lesions because of the extent of the procedure or may be judged to be at too great a medical risk to undergo the procedure. In this situation, external radiation therapy may be used as the sole treatment or in combination with chemotherapy (Rothrock, 2011).

In addition, brachytherapy, a concentrated and localized method of delivering radiation that involves placing a radioactive source into or near the tumour, may be used to treat head and neck cancer. The goal is to deliver high doses of radiation to the target area while limiting exposure of surrounding tissues. Thin, hollow, plastic needles are inserted into the tumour area, and radioactive iridium seeds are placed in the needles. The seeds emit continuous radiation. Brachytherapy can be used alone or combined with external radiation or surgical intervention. (Radiation therapy and brachytherapy are discussed in Chapter 18.)

Nutritional Therapy. After radical neck surgery, the patient may be unable to take in nutrients through the normal route of ingestion because of swelling, the location of sutures, or difficulty with swallowing. Parenteral fluids will be given for the first 24 to 48 hours. Tube feedings are usually given via a nasogastric, nasointestinal, or gastrostomy tube that was placed during surgery. (Nasogastric and gastrostomy feedings are described in Chapter 42.) The nurse must observe for tolerance of the feedings and adjust amount, time, and formula if nausea, vomiting, diarrhea, or distension occurs. The patient is instructed about the tube feedings. When the patient can swallow, small amounts of water are given. Close observation for difficulty swallowing is essential. Suctioning may be necessary to prevent aspiration.

Swallowing problems should be anticipated when the patient resumes eating. The type and degree of difficulty vary, depending on the surgical procedure. When a supraglottic laryngectomy is performed, the surgeon excises the upper portion of the larynx, including the epiglottis and the false vocal cords. The patient can speak because the true vocal cords remain intact. However, a new technique, the supraglottic swallow, must be learned to compensate for removal of the epiglottis and minimize risk of aspiration (Table 29-9). When learning this technique, it may be helpful to start with carbonated beverages because the effervescence provides cues about the liquid's position. With this exception, thin, watery fluids should be avoided because they are difficult to swallow and increase the risk of aspiration. A better choice is nonpourable pureed foods, which are thicker and allow more control during swallowing. Swallowing can be enhanced by thickening liquids through the use of a commercially available thickening agent.

Good nutrition is important during radiation therapy because calories and protein are needed for tissue repair. Antiemetics or analgesics may be given before meals to reduce nausea and mouth pain. Bland foods may be better tolerated. Caloric intake may be increased by adding dry milk to foods during preparation, selecting foods high in calories, and using oral supplements. It is helpful to add sauces and gravies to food, which adds calories and moistens food so it is more easily swallowed. If an adequate intake cannot be maintained, enteral feedings may be used. The patient should always be in a position with the head elevated when eating.

NURSING MANAGEMENT: HEAD AND NECK CANCER

Nursing Assessment

Subjective and objective data that should be obtained from a person with head and neck cancer are presented in Table 29-10.

Nursing Diagnoses

Nursing diagnoses for the patient with head and neck cancer include, but are not limited to, those presented in NCP 29-2.

Planning

The overall goals are that the patient will have (1) a patent airway, (2) no spread of cancer, (3) no complications related to therapy, (4) adequate nutritional intake, (5) minimal to no pain, (6) the ability to communicate, and (7) an acceptable body image.

▪ Nursing Implementation

▪ Health Promotion

Development of head and neck cancer is closely related to personal habits, primarily tobacco use, including the use of cigarettes, cigars, chewing tobacco, and snuff. Prolonged alcohol use has been implicated as a potentiating factor in head and neck cancer. Excessive sun exposure to the lips also increases the risk of oral cancer.

The nurse should include information about risk factors in health teaching. If cancer has been diagnosed, tobacco cessation is still important. The patient with head and neck cancer who continues to smoke during radiation therapy has a lower rate of response and survival than the patient who does not smoke during radiation therapy. In addition, risk of a second primary cancer is significantly increased in patients who continue to smoke.

▪ Acute Intervention

The patient and the family must be taught about the type of therapy to be performed and care required. Assessment of concerns is integral to the plan of care. The patient and family must deal with the psychological impact of the diagnosis of cancer, alteration of physical appearance, and possible need for altered methods of communication (Schiech, 2007). The care plan should include assessment of the patient's support system. The patient may not have someone to provide assistance after discharge, may not be employed, or may be employed in a job that cannot be continued.

▪ **Radiation Therapy.** The nurse can suggest interventions to reduce adverse effects of radiation therapy. Fatigue is common. Patients should be encouraged to take frequent rest periods. Light, regular exercise, such as walking, may be helpful.

NURSING ASSESSMENT

Table 29-10 Head and Neck Cancer

Subjective Data	Objective Data
Important Health Information	**Respiratory**
Past health history: Positive family history; prolonged tobacco use (cigarettes, pipes, cigars, chewing tobacco, smokeless tobacco); prolonged, heavy alcohol use	Hoarseness, chronic laryngitis, nasal voice, palpable neck mass and lymph nodes (tender, hard, fixed), tracheal deviation; dyspnea, stridor (late sign)
Medications: Prolonged use of over-the-counter medication for sore throat, decongestants	**Gastrointestinal**
Symptoms	White (leukoplakia) or red (erythroplakia) patches inside mouth, ulceration of mucosa, asymmetrical tongue, exudate in mouth or pharynx, mass or thickening of mucosa
Mouth ulcer that does not heal, change in fit of dentures, change in appetite, weight loss, swallowing difficulty (e.g., sensation of lump in throat, pain with swallowing, aspiration when swallowing)	**Possible Findings**
Fatigue with minimal exertion	Mass on direct or indirect laryngoscopy; tumour on soft tissue radiographic study, computed tomography scan, magnetic resonance imaging, or positron emission tomography; positive biopsy
Sore throat, hoarseness, change in voice quality, referred ear pain	

NURSING CARE PLAN 29-2

Total Laryngectomy and/or Radical Neck Surgery*

NURSING DIAGNOSIS	*Anxiety related to* lack of knowledge regarding surgical procedure, pain management, and prevention of complications *as evidenced by* questioning about impending surgery, postoperative care, agitation, and restlessness
Expected Patient Outcomes	**Nursing Interventions and *Rationales***
• Reports reduced anxiety and maintains a calm appearance • Verbalizes confidence regarding surgical therapy	• Assess knowledge desired by patient *to allay fears and answer questions.* • Facilitate discussion of expected alterations in physical appearance and function; encourage sharing of feelings and concerns *to begin adjustment and acceptance.* • Provide information about what to expect after surgery (tracheostomy tube, stoma, incisions, alternative communication methods, nasogastric tube, drainage tubes, pain management) *to reduce patient's sense of helplessness and increase sense of control.*
NURSING DIAGNOSIS	*Ineffective tissue perfusion related to* tissue edema and disruption of blood flow and lymphatic drainage *as evidenced by* tissue swelling and serous drainage from wound drainage tubes
Expected Patient Outcomes	**Nursing Interventions and *Rationales***
• Has decreased tissue edema • Has minimal to no drainage from tubes • Displays healing of incision lines	• Maintain head of bed at 30 to 40 degrees *to decrease tissue edema.* • Monitor heart rate, blood pressure, hemoglobin, and hematocrit *to detect excessive bleeding.* • Monitor patency of drainage tubes and amount and colour of drainage *to determine if drainage is excessive.* • Clean incision as prescribed *to prevent infection.*

NURSING CARE PLAN 29-2

Total Laryngectomy and/or Radical Neck Surgery—cont'd

NURSING DIAGNOSIS	*Imbalanced nutrition: less than body requirements* related to surgical procedure, edema, and dysphagia as evidenced by absence of or inadequate oral intake
Expected Patient Outcomes	**Nursing Interventions and *Rationales***
• Maintains normal oral intake • Swallows normally • Maintains body weight	• Provide frequent oral hygiene with saline rinses *to promote comfort and remove drainage.* • Administer tube feedings as ordered *to provide adequate nutrients while wound heals.* • When oral feedings begin, give clear liquids and advance as tolerated *to allow patient time to adjust to initiation of oral intake.* • Monitor caloric intake and weight *to evaluate response.*
NURSING DIAGNOSIS	*Disturbed body image* related to disfiguring surgery and loss of speaking ability as evidenced by withdrawal, depression, isolation, unwillingness to look at self or assist with care, and refusal to see visitors
Expected Patient Outcomes	**Nursing Interventions and *Rationales***
• Acknowledges changes in body image • Communicates feelings about surgical changes • Participates in self-care	• Assess patient's body image *to identify patients at high risk for impaired adjustment.* • Provide privacy *to respect patient's request while adjusting to change in body function and appearance.* • Encourage attention to personal hygiene *because improved appearance can boost self-esteem.* • Encourage socialization with family and friends *because acceptance by significant others is a critical factor in patient's own acceptance.* • Provide information about measures to help improve appearance such as wearing clothes with high collars and wearing accessories *to aid in successful adjustment.* • Answer questions honestly about changes in body image *to convey acceptance and to provide accurate information.* • Involve patient in self-care *because participation in self-care is a sign of successful adjustment.* • Assure patient of self-worth *to increase acceptance of altered physical appearance.*
NURSING DIAGNOSIS	*Acute pain* related to surgical procedure as evidenced by report of discomfort; facial mask of pain; changes in blood pressure, pulse, and respiratory rate
Expected Patient Outcomes	**Nursing Interventions and *Rationales***
• Reports satisfactory pain control	• Assess patient's manifestations of pain (e.g., verbalization and description of pain, facial expression, reluctance to cough or move) *to plan appropriate interventions.* • Administer pain medication as prescribed, and assess response *to determine if it is effective.* • Teach use of nonpharmacological techniques to control pain (e.g., relaxation, distraction, massage therapy) *to manage pain.* • Keep head of bed elevated 30 to 40 degrees *to prevent edema.*
NURSING DIAGNOSIS	*Ineffective therapeutic regimen management* related to lack of knowledge about home care after discharge as evidenced by verbalized concern about ability to manage self-care at home.
Nursing Goals	**Nursing Interventions and *Rationales***
• Demonstrates steps to be used in carrying out self-care	• Provide written instructions for patient and family *because an accurate reference reduces error.* • Teach patient and family about laryngectomy tube and stoma care, allowing them to perform care repeatedly in hospital, *to ensure correct performance of technique.* • Teach patient to cover stoma before performing activities such as shaving, application of makeup *to avoid inhalation of foreign materials.* • Teach patient to report changes, such as stoma narrowing, difficulty swallowing, lump in the throat *to detect possible recurrence of tumour or tracheal stenosis.* • Teach patient to provide adequate humidity at home using a bedside humidifier or sitting in a steamy bathroom. • Teach patient to report changes in mucus production such as colour changes (yellow or green) or blood-tinged secretions *because these may be signs of infection or tracheal irritation.* • Make referral for home health care visit *to evaluate self-care.*

*Also see NCP 29-1: Tracheostomy.

Dry mouth (xerostomia), the most frequent and annoying problem, typically begins within a few weeks of treatment. The patient's saliva decreases in volume and becomes thick. The change may be temporary or permanent. Pilocarpine hydrochloride (Salagen) can be effective in increasing saliva production and should be started before the initiation of radiation therapy and continued for 90 days. Symptom relief can also be obtained by increasing fluid intake, chewing sugarless gum or eating sugarless candy, using nonalcoholic mouth rinses (baking soda or glycerin solutions), and using artificial saliva.

The patient may also complain of stomatitis, especially if the oral cavity is in the field of therapy. Irritation, ulceration, and pain are common complaints. Normal saline mouth rinses after meals and at bedtime can be used to clean and soothe irritated tissues. Commercial mouthwashes and hot or spicy foods should be avoided because they are irritating. If the problem is severe, a mouthwash mixture of equal parts of antacid, diphenhydramine (Benadryl), and topical lidocaine can be used.

Skin over the irradiated area often becomes reddened and sensitive to touch. It is common for patients to require a break from their scheduled radiation program because of altered skin integrity. Only prescribed lotions and products should be used during radiation therapy. All exposure to the sun should be avoided to reduce discomfort.

Surgical Therapy. Preoperative care for the patient who is to have a radical neck dissection involves consideration of the patient's physical and psychosocial needs. Physical preparation is the same as for any major surgery, with special emphasis on oral hygiene. Explanations and emotional support are of special significance and should include postoperative measures relating to communication and feeding. The surgical procedure should be explained to the patient and family or caregivers, and the nurse should make sure that the information is understood.

Teaching must be tailored to the planned surgical procedure. For surgeries that involve a laryngectomy, teaching should include information about expected changes in speech. The nurse or speech pathologist should demonstrate means of communicating other than speaking that can be used temporarily or permanently. This may include some type of communication board.

After surgery, maintenance of a patent airway is essential. The inflammation in the surgical area may compress the trachea. A tracheostomy tube will be in place. The patient will be placed in a semi-Fowler position to decrease edema and limit tension on the suture lines. Vital signs should be monitored frequently because of the risk of hemorrhage and respiratory compromise. Pressure dressings, packing, or drainage tubes (Hemovac, Jackson Pratt) may be used for wound management, depending on the type of surgical procedure. When a radical neck dissection is performed, wound suction using a portable system, such as a Hemovac, is generally used. If skin flaps are employed, dressings are typically not used. This allows better visualization of the incision and helps prevent excessive pressure on tissue (see Figure 29-10). The drainage should be serosanguineous and gradually decrease in volume over 24 hours. Patency of drainage tubes should be monitored every 4 hours to ensure that they are properly removing serous drainage and for the amount and character of drainage. If the tubing becomes obstructed, fluid will accumulate under the skin flap and predispose to impaired wound healing and infection. After drainage tubes are removed, the area should be closely monitored for any swelling. If fluid continues to accumulate, aspiration may be necessary.

Immediately after surgery, the patient with a laryngectomy requires frequent suctioning via the laryngectomy tube. Secre-

tions typically change in amount and consistency over time. The patient may initially have copious blood-tinged secretions that diminish and thicken. Administering saline boluses via the tracheostomy tube to loosen secretions is no longer recommended (Regan & Dallachiesa, 2009). The patient will benefit from the use of a humidifier while hospitalized and at home.

Following a neck dissection, an exercise program should be instituted to maintain strength and movement in the affected shoulder and neck. This is especially important when the spinal accessory nerve and the sternocleidomastoid muscles are removed or damaged. Without exercise, the patient will be left with a "frozen" shoulder and limited range of neck motion. This exercise program should be continued following discharge to prevent future functional disabilities. The patient may need the neck supported to be able to move the head after surgery.

Voice Rehabilitation. A speech therapist should meet with the patient following a total laryngectomy to discuss voice restoration options. The International Association of Laryngectomees, an association of laryngectomy patients, focuses on assisting patients to re-establish speech. Local groups called Lost Cord Clubs often provide member volunteers to visit the patient, preferably before surgery. Several options are available to restore speech. These include use of a voice prosthesis, esophageal speech, and an electrolarynx.

The most commonly used voice prosthesis is the Blom-Singer (Figure 29-11). This soft plastic device is inserted into a fistula made between the esophagus and the trachea. The puncture may be created at the time of surgery or afterward, depending on the preference of the surgeon. A red rubber catheter is placed in the tracheoesophageal puncture and must remain intact until a tract is formed. Once the tract is formed, the voice prosthesis is inserted. This prosthesis allows air from the lungs to enter the esophagus by way of the tracheal stoma. A one-way valve prevents aspiration of food or saliva from the esophagus into the tracheostomy. To produce the voice, the patient manually blocks the stoma with

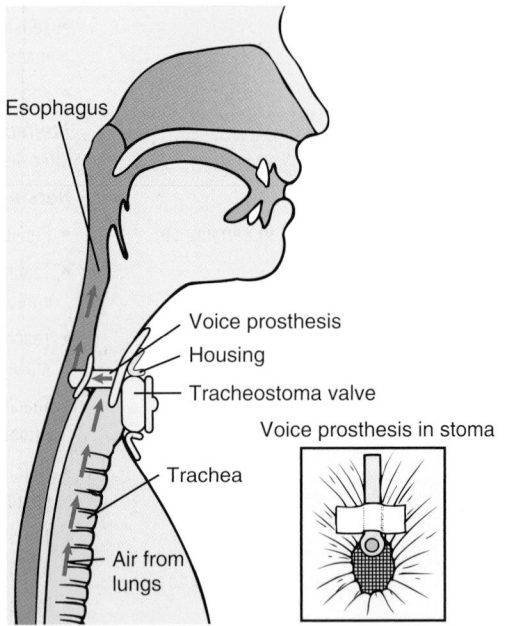

Figure 29-11 Blom-Singer voice prosthesis and tracheostoma valve. With this prosthesis and valve, patients with a laryngectomy can speak normally. *Inset,* laryngectomy stoma and voice prosthesis with tracheostoma valve removed.

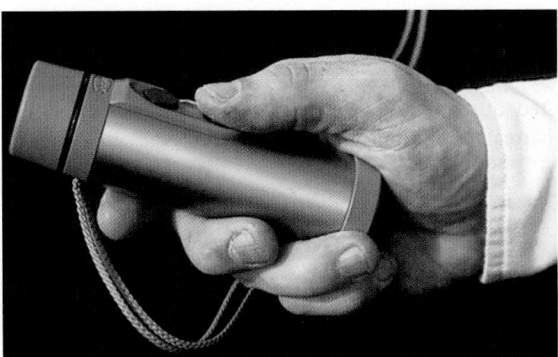

Figure 29-12 Artificial larynx. Battery-powered electronic artificial larynx for a patient who has had a total laryngectomy.

Source: Courtesy CLG Photographics, Inc., St. Louis, Missouri.

the finger. Air moves from the lungs, through the prosthesis, into the esophagus, and out the mouth. The voice is produced by the air vibrating against the esophagus and is formed into words by moving the tongue and lips. A valve may also be used with this device. When the valve is in place, the stoma does not need to be closed with the finger to speak. The prosthesis must be cleaned regularly and replaced when it becomes blocked with mucus.

An electrolarynx is a handheld, battery-powered device that creates speech with the use of sound waves. One device, the Cooper-Rand, uses a plastic tube placed in the corner of the roof of the mouth to create vibrations. To create the most normal sound when using this device, the patient should (1) avoid trying to use the tongue to hold the tube in place; (2) compress the tone generator for short intervals and speak in phrases, rather than full sentences; (3) speak using large movements of the lips, tongue, and jaw, rather than keeping the mouth partially closed; (4) talk face-to-face with the listener; and (5) practise because development of skill takes time.

An artificial larynx is placed against the neck rather than in the mouth. This device is used after surgical healing is complete and no edema remains (Figure 29-12). With experience, the patient can learn to move the lips in ways that create normal-sounding speech. With both devices, voice pitch is low, and the sound is mechanical.

Esophageal speech is a method of swallowing air, trapping it in the esophagus, and releasing it to create sound. The air causes vibration of the pharyngoesophageal segment and sound (which initially is similar to a belch). With practice, 50% of patients develop some speech skills, but only 10% develop fluent speech.

Stoma Care. Before discharge, the patient should be instructed in the care of the laryngectomy stoma. The area around the stoma should be washed daily with a moist cloth. If a laryngectomy tube is in place, the entire tube must be removed at least daily and cleaned in the same manner as a tracheostomy tube. The inner cannula may have to be removed and cleaned more frequently. A scarf, a loose shirt, or a crocheted shield can be used to shield the stoma.

The patient should cover the stoma when coughing (because mucus may be expectorated) and during any activity (e.g., shaving, applying makeup) that might lead to inhalation of foreign materials. Because water can easily enter the stoma, the patient should wear a plastic collar when taking a shower. Swimming is contraindicated. Initially, humidification will be administered via a tracheostomy mask. After discharge, a bedside humidifier can be used. A high oral fluid intake must be maintained, especially in dry weather.

The patient should be told the importance of wearing a medical identification bracelet or other identification that alerts others in an emergency situation of the need for neck breathing. Because the patient no longer breathes through the nose, the ability to smell smoke and food may be lost. Advise the patient to install smoke and carbon monoxide detectors in the home. It is important for food to be colourful, attractively prepared, and nutritious because taste may also be diminished secondary to the loss of smell as well as radiation therapy.

Depression. Depression is common in the patient who has had a radical neck dissection. The patient may not be able to speak because of the laryngectomy and cannot control saliva. The neck and shoulders may be numb because of the transected nerves. The facial appearance may be significantly altered, with swelling, edema, and deformities. The patient must understand that many of the physical changes are reversible as the edema subsides and the tracheostomy tube is removed. Depression may also be related to concern about the prognosis. The nurse can help the patient through the depression by allowing verbalization of feelings, conveying acceptance, and helping the patient regain an acceptable self-concept. Obtain a psychiatric referral for the patient who is experiencing prolonged or severe depression.

Sexuality. Surgery and the presence of foreign attachments such as tracheostomy and gastrostomy tubes may affect body image dramatically. The patient may feel less desirable sexually. The nurse can assist the patient by allowing discussions regarding sexuality and encouraging the patient to discuss this problem with the sexual partner. It may be difficult for the patient to orally discuss sexual problems because of the alteration in communication. The nurse can allow the patient to plan how to communicate with the sexual partner and offer support and guidance to the sexual partner. Helping the patient see that sexuality involves much more than appearance may relieve some anxiety.

Ambulatory and Home Care

The patient is often discharged with a tracheostomy and a nasogastric or gastrostomy feeding tube. Home health care may be needed initially as the family's or the patient's ability to perform self-care activities is evaluated. The patient and the family must be taught how to manage tubes and who to call if there are problems.

The patient can resume exercise, recreation, and sexual activity when able. Most patients can return to work 1 to 2 months after surgery. However, many never return to full-time employment. The changes that follow a total laryngectomy can be upsetting. Loss of speech, loss of the ability to taste and smell, inability to produce audible sounds (including laughing and weeping), and the presence of a permanent tracheal stoma that produces undesirable mucus are often overwhelming to the patient. Although changes are discussed before surgery, the patient may not be prepared for the extent of these changes. If the patient has a significant other, the reaction of this person to the patient's altered appearance is important. Acceptance by another person can promote an improved self-image. Encouraging the patient to participate in self-care is another important part of rehabilitation.

Reconstructive surgery may be performed at the time of the initial surgery or soon after the tumour is removed. Various types of flaps and grafts are used. It may be necessary to rebuild the nose or the mandible or to close oral cutaneous openings. Prosthetic materials, such as Silastic and Plastigel (which is soft), are often used to reconstruct various deformities.

Despite the use of surgical interventions and radiation therapy, the cure rate is disappointingly low for advanced head and neck cancer. Metastatic cancer is often painful, leaving the affected person in a severely debilitated state. If pain is a problem, a pain control regimen should be instituted to provide comfort, and referral should be made to a hospice if indicated.

Evaluation

Expected outcomes for the patient with head and neck cancer who is treated surgically are addressed in NCP 29-2.

CLINICAL DECISION-MAKING EXERCISE

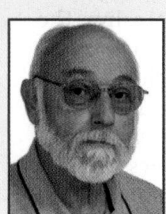

CASE STUDY:
Laryngeal Cancer

Patient Profile

Mr. Carlson, a 60-year-old man, was admitted for evaluation of mild pain on swallowing and a persistent sore throat over the past year.

Subjective Data

- States that his symptoms worsened in the last 2 months
- Has used various cold remedies to relieve symptoms without relief
- Has lost weight because of decrease in appetite and difficulty swallowing
- Has smoked three packs of cigarettes a day for 40 years
- Consumes six cans of beer a day

Objective Data

- Laryngoscopy
- Subglottic mass

Physical Examination
- Enlarged cervical nodes

Computed Tomography Scan
- Subglottic lesion with lymph node involvement
Collaborative Care
- Total laryngectomy with tracheostomy with inflated cuff
- Nasogastric tube

Discussion Questions

1. What information in the assessment suggests that Mr. Carlson might be at risk for cancer of the larynx?
2. What diagnostic tests are typically performed to evaluate the extent of this problem?
3. *Priority Decision:* What are the priority teaching strategies for Mr. Carlson before and after laryngectomy?
4. Discuss methods used to restore speech after laryngectomy.
5. What teaching is required to assist this patient to assume self-care after his surgery? What precautions should the patient take because of his stoma?
6. *Priority Decision:* Based on the assessment data presented, what are the postoperative nursing priorities?

evolve *Answers are available on* **http://evolve.elsevier.com/ Canada/Lewis/medsurg**

REVIEW QUESTIONS

The number of the question corresponds to the same-numbered objective at the beginning of the chapter.

1. A patient was seen in the clinic for an episode of epistaxis, which was controlled by placement of anterior nasal packing. During discharge teaching, what should the nurse instruct the patient to do?
   a. Use aspirin for pain relief.
   b. Remove the packing later that day.
   c. Skip the next dose of antihypertensive medication.
   d. Avoid vigorous nose blowing and strenuous activity.
2. A patient with allergic rhinitis reports severe nasal congestion, sneezing, and watery, itchy eyes and nose at various times of the year. What should the nurse advise the patient to do?
   a. Avoid all intranasal sprays and oral antihistamines.
   b. Limit the duration of use of nasal decongestant spray to 10 days.
   c. Use oral decongestants at bedtime to prevent symptoms during the night.
   d. Keep a diary of when the allergic reaction occurs and what precipitates it.

3. A patient is seen at the clinic with fever, muscle aches, sore throat with yellowish exudate, and headache. Which of the following does the nurse anticipate that the collaborative management will include (*select all that apply*):
   a. antiviral agents to treat influenza.
   b. treatment with antibiotics starting ASAP.
   c. a throat culture or rapid strep antigen test.
   d. supportive care including cool, bland liquids.
   e. comprehensive history to determine possible etiology.
4. What type of tracheostomy tube prevents speech?
   a. Cuffless tracheostomy tube
   b. Fenestrated tracheostomy tube
   c. Tube with an inflated foam cuff
   d. Cuffed tube with the cuff deflated

5. Which nursing action related to the tracheostomy tube cuff pressure would prevent excessive pressure on tracheal capillaries?
   a. Monitor pressure every 2 to 3 days.
   b. Ensure pressure is less than 20 mm Hg or 25 cm H_2O.
   c. Ensure pressure is less than 30 mm Hg or 35 cm H_2O.
   d. Ensure pressure is sufficient to fill the pilot balloon until it is tense.

6. Which of the following is not an early symptom of head and neck cancer?
   a. Hoarseness
   b. Change in fit of dentures
   c. Mouth ulcers that do not heal
   d. Decreased mobility of the tongue

7. While in the recovery room, a patient with a total laryngectomy is suctioned and has bloody mucus with some clots. Which of the following nursing interventions would apply?
   a. Notify the physician immediately.
   b. Place the patient in the prone position to facilitate drainage.
   c. Instill 3 mL of normal saline into the tracheostomy tube to loosen secretions.
   d. Continue the assessment of the patient, including oxygen saturation, respiratory rate, and breath sounds.

8. How should the patient use a voice prosthesis?
   a. Place a vibrating device in the mouth.
   b. Place a speaking valve over the stoma.
   c. Block the stoma entrance with a finger.
   d. Swallow air using Valsalva's manoeuvre.

ANSWERS: 1. d; 2. d; 3. c, d, e; 4. c; 5. b; 6. d; 7. d; 8. c

REFERENCES

Aghababian, R., Bird, S., Braen, G., Kraus, B., McCabe, J., Moorhead, J., …, Volturo, G. (2011). *The essentials of emergency medicine.* Burlington, MA: Jones & Bartlett Learning.

Canadian Cancer Society Steering Committee on Cancer Statistics. (2011). *Canadian cancer statistics 2011.* Toronto, ON: Cancer Society.

Christensen, B., & Kockrow, C. (2011). *Adult health nursing* (6th ed.). St. Louis: Mosby.

Dykewicz, M., & Hamilos, D. (2010). Rhinitis and sinusitis. *Journal of Allergy and Clinical Immunology, 125*(2), S103-S115. doi:10.1016/j.jaci.2009.12.989

Egan, M., & Hickner, J. (2009). Saline irrigation spells relief for sinusitis sufferers. *Journal of Family Practice, 58*(1), 29-32.

Emergency Nurses Association. (2010). *Sheehy's emergency nursing. Principles and practices* (6th ed.). St. Louis: Mosby.

Engels, P., Bayshaw, S. W., Meier, M., & Brindley, P. (2008) Tracheostomy: From insertion to decannulation. *Canadian Journal of Surgery, 52*(5), 427-433.

Goldman, L., & Ausiello, D. (2007). *Cecil medicine* (23rd ed.). Philadelphia: Saunders.

Health Canada. (2009). *It's your health: The flu.* Ottawa: Author. Retrieved from *http://www.hc-sc.gc.ca/iyh-vsv/diseases-maladies/flu-grippe_e.html*

Lynn-McHale Weigand, D. (ed.), (2011). *AACN procedure manual for critical care.* (6th ed.). St. Louis: Saunders.

Monahan, F. (2009). *Mosby's expert physical exam book: Rapid inpatient and outpatient assessments* (3rd ed.). St. Louis: Mosby.

Public Health Agency of Canada (PHAC). (2010). *Canadian pandemic influenza plan.* Ottawa: Author. Retrieved from *http://www.phac-aspc.gc.ca/influenza/pandemicplan_e.html*

Regan, E., & Dallachiesa, L. (2009). How to care for a patient with a tracheostomy. *Nursing, 39*(8), 34-39.

Rothrock, J. (2011). *Alexander's care of the patient in surgery* (14th ed.). St. Louis: Mosby.

Sagrillo, D., & Kunz, S. (2008). Proposed plastic surgery nursing guidelines for care of the rhinoplasty patient. *Plastic Surgery Nursing, 28*(4), 198-200.

Schiech, L. (2007). Looking at laryngeal cancer. *Nursing, 37*(5), 50-55.

Shoup, J. (2011). Management of adult rhinosinusitis. *The Nurse Practitioner, 36*(11), 22-25.

Skillings K., & Curtis B. (2011). Tracheostomy tube care. In D. Lynn-McHale Weigand (ed.), *AACN procedure manual for critical care* (pp. 96-100). St. Louis: Saunders.

Supriya, M., Shakeel, D., Veitch, D. , & Wong, D. (2010). Epistaxis: Prospective evaluation of bleeding site and its impact on patient outcomes. *Journal of Laryngology and Otology, 124,* 744-749. doi:10.1017/S0022215110000411

Thibodeau, G., & Patton, K. (2010). *Anatomy and physiology* (7th ed.). St. Louis: Mosby.

Tickle, J., & Sewell, C. (2007). Managing allergic rhinitis. *Practice Nurse, 33*(8), 15-19.

Urden, L., Stacy, K., & Lough, M. (2010). Thelan's critical care nursing: Diagnosis and management (6th ed.). St. Louis: Mosby.

CANADIAN RESOURCES

Canadian Cancer Society
   http://www.cancer.ca
Canadian Lung Association
   http://www.lung.ca
Canadian Sleep Disorder Centre
   http://sleepdisorders.about.com/cs/canada
Canadian Sleep Society
   http://www.css.to
CHICA Canada—Community and Hospital Infection Control Association
   http://www.chica.org
Health Canada
   http://www.hc-sc.gc.ca
International Association of Laryngectomees
   http://www.larynxlink.com
National Cancer Institute of Canada
   http://www.ncic.cancer.ca
Public Health Agency of Canada
   http://www.phac-aspc.gc.ca
Statistics Canada
   http://www.statcan.gc.ca/start-debut-eng.html
World Health Organization—Avian Influenza
   http://www.who.int/csr/resources/publications/swineflu/surveillance_post_pandemic.pdf

🜁volve   *For additional Internet resources, see the Web site for this book at* **http://evolve.elsevier.com/Canada/Lewis/medsurg**

Nursing Management: Lower Respiratory Problems

Written by Margaret (Peggy) J. Malone

Adapted by Katarzyna (Kat) Moyer

LEARNING OBJECTIVES

1. Describe the pathophysiology, types, clinical manifestations, and collaborative care of pneumonia.
2. Explain the nursing management of the patient with pneumonia.
3. Describe the pathogenesis, classification, clinical manifestations, complications, diagnostic abnormalities, and nursing and collaborative management of tuberculosis.
4. Identify the causes, clinical manifestations, and nursing and collaborative management of pulmonary fungal infections.
5. Explain the pathophysiology, clinical manifestations, and nursing and collaborative management of bronchiectasis and lung abscess.
6. Identify the causative factors, clinical features, and management of environmental lung diseases.
7. Describe the causes, risk factors, pathogenesis, clinical manifestations, and nursing and collaborative management of lung cancer.
8. Identify the mechanisms involved and the clinical manifestations of pneumothorax, fractured ribs, and flail chest.
9. Describe the purpose, methods, and nursing responsibilities related to chest tubes.
10. Explain the types of chest surgery and appropriate preoperative and postoperative care.
11. Compare and contrast extrapulmonary and intrapulmonary restrictive lung disorders in terms of causes, clinical manifestations, and collaborative management.
12. Describe the pathophysiology, clinical manifestations, and management of pulmonary hypertension and cor pulmonale.
13. Discuss the use of lung transplantation as a treatment for pulmonary disorders.

KEY TERMS

acute bronchitis An inflammation of the bronchi in the lower respiratory tract that is usually caused by infection, p. 659

atelectasis A condition of the lungs characterized by collapsed, airless alveoli, p. 699

bronchiectasis A condition of the lungs characterized by permanent, abnormal dilation of one or more large bronchi, p. 676

blebs Air-filled alveolar dilation less than 1 cm in diameter on the edge of the lung at the apex of the upper lobe or superior segment of the lower lobe; usually occurs in young people and can rupture, producing primary pneumothorax, p. 688

chylothorax Presence of lymphatic fluid in the pleural space caused by a leak in the thoracic duct, p. 690

community-acquired pneumonia (CAP) A lower respiratory tract infection of the lung parenchyma with onset in the community or during the first 2 days of hospitalization, p. 660

cor pulmonale Enlargement of the right ventricle secondary to diseases of the lung, the thorax, or the pulmonary circulation, p. 704

empirical therapy Therapy based on observation and experience, implemented when the condition's exact cause is not known, p. 664

empyema A pleural effusion that contains pus, p. 696

flail chest A condition resulting from multiple rib fractures, causing instability of the chest wall, p. 690

hemothorax An accumulation of blood in the intrapleural space, p. 689

hospital-acquired pneumonia (HAP) Pneumonia occurring 48 hours or longer after hospital admission and not incubating at the time of hospitalization, p. 660

lung abscess A pus-containing lesion of the lung parenchyma that gives rise to a cavity, p. 677

pleural effusion A collection of fluid in the pleural space, p. 696

pleurisy (pleuritis) Inflammation of the pleura, p. 699

pneumoconiosis A general term for lung diseases caused by inhalation and retention of dust particles, literally meaning "dust in the lungs," p. 678

pneumonia Acute inflammation of the lung parenchyma caused by a microbial agent, p. 660

pneumothorax Presence of air in the pleural space, p. 688

pulmonary edema An abnormal accumulation of fluid in the alveoli and the interstitial spaces of the lungs, p. 700

pulmonary embolism (PE) The blockage of pulmonary arteries by a thrombus, fat embolus (from fractured long bones), air embolus, bacterial vegetations, amniotic fluid, or tumours, p. 700

pulmonary hypertension Elevated pulmonary pressure resulting from an increase in pulmonary vascular resistance to blood flow through small arteries and arterioles, p. 703

severe acute respiratory syndrome (SARS) A respiratory infection caused by a coronavirus; first appeared in Canada in 2003, p. 668

tension pneumothorax A pneumothorax with rapid accumulation of air in the pleural space causing severely high intrapleural pressures with resultant tension on the heart and great vessels, p. 689

thoracentesis A procedure to remove fluid from the pleural space, p. 697

thoracotomy Surgical opening into the thoracic cavity, p. 695

tuberculosis An infectious disease caused by *Mycobacterium tuberculosis*; usually involves the lungs, but also occurs in the larynx, the kidneys, the bones, the adrenal glands, the lymph nodes, and the meninges and can be disseminated throughout the body, p. 669

ELECTRONIC RESOURCES

Supplemental content related to Chapter 30 can be found…

Evolve Web Site ⊖volve

- Answer Guidelines to Case Study on p. 705
- Clinical Reference: Laboratory Values
- Content Updates
- Customizable Nursing Care Plans:
  - Pneumonia
  - Thoracotomy

- Electronic Calculators
- Examination Review Questions
- Glossary
- Interactive Case Studies:
  - Lung Cancer
  - Pulmonary Embolism
- Key Points (Printable and MP3 Download)

A wide variety of problems affect the lower respiratory system. Lung diseases that are characterized primarily by an obstructive disorder, such as asthma, emphysema, chronic bronchitis, and cystic fibrosis, are discussed in Chapter 31. All other lower respiratory problems are discussed in this chapter.

Respiratory tract infections are common. Lower respiratory tract infections are a common cause of death in the world. In 2004 to 2005, 3% of all Canadian hospitalizations of males and 2.2% of male deaths were attributed to influenza and pneumonia. For females, 2.8% of hospitalizations and 2.8% of deaths were attributed to influenza and pneumonia (Public Health Agency of Canada [PHAC], 2007a). Tuberculosis (TB), although potentially curable and preventable, is a worldwide public health threat of epidemic proportion.

Acute Bronchitis

Acute bronchitis is an inflammation of the bronchi in the lower respiratory tract usually caused by infection. It is one of the most common conditions seen in primary care. It usually occurs as a sequel to an upper respiratory tract infection. A type of acute bronchitis is acute exacerbation of chronic bronchitis (AECB). AECB represents acute infection superimposed on chronic bronchitis. AECB is a potentially serious condition that may lead to respiratory failure. (Chronic bronchitis is discussed in Chapter 31.)

The cause of most cases of acute bronchitis is viral (rhinovirus, influenza). However, bacterial causes are also common both in smokers (e.g., *Streptococcus pneumoniae, Haemophilus influenzae*) and nonsmokers (e.g., *Mycoplasma pneumoniae, Chlamydia pneumoniae*).

In acute bronchitis, persistent cough following an acute upper airway infection (e.g., rhinitis, pharyngitis) is the most common symptom. Cough is often accompanied by production of clear, mucoid sputum, although some patients produce purulent sputum. Associated symptoms include fever, headache, malaise, and shortness of breath on exertion. Physical examination may reveal mildly elevated temperature, pulse, and respiratory rate with either normal breath sounds or expiratory wheezing. Chest radiographic studies can differentiate acute bronchitis from pneumonia because there is no radiographic evidence of consolidation or infiltrates with bronchitis.

Acute bronchitis is usually self-limiting, and the treatment is generally supportive, including fluids, rest, and anti-inflammatory agents. Cough suppressants or bronchodilators may be prescribed for symptomatic treatment of nocturnal cough or wheezing. Antibiotics are generally not prescribed unless the person has a prolonged infection associated with constitutional symptoms, or if the person is a smoker or has chronic obstructive pulmonary disease (COPD).

The patient with AECB is usually treated empirically with broad-spectrum antibiotics. Often, the patient with COPD is taught to recognize symptoms of acute bronchitis and to begin a course of antibiotics when symptoms occur. Many health care providers believe that a more severe infection often results if the patient delays taking antibiotics until after a clinical examination. Early initiation of antibiotic treatment in patients with COPD has resulted in a decrease in relapses and a decrease in hospital admissions.

Pneumonia

Pneumonia is an acute inflammation of the lung parenchyma caused by a microbial agent. The discovery of sulpha drugs and penicillin was pivotal in the treatment of pneumonia. Since that time, there has been remarkable progress in the development of antibiotics to treat pneumonia. However, despite the new antimicrobial agents, pneumonia is still common and is associated with significant morbidity and mortality rates.

Etiology

Normally, the airway distal to the larynx is sterile because of protective defence mechanisms. These mechanisms include the following: filtration of air, warming and humidification of inspired air, epiglottis closure over the trachea, cough reflex, mucociliary escalator mechanism, secretion of immunoglobulin A, and alveolar macrophages (see Chapter 28).

Factors Predisposing to Pneumonia.
Pneumonia is more likely to result when defence mechanisms become incompetent or are overwhelmed by the virulence or quantity of infectious agents. Decreased consciousness depresses the cough and epiglottal reflexes, which may allow aspiration of oropharyngeal contents into the lungs. Tracheal intubation interferes with the normal cough reflex and the mucociliary escalator mechanism. It also bypasses the upper airways in which filtration and humidification of air normally take place. The mucociliary escalator mechanism is impaired by air pollution, cigarette smoking, viral upper respiratory infections (URIs), and normal changes of aging. In the presence of malnutrition, the functions of lymphocytes and polymorphonuclear leukocytes are altered. Certain diseases such as leukemia, alcoholism, and diabetes mellitus are associated with an increased frequency of Gram-negative bacilli in the oropharynx. (Gram-negative bacilli are not normal flora in the respiratory tract.) Altered oropharyngeal flora can also occur secondary to antibiotic therapy given for an infection elsewhere in the body. The factors predisposing to pneumonia are listed in Table 30-1.

Acquisition of Organisms.
Organisms that cause pneumonia reach the lung by three methods:
1. *Aspiration* from the nasopharynx or oropharynx. Many of the organisms that cause pneumonia are normal inhabitants of the pharynx in healthy adults.
2. *Inhalation* of microbes present in the air. Examples include *M. pneumoniae* and fungal pneumonias.
3. *Hematogenous spread* from a primary infection elsewhere in the body. An example is *Staphylococcus aureus*.

Table 30-1 Factors Predisposing to Pneumonia

- Aging
- Air pollution
- Altered consciousness: alcoholism, head injury, seizures, anaesthesia, drug overdose, stroke
- Altered oropharyngeal flora
- Bed rest and prolonged immobility
- Chronic diseases: chronic lung disease, diabetes mellitus, heart disease, cancer, end-stage renal disease
- Debilitating illness
- Human immunodeficiency virus infection
- Immunosuppressive drugs (corticosteroids, cancer chemotherapy, immunosuppressive therapy after organ transplant)
- Inhalation or aspiration of noxious substances
- Intestinal and gastric feedings
- Malnutrition
- Smoking
- Tracheal intubation (endotracheal intubation, tracheostomy)
- Upper respiratory tract infection

Types of Pneumonia

Pneumonia can be caused by bacteria, viruses, *Mycoplasma*, fungi, parasites, and chemicals. Although pneumonia can be classified according to the causative organism, a clinically effective way is to classify pneumonia as community-acquired or hospital-acquired. Classifying pneumonia is important because of differences in the likely causative organisms and the selection of appropriate antibiotics (Table 30-2).

Community-Acquired Pneumonia.
Community-acquired pneumonia (CAP) is defined as a lower respiratory tract infection of the lung parenchyma with onset in the community or during the first 2 days of hospitalization. The incidence of CAP is highest in the winter months. Smoking is an important risk factor. The causative organism in CAP is identified only 50% of the time. Organisms that are commonly implicated in CAP include *S. pneumoniae* and atypical organisms (e.g., *Legionella, Mycoplasma, Chlamydia,* viral). Modifying risk factors include the presence of COPD, recent use of antibiotics, and conditions incurring risk of aspiration.

The Infectious Diseases Society of America/American Thoracic Society (Mandell et al., 2007) consensus guidelines recommend patients be assessed using the CURB-65 score or Pneumonia Severity Index to determine candidates for outpatient treatment. The CURB-65 (Figure 30-1) prognostic model is calculated on the basis of mental *c*onfusion, blood *u*rea (>17 mmol/L), *r*espiratory rate (30 breaths/min), *b*lood pressure (systolic <90 mm Hg or diastolic ≤60 mm Hg), and patient's age (≥65 yr) to indicate severity of pneumonia (Karmakar & Wilsher, 2010). The Pneumonia Severity Index is a more complex assessment tool based on nearly 20 criteria (see Table 30-3). (Antibiotic therapy options for each group are discussed in the later section on drug therapy, p. 665.)

Hospital-Acquired Pneumonia.
Hospital-acquired pneumonia (HAP) is pneumonia occurring 48 hours or longer after

Table 30-2 Epidemiological Conditions and/or Risk Factors Related to Specific Pathogens in Community-Acquired Pneumonia

CONDITION	COMMONLY ENCOUNTERED PATHOGEN(S)
Alcoholism	*Streptococcus pneumoniae*, oral anaerobes, *Klebsiella pneumoniae*, *Acinetobacter* species, *Mycobacterium tuberculosis*
COPD and/or smoking	*Haemophilus influenza*, *Pseudomonas aeruginosa*, *Legionella* species, *S. pneumoniae*, *Moraxella catarrhalis*, *Chlamydophila pneumoniae*
Aspiration	Gram-negative enteric pathogens, oral anaerobes
Lung abscess	CA-MRSA, oral anaerobes, endemic fungal pneumonia, *M. tuberculosis*, atypical mycobacteria
Exposure to bat or bird droppings	*Histoplasma capsulatum*
Exposure to birds	*Chlamydophila psittaci* (if poultry: avian influenza)
Exposure to rabbits	*Francisella tularensis* (tularemia)
Exposure to farm animals or pregnant cats	*Coxiella burnetii* (Q fever)
HIV infection (early)	*S. pneumoniae*, *H. influenzae*, *M. tuberculosis*
HIV infection (late)	The pathogens listed for early infection, plus: *Pneumocystis jiroveci*, *Cryptococcus*, *Histoplasma*, *Aspergillus*, atypical mycobacteria (especially *M. kansasii*), *P. aeruginosa*, *H. influenzae*
Hotel or cruise ship stay in previous 2 wk	*Legionella* species
Travel to or residence in southwestern United States	*Coccidioides* species, Hantavirus
Travel to or residence in Southeast and East Asia	*Burkholderia pseudomallei*, avian influenza, SARS
Influenza active in community	Influenza, *S. pneumonia*, *Staphylococcus aureus*, *H. influenzae*
Cough >2 wk with whoop or post-tussive vomiting	*Bordetella pertussis*
Structural lung disease (e.g., bronchiectasis)	*P. aeruginosa*, *Burkholderia cepacia*, *S. aureus*
Injection drug use	*S. aureus*, anaerobes, *M. tuberculosis*, *S. pneumoniae*
Endobronchial obstruction	Anaerobes, *S. pneumoniae*, *H. influenzae*, *S. aureus*
In context of bioterrorism	*Bacillus anthracis* (anthrax), *Yersinia pestis* (plague), *Francisella tularensis* (tularemia)

CA-MRSA, community-acquired methicillin-resistant *Staphylococcus aureus; COPD,* chronic obstructive pulmonary disease; *HIV,* human immunodeficiency virus; *SARS,* severe acute respiratory syndrome.
Source: Mandell, L. A., Wunderink, R. G., Anzueto, A., Bartlett, J. G., Campbell, G. D., Dean, N. C., . . . Whitney, C. G. (2007). Infectious Diseases Society of America/American Thoracic Society consensus guidelines on the management of community-acquired pneumonia in adults (Table 8, p. S46). *Clinical Infectious Diseases, 44*(Suppl 2), S27-S72. doi:10.1086/511159

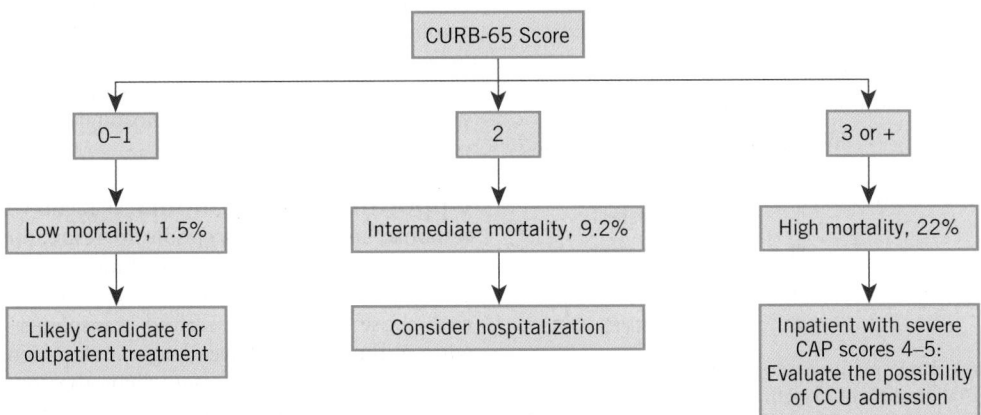

Figure 30-1 CURB-65 score. *CAP,* community-acquired pneumonia; *CCU,* critical care unit; *CURB-65:* mental confusion (C), urea >17 mmol/L (U), respiratory rate 30 breaths/min (R), blood pressure (systolic <90 mm Hg or diastolic ≤60 mm Hg) (B), 65 = age ≥65 years.

Source: Corrêa, R. A, Lundgren, F. L. C., Pereira-Silva, J. L., Silva, R. L. F, Cardoso, A. P., Lemos, A. C. M., ..., da Rocha, R. T. (2009). Brazilian guidelines for community-acquired pneumonia in immunocompetent adults—2009 (Figure 2). *Jornal brasileiro de pneumologia, 35*(6). doi:10.1590/S1806-37132009000600011

Table 30-3 Pneumonia Severity Index

Step 1	Assess arterial oxygenation for all patients.* Is pulse oximetry <90% (usual method) or PO₂ <60 mm Hg? Yes: Inpatient therapy recommended No: Go to step 2
Step 2	Are any of the following present? • Patient ≥51 yr of age • Co-existing conditions listed in Step 3, or • Physical examination findings listed in Step 3 Yes: Go to Step 3 No: Risk class I, go to Step 4
Step 3	Compute Risk Score (sum of applicable points)

RISK FACTOR	POINTS
Demographic Factors	
Age yr (automatically score 10 for women)	
Nursing home resident	10
Coexisting Conditions	
Neoplastic disease	30
Liver disease	20
Heart failure	10
Cerebrovascular disease	10
Renal disease	10
Physical Examination Findings	
Altered mental status	20
Respiratory rate ≥30 breaths/min	20
Systolic blood pressure <90 mm Hg	20
Temperature <35°C or ≥40°C	15
Pulse rate ≥125 beats/min	10
Other Findings	
Arterial pH <7.35	30
Blood urea nitrogen level ≥10.7 mmol/L	20
Sodium <130 mmol/L	20
Glucose ≥13 mmol/L	10
Hematocrit <30%	10
PO₂ <60 mm Hg or O₂ saturation <90%	10
Pleural effusion evident on radiograph	10
Total Score (sum of all points)	

Step 4	Recommended initial site of treatment

RISK SCORE	RISK CLASS	TREATMENT SITE
NA	I	Outpatient
<71	II	Outpatient
71-90	III	Outpatient
91-130	IV	Inpatient
>130	V	Inpatient

NA, not applicable; risk scores are not used to identify these patients (see Step 2); *PO₂*, partial pressure of oxygen.
*Either through ambient pulse oximetry assessment or arterial blood gas analysis (although the latter is not mandatory at this step if the former is available).

Source: Yealy, D. M., Auble, T. E., Stone, R. A., Lave, J. R., Meehan, T. P., Graff, L. G., ..., Fine, M. J. (2004). The emergency department community-acquired pneumonia trial: Methodology of a quality improvement intervention. *Annals of Emergency Medicine, 43*(6), 772. doi:10.1016/j.annemergmed.2003.09.013

hospital admission and not incubating at the time of hospitalization. HAP accounts for 25% of all critical care unit (CCU) infections. It is the second most common hospital-associated infection and has high mortality and morbidity rates (American Thoracic Society, 2005). The microorganisms responsible for HAP are different from those organisms implicated in CAP. Bacteria are responsible for the majority of HAP infections, including *Pseudomonas, Enterobacter, S. aureus,* methicillin-resistant *Staphylococcus aureus* (MRSA), and *S. pneumoniae.* Many of the organisms causing HAP enter the lungs after aspiration of particles from the patient's own pharynx. Immunosuppressive therapy, general debility, and endotracheal intubation may be predisposing factors. Contaminated respiratory therapy equipment is another source of infection.

Fungal Pneumonia. Fungi may also be a cause of pneumonia (see section on pulmonary fungal infections, p. 675).

Aspiration Pneumonia. *Aspiration pneumonia* refers to the sequelae of abnormal entry of secretions or substances into the lower airway. It usually follows aspiration of material from the mouth or the stomach into the trachea and subsequently the lungs. The person who has aspiration pneumonia usually has a history of loss of consciousness (e.g., as a result of seizure, anaesthesia, head injury, stroke, alcohol intake). With loss of consciousness, the gag and cough reflexes are depressed, and aspiration is more likely to occur. Another risk factor is tube feedings. The dependent portions of the lung are most often affected, primarily the superior segments of the lower lobes and the posterior segments of the upper lobes, which are dependent in the supine position.

The aspirated material, food, water, vomitus, or toxic fluids, is the pathological triggering mechanism for the development of this type of pneumonia. There are three distinct forms of aspiration pneumonia. If the aspirated material is an inert substance (e.g., barium), the initial manifestation is usually caused by mechanical obstruction of airways. When the aspirated materials contain toxic fluids such as gastric juices, there is chemical injury to the lung with infection as a secondary event, usually 48 to 72 hours later; this is identified as *chemical (noninfectious) pneumonitis.* The most important form of aspiration pneumonia is bacterial infection. The infecting organism is usually one of the normal oropharyngeal flora, and multiple organisms, including both aerobes and anaerobes, are isolated from the sputum of the patient with aspiration pneumonia. Antibiotic therapy is based on an assessment of the severity of illness, where the infection was acquired (community or hospital), and type of organisms present.

Opportunistic Pneumonia. Patients with altered immune response are highly susceptible to respiratory infections. Individuals considered at risk include those who have severe protein–calorie malnutrition; those who have immune deficiencies; those who have received transplants and been treated with immunosuppressive drugs; and patients who are being treated with radiation therapy, chemotherapy drugs, and corticosteroids (especially for a prolonged period). The individual has a variety of altered conditions, including altered B- and T-lymphocyte function, depressed bone marrow function, and decreased levels or function of neutrophils and macrophages. In addition to the causative agents (especially Gram-negative bacteria), other agents that cause pneumonia in the immunocompromised patient are *Pneumocystis jiroveci* (McLean,

Murray, Schreibman, & Rigsby, 2007), cytomegalovirus (CMV), and fungi.

P. jiroveci is an opportunistic pathogen whose natural habitat is the lung. This organism rarely causes pneumonia in the healthy individual. *P. jiroveci* pneumonia (PCP) affects 70% of human immunodeficiency virus (HIV)–infected individuals and is the most common opportunistic infection in patients with acquired immune deficiency syndrome (AIDS). In this type of pneumonia, the chest radiograph usually shows a diffuse bilateral alveolar pattern of infiltration. In widespread disease, the lungs are massively consolidated.

Clinical manifestations are insidious and include fever, tachypnea, tachycardia, dyspnea, nonproductive cough, and hypoxemia. Pulmonary physical findings are minimal in proportion to the serious nature of the disease. Treatment consists of a course of trimethoprim–sulfamethoxazole (Bactrim) as the primary agent. An alternative medication for the Bactrim-intolerant patient is dapsone–trimethoprim. In populations at risk for development of *P. jiroveci* pneumonitis (e.g., patients with hematological malignancies or AIDS), prophylaxis with trimethoprim–sulfamethoxazole may be advocated. Aerosolized pentamidine (Pneumopent), although less commonly used, is an alternative for prophylaxis in Bactrim-intolerant patients. (PCP is discussed in Chapter 17.)

Cytomegalovirus (CMV) is a cause of viral pneumonia in the immunocompromised patient, particularly in transplant recipients. CMV, a type of herpesvirus, gives rise to latent infections and reactivation with shedding of infectious virus. This type of interstitial pneumonia can be a mild disease, or it can be fulminant and produce pulmonary insufficiency and death. Often, CMV coexists with other opportunistic bacterial or fungal agents in causing pneumonia. Ganciclovir (Cytovene) is recommended for treatment of CMV pneumonia.

Pathophysiology

Pneumococcal pneumonia is the most common cause of bacterial pneumonia. However, regardless of causative factors, pneumonia is characterized by four stages of the disease process:

1. *Congestion.* After the pneumococcus organisms reach the alveoli via droplets or saliva, there is an outpouring of fluid into the alveoli. The organisms multiply in the serous fluid, and the infection is spread. The pneumococci damage the host by their overwhelming growth and interference with lung function.
2. *Red hepatization.* There is massive dilation of the capillaries, and alveoli are filled with organisms, neutrophils, red blood cells (RBCs), and fibrin (Figure 30-2). The lung appears red and granular, similar to the liver, which is why the process is called *hepatization.*
3. *Grey hepatization.* Blood flow decreases, and leukocytes and fibrin consolidate in the affected part of the lung.
4. *Resolution.* Complete resolution and healing occur if there are no complications.

The exudate becomes lysed and is processed by the macrophages. The normal lung tissue is restored, and the person's gas-exchange ability returns to normal.

Clinical Manifestations

Patients with pneumonia usually have a constellation of symptoms including sudden onset of fever, chills, cough productive of purulent sputum, and pleuritic chest pain (in some cases). In the

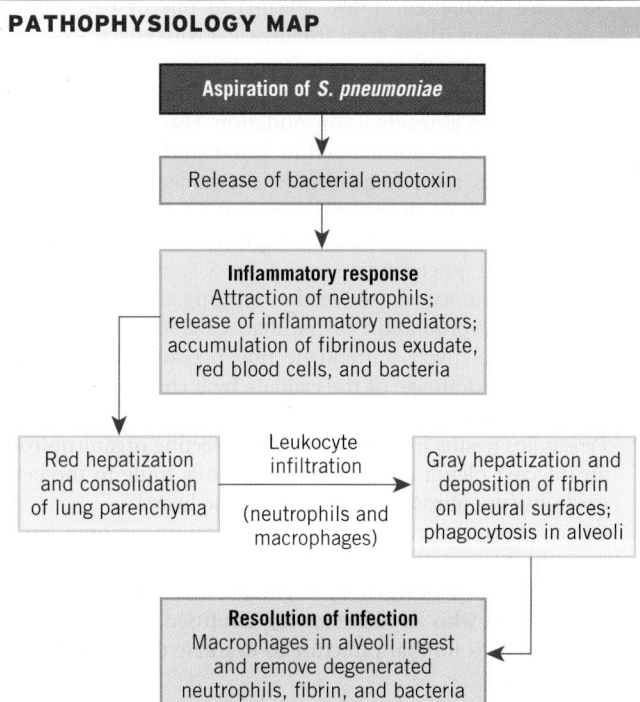

PATHOPHYSIOLOGY MAP

Figure 30-2 Pathophysiological course of pneumococcal pneumonia.

older adult or debilitated patient, confusion or stupor (possibly related to hypoxia) may be the predominant finding. On physical examination, signs of pulmonary consolidation, such as dullness to percussion, increased fremitus, bronchial breath sounds, and crackles, may be found. The typical pneumonia syndrome is usually caused by the most common pathogen in CAP, which is *S. pneumoniae,* but can also be caused by other bacterial pathogens, such as *H. influenzae.*

Pneumonia may also manifest atypically with a more gradual onset, a dry cough, and extrapulmonary manifestations such as headache, myalgias, fatigue, sore throat, nausea, vomiting, and diarrhea. On physical examination, crackles are often heard. This presentation of symptoms is classically produced by *M. pneumoniae* but can also be caused by *Legionella* and *C. pneumoniae.* Patients with hematogenous *S. aureus* pneumonia may have only dyspnea and fever. This necrotizing infection causes destruction of lung tissue, and these patients are usually very sick.

Manifestations of viral pneumonia are highly variable but may be characterized by chills, fever, dry, nonproductive cough, and extrapulmonary symptoms. Viral pneumonia may be found in association with systemic viral diseases such as measles, varicella-zoster, herpes simplex, or influenza virus infection.

Complications

Most cases of pneumonia generally run an uncomplicated course. Complications generally develop more frequently in individuals with underlying chronic diseases and may include the following:

1. *Pleurisy* (inflammation of the pleura) is a relatively common accompanying problem of pneumonia.
2. *Pleural effusion* can occur, and usually, the effusion is sterile and is reabsorbed in 1 to 2 weeks. Occasionally, it necessitates aspiration by means of thoracentesis.

3. *Atelectasis* (collapsed, airless alveoli) of one or part of one lobe may occur. These areas usually clear with effective coughing and deep breathing.

4. *Delayed resolution* results from persistent infection and is seen on radiograph as residual consolidation. Usually, the physical findings return to normal within 2 to 4 weeks. Delayed resolution occurs most frequently in the patient who is older, malnourished, or alcoholic or who has COPD.

5. *Lung abscess* is not a common complication of pneumonia. It is seen with pneumonia caused by *S. aureus* and Gram-negative pneumonias (see section on lung abscess, p. 677).

6. *Empyema* (accumulation of purulent exudate in the pleural cavity) is relatively infrequent but necessitates antibiotic therapy and drainage of the exudate by a chest tube or open surgical drainage.

7. *Pericarditis* results from spread of the infecting organism from an infected pleura or via a hematogenous route to the pericardium (the fibroserous sac around the heart).

8. Bacteremia can occur with pneumococcal pneumonia, more so with older adult patients.

9. *Meningitis* can be caused by *S. pneumoniae.* The patient with pneumonia who is disoriented, confused, or somnolent should have a lumbar puncture to evaluate the possibility of meningitis.

10. *Endocarditis* can develop when the organisms attack the endocardium and the valves of the heart. The clinical manifestations are similar to those of acute infective endocarditis (see Chapter 39).

Diagnostic Studies. The common diagnostic measures for pneumonia are presented in Table 30-4. History, physical examination, and chest radiographic study often provide enough information to make management decisions without costly laboratory tests.

The chest radiograph often shows a typical pattern characteristic of the infecting organism and is an invaluable adjunct in the diagnosis of pneumonia. Lobar or segmental consolidation suggests a bacterial cause, usually *S. pneumoniae* or *Klebsiella.* Diffuse pulmonary infiltrates are most commonly caused by infection with viruses, *Legionella,* or pathogenic fungi. Cavitary shadows

COLLABORATIVE CARE

Table 30-4 Pneumonia	
Diagnostic	**Collaborative Therapy**
• History and physical examination	• Appropriate antibiotic therapy
• Chest radiograph	• Increased fluid intake (at least 3 L/day)
• Gram stain examination of sputum	• Limited activity and rest
• Sputum culture and sensitivity test (if drug-resistant pathogen or organism not covered by empirical therapy)	• Antipyretics
	• Analgesics
	• Oxygen therapy (if indicated)
• Pulse oximetry or ABGs (if indicated)	
• Complete blood count, differential, and routine blood chemistries (if indicated)	
• Blood cultures (if indicated)	

ABGs, arterial blood gases.

suggest the presence of a necrotizing infection with destruction of lung tissue commonly caused by *S. aureus,* Gram-negative bacteria, and *Mycobacterium tuberculosis.* Pleural effusions, which can occur in up to 30% of patients with CAP, can also be seen on radiographic study.

Sputum cultures are recommended if the presence of a drug-resistant pathogen or an organism is suspected that is not covered by the usual **empirical therapy** (therapy based on observation and experience, implemented when the condition's exact cause is not known). A Gram stain examination of the sputum provides information on the predominant causative organism. A sputum culture should be collected before initiating antibiotic therapy (Kleinpell & Elpern, 2004). Because of the poor sensitivity and specificity of sputum cultures, any sputum culture results should be correlated with the predominant organisms found on Gram stain examination results. Before treatment, two blood cultures may be done for patients who are seriously ill. Although microbial studies are expected before treatment, initiation of antibiotics should not be delayed.

Arterial blood gases (ABGs), if obtained, usually reveal hypoxemia. Leukocytosis is found in the majority of patients with bacterial pneumonia, usually with a white blood cell (WBC) count greater than 15×10^9/L with the presence of bands (immature neutrophils).

Collaborative Care

Prompt treatment with the appropriate antibiotic almost always cures bacterial and mycoplasma pneumonia. In uncomplicated cases, the patient responds to drug therapy within 48 to 72 hours. Indications of improvement include decreased temperature, improved breathing, and reduced chest pain. Abnormal physical findings can last for more than 7 days.

In addition to antibiotic therapy, supportive measures may be used, including oxygen therapy to treat hypoxemia, analgesics to relieve the chest pain for patient comfort, and antipyretics such as aspirin or acetaminophen for significantly elevated temperature. During the acute febrile phase, the patient's activity should be restricted, and rest should be encouraged and planned.

Most individuals with mild to moderate illness who have no other underlying disease process can be treated on an outpatient basis. If there is a serious underlying disease or if the pneumonia is accompanied by severe dyspnea, hypoxemia, or other complications, the patient should be hospitalized.

Currently, there is no definitive treatment for viral pneumonia. An antiviral drug, amantadine, is approved for oral use in the treatment of influenza A virus. The new neuraminidase inhibitors, zanamivir (Relenza) and oseltamivir (Tamiflu), are active against both influenza A and B (see Chapter 29). An influenza vaccine is available. It is modified annually to reflect the anticipated strains in the upcoming season. Influenza vaccine is considered a mainstay of prevention and is recommended annually for use in the individual considered to be at risk. Individuals at risk for influenza include older adults, nursing home residents, patients with COPD or diabetes mellitus, and health care workers. For older adults with signs and symptoms of influenza, including those who have received the influenza vaccine, treatment with amantadine or a neuraminidase inhibitor is recommended. During epidemics of influenza A, especially in nursing homes, chemoprophylaxis with these agents is recommended for unvaccinated patients, immunodeficient patients, or those who have received the vaccine within the past 2 weeks.

Pneumococcal Vaccine. Pneumococcal vaccine is indicated primarily for the individual considered at risk who (1) has chronic illnesses such as lung and heart disease and diabetes mellitus, (2) is recovering from a severe illness, (3) is 65 years of age or older, or (4) is in a long-term care facility. This is particularly important because the rate of drug-resistant *S. pneumoniae* infections is increasing. Pneumococcal vaccine can be given simultaneously with other vaccines such as the flu vaccine, but each should be administered in a separate site (PHAC, 2007b).

The current recommendation is that pneumococcal vaccine is good for a person's lifetime (PHAC, 2007b). However, in the immunosuppressed individual at risk for development of fatal pneumococcal infection (e.g., asplenic patient; patient with nephrotic syndrome, renal failure, or AIDS; or transplant recipient), revaccination is recommended every 5 years.

Drug Therapy. The main problems with the use of antibiotics to treat pneumonia are the development of resistant strains of organisms and the patient's hypersensitivity or allergic reaction to certain antibiotics.

Most cases of CAP in otherwise healthy adults do not necessitate hospitalization. The Infectious Diseases Society of America/American Thoracic Society guidelines are aimed to classify patients as follows to determine therapy options (Mandell et al., 2007; see earlier section on community-acquired pneumonia):

1. *Outpatients with no modifying factors* (including presence of COPD, recent antibiotics, and risk of aspiration). The treatment of choice is a macrolide (erythromycin, azithromycin, or clarithromycin).
2. *Outpatients with modifying factors.*
   - Patients with COPD who have not had antibiotics or oral steroids within the past 3 months are at increased risk for *H. influenzae* infection. Therefore, extended-spectrum macrolides (azithromycin or clarithromycin) are recommended.
   - Patients with COPD who have had antibiotics or oral steroids within the past 3 months have an increased risk of infection with Gram-negative rods along with the more common CAP pathogens. Therefore, fluoroquinolones (levofloxacin, moxifloxacin, or gatifloxacin) are recommended. Alternative regimens include a macrolide combined with either amoxicillin–clavulanate or a second-generation cephalosporin (e.g., cefuroxime, cefprozil).
   - Patients who are subject to macroaspiration, such as patients with decreased levels of consciousness, should have antibiotics with enhanced activity against anaerobes. Amoxicillin–clavulanate with or without a macrolide is the first choice. Alternatively, a third-generation fluoroquinolone plus either metronidazole or clindamycin may be used.
3. *Nursing home residents.* Nursing home residents are at risk of enteric Gram-negative rod infections in addition to more common pathogens. Therefore, the first choice of treatment is a fluoroquinolone alone or amoxicillin–clavulanate combined with a macrolide. Alternatively, a second-generation cephalosporin with a macrolide may be used.
4. *Patients hospitalized on medical wards.* For these patients, treatment is directed at bacteremic pneumococcal pneumonia as well as infection with *H. influenzae*, enteric Gram-negative bacilli, or severe atypical infections (*Legionella, Chlamydia*). The treatment of choice is a fluoroquinolone. Alternatively, a macrolide combined with a second-, third-, or fourth-generation cephalosporin may be used.

The oral antibiotic therapy administered is frequently empirical treatment with broad-spectrum antibiotics. Once the patient is assigned a CTS treatment classification, therapy can be based on the likely infecting organism.

For HAP, empirical antibiotic therapy should be based on the likely pathogens in the various patient groups. Even with extensive diagnostic testing, an etiological organism is often not identified. It is important to recognize the nonresponding patient. Therapy may require modification based on the patient's culture results or clinical response. Clinical response is evaluated by factors such as a change in fever, sputum purulence, leukocytosis, oxygenation, or radiographic study patterns. Improvement is often not apparent for the first 48 to 72 hours, and therapy need not be altered during this period unless deterioration is noted or culture results dictate that a different antibiotic should be used. Common antibiotics for HAP include cephalosporins (antipseudomonal third generation [ceftazidime]), β-lactam or β-lactamase inhibitor, vancomycin (for MRSA), aminoglycosides (gentamicin), and antipseudomonal quinolones (ciprofloxacin) (Rotstein et al., 2008).

Patients with ventilator-associated pneumonia may experience rapid deterioration. Patients who deteriorate or fail to respond to therapy will require aggressive evaluation to assess noninfectious etiologies, complications, other coexisting infectious processes, or pneumonia caused by a resistant pathogen (Rotstein et al., 2008). It may be necessary to broaden antimicrobial coverage while awaiting results of cultures and other studies, such as computed tomography (CT) scan, ultrasound, or lung scans.

Nutritional Therapy. Fluid intake of at least 3 L/day is important in the supportive treatment of pneumonia. If the patient has heart failure, fluid intake must be individualized. If oral intake cannot be maintained, intravenous (IV) administration of fluids and electrolytes may be necessary for the acutely ill patient. An intake of at least 1500 calories per day should be maintained to provide energy for the increased metabolic processes in the patient. Small, frequent meals are better tolerated by the patient with dyspnea.

NURSING MANAGEMENT: PNEUMONIA

Nursing Assessment

Subjective and objective data that should be obtained from a patient with pneumonia are presented in Table 30-5.

Nursing Diagnoses

Nursing diagnoses for the patient with pneumonia may include, but are not limited to, those presented in Nursing Care Plan (NCP) 30-1.

Planning

The overall goals are that the patient with pneumonia will have (1) clear breath sounds, (2) normal breathing patterns, (3) no

NURSING ASSESSMENT
Table 30-5 Pneumonia

Subjective Data

Important Health Information

Past health history: Lung cancer, COPD, diabetes mellitus, cigarette smoking, alcoholism; recent upper respiratory tract infection, chronic debilitating disease, malnutrition, altered consciousness, AIDS, exposure to chemical toxins, dust, or allergens; immobility or prolonged bed rest

Medications: Use of antibiotics; corticosteroids, chemotherapy, or any other immunosuppressants

Surgery or other treatments: Recent abdominal or thoracic surgery, splenectomy, endotracheal intubation, general anaesthesia; tube feedings

Symptoms

- Fatigue, weakness, malaise
- Anorexia, nausea, vomiting
- Fever, chills
- Dyspnea, cough (productive or nonproductive); nasal congestion; pain with breathing
- Chest pain, sore throat, headache, abdominal pain, muscle aches

Objective Data

General

Fever, restlessness, or lethargy; splinting of affected area

Respiratory

Tachypnea; dyspnea, nasal congestion, pharyngitis; asymmetrical chest movements or retraction; decreased excursion; nasal flaring; use of accessory muscles (neck, abdomen); grunting; crackles, friction rub on auscultation; dullness on percussion over consolidated areas, increased tactile fremitus on palpation; pink, rusty, purulent, green, yellow, or white sputum (amount may be scant to copious)

Cardiovascular

Tachycardia

Neurological

Changes in mental status, ranging from confusion to delirium

Possible Findings

Leukocytosis; abnormal ABGs with ↓ or normal PaO_2, ↓ $PaCO_2$, and ↑ pH initially, and later ↓ PaO_2, ↑ $PaCO_2$, and ↓ pH; positive sputum Gram stain examination and culture; patchy or diffuse infiltrates, abscesses, pleural effusion, or pneumothorax on chest radiographic study.

ABGs, arterial blood gases; *AIDS,* acquired immune deficiency syndrome; *COPD,* chronic obstructive pulmonary disease; *PaO$_2$,* partial pressure of oxygen in arterial blood; *PaCO$_2$,* partial pressure of carbon dioxide in arterial blood.

signs of hypoxia, (4) normal chest radiograph, and (5) no complications related to pneumonia.

▪ Nursing Implementation

▪ Health Promotion

Many nursing interventions are available to help prevent the occurrence of pneumonia as well as the morbidity associated with it. Teaching a patient to practise good health habits, such as proper diet and hygiene, adequate rest, and regular exercise, can help the patient maintain the natural resistance to infecting organisms. If possible, exposure to URIs should be avoided. If a URI occurs, it should be treated promptly with supportive measures (e.g., rest, fluids). If symptoms persist for more than 7 days, the person should obtain medical care. The individual at risk for pneumonia (e.g., the chronically ill, the older adult) should be encouraged to obtain both influenza and pneumococcal vaccines.

In the hospital, the nursing role involves identifying the patient at risk (see Table 30-1) and taking measures to prevent the development of pneumonia. The patient with altered consciousness should be placed in positions (e.g., side-lying, upright) that will prevent or minimize the risk of aspiration. The patient should be turned and repositioned at least every 2 hours to facilitate adequate lung expansion and to discourage pooling of secretions.

The patient who has a feeding tube generally requires that measures be taken to prevent aspiration (see Chapter 42). Although the feeding tube is small, an interruption in the integrity of the lower esophageal sphincter still exists, which can allow reflux of gastric and intestinal contents. The patient who has difficulty swallowing (e.g., patient who has had a stroke) needs assistance in eating, drinking, and taking medication to prevent aspiration. The patient who has recently had surgery and others who are immobile need assistance with turning and measures to facilitate deep breathing at frequent intervals (see Chapter 22). The nurse must be careful to avoid overmedication with narcotics or sedatives, which can cause a depressed cough reflex and accumulation of fluid in the lungs. Presence of the gag reflex should be ascertained before the administration of fluids or food to the individual who has had local anaesthesia to the throat.

Strict medical asepsis and adherence to infection control guidelines should be practised by the nurse to reduce the incidence of hospital-associated infections. Poor handwashing practices allow spread of pathogens via the hands of the health care worker. Staff should wash their hands, or use hand rubs with 60 to 90% alcohol if hands are not visibly soiled (Community and Hospital Infection Control Association, 2008), before each time they provide care to a patient. Respiratory devices can harbour microorganisms and have been associated with outbreaks of pneumonia. Strict sterile aseptic technique should be used when suctioning the trachea of a patient.

▪ Acute Intervention

Although many patients with pneumonia are treated on an outpatient basis, the NCP for a patient with pneumonia (see NCP 30-1) is applicable to both these individuals as well as in-hospital patients. It is important for the nurse to remember that pneumonia is an acute, infectious disease. Although most cases of pneumonia are potentially completely curable, complications can result. The nurse must be aware of these complications and their manifestations. The infection control nurse can be a valuable resource in assisting with the care of patients with pneumonia.

Therapeutic positioning for patients with pneumonia ensures stable oxygenation status. The "good lung down" position is used for patients with unilateral lung disease, in whom better oxygenation is achieved when the unaffected lung (good lung) is placed in the down (lateral) position to achieve maximum lung expansion. Incentive spirometry, turning, coughing, and deep breathing

NURSING CARE PLAN 30-1

Pneumonia

NURSING DIAGNOSIS	**Ineffective breathing pattern** *related to* inflammation and pain *as evidenced by* rapid respirations, dyspnea, tachypnea, nasal flaring, or altered chest excursion, or some combination
Expected Patient Outcomes	**Nursing Interventions and *Rationales***
• Has normal breathing pattern and rate • Has normal PaO$_2$	• Monitor respiratory and oxygenation status *to provide baseline assessment.* • Auscultate breath sounds, noting areas of decreased or absent ventilation, and presence of adventitious sounds *to assess patient's response to therapy.* • Position to minimize respiratory efforts (e.g., elevate head of bed) *to reduce oxygen needs.* • Monitor effects of position change on oxygenation (SpO$_2$) levels *to assess appropriate position.* • Initiate and maintain supplemental oxygen as prescribed *to improve respiratory status.* • Administer medications (e.g., bronchodilators and inhalers) *that promote airway patency and gas exchange.*
NURSING DIAGNOSIS	**Ineffective airway clearance** *related to* thick secretions *as evidenced by* ineffective cough or thick, tenacious sputum, abnormal breath sounds, or dyspnea, or some combination
Expected Patient Outcomes	**Nursing Interventions and *Rationales***
• Has normal respiratory rate • Has clear breath sounds • Is able to clear sputum	• Monitor rate, rhythm, depth, and effort of respirations *to provide baseline assessment.* • Auscultate breath sounds, noting areas of decreased or absent ventilation and presence of adventitious sounds *to obtain ongoing data on patient's response to therapy.* • Assist patient to a sitting position with head slightly flexed, shoulders relaxed, and knees flexed *to improve respiratory status.* • Encourage use of incentive spirometry as appropriate *to aid in lung expansion and prevent atelectasis.* • Promote systemic fluid hydration as appropriate *to help liquefy secretions.*
NURSING DIAGNOSIS	**Acute pain** *related to* inflammation and ineffective pain management and/or comfort measures *as evidenced by* pleuritic chest pain, pleural friction rub, shallow respirations, or decreased breath sounds, or some combination
Expected Patient Outcomes	**Nursing Interventions and *Rationales***
• Reports satisfactory pain control • Uses pain control measures effectively	• Perform a comprehensive assessment of pain to include location, characteristics, onset and duration, frequency, quality, intensity or severity of pain, and precipitating factors *to create baseline status of pain.* • Consider cultural influences possibly affecting pain response. • Encourage patient to monitor own pain and to intervene appropriately *to allow independence and prepare for discharge.* • Teach the use of nonpharmacological techniques (e.g., biofeedback, hypnosis, relaxation, guided imagery, music therapy, distraction, and massage) before, after, and, if possible, during painful activities; before pain occurs or increases; and along with other pain relief measures *to relieve pain and reduce the need for analgesia.* • Use pain control measures before pain becomes severe *because mild to moderate pain is controlled more quickly.* • Medicate before an activity to increase participation, but evaluate the hazard of sedation, *to help minimize pain that will be experienced.*

Continued

NURSING CARE PLAN 30-1

Pneumonia—cont'd

NURSING DIAGNOSIS	**Imbalanced nutrition: less than body requirements** *related to* increased metabolism, fatigue, and anorexia *as evidenced by* weight loss and patient's statement of foul taste in mouth
Expected Patient Outcomes	**Nursing Interventions and *Rationales***
• Maintains stable weight • Balances intake and output • Has hydrated skin and mucous membranes • Maintains output >30 mL/hr	• Weigh patient at specified intervals *to assess status of weight.* • Schedule treatment and procedures at times other than feeding times *to conserve energy for breathing.* • Monitor food and fluid ingested and calculate daily caloric intake, as appropriate, *to assess if meeting patient's needs.* • Determine food preferences with consideration of cultural and religious preferences *to provide appropriate intake.* • Provide oxygen therapy via nasal cannula if needed during meals *to maintain oxygen status.* • Position patient in high Fowler's position at meal times, if appropriate, *to help relieve dyspnea.* • Provide patient with high-protein, high-calorie, nutritious finger foods and drinks that can be readily consumed, as appropriate, *to provide for nutritional needs.*
NURSING DIAGNOSIS	**Activity intolerance** *related to* interrupted sleep–wake cycle, hypoxia, and weakness *as evidenced by* fatigue, unwillingness or inability to exert self, dyspnea, increased pulse and respiration, or dizziness on exertion, or some combination
Expected Patient Outcomes	**Nursing Interventions and *Rationales***
• Has normal oxygen saturation in response to activity • Has normal pulse rate in response to activity • Performs ADLs	• Determine patient's physical limitations *to establish patient's needs and capabilities.* • Monitor patient's cardiorespiratory and oxygen response to activity (e.g., tachycardia, other dysrhythmias, dyspnea, diaphoresis, pallor, hemodynamic pressures, respiratory rate) *to help establish obtainable goals and create appropriate interventions.* • Plan activities for periods when patient has the most energy and encourage alternate rest and activity periods *to provide activity based on patient's response and promote increased feeling of accomplishment.* • Encourage afternoon nap, if appropriate, *to reduce stress and promote rest.*

ADLs, activities of daily living; *PaO₂,* partial pressure of oxygen in arterial blood; *SpO₂,* oxygen saturation as measured by pulse oximetry.

all increase lung volume, mobilize secretions, and prevent atelectasis. Exercise and early ambulation augment bronchial hygiene and are encouraged as tolerated.

▪ Ambulatory and Home Care

The patient needs to be reassured that complete recovery from pneumonia is possible. It is extremely important to emphasize the need to take all of any drugs prescribed and to return for follow-up medical care and evaluation. The patient needs to be taught about the drug–drug and the food–drug interactions for the prescribed antibiotic. Adequate rest is needed to maintain progress toward recovery and to prevent a relapse. The patient should be told that it may be weeks before the usual vigour and sense of well-being are felt. A prolonged period of convalescence may be necessary for the older adult or chronically ill patient.

The patient considered to be at risk for pneumonia should be told about available vaccines and should discuss them with the health care provider. Deep breathing exercises should be practised for 6 to 8 weeks after the patient is discharged from the hospital.

▪ Evaluation

The expected outcomes for the patient with pneumonia are presented in NCP 30-1.

Severe Acute Respiratory Syndrome

Severe acute respiratory syndrome (SARS) first appeared in China and then spread to other countries. The first cases in Canada were identified in March 2003. These initial cases were in people who had travelled to Hong Kong. SARS is caused by a previously unknown type of coronavirus. (Coronaviruses cause mild to moderate upper respiratory symptoms, such as the common cold.) In addition, factors related to the infected person's immune system and factors in the environment may affect the symptoms and severity of SARS. SARS is spread through close contact with someone who is infected with the SARS coronavirus. Examples of close contact include living in the same household, providing care to someone with SARS, or having direct contact with respiratory secretions and body fluids of someone affected by SARS. To date, it appears that people with SARS are not contagious until they develop symptoms, which may take up to 10 days from the time they were in close contact with someone who has SARS (Health Canada, 2006a).

The symptoms of SARS include a fever higher than 38°C (>100.4°F), followed by respiratory symptoms, such as cough, shortness of breath, and difficulty breathing. Other symptoms may include chills, headaches, muscle aches, sore throat, and diarrhea.

There are no specific tests to diagnose SARS. The diagnosis is based on the presence of the early signs of SARS including fever over 38°C (>100.4°F), a cough or breathing difficulty, and a chest radiographic study that shows a condition consistent with SARS infection, such as pneumonia or respiratory distress syndrome (RDS). For diagnosis of SARS, some risk factors for it must be present and there must be no other cause of illness found.

There is no vaccine or cure for SARS. Patients with SARS receive the same supportive treatment as a patient with serious viral pneumonia, including oxygen therapy. The use of various drugs, such as antiviral drugs, is currently being tested.

The following precautions are recommended to reduce the risk of SARS: (1) ensure good hand hygiene by frequent, thorough, regular handwashing for at least 20 seconds using soap and warm water or by using hand rubs with 60 to 90% alcohol if hands are not visibly soiled (Community and Hospital Infection Control Association, 2008) and (2) check Health Canada travel advisories for information about regions affected by SARS.

Tuberculosis

Tuberculosis (TB) is an infectious disease caused by *M. tuberculosis*. It usually involves the lungs, but it also occurs in the larynx, the kidneys, the bones, the adrenal glands, the lymph nodes, and the meninges and can be disseminated throughout the body. TB kills more people worldwide than any other infectious disease. It is estimated that between 19 and 43% of the world's population is infected with *M. tuberculosis*. In Canada, the number of reported cases of active TB has remained relatively stable with an average of 1623 cases per year. In 2009, foreign-born individuals accounted for 63%, Canadian-born people for 15%, and Canadian-born Aboriginals for 21% of all reported cases (PHAC, 2010). Pulmonary TB continues to be the main diagnostic site of disease, representing 68% of all reported cases (PHAC, 2010).

With the introduction of chemotherapeutic agents (streptomycin, isoniazid [INH]) in the late 1940s and early 1950s, there was a dramatic decrease in the prevalence of TB. However, TB did not disappear by 2000 as was previously anticipated. The major factors for the continued problem include the following (Health Canada, 2007):

1. *Multidrug-resistant (MDR) strains of* M. tuberculosis: MDR strains of TB have developed because of poor adherence to drug therapy leading to treatment failure and the development of resistant strains.
2. *Continued exposure to populations in which TB is more prevalent:* Continued immigration from areas where TB is more prevalent and travel to these countries increases the risk. Canadian immigration laws require that all immigrants older than age 10 be screened for active TB. There are regulations related to the screening results and their implications for entry into Canada and subsequent follow-up.

3. *The presence of pools of high-risk groups.* TB is seen disproportionately in the poor, the underserved, and minorities. Aboriginal peoples (TB rates for Aboriginals remain six times higher than overall Canadian rates of 4.7 [Health Canada, 2009]), homeless people, people who live in long-term care or correctional facilities, people living in inner-city slums, injection drug users, alcoholics, and people working or living with any of these groups have an increased risk of TB infection. Individuals who are immunosuppressed from any etiology (e.g., HIV infection, malignancy), those with diabetes mellitus, those receiving long-term corticosteroid therapy, and smokers are at an increased risk of TB infection. The Tuberculosis Elimination Strategy was introduced in 1992 by Health Canada. Its goals are TB reduction in on-reserve First Nations populations by adopting the Global Stop TB rate reduction targets of 3.6 per 100,000 by 2015. The main objectives of this program are prevention of further occurrence and emergence of drug-resistant TB (Assembly of First Nations, 2011).

DETERMINANTS OF HEALTH
Tuberculosis

Income and Social Status
- Low socioeconomic groups have higher rates of TB (Health Canada, 2009).

Physical Environment
- Overcrowding and homelessness lead to TB (Public Health Agency of Canada/Canadian Lung Association, 2007).

Personal Health Practices and Coping Skills
- Smoking one pack of cigarettes or more per day increases the risk for TB (Health Canada, 2007).
- Alcohol and substance use increases the risk for TB (Public Health Agency of Canada, 2009).

Culture
- TB rates among First Nations peoples are six times higher than overall Canadian rates (Public Health Agency of Canada, 2009).
- Approximately 63% of immigrants to Canada come from countries with high TB incidence (Public Health Agency of Canada, 2009).

TB, tuberculosis.

Etiology and Pathophysiology

M. tuberculosis, a Gram-positive, acid-fast bacillus, is usually spread from person to person via airborne droplets, which are produced when the infected individual with pulmonary or laryngeal TB coughs, sneezes, speaks, or sings. Once released into a room, the organisms are dispersed and can be inhaled. TB is not highly infectious, and transmission usually requires close, frequent, or prolonged exposure. Brief exposure to a few tubercle bacilli rarely causes an infection. The disease cannot be spread by hands, books, glasses, dishes, or other fomites.

The very small droplets, 1 to 5 μm (micrometres) in size, contain *M. tuberculosis*. Because they are so small, the particles remain airborne indoors for minutes to hours. Once inhaled, these small particles lodge in the bronchiole and alveolus. Factors that influence the likelihood of transmission include the (1) number of organisms expelled into the air, (2) concentration of organisms (small spaces with limited ventilation would mean higher concentration), (3) length of time of exposure, and (4) immune system of the exposed person. *M. tuberculosis* replicates slowly and spreads via the lymphatic system. The organisms find favourable environments for growth primarily in the upper lobes of the lungs, kidneys, epiphyses of the bone, cerebral cortex, and adrenal glands.

Healing of the primary lesion usually takes place by resolution, fibrosis, and calcification. The granulation tissue surrounding the lesion may become more fibrous and form a collagenous scar around the tubercle. A *Ghon complex* is formed, consisting of the Ghon tubercle and regional lymph nodes. Calcified Ghon complexes may be seen on chest radiographic studies.

When a TB lesion regresses and heals, the infection enters a latent period in which it may persist without producing clinical symptoms of illness. The infection may develop into clinical disease if the persisting organisms begin to multiply rapidly, or it may remain dormant.

Persons who are infected with *M. tuberculosis*, but who do not have TB disease, cannot spread the infection to other people. TB infection occurs when the bacteria are inhaled but there is an ineffective immune response and the bacteria become inactive. The majority of people mount effective immune responses to encapsulate these organisms for the rest of their lives, preventing primary infection from progressing to disease. TB infection in a person who does not have the active TB disease is not considered a case of TB and is often referred to as *latent tuberculosis infection* (LTBI). If the initial immune response is not adequate, control of the organisms is not maintained and clinical disease results. Dormant but viable organisms persist for years. Reactivation of TB can occur if the host's defence mechanisms become impaired. The reasons for reactivation are not well understood, but they are related to decreased resistance found in older adults, individuals with concomitant diseases, and those who receive immunosuppressive therapy.

Classification

The American Thoracic Association and American Lung Association adopted a classification system that covers the entire population (Table 30-6).

Clinical Manifestations

In the early stages of TB, the person is usually free of symptoms. Many cases are found incidentally when routine chest radiographic studies are done, especially in older adults.

Systemic manifestations may initially consist of fatigue, malaise, anorexia, weight loss, low-grade fevers, and night sweats. The weight loss may not be excessive until late in the disease and is often attributed to overwork or other factors.

A characteristic pulmonary manifestation is a cough that becomes frequent and produces mucoid or mucopurulent sputum. Dyspnea is unusual. Chest pain characterized as dull or tight may be present. Hemoptysis is not a common finding and is usually associated with more advanced cases. Sometimes TB has more acute, sudden manifestations: the patient has high fever, chills, generalized flulike symptoms, pleuritic pain, and a productive cough.

The HIV-infected patient with TB often has atypical physical examination and chest radiographic examination findings. Classical signs such as fever, cough, and weight loss may be attributed to PCP or other HIV-associated opportunistic diseases. Clinical manifestations of respiratory problems in patients with HIV must be carefully investigated to determine the cause.

Complications

Miliary Tuberculosis. If a necrotic Ghon complex erodes through a blood vessel, large numbers of organisms invade the bloodstream and spread to all body organs. This is called *miliary* or *hematogenous* TB. The patient may be either acutely ill with fever, dyspnea, and cyanosis or chronically ill with systemic manifestations of weight loss, fever, and gastrointestinal (GI) disturbance. Hepatomegaly, splenomegaly, and generalized lymphadenopathy may be present.

Pleural Effusion and Empyema. A pleural effusion is caused by the release of caseous material into the pleural space. The bacteria-containing material triggers an inflammatory reaction and a pleural exudate of protein-rich fluid. A form of pleurisy called *dry pleurisy* may result from a superficial tubercular lesion involving the pleura. It appears as localized pleuritic pain on deep inspiration. Empyema is less common than effusion but may

Table 30-6 Classification of Tuberculosis		
CLASS	**DESCRIPTION**	**CHARACTERISTICS**
Class 0	No TB exposure	No TB exposure, not infected (no history of exposure, negative tuberculin skin test)
Class 1	TB exposure, no infection	TB exposure, no evidence of infection (history of exposure, negative tuberculin skin test)
Class 2	Latent TB infection, no disease	TB infection without disease (significant reaction to tuberculin skin test, negative bacteriological studies, no radiographic findings compatible with TB, no clinical evidence of TB)
Class 3	TB clinically active	TB infection with clinically active disease (positive bacteriological studies or both a significant reaction to tuberculin skin test and clinical or radiographic evidence of current disease)
Class 4	TB, but not clinically active	No current disease (history of previous episode of TB or abnormal, stable radiographic findings in a person with a significant reaction to tuberculin skin test; negative bacteriological studies if done; no clinical or radiographic evidence of current disease)
Class 5	TB suspect	TB suspect (diagnosis pending); person should not be in this classification for >3 mo

TB, tuberculosis.
Source: American Thoracic Society. (2000). Diagnostic standards and classification of tuberculosis in adults and children. *American Journal of Respiratory & Critical Care Medicine, 161,* 1376-1395. Retrieved from *http://ajrccm.atsjournals.org/content/161/4/1376.full*

occur from large numbers of organisms spilling into the pleural space, usually from rupture of a cavity.

Tuberculosis Pneumonia. Acute pneumonia may result when large amounts of tubercle bacilli are discharged from the liquefied necrotic lesion into the lung or lymph nodes. The clinical manifestations are similar to those of bacterial pneumonia, including chills, fever, productive cough, pleuritic pain, and leukocytosis.

Other Organ Involvement. Although the lungs are the primary site of TB, other body organs may also be involved. The meninges may become infected. Bone and joint tissue may be involved in the infectious disease process. The kidneys, the adrenal glands, the lymph nodes, and the genital tract (in both females and males) may also be infected.

Diagnostic Studies

Tuberculin Skin Testing. The body's immune response can be demonstrated by hypersensitivity to a tuberculin skin test. A positive reaction occurs 2 to 12 weeks after the initial infection, corresponding to the time needed to mount an immune response.

Purified protein derivative (PPD) of tuberculin is used primarily to detect the delayed hypersensitivity response. (The procedure for performing the tuberculin skin test is described in Chapter 28.) Once acquired, sensitivity to tuberculin tends to persist throughout life. A positive reaction indicates the presence of a TB infection, but it does not show whether the infection is latent or active, that is, causing a clinical illness. Because the response to TB skin testing may be decreased in the immunocompromised patient, induration reactions equal to or greater than 5 mm are considered positive. Sometimes, a repeat PPD can cause an accelerated response (the "booster" effect). Thus, two-step testing is recommended for initial screening of health care workers who will be getting regularly retested in the future and for those who have a decreased response to allergens. This procedure helps identify individuals with past disease and prevent a later positive PPD test from being misinterpreted as a new, infection-related PPD conversion. See Chapter 28, Table 28-12, for guidelines in interpreting TB skin tests. Recent guidelines for targeted tuberculin testing emphasize targeting only high-risk groups and discourage testing low-risk individuals (PHAC/Canadian Lung Association, 2007).

Chest Radiograph Study. Although the findings on chest radiographic examination are important, it is not possible to make a diagnosis of TB solely on the basis of this examination. This is because other diseases can mimic the radiographic appearance of TB. The abnormality most commonly found in TB is multinodular lymph node involvement with cavitation in the upper lobes of the lungs. Calcification of the lung lesions generally occurs within several years of the infection.

Bacteriological Studies. The demonstration of tubercle bacilli bacteriologically is essential for establishing a diagnosis. Microscopic examination of stained sputum smears for acid-fast bacilli (AFB) is usually the first bacteriological evidence of the presence of tubercle bacilli. Three consecutive sputum specimens collected on different days are obtained and sent for smear and culture. In addition to sputum, material for examination can be obtained from gastric washings, cerebrospinal fluid (CSF), or pus from an abscess.

The most accurate means of diagnosis is the culture technique. The major disadvantage of this method is that it may take 6 to 8 weeks for the mycobacterium to grow. The advantage is that it can detect small quantities (as few as 10 bacteria/mL of specimen).

Nucleic acid amplification (NAA) is a rapid diagnostic test for TB. Test results are available in a few hours. They are more sensitive than AFB smears, but less sensitive than TB cultures. NAA does not replace routine sputum smears and cultures, but it offers a health care provider increased confidence in the diagnosis (PHAC/Canadian Lung Association, 2007).

Since 2007, Canada has been testing using QuantiFERON-TB Gold In-Tube. The patient's blood is mixed with mycobacterial antigens and is then measured using an enzyme-linked immunosorbent assay (ELISA). If the patient is infected with TB organisms, the lymphocytes in the blood will recognize the antigens. Guidelines for when to use this rapid diagnostic tool are being developed (PHAC, 2007c).

Collaborative Care

Hospitalization for initial treatment of TB is not necessary in most patients. Most patients are treated on an outpatient basis (Table 30-7), and many can continue to work and maintain their lifestyles with few changes. Hospitalization may be used for diagnostic evaluation, for the severely ill or debilitated, and for those who experience adverse drug reactions or treatment failures.

The mainstay of TB treatment is drug therapy. Drug therapy is used to treat an individual with clinical disease and to prevent disease in an infected person.

Drug Therapy.

Active Disease. Standard therapy has been revised because of the increase in prevalence of MDR TB. MDR TB occurs when resistance develops to two or more anti-TB drugs. The patient with active TB should be managed aggressively; treatment usually consists of a combination of at least four drugs. The reason for combination therapy is to increase the therapeutic effectiveness and decrease the development of resistant strains of *M. tuberculosis*. It has been shown that single-drug therapy can result in rapid development of resistant strains.

The five primary drugs used are INH, rifampin (RMP), pyrazinamide, streptomycin, and ethambutol (Table 30-8). Various drug and dosing regimens are available (Tables 30-9, and 30-10; see also Table 30-8). Fixed-dose combination anti-TB drugs may enhance adherence to treatment recommendations. Combinations of INH and RMP (Rifamate) (Table 30-11) and of INH, RMP, and pyrazinamide (Rifater) are available to simplify therapy. Patients on antiretroviral drugs for HIV cannot take RMP because

COLLABORATIVE CARE

Table 30-7 Tuberculosis

Diagnostic	*Collaborative Therapy*
• History and physical examination	• Long-term treatment with antimicrobial drugs (see Tables 30-8 to 30-11)
• Tuberculin skin test	
• Chest radiograph study	• Follow-up bacteriological studies and chest radiographic examinations
• Bacteriological studies	
• Sputum smear	
• Sputum culture	

it can impair the effectiveness of the antiretroviral drugs. Other drugs are primarily used for treatment of resistant strains or if the patient develops adverse effects to the primary drugs. Many second-line drugs carry a greater risk of adverse effects and necessitate closer monitoring. Other drugs for the treatment of TB that have not been placed in categories of first- or second-line drugs include the quinolones, especially ciprofloxacin (Cipro), ofloxacin (Floxin), and sparfloxacin (Zagam). Rifapentine (Priftin) is an antibiotic that can be used to treat TB in combination with other anti-TB drugs.

In follow-up care for patients on long-term therapy, it is important to monitor the effectiveness of drugs and the development of adverse effects. Usually, sputum specimens are initially obtained weekly and then monthly to assess the effectiveness of the medication. The regimen is considered to be effective if the patient converts to a negative TB sputum status.

Although TB tends to have a rapidly progressive course in the patient co-infected with HIV, it responds well to standard medication. The co-infected patient should receive treatment for TB for at least 6 months beyond the conversion of sputum cultures to negative status.

An important reason for follow-up care in the patient with TB is to ensure adherence to the treatment regimen. Nonadherence is a major factor in the emergence of multidrug resistance and treatment failures. Many individuals do not adhere to the treatment program in spite of understanding the disease process

DRUG THERAPY

Table 30-8 Tuberculosis

DRUG	MECHANISMS OF ACTION	ADVERSE EFFECTS	COMMENTS
First-Line Drugs			
Isoniazid (INH)	Bacteriocidal; interferes with DNA metabolism of tubercle bacillus	Peripheral neuritis, hepatotoxicity, hypersensitivity (skin rash, arthralgia, fever), optic neuritis	Metabolism primarily by liver and excretion by kidneys, pyridoxine (vitamin B$_6$) administration during high-dose therapy as prophylactic measure; use as single prophylactic agent for active TB in individuals whose PPD converts to positive; ability to cross blood–brain barrier; safe in pregnancy
Rifampin/RMP (Rifadin)	Bacteriocidal; has broad-spectrum effects, inhibits RNA polymerase of tubercle bacillus	Hepatitis, febrile reaction, GI disturbance, peripheral neuropathy, hypersensitivity	Most common use with INH; low incidence of adverse effects; suppression of effect of birth control pills; possible orange urine and bodily fluids; safe in pregnancy
Ethambutol	Bacteriostatic; inhibits RNA synthesis	Skin rash, GI disturbance, malaise, peripheral neuritis, optic neuritis	Adverse effects uncommon and reversible with discontinuation of drug; most common use as substitute drug when adverse effects occur with INH or RMP; safe in pregnancy
Pyrazinamide	Bacteriocidal; exact mechanism unknown	Fever, skin rash, hyperuricemia, GI symptoms, jaundice (rare)	High rate of effectiveness when used with streptomycin or capreomycin
Second-Line Drugs			
Rifapentine (Priftin)	Antibiotic; inhibits RNA	GI disturbance	Orange discoloration of bodily fluids; not to be used in patients with porphyria
Rifabutin (Mycobutin)	Inhibits DNA-dependent RNA polymerase activity	Hepatotoxicity, thrombocytopenia, rash, uveitis, nephrotoxicity	Monitor LFTs, CBC; orange discoloration of bodily fluids
Streptomycin	Bacteriocidal; inhibits protein synthesis	Ototoxicity (CN VIII), nephrotoxicity, hypersensitivity	Cautious use in older adults, those with renal disease, and pregnant women; must be given parenterally; check baseline hearing, Romberg's sign, and creatinine levels
Ethionamide (Trecator)	Inhibits protein synthesis	GI disturbance, hepatotoxicity, hypersensitivity	Valuable for treatment of resistant organisms; contraindicated in pregnancy
Capreomycin (Capastat)	Bacteriocidal; inhibits protein synthesis	Ototoxicity, nephrotoxicity	Cautious use in older adults; check baseline hearing, Romberg's sign, and creatinine levels
Kanamycin (Kantrex) and amikacin	Bacteriocidal; interferes with protein synthesis	Ototoxicity, nephrotoxicity	Use in selected cases for treatment of resistant strains; check baseline hearing, Romberg's sign, and creatinine levels
PAS	Bacteriocidal; interferes with metabolism of tubercle bacillus	GI disturbance (frequent), hypersensitivity, hepatotoxicity	Interference with absorption of RMP; infrequent use
Cycloserine (Seromycin)	Bacteriocidal–bacteriostatic; inhibits cell-wall synthesis	Personality changes, psychosis, rash	Contraindicated for use in individuals with a history of psychosis; use in treatment of resistant strains

CBC, complete blood count; *CN,* cranial nerve; *GI,* gastrointestinal; *LFTs,* liver function tests; *PAS,* para-aminosalicylic acid; *PPD,* purified protein derivative; *TB,* tuberculosis.

DRUG THERAPY

Table 30-9 Drug Regimen Options for Treatment of Tuberculosis

| REGIMEN | DURATION (MO) | | | NO. DOSES |
	INTENSIVE	CONTINUING	TOTAL	
INH + RMP + PZA +/- EMB	2	4	6	95
INH + RMP +/- EMB	1-2	7-8	9	120

EMB, ethambutol; *INH*, isoniazid; *PZA*, pyrazinamide; *RMP*, rifampin.
Source: Public Health Agency of Canada/Canadian Lung Association. (2007). *Canadian tuberculosis standards* (6th ed., p. 118, Table 2). Retrieved from *http://www.phac-aspc.gc.ca/tbpc-latb/pubs/pdf/tbstand07_e.pdf*. Reproduced with the permission of the Minister of Public Works and Government Services Canada, 2012.

Table 30-10 Dose-Interval Options for Isoniazid, Rifampin, and Pyrazinamide Regimens

OPTION 1: 95 DOSES	OPTION 2: 60 DOSES
Administer INH, RMP, and PZA daily for 2 mo, followed by INH and RMP daily or 2/wk for 4 mo	Administer INH, RMP, and PZA daily for 2 wk, followed by INH, RMP, and PZA 2/wk for 6 wk, followed by INH and RMP 2/wk for 4 mo

INH, isoniazid; *PZA*, pyrazinamide; *RMP*, rifampin.
Source: Public Health Agency of Canada/Canadian Lung Association. (2007). *Canadian tuberculosis standards* (6th ed., p. 118, Table 3). Retrieved from *http://www.phac-aspc.gc.ca/tbpc-latb/pubs/pdf/tbstand07_e.pdf*. Reproduced with the permission of the Minister of Public Works and Government Services Canada, 2012.

Table 30-11 Dose-Interval Options for Isoniazid and Rifampin Regimens

OPTION 1	OPTION 2	OPTION 3
Administer INH and RMP daily for 2 mo, followed by INH and RMP 2/wk for 7 mo	Administer INH and RMP daily for 1 mo, followed by INH and RMP 2/wk for 8 mo	Administer INH and RMP daily for 9 mo

INH, isoniazid; *RMP*, rifampin.
Source: Public Health Agency of Canada/Canadian Lung Association. (2007). *Canadian tuberculosis standards* (6th ed., p. 119, Table 4). Retrieved from *http://www.phac-aspc.gc.ca/tbpc-latb/pubs/pdf/tbstand07_e.pdf*. Reproduced with the permission of the Minister of Public Works and Government Services Canada, 2012.

and the value of treatment. Directly observed therapy (DOT) is recommended for patients known to be at risk for nonadherence with therapy. DOT is an expensive but essential public health issue. DOT involves observing the ingestion of every dose of medication for the TB patient's entire course of treatment. Completing therapy is important because of the danger of reactivation of TB and the development of MDR TB seen in patients who do not complete the full course of therapy. In many areas, the public health nurse administers DOT at a clinic site. The patient needs to have follow-up visits for 12 months after completion of therapy to check for the presence of resistant strains.

Teaching patients about the adverse effects of these drugs and when to seek medical attention is critical. The major adverse

Table 30-12 Indications for Treatment of Latent Tuberculosis Infection

Treatment is indicated with positive tuberculin skin tests in persons with the following:

- Known or suspected HIV infection
- Recent contact of infectious TB
- Presence of lung scar

Treatment is indicated with significant tuberculin skin test reaction in the following situations:

- Special clinical situations (immunosuppression therapy, use of corticosteroids, diabetes mellitus, silicosis, chronic renal failure, organ transplant, hematological malignancies)
- If the person was born in high-prevalence country or is a resident in communal settings, a health care worker, Aboriginal, or Inuit

HIV, human immunodeficiency virus, *TB*, tuberculosis.
Source: Adapted from Public Health Agency of Canada/Canadian Lung Association. (2007). *Canadian tuberculosis standards* (6th ed., Chapter 4). Retrieved from *http://www.phac-aspc.gc.ca/tbpc-latb/pubs/pdf/tbstand07_e.pdf*

effect of INH, RMP, and pyrazinamide is hepatitis. Liver function tests should be monitored. Baseline liver function tests are done at the start of treatment, and routine monitoring of liver function tests is done if baseline tests are abnormal.

Latent Tuberculosis Infection. Latent TB infection (LTBI) occurs when an individual becomes infected with *M. tuberculosis* but does not become acutely ill. Drug therapy can be used to prevent a TB infection from developing into a clinical disease. Previously used terms such as "preventive therapy" and "chemoprophylaxis" were confusing. Therefore, LTBI is the preferred terminology. The indications for treatment of LTBI are presented in Table 30-12.

The drug generally used in treatment of LTBI is INH. It is effective and inexpensive and can be administered orally.

Vaccine. Immunization with bacille Calmette-Guérin (BCG) vaccine to prevent TB is currently in use in many parts of the world. Although millions of people have been vaccinated with BCG, the efficacy of the vaccine is not clear. BCG vaccination can result in a positive PPD reaction. The BCG vaccine reaction will wane over time, and the mean PPD reaction size among persons who received BCG is less than 10 mm. Because it may be difficult to determine the relevance of increases in individuals who have undergone BCG vaccination, the PHAC/Canadian Lung Association (2007) recommends that a conversion to "positive" be defined as a reaction of 10 mm or greater. Persons who receive BCG are from high-prevalence areas of the world, and it is important that a positive skin reaction be evaluated for TB.

NURSING MANAGEMENT: TUBERCULOSIS

Nursing Assessment

It is important to determine whether the patient was ever exposed to a person with TB. The patient should be assessed for productive cough, night sweats, afternoon temperature elevation, weight loss, pleuritic chest pain, and crackles over the apices of the lungs. If the patient has a productive cough, an early-morning sputum specimen will be required for an AFB smear to detect the presence of mycobacteria.

Nursing Diagnoses

Nursing diagnoses for the patient with TB may include, but are not limited to, the following:
- Ineffective breathing pattern *related to* decreased lung capacity.
- Imbalanced nutrition: less than body requirements *related to* chronic poor appetite, fatigue, and productive cough.
- Noncompliance *related to* lack of knowledge of disease process, lack of motivation, and long-term nature of treatment.
- Ineffective health maintenance *related to* lack of knowledge about the disease process and therapeutic regimen.
- Activity intolerance *related to* fatigue, decreased nutritional status, and chronic febrile episodes.

Planning

The overall goals are that the patient with TB will (1) comply with the therapeutic regimen, (2) have no recurrence of disease, (3) have normal pulmonary function, and (4) take appropriate measures to prevent the spread of the disease.

Nursing Implementation

Health Promotion

The ultimate goal related to TB in Canada is eradication. Selective screening programs in known risk groups are of value in detecting individuals with TB. The person with a positive tuberculin skin test should have a chest radiographic examination to assess for the presence of TB. Another important measure is to identify the contacts of the individual who has TB. These contacts should be assessed for the possibility of infection and the need for prophylactic drug therapy.

When an individual has respiratory symptoms such as cough, dyspnea, or sputum production, especially if accompanied by a history of night sweats or unexplained weight loss, the nurse should assess for exposure to persons with TB. Even if the suspected respiratory problem is something else, such as emphysema, pneumonia, or lung cancer, it is possible that the patient may also have TB.

Acute Intervention

Acute in-hospital care is seldom required for the patient with TB. If hospitalization is needed, it is usually for a brief period. Patients strongly suspected of having TB should (1) be placed in respiratory isolation; (2) receive four-drug therapy; and (3) receive an immediate medical workup, including chest radiographic examination, sputum smear, and culture. Respiratory isolation is indicated for the patient with pulmonary or laryngeal TB until the patient is considered to be noninfectious (effective drug therapy, improving clinically, three negative AFB smears). A negative-pressure isolation room that offers six or more exchanges per hour may be used. Ultraviolet radiation of the air in the upper part of the room is another approach to reduce airborne TB organisms. Ultraviolet lights are commonly seen in clinics and homeless shelters. Masks are needed to filter out droplet nuclei. Use of institution-approved high-efficiency particulate air (HEPA) masks is indicated. The mask must be moulded to fit tightly around the nose and mouth.

The patient should be taught to cover the nose and mouth with paper tissue every time he or she coughs, sneezes, or produces sputum. The tissues should be thrown into a paper bag and disposed of with the trash, burned, or flushed down the toilet. The patient should also be taught careful handwashing techniques to be used after handling sputum and soiled tissues. Special precautions should be taken during high-risk procedures such as sputum induction, aerosolized pentamidine (NebuPent) treatments, intubation, bronchoscopy, or endoscopy.

Ambulatory and Home Care

Patients who have responded clinically are discharged home despite positive smears if their household contacts have already been exposed and the patient is not posing a risk to susceptible persons. Determination of absolute noninfectiousness requires negative cultures. Most treatment failures occur because the patient neglects to take the drug, discontinues it prematurely, or takes it irregularly. On discharge, the physician may order Rifater or Rifamate, a fixed-dose combination drug, to increase the likelihood of adherence, ensure that all drugs are taken, and reduce the risk of developing drug resistance.

It is important for the nurse to develop a therapeutic, consistent relationship with each patient. The nurse must understand the patient's lifestyle and be flexible in planning a program that facilitates the patient's participation in and completion of therapy. The nurse should teach the patient so that the need for dedication to the prescribed regimen is fully understood by the patient. Ongoing reassurance helps the patient understand that adherence can mean cure. If the patient cannot or will not adhere to a self-administered medication regimen, medication may have to be given by a responsible person on a daily or intermittent basis (see the Ethical Dilemmas box). Notification of the public health department is essential if adherence to the drug regimen is questionable so that follow-up of close contacts can be accomplished. In some cases the public health nurse will be responsible for DOT. In other situations, a spouse, grown child, other relative living with the patient, or co-worker may be asked to supervise drug taking.

Some patients may feel that there is a social stigma attached to TB. Many people still remember when TB patients were sent away to TB sanatoriums and isolated from society. These feelings should be discussed, and the patient should be reassured that an individual with TB can be cured if the prescribed regimen is followed. The Canadian Lung Association provides excellent literature for teaching about the disease as well as providing emotional support to the patient and family.

When the chemotherapy regimen has been completed, there is evidence of negative cultures, the patient is improving clinically, and there is radiological evidence of improvement, most individuals can be considered adequately treated. Follow-up care may be indicated during the subsequent 12 months, including bacteriological studies and chest radiographic examinations. Because approximately 5% of individuals experience relapses, the patient should be taught to recognize the symptoms that indicate

- Patient will have complete resolution of the disease.
- Patient will have normal pulmonary function.
- Patient will have absence of any complications.
- Patient will have no transmission of TB.

ETHICAL DILEMMAS
Patient Adherence

Situation

The health clinic for the homeless discovers that a man with tuberculosis has not been adhering to instructions for taking his medication. He tells the nurse that it is hard for him to get to the clinic to obtain the medication, much less to keep on a schedule. The nurse is concerned not only about this patient but also about the risks for the other people at the shelter, in the park, and at the meal sites.

Important Points for Consideration

- Adherence is a complex issue involving a person's culture and values, perceived risk of disease, availability of resources, access to treatment, and perceived consequences of available choices.
- Nurses in the community are concerned not only with providing benefits and supporting decision making for individual patients but also with the health and well-being of the entire community.
- Greater harm may result for the community when more virulent drug-resistant strains of microorganisms develop as a consequence of partial treatment or inability of the patient to complete a course of therapy.
- Advocacy for the patient and the community obliges the nurse to involve other members of the health care team, such as those in social services, to assist in obtaining the necessary resources or support to facilitate completing the course of treatment by the patient.
- If the patient is unable to comply with the treatment program, even with necessary supports in place, concern for the public's health would take priority and necessitate placing him in a supervised living situation until his treatment is completed.

Clinical Decision-Making Questions

1. Under what circumstances are health care providers justified in overriding a patient's autonomy or decision making?
2. How would the nurse determine whether there were cultural beliefs interfering with this man's ability to understand the importance of completing the treatment? What would the nurse do about it?

recurrence of TB. If these symptoms occur, immediate medical attention should be sought.

The patient needs to be instructed about certain factors that could reactivate TB, such as immunosuppressive therapy, malignancy, and prolonged debilitating illness. If the patient experiences any of these events, the health care provider must to be told so that reactivation of TB can be closely monitored. In some situations, it may be necessary to put the patient on anti-TB therapy.

▌ Evaluation

The following are the expected outcomes for the patient with TB:

Atypical Mycobacteria

Pulmonary disease that closely resembles TB may be caused by atypical acid-fast mycobacteria. This type of pulmonary disease is indistinguishable from TB clinically and radiologically but can be differentiated by bacteriological culture. These organisms are not believed to be airborne and, thus, are not transmitted by droplet nuclei.

Atypical mycobacteria may also invade the cervical lymph nodes, causing lymphadenitis. This type of pulmonary disease typically occurs in White men with a history of COPD, cystic fibrosis, or silicosis. *Mycobacterium avium-intracellulare* (MAI) is a common cause of opportunistic infections in the patient with HIV infection (see Chapter 17).

Treatment depends on identification of the causative agent and determination of drug sensitivity. Many of the drugs used in treating TB are used in combating infections from atypical mycobacteria.

Pulmonary Fungal Infections

Pulmonary fungal infections are increasing in incidence. They are found most frequently in seriously ill patients being treated with corticosteroids, antineoplastic and immunosuppressive drugs, or multiple antibiotics. They are also found in patients with AIDS and cystic fibrosis. Types of fungal infections are presented in Table 30-13. These infections are not transmitted from person to person, and the patient does not have to be placed in isolation. The clinical manifestations are similar to those of bacterial pneumonia. Skin and serology tests are available to assist in identifying the infecting organism. However, identification of the organism in a sputum specimen or in other body fluids is the best diagnostic indicator.

Collaborative Care

Amphotericin B is the drug most widely used in treating serious systemic fungal infections. It must be given intravenously to achieve adequate blood and tissue levels because it is poorly absorbed from the GI tract. Amphotericin B is considered a toxic drug with many possible adverse effects, including hypersensitivity reactions, fever, chills, malaise, nausea and vomiting, thrombophlebitis at the injection site, and abnormal renal function. Many of the adverse effects during infusion can be avoided by premedicating with an anti-inflammatory or diphenhydramine (Benadryl) 1 hour before the infusion. Monitoring of renal function and ensuring adequate hydration are essential while a person is receiving this drug. Renal changes are at least partially reversible. Amphotericin infusions are incompatible with most other drugs. Amphotericin is frequently administered every other day after an initial period of several weeks of daily therapy. Total treatment with the drug may range from 4 to 12 weeks.

Oral antifungals such as ketoconazole (Nizoral), fluconazole (Diflucan), and itraconazole (Sporanox), have also been successful in the treatment of fungal infections. Their effectiveness in

Table 30-13 Fungal Infections of the Lung

ORGANISM	CHARACTERISTICS
Histoplasmosis	
Histoplasma capsulatum	Indigenous to soil of the St. Lawrence River valleys; inhalation of mycelia into lungs; infected individual often free of symptoms; generally self-limiting, chronic disease similar to TB
Coccidioidomycosis	
Coccidioides immitis	Indigenous to semi-arid regions of southwestern United States; inhalation of arthrospores into lungs; suppurative and granulomatous reaction in lungs; symptomatic infection in one third of individuals (not normally found in Canada)
Blastomycosis	
Blastomyces dermatitidis	Indigenous to southern Canada; inhalation of fungus into lungs; progression of disease often insidious; possible involvement of skin
Cryptococcosis	
Cryptococcus neoformans	True yeast; indigenous worldwide in soil and pigeon excreta; inhalation of fungus into lungs; possible meningitis
Aspergillosis	
Aspergillus niger or A. fumigatus	True mould inhabiting mouth; widely distributed; invasion of lung tissue resulting in possible necrotizing pneumonia; in individual with asthma, allergic bronchopulmonary aspergillosis may necessitate corticosteroid therapy
Candidiasis	
Candida albicans	Leading cause of mycotic infections in hospitalized and immunocompromised hosts; ubiquitous and frequent colonization of upper respiratory and gastrointestinal tracts; infections often following broad-spectrum antibiotic therapy (systemic or inhaled); possible development of localized pulmonary infiltrate to widespread bilateral consolidation with hypoxemia
Actinomycosis	
Actinomyces israelii	Not a true fungus; anaerobic; Gram-positive bacteria with branching hyphae; presence of necrotizing pneumonia after aspiration; pneumonitis; commonly in lower lobes with abscess or empyema formation
Nocardiosis	
Nocardia asteroides	Not a true fungus; aerobic; soil saprophyte widely distributed in nature; acquisition of infection from nature; rarely present in sputum without accompanying disease
Pneumocystis pneumonia (PCP)	
Pneumocystis jiroveci	Rarely causes pneumonia in healthy individuals; fungus present in the environment; common opportunistic pneumonia in persons with impaired immune systems and/or HIV infection.

HIV, human immunodeficiency virus; *TB*, tuberculosis.

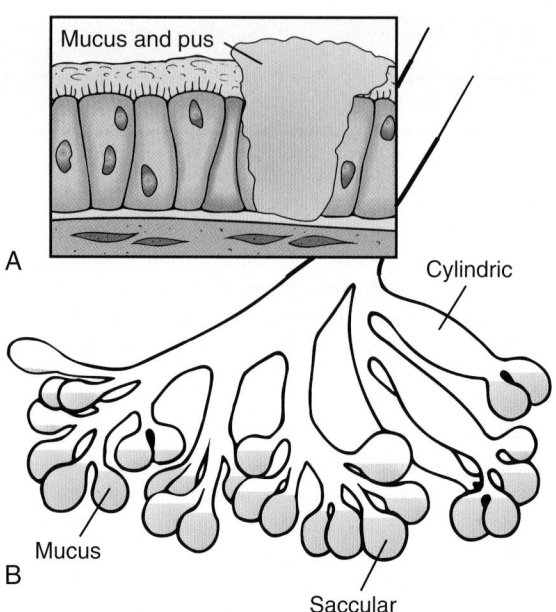

Figure 30-3 Pathological changes in bronchiectasis. **A,** Longitudinal section of bronchial wall where chronic infection has caused damage. **B,** Collection of purulent material in dilated bronchioles, leading to persistent infection.

treatment allows an alternative to the use of amphotericin B in many cases. Effectiveness of therapy can be monitored with fungal serology titres.

Bronchiectasis

Etiology and Pathophysiology

Bronchiectasis is characterized by permanent, abnormal dilation of one or more large bronchi. The pathophysiological change that results in dilation is destruction of the elastic and muscular structures of the bronchial wall. There are two pathological types of bronchiectasis: saccular and cylindrical (Figure 30-3). *Saccular bronchiectasis* occurs mainly in large bronchi and is characterized by cavity-like dilations. The affected bronchi end in large sacs. *Cylindrical bronchiectasis* involves medium-sized bronchi that are mildly to moderately dilated.

Almost all forms of bronchiectasis are associated with bacterial infections. A wide variety of infectious agents can initiate bronchiectasis, including adenovirus, influenza virus, *S. aureus*, *Klebsiella*, and anaerobes. Infections cause the bronchial walls to weaken, and pockets of infection begin to form. When the walls of the bronchial system are injured, the mucociliary mechanism is damaged, allowing bacteria and mucus to accumulate within the pockets. The infection becomes worse and results in bronchiectasis.

The incidence of bronchiectasis has shown a decline in recent years. The emergence of atypical mycobacteria, especially MAI, presents a new threat because MAI can progress to bronchiectasis. MAI is an opportunistic infection found in patients with HIV.

Clinical Manifestations

The hallmark of bronchiectasis is persistent or recurrent cough with production of greater than 20 mL of purulent sputum per day. The cough is paroxysmal and is often stimulated with position changes. Other manifestations include exertional dyspnea, fatigue, weight loss, anorexia, and fetid breath. On auscultation of the lungs, crackle and wheezing may be heard. Sinusitis frequently accompanies diffuse bronchiectasis. The manifestations of advanced, widespread bronchiectasis are generalized wheezing, digital clubbing, and cor pulmonale.

Diagnostic Studies

An individual with a chronic productive cough with copious purulent sputum (which may be blood streaked) should be suspected of having bronchiectasis. Chest radiographic studies are usually done and may show streaky infiltrates or may be normal. High-resolution CT scan of the chest has excellent sensitivity for detecting bronchiectasis, and its availability has made diagnosis easier. Bronchoscopy can also be useful in identifying the source of secretions, in identifying sites of hemoptysis, or for collecting microbiological samples.

Sputum may provide additional information regarding the severity of impairment and the presence of active infection. Pulmonary function studies may be abnormal in advanced bronchiectasis, showing a decrease in vital capacity, expiratory flow, and maximum voluntary ventilation. Complete blood count may be normal or show evidence of leukocytosis or anemia from chronic infection.

Collaborative Care

Bronchiectasis is difficult to treat. Therapy is aimed at treating acute flare-ups and preventing decline in lung function. Antibiotics are the mainstay of treatment and are given on the basis of sputum culture results. Long-term suppressive therapy with antibiotics is occasionally used but is fraught with risks of antibiotic resistance. A form of treatment gaining popularity is the use of nebulized antibiotics. Studies indicate that it is safe and may reduce the number of flare-ups and hospitalizations in bronchiectatic patients (Rubin, 2008). Antipseudomonal antibiotics, such as tobramycin, are commonly used. Concurrent bronchodilator therapy is given to prevent bronchospasm. Other forms of drug therapy may include mucolytic agents and expectorants. Maintaining good hydration is important to liquefy secretions. Chest physiotherapy and other airway clearance techniques are important to facilitate expectoration of sputum. (These techniques are discussed in Chapter 31.) The individual should reduce exposure to excessive air pollutants and irritants, avoid cigarette smoking, and obtain pneumococcal and influenza vaccinations.

Surgical resection of parts of the lungs, although not used as often as previously, may be done if more conservative treatment is not effective. Surgical resection of an affected lobe or segment may be indicated for the patient with repeated bouts of pneumonia, hemoptysis, and disabling complications. Surgery is not advisable when there is diffuse or widespread involvement. For selected patients who are disabled in spite of maximal therapy, lung transplantation is an option. (Lung transplantation is discussed later in this chapter, p. 705.)

NURSING MANAGEMENT: BRONCHIECTASIS

The early detection and treatment of lower respiratory tract infections will help prevent complications such as bronchiectasis. Any obstructing lesion or foreign body should be removed promptly. Other measures to decrease the occurrence or progression of bronchiectasis include avoiding cigarette smoking and decreasing exposure to pollution and irritants.

An important nursing goal is to promote drainage and removal of bronchial mucus. Various airway clearance techniques can be effectively used to facilitate secretion removal. The patient should be taught effective deep-breathing exercises and effective ways to cough (see Chapter 31, Table 31-22). Chest physiotherapy with postural drainage should be done on affected parts of the lung (see Chapter 31, Figure 31-16). Some individuals require elevation of the foot of the bed by 10 to 15 cm to facilitate drainage. Pillows may be used in the hospital and at home to help the patient assume postural drainage positions. A Flutter mucus clearance device is a handheld device that provides airway vibration during the expiratory phase of breathing (see Chapter 31, Figure 31-17). Two to four 15-minute sessions daily by a patient who has been properly trained can provide satisfactory mucus clearance. Positive expiratory pressure therapy is a breathing manoeuvre against an expiratory resistance often used in conjunction with nebulized medications. (Respiratory therapy procedures are explained in Chapter 31.)

Administration of the prescribed antibiotics, bronchodilators, or expectorants is important. The patient needs to understand the importance of taking the prescribed regimen of drugs to obtain maximum effectiveness. The patient should be aware of possible adverse effects or adverse effects that must be reported to the physician.

Health teaching must include information regarding the importance of adequate rest, avoiding excess fatigue, nutrition, hydration, and oral care. Unless there are contraindications such as concomitant congestive heart failure (CHF) or renal disease, the patient should be instructed to drink at least 3 L of fluid daily. Generally, the patient should be counselled to use low-sodium fluids to avoid systemic fluid retention.

Direct hydration of the respiratory system may also prove beneficial in the expectoration of secretions. Usually, a bland aerosol with normal saline solution delivered by a jet-type nebulizer is used. The patient with bronchiectasis should avoid ultrasonic nebulizers because they often induce bronchospasm. At home, a steamy shower can prove effective; expensive equipment that requires frequent cleaning is usually unnecessary. It is important that the patient medicate with an inhaled bronchodilator 10 to 15 minutes before using a bland aerosol to prevent bronchoconstriction.

The patient and caregivers should be taught to recognize significant clinical manifestations to be reported to the health care provider. These manifestations include increased sputum production, grossly bloody sputum, increasing dyspnea, fever, chills, and chest pain.

Lung Abscess

Etiology and Pathophysiology

A **lung abscess** is a pus-containing lesion of the lung parenchyma that gives rise to a cavity. The cavity is formed by necrosis of the lung tissue. In many cases, the causes and pathogenesis of lung abscesses are similar to those of pneumonia. Most lung abscesses are caused by aspiration of material from the oral cavity (the gingival crevices) into the lungs. In general, infectious agents including enteric Gram-negative organisms (e.g., *Klebsiella*), *S. aureus*, and anaerobic bacilli (e.g., *Bacteroides*) are responsible for lung abscesses and the associated infection and necrosis of the lung tissue. A lung abscess can also result from a lung infarct secondary to pulmonary embolus, malignant growth, TB, and various parasitic and fungal diseases of the lung.

The areas of the lung most commonly affected are the superior segments of the lower lobes and the posterior segments of the upper lobes. Fibrous tissue usually forms around the abscess in an attempt to wall it off. The abscess may erode into the bronchial system, causing the production of foul-smelling sputum. It may grow toward the pleura and cause pleuritic pain. Multiple small abscesses can occur within the lung.

Clinical Manifestations and Complications

The onset of a lung abscess is usually insidious, especially if anaerobic organisms are the primary cause. A more acute onset occurs with aerobic organisms. The most common manifestation is cough-producing purulent sputum (often dark brown) that is foul smelling and foul tasting. Hemoptysis is common, especially at the time that an abscess ruptures into a bronchus. Other common manifestations are fever, chills, prostration, pleuritic pain, dyspnea, cough, and weight loss.

Physical examination of the lungs indicates dullness to percussion and decreased breath sounds on auscultation over the segment of lung involved. There may be transmission of bronchial breath sounds to the periphery if the communicating bronchus becomes patent and drainage of the segment begins. Crackles may also be present in the later stages as the abscess drains. Oral examination often reveals dental caries, gingivitis, and periodontal infection.

Complications that can occur include chronic pulmonary abscess, bronchiectasis, and brain abscess as a result of the hematogenous spread of infection, bronchopleural fistula, and empyema from abscess perforation into the pleural cavity.

Diagnostic Studies

A chest radiographic examination will reveal a solitary cavitary lesion with fluid. CT scanning is used if there is suspicion of cavitation not clearly seen. A lung abscess, in contrast to other types of abscesses, does not require assisted drainage, as long as there is drainage via the bronchus. Routine sputum cultures can be collected, but contaminants can confuse the results and it is difficult to isolate anaerobic bacteria. Pleural fluid and blood cultures may be obtained. Bronchoscopy may be used in cases of abscess in which drainage is delayed or in which there are factors that suggest an underlying malignancy.

NURSING AND COLLABORATIVE MANAGEMENT: LUNG ABSCESS

Antibiotics given for a prolonged period (up to 2 to 4 months) are usually the primary method of treatment. Penicillin has historically been the drug of choice because of the frequent presence of anaerobic organisms. However, recent studies suggest that there is β-lactamase production by the anaerobic bacteria involved in abscesses of the lung and that they are resistant to penicillin. Clindamycin has been shown to be superior to penicillin and is the standard treatment for an anaerobic lung infection. Patients with putrid lung abscesses usually show clinical improvement with decreased fever within 3 to 4 days of beginning antibiotics.

Because of the need for prolonged antibiotic therapy, the patient must be aware of the importance of continuing the medication for the prescribed period. The patient needs to know about adverse effects to be reported to the health care provider. Sometimes, the patient is asked to return periodically during the course of antibiotic therapy for repeat cultures and sensitivity tests to ensure that the infecting organism is not becoming resistant to the antibiotic. When antibiotic therapy is completed, the patient is re-evaluated.

The patient should be taught how to cough effectively (see Chapter 31, Table 31-20). Chest physiotherapy and postural drainage are sometimes used to drain abscesses located in the lower or posterior portions of the lung. Postural drainage according to the lung area involved will aid the removal of secretions (see Chapter 31, Figure 31-16). Frequent (every 2 to 3 hours) mouth care is needed to relieve the foul-smelling odour and taste from the sputum. Diluted hydrogen peroxide and mouthwash are often effective.

Rest, good nutrition, and adequate fluid intake are all supportive measures to facilitate recovery. If dentition is poor and dental hygiene is not adequate, the patient should be encouraged to obtain dental care.

Surgery is rarely indicated but occasionally may be necessary when re-infection of a large cavitary lesion occurs or to establish a diagnosis when there is evidence of an underlying neoplasm or chronic associated disease. The usual procedure in such cases is a lobectomy or pneumonectomy. An alternative to surgery is percutaneous drainage, but this has a high risk of contamination of the pleural space.

Environmental Lung Diseases

Environmental or occupational lung diseases result from inhaled dust or chemicals. The duration of exposure and the amount of inhalant have a major influence on whether the exposed individual will have lung damage. Another factor is the susceptibility of the host.

Pneumoconiosis is a general term for lung diseases caused by the inhalation and retention of dust particles. The literal meaning of pneumoconiosis is "dust in the lungs." Examples of this condition are silicosis, asbestosis, and berylliosis. The classical response to the inhaled substance is diffuse parenchymal infiltration with phagocytic cells. This eventually results in diffuse pulmonary fibrosis (excess connective tissue). Fibrosis is the result of tissue repair after inflammation. Pneumoconiosis and other environmental lung diseases are presented in Table 30-14. Hantavirus, a potentially fatal disease with outbreaks reported in Canada and the United States, is transmitted by inhalation of aerosolized rodent excreta particles.

Chemical pneumonitis results from exposures to toxic chemical fumes. Acutely, there is diffuse lung injury characterized as pulmonary edema. Chronically, the clinical picture is that of bronchiolitis obliterans, which is usually associated with a normal chest radiograph or one that shows hyperinflation. An example is silo filler's disease. *Hypersensitivity pneumonitis* or extrinsic allergic alveolitis is the response seen when antigens are inhaled to

Table 30-14 Environmental Lung Diseases

AGENTS AND INDUSTRIES	DESCRIPTION	COMPLICATIONS
Asbestosis		
Asbestos fibres present in insulation, construction material (roof tiling, cement products), shipyards, textiles (for fireproofing), automobile clutch and brake linings	Disease appears 15-35 yr after first exposure. Interstitial fibrosis develops. Pleural plaques, which are calcified lesions, develop on pleura. Dyspnea, basal crackles, and decreased vital capacity are early manifestations.	Diffuse interstitial pulmonary fibrosis; lung cancer, especially in cigarette smokers; mesothelioma (rare type of cancer affecting pleura and peritoneal membrane)
Berylliosis		
Beryllium dust present in aircraft manufacturing, metallurgy, rocket fuels	Formation of noncaseating granulomas is seen. Acute pneumonitis occurs after heavy exposure. Interstitial fibrosis can also occur.	Progress of disease possible even after removal of stimulating inhalant
Bird Fancier's, Breeder's, or Handler's Lung		
Bird droppings or feathers	Hypersensitivity pneumonitis is present.	Progressive fibrosis of lung
Byssinosis		
Cotton, flax, and hemp dust (textile industry)	Airway obstruction is caused by contraction of smooth muscles. Chronic disease results from severe airway obstruction and decreased elastic recoil.	Progression of chronic disease after cessation of dust exposure
Coal Worker's Pneumoconiosis (Black Lung)		
Coal dust	Incidence is high (20-30%) in coal workers. Deposits of carbon dust cause lesions to develop along respiratory bronchioles. Bronchioles dilate because of loss of wall structure. Chronic airway obstruction and bronchitis develop. Dyspnea and cough are common early symptoms.	Progressive, massive lung fibrosis; increased risk of chronic bronchitis and emphysema with smoking
Farmer's Lung		
Inhalation of airborne material from mouldy hay or similar matter	Hypersensitivity pneumonitis occurs. Acute form is similar to pneumonia, with manifestations of chills, fever, and malaise. Chronic, insidious form is type of pulmonary fibrosis.	Progressive fibrosis of lung
Hantavirus Pulmonary Syndrome (HPS)		
Rodent droppings inhaled while in rodent-infested areas	Acute hemorrhagic fever associated with severe pulmonary and cardiovascular collapse and death. Incubation period is 1-4 wk with prodrome (3-5 days) of flulike symptoms. No cure or specific treatment exists.	Critical care unit with careful monitoring of fluid and electrolyte balance and blood pressure; supportive therapy and early intervention vital; research on this virus is done in high-level biocontainment facilities
Siderosis		
Iron oxide present in welding materials, foundries, iron ore mining	Dust deposits are found in lung.	—
Silicosis		
Silica dust present in quartz rock in mining of gold, copper, tin, coal, lead; also present in sandblasting, foundries, quarries, pottery making, masonry	In chronic disease, dust is engulfed by macrophages and may be destroyed, resulting in fibrotic nodules. Acute disease results from intense exposure in short period. Within 5 yr, it progresses to severe disability from lung fibrosis.	Increased susceptibility to tuberculosis; progressive, massive fibrosis; high incidence of chronic bronchitis
Silo Filler's Disease		
Nitrogen oxides from fermentation of vegetation in freshly filled silo	Chemical pneumonitis occurs.	Progressive bronchiolitis obliterans

which an individual is allergic. Examples include bird fancier's lung and farmer's lung.

Although many occupational respiratory diseases have declined, occupational asthma is the occupational lung disease most frequently compensated through workplace compensation (PHAC, 2007d). *Occupational asthma* refers to the development of symptoms of shortness of breath, wheezing, cough, and chest tightness as a result of exposure to fumes or dust that trigger an allergic response. The obstruction may initially be reversible or

intermittent, but continued exposure results in permanent obstructive changes. The best-known causative agent in occupational asthma is toluene di-isocyanate (TDI), which is used in the production of rigid polyurethane foam.

Lung cancer, either squamous cell carcinoma or adenocarcinoma, is the most frequent cancer associated with asbestos exposure. People with more exposure are at a greater risk of disease. There is a minimum lapse of 15 to 19 years between first exposure and development of lung cancer. Mesotheliomas, both pleural and peritoneal, are also associated with asbestos exposure.

Clinical Manifestations

Acute symptoms of pulmonary edema may be seen following early exposures to chemical fumes. However, symptoms of many environmental lung diseases may not occur until at least 10 to 15 years after the initial exposure to the inhaled irritant. Dyspnea and cough are often the earliest manifestations. Chest pain and cough with sputum production usually occur later. Complications that often result are pneumonia, chronic bronchitis, emphysema, and lung cancer. Manifestations of these complications can be the reason the patient seeks health care. Cor pulmonale is a late complication, especially in conditions characterized by diffuse pulmonary fibrosis.

Pulmonary function studies often show reduced vital capacity. A chest radiograph will often reveal lung involvement specific to the primary problem. CT scans have been shown to be useful in detecting early lung involvement.

Collaborative Care

The best approach to management is to try to prevent or decrease environmental and occupational risks. Well-designed, effective ventilation systems can reduce exposure to irritants. Wearing masks is appropriate in some occupations. Periodic inspections and monitoring of workplaces by agencies such as the Canadian Centre for Occupational Health and Safety (CCOHS) reinforce the obligations of employers to provide a safe work environment. In addition, the Canada Labour Code requires that an occupational health and safety committee be established in all workplaces with 20 or more regular employees (Human Resources and Skills Development Canada, 2006).

Cigarette smoking adds increased insult to the lungs, and the person at risk for occupational lung disease should not smoke. In addition, second-hand smoke is an important source of occupational exposure that increases risk for development of lung cancer. This has led to regulations requiring a smoke-free workspace for all employees.

Early diagnosis is essential if the disease process is to be halted. Some places of employment, where there is a known risk of lung disease, may require periodic chest radiographic examinations and pulmonary function studies for exposed employees. These measures can detect pulmonary changes before symptoms develop.

There is no specific treatment for most environmental lung diseases. The best treatment is to decrease or stop exposure to the harmful agent. Strategies are directed toward providing symptomatic relief. If there are coexisting problems, such as pneumonia, chronic bronchitis, emphysema, or asthma, they are treated.

Lung Cancer

Lung cancer, the most preventable cancer, is the leading cause of cancer-related deaths in men and women in Canada. It was estimated that in 2012 there would be 25,600 new cases (13,300 men and 12,300 women) of lung cancer in Canada and 20,100 deaths (10,800 men and 9,400 women) (Canadian Cancer Society's Steering Committee on Cancer Statistics, 2012).

Lung cancer most commonly occurs in individuals older than 50 years who have a long history of cigarette smoking. The disease is found most frequently in persons 40 to 75 years of age, with peak incidence between 55 and 65.

Etiology

Cigarette smoking is the most important risk factor in the development of lung cancer. Smoking is responsible for approximately 80 to 90% of all lung cancers. Tobacco smoke contains 60 carcinogens in addition to substances (carbon monoxide, nicotine) that interfere with normal cell development. Cigarette smoking, a lower airway irritant, causes a change in the bronchial epithelium, which usually returns to normal when smoking is discontinued. The risk of lung cancer is gradually lowered when smoking ceases and continues to decline with time. After 10 years following cessation of smoking, the risk of lung cancer is cut in half (Canadian Lung Association, 2013). From 1999 to 2011, smoking by Canadian teenagers 15 to 19 years decreased from 28 to 12% and in 2011, 17% of all Canadians were smokers (Health Canada, 2012).

The risk of developing lung cancer is directly related to total exposure to cigarette smoke measured by total number of cigarettes smoked in a lifetime, earlier age of smoking onset, depth of inhalation, tar and nicotine content, and the use of unfiltered cigarettes. Sidestream smoke (smoke from burning cigarettes and cigars) contains the same carcinogens found in mainstream smoke (smoke inhaled by smoker). This environmental tobacco smoke (ETS) inhaled by nonsmokers poses a 35% increased risk of the development of lung cancer in nonsmokers (Registered Nurses' Association of Ontario [RNAO], 2007). In 2005, 7.3% of children 12 years and older were exposed to second-hand smoke at home every day or almost every day (RNAO, 2007). Children are more vulnerable to ETS than adults because their respiratory and immune systems are not fully developed. Recent data suggest that childhood exposure to ETS is associated with increased prevalence of asthma among adults and that children exposed to ETS are more likely to become smokers (Health Canada, 2006b).

Compared with nonsmokers, those who smoke pipes and cigars have also been shown to have an increased risk of developing lung cancer. Cigar smokers are at higher risk for lung cancer than pipe smokers. In fact, rates of lung cancer caused by heavy smoking of cigars and inhalation of smoke from small cigars have been shown to correlate with the rates of lung cancer caused by cigarette smoking.

Another major risk factor for lung cancer is inhaled carcinogens. These include asbestos, radon, nickel, iron and iron oxides, uranium, polycyclic aromatic hydrocarbons, chromates, arsenic, and air pollution. Exposure to these substances is common for employees of industries involved in mining, smelting, or chemical or petroleum manufacturing. The cigarette smoker who is also exposed to one or more of these chemicals or to high amounts of air pollution is at significantly higher risk for lung cancer.

There are marked variations in a person's propensity to develop lung cancer (see the Determinants of Health box). To date, no genetic abnormality has conclusively been defined for lung cancer. It is known that the carcinogens in cigarette smoke directly damage DNA. One theory is that people have different genetic carcinogen-metabolizing pathways.

Pathophysiology

The pathogenesis of primary lung cancer is not well understood. More than 90% of cancers originate from the epithelium of the bronchus (bronchogenic). They grow slowly, and it takes 8 to 10 years for a tumour to reach 1 cm in size, which is the smallest detectable lesion on an radiographic study. Lung cancers occur primarily in the segmental bronchi or beyond and have a preference for the upper lobes of the lungs (Figure 30-4). Pathological changes in the bronchial system show nonspecific inflammatory changes with hypersecretion of mucus, desquamation of cells, reactive hyperplasia of the basal cells, and metaplasia of normal respiratory epithelium to stratified squamous cells.

Primary lung cancers are often categorized into two broad subtypes (Table 30-15), non–small cell lung cancer (NSCLC, 75 to 80%) and small cell lung cancer (SCLC, 20 to 25%) (BC Cancer Agency, 2006). Lung cancers metastasize primarily by direct extension and via the blood circulation and the lymph

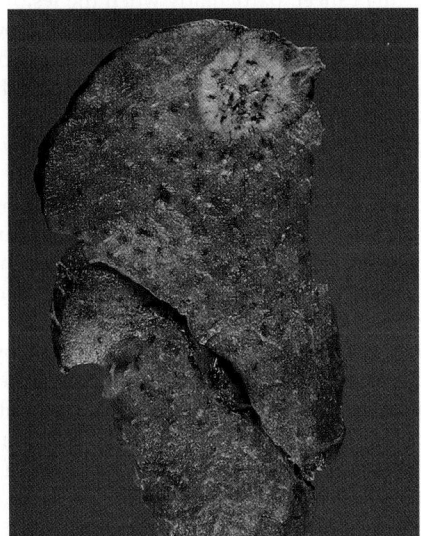

Figure 30-4 Lung cancer. Peripheral adenocarcinoma. The tumour shows prominent black pigmentation, suggestive of having evolved in an anthracotic scar.

Source: Damjanov, I., & Linder, J. (1996). *Anderson's pathology* (10th ed.). St. Louis: Mosby.

DETERMINANTS OF HEALTH
Gender and Lung Cancer

Men

- More men than women are diagnosed with lung cancer.
- More men than women die from lung cancer.
- Men with lung cancer have a worse prognosis than women.
- Lung cancer incidence and deaths are decreasing in men.

Women

- Women who smoke are at a greater risk of developing lung cancer than men who smoke.
- Women develop lung cancer after fewer years of smoking than men do.
- Women develop lung cancer at a younger age than men.
- Women are more likely to develop small cell carcinoma than men.
- Nonsmoking women are at a greater risk of developing lung cancer than nonsmoking men.

Table 30-15 Comparison of the Types of Primary Lung Cancer

CELL TYPE	RISK FACTORS	CHARACTERISTICS	RESPONSE TO THERAPY
Non–Small Cell Lung Cancer (NSCLC)			
Squamous cell (epidermoid) carcinoma	Almost always associated with cigarette smoking; is associated with exposure to environmental carcinogens (e.g., uranium, asbestos)	Accounts for 30% of lung cancers; is more common in men; arises from the bronchial epithelium, produces earlier symptoms because of bronchial obstructive characteristics; does not have a strong tendency to metastasize; metastasizes locally by direct extension; causes cavitating pulmonary lesions	Surgical resection is often attempted; life expectancy is better than for small cell lung cancer
Adenocarcinoma	Has been associated with lung scarring and chronic interstitial fibrosis; is not related to cigarette smoking	Accounts for approximately 40% of lung cancers; is more common in women; often has no clinical manifestations until widespread metastasis is present; metastasizes via bloodstream; is most commonly located in peripheral portions of lungs*	Surgical resection is often attempted; cancer does not respond well to chemotherapy
Large cell undifferentiated carcinoma	High correlation with cigarette smoking and exposure to environmental carcinogens	Accounts for 10% of lung cancers; commonly causes cavitation; is highly metastatic via lymphatics and blood; commonly peripheral rather than central	Surgery is not usually attempted because of high rate of metastases; tumour may be radiosensitive but often recurs
Small Cell Lung Cancer (SCLC)			
Small cell anaplastic undifferentiated (includes oat cell)	Associated with cigarette smoking, exposure to environmental carcinogens	Accounts for 20-25% of lung cancers; is most malignant form; tends to spread early via lymphatics and bloodstream; is frequently associated with endocrine disturbances; predominantly central and can cause bronchial obstruction and pneumonia	Cancer with poorest prognosis; however, chemotherapy advances have been substantial; radiation is used as adjuvant therapy as well as palliative measure; average median survival is 12-18 mo

*See Figure 30-5.

system. The common sites for metastatic growth are liver, brain, bones, scalene lymph nodes, and adrenal glands.

Paraneoplastic Syndrome. Certain lung cancers cause the *paraneoplastic syndrome*, which is characterized by various systemic manifestations caused by factors (e.g., hormones, enzymes, antigens) produced by the tumour cells. SCLCs are most commonly associated with the paraneoplastic syndrome. The systemic manifestations seen are hormonal, dermatological, neuromuscular, vascular, hematological, and connective tissue syndromes. Examples of paraneoplastic syndromes include hypercalcemia, syndrome of inappropriate antidiuretic hormone (SIADH) secretion, anemia, leukocytosis, hypercoagulable disorders, and neurologic syndromes. These syndromes can respond temporarily to symptomatic treatment, but they are impossible to control without successful treatment of the underlying lung cancer.

Clinical Manifestations

Lung cancer is clinically silent for most individuals for the majority of its course. The clinical manifestations of lung cancer are usually nonspecific and appear late in the disease process. Manifestations depend on the type of primary lung cancer, its location, and metastatic spread. Often, there is extensive metastasis before symptoms become apparent. Persistent pneumonitis that is a result of obstructed bronchi may be one of the earliest manifestations, causing fever, chills, and cough.

One of the most significant symptoms, and often the one reported first, is a persistent cough that may be productive of sputum. Blood-tinged sputum may be produced because of bleeding caused by malignancy, but hemoptysis is not a common early symptom. Chest pain may be present and localized or unilateral, ranging from mild to severe. Dyspnea and an auscultatory wheeze may be present if there is bronchial obstruction.

Later manifestations may include nonspecific systemic symptoms such as anorexia, fatigue, weight loss, and nausea and vomiting. Hoarseness may be present as a result of involvement of the recurrent laryngeal nerve. Unilateral paralysis of the diaphragm, dysphagia, and superior vena cava obstruction may occur because of intrathoracic spread of the malignancy. There may be palpable lymph nodes in the neck or the axilla. Mediastinal involvement may lead to pericardial effusion, cardiac tamponade, and dysrhythmias.

Diagnostic Studies

Chest radiographic studies are widely used in the diagnosis of lung cancer. The findings may show the presence of the tumour or abnormalities related to the obstructive features of the tumour such as atelectasis and pneumonitis. The radiograph can also show evidence of metastasis to the ribs or vertebrae and the presence of pleural effusion.

CT scanning is the single most effective noninvasive technique for evaluating lung cancer. CT scans of the brain and bone scans complete the evaluation for metastatic disease. With CT scans, the location and extent of masses in the chest can be identified as well as any mediastinal involvement or lymph node enlargement. Magnetic resonance imaging (MRI) may be used in combination with or instead of CT scans. Positron emission tomography (PET) promises to be a useful diagnostic tool in early clinical staging. PET allows measurement of differential metabolic activity in normal and diseased tissues.

A definitive diagnosis of lung cancer is made by identifying malignant cells. Sputum specimens are usually obtained for cytological studies. An early-morning specimen that has been obtained by having the patient cough deeply provides the most accurate results. However, malignant cells may not be obtained even in the presence of a lung cancer.

The use of the fibreoptic bronchoscope is important in the diagnosis of lung cancer, particularly when the lesions are endobronchial or in close proximity to an airway. It provides direct visualization and allows biopsy specimens to be obtained. A biopsy is usually the best method for establishing the presence of a malignant tumour.

Mediastinoscopy involves the insertion of a scope via a small anterior chest incision into the mediastinum. This is done to examine for metastasis in the anterior mediastinum or the hilum or in the chest extrapleurally. It is also used to determine the stage of the lung cancer, which is important in determining the treatment plan. Video-assisted thoracoscopy (VAT), which involves the insertion of a scope into a small thoracic incision, may be used to explore areas inaccessible by mediastinoscopy.

Pulmonary angiography and lung scans may be performed to assess overall pulmonary status. Fine-needle aspiration (FNA) may be used to obtain a tissue sample to determine tumour histology. FNA is most useful in cases involving a peripheral lesion near the chest wall, and it is usually attempted in an effort to avoid a thoracotomy. If a thoracentesis is performed to relieve a pleural effusion, the fluid should be analyzed for malignant cells. (Table 30-16 summarizes the diagnostic management of lung cancer.)

Staging. Staging of NSCLC is performed according to the tumour–node–metastasis (TNM) staging system in a manner similar to that for other tumours (Tables 30-17 and 30-18). Assessment criteria are T, which denotes tumour size, location, and degree of invasion; N, which indicates regional lymph node involvement; and M, which represents the presence or absence of distant metastases. Depending on the TNM designation, the

COLLABORATIVE CARE

Table 30-16 Lung Cancer

Diagnostic	Collaborative Therapy
• History and physical examination	• Surgery
• Chest radiographic examination	• Radiation therapy
• Sputum for cytological study	• Chemotherapy
• Bronchoscopy	• Biological therapy
• CT scan	• Bronchoscopic laser therapy
• MRI	• Phototherapy
• PET	• Airway stenting
• Spirometry (preoperative)	• Cryotherapy
• Mediastinoscopy	
• VAT	
• Pulmonary angiography	
• Lung scan	
• Fine-needle aspiration	

CT, computed tomography; *MRI,* magnetic resonance imaging; *PET,* positron emission tomography; *VAT,* video-assisted thoracoscopy.

Table 30-17 Lung Cancer Tumour-Node-Metastasis Classifications*

T		PRIMARY TUMOUR
TX		Primary tumour cannot be assessed, or tumour proven by the presence of malignant cells in sputum or bronchial washings but not visualized by imaging or bronchoscopy
T0		No evidence of primary tumour
Tis		Carcinoma in situ
T1		≤3 cm in greatest dimension, surrounded by lung or visceral pleura, without bronchoscopic evidence of invasion more proximal than the lobar bronchus (i.e., not in the main bronchus). This has been subdivided into:
	T1a	Tumour ≤2 cm in greatest dimension
	T1b	Tumour >2 cm but not >3 cm in greatest dimension
T2		Tumour >3 but <7 cm with any of the following features: involves main bronchus, ≥2 cm distal to the carina, invades visceral pleura, associated with atelectasis or obstructive pneumonitis that extends to the hilar region but does not involve the entire lung. T2 >7 cm reclassified as T3. This has been subdivided into:
	T2a	Tumour >3 and ≤5 cm in greatest dimension (or tumour with any of the T2 descriptors, but ≤5 cm)
	T2b	Tumour >5 and ≤7 cm in greatest dimension
T3		Tumour >7 cm or one that directly invades any of the following: chest wall (including superior sulcus tumours), diaphragm, phrenic nerve, mediastinal pleura, parietal pericardium, or tumour in the main bronchus <2 cm distal to the carina but without involvement of the carina; or associated atelectasis or obstructive pneumonitis of the entire lung or separate tumour nodule(s) in the same lobe.
T4		Tumour of any size that invades any of the following: mediastinum, heart, great vessels, trachea, recurrent laryngeal nerve, esophagus, vertebral body, carina, separate tumour nodule(s) in a different ipsilateral lobe. Additional nodule(s) in the same lobe as the primary tumour reclassified as T3. T4 caused by malignant pleural effusion has been reclassified as M1a
N		Node
NX		Regional lymph nodes cannot be assessed
N0		No regional lymph node metastasis
N1		Metastasis in ipsilateral peribronchial and/or ipsilateral hilar lymph nodes and intrapulmonary nodes, including involvement by direct extension
N2		Metastasis in ipsilateral mediastinal and/or subcarinal lymph node(s)
N3		Metastasis in contralateral mediastinal, contralateral hilar, ipsilateral or contralateral scalene or supraclavicular lymph node(s)
M		Distant Metastasis
MX		Distant metastasis cannot be assessed
M0		No distant metastasis
M1		Distant metastasis M1 caused by additional nodule(s) in an ipsilateral lobe other than that of the primary tumour has been reclassified as T4 M1 has been subdivided into:
	M1a	Separate tumour nodule(s) in a contralateral lobe; tumour with pleural nodules or malignant pleural or pericardial effusion
	M1b	Distant metastasis

Source: Khan, B., & Mushtaq, M. (2010). Setting the "stage" for the new TNM lung. *Lung Cancer, 4*(6) (p. 196, Table 1). Retrieved from *http://www.oncologynews.biz/pdf/jan_feb_10/ONJF10_lung.pdf*
*Seventh International Association for the Study of Lung Cancer Staging Project: Tumour–Node–Metastasis Classification.

tumour is then staged, which assists in estimating prognosis and determining the appropriate therapy.

Staging of SCLC has not been useful because the cancer has usually metastasized by the time a diagnosis is made. Instead, SCLC is determined to be limited (confined to one hemothorax and to regional lymph nodes) or extensive (any disease exceeding those boundaries).

Screening for Lung Cancer. Early screening for lung cancer is controversial. No current recommendations exist in Canada or the United States because previous lung cancer screening studies indicated no significant difference in lung cancer deaths between those patients who were screened and those who were not. However, screening studies using sputum cytology, chest radiographic studies, and CT scanning are ongoing (Roberts et al., 2007), and physicians in Canada and the United States may begin to screen their highest-risk patients (i.e., smokers >40 years old with spirometry changes, patients with strong family history of lung cancer). In 2008, an international study discovered a genetic link to lung cancer, which may affect screening practices in the future (Cancer Care Ontario, 2008).

Collaborative Care

Cancer Care Ontario has published evidence-informed clinical guidelines for treating lung cancer. The guidelines can be accessed

Table 30-18 Lung Cancer Staging*			
STAGE		**GROUPING**	
Occult carcinoma	TX	N0	M0
Stage 0	Tis	N0	M0
Stage IA	T1a	N0	M0
	T1b	N0	M0
Stage IB	T2a	N0	M0
Stage IIA	T1a	N1	M0
	T1b	N1	M0
	T2a	N1	M0
	T2b	N0	M0
Stage IIB	T2b	N1	M0
	T3	N0	M0
Stage IIIA	T1	N2	M0
	T2	N2	M0
	T3	N1	M0
	T3	N2	M0
	T4	N0	M0
	T4	N1	M0
Stage IIIB	T4	N2	M0
	Any T	N3	M0
Stage IV	Any T	Any N	M1

Source: Khan, B., & Mushtaq, M. (2010). Setting the "stage" for the new TNM lung. *Lung Cancer, 4*(6) (p. 197, Table 2). Retrieved from *http://www.oncologynews.biz/pdf/jan_feb_10/ONJF10_lung.pdf*
*Seventh International Association for the Study of Lung Cancer Staging Project: Stage Grouping.

at its Web site in the Cancer Care Ontario Toolbox, under Quality Guidelines and Standards. (See the Canadian Resources at the end of the chapter.)

Surgical Therapy.
Surgical resection is considered the treatment of choice in NSCLC Stages I and II because the disease is potentially curable with resection. For other NSCLC stages, surgery may be indicated in conjunction with radiation therapy and/or chemotherapy. In limited-stage SCLC, which is rare, surgical resection, chemotherapy, and radiation therapy may be recommended.

When the tumour is considered operable with a potential for cure, the patient's cardiopulmonary status must be evaluated to determine the ability to withstand surgery. This is done by clinical studies of pulmonary function, ABGs, and others, as indicated by the individual's status. Contraindications for thoracotomy include hypercapnia, pulmonary hypertension, cor pulmonale, and markedly reduced lung function. Coexisting conditions such as cardiac, renal, and liver disease may also be contraindications for surgery.

A tumour may be considered inoperable. If operable, the type of surgery performed is usually a lobectomy (removal of one or more lobes of the lung) and, less often, a *pneumonectomy* (removal of one entire lung).

Radiation Therapy.
Radiation therapy is used as a curative approach in the individual who has a resectable tumour but who

is considered a poor surgical risk. There has been improved survival when radiation therapy is used in combination with surgery and chemotherapy. Adenocarcinomas are the most radioresistant type of cancer cell. Although SCLCs are radiosensitive, radiation (even when used in combination with chemotherapy) does not significantly improve the mortality rate because of the early metastases of this type of cancer.

Radiation therapy is also done as a palliative procedure to reduce distressing symptoms such as cough, hemoptysis, bronchial obstruction, and superior vena cava syndrome. It can be used to treat pain that is caused by metastatic bone lesions or cerebral metastasis. Radiation used as a preoperative or postoperative adjuvant measure has not been found to significantly increase survival in the patient with lung cancer.

Stereotactic Radiotherapy. Stereotactic radiotherapy (SRT), also called stereotactic surgery or radiosurgery, is a new lung cancer treatment. It is a type of radiation therapy that uses high doses of radiation delivered very accurately to the tumour. SRT provides an option to elderly patients, patients with severe lung or heart disease, and other patients with poor health who are not good candidates for surgery. SRT is an outpatient procedure that uses special positioning procedures and radiology techniques so that a higher dose of radiation can be delivered to the tumour, and a smaller part of the healthy lung is exposed.

Chemotherapy. Chemotherapy may be used in the treatment of nonresectable tumours or as adjuvant therapy to surgery in NSCLC with distant metastases. A variety of chemotherapy drugs and multidrug regimens (i.e., protocols) including combination chemotherapy have been used. These drugs include etoposide (VePesid), carboplatin, cisplatin, paclitaxel (Taxol), vinorelbine, cyclophosphamide (Procytox), ifosfamide (Ifex), docetaxel (Taxotere), gemcitabine (Gemzar), topotecan (Hycamtin), and irinotecan (Camptosar). Chemotherapy has improved survival in patients with advanced NSCLC and is now considered standard treatment.

Biological Therapy. Biological (targeted) therapy as adjuvant therapy has been used in individuals with cancer, including malignant lung tumours. (Biological therapy is discussed in Chapter 18.)

Other Therapies
Prophylactic Cranial Radiation. Brain metastasis is a common complication of SCLC. Most chemotherapy drugs do not adequately penetrate the blood–brain barrier. Prophylactic cranial radiation may be used as a potential way to improve the prognosis of patients, especially those who have a complete response to chemotherapy. Toxicity of this therapy may include scalp erythema, fatigue, and alopecia.

Bronchoscopic Laser Therapy. Bronchoscopic laser therapy makes it possible to remove obstructing bronchial lesions. The thermal energy of the laser is transmitted to the target tissue. It is a complicated procedure that often requires general anaesthesia to control the patient's cough reflex. Relief of the symptoms from airway obstruction as a result of thermal necrosis and shrinkage of the tumour can be dramatic. However, it is not a curative therapy for cancer.

Phototherapy. Photodynamic therapy is a safe, nonsurgical therapy for lung cancer. Porfimer (Photofrin) is injected intravenously and selectively concentrates in tumour cells. After a set time (usually 48 hr), the tumour is exposed to laser light, producing a toxic form of oxygen that destroys tumour cells. Necrotic tissue is removed through a bronchoscope.

Airway Stenting. Stents can be used alone or in combination with other techniques for palliation of dyspnea, cough, or respiratory insufficiency. The advantage of an airway stent is that it supports the airway wall against collapse or external compression and can impede extension of the tumour into the airway lumen.

Cryotherapy. Cryotherapy is a technique in which tissue is destroyed as a result of freezing. Bronchoscopic cryotherapy is used to ablate (destroy) bronchogenic carcinomas, especially polypoid lesions. A repeat bronchoscope is performed 8 to 10 days after the first session. The second examination enables assessment of cryodestruction, removal of any slough, and repeat cryotherapy if required for the treatment of large lesions.

NURSING MANAGEMENT: LUNG CANCER

Nursing Assessment

It is important to determine the understanding of the patient and the family concerning the diagnostic tests (those completed as well as those planned), the diagnosis or potential diagnosis, the treatment options, and the prognosis. At the same time, the nurse can assess the level of anxiety experienced by the patient and the support provided and needed by the patient's significant others. Subjective and objective data that should be obtained from a patient with lung cancer are presented in Table 30-19.

Nursing Diagnoses

Nursing diagnoses for the patient with lung cancer may include, but are not limited to, the following:
- Ineffective airway clearance *related to* increased tracheobronchial secretions and presence of tumour.
- Anxiety *related to* lack of knowledge of diagnosis or unknown prognosis and treatments.
- Acute pain *related to* pressure of tumour on surrounding structures and erosion of tissues.
- Imbalanced nutrition: less than body requirements *related to* increased metabolic demands, increased secretions, weakness, and anorexia.
- Ineffective self-health management *related to* lack of knowledge about the disease process and therapeutic regimen.
- Ineffective breathing pattern *related to* decreased lung capacity.

Planning

The overall goals are that the patient with lung cancer will have (1) effective breathing patterns, (2) adequate airway clearance, (3) adequate oxygenation of tissues, (4) minimal to no pain, and (5) a realistic attitude toward treatment and prognosis.

NURSING ASSESSMENT

Table 30-19 Lung Cancer

Subjective Data

Important Health Information

Past health history: Exposure to second-hand smoke; airborne carcinogens (e.g., asbestos, uranium, chromates, hydrocarbons, arsenic) or other pollutants; urban living environment; chronic lung disease, including TB, COPD, bronchiectasis; smoking history; frequent respiratory infections; family history of lung cancer

Medications: Use of cough medicines or other respiratory medications

Symptoms

- Anorexia, nausea, vomiting, dysphagia (late symptom), weight loss
- Persistent cough (productive or nonproductive), dyspnea, hemoptysis (late symptom)
- Fatigue, fever, chills
- Chest pain or tightness, shoulder and arm pain; headache; bone pain (late symptom)

Objective Data

General

Fever, neck and axillary lymphadenopathy, paraneoplastic syndromes (e.g., SIADH secretion)

Integumentary

Jaundice (liver metastasis); edema of neck and face (superior vena cava syndrome), digital clubbing

Respiratory

Wheezing, hoarseness, stridor, unilateral diaphragm paralysis, pleural effusions (late signs)

Cardiovascular

Pericardial effusion, cardiac tamponade, dysrhythmias (late signs)

Neurological

Unsteady gait (brain metastasis)

Musculoskeletal

Pathological fractures, muscle wasting (late sign)

Possible Findings

Observance of lesion on chest radiographic examination, CT scan, lung scan, or PET scan; MRI findings of mediastinal invasion, positive sputum or bronchial washings for cytological studies; positive fibreoptic bronchoscopy and biopsy findings; low serum sodium and hypercalcemia (paraneoplastic syndrome)

COPD, chronic obstructive pulmonary disease; *CT,* computed tomography; *MRI,* magnetic resonance imaging; *PET,* positron emission tomography; *SIADH,* syndrome of inappropriate antidiuretic hormone; *TB,* tuberculosis.

Nursing Implementation

Health Promotion

The best way to halt the epidemic of lung cancer is for people to stop smoking. Important nursing activities to assist in the progress toward this goal include promoting smoking cessation programs and actively supporting education and policy changes related to smoking. Important changes have occurred as the result of the recognition that sidestream smoke is a health hazard. There are now laws that (1) require designation of nonsmoking areas in most public places; (2) prohibit smoking; and (3) ban smoking on airline flights. Other actions aimed at controlling tobacco use include restrictions on tobacco advertising on television and warning label requirements for cigarette packaging. These are examples of beginning steps toward the goal of a smokeless society. Despite the small advances being made, tobacco-producer organizations such as marketing boards and tobacco companies still have strong political influences.

For the individual who does have a smoking habit, efforts should be made to assist the smoker to stop smoking. There are many resources available to help. The RNAO Best Practice Guideline *Integrating Smoking Cessation into Daily Nursing Practice* recommends nurses use the "ask, advise, assist, arrange" protocol to motivate smokers and other tobacco users to quit (RNAO, 2007). The five stages of change identified in smokers attempting to quit include precontemplation, contemplation, preparation, action, and maintenance. (The stages of change in relationship to patient teaching are discussed in Chapter 4, Table 4-3.) Each stage requires specific actions to progress to the next stage. Nurses working with patients at their individual stage of change will help them progress to the next stage. For patients unwilling to quit, motivational interviewing is recommended (discussed in Chapter 11 on p. 212). In Canada, the Canadian Lung Association (2012) has published a report on Canadians' access to counselling, medications, and supports to help Canadians quit smoking, and recommendations for each province, a number of which have been followed to date. The Canadian Cancer Society (2007) has a series of "One Step at a Time" guides for quitting smoking that are available at its Web site. Health Canada (2008) also provides resources via a GoSmokeFree strategy. Tobacco use and dependence and strategies to assist patients to stop smoking are discussed in Chapter 11.

The evidence-informed guideline also offers the five *R*s strategy for motivating smokers to quit: *r*elevance, *r*isk, *r*eward, *r*oadblocks, and *r*epetition. Because some patients relapse months or years after having stopped smoking, nurses must continually provide interactions to prevent relapse.

Nicotine's addictive properties make quitting a difficult task that requires much support. Nicotine replacement significantly lessens the urge to smoke and increases the percentage of smokers who successfully quit smoking. There is no evidence that one product has better results than another, so the choice of agent is dependent on the health care provider and patient preferences.

The advice and motivation of health care providers can be a powerful force in smoking cessation. Nurses are in a unique position to promote smoking cessation because they see large numbers of smokers who may be reluctant to seek help. Support for the smoker includes education that smoking a few cigarettes during a cessation attempt (a slip) is much different from resuming the full smoking habit (a relapse). Despite the slip, smokers should be encouraged to continue the attempt at cessation without viewing the effort as a failure. Measures to assist an individual in quitting should be directed toward the meaning that smoking has to that individual. The nurse must be aware of resources in the community to assist the individual who is interested in quitting.

▮ Acute Intervention

Care of the patient with lung cancer will initially involve support and reassurance during the diagnostic evaluation. (Specific nursing measures related to the diagnostic studies are outlined in Chapter 28.)

Another major responsibility of the nurse is to help the patient and the family deal with the diagnosis of lung cancer. The patient may feel guilty about cigarette smoking having caused the cancer and need to discuss this feeling with someone who has a nonjudgemental attitude. Questions regarding each patient's condition should be answered honestly. Additional counselling from a social worker, psychologist, or member of the clergy may be needed. Specific care of the patient will depend on the treatment plan. Postoperative care for the patient having surgery is discussed later in this chapter. Care of the patient undergoing radiation therapy and chemotherapy is discussed in Chapter 18. The nurse has a major role in providing patient comfort, teaching methods to reduce pain, assessing for signs and symptoms of progressive or recurrent disease, and assessing indications for hospitalization.

▮ Ambulatory and Home Care

Patient teaching needs to include signs and symptoms to report, such as hemoptysis, dysphagia, chest pain, and hoarseness. The patient and caregivers should be encouraged to provide a smoke-free environment. This may include smoking cessation for multiple family members.

If the treatment plan includes the use of home oxygen, part of the teaching plan must include the safe use of oxygen. The patient who has had a surgical resection with intent to cure should be followed up carefully for manifestations of metastasis. The patient and family should be told to contact the physician if symptoms such as hemoptysis, dysphagia, chest pain, and hoarseness develop. For many individuals who have lung cancer, little can be done to significantly prolong their lives. Radiation therapy and chemotherapy can be used to provide palliative relief from distressing symptoms. Constant pain becomes a major problem. (Measures used to relieve pain are discussed in Chapter 10. Care of the patient with cancer is discussed in Chapter 18.) The patient and family or caregivers may need information about palliative care options in the community.

▮ Evaluation

The following are the expected outcomes for the patient with lung cancer:

- Patient will have adequate breathing patterns.
- Patient will have adequate airway clearance.
- Patient will have adequate tissue oxygenation.
- Patient will have minimal to no pain.
- Patient will have realistic attitude about prognosis.

Other Types of Lung Tumours

Other types of primary lung tumours include sarcomas, lymphomas, and bronchial adenomas. Bronchial adenomas are small tumours that arise from the lower trachea or major bronchi and are considered malignant because they are locally invasive and frequently metastasize. Clinical manifestations of bronchial adenomas include hemoptysis, persistent cough, localized obstructive wheezing, and pneumonia. Bronchial adenomas can usually be treated successfully with surgical resection.

The lungs are a common site for secondary metastases and are more often affected by metastatic growth than by primary

Do Noninvasive Interventions Improve Quality of Life in Patients with Lung Cancer?

Clinical Question

In lung cancer patients (P), does receiving noninvasive interventions (I) compared with receiving no additional treatment (C) improve symptoms, psychological functioning, and quality of life (O)?

Best Available Evidence

Systematic review of RCTs or quasi-RCTs

Critical Appraisal and Synthesis of Evidence

- Meta-analysis of 15 clinical trials
- Interventions studied included nursing interventions to manage breathlessness, nursing care programs, nutritional interventions, psychotherapeutic interventions, exercise, and reflexology.

Conclusions

- Nursing interventions to manage breathlessness showed improved symptom control, performance status, and emotional functioning.
- Nursing programs were effective in delaying clinical deterioration, dependency, and symptom distress as well as improving emotional functioning and satisfaction with care.
- Exercise and nutritional interventions had no significant or lasting effects on quality of life.
- Psychological interventions and reflexology had some short-lasting positive effects on quality of life.

Implications for Nursing Practice

- It is important to develop and maintain a supportive and empathetic relationship with the patient with lung cancer.
- Offer patients supportive multidisciplinary interventions that may benefit their emotional, psychological, and physical well-being.
- These interventions may also help patients with other types of cancers.
- Further research is needed to accurately assess the effectiveness of noninvasive nursing interventions on the well-being and quality of life in patients with cancer.

Reference for Evidence

Rueda, J. R., Sola, I., Pascual, A., & Subirana, M., (2011). Non-invasive interventions for improving well-being and quality of life in patients with lung cancer. *Cochrane Database of Systematic Review,* 9. Art. No.: CD004282. doi:10.1002/14651858. CD004282.pub3

PICO: P, Patient population of interest; *I,* intervention or area of interest; *C,* comparison of interest or comparison group; *O,* outcome(s) of interest.
RCTs, randomized controlled trials.

lung tumours. The pulmonary capillaries, with their extensive network, are ideal sites for tumour emboli. In addition, the lungs have an extensive lymphatic network. The primary malignancies that spread to the lungs often originate in the GI or genitourinary tracts and in the breast. General symptoms of lung metastases are chest pain and nonproductive cough.

Benign tumours of the lung are generally classified as *mesenchymal.* Their occurrence is rare, and they have the potential to become malignant. The most common mesenchymal tumours are *chondromas,* which arise in the bronchial cartilage, and *leiomyomas,* which are myomas of smooth, nonstriated muscle fibres. Mesotheliomas may be malignant or benign and originate from the visceral pleura. Benign mesotheliomas are localized lesions.

Hamartomas of the lung are the most common benign tumour. These tumours, composed of fibrous tissue, fat, and blood vessels, are congenital malformations of the connective tissue of the bronchiolar walls. Hamartomas are slow-growing tumours.

Chest Trauma and Thoracic Injuries

Traumatic injuries fall into two major categories: (1) blunt trauma and (2) penetrating trauma. *Blunt trauma* occurs when the body is struck by a blunt object, such as a steering wheel. The external injury may appear minor, but the impact may cause severe, life-threatening internal injuries, such as a ruptured spleen. *Contrecoup trauma,* a type of blunt trauma, is caused by the impact of parts of the body against other objects. This type of injury differs from blunt trauma primarily in the velocity of the impact. Internal organs are rapidly forced back and forth within the bony structures that surround them so that internal injury is sustained not only on the side of the impact but also on the opposite side, where the organ or organs hit bony structures. If the velocity of impact is great enough, organs and blood vessels can literally be torn from their points of origin. This is the shearing injury that can cause transection of the aorta, hemothorax, and diaphragmatic rupture injuries. Compression injury occurs when the body cannot handle the degree of external pressure during blunt trauma, resulting in contusions, crush injuries, and organ rupture.

Penetrating trauma occurs when a foreign body impales or passes through the body tissues (e.g., gunshot wounds, stabbings). Table 30-20 describes selective traumatic injuries as they relate to the categories of trauma and the mechanism of injury.

Table 30-20 Common Traumatic Chest Injuries and Mechanisms of Injury

MECHANISM OF INJURY	COMMON RELATED INJURY
Blunt Trauma	
Blunt steering-wheel injury to chest	Rib fractures, flail chest, pneumothorax, hemopneumothorax, cardiac contusion, pulmonary contusion, cardiac tamponade, great vessel tears
Shoulder-harness seat belt injury	Fractured clavicle, dislocated shoulder, rib fractures, pulmonary contusion, pericardial contusion, cardiac tamponade
Crush injury (e.g., heavy equipment, crushing thorax)	Pneumothorax and hemopneumothorax, flail chest, great vessel tears and rupture, decreased blood return to heart with decreased cardiac output
Penetrating Trauma	
Gunshot or stab wound to chest	Open pneumothorax, tension pneumothorax, hemopneumothorax, cardiac tamponade, esophageal damage, tracheal tear, great vessel tears

Table 30-21 Chest Trauma

ETIOLOGY	ASSESSMENT FINDINGS	INTERVENTIONS
Blunt	**Respiratory**	**Initial**
• Motor vehicle accident	• Dyspnea, respiratory distress	• Ensure patent airway.
• Pedestrian accident	• Cough with or without hemoptysis	• Administer high-flow O_2 with nonrebreather mask.
• Fall	• Cyanosis of mouth, face, nail beds, mucous membranes	• Establish IV access with two large-bore catheters. Begin fluid resuscitation as appropriate.
• Assault with blunt object	• Tracheal deviation	• Remove clothing to assess injury.
• Crush injury	• Audible air escaping from chest wound	• Cover sucking chest wound with nonporous dressing taped on three sides.
• Explosion	• Decreased breath sounds on side of injury	• Stabilize impaling objects with bulky dressings. Do not remove.
Penetrating	• Decreased O_2 saturation	• Assess for other significant injuries and treat appropriately.
• Knife	• Frothy secretions	• Stabilize flail rib segment first with hand and then by application of large pieces of tape horizontal across the flail segment.
• Gunshot	**Cardiovascular**	• Place patient in a semi-Fowler's position or position patient on the injured side if breathing is easier, after cervical spine injury has been ruled out.
• Stick	• Rapid, thready pulse	
• Arrow	• Decreased blood pressure	**Ongoing Monitoring**
• Other missiles	• Narrowed pulse pressure	• Monitor vital signs, level of consciousness, oxygen saturation, cardiac rhythm, respiratory status, and urinary output.
	• Asymmetrical blood pressure values in arms	• Anticipate intubation for respiratory distress.
	• Distended neck veins	• Release dressing if tension pneumothorax develops after sucking chest wound is covered.
	• Muffled heart sounds	
	• Chest pain	
	• Crunching sound synchronous with heart sounds	
	• Dysrhythmias	
	Surface Findings	
	• Bruising	
	• Abrasions	
	• Open chest wound	
	• Asymmetrical chest movement	
	• Subcutaneous emphysema	

IV, intravenous.

Emergency care of the patient with a chest injury is presented in Table 30-21.

Thoracic injuries range from simple rib fractures to life-threatening tears of the aorta, vena cava, and other major vessels. The most common thoracic emergencies and their management are described in Table 30-22.

Pneumothorax

A **pneumothorax** is the presence of air in the pleural space. There is a resultant complete or partial collapse of a lung caused by the accumulation of air in the pleural space. This condition should be suspected after any blunt trauma to the chest wall. Pneumothorax may be closed or open. Pneumothorax associated with trauma may be accompanied by hemothorax, a condition called *hemopneumothorax.*

Types of Pneumothorax

Closed Pneumothorax. *Closed pneumothorax* has no associated external wound. The most common form is a spontaneous pneumothorax, which is accumulation of air in the pleural space without an apparent antecedent event. It is caused by

rupture of small **blebs** (air-filled alveolar dilations <1 cm in diameter on the edge of the lung at the apex of the upper lobe or superior segment of the lower lobe) on the visceral pleural space. The cause of the blebs is unknown. This condition occurs most commonly in underweight male cigarette smokers between 20 and 40 years of age. There is a tendency for this condition to recur.

Other causes of closed pneumothorax include the following:
1. Injury to the lungs from mechanical ventilation
2. Injury to the lungs from insertion of a subclavian catheter
3. Perforation of the esophagus
4. Injury to the lungs from broken ribs
5. Ruptured blebs or bullae in a patient with COPD

Open Pneumothorax. *Open pneumothorax* occurs when air enters the pleural space through an opening in the chest wall (Figure 30-5, *B*). Examples include stab or gunshot wounds and surgical thoracotomies. A penetrating chest wound is often referred to as a *sucking chest wound.*

An open pneumothorax should be covered with a vented dressing. (A vented dressing is one secured on three sides with the fourth side left untaped.) This allows air to escape from the vent and decreases the likelihood of tension pneumothorax developing. If the object that caused the open chest wound is

EMERGENCY MANAGEMENT
Table 30-22 Thoracic Injuries

DEFINITION	CLINICAL MANIFESTATIONS	EMERGENCY MANAGEMENT
Pneumothorax		
Air in pleural space (see Figure 30-5)	Dyspnea, decreased movement of involved chest wall, diminished or absent breath sounds on the affected side, hyperresonance to percussion	Chest tube insertion with chest drainage system; Heimlich (Flutter) valve
Hemothorax		
Blood in the pleural space, usually occurs in conjunction with pneumothorax	Dyspnea, diminished or absent breath sounds, dullness to percussion, shock	Chest tube insertion with chest drainage system; autotransfusion of collected blood, treatment of hypovolemia as necessary
Tension Pneumothorax		
Air in pleural space that does not escape Continued increase in amount of air shifts intrathoracic organs and increases intrathoracic pressure (see Figure 30-6)	Cyanosis, air hunger, violent agitation, tracheal deviation away from affected side, subcutaneous emphysema, neck vein distension, hyperresonance to percussion	Medical emergency: needle decompression followed by chest tube insertion with chest drainage system
Flail Chest		
Fracture of two or more adjacent ribs in two or more places with loss of chest wall stability (see Figure 30-7)	Paradoxical movement of chest wall, respiratory distress, associated hemothorax, pneumothorax, pulmonary contusion	Stabilize flail segment with intubation in some patients and taping in others; oxygen therapy; treat associated injuries; analgesia
Cardiac Tamponade		
Blood rapidly collects in pericardial sac, compresses myocardium because the pericardium does not stretch, and prevents heart from pumping effectively	Muffled, distant heart sounds, hypotension, neck vein distension, increased central venous pressure	Medical emergency: pericardiocentesis with surgical repair as appropriate

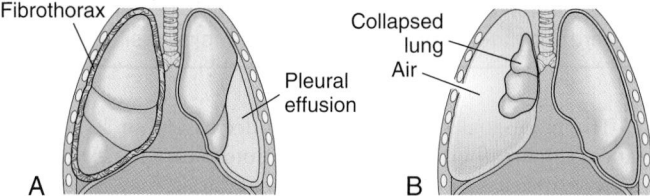

Figure 30-5 Disorders of the pleura. **A,** Fibrothorax resulting from an organization of inflammatory exudate and pleural effusion. **B,** Open pneumothorax resulting from collapse of the lung caused by disruption of the chest wall and outside air entering.

still in place, it should not be removed until a physician is present. The impaling object should be stabilized with a bulky dressing.

Tension Pneumothorax.
Tension pneumothorax is a pneumothorax with rapid accumulation of air in the pleural space causing severely high intrapleural pressures with resultant tension on the heart and great vessels. It may result from either an open or a closed pneumothorax (Figure 30-6). In an open chest wound, a flap may act as a one-way valve; thus, air can enter on inspiration but cannot escape. The intrathoracic pressure increases, the lung collapses, and the mediastinum shifts toward the unaffected side, which is subsequently compressed. As the pressure increases, cardiac output is altered because of decreased venous return and compression of the vena cava and aorta. Tension pneumothorax can occur with mechanical ventilation and resuscitative efforts. It can also occur if chest tubes are clamped or become blocked in a patient with a pneumothorax.

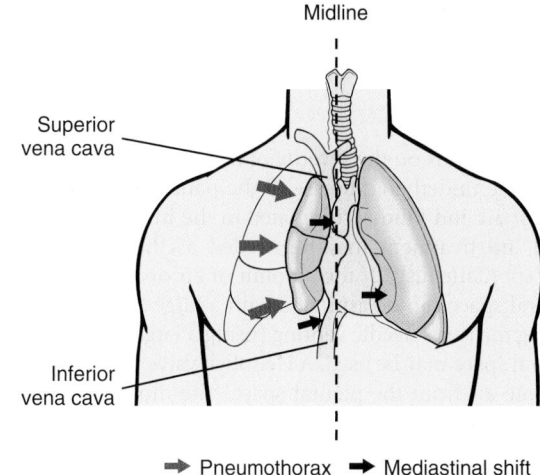

→ Pneumothorax → Mediastinal shift

Figure 30-6 Tension pneumothorax. As pleural pressure on the affected side increases, mediastinal displacement ensues with resultant respiratory and cardiovascular compromise.

Unclamping the tube or relief of the obstruction will remedy this situation.

Tension pneumothorax is a medical emergency with both the respiratory and the circulatory systems affected. If the tension in the pleural space is not relieved, the patient is likely to die from inadequate cardiac output or marked hypoxemia. Nurses and paramedics are now being trained to insert large-bore needles and chest tubes into the chest wall to release the trapped air.

Hemothorax.
Hemothorax is an accumulation of blood in the intrapleural space. It is frequently found in association with

open pneumothorax and is then called a *hemopneumothorax.* Causes of hemothorax include chest trauma, lung malignancy, complications of anticoagulant therapy, pulmonary embolus, and tearing of pleural adhesions.

Chylothorax. **Chylothorax** is the presence of lymphatic fluid in the pleural space because of a leak in the thoracic duct. Causes include trauma, surgical procedures, and malignancy. The thoracic duct is disrupted, and the chylous fluid, milky white with high lipid content, fills the pleural space. Total lymphatic flow through the thoracic duct is 1500 to 2400 mL/day. Fifty percent of those affected will heal with conservative treatment (chest drainage, bowel rest, and total parenteral nutrition). Surgery and pleurodesis are options if conservative therapy fails. *Pleurodesis* is the artificial production of adhesions between the parietal and the visceral pleura, usually done with a chemical sclerosing agent.

Clinical Manifestations

If the pneumothorax is small, mild tachycardia and dyspnea may be the only manifestations. If the pneumothorax is large, respiratory distress may be present, including shallow, rapid respirations; dyspnea; air hunger; and decreased oxygen saturation. Chest pain and a cough with or without hemoptysis may be present. On auscultation, there are no breath sounds over the affected area, and hyperresonance may be present. A chest radiograph shows the presence of air or fluid in the pleural space. If a tension pneumothorax develops, severe respiratory distress, tachycardia, and hypotension occur. Mediastinal displacement occurs, and the trachea shifts to the unaffected side. The patient is hemodynamically unstable.

Collaborative Care

Treatment depends on the severity of the pneumothorax and the nature of the underlying disease. If the patient is stable and the amount of air and fluid accumulated in the intrapleural space is minimal, no treatment may be needed as the pneumothorax resolves spontaneously. If the amount of air or fluid is minimal, the pleural space can be aspirated with a large-bore needle. As a life-saving measure, needle venting (using a large-bore needle) of the pleural space may be used. A Heimlich valve may also be used to evacuate air from the pleural space. The most definitive and common form of treatment of pneumothorax and hemothorax is to insert a chest tube and connect it to water-seal drainage. Repeated spontaneous pneumothorax may have to be treated surgically by a partial pleurectomy, stapling, or pleurodesis to promote adherence of the pleurae to one another.

Fractured Ribs

Rib fractures are the most common type of chest injury resulting from trauma. Ribs 5 through 10 are most commonly fractured because they are least protected by chest muscles. If the fractured rib is splintered or displaced, it may damage the pleura and the lungs.

Clinical manifestations of fractured ribs include pain (especially on inspiration) at the site of injury. The individual splints the affected area and takes shallow breaths to try to decrease the pain. The individual is reluctant to take deep breaths, and the decreased ventilation may cause atelectasis to develop.

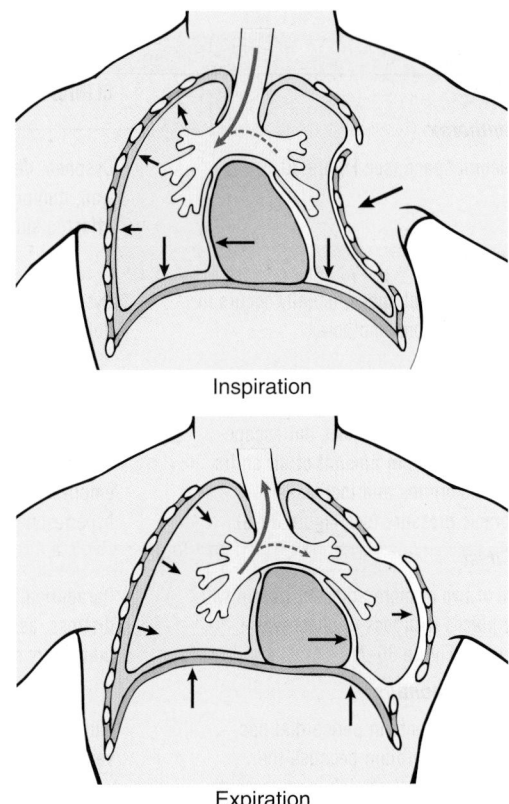

Inspiration

Expiration

Figure 30-7 Flail chest produces paradoxical respiration. On *inspiration*, the flail section sinks in with the mediastinal shift to the uninjured side. On *expiration*, the flail section bulges outward with the mediastinal shift to the injured side.

The main goal in treatment is to decrease pain so that the patient can breathe adequately to promote good chest expansion. Intercostal nerve blocks with local anaesthesia may be used to provide pain relief. The effect of the anaesthesia lasts for a period of hours to days. It must be repeated as necessary to provide pain relief. Narcotic drug therapy must be individualized and used with caution because these drugs can depress respirations. Nonsteroidal anti-inflammatory drugs are used to reduce pain and aid with deep breathing and coughing. Patient teaching should emphasize deep breathing, coughing, use of incentive spirometry, and use of pain medications. Strapping the chest with tape or using a binder is not common practice. Most physicians believe that these measures should be avoided because they reduce lung expansion and predispose the individual to atelectasis.

Flail Chest

Flail chest results from multiple rib fractures, causing instability of the chest wall (Figure 30-7). The chest wall cannot provide the bony structure necessary to maintain bellows action and ventilation. The affected (flail) area will move paradoxically to the intact portion of the chest during respiration. During inspiration, the affected portion is sucked in, and during expiration, it bulges out. This paradoxical chest movement prevents adequate ventilation of the lung in the injured area. The underlying lung may or may not have a serious injury. Associated pain and any lung injury giving rise to loss of compliance will contribute to an alteration in breathing patterns and lead to hypoxemia.

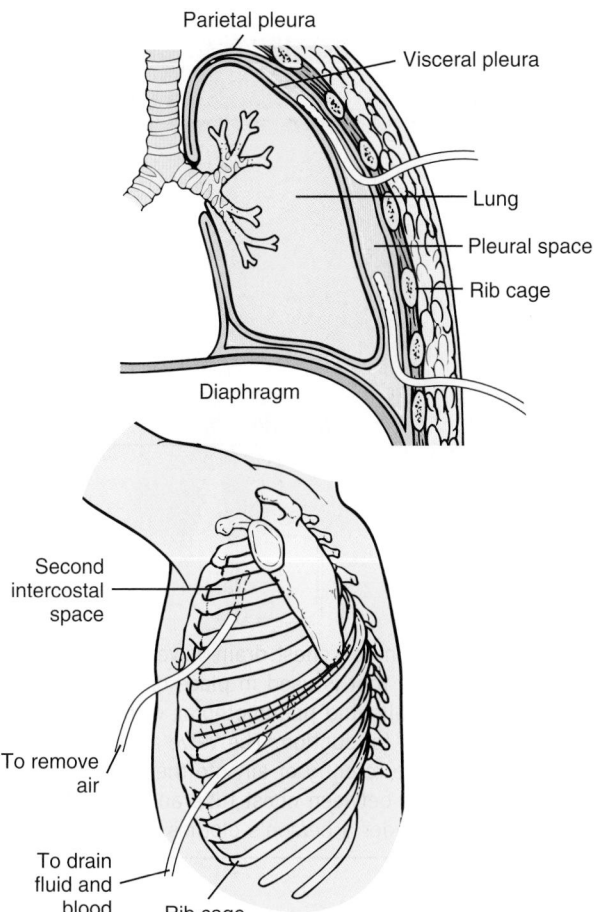

Parietal pleura

Visceral pleura

Lung

Pleural space

Rib cage

Diaphragm

Second
intercostal
space

To remove
air

To drain
fluid and
blood

Rib cage

Figure 30-8 Placement of chest tubes.

A flail chest is usually apparent on visual examination of the unconscious patient. The patient manifests rapid, shallow respirations and tachycardia. A flail chest may not be initially apparent in the conscious patient as a result of splinting of the chest wall. The patient moves air poorly, and movement of the thorax is asymmetrical and uncoordinated. Palpation of abnormal respiratory movements, crepitus of the rib, chest radiography, and ABG assessment assist in the diagnosis.

Initial therapy consists of adequate ventilation, administration of humidified O_2, careful administration of crystalloid IV solutions, and pain control. The definitive therapy is to re-expand the lung and ensure adequate oxygenation. Although many patients can be managed without the use of mechanical ventilation, a short period of intubation and ventilation may be necessary until the diagnosis of the lung injury is complete. The lung parenchyma and fractured ribs will heal with time. Some patients continue to experience intercostal pain after the flail chest has resolved.

Chest Tubes and Pleural Drainage

The purpose of chest tubes and pleural drainage is to remove the air and fluid from the pleural space and to restore normal intrapleural pressure so that the lungs can re-expand. (Intrapleural pressure and the intrapleural space are described in Chapter 28.) Small accumulations of air or fluid in the pleural space may not require removal by thoracentesis or chest tube insertion. Instead, the air and fluid may be reabsorbed over time.

Chest Tube Insertion

Chest tubes can be inserted in the emergency department, at the patient's bedside, or in the operating room, depending on the situation. In the operating room, the chest tube is inserted via the thoracotomy incision. In the emergency department or at the bedside, the patient is placed in a sitting position or is lying down with the affected side elevated. The area is prepared with antiseptic solution, and the site is infiltrated with a local anaesthetic agent. After a small incision is made, one or two chest tubes are inserted into the pleural space. One catheter is placed anteriorly through the second intercostals space to remove air (Figure 30-8). The other is placed posteriorly through the eighth or ninth intercostal space to drain fluid and blood. The tubes are sutured to the chest wall, and the puncture wound is covered with an airtight dressing. During insertion, the tubes are kept clamped. After the tubes are in place in the pleural space, they are connected to drainage tubing and pleural drainage and the clamp is removed. Each tube may be connected to a separate drainage system and suction. More commonly, a Y-connector is used to attach both chest tubes to the same drainage system.

Pleural Drainage

Most pleural drainage systems have three basic compartments, each with its own separate function.

The *first compartment*, or collection chamber, receives fluid and air from the chest cavity. The fluid stays in this chamber while the air vents to the second compartment (Figure 30-9). The *second compartment*, called the water-seal chamber, contains 2 cm of water, which acts as a one-way valve. The incoming air enters from the collection chamber and bubbles up through the water. (The water acts as a one-way valve to prevent backflow of air into the patient from the system.) Initial bubbling of air is seen in this chamber when a pneumothorax is evacuated. Intermittent bubbling can also be seen during exhalation, coughing, or sneezing because of an increase in the patient's intrathoracic pressure. In this chamber, fluctuations, or "tidalling," will be seen that reflect the pressures in the pleural space. If tidalling is not seen, either the lungs have re-expanded or there is a kink or obstruction in the tubing. The air then exits the water seal and enters the suction chamber.

A *third compartment*, the suction control chamber, applies controlled suction to the chest drainage system. The classic suction control chamber uses tubing with one end submerged in a column of water and the other end vented to the atmosphere. It is typically filled with 20 cm of water. When the negative pressure generated by the suction source exceeds 20 cm, the air from the atmosphere enters the chamber through a vent and begins bubbling up through the water. As a result, excess pressure is relieved. The amount of suction applied is regulated by the depth of the suction control tube in the water and not by the amount of suction applied to the system. An increase in suction does not result in an increase in negative pressure to the system because any excess suction merely draws in air through the vented tubing. The suction pressure is usually ordered to be –20 cm H_2O.

Two types of suction control chambers are available on the market: wet and dry. The *wet suction control chamber system* is the classic system outlined previously. Bubbling is one way to tell that suction is functioning. To start the suction, the vacuum source is

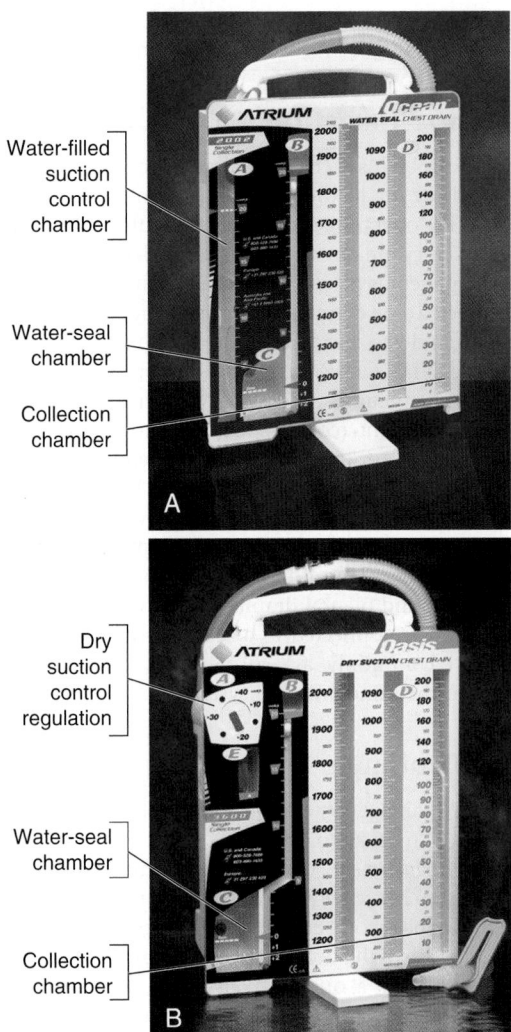

Figure 30-9 caption area:

Figure 30-9 Chest drainage unit. Both units have three chambers: (1) collection chamber; (2) water-seal chamber; and (3) suction control chamber. The suction control chamber requires a connection to a wall suction source that is dialled up higher than the prescribed suction for the suction to work. **A,** Water suction. This unit uses water in the suction control chamber to control the wall suction pressure. **B,** Dry suction. This unit controls wall suction by using a regulator control dial.

Source: Atrium Medical Corporation, Hudson, NH.

turned up until gentle bubbling appears. Turning the vacuum source higher just makes the bubbling more vigorous and makes the water evaporate faster. Even with gentle bubbling, water evaporates in this chamber, and water must be added periodically. The *dry suction control chamber system* contains no water. It uses either a restrictive device or a regulator to dial the desired negative pressure; this is internal to the chest drainage system. The dry system has a visual alert that indicates if the suction is working, so bubbling is not seen in a third chamber. To increase the suction pressures, the dial is turned on the drainage system. Increasing the vacuum suction source will not increase the pressure (see Figure 30-9).

A variety of commercial disposable plastic chest drainage systems are available. The manufacturer's suggestions for use are included with the equipment. The plastic units allow the patient mobility and decrease the risk of breaking or spilling the drainage system.

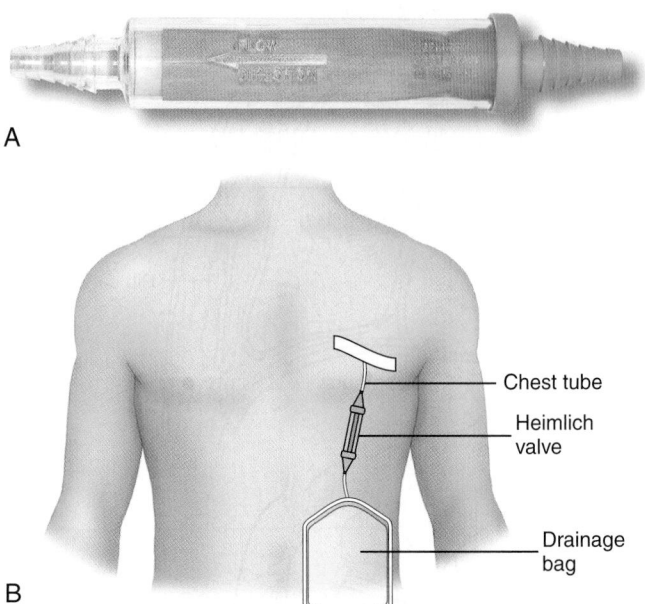

Figure 30-10 A, Heimlich chest drain valve is a specially designed Flutter valve that is used in place of a chest drainage unit for small uncomplicated pneumothorax with little or no drainage and no need for suction. The valve allows for escape of air but prevents the re-entry of air into the pleural space. **B,** Placement of valve between chest tube and drainage bag, which can be worn under a person's clothes.

Heimlich Valves. Another device that may be used to evacuate air from the pleural space is the Heimlich valve (Figure 30-10). This device consists of a rubber Flutter one-way valve within a rigid plastic tube. It is attached to the external end of the chest tube. The valve opens whenever the pressure is greater than atmospheric pressure and closes when the reverse occurs. The Heimlich valve functions like a water seal and is usually used for emergency transport or in special home care situations.

Small Chest Tubes. Small chest tubes ("pigtail catheters") are used in selected patients because they are less traumatic. The drains may be straight catheters or "pigtail" catheters (curled at the distal end to look like a pig's tail). Curled catheters are considered to be less traumatic than straight catheters. These catheters, if occluded, can be irrigated by the physician using sterile water. Chemical pleurodesis can also be performed through this catheter. This system is not suitable for trauma or for drainage of blood. Owing to the smaller size, the tube can become kinked, occluded, or dislodged more easily. Small-bore chest tubes and Heimlich valves should be used with caution in patients on mechanical ventilators because there is a potential for rapid accumulation of air and a tension pneumothorax (Light, 2011).

NURSING MANAGEMENT: CHEST DRAINAGE

Some general guidelines for nursing care of the patient with chest tubes and water-seal drainage systems are presented in Table 30-23. The traditional practice of routine milking and/or

Table 30-23 Clinical Guidelines for Care of Patient With Chest Tubes and Water-Seal Drainage System

1. Keep all tubing loosely coiled below chest level. Tubing should drop straight from bed or chair to drainage unit. Do not let it be compressed.

2. Keep all connections between chest tubes, drainage tubing, and drainage collector tight, and tape at connections.

3. Observe for air fluctuations (tidalling) and bubbling in the water-seal chamber.
   - If no tidalling is observed (rising with inspiration and falling with expiration in the spontaneously breathing patient), the drainage system is blocked, the lungs are re-expanded, or the system is attached to suction.
   - If bubbling increases, there may be an air leak in the drainage system or a leak from the patient (bronchopleural leak).

4. If the chest tube is connected to suction, disconnect from wall suction to check for tidalling.

5. Suspect a system leak when bubbling is continuous.
   - To determine the source of the air leak, momentarily clamp the tubing successively from the chest tube insertion site to the drainage set, observing for the bubbling to cease. When bubbling ceases, the leak is above the clamp.
   - Retape tubing connections.
   - If leak continues, notify physician. It may be necessary to replace the drainage apparatus, or secure the chest tube with an air-occlusive dressing.

6. High fluid levels in the water seal indicate residual negative pressure.
   - The chest system may need to be vented by using the high negativity release valve available on the drainage system to release residual pressure from the system.
   - Do not lower water-seal column when wall suction is not operating or when patient is on gravity drainage.

Patient's Clinical Status

1. Monitor the patient's clinical status. Assess vital signs, lung sounds, pain.

2. Assess for manifestations of reaccumulation of air and fluid in the chest (↓ or absent breath sounds), significant bleeding (>100 mL/hr), chest drainage site infection (drainage, erythema, fever, ↑ white blood cell count), or poor wound healing. Notify physician for management plan. Evaluate for subcutaneous emphysema at chest tube site.

3. Encourage the patient to breathe deeply periodically to facilitate lung expansion, and encourage range-of-motion exercises to the shoulder on the affected side. Incentive spirometry every hour while awake may be necessary to prevent atelectasis or pneumonia.

4. Chest tubes are *not routinely clamped*. A physician order is required. A physician may order clamping for 24 hr to evaluate for reaccumulation of fluid or air before discontinuing the chest tube.

Chest Drainage

1. Never elevate the drainage system to the level of the patient's chest because this will cause fluid to drain back into the lungs. Secure the unit to the drainage stand. If the drainage chambers are full, notify the physician and anticipate changing the system. Do not try to empty it.

2. Mark the time of measurement and the fluid level on the drainage unit according to the unit standards. Report any change in the quantity or characteristics of drainage (e.g., clear yellow to bloody) to the physician and record the change. Notify physician if >100 mL/hr drainage.

3. Check the position of the chest drainage container. If the drainage system is overturned and the water seal is disrupted, return it to an upright position and encourage the patient to take a few deep breaths, followed by forced exhalations and cough manoeuvres.

4. If the drainage system breaks, place the distal end of the chest tubing connection in a sterile water container at a 2-cm level as an emergency water seal.

5. Do not strip chest tubes. This dangerously increases intrapleural pressures. Drainage tubes may be milked on physician order. *Milking:* alternately folding or squeezing and then releasing drainage tubing. Milk only if drainage and evidence of clots/obstruction. Take 15-cm strips of the chest tube and squeeze and release starting close to the chest and repeating down the tube distally.

Monitoring Wet versus Dry Suction Chest Drainage Systems

Suction Control Chamber in Wet Suction System

1. Keep the suction control chamber at the appropriate water level by adding sterile water as needed to replace water lost to evaporation.

2. Keep the muffler covering the suction control chamber in place to prevent more rapid evaporation of water and to decrease the noise of the bubbling.

3. After filling the suction control chamber to the ordered suction amount (generally 20 cm water suction), connect the suction tubing to the wall suction.

4. Dial the wall suction regulator until continuous gentle bubbling is seen in the suction control chamber (generally 80-120 mm Hg). Vigorous bubbling is not necessary and will increase the rate of evaporation.

5. If no bubbling is seen in the suction control chamber, (1) there is no suction, (2) suction is not high enough, or (3) the pleural air leak is so large that suction is not high enough to evacuate it.

Suction Control Chamber in Dry Suction System (see manufacturer's directions)

1. After connecting patient to system, turn the dial on the chest drainage system to amount ordered (generally −20 cm pressure), connect suction tubing to wall suction source, and increase the suction until the correct amount of negative pressure is indicated. There will be a high negative-pressure release valve in the system.

Chest Tube Dressings

1. Dressings are not routinely changed. If there is visible drainage, notify physician for instructions.

2. If orders to change dressings, remove old dressing carefully to avoid removing unsecured chest tube. Assess the site and culture site as indicated.

3. Cleanse the site with sterile normal saline. Apply sterile gauze and tape to secure the dressing. Some physicians may prefer use of petroleum gauze dressing around the tube to prevent air leak. Date the dressing and document dressing change.

Obtaining a Sample From the Chest Tube

1. Form a loop in the tubing in an area to get the most recently drained fluid.

2. Swab the sampling site of the tubing with antiseptic and allow to air dry.

3. Aspirate from the sampling site with syringe; cap syringe; label with patient name, date, time, and source of specimen.

4. Send to laboratory.

Table 30-24 Chest Surgeries

TYPE AND DESCRIPTION	INDICATION	COMMENTS
Lobectomy		
Removal of one lobe of lung	Lung cancer, bronchiectasis, TB, emphysematous bullae, benign lung tumours, fungal infections	Most common lung surgery; postoperative insertion of chest tubes; expansion of remaining lung tissue to fill up space
Pneumonectomy		
Removal of entire lung	Lung cancer (most common), extensive TB, bronchiectasis, lung abscess	Done only when lobectomy or segmental resection will not remove all diseased lung; no drainage tubes (generally), fluid gradually filling space where lung has been removed; position patient on operative side to facilitate expansion of remaining lung
Segmental Resection		
Removal of one or more lung segments	Lung cancer, bronchiectasis, TB	Technically difficult; done to remove lung segment; insertion of chest tubes; expansion of remaining lung tissue to fill space
Wedge Resection		
Removal of small, localized lesion that occupies only part of a segment	Lung biopsy, excision of small nodules	Need for chest tubes after surgery
Decortication		
Removal of thick, fibrous membrane from visceral pleura	Empyema	Use of chest tubes and drainage after surgery
Exploratory Thoracotomy		
Incision into thorax to look for injured or bleeding tissues	Chest trauma	Use of chest tubes and drainage after surgery
Thoracotomy not Involving Lungs*		
Incision into thorax for surgery on other organs	Hiatal hernia repair, open heart surgery, esophageal surgery, tracheal resection, aortic aneurysm repair	
Video-Assisted Thoracscopic Surgery (VATS)		
VATS under general anaesthesia in OR	Procedures performed using VATS include lung biopsy, lobectomy, resection of nodules, repair of fistulas	Video-assisted technique involving insertion of a rigid scope with a distal lens into the pleura with image shown on a monitor screen; allows surgeon to manipulate instruments passed into the pleural space through separate small intercostal incisions
Lung Volume Reduction Surgery (LVRS)		
	Advanced bullous emphysema, α_1-antitrypsin emphysema	Involves reducing lung volume by multiple wedge excisions or VATS (see p. 695)

OR, operating room; *TB*, tuberculosis.
*For comments on thoracotomy not involving the lungs, see discussion of individual diseases in text.

stripping of chest tubes to maintain patency is no longer recommended because it can cause dangerously high intrapleural pressure and damage to pleural tissue. Drainage and blood are not likely to clot inside chest tubes because the newer chest tubes are made with a coating that makes them nonthrombogenic. The nurse should remember that insertion of the chest tube, as well as its continued presence, can be painful to the patient. Dislodgement of the tube may occur if the tube is not stabilized.

Clamping of chest tubes during transport or when the tube is accidentally disconnected is no longer advocated. The danger of rapid accumulation of air in the pleural space causing tension pneumothorax is far greater than that of a small amount of atmospheric air entering the pleural space. Chest tubes may be momentarily clamped to change the drainage apparatus or to check for air leaks. Clamping for more than a few moments is indicated only for assessing how the patient will tolerate chest tube removal. It is done to simulate chest tube removal and identify if there will be negative clinical repercussions with tube removal. Generally,

this is done 4 to 6 hours before the tube is removed, and the patient is monitored closely. If a chest tube becomes disconnected, the most important intervention is re-establishment of the water-seal system immediately and attachment of a new drainage system as soon as possible. In some hospitals, when disconnection occurs, the chest tube is immersed in sterile water (~2 cm) until the system can be re-established. It is important for the nurse to know the unit protocol, individual clinical situation (whether an air leak exists), and physician preference before resorting to prolonged chest tube clamping.

■ Complications

Chest tube malposition is the most common complication. Routine monitoring is done by the nurse to evaluate whether the chest drainage is successful by observing for tidalling in the water-seal chamber, listening for breath sounds over the lung fields, and measuring the amount of fluid drainage. Re-expansion pulmonary edema can occur after rapid expansion of a collapsed lung in patients with a pneumothorax or evacuation of large volumes of pleural fluid (>1 to 1.5 L). A vasovagal response with symptomatic hypotension can occur from too rapid removal of fluid.

Infection at the skin site is also a concern. Meticulous sterile technique during dressing changes can reduce the incidence of infected sites. Other complications include (1) pneumonia from not taking deep breaths, from not using incentive spirometers, and by splinting on the affected side and (2) shoulder disuse ("frozen shoulder") from lack of range of motion exercises. Poor patient adherence or lack of patient teaching can contribute to these complications. Nurses can make a tremendous impact on preventing these complications. As with many procedures, the hospital may have policies and procedures referring to the care of chest tubes. Ensure that these are reviewed and followed.

▌ Chest Tube Removal

The patient with chest tubes may have chest radiographic studies to follow the course of lung expansion. The chest tubes are removed when the lungs are re-expanded and fluid drainage has ceased. Generally, suction is discontinued and the patient is placed on gravity drainage for a period of time before the tubes are removed. The tube is removed by cutting the sutures; applying a sterile petroleum jelly gauze dressing; having the patient take a deep breath, exhale, and bear down (Valsalva's manoeuvre); and then removing the tube. Pain medication is generally given before chest tube removal. The site is covered with an airtight dressing, the pleura seals itself off, and the wound is healed in several days. A chest radiograph is obtained after chest tube removal to evaluate for pneumothorax, reaccumulation of fluid, or both. The wound should be observed for drainage and should be reinforced if necessary. The patient should be observed for respiratory distress, which may signify a recurrent or new pneumothorax.

Chest Surgery

Chest surgery is performed for a variety of reasons, some of which are unrelated to primary lung problems. For example, a thoracotomy may be performed for heart and esophageal surgery. The types of chest surgery are compared in Table 30-24.

Preoperative Care

Before chest surgery, baseline data are obtained on the respiratory and cardiovascular systems. Diagnostic studies performed are pulmonary function, chest radiography, electrocardiogram (ECG), ABGs, blood urea nitrogen (serum urea [nitrogen]), serum creatinine, blood glucose, serum electrolytes, and complete blood count. Additional studies of cardiac function such as cardiac catheterization may be done for the patient who is to undergo a pneumonectomy. A careful physical assessment of the lungs, including percussion and auscultation, should be done. This will allow the nurse to compare preoperative and postoperative findings.

The patient should be encouraged to stop smoking before surgery to decrease secretions and increase O_2 saturation. In the anxious period before surgery, this is not an easy thing for the habitual smoker to do. Chest physiotherapy may be indicated to help drain the lungs of accumulated secretions. This is especially indicated for the patient with a lung abscess or bronchiectasis.

Preoperative teaching should include exercises for effective deep breathing and incentive spirometry. If the patient practises these techniques before surgery, the techniques will be easier to perform after surgery. The patient should be told that adequate medication will be given to reduce the pain, and the patient is helped to splint the incision with a pillow to facilitate deep breathing.

For most types of chest surgery, chest tubes are inserted and connected to water-sealed drainage systems. The purpose of these tubes should be explained to the patient. In addition, O_2 is frequently given the first 24 hours after surgery. Range of motion exercises on the surgical side similar to those for the mastectomy patient should be taught (see Chapter 54).

The thought of losing part of a vital organ is frequently frightening. The patient should be reassured that the lungs have a large degree of functional reserve. Even after the removal of one lung, there is enough lung tissue to maintain adequate oxygenation.

The nurse should be available to deal with the questions asked by the patient and the family. Questions should be answered honestly. The nurse should try to facilitate the expression of concerns, feelings, and questions. (General preoperative care and teaching are discussed in Chapter 20.)

Surgical Therapy

Thoracotomy (surgical opening into the thoracic cavity) surgery is considered major surgery because the incision is large and cuts into bone, muscle, and cartilage. The two types of thoracic incisions are median sternotomy, performed by splitting the sternum, and lateral thoracotomy. The median sternotomy is primarily used for surgery involving the heart. The two types of lateral thoracotomy are posterolateral and anterolateral. The posterolateral thoracotomy is used for most surgeries involving the lung. The incision is made from the anterior axillary line below the nipple level posteriorly at the fourth, fifth, or sixth intercostal space. It is rarely necessary to remove the ribs. Strong mechanical retractors are used to gain access to the lung. The anterolateral incision is made in the fourth or fifth intercostal space from the sternal border to the midaxillary line. This procedure is commonly used for surgery or trauma victims, mediastinal operations, and wedge resections of the upper and middle lobes of the lung.

The extensiveness of the thoracotomy incision often results in severe pain for the patient after surgery. Because muscles have been severed, the patient is reluctant to move the shoulder and arm on the surgical side. Chest tubes are placed in the pleural space except in pneumonectomy surgery. In a pneumonectomy, the space from which the lung was removed gradually fills with serosanguineous fluid.

Video-Assisted Thorascopic Surgery. VATS is a thorascopic surgical procedure that, in many cases, can enable the impact of a full thoracotomy to be avoided. The procedure involves three to four 2.5-cm incisions made on the chest that allow the thorascope (a special fibreoptic camera) and instruments to be inserted and manipulated. Video-assisted thorascopes improve visualization because the surgeon can view the thoracic cavity from the video monitor. The thorascope is equipped with a camera that magnifies the image on the monitor. Thorascopy can be used to diagnose and treat a variety of conditions of the lung, the pleura, and the mediastinum.

The candidate for this type of procedure should not have a prior history of conventional thoracic surgery because the probability of adhesion formation would make access more difficult. The patient whose lesions are in the lung periphery or the mediastinum is a better candidate because of better accessibility. The patient considered for thorascopic surgery should have sufficient pulmonary function before surgery to allow the surgeon to perform conventional thoracotomy if complications occur. Complications that may occur are bleeding, diaphragmatic perforation, air emboli, persistent pleural air leaks, and tension pneumothorax.

There are many benefits of thorascopic surgery when compared with a conventional thoracotomy procedure. These include less adhesion formation, minimal blood loss, less time under anaesthesia, shorter hospitalization, faster recovery, less pain, and no need for postoperative rehabilitation therapy because of minimal disruption of thoracic structures.

Chest tubes are placed at the end of the procedure through one of the incisions. The incisions are closed with sutures or a wound-approximating adhesive bandage. Nursing assessment and care after surgery include monitoring respiratory status and lung re-expansion with the chest tubes and checking the incisions for drainage or dehiscence. The most common complication is prolonged air leak. A return to prior activities should be encouraged as quickly as possible. The hospital stay averages from 1 to 5 days, depending on the type of surgery.

Postoperative Care

Specific measures related to the care after a thoracotomy are presented in NCP 30-2. The specific follow-up care depends on the type of surgical procedure. General postoperative care is discussed in Chapter 22.

Restrictive Respiratory Disorders

Restrictive respiratory disorders are characterized by a restriction in lung volume (caused by decreased compliance of the lungs or chest wall). This is in contrast to obstructive disorders, which are characterized by increased resistance to airflow (see Chapter 1). Pulmonary function tests are the best means of differentiating between restrictive and obstructive respiratory disorders (Table 30-25). Mixed obstructive and restrictive disorders are often manifested. For example, a patient may have both chronic bronchitis (an obstructive problem) and pulmonary fibrosis (a restrictive problem).

Restrictive problems are generally categorized into extrapulmonary and intrapulmonary disorders. Extrapulmonary causes of restrictive lung disease include disorders involving the central nervous system, neuromuscular system, and chest wall (Table 30-26). In these disorders, the lung tissue is normal. Intrapulmonary causes of restrictive lung disease involve the pleura or the lung tissue (Table 30-27).

Pleural Effusion

Types

The pleural space lies between the lung and the chest wall and normally contains a very thin layer of fluid. **Pleural effusion** is a collection of fluid in the pleural space (see Figure 30-5, *A*). It is

Table 30-25 Relationship of Lung Volumes to Type of Ventilatory Disorder			
LUNG VOLUMES	**RESTRICTIVE**	**OBSTRUCTIVE**	**RESTRICTIVE AND OBSTRUCTIVE**
Vital capacity (VC)	↓	Normal or ↓	↓
Total lung capacity (TLC)	↓	↑	Variable
Residual volume (RV)	Normal or ↓	↑	Variable
Forced expiratory volume in 1 sec (FEV₁)	Normal or ↓	↓	↓
FEV₁/Functional vital capacity (FVC)	Normal or ↑	↓	↓

not a disease but rather a sign of a serious disease. Pleural effusion is frequently classified as transudative or exudative according to whether the protein content of the effusion is low or high, respectively. A *transudate* occurs primarily in noninflammatory conditions and is an accumulation of protein- and cell-poor fluid. Transudative pleural effusions (also called *hydrothorax*) are caused by (1) increased hydrostatic pressure found in CHF, which is the most common cause of pleural effusion, or (2) decreased oncotic pressure (from hypoalbuminemia) found in chronic liver or renal disease. In these situations, fluid movement is facilitated out of the capillaries and into the pleural space.

An *exudative effusion* is an accumulation of fluid and cells in an area of inflammation. An exudative pleural effusion results from the increased capillary permeability characteristic of the inflammatory reaction. This type of effusion occurs secondary to conditions such as pulmonary malignancies, pulmonary infections, pulmonary embolization, and GI disease (e.g., pancreatic disease, esophageal perforation).

The type of pleural effusion can be determined from a sample of pleural fluid obtained via **thoracentesis** (a procedure to remove fluid from the pleural space). Exudates have a high protein content (Allibone, 2008), and the fluid is generally dark yellow or amber. Transudates have a low protein content or contain no protein, and the fluid is clear or pale yellow. The fluid can also be analyzed for red and white blood cells, malignant cells, bacteria, and glucose.

An **empyema** is a pleural effusion that contains pus. It is caused by conditions such as pneumonia, TB, lung abscess, and infection of surgical wounds of the chest. Treatment of empyema is generally with chest tube drainage. Appropriate antibiotic therapy is also needed to eradicate the causative organism. A complication of empyema is fibrothorax, in which there is fibrous fusion of the visceral and parietal pleurae (see Figure 30-5, *A*). A condition called *trapped lung* can occur with effusions and empyema. It occurs when the visceral pleura becomes encased with a fibrous peel or rind. The fibrous peel causes severe pulmonary restriction. The pathological process affecting the visceral pleura prevents the lung from expanding and from filling the thoracic cavity. A decortication surgical procedure to remove the pleural peel may be needed.

NURSING CARE PLAN 30-2

Thoracotomy

NURSING DIAGNOSIS	**Impaired gas exchange** related to air and fluid collection in lungs and pleural space as evidenced by chest tube drainage, decreased breath sounds, and abnormal pulse oximetry
Expected Patient Outcomes	**Nursing Interventions and Rationales**
• Achieves full expansion of lungs • Has normal breath sounds bilaterally • Has normal pulse oximetry	• Monitor chest drainage system to ensure adequate ventilation and to detect hemorrhage. • Monitor respiratory rate and pattern and manifestations of hypoxia to allow early recognition of significant changes in respiratory function. • Administer oxygen therapy to treat hypoxemia. • Assist with position changes to increase patient's comfort and facilitate aeration of the lungs.
NURSING DIAGNOSIS	**Ineffective breathing pattern** related to pain, position, and possible complication on affected side as evidenced by shortness of breath, shallow respirations, and use of accessory muscles
Expected Patient Outcomes	**Nursing Interventions and Rationales**
• Has respiratory rate of 12-18 breaths/min • Breathes easily	• Assess respiratory rate and pattern and auscultate lungs every 2-3 hr to evaluate the rate, quality, and depth of patient's respirations and the need for tracheal suctioning. • Observe for manifestations of complications such as pneumothorax or hemothorax with symptoms of acute shortness of breath, shallow rapid respirations, dyspnea, cough, abnormal pulse oximetry, and air hunger to allow early detection. • Assess patency of and drainage from chest tubes to validate proper functioning. • Assist patient with deep breathing to provide encouragement and improve results. • Position patient for comfort and ease of breathing to increase compliance with respiratory treatments. • Encourage use of incentive spirometer every 2-3 hr to provide visual feedback to the patient on effectiveness of respirations. • Use optimal pain control measures to promote deep breathing, turning, and coughing.
NURSING DIAGNOSIS	**Anxiety** related to feelings of dyspnea and pain as evidenced by anxious facial expression and inability to cooperate with instructions to breathe slowly
Expected Patient Outcomes	**Nursing Interventions and Rationales**
• Reports reduced anxiety or is able to manage level of anxiety	• Stay with patient during procedures to provide encouragement and explanations. • Provide feedback about effective breathing to provide encouragement and reduce anxiety. • Administer pain medication as ordered or implement nonpharmacological measures such as distraction and relaxation to control pain because pain increases anxiety and decreases adherence to necessary treatments.
NURSING DIAGNOSIS	**Risk for infection** related to tissue injury, chest tube placement.
Expected Patient Outcomes	**Nursing Interventions and Rationales**
• Shows no indication of infection • Incision and stab wounds heal by first intention	• Monitor for systemic and local signs and symptoms of infection to enable early detection and treatment. • Inspect condition of surgical incisions/wounds to detect early signs of infection. • Encourage early mobility and exercise to increase circulation and promote healing. • Obtain cultures as needed to identify causative organisms and effective antibiotics. **Chest tube care** • Monitor for bubbling of the suction chamber of the chest drainage system and tidalling in water-seal chamber to ensure adequate ventilation. • Ensure all tubing connections are securely attached and taped to prevent air leaks. • Keep the drainage container below chest level to prevent pneumothorax. • Observe volume, shade, colour, and consistency of drainage from lung, and record appropriately, to detect infection. • Clean around the tube insertion site to decrease the exposure to pathogens. • Change dressing around the chest tube every 24-72 hr as needed to monitor site and provide protection.

Clinical Manifestations

Common clinical manifestations of pleural effusion are progressive dyspnea and decreased movement of the chest wall on the affected side. There may be pleuritic pain from the underlying disease. Physical examination of the chest will indicate dullness to percussion and absent or decreased breath sounds over the affected area. The chest radiograph will indicate an abnormality if the effusion is greater than 250 mL. Manifestations of empyema include the manifestations of pleural effusion as well as fever, night sweats, cough, and weight loss. A thoracentesis reveals an exudate containing thick, purulent material.

Thoracentesis

If the cause of the pleural effusion is not known, a diagnostic **thoracentesis** is needed to obtain pleural fluid for analysis (see Chapter 28, Figure 28-15). If the degree of pleural effusion is

Table 30-26 Extrapulmonary Causes of Restrictive Lung Disease

DISEASE OR ALTERATION	DESCRIPTION	COMMENTS
Central Nervous System		
Head injury, CNS lesion (e.g., tumour, stroke)	Injury to or impingement on respiratory centre, causing hypoventilation or hyperventilation; relationship of manifestations to increased intracranial pressure (see Chapters 59 and 60)	Management is directed toward treating the underlying cause, maintaining the airway, using mechanical ventilation for supportive care, and assessing for manifestations of increased intracranial pressure.
Narcotic and barbiturate use	Depression of respiratory centre, respiratory rate of <12 breaths/min	Respiratory depression is caused by drug overdose or inadvertent administration of drugs to a person with respiratory difficulty. These drugs should not be administered to a person with a respiratory rate of <12 breaths/min.
Neuromuscular System		
Spinal cord injury	Complete cervical- and complete upper thoracic–level injuries have restrictive ventilation. The lung volumes are reduced owing to inspiratory muscle weakness	Patient with a cervical injury may need mechanical ventilator support initially.
Guillain-Barré syndrome	Acute inflammation of peripheral nerves and ganglia; paralysis of intercostal nerves leading to diaphragmatic breathing; paralysis of vagal preganglionic and postganglionic fibres leading to reduced ability of bronchioles to constrict, dilate, and respond to irritants	Patient often has to be put on mechanical ventilation for supportive care (see Chapter 63).
Amyotrophic lateral sclerosis	Progressive degenerative disorder of the motor neurons in the spinal cord, brainstem, and motor cortex; respiratory system involvement as a result of interruption of nerve transmission to respiratory muscles, especially diaphragm	See Chapter 61 for clinical manifestations and management.
Myasthenia gravis	Defect in neuromuscular junction; respiratory system involvement as a result of interruption of nerve transmission to respiratory muscles	See Chapter 61 for clinical manifestations and management.
Muscular dystrophy	Hereditary disease; eventual involvement of all skeletal muscles; paralysis of respiratory muscles, including intercostals, diaphragm, and accessory muscles	Pulmonary problems develop late in disease process.
Chest Wall		
Chest-wall trauma (e.g., flail chest, fractured rib)	Rib fracture causing inspiratory pain; voluntary splinting of chest, resulting in shallow, rapid breathing; impaired ventilatory ability caused by paradoxical breathing	Strapping the chest wall to stabilize the fractures is not recommended because this increases the restrictive defect.
Pickwickian syndrome (extreme obesity)	Excess adipose tissue interfering with chest-wall and diaphragmatic excursion, somnolence from hypoxemia and CO_2 retention, polycythemia from chronic hypoxia	Weight loss generally causes reversal of symptoms. Prevention and prompt treatment of respiratory infections is important. Condition is worsened in supine position.
Kyphoscoliosis	Posterior and lateral angulation of the spine; restriction of ventilation as a result of alteration in thoracic excursion; increase in work of breathing; pattern of rapid, shallow breathing; reduction of lung volume; compression of alveoli and blood vessels	Only small number of persons with condition develop severe respiratory problems. Atelectasis and pneumonia are common complications.

CNS, central nervous system.

severe enough to impair breathing, a therapeutic thoracentesis is done to remove fluid as well as to obtain fluid for analysis.

A thoracentesis is performed by having the patient sit on the edge of a bed and lean forward over a bedside table. The puncture site is determined by chest radiograph, and percussion of the chest is used to assess the maximum degree of dullness. The skin is cleaned with an antiseptic solution and anaesthetized locally. The thoracentesis needle is inserted into the intercostal space. Fluid can be aspirated with a syringe, or tubing can be connected to allow fluid to drain into a sterile collection bag. After the fluid is removed, the needle is withdrawn, and a bandage is applied over the insertion site.

Usually, only 1000 to 1200 mL of pleural fluid is removed at one time. Because high volumes are removed, rapid removal can result in hypotension, hypoxemia, or pulmonary edema. A follow-up chest radiograph should be obtained to detect a possible pneumothorax that could have been induced by perforation of the visceral pleura. During and after the procedure, the patient should be observed for any manifestations of respiratory distress.

Collaborative Care

The main goal of management of pleural effusions is to treat the underlying cause. For example, adequate treatment of CHF with

Table 30-27 Intrapulmonary Causes of Restrictive Lung Disease	
DISEASE OR ALTERATION	**DESCRIPTION**
Pleural disorders	Inflammation, scarring, or fluid in the pleural space causing restriction
Pleural effusion	Accumulation of fluid in pleural space secondary to altered hydrostatic or oncotic pressure; fluid collection >250 mL, showing up on chest radiograph
Pleurisy (pleuritis)	Inflammation of pleura; classification as fibrinous (dry) or serofibrinous (wet); wet pleurisy accompanied by an increase in pleural fluid and possibly resulting in pleural effusion
Pneumothorax	Accumulation of air in pleural space with accompanying lung collapse
Parenchymal disorders	Inflammation, collapse, or scarring of the lung tissue
Atelectasis	Condition of lung characterized by collapsed, airless alveoli; possibly acute (e.g., in postoperative patient) or chronic (e.g., in patient with malignant tumour)
Pneumonia	Acute inflammation of lung tissue caused by bacteria, viruses, fungi, chemicals, dusts, and other factors
Interstitial lung diseases (ILDs)	General term that includes a variety of chronic lung disorders characterized by some type of injury, inflammation, and scarring (or fibrosis); this process occurs in the interstitium (tissue between the alveoli) and the lung becomes stiff (fibrotic); can be caused by occupational and environmental exposures (see Table 30-12), infections (e.g., TB), and connective tissue disorders (e.g., rheumatoid arthritis); when all known causes of ILDs are ruled out, the condition is termed *idiopathic pulmonary fibrosis* (IPF)
ARDS*	Atelectasis, pulmonary edema, congestion, and hyaline membrane lining the alveolar wall; result of variety of conditions, including shock lung, O_2 toxicity, Gram-negative sepsis, cardiopulmonary bypass, and aspiration pneumonia

ARDS, acute respiratory distress syndrome; *TB*, tuberculosis.
*See Chapter 70 for clinical manifestations and management.

diuretics and sodium restriction will result in decreased pleural effusions. The treatment of pleural effusions secondary to malignant disease represents a more difficult problem. These types of pleural effusions are frequently recurrent and accumulate quickly after thoracentesis. Chemical pleurodesis may be used to sclerose the pleural space and prevent reaccumulation of effusion fluid. Although doxycycline and bleomycin have been used for sclerosing with good results, talc appears to be the most effective agent for pleurodesis. Thoracoscopy can be used to perform talc pleurodesis after inspection of the pleural space. After instillation of the sclerosing agent, patients are usually instructed to rotate their positions to spread the agent uniformly throughout the pleural space. Chest tubes are left in place after pleurodesis until fluid drainage is less than 150 mL/day and no air leaks are noted.

Pleurisy

Pleurisy (pleuritis) is an inflammation of the pleura. The most common causes are pneumonia, TB, chest trauma, pulmonary infarctions, and neoplasms. The inflammation usually subsides with adequate treatment of the primary disease. Pleurisy can be classified as fibrinous (dry) with fibrinous deposits on the pleural surface or serofibrinous (wet) with increased production of pleural fluid that may result in pleural effusion.

The pain of pleurisy is typically abrupt and sharp in onset and is aggravated by inspiration. The patient's breathing is shallow and rapid to avoid unnecessary movement of the pleura and chest wall. A pleural friction rub may occur, which is the sound over areas where inflamed visceral pleura and parietal pleura rub over one another during inspiration. This sound is usually loudest at peak inspiration but can be heard during exhalation as well.

Treatment of pleurisy is aimed at treating the underlying disease and providing pain relief. Taking analgesics and lying on or splinting the affected side may provide some relief. The patient should be taught to splint the rib cage when coughing. Intercostal nerve blocks may be done if the pain is severe.

Atelectasis

Atelectasis is a condition of the lungs characterized by collapsed, airless alveoli. The most common cause of atelectasis is airway obstruction that results from retained exudates and secretions. This is frequently observed in the postoperative patient. Normally, the pores of Kohn (see Chapter 28, Figure 28-1) provide for collateral passage of air from one alveolus to another. Deep inspiration is necessary to open the pores effectively. For this reason, deep breathing exercises are important in preventing atelectasis in the high-risk patient (e.g., postoperative, immobilized patient). (The prevention and treatment of atelectasis are discussed in Chapter 22.)

Interstitial Lung Disease

Many acute and chronic lung disorders with variable degrees of pulmonary inflammation and fibrosis are collectively referred to as *interstitial lung diseases* (ILDs) or diffuse parenchymal lung diseases. ILDs have been difficult to classify because more than 200 known diseases have diffuse lung involvement, either as the primary condition or as a significant part of a multiorgan process, as may occur in connective tissue disorders (e.g., systemic lupus erythematosus, rheumatoid arthritis).

Among the ILDs of known cause, the largest group comprises occupational and environmental exposures, especially the inhalation of dusts and various fumes or gases. The most common ILDs of unknown etiology are idiopathic pulmonary fibrosis and sarcoidosis.

Idiopathic Pulmonary Fibrosis

Idiopathic pulmonary fibrosis (IPF) is characterized by scar tissue in the connective tissue of the lungs as a sequel to inflammation or irritation. A common risk factor for IPF is environmental or occupational inhalation of organic and inorganic substances (see discussion earlier in this chapter). Other risk factors include cigarette smoking and history of chronic aspiration. There also may be genetic risk factors.

Clinical manifestations of IPF include exertional dyspnea, nonproductive cough, and inspirational crackles with or without clubbing. High-resolution CT scan is the most definitive diagnostic study. Chest radiographic studies show changes characteristic of IPF. Pulmonary function tests show a typical pattern characteristic of restrictive lung disease (see Table 30-25). Open lung biopsy using VATS may help to differentiate the specific pathology.

The clinical course is variable, with a 5-year survival rate of 30 to 50% after diagnosis. Treatment includes corticosteroids, cytotoxic agents (azathioprine [Imuran], cyclophosphamide [Procytox]), and antifibrotic agents (colchicine). However, there is no good evidence that any of these treatments improves survival or quality of life. Lung transplantation is an option that should be considered for those who meet the criteria. (Lung transplantation is discussed later in this chapter, p. 705.)

Sarcoidosis

Sarcoidosis is a chronic, multisystem granulomatous disease of unknown cause that primarily affects the lungs. The disease may also involve skin, eyes, liver, kidney, heart, and lymph nodes. The disease is often acute or subacute and self-limiting, but in many individuals, it is chronic with remissions and exacerbations. Marked pulmonary fibrosis can be present with severe restrictive lung disease. Cor pulmonale and bronchiectasis can develop in the advanced stages.

Corticosteroids are the most commonly used agents for the treatment of pulmonary sarcoidosis. A trial of methotrexate may be considered if the patient does not respond to or cannot tolerate corticosteroid therapy. If this is ineffective or not tolerated, cyclophosphamide (Procytox) or azathioprine (Imuran) may be initiated (King, 2008). Nonsteroidal anti-inflammatory agents, such as ibuprofen (Motrin), may help decrease acute inflammation or relieve symptoms but are not a treatment of sarcoidosis. Disease progression is monitored by pulmonary function tests, chest radiographic studies, and CT scan.

Vascular Lung Disorders

Pulmonary Edema

Pulmonary edema is an abnormal accumulation of fluid in the alveoli and the interstitial spaces of the lungs. It is a complication of various heart and lung diseases (Table 30-28). It is considered a medical emergency and may be life threatening.

Normally, there is a balance between the hydrostatic and the oncotic pressures in the pulmonary capillaries. If the hydrostatic pressure increases or the colloid oncotic pressure decreases, the net effect will be fluid leaving the pulmonary capillaries and entering the interstitial space. This stage is referred to as *interstitial edema*. At this stage, the lymphatic system can usually drain away the excess fluid. If fluid continues to leak from the pulmonary capillaries, it will enter the alveoli. This stage is referred to as *alveolar edema*. Pulmonary edema interferes with gas exchange by causing an alteration in the diffusing pathway between the

Table 30-28 Causes of Pulmonary Edema

- Congestive heart failure
- Overhydration with intravenous fluids
- Hypoalbuminemia: nephrotic syndrome, hepatic disease, nutritional disorders
- Altered capillary permeability of lungs: inhaled toxins, inflammation (e.g., pneumonia), severe hypoxia, near-drowning
- Malignancies of the lymph system
- Respiratory distress syndrome (e.g., O_2 toxicity)
- Unknown causes: neurogenic condition, narcotic overdose, high altitude

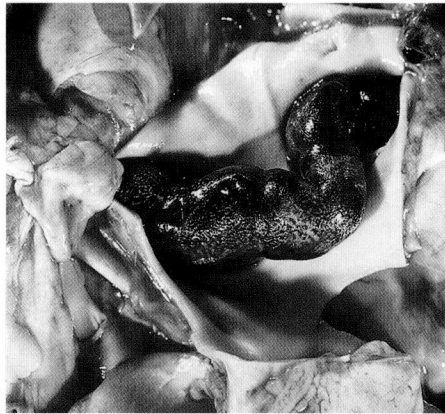

Figure 30-11 Large embolus from the femoral vein lying in the main left and right pulmonary arteries.

Source: From the teaching collection of the Department of Pathology, University of Texas Southwestern Medical School, Dallas.

alveoli and the pulmonary capillaries. The most common cause of pulmonary edema is left-sided CHF. (The clinical manifestations and management of pulmonary edema are described in Chapter 37.)

Pulmonary Embolism

Etiology and Pathophysiology

Pulmonary embolism (PE) is the blockage of pulmonary arteries by a thrombus, fat or air embolus, or tumour tissue. The word *embolus* derives from a Greek word meaning "plug" or "stopper." *Emboli* are mobile clots that generally do not stop moving until they lodge at a narrowed part of the circulatory system. A pulmonary embolus consists of material that gains access to the venous system and then to the pulmonary circulation. The embolus travels with the blood flow through ever-smaller blood vessels until it lodges and obstructs perfusion of the alveoli (Figure 30-11). Because of higher blood flow, the lower lobes of the lung are commonly affected. PE is associated with a mortality rate of up to 30% in patients who are not treated. With diagnosis and anticoagulant therapy, the mortality rate is reduced to 6 to 8% (Hogg, Thomas, Mackway-Jones, Lecky, & Cruickshank, 2011). Most pulmonary emboli arise from deep vein thrombosis (DVT) in the deep veins of the legs. Venous thromboembolism (VTE) is the preferred terminology to describe the spectrum of pathology from DVT to PE (see Table 40-6). Lethal pulmonary emboli most commonly originate in the femoral or iliac veins. Generally, the VTEs that are below the knee have not been considered a risk factor for PE because they rarely migrate to the pulmonary circulation without first extending above the knee. The highest rate of VTE is seen in spinal cord injury patients (67 to 100%) (Perry, 2008).

Other sites of origin of PE include the right side of the heart (especially with atrial fibrillation), the upper extremities (rare), and the pelvic veins (especially after surgery or childbirth). Upper extremity VTE occasionally occurs in the presence of central venous catheters or cardiac pacing wires. These cases may resolve with removal of the catheter. Thrombi in the deep veins can dislodge spontaneously. However, it is more common for mechanical forces (e.g., sudden standing) and changes in the rate of blood flow (e.g., those that occur with the Valsalva manoeuvre) to dislodge the thrombus. The majority of patients with PE caused by VTE have no leg symptoms at the time of diagnosis (Perry, 2008). In addition to dislodged thrombi, less common causes of PE include fat emboli (from fractured long bones), air emboli (from improperly administered IV therapy), bacterial vegetations, amniotic fluid, and tumours. Tumour emboli may originate from primary or metastatic malignancies. The most common risk factors for PE are immobility, surgery within the last 3 months (especially pelvic and lower extremity surgery), stroke, paresis, paralysis, history of DVT, malignancy, obesity in women, heavy cigarette smoking, and hypertension (Perry, 2008).

Clinical Manifestations

The signs and symptoms in PE are varied and nonspecific, making diagnosis difficult. The classic triad—dyspnea, chest pain, and hemoptysis—occurs in only about 20% of patients. Symptoms may begin slowly or suddenly. A mild to moderate hypoxemia with a low $PaCO_2$ is a common finding. Other manifestations are cough, pleuritic chest pain, hemoptysis, crackles, fever, accentuation of the pulmonic heart sound, and sudden change in mental status as a result of hypoxemia. Massive emboli may produce abrupt hypotension, pallor, severe dyspnea, and hypoxemia. Chest pain may or may not be present. ECG may indicate tachycardia and right ventricular strain. The mortality rate of persons with massive PE and shock is approximately 33% (Perry, 2008). Medium-sized emboli often cause pleuritic chest pain, dyspnea, slight fever, and a productive cough with blood-streaked sputum. A physical examination may reveal tachycardia and a pleural friction rub. Small emboli frequently are undetected or produce vague, transient symptoms. The exception to this is the patient with underlying cardiopulmonary disease. In these patients, even small or medium-sized emboli may result in severe cardiopulmonary compromise. However, repeated small emboli gradually cause a reduction in the capillary bed and eventual pulmonary hypertension. An ECG and chest radiography may indicate right ventricular hypertrophy secondary to pulmonary hypertension.

Complications

Pulmonary infarction (death of lung tissue) is most likely when the following factors are present: (1) occlusion of a large or medium-sized pulmonary vessel (>2 mm in diameter), (2) insufficient collateral blood flow from the bronchial circulation, or (3) pre-existing lung disease. Infarction results in alveolar necrosis and hemorrhage. Occasionally, the necrotic tissue becomes infected, and an abscess may develop. Concomitant pleural effusion is

COLLABORATIVE CARE

Table 30-29 Acute Pulmonary Embolism

Diagnostic	Collaborative Therapy
• History and physical examination	• Supplemental oxygen, intubation may be necessary
• Chest radiographic study	• Fibrinolytic agent
• Continuous ECG monitoring	• Unfractionated heparin IV
• ABGs	• Low-molecular-weight heparin (e.g., enoxaparin [Lovenox])
• Venous ultrasound	
• CBC count with WBC differential	• Warfarin (Coumadin) for long-term therapy
• Spiral (helical) CT scan	• Monitoring of aPTT and INR levels
• Ventilation-perfusion ($\dot{V}/\dot{Q}$)	• Limited activity
• Lung scan	• Opioids for pain relief
• D-dimer level	• Inferior vena cava filter
• Troponin level, BNP level	• Pulmonary embolectomy in life-threatening situation
• Pulmonary angiography	

ABGs, Arterial blood gases; *aPTT,* activated partial thromboplastin time; *BNP,* B-type natriuretic peptide; *CBC,* complete blood count; *CT,* computed tomography; *ECG,* electrocardiogram; *INR,* international normalized ratio; *IV,* intravenous; *WBC,* white blood cell.

frequent. *Pulmonary hypertension* results from hypoxemia or from involvement of more than 50% of the area of the normal pulmonary bed. As a single event, an embolus does not cause pulmonary hypertension unless it is massive. Recurrent emboli may result in chronic pulmonary hypertension.

Diagnostic Studies

A *spiral (helical) CT scan* is the most frequently used test to diagnose PE (see Table 30-29). An IV injection of contrast media is required to view the blood vessels. The scanner continuously rotates while obtaining slices and does not start and stop between each slice. This allows visualization of all anatomical regions of the lungs. The computer reconstructs the data to provide a three-dimensional picture and assist in emboli visualization. If a patient cannot have contrast media, a ventilation–perfusion ($\dot{V}/\dot{Q}$) scan is done.

The $\dot{V}/\dot{Q}$ scan has two components and is most accurate when both are performed:
1. Perfusion scanning involves IV injection of a radioisotope. A scanning device images the pulmonary circulation.
2. Ventilation scanning involves inhalation of a radioactive gas such as xenon. Scanning reflects the distribution of gas through the lung. The ventilation component requires the cooperation of the patient and may be impossible to perform in the critically ill patient, particularly if the patient is intubated.

D-dimer is a laboratory test that measures the amount of cross-linked fibrin fragments. These fragments are found in the circulation after clotting events such as VTE, acute myocardial infarction, unstable angina, and acute stroke. This degradation product is rarely found in healthy individuals. The disadvantage of D-dimer is that it is neither specific (other conditions cause elevation) nor sensitive because up to 50% of patients with small pulmonary emboli have normal results. Patients with suspected

PE and an elevated D-dimer level but normal venous ultrasound may need a lung scan or spiral CT.

Pulmonary angiography is a sensitive and specific test for PE. However, it is an invasive procedure that involves the insertion of a catheter through the antecubital or femoral vein, advancement to the pulmonary artery, and injection of contrast medium. This allows visualization of the pulmonary vascular system and location of the embolus. However, with the use of spiral CT, pulmonary angiography is now used less frequently.

ABG analysis is important, but not diagnostic. The PaO_2 is low because of inadequate oxygenation secondary to an occluded pulmonary vasculature preventing matching of perfusion to ventilation. The pH remains normal unless respiratory alkalosis develops as a result of prolonged hyperventilation or to compensate for lactic acidosis caused by shock. Abnormal findings are usually reported on the chest radiograph (atelectasis, pleural effusion) and the ECG (ST-segment and T-wave changes), but they are not diagnostic for PE. Serum troponin levels are elevated in 30 to 50% of patients with PE, and, although not diagnostic, they are predictive of an adverse prognosis. Serum B-type natriuretic peptide levels, although not diagnostic, may be helpful in identifying the severity of the clinical course.

Collaborative Care

Prevention of PE begins with prevention of VTE. VTE prophylaxis includes the use of sequential compression devices, early ambulation, and prophylactic use of anticoagulant medications. To reduce mortality risk, treatment is begun as soon as PE is suspected (see Table 30-29). The objectives are to (1) prevent further growth or multiplication of thrombi in the lower extremities, (2) prevent embolization from the upper or lower extremities to the pulmonary vascular system, and (3) provide cardiopulmonary support if indicated.

Supportive therapy for the patient's cardiopulmonary status varies according to the severity of the PE. The administration of supplemental O_2 by mask or cannula is adequate for some patients. Oxygen is given in a concentration determined by ABG analysis. In some situations, endotracheal intubation and mechanical ventilation are necessary to maintain adequate oxygenation. Respiratory measures such as turning, coughing, deep breathing, and incentive spirometry are important to help prevent or treat atelectasis. If symptoms of shock are present, IV fluids are administered followed by vasopressor agents as needed to support perfusion (see Chapter 69). If heart failure is present, diuretics are used (see Chapter 37). Pain resulting from pleural irritation or reduced coronary blood flow is treated with opioids, usually morphine.

Drug Therapy. Fibrinolytic agents, such as tissue plasminogen activator (tPA) or alteplase (Activase), dissolve the pulmonary embolus and the source of the thrombus in the pelvis or deep leg veins, thereby decreasing the likelihood of recurrent emboli. Indications for thrombolytic therapy in PE include hemodynamic instability and right ventricular dysfunction. (Thrombolytic therapy is discussed in Chapter 40, see Table 40-9.) Because most deaths are caused by recurrent PE, treatment should begin immediately. Properly managed anticoagulant therapy is effective in the prevention of further emboli. Heparin works to prevent future clots but does not dissolve existing clots. Although unfractionated heparin has been traditionally used, low-molecular-weight heparin (e.g., enoxaparin [Lovenox]) is becoming more common. Warfarin (Coumadin) should be

initiated within the first 24 hours and is typically administered for 3 to 6 months. Some health care providers use Factor Xa inhibitors and direct thrombin inhibitors in the treatment of PE. The dosage of heparin is adjusted according to the activated partial thromboplastin time (aPTT), and the dosage of warfarin is determined by the international normalized ratio (INR).

Frequent changes and titrations of heparin doses are needed initially in order to obtain a therapeutic aPTT level. Anticoagulant therapy may be contraindicated if the patient has complicating factors such as blood dyscrasias, hepatic dysfunction causing alteration in the clotting mechanism, injury to the intestine, overt bleeding, a history of hemorrhagic stroke, or neurological conditions.

Surgical Therapy. If the degree of pulmonary arterial obstruction is severe and the patient does not respond to conservative therapy, an immediate embolectomy may be indicated. Pulmonary embolectomy, a rare procedure, has a 50% mortality rate. Preoperative pulmonary angiography is necessary to identify and locate the site of the embolus. When a pulmonary embolectomy is performed, the patient also has placement of a vena cava filter. To prevent further emboli, an inferior vena cava filter may be the treatment of choice in patients who remain at high risk and for patients for whom anticoagulation is contraindicated. This device is placed at the level of the diaphragm in the inferior vena cava via the femoral vein. It prevents migration of large clots into the pulmonary system. Research has shown complications associated with this device include recurrent VTE and post-thrombotic syndrome, in addition to misplacement, migration, and perforation (Sheares, 2011).

NURSING MANAGEMENT: PULMONARY EMBOLISM

Nursing Implementation

Health Promotion

Nursing measures aimed at prevention of PE are similar to those for prophylaxis of VTE (Association of periOperative Registered Nurses [AORN], 2007; see the discussion of venous thrombosis in Chapter 40).

Acute Intervention

The prognosis of a patient with PE is good if therapy is promptly instituted. Keep the patient on bed rest in a semi-Fowler position to facilitate breathing. Maintain an IV line for medications and fluid therapy. Know the adverse effects of medications and observe for them. Administer oxygen therapy as ordered. Careful monitoring of vital signs, cardiac dysrhythmia monitoring, pulse oximetry, ABGs, and lung sounds is critical to assess the patient's status. Monitor laboratory results to ensure normal ranges of aPTT and INR. Nursing care includes assessing for the complications of anticoagulant therapy (e.g., bleeding, hematomas, bruising) and PE (e.g., hypoxia, hypotension). The NCP includes interventions related to immobility and fall precautions. The patient is usually anxious because of pain, a sense of doom, inability to breathe, and fear of death. Carefully explain the situation and provide emotional support and reassurance to help relieve the patient's anxiety.

▪ Ambulatory and Home Care

The patient affected by thromboembolic processes may require emotional support. In addition, some patients may have an underlying chronic illness requiring long-term treatment. To provide supportive therapy, the nurse must understand and differentiate between the various problems caused by the underlying disease and those related to thromboembolic disease. Patient teaching regarding long-term anticoagulant therapy is critical.

Anticoagulant therapy continues for at least 3 to 6 months; patients with recurrent emboli are treated indefinitely. INR levels are drawn at intervals and warfarin dosage is adjusted. Some patients are monitored by nurses in an anticoagulation clinic. Long-term management is similar to that for the patient with VTE (see the discussion of VTE in Chapter 40). Discharge planning is aimed at limiting progression of the condition and preventing complications and recurrence. Reinforce the need for the patient to return to the health care provider for regular follow-up examinations.

▪ Evaluation

The expected outcomes are that the patient who has a PE will have:
- Adequate tissue perfusion and respiratory function
- Adequate cardiac output
- Increased level of comfort
- No recurrence of PE

Pulmonary Hypertension

Pulmonary hypertension comprises a variety of disorders occurring as a primary disease (primary pulmonary hypertension) or as a complication of a large number of respiratory and cardiac disorders (secondary pulmonary hypertension). Pulmonary hypertension is elevated pulmonary pressure resulting from an increase in pulmonary vascular resistance to blood flow through small arteries and arterioles.

Primary Pulmonary Hypertension

Primary pulmonary hypertension (PPH) is a rare, severe, and progressive disease. PPH is characterized by mean pulmonary arterial pressure greater than 25 mm Hg at rest or greater than 30 mm Hg with exercise, in the absence of a demonstrable cause. PPH is associated with a poor prognosis because there is no definitive therapy.

Etiology and Pathophysiology

The exact etiology of PPH is unknown. PPH has been linked to the use of fenfluramine in the drug Fen-Phen, which was used as an appetite suppressant to treat obesity. The drug was withdrawn from the market in 1996. PPH affects more women than men. It may have a genetic component because the incidence is higher in families. It is a rare and potentially fatal disease; the mean age at diagnosis is 36 years.

Normally, the pulmonary circulation is characterized by low resistance and low pressure. In pulmonary hypertension, the pulmonary pressures are elevated. Until recently, the pathophysiol-

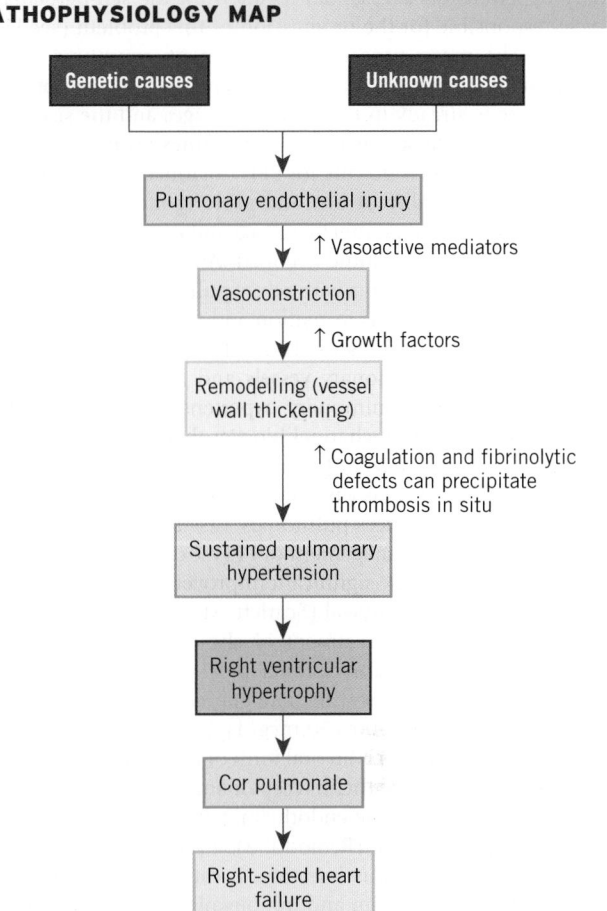

PATHOPHYSIOLOGY MAP

Figure 30-12 Pathogenesis of pulmonary hypertension and cor pulmonale.

ogy of PPH was poorly understood. Recently, it was discovered that a key mechanism involved in PPH is a deficient release of vasodilator mediators from the pulmonary epithelium with a resultant cascade of injury (Figure 30-12).

Clinical Manifestations

Classic symptoms of pulmonary hypertension are dyspnea on exertion and fatigue. Exertional chest pain, dizziness, and exertional syncope are other symptoms. These symptoms are related to the inability of cardiac output to increase in response to increased oxygen demand. Eventually, as the disease progresses, dyspnea occurs at rest. Pulmonary hypertension increases the workload of the right ventricle and causes right ventricular hypertrophy (a condition called *cor pulmonale*) and eventually heart failure. A chest radiograph generally shows enlarged central pulmonary arteries and clear lung fields. An enlarged right heart may be seen. Echocardiogram usually reveals right ventricular hypertrophy.

Collaborative Care

Diagnostic evaluation includes ECG, chest radiographic study, and echocardiogram. CT and cardiac catheterization to measure pulmonary artery pressures can be used. Additional tests may be done to exclude secondary factors. Early recognition of pulmonary hypertension is essential to interrupt the self-perpetuation cycle responsible for the progression of this problem (see Figure 30-12). The mean time between onset of symptoms and the diagnosis is 2 years. By the time patients become symptomatic, the disease is already in the advanced stages and the size of pulmonary artery pressure is two to three times normal.

Although there is no cure for PPH, treatment can relieve symptoms, increase quality of life, and prolong life. Diuretic therapy relieves dyspnea and peripheral edema and may be useful in reducing right ventricular volume overload. Anticoagulation therapy is recommended for patients with severe pulmonary hypertension to prevent in situ thrombus formation and venous thrombosis.

Vasodilator therapy is used to reduce right ventricular overload by dilating pulmonary vessels and reversing remodelling. Many patients with pulmonary hypertension can be effectively managed with calcium channel blocker therapy, such as nifedipine (Adalat) and diltiazem (Cardizem).

Iloprost (Ventavis) is a prostacyclin that promotes pulmonary vasodilation and reduces pulmonary vascular resistance and has revolutionized the management of PPH. Continuous iloprost has been shown to provide significant improvement in clinical symptoms and long-term survival (Scarlett, McGaw, & Aquart-Stewart, 2009). It is now the treatment of choice for selected patients unresponsive to calcium channel blockers. It is a long-acting chemically stable prostacyclin analogue, which is administered in an aerosolized form (100-150 mcg/day).

Bosentan (Tracleer) is an oral form of prostacyclin used to treat PPH. It is an active endothelin receptor antagonist. This drug works by blocking the hormone endothelin, which causes blood vessels to constrict. Treprostinil (Remodulin), a prostacyclin, is used as a continuous subcutaneous injection. It causes vasodilation of the pulmonary arterial system and inhibits platelet aggregation.

Surgical interventions include atrial septostomy, pulmonary thromboendarterectomy, and lung transplantation (Stamm, Risbano, & Mathier, 2011). Lung transplantation is the mainstay of treatment for those patients who do not respond to prostacyclins and progress to severe right-sided heart failure. Recurrence of the disease has not been reported in individuals who have undergone transplantation. A patient education and support site for pulmonary hypertension is located on the Pulmonary Hypertension Association's Web site.

Secondary Pulmonary Hypertension

Secondary pulmonary hypertension (SPH) occurs when a primary disease causes a chronic increase in pulmonary artery pressures. It can develop as a result of parenchymal lung disease, left ventricular dysfunction, intracardiac shunts, chronic pulmonary thromboembolism, or systemic connective tissue disease. The specific primary disease pathology may result in anatomical or vascular changes causing the pulmonary hypertension. Anatomical changes causing increased vascular resistance include (1) loss of capillaries as a result of alveolar wall damage (e.g., COPD), (2) stiffening of the pulmonary vasculature (e.g., pulmonary fibrosis connective tissue disorders), and (3) obstruction of blood flow (chronic emboli).

Vasomotor increases in pulmonary vascular resistance are found in conditions characterized by alveolar hypoxia. Hypoxia causes localized vasoconstriction and shunting of blood away from poorly ventilated alveoli. Alveolar hypoxia can be caused by a wide variety of conditions. It is possible to have a combination of anatomic restriction and vasomotor constriction. This is found in the patient with longstanding chronic bronchitis who has chronic hypoxia in addition to loss of lung tissue.

Symptoms can reflect the underlying disease, but some are directly attributable to the SPH, such as dyspnea, fatigue, lethargy, and chest pain. Physical findings include right ventricular hypertrophy and signs of right ventricular failure (increased pulmonic heart sound, right-sided fourth heart sound, peripheral edema, hepatomegaly). Treatment of pulmonary hypertension caused primarily by pulmonary or cardiac disorders consists mainly of treating the underlying disorder. Treatment of SPH is similar to treatment of PPH.

Cor Pulmonale

Cor pulmonale is enlargement of the right ventricle secondary to diseases of the lung, the thorax, or the pulmonary circulation. Pulmonary hypertension is usually a pre-existing condition in the individual with cor pulmonale. Cor pulmonale may be present with or without overt cardiac failure. The most common cause of cor pulmonale is COPD. Almost any disorder that affects the respiratory system can cause cor pulmonale. The etiology and pathogenesis of pulmonary hypertension and cor pulmonale are outlined in Figure 30-12.

Clinical Manifestations

Clinical manifestations of cor pulmonale include dyspnea, chronic productive cough, wheezing respirations, retrosternal or substernal pain, and fatigue. Chronic hypoxemia leads to polycythemia and increased total blood volume and viscosity of the blood. (Polycythemia is often present in cor pulmonale secondary to COPD.) Compensatory mechanisms that are secondary to hypoxemia can aggravate the pulmonary hypertension. Episodes of cor pulmonale in a person with underlying chronic respiratory problems are frequently triggered by an acute respiratory tract infection.

If heart failure accompanies cor pulmonale, additional manifestations such as peripheral edema; weight gain; distended neck veins; full, bounding pulse; and enlarged liver will also be found. (Heart failure is discussed in Chapter 37.) A chest radiograph will show an enlarged right ventricle and pulmonary artery.

Collaborative Care

The primary management of cor pulmonale is directed at treating the underlying pulmonary problem that precipitated the heart problem (Table 30-30). Long-term low-flow O_2 therapy is used to correct the hypoxemia and reduce vasoconstriction in chronic states of respiratory disorders. If fluid, electrolyte, and acid–base imbalances are present, they must be corrected. Diuretics and a low-sodium diet will help decrease the plasma volume and the load on the heart. Bronchodilator therapy is indicated if the underlying respiratory problem is caused by an obstructive disorder. Digitalis may be used if there is left-sided heart failure. Other treatments include those for pulmonary hypertension and comprise vasodilator therapy, calcium channel blockers, and anticoagulants. Theophylline may help because of its weak inotropic effect on the heart. When medical treatment fails, lung transplantation is an option for some patients.

Chronic management of cor pulmonale resulting from COPD is similar to that described for COPD (see Chapter 31). Continuous low-flow O_2 during sleep; exercise; and small, frequent meals may allow the patient to feel better and be more active.

COLLABORATIVE CARE

Table 30-30 Cor Pulmonale

Diagnostic	Collaborative Therapy
• History and physical examination	• O_2 therapy
• ABGs	• Bronchodilators
• Serum and urine electrolytes	• Diuretics
• Monitoring with ECG	• Low-sodium diet
• Chest radiographic study	• Fluid restriction
	• Antibiotics (if indicated)
	• Digitalis (if left-sided heart failure)
	• Vasodilators (if indicated)
	• Calcium channel blockers (if indicated)

ABGs, arterial blood gases; *ECG,* electrocardiogram.

Table 30-31 Indications for Lung Transplant

• α_1-Antitrypsin deficiency	• Interstitial lung disease
• Bronchiectasis	• Pulmonary fibrosis secondary to other diseases (e.g., sarcoidosis)
• Cystic fibrosis	
• Emphysema	• Pulmonary hypertension
• Idiopathic pulmonary fibrosis	

Lung Transplantation

Lung transplantation has evolved as a viable therapy for patients with end-stage lung disease. A variety of pulmonary disorders are potentially treatable with some type of lung transplantation (Table 30-31). Improved selection criteria, technical advances, and better methods of immunosuppression have resulted in improved survival rates. Various transplant options are available, including single-lung transplant, bilateral-lung transplant, heart–lung transplant, and transplantation of lobes from a living related donor.

Patients being considered for a lung transplant need to undergo extensive evaluation. The candidate for lung transplantation should not have a malignancy or recent history of malignancy (within the last 2 yr), renal or liver insufficiency, or HIV. The typical wait for a lung transplant is longer than 1 year. The candidate and the family undergo psychological screening to determine the ability to cope with a postoperative regimen that requires strict adherence to immunosuppressive therapy, continuous monitoring for early signs of infection, and prompt reporting of manifestations of infection for medical evaluation.

Postoperative care includes ventilatory support, pulmonary clearance measures (bronchodilators, chest physiotherapy, and deep breathing and coughing), fluid and hemodynamic management, immunosuppression, detection of early rejection, and prevention or treatment of infection. Infection is the leading cause of morbidity and mortality. Gram-negative bacterial pneumonia is common. Viral infection with CMV and herpes simplex occur frequently. CMV is a leading cause of mortality, which, if it is going to occur, usually happens 4 to 8 weeks after surgery. Fungal infections are also seen. Empirical antibiotic regimen is routine perioperatively for potential pathogens isolated from donor or recipient.

Immunosuppressive therapy usually includes a triple-drug regimen of cyclosporine, azathioprine (Imuran), and prednisone. Immunosuppressive drugs are discussed in Chapter 16 and Table 16-15.

Acute rejection can be seen as soon as 5 to 7 days after surgery. It is characterized by low-grade fever, fatigue, and oxygen desaturation with exercise. Accurate diagnosis is by transtracheal biopsy. Treatment is bolus corticosteroids, which results in remission of symptoms.

Bronchiolitis obliterans (an obstructive airways disease causing progressive occlusion) is considered to represent chronic rejection in lung transplant patients. The onset is often subacute, with gradual onset of progressive obstructive airflow defect, including cough, dyspnea, and recurrent lower respiratory tract infection. Treatment involves optimum maintenance immunosuppression.

Discharge planning begins in the preoperative phase. Patients are placed in an outpatient rehabilitation program to improve physical endurance. The use of home spirometry has been useful in monitoring trends in lung function. Patients are taught to keep logs of medications, laboratory results, and spirometry. Patients need to be able to perform self-care activities, including medication management and being able to identify when to call the physician. Over the past decade, lung transplantation has become an increasingly important mode of therapy for patients with a variety of end-stage lung diseases.

CLINICAL DECISION-MAKING EXERCISE

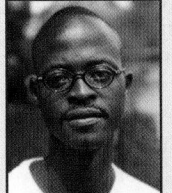

CASE STUDY:
Aspiration Pneumonia

Source: © iStockphoto.com/Will Turner.

Patient Profile

Mr. Jason Lawrence, a 27-year-old man, was admitted to the hospital because of an uncontrollable fever. He was transferred from a long-term care facility. He has a history of a gunshot wound to his left chest. Following a cardiac arrest after the accident, he developed hypoxic encephalopathy. He has a tracheostomy and a gastrostomy tube. He has a history of methicillin-resistant *Staphylococcus aureus* (MRSA) in his sputum.

Subjective Data

• Family says that they visit him regularly and are very devoted to him.

Objective Data

Physical Examination

• Thin, cachectic man in moderate respiratory distress
• Unresponsive to voice, touch, or painful stimuli
• Vital signs: temperature 40° C, heart rate 120, respiratory rate 30, O_2 saturation 90%
• Chest auscultation revealed crackles and scattered wheezes in the left upper lobe

Diagnostic Studies
• Serum albumin 28 g/L
• White blood cell (WBC) count 18×10^9/L
• Sputum specimen: thick, green-coloured, foul smelling; cultures pending
• Arterial blood gases: pH 7.29, PaO_2 80 mm Hg, $PaCO_2$ 40 mm Hg, bicarbonate 16 mmol/L
• Stool culture positive for *Clostridium difficile*
• Chest radiographic examination: infiltrate in left upper lobe; no pleural effusions noted

Discussion Questions

1. What types of infectious disease precautions should be taken related to Mr. Lawrence's hospitalization?
2. What clinical manifestations of aspiration pneumonia did he exhibit? Explain their pathophysiological bases.

3. What antibiotic medication is likely to be prescribed?
4. What is his oxygenation status and metabolic state?
5. What other clinical issues must be addressed in his plan of care?
6. What family interventions would you initiate?
7. *Priority Decision:* Based on the assessment data presented, what are the priority nursing diagnoses? Are there any collaborative problems?
8. *Priority Decision:* What are the priority nursing interventions for Mr. Lawrence?
9. Using the Pneumonia Severity Index (PSI) tool (see Table 30-3), what are Mr. Lawrence's PSI score and risk level?

evolve *Answers are available on* http://evolve.elsevier.com/ Canada/Lewis/medsurg

REVIEW QUESTIONS

The number of the question corresponds to the same-numbered objective at the beginning of the chapter.

1. What clinical manifestations should the nurse expect when assessing a patient with pneumococcal pneumonia?
   a. Fever, chills, and a productive cough with purulent-coloured sputum
   b. Nonproductive cough and night sweats that are usually self-limiting
   c. Gradual onset of nasal stuffiness, sore throat, and purulent productive cough
   d. Abrupt onset of fever, nonproductive cough, and formation of lung abscesses
2. A patient with pneumonia has the nursing diagnosis of ineffective airway clearance related to thick secretions and fatigue. What would be an appropriate nursing intervention?
   a. Promote fluid hydration, as appropriate, to help liquefy secretions.
   b. Provide analgesics as ordered to promote patient comfort.
   c. Administer oxygen as prescribed to maintain optimal oxygen levels.
   d. Teach the patient how to cough effectively to bring secretions to the mouth.
3. A patient with tuberculosis (TB) has a nursing diagnosis of nonadherence. What is the most common etiological factor for this diagnosis in patients with TB?
   a. Fatigue and lack of energy to manage self-care
   b. Lack of knowledge about how the disease is transmitted
   c. Lack of social support systems for the patient and family
   d. Feelings of shame and the response to the social stigma associated with TB
4. A patient has been receiving high-dose corticosteroids and broad-spectrum antibiotics for treatment of serious trauma and infection. Which of the following infections is the patient most susceptible to?
   a. Aspergillosis
   b. Candidiasis
   c. Coccidioidomycosis
   d. Histoplasmosis

5. Which of the following statements best describes the treatment of lung abscess?
   a. It is best treated with surgical excision and drainage.
   b. Antibiotics for a prolonged period is the treatment of choice.
   c. Abscesses are difficult to treat and usually result in pulmonary fibrosis.
   d. Penicillin can effectively eradicate anaerobic organisms.
6. What is a common complication of many types of environmental lung diseases?
   a. Benign tumour growth
   b. Diffuse airway obstruction
   c. Liquefactive necrosis
   d. Pulmonary fibrosis
7. What type of lung cancer is generally associated with the best prognosis because it is potentially surgically resectable?
   a. Adenocarcinoma
   b. Small cell carcinoma
   c. Squamous cell carcinoma
   d. Undifferentiated large cell carcinoma
8. How does the nurse identify a flail chest in a trauma patient?
   a. Multiple rib fractures are determined by radiographic study.
   b. Tracheal deviation to the unaffected side is present.
   c. Paradoxical chest movement occurs during respiration.
   d. Decreased movement of the involved chest wall is apparent.
9. The nurse notes tidalling of the water level in the tube submerged in the water-seal chamber in a patient with closed chest-tube drainage. What should the nurse do?
   a. Continue to monitor this normal finding.
   b. Check all connections for a leak in the system.
   c. Lower the drainage collector further from the chest.
   d. Clamp the tubing at progressively more distal points away from the patient until the tidalling stops.
10. Which nursing measure should be instituted after a pneumonectomy?
    a. Monitor chest-tube drainage and functioning.
    b. Position the patient on the operative side or back.
    c. Perform range of motion exercises on the affected upper extremity.
    d. Auscultate frequently for lung sounds on the affected side.

11. What is the cause of respiratory problems in patients with Guillain-Barré syndrome?
    a. Central nervous system depression
    b. Deformed chest-wall muscles
    c. Paralysis of the diaphragm secondary to trauma
    d. Interruption of nerve transmission to respiratory muscles

12. A patient with chronic obstructive pulmonary disease (COPD) asks why the heart is affected by the respiratory disease. Which of the following statements regarding cor pulmonale is the basis for the nurse's response to the patient?
    a. Pulmonary congestion secondary to left ventricular failure
    b. Excess serous fluid collection in the alveoli caused by retained respiratory secretions
    c. Right ventricular hypertrophy secondary to increased pulmonary vascular resistance
    d. Right ventricular failure secondary to compression of the heart by hyperinflated lungs

13. The patient asks about the possibility of a lung transplant. The nurse's response is based on the knowledge that lung transplantation is contraindicated in which of the following patients?
    a. Those with cor pulmonale
    b. Those who currently smoke
    c. Those older than 50 years
    d. Those with end-stage lung disease

ANSWERS: 1. a; 2. a; 3. d; 4. b; 5. b; 6. d; 7. c; 8. c; 9. a; 10. b; 11. d; 12. c; 13. b.

REFERENCES

Allibone, L. (2008). Assessment and management of patients with pleural effusion. *British Journal of Nursing (BJN), 17*(22), 1382-1388.

American Thoracic Society. (2005). Guidelines for the management of adults with hospital-acquired, ventilator-associated, and healthcare-associated pneumonia. *American Journal of Respiratory Critical Care Medicine, 171*(4), 388-416.

Assembly of First Nations. (2011). Health bulletin. Retrieved from *http://www.afn.ca/uploads/files/health/afn_health_bulletin_-_spring_2011_en.pdf*

Association of Perioperative Registered Nurses (AORN). (2007). Guideline for the prevention of venous stasis. *AORN Journal, 85*, 607.

BC Cancer Agency. (2006). Types of cancer: Lung. Retrieved from *http://www.bccancer.bc.ca/PPI/TypesofCancer/Lung/default.htm*

Canadian Cancer Society. (2007). Quit smoking. Retrieved from *http://www.cancer.ca/ccs/internet/standard/0,3182,3172_12971__langId-en,00.html*

Canadian Cancer Society's Steering Committee on Cancer Statistics. (2012). *Canadian Cancer Statistics 2012.* Toronto, ON: Author. Retrieved from *http://www.cancer.ca/~/media/CCS/Canada%20wide/Files%20List/English%20files%20heading/PDF%20-%20Policy%20-%20Canadian%20Cancer%20Statistics%20-%20English/Canadian%20Cancer%20Statistics%202012%20-%20English.ashx*

Canadian Lung Association (2012). Smoking and tobacco. Retrieved from *http://www.lung.ca/protect-protegez/tobacco-tabagisme/quitting-cesser/index_e.php*

Canadian Lung Association. (2013). Smoking & Tobacco: Benefits of Quitting Smoking. Retrieved from *http://www.lung.ca/protect-protegez/tobacco-tabagisme/quitting-cesser/benefits-bienfaits_e.php*

Cancer Care Ontario. (2008). Research uncovers genetic link to lung cancer. Retrieved from *http://www.cancercare.on.ca/english/about/newsroom/newsreleases/GeneticLinkLung/*

Community and Hospital Infection Control Association. (2008). Information about hand hygiene. Retrieved from *http://www.chica.org/links_handhygiene.html*

Health Canada. (2006a). Severe acute respiratory syndrome (SARS): It's your health. Retrieved from *http://www.hc-sc.gc.ca/hl-vs/iyh-vsv/diseases-maladies/sars-sras-eng.php#ho*

Health Canada. (2006b). It's your health: Second-hand smoke. Retrieved from *http://www.hc-sc.gc.ca/hl-vs/iyh-vsv/life-vie/shs-fs-eng.php*

Health Canada. (2007). It's your health: Tuberculosis. Retrieved from *http://www.hc-sc.gc.ca/iyh-vsv/diseases-maladies/tubercu_e.html*

Health Canada. (2008). GoSmokeFree. Retrieved from *http://www.hc-sc.gc.ca/fniah-spnia/pubs/famil/_preg-gros/2007_radio_smoke-fume/index-eng.php*

Health Canada (2009). A statistical profile on the health of First Nations in Canada: Self-rated health and selected conditions, 2002 to 2005. Retrieved from *http://www.hc-sc.gc.ca/fniah-spnia/pubs/aborig-autoch/2009-stats-profil-vol3/index-eng.php*

Health Canada. (2012). Canadian Tobacco Use Monitoring Survey (CTUMS): Summary of Annual Results for 2011. Retrieved from *http://www.hc-sc.gc.ca/hc-ps/tobac-tabac/research-recherche/stat/_ctums-esutc_2011/ann_summary-sommaire-eng.php*

Hogg, K., Thomas, D., Mackway-Jones, K., Lecky, F., & Cruickshank, K. (2011). Diagnosing pulmonary embolism: a comparison of clinical probability scores. *British Journal of Haematology, 153*(2), 253-258. doi:10.1111/j.1365-2141.2011.08575.x

Human Resources and Skills Development Canada. (2006). Canadian legislation relating to joint occupational health and safety committees. Retrieved from *http://www.hrsdc.gc.ca/en/lp/spila/clli/ohslc/oshcom.pdf*

Karmakar, G., & Wilsher, M. (2010). Use of the "CURB 65" score in hospital practice. *Internal Medicine Journal, 40*(12), 828-832. doi:10.1111/j.1445-5994.2009.02062.x

King, T. (2008). Patient information: Sarcoidosis. *UpToDate.* Retrieved from *http://www.uptodate.com/patients/content/topic.do?topicKey=~z147QGSAZVI5_a*

Kleinpell, R. M., & Elpern, E. H. (2004). Community-acquired pneumonia: Updates in assessment and management. *Critical Care Nursing Quarterly, 27*(3), 231-240.

Light, R. W. (2011). Pleural controversy: Optimal chest tube size for drainage. *Respirology, 16*(2), 244-248. doi:10.1111/j.1440-1843.2010.01913

Mandell, L. A., Wunderink, R. G., Anzueto, A., Bartlett, J. G., Campbell, G. D., Dean, N. C., et al. (2007). Infectious Diseases Society of America/American Thoracic Society consensus guidelines on the management of community-acquired pneumonia in adults. *Clin Infect Dis, 44*(Suppl 2), S27-S72. doi:10.1086/511159

McLean, J., Murray, C., Schreibman, T., & Rigsby, M. (2007). *Pneumocystis jiroveci* pneumonia. *emedicine.* Retrieved from *http://www.emedicine.com/med/topic1850.htm*

Perry, M. (2008). Knowing the early signs of pulmonary embolism. *Practice Nursing, 19*, 620.

Public Health Agency of Canada (PHAC). (2007a). Life and breath: Respiratory disease in Canada. Retrieved from *http://www.phac-aspc.gc.ca/publicat/2007/lbrdc-vsmrc/intro-eng.php#A*

Public Health Agency of Canada (PHAC). (2007b). Part 1: General guidelines timing of vaccine administration. *Canadian immunization guide* (7th ed.). Retrieved from *http://www.phac-aspc.gc.ca/publicat/cig-gci/p01-09-eng.php*

Public Health Agency of Canada (PHAC). (2007c). Interferon gamma release assays for latent tuberculosis infection. *Canada Communicable Disease Report, Vol. 33.* Retrieved from *http://www.phac-aspc.gc.ca/publicat/ccdr-rmtc/07vol33/acs-10/index-eng.html*

Public Health Agency of Canada (PHAC). (2007d). Occupational respiratory disease. Retrieved from *http://www.phac-aspc.gc.ca/publicat/2007/lbrdc-vsmrc/ord-mrp-eng.php*

Public Health Agency of Canada. (2009). Tuberculosis in Canada 2008: Pre-release. Retrieved from *http://intraspec.ca/tbcan2008pre-eng.pdf*

Public Health Agency of Canada. (2010). Tuberculosis in Canada 2009: Pre-release. Retrieved from *http://www.phac-aspc.gc.ca/tbpc-latb/pubs/tbcan09pre/pdf/tbcan2009pre-eng.pdf*

Public Health Agency of Canada (PHAC)/Canadian Lung Association. (2007). *Canadian tuberculosis standards* (6th ed.). Retrieved from *http://www.phac-aspc.gc.ca/tbpc-latb/pubs/pdf/tbstand07_e.pdf*

Registered Nurses' Association of Ontario (RNAO). (2007). *Integrating smoking cessation into daily nursing practice (p. 32). Nursing Best Practice Guidelines.* Toronto: Author. Retrieved from *http://rnao.ca/bpg/guidelines/integrating-smoking-cessation-daily-nursing-practice*

Roberts, H. C., Patsios, D., Paul, N. S., McGregor, M., Weisbrod, G., Chung, T., …, Shepherd F. A. (2007). Lung cancer screening with low-dose computed tomography: Canadian experience. *Canadian Association of Radiologists Journal, 58*(4), 225-235.

Rotstein, C., Evans, G., Born, A., Grossman, R., Light, R. B., Magder, S., & Zhanel, G. G. (2008). Clinical practice guidelines for hospital-acquired pneumonia and ventilator-associated pneumonia in adults. *Canadian Journal of Infectious Diseases & Medical Microbiology, 19*(1), 19-53.

Rubin, B. (2008). Aerosol antibiotics for non-cystic fibrosis bronchiectasis. *Journal of Aerosol Medicine & Pulmonary Drug Delivery, 21*(1), 71-76. doi:10.1089/jamp.2007.0652

Scarlett, M., McGaw, C., & Aquart-Stewart, A. (2009). Pulmonary hypertension: A review of the aetiology, pathophysiology and management. *West Indian Medical Journal, 58*(2), 153-159.

Sheares, K. K. (2011). How do I manage a patient with suspected acute pulmonary embolism? *Clinical Medicine, 11*(2), 156-159.

Stamm, J., Risbano, M. G., & Mathier, M. A. (2011). Overview of current therapeutic approaches for pulmonary hypertension. *Pulmonary Circulation, 1*(2), 138-159. doi:10.4103/2045-8932.83444

CANADIAN RESOURCES

Canadian Cancer Society
http://www.cancer.ca/

Canadian Cancer Society Quit Smoking Guidelines
http://www.cancer.ca/ccs/internet/standard/0,3182,3172_12971__langId-en,00.html

Canadian Lung Association
http://www.lung.ca/

Canadian Tuberculosis Standards (6th ed.)
http://www.phac-aspc.gc.ca/tbpc-latb/pubs/pdf/tbstand07_e.pdf

Cancer Care Ontario
http://www.cancercare.on.ca

Cancer Care Ontario–Lung Cancer Evidence-based Series (EBS) and Practice Guidelines (PG)
http://www.cancercare.on.ca/english/home/toolbox/qualityguidelines/diseasesite/lung-ebs/

Health Canada
http://www.hc-sc.gc.ca

National Cancer Institute of Canada
http://www.ncic.cancer.ca

Public Health Agency of Canada
http://www.phac-aspc.gc.ca

Statistics Canada
http://www.statcan.ca

RELATED RESOURCES

American Cancer Society
http://www.cancer.org

American Lung Association
http://www.lungusa.org

American Society of Clinical Oncology
http://www.asco.org

Centers for Disease Control and Prevention, National Center for Health Statistics
http://www.cdc.gov/nchs/fastats

International Standards for Tuberculosis Care (ISTC)
http://www.nationaltbcenter.edu/international

National Cancer Institute
http://www.nci.nih.gov

Pulmonary Hypertension Association (PHA)
http://www.phassociation.org

Tobacco Information and Prevention Source (TIPS)
http://www.cdc.gov/tobacco

evolve   *For additional Internet resources, see the Web site for this book at* **http://evolve.elsevier.com/Canada/Lewis/medsurg**

Nursing Management: Obstructive Pulmonary Diseases

Written by Lisa Cicutto
Adapted by Shelly W. Hutchinson

LEARNING OBJECTIVES

1. Describe the etiology, pathophysiology, and clinical manifestations of asthma, and describe the collaborative care of patients with asthma.
2. Explain the nursing management of patients with asthma.
3. Describe the etiology, pathophysiology, and clinical manifestations of chronic obstructive pulmonary disease (COPD), and describe the collaborative care of patients with COPD.
4. Explain the effects of cigarette smoking on the lungs.
5. Explain the nursing management of patients with COPD.
6. Identify the indications for oxygen therapy, the methods of delivery, and the complications of oxygen administration.
7. Describe the etiology, pathophysiology, and clinical manifestations of cystic fibrosis, and describe the collaborative care of patients with cystic fibrosis.

KEY TERMS

absorption atelectasis Collapse of the alveoli as a result of airway obstruction when nitrogen is washed out of the alveoli and replaced with oxygen during the administration of high concentrations of oxygen, p. 744

α_1-antitrypsin (AAT) deficiency The only known genetic abnormality that leads to chronic obstructive pulmonary disease (COPD); manifested by lower levels of α1-antitrypsin that result in insufficient inactivation of neutrophil elastase, and the subsequent lysis of lung tissue, which causes emphysema, p. 733

asthma A chronic inflammatory disorder of the airways; hyper-responsiveness or twitchiness of the airways is directly related to the degree of airway inflammation, p. 710

chest physiotherapy Airway clearance technique for reducing mucus; consists of percussion, vibration, and postural drainage, p. 755

chronic bronchitis The presence of chronic productive cough for 3 months in 2 successive years in a patient in whom other causes of chronic cough have been ruled out, p. 732

chronic obstructive pulmonary disease (COPD) A respiratory disorder largely caused by smoking; characterized by progressive, partially reversible airflow obstruction,

systemic manifestations, and increasing frequency and severity of exacerbations, p. 732

cor pulmonale Hypertrophy of the right side of the heart, with or without heart failure, resulting from pulmonary hypertension, p. 736

cough variant asthma Asthma in which cough is the only symptom, p. 714

cystic fibrosis An autosomal recessive, multisystem disease characterized by altered function of the exocrine glands, involving primarily the lungs, the pancreas, and the sweat glands, p. 753

emphysema An abnormal and permanent enlargement of the airspaces distal to the terminal bronchioles, accompanied by destruction of their walls and without obvious fibrosis, p. 732

oxygen toxicity A condition of oxygen overdosage caused by prolonged exposure to a high level of oxygen, p. 744

postural drainage An airway clearance technique in which the principle of gravity is used to assist in bronchial drainage, p. 755

pursed-lip breathing A breathing exercise used to prolong exhalation, prevent bronchiolar collapse and air trapping, and assist with dyspnea, p. 747

ELECTRONIC RESOURCES

Supplemental content related to Chapter 31 can be found …

Evolve Web Site ⊖volve

More than 3 million people in Canada are living with chronic lung disease (Public Health Agency of Canada [PHAC], 2007). Obstructive pulmonary diseases, the most common chronic lung diseases, include conditions characterized by increased airflow resistance as a result of airway obstruction or narrowing. Airway obstruction may result from accumulated secretions, edema, inflammation of the airways, bronchospasm of smooth muscle, or destruction of lung tissue, or some combination. Asthma is a chronic lung condition characterized by variable airflow obstruction caused by airway hyper-responsiveness and airway inflammation. A patient with asthma has variations in airflow over time, often with normal lung function between episodes of worsening symptoms. Another chronic lung condition is chronic obstructive pulmonary disease (COPD), formerly known as emphysema and chronic bronchitis. It is characterized by partially reversible airflow obstruction, lung hyperinflation, systemic manifestations, and exacerbations that increase in frequency and severity as the disease progresses. The limitation in expiratory airflow in patients with COPD is generally more constant in the short term, but it worsens as the disease progresses. Cystic fibrosis, another form of obstructive pulmonary disease, is a genetic disorder that produces airway obstruction because of changes in exocrine glandular secretions.

Asthma

Asthma is a chronic inflammatory disorder of the airways. Inflammation causes varying degrees of obstruction in the airways, which leads to recurrent episodes of wheezing, breathlessness, chest tightness, and cough, particularly at night and in the early morning. The hyper-responsiveness or twitchiness of the airways is directly related to the degree of airway inflammation, in that the more airway inflammation present, the more hyper-responsive the airways are to endogenous or exogenous stimuli or triggers. Asthma occurs as a result of environmental (endogenous or exogenous) effects on the airways that trigger a series of events in the immune system of a genetically predisposed vindividual. These events lead to airway inflammation and bronchoconstriction (airway narrowing). A key characteristic of asthma is the episodic and reversible nature of the airway obstruction and its associated symptoms (cough, wheeze, chest tightness, dyspnea), so that an episode can resolve spontaneously or with treatment.

In the publication *Life and Breath: Respiratory Diseases in Canada Report*, the PHAC (2007) noted that 15.6% (485,700) of children in Canada between the ages of 4 and 11 years have at some time received a diagnosis of asthma and that the prevalence of physician-diagnosed asthma is 8.3% overall (2.2 million) for Canadians older than 12 years of age. The prevalence of asthma is higher in young boys, but the reverse trend is observed in women. Between 1994 and 2005, the prevalence of physician-diagnosed asthma increased by 60% among women 35 to 44 years old and by 80% among women 45 to 64 years old. In contrast, the prevalence increased by 41% among men 35 to 44 years old (PHAC, 2007).

The morbidity associated with asthma is dramatic. Close to 20% of individuals with asthma visit an emergency department one or more times per year. Asthma is a leading cause of hospitalization for children in Canada, accounting for 10% of all admissions of children from infancy to 4 years of age (PHAC, 2007). The PHAC further reports that every day a Canadian dies as a result of asthma, which is unacceptable in view of the fact that this disease is manageable (Lougheed et al., 2010; PHAC, 2007). A national survey revealed that 53% of individuals with asthma have poorly controlled disease (McIvor, Boulet, FitzGerald, Zimmerman, & Chapman, 2007). The high rate of morbidity related to asthma may be attributed to practice that is inconsistent with the Canadian asthma consensus guidelines, inaccurate assessment of disease severity, a delay in seeking help, inadequate medical treatment, nonadherence to prescribed therapy, an increase in allergens in the environment, limited access to health care, and a lack of knowledge on the part of patients and health care professionals.

Triggers of Asthma Attacks

Although the exact mechanisms that cause airway hyper-responsiveness and inflammation remain unknown, multiple stimuli or triggers are involved (Table 31-1, Figure 31-1). Numerous allergens, chemicals, and infectious agents can trigger airway inflammation, which leads to airway narrowing and appearance of symptoms. These triggers are discussed as follows.

Allergens. Some people with asthma have an exaggerated immunoglobulin E (IgE) response to certain allergens (e.g., dust, pollen, grasses, mites, roaches, moulds, animal dander, latex). These allergens attach to IgE receptors on mast cells (Figure 31-2). The IgE–mast cell complexes remain for a long time; thus a second exposure to the allergen triggers mast cell degranulation even years after the initial exposure to the allergen. (Allergic reactions are discussed further in Chapter 14.)

Exercise. Asthma that is induced or exacerbated during physical exertion is called *exercise-induced asthma* (EIA). Typically, EIA occurs after, not during, vigorous exercise and is characterized by bronchospasm (airway smooth muscle contraction) that causes shortness of breath, cough, wheeze, chest tightness, or a combination of these. EIA is pronounced during activities in which the person is exposed to cold, dry air. Airway hyper-responsiveness may result from changes in the airway mucosa caused by the hyperventilation that occurs during exercise with either the cooling or rewarming of air and capillary leakage in the airway wall. Several strategies can be incorporated to prevent EIA: an adequate warm-up period before beginning the activity;

Table 31-1 Triggers of Asthma

Allergens

- Animal dander (e.g., from cats, dogs, horses, mice, guinea pigs)
- Household dust mites
- Cockroaches
- Pollens
- Moulds
- Air pollutants
- Diesel particulates
- Exhaust fumes
- Perfumes
- Ozone
- Sulphur dioxides
- Cigarette smoke
- Aerosol sprays

Viral upper respiratory infection
Sinusitis
Exercise
Cold, dry air
Stress

Hormones or menses
Gastroesophageal reflux disease (GERD)
Drugs

- Aspirin
- Nonsteroidal anti-inflammatory medications
- β-Adrenergic blockers

Occupational exposure

- Agriculture
- Metal salts
- Wood and vegetable dusts
- Industrial chemicals and plastics (isocyanates)
- Pharmaceutical agents

Food additives

- Sulphites (bisulphites and metabisulphites) found in beer, wine, dried fruit, shrimp
- Monosodium glutamate
- Tartrazine

PATHOPHYSIOLOGY MAP

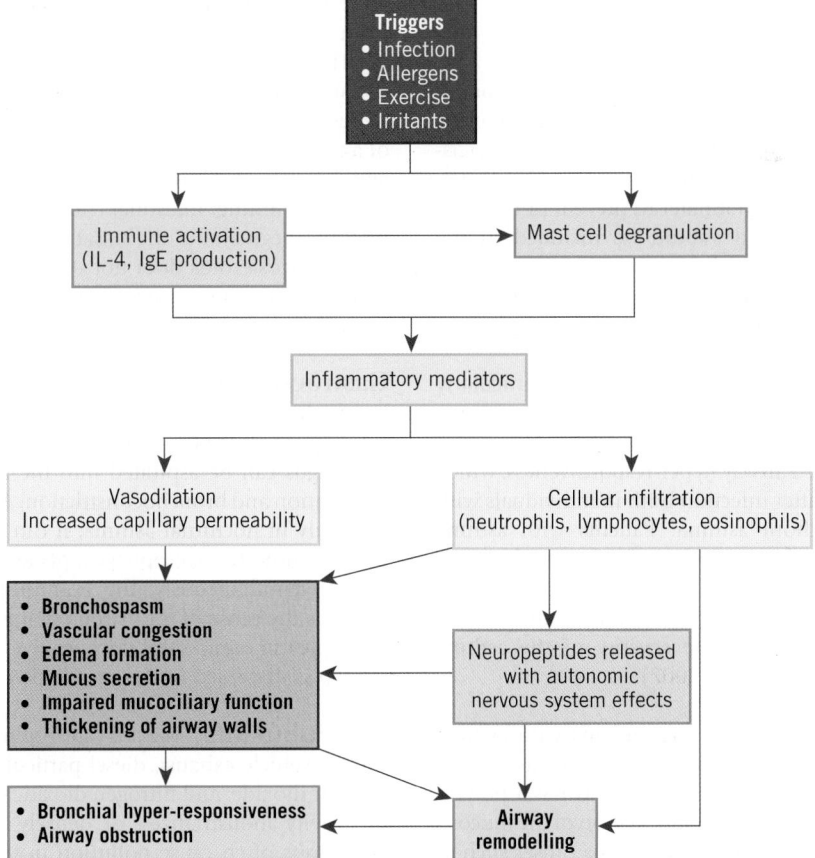

Figure 31-1 Early- and late-phase responses of asthma. *IgE*, immunoglobulin E; *IL-4*, interleukin-4.

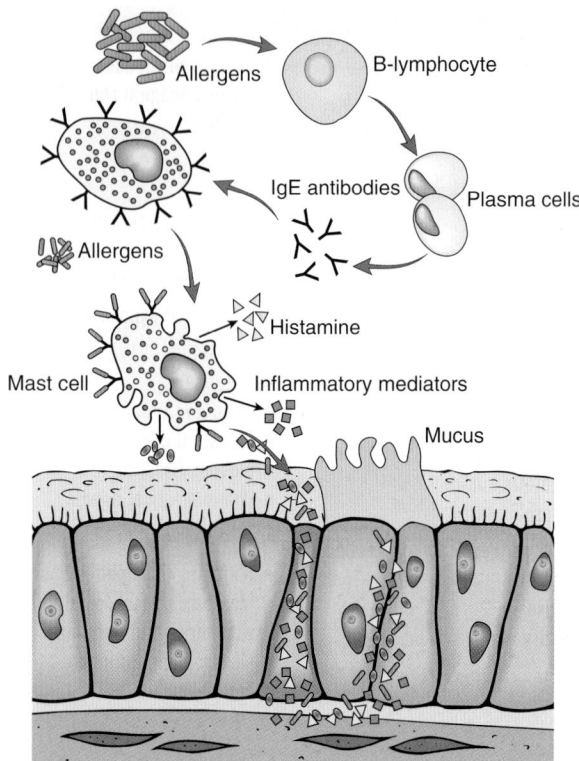

Figure 31-2 The early-phase response in asthma is triggered when an allergen or irritant cross-links immunoglobulin E (IgE) receptors on mast cells, which are then activated to release histamine and other inflammatory mediators.

breathing through a scarf or mask during exercise in a cold or dry climate; and using inhaled short-acting β_2-adrenergic agonists either to relieve the symptoms or, 10 to 20 minutes before exercising, to ward off symptoms. Lougheed and colleagues (2010) suggested that the regular need for an inhaler to prevent or treat EIA signifies suboptimal control and should be included in the weekly limit when control is assessed. Such individuals may need escalation of therapy. (Control criteria and controller therapy are discussed further later in this chapter).

Respiratory Infections. Respiratory infections (particularly viral) are among the most common triggers of worsening asthma. Infections cause increased inflammation in the tracheobronchial system, resulting in increased airway hyper-responsiveness, which can last from 2 to 8 weeks after infection both in individuals with asthma and in those without asthma. Patients with asthma should take steps to reduce the possibility of infections by using proper handwashing techniques and receiving an annual influenza vaccination. Influenza vaccines are safe for children and adults with asthma, regardless of the severity of the asthma (Kmiecik, Arnoux, Kobryn, & Gorski, 2007).

Nose and Sinus Problems. Some patients with asthma have chronic sinus and nasal problems. Nasal problems include allergic rhinitis, either seasonal or perennial, and nasal polyps. Sinus problems are usually related to inflammation of the mucous membranes, most commonly from noninfectious causes such as allergies. However, bacterial sinusitis may also occur. It is important to treat these comorbid conditions because they can often

contribute to poor asthma control (Boulet, 2009; Lougheed et al., 2010). (Sinusitis is discussed further in Chapter 29.)

Drugs and Food Additives. Some patients with asthma, especially those with nasal polyps, may have sensitivity to specific drugs. Some people with asthma have what is termed the *asthma triad*: nasal polyps, asthma, and sensitivity to aspirin and nonsteroidal anti-inflammatory drugs (NSAIDs). Salicylic acid can be found in many over-the-counter (OTC) drugs and some foods, beverages, and flavourings. In some asthmatic patients, wheezing develops within 2 hours after they take aspirin or NSAIDs (e.g., ibuprofen [Motrin]). In addition, most affected patients have profound rhinorrhea, congestion, and tearing. Facial flushing, gastrointestinal symptoms, and angioedema can also occur. Although sensitivity to salicylates persists for many years, the nature and severity of the reaction can change over time. Such patients should avoid aspirin and NSAIDs. However, patients with aspirin sensitivity can, under the care of an allergist, be desensitized by daily administration of the drug (Williams, Simon, Woessner, & Stevenson, 2007). This group of patients may be more likely to benefit from antileukotriene agents.

β-Adrenergic blockers in oral form (e.g., metoprolol) or topical eye drops (e.g., timolol [Timoptic]) may trigger asthma because they induce bronchospasm. Angiotensin-converting enzyme inhibitors (e.g., lisinopril) may induce cough in susceptible individuals, thus worsening asthma symptoms. Other agents that may precipitate asthma symptoms in susceptible patients are tartrazine (yellow dye no. 5, found in many foods) and sulphites (e.g., sodium metabisulphite) widely used in the food and pharmaceutical industries as preservatives and sanitizing agents. Sulphites are commonly found in fruits, beer, and wine and are used extensively in salad bars to protect vegetables from oxidation.

These drugs and food additives are thought to interfere with metabolic pathways, leading to enhanced production of leukotrienes, some of which are potent bronchoconstrictors. The onset of a typical reaction occurs 15 minutes to 3 hours after ingestion and is marked by profuse rhinorrhea, often accompanied by nausea, vomiting, intestinal cramps, and diarrhea. Acute asthma typically begins after the nasal symptoms appear. Pretreatment with corticosteroids does not prevent the reaction. Epinephrine and antihistamines given shortly after the onset usually control the symptoms.

Gastroesophageal Reflux Disease. The exact mechanism by which gastroesophageal reflux disease (GERD) triggers asthma is unknown. It is postulated that reflux of stomach acid into the esophagus can be aspirated into the lungs, causing reflex vagal stimulation and bronchoconstriction. Although GERD is involved primarily in nocturnal asthma, it can trigger daytime asthma as well. By monitoring esophageal pH and peak expiratory flow rate (PEFR) simultaneously, the examiner can determine whether GERD is the cause of the asthma symptoms. H_2-histamine blockers or proton pump inhibitors are given to ameliorate symptoms. (GERD is discussed further in Chapter 44.)

Air Pollutants. Various air pollutants, cigarette or wood smoke, vehicle exhaust, diesel particulate, elevated ozone levels, sulphur dioxide, and nitrogen dioxide can trigger asthma attacks. In heavily industrialized or densely populated areas, climatic conditions often cause pollution in the atmosphere to become concentrated, especially with thermal inversions and stagnant air masses (PHAC, 2007). Ozone alerts are regularly noted on news reports, and patients should minimize outdoor activity during these times.

Emotional Stress. Asthma is not a psychosomatic disease. However, psychological stress that is seen with extremes of emotion such as crying, laughing, anger, and fear can lead to hyperventilation and hypocapnia, which can cause airway narrowing (Global Initiative for Asthma [GINA], 2010). An asthma exacerbation can produce panic and anxiety, which are not unexpected emotions during this experience. Panic is a normal response to not being able to breathe. The extent to which psychological factors contribute to the induction and continuation of any given acute exacerbation is unknown, but it probably varies from patient to patient and in the same patient from episode to episode.

Pathophysiology

The hallmarks of asthma are airway inflammation and hyper-responsiveness. The degree of bronchoconstriction is related to the degrees of airway inflammation, airway hyper-responsiveness, and exposure to endogenous and exogenous triggers (e.g., infections, allergens, histamine, and other cell mediators). Exposure to allergens or irritants initiates an inflammatory cascade involving multiple cell types, mediators, and chemokines. Typically, there are two possible types of asthmatic responses to stimuli: an early-phase response and a late-phase response.

The early-phase response in asthma is characterized by bronchospasm (see Figure 31-1). This response is triggered when an allergen or irritant crosslinks IgE receptors on mast cells found beneath the basement membrane of the bronchial wall (see Figure 31-2). The mast cells become activated, with subsequent release of granules and disruption of the phospholipids' cell membrane. Both processes result in the release of inflammatory mediators, including histamine, bradykinin, leukotrienes, prostaglandins, platelet-activating factor, chemotactic factors, and cytokines (e.g., interleukin-4 and interleukin-5; GINA, 2010). A similar early-phase response process can occur with exercise. These mediators cause intense inflammation in association with bronchial smooth muscle constriction, increased vasodilation and permeability, and epithelial damage. Clinically, the effects are bronchospasm, increased mucus secretion, edema formation, and increased amounts of tenacious sputum (see Figure 31-1), which cause wheeze, cough, chest tightness, shortness of breath, or a combination of these. This immediate response peaks within 30 to 60 minutes after exposure to the trigger (e.g., allergen, irritant) and subsides in another 30 to 90 minutes.

The late-phase response can be more severe than the early-phase response. It peaks 5 to 12 hours after exposure and may last from several hours to days. Its primary characteristic is inflammation, as opposed to bronchial smooth muscle contraction. Eosinophils and neutrophils infiltrate the airways. These cells can subsequently release mediators that can further induce inflammation and cause mast cells to degranulate, thereby releasing histamine and other mediators that set up a self-sustaining cycle. Corticosteroids are effective in preventing and reversing this cycle.

These inflammatory characteristics of a late-phase response increase airway reactivity, which may lower the threshold of exposure necessary to induce a future asthma attack and worsen its symptoms. The person becomes hyper-responsive to allergens and nonspecific stimuli such as air pollution, cold air, and

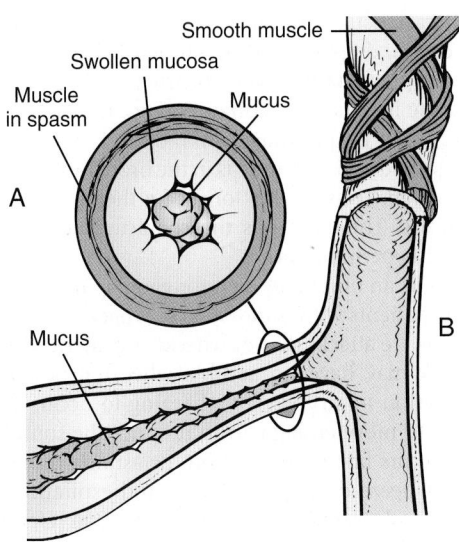

Figure 31-3 Factors causing airway obstruction in asthma. **A,** Cross-section illustration of a bronchiole occluded by muscle spasm, swollen mucosa, and mucus in the lumen. **B,** Longitudinal section illustration of such a bronchiole.

Source: Redrawn from Price, S. A., & Wilson, L. M. (2003). *Pathophysiology: Clinical concepts of disease processes* (6th ed.). St. Louis: Mosby.

dust. In summary, prominent pathophysiological features of asthma are a reduction in airway diameter and an increase in airway resistance that are related to mucosal inflammation, constriction of bronchial smooth muscle, and excess production of mucus (Figure 31-3). Accompanying these changes are hypertrophy of bronchial smooth muscle, thickening of basement membrane, hypertrophy of mucous glands, secretion of thick and tenacious sputum, hyperinflation, and air trapping in the alveoli, all of which increase the work of breathing. As a consequence of these events, respiratory muscle function may be altered, distribution of both ventilation and perfusion may be abnormal, and arterial blood gas (ABG) values may be altered, depending on severity of the disease. Asthma is considered a disease of the airways, but during an asthma attack, eventually all aspects of pulmonary function are compromised. If airway inflammation is not treated or does not resolve, progressive, irreversible lung damage may eventually occur. This irreversible airway obstruction is thought to be the result of inflammation-induced structural changes called *airway remodelling* (GINA, 2010).

Clinical Manifestations

Asthma has an unpredictable, episodic and variable course. Recurrent episodes of wheezing, breathlessness, sensation of chest tightness, coughing, or a combination of these, particularly at night and in the early morning (typically between 2 A.M. and 5 A.M.), are common features. An attack or episode of asthma may have an abrupt onset (minutes) or may be more gradual (1 hour to days). Between attacks, the patient may have no symptoms, with normal or near-normal pulmonary function, depending on the severity of disease. However, in some people, prolonged and uncontrolled asthma may result in compromised pulmonary function and chronic debilitation, resulting in irreversible or fixed airway disease.

The characteristic clinical manifestations of asthma are wheezing, cough, dyspnea, and sensation of chest tightness after exposure to a precipitating factor or trigger. Expiration is often prolonged. The inspiratory–expiratory ratio, instead of being the normal 1:2, may be prolonged to 1:3 or 1:4. As a result of bronchospasm, edema, and mucus in the bronchioles, the airways become narrower. Thus it takes longer for the air to move out of the bronchioles. This produces the characteristic wheezing, air trapping, and hyperinflation.

Wheezing is an unreliable sign for gauging the severity of an attack. Many patients with minor attacks wheeze loudly, whereas others with severe attacks do not wheeze. A patient with a severe asthma attack may have no audible wheezing because of the marked reduction in airflow. For wheezing to occur, the patient must be able to move enough air to produce the sound. Wheezing usually occurs first on exhalation. As asthma progresses, the patient may wheeze during inspiration and expiration. Severely diminished breath sounds or their absence, often referred to as a "silent chest," is an ominous sign of severe obstruction and impending respiratory failure. During an acute attack, the person with asthma usually sits upright or slightly bent forward and uses the accessory muscles of respiration in an attempt to make breathing easier. The more difficult the breathing becomes, the more anxious the patient feels.

SAFETY ALERT

If a patient has been wheezing but the wheeze abruptly disappears (i.e., silent chest) and the patient is obviously in distress, the situation has become life-threatening and may necessitate mechanical ventilation.

In some patients with asthma, cough is the only symptom, which is termed **cough variant asthma.** The bronchospasm may not be severe enough to cause airflow obstruction, but it can increase bronchial tone and cause irritation and stimulation of the cough receptors. The cough may be nonproductive. Mobilizing secretions may be difficult as a result of their thick, tenacious, gelatinous quality.

Examination of patients experiencing an acute attack of moderate or severe asthma usually reveals signs of hypoxemia, which may include restlessness, increased anxiety, inappropriate behaviour, increased pulse and blood pressure, and *pulsus paradoxus* (a drop in systolic pressure during the inspiratory cycle of more than 10 mm Hg). Such a patient's respiratory rate is significantly increased (usually >30 breaths/minute), and the use of accessory muscles is evident. The patient also has difficulty speaking in complete sentences; typically he or she is able to complete only two to five words without requiring another breath. Percussion of the lungs indicates hyper-resonance, and auscultation indicates the presence of inspiratory or expiratory wheezing.

Asthma Control and Severity

A dynamic continuum is used to manage asthma. This approach enables drug therapy to be adapted to the severity of the underlying illness and the current level of asthma control. The concepts of asthma "control" and "severity" are related to each other but not correlated (Taylor et al., 2008). For example, even severe asthma may be well controlled, whereas mild disease may remain out of control. *Optimal asthma* control is defined by the absence

Table 31-2 Asthma Control Criteria

CHARACTERISTIC	FREQUENCY OR VALUE
Daytime symptoms	<4 days/week
Nighttime symptoms	<1 night/week
Physical activity	Normal
Exacerbations	Mild, infrequent
Absence from work or school due to asthma	None
Need for a fast-acting β_2-agonist	<4 doses/week
FEV_1 or PEF	≥90% personal best
PEF diurnal variation*	<10 to 15%

Diurnal variation is calculated as the highest peak expiratory flow (PEF) minus the lowest PEF divided by the highest PEF multiplied by 100 for morning and night (determined over a 2-week period). FEV_1, forced expiratory volume in 1 s.
Source: Adapted from Lougheed, M. D., Lemiere, C., Dell, S. D., Ducharme, F. M., FitzGerald, J. M., Leigh, R., ..., Boulet, L. P. (2010). Canadian Thoracic Society asthma management continuum—2010 Consensus summary for children six years of age and over, and adults. *Canadian Respiratory Journal, 17*(1), 15-24 (Table 2).

of both asthma symptoms and the need for rescue bronchodilator, as well as by normal pulmonary function; however, this is difficult to achieve in all patients with asthma. As a result, according to the Canadian Asthma Consensus Report treatment needs should be based on achieving acceptable asthma control, determined through clinical and physiological criteria (Lougheed et al., 2010) (Table 31-2). Asthma control is obtained through the use of environmental control measures (reduced exposure to triggers), self-management education, written action plans, and pharmacotherapy tailored to the individual (Lougheed, et al.). Asthma control must be assessed regularly and treatment adjusted accordingly.

The severity of asthma is determined from the frequency and duration of symptoms, the presence of persistent airflow limitation, and the medication required to maintain control (Taylor et al., 2008). When asthma is well controlled, severity is gauged by level of treatment required to maintain the state of acceptable control (Table 31-3).

Signs of severe or poorly controlled asthma include a history of a previous near-fatal asthma episode (loss of consciousness, need for intubation); recent hospitalization or recent emergency department visit for asthma; nighttime symptoms; limitations in daily activities; and the need for inhaled β_2-agonists several times each day or night.

Asthma severity levels can change for better or worse over the course of a patient's life. This is particularly true for children with asthma, inasmuch as asthma severity often decreases with age. When asthma control is good, patients have minimal to no symptoms, are able to sleep through the night, and participate in sports, exercise, and strenuous activity. Once asthma control has been maintained for at least a few weeks to months, an attempt should be made to reduce medication dosages and yet maintain acceptable asthma control (Lougheed et al., 2010).

Severe Acute Asthma and Life-Threatening Asthma.
Patients who present with a severe acute asthma attack, or one that is life-threatening, often report a history of progressively worsening of asthma control over days or weeks. Of the people

Table 31-3 Asthma Severity Levels Based on Pharmacotherapy Needed to Achieve Control	
LEVEL OF SEVERITY	**PHARMACOTHERAPY NEEDED TO ACHIEVE CONTROL**
Very mild	None or rare use of short-acting β_2-agonist
Mild	Occasional use of short-acting β_2-agonist and low-dosage inhaled glucocorticosteroid
Moderate	Short-acting β_2-agonist and low- to moderate-dosage inhaled glucocorticosteroid with or without additional therapy
Severe	Short-acting β_2-agonist and high-dosage inhaled glucocorticosteroid with additional therapy
Very severe	Short-acting β_2-agonist and high-dosage inhaled glucocorticosteroid with additional therapy and oral glucocorticosteroid

Source: Reprinted from Cockroft, D. W., & Swystun, V. A. (1996). Asthma control versus asthma severity. *Journal of Allergy & Clinical Immunology, 98*, 1016-1018. Copyright 1996, with permission of the American Academy of Allergy, Asthma, and Immunology.
NOTE: Individuals with very severe asthma may not be able to achieve acceptable asthma control despite high-intensity treatment.

COLLABORATIVE CARE

Table 31-4 Asthma	
Diagnostic	**Collaborative Therapy**
• History and physical examination • Pulmonary function studies (spirometry; methacoline, histamine, exercise challenge test; PEFR) • Chest radiograph • Allergy skin testing • Measurement of oximetry and ABGs during acute episodes when patient is seen in emergency department or hospital	• Establishing partnerships between health care providers and patients and their families • Identification and avoidance or elimination of triggers • Patient and family teaching • Continuous assessment of asthma control and severity • Appropriate pharmacotherapy (see Tables 31-6 and 31-7) • Asthma action plan (see Figure 31-7) • Regular follow-up

ABG, arterial blood gases; *PEFR*, peak expiratory flow rate.

with asthma admitted to the hospital, approximately 10% require monitoring or ventilatory assistance in the critical care unit for severe uncontrolled asthma. Common causes of severe acute attacks include viral illnesses, ingestion of aspirin or other NSAIDs, increases in environmental pollutants or other allergen exposure, and discontinuation of drug therapy (especially corticosteroids). The clinical manifestations of a severe attack are a consequence of increased airway resistance that results from edema, mucous plugging, and bronchospasm with subsequent air trapping and hyperinflation. The clinical manifestations are similar to those of non-severe asthma but are more serious and prolonged. Extreme anxiety, fear of suffocation, severely increased work of breathing, and diaphoresis are common. Absence of diaphoresis may indicate significant dehydration. Sternocleidomastoid, intercostal, and supraclavicular muscle retractions reflect increased work of breathing.

Although wheezing is often audible even without a stethoscope, auscultation may not always be reliable: Airflow obstruction may be so severe and airflow so insufficient that audible wheezing or other abnormal lung sounds may not be produced. Absence of a wheeze (i.e., silent chest) represents a life-threatening situation that may necessitate mechanical ventilation. The chest appears fixed in a hyperinflated position and is often described as "tight," indicating severely decreased movement of air through the constricted bronchial airways.

Forced exhalation with the use of the abdominal musculature can result in increased intrathoracic pressure transmitted to the great vessels and heart. Neck vein distension and pulsus paradoxus with a pressure of 40 mm Hg or higher may result. (Pulsus paradoxus is described in Chapter 39 and Table 39-8.) Hypertension, sinus tachycardia, and ventricular dysrhythmias may occur. These three conditions are related to hypoxemia, the catecholamines present as a result of an endogenous response to hypoxia, and, in older patients, underlying coronary artery disease. An electrocardiogram may show sinus tachycardia or signs of strain on the right side of the heart secondary to pulmonary vasoconstriction, which may appear as cor pulmonale and a right axis deviation.

Hypoxemia with hypocapnia usually occurs initially as the patient attempts to hyperventilate and maintain adequate oxygenation and ventilation. As the severity of the attack increases, the work of breathing increases, making it more difficult for the patient to overcome the increased resistance to breathing. The patient becomes fatigued, which causes more carbon dioxide retention. ABG measurements initially reveal hypocapnia due to increased respiratory rate. Ultimately, these measurements deteriorate to manifest hypercapnia and hypoxemia. The patient must move amounts greater than 150 mL of air to have air participating in gas exchange. A moderate elevation in partial pressure of arterial carbon dioxide ($PaCO_2$) may be tolerated without intubation and mechanical ventilation if the patient remains alert and cooperative and continues to show improvement during the first 2 to 3 hours of treatment (Brenner, Corbridge, & Kazzi, 2009).

Complications of a severe asthma attack may include pneumothorax, pneumomediastinum, acute cor pulmonale with right ventricular failure, and severe respiratory muscle fatigue that leads to respiratory arrest. Respiratory arrest can be fatal.

Diagnostic Studies in Asthma

"A diagnosis of asthma should be considered in individuals of all age groups with recurrent symptoms" (Lougheed et al., 2010, p. 16). Two main features must be considered in the diagnosis of asthma: symptoms and variable airflow obstruction. Several sources of information assist with confirming the diagnosis of asthma along with monitoring severity and control (Table 31-4). A detailed history is important in determining whether a person has had previous attacks of a similar nature, often precipitated by a known cause or trigger as discussed previously in the chapter. Because asthma and allergies commonly coexist, it is also important to determine whether the patient has a history of nonpulmonary symptoms. Rhinitis, eczema, and conjunctivitis are common but not specific to asthma and indicate a predisposition to allergy. Of further value is to determine whether the patient has a family history of asthma, allergies, and eczema because a positive family history increases the likelihood that the patient has asthma. Recurrent symptoms of wheeze, sensation of chest tightness, cough, or breathlessness that improve with treatment are suggestive of asthma. However, wheezing and cough occur with a variety of disorders—COPD, pulmonary embolism, GERD, obesity, vocal cord dysfunction, and heart failure—and their presence can therefore complicate the diagnosis. The Canadian Thoracic Society has acknowledged that differentiating between asthma and COPD can be challenging in a small proportion of patients and suggested that clearly identifying the clinical differences can be of assistance (O'Donnell et al., 2008). This is discussed further in the section on COPD later in this chapter.

In all patients who are able to perform pulmonary testing, clinically suspected asthma should be confirmed with objective lung measurements that demonstrate postbronchodilator reversible obstruction, variable airflow limitation over time, or airway hyper-responsiveness (Lougheed et al., 2010). Spirometry is the preferred test for diagnosing asthma; alternative lung testing includes variations in PEFR and bronchoprovocative challenge testing (Lougheed et al., 2010; Table 31-5).

Spirometry performed before and after bronchodilator treatment can best reveal whether airway obstruction is reversible. Spirometry is the measure of flow rates and volumes during a noninvasive breathing test to determine the forced expiratory volume in 1 second (FEV_1) and the forced vital capacity (FVC). The ratio of FEV_1 to FVC is a measure of airflow obstruction. For spirometry, the patient is asked to refrain from using bronchodilator medication for 6 to 12 hours before the test. The test is then completed both before and after administration of a bronchodilator to determine the degree of response. Most children 6 years of age and older should be able to perform spirometry. (The normal values for pulmonary function tests are discussed in Chapter 28.)

An alternative objective pulmonary measurement, in which variable airflow limitation overtime is measured, is the PEFR, or maximum speed of exhalation, measured by a peak flow meter. The PEFR is a home measurement, which is not as reliable as spirometry but can be used when spirometry or challenge testing is unavailable. To determine an asthma diagnosis through this method, the patient must measure the PEFR four times per day—in the morning and evening both before and after bronchodilator treatment—for several weeks. To determine the PEFR variability, the lowest reading is subtracted from the highest reading, the result is divided by the highest reading, and this answer is then multiplied by 100. Variability in peak expiratory flow of 20% or higher is indicative of asthma.

Determining airway hyper-responsiveness with the use of methacholine, histamine, or exercise challenge testing can be useful in patients with persistent symptoms despite normal spirometry findings and to evaluate work-related asthma (Lougheed et al., 2010). Challenge testing must be performed in a controlled environment with trained staff.

Chest radiographs are not necessary to diagnose asthma; however, they may be used to exclude other diagnoses, such as congenital malformations in children and congestive heart failure in adults (Lougheed et al., 2010). A chest radiograph in an patient with asthma but no symptoms is usually normal but should be used as a baseline on initial diagnosis. A chest radiograph obtained during an acute attack usually shows hyperinflation and may reveal other complications of asthma such as mucoid impaction, pneumothorax, atelectasis, or pneumomediastinum.

Allergy assessment is warranted in a patient with asthma and must be interpreted in view of the patient's history of exposure and symptom experience. Allergy skin testing can be helpful in determining sensitivity to specific allergens (antigens). A positive skin test result does not necessarily mean that the allergen

Table 31-5 Diagnosis of Asthma: Pulmonary Function Criteria

PULMONARY FUNCTION MEASUREMENT	CHILDREN (6 YEARS OF AGE AND OLDER)	ADULTS
Preferred: Spirometry Showing Reversible Airway Obstruction		
Reduced FEV_1/FVC	Less than lower limit of normal based on age, sex, height, and ethnicity (<0.8-0.9)*	Less than lower limit of normal based on age, sex, height, and ethnicity (<0.75-0.8)*
AND	AND	AND
Increase in FEV_1 after a bronchodilator or after a course of controller therapy	≥12%	≥12% (and a minimum ≥200 mL)
Alternative: Peak Expiratory Flow Variability		
Increase after a bronchodilator or after course of controller therapy	≥20%	60 L/min (minimum ≥20%)
OR	OR	OR
Diurnal variation†	Not recommended	>8% based on twice daily readings; >20% based on multiple daily readings
Alternative: Positive Challenge Test		
Methacholine challenge	PC_{20} < 4 mg/mL (4-16 mg/mL is borderline; >16 mg/mL is negative)	
OR	OR	
Exercise challenge	≥10-15% decrease in FEV_1 postexercise	

*Approximate lower limits of normal ratios for children and adults;
†Difference between minimum morning prebronchodilator value in 1 wk and maximum nighttime value as percentage of recent maximum.
Source: Lougheed, M. D., Lemiere, C., Dell, S. D., Ducharme, F. M., FitzGerald, J. M., Leigh, R., …, Boulet, L. P. (2010). Canadian Thoracic Society asthma management continuum—2010 Consensus summary for children six years of age and over, and adults. *Canadian Respiratory Journal, 17*(1), 15-24. Retrieved from *http://www.respiratoryguidelines.ca/ sites/all/files/cts_asthma_consensus_summary_2010.pdf*

(antigen) is causing the asthma attack; however, a negative allergy test result does not mean that asthma is not allergy related. A radioallergosorbent test is sometimes used to identify allergic causes in certain patients whose skin tests results are negative and in those who should not be skin tested (e.g., patients with severe eczema). (Allergy testing is discussed further in Chapter 14.)

If a patient is in acute distress, it is not feasible to obtain a detailed health history (although a family member may supply some pertinent information). During an acute asthma attack, bedside spirometry (FEV_1 and FVC are preferred, but usually PEFR is measured) may be used to monitor obstruction. Serial spirometric parameters, oximetry, and measurement of ABGs help provide information about the severity of the attack and the response to therapy. A complete blood cell count and serum electrolyte measurements are obtained to help monitor the course of therapy because high dosages of inhaled β_2-agonists can cause hypokalemia.

Although it is important to assess the airway for the presence of inflammation, it is not part of routine clinical management of asthma and not yet widely available to diagnose asthma (Lougheed, et al., 2010). Changes in nitric oxide and sputum eosinophil levels may indicate whether treatment for asthma is working. These measurements have been used in adults and children and are becoming more easily available and reliable. However, they continue to be used most frequently in major research centres.

Collaborative Care

In 1990, Canada became the first country to produce asthma practice guidelines. These guidelines provide a medical approach to diagnosing and managing asthma informed by the best available evidence. The Registered Nurses' Association of Ontario (RNAO) also developed asthma best practice guidelines for adults (Cicutto et al., 2007) and children (Olajos-Clow et al., 2008) to provide nurses working in diverse settings with an evidence-informed summary of basic asthma care. The RNAO's *Best Practice Guidelines* build on and complement the Canadian Asthma Consensus Report and remain pertinent with the current Canadian Thoracic Society Asthma Management Continuum (Lougheed et al., 2010). The focus of the nursing guidelines is on promoting asthma control for adults and children affected by asthma. The overall goal of the guidelines is to achieve asthma control with the minimum level of pharmacotherapy while enhancing the quality of lives of individuals living with asthma and reducing the personal and social burdens inflicted by the condition. Existing guidelines acknowledge that successful asthma control involves partnerships among individuals with asthma, their families, and the interdisciplinary health care team.

Education that builds an active partnership with patients remains the cornerstone of asthma management (see the Evidence-Informed Practice box "Adult Asthma Care Guidelines for Nurses"). Education should start at the time of asthma diagnosis and be integrated into every aspect of clinical asthma care. Asthma self-management should be tailored to the needs of each patient; patients' cultural beliefs and practices should be accounted for. Emphasis should be placed on evaluating outcomes in terms of a patient's level of asthma control and perceptions of improvement, especially quality of life and the ability to engage in activities of normal living such as physical activity. A listing of centres that provide asthma education to patients can be accessed through the Canadian Network for Respiratory Care (see the Canadian Resources at the end of this chapter).

General Management Approach.
Several components enable successful management of asthma: (a) establishment of a confirmed diagnosis through the use of objective measures; (b) development of a partnership between health care providers and the patients and families affected by asthma; (c) limited exposure to triggers; (d) education of patients; (e) appropriate pharmacotherapy; (f) continuous assessment and monitoring of asthma control and severity; (g) implementation of a written action plan; and (h) ensuring regular follow-up.

In Canada, asthma treatment is based on the Asthma Management Continuum (Figure 31-4), which reflects the key messages pertaining to asthma diagnosis and management for children 6 years of age and older and for adults. Controlling the disease in order to prevent complications, morbidity, and mortal-

ity is the primary goal of asthma management (Lougheed et al., 2010, 2012). The continuum acknowledges that the level of control and severity of asthma changes over time and that constant assessment and adjustment of therapy is necessary to achieve and maintain control. The general management approach to asthma includes confirming the diagnosis, monitoring the level of asthma control (see Table 31-2), reducing exposure to environmental triggers, providing appropriate medications, providing asthma education, and providing a written action plan.

All individuals with asthma need to have access to either an inhaled short-acting β_2-agonist (SABA)—a bronchodilator—or, in some cases, a combination inhaled corticosteroid (ICS)/long-acting β_2-agonist (LABA) for quick relief of symptoms. If symptoms are infrequent and lung function measurements are normal, a SABA used on an as-needed basis to relieve symptoms is all that is required. However, an ICS is also required if one or more indicators of poor control are identified in a child 6 years of age or older or in an adult (see Table 31-2; Lougheed et al., 2010, 2012). If symptoms persist and are outside the limits of acceptable asthma control, the next step recommended on the asthma management continuum in children 6 to 11 years old is advancement to a moderate-dosage ICS. In children 12 years of age and older and in adults, however, the appropriate second-line therapy is the addition of a LABA in the form of a combination inhaler; the third-line therapy is an increase to a moderate-dosage ICS or addition of leukotriene receptor antagonists (LTRAs). For children 6 to 11 years old in whom asthma is not controlled on a moderate-dosage ICS, the addition of a LABA or LTRA, or both, is recommended. A fourth-line therapy—addition of theophylline—may be considered for adults.

In a minority of patients, symptoms persist despite the use of these therapies. If the FEV_1 is below 60% of predicted levels or of their best value, treatment with an oral corticosteroid (prednisone) should be initiated (Becker et al., 2005; Lemiere et al., 2004). Long-term prednisone use may be indicated and effective for asthma that is difficult to control, but should be avoided, if at all possible, because of its adverse effects. An anti-IgE antagonist, omalizumab (Xolair), may be considered in patients 12 years of age and older with atopic asthma that is poorly controlled despite high-dosage ICS and additional therapies, either with or without prednisone. The asthma management continuum also stresses the importance of assessing symptom control, lung function, inhaler technique, adherence to therapy, avoidance of exposure to asthma triggers, the presence of comorbid conditions and examination of sputum eosinophils (where available) on a regular basis and before therapy is advanced (Lougheed et al., 2012).

Acute Asthma Episode.
Patients with an acute asthma episode often come to the emergency department. The choice of treatment of acute asthma depends on the severity of a patient's condition and the response to initial therapy. The examiner can assess the degree of severity by measuring FEV_1 or PEFR, identifying the degree of change in objective measurements, and evaluating the baseline pulse oximetry value. Inhaled SABA should be administered immediately and supplemental oxygen provided to keep arterial oxygen saturation (SaO_2) above 92%. In more severe cases, ABG measurements may be used. Inhaled β_2-adrenergic agonists are preferably administered through a metered-dose inhaler (MDI) plus spacer giving four to eight puffs every 15 to 20 minutes, usually repeated three times. If the FEV_1 or PEFR is below 40% of predicted, one puff every 30 to 60 seconds (up to 20 puffs) may be administered, depending on the patient's

Adult Asthma Care Guidelines for Nurses: Promoting Control of Asthma

Clinical Question

What are the practice recommendations for nurses caring for adults with asthma?

Best Available Evidence

Multiple systematic reviews of asthma management practices

Synthesis of Best Available Evidence

Recommendations of Clinical Practice Guideline: Assessment of Asthma Control

Recommendation 1.0: All individuals identified as having asthma, or suspected of having asthma, will have their level of asthma control assessed by the nurse.

Recommendation 1.1: Every patient should be screened to identify those most likely to be affected by asthma. As part of the basic respiratory assessment, nurses should ask every patient two questions:

- Have you ever been told by a physician that you have asthma?
- Have you ever used a puffer or inhaler or asthma medication for breathing problems?

Recommendation 1.2: For individuals identified as having asthma or suspected of having asthma, the level of asthma control should be assessed by the nurse. Nurses should be knowledgeable about the acceptable parameters of asthma control, which are as follows:

- Use of inhaled short-acting β_2-agonist <4 times/week
- Experience of daytime asthma symptoms <4 times/week
- Experience of nighttime asthma symptoms <1 time/week
- Normal physical activity levels*
- No absence from work or school
- Infrequent and mild exacerbations

Recommendation 1.3: For individuals identified as potentially having uncontrolled asthma, the level of acuity needs to be assessed by the nurse and an appropriate medical referral provided (i.e., urgent care or follow-up appointment).

Asthma Education

Recommendation 2.0: Asthma education, provided by the nurse, must be an essential component of care.

Recommendation 2.1: The patient's asthma knowledge and skills should be assessed, and when gaps are identified, asthma education should be provided.

Recommendation 2.2: Education should include, as a minimum, the following:

- Basic facts about asthma
- Roles/rationale for medications
- Device technique(s)
- Self-monitoring
- Action plans

Action Plans

Recommendation 3.0: Every patient with asthma should have an individualized written asthma action plan for guided self-management.

Recommendation 3.1: An action plan should be developed in partnership with the health care provider and be based on the evaluation of symptoms with or without peak flow measurement.

Recommendation 3.2: For every patient with asthma, the nurse needs to assess for use and understanding of the asthma action plan. If a patient does not have an action plan, the nurse must provide a sample action plan, explain its purpose and use, and coach the patient to complete the plan with his or her asthma care provider.

Recommendation 3.3: Where deemed appropriate, the nurse should assess, assist, and educate patients in measuring PEFR. A standardized format should be used for teaching patients how to use peak flow measurements.

Medication

Recommendation 4.0: Nurses will understand and be able to discuss with patients their medications.

Recommendation 4.1: Nurses will understand and be able to discuss the two main categories of asthma medications (controllers and relievers) with their patients.

Recommendation 4.2: All asthma patients should have their inhaler/device technique assessed by the nurse to ensure accurate use. Patients with suboptimal technique will be coached in proper inhaler/device use.

Referrals

Recommendation 5.0: The nurse will facilitate referrals as appropriate.

Recommendation 5.1: Patients with poorly controlled asthma should be referred to their physician.

Recommendation 5.2: All patients should be offered links to community resources.

Recommendation 5.3: Patients should be referred to an asthma educator in their community, if appropriate and available.

Reference for Evidence

Registered Nurses' Association of Ontario (RNAO). (2007). Adult asthma care guidelines for nurses: Promoting control of asthma. *Best Practice Guidelines: Shaping the future of nursing.* Toronto: Author. Retrieved from *http://rnao.ca/bpg/guidelines/adult-asthma-care-guidelines-nurses-promoting-control-asthma*

*From Lougheed, M. D., Lemiere, C., Ducharme, F. M., Licskai, C., Dell, S. D., Rowe, B. H., ..., Canadian Thoracic Society Asthma Clinical Assembly (2012). Canadian Thoracic Society 2012 guideline update: Diagnosis and management of asthma in preschoolers, children and adults. *Canadian Respiratory Journal, 19*(2), 127-164.
PEFR, peak expiratory flow rate.

response to and tolerance of treatment (Boulet, Becker, Berube, Beveridge, & Ernst, 1999). Ipratropium bromide (four to eight puffs inhaled every 15 to 20 minutes, repeated three times) may be added to salbutamol during moderate and severe acute asthma episodes. In some emergency departments, bronchodilators are administered via a nebulizer, but a meta-analysis of study results revealed that the MDI plus valved spacer is quicker, less costly, and more effective in reducing hospitalization and improving clinical scores (GINA, 2010).

Oral corticosteroids are indicated for treatment of an acute exacerbation necessitating visit to the emergency department. Intravenous corticosteroids are generally administered to patients

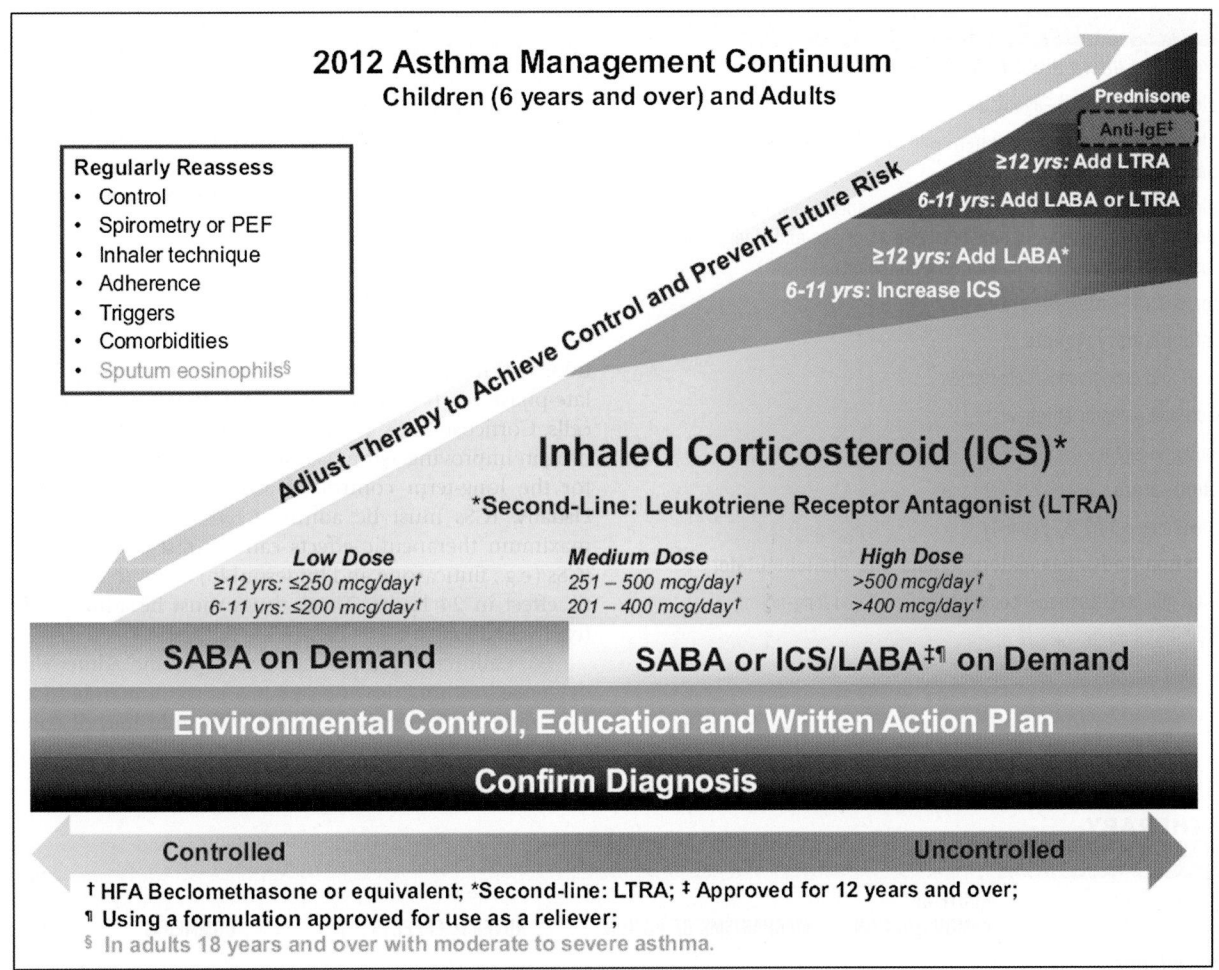

Figure 31-4 The Asthma Management Continuum. *HFA*, hydrofluoroalkane; *IgE*, immunoglobulin E; *LABA*, long-acting β₂-agonst; *PEF*, peak expiratory flow; *SABA*, short-acting β₂-agonist.

Source: Lougheed, M. D., Lemiere, C., Ducharme, F. M., Licskai, C., Dell, S. D. Rowe, B. H., ..., Canadian Asthma Society Asthma Clinical Assembly. (2012). Canadian Thoracic Society 2012 guideline update: Diagnosis and management of asthma in preschoolers, children and adults. *Canadian Respiratory Journal, 19*(2), p. 162, Figure 3. Retrieved from http://www.respiratoryguidelines.ca/guideline/asthma.

who have difficulty with swallowing. Therapy should be continued until the patient is breathing comfortably, wheezing has disappeared, and pulmonary function measurements are near baseline values.

On occasion, an asthma attack is so severe and unresponsive to treatment that the patient requires mechanical ventilation. Indications for mechanical ventilation are persistent or progressive carbon dioxide retention and respiratory acidosis, clinical deterioration (indicated by fatigue, hypersomnolence), metabolic acidosis, and cardiopulmonary arrest. In life-threatening asthma exacerbation, the goals of initiating mechanical ventilation are to achieve a partial pressure of arterial oxygen (PaO_2) of 60 mm Hg or higher, an SaO_2 of 90% or higher, and a normal pH.

Louder wheezing may occur in the airways, indicating a response to therapy as airflow increases. As the patient begins to respond to therapy and symptoms begin to subside, it is important to remember that despite the reversibility of most of the bronchospasm, the edema and cellular infiltration of the airway mucosa and the viscous mucous plugs are still present, and improvement may take several days. Thus intensive therapy includes corticosteroids and must be continued even after clinical improvement has occurred. Patients with moderate or severe acute asthma are typically discharged home with inhaled SABA,

a high-dosage ICS, and an oral corticosteroid (Hodder et al., 2010). In addition, discharge instructions should include an action plan detailing the use of the medications and the criteria for returning to the emergency department for immediate medical assistance. It is important that patients follow up with their primary asthma care professional after an emergency department visit.

Drug Therapy

The Canadian Thoracic Society Asthma Management Continuum 2010 consensus summary recommends using the asthma management continuum approach to drug therapy, with the type and amount of medication dictated by the levels of asthma control and asthma severity (see Table 31-2 and Figure 31-4; Lougheed et al., 2010). The guidelines emphasize that most patients with asthma, unless it is very mild and manifests infrequently, require daily use of ICS in addition to a SABA as necessary (Lougheed et al., 2010). Medications used to treat asthma are divided into two categories: (a) relievers and (b) controllers (Table 31-6). They are available in several forms, and various delivery devices are used to administer them. The inhaled route is preferred because the drug is delivered directly to the lungs, and therefore

Table 31-6 Categories of Asthma Medications

Relievers (for Intermittent Relief of Symptoms)

- Inhaled short-acting β₂-agonists
- Inhaled ipratropium bromide (rarely used except in emergency management)
- Inhaled corticosteroid/long-acting β₂ agonist, specifically budesonide/formoterol (used as relief in patients 12 years of age and older if they are using the combination inhaler as maintenance therapy)

Controllers (Maintenance Therapy)

Anti-inflammatory Agents

- Inhaled and oral glucocorticosteroids
- Leukotriene receptor antagonists
- Antiallergic agents

Bronchodilators

- Inhaled long-acting β₂-agonists

Combination Anti-inflammatory Agents and Bronchodilator

- Inhaled glucocorticosteroid combined with inhaled long-acting β₂-agonist

systemic absorption and thus the number and intensity of adverse events are minimized. Relievers, used to ease asthma symptoms, are also known as "rescue" medication and are used intermittently as required. Controllers are maintenance therapy used on a daily basis, typically twice a day. Because inflammation is considered an early and persistent component of asthma, drug therapy is directed toward long-term suppression of inflammation (Table 31-7).

Anti-inflammatory Drugs

Corticosteroids. Chronic inflammation is a primary component of asthma. Corticosteroids are anti-inflammatory medications that reduce bronchial hyper-responsiveness by blocking the late-phase reaction and that inhibit migration of inflammatory cells. Corticosteroids are more effective than any other long-term drug in improving asthma control. ICSs are the mainstay therapy for the long-term control of asthma (Lougheed et al., 2010). Usually, ICSs must be administered for 1 to 2 weeks before maximum therapeutic effects can be observed. However, some ICSs (e.g., fluticasone and budesonide) begin to have a therapeutic effect in 24 hours. These drugs must be administered on a fixed schedule.

For children 6 years of age and older and adults with newly diagnosed asthma, low-dosage ICS is recommended (see Figure 31-4) and for ICS-naïve patients with mild loss of control (see Table 31-2). In children 6 years of age and older and adults

DRUG THERAPY

Table 31-7 Asthma and Chronic Obstructive Pulmonary Disease

DRUG	ROUTE OF ADMINISTRATION	MECHANISMS OF ACTION	ADVERSE EFFECTS	COMMENTS
Bronchodilators				
Short-Acting β₂-Adrenergic Agonists				
Salbutamol (Airomir, Apo-Salvent, Ventolin)	Diskus DPI, MDI, nebules	Selectively stimulates β₂-receptors on airway smooth muscle, causing relaxation and producing bronchodilation	Tremor, tachycardia, headache, nervousness, palpitations, insomnia; excessive use can cause hypokalemia	Rapid onset of action: 1-3 min Duration of action: up to 6 hr Peak effect: 60-90 min
Terbutaline (Bricanyl)	Turbuhaler DPI	Same as for salbutamol	Same as for salbutamol	Rapid onset of action: within minutes Duration of action: 4-7 hr Peak effect: 15-60 min
Long-Acting β₂-Adrenergic Agonists				
Formoterol (Foradil, Oxeze)	Aerolizer DPI, Turbuhaler DPI	Selectively stimulates β₂-receptors on airway smooth muscle, causing relaxation and producing bronchodilation	Tremor, tachycardia, headache, nervousness, palpitations, insomnia	Rapid onset of action: 1-3 min Duration of protection: 8-12 hr Peak effect: 15 min Typically taken twice daily Oxeze has approval to be used as a reliever in asthma only when used in combination with inhaled steroid
Salmeterol (Serevent)	Diskus DPI	Same as above	Same as above	Onset of action: 10-20 min Duration of action: 8-12 hr Typically taken twice daily; not to exceed 50 mcg q12h Not used for relief of acute exacerbations

DRUG THERAPY

Table 31-7 Asthma and Chronic Obstructive Pulmonary Disease—cont'd

DRUG	ROUTE OF ADMINISTRATION	MECHANISMS OF ACTION	ADVERSE EFFECTS	COMMENTS
Anticholinergics				
Ipratropium bromide (Apo-Ipravent, Atrovent HFA)	MDI, nebulizer	Blocks action of acetylcholine, resulting in bronchodilation; competitive inhibitor of muscarinic receptors	Dry mouth, cough, bad taste, nausea, headache, flushed skin; blurred vision if sprayed in eyes	Onset: 5-15 min Duration: 4-6 hr Peak effect: 1-2 hr Should be used with precaution in individuals with narrow-angle glaucoma, prostatic hyperplasia, or bladder neck obstruction
Ipratropium and salbutamol (Combivent) Ipratropium and fenoterol (Duovent)	Nebulizer	Combination of anticholinergic and β_2-agonist preparations produces bronchodilation	See ipratropium and short-acting β_2-agonists	See ipratropium and short-acting β_2-agonists
Tiotropium bromide (Spiriva)	HandiHaler DPI	Blocks action of acetylcholine, resulting in bronchodilation; competitive inhibitor of muscarinic receptors on bronchial smooth muscle	Dry mouth, cough, bad taste, nausea, headache, constipation, urinary retention	Onset: 30 min Peak: 1-4 hr Duration: 24 hr Should be used only once per day Should be used same time each day Contact with eyes should be avoided Powder capsules sensitive to light and moisture
Anti-Inflammatory Agents				
Steroidal Anti-inflammatory Agents				
Hydrocortisone (Cortef Tab, Solu-Cortef) Methylprednisolone (Medrol, Solu-Medrol) Prednisone (Winpred) Prednisolone (Pediapred) Dexamethasone (Dexasone)	Oral, intravenous Oral, intravenous Oral	Potent anti-inflammatory and immunosuppressive effects; interferes with inflammatory cascade; decreases edema in bronchial airways; increases number and affinity of β_2-receptors; restores and prevents tolerance induced with chronic use of inhaled β_2-agonists; decreases mucus secretion; effective in late-phase reaction of asthma	Short-term use (<2 wk): weight gain, increased appetite, cushingoid appearance, menstrual changes, mood changes, skin changes (acne, striae, bruising) Longer term use (>2 wk): adrenal suppression, immunosuppression, osteoporosis, hyperglycemia, obesity, peptic ulcers, hypertension, hypokalemia, cataracts, glaucoma, muscle weakness, catabolism, growth retardation, avascular necrosis, dysphonia	Onset: Some effects within 2-4 hr In acute severe asthma, 4-12 hr may be required before clinical response noted Reversal of bronchial hyper-responsiveness requires about 1 wk Alternate-day or morning therapy may minimize the intensity of adverse drug events Should be taken with food When drug is given in high doses, patient should be assessed for epigastric pain Histamine (H₂) blockers and antacids may minimize the intensity of GI effects Counsel patient about steps to take to prevent osteoporosis If taken for <2 wk or <2 bursts in 1 year, no tapering of dosage required; otherwise dosage should be tapered gradually If symptoms recur during tapering, asthma care professional should be notified

Continued

DRUG THERAPY

Table 31-7 Asthma and Chronic Obstructive Pulmonary Disease—cont'd

DRUG	ROUTE OF ADMINISTRATION	MECHANISMS OF ACTION	ADVERSE EFFECTS	COMMENTS
Beclomethasone (QVAR, Rivanase AQ)	MDI, nasal spray	Same as for hydrocortisone and others Acts locally in respiratory tract with relatively little systemic absorption at low to medium dosages	Oral candidiasis infection, hoarseness, irritated throat, dry mouth, cough	Mouth should be rinsed after use to reduce the risk for oral fungal infections, hoarseness, and dry mouth If an MDI is used, a spacer should also be used to reduce the intensity of adverse effects Nasal spray form used for allergic rhinitis Typically taken twice daily
Budesonide (Pulmicort, Rhinocort NS)	Turbuhaler DPI, nasal spray, nebulizer	Same as for beclomethasone	Same as for beclomethasone	Mouth should be rinsed after use Nasal spray form used for allergic rhinitis Typically taken twice daily
Ciclesonide (Alvesco, Omnaris NS)	MDI, nasal spray	Same as for beclomethasone	Same as for beclomethasone	Same as for budesonide
Fluticasone (Avamys NS, Flonase NS, Flovent DPI, MDI)	Diskus DPI, MDI, nasal spray	Same as for beclomethasone but with higher potency (about double); as a result, dosages tend to be lower	Same as for beclomethasone; bruising with higher dosages	Mouth should be rinsed after use If an MDI is used, a spacer should also be used to reduce the intensity of adverse effects Nasal spray form used for allergic rhinitis Typically taken twice daily
Mometasone (Nasonex NS)	Metered-dose manual pump spray	Exact mechanism of action unknown	Headache, viral infection, pharyngitis	May require 2 wk of treatment before improvement noted
Combination Inhalers: Inhaled Glucocorticosteroid and Inhaled Long-Acting β_2-Agonist (LABA)				
Budesonide and formoterol (Symbicort) Fluticasone and salmeterol (Advair) Mometasone and formoterol (Zenhale)	Turbuhaler DPI Diskus DPI, MDI	See text sections pertaining to inhaled glucocorticosteroid and inhaled LABAs	See text sections pertaining to inhaled glucocorticosteroid and inhaled LABAs	Commonly used for moderate and severe asthma Combination therapy products may simplify treatment regimen In COPD, ICS is recommended only in combination with LABA and is initiated when a person has had >1 acute exacerbation in a year See text sections pertaining to combination ICS/LABA
Antileukotrienes				
Montelukast (Singulair) Zafirlukast (Accolate)	Oral tablets, chewable tablets for children, granules Oral tablets	Block the action of leukotrienes released by inflammatory cell membranes; have bronchodilator and anti-inflammatory effects	Headache, indigestion, nausea, vomiting, diarrhea, fatigue, abdominal pain, respiratory infections	Prevents exercise-induced asthma Bioavailability of zafirlukast is reduced when it is taken with food Affect metabolism of erythromycin and theophylline Not used to relieve acute asthma episodes

DRUG THERAPY

Table 31-7 Asthma and Chronic Obstructive Pulmonary Disease—cont'd

DRUG	ROUTE OF ADMINISTRATION	MECHANISMS OF ACTION	ADVERSE EFFECTS	COMMENTS
Anti–IgE Antagonist				
Omalizumab (Xolair)	Subcutaneous injection	This binds free IgE and therefore prevents IgE from binding to receptors on its effector cells, primarily mast cells and basophils When IgE does not bind to those cells, allergens are prevented from triggering acute allergic reactions	Reaction at injection site (pain, bruising, redness, warmth)	Only for moderate to severe persistent allergic asthma with symptoms not inadequately controlled by ICS Not for acute bronchospasm Administered under direct medical supervision; patient is observed for a minimum of 2 hr after administration because anaphylaxis has been reported with use
Methylxanthines				
Theophylline (Uniphyl, Theolair) Aminophylline	Oral, intravenous	Relieves bronchoconstriction and its accompanying symptoms by dilating the muscles around the bronchi	Tachycardia, blood pressure changes, dysrhythmias, anorexia, nausea, vomiting, nervousness, irritability, headache, muscle twitching, flushing, epigastric pain, diarrhea, insomnia, palpitations	Wide variety of responses to drug metabolism Half-life: ↓ by smoking and ↑ by heart failure and liver disease Cimetidine, ciprofloxacin, erythromycin, and other drugs may rapidly ↑ theophylline levels The effect of these medications is proportionate to their concentration in the blood To be effective, they must be taken regularly, and blood concentrations should be monitored
Phosphodiesterase 4 Inhibitor				
Roflumilast (Daxas)	Oral	Selective phosphodiesterase 4 inhibitor Nonsteroidal anti-inflammatory drug that targets systemic and pulmonary inflammation associated with COPD	Diarrhea, nausea, anorexia, weight loss, headache, insomnia, anxiety; may resolve after 4 wk of continuous treatment	Indicated for use in severe COPD as an therapeutic addition to long-acting bronchodilators for patients with chronic cough, chronic sputum findings, and history of frequent exacerbations Not currently indicated for asthma Not indicated for acute bronchospasm

COPD, chronic obstructive pulmonary disease; *DPI*, dry powder inhaler; *GI*, gastrointestinal; *ICS*, inhaled corticosteroids; *IgE*, immunoglobulin E; *MDI*, metered-dose inhaler.

presenting with an asthma exacerbation necessitating short-term systemic corticosteroids, a daily low- to moderate-dosage ICS should be initiated as maintenance therapy. In children 6 years of age and older, if low-dosage ICS is not adequate in achieving or maintaining control, then increasing to moderate-dosage ICS (see Figure 31-4) is the preferred approach. To minimize the intensity of adverse effects, however, add-on therapy should be considered in patients 12 years of age and older before ICS therapy is increased to moderate dosages and certainly before high dosages are prescribed adverse events (Lougheed et al., 2010).

When ICSs are administered, asthma can usually be controlled without significant systemic adverse events because little systemic drug absorption occurs from these devices. However, ICSs administered at the highest dosage levels have been associated with adverse events such as easy bruising and accelerated bone loss (Lougheed et al., 2010). Oropharyngeal candidiasis, hoarseness, and dry cough are local adverse effects caused by ICS (Rachelefsky, Liao, & Faruqi, 2007). Occurrence of these oropharyngeal adverse events can be reduced by mouth rinsing and gargling after inhalation. If an MDI is used, absorption can be improved and the intensity of adverse events reduced with the use of a spacer (Figure 31-5). However, newer drugs (e.g., ciclesonide) that are activated in the lungs (not in the pharynx) appear to minimize the intensity of these adverse events without the need for a spacer or mouth rinsing (Lougheed et al., 2010).

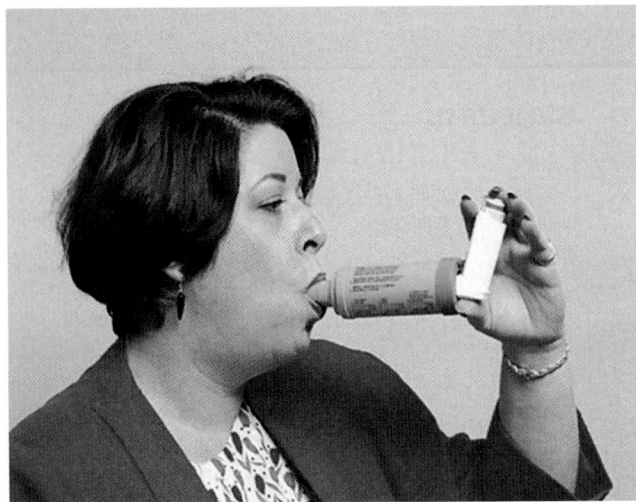

Figure 31-5 Example of an AeroChamber spacer used with a metered-dose inhaler.

In acute asthma exacerbations, short courses of orally administered corticosteroids are indicated for gaining prompt control (Lougheed et al., 2010). In a minority of cases, maintenance dosages of oral corticosteroids are necessary to control severe chronic asthma. However, long-term use should be avoided in all age groups if possible, especially children, because of adverse effects (Lougheed et al., 2010). If long-term use is indicated, a single dose in the morning, to coincide with endogenous cortisol production, and alternate-day dosing should be considered; these schedules are associated with fewer adverse effects. Long-term corticosteroid therapy is discussed further in Chapter 51.

Adults using maintenance oral corticosteroids or high dosages of ICS (>500 mcg fluticasone and beclomethasone; >800 mcg budesonide), or both, should be monitored for osteoporosis with bone densitometry. Patients should take adequate amounts of calcium and vitamin D and participate in regular weight-bearing exercise. (Osteoporosis is discussed in Chapter 66.)

Antileukotrienes. In Canada, two leukotriene receptor antagonists (zafirlukast, montelukast) which block the action of leukotrienes (Lougheed et al., 2010) are available. Leukotrienes are produced from arachidonic acid metabolism (see Chapter 14, Figure 14-7). Some leukotrienes are potent bronchoconstrictors, causing airway edema and inflammation and thus contributing to the symptoms of asthma. The anti-inflammatory action of antileukotrienes is not as potent as that of ICS, and thus they are not recommended as a single agent in the treatment of persistent asthma (Lougheed et al., 2010). These agents are used as adjuvant or add-on therapy for individuals experiencing symptoms (uncontrolled asthma) or significant adverse events while using higher dosage ICS. Antileukotrienes may be considered as an alternative to increasing dosages of ICS. They are not used to reverse bronchospasm in acute asthma attacks. An advantage of these drugs is that they are administered orally.

Anti–Immunoglobulin E Antagonists. Omalizumab (Xolair) is a monoclonal antibody to IgE that decreases circulating free IgE levels (Chapman, Cartier, Hebert, McIvor, & Schellenberg, 2006). Omalizumab prevents IgE from attaching to mast cells, thus preventing the release of chemical mediators. Health Canada

has approved this drug for use by patients who have moderate to severe persistent allergic asthma and are 12 years of age and older. This medication is expensive and therefore should be reserved for specific patients: those with asthma that is difficult to control despite adherence to a regimen of high-dosage ICS plus at least one additional controller therapy, who have objectively confirmed asthma, who have documented allergic perennial asthma, and have a serum IgE level of 30 to 700 IU/mL. The medication is administered subcutaneously every 2 to 4 weeks and should be part of a well-controlled therapeutic trial supervised by an asthma specialist (Lougheed et al., 2010).

Bronchodilators. Three classes of bronchodilator drugs are currently used in asthma therapy: β_2-adrenergic agonists, anticholinergic drugs, and methylxanthines.

β_2-Adrenergic Agonists. These drugs may be SABAs or LABAs. These medications work by binding to β_2-receptors located on airway smooth muscle, causing relaxation of the bronchial smooth muscle and thus bronchodilation. Fast-acting β_2-adrenergic agonists are the drug of choice for relief of acute symptoms of asthma (Lougheed et al., 2010) and are used as rescue or reliever medication for quick relief of symptoms and therefore should be carried by the patient at all times. They are also used to prevent bronchospasm precipitated by exercise with administration 10 to 15 minutes before exercise. In Canada, several SABAs are approved for this indication, including salbutamol and terbutaline (Lougheed et al., 2010). These agents begin to work within a few minutes and cause maximum dilation within 10 to 15 minutes. The duration of effect varies according to the agent, but airflow rates remain significantly elevated for 2 to 6 hours after inhalation. Adverse events from SABAs are few and include mild tremor and tachycardia, which diminish with repeated use without loss of bronchodilator effect. However, frequent daily use of inhaled SABAs may be associated with decreased control of asthma and provides the rationale for as-needed dosage. The frequency of use of reliever medications is a good indicator of a patient's level of asthma control (Lougheed et al., 2010).

LABAs provide sustained bronchodilation (approximately 12 hours) and include formoterol and salmeterol. LABAs should be considered as add-on therapy in adults who have persistent symptoms despite low-dosage ICS and in children 6 to 11 years of age who have persistent symptoms despite use of moderate-dosage ICS (Lougheed et al., 2010). Both formoterol and salmeterol can help patients reduce the amount of ICS required to control asthma and are useful in controlling nocturnal asthma symptoms. However, LABAs are to be used not as monotherapy but rather in combination with an ICS (Lougheed et al., 2010). Neither salmeterol nor formoterol has major adverse events when used in conjunction with ICS. Immediate adverse events are similar to those of SABAs. Salmeterol and formoterol cannot be considered interchangeable. Formoterol has a greater bronchopulmonary protective effect and is rapid acting; thus it can be used as rescue therapy for prompt relief of symptoms when taken in combination with only an ICS (Lougheed et al., 2012). Salmeterol has a narrower therapeutic window, and dosage should stay within the recommended range.

Combination therapy inhalers that contain both a LABA and an ICS are available and commonly used. The three products available in Canada are Advair, which is a combination of salmeterol and fluticasone; Symbicort, which is a combination of formoterol and budesonide; and Zenhale, which is a combination of formoterol and mometasone. Evidence suggests that combination therapy inhalers can replace the two separate inhalers, thus simplifying therapy and probably increasing adherence to the medication regimen. There is no superior effect over using the two inhalers separately; however, using the two medications in a combination inhaler is preferred for asthma, inasmuch as it precludes the use of the LABA without the ICS (Lougheed et al., 2010).

Anticholinergic Drugs. The parasympathetic division of the autonomic nervous system controls airway diameter. The effects of acetylcholine on the airways are increased smooth muscle contraction and mucus secretion, which result in bronchoconstriction. Anticholinergic agents inhibit bronchoconstriction that is related to the parasympathetic nervous system. Anticholinergic bronchodilators are not recommended as first-line therapy in asthma, primarily because their action peaks 30 minutes to 1 hour after ingestion; therefore, they are inferior to SABAs as rescue or reliever inhalers. Anticholinergic drugs, as rescue inhalers, may be useful only in patients who are unable to tolerate SABAs (Lougheed et al., 2010). The combination of ipratropium bromide with salbutamol (Combivent; a nebulized preparation) is commonly used for the emergency management of acute asthma. This combination appears to produce greater bronchodilation than does either agent used alone. The most common adverse effect of anticholinergic drugs is dry mouth. Systemic adverse events are uncommon because it is poorly absorbed.

Methylxanthines. Sustained-release methylxanthines (theophylline) preparations should be used only as controller medication for asthma that is difficult to control, after ICS, LABA, and LTRAs. Methylxanthine is a bronchodilator with mild anti-inflammatory effects. Theophylline should be prescribed only by an asthma specialist because of its narrow toxic/therapeutic ratio and frequent adverse events (Lougheed et al., 2010), which include nausea, headache, insomnia, gastrointestinal distress, tachycardia, dysrhythmias, and seizures. Blood levels must be monitored regularly to determine whether the drug levels are in the therapeutic range.

Patient Education Related to Drug Therapy.
Education about asthma medication is an essential component of asthma care (Cicutto et al., 2007; Lougheed et al., 2010; Olajos-Clow et al., 2008). Information about medications that the patient should know includes name, dosage, method of administration, frequency of use, indications, adverse effects, consequences of improper use, and the importance of adherence. Specifically with regard to asthma, patients need to be taught about the different roles and indications for using relievers and controllers. In addition to providing information, it is essential that the nurse assess a patient's ability to use inhaler devices accurately and provide coaching in the proper use of the device. Thus all nurses should know the correct use of the various devices and feel confident in their ability to assess and coach patients and their families about their proper use.

Most asthma drugs are administered by inhalation. Inhalation of drugs is preferred to oral administration because a lower dosage is required and systemic adverse events are fewer and less intense. The onset of action of bronchodilators is faster when they are delivered via inhalation. Inhalation devices include MDIs with or without spacers, dry powder inhalers (DPIs), and wet nebulizers (see Table 31-7).

Table 31-8 Problems Encountered With Use of Metered-Dose Inhaler (MDI)
1. Failing to coordinate activation with inspiration
2. Activating MDI in the mouth while breathing through nose
3. Inspiring too rapidly
4. Not holding the breath for 10 sec (or as close to 10 sec as possible)
5. Holding MDI upside down or sideways
6. Inhaling more than one puff with each inspiration
7. Not shaking MDI before use
8. Not waiting a sufficient amount of time between each puff
9. Not opening mouth wide enough, which causes medication to bounce off teeth, tongue, or palate
10. Not having adequate strength to activate MDI
11. Being unable to perform all the necessary steps

Wet nebulizers are used primarily to deliver large bronchodilator doses during acute asthma attacks in emergency department and other hospital settings. In the home, they are used as a last resort for patients unable to use other inhalation devices. A trial of wet nebulization in infants and young children at home may be appropriate if an MDI with a spacer is ineffective. In response to the outbreak of severe acute respiratory syndrome (SARS) , the use of wet nebulization has decreased in emergency departments and hospitals because when wet nebulization is used, aerosol is released into the environment, not just to a patient's airways; thus everyone in the room is breathing in the aerosol. MDIs plus spacers are as effective as nebulizers in delivering large doses of bronchodilators during acute asthma attacks, because the amount of drug delivered to the lungs is enhanced with the spacer.

Inadequate technique is widespread among patients using MDIs, and many demonstrate common errors (Table 31-8). If an inhaler technique can be improved and sustained, clinical benefits are likely to result (Table 31-9). Some patients need to add a spacer to the MDI or switch to a DPI to acquire a good technique. Spacers or holding chambers (e.g., AeroChamber, OptiChamber; see Figure 31-5) are used when patients cannot muster the coordination necessary to use a MDI. In addition, spacers enhance the delivery of medication to the airways and decrease the intensity of adverse events from ICS because less medication is delivered to the mouth. MDIs with spacers can be considered for all age groups and should be used when ICSs are delivered via MDI. A spacer with a face mask is recommended for young children and older adults. When spacers with face masks are used in children, however, a conversion to a spacer with a mouthpiece is encouraged as soon as the child is old enough and able to cooperate.

The DPI contains dry, powdered medication and is breath-activated (Figure 31-6). No propellant is used; instead an aerosol is created when the patient inhales quickly and forcefully through a reservoir containing a dose of powder. Patients find DPIs easier to use than MDIs with no spacer. (Table 31-10 describes how to use a DPI.) There are several advantages to using DPIs: (a) Less manual dexterity is required; (b) the patient does not need to coordinate depressing the canister with inhaling; (c) an easily visible colour or number system indicates the number of doses left in the device; and (d) its use does not require a spacer. The biggest problem with DPIs is that the medication may clump if

PATIENT & CAREGIVER TEACHING GUIDE

Table 31-9 How to Use a Metered-Dose Inhaler (MDI) Correctly

The nurse must teach the patient that the key to using all inhaled medications is proper technique. Patients should receive the following instructions to ensure that every puff of the MDI delivers the most medication possible into the lungs, rather than to the back of the throat.

1. Firmly place the metal container into the mouthpiece. Remove the cap, and shake the inhaler vigorously.

2. Breathe out only to the end of a normal breath (not a forced breath).

3. Position the mouthpiece end of the inhaler about 4 cm (1.5 inches) from your mouth.

4. Open your mouth widely and tilt your head back slightly. (Another way of doing this is to close your lips around the mouthpiece, keeping teeth apart and tongue flat so the medication can flow freely into the lungs.)

5. At the same time that you start to breathe in slowly, depress the metal container into the mouthpiece to release one puff of medication.

6. Continue breathing in slowly until your lungs are full (about 5 seconds).

   - Once you have breathed in fully, hold your breath for 10 seconds (or as long as comfortable).
   - If you need a second puff, wait 30-60 seconds before repeating the preceding steps.

Is the Inhaler Full?

The patient needs to know the correct way to determine whether the MDI must be replaced. Shaking the canister is not a reliable method because the patient may be hearing only the propellant move in the canister when the MDI is nearly empty. The only reliable method, if the MDI does not have a counter, is to count each puff. Alternatively, the patient can plan the length of use on the basis of prescribed puffs per day: For example, if the patient uses two puffs, twice-a-day use means that the inhaler must be replaced in 50 days. Most canisters contain 200 doses. It is a good practice to keep a spare inhaler on hand.

Special Instructions for Children

Most children younger than 9 years cannot use an MDI properly. For these children, a spacer should be used with the MDI. Regardless of the child's age, spacers are recommended when a steroid inhaler is used, to reduce the risk of developing a yeast infection in the mouth or the throat and to enhance the distribution of the medication to the small airways.

How to Use a Metered-Dose Inhaler With a Spacer

Some people, no matter how hard they try, still have trouble coordinating an MDI. Fortunately, spacers (holding chambers), which hold the medication for a few seconds after it has been released from the inhaler, are available. The patient's physician or Certified Respiratory Educator may recommend one if the patient has trouble with an MDI or is using ICS.

Spacers may also reduce occurrence of adverse drug events such as a hoarse voice or sore throat if the patient is taking higher dosages of ICS. Spacers can be used with most aerosol inhalers and are very easy to use. Following are instructions for using a spacer with an MDI:

1. Remove the plastic cap from the inhaler mouthpiece and the spacer mouthpiece.

2. Insert the inhaler mouthpiece into the large opening of the spacer.

3. Hold the spacer and inhaler together and shake well.

4. Breathe out.

5. Put the mouthpiece of the spacer into your mouth, close your lips around it; do not cover the small slots.

6. Press the metal canister down into the inhaler to spray the medication into the spacer. Then, breathe in slowly and deeply through your mouth (for about 5 seconds).

7. Hold your breath for as long as you comfortably can (about 10 seconds).

8. Breathe out slowly through your mouth or nose.

9. If more puffs are prescribed, wait 1 minute and then repeat these steps, starting from step 3.

Caring for the Spacer

Spacers require weekly cleaning because powder will collect on the walls of the spacer with repeated use. To clean, agitate the spacer device carefully in warm tap water mixed with dish soap. Shake off excess water, do not rinse, and allow it to air dry overnight; do not dry with a towel. The soap residue left on the chamber, as well as not using a towel to dry, will prevent static cling and therefore prevent medication from clinging to the inside of the chamber.

Source: Adapted from The Asthma Society of Canada, (2011). *How to use your inhaler: Cleaning your spacer.* Retrieved from *www.asthma.ca/adults/treatment/spacers.php.*

exposed to humidity, so they should be stored in a dry place. The care of DPIs involves wiping off the mouthpiece with a dry tissue. Water or other liquids should never be used to clean the device, which could cause clumping of the medication and cause the device to work improperly.

Various inhalation devices are used to deliver medications to the airways. It is important to work with patients individually to identify the inhalation device that best fits their needs.

Poor adherence to asthma therapy regimens is a major challenge in the long-term management of asthma. Patients com-monly rely too heavily on their reliever inhalers because they provide immediate relief of symptoms and gratification, whereas no immediate benefit is felt with anti-inflammatory therapy, which must be sustained on a daily basis. It is impor-tant to explain to patients the importance and purpose of taking controller therapy regularly, emphasizing that maximum improvement may take more than 1 week. It is also important to emphasize that without regular use, the inflammation in the airways may progress and the asthma is likely to worsen over time.

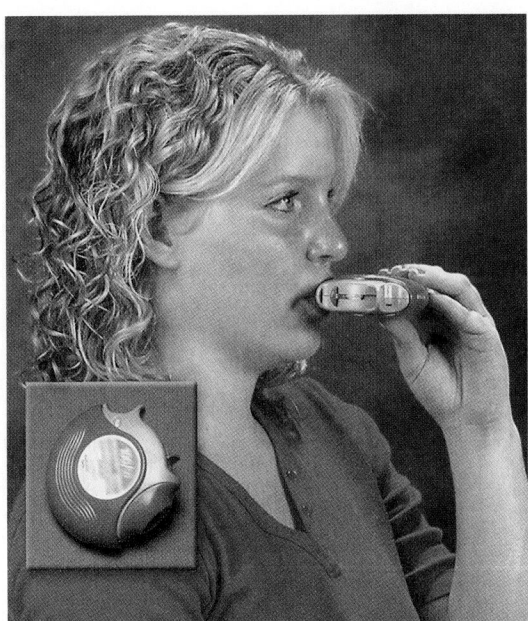

Figure 31-6 Example of a dry powder inhaler (DPI).

Source: Togger, D. A., & Breener, P. S. (2001). Metered dose inhalers. *American Journal of Nursing, 101*(10), 26-32.

PATIENT & CAREGIVER TEACHING GUIDE

Table 31-10 How to Use a Dry Powder Inhaler (DPI)

1. Remove mouthpiece cap. Check for dust or dirt.

2. Load the medicine into the inhaler. A Turbuhaler should be held upright while being loaded. Other types of inhalers can be held sideways or in a horizontal position. A click should be heard to indicate that the device is loaded.

3. Do not shake the inhaler.

4. Breathe out away from the device. Do not breathe into the inhaler because this could affect the dose.

5. Seal your lips around the mouthpiece of the inhaler (see Figure 31-6). Your head should be tilted back slightly to open the airway.

6. Breathe in deeply, forcefully, and quickly. This will ensure that the medication is delivered to your lungs. You may not taste or sense the medicine going into your lungs.

7. Hold your breath for about 10 seconds or as long as possible up to 10 seconds. Breathe out slowly. If a second dose is required, repeat steps 2-7.

Source: Adapted from Registered Nurses' Association of Ontario. (2007). *Adult asthma care guidelines for nurses: Promoting control of asthma* (pp. 78-83, Appendix E). Retrieved from *http://www.rnao.org/ Storage/27/2206_Asthma_Guideline_and_Supplement_-_FINAL_20071.pdf*

NURSING MANAGEMENT: ASTHMA

Nursing Assessment

If a patient can speak and is not in acute distress, a detailed health history, including identification of any precipitating factors and what has helped alleviate attacks in the past, should be documented. If a patient is in acute distress, some of the information may be attainable from the person accompanying the patient. Subjective and objective data to obtain from a patient with asthma are presented in Table 31-11.

Nursing Diagnoses

Nursing diagnoses for the patient with asthma may include, but are not limited to, those presented in Nursing Care Plan 31-1.

Planning

The overall goals are that patients with asthma will (a) be able to participate in activities of normal life (including exercise and other physical activity) with little to no interference; (b) have normal or near-normal pulmonary function; (c) have the asthma under control; (d) experience as few adverse effects from asthma medication as possible while taking the lowest dosage of medication necessary to keep the asthma under control; and (e) possess the knowledge and skills necessary to participate in the management of the asthma.

Nursing Implementation

Asthma Education

Nurses play an essential role in preventing and controlling asthma symptoms by developing a partnership with the patient and family, providing information and education, and helping the patient and family develop the necessary skills for controlling asthma. Education is an essential component of asthma care and should occur at every encounter with patients, families, and caregivers. In order to be effective, asthma education must provide information, help develop and refine asthma-related skills, assist with problem solving, and cause behaviour change. In addition, findings of meta-analyses suggest that self-management asthma education programs can reduce the number of emergency department visits, hospitalizations, urgent care visits, nocturnal awakenings related to asthma, and days of interrupted activity and can improve quality of life (Coffman, Cabana, Halpin, & Yelin, 2008). Asthma education programs can also be cost effective. Table 31-12 details basic asthma education to be provided.

Environmental Control

Environmental control strategies focus on reducing exposure to asthma triggers specific to the individual. Triggers can be divided into two groups: allergens and irritants. Patients should be taught to identify known personal triggers for asthma and to reduce exposure to them (see Table 31-1). Sensitization to environmental allergens is clearly linked to asthma in children and adults (Lougheed et al., 2010). However, before patients and families are advised to use environmental control strategies to reduce or manage exposure to allergens, it is important to know the allergen to which they are sensitized.

House dust mites produce a common allergen that can trigger asthma. House dust mites are sightless, eight-legged microorganisms. They excrete food and digestive enzymes as a fecal particle, which is the major form of mite allergen. House dust mites require dead skin and water to survive, and thus the bed provides

NURSING ASSESSMENT

Table 31-11 Asthma

Subjective Data	Objective Data
Important Health Information	**General**
Current health: Assess the level of asthma control (see Table 31-2); frequency and severity of asthma symptoms (wheeze, cough, chest tightness, dyspnea) in the past week, both during the day and in early morning hours and night; need for reliever medication during the past week; and usual pattern of asthma symptoms. Determine whether the patient experienced a recent worsening of asthma and how it was handled. Identify recent exposure to triggers (e.g., upper respiratory tract infection, pollen, animals, mould, dust, inhaled irritants, weather changes, exercise, smoke).	Restlessness or exhaustion, confusion, upright or forward-leaning body position
	Integumentary
	Eczema, diaphoresis, cyanosis (circumoral, nail beds)
	Respiratory
Past health history: Previous asthma attack(s) and response to treatment; previous emergency department visits or hospitalizations for asthma and the need for CCU admission and intubation; recent exposure to pollen, dander, feathers, mould, dust, inhaled irritants, weather changes, exercise, smoke; allergic rhinitis and eczema; sinus infections; gastroesophageal reflux; family history of asthma and allergies.	Wheezing, crackles, diminishment or absence of breath sounds on auscultation; hyperresonance on percussion; sputum character and quantity; increased work of breathing, demonstrated by use of accessory muscle, intercostal and supraclavicular retractions; tachypnea; prolonged expiration
	Cardiovascular
	Tachycardia, pulsus paradoxus, jugular venous distension, hypertension or hypotension, premature ventricular contractions
Medications: Last time the reliever medication was used, what level of relief was provided, duration of relief, frequency of the reliever use in the past week; pattern of use for controller medications; recent use of antibiotics; use of medications that may precipitate asthma such as aspirin, NSAIDs, β-adrenergic blockers; allergies to medications.	**Possible Diagnostic Findings**
	Abnormal results of pulmonary function tests: decreased flow rates; FVC, FEV_1, PEFR, and FEV_1/FVC ratio that improve with bronchodilators and between exacerbations
Symptoms	↓ O_2 saturation and abnormal ABG values during moderate to life-threatening attacks
• Wheezing, cough, chest tightness, dyspnea	Serum and sputum eosinophilia
• Decreased level of activity or exercise because of symptoms	Positive results of skin tests for allergens and allergies to medication
• Interrupted sleep, fatigue; fear, anxiety, panic, depression, emotional distress	

ABG, arterial blood gas; *CCU,* critical care unit; *FEV₁,* forced expiratory volume in 1 second; *FVC,* forced vital capacity; *NSAIDs,* nonsteroidal anti-inflammatory drugs *PEFR,* peak expiratory flow rate.

NURSING CARE PLAN 31-1

Asthma

NURSING DIAGNOSIS	***Ineffective airway clearance*** *related to* bronchospasm, and airway inflammation, *as evidenced by* bronchoconstriction, increased mucus production, symptom experience (e.g., cough, shortness of breath, heavy chest), and adventitious breath sounds
Expected Patient Outcomes	**Nursing Interventions and *Rationales***
• Maintains open airways	• Position patient to maximize ventilation potential *allowing for adequate chest expansion.*
• Has normal breath sounds and respiratory rate	• Monitor respiratory (including spirometry) and oxygenation status *to determine need for intervention or to note improvement.*
• Has normal or personal best objective lung function measurements (PEFR, FEV_1, FEV_1/FVC)	• Administer medications (e.g., bronchodilators, corticosteroids), as appropriate, *to improve respiratory function.*
• Participates in normal life activities, including exercise and physical activity (helpful to identify activity that is meaningful to the patient)	• Teach patient proper use prescribed inhalers (see Tables 31-9 and 31-10) *to deliver adequate medication to the lungs.*
	• Auscultate lung sounds after treatments *to note improvement.*
	• Regulate fluid intake to optimize fluid balance and liquefy secretions *to facilitate removal.*
	• Provide asthma education *to help patient understand condition and avoid triggers, when possible.*
	• Establish a written asthma action plan with patient to manage exacerbations. Provide education on it *to ensure that patient is prepared for emergency situations.*

NURSING CARE PLAN 31-1

Asthma—cont'd

NURSING DIAGNOSIS	**Anxiety** related to difficulty breathing, perceived or actual loss of control, and fear of suffocation, as evidenced by restlessness; elevated pulse, respiratory rate, and blood pressure

Expected Patient Outcomes	Nursing Interventions and *Rationales*
• Reports reduced anxiety or no anxiety	• Explore patterns of anxiety and feelings, perceptions, and fears *to identify precipitating factors and problem areas so that planning can be concentrated.* • Use a calm, reassuring approach *to provide reassurance.* • Stay with patient *to promote safety and reduce fear.* • Provide factual information concerning diagnosis, treatment, and prognosis *to help patient know what to expect.* • Instruct patient on the use of relaxation techniques *to relieve muscle tension and slow respirations.*

NURSING DIAGNOSIS	**Deficient knowledge, understanding, and skills** related to lack of information and education about asthma and its management, as evidenced by frequent questioning and poor asthma control

Expected Patient Outcomes	Nursing Interventions and *Rationales**
• Demonstrates appropriate use of inhalers, peak flow meters, spacers, and nebulizers (if used) • Maintains good asthma control • Manages personal triggers • Recognizes worsening asthma and initiates early treatment • Actively participates in management decisions with the asthma care team	• Appraise patient's current level of knowledge and skills related to asthma management *to identify learning needs.* • Teach patient to identify and manage triggers *to prevent asthma attacks.* • Encourage patient to verbalize feelings about diagnosis, treatment, and effect on lifestyle *to offer support and increase adherence to medication regimen to improve asthma control.* • Ensure that patient has an asthma action plan and understands its use *to enhance patient's ability to identify worsening asthma and respond appropriately.* • Instruct the patient on the proper administration of each medication* (e.g., inhalers, spacers) *to ensure proper use.* • Evaluate the patient's inhaler techniques *to assess correct technique and ensure maximum benefit.* • Instruct the patient on purpose, action, dosage, indication, and duration of each medication *to promote understanding of effects and use.* • Instruct patient on strategies to decrease the intensity of adverse drug events *to prevent or minimize the intensity of adverse drug events and enhance adherence.* • Assist patient to identify strategies that incorporate taking medications into daily life, for instance, taking inhaled steroids before brushing teeth in the morning and night *to enhance adherence.* • Include the family and significant others as appropriate *to ensure knowledgeable help is available when the patient needs it.*

FEV₁, forced expiratory volume; *FVC*, forced vital capacity; *PEFR*, peak expiratory flow rate.

*Refer to Figures 31-5 and 31-6 and to Patient & Caregiver Teaching Guides (Tables 31-9, 31-10, 31-12, and 31-13)

a perfect environment because when humans sleep, they slough off dead skin and provide humidity. As a result, control strategies focus on the bedroom and include keeping the relative humidity below 50%; encasing the mattress, box springs, and pillows in covers that are impermeable to mites and mite allergens; laundering bed linen in hot water and hot (55°C) air to dry it; and possibly removing carpets (Gotzsche & Johansen, 2008).

Pet dander is another common allergen, and strategies to reduce exposure have been evaluated. The removal of the pet is the most effective means to reduce exposure. However, this is often not a realistic option for patients and families. As a result, numerous alternative strategies have been evaluated to minimize or reduce exposure. These strategies include excluding the pet and its dander from the bedroom by keeping the door and heating register closed; frequent vacuuming (including furniture) with a high-efficiency particulate air (HEPA)–filtered vacuum; removing carpets; and washing the pet at least twice a week (none of these actions to be performed by the allergic person).

Environmental tobacco smoke is the most harmful indoor air irritant and should be avoided. Environmental tobacco smoke is a risk factor for the development of childhood asthma and frequently causes the worsening of asthma in children and adults. Among children with asthma, those whose parents smoke have more severe disease than do those whose parents do not smoke. When parents of children with asthma stop smoking, the child's asthma improves. Nurses must encourage patients and their family members to stop smoking and assist them with identifying

PATIENT & CAREGIVER TEACHING GUIDE

Table 31-12 Basic Asthma Education

Basic Facts About Asthma

- Basic anatomical and physiological characteristics of the lungs
- Pathophysiological changes of asthma
- Relationship of pathophysiological changes to signs and symptoms
- Asthma control criteria (signs and symptoms)

Trigger Control

- Identification of possible triggers and management strategies
- Avoidance of allergens and other triggers

Medications

- Differences between relievers and controllers
- Indications for using reliever as opposed to controller medication
- Establishing medication schedule
- Adverse effects and strategies to reduce their frequency and intensity

Device Technique

- Good inhaler technique
- Good peak flow meter and monitoring technique (if applicable)

Self-Monitoring and Action Plan

- Development of an individualized asthma action plan
- Early recognition of worsening asthma
- Actions to take in response to worsening asthma

Follow-Up Care

- Understanding and accepting the need for regular follow-up care

smoking cessation strategies. Smoking should not be allowed in cars and homes in which individuals with asthma are present.

Exercise and cold air are very common asthma triggers. For many individuals with asthma, exercise and cold air are not troublesome unless they are recovering from a viral infection or have uncontrolled asthma. Under those circumstances, these triggers often provoke asthma symptoms. Strategies to prevent exposure to cold air include using scarves and face masks. Exercise is just as important for individuals with asthma as those without it because it provides multiple health benefits. Asthma is not an excuse for avoiding exercise. If a form of exercise provokes asthma symptoms, the nurse can advise the use of a warm-up period and using an inhaled SABA 10 to 15 minutes before the activity to prevent bronchospasm.

Occupational asthma, defined as asthma symptoms induced by exposure to a specific agent in the workplace, is the most common occupational lung disease. Exposure to agents in the occupational environment has been estimated to cause 25% of adult-onset asthma (Sama et al., 2006). Objective lung function tests, along with a detailed occupational exposure history, are necessary to confirm the diagnosis of occupational asthma. If occupational asthma is suspected, the patient should be referred to his or her primary care provider, a specialist, or an occupational hygienist.

▪ Self-Monitoring and Action Plans

According to the Canadian Asthma Consensus Guidelines (Lougheed et al., 2010), every person with asthma should have an asthma action plan (Figure 31-7). An action plan is a written plan

developed to provide the patient with a framework for monitoring and determining his or her level of asthma control and making treatment changes to achieve and maintain control. Often, action plans are designed according to a traffic-light analogy: green, yellow, and red "zones." The green zone represents good asthma control and signals "go" with current therapy. The yellow zone is a time of worsening or uncontrolled asthma and signals "caution" and the need for enhanced anti-inflammatory therapy. The red zone represents a time of danger during which the asthma is severe enough to necessitate urgent medical attention; the patient must "stop" current activities to address this need.

Nurses must develop a partnership with patients and their families, their primary asthma care provider, and the rest of the asthma care team in order to help patients attain and effectively use an individualized asthma action plan. Systematic reviews concluded that self-management programs that included self-monitoring, either by symptoms or peak flow, combined with a written action plan and regular medical review resulted in reduced use of health care services, fewer days lost from work, and fewer episodes of nocturnal asthma (Zemek, Bhogal, & Ducharme, 2008). Self-monitoring based on symptom experience alone was compared with self-monitoring based on both symptom experience and peak expiratory flow monitoring; comparable outcomes were reported (Zemek et al., 2008). PEFR provides an objective measurement of lung function (Table 31-13). As a result, it has been advocated for detecting asthma exacerbations; however, for most people, asthma symptoms are a more sensitive measure and change earlier in the course of an exacerbation than does PEFR. PEFR monitoring is particularly useful in patients who have difficulty perceiving or recognizing changes in symptoms and require emergency department visits despite the use of a symptom-based action plan. The choice of whether an action plan is based on PEFR or symptom monitoring may be made according to a patient's ability to perceive symptoms and airflow limitation, the availability of peak flow meters, and, of most importance, the patient's preferences.

The level of detail in the plan depends on the patient's understanding of asthma and preferences for monitoring (PEFR or symptoms). Key components for teaching patients and their families how to use an action plan include the signs and symptoms of worsening asthma, knowing the level of asthma control and how to adjust medications, and when to seek medical attention. The green zone represents a time when a patient's asthma is under good control (see Table 31-2). If peak flow rates are used, they are usually 80% or more of predicted or of the patient's personal best (see Table 31-13). When asthma status is in the green zone, the patient should continue with the current therapeutic plan. If asthma status has been in the green zone for a couple of months, an attempt to reduce medication dosages may be warranted. The potential risk of a medication reduction is worsening asthma that necessitates an increase in medications to regain control.

The yellow zone represents a time of uncontrolled asthma as demonstrated by symptom experience, the need for an inhaled short-acting bronchodilator (reliever), and, if measured, PEFR between 50% (some authorities use 60%) and 79% of predicted or personal best (see Table 31-2). In response to worsening asthma, some patients are advised to see their primary asthma care providers, whereas others are advised to increase dosages of anti-inflammatory medication. Typically, this involves initiating the use of an inhaled corticosteroid, doubling, tripling, or quadrupling the dosage of inhaled corticosteroid, or initiating a short burst of oral corticosteroids. Not all patients feel comfort-

THE ✝ LUNG ASSOCIATION

MY ASTHMA ACTION PLAN

Name _____   Doctor _____

Date _____   Doctor's Phone Number _____

GREEN LEVEL   My asthma is under control.

SYMPTOMS
- My breathing is normal.
- I have no trouble sleeping.
- I'm not coughing or wheezing.
- I can do all my normal activities.

PEAK FLOW

_____ to _____ (80 to 100% of your personal best)

WHAT SHOULD I DO?
I should continue using my normal medications as directed by my doctor, and re-measure my peak flow every _____ weeks/months.

Medication	Dose	Take it when?

YELLOW LEVEL   My asthma is getting worse.

SYMPTOMS
- I have symptoms, like wheezing or coughing, with activity or at night. They go away when I use my reliever.
- I'm using my reliever more than ___ times a week/day.
- I can't do many of my usual activities.

PEAK FLOW

_____ to _____ (60 to 80% of your personal best)

WHAT SHOULD I DO?
A problem is beginning. I should increase my medication as specified below until I am in the green level for _____ days or more. **If my symptoms do not improve within 4 days, I will call my doctor.**

Medication	Dose	Take it when?

RED LEVEL   I am having an asthma emergency.

SYMPTOMS
- My breathing is difficult.
- I'm wheezing often when resting.
- I'm having difficulty walking and/or talking.
- My lips and/or fingernails are blue or grey.
- My reliever does not help in 10 minutes OR is needed every 4 hours or more.

PEAK FLOW

_____ to _____ (less than 60% of your personal best)

WHAT SHOULD I DO?

I NEED TO GO TO THE HOSPITAL EMERGENCY RIGHT AWAY.

I SHOULD USE MY RELIEVER AS MUCH AS I NEED TO ON THE WAY THERE.

Figure 31-7 Example of an asthma action plan.

Source: Modified from the Canadian Lung Association. (undated). *Asthma action plan.* Retrieved from *http://www.lung.ca/_resources/asthma_action_plan.pdf.*

able adjusting medications without seeing their asthma care provider, which highlights the importance of tailoring the type of action plan to meet the individual's needs and preferences.

The red zone represents a time of severe asthma and the need for immediate medical assistance. Indications of the red zone are difficulty completing a sentence without needing another breath; incomplete relief from reliever inhaler or use more frequently than every 2 hours; or, if the patient is using a peak flow meter, a PEFR between less than 50 and 60% of pre-

dicted or personal best value. Affected patients are advised to use their short-acting inhaled β_2-agonists on their way to the emergency department.

In developing a management plan, it is important to involve the patient's family. Family members and friends should be taught how to help the patient during an asthma exacerbation. They should know where the patient's inhalers and emergency phone numbers are located. Family members can help patients identify deteriorating levels of asthma control, since they may

Table 31-13 How to Use a Peak Flow Meter

Follow these five steps to use a peak flow meter:

1. Move the indicator to the bottom of the numbered scale.

2. Stand up, or sit upright.

3. Take a deep breath in, and fill your lungs completely.

4. Place the mouthpiece in your mouth and close your lips around it.

5. Blow out as hard and fast as possible in a single blow.

6. Write down the value. If coughing occurred, the value is inaccurate; do not record that value. Repeat the test.

7. Repeat steps 1 through 5 twice more.

8. Record the highest result of the three.

Finding the Personal Best Peak Flow Number

- The patient's personal best peak flow number is the highest peak flow number achieved over a 2- to 3-week period when asthma is under good control.

- Each patient's manifestations of asthma are different, and the "best" peak flow value may be higher or lower than that of another person of the same height, weight, and sex. The action plan must be based on the patient's personal best peak flow value.

- To identify the patient's personal best peak flow number, have the patient take peak flow readings
  - At least twice a day for 2 to 3 weeks
  - Upon awakening and before bed
  - Before and 15 minutes after taking a short-acting inhaled bronchodilator (reliever)

Source: Registered Nurses' Association of Ontario. (2004). *Adult asthma care guidelines for nurses: Promoting control of asthma.* Appendix I: How to use a peak flow meter (p. 94). *Best Practice Guidelines.* Toronto: Author. Retrieved from *http://rnao.ca/sites/rnao-ca/files/Adult_Asthma_Care_Guidelines_for_Nurses_-_Promoting_Control_of_Asthma.pdf* Reprinted with permission of the Registered Nurses' Association of Ontario.

notice an increase in symptoms or avoidance of certain activities before the patient notices.

It appears particularly important to provide asthma education, which should occur at every encounter with the patient and family, during emergency department visits and hospitalization because this is a time when people are highly motivated to learn and do not have to schedule an additional visit. The Canadian Lung Association develops and distributes several excellent resources for individuals affected by asthma. (See the Resources at the end of the chapter.)

▪ Evaluation

The expected outcomes for the patient with asthma are presented in Nursing Care Plan 31-1.

Chronic Obstructive Pulmonary Disease

Chronic obstructive pulmonary disease (COPD) is a respiratory disorder caused largely by smoking and characterized by progressive, partially reversible airflow obstruction, systemic manifestations, and increasing frequency and severity of exacerbations (Global Initiative for Chronic Obstructive Lung Disease [GOLD], 2010; O'Donnell et al., 2007). Cardinal symptoms experienced by patients with COPD are dyspnea, difficulty breathing, or shortness of breath and limitations in activity. Symptoms are usually insidious in onset and progressive. Dyspnea is the subjective experience of shortness of breath and is the most disabling symptom in COPD (Bailey et al., 2010). Initially, COPD is confined to the lungs, but when disease is advanced, skeletal muscle dysfunction, right-sided heart failure, secondary polycythemia, depression, and altered nutrition are commonly observed. Past definitions of COPD included the terms *emphysema* and *chronic bronchitis*. **Emphysema** describes only one pathological change present in COPD: destruction of the alveoli. **Chronic bronchitis,** which is the presence of chronic productive cough for 3 months in 2 successive years, remains a useful epidemiological term but it, too, "does not reflect the major impact of airway limitation in morbidity and mortality in COPD patients" (GOLD, 2010, p. 3). People with COPD often display characteristics of both chronic bronchitis and emphysema (GOLD, 2010; O'Donnell et al., 2007, 2008).

The 2005 Canadian Community Health Survey revealed that 4.4% (754,800) of Canadians older than 35 years probably have COPD (PHAC, 2007). The prevalence among men (4.4%) and women (4.8%) are currently comparable, although rates of COPD and subsequent hospitalization and death are rising more rapidly among women. Hospitalization may be required in the treatment of COPD, particularly when symptoms worsen from infection, which accounts for more than 50% of COPD exacerbations (Mallia et al., 2007). From 2004 to 2005, hospitalization rates for COPD increased steadily, with an average length of stay of 9.6 days (PHAC, 2007). In 2005, approximately 17% of patients with COPD required the use of home care services (PHAC, 2007). Approximately 45% of affected patients report that the disease often causes restriction in their daily activities (PHAC, 2007). COPD accounts for approximately 4% of all deaths in Canada, which is probably an underestimation because the primary cause of death may be listed as pneumonia or congestive heart failure.

Causes

Cigarette Smoking. Exposure to tobacco smoke is the primary cause of 80 to 90% of COPD cases in Canada. In 2010, 18% of Canadians over the age of 15 years were smoking (Health Canada, 2010). Although the prevalence of cigarette smoking has decreased, it is still a major public health concern.

Clinically significant airway obstruction develops in 15 to 20% of smokers. For most Canadians who die of lung diseases related to cigarette smoking, death is preceded by a long period of debilitation characterized by frequent hospitalizations and loss of many years of productivity. Cigarette smoking remains the most preventable cause of premature death in Canada. In addition to being linked with respiratory conditions such as COPD and lung cancer, cigarette smoking has also been implicated as a factor in several other cancers (e.g., mouth, pharynx, larynx, esophagus, pancreas, kidney, stomach) and in cardiac conditions (e.g., hypertension, congestive heart failure, myocardial infarction).

When cigarettes are smoked, approximately 4000 chemicals and gases are inhaled into the lungs. Over 60 carcinogens have been isolated from cigarette smoke, including cyanide, formaldehyde, and ammonia. Nicotine is probably not a carcinogen, but it has deleterious effects. It acts by stimulating the sympathetic nervous system, resulting in increases in heart rate, peripheral vasoconstriction, blood pressure, and cardiac workload. These effects of nicotine compound the problems in a person with coronary artery disease. (The effects of nicotine are discussed further in Chapter 11.)

Cigarette smoke has several direct effects on the respiratory tract. It simulates an inflammatory response in the lung, which is most evident late in the disease. The irritating effect of the smoke causes hyperplasia of goblet cells, which subsequently results in increased production of mucus and is the basis of chronic cough and sputum accumulation. In airways smaller than 2 mm in diameter, injury leads to narrowing and obstruction of the airways. Smoking reduces ciliary activity and accelerates loss of ciliated cells. Smoking also produces abnormal dilation of the distal air space with destruction of alveolar walls. Many cells develop large, atypical nuclei, which is considered a precancerous condition. Removal of the inciting stimulus is of greatest benefit early in the process but may be less effective in late disease. However, smoking cessation can prevent or delay the development of airflow limitation or slow its progression.

Carbon monoxide is a component of tobacco smoke. Carbon monoxide has a high affinity for hemoglobin and combines with it more readily than does oxygen, thereby reducing the smoker's oxygen-carrying capacity. Smokers inhale a lower percentage of oxygen than normal; as a result, less oxygen is available at the alveolar level. The heart's need for oxygen is increased because of the stimulatory effect of nicotine on the sympathetic nervous system. Because the blood's oxygen-carrying capacity is reduced, the heart must pump more rapidly to adequately supply tissues with oxygen. Carbon monoxide also seems to impair psychomotor performance and judgement.

Passive smoking (also known as *environmental tobacco smoke* or *second-hand smoke*) is the exposure of nonsmokers to cigarette smoke. In adults, involuntary smoke exposure is associated with decreased pulmonary function, increased risk for lung cancer, and increased rates of mortality from ischemic heart disease.

Occupational Chemicals and Dusts.
If a person has intense or prolonged exposure to various dusts, vapours, irritants, or fumes in the workplace, COPD can develop independently of cigarette smoking. If the person smokes, the risk of COPD increases (GOLD, 2010).

Infection.
Recurring respiratory tract infections are a major factor contributing to the aggravation and progression of COPD (O'Donnell et al., 2007, 2008). The pathological destruction of lung tissue and the ensuing progression of COPD results from the recurring infections, which impair normal defence mechanisms, making the bronchioles and alveoli more susceptible to injury, and increase inflammation (GOLD, 2010). The most common causative organisms are *Haemophilus influenzae, Streptococcus pneumoniae,* and *Moraxella catarrhalis* (Sethi & Murphy, 2008). Retained secretions constitute a good medium for their proliferation.

Heredity.
α_1-Antitrypsin (AAT) deficiency is currently the only known genetic abnormality that leads to COPD; however, research is ongoing to identify other genes that predispose a person to developing this disease (GOLD, 2010) (see the Genetics in Clinical Practice box). AAT (also termed α_1-*protease inhibitor*) is the major antiprotease in plasma, and its primary function is

to inhibit neutrophil elastase. It is produced by the liver and is normally found in the lungs, where it inhibits the action of proteolytic enzymes from neutrophils (neutrophil elastase) and macrophages. Lower levels of AAT result in insufficient inactivation of neutrophil elastase, and the subsequent lysis of lung tissue causes destruction of the alveoli. Severe AAT deficiency leads to early-onset COPD. Smoking greatly exacerbates the disease process in affected patients (GOLD, 2010; O'Donnell et al., 2007, 2008).

Intravenous or nebulizer-administered AAT (Prolastin) replacement therapy is available for people with AAT deficiency (Kohnlein & Welte, 2008). Infusions are administered weekly. It should be restricted to AAT-deficient patients with a postbronchodilator FEV_1 between 35 and 50% of predicted who do not smoke. Its effectiveness in slowing the progression of the disease continues to be evaluated.

GENETICS IN CLINICAL PRACTICE
α_1-Antitrypsin (AAT) Deficiency

Genetic Basis
- Autosomal recessive disorder
- Gene for AAT is located on chromosome 14
- Several allelic variants of AAT gene

Incidence
- 431,000 Canadians have deficiency alleles and are at risk for adverse health effects
- People of Northern European descent most affected
- Found in equal numbers of male and female patients

Genetic Testing
- DNA testing is available
- Screening of siblings is useful
- Serum assay is available to measure the amount of AAT

Clinical Implications
- Genetic disorder is linked to COPD
- Treatment may include AAT replacement (Prolastin)
- Predisposes to early-onset COPD (in the third or fourth decade of life)
- Participation in AAT Canadian Registry is encouraged

Source: de Serres, F. J., Blanco, I., & Fernandez-Bustillo, E. (2003). Genetic epidemiology of alpha-1 antitrypsin deficiency in North America and Australia/New Zealand: Australia, Canada, New Zealand, and the United States of America. *Clinical Genetics, 64*(5), 382–397.

Aging.
Aging results in changes in the lung structure and respiratory muscles that cause a gradual loss of the elastic recoil of the lung. As a result, the lungs become smaller and stiffer. The number of functional alveoli decreases as a result of the loss of the alveolar supporting structures. Thoracic cage changes result from osteoporosis and calcification of the costal cartilages. The thoracic cage becomes stiff and rigid, and the ribs are less mobile. These changes result in a decreased compliance of the chest wall and an increase in the work of breathing. These changes are similar to those seen in patients with emphysema. With fewer capillaries available for gas exchange, arterial oxygen levels decrease. Clinically significant emphysema is usually not caused by aging alone.

Pathophysiology

COPD is characterized by chronic inflammation found in the airways, lung parenchyma (respiratory bronchioles and alveoli),

PATHOPHYSIOLOGY MAP

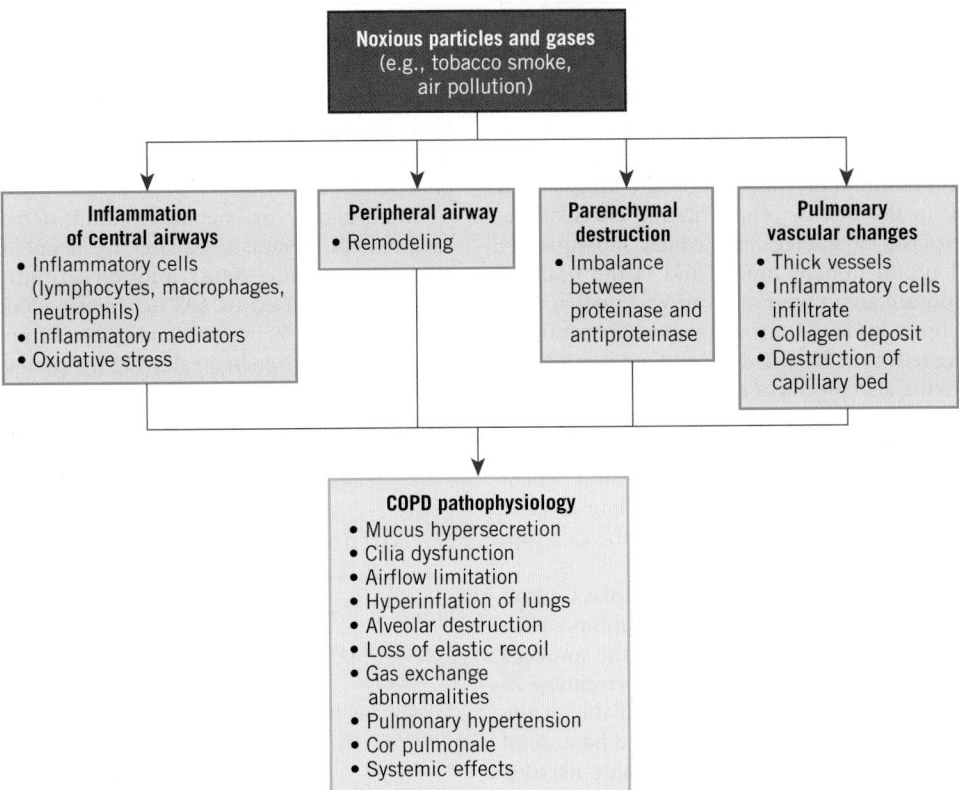

Figure 31-8 Pathophysiological changes of chronic obstructive pulmonary disease (COPD).

and pulmonary blood vessels (Figure 31-8). The pathogenesis of COPD is complex and involves many mechanisms. The defining features of COPD are (a) airflow limitations during forced exhalation caused by loss of elastic recoil and are not fully reversible and (b) airflow obstruction caused by mucus hypersecretion, mucosal edema, and bronchospasm.

In COPD, airflow limitation, air trapping, gas exchange abnormalities, mucus hypersecretion, and, in severe disease, pulmonary hypertension and systemic features are among the various disease processes that occur (see Figure 31-8). COPD results in an uneven distribution of pathological changes, so that severely destroyed lung areas coexist with areas of relatively normal lung (Celli, 2009).

The inflammatory process starts with inhalation of noxious particles and gases (e.g., cigarette smoke) but is magnified in people with COPD. The abnormal inflammatory process causes tissue destruction and disrupts the normal defence mechanisms and repair processes of the lungs.

The predominant inflammatory cells in COPD are neutrophils, macrophages, and lymphocytes. This pattern of inflammatory cells is different from that in asthma. The inflammatory cells in COPD attract other inflammatory mediators (e.g., leukotrienes, interleukins). This cascading inflammatory process results in the activation of proinflammatory cytokines such as tumour necrosis factor. In addition, growth factors are recruited into the area and activated, which results in structural changes in the lungs.

The inflammatory process may also be magnified by oxidative stress. Oxidants are produced by cigarette smoke and other inhaled particles and are released from the inflammatory cells,

such as macrophages and neutrophils, during inflammation. The oxidative stress adversely affects the lungs as it inactivates antiproteases (which prevent the natural destruction of the lungs), stimulates mucus secretion, and increases fluid in the lungs (GOLD, 2010).

After the inhalation of oxidants in tobacco or air pollution, the activity of proteases (which break down the connective tissue of the lungs) increases, and the antiproteases (which protect against the breakdown) are inhibited. Therefore, the natural balance of protease/antiprotease is tipped in favour of destruction of the alveoli and loss of the elastic recoil of the lung (Brashers, 2008; GOLD, 2010).

Inability to expire air is a main characteristic of COPD. The airflow limitation occurs primarily in the smaller airways and is caused by remodelling. As the peripheral airways become obstructed, air is progressively trapped during expiration. The residual air becomes significant in severe disease as alveolar attachments to small airways (similar to rubber bands) are destroyed. The residual air, combined with the loss of elastic recoil, makes passive expiration of air difficult, and air is trapped in the lungs. The chest hyperexpands and becomes barrel-shaped because the respiratory muscles are not able to function effectively. The functional residual capacity is increased, and at this stage, the patient is trying to breathe in when the lungs are in an "overinflated" state; thus the patient appears dyspneic, and exercise capacity is limited (GOLD, 2010).

Abnormal gas exchange resulting in hypoxemia, and hypercapnia (increased carbon dioxide) may be present as the disease progresses. As the air trapping worsens and alveoli are destroyed, bullae (large air spaces in the parenchyma) and blebs (air spaces adjacent to pleurae) can form (Figure 31-9). Bullae and blebs are not effective in gas exchange because the capillary bed that normally surrounds each alveolus does not exist in the bullae and bleb. Therefore, there is a significant ventilation-perfusion ($\dot{V}/\dot{Q}$) mismatch, and hypoxemia results. Peripheral airway obstruction also results in $\dot{V}/\dot{Q}$ imbalance and, in combination with the respiratory muscle impairment, can result in carbon dioxide retention, particularly in severe disease (Brashers, 2008; GOLD, 2010).

Excess mucus production, resulting in a chronic productive cough, is a feature of predominant chronic bronchitis and is not necessarily associated with limitation in airflow. However, not all patients with COPD produce sputum. Excess mucus production is a result of an increased number of mucus-secreting goblet cells and enlarged submucosal glands, which respond to the chronic irritation of smoke or other inhalants. In addition, dysfunction of cilia leads to chronic cough and sputum production. Some of the inflammatory mediators also stimulate mucus production.

Pulmonary vasculature changes that result in mild to moderate pulmonary hypertension may occur late in the course of COPD. The small pulmonary arteries undergo vasoconstriction as a consequence of hypoxemia, and their structure changes, resulting in thickening of the vascular smooth muscle as the disease advances. Because of the loss of alveolar walls and the capillaries surrounding them, the pressure in the pulmonary circulation increases. Affected patients typically do not have difficulty with hypoxemia at rest until late in the disease. However, hypoxemia may develop during exercise, and such patients may benefit from supplemental oxygen.

Pulmonary hypertension may progress and lead to hypertrophy of the right ventricle of the heart or to cor pulmonale, with or without right-sided heart failure. COPD has been shown to have systemic effects, especially in severe disease. These extrapulmonary changes contribute greatly to the clinical findings in affected patients and affect their survival and management. The mechanisms that cause the changes are unclear and are probably multifaceted, but systemic inflammation and inactivity of the patients are probably key factors (Decramer et al., 2008). Cachexia is common with a loss of skeletal muscle mass, and

weakness probably results from increased apoptosis (programmed cell death), muscle disuse (GOLD, 2010), or both. Patients may have weakness in all muscles in the upper and lower extremities (Eisner et al., 2008). They also have exercise intolerance, deconditioning, and osteoporosis. Patients with severe COPD also may develop chronic anemia, anxiety, and depression. The incidence of cardiovascular disease is increased among such patients, probably as a result of an increase in C-reactive protein (another inflammatory marker linked to cardiovascular disease; Decramer et al., 2008).

Clinical Manifestations

Several common aspects of asthma and COPD cause diagnostic confusion. However, there are clinically important differences between COPD and asthma (Table 31-14). In addition, some patients have a mixture of asthma and COPD (e.g., those with asthma who have a significant smoking history), and it is important to identify these people because they may benefit from combination therapy of ICS/LABA and anticholinergic medications. In addition, earlier introduction of ICS may be justified if the asthma component is prominent (O'Donnell et al., 2007).

A diagnosis of COPD should be considered when a person experiences symptoms of cough, sputum production, or dyspnea; has a history of smoking or exposure to risk factors for the disease; or demonstrates both. An intermittent cough, often the earliest symptom, usually occurs in the morning with the expectoration of small amounts of mucus. A productive cough (coughing that brings up mucus) during winter months is also a common early symptom that is often exacerbated by respiratory irritants; cold, damp air; and respiratory infections. Patients usually seek medical help when they have an acute respiratory infection, with dyspnea being the main concern. Dyspnea on exertion may also be one of the earliest symptoms. Dyspnea becomes progressively more severe to the point that it occurs at rest. Patients may dismiss the importance of dyspnea, rationalizing that "I'm just getting older." They change behaviours to avoid dyspnea and adapt, such as by using the elevator instead of stairs. The dyspnea gradually inter-

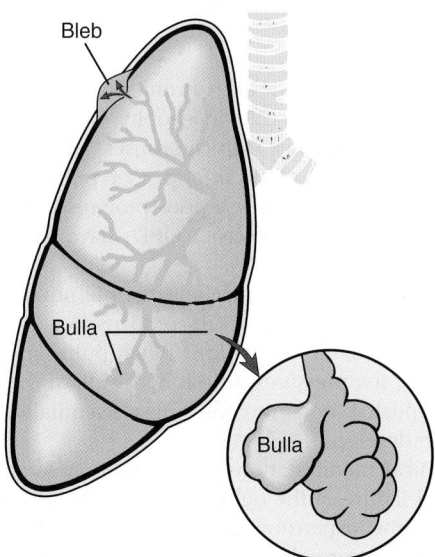

Figure 31-9 Pulmonary blebs and bullae.

Table 31-14 Comparison of Clinical Features of COPD and Asthma		
FEATURE	**COPD**	**ASTHMA**
Age at onset	Usually >40 yr	Usually <40 yr
Smoking history	Usually >10 pack-years	Not causal but can be a trigger
Clinical symptoms	Persistent	Intermittent and variable
Sputum production	Often	Infrequent
Allergies	Infrequent	Often
Spirometry	Findings may improve but never normalize	Findings often normalize
Disease course	Progressive worsening with exacerbations	Stable with exacerbations

Source: Adapted from O'Donnell, D. E., Hernandez, P., Kaplan, A., Aaron, S., Bourbeau, J., Marciniuk, D., ..., Voduc, N. (2008). Canadian Thoracic Society recommendations for the management of chronic obstructive pulmonary disease—2008 Update—Highlights for primary care. *Canadian Respiratory Journal, 15*(Suppl. A), 1-8A.*COPD,* chronic obstructive pulmonary disease.

feres with daily activities, such as carrying grocery bags, bathing, and cooking. People with COPD explain that acute dyspnea is an experience inextricably related to anxiety and emotional functioning. Patients may describe dyspnea in various terms: "My breath does not go out all the way," "It's hard work to breathe," or that breathing feels like "heaviness" or "gasping."

Progressive dyspnea occurs as more alveoli become overdistended, trapping increasing amounts of air. This causes the diaphragm to flatten and the anteroposterior diameter of the chest to increase; as a result, the typical barrel chest. Effective abdominal breathing is decreased because of the flattening of diaphragm, which forces the person to rely on intercostal and accessory muscles. This type of breathing, however, is not very effective because the ribs become fixed in an inspiratory position.

The person with advanced COPD frequently experiences weight loss and anorexia. The exact cause for these developments is not well understood. One possibility is that the patient is in a hypermetabolic state with increased energy requirements, partly because of the increased work of breathing. Even when caloric intake is adequate, weight loss still occurs. The patient with emphysema often has protein-calorie malnutrition with loss of lean muscle mass and subcutaneous fat (Aniwidyaningsih, Varraso, Cano, & Pison, 2008; Odencrants, Ehnfors, & Ehrenberg, 2008). (Malnutrition is discussed in Chapter 42.) Fatigue is a highly prevalent symptom that affects the patient's activities of daily living (ADLs).

During physical examination, a prolonged expiratory phase of respiration, wheezes, or decreased breath sounds, or some combination, are noted in some or all lung fields. The patient may sit upright with arms supported on a fixed surface such as a table (tripod position). The patient may naturally purse lips on expiration (pursed-lip breathing) and use accessory muscles, such as those in the neck, to aid with inspiration. Edema in the ankles may be a clue to right-sided heart involvement.

Over time, hypoxemia ($PaO_2 < 60$ mm Hg or $SaO_2 < 88\%$) may develop with hypercapnia ($PaCO_2 > 45$ mm Hg) later in the disease. The bluish-red colour of the skin results from polycythemia and cyanosis. Polycythemia develops as a result of increased production of red blood cells secondary to the body's attempt to compensate for chronic hypoxemia. Hemoglobin concentrations may reach 200 g/L or more. Cyanosis develops in the presence of at least 50 g/L or more of circulating unoxygenated hemoglobin.

Classification of COPD.

The diagnosis of COPD should be considered in any person with exposure to risk factors such as cigarettes, environmental or occupational pollutants, chronic cough and dyspnea, or a combination of these. The diagnosis of COPD is confirmed by spirometry regardless of whether the patient has chronic symptoms. The FEV_1/FVC ratio of less than 70% establishes the diagnosis of COPD. COPD can be classified as mild, moderate, severe, and very severe (Table 31-15), and this classification is based on the severity of obstruction (as indicated by FEV_1). The management of COPD is based primarily on a patient's symptoms, but the staging provides a general guideline for the type of interventions.

Complications

Cor Pulmonale.

Cor pulmonale is hypertrophy of the right side of the heart, with or without heart failure, that results from pulmonary hypertension. In COPD, pulmonary hypertension is caused primarily by constriction of the pulmonary vessels in response to alveolar hypoxia; acidosis further potentiates the

Table 31-15 Canadian Thoracic Society Chronic Obstructive Pulmonary Disease (COPD) Classification of Severity by Symptoms and Disability,* and Impairment of Lung

FUNCTION CLASSIFICATION BY SYMPTOMS AND DISABILITY	
COPD STAGE	**SYMPTOMS**
Mild	Shortness of breath from COPD† when hurrying on the level or walking up a slight hill (MRC 2)
Moderate	Shortness of breath from COPD† causing the patient to stop after walking approximately 100 m (or after a few minutes) on the level (MRC 3 to 4)
Severe	Shortness of breath from COPD† resulting in the patient being too breathless to leave the house, breathless when dressing or undressing (MRC 5), or the presence of chronic respiratory failure or clinical signs of right heart failure
CLASSIFICATION BY IMPAIRMENT OF LUNG FUNCTION	
COPD STAGE	**SPIROMETRY (POST-BRONCHODILATOR)**
Mild	$FEV_1 >$ or $= 80\%$, $FEV_1/FVC < 0.7$
Moderate	$50\% >$ or $= FEV_1 < 80\%$ predicted, $FEV_1/FVC < 0.7$
Severe	$30\% >$ or $= FEV_1 < 50\%$ predicted, $FEV_1/FVC < 0.7$
Very severe	$FEV_1 < 30\%$ predicted, $FEV_1/FVC < 0.7$

FEV1, forced expiratory volume in one second; *FEV1/FVC*, ratio of FEV1 to forced vital capacity. *MRC*, Medical Research Council dyspnea scale.
*Postbronchodilator forced expiratory volume in 1 s (FEV_1) to forced vital capacity (FVC) ratio less than 0.7 is required for the diagnosis of COPD to be established.
†In the presence of non-COPD conditions that may cause shortness of breath (e.g., cardiac dysfunction, anemia, muscle weakness, metabolic disorders), symptoms may not appropriately reflect COPD disease severity. Classification of COPD severity should be undertaken with care in patients with comorbid disease or other possible contributors to shortness of breath.
Source: O'Donnell, D. E., Aaron, S., Bourbeau, J., Hernandez, P., Marciniuk, D. D., Balter, M., …, Voduc, N. (2007). Canadian Thoracic Society recommendations for management of chronic obstructive pulmonary disease—2007 update. *Canadian Respiratory Journal, 14*(Suppl. B), 5B–32B (Table 3, p. 10B).

vasoconstriction (Figure 31-10). Chronic alveolar hypoxia causes pulmonary arteriolar muscle hypertrophy. Chronic hypoxia also stimulates erythropoiesis, which causes polycythemia and increases the viscosity of the blood. Cor pulmonale is a late manifestation of COPD with a poor prognosis; approximately 40% of patients with severe COPD have cor pulmonale (O'Donnell et al., 2007).

Normally, the right ventricle and the pulmonary circulatory system are low-pressure systems in comparison with the left ventricle and the systemic circulation. When pulmonary hypertension develops, the pressures on the right side of the heart must increase to push blood into the lungs. Eventually, right-sided heart failure develops.

The clinical manifestations of cor pulmonale are related to dilation and failure of the right ventricle with subsequent intravascular volume expansion and systemic venous congestion. Lung sounds are normal, or crackles may be heard in the bases of the lungs. Heart sound changes include accentuation of the pulmonic component of the second heart sound, right-sided ven-

PATHOPHYSIOLOGY MAP

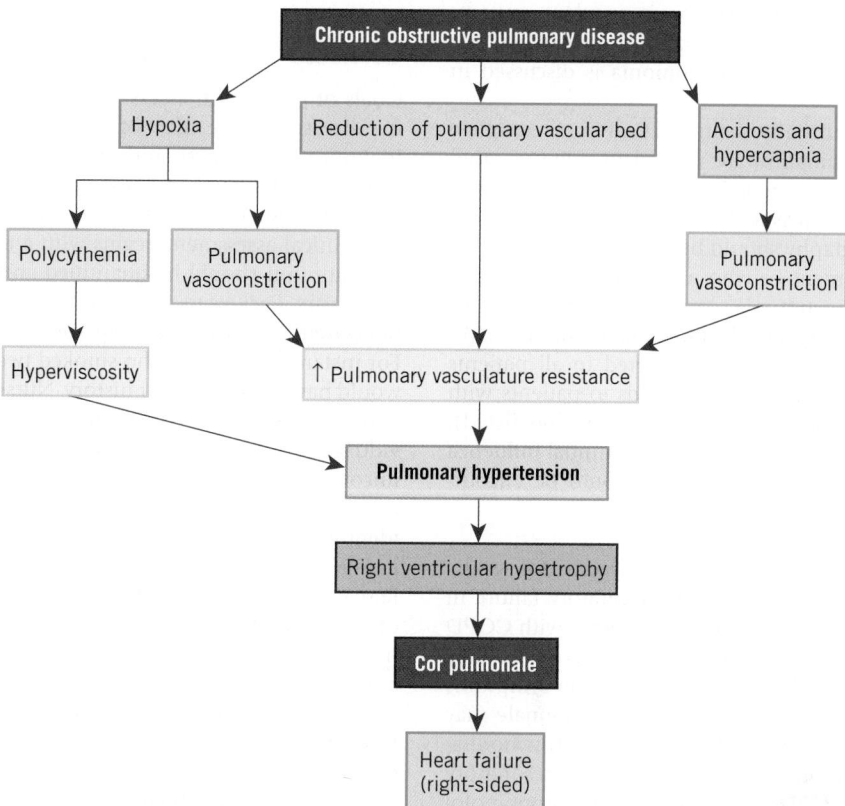

Figure 31-10 Mechanisms involved in the pathophysiological process of cor pulmonale secondary to chronic obstructive pulmonary disease.

tricular diastolic third heart sound gallop, and early systolic ejection click along the left sternal border. Overt manifestations of right-sided heart failure may develop, which include distension of neck veins (jugular venous distension), hepatomegaly with right upper quadrant tenderness, ascites, epigastric distress, peripheral edema, and weight gain.

Management of cor pulmonale includes continuous administration of low-flow oxygen. Long-term oxygen therapy can slow but not reverse the progression of pulmonary hypertension in patients with COPD. Diuretics are generally used, but serum creatinine and blood urea nitrogen must be monitored because diuretics can cause volume depletion. Electrolytes must be monitored because hypokalemia can predispose patients to dysrhythmias. (Cor pulmonale is discussed further in Chapter 30.)

Acute Exacerbations of COPD. Acute exacerbations are the most frequent cause of medical visits, hospitalizations, and death among people with COPD (O'Donnell et al., 2007, 2008). Exacerbations occur on average three times per year in patients with severe COPD (Yende, Newman, & Sin, 2009). Frequent exacerbations contribute to decreases in lung function and deterioration in quality of life. An acute exacerbation of COPD (AECOPD) is defined as a sustained worsening of dyspnea, cough, or sputum production that leads to an increased use of maintenance medications or supplementation with additional medications (O'Donnell et al., 2007, 2008). The term *sustained* implies a change from baseline that lasts 48 hours or longer. Exacerbations should be characterized as purulent or nonpurulent to assist with determining the need for

antibiotic therapy; purulent exacerbations necessitate antibiotic therapy. The frequency of AECOPD is, in part, related to the underlying severity of airflow obstruction, and patients with a history of frequent exacerbations are more likely to continue experiencing frequent exacerbations. The cause of AECOPD is often difficult to determine. Noninfectious triggers for exacerbations include exposure to allergens, irritants, cold air, and air pollution.

At least half of all exacerbations are thought to be infectious in nature; many of these are viral in origin, whereas the remainder are caused by bacterial infection. The most common organisms causing AECOPD are *H. influenzae*, *M. catarrhalis*, and *S. pneumoniae*. As COPD becomes more severe, *Pseudomonas* organisms, *Klebsiella pneumoniae*, and *Escherichia coli* are frequent causes of infection (O'Donnell et al., 2008). Patients with purulent sputum are often given a 7- to 10-day supply of antibiotics. The antibiotics most commonly given are amoxicillin, cefuroxime, cefixime, azithromycin, clarithromycin, trimethoprim-sulphamethoxazole, doxycycline, moxifloxacin, levofloxacin, and amoxicillin with clavulanic acid (O'Donnell et al., 2008). Some patients are provided with a written action plan and instructed to self-manage exacerbations by beginning antibiotics at the first signs of change in sputum production and colour. In concept, the COPD action plan is similar to the action plan used for patients with asthma (see Figure 31-7); however, the COPD action plan is specific to COPD and AECOPD. Many action plans are available. An example of an action plan can be downloaded from the Web site of the Canadian Lung Association (see the Canadian Resources at the end of this chapter).

Pneumonia is a frequent complication of COPD. The most common causative agents are *S. pneumoniae, H. influenzae,* and viruses. The most common manifestation is purulent sputum. Systemic manifestations such as fever, chills, and leukocytosis may not be present. (Treatment of pneumonia is discussed in Chapter 30.)

No diagnostic tests currently define AECOPD. A complete history and physical examination are needed to rule out other causes of increased symptoms. In patients who are very dyspneic, SaO_2 and ABGs should be measured (if oximetry oxygen saturation is low). Chest radiography should be performed for patients in the emergency department or who are admitted to hospital because they may have pneumonia, congestive heart failure, or pneumothorax. Increased inhaled bronchodilator dosages (β_2-agonists and anticholinergics) are administered to all patients with AECOPD, oral or systemic corticosteroids to patients with moderate to severe airflow obstruction ($FEV_1 < 50\%$ of predicted), and antibiotics to those with purulent sputum. Annual influenza vaccination and pneumococcal vaccination should be encouraged unless the patient has a contraindication.

Acute Respiratory Failure.

An acute exacerbation is the event that most commonly leads to acute respiratory failure in COPD (O'Donnell et al., 2007). Frequently, patients with COPD wait too long to contact their health care provider when they develop fever, increased cough and dyspnea, or other symptoms suggestive of AECOPD. An exacerbation of cor pulmonale may also lead to acute respiratory failure. Discontinuing bronchodilator or corticosteroid medication may also precipitate respiratory failure. The use of β-adrenergic blockers (e.g., propranolol [Inderal]) may also exacerbate acute respiratory failure. However, cardioselective β-adrenergic blockers (e.g., atenolol, metoprolol) should not be withheld from patients with mild to moderate diseases because they do not produce clinically significant problems with respiration (Navas & Taylor, 2010).

Indiscriminate use of sedatives and narcotics, especially before or after surgery in the patient who retains carbon dioxide, may suppress ventilatory drive and lead to respiratory failure. The person with COPD who retains carbon dioxide should be treated with low-flow rates of oxygen, and ABG values should be monitored carefully. Surgery or severe, painful illness involving the chest or abdomen may lead to splinting, ineffective ventilation, and respiratory failure. Careful preoperative screening, which includes pulmonary function tests and ABG monitoring, is important in patients with a history of heavy smoking and COPD to prevent postoperative pulmonary complications. (Respiratory failure is defined and discussed in Chapter 70.)

Depression, Anxiety, and Panic.

People with COPD experience higher rates of depression, anxiety, and panic (Hill, Geist, Goldstein, & Lacasse, 2008). Rates of depression range from 20 to 50% among people with COPD and are related to disease severity (O'Donnell et al., 2007). Depression may be related to feelings of loss and grief that accompany the progressive course of the disease. A heightened experience of dyspnea is probably related to anxiety (Bailey et al., 2010), which may precipitate further dyspnea and hyperventilation. When a person is exceptionally dyspneic, particularly if the condition occurs suddenly, the person becomes anxious and tries to breathe faster, which affects oxygenation status. Smoking and nicotine addiction have been identified as factors that predispose people to anxiety and depressive disorders (Hill et al., 2008). Proper screening for anxiety and depression and assessment of coping strate-

gies and supports by health care providers are needed to reduce the intensity of these symptoms and improve quality of life.

Clinical Assessment

Goals of the clinical assessment are to determine the severity of the disease and the effect of disease on a patient's quality of life. Identification of these and other factors enable the health care provider to design an individualized treatment plan (Bailey et al., 2010; O'Donnell et al., 2007, 2008).

Clinical assessment begins with a thorough history. Tobacco consumption should be quantified and is typically expressed in pack-years. Pack-years are calculated by multiplying the number of cigarette packs smoked daily by the number of years smoked. For instance, someone who smoked two packs a day for 30 years would have a 60 pack-year history. Nurses should ask each patient about the experience of symptoms and their impact on the individual's life. A series of probing questions is often necessary to uncover the extent of the patient's breathing difficulty and exercise curtailment. The severity of breathlessness is determined by identifying the magnitude of the task (often an activity of daily living) required to cause discomfort in breathing. The Medical Research Council (MRC) Dyspnea Scale is used to assess the level of shortness of breath and disability in COPD (Figure 31-11). The history also should include an assessment of the frequency and severity of exacerbations because the findings may guide treatment choices. Nurses should also include an assessment of symptoms associated with comorbid conditions or complications of COPD (ankle swelling, weight loss, anxiety, depression) and the current medical treatment.

Physical examination is important for patients with COPD but is not diagnostic. Pulmonary function studies are needed to determine airflow obstruction and therefore to determine a diagnosis of COPD and to assess the severity of lung impairment (O'Donnell et al., 2008). Spirometry is ordered before and after bronchodilator therapy; when the postbronchodilator FEV_1/FVC

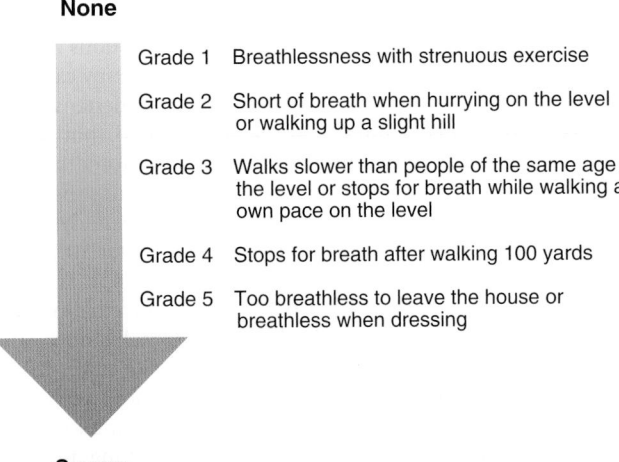

Figure 31-11 Medical Research Council (MRC) Dyspnea Scale. This scale can be used to assess shortness of breath and disability in chronic obstructive pulmonary disease.

Source: O'Donnell, D. E., Aaron, S., Bourbeau, J., Hernandez, P., Marciniuk, D., Balter, M., ..., Weiss, K. (2004). State of the art compendium: Canadian Thoracic Society recommendations for the management of chronic obstructive pulmonary disease. *Canadian Respiratory Journal, 11*(Suppl. B), 1-59B. Reprinted with permission of D. E. O'Donnell.

ratio is less than 70% of the predicted value, it confirms the presence of airway obstruction (O'Donnell et al., 2007).

The FEV$_1$ can provide a guideline to determine the severity of lung impairment and the degree of disease progression (see Table 31-15).

Chest radiographic studies are not diagnostic of COPD but are often necessary to confirm or rule out comorbid conditions. This also applies to high-resolution computed tomography, which is not routinely required. ABG monitoring should be offered to patients with an FEV$_1$ of less than 40% of predicted, patients who have a low SaO$_2$ (<92%) on oximetry, and patients in whom respiratory failure is suspected (O'Donnell et al., 2007). In the later stages of COPD, typical findings are low PaO$_2$, elevated PaCO$_2$, decreased pH, and increased bicarbonate levels. The 6-minute walking test is a useful test of functional disability and provides prognostic information. It includes determination of changes in the SaO$_2$ with exercise.

Collaborative Care

Primary COPD management goals are the following (O'Donnell et al., 2007; O'Donnell et al., 2008):
1. Prevent disease progression (smoking cessation)
2. Reduce the frequency and severity of exacerbations
3. Alleviate breathlessness and other respiratory symptoms
4. Improve exercise tolerance and daily activity
5. Treat exacerbations and complications of the disease
6. Improve health status and quality of life
7. Reduce the risk of mortality

AECOPD and complications such as respiratory failure, pneumonia, and congestive heart failure necessitate hospitalization, but otherwise patients are treated on an outpatient basis and manage their condition at home. Therapy is expected to escalate in intensity as a patient's disability progresses from MRC grade 2 to grade 5; those with an MRC grade of 3 or higher require more intensive management, including pharmacological and nonpharmacological interventions (O'Donnell et al., 2007). Collaborative care guidelines are presented in Table 31-16.

Environmental and occupational irritants and triggers should be assessed for a possible negative effect, and ways to control or avoid them should be determined. Patients with COPD should receive an annual influenza vaccination and a pneumococcal vaccine (pneumococcal revaccination is recommended every 5-10 years) (O'Donnell et al., 2008); see the Evidence-Informed Practice box on COPD and annual influenza vaccination.

Smoking Cessation.
Cessation of cigarette smoking is the most significant factor in slowing the progression of COPD. After a patient stops smoking, not only does the accelerated decline in pulmonary function slow but also pulmonary function usually improves. Thus the sooner the patient stops smoking, the less pulmonary function is lost and the sooner the symptoms decrease, particularly cough and sputum production. (See the RNAO's Best Practice Guideline: *Integrating Smoking Cessation Into Daily Practice* in the Canadian Resources at the end of this chapter.)

Drug Therapy.
Medications for COPD can reduce the intensity of symptoms or abolish them altogether, increase the capacity for exercise, improve overall health, and reduce the number and severity of exacerbations. Bronchodilators are the mainstay of pharmacological therapy for COPD (O'Donnell et al., 2007, 2008). Bronchodilator drug therapy relaxes smooth muscles in the airway, reduces airway resistance and dynamic hyperinflation

COLLABORATIVE CARE

Table 31-16 Chronic Obstructive Pulmonary Disease

Diagnostic
- History and physical examination
- Pulmonary function tests
- Serum α_1-antitrypsin levels
- Chest radiography (if indicated)
- Sputum specimen for Gram stain and culture (if indicated)
- ABG measurements (if indicated)
- Exercise testing with oximetry (if indicated)
- Electrocardiography (if indicated)
- Echocardiography or cardiac nuclear scans (if indicated)

Collaborative Therapy
- Smoking cessation
- Bronchodilator therapy (see Table 31-7)
- β$_2$-adrenergic agonists
- Anticholinergic agents
- Long-acting theophylline preparations (rarely used)
- Prompt treatment of exacerbations
- Corticosteroids (oral for exacerbations)
- Nonsteroidal anti-inflammatory drugs (roflumilast)
- Antibiotics for exacerbations with purulent sputum
- Influenza immunization (yearly)
- Pneumovax immunization (every 5-10 years)
- Pulmonary rehabilitation program
- Progressive plan of exercise, especially walking and upper body strengthening
- Breathing exercises
- Airway clearance techniques
- Hydration of 3 L/day (if not contraindicated)
- Relaxation techniques
- Appropriate pacing and planning of activities
- Patient and family teaching
- Long-term oxygen (if indicated)
- Nutritional supplementation if BMI is low
- Surgery in severe and advanced COPD
  - Lung volume reduction
  - Lung transplantation

ABG, arterial blood gas; *BMI*, body mass index; *COPD*, chronic obstructive pulmonary disease.

of the lungs, and improves the ventilation of the lungs, thus reducing the degree of breathlessness. Although patients with COPD do not respond to bronchodilator therapy as dramatically as do those with asthma, a reduction in dyspnea and an increase in FEV$_1$ are usually achieved. As with asthma, the preferred route of administration is by inhalation because it targets the lungs directly.

Bronchodilator medications commonly used are β$_2$-adrenergic agonists, anticholinergic agents, and methylxanthines (see Table 31-7). Short-acting bronchodilators, both β$_2$-adrenergic agonists and anticholinergic agents, improve pulmonary function, symptoms, and exercise function (O'Donnell et al., 2007, 2008). SABAs and anticholinergics can be used separately, but together they produce superior bronchodilation than does either drug alone. These medications are also available in nebulized combination (salbutamol and ipratropium [Combivent]). For most patients with COPD, bronchodilator therapy is best used as maintenance therapy (three or four times per day) with extra puffs on an as-needed basis for breakthrough symptoms. Bronchodilator therapy for asthma, in contrast, is used on an as-needed basis only during periods of nonexacerbation.

Long-acting bronchodilators also play a role in COPD and are typically indicated for patients with more severe COPD who experience persistent symptoms. Like short-acting

Should People with Chronic Obstructive Pulmonary Disease (COPD) Receive Annual Influenza Vaccination?

Clinical (PICO) Question

In people with COPD (P), in comparison with those who do not have COPD (C), does receiving an annual influenza vaccination (I) prevent exacerbations and reduce the use of urgent health care services (O)?

Best Available Evidence

A systematic review of randomized clinical trials involving people with COPD published in the Cochrane Library.

Critical Appraisal and Evidence

Eleven trials were studied in the review. Inactivated vaccine, given intramuscularly to patients with COPD, resulted in a significant reduction in the total number of exacerbations (>40%) in comparison with those who received placebo. The occurrence of local adverse reactions to vaccines (redness, soreness) was significantly increased, but the effects were generally mild and transient. The inactivated virus vaccine did not cause influenza or any significant worsening of COPD. There was no evidence of an effect of intranasal live attenuated virus when this was added to the inactivated intramuscular vaccination.

Conclusion

The possible risks of the vaccination are outweighed by the long-term benefits.

Implication for Nursing

Nurses should discuss with patients and families the need for annual influenza vaccinations and ensure that these are offered to them every fall.

Reference for Evidence

Poole, P. J., Chacko, E., Wood-Baker, R. W. B., & Cates, C. J. (2006). Influenza vaccine for clients with chronic obstructive pulmonary disease. *Cochrane Database of Systematic Reviews*, (1), CD002733. doi:10.1002/14651858.CD002733.pub2

PICO: P, Patient population of interest; I, intervention or area of interest; C, comparison of interest or comparison group; O, outcome(s) of interest.

and decrease diaphragmatic fatigue. The addition of theophylline to inhaled bronchodilator therapy may provide some benefit in some patients. However, the benefits and the risks need to be weighed because theophylline produces serious cardiovascular and neurological adverse effects. (Bronchodilator drugs are described in Table 31-7.)

The use of ICS monotherapy in COPD is very controversial (O'Donnell et al., 2008). ICS monotherapy does not have consistent effects on important outcomes (e.g., pulmonary function, symptoms, exacerbations). However, ICS in combination with a LABA has been found to reduce the frequency of exacerbations and to improve lung function and health status (O'Donnell et al., 2007). In Canada, two ICS and LABA combination products are currently used in the management of COPD: budesonide-formoterol (Symbicort) and fluticasone-salmeterol (Advair). The Canadian Thoracic Society Guidelines (O'Donnell et al., 2007) suggest the addition of an ICS in combination with a LABA when the patient has moderate to severe lung impairment and has frequent AECOPD (defined as one or more per year) (O'Donnell et al., 2007).

A new medication, approved for the treatment of COPD in 2011, is a phosphodiesterase 4 inhibitor, roflumilast (Daxas). This drug is indicated as add-on therapy with bronchodilators for the maintenance of COPD in patients with chronic cough and sputum and frequent exacerbations.

Oral or parenteral corticosteroids are used for the treatment of AECOPD. They speed recovery time, reduce relapse rates, reduce the need for hospitalization, and improve FEV_1 and partial pressure of oxygen. The dosage and duration should be individualized, but treatment periods between 7 and 14 days are recommended for people with moderate to severe COPD (O'Donnell et al., 2007, 2008). Continuous use of oral corticosteroids is not recommended for routine use in managing COPD because it can produce deleterious effects.

Oxygen Therapy. Oxygen therapy is frequently used in the treatment of COPD and other problems associated with hypoxemia. Oxygen is a colourless, odourless, tasteless gas that constitutes 20.95% of the atmosphere. Administering supplemental oxygen raises the partial pressure of oxygen in inspired air.

Indications for Use. Oxygen is usually administered to treat hypoxemia caused by respiratory disorders such as COPD, acute exacerbations of COPD, cor pulmonale, pneumonia, atelectasis, and lung cancer. Long-term oxygen therapy (15 hr/day or more to achieve an oxygen saturation of 90% or greater) prolongs life in patients with hypoxemia. Hypoxemia is defined as a PaO_2 lower than 55 mm Hg or lower than 60 mm Hg in the presence of cor pulmonale with a hematocrit higher than 56%. Patients with COPD are at risk of developing hypoxemia during an exacerbation.

Methods of Administration. The goal of oxygen administration is to supply the patient with adequate oxygen to maximize the oxygen-carrying ability of the blood. There are various methods of oxygen administration (Table 31-17, Figures 31-12 through 31-15). The method selected depends on factors such as the fraction of inspired oxygen, mobility of the patient, humidification required, patient cooperation, comfort, cost, and available financial resources.

Oxygen delivery systems are classified as low- or high-flow systems. Most methods of oxygen administration are low-flow devices that deliver oxygen in concentrations that vary with the

bronchodilators, long-acting bronchodilators include both β₂-adrenergic agonists (formoterol [Oxeze; Foradil], salmeterol [Serevent]), and anticholinergic agents (tiotropium [Spiriva]). The long-acting anticholinergic agents and LABAs produce more sustained improvements in pulmonary function, activity-related dyspnea, and quality of life than do the short-acting bronchodilators. Tiotropium reduces the frequency of hospitalization and exacerbation, improves health status and hyperinflation, and is taken only once daily. In comparison with LABAs, tiotropium provides greater improvements in dyspnea and health status (O'Donnell et al., 2007, 2008). These two classes of long-acting bronchodilators can be used separately or in combination.

The use of theophylline in the treatment of COPD is controversial. Although it has some weak bronchodilator effects, its main value may be to improve contractility of the diaphragm

Table 31-17 Methods of Oxygen Administration

ADVANTAGES	DISADVANTAGES	NURSING INTERVENTIONS
Low-Flow Delivery Devices		
Nasal Cannula		
May be used by a mobile or restless patient.	Difficult to maintain in position and can be easily dislodged.	Stabilize cannula during care for a restless patient.
Safe and simple method that is relatively comfortable and acceptable.	Patient needs to be alert to keep cannula in proper place.	Flow rate of 2 L/min produces an O_2 concentration of approximately 28%.
Used for patients requiring low O_2 concentrations.	High flow rates (>5 L/min) dry nasal membranes and may cause pain in frontal sinuses.	Amount of O_2 inhaled depends on room air and patient's breathing pattern.
Patient can eat, talk, or cough while wearing device (see Figure 31-12, *E*).	Can cause pressure necrosis or excoriation of nares.	Most patients with COPD can tolerate 2 L/min via cannula.
Simple Face Mask		
Delivers O_2 quickly for short periods.	Not as well tolerated as nasal cannula; lack of patient tolerance results in inadequate therapy.	Wash and dry under mask q2h.
O_2 concentrations of 35-50% can be achieved with flow rates of 6-12 L/min.	Mask may be uncomfortable because a tight seal must be maintained between face and mask.	Mask must fit snugly.
Mask provides adequate humidification of inspired air (see Figure 31-12, *A*).	Mask may produce pressure necrosis of the skin and confines heat radiating from the face about nose and mouth.	Nasal cannula may be provided while patient is eating.
	Must be removed to eat or drink.	Watch for pressure necrosis at the top of ears from elastic straps. (Gauze or other padding may be used to alleviate this problem.)
		Method requires at least 5 L/min flow to prevent accumulation of expired air in the mask.
Nasal Catheter		
Allows continuous, uninterrupted O_2 therapy.	Inserted into nasopharynx through a nostril and can produce excoriation of the nostril.	Should be changed q8h, alternating the nostrils.
Delivers O_2 even if patient is a mouth breather.	High flow rates (>6 L/min) cause drying of nasal membranes.	Distance that catheter is to be inserted is measured from distance between tip of nose and earlobe.
Does not interfere with patient care.	Inadvertent gas flow distends the stomach.	A flow rate of 5-6 L/min produces O_2 concentration of about 30%.
Rarely used except for short-term procedures (e.g., bronchoscopy).	Cannula does not enable a high degree of humidification and must be taped to patient's face.	Best for short-term therapy.
Partial Rebreathing Mask		
Light weight and easy to use.	Cannot be used when a high degree of humidity is required by the patient.	Useful when blood O_2 concentrations must be raised.
Reservoir bag conserves O_2.		Not recommended for patient with COPD and should never be used with a nebulizer.
Concentrations of 40-60% can be achieved with flow rates of 6-10 L/min.		Bag should not be allowed to deflate during inspiration.
Non-rebreathing Mask		
High concentrations of O_2 can be delivered accurately.	Cannot be used when a high degree of humidity is required by the patient.	Mask should fit snugly.
O_2 flows into bag and mask during inhalation.		Flow rate must be sufficient to keep bag from collapsing during inspiration.
Valve prevents expired air from flowing back into bag.		Bag should not be allowed to deflate during inspiration.
Concentrations of 60-90% can be achieved.		
Oxygen-Conserving Cannula		
Has a built-in reservoir that increases O_2 concentration delivered and allows patient to use lower flow rates, usually 30-50%, which increases comfort and lowers cost.	Cannot be cleaned: manufacturer changing cannula qwk is recommended.	Generally indicated when long-term O_2 therapy is used at home rather than during hospitalization.
Reported to be more comfortable than standard nasal cannulas (see Figure 31-12, *E*).	More expensive than standard cannulas and requires evaluation with measurement of ABGs and oximetry to determine correct flow.	It may be "moustache" or "pendant" type.
	Highly visible and heavy on ears.	May cause necroses over the tops of the ears; can be padded.

Continued

Table 31-17 Methods of Oxygen Administration—cont'd		
ADVANTAGES	**DISADVANTAGES**	**NURSING INTERVENTIONS**
Transtracheal Catheter		
Less visible than cannula. Flow requirement may be reduced 60-80%, which greatly increases amount of time available from portable source of O_2. Less nasal irritation occurs (see Figure 31-13).	Patient and family must learn entire program of care for tracheostoma and how to replace catheter. Procedure is invasive. Equipment is more costly.	Method may not be appropriate for patient with excessive mucus production from mucous plugging.
Tracheostomy Collar		
Collar can deliver high humidity and O_2 via tracheostomy.	Condensed fluid in tubing may drain into tracheostomy. Water traps are usually inserted. Secretions collect inside collar and around tracheostomy. O_2 concentration is lost into atmosphere because collar does not fit tightly.	Collar attaches to neck with elastic strap and should be removed and cleaned at least q4h to prevent aspiration of fluid and infection.
Low-Flow Delivery Devices		
Tracheostomy T Bar		
Tight fit allows better O_2 and humidity delivery than does tracheostomy collar.	Condensed fluid in tubing may drain into tracheostomy. Water traps are usually inserted.	T bar must be removed for suctioning. Mörch swivel may be used to eliminate the need for removal. It should be emptied as necessary.
Tent or Incubator		
Has ability to control temperature and humidity.	Limited usefulness. Difficult to maintain adequate concentrations of O_2. Isolates patient from environment.	Tent should be flushed with O_2 every time it is opened. Nurse should assess for leaks around canopy.
High-Flow Delivery Devices		
Venturi Mask		
Delivers precise, high flow rates of O_2. Lightweight, cone-shaped plastic device is fitted to face. Available for delivery of 24%, 28%, 31%, 35%, 40%, and 50% O_2. Adaptors can be applied to increase humidification (see Figure 31-12, *C*).	Uncomfortable and must be removed when patient eats. Patient can talk while wearing mask, but voice may be muffled. Other disadvantages are the same as those for the simple face mask.	Entrainment device on mask must be changed to deliver higher concentrations of O_2. Method is especially helpful for administering low, constant O_2 concentrations to patients with COPD. Air entrainment ports must not be occluded.

ABGs, arterial blood gases; *COPD*, chronic obstructive pulmonary disease.

person's respiratory pattern. In contrast, the Venturi mask is a high-flow device that delivers fixed concentrations of oxygen independent of a patient's respiratory pattern. With the Venturi mask, oxygen is delivered to a small jet (Venturi device) in the centre of a wide-based cone (see Figure 31-12, *C*). Air is entrained (pulled) through openings in the cone as oxygen flows through the small jet. The mask has large vents through which exhaled air can escape. The degree of restriction, or narrowness, of the jet determines the amount of entrainment and the dilution of pure oxygen with room air and thus the concentration of oxygen. Mechanical ventilators are another example of a high-flow oxygen delivery system. Because room air is mixed with oxygen, the percentage of oxygen delivered to the patient is not as precise in low-flow systems as in high-flow systems.

Humidification. Oxygen obtained from cylinders or wall systems is dry. Dry oxygen has an irritating effect on mucous membranes and dries secretions. Therefore, it is important that

oxygen be humidified when administered, either by humidification or nebulization. A device commonly used for humidification when the patient has a catheter, cannula, or low-flow mask is a bubble-through humidifier. It is a small plastic jar filled with sterile distilled water that is attached to the oxygen source by means of a flow meter. Oxygen passes into the jar, bubbles through the water, and then goes through tubing to a patient's catheter, cannula, or mask. The purpose of the bubble-through humidifier is to restore the humidity conditions of room air. However, the need for bubble-through humidifiers at flow rates between 1 and 4 L/min is debatable when humidity in the environment is adequate.

Complications

Combustion. Oxygen supports combustion and increases the rate of burning; thus it is important that smoking be prohibited in an area where oxygen is being used. A "No Smoking" sign should be prominently displayed on patients' doors and in their

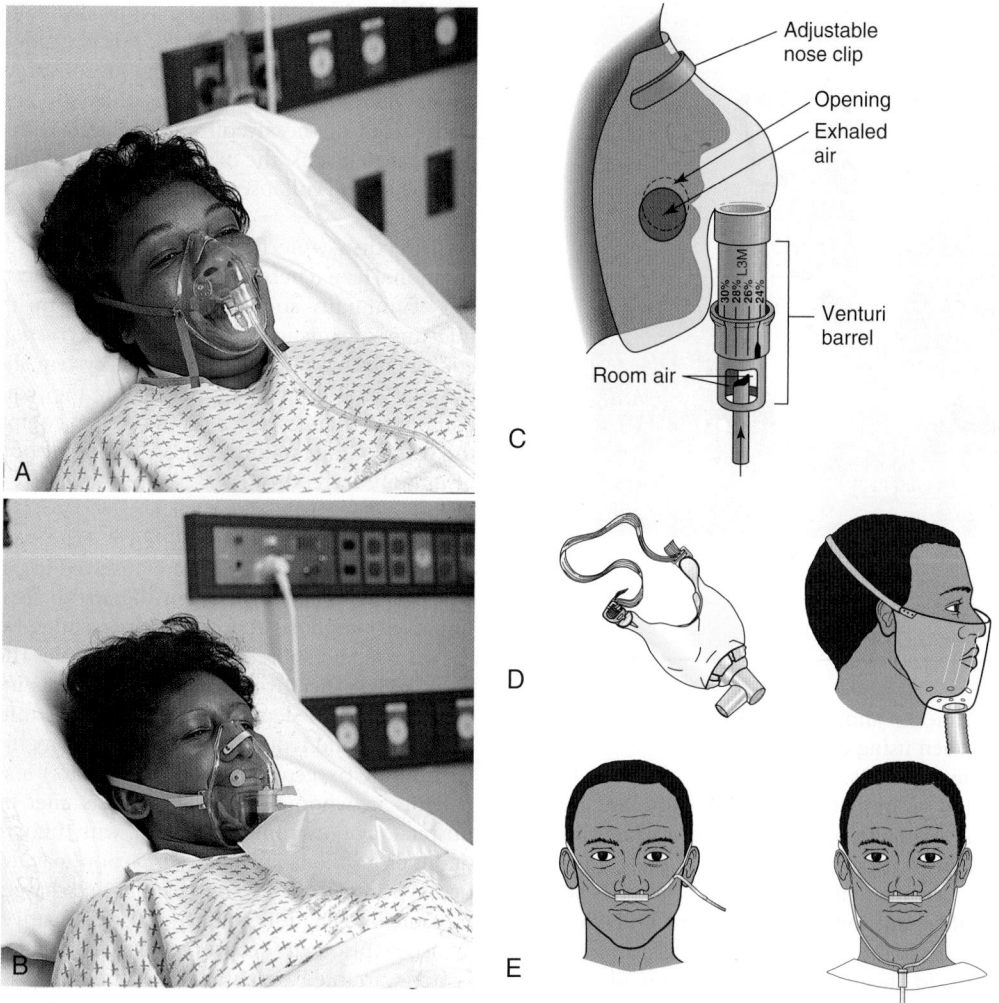

Figure 31-12 Methods of oxygen administration. **A,** Simple face mask. **B,** Plastic face mask with reservoir bag. **C,** Venturi mask. **D,** Tracheostomy mask. **E,** Standard nasal cannulas.

Source: Adapted from Potter, P. A., & Perry, A. G. (2009). *Fundamentals of nursing* (7th ed., pp. 958-59, Figs 40-15, 40-16, 40-17). St. Louis: Mosby.

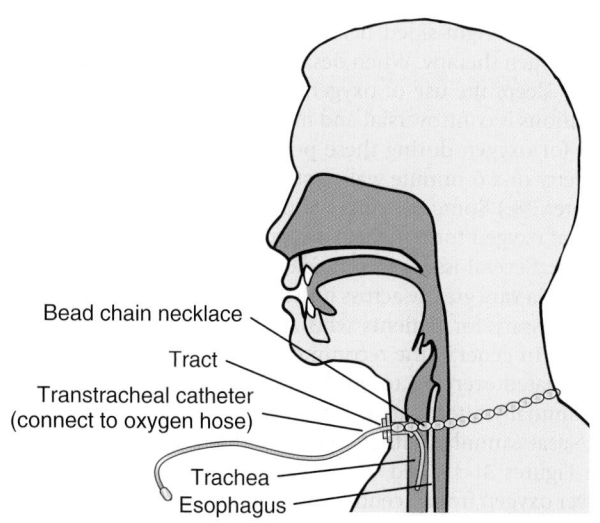

Figure 31-13 Transtracheal catheter for oxygen administration.

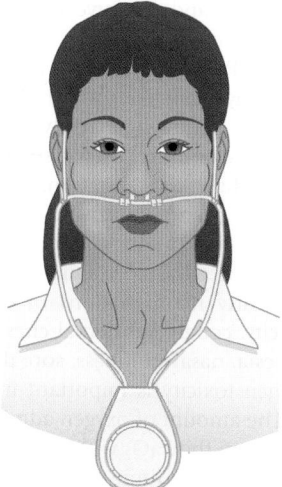

Figure 31-14 Pendant type of oxygen-conserving cannula.

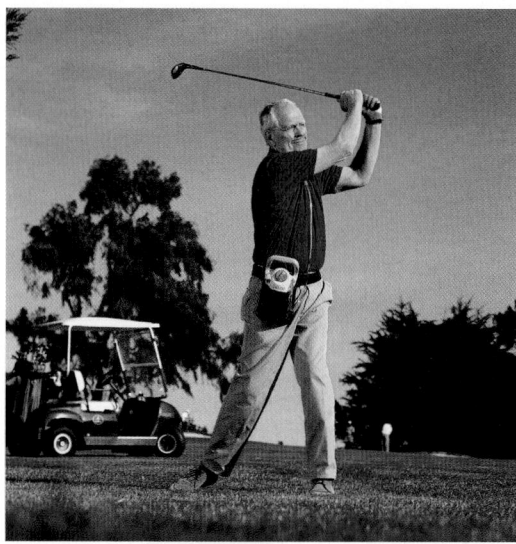

Figure 31-15 Golfer using Helios liquid portable oxygen system.

Source: Nellcor Puritan Bennett, Inc., Pleasanton, California.

homes and cars. Patients should also be cautioned against smoking cigarettes when using oxygen.

Carbon Dioxide Narcosis. The two chemoreceptors in the respiratory centre that control the drive to breathe are carbon dioxide and oxygen. Normally, accumulation of carbon dioxide is the major stimulant of the respiratory centre. Over time, the respiratory centre loses its sensitivity to the elevated carbon dioxide levels in COPD, and some patients with COPD develop a tolerance for high carbon dioxide levels. Theoretically, for these individuals the "drive" to breathe is hypoxemia. Thus administering oxygen to patients with COPD has been thought to weaken their drive to breathe. This has been a pervasive myth but is not a serious threat. In fact, not providing adequate oxygen to these patients is much more detrimental. Although oxygen administration should be titrated to the lowest effective dosage, many patients who have end-stage COPD require high-flow rates. They may, in fact, exhibit higher-than-normal levels of carbon dioxide in their blood, but this is of little concern. What is important is careful, ongoing physical and cognitive assessment when providing oxygen to these patients.

Oxygen toxicity. Pulmonary **oxygen toxicity,** a condition of oxygen overdosage, may result from prolonged exposure to a high level of oxygen (PaO_2). Although relatively rare, the development of oxygen toxicity is determined by patient tolerance, exposure time, and dosage. High concentrations of oxygen damage alveolar–capillary membranes, inactivate pulmonary surfactant, cause interstitial and alveolar edema, and decrease lung compliance, ultimately leading to acute respiratory distress syndrome (see Chapter 70). Early manifestations of oxygen toxicity are reduced vital capacity, cough, substernal chest pain, nausea and vomiting, paraesthesia, nasal stuffiness, sore throat, and malaise. Prevention of oxygen toxicity is important in patients who are receiving oxygen. The amount of oxygen administered should be just enough to maintain the PaO_2 within a normal or acceptable range for each patient. A safe limit of oxygen concentrations has not yet been established. All levels above 50% and supplemental oxygen used for longer than 24 hours should be considered potentially toxic. Levels of 40% and below may be regarded as relatively nontoxic if the exposure period is short.

Absorption Atelectasis. Normally, nitrogen constitutes 79% of the air that is breathed, but it is not absorbed into the bloodstream. Its presence in the alveoli prevents alveolar collapse. When high concentrations of oxygen are given, nitrogen is washed out of the alveoli and replaced with oxygen. If airway obstruction occurs, the oxygen is absorbed into the bloodstream and the alveoli collapse. This process is called **absorption atelectasis.**

Infection. Infection can be a major hazard of oxygen administration. Heated nebulizers present the highest risk. The constant use of humidity supports bacterial growth, the most common infecting organism being *Pseudomonas aeruginosa.* Disposable equipment that operates as a closed system should be used. The hospital should have a policy stating the required frequency of equipment changes based on the type of equipment used and for the use of Gram staining and culturing of both equipment and respiratory secretions.

Long-Term Oxygen Therapy at Home. Improved survival and enhanced quality of life are observed in patients with COPD who receive long-term oxygen therapy to treat hypoxemia. The improved prognosis results from preventing both progression of the disease and subsequent cor pulmonale. The benefits of long-term oxygen therapy include improvements in neuropsychological function and sleep, increase in exercise tolerance, decrease in hematocrit, and reduced rates of pulmonary hypertension. Short-term home oxygen therapy (1 to 30 days) may be indicated for patients in whom hypoxemia persists after discharge from the hospital. For example, a patient with underlying COPD who develops a serious respiratory infection may demonstrate continued hypoxemia for 4 to 6 weeks after discharge. It is important to measure oxygenation status by pulse oximetry 2 to 3 months after an acute episode to determine whether long-term oxygen therapy is still warranted because, at that point, up to 50% of patients requiring oxygen during an exacerbation no longer meet the requirements for long-term oxygen therapy (O'Donnell et al., 2007).

Patients whose disease is stable with a PaO_2 of 55 mm Hg or lower (corresponding to an SaO_2 of 88% or lower) should receive long-term oxygen therapy. A patient whose PaO_2 is between 55 and 59 mm Hg (SaO_2 of 89%) and who exhibits signs of tissue hypoxia, such as cor pulmonale, erythrocytosis, and peripheral edema from right-sided heart failure, should also receive long-term oxygen therapy. When desaturation occurs only during exercise or sleep, the use of oxygen therapy specifically under those conditions is controversial and must be assessed individually. The need for oxygen during these periods should be evaluated with oximetry or a 6-minute walk test. (Pulse oximetry is discussed in Chapter 28.) Some provinces and jurisdictions do not cover the costs of oxygen for patients who exhibit hypoxia during sleep or exercise. Several issues in Canada related to funding and eligibility criteria vary greatly across jurisdictions. Periodic re-evaluations are necessary for patients who are using chronic supplemental oxygen. In general, the recommendation is that such patients be re-evaluated every 30 to 90 days during the first year of therapy and annually after that, as long as patients remain stable.

Nasal cannulas, either regular or the oxygen-conserving type (see Figures 31-14 and 31-15, Table 31-17) are usually used to deliver oxygen from a central source in the home. The source may be a liquid oxygen storage system, compressed oxygen in tanks, or an oxygen concentrator or extractor, depending on home environment, insurance coverage, activity level, and proximity to an oxygen supply company (Table 31-18). To increase mobility in

Table 31-18 Home Oxygen Delivery Systems

ADVANTAGES	DISADVANTAGES	COMMENTS
Liquid Oxygen		
Portable unit* can be refilled by patient from reservoir. Portable unit holds 6- to 8-hr supply at 2 L/min; reservoir will last approximately 7-10 days when 2 L/min is used continuously.	Liquid system slightly more expensive, depending on location; not available everywhere; generally limited to urban areas.	As liquid warms to gas, some is vented from the system. In summer, evaporation is accelerated and may decrease reservoir duration to <1 wk.
Compressed O_2 Tanks or Cylinders		
Good availability in most areas. Portability possible with cart. Aluminum cylinders available in varying sizes (e.g., D, E, M, H, J) that are markedly lighter than steel and easier to manoeuvre.	Duration of large (H or J) tank at 2 L/min flow about 50 hr; storage of four or five large cylinders in the home necessary to have 7- to 10-day supply; portable cylinder on cart is cumbersome and heavy. Duration of E cylinder when 2 L/min is used is approximately 4-5 hr.	Some smaller tanks (D or M) may be used; these can be refilled from large cylinders and weigh about 4.5 kg (10 lb). Tank can be carried on shoulder strap, backpack, or fanny pack or placed on portable cart.
Concentrator or Extractor		
Because the O_2 supply is made from room air, they never need to be "filled." On wheels, movable from room to room. Compact, excellent system for rural or homebound patients. Convenient, safe, and reliable (assuming electricity source is reliable).	—	Concentrator should be kept in room other than bedroom if noise disturbs sleep.
Portable Oxygen Concentrator		
Light-weight devices (3.9-17.7 kg [8.5-17 lb]) that are portable via carts or shoulder straps. Batteries last up to 8 hr with recharging in either AC or DC (e.g., car) outlets. Provides the patient with exceptional freedom and is beneficial to the active patient who may use more than their allotted requirement of O_2 cylinders each month.	Can be costly. Patient must meet qualifications of O_2 company to use.	—
Pulse or Demand Delivery System (Oxygen-Conserving Device)		
Delivers a pulse of O_2 only during inhalation to conserve O_2. Attaches to cylinders. Increases duration of O_2 supply. Less drying or irritation to nasal mucosa. Saves O_2.	May not be able to provide sufficient oxygen during exertion; audible pulses may be annoying; costly; less efficient at higher O_2 flow rates; best for low activity levels. Patient must be a nose-breather to trigger the flow of O_2.	Monitor O_2 saturation during rest and exercise to determine whether oxygenation is acceptable. Consult with vendor or respiratory therapist if O_2 saturation is below desired level.

*Portable usually refers to units weighing more than 4.5 kg (10 lb); ambulatory units weigh less than 4.5 kg (10 lb).

the home, the patient can use extension tubing (up to 15 m [50 ft]) without adversely affecting the oxygen flow delivery if the flow meter is the back pressure–compensated type. Small portable systems, such as that for liquid oxygen, may be provided for the patient who remains active outside the home.

Reservoir cannulas operate on the principle of storing oxygen in a small reservoir during exhalation. The oxygen is then delivered to the patient during the subsequent inhalation, in a manner similar to a bolus effect. The reservoir cannulas can reduce flow requirements by approximately 50%. A pendant type is available (see Figure 31-14). Other delivery devices for chronic oxygen therapy include transtracheal oxygen delivery and intermittent-demand oxygen delivery systems. Transtracheal oxygen delivery necessitates a surgical procedure to insert the small oxygen catheter into the patient's trachea (see Figure 31-13). Nursing care involves teaching the patient and caregivers how to care for the

stoma and the transtracheal catheter. The transtracheal catheter is less visible than nasal cannulas, and there is no nasal irritation. It also reduces the oxygen flow requirement by 30 to 50%.

Intermittent-demand delivery systems or conserver devices are mechanically complex devices that most commonly attach to the oxygen cylinders. They deliver "pulses" of oxygen to the patient, usually during inspiration, and thus eliminate waste of oxygen during exhalation, as is experienced during continuous flow.

Home oxygen systems are usually rented from a company that sends a respiratory therapist or respiratory nurse specialist to the patient's home to teach how to use and care for the oxygen system and how to recognize when the supply is running low and must be reordered. A patient and caregiver teaching guide for the use of oxygen at home is presented in Table 31-19.

A patient who uses home oxygen should be encouraged to remain active and to travel. If long-distance travel is by automo-

PATIENT & CAREGIVER TEACHING GUIDE

Table 31-19 Home Oxygen Use

Mask or Cannula

- Ensure that the straps are not too tight.
- Remove two or three times per day to wash and dry skin where straps are placed.
- Pad any pressure points.
- Observe tops of ears for skin breakdown from pressure points.

Oral and Nasal Mucous Membranes

- Assess oral and nasal mucous membranes two or three times per day.
- Use water-based gel on lips and nasal mucosa.
- Practise frequent oral hygiene.
- Avoid dry ambient air; humidity is required whenever oxygen is used.

Decreasing Risk for Infection

- Remove mask or collar, and clean with water two or three times per day.
- Clean skin carefully and observe for cuts, scratches, and bruises.
- Change disposable equipment frequently.
- Remove secretions that are expectorated.

Decreasing Risk of Fire Injuries

- Post "No Smoking" warning signs in home where they can be seen.
- Do not use electric razors, portable radios, open flames, wool blankets, or mineral oils in the area where oxygen is in use.
- Do not allow smoking in the home or car.

NOTE: The Canadian Lung Association has good resources for patients using oxygen at home. See the Resources at the end of the chapter.

bile, arrangements can be made for oxygen to be available at the destination point. Oxygen-supply companies can often assist with these arrangements. If a patient wishes to travel by bus, train, or airplane, these parties require notification of the need for oxygen during travel when reservations are made. A high-altitude simulation test (HAST) may be performed or a mathematical formula calculated in a hospital pulmonary function laboratory to determine the oxygen prescription required. Because airplane cabins are pressurized to an elevation of 2100 or 2400 m (7000 or 8000 ft), the patient who uses supplemental oxygen should have oxygen provided during flight. The plane's oxygen system must be used. Patients may not use their own oxygen system during flight because it is not properly pressurized. Airlines allow patients to bring their oxygen system to be carried in the baggage compartment for use at the point of destination, but the reservoirs (liquid or tank) must be empty and the valves left open. Some patients may need to avoid prolonged exposure to high elevations during travel unless they are instructed by their health care provider how to adjust their oxygen flow to attempt to compensate for altitude.

Surgical Therapy.

Two different surgical procedures have been used in management of severe COPD. One type of surgery is *lung volume reduction surgery* (O'Donnell et al., 2007). The rationale for the surgery is that by reducing the size of the hyperinflated emphysematous lungs, airway obstruction is decreased and room for the remaining normal alveoli to function is increased. The procedure reduces volume by approximately 20 to 35% of the most emphysematous lungs and improves lung and chest wall mechanics. The most common postoperative complication is pneumonia. However, lung volume reduction surgery may offer benefit to a subgroup of patients with severe COPD in terms of improvements in lung function, exercise capacity, quality of life, and possibly survival. However, the procedure is very expensive and appropriate only for a select group of patients with severe COPD (Miller et al., 2006; O'Donnell et al., 2007).

The second surgical procedure is *lung transplantation* for selected patients with advanced, severe COPD. In Canada between 1995 and 2004, 291 lung transplantations (double-lung, single-lung, or heart-lung) were performed for patients with COPD. Survival rates for patients following lung transplant who have AAT deficiency and COPD are in the range of 79 to 80% at 1 year and 60 to 62% at 5 years (Canadian Institute for Health Information, 2006). However, recipients of lung transplants who have COPD tend to have better outcomes than do those with other conditions (O'Donnell et al., 2007). The major complication affecting long-term morbidity and mortality is chronic graft dysfunction associated with obliterative bronchiolitis, which is present in approximately half of all long-term survivors (Whitson et al., 2007). Patients with COPD who receive lung transplants can achieve substantial improvements in exercise capacity and improved quality of life, and most are free of supplemental oxygen. (Lung transplantation is discussed in Chapter 30.)

Pulmonary Rehabilitation Programs.

All patients with COPD should be encouraged to maintain an active lifestyle. Pulmonary rehabilitation programs (PRPs) are used to optimize the functional status of patients with COPD—as well as their quality of life, experience of dyspnea, exercise endurance, psychosocial functioning, and overall autonomy—and to reduce their use of health care services and exacerbations of their condition (Lacasse, Goldstein, Lasserson, & Martin, 2006; Marciniuk et al., 2010, 2011; O'Donnell et al., 2007, 2008). The benefits observed with PRPs are often superior to the benefits of pharmacological therapy. These benefits are largely attributable to exercise. Specific components of a PRP can include exercise conditioning (aerobic and upper and lower body conditioning), breathing exercises, energy conservation, nutrition, smoking cessation, environmental factors, health promotion, patient education and self-management, psychological support, psychological counselling, and vocational rehabilitation. PRPs can be provided as inpatient or outpatient or in-home programs. The duration of the program is typically 4 to 12 weeks. However, PRPs lasting longer than 12 weeks and those that are ongoing may have even better benefits (Marciniuk et al., 2010). If patients are clinically stable and experience exercise or activity limitation and dyspnea, they should receive a supervised PRP. In addition, those patients who attend a PRP within 1 month of an exacerbation are shown to have improved outcomes (Marciniuk et al., 2011).

Exercise training involves both lower and upper extremity training and improves dyspnea and exercise performance. Lower extremity training focuses on aerobic training and includes walking, treadmill walking, bicycling, and cycling ergometry. Upper extremity training focuses on improving arm strength and endurance. Peripheral muscle wasting and weakness affects about 25% of patients with COPD. Exercise training should be performed more than three times per week. Health care providers working in PRPs assess the individual's limitations and conditioning status and develop a customized exercise program that is monitored over the length of the rehabilitation program.

Breathing Exercises. In patients with COPD, the respiratory rate increases and expiration is prolonged, to compensate for airflow obstruction and dyspnea. The accessory muscles of breathing, located in the neck and the upper part of the chest, are used excessively to promote chest wall movement. These muscles are not adapted to long-term use for breathing and, as a result, become fatigued. Breathing exercises can assist the patient during rest and activity (e.g., lifting, walking, stair climbing). The main types of breathing exercises are (a) pursed-lip breathing and (b) diaphragmatic breathing.

Pursed-lip breathing is used to prolong exhalation, prevent bronchiolar collapse and air trapping, and assist with dyspnea. Exhalation should be at least three times longer than inhalation. It is important to demonstrate and teach patients how to use this technique and for them to practise until it works for them and they feel comfortable using it. Patients should be instructed to follow this sequence:

1. Relax neck and shoulder muscles.
2. Inhale slowly through the nose to the count of 2.
3. Pucker lips as if whistling.
4. Exhale slowly and gently through the lips while mentally counting to 6.
5. Always exhale longer than they inhale.

Diaphragmatic (abdominal) breathing focuses on using the diaphragm instead of accessory muscles to achieve maximum inhalation and to slow the respiratory rate. Currently, the evidence from controlled studies does not support the use of diaphragmatic breathing in patients with COPD (Nici, et al., 2006).

Effective Coughing. Many patients with COPD have developed ineffective coughing patterns that do not adequately clear their airways of sputum. In addition, they fear they may develop spastic coughing, which would increase dyspnea. *Huff coughing* is an effective technique that the patient can be taught easily; guidelines are presented in Table 31-20. The main goals of effective coughing are to conserve energy, reduce fatigue, and facilitate removal of secretions.

Nutritional Therapy. Weight loss and malnutrition are common among people with severe COPD and are a result of multiple factors. In these patients, energy expenditure related is increased as a result of increased work of breathing (30 to 50% more energy is spent on breathing than in the average person); oxygen consumption is increased; gas exchange is inefficient; and dead space ventilation is increased. Other factors contributing to weight loss and malnutrition are decreased food intake, the effects of certain drugs, and a high systemic inflammatory response (Batres, Leon, & Rodolfo, 2007). Other factors further affecting patients' nutritional status may be dyspnea, dysphagia, dyspepsia, depression, anxiety, physical limitations, social or financial considerations, decreased sense of smell and taste, and drug and alcohol consumption. Eating becomes an effort as a result of dyspnea, especially in the later stages of COPD. In addition, a full stomach presses up on the flattened diaphragm, further increasing dyspnea and causing discomfort. It is difficult for some patients to eat and breathe at the same time; therefore, they eat inadequate amounts of food. The role of a registered dietitian is critical for nutritional screening and intervention.

Patients with COPD should try to keep body mass index (BMI) between 21 and 25 kg/m^2. Being either overweight or underweight can cause further problems in conjunction with COPD. However, a reduced BMI or weight loss is especially associated with poor outcomes in acute exacerbations and with increased rates of morbidity and mortality among patients with COPD. To decrease dyspnea and conserve energy, patients may need to rest (30 minutes) before eating, use a bronchodilator before meals, and select foods that can be prepared in advance. Eating five to six small meals per day helps avoid feelings of bloating and early satiety. Patients may want to avoid foods that form intestinal gas, such as cabbage, Brussels sprouts, and beans. Cold foods produce less of a sense of fullness than do hot foods. Foods that require a great deal of chewing can be served in another manner (e.g., grated, pureed). The use of frozen foods and a microwave oven may help conserve a patient's energy in food preparation. Exercises should be avoided for at least 1 hour before and after eating. In patients with late-stage or severe COPD, nutritional requirements for protein and calories may be greater than normal. They may need 1.2 to 1.3 times the normal kilocalorie requirement to even maintain their weight. A high-calorie, high-protein diet is recommended. High-protein, high-calorie nutritional supplements can be offered between meals. (Nutritional supplements are discussed in Chapter 42.)

Fluid intake should be at least 2 to 3 L per day unless contraindicated for other medical conditions, such as heart failure. Fluids should be taken between meals (rather than with them) to prevent excess stomach distension and to decrease pressure on the diaphragm. Sodium restriction may be indicated if a patient also has heart failure. In older patients, corticosteroid use increases the risk of or leads to osteoporosis. As a result, it is important to stress the necessity for adequate calcium and vitamin D intake.

PATIENT & CAREGIVER TEACHING GUIDE

Table 31-20 Huff Coughing

1. Patient assumes a sitting position with neck slightly flexed, shoulders relaxed, knees flexed, and forearms supported by pillow and, if possible, with feet on the floor.
2. Patient then drops head and bends forward while using slow, pursed-lip breathing to exhale.
3. Sitting up again, patient uses diaphragmatic breathing to inhale slowly and deeply.
4. Patient repeats steps 2 and 3 another three or four times to facilitate mobilization of secretions.
5. Before initiating a cough, patient should take a deep abdominal breath, bend slightly forward, and then cough three or four times on exhalation (huff coughing). Patient may need to support or splint the thorax or the abdomen to achieve a cough of maximum effectiveness.

NURSING MANAGEMENT: CHRONIC OBSTRUCTIVE PULMONARY DISEASE

Nursing Assessment

Subjective and objective data that should be obtained from a person with COPD are presented in Table 31-21.

Nursing Diagnoses

Nursing diagnoses for patients with COPD may include, but are not limited to, those presented in Nursing Care Plan 31-2.

NURSING ASSESSMENT

Table 31-21 Chronic Obstructive Pulmonary Disease (COPD)

Subjective Data	Objective Data
Important Health Information	**General**
Present health: Assess experience of dyspnea (with activity and at rest) and cough. If cough is productive, determine colour, consistency, and quantity of secretions. Current dyspnea should be measured on a quantitative scale such as a visual analogue or a numeric rating scale. (See Chapter 28 with regard to dyspnea.) The usual level of dyspnea that a patient experiences should be measured against the Medical Research Council Dyspnea Scale (see Figure 31-11)	Height, weight, BMI
	Distress, increased work of breathing, use of compensatory mechanisms for breathing (upright position, pursed-lip breathing), anxiety, depression, restlessness
	Integumentary
	Cyanosis (bronchitis), pallor or ruddy colour, poor skin turgor, thin skin, easy bruising, peripheral edema (cor pulmonale)
Past health history: Long-term exposure to chemical pollution, respiratory irritants, occupational fumes, and dust; history and frequency of respiratory infections; previous hospitalizations and emergency department visits related to breathing and cardiac problems; smoking exposure (pack-years, exposure to secondary smoke, previous attempts at cessation); personal and family history of respiratory and cardiac conditions	**Respiratory**
	Rapid, shallow breathing; accessory muscle use; inability to speak at all; prolonged expiratory phase; pursed-lip breathing; wheezing, crackles, diminished breath sounds; ↓ chest excursion and diaphragmatic movement; use of accessory muscles; hyper-resonant or dull chest sounds on percussion
Medications: Use and duration of supplemental O_2, bronchodilators, anticholinergics, corticosteroids, antibiotics, OTC drugs, complementary therapies; effectiveness of bronchodilators and experience of adverse effects	**Cardiovascular**
	Tachycardia, dysrhythmias, jugular vein distension, right-sided third heart sound (cor pulmonale), edema (especially in feet)
Symptoms	**Gastrointestinal**
• Anorexia, weight loss or gain, early satiety, difficulty eating	Ascites, hepatomegaly (cor pulmonale)
• Decreased level of activity and ability to perform ADLs or exercise. Dyspnea, palpitations, recurrent cough, use of sitting-up position for sleeping, paroxysmal nocturnal dyspnea, orthopnea, swelling of feet	**Musculoskeletal**
	Muscle atrophy, ↑ anteroposterior diameter (barrel-chest)
• Constipation, gas, bloating	**Possible Diagnostic Findings**
• Headache, loss of memory, inability to concentrate	Pulmonary function test results demonstrating airflow obstruction (e.g., decreased FEV_1, FEV_1/FVC, PEFR; increased RV), decreased SaO_2 measured by pulse oximetry, abnormal arterial blood gas values, polycythemia
• Fatigue, insomnia, depression, anxiety, panic	Chest radiograph showing flattened diaphragm and hyperinflation or infiltrates
	ECG showing dysrhythmias

ADLs, activities of daily living; *BMI,* body mass index; *ECG,* electrocardiogram; *FEV₁,* forced expiratory volume in one second; *FVC,* forced vital capacity; *OTC,* over-the-counter; *PEFR,* peak expiratory flow rate; *RV,* residual volume; *SaO₂,* arterial oxygen saturation.

NURSING CARE PLAN 31-2

Chronic Obstructive Pulmonary Disease (COPD)

NURSING DIAGNOSIS	***Ineffective airway clearance*** *related to* expiratory airflow obstruction, ineffective cough, increased mucus production, decreased cilia, and infection in airways, *as evidenced by* the presence of abnormal breath sounds (wheeze) or absence of breath sounds and dyspnea
Expected Patient Outcomes	**Nursing Interventions and *Rationales***
• Has normal breath sounds for patient	• Facilitate deep breathing by sitting patient up *to maximize use of diaphragm and prolong expiratory phase.*
• Demonstrates effective coughing	• Ensure adequate hydration (oral intake approximately 2-3 L/day, humidified ambient air) *to liquefy secretions for easier expectoration.*
• Reports decreased dyspnea	
• Maintains clear airway	• Teach effective cough techniques *to minimize the extent of airway collapse and to enhance airway clearance.*
	• Assist with inhaled bronchodilator administration *to facilitate clearance of retained secretions.*

NURSING CARE PLAN 31-2

Chronic Obstructive Pulmonary Disease (COPD)—cont'd

NURSING DIAGNOSIS	*Impaired gas exchange* related to alveolar hypoventilation, *as evidenced by* headache on awakening, $PaCO_2 \geq 45$ mm Hg and abnormal for patient's baseline, $PaO_2 < 60$ mm Hg, or $SaO_2 < 90\%$ at rest
Expected Patient Outcomes	**Nursing Interventions and *Rationales***
• Has $PaCO_2$ of 35-45 mm Hg or usual compensated baseline value • Experiences return of PaO_2 to normal range for patient • Reports improved mental status • Reports decreased dyspnea • Performs ADLs	• Monitor respiratory and oxygenation status *to assess need for intervention.* • Teach pursed-lip breathing *to prolong expiratory phase and slow respiratory rate.* • Assist patient to assume position of comfort (e.g., tripod position, elevated back rest, support of upper extremities to fix shoulder girdle) *to maximize respiratory excursion.* • Administer and teach appropriate use of bronchodilators *to open the airways.* • Teach signs, symptoms, and consequences of hypercapnia (e.g., confusion, somnolence, headache, irritability, decrease in mental acuity, increase in respiration, facial flush, diaphoresis) *to recognize problem early and initiate treatment.* • Teach avoidance of central nervous system depressants *because they further depress respirations.* • Administer O_2 if appropriate *to increase SaO_2 saturation.* • Select O_2 supply systems and devices (e.g., nasal cannula, mask) that are appropriate for patient's ADLs (rest, sleep, exercise) *to minimize effect on preferred lifestyle.*
NURSING DIAGNOSIS	*Imbalanced nutrition: less than body requirements* related to poor appetite, lowered energy level, shortness of breath, gastric distension, sputum production, and depression, *as evidenced by* weight loss of >10% of ideal body weight, serum albumin level below normal laboratory values, or lack of interest in food
Expected Patient Outcomes	**Nursing Interventions and *Rationales***
• Maintains body weight within normal range for sex, height, and age • Has normal serum protein and albumin levels	• Monitor caloric intake, weight, and serum albumin and protein *to determine adequacy of intake.* • Provide menu suggestions for high-protein, high-calorie foods *to ensure maintenance of weight.* • Give patient high-protein, high-calorie liquid supplements if necessary *to provide adequate calories and protein to prevent weight loss and muscle wasting.* • Plan periods of rest before and after food intake *to assist with controlling fatigue and to compensate for blood flow diversion to the gastrointestinal tract for digestion.* • Refer to agency for financial or nutritional assistance as necessary (e.g., Meals-On-Wheels, home care) *to ensure nutritional adequacy after discharge.* • Discuss benefit of five to six small meals throughout the day *because this reduces bloating.*
NURSING DIAGNOSIS	*Disturbed sleep pattern* related to dyspnea, depression, anxiety, hypoxemia, or hypercapnia, *as evidenced by* insomnia, lethargy, fatigue, restlessness, irritability, orthopnea, or paroxysmal nocturnal dyspnea
Expected Patient Outcomes	**Nursing Interventions and *Rationales***
• Sleeps at least 5 hr over a 24-hr period • Reports improved sleep pattern • Reports feeling rejuvenated on awakening	• Identify usual sleep habits and elicit reasons for difficulty sleeping *to provide baseline data.* • Monitor patient's sleep pattern, and note physical circumstances (e.g., pain or discomfort and urinary frequency) and psychological circumstances (e.g., fear or anxiety) that interrupt sleep *to initiate appropriate interventions.* • Observe for signs and symptoms of sleep apnea such as frequent awakenings at night, excessive daytime sleepiness, or a partner that complains of the patient's snoring or gasping for air *to initiate appropriate diagnostic tests and interventions.* • Identify patient-specific methods of relaxation, and teach patient relaxation methods *to foster sleep.* • Encourage exercise and activity during daylight hours *to ensure improved sleep at night.* • Provide patient with activity that promotes wakefulness *to limit daytime sleep.* • Instruct patient in arranging surroundings (e.g., clothing, temperature, position, noise level) *to produce an environment conducive to sleep.* • Teach patient to avoid alcoholic beverages, caffeine products, or other stimulants before bedtime *to reduce interference with sleep.*

Continued

NURSING CARE PLAN 31-2

Chronic Obstructive Pulmonary Disease (COPD)—cont'd

NURSING DIAGNOSIS	**_Risk for infection_** _related to_ increased mucus production and ciliary dyskinesia and denudation, possible corticosteroid therapy, and lack of knowledge regarding signs and symptoms of infection and preventive measures, _as evidenced by_ signs and symptoms of an exacerbation
Expected Patient Outcomes	**Nursing Interventions and _Rationales_**
• Uses behaviours that minimize risk of infection • Experiences fewer or no respiratory infections	• Monitor for systemic and localized signs and symptoms of infection _to determine whether an infection is present._ • Teach patient to assess indicators of infection: change in sputum colour, quantity, odour, and viscosity; increase in cough and dyspnea; experience of fever, chills, diaphoresis, excessive fatigue; increase in respiratory rate; and abnormal breath sounds (gurgles, wheezing) _to determine whether an infection is present._ • Teach patient to use good handwashing and hygiene techniques and to avoid contact (when possible) with people with respiratory infections _to minimize sources of infection._ • Encourage patient to obtain vaccination for influenza and pneumococcal pneumonia _to decrease occurrence or severity of influenza or pneumonia._ • Teach proper care and cleaning of home respiratory equipment _to eliminate this source of infection._ • Instruct patient to seek medical attention for manifestations of early infection _to initiate treatment promptly._ • Teach patient to follow plan of care for managing exacerbations (e.g., increase fluid intake, initiate antibiotics and oral corticosteroid) _to initiate appropriate self-care promptly._

ADLs, activities of daily living; _PaCO₂,_ partial pressure of arterial carbon dioxide; _PaO₂,_ partial pressure of arterial oxygen; _SaO₂,_ arterial oxygen saturation.

▪ Planning

Overall goals for patients with COPD include (a) the prevention of disease progression, (b) the ability to perform ADLs, (c) relief from breathlessness and other respiratory symptoms, (d) improvement in exercise tolerance, (e) the prevention and treatment of exacerbations, (f) improved overall quality of life, and (g) reduction in premature mortality.

▪ Nursing Implementation

▪ Health Promotion

The best prevention for COPD is never to smoke, and the next best step is to stop smoking immediately. (See section on nursing management of lung cancer in Chapter 30.) Avoiding or controlling exposure to occupational and environmental pollutants and irritants is another preventive measure to maintain healthy lungs. (These factors are discussed in the section on environmental lung diseases in Chapter 30.) Early detection of airway disease is important and is the rationale for the use of spirometry or pulmonary function tests. Early identification and treatment of respiratory tract infections is important for improving the long-term prognosis of COPD. Avoiding exposure to large crowds in the peak influenza periods may be necessary, especially for older adults and patients with a history of respiratory problems. Patients should also be taught good handwashing technique, to avoid sharing food and drinks, and to keep their hands away from their nose, mouth, and ears. Influenza and pneumococcal pneumonia vaccinations are recommended.

Families with a history of both COPD and AAT deficiency should be aware of the genetic nature of the disease. Genetic counselling may be appropriate for patients and their families with a history of AAT deficiency.

▪ Education

An important aspect in the long-term care of the patient with COPD is education (Table 31-22). (Patient teaching is discussed in Chapter 4.) One component of education may involve preparation of an advance care plan (see the Ethical Dilemmas box on p. 753).

▪ Exercise

Walking is by far the best physical exercise for the patient with COPD. Coordinated walking with slow, pursed-lip breathing without breath holding is a difficult task that requires conscious effort and frequent reinforcement. During coordinated walking and breathing, the patient is taught to breathe in through the nose while taking one step, then to breathe out through pursed lips while taking two to four steps (the number depends on a patient's tolerance). Walking should occur at a slow pace with rest periods when necessary. Many patients need to sit or lean against an object such as a tree or post. If a patient has been prescribed supplemental oxygen, he or she needs to use oxygen while walking or exercising. Walking with the patient helps decrease anxiety and helps maintain an appropriate pace. It also enables the nurse to observe the patient's actions and physiological responses to the activity. Many patients with moderate or severe COPD are anxious and fearful of walking or performing exercise. These patients and their families require much support while they build the confidence they need to walk or to perform daily exercises (Cicutto & Brooks, 2006).

Patients should be encouraged to walk 15 to 20 minutes a day and gradually increase this time. Patients can begin at a

PATIENT & CAREGIVER TEACHING GUIDE

Table 31-22 Chronic Obstructive Pulmonary Disease

Goal: To assist patient and caregivers in improving quality of life through education and to promote lifestyle practices that support successful living with chronic obstructive pulmonary disease (COPD).

TEACHING TOPIC	STRATEGIES AND RESOURCES
• Overall guide to COPD, including topics listed below	Global Initiative for Chronic Obstructive Lung Disease (GOLD): *Patient guide: What you can do about a lung disease called COPD*, available at http://www.goldcopd.org
	Canadian Lung Association: The Breathworks Plan: toll-free helpline at 1-866-717-COPD (2673)
	Living Well With COPD program: available online (see the Resources at the end of this chapter)
	Bailey et al. (2010): *Nursing care of dyspnea: The 6th vital sign in individuals with chronic obstructive pulmonary disease (COPD)*, available online (see references)
What is COPD?	
• Basic anatomy and physiology of lung	Models and posters of the lungs
• Basic pathophysiological changes of COPD	
• Signs and symptoms of COPD, exacerbations, cold, flu, pneumonia	
• Tests to assess breathing	
Nonpharmacological Therapy	
• Breathing exercises	Demonstration and return demonstration
• Pursed-lip breathing	RNAO dyspnea guidelines
• Relaxation techniques	Developing and using a schedule of daily and weekly activities
• Energy conservation techniques	Pulmonary rehabilitation program
Pacing and planning throughout the day for ADLs (pacing activity and using pursed-lip breathing with activities)	
• Regular exercise (upper and lower extremity)	
• Smoking cessation	See Chapter 11
	Smoking cessation guidelines for nurses (e.g., the RNAO's Best Practice Guideline *Integrating Smoking Cessation into Daily Practice*); Quit smoking helplines

TEACHING TOPIC	STRATEGIES AND RESOURCES
Medications	
Types (include mechanism of action)	Written medication list and schedule
• β_2-adrenergic agonists	Having patients explain purpose of the medication and show the medication they are referring to
• Anticholinergics	
• Corticosteroids	Knowing the various colours of the inhalers because patients typically refer to them by colour
• Methylxanthines	
• Phosphodiesterase 4 inhibitor	
• Antibiotics	
Review medication schedule and indications for use	
Adverse drug events	
Correct Use of Inhalation Devices	
• Metered-dose inhalers with and without spacers	See Figures 31-5 and 31-6
• Dry powder inhalers	Canadian Lung Association
	• Handouts
	• DVD: Inhalation Devices: Techniques and Procedures
	Placebo and demonstration units (provided by pharmaceutical companies) to assist with hands-on training
	Having patients demonstrate inhaler technique, and providing feedback about technique
	Checking periodically to ensure maintenance of proper technique
	Repeating process until accurate technique is demonstrated
	Exploring alternative delivery devices for patients who cannot demonstrate accurate technique
Home Oxygen	
• Explain need for O_2	Canadian Lung Association Web site (see Resources)
• Explain equipment and rationale for use	See Tables 31-17 through 31-19
• Guide for home O_2 and ambulatory use	
• Care of oxygen equipment	
Psychosocial/Emotional Issues	
Concerns about interpersonal relationships	Canadian Lung Association Web site (see Resources at the end of this chapter)
• Dependency	Open discussion (sharing with patient, significant other, and family)
• Intimacy	
Emotional difficulties	Exploring idea of attending social support groups or speaking to another person with COPD
• Depression	
• Anxiety and panic	
Treatment decisions	
• Support and rehabilitation groups	

Continued

PATIENT & CAREGIVER TEACHING GUIDE

Table 31-22 Chronic Obstructive Pulmonary Disease—cont'd

TEACHING TOPIC	STRATEGIES AND RESOURCES	TEACHING TOPIC	STRATEGIES AND RESOURCES
COPD Management Plan		**Healthy Nutrition**	
• Focus on self-management • Need for a written action plan • Monitoring signs and symptoms • Reporting changes in symptoms • Causes of flares or exacerbations • Recognition of signs and symptoms of respiration infection, heart failure • Reduce the number of risk factors, especially smoking • Pulmonary rehabilitation program • Yearly follow-up	COPD management plan, developed and agreed upon by nurse and patient, that meets individual needs Assessment of patient's confidence level in managing COPD, and enhancement of skill development and confidence as necessary	• Strategies to lose weight (if patient is overweight) • Strategies to gain weight (if patient is underweight)	Consultation with dietitian
		End-of-Life and Advance Planning	
		• Identifying concerns and preferences for end-of-life care • Support problem solving, decision making, and planning	End-of-life planning module in the Living Well With COPD program (see the Resources at the end of this chapter) Open discussion (health care team, patient, and family)

slower pace by walking for 2 to 5 minutes three times a day and slowly building up to 20 minutes a day, if possible. Adequate rest periods should be allowed. Some patients benefit from using a SABA (see Table 31-7) approximately 10 minutes before exercise. Parameters to monitor with exercise include resting pulse and pulse rate after activity. Pulse rate after exercise should not exceed 75 to 80% of the maximum heart rate (maximum heart rate = 220 − Age in years). Dyspnea is usually the limiting factor, rather than increased heart rate, for exercise; therefore, the patient's perceived sense of dyspnea should be used as an indication of exercise tolerance. The patient can use the MRC scale (see Figure 31-11) to determine the intensity of dyspnea.

Patients should be informed that shortness of breath often increases during exercise (as it does for a healthy individual). The activity is not being overdone unless the increased dyspnea does not return to baseline within 5 minutes after the cessation of exercise. Patients should wait about 5 minutes after completion of exercise, and if the dyspnea has not returned to baseline levels, then a SABA should be used. During the recovery time, slow, pursed-lip breathing should be used. If dyspnea takes longer than 5 minutes to return to baseline levels, the patient has probably overdone the exercise and should proceed at a slower pace during the next exercise period. Keeping a diary or log of the exercise program may be beneficial. Diaries provide a realistic evaluation of progress, help motivate, and add to a sense of accomplishment. Stationary bicycles and treadmills can also be used and are particularly valuable when weather prevents walking outside.

Energy-Conserving Strategies. Energy conservation is another important component in COPD rehabilitation. Exercise training of the upper extremities improves function and reduces dyspnea. Many patients have already adapted alternative energy-saving practices for ADLs. Alternative or modified methods of hair care, shaving, showering, and other activities that necessitate over-the-head reaching must be explored. Assuming a tripod posture (elbows supported on a table, chest in fixed position) and

placing a mirror on the table while using an electric razor or hair dryer conserves energy in comparison with standing in front of a mirror to perform these activities. If the patient uses home oxygen therapy, it must be used during activities of hygiene because these activities consume energy. Another energy-saving tip is to exhale when pushing, pulling, or exerting effort during an activity and to inhale during rest. Patients should also try to sit as much as possible when performing activities.

Sexual Activity. Modifying but not abstaining from sexual activity can contribute to a feeling of well-being. Using a SABA before sexual activity can help control dyspnea. Patients with COPD also need less energy if these guidelines are followed: (a) have sexual activity during the part of the day when breathing is best, (b) use slow pursed-lip breathing, (c) refrain from sexual activity after eating or other strenuous activity, (d) do not assume a dominant position, and (e) do not prolong foreplay. These aspects of sexual activity require open communication between partners regarding their needs and expectations and the changes that may be necessary as the result of a chronic disease (e.g., changes in body image, role reversal).

Sleep. Adequate sleep is extremely important. Getting adequate amounts of sleep can be difficult for patients with COPD. Medications may cause restlessness and insomnia. If patients experience cough during the night, the use of long-acting bronchodilators may help. Postnasal drip may cause coughing at night and can be treated with nasal saline sprays or rinses or nasal steroids, or both, before sleep and in the morning. If a patient snores, stops breathing, or makes gasping breaths while sleeping and has a tendency to fall asleep during the day, the patient may need to be tested for sleep apnea (see Chapter 29).

Psychosocial Considerations. Healthy coping is often challenging for patients with COPD. Such patients frequently have to deal with many lifestyle changes that may involve a decreased ability to care for themselves and their condition, decreased energy for performing day-to-day activities and social activities, and the loss of a job.

When a patient first receives a diagnosis of COPD or experiences complications, the nurse should expect a variety of emotional responses. Emotions frequently encountered include guilt, depression, anxiety, social isolation, denial, and dependence. Guilt may result from the knowledge that the disease was caused largely by cigarette smoking. The patient may experience depression as he or she realizes the severity and chronicity of the disease. The nurse should convey a sense of understanding and caring to the patient. Relaxation techniques may provide benefit in terms of relief of dyspnea for some patients, but the evidence for this is unclear. Relaxation techniques include progressive muscular relaxation, positive thinking and visualization, use of music, yoga, massage, and humour (see Chapters 8 and 12; Bailey et al., 2010). Progressive relaxation techniques are performed by having the patient listen to music, or to his or her own or another voice, and then gradually begin to slowly tense and relax muscle groups. Have the patient start with the toes and work all the way up to the scalp. Support groups at local Canadian Lung Associations, hospitals, and clinics can also be helpful.

▮ **End-of-Life Issues.** Nurses have a responsibility to discuss with and plan for end-of-life care with patients and their families or caregivers to make sure that the necessary supports are in place to assist them through this critical terminal phase. Patients, their families, and health care providers should be involved in writing advance directives. Nurses must explore and understand the issues facing patients and their families through empathic, honest, and informative conversations. Discussions that highlight the importance of palliative care services and alleviation of terminal dyspnea lessen anticipatory fear and anxiety. The Ethical Dilemmas box discusses advance directives.

▮ Evaluation

The expected outcomes for the patient with COPD are presented in Nursing Care Plan 31-2.

Cystic Fibrosis

Cystic fibrosis (CF) is an autosomal recessive, multisystem disease characterized by altered function of the exocrine glands involving primarily the lungs, the pancreas, and the sweat glands (Boyle, 2007). (Autosomal recessive disorders are discussed in Chapter 15.) Abnormally thick, abundant secretions from mucous glands leads to a chronic, diffuse, obstructive pulmonary disorder in almost all patients. Exocrine pancreatic insufficiency is associated with most cases of CF. Sweat glands excrete increased amounts of sodium and chloride.

A chronic fatal respiratory disease, CF is the most common genetic disease among White people in Canada (PHAC, 2007). According to the Canadian Cystic Fibrosis Patient Data Registry, more than 3800 Canadians have cystic fibrosis, and the numbers of male and female patients are roughly equal (Cystic Fibrosis Canada, 2010). The disease occurs primarily in White people, with a frequency of 1 per 2000 births. This autosomal recessive disease has a carrier rate of 1 per 25. If both parents carry the gene, the chance that their offspring will have the disease is 25%. The first signs and symptoms typically occur in early childhood,

---

ETHICAL DILEMMAS
Advance Directives

Situation

A 79-year-old man with chronic obstructive pulmonary disease is admitted to the hospital in respiratory failure. He is placed on a ventilator and responds occasionally by opening his eyes. His living will was written 5 years ago, and a copy was given to his wife and health care provider at that time. The wife brings the document to the critical care unit and tells the nurse that the hospital must stop treating her husband and allow him to die as he requested. However, the oldest son is threatening the hospital with a lawsuit if the staff does not provide full care to his father.

Important Points for Consideration

- A living will is one type of an advance directive.
- A living will is prepared by the person in advance, indicating the person's treatment wishes should he or she become terminally ill or in a situation in which there is no hope of recovery.
- Health care providers must determine whether this respiratory crisis is reversible.
- Power of attorney for health care is another form of advance directive in which one person names another person to make health care decisions in the event that the first person is no longer able to do so.
- An advance directive respects the patient's autonomy: that is, the right to self-determination regarding health care at the end of life.
- A legally written living will is legally binding.
- Health care providers are obligated to follow the patient's advance directive when the patient is no longer able to speak for himself or herself.
- Health care providers are protected from liability when they adhere to advance directives.

Clinical Decision-Making Questions

1. What should the nurse do next with the information provided by the wife?
2. How should the nurse address the needs of each member of this family in the patient's plan of care?
3. What resources can the nurse use to facilitate decision making in this situation?

---

and in most patients, the disease is diagnosed by the age of 5 years. However, some patients tend to have less severe disease, and their cases are not diagnosed until they are adults.

The severity and the progression of the disease vary from person to person. In the past two decades, the prognosis of this disease has improved dramatically as a result of early diagnosis and improvements in therapy. In 1998, 81% of patients with CF lived at least to the age of 20 years, in comparison with 46% just 10 years earlier. The biggest changes were an increase in life span past age 40, and a decrease in deaths before age 10 (PHAC, 2007). Of the 40 patients with CF that died in Canada in 2010, half were over 26 years old (Cystic Fibrosis Canada, 2012) and the median age of survival for Canadians with CF is currently estimated to be 48.1 years of age (Cystic Fibrosis Canada, 2010). The biggest changes were an increase in life span past age 40 and a decrease in deaths before age 10 (PHAC, 2007).

Etiology and Pathophysiology

CF results from mutations in a gene located on chromosome 7. The most common genetic mutation in CF occurs in what is known as the cystic fibrosis transmembrane regulator (CFTR) gene. The CFTR protein localizes to the lining of the exocrine portion of particular organs such as airways, pancreatic duct, sweat gland duct, and reproductive tract. The CFTR gene regulates sodium and chloride channels. Mutations in the CFTR gene alter this protein in such a way that the channels are blocked (Yankaskas, 2004). As a result, cells that line the passages of the lungs, the pancreas, and other organs produce abnormally thick, sticky mucus. This mucus obstructs the airways and glands. The glands distal to the duct eventually undergo fibrosis. The high concentrations of sodium and chloride in the sweat of the patient with CF result from decreased chloride resorption in the sweat duct.

In the respiratory system, both upper and lower respiratory tracts can be affected. Upper respiratory tract manifestations include chronic sinusitis and nasal polyposis. The hallmark of respiratory involvement in CF is its effect on the airways. From being a disease of the small airways (chronic bronchiolitis), CF progresses to an entity that eventually involves the larger airways and finally causes destruction of lung tissue. Thick secretions obstruct bronchioles and lead to air trapping and hyperinflation of the lungs. The stasis of mucus provides an excellent growth medium for bacteria, making the airways more susceptible to serious lower respiratory tract infections. CF is thus characterized by chronic airway infection. The most common organisms cultured from the sputum of a patient with CF are *Staphylococcus aureus, H. influenzae,* and *P. aeruginosa* (Flume et al., 2009). These infections increase the rate of lung destruction through inflammatory mediators such as interleukins, tumour necrosis factor, and leukotrienes.

Lung disorders that can result from this pathological process include pneumonia, bronchiolitis, bronchitis, bronchiectasis, atelectasis, and emphysema. Lung tissue is progressively destroyed by inflammation and scarring, and the resultant chronic hypoxia leads to pulmonary hypertension and cor pulmonale. Blebs and large cysts in the lung are further severe manifestations of lung destruction. Other pulmonary complications include hemoptysis, which can sometimes be fatal, and pneumothorax. The degree of hemoptysis may range from scant streaking to major bleeding.

Initially, CF is an obstructive lung disease caused by the overall obstruction of the airways with mucus. Later, CF also progresses to a restrictive lung disease because of the fibrosis, lung destruction, and thoracic wall changes. Death usually results from loss of pulmonary function. Cor pulmonale is a common late complication caused by extensive loss of lung tissue and chronic hypoxia.

Pancreatic insufficiency is caused primarily by mucous plugging of the pancreatic duct and its branches, which results in fibrosis of the acinar glands of the pancreas and leads to the loss of exocrine function. Pancreatic enzymes such as trypsinogen, lipase, and amylase do not reach the intestine to digest ingested nutrients. Fat, protein, and fat-soluble vitamins (vitamins A, D, E, and K) are malabsorbed. Fat malabsorption results in steatorrhea, and protein malabsorption results in malnutrition, failure to grow, and failure to gain weight.

Diabetes mellitus may occur if the islets of Langerhans become fibrotic. CF-related diabetes mellitus affects approximately 15% of all patients with CF. It differs from type 1 diabetes in that some insulin is secreted, it is nonketotic, and it is slow in onset. It differs from type 2 diabetes in that individuals are underweight (as opposed to being obese), the onset is in a younger age population, and the individual is hypoinsulinemic. Routine screening of serum glucose levels is recommended. Insulin may be required for treatment of CF-related diabetes.

The sweat glands of the patient with CF secrete normal volumes of sweat but are unable to absorb sodium and chloride from sweat as it moves through the sweat duct. Therefore, these patients excrete four times the normal amount of sodium and chloride in sweat. This abnormality does not seem to affect the general health of the person, but it is useful as a diagnostic indicator.

Individuals with CF often have gastrointestinal problems. Intestinal obstruction resulting in meconium ileus is seen in newborns with CF. However, GERD, distal intestinal obstructive syndrome (DIOS), and constipation are common. GERD is a major problem in individuals with CF. The relationship between reflux and exacerbation of respiratory disease is not known, but it is known that these two entities enhance each other.

DIOS is a syndrome that results from intermittent obstruction in the ileocecal area in patients with pancreatic insufficiency. The degree to which the bowel is obstructed may vary with each episode, and a partial obstruction may progress to a complete obstruction. Complete obstruction necessitates gastric decompression and a surgical consultation; partial and uncomplicated episodes of DIOS are treated with ingestion of a balanced polyethylene glycol electrolyte solution. Constipation develops in the sigmoid colon and progresses proximally, whereas DIOS develops in the ileocecal area and progresses distally. Careful monitoring of bowel habits and patterns is essential.

The liver may become involved. Biliary cirrhosis may not be recognized until late in the disease. Hepatobiliary disease is common in adult patients with CF. Chronic cholestasis, inflammation, fibrosis, and portal hypertension can occur.

Clinical Manifestations

The clinical manifestations of CF vary depending on the severity of the disease. Meconium ileus is present in 10 to 15% of newborns with CF. Early childhood manifestations are failure to grow, digital clubbing, persistent cough with mucus production, tachypnea, and large, frequent bowel movements. The abdomen may become large and protuberant, and the extremities may develop an emaciated appearance.

The first symptom of CF in the adult is frequently cough. With time, the cough becomes persistent and produces viscous, purulent, and often greenish sputum. Other respiratory problems that may be indicative of CF are recurring lung infections such as bronchiolitis, bronchitis, and pneumonia. As the disease progresses, periods of clinical stability are interrupted by exacerbations characterized by increased cough and sputum production, weight loss, and decreases in pulmonary function. Over time, the exacerbations become more frequent and lost lung function is less completely recovered, which ultimately leads to respiratory failure.

DIOS causes pain in the right lower quadrant, loss of appetite, and emesis, and a mass is often palpable. Insufficient pancreatic enzyme release causes the typical pattern of protein and fat malabsorption with frequent, bulky, foul-smelling stools.

The function of the reproductive system is altered. This finding is important because increasing numbers of people with CF are living to adulthood. Nearly all men with CF have reproductive issues because they have congenital absence of the vas deferens, which transports the sperm from the storage in the testes to the penile urethra. However, they make sperm normally and thus, with assisted reproductive technology, have the capability of fathering a child. In women with CF, menarche is usually delayed. During exacerbations, menstrual irregularities and secondary amenorrhea are fairly common. Affected women may be unable to become pregnant because of the increased viscosity of the cervical mucus. Many women with CF do have children, but the fertility rate is lower than among healthy women (Hodges, Palmert, & Drumm, 2008). The baby of such a patient is heterozygous for CF (and hence a carrier of the CFTR gene) if the father is not a carrier. If the father is a carrier, the baby has a 50% chance of having CF. Genetic counselling can assist couples in deciding whether they want to have children and whether they want to use assisted reproductive technology to have a baby without the risk of CF. Screening of newborns can identify who will develop CF. Debate about the usefulness of this technology continues. (See Chapter 15, Figures 15-7 and 15-8, for an explanation of genetic transmission of CF.)

Complications

Pneumothorax is common among patients with CF, occurring in 3.4% of patients overall (Flume et al., 2005). The presence of small amounts of blood in the sputum is common in patients with CF who have lung infection. Massive hemoptysis is life-threatening. With advanced lung disease, digital clubbing becomes evident. Respiratory failure and cor pulmonale are late complications of CF.

Diagnostic Studies

Diagnostic criteria for CF are evidence of CFTR protein malfunction assessed by the sweat chloride test and characteristic respiratory or gastrointestinal symptoms. The sweat chloride test is performed with the pilocarpine iontophoresis method, which yields abnormal results in more than 90% of adults with CF. Pilocarpine carried by a small electric current is used to stimulate sweat production. The sweat is collected on filter paper or gauze and then analyzed for sodium and chloride concentrations. The test takes approximately 40 to 60 minutes. Values higher than 65 mEq/L for both sodium and chloride are suggestive of CF, especially in a person who has other clinical features of the disease. A second sweat chloride test is recommended to confirm the diagnosis unless two CF mutations have been identified by genetic testing (Farrell et al., 2008). The degree of sodium and chloride elevation is not necessarily correlated with the severity of the disease. Other diagnostic studies include chest radiography, pulmonary function tests, fecal analysis for fat, and duodenoscopy for quantitative determination of pancreatic enzymes.

Because of the large number of CF mutations, DNA analysis is not used for the primary diagnostic test. DNA analysis does, however, corroborate the diagnosis. Fetal diagnosis can be performed from specimens obtained by amniocentesis or chorionic villus sampling.

Collaborative Care

A multidisciplinary team should be involved in patients' care and should include nurses, physicians, respiratory and physical therapists, dietitians, pharmacists, and social workers. The major objectives of therapy in CF are to (a) promote clearance of secretions, (b) control infection in the lungs, and (c) provide adequate nutrition. Management of pulmonary problems in CF is directed at relieving airway obstruction and controlling infection. Drain-

age of thick bronchial mucus is assisted by aerosol and nebulized forms of medications to liquefy mucus and to facilitate coughing. The abnormal viscosity of CF secretions results primarily from mucus glycoproteins and DNA from degenerated neutrophils. Agents that degrade the high concentrations of DNA in CF sputum (e.g., DNase [Pulmozyme]) decrease sputum viscosity and increase airflow. Bronchodilators (e.g., β_2-adrenergic agonists, theophylline), hypertonic saline, and mucolytic agents may be used (Flume et al., 2007).

Airway clearance techniques are critical in reducing mucus. These techniques include chest physiotherapy (CPT), postural drainage, and positive expiratory pressure breathing. **Chest physiotherapy** consists of percussion, vibration, and postural drainage. Percussion and vibration are manual or mechanical techniques used to augment postural drainage. In **postural drainage,** the principle of gravity is used to assist in bronchial clearance (Figure 31-16). Percussion and vibration are used after the patient has assumed a postural drainage position to assist in loosening the mobilized secretions. Percussion, vibration, and postural drainage may assist in bringing secretions into larger, more central airways. Effective coughing is then necessary to help raise these secretions. After each drainage position change, the patient should be given time to cough and breathe deeply. These techniques are individualized on the basis of the patient's pulmonary condition and response to the initial treatment. Sometimes it takes several hours after CPT for secretions to be expectorated. It is important to evaluate the effectiveness of CPT and its relief of symptoms; a physiotherapist who is trained in the proper technique often performs CPT. Complications associated with improperly performed CPT include fractured ribs, bruising, hypoxemia, and discomfort. CPT may not be beneficial and can be stressful for some patients. Some patients may develop hypoxemia and bronchospasm with CPT.

The Flutter mucus clearance device is also effective in promoting mucus removal (Figure 31-17). It is a handheld device that provides positive expiratory pressure. The Flutter valve works by (a) causing the airways to vibrate, which loosens mucus from airway walls; (b) intermittently increasing the endobronchial pressure, which helps maintain the patency of the airway; and (c) accelerating expiratory airflow. It helps move mucus up through the airways to the mouth, where the mucus can be expectorated.

It is important to work collaboratively with families and patients because individuals with CF may have a preference for a certain technique that works well for them. Aerobic exercise seems to be effective in clearing the airways. Important needs to consider in planning an aerobic exercise program for a patient with CF are (a) frequent rest periods interspersed throughout the exercise regimen, (b) meeting increased nutritional demands of exercise, (c) being alert for manifestations of hyperthermia, and (d) drinking large amounts of fluid and replacing salt losses.

Most CF patients die of complications resulting from lung infection. Antimicrobial treatment is used for prophylaxis and early treatment of infections (Flume et al., 2007). For patients who have moderate to severe lung disease and whose sputum cultures persistently manifest *P. aeruginosa,* the chronic use of inhaled tobramycin can improve lung function and reduce the frequency of exacerbations. The use of antibiotics is often guided by sputum culture results. Early intervention with antibiotics is important, and long courses of antibiotics are the usual treatment (Smyth & Tan, 2006). Prolonged high-dosage therapy may be necessary because many drugs are abnormally metabolized and rapidly excreted in patients with CF. Results of pharmacokinetic and kidney function studies should be monitored closely. Oral

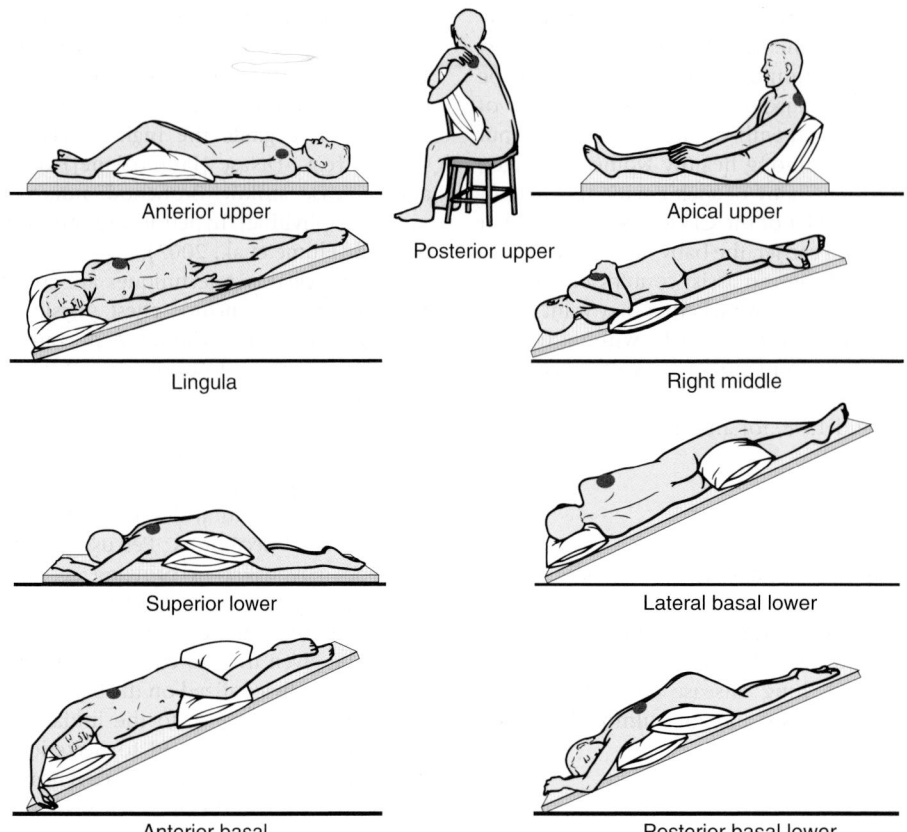

Figure 31-16 Representative positions for postural drainage. *Shaded areas* in each illustration indicate the segment of the lung in which drainage is promoted.

agents commonly used are trimethoprim-sulphamethoxazole, tetracycline, chloramphenicol, cephalosporins, antistaphylococcal penicillins, and oral quinolones, especially ciprofloxacin.

Although oral and aerosolized antimicrobial therapy is usually adequate, some patients require a 2- to 4-week course of IV antimicrobial therapy. If home care supports are adequate, the patient and family may choose parenteral therapy at home. The usual treatment for an acute infectious exacerbation is either an aminoglycoside combined with penicillin or a third-generation cephalosporin. Aerosolized bronchodilators may be used in selected patients, particularly before CPT. Patients with cor pulmonale or hypoxemia may require oxygen therapy. (Oxygen therapy is discussed earlier in this chapter.) Sclerosing of the pleural space or partial pleural stripping and pleural abrasion performed surgically are usually indicated for recurrent episodes of pneumothorax. (See the section on collaborative care of pleural effusions in Chapter 30.)

CF has become a leading indication for bilateral lung transplantation, accounting for 32% of these operations. In 2009, 44 people with cystic fibrosis—a number that had doubled since 10 years earlier (Cystic Fibrosis Canada, 2011)—received bilateral lung transplants. (Lung transplantation is discussed in Chapter 30.) Lung transplantation for people with CF has resulted in significant improvements in pulmonary function and quality of life, as well as longer life expectancy. The rate of survival after lung transplantation is higher for people with CF than for those with other pulmonary diseases such as COPD. The survival rate is 87% at 1 year, and 89% of those at 5 years. Recent cost estimates for the initial hospitalization for lung transplantation range from C$100,000 to C$150,000 (PHAC, 2007).

The management of pancreatic insufficiency includes pancreatic enzyme replacement of lipase, protease, and amylase (e.g., pancrelipase [Cotazym, Creon, Ultrase, Viokase] and zymase, an enzyme complex) administered before each meal and snack. A high-calorie, high-protein diet and multivitamin supplementation are recommended. Fat restriction usually is not necessary. Fat-soluble vitamin supplementation (vitamins A, D, E, and K) is necessary. Use of caloric supplements improves nutritional status. Added dietary salt is indicated whenever sweating is excessive, such as during hot weather, in the presence of fever, or from intense physical activity.

Gene therapy has been used as an experimental therapy for treating CF, but more research is still required (Mitomo et al., 2010). (Gene therapy is discussed in Chapter 15.)

NURSING MANAGEMENT: CYSTIC FIBROSIS

▪ Nursing Assessment

Subjective and objective data that should be obtained from the patient with cystic fibrosis are presented in Table 31-23.

▪ Nursing Diagnoses

Nursing diagnoses for the patient with CF may include, but are not limited to, the following:

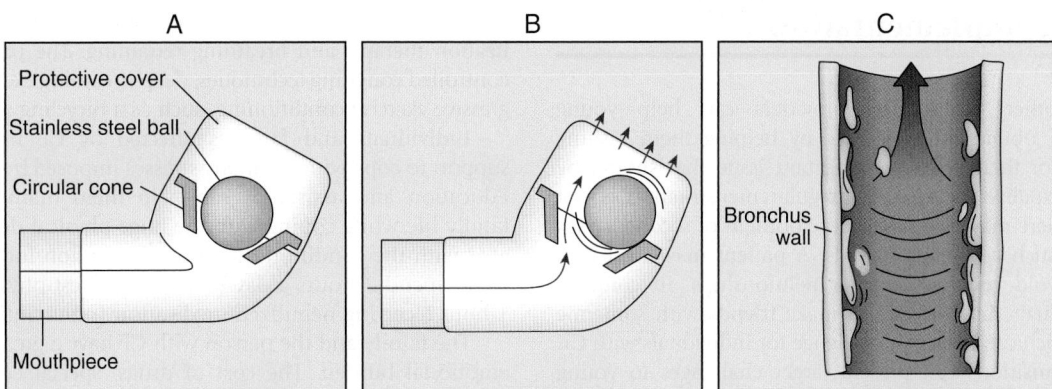

Figure 31-17 The Flutter mucus clearance device is a small, handheld device that provides positive expiratory pressure therapy. It is used to facilitate removal of mucus from the lungs. **A,** It consists of a hard plastic mouthpiece, a plastic perforated cover, and a high-density stainless steel ball resting in a circular cone. **B,** The Flutter effect occurs during expiration. Before exhalation, the steel ball blocks the conical canal of the Flutter. During exhalation, the position the steel ball occupies is the result of equilibrium between the pressure of the exhaled air, the force of gravity on the ball, and the angle of the cone where the contact with the ball occurs. As the steel ball rolls and moves up and down, it creates an opening-and-closing cycle that repeats itself many times throughout each exhalation. The net result is that vibrations occur in the airways, resulting in the "fluttering" sensation. **C,** These vibrations loosen mucus from the airway walls and facilitate its movement up the airways.

Source: Axcan Scandipharm, Inc., Birmingham, Alabama.

NURSING ASSESSMENT

Table 31-23 Cystic Fibrosis (CF)

Subjective Data	*Objective Data*
Important Health Information	**General**
Present health: Experience of cough and mucus production (quantity, colour, consistency), dyspnea, and wheeze	Restlessness, failure to thrive
	Integumentary
Past health history: Past respiratory and sinus infections: typical pattern, how treated, how responded to treatment; past hospitalizations and emergency department visits; when CF was diagnosed; family history of CF	Cyanosis (circumoral, nail beds), digital clubbing, salty skin
	Eyes
	Scleral icterus
Medications: Use of bronchodilators, antibiotics, enzymes, herbs, and complementary therapies; adverse effects experienced; and adherence to treatment regimen	**Respiratory**
	Runny nose, diminished breath sounds, sputum (amount, colour, tenacious), hemoptysis, increased work of breathing evidenced by use of accessory muscles of respiration, barrel chest
Nonpharmacological therapies: Use of postural drainage, percussion, and vibration	
Symptoms	**Cardiovascular**
• Runny nose; increased work of breathing; thick, tenacious sputum	Tachycardia
	Gastrointestinal
• Dietary intolerances, voracious appetite, weight loss, intestinal gas, bulky and foul-smelling stools, abdominal pain	Assess for protuberant abdomen and abdominal distension and for foul, fatty stools
• Fatigue, restlessness, decreased exercise tolerance	**Possible Diagnostic Findings**
• Anxiety, depression	Abnormal results of the following: pulmonary function tests, sweat chloride test, chest radiography, fecal fat analysis for fatty stools
• Delayed menarche, menstrual irregularities, and secondary amenorrhea; fertility issues	

• Ineffective airway clearance related to abundant, thick bronchial mucus; and fatigue related to increased work of breathing and malnutrition
• Ineffective breathing pattern related to bronchoconstriction, airway obstruction, anxiety, and fatigue
• Impaired gas exchange related to recurring lung infections
• Imbalanced nutrition: less than body requirements related to dietary intolerances, intestinal gas, and altered pancreatic enzyme production

▌ Planning

Overall goals for patients with CF include (a) adequate airway clearance, (b) reduction in number of risk factors associated with respiratory infections, (c) the ability to perform ADLs, (d) experiencing as few complications related to CF as possible, (e) adequate nutritional support to maintain appropriate BMI, and (f) active participation in planning and implementing a therapeutic regimen.

Nursing Implementation

Nurses and other health care providers can help young adults with CF obtain independence by helping them assume responsibility for their care. An important issue that should be discussed is sexuality. Delayed or irregular menstruation is not uncommon. There may be delayed development of secondary sex characteristics such as breasts in girls. A patient may use CF as a reason to avoid certain events or relationships. In contrast, healthy individuals may hesitate to make friends with someone who is sick, which can present a challenge for individuals with CF. Normal life transitions can present larger challenges to young adults with CF, such as building confidence and self-respect on the basis of achievements, persevering with employment goals and opportunities, developing motivation to set and achieve goals, learning to cope with the intensity and chronicity of the treatment program, and adjusting to losing independence when health fails. Disclosing the CF diagnosis to friends, potential spouses, or employers may pose challenges emotionally and financially.

Respiratory intervention for the patient with CF targets relief of bronchoconstriction, airway obstruction, and airflow limitation through the use of aggressive chest physiotherapy, antibiotics, and bronchodilators. Good nutrition, nutritional supplements, and pancreatic enzymes are also important. Advances in long-term vascular access (e.g., implanted ports) have made intravenous access and administration of medication much easier and has eased the transition for intravenous treatment from hospital to home.

Chest physiotherapy is the mainstay of intervention for airway clearance. Home management of CF includes an aggressive plan of postural drainage with percussion and vibration, aerosol nebulization therapy, and breathing retraining. The patient is taught controlled coughing techniques, deep-breathing exercises, and progressive exercise conditioning, such as a bicycling program.

Individuals and families affected by CF need significant support to cope with the many stresses imposed by the condition. Education and assistance can help them maintain a normal family life while coping with the huge physical demands associated with the condition. It is not uncommon for a person with CF to spend 2 hours a day performing chest physiotherapy and 1 hour receiving nebulized medication (often antibiotics).

The family and the person with CF have a great financial and emotional burden. The cost of drugs, special equipment, and health care is often a financial hardship. Financial support for medications varies considerably across provinces. Some provinces provide complete support, whereas others have much lower levels of subsidy. In addition, some provinces cover only the cost of medications in childhood but stop coverage when the patient becomes an adult. Because the majority of people with CF are now surviving into adulthood, this is a serious problem. The Canadian Cystic Fibrosis Foundation has established cystic fibrosis centres across the country to provide a comprehensive range of services to patients and families. A major advantage of the centres is the multidisciplinary team of nurses, physiotherapists, respiratory therapists, nutritionists, and doctors who work very closely with the family to tailor care to meet the family's needs.

As the person continues toward and into adulthood, the nurse and other skilled health professionals should be available to help the patient and family cope with complications resulting from the disease.

CLINICAL DECISION-MAKING EXERCISE

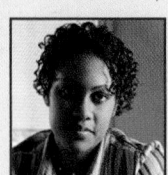

CASE STUDY:
Asthma
Source: © iStockphoto.com/Sandy Jones.

Patient Profile
Mrs. Hookong, a 30-year-old mother of two preschoolers, returns to the emergency department with severe wheezing, dyspnea, and anxiety. She was in the emergency department only 6 hours earlier with an acute asthma attack.

Subjective Data
- Treated in the emergency department previously with inhaled salbutamol MDI (via a spacer) and responded quickly
- Can speak only one- to three-word sentences
- Her asthma is triggered by cigarette smoke
- Began to experience increased shortness of breath and tightness in her chest when she returned home
- Used salbutamol MDI (without a spacer) repeatedly at home with no relief

Objective Data
Physical Examination
- Uses accessory muscles to breathe
- Has audible wheezing

- Respiratory rate: 34/min
- Auscultation reveals no air movement in lower lobes
- Heart rate: 126 beats/min

Diagnostic Studies
- ABG measurements: PaO_2, 80 mm Hg; $PaCO_2$, 35 mm Hg; pH, 7.46
- PEFR: 150 L/min (personal best: 400 L/min)

Discussion Questions
1. Why did Mrs. Hookong return to the emergency department? Explain the pathophysiological processes of this exacerbation of asthma.
2. *Priority decision:* What are the nursing care priorities for Mrs. Hookong?
3. What are the complications that the nurse must be ready for based on the nurse's assessment of Mrs. Hookong?
4. *Priority decision:* What nursing priorities should be included in Mrs. Hookong's discharge plan of care?
5. *Priority decision:* On the basis of the assessment data presented, what are the priority nursing diagnoses? Are there any collaborative problems?

evolve *Answers are available at* **http://evolve.elsevier.com/ Canada/Lewis/medsurg**

REVIEW QUESTIONS

The number of the question corresponds to the same-numbered objective at the beginning of the chapter.

1. How is asthma best characterized?
   a. As an inflammatory disease
   b. As a steady progression of bronchoconstriction
   c. As an obstructive disease with loss of alveolar walls
   d. As a chronic obstructive disorder characterized by mucus production

2. In assessing the knowledge of self-care of a patient with asthma, the nurse recognizes that additional instruction is needed when the patient makes which of the following statements?
   a. "I use my corticosteroid inhaler when I feel short of breath."
   b. "I get a flu shot every year and see my health care professional if I have an upper respiratory infection."
   c. "I use my bronchodilator inhaler before I visit my aunt who has a cat, but I only visit for a few minutes because of my allergies."
   d. "I walk 30 minutes every day but sometimes I have to use my bronchodilator inhaler before walking to prevent me from getting short of breath."

3. Which of the following elements should a plan of care for the patient with COPD include?
   a. Chronic corticosteroid therapy
   b. Reduction of risk factors for infection
   c. High-flow oxygen administration
   d. Lung exercises that involve inhaling longer than exhaling

4. What are the common effects of cigarette smoking on the respiratory system?
   a. Increased proliferation of ciliated cells
   b. Hypertrophy of the alveolar membrane
   c. Destruction of all alveolar macrophages
   d. Hyperplasia of goblet cells and increased production of mucus

5. Which of the following is one of the most important things that a nurse can teach a patient with COPD?
   a. Move to a hot, dry climate.
   b. Perform chest physiotherapy.
   c. Obtain adequate rest in the supine position.
   d. Know the early signs of respiratory infection.

6. What is the major advantage of a Venturi mask?
   a. It can deliver up to 80% oxygen.
   b. It can provide continuous 100% humidity.
   c. It can deliver a precise concentration of oxygen.
   d. It can be used while a patient eats and sleeps.

7. What studies are used to diagnose cystic fibrosis?
   a. Insulin tolerance and blood glucose
   b. Pancreatic enzymes and hormones
   c. Sweat test and vitamin B tolerance test
   d. Pulmonary function test and sweat test

ANSWERS: 1. a; 2. a; 3. b; 4. d; 5. d; 6. c; 7. d

REFERENCES

Aniwidyaningsih, W., Varraso, R., Cano, N., & Pison, C. (2008). Impact of nutritional status on body functioning in chronic obstructive pulmonary disease and how to intervene. *Current Opinion in Clinical Nutrition and Metabolic Care, 11*(4), 435-442. doi:10.1097/MCO.0b013e3283023d37

Bailey, P. H., Bartlett, A., Beatty, G., Bissonnette, J., Dabrowski, B., Manji, M., …, Pollock, R. (2010). *Nursing care of dyspnea: The 6th vital sign in individuals with chronic obstructive pulmonary disease (COPD).* Toronto: Registered Nurses' Association of Ontario. Retrieved from *http://rnao.ca/bpg/guidelines/nursing-care-dyspneathe-6th-vital-sign-individuals-chronic-obstructive-pulmonary-dise*

Batres, S. A., Leon, J. V., & Rodolfo, A. S. (2007). Nutritional status in COPD. *Archivos de Bronconeumologia (English edition), 43*(5), 283-288. doi:10.1016/S1579-2129(07)60068-8

Becker, A., Lemiere, C., Berube, D., Boulet, L. P., Ducharme, F. M., FitzGerald, M., & Kovesi, T. (2005). Summary of recommendations from the Canadian asthma consensus guidelines, 2003. *Canadian Medical Association Journal, 173*(6 Suppl.), S3-S11.

Boulet, L. P. (2009). Influence of co-morbid conditions on asthma. *European Respiratory Journal, 33*(4), 897-906. doi:10.1183/09031936.00121308

Boulet, L. P., Becker, A., Berube, D., Beveridge, R., & Ernst, P. (1999). Summary of the recommendations of the Canadian consensus conference on asthma 1999. Canadian Asthma Consensus Group. *Canadian Medical Association Journal, 161*(11 Suppl. Resume), SF1-SF14.

Boyle, M. P. (2007). Adult cystic fibrosis. *Journal American Medical Association, 298,* 1787-1793. doi:10.1001/jama.298.15.1787

Brashers, V. L. (2008). Alterations of pulmonary function. In S. E. Huether & K. L. McCance (Eds.), *Understanding pathophysiology* (4th ed.). St. Louis: Mosby.

Brenner, B., Corbridge, T., & Kazzi, A. (2009). The intubation and mechanical ventilation of the asthmatic patient in respiratory failure. *Proceedings of the American Thoracic Society, 6,* 371-379. doi:10.1513/pats.P09ST4

Canadian Institute for Health Information. (2006). Treatment of end-stage organ failure in Canada, 1995 to 2004. *2006 Annual Report.* Ottawa: Author.

Celli, B. R. (2009). Pathophysiology of chronic obstructive pulmonary disease. In J. E. Hodgkin, B. R. Celli, & G. L. Conners (Eds.), *Pulmonary rehabilitation: Guidelines to success* (4th ed.). St. Louis: Mosby.

Chapman, K. R., Cartier, A., Hebert, J., McIvor, R. A., & Schellenberg, R. R. (2006). The role of omalizumab in the treatment of severe allergic asthma. *Canadian Respiratory Journal, 13*(Suppl. B), 1B-9B.

Cicutto, L., Bailey, P. H., Bartlett, A., Bissonnette, J., Cornelius, N., Duff Cloutier, J., …, McConnell, H. (2007). *Adult asthma care guidelines for nurses—Promoting control of asthma. Best Practice Guidelines: Shaping the future of nursing.* Toronto: Registered Nurses' Association of Ontario. Retrieved from *http://rnao-ca.rnao-*

dev.org/bpg/guidelines/adult-asthma-care-guidelines-nurses-promoting-control-asthma

Cicutto, L., & Brooks, D. (2006). Self-care approaches to managing chronic obstructive pulmonary disease: A provincial survey. *Respiratory Medicine, 100*(9), 1540-1546.

Coffman, J. M., Cabana, M. D., Halpin, H. A., & Yelin, E. H. (2008). Effects of asthma education on children's use of acute care services: A meta-analysis. *Pediatrics, 121*(3), 575-586.

Cystic Fibrosis Canada. (2010). *Canadian CF Patient Data Registry—2010 Report.* Retrieved from *http://www.cysticfibrosis.ca/assets/files/pdf/CPDR_ReportE.pdf*

Cystic Fibrosis Canada. (2011). *Cystic fibrosis in Canada: About cystic fibrosis.* Retrieved from *http://www.cysticfibrosis.ca/en/aboutCysticFibrosis/CfStatistics.php*

Cystic Fibrosis Canada. (2012). *The Canadian Facts & Figures on Cystic Fibrosis.* Retrieved from *http://www.cysticfibrosis.ca/en/aboutCysticFibrosis/CfStatistics.php*

Decramer, M., Rennard, S., Troosters, T., Mapel, D. W., Giardino, N., Mannino, D., …, Cooper, C. B. (2008). COPD as a lung disease with systemic consequences—clinical impact, mechanisms, and potential for early interventions. *COPD, 5*(4), 235-256. doi:10.1080/15412550802237531

Eisner, M. D., Blanc, P. D., Yelin, E. H., Sidney, S., Katz, P. P., Ackerson, L., …, Iribarren, C. (2008). COPD as a systemic disease: Impact on physical functional limitations. *American Journal of Medicine, 121*(9), 789-796. doi:10.1016/j.amjmed.2008.04.030

Farrell, P. M., Rosenstein, B. J., White, T. B., Accurso, F. J., Castellani, C., Cutting, G. R., …, Campbell, P. W. (2008). Guidelines for diagnosis of cystic fibrosis in newborns through older adults: Cystic Fibrosis Foundation consensus report. *Journal of Pediatrics, 153*(2), S4-S14. doi:10.1016/j.jpeds.2008.05.005

Flume, P. A., Mogayzel, P. J., Robinson, K. A., Goss, C. H., Rosenblatt, R. L., Kuhn, R. J., & Marshall, B. C. (2009). Cystic fibrosis pulmonary guidelines. *American Journal of Respiratory & Critical Care Medicine, 180*, 802-808. doi:10.1164/rccm.200812-1845pp

Flume, P. A., O'Sullivan, B. P., Robinson, K. A., Goss, C. H., Mogayzel, P. J., Willey-Courand, D. B., …, Marshall, B. (2007). Cystic fibrosis pulmonary guidelines: Chronic medications for maintenance of lung health. *American Journal of Respiratory and Critical Care Medicine, 176*(10), 957-969. doi:10.1164/rccm.200705-664OC

Flume, P. A., Strange, C., Ye, X., Ebeling, M., Hulsey, T., & Clark, L. L. (2005). Pneumothorax in cystic fibrosis. *Chest, 128*(2), 720-728. doi:10.1378/chest.128.2.720

Global Initiative for Asthma (GINA). (2010). *Global strategy for asthma management and prevention.* Retrieved from *http://www.ginasthma.org/Guidelines/guideline-report-2010.html*

Global Initiative for Chronic Obstructive Lung Disease (GOLD). (2010). Global strategy for the diagnosis, management and prevention of COPD. Retrieved from *http://www.goldcopd.org/Guidelines/guideline-2010-gold-report.html*

Gotzsche, P. C., & Johansen, H. K. (2008). House dust mite control measures for asthma: Systematic review. *Allergy, 63*(6), 646-659. doi:10.1111/j.1398-9995.2008.01690.x

Health Canada. (2010). *Canadian tobacco use monitoring survey (CTUMS).* Retrieved from *http://www.hc-sc.gc.ca/hc-ps/tobac-tabac/research-recherche/stat/ctums-esutc_2010-eng.php*

Hill, K., Geist, R., Goldstein, R. S., & Lacasse, Y. (2008). Anxiety and depression in end-stage COPD. *European Respiratory Journal, 31*(3), 667-677. doi:10.1183/09031936.00125707

Hodder, R., Lougheed, D. M., Rowe, B. H., FitzGerald, J. M., Kaplan, A. G., & McIvor, A. R. (2010). Management of acute asthma in adults in the emergency department: Non-ventilatory management. *Canadian Medical Association Journal, 182*(2), E55-E67. doi:10.1503/cmaj.080072

Hodges, C. A., Palmert, M. R., & Drumm, M. L. (2008). Infertility in females with cystic fibrosis is multifactorial: Evidence from mouse models. *Endocrinology, 149*, 2790-2797. doi:10.1210/en.2007-1581

Kmiecik, T., Arnoux, S., Kobryn, A., & Gorski, P. (2007). Influenza vaccination in adults with asthma: Safety of an inactivated trivalent influenza vaccine. *Journal of Asthma, 44*, 817-822. doi:10.1080/02770900701539723

Kohnlein, T., & Welte, T. (2008). Alpha-1 antitrypsin deficiency: Pathogenesis, clinical presentation, diagnosis, and treatment. *American Journal of Medicine, 121*(1), 3-9. doi:10.1016/j.amjmed.2007.07.025

Lacasse, Y., Goldstein, R., Lasserson, T. J., & Martin, S. (2006). Pulmonary rehabilitation for chronic obstructive pulmonary disease. *Cochrane Database of Systematic Reviews 2006,* (2), CD003793. doi:10.1002/14651858.CD003793.pub2

Lemiere, C., Bai, T., Balter, M., Bayliff, C., Becker, A., Boulet, L. P., …, White Markham, A. (2004). Adult asthma consensus guidelines update 2003. *Canadian Respiratory Journal, 11*(Suppl. A), 9A-18A.

Lougheed, M. D., Lemiere, C., Dell, S. D., Ducharme, F. M., FitzGerald, J. M., Leigh, R., …, Boulet, L. P. (2010). Canadian Thoracic Society asthma management continuum—2010 consensus summary for children six years of age and over, and adults. *Canadian Respiratory Journal, 17*(1), 15-24.

Lougheed, M. D., Lemiere, C., Ducharme, F. M., Licskai, C., Dell, S. D., Rowe, B. H., …, Canadian Thoracic Society Asthma Clinical Assembly (2012). Canadian Thoracic Society 2012 guideline update: Diagnosis and management of asthma in preschoolers, children and adults. *Canadian Respiratory Journal, 19*(2), 127-164.

Mallia, P., Contoli, M., Caramori, G., Pandit, A., Johnston, S. L., & Papi, A. (2007). Exacerbations of asthma and chronic obstructive pulmonary disease (COPD): Focus on virus induced exacerbations. *Current Pharmaceutical Design, 13*(1), 73-97.

Marciniuk, D. D., Brooks, D., Butcher, S., Debigare, R., Dechman, G., Ford, G., …, Muthuri, S. K. (2010). Optimizing pulmonary rehabilitation in chronic obstructive pulmonary disease—practical issues: A Canadian Thoracic Society clinical practice guideline. *Canadian Respiratory Journal, 17*(4), 159-168.

Marciniuk, D. D., Goodridge, D., Hernandez, P., Rocker, G., Balter, M., Bailey, P., …, Brown, C. (2011). Managing dyspnea in patients with advanced chronic obstructive pulmonary disease: A Canadian Thoracic Society clinical practice guideline. *Canadian Respiratory Journal, 18*(2), 1-10.

McIvor, R. A., Boulet, L. P., FitzGerald, J. M., Zimmerman, S., & Chapman, K. R. (2007). Asthma control in Canada: No improvement since we last looked in 1999. *Canadian Family Physician, 53*(4), 673-677.

Miller, J. D., Malthaner, R. A., Goldsmith, C. H., Goeree, R., Higgins, D., Cox, P. G., …, Road, J. D. (2006). A randomized clinical trial of lung volume reduction surgery versus best medical care for patients with advanced emphysema: A two-year study from Canada. *Annals of Thoracic Surgery, 81*(1), 314-321.

Mitomo, K., Griesenbach, U., Inoue, M., Somerton, L., Meng, C., Akiba, E., …, Alton, E. W. (2010). Toward gene therapy for cystic fibrosis using a lentivirus pseudotyped with Sendai virus envelopes. *Molecular Therapy, 18*(6), 1173-1182. doi:10.1038/mt.2010.13

Navas, E. V., & Taylor, D. O. (2010). Canadian patients with COPD or asthma take a beta-blocker? *Cleveland Clinic Journal of Medicine, 77*(8), 498-499. doi:10.3949/ccjm.77a.09133

Nici, L., Donner, C., Wouters, E., Zuwallack, R., Ambrosino, N., Bourbeau, J., …, Troosters, T. (2006). American Thoracic Society/European Respiratory Society statement on pulmonary rehabilitation. *American Journal of Respiratory and Critical Care Medicine, 173*, 1390-1413. doi:10.1164/rccm.200508-1211st

Odencrants, S., Ehnfors, M., & Ehrenberg, A. (2008). Nutritional status and patient characteristics for hospitalised older patients with chronic obstructive pulmonary disease. *Journal of Clinical Nursing, 17*(13), 1771-1778. doi:10.1111/j.1365-2702.2008.02292.x

O'Donnell, D. E., Aaron, S., Bourbeau, J., Hernandez, P., Marciniuk, D. D., Balter, M., …, Voduc, N. (2007). Canadian Thoracic Society recommendations for management of chronic obstructive pulmonary disease—2007 update. *Canadian Respiratory Journal, 14*(Suppl. B), 5B-32B.

O'Donnell, D. E., Hernandez, P., Kaplan, A., Aaron, S., Bourbeau, J., Marciniuk, D., ..., Voduc, N. (2008). Canadian Thoracic Society recommendations for management of chronic obstructive pulmonary disease—2008 update—Highlights for primary care. *Canadian Respiratory Journal, 15*(Suppl. A), 1A-8A.

Olajos-Clow, J., Cicutto, L., Duff Cloutier, J., Fleming-Carroll, B., Lacroix, H., Martin, L., ..., Chiu, E. (2008). *Promoting asthma control in children. Nursing best practice guidelines.* Toronto: Registered Nurses' Association of Ontario. Retrieved from http://rnao.ca/bpg/guidelines/promoting-asthma-control-children

Public Health Agency of Canada (PHAC). (2007). *Life and breath: Respiratory diseases in Canada.* Ottawa: Author. (Cat. No: HP35-8/2007E-PDF); ISBN: 978-0-662-47060-1. Retrieved from http://www.phac-aspc.gc.ca/publicat/2007/lbrdc-vsmrc/index-eng.php

Rachelefsky, G. S., Liao, Y., & Faruqi, R. (2007). Impact of inhaled corticosteroid-induced oropharyngeal adverse events: Results from a meta-analysis. *Annals of Allergy, Asthma and Immunology, 98*(3), 225-238. doi:10.1016/S1081-1206(10)60711-9

Sama, S. R., Milton, D. K., Hunt, P. R., Houseman, E. A., Henneberger, P. K., & Rosiello, R. A. (2006). Case-by-case assessment of adult-onset asthma attributable to occupational exposures among members of a health maintenance organization. *Journal of Occupational Environmental Medicine, 48,* 400-407. doi:10.1097/01.jom.0000199437.33100.cf

Sethi, S., & Murphy, T. F. (2008). Infection in the pathogenesis and course of chronic obstructive pulmonary disease. *New England Journal of Medicine, 359*(22), 2355-2365. doi:10.1056/NEJMra0800353

Smyth, A. R., & Tan, K. H. (2006). Once-daily versus multiple-daily dosing with intravenous aminoglycosides for cystic fibrosis. *Cochrane Database of Systematic Review, 3,* Issue 3. Art. No.: CD002009. doi:10.1002/14651858.CD002009.pub2

Taylor, D. R., Bateman, E. D., Boulet, L. P., Boushey, H. A., Busse, W. W., Casale, T. B., ..., Reddel, H. K. (2008). A new perspective on concepts of asthma severity and control. *European Respiratory Journal, 32,* 545-554. doi:10.1183/09031936.00155307

Whitson, B. A., Prekker, M. E., Herrington, C. S., Whelan, T. P., Radosevich, D. M., Hertz, M. I., & Dahlberg, P. S. (2007). Primary graft dysfunction and long-term pulmonary function after lung transplantation. *Journal of Heart and Lung Transplantation, 26*(10), 1004-1011.

Williams, A. N., Simon, R. A., Woessner, K. M., & Stevenson, D. D. (2007). The relationship between historical aspirin-induced asthma and severity of asthma induced during oral aspirin challenges. *Journal of Allergy and Clinical Immunology, 120*(2), 273-277. doi:10.1016/j.jaci.2007.03.020

Yankaskas, J. R. (2004). Cystic fibrosis. In J. D. Crapo, J. L. Glassroth, J. B. Karlinsky, & T. E. King (Eds.), *Baum's textbook of pulmonary diseases* (7th ed.). Philadelphia: Lippincott Williams & Wilkins.

Yende, S., Newman, A. B., & Sin, D. (2009). Chronic obstructive pulmonary disease. In J. B. Halter, J. G. Ouslander, M. E. Tinetti, S. Studenski, K. P. High, & S. Asthana (Eds.), *Hazzard's geriatric medicine and gerontology* (6th ed., pp. 987-1001). New York: McGraw-Hill.

Zemek, R. L., Bhogal, S. K., & Ducharme, F. M. (2008). Systematic review of randomized controlled trials examining written action plans in children: What is the plan? *Archives of Pediatrics & Adolescent Medicine, 162*(2), 157-163.

CANADIAN RESOURCES

Allergy/Asthma Information Association (AAIA)
www.aaia.ca/
Alpha 1 Canadian Registry
http://www.alpha1canadianregistry.com
Asthma Society of Canada
http://www.asthma.ca
Canadian Cancer Society
http://www.cancer.ca
Canadian Network for Respiratory Care
http://cnrchome.net/
Canadian Respiratory Health Professionals
http://www.lung.ca/crhp-pcsr/home-accueil_e.php
Canadian Thoracic Society Asthma Management Continuum – 2010 Consensus Summary for children six years of age and over, and adults
http://www.respiratoryguidelines.ca/sites/all/files/cts_asthma_consensus_summary_2010.pdf
Canadian Thoracic Society Guidelines
The Canadian Respiratory Guidelines (CRGC) Site
http://www.respiratoryguidelines.ca/
Cystic Fibrosis Canada
http://www.cysticfibrosis.ca
Living Well With COPD Program
http://livingwellwithcopd.com/english/home/default.asp?s=1
Lung Association*
http://www.lung.ca
Downloadable Action Plan
http://www.lung.ca/_resources/asthma_action_plan.pdf
Fact Sheet: What you need to know about oxygen
http://www.lung.ca/diseases-maladies/copd-mpoc/breathworks-actionair/pdf/Factsheet_oxygen_EN.pdf
Oxygen and COPD
http://www.lung.ca/_resources/Oxygen_COPD_LungAssoc.pdf
Public Health Agency of Canada
Includes Canadian Communicable Disease Reports
http://www.phac-aspc.gc.ca/
Registered Nurses' Association of Ontario
Adult Asthma Guidelines
http://rnao.ca/bpg/guidelines/adult-asthma-care-guidelines-nurses-promoting-control-asthma
Best Practice Guideline
Integrating Smoking Cessation Into Daily Practice
http://rnao.ca/bpg/guidelines/integrating-smoking-cessation-daily-nursing-practice

RELATED RESOURCES

Alpha-1 Association (United States)
http://www.alpha1.org/
Cystic Fibrosis Foundation (United States)
http://www.cff.org
Global Initiative for Asthma (GINA)
http://www.ginasthma.com
Global Initiative for Chronic Obstructive Lung Disease (GOLD)
http://www.goldcopd.com

Θvolve   *For additional Internet resources, see the Web site for this book at http://evolve.elsevier.com/Canada/Lewis/medsurg*

---

*Most provinces have their own Lung Association and Web site.

Problems of Oxygenation: Transport

SECTION

6

SECTION OUTLINE

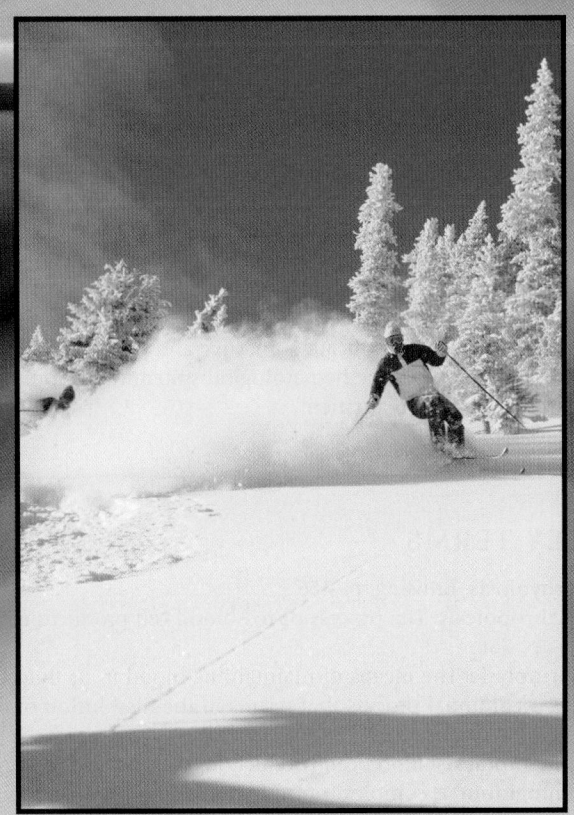

Karl Weatherly/Digital Vision/Thinkstock

Nursing Assessment: Hematological System

Written by Sandra Irene Rome
Adapted by Bridgette Lord

LEARNING OBJECTIVES

1. Describe the structures and functions of the hematological system.
2. Differentiate among the different types of blood cells and their functions.
3. Explain the process of hemostasis.
4. Understand how age-related changes in the hematological system may result in differences in findings of hematological studies.
5. Describe the significant subjective and objective assessment data related to the hematological system that should be obtained from a patient.
6. Describe how to conduct a physical assessment of the hematological system.
7. Differentiate normal from common abnormal physical findings in the hematological system.
8. Describe the purpose, the significance of results, and the nursing responsibilities related to diagnostic studies of the hematological system.

KEY TERMS

ecchymosis Bruising, p. 776
erythropoiesis The process of red blood cell production, p. 766
fibrinolysis The means of maintaining blood in its fluid form, a continual process that results in the dissolution of fibrin, p. 770
hematopoiesis Blood cell production, p. 765
hemoglobin A complex, protein–iron compound composed of heme (an iron compound) and globin (a simple protein) that binds with oxygen and carbon dioxide, p. 765
hemolysis Destruction of erythrocytes, p. 767
leukopenia An abnormal decrease in the number of total white blood cells to less than $4 \times 10^9/L$, p. 776
neutropenia An abnormal reduction of the neutrophil count to less than 1 to $1.5 \times 10^9/L$, p. 776

pancytopenia Marked decrease in the number of red blood cells, white blood cells, and platelets, p. 776
petechiae Small, purplish-red lesions, p. 776
phagocytosis A process by which white blood cells ingest or engulf an unwanted organism and subsequently digest it, p. 767
polycythemia An abnormal condition characterized by excessive levels of red blood cells, p. 774
stem cell A nondifferentiated immature blood cell found in the bone marrow, p. 765
thrombocytopenia A reduction of the platelet count to less than $10 \times 10^9/L$, p. 776
thrombocytosis A condition characterized by excessive levels of platelets; a disorder that occurs with inflammation and some malignant diseases, p. 776

ELECTRONIC RESOURCES

Supplemental content related to Chapter 32 can be found ...

Evolve Web Site ⊝volve

http://evolve.elsevier.com/Canada/Lewis/medsurg
- Assessment Case Study
- Clinical Reference: Laboratory Values
- Content Updates
- eFigure 32-1: Lymphatic Drainage
- Electronic Calculators
- Examination Review Questions

- Glossary
- Key Points (Printable and MP3 Download)
- Physical Examination Video Clips:
  - Precordium and Jugular Veins
  - Neck
  - Upper Extremities
  - Anterior Chest
  - Abdominal Reflexes, Abdominal Muscles, and Inguinal Area

---

*H*ematology is the study of blood and blood-forming tissues. Hematological structures include the bone marrow, the blood, the spleen, and the lymph system. A basic knowledge of hematology is useful in clinical settings to evaluate a patient's ability to transport oxygen and carbon dioxide, coagulate blood, and combat infections. Assessment of the hematological system is based on the patient's health history, physical examination, and results of diagnostic studies.

Structures and Functions of the Hematological System

Bone Marrow

Blood cell production (**hematopoiesis**) occurs within the bone marrow. *Bone marrow* is the soft material that fills the central core of bones. There are two types of bone marrow (yellow [adipose] and red [hematopoietic]), and it is the red marrow that actively produces blood cells. In adults, the red marrow is located primarily in the flat and the irregular bones, such as the ends of long bones, pelvic bones, vertebrae, sacrum, sternum, ribs, flat cranial bones, and scapulae.

All three types of blood cells develop from a common hematopoietic stem cell within the bone marrow. The hematopoietic **stem cell** is best described as a nondifferentiated, immature blood cell found in the bone marrow. As the blood cells mature and differentiate, several different types of cells are formed (Figure 32-1). The marrow is able to respond to increased demands for various types of blood cells by increasing production by means of a negative feedback system. The bone marrow is stimulated by various factors (e.g., erythropoietin) that cause differentiation of the stem cells into one type of the committed hematopoietic cells (e.g., RBC).

Blood

Blood is a type of connective tissue that performs three major functions: transportation, regulation, and protection (Table 32-1). Blood is responsible for the *transportation* of oxygen, nutrients, hormones, and waste products around the body. Blood also

plays a role in the *regulation* of fluid, electrolyte, and acid–base balance. Finally, blood plays a *protective* role in its ability to coagulate (or clot) and combat infections. Blood has two major components: plasma and blood cells.

Plasma. Approximately 55% of blood is plasma (Figure 32-2). Plasma is composed primarily of water, but it also contains proteins, electrolytes, gases, nutrients, and waste. Plasma proteins include albumin, globulin, and clotting factors, mostly fibrinogen (McCance & Huether, 2010). The term *serum* refers to plasma without its clotting factors.

Blood Cells. About 45% of the blood (see Figure 32-2) is composed of formed elements, or blood cells. There are three types of blood cells: *erythrocytes*, or red blood cells (RBCs); *leukocytes*, or white blood cells (WBCs); and *thrombocytes*, or platelets. The primary function of erythrocytes is oxygen transportation, whereas the leukocytes are involved in protection of the body from infection. Platelets mainly function to promote blood coagulation.

Erythrocytes. The primary functions of erythrocytes (RBCs) include transport of gases (both oxygen and carbon dioxide) and assistance in maintaining acid–base balance. The composition and features of an erythrocyte are ideal for its role in gas transportation. It is a flexible cell with a unique biconcave shape. Flexibility enables the cell to alter its shape so that it can easily pass through tiny capillaries. The cell membrane is also very thin, which facilitates the diffusion of gases. Erythrocytes are composed primarily of a large molecule called **hemoglobin,** a complex compound composed of heme (an iron compound) and globin (a simple protein), which functions to bind with oxygen and carbon dioxide. As erythrocytes circulate through the capillaries surrounding alveoli within the lungs, oxygen attaches to the iron on the hemoglobin. The oxygen-bound hemoglobin is referred to as *oxyhemoglobin* and is responsible for the bright red appearance of arterial blood. As erythrocytes flow to body tissues, oxygen detaches from the hemoglobin and diffuses from the capillary into tissue cells. Carbon dioxide diffuses from tissue cells into the capillary, attaches to the globin portion of hemoglobin, and is transported to the lungs for removal. Hemoglobin also acts as a buffer and plays a role in maintaining

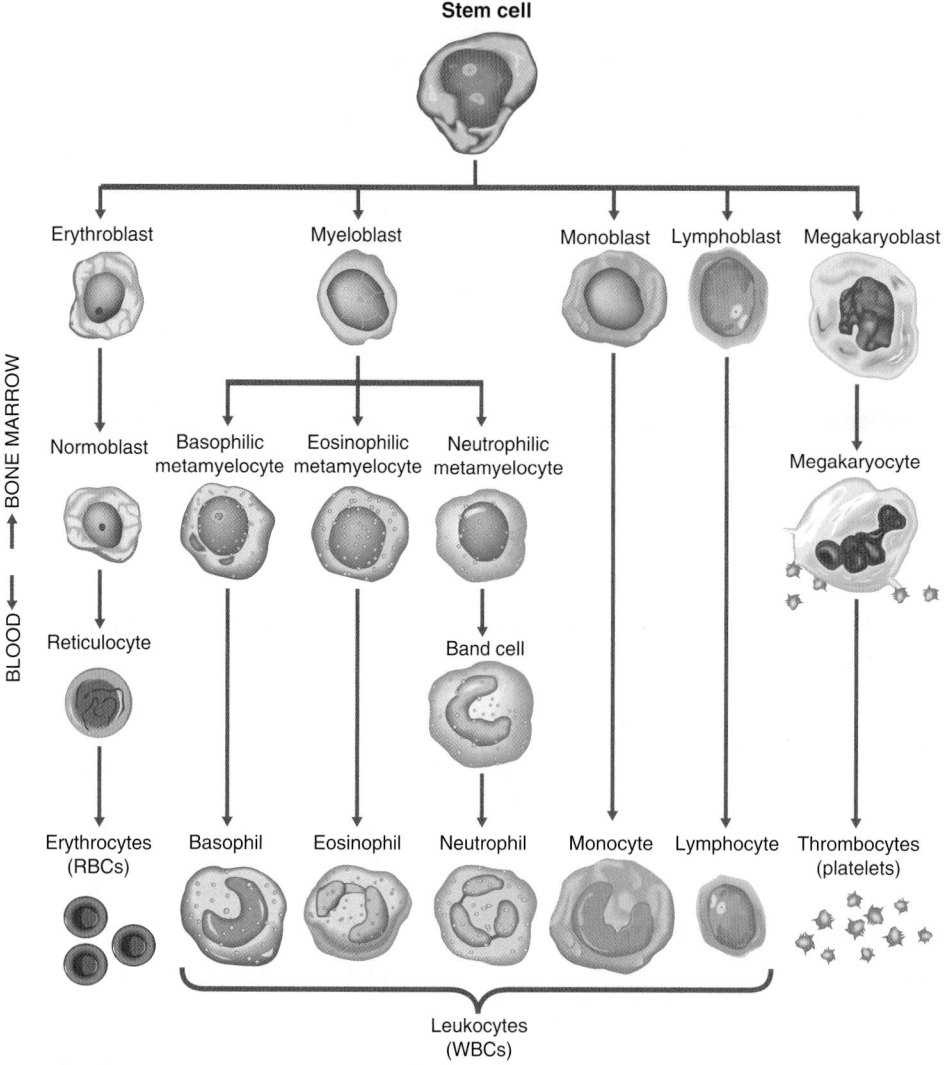

Figure 32-1 Development of blood cells. *RBCs*, red blood cells; *WBCs*, white blood cells.

Table 32-1	Functions of Blood
FUNCTION	**EXAMPLES**
Transportation	• Oxygen from lungs to cells
	• Nutrients from gastrointestinal tract to cells
	• Hormones from endocrine glands to tissues and cells
	• Metabolic waste products (e.g., CO_2, NH_3, urea) from cells to lungs, liver, and kidneys
Regulation	• Fluid and electrolyte balance
	• Acid–base balance
	• Body temperature
Protection	• Combating invasion of pathogens and other foreign substances
	• Maintaining homeostasis of blood coagulation

acid–base balance. This buffering function is described further in Chapter 19.

Erythropoiesis (the process of RBC production) is regulated by cellular oxygen requirements and general metabolic activity. Erythropoiesis is stimulated by hypoxia and controlled by *erythropoietin*, a glycoprotein growth factor synthesized and released by the kidneys. Erythropoietin stimulates the bone marrow to increase erythrocyte production. Normally, the bone marrow releases 3×10^9 RBCs per kilogram of body weight per day. Erythropoiesis is also influenced by the availability of nutrients. Many essential nutrients are necessary for erythropoiesis, including protein, iron, folate (folic acid), cobalamin (vitamin B_{12}), riboflavin (vitamin B_2), and pyridoxine (vitamin B_6) (McCance & Huether, 2010). Erythrocyte production is also affected by endocrine hormones, such as thyroxine, corticosteroids, and testosterone. For example, hypothyroidism is often associated with anemia (Jafarzadeh, Poorgholami, Izadi, Nemati, & Rezayati, 2010).

Several distinct cell types evolve during erythrocyte maturation (see Figure 32-1). The *reticulocyte* is an immature erythrocyte. The reticulocyte count is a measure of the rate at which new RBCs

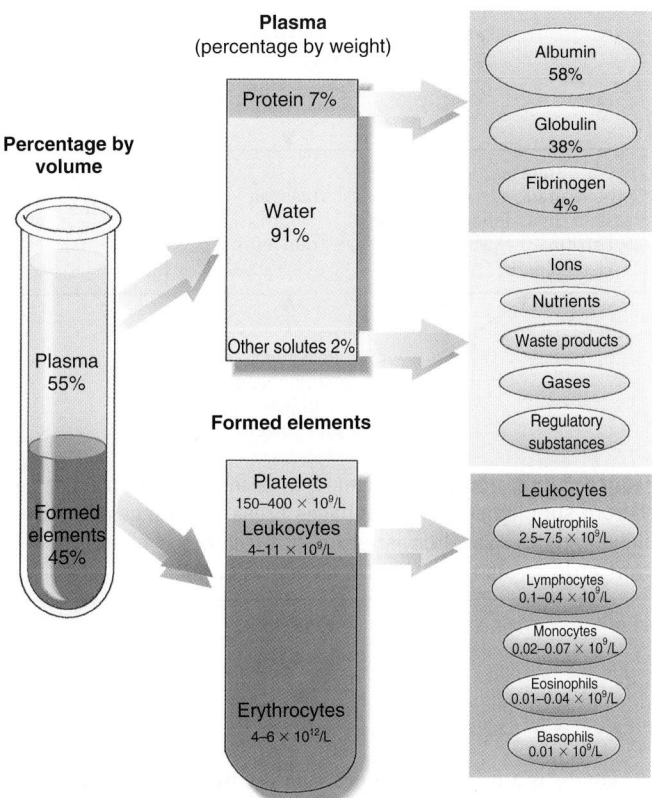

Figure 32-2 Approximate values for the components of blood in the adult. Normally, 45% of the blood is composed of blood cells, and 55% is composed of plasma.

Source: Adapted from Patton, K. T., & Thibodeau, G.A. (2010). *Anatomy and physiology* (7th ed., p. 583, Figure 17-1). St Louis: Mosby.

Table 32-2 Types and Functions of Leukocytes	
TYPE	**CELL FUNCTION**
Granulocytes	
Neutrophil	Phagocytosis, especially during the early phase of inflammation
Basophil	Inflammatory response and allergic response; release of bradykinin, heparin, histamine, serotonin; limited phagocytosis
Eosinophil	Phagocytosis (not as effective as neutrophil); allergic response; protection from parasitic infections
Agranulocytes	
Lymphocyte	Cellular and humoral immune response
Monocyte	Phagocytosis; cellular immune response

Granulocytes. The primary function of the granulocytes is **phagocytosis,** a process by which WBCs ingest or engulf any unwanted organism and then digest and kill it. The *neutrophil* is the most common type of granulocyte, accounting for 50 to 70% of all WBCs. Neutrophils are the primary phagocytic cells involved in acute inflammatory responses. Neutrophil production and maturation is stimulated by hematopoietic growth factors (e.g., granulocyte colony–stimulating factor and granulocyte-macrophage colony–stimulating factor; Mughal, Goldman, & Mughal, 2010).

A mature neutrophil is called a *segmented neutrophil* ("seg") because the nucleus is segmented into two to five lobes connected by strands. An immature neutrophil is called a *band* (for the bandlike or rodlike appearance of the nucleus). Although band cells are sometimes found in the peripheral circulation of normal people and are capable of phagocytosis, the mature neutrophils are more effective. An increase in neutrophils in the blood is a common diagnostic indicator of infection or tissue injury (Kumar & Sharma, 2010). The existence of many immature cells is termed a *shift to the left* and may be indicative of active infection or inflammation. (Shift to the left is explained further in the "White Blood Cells" section on p. 776.)

Eosinophils account for only 2 to 4% of all WBCs. They have a similar but reduced ability for phagocytosis. One of their primary functions is to engulf antigen–antibody complexes formed during an allergic response. The level of eosinophils is also elevated in some neoplastic disorders, such as Hodgkin's lymphoma, as well as in various skin diseases and connective tissue disorders (Howard & Hamilton, 2008). Eosinophils are able to defend against parasitic infections.

Basophils constitute less than 2% of all leukocytes. They have a limited role in phagocytosis. These cells have cytoplasmic granules that contain heparin, serotonin, and histamine. If a basophil is stimulated by an antigen or by tissue injury, it will respond by releasing substances within the granules. This is part of the response in allergic and inflammatory reactions.

Agranulocytes. Agranulocytes differ from granulocytes in that their cytoplasm does not contain lysosomal granules. *Lymphocytes,* one type of agranular leukocyte, constitute 20 to 40% of the WBCs. Lymphocytes originate from stem cells in the bone marrow, and their main function is related to the immune response (see Chapter 14). Two lymphocyte subtypes are B cells and T cells. Although T cell precursors originate in the bone

appear in the circulation. Reticulocytes can develop into mature erythrocytes within 48 hours of their release into circulation. Therefore, assessing the number of reticulocytes is a useful means of evaluating the rate and adequacy of erythrocyte production.

Hemolysis (destruction of RBCs) by monocytes and macrophages removes abnormal, defective, damaged, and old RBCs from circulation. Hemolysis occurs in the bone marrow, the liver, and the spleen and results in increased levels of bilirubin that must be processed by the body. When hemolysis occurs under normal conditions, the liver is able to conjugate and excrete the bilirubin produced. The normal lifespan of an erythrocyte is 120 days.

Leukocytes. Leukocytes (WBCs) appear white when separated from blood. Like erythrocytes, leukocytes originate from stem cells within the bone marrow (see Figure 32-1). There are five different types of leukocytes, each of which has a different function. Leukocytes that contain granules within the cytoplasm are called *granulocytes* (also known as *polymorphonuclear leukocytes*). Granulocytes include three types: neutrophils, basophils, and eosinophils. Leukocytes that do not have granules within the cytoplasm are called *agranulocytes* and include lymphocytes and monocytes (Table 32-2). Lymphocytes and monocytes are also referred to as *mononuclear cells* because they have only one discrete nucleus. The life span of leukocytes varies widely: Granulocytes may live for only a few hours, whereas some lymphocytes may live for many years.

marrow, these cells migrate to the thymus gland for further differentiation into T cells. (Details of lymphocyte function are presented in Chapter 14.)

Monocytes are the other type of agranular leukocyte. These cells are usually larger than other WBCs and account for approximately 4 to 8% of all WBCs. Monocytes are potent phagocytic cells. They can ingest small or large masses of matter, such as bacteria, dead cells, tissue debris, and old or defective RBCs. Monocytes are the second type of WBC to arrive at the scene of an injury. These cells are present in the bone marrow for only a short time before they migrate into the tissues and become macrophages. In addition to macrophages that have differentiated from monocytes, resident macrophages can also be found in tissues. These resident macrophages are further differentiated; they include Kupffer's cells in the liver, osteoclasts in the bone, and alveolar macrophages in the lung. These macrophages protect the body from pathogens at these entry points and are more phagocytic than monocytes. Macrophages also interact with lymphocytes to facilitate the humoral and cellular immune responses.

Thrombocytes. The primary function of thrombocytes (platelets) is to initiate the clotting process by producing an initial "platelet plug" in the early phases of the clotting process. Platelets must be available in sufficient numbers and must be structurally and metabolically sound for blood clotting to occur. When capillaries are damaged, platelets adhere to the damaged capillary wall, and platelet activation is initiated. Increasing numbers of platelets accumulate to form the platelet plug, which is stabilized with clotting factors. Platelets are also important in the process of clot shrinkage and retraction.

Platelets, like other blood cells, originate from stem cells within the bone marrow (see Figure 32-1). The stem cell undergoes differentiation by transforming into a *megakaryocyte*, which produces platelets. Platelet production is partly regulated by *thrombopoietin*, a growth factor that acts on bone marrow to stimulate platelet production (Shaheen & Broxmeyer, 2009). Thrombopoietin is produced in the liver, kidneys, smooth muscle, and bone marrow. Typically, platelets have a lifespan of 5 to 9 days.

Iron Metabolism

Iron is obtained from foods and dietary supplements. On average, only 5 to 10% of the dietary iron that is consumed is absorbed by the body. Absorption primarily takes place in the duodenum and the upper jejunum.

Iron is present in the body within RBCs and in a stored form. Approximately two thirds of the body's iron is found as the heme part of the hemoglobin molecule in RBCs. The other third of iron is stored as ferritin and hemosiderin in the bone marrow, spleen, liver, and macrophages (Figure 32-3). When stored iron is not replaced, hemoglobin production is reduced.

Transferrin, which is synthesized in the liver, serves as a carrier plasma protein for iron. The degree to which transferrin is saturated with iron is a reliable indicator of the iron supply for developing RBCs.

Iron is recycled in the body after old and damaged RBCs are phagocytized (ingested and destroyed) by macrophages in the liver and spleen. Iron is released into the plasma and transported by transferrin to the bone marrow for RBC production. Alternatively, iron may be stored as ferritin or hemosiderin (see Figure 32-3).

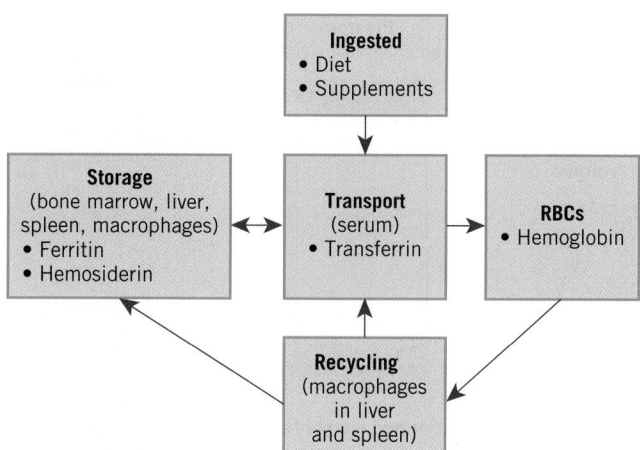

Figure 32-3 Iron metabolism. Iron is ingested in the diet or from supplements. Macrophages break down ingested red blood cells (RBCs). Iron is returned to the blood bound to transferrin or stored as ferritin or hemosiderin.

Clotting Mechanisms

Hemostasis is a term used to describe the blood clotting process. This process is important in minimizing blood loss when body structures are injured. Four components contribute to normal hemostasis: (a) vascular response, (b) platelet plug formation, (c) fibrin clot development, and (d) clot dissolution.

Vascular Response. When a blood vessel is injured, an immediate local vasoconstrictive response occurs. Vasoconstriction reduces the leakage of blood from the vessel not only by restricting the vessel size but also by pressing the endothelial surfaces together. The latter reaction enhances vessel wall stickiness and maintains closure of the vessel even after the vasoconstriction subsides. Vascular spasm may last for 20 to 30 minutes, allowing time for the platelet response and plasma clotting factors to be activated. The platelet response and plasma clotting factors are triggered by endothelial injury and the release of substances such as tissue factor (Owens & Mackman, 2011).

Platelet Plug Formation. Platelets are activated when they are exposed to interstitial collagen from injured blood vessels. Platelets stick to one another and form clumps. The stickiness is termed *adhesiveness*, and the formation of clumps is termed *aggregation* or *agglutination*. When a blood vessel is injured, the circulating platelets are exposed to the collagen from the inner lining of the vessel. This interaction causes the platelets to release substances such as platelet factor 3 and serotonin, which facilitate coagulation. At the same time, platelets release adenosine diphosphate, which increases platelet adhesiveness and aggregation, thereby enhancing the formation of a platelet plug. In addition, von Willebrand's factor is important in forming an adhesive bridge between platelets and vascular subendothelial structures. It is synthesized in endothelial cells and megakaryocytes and acts as a carrier for factor VIII (Ginsburg & Wagner, 2009).

In addition to their contribution to clotting, platelets also facilitate the reactions of the plasma clotting factors within the coagulation cascade. Platelet lipoproteins stimulate necessary conversions in the clotting process (Figure 32-4).

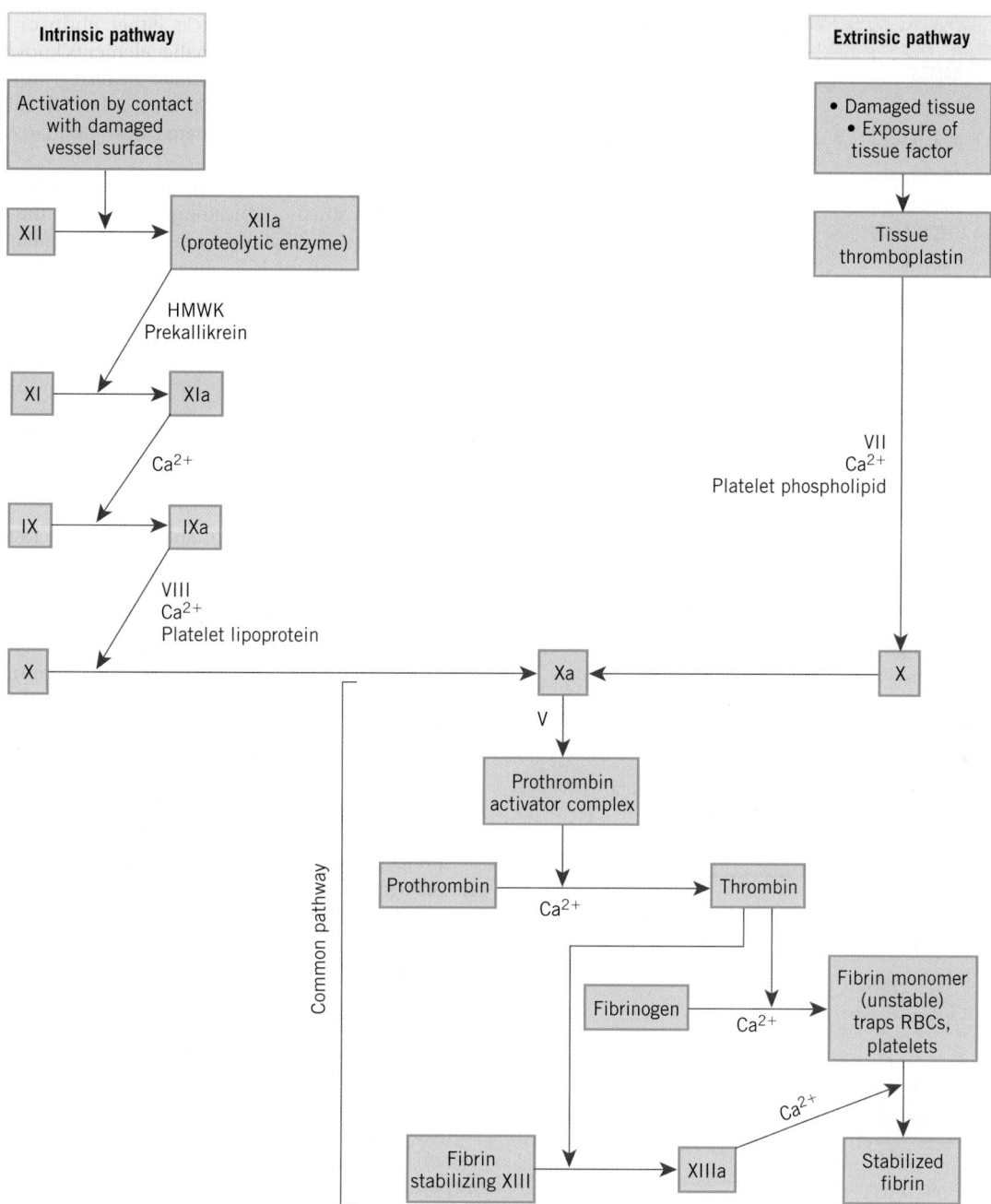

Figure 32-4 Coagulation mechanism showing steps in the intrinsic and the extrinsic pathways as they would occur in the test tube. *Ca²⁺*, calcium ion; *HMWK*, high-molecular weight kininogen; *RBCs*, red blood cells.

Fibrin Clot Development. The formation of a fibrin clot interlaced with the platelet plug is the conclusion of a complex series of reactions involving different clotting factors. The plasma clotting factors are labelled with both names and Roman numerals (Table 32-3). Plasma proteins circulate in inactive forms until stimulated to initiate clotting through one of two pathways, intrinsic or extrinsic. The *intrinsic pathway* is activated by collagen exposure from endothelial injury when the blood vessel is damaged. The *extrinsic pathway* is initiated when tissue thromboplastin is released extravascularly from injured tissues.

Regardless of whether clotting is initiated by substances inside or outside the blood vessel, coagulation ultimately follows the same final common pathway of the clotting cascade. Thrombin, in the common pathway, is the most powerful enzyme in the coagulation process (Figure 32-5). It converts fibrinogen to fibrin, which is an essential component of a blood clot.

Clot Dissolution. Just as some blood elements foster coagulation *(procoagulants)*, others interfere with clotting *(anticoagulants)*. This countermechanism to blood clotting serves to keep blood in its fluid state. Anticoagulation may be achieved by two means: antithrombin activity and fibrinolysis. As the name implies, antithrombins keep blood fluid by antagonizing thrombin, a powerful coagulant. Endogenous heparin, protein C, and protein S are examples of anticoagulants.

Table 32-3 Coagulation Factors	
FACTOR	**NAMES**
I	Fibrinogen
II	Prothrombin
III	Thromboplastin Thrombokinase Tissue factor
IV	Calcium
V	Proaccelerin Labile factor AC globulin
VI	—
VII	Prothrombin conversion accelerator
VIII	Antihemophilic globulin Antihemophilic factor
IX	Plasma thromboplastin component Antihemophilic factor B
X	Stuart factor
XI	Plasma thromboplastin antecedent Antihemophilic factor C
XII	Hageman factor
XIII	Fibrin-stabilizing factor

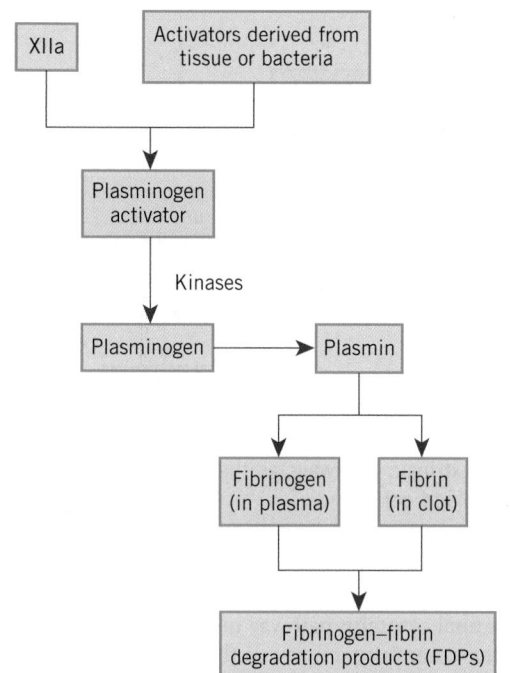

Figure 32-5 Fibrinolytic system.

The second method of maintaining blood in its fluid form is **fibrinolysis,** a continual process resulting in the dissolution of fibrin and thus clots. The fibrinolytic system is initiated when conversion of plasminogen to plasmin is activated (see Figure 32-5). Thrombin is one of the substances that can activate the conversion of plasminogen to plasmin, thereby propagating

fibrinolysis. The plasmin attacks either fibrin or fibrinogen by splitting the molecules into smaller elements known as *fibrin split products* (FSPs) or *fibrin degradation products.* (More information about FSPs can be found in Table 32-9 later in this chapter and in the discussion of disseminated intravascular coagulation in Chapter 33.)

If fibrinolysis is excessive, the patient is predisposed to bleeding. In such a situation, bleeding results from the destruction of fibrin in platelet plugs or from the anticoagulation effects of increased amounts of FSPs. Increased amounts of FSPs lead to impairment in platelet aggregation, reduction in prothrombin, and an inability to stabilize fibrin.

Spleen

Another component of the hematological system is the spleen, which is located in the upper left quadrant of the abdomen. The role of the spleen can be classified into the following four general functions:

1. *Hematopoietic function:* The spleen produces RBCs during fetal development.
2. *Filter function:* The splenic structure provides an ideal filter mechanism for cleansing the blood. For example, the spleen removes old and defective RBCs from circulation by means of the mononuclear phagocyte system. Filtration also involves the reuse of iron. The spleen is able to catabolize hemoglobin released by hemolysis and return the iron component of the hemoglobin to the bone marrow for reuse. The spleen also plays an important role in filtering circulating bacteria, especially encapsulated organisms such as gram-positive cocci.
3. *Immune function:* The spleen contains a rich supply of lymphocytes, monocytes, and stored immunoglobulins.
4. *Storage function:* The spleen serves as a storage site for platelets and RBCs.

Lymph System

The lymph system—consisting of lymph fluid, lymphatic capillaries, lymphatic ducts, and lymph nodes—carries fluid from the interstitial spaces to the blood. It is by means of the lymph system that proteins and fat from the gastrointestinal tract and certain hormones are able to return to the circulatory system. The lymph system also returns excess interstitial fluid to the blood, which is important in preventing the development of edema.

Lymph fluid is a pale yellow fluid that has diffused through capillary walls. This fluid is formed when interstitial fluid (the fluid that bathes and surrounds cells) is collected through lymph capillaries. It circulates through a special vasculature, much as blood moves through blood vessels. The formation of lymph fluid increases when interstitial fluid increases, thereby forcing more fluid into the lymph system. When too much interstitial fluid forms or when something interferes with the reabsorption of lymph, lymphedema develops. Lymphedema may occur as a complication of a mastectomy or lumpectomy when axillary lymph nodes are removed and the lymph drainage is disrupted. Lymphedema may also be associated with disruption of the lymphatic drainage in the abdomen after surgical procedures such as a hysterectomy or a bowel resection.

The lymphatic capillaries are thin-walled vessels that have an irregular diameter. They are somewhat larger than blood capillaries and do not contain valves. Lymphatic capillaries unite to form lymphatic vessels that carry all lymph fluid to either the right lymphatic duct or the thoracic duct. These large lymphatic ducts drain into the subclavian veins of the neck (eFigure 32-1 shows the lymph drainage throughout the body, and is available on the Evolve Web site for this chapter).

The lymph nodes are round, oval, or bean-shaped and vary in size according to their location. Structurally, the lymph nodes are small clumps of lymphatic tissue and are found in groups along lymph vessels at various sites in the body. There are more than 200 lymph nodes throughout the body; the greatest amount are in the abdomen, surrounding the gastrointestinal tract. Lymph nodes are situated both superficially and deep. The superficial nodes can be palpated, but evaluation of the deep nodes requires radiological examination. A primary function of lymph nodes is the filtration of pathogens and foreign particles that are carried by lymph fluid to the nodes.

Liver

The liver functions as a filter. It also produces procoagulants that are essential for hemostasis and blood coagulation. In addition, when the amount of iron exceeds tissue needs (which can occur with frequent blood transfusions or diseases that cause iron overload), the excess is stored in the liver. *Hepcidin*, a protein produced by the liver, is a key regulator of iron balance. The synthesis of hepcidin is stimulated by iron overload or inflammation (Gardenghi, Grady, & Rivella, 2010). Hepcidin reduces the release of stored iron from enterocytes (in the intestines) and macrophages (Andrews, 2009). Other functions of the liver are described in Chapter 46.

AGE-RELATED DIFFERENCES IN ASSESSMENT

Table 32-4 Effects of Aging on Hematological Studies	
STUDY	**CHANGES**
CBC Studies	
Hemoglobin	Normal; possibly slightly decreased in men
MCV	May be slightly increased
MCHC	May be slightly decreased
WBC count	Diminished response to infection
Platelets	Unchanged
Clotting Studies	
Partial thromboplastin time	Decreased
Fibrinogen	Level may be elevated
Factors V, VII, VIII, IX	Levels may be elevated
ESR	Increased significantly
Iron Studies	
Serum iron	Level decreased
Total iron-binding capacity	Decreased
Ferritin	Level increased
Erythropoietin	Level may be decreased

CBC, complete blood count; *ESR*, erythrocyte sedimentation rate; *MCHC*, mean corpuscular hemoglobin concentration; *MCV*, mean corpuscular volume; *WBC*, white blood cell.

AGE-RELATED CONSIDERATIONS: HEMATOLOGICAL SYSTEM

Physiological aging is a gradual process that involves cell loss and organ atrophy. The amount of red marrow and the number of stem cells decrease with age. However, the depletion does not appear to be complete even in very old adults (Ershler & Longo, 2010). The remaining stem cells maintain their functional capacity to divide, but the percentage of marrow space occupied by hematopoietic tissue declines progressively after about age 70. Although older adults are still capable of maintaining adequate blood cell levels, the lower reserve capacity leaves them more vulnerable to possible problems with clotting, oxygen transport, and fighting infection. This results in a diminished ability to compensate for an acute or chronic illness.

Hemoglobin levels begin to decrease in both men and women after middle age; levels are low-normal in most older people. Although iron deficiency is usually responsible for the low hemoglobin levels, the cause of anemia in many older patients is unknown. Healthy older patients are not able to produce reticulocytes in response to hemorrhage or hypoxemia as well as are younger adults. Whether this is because of ineffective erythropoiesis, changes in the bone marrow and hematopoietic elements, or changes in growth factors is not known.

Iron absorption is not impaired in older patients, but adequate nutritional intake of iron may be decreased. It is essential for the examiner to assess for signs of disease processes such as gastrointestinal bleeding before concluding that decreased hemoglobin levels are solely related to age. Thus iron-deficiency anemia is a diagnosis that should be made after other causes have been ruled out.

The osmotic fragility of RBCs (susceptibility of RBCs to burst in hypotonic solutions) is increased in older people. This may account for a slight increase in mean corpuscular volume (measure of the average volume or size of a single RBC) and a slight decrease in mean corpuscular hemoglobin concentration (concentration of hemoglobin in a given volume of RBCs, derived from the ration of the hemoglobin to the hematocrit) in some older individuals.

The total WBC count and differential are generally not affected by aging (Ershler & Longo, 2010). However, humoral antibody response and T cell function may decrease (Wu & Meydani, 2008). During an infection, an older adult may have only a minimal elevation in the total WBC count. This laboratory finding suggests that the bone marrow reserve of granulocytes is diminished in older adults and reflects the possible impairment in stimulation of hematopoiesis. Platelets are unaffected by the aging process. However, changes in vascular integrity from aging can manifest as easy bruising. The effects of aging on hematological studies are presented in Table 32-4. Immune changes related to aging are described in Chapter 16.

Assessment of the Hematological System

Much of the evaluation of the hematological system is based on a thorough health history. Key questions to ask a patient with a hematological problem are presented in Table 32-5.

Table 32-5   Hematological System: Subjective Data

Past History

- Have you had any previous problems with anemia, bleeding disorders, and blood diseases such as leukemia?*
- Have you ever received a blood transfusion?*
- Have you undergone any surgical procedures?

Family History

- Has anyone in your family had anemia, kidney problems, cancer, bleeding, or clotting problems?*

Social and Occupational History

- Does your occupation bring you into contact with hazardous substances?*
- Have you had any past or current occupational or household exposures to radiation or chemicals?*
- Have you had any past exposure to radiation as a medical treatment?
- Do you have a support system to assist you when needed?
- What coping strategies do you use when your symptoms get worse?

Self-Care History

- Do you smoke or drink alcohol?*
- Do you take any prescribed or over-the-counter medications?*
- Are you having or have you ever had chemotherapy?*
- Do you take any herbal products?* Home remedies?*
- Have you in the past or are you currently consuming illegal drugs? What agents? What route? How frequently? When did you last use?

Activities of Daily Living

- Do you have any difficulty performing daily activities because of a lack of energy?*
- Have you experienced excessive fatigue recently?*
- Do you have any shortness of breath at rest? With activity?*

Nutrition–Metabolic History

- Do you have any difficulties with eating, chewing, or swallowing?*
- Have you had a sore tongue or any mouth sores, swollen or sore gums, or excessive oral bleeding?
- How has your appetite been?
- What kind of diet do you follow? If vegetarian, do you eat eggs, milk products, fish or chicken? Do you follow a vegan diet?
- Do you take any vitamins, nutritional supplements, or iron?*
- Have you had any changes in your weight in the past year?*
- Are nausea and vomiting a problem for you?*
- Have you ever experienced any unusual bleeding or bruising?*
- Have there been recent changes in the condition of your skin?*
- Have you noticed any swelling in your armpits, neck, or groin?*
- Have you experienced night sweats or cold intolerance?*

Elimination

- Have you had black or tarry stools?* Have you had light or clay-coloured stools?
- Do you ever have diarrhea or a change in your bowel habits?*
- Have you noticed any blood or a dark tea colour in your urine?*
- Have you been urinating less?*
- Has your urine had a foul odour or cloudiness?

Neurological History

- Do you have any pain, such as bone, joint, or abdominal pain, or abdominal fullness?*
- Do you have pain when moving your joints?*
- Have your muscles been sore or achy recently?*
- Do you have any limitations in joint motion?*
- Do you have a problem with unsteady gait?*
- Have you experienced any numbness or tingling?*
- Have you had any problems with your vision, hearing, or taste?*
- Have you noticed any changes in your mental functions?*

Sleep History

- Do you feel fatigued? Are you more fatigued than usual?*
- Do you feel rested on awakening? If no, explain.

Sexual–Reproductive History

- Has your hematological problem caused any sexual problems that concern you?*
- Women: When was your last menses? Do you consider your cycle normal? How long does your bleeding usually last? Have you had any increase in cramping or clotting?* Have there been any changes in the amount of flow?
- Men: Do you experience erectile dysfunction?*
- Have you had unprotected sex in the past 6 months?* Was your partner someone new or a person with whom you have had a long-term sexual relationship?

Other

- Has your current illness caused a change in your roles and relationships?*
- Does your health problem make you feel differently about yourself?*
- Do you have any other physical changes that cause you distress?*
- Do you have any conflicts between your planned therapy and your value-belief system?*

*If yes, describe.

Subjective Data

Important Health Information

Past Health History. It is important to learn whether the patient has had prior hematological problems or whether the patient's family has any hereditary disorders (e.g., hemophilia, sickle cell disease). Specifically, the nurse should ask about previous problems with anemia, bleeding disorders, and blood diseases such as leukemia. The nurse should also document other related medical conditions such as mononucleosis, malabsorption, and liver disorders (e.g., hepatitis, cirrhosis), as well as kidney or spleen disorders. A patient may have received a kidney transplant, may have lost a spleen to traumatic injury, or may have a history of intravenous drug use that may affect a patient's risk for hematological disorders. A history of recurrent infection or problems with blood clotting is also important to note.

Table 32-6 Drugs Affecting Hematological Function and Laboratory Values*

DRUG CLASS	HEMATOLOGICAL EFFECTS
Antidysrhythmics (e.g., procainamide [Procan SR], quinidine)	Agranulocytosis, anemia, hemolytic anemia, thrombocytopenia
Antihypertensives (e.g., methyldopa)	Hemolytic anemia
Antimicrobials	
• Aminoglycosides	Interference with platelet function
• Amphotericin B	Anemia
• Chloramphenicol (Chloromycetin)	Anemia, neutropenia, thrombocytopenia
• Isoniazid (INH)	Neutropenia
• Trimethoprim-sulphamethoxazole (Septra)	Anemia, leukopenia, neutropenia, thrombocytopenia
Antineoplastics (e.g., alkylating agents, antitumour antibiotics, platinol agents)	Anemia, neutropenia, leukopenia, thrombocytopenia
Antiplatelet agents (e.g., clopidogrel [Plavix])	Interference with platelet function, thrombocytopenia
Antiretrovirals (e.g., zidovudine [AZT, Retrovir])	Neutropenia, anemia
Antiseizure agents (e.g., phenytoin [Dilantin], carbamazepine [Tegretol])	Anemia
Corticosteroids (e.g., dexamethasone, hydrocortisone, prednisolone)	Lymphopenia, neutrophilia
Diuretics (e.g., loop diuretics, thiazide diuretics)	Interference with platelet function
Histamine H₂–blocking agents (e.g., ranitidine [Zantac], cimetidine)	Interference with platelet production
Hormonal agents (e.g., diethylstilbestrol [DES], megestrol acetate, oral contraceptives)	Increase in factors II, V, VII, VIII, IX, X; increase in fibrinogen; increase in thrombin; decrease in prothrombin and partial thromboplastin times; increase in coagulation and thromboemboli formation
Immunosuppressants (e.g., azathioprine [Imuran], cyclosporine, tacrolimus [Prograf])	Lymphopenia
Nonsteroidal anti-inflammatory agents (e.g., ibuprofen [Motrin, Advil], phenylbutazone)	Anemia, leukopenia, neutropenia, thrombocytopenia, inhibit platelet aggregation
Phenothiazines (e.g., chlorpromazine, prochlorperazine)	Interference with platelet function
Salicylates (e.g., aspirin and aspirin-containing compounds	Interference with platelet function
Sympathomimetics (e.g., dopamine, epinephrine)	Leukocytosis
Tricyclic antidepressants	Interfere with platelet function
Miscellaneous	
• Allopurinol	Neutropenia
• Dextran	Interference with platelet function

*This represents only a partial listing of drugs that affect the hematological system.

Medications. A complete medication history of prescription and over-the-counter drugs is an important component of a hematological assessment. The use of vitamins, herbal products, or dietary supplements should specifically be addressed because many patients may not consider these to be drugs. Many drugs or supplements interfere with normal hematological functions (Table 32-6). For example, herbal therapy can interfere with clotting. Antineoplastic agents used to treat malignant disorders and antiretroviral agents used to treat human immunodeficiency virus (HIV) infection may cause bone marrow depression (see Chapter 18). A patient previously treated with chemotherapy agents, particularly alkylating agents, is at a higher risk of developing a secondary malignancy such as leukemia or lymphoma. A patient receiving long-term anticoagulation therapy (e.g., warfarin [Coumadin]) may be at increased risk for bleeding.

Surgery or Other Treatments. The patient should be asked about specific past surgical procedures: splenectomy, tumour removal, prosthetic heart valve placement, surgical excision of the duodenum (in which iron absorption occurs), partial or total gastrectomy (in which parietal cells are removed, thus reducing

intrinsic factor needed for the absorption of cobalamin [vitamin B₁₂]), and resection of the ileus (in which cobalamin absorption takes place). The nurse should also ascertain how wound healing progressed postoperatively and whether and when any bleeding problems occurred in relation to the surgery. Wound healing and bleeding as responses to past injuries (including minor trauma) and to dental extractions should be documented. The date and number of previous blood transfusions and any transfusion-related adverse events should be ascertained and documented.

Approach to Obtaining a Hematological History

Social and Occupational History. The patient should be questioned about any past or current occupational or household exposures to radiation or chemicals. If such exposure has occurred, the type, amount, and duration of the exposure should be determined. A person who has been exposed to radiation, as a treatment modality or by accident, has a higher incidence of certain hematological problems (see Table 18-16). The same is true of a person who has been exposed to chemicals (e.g., benzene, lead, naphthalene, phenylbutazone). These chemicals are commonly used by potters, dry cleaners, and individuals involved with occupations involving the use of adhesives. The nurse should assess the effect of the current illness on a patient's usual roles and responsibilities. The patient's support systems and coping skills should also be assessed.

Self-Care History. Risk factors that might disrupt the hematological system, such as alcohol and cigarette use, must be assessed. Alcohol is a caustic agent, and damage to the gastrointestinal tract secondary to alcohol can cause bleeding. *Hematemesis* (bright red, brown, or black vomit) can be a symptom of this problem and should be investigated. Alcohol also exerts a damaging effect on platelet function and the liver, in which clotting factors are produced. Consequently, bleeding problems can develop and should be anticipated in cases of known alcohol abuse. Cigarette smoking increases low-density lipoprotein cholesterol and levels of carbon dioxide, leading to hypoxia and altering the anticoagulant properties of the endothelium. Smoking also increases platelet reactivity, plasma fibrinogen, hematocrit, and blood viscosity, which increases the risk for developing blood clots. Chemicals in cigarettes, such as benzene, are also linked to an increased risk of leukemia (Huff, 2007). Illegal drug use should also be documented because many illegal drugs may affect hematopoiesis.

Activities of Daily Living. Because fatigue is a prominent symptom in many hematological disorders, the patient should be asked about feelings of tiredness. The nurse should also ask whether the patient experiences weakness and complains of heavy extremities. Symptoms of apathy, malaise, dyspnea, or palpitations should be documented. Any change in a patient's ability to perform activities of daily living should be noted.

Nutritional–Metabolic History. During the patient interview and assessment, the nurse should measure the patient's weight and determine whether the patient has experienced any anorexia, nausea, vomiting, or oral discomfort. A dietary history may provide clues about the cause of anemia. Iron, cobalamin, and folic acid are necessary for the development of RBCs. Iron and folic acid deficiencies are associated with inadequate dietary intake; foods containing these substances include liver, meat, eggs, whole-grain and enriched breads and cereals, potatoes, leafy green vegetables, dried fruits, legumes, and citrus fruits. Folic acid deficiencies may be offset by a diet that includes foods that are also high in iron (Alpers, Stenson, Taylor, & Bier, 2008).

Any changes in the skin's texture or colour should be explored. The patient should be asked about any bleeding of gum tissue. Any *petechiae* or *ecchymotic* areas on the skin should be noted; if they are present, the frequency, size, and cause should be documented. The location of petechiae can indicate an accumulation of blood in the skin or mucous membranes. Small vessels leak under pressure, and if platelet numbers are insufficient to stop the bleeding, petechiae may result. Petechiae may also occur in areas where clothing constricts the circulation.

The patient should also be questioned about any lumps or swelling in the neck, the armpits, or the groin. Specifically, the patient must be asked what the lumps feel like (i.e., hard or soft, tender or nontender) and if they are mobile or fixed. Primary lymph tumours are usually not painful. A nontender swollen lymph node may be a sign of Hodgkin's disease or non-Hodgkin's lymphoma. Lymph nodes that are enlarged and tender are usually associated with an acute infection. Any incidents of fever should be explored thoroughly. It should be determined whether the patient currently has a fever, recurring fevers, chills, or night sweats.

Patients should be asked whether they have a history of cardiac or pulmonary diseases. Cardiovascular disorders such as valvular disease or hypertension may predispose patients to hemolysis. Many of the medications used to treat cardiovascular disease can also cause abnormalities in hematopoietic cell production or coagulation. Pulmonary disorders that lead to hypoxemia may cause chronic stimulation of erythropoietin and result in **polycythemia** (excessive RBCs).

Elimination Pattern. The patient should be asked whether blood has been noted in the urine or stool or whether stools have been black and tarry. The patient should indicate whether he or she has had a recent stool Hemoccult (blood) test or colonoscopy. Also, any decrease in urinary output or diarrhea should be documented.

Neurological History. *Arthralgia* (joint pain) may be caused by a hematological problem and should be assessed. Pain in the joint may be indicative of an autoimmune disorder or may be caused by gout secondary to increased uric acid production, which in turn may be secondary to a hematological malignancy or hemolytic anemia. Aching bones may result from pressure of expanding bone marrow with diseases such as leukemia. *Hemarthrosis* (blood in a joint) can occur in patients with bleeding disorders and can be painful.

Paraesthesias, numbness, and tingling may be related to a hematological disorder and should be noted. Any changes in vision, hearing, taste, or mental status should also be assessed carefully.

Sleep History. The patient's feeling of being rested after a night's sleep should be determined. Fatigue secondary to a hematological problem often does not resolve after sleep.

Sexual–Reproductive History. A careful gynecological history should be obtained from women, including the ages at menarche and menopause, duration and amount of bleeding, incidence of clotting and cramping, and any associated problems. Any intrapartum or postpartum bleeding problems should also be documented. Men should be asked whether they have any problems related to erectile dysfunction because this is common in men with hematological problems. Patients should also be questioned about sexual behaviour because HIV infection is potentially a concern, particularly among populations at high risk for acquiring this disease.

Values and Beliefs. Some hematological problems are treated with blood transfusions or bone marrow transplantation. Determine whether any treatment plans may conflict with a patient's values or beliefs.

Objective Data

Physical Examination. A complete and thorough physical examination is necessary to assess all the body systems that affect or are affected by the hematological system (see Chapter 3). Disorders of the hematological system can manifest in various ways; thus a patient's presenting symptoms may not immediately point to a hematological problem. For example, paraesthesias of the lower extremities may not appear to reflect a hematological problem, but when they are accompanied by other clinical

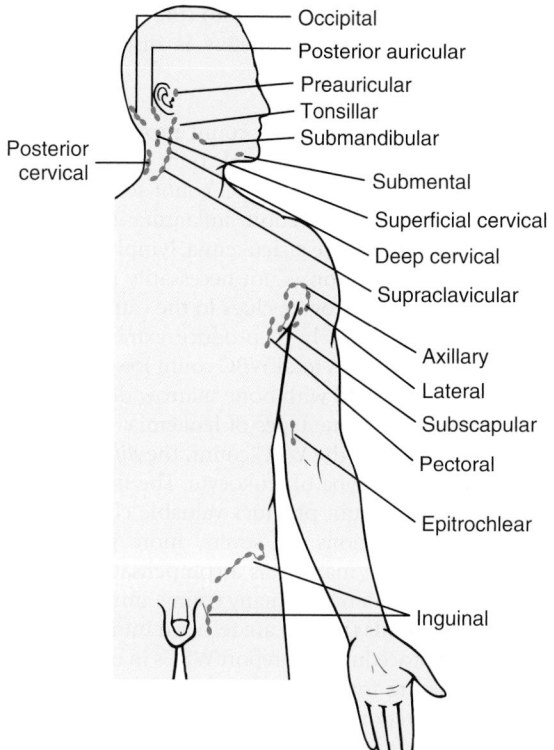

Occipital
Posterior auricular
Preauricular
Tonsillar
Submandibular
Posterior cervical
Submental
Superficial cervical
Deep cervical
Supraclavicular
Axillary
Lateral
Subscapular
Pectoral
Epitrochlear
Inguinal

Figure 32-6 Palpable superficial lymph nodes.

findings or risk factors, cobalamin deficiency and resulting pernicious anemia may be suspected. Although a full examination should be performed on patients suspected of a hematological disorder, certain aspects of the physical examination are specifically relevant in hematological disorders; these include the skin, the lymph nodes, the spleen, and the liver. Examination of the skin is discussed in Chapter 25; spleen and liver examination is described in Chapter 41.

Lymph Node Assessment. Lymph nodes are distributed throughout the body. Superficial lymph nodes can be evaluated by light palpation (Figure 32-6). Deep lymph nodes cannot be palpated and are best evaluated with radiological examination. Lymph nodes should be assessed with regard to symmetry in location, size (in centimetres), degree of fixation (e.g., movable, fixed), tenderness, and texture. To assess superficial lymph nodes, the examiner lightly palpates the nodes with the pads of his or her fingers and then gently rolls the skin over the area and concentrates on feeling for possible lymph node enlargement. If a node is palpable, it should be small (0.5 to 1 cm), mobile, firm, and nontender to be considered normal. A node that is tender, hard, fixed, or enlarged (regardless of whether it is tender or not) is abnormal and warrants further investigation. Tender nodes are usually a result of inflammation, whereas hard or fixed nodes are suggestive of malignancy (Bickley, 2008).

It is important to develop a sequence for examining the lymph nodes. A convenient sequence for examination is to start at the head and neck. First preauricular, posterior auricular, occipital, tonsillar, submaxillary, submental, superficial cervical, posterior cervical chain, deep cervical chain, and supraclavicular nodes are palpated. Next, the axillary lymph nodes and pectoral, subscapular, and lateral groups of nodes are palpated. The

epitrochlear nodes, located in the antecubital fossa between the biceps and triceps muscles, are then examined. The inguinal lymph nodes, found in the groin, are palpated last.

A focused assessment of the hematology system is used to evaluate previously identified hematological problems and to monitor for signs of new problems. An example of such an assessment is presented in the Focused Assessment box "Hematological System."

FOCUSED ASSESSMENT
Hematological System

Use this checklist to make sure the key assessment steps have been performed.

Subjective
Ask the patient about any of the following and note the responses

Unusual bleeding or bruising	Y	N
Black, tarry stool	Y	N
Blood in vomit	Y	N
Swelling in neck, armpits, groin	Y	N
Dark-coloured urine	Y	N
Fatigue	Y	N
Heart palpitations	Y	N

Objective: Diagnostic
Check the following laboratory results for critical values

CBC	✓
Clotting: PT, INR, aPTT, platelets	✓
Hematocrit and hemoglobin	✓

Objective: Physical Examination
Inspect

Skin for lesions or colour changes	✓

Auscultate

Blood pressure for alteration or othostasis	✓

Palpate

Pulse for tachycardia	✓
Liver and spleen for enlargement	✓
Lymph nodes for lymphadenopathy	✓

aPTT, activated partial thromboplastin time; *CBC*, complete blood count; *INR*, international normalized ratio; *PT*, prothrombin time.

Palpation of the Liver or the Spleen. Both the liver and the spleen are normally not detectable through palpation of the abdomen. When they are enlarged, they may be detectable through percussion or palpation. The degree of enlargement of the liver is measured by the number of fingerbreadths it extends below the rib border. The spleen may be more difficult to palpate because of its deep location in the abdomen.

Skin Assessment. In hematological disorders, assessment of the skin may yield valuable information about the hematological system. The skin should be examined over the entire body in a systematic manner (e.g., starting with the face and oral cavity and moving downward over the body). In patients with RBC disorders, the skin may be pale, have a pasty colour, or, in severe anemia, have a cyanotic tinge. Erythrocytosis often produces small vessel occlusions, causing a purple, mottled appearance of the face, the nose, the fingers, or the toes. Digital clubbing can occur with conditions of chronic anemia, such as sickle cell disease. Leukocyte disorders may cause infectious skin lesions or malignant nodular lesions. These lesions may occur anywhere and have a variable distribution pattern. During the physical assessment of the skin, the nurse must look carefully for **petechiae** (small, purplish-red lesions), **ecchymosis** (bruising), and *spider nevus* (a form of *telangiectasia*; Table 32-7) because these can indicate bleeding disorders.

Diagnostic Studies of the Hematological System

The most direct means of evaluating the hematological system is through laboratory analysis and other diagnostic studies. Diagnostic tests of the hematological system are presented in Tables 32-8 through 32-12.

Laboratory Studies

Complete Blood Cell Count.
The complete blood cell count (CBC) involves several laboratory tests (Table 32-8), each of which serves to assess the three major blood cells formed in the bone marrow. In addition to the CBC, a *peripheral blood smear* may be ordered. The smear is used to look at the morphological features (shape and appearance) of the blood cells and may assist with the diagnosis. For example, a large number of immature *blast* WBCs may indicate acute leukemia (Howard & Hamilton, 2008).

Although the status of each cell type is important, the entire system may be disrupted by diseases, as well as by the treatment of diseases. Suppression of the entire CBC is termed **pancytopenia** (marked decrease in the number of RBCs, WBCs, and platelets). In such cases, care is directed toward the management of anemia, infection, and hemorrhage (see Chapter 33).

Red Blood Cells.
Normal values of some RBC tests are reported separately for men and for women because normal values are based on body mass and men usually have a larger body mass than do women.

The *hemoglobin* value is reduced in cases of anemia, hemorrhage, and states of hemodilution, such as those that occur when the fluid volume is excessive. Hemoglobin is increased in polycythemia or in states of hemoconcentration, which can develop from volume depletion (dehydration).

The *hematocrit* value is determined by spinning blood in a centrifuge, which causes erythrocytes (RBCs) and plasma to separate. The RBCs, being the heavier elements, settle to the bottom. The hematocrit value represents the percentage of RBCs in comparison with the total blood volume. The hematocrit value is reduced and elevated in the same conditions that raise and lower the hemoglobin value.

The total RBC count is reported as RBC × 10^{12}/L. However, total RBC count is not always reliable in determining the adequacy of RBC function. Consequently, other data, such as hemoglobin, hematocrit, and RBC indices, must also be evaluated. The RBC count is altered by the same conditions that raise and lower the hemoglobin and hematocrit values.

RBC indices are special indicators that reflect RBC volume, colour, and hemoglobin saturation (see Table 32-8). These

parameters may provide insight into the cause of anemia. (The significance of these parameters is discussed further in Chapter 33.)

White Blood Cells. The WBC count provides two different sets of information. The first is a total count of WBCs per litre of peripheral blood. Elevations in WBC count to more than 11 × 10^9/L are associated with infection, inflammation, tissue injury or death, and malignancies (e.g., leukemia, lymphoma). Although the degree of WBC elevation is not necessarily predictive of the severity of illness, it can provide clues to the cause. Certain types of leukemias are more likely to produce extremely high WBC counts (e.g., >25 × 10^9/L). A total WBC count lower than 4 × 10^9/L **(leukopenia)** is associated with bone marrow depression, severe or chronic illness, and some types of leukemia.

The second aspect of the WBC count, the *differential count*, is the percentage of each type of leukocyte. The information from the WBC differential count provides valuable clues to the cause of illness. When infections are severe, more granulocytes are released from the bone marrow as a compensatory mechanism. To meet the increased demand, many young, immature polymorphonuclear neutrophils (bands) are released into circulation. The usual laboratory procedure is to report WBCs in order of maturity, with the less mature forms (i.e., band neutrophils) on the left side of the written report; hence, the existence of many immature cells is termed a *shift to the left*. A shift to the left may be indicative of active infection or inflammation (e.g., postsurgically). The WBC differential count is of considerable significance because it is possible for the total WBC count to remain essentially normal despite a marked change in one type of leukocyte. For example, a patient may have a normal WBC count of 8.8 × 10^9/L, whereas the differential count may reveal a relative proportion of lymphocytes to be reduced to 10%. This is an abnormal finding that warrants further investigation.

When the lymphocyte count is low, an absolute lymphocyte count may be tabulated. If this count is low, other diagnostic tests may be performed to investigate for an underlying reason.

When the bone marrow does not produce enough neutrophils, neutropenia occurs. **Neutropenia** is a condition associated with a neutrophil count (absolute neutrophil count) lower than 1 × 10^9/L to 1.5 × 10^9/L; severe neutropenia is associated with a neutrophil count lower than 0.5 × 10^9/L. The absolute neutrophil count is determined as the total WBCs multiplied by the percentage of neutrophils. Neutropenia results from a number of disease processes, such as leukemia, or from bone marrow depression (see Chapter 33) and is associated with an increased risk of infection and death from sepsis.

Platelet Count. The platelet count is the number of platelets per microlitre of blood. Normal platelet counts are between 150 × 10^9/L and 400 × 10^9/L; counts lower than 10 × 10^9/L signify a condition termed **thrombocytopenia.** Bleeding may occur with thrombocytopenia. Spontaneous hemorrhage is probable once platelet counts fall below 10 × 10^9/L. A more extensive description of clotting studies is presented in Table 32-9. **Thrombocytosis,** in contrast, is an excess of platelets, a disorder that occurs with inflammation and some malignant disorders. The complication related to thrombocytosis that is most likely to occur is excessive clotting.

Erythrocyte Sedimentation Rate. Erythrocyte sedimentation rate (ESR, or "sed rate") measures the sedimentation, or settling,

Text continued on p. 780

COMMON ASSESSMENT ABNORMALITIES

Table 32-7 Hematological System

FINDING	DESCRIPTION	POSSIBLE ETIOLOGY AND SIGNIFICANCE
Skin		
Pallor of skin or nail beds	Paleness; decrease in or absence of skin coloration	Low Hb level (anemia)
Flushing	Transient, episodic redness of skin (usually around face and neck)	Increase in Hb (polycythemia), congestion of capillaries Flushing of the palms of the hands or the soles of the feet may indicate anemia
Jaundice	Yellow appearance of skin and mucous membranes	Accumulation of bile pigment caused by rapid or excessive hemolysis or liver damage
Cyanosis	Bluish discoloration of skin and mucous membranes	Reduced Hb Excessive concentration of deoxyhemoglobin in blood
Excoriation	Scratch or abrasion of skin	Scratching from intense pruritus
Pruritus	Unpleasant cutaneous sensation that provokes the desire to rub or scratch the skin	Hodgkin's lymphoma Cutaneous lymphomas Infiltrative leukemias Increased bilirubin level
Leg ulcers	Prominent on the malleoli on the ankles	Sickle cell disease
Angioma	Benign tumour consisting of blood or lymph vessels	Most are congenital; some may disappear spontaneously
Telangiectasia	Small angioma with tendency to bleed; focal red lesions, coarse or fine red lines	Dilation of small vessels
Spider nevus	Form of telangiectasia characterized by a round red central portion and branching radiations resembling the profile of a spider; usually develop on face, neck, or chest	Elevated estrogen levels as in pregnancy or liver disease
Purpura	Any of a small group of conditions characterized by ecchymosis or other small hemorrhages in skin and mucous membranes	Decreased numbers of platelets or clotting factors, resulting in hemorrhage into the skin Vascular abnormalities Break in blood vessel walls as a result of trauma
Petechiae	Pinpoint, nonraised, perfectly round area >2 mm; purple, dark red, or brown in colour	Same as for purpura
Ecchymosis (bruise)	Small hemorrhagic spot, larger than petechiae; nonelevated; round or irregular	Same as for purpura
Hematoma	A localized collection of blood, usually clotted	Same as for purpura
Chloroma	A tumour arising from myeloid tissue and containing a pale green pigment	Acute myelogenous leukemia that has infiltrated the skin
Plasmacytoma	A tumour arising from abnormal plasma cells	Multiple myeloma that has infiltrated tissue
Eyes		
Jaundiced sclera	Yellow appearance of the sclera	Accumulation of bile pigment resulting from rapid or excessive hemolysis or liver disease or infiltration
Conjunctival pallor	Paleness; decreased or absence of coloration in the conjunctiva	Low Hb level (anemia)
Blurred vision, diplopia, visual field cuts	Decreased visual acuity or areas of blindness (field cuts)	Anemia, extreme leukocytosis, and polycythemia may cause visual abnormalities Thrombocytopenia may cause intraocular hemorrhage with visual abnormalities Excessive clotting may cause thromboses in the circulation to the brain that cause visual field cuts
Nose		
Epistaxis	Spontaneous bleeding from the nares	May occur with low platelet counts, especially if the patient bends down for a long period, tries to lift a heavy item, or attempts an intense Valsalva manoeuvre

Continued

Table 32-7 Hematological System—cont'd

FINDING	DESCRIPTION	POSSIBLE ETIOLOGY AND SIGNIFICANCE
Mouth		
Gingival and mucous membrane changes	Pallor	Low Hb level (anemia)
	Gingival or mucosal ulceration, swelling, or bleeding	Neutropenia; inability of impaired leukocytes to combat oral infections; thrombocytopenia
		Gingival hyperplasia may be present with some types of leukemia
Smooth tongue	Tongue surface is smooth and shiny; mucosa is thin and red from decreased papillae	Pernicious anemia, iron-deficiency anemia
Lymph Nodes		
Lymphadenopathy	Lymph nodes are enlarged (>1 cm diameter)	Infection, foreign infiltrations, or systemic disease such as leukemia, lymphoma, Hodgkin's lymphoma, and metastatic cancer
Heart and Chest		
Tachycardia	Heart rate >100 beats/min	Compensatory mechanism in anemia to increase cardiac output
Palpitations	Sensation of feeling the heart beat, flutter, or pound in the chest	Anemia, fluid volume overload, hypotension with impending syncope, hypertension, and dysrhythmias may cause palpitations
Altered blood pressure	Orthostasis: >20/min increase in heart rate or >20 mm Hg decrease in blood pressure from baseline value when moving from a lying position to either sitting or standing	Orthostasis is a common manifestation in anemia, especially if accompanied by low blood volume
	Hypotension: <90 mm Hg systolic or >40 mm Hg drop in systolic reading from baseline BP	Hypotension may indicate an infectious process, blood loss, or compromised cardiovascular compensatory mechanisms
	Hypertension: >130/90 mm Hg	In anemia, hypertension may occur initially as a compensatory mechanism for anemia
Sternal tenderness	Abnormal sensitivity to touch or pressure on sternum	Leukemia, as a result of increased bone marrow cellularity, which causes increase in pressure and bone erosion; multiple myeloma, as a result of stretching of periosteum
Low oxygen saturation	Oxygen-carrying capacity is reflected by the oxygen saturation as measured with pulse oximetry	Oxygen saturation may be decreased in cases of severe anemia
Abdomen		
Hepatomegaly	Palpable liver	Leukemia, cirrhosis, or fibrosis secondary to iron overload from sickle cell disease or thalassemia
Splenomegaly	Palpable spleen	Anemia, thrombocytopenia, leukemia, lymphomas, leukopenia, mononucleosis, malaria, cirrhosis, trauma, portal hypertension
Distended abdomen	Distended abdomen is an abdominal profile that is larger than normal; it may be soft or firm, tender or nontender, and accompanied by other symptoms such as nausea, vomiting, or rebound tenderness	Lymphoma may manifest as abdominal adenopathy, one or more masses, or bowel obstruction
Nervous System		
Paraesthesias of feet and hands; ataxia	Numbness sensation and extreme sensitivity experienced in central and peripheral nerves; impaired muscle movement	Cobalamin (vitamin B_{12}) deficiency or folate deficiency
Weakness	Lacking physical strength or energy	Low Hb level (anemia)
Headache, nuchal rigidity	Pain in the cranium, potentially involving one area or extending from the frontal area to the back of the neck	Generalized headache is a common manifestation of mild to moderate anemia
		Severe headache with or without visual disturbances may signal intracranial hemorrhage caused by thrombocytopenia
Musculoskeletal System		
Bone pain	Pain in pelvis, ribs, spine, sternum	Multiple myeloma, in relation to enlarged tumours that stretch periosteum
		Bone invasion by leukemia cells
		Bone demineralization that results from various malignancies
		Sickle cell disease
Joint swelling	Fluid-filled spaces surrounding the joints	Occurs with sickle cell anemia as bleeding into the joint (hemarthrosis) causes inflammation
Arthralgia	Joint pain	Sickle cell disease, as a result of hemarthrosis

Hb, hemoglobin.

Table 32-8 Complete Blood Cell Count Studies

STUDY	DESCRIPTION AND PURPOSE	NORMAL VALUES
Hb	Measurement of gas-carrying capacity of RBCs	Women: 120-160 g/L Men: 140-180 g/L
Hct	Measurement of packed cell volume of RBCs, expressed as a percentage of the total blood volume	Women: 0.37-0.47 Men: 0.42-0.52
Total RBC count	Count of number of circulating RBCs	Women: $4.2\text{-}5.4 \times 10^{12}$/L Men: $4.7\text{-}6.1 \times 10^{12}$/L
RBC indices		
• MCV (Hct/RBC)	Determination of relative size of RBC; low MCV reflection of microcytosis, high MCV reflection of macrocytosis	80-95 fL
• MCH (Hb/RBC)	Measurement of average weight of Hb/RBCs; low MCH is indication of microcytosis or hypochromia, high MCH is indication of macrocytosis	27-31 pg
• MCHC	Evaluation of RBC saturation with Hb; low MCHC is indication of hypochromia, high MCHC is evident in spherocytosis	320-360 g/L
• RBC morphology	Examination of the shape and size of RBCs	No variation in RBC structure
• WBC count	Measurement of total number of leukocytes	$5\text{-}10 \times 10^9$/L
• WBC differential	Determination of whether each kind of WBC is present in proper proportion; absolute value is determined by multiplying percentage of cell type by total WBC count and dividing by 100	Neutrophils: $2.5\text{-}7.5 \times 10^9$/L Eosinophils: $0.01\text{-}0.04 \times 10^9$/L Basophils: $0\text{-}0.01 \times 10^9$/L Lymphocytes: $0.1\text{-}0.4 \times 10^9$/L Monocytes: $0.02\text{-}0.07 \times 10^9$/L
• Platelet count	Measurement of number of platelets available to maintain platelet clotting functions (not measurement of quality of platelet function)	$150\text{-}400 \times 10^9$/L

Hb, hemoglobin; *Hct*, hematocrit; *MCH*, mean corpuscular hemoglobin; *MCHC*, mean corpuscular hemoglobin concentration; *MCV*, mean corpuscular volume; *RBC*, red blood cell; *WBC*, white blood cell.

Table 32-9 Clotting Studies

STUDY	DESCRIPTION AND PURPOSE	NORMAL VALUES
Activated clotting time (ACT)	Evaluation of intrinsic coagulation status; more accurate than aPTT; used during dialysis, coronary artery bypass procedure, arteriography	70-120 sec
Activated partial thromboplastin time (aPTT)	Assessment of intrinsic coagulation by measuring factors I, II, V, VIII, IX, X, XI, and XII; longer with the use of heparin	30-40 sec
Antithrombin	Naturally occurring protein synthesized by the liver that inhibits coagulation through inactivation of thrombin and other factors; is depleted in DIC	220-300 mg/L or 0.85-1.15 of standard
Bleeding time	Measurement of timed small skin incision bleeds; reflection of ability of small blood vessels to constrict	60-540 sec (1-9 min)
Capillary fragility test (tourniquet test, Rumpel-Leede test)	Reflection of capillary integrity when positive or negative pressure is applied to various areas of the body; positive result is indication of thrombocytopenia, toxic vascular reactions	No petechiae, or negative
Clot retraction	Reflection of clot shrinkage or retraction from sides of test tube after 24 hr; used to confirm a platelet problem	50-100% in 1-2 hr, complete retraction in 24 hr
D-Dimer	Assay to measure a fragment of fibrin that is formed as a result of fibrin degradation and clot lysis; used in diagnosis of hypercoagulable conditions	<250 mcg/L
Fibrin split products (FSP) or fibrin degradation products	Reflection of degree of fibrinolysis and predisposition to bleed (if present); screening test for DIC; elevated levels associated with DIC, advanced malignancy, severe inflammation	<10 mg/L
Fibrinogen	Reflection of level of fibrinogen; increase in fibrinogen may indicate enhancement of fibrin formation, which renders patient hypercoagulable; decrease in fibrinogen indicates that patient may be predisposed to bleeding	2-4 g/L
International normalized ratio (INR)	Standardized system of reporting PT that is based on a reference calibration model and calculated by comparison of the patient's PT with a control value	0.8-1.2
Platelet count	Count of number of circulating platelets	150×10^9/L to 400×10^9/L
Prothrombin time (PT)	Assessment of extrinsic coagulation by measurement of factors I, II, V, VII, and X	11-12.5 sec
Thrombin time	Reflection of adequacy of thrombin; prolonged thrombin time indicates that coagulation is inadequate secondary to decreased thrombin activity	8-12 sec

DIC, disseminated intravascular coagulation.

Table 32-10 ABO Blood Group Names and Patient/Donor Compatibilities*

RECIPIENT'S BLOOD GROUP	RBC ANTIGEN	PLASMA/SERUM ANTIBODY	COMPATIBLE DONOR FOR RBC TRANSFUSIONS	COMPATIBLE DONOR FOR PLASMA TRANSFUSIONS
A	A	Anti-B	A and O	A and AB
B	B	Anti-A	B and O	B and AB
AB (universal recipient)	Both A and B	Neither anti-A nor anti-B	A, B, AB, and O	AB
O	Neither A nor B	Both anti-A and anti-B	O (universal donor)	A, B, AB, and O

*ABO blood groups are named for the antigen found on the RBCs. Donor compatibility is based on the antibodies present in the serum.
RBC, red blood cell.

of RBCs and is used as a nonspecific measure of many diseases, especially inflammatory conditions. ESR commonly increases during acute and chronic inflammatory reactions when cell destruction is increased. ESR is also increased with malignancy, myocardial infarction, and end-stage renal disease. Although the ESR is a nonspecific test, it is often used as a routine screening procedure.

Blood Typing and Rh Factor.

Blood group antigens (A and B) are found only on RBC membranes and form the basis for the ABO blood typing system. The presence or absence of one or both of the two inherited antigens is the basis for the four blood groups: *A, B, AB,* and *O*. People with blood group A have A antigens, those with group B have B antigens, those with group AB have both A and B antigens, and those with group O have neither A nor B antigens. People with blood types A, B, or O have antibodies in the serum termed *anti-A* and *anti-B* that react with A or B antigens. These antibodies are found when the corresponding antigen is absent from the RBC membrane. For example, anti-B antibodies are found in the plasma of people with blood group A (Table 32-10).

Blood reactions caused by ABO incompatibilities result in intravascular hemolysis of the RBCs. RBCs *agglutinate* (or clump) when a serum antibody that reacts with the antigens on the RBC membrane is present. For example, agglutination would occur in the blood of a person with type A blood if he or she received blood from a donor with B antigens (i.e., type B or AB). The anti-B antibodies in the serum of the person with type A blood would react with the B antigens on the donor RBCs, thus initiating the process that results in RBC hemolysis.

The Rhesus (Rh) system is based on a third antigen, D, which is also found on the RBC membrane. Rh-positive people have the D antigen, whereas Rh-negative people do not. Rh-positive blood is indicated with a plus sign after the ABO group name (e.g., "AB+"). A Coombs test is used to evaluate the person's Rh status (Table 32-11).

As a result of transfusion therapy or during childbirth, an Rh-negative person may be exposed to Rh-positive blood. If an Rh-negative mother gives birth to an Rh-positive infant, the mother forms an antibody, anti-D, which acts against Rh antigens. (Rh-positive people normally have no anti-D antibody.) In subsequent pregnancies, the mother's anti-D antibodies can cross the placenta and attack the RBCs of a fetus who is Rh-positive, thus causing hemolysis of the RBCs. A pregnant Rh-negative woman should receive RhoGAM injections during pregnancy to prevent anti-D antibodies from forming.

Iron Metabolism.

The laboratory tests used in evaluating iron metabolism include serum iron, total iron-binding capacity (TIBC), serum ferritin, and transferrin saturation. Additional tests for nutritional deficiencies leading to defective RBC production may also be performed (see Table 32-11).

Serum iron is a measurement of the amount of protein-bound iron circulating in the serum. TIBC provides a measurement of all proteins that bind or transport iron between the tissues and the bone marrow. Although this indirect measurement is a general reflection of the amount of transferrin present in the circulation, it overestimates transferrin levels by 16 to 20% because it also measures other proteins that can bind iron. These alternative proteins bind iron only when transferrin is more than half saturated. Also, TIBC varies inversely with tissue iron stores; it is higher when iron stores are low and lower when iron stores are high.

Transferrin saturation is a better indicator of the availability of iron for erythropoiesis than is serum iron because, unlike serum iron, the iron bound to transferrin is readily available for the body to use. To calculate transferrin saturation, the serum iron value is divided by TIBC, and the result is multiplied by 100. For example, a patient with a serum iron level of 100 mcg/dL and a TIBC of 300 mcg/dL would have a transferrin saturation of about 33%. Under normal conditions, the serum ferritin concentration is correlated closely with body iron stores.

Radiological Studies

Radiological studies for the hematology system involve primarily the use of computed tomography or magnetic resonance imaging for evaluating the spleen, the liver, and the lymph nodes. Nursing responsibilities related to these studies are presented in Table 32-12.

Biopsy

Biopsy procedures specific to hematological assessment are bone marrow examination and lymph node biopsy. In general, these procedures are performed because a peripheral blood smear yields nonspecific results and a diagnosis cannot usually be established from a peripheral blood smear. Furthermore, a biopsy provides additional information about a hematological problem; such information is needed for diagnostic purposes, as well as for planning treatment options.

Bone Marrow Examination.

Bone marrow examination is important in the evaluation of many hematological disorders. The examination of the marrow may involve aspiration alone or aspiration with biopsy. The benefits of bone marrow examination include the ability to (a) fully evaluate hematopoiesis and (b) obtain specimens for cytopathological study and evaluation for chromosomal abnormalities.

The preferred site for both aspiration and biopsy of bone marrow is the posterior superior iliac crest (Pagana & Pagana, 2011). In adults, the anterior superior iliac crest is an alternative site. Bone marrow aspiration and biopsy are performed by a physician or by a nurse with special credentials. Conscious seda-

Table 32-11 Miscellaneous Laboratory Blood Studies

STUDY/SUBSTANCE STUDIED	DESCRIPTION AND PURPOSE	NORMAL VALUES
Bilirubin	Measurement of degree of RBC hemolysis or liver's inability to excrete normal quantities of bilirubin Increase in indirect bilirubin with hemolytic problems	Total: 5.1-17 mcmol/L Direct: 1.7-5.1 mcmol/L Indirect: 3.4-12 mcmol/L
Coombs test	Differentiation among types of hemolytic anemias; detection of immune antibodies; detection of Rh factor	Negative finding (no agglutination)
• Direct	Detection of antibodies that are attached to RBCs	Negative finding
• Indirect	Detection of antibodies in serum	Negative finding
Cobalamin (vitamin B$_{12}$)	Level of vitamin B$_{12}$ available for production of new RBCs	118-701 pmol/L
Erythropoietin	Measurement of degree of hormonal stimulation of the bone marrow to release RBCs	5-36 IU/L
Erythrocyte sedimentation rate (ESR)	Measurement of sedimentation, or settling, of RBCs in 1 hr Inflammatory process causes an alteration in plasma proteins, resulting in aggregation of RBCs and making them heavier; the faster the RBCs settle, the higher the ESR is	Female • <50 yr: <20 mm/hr • >50 yr: <30 mm/hr Male • <50 yr: <15 mm/hr • >50 yr: <20 mm/hr
Ferritin	Major iron storage protein; is normally present in blood in concentrations directly related to iron storage	Female: 10-150 mcg/L Male: 12-300 mcg/L
Folic acid (folate)	Amount of folic acid or folate available for RBC production	11-57 nmol/L
Hemoglobin (Hb) electrophoresis	Proteins involved in development of the hemoglobin molecule have a definitive pattern of separation on electrophoresis; this pattern is altered with abnormal Hb synthesis, as occurs in thalassemia or in sickle cell anemia, in which sickle Hb (HbS) is increased	Normal HbA$_1$: 95-98% HbA$_2$: 2-3% HbF: 0.8-2% HbS: 0% HbC: 0%
Homocysteine	An amino acid formed from methionine Rapidly metabolized through pathways that require cobalamin (vitamin B$_1$) and folic acid; increased in deficiencies of cobalamin and folic acid	4-14 mcmol/L
Iron		
• Serum iron	Reflection of amount of iron combined with proteins in serum; accurate indication of status of iron storage and use	9-26.9 mcmol/L
• Total iron-binding capacity (TIBC)	Measurement of all proteins available for binding iron Transferrin represents the largest quantity of iron-binding proteins; therefore, TIBC is an indirect measure of transferrin	45-82 mcmol/L
Methylmalonic acid (MMA)	Indirect test for cobalamin: MMA metabolism requires cobalamin; test helps differentiate cobalamin deficiency from folic acid deficiency	80-560 mcmol/L
Reticulocyte count	Measurement of immature RBCs; reflection of bone marrow activity in producing RBCs	0.5-2% of RBC count (0.005-0.015 of RBC count)
Serum protein electrophoresis	Separates proteins in the blood on basis of electrical charge; helps detect hyperglobulinemic states, as in multiple myeloma or some lymphomas	Normal banding pattern of albumin and globulins; an increase in any protein ("protein spike") is abnormal
Transferrin	The largest of proteins that bind to iron; increased in majority of people with iron-deficiency anemia	2.15-3.18 g/L
Transferrin saturation (%)	Decreased in iron-deficiency anemia and increased in hemolytic and megaloblastic anemia	15-50%

RBCs, red blood cells.

Table 32-12 Hematological System

STUDY/SUBSTANCE STUDIED	DESCRIPTION AND PURPOSE	NURSING RESPONSIBILITY
Urine Studies		
Bence Jones protein	An electrophoretic measurement is used to detect the presence of the Bence Jones protein, which is found in most cases of multiple myeloma. Negative finding is considered normal.	Acquire random urine specimen.
Radioisotope Studies		
Liver–spleen scan	Radioactive isotope is injected intravenously. Images from the radioactive emissions are used to evaluate the structure of the spleen and the liver. Patient is not a source of radioactivity.	No specific nursing responsibilities.
Bone scan	Same procedure as for the spleen scan except used for evaluating the structure of the bones.	Intravenous access is required.
Radiological Studies		
Skeletal radiography	Radiographic studies performed as a bone survey to determine the presence of lytic lesions associated with multiple myeloma. Bone scans do not identify lesions in this condition: Because of lack of blood supply, there is no uptake of radioactive isotopes.	No specific nursing responsibilities.
Liver, spleen, or abdominal ultrasonography	Noninvasive probe is lubricated and slid across the abdomen to detect the density and borders of the abdominal organs. Irregular borders, masses, vascular structure, and biliary tree can be detected.	Patients must be comfortable lying flat, and the probe must compress the abdomen.
Positron emission tomography (PET)	A nuclear tracer substance is injected and is taken up by metabolically active cells. The follow-up scan shows tissues in different colours that are based on the metabolic rate. "Hot spots" reflect increased glucose consumption that may reflect tumours.	Intravenous access is required for injection of the tracer substance. Patients should ingest nothing by mouth, except water and medications, for at least 4 hr before the test. IV solutions containing glucose may be held. Patients who are glucose intolerant or diabetic may need adjustments in their medications. Bowel preparation may also be needed, depending on the area being studied.
Computed tomography (CT)	Noninvasive examination in which computer-assisted radiography is used to evaluate the lymph nodes. Contrast medium often is used in abdominal studies of the liver or the spleen. Spiral CT is used to evaluate lymph nodes.	If contrast medium is used, investigate whether patient has iodine sensitivity.
Magnetic resonance imaging (MRI)	Noninvasive procedure that produces sensitive images of soft tissue without the use of contrast medium. No ionizing radiation is required. Technique is used to evaluate spleen, liver, and lymph nodes.	Instruct patient to remove all metal objects and ask about any history of surgical insertion of staples, plates, or other metal appliances. Inform patient of need to lie still in small chamber.
Biopsy		
Bone marrow	Removal of bone marrow through a locally anaesthetized site to evaluate the status of the blood-forming tissue. Used to diagnose multiple myeloma, leukemia, some lymphomas and to stage some solid tumours. Also performed to assess efficacy of leukemia therapy.*	Explain procedure to patient. Obtain signed consent form. Consider preprocedure analgesic administration to enhance patient comfort and cooperation. Apply pressure dressing after procedure. Assess biopsy site for bleeding.
Lymph node biopsy	Excision of lymph tissue for histological examination to determine diagnosis and therapy.	Explain procedure to patient. Obtain signed consent form. Use sterile technique in dressing changes after procedure.
• Open	Excision of lymph node and surrounding tissue through an incision. Performed in the operating room or procedure area; either local or general anaesthesia is administered.	Observe site for bleeding, and monitor vital signs, especially if the platelet count is low. The sterile dressing should be changed as ordered, and the wound should be inspected for healing and infection.
• Closed (needle) or fine needle	Performed at patient's bedside or in an outpatient area.	—
Molecular, Cytogenic, and Gene Analysis Studies		
Fluorescent in situ hybridization (FISH) Comparative genomic hybridization (CGH) Spectral karyotyping (SKY)	Tests performed on malignant cells, either peripheral blood (e.g., leukemia) or biopsy specimen (bone marrow, lymph node), to assess genetic or chromosomal abnormalities of cancer cells. May be useful in confirming diagnosis and determining treatment modalities and prognosis.	No specific nursing responsibilities. Explain purpose of testing to patient.
Blood Studies†		

*See Chapter 33.
†See Tables 32-8, 32-9, and 32-11.
IV, intravenous.

tion may be induced in the patient to minimize anxiety and pain. For bone marrow aspiration, the skin over the puncture site is cleansed with a bactericidal agent. The skin, subcutaneous tissue, and periosteum are infiltrated with a local anaesthetic agent (Figure 32-7). The patient may be uncomfortable when the periosteum is penetrated. Once the area is anaesthetized, a bone marrow needle is inserted through the cortex of the bone. The stylet of the needle is then removed, the hub is attached to a 10-mL syringe, and 0.2 to 0.5 mL of the marrow fluid is aspirated. The patient may experience pain with aspiration. Although it generally lasts for only a few seconds, the pain may be quite uncomfortable. After the marrow aspiration, the needle is removed. Pressure is applied over the aspiration site to ensure hemostasis. If the patient is thrombocytopenic, pressure may be required for 5 to 10 minutes or longer. With severe thrombocytopenia, platelets may be infused before the procedure. If a bone biopsy is required, the preparatory procedure remains the same, but a different needle is used. The needle has a cutting blade that allows a specimen of the bone to be removed.

Although complications of bone marrow aspiration are minimal, there is a possibility of penetrating the bone and damaging underlying structures. Other complications include hemorrhage (particularly if the patient is thrombocytopenic) and infection (particularly if the patient is leukopenic).

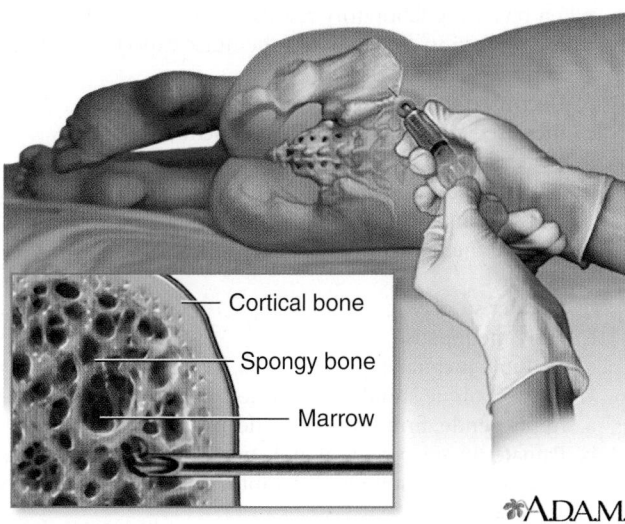

Figure 32-7 Bone marrow aspiration from the posterior superior iliac crest.

Source: A.D.A.M., Inc.

Lymph Node Biopsy.
Lymph node biopsy involves obtaining lymph tissue for histological examination to determine the diagnosis and to help plan for therapy. This may be accomplished through either an open biopsy or a closed (needle) biopsy. Negative results from a needle biopsy may indicate only that the cancer cells were not part of tissue specimen obtained. A repeated needle biopsy or a larger tissue specimen (open biopsy) may be subsequently required.

Molecular Cytogenetics and Gene Analysis

Testing for specific genetic or chromosomal variations in hematological conditions is often helpful in diagnosis, in determining the treatment options, and in determining prognosis. If a large number of abnormal cells are circulating in the blood, as in acute leukemia, these tests may be performed with peripheral blood samples. However, testing is usually performed on samples from bone marrow and from lymph node biopsy. For example, fluorescent in situ hybridization can be used to identify specific areas: A probe attached to a targeted region of DNA can reveal an abnormal extra chromosome 8 that is common in certain leukemias. Spectral karyotyping allows for each set of chromosomes to be coloured individually. It can be used to identify the 9;2 translocation in the Philadelphia chromosome of chronic myelogenous leukemia. More information on genetics is available in Chapter 15.

---

evolve   *An assessment case study of the hematological system is available at* **http://evolve.elsevier.com/Canada/Lewis/medsurg**

REVIEW QUESTIONS

The number of the question corresponds to the same-numbered objective at the beginning of the chapter.

1. Why might an individual who lives at a high altitude normally have an increased RBC count?
   a. High altitudes cause vascular fluid loss, leading to hemoconcentration.
   b. Hypoxia caused by decreased atmospheric oxygen stimulates erythropoiesis.
   c. The function of the spleen in removing old erythrocytes is impaired at high altitudes.
   d. Impaired production of leukocytes and platelets leads to proportionally higher RBC counts.

2. What would be the primary effect of a malignant disorder that arises from granulocytic cells in the bone marrow?
   a. Risk for hemorrhage
   b. Altered oxygenation
   c. Decreased production of antibodies
   d. Decreased phagocytosis of bacteria

3. When will an anticoagulant such as warfarin (Coumadin), which interferes with the production of prothrombin, alter the clotting mechanism?
   a. During platelet aggregation
   b. During activation of thrombin
   c. During the release of tissue thromboplastin
   d. During stimulation of factor activation complex

4. When reviewing laboratory results of an 83-year-old patient with an infection, what should the nurse expect to find?
   a. Minimal leukocytosis
   b. Decreased platelet count
   c. Increased hemoglobin and hematocrit levels
   d. Decreased ESR

5. Which of the following information, obtained from a patient's health history, would be considered significant in relation to the hematological system?
   a. Jaundice
   b. Bladder surgery
   c. Early menopause
   d. Multiple pregnancies

6. Which technique should be used to assess lymph nodes?
   a. Apply gentle, firm pressure to deep lymph nodes.
   b. Palpate the deep cervical and supraclavicular nodes last.
   c. Lightly palpate superficial lymph nodes with the pads of the fingers.
   d. Use the tips of the second, third, and fourth fingers to apply deep palpation.

7. When a lymph node is palpated, which of the following is a normal finding?
   a. Hard, fixed nodes
   b. Firm, mobile nodes
   c. Enlarged, tender nodes
   d. Hard, nontender nodes

8. Nursing care for a patient immediately after a bone marrow biopsy and aspiration includes which of the following?
   a. Administering analgesics as necessary
   b. Preparing to administer a blood transfusion
   c. Administering postprocedure antibiotics
   d. Cleansing the site immediately with povidone-iodine

ANSWERS: 1. b; 2. d; 3. b; 4. a; 5. a; 6. c; 7. b; 8. a.

REFERENCES

Alpers, D. H., Stenson, W. F., Taylor, B. E., & Bier, D. M. (2008). *Manual of nutritional therapeutics* (5th ed.). Philadelphia: Lippincott Williams & Wilkins.

Andrews, N. C. (2009). Pathology of iron metabolism. In R. Hoffman, R. Benz, S. Shattil, B. Furie, H. J. Cohen, L. E. Silberstein, & P. McGlave (Eds.), *Hematology: Basic principles and practice* (5th ed.). Philadelphia: W. B. Saunders.

Bickley, L. S. (2008). *Bates' guide to physical examination and history taking* (10th ed.). Philadelphia: Lippincott Williams & Wilkins.

Ershler, W. B., & Longo, D. L. (2010). Hematology in older persons. In K. Kaushansky, M. Lichtman, E. Beutler, T. Kipps, J. Prchal, & U. Seligsohn (Eds.), *Williams hematology* (8th ed.). New York: McGraw-Hill.

Gardenghi, S., Grady, R. W., & Rivella, S. (2010). Anemia, ineffective erythropoiesis, and hepcidin: Interacting factors in abnormal iron metabolism leading to iron overload β-thalassemia. *Hematology Oncology Clinics of North America, 24*, 1089-1107. doi:10.1016/j.hoc.2010.08.003

Ginsburg, D., & Wagner, D. D. (2009). Structure, biology, and genetics of von Willebrand factor. In R. Hoffman, R. Benz, S. Shattil, B. Furie, H. J. Cohen, L. E. Silberstein, & P. McGlave (Eds.), *Hematology: Basic principles and practice* (5th ed.). Philadelphia: W. B. Saunders.

Howard, M. R., & Hamilton, P. J. (2008). *Haematology: An illustrated colour text* (3rd ed.). Edinburgh: Churchill Livingstone.

Huff, J. (2007). Benzene-induced cancers: Abridged history and occupational health impact. *International Journal of Occupational and Environmental Health, 13*, 213-221.

Jafarzadeh, A., Poorgholami, M., Izadi N., Nemati, M., & Rezayati, M. (2010). Immunological and haematological changes in patients with hyperthyroidism and hypothyroidism. *Clinical & Investigative Medicine, 33*, 271-279.

Kumar, V., & Sharma, A. (2010). Neutrophils: Cinderella of innate immune system. *International Immunopharmacology, 10*, 1325-1334. doi:10.1016/j.intimp.2010.08.012

McCance, K. L., & Huether, S. E. (Eds.). (2010). *Pathophysiology: The biologic basis for disease in adults and children* (6th ed.). St. Louis: Mosby.

Mughal, T. I., Goldman, J. M. & Mughal, S. T. (2010). *Understanding leukemias, lymphomas, and myelomas*. London, England: Informa UK.

Owens, A. P., & Mackman, N. (2011). Microparticles in hemostasis and thrombosis. *Circulation Research, 108*, 1284-1297. doi:10.1161/CIRCRESAHA.110.233056

Pagana, K. D., & Pagana, K. J. (2011). *Mosby's diagnostic and laboratory test reference* (11th ed.). St. Louis: Elsevier Mosby.

Shaheen, M., & Broxmeyer, H. D. (2009). The humoral regulation of hematopoiesis. In R. Hoffman, R. Benz, S. Shattil, B. Furie, H. J. Cohen, L. E. Silberstein, & P. McGlave (Eds.), *Hematology: Basic principles and practice* (5th ed.). Philadelphia: Saunders.

Wu, D., & Meydani, S. N. (2008). Age-associated changes in the immune and inflammatory responses: Impact of vitamin E intervention. *Journal of Leukocyte Biology, 84*, 900-914. doi:10.1189/jlb.0108023

RESOURCES

Resources for this chapter are listed in Chapter 33 on page 839.

Nursing Management: Hematological Problems

Written by Sandra Irene Rome
Adapted by Bridgette Lord

LEARNING OBJECTIVES

1. Describe the general clinical manifestations and complications of anemia.
2. Describe the etiologies, clinical manifestations, diagnostic findings, and nursing and collaborative management of iron-deficiency, megaloblastic, and aplastic anemias and anemia of chronic disease.
3. Explain the nursing management of patients with anemia secondary to blood loss.
4. Describe the pathophysiology, clinical manifestations, and nursing and collaborative management of anemia caused by increased erythrocyte destruction, including sickle cell disease and acquired hemolytic anemias.
5. Describe the pathophysiology and nursing and collaborative management of polycythemia.
6. Explain the pathophysiology, clinical manifestations, and nursing and collaborative management of various types of thrombocytopenia.
7. Describe the types, clinical manifestations, diagnostic findings, and nursing and collaborative management of hemophilia and von Willebrand's disease.
8. Explain the pathophysiology, diagnostic findings, and nursing and collaborative management of disseminated intravascular coagulation.
9. Describe the etiology, clinical manifestations, and nursing and collaborative management of neutropenia.
10. Describe the pathophysiology, clinical manifestations, and nursing and collaborative management of myelodysplastic syndrome.
11. Compare and contrast the major types of leukemia in terms of age of onset, clinical manifestations, and diagnostic findings.
12. Explain the nursing and collaborative management of patients with acute and chronic leukemias.
13. Compare Hodgkin's lymphoma and non-Hodgkin's lymphoma in terms of clinical manifestations, staging, and nursing and collaborative management.
14. Describe the pathophysiology, clinical manifestations, and nursing and collaborative management of multiple myeloma.
15. Describe the care of patients with spleen disorders and related collaborative care.
16. Describe the nursing management of the patient receiving transfusions of blood and blood products.

KEY TERMS

anemia A deficiency in the number of erythrocytes (red blood cells [RBCs]), the quantity of hemoglobin, and/or the volume of packed RBCs (hematocrit), p. 786

aplastic anemia A disease in which the patient has peripheral blood pancytopenia (decrease of all blood cell types—RBCs, white blood cells [WBCs], and platelets) and hypocellular bone marrow, p. 795

disseminated intravascular coagulation (DIC) A grave coagulopathy resulting from the abnormally initiated and accelerated clotting and anticlotting processes that occur in response to disease or injury, p. 812

hemochromatosis An autosomal recessive disease characterized by increased intestinal iron absorption and, as a result, increased tissue iron deposition, p. 801

hemolytic anemia A condition caused by the destruction or hemolysis of RBCs at a rate that exceeds production, p. 797

hemophilia A sex-linked recessive genetic disorder caused by defective or deficient coagulation factor, p. 809

Hodgkin's lymphoma A malignant condition characterized by proliferation of abnormal giant, multinucleated cells, called *Reed-Sternberg cells*, which are located in lymph nodes, p. 825

iron-deficiency anemia A microcytic hypochromic anemia caused by inadequate supplies of the iron needed to synthesize hemoglobin, p. 790

leukemia A broad term given to a group of malignant diseases characterized by diffuse replacement of bone marrow with proliferating leukocyte precursors, p. 819

lymphomas Malignant neoplasms originating in the bone marrow and lymphatic structures resulting in the proliferation of lymphocytes, p. 825

megaloblastic anemias A group of disorders caused by impaired DNA synthesis and characterized by the presence of large RBCs, p. 793

multiple myeloma A condition in which neoplastic plasma cells infiltrate the bone marrow and destroy bone, p. 829

myelodysplastic syndrome (MDS) A group of related hematological disorders characterized by a change in the quantity and the quality of bone marrow elements, p. 818

neutropenia An abnormal reduction of the neutrophil count to less than 1 to 1.5×10^9/L, p. 815

non-Hodgkin's lymphomas (NHLs) A heterogeneous group of malignant neoplasms of primarily B- or T-cell origin, affecting all ages, p. 827

pernicious anemia A disease in which the gastric mucosa does not secrete intrinsic factor (IF) because of antibodies being directed against the gastric parietal cells and/or IF itself, p. 793

polycythemia The production and presence of increased numbers of RBCs, p. 802

sickle cell disease (SCD) A group of inherited, autosomal recessive disorders characterized by the presence of an abnormal form of hemoglobin in the erythrocyte, p. 797

thalassemia An autosomal recessive genetic disorder in which there is inadequate production of normal hemoglobin, p. 792

thrombocytopenia A reduction of platelets to an amount below 150×10^9/L, p. 803

ELECTRONIC RESOURCES

Supplemental content related to Chapter 33 can be found …

Evolve Web Site ⊖volve

http://evolve.elsevier.com/Canada/Lewis/medsurg
- Answer Guidelines for Case Study on p. 836
- Clinical Reference: Laboratory Values
- Content Updates
- Customizable Nursing Care Plans:
  - Anemia
  - Neutropenia
  - Thrombocytopenia

- Electronic Calculators
- Examination Review Questions
- Glossary
- Interactive Case Studies
  - Chronic Myelogenous Leukemia Including End-of-Life Care
  - Sickle Cell Anemia
- Key Points (Printable and MP3 Download)

Anemia

Definition and Classification

Anemia is a deficiency in the number of erythrocytes (red blood cells [RBCs]), the quantity of hemoglobin (Hb), and the volume of packed RBCs (hematocrit [Hct]). It is a prevalent condition with many diverse causes such as blood loss, impaired production of erythrocytes, or increased destruction of erythrocytes (Figure 33-1). Because RBCs transport oxygen (O_2), erythrocyte disorders can lead to tissue hypoxia; this accounts for many of the signs and symptoms of anemia. Anemia is not a specific disease: it is a manifestation of a pathological process.

Anemia is identified by a thorough history and physical examination, and then classified based on laboratory review of the complete blood count, reticulocyte count, and peripheral blood smear. Once anemia is identified, further investigation is done to determine its cause (Marks & Glader, 2009).

Anemia can result from primary hematological problems or can develop as a secondary consequence of defects in other body systems. There are also biological and genetic factors (see the Determinants of Health box). The various types of anemia can be grouped according to either a morphological classification (by cellular characteristics) or an etiological one (by underlying cause). Morphological classification is based on descriptive, objective laboratory information about erythrocyte size and colour (Table 33-1). Etiological classification is related to the clinical conditions causing the anemia (Table 33-2). Although the morphological system is the most accurate means of classifying anemias, it is easier to discuss patient care by focusing on the cause or etiology of the anemia.

Clinical Manifestations

The clinical manifestations of anemia are caused by the body's response to tissue hypoxia. Specific manifestations vary depending on the severity of the anemia and the presence of coexisting disease. Hb levels are often used to determine the severity of anemia. Mild states of anemia (Hb 100-120 g/L) may exist without causing symptoms. If symptoms develop, it is because the patient has an underlying disease or is experiencing a compensatory response to heavy exercise. Symptoms include palpitations, dyspnea, and diaphoresis. In cases of moderate anemia (Hb 60-100 g/L), the cardiopulmonary symptoms are increased and the patient may experience them while resting as well as with activity. The patient with severe anemia (Hb <60 g/L) displays

DETERMINANTS OF HEALTH
Biology and Genetic Endowment

- Sickle cell disease has a high incidence among people of African descent but may also affect people of Latin American, Caribbean, Arabian, Indian, and Mediterranean descent.
- Thalassemia has a higher incidence among people of North African, East Asian, and Mediterranean origin.
- Pernicious anemia has a high incidence among people of African and Scandinavian descent.
- Indigenous people have a much higher incidence of iron-deficiency anemia, primarily caused by inadequate diet, poor living conditions, and high infection rates (Khambalia, Aimone, & Zlotkin, 2011).

Table 33-1 Relationship of Morphological Classification and Etiologies of Anemia

MORPHOLOGY	ETIOLOGY
Normocytic, normochromic (normal size and colour) MCV 80-95 fL, MCH 27-31 pg	Acute blood loss, hemolysis, chronic renal disease, chronic disease, cancers, sideroblastic anemia, refractory anemia, diseases of endocrine dysfunction, aplastic anemia, pregnancy
Macrocytic (megaloblastic), normochromic (large size, normal colour) MCV >95 fL, MCH >31 pg	Vitamin B_{12} deficiency, folate deficiency, liver disease (including effects of alcohol abuse), medications that impair DNA synthesis, hypothyroidism
Microcytic, hypochromic (small size, pale colour) MCV <80 fL, MCH <27 pg	Iron-deficiency anemia, thalassemia, anemia of chronic disease, sideroblastic anemia, lead poisoning

MCH, mean corpuscular hemoglobin; *MCV*, mean corpuscular volume.

Decreased RBC Production

Deficient nutrients	Decreased erythropoietin	Decreased iron availability
• Iron		
• Cobalamin		
• Folic acid		

Blood Loss

Chronic hemorrhage
- Bleeding duodenal ulcer
- Colorectal cancer
- Liver disease

- Acute trauma
- Ruptured aortic aneurysm
- GI bleeding

Increased RBC Destruction

Hemolysis
- Sickle cell disease
- Medication (e.g., methyldopa)
- Incompatible blood
- Trauma (e.g., cardiopulmonary bypass)

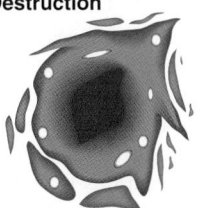

Figure 33-1 Causes of anemia. *RBC*, red blood cell.

Table 33-2 Etiological Classification of Anemia

Decreased Red Blood Cell Production

Decreased Hemoglobin Synthesis
- Iron deficiency
- Thalassemias (decreased globin synthesis)
- Sideroblastic anemia (decreased porphyrin)

Defective DNA Synthesis
- Cobalamin (vitamin B_{12}) deficiency
- Folic acid deficiency

Decreased Number of Erythrocyte Precursors
- Aplastic anemia
- Anemia of myeloproliferative disorders and myelodysplasia
- Chronic diseases or disorders
- Medications (e.g., chemotherapy)

Blood Loss

Acute
- Trauma
- Blood vessel rupture

Chronic
- Gastritis
- Menstrual flow
- Hemorrhoids

Increased Red Blood Cell Destruction

Intrinsic
- Abnormal hemoglobin (hemoglobin S—sickle cell anemia)
- Enzyme deficiency (G6PD)
- Membrane abnormalities (paroxysmal nocturnal hemoglobinuria, hereditary spherocytosis)

Extrinsic
- Physical trauma (prosthetic heart valves, extracorporeal circulation)
- Antibodies (isoimmune and autoimmune)
- Infectious agents, medications and toxins (malaria)

G6PD, glucose-6-phosphate dehydrogenase.

Table 33-3 Clinical Manifestations of Anemia

| BODY SYSTEM* | SEVERITY OF ANEMIA | | |
	MILD (HB 100-120 g/L) 6.2-8.7 mmol/L	MODERATE (HB 60-100 g/L) 3.7-6.2 mmol/L	SEVERE (HB <60 g/L) <3.7 mmol/L
Integument	None	None	Pallor, jaundice,† pruritus†
Eyes	None	None	Icteric conjunctiva and sclera,* retinal hemorrhage, blurred vision
Mouth	None	None	Glossitis, smooth tongue
Cardiovascular	Palpitations	Increased palpitations, "bounding pulse"	Tachycardia, increased pulse pressure, systolic murmurs, intermittent claudication, angina, HF, MI
Pulmonary	Exertional dyspnea	Dyspnea	Tachypnea, orthopnea, dyspnea at rest
Neurological	None	"Roaring in the ears"	Headache, vertigo, irritability, depression, impaired thought processes
Gastrointestinal	None	None	Anorexia, hepatomegaly, splenomegaly, difficulty swallowing, sore mouth
Musculoskeletal	None	None	Bone pain
General	None	Fatigue	Sensitivity to cold, weight loss, lethargy

Hb, hemoglobin; *HF*, heart failure; *MI*, myocardial infarction.
*Applies to female values; will be slightly higher in males.
†Caused by hemolysis.

many clinical manifestations involving multiple body systems (Table 33-3).

Integumentary Changes

Integumentary changes include pallor, jaundice, and pruritus. Pallor results from reduced amounts of Hb and reduced blood flow to the skin. Jaundice occurs when hemolysis of RBCs results in an increased concentration of serum bilirubin. Pruritus occurs because of increased serum and skin bile salt concentrations. In addition to the skin, the sclera of the eyes and the mucous membranes should be evaluated for jaundice because they reflect the integumentary changes more accurately, especially in dark-skinned individuals.

Cardiopulmonary Manifestations

Cardiopulmonary manifestations of severe anemia result from additional attempts by the heart and lungs to provide adequate amounts of O_2 to the tissues. Cardiac output is maintained by increasing the heart rate and the stroke volume. The low viscosity of the blood contributes to the development of systolic murmurs and bruits. In extreme cases or when concomitant heart disease is present, angina pectoris and myocardial infarction (MI) may occur if myocardial O_2 needs cannot be met. Heart failure (HF), cardiomegaly, pulmonary and systemic congestion, ascites, and peripheral edema may develop if the heart is overworked for an extended period.

NURSING MANAGEMENT: ANEMIA

This section discusses general nursing management of anemia. Specific care related to various types of anemia is discussed later in this chapter.

▌ Nursing Assessment

Subjective and objective data that should be obtained from a patient with anemia are presented in Table 33-4.

▌ Nursing Diagnoses

Nursing diagnoses for the patient with anemia include, but are not limited to, those presented in NCP 33-1.

▌ Planning

The overall goals are that the patient with anemia will (1) assume normal activities of daily living, (2) maintain adequate nutrition, and (3) develop no complications related to anemia.

▌ Nursing Implementation

The numerous causes of anemia necessitate different nursing interventions specific to the needs of the patient. Nevertheless, there are certain general components of care for all patients with anemia that are presented in NCP 33-1.

Correcting the cause of anemia is ultimately the goal of therapy. Acute interventions may include blood or blood product transfusions, drug therapy, volume replacement, and O_2 therapy to stabilize the patient's condition. Dietary and lifestyle changes can reverse some types of anemias so that the patient can return to the former state of health. Ongoing assessment should be included in the plan of care regarding the patient's knowledge regarding adequate nutritional intake and drug therapies as well as the patient's compliance with safety precautions to prevent falls and injury.

NURSING ASSESSMENT
Table 33-4 Anemia

Subjective Data	*Objective Data*
Important Health Information	**General**
Past health history: Recent blood loss or trauma; chronic liver, endocrine, or renal disease (including dialysis); GI disease (malabsorption syndrome, ulcers, gastritis, or hemorrhoids); inflammatory disorders (especially Crohn's disease); smoking, exposure to radiation or chemical toxins (arsenic, lead, benzenes, copper); infectious disease (HIV) or recent travel suggesting exposure to infection; angina, myocardial infarction; history of falling; family history of anemia	Lethargy, apathy, general lymphadenopathy, fever
	Integumentary
	Pale skin and mucous membranes; blue, pale white, or icteric sclera; cheilitis; poor skin turgour; brittle, spoon-shaped fingernails; jaundice; petechiae; ecchymoses; nose or gingival bleeding; poor healing; dry, brittle, thinning hair
Medications: Use of vitamin and iron supplements, aspirin, anticoagulants, oral contraceptives, phenobarbital, penicillins, nonsteroidal anti-inflammatory drugs, phenacetin, quinine, quinidine, phenytoin (Dilantin), methyldopa, sulphonamides, herbal products	**Respiratory**
	Tachypnea
	Cardiovascular
Surgery or other treatments: Recent surgery, small bowel resection, gastrectomy, prosthetic heart valves, chemotherapy, radiation therapy	Tachycardia, systolic murmur, dysrhythmias; postural hypotension, widened pulse pressure, bruits (especially carotid); intermittent claudication, ankle edema
Dietary history: General dietary patterns, consumption of alcohol, pica	**Gastrointestinal**
Symptoms	Hepatosplenomegaly; glossitis; beefy, red tongue; stomatitis; abdominal distension; anorexic
• Nausea, vomiting, anorexia, dysphagia, dyspepsia, heartburn, painful tongue	**Neurological**
• Night sweats, cold intolerance, weight loss, pruritus, pain	Headache, roaring in the ears, confusion, impaired judgement, irritability, ataxia, unsteady gait, paralysis, loss of vibration noise.
• Hematuria, decreased urinary output, diarrhea, constipation, flatulence, tarry stools, bloody stools	**Possible Diagnostic Findings**
• Fatigue, muscle weakness, and decreased strength	↓ RBCs; ↓ Hb; ↓ Hct; ↓ or ↑ reticulocytes, MCV, serum iron, ferritin, folate, or cobalamin (vitamin B$_{12}$); heme (guaiac)-positive stools; ↓ serum erythropoietin level; ↓ or ↑ LDH, bilirubin, transferrin (see Table 33-6)
• Dyspnea, orthopnea, cough, hemoptysis, palpitations, shortness of breath with activity	
• Headache; paresthesias of feet and hands; disturbances in vision, taste, or hearing, vertigo	
• Menorrhagia, metrorrhagia, recent or current pregnancy in women; male erectile dysfunction in men	

GI, gastrointestinal; *Hb,* hemoglobin; *Hct,* hematocrit; *HIV,* human immunodeficiency virus; *LDH,* lactate dehydrogenase; *MCV,* mean corpuscular volume; *RBCs,* red blood cells.

NURSING CARE PLAN 33-1
Anemia

NURSING DIAGNOSIS	**Fatigue** *related to* inadequate oxygenation of the blood *as evidenced by* increased pulse and blood pressure in response to activity and patient verbalization of lack of energy
Expected Patient Outcomes	**Nursing Interventions and *Rationales***
• Participates in activities of daily living (e.g., bathing, dressing, grooming, feeding) without abnormal increases in pulse and blood pressure. • Reports increased endurance of activity	• Correct physiological status deficits (e.g., chemotherapy-induced anemia) *to help mitigate the underlying cause of anemia.* • Encourage alternate periods of rest and activity *to provide activity without tiring the patient.* • Monitor cardiovascular response to activity *to evaluate activity intolerance.* • Limit environmental stimuli *to reduce demands placed on patient.* • Assist the patient in assigning priority to activities *to allow for the completion of important activities.* • Assist patient with activities of daily living as needed *to limit physical demands placed on the patient.*
NURSING DIAGNOSIS	**Altered nutrition: less than body requirements** *related to* inadequate nutritional intake, and anorexia *as evidenced by* weight loss, low serum albumin, decreased iron levels, and vitamin deficiencies
Expected Patient Outcomes	**Nursing Interventions and *Rationales***
• Maintains dietary intake that provides minimum daily requirements of nutrients. • Experiences normal blood values of nutrients necessary to prevent anemia.	• Determine, in collaboration with dietitian, number of calories and type of nutrients needed to meet nutritional requirements *to plan interventions.* • Teach patient how to use a food diary *to help evaluate nutritional intake.* • Monitor recorded intake for nutritional content and calories *to evaluate nutritional status.* • Encourage increased intake of protein, iron, and vitamin C *to provide nutrients needed for hematopoiesis.* • Suggest eating small, frequent meals with snacks throughout the day *to increase patient's dietary intake.*

AGE-RELATED CONSIDERATIONS: ANEMIA

Modest changes in RBC mass occur in older adults. In healthy older men, there is a modest decline in Hb of about 10 g/L between ages 70 and 88 years, in part because of the decreased production of androgens. Only a minimal decrease in Hb occurs between these ages in healthy women (~2 g/L) (Marks & Glader, 2009).

For older adults with anemia, about one third have a nutritional type of anemia (e.g., folate or iron deficiency), another third have renal insufficiency and/or chronic inflammation, and the final third have anemia that is unexplained (den Elzen et al., 2009). Cobalamin (vitamin B_{12}) deficiency may occur in up to 15% of older adults because of pernicious anemia, insufficient dietary intake, and malabsorption (Andrès, Fothergill, & Mecili, 2010). Multiple co-morbid conditions in older adults increase the likelihood of occurrence of many types of anemia.

Signs and symptoms of anemia in the older adult may include pallor, confusion, ataxia, fatigue, worsening angina, and HF. Unfortunately, anemia may go unrecognized in the older adult because manifestations of anemia may be mistaken as normal aging changes or overlooked because of another health problem. By recognizing signs of anemia, the nurse can play a pivotal role in appropriate health assessment and related interventions for older adults.

Anemia Caused by Decreased Erythrocyte Production

Normally, RBC production (termed *erythropoiesis*) is in equilibrium with RBC destruction and loss. This balance ensures that an adequate number of erythrocytes are available at all times. The normal lifespan of an RBC is 120 days. Three alterations in erythropoiesis may occur that decrease RBC production: (1) decreased Hb synthesis may lead to iron-deficiency anemia, thalassemia, and sideroblastic anemia; (2) defective DNA synthesis in RBCs (e.g., cobalamin or folic acid deficiency) may lead to megaloblastic anemias; and (3) diminished availability of erythrocyte precursors may result in aplastic anemia and anemia of chronic disease (see Table 33-1).

Iron-Deficiency Anemia

Iron-deficiency anemia, one of the most common chronic hematological disorders, is found in 30% of the world's population (World Health Organization [WHO], 2012). In Canada, those most susceptible to iron-deficiency anemia are the very young, those with poor diets, and women in their reproductive years. Normally, 1 mg of iron is lost daily through feces, sweat, and urine in the adult male and 1.5 mg/day in normal menstruating women.

Etiology

Iron deficiency may develop from inadequate dietary intake, malabsorption, blood loss, or hemolysis. Iron is obtained from food and dietary supplements. Dietary iron is adequate to meet the needs of men and older women, but it may be inadequate for individuals with higher iron needs (e.g., menstruating or pregnant women). Table 33-5 lists nutrients needed for erythropoiesis (Alpers, Stenson, Taylor, & Bier, 2008). Malabsorption of iron may occur after certain types of gastrointestinal (GI) surgery and in malabsorption syndromes. Surgical procedures may involve removal or bypass of the duodenum (see Chapter 44). Because iron absorption occurs primarily in the duodenum, malabsorption syndromes may involve disease of the duodenum in which the absorptive surface is altered or destroyed.

Blood loss is a major cause of iron deficiency in adults. Two millilitres of whole blood contain 1 mg of iron. The major sources of chronic blood loss are from the GI and genitourinary (GU) systems. GI bleeding is often not apparent and, therefore, may be present for a considerable time before the problem is identified. Loss of 50 to 75 mL of blood from the upper GI tract is required for stools to appear black *(melena)*. The black colour results from the iron in the RBCs. Common causes of GI blood loss are peptic ulcer, gastritis, esophagitis, diverticuli, hemorrhoids, and neoplasia. GU blood loss occurs primarily from menstrual bleeding. The average monthly menstrual blood loss is about 45 mL and causes the loss of about 22 mg of iron. Postmenopausal bleeding can contribute to anemia in a susceptible older woman. Pregnancy contributes to

NUTRITIONAL THERAPY

Table 33-5 Nutrients Needed for Erythropoiesis

NUTRIENT	ROLE IN ERYTHROPOIESIS	FOOD SOURCES
Cobalamin (vitamin B_{12})	RBC maturation	Red meats (especially liver), eggs, enriched grain products
Folic acid	RBC maturation	Green leafy vegetables, liver, meat, fish, legumes, whole grains
Iron	Hemoglobin synthesis	Liver and muscle meats, eggs, dried fruits, legumes, dark green leafy vegetables, whole-grain and enriched bread and cereals, potatoes
Pyridoxine (vitamin B_6)	Hemoglobin synthesis	Meats, wheat germ, legumes, potatoes, cornmeal, bananas
Amino acids	Synthesis of nucleoproteins	Eggs, meat, milk and milk products, poultry, fish, legumes, nuts
Ascorbic acid (vitamin C)	Conversion of folic acid to its active forms; aids in iron absorption	Citrus fruits, leafy green vegetables, strawberries, cantaloupe

RBC, red blood cell.

iron deficiency because of the diversion of iron to the fetus for erythropoiesis, blood loss at delivery, and lactation (Lee & Okam, 2011). In addition to anemia of chronic renal failure, dialysis treatment may induce iron-deficiency anemia because of the blood lost in the dialysis equipment and frequent blood sampling.

Clinical Manifestations

In the early course of iron-deficiency anemia, the patient may be free of symptoms. As the disease becomes chronic, any of the general manifestations of anemia may develop (see Table 33-3). In addition, specific clinical symptoms may occur related to iron-deficiency anemia. Pallor is the most common finding, and *glossitis* (inflammation of the tongue) is the second most common (Figure 33-2); another finding is *cheilitis* (inflammation of the lips). In addition, the patient may report headache, paresthesias, and a burning sensation of the tongue, all of which are caused by a lack of iron in the tissues.

Diagnostic Studies

Iron-deficiency anemia will lead to a number of characteristic laboratory abnormalities (Table 33-6). Other diagnostic studies are done to determine the cause of the iron deficiency (e.g., stool guaiac test). Endoscopy and colonoscopy may be used to detect GI bleeding. A bone marrow biopsy may be done if other tests are inconclusive.

Collaborative Care

The main goal of the collaborative care of iron-deficiency anemia is to treat the underlying disease that is causing reduced intake or absorption of iron. In addition, efforts are directed toward replacing iron (Table 33-7). The patient should be taught which foods are good sources of iron (see Table 33-5). If nutrition is already adequate, increasing iron intake by dietary means may

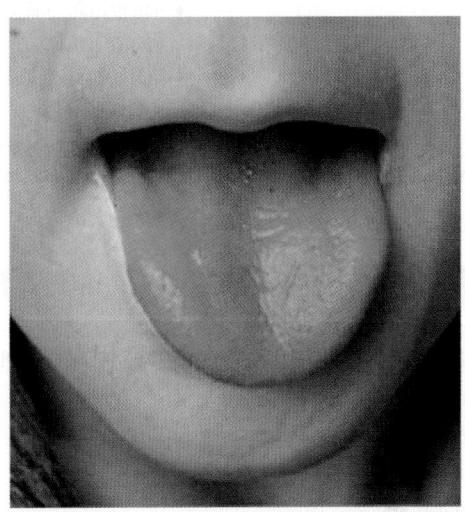

Figure 33-2 Glossitis in a patient with iron-deficiency anemia.

Source: Forbes, C. F., & Jackson, W. F. (2003). *Color atlas and text of clinical medicine* (3rd ed., p. 406). London: Mosby.

Table 33-6 Laboratory Study Findings in Anemias

HB, HCT	MCV	RETICULOCYTES	SERUM IRON	TIBC	TRANSFERRIN	FERRITIN	BILIRUBIN
Iron Deficiency							
↓	↓	N or slight ↓ or ←↑	↓	←↑	N or ↓	↓	N or ↓
Thalassemia Major							
↓	N or ↓	←↑	←↑	↓	↓	N or ←↑	←↑
Cobalamin Deficiency							
↓	←↑	N or ↓	N or ←↑	N	Slight ←↑	←↑	N or slight ←↑
Folic Acid Deficiency							
↓	←↑	N or ↓	N or ←↑	N	Slight ←↑	←↑	N or slight ←↑
Aplastic Anemia							
↓	N or slight ←↑	↓	N or ←↑	N or ←↑	N	N	N
Chronic Disease							
↓	N or ↓	N or ↓	N or ↓	↓	N or ↓	N or ←↑	N
Acute Blood Loss							
↓	N or ↓	N or ←↑	N	N	N	N	N
Chronic Blood Loss							
↓	↓	N or ←↓	↓	↓	N	N	N or ↓
Sickle Cell Anemia							
↓	N	←↑	N or ←↑	N or ↓	N	N	←↑
Hemolytic Anemia							
↓	N or ←↑	←↑	N or ←↑	N or ↓	N	N or ←↑	←↑

Hb, hemoglobin; *Hct*, hematocrit; *MCV*, mean corpuscular volume; *N*, normal; *TIBC*, total iron-binding capacity; ↓ decreased; ↑ increased; ← unchanged.

COLLABORATIVE CARE

Table 33-7 Iron-Deficiency Anemia

Diagnostic	Collaborative Therapy
• History and physical examination	• Identification and treatment of underlying cause
• Hct and Hb levels	
• RBC count, including morphology	• Ferrous sulphate or ferrous gluconate
• Reticulocyte count	
• Serum iron	• Iron dextran, iron sucrose, sodium ferrous gluconate
• Serum ferritin	
• Total iron-binding capacity (TIBC)	• Nutritional and diet therapy (see Table 33-5)
• Stool examination for occult blood	
• Bone marrow aspirate	• Transfusion of packed RBCs (symptomatic patient only)

Hb, hemoglobin; *Hct*, hematocrit; *RBC*, red blood cell.

Table 33-8 Common Iron Preparations and Elemental Iron Provided

IRON PREPARATION	AMOUNT OF ELEMENTAL IRON (mg)
Ferrous sulphate (300-mg tablet)	60
Ferrous gluconate (300-mg tablet)	35
Ferrous fumarate (300-mg tablet)	99
Heme iron polypeptide	11
Polysaccharide-iron complex	150

Source: Adapted from Canadian Pharmacists Association. (2011). *Iron preparations: Oral*. Retrieved from *https://www.e-therapeutics.ca/ cps.showMonograph.action?newSearch=true&simpleIndex=BrandGeneric&sim pleQuery=Iron+Preparations%3A+Oral&=#m267400n00027*

not be practical. Consequently, oral or occasionally parenteral iron supplements are used. If the iron deficiency is from acute blood loss, the patient may require a transfusion of packed RBCs.

Drug Therapy. Oral iron should be used whenever possible because it is inexpensive and convenient. Many iron preparations are available. The following five factors should be considered in the administration of iron:

1. Iron is absorbed best from the duodenum and the proximal jejunum. Therefore, enteric-coated or sustained-release capsules, which release iron farther down in the GI tract, are counterproductive.
2. The daily dosage should provide 150 to 200 mg of elemental iron. This can be ingested in three or four daily doses, with each tablet or capsule of the iron preparation containing between 50 and 100 mg of iron. Common iron preparations and amounts of elemental iron are provided in Table 33-8.
3. Iron is best absorbed as ferrous sulphate (Fe^{2+}) in an acidic environment. For this reason and to avoid binding the iron with food, iron should be taken about an hour before meals when the duodenal mucosa is most acidic. Taking iron with vitamin C (ascorbic acid) or orange juice, which contains ascorbic acid, also enhances iron absorption. Gastric adverse effects, however, may necessitate ingesting iron with meals.
4. Undiluted liquid iron may stain the patient's teeth; therefore, it should be diluted and ingested through a straw.
5. GI adverse effects of iron administration may occur, including heartburn, constipation, and diarrhea. If adverse effects develop, the dosage and type of iron supplement may be adjusted. For example, many individuals who need

supplemental iron cannot tolerate Fe^{2+} because of the effects of the sulphate base. However, ferrous gluconate may be an acceptable substitute. All patients should know that the use of iron preparations will cause their stools to become black because the GI tract excretes excess iron. Constipation is common, and patients should be started on stool softeners and laxatives, if needed, when taking iron.

In some situations, it may be necessary to administer iron parenterally. Parenteral use of iron is indicated for malabsorption, intolerance of oral iron, a need for iron beyond oral-intake limits, or poor patient compliance in taking the oral preparations of iron. Parenteral iron may be given intramuscularly or intravenously. Because IM iron solutions may stain the skin, separate needles should be used for drawing up the solution and for injecting the medication. A Z-track technique should be used for injection to prevent leakage of the iron solution to the subcutaneous tissue. Some preparations of IV iron have a high risk of an allergic reaction, and the patient should be monitored accordingly.

NURSING MANAGEMENT: IRON-DEFICIENCY ANEMIA

It is important to recognize groups of individuals who are at an increased risk for the development of iron-deficiency anemia. These include premenopausal and pregnant women, people from low socioeconomic backgrounds, older adults, and individuals experiencing blood loss. Nutritional education, with an emphasis on foods high in iron and how to maximize absorption, is important for these groups. Appropriate nursing measures are presented in NCP 33-1. Discuss with the patient the need for diagnostic studies to identify the cause. Reassess the Hb and RBC counts to evaluate the response to therapy. Emphasize compliance with dietary and drug therapy. To replenish the body's iron stores, the patient needs to continue to take iron therapy for 2 to 3 months after the Hb level returns to normal. Patients who require lifelong iron supplementation should be monitored for potential liver problems related to the iron storage.

Thalassemia

Etiology

Another cause of decreased erythrocyte production is thalassemia. **Thalassemia** is a group of diseases that have an autosomal recessive genetic basis involving inadequate production of normal Hb. Hemolysis also occurs in thalassemia, but insufficient production of normal Hb is the predominant problem. In contrast to iron-deficiency anemia, in which heme synthesis is the problem, thalassemia is caused by an absent or reduced globulin protein. α-Globulin chains are absent or reduced in α-thalassemia, and β-globin chains are absent or reduced in β-thalassemia. Therefore, the basic defect of thalassemia is the synthesis of abnormal Hb.

Thalassemia is commonly found in members of ethnic groups whose origins are near the Mediterranean Sea and equatorial or near-equatorial regions of Asia and Africa. An individual with thalassemia may have a heterozygous or homozygous form of the disease. A person who is heterozygous has one thalassemic gene and one normal gene and is said to have *thalassemia minor* (or thalassemic trait), a mild form of the disease. A homozygous person has two thalassemic genes, causing a severe condition known as *thalassemia major* (Howard & Hamilton, 2008).

Clinical Manifestations

Thalassemia major is a life-threatening disease in which growth, both physical and mental, is often retarded. The person who has thalassemia major is pale and displays other general symptoms of anemia (see Table 33-3). The symptoms develop in childhood by 2 years of age and can cause growth and development deficits. In addition, the person has pronounced splenomegaly and hepatomegaly. Jaundice from RBC hemolysis is prominent. As the bone marrow responds to the blood's deficient O_2-carrying capacity, RBC production is stimulated and the marrow becomes packed with immature erythroid precursors that die. This stimulates further erythropoiesis, leading to chronic bone marrow hyperplasia and expansion of the marrow space. This may cause thickening of the cranium and the maxillary cavity. The patient with thalassemia minor is frequently asymptomatic. The patient has mild to moderate anemia with *microcytosis* (small cells) and *hypochromia* (pale cells).

Collaborative Care

The laboratory abnormalities of thalassemia major are summarized in Table 33-6. No specific drug or diet therapies are effective in treating thalassemia. Although thalassemia minor does not necessitate treatment because the body adapts to the reduction of normal Hb, genetic counselling is advised. The symptoms of thalassemia major are managed with life-long blood transfusions in conjunction with IV deferoxamine (Desferal) (a chelating agent that binds to iron) to reduce the risk of iron overload associated with RBC transfusion. Transfusions are administered to keep the Hb level at approximately 100 g/L. This level is low enough to foster the patient's own erythropoiesis without enlarging the spleen. Zinc supplementation may be needed (it is reduced with chelation therapy) as well as ascorbic acid supplementation during the chelation therapy (increases urine excretion of iron; it should not be taken otherwise because it increases the absorption of dietary iron). Regular folic acid may be given if diet is poor. Iron supplements should not be given.

Death from cardiac failure is the most common clinical consequence of iron excess; however, other organs and tissues can be affected such as the liver, heart, and endocrine glands (Gardenghi, Grady, & Rivella, 2010). Thus, hepatic, cardiac, and endocrine functions should be monitored appropriately. In addition, thrombosis may be a complication of the disease (Hoffbrand & Moss, 2011). With proper iron chelation therapy, patients are living longer (Lucarelli & Gaziev, 2008).

For some patients, allogeneic bone marrow transplantation offers the prospect of a cure; however, the risks may outweigh the benefits. New approaches to treatment/cure are being developed such as gene therapy (Gardenghi et al., 2010).

Megaloblastic Anemias

Megaloblastic anemias are a group of disorders caused by impaired DNA synthesis and characterized by the presence of large RBCs. When DNA synthesis is impaired, defective RBC maturation results. The RBCs are large (macrocytic) and abnormal

Table 33-9 Classification of Megaloblastic (Macrocytic) Anemias

Cobalamin (Vitamin B₁₂) Deficiency	• Increased requirement
• Dietary deficiency	• Alcohol abuse
• Deficiency of gastric intrinsic factor	• Anorexia
• Pernicious anemia	• Hemodialysis patients
• Gastrectomy	***Drug-Induced Suppression of DNA Synthesis***
• Intestinal malabsorption	• Folate antagonists (e.g., 5-fluorouracil)
• Increased requirement	• Metabolic inhibitors
• Chronic alcoholism	• Alkylating agents
Folic Acid Deficiency	***Inborn Errors***
• Dietary deficiency	• Defective folate metabolism
• Malabsorption syndromes	• Defective transport of cobalamin
• Drugs interfering with absorption/use of folic acid (e.g., methotrexate, phenobarbital)	***Erythroleukemia***

and are referred to as *megaloblasts*. Macrocytic RBCs are easily destroyed because they have fragile cell membranes. Although the overwhelming majority of megaloblastic anemias result from cobalamin (vitamin B_{12}) and folic acid deficiencies, this type of RBC deformity can also occur from suppression of DNA synthesis by drugs, inborn errors of cobalamin and folic acid metabolism, and *erythroleukemia* (malignant blood disorder characterized by a proliferation of erythropoietic cells in bone marrow) (Table 33-9).

Cobalamin (Vitamin B₁₂) Deficiency

Normally, a protein termed *intrinsic factor* (IF) is secreted by the parietal cells of the gastric mucosa. IF is required for cobalamin (extrinsic factor) absorption. Thus, if IF is not secreted, cobalamin will not be absorbed. (Cobalamin is normally absorbed in the distal ileum.) There are many causes of cobalamin deficiency. The most common is **pernicious anemia,** a disease in which the gastric mucosa is not secreting IF because of antibodies being directed against the gastric parietal cells and/or IF itself. Other causes of cobalamin deficiency include gastrectomy, gastritis, nutritional deficiency, chronic alcoholism, and hereditary enzymatic defects of cobalamin utilization (see Table 33-9).

Pernicious anemia is a disease of insidious onset that begins in middle age or later (usually after age 40), with 60 years being the most common age at diagnosis. Pernicious anemia occurs frequently in people of African or Northern European ancestry (particularly Scandinavians). In people of African descent, the disease tends to begin early, occurs with higher frequency in women, and is often severe.

Etiology

Cobalamin deficiency can occur in patients who have had GI surgery such as gastrectomy; patients who have had a small bowel resection involving the ileum; and patients with Crohn's disease, ileitis, celiac disease, diverticulitis of the small intestine, and/or chronic atrophic gastritis. In these cases, cobalamin deficiency results from the loss of IF-secreting gastric mucosal cells or impaired absorption of cobalamin in the distal ileum. Cobalamin deficiency is also found in long-term users of histamine (H_2)-receptor blockers and proton pump inhibitors and those who are strictly vegetarians (Antony, 2009).

Pernicious anemia is caused by an absence of IF, from either gastric mucosal atrophy or autoimmune destruction of parietal cells. This results in a decrease of hydrochloric acid secretion by the stomach. An acid environment in the stomach is required for the secretion of IF.

Clinical Manifestations

General symptoms of anemia related to cobalamin deficiency develop because of tissue hypoxia (see Table 33-3). GI manifestations include a sore, red, shiny tongue; anorexia; nausea, vomiting; and abdominal pain. Typical neuromuscular manifestations include weakness, paresthesias of the feet and hands, reduced vibratory and position senses, ataxia, muscle weakness, and impaired thought processes ranging from confusion to dementia. Because cobalamin deficiency–related anemia has an insidious onset, it may take several months for these manifestations to develop.

Diagnostic Studies

Laboratory data reflective of cobalamin deficiency anemia are presented in Table 33-6. The RBCs appear large (macrocytic) and have abnormal shapes. This structure contributes to erythrocyte destruction because the cell membrane is fragile. Serum cobalamin levels are reduced. It is important to know serum folate levels because, if they are normal and cobalamin levels are low, it suggests that megaloblastic anemia is caused by a cobalamin deficiency. Because the potential for gastric cancer is increased in patients with pernicious anemia, a gastroscopy and biopsy of the gastric mucosa may also be done.

Another means of assessing parietal cell function is a Schilling test. After radioactive cobalamin is administered to the patient, the amount of cobalamin excreted in the urine is measured. An individual who cannot absorb cobalamin excretes only a small amount of this radioactive form. The same procedure may be followed with the parenteral administration of IF. Absorption of cobalamin when IF is added is diagnostic of pernicious anemia.

Collaborative Care

Regardless of how much is ingested, the patient is not able to absorb cobalamin if IF is lacking or if there is impaired absorption in the ileum. For this reason, increasing dietary cobalamin does not correct the anemia. However, the patient should be instructed on adequate dietary intake to maintain good nutrition (see Table 33-5). Parenteral or intranasal administration of cobalamin (cyanocobalamin or hydroxocobalamin) is the treatment of choice. Without cobalamin administration, these individuals will die in 1 to 3 years. The dosage and frequency of cobalamin administration may vary. A typical treatment schedule consists of 1000 mg of cobalamin intramuscularly daily for 2 weeks and then weekly until the Hct is normal, then monthly for life. High-dose oral cobalamin and sublingual cobalamin are also available for those whose GI absorption is intact. As long as supplemental cobalamin is used, the anemia can be reversed. However, if the person has had longstanding neuromuscular complications, these may not be reversible.

Folic Acid Deficiency

Folic acid (folate) deficiency also causes megaloblastic anemia. Folic acid is required for DNA synthesis leading to RBC formation and maturation. Common causes of folic acid deficiency are listed in Table 33-9.

The clinical manifestations of folic acid deficiency are similar to those of cobalamin deficiency. The disease develops insidiously, and the patient's symptoms may be attributed to other, coexisting problems such as cirrhosis or esophageal varices. GI disturbances include dyspepsia and a smooth, beefy-red tongue. The absence of neurological problems is an important diagnostic finding. This lack of neurological involvement differentiates folic acid deficiency from cobalamin deficiency (Milman, 2011).

The diagnostic findings for folic acid deficiency are presented in Table 33-6. In addition, the serum folate level is low (normal is 11-57 mmol/L) and the serum cobalamin level is normal. Folic acid deficiency is treated by replacement therapy. The usual dose is 1 mg/day by mouth. In malabsorption states, up to 5 mg/day may be required. The duration of treatment depends on the reason for the deficiency. In addition to supplements, the patient should be encouraged to eat foods containing large amounts of folic acid (see Table 33-5).

NURSING MANAGEMENT: MEGALOBLASTIC ANEMIA

Because there is a familial predisposition for pernicious anemia (the most common type of cobalamin deficiency), patients who have a positive family history of pernicious anemia should be evaluated for symptoms. Although disease development cannot be prevented, early detection and treatment can help reverse symptoms more easily. Signs and symptoms of other possible causes of megaloblastic anemia should be brought to the attention of the primary health care provider.

The nursing measures presented in the NCP for the patient with anemia (see NCP 33-1) are appropriate for the patient with cobalamin-deficiency anemia. In addition to these measures, the nurse should ensure that injuries are not sustained because of the diminished sensations to heat and pain resulting from the neurological impairment. Protect the patient from falls, burns, and trauma. If heat therapy is required, the patient's skin must be evaluated at frequent intervals to detect redness.

Ongoing care is focused on ensuring good patient compliance with treatment. There must also be careful follow-up to assess for neurological difficulties that were not fully corrected by adequate cobalamin replacement therapy. Because the potential for gastric cancer may be increased in patients with atrophic gastritis–related pernicious anemia, the patient should have frequent and appropriate screening.

Anemia of Chronic Disease

Chronic inflammation, autoimmune, infectious, or malignant diseases can lead to anemia of chronic disease. *Anemia of chronic disease* is associated with an underproduction of RBCs and mild shortening of RBC survival. The RBCs are usually normocytic, normochromic, and hypoproliferative. The anemia is usually mild, but it can be more severe. This type of anemia is primarily immune driven. Cytokines released with inflammatory, autoimmune, infectious, or malignant disease cause an increased uptake and retention of iron within macrophages. This leads to a diversion of iron from the circulation into storage sites and subsequent limitation of the availability of iron for erythroid progenitor cells. For any chronic disease, there may also be additional factors. For example, with renal disease, the primary factor causing anemia is decreased erythropoietin, a hormone made in the kidneys that is necessary for erythropoiesis. With impaired renal function, erythropoietin production is decreased (see Chapter 49).

Any condition that causes increased RBC destruction (e.g., autoimmune hemolysis) accompanied by the failure to augment erythropoiesis will contribute to anemia. Myelosuppression and decreased erythropoiesis caused by disease, medications (e.g., chemotherapy), or radiation will contribute to the anemia of chronic disease. Human immunodeficiency virus (HIV) and its treatments, hepatitis, malaria, and bleeding episodes are other contributors to this type of anemia (Adamson, 2008).

Hypopituitary and hypothyroid states both lead to reduced tissue metabolism; therefore, tissue O_2 needs are diminished, leading to a reduced production of erythropoietin by the kidneys. Adrenal dysfunction caused by either adrenalectomy or Addison's disease also results in anemia.

Anemia of chronic disease must first be recognized and differentiated from anemias of other etiologies. Findings of elevated serum ferritin and increased iron stores distinguish it from iron-deficiency anemia. Normal folate and cobalamin blood levels distinguish it from deficiency anemias of those substances. The best treatment of anemia of chronic disease is correction of the underlying disorder. Unless the anemia is severe, blood transfusions are rarely indicated. Erythropoietin therapy given parenterally is used for anemia related to renal disease or anemia related to cancer therapies (see Chapter 49). However, it is used conservatively because there is increased risk of thromboembolism and mortality in some patients (Dronca & Steensma, 2008).

Aplastic Anemia

Aplastic anemia is a disease in which the patient has peripheral blood *pancytopenia* (decrease of all blood cell types—RBCs, white blood cells [WBCs], and platelets) and hypocellular bone marrow. The signs and symptoms can range from a chronic condition managed with erythropoietin or blood transfusions to a critical condition with hemorrhage and sepsis.

Etiology

The incidence of aplastic anemia is low, affecting approximately 4 of every 1 million people. There are various etiological classifications for aplastic anemia, but they can be divided into two major groups: *congenital* and *acquired* (Table 33-10). Approximately 70% of the acquired aplastic anemias are idiopathic and thought to be autoimmune (Dokal & Vulliamy, 2008).

Clinical Manifestations

Aplastic anemia can manifest acutely (over days) or insidiously over weeks to months and can vary from mild to severe. Clinically, the patient may have symptoms caused by suppression of any or all bone marrow elements. General manifestations of

Table 33-10 Causes of Aplastic Anemia	
Congenital (Chromosomal Alterations)	**Acquired**
• Fanconi's syndrome • Congenital dyskeratosis • Amegakaryocytic thrombocytopenia • Schwachman-Diamond syndrome	• Chemical agents and toxins (e.g., benzene, arsenic) • Drugs (e.g., gold, antimicrobials) • Idiopathic/autoimmune • Radiation • Viral and bacterial infections

anemia, such as fatigue and dyspnea, as well as cardiovascular and cerebral responses may be seen (see Table 33-3). Patients with neutropenia (low neutrophil count) are susceptible to infection and may be febrile. Thrombocytopenia is manifested by a predisposition to bleeding (e.g., petechiae, ecchymosis, epistaxis).

Diagnostic Studies

The diagnosis is confirmed by laboratory studies. Because all marrow elements are affected, Hb, WBC, and platelet values are often decreased in the patient with aplastic anemia. Other RBC indexes are generally normal (see Table 33-6). The condition is, therefore, classified as a normocytic, normochromic anemia. The reticulocyte count is low. Bleeding time is prolonged.

Aplastic anemia can be further evaluated by assessing various iron studies. The serum iron and total iron-binding capacity (TIBC) may be elevated as initial signs of erythropoiesis suppression. Bone marrow biopsy, aspiration, and pathological examination may be done for any anemic state. However, the findings are especially important in aplastic anemia because the marrow is hypocellular, with increased yellow marrow (fat content).

NURSING AND COLLABORATIVE MANAGEMENT: APLASTIC ANEMIA

Management of aplastic anemia is based on identifying and removing the causative agent (when possible) and providing supportive care until the pancytopenia reverses. Nursing interventions appropriate for the patient with pancytopenia from aplastic anemia are presented in the NCP for the patient with anemia (see NCP 33-1) earlier in this chapter and the NCPs for thrombocytopenia (NCP 33-2) and neutropenia (NCP 33-3) later in this chapter. Nursing actions are directed at preventing complications from infection and hemorrhage.

The prognosis for severe untreated aplastic anemia is poor (~70% fatal). However, advances in medical management, including immunosuppressive therapy with antithymocyte globulin (ATG) and cyclosporine and bone marrow transplantation, have improved outcomes significantly. ATG is a horse or rabbit serum that contains polyclonal antibodies against human T cells. The rationale for this therapy is that aplastic anemia is an immune-mediated disease resulting from the upregulation of T cells actively targeting and destroying the patient's own hematopoietic stem cells. ATG can cause anaphylaxis, but with premedications and careful infusion, most patients can complete the prescribed course of treatment. The treatment of choice for adults younger than 40 years of age who have a human leukocyte antigen (HLA)–matched donor is bone marrow transplantation. The best results occur in younger patients (Bacigalupo & Passweg, 2009). Prior transfusions increase the risk of graft rejection. (Bone marrow transplants are discussed in Chapter 18.)

For the older adult or the patient without an HLA-matched donor, the treatment of choice is immunosuppression with ATG or cyclosporine. Although this therapy may be only partially beneficial, transfusions usually can be avoided.

Anemia Caused by Blood Loss

Anemia resulting from blood loss may be caused by either acute or chronic problems.

Acute Blood Loss

Acute blood loss occurs as a result of sudden hemorrhage. Causes of acute blood loss include trauma, complications of surgery, and conditions or diseases that disrupt vascular integrity. There are two clinical concerns in such situations. First, there is a sudden reduction in the total blood volume that can lead to hypovolemic shock. Second, if the acute loss is more gradual, the body maintains its blood volume by slowly increasing the plasma volume. Although the circulating fluid volume is preserved, the number of RBCs available to carry O_2 is significantly diminished.

Clinical Manifestations

The clinical manifestations of anemia from acute blood loss are caused by the body's attempts to maintain an adequate blood volume and meet O_2 requirements. Table 33-11 summarizes the clinical manifestations of patients with varying degrees of blood volume loss. It is essential to understand that the clinical signs and symptoms the patient is experiencing are more important than the laboratory values. For example, an adult with a bleeding peptic ulcer who had a 750-mL hematemesis (15% of a normal total blood volume) within the past 30 minutes may have postural hypotension but have normal values for Hb and Hct. Over the ensuing 36 to 48 hours, most of the volume deficit will be repaired by the movement of fluid from the extravascular into the intravascular space. Only at these later times will the Hb and Hct reflect the blood loss.

The nurse should be alert to the patient's expression of pain. Internal hemorrhage may cause pain because of tissue distension, organ displacement, and nerve compression. Pain may be localized or referred. In the case of retroperitoneal bleeding, the patient may not experience abdominal pain. Instead, the patient may have numbness and pain in a lower extremity secondary to compression of the lateral cutaneous nerve, which is located in the region of the first to third lumbar vertebrae. The major complication of acute blood loss is shock. (Shock and its management are discussed in Chapter 69.)

Diagnostic Studies

When blood volume loss is sudden, plasma volume has not yet had a chance to increase, the loss of RBCs is not reflected in laboratory data, and values may seem normal or high for 2 to 3 days. However, once the plasma is replaced by endogenous and exogenous means, the RBC mass is less concentrated. At this time, RBC, Hb, and Hct levels are low and reflect the actual blood loss.

Collaborative Care

Collaborative care is initially concerned with (1) replacing blood volume to prevent shock and (2) identifying the source of the hemorrhage and stopping the blood loss. IV fluids used in emergencies include dextran, hetastarch, albumin, crystalloid electrolyte solutions such as lactated Ringer's, or some combination of these. The amount of infusion varies with the solution used. (Management of shock is discussed in Chapter 69.)

Once volume replacement is under way, attention can be directed to correcting RBC loss. The body needs 2 to 5 days to manufacture more RBCs in response to increased erythropoietin. Consequently, blood transfusions (packed RBCs) may be needed if the blood loss is significant. In addition, if the bleeding is related to a platelet or clotting disorder, replacement of that deficiency must be addressed.

The patient may also need supplemental iron because the availability of iron affects the marrow production of erythrocytes. When anemia exists after acute blood loss, dietary sources of iron will probably not be adequate to maintain iron stores. Therefore, oral or parenteral iron preparations are administered.

Table 33-11 Clinical Manifestations of Acute Blood Loss	
VOLUME LOST (%)	**CLINICAL MANIFESTATIONS**
10	None
20	No detectable signs of symptoms at rest, tachycardia with exercise and slight postural hypotension
30	Normal supine blood pressure and pulse at rest, postural hypotension and tachycardia with exercise
40	Blood pressure, central venous pressure, and cardiac output below normal at rest; rapid, thready pulse and cold, clammy skin
50	Shock and potential death

NURSING MANAGEMENT: ACUTE BLOOD LOSS

In the case of trauma, it may be impossible to prevent the situation leading to the blood loss. For the postoperative patient, carefully monitor the blood loss from various drainage tubes and dressings and implement appropriate actions. The NCP for the patient with anemia resulting from acute blood loss will most likely include administration of blood products (described at the end of this chapter).

Once the source of hemorrhage is identified, blood loss is controlled, and fluid and blood volumes are replaced, the anemia should begin to correct itself. There should be no need for long-term treatment of this type of anemia.

Chronic Blood Loss

The sources of chronic blood loss are similar to those of iron-deficiency anemia (e.g., bleeding ulcer, hemorrhoids, menstrual and postmenopausal blood loss). The effects of chronic blood loss are usually related to the depletion of iron stores and are usually considered as iron-deficiency anemia. Management of chronic blood loss anemia involves identifying the source and stopping the bleeding. Supplemental iron may be required. The nursing measures presented in NCP 33-1 are relevant to anemia of chronic blood loss.

Anemia Caused by Increased Erythrocyte Destruction

The third major cause of anemia is termed **hemolytic anemia,** a condition caused by the destruction or hemolysis of RBCs at a rate that exceeds production. Hemolysis can occur because of problems intrinsic or extrinsic to the RBCs. Intrinsic hemolytic anemias result from defects in the RBCs themselves caused by abnormal Hb (e.g., sickle cells), enzyme deficiencies that alter glycolysis (glucose-6-phosphate dehydrogenase [G6PD] deficiency), or RBC membrane abnormalities. Intrinsic hemolytic anemias are usually hereditary. More common are the extrinsic hemolytic anemias, which are acquired. In this type of anemia, the patient's RBCs are normal; damage is caused by external factors (see Table 33-2). The spleen is the primary site of the destruction of RBCs that are old, defective, or moderately damaged. Figure 33-3 indicates the sequence of events involved in extravascular hemolysis.

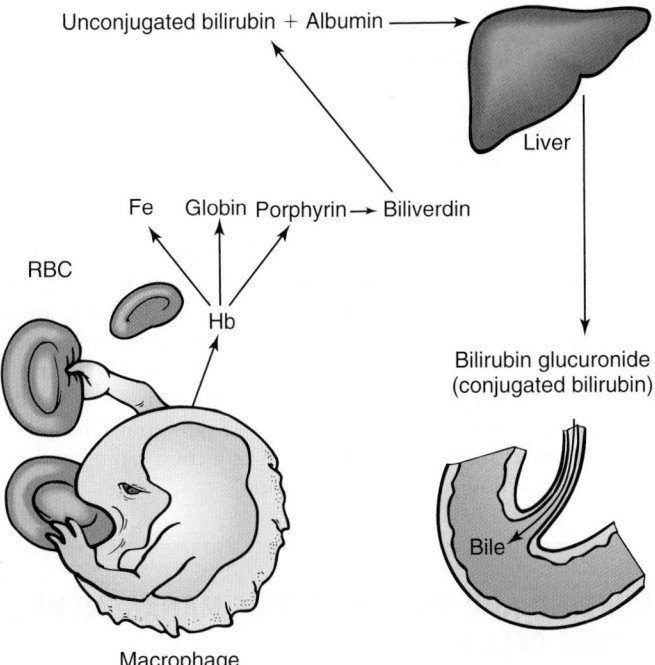

Figure 33-3 Sequence of events in extravascular hemolysis. *Fe,* iron; *Hb,* hemoglobin; *RBC,* red blood cell.

The patient with hemolytic anemia manifests the general symptoms of anemia and clinical manifestations specific to this type of anemia (see Table 33-3). Jaundice is likely because the increased destruction of RBCs causes an elevation in bilirubin levels. The spleen and the liver may enlarge because of their hyperactivity, which is related to macrophage phagocytosis of the defective erythrocytes.

In all causes of hemolysis, a major focus of treatment is to maintain renal function. When an RBC is hemolyzed, the Hb molecule is released and filtered by the kidneys. The accumulation of Hb molecules can obstruct the renal tubules and lead to acute tubular necrosis (see Chapter 49).

Sickle Cell Disease

Sickle cell disease (SCD) is a group of inherited, autosomal recessive disorders characterized by the presence of an abnormal form of Hb in the erythrocyte. (Autosomal recessive genetic disorders are discussed in Chapter 15.) This abnormal Hb, *hemoglobin S* (HbS), causes the erythrocyte to stiffen and elongate and take on a sickle shape in response to low levels of oxygen in the blood. HbS results from substitution of valine for glutamic acid on the β-globin chain of Hb. Because this is a genetic disorder, SCD is usually identified during infancy or early childhood. It is an incurable disease that is often fatal by the time the affected individual reaches middle age. Death usually results from renal and pulmonary failure and/or stroke (Gladwin & Vichinsky, 2008).

SCD is common in the African-descended population of Canada. It affects millions of people around the world, mainly those whose ancestors come from sub-Saharan Africa, Spanish-speaking regions (South America, Cuba, Central America), Saudi Arabia, India, and Mediterranean countries.

Etiology and Pathophysiology

Types of Sickle Cell Disease. Types of SCD disorders include sickle cell anemia, sickle cell–thalassemia, sickle cell–HbC disease, and sickle cell trait. *Sickle cell anemia,* the most severe of the SCD syndromes, occurs when a person is homozygous for HbS (HbSS); the person has inherited HbS from both parents. *Sickle cell–thalassemia* and *sickle cell–HbC* occur when a person inherits HbS from one parent and another type of abnormal Hb (such as thalassemia or HbC) from the other parent. Both of these forms of SCD are less common and less severe than sickle cell anemia. *Sickle cell trait* occurs when a person is heterozygous for hemoglobin S (HbAS); the person has inherited HbS from one parent and normal Hb (HbA) from the other parent. Sickle cell trait is typically a very mild or even asymptomatic condition.

Sickling Episodes. The major pathophysiological event of SCD is the sickling of RBCs. Sickling episodes are most commonly triggered by low O$_2$ tension in the blood. Hypoxia or deoxygenation of the RBCs can be caused by viral or bacterial infection, high altitude, emotional or physical stress, surgery, and blood loss. Infection is the most common precipitating factor. Other events that can trigger or sustain a sickling episode include dehydration, increased hydrogen ion concentration (acidosis), increased plasma osmolality, decreased plasma volume, and low body temperature. A sickling episode can also occur without an obvious cause.

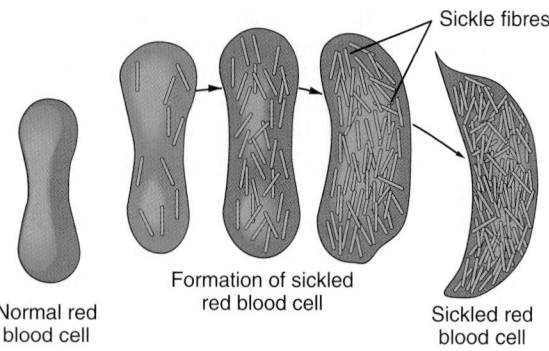

Figure 33-4 Sickle cell hemoglobin aggregates into long chains and alters the shape of the red blood cell.

Source: Redrawn from Raven, P. H., & Johnson, G. B. (1991). *Biology* (2nd ed.). St. Louis: Mosby.

Sickled RBCs become rigid and take on an elongated, crescent shape (Figure 33-4). Sickled cells cannot easily pass through capillaries or other small vessels and can cause vascular occlusion, leading to acute or chronic tissue injury. The resulting hemostasis promotes a self-perpetuating cycle of local hypoxia, deoxygenation of more erythrocytes, and more sickling. Circulating sickled cells are hemolyzed by the spleen, leading to anemia. Initially, the sickling of cells is reversible with reoxygenation, but it eventually becomes irreversible owing to cell membrane damage from recurrent sickling.

Sickle cell crisis is a severe, painful, acute exacerbation of RBC sickling causing a vaso-occlusive crisis. As blood flow is impaired by sickled cells, vasospasm occurs, further restricting blood flow. Severe capillary hypoxia causes changes in membrane permeability, leading to plasma loss, hemoconcentration, the development of thrombi, and further circulatory stagnation. Tissue ischemia, infarction, and necrosis eventually occur from lack of O_2. Shock is a possible life-threatening consequence of sickle cell crisis owing to severe O_2 depletion of the tissues and a reduction of the circulating fluid volume. Sickle cell crisis can begin suddenly and persist for days to weeks.

The frequency, extent, and severity of sickling episodes are highly variable and unpredictable, but are largely dependent on the percentage of HbS present. Individuals with sickle cell anemia have the most severe form because the erythrocytes contain a high percentage of HbS.

Clinical Manifestations

The effects of SCD vary greatly from person to person, the severity of which may be because of genetic polymorphisms. Many people with sickle cell anemia are in reasonably good health the majority of the time. However, they may have chronic health problems and pain because of organ tissue hypoxia and damage (e.g., involving the kidneys or liver, or both). The typical patient is anemic but asymptomatic except during sickling episodes. Because most individuals with sickle cell anemia have dark skin, pallor is more readily detected by examining the mucous membranes. The skin may have a greyish cast. Because of the hemolysis, jaundice is common and patients are prone to gallstones (cholelithiasis).

The primary symptom associated with sickling is pain. The pain can range from mild to excruciating because of tissue ischemia. The episodes can affect any area of the body or several sites simultaneously, with the back, chest, extremities, and abdomen most commonly affected. Pain episodes are often accompanied by objective clinical signs such as fever, swelling, tenderness, tachypnea, hypertension, nausea, and vomiting.

Complications

With repeated episodes of sickling, there is gradual involvement of all body systems, especially the spleen, lungs, kidneys, and brain. Organs that have a high need for O_2 are most often affected, and their involvement forms the basis for many of the complications of SCD (Figure 33-5). Infection is a major cause of morbidity and mortality in patients with SCD. One reason for this is the failure of the spleen to phagocytize foreign substances as it becomes infarcted and dysfunctional (usually by 2-4 yr of age) from the sickled RBCs. The spleen becomes small because of repeated scarring, a phenomenon termed *autosplenectomy*.

Pneumonia is the most common infection and often is of pneumococcal origin. Infections can be so severe that they can cause an aplastic and hemolytic crisis and gallstones. *Acute chest syndrome* is a term used to describe acute pulmonary complications that include pneumonia, tissue infarction, and fat embolism. It affects 30% of patients with SCD; is characterized by fever, chest pain, cough, pulmonary infiltrates, and dyspnea; and may be life-threatening. Pulmonary infarctions may cause pulmonary hypertension, MI, HF, and ultimately cor pulmonale (right-sided HF). The heart may become ischemic and enlarged, leading to HF. Retinal vessel obstruction may result in hemorrhage, scarring, retinal detachment, and blindness. The kidneys may be injured from the increased blood viscosity and the lack of O_2, which can lead to renal failure. Stroke can result from thrombosis and infarction of cerebral blood vessels. Bone changes may include osteoporosis and osteosclerosis after infarction. Chronic leg ulcers can result from the hypoxia and are especially prevalent around the ankles. *Priapism* (persistent penile erection) may occur if penile veins become occluded.

Diagnostic Studies

A peripheral blood smear may reveal sickled cells and abnormal reticulocytes. The presence of sickle Hb can be diagnosed by the sickling test, which uses RBCs (in vitro) and exposes them to a deoxygenation agent. As a result of the accelerated RBC breakdown, the patient has characteristic clinical findings of hemolysis (jaundice, elevated serum bilirubin levels) and abnormal laboratory test results. Hb electrophoresis may be done to determine the proportion of HbS and other variants. Skeletal radiographic studies will demonstrate bone and joint deformities and flattening. Magnetic resonance imaging (MRI) may be used to diagnose a stroke caused by blocked cerebral vessels from sickled cells. Doppler studies may be used to assess for deep venous thrombosis. Other tests may be indicated, such as a chest radiograph, to diagnose infection or organ malfunction.

NURSING AND COLLABORATIVE MANAGEMENT: SICKLE CELL DISEASE

Collaborative care for a patient with SCD is directed toward alleviating the symptoms from the complications of the disease,

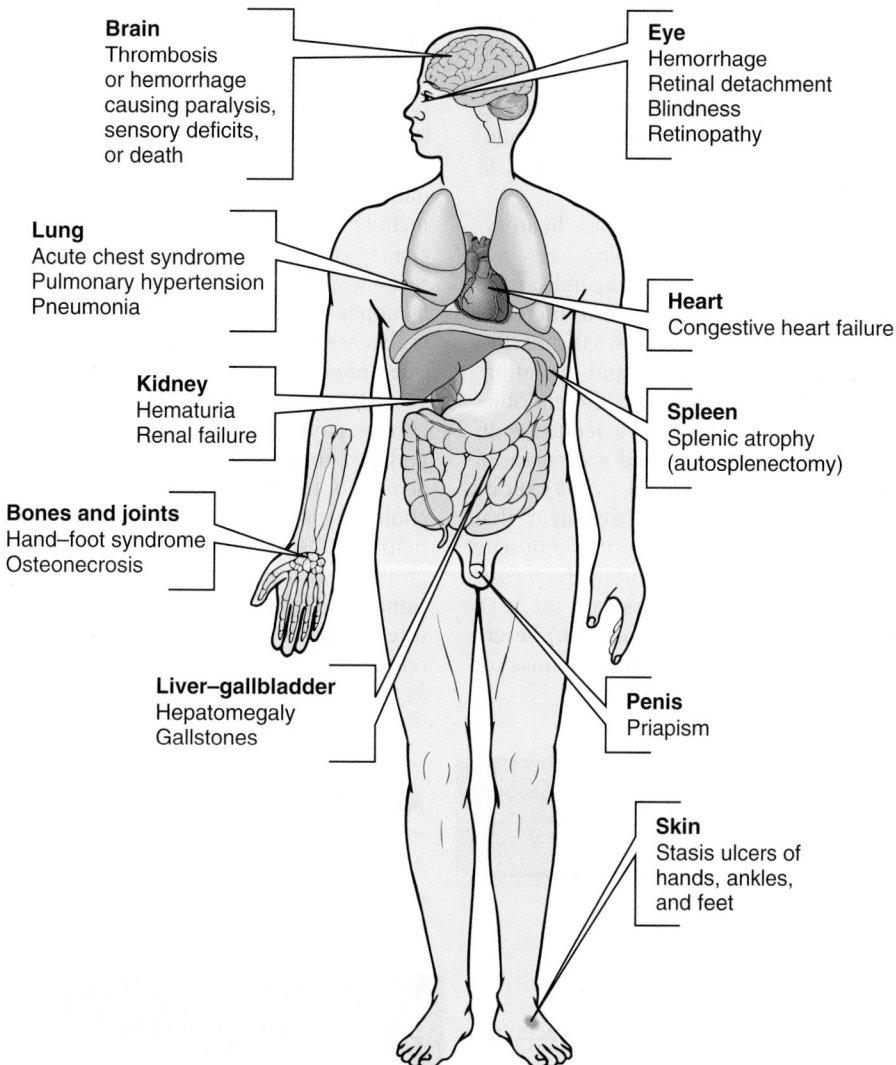

Brain
Thrombosis
or hemorrhage
causing paralysis,
sensory deficits,
or death

Eye
Hemorrhage
Retinal detachment
Blindness
Retinopathy

Lung
Acute chest syndrome
Pulmonary hypertension
Pneumonia

Heart
Congestive heart failure

Kidney
Hematuria
Renal failure

Spleen
Splenic atrophy
(autosplenectomy)

Bones and joints
Hand–foot syndrome
Osteonecrosis

Liver–gallbladder
Hepatomegaly
Gallstones

Penis
Priapism

Skin
Stasis ulcers of
hands, ankles,
and feet

Figure 33-5 Clinical manifestations and complications of sickle cell disease.

Source: Adapted from McCance, K. L., & Huether, S. E. (2010). *Pathophysiology: The biologic basis for disease in adults and children* (6th ed., p. 1075, Figure 28-8). St. Louis: Mosby.

minimizing end–target organ damage, and promptly treating serious sequelae, such as acute chest syndrome. Teach patients to avoid high altitudes, maintain adequate fluid intake, and treat infections promptly. Pneumovax, *Haemophilus influenzae*, influenza, and hepatitis immunizations should be administered. Chronic leg ulcers may be treated with bed rest, antibiotics, warm saline soaks, mechanical or enzyme debridement, and grafting if necessary. Priapism is managed with pain medication and nifedipine.

Sickle cell crises may necessitate hospitalization. O_2 may be administered to treat hypoxia and control sickling. Because respiratory failure is the most common cause of death, the nurse should be vigilant in assessing for any changes in respiratory status. Rest may be encouraged to reduce metabolic requirements. Fluids and electrolytes are administered to reduce blood viscosity and maintain renal function. Transfusion therapy is indicated when an aplastic crisis occurs; aggressive total RBC exchange transfusion programs may be implemented for patients who have frequent crises and/or serious complications such as acute chest syndrome. These patients, like those with thalassemia major, may

require chelation therapy to reduce transfusion-produced iron overload.

Undertreatment of sickle cell pain is a major problem. Lack of understanding can lead health care providers to underestimate how much pain these patients suffer. During an acute crisis, optimal pain management usually includes large doses of continuous (rather than as-needed [PRN]) opioid analgesics along with breakthrough analgesia, often in the form of patient-controlled analgesia (PCA). (PCA is discussed in Chapter 10.) Because patients may be experiencing different types and sites of pain, a multimodal and multidisciplinary approach to pain management is often needed. Adjunctive measures, such as nonsteroidal anti-inflammatory agents, antineuropathic pain medications (e.g., tricyclic antidepressants, antiseizure medications), local anesthetics, nerve blocks, transelectrodermal nerve stimulator (transcutaneous electrical nerve stimulation [TENS]), acupuncture, or some combination of these strategies may be used.

Although pain is the most common symptom of patients with SCD seeking medical care, infection is a frequent complication and must be treated. Patients with acute chest syndrome are treated with broad-spectrum antibiotics, O_2 therapy, fluid therapy, and possibly exchange transfusion. Blood transfusions have little, if any, role in the treatment between crises because patients develop antibodies to RBCs and iron overload. However, because chronic hemolysis results in increased utilization of folic acid stores, routine folic acid should be taken.

Although many antisickling agents have been tried, hydroxyurea (Hydrea) is the only one that has been shown to be clinically beneficial (McGann & Ware, 2011). However, the indications as to when to start have yet to be determined. This drug increases the production of fetal hemoglobin (HbF), decreases the reactive neutrophil count, increases erythrocyte volume and hydration, and alters the adhesion of sickle erythrocytes to the endothelium. The increase in HbF is accompanied by a reduction in hemolysis, an increase in Hb concentration, and a decrease in sickled cells and painful crises (Lanzkron et al., 2008). Bone marrow transplantation is the only available treatment that can cure some patients with SCD. The selection of appropriate recipients, scarcity of appropriate donors, risk, and the high cost/benefit ratio limit the use of bone marrow transplant for SCD. (Bone marrow transplants are discussed in Chapter 18.) Recent advances in gene therapy technology provide some promise for the future treatment of SCD. (Gene therapy is discussed in Chapter 15.)

Patient teaching and support are important in the long-term care of the patient. The patient and family must understand the basis of the disease and the reasons for supportive care and ongoing screening pertinent to SCD patients, such as eye examinations. The patient must be taught ways to avoid crises, which include taking steps to avoid dehydration and reducing the chance of developing hypoxia by avoiding high altitudes and seeking medical attention quickly to counteract problems such as upper respiratory tract infections. Education on pain control is also needed because the pain during a crisis may be severe and often requires considerable analgesia.

Recurrent episodes of severe acute pain and unrelenting chronic pain can be profoundly disabling and depressing. Occupational therapists and physiotherapists can help the patient achieve optimum physical functioning and independence; a psychologist may be able to use cognitive–behavioural therapy to help patients with SCD cope with anxiety and depression; support groups may also be helpful. Because there are often such additional quality-of-life issues, the nurse can play an important role in ensuring that these needs are met through appropriate referrals.

GENETICS IN CLINICAL PRACTICE
Sickle Cell Disease

Genetic Basis
- Autosomal recessive disorder
- Mutation in β-globin gene; sickle hemoglobin (HbS) on chromosome 11
- HbS variant involves substitution of valine for glutamic acid in the β-globin gene

Incidence
- More commonly affects people of African descent
- Also affects people of Mediterranean, Caribbean, South and Central American, Arabian, and East Indian descent
- Affects 8 of every 100,000 people

Genetic Testing
- DNA testing is available.
- Electrophoresis of hemoglobin and sickling screening test are more commonly used.

Clinical Implications
- SCD requires ongoing continuity of care and extensive patient education.
- Sickle cell trait is the carrier state for sickle cell disease and represents a mild type of sickle cell disease.
- If both parents have the trait, there is a 1 in 4 chance that their child will have SCD.
- Management of SCD should focus on the prevention of sickle cell crisis.
- Genetic counselling is recommended for individuals with a family history of SCD. Individuals should understand the risks of transmitting the genetic mutation.

SCD, sickle cell disease.

Acquired Hemolytic Anemia

Acquired hemolytic anemia results from hemolysis of RBCs from extrinsic factors. These factors can be separated into three catego-

ETHICAL DILEMMAS
Pain Management

Situation
A 21-year-old man is admitted to the emergency department in sickle cell crisis with complaints of excruciating pain. He is known to several of the nurses and physicians in the department. One of the nurses remarks to the nurse that it must be time for his "fix" of pain medications.

Important Points for Consideration
- The experience of pain is subjective, and experts in pain management agree that "pain is what the patient says it is." The single most reliable indicator of pain is self-report.
- Acute or chronic pain can have serious and debilitating physical and psychological effects.
- Chronic pain can alter physiological and psychological responses to pain and to pain medication.
- People with chronic pain are often stigmatized because of health care providers' lack of knowledge about pain and/or long-term use of opioids or other pain medications.

Clinical Decision-Making Questions
1. How can the nurse educate peers regarding pain assessment and management?
2. What important factors would need to be included in the nurse's assessment and management of this patient?

ries: (1) physical factors, (2) immune reactions, and (3) infectious agents and toxins (see Table 33-2)

Physical destruction of RBCs results from the exertion of extreme force on the cells. Traumatic events causing disruption of the RBC membrane include use of hemodialysis, extracorporeal circulation used in cardiopulmonary bypass, and prosthetic heart valves. In addition, the force needed to push blood through abnormal vessels, such as those that have been burned or affected by angiopathic disease (e.g., diabetes mellitus), may also physically damage RBCs.

Antibodies may destroy RBCs by the mechanisms involved in antigen–antibody reactions. The reactions may be of an isoimmune or autoimmune type. *Isoimmune reactions* occur when antibodies develop against antigens from another individual of the same species—in the case of humans, that is, from another person. Blood transfusion reactions typify this response, when the recipient's antibodies hemolyze donor cells.

Autoimmune reactions result when individuals develop antibodies against their own RBCs. Autoimmune hemolytic reactions may be idiopathic, developing with no prior hemolytic history as a result of the immunoglobulin G (IgG) covering the RBCs, or secondary to other autoimmune diseases (e.g., systemic lupus erythematosus), leukemia, or lymphoma, or reactions to drugs (penicillin, indomethacin, quinidine, quinine, and methyldopa).

Infectious agents and toxins constitute the third category of acquired hemolytic disorders. Infectious agents foster hemolysis in four ways: (1) by invading the RBC and destroying its contents (e.g., parasites such as in malaria); (2) by releasing hemolytic substances (e.g., *Clostridium perfringens*); (3) by generating an antigen–antibody reaction; and (4) by contributing to splenomegaly as a means of increasing removal of damaged RBCs from the circulation. Various agents may be toxic to RBCs and cause hemolysis. These hemolytic toxins involve chemicals such as oxidative drugs, arsenic, lead, copper, and snake venom.

Laboratory findings in hemolytic anemia are presented in Table 33-6. Treatment and management of acquired hemolytic anemias involve general supportive care until the causative agent can be eliminated or at least rendered less injurious to the RBCs. Because a hemolytic crisis is a potential consequence, the nurse must be ready to institute appropriate emergent therapy. Supportive care may include administering corticosteroids and blood products or removing the spleen.

Hemochromatosis

Hemochromatosis is an iron overload disorder. Although it is primarily caused by a genetic defect, hemochromatosis occurs secondary to diseases such as thalassemia and sideroblastic anemia. It may also be caused by liver disease and multiple blood transfusions.

The genetic disorder is autosomal recessive characterized by increased intestinal iron absorption and, as a result, increased tissue iron deposition (see the Genetics in Clinical Practice box). In Canada, it is one of the most common genetic disorders (Canadian Hemochromatosis Society, 2012). It is most common among Canadians of Northern European descent, with an incidence of 1 in 300. One in 250 to 300 Canadians are at risk of developing the full-blown disease (homozygous with two recessive genes), and approximately 1 in 9 are potential carriers with one recessive gene (Canadian Hemochromatosis Society, 2012).

GENETICS IN CLINICAL PRACTICE
Hemochromatosis

Genetic Basis
- Autosomal recessive trait
- Most common mutations: C282Y and H63D
- Genetic defect located in close proximity to the major histocompatibility complex on chromosome 6

Incidence
- Most common genetic disease in people of European ancestry
- Affects approximately 1 in 300 Canadians of Northern European ancestry
- Very low prevalence in other ethnic populations

Genetic Testing
- Genetic testing is recommended for all first-degree relatives of people with disease.
- Useful diagnostic tests include serum iron concentration, total iron-binding capacity, and transferrin saturation.
- Liver biopsy, once considered the gold standard diagnostic test, is primarily used to quantify iron deposition and estimate the prognosis and extent of disease.

Clinical Implications
- Early treatment can prevent serious complications.
- Clinical expression is variable depending on dietary iron, blood loss, and other modifying factors.
- If untreated, progressive iron deposits can lead to multiple organ failure.

The normal range for total body iron is 2 to 6 g. Individuals with hemochromatosis accumulate iron at a rate of 0.5 to 1.0 g each year and may accumulate total iron concentrations exceeding 50 g. Symptoms of hemochromatosis usually develop between 40 and 60 years of age. Early symptoms are nonspecific and include fatigue, arthralgia, erectile dysfunction, abdominal pain, and weight loss. Later, the excess iron accumulates in the liver and causes liver enlargement and eventually cirrhosis. Patients with hemochromatosis are at increased risk for hepatocellular carcinoma (Villanueva, Newell, & Hoshida, 2010). Other organs also become affected, resulting in diabetes mellitus, skin pigment changes (bronzing), cardiac changes (e.g., cardiomyopathy), arthritis, and testicular atrophy. Physical examination reveals an enlarged liver and spleen and pigmentation changes in the skin. Laboratory values demonstrate an elevated serum iron, TIBC, and serum ferritin. A liver biopsy can quantify the amount of iron and is the definitive way to establish the diagnosis.

The goal of treatment is to remove excess iron from the body and minimize any symptoms the patient may have. Iron removal is achieved by removing 500 mL of blood each week for 2 to 3 years until the iron stores in the body are depleted. Then, less frequent removal of blood is needed to maintain iron levels within normal limits. Management of organ involvement (e.g., diabetes mellitus, HF) is the same as conventional treatment for these problems. Dietary modifications, such as avoidance of vitamin C and iron supplements, uncooked seafood, and iron-rich foods, may also assist in the reduction of iron accumulation. The most common causes of death are cirrhosis, liver failure, hepatic carcinoma, and cardiac failure. With early diagnosis and treatment, life expectancy is normal. However, many cases go undetected and untreated.

Polycythemia

Polycythemia is the production and presence of increased numbers of RBCs. The increase in RBCs can be so great that blood circulation is impaired as a result of the increased blood viscosity *(hyperviscosity)* and volume *(hypervolemia)*.

Etiology and Pathophysiology

The two types of polycythemia are primary polycythemia, or polycythemia vera, and secondary polycythemia (Figure 33-6). Their etiologies and pathogenesis differ, although their complications and clinical manifestations are similar. *Polycythemia vera* is considered a myeloproliferative disorder arising from a chromosomal mutation in a single pluripotent stem cell. Therefore, not only are RBCs involved but also granulocytes and platelets, leading to increased production of each of these blood cells. The disease develops insidiously and follows a chronic, vacillating course. The median age at diagnosis is 60 years old with a slight male predominance. With this myeloproliferative disorder, the patient has enhanced blood viscosity and blood volume and congestion of organs and tissues with blood. These patients have hypercoagulopathies that predispose them to clotting. Splenomegaly and hepatomegaly are common.

Secondary polycythemia can be either hypoxia driven or hypoxia independent. In the former, hypoxia stimulates erythropoietin (EPO) production in the kidney, which in turn stimulates erythrocyte production. The need for O_2 may be because of high altitude, pulmonary disease, cardiovascular disease, alveolar hypoventilation, defective O_2 transport, or tissue hypoxia. EPO levels may return to normal once the Hb is stabilized at a higher level. In this situation, secondary polycythemia is a physiological response in which the body tries to compensate for a problem rather than a pathological response. (Hypoxia-driven polycythemia is discussed in the section on chronic obstructive pulmonary disease in Chapter 31.) In hypoxia-independent secondary polycythemia, EPO is produced by malignant or benign tumour tissue. Serum EPO levels often remain elevated in these situations.

Clinical Manifestations and Complications

Circulatory manifestations of polycythemia vera occur because of the hypertension caused by hypervolemia and hyperviscosity. They are often the first symptoms and include subjective complaints of headache, vertigo, dizziness, tinnitus, and visual disturbances. Generalized pruritus (often exacerbated by a hot bath) may be a striking symptom and is related to histamine release from an increased number of basophils. Paresthesias and *erythromelalgia* (painful burning and redness of the hands and feet caused by paroxysmal peripheral dilation of peripheral blood vessels) may also be present. In addition, the patient may experience angina, HF, intermittent claudication, and thrombophlebitis, which may be complicated by embolization. These manifestations are caused by blood vessel distension, impaired blood flow, circulatory stasis, thrombosis, and tissue hypoxia caused by the hypervolemia and hyperviscosity. The most common serious complication is stroke secondary to thrombosis (Tefferi, 2008).

Hemorrhagic phenomena caused by either vessel rupture from overdistension or inadequate platelet function may result in petechiae, ecchymoses, epistaxis, or GI bleeding. Hemorrhage can be acute and catastrophic. Hepatomegaly and splenomegaly from organ engorgement may contribute to patient complaints of satiety and fullness. The patient may also experience pain from peptic ulcer caused by either increased gastric secretions or liver and spleen engorgement. *Plethora* (ruddy complexion) may also be present. Because uric acid is one of the products of cell destruction, the increase in RBC destruction that accompanies excessive RBC production causes a similar increase in uric acid production,

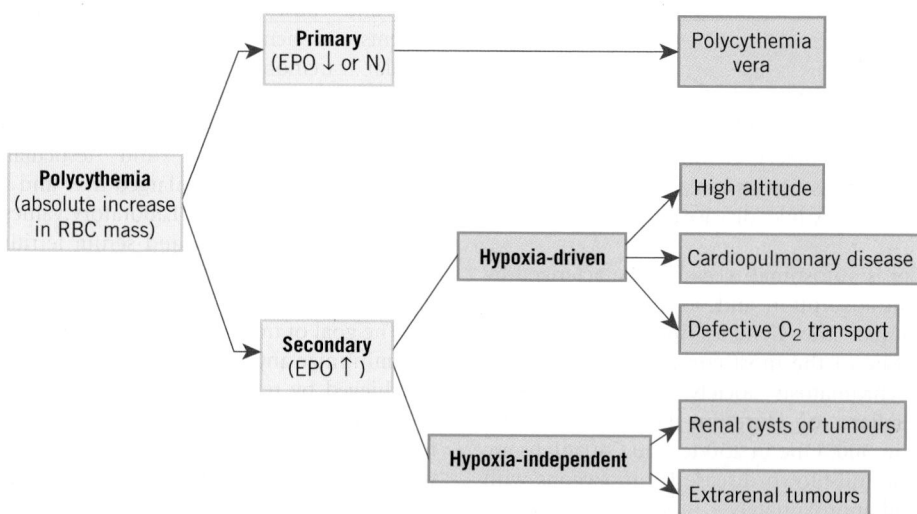

Figure 33-6 Differentiating between primary and secondary polycythemia. *EPO,* erythropoietin; *N,* normal; *RBC,* red blood cell.

thus leading to hyperuricemia. This problem may cause a form of gout.

Diagnostic Studies

The following laboratory manifestations are seen in a patient with polycythemia vera: (1) elevated Hb and RBC count with microcytosis; (2) low to normal EPO level (secondary polycythemia will have a high level); (3) elevated WBC count with basophilia; (4) elevated platelets (thrombocytosis) and platelet dysfunction; (5) elevated leukocyte alkaline phosphatase, uric acid, and cobalamin levels; and (6) elevated histamine levels. Bone marrow examination in polycythemia vera shows hypercellularity of RBCs, WBCs, and platelets. Splenomegaly is found in 90% of patients with primary polycythemia but does not accompany secondary polycythemia.

Collaborative Care

Treatment is directed toward reducing blood volume and viscosity and bone marrow activity. Phlebotomy is the mainstay of treatment. The aim of phlebotomy is to reduce the Hct and keep it less than 45 to 48%. Generally, from the time of diagnosis, 300 to 500 mL of blood may be removed every other day until the Hct is reduced to normal levels. An individual managed with repeated phlebotomies eventually becomes deficient in iron, although this effect is rarely symptomatic. Iron supplementation should be avoided. Hydration therapy is used to reduce the blood's viscosity. Myelosuppressive agents such as busulphan (Myleran) and hydroxyurea (Hydrea) may be given to inhibit bone marrow activity. Newer, targeted therapies (targeting the *JAK2* mutation) are being studied (Tefferi, 2008). Antiplatelet agents, such as aspirin, may be used for erythromelalgia and/or antithrombotic primary prophylaxis. Allopurinol may reduce the number of acute gouty attacks and antihistamines may be used to alleviate pruritus.

NURSING MANAGEMENT: POLYCYTHEMIA VERA

Primary polycythemia vera is not preventable. However, because secondary polycythemia is generated by any source of hypoxia, maintaining adequate oxygenation may prevent problems. Therefore, controlling chronic pulmonary disease, stopping smoking, and avoiding high altitudes may be important.

When acute exacerbations of polycythemia vera develop, the nurse has several responsibilities. Depending on the institution's policies, the nurse may assist with or perform the phlebotomy. Fluid intake and output must be evaluated during hydration therapy to avoid fluid overload (which further complicates the circulatory congestion) and underhydration (which can cause the blood to become even more viscous). If myelosuppressive agents are used, the nurse must administer the drugs as ordered, observe the patient, and teach the patient about medication adverse effects.

Assessment of the patient's nutritional status in collaboration with the dietitian may be necessary to offset the inadequate food intake that can result from GI symptoms of fullness, pain, and dyspepsia. Activities and/or medications must be instituted to decrease thrombus formation. Active or passive leg exercises and ambulation, when possible, should be initiated.

Because of its chronic nature, polycythemia vera requires ongoing evaluation. Phlebotomy may need to be done every 2 to 3 months, reducing the blood volume by about 500 mL each time. The nurse must evaluate the patient for the development of complications.

Although the incidence is low, myelofibrosis and leukemia develop in some patients with polycythemia vera (10% and 5%, respectively). These occurrences may be caused by the chemotherapeutic drugs used to treat the disease, or they may be secondary to a disorder in the stem cells that progresses to erythroleukemia. The major cause of morbidity and mortality from polycythemia vera is related to thrombosis (e.g., stroke).

Problems of Hemostasis

The homeostatic process involves the vascular endothelium, platelets, and coagulation factors, which normally function together to arrest hemorrhage and repair vascular injury. (These mechanisms are described in Chapter 32.) Disruption in any of these components may result in bleeding or thrombotic disorders.

Three major disorders of hemostasis discussed in this section are (1) thrombocytopenia (low platelet count), (2) hemophilia and von Willebrand's disease (inherited disorders of specific clotting factors), and (3) disseminated intravascular coagulation (DIC).

Thrombocytopenia

Etiology and Pathophysiology

Thrombocytopenia is a reduction of platelets to an amount below $150 \times 10^9/L$ or 150,000 per microlitre. Acute, severe, or prolonged decreases from this normal range can result in abnormal hemostasis whose manifestations range from prolonged bleeding from minor trauma to spontaneous bleeding without injury.

Platelet disorders can be inherited (e.g., Wiskott-Aldrich syndrome), but the vast majority are acquired (see Table 33-11). A common cause of acquired abnormalities is the ingestion of certain foods, herbs, or drugs (Table 33-12). Although some agents are directly myelosuppressive (e.g. chemotherapy, ganciclovir [Cytovene]), the usual mechanism of thrombocytopenia caused by foods, herbs, or drugs is accelerated platelet destruction caused by drug-dependent antibodies. Antibodies attack the platelets when the offending agent binds to a platelet surface glycoprotein. A careful review of the patient's history helps distinguish these causes from one of the causes mentioned in Table 33-13. For example, quinine may cause thrombocytopenia and is found in tonic water and in many herbal preparations. In addition, some drugs can affect platelet aggregation. Aspirin doses as low as 81 mg (a baby aspirin) can alter the function of circulating platelets. Normal function is restored with the generation of newly formed platelets.

Immune Thrombocytopenic Purpura. The most common acquired thrombocytopenia is a syndrome of abnormal destruction of circulating platelets termed *immune thrombocytopenic purpura* (ITP). It was originally termed *idiopathic thrombocytopenic purpura* because its cause was unknown. However, it is now known that ITP is an autoimmune disease. In ITP, platelets are

Table 33-12 Food, Drug, and Herbal Causes of Thrombocytopenia*

- Thiazide diuretics
- Alcohol
- Estrogen
- Chemotherapeutic drugs
- Digoxin
- Nonsteroidal anti-inflammatory drugs: ibuprofen (Advil), indomethacin, naprosen (Naprelan, Aleve)
- Antibiotics: penicillins, cephalosporins, sulphonamides
- Other anti-infectives: rifampin (Rifadin), ganciclovir (Cytovene), amphotericin B
- Analgesics: aspirin and aspirin-containing drugs, acetaminophen
- Antipsychotics and antiseizures: haloperidol, lithium
- Platelet glycoprotein inhibitors: abciximab (ReoPro), tirofiban (Aggrastat), clopidogrel (Plavix)
- H_2 antagonists: cimetidine, ranitidine (Zantac)
- Gold compounds: auranofin (Ridaura)
- Spices: ginger, cumin, turmeric, cloves
- Vitamins: C, E
- Heparin
- Herbs: angelica, bilberry, evening primrose, feverfew, garlic, ginger, *Ginkgo biloba*, ginseng, goldenseal
- Quinine compounds: tonic water, china bark, Peruvian bark, yellow cinchona

*List is not all-inclusive.

Table 33-13 Causes of Thrombocytopenia

Inherited

- Fanconi's syndrome (pancytopenia)
- Hereditary thrombocytopenia

Acquired

Immune

- Immune thrombocytopenic purpura (ITP)
- Neonatal alloimmune thrombocytopenia

Nonimmune

- Shortened circulation
  - Thrombotic thrombocytopenic purpura (TTP)
  - Disseminated intravascular coagulation (DIC)
  - Heparin-induced thrombocytopenia (HIT)
  - Splenomegaly, splenic sequestration
- Turbulent blood flow (hemangiomas, abnormal cardiac valves, intra-aortic balloon pumps)
- Decreased production
  - Drug-induced marrow suppression
  - Chemotherapy
  - Viral infections (hepatitis C virus, HIV, cytomegalovirus)
  - Bacterial infection (sepsis)
  - Alcoholism/bone marrow suppression
  - Myelodysplastic syndrome (MDS)
  - Myelofibrosis
  - Aplastic anemia
  - Hematological malignancy (leukemias, lymphomas, myeloma)
  - Solid tumour infiltrating bone marrow
  - Radiation to the bone

HIV, human immunodeficiency virus.

coated with antibodies. Although these platelets function normally, when they reach the spleen, the antibody-coated platelets are recognized as foreign and are destroyed by macrophages.

Platelets normally survive 8 to 10 days. However, in ITP, survival of platelets is only 1 to 3 days. Chronic ITP occurs most commonly in women between 20 and 40 years of age and has a gradual onset; transient remissions occur.

Thrombotic Thrombocytopenic Purpura.

Thrombotic thrombocytopenic purpura (TTP) is an uncommon syndrome characterized by hemolytic anemia, thrombocytopenia, neurological abnormalities, fever (in the absence of infection), and renal abnormalities. Not all features are present in all patients. Because it is almost always associated with hemolytic–uremic syndrome (HUS), it is often referred to as TTP–HUS. The disease is associated with enhanced agglutination of platelets, which form microthrombi that deposit in arterioles and capillaries. In most cases, the syndrome is due to the deficiency of a plasma enzyme (ADAMTS-13) that usually breaks down the von Willebrand's clotting factor (vWF) into normal size. (vWF is the most important protein mediating platelet adhesion to damaged endothelial cells.) Without the enzyme, unusually large vWF multimers attach to activated platelets, thereby promoting platelet aggregation.

TTP is seen primarily in adults between 20 and 50 years of age, with a slight female predominance. The syndrome may be idiopathic (thought to be due to an autoimmune disorder against ADAMTS-13), may be caused by certain drug toxicities, pregnancy, or infection or may be the result of a known autoimmune disorder such as systemic lupus erythematosus or scleroderma. TTP is a medical emergency because bleeding and clotting occur simultaneously (Kremer Hovinga & Meyer, 2008).

Heparin-Induced Thrombocytopenia and Thrombosis Syndrome.

One of the risks associated with the broad and increasing use of heparin is the development of the life-threatening condition called *heparin-induced thrombocytopenia* (HIT), also called *heparin-induced thrombocytopenia and thrombosis syndrome* (HITTS). An estimated 5 to 25% of patients on heparin therapy develop HITTS (Baldwin, Spitzer, Ng, & Harken, 2008). The major clinical problem of HITTS is venous thrombosis; arterial thrombosis can also develop. Deep venous thromboses and pulmonary emboli most commonly result as a complication of the thromboses. Additional complications may include arterial vascular infarcts resulting in skin necrosis, stroke, and end-organ damage, such as to the kidneys. There are rarely symptoms of bleeding because the platelet count rarely drops below 60×10^9/L or 60,000 per microlitre.

In HIT, platelet destruction and vascular endothelial injury are the two major responses to what is believed to be an immune-mediated response to heparin. Platelet factor 4 (PF4) binds to heparin. This complex then binds to the platelet surface, leading to further platelet activation and release of more PF4, thus creating a positive feedback loop. Antibodies are created against this complex, and they are removed prematurely from circulation, leading to thrombocytopenia and platelet-fibrin thrombi. Platelet aggregation also induces heparin to be neutralized. Thus, more

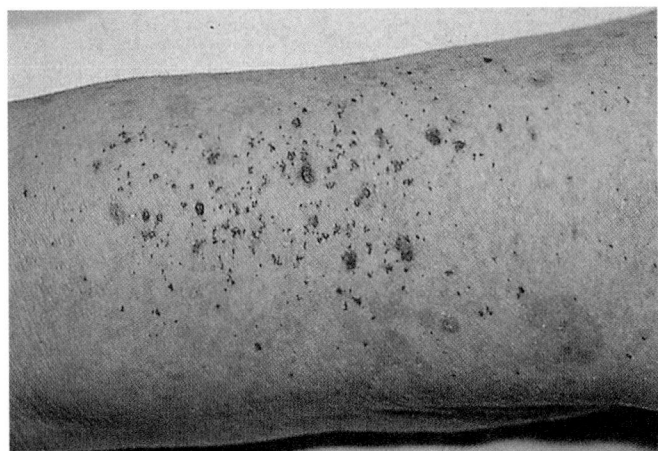

Figure 33-7 Acute idiopathic thrombocytopenic purpura commonly manifests with purpuric lesions of this kind, although they may often be widespread by the time medical attention is sought.

Source: Forbes, C. D., & Jackson, W. F. (2003). *Color atlas and text of clinical medicine* (3rd ed., p. 437, Figure 10.96). London: Mosby.

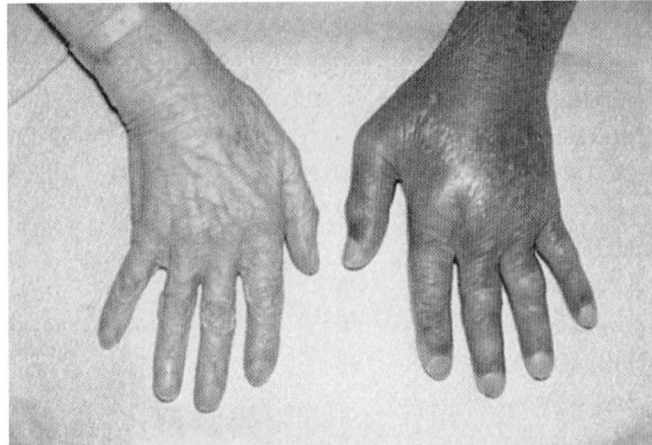

Figure 33-8 Severe ecchymosis of the left hand.

heparin is required to maintain therapeutic activated partial thromboplastin times (aPTT).

Clinical Manifestations. Many patients with thrombocytopenia are asymptomatic. The most common symptom is bleeding, usually mucosal or cutaneous. Mucosal bleeding may manifest as epistaxis and gingival bleeding, and large bullous hemorrhages may appear on the buccal mucosa owing to the lack of vessel protection afforded by the submucosal tissue. Bleeding into the skin is manifested as petechiae or superficial ecchymoses (Figure 33-7).

Petechiae are small, flat, pinpoint, red or reddish-brown microhemorrhages. When the platelet count is low, RBCs may leak out of the blood vessels and into the skin to cause petechiae. When petechiae are numerous, the resulting reddish skin bruise is called *purpura* (see Figure 33-7). Larger purplish lesions caused by hemorrhage are termed *ecchymoses* (Figure 33-8). Ecchymoses may be flat or raised; pain and tenderness sometimes are present.

Prolonged bleeding after routine procedures such as venipuncture or IM injection may also indicate thrombocytopenia. Because the bleeding may be internal, the nurse must be aware of manifestations that reflect this type of blood loss, including weakness, fainting, dizziness, tachycardia, abdominal pain, and hypotension.

The major complication of thrombocytopenia is hemorrhage. The hemorrhage may be insidious or acute and internal or external. It may occur in any area of the body, including the joints, retina, and brain. Cerebral hemorrhage may be fatal in people with ITP. Insidious hemorrhage may first be detected by discovering the anemia that accompanies blood loss.

Diagnostic Studies

The platelet count is decreased in cases of thrombocytopenia. Any reduction below 150×10^9/L or 150,000 per microlitre may be termed *thrombocytopenia*. However, prolonged bleeding from trauma or injury does not usually occur until platelet counts are less than 50×10^9/L or 50,000 per microlitre. When the count drops below 10×10^9/L or 10,000 per microlitre, spontaneous,

life-threatening hemorrhages (e.g., intracranial bleeding) can occur. Platelet transfusions are generally not recommended until the count is below 10×10^9/L unless the patient is actively bleeding or critically ill with fever or sepsis. Laboratory tests that assess secondary hemostasis or coagulation, such as the prothrombin time (PT) and aPTT, can yield normal results even in severe thrombocytopenia. If they are elevated, this may point toward *disseminated intravascular coagulation* (DIC). Specific assays, such as the ITP antigen-specific assay, ^{14}C-serotonin release assay, or enzyme-linked immunoassay (ELISA) for PF4-heparin complex for HIT, can be done to assist with the diagnosis. In TTP, testing for deficiency of ADAMTS-13 is not widely available, so an increase of lactic dehydrogenase (LDH) is used to help establish the diagnosis (Table 33-14).

Examination of the peripheral blood smear may help distinguish acquired disorders such as ITP and TTP from congenital disorders, which may be indicated by abnormally sized platelets. Bone marrow examination is done to rule out production problems as the cause of thrombocytopenia (e.g., leukemia, aplastic anemia, other myeloproliferative disorders). It is performed if the other tests are inconclusive, especially in older patients with a suspicion of an underlying bone marrow disorder. When destruction of circulating platelets is the cause, bone marrow analysis shows *megakaryocytes* (precursors of platelets) to be normal or increased, even though circulating platelets are reduced. The absence or decreased numbers of megakaryocytes on bone marrow biopsy is consistent with thrombocytopenia caused by decreased bone marrow production (e.g., aplastic anemia).

The nurse must closely monitor the platelet count and other coagulation studies. Together, these provide clinical information regarding potential or actual bleeding. When thrombocytopenia occurs with anemia, characterized by altered RBC morphology, including *spherocytes* (small globular, completely hemoglobinated erythrocytes), fragmented cells (*schistocytes*), and pronounced reticulocytosis, a diagnosis of TTP should be suspected. These findings are partially a result of intravascular fibrin deposition causing a "slicing" of RBCs. In TTP, thrombocytopenia may be severe but the results of coagulation studies are normal.

Collaborative Care

Collaborative care of thrombocytopenia differs according to the etiology of the thrombocytopenia. Discussion of management strategies for these different etiologies follows (Table 33-15).

Table 33-14 Comparison of Disorders Causing Thrombocytopenia

LABORATORY TEST	ITP	TTP	HIT	DIC
Platelets	↓↓↓	↓↓↓	↓↓	↓↓↓
Hemolysis				
Hb	N	↓↓	N	N, ↓
LDH	N	↑↑↑	N	↑
Reticulocytes	N	↑	N	N, ↑
Haptoglobin	N	↓	N	↓
Indirect bilirubin	N	↑	N	N, ↑
Schistocytes	N	↑↑↑	N, ↑	N, ↑
Coagulopathy				
PT	N	N	N	↑
aPTT	N	N	N	↑
D-dimer	N	N, ↑	↑	↑↑
Other Tests	ITP antigen-specific assay; ^{14}C-serotonin release assay; *Helicobacter pylori*	ADAMTS-13	^{14}C-serotonin release assay; ELISA for PF4-heparin complex	

aPTT, activated partial thromboplastin time; *DIC*, disseminated intravascular coagulation; *ELISA*, enzyme-linked immunoassay; *Hb*, hemoglobin; *HIT*, heparin-induced thrombocytopenia; *ITP*, idiopathic thrombocytopenic purpura; *LDH*, lactic dehydrogenase; *N*, normal; *PF4*, platelet factor 4; ↑, increased; ↓, decreased; *PT* , prothrombin time; *TTP*, thrombotic thrombocytopenic purpura.

Immune Thrombocytopenic Purpura. Multiple therapies are used to manage the patient with ITP. If the patient is asymptomatic, therapy may not be used unless the patient's platelet count is less than 30×10^9/L or 30,000 per microlitre. Corticosteroids (e.g., prednisone) are used to treat ITP because of their ability to suppress the phagocytic response of splenic macrophages. This alters the spleen's recognition of platelets and increases the lifespan of the platelets. In addition, corticosteroids depress antibody formation. Corticosteroids also reduce capillary fragility and bleeding time. The mechanism of action for this response is poorly understood. If there are neurological manifestations related to intracranial bleeding, high-dose methylprednisolone (Solu-Medrol) can be administered by IV route. Methylprednisolone has also been used in patients whose disease is resistant to prednisone.

Splenectomy is indicated if the patient does not respond to prednisone initially or requires unacceptably high doses to maintain an adequate platelet count. Approximately 80% of patients benefit from splenectomy, resulting in a complete or partial remission. The effectiveness of splenectomy is based on four factors. First, the spleen contains an abundance of the macrophages that sequester and destroy platelets. Second, structural features of the spleen enhance the interaction between antibody-coated platelets and macrophages. Third, some antibody synthesis occurs in the spleen; thus, antiplatelet antibodies decrease after splenectomy. Fourth, the spleen normally sequesters approximately one third of the platelets, so its removal increases the number of platelets in circulation.

High doses of IV immunoglobulin (IVIG) and a component of IVIG, anti-Rh$_o$(D) (anti-D, WinRho), may be used to treat the patient who is unresponsive to corticosteroids or splenectomy. These agents work by competing with the antiplatelet antibodies for macrophage receptors. They effectively raise the platelet count, but the beneficial effects are temporary.

Danazol (Cyclomen), an androgen, may also be used along with steroids in some patients. Although the mechanism is not totally understood, it is suggested that danazol increases CD4$^+$ T cells, thereby reducing the immune response. Immunosuppressive therapy may be used in refractory cases (see Table 33-15).

Platelet transfusions may be used to increase platelet counts in cases of life-threatening hemorrhage. Platelets should not be given prophylactically because of the possibility of antibody formation. The usual indication for administering platelets is a platelet count less than 10×10^9/L or 10,000 per microlitre or if there is bleeding before a procedure. Several studies indicate that the risk of bleeding may not be substantial until the count is less than 5×10^9/L or 5000 per microlitre. ABO compatibility is not a necessary prerequisite for platelet transfusions. However, after multiple platelet transfusions, a patient may develop anti-HLA antibodies to the transfused platelets. HLA matching of the donor and the recipient may help patients who have recurrent minor allergic reactions. The patient may also be ordered premedication, such as antihistamines (e.g., diphenhydramine [Benadryl]) and hydrocortisone, to decrease the possibility of reacting to platelet transfusions. Aspirin and aspirin-containing compounds should be avoided in the patient with thrombocytopenia.

Thrombotic Thrombocytopenic Purpura. TTP may be treated in a variety of ways. The first step is to treat the underlying disorder (e.g., infection) or remove the causative agent, if identified. If untreated, TTP usually results in irreversible renal failure and death. Plasma exchange or plasmapheresis (see Chapter 16) is used to aggressively reverse platelet consumption by supplying the appropriate vWF and enzyme (ADAMTS-13) and removing the large vWF molecules binding with platelets. Treatment should be continued daily until the patient's counts normalize and hemolysis has ceased. Corticosteroids may be added to this treatment. Monoclonal antibody therapy (e.g., rituximab), immunosuppressants (e.g., cyclosporine or cyclophosphamide), and splenectomy have also been used with success. The administration of platelets is generally contraindicated because this may lead to new vWF-platelet complexes and increased clotting.

Heparin-Induced Thrombocytopenia and Thrombosis Syndrome.

Heparin must be discontinued when HITTS is first recognized, which is usually if the patient's platelet count has fallen 50% or more from its baseline or if a thrombus forms while the patient is receiving heparin therapy. Heparin flushes for vascular catheters should be stopped.

To maintain anticoagulation, the patient should be started on a direct thrombin inhibitor, such as lepirudin (Refludan) or argatroban. If clotting is severe, the most commonly used treatment modalities are plasmapheresis to clear the platelet-aggregating IgG from the blood, protamine sulphate to interrupt the circulating heparin, thrombolytic agents to treat the thromboembolic events, and surgery to remove clots. Platelet transfusions are not effective because they may enhance thromboembolic events. Patients who have had HITTS should never be given heparin or low–molecular weight heparin.

COLLABORATIVE CARE

Table 33-15 Thrombocytopenia

Diagnostic	Thrombotic Thrombocytopenic Purpura
• History and physical examination	• Identification and treatment of cause
• Bone marrow aspiration and biopsy	• Plasmapheresis (plasma exchange)
• CBC including platelet count	• High-dose prednisone
• Specific studies (see Table 33-14)	• Splenectomy
Collaborative Therapy	• Dextran
Immune Thrombocytopenic Purpura	• Chemotherapy (e.g., vincristine, vinblastine)
• Corticosteroids	• Immunosuppressives (e.g., cyclophosphamide [Procytox], rituximab [Rituxan])
• Intravenous immunoglobulin (IVIG)	**Heparin-Induced Thrombocytopenia**
• Anti-Rh$_0$ (D)	• Discontinuation of heparin
• Romiplostim (Nplate)	• Direct thrombin inhibitor (e.g., lepirudin [Refludan])
• Eltrombopag (Revolade)	• Indirect thrombin inhibitor (e.g., fondaparinux [Arixtra])
• Tranexamic acid	• Plasmapheresis (plasma exchange)
• Platelet transfusions (if life-threatening)	• Protamine sulphate
• Vaccination (pneumococcal, meningococcal, *Haemophilus influenzae* B)	• Warfarin (Coumadin)
• Danazol	• Thrombolytic agents
• Immunosuppressives (e.g., rituximab [Rituxan], cyclosporine)	**Decreased Platelet Production**
• High-dose cyclophosphamide or combination chemotherapy	• Identification and treatment of cause
• Splenectomy	• Corticosteroids
	• Platelet transfusions
	• Romiplostim (Nplate)
	• Eltrombopag (Revolade)

CBC, complete blood count.

Acquired Thrombocytopenia From Decreased Platelet Production.

The management of acquired thrombocytopenia is based on identifying the cause and treating the disease or removing the causative agent. If the precipitating factor is unknown, the patient may receive corticosteroids. Platelet transfusions are given if life-threatening hemorrhage develops. Splenectomy is not used because the spleen does not contribute to this type of thrombocytopenia.

Often, acquired thrombocytopenia is caused by another underlying condition (e.g., aplastic anemia, leukemia) or therapy used to treat another problem. For example, in acute leukemia, all blood cell types may be depressed. In addition, the patient may receive chemotherapeutic drugs that cause bone marrow suppression. If the patient can be adequately supported throughout the course of chemotherapy-induced thrombocytopenia, the thrombocytopenia will also resolve.

NURSING MANAGEMENT: THROMBOCYTOPENIA

▪ Nursing Assessment

Subjective and objective data that should be obtained from a patient with thrombocytopenia are presented in Table 33-16.

NURSING ASSESSMENT

Table 33-16 Thrombocytopenia

Subjective Data

Important Health Information

Past health history: Recent hemorrhage, excessive bleeding, or viral illness; HIV infection; cancer (especially leukemia or lymphoma); aplastic anemia; systemic lupus erythematosus; cirrhosis; exposure to radiation or toxic chemicals; disseminated intravascular coagulation; family history of bleeding problems

Medications: See Table 33-12

Surgeries or other treatments: Recent surgery, splenectomy

Symptoms

• Bleeding gingiva; coffee-ground or bloody vomitus; epistaxis; hemoptysis; easy bruising, hematuria; dark or bloody stools; menorrhagia, metrorrhagia

• Headache; fatigue, weakness, fainting, general malaise

• Dyspnea

• Fever

Objective Data

General

Fever, lethargy

Integumentary

Petechiae, ecchymoses, purpura

Gastrointestinal

Splenomegaly, abdominal distension, guaiac-positive stools

Possible Findings

Platelet count $< 150 \times 10^9$ (150,000 per microlitre) or prolonged bleeding time, decreased hemoglobin and hematocrit; normal or increased megakaryocytes in bone marrow examination

HIV, human immunodeficiency virus.

NURSING CARE PLAN 33-2

Thrombocytopenia

NURSING DIAGNOSIS	**Impaired oral mucous membrane** *related to* low platelet counts and/or effects of pathological conditions and treatment *as evidenced by* oral bleeding and blood-filled bullae
Expected Patient Outcomes	**Nursing Interventions and *Rationales***
• Experiences lesion-free oral mucosa without bleeding	• Monitor lips, tongue, mucous membranes, tonsillar fossae, and gums for moisture, colour, texture, and presence of debris and infection using good lighting and a tongue blade *to provide information for planning interventions.*
	• Assist the patient to select soft, bland, and nonacidic foods *to decrease irritation of oral mucosa.*
	• Provide oral hygiene with minimal friction: use soft-bristle toothbrush, cotton swabs, mild mouthwash, or irrigating syringe *to gently cleanse mouth without trauma.*
	• Instruct and assist patient to perform oral hygiene after eating and as often as needed *to avoid breakdown of oral mucosa.*
NURSING DIAGNOSIS	**Risk for bleeding** *related to* low platelet count and treatments
Expected Patient Outcomes	**Nursing Interventions and *Rationales***
• Maintains tissue integrity • Has no evidence of bleeding or bruising	• Monitor for signs and symptoms of persistent bleeding (e.g., check all secretions for frank or occult blood) *to detect internal bleeding.*
	• Monitor coagulation studies, including prothrombin time (PT) and international normalized ratio (INR), partial thromboplastin time (PTT), fibrinogen, fibrin degradation or fibrin split products, and platelet counts *to determine bleeding risk.*
	• Avoid injections (IV, IM, and subcut) when possible *to prevent bleeding into tissue surrounding puncture site.*
	• Use electric razor for shaving *to reduce potential for skin nicks.*
	• Protect patient from trauma *to reduce tissue trauma and subsequent bleeding into tissue.*
	• Administer blood products (e.g., platelets, fresh-frozen plasma) *to replace coagulation factors.*
	• Teach patient to avoid aspirin or other anticoagulants *to prevent additional bleeding risk.*

IM, intramuscular; *IV,* intravenous; *subcut,* subcutaneous.

■ Nursing Diagnoses

Nursing diagnoses for the patient with thrombocytopenia may include, but are not limited to, those presented in NCP 33-2.

■ Planning

The overall goals are that the patient with thrombocytopenia will (1) have no gross or occult bleeding, (2) maintain vascular integrity, and (3) manage home care to prevent any complications related to an increased risk for bleeding.

■ Nursing Implementation

■ Health Promotion

It is important for the nurse to discourage excessive use of over-the-counter medications known to be possible causes of acquired thrombocytopenia. Many medications contain aspirin as an ingredient. Aspirin reduces platelet adhesiveness, thus contributing to bleeding. It is also important for the nurse to encourage people to have a complete medical evaluation if manifestations of bleeding tendencies (e.g., prolonged epistaxis, petechiae) develop. In addition, the nurse must observe for early signs of thrombocytopenia in the patient receiving cancer chemotherapy drugs.

■ Acute Intervention

The goal during acute episodes of thrombocytopenia is to prevent or control hemorrhage (see NCP 33-2). In the patient with thrombocytopenia, bleeding is usually from superficial sites; deep bleeding (into muscles, joints, and abdomen) usually occurs only when clotting factors are diminished. It is important to emphasize to the patient that a seemingly minor nosebleed or new petechiae may indicate potential hemorrhage and that the health care provider should be notified. Bleeding from the posterior nasopharynx may be difficult to detect because the blood may be swallowed. If a subcutaneous injection is unavoidable, a small-gauge needle should be used and direct pressure applied for at least 5 to 10 minutes after injection; application of an ice pack may also be helpful; IM injections should be avoided. The patient needs to understand the importance of adherence to self-care measures that reduce the risk of bleeding (Table 33-17).

In a woman with thrombocytopenia, the amount and duration of menstrual blood loss may exceed the usual. Counting sanitary napkins used during menses is another important intervention to detect excess blood loss. Fifty millilitres of blood will completely soak a sanitary napkin. Suppression of menses with hormonal agents may be indicated during predictable periods of thrombocytopenia to reduce blood loss from menses (e.g., during chemotherapy and bone marrow transplantation).

The proper administration of platelet transfusions is an important nursing responsibility. This is discussed under Blood Component Therapy later in this chapter.

PATIENT & CAREGIVER TEACHING GUIDE
Table 33-17 Thrombocytopenia

This instruction sheet explains precautions you should take to protect yourself when your platelet count is low. Please make sure to ask your health care provider about specific precautions you should take that relate to your bleeding risk factors.

• Notify your health care provider of any manifestations of bleeding.

These include the following:

• Black, tarry, or bloody bowel movements
• Black or bloody vomit, sputum, or urine
• Bruising or small red or purple spots on the skin
• Bleeding from the mouth or anywhere in the body
• Headache or changes in how well you can see
• Difficulty talking, sudden weakness of an arm or leg, or feeling confused

• Ask your health care provider regarding restrictions in your normal activities, such as vigorous exercise, lifting weights, and so on. Generally, walking can be done safely and should be done while wearing sturdy shoes or slippers. If you are weak and at risk for falling, get help or supervision when getting out of bed.

• Do not blow your nose forcefully; gently pat it with a tissue if needed. For a nosebleed, keep your head up and apply firm pressure to the nostrils and the bridge of your nose. If bleeding continues, place an ice bag over the bridge of your nose and the nape of your neck. If you are unable to stop a nosebleed after 10 min, call your health care provider.

• Do not bend down with your head lower than your waist.

• Prevent constipation by drinking plenty of fluids, and do not strain when having a bowel movement. Your health care provider may prescribe a stool softener. Do not use a suppository, an enema, or a rectal thermometer without the permission of your health care provider.

• Shave only with an electric razor; do not use blades.

• Do not pluck your eyebrows or other body hair.

• Do not puncture your skin, such as by getting tattoos or body piercing.

• Avoid using any medication (e.g., aspirin) or herbal product that can prolong clotting time. If you are unsure about a connection between any medication or herbal product and your thrombocytopenia, check with your health care provider or pharmacist.

• Use a soft-bristle toothbrush to prevent injuring the gums. Flossing is also usually safe if it is done gently using the thin tape floss. Do not use alcohol-based mouthwashes because they can dry your gums and increase bleeding.

• Women who are menstruating should keep track of the number of pads that are used per day. When you start using more pads per day than usual or bleed more days, notify your health care provider. Do not use tampons; use sanitary pads only.

• Ask your health care provider before you have any invasive procedures done, such as a dental cleaning, manicure, or pedicure.

■ Ambulatory and Home Care

The patient with ITP who is receiving treatment should be monitored for response to therapy. The person with acquired thrombocytopenia must be taught to avoid causative agents when possible (see Table 33-12). If the causative agents cannot be avoided (e.g., chemotherapy), the patient should learn to avoid injury or trauma during these periods and to detect the clinical signs and symptoms of bleeding caused by thrombocytopenia (see Table 33-17). Patients with either ITP or acquired thrombocytopenia should have periodic medical evaluations so the health care provider can assess the patient's status and intercede in situations in which exacerbations and bleeding are likely to occur.

■ Evaluation

The expected outcomes for the patient with thrombocytopenia are presented in NCP 33-2.

Hemophilia and von Willebrand's Disease

Hemophilia is an X-linked recessive genetic disorder caused by defective or deficient coagulation factor (see the Genetics in Clinical Practice box later and Figure 15-9). (X-linked genetic disorders are discussed in Chapter 15.) The two major forms of hemophilia, which can occur in mild to severe forms, are hemophilia A (classic hemophilia, Factor VIII deficiency) and hemophilia B (Christmas disease, Factor IX deficiency); von Willebrand's disease is a related disorder involving a deficiency of the von Willebrand's coagulation protein. Factor VIII is synthesized in the liver and circulates as a complex with vWF (Lenting, Pegon, Christophe, & Denis, 2010).

Hemophilia A is the most common form of hemophilia, accounting for approximately 80% of all cases. In Canada, both

GENETICS IN CLINICAL PRACTICE
Hemophilia A and B

Genetic Basis
• X-linked recessive disorder
• Mutations in gene that encodes clotting Factor VIII (hemophilia A) or IX (hemophilia B)

Incidence
• 1 in 5000 to 10,000 male births (hemophilia A)
• 1 in 30,000 to 50,000 male births (hemophilia B)

Genetic Testing
• Possible with DNA technology

Clinical Implications
• Female carriers will transmit the genetic defect to 50% of their sons, and 50% of their daughters will be carriers.
• Men with hemophilia will not transmit the genetic defect to their sons, but all of their daughters will be carriers.
• Female hemophilia can occur if a man with hemophilia mates with a female carrier. However, this is a rare occurrence.
• Clinical manifestations of hemophilias A and B are very similar.
• Replacement therapy is available for Factors VIII and IX (see Table 33-19).

Table 33-18 Comparison of Types of Hemophilia		
DISORDER	**DEFICIENCY**	**INHERITANCE PATTERN**
Hemophilia A	Factor VIII	Recessive X-linked (transmitted by female carriers, displayed almost exclusively in men)
Hemophilia B	Factor IX	Recessive X-linked (transmitted by female carriers, displayed almost exclusively in men)
von Willebrand's disease	vWF; variable Factor VIII deficiencies and platelet dysfunction	Autosomal dominant, seen in both sexes Recessive (in severe forms of the disease)

vWF, von Willebrand's factor.

hemophilia A and hemophilia B are rare disorders. About 2500 Canadians are known to be affected by hemophilia A and about 500 Canadians by hemophilia B. von Willebrand's disease is considered the most common congenital bleeding disorder and is estimated to affect as many as 1 in 1000 Canadians (Canadian Hemophilia Society, 2012). This disease can exist in mild to severe forms; however, life-threatening hemorrhage is rare. The deficiency and inheritance patterns of these three forms of inherited coagulopathies are compared in Table 33-18.

Clinical Manifestations and Complications

Clinical manifestations and complications related to hemophilia include (1) slow, persistent, prolonged bleeding from minor trauma and small cuts; (2) delayed bleeding after minor injuries (the delay may be several hours or days); (3) uncontrollable hemorrhage after dental extractions or irritation of the gingiva with a hard-bristle toothbrush; (4) epistaxis, especially after a blow to the face; (5) GI bleeding from ulcers and gastritis; (6) hematuria from GU trauma and splenic rupture resulting from falls or abdominal trauma; (7) ecchymoses and subcutaneous hematomas (Figure 33-9); (8) neurological signs, such as pain, anaesthesia, and paralysis, that may develop from nerve compression caused by hematoma formation; and (9) hemarthrosis (bleeding into the joints) (Figure 33-10), which may lead to joint deformity severe enough to cause crippling (most commonly in knees, elbows, shoulders, hips, and ankles).

These symptoms in children may lead to diagnosis during childhood. In adults, these developments may be the first sign of a mild form of the disease that escaped detection because of a childhood free of major injuries, dental procedures, or surgeries. All clinical manifestations relate to bleeding, and any bleeding episode in people with hemophilia may lead to a life-threatening hemorrhage.

Historically, hemophilia was a disease of childhood because of early death from complications. In the early 1900s, the average life expectancy was 11 years. By the 1970s, advances in treatment enabled people with hemophilia to have an average life expectancy of 68 years. Unfortunately, the acquired immune deficiency syndrome (AIDS) epidemic and the HIV contamination of blood products reduced average life expectancy to 49 years in the late

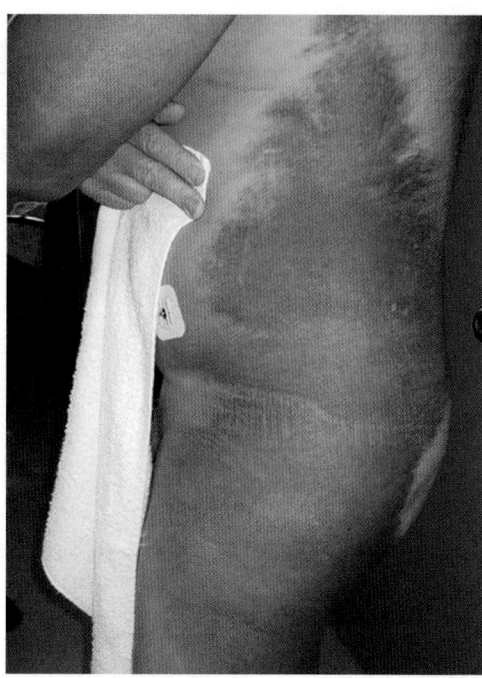

Figure 33-9 Severe ecchymoses in a person with hemophilia following a fall.

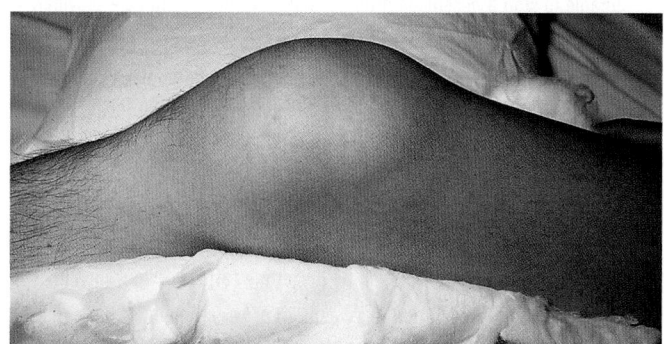

Figure 33-10 Acute hemarthrosis of the knee is a common complication of hemophilia.

Source: Forbes, C. D., & Jackson, W. F. (2003). *Color atlas and text of clinical medicine* (3rd ed., p. 441, Figure 10.106). London: Mosby.

1980s. However, longer-term survival (≤72 yr of age) is now being observed because of improved preparation of replacement products, improved screening of donor populations, and use of recombinant replacement factors.

Diagnostic Studies

Laboratory studies are used to determine the type of hemophilia present. Any factor deficiency within the intrinsic system (Factors VIII, IX, XI, or XII or vWF) will yield the laboratory results presented in Table 33-19.

Collaborative Care

The goals of collaborative care are to prevent and treat bleeding. Collaborative care for people with hemophilia or von Wille-

Table 33-19 Laboratory Results in Hemophilia

TEST	COMMENTS
Prothrombin time	No involvement of extrinsic system
Thrombin time	No impairment of thrombin–fibrinogen reaction
Platelet count	Adequate platelet production
Partial thromboplastin time	Prolonged because of deficiency in any intrinsic clotting system factor
Bleeding time	Prolonged in von Willebrand's disease because of structurally defective platelets; normal in hemophilias A and B because platelets not affected
Factor assays	Reduction of Factor VIII in hemophilia A; vWF in von Willebrand's disease; Factor IX in hemophilia B

vWF, von Willebrand's factor.

DRUG THERAPY

Table 33-20 Replacement Factors Used in Treating Hemophilia

Advate	Immunine
BeneFix	Kogenate FS
Helixate FS	Mononine
Humate P	Xyntha

Source: Adapted from Canadian Hemophilia Society. (2010). *Clotting factor concentrates.* Retrieved from *http://www.hemophilia.ca/en/bleeding-disorders/clotting-factor-concentrates/*

brand's disease calls for the provision of preventive care, the use of replacement therapy during acute bleeding episodes and as prophylaxis, and the treatment of the complications of the disease and its therapy.

Replacement of deficient clotting factors is the primary means of supporting a patient with hemophilia. In addition to treating acute crises, replacement therapy may be given before surgery and dental care as a prophylactic measure. Examples of replacement therapy are listed in Table 33-20. Fresh-frozen plasma, once commonly used for replacement therapy, is rarely used today.

For mild hemophilia A and certain subtypes of von Willebrand's disease, desmopressin acetate (also known as DDAVP), a synthetic analog of vasopressin, may be used to stimulate an increase in Factor VIII and vWF. This drug acts on endothelial cells to cause the release of vWF, which subsequently binds with Factor VIII, thus increasing their concentration. It can be administered intravenously, subcutaneously, or intranasally. Beneficial effects (e.g., decreased bleeding time) of DDAVP, when administered by IV, are seen within 30 minutes and can last for more than 12 hours. Because the effect of DDAVP is relatively short-lived, the patient must be closely monitored and repeated doses may be necessary. It is an appropriate therapy for minor bleeding episodes and dental procedures. The intranasal form may be indicated for home therapy for some patients with mild to moderate forms of the disease.

Antifibrinolytic therapy (e.g., tranexamic acid [Cyklokapron]) inhibits fibrinolysis by inhibiting plasminogen activation in the fibrin clot, thereby enhancing clot stability. These agents are useful therapeutic adjuncts to stabilize clots in areas of increased fibrinolysis, such as the oral cavity, and in patients with difficult-to-manage episodes of epistaxis and menorrhagia. Complications of treatment of hemophilia include development of inhibitors to Factors VIII or IX, transfusion-transmitted infectious disorders, allergic reactions, and with the use of Factor IX, thrombotic complications, because it contains activated coagulation factors. Patients with vWF may also develop alloantibodies against vWF, the infusion of which could cause life-threatening anaphylaxis; thus, replacement factors for these patients should be devoid of vWF. Because of the improved viral-detecting processes and donor screening practices, the risk of HIV and hepatitis B and C transmission is greatly reduced.

The most common difficulties with acute management are starting factor replacement therapy too late and stopping it too soon. Generally, minor bleeding episodes should be treated for at least 72 hours. Surgery and traumatic injuries may need more prolonged therapy. Chronically, development of inhibitors to the factor products has occurred and necessitates individualized expert patient management by the health care team.

Designated treatment centres have been established in Canada as well as many other countries to provide multidisciplinary care of hemophilia and related disorders. Gene therapy has been used on an experimental basis to treat hemophilia. These clinical trials have involved (1) removing cells from the patient and genetically modifying them to secrete Factor VIII or IX and (2) injecting vectors with the genes for Factors VIII and IX (Ragni, Kessler, & Lozier, 2009). (Gene therapy is discussed in Chapter 15.)

NURSING MANAGEMENT: HEMOPHILIA

Nursing Implementation

Health Promotion

Genetic counselling referral is especially important now that many people with hemophilia live into adulthood. Reproductive concerns and long-term effects are issues that the nurse should include in the patient's care plan.

Acute Intervention

Interventions are related primarily to controlling bleeding and include the following:

1. Stop the topical bleeding as quickly as possible by applying direct pressure or ice, packing the area with Gelfoam or fibrin foam, and applying topical hemostatic agents such as thrombin.
2. Administer the specific coagulation factor to raise the patient's level of the deficient coagulation factor. Monitor the patient for signs and symptoms, such as hypersensitivity.
3. When joint bleeding occurs, in addition to administering replacement factors, it is important to totally rest the involved joint to prevent crippling deformities from hemarthrosis. The joint may be packed in ice. Analgesics (e.g., acetaminophen, codeine) are given to reduce severe pain. However, aspirin and aspirin-containing compounds should never be used. As soon as bleeding ceases, it is important to

encourage mobilization of the affected area through range of motion exercises and physical therapy. Weight bearing is avoided until all swelling has resolved and muscle strength has returned.

4. Manage any life-threatening complication that may develop as a result of hemorrhage or adverse effects from coagulation factors or other medications, such as hyponatremia from use of desmopressin. Examples include nursing interventions to prevent or treat airway obstruction from hemorrhage into the neck and pharynx as well as early assessment and treatment of intracranial bleeding.

■ Ambulatory and Home Care

Home management is a primary consideration for the patient with hemophilia because the disease follows a progressive, chronic course. The quality and the length of life may be significantly affected by the patient's knowledge of the illness and how to live with it. The patient and family can be referred to a local treatment centre or the provincial chapter of the Canadian Hemophilia Society to encourage associations with other individuals who are dealing with the problems of hemophilia. The nurse must provide ongoing assessment of the patient's adaptation to the illness. Psychosocial support and assistance should be readily available as needed.

Most of the needed long-term care measures are related to patient teaching. The patient with hemophilia must be taught to recognize disease-related problems and to know which problems can be resolved at home and which necessitate hospitalization. Immediate medical attention is required for severe pain or swelling of a muscle or joint that restricts movement or inhibits sleep and for a head injury, a swelling in the neck or the mouth, abdominal pain, hematuria, melena, and skin wounds in need of suturing.

Daily oral hygiene must be performed without causing trauma. Understanding how to prevent injuries is another consideration. The patient can learn to participate in noncontact sports (e.g., golf) and wear gloves when doing household chores to prevent cuts or abrasions from knives, hammers, and other tools. The patient should wear medical alert identification to ensure that health care providers know about the hemophilia in case of an accident.

The patient needs information about routine follow-up care, and the compliance with scheduled visits must be assessed. A reliable person can be taught to self-administer some of the factor replacement therapies at home.

■ Evaluation

The overall expected outcomes are similar to those for the patient with thrombocytopenia and are presented in NCP 33-2.

Disseminated Intravascular Coagulation

Disseminated intravascular coagulation (DIC) is a serious bleeding and thrombotic disorder. It results from the abnormally initiated and accelerated clotting and anticlotting processes that occur in response to disease or injury. The term *disseminated*

intravascular coagulation can be misleading because it suggests that blood is clotting. In fact, the paradox of this condition is that it is characterized by the profuse bleeding that results from the depletion of platelets and clotting factors. An underlying disease or condition always causes DIC. The underlying disease must be treated for the DIC to resolve.

Etiology and Pathophysiology

DIC is not a disease; it is an abnormal response of the normal clotting cascade stimulated by a disease process or disorder. The diseases and disorders known to predispose a patient to DIC are listed in Table 33-21. DIC can occur as an acute, catastrophic condition, or it may exist at a subacute or chronic level. Each condition may have one or multiple triggering mechanisms to start the clotting cascade. For example, tumours and traumatized or necrotic tissue release tissue factors into circulation. Endotoxin from Gram-negative bacteria activates several steps in the coagulation cascade (Opal, 2010).

Tissue factor is released at the site of tissue injury and by some malignancies, such as leukemia, and causes normal coagulation mechanisms to be enhanced. Abundant intravascular thrombin, the most powerful coagulant, is produced (Figure 33-11). It catalyzes the conversion of fibrinogen to fibrin and enhances platelet aggregation. There is widespread fibrin and platelet deposition in capillaries and arterioles, resulting in thrombosis; this can lead to multiorgan failure. In addition, clotting inhibitory

Table 33-21 Predisposing Conditions to Development of Disseminated Intravascular Coagulation	
Acute Disseminated Intravascular Coagulation	• Tissue damage
• Shock	• Extensive burns and trauma
• Hemorrhagic	• Heatstroke
• Cardiogenic	• Severe head injury
• Anaphylactic	• Transplant rejections
• Septicemia	• Postoperative damage, especially after extracorporeal membrane oxygenation
• Hemolytic processes	• Fat and pulmonary emboli
• Transfusion of mismatched blood	• Snakebites
• Acute hemolysis from infection or immunological disorders	• Glomerulonephritis
	• Acute anoxia (e.g., after cardiac arrest)
• Obstetric conditions	• Prosthetic devices
• Abruptio placentae	• Fulminant hepatitis
• Amniotic fluid embolism	**Subacute Disseminated Intravascular Coagulation**
• Septic abortion	• Malignant disease
• Malignancies	• Myeloproliferative and lymphoproliferative malignancies
• Acute leukemia	• Metastatic cancer
• Lymphoma	• Obstetric: retained dead fetus
• Tumour lysis syndrome	**Chronic Disseminated Intravascular Coagulation**
	• Liver disease
	• Systemic lupus erythematosus
	• Localized malignancy

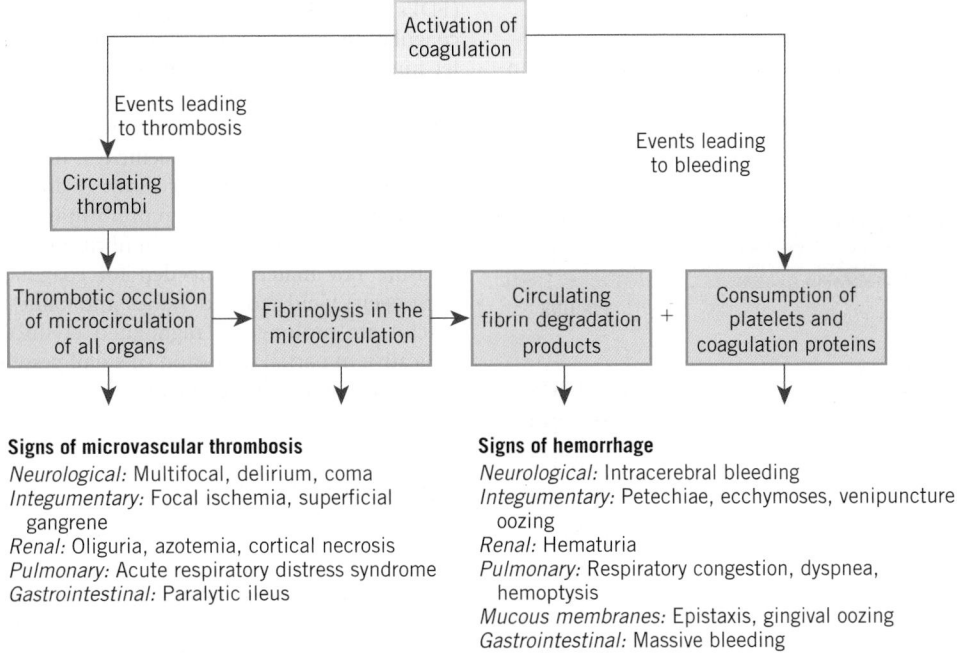

Signs of microvascular thrombosis
Neurological: Multifocal, delirium, coma
Integumentary: Focal ischemia, superficial gangrene
Renal: Oliguria, azotemia, cortical necrosis
Pulmonary: Acute respiratory distress syndrome
Gastrointestinal: Paralytic ileus

Signs of hemorrhage
Neurological: Intracerebral bleeding
Integumentary: Petechiae, ecchymoses, venipuncture oozing
Renal: Hematuria
Pulmonary: Respiratory congestion, dyspnea, hemoptysis
Mucous membranes: Epistaxis, gingival oozing
Gastrointestinal: Massive bleeding

Figure 33-11 The sequence of events that occur during disseminated intravascular coagulation.

mechanisms, such as antithrombin III (AT III) and protein C, are depressed. This excessive clotting activates the fibrinolytic system, which in turn breaks down the newly formed clot, creating fibrin split products (FSPs; fibrin degradation products [FDPs]). These products have anticoagulant properties and inhibit normal blood clotting. Ultimately, with FSPs accumulating and clotting factors being depleted, the blood loses its ability to clot. Therefore, a stable clot cannot be formed at injury sites. This situation predisposes the patient to hemorrhage.

Chronic and subacute DIC are most commonly seen in patients with longstanding illnesses such as malignant disorders or autoimmune diseases. The incidence of DIC associated with malignancy ranges from 10 to 75%. Occasionally, these patients have subclinical disease manifested only by laboratory abnormalities. However, the clinical spectrum ranges from easy bruising to hemorrhage and from hypercoagulability to thrombosis.

Clinical Manifestations

There is no well-defined sequence of events in acute DIC. Bleeding in a person with no previous history or obvious cause should be questioned because it may be one of the first manifestations of acute DIC. Other nonspecific manifestations can include weakness, malaise, and fever.

There are both bleeding and thrombotic manifestations in DIC. Bleeding manifestations of DIC are multifactorial (see Figure 33-11) and result from consumption and depletion of platelets and coagulation factors as well as from clot lysis and formation of FSPs that have anticoagulant properties. Bleeding manifestations include (1) integumentary manifestations, such as pallor, petechiae, purpura (Figure 33-12), oozing blood, venipuncture site bleeding, hematomas, and occult hemorrhage; (2) respiratory manifestations, such as tachypnea, hemoptysis, and orthopnea; (3) cardiovascular manifestations, such as tachycardia and hypotension; (4) GI manifestations, such as upper and lower GI bleeding, abdominal distension, and bloody stools;

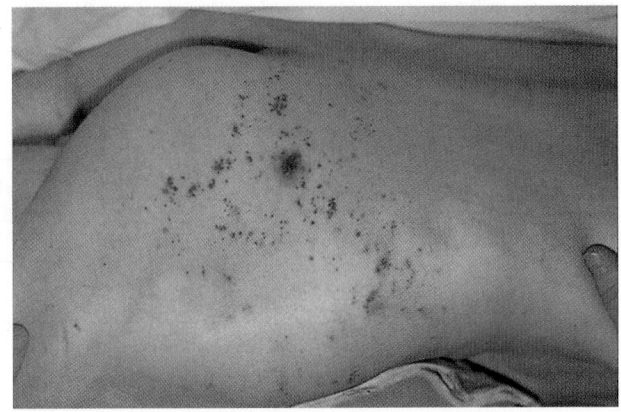

Figure 33-12 Disseminated intravascular coagulation resulting from staphylococcal septicemia. Note the characteristic skin hemorrhage ranging from small purpuric lesions to larger ecchymoses.

Source: Forbes, D. D., & Jackson, W. F. (2003). *Color atlas and text of clinical medicine* (3rd ed., p. 443, Figure 10.110). London: Mosby.

(5) urinary manifestations, such as hematuria; (6) neurological changes, such as vision changes, dizziness, headache, changes in mental status, and irritability; and (7) musculoskeletal complaints, such as bone and joint pain.

Thrombotic manifestations are a result of fibrin or platelet deposition in the microvasculature (see Figure 33-11) and include integumentary changes, such as cyanosis, ischemic tissue necrosis (e.g., gangrene), and hemorrhagic necrosis; respiratory changes, such as tachypnea, dyspnea, pulmonary emboli, and acute respiratory distress syndrome (ARDS); cardiovascular changes, such as electrocardiogram (ECG) changes and venous distension; GI changes, such as abdominal pain and paralytic ileus; and urinary changes, such as oliguria, leading to renal failure.

Diagnostic Studies

Tests used to diagnose acute DIC and their findings are listed in Table 33-22. As more clots are made in the body, more breakdown products from fibrinogen and fibrin are also formed. These are termed *fibrin split products* (FSPs) or *fibrin degradation products*

Table 33-22 Laboratory Abnormalities of Acute Disseminated Intravascular Coagulation	
TEST	**FINDING**
Screening Tests	
Prothrombin time (PT)	Prolonged
Partial thromboplastin time (PTT)	Prolonged
Activated partial thromboplastin time (aPTT)	Prolonged
Thrombin time	Prolonged
Fibrinogen	Reduced
Platelets	Reduced
Special Tests	
Fibrin split products (FSPs)	Elevated
Factor assays (for Factors V, VII, VIII, X, XIII)	Reduced
D-dimers (cross-linked fibrin fragments)	Elevated
Euglobin lysis time (ELT)	Elevated
Antithrombin III (AT III)	Reduced
Protein S	Reduced
Protein C	Reduced

(FDPs), and they work in three ways to interfere with blood coagulation. First, they coat the platelets and interfere with platelet function. Second, they interfere with thrombin and thereby disrupt coagulation. Third, the FSPs attach to fibrinogen, which interferes with the polymerization process necessary to form a stable clot. A much more specific test that is replacing measurement of FSP is the D-dimer assay. D-dimer, a specific polymer resulting from the breakdown of fibrin (and not fibrinogen), is a specific marker for the degree of fibrinolysis. In general, tests that measure raw materials needed for coagulation (e.g., platelets, fibrinogen) yield reduced values and values that indicate times to clot are prolonged. Fragmented erythrocytes (schistocytes), indicative of partial occlusion of small vessels by fibrin thrombi, may be found on blood smears.

Collaborative Care

It is important to diagnose DIC quickly, stabilize the patient's condition if needed, institute therapy that will resolve the underlying causative disease or problem, and provide supportive care for the manifestations resulting from the pathology of DIC itself. The treatment of DIC remains controversial and under investigation as researchers attempt to determine the most suitable means of managing this dangerous syndrome. Consequently, it is imperative that the nurse maintain an ongoing awareness of current modes of therapy. Diagnosing and treating the primary disease process is essential to the resolution of DIC.

Depending on its severity, a variety of different methods are used to provide supportive and symptomatic management of DIC (Figure 33-13). First, if chronic DIC is diagnosed in a patient

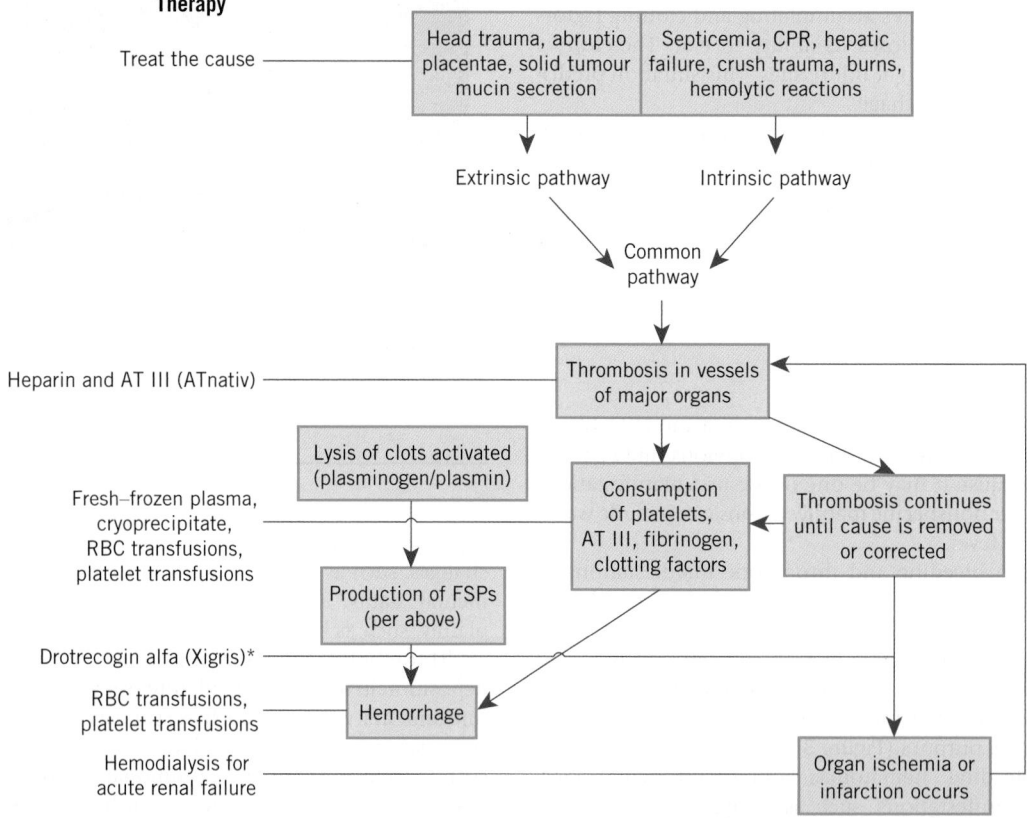

Figure 33-13 Intended sites of action for therapies in disseminated intravascular coagulation (DIC). *AT III*, antithrombin III; *CPR*, cardiopulmonary resuscitation; *FSPs*, fibrin split products; *RBC*, red blood cell. *Recombinant form of activated protein C.

who is not bleeding, no therapy for DIC is necessary. Treatment of the underlying disease may be sufficient to reverse the DIC (e.g., chemotherapy when DIC is caused by malignancy). Second, when the patient with DIC is bleeding, therapy is directed toward providing support with necessary blood products while treating the primary disorder. The blood products are administered on the basis of specific component deficiencies. Blood product support with platelets, cryoprecipitate, and fresh-frozen plasma is usually reserved for a patient with life-threatening hemorrhage. The concern is that one is adding "fuel to the fire" of already activated coagulation. However, it may be the only method to prevent death in some patients with severe hemorrhage. Therapy will stabilize a patient, prevent exsanguination or massive thrombosis, and permit institution of definitive therapy to treat the underlying cause.

A patient with manifestations of thrombosis is often treated by anticoagulation with heparin or low–molecular weight heparin. However, the use of heparin in the treatment of DIC remains controversial. AT III (ATnativ) is sometimes used in fulminant DIC, although it increases the risk of bleeding. Chronic DIC does not respond to oral anticoagulants, but it can be controlled with long-term use of heparin.

NURSING MANAGEMENT: DISSEMINATED INTRAVASCULAR COAGULATION

Nursing Diagnoses

Nursing diagnoses for the patient with DIC may include, but are not limited to, the following:
- Ineffective peripheral tissue perfusion *related to* bleeding and sluggish or diminished blood flow secondary to thrombosis
- Acute pain *related to* bleeding into tissues and diagnostic procedures
- Decreased cardiac output *related to* fluid volume deficit and hypotension
- Anxiety *related to* fear of the unknown, disease process, diagnostic procedures, and therapy

Nursing Implementation

Nurses must be alert to the possible development of DIC and especially to the precipitating factors listed in Table 33-21. This may be difficult because the nurse is focusing on the complex care often required by the primary problem that precipitated the DIC. The nurse must also remember that, because DIC is secondary to an underlying disease, appropriate care for managing the causative problem must be provided while providing supportive care related to the manifestations of DIC (Wada et al., 2010)

Appropriate nursing interventions are essential to the survival of a patient with acute DIC. Astute, ongoing assessment, active attention to manifestations of the syndrome, and institution of appropriate treatment measures are challenging and sometimes counterintuitive nursing responsibilities (e.g., administering heparin to a bleeding patient). Early detection of bleeding, both occult and overt, must be a primary goal. Table 33-15 and NCP 33-2 provide assessments and interventions appropriate for the patient with DIC. Early detection of bleeding, both occult and overt, must be a primary goal. Assess for signs of external bleeding (e.g., petechiae, oozing at IV or injection sites) and signs of internal bleeding (e.g., increased heart rate, changes in mental status, increasing abdominal girth, pain) as well as indications that microthrombi may be causing significant organ damage (e.g., decreased urinary output). Tissue damage should be minimized and the patient protected from additional foci of bleeding.

An additional nursing responsibility is to administer blood products and medications correctly. (Blood product transfusion is discussed later in this chapter.)

Neutropenia

Leukopenia refers to a decrease in the total WBC count (granulocytes, monocytes, and lymphocytes). *Granulocytopenia* is a deficiency of granulocytes, which include neutrophils, eosinophils, and basophils. The neutrophilic granulocytes, which play a major role in phagocytizing pathogenic microbes, are closely monitored in clinical practice as an indicator of a patient's risk for infection. A reduction in neutrophils is termed *neutropenia*. (Some clinicians use the terms *granulocytopenia* and *neutropenia* interchangeably because neutrophils constitute the largest proportion of granulocytes.) The *absolute neutrophil count* (ANC) is determined by multiplying the total WBC count by the percentage of neutrophils. **Neutropenia** is defined as a neutrophil count of less than 1 to 1.5×10^9/L or 1000 to 1500 per microlitre. Normally, neutrophils range from 2.5 to 7.5×10^9/L. However, in considering the clinical significance of neutropenia, it is important to know the rate of the decrease in the neutrophil count (gradual or rapid) and the degree and duration of neutropenia. The faster the drop and the longer it persists, the greater the likelihood of developing life-threatening infection, sepsis, and death. Other factors and co-morbid conditions— such as being older than 60 years of age, the presence of an existing infection, being in a hospital, having diabetes, and other factors—can increase the risk of a serious infection (Lukaszewicz & Payen, 2010).

Neutropenia is not a disease; it is a clinical consequence that occurs with a variety of conditions or diseases (Table 33-23). It can also be a predictable or an unanticipated adverse effect of taking certain drugs. The most common cause of neutropenia is iatrogenic, resulting from widespread use of chemotherapeutic and immunosuppressive therapy in the treatment of malignancies and autoimmune diseases.

Clinical Manifestations

The patient with neutropenia is predisposed to infection with nonpathogenic organisms that constitute normal body flora as well as opportunistic pathogens. When the WBC count is depressed or immature WBCs are present, normal phagocytic mechanisms are impaired. Also, because of the diminished phagocytic response, the classic signs of inflammation—redness, heat, and swelling—may not occur. WBCs are the major component of pus. Therefore, in the patient with neutropenia, pus formation (e.g., as a visible skin lesion or as pulmonary infiltrates on a chest radiograph) is also absent.

Table 33-23 Causes of Neutropenia

Drug Therapy

- Antitumour antibiotics (daunorubicin [Cerubidine], doxorubicin)
- Alkylating agents (nitrogen mustards, busulfan [Myleran])
- Antimetabolites (methotrexate, 6-mercaptopurine)
- Anti-inflammatory drugs (phenylbutazone)
- Psychotropics and antidepressants (clozapine, imipramine)
- Miscellaneous (gold, penicillamine, mepacrine, amodiaquine)
- Antimicrobial agents (zidovudine [Retrovir], trimethoprim–sulphamethoxazole)

Hematological Disorders

- Idiopathic neutropenia
- Fanconi's anemia
- Congenital (cyclical neutropenia)
- Aplastic anemia
- Leukemia
- Myelodysplastic syndrome

Autoimmune Disorders

- Systemic lupus erythematosus
- Felty's syndrome
- Rheumatoid arthritis

Infections

- Viral (e.g., hepatitis, influenza, HIV, measles)
- Fulminant bacterial infection (e.g., typhoid fever, miliary tuberculosis)
- Parasitic
- Rickettsial

Miscellaneous

- Severe sepsis
- Bone marrow infiltration (e.g., carcinoma, tuberculosis, lymphoma)
- Hypersplenism (e.g., portal hypertension, Felty's syndrome, storage diseases [e.g., Gaucher's disease])
- Nutritional deficiencies (cobalamin, folic acid)
- Transfusion reaction
- Hemodialysis

HIV, human immunodeficiency virus.

SAFETY ALERT

- Presence of a low-grade fever in neutropenic patients is of great significance because it may indicate infection and quickly lead to septic shock and death.
- A fever greater than 38°C and a neutrophil count less than 0.5×10^9/L is a medical emergency.

When fever occurs in a neutropenic patient, it is assumed to be caused by infection and calls for immediate attention. The immunocompromised, neutropenic patient has little or no ability to fight infection. Thus, minor infections can lead rapidly to sepsis. The mucous membranes of the throat and mouth, skin, perianal area, and pulmonary system are common entry points for pathogenic organisms in susceptible hosts. Clinical manifestations related to infection at these sites include

COLLABORATIVE CARE

Table 33-24 Neutropenia

Diagnostic	Collaborative Therapy
• History and physical examination • WBC count with differential • WBC morphology • Hct and Hb values • Reticulocyte and platelet count • Bone marrow aspiration or biopsy • Cultures of nose, throat, sputum, urine, stool, obvious lesions, blood (as indicated) • Chest radiograph	• Identification and removal of cause of neutropenia (if possible) • Identification of site of infection (if present) and causative organism • Antibiotic therapy • Hematopoietic growth factors (G-CSF, GM-CSF, pegfilgrastim [Neulasta]) • Strict adherence to handwashing and patient hygiene protocols • Single-patient room, positive-pressure or HEPA filtration, depending on risk • Community isolation and home precautions if outpatient

G-CSF, granulocyte colony–stimulating factor; *GM-CSF,* granulocyte-macrophage colony–stimulating factor; *Hb,* hemoglobin; *Hct,* hematocrit; *HEPA,* high-efficiency particulate air; *WBC,* white blood cell.

complaints of sore throat and dysphagia, appearance of ulcerative lesions of the pharyngeal and the buccal mucosa, diarrhea, rectal tenderness, vaginal itching or discharge, shortness of breath, and nonproductive cough. Any minor complaint by the patient of pain or any other symptom should be taken seriously. These seemingly minor complaints can progress to fever, chills, sepsis, and septic shock if not recognized and treated in the early stages.

Systemic infections caused by bacterial, fungal, and viral organisms are common in patients with neutropenia. The patient's own flora (normally nonpathogenic) contributes significantly to life-threatening infections such as pneumonia. Organisms that are known to be common sources of infection include Gram-positive *Staphylococcus aureus* and aerobic Gram-negative organisms. Fungi that are involved include *Candida* (usually *C. albicans*) and *Aspergillus*. Viral infections caused by reactivation of herpes simplex and herpes zoster are common following prolonged periods of neutropenia, such as in bone marrow transplant patients.

Diagnostic Studies

The primary diagnostic tests for assessing neutropenia are the peripheral WBC count and bone marrow aspiration and biopsy (Table 33-24). A total WBC count of 4×10^9/L or 4000/mcL reflects leukopenia. However, only a differential count can confirm the presence of neutropenia (ANC of $1\text{-}1.5 \times 10^9$/L or 1000-1500/mcL). If the differential WBC count reflects an ANC of 0.5 to 1×10^9/L or 500 to 1000/mcL, the patient is at moderate risk for a bacterial infection. An ANC less than 0.5 to 1×10^9/L or 500 to 1000/mcL places the patient at severe risk.

A peripheral blood smear is used to assess for immature forms of WBCs (e.g., bands). The Hct level, the reticulocyte count, and the platelet count are performed to evaluate bone marrow function. A review of the patient's recent past and current drug history should also be done. If the cause of neutropenia is unknown, bone marrow aspirations and biopsies are performed to examine cellularity and cell morphology. Additional studies may be done as indicated to assess spleen and liver function.

NURSING AND COLLABORATIVE MANAGEMENT: NEUTROPENIA

The factors involved in the nursing and collaborative care of neutropenia include (1) determining the cause of the neutropenia; (2) identifying the offending organisms if an infection has developed; (3) instituting prophylactic, empirical, or therapeutic antibiotic therapy; (4) administering hematopoietic growth factors (e.g., granulocyte colony–stimulating factor [G-CSF] and granulocyte-macrophage colony–stimulating factor [GM-CSF]); and (5) instituting protective isolation practices, such as strict handwashing, visitor restrictions, and a private room if hospitalized; a positive-pressure or high-efficiency particulate air (HEPA) filtration may be used for patients undergoing hematopoietic stem cell transplantation (HSCT) (see Table 33-24).

Occasionally, the cause of the neutropenia can be easily treated (e.g., nutritional deficiencies). However, neutropenia can also be an adverse effect that must be tolerated as a necessary step in therapy (e.g., chemotherapy, radiation therapy). In some situations, the neutropenia resolves when the primary disease is treated (e.g., tuberculosis).

The nurse must monitor the neutropenic patient for signs and symptoms of infection (any fever ≥38°C) and early septic shock. Early identification of a potentially infective organism depends on acquiring cultures from various sites. Serial blood cultures (at least two) or one from a peripheral site and one from a venous access device should be done promptly and antibiotics started immediately. In addition, cultures of sputum, throat, lesions, wounds, urine, and feces may be required. It may also be necessary to do a tracheal aspiration, bronchoscopy with bronchial brushings, or lung biopsy to diagnose the cause of pneumonic infiltrates. Despite these many tests, the causative organism is identified in only approximately half of patients with neutropenia.

When a febrile episode occurs in a patient with neutropenia, antibiotic therapy must be initiated immediately (within 1 hr), even before the determination by culture of a specific causative organism. Broad-spectrum antibiotics are usually ordered by the IV route because of the potential lethal effects of infection. However, some oral antibiotics are highly effective and routinely used for prophylaxis against infection in some patients with neutropenia. Antibiotics are often used in combinations because of their synergistic effects and in the event that multiple organisms are responsible for the infectious symptoms. Regardless of the combination, the nurse must initiate therapy promptly and observe for adverse effects of antimicrobial agents. Adverse effects common to aminoglycosides include nephrotoxicity and ototoxicity; adverse effects common to cephalosporins include rashes, fever, and pruritus.

The extended duration of neutropenia increases the infection risk of the patient. The longer the neutropenia lasts, the greater

NURSING CARE PLAN 33-3

Neutropenia	
NURSING DIAGNOSIS	**Risk for infection** related to decreased neutrophils, altered response to microbial invasion, and presence of environmental pathogens
Expected Patient Outcomes	**Nursing Interventions and *Rationales***
• Adheres to infection control and protection practices • Experiences no signs and symptoms of infection	**Infection Control** • Institute designated isolation precautions *to reduce exposure to environmental pathogens.* • Wash hands with antimicrobial soap before and after each patient care activity *to prevent transmission of pathogens.* • Instruct visitors to wash hands on entering and leaving patient's room *to prevent the transmission of harmful pathogens to patient.* • Teach patient how to avoid infections (e.g., handwashing, oral care, skin hygiene, and pulmonary hygiene) *to reduce infection risk.* • Teach patient and caregivers about the signs and symptoms of infection, and when to report them to the health care provider *to receive early treatment of infection.* • Instruct patient to take antibiotics as prescribed *to prevent microbial resistance.* **Infection Protection** • Monitor for systemic and localized signs and symptoms of infection *to promote early detection of infection.* • Monitor absolute neutrophil count, WBC count, and differential results *to identify signs of and potential for infection.* • Inspect skin and mucous membranes for redness, extreme warmth, or drainage *to identify signs of infection.* • Follow neutropenic precautions *to avoid introduction of pathogens.* • Remove fresh flowers and plants from patient areas *to avoid introduction of pathogens.* • Report suspected infections to infection control personnel *to promptly initiate antibiotic therapy because of the rapidly lethal effects of infection.*

WBC, white blood cell.

the risk of a fungal infection. Antifungal therapy is initiated whenever a culture is positive or in patients who do not become afebrile with broad-spectrum antibiotic coverage.

G-CSF (filgrastim [Neupogen] and pegfilgrastim [Neulasta]) and GM-CSF can be used to prevent neutropenia or to reduce the severity and/or duration of neutropenia. They should be considered for patients after chemotherapy based on their risk factors for neutropenia. G-CSF stimulates the production and function of neutrophils. GM-CSF stimulates the production and function of neutrophils and monocytes. These agents can be given by intravenously or subcutaneously. Keratinocyte growth factor (palifermin) may also be used to reduce the duration and severity of mucositis, which may contribute to infection (Weigelt, Haas, & Kobbe, 2011). An important consideration in the care of a patient with neutropenia is the determination of the best means to protect the patient, whose own defences against infection are compromised. To accomplish this goal, the following principles must be kept in mind: (1) the patient's normal flora is the most common source of microbial colonization and infection; (2) transmission of organisms from humans most commonly occurs by direct contact with the hands; (3) air, food, water, and equipment provide additional opportunities for infection transmission; and (4) health care providers with transmissible illnesses and other patients with infections can also be sources of infection under certain conditions.

Handwashing is the single most important preventive measure in minimizing the risk of infection in the patient with neutropenia. Strict adherence to handwashing protocol by all people coming in contact with the compromised patient is the major method to prevent transmission of harmful pathogens. Immunocompromised patients should be separated from those who are infected or who have conditions that increase the probability of transmitting infections. Often, patients can be managed on an outpatient basis if the patient and caregivers can astutely monitor for fevers and other signs of infection and then report promptly to a nearby health care facility (Table 33-25). If the patient is hospitalized, private rooms should be used. HEPA filtration is an air-handling method with a high-flow filtering system that can reduce or eliminate the number of aerosolized pathogens in the environment. Although it is expensive to install, it is often used for a patient with severe, prolonged neutropenia (e.g., patients who have undergone bone marrow transplant). Care routines in a HEPA environment are essentially the same as care in any other private room. Prophylactic antibiotics and antifungals may also be used for severely immunocompromised patients.

Quality-of-life issues for the patient with neutropenia should not be overlooked. Potential patient experiences of fatigue, malaise, decrease in functioning, social isolation, and depression and perceived lack of support require appropriate interventions. In addition, the value of effective nursing care in reducing the development of infection or limiting its extent cannot be overemphasized. Regular assessment and early detection of infectious sources are key roles for the nurse in reducing morbidity and mortality rates from infection.

AGE-RELATED CONSIDERATIONS: THROMBOCYTOPENIA AND NEUTROPENIA

About 55 to 60% of cancers are currently diagnosed in individuals older than 65 years. This proportion is expected to further

PATIENT & CAREGIVER TEACHING GUIDE
Table 33-25 Neutropenia

This instruction sheet explains precautions you should take to protect yourself when your neutrophil count is low. Please make sure to ask your health care provider about specific precautions you should take that relate to your particular risk factors for infection.

- *Wash your hands* frequently and make sure those around you wash their hands frequently, particularly if they help with your care. An antibacterial hand gel may also be used.

- Notify your nurse or health care provider if you have any of the following:
  - A fever greater than 38°C
  - Chills, or you feel hot
  - Redness, swelling, discharge, or new painful area either on the skin or deeper in your body
  - Changes in urination or bowel movements
  - A cough, sore throat, mouth sores, or blisters

- If you are at home, take your temperature as directed and follow instructions on what to do if you have a fever.

- Avoid crowds and people with colds, flu, or infections. If you are in a public area, wear a mask.

- Avoid uncooked meats, seafood, eggs, and unwashed fruits and vegetables. Ask your health care provider about specific dietary guidelines for you.

- Bathe or shower daily. A moisturizer may be used to prevent skin from drying and cracking.

- Do not perform gardening or clean up after pets. Feeding and petting your dog or cat is fine as long as you wash your hands well after handling.

increase in the next 2 decades as the Baby Boomers move into this age group. Age-related changes of bone marrow function are rather subtle and probably not significant for the hematopoietic function of normal older individuals. These changes, however, may become clinically evident under conditions of severe hematopoietic stress, such as the administration of repeated courses of chemotherapy and/or radiation therapy and the resultant sequelae of myelosuppression (Gazit, Weissman, & Rossi, 2008). The use of supportive therapies, such as hematopoietic growth factors, increases the likelihood that older individuals will be treated with standard and even aggressive therapies, leading to neutropenia and thrombocytopenia. The nurse also needs to be aware that older individuals may have signs and symptoms different from those of a younger individual. For example, the older adult may have delirium as compared with cough as a clinical manifestation of pneumonia.

Myelodysplastic Syndrome

Myelodysplastic syndrome (MDS) is a group of related hematological disorders characterized by a change in the quantity and quality of bone marrow elements. Peripheral blood cytopenias in combination with a hypercellular bone marrow exhibiting dysplastic changes is the hallmark of MDS. Although it can occur in all age groups, the median age at diagnosis is 71 years (Barzi & Sekeres, 2010).

Etiology and Pathophysiology

The etiology of MDS is unknown. Its manifestations result from neoplastic transformation of the pluripotent hematopoietic stem cells within the bone marrow. Occasionally, one type of MDS transforms into another. In one third of patients, MDS progresses to acute myelogenous leukemia (AML) (Barzi & Sekeres, 2010). MDS is referred to as a clonal disorder because some bone marrow stem cells continue to function normally whereas others (a specific clone) do not. The abnormal clone of the stem cells is usually found in the bone marrow but eventually may be found in circulation. In contrast to AML, in which the leukemic cells show little normal maturation, the clonal cells in MDS always display some degree of maturity. Disease progression is slower than in AML. However, eventually, the abnormal cells replace the bone marrow. Typically, life-threatening anemia, thrombocytopenia, and neutropenia occur during the advanced stage of MDS.

Clinical Manifestations

MDS commonly manifests as infection and bleeding caused by inadequate numbers of ineffectively functioning circulating granulocytes or platelets. MDS is often discovered in the older adult in the course of investigating symptoms of anemia, thrombocytopenia, or neutropenia. It may also be diagnosed incidentally from a routine complete blood count.

Diagnostic Studies

Bone marrow biopsy with aspirate analysis is essential for both the diagnosis and the classification of the specific types of myelodysplasia. In MDS, the bone marrow is normocellular, hypocellular, or hypercellular, and the patient has peripheral cytopenia. Laboratory data and bone marrow studies will help rule out other causes of the dysplasia, such as nonmalignant disorders, cobalamin and folate deficiencies, and infectious causes. MDS is staged according to clinical and laboratory findings. The relationship between the number of circulating blast cells and the number of blast cells in the bone marrow serves as the main indicator of prognosis in this disease, as well as chromosomal aberrations, such as partial or total loss of chromosomes 5, 7, and Y or trisomy 8 (Haase, 2008).

NURSING AND COLLABORATIVE MANAGEMENT: MYELODYSPLASTIC SYNDROME

Supportive treatment of MDS is based on the premise that the aggressiveness of treatment should match the aggressiveness of the disease. Supportive treatment consists of hematological monitoring (serial bone marrow and peripheral blood examinations), antibiotic therapy, or transfusions with blood products. Adverse effects and toxicities from supportive treatment include anemia, thrombocytopenia, and blood transfusion reactions. The overall goal is to improve hematopoiesis and safeguard quality of life as far as possible.

Low-risk patients (<5% blasts in marrow) can often be treated with transfusions, antibiotics, antifungals, EPO, and hematopoietic growth factors. High-risk patients (>5% blasts in marrow) may be treated with single-agent chemotherapy (e.g., hydroxyurea) or intensive chemotherapy as in AML. Only about one third of high-risk patients are treated with intensive chemotherapy and/or bone marrow transplants.

Nursing care of a patient with MDS is similar to that of a patient with manifestations of anemia (see the NCPs for patients with anemia [NCP 33-1]), thrombocytopenia [NCP 33-2]), and neutropenia [NCP 33-3]).

Leukemia

Leukemia is a broad term given to a group of malignant diseases that affect the blood and blood-forming tissues of the bone marrow, lymph system, and spleen. Leukemia occurs in all age groups. It is characterized by diffuse replacement of bone marrow with proliferating leukocyte precursors. This loss of regulation in cell division results in an accumulation of dysfunctional cells. Leukemia follows a progressive course that is eventually fatal if untreated. In Canada, males account for 65% of the incidence of leukemia. In 2010, it was estimated that there would be 4800 new cases and 2500 deaths due to leukemia in Canada, and that males would account for more than 58% of new cases (Leukemia and Lymphoma Society of Canada, 2011). Although often thought of as a disease of children, the number of adults affected with leukemia is 10 times that of children (Siegel, Ward, Brawley, & Jemal, 2011).

Etiology and Pathophysiology

Regardless of the specific type of leukemia, there is generally no single causative agent in the disease's development. Most leukemias result from a combination of factors, including genetic and environmental influences. Chromosomal changes, first recognized in chronic myelogenous leukemia, have led to discoveries of how normal genes, once transformed, can result in abnormal genes (*oncogenes*) capable of causing many types of cancers, including leukemias (see Chapter 18). Chemical agents (e.g., benzene), chemotherapeutic agents (e.g., alkylating agents), viruses, radiation, and immunological deficiencies have all been associated with the development of leukemia in susceptible hosts. There is an increased incidence of leukemia in radiologists, people who have lived near nuclear bomb test sites or nuclear reactor accidents (e.g., Chernobyl), survivors of the bombing of Nagasaki and Hiroshima, and people previously treated with radiation therapy or chemotherapy. Although RNA retroviruses cause a number of leukemias in animals, a viral cause for a human leukemia has been established only for some patients with adult T-cell leukemia. This form of leukemia is endemic in southwestern Japan and parts of the Caribbean and central Africa and is caused by the human T-cell leukemia virus type 1 (HTLV-1).

Classification

Leukemia can be classified as either acute or chronic. The terms *acute* and *chronic* refer to cell maturity and the nature of disease's onset. *Acute leukemia* is characterized by the clonal proliferation of immature hematopoietic cells. The leukemia develops following malignant transformation of a single type of immature hematopoietic cell, followed by cellular replication and expansion of that malignant clone. *Chronic leukemias* involve more mature forms of WBCs, and the disease onset is more gradual.

Table 33-26 Types of Leukemia

TYPE	AGE OF ONSET	CLINICAL MANIFESTATIONS	DIAGNOSTIC FINDINGS
Acute myelogenous leukemia (AML)	Increase in incidence with advancing age; peak incidence between 60 and 70 yr of age	Fatigue and weakness, headache, mouth sores, anemia, bleeding, fever, infection, sternal tenderness, gingival hyperplasia, minimal hepatosplenomegaly and lymphadenopathy	Low RBC count, Hb, Hct; low platelet count; low to high WBC count with myeloblasts; high LDH, greatly hypercellular bone marrow with myeloblasts
Acute lymphocytic leukemia (ALL)	Before 14 yr of age, peak incidence between 2 and 9 yr of age; also in older adults	Fever; pallor; bleeding; anorexia; fatigue and weakness; bone, joint, and abdominal pain; generalized lymphadenopathy; infections; weight loss; hepatosplenomegaly; headache; mouth sores; neurological manifestations, including CNS involvement, increased intracranial pressure, secondary to meningeal infiltration	Low RBC count, Hb, Hct; low platelet count; low, normal, or high WBC count; high LDH; transverse lines of rarefaction at ends of metaphysis of long bones on radiograph; hypercellular bone marrow with lymphoblasts; lymphoblasts also possible in cerebrospinal fluid; presence of Philadelphia chromosome (20-25% of patients)
Chronic myelogenous leukemia (CML)	25-60 yr of age; peak incidence around 45 yr of age	No symptoms early in disease; then fatigue and weakness, fever, sternal tenderness, weight loss, joint pain, bone pain, massive splenomegaly, increase in sweating	Low RBC count, Hb, Hct; high platelet count early, lower count later; increase in polymorphonuclear neutrophils, normal number of lymphocytes, and normal or low number of monocytes in WBC differential; low leukocyte alkaline phosphatase; presence of Philadelphia chromosome (90% of patients)
Chronic lymphocytic leukemia (CLL)	50-70 yr of age; rare below 30 yr of age; predominance in men	No symptoms frequently; detection of disease often during examination for unrelated condition; chronic fatigue, anorexia, splenomegaly and lymphadenopathy and hepatomegaly; may progress to fever, night sweats, weight loss, fatigue, and frequent infections	Mild anemia and thrombocytopenia with disease progression; total WBC count > 100×10^9/L; increase in peripheral lymphocytes; increase in presence of lymphocytes in bone marrow; hypogammaglobulinemia; may have autoimmune hemolytic anemia (4-11%), idiopathic thrombocytopenia purpura (2-4%)

CNS, central nervous system; *Hb*, hemoglobin; *Hct*, hematocrit; *LDH*, lactic dehydrogenase; *RBC*, red blood cell; *WBC*, white blood cell.

Leukemia can also be classified by identifying the type of leukocyte involved, that is, whether it is of myelogenous origin or of lymphocytic origin. By combining the acute and chronic categories with the cell type involved, specific types of leukemia can be identified. Four major types of leukemia are acute lymphocytic leukemia (ALL), acute myelogenous leukemia (AML), chronic myelogenous (granulocytic) leukemia (CML), and chronic lymphocytic leukemia (CLL). Other defining features of these leukemic subtypes are presented in Table 33-26.

Acute Myelogenous Leukemia. AML represents only one fourth of all leukemias, but it makes up approximately 85% of the acute leukemias in adults. Its onset is often abrupt and dramatic. A patient may have serious infections and abnormal bleeding from the onset of the disease (Figure 33-14).

AML is characterized by uncontrolled proliferation of myeloblasts, the precursors of granulocytes. There is hyperplasia of the bone marrow and the spleen. The clinical manifestations are usually related to replacement of normal hematopoietic cells in the marrow by leukemic myeloblasts and, to a lesser extent, to infiltration of other organs (see Table 33-26.)

Acute Lymphocytic Leukemia. ALL is the most common type of leukemia in children and accounts for about 15% of acute leukemia in adults. Over the last several decades, the 5- and 10-year overall survival rates for ALL have improved in all ages, except for those patients older than 60 years (Schafer, Hunger, &

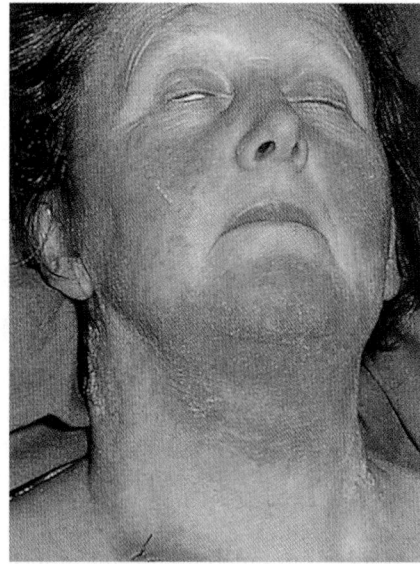

Figure 33-14 Complications of acute leukemia. Spreading cellulitis of the neck and chin in this woman with acute myelogenous leukemia results from streptococcal and candidal infection. She is at risk because of previous chemotherapy and prolonged neutropenia.

Source: Skarin, A. T. (1996). *Atlas of diagnostic oncology* (2nd ed.). London: Mosby-Wolfe.

Stephen, 2011). In ALL, immature lymphocytes proliferate in the bone marrow; most are of B-cell origin. Fever is present in the majority of patients at the time of diagnosis. Signs and symptoms may appear abruptly with bleeding or fever, or they may be insidious with progressive weakness, fatigue, and bleeding tendencies.

Central nervous system (CNS) manifestations are especially common in ALL and represent a serious problem. Leukemic meningitis caused by arachnoid infiltration occurs in many patients with ALL (Seif, Reilly, & Rheingold, 2010).

Chronic Myelogenous Leukemia.
CML is caused by excessive development of mature neoplastic granulocytes in the bone marrow. The excess neoplastic granulocytes move into the peripheral blood in massive numbers and ultimately infiltrate the liver and the spleen. These cells contain a distinctive cytogenetic abnormality, the *Philadelphia chromosome*, which serves as a disease marker and results from translocation of genetic material between chromosomes 9 and 22.

The natural history of CML is a chronic stable phase followed by the development of a more acute, aggressive phase referred to as the *blastic phase*. The chronic phase of CML can last for several years and can usually be well controlled with treatment. Even with treatment, the chronic phase of the disease will eventually progress to the accelerated phase, ending in a blastic phase. Once CML transforms to an acute or blastic phase, it is often refractory to therapy, and the patient may live for only a few months.

Chronic Lymphocytic Leukemia.
CLL is the most common leukemia in adults. CLL is characterized by the production and accumulation of functionally inactive but long-lived, mature-appearing lymphocytes. The type of lymphocyte involved is usually the B cell. The lymphocytes infiltrate the bone marrow, spleen, and liver. Lymph node enlargement (lymphadenopathy) is present throughout the body, and there is an increased incidence of infection because of T-cell deficiencies or hypogammaglobulinemia. B-cell CLL is considered to be identical to the mature B-cell small lymphocytic lymphoma, a type of non-Hodgkin's lymphoma. Complications from early-stage CLL are rare but may develop as the disease advances. Pressure on nerves from enlarged lymph nodes causes pain and even paralysis. Mediastinal node enlargement leads to pulmonary symptoms. Because CLL is usually a disease of older adults, treatment decisions must be made by considering the progression of the disease and the adverse effects of treatment. Many individuals in the early stages of CLL require no treatment. Others may be followed closely and receive treatment only when the disease progresses.

Other Leukemias.
Occasionally, the subtype of leukemia cannot be identified. The malignant leukemic cells may have lymphoid, myeloid, or mixed characteristics. Frequently, these patients do not respond to treatment and have a poor prognosis. Other rare types include hairy cell and biphenotypic leukemias.

Clinical Manifestations

The clinical manifestations of leukemia are varied (see Table 33-26). Essentially, they relate to problems caused by bone marrow failure and the formation of leukemic infiltrates. Bone marrow failure results from (1) bone marrow overcrowding by abnormal cells and (2) inadequate production of normal marrow elements. The patient is predisposed to anemia, thrombocytopenia, and decreased number and function of WBCs.

As leukemia progresses, fewer normal blood cells are produced. The abnormal WBCs continue to accumulate because they do not go through the normal cell life cycle to death *(apoptosis)*. The leukemic cells infiltrate the patient's organs, leading to problems such as splenomegaly, hepatomegaly, lymphadenopathy, bone pain, meningeal irritation, and oral lesions. Solid masses resulting from collections of leukemic cells called *chloromas* can also occur.

Diagnostic Studies

Peripheral blood evaluation and bone marrow examination are the primary methods of diagnosing and classifying the subtypes of leukemia. Morphological, histochemical, immunological, and cytogenetic methods are all used to identify cell subtypes and the stage of development of leukemic cell populations. This is important because different subtypes have different natural histories, prognoses, and chemotherapeutic regimens. Other studies such as lumbar puncture and computed tomography (CT) scan can determine the presence of leukemic cells outside of the blood and the bone marrow.

The malignant cells in most patients with AML and ALL have chromosomal abnormalities. In some cases, specific cytogenetic abnormalities are associated with distinct subsets of the disease. In addition to establishing the type of AML or ALL, specific cytogenetic abnormalities have diagnostic, prognostic, and therapeutic importance. In CML, the finding of the Philadelphia chromosome has diagnostic value.

Collaborative Care

Once a diagnosis of leukemia has been made, collaborative care is focused on the initial goal of attaining remission. Age and chromosome analysis often help form the basis of important treatment decisions. Because cytotoxic chemotherapy is the mainstay of the treatment, the nurse must understand the principles of cancer chemotherapy, including cellular kinetics, the use of multiple drugs rather than single agents, and the cell cycle. (See the section on chemotherapy in Chapter 18.)

In some cases, such as with asymptomatic patients who have CLL, watchful waiting with active supportive care may be appropriate. Although a patient may not be cured, attaining remission or disease control is a realistic option for the majority of patients. In *complete remission*, there is no evidence of overt disease on physical examination, and the bone marrow and peripheral blood appear normal. A lesser state of control is known as partial remission. *Minimal residual disease* is defined as tumour cells that cannot be detected by morphological examination, but can be detected by molecular testing. *Partial remission* is characterized by a lack of symptoms and a normal peripheral blood smear, but there is still evidence of disease in the bone marrow. *Molecular remission* indicates that all molecular studies are negative for residual leukemia. The patient's prognosis is directly related to the ability to maintain a remission and becomes more unfavourable with each relapse. Each time there is a relapse, the succeeding remission may be more difficult to achieve and shorter in duration.

Sometimes patients have such a high WBC count that initial emergent treatment may employ the use of leukapheresis and hydroxyurea administration. The purpose of these treatments is to reduce the WBC count and the risk of leukemia-induced thrombosis.

The chemotherapeutic treatment of acute leukemia is divided into stages. The first stage, induction therapy, is the attempt to induce or bring about a remission. *Induction* is aggressive treatment that seeks to destroy leukemic cells in the tissues, peripheral blood, and bone marrow in order to eventually restore normal hematopoiesis on bone marrow recovery. During induction therapy, a patient may become critically ill because the bone marrow is severely depressed by the chemotherapeutic agents. Throughout the induction phase, nursing interventions focus on neutropenia, thrombocytopenia, and anemia as well as providing psychosocial support to the patient and family. Common chemotherapy agents for induction of AML include cytarabine (Cytosar) and antitumour antibiotics (anthracyclines) such as daunorubicin (Cerubidine), doxorubicin (Adriamycin), idarubicin (Idamycin), or mitoxantrone. After one course of induction therapy, approximately 70% of newly diagnosed patients achieve complete remission. There is one subtype of AML, called *promyelocytic leukemia* (M3), in which tretinoin (Vesanoid) is used along with chemotherapy to induce a remission (Sanz & Lo Coco, 2011). It is generally assumed that leukemia cells persist undetected after induction therapy. This could lead to relapse within a few months if no further therapy is administered.

Terms used to describe postinduction or postremission chemotherapy include intensification, consolidation, and maintenance. *Intensification therapy*, or high-dose therapy, may be given immediately after induction therapy for several months. This therapy may use the same drugs as those used in induction, but at higher dosages. Other drugs that target the cell in a different way than those administered during induction may also be added.

Consolidation therapy is started after a remission is achieved. It may consist of one or two additional courses of the same drugs given during induction or involve high-dose therapy (intensive consolidation). The purpose of consolidation therapy is to eliminate remaining leukemic cells that may not be clinically or pathologically evident.

Maintenance therapy is treatment with lower doses of the same drugs used in induction or other drugs given every 3 to 4 weeks for a prolonged period of time. Like consolidation or intensification, the goal is to keep the body free of leukemic cells. Each leukemia calls for different maintenance therapy. In AML, maintenance therapy is rarely effective and, therefore, rarely administered.

In addition to chemotherapy, corticosteroids and radiation therapy can also have a role in the complex therapeutic plans for the patient with leukemia. Total body radiation may be used to prepare a patient for bone marrow transplantation, or it may be restricted to certain areas (fields) such as the liver and spleen or other organs affected by infiltrates. In ALL, prophylactic intrathecal methotrexate is given to decrease the chance of CNS involvement, which is common in this particular type of leukemia. When CNS leukemia does occur, cranial radiation may be given. Biological therapy may be indicated for specific leukemias. (Biological therapy is discussed in Chapter 18.)

Drug Therapy Regimens.

The mechanisms of action and the therapeutic agents used to treat leukemia are listed in Tables 33-27 and 33-28.

Combination chemotherapy is the mainstay of treatment for leukemia. The three purposes for using multiple drugs are to (1) decrease drug resistance, (2) minimize the drug toxicity to the patient by using multiple drugs with varying toxicities, and (3) interrupt cell growth at multiple points in the cell cycle.

DRUG THERAPY

Table 33-27 Chemotherapeutic Classes and Mechanisms of Action for Drugs Used to Treat Leukemia

DRUG CLASSIFICATION	DRUG NAME	MECHANISM OF ACTION
Alkylating agents	Busulfan (Myleran)	Damages DNA via alkylation of base pairs, leads to cross-linking of bases, abnormal base pairing, DNA breakage
	Chlorambucil (Leukeran), cyclophosphamide (Procytox)	
	Carboplatin, Cisplatin	
	Dacarbazine, Procarbazine	
Antitumour antibiotics	Daunorubicin (Cerubidine)	Interferes with DNA and RNA synthesis
	Doxorubicin (Adriamycin)	
	Bleomycin	
	Mitomycin C	
	Mitoxantrone	
	Idarubicin (Idamycin)	
Antimetabolites	Methotrexate	Inhibits DNA synthesis
	5-FU	
	Cytarabine (Cytosar)	
	6-Mercaptopurine (Purinethol)	
	Fludarabine	
	Hydroxyurea	
	6-Thioguanine	
Taxanes	Paclitaxel	Stabilizes microtubules against breakdown once cell division complete
	Docetaxel	
Vinca-alkaloids	Vincristine	Inhibits microtubule formation preventing cell division
	Vinorelbine	
	Vinblastine	
Monoclonal antibodies	Rituximab (Rituxan)	Binds to B-cell antigen CD20
Podophyllotoxin (Topoisomerase inhibitors)	Etoposide (VePesid)	Interferes with DNA unwinding necessary for normal replication and transcription
Small molecule inhibitors	Imatinib (Gleevec)	Bcr-Abl tyrosine kinase inhibitor

Newer therapeutic drugs are aimed at affecting small molecules that promote the growth and differentiation of leukemic cells. For example, imatinib mesylate (Gleevec) represents a new class of drugs that specifically target an abnormal cell. Imatinib targets an abnormal version of a normal cell protein (the Bcr-Abl protein) that is present in nearly all patients with CML. This abnormal protein is probably the cause of the disease. The *Bcr-Abl* gene is located on the Philadelphia chromosome. Thus, this drug kills only cancer cells, leaving healthy cells alone.

The use of specific targeted therapy in the form of monoclonal antibodies is an exciting new treatment modality in hematopoietic malignancies, but cures with these therapies alone are

DRUG THERAPY

Table 33-28 Treatments Used in Leukemia*

DRUG THERAPY	OTHER THERAPY
Acute Myelogenous Leukemia Cytarabine (Cytosar), daunorubicin (Cerubidine), idarubicin (Idamycin), thioguanine (Lanvis), mitoxantrone, † tretinoin (Vesanoid), † etoposide (Vepesid), clofarabine (Clolar) Combination chemotherapy of cytarabine and antitumour antibiotic (most common)	Autologous or allogeneic hematopoietic stem cell transplant (see Chapter 18)
Acute Lymphocytic Leukemia Daunorubicin, doxorubicin (Adriamycin), vincristine, prednisone, dexamethasone, L-asparaginase (Kidrolase) dasatinib (Sprycel), cyclophosphamide (Procytox), methotrexate, 6-mercaptopurine (Purinethol), cytarabine, nelarabine (Atriance), imatinib (Gleevec), clofarabine (Clolar) Combination chemotherapy of several agents is common	Cranial radiation therapy, intrathecal methotrexate or cytarabine, allogeneic hematopoietic stem cell transplant (see Chapter 18)
Chronic Myelogenous Leukemia Imatinib, dasatinib, nilotinib (Tasigna), hydroxyurea (Hydrea) *Combination chemotherapy including any of the following:* cytarabine, thioguanine, daunorubicin, methotrexate, prednisone, vincristine, L-asparaginase, carmustine (BiCNU), 6-mercaptopurine	Radiation, hematopoietic stem cell transplant, α-interferon, leukapheresis
Chronic Lymphocytic Leukemia Chlorambucil (Leukeran), cyclophosphamide, prednisone, vincristine, fludarabine , rituximab (Rituxan), alemtuzumab (Campath)	Radiation, splenectomy, colony-stimulating factors, allogeneic hematopoietic stem cell transplant

*The classification and mechanisms of action of these drugs are presented in Tables 18-8 and 18-16.
†Used for acute promyelocytic leukemia.

rare. Rituximab (Rituxan) binds to the B-cell antigen (CD20) and has been used with CLL.

Hematopoietic Stem Cell Transplantation. HSCT is another type of therapy used for patients with different forms of leukemia. The goal of HSCT is to totally eliminate leukemic cells from the body using combinations of chemotherapy with or without total body irradiation. This treatment also eradicates the patient's hematopoietic stem cells, which are then replaced with those of an HLA-matched sibling or volunteer donor (allogeneic), with those of an identical twin (syngeneic), or with the patient's own (autologous) stem cells that were removed (harvested) before the intensive therapy. (HSCT is discussed in Chapter 18.)

The primary complications of patients with allogeneic HSCT are graft–versus–host disease (GVHD), relapse of leukemia (especially ALL), and infection (especially interstitial pneumonia). GVHD is discussed in Chapter 16. Because HSCT has serious

associated risks, the patient must weigh the significant risks of treatment-related death or treatment failure (relapse) with the hope of cure.

NURSING MANAGEMENT: LEUKEMIA

Nursing Assessment

Subjective and objective data that should be obtained from a patient with leukemia are presented in Table 33-29.

Nursing Diagnoses

Nursing diagnoses for the patient with leukemia include those appropriate for anemia, thrombocytopenia, and neutropenia (see the respective NCPs [33-1, 33-2, and 33-3] in this chapter).

Planning

The overall goals are that the patient with leukemia will (1) understand and follow the treatment plan, (2) experience minimal adverse effects and complications associated with both the disease and its treatment, and (3) feel hopeful and supported during the periods of treatment, relapse, or remission.

Nursing Implementation

Acute Intervention

The nursing role during acute phases of leukemia is extremely challenging because the patient has many physical and psychosocial needs. As with other forms of cancer, the diagnosis of leukemia can evoke great fear and be equated with death. It may be viewed as a hopeless, horrible disease with many painful and undesirable consequences. For each patient, it is important that the nurse has an understanding of the patient's type of leukemia, prognosis, treatment plan, and goals. By doing this, the nurse can help the patient realize that, although the future may be uncertain, one can have a meaningful quality of life while in remission or with disease control and that, in some cases, there is reasonable hope for cure. The family also needs help in adjusting to the stress of this abrupt onset of serious illness (e.g., dependence, withdrawal, changes in role responsibilities, alterations in body image) and the losses imposed by the sick role. The diagnosis of leukemia often brings with it the need to make difficult decisions at a time of profound stress for the patient and family. Because the majority of patients are older than 65 years, patients may have co-morbid conditions that affect treatment decisions. In addition, although older adults have often learned to live with the hardships, disappointments, and loss experienced in various periods of their lives, health care providers must assess all patients for potential symptoms of depression and provide appropriate care and referrals.

The nurse is an important advocate in helping the patient and family understand the complexities of treatment decisions and manage the adverse effects and toxicities. A patient empowered by knowledge of the disease and treatment can have a more

NURSING ASSESSMENT

Table 33-29 Leukemia

Subjective Data

Important Health Information

Past health history: Exposure to chemical toxins (e.g., benzene, arsenic), radiation, or viruses (Epstein-Barr, HTLV-1); chromosome abnormalities (Down, Klinefelter's, and Fanconi's syndromes), immunological deficiencies; organ transplantation; frequent infections; bleeding tendencies; family history of leukemia

Medications: Use of chloramphenicol, chemotherapy

Surgery or other treatments: Radiation exposure; prior radiation and chemotherapy for cancer

Symptoms

- Weight loss, chills, night sweats
- Fatigue with progressive weakness; bone pain, joint pain; muscle cramps
- Dyspnea, cough
- Nausea, vomiting, anorexia, dysphagia, early satiety; mouth sores, sore throat
- Hematuria, decreased urine output
- Diarrhea, dark or bloody stools
- Headaches, confusion, numbness, tingling, visual disturbances; bone pain, joint pain
- Easy bruising; epistaxis; prolonged menses; menorrhagia; erectile dysfunction

Objective Data

General

Fever, generalized lymphadenopathy, lethargy

Integumentary

Pallor or jaundice; petechiae, ecchymoses, purpura, reddish-brown to purple cutaneous infiltrates, macules, and papules

Cardiovascular

Tachycardia, systolic murmurs

Gastrointestinal

Gingival bleeding and hyperplasia; oral ulcerations, herpes and *Candida* infections; perirectal irritation and infection; hepatomegaly, splenomegaly

Neurological

Seizures, disorientation, confusion, decreased coordination, cranial nerve palsies, papilledema

Musculoskeletal

Muscle wasting, bone pain, joint pain

Possible Findings

Low, normal, or high WBC count with shift to the left (blast cells); anemia, ↓ hematocrit and hemoglobin, thrombocytopenia, Philadelphia chromosome; hypercellular bone marrow aspirate or biopsy with myeloblasts, lymphoblasts, and markedly ↓ normal cells

HTLV-1, human T-cell leukemia virus, type 1; *WBC,* white blood cell.

positive outlook and improved quality of life. A patient may require isolation or may need to temporarily relocate to an appropriate treatment centre. These situations can lead a patient to feel deserted and isolated at a time when support is most needed.

The intense psychosocial needs of the patient and family are best met by a multidisciplinary team (e.g., psychiatric and oncology clinical nurse specialists, case managers, dietitians, chaplains, and social workers).

From a physical care perspective, the challenge is to make astute assessments and plan care to help the patient manage the severe adverse effects of chemotherapy. The life-threatening results of bone marrow suppression (neutropenia, thrombocytopenia, and anemia) require aggressive nursing interventions (see NCPs 33-1, 33-2, and 33-3). Additional complications of chemotherapy may affect the patient's GI tract, nutritional status, skin and mucosa, cardiopulmonary status, liver, kidneys, and neurological system. (Nursing interventions related to chemotherapy are discussed in Chapter 18.)

The nurse must be knowledgeable about all drugs being administered. This includes mechanism of action, purpose, routes of administration, usual doses, potential adverse effects, safe-handling considerations, and toxic effects of the drugs. In addition, the nurse must know how to assess laboratory data reflecting the effects of the drugs. Patient survival and comfort during aggressive chemotherapy are significantly affected by the quality of nursing care.

■ Ambulatory and Home Care

Ongoing care for the patient with leukemia is necessary to monitor for signs and symptoms of disease control or relapse. For a patient requiring long-term or maintenance chemotherapy, long-term chronic disease management can become arduous and discouraging. Therefore, a patient and the significant other must be taught to understand the importance of the continued diligence in disease management and the need for follow-up care. The patient and significant other must be taught about the drugs, self-care measures, and when to seek medical attention.

The goals of rehabilitation for long-term survivors of childhood and adult leukemia are to manage the physical, psychological, social, and spiritual consequences and delayed effects from the disease and its treatment. (Delayed effects are discussed in Chapter 18.) Assistance may be needed to re-establish the various relationships that are a part of the patient's life. Friends and family may not know how to interact with the patient. The patient and the family must learn to regain attitudes of health and life while facing the real fear of relapse of disease. Involving the patient in survivor networks and support groups may help the patient adapt to living after a life-threatening illness. Exploring community resources (e.g., Canadian Cancer Society) may reduce the financial burden and the feelings of dependence. Spiritual support may give the patient inner strength and peace.

The patient will need support in adapting to any physical limitations or changes imposed by the illness. Vigilant follow-up care by providers who are aware of the unique needs of a cancer survivor is of the utmost importance for early recognition and treatment of long-term or delayed physical, psychological, and social effects. Often, these needs may require the initiation of a referral or consultation. For example, physiotherapy personnel may be asked to develop an exercise program to prevent post-treatment deficits caused by drug-induced peripheral neuropathy. These needs can also include other concerns such as growth and development concerns for childhood survivors, vocational retraining, and reproductive concerns for a patient of child-bearing age. The long-term recovery following treatment for leukemia affects the quality of the patient's life.

Evaluation

The expected outcomes are that the patient with leukemia will (1) cope effectively with diagnosis, treatment regimen, and prognosis; (2) attain and maintain adequate nutrition; (3) experience no complications related to the disease or its treatment; and (4) feel comfortable and supported throughout treatment.

Lymphomas

Lymphomas are malignant neoplasms originating in the bone marrow and lymphatic structures resulting in the proliferation of lymphocytes. Two major types of lymphoma—Hodgkin's disease and non-Hodgkin's lymphoma (NHL)—are discussed in this chapter. NHLs are the fifth most common type of cancer in Canada (Canadian Cancer Society/National Cancer Institute of Canada/Public Health Agency of Canada/Statistics Canada, 2008). A comparison of these two types of lymphoma is presented in Table 33-30.

Hodgkin's Lymphoma

Hodgkin's lymphoma, also called *Hodgkin's disease*, makes up about 12% of all lymphomas. It is a malignant condition characterized by proliferation of abnormal giant, multinucleated cells, called *Reed-Sternberg cells*, which are located in lymph nodes. The disease has a bimodal age-specific incidence, occurring most frequently in people from 15 to 35 years of age and older than 50 years. In adults, it is twice as prevalent in men as in women. In 2012, it was estimated that 940 people would be diagnosed with Hodgkin's lymphoma in Canada (Canadian Cancer Society's Steering Committee on Cancer Statistics, 2012).

Etiology and Pathophysiology

Although the cause of Hodgkin's lymphoma remains unknown, several key factors are thought to play a role in its development. The main interacting factors include infection with Epstein-Barr virus (EBV), genetic predisposition, and exposure to occupational toxins. The incidence of Hodgkin's lymphoma is increased in patients with HIV (Howard & Hamilton, 2008).

Normally, the lymph nodes are composed of connective tissues that surround a fine mesh of reticular fibres and cells. In Hodgkin's lymphoma, the normal structure of lymph nodes is destroyed by hyperplasia of monocytes and macrophages. The main diagnostic feature of Hodgkin's disease is the presence of Reed-Sternberg cells in lymph node biopsy specimens. The disease is believed to arise in a single location (it originates in lymph nodes in 90% of patients) and then spreads along adjacent lymphatics. However, in recurrent disease, it may be more diffuse, and not necessarily contiguous. It eventually infiltrates other organs, especially the lungs, spleen, and liver. In approximately two thirds of patients, the cervical lymph nodes are the first to be affected. When the disease begins above the diaphragm, it remains confined to lymph nodes for a time, which is variable. Disease originating below the diaphragm frequently spreads to extralymphoid sites such as the liver.

Clinical Manifestations

The onset of symptoms in Hodgkin's lymphoma is usually insidious. The initial development is most often enlargement of cervical, axillary, or inguinal lymph nodes (Figure 33-15); a mediastinal node is the second most common location for a mass. This lymphadenopathy affects discrete nodes that remain movable and nontender. The enlarged nodes are not painful unless they exert pressure on adjacent nerves.

The patient may notice weight loss, fatigue, weakness, fever, chills, tachycardia, or night sweats. A group of initial findings including fever, night sweats, and weight loss (termed *B symptoms*) correlates with a worse prognosis. After the ingestion of even small amounts of alcohol, individuals with Hodgkin's disease may complain of a rapid onset of pain at the site of disease. The cause for the alcohol-induced pain is unknown. Generalized pruritus without skin lesions may develop. Cough, dyspnea, stridor, and dysphagia may all reflect mediastinal node involvement.

In more advanced disease, there is hepatomegaly and splenomegaly. Anemia results from increased destruction and decreased production of erythrocytes. Other physical signs vary depending on where the disease is located; for example, (1) intrathoracic involvement may lead to superior vena cava syndrome, (2) enlarged retroperitoneal nodes may cause palpable abdominal

	HODGKIN'S DISEASE	NON-HODGKIN'S LYMPHOMA
Cellular origin	B lymphocytes	B lymphocytes (90%)
		T lymphocytes (10%)
Extent of disease	Localized to regional, but may be bulky	Disseminated
B symptoms*	Common	Less common (40%)
Extranodal involvement	Rare	Common

Table 33-30 Comparison of Hodgkin's Disease and Non-Hodgkin's Lymphoma

*B symptoms include fever, night sweats, and weight loss.

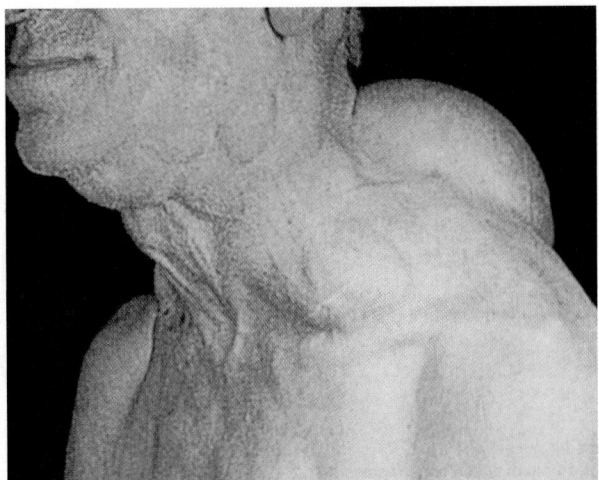

Figure 33-15 Hodgkin's lymphoma (Stage IIA). This patient has enlargement of the cervical lymph nodes.

Source: Skarin, A. T. (1996). *Atlas of diagnostic oncology* (2nd ed.). London: Mosby-Wolfe.

masses or interfere with renal function, (3) jaundice may occur from liver involvement, and (4) spinal cord compression leading to paraplegia may occur with extradural involvement. Bone pain occurs as a result of bone involvement.

Diagnostic and Staging Studies

Peripheral blood analysis, excisional lymph node biopsy, bone marrow examination, and radiological evaluation are important means of evaluating Hodgkin's lymphoma. Peripheral blood analysis often reveals a microcytic hypochromic anemia, neutrophilic leukocytosis ($15\text{-}28 \times 10^9/L$), which may be associated with lymphopenia and an increased platelet count. Leukopenia and thrombocytopenia may develop, but they are usually a consequence of treatment, advanced disease, or superimposed hypersplenism. Other blood studies may show hypoferremia caused by excessive iron uptake by the liver and spleen, elevated leukocyte alkaline phosphatase from liver and bone involvement, hypercalcemia from bone involvement, and hypoalbuminemia from liver involvement.

Excisional lymph node biopsy offers a definitive means of diagnosis. The removed peripheral lymph node is examined for the presence of the diagnostic Reed-Sternberg cells. Bone marrow biopsy is performed as an important aspect of staging. Reed-Sternberg cells may also be found in the patient's bone marrow.

Radiological evaluation can help define all sites and determine the clinical stage of the disease. CT or MRI scans are used as initial staging tools. These scans may show mediastinal lymphadenopathy, renal displacement caused by retroperitoneal node enlargement; abdominal lymph node enlargement; and liver, spleen, bone, and brain infiltration. Gallium scans may also be used to monitor response to treatment.

NURSING AND COLLABORATIVE MANAGEMENT: HODGKIN'S LYMPHOMA

Using all of the information from the various diagnostic studies, the stage of the disease is determined (Figure 33-16). The final staging is based on the clinical stage (extent of the disease) as well as the absence or presence of B symptoms (A or B classification). The absence of constitutional or B-type symptoms (i.e., fever, night sweats, and weight loss) is denoted by adding

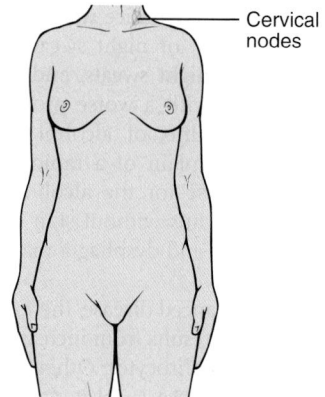

Stage I
Involvement of a single lymph node or a single extranodal site

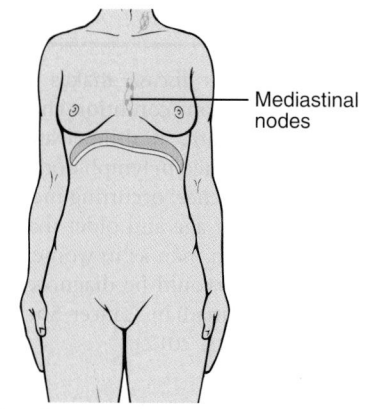

Stage II
Involvement of two or more lymph node regions on the same side of the diaphragm or localized involvement of an extranodal site and one or more lymph node regions of the same side of diaphragm

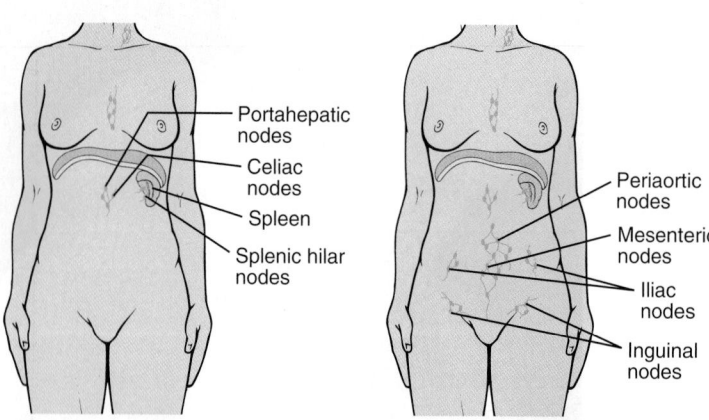

Stage III
Involvement of lymph node regions on both sides of the diaphragm. May include a single extranodal site, the spleen, or both; now subdivided into lymphatic involvement of the upper abdomen in the spleen (splenic, celiac, and portal nodes) (*Stage III₁*) and the lower abdominal nodes in the para–aortic, mesenteric, and iliac regions (*Stage III₂*)

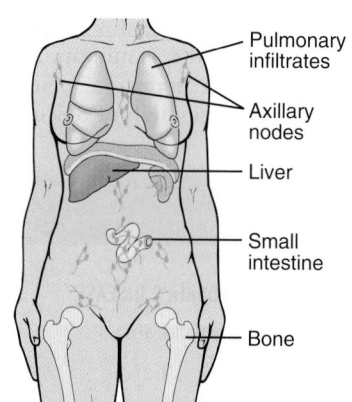

Stage IV
Diffuse or disseminated disease of one or more extralymphatic organs or tissues with or without associated lymph node involvement; the extranodal site is identified as *H*, hepatic; *L*, lung; *P*, pleura; *M*, marrow; *D*, dermal; or *O*, osseous

Figure 33-16 Staging system for Hodgkin's lymphoma and non-Hodgkin's lymphoma.

an A to the stage; the presence is denoted by adding a B to the stage. Treatment depends on the nature and the extent of the disease. Additional features, such as an elevated sedimentation rate; age 50 years or older; and the presence of a large mediastinal mass and low serum albumin, Hb, and lymphocyte counts may indicate an unfavourable prognosis, even in a patient with early Stage I or II disease, warranting more aggressive therapy.

Once the stage of Hodgkin's lymphoma is established, management focuses on selecting a treatment plan. The standard for chemotherapy is the ABVD regimen: doxorubicin (*A*driamycin), *b*leomycin, *v*inblastine, and *d*acarbazine. Patients with early-stage disease with favourable characteristics will receive two to four cycles of chemotherapy. Patients with early-stage but unfavourable prognostic features (e.g., the presence of B symptoms) or intermediate-stage disease will be treated with four to six cycles of chemotherapy. Advanced-stage Hodgkin's lymphoma is treated more aggressively using six to, potentially, eight cycles of chemotherapy. A more aggressive chemotherapy regimen is BEACOPP (*b*leomycin, *e*toposide, doxorubicin (*A*driamycin), *c*yclophosphamide, vincristine (former trade name *O*ncovin), *p*rocarbazine, and *p*rednisone) (Cashen & Bartlett, 2008). The role of radiation as a supplement to chemotherapy varies depending on sites of disease and the presence of resistant disease after chemotherapy.

Intensive chemotherapy with or without the use of autologous or allogeneic HSCT and hematopoietic growth factors is the treatment of choice for advanced Hodgkin's lymphoma (Stages IIIB and IV). HSCT has allowed patients to receive higher, potentially curative doses of chemotherapy while reducing life-threatening leukopenia. Combination chemotherapy works well because, as in leukemia, drugs are used that have an additive antitumour effect without increasing adverse effects. As with leukemia, therapy must be aggressive. Thus, potentially life-threatening problems are risked for the sake of attempting to achieve a remission.

Maintenance chemotherapy does not contribute to increased survival once a complete remission is achieved. Occasionally, single drugs may be administered palliatively to patients who cannot tolerate intensive combination therapy. A serious consequence of the treatment for Hodgkin's lymphoma is the later development of secondary malignancies (see Chapter 18) as well as potential long-term toxicities from the treatment, such as endocrine, cardiac, and pulmonary dysfunction (Mughal, Goldman, & Mughal, 2010). The nursing care for Hodgkin's lymphoma is largely based on managing problems related to the disease (e.g., pain caused by the tumour), pancytopenia, and other adverse effects of therapy. Because the survival of patients with Hodgkin's lymphoma depends on their response to treatment, supporting the patient through the immunosuppressive state is extremely important.

Psychosocial considerations are just as important as they are with leukemia. However, the prognosis for Hodgkin's lymphoma is better than that for many forms of cancer or leukemia. Early-stage Hodgkin's lymphoma has a 10-year survival rate near 90%, and advanced-stage Hodgkin's lymphoma has a 10-year survival rate of more than 50%. The physical, psychological, social, and spiritual consequences of the patient's disease must be addressed. Fertility issues may be of particular concern because this disease is frequently seen in adolescents and young adults. The nurse must help ensure that these issues have been addressed soon after diagnosis. Evaluation of patients for long-term effects of therapy is important because delayed consequences of disease and treatment may not be apparent for many years. (Secondary malignancies and delayed effects are discussed in Chapter 18.)

Non-Hodgkin's Lymphoma

Non-Hodgkin's lymphomas (NHLs) are a heterogeneous group of malignant neoplasms of primarily B- or T-cell origin affecting all ages. B-cell lymphomas constitute about 90% of all NHLs. They are classified according to different cellular and lymph node characteristics. A variety of clinical presentations and courses are recognized, from indolent (slowly developing) to rapidly progressive disease. NHL is the most commonly occurring hematological cancer and the fifth leading cause of cancer death. In 2012, it was estimated there would be 7800 new cases of NHL diagnosed in Canada, and approximately 2800 deaths due to NHL (Canadian Cancer Society's Steering Committee on Cancer Statistics, 2012).

Etiology and Pathophysiology

As with Hodgkin's lymphoma, the cause of NHL is usually unknown. However, as the population has aged and the incidence of HIV infection has increased, the incidence of NHL has increased 2 to 3% per year for at least the past 30 years. It is also more common in individuals who have used immunosuppressive medications (e.g., to prevent rejection following an organ transplant or to treat autoimmune disorders) or received chemotherapy or radiation therapy. EBV is associated with Burkitt's lymphoma, Hodgkin's lymphoma, immunoblastic lymphoma, and some carcinomas, but not all individuals with EBV get these malignancies.

There is no hallmark feature in NHL that parallels the Reed-Sternberg cell of Hodgkin's lymphoma. However, all NHLs involve lymphocytes arrested in various stages of development. For example, lymphoblastic lymphoma and lymphoblastic leukemia (which has a majority of disease within the bone marrow rather than the lymph nodes) result from malignant proliferation of small, immature B lymphocytes. Diffuse large B-cell lymphoma, the most common aggressive lymphoma in adults, is a neoplasm that originates in the lymph nodes. Burkitt's lymphoma is a highly aggressive disease thought to originate from B-cell blast cells in the lymph nodes.

Clinical Manifestations

NHLs can originate outside the lymph nodes, the method of spread can be unpredictable, and the majority of patients have widely disseminated disease at the time of diagnosis (Figure 33-17). The primary clinical manifestation is painless lymph node enlargement. Because the disease is usually disseminated when it is diagnosed, other symptoms will be present depending on where the disease has spread (e.g., hepatomegaly with liver involvement or neurological symptoms with CNS disease). NHL can also manifest in nonspecific ways, such as an airway obstruction, hyperuricemia, and renal failure or acute kidney injury from tumour lysis syndrome, pericardial tamponade, and GI complaints.

Patients with high-grade lymphomas may have lymphadenopathy and constitutional symptoms (B symptoms) such as fever, night sweats, and weight loss. The peripheral blood is usually normal, but some lymphomas manifest in a "leukemic" phase.

Diagnostic and Staging Studies

Diagnostic studies used for NHL resemble those used for Hodgkin's disease. However, because NHL is more often in extranodal sites, more diagnostic studies may be done, such as an MRI to rule out CNS or bone marrow infiltration or a barium enema or CT to visualize suspected GI involvement. Clinical staging, as described for Hodgkin's lymphoma, is used to help guide therapy (see Figure 33-16), but establishment of the precise histological subtype is extremely important. Lymph node biopsy establishes the cell type and the pattern. NHL is classified based on morphological, genetic, immunophenotypic (cell surface antigens, CD20, CD52), and clinical features (Matasar & Zelenetz, 2008).

A useful system for classifying NHL is the International Working Formulation (IWF), which divides each subtype of lymphoma into low grade (indolent), intermediate grade (aggressive), and high grade (very aggressive) (Table 33-31). Additional factors, known as the *International Prognostic Index* (IPI), may be

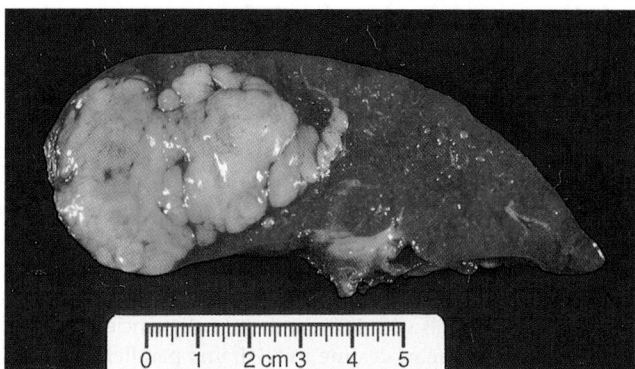

Figure 33-17 Non-Hodgkin's lymphoma involving the spleen. The presence of an isolated mass is typical.

Source: Kumar, V., Abbas, A. K., Fausto, N., & Aster, J. C. (2010). *Robbins and Cotran pathologic basis of disease* (8th ed., p. 607, Figure 13-14). Philadelphia: Saunders.

considered to help select the appropriate treatment for these patients. Factors considered may include the clinical stage, number of extranodal sites, age, serum LDH level, WBC count, Hb, and performance status. Immunological, cytogenetic, and molecular studies are also useful for making therapeutic decisions and assessing prognosis. The prognosis for NHL is generally not as good as that for Hodgkin's lymphoma.

NURSING AND COLLABORATIVE MANAGEMENT: NON-HODGKIN'S LYMPHOMA

Treatment for NHL involves radiation therapy and chemotherapy (Table 33-32). Ironically, more aggressive lymphomas are more responsive to treatment and more likely to be cured. In contrast, indolent lymphomas have a naturally long course but are difficult to treat effectively.

Patients with low-grade (indolent) lymphoma have a median overall survival of 9 years. However, most patients relapse several times, and cure is very unlikely. A previous approach was that patients who were asymptomatic were followed with "watchful waiting" to assess the progress of the disease. However, some initial therapies can be well tolerated and have been shown to extend the time to progression of the disease. Therapy would be indicated if the patient has local symptoms from progressive, bulky, or painful disease or a compromise of normal organ function. An option for these patients is rituximab every week and then every 2 months as maintenance therapy. Rituximab, a genetically engineered monoclonal antibody against the CD20 antigen on the surface of normal and malignant B lymphocytes, is used to treat NHL. Once bound to the cells, rituximab causes lysis and cell death. Once the disease is symptomatic, rituximab with chemotherapy, such as cyclophosphamide with or without prednisone or even the CHOP regimen (cyclophosphamide, doxorubicin [Adriamycin], vincristine, and prednisone) or the CHOP-R (CHOP plus rituximab [Rituxan]), may be used. Complete remissions are uncommon, but the majority of patients will respond with improvement in adenopathy and symptoms. Numerous

Table 33-31 Non-Hodgkin's Lymphoma Classification*

B-Cell Lymphomas

Low-Grade (Indolent) Lymphomas
- Small lymphocytic, plasmacytoid
- Follicular
- Marginal sone (MALT) splenic, nodal

Intermediate-Grade (Aggressive) Lymphomas
- Follicular, predominantly large cell
- Diffuse, small cleaved cell
- Diffuse, mixed, small and large cell
- Diffuse, large cell; cleaved cell
- Peripheral T cell

High-Grade (Very Aggressive) Lymphomas
- Large cell immunoblastic
- Lymphoblastic
- Small noncleaved cell; Burkitt's

B-Cell Lymphomas
- Peripheral T-cell lymphoma
- Mycosis fungoides/Sézary syndrome

MALT, mucosa-associated lymphoid tissue.
*Partial listing.

Table 33-32 Guidelines for Treatment of Non-Hodgkin's Lymphoma

	RECOMMENDED THERAPY	
GRADE	**STAGES I, II,***	**STAGES II₂,† III, IV**
Low (indolent)	Localized irradiation	Observation until disease progression, then palliative irradiation or single-agent or combination chemotherapy
Intermediate (aggressive)	Combination chemotherapy with localized radiation	Combination chemotherapy
High (very aggressive)	Combination chemotherapy (high dose) with localized radiation	Combination chemotherapy (high dose)

*Stage II₁ = nonbulky disease.
†Stage II₂ = bulky disease > 10 cm or one third the diameter of the chest.

chemotherapy combinations have been used to try to overcome the resistant nature of this disease.

Intermediate-grade (aggressive) and high-grade (very aggressive) lymphomas may be treated similarly, depending on the extent of the disease and the patient's prognostic factors. Diffuse large B-cell NHL is the most common high-grade lymphoma and the most common subtype. The most common standard chemotherapeutic regimen is CHOP-R. Other combination therapies may be used for very aggressive or refractory disease. These include rituximab, ifosfamide, carboplatin, and etoposide (RICE); etoposide, prednisone, vincristine (former trade name Oncovin), doxorubicin, and cyclophosphamide (EPOCH); dexamethasone, cytarabine (former trade name Ara C), and cisplatin (which contains platinum) (DHAP); and etoposide, methylprednisolone, and cisplatin (which contains platinum) (ESHAP). Dose-dense (intensified) treatment with CHOP-14 every 2 weeks (as opposed to every 3-4 wk) with hematopoietic growth factor support may be used in patients with aggressive disease. High-dose chemotherapy with autologous HSCT has shown a better outcome than conventional chemotherapy in the treatment of patients with relapsed, aggressive NHL who are still responding to salvage chemotherapy. The role of allogeneic transplant in NHL is uncertain, but it is thought that it may have some benefit in certain subtypes with aggressive or refractory lymphoma.

Because NHL represents a large variety of neoplasms, some subtypes may be treated differently from the general standards described previously. For example, cutaneous T-cell lymphoma may be treated with topical corticosteroids or topical chemotherapy for limited-stage disease. For more diffuse disease, treatment may include phototherapy, α-interferon, a retinoid, or a novel fusion protein consisting of interleukin-2 (IL-2) and diphtheria toxin. (Biological and targeted therapy are discussed in Chapter 18.)

SAFETY ALERT

- Monitor patients for signs of severe hypersensitivity infusion reactions when infusing rituximab (Rituxan), especially with the first infusion.
- Manifestations may include hypotension, bronchospasm, dysrhythmias, angioedema, and cardiogenic shock.
- Screen patients for history of hepatitis because rituximab may reactivate the disease.

Other therapies for NHL include the monoclonal antibodies ibritumomab tiuxetan (Zevalin) and tositumomab (Bexxar). These antibodies are linked to a radioactive isotope (yttrium-90 and iodine-131, respectively) (see Chapter 18, Table 18-16). The monoclonal antibody targets the CD20 antigen, which is on the surface of mature B cells and B-cell tumours. This allows for the delivery of radiation directly to the malignant cells. Adverse effects of these medications include pancytopenia. The nurse must be aware of the necessary precautions in caring for these patients, both to educate patients about safety issues and to minimize the risk of radiation exposure to staff and others. The nursing care for NHL is similar to that for Hodgkin's lymphoma. Nursing care is largely based on managing problems related to the disease (e.g., pain caused by the tumour, spinal cord compression, tumour lysis syndrome), pancytopenia, and other adverse effects of therapy. However, because NHL can be more extensive and involve specific organs (e.g., CNS, spleen, liver, GI tract, bone marrow), it is important that the nurse have an understanding of

the subtype and the extent of the disease. For example, a patient with known involvement of the colon may complain of acute abdominal pain. The patient most likely would have abdominal guarding and an enlarged and tympanic abdomen. This could indicate a bowel perforation and be considered a medical emergency. A patient with a Burkitt NHL starting chemotherapy would be at high risk for tumour lysis syndrome, and would have to have frequent specimens drawn for the monitoring of laboratory parameters as well as being on strict intake and output monitoring. For oncological problems, refer to Chapter 18. Because most of these patients receive therapy that is potentially myelosuppressive, NCPs 33-1, 33-2, and 33-3 would apply to these patients as well.

The patient undergoing radiation therapy has special nursing needs. The skin in the radiation field requires attention. In addition, the nurse must understand the concepts related to administration of and safety issues regarding radiation therapy (see Chapter 18).

Psychosocial considerations are very important. Helping the patient and the family understand the disease, the treatment, and expected and potential untoward adverse effects is paramount in enlisting their help in the patient's well-being and safety. Fertility issues may be of concern in young patients. As in Hodgkin's lymphoma, evaluation of patients with NHL for long-term effects of therapy is important because delayed consequences of disease and treatment may not be apparent for many years. (Secondary malignancies and delayed effects are discussed in Chapter 18.)

Multiple Myeloma

Multiple myeloma, or *plasma cell myeloma*, is a condition in which neoplastic plasma cells infiltrate the bone marrow and destroy bone. The disease is more common in men than in women and usually develops after 40 years of age, with an average age at onset of 70 years. Myeloma has a higher incidence in Afro-Caribbean ethnic groups than in Whites (Bird et al., 2011). In 2012, it was estimated that 2400 new cases of multiple myeloma would be diagnosed in Canada that year (Canadian Cancer Society's Steering Committee on Cancer Statistics, 2012).

Etiology and Pathophysiology

The cause of multiple myeloma is unknown. Exposure to radiation, organic chemicals (such as benzene), herbicides, and insecticides may play a role. Genetic factors and viral infection may also influence the risk of developing multiple myeloma. The disease process involves excessive production of plasma cells. Plasma cells are activated B cells, which produce immunoglobulins (antibodies) that normally serve to protect the body. However, in multiple myeloma, the malignant plasma cells infiltrate the bone marrow and produce abnormal and excessive amounts of immunoglobulin (usually IgG [most common], IgA, IgD, or IgE). This abnormal immunoglobulin is termed a *myeloma protein* or *monoclonal (M) protein*. Furthermore, plasma-cell production of excessive and abnormal amounts of cytokines (IL-4, IL-5, and IL-6) also plays an important role in the pathological process of bone destruction. As myeloma protein increases, normal plasma cells are reduced, which further compromises the body's normal immune response. In some patients, excessive production and secretion of free light-chain proteins (called *Bence Jones* proteins) from the myeloma cell also occurs; these can be detected in the urine (Tariman, 2010). Proliferation of malignant plasma cells and the overproduction of immunoglobulin and proteins result in the end-organ effects of myeloma to the bone marrow, bone, and kidneys and possibly the spleen, lymph nodes, liver, and even heart muscle.

Clinical Manifestations

Multiple myeloma develops slowly and insidiously. The patient often does not manifest symptoms until the disease is advanced, at which time skeletal pain is the major manifestation. Pain in the pelvis, spine, and ribs is particularly common and is triggered by movement. Diffuse osteoporosis develops as the myeloma protein destroys bone. Osteolytic lesions are seen in the skull, vertebrae, and ribs (Figure 33-18). Vertebral destruction can lead to collapse of vertebrae with ensuing compression of the spinal cord. Loss of bone integrity can lead to the development of pathological fractures; about 30% of patients have pathological fractures.

Bony degeneration also causes calcium to be lost from bones, eventually causing hypercalcemia. Hypercalcemia may cause renal, GI, or neurological manifestations such as polyuria, anorexia, confusion, and ultimately seizures, coma, and cardiac problems. High protein levels caused by the presence of the myeloma protein can result in renal failure from renal tubular obstruction by the myeloma protein and interstitial nephritis. The patient may also display manifestations of anemia, thrombocytopenia, and granulocytopenia (recurrent infections), all of which are related to the replacement of normal bone marrow with plasma cells.

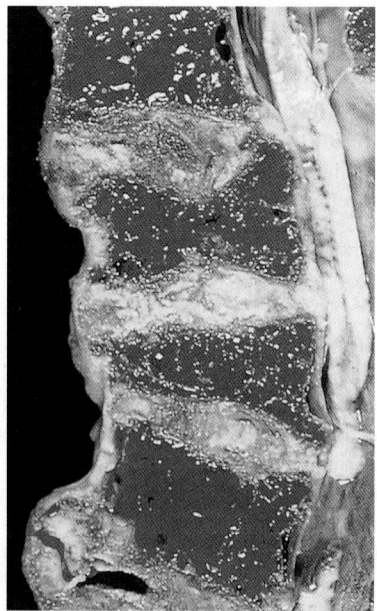

Figure 33-18 Multiple myeloma. This segment of the lower thoracic spine has been sectioned to show the extensive replacement of the bone and the marrow with red gelatinous tissue.

Source: Skarin, A. T. (1996). *Atlas of diagnostic oncology* (2nd ed.). London: Mosby-Wolfe.

Diagnostic Studies

Evaluating multiple myeloma involves laboratory, radiological, and bone marrow examination. The presence of an M protein can be noted in the blood and urine. Pancytopenia, hypercalcemia, the presence of Bence Jones protein in the urine, and an elevated serum creatinine are possible findings.

Radiographic studies show distinct lytic areas of bone erosions, generalized thinning of the bones, and/or fractures, especially in vertebrae, ribs, pelvis, and bones of the thigh and the upper arms. Bone marrow analysis shows significantly increased numbers of plasma cells in the bone marrow. The simplest criteria for prognosis in multiple myeloma are the blood levels of two markers: β_2-microglobulin and albumin. In general, higher levels of β_2-microglobulin and lower levels of albumin are associated with a poorer prognosis.

Collaborative Care

Collaborative care involves managing both the disease and its symptoms. The current treatment options include watchful waiting (for early multiple myeloma), corticosteroids, chemotherapy, biological therapy, and HSCT (Bird et al., 2011). Multiple myeloma is seldom cured, but treatment can relieve symptoms, produce remission, and prolong life. Ambulation and adequate hydration are used to treat hypercalcemia, dehydration, and potential renal damage. Weight bearing helps the bones reabsorb some calcium, and fluids dilute calcium and prevent protein precipitates from causing renal tubular obstruction. Control of pain and prevention of pathological fractures are other goals of management. Analgesics, orthopedic supports, and localized radiation help reduce the skeletal pain.

Bisphosphonates, such as pamidronate (Aredia) and zoledronic acid (Zometa), inhibit bone breakdown and are used for the treatment of skeletal pain and hypercalcemia. They inhibit bone resorption without inhibiting bone formation and mineralization. They are given monthly by IV infusion and are recommended for all patients with symptomatic multiple myeloma.

Radiation therapy is another component of treatment, primarily because of its effect on localized lesions. Surgical procedures, such as vertebroplasty, may be done to support degenerative vertebrae.

SAFETY ALERT

- Patients must be adequately hydrated prior to administering zoledronic acid (Zometa).
- Renal toxicity may occur if IV zoledronic acid is infused in less than 15 minutes.

Chemotherapy is often recommended for multiple myeloma. It is used to reduce the number of plasma cells. Three regimes commonly used are MPT (*m*elphalan, *p*rednisone, and *t*halidomide), MPV (*m*elphalan, *p*rednisone, and bortezomib [*V*elcade], and MPR (*m*elphalan, *p*rednisone, and lenalidomide [*R*evlimid]). High-dose chemotherapy followed by autologous HSCT has evolved as the standard of care in eligible patients. Drugs may be used to treat complications of multiple myeloma. For example, allopurinol (Zyloprim) may be given to reduce hyperuricemia, and IV furosemide (Lasix) promotes renal excretion of calcium. Antibiotics may be used prophylactically and erythropoietin may be given for anemia.

NURSING MANAGEMENT: MULTIPLE MYELOMA

A major focus of care relates to the bone involvement and the sequelae from bone breakdown. Maintaining adequate hydration is a primary nursing consideration to minimize problems from hypercalcemia. Fluids are administered to attain a urinary output of 1.5 to 2 L/day. This may require an intake of 3 to 4 L. In addition, weight bearing helps bones reabsorb some of the circulating calcium, and corticosteroids may augment the excretion of calcium. Once chemotherapy is initiated, the uric acid levels may rise because of the increased cell destruction. Hyperuricemia is treated by ensuring adequate hydration and using allopurinol to prevent any renal damage. Because of the myeloma proteins, the patient is at additional risk of renal dysfunction. The nurse must monitor electrolytes and fluid balance.

Because of the potential for pathological fractures, the nurse must be careful when moving and ambulating the patient. A slight twist or strain in the wrong area (e.g., a weak area in the patient's bones) may be sufficient to cause a fracture. In addition, the development of peripheral neuropathy is common with several therapies for multiple myeloma and can contribute to discomfort, the inability to perform basic activities of daily living, and the risk of injury from falling.

Pain management requires innovative and knowledgeable nursing interventions. Analgesics, such as nonsteroidal anti-inflammatory drugs, acetaminophen, or an acetaminophen–opioid combination, may be more effective than opioids alone in diminishing bone pain. Braces, especially for the spine, may also help control pain. As in any situation in which pain management enters in, the nurse is responsible for assessing the patient and for implementing necessary measures to alleviate the pain. (Pain management is discussed in Chapter 10.) Patients may also be at risk for deep vein thrombosis related to chemotherapy and immobility and should have preventive measures employed (Bird et al., 2011).

Assessment and prompt treatment of infection are important in the care of patients with multiple myeloma. Recurrent infections may be caused by a decrease in the production of normal immunoglobins, the ineffectiveness of the overproduced and abnormal immunoglobins, and/or neutropenia that results from the bone marrow infiltration or is an adverse effect of treatment. NCPs for anemia (NCP 33-1), thrombocytopenia (NCP 33-2), and neutropenia (NCP 33-3) apply to the patient with multiple myeloma.

The patient's psychosocial needs require sensitive, skilled management. It is important to help the patient and significant others adapt to changes fostered by chronic sickness and adjust to the losses related to the disease process while helping to maximize functioning and quality of life. The symptoms of multiple myeloma go through remission and exacerbation periods. Consequently, acute care is needed at various times during the course of the illness. The final, acute phase is unresponsive to treatment and usually short. The way in which patients and families deal with confronting death may be affected by the manner in which they learned to accept and live with the chronic nature of the disease.

Disorders of the Spleen

The spleen can be affected by many illnesses, most of which cause some degree of *splenomegaly* (enlarged spleen) (Table 33-33). The

Table 33-33 Causes of Splenomegaly	
Hereditary Hemolytic Anemias	• Fungal infections: histoplasmosis
• Sickle cell disease	• Systemic lupus erythematosus, rheumatoid arthritis
• Thalassemia	
Autoimmune Cytopenias	***Infiltrative Diseases***
• Acquired hemolytic anemia	• Acute and chronic leukemia
• Immune thrombocytopenia	• Lymphomas
Infections and Inflammations	• Polycythemia vera
• Bacterial infections: endocarditis	• Multiple myeloma, amyloidosis
• Mycobacterial infections: tuberculosis	• Other primary or secondary neoplasms and cysts
• Spirochetes: syphilis, Lyme disease	• Sarcoidosis
• Viral infections: hepatitis, human immunodeficiency virus, cytomegalovirus, mononucleosis	***Congestion***
	• Cirrhosis of the liver
• Parasitic infections: malaria, trypanosomiasis, schistosomiasis, leishmaniasis, toxoplasmosis,	• Heart failure
	• Portal or splenic vein thrombosis
• Rickettsial infections: Rocky Mountain spotted fever, typhoid fever	

term *hypersplenism* refers to the occurrence of splenomegaly and peripheral cytopenias (anemia, leukopenia, and thrombocytopenia). The degree of splenic enlargement varies with the disease. For example, massive splenic enlargement occurs with chronic myelogenous leukemia, hairy cell leukemia, and thalassemia major. Mild splenic enlargement occurs with HF and systemic lupus erythematosus.

When the spleen enlarges, its normal filtering and sequestering capacity increases. Consequently, there is often a reduction in the number of circulating blood cells. In addition, there are unusual findings in the peripheral smear, such as pitted or pocked erythrocytes or Howell-Jolly bodies. These findings assist with diagnosing a malfunctioning spleen. A slight to moderate enlargement of the spleen is usually asymptomatic and found during a routine examination of the abdomen. Even massive splenomegaly can be well tolerated, but the patient may complain of abdominal discomfort and early satiety. In addition to physical examination, other techniques to assess the size of the spleen include technetium-99m (^{99m}Tc)-sulphur colloid liver–spleen scan, CT scan, MRI, and ultrasound scan.

Occasionally, laparotomy and splenectomy are indicated in the evaluation or treatment of splenomegaly. Splenectomy can have a dramatic effect in increasing peripheral RBC, WBC, and platelet counts. Another major indication for splenectomy is splenic rupture. The spleen may rupture from trauma, inadvertent tearing during other surgical procedures, and diseases such as mononucleosis, malaria, and lymphoid neoplasms.

Nursing responsibilities for the patient with spleen disorders vary depending on the nature of the problem. Splenomegaly may be painful and may necessitate analgesic administration; care in moving, turning, and positioning; and evaluation of lung expansion because spleen enlargement may impair diaphragmatic excursion. If anemia, thrombocytopenia, or leukopenia develops from splenic enlargement, nursing measures must be instituted to support the patient and prevent life-threatening complications. If splenectomy is performed, the nurse must provide the meticulous care warranted after any surgery. In addition, there must be special observation for hemorrhage, which could lead to shock, fever, and abdominal distension.

After splenectomy, immunological deficiencies may develop. IgM levels are reduced, and IgG and IgA values remain within normal limits. Patients who have had splenectomy have a lifelong risk for infection, especially from encapsulated organisms such as pneumococcus. This risk is reduced by immunization with pneumococcal vaccine (e.g., Pneumovax).

Blood Component Therapy

Blood component therapy is frequently used in managing hematological diseases. Many therapeutic and surgical procedures depend on blood product support. However, blood component therapy only temporarily supports the patient and is used in the interim until the underlying problem is resolved. Because transfusions are not free from hazards, they should be used only if necessary. The research regarding RBC substitutes is ongoing. To reduce the use of blood products, antifibrinolytic agents and other products may be used in some situations. Nurses must be careful to avoid developing a complacent attitude about this common but potentially dangerous therapy. The nurse also must make sure that the physician has discussed the risks and benefits and alternatives with the patient and that this is documented in the patient's medical record.

Traditionally, the term *blood transfusion* meant the administration of whole blood. Blood transfusion now has a broader meaning because of the ability to administer specific components of blood such as platelets, packed red blood cells (PRBCs), or plasma. Usually, a specific component is ordered, although whole blood may be used rarely with massive hemorrhage or for an exchange transfusion (Table 33-34).

After the Canadian blood supply was found to be tainted with viruses in the 1980s, a government inquiry known as the Krever Commission (1997) led to a new federally mandated and regulated system (Ministry of Health, 1997). For example, in Canada, all blood is tested for viruses such as HIV and hepatitis as well as other infectious organisms. Strict donor screening now takes place to reduce risk of transfusion-transmitted infection. Although the blood supply in Canada is very safe, the Krever Commission recommended recipients be informed of the benefits, risks, and alternatives to receiving donor blood products. The new federal standards on blood and blood components are relevant to nursing policy and practice because they highlight critical areas such as proper patient and product identification as well as careful monitoring of patients receiving blood products.

Administration Procedure

Blood components are usually administered with at least a 19-gauge needle. Larger needles (e.g., 18- or 16-gauge) may be preferred if rapid transfusions are given. Smaller needles can be used for platelets, albumin, and clotting factor replacement. Whatever type of venous access used, it is important to assess patency prior to requesting the blood component from the blood bank. Most blood product administration tubing is of a "Y type" with a microaggregate filter (filters out particulate) with one branch of the Y for the isotonic saline solution and the other branch for the blood product.

> **SAFETY ALERT**
> - Do not use dextrose solutions or lactated Ringer's solution for administering blood because they will cause RBC hemolysis.
> - Do not give any additives (including medications) via the same tubing as the blood unless the tubing is first cleared with saline solution.

When the blood or blood components have been obtained from the blood bank, positive identification of the blood donor and the recipient must be made. Improper product–to–patient identification causes 90% of hemolytic transfusion reactions, thus placing a great responsibility on nursing personnel to carry out the identification procedure appropriately. The nurse must follow the policy and procedures of the institution where care is being provided; many institutions have implemented a dual-checking system with two licensed individuals checking patient identification with the labelled blood component. The blood bank is responsible for typing and crossmatching the donor's blood with the recipient's blood; the result of the compatibility testing should be noted on the product bag or tag, if pertinent. The nurse must make sure that the patient understands the procedure and the signs and symptoms to report and that he or she agrees with the treatment plan. The nurse takes the patient's vital signs before the beginning of the transfusion to obtain a baseline measure; if the patient has abnormal vital signs, such as an elevated fever, the clinician is called to clarify when the blood component may be administered. The blood should be administered as soon as it is brought to the patient. No blood products are to be refrigerated on the nursing unit in food or drug refrigerators because the temperature does not meet the temperature-range requirements for safe storage. If products are not used right away (i.e., within 30 minutes of being issued), they should be returned to the blood bank. During the first 15 minutes or 50 mL of blood infusion, the nurse should remain with the patient. If there are any untoward reactions, they are most likely to occur at this time. The rate of infusion during this period should be no more than 2 mL/min. PRBCs should not be infused quickly unless an emergency exists. Rapid infusion of cold blood may cause the patient to become chilled. If rapid replacement of large amounts of blood is necessary, a blood-warming device may be used. Other blood components, such as fresh-frozen plasma and platelets, may be infused over 15 to 30 minutes.

After the first 15 minutes, vital signs are usually retaken, and the rate of infusion is governed by the clinical condition of the patient and the product being infused. Observe the patient periodically throughout the transfusion (e.g., every 30 minutes) and up to 1 hour after the transfusion. Most patients not in danger of fluid overload can tolerate the infusion of 1 unit of PRBCs over 2 hours. The transfusion should not take more than 4 hours to administer because of the increased risk of bacterial growth in the product once it is out of refrigeration. Blood left unrefrigerated for 4 hours or longer should not be infused and should be returned to the blood bank.

Blood Transfusion Reactions

A *blood transfusion reaction* is an adverse reaction to blood transfusion therapy that can range in severity from mild symptoms to a

Table 33-34 Blood Products*

DESCRIPTION	SPECIAL CONSIDERATIONS	INDICATIONS FOR USE
Packed Red Blood Cells		
Packed RBCs are prepared from whole blood by sedimentation or centrifugation. One unit contains 250-350 mL.	• Use of RBCs for treatment allows remaining components of blood (e.g., platelets, albumin, plasma) to be used for other purposes. There is less danger of fluid overload. • Leukocyte depletion (by the blood bank or with a filter) may be used to reduce hemolytic febrile reactions in patients who receive frequent transfusion.	Severe or symptomatic anemia; acute blood loss. In general, 1 unit of packed red blood cells can be expected to increase a patient's hemoglobin level by 10 g/L or the Hct by 30%
Frozen Red Blood Cells		
Frozen RBCs are prepared from RBCs using glycerol for protection and frozen.	They must be used within 24 hr of thawing. Successive washings with saline solution remove the majority of WBCs and plasma proteins.	Autotransfusion; stockpiling or rare donors for patients with allobodies. Infrequently used because filters remove most WBCs.
Platelets		
Platelets are prepared from fresh whole blood within 4 hr after collection. One unit contains 30-60 mL of platelet concentrate.	Multiple units of platelets can be obtained from one donor by platelet pheresis. Expected increase is 10,000 microlitres per unit. Failure to obtain a rise may be caused by fever, sepsis, splenomegaly, or DIC. For patients who receive frequent transfusions or who have not responded to previous platelet transfusions, platelets that are leukocyte-reduced or HLA- or type-specific may be given to prevent alloimmunization to HLA antigens.	Bleeding caused by thrombocytopenia or platelet levels $<10\text{-}20 \times 10^9$/L; use may be contraindicated in the presence of thrombocytopenic purpura, thrombotic thrombocytopenic purpura, and heparin-induced thrombocytopenia except for life-threatening hemorrhage
Fresh-Frozen Plasma		
Liquid portion of whole blood is separated from cells and frozen. One unit contains 200-250 mL. Plasma is rich in clotting factors but contains no platelets. It must be used within 2 hr after thawing.	Use of plasma in treating hypovolemic shock is being replaced by use of pure preparations such as albumin plasma expanders.	Bleeding caused by deficiency in clotting factors (e.g., DIC, hemorrhage, massive transfusion, liver disease, vitamin K deficiency, excess warfarin)
Albumin		
Albumin is prepared from plasma. It is available in 5% or 25% solution.	Albumin 25 g/100 mL is osmotically equal to 500 mL of plasma. Hyperosmolar solution acts by moving water from extravascular to intravascular space. It is heat treated and does not transmit viruses.	Hypovolemic shock, hypoalbuminemia
Cryoprecipitates and Commercial Concentrates		
Cryoprecipitate is prepared from fresh-frozen plasma, with 10-20 mL/bag. Once thawed, it must be used.	See Table 33-19.	Replacement of clotting factors, especially Factor VIII and fibrinogen

DIC, disseminated intravascular coagulation; *Hct,* hematocrit; *HLA,* human leukocyte antigen; *RBCs,* red blood cells; *WBCs,* white blood cells.
*Component therapy has replaced the use of whole blood, which accounts for < 10% of all transfusions. Granulocyte transfusions are not included here because they are rarely used.

life-threatening condition. Because complications of transfusion therapy may be significant, judicious evaluation of the patient is required. Blood transfusion reactions can be classified as acute or delayed (Tables 33-35 and 33-36).

If an *acute transfusion reaction* occurs, the following steps should be taken: (1) stop the transfusion; (2) maintain a patent IV line with saline solution; (3) notify the blood bank and the health care provider immediately; (4) recheck identifying tags and numbers; (5) monitor vital signs and urine output; (6) treat symptoms as per physician order; (7) save and return the blood bag and tubing to the blood bank for examination; (8) collect blood and urine samples at intervals as stipulated by hospital policy to evaluate for hemolysis; and (9) document the incident (and Steps 1-8) on a transfusion reaction form and the patient chart. The blood bank and laboratory are responsible for identifying the type of reaction.

Acute Transfusion Reactions

Acute Hemolytic Reactions. The most common cause of hemolytic reactions is transfusion of ABO-incompatible blood (see Table 33-36). This is an example of a Type II cytotoxic hypersensitivity reaction (see Chapter 16). Severe hemolytic reactions are rare. Mislabelling specimens and administering blood to the wrong individual cause most acute hemolytic reactions. This again points to the importance of the use of proper patient identifiers when drawing blood samples and when administering medications and blood products.

When an acute hemolytic reaction occurs, antibodies in the recipient's serum react with antigens on the donor's RBCs. This results in agglutination of cells, which can obstruct capillaries and block blood flow. Hemolysis of the RBCs releases free Hb into the plasma. The Hb is filtered by the kidney and may be found

Table 33-35 Acute Transfusion Reactions

CAUSE	CLINICAL MANIFESTATIONS	MANAGEMENT	PREVENTION
Acute Hemolytic Reaction			
Infusion of ABO-incompatible whole blood, RBCs, or components containing 10 mL or more of RBCs Antibodies in the recipient's plasma attach to antigens on transfused RBCs causing RBC destruction	Chills, fever, low back pain, flushing, tachycardia, tachypnea, hypotension, vascular collapse, hemoglobinuria, acute jaundice, dark urine, bleeding, acute renal failure, shock, cardiac arrest, death	Treat shock and DIC if present. Draw blood samples for serological testing slowly to avoid hemolysis. Send urine specimen to the laboratory. Maintain BP with IV colloid solutions. Give diuretics as prescribed to maintain urine flow. Insert in-dwelling urinary catheter or measure voided amounts to monitor hourly urine output. Dialysis may be required if renal failure or AKI occurs. Do not transfuse additional RBC-containing components until blood bank has provided newly crossmatched units.	Meticulously verify and document patient identification at each step from sample collection to component infusion.
Febrile, Nonhemolytic Reaction (Most Common)			
Sensitization to donor WBCs, platelets, or plasma proteins	Sudden chills and fever (rise in temperature of >1°C), headache, flushing, anxiety, vomiting, muscle pain	Give antipyretics as prescribed—avoid aspirin in patients with thrombocytopenia. *Do not restart transfusion* unless physician so orders.	Consider leukocyte-poor blood products (filtered, washed, or frozen) for patients with a history of two or more such reactions.
Mild Allergic Reaction			
Sensitivity to foreign plasma proteins	Flushing, itching, urticaria (hives)	Give antihistamine as directed. If symptoms are mild and transient, transfusion may be restarted slowly. Do not restart transfusion if fever or pulmonary symptoms develop.	Treat prophylactically with antihistamines. Consider using washed RBCs and platelets.
Anaphylactic and Severe Allergic Reaction			
Sensitivity to donor plasma proteins Infusion of IgA proteins to IgA-deficient recipient who has developed IgA antibody	Anxiety, urticaria, dyspnea, wheezing, progressing to cyanosis, bronchospasm, hypotension, shock, and possible cardiac arrest	Initiate CPR, if indicated. *Do not restart transfusion.*	Transfuse extensively washed RBC products, from which all plasma has been removed. Use blood from IgA-deficient donor. Use autologous components.
Circulatory Overload Reaction			
Fluid administered faster than the circulation can accommodate.	Cough, dyspnea, pulmonary congestion, headache, hypertension, tachycardia, distended neck veins	Place patient upright with feet in dependent position. Administer prescribed diuretics, oxygen, and/or morphine.	Adjust transfusion volume and flow rate based on patient size and clinical status. Have blood bank divide unit into smaller aliquots for better spacing of fluid input.
Sepsis Reaction			
Transfusion of bacterially infected blood components	Rapid onset of chills, high fever, vomiting, diarrhea, marked hypotension, or shock	Obtain culture of patient's blood and send bag with remaining blood and tubing to blood bank for further study. Treat septicemia as directed—administration of antibiotics, IV fluids, and/or vasopressors.	Collect, process, store, and transfuse blood products according to blood banking standards, and infuse within 4 hr of starting time.
Transfusion-Related Acute Lung Injury (TRALI) Reaction			
Reaction between transfused antileukocyte antibodies and recipient's leukocytes, causing pulmonary inflammation and capillary leak	Fever, hypotension, tachypnea, dyspnea, decreased oxygen saturation, frothy sputum	Send bag with remaining blood and tubing to blood bank for further study; draw blood to analyse arterial blood gases and HLA or antileukocyte antibodies; obtain chest radiograph. Provide oxygen and administer corticosteroids (diuretics of no value). Initiate CPR if needed, and provide ventilatory and blood pressure support if needed.	Provide leukocyte-reduced products. Identify donors who are implicated in TRALI reactions, and do not allow them to donate.

AKI, acute kidney injury; *BP*, blood pressure; *CPR*, cardiopulmonary resuscitation; *DIC*, disseminated intravascular coagulation; *HLA*, human leukocyte antigen; *IgA*, immunoglobulin A; *IV*, intravenous; *RBC*, red blood cell; *WBC*, white blood cell.

Table 33-36 Delayed Transfusion Reactions

REACTION	CLINICAL MANIFESTATIONS
Delayed hemolytic	Fever, mild jaundice, decreased hematocrit. Occurs as early as 3 days or as late as several months, but usually 5-10 days post-transfusion as the result of destruction of transfused RBCs by alloantibodies not detected during crossmatch. Generally, no acute treatment is required, but hemolysis may be severe enough to warrant further transfusions.
Hepatitis B*	Elevated liver enzymes (AST and ALT), anorexia, malaise, nausea and vomiting, fever, dark urine, jaundice. Usually resolves spontaneously within 4-6 wk. Chronic carrier state can develop and can result in permanent liver damage. Treat symptomatically. (See Chapter 46.)
Hepatitis C*	Similar to hepatitis B, but symptoms are usually less severe. Chronic liver disease and cirrhosis may develop. Before introduction of anti-HCV test, accounted for 90-95% of all post-transfusion hepatitis. Treat symptomatically. (See Chapter 46.)
Iron overload	Excess iron is deposited in the heart, liver, pancreas, and joints, causing dysfunction. Heart failure, dysrhythmias, impaired thyroid and gonadal function, diabetes, arthritis, and cirrhosis can occur. Commonly occurs in patients receiving >100 units for chronic anemia (e.g., sickle cell) over a period of time. Treat symptomatically. Deferoxamine (Desferal), which chelates and removes accumulated iron via the kidneys, may be administered by IV or subQ route.
Other	Other infectious diseases and agents may be transmitted via transfusion, including cytomegalovirus, HTLV-1, and those causing malaria.

ALT, alanine aminotransferase; *AST,* aspartate aminotransferase; *HCV,* hepatitis C virus; *HTLV-1,* human T-cell leukemia virus, type 1; *IV,* intravenous; *RBCs,* red blood cells; *subQ,* subcutaneous.
*New cases of transfusion-related hepatitis B and C are not common.

in the urine (hemoglobinuria). Hb may obstruct the renal tubules, leading to acute kidney injury, DIC, and death (see Chapter 49).

The clinical manifestations of an acute hemolytic reaction may be mild or severe and usually develop within the first 15 minutes of transfusion. Free Hb in blood and urine specimens obtained at the onset of the reaction will provide evidence of an acute hemolytic reaction. Delayed transfusion reactions are defined as those occurring 24 hours to 14 days after the administration of blood.

Febrile Reactions. Febrile reactions are most commonly caused by leukocyte incompatibility. Many individuals who receive five or more transfusions develop circulating antibodies to the small amount of WBCs in the blood product. Febrile reactions can often be prevented by using additional filters in the tubing to leukocyte-deplete RBCs and platelets. Donated blood in Canada is processed to reduce the number of circulating WBCs (i.e., leukodepleted), which has helped reduce the incidence of the febrile nonhemolytic and minor allergic reactions. Medications may be ordered before blood administration to reduce these reactions. Generally, this includes acetaminophen and diphenhydramine (Benadryl) given 30 minutes before the transfusion.

Allergic Reactions. Allergic reactions result from the recipient's sensitivity to plasma proteins of the donor's blood. These reactions are more common in an individual with a history of allergies. Antihistamines may be used to prevent allergic reactions. Epinephrine or corticosteroids may be used to treat a severe reaction.

Circulatory Overload. An individual with cardiac or renal insufficiency is at risk for developing circulatory overload. This is especially true if a large quantity of blood is infused in a short period, particularly in an older adult. PRBCs can be split by the blood bank, allowing for one half of a unit to be given over a time frame of up to 4 hours. A fluid balance assessment, including baseline auscultation of the patient's lungs, is performed. Complaints of shortness of breath and the presence of adventitious breath sounds may indicate fluid overload in any patient.

Sepsis. Blood products can become infected from improper handling and storage. Bacterial contamination of blood products can result in bacteremia, sepsis, or septic shock.

Transfusion-related Acute Lung Injury. Transfusion-related acute lung injury (TRALI) is characterized by the sudden development of noncardiogenic pulmonary edema (acute lung injury). It usually occurs within hours of the transfusion of blood products (Gilliss, Looney, & Gropper, 2011). With the reduction of clerical errors, leukocyte-reduced products, more effective screening, and the prevention of the transmission of infectious agents, TRALI has surpassed hemolytic reactions as the leading cause of transfusion-related death. It is thought to be caused by an antibody-mediated reaction between the recipient's leukocytes and antileukocyte antibodies from donors who were sensitized during pregnancy or by previous transfusions. This causes pulmonary capillary inflammation and increased permeability, leading to respiratory distress and potentially death.

Massive Blood Transfusion Reaction. An acute complication of transfusing large volumes of blood products is termed *massive blood transfusion reaction.* Massive blood transfusion reactions can occur when replacement of RBCs or blood exceeds the total blood volume within 24 hours. In this situation, an imbalance of normal blood elements results because clotting factors, albumin, and platelets are not found in RBC transfusions. Thus, appropriate monitoring of hemostatic laboratory parameters must be done concurrently.

Additional problems such as hypothermia, citrate toxicity, hypocalcemia, and hyperkalemia may occur when massive blood transfusions are given. Hypothermia and cardiac dysrhythmias can result from rapid infusion of large quantities of cold blood. Blood-warming equipment prevents this problem. Citrate toxicity can occur when large quantities of blood products are used because citrate is part of the storage solution; calcium binds to the citrate (Sihler & Napolitano, 2010). Citrate toxicity is likely to develop when blood is transfused at a rate of 1 unit in 10 minutes (or 8-10 units of RBCs within a few hours). Manifestations such as muscle tremors and ECG changes may be observed with hypocalcemia but can be prevented or reversed by the infusion of 10% calcium gluconate (10 mL with every litre of citrated blood). Hyperkalemia results when potassium leaks from RBCs in stored blood. Mild to severe signs and symptoms can occur, including nausea, muscle weakness, diarrhea, paresthesias, flaccid paralysis of the cardiac or respiratory muscles, and cardiac arrest. Electrolyte monitoring is an important aspect of the care of the patient receiving massive transfusions of blood products.

Delayed Transfusion Reactions.
Delayed transfusion reactions include delayed hemolytic reactions (discussed previously), infections, and iron overload (see Table 33-36).

Infection. Infectious agents transmitted by blood transfusion include hepatitis B and C viruses, HIV, human herpesvirus type 6 (HSV-6), EBV, HTLV-1, cytomegalovirus (CMV), and malaria. Hepatitis is still the most common viral infection transmitted, although its incidence is decreasing. Hepatitis B virus can be detected in the blood by the presence of hepatitis B surface antigen (HBsAg). A test for hepatitis C antibodies in donor blood is used to exclude the use of any donated blood testing positive for hepatitis C. Therefore, the risk of transmission of hepatitis C has been reduced. Leukocyte-reduced blood products drastically reduce the risk of blood transfusion–associated viral infections, including CMV.

In the past, HIV was transmitted by contaminated blood and blood products. This posed a serious problem for an individual who received infected transfusions. Patients with hemophilia who received antihemophilic factors that had been prepared from pooled plasma of a large number of donors, of whom some donors were infected, have a high rate of HIV infection from transfusion sources. At present, the use of recombinant antihemophilic factors, donor education, donor screening, and HIV-antibody testing has greatly reduced the transmission of HIV by blood transfusion or factor replacement therapy.

Autotransfusion

Autotransfusion, or autologous transfusion, consists of removing whole blood from a person and transfusing that blood back into the same person. The problems of incompatibility, allergic reactions, and transmission of disease can be avoided. Methods of autotransfusion include the following:

- *Autologous donation or elective phlebotomy* (predeposit transfusion). A person donates blood before a planned surgical procedure. The blood can be frozen and stored for up to 10 years. Usually, the blood is stored without being frozen and is given to the person within a few weeks of donation. This technique is especially beneficial to the patient with a rare blood type or for any patient who might be expected to require limited blood product support during a major surgical procedure (e.g., elective orthopedic surgery).

- *Autotransfusion.* A newer method for replacing blood volume involves safely and aseptically collecting, filtering, and returning the patient's own blood that is lost during a major surgical procedure or from a traumatic injury. This system was originally developed in response to patients' concerns about the safety of blood from blood products. However, today it provides an important way to safely replace volume and stabilize the condition of bleeding patients. Collection devices are most often used during surgeries. Some systems allow blood to be automatically and continuously reinfused; others require collection for some period (usually no longer than 4 hours), after which the blood is reinfused. Hospitals in Canada are now required to have a blood conservation program in place.

CLINICAL DECISION-MAKING EXERCISE

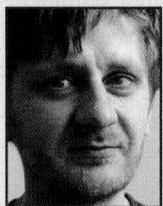

CASE STUDY:
Leukemia
Source: ©iStockphoto.com/Beata Pastuszek.

Patient Profile
Viktor Varga, a 35-year-old White man, went to the emergency department because of severe bruising caused by a fall while hiking.

Subjective Data
- Complains of oral pain and white patches covering his tongue
- Has had a 2-month history of fatigue, malaise, and flu symptoms
- Complains of shortness of breath and while doing activities that previously required no exertion
- Has taken numerous prescribed antibiotics and increased rest and sleep in the past 2 months without relief of symptoms

Objective Data
Physical Examination
- Has bruises and ecchymoses from fall
- Gingiva has petechiae and patchy white spots
- Temperature 39°C, respiratory rate 26/min, pulse 110
- Has splenomegaly

Laboratory Results
- Hematocrit 0.2
- White blood cell (WBC) count 120×10^9/L
- Hemoglobin (Hb) 6.9 mmol/L
- Platelet count 25×10^9/L

Bone Marrow Biopsy
- Multiple myeloblasts (>50%)

Discussion Questions
1. What components of the laboratory test results suggest acute leukemia?
2. How is acute myelogenous leukemia treated?
3. What is the prognosis for Viktor?
4. What are the life-threatening problems that can occur as a result of this disease and treatment? How can the nurse anticipate and assess for these problems?
5. *Priority Decision:* What are the priority nursing interventions?
6. *Priority Decision:* What are the priorities for patient teaching with a newly diagnosed young adult with leukemia?
7. *Priority Decision:* Based on the assessment data presented, what are the priority nursing diagnoses? Are there any collaborative problems?

ⓔvolve *Answers are available at* **http://evolve.elsevier.com/ Canada/Lewis/medsurg**

REVIEW QUESTIONS

The number of the question corresponds to the same-numbered objective at the beginning of the chapter.

1. What signs and symptoms would the nurse expect to find in a severely anemic patient?
   a. Dyspnea and tachycardia
   b. Cyanosis and pulmonary edema
   c. Cardiomegaly and pulmonary fibrosis
   d. Ventricular dysrhythmias and wheezing

2. When obtaining assessment data from a patient with a microcytic, normochromic anemia, what would the nurse question the patient about?
   a. Folic acid intake
   b. Dietary intake of iron
   c. A history of gastric surgery
   d. A history of sickle cell anemia

3. Which of the following is a nursing intervention for a patient with severe anemia related to chronic kidney disease?
   a. Monitoring stools for guaiac
   b. Instructions in high-iron diet
   c. Monitoring urine intake and output
   d. Teaching self-injection of erythropoietin

4. Which of the following is included in the nursing management of a patient in sickle cell crisis?
   a. Bed rest and heparin therapy
   b. Blood transfusions and iron replacement
   c. Aggressive analgesic and oxygen therapy
   d. Platelet administration and monitoring of complete blood count

5. What is a complication of the hyperviscosity of polycythemia?
   a. Thrombosis
   b. Cardiomyopathy
   c. Pulmonary edema
   d. Disseminated intravascular coagulation (DIC)

6. What instructions does the nurse give the patient with thrombocytopenia?
   a. Wipe her or his nose gently instead of blowing.
   b. Be careful when shaving with a safety razor.
   c. Continue with physical activities to stimulate thrombopoiesis.
   d. Avoid aspirin because it may mask the fever that occurs with thrombocytopenia.

7. The nurse would anticipate that a patient with von Willebrand's disease who is undergoing surgery would be treated with administration of von Willebrand's factor (vWF) as well as which of the following?
   a. Thrombin
   b. Factor VI
   c. Factor VII
   d. Factor VIII

8. Which of the following best describes DIC?
   a. The coagulation pathway is genetically altered, leading to thrombus formation in all major blood vessels.
   b. An underlying disease depletes hemolytic factors in the blood, leading to diffuse thrombotic episodes and infarcts.
   c. A disease process stimulates coagulation processes with resultant depletion of clotting factors, leading to diffuse clotting and hemorrhage.
   d. An inherited predisposition causes a deficiency of clotting factors that leads to overstimulation of coagulation processes in the vasculature.

9. Which of the following are appropriate nursing actions when caring for a hospitalized patient with severe neutropenia?
   a. Perirectal care and platelet administration
   b. Oral care and red blood cell administration
   c. Monitoring lung sounds and invasive monitoring of blood pressure
   d. Strict adherence to handwashing practices and frequent temperature assessment

10. Because myelodysplastic syndrome arises from the pluripotent hematopoietic stem cell in the bone marrow, what laboratory results would the nurse expect to find?
    a. An excess of T cells
    b. An excess of platelets
    c. A deficiency of granulocytes
    d. A deficiency of all cellular blood components

11. Which is the most common type of leukemia in older adults?
    a. Acute myelocytic leukemia
    b. Acute lymphocytic leukemia
    c. Chronic lymphocytic leukemia
    d. Chronic granulocytic leukemia

12. Why are multiple drugs primarily used in combinations to treat leukemia and lymphoma?
    a. There are fewer toxic and adverse effects.
    b. The chance that one drug will be effective is increased.
    c. They can interrupt cell growth at multiple points in the cell cycle.
    d. They are more effective and have fewer exacerbating adverse effects.

13. What is a major difference between Hodgkin's lymphoma and non-Hodgkin's lymphoma?
    a. Hodgkin's lymphoma occurs only in young adults.
    b. Hodgkin's lymphoma is considered potentially curable.
    c. Non-Hodgkin's lymphoma can manifest in multiple organs.
    d. Non-Hodgkin's lymphoma is treated only with radiation therapy.

14. A patient with multiple myeloma becomes confused and lethargic. Which of the following explain these clinical manifestations?
    a. Hyperkalemia
    b. Hyperuricemia
    c. Hypercalcemia
    d. Central nervous system myeloma

15. What would the nurse expect to find when reviewing the patient's hematological laboratory values after a splenectomy?
    a. Leukopenia
    b. Red blood cell abnormalities
    c. Decreased hemoglobin
    d. Increased platelet count

16. Which of the following complications of transfusions can be decreased by the use of leukocyte reduction filters for red blood cells and platelets?
    a. Chills, rigors, back pain
    b. Leukostasis and neutrophilia
    c. Fluid overload and pulmonary edema
    d. Transmission of cytomegalovirus and alloimmunization

ANSWERS: 1. a; 2. b; 3. d; 4. c; 5. a; 6. a; 7. d; 8. c; 9. d; 10. d; 11. c; 12. c; 13. b; 14. c; 15. d; 16. d.

REFERENCES

Adamson, J. W. (2008). The anemia of inflammation/malignancy: Mechanisms and management. *Hematology: American Society of Hematology Education Program Book, 1*, 159-165.

Alpers, D. H., Stenson, W. F., Taylor, B. E., & Bier, D. M. (2008). *Manual of nutritional therapeutics* (5th ed.). Philadelphia: Lippincott Williams & Wilkins.

Andrès, E., Fothergill, H., & Mecili, M. (2010). Efficacy of oral cobalamin (vitamin B_{12}) therapy. *Expert Opinion on Pharmacotherapy, 11*(2), 249-256. doi:10.1517/14656560903456053

Antony, A. C. (2009). Megaloblastic anemias. In R. Hoffman, E. Benz, S. J. Shattil, B. Furie, H. J. Cohen, L. E. Silberstein, ..., J. Anastasi (Eds.), *Hematology: Basic principles and practice* (5th ed.). Philadelphia: Churchill Livingstone.

Bacigalupo, A., & Passweg, J. (2009). Diagnosis and treatment of acquired aplastic anemia. *Hematology Oncology Clinics of North America, 23*, 159-170. doi:10.1016/j.hoc.2009.01.005

Baldwin, Z. K., Spitzer, A. L., Ng, V. L., & Harken, A. H. (2008). Contemporary standards for the diagnosis and treatment of heparin-induced thrombocytopenia (HIT). *Surgery, 143*(3), 305-312. doi:10.1016/j.surg.2007.09.036

Barzi, A., & Sekeres, M. A. (2010). Myelodysplastic syndromes: A practical approach to diagnosis and treatment. *Cleveland Clinic Journal of Medicine, 77*(1), 37-44. doi:10.3949/ccjm.77a.09069

Bird, J. M., Owen, R. G., D'Sa, S., Snowden, J. A., Pratt, G., Ashcroft, J., ..., Behrens, J. (2011). Guidelines for the diagnosis and management of multiple myeloma 2011. *British Journal of Hematology, 154*, 32-75. doi:10.1111/j.1365-2141.2011.08573.x

Canadian Cancer Society/National Cancer Institute of Canada/Public Health Agency of Canada/Statistics Canada. (2008). *Canadian cancer statistics*. Retrieved from *http://www.cancer.ca*

Canadian Cancer Society's Steering Committee on Cancer Statistics. (2012). *Canadian Cancer Statistics 2012*. Toronto, ON: Canadian Cancer Society.

Canadian Hemochromatosis Society. (2012). *Hemochromatosis—Canada's most common genetic disorder*. Retrieved from *http://www.cdnhemochromatosis.ca*

Canadian Hemophilia Society. (2012). An introduction to von Willebrand disease. Retrieved from *http://www.hemophilia.ca/en/bleeding-disorders/von-willebrand-disease/an-introduction-to-von-willebrand-disease/*

Cashen, A. F., & Bartlett, N. L. (2008). Salvage regimens of Hodgkin lymphoma. *Clinical Advances in Hematology & Oncology, 6*(7), 517-524.

den Elzen, W. P., Willems, J. M., Westendorp, R. G., de Craen, A. J., Assendelft, W. J., & Gussekloo, J. (2009). Effect of anemia and comorbidity on functional status and mortality in old age: Results from the Leiden 85-plus Study. *CMAJ 181*(3-4), 151-157. doi:10.1503/cmaj.090040

Dokal, I., & Vulliamy, T. (2008). Inherited aplastic anaemias/bone marrow failure syndromes. *Blood Review, 22*(3), 141-153. doi:10.1002/9781444323160.ch12

Dronca, R. S., & Steensma, D. P. (2008). VTE and mortality associated with erythropoiesis-stimulation agents in cancer-associated anemia. *Nature Reviews Clinical Oncology, 5*(9), 504-505. doi:10.1038/ncponc1202

Gardenghi, S., Grady, R. W., & Rivella, S., (2010). Anemia, ineffective erythropoiesis, and hepcidin: Interacting factors in abnormal iron metabolism leading to iron overload in B-thalassemia. *Hematology Oncology Clinics of North America, 24*, 1089-1107. doi:10.1016/j.hoc.2010.08.003

Gazit, R., Weissman, I. L., & Rossi, D. J. (2008). Hematopoietic stem cells and the aging hematopoietic system. *Seminars in Hematology, 45*, 218. doi:10.1053/j.seminhematol.2008.07.010

Gilliss, B. M., Looney, M. R., & Gropper, M. A. (2011). Reducing non-infectious risks of blood transfusion. *Anesthesiology, 115*(3), 635-649. doi:10.1097/ALN.0b013e31822a22d9

Gladwin, M. T., & Vichinsky, E. (2008). Pulmonary complications of sickle cell disease. *New England Journal of Medicine, 359*, 2254-2265. doi:10.1056/NEJMra0804411

Haase, D. (2008). Cytogenetic features in myelodysplastic syndromes (MDS). *Seminars in Oncology, 87*, 515-526.

Hoffbrand, A. V., & Moss, P. A. H. (2011). *Essential haematology* (6th ed.). Malden, MA: Wiley-Blackwell.

Howard, M. R., & Hamilton, P. J. (2008). *Haematology: An illustrated colour text* (3rd ed.). Edinburgh: Churchill Livingstone.

Khambalia, A. Z., Aimone, A. M., & Zlotkin, S. H. (2011). Burden of anemia among indigenous populations. *Nutrition Reviews, 69*(12), 693-719. doi:10.1111/j.1753-4887.2011.00437.x

Kremer Hovinga, J. A., & Meyer, S. C. (2008). Current management of thrombotic thrombocytopenic purpura. *Current Opinion in Hematology, 15*(5), 445-450. doi:10.1097/MOH.0b013e328309ec62

Lanzkron, S., Strouse, J. J., Wilson, R., Beach, M. C., Haywood, C., Park, H., ..., Segal, J. B. (2008). Systematic review: Hydroxyurea for the treatment of adults with sickle cell disease. *Annals of Internal Medicine, 148*(12), 939-955.

Lee, A. I., & Okam, I. (2011). Anemia in pregnancy. *Hematology Oncology Clinics of North America, 25*(2), 241-259. doi:10.1016/j.hoc.2011.02.001

Lenting, P. J., Pegon, J. N., Christophe, O. D., & Denis, C. V. (2010). Factor VIII and von Willebrand factor—Too sweet for their own good. *Haemophilia, 16*(Suppl 5), 194-199. doi:10.1111/j.1365-2516.2010.02320.x

Leukemia and Lymphoma Society of Canada. (2011). *Leukemia*. Retrieved from *http://www.llscanada.org/diseaseinformation/getinformationsupport/factsstatistics/leukemia/*

Lukaszewicz, A. C., & Payen, D. (2010). The future is predetermined in severe sepsis, so what are the implications? *Critical Care Medicine, 38*(10), S512-17. doi:10.1097/CCM.0b013e3181f23dc4

Lucarelli, G., & Gaziev, J. (2008). Advances in the allogeneic transplantation for thalassemia. *Blood Reviews, 22*(2), 53-63. doi:10.1016/j.blre.2007.10.001

Marks, P. W., & Glader, B. (2009). Approach to anemia in the adult and child. In R. Hoffman, E. Benz, S. J. Shattil, B. Furie, H. J.

Cohen, L. E. Silberstein, …, J. Anastasi (Eds.), *Hematology: Basic principles and practice* (5th ed.). Philadelphia: Churchill Livingstone.

Matasar, M. J., & Zelenetz, A. D. (2008). Overview of lymphoma diagnosis and management. *Radiology Clinics of North America, 46*(2), 175-198. doi:10.1016/j.rcl.2008.03.005

McGann, P. T., & Ware, R. E. (2011). Hydroxyurea for sickle cell anemia: What have we learned and what questions still remain? *Current Opinion in Hematology 18*(3), 158-165. doi:10.1097/MOH.0b013e32834521dd

Milman, N. (2011). Anemia—Still a major health problem in many parts of the world! *Annals of Hematology, 90*(4), 369-377. doi:10.1007/s00277-010-1144-5

Ministry of Health. (1997). *Commission of inquiry on the blood system in Canada.* Ottawa: Canadian Government Publishing.

Mughal, T., Goldman, J. M., & Mughal, S. T. (2010). *Understanding leukemias, lymphomas, and myelomas* (2nd ed.). London: Informa Healthcare.

Opal, S. M. (2010). Endotoxins and other sepsis triggers. *Contributions to Nephrology, 167,* 14-24.

Ragni, M. V., Kessler, C. M., & Lozier, J. N. (2009). Clinical aspects and therapy for haemophilia. In R. Hoffman, E. Benz, S. J. Shattil, B. Furie, H. J. Cohen, L. E. Silberstein, …, J. Anastasi (Eds.), *Hematology: Basic principles and practice* (5th ed.). Philadelphia: Churchill Livingstone.

Sanz, M. A., & Lo Coco, F. (2011). Modern approaches to treating acute promyelocytic leukemia. *Journal of Clinical Oncology, 29*(5), 495-503. doi:10.1200/JCO.2010.32.1067

Schafer, E., Hunger, S., & Stephen, P. (2011). Optimal therapy for acute lymphoblastic leukemia in adolescents and young adults. *Nature Reviews Clinical Oncology, 8*(7), 417-424. doi:10.1038/nrclinonc.2011.77

Seif, A. E., Reilly, A. F., & Rheingold, S. R. (2010). Intrathecal liposomal cytarabine in relapsed or refractory infant and pediatric leukemias: The Children's Hospital of Philadelphia experience and review of the literature. *Journal of Pediatric Hematology/Oncology, 32*(8), 349-352. doi:10.1097/MPH.0b013e3181ec0c25

Siegel, R., Ward, E., Brawley, O., & Jemal, A. (2011). Cancer statistics, 2011. *CA: A Cancer Journal for Clinicians, 61*(4), 212-236. doi:10.3322/caac.20121

Sihler, K., & Napolitano, L. M. (2010). Complications of massive transfusion. *Chest, 137*(1), 209-220. doi:10.1378/chest.09-0252

Tariman, J. D. (2010). *Multiple myeloma: A textbook for nurses.* Philadelphia: Oncology Nursing Society.

Tefferi, A. (2008). Essential thrombocythemia, polycythemia vera, and myelofibrosis: Current management and the prospect of targeted therapy. *American Journal of Hematology, 83,* 491-497. doi:10.1002/ajh.21183

Villanueva, A., Newell, P., & Hoshida, Y. (2010). Inherited hepatocellular carcinoma. *Best Practice & Research in Clinical Gastroenterology, 24*(5), 725-734. doi:10.1016/j.bpg.2010.07.008

Wada, H., Asakura, H., Okamoto, K., Iba, T., Uchiyama, T., Kawasugi, K., …, Japanese Society of Thrombosis Hemostasis/DIC subcommittee. (2010). Expert consensus for the treatment of disseminated intravascular coagulation in Japan. *Thrombosis Research, 125*(1), 6-11. doi:10.1016/j.thromres.2009.08.017

Weigelt, C., Haas, R., & Kobbe, G. (2011). Pharmacokinetic evaluation of palifermin for mucosal protection from chemotherapy and radiation. *Expert Opinion on Drug Metabolism & Toxicology, 7*(4), 505-515. doi:10.1517/17425255.2011.566556

World Health Organization (WHO). (2012). *Micronutrient deficiencies: Iron deficiency anaemia.* Retrieved from *http://www.who.int/nutrition/topics/ida/en/index.html*

CANADIAN RESOURCES

BC Cancer Agency
http://www.bccancer.bc.ca
Canadian Blood Services
http://www.bloodservices.ca
Canadian Cancer Society
http://www.cancer.ca
Canadian Hemochromatosis Society
http://www.cdnhemochromatosis.ca
Canadian Hemophilia Society
http://www.hemophilia.ca
Cancer Care Ontario
http://www.cancercare.on.ca
Childhood Cancer Foundation Canada
http://www.childhoodcancer.ca
Fanconi Canada
http://www.fanconicanada.org
Leukemia and Lymphoma Society of Canada
http://www.leukemia.ca
Lymphoma Foundation of Canada
http://www.lymphoma.ca
Sickle Cell Association of Ontario
http://www.sicklecellontario.com
Thalassemia Foundation of Canada
http://www.thalassemia.ca

RELATED RESOURCES

National Cancer Institute
http://www.cancer.gov
National Heart, Lung, and Blood Institute
http://www.nhlbi.nih.gov
National Hemophilia Foundation
http://www.hemophilia.org

evolve *For additional Internet resources, see the Web site for this book at* **http://evolve.elsevier.com/Canada/Lewis/medsurg**

Problems of Oxygenation: Perfusion

SECTION OUTLINE

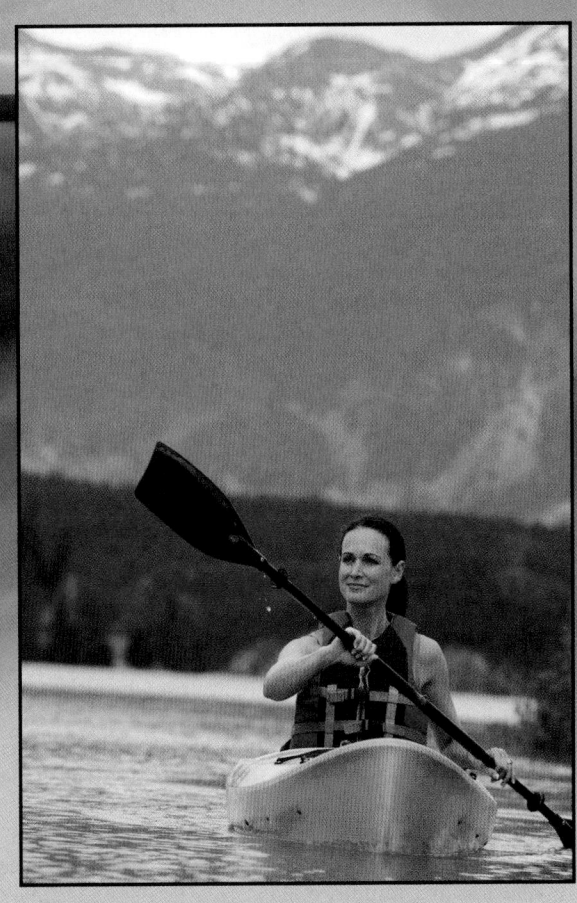

Noel Hendrickson/Digital Vision/Thinkstock

Nursing Assessment: Cardiovascular System

Written by Angela J. DiSabatino and Linda Bucher

Adapted by Sandra Goldsworthy

LEARNING OBJECTIVES

1. Describe the anatomical location and function of the following cardiac structures: pericardial layers, atria, ventricles, semilunar valves, and atrioventricular valves.
2. Describe coronary circulation and the areas of heart muscle supplied by each blood vessel.
3. Explain the normal sequence of events involved in the conduction pathway of the heart.
4. Describe the structure and function of arteries, capillaries, and veins.
5. Define blood pressure and the mechanisms involved in its regulation.
6. Identify the significant subjective and objective assessment data related to the cardiovascular system that should be obtained from a patient.
7. Describe the appropriate techniques used in the physical assessment of the cardiovascular system.
8. Differentiate normal from common abnormal findings of a physical assessment of the cardiovascular system.
9. Describe the age-related changes of the cardiovascular system and differences in assessment findings.
10. Describe the purpose and the significance of results of diagnostic studies of the cardiovascular system and the nursing responsibilities associated with them.
11. Identify waveforms and the associated cardiac events represented on the normal electrocardiogram.

KEY TERMS

afterload The peripheral resistance against which the left ventricle must pump, p. 846

arterial blood pressure (BP) A measure of the pressure exerted by blood against the walls of the arterial system, p. 847

cardiac index (CI) A measure of the cardiac output of a patient per square metre of body surface area, p. 845

cardiac output (CO) The amount of blood pumped by each ventricle in 1 minute, p. 845

cardiac reserve The ability to respond to physiological demands (exercise, stress, hypovolemia) by increasing or decreasing cardiac output as much as three-fold or four-fold, p. 846

diastole Relaxation of the myocardium, p. 845

diastolic blood pressure (DBP) The residual pressure of the arterial system during ventricular relaxation, p. 847

ejection fraction (EF) The percentage of end-diastolic blood volume that is ejected during systole, p. 860

mean arterial pressure (MAP) A measurement related to BP; calculated by adding the diastolic pressure to one third of the pulse pressure, p. 847

murmurs Sounds produced by turbulent blood flow through the heart or the walls of large arteries, p. 853

point of maximal impulse (PMI) The site on the chest wall at the fifth intercostal space at which the thrust or pulsation of the left ventricle is most prominent, p. 843

preload The volume of blood in the ventricles at the end of diastole, before the next contraction, p. 846

pulse pressure The difference between the systolic and the diastolic pressures, p. 847

systole Contraction of the myocardium, p. 845

systolic blood pressure (SBP) The peak pressure exerted against the arteries when the heart contracts, p. 847

ELECTRONIC RESOURCES

Supplemental content related to Chapter 34 can be found ...

Evolve Web Site ⊖volve

http://evolve.elsevier.com/Canada/Lewis/medsurg

- Animations:
  - Auscultation of Heart Valves
  - Blood Flow: Circulatory System
  - Cardiac Cycle During Systole and Diastole
  - Pulse Variations
- Assessment Case Study
- Audio Clips:
  - Diastolic Murmur
  - Fourth Heart Sound (S4)
  - Murmurs: Blowing, Harsh or Rough, and Rumble
  - Murmurs: High, Medium, and Low
  - First Heart Sound (S1) at Various Locations
  - Second Heart Sound (S2) at Various Locations
  - Single S1
  - Single S2
  - Systolic Murmur
  - Third Heart Sound (S3)
- Clinical Reference: Laboratory Values
- Content Updates
- eFigures:
  - eFigure 34-1: Types of Serum Lipids
  - eFigure 34-2: Cholesterol Delivery
- Electronic Calculators
- Examination Review Questions
- Glossary
- Key Points (Printable and MP3 Download)
- Physical Examination Video Clips:
  - Anterior Chest, Lungs, and Heart
  - Neck
  - Precordium and Jugular Veins
  - Upper Extremities
- Video Clips:
  - Auscultation: Cardiac, with Bell
  - Auscultation: Cardiac, with Diaphragm
  - Auscultation: Cardiac, with Diaphragm and Bell
  - Auscultation: Carotid Artery
  - Inspection and Palpation: Cardiac Auscultatory Landmarks
  - Inspection and Palpation: Cardiac, Anterior Chest
  - Inspection and Palpation: Pulses, Lower Extremities

Structures and Functions of the Cardiovascular System

Heart

Structure. The heart is a four-chambered, hollow, muscular organ approximately the size of a fist. The heart lies within the thorax between the lungs in the mediastinal space. Its beating is often palpable at the fifth intercostal space (ICS) approximately 5 cm left of the midline. The site of this pulsation, arising at the apex of the heart, is termed the **point of maximal impulse (PMI)** and is located on the chest wall at the fifth ICS, where the thrust or pulsation of the left ventricle is most prominent.

The heart is composed of three layers: a thin inner lining, the *endocardium;* a layer of muscle, the *myocardium;* and a fibrous outer layer, the *epicardium.* The heart is surrounded by the pericardium. The inner (visceral) layer of the pericardium is in contact with the epicardium, and the outer (parietal) layer is in contact with the mediastinum. A small amount of pericardial fluid lubricates the space between the pericardial layers *(pericardial space)* and prevents friction between the surfaces as the heart beats.

The heart is divided vertically by the septum. This creates a right and left atrium and a right and left ventricle. The thickness of the wall of each chamber is different. The atrial myocardium is thinner than that of the ventricles, and the left ventricular wall is three times thicker than the right ventricular wall (Drake, Vogl, & Mitchell, 2010). The thickness of the ventricle provides the force to pump the blood into the systemic circulation.

Blood Flow Through the Heart. The right atrium receives venous blood from the inferior and superior venae cavae and the coronary sinus. The blood then passes through the tricuspid valve into the right ventricle. With each contraction, the right ventricle pumps blood through the pulmonic valve into the pulmonary artery.

Blood flows to the left atrium by way of the pulmonary veins. It then passes through the mitral valve and into the left ventricle. As the heart contracts, blood is ejected through the aortic valve into the aorta and thus enters the high-pressure systemic circulation (Figure 34-1).

Cardiac Valves. The four valves of the heart serve to keep blood flowing in a forward direction. The cusps of the mitral and tricuspid valves are attached to thin strands of fibrous tissue termed *chordae tendineae* (Figure 34-2). Chordae are anchored in the papillary muscles of the ventricles. This support system prevents the eversion of the leaflets into the atria during ventricular contraction. The pulmonic and aortic valves (also known as *semilunar valves*) prevent blood from regurgitating into the ventricles at the end of each ventricular contraction.

Blood Supply to the Myocardium. The myocardium has its own blood supply, the *coronary circulation* (Figure 34-3). Blood flow into the coronary arteries occurs primarily during diastole. The right coronary artery and its branches usually supply the right atrium, the right ventricle, and a portion of the posterior wall of the left ventricle. The left coronary artery and its branches (left anterior descending artery and left circumflex artery) supply the left atrium and the left ventricle. In 90% of people, the atrioventricular (AV) node and the bundle of His (part of the cardiac conduction system) receive blood supply from the right coronary artery. For this reason, obstruction of this artery often causes serious defects in cardiac conduction.

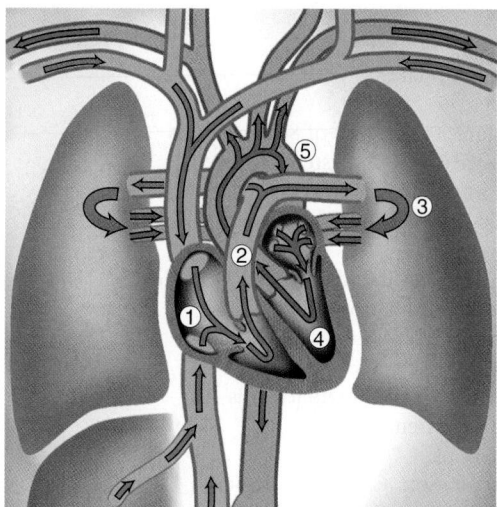

Figure 34-1 Schematic representation of blood flow through the heart. *Arrows* indicate direction of flow. *1,* The right atrium receives venous blood from the inferior and superior venae cavae and the coronary sinus. The blood then passes through the tricuspid valve into the right ventricle. *2,* With each contraction, the right ventricle pumps blood through the pulmonic valve into the pulmonary artery and to the lungs. *3,* Oxygenated blood flows from the lungs to the left atrium by way of the pulmonary veins. *4,* It then passes through the mitral valve and into the left ventricle. *5,* As the heart contracts, blood is ejected through the aortic valve into the aorta and thus enters the systemic circulation.

Source: Adapted from Jarvis, C. (2008). *Physical examination and health assessment* (5th ed., p. 485, Figure 19-5). St. Louis: Saunders.

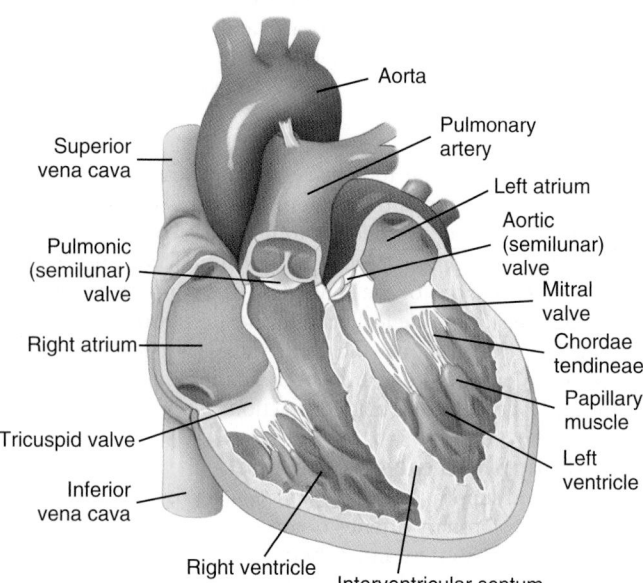

Figure 34-2 Anatomic structures of the atrioventricular valves.

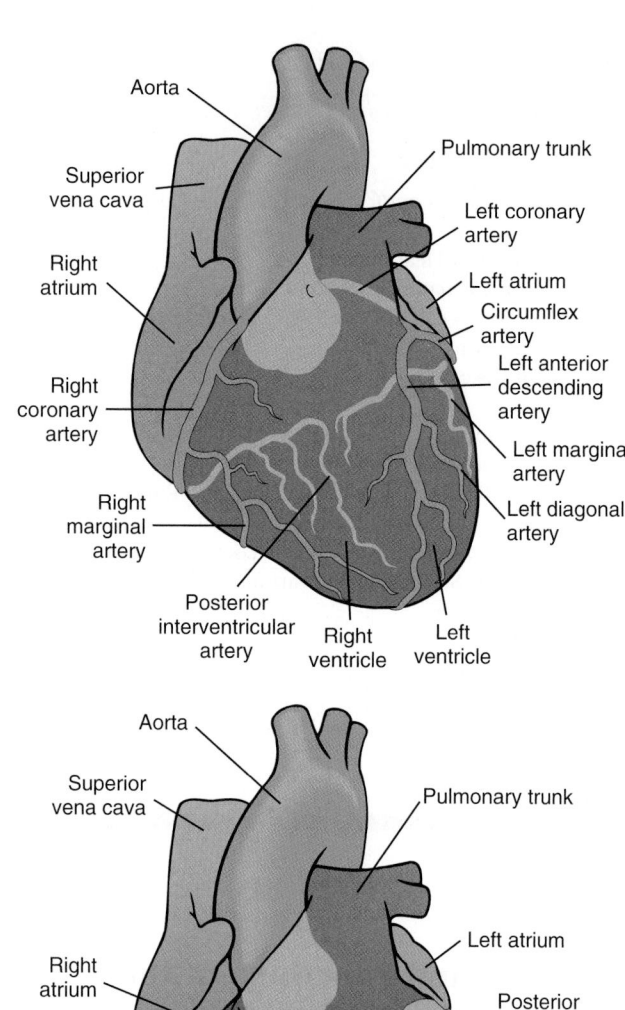

Figure 34-3 Coronary arteries and veins.

The divisions of coronary veins parallel the coronary arteries. Most of the blood from the coronary system drains into the coronary sinus, which empties into the right atrium near the entrance to the inferior vena cava (see Figure 34-3).

Conduction System. The conduction system is specialized nerve tissue responsible for creating and transporting the electrical impulse, or action potential. This impulse initiates depolarization and, subsequently, cardiac contraction. The electrical impulse is initiated by the sinoatrial (SA) node (the pacemaker of the heart) (Figure 34-4). Each impulse generated at the SA node travels swiftly through the muscle fibres of the atria by internodal pathways and cell–to–cell conduction. Mechanical contraction of the atria follows the depolarization of the cells.

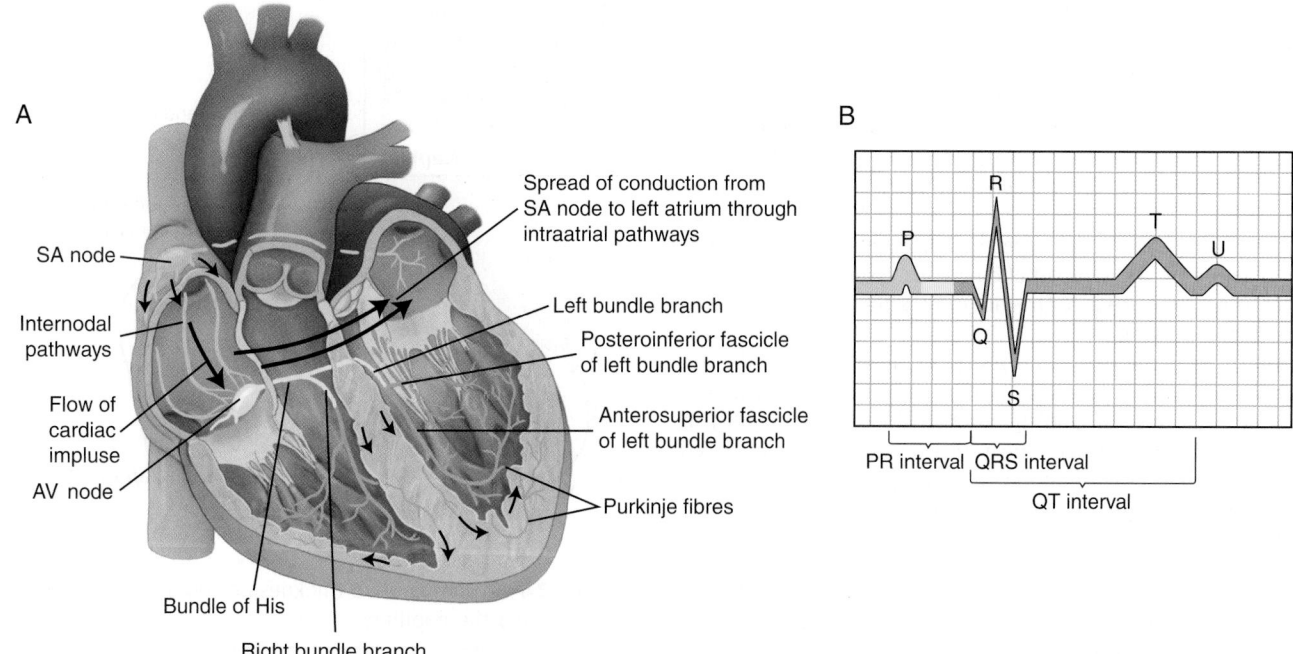

Figure 34-4 A, Conduction system of the heart. *AV*, atrioventricular; *SA*, sinoatrial. **B,** The normal electrocardiogram pattern. The P wave represents depolarization of the atria. The QRS complex indicates depolarization of the ventricles. The T wave represents repolarization of the ventricles. The U wave, if present, may represent repolarization of the Purkinje fibres or may be associated with hypokalemia. The PR, QRS, and QT intervals reflect the length of time it takes for the impulse to travel from one area of the heart to another.

The electrical impulse travels from the atria to the AV node. The excitation then moves through the bundle of His and the left and right bundle branches. The left bundle branch has two fascicles, an anterior and a posterior. The action potential diffuses widely through the walls of both ventricles by means of *Purkinje fibres*. The efficient ventricular conduction system delivers the impulse within 0.12 second. This triggers a uniform ventricular contraction.

The cardiac cycle starts with depolarization of the SA node. The cycle's climax is ejection of blood into the pulmonary and systemic circulations. It ends with repolarization, when the contractile fibre cells and the conduction pathway cells regain their resting polarized condition. Cardiac muscle cells have a compensatory mechanism that makes them unresponsive or refractory to restimulation during the action potential. During systole, there is an absolute refractory period during which cardiac muscle does not respond to any stimuli. After this period, cardiac muscle gradually recovers its excitability and a relative refractory period occurs by early diastole.

Electrocardiogram. The electrical activity of the heart can be detected on the body surface and recorded on an electrocardiogram (ECG). The letters *P, QRS, T,* and *U* are used to identify the separate waveforms (see Figure 34-4, *B*). The first wave, P, begins with the firing of the SA node and represents depolarization of the fibres of the atria. The QRS wave represents depolarization from the AV node throughout the ventricles. There is a delay of impulse transmission through the AV node that accounts for the time sequence between the end of the P wave and the beginning of the QRS wave. The T wave represents repolarization of the ventricles. The U wave, if seen, represents delayed ventricular

repolarization and may be associated with electrolyte imbalance (i.e., hypokalemia, hypomagnesemia, hypercalcemia) and is most typically seen in bradycardias.

Intervals between these waves (PR, QRS, and QT intervals) reflect the length of time it takes for the impulse to travel from one area of the heart to another. These time intervals can be measured and deviations from these time references often indicate pathological conditions (Aehlert, 2011).

Mechanical System. Depolarization triggers mechanical activity. **Systole,** contraction of the myocardium, results in ejection of blood from the cardiac chamber. Relaxation of the myocardium, **diastole,** allows for filling of the chamber. **Cardiac output (CO)** is the measurement of mechanical efficiency. CO is the amount of blood pumped by each ventricle in 1 minute. It is calculated by multiplying the amount of blood ejected from the ventricle with the heartbeat, the stroke volume (SV), by the heart rate (HR) per minute:

$$CO = SV \times HR$$

For the normal adult at rest, CO is maintained in the range of 4 to 8 L/min. **Cardiac index (CI)** is the CO divided by the body mass index (BMI). A measure of the CO of a patient per square metre of body surface area, the CI adjusts the CO to the body size. The normal CI is 2.8 to 4.2 L/min/m².

Factors Affecting Cardiac Output. Numerous factors can affect either the HR or the SV and, thus, the CO. The HR is regulated primarily by the autonomic nervous system. The factors affecting the SV are preload, contractility, and afterload (Huether & McCance, 2007). Increasing preload, contractility, and afterload increases the workload of the myocardium, resulting in increased oxygen demand.

The volume of blood in the ventricles at the end of diastole, before the next contraction, is called **preload.** Preload determines the amount of stretch placed on myocardial fibres. Starling's Law states that, to a point, the more the fibres are stretched (i.e., the greater the preload), the greater their force of contraction, or contractility.

Contractility can be increased by administering norepinephrine, released by the sympathetic nervous system, as well as by epinephrine. Increasing contractility raises the SV by increasing ventricular emptying.

Afterload is the peripheral resistance against which the left ventricle must pump. Afterload is affected by the size of the ventricle, the wall tension, and the arterial blood pressure (BP). If the arterial BP is elevated, the ventricles will meet increased resistance to ejection of blood, increasing the work demand. Eventually, this results in ventricular hypertrophy (enlargement of the cardiac muscle tissue without an increase in the size of cavities).

Cardiac Reserve. The cardiovascular system must respond to numerous situations in health and illness (e.g., exercise, stress, hypovolemia). The ability to respond to these demands by increasing CO as much as three-fold or four-fold is termed **cardiac reserve.**

The increase in CO results from an increase in HR or SV. The HR can increase to as high as 180 beats per minute (bpm) for short periods without deleterious effects. The SV can be increased by increasing either preload or contractility.

Vascular System

Blood Vessels. The three major types of blood vessels in the vascular system are the arteries, the veins, and the capillaries. Arteries carry blood away from the heart and, except for the pulmonary artery, carry oxygenated blood. Veins carry blood toward the heart and, except for the pulmonary veins, carry deoxygenated blood. Small branches of arteries and veins are arterioles and venules, respectively. Blood circulates from the heart into arteries, arterioles, capillaries, venules, and veins and back to the heart.

Arteries and Arterioles. The arterial system differs from the venous system by the amount and type of tissue that makes up arterial walls (Figure 34-5). The large arteries have thick walls that are composed mainly of elastic tissue. This elastic property cushions the impact of the pressure created by ventricular contraction and provides recoil that propels blood forward into the circulation. Large arteries also contain some smooth muscle. Examples of large arteries are the aorta and the pulmonary artery.

Arterioles have relatively little elastic tissue and more smooth muscle. Arterioles serve as the major control of arterial BP and distribution of blood flow. They respond readily to local conditions such as low O_2 and increasing levels of CO_2 by dilating or constricting.

Capillaries. The thin capillary wall is made up of endothelial cells, with no elastic or muscle tissue (see Figure 34-5). There are many kilometres of capillaries in an adult. The exchange of cellular nutrients and metabolic end products takes place through these thin-walled vessels.

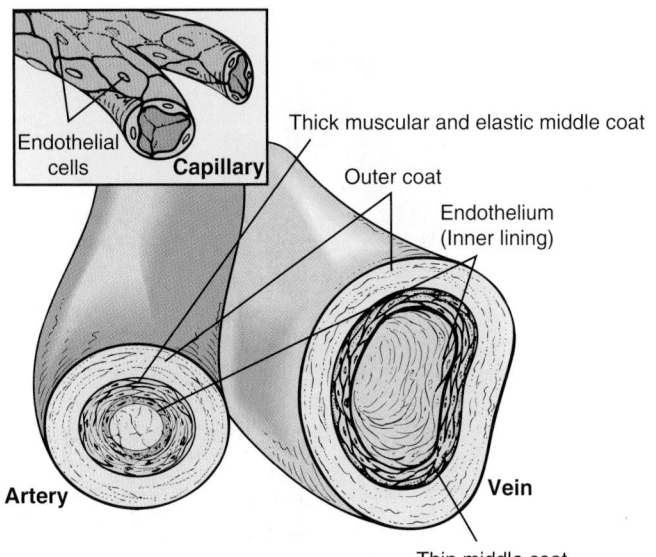

Figure 34-5 Comparative thickness of layers of the artery, the vein, and the capillary.

Veins and Venules. Veins are large-diameter, thin-walled vessels that return blood to the right atrium (see Figure 34-5). The venous system is a low-pressure, high-volume system. The larger veins contain semilunar valves at intervals to maintain the blood flow toward the heart and to prevent backward flow. The amount of blood in the venous system is affected by a number of factors, including arterial flow, compression of veins by skeletal muscles, alterations in thoracic and abdominal pressures, and right atrial pressure.

The largest veins are the superior vena cava, which returns blood to the heart from the head, neck, and arms, and the inferior vena cava, which returns blood to the heart from the lower part of the body. These large-diameter vessels are affected by the pressure in the right side of the heart. Elevated right atrial pressure can cause distended neck veins or liver engorgement as a result of resistance to blood flow.

Venules are relatively small vessels made up of a small amount of muscle and connective tissue. Venules collect blood from various capillary beds and channel it to the larger veins.

Regulation of the Cardiovascular System

Autonomic Nervous System. The autonomic nervous system consists of the sympathetic nervous system and the parasympathetic nervous system.

Effect on the Heart. Stimulation of the sympathetic nervous system increases the HR, the speed of impulse conduction through the AV node, and the force of atrial and ventricular contractions. This effect is mediated by specific sites in the heart called *β-adrenergic receptors* that are receptors for norepinephrine and epinephrine.

In contrast, stimulation of the parasympathetic system (mediated by the vagus nerve) causes a decrease in HR by the action on the SA node and slows conduction through the AV node.

Effect on the Blood Vessels. The source of neural control of blood vessels is the sympathetic nervous system. The α-adrenergic receptors are located in vascular smooth muscles. Stimulation of the α-adrenergic receptors results in vasoconstriction. Decreased stimulation to the α-adrenergic receptors causes vasodilation. (Sympathetic nervous system receptors that influence BP are presented in Chapter 35, Table 35-2.)

The parasympathetic nerves have selective distribution in the blood vessels. Blood vessels in skeletal muscle do not receive parasympathetic input.

Baroreceptors. *Baroreceptors* in the aortic arch and the carotid sinus (at the origin of the internal carotid artery) are sensitive to stretch or pressure within the arterial system. Stimulation of these receptors sends information to the vasomotor centre in the brainstem. This results in temporary inhibition of the sympathetic nervous system and enhancement of the parasympathetic influence, causing a decreased HR and peripheral vasodilation. Decreased arterial pressure causes the opposite effect.

Chemoreceptors. *Chemoreceptors* are located in the aortic arch and the carotid body. They are capable of initiating changes in HR and arterial pressure in response to decreased arterial O_2 pressure, increased arterial CO_2 pressure, and decreased plasma pH. When the chemoreceptor reflexes are stimulated, they stimulate the vasomotor centre, in turn, to increase cardiac activity.

Blood Pressure

The **arterial blood pressure (BP)** is a measure of the pressure exerted by blood against the walls of the arterial system. The **systolic blood pressure (SBP)** is the peak pressure exerted against the arteries when the heart contracts. The **diastolic blood pressure (DBP)** is the residual pressure of the arterial system during ventricular relaxation. BP is usually expressed as the ratio of SBP to DBP.

The two main factors influencing BP are CO and systemic vascular resistance (SVR):

$$BP = CO \times SVR$$

SVR is the force opposing the movement of blood. This force is created primarily in small arteries and arterioles.

Measurement of Arterial Blood Pressure. BP can be measured by invasive and noninvasive techniques. The invasive technique consists of catheter insertion into an artery. The catheter is attached to a recording device and the pressure is measured directly (see Chapter 68).

Noninvasive, indirect measurement of BP can be done with a sphygmomanometer and a stethoscope. The sphygmomanometer consists of an inflatable cuff and a pressure gauge or an electronic cuff. The BP is measured externally by listening for sounds of turbulent blood flow through a compressed artery (termed *Korotkoff sounds*). The brachial artery is the usual site for taking a BP.

After placing the appropriate size cuff on the extremity, the cuff is inflated to a pressure in excess of the SBP. This causes blood flow in the artery to cease. As the pressure in the cuff is lowered, the artery is auscultated for Korotkoff sounds. There are five phases of Korotkoff sounds. The first phase is a tapping sound caused by the spurt of blood into the constricted artery as the pressure in the cuff is gradually deflated. The pressure when this sound is heard is considered the SBP. The fifth phase occurs when the sound disappears, and this pressure is known as the DBP (Jarvis, 2011). Clinically, the BP is recorded as SBP/DBP

(120/80 mm Hg). Occasionally, an auscultatory gap is heard. An auscultatory gap is a loss of sound between the SBP and the DBP. The BP could be measured incorrectly if the cuff is not inflated to exceed the true SBP.

In addition to the manual technique, another noninvasive way to measure BP indirectly is to use automatic BP monitors (see Chapter 35). The monitor consists of a BP cuff and a lightweight microprocessing unit. This system, which records a patient's BP at preset intervals during routine activities over 24 to 48 hours, permits ambulatory BP monitoring and may diagnose hypertension more accurately in some patients.

Pulse Pressure and Mean Arterial Pressure. **Pulse pressure** is the difference between the SBP and the DBP. It is normally about one third of the SBP. If the BP is 120/80 mm Hg, the pulse pressure is 40 mm Hg. An increased pulse pressure may occur during exercise or in individuals with atherosclerosis of the larger arteries because of increased SBP. A decreased pulse pressure may be found in cardiac failure or hypovolemia.

Another measurement related to BP is **mean arterial pressure (MAP)**. It is not the average of the DBP and SBP because the duration of diastole exceeds that of systole at normal HRs. MAP is calculated by adding the DBP to one third of the pulse pressure:

$$MAP = DBP + 1/3 \text{ pulse pressure}$$

A person with a BP of 120/60 mm Hg has an MAP of 80 mm Hg.

AGE-RELATED CONSIDERATIONS: EFFECTS OF AGING ON THE CARDIOVASCULAR SYSTEM

In Canada, 9 out of 10 people older than 20 years have at least one risk factor for cardiovascular disease and cardiovascular disease continues to be the leading cause of hospitalization in Canada (Public Health Agency of Canada [PHAC], 2009). The most common cardiovascular problem is coronary artery disease (CAD) secondary to atherosclerosis. It is difficult to separate normal aging changes from the pathophysiological changes of atherosclerosis. Current thinking suggests that many of the physiological changes in the cardiovascular system of the older adult are a result of the combined effects of the aging process, disease, environmental factors, and lifetime health behaviours rather than age alone (Ebersole et al., 2011; Jarvis, 2011).

With increased age, the amount of collagen in the heart increases and the amount of elastin decreases. These changes affect the contractile and distensible properties of the myocardium. One of the major age-associated alterations in the cardiovascular response to physical or emotional stress is a decrease in CO and SV, which is caused by the combination of decreased contractility and a reduced HR response to stress. The resting HR is not markedly affected by aging.

Cardiac valves become thicker and stiffer from lipid accumulation, degeneration of collagen, and fibrosis (Ebersole et al., 2011). The aortic and mitral valves are most frequently affected. These changes result in either regurgitation of blood when the valve should be closed or narrowing of the orifice of the valve (stenosis) when the valve should be open. The turbulent blood flow across the affected valve results in a murmur.

The number of pacemaker cells in the SA node decreases with age. By age 75, a person may have only 10% of the normal number of pacemaker cells, although this is compatible with normal SA node function (Woods, Froelicher, Motzer, & Bridges, 2009). Similar decreases in the number of conduction cells in the AV node, the bundle of His, and the bundle branches also occur with aging. Fibrosis of the bundle branches has been shown to precipitate chronic heart block in people aged 65 years and older (Woods et al., 2009). A normal ECG of an aging patient may show small, inconspicuous increases in PR, QRS, and QT intervals.

The autonomic nervous system control of the cardiovascular system is altered with aging. The number and function of β-adrenergic receptors in the heart decrease with age. Therefore, the older adult not only has a decreased response to physical and emotional stress but also is less sensitive to β-adrenergic agonist drugs.

Arterial blood vessels thicken and become less elastic with age (Huether & McCance, 2007). Arteries increase their sensitivity to vasopressin (antidiuretic hormone). Both of these changes contribute to a progressive increase in SBP and a decrease or no change in DBP with age. Consequently, an increase in the pulse pressure is found. Hypertension is not considered a normal consequence of aging and should be treated.

Orthostatic hypotension is estimated to be present in more than 30% of patients older than age 70 with systolic hypertension (Libby, Bonow, Mann, & Zipes, 2008). Despite the changes associated with aging, the heart is able to function adequately under most circumstances.

Age-related changes in the cardiovascular system and differences in assessment findings are presented in Table 34-1.

Assessment of the Cardiovascular System

Subjective Data

Important Health Information

A careful health history and physical examination (Table 34-2) should aid the nurse in differentiating symptoms that reflect a cardiovascular problem from problems of other body systems. For instance, it is important to determine whether weight gain is because of overeating or a manifestation of fluid retention.

Important Health Information

Past Health History. Many illnesses affect the cardiovascular system directly or indirectly. The patient should be questioned about a history of chest pain, shortness of breath, alcoholism or excessive drinking, anemia, rheumatic fever, streptococcal sore throat, congenital heart disease, stroke, syncope, hypertension, thrombophlebitis, intermittent claudication, varicosities, obesity, and edema.

Medications. An assessment of the patient's current and past use of medications should be made. This includes both over-the-counter (OTC) drugs and prescription drugs. For example, aspirin, which prolongs the blood clotting time, is contained in many drugs used to alleviate cold symptoms.

A medication assessment should list the name of the drug and the patient's understanding of its purpose and adverse effects. Drugs that may adversely affect the cardiovascular system should also be assessed. Some of these, and examples of their effect on the cardiovascular system, follow.

AGE-RELATED DIFFERENCES IN ASSESSMENT

Table 34-1 Cardiovascular System

CHANGES	DIFFERENCES IN ASSESSMENT FINDINGS
Chest Wall	
Kyphosis	Altered chest landmarks for palpation, percussion, and auscultation; distant heart sounds
Heart	
Myocardial hypertrophy, ↑ collagen and scarring, ↓ elastin	↓ Cardiac reserve, slight ↓ HR
Downward displacement	Difficulty in isolating apical pulse
↓ CO, HR, SV in response to exercise or stress	Slowed, ↓ response to stress; slowed recovery from activity
Cellular aging changes and fibrosis of conduction system	↓ Amplitude of QRS complex and lengthening of PR, QRS, and QT intervals; left axis deviation; irregular cardiac rhythms
Valvular rigidity from calcification, sclerosis, or fibrosis, impeding complete closure of valves	Systolic murmur (aortic or mitral) possible without being indication of cardiovascular pathology
Blood Vessels	
Arterial stiffening caused by loss of elastin in arterial walls, thickening of intima of arteries and progressive fibrosis of media	Elevation in systolic and possibly diastolic BP (e.g., 160/90 mm Hg); possibly, widened pulse pressures; more pronounced arterial pulses; pedal pulses diminished

BP, blood pressure; *CO,* cardiac output; *HR,* heart rate; *SV,* stroke volume.

- Tricyclic antidepressants: dysrhythmias
- Phenothiazines: dysrhythmias and hypotension
- Oral contraceptives: thrombophlebitis
- Doxorubicin (Adriamycin): cardiomyopathy
- Lithium: dysrhythmias
- Corticosteroids: sodium and fluid retention
- Theophylline preparations: tachycardia and dysrhythmias
- Recreational or abused drugs: tachycardia and dysrhythmias

Surgery or Other Treatments. The patient should also be asked about specific treatments, past surgeries, and hospital admissions related to cardiovascular problems. Any hospitalizations for diagnostic workups or cardiovascular symptoms should be explored. It should be noted whether an ECG or a chest radiograph was taken for baseline data.

Objective Data

Physical Examination

Vital Signs. After the patient's general appearance has been observed, vital signs, including BP, heart and respiratory rate, and temperature, are taken. The BP should be measured while the patient is sitting, lying, and standing. An appropriate cuff size should be used for accurate readings. Normally, there is a reduction of up to 15 mm Hg in the SBP and 3 to 5 mm Hg in the DBP

HEALTH HISTORY

Table 34-2 Cardiovascular System: Questions for Obtaining Subjective Data

Chest Pain

- Do you have any chest pain or discomfort? Please show me where it is.
- Is the pain in one spot or does it move around?
- How long have you had this pain?
- Does it come and go or is it constant? Does it get worse before or after meals? When is the pain worst (e.g., with a certain position or activity, with stress)?
- Can you describe how it feels (e.g., burning, stabbing, aching, heaviness, squeezing)?
- What brings the pain on (e.g., activity, stress)?
- Any other symptoms that occur when you get the pain (e.g., shortness of breath, weakness, nausea, vomiting)?*
- What works to relieve the pain (e.g., rest, change of position, medication)?*

Dyspnea

- Have you experienced any shortness of breath? If yes, what kind of activity precipitates your shortness of breath?
- Is your shortness of breath dependent on your position (e.g., lying down)?*
- How does the shortness of breath affect your daily activities?*

Orthopnea

- How many pillows do you sleep on at night? Has this changed recently?*

Cough

- Do you have a cough? If yes, describe the duration, the frequency, and the kind of cough (e.g., dry, hoarse, congested).
- Do you cough up mucus? If yes, describe the colour and the amount.
- Is coughing associated with any activity such as talking, lying down, stress, and so on?*
- Is the coughing relieved by anything (e.g., walking, exercise, rest, medication)?*

Fatigue

- Do you tire easily?* If yes, when did you notice a change in your level of fatigue?
- Is your energy level related to the time of the day?*

Cyanosis or Pallor

- Have you ever noticed a bluish or ashen colour to your face?*

Edema

- Have you ever noticed any swelling in your feet and legs?*
- When did you first experience swelling and have there been any recent changes?*
- Are both feet swollen to the same degree?*

Nocturia

- How many times a night do you awaken to urinate?*

Cardiac History

- Do you have any past history of hypertension, elevated cholesterol or triglycerides, heart murmur, congenital heart diseases, rheumatic fever or unexplained joint pains in your youth, recurrent tonsillitis, or anemia?
- Do you have any history of heart disease?*
- When was your last ECG, serum cholesterol blood work, or other heart-related tests?*

Family History

- Do you have any family history of heart disease, high blood pressure, obesity, diabetes, or sudden death at a young age?*

Self-Care History

- Describe your usual daily diet including sodium and fluid intake. What is your present weight? What was your weight 1 year ago?
- Have you ever used tobacco? If yes, in what form, how much, and for how long? Have you ever tried to quit? If yes, what methods have you tried?
- How often and how much alcohol do you drink? Have you ever been told that you have a problem with alcohol?*
- What is your usual amount of exercise per week?
- Do you take any cardiac medications (e.g., antihypertensives, diuretics, aspirin, anticoagulants), over-the-counter medications, herbal products, or street drugs?*

ECG, electrocardiogram.
*If yes, describe.
Source: Adapted from Jarvis, C., Browne, A. J., MacDonald-Jenkins, J., & Luktar-Flude, M. (2009). *Physical examination and health assessment* (1st Canadian ed., pp. 492-494). Toronto: Elsevier Canada.

in the standing position. BP measurements should be taken in both arms. These readings may vary from 5 to 15 mm Hg. A greater variance indicates pathological findings. BP in the lower extremities is expected to be about 10 mm Hg higher than in the upper extremities.

Peripheral Vascular System

Inspection. Inspection of the skin colour, hair distribution, and venous blood flow provides information about arterial blood flow and venous return. The extremities should be inspected for conditions such as edema, thrombophlebitis, varicose veins, and lesions such as stasis ulcers. Edema in the extremities can be caused by gravity, interruption of venous return, or elevation of right atrial pressure.

A measure used for assessing arterial flow to the extremities is the *capillary filling time*. The patient's nail beds are squeezed to produce blanching and observed for the return of colour. With normal arterial capillary perfusion, the colour will return within 3 seconds.

The large veins in the neck (internal and external jugular) should be inspected while the patient is gradually elevated to an upright position. Distension and prominent pulsations of these neck veins can be caused by right atrial pressure elevation.

Palpation. Palpation of the pulses in the neck and extremities also provides information on arterial blood flow. The pulses should be palpated to assess the volume and pressure within each vessel. Characteristics of the arteries on the right and left sides of the body should be compared. It is important to palpate each carotid pulse separately to avoid vagal stimulation and subsequent dysrhythmias.

When palpating the arteries identified in Figure 34-6, the assessor should note the pressure of the pulse wave, or how far the vessel wall distends when the pulse occurs. This judgement of the pulsation volume is recorded as normal, bounding, thready,

or absent. A scale may be used to document pulse volume or amplitude (Jarvis, 2011).

0   Absent
1+   Weak, thready
2+   Normal
3+   Full, bounding

The *rigidity* (hardness) of the vessel should also be noted. The normal pulse will feel like it is tapping, whereas a vessel wall that is narrowed or bulging will vibrate. A term for a palpable vibration is *thrill*.

Auscultation. An artery that has a narrowed or bulging wall may create turbulent blood flow. This abnormal flow can create a buzzing or humming termed a *bruit*. It can be heard with a stethoscope placed over the vessel. Auscultation of major arteries such as the carotid arteries, the abdominal aorta, and the femoral arteries should be part of the initial cardiovascular assessment. Abnormalities of the cardiovascular system are described in Table 34-3.

Thorax

Inspection and Palpation. An overall inspection and palpation of the bony structures of the thorax is the initial step in the examination.

Next, the areas where the cardiac valves project their sounds are inspected and palpated by identifying the ICSs. The raised notch, the angle of Louis, that is created where the manubrium and the body of the sternum are joined, is readily palpable in the midline of the sternum. The angle of Louis is at the level of the second rib and can, therefore, be used to count ICSs and locate specific auscultatory areas.

The following auscultatory areas can be located (Figure 34-7): the aortic area in the second ICS to the right of the sternum, the pulmonic area in the second ICS to the left of the sternum, the tricuspid area in the fifth left ICS close to the sternum, and the mitral area in the left midclavicular line (MCL) at the level of the fifth ICS. A fifth auscultatory area is Erb's point, located at the

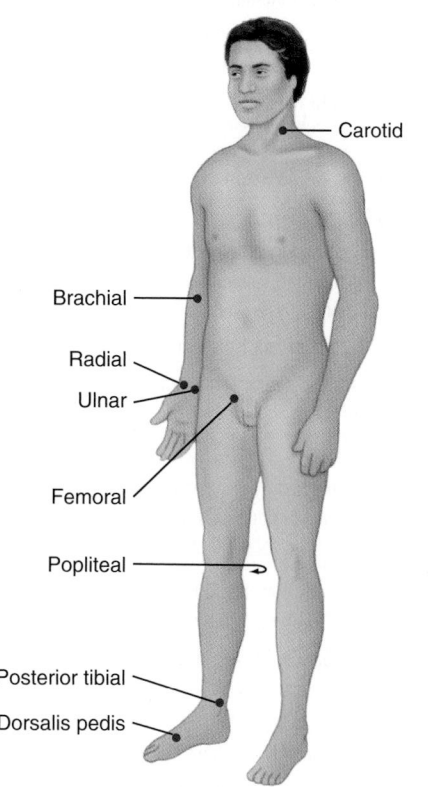

Figure 34-6 Common sites for palpating arteries.

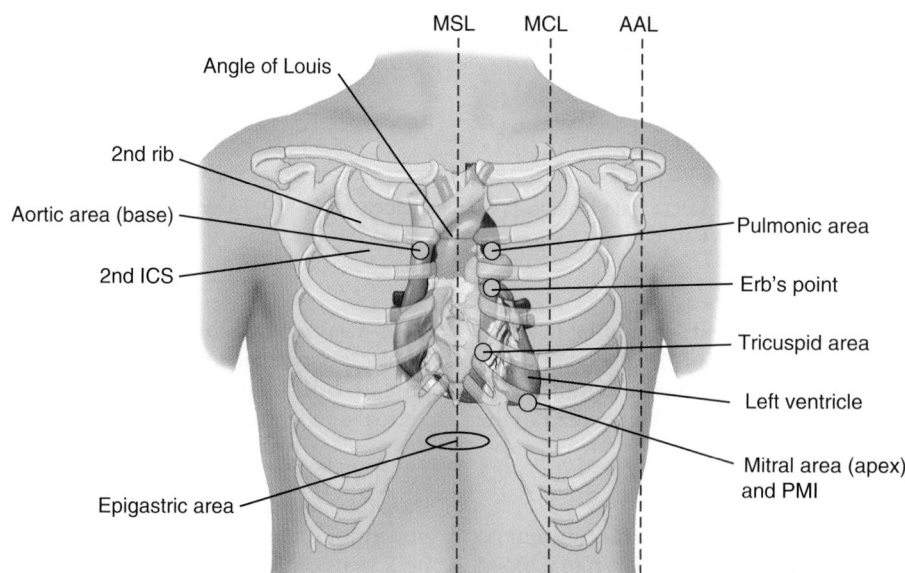

Figure 34-7 Orientation of the heart within the thorax and cardiac auscultatory areas. *Red lines* indicate the midsternal line *(MSL)*, midclavicular line *(MCL)*, and anterior axillary line *(AAL)*. *ICS*, intercostal space; *PMI*, point of maximal impulse.

Source: Adapted from Price, S. A., & Wilson, L. M. (2003). *Pathophysiology: Clinical concepts of disease processes* (6th ed.). St. Louis: Mosby; and Kinney, M. R., & Packa, D. R. (Eds.). (1996). *Andreoli's comprehensive cardiac care* (8th ed.). St. Louis: Mosby.

COMMON ASSESSMENT ABNORMALITIES

Table 34-3 Cardiovascular System

FINDING	DESCRIPTION	POSSIBLE ETIOLOGY AND SIGNIFICANCE*
Inspection		
Distended neck veins	Vertical distance between intersection of angle of Louis and level of jugular distension >3 cm with patient sitting at 30- to 45-degree angle	Elevated right atrial pressure; right-sided heart failure
Central cyanosis	Bluish or purplish tinge in central areas such as tongue, conjunctivae, inner surface of lips	Inadequate O_2 saturation of arterial blood caused by pulmonary or cardiac disorders (e.g., congenital defects)
Peripheral cyanosis	Bluish or purplish tinge in extremities or nose and ears	Reduced blood flow because of heart failure, vasoconstriction, cold environment
Splinter hemorrhages	Small red to black streaks under fingernails	Infective endocarditis (infection of endocardium, usually in area of cardiac valves)
Clubbing of nail beds	Obliteration of normal angle between base of nail and skin	Endocarditis, congenital defects, prolonged O_2 deficiency
Colour changes in extremities with postural change	Pallor, cyanosis, mottling of skin after limb elevation; glossy skin	Chronic decreased arterial perfusion
Ulcers	*Venous:* necrotic crater-like lesion usually found on lower leg at medial malleolus; characterized by slow wound healing *Arterial:* pale ischemic base, well-defined edges usually found on toes, heels, lateral malleoli	Poor venous return, varicose veins, incompetent venous valves; arteriosclerosis, diabetes
Varicose veins	Visible dilated, tortuous vessels in lower extremities	Incompetent valves in vein
Palpation		
Pulse		
Bounding	Sharp, brisk, pounding pulse	Hyperkinetic states (anxiety, fever), anemia, hyperthyroidism
Thready	Weak, slowly rising pulse; easily obliterated by pressure	Blood loss, decreased cardiac output, aortic valve disease, peripheral arterial disease
Irregular	Regularly irregular or irregularly irregular; skipped beats	Cardiac dysrhythmias
Pulsus alternans	Regular rhythm but strength of pulse varies with each beat	Heart failure
Absent	Lack of pulse	Atherosclerosis, thrombus, trauma, embolus
Thrill	Vibration of vessel or chest wall	Aneurysm, aortic regurgitation, arteriovenous fistula
Rigidity	Stiffness or inflexibility of vessel wall	Atherosclerosis
>100 bpm	Tachycardia	May be exercise-induced; anxiety, shock, need for increased cardiac output, hyperthyroidism
<60 bpm	Bradycardia	May be rest-induced; SA or AV node damage, athletic conditioning, adverse effect of drugs (e.g., β-adrenergic blockers), hypothyroidism
Displaced point of maximal impulse (apical pulse)	Point of maximal impulse is palpated (or auscultated) below the fifth ICS and to the left of the MCL	Left ventricular dilation
Extremities		
Unusually warm extremities	Hands and feet warmer than normal	Possible thyrotoxicosis
Cold extremities	Hands and/or feet cold to touch, external covering necessary for comfort	Intermittent claudication, peripheral arterial obstruction, low cardiac output, severe anemia
Pitting edema of lower extremities or sacral area	Visible finger indentation after application of firm pressure	Interruption of venous return to heart, fluid in tissues
Positive Homans' sign	Presence of calf pain during sharp dorsiflexion of foot	Thrombophlebitis
Abnormal capillary filling time	Blanching of nail bed for >3 sec after release of pressure	Reduced arterial capillary perfusion, anemia
Asymmetry in limb circumference	Measurable swelling of involved limb	Thrombophlebitis, varicose veins, lymphedema

AV, atrioventricular; *bpm,* beats per minute; *ICS,* intercostal space; *MCL,* midclavicular line; *SA,* sinoatrial.

Continued

COMMON ASSESSMENT ABNORMALITIES

Table 34-3 Cardiovascular System—cont'd

FINDING	DESCRIPTION	POSSIBLE ETIOLOGY AND SIGNIFICANCE*
Percussion		
Abnormal cardiac borders	Left border of cardiac dullness extends beyond MCL in fifth ICS; right border of cardiac dullness extends beyond sternal border	Cardiac enlargement due to coronary heart disease, heart failure, cardiomyopathy
Auscultation		
Pulse deficit	Apical heart rate exceeds the peripheral pulse rate	Cardiac dysrhythmias
Arterial bruit	Turbulent flow sound in peripheral artery	Arterial obstruction or aneurysm
Third heart sound (S3)	Extra heart sound, low-pitched, heard in early diastole, similar to sound of a gallop	Left ventricular failure; volume overload; mitral, aortic, or tricuspid regurgitation; hypertension (possible)
Fourth heart sound (S4)	Extra heart sound, low-pitched, heard in late diastole, similar to sound of a gallop	Forceful atrial contraction from resistance to ventricular filling (e.g., in left ventricular hypertrophy, aortic stenosis, hypertension, coronary artery disease)
Cardiac murmurs	Turbulent sounds occurring between normal heart sounds; characterized by loudness, pitch, shape, quality, duration, timing	Cardiac valve disorder, abnormal blood flow patterns
Pericardial friction rub	High-pitched, scratchy sound heard during S1 and/or S2 at the apex. Heard best with patient sitting and leaning forward, and at the end of expiration	Pericarditis

*Limited to common etiological factors. (Further discussion of conditions listed may be found in Chapters 35 through 40 and 68.)

third left ICS near the sternum. Normally, no pulsations are felt in these areas unless the patient has a thin chest wall.

A valvular disorder may be suspected if abnormal pulsations or thrills are felt. Next, the epigastric area, which lies on either side of the midline just below the xyphoid process, is inspected and palpated. In a thin person, the pulsation of the abdominal aorta may be visible and can normally be palpated here. Next, the precordium, which is located between the apex and the sternum, is inspected for heaves. *Heaves* are sustained lifts of the chest wall in the precordial area that can be seen or palpated. They may be caused by left ventricular enlargement. Normally, no pulsations are seen or felt here.

When the patient is recumbent, the mitral valve area at the apex of the heart is inspected and palpated for the PMI, the site of strongest pulsation. This pulsation or ventricular thrust lies within the MCL in the fifth ICS. If the PMI is palpable, its position is recorded in relation to the MCL and ICSs. When the PMI is to the left of the MCL, the heart may be enlarged.

Percussion. The borders of the right and left sides of the heart can be estimated by percussion. The nurse stands to the right of the recumbent patient and percusses along the curve of the rib in the fourth and fifth ICSs, starting at the midaxillary line. The percussion note over the heart is dull in comparison with the resonance over the lung and is recorded in relation to the MCL.

Auscultation. The movement of the cardiac valves creates some turbulence in the blood flow, resulting in normal heart sounds (Figure 34-8). These sounds can be heard through a stethoscope placed on the chest wall. The first heart sound (S1), which is associated with the closure of the tricuspid and mitral (AV) valves, has a soft lubb sound. The second heart sound (S2), which is associated with the closure of the aortic and pulmonic (semilunar) valves, has a sharp dupp sound. S1 signals the beginning of systole. S2 signals the beginning of diastole (Figure 34-9).

The nurse should listen to the auscultatory areas in sequence with both the diaphragm and the bell of the stethoscope.

S1 and S2 are heard best with the diaphragm of the stethoscope because they are high pitched. Extra heart sounds (S3 or S4), if present, are heard best with the bell of the stethoscope because they are low pitched. Having the patient leaning forward while sitting accentuates sounds from the second ICSs (aortic and pulmonic areas), whereas the left lateral decubitus position accentuates sounds produced at the mitral area.

The nurse listens at the apical area with the diaphragm of the stethoscope while simultaneously palpating the radial pulse. If fewer radial than apical pulses are counted, a pulse deficit is present. A judgement about the rhythm (regular or irregular) is also made when listening at the apex.

Palpating one carotid artery while auscultating it allows differentiation of S1 from S2 and systole from diastole. Because S1 (lubb) occurs almost simultaneously with ventricular ejection, it is heard when the carotid pulse is felt.

Normally, no sound is heard between S1 and S2 during the periods of systole and diastole. Sounds that are heard during these periods may represent abnormalities and should be described. An exception to this is a normal splitting of S2, which is best heard at the pulmonic area during inspiration. Splitting of this heart sound can be abnormal if it is heard during expiration or if it is constant (fixed) during the respiratory cycle.

S3 is a low-intensity vibration of the ventricular walls usually associated with ventricular filling. S3 may occur in patients with left ventricular failure or mitral valve regurgitation. It is heard closely after S2 and is known as a *ventricular gallop*. S4 is a low-frequency vibration caused by atrial contraction. It precedes S1 of the next cycle and is known as an *atrial gallop*. S4 may occur in patients with CAD, left ventricular hypertrophy, or aortic stenosis.

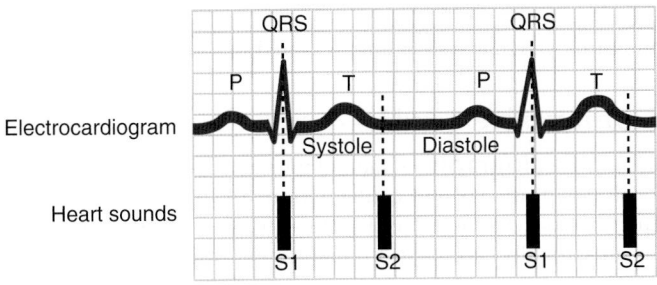

Figure 34-8 Relationship of electrocardiogram, cardiac cycle, and heart sounds (S1, S2).

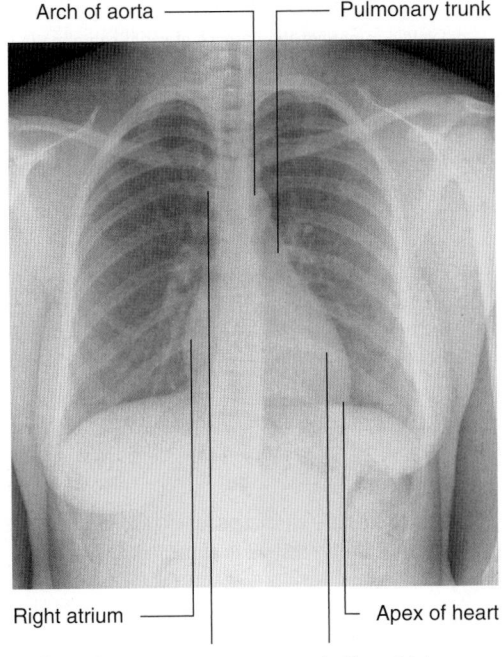

Figure 34-9 Chest radiograph: Standard posteroanterior view.

Murmurs are sounds produced by turbulent blood flow through the heart or the walls of large arteries. Most murmurs are the result of cardiac abnormalities, but some occur in normal cardiac structures. Murmurs are graded on a six-point scale of loudness and recorded as a Roman numeral ratio: the numerator is the intensity of the murmur and the denominator is always VI, which indicates that the six-point scale is being used. An I/VI indicates a soft, faint murmur; a VI/VI indicates a murmur that can be heard without a stethoscope.

If an abnormal sound is heard, it should be documented. This description should include the timing (during systole or diastole), the location (the site on the chest where it is heard the loudest), the pitch (heard best with the diaphragm or the bell of the stethoscope), the position (heard best when patient is recumbent, sitting and leaning forward, or in the left lateral decubitus position), the characteristic (harsh, musical, soft, short, long), and any other abnormal findings (irregular cardiac rhythms or palpable chest wall heaves) associated with the sound.

Table 34-4 Normal Physical Assessment of the Cardiovascular System	
Inspection	Normal skin colour with capillary refill <3 sec; thorax symmetrical with no visible PMI; no JVD with patient at 45-degree angle
Palpation	PMI palpable in fifth ICS at MCL; no forceful pulsations, thrills, or heaves; slight palpable pulsations of abdominal aorta in epigastric area; carotid and extremity pulses 2+ and equal bilaterally; no evidence of impaired arterial flow or venous return in lower extremities
Percussion	Unable to distinguish right-sided heart border
Auscultation	S1 and S2 heard; HR 72 and regular; no murmurs or extra heart sounds

HR, heart rate; *ICS*, intercostal space; *JVD*, jugular venous distension; *MCL*, midclavicular line; *PMI*, point of maximal impulse.

The most common abnormal sounds and abnormal assessment findings are described in Table 34-3. A method of recording data from the cardiovascular assessment is presented in Table 34-4.

A focused assessment is used to evaluate the status of previously identified cardiovascular problems and to monitor for signs of new problems (see Table 3-6). A focused assessment of the cardiovascular system is presented in the box below.

FOCUSED ASSESSMENT
Cardiovascular System

Use this checklist to make sure the key assessment steps have been done.

Subjective

Ask the patient about any of the following and note responses

Chest pain	Y	N
Shortness of breath (especially when lying down)	Y	N
Edema in legs or any part of body	Y	N
Leg pain during exercise	Y	N
Excess urination at night	Y	N
Palpitations	Y	N

Objective: Diagnostic

Check the following laboratory tests for critical values

Hematocrit and hemoglobin	✓
Cardiac biomarkers (CK-MB, troponin)	✓
Electrocardiogram	✓

Objective: Physical Examination

Inspect and Palpate

Anterior chest wall for contour, lifts, and heaves	✓
Check pulses for symmetry, quality, and rhythm	✓

Auscultate

Blood pressure	✓
Heart for rate, rhythm, and sounds	✓

CK-MB, MB isoenzyme of creatine kinase.

Diagnostic Studies of the Cardiovascular System

Numerous diagnostic procedures add to the information obtained from the history and physical examination of the cardiovascular system. These procedures are usually classified as noninvasive or invasive. If only needle insertion for withdrawal of blood or injection of contrast media is used, these studies are usually considered noninvasive. Catheter insertion for angiography is considered

an invasive procedure. The most common studies used to assess the cardiovascular system are presented in Table 34-5.

Noninvasive Studies

Chest Radiograph. A radiographic picture can depict cardiac contours, heart size and configuration, and anatomical changes in individual chambers (see Figure 34-9). The radiographic image records any displacement or enlargement of the heart, the pres-

Text continued on p. 859

DIAGNOSTIC STUDIES

Table 34-5 Cardiovascular System

STUDY	DESCRIPTION AND PURPOSE	NURSING RESPONSIBILITY
Blood Studies*		
CK-MB	Cardiospecific isoenzyme that is released in the presence of myocardial tissue injury. Concentrations >4-6% of total CK are highly indicative of MI. Serum levels increase within 4-6 hr after MI.	Explain to patient the purpose of serial sampling (e.g., q6-8h ×3) in conjunction with serial ECGs.
Troponin (cardiac)	Contractile proteins that are released following an MI. Both troponin T and troponin I are highly specific to cardiac tissue. *Reference intervals* **Troponin I (cTnI)** Negative: <0.5 mcg/L Indeterminate or suspicious for injury to myocardium: 0.5-2.3 mcg/L Positive for myocardial injury: >2.3 mcg/L (2.3 mcg/L) **Troponin T (cTnT)** <0.1 mcg/L	Rapid point of care (bedside) assays are available. Serial sampling often done in conjunction with CK-MB and ECGs.
Myoglobin	Low-molecular-weight protein that is 99-100% sensitive for myocardial injury. Serum concentrations rise 30-60 min after MI. *Male:* 15.2-91.2 mcg/L *Female:* 11.1-57.5 mcg/L	Cleared from the circulation rapidly and most diagnostic if measured within first 12 hr of onset of chest pain.
C-reactive protein (CRP)	Marker of inflammation that can predict risk of cardiac disease and cardiac events, even in patients with normal lipid values. High-sensitivity CRP assay used. *Lowest risk:* <1 mg/L *Moderate risk:* 1-3 mg/L *High risk:* >3 mg/L	Stable levels that can be measured nonfasting and any time during the day. May be more predictive risk factor of cardiac disease than LDLs for women.
Homocysteine	Amino acid produced during protein catabolism that has been identified as a risk factor for cardiovascular disease. Homocysteine may cause damage to the endothelium or have a role in formation of thrombi. *Male:* 5.2-12.9 micromol/L *Female:* 3.7-10.4 micromol/L	Hyperhomocysteinemia resulting from dietary deficiencies is treated with folic acid, vitamin B_6, and vitamin B_{12} supplements.
B-type natriuretic peptide (BNP)	Peptide that causes natriuresis. Elevation indicates presence of heart failure and may help distinguish cardiac vs. respiratory cause of dyspnea. *Reference intervals:* *BNP* (diagnostic for heart failure) <100 ng/L	Continue to monitor for signs and symptoms of heart failure.
NT-Pro-BNP	≤74 yr: 124 pg/mL >75 yr: 449 pg/mL	

DIAGNOSTIC STUDIES

Table 34-5 Cardiovascular System—cont'd

STUDY	DESCRIPTION AND PURPOSE	NURSING RESPONSIBILITY
Serum Lipids		
Cholesterol	Cholesterol is a blood lipid. Elevated cholesterol is considered a risk factor for atherosclerotic heart disease. *Reference interval:* <5.18 mmol/L (varies with age and gender)	Cholesterol levels can be obtained in a nonfasting state.
Triglycerides	Triglycerides are mixtures of fatty acids. Elevations are associated with cardiovascular disease and diabetes. *Reference interval:* <1.7 mmol/L (varies with age)	Triglyceride levels and lipoproteins must be obtained in a fasting state (at least 12 hr, except for water); alcohol should be withheld for 24 hr before testing.
Lipoproteins† (HDL, LDL)	Electrophoresis is done to separate lipoproteins into HDL and LDL. There are marked day-to-day fluctuations in serum lipid levels. More than one determination is needed for accurate diagnosis and treatment. *Reference intervals* (vary with age): **HDL** *Recommended* *Male:* >1.04 mmol/L *Female:* >1.3 mmol/L *Low risk for CAD:* >1.55 mmol/L *High risk for CAD:* <1.04 mmol/L **LDL** *Recommended:* <2.6 mmol/L *Near optimal:* 2.6-3.34 mmol/L *Moderate risk for CAD:* 3.37-4.12 mmol/L *High risk for CAD:* >4.14 mmol/L	Risk for cardiac disease is assessed by dividing the total cholesterol level by the HDL level and obtaining a ratio. *Low risk:* Ratio <3 *Average risk:* Ratio 3-5 *Increased risk:* Ratio >5
Lipoprotein (a) (Lp[a])	Increased levels are associated with an increased risk of premature CAD and stroke. *Reference interval:* <0.3 g/L	Lp(a) levels can be obtained in a nonfasting state.
Lipoprotein-associated phospholipase A2 (Lp-PLA2)	Elevated levels of Lp-PLA2 are associated with vascular inflammation and increased risk for CAD. *Reference intervals:* *Male:* 131-376 ng/mL *Female:* 120-342 ng/mL	Lp-PLA2 levels can be obtained in a nonfasting state.
Chest radiograph	Patient is placed in two upright positions to examine the lung fields and size of the heart. The two common positions are PA and lateral. Normal heart size and contour for the individual's age, sex, and size are noted.	Inquire about frequency of recent radiographic studies and possibility of pregnancy. Provide lead shielding to areas not being viewed. Remove any jewellery or metal objects that may obstruct the view of the heart and lungs.
ECG	Electrodes are placed on the chest and extremities, allowing the ECG machine to record cardiac electrical activity from different views. Can detect rhythm of heart, activity of pacemaker, conduction abnormalities, position of heart, size of atria and ventricles, presence of injury, and history of MI.	Prepare skin and apply electrodes and leads. Inform patient that no discomfort is involved. Instruct to avoid moving to decrease motion artifact.
Signal-averaged electrocardiogram (SAECG)	Signal-averaged ECG is a high-resolution ECG that can identify electrical activity called late potentials indicating a patient is at risk for developing ventricular dysrhythmias (e.g., ventricular tachycardia).	Same as for ECG.
Ambulatory ECG Monitoring		
Holter monitoring	Recording of ECG rhythm for 24-48 hr and then correlating rhythm changes with symptoms recorded in diary. Normal patient activity is encouraged to simulate conditions that produce symptoms. Electrodes are placed on chest and a recorder is used to store information until it is recalled, printed, and analyzed for any rhythm disturbance. It can be performed on an inpatient or outpatient basis.	Prepare skin and apply electrodes and leads. Explain importance of keeping an accurate diary of activities and symptoms. Tell patient that no bath or shower can be taken during monitoring. Skin irritation may develop from electrodes.

Continued

DIAGNOSTIC STUDIES

STUDY	DESCRIPTION AND PURPOSE	NURSING RESPONSIBILITY
Table 34-5 Cardiovascular System—cont'd		
Ambulatory ECG Monitoring—cont'd		
Event monitor or loop recorder	Records rhythm disturbances that are not frequent enough to be recorded in one 24-hr period. It allows more freedom than a regular Holter monitor. Some units have electrodes that are attached to the chest and have a loop of memory that captures the onset and end of an event. Other types are placed directly on patient's wrist, chest, or fingers and have no loop of memory, but record the patient's ECG in real time. Recordings may be transmitted over the phone to a receiving unit.	Instruct in the use of equipment for recording and transmitting (if appropriate) of transient events. Teach patient about skin preparation for lead placement or steady skin contact for units not requiring electrodes. This will ensure the reception of optimal ECG tracings for analysis. Instruct patient to initiate recording as soon as symptoms begin or as soon thereafter as possible.
Exercise or stress testing	Various protocols are used to evaluate the effect of exercise tolerance on cardiovascular function. A common protocol uses 3-min stages at set speeds and elevation of the treadmill belt. The patient can exercise to either predicted peak HR (calculated by subtracting the person's age from 220) or to peak exercise tolerance, at which time the test is terminated. The test is also terminated for chest discomfort, significant increase or decrease in vital signs from baseline, or significant ECG changes indicating cardiac ischemia. Vital signs and ECG are monitored. The ECG is monitored after exercise for rhythm disturbances or, if ECG changes occurred with exercise, for return to baseline. Continual monitoring of vital signs and ECG rhythms for ischemic changes is important in the diagnosis of CAD. An exercise bike may be used if the patient is unable to walk on the treadmill.	Instruct patient to wear comfortable clothes and shoes that can be used for walking and running. Instruct patient about procedure and importance of reporting any symptoms that may occur. Monitor vital signs and obtain 12-lead ECG before exercise, during each stage of exercise, and after exercise until all vital signs and ECG changes have returned to normal. Monitor patient's response throughout procedure. Contraindications include any reasons patient is unable to reach peak exercise. β-Adrenergic blockers may be held 24 hr before the test because they will blunt the heart rate and limit the patient's ability to achieve maximal heart rate. Caffeine-containing food and fluids are held for 24 hr. Patients must refrain from smoking and strenuous exercise for 3 hr before test.
6-Minute walk test	Distance patient is able to walk on a flat surface in 6 min. Used to measure response to treatments and determine functional capacity for activities of daily living. Useful in people who are unable to perform treadmill or exercise bike testing.	Instruct patient to wear comfortable shoes. Inform patient to carry or pull oxygen if used routinely. Patient should be encouraged to walk as quickly as possible.
Echocardiogram • Contrast • M-mode • Two-dimensional • Colour-flow imaging (duplex) • Real-time three-dimensional	Transducer that emits and receives ultrasound waves is placed in four positions on the chest above the heart. Transducer records sound waves that are bounced off the heart. Also records direction and flow of blood through the heart and transforms it to audio and graphic data that measure valvular abnormalities, congenital cardiac defects, wall motion, ejection fraction, and cardiac function. IV contrast agent may be used to enhance images.	Place patient in a supine position on left side facing equipment. Instruct patient about procedure and sensations (pressure and mechanical movement from head of transducer). No contraindications to procedure exist.
Stress echocardiogram	Combination of exercise test and echocardiogram. Resting images of the heart are taken with ultrasound and then the patient exercises. Postexercise images are taken immediately after exercise (within 1 min of stopping exercise). Differences in left ventricular wall motion and thickening before and after exercise are evaluated.	Instruct and prepare patient for treadmill or exercise bicycle. Inform patient of importance of timely return to examination table for imaging after exercise. Contraindications include any reasons patient is unable to reach peak exercise.
Pharmacological echocardiogram	Used as a substitute for the exercise stress test in individuals unable to exercise. Dobutamine (a positive inotropic agent) or dipyridamole is infused intravenously and dosage is increased in 5-min intervals while echocardiogram is performed to detect wall motion abnormalities at each stage.	Start IV infusion. Administer medication per protocol. Monitor vital signs before, during, and after test until baseline achieved. Monitor patient for signs and symptoms of distress during procedure. Observe patient for adverse effects (e.g., shortness of breath, dizziness, nausea). Aminophylline may be given to prevent or reverse adverse effects of dipyridamole. Contraindications include any known allergies to medications.

DIAGNOSTIC STUDIES

Table 34-5 Cardiovascular System—cont'd

STUDY	DESCRIPTION AND PURPOSE	NURSING RESPONSIBILITY
Transesophageal echocardiogram (TEE)	A probe with an ultrasound transducer at the tip is swallowed while the physician controls angle and depth. As it passes down the esophagus, it sends back clear images of heart size, wall motion, valvular abnormalities, endocarditis vegetation, and possible source of thrombi without interference from lungs or chest ribs. A contrast medium may be injected intravenously for evaluating direction of blood flow if an atrial or ventricular septal defect is suspected. Doppler ultrasound and colour-flow imaging can also be used concurrently.	Instruct patient to be NPO for at least 6 hr before test. Remove dentures. A bite block is placed in the mouth. IV sedation is administered and throat locally anesthetized. A designated driver is needed if test is done in the outpatient department. Monitor vital signs and oxygen saturation levels and perform suctioning as needed during procedure. Assist patient to relax. Patient may not eat or drink until gag reflex returns. Sore throat is temporary.
Nuclear cardiology	Study involves IV injection of radioactive isotopes (99m technetium-sestamibi). Radioactive uptake is counted over the heart by scintillation camera. It supplies information about myocardial contractility, myocardial perfusion, and acute cell injury.	Explain procedure to patient. Establish IV line for injection of isotopes. Explain that radioactive isotope used is a small, diagnostic amount and will lose most of its radioactivity in a few hours. Inform the patient that he or she will be lying still on back with arms extended overhead for 20 min. Repeat scans are performed within a few minutes to hours after the injection.
Multigated acquisition (MUGA) (cardiac blood pool) scan	A small amount of the patient's blood is removed, mixed with a radioactive isotope (e.g., 99m technetium-sestamibi [Cardiolite]), and reinjected intravenously. Using the ECG for timing, images are acquired during the cardiac cycle. Indicated for patients with MI, heart failure, or valvular heart disease. It also can be used to evaluate the effect of various cardiac or cardiotoxic medications on the heart.	Explain procedure to patient. Establish IV line for removal of blood sample and reinjection of isotope. Establish ECG monitoring. Inform patient that procedure involves little risk.
Single-photon emission computed tomography (SPECT)	Used to evaluate myocardium at risk of infarction and to determine infarction size. Small amounts of a radioactive isotope (e.g., 99m technetium-tetrofosmin [Myoview], thallium-201) are injected intravenously and recordings are made of the radioactivity emitted over a specific area of the body. Circulation of the isotope can be used to detect coronary artery blood flow, intracardiac shunts, motion of ventricles, EF, and size of the heart chambers.	Explain procedure to patient. Establish IV line for injection of isotope. Establish ECG monitoring. Inform patient that procedure involves little risk.
Exercise (stress) nuclear imaging	Nuclear imaging images are taken at rest and after exercise. The injection is given at maximum heart rate on bicycle or treadmill. Patient is then required to continue exercise for 1 min to circulate the radioactive isotope. Scanning is done 15-60 min after exercise. A resting scan is performed 60-90 min after initial infusion or 24 hr later.	Explain procedure to patient. Instruct patient to eat only a light meal between scans. Certain medications may need to be held for 1-2 days before the scan.
Pharmacological nuclear imaging	Dipyridamole or adenosine is used to produce vasodilation when patients are unable to tolerate exercise. Vasodilation will increase blood flow to well-perfused coronary arteries. Scanning procedure is same. Aminophylline may be given to prevent or reverse adverse effects of dipyridamole (e.g., shortness of breath, dizziness, nausea). Dobutamine is used if vasodilators are contraindicated.	Explain procedure to patient. Instruct patient to hold all caffeine products for 12 hr before procedure. Calcium channel blockers and β-adrenergic blockers should be held 24 hr before the test. Observe patient for adverse effects (e.g., shortness of breath, dizziness, nausea).
Positron emission tomography (PET)	Highly sensitive in distinguishing viable and nonviable myocardial tissue. Uses two radionuclides. Nitrogen-13-ammonia is injected intravenously first and scanned to evaluate myocardial perfusion. A second radioactive isotope, fluoro-18-deoxyglucose, is then injected and scanned to show myocardial metabolic function. In the normal heart, both scans will match, but in an ischemic or damaged heart, they will differ. The patient may or may not be stressed. A baseline resting scan is usually obtained for comparison.	Instruct patient on procedure. Explain that patient will be scanned by a machine and will need to stay still for a period of time. Patient's glucose level must be between 3.3 and 7.8 μmol/L for accurate glucose metabolic activity. If exercise is included as part of testing, patient will need to be NPO and refrain from tobacco and caffeine for 24 hr before test.

Continued

DIAGNOSTIC STUDIES

Table 34-5 Cardiovascular System—cont'd

STUDY	DESCRIPTION AND PURPOSE	NURSING RESPONSIBILITY
Magnetic resonance imaging (MRI)	Noninvasive imaging technique obtains information about cardiac tissue integrity, aneurysms, ejection fractions, cardiac output, and patency of proximal coronary arteries. It does not involve ionizing radiation and is an extremely safe procedure. It provides images in multiple planes with uniformly good resolution.	Explain procedure to patient. Inform patient that the small diameter of the cylinder, along with loud noise of the procedure, may cause panic or anxiety. Antianxiety drugs and distraction strategies (e.g., music) may be recommended. Patient must lie still during MRI. Contraindicated for people with implanted metallic devices or other metal fragments. Discuss any implants before scan.
Magnetic resonance angiography (MRA)	Used for imaging vascular occlusive disease and abdominal aortic aneurysms. Same as MRI but with use of gadolinium as IV contrast medium.	Contraindications include any known allergies to contrast medium and people with implanted metallic devices or other metal fragments.
Cardiac CT	Cardiac CT is heart-specific CT imaging technology with or without IV contrast media used to visualize heart anatomy, coronary circulation, and blood vessels.	
Computed tomography angiography (CTA)	Use of CT with injected IV contrast medium to obtain images of blood vessels and diagnose CAD.	Explain procedure to patient. Metal objects should be removed before examination. The patient may be asked not to eat or drink for several hours before the procedure.
Calcium-scoring CT scan • Electron beam computed tomography (EBCT)	EBCT, also known as ultrafast CT, uses a scanning electron beam to quantify calcification in coronary arteries and heart valves (see Figure 34-12). Primarily used for risk assessment in asymptomatic patients and to assess for heart disease in patients with atypical symptoms potentially caused by cardiac causes.	Explain procedure to patient. Inform patient that procedure is quick and involves little or no risk.
Cardiac catheterization	Involves insertion of catheter into heart to obtain information about O_2 levels and pressure readings within heart chambers. Contrast medium is injected to assist in examining structure and motion of heart. Procedure is done by inserting a catheter into the artery.	Check for iodine sensitivity. Withhold food and fluids for 6-18 hr before procedure. Give sedative and other drugs, if ordered. Inform patient about use of local anaesthesia, insertion of catheter, and feeling of warmth when dye is injected and possible fluttering sensation of heart as catheter is passed. Note that patient may be instructed to cough or take a deep breath when dye is injected and that patient is monitored by ECG throughout procedure. After procedure, assess circulation to extremity used for catheter insertion. Check peripheral pulses, colour, and sensation of extremity every 15 min for 1 hr and then with decreasing frequency. Observe puncture site for hematoma and bleeding. Place compression device over arterial site to achieve hemostasis, if indicated. Monitor vital signs and ECG. Assess for hypotension or hypertension, abnormal HR, dysrhythmias, and signs of pulmonary emboli (e.g., respiratory difficulty).
Coronary angiography	During a cardiac catheterization contrast medium is injected directly into coronary arteries. Used to evaluate patency of coronary arteries and collateral circulation.	Same as for cardiac catheterization.
Noninvasive coronary computed tomography angiography (CCTA)	CCTA is a noninvasive imaging modality which can be used to evaluate the anatomy of the coronary arteries. Unlike coronary artery calcium scoring, which utilizes noncontrast CT to assess atherosclerotic disease burden, CCTA allows direct visualization of the coronary artery wall and lumen with the administration of IV contrast.	Same as for cardiac catheterization.
Intracoronary ultrasound	During cardiac catheterization a small ultrasound probe is introduced into coronary arteries. Data are used to assess size and consistency of plaque, arterial walls, and effectiveness of intracoronary artery treatment.	Same as for cardiac catheterization.

DIAGNOSTIC STUDIES

Table 34-5 Cardiovascular System—cont'd

STUDY	DESCRIPTION AND PURPOSE	NURSING RESPONSIBILITY
Fractional flow reserve	During cardiac catheterization, a special wire is inserted into the coronary arteries to measure pressure and flow. Information is used to determine need for angioplasty or stenting on nonsignificant blockages.	Same as for cardiac catheterization.
Electrophysiology study (EPS)	Invasive study used to record intracardiac electrical activity using catheters (with multiple electrodes) inserted via the femoral and jugular veins into the right side of the heart. The catheter electrodes record the electrical activity in different cardiac structures. In addition, dysrhythmias can be induced and terminated.	Antidysrhythmic medications may be discontinued several days before study. Keep patient NPO 6-8 hr before test. Give premedication to promote relaxation if ordered. IV sedation often used during procedure. Patient must have frequent vital signs and continuous ECG monitoring after the procedure.
Peripheral arteriography and venography‡	Involves injection of radiopaque contrast medium into either arteries or veins. Serial radiographs taken to detect and visualize any atherosclerotic plaques, occlusion, aneurysms, or traumatic injury.	Check for iodine allergy. Give mild sedative, if ordered. Check extremity with puncture site for pulsation, warmth, colour, and motion after procedure. Inspect insertion site for bleeding or swelling. Observe patient for allergic reactions to dye.
Hemodynamic monitoring	Hemodynamic monitoring of arterial blood pressures, pulmonary artery pressure, pulmonary artery wedge pressure, and cardiac output is done to evaluate cardiovascular status and response to treatment.	Patients requiring hemodynamic monitoring are critically ill and are monitored in critical care units. See Chapter 68 for complete information on hemodynamic monitoring.

CAD, coronary artery disease; *CK*, creatine kinase; *CK-MB*, MB isoenzyme of creatine kinase; *CT*, computed tomography; *ECGs*, electrocardiograms; *EF*, ejection fraction; *HDL*, high-density lipoprotein; *HR*, heart rate; *IV*, intravenous; *LDLs*, low-density lipoproteins; *MI*, myocardial infarction; *NPO*, nothing by mouth; *NT-pro-BNP*, N-terminal–pro b-type natriuretic peptide; *O₂*, oxygen; *PA*, posteroanterior.

*Reference ranges for the laboratory tests vary by institution because of differences in equipment and reagents used.
†Source: American Heart Association. (2011). *What your cholesterol levels mean.* Retrieved from *http://www.heart.org/HEARTORG/Conditions/What-Your-Cholesterol-Levels-Mean_UCM_305562_Article.jsp*
‡Additional peripheral vascular diagnostic studies are found in Table 40-8.

ence of extra fluid around the heart (pericardial effusion), and pulmonary congestion.

Electrocardiogram. The basic P, QRS, and T waveforms (see Figure 34-4) are used to assess cardiac function. Deviations from the normal sinus rhythm can indicate abnormalities in heart function. There are many types of electrocardiographic monitoring, including resting ECG, ambulatory ECG monitoring, and exercise or stress testing.

A resting ECG helps identify at one point in time primary conduction abnormalities, cardiac dysrhythmias, cardiac hypertrophy, pericarditis, myocardial ischemia, site and extent of myocardial infarction (MI), pacemaker performance, and effectiveness of drug therapy. It is also used to monitor recovery from an MI. (See Chapter 38 for a complete discussion of ECG monitoring.)

Ambulatory Electrocardiogram Monitoring. Continuous ambulatory ECG (Holter monitoring) can provide diagnostic information over a greater period than a standard resting ECG. In Holter monitoring, a recorder is worn by the patient for 24 to 48 hours, and the resulting ECG information is then stored until it is played back for printing and evaluation. Holter monitoring gives the patient freedom to perform usual activities of daily living and those that may be associated with cardiovascular symptoms. The patient maintains a record of activities, symptoms, and sleep and this record is correlated with the ECG events recorded by the device (see Table 34-5).

Transtelephonic Event Recorders. This type of recorder is helpful for monitoring less frequent ECG events. The monitor is a portable unit that uses electrodes to transmit a limited ECG over the phone to a receiving device. A disadvantage of this type of monitoring is that, if the event occurs for only a short duration, the symptoms may pass before the patient puts on the device and calls the assigned number. Likewise, if patients are extremely symptomatic (e.g., syncopal), they may not be physically able to transmit the ECG.

Exercise or Stress Testing. Cardiac symptoms frequently occur only with activity as a result of the demand on the coronary arteries to provide additional oxygen. Exercise testing is a method used to evaluate the cardiovascular response to physical stress. This is helpful in assessing cardiovascular disease and defining limits for exercise programs. Patient selection for exercise testing is appropriate for individuals who do not have limitations related to walking or using a bicycle and those without abnormal ECGs that limit diagnostic interpretation (e.g., pacemakers, left bundle branch block). β-Adrenergic blockers may be held 24 hours before the test because they will blunt the HR and not allow the patients to achieve maximal HR. Patients should be instructed to refrain from eating, drinking caffeine-containing drinks, smoking, and participating in strenuous exercise for 3 hours before the test.

The placement of electrodes is similar to that of a regular 12-lead placement (see Chapter 38). Resting BPs and ECGs are performed in the supine position, while standing, and after hyperventilation to provide a baseline for comparison of any changes during exercise.

As the patient exercises on a treadmill or stationary bicycle, the BP, the ECG, and often the oxygen saturation level are measured and monitored. The patient exercises to either peak HR

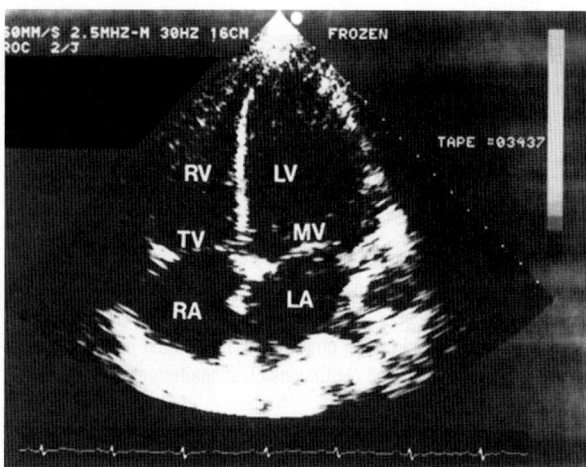

Figure 34-10 Apical four-chamber two-dimensional echocardiographic view in a normal patient. *LA*, left atrium; *LV*, left ventricle; *MV*, mitral valve; *RA*, right atrium; *RV*, right ventricle; *TV*, tricuspid valve.

Source: Adapted from Kinney, M. R., & Packa, D. R. (Eds.). (1996). *Andreoli's comprehensive cardiac care* (8th ed.). St Louis: Mosby.

(calculated by subtracting the person's age from 220) or peak exercise tolerance, at which time the test is terminated and the treadmill is slowed while the patient continues walking. The test is also terminated for moderate to severe chest discomfort, significant increase or decrease in BP from baseline, or significant ECG changes indicating ischemia associated with CAD. The ECG is monitored after exercise for rhythm disturbances or, if ECG changes occurred with exercise, for return to baseline.

Echocardiogram. The echocardiogram uses ultrasound waves to record the movement of the structures of the heart. In the normal heart, ultrasonic sound waves directed at the heart are reflected back in typical configurations (Figure 34-10). The echocardiogram provides information about abnormalities of (1) valvular structure and motion, (2) cardiac chamber size and contents, (3) ventricular muscle and septal motion and thickness, (4) the pericardial sac, and (5) the ascending aorta. The **ejection fraction (EF),** or the percentage of end-diastolic blood volume that is ejected during systole, can also be measured. The EF provides information about the function of the left ventricle during systole.

Two commonly used types are the M-mode (motion mode) and the two-dimensional echocardiogram. In the M-mode type, a single ultrasound beam is directed toward the heart, recording the motion of the intracardiac structures as well as detecting wall thickness and chamber size. The two-dimensional echocardiogram sweeps the ultrasound beam through an arc, producing a cross-sectional view, and shows correct spatial relationships among the structures.

Doppler technology allows for sound evaluation of the flow or motion of the scanned object (heart valves, ventricular walls, blood flow). Colour-flow imaging (duplex) is the combination of two-dimensional echocardiography and Doppler technology. It uses colour changes to demonstrate the velocity and direction of blood flow. Pathological conditions, such as valvular leaks and congenital defects, can be diagnosed more effectively. Stress echocardiography, a combination of treadmill test and ultrasound images, evaluates segmental wall motion abnormalities (Pagana & Pagana, 2010). Using a digital computer system to compare

images before and after exercise, wall motion and segmental function can be clearly seen. This diagnostic test provides the information of an exercise stress test combined with that gained from an echocardiogram. For those individuals unable to exercise, infusion of a pharmacological agent—usually dobutamine (Dobutrex) or dipyridamole (Persantine)—induces stress on the heart while the patient is resting. The same ultrasound technology is used.

Transesophageal echocardiography (TEE) is used to provide more precise echocardiography of the heart than surface two-dimensional echocardiography by eliminating interference from the chest wall and the lungs. The TEE uses a modified, flexible endoscope probe with an ultrasound transducer in the tip for imaging of the heart and great vessels. The probe is introduced into the esophagus to the level of the heart, and M-mode, two-dimensional, pulsed Doppler, and colour-flow imaging can be obtained.

TEE is used frequently in an outpatient setting primarily for evaluation of mitral regurgitation, the presence of thrombus before performing cardioversion, or the source of cardiac emboli. In addition, TEE has applications in the operating room to assess presurgical and postsurgical cardiac function and in the emergency department for suspicion of aortic dissection.

The risks of TEE are minimal. However, complications may include perforation of the esophagus, hemorrhage, dysrhythmias, vasovagal reactions, and transient hypoxemia. TEE is contraindicated if the patient has a history of esophageal disorders, dysphagia, or radiation therapy to the chest wall. Patients must be sedated during a TEE.

Contrast echocardiography uses intravenous contrast agents (e.g., albumin microbubbles, agitated saline) to assist in delineation of the images, especially in patients presenting technical difficulties (Pagana & Pagana, 2010). When these agents are injected into the cardiac blood pool, they greatly enhance reflectivity for the ultrasound procedure.

Real-time three-dimensional ultrasound is a new technology that uses multiple two-dimensional echo images with computer technology to provide a reconstruction of the heart. This technique generates precise information about the structures of the heart and how these structures change during the cardiac cycle (Pagana & Pagana, 2010). It is useful for the detection of congenital heart defects and endocarditis as well as for the calculation of ventricular volumes.

Nuclear Cardiology. One of the most common nuclear imaging tests is the multigated acquisition (MUGA) or cardiac blood pool scan. This test provides information on wall motion during systole and diastole, cardiac valves, and EF. A small amount of the patient's blood is removed, mixed with a radioactive isotope (e.g., technetium-99m [^{99m}Tc] sestamibi [Cardiolite]), and reinjected. Using the ECG for timing, images are acquired during the cardiac cycle.

Single-photon emission computed tomography (SPECT) is used for the evaluation of the myocardium at risk of infarction and to determine infarction size. Small amounts of a radioactive isotope (e.g., ^{99m}Tc tetrofosmin [Myoview] or thallium-201) are injected intravenously, and recordings are made of the radioactivity emitted over a specific area of the body. The total radiation exposure is minimal. The circulation of this tagged material can be used to detect coronary artery blood flow, intracardiac shunts, motion of ventricles, EF, and size of the heart chambers.

Positron emission tomography (PET) scanning uses two isotopes (see Table 34-5). PET scans are highly sensitive in distinguishing viable and nonviable myocardial tissue. Equipment costs limit the widespread use of PET scanning (Pagana & Pagana, 2010).

Perfusion imaging is also used with exercise testing to determine whether the coronary blood flow changes with increased activity. Stress perfusion imaging may show an abnormality even when a resting image is normal. This procedure is indicated to diagnose CAD, determine the prognosis in already diagnosed CAD, assess the physiological significance of a known coronary lesion, and assess the effectiveness of various therapeutic modalities such as coronary artery bypass surgery or percutaneous coronary intervention (see Chapter 36). Technetium pyrophosphate imaging can also provide an estimate of the magnitude of myocardial salvage at the time of acute MI. Because Cardiolite remains in the myocardium for several hours after injection, a patient can be injected before treatment and later scanned to obtain a picture of the potential infarct size before treatment. A second injection later will determine the final infarct size, and the change between the two images demonstrates myocardial salvage.

Stress perfusion imaging is always preferred but, if a patient is unable to tolerate exercise, intravenous dipyridamole or adenosine (Adenocard) may be given to dilate the coronary arteries and simulate the effect of exercise. After the vasodilator takes effect, the isotope is injected and the nuclear procedure proceeds. All caffeine and theophylline products must be held 12 hours before the study because they counteract the vasodilator effects of the stress agents. Calcium channel blockers and β-adrenergic blockers should be held 24 hours before the test. Patients may be given aminophylline either prophylactically at the end of the test or in response to symptoms because it is a specific blocker of the vasodilators and will eliminate or reduce adverse effects (e.g., bronchospasm). Dobutamine is used as a pharmacological adrenergic stress agent for patients who have contraindications to vasodilator stress agents. The protocol for its use is similar for the vasodilator stress tests, and adverse effects are rare (Wackers, Bruni, & Zaret, 2007).

Magnetic Resonance Imaging.
Although not widely used because of equipment size and access, magnetic resonance imaging (MRI) allows detection and localization of areas of MI in a three-dimensional view. It is sensitive enough to gauge even small MIs not apparent with SPECT imaging and can assist in the final diagnosis of MI. It is also beginning to play a role in prediction of viability and recovery from MI. Its utility for diagnosis of presence and severity of CAD is still being studied (Wackers et al., 2007).

Magnetic resonance angiography (MRA) is used for imaging vascular occlusive disease and abdominal aortic aneurysms. The contrast material is non–iodine based and is injected through an intravenous line. The MRA images compare favourably to duplex ultrasound of arterial stenosis (Debrey et al., 2008).

Computed Tomography.
Computed tomography (CT) with spiral technology is a noninvasive scan used to quantify calcium deposits in coronary arteries. It has been limited by the difficulty of imaging the constantly moving heart and the need for patients to hold their breath for each set of image acquisitions (Libby et al., 2008). Electron beam computed tomography (EBCT), also known as *ultrafast CT,* uses a scanning electron beam to allow quantification of calcification in the coronary arteries and the heart valves. A calcium score can be formulated for a segment of a coronary artery, a specific coronary artery, or

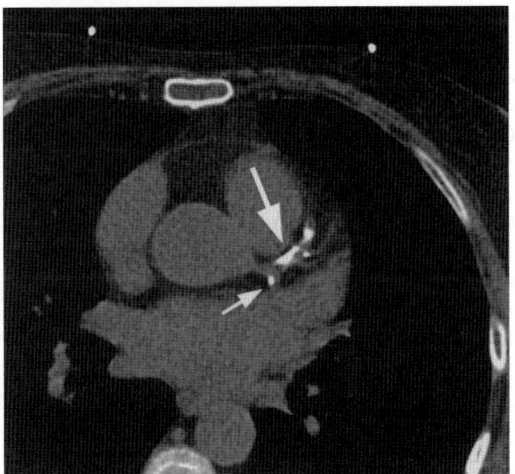

Figure 34-11 Examples of coronary calcification of the left anterior descending coronary artery *(large arrow)* and left circumflex artery *(small arrow)* as seen on electron beam computed tomography.

Source: Braunwald, E. (2005). In D. Zipes, D. Libby, & R. Bonow (Eds.), *Braunwald's heart disease: A textbook of cardiovascular medicine,* Vol. 1 (7th ed., p. 363, Figure 15-14, A). St. Louis: Saunders.

the entire coronary system (Pagana & Pagana, 2010). The test is rapid and noninvasive and may have clinical applications for screening in patients with and without symptoms of cardiac disease (Figure 34-11).

Blood Studies. Numerous diagnostic procedures add to the information obtained from the history and the physical examination of the cardiovascular system. The most common studies used to assess the cardiovascular system are presented in Table 34-5.

Cardiac Markers. When myocardial cells are injured, they release their contents, including enzymes and other proteins, into the circulation. These biochemical markers are useful in the diagnosis of myocardial injury and necrosis. The enzymes characteristic of cardiac injury are creatine kinase (CK), lactate dehydrogenase (LDH), and serum aspartate aminotransferase (AST), formerly called serum glutamic–oxaloacetic transaminase (SGOT). Because these enzymes are found in a variety of body tissues, they can be elevated as a result of injury to the muscles, the liver, the brain, and other organs. LDH and AST levels are no longer used as markers of myocardial injury. CK is present in heart muscle, skeletal muscle, and brain tissue. The MM isoenzyme of creatine kinase (CK-MM) is found primarily in the skeletal muscle, and the BB isoenzyme of creatine kinase (CK-BB) is found in the brain and nervous tissue. MB isoenzyme of creatine kinase (CK-MB) elevation is specific for myocardial tissue injury. CK-MB levels rise 4 to 6 hours after symptom onset, peak in 18 to 24 hours, and return to baseline within 3 days after MI (Screiber, 2011).

Cardiac-specific troponin is a myocardial muscle protein released into circulation after injury. There are two subtypes, cardiac-specific troponin T (cTnT) and cardiac-specific troponin I (cTnI), that are specific to myocardial tissue. Normally, there is no circulating troponin, so a rise in its level is diagnostic of myocardial injury. cTnT and cTnI are detectable within 1 hour of myocardial injury, have high specificity at 3 to 6 hours following the onset of symptoms, and reach peak levels within 12 hours (Screiber, 2011).

Myoglobin is a low-molecular-weight heme protein found in cardiac and skeletal muscle. Myoglobin elevation is a sensitive indicator of early myocardial injury, and serum elevations occur within 30 to 60 minutes after injury but decline rapidly after 7 hours. Its clinical value is limited owing to the nonspecificity of myoglobin for MI and its brief presence following infarction (Screiber, 2011).

Correct interpretation of diagnostic tests requires consideration of the time frame from the onset of symptoms together with the time frame of the expected presence and elevated levels of the biomarkers. The additional data (patient symptoms, history, and ECG changes) complete the diagnostic picture for the patient with a suspected MI (Aehlert, 2011).

Serum Lipids. Serum lipids consist of triglycerides, cholesterol, and phospholipids. They circulate in the blood bound to protein. Thus, they are often referred to as *lipoproteins* (see Chapter 36, Figure 36-5). (Types of serum lipids are depicted in eFigure 34-1, available on the Evolve website for this chapter.)

Triglycerides are the main storage form of lipids and constitute approximately 95% of fatty tissue. Cholesterol, a structural component of cell membranes and plasma lipoproteins, is a precursor of corticosteroids, sex hormones, and bile salts. In addition to being absorbed from food in the gastrointestinal tract, cholesterol can also be synthesized in the liver. Phospholipids contain glycerol, fatty acids, phosphates, and a nitrogenous compound. Although formed in most cells, phospholipids usually enter the circulation as lipoproteins synthesized by the liver. Apoproteins are water-soluble proteins that combine with most lipids to form lipoproteins.

Different classes of lipoproteins contain varying amounts of the naturally occurring lipids. These include the following:

1. Chylomicrons: primarily exogenous triglycerides from dietary fat.
2. Low-density lipoproteins (LDLs): mostly cholesterol with moderate amounts of phospholipids.
3. High-density lipoproteins (HDLs): about one-half protein and one-half phospholipids and cholesterol.
4. Very low density lipoproteins (VLDLs): primarily endogenous triglycerides with moderate amounts of phospholipids and cholesterol.

A lipid profile test usually consists of cholesterol, triglyceride, LDL, and HDL measurements. An elevation in LDL level has a strong and direct association with CAD; an increased HDL level has been associated with a decreased risk of CAD (Woods et al., 2009). High levels of HDLs serve a protective role by mobilizing cholesterol from tissues. (This is illustrated in eFigure 34-2, available on the Evolve Web site for this chapter.)

Increased triglyceride levels are also linked to the progression of CAD. Although the association between elevated serum cholesterol levels and CAD exists, determination of the total cholesterol level alone is not sufficient for an assessment of coronary risk. A risk assessment for CAD is determined by comparing the total cholesterol with the HDL ratio over time (Mudd et al., 2007). An increase in the ratio indicates increased risk. This combination provides more information than either value alone. The patient must fast for 12 to 14 hours before the blood draw to eliminate the effects of a recent meal. A specimen should not be drawn if the patient is having acute stress.

Plasma levels of apolipoprotein A-1 (apo A-1) (the major HDL protein) and apolipoprotein B (apo B) (the major LDL protein) may be better predictors of CAD than HDLs or LDLs. Measurements of these lipoproteins may replace cholesterol–lipoprotein determinations in assessing the risk of CAD but typically are used for patients with known CAD, suspected familial hypercholesterolemia, or other lipid disorders (Woods et al., 2009).

Lipoprotein (a), or Lp(a), has been associated with cardiovascular disease in a number of studies and more evidence is emerging demonstrating the interaction with Lp(a) and other cardiac risk factors (Berglund & Anuurad, 2008). Increased levels of Lp(a), especially with increased levels of LDH, have been associated with the progression of atherosclerosis. In addition, Lp(a) has been found to have thrombogenic properties that increase the risk of clot formation at the site of intravascular lesions.

Lipoprotein-Associated Phospholipase A2. Lipoprotein-associated phospholipase A2 (Lp-PLA2) is an enzyme made by macrophages. Lp-PLA2 promotes vascular inflammation through the hydrolysis of oxidized LDLs within the intima of blood vessels, thus contributing directly to the development of atherosclerosis. Elevated levels of Lp-PLA2 are indicative of the vascular inflammation that is associated with the formation of plaque within the arteries.

Serum levels of Lp-PLA2 are measured by the PLAC® test. An elevated Lp-PLA2 level, even without an elevation in the LDL cholesterol level, has been related to an increased risk of having CAD. The PLAC® blood test can be included in a normal clinical evaluation to better determine a patient's risk for developing CAD.

C-Reactive Protein. C-reactive protein (CRP) is a protein produced by the liver during periods of acute inflammation. It is emerging as an independent risk factor for CAD and a predictor of cardiac events. In one large study of women, it was found to be more predictive of cardiac events than LDLs (Woods et al., 2009).

Homocysteine. Homocysteine (Hcy) is an amino acid that is produced during protein catabolism. Elevated Hcy levels can be either hereditary or acquired from dietary deficiencies of vitamins B_6 or B_{12} or folate. Elevated levels of Hcy have been linked to an increased risk of a first cardiac event. They have also been identified as a predictor of CAD, stroke, and thromboembolism even in the presence of normal lipid levels. It is recommended that Hcy testing be performed in those patients with a familial predisposition for early cardiovascular disease (Woods et al., 2009). "Evidence suggests that homocysteine may promote atherosclerosis (fatty deposits in blood vessels) by damaging the inner lining of arteries and promoting blood clots. However, a causal link hasn't been established" (American Heart Association, 2008).

Cardiac Natriuretic Peptide Markers. There are three natriuretic peptides: atrial natriuretic peptide (ANP) originates in the atrium, B-type natriuretic peptide (BNP) in the ventricles, and C-type natriuretic peptide in endothelial and renal epithelial cells. BNP has emerged as the marker of choice for distinguishing a cardiac or respiratory cause of dyspnea. N-terminal pro–brain natriuretic peptide (NT-pro-BNP) is also secreted in the ventricles and is more sensitive but less specific than BNP for heart failure (Olsson et al., 2007). When DBP increases (e.g., heart failure), BNP and NT-pro-BNP are released and increase natriuresis.

Invasive Studies

Invasive studies are performed if definitive information is required. These studies include cardiac catheterization, coronary angiography, electrophysiology, and intracoronary ultrasound.

Cardiac Catheterization and Coronary Angiography. Cardiac catheterization is a common outpatient procedure. It provides a means of obtaining information about CAD, congenital heart disease, valvular heart disease, and ventricular function. Cardiac catheterization can be used to measure intracardiac pressures and O_2 levels in various parts of the heart, as well as CO. With injection of contrast media and fluoroscopy, the coronary arteries can be visualized, chambers of the heart can be outlined, and wall motion can be observed.

Cardiac catheterization is performed by insertion of a radiopaque catheter into the right or left side of the heart. For the right side of the heart, a catheter is inserted through an arm vein (basilica or cephalic) or a leg vein (femoral). The catheter is advanced into the vena cava, the right atrium, and the right ventricle. The catheter is further inserted into the pulmonary artery, and pressures are recorded. The catheter is then advanced until it is wedged or lodged in position. This position is called the *pulmonary artery wedge position*. The pulmonary artery wedge position (wedge pressure) obstructs the flow and the pressure from the right side of the heart and looks forward through the pulmonary capillary bed to the pressure in the left side of the heart. The wedge pressure is used to determine the function of the left side of the heart.

The left heart catheterization is performed by insertion of a catheter into a femoral or brachial artery. The catheter is passed in a retrograde manner up the aorta, across the aortic valve, and into the left ventricle. Coronary angiography can be done with a left heart catheterization (Figure 34-12).

Patients frequently feel a temporary hot and flushed sensation with contrast media injection. (See Table 34-5 for the nursing responsibilities related to cardiac catheterization.)

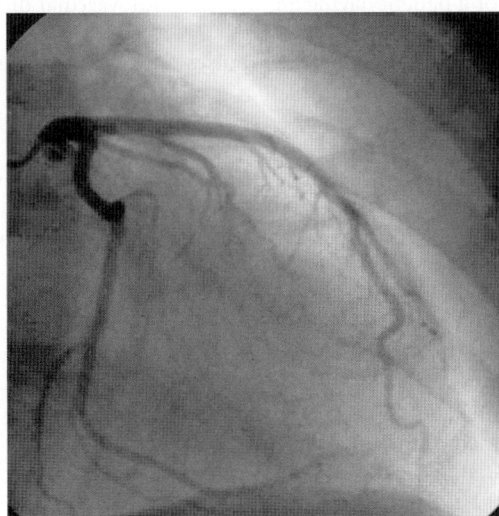

Figure 34-12 Normal left coronary artery angiogram.

Complications of cardiac catheterization include looping, kinking, or breaking off of the catheter; blood loss; allergic reaction to the contrast media; infection; thrombus formation; air or blood embolism; dysrhythmias; MI; stroke; puncture of the ventricles, cardiac septum, or lung tissue; and rarely, death (Dixon, Grines, & O'Neill, 2008).

Coronary computed tomography angiography (CCTA) is a noninvasive imaging modality that can be used to evaluate the anatomy of the coronary arteries. This study allows direct visualization of the coronary artery wall and lumen with the administration of intravenous contrast. Improvements in this noninvasive technology allow reliable noninvasive detection of obstructive CAD (Raff, Gallagher, O'Neill, & Goldstein, 2005).

Electrophysiology Study. Electrophysiology study (EPS) is the direct study and manipulation of the electrical activity of the heart using electrodes placed inside the cardiac chambers. It provides information on SA node function, AV node conduction, and ventricular conduction. It is particularly helpful in diagnosing the source of dysrhythmias. Patients with a history of symptomatic supraventricular or ventricular tachycardias may obtain an accurate diagnosis and treatment with this technique (Josephson, 2008).

Catheters are inserted in a method similar to that used for right and left heart catheterization. These catheters are placed at specific anatomical sites within the heart to record electrical activity. Nursing care for patients after EPS includes close ECG monitoring, puncture site assessment, vital signs, and other responsibilities related to care following a cardiac catheterization.

Intracoronary Ultrasound. Intracoronary ultrasound (ICUS), also known as intravascular ultrasound (IVUS), is an invasive procedure performed in the catheterization laboratory. The two-dimensional or three-dimensional ultrasound images provide a cross-sectional view of the arterial walls of the coronary arteries.

A miniature transducer attached to a small catheter is introduced through a peripheral artery and advanced to the artery to be studied. Once in the artery, ultrasound images are obtained. The health of the arterial layers is assessed, as are the composition, the location, and the thickness of plaque.

ICUS is currently used in conjunction with coronary angiography to diagnose severity of CAD. It may also evaluate the vessel response to treatments such as stent placement and atherectomy.

Because the patient will most often have ICUS in addition to angiography or an invasive treatment, nursing care of the patient following ICUS is similar to that following cardiac catheterization (see Table 34-5).

Blood Flow and Pressure Measurements

Peripheral Vessel Blood Flow. Duplex imaging is useful in the diagnosis of occlusive disease in the peripheral blood vessels and for the diagnosis of thrombophlebitis. Peripheral vessel blood flow can be assessed by injection of contrast media into the appropriate arteries or veins (arteriography and venography). With these tests, arterial occlusions and venous abnormalities can be located. (Additional studies of peripheral blood vessels are discussed in Chapter 40 and Table 40-8.)

Hemodynamic Monitoring. Bedside hemodynamic monitoring of pressures of the cardiovascular system is frequently used to assess cardiovascular status. Invasive hemodynamic monitoring using intra-arterial and pulmonary artery catheters can be used to monitor arterial BP, intracardiac pressures, and CO (see Chapter 68). The central venous pressure (CVP) is a measurement of preload and can be used to monitor the pressure in the right atrium and right ventricle. The CVP reading is influenced by the function of the left side of the heart, pressures in the pulmonary vessels, venous return to the heart, and the position of the patient when the reading is taken. The last factor must be kept in mind to obtain an accurate reading. The CVP can be used as a guide in fluid volume management of overhydration or dehydration.

CVP can be measured with a pulmonary artery catheter (see Chapter 68) or a central venous line threaded through the jugular or the subclavian vein into the superior vena cava. The normal CVP is 2 to 9 mm Hg.

⊖volve *An assessment case study of the cardiovascular system is available at* **http://evolve.elsevier.com/Canada/Lewis/medsurg**

REVIEW QUESTIONS

The number of the question corresponds to the same-numbered objective at the beginning of the chapter.

1. A patient has a tricuspid valve disorder. Between which of the following will the blood flow be impaired?
   a. Vena cava and right atrium
   b. Left atrium and left ventricle
   c. Right atrium and right ventricle
   d. Right ventricle and pulmonary artery
2. When a patient has a myocardial infarction (MI) of the anterior wall, which vessel is likely occluded?
   a. Right marginal artery
   b. Left circumflex artery
   c. Left anterior descending artery
   d. Right anterior descending artery
3. Where is the conduction impairment when the Purkinje system is damaged?
   a. Atria
   b. Atrioventricular (AV) node
   c. Ventricles
   d. Bundle of His
4. Why does prolonged pressure on the skin cause reddened areas at the point of contact?
   a. Arterial vasodilation from smooth muscle relaxation
   b. Compression of veins resulting in venous engorgement
   c. Occlusion of major arteries causing infarction of the tissue
   d. Tissue damage and inflammation resulting from impaired capillary blood flow
5. When a person's blood pressure rises, which compensatory homeostatic mechanism is stimulated?
   a. Chemoreceptors that inhibit the sympathetic nervous system, causing vasodilation
   b. Baroreceptors that inhibit the parasympathetic nervous system, causing vasodilation
   c. Baroreceptors that inhibit the sympathetic nervous system, causing a decreased heart rate
   d. Chemoreceptors that stimulate the sympathetic nervous system, causing an increased heart rate
6. If a patient's capillary refill assessment shows that the colour returns in 10 seconds, what does this indicate?
   a. A normal response
   b. Thrombus formation in the veins
   c. Lymphatic obstruction of venous return
   d. Impaired arterial flow to the extremities
7. Which auscultatory area is found at the left midclavicular line at the level of the fifth intercostal space (ICS)?
   a. Aortic area
   b. Mitral area
   c. Tricuspid area
   d. Pulmonic area
8. When a palpable precordial thrill is found upon assessment, what could this indicate?
   a. Heart murmurs
   b. Gallop rhythms
   c. Pulmonary edema
   d. Right ventricular hypertrophy
9. Which of the following may be found on assessment of a 79-year-old patient?
   a. A narrowed pulse pressure
   b. Diminished carotid artery pulses
   c. Difficulty in isolating the apical pulse
   d. An increased heart rate in response to stress
10. Which of the following is an important nursing responsibility for a patient having an invasive cardiovascular diagnostic study?
    a. Checking the peripheral pulses and percutaneous insertion site
    b. Instructing the patient about radioactive isotope injection
    c. Informing the patient that general anaesthesia will be given
    d. Assisting the patient to do a surgical scrub of the insertion site
11. Which of the following statements best describe the P-wave impulse?
    a. Arising at the sinoatrial (SA) node and repolarizing the atria
    b. Arising at the SA node and depolarizing the atria
    c. Arising at the AV node and depolarizing the atria
    d. Arising at the AV node and spreading to the bundle of His

ANSWERS: 1. c; 2. c; 3. c; 4. d; 5. c; 6. d; 7. b; 8. a; 9. c; 10. a; 11. b.

REFERENCES

Aehlert, B. (2011). *ECGs made easy* (4th ed.). St. Louis: Mosby.

American Heart Association. (2008). Homocysteine, folic acid and cardiovascular disease. Retrieved from *http://www.heart.org/HEARTORG/GettingHealthy/NutritionCenter/Homocysteine-Folic-Acid-and-Cardiovascular-Disease_UCM_305997_Article.jsp*

Berglund, L., & Anuurad, E. (2008). Role of lipoprotein(a) in cardiovascular disease. *Journal of the American College of Cardiology, 52,* 132-134. doi:10.1016/j.jacc.2008.04.008

Debrey, S., Yu, H., Lynch, J., Lövblad, K. O., Wright, V. L., Janket, S. D., & Baird, A. E. (2008). Diagnostic accuracy of magnetic resonance angiography for internal carotid artery disease. A systematic review and meta-analysis. *Stroke, 39*(8):2237-2248. doi:10.1161/STROKEAHA.107.509877

Dixon, S., Grines, C., & O'Neill, W. (2008). The year in interventional cardiology. *Journal of American College of Cardiology, 51,* 2355-2369. doi:10.1016/j.jacc.2008.03.021

Drake, R., Vogl, W., & Mitchell, A. (2010). *Gray's anatomy for students* (2nd ed.). Philadelphia: Churchill Livingstone, Elsevier.

Ebersole, P., Hess, P., Touhy, T., Jett, K., Boscart, V., & McCleary, L. (2011). *Ebersole and Hess' gerontological nursing and healthy aging* (1st Canadian ed.). Toronto: Elsevier Canada.

Huether, S., & McCance, K. (2007). *Understanding pathophysiology* (4th ed.). St. Louis: Elsevier.

Jarvis, C. (2011). *Physical examination and health assessment* (6th ed.). St. Louis: Saunders.

Josephson, M. (2008). *Clinical cardiac electrophysiology: Techniques and interpretations* (4th ed.). Philadelphia: Lippincott Williams & Wilkins.

Libby, D., Bonow, R., Mann, D., & Zipes, D. (2008). *Braunwald's heart disease: A textbook of cardiovascular medicine* (8th ed.). Philadelphia: Saunders.

Mudd, J., Borlaug, B., Johnston, P., Kral, B. G., Rouf, R., Blumenthal, R. S., & Kwiterovich, Jr., P. O. (2007). Beyond low-density lipoprotein cholesterol—Defining the role of low density lipoprotein heterogeneity in coronary artery disease. *Journal of American College of Cardiology, 50,* 1735-1741. doi:10.1016/j.jacc.2007.07.045

Olsson, L., Swedberg, K., Cleland, J., Spark, P. A., Komajda, M., Metra, M., Poole-Wilson, P. (2007). Prognostic importance of plasma NT-pro BNP in chronic heart failure in patients treated with a β-blocker: Results from the Carvedilol or Metoprolol European Trial (COMET). *European Journal of Heart Failure, 9*(8), 795–801. doi:10.1016/j.ejheart.2007.07.010

Pagana, K., & Pagana, T. (2010). *Mosby's manual of diagnostic and laboratory tests* (4th ed.). St. Louis: Mosby.

Public Health Agency of Canada (PHAC). (2009). Tracking heart disease and stroke in Canada. Retrieved from *http://www.phac-aspc.gc.ca/publicat/2009/cvd-avc/pdf/CVD_report-eng.pdf*

Raff, G., Gallagher, M., O'Neill, W., & Goldstein, J. (2005). Diagnostic accuracy of non-invasive coronary angiography using 64-slice spiral computed tomography. *Journal of American College of Cardiology, 46*(3), 552-557. doi:10.1016/j.jacc.2005.05.056

Screiber, D. (2011). Use of cardiac markers in the emergency department. Retrieved from *http://emedicine.medscape.com/article/811905-overview*

Wackers, F., Bruni, W., & Zaret, B. (2007). *Nuclear cardiology: The basics: How to set up a laboratory.* Totowa, NJ: Humana.

Woods, S. L., Froelicher, E., Motzer, S., & Bridges, E. (2009). *Cardiac nursing* (6th ed.). Philadelphia: Lippincott Williams & Wilkins.

RESOURCES

Resources for this chapter are listed in Chapter 36 on p. 927.

Nursing Management: Hypertension

Written by Elisabeth G. Bradley

Adapted by Beth Swart

LEARNING OBJECTIVES

1. Describe the mechanisms involved in the regulation of blood pressure.
2. Explain the pathophysiological mechanisms associated with primary hypertension.
3. Describe the clinical manifestations and the complications of hypertension.
4. Describe strategies for the prevention of primary hypertension.
5. Describe the collaborative care for hypertension, including drug and nutritional therapy.
6. Discuss the collaborative care of the older adult patient with hypertension.
7. Describe the nursing management of the patient with hypertension, emphasizing patient teaching.
8. Describe the clinical manifestations and the collaborative care of hypertensive crisis.

KEY TERMS

baroreceptors Specialized nerve cells located in the carotid sinus and in the arch of the aorta that are sensitive to stretching and, when stimulated by an increase in blood pressure, send inhibitory impulses to the sympathetic vasomotor centre in the brainstem, p. 868

blood pressure (BP) The force exerted by the blood against the walls of the blood vessel; must be adequate for tissue perfusion to be maintained during activity and rest, p. 868

cardiac output (CO) The total blood flow through the systemic or pulmonary circulation per minute; can be described as the stroke volume (amount of blood pumped out of the left ventricle per beat [~70 mL]) multiplied by the heart rate (HR) over 1 minute, p. 868

hypertension (HTN) Sustained elevation of blood pressure over more than one reading; in adults, exists when systolic blood pressure (SBP) is equal to or greater than 140 mm Hg or diastolic blood pressure (DBP) is equal to or greater than 90 mm Hg, p. 867

hypertensive crisis A severe and abrupt elevation in blood pressure, arbitrarily defined as a diastolic blood pressure above 120 to 130 mm Hg, p. 887

isolated systolic hypertension (ISH) Defined as a sustained elevation in systolic blood pressure equal to or greater than 160 mm Hg with a diastolic blood pressure less than 90 mm Hg, p. 871

orthostatic hypotension A decrease of 20 mm Hg (or more) in systolic pressure or a decrease of 10 mm Hg (or more) in the diastolic pressure that occurs when an individual assumes a standing position, p. 885

primary (essential) hypertension Elevated blood pressure without an identified cause; accounts for about 90 to 95% of all cases of hypertension, p. 871

secondary hypertension Hypertension for which there is a known cause; accounts for about 5 to 10% of all hypertension cases, p. 871

systemic vascular resistance (SVR) The force opposing the movement of blood within the blood vessels; the radius of the small arteries and arterioles is the principal factor determining vascular resistance, p. 868

ELECTRONIC RESOURCES

Supplemental content related to Chapter 35 can be found...

Evolve Web Site ⊝volve

http://evolve.elsevier.com/Canada/Lewis/medsurg
• Answer Guidelines for Case Study on p. 888
• Clinical Reference: Laboratory Values
• Content Updates
• Electronic Calculators

• eTables:
  • eTable 35-1: Recommended Intake for Sodium
  • eTable 35-2: Dietary Management of Hypertension
• Examination Review Questions
• Glossary
• Interactive Case Study: Hypertension and Stroke
• Key Points (Printable and MP3 Download)

Hypertension (HTN) is sustained elevation of systemic arterial blood pressure (BP) and is the leading cause for visits to primary care physicians. High BP is the most significant modifiable risk factor for cardiovascular disease and mortality in Canada (McAlister et al., 2011) and is predicted to become the leading cause of death and disability worldwide by 2020 (Sliwa, Stewart, & Gersh, 2011). Ninety-one percent of Canadians with HTN have at least one additional cardiovascular risk factor (Campbell et al., 2011). Consequently, global risk assessment is a new recommendation in the 2011 Canadian Hypertension Education Program (CHEP) guidelines. The CHEP is Hypertension Canada's "knowledge translation program that targets various healthcare providers in clinical and community settings, provides annually updated standardized recommendations and clinical practice guidelines to detect, treat and control hypertension" (Hypertension Canada, 2012).

HTN is defined as a systolic blood pressure (SBP) equal to or greater than 140 mm Hg or a diastolic blood pressure (DBP) equal to or greater than 90 mm Hg. This is the established level at which antihypertensive therapy is effective at decreasing cardiovascular morbidity and mortality. Canadian targets for blood pressure are shown in Table 35-1. The American Joint National Committee 7 (JNC-7) defines normal BP as an SBP less than 120 mm Hg and a DBP less than 80 mm Hg. Based on JNC-7, patients with sustained HTN are further divided into Stage 1 HTN (SBP 140-159 or DBP 90-99 mm Hg), and Stage 2 HTN (SBP =160 or DBP =100 mm Hg).

According to the Canadian Health Measures Survey (CHMS), approximately 19% of adults ages 20 to 79 years have HTN, with the rates increasing with age. Older women have higher rates of HTN than older men. Women with high BP have three and one half times greater risk of developing cardiovascular disease than women with normal BP (Heart and Stroke Foundation, 2012). See the Determinants of Health box for statistics on HTN in selected ethnic groups.

Canada has impressive statistics in the awareness and treatment of HTN compared with other developed countries. According to McAlister and colleagues (2011), the status of HTN control improved considerably between 1992 and 2009. Large-scale education programs, such as the CHEP, provided by various organizations have increased awareness of HTN. McAlister and colleagues (2011) found that 83% of those with HTN are aware of their condition and 17% remain unaware. Eighty percent are treated, and of these, 66% have their BP under control (Heart and Stroke Foundation, 2012). Despite these statistics, HTN is on the rise in Canada, with more than 25% of adults expected to be diagnosed by 2012 to 2013. In addition, individuals ages 20 to 49 years with

DETERMINANTS OF HEALTH
Hypertension

Ethnicity

• In Canada, Blacks and people of South Asian descent are three times more likely to be hypertensive than Canadians of East Asian descent or Whites, and they are likely to develop it at a younger age.
• Almost 50% of Blacks have already developed hypertension in their 40s and 50s.
• Blacks in Canada have a higher mortality rate related to hypertension than Whites.
• Female Black Canadians have a disproportionately high prevalence of hypertension.
• Hypertension is more prevalent among First Nations adults than the general population of Canada.
• Hypertension is more aggressive in Blacks and Aboriginals and results in more severe end-organ damage.

Source: Heart and Stroke Foundation. (2012). *Pressure rising: High blood pressure rates still very high, particularly for some ethnic groups, warns Heart and Stroke Foundation.* Retrieved from *http://www.heartandstroke.on.ca/site/apps/nlnet/content2.aspx?c=pvI3leNWJwE&b=3582275&ct=5365013*; Leenen, F. H., Dumais, J., McInnis, N. H., Turton, P., Stratychuk, L., Nemeth, K., Fodor, G. (2008). Results of the Ontario survey on the prevalence and control of hypertension. *Canadian Medical Association Journal, 178*(11), 1441-1449.

HTN are two to four times more likely to die than those without HTN (Robitaille et al., 2012).

One in five adult Canadians has high-normal BP (130-139/85-89 mm Hg), and up to 60% of them will develop HTN within 4 years (Padwal et al., 2008). Adults with high-normal BP (also called *prehypertension*) require annual BP assessment. Health care providers who have been specifically trained to measure BP accurately should assess BP in all adult patients, at all appropriate visits, to determine cardiovascular risk and monitor antihypertensive treatment. Home measurement of BP has been recommended since the 2008 CHEP guidelines (Padwal et al., 2008) to encourage patient self-efficacy. Home BP readings have a stronger association with cardiovascular outcomes than readings taken in a health care provider's office (Padwal et al., 2008). Patient instructions for purchasing and using home BP measurement devices are available at both the Hypertension Canada and the Heart and Stroke Foundation of Canada Web sites. A comprehensive instructional DVD on home measure-

Table 35-1 Target Values for Blood Pressure*	
SETTING	**TARGET (mm Hg)**
Home	
Home blood pressure and daytime ambulatory blood pressure measurement*	Awake <135/85
Office	
Diastolic and/or systolic hypertension	<140/90
Isolated systolic hypertension	<140
Diabetes	<130/80
Chronic kidney disease	
Automated Office Oscillometric Device	
Awake	<135/85
24-hr	<130/80

*The target value readings taken by home measurement and ambulatory blood pressure measurement in those with diabetes or chronic kidney disease have not been established.
Source: Adapted from Canadian Hypertension Education Program (CHEP). (2012). *2012 Canadian Recommendations for the Management of Hypertension. What's new? What's still really important?* (Summary document.) Markham, ON: Hypertension Canada. Retrieved from *http://www.hypertension.ca/images/stories/dls/2011gl/2012_CHEPRecommendationsBooklet_EN_HCP1030.pdf*

ment of BP was developed in 2009 and can be downloaded from the Hypertension Canada Web site.

The 2011 CHEP recommendations for diagnosis of HTN and follow-up are shown in Figure 35-1. It should be emphasized that when using BPs recorded during office visits to diagnose HTN, the thresholds given refer to readings averaged over a specified range of visits and are not one-time measurements from the last visit.

Normal Regulation of Blood Pressure

Blood pressure (BP) is the force exerted by the blood against the walls of the blood vessel and must be adequate for tissue perfusion to be maintained during activity and rest. The maintenance of normal BP and tissue perfusion requires the integration of both systemic factors and local peripheral vascular effects. Arterial BP is primarily a function of cardiac output (CO) and systemic vascular resistance (SVR). The relationship is summarized by the following equation:

$$\text{Arterial BP} = \text{CO} \times \text{SVR}$$

Cardiac output (CO) is the total blood flow through the systemic or pulmonary circulation per minute. CO can be described as the stroke volume (SV, or the amount of blood pumped out of the left ventricle per beat [~70 mL]) multiplied by the heart rate (HR) for 1 minute. **Systemic vascular resistance (SVR)** is the force opposing the movement of blood within the blood vessels. The radius of the small arteries and arterioles is the principal factor determining vascular resistance. A small change in the radius of the arterioles creates a major change in the SVR. If SVR is increased and CO remains constant or increases, arterial BP will increase.

The mechanisms that regulate BP can affect either CO or SVR, or both. Regulation of BP is a complex process involving

nervous, cardiovascular, renal, and endocrine functions (Figure 35-2). BP is regulated by both short-term (over seconds to hours) and long-term (over days to weeks) mechanisms. Short-term mechanisms, including the effects exerted by the sympathetic nervous system (SNS) and the vascular endothelium, are active within a few seconds. Long-term mechanisms include renal and hormonal processes that regulate arteriolar resistance and blood volume.

Sympathetic Nervous System

The nervous system, which reacts within seconds after a decrease in arterial pressure, increases BP primarily by activation of the SNS. Increased SNS activity increases HR and cardiac contractility, produces widespread vasoconstriction in the peripheral arterioles, and promotes the release of renin from the kidneys. The net effect of SNS activation is to increase arterial pressure by increasing both CO and SVR.

Changes in BP are sensed by specialized nerve cells called *baroreceptors* and transmitted to the vasomotor centres in the brainstem. Information received in the brainstem is relayed throughout the brain by complex networks of interneurons that excite or inhibit efferent nerves, thereby influencing cardiovascular function. Sympathetic efferent nerves innervate cardiac and vascular smooth muscle cells. Under normal conditions, a low level of continuous sympathetic activity maintains tonic vasoconstriction. BP may be reduced by withdrawal of SNS activity or by stimulation of the parasympathetic nervous system, which decreases the HR (via the vagus nerve) and thereby decreases CO.

The neurotransmitter norepinephrine (NE) is released from sympathetic nerve endings. NE activates receptors located in the sinoatrial node, the myocardium, and vascular smooth muscle. The response to NE depends on the type and the density of receptors present. SNS receptors are classified as α_1, α_2, β_1, and β_2 (Table 35-2). α-Adrenergic receptors located in peripheral vasculature cause vasoconstriction when stimulated by NE. β_1-Adrenergic receptors in the heart respond to NE with increased HR (chronotropic effect), increased force of contraction (inotropic effect), and increased speed of conduction (dromotropic effect). Diminished responsiveness of cardiovascular cells to sympathetic stimulation is one of the most significant cardiovascular effects of aging. The smooth muscle of the blood vessels has β_1-adrenergic and β_2-adrenergic receptors. β_2-Adrenergic receptors are activated primarily by epinephrine released from the adrenal medulla and cause vasodilation.

The sympathetic vasomotor centre, located in the medulla, interacts with many areas of the brain to maintain normal BP under various conditions. During exercise, the motor area of the cortex is stimulated, activating the vasomotor centre and the SNS through neuronal connections. This causes an appropriate increase in BP to accommodate the increased oxygen demand of the exercising muscles. During postural change from lying to standing, there is a transient decrease in BP. The vasomotor centre is stimulated and activates the SNS, causing peripheral vasoconstriction and increased venous return to the heart. If this response did not occur, there would be inadequate blood flow to the brain, resulting in dizziness. Cerebral cortical perceptions such as pain and stress activate the vasomotor centres through the neuronal connections.

Baroreceptors. Baroreceptors (pressoreceptors) are specialized nerve cells located in the carotid sinus at the bifurcation of the external and internal carotid arteries and the arch of the aorta.

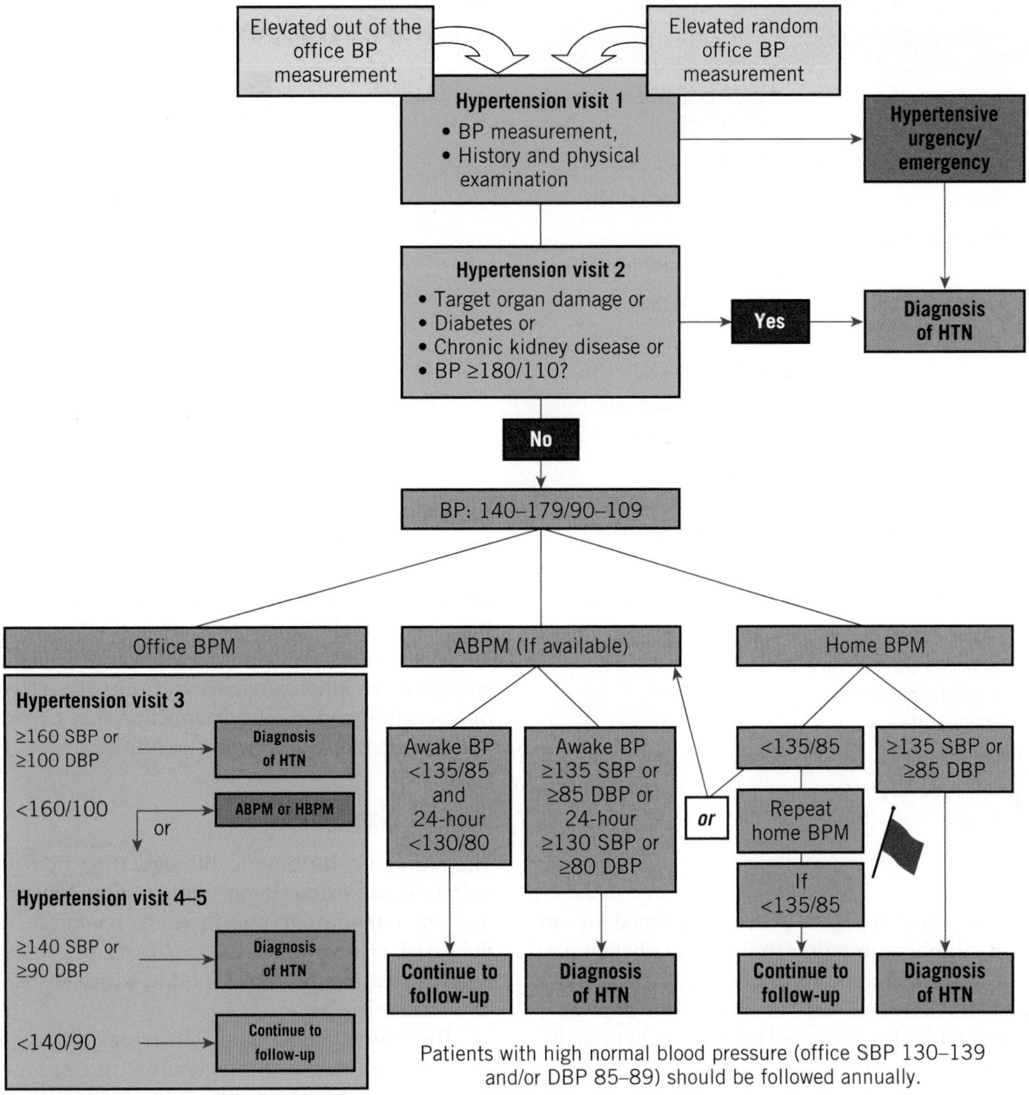

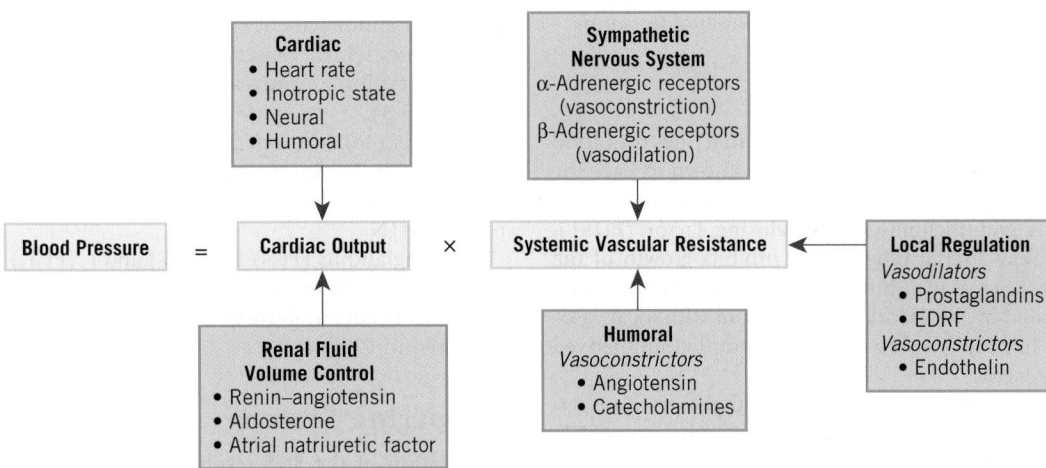

Figure 35-1 Criteria for the diagnosis of hypertension *(HTN)* and recommendations for follow-up. The thresholds shown here are blood pressure *(BP)* values that are averaged across the corresponding number of visits and are not one-time measurements taken at the most recent office visit. All BP measurements are in millimetres of mercury. *ABPM,* ambulatory blood pressure monitoring; *BPM,* blood pressure monitoring; *DBP,* diastolic blood pressure; *HBPM,* home blood pressure monitoring; *SBP,* systolic blood pressure.

Source: Canadian Hypertension Education Program (CHEP). (2012). *2012 CHEP recommendations: Part 1: Recommendations for hypertension diagnosis and follow-up* (Slides 20 and 21). Retrieved from *http://www.hypertension.ca/chep-recommendations*

Figure 35-2 Factors influencing blood pressure. *EDRF,* endothelium-derived relaxing factor.

Source: Redrawn from West, J. B. (1991). *Physiological basis of medical practice* (12th ed.). Baltimore: Williams & Wilkins.

Table 35-2 Sympathetic Nervous System Receptors Influencing Blood Pressure		
RECEPTOR	**LOCATION**	**RESPONSE WHEN ACTIVATED**
α_1	Vascular smooth muscle	Vasoconstriction
	Heart	Increased contractility
α_2	Presynaptic membrane	Inhibition of norepinephrine release
	Vascular smooth muscle	Vasoconstriction
β_1	Heart	Increased contractility (positive inotropic effect)
		Increased heart rate (positive chronotropic effect)
		Increased conduction (positive dromotropic effect)
	Juxtaglomerular cells	Increased renin secretion
β_2	Smooth muscle of peripheral blood vessels in skeletal muscle and coronary arteries	Vasodilation
Dopaminergic receptors	Primarily kidney and mesenteric blood vessels	Vasodilation

They are sensitive to stretching and, when stimulated by an increase in BP, send inhibitory impulses to the sympathetic vasomotor centre in the brainstem. Inhibition of sympathetic activity results in decreased HR, decreased force of contraction, and vasodilation in peripheral arterioles. Increased parasympathetic activity (vagus nerve) also reduces HR.

A fall in BP, sensed by the baroreceptors, leads to activation of the SNS. The result is constriction of the peripheral arterioles, increased HR, and increased contractility of the heart. The baroreceptors have an important role in the maintenance of BP stability during normal activities. In the presence of longstanding HTN, the baroreceptors become adjusted to elevated levels of BP and recognize this level as "normal." Consequently, the long-term regulation of arterial pressure requires activation of other mechanisms (primarily hormonal and renal) to maintain normal BP. The baroreceptor reflex is less responsive in some older adults.

Vascular Endothelium

The vascular endothelium is a single cell layer that lines the blood vessels. Previously considered inert, it is now known to have the ability to produce vasoactive substances and growth factors. Nitric oxide, an endothelium-derived relaxing factor (EDRF), helps maintain low arterial tone at rest, inhibits growth of the smooth muscle layer, and inhibits platelet aggregation. Other substances released by the vascular endothelium with local vasodilator effects include prostacyclin and endothelium-derived hyperpolarizing factor.

Endothelin (ET), produced by the endothelial cells, is an extremely potent vasoconstrictor. There are three subclasses of ETs (ET-1, ET-2, and ET-3). ET-1 is the most potent ET in producing vasoconstriction. ET-1 also causes adhesion and aggregation of

PATHOPHYSIOLOGY MAP

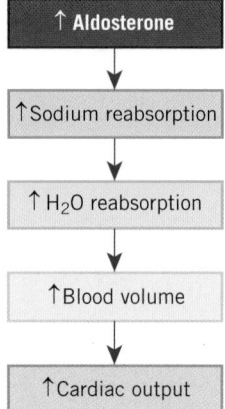

Figure 35-3 Mechanism of action of aldosterone.

neutrophils and stimulates smooth muscle growth. Endothelial function and dysfunction is an area of ongoing investigation. There is some evidence that vascular endothelial dysfunction may contribute to atherosclerosis and primary HTN. The prevention or reversal of endothelial dysfunction may become important for therapeutic interventions in the future.

Renal System

The kidneys contribute to BP regulation by controlling sodium excretion and extracellular fluid (ECF) volume (see Chapter 47). Sodium retention results in water retention, which causes an increased ECF volume. This increases the venous return to the heart, increasing the stroke volume, which elevates the BP through an increase in CO.

The renin–angiotensin–aldosterone system (RAAS) also plays an important role in BP regulation. In response to sympathetic stimulation, decreased blood flow through the kidneys, or decreased serum sodium concentration, renin is secreted from the juxtaglomerular apparatus in the kidney. Renin is an enzyme that converts angiotensinogen to angiotensin I. Angiotensin-converting enzyme (ACE) converts angiotensin I into angiotensin II (A-II), which can increase BP by two different mechanisms (see Chapter 47, Figure 47-6). First, A-II is a potent vasoconstrictor and increases vascular resistance, resulting in an immediate increase in BP. Second, over a period of hours or days, A-II increases BP indirectly by stimulating the adrenal cortex to secrete aldosterone, which causes sodium and water retention by the kidneys, resulting in increased blood volume and increased CO (Figure 35-3).

A-II also functions at a local level within the heart and the blood vessels. The local vasoactive effects of A-II (vasoconstriction and growth promotion) may contribute to atherosclerosis and primary HTN.

Prostaglandins (PGs) E_2 (PGE$_2$) and I_2 (PGI$_2$) secreted by the renal medulla have a vasodilator effect on the systemic circulation. This results in decreased SVR and lowering of BP. (PGs are discussed in Chapter 14.)

Endocrine System

Stimulation of the SNS results in release of epinephrine along with a small fraction of NE by the adrenal medulla. Epinephrine

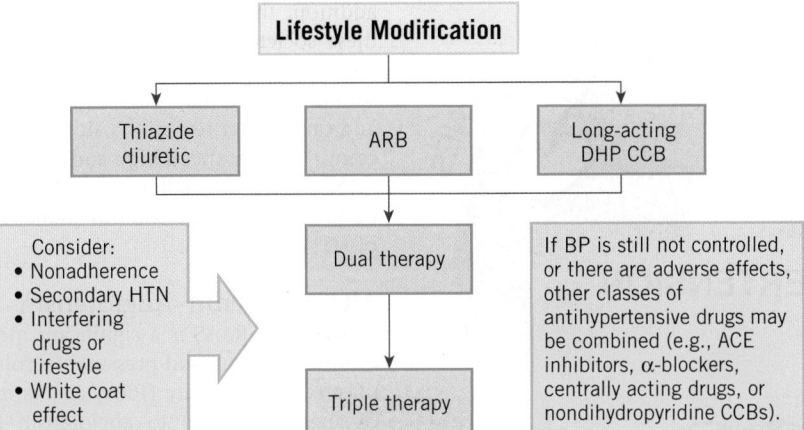

Figure 35-4 Treatment of isolated systolic hypertension *(HTN)* without other compelling indications. *ACE*, angiotensin-converting enzyme; *ARB*, angiotensin II receptor blocker; *BP*, blood pressure; *CCBs*, calcium channel blockers; *DHP*, dihydropyridine.

Source: Adapted from Canadian Hypertension Education Program (CHEP). (2012). *Part 2: Recommendations for hypertension treatment. 2012 Canadian Hypertension Education Program recommendations* (Slides 41 and 42). Retrieved from *http://www.hypertension.ca/chep-recommendations*

increases CO by increasing HR and myocardial contractility. Epinephrine activates β_2-adrenergic receptors in peripheral arterioles of skeletal muscle, causing vasodilation. In peripheral arterioles with only α_1-adrenergic receptors (skin and kidneys), epinephrine causes vasoconstriction.

The adrenal cortex is stimulated by A-II to release aldosterone. (Release of aldosterone is also regulated by other factors, such as low sodium levels [see Chapters 50 and 51].) Aldosterone stimulates the kidneys to retain sodium and, therefore, water. This increases BP by increasing CO (see Figure 35-3).

An increased blood sodium osmolarity level stimulates the release of antidiuretic hormone (ADH) from the posterior pituitary gland. ADH increases the ECF volume by promoting the reabsorption of water in the distal and the collecting tubules of the kidneys. The resulting increase in blood volume can cause an elevation in BP.

In the healthy person, these regulatory mechanisms function in response to the demands of the body. When HTN develops, one or more of the BP-regulating mechanisms are defective.

Hypertension

Subtypes of Hypertension

Isolated systolic hypertension (ISH) is defined as a sustained elevation in SBP equal to or greater than 140 mm Hg with a DBP less than 90 mm Hg. (A one-time isolated reading of increased SBP is not classified as ISH.) Arterial BP increases with advancing age.

An increase of the SDP without an increase of the DBP, as occurs in ISH, increases the pulse pressure. The *pulse pressure* is the difference between the SBP and the DBP. Loss of elasticity of the large arteries contributes to this widening of the pulse pressure. Once considered to be harmless, a high pulse pressure is now considered an independent risk factor for cardiovascular disease and end-organ damage. ISH is associated with a two- to four-fold increased future risk of cardiomegaly, myocardial infarction, or stroke. There is compelling evidence that treatment of ISH with a reduction in the SBP of 20 to 30 mm Hg results in

significant cardiovascular benefits. See Figure 35-4 for the treatment algorithm for ISH.

Etiology

HTN can be classified etiologically as either primary or secondary.

Primary Hypertension. **Primary (essential) hypertension** is elevated BP and accounts for 90 to 95% of all cases of HTN (Riaz, Dreisbach, Madhur, & Harrison, 2012). Although the exact cause of primary HTN has not been identified, it is considered to be a complex interaction between genes and the environment (Singh, Mensha, & Bakris, 2010) (Figure 35-5). Several contributing factors, including increased SNS activity, overproduction of sodium-retaining hormones and vasoconstrictors, increased sodium intake, greater than ideal body weight, diabetes mellitus, and excessive alcohol intake, have been identified. Primary HTN is the focus of this chapter because of its prevalence in clinical practice.

Secondary Hypertension. **Secondary hypertension** is elevated BP with a specific cause that often can be identified and corrected. This type of HTN accounts for 5 to 10% of HTN in adults and more than 80% of HTN in children. If a person younger than age 20 or older than age 50 suddenly develops HTN, especially if it is severe, a secondary cause should be suspected. Clinical findings that suggest secondary HTN include unprovoked hypokalemia; abdominal bruit; variable pressures with history of tachycardia, sweating, and tremor; or a family history of renal disease.

Causes of secondary HTN include the following: (1) coarctation or congenital narrowing of the aorta; (2) renal disease such as renal artery stenosis and parenchymal disease (see Chapter 48); (3) endocrine disorders such as pheochromocytoma, Cushing's syndrome, and hyperaldosteronism (see Chapter 51); (4) neurological disorders such as brain tumours, quadriplegia, and head injury; (5) sleep apnea; (6) medications such as sympathetic stimulants (including cocaine), monoamine oxidase inhibitors taken with tyramine-containing foods, estrogen replacement therapy, oral contraceptive pills, and nonsteroidal

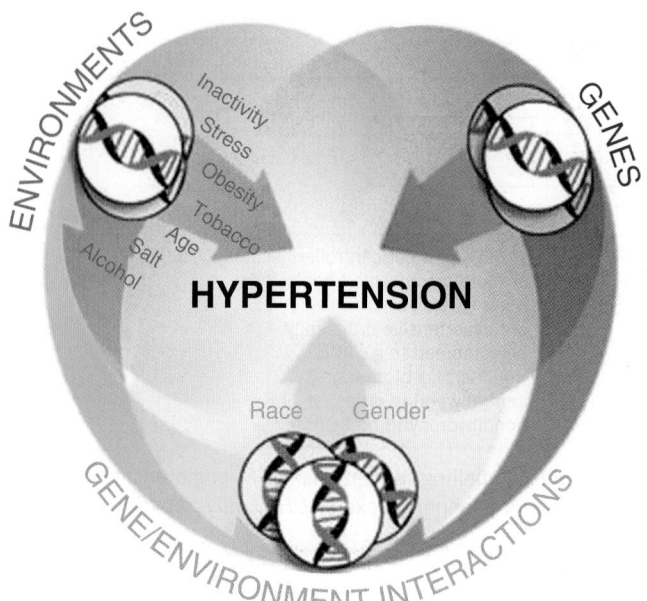

Figure 35-5 Interrelationship of factors resulting in primary hypertension.

Source: Stroke Survivors Association of Ottawa.

anti-inflammatory drugs (NSAIDs); and (7) pregnancy-induced HTN. Treatment of secondary HTN is directed at eliminating the underlying cause. Secondary HTN is a contributing factor to hypertensive urgency (see section at end of this chapter).

Pathophysiology of Primary Hypertension

For arterial pressure to rise, there must be an increase in either CO or SVR. Increased CO is sometimes found in the early and the borderline hypertensive person. Later in the course of HTN, SVR rises and the CO returns to normal. The hemodynamic hallmark of HTN is persistently increased SVR. This persistent elevation in SVR may come about in various ways. Factors that are known to be related to the development of primary HTN or contribute to its consequences are presented in Table 35-3.

Genes. Genetic observations to date suggest that primary HTN is polygenic and also involves numerous environmental influences. Genetic factors are thought to account for a 30 to 60% variability in BP in individuals (Singh et al., 2010) and vary depending on the study population from 15 to 20% or from 65 to 70%. Familial heritability is a significant factor. A child with both parents and a sibling with HTN has a 40 to 60% chance of developing HTN. This risk increases to 80% if the child is a monozygotic twin. It is unlikely that this risk is from a single genetic locus but, rather, from multiple genes. Similarities across populations have not been established; ongoing research is needed in the area of genetic susceptibility to HTN.

Sodium and Water Retention. Excessive dietary intake of sodium is the most studied environmental factor and is strongly linked to the initiation of HTN in some people. Studies of populations with a low sodium intake (usually primitive hunter–gatherer societies) show little or no HTN and no progressive increase in BP with age as is found in industrialized societies. In addition, the prevalence of HTN increases when people from these societies adopt industrialized lifestyles. When sodium is restricted in many hypertensive people, their BP falls. A high sodium intake may alter the pressure–natriuresis relationship and cause water retention. Although almost everyone in Western countries consumes a high-sodium diet, only about 20% develop HTN. This indicates that some degree of sodium sensitivity must be present for high sodium intake to trigger the development of HTN.

Altered   Renin–Angiotensin–Aldosterone   Mechanism. The RAAS is a significant mechanism in the regulation of blood volume and pressure. Its role in HTN is complex. High plasma renin activity (PRA) results in the increased conversion of angiotensinogen to angiotensin I (see Chapter 47, Figure 47-6). A-II causes direct arteriolar constriction, promotes vascular hypertrophy, and induces aldosterone secretion. Thus, altered renin–angiotensin mechanisms may contribute to the development and maintenance of HTN. However, only about 20% of patients with primary HTN have high PRA.

Stress and Increased Sympathetic Nervous System Activity. The SNS also has a critical role in BP control. It has long been recognized that arterial pressure is influenced by factors such as anger, fear, and pain. Physiological responses to stress, which are normally protective, may persist to a pathological degree, resulting in prolonged increase in SNS activity. Increased sympathetic stimulation produces increased vasoconstriction, increased HR, and increased renin release. Increased renin activates the angiotensin mechanism and increases aldosterone secretion, both leading to elevated BP. People exposed to high levels of repeated psychological stress develop HTN to a greater extent than those who do not experience as much stress.

Insulin Resistance and Hyperinsulinemia. Abnormalities of glucose, insulin, and lipoprotein metabolism are common in primary HTN. Insulin resistance is present in 50% of patients with primary HTN; a strong genetic component is associated with hyperinsulinemia-associated HTN. Insulin resistance is associated with endothelial dysfunction. High insulin concentration in the blood stimulates SNS and RAAS activity and impairs nitric oxide–mediated vasodilation. Additional pressor effects of insulin include vascular hypertrophy and increased renal sodium reabsorption.

Endothelial Cell Dysfunction. Vascular endothelial cells are known to be a source of multiple vasoactive substances such as nitric oxide and ET. Some hypertensive people have a reduced vasodilator response to nitric oxide. ET produces pronounced and prolonged vasoconstriction. The role of endothelial dysfunction in the pathogenesis and treatment of HTN is an area of ongoing investigation.

Obesity. Obesity is a well-known risk factor for HTN. Hypertension and central (visceral) obesity are major components of the cardiometabolic syndrome. The relationship between HTN and obesity is multifaceted; the etiology is complex, and it is not well elucidated. Several hormone abnormalities that are associated with obesity are linked to the development of HTN. Enlarged adipocytes or fat cells secrete leptin, proinflammatory cytokines, and reactive oxygen species. This dysfunctional adipose tissue may induce activation of the SNS and RAAS.

Table 35-3 Risk Factors for Primary Hypertension

Advancing age	• BP rises progressively with increasing age. • Elevated BP is present in approximately 50% of people >65 yr, with 90% of the remainder developing hypertension during their lifespan.
Heavy alcohol consumption	• Excessive alcohol intake is strongly linked to hypertension. • Canadians with hypertension should limit their daily intake to 30 mL of alcohol.
Cigarette smoking	• The incidence of hypertension is increased among those who smoke ≥15 cigarettes/day. • Canadians with hypertension and who smoke have a greater risk of secondary cardiovascular disease.
Glucose intolerance (diabetes mellitus)	• Hypertension is diagnosed three times more often in individuals diagnosed with diabetes. • When hypertension and diabetes coexist, hypertension augments the already raised risk of cardiovascular diseases and worsens outcomes.
Elevated serum lipids	• Elevated levels of cholesterol and triglycerides are primary risk factors in atherosclerosis. • Hyperlipidemia is more common in Canadians with hypertension.
High dietary sodium intake	• High sodium intake can contribute to hypertension in some patients and can decrease the efficacy of certain antihypertensive medications. • For prevention of hypertension, the daily recommended dietary sodium intake is 1500 mg for adults ages 14-50 yr of age; 1300 mg for adults ages 50-70 yr; and 1200 mg for adults >70 yr.
Gender	• Hypertension is more prevalent in men in young adulthood and early middle age. • After age 55, hypertension is more prevalent in women.
Family history	• Level of BP is strongly familial. • Risk of hypertension increases for those with a close relative having hypertension.
Obesity	• Weight gain is associated with increased risk of hypertension. • According to Statistics Canada, 59% of Canadian adults are at a weight that increases their risk of hypertension. • Risk is greatest with central abdominal obesity. Waist circumference recommendation for European/Caucasian, sub-Saharan Africans, Eastern Mediterranean, and Middle Eastern men is 102 cm, and for women, 88 cm; South Asian, Malaysian, Asian, Chinese, Japanese, Ethnic South and Central American men is 90 cm; for women, 80 cm. • Maintenance of a healthy weight and BMI of 18.5-24.9 kg/m² is recommended.*
Ethnicity	• Blacks or people of South Asian descent are three times more likely to be hypertensive than the general population. • Almost 50% of Blacks have already developed hypertension in their 40s and 50s.
Sedentary lifestyle	• Physical activity may decrease BP. • Regular physical activity can help control weight and reduce cardiovascular risk. • Daily accumulation of 30-60 min of moderate-intensity dynamic exercise (walking, jogging, cycling, or noncompetitive swimming) 4-7 days/wk is recommended. • Higher intensities of exercise are no more effective.
Socioeconomic status	• Canadians living in low-income neighbourhoods have higher rates of hypertension.
Psychosocial stress	• Canadians exposed to repeated stress may develop hypertension more frequently than others. • Canadians who become hypertensive may respond differently to stress than those who do not become hypertensive.

BP, blood pressure; *BMI*, body mass index.
*Heart and Stroke Foundation. (2010). *Healthy waists*. Retrieved from *http://www.heartandstroke.com/site/c.ikIQLcMWJtE/b.3876195/*

Clinical Manifestations

HTN is a lanthanic or silent disease because it is frequently asymptomatic until it becomes severe and target-organ disease has occurred. A patient with severe HTN may experience a variety of symptoms secondary to effects on blood vessels in the various organs and tissues or to the increased workload of the heart. These secondary symptoms include fatigue, reduced activity tolerance, dizziness, palpitations, angina, and dyspnea. In the past, symptoms of HTN were thought to include headache, nosebleeds, and dizziness. However, unless BP is extremely high or low, these symptoms are not more frequent in people with HTN than in the general population.

Complications

The most common complications of HTN are *target-organ diseases* (Table 35-4) occurring in the heart (hypertensive heart disease), the brain (cerebrovascular disease), the peripheral vasculature (peripheral vascular disease), the kidneys (nephrosclerosis), and the eyes (retinal damage).

Hypertensive Heart Disease

Coronary Artery Disease. HTN is an established major risk factor for coronary artery disease, almost doubling the risk. The mechanisms by which HTN contributes to the development of atherosclerosis are multifactorial. The shear stress (response-to-

Table 35-4 Pathological Effects of Sustained, Complicated Primary Hypertension

SITE OF INJURY	MECHANISM OF INJURY	POTENTIAL PATHOLOGICAL EFFECT
Heart		
Myocardium	Increased workload combined with diminished blood flow through coronary arteries	Left ventricular hypertrophy, myocardial ischemia, left heart failure
Coronary arteries	Accelerated atherosclerosis (coronary artery disease)	Myocardial ischemia, myocardial infarction, sudden death
Aorta	Weakened vessel wall	Aneurysms, acute aortic syndromes
Kidneys	Renin and aldosterone secretion stimulated by reduced blood flow	Retention of sodium and water, leading to increased blood volume and perpetuation of hypertension
	Inflammation and ischemia	Tissue damage that compromises filtration
	High pressures in renal arterioles	Nephrosclerosis leading to renal failure
Brain	Reduced blood flow and oxygen supply; weakened vessel walls, accelerated atherosclerosis	Transient ischemic attacks, cerebral thrombosis, aneurysm, hemorrhage, acute brain infarction
Eyes (retinas)	Reduced blood flow	Retinal vascular sclerosis
	High arteriolar pressure	Exudation, hemorrhage
Arterial vessels of lower extremities	Reduced blood flow and high pressures in arterioles, accelerated atherosclerosis	Intermittent claudication, arterial thrombosis, gangrene

Source: McCance, K. L., & Huether, S. E. (2010). *Pathophysiology: The biologic basis for disease in adults and children* (6th ed., p. 1155). St. Louis: Mosby.

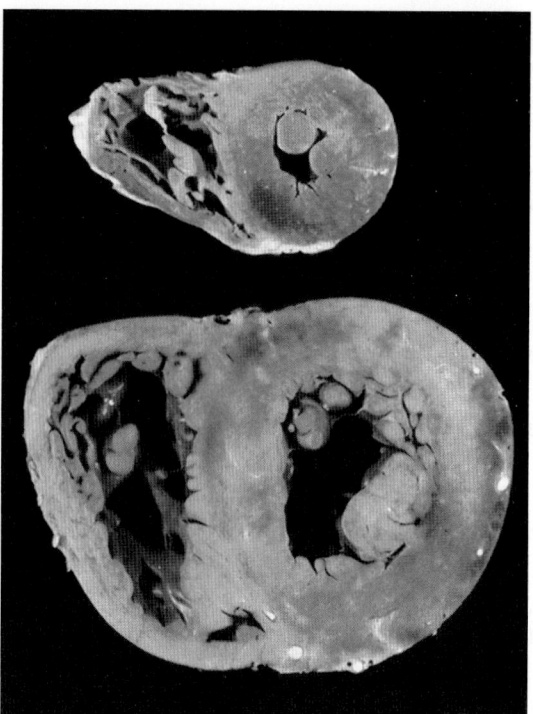

Figure 35-6 Massively enlarged heart caused by hypertrophy of both ventricles. The normal heart weighs 325 g. The heart with biventricular hypertrophy weighs 1100 g. The patient had suffered from severe systemic hypertension.

Source: Kissane, J. M. (1990). *Anderson's pathology* (9th ed.). St Louis: Mosby.

injury hypothesis of atherogenesis) results in endothelial dysfunction causing impairment in the synthesis and release of the potent vasodilator nitric oxide. A decreased nitric oxide level promotes the development and acceleration of atherosclerosis and plaque formation.

The intimal layer is exposed to activated white blood cells and platelets. Growth factors released by the vascular endothelium and platelets may induce smooth muscle proliferation within the lesion. These arteriolar changes may account for a high incidence of coronary artery disease and the resulting problems of angina and myocardial infarction (MI).

Left Ventricular Hypertrophy. Sustained high BP increases the cardiac workload and produces left ventricular hypertrophy (LVH) (Figure 35-6). The risk of LVH doubles with associated obesity. Initially, LVH is an adaptive or compensatory mechanism that strengthens cardiac contraction and increases CO. However, increased contractility increases myocardial work and oxygen consumption. When the heart can no longer meet the demands for myocardial oxygen, heart failure develops. Progressive LVH, especially in association with coronary artery disease, is associated with the development of heart failure.

Heart Failure. Heart failure is a common complication of a chronically elevated BP and occurs when the heart's compensatory adaptations are overwhelmed and the heart can no longer pump enough blood to meet the metabolic needs of the body (see Chapter 37). Contractility is depressed, and SV and CO are decreased. The patient may complain of shortness of breath on exertion, paroxysmal nocturnal dyspnea, and fatigue. Signs of an enlarged heart may be present on radiograph, and an electrocardiogram (ECG) may show electrical changes indicative of LVH.

Cerebrovascular Disease. Atherosclerosis is the most common cause of cerebrovascular disease. HTN is a major risk factor for cerebral atherosclerosis and stroke. Even in mildly hypertensive people, the risk of stroke is four times higher than in normotensive people. Adequate control of BP effectively diminishes the risk of stroke.

Atherosclerotic plaques are commonly distributed at the bifurcation of the common carotid artery into the internal and external carotid arteries. Portions of the atherosclerotic plaque, or the blood clot that forms on the plaque, may break off and travel to intracerebral vessels, producing a thromboembolism. The patient may experience transient ischemic attacks or a stroke. (These conditions are discussed in Chapter 60.)

Hypertensive encephalopathy may occur after a marked rise in BP if the cerebral blood flow is not decreased by autoregulation. *Autoregulation* is a physiological process that maintains constant cerebral blood flow despite fluctuations in arterial BP. Normally, as pressure in the cerebral blood vessels rises, the vessels constrict to maintain constant flow. When arterial BP exceeds the body's ability to autoregulate, the cerebral vessels suddenly dilate and cerebral edema develops, producing a rise in intracranial pressure. If left untreated, patients die quickly from brain damage. (Cerebral blood flow and autoregulation are discussed in Chapter 59.)

Peripheral Vascular Disease. As it does with other vessels, HTN speeds up the process of atherosclerosis in the peripheral arterial blood vessels, leading to the development of aortic aneurysm, aortic dissection, and peripheral vascular disease (see Chapter 40). *Intermittent claudication* (ischemic muscle pain precipitated by activity and relieved with rest) is a classical symptom of peripheral vascular disease.

Nephrosclerosis. HTN is one of the leading causes of end-stage renal disease (ESRD), especially among Blacks. Aboriginals have a high incidence of ESRD as well, but this is more commonly caused by complications of diabetes, although HTN does play a significant role (Sood et al., 2010). Some degree of kidney dysfunction is usually present in the patient with HTN, even one with a minimally elevated BP. One of the earliest markers of nephropathy is microalbuminuria, the presence of protein in the urine. Kidney dysfunction is the direct result of ischemia caused by the narrowed lumen of the intrarenal blood vessels. Gradual narrowing of the arteries and arterioles leads to atrophy of the tubules, destruction of the glomeruli, and eventual death of nephrons. Initially intact nephrons can compensate, but these changes may eventually lead to kidney failure. Common laboratory indications of kidney dysfunction are microalbuminuria, macroalbuminuria, elevated blood urea nitrogen (BUN), serum creatinine levels, and microscopic hematuria.

Retinal Damage. The appearance of the retina provides important information about how severe and longstanding the hypertensive process has been. The retina is the only place in the body where the blood vessels can be directly visualized. Damage seen to have occurred to retinal vessels thus provides an indication of vessel damage in the heart, the brain, and the kidney. An ophthalmoscope is used to visualize the blood vessels of the eye. Manifestations of severe retinal damage include blurring of vision, retinal hemorrhage, and loss of vision.

Diagnostic Studies

The diagnosis of HTN is not based on a single elevated reading (if <180/110 mm Hg) but requires several elevated readings over several weeks (see Figure 35-1). (Measurement of BP is discussed in Chapter 34 on p. 847 and p. 863.)

Table 35-5 is a list of basic laboratory studies that are performed in a person with sustained HTN. Routine urinalysis and serum creatinine levels are used to screen for kidney involvement and to provide baseline information about kidney function. (Serum creatinine is discussed in Chapters 47 and 49.)

Measurement of serum electrolytes, especially potassium levels, is important to detect hyperaldosteronism, a cause of secondary HTN. Blood glucose levels should be assessed to assist in the diagnosis of diabetes mellitus. Serum cholesterol and

COLLABORATIVE CARE

Table 35-5 Hypertension

Diagnosis

History and Physical Examination

- Routine laboratory tests should be performed for the investigation of all patients with hypertension, including the following:
  - Urinalysis
  - Blood chemistry (potassium, sodium, and creatinine)
  - Fasting blood glucose
  - Fasting total cholesterol and high-density lipoprotein cholesterol, low-density lipoprotein cholesterol, and triglycerides
  - Standard 12-lead electrocardiography
- Assess urinary albumin excretion in patients with diabetes
- All patients with treated hypertension need to be monitored for the appearance of diabetes according to the Current Diabetes Association (CDA) guidelines (available at *www.diabetes.ca/for-professionals/resources/2008-cpg/*)

Collaborative Therapy

- Periodic monitoring of BP
- Home BP monitoring
- Ambulatory BP monitoring
- Every 3-6 mo once BP is stabilized

Nutritional Therapy (see Tables 35-7 and 35-8)

- Restrict sodium
- Reduce weight (if indicated)
- Restrict cholesterol and saturated fats
- Maintain adequate intake of potassium
- Maintain adequate intake of calcium and magnesium
- Regular, moderate physical activity
- Cessation of smoking
- Moderation of alcohol consumption
- Antihypertensive drugs (see Table 35-8)

NOTE: During the maintenance phase of hypertension management, tests (including those for electrolytes, creatinine, and fasting lipids) should be repeated with a frequency reflecting the clinical situation. *BP*, blood pressure.

triglyceride levels provide information about additional risk factors that predispose to atherosclerosis. An ECG provides baseline information about the cardiac status. It is helpful in identifying the presence of LVH and myocardial ischemia. If the patient's age, history, physical examination findings, or severity of HTN points to a secondary cause, further diagnostic tests may be indicated.

Ambulatory Blood Pressure Monitoring. Twenty-four–hour ambulatory BP readings are useful in the diagnosis of uncomplicated mild-to-moderate HTN and are more accurate in predicting cardiovascular risk than office BP. It is incorporated into the CHEP diagnostic algorithm to facilitate more rapid diagnosis of HTN and reduce the risk of patients left untreated for long periods of time while a diagnosis is being made over numerous office visits.

A fully automated system that measures BP at preset intervals over a 24-hour period is used. The equipment includes a BP cuff and a small microprocessing unit that fits into a pouch worn on a shoulder strap or belt. Patients are asked to maintain a diary of activities that may affect BP. This procedure may be helpful in patients with suspected white coat HTN, masked HTN, apparent drug resistance, hypotensive symptoms with hypertensive medications, episodic HTN, or autonomic nervous system dysfunction.

Some patients have elevated BP readings in a clinical setting and normal readings when BP is measured elsewhere. This phenomenon is referred to as *white coat hypertension*. Other patients have normal BP in the office and elevated BP at home. This condition is called *masked hypertension*.

As with most physiological phenomena, BP demonstrates diurnal variability expressed as sleep–wakefulness difference. For day-active people, BP is highest in the early morning, decreases during the day, and is lowest at night. Some patients with HTN do not show a normal, nocturnal fall in BP. They are called "non-dippers." A decrease in nocturnal BP of less than 10% is associated with increased risk of cardiovascular events. The presence or absence of diurnal variability can be determined by continuous ambulatory BP monitoring.

Canadians with HTN should be encouraged to use an approved BP-measuring device and use proper technique to assess BP at home. BP measured at home is a stronger predictor of cardiovascular events than office-based readings. Home measurement can help to confirm the diagnosis of HTN, improve BP control, reduce the need for medications, help to identify white coat and masked HTN, and improve medication adherence in nonadherent patients. An Internet-based toolbox to assist patient self-management for home BP measurement and lifestyle change can be found at the Heart and Stroke Foundation of Canada's Web site.

Canadian adults with high-normal BP require annual BP assessment. All Canadian adults need to have BP assessed at all appropriate clinical visits. One in five adult Canadians has HTN, and for those age 55 with normal BP, 90% will develop HTN if they live to an average age. All adults require ongoing assessment of BP throughout their lives.

Collaborative Care

Each year the Canadian Hypertension Education Program (CHEP), established in 1999, updates evidence-informed recommendations for the management of HTN. In 2011, CHEP joined with Hypertension Canada and Blood Pressure Canada with the goal of providing a stronger, united approach to the prevention and control of HTN. Each year, CHEP reviews the new evidence and integrates it into previous evidence-informed guidelines to develop new guidelines, where appropriate. Guidelines can be retrieved from the Hypertension Canada Web site. In order for health care providers to keep informed of CHEP recommendations, HTN resources are available at the CHEP Web site.

Risk Stratification. The risk of cardiovascular disease in people with HTN is determined by the level of BP; the presence of target-organ damage; risk factors such as diabetes, dyslipidemia, smoking, and obesity; and other exogenous, potentially modifiable factors that can induce or aggravate HTN (Table 35-6). Over 90% of hypertensive Canadians have other cardiovascular risks. The CHEP recommended that global cardiovascular risk should be assessed in all patients. Simply counting risk factors may lead to underestimating risk.

Follow-up monitoring of BP is important. The frequency of monitoring varies initially with the level of BP. After the BP has stabilized, follow-up visits should be scheduled every 3 to 6

Table 35-6 Assessment of the Overall Cardiovascular Risk	
Search for Target-Organ Damage	**Modifiable**
• Cerebrovascular disease	• Sedentary lifestyle
• Transient ischemic attacks	• Poor dietary habits
• Ischemic or hemorrhagic stroke	• Abdominal obesity
• Vascular dementia	• Dysglycemia
• Hypertensive retinopathy	• Smoking
• Left ventricular dysfunction	• Dyslipidemia
• Left ventricular hypertrophy	• Stress
• Coronary artery disease	• Nonadherence
• Myocardial infarction	***Search for Exogenous, Potentially Modifiable Factors That Can Induce or Aggravate Hypertension***
• Angina pectoris	
• Congestive heart failure	
• Chronic kidney disease	• Prescription drugs
• Hypertensive nephropathy (GFR <60 mL/min/1.73 m^2)	• NSAIDs, including "coxibs"
• Albuminuria	• Corticosteroids and anabolic steroids
• Peripheral artery disease	• Oral contraceptive and sex hormones
• Intermittent claudication	• Vasoconstricting/ sympathomimetic decongestants
• Ankle brachial index <0.9	• Calcineurin inhibitors (cyclosporin, tacrolimus)
Search for Key Cardiovascular Risk Factors for Atherosclerosis	• Erythropoietin and analogues
	• Antidepressants: MAOIs, SNRIs, SSRIs
Non-Modifiable	• MAOIs
	• Midodrine
• Age ≥55 yr	• Other
• Male	• Licorice root
• Family history of premature cardiovascular disease (<55 yr in men and <65 yr in women)	• Stimulants including cocaine
	• Salt
	• Excessive alcohol use

GFR, glomerular filtration rate; *MAOIs,* monoamine oxidase inhibitors; *NSAIDs,* nonsteroidal anti-inflammatory drugs; *SNRIs,* serotonin–norepinephrine reuptake inhibitors; *SSRIs,* selective serotonin reuptake inhibitors.
Source: Adapted from Canadian Hypertension Education Program (CHEP). (2011). *2011 CHEP recommendations for the management of hypertension* (pp 13-16, Tables 3, 4, 5). Markham, ON: Hypertension Canada. Retrieved from *http://www.hypertension.ca/images/stories/dls/2011gl/FullCHEPRecommendations_EN_2011.pdf* Reprinted with the permission of the Canadian Hypertension Program.

months to ensure continued control of BP, provide support for lifestyle changes, assess for target-organ damage, and detect adverse effects of medications.

Lifestyle Modifications. Lifestyle modifications should be used in all hypertensive patients as either definitive or adjunctive therapy. Lifestyle modifications are directed toward reducing BP and overall cardiovascular risk factors. Modifications include (1) dietary changes including reduced sodium intake, (2) limitation of alcohol intake, (3) regular physical activity, (4) avoidance of tobacco use (smoking and chewing), (5) stress management, and (6) weight reduction (see Figure 35-8 on p. 882).

NUTRITIONAL THERAPY

Table 35-7 Hypertension

FOOD GROUP	DAILY SERVINGS	EXAMPLES	SIGNIFICANCE TO DASH EATING PATTERN
Whole grains	6-8	Whole wheat breads, cereals; oatmeal; brown rice; pasta; quinoa; barley; low-fat, low-sodium crackers	Major sources of energy and fibre
Vegetables	4-5	Dark green and orange fresh or frozen vegetables, tomatoes, leafy greens, carrots, peas, squash, spinach, peppers, broccoli, sweet potatoes	Rich sources of potassium, magnesium, and fibre
Fruits	4-5	Have fruit more often than juice: apples, apricots, bananas, dates, grapes, oranges, grapefruit, melons, peaches, berries, pineapple	Important sources of potassium, magnesium, and fibre
Low-fat or fat-free dairy foods or alternatives	2-3	Skim, 1% milk, fortified soy beverage or yogurt, 6-18% modified-fat cheese	Major sources of calcium and protein
Meat, poultry, and fish	≤2	Lean meats. Choose fish such as char, herring, mackerel, salmon, sardines, and trout. Trim fat. Broil, roast, or boil. No frying. Remove skin from poultry. Low-sodium, low-fat deli meats.	Rich sources of protein and magnesium
Nuts, seeds, and dry beans	4-5/wk	—	Rich sources of energy, magnesium, potassium, protein, and fibre
Fats and oils	2-3 tsp	Soft margarine, mayonnaise, vegetable oil (olive, corn, canola, or safflower), salad dressing	Added fat and high-fat sources should be minimal. DASH has 27% of calories as fat, including fat in or added to foods.
Sweets	5 tbsp/wk	Sugar, jelly, jam, hard candy, syrups, sorbet, chocolate	Sweets should be low in fat.

DASH, Dietary Approaches to Stop Hypertension. The DASH eating plan is based on ~2000 calories/day. The number of daily servings in a food group may vary from those listed, depending on specific caloric needs.
Source: National Heart, Lung, and Blood Institute. (2006). *The DASH diet*. NIH Publication No. 06-4082. Washington, DC: National Institutes of Health. Retrieved from *http://www.nhlbi.nih.gov/health/public/heart/hbp/dash/new_dash.pdf*

Nutritional Therapy. The CHEP and the Heart and Stroke Foundation of Canada recommend the consumption of a diet that emphasizes fruits, vegetables, and low-fat dairy products; dietary and soluble fibre; and whole grains and protein from plant sources and that is reduced in saturated fat and cholesterol (Dietary Approaches to Stop Hypertension [DASH] diet) for hypertensive patients and normotensive individuals at increased risk of developing HTN. Dietary management of HTN consists of restriction of sodium; maintenance of dietary potassium, calcium, and magnesium intake; and calorie restriction if the patient is overweight (Table 35-7). (See eTable 35-1, Recommended Intake for Sodium, and eTable 35-2, Dietary Management of Hypertension, available on the Evolve Web site for this chapter.)

The CHEP 2010 recommendations included the reduction in salt intake for the prevention and treatment of HTN in accordance with the recommendations of Health Canada. It is estimated that lower sodium consumption could decrease the prevalence of HTN by 30% with a savings of approximately $430 million per year to Canada's health care system (Joffres, Campbell, Manns, & Tu, 2007).

About 1 million Canadians who currently have HTN would have normal BP if their diet contained a healthy amount of sodium (Joffres, Campbell, Manns, & Tu, 2007). The daily adequate intake (AI) for sodium is 1200 (52 mmol) to 1500 mg (65 mmol) for healthy adults, decreasing with age. The Upper Tolerable Intake Level (UL) for sodium is 2300 mg/day (see eTable 35-1, available on the Evolve Web site for this chapter). There is a large discrepancy between recommended levels of sodium intake and actual sodium intake levels by Canadians. The average sodium consumption in Canada is 3500 mg/day. Eighty

percent of sodium intake comes from processed and restaurant foods whereas only 10% is added at the table or in cooking. See "Sodium 101" and Health Canada's "Sodium – It's Your Health" in the Resources at the end of this chapter for more educational resources about salt. See also Chapter 37, Tables 37-11, 37-12, and 37-13.)

The patient and caregivers, especially those who prepare the meals, should be taught about sodium-restricted diets. Instruction should include reading labels of over-the-counter drugs, packaged foods, and health products (e.g., baking soda–containing toothpaste) to identify hidden sources of sodium. It is helpful to review the patient's normal diet and to identify foods high in sodium. Analysis of a 3-day diet history will help identify foods high in sodium in the patient's usual diet.

Sodium restriction may be enough to control BP in some patients with Stage 1 HTN. If drug therapy is needed, a lower dose may be effective if the patient also restricts sodium intake. Furthermore, moderate sodium restriction lessens the risk of hypokalemia associated with diuretic therapy. However, people with HTN respond differently to salt restriction. This heterogeneity of response has led to attempts to define subgroups of people with HTN as "salt sensitive" or "salt resistant." Patients with low renin activity are more likely to respond to salt restriction with a reduction in BP.

The significance of other dietary elements for the control of HTN is not certain. There is evidence that greater levels of dietary potassium, calcium, and vitamin D are associated with lower BP in the general population and in those with HTN. Based on available data, the CHEP 2011 recommendations (Rabi et al., 2011) advise the maintenance of adequate potassium, magnesium, and calcium intake from food sources. Supplementation of potassium, calcium, and magnesium is not recommended for the prevention or treatment of HTN. Caffeine may raise BP acutely, but there is no long-term relationship between caffeine intake and elevated BP.

Weight Reduction. Overweight individuals have an increased incidence of HTN and increased cardiovascular disease risk. Height, weight, and waist circumference should be measured and body mass index (BMI) calculated for all adults. Maintenance of a healthy body weight (BMI 18.5-24.9 kg/m^2 and waist circumference <102 cm for men and <88 cm for women) is recommended for individuals who are normotensive to prevent HTN and for Canadians with HTN to reduce BP. All overweight hypertensive individuals should be advised to lose weight. Weight reduction has a significant effect on lowering BP, and the effect is seen with even moderate weight loss. When a person decreases caloric intake, sodium and fat intake may also be reduced. Although reducing the fat content of the diet has not been shown to produce sustained benefits in BP control, it may slow the progress of atherosclerosis and reduce overall cardiovascular disease risk (see Chapter 36). Weight loss strategies should employ a multidisciplinary approach that includes dietary education, increased physical activity, and behavioural intervention.

Modification in Alcohol Consumption. Excessive alcohol consumption is strongly associated with HTN. To reduce BP, alcohol consumption should be in accordance with Canadian low-risk drinking guidelines for both normotensive and hypertensive adults. Healthy adults should limit alcohol consumption to 2 drinks or fewer per day, and consumption should not exceed 14 standard drinks per week for men and 9 standard drinks per week for women. (According to CHEP, 1 standard drink is considered 13.6 g or 17.2 mL of ethanol, or ~44 mL of 80-proof [40%] spirits, 148 mL of 12% wine, or 355 mL of 5% beer.)

Physical Activity. CHEP recommendations for nonhypertensive individuals (to reduce the possibility of becoming hypertensive) or for patients with HTN (to reduce their BP) include the accumulation of 30 to 60 minutes of moderate-intensity dynamic exercise (such as walking, jogging, cycling, or swimming) 4 to 7 days per week in addition to the routine activities of daily living. Higher intensities of exercise are no more effective.

Moderately intense activity can lower BP, promote relaxation, and decrease or control body weight. Regular activity of this type can reduce SBP in the patient with HTN by approximately 10 mm Hg. Sedentary people should be advised to increase activity levels gradually. People with heart disease or other serious health problems need a thorough examination, possibly including a stress test, before beginning an exercise program.

Avoidance of Tobacco Products. Nicotine contained in tobacco causes vasoconstriction and increases BP in hypertensive people. In addition, smoking tobacco is a major risk factor for cardiovascular disease. The cardiovascular benefits of discontinuing tobacco use can be seen within 1 year in all age groups. Everyone, especially a patient with HTN, should be strongly advised to avoid tobacco use. The lower amounts of nicotine contained in smoking cessation aids usually will not raise BP and may be used as indicated. People who continue to use tobacco products should be advised to monitor their BP during use. (See Chapter 11 and the Resources at the end of this chapter for links to smoking cessation materials.)

Stress Management. In hypertensive patients in whom stress may be contributing to BP elevation, stress management should be considered as an intervention. Individualized cognitive-behavioural interventions are more likely to be effective when relaxation techniques are used.

Drug Therapy. The implementation of the CHEP recommendations resulted in an increased use of antihypertensive medications, increased use of multiple antihypertensive medications, and improved persistence with medication use. The general goal of drug therapy is to achieve a BP of less than 140/90 mm Hg. For patients with chronic kidney disease or diabetes, target BP is less than 130/80 mm Hg. The drugs currently available for treating HTN have two main actions: (1) to reduce SVR and (2) to decrease the volume of circulating blood (Table 35-8). The drugs used in the treatment of HTN include diuretics, adrenergic (sympathetic) inhibitors, direct vasodilators, angiotensin inhibitors, and calcium channel blockers. The sites where the drugs exert their action and the methods of action are shown in Figure 35-7.

Although the precise action of diuretics in the reduction of BP is unclear, it is known that they promote sodium and water excretion, reduce plasma volume, decrease sodium in the arteriolar walls, and reduce the vascular response to catecholamines. Adrenergic-inhibiting drugs act by diminishing the sympathetic effects that increase BP. Adrenergic inhibitors include drugs that act centrally on the vasomotor centre and peripherally to inhibit NE release or to block the adrenergic receptors on blood vessels. Direct vasodilators decrease the BP by relaxing vascular smooth muscle and reducing SVR. Calcium channel blockers increase sodium excretion and cause arteriolar vasodilation by preventing the movement of extracellular calcium into cells.

There are two types of angiotensin inhibitors. The first type is ACE inhibitors, which prevent the conversion of angiotensin I to A-II and thus reduce A-II–mediated vasoconstriction and sodium and water retention. The second type is A-II receptor blockers (ARBs), which prevent A-II from binding to its receptors in the walls of the blood vessels.

Drug therapy is recommended for all patients at low risk with Stage 1 HTN (140-159/90-99 mm Hg), although lifestyle management may be the sole therapy. For clients with diabetes or chronic kidney disease, target blood pressure is <130/80 mm Hg. Many younger Canadians with HTN have multiple cardiovascular risks and are not treated with antihypertensive drugs. Currently, this is a gap in treatment. See CHEP's treatment algorithm of systolic-diastolic HTN without other compelling indications in Figure 35-8 and Tables 35-9 and 35-10.

The initial drug may be started at a low dosage for several weeks. The full effects of antihypertensive medication may not be apparent for up to 6 weeks. If the BP is not controlled, the dosage of the first-line drug can be increased. A second drug from a different class can be substituted, or a second drug from a different class can be added if the initial drug was ineffective or there were adverse effects to the initial drug. For most patients, at least two medications (probably taken in a single tablet) will be necessary in addition to lifestyle changes. Before proceeding with the addition or substitution of medication, consideration should be given to possible reasons for the lack of response to drug therapy.

A new drug therapy has been marketed recently in Canada. Although long-term mortality and morbidity studies have yet to be published, it has been authorized for use in Canada. Aliskiren fumarate (Rasilez) is an oral direct renin inhibitor (DRI). Renin

Text continued on p. 883

DRUG THERAPY

Table 35-8 Hypertension

DRUG	MECHANISM OF ACTION	ADVERSE EFFECTS	NURSING CONSIDERATIONS
Diuretics			
Thiazide and Related Diuretics			
Chlorthalidone hydrochlorothiazide indapamide (Lozide) Metolazone (Zaroxolyn)	Inhibit NaCl reabsorption in the distal convoluted tubule; increases excretion of Na⁺ and Cl⁻. Initial decrease in ECF; sustained decrease in SVR. Lower BP moderately in 2-4 wk.	Fluid and electrolyte imbalances (volume depletion, hypokalemia, hyponatremia, hypochloremia, hypomagnesemia, hypercalcemia, hyperuricemia, metabolic alkalosis); CNS effects (vertigo, headache, weakness); GI effects (anorexia, nausea, vomiting, diarrhea, constipation, pancreatitis); sexual problems (impotence and decreased libido); blood dyscrasias; and dermatological (photosensitivity, skin rash) effects; decreased glucose tolerance	Monitor for orthostatic hypotension, hypokalemia, and alkalosis. Thiazides may potentiate cardiotoxicity of digoxin by producing hypokalemia. Dietary sodium restriction reduces the risk of hypokalemia. NSAIDs can decrease diuretic and antihypertensive effect of thiazide diuretics. Advise patient to supplement with potassium-rich foods. Current doses are lower than previously recommended. Indapamide should be administered with caution to patients with kidney failure.
Loop Diuretics			
Bumetanide (Burinex) Ethacrynic acid (Edecrin) Furosemide (Lasix)	Inhibit NaCl reabsorption in the thick ascending limb of the loop of Henle. Increase excretion of Na⁺ and Cl⁻. More potent diuretic effect than thiazides, but shorter duration of action, less effective for hypertension.	Fluid electrolyte imbalance as with thiazides, except no hypercalcemia; ototoxicity (hearing impairment, deafness, vertigo) that is usually reversible; metabolic effects, including hyperuricemia, hyperglycemia, increased LDL cholesterol and triglycerides with decreased HDL cholesterol	Monitor for orthostatic hypotension and electrolyte abnormalities. Loop diuretics remain effective despite renal insufficiency. Diuretic effect of drug increases at higher doses.
Potassium-Sparing Diuretics			
Amiloride hydrochloride (Midamor, Novamilor)	Reduce K⁺ and Na⁺ exchange in the distal and collecting tubules. Reduces excretion of K⁺, H⁺, Ca²⁺, and Mg²⁺.	Hyperkalemia, nausea, vomiting, diarrhea, headache, leg cramps, and dizziness	Monitor for orthostatic hypotension and hyperkalemia. Potassium-sparing diuretics are contraindicated for use in patients with renal failure and used with caution in patients on ACE inhibitors or angiotensin II blockers. Avoid potassium supplements.
Spironolactone (Aldactone)	Inhibit the Na⁺–retaining and K⁺–excreting effects of aldosterone in the distal and collecting tubules.	Same as amiloride; may cause gynecomastia, impotence, decreased libido, and menstrual irregularities	
Adrenergic Inhibitors			
Central-Acting Adrenergic Antagonists			
Clonidine hydrochloride (Catapres)	Reduce sympathetic outflow from CNS. Reduce peripheral sympathetic tone, produces vasodilation; decreases SVR and BP.	Dry mouth, sedation, impotence, nausea, dizziness, sleep disturbance, nightmares, restlessness, and depression; symptomatic bradycardia in patients with conduction disorder	Sudden discontinuation may cause withdrawal syndrome including rebound hypertension, tachycardia, headache, tremors, apprehension, and sweating. Chewing gum or hard candy may relieve dry mouth. Alcohol and sedatives increase sedation. May be given transdermally with fewer adverse effects and better patient adherence.
Methyldopa	Same as clonidine.	Sedation, fatigue, orthostatic hypotension, decreased libido, impotence, dry mouth, hemolytic anemia, hepatotoxicity, sodium and water retention, psychological depression	Instruct patient about daytime sedation and avoidance of hazardous activities. Administration of a single daily dose at bedtime minimizes sedative effect.

Continued

DRUG THERAPY

Table 35-8 Hypertension—cont'd

DRUG	MECHANISM OF ACTION	ADVERSE EFFECTS	NURSING CONSIDERATIONS
α_1-Adrenergic Blockers			
Doxazosin mesylate (Cardura) Prazosin hydrochloride (Minipress) Terazosin hydrochloride (Hytrin)	Block α_1-adrenergic effects producing peripheral vasodilation (decreases SVR and BP).	Variable amount of postural hypotension depending on the plasma volume; may see profound orthostatic hypotension with syncope within 90 min after initial dose; retention of salt and water	Reduced resistance to the outflow of urine in benign prostatic hyperplasia. Taking drug at bedtime reduces risks associated with orthostatic hypotension. Has beneficial effects on lipid profile.
Phentolamine mesylate (Rogitine)	Block α_1-adrenergic receptors, resulting in peripheral vasodilation (decrease SVR and BP).	Acute, prolonged hypotension, cardiac dysrhythmias, tachycardia, weakness, flushing; abdominal pain, nausea, and exacerbation of peptic ulcer	Used in short-term management of pheochromocytoma. Also used locally to prevent necrosis of skin and subcutaneous tissue after extravasation of an α-adrenergic drug. No oral formulation.
β-Adrenergic Blockers			
Acebutolol hydrochloride (Sectral) Atenolol (Tenormin) Betaxolol hydrochloride Bisoprolol fumarate Carvedilol Metoprolol tartrate (Lopressor) Nadolol pindolol (Visken) Propranolol hydrochloride Timolol maleate	Reduce BP by antagonizing β_1-adrenergic effects. Decrease CO and reduce sympathetic vasoconstrictor tone. Decrease renin secretion by kidney.	Bronchospasm, atrioventricular conduction block, impaired peripheral circulation; nightmares, depression, weakness, reduced exercise capacity; may induce or exacerbate heart failure in susceptible patients; sudden withdrawal of β-adrenergic blockers may cause rebound hypertension and exacerbate symptoms of ischemic heart disease	β-Adrenergic blockers vary in lipid solubility, selectivity, and presence of partial sympathomimetic effect, which explains different therapeutic and adverse effect profiles of specific agents. Monitor pulse regularly. Use with caution in patients with diabetes mellitus because drug may mask signs of hypoglycemia.
Esmolol hydrochloride (Brevibloc)	Reduce BP by antagonizing β_1-adrenergic effects.	—	IV administration; has rapid onset and brief duration of action.
Combined α- and β-Adrenergic Blocker			
Labetalol hydrochloride (Trandate)	α_1-, β_1-, and β_2-Adrenergic blocking properties producing peripheral vasodilation and decreased heart rate. Reduce CO, SVR, and BP.	Dizziness, fatigue, nausea, vomiting, dyspepsia, paresthesia, nasal stuffiness, impotence, edema; hepatic toxicity	Same as β-adrenergic blockers. IV form available for hypertensive crisis in hospitalized patients. Patients must be kept supine during IV administration. Assess patient tolerance of upright position (severe postural hypotension) before allowing upright activities (e.g., commode).
Direct Vasodilators			
Diazoxide (Proglycem)	Reduce SVR and BP by direct arterial vasodilation.	Reflex sympathetic activation producing increased HR, CO, and salt and water retention; hyperglycemia, especially in patients with type 2 diabetes	IV use only for hypertensive crisis in hospitalized patients. Administer only into peripheral vein.
Hydralazine hydrochloride (Apresoline)	Reduce SVR and BP by direct arterial vasodilation.	Headache, nausea, flushing, palpitation, tachycardia, dizziness, and angina; hemolytic anemia, vasculitis, and rapidly progressive glomerulonephritis	IV use for hypertensive crisis in hospitalized patients. Twice-daily oral dosage. Not used as monotherapy because of adverse effects. Contraindicated for use in patients with coronary artery disease; used with caution in patients >40 yr of age.

DRUG THERAPY

Table 35-8 Hypertension—cont'd

DRUG	MECHANISM OF ACTION	ADVERSE EFFECTS	NURSING CONSIDERATIONS
Minoxidil (Loniten)	Reduce SVR and BP by direct arterial vasodilation.	Reflex tachycardia, marked sodium and fluid retention (may require loop diuretics for control), and hirsutism; may cause ECG changes (flattened and inverted T waves) not related to ischemia	Reserved for treatment of severe hypertension associated with kidney failure and resistant to other therapy. Once- or twice-daily dosage.
Nitroglycerin	Relax arterial and venous smooth muscle reducing preload and SVR. At low dose, venous dilation predominates; at higher dose, arterial dilation is present.	Hypotension, headache, vomiting, flushing IV use for hypertensive crisis in hospitalized patients with myocardial ischemia	Administered by continuous IV infusion with pump or control device.
Sodium nitroprusside (Nipride)	Direct arterial vasodilation reduces SVR and BP.	Acute hypotension, nausea, vomiting, muscle twitching; signs of thiocyanate toxicity include anorexia, nausea, fatigue, disorientation	IV use for hypertensive crisis in hospitalized patients. Administered by continuous IV infusion with pump or control device. Use intra-arterial monitoring of BP. Light-resistant bags, bottles, and administration sets must be used; stable for 24 hr. Monitor thiocyanate levels with prolonged (>24-48 hr) use.

Angiotensin Inhibitors

Angiotensin-Converting Enzyme (ACE) Inhibitors

Benazepril hydrochloride (Lotensin) Captopril Enalapril sodium (Vasotec) Fosinopril sodium (Monopril) Lisinopril (Prinivil, Zestril) Perindopril erbumine (Coversyl) Quinapril hydrochloride (Accupril) Ramipril (Altace) Trandolapril (Mavik, Tarka) Enalaprilat injection (Vasotec IV)	Inhibit ACE; reduce conversion of angiotensin I to angiotensin II (A-II); prevent A-II–mediated vasoconstriction. Inhibit ACE when oral drugs not appropriate.	Hypotension, loss of taste, cough, hyperkalemia, acute renal failure, skin rash, angioneurotic edema; same as oral forms	Aspirin and NSAIDs may reduce drug effectiveness. Addition of diuretic enhances drug effect. Should not be used with potassium-sparing diuretics. Can cause fetal morbidity or mortality. Captopril may be given orally for hypertensive crisis. Given by IV route over 5 min; may be given every 6 hr.

Angiotensin II Receptor Blockers

Candesartan cilexetil (Atacand) Eprosartan mesylate (Teveten) Irbesartan (Avapro) Losartan potassium (Cozaar) Telmisartan (Micardis) Valsartan (Diovan)	Prevent action of angiotensin II and produce vasodilation and increased salt and water excretion.	Hyperkalemia, decreased kidney function	Full effect on BP may not be seen for 3-6 wk.

Calcium Channel Blockers

Amlodipine besylate (Caduet, Norvasc) Diltiazem hydrochloride (Tiazac) Felodipine (Plendil, Renedil) Nifedipine (Adalat) Verapamil hydrochloride (Covera, Isoptin)	Block movement of extracellular calcium into cells, causing vasodilation and decreased SVR.	Nausea, headache, dizziness, peripheral edema; reflex tachycardia (with dihydropyridines); reflex decrease HR (with diltiazem); constipation (with verapamil)	Use with caution in patients with heart failure. Contraindicated for use in patients with second- or third-degree heart block. Sustained-release formulations for some drugs. Avoid grapefruit consumption when on nifedipine.

ACE, angiotensin-converting inhibitor; *BP*, blood pressure; *CNS*, central nervous system; *CO*, cardiac output; *ECF*, extracellular fluid; *ECG*, electrocardiogram; *GI*, gastrointestinal; *HDL*, high-density lipoprotein; *HR*, heart rate; *IV*, intravenous; *LDL*, low-density lipoprotein; *NSAIDs*, nonsteroidal anti-inflammatory drugs; *SVR*, systemic vascular resistance.

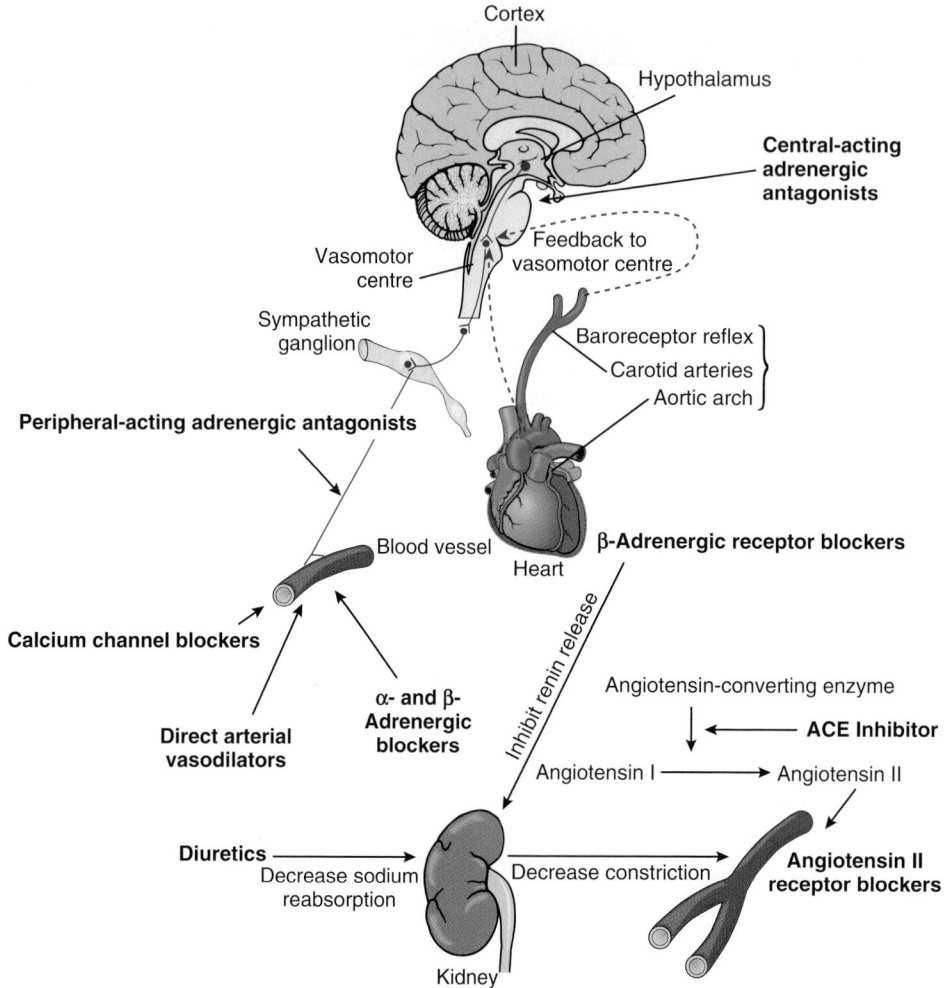

Figure 35-7 Site and method of action of various antihypertensive drugs. *ACE,* angiotensin-converting enzyme.

Source: U.S. Department of Health and Human Services. (2003). The seventh report of the Joint National Committee on Detection, Evaluation, and Treatment of High Blood Pressure (JNC-7). Washington, DC: National Institutes of Health.

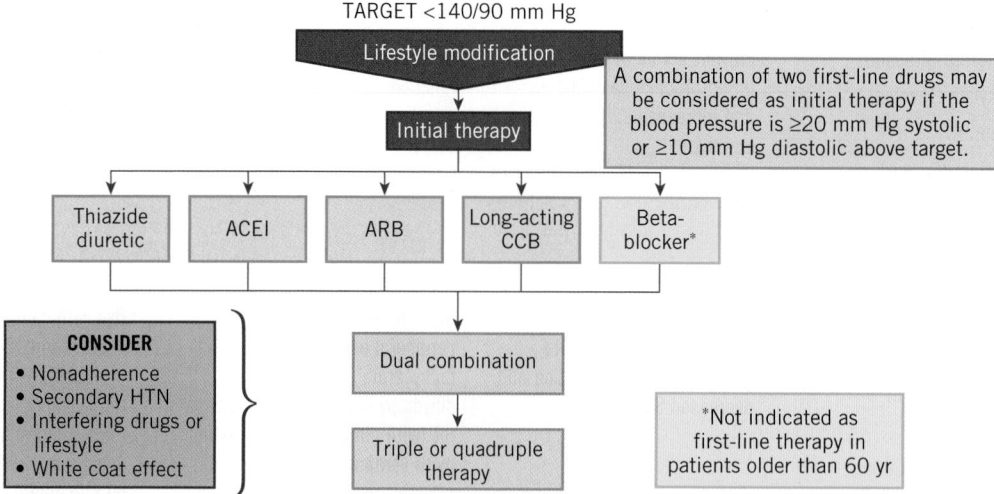

Figure 35-8 Treatment of systolic–diastolic hypertension *(HTN)* without other compelling indications. *ACEI,* angiotensin-converting enzyme inhibitor; *ARB,* angiotensin II receptor blocker; *CCB,* calcium channel blocker.

Source: Canadian Hypertension Education Program (CHEP). (2011). *2011 Canadian Hypertension Education Program recommendations: Part 2, Recommendations for hypertension treatment* (Slide 50). Retrieved from *http://www.hypertension.ca*

Table 35-9 Considerations Regarding the Choice of First-Line Therapy
• Use caution in initiating therapy with two drugs in patients in whom adverse events are more likely (e.g., frail elderly, those with postural hypotension or who are dehydrated).
• ACE inhibitors, renin inhibitors, and ARBs are contraindicated in pregnancy and caution is required in prescribing to women of child-bearing potential.
• β-Adrenergic blockers are not recommended for patients ≥60 yr without another compelling indication.
• Diuretic-induced hypokalemia should be avoided through the use of potassium-sparing agents if required.
• The use of dual therapy with an ACE inhibitor and an ARB should be considered only in selected and closely monitored people with advanced heart failure or proteinuric nephropathy.
• ACE inhibitors are not recommended (as monotherapy) for Black patients without another compelling indication.

ACE, angiotensin-converting enzyme; *ARB,* angiotensin II receptor blocker.
Source: Canadian Hypertension Education Program (CHEP). (2011). *2011 Canadian Hypertension Education Program recommendations. Part 2, Recommendations for hypertension treatment* (Slide 43). Available at *http://www.hypertension.ca*

Table 35-10 Drug Combinations
When combining drugs, use first-line therapies.
• Two-drug combinations of β-blockers, ACEIs, and ARBs have not been proved to have additive hypotensive effects. Therefore, these potential two-drug combinations should not be used unless there is a compelling (non–blood pressure-lowering) indication.
• Combinations of an ACEI with an ARB do not reduce cardiovascular events more than the ACEI alone and have more adverse effects; therefore, they are not generally recommended.
• Caution should be exercised in combining a nondihydropyridine CCB and a β-blocker to reduce the risk of bradycardia or heart block.
• Monitor serum creatinine and potassium when combining potassium-sparing diuretics, ACEIs and/or ARBs.
• If a diuretic is not used as first- or second-line therapy, triple-dose therapy should include a diuretic, when not contraindicated.

ACEIs, angiotensin-converting enzyme inhibitors; *ARBs,* angiotensin II receptor blockers; *CCB,* calcium channel blocker.
Source: Canadian Hypertension Education Program (CHEP). (2011). *2011 Canadian Hypertension Education Program recommendations. Part 2, Recommendations for hypertension treatment* (Slides 45-46). Markham, ON: Hypertension Canada. Retrieved from *http://www.hypertension.ca*

inhibition acts on the conversion of angiotensinogen to angiotensin I. This is the rate-limiting step in the production of A-II, which is a key mediator of BP, body fluid volume, and vascular remodelling. DRIs may be more effective in inhibiting RAAS when compared with ACE inhibitors or ARBs.

The addition of a third or fourth drug may be necessary, but only after the maximum doses of the first and second drugs have been achieved.

After 1 year of optimum BP control, step-down therapy may be tried. The number of medications and their dosages are gradually decreased to the lowest amount that controls the BP. Regular follow-up is needed to detect any elevation of BP.

Adverse effects of antihypertensive drugs may be so severe or undesirable that the patient does not adhere to therapy. Table 35-8 describes the major adverse effects of antihypertensive drugs. Hyperuricemia, hyperglycemia, and hypokalemia are common adverse effects with both thiazide and loop diuretics. ACE inhibitors can lead to high levels of bradykinin, which can cause coughing. An individual who develops a cough with the use of ACE inhibitors may be switched to an A-II receptor blocker. Hyperkalemia can be a serious adverse effect of the potassium-sparing diuretics and ACE inhibitors. Impotence may occur with some of the diuretics. Orthostatic hypotension and sexual dysfunction are two undesirable effects of adrenergic-inhibiting agents. Tachycardia and orthostatic hypotension are potential adverse effects of both vasodilators and angiotensin inhibitors.

Patient Teaching Related to Drug Therapy. Patient and caregiver teaching related to drug therapy is needed to identify and minimize adverse effects and to cope with therapeutic effects. Adverse effects of antihypertensive drug therapy are common. Adverse effects may be an initial response to a drug and may decrease with continued use of the drug. Informing the patient that adverse effects may lessen with time may enable the individual to continue taking the drug. The number or severity of adverse effects may be related to the dosage, and it may be neces-

sary to change the drug or decrease the dosage. In this case, the patient should be advised to report the adverse effects to the health care provider who prescribed the medication.

A common adverse effect of several of these drugs is orthostatic hypotension. This condition is caused by an alteration of the autonomic nervous system's mechanisms for regulating pressure, which are required for position changes. Consequently, the patient may feel dizzy, weak, and faint when assuming an upright position after sitting or lying down. (Specific measures to control or decrease orthostatic hypotension are presented in Table 35-14.)

Sexual dysfunction may occur with many of the antihypertensive drugs (see Table 35-8) and can be a major reason for nonadherence to the treatment plan. Often, the nurse must approach the patient on this sensitive subject and encourage discussion of any sexual dysfunction that may be experienced. The sexual problems may be easier for the patient to discuss once it has been explained that the drug may be the source of the problem and the adverse effects can be decreased or eliminated by changing to another antihypertensive drug. The patient should be encouraged to discuss adverse effects with the person who prescribed the medication. If the patient is reluctant to do so, the nurse may offer to alert the health care provider to the sexual adverse effect that the patient is experiencing. There are many options for treating HTN; a plan that is acceptable to the patient should be achievable.

Some unpleasant effects of drugs result from their therapeutic effect, but the impact can be minimized. For example, dry mouth and frequent voiding are unpleasant effects of diuretics. Sugarless gum or candy may relieve the dry mouth. The nurse can assist the patient to develop a medication schedule to minimize unpleasant effects. When frequent urination interrupts sleep, taking the diuretic earlier in the day may be beneficial. Adverse effects of vasodilators and adrenergic inhibitors decrease if the drugs are taken in the evening. BP is lowest during the night and highest shortly after awakening; therefore, drugs with 24-hour duration of action should be taken as early in the morning as possible (e.g., 0400 or 0500 if the patient awakens to void).

NURSING MANAGEMENT: PRIMARY HYPERTENSION

▪ Nursing Assessment

Subjective and objective data that should be obtained from a patient with HTN are presented in Table 35-11.

▪ Nursing Diagnoses

Nursing diagnoses and collaborative problems for the patient with HTN include, but are not limited to, those presented in Table 35-12.

NURSING ASSESSMENT

Table 35-11 Hypertension Data
Subjective Data
Important Health Information
Current health history: Family history of hypertension or cardiovascular disease; smoking or other tobacco use, alcohol use; sedentary lifestyle; usual salt and fat intake; weight gain or loss
Past health history: Known duration and past workup of high BP; cardiovascular, cerebrovascular, renal, or thyroid disease; diabetes; pituitary disorders; obesity; dyslipidemia; menopause or hormone replacement status
Medications: Use of any prescription or over-the-counter, illicit, or natural health products; previous use of antihypertensive drug therapy
Symptoms
• Dyspnea on exertion, palpitations on exertion, anginal chest pain
• Fatigue
• Intermittent claudication, muscle cramps
• Nocturia
• Dizziness; blurred vision, paresthesias
• Erectile dysfunction, decreased libido
Objective Data
Cardiovascular
BP consistently >140 mm Hg systolic or 90 mm Hg diastolic, orthostatic change in BP and pulse; abnormal heart sounds; laterally displaced, sustained, forceful, apical pulse; diminished or absent peripheral pulses; carotid, kidney, ischial, or femoral bruits; presence of edema
Musculoskeletal
Truncal obesity
Neurological
Mental status changes
Possible Findings
Abnormal serum electrolytes (especially potassium); increased creatinine, glucose, cholesterol, and triglyceride levels; proteinuria, microalbuminuria; evidence of ischemic heart disease and left ventricular hypertrophy on ECG

BP, blood pressure; *ECG,* electrocardiogram.

▪ Planning

The overall goals for the patient with HTN are that the patient will (1) achieve and maintain the individually determined target BP; (2) understand, accept, and implement the therapeutic plan; (3) experience minimal or no unpleasant adverse effects of therapy; and (4) be confident of ability to manage and cope with this condition.

▪ Nursing Implementation

▪ Health Promotion

Primary prevention of HTN provides an attractive alternative to the costly cycle of managing HTN and its complications. Current recommendations for primary prevention are based on lifestyle modifications that have been shown to prevent or delay the expected rise in BP in susceptible people. A diet rich in fruits, vegetables, and low-fat dairy foods, with reduced saturated and total fats, significantly lowers BP (see Table 35-7). This diet has been recommended for primary prevention in the general population. Dietary modifications that do not require active participation of the individual, such as a reduction in the amount of salt added to processed foods, may be even more effective.

▪ **Individual Patient Evaluation.** The majority of cases of HTN are identified through routine screening procedures such as insurance and pre-employment or premilitary physical

NURSING ASSESSMENT

Table 35-12 Hypertension
Nursing Diagnoses
• Ineffective health maintenance related to lack of knowledge of pathology, complications, and management of hypertension
• Anxiety related to complexity of management regimen, possible complications, and lifestyle changes associated with hypertension
• Sexual dysfunction related to effects of antihypertensive medication
• Ineffective self-health management related to:
• Lack of knowledge
• Unpleasant adverse effects of medication
• Return of blood pressure to normal while on medication
• High cost of some medications
• Inconvenient schedule for taking medications
• Lack of trusting relationship with health care provider
• Disturbed body image related to diagnosis of hypertension
• Ineffective tissue perfusion related to complications of hypertension *(specify)*
• Cerebral
• Cardiovascular
• Renal
Collaborative Problems
• Potential complication: adverse effects from antihypertensive therapy
• Potential complication: hypertensive crisis
• Potential complication: stroke

examinations. The nurse in these settings, as well as in most other practice settings, is in an ideal position to assess for the presence of HTN, identify the risk factors for HTN and coronary artery disease, and teach the patient about these conditions. In addition to BP determination, a complete health assessment should include such factors as age, sex, and race; diet history (including sodium and alcohol intake); weight patterns; and family history of heart disease, stroke, renal disease, and diabetes mellitus. Medications taken, both prescribed and over-the-counter, should be noted. The patient should be asked about a previous history of high BP and the results of treatment (if any) (see Table 35-11).

Initially, the BP is taken two or three times, at least 2 minutes apart, with the average pressure recorded as the value for that visit. Waiting for at least 2 minutes between readings allows the venous blood to drain from the arm and prevents inaccurate readings. Size and placement of BP cuff are important considerations for accurate measurement. The width of the inflatable bladder should be 40% and length should be 80% of the upper arm circumference. Use of a cuff that is too small or too large will result in readings that are falsely high or low, respectively.

BP measurements of both arms should be performed initially to detect any differences between arms. Atherosclerotic narrowing of the subclavian artery can cause a falsely low reading on the side where the narrowing occurs. Therefore, the arm with the higher reading should be used for all subsequent BP measurements. The patient's arm is uncovered and placed at the level of the heart. The cuff should be inflated until no pulse is felt in the brachial artery located in the antecubital fossa of the arm being used. The cuff is then inflated an additional 10 to 20 mm Hg to ensure vascular occlusion. The pressure is released at 2 mm Hg/sec. Releasing any more slowly or quickly may create inaccurate readings. Both SBP and DBP should be recorded, with the DBP recorded as the disappearance of sound (Table 35-13).

The BP and the pulse are initially measured with the patient in either the supine or the sitting position after at least 5 minutes of rest. BP and pulse should be measured again after 2 minutes in the standing position. Usually, the SBP decreases on standing, whereas the DBP and the pulse increase. A decrease of more than 10 mm Hg in SBP or any decrease in DBP when standing is abnormal and should prompt further investigation. Common causes of abnormal postural BP values include intravascular volume loss (e.g., with diuretic therapy or dehydration) and inadequate vasoconstrictor mechanisms related to disease or medications. Postural changes in BP and pulse should be measured in older adults, people taking antihypertensive drugs, and when orthostatic hypotension is suspected. The common definition for **orthostatic hypotension** is a decrease of 20 mm Hg (or more) in SBP or a decrease of 10 mm Hg (or more) in the DBP that occurs when an individual assumes a standing position.

▌ Screening Programs.
Screening programs in the community are widely used to assess BP. At the time of the BP measurement, each person should be informed in writing of the numerical value of the reading and, if necessary, why further evaluation is important. Effort and resources should be focused on controlling BP in the person already identified as having HTN; identifying and controlling BP in high-risk groups such as Blacks, Southeast Asians, people who are obese, and blood relatives of people with HTN; and screening those with limited access to the health care system.

Table 35-13 Appropriate Technique for Measuring Blood Pressure

1. The use of a sphygmomanometer known to be accurate. Patient should be seated with the arm bared, supported, and positioned at heart level. The patient should have neither smoked nor ingested caffeine within 30 min before measurement nor used substances containing adrenergic stimulants, such as phenylephrine or pseudoephedrine and that may be found in decongestants or ophthalmic drops.

2. The bowel and the bladder should be comfortable. Provide a quiet environment at a comfortable room temperature.

3. The patient should stay quiet before and during the procedure.

4. For initial readings, take the blood pressure in both arms, and subsequently measure in the arm with the highest reading. Thereafter, take two measurements on the side where the BP is highest.

5. The appropriate cuff size must be used to ensure an accurate measurement. The rubber bladder should reach nearly around (at least 80% of the circumference) or completely encircle the arm. Cuff width should be at least 40% of the arm circumference. Several sizes of cuffs (e.g., child, adult, and large adult) should be available.

6. Measurements should be taken with a mercury sphygmomanometer, a recently calibrated aneroid manometer, or a calibrated electronic device.

7. Both systolic and diastolic pressures should be recorded. The disappearance of sound should be used for the diastolic reading.

8. Two or more readings (taken at least 2 min apart) should be averaged. If the first two readings differ by >5 mm Hg, additional readings should be obtained.

9. The patient should be informed of the reading and advised of the need for periodic remeasurement.

BP, blood pressure.
Source: Adapted from Canadian Hypertension Education Program (CHEP). (2011). *2011 CHEP recommendations for the management of hypertension* (pp. 9-11, Table 1). Markham, ON: Hypertension Canada. Retrieved from *http://www.docvadis.it/eugenio.greco/document/eugenio.greco/canadian_hypertension_education_program/fr/metadata/files/0/file/CanadianHypertensionEducationProgram.pdf*

▌ Cardiovascular Risk Factor Modification.
Education regarding cardiovascular risk factors is appropriate for individual and targeted screening programs. Modifiable cardiovascular risk factors include HTN, obesity, diabetes mellitus, elevated serum lipids, tobacco use, and physical inactivity. Risk factors can easily be identified and modification discussed with the patient. (Health-promoting behaviours for cardiovascular risk factors are presented in Chapter 36, Table 36-4.)

▌ Ambulatory and Home Care

The primary nursing responsibilities for long-term management of HTN are to assist the patient in reducing BP and adhering to the treatment plan. Nursing actions include patient and family teaching, detection and reporting of adverse treatment effects, adherence assessment and enhancement, and evaluation of therapeutic effectiveness (Table 35-14). Patient and caregiver teaching includes the following: (1) nutritional therapy, (2) drug therapy, (3) physical activity, (4) home monitoring of BP (if appropriate), (5) tobacco cessation (if applicable), and (6) stress management.

When presenting information to the patient or caregiver, the nurse should do the following:

1. Provide the numerical value of the patient's BP and explain what it means.
2. Inform the patient that hypertension is usually asymptomatic and symptoms do not reliably indicate BP levels.
3. Explain that hypertension means elevated BP and does not relate to a "hyper" personality.
4. Explain that long-term follow-up and therapy are necessary to treat hypertension.
5. Explain that therapy will not cure, but should control, hypertension.
6. Tell patient that controlled hypertension is usually compatible with an excellent prognosis and a normal lifestyle.
7. Explain the potential dangers of uncontrolled hypertension.
8. Be specific about the names, the actions, the dosages, and the adverse effects of prescribed medications.
9. Tell the patient to plan regular and convenient times for taking medications.
10. Tell the patient not to discontinue drugs abruptly because withdrawal may cause a severe hypertensive reaction.
11. Tell the patient not to double up on doses when a dose is missed.
12. Inform the patient that, if BP increases, the patient should not take an increased medication dosage before consulting with the health care provider.
13. Tell the patient not to take a medication belonging to someone else.
14. Inform the patient that adverse effects of medication often diminish with time.
15. Tell the patient to consult with the health care provider about changing drugs or dosages if impotence or other sexual problems develop.
16. Tell the patient to supplement diet with foods high in potassium (e.g., citrus fruits and green leafy vegetables) if taking potassium-losing diuretics.
17. Tell the patient to avoid hot baths, excessive amounts of alcohol, and strenuous exercise within 3 hr of taking medications that promote vasodilation.
18. Explain that, to decrease orthostatic hypotension, the patient should arise slowly from bed, sit on the side of the bed for a few minutes, stand slowly, not stand still for prolonged periods, do leg exercises to increase venous return, sleep with the head of the bed raised or on pillows, and lie or sit down when dizziness occurs.
19. Caution about potentially high-risk over-the-counter medications, such as high-sodium antacids, appetite suppressants, and cold and sinus medications. Advise the patient to read warning labels and to consult with pharmacist.

BP, blood pressure.

Physical Activity. Physical activity is bodily movement produced by skeletal muscles that requires energy expenditure. Health benefits from physical activity can be achieved with moderate-intensity activities. The goal for all adults is to accumulate 30 minutes of moderate-intensity activity daily. Generally, physical activity is more likely to be sustained if it is safe and enjoyable, fits easily into the daily schedule, and does not generate financial or social costs.

Shopping malls in many communities are open early in the morning (before shopping hours) and provide a warm, safe, flat area for walking. In some communities, health clubs offer special "off-peak" rates to encourage physical activity among older adults. Cardiac rehabilitation programs offer supervised exercise with education about reduction of cardiovascular risk factors. Nurses can assist people with HTN to increase their physical activity by identifying and communicating the need for increased activity, explaining the difference between physical activity and exercise, assisting in initiating activity, and following up appropriately.

Home Blood Pressure Monitoring. Some patients benefit from regularly monitoring their BP at home. Home BP measurement may give a more valid indication of the BP because the patient is more relaxed. It is important to emphasize to the patient that a single reading is not as important as a series of readings over time. The patient should be instructed to take BP readings weekly (unless otherwise instructed) once the BP has stabilized. A log of the BP measurements should be maintained by the patient and brought to office visits.

Home BP readings may help achieve patient adherence by reinforcing the need to continue therapy. A patient may become excessively concerned with the BP readings when using home monitoring. Generally, however, this practice should reassure the patient that the treatment is effective.

Patient Adherence. A major challenge in the long-term management of the patient with HTN is poor adherence with the prescribed treatment plan. The reasons are many and include inadequate patient teaching, unpleasant adverse effects of drugs, return of BP to normal range while on medication, lack of motivation, high cost of drugs, and lack of a trusting relationship between the patient and the health care provider. In addition to using BP determinations as an indicator of adherence, the nurse should also assess the patient's diet, activity level, and lifestyle.

Individual assessment to determine the reasons the patient does not adhere to the treatment plan and the development of an individualized plan with the patient's assistance are essential. The plan should be compatible with the patient's personality, habits, and lifestyle. Active patient participation increases the likelihood of adherence to the treatment plan. Measures such as involving the patient in scheduling medication convenient to a daily routine, helping the patient link pill-taking with another daily activity, and involving family members (if necessary) help increase patient adherence. Substituting combination tablets for multiple drugs once the BP is stabilized may also facilitate adherence because the patient has to take fewer drugs each day and the cost may be less. It is important to help the patient and the family understand that HTN is a chronic condition that cannot be cured but can be controlled with drug therapy, diet therapy, physical activity, periodic evaluation, and other relevant lifestyle changes (Table 35-15).

Evaluation

The overall expected outcomes are that the patient with HTN will (1) achieve and maintain desired BP as defined for the individual;

Table 35-15 Recommendations to Improve Adherence to Antihypertensive Prescriptions

Adherence can be improved by a multipronged approach:

- Assess adherence to pharmacological and nonpharmacological therapy at every physician visit.
- Simplify medication regimens to once-daily administration and utilize electronic medication adherence aids. Use fixed-dose combinations where available and appropriate.
- Tailor pill-taking to fit patient's daily habits.
- Encourage greater patient responsibility and autonomy in monitoring blood pressure and adjusting prescriptions.
- Coordinate with work-site health care providers to improve monitoring of adherence to pharmacological and lifestyle modification prescriptions.
- Educate patients and families about disease or treatment regimens.

(2) understand, accept, and implement the therapeutic plan; and (3) experience minimal or no unpleasant adverse effects of therapy.

AGE-RELATED CONSIDERATIONS: HYPERTENSION

HTN is common in people 60 years of age and older in industrialized countries. The SBP rises throughout the lifespan and DBP rises until age 55 or 60 years and then levels off. The following age-related physical changes play a role in the pathophysiology of HTN in the older adult: (1) loss of tissue elasticity; (2) increased collagen content and stiffness of the myocardium; (3) increased peripheral vascular resistance; (4) decreased β-adrenergic receptor sensitivity; (5) blunting of baroreceptor reflexes; (6) decreased kidney function; and (7) decreased renin response to sodium and water depletion (Acelajado & Oparil, 2009).

In the older adult taking antihypertensive medication, absorption of some drugs may be altered as a result of decreased splanchnic blood flow. Metabolism and excretion of drugs may also be prolonged.

Careful technique is important in assessing BP in older adults. In some older people, there is a wide gap between the first Korotkoff sound and subsequent beats. This is called the *auscultatory gap.* Failure to inflate the cuff high enough may result in seriously underestimating the SBP. This problem can be avoided by palpating the brachial or radial artery while inflating the cuff to a level above the disappearance of the pulse.

Older adults are sensitive to BP changes; therefore, reducing SBP to less than 120 mm Hg in a person with longstanding HTN could lead to inadequate cerebral blood flow. Older adults also produce less renin and are more resistant to the effects of ACE inhibitors and A-II receptor blockers (Acelajado & Oparil, 2009).

Because of varying degrees of impaired baroreceptor reflex mechanisms, postural or orthostatic hypotension occurs often in older adults, especially in those with ISH. Postural hypotension in this age group is often associated with volume deple-

tion or chronic disease states, such as decreased renal and hepatic function or electrolyte imbalance. To reduce the likelihood of postural hypotension, antihypertensive drugs should be started at low doses and increased cautiously. BP and pulse should be measured in the sitting and standing positions at every visit.

Hypertensive Crisis

Hypertensive crisis is a severe and abrupt elevation in BP, arbitrarily defined as a DBP above 120 to 130 mm Hg. The rate of the rise of BP is more important than the absolute value in determining the need for emergency treatment. Patients with chronic HTN can tolerate much higher BP than previously normotensive people (Drouin & Milot, 2007). Prompt recognition and management of hypertensive crisis is essential to decrease the threat to organ function and life.

Hypertensive crisis occurs most commonly in patients with a history of HTN who have failed to adhere to their prescribed medication regimen or who have been undermedicated. In this setting, rising BP is thought to trigger endothelial damage and the release of vasoconstrictor substances. A vicious cycle of BP elevation ensues leading to life-threatening damage to target organs. Hypertensive crisis related to cocaine or crack use is becoming a more frequent problem. Other drugs such as amphetamines, phencyclidine (PCP), and lysergic acid diethylamide (LSD) may also precipitate hypertensive crisis that may be complicated by drug-induced seizures, stroke, MI, or encephalopathy. Hypertensive crisis is classified by the degree of organ damage and the rapidity with which the BP must be lowered. *Hypertensive emergency,* which develops over hours to days, is a situation in which a patient's BP is severely elevated with evidence of acute target-organ damage, especially damage to the central nervous system. Hypertensive emergencies include hypertensive encephalopathy, intracranial or subarachnoid hemorrhage, acute left ventricular failure with pulmonary edema, MI, kidney failure, and dissecting aortic aneurysm. *Hypertensive urgency,* which develops over days to weeks, is a situation in which a patient's BP is severely elevated but there is no clinical evidence of target-organ damage.

Clinical Manifestations. A hypertensive emergency may be manifested as *hypertensive encephalopathy,* a syndrome in which a sudden rise in BP is associated with headache, nausea, vomiting, seizures, confusion, stupor, and coma. Other common manifestations are blurred vision and transient blindness. The manifestations of encephalopathy are probably the results of cerebral edema and spasms of cerebral vessels.

Renal insufficiency ranging from minor impairment to complete renal shutdown may occur. Rapid cardiac decompensation ranging from unstable angina to infarction and pulmonary edema is also possible with chest pain and dyspnea. Aortic dissection causes excruciating chest and back pain often accompanied by diaphoresis and the loss of pulses in an extremity.

Patient assessment is extremely important, especially monitoring for signs of neurological dysfunction, retinal damage, heart failure, pulmonary edema, and renal failure. The neurological manifestations are often similar to the presentation of a stroke. However, a hypertensive crisis does not show the focal or lateralizing signs often seen with a stroke.

NURSING AND COLLABORATIVE MANAGEMENT: HYPERTENSIVE CRISIS

BP level alone is a poor indicator of the seriousness of the patient's condition and is not the major factor in deciding the treatment for a hypertensive crisis. The association between elevated BP and signs of new or progressive end-organ damage (e.g., cerebrovascular, cardiac, retinal, or renal involvement) determines the seriousness of the situation.

Hypertensive emergencies necessitate hospitalization, parenteral administration of antihypertensive drugs, and intensive care monitoring. Generally, the initial treatment goal is to decrease mean arterial pressure (MAP) 10 to 20% in the first one to two hours with further gradual reduction over the next 24 hours. Lowering the BP too far or too fast may decrease cerebral perfusion and could precipitate a stroke. A patient who has aortic dissection, unstable angina, or signs of MI must have the SBP lowered to 100 to 120 mm Hg as quickly as possible.

The intravenous (IV) drugs used for hypertensive emergencies include vasodilators (e.g., sodium nitroprusside, nitroglycerin, diazoxide [Proglycem], and hydralazine hydrochloride [Apresoline]), adrenergic inhibitors (e.g., phentolamine mesylate [Rogitine], labetalol [Trandate], and esmolol hydrochloride [Brevibloc]), and the ACE inhibitor enalaprilat sodium (Vasotec). Sodium nitroprusside is the most effective parenteral drug for the treatment of hypertensive emergencies. Oral agents may be administered in addition to the parenteral drugs to help make an earlier transition to long-term therapy. The mechanisms of action and the adverse effects of these drugs are shown in Table 35-8.

Administered intravenously, the drugs have a rapid (within seconds to minutes) onset of action. The patient's BP and pulse should be taken every 2 to 3 minutes during the initial administration of these drugs. The use of an arterial line (see Chapter 68) or an automated BP monitoring machine (e.g., Dynamap) to monitor the BP is ideal. The rate of drug administration is titrated according to the level of BP. It is important to prevent hypotension and its effects in a person whose body has adjusted to hypertension. An excessive reduction in BP may cause stroke, MI, or visual changes. Continual ECG monitoring is frequently done to observe for cardiac dysrhythmias. Extreme caution is needed in treating the patient with coronary artery disease or cerebrovascular insufficiency. Hourly urinary output should be measured to assess renal perfusion. Careful monitoring of vital signs and urinary output provides information regarding the effectiveness of these drugs and the patient's response to therapy. Patients receiving IV antihypertensive drugs may be restricted to bed; getting up (e.g., to use the commode) may cause severe cerebral ischemia and fainting.

Regular, ongoing assessment is essential to evaluate the patient with severe hypertension. Frequent neurological checks, including level of consciousness, pupillary size and reaction, movement of extremities, and reactions to stimuli, help detect any changes in the patient's condition. Cardiac, pulmonary, and renal systems should be monitored for decompensation caused by the severe elevation in BP (e.g., pulmonary edema, congestive heart failure, angina, renal failure).

Hypertensive urgencies usually do not necessitate IV administration of medications but can be managed with oral agents. The patient with a hypertensive urgency may not need hospitalization, but requires frequent follow-up. The oral drugs most frequently used for hypertensive urgencies are captopril and clonidine (Catapres) (see Table 35-8). The disadvantage of oral medications is the inability to regulate the dosage from moment to moment, as can be done with IV medications. If a patient with a hypertensive urgency is not hospitalized, outpatient follow-up should be arranged within 24 hours.

A patient with severe elevation of BP but without target-organ damage may not require emergent drug therapy or hospitalization. Allowing the patient to sit for 20 or 30 minutes in a quiet environment may significantly reduce BP. Oral drugs may then be instituted or adjusted. Additional nursing interventions include encouraging the patient to verbalize fears, answering questions concerning the hypertension, and eliminating excess noise in the patient's environment.

Once the hypertensive crisis is resolved, it is important to determine the cause. The patient will need appropriate management and extensive education to avoid future crises.

CLINICAL DECISION-MAKING EXERCISE

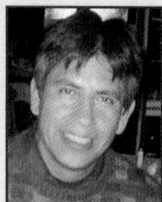

CASE STUDY:
Primary Hypertension

© iStockphoto.com/Juanmonino.

- Smokes one pack of cigarettes daily
- Drinks a six-pack of beer on Friday and Saturday nights
- Does not enjoy physical activity
- Has been diagnosed with type 2 diabetes for 5 years and is nonadherent to his diabetic treatment plan
- Has been told that some medications interfere with sexual relationships

Patient Profile

Mr. Windsong is a 45-year-old man of Aboriginal descent who has no previous history of hypertension. At a screening clinic, his BP was found to be 180/120 mm Hg.

Objective Data

Physical Examination
- Moderately obese male
- Sustained apical impulse palpable in the fourth intercostals space just lateral to the midclavicular line

Subjective Data

- Father died of stroke at age 60
- Mother is alive but has type 2 diabetes
- States that he feels fine and is not a "hyper" person

Diagnostic Studies
- ECG: left ventricular hypertrophy
- Urinalysis: protein 0.3 g/L
- Serum creatinine level: 141 mmol/L

Collaborative Care

- Low-sodium diet
- Hydrochlorothiazide (HCTZ) 12.5 mg daily PO
- Enalapril sodium (Vasotec) 5 mg daily PO

Discussion Questions

1. What risk factors for hypertension does Mr. Windsong have?
2. What evidence of target-organ damage is present?
3. What misconceptions about hypertension should be corrected?

4. What are the nursing priorities for Mr. Windsong? What resources are available to assist you with promoting health for Mr. Windsong?
5. *Priority Decision:* Based on the assessment data presented, what are the priority nursing diagnoses? Are there any collaborative problems? How will they affect Mr. Windsong's treatment?

e**volve** *Answers are available at* http://evolve.elsevier.com/ Canada/Lewis/medsurg

REVIEW QUESTIONS

The number of the question corresponds to the same-numbered objective at the beginning of the chapter.

1. If a patient has decreased cardiac output caused by fluid volume deficit and marked vasodilation, what regulatory mechanism will increase the blood pressure by improving both of these?
   a. Release of antidiuretic hormone (ADH)
   b. Secretion of prostaglandins PGE_2 and PGI_2
   c. Stimulation of the sympathetic nervous system
   d. Activation of the renin–angiotensin–aldosterone system
2. While obtaining subjective assessment data from a patient with hypertension, the nurse recognizes which of the following as a modifiable risk factor for the development of hypertension?
   a. Hyperlipidemia
   b. Excessive alcohol intake
   c. A family history of hypertension
   d. Consumption of a high-carbohydrate, high-calcium diet
3. Target-organ damage that can occur from hypertension includes which of the following?
   a. Headache and dizziness
   b. Retinopathy and diabetes
   c. Hypercholesterolemia and renal dysfunction
   d. Renal dysfunction and left ventricular hypertrophy
4. Which of the following is a high-risk population that should be targeted in the primary prevention of hypertension?
   a. Smokers
   b. Blacks
   c. Business executives
   d. Middle-aged women
5. The nurse includes which of the following ideas in teaching a patient with hypertension about controlling the condition?
   a. All patients with elevated BP require medication.
   b. It is not necessary to limit salt in the diet if taking a diuretic.
   c. Obese people must achieve a normal weight in order to lower BP.
   d. Lifestyle modifications are indicated for all people with elevated BP.

6. What is a major consideration in the management of the older adult with HTN?
   a. Prevent pseudohypertension from converting to true HTN.
   b. Recognize that the older adult is less likely to adhere to the drug therapy than a younger adult.
   c. Ensure that the patient receives larger initial doses of antihypertensive drugs because of impaired absorption.
   d. Use careful technique in assessing the BP of the patient because of the possible presence of an auscultatory gap.
7. A patient with newly diagnosed HTN has a blood pressure of 158/98 mm Hg after 12 months of exercise and diet modifications. How does the nurse advise the patient?
   a. Medication may be required because the BP is still not within the normal range.
   b. Continued monitoring of the BP every 3 to 6 months is all that will be necessary for treatment.
   c. Because lifestyle modifications were not effective, they do not need to be continued and drugs will be used.
   d. The patient will have to make more vigorous changes in lifestyle if the patient wants to stay off medication for HTN.
8. A patient is admitted to the hospital in hypertensive crisis. By which criterion does the nurse recognize that the hypertensive urgency differs from hypertensive emergency?
   a. The BP is always higher in a hypertensive emergency.
   b. Hypertensive emergencies are associated with evidence of target-organ damage.
   c. Hypertensive urgency is treated with rest and tranquillizers to lower the BP.
   d. Hypertensive emergencies require intra-arterial catheter measurement of the BP.

REFERENCES

Acelajado, M. C., & Oparil, S. (2009). Hypertension in the elderly. *Clinics in Geriatric Medicine, 25*(3), 391-412. doi:10.1016/j.cger.2009.06.001

Campbell, N. R. C., Poirier, L., Tremblay, G., Lindsay, P., Reid, D., & Tobe, S. W. (2011). The science supporting new 2011 CHEP recommendations with an emphasis on health advocacy and knowledge translation. *Canadian Journal of Cardiology, 27*(4), 407-414.

Drouin, D., Milot, A., Campbell, N. R., (Eds.). (2007). Hypertension—Therapeutic Guide Quebec: Canadian Hypertension Society and Société Québécoise d'Hypertension Artérielle, 99-115.

Heart and Stroke Foundation. (2012). Statistics. Retrieved from *http://www.heartandstroke.bc.ca/site/c.kpIPKXOyFmG/b.3644453/k.3454/Statistics.htm#riskfactors*

Hypertension Canada. (2012). Recommendations. Retrieved from *http://www.hypertension.ca/chep-recommendations*

Joffres, M. R., Campbell, N. R. C., Manns, B., & Tu, K. (2007). Estimate of the benefits of a population-based reduction in dietary sodium additives on hypertension and its related health care costs in Canada. *Canadian Journal of Cardiology, 23*(6), 437-443. doi:10.1016/S0828-282X(07)70780-8

McAlister, F. A., Wilkins, K., Joffres, M., Leenen, F. H. H., Fodor, G., Gee, M., …, Campbell, N. (2011). Changes in the rates of awareness, treatment and control of hypertension in Canada over the past two decades. *Canadian Medical Association Journal, 183*(9), 1007-1013. doi:10.1503/cmaj.101767

Padwal, R. S., Hemmelgarn, B. R., Khan, N. A., Grover, S., McAlister, F. A., McKay, D. W., …, Tobe, S. W. (2008). The 2008 Canadian Hypertension Education Program (CHEP) recommendations for the management of hypertension. Part I: Blood pressure measurement, diagnosis, and assessment of risk. *Canadian Journal of Cardiology, 24*(6), 455-463. doi:10.1016/S0828-282X(08)70619-6

Rabi, D. M., Daskalopoulou, S. S., Padwal, R. S., Khan, N. A., Grover, S. A., Hackam, D. G., …, Tobe, S. W. (2011). The 2011 Canadian Hypertension Education Program recommendations for the management of hypertension: Blood pressure measurement, diagnosis, assessment of risk, and therapy. *Canadian Journal of Cardiology, 27*(4), 415-433. doi:10.1016/j.cjca.2011.03.015

Riaz, K., Dreisbach, A. W., Madhur, M. S., & Harrison, D. G. (2012). Hypertension. Retrieved from *http://emedicine.medscape.com/article/241381-overview*

Robitaille, C., Dai, S., Waters, C., Loukine, L., Bancej, C., Quach, S., …, Quan, H. (2012). Diagnosed hypertension in Canada: Incidence, prevalence, and associated mortality. *Canadian Medical Association Journal, 184*(1), E49-E56. doi:10.1503/cmaj.101863

Singh, M., Mensah, G. A., Bakris, G. (2010). Pathogenesis and clinical physiology of hypertension. *Cardiology Clinics, 28*(4):545-559. doi:10.1016/j.ccl.2010.07.001

Sliwa, K., Stewart, S., & Gersh, B. (2011). Hypertension: A global perspective. *Circulation, 123*, 2892-6. doi:10.1161/CIRCULATIONAHA.110.992362

Sood, M., Komenda, P., Sood, A. R., Reslerova, M., Verrelli, M., Sathianathan, C., …, Rigatto, C. (2010). Adverse outcomes among Aboriginal patients receiving peritoneal dialysis. *Canadian Medical Association Journal, 182*(13). doi:10.1503/cmaj.100105

CANADIAN RESOURCES

Canadian Hypertension Education Program (CHEP) Recommendations

The full CHEP recommendations are available at *http://www.hypertension.ca*. Summary documents, including downloadable slide kits, are available free of charge on the Hypertension Canada Web site. Health care providers can enroll on the home page for automated e-mail notices when new or updated hypertension resources are available for them or for their patients. Current resources are available at *http://www.hypertension.ca/tools*.

A case-based interactive lecture series on clinically important hypertension topics will also be launched on the Internet so that health care providers can learn and interact with national hypertension experts, ask questions and make comments. Those who sign up at *http://www.hypertension.ca* will be notified when these lectures begin. The CHEP is also developing a program to train community leaders in hypertension.

The CHEP team plans to develop a hypertension association for Canadians with high blood pressure. Currently, individuals can register at *http://www.hypertension.ca/measuring-blood-pressure* to receive notices of updated and new educational resources, a regular newsletter, discount coupons to encourage a healthy lifestyle and access to lectures. A future goal is to provide personalized advice from health care providers.

Programs that compare risk by using terms such as "cardiovascular age," "vascular age," and "heart age" have been shown to improve risk perception by patients and risk factor management by physicians and can be accessed at *http://www.myhealthcheckup.com* and *http://www.monbilansante.com*. The SCORE risk calculator uses Canadian data and is available at *http://www.score-Canada.ca*.

Education Resources for Sodium
http://www.lowersodium.ca

Health Canada: Sodium—It's Your Health
http://www.hc-sc.gc.ca/hl-vs/iyh-vsv/food-aliment/sodium-eng.php

Heart and Stroke Foundation Blood Pressure Action Plan
https://ehealth.heartandstroke.ca/heartstroke/bpap.net/?pgSrc=bpvanity

Heart and Stroke Foundation of Canada
http://www.heartandstroke.ca

Hypertension Canada
www.hypertension.ca
www.hypertension.qc.ca

Registered Nurses' Association of Ontario
Nursing management of hypertension. (2005). *Best Practice Guideline*. Available at *www.rnao.org/Storage/11/607_BPG_Hypertension.pdf*

Sodium 101
http://www.sodium101.ca/

Tobacco Free RNAO
http://tobaccofreernao.ca/en
http://tobaccofreernao.ca/en/treatment/intervention-strategies

ⓔvolve For additional Internet resources, see the Web site for this book at **http://evolve.elsevier.com/Canada/Lewis/medsurg**

CHAPTER

36

Nursing Management:
Coronary Artery Disease and
Acute Coronary Syndrome

Written by Linda Bucher and Deborah Castellucci
Adapted by Sandra Goldsworthy

LEARNING OBJECTIVES

1. Describe the prevalence of heart disease in Canada.
2. Describe the etiology and the pathophysiology of coronary artery disease, angina, and acute coronary syndrome.
3. Identify risk factors for coronary artery disease and the nursing role in the promotion of therapeutic lifestyle changes for patients at risk.
4. Compare and contrast the precipitating factors, the clinical manifestations, and the collaborative care and nursing management of patients with coronary artery disease and chronic stable angina.
5. Describe the clinical manifestations, the complications, the diagnostic study results, and the collaborative care of patients with acute coronary syndrome.
6. Describe the pathophysiology of myocardial infarction from the onset of injury through the healing process.
7. Identify drug therapy commonly used in treating patients with coronary artery disease and acute coronary syndrome.
8. Identify key issues to include in the rehabilitation of patients recovering from acute coronary syndrome and coronary revascularization procedures.
9. Describe the precipitating factors, the clinical presentation, and the collaborative care of patients who are at risk for or have experienced sudden cardiac death.

KEY TERMS

acute coronary syndrome (ACS) Condition consisting of unstable angina, non–ST-segment elevation myocardial infarction, and ST-segment elevation myocardial infarction; develops when the oxygen supply to the myocardium is diminished (myocardial ischemia) and not immediately reversible, p. 908

angina Chest pain that is the clinical manifestation of reversible myocardial ischemia, p. 903

atherosclerosis Formation of the focal deposits of cholesterol and lipids known as atheromas or plaque, primarily within the intimal wall of arteries, that obstruct circulation, p. 893

chronic stable angina Chest pain that occurs intermittently over a long period with the same pattern of onset, duration, and intensity of symptoms, p. 903

collateral circulation Arterial branching within the coronary circulation; development depends on (a) the inherited predisposition to develop new blood vessels and (b) the presence of chronic ischemia that results when, over a long period, an atherosclerotic plaque occludes the normal flow of blood through a coronary artery, p. 895

coronary artery disease (CAD) An abnormal condition that may affect the heart's arteries and produce various pathological effects, especially the reduction in flow of oxygen and nutrients to the myocardium, p. 893

coronary revascularization An intervention that restores blood flow to the affected myocardium; the coronary lesion must be amenable to this procedure, p. 915

myocardial infarction (MI) Irreversible cardiac cellular death caused by sustained myocardial ischemia, p. 909

percutaneous coronary intervention (PCI) An intervention to treat coronary artery disease in which a catheter equipped with an inflatable balloon tip is inserted into a narrowed coronary artery and the balloon is inflated; common as elective procedure and also used in emergent situations, p. 912

Prinzmetal's angina Variant angina; occurs at rest, usually in response to reversible, severe spasm of a major coronary artery, p. 905

silent ischemia Ischemia that occurs in the absence of any subjective symptoms, p. 904

stent Expandable meshlike structure designed to maintain vessel patency by compressing the arterial walls and resisting vasoconstriction, p. 915

sudden cardiac death (SCD) Unexpected death from cardiac causes, p. 924

unstable angina (UA) Angina that is new in onset, occurs at rest, or has a worsening pattern, p. 908

ELECTRONIC RESOURCES

Supplemental content related to Chapter 36 can be found...

Evolve Web Site ⊖volve

http://evolve.elsevier.com/Canada/Lewis/medsurg
- Answer Guidelines for Case Study on p. 925
- Audio Lecture: Risk Factors for Coronary Artery Disease
- Clinical Reference: Laboratory Values
- Content Updates
- Customizable Nursing Care Plan: Acute Coronary Syndrome
- Electronic Calculators

- Examination Review Questions
- Glossary
- Interactive Case Study: Client with Coronary Artery Disease and Acute Coronary Syndrome
- Key Points (Printable and MP3 Download)
- Patient & Caregiver Teaching Guides:
  - Decreasing Risk Factors for Coronary Artery Disease
  - FITT Physical Activity Guidelines After Acute Coronary Syndrome

Cardiovascular disease is the major cause of death in Canada, accounting for 29% (69,648) of all deaths (Heart and Stroke Foundation of Canada [HSF], 2012). Of all cardiovascular deaths in 2008 (the most recent year for which data are available), 54% resulted from ischemic heart disease, 23% from myocardial infarction, and 20% from stroke (HSF, 2012). Trends for younger and older Canadians between 1994 and 2005 show alarming increases in cardiac disease that include a 77% increase in rates of high blood pressure, a 45% increase in the incidence of diabetes, and an 18% increase in the rate of obesity (HSF, 2010a).

Patients with coronary artery disease (CAD) can be asymptomatic or develop chronic stable angina. Unstable angina and myocardial infarction (MI) are more serious manifestations of CAD and are termed *acute coronary syndrome* (ACS). The HSF estimates that more than 72,000 Canadians have an MI annually, and about 25% of these patients die in an emergency department (ED) or before reaching a hospital (HSF, 2012). Cardiovascular disease is the most common reason for hospitalization in Canada (HSF, 2012). Circulatory diseases are the leading cause of death among First Nations people in Canada (HSF, 2012). Another population at risk for CAD is Canadian children. The rate of childhood obesity has tripled over the last 25 years and it continues to increase (HSF, 2010b). More than 25% of Canadian children between the ages of 2 and 17 years are overweight or obese, and the health risks for these children include the development of heart disease, high blood pressure, and type 2 diabetes. Furthermore, more than 250,000 Canadians age 20 to 34 have high blood pressure; 3 million of these young adults are inactive, and 2.5 million are obese (HSF, 2010b).

Heart disease is no longer just a disease primarily affecting White men. Canadians of South Asian, African, and Caribbean descent have a greater risk of heart disease and stroke because they have an increased risk for developing high blood pressure

and diabetes. In particular, Canadians of South Asian descent can develop heart disease 5 to 10 years earlier than Canadians of other ethnic groups (HSF, 2010a). (The Determinants of Health box on this page discusses culture and social status as determinants of cardiovascular disease in Canada.)

DETERMINANTS OF HEALTH
Coronary Artery Disease in Canada

Culture
- Immigrants to Canada tend to have better cardiovascular health than do native-born Canadians.
- Canadian research also demonstrates that immigrants from South Asia have a particularly high risk for cardiovascular disease, whereas immigrants from China have particularly low rates.
- Regardless of where they live, Asian Indians appear to suffer high rates of cardiovascular disease.

Income and Social Status
- Members of minority and low-income populations experience a disproportionate burden of death and disability from cardiovascular disease.

Source: Beiser, M. (2005). The health of immigrants and refugees in Canada. *Canadian Journal of Public Health, 96*(Suppl. 2), S30-S44. Retrieved from *http://journal.cpha.ca/index.php/cjph/article/download/1494/1683*

Table 36-1 shows the ranking of provinces and territories with regard to heart-related health behaviours in the period 2007 to 2008.

Table 36-1 2007-2008 Ranking of Provinces and Territories on Heart-Related Health Behaviours

PROVINCE OR TERRITORY	COMBINED HEALTH BEHAVIOURS RANK	SMOKE-FREE RANK (%)	PHYSICAL ACTIVITY RANK (%)	HEALTHY WEIGHT RANK (%)	ADEQUATE VEGETABLE AND FRUIT CONSUMPTION RANK (%)
BC	1st (best)	1st (81.8)	2nd (53.7)	1st (49.7)	2nd (tie: 43.4)
ALTA	2nd	4th (77.7)	3rd (53.4)	5th (42.9)	2nd (tie: 43.4)
ONT	3rd	2nd (78.7)	6th (48.8)	4th (43.6)	4th (41.4)
QUE	4th	8th (75.8)	10th (tie: 45.7)	2nd (46.8)	1st (52.6)
Yukon	5th	11th (68.2)	1st (55.4)	3rd (44.6)	7th (38.7)
MAN	6th	5th (76.7)	4th (51.8)	7th (40.4)	9th (35.9)
PEI	7th	3rd (78.8)	8th (47.3)	12th (36.5)	8th (36.7)
SASK	8th	10th (74.3)	9th (46.1)	8th (39.2)	5th (tie: 38.8)
NS	9th	7th (76.0)	7th (47.6)	9th (38.4)	10th (35.8)
NB	10th (tie)	6th (76.6)	12th (42.7)	10th (37.4)	5th (tie: 38.8)
NWT	10th (tie)	12th (64.8)	5th (49.3)	11th (36.8)	12th (24.6)
NFLD/LAB	12th	9th (75.1)	10th (tie: 45.7)	13th (33.3)	11th (30.8)
Nunavut	13th (worst)	13th (42.1)	13th (40.5)	6th (42.7)	13th (24.2)
National (Canadian) Average		78.3	49.0	44.4	43.8

Source: Heart and Stroke Foundation of Canada. (2010). *A perfect storm of heart disease looming on our horizon: 2010 Heart and Stroke Foundation Annual Report on Canadians' Health* (p. 6). Ottawa: Author. Retrieved from *http://www.heartandstroke.com/atf/cf/%7B99452D8B-E7F1-4BD6-A57D-B136CE6C95BF%7D/Jan23_EN_ReportCard.pdf*

Coronary Artery Disease

Coronary artery disease (CAD) is a type of blood vessel disorder that is included in the general category of atherosclerosis; it may affect the heart's arteries and produce various pathological effects, especially the reduced flow of oxygen and nutrients to the myocardium. The term *atherosclerosis* is derived from two Greek words: *athere,* meaning "fatty mush," and *skleros,* meaning "hard." This word combination indicates that atherosclerosis begins as soft deposits of fat that harden with age. Atherosclerosis is often referred to as "hardening of the arteries." Although this condition can occur in any artery in the body, the atheromas have a preference for the coronary arteries. *Arteriosclerotic heart disease (ASHD), cardiovascular heart disease (CVHD), ischemic heart disease (IHD),* and *coronary heart disease (CHD)* are synonymous terms used to describe CAD.

Etiology and Pathophysiology

Atherosclerosis is the major cause of CAD. It is characterized by a focal deposit of cholesterol and lipids, primarily within the intimal wall of the artery. Plaque formation is the result of complex interactions between the components of the blood and the elements that form the vascular wall (Huether & McCance, 2011). Inflammation and endothelial injury play a central role in the development of atherosclerosis. Figure 36-1 depicts the progression of atherosclerosis.

Intact normal endothelium is more than a simple barrier between the vessel wall and the lumen of the vessel. Normally, it is nonreactive to platelets and leukocytes, as well as coagulation, fibrinolytic, and complement factors. However, the endothelial lining can be injured as a result of tobacco use, hyperlipidemia, hypertension, diabetes, hyperhomocysteinemia, and infection

(e.g., *Chlamydia pneumoniae,* herpes), which causes a local inflammatory response (Huether & McCance, 2008; see Figure 36-1, *A*).

C-reactive protein (CRP), which is produced by the liver, is a nonspecific marker of inflammation. The level of CRP rises with systemic inflammation and is increased in many patients with CAD. Chronic elevations of CRP are associated with unstable plaques and the oxidation of low-density lipoprotein (LDL) cholesterol, leading to increased uptake by macrophages in the endothelial lining (see Table 34-5).

Developmental Stages

CAD is a progressive disease that takes many years to develop. When it becomes symptomatic, the disease process is usually well advanced. The stages of development in atherosclerosis are (a) fatty streak, (b) fibrous plaque resulting from smooth muscle cell proliferation, and (c) complicated lesion.

Fatty Streak. *Fatty streaks,* the earliest lesions of atherosclerosis, are characterized by lipid-filled smooth muscle cells. As streaks of fat develop within the smooth muscle cells, a yellow tinge appears. Fatty streaks can be observed in the coronary arteries by age 15 and involve an increasing amount of surface area as the patient ages. Treatment that lowers LDL cholesterol may reverse this process (see Figure 36-1, *B*).

Fibrous Plaque. The *fibrous plaque stage* is the beginning of progressive changes in the endothelium of the arterial wall. These changes can appear in the coronary arteries by age 30 and increase with age. Normally the endothelium repairs itself immediately; however, this does not happen in individuals with CAD. LDLs and growth factors from platelets stimulate smooth muscle proliferation and thickening of the arterial wall. Once endothelial injury has occurred, lipoproteins (carrier proteins within the bloodstream) transport cholesterol and other lipids into the arte-

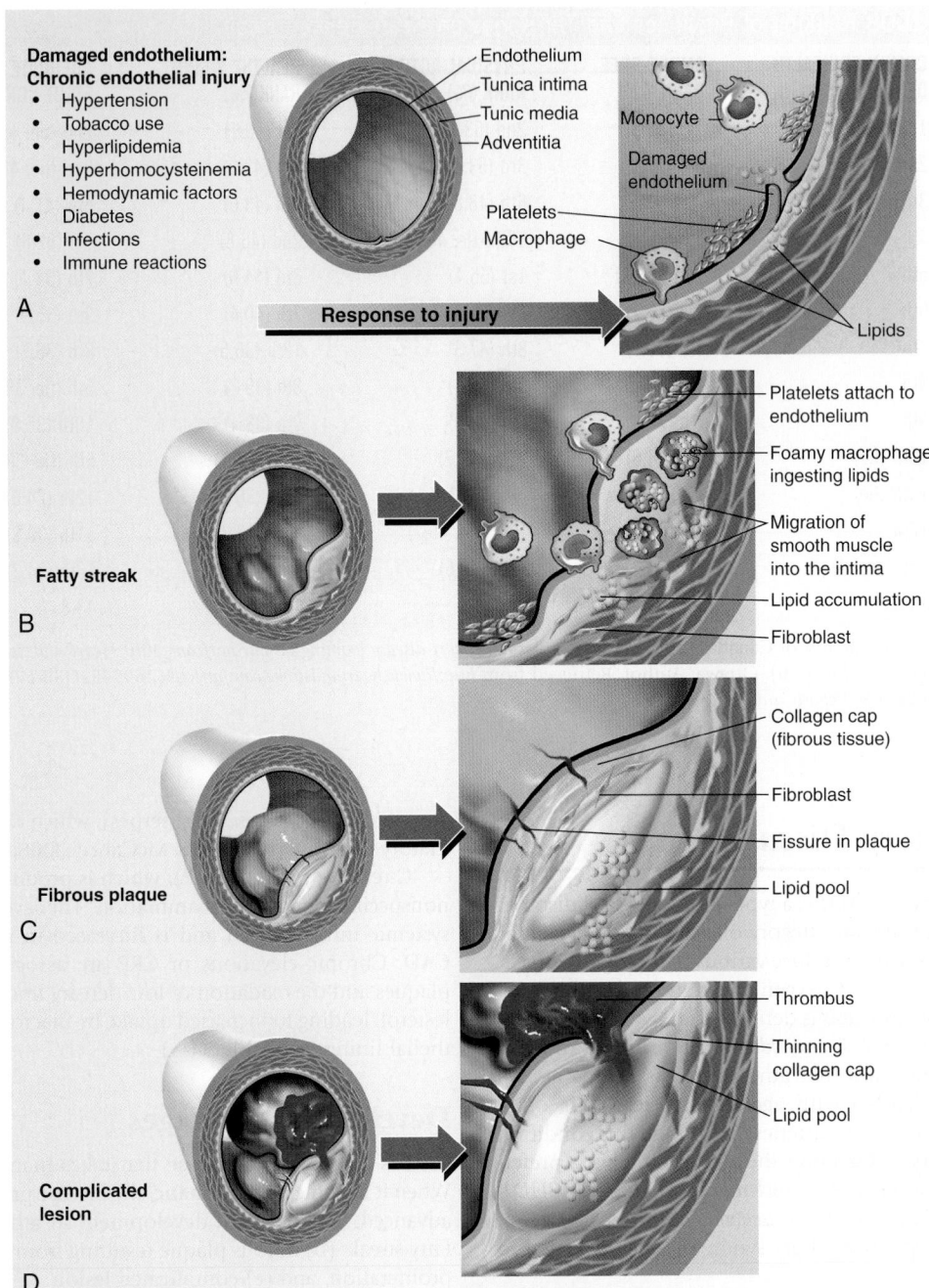

Figure 36-1 Diagrams of the progression of atherosclerosis. **A,** Damaged endothelium. **B,** Fatty streak and lipid core formation. **C,** Fibrous plaque. Raised plaques are visible: Some are yellow, and others are white. **D,** Complicated lesion: Thrombus is red, and collagen is blue. Plaque is complicated by red thrombus deposition.

Source: McCance, K. L., & Huether, S. E. (2010). *Understanding pathophysiology* (6th ed., p. 1158, Fig. 30-11). St Louis: Mosby.

rial intima. Collagen covers the fatty streak and forms a fibrous plaque with a greyish or whitish appearance. These plaques can form on one portion of the artery or in a circular manner that involves the entire lumen. The borders can be smooth or irregular with rough, jagged edges. The result is a narrowing of the vessel lumen and a reduction in blood flow to the distal tissues (see Figure 36-1, *C*).

Complicated Lesion. The final stage in the development of the atherosclerotic lesion is the most dangerous. As the fibrous

plaque grows, continued inflammation can result in plaque instability, ulceration, and rupture. Once the integrity of the artery's inner wall is compromised, platelets accumulate in large numbers and form a thrombus. The thrombus may adhere to the wall of the artery, causing further narrowing or total occlusion of the artery. Activation of the exposed platelets causes expression of glycoprotein IIb/IIIa receptors that bind fibrinogen. This, in turn, leads to further platelet aggregation and adhesion, further enlarging the thrombus. At this stage, the plaque is referred to as a *complicated lesion* (see Figure 36-1, *D*).

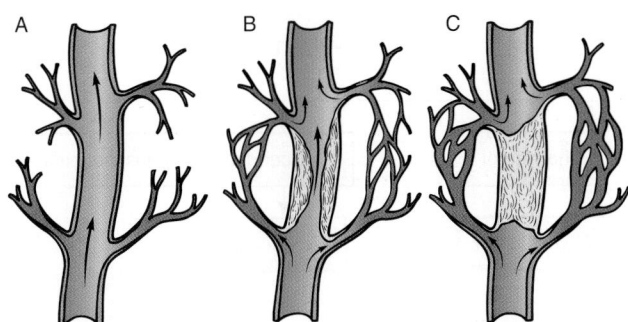

Figure 36-2 Vessel occlusion with collateral circulation. **A,** Open, functioning coronary artery. **B,** Partial coronary artery closure with collateral circulation being established. **C,** Total coronary artery occlusion with collateral circulation bypassing the occlusion to supply the myocardium.

Table 36-2 Risk Factors for Coronary Artery Disease	
NONMODIFIABLE RISK FACTORS	**MODIFIABLE RISK FACTORS**
Increasing age	**MAJOR**
Gender (men > women until 65 yr of age)	Serum lipids alterations: elevated triglyceride and LDL cholesterol levels, decreased HDL levels
Ethnicity (Whites > Blacks)	Blood pressure ≥140/90 mm Hg
Genetic predisposition and family history of heart disease	Diabetes mellitus
	Tobacco use
	Physical inactivity
	Obesity: Waist circumference ≥102 cm (40 inches) in men and ≥88 cm (35 inches) in women
	CONTRIBUTING
	Fasting blood glucose level >10 mmol/L
	Psychosocial risk factors (e.g., depression, hostility and anger, stress)
	Elevated homocysteine levels

HDL, High-density lipoprotein; *LDL,* low-density lipoprotein.

Collateral Circulation. Normally some arterial anastomoses or connections, termed **collateral circulation,** exist within the coronary circulation. Two factors contribute to the growth and extent of collateral circulation: (a) the inherited predisposition to develop new blood vessels *(angiogenesis)* and (b) the presence of chronic ischemia. When an atherosclerotic plaque occludes the normal flow of blood through a coronary artery and the resulting ischemia is chronic, increased collateral circulation develops (Figure 36-2). When occlusion of the coronary arteries occurs slowly over a long period, there is a greater chance that adequate collateral circulation will gradually develop, and the myocardium may continue receiving an adequate amount of blood and oxygen.

However, when CAD has a rapid onset (as in familial hypercholesterolemia) or coronary spasm occurs, the amount of time is inadequate for collateral circulation development, and the diminished arterial blood flow results in more severe ischemia or infarction.

CAD usually develops over many years, and clinical manifestations are not apparent in the early stages of the disease. Therefore, it is extremely important to identify people at risk and initiate therapeutic lifestyle changes and treatment strategies early.

Risk Factors for Coronary Artery Disease

Risk factors are characteristics or conditions that are statistically associated with a high incidence of a disease. Many risk factors have been associated with CAD. In a study of risk factors in 52 countries, researchers found that the following nine common risk factors accounted for 90% of population-attributable risks, regardless of sex and age, in all regions of the world: tobacco use, elevated blood levels of apolipoprotein B or A-1 (apo B, apo A-1), history of hypertension, diabetes mellitus, abdominal obesity, psychosocial factors, lack of fruit and vegetable intake, alcohol consumption, and physical inactivity (Yusuf, Hawkem, Ounpuu, & Dans, 2004).

Cardiac risk factors are categorized as either nonmodifiable or modifiable (Table 36-2). *Nonmodifiable risk factors* are age, gender, ethnicity, family history, and genetic inheritance. *Modifi-* *able risk factors* include elevated serum lipid levels, elevated blood pressure, tobacco use, physical inactivity, obesity, diabetes, metabolic syndrome, psychological states, and elevated homocysteine level (Anderson et al., 2007). Data on risk factors for CAD come from several major studies. In the Framingham Heart Study (one of the most widely known), 5209 men and women were observed for 20 years. Over time, the researchers noted that elevated serum cholesterol levels (>6.2 mmol/L), elevated systolic blood pressure (BP) (>160 mm Hg), and cigarette smoking (one or more packs a day) were positively correlated with an increased incidence of CAD.

The degree of coronary artery calcification correlates with the severity of CAD. Calcification is detected by noninvasive means such as cardiac computed tomography (CT). This technology is often referred to as *multidetector CT* (MDCT) scanning. One type of CT scan is the calcium-score screening heart scan used to detect calcium deposits found in atherosclerotic plaque in the coronary arteries. The most common method used is *electron beam CT* (EBCT) (see Figure 34-11).

Measurement of coronary calcification can be useful for predicting adverse cardiovascular events (Rubenstein et al., 2007). A person with a calcium score above 400 has a high probability of having a significant lesion in at least one coronary artery. However, additional testing (e.g., stress testing) is needed to demonstrate the impact of the lesion on coronary blood flow.

Nonmodifiable Risk Factors

Age and Sex. Even though women are generally protected from developing heart disease until midlife, heart disease still kills more women every year than all forms of cancer combined (HSF, 2010a). Heart disease is the number one cause of death in Canada for women older than 55. Women are more likely to die from heart disease than from any other disease (Public Health Agency of Canada [PHAC], 2009a).

Women tend to manifest CAD 10 years later in life than men (PHAC, 2009b). This is thought to be related to the loss of the cardioprotective effects of natural estrogen with the onset of menopause.

Family History and Genetics. Genetic predisposition is an important factor in the occurrence of CAD, although the exact mechanism of inheritance is not fully understood. Some congenital defects in coronary artery walls predispose the person to the formation of plaques. Familial hypercholesterolemia, an autosomal dominant disorder, has been strongly associated with CAD at early ages (see the Genetics in Clinical Practice box). In most cases, patients with angina or MI can identify a parent or sibling who has died of CAD.

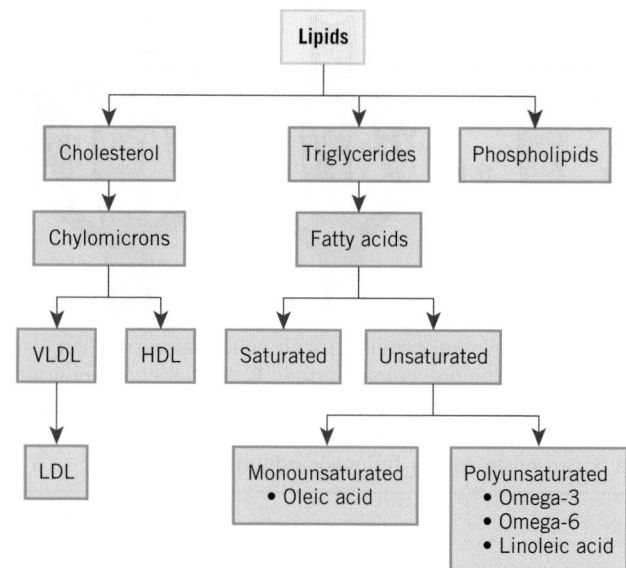

Figure 36-3 Types of serum lipids. *HDL*, high-density lipoprotein; *LDL*, low-density lipoprotein; *VLDL*, very low density lipoprotein.

GENETICS IN CLINICAL PRACTICE
Familial Hypercholesterolemia

Genetic Basis
- Autosomal dominant disorder
- Mutation in gene coding for the LDL receptor
- Multiple mutant alleles

Incidence
- Heterozygotes: 1 per 500
- Homozygotes: rare

Genetic Testing
- Disorder characterized by elevated serum LDL level
- Serum lipid profile can be used to measure total cholesterol, triglyceride, LDL, and HDL levels
- DNA testing available

Clinical Implications
- Common genetic disease
- Leading cause of coronary artery disease
- High cholesterol levels are a result of defective function of the LDL receptors
- Plasma levels of LDL remain elevated throughout life
- Those affected develop severe atherosclerosis in early to middle years

HDL, high-density lipoprotein; *LDL*, low-density lipoprotein.

Modifiable Major Risk Factors

The HSF has classified modifiable risk factors as *major* and *contributing* risk factors. Major risk factors are those that research has shown to be definitely associated with a significant increase in the risk of the development of CAD. Contributing risk factors are those associated with increased risk of CAD, but their significance and prevalence have not been precisely determined (PHAC, 2009b). Nine in 10 Canadians (90%) have at least one risk factor for heart disease or stroke (smoking, alcohol, physical inactivity, obesity, high blood pressure, high blood cholesterol, diabetes (PHAC, 2009b).

Elevated Serum Lipid Levels. An elevated serum lipid level is one of the four most firmly established risk factors for CAD (Grundy et al., 2004; Libby et al., 2008). The various types

of serum lipids are presented in Figure 36-3. Approximately 40% of Canadians have high blood cholesterol (>5.2 mmol/L; HSF, 2012). There has been a gradual decline in the rate of cardiac mortality, and this has been related to improvements in control of risk factors such as cholesterol levels, smoking, and blood pressure (Genest et al., 2009). In Canada, clinical practice guidelines for the diagnosis, treatment, and prevention of dyslipidemia are available (Genest et al., 2009). These guidelines incorporate (a) a description of patients whose lipid profile should be screened and (b) a classification of metabolic syndrome to evaluate central obesity (waist circumference plus two of the following: plasma triglyceride levels, high-density lipoprotein [HDL] cholesterol level, blood pressure, and fasting plasma glucose level).

The current Canadian guidelines for treating dyslipidemia include a description of patients whose plasma lipid profile should be screened (Table 36-3) and target lipid levels associated with risk level (Genest et al., 2009). In the summary of these 2009 guidelines, recommended treatment includes smoking cessation, diet modification (reduced consumption of both saturated fats and refined sugars), weight reduction and maintenance, daily exercise, stress management, and (in patients at high risk) pharmacological therapy.

Hypertension. Another major risk factor in CAD is hypertension, which is defined as a BP of 140/90 mm Hg or higher. Hypertension was first identified as a major risk factor for heart disease in the Framingham Heart Study (Rabi et al., 2011). In postmenopausal women, hypertension is associated with a higher incidence of CAD than in men and in premenopausal women. Hypertension increases the risk of death from CAD ten-fold in all people. The 2012 Canadian Health Education Plan (CHEP) recommendations for diagnosis of hypertension and follow-up are presented in Figure 35-1 in Chapter 35.

The stress of a constantly elevated BP increases the rate of atherosclerotic development. This is related to the shearing stress that causes endothelial injury. Atherosclerosis, in turn, causes

Table 36-3 Patients Whose Plasma Lipid Profile Should Be Screened

Men ≥40 yr of age and women ≥50 yr of age or postmenopausal
All patients with the following conditions, regardless of age:
- Diabetes
- Hypertension
- Current cigarette smoking
- Obesity (Obesity Canada guidelines)
- Family history of premature CAD (onset at <60 yr of age in first-degree relatives)
- Inflammatory diseases* (systemic lupus erythematosus, rheumatoid arthritis, psoriasis)
- Chronic renal diseases (eGFR <60 mL/min/1.73 m^2)
- Evidence of atherosclerosis
- HIV infection treated with highly active antiretroviral therapy
- Clinical manifestations of hyperlipidemias (xanthomas, xanthelasmas, premature arcus cornealis)
- Erectile dysfunction

Children with a family history of hypercholesterolemia or chylomicronemia

Source: Genest, J., Macpherson, R., Frohlich, J., Anderson, T., Campbell, N., Carpentier, A., ..., Ur, E. (2009). 2009 Canadian Cardiovascular Society/Canadian Guidelines for the diagnosis and treatment of dyslipidemia and prevention of cardiovascular disease in the adult—2009 Recommendations, *Canadian Journal of Cardiology, 25*(10) (p. 568, Table 1). doi:10.1016/S0828-282X(09)70715-9
*Data on inflammatory bowel diseases are lacking.
CAD, coronary artery disease; *eGFR*, estimated glomerular filtration rate; *HIV*, human immunodeficiency virus.

narrowing and thickening of the arterial walls and decreases the distensibility and elasticity of vessels. More force is required to pump blood through diseased arterial vasculature, and this increased force is reflected in a higher BP. This increased workload is also manifested by left ventricular hypertrophy and decreased stroke volume with each contraction. Salt intake is positively correlated with elevated BP, adding volume and increasing systemic vascular resistance (SVR) to the cardiac workload. (See Chapter 35 for a complete discussion of hypertension.) Lifestyle modifications are a critical component of hypertension management. Lifestyle factors that increase risk of hypertension include obesity, poor dietary habits, high sodium intake, sedentary activity levels, high alcohol consumption, and high stress levels (Rabi et al., 2011).

Tobacco Use. A third major risk factor in CAD is tobacco use. The risk of developing CAD is two to six times higher in people who smoke tobacco or use smokeless tobacco than in those who do not. Furthermore, tobacco smoking decreases estrogen levels, which increases premenopausal women's risk for CAD. Risk is proportional to the number of cigarettes smoked. Changing to lower nicotine or filtered cigarettes does not affect risk. Studies have yielded strong evidence that chronic exposure to environmental tobacco (second-hand) smoke also increases the risk of CAD (Lloyd-Jones et al., 2009). Pipe and cigar smokers, who often do not inhale, have an increased risk of CAD similar to that in people exposed to environmental tobacco smoke. Nicotine in tobacco smoke causes catecholamine (i.e., epinephrine, norepinephrine) release. These neurohormones cause an increase in heart rate, peripheral vasoconstriction, and an increase in BP. These changes increase the cardiac workload, necessitating greater myocardial oxygen consumption. Nicotine also increases platelet

adhesion, which increases the risk of emboli formation (Quinn, 2008).

Carbon monoxide, a by-product of combustion found in tobacco smoke, affects the oxygen-carrying capacity of hemoglobin by reducing the sites available for oxygen transport. Thus the effects of an increased cardiac workload, combined with the oxygen-depleting effect of carbon monoxide, significantly decrease the oxygen available to the myocardium. There is also some indication that carbon monoxide is a chemical irritant, thus causing injury to the endothelium. The benefits of smoking cessation are dramatic and almost immediate. CAD mortality rates drop to those of nonsmokers within 12 months. However, nicotine is highly addictive, and intensive intervention is often needed to assist people to quit. Individual and group counselling sessions, nicotine replacement therapy, smoking cessation medications (e.g., bupropion [Zyban], varenicline [Champix]), and hypnosis are examples of smoking cessation strategies.

Overall, smoking rates in Canada have decreased; however, 20-year-olds continue to be the heaviest smokers, which increases their risk of heart disease (HSF, 2010a). (See Chapter 11 for information on smoking cessation.)

Physical Inactivity. Physical inactivity is a fourth major modifiable risk factor. Physical inactivity implies a lack of adequate physical exercise on a regular basis. The Canadian Physical Activity Guidelines recommend a minimum of 150 minutes per week of moderate to vigorous exercise and to also add muscle and bone strengthening activities at least twice per week to improve health and reduce cardiac disease risk (Canadian Society for Exercise Physiology, n.d.). The mechanism by which physical inactivity predisposes to CAD is mostly still unknown. Physically active people have increased HDL levels, and exercise enhances fibrinolytic activity, thus reducing the risk of clot formation. Exercise may also encourage the development of collateral circulation in the heart. Exercise training for people who are physically inactive decreases the risk of CAD through more efficient lipid metabolism, increased production of HDL2 (a subfraction of HDL), and more efficient oxygen extraction by the working muscle groups, thereby decreasing the cardiac workload. For individuals with CAD, regular physical activity reduces symptoms, improves functional capacity, and reduces other risk factors such as insulin resistance and glucose intolerance.

Obesity. The mortality rate from CAD is statistically higher among obese individuals. Obesity is defined as a body mass index (BMI) of more than 30 kg/m^2 and a waist circumference of 102 cm (40 inches) or larger for men and 88 cm (35 inches) or larger for women. BMI is a calculation of body fat based on height and weight and can be calculated online (see the Resources section at the end of this chapter). The increased risk for CAD is proportional to the degree of obesity. Between 2007 and 2009, only 38% of Canadians were at a healthy weight and almost 25% of Canadians were obese; among adults, more men than women were overweight. Typically, BMI was the key indicator of health risk related to obesity, but beyond the BMI, waist circumference is now regarded as the factor that indicates the greatest health risk related to obesity (Statistics Canada, 2010).

Almost half of all Canadians are overweight. Obesity is often associated with hypertension, which is three times more likely to develop in an obese person than in a person of normal weight. There is also some evidence that individuals who tend to store fat in the abdomen (an "apple" shape, thus a greater waist-to-hip ratio) have a higher incidence of CAD than those who tend to store more fat in the hips and buttocks (a "pear" shape; Després, 2005). As obesity increases, the heart becomes enlarged, which causes increased myocardial oxygen consumption. In addition, the incidence of type 2 diabetes mellitus is higher among obese individuals.

Modifiable Contributing Risk Factors

Diabetes Mellitus. The incidence of CAD is two to four times higher among people who have diabetes, even those with well-controlled blood glucose levels, than among the general population. Patients with diabetes manifest CAD not only more frequently but also at an earlier age. The age at onset of manifestations of CAD does not differ between male and female patients with diabetes. Although the incidence of CAD is generally low in premenopausal women, it is much higher among those with diabetes. In general, women with diabetes in general have higher risk for CAD than other women (Huang, 2009). Undiagnosed diabetes is frequently discovered at the time of MI. People with diabetes have an increased tendency for connective tissue degeneration and endothelial dysfunction. This may account for the tendency toward atheroma development observed in patients with diabetes. Diabetic patients also have alterations in lipid metabolism and tend to have high cholesterol and triglyceride levels. Management of diabetes should include lifestyle changes and drug therapy to achieve a hemoglobin A_{1C} (HbA_{1C}) level lower than 7% (Smith et al., 2006).

Metabolic Syndrome. *Metabolic syndrome* is a cluster of risk factors for CAD whose underlying pathophysiological processes may be related to insulin resistance. These risk factors include obesity, as defined by increased waist circumference; hypertension; abnormal serum lipid levels; and an elevated fasting blood glucose level (Grassi et al, 2009; see Table 43-10). These interrelated risk factors of metabolic origin appear to promote the development of CAD. (Metabolic syndrome is further discussed in Chapter 43.)

Psychological States. The Framingham Heart Study provided early evidence that certain behaviours and lifestyles contribute to the development of CAD. Several behaviour patterns were correlated with the development of CAD. However, the study of these behaviours remains controversial and complex. One type of behaviour, referred to as *type A*, includes perfectionism and a hardworking, driving personality. People with so-called type A personality often suppress anger and hostility, have a sense of time urgency, are impatient, and often creates stress and tension. These people may be more prone to MIs than people with type B personality, who are more easygoing, take upsets in stride, know personal limitations, take time to relax, and are not overachievers. However, findings from studies regarding these relationships are inconsistent.

Studies now are focusing on specific psychological risk factors thought to increase risk of CAD. These include depression, acute and chronic stress (e.g., poverty, serving as a caregiver), anxiety, hostility and anger, and lack of social support (Lippi, Montagnana, Favaloro, & Franchini, 2009; Thombs et al., 2008). In particular, depression is a risk factor for both the development and worsening of CAD. Depressed patients have elevated levels of circulating catecholamines, which may contribute to endothelial injury and inflammation, and increased platelet activation (Lippi et al., 2009). Higher levels of depression are also associated with an increased number of adverse cardiac events (Lippi et al., 2009; Thombs et al., 2008). More research on the treatment of depression and other negative psychological states (e.g., anger) in patients with or at risk for CAD is needed to improve the emotional and physical health of these patients (Delville & McDougall, 2008).

Stressful states are indeed correlated with the development of CAD. Stimulation of the sympathetic nervous system (SNS) and its effect on the heart are the physiological mechanism by which stress predisposes to the development of CAD. SNS stimulation causes an increased release of catecholamines (i.e., epinephrine, norepinephrine), increased HR, and intensification of the force of myocardial contraction, leading to increased myocardial oxygen demand. Also, stress-induced mechanisms can cause elevated lipid and glucose levels and alterations in blood coagulation, which can lead to increased atherogenesis.

Homocysteine. High blood levels of homocysteine have been linked to an increased risk for CAD and other cardiovascular diseases (Humphrey, Fu, Rogers, Freeman, & Helfand, 2008). Homocysteine is produced by the breakdown of the essential amino acid methionine, which is found in dietary protein. High homocysteine levels possibly contribute to atherosclerosis by (a) damaging the inner lining of blood vessels, (b) promoting plaque buildup, and (c) altering the clotting mechanism so that clots are more likely to occur (see Table 34-5). Research is ongoing to determine whether a decline in homocysteine can reduce the risk of heart disease. B-complex vitamins (B_6, B_{12}, folic acid) have been shown to lower blood levels of homocysteine. In general, a screening test for homocysteine is limited to people suspected of having elevated levels, such as older patients with pernicious anemia or people who develop CAD at an early age.

Substance Use. The use of illicit drugs, such as cocaine and methamphetamine, can produce coronary spasm resulting in myocardial ischemia and chest pain. Most individuals who are seen in the ED with drug-induced chest pain are initially indistinguishable from patients with CAD. Although MI can occur, patients with drug-induced chest pain more often have sinus tachycardia, high BP, angina, and anxiety (Chen, 2007; Hollander & Henry, 2006).

The U.S. Food and Drug Administration prohibited the sale of dietary supplements containing ephedrine alkaloids. In Canada, the ephedrine alkaloid is limited to levels well below the excessive amounts seen in U.S. products, a policy that allows the continued sale of traditional Chinese ephedra products. Although Health Canada has approved certain oral products containing low doses of ephedra for short-term use as nasal decongestants, products that contain a combination of ephedra and a stimulant, such as caffeine, or other ingredients that might increase the effects of ephedra are not approved for use in Canada. Ephedra products that are marketed for weight loss, body building, or increased energy are also not allowed to be sold in Canada (Health Canada, 2008). Because these compounds cause high BP, MI, and stroke, they should be avoided.

Health Promotion

The appropriate management of risk factors in CAD may prevent, modify, or retard the progression of the disease. Emphasis on prevention and early treatment of heart disease must be ongoing.

Identification of People at High Risk.
In both the acute care setting and the community, the nurse should identify people at risk for CAD. Risk screening involves obtaining personal and family health histories. Each person should be questioned about a family history of heart disease in parents, grandparents, and siblings. The presence of any cardiovascular symptoms should be noted. Environmental factors, such as eating habits, type of diet, and level of exercise, are assessed to identify lifestyle patterns. A psychosocial history is included to determine smoking habits, alcohol ingestion, type A behaviours, recent stressful life events, sleeping habits, and the presence of anxiety or depression. Details about the workplace and the type of work can provide important information on the kind of activity performed; work-related exposure to pollutants, allergens, or noxious chemicals; and the degree of emotional stress associated with employment.

The nurse should identify the person's attitudes and beliefs about health and illness. This information can give some indication of how disease and lifestyle changes may affect the person and can reveal possible misconceptions about heart disease. Knowledge of the person's educational background is frequently helpful in deciding at what level to begin teaching. If the person is taking medications, it is important to know what the medications are, when they are taken, the person's adherence to the medication regimen, and the person's attitudes toward the taking of medications.

Management of People at High Risk.
Once a person is identified as being at high risk, preventive measures can be taken. Risk factors such as age, sex, and genetic inheritance cannot be modified. However, the person with any of these risk factors can modify the risk of CAD by controlling or changing the additive effects of modifiable risk factors. For example, a young man with a family history of heart disease can decrease the risk of an MI by maintaining an ideal weight, getting adequate physical exercise, reducing intake of saturated fats, and not smoking.

The person who has modifiable risk factors should be encouraged and motivated to make changes in lifestyle to reduce the risk of heart disease. The nurse can play a major role in teaching health-promoting behaviours to the person at risk for CAD (Table 36-4). For highly motivated people, knowing how to reduce this risk may be the only information needed to induce them to make changes. (The Nursing Research box on this page examines additional factors that can affect people's management of their CAD risk.)

For people who are less motivated to assume responsibility for health, the idea of risk factor reduction may be so remote that they are unable to perceive a threat of CAD in their life. Especially in the absence of symptoms, few people desire to make lifestyle changes. The nurse should first assist such a person in clarifying personal values. Then, by explaining the risk factors and having the person identify vulnerability to various risks, the nurse may help the person recognize susceptibility to CAD. The nurse may also help the person set realistic goals and allow the person to choose which risk factor to change first. Some people are reluctant to change until they begin to manifest overt symptoms or actually suffer an MI. Others, having suffered an MI, may find the idea of changing lifelong habits totally unacceptable. The nurse must be able to identify such attitudes and respect them.

PATIENT & CAREGIVER TEACHING GUIDE

Table 36-4 Decreasing Risk Factors for Coronary Artery Disease

RISK FACTOR	HEALTH-PROMOTING BEHAVIOURS
Hypertension	• Have regular BP checkups • Take prescribed medications for BP control • Reduce salt intake • Never smoke or stop smoking • Control or reduce weight • Exercise regularly
Elevated serum lipids	• Reduce total fat intake • Reduce animal (saturated) fat intake • Adjust total caloric intake to achieve and maintain ideal body weight • Engage in regular exercise program • Increase amount of complex carbohydrates and vegetable proteins in diet
Smoking*	• Enroll in program to stop smoking • Change daily routines associated with smoking to reduce desire to smoke • Substitute other activities for smoking • Ask family members to support efforts to stop smoking
Physical inactivity	• Develop and maintain routine for physical activity that is performed at least three or four times a week • Increase activities to a level compatible with physical fitness
Stressful lifestyle	• Increase awareness of behaviours that are detrimental to health • Alter patterns that are conducive to stress and rushing (e.g., get up 30 min earlier so that breakfast is not eaten on way to work) • Set realistic goals for self • Reassess priorities in view of health needs • Learn effective coping strategies • Avoid excessive and prolonged stress • Take 20 min/day to meditate • Plan time for adequate rest and sleep
Obesity	• Change eating patterns and habits • Reduce caloric intake • Exercise regularly to increase caloric expenditure • Avoid fad and crash diets, which are not effective over the long term • Avoid large, heavy meals
Diabetes mellitus†	• Follow the recommended diet • Reduce weight and control diet • Monitor blood glucose levels regularly

*See Registered Nurses' Association of Ontario (RNAO). (2007). *Integrating smoking cessation into daily nursing practice: Nursing Best Practices Guideline.* Toronto: RNAO. Available at *http://rnao.ca/bpg/guidelines/integrating-smoking-cessation-daily-nursing-practice*
†See Chapter 52 for additional health-promoting behaviours.
BP, blood pressure.

NURSING RESEARCH

Men and Women Managing Coronary Artery Risk: Urban–Rural Contrasts

Citation

King, K. M., Thomlinson, E., Sanguins, J., & LeBlanc, P. (2006). Men and women managing coronary artery disease risk: Urban–rural contrasts. *Social Science & Medicine, 62*(5), 1091-1102.

Purpose

To describe how gender and ethnocultural affiliation influence the process that people undergo when faced with making lifestyle changes related to coronary artery disease (CAD) risk.

Methods

This qualitative study was conducted in Alberta, Canada, and data were collected through recorded interviews. The sample consisted of men and women from five ethnocultural groups ($n = 42$) who received a diagnosis of CAD.

Results and Conclusions

The investigators found that intrapersonal, interpersonal, extrapersonal, and sociodemographic factors influenced the participants' capacity to manage their CAD risk.

Implications for Nursing Practice

When health care providers develop a better understanding of the gender- and ethnocultural-based components that influence individuals' decision making around their CAD risk management, secondary interventions will become more appropriate, and health outcomes will be positive.

NUTRITIONAL THERAPY

Table 36-5 Coronary Artery Disease: Comparison of Step 1 and Step 2 Low-Fat Diets	
PRINCIPLES OF STEP 1 DIET	**PRINCIPLES OF STEP 2 DIET**
• Between 8 and 10% of total calories come from saturated fat; ≤30% of total calories come from fat. • Visible fat (e.g., butter, cream, margarine, salad dressing, cooking oil) is restricted to 1 tsp per meal. • When oil is used, it should be in the form of unsaturated vegetable oil. • Lean meats, skim milk or 1% milk, and no more than three egg yolks per week are used. • Food high in fat content (e.g., avocados, fatty meat, olives, nuts) are avoided. • Cooking methods such as steaming, baking, broiling, grilling, or stir-frying in small amounts of fat are recommended.	• Less than 7% of total calories come from saturated fat; ≤30% of total calories come from fat. • Meat: Only leanest cuts are allowed. • Organ meats and shrimp are restricted because they are high in cholesterol although low in total fat. • Eggs: Only one egg yolk per week is used because egg yolk is high in cholesterol. Egg whites or egg substitutes may be used as desired. • Vegetable oils are used in cooking and food preparation. Coconut and palm oils are not allowed because of their high content of saturated fats. Choose margarine that contains ≤2 g of saturated fat per Tbsp. • Skim milk is highly recommended. Low-fat yogourt and low-fat cheeses may be used, as may low-fat ice milk, frozen yogourt, or sherbet.

Physical Activity. In Canada, the interest in attaining and maintaining health has made physical activity a field of major importance. Communities are developing exercise programs for people of all ages and with all health needs, ranging from aerobic exercise classes to cardiac walking and jogging programs. Local YMCAs often sponsor exercise jogging, bicycling, and related courses. Many shopping malls open their doors in the early morning to allow people to walk indoors. The HSF organizes many events to promote health that emphasize the need for physical activity. Many large corporations provide gymnasiums in which their employees can exercise. For many people, running may be inadvisable; such people should be encouraged to pursue walking, swimming, or whatever exercise will accommodate their individual physical abilities.

Health Education in Schools. Awareness of the body and physical health is also present in school systems. Schoolteachers have an important role in teaching good health practices. Besides teaching physical fitness topics, teachers can instruct students in how the body functions and responds to daily living. Lifestyle habits can be positively influenced at an early age to decrease the need for drastic changes later in life, such as those that confront the students' parents. Teachers should take advantage of the social climate that promotes health and health practices and find innovative ways to present these values to a receptive youthful

audience before their habits become ingrained. The HSF has established school programs such as "Heart Smart," which provides teaching materials for teachers to incorporate into their curriculum. Printed and electronic materials are also available to help teachers educate children in their schools about healthy habits for better cardiac health.

Nutritional Therapy

The Adult Treatment Panel III of the National Heart, Lung, and Blood Institute has recommended *therapeutic lifestyle changes* for all people to reduce the risk of CAD by lowering LDL cholesterol. These recommendations provide guidelines that emphasize a decrease in saturated fat and cholesterol and an increase in complex carbohydrates (e.g., whole grains, fruit, vegetables) (Gidding et al., 2009; Grundy et al., 2004; Table 36-5). Fat intake should constitute about 30% of calories, with most coming from monounsaturated fats (Figure 36-4). Red meats, eggs, and whole milk products are major sources of saturated fat and cholesterol and should be reduced or eliminated from the diet. If the serum triglyceride level is elevated, the guidelines recommend reducing or eliminating the consumption of alcohol and simple sugars.

Omega-3 fatty acids reduce the risks associated with CAD when consumed regularly. For individuals without CAD, the American Heart Association (AHA) recommends eating fatty fish such as salmon and tuna twice a week because fatty fish contain

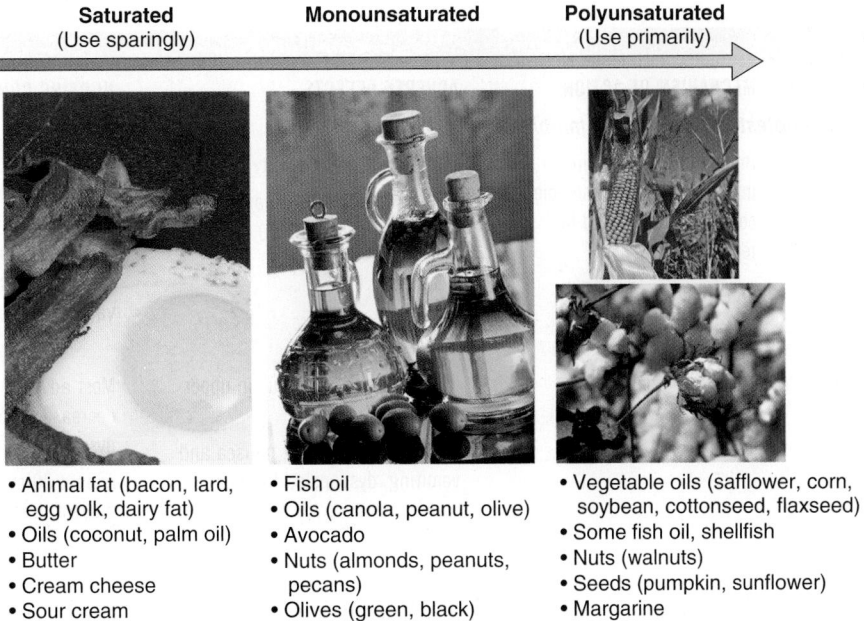

Figure 36-4 Types of dietary fat.

Source: Photos © 2011 JupiterImages Corporation. (Bacon and eggs, Hemera/Thinkstock; corn, iStockphoto/Thinkstock; cotton plant, JupiterImages.)

two types of omega-3 fatty acids: eicosapentaenoic acid and docosahexaenoic acid. Patients with CAD are encouraged to take supplements of these fatty acids with their diet. The AHA also recommends eating tofu and other forms of soybeans, canola oil, walnuts, and flaxseed because these products contain α-linolenic acid, which is converted to omega-3 fatty acid in the body. For more information on the AHA's nutritional recommendations, see their Web site (in the Related Resources at the end of this chapter). Several studies have demonstrated regression in coronary atherosclerosis and reduction in coronary events by lifestyle changes, including a low-saturated-fat diet, avoidance of tobacco, and increase in physical activity. Many of these studies included cholesterol-lowering drug therapy as well (Grundy et al., 2004; Smith et al., 2006).

Cholesterol-Lowering Drug Therapy

An estimated 10 million Canadians have high cholesterol levels (≥5.2 mmol/L) (HSF, 2012). A complete lipid profile should be obtained every 5 years beginning at age 20. A person with a serum cholesterol level exceeding 5.2 mmol/L is at risk for CAD and should be treated. The Canadian guidelines for treatment focus on LDL levels (Table 36-6). Treatment usually begins with smoking cessation, dietary caloric restriction (if overweight), decreased dietary fat and cholesterol intake, increased physical activity, and stress management (Genest et al., 2009). Serum cholesterol levels are reassessed after 6 months of diet therapy. If they remain elevated, additional dietary options (see the Complementary & Alternative Therapies boxes on pp. 902 and 903) or drug therapy may be started (Table 36-7).

Drugs That Restrict Lipoprotein Production. The

"statin" drugs are the most widely used and studied lipid-lowering drugs. Examples include lovastatin (Mevacor), pravastatin (Pravachol), simvastatin (Zocor), atorvastatin (Lipitor), and rosuvastatin (Crestor). These drugs inhibit the synthesis of cholesterol in

Table 36-6 Treatment Decisions for High Blood Cholesterol, Based on Low-Density Lipoprotein Levels

RISK LEVEL	PRIMARY TARGET LDL-C	CLASS, LEVEL
High		
• CAD, PVD, atherosclerosis, most cases of diabetes • FRS ≥20% • RRS ≥20%	<2 mmol/L *or* ≥50% ↓ LDL-C Apo B <0.80 g/L	Class I, Level A
Moderate		
• FRS = 10-19% • LDL-C >3.5 mmol/L • TC/HDL-C >5.0 • hs-CRP >2 mg/L in men age 50 years and women age >60 years • Family history and hs-CRP modulate risk	<2 mmol/L *or* ≥50% ↓ LDL-C Apo B <0.80 g/L	Class II A, Level A
Low		
• FRS <10%	≥50% ↓ LDL-C	Class II A, Level A

Source: Adapted from Genest, J., Macpherson, R., Frohlich, J., Anderson, T., Campbell, N., Carpentier, A., ..., Ur, E. (2009). 2009 Canadian Cardiovascular Society/Canadian Guidelines for the diagnosis and treatment of dyslipidemia and prevention of cardiovascular disease in the adult—2009 Recommendations, *Canadian Journal of Cardiology,* 25(10), p. 569 (Table 3). doi:10.1016/S0828-282X(09)70715-9
Apo B, apolipoprotein B; *FRS,* Framingham risk score; *HDL-C,* high-density lipoprotein cholesterol; *hs-CRP,* high-sensitivity C-reactive protein; *LDL-C,* low-density lipoprotein cholesterol; *PVD,* peripheral vascular disease; *RRS,* Reynolds Risk Score; *TC,* total cholesterol.

DRUG THERAPY

Table 36-7 Hyperlipidemia

TYPE AND NAME	MECHANISM OF ACTION	ADVERSE EFFECTS	NURSING CONSIDERATIONS
Bile Acid Sequestrants and Cholesterol Absorption Inhibitors			
Cholestyramine Colestipol (Colestid) Ezetimibe (Ezetrol)	Bind with bile acids in intestine, forming insoluble complex and excreted in feces	Unpleasant gritty quality to taste GI disturbances (e.g., nausea, dyspepsia, constipation)	Effective and safe for long-term use; adverse effects diminish with time; interfere with absorption of digoxin, thiazides, β-adrenergic blockers, fat-soluble vitamins, folic acid, vancomycin (Vancocin)
Niacin			
Nicotinic acid (niacin, Niaspan)	Inhibits synthesis and secretion of VLDL and LDL ↑ HDL level	Hot flashes and pruritus in upper torso and face GI disturbances (e.g., nausea and vomiting, dyspepsia, diarrhea)	Most adverse effects subside with time; decreased liver function and dysrhythmias may occur with high doses Aspirin 30 min to 1 hr before niacin may prevent flushing; niacin should be taken with food
Fibrates			
Bezafibrate (Bezalip) Fenofibrate (Lipidil) Gemfibrozil (Lopid)	↓ Triglycerides by ↓ VLDL level ↓ Hepatic synthesis and secretion of VLDL ↑ HDL level	Mild GI disturbances (e.g., nausea, diarrhea)	May ↑ effects of anticoagulants and hypoglycemics
Statins			
Atorvastatin (Lipitor) Fluvastatin (Lescol) Lovastatin (Mevacor) Pravastatin (Pravachol) Rosuvastatin (Crestor) Simvastatin (Zocor)	Block synthesis of cholesterol ↓ LDL and triglyceride levels ↑ HDL level	Rash, mild GI disturbances, insomnia, elevated liver enzyme levels, lens opacities, rhabdomyolysis (specifically with lovastatin)	Well tolerated with few adverse effects Monitor patient with liver function tests and eye examinations

GI, gastrointestinal; *HDL*, high-density lipoprotein; *LDL*, low-density lipoprotein; *VLDL*, very low–density lipoprotein.

COMPLEMENTARY & ALTERNATIVE THERAPIES

Garlic

Clinical Uses

High blood cholesterol and hypertension

Effects

Antihyperlipidemic, antihypertensive, antioxidant, antithrombotic, and hypoglycemic activity. Because of garlic's hypoglycemic effect, blood glucose levels should be monitored closely when it is used. Moderate garlic consumption has few adverse effects other than a peculiar odour on the breath and the body.

Nursing Implications

Relatively safe herb, but use may be contraindicated in people with bleeding disorders, gastrointestinal infection, diabetes, and inflammation. Enhances the effects of warfarin and should not be used with anticoagulant or antiplatelet drugs. Odour-modified garlic preparations are just as effective as fresh garlic, but dried garlic has little to no effect.

the liver by blocking 3-hydroxy-3-methylglutaryl coenzyme A (HMG-CoA) reductase. An unexplained result of the inhibition of cholesterol synthesis is an increase in hepatic LDL receptors. Consequently, the liver is able to remove more LDLs from the blood. In addition, levels of HDLs also increase slightly with the use of statins (Lehne, 2012). Serious adverse effects of these drugs can include liver damage and myopathy that can progress to rhabdomyolysis (breakdown of skeletal muscle), but these are rare. Liver enzymes (e.g., aspartate aminotransferase, alanine aminotransferase) must be monitored regularly and checked any time dosage is increased. Creatine kinase (CK) enzymes are assessed if symptoms of myopathy (e.g., muscle aches, weakness) occur (Lehne, 2012).

Drugs That Increase Lipoprotein Removal.

The major process of cholesterol elimination begins with its conversion to bile acids in the liver. Bile acid sequestrants such as cholestyramine and colestipol (Colestid) increase conversion of cholesterol to bile acids and decrease hepatic content of total cholesterol and LDLs.

Complaints associated with these drugs are related to palatability and a variety of upper and lower GI symptoms, including belching, heartburn, nausea, abdominal pain, and constipation. Bile acid sequestrants may interfere with absorption of other

Natural Lipid-Lowering Agents*

Agent	Comments
Niacin (nicotinic acid)	• Inhibits synthesis and secretion of LDLs • Increases HDL levels
Garlic	• See Complementary & Alternative Therapies box "Garlic"
Omega-3 fatty acids	• Found in fish oil and flaxseed oil • Fish with high levels include cold-water ocean fish such as salmon, herring, mackerel, halibut, and sardines • ↓ Triglyceride levels and ↑ HDL levels
Milk thistle	• Silymarin, active part of milk thistle, has a cholesterol-lowering effect • ↑ HDL levels
Fibre	• Soluble fibre (e.g., pectin, oat bran, psyllium husk, fruits, beans) • ↓ Cholesterol and LDL levels by binding bile acids and slowing rate of lipid absorption
Phytosterols (plant sterols and stanols)	• Plant sterols are found in nuts, seeds, soybeans, and vegetable oils • Natural plant alcohols ↓ serum cholesterol
Soy	• ↓ Cholesterol, LDL, and triglyceride levels and ↑ HDL levels • Acts by ↓ absorption of cholesterol from GI tract
Coenzyme Q₁₀	• HMG-CoA reductase inhibitors (e.g., (ubiquinone) lovastatin [Mevacor]) decrease plasma levels of coenzyme Q₁₀

GI, gastrointestinal; *HDL,* high-density lipoprotein; *HMG-CoA,* 3-hydroxy-3-methylglutaryl coenzyme A; *LDL,* low-density lipoprotein.

*Cardiovascular disease is a serious health problem. Herbal or other natural therapy should not be initiated without consultation with a health care professional. This is especially important when conventional drug therapy for cardiovascular disease is also being used.

drugs (e.g., warfarin [Coumadin], thiazides, thyroid hormones, β-adrenergic blockers). Administering these drugs at a different time than other drugs may decrease this adverse effect (Lehne, 2012).

Drugs That Decrease Cholesterol Absorption.
Drug therapy for hyperlipidemia is likely to be prolonged, perhaps continuing for a lifetime. It is essential that diet be modified in order to minimize the need for drug therapy. The patient must fully understand the rationale and goals of treatment, as well as the safety and adverse effects of lipid-lowering drug therapy (Lehne, 2012).

Chronic Stable Angina

CAD is a progressive disease, and patients may be asymptomatic for many years, or they may develop chronic but stable chest pain syndromes. When the demand for myocardial oxygen exceeds the ability of the coronary arteries to supply the heart with oxygen, myocardial ischemia occurs. **Angina,** or chest pain, is the clinical

Table 36-8 Factors Determining Myocardial Oxygen Needs

DECREASED OXYGEN SUPPLY	INCREASED OXYGEN DEMAND OR CONSUMPTION
Noncardiac Factors	
Anemia	Anxiety
Hypoxemia	Cocaine use
Pneumonia	Hypertension
Asthma	Hyperthermia
Chronic obstructive pulmonary disease	Hyperthyroidism
Low blood volume	Physical exertion
Cardiac Factors	
Coronary artery spasm	Aortic stenosis
Coronary artery thrombosis	Cardiomyopathy
Dysrhythmias	Dysrhythmias
Heart failure	Tachycardia
Valve disorders	

manifestation of reversible myocardial ischemia. Either an increased demand for oxygen or a decreased supply of oxygen can lead to myocardial ischemia (Table 36-8). The primary reason for insufficient blood flow is narrowing of coronary arteries by atherosclerosis (Libby et al., 2008). For ischemia secondary to atherosclerosis to occur, the artery is usually 75% or more obstructed (stenosed).

On the cellular level, the myocardium becomes hypoxic within the first 10 seconds of coronary occlusion. With total occlusion of the coronary arteries, contractility ceases after several minutes, depriving the myocardial cells of oxygen and glucose for aerobic metabolism. Anaerobic metabolism begins, and lactic acid accumulates. Myocardial nerve fibres are irritated by the increased lactic acid and transmit a pain message to the cardiac nerves and the upper thoracic posterior nerve roots. This is the reason for referred cardiac pain to the left shoulder and arm. In ischemic conditions, cardiac cells are viable for approximately 20 minutes. With restoration of blood flow, aerobic metabolism resumes, contractility is restored, and cellular repair begins.

Chronic stable angina refers to chest pain that occurs intermittently over a long period with the same pattern of onset, duration, and intensity of symptoms. When questioned (Table 36-9), some patients may deny feeling pain but describe a pressure or ache in the chest. It is an unpleasant feeling, often described as a constrictive, squeezing, heavy, choking, or suffocating sensation. Angina is rarely sharp or stabbing, and it usually does not change with position or breathing. Many people with angina complain of indigestion or a burning sensation in the epigastric region. Although most of the pain experienced by people with angina is substernal, the sensation may occur in the neck or radiate to various locations, including the jaw, the shoulders, and down the arms (Figure 36-5). Sometimes the person may complain of pain between the shoulder blades and dismiss it as not being related to their heart.

The pain is usually brief (lasting 3 to 5 minutes) and commonly subsides when the precipitating factor is relieved (Table 36-10). Pain at rest is unusual. Electrocardiography usually reveals transient ST segment depression, indicative of ischemia (see Chapter 38).

Table 36-9 "PQRST" Assessment of Angina

"PQRST" can be used as a mnemonic to assist in obtaining information from the patient who has chest pain, as follows:

FACTOR		QUESTIONS TO ASK PATIENT
P	Precipitating events	What events or activities precipitated the pain (e.g., argument, exercise, resting)?
Q	Quality of pain	What does the pain feel like (e.g., pressure, dull, aching, tight, squeezing)?
R	Radiation of pain	Where is the pain located? Does the pain radiate to other areas (e.g., back, arms, jaw, teeth, shoulder, elbow)?
S	Severity of pain	On a scale of 0 to 10, with 10 being the most severe pain you could imagine, how would you rate the pain?
T	Timing	When did the pain begin? Has the pain changed since this time? Have you had pain like this before?

Table 36-10 Factors Precipitating Angina

Physical Exertion
- Increased HR reduces the time the heart spends in diastole (the time of greatest coronary blood flow) and results in an increase in myocardial oxygen demand.
- Isometric exercise of the arms (e.g., raking, lifting heavy objects, or shovelling snow) can cause exertional angina.

Temperature Extremes
- Workload of the heart is increased.
- Blood vessels constrict in response to a cold stimulus.
- Blood vessels dilate and blood pools in the skin in response to a hot stimulus.

Strong Emotions
- The sympathetic nervous system is stimulated.
- The workload of the heart is increased.

Consumption of Heavy Meal
- The workload of the heart may be increased.
- During the digestive process, blood is diverted to the GI system, which reduces blood flow in the coronary arteries.

Tobacco Use
- Nicotine stimulates catecholamine release, causing vasoconstriction and an increase in HR.
- Tobacco diminishes available oxygen by increasing the level of carbon monoxide.

Sexual Activity
- The cardiac workload and sympathetic stimulation are increased.
- In a person with CAD, the extra cardiac workload may precipitate angina.

Stimulants*
- HR and subsequent myocardial oxygen demand are increased.

Circadian Rhythm Patterns
- These patterns are related to the occurrence of chronic stable angina, Prinzmetal's angina, myocardial infarction, and sudden cardiac death.
- Manifestations of CAD tend to occur in the early morning after the patient awakens.

CAD, coronary artery disease; *GI*, gastrointestinal; *HR*, heart rate.
*For example, cocaine and amphetamines.

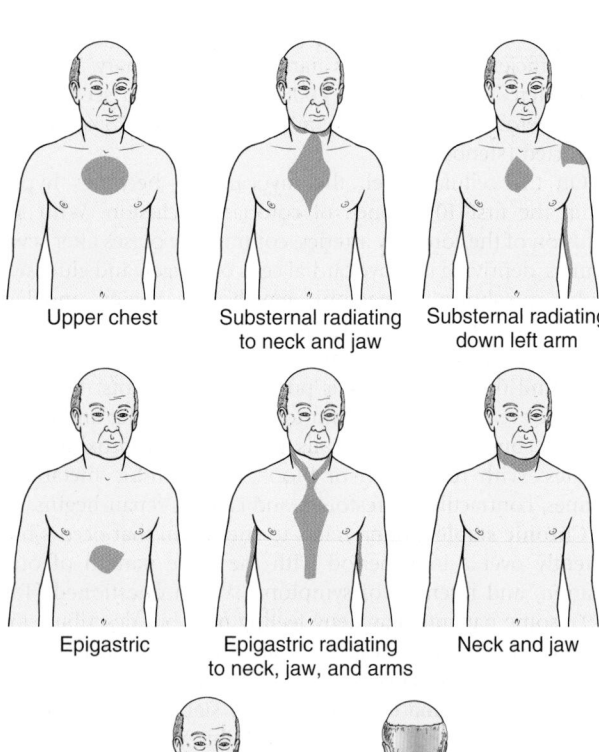

Upper chest | Substernal radiating to neck and jaw | Substernal radiating down left arm

Epigastric | Epigastric radiating to neck, jaw, and arms | Neck and jaw

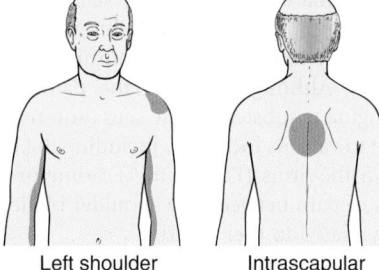

Left shoulder and down both arms | Intrascapular

Figure 36-5 Locations of pain during angina or myocardial infarction.

Chronic stable angina can be controlled with medications on an outpatient basis. Because episodes of chronic stable angina are often predictable, medications can be timed to provide peak effects during the time of day when angina is likely to occur. For example, if angina occurs on arising, the patient can take medication upon awakening and wait 30 minutes to 1 hour before engaging in activity. (The different types of angina are compared in Table 36-11.)

Silent Ischemia

Silent ischemia refers to ischemia that occurs in the absence of any subjective symptoms (Libby et al., 2008). Patients with diabetes have an increased prevalence of silent ischemia, possibly related to diabetic neuropathy affecting the nerves that innervate the cardiovascular system. (Vinik, Maser, Mitchell, & Freeman,

Table 36-11 Comparison of Types of Angina

FEATURE	CHRONIC STABLE ANGINA	PRINZMETAL'S ANGINA	UNSTABLE ANGINA
Etiology	Myocardial ischemia, usually secondary to CAD	Coronary vasospasm	Rupture of thickened plaque, exposing thrombogenic surface
Characteristics	Episodic pain lasting 5-15 min	Occurs primarily at rest	New-onset angina
	Provoked by exertion	Triggered by smoking	Angina of increasing frequency, duration, or severity
	Relieved by rest or nitroglycerin	May occur in presence or absence of CAD	Occurs at rest or with minimal exertion
			Pain refractory to nitroglycerin

CAD, coronary artery disease.

2003). When patients are monitored (e.g., Holter monitor) and silent ischemia occurs, ECG changes are revealed. Ischemia—with or without pain—has the same prognosis.

Nocturnal Angina and Angina Decubitus. Nocturnal angina occurs only at night but not necessarily when the person is in the recumbent position or during sleep. Angina decubitus is chest pain that occurs only while the person is lying down and is usually relieved by standing or sitting.

Prinzmetal's Angina. Prinzmetal's angina (variant angina) often occurs at rest, usually in response to spasm of a major coronary artery. It is a rare form of angina and occurs in many patients with a history of migraine headaches and Raynaud's phenomenon. The spasm may occur in the absence of CAD, as well as with documented disease. Prinzmetal's angina is not usually precipitated by increased physical demand. Coronary spasm can be described as a strong contraction of smooth muscle in the coronary artery caused by an increase in intracellular calcium.

Factors that may precipitate coronary artery spasm include increased myocardial oxygen demand and increased levels of certain substances (e.g., histamine, angiotensin, epinephrine, norepinephrine, prostaglandins). When spasm occurs, the patient experiences angina, and the ECG demonstrates transient ST-segment elevation (see Chapter 38). The pain may occur during rapid eye movement (REM) sleep, when myocardial oxygen consumption increases. The pain may be relieved by moderate exercise, or it may disappear spontaneously. Cyclic, short bursts of pain at a consistent time each day may also occur with this type of angina. It is usually treated with calcium channel blockers, nitrates, or both.

Collaborative Management

The treatment of chronic stable angina is aimed at decreasing oxygen demand or increasing oxygen supply, or both. Continued emphasis on the reduction of risk factors is a priority and should include those strategies discussed for patients with CAD (see pp. 895-900). In addition to antiplatelet and cholesterol-lowering drug therapy, the most common therapeutic intervention for the management of chronic stable angina is the use of nitrate therapy to enhance coronary blood flow (Gluckman, Sachdev, Schulman, & Blumenthal, 2005; Table 36-12, Figure 36-6.)

Drug Therapy

Drug therapy for chronic stable angina is aimed at preventing MI and death and reducing symptoms. Aspirin (previously dis-

Table 36-12 Major Treatment Elements of Chronic Stable Angina

Strategies for the patient with chronic stable angina should address all of the treatment elements in the "ABCDEF" mnemonic:

A	Antiplatelet agent
	Antianginal therapy
	ACE inhibitor*
B	β-Adrenergic blocker
	Blood pressure
C	Cigarette smoking
	Cholesterol
D	Diet
	Diabetes
E	Education
	Exercise
F	Flu vaccination*

*Source: Smith, S. C., Allen, J., Blair, S. N., Bonow, R., Brass, L, Fonarow, G., …, Taubert, K. (2006). American Heart Association/American College of Cardiology guidelines for secondary prevention for patients with coronary and other atherosclerotic vascular disease: 2006 Update. *Circulation, 113,* 2363-2372. doi:10.1161/CIRCULATIONAHA. 106.174516
ACE, angiotensin-converting enzyme.

cussed) is recommended in the absence of contraindications (Table 36-13).

Short-Acting Nitrates. Short-acting nitrates are first-line therapy for the treatment of angina. Nitrates produce their principal effects by the following mechanisms:

1. Dilating peripheral blood vessels. This results in decreased systemic vascular resistance (SVR), venous pooling, and decreased venous blood return to the heart. Because of the reduced cardiac workload, myocardial oxygen demand is decreased.
2. Dilating coronary arteries and collateral vessels. This may increase blood flow to the ischemic areas of the heart. However, when the coronary arteries are severely atherosclerotic, coronary dilation is difficult to achieve.

Sublingual Nitroglycerin. Nitroglycerin administered sublingually (Nitrostat) or by translingual spray (Nitrolingual) usually relieves pain in approximately 3 minutes, and its action has a duration of approximately 30 to 60 minutes. The recommended dosage for symptoms of angina is one tablet taken sub-

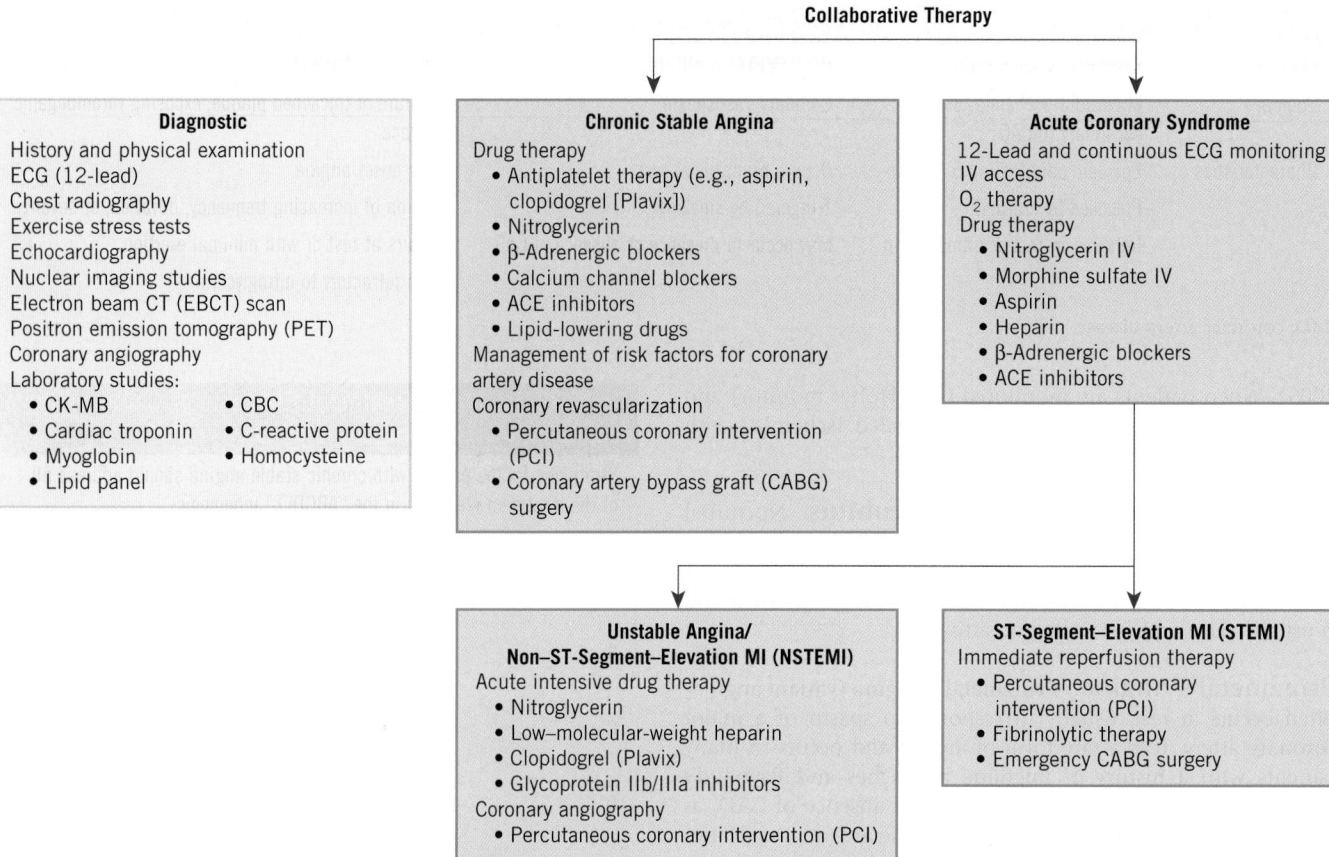

Figure 36-6 Collaborative care: Chronic stable angina and acute coronary syndrome. *ACE*, angiotensin-converting enzyme; *CBC*, complete blood count; *CK-MB*, MB isoenzyme of creatine kinase; *CT*, computed tomography; *ECG*, electrocardiogram; *IV*, intravenous; *MI*, myocardial infarction.

lingually (SL) or one metered spray. If symptoms are unchanged or worse after 5 minutes, the patient should be instructed to contact the emergency medical services (EMS) system (Kushner et al., 2009).

The patient must be instructed in the proper use of nitroglycerin. It should be easily accessible to the patient at all times. For protection from degradation, tablets should be kept in a tightly closed dark glass bottle. The patient should be instructed to place a nitroglycerin tablet under the tongue and allow it to dissolve. The spray should be directed under the tongue, not inhaled. Nitroglycerin should cause a tingling sensation. If tingling is not felt and chest pain still persists, the patient should contact EMS. The patient should be warned that HR may increase and a pounding headache, dizziness, or flushing may occur. The patient should be cautioned against quickly rising to a standing position because orthostatic hypotension may occur after nitroglycerin use.

Nitroglycerin tablets are marketed in light-resistant bottles with metal caps. Because they tend to lose potency once a bottle has been opened, the patient should be advised to purchase a new supply every 6 months.

Long-Acting Nitrates. Nitrates, such as isosorbide dinitrate and isosorbide mononitrate (Imdur), are longer acting than SL or translingual nitroglycerin and can be used to reduce the incidence of anginal attacks (Lehne, 2012). The predominant adverse effect of all nitrates is headache from the dilation of cerebral blood vessels. Patients can be advised to take acetaminophen

(Tylenol) with their nitrate to relieve the headache. Over time, the headaches may decrease, but the principal antianginal effect remains the same.

Orthostatic hypotension is a complication of all nitrates. Nurses should monitor BP after the initial dose because the venous dilation that occurs may cause a drop in BP, especially in volume-depleted patients. In addition, tolerance to nitroglycerin-induced vasodilation can develop. It is recommended that patients schedule an 8-hour nitrate-free period every day, usually during the night, unless a patient experiences nocturnal angina (Lehne, 2012).

Transdermal Controlled-Release Nitrates. Currently, two systems are available for transdermal nitroglycerin drug administration: reservoir and matrix. The reservoir system delivers the drug using a rate-controlled permeable membrane. The matrix system provides for a slow delivery of the drug through a polymer matrix. Both reservoir and matrix delivery systems offer the advantages of steady plasma levels within the therapeutic range during 24 hours; thus only one application a day is necessary. The reservoir system has the disadvantage of dose dumping if the reservoir seal is punctured or broken; the matrix system, in contrast, avoids this problem. Both systems achieve steady-state plasma drug levels by 2 hours.

β-Adrenergic Blockers. β-Adrenergic blockers are the preferred drugs for the management of chronic stable angina

DRUG THERAPY

Table 36-13 Chronic Stable Angina and Acute Coronary Syndrome

DRUG CLASSIFICATION	MECHANISM OF ACTION AND COMMENTS	DRUG CLASSIFICATION	MECHANISM OF ACTION AND COMMENTS
Antiplatelet Agents		**Angiotensin-Converting Enzyme (ACE) Inhibitors***	
Aspirin	• Inhibit cyclooxygenase (which produces thromboxane A₂, a potent platelet activator) • Should be administered as soon as acute coronary syndrome is suspected	Captopril Enalapril (Vasotec)	• Prevent conversion of angiotensin I to angiotensin II • Decrease endothelial dysfunction • Useful in treatment of heart failure, tachycardia, MI, hypertension, diabetes, and chronic kidney disease
Adenosine Diphosphate Receptor Antagonists		**Unfractionated Heparins†**	
Clopidogrel (Plavix)	• Inhibit platelet aggregation • Alternative for patient who cannot use aspirin • Oral clopidogrel (Plavix), 75 mg/day, should be added to aspirin therapy in patients with STEMI, regardless of whether they undergo reperfusion therapy (Kushner et al., 2009)	Heparin	• Prevent conversion of fibrinogen to fibrin and of prothrombin to thrombin
		Low–Molecular Weight Heparins†	
		Dalteparin (Fragmin) Enoxaparin (Lovenox)	• Bind to antithrombin III, enhancing its effect • Heparin–antithrombin III complex inactivates activated Factor X and thrombin • Prevent conversion of fibrinogen to fibrin
Nitrates			
Sublingual nitroglycerin (Nitrostat) Translingual spray nitroglycerin (Nitrolingual) Transdermal nitroglycerin (Transderm-Nitro, Minitran) Extended-release buccal tablets Isosorbide dinitrate Isosorbide mononitrate (Imdur) IV nitroglycerin (Nitroject)	• Promote peripheral vasodilation, decreasing preload and afterload • Promote coronary artery vasodilation	**Glycoprotein IIB and IIIA Inhibitors**	
		Abciximab (ReoPro) Eptifibatide (Integrilin) Tirofiban (Aggrastat)	• Prevent the binding of fibrinogen to platelets, thereby blocking platelet aggregation • Standard antiplatelet therapy in combination with aspirin for patients at high risk for unstable angina
β-Adrenergic Blockers*		**Opioid Analgesics**	
Atenolol (Tenormin) Carvedilol Esmolol (Brevibloc) Metoprolol (Lopressor) Nadolol Propranolol (Inderal)	• Inhibit sympathetic nervous stimulation of the heart • Reduce both heart rate and contractility • Decrease afterload	Morphine, morphine sulphate	• Function as analgesic and sedative • Act as vasodilator to reduce preload and myocardial O₂ consumption
Calcium Channel Blockers*		**Fibrinolytic Therapy**	
Amlodipine (Norvasc) Diltiazem (Cardizem) Felodipine (Plendil) Nifedipine Verapamil (Isoptin)	• Prevent calcium entry into vascular smooth muscle cells and myocytes (cardiac cells) • Promote coronary and peripheral vasodilation • Reduce both heart rate and contractility	Recombinant plasminogen activator (r-PA; reteplase [Retavase]) Tissue plasminogen activator (t-PA; alteplase [Activase]) Tenecteplase (TNK, TNKase)	• Break up fibrin meshwork in clots • Used only in STEMI

*See Chapter 35, Table 35-8.
†See Chapter 40, Table 40-9.
IV, intravenous; *MI,* myocardial infarction; *STEMI,* ST-segment–elevation myocardial infarction.

(Lehne, 2012). Examples include propranolol (Inderal), metoprolol (Lopressor), nadolol, atenolol (Tenormin), and carvedilol. These drugs cause decreases in myocardial contractility, HR, SVR, and BP, all of which reduces the myocardial oxygen demand. β-Adrenergic blockers also have been shown to

decrease the rates of morbidity and mortality in patients with CAD, especially following MI (Adler & Greenberg, 2004).

β-Adrenergic blockers have many adverse effects and are sometimes poorly tolerated. Adverse effects may include bradycardia, hypotension, wheezing, and GI complaints. Many patients also complain of weight gain, depression, and sexual dysfunction. β-Adrenergic blockers should be avoided by patients with asthma and used cautiously by patients with diabetes because their effects mask signs of hypoglycemia. β-Adrenergic blockers should not be discontinued abruptly without medical supervision because this may precipitate an increase in the frequency and intensity of angina attacks (Lehne, 2012).

Calcium Channel Blockers. If use of β-adrenergic blockers is contraindicated or if they are poorly tolerated or do not control anginal symptoms, calcium channel blockers are used (e.g., nifedipine, verapamil, diltiazem [Cardizem]) (Lehne, 2012). These drugs are also used to manage Prinzmetal's angina. Most of these agents are available in sustained-release formulations for longer action, which has the advantages of helping increase patient adherence to therapy and stabilizing blood levels of the drug. The three primary effects of calcium channel blockers are (a) systemic vasodilation with decreased SVR, (b) decreased myocardial contractility, and (c) coronary vasodilation.

Cardiac muscle and vascular smooth muscle cells are more dependent on extracellular calcium than are skeletal muscles and are therefore more sensitive to calcium channel blockers. Calcium channel blockers cause smooth muscle relaxation and relative vasodilation of coronary and systemic arteries, thus increasing blood flow.

Calcium channel blockers potentiate the action of digoxin by increasing serum digoxin levels during the first week of therapy. Therefore, serum digoxin levels should be closely monitored after starting this therapy. The patient should be taught the signs and symptoms of digoxin toxicity.

Angiotensin-Converting Enzyme Inhibitors. Certain high-risk patients with chronic stable angina may benefit from the addition of an angiotensin-converting enzyme (ACE) inhibitor (e.g., captopril) to the drug regimen (Lehne, 2012). Such patients include those with diabetes, significant CAD as determined by coronary angiography (e.g., multivessel disease), and/or previous history of MI with left ventricular dysfunction. (ACE inhibitors are discussed later in this chapter and in Chapter 35 and Table 35-8.)

Diagnostic Studies

When a patient has a history of CAD or if CAD is suspected, the physician orders a variety of studies (see Figure 36-7). After a detailed health history is documented and a physical examination is performed, a chest radiograph is usually taken to look for cardiac enlargement, aortic calcifications, and pulmonary congestion. A 12-lead ECG is obtained and, when possible, compared with an earlier tracing. Certain laboratory tests (e.g., lipid profile) and diagnostic studies (e.g., Holter monitoring, echocardiography) are ordered to confirm CAD and identify specific risk factors for CAD.

For patients with known CAD and chronic stable angina, common diagnostic studies include 12-lead ECG, echocardiography, exercise stress testing, pharmacological nuclear imaging, and coronary angiography (Pagana & Pagana, 2009). (See Chapter 34 and Table 34-5 for a discussion of these studies, including nursing considerations.) Electrocardiography and coronary angiography are discussed in further detail in the section on diagnostic tests.

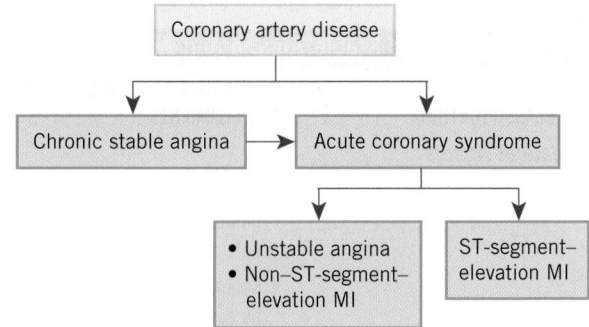

Figure 36-7 Relationships among coronary artery disease, chronic stable angina, and acute coronary syndrome. *MI*, myocardial infarction.

Source: Braunwald, E., Zipes, D., Libby, D., & Bonow, R. (Eds.), (2005). *Braunwald's heart disease: A textbook of cardiovascular medicine* (7th ed.). St. Louis: W. B. Saunders.

Acute Coronary Syndrome

When myocardial ischemia is prolonged and not immediately reversible, **acute coronary syndrome (ACS)** develops; this syndrome encompasses the spectrum of unstable angina, non–ST-segment–elevation myocardial infarction (NSTEMI), and ST-segment–elevation myocardial infarction (STEMI; Figure 36-7). Although each remains a distinct diagnosis, this nomenclature (ACS) reflects the relationships among pathophysiology, diagnosis, prognosis, and interventions for these disorders.

Etiology and Pathophysiology

ACS is associated with deterioration of an atherosclerotic plaque that was once stable. The plaque ruptures, exposing the intima to blood and stimulating platelet aggregation and local vasoconstriction with thrombus formation. This unstable lesion may be partially occluded by a thrombus (manifesting as unstable angina or NSTEMI) or totally occluded by a thrombus (manifesting as STEMI; Libby et al., 2008). What causes a coronary plaque to suddenly become unstable is not well understood, but systemic inflammation (described earlier) is thought to play a role. Patients with suspected ACS require immediate hospitalization.

Manifestations of Acute Coronary Syndrome

Unstable Angina

Chest pain that is new in onset, occurs at rest, or has a worsening pattern is called **unstable angina (UA)**. The patient with chronic stable angina may develop UA, or UA may be the first clinical manifestation of CAD. Unlike chronic stable angina, UA is unpredictable and represents an emergency. Patients with previously diagnosed chronic stable angina describe a significant change in the pattern of angina. It occurs with increasing frequency and is easily provoked by minimal or no exertion, during sleep, or even at rest. Patients without previously diagnosed angina describe

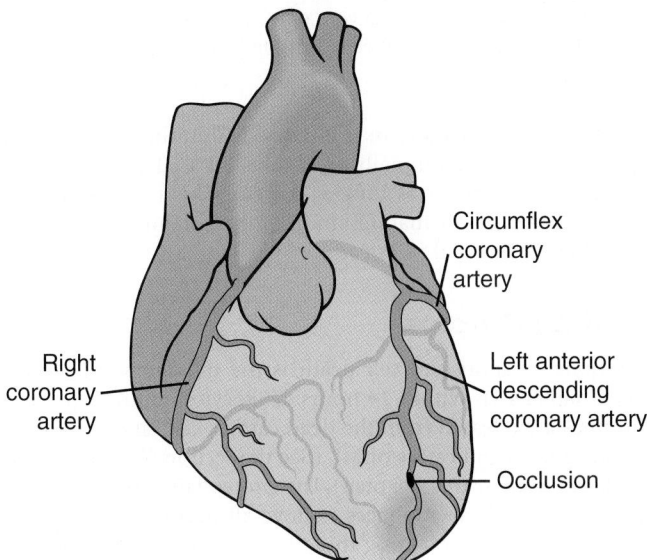

Figure 36-8 Diagram of occlusion of the left anterior descending coronary artery, which results in a myocardial infarction.

Source: Courtesy Mayo Clinic, Rochester, Minnesota.

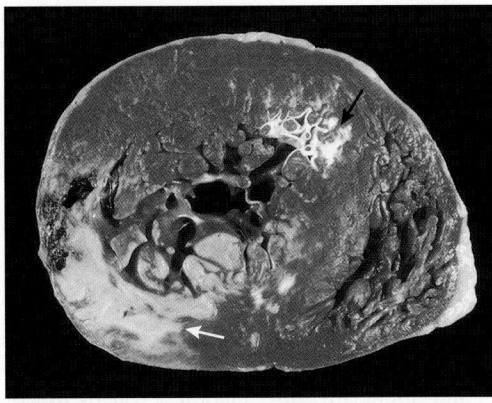

Figure 36-9 Acute myocardial infarction in the posterolateral wall of the left ventricle. This is demonstrated by the absence of staining in the areas of necrosis *(white arrow)*. Note the scarring from a previous anterior wall myocardial infarction *(black arrow)*.

Source: Kumar, V., Abbas, A. K., Fausto, N., & Aster, J. C. (2010). *Robbins and Cochran pathologic basis of disease* (8th ed., p. 6, from Figure 1-2). Philadelphia: W. B. Saunders.

anginal pain that has progressed rapidly in the past few hours, days, or weeks, often culminating in pain at rest (Libby et al., 2008).

Women with symptoms of UA seek medical attention more often than do men. Studies have shown that women have prodromal symptoms that are early manifestations of CAD, but because they are not recognized as such, what brings these women to first seek care is UA, before CAD is diagnosed (McSweeney et al., 2003). These symptoms include fatigue, shortness of breath, indigestion, and anxiety. Fatigue is the most prominent symptom. Because fatigue can be a symptom of many different diseases and syndromes, a thorough history of CAD risk factors should be obtained to identify these women.

Myocardial Infarction

A **myocardial infarction (MI)** occurs as a result of sustained ischemia, causing irreversible myocardial cell death (necrosis; Figures 36-8 and 36-9). Between 80 and 90% of all acute MIs occur secondary to thrombus formation (Libby et al., 2008). When a thrombus develops, perfusion to the myocardium distal to the occlusion is halted, resulting in necrosis. Contractile function of the heart stops in the necrotic areas. The degree of altered function depends on the area of the heart involved and the size of the infarction. Most MIs involve some portion of the left ventricle.

The acute MI process takes time. Cardiac cells can withstand ischemic conditions for approximately 20 minutes before cellular death begins. The tissue to become ischemic earliest is the subendocardium (the innermost layer of tissue in the cardiac muscle). If ischemia persists, the entire thickness of the heart muscle becomes necrosed in approximately 5 to 6 hours (Figure 36-10).

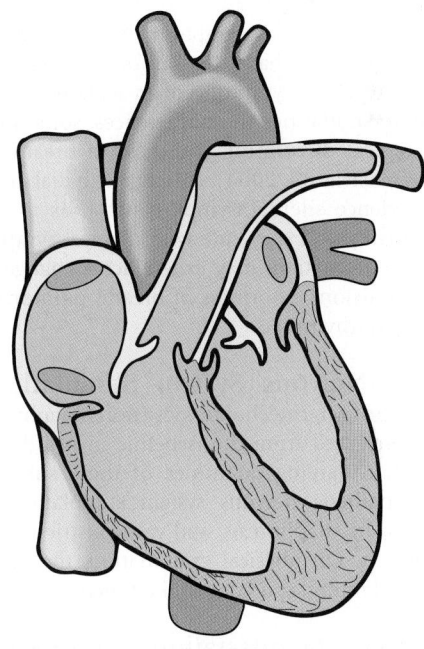

Figure 36-10 Diagram of myocardial infarction involving the full thickness of the left ventricular wall *(grey area)*.

Source: Courtesy Mayo Clinic, Rochester, Minnesota.

Descriptions of infarctions are usually based on the location of damage (e.g., anterior, inferior, lateral, or posterior wall infarction). Damage can occur in more than one location (e.g., anterolateral MI, anteroseptal MI). The location of the infarction correlates with the involved coronary circulation. For example, inferior wall infarctions result from occlusions in the right coronary artery. Anterior wall infarctions result from occlusions in the left anterior descending artery. Occlusions in the left circumflex artery usually cause MIs in the lateral or posterior wall or both.

The degree of pre-established collateral circulation also influences the severity of infarction (see Figure 36-2). In an individual with a history of CAD, collateral circulation may be established, and so the area surrounding the infarction site has developed a blood supply. This is one explanation why a younger person who has an MI is often likely to have a more serious impairment than an older person with the same degree of occlusion.

Clinical Manifestations of Myocardial Infarction

Pain. Severe, immobilizing chest pain not relieved by rest, position change, or nitrate administration is the hallmark of an MI. Persistent and unlike any other pain, it is usually described as a feeling of heaviness, pressure, tightness, burning, or constriction or as a crushing sensation. Common locations are substernal, retrosternal, and epigastric areas. The pain may radiate to the neck, the jaw, and the arms or to the back (see Figure 36-6). It may occur while the patient is active or at rest or when the patient is asleep or awake. However, it commonly occurs in the early morning hours. It usually lasts for 20 minutes or more and is described as more severe than usual anginal pain. When epigastric pain is present, the patient may relate it to indigestion and take antacids without relief.

Not everyone has classic symptoms. Some patients may not experience pain but may have "discomfort," weakness, or shortness of breath. Although symptoms of an acute MI in women and men have more similarities than differences, some women may experience atypical discomfort, shortness of breath, or fatigue (Deaton & Namasivayam, 2004). Patients with diabetes are more likely to experience silent (asymptomatic) MIs as a result of cardiac neuropathy and seek care with atypical symptoms (e.g., dyspnea). An older patient may experience a change in mental status (e.g., confusion), shortness of breath, pulmonary edema, dizziness, or a dysrhythmia.

Sympathetic Nervous System Stimulation. During the initial phase of MI, catecholamines (norepinephrine and epinephrine) are released from the ischemic myocardial cells that normally contain varying quantities of these substances. The increased sympathetic nervous system stimulation results in release of glycogen, diaphoresis, and vasoconstriction of peripheral blood vessels. On physical examination, the patient's skin may be ashen, clammy, and cool to the touch.

Cardiovascular Manifestations. In response to the release of catecholamines, the BP and HR may initially be elevated. Later, the BP may drop because of decreased cardiac output (CO). If the drop is severe enough, renal perfusion and urine output may decrease. Crackles may be noted in the lungs, persisting for several hours to several days, which are suggestive of left ventricular dysfunction. Jugular venous distension, hepatic engorgement, and peripheral edema may indicate right ventricular dysfunction.

Cardiac examination may reveal abnormal heart sounds that may seem distant. Careful auscultation may reveal splitting of heart sounds. Other abnormal sounds suggestive of ventricular dysfunction are S3 and S4. In addition, a loud holosystolic murmur may develop and may indicate a septal defect or mitral valve dysfunction.

Nausea and Vomiting. The patient may be nauseated and vomit. Nausea and vomiting can result from reflex stimulation of the vomiting centre by the severe pain. These symptoms can also result from vasovagal reflexes initiated from the area of the infarcted myocardium.

Fever. The temperature may increase within the first 24 hours up to 38°C and occasionally as high as 39°C. The temperature elevation may last for as long as 1 week. This increase in temperature is a systemic manifestation of the inflammatory process caused by myocardial cell death.

Healing Process

The body's response to cell death is the inflammatory process (see Chapter 14). Within 24 hours, leukocytes infiltrate the area. Enzymes are released from the dead cardiac cells and are important diagnostic indicators of MI. (See the section "Serum Cardiac Markers" later in this chapter.) The proteolytic enzymes of the neutrophils and macrophages remove all necrotic tissue by the second or third day. During this time, the necrotic muscle wall is thin. The development of collateral circulation improves areas of poor perfusion and may limit the zones of injury and infarction. Once infarction takes place, catecholamine-mediated lipolysis and glycogenolysis occur. These processes allow the increased amounts of plasma glucose and free fatty acids to be used by the oxygen-depleted myocardium for anaerobic metabolism. For this reason, serum glucose levels are frequently elevated after MI.

The necrotic zone is identifiable by ECG changes (e.g., ST-segment elevation, pathological Q wave) and on nuclear scanning after the onset of symptoms. At this point, the neutrophils and monocytes have cleared the necrotic debris from the injured area, and the collagen matrix that will eventually form scar tissue is laid down.

Ten to 14 days after MI, the scar tissue beginning to form is still weak. The myocardium is considered to be especially vulnerable to increased stress because of the unstable state of the healing heart wall. It is also at this time that the patient's activity level may be increasing, and so special caution and assessment is necessary. By 6 weeks after MI, scar tissue has replaced necrotic tissue. At this time, the injured area is said to be healed. The scarred area is often less malleable than the surrounding fibres. This condition may be manifested by uncoordinated wall motion, ventricular dysfunction, or pump failure (Libby et al., 2008).

These changes in the infarcted muscle also cause changes in the unaffected myocardium. In an attempt to compensate for the infarcted muscle, the normal myocardium hypertrophies and dilates. This process is called *ventricular remodelling*. Remodelling of normal myocardium can lead to the development of late heart failure (HF), especially in individuals with atherosclerosis of other coronary arteries, an anterior MI, or both.

Complications of Myocardial Infarction

Dysrhythmias. The most common complication after an MI is a dysrhythmia, which is present in 80% of patients who have had an MI. Dysrhythmias are the most common cause of death in patients in the prehospitalization period. Dysrhythmias are caused by any condition that affects the myocardial cell's sensitivity to nerve impulses, such as ischemia, electrolyte imbalances, and sympathetic nervous system stimulation. The intrinsic rhythm of the heartbeat is disrupted, causing a fast HR (tachycardia), a slow HR (bradycardia), or an irregular beat, all of which adversely affect the ischemic myocardium.

Life-threatening dysrhythmias occur most often with anterior wall infarction, HF, or shock. Complete heart block can occur in massive infarction. Ventricular fibrillation, a common cause of sudden cardiac death, is a lethal dysrhythmia that most often occurs within the first 4 hours after the onset of pain. Premature ventricular contractions (PVCs) may precede ventricular tachycardia and fibrillation. Life-threatening ventricular dysrhythmias must be treated immediately. (See Chapter 38 for a detailed description of dysrhythmias and their management.)

Heart Failure. Heart failure is a complication of MI in which the pumping power of the heart has diminished. Depending on the severity and extent of the injury, HF occurs initially with subtle signs such as mild dyspnea, restlessness, agitation, or slight tachycardia. Other signs indicating the onset of HF include pulmonary congestion, seen on chest radiograph; S3 or S4 heart sounds, heard on auscultation, crackles, heard on auscultation of breath sounds; and jugular vein distension, caused by right-sided HF. (The treatment of acute decompensated HF is discussed in Chapter 37.)

Cardiogenic Shock. Cardiogenic shock is a condition in which inadequate oxygen and nutrients are supplied to the tissues because of severe left ventricular failure. Cardiogenic shock has occurred less often since the advent of early and rapid treatment of MI with percutaneous coronary intervention (PCI) and fibrinolytic therapy. The rate of mortality from cardiogenic shock is high. Cardiogenic shock necessitates aggressive management, including control of dysrhythmias, intra-aortic balloon pump (IABP) therapy, and support of contractility with the use of vasoactive drugs. The goal of therapy is to maximize oxygen delivery, reduce oxygen demand, and prevent complications such as acute renal failure (Libby et al., 2008). (Cardiogenic shock is discussed in Chapter 69.)

Papillary Muscle Dysfunction. Papillary muscle dysfunction may occur if the infarcted area includes or is adjacent to the papillary muscle that attaches to the mitral valve (see Figure 34-2). Papillary muscle dysfunction causes mitral valve regurgitation, which increases the volume of blood in the left atrium. This condition aggravates an already compromised left ventricle by reducing CO even further. Papillary muscle dysfunction is detected by a systolic murmur at the cardiac apex radiating toward the axilla.

Papillary muscle rupture is a rare but life-threatening complication that causes massive mitral valve regurgitation, which results in dyspnea, pulmonary edema, and decreased CO. The patient's condition deteriorates rapidly. Treatment consists of rapid afterload reduction with nitroprusside, IABP therapy and immediate open heart surgery with mitral valve replacement, or both. (See Chapter 39 for discussion of valve disorders.)

Ventricular Aneurysm. Ventricular aneurysm results when the infarcted myocardial wall becomes thinned and bulges out during contraction. The patient with a ventricular aneurysm may experience refractory HF, dysrhythmias, and angina. Besides ventricular rupture, which is fatal, ventricular aneurysms harbour thrombi, which can cause an embolic stroke.

Pericarditis. Acute pericarditis—an inflammation of the visceral or parietal pericardium or both—may result in cardiac compression, decreased ventricular filling and emptying, and HF.

It may occur 2 to 3 days after an acute MI as a common complication. Pericarditis is characterized by chest pain, which may vary from mild to severe and is aggravated by inspiration, coughing, and movement of the upper body. The pain may be relieved by sitting in a forward position. The pain is usually different from the pain associated with an MI.

Assessment of the patient with pericarditis may reveal a friction rub over the pericardium. The sound may be best heard with the diaphragm of the stethoscope at the midsternal to lower sternal border. It may be persistent or intermittent. Fever may also be present.

Diagnosis of pericarditis can be made with serial 12-lead ECGs. Characteristic ECG changes are diffuse and reflect the inflammation of the pericardium. Treatment may include pain relief by aspirin, corticosteroids, or NSAIDs. (Pericarditis is discussed further in Chapter 39.)

Dressler's Syndrome. Dressler's syndrome is characterized by pericarditis with effusion and fever that develops 4 to 6 weeks after MI. It may also occur after open heart surgery. It is thought to be caused by an antigen–antibody reaction to the necrotic myocardium. The patient experiences pericardial pain, fever, a friction rub, pleural effusion, and arthralgia. Laboratory findings include an elevated white blood cell count and an elevated sedimentation rate. Short-term courses of corticosteroids are used to treat this condition. (Dressler's syndrome is discussed further in Chapter 39.)

Diagnostic Studies

Unstable Angina and Myocardial Infarction

In addition to the patient's history of pain, risk factors, and health history, the primary diagnostic studies used to determine whether a person has UA or an MI include an ECG and measurement of serum cardiac markers (see Figure 36-6).

Electrocardiographic Findings. ECG is the primary tool to rule out or confirm UA or an MI. Changes in the QRS complex, the ST segment, and the T wave caused by ischemia and infarction can develop quickly with UA and MI. For diagnostic and treatment purposes, it is important to distinguish among STEMI, UA and NSTEMI. Patients with STEMI tend to have a more extensive MI associated with prolonged and complete coronary occlusion and the development of a pathological Q wave on the ECG. Patients with UA or NSTEMI usually have transient thrombosis or incomplete coronary occlusion and usually do not develop pathological Q waves. Areas of ischemia or infarction may be noted on the ECG. Because MI is a dynamic process that evolves with time, the ECG often reveals the time sequence of ischemia, injury, infarction, and resolution of the infarction.

The ECG may also be normal or nondiagnostic when the patient comes to the ED with a complaint of chest pain. Within a few hours, the ECG may change to reflect the infarction process. These changes take place when cellular damage has occurred, interrupting the normal electrical depolarization of the ventricles. When the initial ECG is nondiagnostic, serial ECGs are obtained every 2 to 4 hours (Aehlert, 2011). (See Chapter 38 for discussion of ECG changes associated with ischemia and MI.)

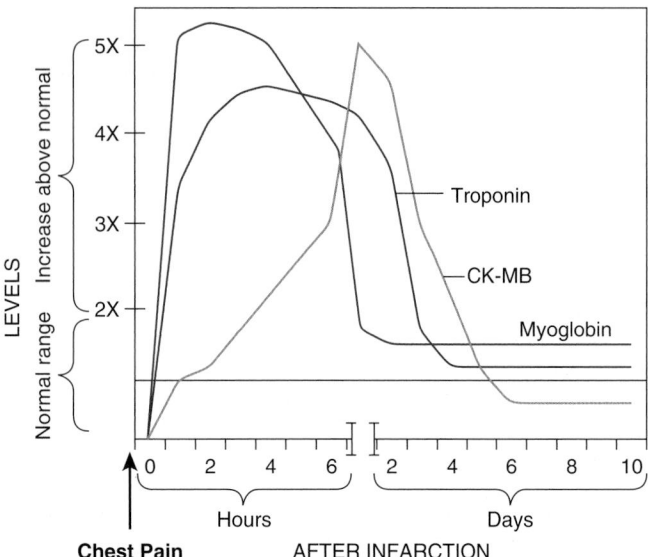

Figure 36-11 Levels of serum cardiac markers in the blood after myocardial infarction. *CK-MB*, MB isoenzyme of creatine kinase.

Serum Cardiac Markers. Certain proteins called *serum cardiac markers* are released into the blood in large quantities from necrotic heart muscle after an MI. These markers, specifically serum cardiac enzymes and troponin, are important in the diagnosis of MI. When cardiac cells die, their intracellular enzymes are released into circulation. The increase in serum cardiac markers that occurs after cellular death can indicate whether cardiac damage is present and the approximate extent of the damage. Creatine kinase (CK) and troponin are typically measured to diagnose an MI. (Figure 36-11 indicates the peak levels and durations of these markers in the presence of MI.)

CK levels begin to rise approximately 3 to 12 hours after an MI, peak in 24 hours, and return to normal within 2 to 3 days. The CK enzymes may be fractionated into bands, including the MB band. The MB isoenzyme of creatine kinase (CK-MB) band is specific to myocardial cells and can help quantify myocardial damage.

Cardiac-specific troponin is a myocardial muscle protein released into circulation after myocardial injury. In the heart, there are two subtypes: cardiac-specific troponin T (cTnT) and cardiac-specific troponin I (cTnI). These markers are highly specific indicators of MI and their tests have greater sensitivity and specificity for myocardial injury than that for CK-MB (Pagana & Pagana, 2009). The troponin level rises as quickly as the CK level. Troponins are usually measured for diagnostic purposes in conjunction with total CK and the MB fraction. Serum levels of cTnI and cTnT increase 3 to 12 hours after the onset of MI, peak at 24 to 48 hours, and return to baseline over 5 to 14 days.

Myoglobin is released into circulation within a few hours after an MI. Although it is one of the first serum cardiac markers whose levels increase after an MI, it lacks cardiac specificity. In addition, it is rapidly excreted in urine so that blood levels return to normal range within 24 hours after an MI (see Chapter 34, Table 34-5).

Coronary Angiography. The patient with UA or NSTEMI may undergo coronary angiography to evaluate the extent of the

disease and to determine the most appropriate therapeutic modality. If appropriate, percutaneous coronary intervention (PCI) may be performed at this time. Other patients may be treated with conservative medical management. Coronary angiography is the only way to confirm the diagnosis of Prinzmetal's angina.

Other Measures

When the ECG and serum cardiac marker levels do not confirm MI, other measures for diagnosing UA may be considered (see Chapter 34, Table 34-5). Exercise stress testing and echocardiography may be conducted when a patient has an abnormal but nondiagnostic baseline ECG. Dobutamine stress echocardiography can be performed in patients unable to exercise. (See Chapter 34 for additional information on cardiac assessment.)

Collaborative Care

It is extremely important that ACS be rapidly diagnosed and treated to preserve cardiac muscle. Initial management of chest pain most often occurs in the ED. Emergency care of the patient with chest pain is described in Table 36-14. An IV route is established to provide an accessible means for emergency drug therapy. Sublingual nitroglycerin and aspirin (chewable) are administered if this was not done by emergency medical personnel before arrival at the ED. Morphine sulphate is given by IV route for pain unrelieved by nitroglycerin. Oxygen is administered by nasal cannula at a rate of 2 to 4 L/min. Patients usually receive ongoing care in a critical care unit or telemetry unit, in which continuous ECG monitoring is available. Dysrhythmias may be detected, and appropriate treatment can be instituted. The collaborative care of ACS is described in Figure 36-6.

Vital signs, including pulse oximetry, are monitored frequently during the first few hours after admission and are monitored closely thereafter. Bed rest and limitation of activity for 12 to 24 hours are initially ordered, with a gradual increase in activity unless it is contraindicated.

For patients with UA or NSTEMI who have increased levels of cardiac markers and ongoing angina, a combination of aspirin, heparin (unfractionated [UH] or low–molecular weight [LMWH]), and a glycoprotein IIb and IIIa inhibitor (e.g., abciximab [ReoPro], eptifibatide [Integrilin], tirofiban [Aggrastat]) is recommended. **Percutaneous coronary intervention (PCI)**—an intervention to treat CAD in which a catheter equipped with an inflatable balloon tip is inserted into a narrowed coronary artery and the balloon is inflated—is a common elective procedure considered once the patient is stabilized and angina is controlled, or if angina returns or increases in severity.

For patients with STEMI or NSTEMI with elevated levels of cardiac markers, reperfusion therapy is initiated (see Figure 36-6). Reperfusion therapy can include emergent PCI or fibrinolytic (thrombolytic) therapy. The goal in the treatment of MI is to salvage as much myocardial muscle as possible.

Emergent Percutaneous Coronary Intervention

In centres performing at least 200 PCI procedures a year and that have trained interventional cardiologists and cardiac surgical capability, emergent PCI is recommended as the first

EMERGENCY MANAGEMENT

Table 36-14 Chest Pain

ETIOLOGY	ASSESSMENT FINDINGS	INTERVENTIONS
Cardiovascular	• Pain in chest, neck, arm, or shoulder	**Initial**
• Angina	• Cold, clammy skin	• Ensure patent airway.
• Myocardial infarction	• Diaphoresis	• Administer O₂ by nasal cannula or non-rebreather mask.
• Dysrhythmia	• Nausea and vomiting	• Obtain 12-lead ECG.
• Pericarditis	• Epigastric pain	• Insert two IV catheters.
• Aortic aneurysm	• Indigestion or heartburn	• Assess pain, using "PQRST" mnemonic (see Table 36-10).
• Aortic valve disease	• Dyspnea	• Medicate for pain as ordered (e.g., morphine, nitroglycerin).
Respiratory	• Weakness	• Initiate continuous ECG monitoring and identify underlying rhythm.
• Costochondritis	• Anxiety	• Obtain baseline blood test results (e.g., cardiac markers).
• Pleurisy	• Feeling of impending doom	• Obtain portable chest radiograph.
• Pneumonia	• Tachycardia	• Assess for antiplatelet, anticoagulation, or fibrinolytic therapy or for PCI as appropriate.
• Pneumothorax	• Irregular HR, murmurs	• Administer aspirin and β-adrenergic blockers for cardiac-related chest pain unless contraindicated.
• Pulmonary edema	• Palpitations	• Administer antidysrhythmic drugs as indicated.
• Pulmonary embolus	• Dysrhythmias	
Chest Trauma	• Decreased BP	**Ongoing Monitoring**
• Rib or sternal fracture	• Narrowed pulse pressure	• Monitor vital signs, level of consciousness, cardiac rhythm, and O₂ saturation.
• Flail chest	• Unequal BP readings in upper extremities	• Monitor response to medications (e.g., decrease in chest pain) and readminister or titrate medications (e.g., nitroglycerin) as needed.
• Cardiac tamponade	• Syncope, loss of consciousness	• Provide reassurance and emotional support to patient and family.
• Pneumothorax	• Decreased O₂ saturation	• Explain all interventions and procedures to patient in simple terms.
• Pulmonary contusion	• Decreased or absent breath sounds	• Anticipate need for intubation if respiratory distress is evident.
• Great vessel injury	• Crackles, wheezes	• Prepare for CPR, defibrillation, transcutaneous pacing, or cardioversion.
Gastrointestinal	• Pericardial friction rub	
• Esophagitis		
• GERD		
• Hiatal hernia		
• Peptic ulcer		
• Cholecystitis		
Others		
• Stress		
• Strenuous exercise		
• Drugs		
• Acute anxiety		

BP, blood pressure; *CPR*, cardiopulmonary resuscitation; *GERD*, gastroesophageal reflux disease; *HR*, heart rate; *IV*, intravenous; *PCI*, percutaneous coronary intervention.

line of treatment for patients with confirmed MI (i.e., definitive ECG changes, presence of cardiac markers, or both). The goal is to open the affected artery within 90 minutes of the patient's arrival at the ED. In this situation, the patient undergoes cardiac catheterization to locate the blockage or blockages, to assess the severity of the blockages, to determine the presence of collateral circulation, and to evaluate left ventricular function. With actual visualization of the coronary artery system and left ventricular function, treatment modalities most beneficial to the patient can be selected. Usually PCI with the placement of one or more drug-eluting stents will be performed. Patients with severe left ventricular dysfunction may require the addition of IABP therapy, and a small percentage of patients

may require emergency coronary artery bypass graft (CABG) surgery.

The advantages of PCI are that (a) it is an alternative to surgical intervention; (b) it is performed with the use of local anaesthetic; (c) the patient is ambulatory 24 hours after the procedure; (d) the length of hospital stay is approximately 1 to 3 days compared with the 4- to 6-day stay necessary with CABG surgery, thus reducing hospital costs; and (e) the patient can make a rapid return to work (approximately 5 to 7 days after PCI) instead of the 2- to 8-week convalescence period after CABG.

PCI is performed more frequently than CABG surgery. Techniques have been developed to provide blood flow to the distal myocardium during balloon inflation, which increases the safety of the procedure. Dilation may also be performed for stenotic grafts from previous CABG surgery.

The most serious complication of PCI is dissection of the newly dilated coronary artery. If the damage is extensive, the coronary artery could rupture, which would cause cardiac tamponade, ischemia and infarction, decreased CO, and possibly death. There is also danger of infarction if the lesion is calcified and a portion of the plaque becomes dislodged and occludes the vessel distal to the catheter. Coronary spasm can occur from the mechanical irritation of the catheter or the balloon or from chemical irritation by the contrast medium used to visualize the artery. Abrupt closure is a complication that can occur in the first 24 hours after PCI. Re-stenosis after PCI can also occur, and risk is greatest in the first 30 days after the procedure. Nursing care of the patient after PCI is similar to that of cardiac catheterization (see Chapter 34, Table 34-5).

Fibrinolytic Therapy

Fibrinolytic therapy offers the advantages of availability and rapid administration in facilities that do not have an interventional cardiac catheterization laboratory or when the nearest one is too far away for safe transfer of the patient. Treatment of MI with fibrinolytic therapy is aimed at stopping the infarction process by dissolving the thrombus in the coronary artery and reperfusing the myocardium. To be of most benefit, fibrinolytic therapy must be given as soon as possible, ideally within the first hour, and preferably within the first 6 hours, after the onset of symptoms. When reperfusion occurs within 6 hours, the mortality rate is reduced by 25%.

Indications and Contraindications.

All fibrinolytics are given by IV (see Table 36-13). The choice of a thrombolytic agent is guided by considerations of cost, efficacy, and ease of administration. Although these drugs have different mechanisms of action and different pharmacokinetics, they all open the artery by lysis of the thrombus in the coronary artery. Administration of a fibrinolytic is targeted to occur within 30 minutes of the patient's arrival at the ED. Optimal outcomes can be achieved if the fibrinolytic is administered within 60 minutes after onset of symptoms (Lehne, 2012).

Because all the fibrinolytics produce lysis of the pathological clot, they may also lyse other clots (e.g., a postoperative site). Therefore, patients selection is important because minor or major bleeding can be a complication of therapy (Lehne, 2012). Inclusion criteria for fibrinolytic therapy include (a) chest pain typical of acute MI and less than 6 hours in duration, (b) 12-lead ECG findings consistent with acute MI, and (c) no absolute contraindications (Table 36-15).

Procedure.

Each hospital has its own protocol to follow for administration of fibrinolytic therapy. However, all protocols have several common factors. Blood for baseline laboratory studies is collected, two to three lines for IV therapy are started, and all other invasive procedures are performed before the fibrinolytic agent is given. This sequence reduces the possibility of bleeding in the patient.

Depending on the drug selected, therapy may be administered in one IV bolus or over time (30 to 90 minutes). The time at which therapy begins is noted, and the patient is monitored during and after administration. ECG, vital sign measurement, pulse oximetry, and heart and lung assessments are

Table 36-15 Contraindications for the Use of Fibrinolytic Therapy	
ABSOLUTE CONTRAINDICATIONS	**RELATIVE CONTRAINDICATIONS**
• Active internal bleeding or bleeding diathesis (except for menstruation)	• Active peptic ulcer disease
	• Current use of anticoagulants
• Known history of cerebral aneurysm or arteriovenous malformation	• Pregnancy
	• Prior ischemic stroke not within past 3 mo; dementia; or known intracranial disease not covered under absolute contraindications
• Known intracranial neoplasm (primary or metastatic)	
• Previous cerebral hemorrhage	• Surgery (including eye laser surgery) or puncture of noncompressible vessel within past 3 wk
• Ischemic stroke within past 3 mo	• Internal bleeding within past 2-4 wk
• Significant closed-head or facial trauma within past 3 mo	• Serious systemic disease (e.g., advanced or terminal cancer, severe liver or kidney disease)
• Suspected aortic dissection	• Severe uncontrolled hypertension (BP >180/110 mm Hg) on patient's arrival for care or chronic severe, poorly controlled hypertension
	• Traumatic or prolonged (>10 min) cardiopulmonary resuscitation

BP, blood pressure.

completed frequently to evaluate the patient's response to therapy. When reperfusion occurs (i.e., the coronary artery that was occluded is opened, and blood flow is restored to the myocardium), several clinical markers may change. The most reliable marker is the return of the ST segment to baseline values on the ECG. Other markers include a resolution of chest pain and a rapid rise of the CK-MB enzyme levels that occurs within 3 hours of therapy and peaks within 12 hours. The CK-MB levels increase as the necrotic myocardial cells release CK-MB enzymes into the circulation after perfusion has been restored to the area. The presence of reperfusion dysrhythmias (e.g., accelerated idioventricular rhythm) is a less reliable marker of reperfusion. These dysrhythmias are generally self-limiting and do not necessitate aggressive treatment. (See Chapter 38 for management of dysrhythmias.)

A major concern with fibrinolytic therapy is reocclusion of the artery. The site of the thrombus is unstable, and another clot may form or spasm of the artery may occur. Because of this possibility, most physicians begin IV heparin therapy. If another clot develops, the patient reports similar complaints of chest pain, and ECG changes return. The patient is re-evaluated and may receive a second dose of the fibrinolytic or be transferred to a cardiac catheterization laboratory for rescue PCI.

The major complication with fibrinolytic therapy is bleeding. Ongoing nursing assessment is essential. Minor bleeding (e.g., surface bleeding from IV sites or gingival bleeding) is expected and can be controlled by applying a pressure dressing or ice packs. If signs and symptoms of major bleeding occur (e.g., a drop in BP, an increase in HR, a sudden decrease in the patient's level of consciousness, blood in the urine or stool), the physician should be notified, and the therapy should be stopped.

Drug Therapy

IV nitroglycerin, aspirin, β-adrenergic blockers, and systemic anticoagulation with either subcutaneous LMWH or IV UH are the initial drug treatments of choice for ACS (Lehne, 2012). IV antiplatelet agents (e.g., glycoprotein IIb and IIIa inhibitor) may also be used if PCI is anticipated. ACE inhibitors are added for select patients after MI (discussed in the section on Angiotensin-Converting Enzyme Inhibitors). Calcium channel blockers or long-acting nitrates can be added if the patient is already receiving adequate doses of β-adrenergic blockers or cannot tolerate β-adrenergic blockers, or if the patient has Prinzmetal's angina (Lehne, 2012).

Drug therapy for patients with ACS is described in Table 36-13 and Figure 36-7. These drugs are discussed on pp. 905 to 908. ACS-specific drugs are discussed in the following sections.

Intravenous Nitroglycerin.

IV nitroglycerin is used in the initial treatment of patients with ACS. The goal of therapy is to reduce anginal pain and improve coronary blood flow. Nitroglycerin has an immediate onset of action and can be titrated to prevent, treat, and stop UA (Lehne, 2012).

IV nitroglycerin is used to decrease preload and afterload while increasing the myocardial oxygen supply. The dose is usually titrated to relieve pain. Because hypotension is a common adverse effect, BP is closely monitored during this time. Tolerance is another adverse effect of IV nitroglycerin therapy. An effective strategy to manage this phenomenon is to administer a lower dosage at night and during sleep and a higher dosage during the day.

Morphine Sulphate.

Morphine is given for chest pain that is unrelieved by nitroglycerin. As a vasodilator, it decreases cardiac workload by lowering myocardial oxygen consumption, reducing contractility, and decreasing BP and HR. In addition, morphine can help reduce anxiety and fear. In rare situations, morphine can depress respiration. Patients should be monitored for signs of bradypnea or hypoxia, a condition to be prevented when at all possible in myocardial ischemia and infarction.

β-Adrenergic Blockers.

IV β-adrenergic blockers should not be given to patients with STEMI. They may be considered for treatment of hypertension if patients have no contraindications such as heart failure or low cardiac output. Oral β-adrenergic blocker therapy should be initiated within 24 hours of STEMI in patients with no contraindications. β-Adrenergic blockers are used to decrease myocardial oxygen demand by reducing HR, BP, and contractility. (See Table 36-13 and Chapter 35, Table 35-8 for a discussion of β-adrenergic blockers.)

Angiotensin-Converting Enzyme Inhibitors.

ACE inhibitors (e.g., captopril) are recommended after anterior wall MIs or MIs that result in decreased left ventricular function (ejection fraction <40%) or pulmonary congestion (Libby et al., 2008). The use of ACE inhibitors can help prevent ventricular remodelling and prevent or slow the progression of HF. ACE inhibitor therapy should be continued indefinitely. For patients who cannot tolerate ACE inhibitors, angiotensin receptor blockers (e.g., losartan [Cozaar]) should be considered (Antman et al., 2004). (See Table 36-13 and Chapter 35, Table 35-8.)

Antidysrhythmia Medications.

Dysrhythmias are the most common complications after an MI. In general, they are not treated aggressively unless they are life-threatening. (The medications used in the treatment of dysrhythmias are discussed in Chapter 38.)

Cholesterol-Lowering Drugs.

A fasting lipid panel should be obtained for all patients admitted with ACS. Cholesterol-lowering drugs are recommended for all patients with elevated LDL cholesterol levels (see Tables 36-6 and 36-7).

Stool Softeners.

After an MI, the patient may be predisposed to constipation as a result of bed rest and opioid administration. Stool softeners such as docusate sodium (Colace) are given to facilitate and promote the comfort of bowel evacuation. This prevents straining and the resultant vagal stimulation from Valsalva's manoeuvre. Vagal stimulation produces bradycardia and can provoke dysrhythmias.

Nutritional Therapy

Initially, patients may be kept NPO (nothing by mouth) except for sips of water until stable (e.g., pain alleviated, nausea resolved). Diet is advanced as tolerated to one of low salt, low saturated fats, and low cholesterol.

Coronary Surgical Revascularization

Coronary revascularization with PCI or CABG surgery is performed, when a coronary lesion is amenable to these procedures, to allow blood flow to the affected myocardium. CABG is recommended for patients (a) who do not achieve satisfactory improvement with medical management, (b) who have left main coronary artery or three-vessel disease, (c) who are not candidates for PCI (e.g., lesions are long or difficult to access), or (d) in whom PCI has failed and chest pain is ongoing (Eagle et al., 2004).

Coronary Artery Bypass Graft Surgery.

CABG surgery consists of the construction of new conduits (vessels to transport blood) between the aorta, or other major arteries, and the myocardium distal to the obstructed coronary artery (or arteries). The procedure involves one or more grafts from the internal mammary artery, the saphenous vein, the radial artery, the gastroepiploic artery, the inferior epigastric artery, or some combination.

CABG surgery necessitates a sternotomy (opening of the chest cavity) and the use of cardiopulmonary bypass (CPB). CPB involves diverting (bypassing) the patient's blood from the heart to the CPB machine. Blood is oxygenated in the machine and then returned (via a pump) to the patient. In this way, vital organs are perfused while the surgeon operates on a nonbeating, bloodless heart.

The internal mammary artery (IMA) is the most common artery used for bypass graft. The left or the right IMA (or both) is left attached to its origin (the subclavian artery) and dissected from the chest wall. It is then anastomosed (connected with sutures) to the coronary artery distal to the stenosis. The long-term patency rate for IMA grafts is 90% after 10 years (Eagle et al., 2004; Figure 36-12).

The saphenous vein is also used for bypass grafts. It is removed from one or both legs, and sections are anastomosed proximally to the ascending aorta and to a coronary artery distal to the blockage. Saphenous vein grafts do develop diffuse intimal hyperplasia, which contributes to future stenosis and graft occlusions. The use of antiplatelet therapy and statins after surgery has improved vein graft patency. The patency rate of saphenous vein grafts is 66% at 10 years. When vein grafts do become stenosed, a **stent**

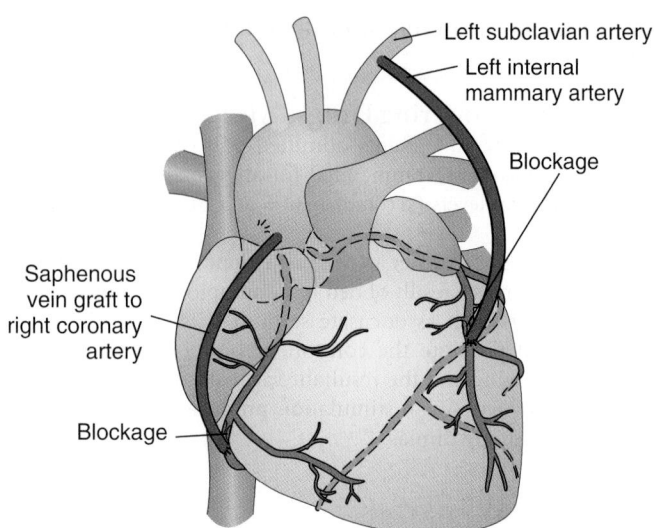

Figure 36-12 The distal end of the left internal mammary artery is grafted below the area of blockage in the left anterior descending artery. The proximal end of the saphenous vein is grafted to the aorta, and the distal end is grafted below the area of blockage in the right coronary artery.

Source: Bucher, L., & Melander, S. (1999). *Critical care nursing*. Philadelphia: Saunders.

may be used to open occlusions; these are expandable, meshlike structures designed to maintain vessel patency by compressing the arterial walls and resisting vasoconstriction.

Use of the radial artery for bypass graft has become of interest. The radial artery is a thick, muscular artery that is prone to spasm when mechanically stimulated. Perioperative calcium channel blockers and long-acting nitrates are used to control this complication. Early studies show patency rates at 5 years to be as high as 84%. There have been no reports of extremity complications (e.g., hand ischemia, wound infection) after the dissection of this artery (Eagle et al., 2004).

For patients who have previously undergone CABG surgery, the gastroepiploic or inferior epigastric artery can be used. These arteries are excellent conduits. However, the dissection of the arteries is extensive, increasing the length of surgery and the risk for wound complications at the harvest site, especially in obese or diabetic patients. Many patients require reoperation; therefore, research on the use of alternative arteries (e.g., bovine IMAs) and veins (e.g., umbilical veins) and synthetic grafts (e.g., Dacron grafts), will become increasingly important (Eagle et al., 2004).

CABG surgery remains a palliative treatment for CAD and not a cure. Studies have demonstrated improved patient outcomes, quality of life, and survival rates after CABG surgery. However, postoperative complications and the rate of mortality increases as a function of age. The operative mortality rate is higher among women than among men. This has been attributed to the delay in treatment of CAD in women: Women seek care at an older age and when they are already more ill (e.g., have decreased left ventricular function) at the time of surgery. Other possible causes include the fact that women's coronary vessels have smaller diameters and the less frequent use of the IMA.

Minimally Invasive Direct Coronary Artery Bypass.

With efforts to reduce cost, length of hospital stay, and morbidity, newer approaches to CABG surgery have been developed. Minimally invasive direct coronary artery bypass (MIDCAB) is a technique that offers the patient with single-vessel disease (i.e., left anterior descending or right-sided CAD) an approach to surgical treatment that does not involve a sternotomy and CPB.

The technique entails several small incisions between the ribs. A thoracoscope is used to dissect the IMA. The heart is slowed by means of a β-adrenergic blocker (e.g., esmolol [Brevibloc]) or stopped temporarily with adenosine (Adenocard), and a mechanical stabilizer is used to immobilize the anastomosis site. The IMA is then sutured to the left anterior descending artery or the right coronary artery. A radial artery or saphenous vein graft may be used if the IMA is not available.

Off-Pump Coronary Artery Bypass. In the off-pump coronary artery bypass (OPCAB) procedure, full or partial sternotomy enables access to all coronary vessels. OPCAB is also performed on a beating heart with the use of mechanical stabilizers and without CPB.

NURSING MANAGEMENT: CHRONIC STABLE ANGINA AND ACUTE CORONARY SYNDROME

▪ Nursing Assessment

Subjective and objective data that should be obtained from a patient with ACS are listed in Table 36-16.

▪ Nursing Diagnoses

Nursing diagnoses for the patient with ACS may include, but are not limited to, those presented in Nursing Care Plan 36-1.

▪ Planning

The overall goals for a patient with ACS include (a) relief of pain, (b) preservation of the myocardium, (c) immediate and appropriate treatment of ischemia, (d) effective coping with illness-associated anxiety, (e) participation in a rehabilitation plan, and (f) reduction of risk factors.

▪ Nursing Implementation: Chronic Stable Angina

▪ Health Promotion

Behaviours to reduce the risk for CAD are presented in Table 36-4 and discussed on pp. 899 to 903.

▪ Acute Intervention

If a nurse is present during an anginal attack, the following measures should be instituted: (a) administration of supplemental oxygen; (b) measurement of vital signs; (c) 12-lead ECG; (d) prompt pain relief, first with a nitrate and, if necessary, followed by an opioid analgesic; (e) auscultation of heart sounds; and (f)

NURSING ASSESSMENT

Table 36-16 Acute Coronary Syndrome

Subjective Data

Important Health Information

Current health history: Family history of heart disease; sedentary lifestyle; tobacco use

Past health history: Previous history of CAD, angina, MI, aortic stenosis, HF, or cardiomyopathy; hypertension; diabetes; anemia; lung disease; hyperlipidemia

Medications: Use of aspirin, nitrates, β-adrenergic blockers, calcium channel blockers, angiotensin-converting enzyme inhibitors; antihypertensive drugs; cholesterol-lowering drugs; vitamin or herbal supplements

Symptoms

- Substernal chest pain or pressure (squeezing, constricting, aching, sharp, tingling), possible radiation to jaw, neck, shoulders, back, or arms

- Indigestion, heartburn, nausea, belching, vomiting

- Palpitations, dyspnea, dizziness, weakness

- Fatigue, anxiety, feeling of impending doom

Objective Data

General

Anxiety, fear, restlessness

Integumentary

Cool, clammy, pale skin

Cardiovascular

Tachycardia or bradycardia, pulsus alternans (alternating weak and strong heartbeats), dysrhythmias (especially ventricular), S3, S4, higher or lower BP, murmur

Possible Findings

Elevated or nonelevated levels of serum cardiac markers, increased levels of serum lipids; increased WBC count; positive results of exercise stress test and thallium scans; ST-segment and T-wave abnormalities on ECG; cardiac enlargement, calcifications, or pulmonary congestion on chest radiograph; evidence of abnormal wall motion on stress echocardiogram; positive findings on coronary angiogram

BP, blood pressure; *CAD,* coronary artery disease; *ECG,* electrocardiogram; *HF,* heart failure; *MI,* myocardial infarction; *WBC,* white blood cell.

comfortable positioning of the patient. The patient is likely to appear distressed and to have pale, cool, clammy skin. The BP and HR are probably elevated, and an atrial gallop sound (S4) may be heard. A ventricular gallop sound (S3) may indicate left ventricular dysfunction. A murmur heard during an anginal attack may be secondary to ischemia of a papillary muscle of the mitral valve. The murmur is likely to be transient and to disappear with the cessation of symptoms.

The nurse should ask the patient to rate the pain on a scale of 0 to 10 before and after treatment, to evaluate the effectiveness of the interventions. It is important to use the same words that patients use to describe their pain. Some patients may not always verbalize pain. The nurse must be attuned to other manifestations of pain, such as restlessness; elevated HR, respiratory rate, or BP; clutching of the bedclothes; or other nonverbal cues. Supportive and realistic reassurance and a calm, soothing

manner help reduce the patient's anxiety during an anginal attack.

■ Ambulatory and Home Care

The patient with a history of angina should be reassured that a long, productive life is possible. Prevention of angina is preferable to its treatment, and this is why teaching is important. The patient should be provided information regarding CAD, angina, precipitating factors for angina, risk factor reduction, and medications.

Patient teaching can be handled in a variety of ways. One-to-one contact between the nurse and the patient is often the most effective strategy. The time spent in providing daily care is often an ideal teaching period. Teaching tools such as pamphlets, video recordings, heart models, and especially written information are necessary components of patient and family teaching (see Chapter 4).

The patient should be assisted in identifying factors that precipitate angina (see Table 36-10). The patient should be given instruction on how to avoid or control precipitating factors. For example, the patient should be taught to avoid exposure to extremes of weather and the consumption of large, heavy meals. If a heavy meal is ingested, adequate rest should be planned for 1 to 2 hours after the meal because blood is shunted to the GI tract to aid in digestion and absorption.

The patient should be assisted in identifying personal risk factors in CAD. Once these are known, various methods of decreasing any modifiable risk factors should be discussed (see Table 36-4).

Teaching the patient and the family or caregivers about diets with low sodium and saturated fat content may be appropriate. Maintaining ideal body weight is important in controlling angina because weight above this level increases the myocardial workload.

Adhering to a regular, individualized program of physical activity that conditions the heart rather than overstressing the myocardium is important. Most patients can be advised to walk briskly on a flat surface at least 30 minutes a day, 5 or more days a week (Haskell, 2003). It is important to instruct the patient and the caregivers in the proper use of nitroglycerin (see pp. 905-906). Nitroglycerin tablets or ointments may be used prophylactically before an emotionally stressful situation, sexual intercourse, or physical exertion (e.g., climbing a long flight of stairs).

Counselling should be provided to assess the psychological adjustment of the patient and the family to the diagnosis of CAD and the resulting angina. Many patients feel a threat to their identity and self-esteem and may be unable to fill their usual roles in society. These emotions are normal and real.

■ Nursing Implementation: Acute Coronary Syndrome

■ Acute Intervention

Priorities for nursing interventions in the initial phase of ACS include pain assessment and relief, physiological monitoring, promotion of rest and comfort, alleviation of stress and anxiety, and understanding of the patient's emotional and behavioural reactions. Research has shown that patients with increased

NURSING CARE PLAN 36-1

Acute Coronary Syndrome

NURSING DIAGNOSIS	*Acute pain* related to myocardial ischemia *as evidenced by* severe chest pain and tightness, radiation of pain to the neck and arms

Expected Patient Outcomes	Nursing Interventions and *Rationales*
• Reports relief of pain	**Cardiac care: acute**
	• Evaluate chest pain (e.g., intensity, location, radiation, duration, and precipitating and alleviating factors) *to accurately evaluate, treat, and prevent further ischemia.*
	• Monitor effectiveness of oxygen therapy *to increase oxygenation of myocardial tissue and prevent further ischemia.*
	• Administer medications to relieve or prevent pain and ischemia *to decrease anxiety and cardiac workload.*
	• Obtain 12-lead ECG during pain episode *to help differentiate angina from extension of MI or pericarditis.*
	• Monitor cardiac rhythm and rate, trends in blood pressure, and trends in hemodynamic parameters (e.g., central venous pressure and pulmonary artery wedge pressure) *to monitor for hypotension and bradycardia, which may lead to hypoperfusion.*

NURSING DIAGNOSIS	*Decreased cardiac output* related to myocardial injury *as evidenced by* decrease in BP, elevation in HR, dyspnea, dysrhythmias, peripheral edema, and pulmonary edema

Expected Patient Outcomes	Nursing Interventions and *Rationales*
• Maintains stable signs of effective cardiac perfusion	**Cardiac care**
	• Monitor vital signs frequently *to determine baseline and ongoing changes.*
	• Monitor for cardiac dysrhythmias, including disturbances of both rhythm and conduction, *to identify and treat significant dysrhythmias.*
	• Monitor respiratory status for symptoms of heart failure *to maintain appropriate levels of oxygenation and to detect signs of pulmonary edema.*
	• Monitor fluid balance (e.g., intake and output, daily weight) *to monitor renal perfusion and observe for fluid retention.*
	• Arrange exercise and rest periods *to prevent fatigue and decrease the oxygen demand on myocardium.*

NURSING DIAGNOSIS	*Anxiety* related to perceived or actual threat of death, pain, possible lifestyle changes *as evidenced by* restlessness, agitation, and verbalization of concern over lifestyle changes and prognosis, such as "What is going to happen when I die? Everyone relies on me."

Expected Patient Outcomes	Nursing Interventions and *Rationales*
• Reports decreased anxiety and increased sense of self-control	**Anxiety reduction**
	• Observe for verbal and nonverbal signs of anxiety.
	• Identify changes in level of anxiety *because anxiety increases the need for oxygen.*
	• Use a calm, reassuring approach *so as not to increase patient's anxiety.*
	• Instruct patient in use of relaxation techniques (e.g., relaxation breathing, imagery) *to enhance the patient's self-control.*
	• Encourage family members to stay with patient *to provide comfort.*
	• Encourage verbalization of feelings, perceptions, and fears *to decrease anxiety and stress.*
	• Provide factual information concerning diagnosis, treatment, and prognosis *to decrease fear of the unknown.*

NURSING DIAGNOSIS	*Activity intolerance* related to fatigue secondary to decreased cardiac output and poor lung and tissue perfusion *as evidenced by* fatigue with minimal activity, inability to care for self without dyspnea, and increased heart rate

Expected Patient Outcomes	Nursing Interventions and *Rationales*
• Achieves a realistic program of activity that balances physical activity with energy-conserving activities	**Cardiac care**
	• Monitor patient's response to antidysrhythmic medications before activity *because these medications affect blood pressure and pulse.*
	• Arrange exercise and rest periods *to prevent fatigue and to increase activity tolerance without rapidly increasing cardiac workload.*
	Energy management
	• Assist patient to understand energy conservation principles (e.g., the requirement for restricted activity) *to conserve energy and promote healing.*
	• Teach patient and significant others techniques of self-care that will minimize oxygen consumption (e.g., self-monitoring and pacing techniques for performance of activities of daily living) *to promote independence as well as minimize O_2 consumption.*

NURSING CARE PLAN 36-1

Acute Coronary Syndrome—cont'd

NURSING DIAGNOSIS	*Ineffective self-health management* related to lack of knowledge of risk factors, disease process, rehabilitation, home activities, and medications *as evidenced by* frequent questioning about illness, management, and care after discharge
Expected Patient Outcomes	**Nursing Interventions and *Rationales***
• Describes risk factors, the disease process, and rehabilitation activities necessary to manage the therapeutic regimen	**Teaching: disease process** • Appraise the patient's current level of knowledge related to myocardial infarction *to obtain information about patient's teaching needs.* • Explain the pathophysiological features of the disease and how they are related to anatomy and physiology *to individualize the information and to increase understanding.* • Discuss lifestyle changes that may be necessary to prevent further complications or to control the disease process *to obtain the cooperation of the patient's significant support system.* • Refer the patient to local community agencies and support groups *so that the patient and family have resources and support available.* **Teaching: prescribed medication** • Instruct the patient about the purpose and action of each medication. • Instruct the patient about the dosage, the route, and the duration of action of each medication *so that the patient understands the reason for taking the medication and will be less likely to refuse to take medications.*

anxiety levels have a greater risk for adverse outcomes such as recurrent ischemic events and dysrhythmias (Deaton & Namasivayam, 2004). Proper management of these priorities decreases the oxygen needs of a compromised myocardium and reduces the risk of complications. In addition, the nurse should institute measures to avoid the hazards of immobility and yet encourage rest.

▊ **Pain.** Nitroglycerin, morphine sulphate, and supplemental oxygen should be provided as needed to eliminate or reduce chest pain. Ongoing evaluation and documentation of the effectiveness of the interventions is important. Once pain is relieved, the nurse may have to deal with denial in a patient who interprets the absence of pain as an absence of cardiac disease.

▊ **Monitoring.** A patient has continuous ECG monitoring while in the ED and the critical care unit and usually after transfer to a stepdown or general unit. The nurse should be educated in interpretation of the ECG so that dysrhythmias causing further deterioration of the cardiovascular status can be identified and treated. During the initial period after MI, ventricular fibrillation is the most common lethal dysrhythmia. In many patients, this dysrhythmia is often preceded by premature ventricular contractions (PVCs) or ventricular tachycardia. The nurse should also monitor the patient for the presence of silent ischemia by monitoring the ST segment for shifts above or below the baseline of the ECG. Silent ischemia occurs without clinical symptoms such as chest pain, but its presence places a patient at higher risk for adverse outcomes and even death (Deaton & Namasivayam, 2004). If episodes of silent ischemia are observed, the physician should be notified. (See Chapter 38 for a complete discussion of ECG monitoring.)

In addition to frequent assessment of vital signs, intake and output should be evaluated at least once per shift, and physical assessment should be carried out to detect deviations from the patient's baseline parameters. Included is an assessment of lung sounds and heart sounds and inspection for evidence of early HF (e.g., dyspnea, tachycardia, pulmonary congestion, distended neck veins).

Assessment of the patient's oxygenation status is important, especially if the patient is receiving oxygen. Also, the nares should be checked for irritation or dryness, which can cause considerable discomfort if the nasal route is used for oxygen administration.

▊ **Rest and Comfort.** With a severe insult to the myocardium, as in the case of ACS, it is important for the nurse to promote rest and comfort. Bed rest may be ordered for the first few days after an MI involving a large portion of the ventricle. A patient with an uncomplicated MI (e.g., angina resolved, no signs of complications) may rest in a chair within 8 to 12 hours after the event. The use of a commode or bedpan is based on patient preference.

When sleeping or resting, the body requires less work from the heart than it does when active. It is important to plan nursing and therapeutic actions to ensure adequate rest periods free from interruption. Comfort measures that can promote rest include frequent oral care, adequate warmth, a quiet atmosphere, use of relaxation therapy (e.g., guided imagery), and assurance that personnel are nearby and responsive to the patient's needs.

It is important that the patient understand the reasons why activity is limited. However, in spite of this limitation, the patient is not completely restricted. Gradually the cardiac workload is increased through more demanding physical tasks so that the patient can achieve a discharge activity level adequate for home care. Phases of cardiac rehabilitation are outlined in Table 36-17.

▊ **Anxiety.** Anxiety is present to various degrees in all patients with ACS. The nurse's role is to identify the source of anxiety and assist the patient in reducing anxiety. If the patient is afraid of being alone, a family member should be allowed to sit quietly by the bedside or to check in with the patient frequently. If a source of anxiety is fear of the unknown, the nurse should explore these concerns with the patient and help with appropriate reality testing.

Table 36-17 Phases of Rehabilitation After Acute Coronary Syndrome

Phase I: Hospital

- Occurs while the patient is still hospitalized.
- Activity level depends on severity of angina or MI.
- Patient may initially sit up in bed or chair, perform range-of-motion exercises and self-care (e.g., washing, shaving), and progress to ambulation in hallway and limited stair climbing.
- Attention focuses on management of pain, anxiety, dysrhythmias, and complications.

Phase II: Early Recovery

- Phase begins after the patient is discharged.
- Phase usually lasts from 2-12 wk and is conducted in an outpatient facility.
- Activity level is gradually increased under the supervision of the cardiac rehabilitation team and with electrocardiographic monitoring.
- Team may suggest that physical activity (e.g., walking) be initiated at home.
- Information regarding risk-factor reduction is provided at this time.

Phase III: Late Recovery

- Long-term maintenance program is followed.
- Individual physical activity programs are designed and implemented at home, a local gym, or the rehabilitation centre.
- Patient and family may restructure lifestyles and roles as possible.
- Lifestyle changes should become lifelong habits.
- Medical supervision is still recommended.

MI, myocardial infarction.

Table 36-18 Emotional and Behavioural Responses to Acute Coronary Syndrome

Denial

- May have history of ignoring symptoms related to heart disease
- Minimizes severity of medical condition
- Ignores activity restrictions
- Avoids discussing illness or its significance

Anger

- Is commonly expressed as, "Why did this happen to me?"
- Possibly directed at family, staff, or medical regimen

Anxiety and Fear

- Fears long-term disability and death
- Overtly manifests apprehension, restlessness, insomnia, tachycardia
- Less overtly manifests increased verbalization, projection of feelings to others, hypochondriasis
- Fears activity
- Fears recurrent angina, heart attacks, and sudden death

Dependency

- Is totally reliant on staff
- Is unwilling to perform tasks or activities unless approved by health care provider
- Wants to be monitored by ECG at all times
- Is hesitant to leave the critical care unit or hospital

Depression

- Mourns loss of health, altered body function, and changes in lifestyle
- Realizes seriousness of situation
- Begins to worry about future implications of health problem
- Shows manifestations of withdrawal, crying, apathy
- May be more evident after hospital discharge

Realistic Acceptance

- Focuses on optimum rehabilitation
- Plans changes compatible with altered cardiac function

If anxiety is caused by lack of information, the nurse should provide teaching appropriate to the patient's stated need and level. The nurse should answer the patient's questions with clear, simple explanations sufficient to reduce the patient's anxiety.

It is important to start teaching at the patient's level rather than to present a prepackaged protocol. Many patients are not yet ready to hear about the pathogenesis of CAD. The earliest questions usually relate to how the disease affects perceived control and independence. These questions include the following:

- When will I leave the critical care unit?
- When can I be out of bed?
- When will I be discharged?
- When can I return to work?
- How much change will I have to make in my life?
- Will this happen again?

The nurse should advise patients to begin a more complete teaching program once they are feeling stronger. Many patients may not be able to consciously examine the most pervasive and typical concern: "Am I going to die?" Even if a patient denies this concern, it is helpful for the nurse to initiate conversation by remarking that fear of dying is a common concern reported by most patients who have experienced ACS. This gives the patient "permission" to talk about an uncomfortable and frightening topic (see Table 36-18).

▌ Emotional and Behavioural Reactions. The emotional and behavioural reactions of a patient are varied and frequently follow a predictable response pattern (Table 36-18). The role of the nurse is to understand what the patient is currently experiencing, to assist the patient in testing reality, and to support the use of constructive coping styles. Denial may be a positive coping style in the early phase of recovery from ACS.

The nurse has a duty to maximize and enhance the patient's social support systems. This entails assessing the support structure of the patient and family and allowing it to function. Often the patient is separated from the most significant support system at the time of hospitalization. The nurse's role can include talking with the family members, informing them of the patient's progress, allowing the patient and the family to interact as necessary, and supporting the family members who will be able to provide the necessary support to the patient. Open visitation is helpful in decreasing anxiety and increasing support for the patient with ACS. Social isolation has been associated with negative outcomes after MI in both men and women (McSweeney & Coon, 2004). It is important for the nurse to help the patient identify additional support systems (e.g., spiritual care, Mended Hearts) that can help the patient after discharge.

Coronary Revascularization

Patients with ACS may undergo coronary revascularization with PCI or CABG surgery. The major nursing responsibilities for the care of the patient after PCI involve monitoring for signs of recurrent angina; frequent assessment of vital signs, including HR and rhythm; evaluation of the groin site for signs of bleeding; and maintenance of bed rest per institution policy (see Chapter 34 and Table 34-5).

For patients undergoing CABG surgery, care is provided in the critical care unit for the first 24 to 36 hours. Ongoing and intensive monitoring of patients' hemodynamic status is critical. For such patients, much invasive equipment for monitoring cardiac status and other vital organs is present (see Chapter 68). This equipment includes a pulmonary artery catheter for measuring cardiac output and other hemodynamic parameters, an intra-arterial line for continuous BP monitoring, pleural and mediastinal chest tubes for chest drainage, ECG leads for continuous monitoring to detect dysrhythmias, an endotracheal tube connected to mechanical ventilation, epicardial pacing wires for emergency pacing of the heart, a urinary catheter to monitor urine output, and a nasogastric tube for gastric decompression. Most patients are extubated within 12 hours after surgery and transferred to a stepdown unit within 24 hours for continued monitoring of cardiac status.

Many of the postoperative complications that develop after CABG surgery are related to the use of CPB. Major consequences of CBP include bleeding and anemia from damage to red blood cells and platelets, fluid and electrolyte imbalances, and hypothermia because blood is cooled as it passes through the CPB machine. Nursing care is focused on assessing the patient for bleeding (e.g., chest tube drainage, incision sites), monitoring fluid status, replacing electrolytes as needed, and restoring temperature (e.g., with use of warming blankets).

Postoperative dysrhythmias, specifically atrial dysrhythmias, are common in the first 3 days after CABG surgery. Between 20 and 40% of patients develop postoperative atrial fibrillation. Discharge is often delayed in these patients as a result of the need for anticoagulation. (See Chapter 38 for information on treatment of atrial fibrillation.)

Nursing care for the patient with a CABG also involves caring for the surgical sites: the chest, the arm, the leg, the abdomen, or some combination of these. Care of the radial artery harvest site includes careful observation of the incision site, as well as monitoring sensory and motor function of the distal thumb and fingers. The patient with radial artery harvest should receive therapy with a calcium channel blocker for approximately 3 months to decrease the incidence of arterial spasm at the arm or the anastomosis site.

The care of the leg wound is similar to the postoperative care after the stripping of varicose veins (see Chapter 40). The management of the chest wound, which involves a sternotomy, is similar to that for other chest surgical procedures (see Chapter 30).

Elective CABG is generally well tolerated by older patients. However, the incidence of postoperative complications—including dysrhythmias, stroke, and infection—is high. The nurse caring for older adults must be aware that although the benefits of treatment may outweigh risks in this population, the incidence of complications is higher than in younger individuals.

Postoperative nursing care of patients who have undergone a MIDCAB or OPCAB procedure is similar to that of patients who have undergone CABG surgery. Pain management is essential because patients report higher levels of pain with thoracotomy incisions than with a sternotomy incision. The recovery time is somewhat shorter with these procedures, and patients often resume routine activities sooner than do patients who have CABG surgery.

Ambulatory and Home Care

Rehabilitation may be defined as the process of helping the patient adjust to a disability by teaching integration of all resources and concentrating more on existing abilities than on permanent disabilities. Cardiac rehabilitation is the restoration of a person to an optimal state of function in six areas: physiological, psychological, mental, spiritual, economic, and vocational. Many people recover from ACS physically, but they may never attain psychological well-being because of misconceptions about the illness or a need to practise illness behaviours. Returning to work and resuming all activities have long been outcome measures of cardiac rehabilitation and are important in terms of the cost effectiveness of cardiac care and rehabilitation. (See the Evidence-Informed Practice box "What Is the Most Effective Cardiac Rehabilitation Program?")

In considering rehabilitation, the nurse and the patient must recognize that CAD is a chronic disease. It will not be cured, nor will it disappear by itself. Therefore, basic changes in lifestyle must be made to promote recovery and health. In many cases, these changes must be made at a time when the patient is middle-aged or older. The patient must also realize that recovery takes time. Resumption of physical activity after ACS or CABG surgery is slow and gradual. However, with appropriate and adequate supportive care, recovery is more likely to occur.

Patient Teaching

Patient teaching begins with the nurse in the ED, progresses through the care provided by the staff nurse, and continues with the community health nurse. The purpose of teaching is to give the patient and the family the tools they need to make informed decisions about attainment of health. For teaching to be meaningful, the patient must be aware of the need to learn. Careful assessment of the patient's learning needs helps the nurse set goals and objectives that are realistic.

The timing of the teaching is important. When patients or families are in crisis (either physiological or psychological), they may not be able to learn new information. It is important to remember that early questions should be answered initially in simple, brief terms, without detailed elaboration, and that the answers to these questions often require repetition and elaboration. When the shock and disbelief accompanying a crisis subside, the patient and the family are better able to focus on new information.

In addition to teaching the patient and the family what they wish to know, several types of information are considered necessary for achieving optimal health. A teaching guide for the patient with ACS is presented in Table 36-19.

When medical terminology is used, its meaning should be explained in lay terms. For example, it can be explained that the heart, a four-chambered pump, is a muscle that, like all other muscles, needs oxygen to work properly. When blood vessels supplying the heart muscle with oxygen become narrowed by atherosclerosis, less oxygen reaches the heart muscle. It is a good idea for the nurse to have a model of the heart or to use a pad and pencil to sketch what is being explained. Literature written

EVIDENCE-INFORMED PRACTICE

What Is the Most Effective Cardiac Rehabilitation Program?

Clinical (PICO) Question

In patients with coronary CAD (P), are comprehensive cardiac rehabilitation programs (I) more effective than exercise-only cardiac rehabilitation programs (C) in reducing mortality (O)?

Best Available Evidence

Systematic review of randomized controlled trials

Critical Appraisal and Synthesis of Evidence

- 47 randomized controlled trials ($n = 10{,}794$)
- Reduction in overall and cardiovascular mortality.
- Reduction in hospital readmissions.
- Comprehensive cardiac rehabilitation (e.g., exercise in addition to psychosocial and educational interventions): 13%
- Of 10 trials, 7 revealed significantly higher quality of life with exercise-based cardiac rehabilitation than with usual care.

Conclusions

- Exercise-based cardiac rehabilitation is effective in reducing cardiac deaths and other causes of mortality in patients with CAD.
- A broader sample is needed for subsequent studies that would include more women and is more ethnically diverse.

Implications for Nursing Practice

- Counsel patients at risk for CAD on the benefits of exercise.
- Include an exercise component in health and wellness programs for patients with CAD and those who have suffered a cardiac event.

Reference for Evidence

Heran, B., Ebrahim, S., Moxham, T., Oldridge, N., Rees, K., Thompson, D., & Taylor, R. (2011). Exercise-based rehabilitation for coronary heart disease, Cochrane Heart Group. *Cochrane Database of Systematic Reviews*, (7), CD001800. doi:10.1002/14651858.CD001800.pub2

CAD, coronary artery disease; *PICO: P*, patient population of interest; *I*, intervention or area of interest; *C*, comparison of interest or comparison group; *O*, outcome(s) of interest.

Table 36-19 Acute Coronary Syndrome

The nurse must teach the following to the patient and the caregivers:

- Signs and symptoms of angina and MI and reasons why they occur*
- Anatomy and physiology of the heart and vessels
- Cause and effect of atherosclerosis
- Definition of terms (e.g., CAD, angina, MI, sudden cardiac death, HF)
- Healing after MI
- Identification of and decreasing risk factors* (see Table 36-4)
- Rationale for tests and treatments, including ECG, blood tests, and angiography, and for monitoring, rest, diet, and medications*
- Appropriate expectations about recovery and rehabilitation (anticipatory guidance)
- Resumption of work, physical activity, sexual activity
- Measures to take to promote recovery and health
- Importance of the gradual, progressive resumption of activity*
- When and how to seek help (e.g., contact EMS)

CAD, coronary artery disease; *ECG*, electrocardiogram; *EMS*, emergency medical services; *HF*, heart failure; *MI*, myocardial infarction.
*Identified by patients as most important to learn before discharge.

---

for a nonmedical audience is available through the HSF. Video recordings are also helpful tools that can be used to teach patients.

Anticipatory guidance involves preparing the patient and the family for what to expect in the course of recovery and rehabilitation. By learning what to expect during treatment and recovery, the patient gains a sense of control over life. This sense of perceived control allows the patient to consciously consider stressors and thus possibly to promote recovery.

■ **Physical Activity.** Physical activity is an integral part of the rehabilitation program. It is necessary for optimal physiological functioning and psychological well-being. It has a direct, positive effect on maximal oxygen uptake, increasing CO, decreasing blood lipids, decreasing BP, increasing blood flow through the coronary arteries, increasing muscle mass and flexibility, improving the psychological state, and assisting in weight loss and control. A regular schedule of physical activity, even when begun after many years of sedentary living, is beneficial. The Canadian Guidelines for Physical Activity outline recommended activities and duration for all ages (CSEP, n.d.).

In the hospital, the activity level is gradually increased so that by the time of discharge, the patient can tolerate moderate-energy activities of 3 to 6 metabolic equivalents (METs). Many patients with UA that has resolved or with an uncomplicated MI are in the hospital for approximately 3 to 4 days. By day 2, patients can ambulate in the hallway and begin limited stair climbing (e.g., three to four steps). Because of the short hospital stay, it is critical to give patients specific guidelines for physical activity so that overexertion will not occur. It is important to stress that patients should "listen to what the body is saying"—the most important facet of recovery.

Teaching the patient to check the pulse rate is a nursing responsibility. The patient should be taught the parameters within which to exercise. The patient should be told the maximum rate that the heart should beat at any point. If the heart rate exceeds this level or does not return to the rate of the resting pulse within a few minutes, the patient should stop and rest. The patient should also be instructed to stop exercising if angina or dyspnea occurs. Basic physical activity guidelines for patients after ACS are based on the formula for frequency, intensity, time, and type (FITT) and are presented in Table 36-20.

The basic categories of physical activity are static (isometric) and dynamic (isotonic). Most daily activities are a mixture of the two. Static activities involve the development of tension during muscular contraction but produce little or no change in muscle length or joint movement. Lifting, carrying, and pushing heavy objects are primarily isometric activities. Because the HR and BP increase rapidly during isometric work, exercise programs involving isometric exercises should be limited.

Isotonic activities involve changes in muscle length and joint movement with rhythmic contractions at relatively low muscular

PATIENT & CAREGIVER TEACHING GUIDE

Table 36-20 FITT Physical Activity Guidelines After Acute Coronary Syndrome

Warm-up and Cool-down

Mild stretching for 3-5 min before the physical activity and 5 min after the activity is important. Activity should not be started or stopped abruptly.

Frequency

The patient should perform physical activity five or more times per week.

Intensity

Activity intensity should be determined by the patient's HR. If a treadmill test has not been performed, the person recovering from MI should not exceed 20 beats/min over the resting HR.

Type of Physical Activity

Physical activity should be regular, rhythmic, and repetitive; large muscles should be used to build up endurance (as in walking, cycling, swimming, and rowing).

Time

Duration of physical activity can be from 30-60 min. It is important to begin slowly according to personal tolerance (perhaps only 5-10 min) and build up to 30 min.

FITT, frequency, intensity, time, and type; *HR,* heart rate; *MI,* myocardial infarction.

Table 36-21 Sexual Activity After Acute Coronary Syndrome

- When planning for resumption of sexual activity, the goal should correspond to sexual activity before hospitalization for acute coronary syndrome.
- Physical training seems to improve the physiological response to coitus; therefore, daily physical activity during recovery should be encouraged.
- Consumption of food and alcohol should be reduced before intercourse is anticipated (e.g., waiting 3 to 4 hr after ingesting a large meal before engaging in sexual activity).
- Familiar surroundings and a familiar partner reduce anxiety.
- Masturbation may be a useful sexual outlet and may reassure the patient that sexual activity is still possible.
- Hot or cold showers should be avoided just before and just after intercourse.
- Foreplay is desirable because it allows a gradual increase in heart rate before orgasm.
- Positions during intercourse are a matter of individual choice.
- Orogenital sex places no undue strain on the heart.
- A relaxed atmosphere free of fatigue and stress is optimal.
- Prophylactic use of nitrates is effective in decreasing angina during sexual activity.
- Use of erectile agents (e.g., sildenafil [Viagra]) is contraindicated if the patient is taking nitrates in any form.
- Anal intercourse may cause undue cardiac stress because of the possibility of inducing a vasovagal response.

tension. Walking, jogging, swimming, bicycling, and jumping rope are examples of activities that are predominantly isotonic. Isotonic exercise can put a safe, steady load on the heart and lungs and improve the circulation in many organs.

Many patients are referred to an outpatient cardiac rehabilitation program (see Table 36-17). These programs have been found to be beneficial to patients, but not all patients choose or are able to participate in them. Home-based cardiac rehabilitation programs have been developed as an alternative. Maintaining contact with patients appears to be the key to the success of these programs.

Research has shown that older women (≥65 years) who experience MI tend to have poor adherence to a regular physical activity program. Many of the women described continued fatigue after MI that is poorly understood (Crane, 2005). One study found that home-based cardiac rehabilitation programs were more successful than traditional outpatient programs for older women (Deaton & Namasivayam, 2004).

Another factor that has been linked to poor adherence to a physical activity program after MI is depression (Crane, 2005). Both men and women typically experience mild to moderate depression after MI that takes about 1 to 4 months to resolve (Deaton & Namasivayam, 2004). If depression persists after this period, patients should be referred for appropriate treatment (e.g., counselling, medication).

The Evidence-Informed Practice box on p. 922 outlines recent research on the most effective type of cardiac rehabilitation program.

■ **Resumption of Sexual Activity.** It is important to include sexual counselling in the treatment for patients with cardiac disease and their partners. Engaging in this often-neglected area of discussion may be difficult for both patients and health care providers. However, the patient's concern about resumption of sexual activity after hospitalization for ACS

often produces more stress than the physiological act itself. About one third of men and women do not resume sexual activity or have a decrease in sexual activity after MI (Deaton & Namasivayam, 2004).

The majority of these patients change their sexual behaviour not because of physical problems but because of concerns about sexual inadequacy, death during coitus, and impotence. These misconceptions can be clarified with specific counselling by a concerned and knowledgeable health care provider.

Before the nurse provides guidelines on resumption of sexual activity, it is important to know the physiological status of the patient and to understand the physiological effects of sexual activity and the psychological effects of having a heart attack. Sexual activity for middle-aged men and women with their usual partners is no more strenuous than climbing two flights of stairs. Common guidelines are presented in Table 36-21.

It is not uncommon for a patient who experiences chest pain on physical exertion to have some angina during sexual stimulation or intercourse. The patient should be instructed to take nitroglycerin prophylactically. It is also helpful to have the patient avoid sex soon after a heavy meal or after excessive ingestion of alcohol, when extremely tired or stressed, or with unfamiliar partners. Anal intercourse is to be avoided because of the likelihood of eliciting a vasovagal response.

The patient should be counselled that resumption of sex depends on the patient and his or her partner's emotional readiness and on the physician's assessment of the extent of recovery. It is now known that it is safe to resume sexual activity 7 to 10 days after an uncomplicated MI (Antman et al., 2004). Some physicians believe that the patient should decide when he or she is ready to resume sex. Others say that a patient must be able to climb two flights of stairs briskly without dyspnea or angina before sexual activity can be resumed.

▪ Evaluation

The expected outcomes for the patient with an ACS are presented in Nursing Care Plan 36-1.

Sudden Cardiac Death

Sudden cardiac death (SCD) is unexpected death resulting from various causes, including cardiac arrest. In many cases, SCD is not actually sudden. Teaching people about the symptoms of impending cardiac arrest and the actions to take can save lives. Rapid cardiopulmonary resuscitation (CPR) and defibrillation with an automated external defibrillator (AED), in combination with early advanced cardiac life support, can enhance the chances for long-term survival after a witnessed arrest.

Etiology and Pathophysiology

In SCD, cardiac function is disrupted abruptly, which causes immediate loss of CO and cerebral blood flow. The affected person may or may not have a known history of CAD. SCD is the first sign of illness for 25% of people who die of heart disease (Mudawi, Albouaini, & Kaye, 2009). Death usually occurs within 1 hour of the onset of acute symptoms (e.g., angina, palpitations).

Acute ventricular dysrhythmias (e.g., ventricular tachycardia, ventricular fibrillation) cause the majority of cases of SCD. Less commonly, SCD occurs because of a primary left ventricular outflow obstruction (e.g., aortic stenosis, hypertrophic cardiomyopathy) or extreme slowing of the heart (bradycardia).

People who experience SCD because of CAD are categorized as (a) those who did not have an acute MI and (b) those who did have an acute MI. The first group accounts for the majority of cases of SCD. In this instance, victims usually have no warning signs or symptoms. Patients who survive are at risk for another episode of SCD because of the continued electrical instability of the myocardium that led to the initial event.

The second, smaller group of patients includes those who have had an MI and have suffered SCD. In these cases, patients usually do have prodromal symptoms, such as chest pain, palpitations, and dyspnea.

It is difficult to predict who is at risk for SCD. However, left ventricular dysfunction (EF <30%) and ventricular dysrhythmias after MI have been found to be the strongest predictors (Mudawi

et al., 2009). Other risk factors for SCD include (a) male gender (especially Black men), (b) family history of premature atherosclerosis, (c) tobacco use, (d) diabetes mellitus, (e) hypercholesterolemia, (f) hypertension, and (g) cardiomyopathy.

NURSING AND COLLABORATIVE MANAGEMENT

▪ Sudden Cardiac Death

People who survive an episode of SCD generally require a diagnostic workup to determine whether they have had an MI. Thus serial analyses of cardiac markers and ECGs are done, and treatment is planned accordingly. (See section on collaborative care of ACS.) In addition, because most people with SCD have CAD, cardiac catheterization is indicated to determine the possible location and extent of coronary artery occlusion. PCI or CABG surgery may also be indicated.

Most patients with SCD have a lethal ventricular dysrhythmia that has a high incidence of recurrence. Thus it is useful to know when those people are most likely to have a recurrence and what drug therapy is the most effective treatment. Assessment of dysrhythmias in these patients includes 24-hour Holter monitoring or other type of event recorder, exercise stress testing, signal-averaged ECG, and electrophysiological study (EPS) performed with fluoroscopy. Pacing electrodes are placed in selected intracardiac areas, and stimuli are selectively used to attempt to produce dysrhythmias. The patient's response to various antidysrhythmic medications is determined and monitored in a controlled environment. (EPS is discussed in Chapters 34 and 38.)

The most common approach to preventing a recurrence is the use of an implantable cardioverter-defibrillator (ICD). Research has shown survival rates are better with an ICD than with drug therapy alone (Mudawi et al., 2009; Exner, 2009). (ICDs are discussed further in Chapter 38.) Drug therapy with amiodarone (Cordarone) may be used in conjunction with an ICD to decrease episodes of ventricular dysrhythmias.

When caring for these patients, the nurse should be alert to the patient's psychosocial adaptation to this sudden "brush with death." Many of these patients develop a "time bomb" mentality. They fear the recurrence of cardiopulmonary arrest and may become anxious, angry, and depressed. Their caregivers are likely to experience the same feelings. This fear often interferes with resumption of normal activities such as sexual and recreational activities (Shea, 2004).

Patients and caregivers also may need to deal with additional issues such as possible driving restrictions and change in occupation. The grief response varies among patients and caregivers. The nurse should be attuned to the specific needs of the patient and caregiver and teach them accordingly while providing appropriate emotional support.

CLINICAL DECISION-MAKING EXERCISE

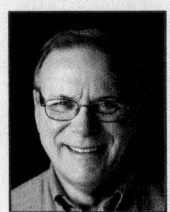

CASE STUDY:
Myocardial Infarction

Source: © iStockphoto.com/Floyd Anderson.

Patient Profile

Mr. Matthews, a 51-year-old, White, successful executive, is rushed to the hospital by ambulance after experiencing crushing substernal chest pain that radiates down his left arm. He also complains of dizziness and nausea.

Subjective Data

- Has a history of chronic stable angina and hypertension
- States that he is "borderline diabetic"
- Overweight but recently lost 10 pounds
- Rarely exercises
- Has three teenage children who are causing "problems"
- Recently experienced loss of best friend and business partner, who died from cancer

Objective Data

Physical Examination
- Diaphoresis, shortness of breath, nausea
- BP, 165/100 mm Hg; pulse rate, 120; respiratory rate, 26/min

Diagnostic Studies
- ECG shows occasional premature ventricular contractions and ST elevation in leads II, III, aV_F, V_5, and V_6.
- Cardiac-specific troponin I level are elevated.
- Cholesterol level is 9.1 mmol/L.
- HbA_{1C} level is 9.0%.
- Inferolateral wall MI is diagnosed.

Collaborative Care

Emergency Department
- Oxygen, 2 L/min via nasal cannula, titrated to keep O_2 saturation >93%
- Continuous ECG monitoring
- Aspirin, 324 mg (chewable)
- Eptifibatide (Integrilin), IV
- Weight-based heparin, IV
- Nitroglycerin intravenously, titrated to relieve chest pain; withheld for systolic BP <100 mm Hg
- Morphine, 2 to 4 mg, IV q5min PRN for chest pain unrelieved by nitroglycerin
- Metoprolol (Lopressor), 5 mg IV q5min × 3 doses
- Vital sign measurements and pulse oximetry q10min
- Preparation of patient for transfer to cardiac catheterization laboratory for possible PCI

Discussion Questions

1. Which coronary arteries are probably occluded in Mr. Matthews' coronary circulation?
2. What is the pathogenesis of CAD? What risk factors contribute to its development? What risk factors were present in Mr. Matthews' life?
3. What is angina? How does chronic stable angina differ from angina associated with ACS?
4. What is the pathophysiological basis for the clinical manifestations that Mr. Matthews exhibited?
5. What is the significance of the results of the laboratory tests and ECG findings?
6. What is the rationale for each treatment measure ordered for Mr. Matthews?
7. *Priority decision:* What are the priority nursing interventions for Mr. Matthews immediately after his MI?
8. *Priority decision:* Based on the assessment data presented, what are the priority nursing diagnoses? Identify any collaborative problems.

evolve *Answers are available at* **http://evolve.elsevier.com/Canada/Lewis/medsurg**

REVIEW QUESTIONS

The number of the question corresponds to the same-numbered objective at the beginning of the chapter.

1. What number of people in Canada will experience a myocardial infarction in a given year?
   a. 20,000
   b. 50,000
   c. 80,000
   d. 100,000
2. What changes occur in the development of CAD?
   a. Diffuse involvement of plaque formation in coronary veins
   b. Formation of fibrous tissue around coronary artery orifices
   c. Accumulation of lipid and fibrous tissue within the coronary arteries
   d. Chronic vasoconstriction of coronary arteries, which leads to permanent vasospasm

3. Which statement indicates that the patient requires additional instruction in reducing cardiac risk factors?
   a. "I would like to add weightlifting to my exercise program."
   b. "I can't keep my blood pressure normal without medication."
   c. "I can change my diet to decrease my intake of saturated fats."
   d. "I will change my lifestyle to reduce activities that increase my stress."
4. A hospitalized patient with angina tells the nurse that she is having chest pain. What best describes the nature of anginal pain?
   a. Will be relieved by rest, nitroglycerin, or both
   b. Is less severe than pain of a myocardial infarction
   c. Indicates that irreversible cellular damage is occurring
   d. Is frequently associated with vomiting and extreme fatigue

5. What does the clinical spectrum of ACS include?
   a. Unstable angina and STEMI
   b. Unstable angina and NSTEMI
   c. Stable angina and sudden cardiac death
   d. Unstable angina, STEMI, and NSTEMI

6. In a patient recovering from an MI, in which period is the heart most vulnerable to stress?
   a. 3 weeks after the infarction
   b. 4 to 6 days after the infarction
   c. 10 to 14 days after the infarction
   d. When healing is complete at 6 to 8 weeks

7. A patient is admitted to the ED with chest pain of 2 hours' duration, ECG findings consistent with an acute MI, and occasional ventricular dysrhythmias. With what pharmacological therapy would the nurse expect the patient to be managed initially?
   a. Diuretics
   b. Nitroglycerin spray
   c. β-Adrenergic blockers
   d. Thrombolytic therapy with tissue plasminogen activator

8. Five days after MI, a patient is restless and apprehensive. How can the nurse assist the patient?
   a. Providing all care by doing everything for the patient
   b. Structuring the environment and the routine so that the patient can rest
   c. Allowing the patient to participate in planning and carrying out activities
   d. Encouraging the family to provide for the patient's physical care and give emotional support

9. What is the most common pathological finding in individuals experiencing SCD?
   a. Cardiomyopathies
   b. Mitral valve disease
   c. Atherosclerotic heart disease
   d. Left ventricular hypertrophy

ANSWERS: 1. c; 2. c; 3. a; 4. a; 5. d; 6. c; 7. b; 8. c; 9. c.

REFERENCES

Adler, A., & Greenberg, B. (2004). Use of beta blockers in patients with post-MI left ventricular dysfunction. *Current treatment options in cardiovascular medicine, 6*(4), 335-343. doi:10.1007/s11936-004-0035-2

Aehlert, B. (2011). *ECGs made easy* (4th ed.). St. Louis: Elsevier.

Anderson, J., Adams, C., Antman, E., Bridges, C. R., Califf, R. M., Casey, Jr., D.E., …, Wright, R. S. (2007). ACC/AHA 2007 guidelines for the management of patients with unstable angina/non ST-elevation myocardial infarction: Executive summary, *Circulation: Journal of American College of Cardiology, 50*, 652. doi:10.1161/CIRCULATIONAHA.107.185752

Antman, E. M., Anbe, D. T., Armstrong, P. W., Bates, E. R., Green, L. A., Hand, M., …, Ornato, J. P. (2004). ACC/AHA guidelines for the management of patients with ST elevation myocardial infarction—Executive summary: A report of the ACC/AHA Task Force on Practice Guidelines. *Circulation, 110*, 588. doi:10.1161/01.CIR.0000134791.68010.FA

Canadian Society for Exercise Physiology. (n.d.) Canadian Physical Activity Guidelines: For adults—18-64 years. Retrieved from *http://www.csep.ca/CMFiles/Guidelines/CSEP-InfoSheets-adults-ENG.pdf*

Chen, J. (2007). Methamphetamine-associated acute myocardial infarction and cardiogenic shock with normal coronary arteries: Refractory global coronary microvascular spasm. *Journal of Invasive Cardiology, 19*(4), e89-e92. doi:10.1016/S0167-5273(08)70628-4

Crane, P. B. (2005). Fatigue and physical activity in older women after myocardial infarction. *Heart & Lung, 34*, 30. doi:10.1016/j.hrtlng.2004.08.007

Deaton, C., & Namasivayam, S. (2004). Nursing outcomes in coronary heart disease. *Journal of Cardiovascular Nursing, 19*, 308.

Delville, C. L., & McDougall, G. (2008). A systematic review of depression in adults with heart failure: Instruments and incidence. *Issues in Mental Health Nursing, 29*(9): 1002-1017. doi:10.1080/01612840802274867

Després, J. (2005). Our passive lifestyle, our toxic diet and the atherogenic/diabetogenic metabolic syndrome: Can we afford to be sedentary and unfit? *Circulation, 112*, 453. doi:10.1161/CIRCULATIONAHA.105.553289

Eagle, K. A., Guyton, R. A., Davidoff, R., Edwards, F. H., Ewy, G. A., Gardner, T. J., …, Ornato, J. P. (2004). ACC/AHA 2004 guideline update for Coronary Artery Bypass Graft surgery: A report of the ACC/AHA Task Force on Practice Guidelines (Committee to Update 1999 CABG Guidelines). *Circulation, 110*, 1168-1176. doi:10.1161/01.CIR.0000138790.14877.7D

Exner, D. (2009). Implantable cardioverter defibrillator therapy for patients with less severe left ventricular dysfunction. *Current Opinions in Cardiology, 24*(1), 61-67. doi:10.1097/HCO.0b013e32831c4cc5

Genest, J., Macpherson, R., Frohlich, J., Anderson, T., Campbell, N., Carpentier, A., …, Ur, E. (2009). 2009 Canadian Cardiovascular Society/Canadian Guidelines for the diagnosis and treatment of dyslipidemia and prevention of cardiovascular disease in the adult—2009 Recommendations. *Canadian Journal of Cardiology, 25*(10), 567-579. doi:10.1016/S0828-282X(09)70715-9

Gidding, S. S., Lichtenstein, A. H., Faith, M. S., Karpyn, A., Mennella, J. A., Popkin, B., …, Whitsel, L. (2009). Implementing American Heart Association pediatric and adult nutrition guidelines: A scientific statement from the American Heart Association Nutrition Committee of the Council on Nutrition, Physical Activity and Metabolism, Council on Cardiovascular Disease in the Young, Council on Arteriosclerosis, Thrombosis and Vascular Biology, Council on Cardiovascular Nursing, Council on Epidemiology and Prevention, and Council for High Blood Pressure Research. *Circulation, 119*(8), 1161-1175. doi:10.1161/CIRCULATIONAHA.109.191856

Gluckman, T. J., Sachdev, M., Schulman, S. P., & Blumenthal, R. S. (2005). A simplified approach to the management of non-ST-segment elevation acute coronary syndromes. *JAMA, 293*, 349. doi:10.1001/jama.293.3.349

Grassi, G., Seravalle, G., Quarti-Trevano, F., Dell'Oro, R., Bombelli, M., & Mancia, G. (2009). Metabolic syndrome and cardiometabolic risk: An update. *Blood Pressure, 18*(1-2), 7-16.

Grundy, S. M., Cleeman, J. I., Merz, M. B., Brewer, H. B., Jr., Clark, L. T., Hunninghake, D. B., …, American Heart Association. (2004). Implications of recent clinical trials for the National Cholesterol Education Program Adult Treatment Panel III Guidelines. *Circulation, 110*, 227. doi:10.1161/01.CIR.0000133317.49796.0E

Haskell, W. L. (2003). Cardiovascular disease prevention and lifestyle interventions: Effectiveness and efficacy. *Journal of Cardiovascular Nursing, 18*, 245.

Health Canada. (2008). Health Canada reminds Canadians not to use ephedra/ephedrine products. Retrieved from *http://*

www.hc-sc.gc.ca/ahc-asc/media/advisories-avis/_2008/2008_41-eng.php

Heart and Stroke Foundation of Canada. (2010a). *A perfect storm of heart disease looming on our horizon.* Ottawa: Author. Retrieved from *http://www.heartandstroke.com/atf/cf/%7B99452D8B-E7F1-4BD6-A57D-B136CE6C95BF%7D/Jan23_EN_ReportCard.pdf*

Heart and Stroke Foundation of Canada. (2010b). *Reverse fountain of youth? Obese children have signs of heart disease typically seen in middle aged adults* [News release from the Canadian Cardiovascular Congress 2010]. Retrieved from *http://www.heartandstroke.on.ca/site/apps/nlnet/content2.aspx?c=pvI3IeNWJwE&b=6349253&ct=8829227*

Heart and Stroke Foundation of Canada. (2012). *Statistics.* Ottawa: Author. Retrieved from *http://www.heartandstroke.com/site/c.ikIQLcMWJtE/b.3483991/k.34A8/Statistics.htm*

Hollander, J., & Henry, T. (2006). Evaluation and management of the patient who has cocaine induced chest pain. *Cardiology Clinics, 24*(1), 103-114. doi:10.1016/j.ccl.2005.09.003

Huang, P. (2009). A comprehensive definition for metabolic syndrome. *Disease Models and Mechanisms, 2*(5-6), 231-237. doi:10.1242/dmm.001180

Huether, S. E., & McCance, K. L. (2011). *Understanding pathophysiology* (5th ed.). St. Louis: Elsevier.

Huether, S. E., & McCance, K. L. (2008). *Understanding pathophysiology* (4th ed.). St. Louis: Mosby.

Humphrey, L., Fu, R., Rogers, K., Freeman, M., & Helfand, M. (2008). Homocysteine level and coronary artery disease incidence: A systematic review and meta-analysis. *Mayo Clinic Proceedings, 83*(11), 1203-1212. doi:10.4065/83.11.1203

Kushner, F., Hand, M., Smith, S., King, S., Anderson, J., Antman, E., …, Williams, D. O. (2009). 2009 Focused Updates: ACC/AHA Guidelines for the Management of Patients With ST-Elevation Myocardial Infarction (updating the 2004 Guideline and 2007 Focused Update) and ACC/AHA/SCAI Guidelines on Percutaneous Coronary Intervention (updating the 2005 Guideline and 2007 Focused Update): A report of the American College of Cardiology Foundation/American Heart Association Task Force on Practice Guidelines. *Circulation, 120*, 2271-2306. doi:10.1161/CIRCULATIONAHA.109.192663

Lehne, R.A. (2012). *Pharmacology for nursing care* (8th ed.). St. Louis: Saunders.

Libby, D., Bonow, R., Mann, D., & Zipes, D. (2008). *Braunwald's heart disease: A textbook of cardiovascular medicine* (8th ed.). Philadelphia: Saunders.

Lippi, G., Montagnana, M., Favaloro E., & Franchini, M. (2009). Mental depression and cardiovascular disease: A multifaceted, bidirectional association. *Seminars in Thrombosis and Hemostasis, 35*(3), 325-336. doi:10.1055/s-0029-1222611

Lloyd-Jones, D., Adams, R., Carnethon, M., De Simone, G., Ferguson, T. B., Flegal, K., …, Hong, Y. (2009). Heart disease and stroke statistics—2009 Update. *Circulation, 119*, e21-e181. doi:10.1161/CIRCULATIONAHA.108.191261

McSweeney, J. C., Cody, M., O'Sullivan, P., Elberson, K., Moser, D., & Garvin, B. (2003). Women's early warning symptoms of acute myocardial infarction. *Circulation, 108*, 2619. doi:10.1161/01.CIR.0000097116.29625.7C

McSweeney, J. C., & Coon, S. (2004). Women's inhibitors and facilitators associated with making behavioral changes after myocardial infarction. *Medsurg Nursing, 13*, 49.

Mudawi, T., Albouaini, K., & Kaye, G. (2009). Sudden cardiac death: History, aetiology and management. *British Journal of Hospital Medicine, 70*(2), 89-94.

Pagana, K., & Pagana, T. (2009). *Mosby's manual of diagnostic and laboratory tests* (4th ed.). St. Louis: Elsevier.

Public Health Agency of Canada. (2009a). Are women at risk for heart disease? Retrieved from *http://www.phac-aspc.gc.ca/cd-mc/cvd-mcv/women-femmes_01-eng.php*

Public Health Agency of Canada. (2009b). Tracking heart disease and stroke in Canada. Retrieved from *http://www.phac-aspc.gc.ca/publicat/2009/cvd-avc/pdf/cvd-avs-2009-eng.pdf*

Quinn, J. (2008). Update on women and heart disease. *Nursing Management, 39*, 22-27. doi:10.1097/01.NUMA.0000333719.42615.d8

Rabi, D. M., Daskalopoulou, S. S., Padwal, R. S., Khan, N. A., Grover, S. A., Hackam, D. G., …, Tobe, S. W. (2011). The 2011 Canadian Hypertension Education Program Recommendations for the Management of Hypertension: Blood Pressure Measurement, Diagnosis, Assessment of Risk, and Therapy. *Canadian Journal of Cardiology, 27*(4), 415-433e2. doi:10.1016/j.cjca.2011.03.015

Rubenstein, R., Halon, D., Gaspar, T., Jaffe, R., Karkabi, B., Flugelman, M. Y., …, Lewis, B. S. (2007). Usefulness of 64-slice cardiac computed tomographic angiography for diagnosing acute coronary syndrome and predicting clinical outcomes in emergency department patients with chest pain of uncertain origin. *Circulation, 115*, 1762. doi:10.1161/CIRCULATIONAHA.106.618389

Shea, J. (2004). Quality of life issues in patients with implantable cardioverter defibrillators. *AACN Clinical Issues, 15*, 478-489. doi:10.1097/00044067-200407000-00013

Smith, S. C., Allen, J., Blair, S. N., Bonow, R., Brass, L., Fonarow, G., …, Taubert, K. (2006). American Heart Association/American College of Cardiology guidelines for secondary prevention for patients with coronary and other atherosclerotic vascular disease: 2006 Update. *Circulation, 113*, 2363-2372. doi:10.1161/CIRCULATIONAHA.106.174516

Statistics Canada. (2010). Canadian Health Measures Survey: Body composition and fitness. Retrieved from *http://www.statcan.gc.ca/daily-quotidien/100113/dq100113a-eng.htm*

Thombs, B., de Jonge, P., Coyne, J., Whooley, M. A., Frasure-Smith, N., Mitchell, A. J., …, Ziegelstein, R. C. (2008). Depression screening and patient outcomes in cardiovascular care: A systematic review. *JAMA, 300*(18), 2161-2171. doi:10.1001/jama.2008.667

Vinik, A. I., Maser, R. E., Mitchell, B. D., & Freeman, R. (2003). Diabetic autonomic neuropathy. *Diabetes Care, 26*, 1553-79. doi:10.2337/diacare.26.5.1553

Yusuf, S., Hawkem, S., Ounpuu, S., & Dans, T. (2004). Effect of potentially modifiable risk factors associated with MI in 52 countries (the INTERHEART Study). *Lancet, 364*, 9438.

CANADIAN RESOURCES

Canadian Association of Critical Care Nurses
http://www.caccn.ca
Canadian Council of Cardiovascular Nurses
http://www.cccn.ca
Canadian Lipid Nurse Network
http://www.lipidnurse.ca
Cardiac Arrest Survivor Network
http://www.early-defib.org/survivors.asp
Heart and Stroke Foundation of Canada
http://ww2.heartandstroke.ca
Pacemaker and defibrillator site with patient support forums
http://www.implantable.com

RELATED RESOURCES

American College of Cardiovascular Nurses (ACCN)
http://www.accn.net
American Heart Association
http://www.heart.org/
Framingham Heart Study
http://www.framingham.com/heart/index.htm
Heartinfo.org
http://www.heartinfo.org
National Heart, Lung, and Blood Institute: BMI Calculator
http://nhlbisupport.com/bmi/bmicalc.htm

ℰvolve *For additional Internet resources, see the Web site for this book* at **http://evolve.elsevier.com/Canada/Lewis/medsurg**

Nursing Management: Heart Failure

Written by Lynne Dantino Bouffard
Adapted by Annemarie F. Kaan

LEARNING OBJECTIVES

1. Compare the pathophysiology of systolic and diastolic heart failure (HF).
2. Relate the compensatory mechanisms involved in HF to the development of acute decompensated heart failure (ADHF) and chronic HF.
3. Select the appropriate nursing and collaborative interventions to manage the patient with ADHF and pulmonary edema.

4. Select the appropriate nursing and collaborative interventions to manage the patient with chronic HF.
5. Describe the indications for cardiac transplantation and the nursing management of cardiac transplant recipients.

KEY TERMS

cardiac transplantation Transfer of a heart from one person to another, p. 944

diastolic heart failure Often referred to as heart failure with preserved systolic function, it is an impaired ability of the ventricles to fill during diastole, p. 930

heart failure (HF) An abnormal clinical condition that describes impaired cardiac pumping resulting in the characteristic pathophysiological changes of vasoconstriction and fluid retention, p. 929

paroxysmal nocturnal dyspnea A disorder characterized by sudden attacks of respiratory distress that occur when the

patient is asleep, usually after several hours of being in a recumbent position, p. 932

pulmonary edema An acute, life-threatening situation in which the lung alveoli become filled with serous or serosanguineous fluid; caused most commonly by acute left ventricular failure secondary to acute myocardial ischemia, p. 931

systolic heart failure The most common type of heart failure, it is caused by a defect in the ability of the ventricles to contract (pump), increased afterload, or mechanical abnormalities, p. 929

ELECTRONIC RESOURCES

Supplemental content related to Chapter 37 can be found ...

Evolve Web Site ⒺVOLVE

http://evolve.elsevier.com/Canada/Lewis/medsurg
- Answer Guidelines to Case Study on p. 947
- Clinical Reference: Laboratory Values
- Content Updates

- Customizable Nursing Care Plan: Heart Failure
- Electronic Calculators
- Examination Review Questions
- Glossary
- Interactive Case Study: Heart Failure
- Key Points (Printable and MP3 Download)
- Patient & Caregiver Teaching Guide: Heart Failure

Heart Failure

Heart failure (HF) is an abnormal clinical syndrome involving impaired cardiac pumping and/or filling. *Heart failure*, formerly called congestive HF, is the terminology preferred today because not all patients with HF will have pulmonary congestion or volume overload. HF is associated with numerous types of cardiovascular diseases, particularly longstanding hypertension, coronary artery disease (CAD), and myocardial infarction (MI) (Table 37-1). HF is characterized by ventricular dysfunction, reduced exercise tolerance, diminished quality of life, and shortened life expectancy.

In most industrial nations, HF has become a major health problem. In contrast to other cardiovascular diseases, HF is projected to increase in incidence. This increase is caused, in part, by the rapidly expanding aging population (Lee et al., 2004).

In Canada, it is estimated that there are 500,000 people living with HF and 50,000 new cases are diagnosed each year (Ross et al., 2006). Depending on the severity of symptoms, heart dysfunction, age, and other factors, HF can be associated with an annual mortality of between 5 and 50% (Arnold et al., 2006).

HF is associated with high rates of mortality and economic costs. It is estimated that as many as 33% of people with HF will be dead in 1 year. Readmissions to hospital are common—as many as 50% of patients with HF are readmitted within 1 year (Lee et al., 2004). Multiple hospitalizations translate to a significant economic burden on communities.

Etiology and Pathophysiology

Hypertension is a major contributing factor for the development of HF, increasing the risk approximately three-fold. The risk of HF increases progressively with the severity of hypertension, and systolic and diastolic hypertension equally predict risk. By age 65, 50% of Canadians will have hypertension and over 90% will develop it within their lifespan (Hypertension Canada, 2012).

Diabetes mellitus predisposes an individual to HF regardless of the presence of concomitant CAD or hypertension. The etiology is thought to be complex and related in part to microvascular pathology caused by diabetes (Cheung et al., 2008). Other risk factors for the development of HF include cigarette smoking, obesity, and high serum cholesterol (Arnold et al., 2007).

HF may be caused by any interference with the normal mechanisms regulating cardiac output (CO). CO depends on (1) preload, (2) afterload, (3) myocardial contractility, (4) heart rate (HR), and (5) metabolic state of the individual. (Preload and afterload are discussed in Chapter 34.) Any alteration in these factors can lead to decreased ventricular function and the resultant manifestations of HF. In general, major causes of HF may be divided into two subgroups: (1) primary causes (see Table 37-1) and (2) precipitating causes (Table 37-2). Precipitating causes often increase the workload of the ventricles, causing a decompensated condition that leads to decreased myocardial function.

Pathology of Ventricular Failure. HF can be described as systolic or diastolic.

Systolic Heart Failure. **Systolic heart failure,** the most common type of HF, results from an inability of the heart to pump blood. It is caused by a defect in the ability of the ventricles to contract (pump) or by increased afterload or mechanical abnormalities. The left ventricle (LV) loses its ability to generate enough pressure to eject blood forward through the high-pressure aorta. The hallmark of systolic HF is a decrease in the left ventricular ejection fraction (the fraction or percentage of total amount of blood in the LV that is ejected during each ventricular contraction). Normal ejection fraction (EF) is greater than 55% of the ventricular volume. Systolic HF is caused by impaired contractile function (e.g., MI), increased afterload (e.g., hypertension), cardiomyopathy, and mechanical abnormalities (e.g., valvular heart disease).

Table 37-1 Common Causes of Heart Failure

CHRONIC	ACUTE
• Coronary artery disease	• Acute myocardial infarction
• Hypertension	• Dysrhythmias
• Rheumatic heart disease	• Pulmonary embolus
• Congenital heart disease	• Thyrotoxicosis
• Pulmonary disease	• Hypertensive crisis
• Cardiomyopathy	• Rupture of papillary muscle
• Anemia	• Ventricular septal defect
• Bacterial endocarditis	• Myocarditis
• Valvular disorders	

Table 37-2 Precipitating Causes of Heart Failure

CAUSE	MECHANISM
Anemia	↓ O$_2$-carrying capacity of the blood stimulating ↑ in CO to meet tissue demands
Infection	↑ O$_2$ demand of tissues, stimulating ↑ CO
Thyrotoxicosis	Changes the tissue metabolic rate; ↑ HR and workload of the heart
Hypothyroidism	Indirectly predisposes to ↑ atherosclerosis; severe hypothyroidism decreases myocardial contractility
Dysrhythmias	May ↓ CO and ↑ workload and O$_2$ requirements of myocardial tissue
Bacterial endocarditis	*Infection:* ↑ metabolic demands and O$_2$ requirements *Valvular dysfunction:* causes stenosis and regurgitation
Myocarditis	↑ HR, ↓ CO, acute RV and LV failure
Pulmonary embolism	↑ Pulmonary pressure and exerts pressure on the RV, leading to RV hypertrophy and failure
Pulmonary disease	↑ Pulmonary pressure and exerts a pressure load on the RV, leading to RV hypertrophy and failure
Paget's disease	↑ Workload of the heart by ↑ vascular bed in the skeletal muscle
Nutritional deficiencies	May ↓ cardiac function by ↓ myocardial muscle mass and myocardial contractility
Hypervolemia	↑ Preload and causes volume load on the RV

CO, cardiac output; *HR,* heart rate; *LV,* left ventricle/ventricular; *RV,* right ventricle/ventricular.

Diastolic Heart Failure. **Diastolic heart failure**—often referred to as HF with preserved systolic function—is an impaired ability of the ventricles to fill during diastole. Decreased filling of the ventricles will result in decreased stroke volume. Diastolic HF is characterized by high filling pressures and the resultant venous engorgement in both the pulmonary and the systemic vascular systems. The diagnosis of diastolic HF is made on the basis of the presence of pulmonary congestion, pulmonary hypertension, ventricular hypertrophy, and a normal EF (Huether & McCance, 2008).

Diastolic HF is usually the result of left ventricular hypertrophy from chronic systemic hypertension, aortic stenosis, or hypertrophic cardiomyopathy. Diastolic HF is commonly seen in older adults, and predominantly women (see the Determinants of Health box), as a result of myocardial fibrosis and hypertension. However, the majority of patients who are seen with HF and normal systolic function do not have an identifiable heart disease.

Mixed Systolic and Diastolic Heart Failure. HF of mixed origin is seen in disease states such as dilated cardiomyopathy. Dilated cardiomyopathy is a condition in which poor systolic function (weakened muscle function) is further compromised by dilated left ventricular walls that are unable to relax effectively.

DETERMINANTS OF HEALTH
Heart Failure

Sex

Women comprise 51% of all new HF cases in Canada. Women tend to be older than men when diagnosed, and are more likely to be diabetic and have high blood pressure. Women are more likely to have HF with preserved systolic function (diastolic HF).

HF, heart failure.
Source: Pilote, L., Dasgupta, K., Guru, V., Humphries, K. H., McGrath, Jennifer, Norris, C., …, Tagalakis, V. (2007). A comprehensive view of sex-specific issues related to cardiovascular disease. *Canadian Medical Association Journal, 176* (6 Suppl.), S1-S44. doi:10.1503/cmaj.051455

These patients often have extremely poor EF (<35%), high pulmonary pressures, and biventricular failure (both ventricles may be dilated and have poor filling and emptying capacity).

The patient with HF of any type has low systemic arterial blood pressure (BP), low CO, and poor renal perfusion. Poor exercise tolerance and ventricular dysrhythmias are also common. Whether a patient arrives at this point acutely as a result of an MI or chronically from worsening cardiomyopathy or hypertension, the body's response to this low CO is to mobilize its compensatory mechanisms to maintain CO and BP.

Compensatory Mechanisms. HF can have an abrupt onset, as with acute MI, or it can be an insidious process resulting from slow, progressive changes. The overloaded heart resorts to certain compensatory mechanisms to try to maintain adequate CO. The main compensatory mechanisms include (1) ventricular dilation, (2) ventricular hypertrophy, (3) increased sympathetic nervous system (SNS) stimulation, and (4) neurohormonal responses.

Dilation. Dilation is an enlargement of the chambers of the heart. It occurs when pressure in the heart chambers (usually the LV) is elevated over time. The muscle fibres of the heart stretch in response to the volume of blood in the heart at the end of diastole. The degree of stretch is directly related to the force of the contraction (systole) (Starling's law). Initially, dilation is an adaptive mechanism to cope with increasing blood volume, and this increased contraction leads to increased CO and maintenance of arterial BP and perfusion. Eventually, this mechanism becomes inadequate because the elastic elements of the muscle fibres are overstretched and can no longer contract effectively, and CO diminishes (Figure 37-1).

Hypertrophy. Hypertrophy is an increase in the muscle mass and cardiac wall thickness in response to the overwork and strain of chronic HF. It occurs slowly because it takes time for this increased muscle tissue to develop. Hypertrophy generally follows persistent or chronic dilation and, thus, further increases the contractile power of the muscle fibres. This will lead to an increase

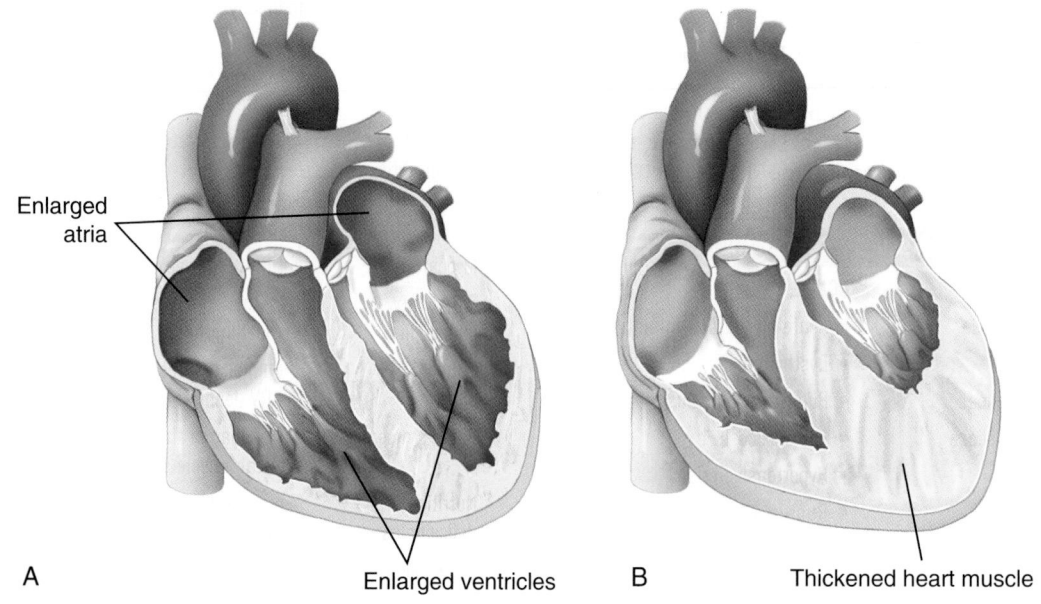

Figure 37-1 A, Dilated heart chambers. **B,** Hypertrophied heart chambers.

in CO and maintenance of tissue perfusion. However, hypertrophic heart muscle has poor contractility, requires more oxygen to perform work, has poor coronary artery circulation (tissue becomes more easily ischemic), and is prone to ventricular dysrhythmias.

Sympathetic Nervous System Activation.

SNS stimulation is often the first mechanism triggered in low-CO states. However, it is the least effective compensatory mechanism. Because there is inadequate stroke volume and CO, there is increased SNS activation, resulting in the increased release of epinephrine and norepinephrine. This results in an increased HR, myocardial contractility, and peripheral vascular constriction. Initially, this increase in HR and contractility improves CO. However, over time, these factors are counterproductive, increasing the myocardium's need for oxygen and the workload of the already failing heart. The vasoconstriction causes an immediate increase in preload, which may initially increase CO. However, an increase in venous return to the heart, which is already volume-overloaded, actually worsens ventricular performance.

Neurohormonal Response.

As the CO falls, blood flow to the kidneys decreases. This is sensed by the juxtaglomerular apparatus in the kidney as decreased volume. In response, the kidneys release renin, which converts angiotensinogen to angiotensin I (see Chapter 47 and Figure 47-6). Angiotensin I is subsequently converted to angiotensin II by a converting enzyme made in the lungs. Angiotensin II causes (1) the adrenal cortex to release aldosterone, which results in sodium and water retention, and (2) increased peripheral vasoconstriction, which increases BP. This response is known as the *renin–angiotensin–aldosterone system.*

Other neurohormonal factors contribute to the development of HF. The production of *endothelin* produced by the vascular endothelial cells is stimulated by antidiuretic hormone, catecholamines, and angiotensin II. Endothelin results in further arterial vasoconstriction and an increase in cardiac contractility and hypertrophy (Carlson, 2009). Locally, proinflammatory cytokines are released by cardiac myocytes in response to various forms of cardiac injury (e.g., MI). Two cytokines, tumour necrosis factor and interleukin, further depress cardiac function by causing cardiac hypertrophy, contractile dysfunction, and myocyte cell death. Over time, a systemic inflammatory response is also mounted and accounts for the cardiac wasting, muscle myopathy, and fatigue that accompany advanced HF.

The body's ability to try to maintain balance is demonstrated by several counterregulatory processes. Natriuretic peptides (atrial natriuretic peptide and brain—or B-type—natriuretic peptide [BNP]) are hormones produced by the heart muscle that promote venous and arterial vasodilation (thus reducing afterload and preload). Natriuretic peptides are endothelin and aldosterone antagonists and enhance diuresis by increasing glomerular filtration rates (thus reducing preload and volume stress) and blocking the effects of the renin–angiotensin–aldosterone system. In addition, they inhibit the development of cardiac hypertrophy and may have anti-inflammatory effects. Atrial natriuretic peptide is produced by the atrium, and BNP is produced by the ventricles. Release of BNP into the circulation is primarily triggered by increased ventricular distension and, thus, serves as a sensitive marker of fluid overload (Silver et al., 2004).

Cardiac compensation occurs when compensatory mechanisms succeed in maintaining a CO that is adequate for essential tissue perfusion. *Cardiac decompensation* occurs when these mechanisms

can no longer maintain adequate CO and insufficient tissue perfusion results.

Ventricular Remodelling.

The mechanisms discussed in the preceding paragraphs contribute to ventricular remodelling. This involves hypertrophy of the cardiac myocytes, resulting in large, abnormal cells. This eventually leads to increased ventricular mass, changes in ventricular shape, and impaired contractility. Although the ventricles become larger, they are a less effective pump.

Types of Heart Failure

HF is usually as evidenced by biventricular failure, although one ventricle may precede the other in dysfunction. Normally, the pumping actions of the left and right sides of the heart complement each other, producing a continuous flow of blood. However, as a result of pathological conditions, one side may fail while the other side continues to function normally for a time. Because of the prolonged strain, both sides of the heart will eventually fail, resulting in *biventricular failure.*

Left-Sided Heart Failure.

The most common form of initial heart failure is left-sided failure (Figure 37-2). Left-sided failure results from left ventricular dysfunction, which causes blood to back up through the left atrium and into the pulmonary veins. The increased pulmonary pressure causes fluid extravasation from the pulmonary capillary bed into the interstitium and then the alveoli, which is manifested as pulmonary congestion and edema.

Right-Sided Heart Failure.

Right-sided heart failure causes backward blood flow to the right atrium and venous circulation. Venous congestion in the systemic circulation results in peripheral edema, hepatomegaly, splenomegaly, vascular congestion of the gastrointestinal (GI) tract, and jugular venous distension. The primary cause of right-sided failure is left-sided failure. In this situation, left-sided failure results in pulmonary congestion and increased pressure in the blood vessels of the lung (pulmonary hypertension). Eventually, chronic pulmonary hypertension results in right-sided hypertrophy and failure. *Cor pulmonale* (right ventricular dilation and hypertrophy caused by pulmonary pathology) can also cause right-sided failure. (Cor pulmonale is discussed in Chapter 30.) Right ventricular infarction may also cause right ventricular failure.

Clinical Manifestations of Heart Failure

Regardless of etiology, acute decompensated heart failure (ADHF) typically manifests as **pulmonary edema,** an acute, life-threatening situation in which the lung alveoli become filled with serous or serosanguineous fluid (Figure 37-3). The most common cause of pulmonary edema is acute left ventricular failure secondary to acute myocardial ischemia. (Other etiological factors for pulmonary edema are listed in Chapter 30, Table 30-26.)

In most cases of ADHF, there is an increase in the pulmonary venous pressure caused by decreased efficiency of the LV. This results in engorgement of the pulmonary vascular system. As a result, the lungs become less compliant, and there is increased resistance in the small airways. In addition, the lymphatic system increases its flow to help maintain a constant volume of the pulmonary extravascular fluid. This early stage is clinically

PATHOPHYSIOLOGY MAP

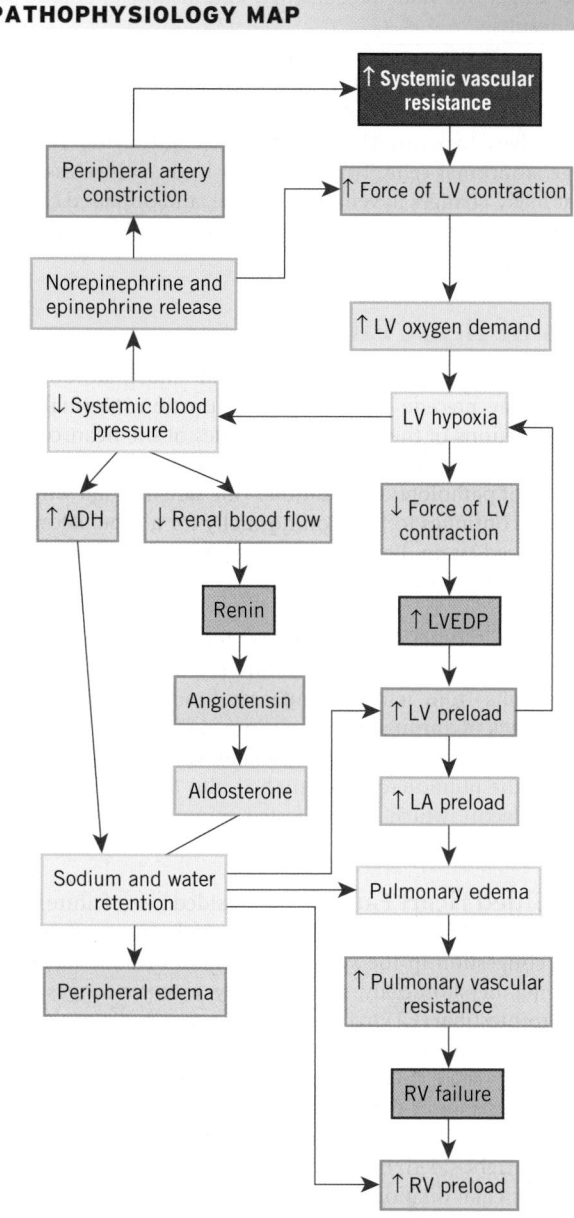

Figure 37-2 Left-sided heart failure from elevated systemic vascular resistance. Left-sided heart failure leads to right-sided heart failure. Systemic vascular resistance and preload are exacerbated by renal and adrenal mechanisms. *ADH*, antidiuretic hormone; *LA*, left atrial; *LV*, left ventricle/ventricular; *LVEDP*, left ventricular end-diastolic pressure; *RV*, right ventricle/ventricular.

Source: Adapted from Huether, S. E., & McCance, K. L. (2004). *Understanding pathophysiology* (3rd ed.). St Louis: Mosby.

associated with a mild increase in the respiratory rate and a decrease in arterial partial pressure of oxygen (PaO₂).

If pulmonary venous pressure continues to increase, the increase in intravascular pressure causes more fluid to move into the interstitial space than the lymphatics can drain. *Interstitial edema* occurs at this point. Tachypnea develops, and the patient becomes symptomatic (short of breath out of proportion to activity level). If the pulmonary venous pressure increases further, the tight alveoli lining cells are disrupted and a fluid containing red

blood cells moves into the alveoli (alveolar edema). As the disruption becomes worse from further increases in the pulmonary venous pressure, the alveoli and the airways are flooded with fluid (see Figure 37-3). This is accompanied by a worsening of the blood gas values (i.e., lower PaO₂ and possible increased arterial partial pressure of carbon dioxide [PaCO₂] and progressive respiratory acidemia).

Clinical manifestations of pulmonary edema are unmistakable. The patient is usually anxious, pale, and possibly cyanotic. The skin is clammy and cold from vasoconstriction caused by stimulation of the SNS. The patient has severe dyspnea, as evidenced by the use of accessory muscles of respiration, a respiratory rate greater than 30 breaths/min, and orthopnea. There may be wheezing and coughing with the production of frothy, blood-tinged sputum. Auscultation of the lungs may reveal crackles, wheezes, and rhonchi throughout the lungs. The patient's HR is rapid, and BP may be elevated or decreased depending on the severity of the HF.

Clinical Manifestations of Chronic Heart Failure

The clinical manifestations of chronic HF depend on the patient's age, the underlying type and extent of heart disease, and which ventricle is failing to pump effectively. Table 37-3 lists the manifestations of right-sided HF and left-sided HF. The patient with chronic HF will probably have manifestations of biventricular failure.

Fatigue. Fatigue is one of the earliest symptoms of chronic HF. The patient notices fatigue after activities that normally are not tiring. The fatigue is caused by decreased CO, impaired perfusion to vital organs, decreased oxygenation of the tissues, and anemia. Anemia can result from poor nutrition, renal disease, or drug therapy (e.g., angiotensin-converting enzyme [ACE] inhibitors).

Dyspnea. *Dyspnea* (shortness of breath) is a common manifestation of chronic HF. It is caused by increased pulmonary pressures secondary to interstitial and alveolar edema. Dyspnea can occur with mild exertion or at rest. *Orthopnea* is shortness of breath that occurs when the patient is in a recumbent position. **Paroxysmal nocturnal dyspnea** is a disorder characterized by sudden attacks of respiratory distress that occur when the patient is asleep. It is caused by the resorption, usually after several hours of being in a recumbent position, of fluid accumulated in dependent body areas. The patient awakens in a panic, has feelings of suffocation, and has a strong desire to seek relief by sitting up. Careful questioning of patients often reveals adaptive behaviour such as sleeping with two or more pillows to aid breathing. Because there are increased pulmonary pressures and fluid accumulation in the lung tissues, the patient may have a persistent, dry cough, unrelieved with position or over-the-counter cough suppressants. A dry, hacking cough may be the first clinical symptom of HF.

Tachycardia. Tachycardia is an early clinical sign of HF. One of the body's first mechanisms to compensate for a failing ventricle is to increase the HR. Because of diminished CO, there is increased SNS stimulation, which increases HR. However, many patients with chronic HF take β-blocker medications and may not show an increase in response to SNS stimulation.

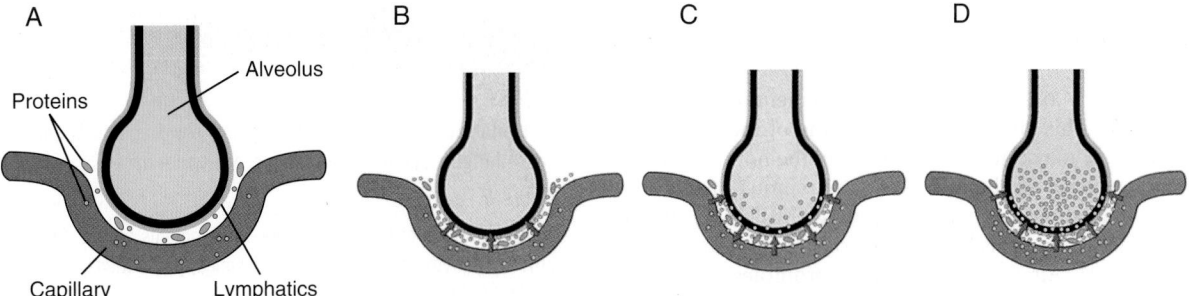

Figure 37-3 As pulmonary edema progresses, it inhibits oxygen and carbon dioxide exchange at the alveolar capillary interface. **A,** Normal relationship. **B,** Increased pulmonary–capillary hydrostatic pressure causes fluid to move from the vascular space into the pulmonary interstitial space. **C,** Lymphatic flow increases in an attempt to pull fluid back into the vascular or lymphatic space. **D,** Failure of lymphatic flow and worsening of left-sided heart failure result in further movement of fluid into the interstitial space and into the alveoli.

Source: Redrawn from Urden, L. D., Stacy, K. M., & Lough, M. E. (2010). *Critical care nursing: Diagnosis and management* (6th ed., p. 462, Figure 19-17). St. Louis: Mosby.

Table 37-3 Clinical Manifestations of Heart Failure

RIGHT-SIDED HEART FAILURE	LEFT-SIDED HEART FAILURE
Signs	
• RV heaves	• LV heaves
• Murmurs	• Cheyne-Stokes respirations
• Peripheral edema	• Pulsus alternans (alternating pulses: strong, weak)
• Weight gain	
• ↑ HR	• ↑ HR
• Edema of dependent body parts (sacrum, anterior tibias, pedal edema)	• PMI displaced inferiorly and posteriorly (LV hypertrophy)
• Ascites	• ↓ PaO$_2$, slight ↑ PaCO$_2$ (poor O$_2$ exchange)
• Anasarca (massive generalized body edema)	• Crackles (pulmonary edema)
• Jugular venous distension	• S3 and S4 (see Easy Auscultation Web site listed in the Resources at the end of this chapter)
• Hepatomegaly (liver enlargement)	
• Right-sided pleural effusion	
Symptoms	
• Fatigue	• Fatigue
• Dependent edema	• Dyspnea (shallow respirations ≤32-40/min)
• Right upper quadrant pain	• Orthopnea (shortness of breath in recumbent position)
• Anorexia and GI bloating	
• Nausea	• Dry, hacking cough
	• Pulmonary edema
	• Nocturia
	• Paroxysmal nocturnal dyspnea

GI, gastrointestinal; *HR,* heart rate; *LV,* left ventricle/ventricular; *PaO$_2$,* arterial partial pressure of oxygen; *PaCO$_2$,* arterial partial pressure of carbon dioxide; *PMI,* point of maximal impulse; *RV,* right ventricle/ventricular; *S3, S4,* third and fourth heart sounds.

Edema. Edema is a common sign of HF. It may occur in dependent body areas (peripheral edema), liver (hepatomegaly), abdominal cavity (ascites), and lungs (pulmonary edema and pleural effusion). If the patient is in bed, sacral and scrotal edema may develop. Pressing the edematous skin with the finger may leave a transient indentation (pitting edema). The development of dependent edema or a sudden weight gain of more than 2 kg in 2 days is often indicative of exacerbated HF.

Nocturia. A person with chronic HF who has decreased CO will also have impaired renal perfusion and decreased urinary output during the day. However, when the person lies down at night, fluid movement from interstitial spaces back into the circulatory system is enhanced. This causes increased renal blood flow and diuresis. The patient may complain of having to void six or seven times during the night.

Skin Changes. Because tissue capillary oxygen extraction is increased in a person with chronic HF, the skin may appear dusky. It is also cool and may be cool to the touch from diaphoresis. Often, the lower extremities are shiny and swollen, with diminished or absent hair growth. Chronic swelling may result in pigment changes, causing the skin of the ankles and lower legs to appear brown.

Behavioural Changes. Cerebral circulation may be impaired with chronic HF secondary to decreased CO. The patient or family may report unusual behaviour, including restlessness, confusion, and decreased attention span or memory. This may also be secondary to poor gas exchange and worsening renal failure.

Chest Pain. HF can precipitate chest pain because of decreased coronary perfusion from decreased CO and increased myocardial work. Pain of the anginal type may accompany either acute or chronic HF.

Weight Changes. Many factors contribute to weight changes. Initially, there may be a progressive weight gain from fluid retention. However, over time, the patient is often too sick to eat. Abdominal fullness from ascites and hepatomegaly frequently causes anorexia and nausea. Renal failure may also contribute to fluid retention. In many cases, the muscle and fat loss is masked by the patient's edematous condition. The actual weight loss may not be apparent until after the edema subsides.

Complications of Heart Failure

Pleural Effusion. Pleural effusion results from increasing pressure in the pleural capillaries. A transudation of fluid occurs from these capillaries into the pleural space. (Pleural effusion is discussed in Chapter 30.)

Dysrhythmias. Chronic HF causes enlargement of the chambers of the heart. This enlargement (stretching of the atrial and ventricular tissues) may cause an alteration in the normal electrical pathway, especially in the atria. When numerous sites in the atria fire spontaneously and rapidly (atrial fibrillation), atrial systole no longer occurs. This loss of atrial contraction can reduce CO by 10 to 20%. Atrial fibrillation also promotes thrombus formation within the atria, which may break loose and form emboli. Patients with atrial fibrillation are at risk for stroke and require treatment with cardioversion, antidysrhythmics, anticoagulants, or some combination. (Dysrhythmias are discussed in Chapter 38.)

Patients with HF (those with an EF <35%) have a high risk of fatal dysrhythmias; nearly one half experience sudden cardiac death, usually because of ventricular tachydysrhythmias. (Sudden cardiac death is discussed in Chapter 36.)

Left Ventricular Thrombus. With acute or chronic HF, the enlarged LV and the decreased CO combine to increase the chance of thrombus formation in the LV. Current guidelines of the CCS recommend anticoagulation in patients with HF and atrial fibrillation or with documented or suspected left ventricular thrombus (Arnold et al., 2006). Once a thrombus has formed, it may also decrease left ventricular contractility, decrease CO, and further worsen the patient's perfusion. The development of emboli from the thrombus is also a possibility and can result in a stroke.

Hepatomegaly. HF can lead to severe hepatomegaly, especially with right ventricular failure. The liver lobules become congested with venous blood. The hepatic congestion leads to impaired liver function. Eventually, liver cells die, fibrosis occurs, and cirrhosis can develop (see Chapter 46).

Renal Failure. The decreased CO that accompanies acute and chronic HF results in decreased perfusion to the kidneys and can lead to renal insufficiency or failure.

Classification of Heart Failure

The New York Heart Association (NYHA) has developed functional guidelines for classifying symptoms experienced by patients with HF. The classification is based on the person's tolerance of physical activity (Table 37-4).

Diagnostic Studies

Diagnosing HF is often difficult because neither patient signs nor symptoms are highly specific, and both may mimic many other medical conditions, such as anemia or lung disease. The primary goal in diagnosis is to determine the underlying etiology of HF. Measures to assess the cause and degree of HF include a thorough history, physical examination, chest radiograph, electrocardiogram (ECG), laboratory data (cardiac enzymes, BNP, serum chemistries, liver function studies, thyroid function studies, and complete blood count), hemodynamic assessment, echocardiogram, stress testing, and cardiac catheterization. EF can be measured using echocardiography or nuclear imaging studies, or both. Echocardiography and measurement of EF can be used to differentiate between systolic and diastolic HF, an important dis-

Table 37-4 New York Heart Association Functional Classification of People With Cardiac Disease

Class I

No limitation of physical activity. Ordinary physical activity does not cause fatigue, dyspnea, palpitations, or anginal pain.

Class II

Slight limitation of physical activity. No symptoms at rest. Ordinary physical activity results in fatigue, dyspnea, palpitations, or anginal pain.

Class III

Marked limitation of physical activity. Usually comfortable at rest. Ordinary physical activity causes fatigue, dyspnea, palpitations, or anginal pain.

Class IV

Inability to carry on any physical activity without discomfort. Symptoms of cardiac insufficiency or of angina may be present even at rest. If any physical activity is undertaken, discomfort is increased.

Source: Heart Failure Society of America. (2002). Retrieved from *http://www.abouthf.org/questions_stages.htm*

Table 37-5 Plasma B-type or Brain Natriuretic Peptide Levels*

BNP < 100 ng/L	BNP 100-500 ng/L	BNP > 500 ng/L
HF very improbable	HF probable	HF very probable

BNP, B-type or brain natriuretic peptide; *HF,* heart failure.
*Levels can be increased in the presence of renal dysfunction or sepsis and be decreased in obese patients.

tinction to make in the early treatment of HF. BNP levels are used to assist in the diagnosis of HF; in general, levels correlate positively with the degree of left ventricular dysfunction and can help to differentiate dyspnea caused by HF from other causes of dyspnea (Arnold et al., 2007) (Table 37-5). Diagnostic studies used for the patient with ADHF are presented in Table 37-6, and those for the patient with chronic HF are presented in Table 37-7.

NURSING AND COLLABORATIVE MANAGEMENT: ACUTE DECOMPENSATED HEART FAILURE AND PULMONARY EDEMA

The goal of therapy is to improve left ventricular function by decreasing intravascular volume, decreasing venous return (preload), decreasing afterload, improving gas exchange and oxygenation, increasing CO, and reducing anxiety. Table 37-6 lists the major components of the therapeutic approach.

Decreasing Intravascular Volume

Decreasing intravascular volume with the use of diuretics reduces venous return. A loop diuretic (e.g., furosemide [Lasix]) may be used to decrease volume because it may be administered by intravenous (IV) push, and its action within the kidney occurs rapidly. By decreasing venous return to the LV and thereby reducing

COLLABORATIVE CARE

Table 37-6 Acute Decompensated Heart Failure and Pulmonary Edema

Diagnostic	Collaborative Therapy
• History and physical examination	• Treatment of underlying cause
• ABGs, serum chemistries, liver function tests, BNP	• Place patient in high Fowler's position
• Chest radiographic examination	• O_2 by mask or nasal catheter
• Hemodynamic monitoring	• Cardiac monitoring and pulse oximetry
• 12-lead ECG	• BP, HR, RR, urinary output at least q1h
• Echocardiogram	• Hemodynamic monitoring (e.g., intra-arterial BP, PAOP, CO)
• Nuclear imaging studies	• Daily measurement of weight
• Cardiac catheterization	• Drug therapy: morphine IV; diuretics IV (furosemide [Lasix]); nitroglycerin IV; inotropic therapy (see Table 37-8)
	• Cardioversion
	• Endotracheal intubation and mechanical ventilation
	• Circulatory assist devices (e.g., intra-aortic balloon pump, ventricular assist device)

ABGs, arterial blood gases; *BNP*, B-type or brain natriuretic peptide; *BP*, blood pressure; *CO*, cardiac output; *ECG*, electrocardiogram; *HR*, heart rate; *IV*, intravenously; *PAOP*, pulmonary artery occlusive pressure; *RR*, respiratory rate.

COLLABORATIVE CARE

Table 37-7 Chronic Heart Failure

Diagnostic	Collaborative Therapy
• History and physical examination	• Treatment of underlying cause
• Determination of underlying cause	• Drug therapy (see Table 37-8)
• Serum chemistries, BNP, liver function tests	• Daily measurement of weight
	• Sodium- and fluid-restricted diet
• Chest radiographic examination	• Oxygen therapy if O_2 saturation <95%
• 12-lead ECG	• Regular activity and rest periods
• Echocardiography	
• Exercise stress testing	• Cardiac resynchronization therapy (biventricular pacemaker)
• Nuclear imaging studies (e.g., cardiac MRI, cardiac CT scan)	• Implantable cardioverter–defibrillator
• Cardiac catheterization	• Cardiac transplantation
• Sleep study	• Consider circulatory assist device (intra-aortic balloon pump, ventricular assist device)

BNP, B-type or brain natriuretic peptide; *CT*, computed tomography; *ECG*, electrocardiogram; *MRI*, magnetic resonance imaging.

preload, the overfilled LV may contract more efficiently and thus contribute to improving CO. This improves left ventricular function, decreases pulmonary vascular pressures, and improves gas exchange.

Ultrafiltration is an option for the patient with volume overload. Ultrafiltration has generally been achieved through hemodialysis or with ultrafiltration by way of central venous access. Newer technology allows removal of up to 500 mL/hr of fluid through either a peripheral or a central venous line without significantly changing mean arterial pressure. When ultrafiltration is performed, only fluid volume is removed using a technique similar to hemodialysis. This therapeutic modality may be an appropriate therapy for patients with HF who are resistant to standard diuretic therapy or who cannot tolerate these medications. Research shows that more fluid can be removed in the setting of diuretic resistance, resulting in a lower rehospitalization rate (Costanzo et al., 2007). (Ultrafiltration is discussed in Chapter 49.)

Decreasing Venous Return

Decreasing venous return (preload) reduces the amount of volume returned to the LV during diastole. This can be accomplished by placing the patient in a high Fowler's position with the feet horizontal in the bed or dangling at the bedside. This position helps decrease venous return because of the pooling of blood in the extremities. This position also increases the thoracic capacity, allowing for improved ventilation. IV nitroglycerin is a vasodilator used in the treatment of ADHF. It reduces circulating volume by decreasing preload and also increases coronary artery circulation by dilating the coronary arteries. In addition to reducing preload, it slightly reduces afterload (in high doses) and increases myocardial oxygen supply.

Decreasing Afterload

Afterload is the resistance against which the LV must pump; that is, it is the amount of work it takes for the LV to eject blood into the systemic circulation. Systemic vascular resistance (SVR) is a determinant of afterload, as is left ventricular filling. If afterload is reduced, the CO of the LV improves and thereby decreases pulmonary congestion.

IV nitroprusside (Nipride) is a potent vasodilator that reduces preload and afterload. Because of its potent effects on the vascular system, it should be considered only if the systolic BP is greater than 100 mm Hg (Arnold et al., 2007). By reducing both preload and afterload (by arteriolar and venous dilation), myocardial contraction improves, increasing CO and reducing pulmonary congestion (Mullens et al., 2008). Complications of IV nitroprusside include (1) severe hypotension (continuous BP monitoring is required) and (2) thiocyanate toxicity, which can develop after 48 hours of use.

Morphine also reduces preload and afterload. It dilates both the pulmonary and the systemic blood vessels, a goal in decreasing pulmonary pressures and improving the exchange of gases.

Improving Gas Exchange and Oxygenation

Gas exchange may be improved by several measures. IV morphine decreases oxygen demands, which may be raised as a result of anxiety and subsequent increased musculoskeletal and respiratory activity. Administration of oxygen if the O_2 saturation is below 95% (Arnold et al., 2007) helps increase the percentage of oxygen in inspired air. (Oxygen therapy is discussed in Chapter 31.) In severe pulmonary edema, the patient may need noninvasive ventilatory support (e.g., bilevel positive airway pressure) or intubation and mechanical ventilation. (Ventilatory support is discussed in Chapter 68.)

Improving Cardiac Function

In a patient who is or becomes hemodynamically unstable—that is, becomes progressively hypotensive, has an HR that is abnormally fast or slow, develops dysrhythmias, or becomes hypoxic with cool and clammy skin—nursing care becomes more urgent, and treatment protocols may call for aggressive, complex therapies. The use of diuretics, morphine sulphate, and vasodilators may not be sufficient to control symptoms. The addition of positive inotropic therapy may be warranted as well as the initiation of hemodynamic monitoring to evaluate the effectiveness of interventions. Once a pulmonary artery catheter is in position, accurate measurement of CO, pulmonary artery pressure (PAP), and PAOP may be made and therapy instituted and titrated to maximize CO. A PAOP of 14 to 18 mm Hg will generally achieve the goal of increasing CO. (Hemodynamic monitoring is discussed in Chapter 68.)

Inotropic drugs (e.g., dobutamine, milrinone) that increase myocardial contractility without increasing oxygen consumption are also effective. Dobutamine and milrinone also cause increased peripheral vasodilation. In patients with systolic BP less than 90 mm Hg, dobutamine should be used instead of milrinone (Arnold et al., 2007).

Reducing Anxiety

Reduction of anxiety is facilitated by the sedative action of morphine administered intravenously. When morphine is used, the patient must be watched closely for respiratory depression. In addition, a calm approach in providing care helps reduce anxiety.

Once the patient is more stable, determination of the cause of pulmonary edema is important. Diagnosis of systolic or diastolic failure will then determine further management protocols. Aggressive drug therapy may continue with IV forms of inotropic drugs, vasodilators, and ACE inhibitors. Nursing care focuses on continual physical assessment, hemodynamic monitoring, and monitoring the patient's response to treatment.

Collaborative Care: Chronic Heart Failure

The main goal in the management of HF is to treat the underlying cause and contributing factors, maximize CO, and provide treatment to alleviate symptoms (see Table 37-6). The management of dysrhythmias is discussed in Chapter 38, hypertension in Chapter 35, valvular disorders in Chapter 39, and coronary artery disease in Chapter 36.

In a person with HF, oxygen saturation of the blood is reduced because the blood is not adequately oxygenated in the lungs.

Administration of oxygen, if the O_2 saturation is less than 95%, improves tissue oxygenation. Thus, oxygen therapy helps relieve dyspnea and fatigue. Pulse oximetry should be used to monitor the effectiveness of oxygen therapy.

Regular exercise periods should be prescribed for all patients with stable chronic HF. Even patients with NYHA Class III symptoms (see Table 37-4) should exercise three to five times per week for 30 to 45 minutes at a time. A graded exercise test should be performed first, and involvement in a cardiac rehabilitation program will provide the patient with an individualized exercise regimen (Arnold et al., 2006).

Other nonpharmacological therapies are used in the management of patients with HF who are receiving maximum medical therapy, continue to have NYHA functional Class III or IV symptoms (see Table 37-4), and have a widened QRS interval. One therapy is biventricular pacing. Traditional pacemakers pace one or two chambers (e.g., atrium or ventricle, or both). Cardiac resynchronization therapy (CRT) coordinates right ventricle (RV) and LV contractility through biventricular pacing. The ability to have normal electrical conduction within the RV and LV improves left ventricular performance and CO. This additional therapy allows patients to increase their exercise capacity and decrease their overall symptoms. CRT has been shown to prolong life and improve quality of life in patients with NYHA functional Class III and IV HF (Howlett et al., 2009). CRT can be combined with traditional pacing capability as well as defibrillator technology. If the patient has HF, has NYHA functional Class II or III, is on optimal medical therapy, and has an EF of less than 35%, the implementation and use of an implantable cardioverter–defibrillator (ICD) with CRT may be warranted. Life-threatening ventricular dysrhythmias (e.g., ventricular tachycardia) are a complication of the ischemic myocardium and can cause sudden cardiac death. The addition of the ICD in these patients has reduced the overall mortality from sudden death (Arnold et al., 2006). (Pacemakers and defibrillators are discussed in Chapter 38.)

Cardiac transplantation is often the treatment of choice. However, the lack of donor hearts makes it an option for only a small number of patients with HF. (Heart transplants are discussed later in this chapter.)

Several mechanical options are available to sustain HF patients with deteriorating conditions, especially those awaiting cardiac transplantation. The intra-aortic balloon pump (IABP) is used for short-term support for HF patients with acute decompensation. However, the limitations of bed rest, infection, and vascular complications preclude its long-term use. Ventricular assist devices (VADs) (Figure 37-4) provide highly effective long-term support for more than 2 years and have become standard care for acutely decompensated transplant candidates. (IABPs and VADs are discussed further in Chapter 68.)

Drug Therapy: Chronic Heart Failure

General therapeutic objectives for drug management of chronic HF include the following: (1) identification of the type of HF and the underlying causes, (2) correction of sodium and water retention and volume overload, (3) reduction of cardiac workload, (4) improvement of myocardial contractility, and (5) control of precipitating and complicating factors. The aims of treating HF are to improve symptoms, minimize adverse effects of treatment, prevent morbidity, and prolong survival. Current therapeutic approaches stress the importance of ACE inhibitors and β-adrenergic blockers (Arnold et al., 2006) (Table 37-8).

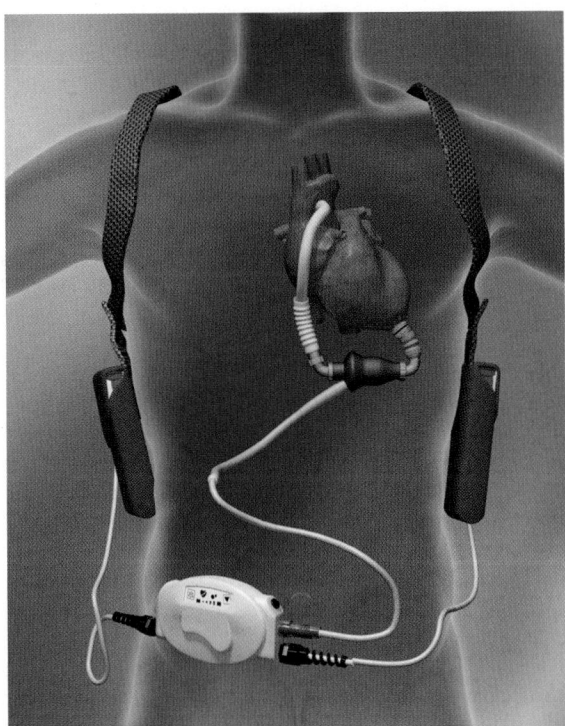

Figure 37-4 The HeartMate II ventricular assist device (Thoratec Corp., Pleasanton, CA), now used in many transplant centres across Canada as a bridge to heart transplantation.

Source: Reprinted with permission from Thoratec Corporation. Retrieved from *http://www.thoratec.com/about-us/media-room/index.aspx*

Diuretics

Diuretics are used in HF to mobilize edematous fluid, reduce pulmonary venous pressure, and reduce preload (see Chapter 35, Table 35-8). If excess extracellular fluid is excreted, blood volume returning to the heart can be reduced and cardiac function improved.

Diuretics act on the kidney by promoting excretion of sodium and water. Many varieties of diuretics are available, and some have specific indications for use. Thiazide diuretics may be the first choice in chronic HF because of their convenience, safety, low cost, and effectiveness. They are particularly useful in treating edema secondary to HF and in controlling hypertension. The thiazides inhibit sodium reabsorption in the distal tubule, thus promoting excretion of sodium and water.

Loop diuretics (e.g., furosemide [Lasix], bumetanide [Burinex]) are potent diuretics. These drugs act on the ascending loop of Henle to promote sodium, chloride, and water excretion. Furosemide is more commonly used in acute HF and pulmonary edema because it is slightly more predictable in its response. Problems in using loop diuretics include reduction in serum potassium levels, ototoxicity, and possible allergic reaction in the patient who is sensitive to sulpha-type drugs.

Spironolactone (Aldactone) is a potassium-sparing diuretic that promotes sodium and water excretion but blocks potassium excretion by blocking the action of aldosterone. The drug is effective in patients with advanced heart failure (Arnold et al., 2006). Spironolactone appears to be additive to the benefits of ACE inhibitors, and careful monitoring of renal function and potassium levels is important.

In patients who are not responsive to high-dose loop diuretics, metolazone (Zaroxolyn) or a thiazide diuretic can be used

DRUG THERAPY
Table 37-8 Heart Failure

DRUG	BOTH ADHF AND CHRONIC HF	ADHF	CHRONIC HF
Diuretics (see Table 35-8)			
• Loop: furosemide (Lasix), bumetanide (Burinex)	X*	—	—
• *Thiazides:* hydrochlorothiazide	—	—	X
Inhibitors of renin–angiotensin–aldosterone system (see Table 35-8)			
• *ACE inhibitors:* captopril, benazepril (Lotensin), enalapril (Vasotec)	X	—	—
• *Angiotensin II receptor blockers:* losartan (Cozaar), valsartan (Diovan)	X	—	—
• *Aldosterone antagonists:* spironolactone (Aldactone), eplerenone (Inspra)	X	—	—
Morphine	—	X†	—
Vasodilators			
• Nitroprusside (Nipride)	—	X†	—
• Nitrates (e.g., nitroglycerin, isosorbide dinitrate)	X*	—	—
• Hydralazine (Apresoline)	—	—	X
β-Adrenergic blockers (see Table 35-8)			
• Metoprolol (Lopressor)	—	—	X
• Bisoprolol	—	—	—
• Carvedilol	—	—	—
Positive inotropes			
• Digitalis glycoside: digoxin (Lanoxin)	—	—	X
• β-Adrenergic agonists: dopamine, dobutamine	—	X†	—
• Phosphodiesterase inhibitors: milrinone	—	X†	—
Antidysrhythmic drugs (see Table 38-9)	X	—	—
Anticoagulants	X‡	—	—

ACE, angiotensin-converting enzyme; *ADHF,* acute decompensated heart failure; *HF,* heart failure.
*Administered intravenously or orally.
†Administered intravenously.
‡Recommended for patients with an ejection fraction <20% and/or atrial fibrillation.

(Arnold et al., 2006). A combination of diuretics may be administered for maximum effect.

Angiotensin-Converting Enzyme Inhibitors

ACE inhibitors are useful in both systolic and diastolic HF, and they are the first-line therapy in the treatment of HF. Examples of

ACE inhibitors include ramipril (Altace) and enalapril (Vasotec). Other examples of ACE inhibitors are discussed in Chapter 35 and listed in Table 35-8.

The conversion of angiotensin I to the potent vasoconstrictor angiotensin II requires the presence of ACE (see Chapter 47, Figure 47-6). ACE inhibitors exert their effects through blocking this enzyme, resulting in decreased levels of angiotensin II. As a result, plasma aldosterone levels are also reduced.

Because CO is dependent on afterload in chronic HF, the reduction in SVR seen with the use of ACE inhibitors produces a significant increase in CO. Furthermore, the improvement of CO and the redistribution of regional blood flow that result from the use of ACE inhibitors help maintain tissue perfusion, even though BP may be decreased. Other hemodynamic changes include a reduction in (1) PAP, (2) right arterial pressure, and (3) left ventricular filling pressure. Adverse effects of ACE inhibitors include symptomatic hypotension, chronic cough, and renal insufficiency (when used in high doses). Aging and baseline renal insufficiency slow the metabolism of ACE inhibitors and may, therefore, lead to increased toxicity (Arnold et al., 2006). It is recommended that these drugs be started at the lowest dose and slowly increased over a 2- to 3-month period and that BP and renal function be monitored at regular intervals. Overall, ACE inhibitors are well tolerated by patients.

In patients who are unable to tolerate the ACE inhibitors because of angioedema or cough, angiotensin II receptor blockers (ARBs) such as losartan (Cozaar) or valsartan (Diovan) may be used (see Chapter 35, Table 35-8). If a patient is already on an ACE inhibitor and a β-adrenergic blocker, an ARB can be added to the combination (Arnold et al., 2006).

β-Adrenergic Blockers

The use of β-adrenergic blockers (or β-blockers) in combination with ACE inhibitors in the management of HF has become standard therapy for most patients. Examples include carvedilol and metoprolol (Lopressor). Marked improvement in patient survival has been shown with the use of β-adrenergic blockers. β-Adrenergic blockers directly block the negative effects of the SNS on the failing heart, such as increased HR. Because β-adrenergic blockade can reduce myocardial contractility, care must be taken to start gradually, increasing the dosage slowly (typically every 2 wk) as tolerated by the patient, until a maximum dose is achieved. Major adverse effects include edema, hypotension, fatigue, asthma exacerbations, and bradycardia (Lehne, 2007).

Inotropic Drugs

The use of inotropic drugs in the patient with HF is directed at improving cardiac contractility to increase CO, decrease left ventricular diastolic pressure, and decrease SVR. Types of inotropic agents are listed in Table 37-8.

Sympathomimetic Agents.
Sympathomimetic agents (or β-adrenergic agonists) include dopamine, dobutamine, epinephrine (Adrenalin), and norepinephrine (Levophed). Stimulation of β-adrenergic receptors results in an increase in cyclic adenosine monophosphate within the myocardial cells and an increase in contractility (inotropic effect). The β-adrenergic agents are typically used as a short-term treatment of acute exacerbations of HF in the critical care environment. However, their role in long-term therapy of HF is controversial (Arnold et al.,

2007). Potential problems related to long-term treatment with these agents include tolerance (tachyphylaxis), increased ventricular irritability, limb ischemia, and increased myocardial oxygen demand.

Phosphodiesterase Inhibitors.
Inhibition of phosphodiesterase enhances calcium entry into the cell and improves myocardial contractility. Phosphodiesterase inhibitors are also potent vasodilators. They increase CO and reduce arterial pressure (decrease afterload). These drugs are not currently available in oral form. Therefore, they are limited to short-term use in the critical care setting.

Milrinone increases myocardial contraction, increases CO, promotes peripheral vasodilation, and decreases SVR, thus augmenting performance of the LV. Adverse reactions include dysrhythmias, thrombocytopenia, and GI effects. As for other inotropes, there is little evidence that these drugs offer a beneficial effect on mortality. Therefore, their use should be confined for short-term therapy only to patients in cardiogenic shock with volume overload and who have diuretic resistance (Arnold et al., 2007) (Table 37-9).

Digitalis Preparations.
Cardiac glycosides (e.g., digoxin [Lanoxin]) have been used for more than 200 years and remain important in the treatment of advanced HF. However, patients receiving digoxin should be closely monitored for signs of toxicity. Digoxin has been shown to reduce both symptoms and hospitalizations for HF. Digoxin can be useful in the treatment of HF with atrial fibrillation and rapid ventricular rate despite use of β-adrenergic blockers (Arnold et al., 2006). Digoxin has positive inotropic effects as well as decreasing the conduction speed within the myocardium to slow the HR (negative chronotropic action). These actions allow for more complete emptying of the ventricles, thus diminishing the volume remaining in the ventricles during diastole. CO increases because of an increased stroke volume from improved contractility.

An individual receiving a digitalis preparation should be closely monitored for signs and symptoms of digitalis toxicity. The incidence of digitalis toxicity can be increased in the presence of hypokalemia, renal dysfunction, and dehydration. Care should also be taken when introducing medications that may alter digoxin levels.

Vasodilator Drugs.
Vasodilator drugs are a class of drugs clearly shown to improve survival in overt HF. The goals of vasodilator therapy in the treatment of HF include (1) increasing venous capacity, (2) improving EF through improved ventricular contraction, (3) slowing the process of ventricular dysfunction, (4) decreasing heart size, and (5) avoiding stimulation of the neurohormonal responses initiated by the compensatory mechanisms of HF.

Nitrates.
Nitrates cause vasodilation by acting directly on the smooth muscle of the vessel wall. Their effects primarily involve increasing venous capacitance, dilating the pulmonary vasculature, and improving arterial compliance. Therefore, the major hemodynamic effect of nitrates is to decrease preload. Nitrates are of particular benefit in the management of myocardial ischemia related to HF because they promote vasodilation of the coronary arteries. Men with HF who take nitrates should not also take an erectile agent (e.g., sildenafil [Viagra]) to manage erectile dysfunction because together these drugs could precipitate profound hypotension.

Table 37-9 Intravenous Medications Used in the Management of Acute Decompensated Heart Failure

CHARACTERISTIC	NITROGLYCERIN	NITROPRUSSIDE	MILRINONE	DOBUTAMINE
Typical dose range	10-200 mcg/min	0.1-5 mcg/kg/min	Bolus 50 mcg/kg* then 03.75-0.75 mcg/kg/min	2.5-15 mcg/kg/min
Action				
Venodilator	X	X	—	—
Arterial vasodilator	X (coronary)	X	X	—
Diuretic	—	—	—	—
Inotropic	—	—	X	X
Indication	Myocardial ischemia, elevated PAOP, hypertension	Hypertensive crisis, elevated PAOP, acute aortic or mitral regurgitation	Very low cardiac output, high PAOP, pulmonary hypertension	Very low cardiac output with or without congestion or hypotension
Primary Effect				
Preload	↓	↓	↓	—
Afterload	Mild ↓	↓↓	↓	—
Diuresis	—	—	—	—
Natriuresis	—	—	—	—
Cardiac output	—	↑ (indirectly)	↑	↑
Stroke volume	—	—	—	↑
Comments	Rapid onset	Risk of cardiac ischemia from hypotension; assess for thiocyanate poisoning	Long half-life; risk of hypotension, prodysrhythmia	Assess for tachyphylaxis, tachycardia, ischemia, prodysrhythmia

PAOP, pulmonary artery occlusive pressure.
NOTE: X denotes that the drug has the specified action; ↓ denotes decrease; ↑ denotes increase. No entry indicates action or effect does not occur.
*Consider eliminating the bolus dose when systolic blood pressure ≤100 mm Hg; just begin infusion and wait 2 hours to assess patient for desired effects (there is a delay to peak effect if bolus omitted).
Source: Albert, N., Eastwood, C., & Edwards, M. (2004). Evidence-based practice for acute decompensated heart failure. *Critical Care Nurse, 24*(6), 14-29. Reprinted with permission.

Sodium Nitroprusside. Nitroprusside is a vasodilator used in the management of acute HF and pulmonary edema (see discussion earlier in this chapter).

Nutritional Therapy: Chronic Heart Failure

Diet education and weight management are critical to the patient's control of chronic HF. The nurse or the dietitian should obtain a detailed diet history, determining not only what foods the patient eats and when but also the sociocultural value of food for the patient. The nurse can use this information to assist the patient in solving problems and working with a dietitian to develop an individualized diet plan. The patient should be taught what foods are low and which are high in sodium and ways to enhance food flavours without the use of salt (e.g., substituting lemon juice and various spices).

The edema of chronic HF is often treated by dietary restriction of sodium. The degree of sodium restriction depends on the severity of the HF and the effectiveness of diuretic therapy. Diets that are severely restricted in sodium are rarely prescribed because they are unpalatable and patient adherence is poor. The Dietary Approach to Stop Hypertension (DASH) diet is effective as a first-line therapy for many individuals with isolated systolic hypertension (see Chapter 35, Table 35-7). The average daily dietary intake of sodium ranges from 3 to 7 g. A commonly prescribed diet for a patient with mild HF is a 2-g sodium diet. All foods high in

sodium should be eliminated. For more severe HF, sodium intake is restricted to 1 g (Arnold et al., 2006). With this diet, milk, cheese, bread, cereals, canned soups, and some canned vegetables must be eliminated. The patient and caregivers should be instructed on how to read labels to look for sodium as an ingredient (Table 37-10).

Typically, a low-sodium diet is unpalatable. In order to increase compliance with a low-sodium diet, the Canadian Heart Failure Network (CHFN) (2012) recommends that patients should be advised to do the following:

- Stop using the salt shaker (remove it from the dinner table).
- Do not add salt to food during preparation.
- Read food labels carefully.
- Stop eating processed and high-sodium foods: the greatest source of sodium (≤80%) is the salt and other sodium compounds added to food during processing.
- Be aware of "hidden" sources of sodium: for example, one slice of bread contains only 150 mg of sodium; however, the quantity of bread eaten during 1 day could cause total daily sodium intake to be high.

The CCS recommends that all patients with fluid retention or congestion not responsive to diuretic therapy, or patients with renal dysfunction or hyponatremia, should restrict fluid intake to 1.5 to 2 L/day (Arnold et al., 2006). That equates to six to eight glasses of fluid per day. Patients should be reminded that fluid is hidden in foods such as fruits and ice cream. In practice, most Canadian HF clinics advise fluid restriction for all HF patients.

NUTRITIONAL THERAPY

Table 37-10 Sodium Label Language*

CLAIM	WHAT IT MEANS
a. Free of sodium or salt	<5 mg of sodium per serving
b. Low in sodium or salt	≤140 mg of sodium per serving (or per 100 g, if the food is a prepackaged meal)
c. Reduced or lower in sodium or salt	The food is processed, formulated, reformulated, or otherwise modified so that it contains at least 25% less sodium than regular foods of its type
d. No added sodium or salt	The food contains no added salt, other sodium salts, or ingredients that contain sodium that functionally substitute for added salt
e. Lightly salted	The food contains at least 50% less sodium added than the sodium added to the similar reference food
f. Words to the effect that the food is "for use in a sodium-restricted diet"	The food meets the criteria for item a, b, or c, above
g. Words to the effect that the food is "for special dietary use" with respect to the sodium (salt) content	The food meets the criteria for either item a or b above

*Use caution with products advertised as salt replacements. They may contain high quantities of potassium.
Source: Adapted from Canadian Food Inspection Agency. (2011). *Summary table for sodium (salt) claims.* Retrieved from *http://www.inspection.gc.ca/english/fssa/labeti/guide/ch7be.shtml#tab7-10*

NUTRITIONAL THERAPY

Table 37-11 Sodium Content in Different Food Groups

FOOD GROUPS	SODIUM (mg)
Grains and Grain Products	
Cooked cereal, rice, pasta, unsalted, ½ cup	0-5
Ready-to-eat cereal, 1 cup	100-360
Bread, 1 slice	110-175
Vegetables	
Fresh or frozen, cooked without salt, ½ cup	1-70
Canned or frozen with sauce, ½ cup	140-460
Tomato juice, canned, ¾ cup	820
Fruit	
Fresh, frozen, canned, ½ cup	0-5
Low-Fat or Fat-Free Dairy Foods	
Milk, 1 cup	120
Yogurt, 250 mL	160
Natural cheeses, 45 g	110-450
Processed cheeses, 45 g	600
Nuts, Seeds, and Dry Beans	
Peanuts, salted, ⅓ cup	120
Peanuts, unsalted, ⅓ cup	0-5
Beans, cooked from dried or frozen, without salt, ½ cup	400
Meats, Fish, and Poultry	
Fresh meat, fish, poultry, 85 g	30-90
Tuna, canned, water pack, no salt added, 85 g	34-45
Tuna, canned, water pack, 85 g	250-350
Ham (lean) roasted, 85 g	1020

It is vital that patients weigh themselves daily to monitor fluid retention. Patients should be instructed to weigh themselves at the same time each day, preferably before breakfast, while wearing the same type of clothing. This helps ensure valid comparisons from day to day and helps identify early signs of fluid retention. If a patient experiences a weight gain of 2 kg over a 2- to 5-day period, the primary care provider should be called.

General Principles

Eating Well with Canada's Food Guide (Health Canada, 2011), containing dietary recommendations endorsed by Health Canada in 2011, advises a diet low in sodium for all Canadians. The guide recommends that, before purchasing foods, the patient should read the "Nutrition Facts" label, which is mandatory on all packaged foods (see Chapter 42, Figure 42-3).

Only a small amount of sodium occurs naturally in foods. Most sodium is added during processing. Table 37-11 gives examples of varying amounts of sodium that occur in Western foods before and after processing.

The Chinese diet is usually very high in sodium. Patients with HF who adhere to a Chinese diet should be taught to consider the advice in Table 37-12. When teaching the patient with HF who adheres to an East Indian diet, the nurse should take into account the considerations presented in Table 37-13.

NURSING MANAGEMENT: CHRONIC HEART FAILURE

Nursing Assessment

Subjective and objective data that should be obtained from a patient with HF include those presented in Table 37-14.

Nursing Diagnoses

Nursing diagnoses for the patient with HF include, but are not limited to, those presented in Nursing Care Plan (NCP) 37-1.

Planning

The overall goals are that the patient with HF will have (1) decreased peripheral edema, (2) decreased shortness of breath, (3) increased exercise tolerance, (4) adherence to drug regimen, and (5) no complications related to HF.

Table 37-12 Considerations for Sodium Intake in the Chinese Diet

	HIGH IN SODIUM	INSTEAD CHOOSE
Protein	Barbecued meats, Chinese sausages, salted fish, dried shrimp, salted eggs, century eggs, canned fish with black beans	Fresh or frozen unsalted meats, fish, poultry, seafood, eggs, tofu
Condiments and sauces	Monosodium glutamate (MSG), soy sauce, oyster sauce, fish sauce, shrimp paste, Hoisin sauce, Teriyaki sauce, Chinese cooking wine, bean paste, miso, fermented tofu, ketchup	Fresh herbs and spices, such as ginger, onion, garlic, garlic powder, green onion, curry powder, pepper, lemon, vinegar, honey, sesame oil, low-sodium soy sauce
Other foods	Instant noodles, instant rice with seasonings, salty soups, bouillon (cubes or powder)	Unprocessed grain products (e.g., fresh rice, rice noodles, udon noodles, congee, pasta, bread), low-sodium soups
Dining-out tips	Most food served in Chinese restaurants is high in sodium; eat in restaurants only occasionally	Choose plain rice rather than rice or noodles mixed with sauces (especially soy sauce or teriyaki sauce)

Table 37-13 Considerations for Sodium Intake in the East Indian Diet

	HIGH IN SODIUM	INSTEAD TRY THIS
Protein	Canned beans and lentils	Use fresh beans and lentils to make daal
Condiments and sauces	Achaars (pickles); chutneys (made with salt); relish; tomato, curry, or mustard paste; black salt	Fresh herbs and spices: curry powder, turmeric, chili powder, mustard seeds, ginger, garlic, pepper, cumin, fenugreek (methi), garam masala
Dining out tips	Most food served in East Indian restaurants is high in sodium; eat in restaurants only occasionally	Ask for foods prepared without salt / Avoid salty chutneys or relishes

▪ Nursing Implementation

▪ Health Promotion

An important measure used to prevent HF is the treatment or control of the underlying heart disease. For example, in valvular disease, valve replacement should be planned before lung congestion develops. Coronary revascularization procedures should be performed in patients with CAD. Another important preventive

NURSING ASSESSMENT
Table 37-14 Heart Failure

Subjective Data

Important Health Information

Past health history: CAD (including recent MI), hypertension, cardiomyopathy, valvular or congenital heart disease, diabetes mellitus, thyroid or lung disease, rapid or irregular heart rate

Medications: Use of and adherence to any cardiac medications; use of diuretics, estrogens, corticosteroids, nonsteroidal anti-inflammatory drugs, over-the-counter drugs, herbal supplements

Symptoms

- Fatigue, depression, anxiety
- Nausea, vomiting, anorexia, stomach bloating
- Weight gain, ankle swelling, nocturia, decreased daytime urinary output
- Dyspnea, orthopnea, cough
- Chest pain or heaviness; palpitations, dizziness, fainting
- RUQ pain, abdominal discomfort, constipation
- Behavioural changes, visual changes

Objective Data

Integumentary

Cool, diaphoretic skin; cyanosis or pallor, peripheral edema (right-sided heart failure)

Respiratory

Tachypnea, crackles, rhonchi, wheezes; frothy, blood-tinged sputum

Cardiovascular

Tachycardia, S3, S4, murmurs; pulsus alternans, PMI displaced inferiorly and posteriorly, jugular vein distension

Gastrointestinal

Abdominal distension, hepatosplenomegaly, ascites

Neurological

Restlessness, confusion, decreased attention or memory

Possible Findings

Altered serum electrolytes (especially Na^+ and K^+), ↑ BUN (serum urea [nitrogen]), ↑ BNP, creatinine, or liver function tests; chest radiograph demonstrating cardiomegaly, pulmonary congestion, and interstitial pulmonary edema; echocardiogram showing increased chamber size and decreased wall motion; ECG showing atrial and ventricular enlargement; ↓ O_2 saturation

BNP, brain or B-type natriuretic peptide; *BUN,* blood urea nitrogen; *CAD,* coronary artery disease; *ECG,* electrocardiogram; *MI,* myocardial infarction; *PMI,* point of maximal impulse; *RUQ,* right upper quadrant; *S3, S4,* third and fourth heart sounds.

measure concerns early and continued treatment of hypertension. Hyperlipidemic states in people with CAD should be managed with diet, exercise, and medication. The use of antidysrhythmic agents or an ICD–pacemaker is indicated for people with continuing low EF even if they are receiving optimal medical therapy or are at risk for sudden cardiac death. In addition, patients with HF should be counselled to quit smoking and obtain yearly vaccinations against the flu.

When a patient is diagnosed with HF, preventive care should focus on slowing the progression of the disease. Knowledge of the importance of following the medication, diet, and

Does Patient Discharge Education Improve Clinical Outcomes in Chronic Heart Failure Patients?

Clinical Question

For patients with chronic heart failure (P), will a 1-hr patient education session at discharge (I) improve clinical outcomes (O) compared with patients who receive no education (C)?

Best Available Evidence

RCT

Critical Appraisal and Synthesis of Evidence

- RCT (n = 223) of patients with chronic heart failure.
- Patients received a 1-hr one-on-one teaching session with a nurse educator upon hospital discharge.
- Patients who received the education had improved adherence to self-care, lower risk of rehospitalization and death, and lower cost of care.

Conclusion

Adding a 1-hr patient education session at time of discharge improves clinical outcomes, increases self-care adherence, and reduces cost of care for patients with heart failure.

Implications for Nursing Practice

- Planning for patient discharge is essential to improve clinical outcomes.
- Discharge education should include information about the cause of heart failure, drug therapy, dietary limitations, and importance of self-care behaviours (e.g., smoking cessation, daily weight monitoring).

Reference for Evidence

Koelling, T. M., Johnson, M. L., Cody, R. J., & Aaronson, K. D. (2005). Discharge education improves clinical outcomes in patients with chronic heart failure. *Circulation, 111*, 179.

PICO: P, patient population of interest; *I,* intervention or area of interest; *C,* comparison of interest or comparison group; *O,* outcome(s) of interest; *RCT,* randomized controlled trial.

exercise regimens is essential. Exercise training (e.g., cardiac rehabilitation) improves symptoms of chronic HF but is often underprescribed.

The registered nurse may request home nursing care for the patient and family or caregivers to provide for follow-up care and counselling. When the patient learns to identify signs and symptoms of worsening HF, it may help prevent an acute episode requiring an emergency department visit and possible rehospitalization (Koelling, Johnson, Cody, & Aaronson, 2005).

■ Acute Intervention

Successful HF management depends on several important principles: (1) HF is a progressive disease, and treatment plans are established with quality-of-life goals; (2) symptoms are managed by the patient with self-management tools (daily weights, drug regimens, exercise plans); (3) salt and water must be restricted; (4) a regular, prescribed level of exercise should be maintained; and (5) use of support systems is essential to the success of the entire treatment plan (Arnold et al., 2006).

Many people with HF experience one or more episodes of acute decompensation. When they do, they may be initially managed in a critical care area and later transferred to a general medical or cardiology unit when their condition has stabilized. The NCP for the patient with HF (see NCP 37-1) applies to the patient with stabilized acute or chronic HF.

■ Ambulatory and Home Care

HF is almost always a chronic illness. Important nursing responsibilities are (1) teaching the patient about the physiological changes that have occurred, (2) assisting the patient to adapt to both the physiological and the psychological changes, and (3) integrating the patient and the patient's family or support system in the overall care plan (Arnold et al., 2006). Research has revealed that patients with HF are at risk for depression (Rutledge, Reis, Linke, Greenberg, & Mills, 2006). Research shows that HF patients who are depressed are more likely to be rehospitalized and die prematurely (Sherwood et al., 2007). Depression should be treated appropriately in order for patients to adhere to medical therapy. It must be emphasized to the patient and the patient's caregivers that it is possible to live productively with this chronic illness. Managing patients with HF in their own communities is a priority of care. A patient and caregiver teaching guide for the patient with HF is presented in Table 37-15.

Patients with chronic HF are required to take medication for the rest of their lives. This often becomes difficult because a patient may be asymptomatic when HF is under control. It must be stressed that the disease is chronic and that medication administration must be continued even through stable periods to prevent acute decompensation of their HF.

The patient and caregivers should learn to evaluate how the patient is feeling and recognize symptoms of possible decompensation and to report them early. They need to understand that the medications the patient is taking may cause adverse effects that—especially in the initiation phase—can make the patient feel worse for some weeks after initiation and up-titration. The patient, caregivers, and primary health providers need to know that simply stopping some HF medications may not be appropriate. For example, a reported pulse rate of 50 bpm (especially in a patient who is also taking β-adrenergic blockers) may be acceptable and does not necessarily mean that the patient should stop taking the prescribed medication.

The home health nurse, the physiotherapist, or the occupational therapist can instruct the patient in energy-saving and energy-efficient behaviours after an evaluation of daily activities has been done. The nurse can help link the patient with a cardiac rehabilitation or chronic disease program in the community to facilitate the recommended weekly exercise (30-40 min, three to five times per week, including aerobic activity and resistance training).

Using home health care services is essential in the care of HF patients and their caregivers. Often, multiple co-morbidities exist, and a degree of cognitive impairment is common. Frequent physical assessments, including vital signs and weight, are extremely important. The home care nurse can coach the patient and the patient's caregivers to implement systems to remember

NURSING CARE PLAN 37-1

Heart Failure

NURSING DIAGNOSIS	*Activity intolerance* related to fatigue secondary to cardiac insufficiency and pulmonary congestion *as evidenced by* dyspnea, shortness of breath, weakness, increase in heart rate on exertion, and patient's statement, "I feel too weak to do anything."
Expected Patient Outcomes	**Nursing Interventions and *Rationales***

- Achieves a realistic program of activity that balances physical activity with energy-conserving activities
- Vital signs, O₂ saturation, and colour are within normal limits in response to activity

Energy management

- Encourage alternate rest and activity periods *to reduce cardiac workload.*
- Provide calming diversionary activities to promote relaxation *to reduce O₂ consumption and to relieve dyspnea and fatigue.*
- Monitor patient's oxygen response (e.g., pulse rate, cardiac rhythm, colour, O₂ saturation, and respiratory rate) to self-care or nursing activities *to determine level of activity that can be performed.*
- Teach patient and significant other techniques of self-care *to minimize oxygen consumption (e.g., self-monitoring and pacing techniques for performance of activities of daily living).*

Activity therapy

- Assist to choose activities consistent with physical, psychological, and social capabilities *to determine level of activity that can be performed.*
- Collaborate with occupational, physical, and/or recreational therapists *to plan and monitor activity and exercise program.*
- Determine patient's commitment to increasing frequency and/or range of activities and exercise *to provide patient with obtainable goals.*

NURSING DIAGNOSIS	*Excess fluid volume* related to cardiac failure *as evidenced by* edema, dyspnea on exertion, increased weight gain, and patient's statement, "I'm short of breath and my ankles are so big and puffy!"
Expected Patient Outcomes	**Nursing Interventions and *Rationales***

- Experiences reduced edema or absence of edema

Fluid and electrolyte management

- Weigh patient daily, and monitor trends *to evaluate fluid retention or diuresis and weight reduction.*
- Monitor for abnormal serum electrolyte levels *to assess response to treatment.*

Hypervolemia management

- Monitor respiratory pattern for symptoms of respiratory difficulty *for early recognition of pulmonary congestion.*
- Monitor hemodynamic status, including CVP, MAP, PAOP, if available, *to evaluate effectiveness of therapy.*
- Monitor renal function and intake and output *to monitor fluid balance.*
- Monitor for therapeutic effect of diuretic (↑ urine output, ↑ CVP, improvement of breath sounds) *to assess response to treatment.*

NURSING DIAGNOSIS	*Impaired gas exchange* related to increased preload, mechanical failure, or immobility *as evidenced by* increased respiratory rate, shortness of breath, dyspnea on exertion, and patient's statement, "I just can't seem to catch my breath."
Expected Patient Outcomes	**Nursing Interventions and *Rationales***

- Maintains adequate respiratory rate and rhythm for activities of daily living

Respiratory monitoring

- Monitor rate, rhythm, depth, and effort of respirations *to evaluate changes in respiratory status.*
- Auscultate breath sounds, noting areas of decreased or absent ventilation and presence of adventitious sounds, *to assess congestion.*
- Monitor for dyspnea and events that improve and worsen it *to detect events that can influence ADLs.*

Oxygen therapy

- Administer supplemental O₂ as ordered *to maintain O₂ levels.*
- Change O₂ delivery device from mask to nasal prongs during meals as tolerated *to sustain O₂ levels while doing ADLs.*
- Monitor the effectiveness of O₂ therapy *to identify hypoxemia and establish range of O₂ saturation.*

Positioning

- Position to alleviate dyspnea (e.g., semi-Fowler's position), as appropriate, to improve ventilation by decreasing venous return to the heart and increasing thoracic capacity.

Continued

NURSING CARE PLAN 37-1

Heart Failure—cont'd

NURSING DIAGNOSIS	*Anxiety* *related to* dyspnea or perceived threat of death *as evidenced by* restlessness, irritability, expression of feelings of life threat, and patient's statement, "Don't leave me alone, I'm afraid I might die."
Expected Patient Outcomes	**Nursing Interventions and *Rationales***
• Verbalizes less anxiety about condition and prognosis	**Anxiety reduction**
	• Use a calm, reassuring approach *to increase confidence in caregiver and relieve anxiety.*
	• Explain all procedures, including sensations likely to be experienced during a procedure, *to promote sense of security.*
	• Help patient identify situations that precipitate anxiety *to plan appropriate use of anxiety-reducing techniques.*
	• Create an atmosphere to facilitate trust (e.g., answer call bell promptly and make frequent checks) *to promote sense of security.*
	• Instruct patient in use of relaxation techniques (e.g., imagery) *to help alleviate anxiety.*
NURSING DIAGNOSIS	*Deficient knowledge* *related to* disease process *as evidenced by* questions about the disease and patient's statement, "I don't know why I keep getting sick."
Expected Patient Outcomes	**Nursing Interventions and *Rationales***
• Describes disease process and rationales for dietary and medication regimen	**Teaching: disease process**
	• Appraise the patient's current level of knowledge related to specific disease process *to identify needed areas of teaching.*
	• Describe common signs and symptoms of the disease so patient will know signs and symptoms *to report to health care provider.*
	• Instruct the patient on measures to prevent or minimize adverse effects of treatment for the disease *so patient may be able to decrease number of acute episodes of HF.*
	Teaching: prescribed diet
	• Appraise the patient's current level of knowledge about prescribed diet *to assess areas needing additional instruction.*
	Teaching: prescribed medication
	• Review patient's knowledge of medications *to determine where further teaching is needed.*
	• Include the family and significant others *to provide support for the patient.*

ADLs, activities of daily living; *CVP,* central venous pressure; *HF,* heart failure; *MAP,* mean arterial pressure; *PAOP,* pulmonary artery occlusive pressure.

medications and times; identify problems, such as an increase in weight as evidence of worsening failure; and institute interventions to prevent hospitalization. This may include altering medications and fluid restrictions. The home care nurse can also help identify the need for respite services to reduce caregiver burden.

◾ Evaluation

The expected outcomes for the patient with HF are presented in NCP 37-1.

Cardiac Transplantation

The first heart transplant was performed in 1967. Since that time, **cardiac transplantation** (transfer of a heart from one person to another) has become the treatment of choice for carefully selected patients with end-stage HF. Patients with dilated cardiomyopathy account for almost 45% of cardiac transplant recipients. HF secondary to ischemic heart disease is the second most common indication for transplantation, accounting for 38% of candidates

(Taylor et al., 2007). See Table 37-16 for more detailed indications and contraindications to heart transplant.

Once an individual meets the criteria for cardiac transplantation, the goal of the evaluation process is to identify patients who would most benefit from a new heart. After a complete physical examination and diagnostic workup, the patient and family undergo a comprehensive psychological profile that includes assessing coping skills, family support systems, and motivation to follow the rigorous regimen that is essential to a successful transplantation. The complexity of the transplant process may be overwhelming to a patient with inadequate support systems and a poor understanding of the lifestyle changes required after transplant.

Once an individual is accepted as a transplant candidate (this may happen rapidly during an acute illness or over a longer period, depending on the patient's condition), he or she is placed on a transplant list. Patients may wait at home and receive ongoing medical care if their medical condition is stable. If their condition is not stable, they may require hospitalization for more intensive therapy including long-term mechanical cardiac support with a VAD. Unfortunately, the overall waiting period for a transplant is difficult to define and ranges from a few minutes to years.

What Is Heart Failure?

1. Provide individually tailored information about what HF is and how it is treated.
2. Discuss how people make the most of life with a chronic illness.

Health Promotion

1. Obtain annual flu vaccination.
2. Obtain pneumococcal vaccine (e.g., Pneumovax) and revaccination after 5 yr (for people at high risk of infection or serious disease).
3. Provide counselling regarding smoking cessation and weight reduction, if relevant.

Exercise and Rest

1. Once cleared by physician, discuss the benefits of regular exercise and dispel myths.
2. Plan a regular activity program and scheduled rest periods throughout the day.
3. Encourage communication of concerns and fears and provide encouragement.

Drug Therapy

1. Take each drug as prescribed by the physician or nurse practitioner.
2. Develop a system (e.g., daily chart) to ensure medications have been taken.
3. Take pulse and BP each day before taking medications. Know what is normal for the patient.
4. Know signs and symptoms of orthostatic hypotension and how to prevent them.
5. Know own INR if taking warfarin (Coumadin) and how often to have blood monitored.
6. If relevant, know signs and symptoms of overadministration of anticoagulation agents.

Dietary Therapy

1. Consult the written diet plan and list of permitted and restricted foods.
2. Examine labels to determine sodium content. Also examine the labels of over-the-counter drugs such as laxatives, cough medicines, and antacids.
3. Do not use salt in cooking or at the table.
4. Weigh yourself in the early morning every day after emptying your bladder. Use the same scale, and wear similar clothes.
5. Keep track of your daily weight and report weight gain of more than 2 kg (or ~4 lb) in the course of 2 to 5 days.
6. Restrict fluid to no more than 6 to 8 cups per day, and remember that fluid can be hidden in many foods. These hidden fluids should be counted in the daily restriction.

Other Topics

1. If adverse effects are bothersome, discuss ways in which timing of medications may help to manage them.
2. Avoid extremes of heat and cold.
3. Keep regular appointments with health care provider.
4. Discuss end-of-life planning and the importance of advance directives.

Ongoing Monitoring

1. Know the signs and symptoms of recurring or progressing heart failure.
2. Report immediately to health care provider development or worsening of any of the following:
   - Difficulty breathing, especially with exertion or when lying flat
   - Waking up breathless at night
   - Frequent dry, hacking cough, especially when lying down
   - Fatigue, weakness
   - Swelling of ankles, feet, or abdomen
   - Nausea with abdominal swelling, pain, and tenderness
   - Dizziness or fainting
3. Join local support networks such as cardiac rehabilitation or "Chronic Disease Management" programs.
4. Recognize depression as a major issue, and seek treatment should signs and symptoms of depression occur.
5. Caregivers should be able to recognize signs of cognitive impairment.

BP, blood pressure; *HF,* heart failure; *INR,* international normalized ratio.

Donor and recipient matching is based on body and heart size and ABO type. Negative lymphocyte crossmatch (explained in Chapter 16) is also important.

Most donor hearts are obtained at sites away from the institution performing the transplant. The maximum acceptable ischemic time for cardiac transplant is 4 to 6 hours.

The recipient is prepared for surgery, and cardiopulmonary bypass is used. The usual surgical procedure involves removing the recipient's heart, except for the posterior right and left atrial walls and their venous connections. The recipient's heart is then replaced with the donor heart, which has been trimmed to match. Care is taken to preserve the integrity of the donor sinoatrial node so that a sinus rhythm may be achieved postoperatively.

Immunosuppressive therapy begins in the operating room. Some transplant centres administer drugs to rapidly induce immunosuppression in the operating room and critical care area because the regimens most commonly used are nephrotoxic and, hence, cannot be started for a few days after the surgery. This induction therapy (usually with a monoclonal antibody) buys time to allow the kidneys to recover from the insult of surgery. (The mechanisms of action and adverse effects of these and other immunosuppressants are discussed in Chapter 16 and Table 16-15.) Regimens vary, but currently, cyclosporine (Neoral) is most often used (or, alternatively, tacrolimus [Prograf]) with mycophenolate mofetil (Cellcept) and prednisolone for maintenance immunosuppression. Many Canadian programs wean prednisolone over a number of months, and after a year, it is uncommon to see patients receiving prednisolone. The use of today's immunosuppression has resulted not only in reduced rejection but also in slowing the rejection process so that early treatment can be instituted. Because of the use of immunosuppressants, infection is a major complication following transplant.

EVIDENCE-INFORMED PRACTICE

Telemonitoring or Telephone Support for Patients With Heart Failure

Clinical Question

For patients with chronic HF (P), does remote monitoring of patients using the telephone or other available systems (I), as opposed to usual care (C), decrease all-cause mortality, hospital readmissions, and costs, and increase patient's quality of life (O)?

Best Available Evidence

Meta-analysis

Critical Appraisal and Synthesis of Evidence

- 14 randomized controlled trials (*n* = 4264 patients).
- Patients received structured telephone support or other forms of telemonitoring that transfers physiological data electronically to a centralized point.
- Readmission rates for HF were significantly reduced by 21%, and all-cause mortality was significantly reduced by 20%. Quality-of-life improvements were seen in some, but not all, studies reviewed, and three of four studies reported significant cost savings.

Conclusion

Remote monitoring of patients with HF improves outcomes in patients living in the community.

Implications for Nursing Practice

- HF is a chronic disease, and patients benefit from ongoing education and support once they leave hospital.
- Nurses must understand the emerging importance of telemanagement and telephone support, because this is a rapidly expanding area of nursing care.

Reference for Evidence

Clark, R. A., Inglis, S. C., McAlister, F. A., Cleland, J. G. F., & Stewart, S. (2007). Telemonitoring or structured telephone support programmes for patients with chronic heart failure: Systematic review and meta-analysis. *BMJ, 334*(7600), 942.

HF, heart failure; *PICO: P*, patient population of interest; *I*, intervention or area of interest; *C*, comparison of interest or comparison group; *O*, outcome(s) of interest.

Table 37-16 Indications and Contraindications for Cardiac Transplantation

Indications: Transplant Centre–Specific

- End-stage heart disease refractory to medical therapy
- Refractory, life-threatening cardiac dysrhythmias
- Functional Class III or IV status (NYHA) with demonstrated poor exercise capacity

Contraindications*

- Pulmonary hypertension unrelieved with medication
- Primary systemic disease that will limit survival (e.g., pulmonary or hepatic diseases)
- Renal dysfunction (creatinine >200 mmol/L)—could be considered for combined transplant
- Active infection
- Technical issues
- Current tobacco use (3 mo abstinence required)
- Illicit drug or excessive alcohol use (3 mo abstinence required)
- Unstable or chronic psychiatric conditions
- Documented life-threatening nonadherence
- Malignancy (generally must be cancer-free for 5 yr)
- Severe osteoporosis
- Significant vascular disease
- Diabetes mellitus with end-organ damage

NYHA, New York Heart Association.
*Contraindications may vary at different cardiac transplant centres.
Source: Ross, H., Hendry, P., Dipchand, A., Giannetti, N., Hirsch, G., Isaac, D., …, White, M. (2001). 2001 Canadian Cardiovascular Society Consensus Conference on Cardiac Transplantation. *Canadian Journal of Cardiology, 19,* 620-654.

transplantation, the major causes of death are acute rejection and infection. Later on, malignancy (especially lymphoma) and graft vasculopathy are major causes of death. Nursing management throughout the post-transplant period focuses on promoting patient adaptation to the transplant process, monitoring, managing lifestyle changes, and ongoing teaching of the patient and caregivers.

Mechanical Cardiac Support Devices

Temporary support of one or both failed ventricles has been available for many years in the form of IABP or extracorporeal membrane oxygenation. These circulatory support devices are designed for short-term use (days to weeks).

More recently, longer-term devices (for use over months to years) are being used in Canada as a "bridge" to heart transplant or recovery of the native heart. These pumps are called *ventricular assist devices* (VADs). A number of devices are available in Canada. Some examples include the HeartMate II (made by Thoratec Corp in California) (see Figure 37-4) and HeartWare HVAD (made by HeartWare Inc., based in Massachusetts) electronic devices. These pumps are designed to support the LV. In many patients, if carefully selected, support of the LV alone will alleviate symptoms of right-sided HF by unloading the left side.

Patients carry a battery pack with a small computer attached to their belt around with them. With adequate social support, patients are able to live at home with these devices and, in some

Endomyocardial biopsies via the right internal jugular vein are performed at repeated intervals to detect rejection in the first year. After 3 months, the incidence of acute rejection decreases dramatically; however, a type of CAD known as graft vasculopathy develops in a significant proportion of heart transplant recipients over the long term. This is also known as chronic rejection. As a result, regular surveillance of the transplanted heart by means of diagnostic tests such as coronary angiography and echocardiography is performed for the rest of the recipient's life.

Advances in surgical technique and postoperative care have improved survival rates after cardiac transplantation. It is estimated that 50% of transplant recipients will be living after 10 years. This number is an overall average and varies greatly depending on age at transplant, severity of illness, adherence to medication regimens and risk factor modification, and social support systems, to name a few factors. In the first year after

ETHICAL DILEMMAS
Competence

Situation

A 60-year-old man has been awaiting heart transplantation for 6 months. He has been in intensive care for 1 month since receiving a VAD for his failing heart. He recently suffered a stroke—a complication of the device—that left him paralyzed on his right side and requiring ventilation. He is only able to answer yes–no questions by nodding or shaking his head. For the past 2 weeks, he has needed hemodialysis because of renal failure. In recent days, he has tried to prevent the nurses from reconnecting the ventilator tube after suctioning by turning his head or by pushing it away with his left hand. Although he does not have any advance directives, his wife and daughter state that before these events occurred, he had often expressed that he would not want to live if he lost his independence. They have requested that the mechanical ventilator be withdrawn.

Important Points for Consideration

- Informed consent related to treatment decisions entails four elements: (1) information provided about possible treatment options must be understandable to the patient; (2) possible outcomes of the various treatment options must be explained; (3) the patient must have the capacity to deliberate about the treatment choices and their consequences; and (4) the patient's treatment decision must be freely chosen or made without coercion.
- It may be difficult under certain circumstances, such as with impaired communication, to determine a patient's capacity to make an informed treatment decision.
- The patient—if deemed competent—is the decision maker in the patient's care. If any doubt about competence exists, a formal evaluation should take place.
- The wife, acting as the patient's surrogate decision maker, is using substituted judgement to indicate what the patient would want based on what she says are his previously expressed wishes.

Clinical Decision-Making Questions

1. What would the nurse do next given the patient's behaviour and the information that the nurse has obtained from the patient's wife?
2. What might be the nurse's feelings about participating in the care of a patient in whom withdrawal of treatment will result in death?

cases, return to work while waiting for a heart transplant. This improved mobility—the ability to live out of the hospital—and the improvement that results in the patient's nutritional state allow the patient to undergo transplantation in much improved physical condition. These devices are being used in the United States and Europe instead of a transplant. This is commonly referred to as "destination therapy."

A totally artificial heart is available; however, it is not currently in use in Canada. For more information on mechanical cardiac support, see Chapter 68.

CLINICAL DECISION-MAKING EXERCISE

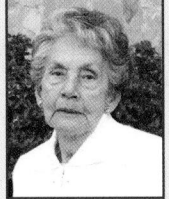

CASE STUDY:
Heart Failure

Source: © iStockphoto.com/Andres Rodriguez.

Patient Profile

Mrs. Estrela, a 70-year-old Portuguese Canadian woman, was admitted to the medical unit with complaints of increasing dyspnea on exertion.

Subjective Data

- Had a severe myocardial infarction (MI) at 58 years of age
- Has experienced increasing dyspnea on exertion during the last 2 years
- Recently had a respiratory tract infection, has frequent cough, and had edema in legs 2 weeks ago
- Cannot walk two blocks without getting short of breath
- Has to sleep with head elevated on three pillows
- Does not always remember to take medication
- 5-kg weight gain

Objective Data

Physical Examination
- In respiratory distress, use of accessory muscles, respiratory rate 36 breaths/min
- Systolic heart murmur
- Moist crackles in both lungs
- Cyanotic lips and extremities
- Skin cool and diaphoretic

Diagnostic Studies
- Chest radiographic examination results: cardiomegaly with right and left ventricular hypertrophy; fluid in lower lung fields
- Echocardiogram results: ejection fraction (EF) 20%

Collaborative Care

- Enalapril 5 mg PO daily
- Digoxin 0.25 mg PO daily
- Furosemide (Lasix) 40 mg IV bid
- Potassium 40 mEq PO bid
- 2-g sodium diet
- Oxygen 6 L/min
- Daily weight measurements

- Daily 12-lead electrocardiogram (ECG), cardiac enzymes q8h × 3
- Continuous cardiac monitoring
- Cardiac enzyme levels prn with chest pain

Discussion Questions

1. Explain the pathophysiology of Mrs. Estrela's heart disease.
2. What clinical manifestations of heart failure did Mrs. Estrela exhibit?
3. What is the significance of the findings of the diagnostic studies?
4. Explain the rationale for each of the medical orders prescribed for Mrs. Estrela.

5. *Priority Decision:* What are the nurse's priority nursing interventions for Mrs. Estrela?
6. *Priority Decision:* What priority patient teaching measures should be instituted to prevent recurrence of an acute episode of heart failure?
7. *Priority Decision:* Based on the assessment data presented, write one or more appropriate nursing diagnoses. Are there any collaborative problems?

evolve *Answers are available at* http://evolve.elsevier.com/
Canada/Lewis/medsurg

REVIEW QUESTIONS

The number of the question corresponds to the same-numbered objective at the beginning of the chapter.

1. What are the manifestations of systolic heart failure (HF) that the nurse should recognize?
   a. ↓ Afterload and ↓ left ventricular end-diastolic pressure (LVEDP)
   b. ↓ Ejection fraction (EF) and ↑ pulmonary artery occlusive pressure (PAOP)
   c. ↓ PAOP and ↑ left ventricular EF
   d. ↑ Pulmonary hypertension associated with normal EF
2. Which compensatory mechanism leads to inappropriate sodium and fluid retention?
   a. Ventricular dilation
   b. Ventricular hypertrophy
   c. Neurohormonal response
   d. Sympathetic nervous system activation

3. Which drug used in the management of a patient with acute pulmonary edema will decrease both preload and afterload and provide relief of anxiety?
   a. Morphine
   b. Amiodarone
   c. Dobutamine
   d. Aminophylline
4. How can a patient with chronic HF best decrease the chances of having an acute decompensation?
   a. Resting and not making any exertions except under medical supervision
   b. Documenting fluid intake and urinary output each day
   c. Monitoring weight daily and reporting changes outside of recommended parameters
   d. Taking extra furosemide when shortness of breath occurs
5. In the first year after heart transplant, what are the two primary causes of death?
   a. Infection and rejection
   b. Rejection and dysrhythmias
   c. Dysrhythmias and infection
   d. Myocardial infarction and lymphoma

ANSWERS: 1. b; 2. c; 3. a; 4. c; 5. a.

REFERENCES

Arnold, J. M. O., Howlett, J. G., Dorian, P., Ducharme, A., Giannetti, N., Haddad, H., …, White, M. (2007). Canadian Cardiovascular Society Consensus Conference recommendations on heart failure update 2007: Prevention, management during intercurrent illness or acute decompensation, and use of biomarkers. *Canadian Journal of Cardiology, 23*(1), 21-45. doi:10.1016/S0828-282X(07)70211-8

Arnold, J. M. O., Liu, P., Demers, C., Dorian, P., Giannetti, N., Haddad, H., …, White, M. (2006). Canadian Cardiovascular Society consensus conference recommendations on heart failure 2006: Diagnosis and management. *Canadian Journal of Cardiology, 22*(1), 23-45. doi:10.1016/S0828-282X(06)70237-9

Canadian Heart Failure Network (CHFN). (2012). *Dietary considerations.* Retrieved from http://www.chfn.ca/patient-education/health-professional-patient-education/dietary-considerations

Carlson, K. K. (2009). *Advanced critical care nursing.* St. Louis: Saunders.

Cheung, N., Wang, J. J., Rogers, S. L., Brancati, F., Klein, R., Sharrett, A. R., & Wong, T. Y. (2008). Diabetic retinopathy and risk of heart failure. *Journal of the American College of Cardiology, 51*, 1573-1578. doi:10.1016/j.jacc.2007.11.076

Costanzo, M. R., Guglin, M. E., Saltzberg, M. T., Jessup, M. L., Bart, B. A., Teerlink, J. R., …, Sobotka, P. A. (2007). Ultrafiltration versus intravenous diuretics for patients hospitalized for acute decompensated heart failure. *Journal of the American College of Cardiology, 49*, 675-683. doi:10.1016/j.jacc.2006.07.073

Health Canada. (2011). *Eating well with Canada's food guide.* Ottawa: Author. Retrieved from www.hc-sc.gc.ca/fn-an/alt_formats/hpfb-dgpsa/pdf/food-guide-aliment/view_eatwell_vue_bienmang-eng.pdf

Howlett, J. G., McKelvie, R. S., Arnold, J. M. O., Costigan J., Dorian, P., Ducharme, A., …, White, M. (2009). Canadian Cardiovascular Society Consensus Conference guidelines on heart failure, update 2009: Diagnosis and management of right-sided heart failure, myocarditis, device therapy and recent important clinical trials. *Canadian Journal of Cardiology, 25*(2), 85-105.

Huether, S. E., & McCance, K. L. (2008). *Understanding pathophysiology* (4th ed.). St Louis: Mosby.

Hypertension Canada. (2012). *What is hypertension?* Markham, ON: Author. Retrieved from *http://www.hypertension.ca/what-is-hypertension-dp1*

Koelling, T. M., Johnson, M. L., Cody, R. J., & Aaronson, K. D. (2005). Discharge education improves clinical outcomes in patients with chronic heart failure. *Circulation, 111,* 179. doi:10.1161/01.CIR.0000151811.53450.B8

Lee, D. S., Johansen, H., Gong, Y., Hall, R. E, Tu, J. V., & Cox, J. L., for the Canadian Cardiovascular Outcomes Research Team. (2004). Regional outcomes of heart failure in Canada. *Canadian Journal of Cardiology, 20,* 599-607.

Lehne, R. A. (2007). *Pharmacology for nursing care* (6th ed.). St Louis: Saunders.

Mullens, W., Abahams, Z., Francis, G., Skouri, H. N., Starling, R. C., Young, J. B., …, Tang, W. H. W. (2008). Sodium nitroprusside for advanced low-output heart failure. *Journal of the American College of Cardiologists, 52*(3), 200-207. doi:10.1016/j.jacc.2008.02.083

Ross, H., Howlett, J., Arnold, J. M. O., Liu, P., O'Neill, B. J., Brophy, J. M., …, Glasgow, K. (2006). Treating the right patient at the right time: Access to heart failure care. *Canadian Journal of Cardiology, 22*(9), 749-54. doi:10.1016/S0828-282X(06)70290-2

Rutledge, T., Reis, V. A., Linke, S. E., Greenberg, B. H., & Mills, P. J. (2006). Depression in heart failure: A meta-analytic review of prevalence, intervention effects, and associations with clinical outcomes. *Journal of the American College of Cardiologists, 48,* 1527-1537. doi:10.1016/j.jacc.2006.06.055

Sherwood, A., Blumenthal, J. A., Trivedi, R., Johnson, K. S., O'Connor, C. M., Adams, K. F., …, Hinderliter, A. L. (2007). Relationship of depression to death or hospitalization in patients with heart failure. *Archives of Internal Medicine, 167,* 367-373. doi:10.1001/archinte.167.4.367

Silver, M. A., Maisel, A., Yancy, C. W., McCullough, P., Burnett, J., Francis, G., …, Hollander, J. (2004). BNP Consensus Panel 2004: A clinical approach for the diagnostic, prognostic, screening, treatment monitoring, and therapeutic roles of natriuretic peptides in cardiovascular diseases. *Congestive Heart Failure, 10*(Suppl. 3), 1-30. doi:10.1111/j.1527-5299.2004.03271.x

Taylor, D. O., Edwards, L. B., Boucek, M. M., Trulock, E. P., Aurora, P., Christie, J., …, Hertz, M. I. (2007). Registry of the International Society for Heart and Lung Transplantation: Twenty-Fourth Official Adult Heart Transplant Report. *Journal of Heart and Lung Transplantation, 26,* 769-781. doi:10.1016/j.healun.2007.06.004

CANADIAN RESOURCES

Canadian Association of Cardiac Rehabilitation (CACR)
http://www.cacr.ca

Canadian Cardiovascular Society (CCS)
http://www.ccs.ca

Canadian Council of Cardiovascular Nurses
http://www.cccn.ca

Easy Auscultation S3 and S4 Sounds
http://www.easyauscultation.com/cases.aspx?CourseCaseOrder=3&CourseID=25

Heart and Stroke Foundation of Canada
http://ww2.heartandstroke.ca

evolve *For additional Internet resources, see the Web site for this book at* **http://evolve.elsevier.com/Canada/Lewis/medsurg**

Nursing Management: Dysrhythmias

Written by Linda Bucher

Adapted by Sandra Goldsworthy

LEARNING OBJECTIVES

1. Describe the nursing management of patients requiring continuous electrocardiographic (ECG) monitoring.
2. Identify the clinical characteristics and ECG patterns of normal sinus rhythm, common dysrhythmias, and acute coronary syndrome (ACS).
3. Describe the nursing and collaborative management of patients with common dysrhythmias and ECG changes associated with ACS.
4. Differentiate between defibrillation and cardioversion, identifying indications for their use and nursing implications.
5. Describe the management of patients with temporary and permanent pacemakers.
6. Describe the management of patients with implantable cardioverter–defibrillators.
7. Explain the management of patients undergoing electrophysiological testing and radiofrequency catheter ablation therapy.

KEY TERMS

asystole The total absence of ventricular electrical activity, p. 965

atrial fibrillation A cardiac dysrhythmia characterized by a total disorganization of atrial electrical activity without effective atrial contraction, p. 961

atrial flutter An atrial tachydysrhythmia identified by recurring, regular, sawtooth-shaped flutter waves, p. 960

automatic external defibrillators (AEDs) Defibrillators that have rhythm detection capability and the ability to advise the operator to deliver a shock by means of hands-free defibrillator pads, p. 967

automaticity A property of specialized cells of the heart found in the sinoatrial (SA) node, parts of the atria, the atrioventricular (AV) node, and the His-Purkinje system that are able to discharge spontaneously, p. 956

cardiac pacemaker An electronic device used to pace the heart when the normal conduction pathway is damaged or diseased, p. 968

complete heart block Third-degree AV heart block in which no impulses from the atria are conducted to the ventricles, p. 963

dysrhythmias Abnormal cardiac rhythms, p. 951

electrocardiogram (ECG) A graphic tracing of the electrical impulses produced in the heart, p. 951

premature atrial contraction (PAC) Contraction originating from an ectopic focus in the atrium (in a location other than the sinus node), p. 959

premature ventricular contraction (PVC) A contraction originating in an ectopic focus in the ventricles, p. 963

ventricular fibrillation A severe derangement of the heart rhythm characterized on ECG by irregular undulations of varying shapes and amplitude, p. 965

ventricular tachycardia (VT) Occurrence of three or more PVCs in succession; occurs when an ectopic focus or foci fire repetitively, and the ventricle takes control as the pacemaker, p. 964

ELECTRONIC RESOURCES

Supplemental content related to Chapter 38 can be found...

Evolve Web Site ⊖volve

http://evolve.elsevier.com/Canada/Lewis/medsurg
- Algorithms for Treatment of Dysrhythmias
- Answer Guidelines for Case Study on p. 973

- Content Updates
- Electronic Calculators
- Examination Review Questions
- Glossary
- Interactive Case Study: Atrial Fibrillation
- Key Points (Printable and MP3 Download)

Rhythm Identification and Treatment

The ability to recognize normal and abnormal cardiac rhythms is an essential nursing skill. Cardiac monitoring is now used in a wide range of hospital, clinic, and home settings. Prompt assessment of abnormal cardiac rhythms, called **dysrhythmias,** and of the patient's response to them is critical. This chapter describes basic principles of electrocardiographic (ECG) monitoring and recognition of common dysrhythmias, as well as ECG changes that are associated with acute coronary syndrome (ACS). For more detailed information on ECG interpretation, the reader should refer to dedicated texts on this topic (Aehlert, 2011).

Conduction System

Four properties of cardiac cells enable the conduction system to initiate an electrical impulse, which is transmitted through the cardiac tissue and stimulates muscle contraction (Table 38-1). The conduction system of the heart is made up of specialized neuromuscular tissue located throughout the heart (see Chapter 34, Figure 34-4). A normal cardiac impulse begins in the sinoatrial (SA) node in the upper right atrium. It is transmitted over the atrial myocardium via the bundle of Bachmann and internodal pathways, which causes atrial contraction. The impulse then travels to the atrioventricular (AV) node through the bundle of His and down the left and right bundle branches, ending in the Purkinje fibres, which transmit the impulse to the ventricles.

Conduction to the point just before the impulse leaves the Purkinje fibres takes place within the time of the PR interval of the ECG. When the impulse emerges from the Purkinje fibres, ventricular depolarization occurs, producing mechanical contraction of the ventricles and the QRS complex on the ECG. The electrical activity of the heart is illustrated in Chapter 34, Figure 34-4.

Nervous Control of the Heart

The autonomic nervous system plays an important role in the rate of impulse formation, the speed of conduction, and the strength of cardiac contraction. The components of the autonomic nervous system that affect the heart are the right and left vagus nerve fibres of the parasympathetic nervous system and the fibres of the sympathetic nervous system.

Stimulation of the vagus nerve causes a decrease in the rate of firing of the sinoatrial node, a slowing of impulse conduction of the atrioventricular node, and a decrease in the force of cardiac

Table 38-1 Properties of Cardiac Cells	
Automaticity	Ability to initiate an impulse spontaneously and continuously
Contractility	Ability to respond mechanically to an impulse
Conductivity	Ability to transmit an impulse along a membrane in an orderly manner
Excitability	Ability to be electrically stimulated

muscle contraction. Stimulation of the sympathetic nerves that supply the heart has essentially the opposite effect on the heart (Standring, 2009).

Electrocardiographic Monitoring

The **electrocardiogram (ECG)** is a graphic tracing of the electrical impulses produced in the heart. The waveforms on the ECG are produced by the movement of charged ions across the membranes of myocardial cells, representing depolarization and repolarization.

The membrane of a cardiac cell is semipermeable, allowing the intracellular concentration of potassium to remain high and the intracellular concentration of sodium to remain low. A high concentration of sodium and a low concentration of potassium are maintained outside the cell. The inside of the cell, when the cell is at rest or in the polarized state, is negative compared with the outside. When a cell or groups of cells are stimulated, each cell membrane changes its permeability and allows sodium to move rapidly into the cell, making the inside of the cell positive compared with the outside (*depolarization*). A slower movement of ions across the membrane restores the cell to the polarized state; this restoration is called *repolarization*. In Figure 38-1, the phases of the cardiac action potential are as follows: phase 0 is the upstroke of rapid depolarization; phases 1, 2, and 3 represent repolarization; and phase 4 is a polarized state. Antidysrhythmia drugs have a direct effect on the various phases of the action potential. When antidysrhythmia drugs are used in a clinical setting, it is important to understand the ionic shifts in the cardiac cell and the action potential mechanism (Aehlert, 2011).

Conventionally, there are 12 recording leads in the ECG. Six of the 12 ECG leads (leads I, II, III, aV_R, aV_L, and aV_F) measure electrical forces in the frontal plane (Figure 38-2). The remaining six leads (V_1 through V_6) measure the electrical forces in the

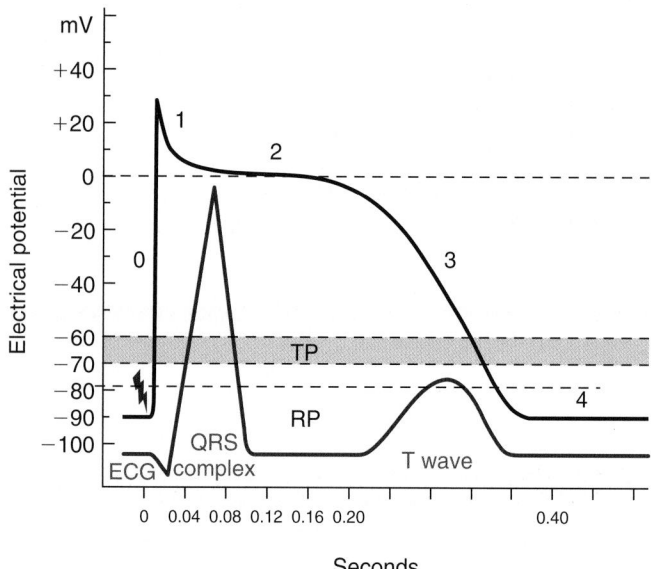

Figure 38-1 Phases of the cardiac action potential on an electrocardiogram (ECG). The electrical potential, measured in millivolts, is indicated along the vertical axis of the graph. Time, measured in milliseconds, is indicated along the horizontal axis. The action potential has five phases, labelled *phase 0* through *phase 4*. Each phase represents a particular electrical event or combination of electrical events. Phase 0 is the upstroke of rapid depolarization and corresponds with ventricular contraction. Phases 1, 2, and 3 represent repolarization. Phase 4 is known as *complete repolarization* (or the polarized state) and corresponds to diastole. *RP*, resting membrane potential; *TP*, threshold membrane potential.

Source: Adapted from Wesley, K. (2011). *Huszar's basic dysrhythmias and acute coronary syndromes: Interpretation and management* (4th ed., p. 10, Figure 1-10). St. Louis: Mosby.

horizontal plane (precordial leads). The 12-lead ECG may show changes that are indicative of structural changes or damage such as ischemia, infarction, enlarged cardiac chambers, electrolyte imbalance, or drug toxicity (Aehlert, 2011). Obtaining 12 ECG views of the heart is also helpful in the assessment of dysrhythmias. An example of a normal 12-lead ECG appears in Figure 38-3.

When a patient's ECG is being continuously monitored, between 1 and 12 ECG leads may be used. The leads most commonly selected are leads II, V_1, and a modified chest lead, MCL_1 (Figure 38-4), which is similar to V_1 and is used when only three leads are available for monitoring.

The ECG can be visualized continuously on a monitor oscilloscope. A recording of the ECG (i.e., rhythm strip) is obtained on ECG paper attached to the monitor. The recording provides documentation of the patient's rhythm. It also allows for measurement of complexes and intervals and for assessment of dysrhythmias.

To correctly interpret an ECG, the nurse must know how to measure time and voltage on the ECG paper. ECG paper consists of large squares (heavy lines) and small squares (light lines; Figure 38-5). Each large square incorporates 25 smaller squares (five horizontal and five vertical). Each small square represents 0.04 sec horizontally and 0.1 millivolt (mV) vertically. This means that the large square represents 0.20 sec and that 300 large squares represent 1 min. Vertically, one large square is equal to 0.5 mV. These squares are used to calculate the heart rate (HR) and intervals between different ECG complexes.

A variety of methods can be used to calculate the HR from an ECG. Probably the most accurate way is to count the number of QRS complexes in 1 minute. However, this method is time consuming. If the rhythm is regular, a simpler process can be used: Every 3 sec, a marker appears on the ECG paper. An R wave is the first upward (or positive) deflection of the QRS complex. The nurse can count the number of R–R intervals in 6 sec and

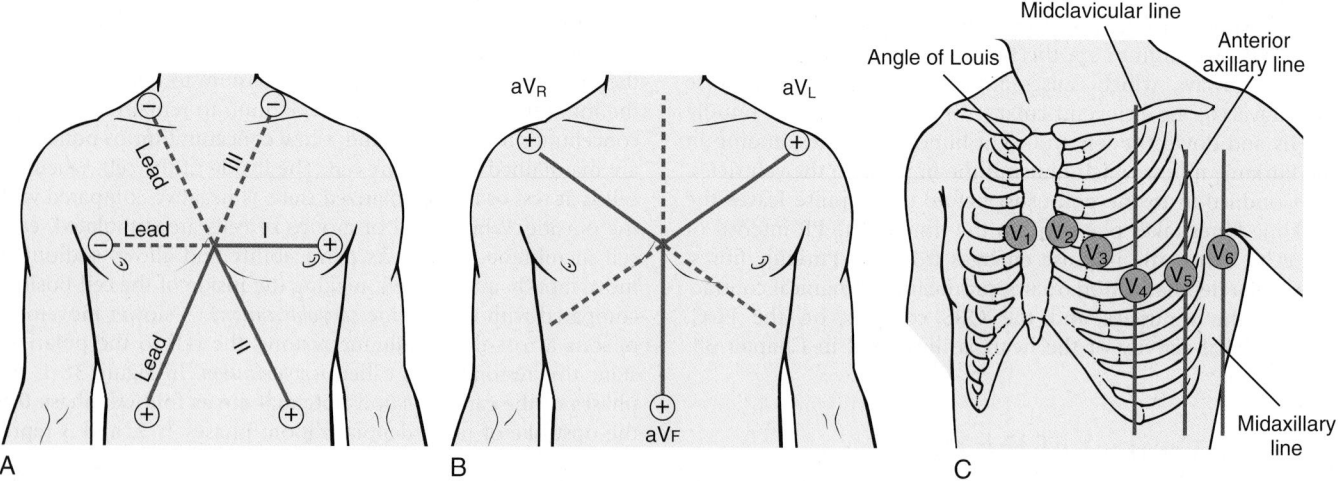

Figure 38-2 A, Placement of limb leads I, II, and III, which are located on the extremities. Illustrated are the angles from which these leads "view" the heart. **B,** Placement of limb leads aV_R, aV_L, and aV_F. For these unipolar leads, the calculated centre of the heart is used as their negative electrode. **C,** Lead placement for the chest electrodes: V_1, at the fourth intercostal space at the right sternal border; V_2, at the fourth intercostal space at the left sternal border; V_3, equidistant between V_2 and V_4; V_4, at the fifth intercostal space at the left midclavicular line; V_5, at the anterior axillary line and on the same horizontal level as V_4; V_6, at the midaxillary line and on the same horizontal level as V_4.

Source: Adapted from Goldberger, A. L. (2006). *Clinical electrocardiography: A simplified approach* (7th ed.). St. Louis: Mosby.

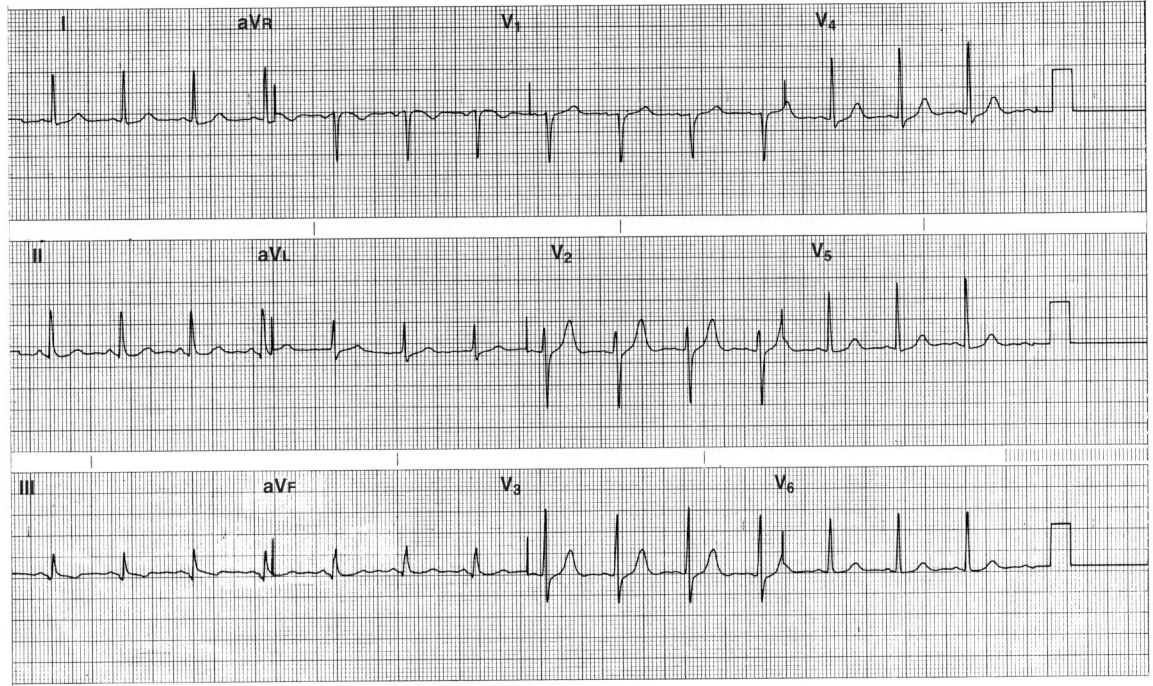

Figure 38-3 Twelve-lead electrocardiogram showing a normal sinus rhythm.

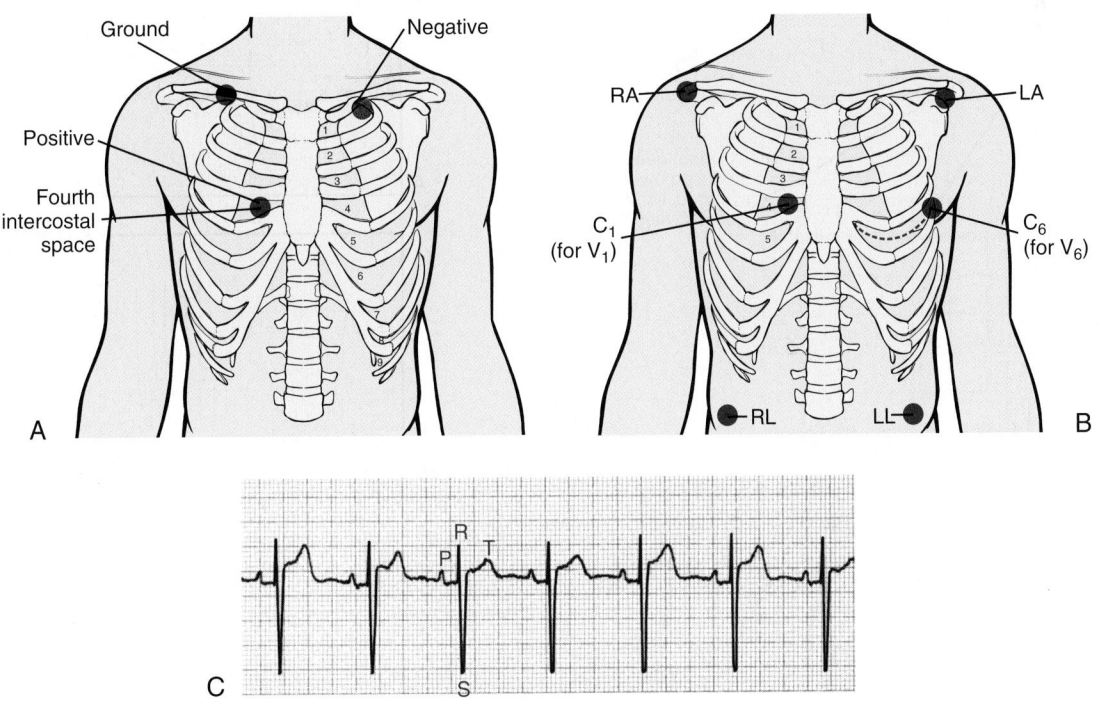

Figure 38-4 A, Lead placement for MCL₁ when a three-lead system is used. **B,** Lead placement for V₁ or V₆ when a five-lead system is used. **C,** Typical electrocardiographic tracing for lead MCL₁. *C,* chest; *LA,* left arm; *LL,* left leg; *RA,* right arm; *RL,* right leg.

Source: Adapted from Urden, L. D., Stacy, K. M., & Lough, M. E. (2010). *Critical care nursing: Diagnosis and management* (6th ed., p. 370, Figure 18-34). St. Louis: Mosby.

multiply that number by 10. This calculation yields the approximate number of beats per minute (Figure 38-6).

Another rapid method for calculating the HR when the rhythm is regular is to count the number of small squares between one R–R interval. Dividing this number by 1500 yields the HR. The number of large squares between one R–R interval can also

be counted and divided by 300 (see Figure 38-6). These methods are accurate only if the rhythm is regular.

An additional way to measure distances on the ECG strip is to use calipers. Calipers are used for fine measurements, especially for points of a specific wave or interval. Many times a P or R wave does not fall directly on a light or heavy line. The fine points of the calipers can be placed exactly on the components to be measured and then moved to another part of the strip for time measurement.

ECG leads are attached to the patient's chest wall by means of an electrode pad fixed with electrical conductive gel. Before placing these on a patient, the nurse must properly prepare the patient's skin. Excessive hair on the chest wall should be clipped with scissors. The nurse should prepare the skin by rubbing gently with dry gauze until the skin is slightly pink. If the skin is oily, alcohol may be used first. In the case of a diaphoretic patient, a skin protectant should be applied before the electrode is placed. If leads and electrodes are not firmly placed, or if there is muscle activity or electrical interference from an outside source, an artifact may be seen on the monitor. An artifact is a distortion of the baseline and waveforms seen on the ECG (Figure 38-7). Accurate interpretation of cardiac rhythm is difficult when an artifact is present. If artifacts occur, the nurse should check for loose connections in the equipment. The electrodes on the patient may need to be removed and replaced more securely or moved to areas that are less affected by movement (Aehlert, 2011).

Telemetry Monitoring. Telemetry monitoring is the observation of a patient's HR and rhythm to rapidly diagnose dysrhythmias, ischemia, or infarction. Two types of systems are used for telemetry monitoring. The first type, a centralized monitoring system, requires a nurse or telemetry technician to continuously observe all patients' rhythms at a central location. The second system of telemetry monitoring does not require constant surveillance by the nurse or technician. These systems have the capability of detecting and storing data. Sophisticated alarm systems provide different levels of detection of dysrhythmias, ischemia, or infarction, depending on the severity of each. However, computerized monitoring systems are not fail-proof. Frequent nursing assessment is important in caring for monitored patients.

Assessment of Cardiac Rhythm

When assessing the cardiac rhythm, the nurse must make an accurate interpretation and immediately evaluate the consequences of the findings for an individual patient. Assessment of the patient's hemodynamic response to any change in rhythm is essential because this information guides the selection of therapeutic interventions. Determination of the cause of dysrhythmias

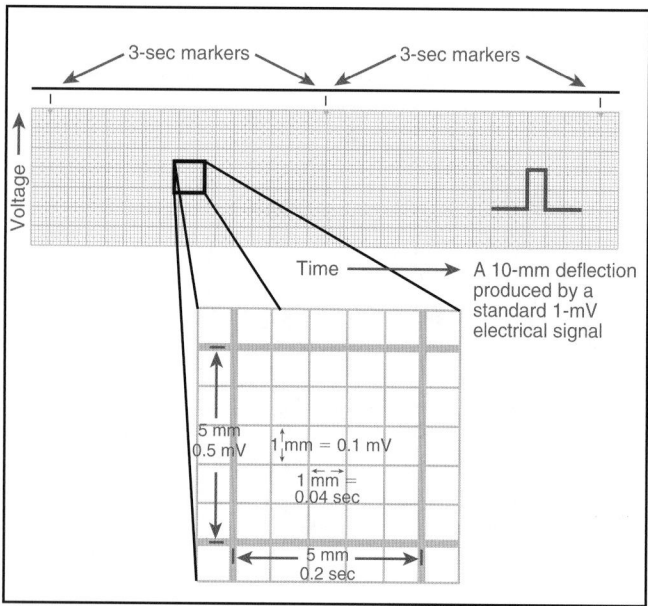

Figure 38-5 Time and voltage on the electrocardiogram.

Source: Adapted from Wesley, K. (2011). *Huszar's basic dysrhythmias and acute coronary syndromes: Interpretation and management* (4th ed., p. 19, Figure 2-2). St. Louis: Mosby.

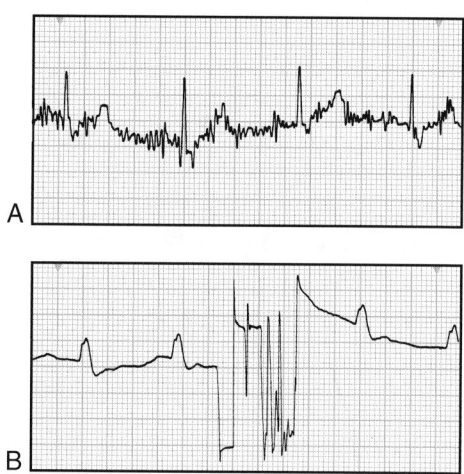

Figure 38-7 A, Electrocardiogram (ECG) demonstrating muscle tremor. **B,** ECG reflecting loose electrodes.

Source: Adapted from Wesley, K. (2011). *Huszar's basic dysrhythmias and acute coronary syndromes: Interpretation and management* (4th ed., p. 24, Figure 2-11, and p. 25, Figure 2-13). St. Louis: Mosby.

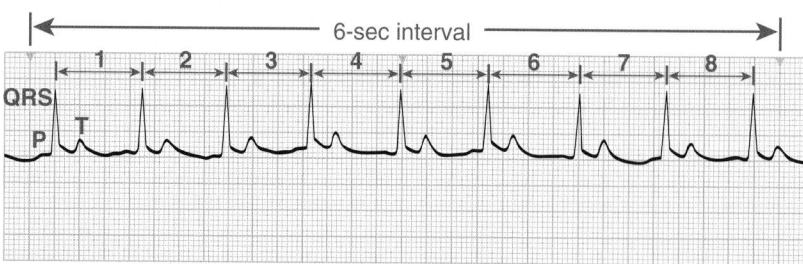

Figure 38-6 The heart rate is calculated according to the interval between first upward (or positive) deflection (R wave) of one QRS complex to the R wave of the next. When the rhythm is regular, heart rate can be determined at a glance. The estimated heart rate is 80. The actual heart rate is 86.

Source: Adapted from Wesley, K. (2011). *Huszar's basic dysrhythmias and acute coronary syndromes: Interpretation and management* (4th ed., p. 56, Figure 4-2). St. Louis: Mosby.

should be a priority. For example, tachycardias may be the result of fever and possibly may cause a decrease in cardiac output (CO) and hypotension. Certain dysrhythmias may be a result of electrolyte disturbances and may lead to a life-threatening dysrhythmia (Aehlert, 2011; Palatnik, 2011). At all times, the patient must be assessed and abnormalities treated.

Normal sinus rhythm is a rhythm that originates in the SA node and follows the normal conduction pattern of the cardiac cycle (Figure 38-8). Figure 38-9 shows the normal electrical pattern of the cardiac cycle. Table 38-2 provides a description of ECG waveforms and intervals and possible sources of disturbances in these features. The P wave represents the depolarization of the atria (passage of an electrical impulse through the atria), causing atrial contraction. The PR interval represents the period when the impulse spreads through the atria, the AV node, the bundle of His, and the Purkinje fibres. The QRS complex represents depolarization of the ventricles (ventricular contraction), and the QRS interval represents the time it takes for depolarization. The ST segment represents the time between ventricular depolarization and repolarization. This segment should be flat, or isoelectric, representing the absence of any electrical activity

between these two events. The T wave represents repolarization of the ventricles. The QT interval represents the total time for depolarization and repolarization of the ventricles.

Electrophysiological Mechanisms of Dysrhythmias

Disorders of impulse formation can cause dysrhythmias. The heart has specialized cells found in the SA node, parts of the atria, the AV node, and the bundle of His and Purkinje fibres (His-

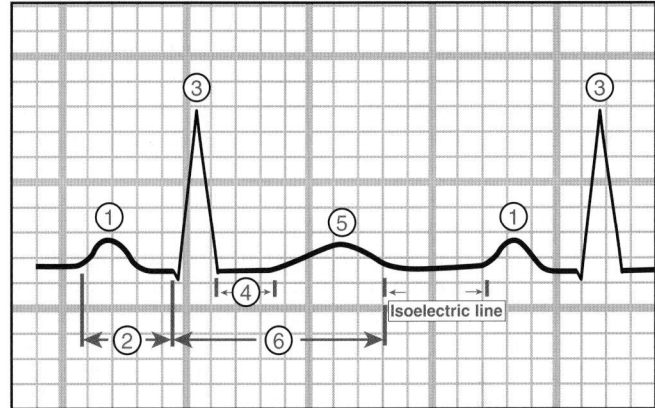

Figure 38-9 The electrocardiographic complex as seen in a normal sinus rhythm. Isoelectric (flat) line represents the absence of electrical activity in the cardiac cells. *1*, P wave (normal is 0.06-0.12 sec); *2*, PR interval (normal is 0.12-0.20 sec); *3*, QRS complex (normal is 0.04-0.12 sec); *4*, ST segment (normal is 0.12 sec); *5*, T wave (normal is 0.16 sec); *6*, QT interval (normal is 0.34-0.43 sec).

Source: Huszar, R. J. (2002). *Basic dysrhythmias: Interpretation and management* (3rd ed.). St. Louis: Mosby.

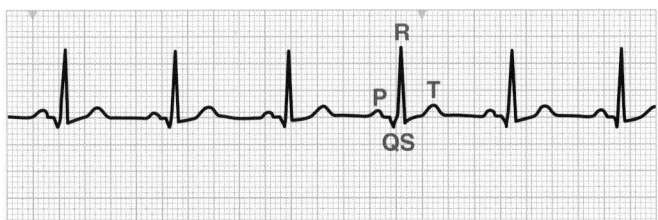

Figure 38-8 Electrocardiogram depicting normal sinus rhythm in lead II.

Source: Huszar, R. J. (2002). *Basic dysrhythmias: Interpretation and management* (3rd ed.). St. Louis: Mosby.

Table 38-2 Definition and Sources of Variation in ECG Waveforms and Intervals*

DESCRIPTION	NORMAL DURATION (SEC)	SOURCE OF POSSIBLE VARIATION
P wave: Represents time for the electrical impulse that causes atrial depolarization (contraction) to pass through the atrium; should be upright	0.06-0.12	Disturbance in conduction within atria
PR interval: Measured from beginning of P wave to beginning of QRS complex; represents time taken for impulse to spread through the atria, the AV node and bundle of His, the bundle branches, and Purkinje fibres, to a point immediately before ventricular contraction	0.12-0.20	Disturbance in conduction usually in AV node, bundle of His, or bundle branches but can be in atria as well
QRS interval: Measured from beginning to end of QRS complex; represents time taken for depolarization (contraction) of both ventricles (systole)	0.06-0.10	Disturbance in conduction in bundle branches or in ventricles
ST segment: Measured from the S wave of the QRS complex to the beginning of the T wave; represents the time between ventricular depolarization and repolarization (diastole); should be isoelectric (flat)	N/A	Disturbances usually caused by ischemia, injury, or infarction
T wave: Represents time for ventricular repolarization; should be upright	N/A	Disturbances usually caused by electrolyte imbalances, ischemia, or infarction
QT interval: Measured from beginning of QRS complex to end of T wave; represents time taken for entire electrical depolarization and repolarization of the ventricles	0.34-0.43	Disturbances usually affecting repolarization more than depolarization and caused by drugs, electrolyte imbalances, and changes in heart rate

*Heart rate influences the duration of these intervals, especially those of the PR and QT intervals (e.g., QT interval decreases in duration as heart rate increases).

AV, atrioventricular; *ECG,* electrocardiogram; *N/A,* not applicable.

Table 38-3 Rates of the Conduction System	
SA node	60-100 times/min
AV junction	40-60 times/min
Purkinje fibres	20-40 times/min

AV, atrioventricular; *SA,* sinoatrial.

Table 38-4 Common Causes of Dysrhythmias	
Cardiac Conditions	**Other Conditions**
• Accessory pathways	• Acid–base imbalances
• Conduction defects	• Alcohol
• Congestive heart failure	• Coffee, tea, tobacco
• Hypertrophy of cardiac muscle	• Connective tissue disorders
• Myocardial cell degeneration	• Drug effects or toxicity
• Myocardial infarction	• Electric shock
	• Electrolyte imbalances
	• Emotional crisis
	• Hypoxia, shock
	• Metabolic conditions (e.g., thyroid dysfunction)
	• Near-drowning
	• Poisoning

Purkinje system) that are able to discharge spontaneously. This situation is termed **automaticity.** Normally, the main pacemaker of the heart is the SA node, which spontaneously discharges 60 to 100 times per minute (Table 38-3). A pacemaker from another site may be discharged in two ways. If the SA node discharges more slowly than a secondary pacemaker, the electrical discharges from the secondary pacemaker may passively "escape." The secondary pacemaker then discharges automatically at its intrinsic rate. These secondary pacemakers may originate from the AV node or the His-Purkinje system at rates of 40 to 60 times per minute and 20 to 40 times per minute, respectively.

Another way that secondary pacemakers can originate is when they discharge more rapidly than the normal pacemaker of the SA node. Early or late beats may be triggered at an ectopic focus (area outside the normal conduction pathway) in the atria, the AV node, or the ventricles. This may result in a dysrhythmia, which replaces the normal sinus rhythm.

The impulse started by the SA node or an ectopic focus must be conducted to the entire heart chamber. The property of myocardial tissue that allows it to be depolarized by a stimulus is called *excitability.* This is an important part of the transmission of the impulse from one fibre to another. The level of excitability is determined by the length of time after depolarization that the tissues can be restimulated. The recovery period after stimulation is called the *refractory phase* or *refractory period.* The absolute refractory phase or period occurs when excitability is zero and heart tissue cannot be stimulated. The relative refractory period occurs slightly later in the cycle, and excitability is more likely to occur. In states of full excitability, the heart is completely recovered. Figure 38-10 shows the relationship between the refractory period and the ECG.

If conduction is depressed, and if some areas of the heart are blocked (e.g., by necrosis), the unblocked areas are activated earlier than the blocked areas. When the block is unidirectional, this uneven conduction may allow the initial impulse to re-enter areas that were previously not excitable but have recovered. The re-entering impulse may be able to depolarize the atria and ventricles, causing a premature beat. If the re-entrant excitation continues, tachycardia occurs (Aehlert, 2011).

Evaluation of Dysrhythmias

Dysrhythmias occur as the result of various abnormalities and disease states (Aehlert, 2011). The cause of a dysrhythmia influences the treatment of the patient. Common causes of dysrhythmias are listed in Table 38-4. In Table 38-5, a systematic approach to assessing a cardiac rhythm is presented.

Dysrhythmias occurring in out-of-hospital settings present problems of management. Determination of the rhythm by cardiac monitoring is a high priority. If indicated, the emergency medical services (EMS) system is contacted after the patient has been assessed. Emergency care of the patient with a dysrhythmia is outlined in Table 38-6.

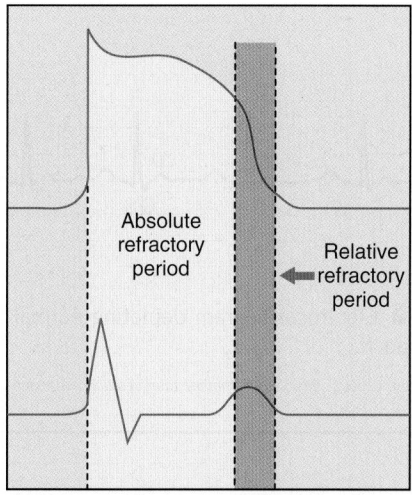

Figure 38-10 Diagram of absolute and relative refractory periods correlated with the cardiac muscle's action potential and with an ECG tracing.

Source: Adapted from Urden, L. D., Stacy, K. M., & Lough, M. E. (2010). *Critical care nursing: Diagnosis and management* (6th ed., p. 368, Figure 18-32). St. Louis: Mosby.

In addition to continuous ECG monitoring during hospitalization, several other methods are used to evaluate cardiac dysrhythmias and the effectiveness of antidysrhythmia drug therapy. An electrophysiological test (an invasive method) and Holter monitoring, event recorder monitoring, exercise treadmill testing, and signal-averaged ECG (all noninvasive methods) can be performed on both an inpatient and an outpatient basis.

An electrophysiological study (EPS) is performed to identify different mechanisms of tachydysrhythmias (dysrhythmias with rates >100), as well as heart blocks, bradydysrhythmias (dysrhythmias with rates <100), and causes of syncope. It can also be used to identify locations of accessory pathways and to determine the effectiveness of antidysrhythmia drugs. It involves introducing several electrode catheters transvenously through the femoral vein to the right side of the heart with fluoroscopic guidance. Electrical stimulation to various areas of the atrium and the

Table 38-5 Systematic Approach to Assessing Cardiac Rhythms

When assessing a cardiac rhythm, always assess the patient first, and then proceed with a systematic approach to interpreting the rhythm. A recommended approach is as follows:

1. Evaluate the rhythm (ventricular and atrial).
2. Determine the rate (ventricular and atrial).
3. Assess the presence and configuration of P waves.
4. Calculate the duration of the PR interval.
5. Calculate the QRS duration.
6. Calculate the QT interval.
7. Assess for changes in ST segment, T wave, or both.
8. Interpret the rhythm (e.g., atrial fibrillation).
9. Determine the clinical significance of this rhythm. Is the patient stable or unstable?
10. Determine the treatment for the rhythm.

Table 38-6 Emergency Management: Dysrhythmias

ETIOLOGY	ASSESSMENT FINDINGS	INTERVENTIONS
See Table 38-4	• Irregular rate and rhythm, palpitations • Chest, neck, shoulder, or arm pain • Dizziness, syncope • Dyspnea • Extreme restlessness • Decreased level of consciousness • Feeling of impending doom • Numbness, tingling of arms • Weakness and fatigue • Cold, clammy skin • Diaphoresis • Pallor • Nausea and vomiting • Decreased blood pressure • Decreased O₂ saturation	**Initial** • Ensure patent airway • Administer O₂ via nasal cannula • Establish IV access • Apply cardiac monitoring electrodes • Identify underlying rhythm • Identify ectopic beats **Ongoing Monitoring** • Monitor vital signs, level of consciousness, O₂ saturation, and cardiac rhythm • Anticipate need for intubation if respiratory distress is evident • Prepare to initiate CPR or defibrillation, or both

CPR, cardiopulmonary resuscitation; *IV,* intravenous.

ventricle is performed to induce the dysrhythmia. Immediate cardioversion or defibrillation may be required because serious dysrhythmias can be provoked during the procedure.

Preprocedure anxiety is common for patients undergoing EPS. Emotional support from the nurse is important. Patients should be instructed that they will be sedated but conscious during the procedure. Nursing care before and after the procedure is similar to that for cardiac catheterization (see Chapter 34). (EPS is also discussed in Chapter 34.)

The Holter monitor is a device that records the ECG while the patient is ambulatory. The device can record heart rhythm for 24 to 48 hours while the patient performs daily activities. The patient maintains a diary in which activities and any symptoms are recorded. Events in the diary can later be correlated with any dysrhythmias observed on the recording. The monitor is generally a useful device for detecting significant dysrhythmias and evaluating the effects of drugs during a patient's normal activities. It can also be used for detecting ischemia by analyzing ST segments. A limitation of the device is that patients who have frequent ventricular dysrhythmias, some of which may be lethal, may not have these dysrhythmias during the monitored time. (Holter monitoring is also discussed in Chapter 34.)

Use of event monitors has greatly improved the evaluation of outpatient dysrhythmias. Event monitors are recorders that are activated by the patient and can be used only at the time the patient experiences symptoms. The recorder is placed over the patient's chest during symptoms. The patient then transmits the rhythm to a central monitoring company via telephone. This is an easier method of documenting a dysrhythmia than the 24-hour monitor, especially if symptoms are not occurring daily. (Ambulatory ECG monitoring is discussed in Chapter 34.)

Exercise treadmill testing is used for evaluation of cardiac rhythm response to exercise. Exercise-induced dysrhythmias can be reproduced and analyzed, and drug therapy can be evaluated. These tests are performed with routine treadmill testing protocols. Diagnostic procedures for assessment of the cardiovascular system are presented in Chapter 34, Table 34-5.

Types of Dysrhythmias

Examples of the ECG tracings of common dysrhythmias are presented in Figures 38-11 through 38-19. Descriptive characteristics of common dysrhythmias are presented in Table 38-7.

Sinus Bradycardia. In sinus bradycardia, the conduction pathway is the same as that in sinus rhythm, but the SA node fires at a rate less than 60 beats/min. This is referred to as *absolute bradycardia* (Figure 38-11, *A*). Relative bradycardia is an HR that is less than expected for the patient's condition, causing symptoms (Aehlert, 2011).

Clinical Associations. Sinus bradycardia may be a normal sinus rhythm in aerobically trained athletes and in other individuals during sleep. It also occurs in response to carotid sinus massage, Valsalva's manoeuvre, hypothermia, increased intraocular pressure, increased vagal tone, and administration of parasympathomimetic drugs (e.g., bethanechol [Duvoid]). Disease states associated with sinus bradycardia are hypothyroidism, increased intracranial pressure, obstructive jaundice, and inferior wall myocardial infarction (MI).

Electrocardiographic Characteristics. In sinus bradycardia, the HR is less than 60 beats/min, and the rhythm is regular. The P wave precedes each QRS complex and has a normal shape and duration. The PR interval is normal, and the QRS complex has a normal shape and duration.

Clinical Significance. The clinical significance of sinus bradycardia depends on how the patient tolerates it hemodynami-

Table 38-7 Characteristics of Common Dysrhythmias

PATTERN	RATE AND RHYTHM	P WAVE	PR INTERVAL	QRS COMPLEX
Normal sinus rhythm	60-100 beats/min and regular	Normal	Normal	Normal
Sinus bradycardia	<60 beats/min and regular	Normal	Normal	Normal
Sinus tachycardia	>100 beats/min and regular	Normal	Normal	Normal
Premature atrial contraction	Usually 60-100 beats/min and irregular	Abnormal shape	Normal or variable	Normal (usually)
Paroxysmal supraventricular tachycardia	150-250 beats/min and regular	Abnormal shape, may be hidden	Variable	Normal (usually)
Atrial flutter	*Atrial:* 250-350 beats/min and regular *Ventricular:* >100 beats/min and irregular	Sawtooth shape	Variable	Normal (usually)
Atrial fibrillation	*Atrial:* 350-600 beats/min and irregular *Ventricular:* >100 beats/min and irregular or possibly any rate	Chaotic, fibrillatory	Not present	Normal (usually)
Junctional rhythms	40-140 beats/min and regular	Inverted (may be hidden)	Variable	Normal (usually)
First-degree AV heart block	Normal and regular	Normal	>0.20 sec, constant	Normal
Second-degree AV heart block				
Type I (Mobitz I, Wenckebach)	*Atrial:* Normal and regular *Ventricular:* Slower and irregular	Normal	Progressively lengthened	Normal width, with pattern of one nonconducted QRS complex
Type II (Mobitz II)	*Atrial:* Usually normal and regular or irregular *Ventricular:* Slower and regular or irregular	More P waves than QRS complexes	Normal or prolonged	Widened, preceded by two or more P waves
Third-degree AV heart block	Ventricular rate 20-40 beats/min and regular	Normal, but no connection with QRS complex	None; PR interval not related to QRS complex; more P waves than QRS complexes	Normal or widened; no connection with P waves
Premature ventricular contraction	60-100 beats/min and irregular	None	Not present	Wide and distorted
Ventricular tachycardia	100-250 beats/min and regular or irregular	None	None	Wide and distorted
Ventricular fibrillation	Not measurable and irregular	Absent	Not present	Not measurable

AV, atrioventricular.

cally. Signs of symptomatic bradycardia can include pale, cool skin; hypotension; weakness; angina; dizziness or syncope; confusion or disorientation; and shortness of breath.

Treatment. Treatment consists of administration of atropine (an anticholinergic drug) for the patient with symptoms. Pacemaker therapy may be required.

Sinus Tachycardia. The conduction pathway is the same in sinus tachycardia as that in normal sinus rhythm. The discharge rate from the sinus node is increased as a result of vagal inhibition or sympathetic stimulation. The sinus rate is greater than 100 beats/min (see Figure 38-11, *B*).

Clinical Associations. Sinus tachycardia is associated with physiological and psychological stressors such as exercise, fever, pain, hypotension, hypovolemia, anemia, hypoxia, hypoglycemia, myocardial ischemia, heart failure (HF), hyperthyroidism, anxiety, and fear. It can also be an effect of drugs such as epinephrine (Epi-Pen), norepinephrine (Levophed), atropine, caffeine, theophylline, nifedipine, or hydralazine (Apresoline). In addition, many over-the-counter cold remedies have active ingredients (e.g., pseudoephedrine [Sudafed]) that can cause tachycardia.

Electrocardiographic Characteristics. In sinus tachycardia, the HR is greater than 100 beats/min and the rhythm is regular.

The P wave is normal, precedes each QRS complex, and has a normal shape and duration. The PR interval is normal, and the QRS complex has a normal shape and duration.

Clinical Significance. The clinical significance of sinus tachycardia depends on the patient's tolerance of the increased HR. The patient may have symptoms of dizziness, dyspnea, and hypotension. Increased myocardial oxygen consumption is associated with an increased HR. Angina or an increase in infarction size may accompany persistent sinus tachycardia in the patient with an acute MI.

Treatment. Treatment is based on the underlying cause. If the patient is experiencing tachycardia from pain, tachycardia should resolve with effective pain management. Treating hypovolemia should resolve any associated tachycardia.

Premature Atrial Contraction. A **premature atrial contraction (PAC)** is a contraction originating from an ectopic focus in one atrium in a location other than the sinus node. The ectopic signal originates in the left or the right atrium and travels across both atria by an abnormal pathway, causing the P wave to be distorted (Figure 38-12). At the AV node, it may be stopped (nonconducted PAC), delayed (lengthened PR interval), or conducted normally. If the signal moves through the AV node, in most cases it is conducted normally through the ventricles.

Clinical Associations. In a normal heart, a PAC can result from emotional stress, physical fatigue, or the use of caffeine, tobacco, or alcohol. A PAC can also result from hypoxia, electrolyte imbalances, and disease states such as hyperthyroidism, chronic obstructive pulmonary disease (COPD), and heart disease, including coronary artery disease (CAD) and valvular disease.

Electrocardiographic Characteristics. Heart rate varies with the underlying rate and frequency of the PAC, and the rhythm is irregular. The P wave has a different shape from that of the P wave originating from the SA node. It may be notched or have downward (or negative) deflection, or it may be hidden in the preceding T wave. The PR interval may be shorter or longer than the PR interval originating from the SA node, but its length is within normal limits. The QRS complex is usually normal. If the QRS interval is 0.12 sec or longer, conduction through the ventricles is abnormal.

Clinical Significance. In people with healthy hearts, isolated PACs are not significant. In people with heart disease, frequent PACs may indicate enhanced automaticity of the atria or a re-entry mechanism. Such PACs may warn of or initiate more serious dysrhythmias (e.g., supraventricular tachycardia).

Treatment. Treatment depends on the patient's symptoms. Withdrawal of sources of stimulation such as caffeine or sympathomimetic drugs may be warranted. β-Adrenergic blockers may be used to decrease PACs.

Paroxysmal Supraventricular Tachycardia. Paroxysmal supraventricular tachycardia (PSVT) is a dysrhythmia originating in an ectopic focus anywhere above the bifurcation of the bundle of His (Figure 38-13). Identification of the ectopic focus is often difficult even with 12-lead ECG because the dysrhythmia must be recorded as it is initiated.

PSVT occurs because of a re-entrant phenomenon (re-excitation of the atria when there is a one-way block). Usually a PAC triggers a run of repeated premature beats. *Paroxysmal* refers to an abrupt onset and termination. Termination is sometimes followed by a brief period of asystole. Some degree of AV block may be present. PSVT can occur in the presence of Wolff-Parkinson-White (WPW) syndrome, or "pre-excitation." In this syndrome, extra conduction pathways or accessory pathways are present.

Clinical Associations. In the normal heart, PSVT is associated with overexertion, emotional stress, deep inspiration, and stimulants such as caffeine and tobacco. PSVT is also associated with rheumatic heart disease, digitalis toxicity, CAD, and cor pulmonale.

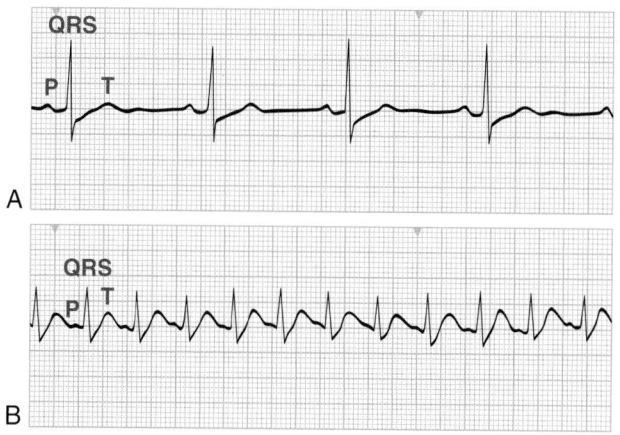

Figure 38-11 A, ECG demonstrating sinus bradycardia. **B,** ECG demonstrating sinus tachycardia.

Source: Wesley, K. (2011). *Huszar's basic dysrhythmias and acute coronary syndromes: Interpretation and management* (4th ed., p. 83, Figure 5-3, *A*, and p. 87, Figure 5-5, *A*). St Louis: Mosby.

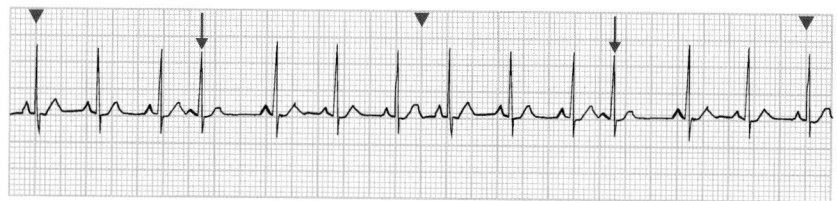

Figure 38-12 ECG demonstrating premature atrial contractions *(arrows)*.

Source: Bucher, L., & Melander, S. (1999). *Critical care nursing.* Philadelphia: W. B. Saunders.

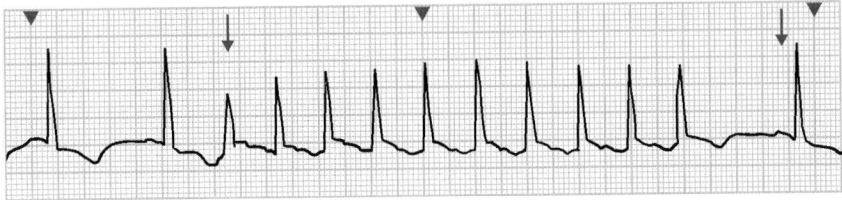

Figure 38-13 Electrocardiogram demonstrating paroxysmal supraventricular tachycardia (PSVT). *Arrows* indicate beginning and ending of PSVT.

Source: Bucher, L., & Melander, S. (1999). *Critical care nursing.* Philadelphia: W. B. Saunders.

Electrocardiographic Characteristics. In PSVT, the HR is 100 to 300 beats/min, and rhythm is regular or slightly irregular. The P wave is often hidden in the preceding T wave, but if seen, it may have an abnormal shape. The PR interval may be shortened or normal, and the QRS complex is usually normal.

Clinical Significance. The clinical significance of PSVT depends on symptoms and HR. A prolonged episode and heart rate greater than 180 beats/min may precipitate a decrease in CO, resulting in hypotension, dyspnea, and angina.

Treatment. Treatment for PSVT includes vagal stimulation and drug therapy. Common vagal manoeuvres include Valsalva's manoeuvres and coughing. IV adenosine is the drug of first choice to convert PSVT to a normal sinus rhythm. This drug has a short half-life (1.5-10 sec) and is well tolerated by most patients (Lehne, 2013). IV β-adrenergic blockers, calcium channel blockers (e.g., diltiazem [Cardizem]), and amiodarone (Cordarone) can also be used. For a patient with WPW syndrome, amiodarone should be used. If vagal stimulation and drug therapy are ineffective and the patient becomes hemodynamically unstable, direct-current (DC) cardioversion may be used. (Cardioversion is discussed on p. 967.) If PSVT recurs in patients with WPW syndrome, they may ultimately be treated with radiofrequency catheter ablation of the accessory pathway (Woods et al., 2005). (Catheter ablation therapy is discussed on p. 971.)

Atrial Flutter. **Atrial flutter** is an atrial tachydysrhythmia identified by recurring, regular, sawtooth-shaped flutter (F) waves that originate from a single ectopic focus in the right atrium (Figure 38-14, *A*).

Clinical Associations. Atrial flutter rarely occurs in a normal heart. It is associated with disease states such as CAD, hypertension, mitral valve disorders, pulmonary embolus, chronic lung disease, cor pulmonale, cardiomyopathy, and hyperthyroidism and with the use of drugs such as digoxin, quinidine, and epinephrine.

Electrocardiographic Characteristics. Atrial rate is 250 to 350 beats/min. The ventricular rate varies according to the conduction ratio. In 2:1 conduction, the ventricular rate is typically found to be approximately 150 beats/min. Atrial rhythm is regular, and ventricular rhythm is usually regular. The atrial flutter waves represent atrial depolarization followed by repolarization. The PR interval is variable and cannot be measured. The QRS complex is usually normal. Because of the ability of the AV node to delay signals from the atria, there is usually some AV block in a fixed ratio of flutter waves to QRS complexes (e.g., 2:1, 3:1).

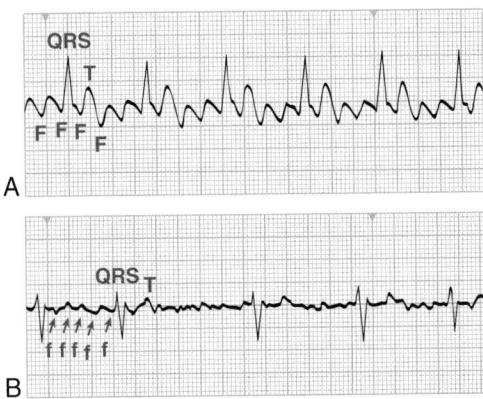

Figure 38-14 A, ECG demonstrating atrial flutter with a 4:1 conduction (four flutter *[F]* waves to each QRS complex). **B,** ECG demonstrating atrial fibrillation. Note the chaotic fibrillatory *(f)* waves between the QRS complexes.

Source: Huszar, R. J. (2002). *Basic dysrhythmias: Interpretation and management* (3rd ed.). St. Louis: Mosby.

Clinical Significance. The high ventricular rates (>100 beats/min) and loss of the atrial "kick" (atrial contraction reflected by a sinus P wave) that are associated with atrial flutter can decrease CO and cause serious consequences such as HF, especially in the patient with underlying heart disease. Patients with atrial flutter are at increased risk of stroke because of the risk of thrombus formation in the atria from the stasis of blood. Warfarin (Coumadin) is used to prevent stroke in patients with atrial flutter of longer than 48 hours' duration (Woods et al., 2005).

Treatment. The primary goal in treatment of atrial flutter is to slow the ventricular response by increasing AV block. Drugs used to control ventricular rate include calcium channel blockers and β-adrenergic blockers. Electrical cardioversion may be used to convert the atrial flutter to sinus rhythm in an emergency situation (i.e., the patient is hemodynamically unstable) and electively. Antidysrhythmia drugs used to convert atrial flutter to sinus rhythm or to maintain sinus rhythm include amiodarone, propafenone (Rythmol), and ibutilide (Corvert) (Lehne, 2013).

Radiofrequency catheter ablation is increasingly being used as curative therapy for atrial flutter. The procedure is performed in the electrophysiology laboratory and involves positioning a catheter in the right atrium between the inferior vena cava and the tricuspid valve. With the use of a low-voltage, high-frequency form of electrical energy, the tissue is ablated (or destroyed), the dysrhythmia is terminated, and normal sinus rhythm is restored in most cases (Greenberg & Chandrakantan, 2011). (Catheter ablation in discussed on p. 971.)

Atrial Fibrillation.

Atrial fibrillation is characterized by a total disorganization of atrial electrical activity caused by multiple ectopic foci, resulting in loss of effective atrial contraction (see Figure 38-14, *B*). Atrial fibrillation is the most common dysrhythmia encountered in the emergency department, and the focus of treatment is the rapid assessment of potential hemodynamic instability and identification and treatment of the underlying cause (Steill & Macle, 2011). The dysrhythmia may be chronic or intermittent. Atrial fibrillation is the most common dysrhythmia in Canada and the United States, affecting approximately 1 per 136 adults. Its prevalence increases with age. As the older adult population increases, a 60% increase in this dysrhythmia is predicted by 2020 (Woods et al., 2005).

Clinical Associations. Atrial fibrillation usually occurs in patients with underlying heart disease, such as CAD, rheumatic heart disease, cardiomyopathy, hypertensive heart disease, HF, and pericarditis. It is often acutely caused by factors such as thyrotoxicosis, alcohol intoxication, caffeine use, electrolyte disturbances, stress, and cardiac surgery.

Electrocardiographic Characteristics. During atrial fibrillation, the atrial rate may be as high as 600 beats/min. Ventricular rate can vary from as low as 50 beats/min to as high as 180 beats/min. Atrial fibrillation with ventricular rates greater than 100 are described as atrial fibrillation with a rapid ventricular response. When ventricular rates are less than 100, the condition is described as atrial fibrillation with a slow or controlled ventricular response. P waves are replaced by chaotic, fibrillatory waves in atrial fibrillation. The ventricular rhythm is usually irregular. The PR interval is not measurable, but the QRS complex usually has a normal shape and duration. At times, atrial flutter and atrial fibrillation may coexist.

Clinical Significance. Atrial fibrillation can often result in a decrease in CO because of ineffective atrial contractions or loss of atrial kick, a rapid ventricular response, or both. Thrombi may form in the atria as a result of blood stasis. An embolized clot may develop and travel to the brain, causing a stroke. Overall risk of stroke increases five-fold with atrial fibrillation. Risk of stroke is even higher in patients with structural heart disease, those with hypertension, and those older than 65 years (Woods et al., 2005).

Treatment. The goals of treatment include a decrease in ventricular response (to <100) and prevention of cerebral embolic events (Steill & Macle, 2011). Ventricular rate control is a priority for patients with atrial fibrillation. Drugs used for rate control include calcium channel blockers (e.g., diltiazem) and β-adrenergic blockers (e.g., metoprolol).

For some patients, conversion of atrial fibrillation to a normal sinus rhythm may be a consideration (e.g., reduced exercise tolerance with rate control drugs, contraindications to warfarin). Antidysrhythmia drugs used for conversion to and maintenance of sinus rhythm include medications such as amiodarone (Aehlert, 2011). In patients with severe left ventricular dysfunction or HF, amiodarone or DC cardioversion should be used (Aehlert, 2011).

Cardioversion may be used to convert atrial fibrillation to a normal sinus rhythm. Before proceeding to cardioversion, in the absence of systemic anticoagulation, the nurse must determined

that the patient has had atrial fibrillation or atrial flutter for less than 48 hours (Steill & Macle, 2011). The cardioversion procedure can cause the clots to dislodge, which increases the patient's risk for stroke. If clots are present, the procedure is contraindicated.

If drugs or cardioversion do not convert atrial fibrillation to normal sinus rhythm, long-term anticoagulation therapy is required. Long-term follow-up with patients experiencing atrial fibrillation or flutter is recommended to assess the need for long term antithrombotic therapy or antiarrhythmic therapy. (See Chapter 40 for discussion of anticoagulation therapy.)

Other treatment strategies exist for drug-refractory atrial fibrillation and for patients who cannot or choose not to have long-term anticoagulation. These include the use of radiofrequency catheter ablation, which is similar to the procedure for atrial flutter (Canadian Cardiovascular Society, 2011).

Junctional Dysrhythmias.

Junctional dysrhythmias are dysrhythmias that originate in the area of the AV node, primarily because the SA node has failed to fire or the signal has been blocked. In this situation, the AV node becomes the pacemaker of the heart. The impulse from the AV node usually moves in a retrograde (backward) manner that produces an abnormal P wave occurring just before or after the QRS complex or that is hidden in the QRS complex. The impulse usually moves normally through the ventricles. Junctional premature beats may occur, and they are treated in a manner similar to that for PACs. Other junctional dysrhythmias include junctional escape rhythm (Figure 38-15), accelerated junctional rhythm, and junctional tachycardia. These dysrhythmias are treated according to the patient's tolerance of the rhythm and the patient's clinical condition.

Clinical Associations. Junctional dysrhythmias are often associated with CAD, HF, cardiomyopathy, electrolyte imbalances, inferior MI, and rheumatic heart disease. Certain drugs (e.g., digoxin, amphetamines, caffeine, nicotine) can also cause junctional dysrhythmias (Aehlert, 2011).

Electrocardiographic Characteristics. In junctional escape rhythm, the HR is 40 to 60 beats/min; in accelerated junctional rhythm, it is 61 to 100 beats/min; and in junctional tachycardia, it is 101 to 150 beats/min. Rhythm is regular. The P wave is abnormal in shape and inverted, or it may be hidden in the QRS complex (see Figure 38-15). The PR interval is less than 0.12 sec when the P wave precedes the QRS complex. The QRS complex is usually normal.

Clinical Significance. Junctional escape rhythms serve as a safety mechanism for when the SA node has not been

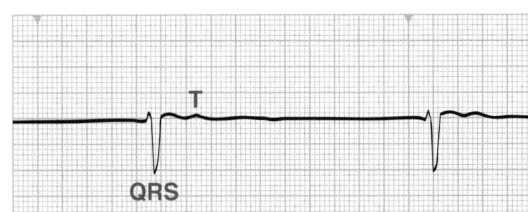

Figure 38-15 Electrocardiogram demonstrating junctional escape rhythm. The P wave is hidden in the QRS complex.

Source: Huszar, R. J. (2002). *Basic dysrhythmias: Interpretation and management* (3rd ed.). St. Louis: Mosby.

effective in firing. Escape rhythms such as this should not be suppressed. Accelerated junctional rhythm and junctional tachycardia, however, indicate a more serious problem with the sinoatrial node. These rhythms may result in a reduction of CO, causing the patient to become hemodynamically unstable (e.g., hypotensive).

Treatment. Treatment varies according to the type of junctional dysrhythmia. If a patient has symptoms with an escape junctional rhythm, atropine can be administered. In accelerated junctional rhythm and junctional tachycardia caused by digoxin toxicity, the digoxin is withheld. In the absence of digoxin toxicity, β-adrenergic blockers, calcium channel blockers, and amiodarone are used for rate control. Direct-current cardioversion should not be used.

First-Degree Atrioventricular Block.

First-degree AV block is a type of AV block in which every impulse is conducted to the ventricles but the duration of AV conduction is prolonged (Figure 38-16, *A*). After the impulse moves through the AV node, it is usually conducted normally through the ventricles.

Clinical Associations. First-degree AV block is associated with MI, CAD, rheumatic fever, hyperthyroidism, vagal stimulation, and drugs such as digoxin, β-adrenergic blockers, calcium channel blockers, and flecainide.

Electrocardiographic Characteristics. In first-degree AV block, the HR is normal, and the rhythm is regular. The P wave is normal, the PR interval is prolonged to more than 0.20 sec, and the QRS complex usually has a normal shape and duration.

Clinical Significance. First-degree AV block is usually not serious but can be a precursor of higher degrees of AV block. Patients with first-degree AV block have no symptoms.

Treatment. There is no treatment for first-degree AV block. Modifications to causative medications may be considered. Patients should continue to be monitored for any new changes in heart rhythm.

Second-Degree Atrioventricular Block, Type I.

Type I second-degree AV block (Mobitz I or Wenckebach's heart block) includes a gradual lengthening of the PR interval. It occurs because of a prolonged AV conduction time until an atrial impulse is not conducted and a QRS complex is blocked (missing) (see Figure 38-16, *B*). Type I AV block most commonly occurs in the AV node, but it can also occur in the His-Purkinje system.

Clinical Associations. Type I AV block may result from use of drugs such as digoxin or β-adrenergic blockers. It may also be associated with CAD and other diseases that can slow AV conduction.

Electrocardiographic Characteristics. The atrial rate is normal, but the ventricular rate may be slower as a result of nonconducted atrial impulses or blocked QRS complexes. Once a ventricular beat is blocked, the cycle repeats itself with progressive lengthening of the PR intervals until another QRS complex is blocked. The rhythm appears on the ECG in a pattern of grouped beats. Ventricular rhythm is irregular. The P wave has a normal shape. The QRS complex has a normal shape and duration.

First-degree AV block

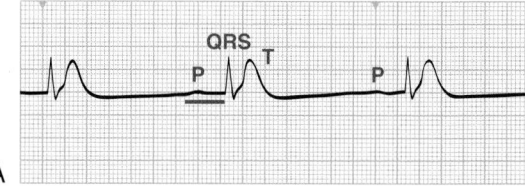

A

Second-degree AV block
(type I AV block [Wenckebach's])

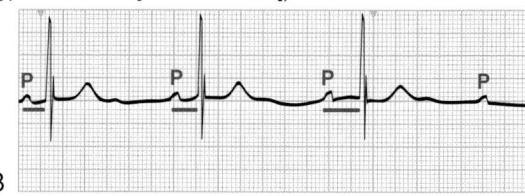

B

Second-degree AV block
(type II AV block)

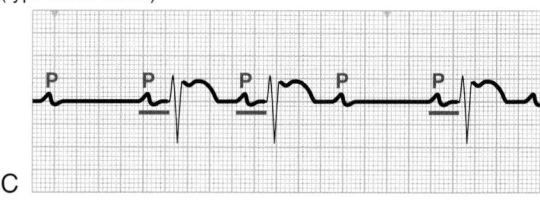

C

Third-degree AV block
(complete AV block)

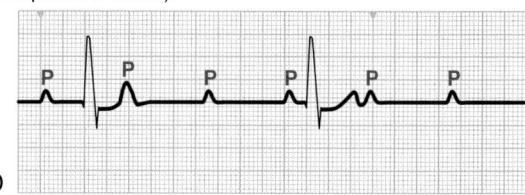

D

Figure 38-16 ECGs demonstrating heart block. **A,** First-degree AV heart block. **B,** Second-degree AV heart block, type I (Wenckebach's). *Red line* indicates PR interval. **C,** Second-degree AV heart block, type II. *Red line* indicates PR interval. **D,** Third-degree (complete) AV block.

Source: Wesley, K. (2011). *Huszar's basic dysrhythmias and acute coronary syndromes: Interpretation and management* (4th ed.). St. Louis: Mosby.

Clinical Significance. Type I AV block is usually a result of myocardial ischemia or infarction. It is almost always transient and is usually well tolerated. However, in some patients (e.g., after MI), it may be a warning signal of a more serious AV conduction disturbance.

Treatment. If the patient has symptoms, atropine is used to increase the HR, or a temporary pacemaker may be needed, especially if the patient has experienced an MI. If the patient has no symptoms, the rhythm should be closely observed with a transcutaneous pacemaker on standby. Bradycardia is more likely to become symptomatic when one or more of the following are present: (a) hypotension, (b) HF, or (c) shock.

Second-Degree Atrioventricular Block, Type II.

In *type II second-degree AV block (Mobitz II heart block)*, a P wave is not conducted without progressive antecedent PR lengthening.

This almost always occurs when a block in one of the bundle branches is present (see Figure 38-16, C). On conducted beats, the PR interval is constant. Type II second-degree AV block is a more serious type of block in which a certain number of impulses from the SA node are not conducted to the ventricles. This occurs in ratios of 2:1, 3:1, and so on (i.e., two P waves to one QRS complex, three P waves to one QRS complex). It may occur with varying ratios. Type II AV block almost always originates in the His-Purkinje system.

Clinical Associations. Type II AV block is associated with rheumatic heart disease, CAD, anterior MI, and digitalis toxicity.

Electrocardiographic Characteristics. The atrial rate is usually normal. The ventricular rate depends on the intrinsic rate and the degree of AV block. The atrial rhythm is regular, but the ventricular rhythm may be irregular. The P wave has a normal shape. The PR interval may be normal or prolonged in duration and remains constant on conducted beats. The QRS complex is usually more than 0.12 sec because of bundle-branch block.

Clinical Significance. Type II AV block often progresses to third-degree AV block and is associated with a poor prognosis. The reduced HR often results in decreased CO with subsequent hypotension and myocardial ischemia. Type II AV block is an indication for therapy with a permanent pacemaker.

Treatment. Temporary treatment before the insertion of a permanent pacemaker may be necessary if the condition becomes symptomatic (e.g., hypotension, angina). Such treatment involves the use of a temporary transvenous or transcutaneous pacemaker (Aehlert, 2011).

Third-Degree Atrioventricular Block.
Third-degree AV block, or **complete heart block,** constitutes one form of AV dissociation in which no impulses from the atria are conducted to the ventricles (see Figure 38-16, D). The atria are stimulated and contract independently of the ventricles. The ventricular rhythm is an escape rhythm, and the ectopic pacemaker may be above or below the bifurcation of the bundle of His.

Clinical Associations. Third-degree AV block is associated with severe heart disease, including CAD, MI, myocarditis, cardiomyopathy, and some systemic diseases such as amyloidosis and progressive systemic sclerosis (scleroderma). Some medications can also cause third-degree AV block, such as digoxin, β-adrenergic blockers, and calcium channel blockers.

Electrocardiographic Characteristics. The atrial rate is usually a sinus rate of 60 to 100 beats/min. The ventricular rate depends on the site of the block. If it is in the AV node, the rate is 40 to 60 beats/min, and if it is in the His-Purkinje system, it is 20 to 40 beats/min. Atrial and ventricular rhythms are regular but unrelated to each other. The P wave has a normal shape. The PR interval is variable, and there is no time relationship between the P wave and the QRS complex. The QRS complex is normal if an escape rhythm is initiated at the bundle of His or above. It is widened if an escape rhythm is initiated below the bundle of His.

Clinical Significance. Third-degree AV block almost always results in reduced CO with subsequent ischemia, HF, and shock. Syncope from third-degree AV block may result from severe bradycardia or even periods of asystole.

Treatment. When patients have symptoms, a transcutaneous pacemaker is used until a temporary transvenous pacemaker can be inserted (Aehlert, 2011). The use of drugs such as atropine, epinephrine, isoproterenol, and dopamine is a temporary measure to increase the HR and support blood pressure (BP) until temporary pacing is initiated. Patients need a permanent pacemaker implanted as soon as possible.

Premature Ventricular Contractions.
A **premature ventricular contraction (PVC)** is a contraction originating in an ectopic focus in the ventricles. It is the premature occurrence of a QRS complex, which is wide and whose shape is distorted in comparison with a QRS complex initiated from the normal conduction pathway (Figure 38-17). PVCs that are initiated from different foci appear different in shape from each other and are called *multifocal* PVCs. PVCs that appear to have the same shape are called *unifocal* PVCs. When every other beat is a PVC, it is called *ventricular bigeminy.* When every third beat is a PVC, it is called *ventricular trigeminy.* Two consecutive PVCs are called a *couplet.* When three or more consecutive PVCs occur, it is called *ventricular tachycardia.* A PVC that falls on the T wave of a preceding beat is called *R-on-T phenomenon.* This is considered especially dangerous because the PVC is occurring during the relative refractory phase of ventricular repolarization. Excitability of the cardiac cells is increased during this time, and the risk for the PVC to initiate ventricular tachycardia or ventricular fibrillation is high.

Clinical Associations. PVCs are associated with stimulants such as caffeine, alcohol, nicotine, aminophylline, epinephrine, isoproterenol, and digoxin. They are also associated with electrolyte imbalances, hypoxia, fever, exercise, and emotional stress.

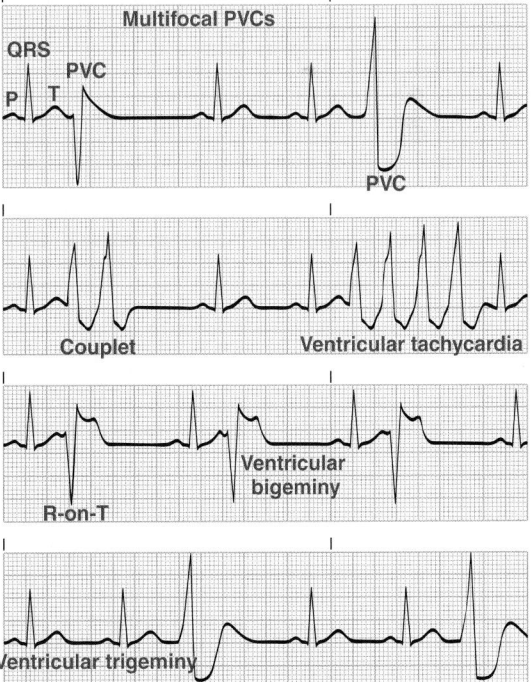

Figure 38-17 Various forms of premature ventricular contractions (PVCs). All were recorded from lead II.

Source: Wesley, K. (2011). *Huszar's basic dysrhythmias and acute coronary syndromes: Interpretation and management* (4th ed., p. 119, Figure 8-1, *H-K*). St. Louis: Mosby.

Disease states associated with PVCs include MI, mitral valve prolapse, HF, and CAD.

Electrocardiographic Characteristics. HR varies according to intrinsic rate and number of PVCs. The rhythm is irregular because of premature beats. The P wave is rarely visible and is usually hidden in the QRS complex of the PVC. Retrograde conduction may occur, and the P wave may occur after the ectopic beat. The PR interval is not measurable. The QRS complex is wide and distorted in shape, lasting more than 0.12 sec. The T wave is generally large and opposite in direction to the major direction of the QRS complex.

Clinical Significance. PVCs are usually a benign finding in the patient with a normal heart. In heart disease, depending on frequency, PVCs may reduce the CO and precipitate angina and HF. Because PVCs in CAD or acute MI represent ventricular irritability, the patient's physiological response to PVCs must be monitored. It is important to assess the patient's apical–radial pulse rate because PVCs often do not generate a sufficient ventricular contraction to result in a peripheral pulse. This may lead to a pulse deficit.

Treatment. Treatment is often based on the cause of the PVCs (e.g., oxygen therapy for hypoxia, electrolyte replacement). Assessment of the patient's hemodynamic status is important to determine whether treatment with drug therapy is indicated. Drugs that should be considered include β-adrenergic blockers, procainamide, amiodarone, or lidocaine (Xylocaine).

Ventricular Tachycardia. The diagnosis of **ventricular tachycardia (VT)** is made when a run of three or more PVCs occurs. It occurs when an ectopic focus or foci fire repetitively and the ventricle takes control as the pacemaker. VT appears in different forms, depending on the QRS configuration. Monomorphic VT (Figure 38-18, *A*) has QRS complexes that are the same in shape, size, and direction. In polymorphic VT, the QRS complexes gradually change back and forth from one shape, size, and direction to another over a series of beats. *Torsades de pointes* (French, "twisting of the points") is polymorphic VT associated with a prolonged QT interval of the underlying rhythm (see Figure 38-18, *B*).

Ventricular tachycardia may be sustained or nonsustained. Sustained VT lasts for more than 30 sec. Nonsustained VT lasts for 30 sec or less. The development of ventricular tachycardia is an ominous sign. It is considered to be a life-threatening dysrhythmia because of decreased CO and the possibility of deterioration to ventricular fibrillation, which is a lethal dysrhythmia.

Clinical Associations. Ventricular tachycardia is associated with MI, CAD, significant electrolyte imbalances, cardiomyopathy, mitral valve prolapse, long QT syndrome, digitalis toxicity, and central nervous system disorders. This dysrhythmia has also been observed in patients who have no evidence of cardiac disease.

Electrocardiographic Characteristics. The ventricular rate is 150 to 250 beats/min. The rhythm may be regular or irregular. AV dissociation may be present, with P waves occurring independently of the QRS complex. The atria may also be depolarized by the ventricles in a retrograde manner. The P wave is usually hidden in the QRS complex, and the PR interval is not measurable.

The QRS complex is distorted in appearance, with a duration exceeding 0.12 sec and with the ST–T wave in the opposite direction of the QRS complex (see Figure 38-18). The R–R interval may be irregular or regular.

Clinical Significance. Ventricular tachycardia can be stable (patient has a pulse) or unstable (patient is pulseless). Sustained ventricular tachycardia causes a severe decrease in CO as a result of decreased ventricular diastolic filling times and loss of atrial contraction. Results include hypotension, pulmonary edema, decreased cerebral blood flow, and cardiopulmonary arrest. The dysrhythmia must be treated quickly, even if it occurs only briefly and stops abruptly, because episodes may recur if prophylactic treatment is not begun. Ventricular fibrillation may also develop.

Treatment. Precipitating causes must be identified and treated (e.g., electrolyte imbalances, ischemia). If the VT is monomorphic and the patient is hemodynamically stable (e.g., pulse is present) and has preserved left ventricular function, IV amiodarone or lidocaine is typically used. If the patient becomes hemodynamically unstable or has poor left ventricular function, IV amiodarone or lidocaine is given, followed by cardioversion if the original drug therapy alone is ineffective.

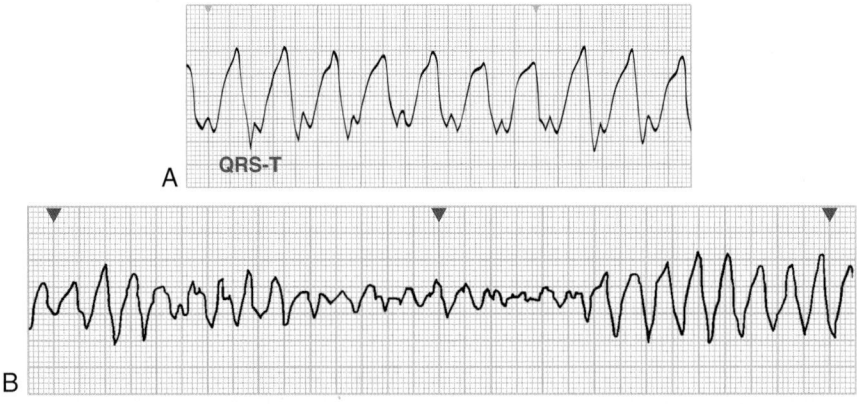

Figure 38-18 ECGs demonstrating ventricular tachycardia. **A,** Monomorphic. **B,** Torsades de pointes (polymorphic).

Source: Bucher, L., & Melander, S. (1999). *Critical care nursing.* Philadelphia: W. B. Saunders.

If the VT is polymorphic with a normal baseline QT interval, any one of the following medications is used: β-adrenergic blockers, lidocaine, amiodarone, procainamide, or sotalol. Cardioversion is performed if drug therapy is ineffective.

If the VT is polymorphic with a prolonged baseline QT interval, therapies include IV magnesium, lidocaine, and antitachycardia pacing (discussed later in this chapter). Drugs that prolong the QT interval should be discontinued. If the rhythm is not converted, cardioversion may be needed.

VT without a pulse is a life-threatening situation and is treated in the same manner as ventricular fibrillation. Cardiopulmonary resuscitation (CPR) and rapid defibrillation are the first lines of treatment, followed by the administration of epinephrine if defibrillation is unsuccessful (American Heart Association [AHA], 2010).

An *accelerated idioventricular rhythm* (AIVR) can develop when the intrinsic pacemaker rate (SA node or AV node) becomes lower than that of a ventricular ectopic pacemaker. The rate is between 40 and 100 beats/min. It is most commonly associated with acute MI and reperfusion of the myocardium after fibrinolytic therapy or angioplasty of coronary arteries. It can also occur with digitalis toxicity. In the setting of acute MI, AIVR is usually self-limiting and well tolerated and necessitates no treatment. If it becomes symptomatic (e.g., hypotension, angina), atropine can be considered. Temporary pacing may be required. Drugs that suppress ventricular rhythms (e.g., lidocaine) should not be used because they can terminate the ventricular rhythm and further reduce the HR.

Ventricular Fibrillation.
Ventricular fibrillation is a severe derangement of the heart rhythm characterized on the ECG by irregular undulations of varying shapes and amplitude (Figure 38-19). This represents the firing of multiple ectopic foci in the ventricle. Mechanically the ventricle is simply "quivering," and no effective contraction, and consequently no cardiac output, occurs.

Clinical Associations. Ventricular fibrillation occurs in acute MI and myocardial ischemia and in chronic diseases such as CAD and cardiomyopathy. It may occur during cardiac pacing or cardiac catheterization procedures as a result of catheter stimulation of the ventricle. It may also occur with coronary reperfusion after fibrinolytic therapy. Other clinical associations are accidental electric shock, hyperkalemia, hypoxemia, acidosis, and drug toxicity.

Electrocardiographic Characteristics. The HR is not measurable. The rhythm is irregular and chaotic. The P wave is not detectable, and the PR and the QRS intervals are not measurable.

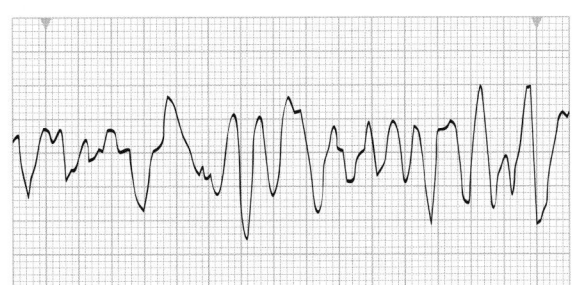

Figure 38-19 ECG demonstrating ventricular fibrillation.

Source: Wesley, K. (2011). *Huszar's basic dysrhythmias and acute coronary syndromes: Interpretation and management* (4th ed., p. 127, Figure 8-5, *B*). St. Louis: Mosby.

Clinical Significance. Ventricular fibrillation results in an unresponsive, pulseless, and apneic state. If it is not rapidly treated, the patient will die.

Treatment. Treatment consists of assessment of circulation, airway, and breathing (CAB) and if no pulse is found, CPR and advanced cardiac life support (ACLS) measures are initiated immediately with the use of defibrillation and definitive drug therapy. If a defibrillator is immediately available, it must be used without delay (AHA, 2010).

Asystole.
Asystole represents the total absence of ventricular electrical activity. On occasion, P waves are detected. No ventricular contraction occurs because depolarization does not occur. Patients are unresponsive, pulseless, and apneic. This is a lethal dysrhythmia that necessitates immediate treatment. Ventricular fibrillation may masquerade as asystole; thus the rhythm should be assessed in more than one lead. The prognosis of a patient with asystole is extremely poor.

Clinical Associations. Asystole is usually a result of advanced cardiac disease, a severe cardiac conduction system disturbance, or end-stage HF.

Clinical Significance. In general, patients with asystole have end-stage cardiac disease or have a prolonged cardiac arrest and cannot be resuscitated.

Treatment. Treatment consists of CPR with initiation of ACLS measures, which include intubation, transcutaneous pacing, and IV therapy with epinephrine and atropine.

Pulseless Electrical Activity.
Pulseless electrical activity (PEA) is a situation in which electrical activity can be observed on the ECG, but there is no mechanical activity of the ventricles and the patient has no pulse. The prognosis is poor unless the underlying cause can be identified and quickly corrected. The most frequent causes of PEA include hypovolemia, hypoxia, metabolic acidosis, hyperkalemia or hypokalemia, hypothermia, drug overdose, cardiac tamponade, MI, tension pneumothorax, and pulmonary embolus. Treatment begins with assessment of CAB and if no pulse is detected, CPR is initiated and followed by intubation and IV therapy with epinephrine. Atropine is also used if the ventricular rate is slow. Treatment is directed toward correction of the underlying cause.

Sudden Cardiac Death.
The term *sudden cardiac death (SCD)* refers to death from a cardiac cause. The majority of SCDs result from ventricular dysrhythmias, specifically ventricular tachycardia or fibrillation. (SCD is discussed further in Chapter 36.)

Prodysrhythmia.
Antidysrhythmia drugs may cause life-threatening dysrhythmias similar to those for which they are administered. This concept is termed *prodysrhythmia*. Patients who have severe left ventricular dysfunction are the most susceptible to prodysrhythmias. Digoxin and classes IA, IC, and III antidysrhythmia drugs can cause a prodysrhythmic response (Table 38-8). The first several days of drug therapy are period in which the risk for developing prodysrhythmias is highest. For this reason, many oral antidysrhythmia drug regimens are initiated in a monitored hospital setting.

DRUG THERAPY

Table 38-8 Antidysrhythmia Drugs: Classifications, Actions, and Effects on ECG

CLASSIFICATION	ACTIONS	EFFECTS ON ECG
Class I: sodium channel blockers	Decrease conduction velocity in the atria, ventricles, and His-Purkinje system	—
Class IA Disopyramide (Rythmodan) Procainamide (Procan) Quinidine	Delay repolarization	Widened QRS and prolonged QT interval
Class IB Lidocaine (Xylocaine) Mexiletine Phenytoin (Dilantin)	Accelerate repolarization	Little or none
Class IC Flecainide (Tambocor) Propafenone (Rythmol)	Decrease impulse conduction	Pronounced prodysrhythmic actions, widened QRS, prolonged QT interval
Class II: β-adrenergic blockers Atenolol (Tenormin) Carvedilol Esmolol (Brevibloc) Metoprolol (Lopressor) Sotalol*	Decrease automaticity of the SA node; decrease conduction velocity in AV node; reduce atrial and ventricular contractility	Bradycardia, prolonged PR interval, AV block
Class III: potassium channel blockers Amiodarone (Cordarone) Bretylium Ibutilide (Corvert) Sotalol*	Delay repolarization, which results in prolonged duration of action potential and prolonged refractory period	Prolonged PR and QT intervals, widened QRS, bradycardia
Class IV: calcium channel blockers Diltiazem (Cardizem) Verapamil	Decrease automaticity of SA node; delay AV node conduction; reduce myocardial contractility	Bradycardia, prolonged PR interval, AV block
Other antidysrhythmia drugs Adenosine (Adenocard) Digoxin (Lanoxin) Magnesium	Decrease conduction through AV node; reduce automaticity of SA node	Prolonged PR interval, AV block

*Sotalol has both class II and class III properties.
AV, atrioventricular; *ECG*, electrocardiogram; *SA*, sinoatrial.

Antidysrhythmia Drugs

An increasing number of antidysrhythmia drugs have become available. Table 38-8 categorizes major drug classes by primary effects on the cardiac cells.

Defibrillation

Defibrillation is the most effective method of terminating ventricular fibrillation and pulseless VT. It is most effective when the myocardial cells are not anoxic or acidotic, making rapid defibrillation crucial for a successful patient outcome. Defibrillation is accomplished by the passage of a DC electric shock through the heart that is sufficient to depolarize the cells of the myocardium. The intent is that subsequent repolarization of myocardial cells allows the SA node to resume the role of pacemaker (AHA, 2010).

Defibrillators deliver energy by means of a monophasic or biphasic waveform. Monophasic defibrillators deliver energy in one direction, and biphasic defibrillators deliver energy in two directions (Figure 38-20). Research has shown that biphasic defibrillators deliver successful shocks at lower energies and with fewer postshock ECG abnormalities than monophasic defibrillators (AHA, 2010).

The output of a defibrillator is measured in joules, or watts per second. The recommended energy for initial shocks in defibrillation depends on the type of defibrillator. Biphasic defibrillators deliver all shocks of 150 to 200 joules (J). Recommendations for monophasic defibrillators include an initial shock at 360 J. After the initial shock, CPR should be started immediately, beginning with chest compressions.

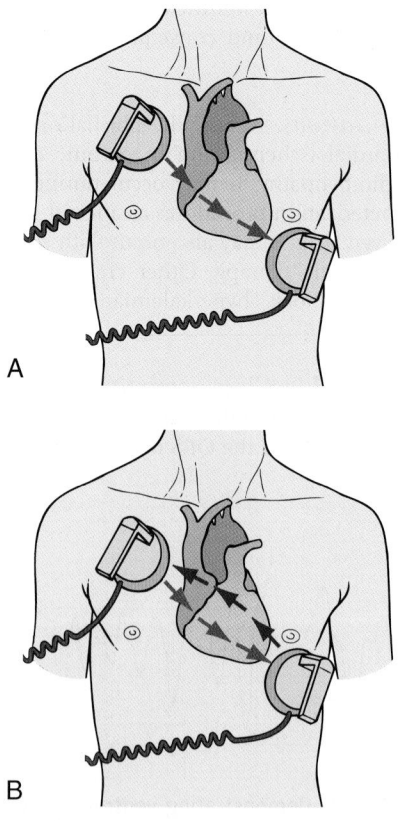

Figure 38-20 Paddle placement and current flow in monophasic defibrillation **(A)** and biphasic defibrillation **(B)**.

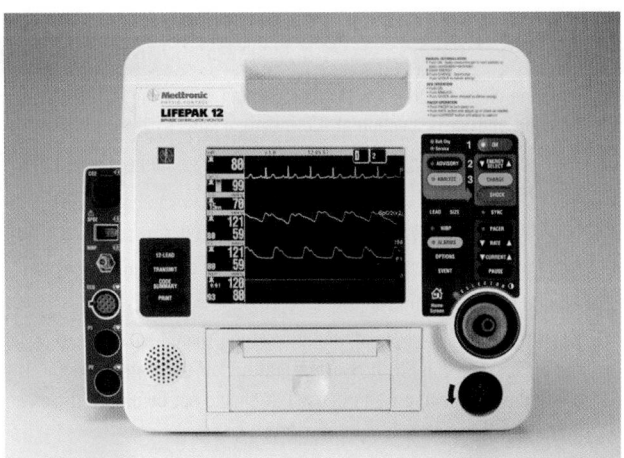

Figure 38-21 The LifePak device contains a monitor, a defibrillator, and a transcutaneous pacemaker.

Source: Courtesy Medtronic Physio-Control, Redmond, Washington.

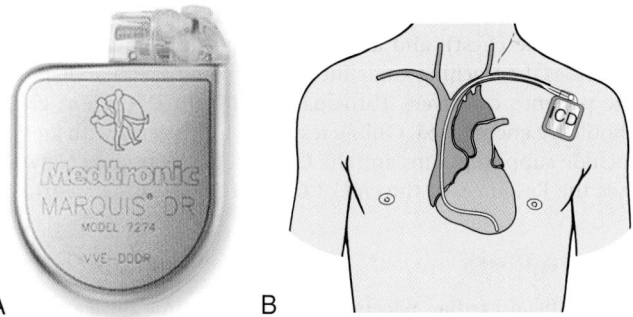

A   B

Figure 38-22 A, The implantable cardioverter–defibrillator (ICD) pulse generator from Medtronic, Inc. **B,** Diagram of ICD placement. The ICD is placed in a subcutaneous pocket over the pectoralis muscle. A single-lead system is placed transvenously from the pulse generator to the endocardium. The single lead detects dysrhythmias and delivers an electrical shock to the heart muscle.

Source: **A,** Courtesy Medtronic, Inc., Minneapolis, Minnesota.

Rapid defibrillation can be performed with a manual or automatic device (Figure 38-21). Manual defibrillators require health care providers to interpret cardiac rhythms, determine the need for a shock, and deliver a shock. **Automatic external defibrillators (AEDs)** are defibrillators that have rhythm detection capability and the ability to advise the operator to deliver a shock with hands-free defibrillator pads. Proficiency in use of the AED is incorporated in the basic life support course for health care providers (AHA, 2010). The nurse should be familiar with the operation of the type of defibrillator that is used in the clinical setting and must be certified to use this equipment. The Heart and Stroke Foundation of Ontario has implemented a public access defibrillation (PAD) program in communities in order to enhance the provision of early advanced cardiac care to save lives (Heart and Stroke Foundation, 2012). Through this program, AEDs are placed in public places such as arenas, pools, and community centres.

Upon defibrillation, the operator calls, "All clear" and looks to see that personnel are not touching the patient or the bed at the time of defibrillator discharge. It is essential that the operator ensures that all personnel are clear before the defibrillator is discharged.

Synchronized Cardioversion.
Synchronized cardioversion is the therapy of choice for the patient with hemodynamically unstable ventricular or supraventricular tachydysrhythmias. A synchronized circuit in the defibrillator is used to deliver a countershock that is programmed to occur on the R wave of the QRS complex. The synchronizer switch must be turned on when cardioversion is planned.

The procedure for synchronized cardioversion is the same as for defibrillation, with the following exceptions. If synchronized cardioversion is performed on a nonemergency basis (i.e., the patient is awake and hemodynamically stable), the patient is sedated (e.g., IV midazolam) before the procedure. Strict attention to maintenance of a patent airway is important in this situation. When a patient with supraventricular tachycardia or VT with a pulse is hemodynamically unstable, synchronized cardioversion is performed as quickly as possible. In addition, the energy needed for synchronized cardioversion is generally less

than the energy needed for defibrillation. Energy levels are started at 50 J on a monophasic defibrillator and increased (e.g., 100 J, 200 J) if needed.

Implantable Cardioverter–Defibrillator.
The implantable cardioverter–defibrillator (ICD) is important technology for patients who (a) have survived SCD, (b) have spontaneous sustained VT, (c) demonstrate syncope with inducible ventricular tachycardia or fibrillation during EPS, and (d) are at high risk for future life-threatening dysrhythmias (e.g., have cardiomyopathy). Use of the ICD has significantly decreased cardiac mortality rates among such patients and has added a new dimension to the management of life-threatening dysrhythmias and the prevention of SCD (AHA, 2010).

The ICD consists of a lead system placed via a subclavian vein to the endocardium. A battery-powered pulse generator is implanted subcutaneously, usually over the pectoral muscle on the patient's nondominant side. The pulse generator is similar in size to a cardiac pacemaker. The newest systems are single-lead systems instead of earlier multilead or patch systems (Figure 38-22). The ICD sensing system monitors the HR and the rhythm and identifies ventricular tachycardia or ventricular fibrillation. Approximately 25 sec after the sensing system detects a lethal dysrhythmia, the defibrillating mechanism delivers a 25-J or milder shock to the patient's heart. If the first shock is unsuccessful, the generator recycles and can continue to deliver shocks.

In addition to defibrillation capabilities, ICDs are equipped with antitachycardia and antibradycardia pacemakers. These sophisticated devices use dysrhythmia algorithms that detect dysrhythmias and determine the appropriate programmed response. These devices can initiate overdrive pacing of supraventricular and ventricular tachycardias, sparing the patient painful defibrillator shocks. They also provide backup pacing for bradydysrhythmias that may occur after defibrillation discharges. Preprocedure and postprocedure nursing care of patients undergoing ICD placement is similar to the care of patients undergoing permanent pacemaker implantation (see pp. 968 to 969).

Education of patients who receive an ICD is of extreme importance. Patients experience a variety of emotions, including fear of body image change, fear of recurrent dysrhythmias, expectation of pain with ICD discharge (described as a feeling of a blow to the chest), and anxiety about going home. Table 38-9 describes the teaching guidelines for the patient with an ICD and the patient's caregivers. Participation in an ICD support group should be encouraged. Online resources for patients with an ICD include support groups and the Cardiac Arrest Survivor Network (see the Resources at the end of Chapter 36.)

Pacemakers

The artificial **cardiac pacemaker** is an electronic device used to pace the heart when the normal conduction pathway is damaged or diseased. The basic pacing circuit consists of a power source (battery-powered pulse generator), one or more conducting leads (pacing leads), and the myocardium. The electrical signal (stimulus) travels from the pacemaker, through the leads, to the wall of the myocardium. The myocardium is "captured" and stimulated to contract (Figure 38-23).

Advances in technology have been applied extensively to pacemakers. This has resulted in sophisticated, noninvasive, programmable single- and dual-chambered pacemakers with specialized circuits. The newer pacemakers are more physiologically accurate, pacing the atrium and one or both of the ventricles (Aehlert, 2011). Pacemakers were initially indicated for symptomatic bradydysrhythmias. However, advances now include pacing for antitachycardia and overdrive pacing. Antitachycardia pacing involves the delivery of a stimulus to the ventricle to terminate tachydysrhythmias (e.g., VT). Overdrive pacing involves pacing the atrium at rates of 200 to 500 impulses per minute in an attempt to terminate atrial tachycardias (e.g., atrial flutter, atrial fibrillation). Multiple other indications for pacemakers have evolved. A permanent pacemaker is one that is implanted totally within the body (Figure 38-24). The permanent pacemaker power source is implanted subcutaneously, usually over the pectoral muscle on the patient's nondominant side. It is attached to pacing leads, which are threaded transvenously to the right atrium and one or both ventricles. Indications for insertion of permanent pacemakers are listed in Table 38-10.

A specialized type of cardiac pacing has been developed for the management of HF. More than 50% of patients with HF have intraventricular conduction delays that cause abnormal ventricular activation and contraction and subsequent asynchrony between the right and left ventricles. This can result in reduced systolic function, pump inefficiency, and worsened HF. Cardiac

PATIENT & CAREGIVER TEACHING GUIDE

Table 38-9 Implantable Cardioverter–Defibrillator

1. Maintain close follow-up with the physician for testing of ICD function and for inspection of ICD insertion site.

2. Watch for signs of infection at incision site (e.g., redness, swelling, drainage).

3. Keep the incision dry for 1 wk after ICD insertion.

4. Avoid lifting the operative-side arm above the shoulder for 1 wk.

5. Avoid direct blows to ICD site.

6. When travelling by airplane, airport security should be informed of the presence of the ICD because it may set off the metal detector. If a handheld screening wand is used, it should not be placed directly over the ICD.

7. When the ICD fires:
   - The patient should lie down.
   - If the patient loses consciousness or if there is repetitive firing, 911 should be called.
   - If the patient is feeling well and there is repetitive firing, the patient should contact the physician's office for ICD interrogation, including battery checks and safety and diagnostic checks.

8. Routine ICD check with interrogator–programmer device is needed every 2 to 3 months.

9. Medical alert identification (e.g., bracelet) should be worn at all times.

10. An information card about the ICD should be easily accessible in the patient's wallet.

11. Family members should learn CPR.

12. The nurse should assist the patient with the development of positive coping strategies to reduce stress.

13. Avoid large electromagnetic and vibratory forces because they may turn off the device.

14. In general, patients should not drive until cleared by the physician. The approval to drive is based on the presence of dysrhythmias, the frequency of ICD firings, the patient's overall health, and provincial laws regarding drivers with ICDs.

CPR, cardiopulmonary resuscitation; *ICD,* implantable cardioverter–defibrillator.

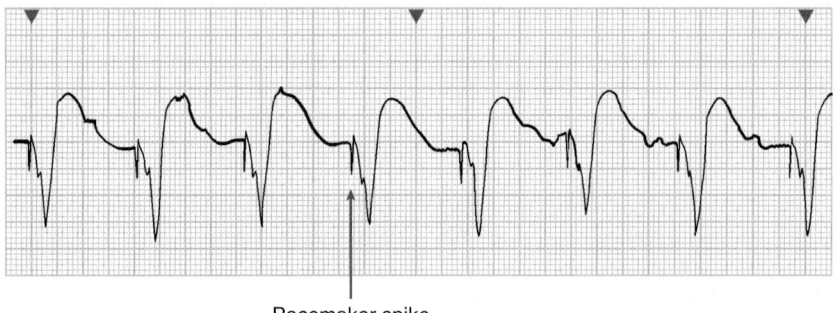

Pacemaker spike

Figure 38-23 ECG demonstrating ventricular capture (depolarization) secondary to signal (pacemaker spike) from pacemaker lead in the right ventricle.

Source: Bucher, L., & Melander, S. (1999). *Critical care nursing.* Philadelphia: W. B. Saunders.

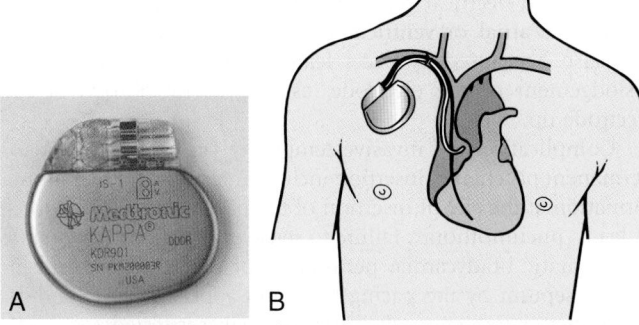

Figure 38-24 A, Dual-chamber rate-responsive pacemaker from Medtronic, Inc., designed to treat patients with chronic heart problems in which the heart beats too slowly to adequately support the body's circulation needs. **B,** Diagram of pacemaker placement. Pacing leads in both the atrium and the ventricle enable a dual-chamber pacemaker to sense rhythm and pace in both heart chambers.

Source: **A,** Courtesy Medtronic, Inc., Minneapolis, Minnesota.

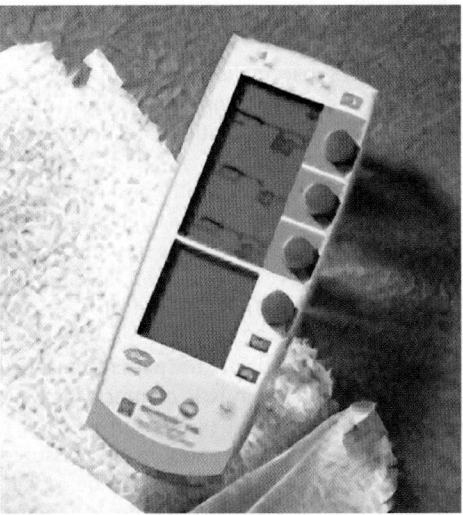

Figure 38-25 Temporary external, dual-chamber demand pacemaker.

Source: Courtesy Medtronic, Inc., Minneapolis, Minnesota.

Table 38-10 Indications for Permanent Pacemaker Therapy
• Chronic atrial fibrillation with slow ventricular response
• Fibrosis or sclerotic changes of cardiac conduction system
• Hypersensitive carotid sinus syndrome
• Sick sinus syndrome
• Sinus node dysfunction
• Tachydysrhythmias
• Third-degree AV block

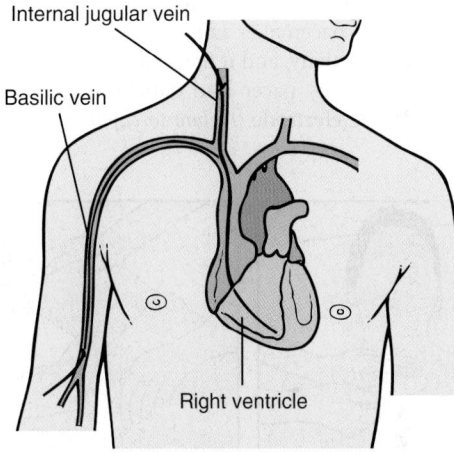

Figure 38-26 Diagram of temporary transvenous pacemaker catheter insertion. A single lead is positioned in the right ventricle.

resynchronization therapy (CRT) is a pacing technique that resynchronizes the cardiac cycle by pacing both ventricles, thus promoting improvement in ventricular function. Several devices are available in which cardiac resynchronization therapy is combined with an ICD for maximum therapy. (HF is discussed in Chapter 37.)

Temporary Pacemaker. A temporary pacemaker is one whose the power source is outside the body (Figure 38-25). There are three types of temporary pacemakers: transvenous, epicardial, and transcutaneous. Indications for temporary pacing are listed in Table 38-11.

A transvenous pacemaker consists of a lead or leads that are threaded transvenously to the right atrium, the right ventricle, or both and attached to the external power source (Figure 38-26). Most temporary transvenous pacemakers are inserted in critical care units in emergency situations. They are used until a permanent pacemaker can be inserted or the underlying cause of the dysrhythmia has been resolved.

To achieve epicardial pacing, an atrial pacing lead and a ventricular pacing lead are attached to the epicardium during heart surgery. The leads are passed through the chest wall and attached to the external power source. Epicardial pacing leads are placed prophylactically in case any bradydysrhythmias or tachydysrhythmias occur postoperatively.

Table 38-11 Indications for Temporary Pacing
• Maintenance of adequate HR and rhythm during special circumstances such as surgery and postoperative recovery, cardiac catheterization, or coronary angioplasty; during drug therapy that may cause bradycardia; and before implantation of a permanent pacemaker
• As prophylaxis after open heart surgery
• Acute anterior MI with second- or third-degree AV block or bundle-branch block
• Acute inferior MI with symptomatic bradycardia and AV block
• Termination of AV nodal re-entry or reciprocating tachycardia associated with WPW syndrome, atrial flutter, or ventricular tachycardia
• Suppression of ectopic atrial or ventricular rhythm
• EPS to evaluate patient with bradydysrhythmias and tachydysrhythmias

AV, atrioventricular; *EPS,* electrophysiology study; *MI,* myocardial infarction; *WPW,* Wolff-Parkinson-White.

A transcutaneous pacemaker (TCP) is used to maintain adequate HR and rhythm in an emergency situation. Placement of the transcutaneous pacemaker is a noninvasive procedure, and this pacemaker is used temporarily until a transvenous pacemaker can be inserted or until more definitive therapy is available.

The TCP consists of a power source and a rate- and voltage-control device that is attached to two large, multifunction electrode pads. One pad is positioned on the anterior part of the chest, usually at the V_2 or V_5 lead position, and the other pad is placed on the back between the spine and the left scapula at the level of the heart (Figure 38-27).

Before TCP therapy is initiated, the patient must be told what to expect. The uncomfortable muscle contractions that the pacemaker creates when the current passes through the chest wall should be explained. The patient should be reassured that the therapy is temporary and that the TCP will be replaced with a transvenous pacemaker as soon as possible. Whenever possible, an analgesic, sedative, or both should be provided.

Patient Monitoring.

Patients with temporary or permanent pacemakers are monitored by ECG to evaluate the status of the pacemaker. Pacemaker malfunction is manifested primarily by a failure to sense or a failure to capture. *Failure to sense* is the situation in which the pacemaker fails to recognize spontaneous atrial or ventricular activity, and it fires inappropriately. Failure to sense may be caused by pacer lead damage, battery failure, or dislodgement of the electrode. *Failure to capture* is the situation in which the electrical charge to the myocardium is insufficient to produce atrial or ventricular contraction. Failure to capture may also be caused by pacer lead damage, battery failure, or dislodgement of the electrode, as well as by fibrosis at the electrode tip.

Complications of invasive temporary (i.e., transvenous) or permanent pacemaker insertion include infection and hematoma formation at the site of insertion of the pacemaker power source or leads; pneumothorax; failure to sense or capture with possible symptomatic bradycardia; perforation of the atrial or the ventricular septum by the pacing lead; and appearance of "end-of-life" battery parameters when the pacemaker is tested.

Several measures are taken to prevent or assess for complications, including prophylactic IV antibiotic therapy before and after insertion, postinsertion chest radiographic study to check lead placement and to rule out the presence of a pneumothorax; careful observation of insertion site; and continuous ECG monitoring of the patient's rhythm. After pacemaker insertion, the patient is permitted out of bed once the HR and rhythm are stable. Arm and shoulder activity is limited to prevent dislodgement of the newly implanted pacing leads. The nurse observes the insertion site for signs of bleeding and to check that the incision is intact. Any temperature elevation should be noted, and pain at the insertion site should be treated. Most patients are discharged the next day if the HR and rhythm are stable.

The nurse must provide patient teaching in addition to observing for complications after pacemaker insertion. The patient with a newly implanted pacemaker may have questions about activity restrictions and concerns about body image after the procedure. The goal of pacemaker therapy should be to enhance physiological functioning and the quality of life. This should be emphasized to the patient, and the nurse should give specific advice about activity restrictions. Patient and caregiver teaching for the patient with a pacemaker is outlined in Table 38-12.

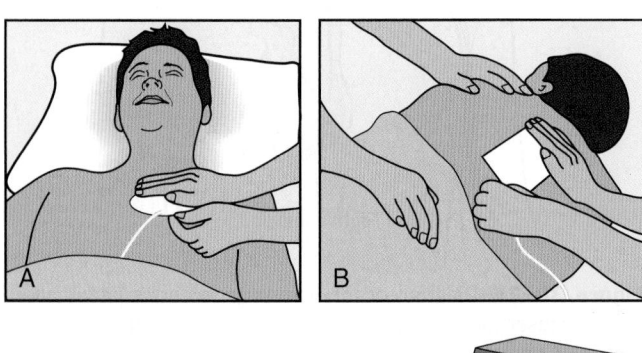

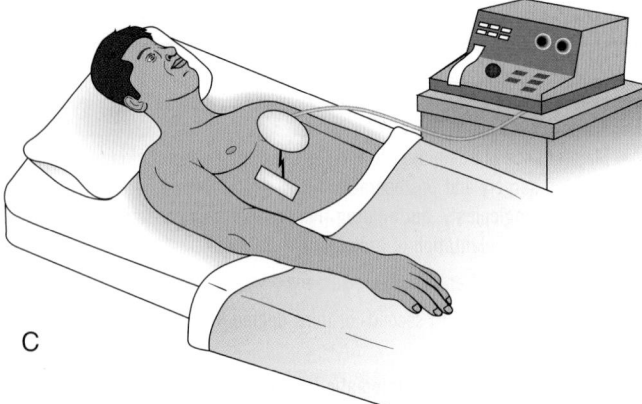

Figure 38-27 Diagram of placement of transcutaneous pacemaker. Pacing electrodes are placed on the patient's anterior (**A**) and posterior (**B**) chest walls and attached to an external pacing unit (**C**).

Sources: **A** and **B** from Craig, K. (2005). How to provide transcutaneous pacing. *Nursing, 35,* 10; **C** from Woods, S. L., Sivarajan Froelicher, E. S., Underhill Motzer, S., & Bridges, E. J. (Eds.). [2005]. *Cardiac nursing* (5th ed.). Philadelphia: Lippincott, Williams & Wilkins.

PATIENT & CAREGIVER TEACHING GUIDE

Table 38-12 Pacemaker

1. Maintain follow-up care plan with a physician to check the pacemaker site and begin regular pacemaker function checks with interrogator or programmer device.
2. Watch for signs of infection at incision site: redness, swelling, or drainage.
3. Keep the incision dry for 1 wk after pacemaker implantation.
4. Avoid lifting operative-side arm above shoulder level for 1 wk.
5. Avoid direct blows to generator site.
6. Avoid close proximity to high-output electrical generators or to large magnets such as an MRI scanner. These devices can reprogram a pacemaker.
7. Microwave ovens are safe to use and do not threaten pacemaker function.
8. Travel without restrictions is allowed. The small metal case of an implanted pacemaker rarely sets off an airport security alarm.
9. The patient should be taught how to take the pulse.
10. Carry a pacemaker information card at all times.
11. Watch for return of preimplantation symptoms (i.e., chest pain, diaphoresis, dizziness).

MRI, magnetic resonance imaging.

After discharge, pacemaker function should be checked regularly during outpatient visits to a pacemaker interrogator or programmer or by home monitoring using telephone transmitter devices. Another method to evaluate pacemaker performance is noninvasive program stimulation, which is done on an outpatient basis in the electrophysiology laboratory.

Radiofrequency Catheter Ablation Therapy

Radiofrequency catheter ablation therapy is a relatively new development in the area of antidysrhythmia therapy. Radiofrequency energy (produced by a low-voltage, high-frequency form of electrical energy) is used to "burn" or ablate areas of the conduction system as definitive treatment of tachydysrhythmias.

Ablation therapy is performed after EPS has identified the source of the dysrhythmia. An electrode-tipped ablation catheter is used to ablate accessory pathways or ectopic sites in the atria, the AV node, and the ventricles. Catheter ablation is considered the nonpharmacological treatment of choice for AV nodal re-entrant tachycardia or for re-entrant tachycardia related to accessory bypass tracts, and to control the ventricular response of certain tachydysrhythmias. In some cases of uncontrolled ventricular response in atrial fibrillation or of atrial flutter that is unresponsive to medical therapy, the AV node or bundle of His may be ablated completely. If this is done, the patient must have a permanent pacemaker inserted at the same time. The ablation procedure is a successful therapy with a low complication rate. Care of the patient undergoing ablation therapy is similar to that of a patient undergoing cardiac catheterization (see Chapter 34).

Electrocardiographic Changes Associated With Acute Coronary Syndrome

The 12-lead ECG is the primary diagnostic tool used to evaluate patients receiving care for acute coronary syndrome (ACS). Many treatment decisions are directed by the ECG changes that occur with ACS. These definitive changes are in response to ischemia, injury, or infarction of myocardial cells and are detected in the leads that face the area of involvement (Figure 38-28). Reciprocal (opposite) ECG changes are often detected in the leads facing opposite the area involved in ACS. In addition, the pattern of ECG changes provides information on the coronary artery involved in ACS (Table 38-13).

Ischemia

Typical ECG changes that are seen in myocardial ischemia include ST-segment depression, T-wave inversion, or both (Figure 38-29, A). ST-segment depression is significant if it is at least 1 mm (one small box) below the isoelectric line (see Figure 38-5). The isoelectric line is flat and represents the normal times in the cardiac cycle when the ECG is not recording any electrical activity in the heart. These times are as follows: (a) from the end of the P wave to the start of the QRS complex, (b) the entire ST segment, and (c) from the end of the T wave to the start of the next P wave (see Figure 38-9). ST-segment depression, T-wave inversion, or both occur in response to the electrical disturbance in the myocardial cells that is caused by an inadequate supply of blood and oxygen.

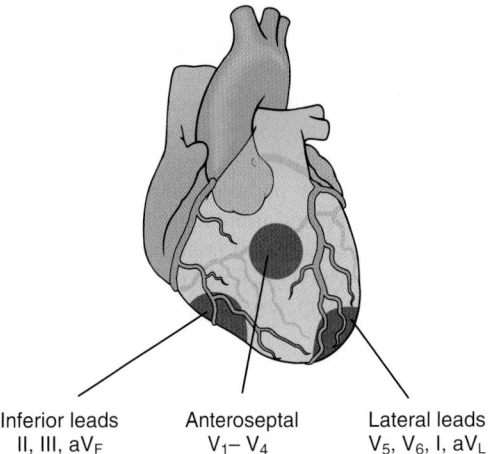

| Inferior leads | Anteroseptal | Lateral leads |
| II, III, aV$_F$ | V$_1$– V$_4$ | V$_5$, V$_6$, I, aV$_L$ |

Figure 38-28 Diagram showing where leads detect ECG changes. Definitive ECG changes occur in leads that face the area of ischemia, injury, or infarction. Reciprocal changes may occur in leads facing opposite the area of ischemia, injury, or infarction.

Table 38-13 ECG Evidence and Associated Coronary Artery in Acute Coronary Syndrome

| AREA OF INVOLVEMENT OF LEFT VENTRICLE | ECG EVIDENCE | | ASSOCIATED CORONARY ARTERY |
	LEADS FACING AREA	LEADS OPPOSITE AREA	
Septal wall	V$_1$, V$_2$	II, III, aV$_F$	Left anterior descending
Anterior wall	V$_2$, V$_3$, V$_4$	II, III, aV$_F$	Left anterior descending
Lateral wall, low	V$_5$, V$_6$	II, III, aV$_F$	Left anterior descending or circumflex
Lateral wall, high	I, aV$_L$	II, III, aV$_F$	Circumflex
Inferior wall	II, III, aV$_F$	I, aV$_L$, V$_5$, V$_6$	Right coronary artery

Once the cause of the disturbance is treated (adequate blood flow is restored), the ECG changes resolve, and the ECG returns to the patient's baseline. (See Chapter 36 for a complete discussion of ACS.)

Injury and Infarction

Myocardial injury represents a stage of worsening ischemia that is potentially reversible but may evolve to infarction (necrosis) of myocardial cells. The typical ECG change seen during injury is ST-segment elevation. ST-segment elevation is significant if it is at least 1 mm above the isoelectric line (see Fig. 38-29, B). If treatment is prompt and effective, it is possible to restore oxygen to the myocardium and avoid infarction. This is confirmed by the absence of serum cardiac markers. If serum cardiac markers are present, infarction has occurred and is referred to as an *ST-segment–elevation myocardial infarction* (STEMI).

In addition to ST-segment elevation, a pathological Q wave may be seen on the ECG with infarction (see Figure 38-29, *C*). A physiological Q wave is the first negative deflection (wave) after the P wave (see Figure 38-9). It is normally very small and narrow (<0.04 sec in duration). A pathological Q wave that develops during infarction is deep and more than 0.03 sec in duration. If it does appear, it indicates that at least half the thickness of the heart wall is involved, which is referred to as a *Q-wave MI* (Aehlert, 2011). The pathological Q wave may be present on the ECG indefinitely.

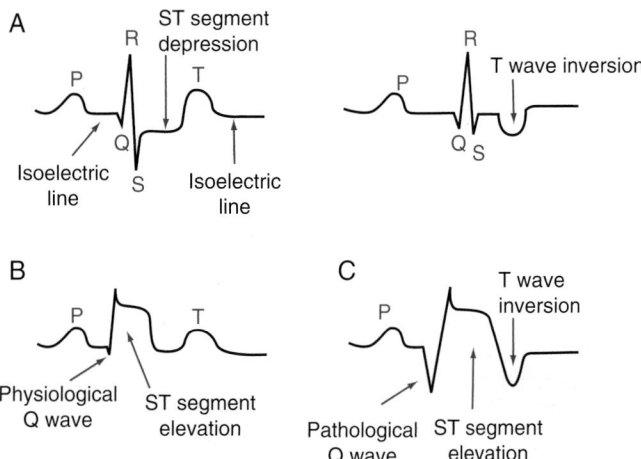

Figure 38-29 Diagrams of changes in ST segment, T wave, and Q wave in association with myocardial ischemia **(A)**, injury **(B)**, and infarction **(C)**.

T-wave inversion related to infarction occurs within hours after an infarction and may persist for months. The ECG changes seen in injury and infarction reflect electrical disturbances in the myocardial cells that are caused by a prolonged lack of blood and oxygen leading to necrosis (Figure 38-30).

Patient Monitoring

Monitoring guidelines for patients with suspected ACS include continuous, multilead ECG and ST-segment monitoring (Drew et al., 2004). The leads selected for monitoring should minimally include the leads that reflect the area of ischemia, injury, or infarction.

Syncope

Syncope—a brief lapse in consciousness accompanied by a loss in postural tone (fainting)—is a common diagnosis in the emergency department and the hospital. The causes of syncope can be categorized as cardiovascular or noncardiovascular. The most common cardiovascular causes of syncope include (a) neurocardiogenic syncope or "vasovagal" syncope (e.g., carotid sinus sensitivity) and (b) primary cardiac dysrhythmias (e.g., tachycardias, bradycardias). Others causes can be related to prosthetic valve malfunction, pulmonary emboli, aortic dissection, and hypertrophic cardiomyopathy. Noncardiovascular causes are varied and can include hypoglycemia, hysteria, unwitnessed seizure, and vertebrobasilar transient ischemic attack (Woods et al., 2005).

A diagnostic workup for a patient with syncope from a suspected cardiac cause begins with ruling out structural or ischemic heart disease, or both. This is done with echocardiography and stress testing. In older patients, who are more likely to have ischemic and structural heart disease, EPS is used to diagnose atrial and

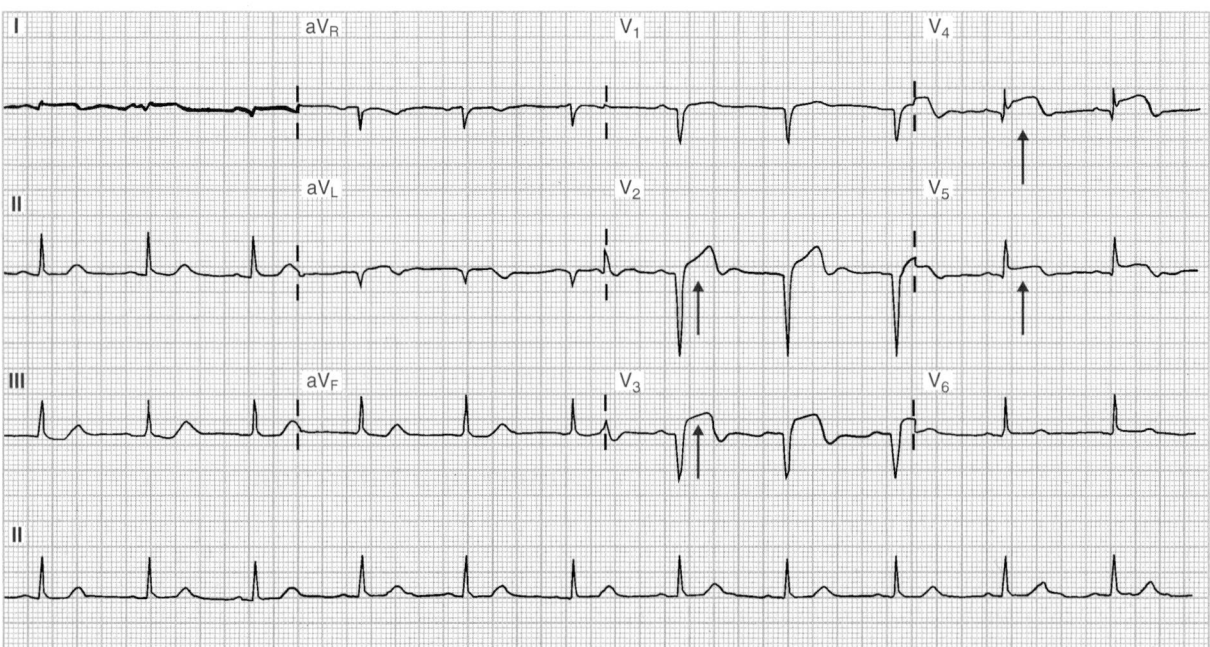

Figure 38-30 ECG findings with anterolateral wall myocardial infarction. Note the pathological Q waves in leads V_1, V_2, V_3, I, and aV_L and the ST-segment elevation in leads V_2 to V_5 *(arrows)*.

ventricular tachydysrhythmias, as well as conduction system disease causing bradydysrhythmias, all of which can cause syncope. These problems can be treated with antidysrhythmia drug therapy, pacemakers, ICDs, catheter ablation therapy, or a combination.

In patients without structural heart disease or in whom the results of EPS testing are not diagnostic, head-upright tilt-table testing may be performed. Normally, an upright position results in gravity displacing 300 to 800 mL of blood to the lower extremities. Specialized nerve fibres called *mechanoreceptors* are located throughout the vascular system. These receptors respond to the increased blood volume by initiating a reflex increase in sympathetic stimulation and decrease in parasympathetic output. The end results are slight increases in HR and diastolic BP, and a slight decrease in systolic BP.

In neurocardiogenic syncope, the increase in venous pooling that occurs in the upright position reduces venous return to the heart. This results in a sudden, compensatory increase in ventricular contraction. This is misinterpreted by the brain as a hypertensive state, and sympathetic stimulation is consequently withdrawn. This produces a paradoxical vasodilation and bradycardia (vasovagal response). The end results are bradycardia, hypotension, cerebral hypoperfusion, and syncope.

In the head-upright tilt-table test, the patient is placed supine on a table and supported by belts across the torso and the feet. Baseline ECG, BP, and HR are obtained in the horizontal position. Next, the table is tilted 60 to 80 degrees, and the patient is maintained in this upright position for 20 to 60 min. The ECG and HR are recorded continuously, and BP is measured every 3 min throughout the test. In healthy individuals, venous pooling activates the mechanoreceptors, resulting in the normal response just described.

If the patient's BP and HR responses are abnormal and clinical symptoms are reproduced (e.g., faintness), the test result is considered positive. If after 30 min there is no response, the table is returned to the horizontal position and an intravenous infusion of low-dose isoproterenol may be started in an attempt to provoke a response. Neurocardiogenic syncope that recurs frequently and interferes with normal activities can be treated with a variety of drugs (e.g., metoprolol).

Other diagnostic tests for syncope include various recording devices. Holter monitors and event monitors are used, and are discussed in this chapter and Chapter 34. A subcutaneously implanted loop-recording device can also be used to record the ECG during presyncopal and syncopal events. The device can be interrogated after a syncopal event in order to determine the ECG rhythm at the time of the event. Patients with a cardiovascular cause of syncope have a 1-year mortality rate as high as 30% (Woods et al., 2005).

CLINICAL DECISION-MAKING EXERCISE

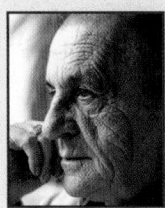

CASE STUDY:
Dysrhythmia

Source: © iStockphoto.com/Joseph Jean Rolland Dubé.

Patient Profile

Mr. Singer, a 68-year-old retired postal worker, is admitted to the cardiac care unit after cardiac arrest. Defibrillation was performed by paramedics at his home. Mr. Singer is awake and lethargic but responding appropriately.

Subjective Data

- Has had two MIs and a history of HF
- Has shortness of breath, even in a sitting position

Objective Data

Physical Examination
- Appears anxious
- BP 92/60 mm Hg, pulse 98/min, respirations 28/min
- Lungs: bilateral coarse crackles
- Heart: S3 gallop at apex

Diagnostic Studies
- ECG: frequent PVCs
- Echocardiogram: severe left ventricular dysfunction with ejection fraction (EF) of 20%
- Serum potassium level: 2.9 mmol/L

Collaborative Care

- Amiodarone (Cordarone) infusion
- Scheduled for electrophysiology study (EPS)

Discussion Questions

1. Why is Mr. Singer at risk for ventricular fibrillation?
2. Why is amiodarone used after ventricular fibrillation?
3. What methods may be used to assess the effectiveness of an antidysrhythmia drug?
4. Would Mr. Singer be a candidate for an ICD?
5. If ventricular fibrillation recurred while Mr. Singer was receiving amiodarone infusion, what other IV medications would be tried?
6. What is the significance of the serum potassium value?
7. *Priority Decision:* On the basis of these nursing diagnoses, what are the priority nursing interventions for Mr. Singer?

evolve Answers are available at **http://evolve.elsevier.com/ Canada/Lewis/medsurg**

REVIEW QUESTIONS

The number of the question corresponds to the same-numbered objective at the beginning of the chapter.

1. A patient with a stable blood pressure and no symptoms has the following ECG characteristics: atrial rate, 74 beats/min and regular; ventricular rate, 62 beats/min and irregular; P wave, normal contour; PR interval, lengthens progressively until a P wave is not conducted; QRS complex, normal contour. What would be the appropriate treatment for this rhythm?
   a. Epinephrine, 1 mg IV push
   b. Isoproterenol, IV continuous drip
   c. Immediate insertion of a temporary pacemaker
   d. Careful observation for signs of further heart block

2. The nurse is monitoring the ECG of a patient admitted with ACS. Which of the following ECG characteristics would be most suggestive of ischemia?
   a. Sinus rhythm with a pathological Q wave
   b. Sinus rhythm with an elevated ST segment
   c. Sinus rhythm with a depressed ST segment
   d. Sinus rhythm with premature atrial contractions

3. The cardiac monitor of a patient in the cardiac care unit after an acute myocardial infarction indicates ventricular bigeminy. What would be the most appropriate intervention from the following list?
   a. Performing defibrillation
   b. Treatment with intravenous amiodarone
   c. Insertion of a temporary pacemaker
   d. Continue monitoring and attempt to determine the underlying cause

4. How does defibrillation differ from cardioversion?
   a. Defibrillation requires a greater dose of electrical current.
   b. Defibrillation is synchronized to countershock during the QRS complex.
   c. Cardioversion is indicated only for treatment of atrial tachydysrhythmias.
   d. Cardioversion may be done on a nonemergency basis with sedation of the patient.

5. Which of the following discharge instructions would be appropriate in teaching a patient with a new permanent pacemaker?
   a. Take and record a daily pulse rate.
   b. Request special hand scanning at airport and other security gates.
   c. Immobilize the arm and shoulder on the side of the pacemaker insertion for 6 wk.
   d. Avoid microwave ovens because they emit radio waves that alter pacemaker function.

6. Which of the following is true when the patient has an implantable cardiac defibrillator?
   a. Antidysrhythmia drugs can be discontinued.
   b. All members of the patient's family should learn CPR.
   c. The patient should not drive until the physician approves it after the ICD has been implanted.
   d. The patient is usually relieved to have the device implanted to prevent dysrhythmias.

7. Which of the following would be essential to teach a patient about before electrophysiological monitoring?
   a. A catheter will be placed in each of the femoral arteries to allow double-catheter use.
   b. The patient will be given a general anaesthetic to prevent the awareness of "near-death" experiences.
   c. Ventricular tachycardia and ventricular fibrillation may be induced and treated during the procedure.
   d. The procedure is used to "burn" or ablate areas of the conduction system that are causing tachydysrhythmias.

ANSWERS: 1. d; 2. c; 3. d; 4. d; 5. a; 6. c; 7. d.

REFERENCES

Aehlert, B. (2011). *ECGs made easy* (4th ed.). St. Louis: Mosby.
American Heart Association. (2010). 2010 American Heart Association Guidelines for cardiopulmonary resuscitation and emergency cardiovascular care science. *Circulation, 122*(18), S639. doi:10.1161/CIR.0b013e3181fdf7aa
Canadian Cardiovascular Society. (2011). Canadian Cardiovascular Society atrial fibrillation guidelines 2010. *Canadian Journal of Cardiology, 27*(2011), 27-97. doi:10.1016/j.cjca.2010.11.003
Drew, B., Califf, R., Funk, M., Kaufman, E. S., Krucoff, M. W., Laks, M. M., …, Van Hare, G. F. (2004). Practice standards for electrocardiographic monitoring in hospital settings. *Circulation, 110,* 2721. doi:10.1161/01.CIR.0000145144.56673.59
Greenberg, M. L., & Chandrakantan, A. (2011). *Catheter ablation.* New York: eMedicine. Retrieved from *http://www.emedicine.com/med/topic2957.htm.*
Heart and Stroke Foundation. (2012). Public access defibrillation (PAD) programs. Retrieved from *http://restart.heartandstroke.ca/public-access-defibrillation-pad-programs.*
Lehne, R. (2013). *Pharmacology for nursing care* (8th ed.). St. Louis: Elsevier.
Palatnik, A. (2011). Too fast, too slow, too ugly: Dangerous dysrhythmias. *Nursing Management, 4*(2), 26-35.
Standring, S. (Ed.) (2009). *Gray's anatomy* (40th ed.). Philadelphia: Churchill Livingstone.
Steill, I., Macle, L. (2011). Canadian Cardiovascular Society Atrial Fibrillation Guidelines 2010: Management of recent-onset atrial fibrillation and flu in the emergency department. *Canadian Journal of Cardiology, 27*(1), 38-46. doi:10.1016/j.cjca.2010.11.014
Woods, S. L., Sivarajan Froelicher, E. S., Underhill Motzer, S., & Bridges, E. J. (Eds.). (2005). *Cardiac nursing* (5th ed.). Philadelphia: Lippincott, Williams & Wilkins.

RESOURCES

Resources for this chapter are listed in Chapter 36 on p. 927.

Nursing Management: Inflammatory and Structural Heart Disorders

Written by Nancy Kupper and De Ann Fisher Mitchell

Adapted by Sheila Rizza

LEARNING OBJECTIVES

1. Describe the etiology, pathophysiology, and clinical manifestations of infective endocarditis and pericarditis.
2. Discuss the collaborative care and nursing management of infective endocarditis and pericarditis.
3. Explain the importance of prophylactic antibiotic therapy in infective endocarditis.
4. Explain the etiology, clinical manifestations, collaborative care, and nursing management of myocarditis.
5. Describe the etiology, pathophysiology, and clinical manifestations of rheumatic fever and rheumatic heart disease.
6. Discuss the collaborative care and nursing management of the patient with rheumatic fever and rheumatic heart disease.
7. Identify the etiologies of congenital and acquired valvular heart diseases.
8. Discuss the pathophysiology and clinical manifestations of the various types of valvular heart problems and the diagnostic studies used in connection with them.
9. Describe the collaborative care and nursing management of the patient with valvular heart disease.
10. Describe surgical interventions used in management of the patient with valvular heart problems.
11. Describe the pathophysiology and clinical manifestations of the different types of cardiomyopathies.
12. Discuss the nursing and collaborative management of patients with different types of cardiomyopathies.

KEY TERMS

acute rheumatic fever (ARF) A complication that occurs as a delayed sequelae (usually after 2-3 wk) of group A streptococcal pharyngitis, p. 987

aortic stenosis A narrowing or stricture of the aortic valve resulting in obstruction of the flow from the left ventricle to the aorta during systole; causes left ventricular hypertrophy and increased myocardial oxygen consumption, p. 992

aortic valve regurgitation (AR) Retrograde blood flow from the ascending aorta into the left ventricle when the valve should be closed, resulting in volume overload, p. 993

Aschoff's bodies Tiny rounded or spindle-shaped nodules formed by a reaction to myocardial inflammation with accompanying swelling and fragmentation of collagen fibres, p. 987

cardiac tamponade Develops as fluid accumulates in the pericardial sac (pericardial effusion), causing an increase in intrapericardial pressure and producing compression of the heart, p. 982

cardiomyopathy (CMP) A group of diseases that directly affect the structural or functional ability of the myocardium, p. 996

dilated cardiomyopathy Characterized by a diffuse inflammation and rapid degeneration of myocardial fibres that results in ventricular dilation, impairment of systolic function, atrial enlargement, and stasis of blood in the left ventricle, p. 998

endomyocardial biopsy (EMB) A technique that involves removing several small pieces of myocardial tissue percutaneously from the right ventricle and microscopically examining the samples, p. 985

hypertrophic cardiomyopathy (HCM) Asymmetrical left ventricular hypertrophy without ventricular dilation, p. 1000

infective endocarditis (IE) An infection of the heart valves or the endocardial surface of the heart, p. 976

Janeway's lesions Flat, painless, small, red spots that may be found on the palms and the soles in patients with infective endocarditis, p. 978

mitral valve prolapse (MVP) A structural abnormality of the mitral valve leaflets and the papillary muscles or chordae that allows the leaflets to prolapse, or buckle, back into the left atrium during ventricular systole, p. 991

myocarditis A focal or diffuse inflammation of the myocardium, p. 985

Osler's nodes Painful, tender, red or purple, pea-size lesions that may be found on the fingertips or the toes in patients with infective endocarditis and usually last only 1 or 2 days, p. 978

pericardial effusion An accumulation of excess fluid in the pericardial space, p. 982

pericardial friction rub A scratching, grating, high-pitched sound believed to arise from friction between the roughened pericardial and the epicardial surfaces, p. 982

pericardiocentesis Procedure in which a 16- to 18-gauge needle is inserted into the pericardial space to remove fluid for analysis and to relieve cardiac pressure, p. 984

pericarditis A condition caused by inflammation of the pericardial sac, p. 981

regurgitation Incomplete closure of the valve leaflets results in the backward flow of blood, p. 990

rheumatic fever An inflammatory disease that may affect several connective tissues of the body, especially those of the heart, the brain, the joints, or the skin; potentially involves all layers of the heart (endocardium, myocardium, and pericardium), p. 985

rheumatic heart disease The resulting damage to the heart muscle and heart valves from rheumatic fever; a chronic condition characterized by scarring and deformity of the heart valves, p. 987

ELECTRONIC RESOURCES

Supplemental content related to Chapter 39 can be found . . .

Evolve Web Site ⊖volve

http://evolve.elsevier.com/Canada/Lewis/medsurg
- Answer Guidelines for Case Study on p. 1002
- Audio Clip: Pericardial Friction Rub
- Clinical Reference: Laboratory Values

- Customizable Nursing Care Plan: Valvular Heart Disease
- Electronic Calculators
- eNCP 39-1: Infective Endocarditis
- Examination Review Questions
- Glossary
- Interactive Case Study: Rheumatic Fever and Heart Disease
- Key Points (Printable and MP3 Download)

Inflammatory Disorders of the Heart

Infective Endocarditis

Infective endocarditis (**IE**; also known as *bacterial endocarditis*) is an infection of the heart valves or the endocardial surface of the heart. The name of this disorder has changed because it is now recognized that other organisms besides bacteria may cause the disease (Heart and Stroke Foundation of Canada [HSF], 2011a). The endocardium, the inner layer of the heart (Figure 39-1), is contiguous with the valves of the heart. Therefore, inflammation from IE affects the cardiac valves.

Before the era of antibiotics, IE was almost always fatal. The advent of penicillin therapy changed the prognosis dramatically, and mortality rates decreased appreciably.

Classification

Four different categories of IE are identified that describe the site of infection, the presence of cardiovascular devices, and how the individual acquired the infection: left-sided native valve IE, left-sided prosthetic valve IE, right-sided IE (includes intravenous [IV] drug use), and intracardiac devices (e.g., pacemaker/defibrillator wires). Acquisition of IE is identified as being community-acquired IE or health care–associated IE (nosocomial and non-nosocomial) (Habib et al., 2009; Que & Moreillon, 2011).

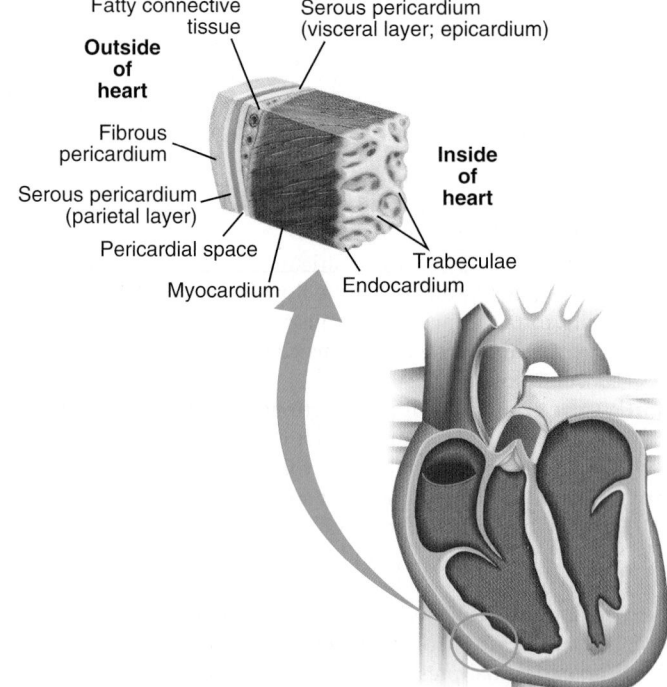

Figure 39-1 Layers of the heart.

Source: Adapted from Thibodeau, G. A., & Patton, K. T. (2010). *The human body in health and disease* (5th ed., p. 375, Figure 13-2). St Louis: Mosby.

Table 39-1 Causative Organisms Associated With Infective Endocarditis

Bacteria	
• *Bartonella quintana*	• *Staphylococcus epidermidis*
• Chlamydiae	• *Streptococcus bovis*
• Coagulase-negative staphylococci	• Streptococcus groups A, B, and C
• Enterococci	• *Streptococcus pneumoniae*
• HACEK group (*Haemophilus, Actinobacillus, Cardiobacterium, Eikenella, Kingella* species)	• *Streptococcus viridans*
	• *Tropheryma whipplei*
	Fungi
• Methicillin-resistant *Staphylococcus aureus*	• *Candida albicans*
	• *Candida parapsilosis*
• Rickettsiae	**Viruses**
• *S. aureus*	• Coxsackie B virus

Table 39-2 Predisposing Conditions for the Development of Infective Endocarditis

Cardiac Conditions

- Prior endocarditis
- Prosthetic valves
- Cardiac transplant recipients who have cardiac valvulopathy
- Rheumatic heart disease (e.g., mitral valve regurgitation)
- Unrepaired cyanotic congenital heart disease, including palliative shunts and conduits
- Repaired congenital heart defect with prosthetic material or device, surgically or through catheterization, during the first 6 months when endothelialization occurs

Noncardiac Conditions

- Intravenous drug abuse
- Nosocomial bacteremia

Procedure-Associated Risks

- Intravascular devices (e.g., hemodialysis catheters)
- Procedures listed in Table 39-3

Etiology and Pathophysiology

The most common causative organisms of IE, *Staphylococcus aureus,* oral *Streptococcus,* and Enterococci are Gram-positive bacterial organisms responsible for more than 80% of IE cases (Table 39-1). Other possible pathogens include fungi and viruses. Newly identified pathogens, which are difficult to cultivate (e.g., *Bartonella, Tropheryma whipplei*), have been found to cause IE. Resistant organisms (e.g., methicillin-resistant *S. aureus*) also cause IE and are challenging conventional antibiotic therapy (Que & Moreillon, 2011).

IE occurs when blood flow turbulence within the heart allows the causative organism to infect previously damaged valves or other endothelial surfaces. This can occur in individuals with a variety of underlying cardiac conditions. The principal risk factors for IE are prior endocarditis, prosthetic valves, acquired valvular disease, and cardiac lesions. Several noncardiac conditions and procedures also can allow large numbers of organisms to enter the bloodstream and initiate the infectious process (Tables 39-2 and 39-3).

Vegetations, the primary lesions of IE, consist of fibrin, leukocytes, platelets, and microbes that adhere to the valve surface or the endocardium (Figure 39-2). The loss of portions of these friable vegetations into the circulation results in embolization. As many as 22 to 50% of patients with IE will experience systemic embolization. These emboli arise from left-sided heart vegetation and progress to various organs (particularly the brain, the kidneys, and the spleen), where they cause infarction, and to the extremities, causing limb infarction. Right-sided heart lesions embolize to the lungs. The risk of embolization is greatest within the first few days of commencing antimicrobial therapy (Habib et al., 2009).

The infection may spread locally to cause damage to the valves or to their supporting structures. This results in dysrhythmias, valvular incompetence, and eventual invasion of the myocardium, leading to heart failure (HF), sepsis, and heart block (Figure 39-3).

Rheumatic heart disease was, at one time, the most common cause of IE; it now accounts for fewer than 20% of cases. Currently, the main contributing factors include (1) degenerative

Table 39-3 Procedures Necessitating Antibiotic Prophylaxis to Prevent Endocarditis*

Oropharyngeal

- All dental procedures likely to produce gingival or mucosal bleeding (not simple adjustment of orthodontic appliances or shedding of deciduous teeth), including professional cleaning
- Tonsillectomy or adenoidectomy

Respiratory

- Surgical procedures or biopsy involving respiratory mucosa

Integument

- Procedures on infected skin, skin structures, or musculoskeletal tissues with incision of the tissue
- Prophylactic administration of antimicrobial agents to prevent infective endocarditis in patients undergoing genitourinary or gastrointestinal procedures no longer recommended (Wilson et al., 2007)

*This table lists selected procedures and is not all-inclusive.

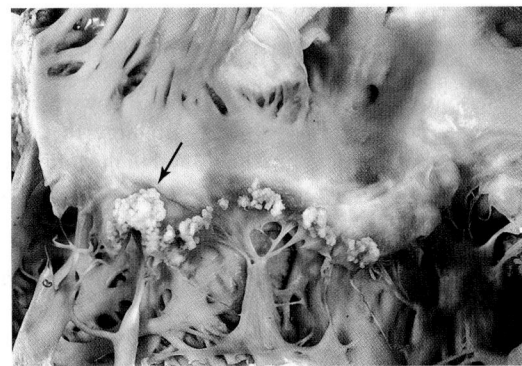

Figure 39-2 Bacterial endocarditis of the mitral valve. The valve is covered with large, irregular vegetations *(arrow).*

Source: Damjanov, I., & Linder, J. (1999). *Pathology: A color atlas.* St. Louis: Mosby.

PATHOPHYSIOLOGY MAP

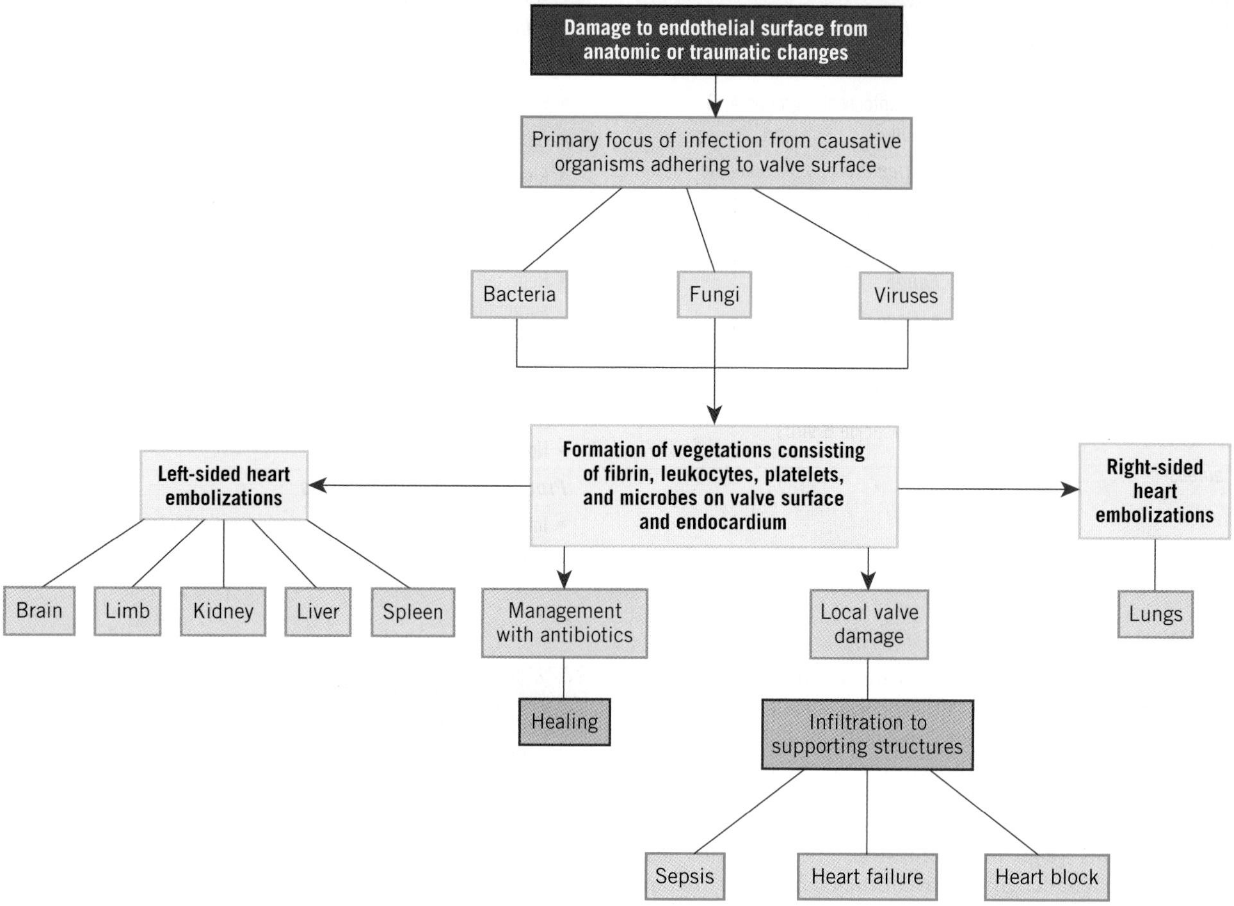

Figure 39-3 Sequence of events in infective endocarditis.

valve sclerosis; (2) IV drug use; (3) use of prosthetic valves; (4) proliferation of intravascular device placement, resulting in nosocomial infections; and (5) renal dialysis (Habib et al., 2009). Left-sided endocarditis is more common in patients with bacterial infections and underlying heart disease. The primary cause of right-sided endocarditis is IV drug use. However, the incidence of left-sided valves being affected has increased, especially with cocaine abuse. *S. aureus* is the most common causative organism in IV drug use IE.

Clinical Manifestations

The findings in IE are nonspecific and can involve multiple organ systems. Low-grade fever occurs in more than 90% of patients. Fever may absent in the elderly and in the immunocompromised patient. Other nonspecific manifestations include chills, weakness, malaise, fatigue, and anorexia. Arthralgias, myalgias, back pain, abdominal discomfort, weight loss, headache, and clubbing of fingers may occur in subacute forms of endocarditis.

Vascular manifestations of IE include splinter hemorrhages (longitudinal black streaks) that may occur in the nail beds. Petechiae may occur as a result of fragmentation and microembolization of vegetative lesions and are common in the conjunctivae, the lips, the buccal mucosa, the palate, and over the ankles,

the feet, and the antecubital and popliteal areas. **Osler's nodes** (painful, tender, red or purple, pea-size lesions) may be found on the fingertips or the toes. **Janeway's lesions** (flat, painless, small red spots) may be found on the palms and the soles. Funduscopic examination may reveal hemorrhagic retinal lesions called *Roth's spots*.

The onset of a new murmur or a changing murmur is noted in most patients with IE, with the aortic and mitral valves most commonly affected. The mitral murmur of endocarditis is generally a mid-to-late systolic regurgitant type. The aortic murmur may be early diastolic. Murmurs are often absent in tricuspid endocarditis because right-sided heart pressures are too low to be heard. HF is observed in 50 to 60% of patients with IE, more often in those with aortic valve endocarditis (29%) than in patients with mitral valve endocarditis (20%) (Habib et al., 2009).

Clinical manifestations secondary to embolization in various body organs may also be present. Embolization to the spleen may result in sharp, left upper quadrant pain and splenomegaly. Local tenderness and abdominal rigidity may be present. Embolization to the kidneys may cause pain in the flank, hematuria, and azotemia. Emboli may lodge in small peripheral blood vessels of arms and legs and may cause gangrene. Embolization to the brain may cause neurological problems such as hemiplegia, ataxia, aphasia, visual changes, and change in the level of consciousness. Pulmonary emboli may occur in right-sided endocarditis.

Diagnostic Studies

Obtaining the patient's recent health history is important in assessing IE. Inquiry should be made regarding any recent (within the past 3-6 mo) dental, urological, surgical, or gynecological procedures, including normal or abnormal obstetrical delivery. Previous history of IV drug use, previous valvular or congenital heart disease, intracardiac prosthetic device, recent cardiac catheterization, and skin, respiratory, or urinary tract infections should be documented.

Laboratory data, especially blood cultures, should also be assessed. Two blood cultures drawn 30 minutes apart will be positive in more than 90% of patients. Culture-negative endocarditis is often associated with antibiotic usage within the previous 2 weeks or caused by a pathogen not easily detected by standard culture procedures (e.g., *Bartonella* species). Negative cultures should be kept for 3 weeks if the clinical diagnosis remains endocarditis because of the possibility that a slow-growing causative organism may be detected.

A mild leukocytosis occurs in acute endocarditis (uncommon in the subacute form) with average white blood cell (WBC) counts ranging from 10 to $11 \times 10^9/L$. Erythrocyte sedimentation rate (ESR) and C-reactive protein (CRP) levels may be elevated.

Echocardiography is valuable in the diagnostic workup for a patient with IE when the blood cultures are negative or for the patient who is a surgical candidate and has an active infection. Transesophageal echocardiograms and digital imaging using two-dimensional transthoracic echocardiograms can detect vegetation, destructive lesions, and abscesses on valves (Habib et al., 2010). A chest radiograph is done to detect the presence of an enlarged heart. An electrocardiogram (ECG) may show first- or second-degree atrioventricular (AV) block because the cardiac valves lie in proximity to cardiac conductive tissue, especially the AV node. Cardiac catheterization may be used to evaluate coronary artery patency and valvular function when surgical intervention is being considered for patients with IE.

Collaborative Care

Prophylactic Treatment. Antibiotic prophylaxis is recommended for patients with specific cardiac conditions before they undergo certain dental or surgical procedures (Wilson et al., 2007). Procedures that require endocarditis prophylaxis are summarized in Table 39-4. Specific antibiotic regimens are recommended for dental procedures that require manipulation of the gingival or periapical region of the teeth or perforation of the oral mucosa and respiratory tract. Current guidelines suggest that routine activities of oral hygiene contribute to bacteremia that may result in IE (Habib et al., 2009).

Drug Therapy. Accurate identification of the infecting organism is the key to successful treatment of IE. Long-term treatment is necessary to kill dormant bacteria clustered within the valvular vegetations. Complete eradication of the organism generally takes weeks to achieve, and relapses are common. Initially, patients are hospitalized and IV antibiotic therapy is started. Table 39-5 outlines suggested antibiotic regimens for patients

COLLABORATIVE CARE

Table 39-4 Cardiac Conditions* Necessitating Antibiotic Prophylaxis to Prevent Infective Endocarditis

- Prosthetic cardiac valves
- History of endocarditis
- Surgically constructed systemic–pulmonary shunts
- Complex cyanotic congenital heart disease
- Vascular grafts (first 6 mo after implantation)
- Cardiac transplantation requiring valvulopathy

*This table lists common cardiac conditions associated with high risk for infective endocarditis and is not all-inclusive.
Source: Habib, G., Hoen, B., Tornos, P., Thuny, F., Prendergast, B., Vilacosta, I., …, Zamorano, J. (2009). Guidelines on the prevention, diagnosis, and treatment of infective endocarditis. *European Heart Journal, 30,* 2369-2413.

DRUG THERAPY

Table 39-5 Treatment of Infective Endocarditis With Outpatient Antibiotic Therapy*

CAUSATIVE AGENT	ANTIBIOTIC REGIMEN OPTIONS
Streptococcal endocarditis involving native valve	IV penicillin G (Pfizerpen) or IV or IM ceftriaxone; IV penicillin G or IV or IM ceftriaxone plus IV or IM gentamicin (Garamycin); or IV vancomycin (Vancocin)
Enterococcal endocarditis involving native or prosthetic valve	IV ampicillin (Omnipen) plus IV or IM gentamicin; or IV penicillin G plus IV or IM gentamicin; or IV vancomycin plus IV or IM gentamicin
Staphylococcal endocarditis in absence of prosthetic materials	IV vancomycin with IV gentamicin and IV rifampin
Fungal endocarditis in native or prosthetic valves	IV amphotericin B (Fungizone)

IM, intramuscular; *IV,* intravenous.
*This table lists common drug regimens but is not all-inclusive.

with IE from various causative organisms and with different clinical circumstances (Wilson et al., 2007).

Subsequent blood cultures may be performed to evaluate the effectiveness of antibiotic therapy. Blood cultures that remain positive indicate inadequate or inappropriate antibiotic administration, aortic root or myocardial abscess, or the wrong diagnosis (e.g., an infection elsewhere). Serum antibiotic drug levels are often monitored to establish therapeutic dosages. Finally, renal function is monitored when antibiotics are used that are nephrotoxic (e.g., vancomycin [Vancocin]) and/or for patients with poor kidney function.

Fungal infection and prosthetic valve endocarditis are most frequently observed in IV drug users and immunocompromised patients and respond poorly to antibiotic therapy alone. Early valve replacement followed by prolonged ($\geq$6 wk) drug therapy is recommended in these situations (Habib et al., 2009). Valve replacement has become an important adjunct procedure in the management of IE. It is used in more than 25% of cases. (Valve replacement is discussed later in this chapter.)

Fever may persist for 5 to 10 days after treatment has been started and can be treated with aspirin, acetaminophen (Tylenol), ibuprofen (Motrin), fluids, and rest. Complete bed rest is usually not indicated unless the temperature remains elevated or there are signs of HF. Endocarditis coupled with HF responds poorly to both drug therapy and valve replacement and is often life threatening.

NURSING MANAGEMENT: INFECTIVE ENDOCARDITIS

▪ Nursing Assessment

Subjective and objective data that should be obtained from a patient with IE are presented in Table 39-6. Heart sounds should be assessed together with vital signs to detect a murmur or a change in the character of a pre-existing murmur and the presence of extradiastolic sounds. Arthralgia is common, may involve multiple joints, and may be accompanied by myalgias. The patient should be assessed for joint tenderness, decreased range of motion, and muscle tenderness. The oral mucosa, conjunctivae, upper chest, and lower extremities should be examined for petechiae. A general systems assessment should be completed to facilitate recognition of hemodynamic and embolic complications.

▪ Nursing Diagnoses

Nursing diagnoses for the patient with IE may include, but are not limited to:

- Decreased cardiac output *related to* altered rhythm, valvular insufficiency, and fluid overload
- Activity intolerance *related to* generalized weakness, arthralgia, and alteration in O_2 transport secondary to valvular dysfunction
- Hyperthermia *related to* infection of cardiac tissue

Additional information on nursing diagnoses is presented in a nursing care plan (eNCP-1) for the patient with IE, available at the Evolve Web site for this chapter.

▪ Planning

The overall goals are that the patient with IE will (1) have normal or baseline cardiac function, (2) perform activities of daily living without fatigue, and (3) have knowledge of the therapeutic regimen to prevent recurrence of endocarditis.

▪ Nursing Implementation

▪ Health Promotion

The incidence of IE can be decreased by identifying individuals who are at risk for the development of endocarditis (see Tables 39-2 and 39-4). Assessment of the patient's history and an understanding of the disease process are crucial for planning and implementing appropriate health promotion strategies. Teaching

NURSING ASSESSMENT
Table 39-6 Infective Endocarditis

Subjective Data

Important Health Information

Past health history: Valvular, congenital, or syphilitic cardiac disease (including valve repair or replacement); previous endocarditis, childbirth, staphylococcal or streptococcal infections, hospital-associated bacteremia

Medications: Immunosuppressive therapy, IV drug abuse

Surgery or other treatments: Recent obstetrical or gynecological procedures; invasive techniques including catheterization, cystoscopy, intravascular procedures; recent dental or surgical procedure

Symptoms

- Exercise intolerance, generalized weakness, fatigue, malaise
- Cough, dyspnea on exertion, orthopnea
- Palpitations, night sweats
- Chest, back, or abdominal pain
- Headache, joint tenderness, muscle tenderness
- Weight gain or loss; anorexia
- Chills, diaphoresis
- Bloody urine

Objective Data

General

Fever

Integumentary

Osler's nodes on extremities; splinter hemorrhages under nail beds; Janeway's lesions on palms and soles; petechiae of skin, mucous membranes, or conjunctivae; purpura; peripheral edema, finger clubbing

Respiratory

Tachypnea, crackles

Cardiovascular

Dysrhythmias, tachycardia, new or enhanced murmurs, S3, S4, retinal hemorrhages

Possible Findings

Leukocytosis, anemia, ↑ ESR and serum cardiac enzymes; positive blood cultures; microscopic hematuria; echocardiogram showing chamber enlargement, valvular dysfunction, and vegetations; chest radiograph showing cardiomegaly and pulmonary infiltrates; ECG demonstrating ischemia and conduction defects

ECG, electrocardiogram; *ESR,* erythrocyte sedimentation rate; *IV,* intravenous; *S3,* third heart sound; *S4,* fourth heart sound.

the patient who is at risk for or has had IE helps reduce the incidence and recurrence of the disease. Teaching is crucial for the patient's understanding of and adherence to the planned treatment regimen. The patient should understand the need to avoid people with infection, especially upper respiratory infection, and to report cold, flu, and cough symptoms. The importance of avoiding excessive fatigue and the need to plan rest periods before and after activity should be carefully explained to the patient. Good oral hygiene, including daily care and regular dental visits, is also important. The patient must inform all health care providers performing dental, medical, or surgical procedures of the history of IE. The patient should understand the significance of the prescribed prophylactic antibiotic therapy before any invasive procedure. The patient with a history of IV drug use should be referred for drug treatment.

▪ Ambulatory and Home Care

A patient with IE will require nursing management (see eNCP 39-1, available on the Evolve Web site for this chapter). IE generally requires treatment with antibiotics for 4 to 6 weeks, depending on the results of blood cultures. After initial treatment in the hospital, the patient may continue treatment in the home setting if hemodynamically stable and compliant. The adequacy of the home environment in terms of in-home support and hospital access must be determined for successful management. Patients who receive outpatient IV antibiotics will require vigilant home nursing care.

Assessment findings are often nonspecific (see Table 39-6) but can help assist with the treatment plan. Fever, chronic or intermittent, is a common early sign. The patient or the caregiver needs instructions about the importance of monitoring body temperature because persistent, prolonged temperature elevations may mean that the drug therapy is ineffective. Patients with IE are at risk for life-threatening complications, such as cerebral emboli, pulmonary edema, and HF. Patients and caregivers must be taught to recognize signs and symptoms of these complications (e.g., change in mental status, dyspnea, chest pain).

The patient with IE needs adequate periods of physical and emotional rest. Bed rest may be necessary when fever is present or when there are complications (e.g., heart damage). Otherwise, the patient may ambulate and perform moderate activity. To prevent problems because of immobility, the patient should wear elastic compression stockings, perform range of motion exercises, and cough and deep breathe every 2 hours. The patient may experience anxiety and fear associated with the illness. The nurse must recognize this and implement strategies to help the patient cope with the illness.

Laboratory data should be monitored to determine the effectiveness of the antibiotic therapy. Ongoing monitoring of the patient's blood cultures is necessary to ensure eradication of the infecting organism. IV lines should be monitored for patency, and antibiotics should be given according to schedule. The patient should be monitored continuously for adverse drug reactions.

During the course of therapy in either the home or the hospital setting, management will also focus on teaching the patient about the nature of the disease and on reducing the risk of reinfection. The nurse must explain to the patient the relationship of follow-up care, good nutrition, and early treatment of common infections (e.g., colds) to maintain good health. The patient should be instructed about symptoms that may indicate recurrent infection, such as fever, fatigue, malaise, and chills. If any of these symptoms occur, the patient should be aware of the importance of notifying the health care provider. Finally, the patient must be instructed about the need for and importance of prophylactic antibiotic therapy before invasive procedures (see Table 39-3).

▪ Evaluation

Expected outcomes for the patient with IE are presented in eNCP 39-1.

Acute Pericarditis

Pericarditis, which may occur on an acute basis, is a condition caused by inflammation of the pericardial sac (the pericardium). The pericardium is composed of the inner serous membrane (visceral pericardium) that closely adheres to the epicardial surface of the heart and the outer fibrous (parietal) layer (see Figure 39-1). The pericardial space is the cavity between these two layers, and in the normal state, it contains 10 to 30 mL of serous fluid. Although the pericardium may be congenitally absent or surgically removed, it serves a useful anchoring function, provides lubrication to decrease friction during systolic and diastolic heart movements, and assists in preventing excessive dilation of the heart during diastole.

Etiology and Pathophysiology

The common causes of acute pericarditis are listed in Table 39-7. Acute pericarditis most often is idiopathic (80-85%), with a variety of suspected viral causes. The coxsackievirus B group is the most commonly identified virus. In addition to idiopathic or viral pericarditis, causes of this syndrome include bacterial infection, fungal infection, acute myocardial infarction (MI),

---

Table 39-7 Etiologies of Pericarditis

Infectious

- Viral: Coxsackievirus A and B, echovirus, adenovirus, mumps, rubella, Epstein-Barr, varicella-zoster, hepatitis B, hepatitis C, human immunodeficiency virus, cytomegalovirus
- Bacterial: Tuberculosis (most common; 4-5%); rarely other bacteria; pneumococci, staphylococci, streptococci, *Neisseria gonorrhoeae*, *Legionella pneumophila*, septicemia from Gram-negative organisms
- Fungal: *Histoplasma, Candida* species
- Infections: Toxoplasmosis, Lyme disease

Metabolic

- Uremia
- Myxedema
- Acute myocardial infarction
- Neoplasms: Lung cancer, breast cancer, leukemia, Hodgkin's disease, lymphoma
- Trauma: Thoracic surgery, pacemaker insertion, cardiac diagnostic procedures
- Radiation
- Dissecting aortic aneurysm

Hypersensitive or Autoimmune

- Delayed post–myocardial-pericardial injury
- Post–myocardial infarction (Dressler's) syndrome
- Postpericardiotomy syndrome
- Rheumatic fever
- Drug reactions: Procainamide, hydralazine [Apresoline], isoniazid, doxorubicin, and daunorubicin (often associated with cardiomyopathy)
- Rheumatological diseases: Rheumatoid arthritis, systemic lupus erythematosus, systemic sclerosis (scleroderma), ankylosing spondylitis, sarcoidosis

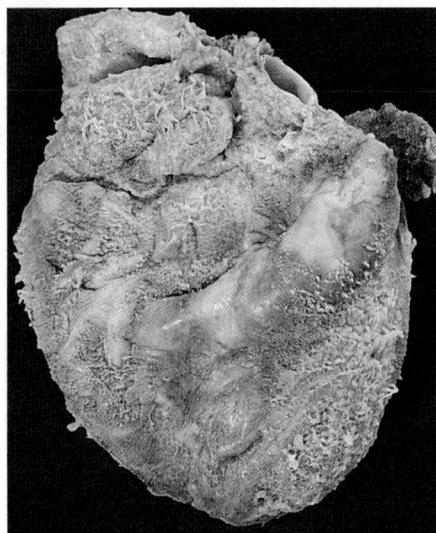

Figure 39-4 Acute pericarditis. Note the shaggy coat of fibrin covering the surface of the heart.

Source: Damjanov, I., & Linder, J. (1999). *Pathology: A color atlas.* St. Louis: Mosby.

Table 39-8 Measurement of Pulsus Paradoxus

1. Make determination during quiet breathing with stable rhythm.
2. Determine systolic blood pressure.
3. Inflate blood pressure cuff until no sounds are heard with stethoscope.
4. Deflate cuff slowly until systolic sounds are heard on expiration, and note the pressure.
5. Deflate cuff until systolic sounds are heard throughout the respiratory cycle, and note the pressure.
6. Determine the difference between the measurements taken in Steps 4 and 5. This will equal the amount of paradox:

Sounds heard in expiration at	110 mm Hg
Sounds heard throughout cycle at	82 mm Hg
Amount of paradox	28 mm Hg

The difference is usually <10 mm Hg. If the difference >10 mm Hg, cardiac tamponade may be present.

tuberculosis, neoplasm, autoimmune, drug, metabolic, and trauma (Imazio, 2011).

Pericarditis in the acute MI patient may be described as two distinct syndromes. The first is *acute pericarditis,* which may occur within the initial 48 to 72 hours after an MI. The second is *Dressler's syndrome* (late pericarditis), which appears 4 to 6 weeks after an MI (see Chapter 36).

An inflammatory response is the characteristic pathological finding in acute pericarditis. There is an influx of neutrophils, increased pericardial vascularity, and eventually fibrin deposition on the visceral pericardium (Figure 39-4).

Clinical Manifestations

Characteristic clinical manifestations found in acute pericarditis include progressive, frequently severe chest pain that is sharp and pleuritic in nature. The pain is generally worse with deep inspiration and when lying supine. It is relieved by sitting. The pain may radiate to the neck, arms, or left shoulder, making it difficult to differentiate from angina. One distinction is that the pain from pericarditis can be referred to the trapezius muscle (shoulder, upper back) because the phrenic nerve innervates these two regions. Pericarditis is diagnosed in 5% of people presenting to the emergency department with chest pain (Imazio, 2011; Futterman & Lemberg, 2006). The dyspnea that accompanies acute pericarditis is related to the patient's need to breathe in rapid, shallow breaths to avoid chest pain and may be aggravated by fever and anxiety.

The hallmark finding in acute pericarditis is the **pericardial friction rub.** The rub is a scratching, grating, high-pitched sound believed to arise from friction between the roughened pericardial and epicardial surfaces. It is best heard with the stethoscope diaphragm firmly placed at the lower left sternal border of the chest. The pericardial friction rub does not radiate widely or vary in timing from the heartbeat, but it may require frequent auscultation to identify because it may be elusive and transient. Timing the pericardial friction rub with the pulse

(and not respirations) will help distinguish it from pleural rub (e.g., from pleurisy).

Complications

Two major complications that may result from acute pericarditis are pericardial effusion and cardiac tamponade. **Pericardial effusion** is an accumulation of excess fluid in the pericardium. It can occur rapidly (e.g., chest trauma) or slowly (e.g., tuberculous pericarditis). Large effusions may compress adjoining structures. Pulmonary tissue compression can cause cough, dyspnea, and tachypnea. Phrenic nerve compression can induce hiccups, and compression of the recurrent laryngeal nerve may result in hoarseness. Heart sounds are generally distant and muffled, although blood pressure (BP) is usually maintained by compensatory mechanisms.

Cardiac tamponade, also referred to as *pericardial tamponade,* develops as fluid accumulates in the pericardial sac (pericardial effusion), causing an increase in intrapericardial pressure and producing compression of the heart. The speed of fluid accumulation affects the severity of clinical manifestations. Cardiac tamponade can occur acutely (e.g., rupture of heart, trauma) or subacutely (e.g., secondary to uremia, malignancy). The patient with cardiac tamponade may report chest pain and is often confused, anxious, and restless. As the compression of the heart increases, heart sounds become muffled and the pulse pressure is narrowed. The patient will develop tachypnea, tachycardia, and a decreased cardiac output (CO). The neck veins are usually markedly distended because of jugular venous pressure elevation, and a significant pulsus paradoxus is present. Pulsus paradoxus is a decrease in systolic BP with inspiration that is exaggerated in cardiac tamponade. (Table 39-8 shows measurement technique.) In a patient with a slow onset of a cardiac tamponade, dyspnea may be the only clinical manifestation.

Diagnostic Studies

The ECG may be normal or may exhibit nonspecific or specific and diffuse changes. If specific ECG changes do develop, they will evolve over a period of hours to days or weeks and can include PR-segment depression, ST-segment elevation, and T-wave flattening and inversion. These changes are believed to be caused

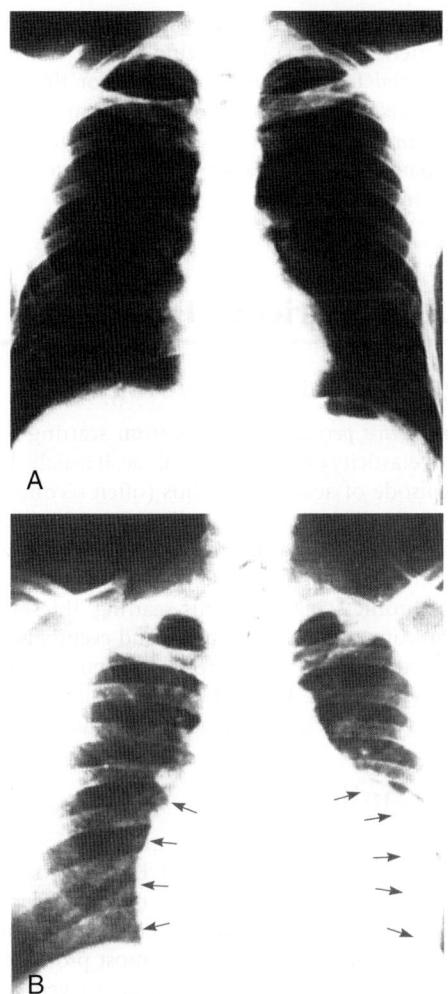

Figure 39-5 A, Radiograph of a normal chest. **B,** Pericardial effusion is present and the cardiac silhouette is enlarged with a globular shape *(arrows).*

Source: Guzetta, C. E., & Dossey, B. M. (1992). *Cardiovascular nursing: Holistic practice.* St. Louis: Mosby.

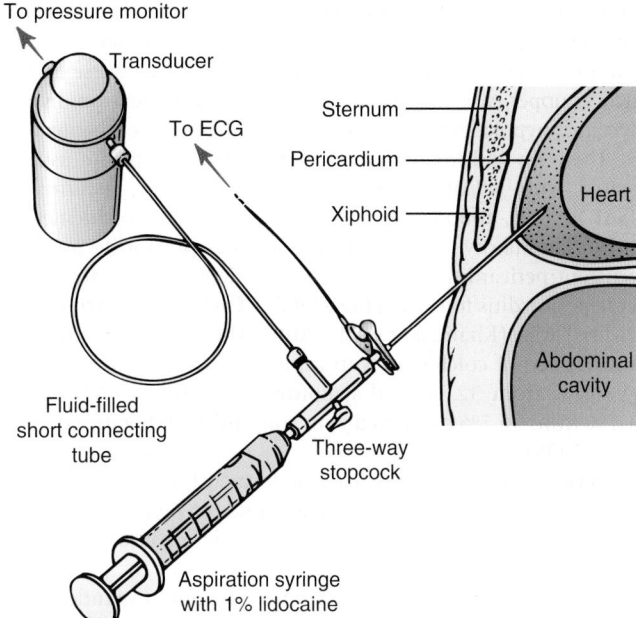

Figure 39-6 Pericardiocentesis is performed under sterile conditions in conjunction with electrocardiogram (ECG) and hemodynamic measurements.

Source: Redrawn from Braunwald, E. (1988). *Heart disease: A textbook of cardiovascular medicine* (3rd ed.). Philadelphia: Saunders.

COLLABORATIVE CARE

Table 39-9 Acute Pericarditis

Diagnostic	*Collaborative Therapy*
• History and physical examination	• Treatment of underlying disease
• Auscultation of chest	• Bed rest
• ECG	• Aspirin
• BUN,* serum creatinine	• NSAIDs
• TB test	• Colchicine
• Chest radiographic examination	• Corticosteroids
• Echocardiogram	• Pericardiocentesis (for large pericardial effusion or tamponade)
• Pericardiocentesis	
• Pericardial biopsy	
• CT scan	
• Cardiac nuclear scan	

BUN, blood urea nitrogen; *CT,* computed tomography; *ECG,* electrocardiogram; *NSAIDs,* nonsteroidal anti-inflammatory drugs; *TB,* tuberculosis.
*Serum urea (nitrogen).

by superficial myocardial inflammation under the pericardium. (See Chapter 38 for more information on ECG monitoring.) The chest radiographic findings are generally normal, but cardiomegaly may be seen in a patient who has a large pericardial effusion (Figure 39-5). Echocardiographic findings are more useful in determining the presence of a pericardial effusion or cardiac tamponade. Newer methods such as tissue Doppler imaging and colour M-mode of early left ventricular flow help to assess diastolic function and diagnose constrictive pericarditis (discussed later in the chapter). Computed tomography (CT) and cardiac magnetic resonance imaging (CMRI) provide for visualization of the pericardium and pericardial space (Imazio, 2011; Khandaker et al., 2010).

Common laboratory findings include leukocytosis and elevation of CRP and ESR. Troponin levels may be elevated in patients with ST-segment elevation and acute pericarditis, which would indicate concurrent myocardial damage. The fluid obtained during pericardiocentesis (Figure 39-6) or the tissue from a pericardial biopsy may also be analyzed to determine the cause of the pericarditis.

Collaborative Care

Management of acute pericarditis is directed toward identification and treatment of the underlying problem (Table 39-9). Antibiotics should be used to treat bacterial pericarditis. Corticosteroids are generally reserved for patients with pericarditis secondary to systemic lupus erythematosus, patients already taking corticosteroids for a rheumatological or other immune system condition, or patients who do not respond to nonsteroidal anti-inflammatory drugs (NSAIDs). When necessary, prednisone is usually given according to a tapering dosage schedule. Corticosteroids are administered cautiously because of their numerous adverse effects, such as upper gastrointestinal bleeding, sodium retention, hyperglycemia, hypokalemia, and Cushing's syndrome (see Chapter 51).

The pain and inflammation of acute pericarditis are usually treated with NSAIDs. High-dose salicylates (e.g., aspirin) or NSAIDs, (e.g., ibuprofen) are commonly used. Colchicine, an anti-inflammatory agent used for gout, and previously used for recurrent pericarditis, is now recommended in the treatment of acute pericarditis following the COPE (COlchicine for acute PEricarditis) trial (Khandaker et al., 2010). The study demonstrated that the use of colchicine with aspirin reduced recurrence rates by 10.7% from 32.3% and symptom reduction at 72 hours to 11.7% from 36.7% compared with conventional therapy (Imazio et al., 2005).

Pericardiocentesis is usually performed for pericardial effusion with acute cardiac tamponade, purulent pericarditis, and a high index of suspicion of neoplasm (see Figure 39-6). Hemodynamic support for the patient being prepared for the pericardiocentesis may include administration of volume expanders and inotropic agents (e.g., dopamine) and the discontinuation of any anticoagulants. The procedure is performed rapidly and safely using a percutaneous approach that is guided by ECG and echocardiography. If surgical drainage is necessary, a 16- to 18-gauge needle is inserted into the pericardial space to remove fluid for analysis and to relieve cardiac pressure. Complications from pericardiocentesis include dysrhythmias, further cardiac tamponade, pneumomediastinum, pneumothorax, myocardial laceration, and coronary artery laceration.

NURSING MANAGEMENT: ACUTE PERICARDITIS

The management of the patient's pain and anxiety during acute pericarditis is a primary nursing consideration. Assessment of the amount, the quality, and the location of the pain is important, particularly in distinguishing the pain of myocardial ischemia (angina) from the pain of pericarditis. Pericarditic pain is usually located in the precordium or left trapezius ridge and has a sharp, pleuritic quality that increases with inspiration. Pain is often relieved by sitting or leaning forward, and the pain is worsened when lying supine. ECG monitoring can aid in distinguishing these types of pain because ischemia usually involves localized ST-segment changes, as compared with the diffuse ST-segment changes present in acute pericarditis.

Pain relief measures include maintaining the patient on bed rest with the head of the bed elevated to 45 degrees and providing an overbed table for support. Anti-inflammatory medications help alleviate the patient's pain. However, because of the potential for upper gastrointestinal bleeding with the use of high doses of these medications, nursing interventions should be directed toward management of this potential problem. Specific interventions include the administration of these drugs with food or milk and instructing the patient to avoid any alcoholic beverages while taking the medications.

Other drugs, such as misoprostol, or a proton pump inhibitor, may be ordered to protect the gastric mucosa. Anxiety-reducing measures for the patient with acute pericarditis include providing simple, complete explanations of all procedures performed and the possible cause of the pain. These explanations are particularly important for the patient whose diagnosis of

acute pericarditis is being established and for the patient who has already experienced angina or an acute MI.

The potential for decreased CO exists for the patient with acute pericarditis because of the possibility of cardiac tamponade. Monitoring for the signs and symptoms of tamponade and making preparations for possible pericardiocentesis are important nursing responsibilities.

Chronic Constrictive Pericarditis

Etiology and Pathophysiology

Chronic constrictive pericarditis results from scarring with consequent loss of elasticity of the pericardial sac. It usually begins with an initial episode of acute pericarditis (often secondary to idiopathic causes, cardiac surgery, or radiation) and is characterized by fibrin deposition with a clinically undetected pericardial effusion. Resorption of the effusion slowly follows with progression toward the chronic stage of fibrous scarring, thickening of the pericardium from calcium deposition, and eventual obliteration of the pericardial space. The fibrotic, thickened, and adherent pericardium encases the heart, thereby impairing the ability of the atria and ventricles to stretch adequately during diastole.

Clinical Manifestations

Manifestations of chronic constrictive pericarditis occur over an extended period and mimic those of HF and cor pulmonale. Many of the clinical manifestations are related to decreased CO. They include dyspnea on exertion, peripheral edema, ascites, fatigue, anorexia, and weight loss. The most prominent finding upon physical examination is elevated jugular venous pressure. Unlike with cardiac tamponade, the presence of significant pulsus paradoxus is uncommon. Auscultatory findings include a *pericardial knock*, which is a loud early diastolic sound often heard along the left sternal border.

Diagnostic Studies

ECG results are often nonspecific in chronic constrictive pericarditis. The cardiac silhouette on the chest radiograph may be normal or enlarged depending on the degree of pericardial thickening and the presence of a coexisting pericardial effusion. Two-dimensional echocardiographic is insensitive for determining pericardial thickness but may inform the practitioner about the physiology (Howlett et al., 2009). Colour M-mode and tissue Doppler imaging are used to confirm constrictive pericarditis. CT and MRI provide measurement of pericardial thickness and assessment of diastolic filling patterns.

NURSING AND COLLABORATIVE MANAGEMENT: CHRONIC CONSTRICTIVE PERICARDITIS

Unless the patient is free of symptoms or the condition is inoperable, the treatment of choice for chronic constrictive pericarditis is a *pericardiectomy*. The pericardiectomy usually involves complete resection of the pericardium through a median sternotomy with the use of cardiopulmonary bypass. Some patients show immediate improvement after surgery, but others may take weeks.

The postoperative prognosis is improved when the surgery is performed before the development of severe clinical disability.

Myocarditis

Etiology and Pathophysiology

Myocarditis is a focal or diffuse inflammation of the myocardium. Possible causes include viruses, bacteria, fungi, parasites, radiation therapy, and pharmacological and chemical factors. Viruses, particularly coxsackievirus types A and B, are the most common causative agents of myocarditis in Canada and the United States. Autoimmune disorders (e.g., polymyositis) also have been associated with the development of myocarditis. Myocarditis may also occur when no causative agent or factor can be identified (i.e., idiopathic). Myocarditis is frequently associated with acute pericarditis, particularly when it is caused by coxsackievirus B strains or echoviruses (Cooper, 2009). When the myocardium becomes infected, the causative agent invades the myocytes and causes cellular damage and necrosis. The immune response is activated, and cytokines and oxygen free radicals are released. As the infection progresses, an autoimmune response is activated, leading to further destruction of myocytes (Figure 39-7). Myocarditis results in cardiac dysfunction and has been linked to the development of dilated cardiomyopathy (CMP) (discussed later in this chapter).

Clinical Manifestations

The clinical features of myocarditis are variable, ranging from a benign course without any overt manifestations to severe heart involvement or sudden cardiac death (SCD). Fever, fatigue, malaise, myalgias, pharyngitis, dyspnea, lymphadenopathy, and nausea and vomiting are early systemic manifestations of the viral illness.

Early cardiac manifestations appear 7 to 10 days after viral infection. These include pleuritic chest pain with a pericardial friction rub and effusion because pericarditis often accompanies myocarditis. Late cardiac signs relate to the development of congestive heart failure (CHF) and may include a third heart sound (S3), crackles, jugular venous distension, syncope, peripheral edema, and angina.

Diagnostic Studies

The ECG changes for a patient with myocarditis are often non-specific and reflect associated pericardial involvement (e.g., diffuse ST-segment abnormalities). Dysrhythmias and conduction disturbances may be present. Laboratory findings are also often inconclusive. They may include mild to moderate leukocytosis and atypical lymphocytes, increased ESR and CRP levels, elevated levels of myocardial markers such as troponin, and elevated viral titres (virus is generally only present in tissue and fluid samples during the initial 8-10 days of illness). Histological confirmation of myocarditis is done through **endomyocardial biopsy (EMB).** This technique involves removing several small pieces of myocardial tissue percutaneously from the right ventricle with a special instrument called a *bioptome* and microscopically examining the samples (Cooper, 2009). A biopsy done during the initial 6 weeks of acute illness is most diagnostic because this is the period in which lymphocytic infiltration and myocyte damage

indicative of myocarditis are present. Other studies include the use of echocardiography, nuclear scans, and MRI to evaluate cardiac function.

Collaborative Care

The treatment for myocarditis in the patient with fulminant heart failure will require cardiovascular support with inotropic and/or vasopressor therapy and mechanical circulatory support (e.g., left ventricular assist device [LVAD]). Care of the patient with myocarditis and HF is usual care for HF patients with β-blockers, angiotensin-converting enzyme inhibitors (ACEIs), and diuretic therapy, which may help to reduce fluid volume and decrease preload (Howlett et al., 2009). Immunosuppressive therapy with agents such as prednisone, azathioprine (Imuran), and cyclosporine is not routinely recommended in the management of the patient with myocarditis but may be trialed in patients with an autoimmune disorder and those who are severely hemodynamically compromised and not responding to treatment. Intravenous immunoglobulin (IVIG) has not demonstrated improved incomes but may be of use in the pediatric population (Cooper, 2009). Antiviral therapy with ribavirin and interferon is undergoing clinical investigation for the treatment of acute viral myocarditis in which a reduction in myocardial lesion and mortality has been seen in animal studies (Cooper, 2009). Oxygen therapy, bed rest, restricted activity, and maintenance of standby emergency equipment are general supportive measures used for management of myocarditis.

NURSING MANAGEMENT: MYOCARDITIS

Decreased CO is an ongoing nursing diagnosis in the care of the patient with myocarditis. Interventions focus on assessment for the signs and symptoms of HF. Important nursing measures to decrease cardiac workload include the use of the semi-Fowler position, spacing of activity and rest periods, and provisions for a quiet environment. Prescribed medications that increase the heart's contractility and decrease the preload, the afterload, or both require careful monitoring. Ongoing evaluation of the effectiveness of these interventions is necessary.

The patient may be anxious about the diagnosis of myocarditis, recovery from myocarditis, and the therapeutic plan. Nursing measures include assessing the level of anxiety, instituting measures to decrease anxiety, and keeping the patient and caregivers informed about therapeutic measures.

The patient who receives immunosuppressive therapy has additional problems of alterations in the immune response with the potential for infection and complications related to the therapy. Guidelines for care include monitoring for complications and providing the patient with a clean, safe environment by following proper infection control procedures. Most patients with myocarditis recover spontaneously, although some may develop dilated CMP. If severe HF occurs, the patient may require heart transplantation.

Rheumatic Fever and Heart Disease

Rheumatic fever is defined by the Heart and Stroke Foundation of Canada (HSF, 2011b) as an inflammatory disease that may

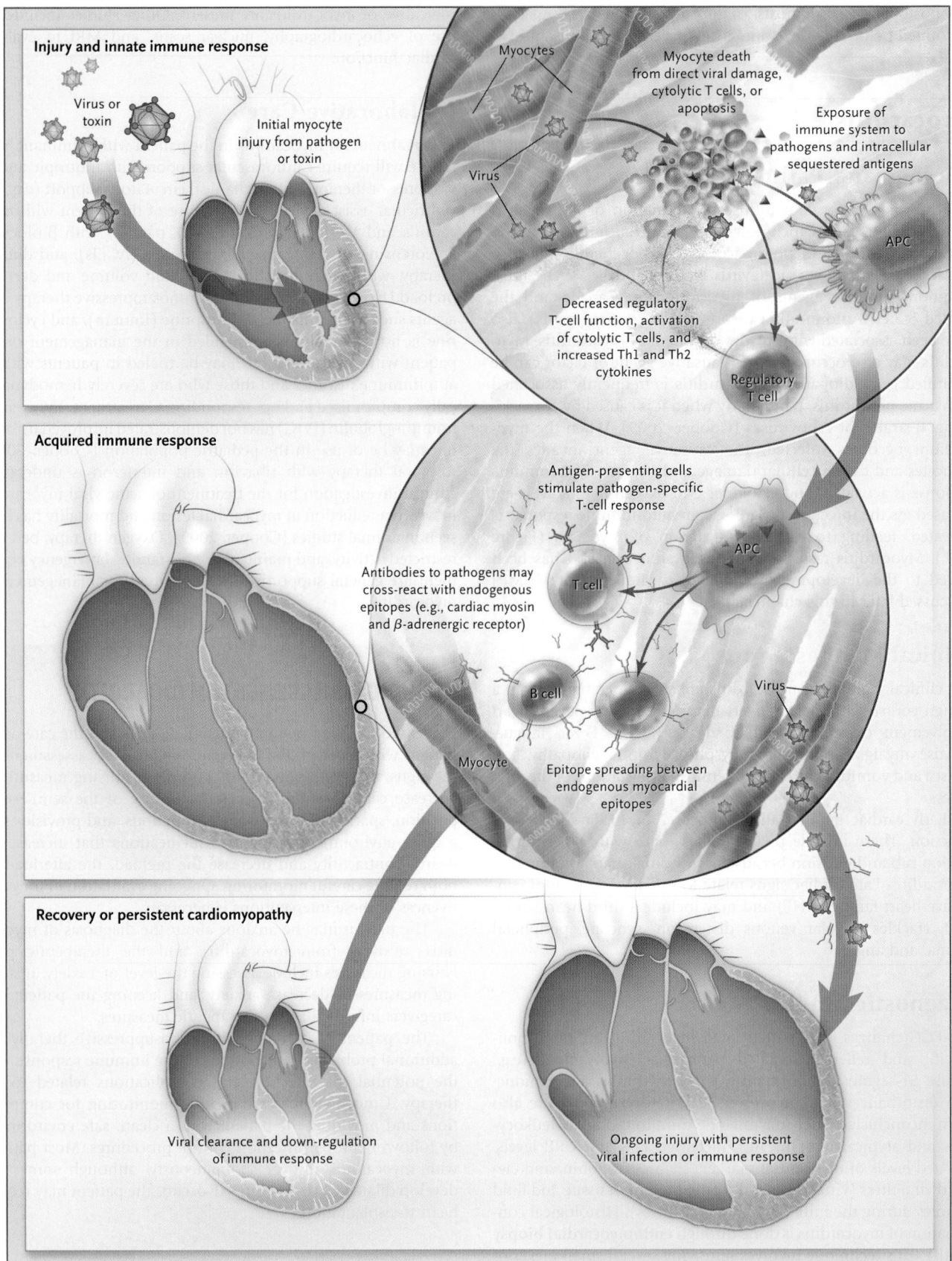

Figure 39-7 Myocarditis. *Th1, Th2,* T helper cells.

Source: Cooper, L. T. (2009). Myocarditis. *New England Journal of Medicine, 360,* 1531. doi:10.1056/NEJMra0800028. Copyright © 2009 Massachusetts Medical Society. All rights reserved.

affect several connective tissues of the body, especially those of the heart, brain, joints, or skin. Rheumatic fever potentially involves all layers of the heart (endocardium, myocardium, and pericardium). **Rheumatic heart disease** is a chronic condition resulting from rheumatic fever that is characterized by scarring and deformity of the heart valves.

Etiology and Pathophysiology

Acute rheumatic fever (ARF) is a complication that occurs as a delayed sequel (usually after 2-3 wk) of group A streptococcal pharyngitis (Mayo Foundation for Medical Education and Research [MFMER], 2007). Manifestations of ARF appear to be related to an abnormal immunological response to group A streptococcal cell membrane antigens. ARF has declined in developed countries as a result of the effective use of antibiotics to treat streptococcal infections. It remains an important public health problem in developing countries. The sequelae of ARF, rheumatic heart disease, is found primarily in young adults.

Cardiac Lesions and Valvular Deformities.
About 40% of ARF episodes are marked by carditis, and all layers of the heart (endocardium, myocardium, and pericardium) may be involved. This generalized involvement gives rise to the term *rheumatic pancarditis.*

Rheumatic endocarditis is found primarily in the valves, with swelling and erosion of the valve leaflets. Vegetations form from deposits of fibrin and blood cells in areas of erosion (Figure 39-8). The lesions initially create fibrous thickening of the valve leaflets, fusion of commissures and chordae tendineae, and fibrosis of the papillary muscle. Valve leaflets may fuse and become thickened or even calcified, resulting in stenosis. Reduction in the mobility of valve leaflets may occur with failure of the leaflets, resulting in regurgitation. The mitral and aortic valves are most commonly affected.

Myocardial involvement is characterized by **Aschoff's bodies,** which are tiny, rounded or spindle-shaped nodules formed by a reaction to inflammation with accompanying swelling and fragmentation of collagen fibres. As the Aschoff's bodies age, they become more fibrous, and scar tissue is formed in the myocardium. In addition to Aschoff's bodies, a diffuse cellular infiltrate

is present in interstitial tissues. Rheumatic pericarditis affects both layers of the pericardium, which become thickened and covered with a fibrinous exudate, and a serosanguineous pericardial effusion may develop. When healing occurs, fibrosis and adhesions develop that partially or completely obliterate the pericardial sac, but constrictive pericarditis does not occur.

These pathophysiological changes in the heart may occur as a result of an initial attack of rheumatic fever. However, recurrent infections may cause further structural damage.

Extracardiac Lesions. The lesions of rheumatic fever are systemic, involving the connective tissue especially. The joints (polyarthritis), skin (subcutaneous nodules), and central nervous system may be involved in rheumatic fever.

Clinical Manifestations

Symptoms of ARF can include chest pain, excessive fatigue, heart palpitations (when the heart flutters or misses beats), a thumping sensation in the chest, shortness of breath, and swollen ankles, wrists, or stomach (HSF, 2011a). The diagnosis of ARF is suggested by a clustering of signs and symptoms as well as from laboratory findings. When not observed in its most severe form, the disease may be difficult to differentiate from many illnesses with similar clinical manifestations. Criteria established by T. D. Jones in 1944 were revised by the American Heart Association and modified by the World Health Organization (WHO) to provide a basis for diagnosis (WHO, 2004; Dajani et al., 1992) (Table 39-10). The presence of two major criteria or one major and two minor criteria plus evidence of a preceding group A streptococcal infection indicates a high probability of ARF.

Major Criteria.
Carditis is the most important manifestation of ARF and results in three signs: (1) an organic heart murmur or murmurs of mitral or aortic regurgitation or mitral stenosis; (2) cardiac enlargement and HF occurring secondary to myocarditis; and (3) pericarditis resulting in muffled heart sounds, chest pain, a pericardial friction rub, or signs of effusion. *Monoor polyarthritis* is the most common finding in rheumatic fever. The inflammatory process affects the synovial membranes of the joints, causing swelling, heat, redness, tenderness, and limitation

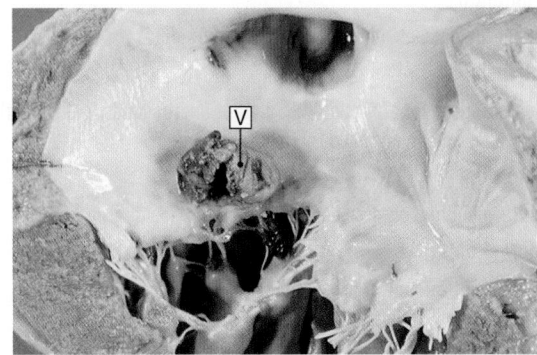

Figure 39-8 Mitral stenosis and clumps of vegetation *(V)* containing platelets and fibrin. Mitral leaflets are thickened and fused and have clumps of vegetation containing platelets and fibrin.

Source: Stevens, A., & Lowe, J. (2000). *Pathology: Illustrated review in color* (2nd ed.). St. Louis: Mosby.

Table 39-10 Modified Jones Criteria for Acute Rheumatic Fever		
MAJOR CRITERIA	**MINOR CRITERIA**	**EVIDENCE OF GROUP A STREPTOCOCCAL INFECTION**
Carditis	Clinical findings: fever, polyarthralgia	Laboratory findings: antistreptolysin-O titre, positive throat culture, positive rapid antigen test for group A streptococci
Mono- or polyarthritis		
Chorea	Laboratory findings: ESR, WBC count, CRP	
Erythema marginatum		
Subcutaneous nodules		ECG findings: Prolonged PR interval

CRP, C-reactive protein; *ECG,* electrocardiogram; *ESR,* erythrocyte sedimentation rate; *WBC,* white blood cell.

of motion. The larger joints are most frequently affected, particularly knees, ankles, elbows, and wrists. *Chorea (Sydenham's chorea)* is the major central nervous system manifestation of ARF, often a delayed sign occurring several months after the initial infection. It is characterized by involuntary movements, especially of the face and the limbs, muscle weakness, and disturbances of speech and gait. *Erythema marginatum* lesions are a less common feature of ARF. The bright pink maplike macular lesions occur mainly on the trunk and the proximal extremities and may be exacerbated by heat (e.g., warm bath). Subcutaneous nodules, usually associated with severe carditis, are firm, small, hard, painless swellings located over extensor surfaces of the joints, particularly knees, wrists, and elbows.

Minor Criteria. Minor clinical manifestations (see Table 39-10) are frequently present and are helpful in diagnosing the disease. The minor criteria are used as supplemental data to confirm the presence of rheumatic fever when only one major criterion is present.

Complications

A complication that can result from ARF is chronic rheumatic carditis. It results from changes in valvular structure that may occur months to years after an episode of ARF. Rheumatic endocarditis can result in fibrous tissue growth in valve leaflets and chordae tendineae with scarring and contractures. The mitral valve is most frequently involved. Other valves that may be affected are the aortic and the tricuspid.

Diagnostic Studies

No single diagnostic test exists for rheumatic fever (see Table 39-10). An echocardiogram may show valvular insufficiency and pericardial fluid or thickening. A chest radiographic study may show an enlarged heart if HF is present. The most consistent ECG change is delayed AV conduction as evidenced by prolongation of the PR interval.

Collaborative Care

Treatment consists of drug therapy and supportive measures (Table 39-11). Antibiotic therapy does not modify the course of

COLLABORATIVE CARE

Table 39-11 Rheumatic Fever	
Diagnostic	*Collaborative Therapy*
• History and physical examination	• Bed rest (modified)
• ASO titre	• Benzathine penicillin (1.2 million units IM) or procaine penicillin (600,000 units IM) daily for 10 days
• Throat culture	
• ESR	• Acetylsalicylic acid
• C-reactive protein	• Corticosteroids
• WBC count	• Codeine
• Chest radiograph	• Carbamazepine, valproic acid, phenobarbital
• Echocardiogram	
• ECG	

ASO, antistreptolysin O; *ECG,* electrocardiogram; *ESR,* erythrocyte sedimentation rate; *IM,* intramuscularly; *WBC,* white blood cell.

the acute disease or the development of carditis. It does eliminate residual group A streptococci remaining in the tonsils and the pharynx and prevent the spread of organisms to close contacts. Salicylates, NSAIDs, and corticosteroids are the anti-inflammatory agents most widely used in the management of ARF. All are effective in controlling the fever and joint manifestations. Salicylates or NSAIDs are used when arthritis is the main manifestation, and corticosteroids are used if severe carditis is present.

NURSING MANAGEMENT: RHEUMATIC FEVER AND HEART DISEASE

Nursing Assessment

Subjective and objective data that should be obtained from a patient with rheumatic fever and heart disease are presented in Table 39-12. It is important to note that rheumatic fever is more

NURSING ASSESSMENT

Table 39-12 Rheumatic Fever and Rheumatic Heart Disease

Subjective Data

Important Health Information

Past health history: Recent β-hemolytic streptococcal infection, previous rheumatic fever or rheumatic heart disease, family history of rheumatic fever

Symptoms

• Malaise, generalized weakness, fatigue

• Anorexia; weight loss

• Palpitations

• Ataxia; migratory joint pain and tenderness (especially large joints)

• Chest pain; abdominal pain

Objective Data

General

Low-grade fever

Integumentary

Subcutaneous nodules and erythema marginatum

Cardiovascular

Tachycardia, pericardial friction rub, distant heart sounds; gallop rhythm, diastolic and systolic murmurs, peripheral edema

Neurological

Chorea (involuntary, purposeless, rapid motions; facial grimaces)

Musculoskeletal

Signs of polyarthritis including swelling, heat, redness, limitation of motion (especially of knees, ankles, elbows, shoulders, and wrists)

Possible Findings

Cardiomegaly on chest radiographic study; delayed AV conduction on ECG; valve abnormalities, chamber dilation, and pericardial effusion on echocardiogram; ↑ ASO titre, ↑ ESR, positive C-reactive protein, leukocytosis, ↓ RBC, hemoglobin, and hematocrit

ASO, antistreptolysin O; *AV,* atrioventricular; *ECG,* electrocardiogram; *ESR,* erythrocyte sedimentation rate; *RBC,* red blood cell.

likely to reoccur in a person with a previous history of rheumatic fever than in the general population. The skin of the patient should be assessed for subcutaneous nodules and erythema marginatum. The procedure involves palpation for subcutaneous nodules over all bony surfaces and along extensor tendons of the hands and feet. The nodules range in size from 1 to 4 cm and are hard, painless, and freely movable. Erythema marginatum can occur on the trunk and the inner aspects of the upper arm and the thigh. The erythematous maplike macules do not itch and are not raised. The possible presence of these bright pink macules should be assessed in good light because the rash is difficult to observe, especially if the patient is dark skinned.

Nursing Diagnoses

Nursing diagnoses for the patient with rheumatic fever and heart disease may include, but are not limited to, the following:
- Activity intolerance *related to* arthralgia secondary to joint pain, pain from pericarditis, and HF.
- Ineffective self-health management *related to* lack of knowledge concerning the need for long-term prophylactic antibiotic therapy and possible disease sequelae.

Planning

The overall goals for a patient with rheumatic fever include (1) normal or baseline heart function, (2) resumption of daily activities without joint pain, and (3) verbalization of the ability to manage the disease.

Nursing Implementation

Health Promotion

Rheumatic fever is a preventable cardiovascular disease. Prevention involves early detection and immediate treatment of group A β-hemolytic streptococcal pharyngitis. Adequate treatment of streptococcal pharyngitis prevents initial attacks of rheumatic fever. Treatment consists of intramuscular injection of penicillin G benzathine (Bicillin L-A) or oral penicillin V potassium. If the patient is allergic to penicillin, erythromycin or azithromycin (Zithromax) may be substituted. Oral therapy requires faithful adherence to the full course of treatment. The nurse's role is to educate people in the community to seek medical attention for symptoms of streptococcal pharyngitis and to emphasize the need for adequate treatment of this infection.

Acute Intervention

The primary goals of managing a patient with ARF are to control and eradicate the infecting organism; prevent cardiac complications; relieve joint pain, fever, and other symptoms; and support the patient psychologically and emotionally. The nurse should administer antibiotics as ordered to treat the streptococcal infection and should teach the patient that oral antibiotic therapy requires faithful adherence to the full course of therapy. Antipyretics, NSAIDs, and corticosteroids should be administered as

prescribed and fluid intake monitored. Promotion of optimal rest is essential to reduce the cardiac workload and to diminish the metabolic needs of the body. Relief of joint pain is an important nursing goal. Painful joints should be positioned for comfort and proper alignment. Heat may be applied and salicylates or NSAIDs administered to relieve joint pain. After the acute symptoms have subsided, the patient without carditis should ambulate. If the patient has carditis with HF, bed rest restrictions should be applied. (See Chapter 37 for care of a patient with HF.) Nonstrenuous activities should be encouraged once recovery has begun.

Ambulatory and Home Care

Secondary prevention aims at preventing the recurrence of rheumatic fever. The patient with a previous history of rheumatic fever should be taught about the disease process, possible sequelae, and the ongoing or permanent need for prophylactic antibiotics. Prior history of rheumatic fever makes the patient more susceptible to a second attack after a streptococcal infection. The best prevention is monthly injections of long-acting penicillin. Alternative treatment is administration of oral penicillin or erythromycin one or two times a day. Rheumatic fever without carditis after age 18 may require only 5 years of prophylactic antibiotic therapy, or therapy may continue indefinitely in patients with frequent exposure to group A streptococcus. Prophylactic treatment should continue for 10 years or until the age of 40 in individuals who develop rheumatic heart disease (Gerber et al., 2009).

The dosage of antibiotics used in maintenance prophylaxis of rheumatic fever is not adequate to prevent IE when invasive procedures are performed. Additional prophylaxis is necessary if a patient with known rheumatic heart disease has dental or surgical procedures involving the upper respiratory tract that involves perforation of the mucosa (see Table 39-3). The nurse must explain the difference between these two prophylactic programs.

Patient teaching should encourage good nutrition, hygienic practices, and the importance of receiving adequate rest. The patient should also be cautioned about the possibility of developing valvular heart disease. The nurse should teach the patient to seek medical attention if symptoms such as excessive fatigue, dizziness, palpitations, or exertional dyspnea develop.

Evaluation

The following include expected outcomes for the patient with rheumatic fever and heart disease:
- Ability to perform activities of daily with minimal fatigue and pain
- Adherence to treatment regimen
- Expression of confidence in managing disease

Valvular Heart Disease

The heart contains two AV valves, the mitral and the tricuspid, and two semilunar valves, the aortic and the pulmonic, that are located in four strategic locations to control unidirectional blood flow (see Figure 34-2). Valvular heart disease is defined according to the valve or valves affected and the types of functional alteration: stenosis or regurgitation.

The pressure on either side of an open valve is normally equal. However, in a stenotic valve, the valve orifice is restricted, impeding the forward flow of blood and creating a pressure gradient across an open valve. The degree of stenosis (constriction or narrowing) is reflected in the degree of the pressure gradient (i.e., the higher the gradient, the greater the stenosis). In **regurgitation** (also called *valvular incompetence* or *insufficiency*), incomplete closure of the valve leaflets results in the backward flow of blood.

Valvular disorders occur in children and adolescents primarily from congenital conditions such as tricuspid atresia, pulmonary stenosis, and aortic stenosis. Valvular heart disease has remained prevalent because of an increase in the number of older adults, many of whom have some form of cardiovascular disease. Aortic stenosis and mitral regurgitation (MR) are common valvular disorders in older adults. Other causes of valvular diseases in adults include disorders related to acquired immune deficiency syndrome and the use of some antiparkinsonian drugs (e.g., pergolide [Permax]) (Steiger, Jost, Grandas, & Van Camp, 2009).

Mitral Valve Stenosis

Etiology and Pathophysiology

Most cases of adult mitral valve stenosis result from rheumatic heart disease; rheumatic mitral stenosis is more prevalent in developing countries (Lung & Vahanian, 2011). Less common causes include congenital mitral stenosis, rheumatoid arthritis, and systemic lupus erythematosus. Rheumatic endocarditis causes scarring of the valve leaflets and the chordae tendineae. Contractures and adhesions develop between the commissures (the junctional areas) of the two leaflets (Figure 39-9). These structural deformities cause obstruction of blood flow and create a pressure difference between the left atrium and the left ventricle during diastole. Left atrial pressure and volume elevations cause

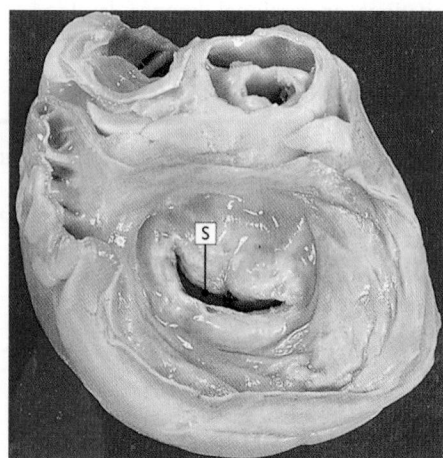

Figure 39-9 Mitral stenosis *(S)* with classic "fish mouth" orifice.

Source: Stevens, A., & Lowe, J. (2000). *Pathology: Illustrated review in color* (2nd ed.). St. Louis: Mosby.

increased pulmonary vasculature pressure and subsequent hypertrophy of the pulmonary vessels. In chronic mitral stenosis, pressure overload occurs in the left atrium, the pulmonary bed, and the right ventricle.

Clinical Manifestations

The primary symptom of mitral stenosis is exertional dyspnea owing to reduced lung compliance (Table 39-13). Fatigue and palpitations from atrial fibrillation may occur. Heart sounds include a loud first heart sound and a low-pitched, rumbling diastolic murmur (best heard at the apex with the stethoscope bell). Less frequently, patients may have hoarseness (from atrial enlargement pressing on the laryngeal nerve), hemoptysis (from pulmonary hypertension), chest pain (from decreased CO), and seizures or a stroke (from emboli). Emboli can arise from blood stasis in the left atrium.

Mitral Valve Regurgitation

Etiology and Pathophysiology

Mitral valve function depends on intact mitral leaflets, mitral annulus, chordae tendineae, papillary muscles, left atrium, and left ventricle. Any defect in any of these structures can result in regurgitation. Most cases of MR are caused by MI, chronic rheumatic heart disease, mitral valve prolapse (MVP), ischemic papillary muscle dysfunction, and IE. MI with left ventricular failure increases the risk for rupture of the chordae tendineae and acute MR.

MR allows blood to flow backward from the left ventricle to the left atrium because of incomplete valve closure during systole. The left ventricle and the left atrium both work harder to preserve an adequate CO. In chronic MR, the additional volume load results in atrial enlargement, ventricular dilation, and eventual ventricular hypertrophy. In acute MR, the left atrium and ventricle do not abruptly dilate. The sudden increase in pressure and volume is transmitted to the pulmonary bed, resulting in pulmonary edema and shock.

Clinical Manifestations

The clinical course of MR is determined by the nature of its onset (see Table 39-13). Patients with acute MR will have thready, peripheral pulses and cool, clammy extremities. A low CO may obscure a new systolic murmur. Rapid assessment (e.g., cardiac catheterization) and intervention (e.g., valve repair or replacement) are critical for a positive outcome.

Patients with chronic MR may remain asymptomatic for many years until the development of some degree of left ventricular failure. Initial symptoms of left ventricular failure may include weakness, fatigue, palpitations, and dyspnea that gradually progress to orthopnea, paroxysmal nocturnal dyspnea, and peripheral edema. Accentuated left ventricular filling leads to an audible S3, even with normal left ventricular function. The murmur is a loud holosystolic or pansystolic murmur at the apex radiating to the left axilla. Patients with asymptomatic MR should be monitored carefully because the natural history for MR can be variable and surgery (valve repair or replacement) should be considered before significant left ventricular failure or pulmonary hypertension develops (Bonow et al., 2008).

Table 39-13 Clinical Manifestations and Diagnostic Findings of Valvular Heart Diseases

	CLINICAL MANIFESTATIONS	ELECTROCARDIOGRAM	ECHOCARDIOGRAM	CARDIAC CATHETERIZATION
Mitral valve stenosis	Dyspnea, hemoptysis; fatigue; palpitations; loud, accentuated S1; opening snap; low-pitched, rumbling diastolic murmur	Right axis deviation, left atrial enlargement, right ventricular hypertrophy, P mitrale (wide, M-shaped P wave), atrial flutter or fibrillation	Restricted movement of mitral valve leaflets; decreased size of orifice; diastolic turbulence	Left atrial pressure increased at end of diastole, reduction in CO
Mitral valve regurgitation	*Acute:* generally poorly tolerated with fulminating pulmonary edema and shock developing rapidly; systolic murmur	Left atrial enlargement, atrial fibrillation	Hyperdynamic left ventricular contraction in association with shock; regurgitant jets and flail* chordae or leaflets	Contrast medium injection in left ventricle showing regurgitation of blood into left atrium
	Chronic: weakness, fatigue, exertional dyspnea, palpitations; an S3 gallop, holosystolic or pansystolic murmur	P mitrale, left ventricular hypertrophy, atrial flutter or fibrillation	Left atrial enlargement; left ventricular hypertrophy; flail leaflets	Contrast medium injection in left ventricle showing regurgitation of blood into left atrium
Mitral valve prolapse	Palpitations, dyspnea, chest pain, activity intolerance, syncope; mobile midsystolic nonejection click and a late or holosystolic murmur	Usually normal; occasionally T-wave inversion or biplasticity in leads II, III, and aVf are noted; PVCs and tachydysrhythmias possible	On the M-mode echo, late systolic posterior motion or holosystolic billowing of the mitral leaflets; on two-dimensional echo, systolic billowing of the mitral leaflets	Left ventricular angiogram reveals mitral leaflets with prominent scalloping as the leaflets billow into the left atrium during systole
Aortic valve stenosis	Angina pectoris, syncope, heart failure, normal or soft S1, prominent S4, crescendo–decrescendo murmur	Left ventricular hypertrophy, left bundle branch block, complete atrioventricular heart block	Restricted movement of aortic valve; diminished orifice; systolic turbulence	Left ventricular systolic pressure increased, reduction in CO
Aortic valve regurgitation	*Acute:* abrupt onset of profound dyspnea, transient chest pain, progression to shock	Left ventricular strain	Normal-sized left ventricle with hyperdynamic systolic contraction; aortic dissection can be seen, if cause of acute process	Significant elevation of left ventricular diastolic pressure
	Chronic: fatigue, exertional dyspnea; Corrigan's pulse; heaving precordial impulse; diastolic high-pitched soft decrescendo diastolic murmur, characteristic Austin Flint murmur at diastolic rumble, systolic ejection click	Left ventricular hypertrophy	Enlarged left ventricle and dilated aortic root	Increase in left ventricular diastolic pressure, aortic root contrast medium injection demonstrating regurgitation of blood into left ventricle
Tricuspid stenosis and regurgitation	Peripheral edema, ascites, hepatomegaly; diastolic low-pitched, decrescendo murmur with increased intensity during inspiration (stenosis), pansystolic murmur with increased intensity at inspiration (regurgitation)	Tall, peaked P waves; atrial fibrillation	Right ventricular dilation and paradoxical septal motion, usually poor visualization of tricuspid valve itself	Pressure gradient across tricuspid valve and increased right atrial pressure (stenosis), reflux of contrast medium into right atrium (regurgitation)

CO, cardiac output; *PVCs*, premature ventricular contractions; *S1*, first heart sound; *S3*, third heart sound; *S4*, fourth heart sound.
*Flail mitral leaflet is a complication of mitral valve prolapse, which can lead to severe mitral regurgitation and left ventricular dysfunction.

Mitral Valve Prolapse

Etiology and Pathophysiology

Mitral valve prolapse (MVP) is an abnormality of the mitral valve leaflets and the papillary muscles or chordae that allows the leaflets to prolapse, or buckle, back into the left atrium during systole (Figure 39-10). The etiology of MVP is unknown but is related to diverse pathogenic mechanisms of the mitral valve apparatus. The use of the term *prolapse* is unfortunate because it is used even when the valvular anomaly permits normal function. MVP is one of the most common forms of valvular heart disease.

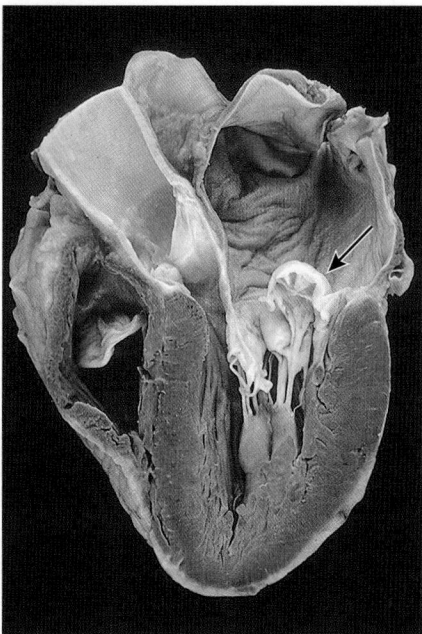

Figure 39-10 Mitral valve prolapse. In this valvular abnormality, the mitral leaflets have prolapsed back into the left atrium. They also demonstrate hooding *(arrow)*. The left ventricle is on the right.

Source: Kumar, V., Abbas, A. K., Fausto, N., & Aster, J. (2010). *Robbins and Cotran pathologic basis of disease* (8th ed., p. 564, Figure 12-23, *A*). Philadelphia: Saunders.

MVP is usually benign, but serious complications can occur, including MR, IE, SCD, and cerebral ischemia. There is an increased familial incidence (autosomal dominant) in some patients.

MVP in this group results from a connective tissue defect affecting only the valve or as part of Marfan syndrome or other hereditary conditions that affect the structure of collagen in the body. In many patients, the abnormality detected by echocardiography is not accompanied by any other clinical manifestations of cardiac disease, and the significance of the finding is unclear.

Clinical Manifestations

MVP covers a broad spectrum of severity. Most patients are asymptomatic and remain so for their entire lives. A characteristic of MVP is a murmur from regurgitation that gets more intense through systole. This could be a late or holosystolic murmur. Another major sign is one or more clicks usually heard in mid-systole to late systole. MVP does not alter the first (S1) or second (S2) heart sounds. Severe MR is an uncommon complication of MVP.

M-mode echocardiography confirms MVP by demonstrating late-systolic prolapse, and two-dimensional echocardiography reveals leaflet billowing into the left atrium. Dysrhythmias, most commonly ventricular premature contractions, paroxysmal supraventricular tachycardia, and ventricular tachycardia, may cause palpitations, light-headedness, and dizziness. IE may occur in patients with MR associated with MVP.

Patients may or may not have chest pain. The cause of the chest pain is not known, but it may be caused by abnormal tension on the papillary muscles. If chest pain occurs, it tends to occur in clusters, especially during periods of emotional stress.

Dyspnea, palpitations, and syncope may occasionally accompany the chest pain and do not respond to antianginal treatment (e.g., nitrates). β-Adrenergic blockers may be prescribed to control palpitations and chest pain. Patients with MVP generally have a benign, manageable course unless problems associated with MR are present. A teaching plan for patients with MVP is presented in Table 39-14.

Aortic Valve Stenosis

Etiology and Pathophysiology

Congenitally abnormal stenotic aortic valves are generally discovered in childhood, adolescence, or young adulthood. In older patients, aortic stenosis is a result of calcification of a tricuspid valve or a congenital bicuspid valve that may have an etiology similar to that of coronary artery disease or from scarring owing to rheumatic fever (Bonow et al., 2008). In rheumatic valvular disease, fusion of the commissures and secondary calcification cause the valve leaflets to stiffen and retract, resulting in stenosis. If aortic stenosis does occur owing to rheumatic heart disease, mitral valve disease accompanies it. Isolated aortic valve stenosis is almost always nonrheumatic in origin. The incidence of rheumatic aortic valvular disease has been decreasing, but senile or degenerative stenosis is expected to increase as the population ages.

A narrowing or stricture of the aortic valve resulting in obstruction of the flow from the left ventricle to the aorta during systole, **aortic stenosis** causes obstruction of flow from the left ventricle to the aorta during systole. The effect is left ventricular hypertrophy and increased myocardial oxygen consumption because of the increased myocardial mass. As the disease course progresses and compensatory mechanisms fail, reduced CO leads to pulmonary hypertension and HF.

Clinical Manifestations

Symptoms of aortic stenosis (see Table 39-13) develop when the valve orifice becomes approximately one third its normal size. Symptoms include the classic triad of angina, syncope, and exertional dyspnea, reflecting left ventricular failure. The prognosis is poor for a patient with symptoms and whose valve obstruction is not relieved. Use of nitroglycerin is contraindicated for the patient with significant aortic stenosis because it would reduce preload, and preload is necessary to help open the stiffened aortic valve. Auscultation of aortic stenosis typically reveals a normal or soft S1; a diminished or absent S2; a systolic, crescendo–decrescendo murmur that ends before S2; and a prominent fourth heart sound (S4).

Aortic Valve Regurgitation

Etiology and Pathophysiology

Aortic valve regurgitation (AR) may be the result of a primary disease of the aortic valve leaflets, the aortic root, or both. Acute AR is caused by IE, trauma, or aortic dissection and constitutes a life-threatening emergency. Chronic AR is generally the result of rheumatic heart disease, a congenital bicuspid aortic valve, syphilis, or chronic rheumatic conditions such as ankylosing spondylitis or Reiter's syndrome.

AR entails retrograde blood flow from the ascending aorta into the left ventricle resulting in volume overload. The left ventricle initially compensates for chronic AR by dilation and hypertrophy. Myocardial contractility eventually declines, and blood volumes increase in the left atrium and the pulmonary bed. This results in pulmonary hypertension and right ventricular failure.

Clinical Manifestations

Patients with acute AR have sudden clinical manifestations of cardiovascular collapse (see Table 39-13). The left ventricle is exposed to aortic pressure during diastole. The patient develops severe dyspnea, chest pain, hypotension (indicating left ventricular failure), and shock, all of which constitute a medical emergency.

Patients with chronic, severe AR develop a water-hammer pulse (a strong, quick beat that collapses immediately). Heart sounds may include a soft or absent S1, presence of S3 or S4, and a soft, decrescendo high-pitched diastolic murmur. A systolic ejection click may also be heard as well as a low-frequency diastolic murmur known as an *Austin Flint murmur*.

The patient with chronic AR generally remains asymptomatic for years and is seen with exertional dyspnea, orthopnea, and paroxysmal nocturnal dyspnea only after considerable myocardial dysfunction has occurred (see Table 39-13). Angina occurs less frequently than in aortic stenosis.

Tricuspid and Pulmonic Valve Disease

Etiology and Pathophysiology

Diseases of the tricuspid and pulmonic valves are uncommon, with stenosis occurring more frequently than regurgitation. Tricuspid valve stenosis occurs almost exclusively in patients with rheumatic fever, in IV drug users, or in patients who have had multiple myocardial biopsies, radiation treatment, anorectic drugs and who were treated with a dopamine receptor agonist (e.g., pergolide) (Bonow et al., 2008). Pulmonary stenosis is almost always congenital.

Tricuspid and pulmonic stenosis both result in an increase in blood volume in the right atrium and the right ventricle, respectively. Tricuspid stenosis results in right atrial enlargement and elevated systemic venous pressures. Pulmonic stenosis results in right ventricular hypertension and hypertrophy (see Table 39-13).

Diagnostic Studies for Valvular Heart Disease

Diagnosis of valvular heart disease is generally based on the results of history, physical examination, echocardiogram, and cardiac catheterization (especially if surgery is considered) (Table 39-15). Chest radiograph results, ECG findings, and the clinical manifestations exhibited by the patient also aid in establishing the correct diagnosis.

An echocardiogram reveals valve structure, function, and chamber size. Transesophageal echocardiography and Doppler colour-flow imaging are valuable in diagnosing and monitoring the progression of valvular heart disease. Real-time three-dimensional echocardiography may be helpful in qualitative assessments of mitral valve and congenital heart disease (Hung et al., 2007). Cardiac catheterization detects pressure changes in the cardiac chambers, measures pressure gradients across the valves, and quantifies the size of valve openings. An ECG shows heart rate and rhythm and provides information about any ischemia or chamber enlargement. Chest radiograph reveals the heart size, alterations in pulmonary circulation, and calcification of valves.

Collaborative Care of Valvular Heart Disease

Conservative Therapy. An important aspect of conservative management of valvular heart disease is prevention of recurrent

COLLABORATIVE CARE

Table 39-15 Valvular Heart Disease

Diagnostic	• Antidysrhythmic drugs (see Chapter 38, Table 38-8)
• History and physical examination	• Oral nitrates†
• Chest radiograph	• β-Adrenergic blockers (see Chapter 35, Table 35-8)
• ECG	• Percutaneous transluminal balloon valvuloplasty
• Echocardiogram	
• Cardiac catheterization	**Surgical**
Collaborative Therapy	• Valvuloplasty
Nonsurgical	• Closed commissurotomy (valvulotomy)
• Prophylactic antibiotic therapy*	• Open commissurotomy (valvulotomy)
• Rheumatic fever	• Annuloplasty
• Digitalis	• Valve replacement
• Diuretics (see Chapter 35, Table 35-8)	
• Sodium restriction	
• Anticoagulant agents	
• Warfarin (Coumadin)	
• Dipyridamole (Persantine)	
• Aspirin	

ECG, electrocardiogram.
*See Tables 39-4 and 39-5.
†Sublingual nitroglycerin is contraindicated for use in aortic stenosis.

rheumatic fever and IE (see Table 39-15). Treatment depends on the valve involved and the severity of the disease. It focuses on preventing exacerbations of HF, acute pulmonary edema, thromboembolism, and recurrent endocarditis. If manifestations of HF develop, vasodilators, positive inotropes, β-adrenergic blockers, diuretics, and a low-sodium diet are recommended (see Chapter 37). Anticoagulant therapy is used to prevent and treat systemic or pulmonary embolization, and it is also used prophylactically in patients with atrial fibrillation. Atrial dysrhythmias are common and are treated with digoxin, antidysrhythmia drugs, or electrical cardioversion. β-Adrenergic blockers may be used to slow the ventricular response in patients with atrial fibrillation. (Dysrhythmias are discussed in Chapter 38.)

Percutaneous Aortic Valve Replacement. Percutaneous aortic valve replacement is an alternative for selected patients with severe symptomatic aortic stenosis who are at high risk and cannot be treated with traditional surgical intervention. Canada has been a world leader in this technique (Wilson & Webb, 2011). The procedure, performed in the cardiac catheterization laboratory, involves inserting a bioprosthetic valve, which is advanced over a stiff guidewire using a femoral arterial approach.

Percutaneous Transluminal Balloon Valvuloplasty. An alternative treatment for some patients with valvular heart disease is the percutaneous transluminal balloon valvuloplasty (PTBV) procedure, which splits open the fused commissures. PTBV is used for mitral, tricuspid, and pulmonic stenosis, and less often for aortic stenosis. The procedure, performed in the cardiac catheterization laboratory, involves threading a balloon-tipped catheter from the femoral artery or vein to the stenotic valve so that the balloon may be inflated in an attempt to separate the valve leaflets. A single- or double-balloon technique may be used for the PTBV procedure. Currently, the use of a single Inoue balloon with hourglass configuration allows sequential inflation. This technique is the most popular because it is easy, has good results, and has fewer complications (e.g., left ventricular perforation) (Bonow et al., 2008). The PTBV procedure is generally indicated for older adult patients and for patients who are poor surgery candidates. PTBV has fewer complications than valve replacement. The long-term results of PTBV are similar to those of surgical commissurotomy (Bonow et al., 2008).

Surgical Therapy. The decision for surgical intervention is based on the clinical state of the patient. The type of surgery used for a particular patient depends on the valves involved, the valvular pathology, the severity of the disease, and the patient's clinical condition. All types of valve surgery are palliative, not curative, and patients will require lifelong health care. Valve repair is typically the surgical procedure of choice. It is often used in mitral or tricuspid valvular heart disease and has a lower operative mortality rate than replacement. Mitral commissurotomy (valvulotomy) is the procedure of choice for patients with pure mitral stenosis. The less precise closed method of commissurotomy has generally been replaced by the open method in Canada, the United States, and Western Europe. The direct vision, or open, procedure requires the use of cardiopulmonary bypass, removal of thrombi from the atrium, excision of the left atrial appendage, commissure incision, and as indicated, separation of fused chordae, splitting of underlying papillary muscle, and debriding of calcification of the valve. In contrast, the closed procedure is usually performed with the aid of a transventricular dilator inserted through the apex of the left ventricle into the ostium of the mitral valve.

Open surgical valvuloplasty involves repair of the valve by suturing the torn leaflets, chordae tendineae, or papillary muscles. It is primarily used to treat mitral or tricuspid regurgitation. Valve repair avoids the risks of replacement but may not establish total valvular competence. Minimally invasive valvuloplasty surgery, using mini-sternotomy or parasternal approaches, has shown results comparable with those of the open procedure in addition to decreasing length of stay, use of blood transfusions, and postoperative atrial fibrillation (Schmitto, Mokashi, & Cohn, 2010).

Further repair or reconstruction of the valve may be necessary and can be achieved by annuloplasty, a procedure also used in cases of mitral or tricuspid regurgitation. Annuloplasty entails reconstruction of the annulus, with or without the aid of prosthetic rings (e.g., a Carpentier ring).

Prosthetic valves. Valvular replacement may be required for mitral, aortic, tricuspid, and occasionally pulmonic valvular disease. The surgical treatment of choice for combined aortic stenosis and AR is valvular replacement.

A wide variety of prosthetic valves are available for use. Desirable valves are nonthrombogenic and durable and create minimal stenosis. Prosthetic valves are categorized as mechanical or biological (tissue) valves (Table 39-16 and Figure 39-11).

Mechanical valves are manufactured from artificial materials and consist of combinations of metal alloys, Pyrolite carbon, and Dacron. *Biological valves* are constructed from bovine, porcine, and human cardiac tissue and usually contain some artificial

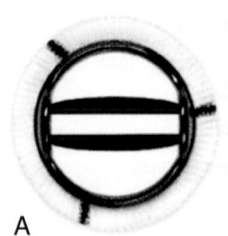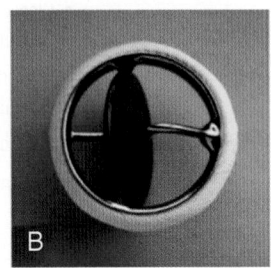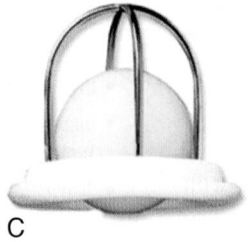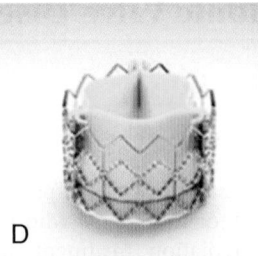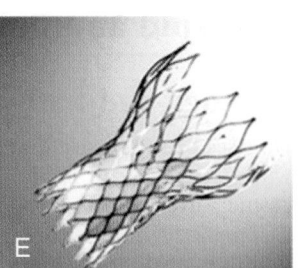

Figure 39-11 Different types of prosthetic heart valves. **A,** Bileaflet mechanical valve (St. Jude Medical, West Berlin, NJ). **B,** Monoleaflet mechanical valve (Medtronic-Hall, Medtronic, Minneapolis). **C,** Caged ball valve (Starr-Edwards). **D,** Transcatheter bioprosthesis expanded over a balloon (Edwards SAPIEN). **E,** Self-expandable percutaneous bioprosthesis (CoreValve, Medtronic).

Source: Pibarot, P., Dumesnil, J. G. (2009). Prosthetic heart valves: Selection of the optimal prosthesis and long-term management. *Circulation, 119,* 1034-1048. doi:10.1161/CIRCULATIONAHA.108.778886

Table 39-16 Types of Cardiac Prosthetic and Tissue Valves

TYPE	DESCRIPTION	ADVANTAGES	DISADVANTAGES
Mechanical			
Caged-ball valve (Starr-Edwards, Sutter, Magovern-Cromie)	Metal cage with several struts mounted on a circular ring; hollow metal or plastic ball (poppet) inside of cage	High durability (≤20 yr)	Possibility of blood clots forming on or around valve (thrombogenic) with risk of embolism Need for long-term anticoagulation therapy Is very large
Tilting-disc valve (Lillehei-Kaster therapy, Hall-Medtronic)	Mobile, lens-shaped disc attached to a circular sewing ring by two offset transverse struts; pyrolytic carbon composition	Hemodynamic efficiency High durability Low thrombogenicity	Need for long-term anticoagulation
Bileaflet valve (St. Jude Medical, Duromedics, CarboMedic)	Two pivoting semicircular discs that open centrally, mounted directly onto a sewing ring	Is compact; successful use in children and patients with small aortic roots	Possibility of thrombogenicity and embolism Need for long-term anticoagulation therapy
Biological			
Porcine heterograft (Hancock, Carpentier-Edwards, Medtronic)	Harvested aortic valve of pig that is preserved in glutaraldehyde and mounted on specially designed sewing ring	Low thrombogenicity Need for anticoagulation therapy for only 3 mo after placement	Limited durability (failure rate increases sharply after 5-7 yr) Cumbersome structural design
Pericardial heterograft (Carpentier-Edwards, Ionescu-Shiley)	Three leaflets composed of pericardium from 16- to 18-mo-old calves that are preserved in glutaraldehyde and mounted on a Dacron-covered frame	Low thrombogenicity Need for only short-term anticoagulation therapy Less resistance to blood flow; useful in patients with small aortic roots; outstanding durability	Early valve failure secondary to calcification and degeneration
Homograft (cadaver valve)	Harvested aortic valve from human cadaver that is initially frozen until needed for valve replacement; then thawed, trimmed, and sewn into place with special mounting material	Excellent hemodynamics No hemolysis and low risk for embolism Only rare need for anticoagulation therapy	Limited durability Not useful for mitral or tricuspid valve replacement

materials. Innovations in freezing and thawing techniques have enabled human grafts to be preserved for extensive periods while retaining viability. Mechanical prosthetic valves are more durable and last longer than biological valves. However, they have an increased risk of thromboembolism, necessitating long-term anticoagulation therapy. The main complication of mechanical valves is hemorrhage from the use of anticoagulants (Bonow et al., 2008). Biological valves do not necessitate anticoagulation therapy thanks to their low thrombogenicity. However, they are less durable because of the tendency for early calcification, tissue degeneration, and stiffening of the leaflets. Problems with either type of prosthetic valves include paravalvular leaks and endocarditis.

Long-term anticoagulation is recommended for all patients with mechanical valves and for those with biological valves who have atrial fibrillation. Some patients with biological valves or annuloplasty with prosthetic rings may need anticoagulation the first few months after surgery until the suture lines are covered by endothelial cells (endothelialized).

The choice of valves depends on many factors. For example, if a patient cannot take an anticoagulant (e.g., women of child-bearing age), a biological valve may be considered. A mechanical valve may be best for a younger patient because it is more durable. For patients older than age 65, durability is less important than the risks of hemorrhage from anticoagulants.

NURSING MANAGEMENT: VALVULAR DISORDERS

Nursing Assessment

Subjective and objective data should be obtained from an individual with valvular disease and are presented in Table 39-17.

Nursing Diagnoses

Nursing diagnoses for the patient with valvular disease may include, but are not limited to, those presented in NCP 39-1.

NURSING ASSESSMENT

Table 39-17 Valvular Heart Disease

Subjective Data

Important Health Information

Past health history: Rheumatic fever, endocarditis, congenital defects, myocardial infarction, chest trauma, cardiomyopathy, syphilis, Marfan syndrome, staphylococcal or streptococcal infections, HIV status or immunocompromised.

Medications

IV drug abuse

Symptoms

- Fatigue, generalized weakness, activity intolerance
- Palpitations, dizziness, fainting
- Dyspnea on exertion, cough, hemoptysis, orthopnea, paroxysmal nocturnal dyspnea
- Anginal or atypical chest pain

Objective Data

General

Fever

Integumentary

Diaphoresis, flushing, cyanosis, clubbing; peripheral edema

Respiratory

Crackles, wheezes, hoarseness

Cardiovascular

Abnormal heart sounds, including opening snaps, clicks, thrills, systolic and diastolic murmurs, S3, and S4; dysrhythmias, including premature atrial contraction, atrial fibrillation; tachycardia; ↑ or ↓ in pulse pressure; hypotension, water-hammer or thready peripheral pulses, brisk carotid pulses

Gastrointestinal

Ascites, hepatomegaly

HIV, human immunodeficiency virus; *IV,* intravenous; S3, third heart sound; S4, fourth heart sound.

◼ Planning

The overall goals for the patient with valvular heart disease include (1) normal cardiac function, (2) improved activity tolerance, and (3) an understanding of the disease process and health maintenance measures.

◼ Nursing Implementation

◼ Health Promotion

Diagnosing and treating streptococcal infections and providing prophylactic antibiotics for patients with a history of rheumatic fever are critical to prevent acquired rheumatic valvular disease. The patient at high risk for endocarditis and any patient with valvular prosthesis must also be treated with prophylactic antibiotics (see Table 39-4).

The patient must adhere to recommended therapies. The individual with a history of rheumatic fever, endocarditis, and congenital heart disease should know the symptoms suggestive of valvular heart disease so that early medical treatment may be obtained.

◼ Acute Intervention and Ambulatory and Home Care

A patient with progressive valvular heart disease may require hospitalization or outpatient care for management of HF, endocarditis, embolic disease, or dysrhythmias. HF is the most common reason for an ongoing need for medical care.

The role of the nurse is to implement and evaluate the effectiveness of therapeutic management. Activity should be designed after considering the patient's limitations. An appropriate exercise plan can increase cardiac tolerance. However, activities that regularly produce fatigue and dyspnea should be restricted, and an explanation should be provided to the patient. Smoking cessation should be discussed and encouraged. Strenuous physical exercise should be avoided because damaged valves may not be able to handle the required increase in CO. The patient should be assisted in planning activities of daily living, with an emphasis on conserving energy, setting priorities, and taking planned rest periods. Referral to a vocational counsellor may be necessary if the patient has a physically or emotionally demanding job.

Auscultation of the heart should be performed to monitor the effectiveness of digoxin, β-adrenergic blockers, and antidysrhythmic drugs. Teaching regarding the actions and adverse effects of drugs is important to achieve compliance. The patient must understand the importance of prophylactic antibiotic therapy to prevent IE (see Table 39-3). If the valve disease was caused by rheumatic fever, ongoing prophylaxis to prevent recurrence is necessary.

When valvular heart disease can no longer be managed medically, surgical intervention is necessary. The patient who is on anticoagulation therapy after surgery for valve replacement must have the international normalized ratio (INR) checked regularly (usually monthly) to assess the adequacy of therapy. The INR is a standardized system of reporting prothrombin time. Values of 2.5 to 3.5 are therapeutic for patients with mechanical valves.

The patient must realize that valve surgery is not a cure and that regular follow-up examinations by the health care provider will be required. The nurse also must teach the patient about when to seek medical care. Any manifestations of infection or HF, any signs of bleeding, and any planned invasive or dental procedures require the patient to notify the health care provider. Finally, patients should be encouraged to wear medical alert identification (e.g., bracelet).

◼ Evaluation

The expected outcomes for a patient with valvular heart disease are addressed in NCP 39-1.

Cardiomyopathy

Cardiomyopathy (CMP) constitutes a group of diseases that directly affect the structural or functional ability of the myocardium. A diagnosis of CMP is made based on the patient's clinical manifestations and noninvasive and invasive diagnostic procedures.

CMP can be classified as primary or secondary. *Primary CMP* refers to those conditions in which the etiology of the heart disease is unknown (idiopathic). The heart muscle in this case is the only portion of the heart involved; other cardiac structures are unaffected. In *secondary CMP,* the cause of the myocardial disease is

NURSING CARE PLAN 39-1

Valvular Heart Disease

NURSING DIAGNOSIS	**Activity intolerance** *related to* insufficient oxygenation secondary to decreased cardiac output and pulmonary congestion *as evidenced by* weakness, fatigue, shortness of breath, increase or decrease in pulse rate, and BP changes
Expected Patient Outcomes	**Nursing Interventions and *Rationales***
• Demonstrates cardiac tolerance to increased activity (e.g., stable pulse, respirations, and BP)	• Assess and monitor patient responses to activity (e.g., pulse rate, respirations, BP) *to plan appropriate interventions.* • Plan rest periods between activities *to conserve energy and decrease cardiac demands.* • Organize care *to minimize unnecessary disturbance.* • Progressively increase activity *to increase cardiac tolerance.*
NURSING DIAGNOSIS	**Excess fluid volume** *related to* cardiac failure secondary to incompetent valves *as evidenced by* peripheral edema, weight gain, increased BP and pulse, and adventitious breath sounds
Expected Patient Outcomes	**Nursing Interventions and *Rationales***
• Has normal BP and pulse • Has normal breath sounds • Exhibits no peripheral edema	• Monitor for manifestations of hypervolemia such as peripheral edema; taut, shiny skin; and adventitious breath sounds *to detect hypervolemia.* • Assess vital signs, auscultate breath sounds, assess for jugular distension, measure intake and output, palpate for edema, and assess for weight gain (>0.9 kg/day or >2.3 kg/wk) *to monitor indicators of hypervolemia.* • Restrict sodium as ordered *to prevent fluid retention.*
NURSING DIAGNOSIS	**Decreased cardiac output** *related to* valvular incompetence *as evidenced by* heart murmurs, dyspnea, tachycardia, or dysrhythmias
Expected Patient Outcomes	**Nursing Interventions and *Rationales***
• Reports no fatigue • Has normal heart rate and rhythm • Has normal breath sounds	• Monitor BP, apical pulse, respirations, breath and heart sounds *to assess for signs of decreased cardiac output such as fatigue, malaise, shortness of breath, dyspnea on exertion, palpitations, angina, vertigo, heart murmur, and widened pulse pressure.* • Maintain rest as ordered *to decrease cardiac workload and O₂ demands.* • Elevate head of bed 30 to 40 degrees *to reduce venous return, reduce O₂ demand, and maximize chest excursion.* • Administer O₂ as ordered *to improve O₂ saturation.* • Monitor cardiac rhythm *to detect changes from baseline.* • Administer inotropic medication as ordered *to increase myocardial contractility.*
NURSING DIAGNOSIS	**Ineffective self-health management** *related to* lack of knowledge about disease process and prevention and treatment strategies *as evidenced by* lack of compliance with therapeutic regimen
Expected Patient Outcomes	**Nursing Interventions and *Rationales***
• Knows signs and symptoms that indicate a need to seek health care • Recognizes needs and knows when to use prophylactic antibiotics • Adheres to therapeutic regimen	• Explain nature and cause of disease process *to ensure patient has adequate knowledge base.* • Teach signs and symptoms of heart failure and infective endocarditis *to ensure early reporting and treatment of complications.* • Teach the need to avoid all invasive surgical or diagnostic procedures *that may predispose to bacteremia until prophylactic antibiotics have been given.* • Explain the importance of notifying dentist, urologist, gynecologist, and other health care providers of valvular disease *so prophylactic antibiotic treatment can be initiated.* • Discourage smoking *to prevent an increased cardiac workload and the oxygen-depleting effect of carbon monoxide from decreasing the O₂ available to all tissues.* • Discuss the name of prescribed medication and dosage, purpose, and adverse effects *to promote safe and accurate self-medication.* • Instruct patient to wear medical identification.

BP, blood pressure.

ETHICAL DILEMMAS
Do Not Resuscitate

Situation

A 68-year-old man has been admitted for a second mitral valve surgery and possible coronary artery bypass graft surgery. He did not adhere to the treatment plan following his original surgery 7 years ago. The nurse is worried about his future adherence to medication, diet, and exercise regimens. His kidneys are failing and he is on dialysis, but not tolerating it well. Both the patient and the family want complete therapeutic treatment and refuse to discuss do not resuscitate (DNR) orders.

Important Points for Consideration

- Nonadherence to the treatment plan in the past does not always indicate the patient will not follow the plan of care in the future.
- A competent patient can decide whether he wants continued treatment to be able to fight to live. This is even more important when family members support the patient's decision.
- Health care providers have an obligation to respect the patient's request for treatment unless there is no clear benefit to continued treatment. Patients' choices to continue or end treatment are based on their values and beliefs, which may not always coincide with those of the health care provider or team.
- DNR orders should reflect the patient's expressed wishes either through conversation, advance directives, or a surrogate decision maker.
- DNR orders should be re-evaluated periodically with the patient and family, especially before major diagnostic procedures or treatments.
- If a health care provider does not agree with a patient's treatment choice, the nurse should respect the patient's choice and ask the patient to "tell me more about your situation and decision" (Registered Nurses' Association of Ontario, *Best Practice Guideline: Client Centred Care*, 2006). The nurse should communicate the patient's choice to the health care team and a referral should be made to an Ethics Committee or similar group as appropriate.

Clinical Decision-Making Questions

1. What type of information should be provided to a patient and family in discussions about DNR orders? Who should provide this information?
2. What measures or strategies would be beneficial to assist the patient to better adhere to the treatment plan?

Table 39-18 Causes of Secondary Cardiomyopathy

Dilated	Hypertrophic
- Cardiotoxic agents—alcohol, cocaine, doxorubicin (Adriamycin)	- Aortic stenosis
	- Genetic (autosomal dominant)
- Genetic (autosomal dominant) or familial	- Hypertension
	Restrictive
- Hypertension	- Amyloidosis
- Ischemia (coronary artery disease)	- Endomyocardial fibrosis
- Metabolic disorders	- Neoplastic tumour
- Muscular dystrophy	- Post–radiation therapy
- Myocarditis	- Sarcoidosis
- Pregnancy	- Ventricular thrombus
- Valve disease	

Table 39-19 Comparison of Cardiomyopathies

DILATED	HYPERTROPHIC	RESTRICTIVE
Major Manifestations		
Fatigue, weakness, palpitations, dyspnea	Exertional dyspnea, fatigue, angina, syncope, palpitations	Dyspnea, fatigue
Cardiomegaly: moderate to marked	Mild to moderate	Mild
Contractility		
↓	↑ or ↓	Normal or ↓
Valvular Incompetence		
Atrioventricular valves, particularly mitral	Mitral valve	Atrioventricular valves
Dysrhythmias		
Sinoatrial tachycardia, atrial and ventricular dysrhythmias	Atrial and ventricular dysrhythmias	Atrial and ventricular dysrhythmias
Cardiac Output		
↓	Normal or ↓	Normal or ↓
Outflow Tract Obstruction		
None	↑	None

known and is secondary to another disease process. Common causes of secondary CMP are listed in Table 39-18. Each type has its own pathogenesis, clinical presentation, and treatment protocols (Tables 39-19 and 39-20). CMPs can lead to cardiomegaly and CHF and are the leading reason for heart transplantation.

Dilated Cardiomyopathy

Etiology and Pathophysiology

Dilated cardiomyopathy is the most common type of CMP. It causes HF in 25 to 40% of cases and has a genetic link in 25 to 35% of cases (Luk, Ahn, Soor, & Butany, 2009). Dilated CMP is characterized by a diffuse inflammation and rapid degeneration of myocardial fibres that results in ventricular dilation, impairment of systolic function, atrial enlargement, and stasis of blood in the left ventricle. Cardiomegaly results from ventricular dilation (Figure 39-12) and causes contractile dysfunction in spite of an enlarged chamber size. In contrast to HF, the walls of the ventricles do not hypertrophy (Figure 39-13).

Dilated CMP often follows an infectious myocarditis. Other common causes of dilated CMP are listed in Table 39-18.

Clinical Manifestations

The signs and symptoms of dilated CMP may develop acutely after an infectious process or insidiously over time. Most people eventually develop HF. Symptoms can include decreased exercise

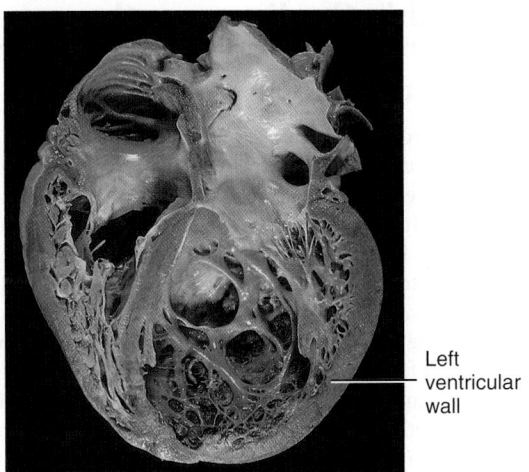

Figure 39-12 Dilated cardiomyopathy. The dilated left ventricular wall has thinned, and the chamber size and volume are increased.

Source: Kumar, V., Abbas, A. K., Fausto, N., & Aster, J. (2010). *Robbins and Cotran pathologic basis of disease* (8th ed., p. 572, Figure 12-31, *A*). Philadelphia: Saunders.

COLLABORATIVE CARE

Table 39-20 Cardiomyopathy

Diagnostic	*Collaborative Therapy*
• History and physical examination	• Treatment of underlying cause
• Electrocardiogram	• Drug therapy
• Serum laboratory tests	• Nitrates (except in HCM)
• Chest radiograph	• β-Adrenergic blockers
• Echocardiogram	• Antidysrhythmics
• Nuclear imaging studies	• ACE inhibitors
• Cardiac catheterization	• Diuretics
• Endocardial biopsy	• Digitalis (except in HCM with normal sinus rhythm)
	• Anticoagulants (if indicated)
	• Ventricular assist device
	• Cardiac resynchronization therapy
	• Implantable cardioverter–defibrillator
	• Surgical correction
	• Cardiac transplant

ACE, angiotensin-converting enzyme; *HCM,* hypertrophic cardiomyopathy.

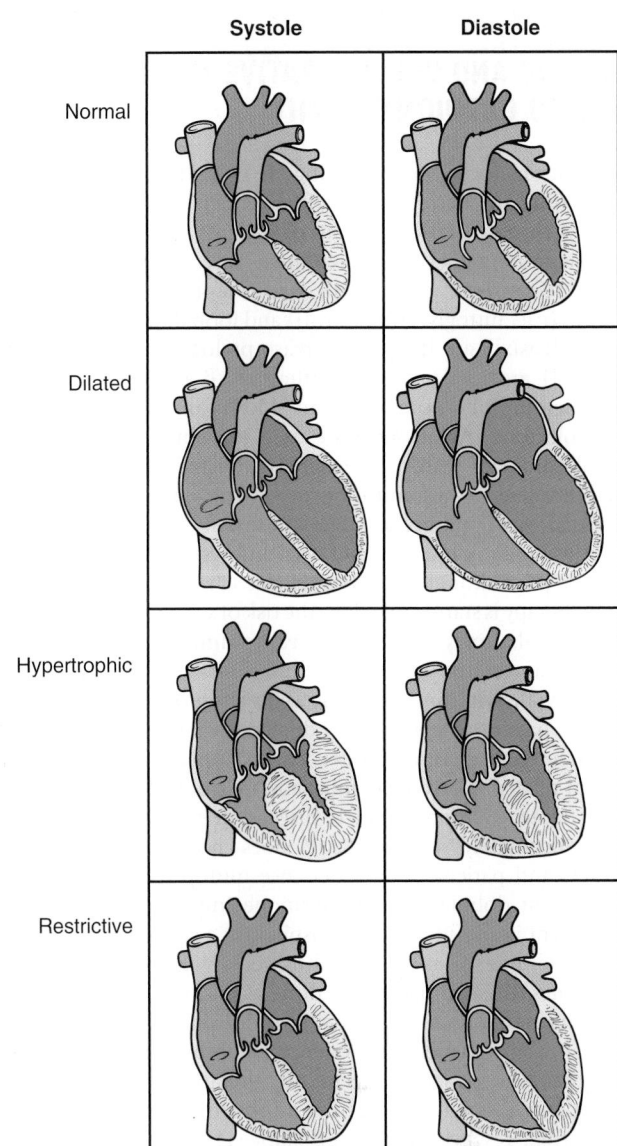

Figure 39-13 Types of cardiomyopathies and the differences in ventricular diameter during systole and diastole, compared with a normal heart.

Source: Adapted from Urden, L. D., Stacy, K. M., & Lough, M. E. (2010). *Critical care nursing: Diagnosis and management* (6th ed., p. 466, Figure 19-18). St. Louis: Mosby.

capacity, fatigue, dyspnea at rest, paroxysmal nocturnal dyspnea, and orthopnea. As the disease progresses, the patient may experience dry cough, palpitations, abdominal bloating, nausea, vomiting, and anorexia. Signs can include an irregular heart rate with an abnormal S3 and/or S4, tachycardia or bradycardia, pulmonary crackles, edema, weak peripheral pulses, pallor, hepatomegaly, and jugular venous distension. Heart murmurs and dysrhythmias are common. Decreased blood flow through an enlarged heart promotes stasis and blood clot formation and may lead to systemic embolization.

Diagnostic Studies

The diagnosis of dilated CMP is made on the basis of the patient's history and by ruling out other conditions that cause CHF.

Doppler echocardiography provides the basis for the diagnosis of dilated CMP in the majority of patients and distinguishes dilated CMP from other structural abnormalities. The chest radiograph may show cardiomegaly with signs of pulmonary venous hypertension as well as pleural effusion. The ECG may reveal tachycardia, bradycardia, and dysrhythmias with conduction disturbances. Laboratory studies may reveal elevated serum levels of B-type natriuretic peptide (BNP or NT-Pro-BNP) in the presence of HF.

Cardiac catheterization is done to confirm or rule out coronary artery disease, and multigated acquisition radionuclide angiocardiographies (MUGAs) are done to determine ejection fraction (EF). EFs of less than 20% are associated with a 50% mortality within 1 year. EMB may be done at the time of the right-sided heart catheterization to detect viral antigens in myocardial tissue.

NURSING AND COLLABORATIVE MANAGEMENT: DILATED CARDIOMYOPATHY

Interventions focus on controlling HF by enhancing myocardial contractility and decreasing afterload. This is similar to the treatment of chronic CHF. Treatment of patients with Class IV, Stage D HF is more palliative than curative. Several different types of drugs are used to manage HF (see Chapter 37, Table 37-9). Nitrates (e.g., nitroglycerin [Nitrol]) and loop diuretics (e.g., furosemide [Lasix]) are used to decrease preload, and ACEIs (e.g., captopril) are used to reduce afterload. β-Adrenergic blockers (e.g., metoprolol [Lopressor]) and aldosterone antagonists (e.g., spironolactone [Aldactone]) are used to control the neurohormonal stimulation that occurs in HF. Digoxin is used to treat atrial fibrillation but must be used with caution because of increased susceptibility to digoxin toxicity in these patients. Other dysrhythmias are treated with antidysrhythmics (e.g., amiodarone [Cordarone]) as indicated (see Chapter 38). Anticoagulation therapy is started to reduce the risk of systemic embolization from clots that may form in the heart chambers.

Drug and nutritional therapy and cardiac rehabilitation may help alleviate symptoms of HF as well as improve CO and quality of life. A patient with secondary dilated CMP must be treated for the underlying disease process. For example, the patient with alcohol-related dilated CMP must abstain from all alcohol intake. (See Chapter 37 for a complete discussion of HF.)

Unfortunately, dilated CMP does not respond well to therapy, and patients may experience multiple episodes of HF. Intermittent dobutamine or milrinone infusions can be used. The patient is admitted to the hospital for a continuous infusion of dobutamine or milrinone followed by aggressive diuresis. Sometimes, these infusions are done as an outpatient treatment or in the home under supervision of a home care nurse. After infusion, many patients experience an improvement in symptoms that lasts for several weeks after therapy.

Patients also may benefit from nonpharmacological therapies such cardiac resynchronization therapy (Howlett et al., 2009) or a ventricular assist device (VAD) that may allow the heart to rest and recover from acute HF or as a bridge to heart transplantation. The patient with terminal end-stage CMP may be considered for heart transplantation or destination therapy with a permanent or implantable VAD (see Chapter 37). Currently, approximately 50% of heart transplantations are performed for treatment of CMP. Cardiac transplant recipients have a good prognosis for survival. However, donor hearts are difficult to obtain, and many patients with dilated CMP die while awaiting heart transplantation.

Patients with dilated CMP are very ill people with a grave prognosis who need expert nursing care. The patient's family must learn cardiopulmonary resuscitation (CPR) and how to access emergency care. The nurse should include family members and other support systems when planning a patient's care.

Home health and hospice nursing can provide the patient and the family with the continuous assessments and therapeutic interventions that are required to maximize and maintain functional status or prepare for a peaceful death. Observing for signs and symptoms of worsening HF, dysrhythmias, and embolic formation is paramount in this patient, as is monitoring drug responsiveness. The goal of therapy is to keep the patient at an optimal level of function and out of the hospital.

Hypertrophic Cardiomyopathy

Etiology and Pathophysiology

Hypertrophic cardiomyopathy (HCM), formerly called *idiopathic hypertrophic subaortic stenosis or asymmetrical septal hypertrophy* (ASH), is asymmetrical left ventricular hypertrophy without ventricular dilation. In one form of the disease, the septum between the two ventricles becomes enlarged and obstructs the blood flow from the left ventricle. Historically, HCM has been termed *hypertrophic obstructive cardiomyopathy* (HOCM), which may be misleading because one third of all patients with HCM have a nonobstructive left ventricular outflow tract (LVOT) at rest or with exertion. HCM can be idiopathic, although about one half of all cases have a genetic basis characterized by inappropriate myocardial hypertrophy (see Table 39-18). HCM occurs less commonly than dilated CMP and is more common in men ages 30 to 40 than in women. In one review, HCM occurred more frequently in young Black male athletes than in young White male athletes. The four main characteristics of HCM are (1) massive ventricular hypertrophy; (2) rapid, forceful contraction of the left ventricle; (3) impaired relaxation (diastolic dysfunction); and (4) obstruction of LVOT (not present in all patients). Ventricular hypertrophy is associated with a thickened intraventricular septum and ventricular wall (Figure 39-14). The end result is impaired ventricular filling as the ventricle becomes noncompliant and unable to relax. The primary defect of HCM is diastolic dysfunction from left ventricular stiffness. Decreased ventricular filling and obstruction to outflow can result in decreased CO, especially during exertion. HCM is the most common cause of SCD in otherwise healthy young people. It is usually diagnosed in young adulthood and is often seen in active, athletic individuals (Maron, Doerer, Haas, Tierney, & Mueller, 2009; Cross, Estes, & Link, 2011).

Clinical Manifestations

Patients with HCM may be asymptomatic or may have exertional dyspnea, fatigue, angina, and syncope. The most common

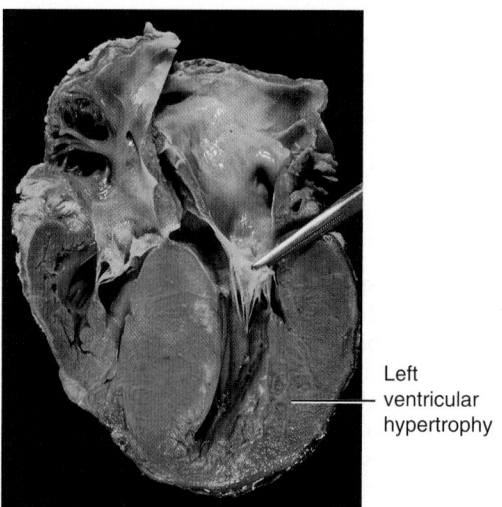

Left ventricular hypertrophy

Figure 39-14 Hypertrophic cardiomyopathy. There is marked left ventricular hypertrophy, and the chamber size and volume are decreased.

Source: Kumar, V., Abbas, A. K., Fausto, N., & Aster, J. (2010). *Robbins and Cotran pathologic basis of disease* (8th ed., p. 576, Figure 12-35, *A*). Philadelphia: Saunders.

symptom is dyspnea, which is caused by an elevated left ventricular diastolic pressure. Fatigue occurs because of the resultant decrease in CO and in exercise-induced flow obstruction. Angina can occur and is most often caused by the increased left ventricular muscle mass or compression of the small coronary arteries by the hypercontractile ventricular myocardium. The patient may also have syncope, especially during exertion. Syncope is most often caused by an increase in obstruction to aortic outflow during increased activity, resulting in decreased CO and cerebrovascular circulation. Syncope can also be caused by dysrhythmias. Common dysrhythmias include supraventricular tachycardia, atrial fibrillation, ventricular tachycardia, and ventricular fibrillation. Any of these dysrhythmias may lead to loss of consciousness or SCD (see Chapter 36).

Diagnostic Studies

Clinical findings on examination may be unremarkable. However, on palpation of the chest, there may be a forced apical impulse that may be displaced laterally. Auscultation may reveal an S4 and a systolic ejection murmur between the apex and the sternal border at the fourth intercostal space. ECG findings usually indicate ventricular hypertrophy, ST-T–wave abnormalities, prominent Q waves in the inferior or precordial leads, left axis deviation, and ventricular and atrial dysrhythmias (see Chapter 38).

The echocardiogram is the primary diagnostic tool to confirm the classic feature of HCM, which is left ventricular hypertrophy. The echocardiogram may also demonstrate wall motion abnormalities and diastolic dysfunction. Cardiac catheterization may also be helpful in the diagnosis of HCM.

NURSING AND COLLABORATIVE MANAGEMENT: HYPERTROPHIC CARDIOMYOPATHY

Goals of intervention are to improve ventricular filling by reducing ventricular contractility and relieving LVOT obstruction. These can be accomplished with the use of β-adrenergic blockers, such as metoprolol (Lopressor), or calcium channel blockers, such as verapamil. Use of digitalis preparations is contraindicated unless they are used to treat atrial fibrillation. Antidysrhythmics, such as amiodarone or sotalol, are effective medications for dysrhythmias. However, their use has not been shown to prevent SCD. For patients at risk for SCD, the implantation of a cardioverter–defibrillator is recommended (see Chapter 38).

It has been found that AV pacing can be beneficial for patients with HCM and LVOT obstruction. By pacing the ventricles from the apex of the right ventricle, septal depolarization occurs first, allowing the septum to move away from the left ventricular wall and reducing the degree of obstruction of the LVOT.

Some patients may be candidates for surgical treatment of their hypertrophied septum. The indications for surgery include severe symptoms refractory to therapy with marked obstruction at rest to aortic outflow (>50 mm Hg). The surgery is termed a *ventriculomyotomy and myectomy*. It involves incision of the hypertrophied septal muscle and resection of some of the hypertrophied ventricular muscle. Most patients have good symptomatic improvement and improved exercise tolerance after surgery.

An alternate, nonsurgical procedure to reduce symptoms and the LVOT obstruction is alcohol-induced, percutaneous transluminal septal myocardial ablation (PTSMA). This procedure consists of administering alcohol into the first septal artery branching off the left anterior descending artery, which causes ischemia and septal wall myocardial infarction. Ablation of the septal wall will decrease the flow obstruction, and the patient's symptoms will decrease. The procedure improves HF symptoms and exercise capacity 3 months after ablation. Mortality rates for the procedure are approximately 1% depending on the age and condition of the patient. Information on long-term effects of PTSMA in treated patients is lacking because of the newness of the procedure. Potential complications of PTSMA include conduction disturbances (e.g., heart block) and MI beyond the intended septum.

Nursing interventions for HCM focus on relieving symptoms, observing for and preventing complications, and providing emotional and psychological support. Teaching should focus on helping patients adjust their lifestyle to avoid strenuous activity and dehydration. Any activity or procedure that causes an increase in systemic vascular resistance (thus increasing the obstruction to forward flow) is dangerous and should be avoided. HCM patients who experience chest pain are managed by rest and elevation of the feet to improve venous return to the heart. Vasodilators such as nitroglycerin may worsen the chest pain by decreasing venous return to the heart, which would further increase obstruction of blood flow from the heart.

Restrictive Cardiomyopathy

Etiology and Pathophysiology

Restrictive CMP is the least common of the cardiomyopathic conditions. It is a disease of the heart muscle that impairs diastolic filling and stretch (see Figure 39-13). Systolic function remains unaffected. Although the specific etiology of restrictive CMP is unknown, a number of pathological processes may be involved in its development. Myocardial fibrosis, hypertrophy, and infiltration produce stiffness of the ventricular wall with loss of ventricular compliance. Secondary causes of restrictive CMP include amyloidosis, endocardial fibrosis, sarcoidosis, fibrosis of different etiology, and radiation to the thorax. With restrictive CMP, the ventricles are resistant to filling and, therefore, demand high diastolic filling pressures to maintain CO.

Clinical Manifestations

Classic symptoms of restrictive CMP are fatigue, exercise intolerance, and dyspnea because the heart cannot increase CO by increasing the heart rate without further compromising ventricular filling. Additional symptoms may include angina, orthopnea, syncope, and palpitations. The patient may have signs of HF, including dyspnea, peripheral edema, ascites, hepatomegaly, and jugular venous distension.

Diagnostic Studies

The chest radiograph may be normal, or it may show cardiomegaly from right and left atrial enlargement. Pleural effusions and pulmonary congestion may be evident in the patient with progression to HF. The ECG may reveal a mild tachycardia at rest. The most common dysrhythmias are supraventricular (atrial fibrillation) or AV block. Echocardiography may reveal a left ventricle that is of normal size with a thickened wall, slightly dilated right ventricle, and dilated atria. EMB, CT, and nuclear imaging may be helpful in the diagnosis.

NURSING AND COLLABORATIVE MANAGEMENT: RESTRICTIVE CARDIOMYOPATHY

Currently, no specific treatment for restrictive CMP exists. Interventions are aimed at improving diastolic filling and the underlying disease process. Treatment includes conventional therapy for HF and dysrhythmias. Heart transplant may also be a consideration. Nursing care is similar to the care of a patient with HF. As in the treatment of patients with HCM, the patient should be taught to avoid situations that impair ventricular filling, such as strenuous activity, dehydration, and increases in systemic vascular resistance.

Nursing care of a patient with CMP includes individualized teaching based on the patient's clinical manifestations. All patients with CMP are at risk for IE from any procedure that may cause bacteremia and should be instructed on the need for prophylactic antibiotics (see Table 39-3). A general patient and caregiver teaching guide is presented in Table 39-21.

PATIENT & CAREGIVER TEACHING GUIDE
Table 39-21 Cardiomyopathy

- Instruct patient to take all medications as prescribed and to follow up with health care provider.
- Encourage patient to use a low-sodium diet (if ordered) and to read all product labels (food and over-the-counter drugs) for sodium content.
- Unless fluids are restricted, patient should be encouraged to drink 6 to 8 glasses of water a day.
- Encourage patient to achieve and maintain a reasonable weight and avoid large meals.
- Advise patient to avoid alcohol, caffeine, diet pills, and over-the-counter cold medicines that may contain stimulants.
- Teach patient to balance activity and rest periods.
- Instruct patient to avoid heavy lifting or vigorous isometric exercises and to check with health care provider for exercise guidelines.
- Encourage the use of stress reduction activities: relaxation to relieve tension, guided imagery, diversional activities (see Chapter 8).
- Instruct patient to report any signs of heart failure to health care provider, including weight gain, edema, shortness of breath, and increased fatigue.
- Suggest that family members learn CPR because of the potential of sudden cardiac arrest.
- Instruct patient to notify health care provider or dentist before any invasive medical or dental procedures since patients with cardiomyopathy are at risk for endocarditis (see Table 39-3).

CPR, cardiopulmonary resuscitation.

CLINICAL DECISION-MAKING EXERCISE

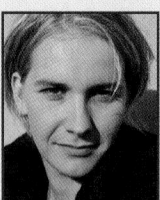

CASE STUDY:
Valvular Heart Disease

Source: © iStockphoto.com/Kati Neudert.

Patient Profile
Ms. Halderson, a 35-year-old woman, is admitted to the hospital for valvular heart disease.

Subjective Data
- Reports history of IV drug use
- Prior hospital admission for IE
- Must sleep sitting up
- Shortness of breath, even with dressing self
- Takes "water pill" for her "pressure"
- Smokes a pack of cigarettes a day

Objective Data
Physical Examination
- S3
- Loud holosystolic murmur of MR
- Pitting pretibial and pedal edema
- Irregular pulse; apical pulse rate and radial pulse rate

Diagnostic Studies
- Two-dimensional echocardiogram shows left atrial and ventricular enlargement and flail valve leaflets.
- ECG shows atrial fibrillation and enlarged left ventricle and atrium.
- Chest radiograph reveals pulmonary congestion.

Discussion Questions
1. Identify the cause and course of Ms. Halderson's disease based on her history and current examination.
2. Differentiate between acute and chronic MR.
3. What surgical procedure will Ms. Halderson probably require as her condition worsens?
4. *Priority Decision:* Identify three priority nursing interventions for Ms. Halderson.
5. *Priority Decision:* On the basis of the assessment data provided, identify at least three priority nursing diagnoses.

ⓔvolve *Answers are available at* **http://evolve.elsevier.com/ Canada/Lewis/medsurg**

REVIEW QUESTIONS

The number of the question corresponds to the same-numbered objective at the beginning of the chapter.

1. A patient with a history of intravenous (IV) cocaine use has acute infective endocarditis (IE). For signs and symptoms of which of the following does the nurse closely assess the patient?
   a. Weight gain
   b. A new murmur
   c. A distended abdomen
   d. Red spots on the chest

2. Nursing assessment findings for acute pericarditis include which of the following?
   a. Wheezing and dull precordial pain
   b. Bradycardia, tachypnea, and murmur
   c. Chest pain, dyspnea, and pericardial friction rub
   d. Respiratory stridor, dull chest pain, and abdominal discomfort

3. Prophylactic antibiotics are indicated to prevent IE for which of the following at-risk individuals?
   a. Those with a history of IE.
   b. Those having a viral respiratory infection.
   c. Those entering the third trimester of pregnancy.
   d. Those exposed to human immunodeficiency virus.

4. What is the most common cause of myocarditis?
   a. Heart failure
   b. A viral infection
   c. A bacterial infection
   d. A myocardial infarction

5. Teaching the patient with rheumatic fever about the disease, the nurse explains that rheumatic fever is which of the following?
   a. A *Streptococcus viridans* infection
   b. A viral infection of endocardium and valves
   c. A sequel of β-hemolytic streptococcal infection
   d. Frequently triggered by immunosuppressive therapy

6. A patient with rheumatic fever should be taught about the need for which of the following?
   a. Regular exercise
   b. Antibiotic therapy
   c. A high-protein diet
   d. Anticoagulant therapy

7. What is a common cause of aortic valve stenosis in older adults?
   a. Rheumatic fever
   b. Cardiomyopathy
   c. Congenital heart disease
   d. Acute infective endocarditis

8. Which of the following findings is indicative of left ventricular overload in a patient with chronic aortic regurgitation?
   a. Dehydration and a pericardial friction rub
   b. An audible third heart sound and a midsystolic murmur
   c. Exertional dyspnea and a diastolic high-pitched murmur
   d. An audible third heart sound and a pansystolic or holosystolic murmur

9. A patient hospitalized with aortic stenosis has a nursing diagnosis of activity intolerance related to insufficient oxygen secondary to decreased cardiac output. Which of the following is an appropriate nursing intervention for this patient?
   a. Monitor electrocardiogram to assess cardiac output.
   b. Maintain on bed rest to reduce tissue oxygen demands.
   c. Progressively increase activity to increase cardiac tolerance.
   d. Use semi-Fowler's position to decrease venous return and increase respiratory excursion.

10. What does the nurse caring for a patient scheduled for a mitral valve replacement with a mechanical valve understand about this procedure?
    a. It is similar to a commissurotomy.
    b. It requires long-term anticoagulation therapy.
    c. It is the treatment of choice for an older adult patient with a history of falling.
    d. It involves the insertion of a transventricular dilator into the opening of the valve.

11. Which of the following assessment findings would the nurse expect in a patient with dilated cardiomyopathy?
    a. Dyspnea and fatigue
    b. Wheezing and epigastric pain
    c. Palpitations and left lower quadrant tenderness
    d. Excessive sputum and lower abdominal cramping

12. The nurse plans care for the patient with dilated cardiomyopathy based on knowledge of which of the following?
    a. Family members may be at risk because of the infectious nature of the disease.
    b. Medical management of the disorder focuses on treatment of the underlying cause.
    c. The prognosis of the patient is poor, and emotional support is a high priority of care.
    d. The condition may be successfully treated with surgical ventriculomyotomy and septal ablation.

ANSWERS: 1. b; 2. c; 3. a; 4. b; 5. c; 6. b; 7. a; 8. c; 9. c; 10. b; 11. a; 12. c.

REFERENCES

Bonow, R., Carabello, B., Chatterjee, K., de Leon, A., Fraxon, P., & Freed, M. (2008). Focused update incorporated into the ACC/AHA 2006 guidelines for the management of patients with valvular heart disease: A report of the American College of Cardiology/American Heart Association Task Force on Practice Guidelines (Writing Committee to Develop Guidelines for the Management of Patients With Valvular Heart Disease). *Circulation, 118*, e523-e661. doi:10.1161/CIRCULATIONAHA.108.190748

Cooper, L. (2009). Myocarditis. *New England Journal of Medicine, 360*(15), 1526-1538. doi:10.1056/NEJMra0800028

Cross, B., Estes, N., & Link, M. (2011). Sudden cardiac death in young athletes and nonathletes. *Current Opinion in Critical Care, 17*(4), 328-334. doi:10.1097/MCC.0b013e328348bf84

Dajani, A., Ayoub, E., Bierman, F., Bisno, A., Denny, F., Durack, D., ..., Wilson, W. (1992). Guidelines for the diagnosis of rheumatic fever. Jones Criteria, 1992 update. *Journal of the American Medical Association, 268*(15), 2069-2073. doi:10.1001/jama.1992.03490150121036

Futterman, L., & Lemberg, L. (2006). Pericarditis. *American Journal of Critical Care, 15*(6), 626.

Gerber, M., Baltimore, R., Eaton, C., Gewitz, M., Rowley, A. H., Stanford, T. S, & Taubert, K. A. (2009). Prevention of rheumatic fever and diagnosis and treatment of acute streptococcal pharyngitis, *Circulation, 119*(11), 1541-1551. doi:10.1161/CIRCULATIONAHA.109.191959

Habib, G., Badano, L., Tribouilloy, C., Vilacosta, I., Zamorano, J. (2010). Recommendations for the practice of echocardiography in infectious endocarditis. *European Journal of Echocardiography, 11*(2), 202-219. doi:10.1093/ejechocard/jeq004

Habib, G., Hoen, B., Tornos, P., Thuny, F., Prendergast, B., Vilacosta, I., ..., Zamorano, J. (2009). Guidelines on prevention, diagnosis and treatment of infective endocarditis. *European Heart Journal, 30*, 2369-2413. doi:10.1093/eurheartj/ehp285

Heart and Stroke Foundation of Canada (HSF). (2011a). Heart disease conditions. Infective endocarditis. Retrieved from *http://www.heartandstroke.com/site/c.ikIQLcMWJtE/b.3484071/k.891C/Heart_disease__Infective_endocarditis.htm*

Heart and Stroke Foundation of Canada (HSF). (2011b). What is rheumatic heart disease? Retrieved from *http://www.heartandstroke.com/site/c.ikIQLcMWJtE/b.3484081/k.5BE1/Heart_disease__What_is_rheumatic_heart_disease.htm*

Howlett, J., McKelvie, R., Arnold, J., Costigan, J., Dorian, P., Ducharme, A., ..., White, M. (2009). Canadian Cardiovascular Society Consensus Conference guidelines on heart failure, update 2009: Diagnosis and management of heart failure, myocarditis, device therapy and recent important clinical trials. *Canadian Journal of Cardiology, 25*(2), 85-105. doi:10.1016/S0828-282X(09)70477-5

Hung, J., Lang, R., Flachskampf, F., Shernan, S., McCulloch, M., Adams, P., ..., Ryan, T. (2007). 3D echocardiography: A review of the current status and future directions. *Journal of Society of Echocardiography, 20*(3), 213-233. doi:10.1016/j.echo.2007.01.010

Imazio, M. (2011). Pericarditis: Pathophysiology, diagnosis and management. *Current Infectious Diseases, 13*(4), 308-316. doi:10.1007/s11908-011-0189-5

Imazio, M., Bobbio, M., Cecchi, E., Demarie, D., Demichelis, B., & Pomari, F. (2005). Colchicine in addition to conventional therapy for acute pericarditis: Results of the Colchicine for acute pericarditis trial (COPE). *Circulation, 112*, 2012-2016. doi:10.1161/CIRCULATIONAHA.105.542738

Khandaker, M., Espinosa, R., Nishimura, R., Sinak, L., Sharonne, H., Melduni, R., Oh, J. (2010). Pericardial disease: Diagnosis and management. *Mayo Clinic Proceedings, 85*(6), 572-593. doi:10.4065/mcp.2010.0046

Lung, B., & Vahanian, A. (2011). Epidemiology of valvular heart disease in the adult. *Nature Reviews in Cardiology, 8*, 162-172. doi:10.1038/nrcardiology.2010.202

Luk, A., Ahn, E., Soor, G., & Butany, J. (2009). Dilated cardiomyopathy: A review. *Journal of Clinical Pathology, 62*(3), 219-225. doi:10.1136/jcp.2008.060731

Maron, B., Doerer, H., Haas, T., Tierney, D., & Mueller, F. (2009). Sudden deaths in young competitive athletes: Analysis of 1866 deaths in the United States, 1980-2006, *Circulation, 119*(8), 1085-1092. doi:10.1161/CIRCULATIONAHA.108.804617

Mayo Foundation for Medical Education and Research (MFMER). (2007). *Rheumatic fever overview.* Rochester, MN: Mayo Clinic. Retrieved from *http://www.mayoclinic.com/health/rheumatic-fever/DS00250*

Que, Y., & Moreillon, P. (2011). Infective endocarditis. *Nature Reviews: Cardiology, 8*(6), 322-336. doi:10.1038/nrcardio.2011.43

Schmitto, J., Mokashi, S., & Cohn, L. (2010). Minimally-invasive valve surgery. *Journal of the American College of Cardiology, 56*(6), 455-462. doi:10.1016/j.jacc.2010.03.053

Steiger, M., Jost, W., Grandas, F., & Van Camp, G. (2009). Risk of valvular heart disease associated with the use of dopamine agonists in Parkinson's disease: A systematic review. *Journal of Neural Transmission, 116*(2), 179-191. doi:10.1007/s00702-008-0179-4

Willson, A., & Webb, J. (2011). Transcatheter treatment approach for aortic valve disease. *The International Journal of Cardiovascular Imaging, 27*(8), 1123-1132. doi:10.1007/s1055-011-9803-8

Wilson, W., Taubert, K., Gewitz, M., Lockhart, P., Baddour, L., Levison, M., ..., Durack, D. (2007). Prevention of infective endocarditis: Guidelines from the American Heart Association: A guideline from the American Heart Association Rheumatic Fever, Endocarditis, Kawasaki Disease Committee, Council on Cardiovascular Disease in the Young, and the Council on Clinical Cardiology, Council on Cardiovascular Surgery and Anesthesia, and the Quality of Care and Outcomes Research Interdisciplinary Working Group, *Circulation, 116*(15), 1736-1754. doi:10.1161/CIRCULATIONAHA.106.183095

World Health Organization (WHO). (2004). *Rheumatic fever and rheumatic heart disease: Report of a WHO expert consultation study group* (Technical Report Series No. 923). Geneva: Author.

RESOURCES

Resources for this chapter are listed in Chapter 36 on p. 927 and Chapter 37 on p. 949.

Nursing Management: Vascular Disorders

Written by **Deidre D. Wipke-Tevis** and **Kathleen Rich**

Adapted by **Renée Chauvin**

LEARNING OBJECTIVES

1. Explain the major risk factors to the etiology and pathophysiology of peripheral arterial disease.
2. Differentiate the pathophysiology, clinical manifestations, and collaborative care of different types of aortic aneurysms.
3. Select appropriate nursing interventions for the patient undergoing an aortic aneurysm repair.
4. Describe the pathophysiology, clinical manifestations, collaborative care, and nursing management of aortic dissection.
5. Describe the clinical manifestations, collaborative care, surgical management, and nursing management of peripheral artery disease of the lower extremities.
6. Plan appropriate nursing care for the patient with acute arterial ischemic disorders of the lower extremities.
7. Differentiate the pathophysiology, clinical manifestations, collaborative care, and nursing management of thromboangiitis obliterans (Buerger's disease) and Raynaud's phenomenon.
8. Evaluate the risk factors predisposing to the development of superficial vein thrombosis and venous thromboembolism.
9. Discriminate between the clinical characteristics of superficial vein thrombosis and those of venous thromboembolism.
10. Compare and contrast the collaborative care and nursing management of patients with superficial vein thrombosis and venous thromboembolism.
11. Prioritize the key aspects of nursing management of the patient receiving anticoagulant therapy.
12. Explain the pathophysiology and clinical manifestations to the collaborative care of patients with varicose veins, chronic venous insufficiency, and venous leg ulcers.

KEY TERMS

acute arterial ischemia Sudden interruption in the arterial blood supply to a tissue, organ, or extremity, p. 1020

aneurysm Outpouching or dilation of the arterial wall; a common problem involving the aorta, p. 1006

aortic dissection The result of a tear in the intimal (innermost) lining of the arterial wall that allows blood to enter between the intima and the media, thus creating a false lumen; occurs most commonly in the thoracic aorta, p. 1011

critical limb ischemia Characterized by pain at rest or at night, tissue loss such as ulcerations and or gangrene of the leg attributed to peripheral artery disease, p. 1016

deep vein thrombosis (DVT) A disorder involving a thrombus in a deep vein, most commonly the iliac and femoral veins, p. 1022

intermittent claudication Ischemic muscle ache or pain that is precipitated by a consistent level of exercise, resolves within 10 minutes or less with rest, and is reproducible, p. 1014

peripheral artery disease (PAD) Progressive narrowing and degeneration of the arteries of the neck, the abdomen, and the extremities, p. 1006

Raynaud's phenomenon An episodic vasospastic disorder of small cutaneous arteries, most frequently involving the fingers and toes, p. 1021

superficial vein thrombosis (SVT) The formation of a thrombus in a superficial vein, p. 1022

thromboangiitis obliterans (Buerger's disease) A somewhat rare nonatherosclerotic, segmental inflammatory disorder of the medium-sized arteries, veins, and nerves of the upper and lower extremities, p. 1021

varicose veins Dilated, tortuous subcutaneous veins most frequently found in the saphenous system, p. 1031

venous thromboembolism (VTE) Thromboembolic event in the venous system comprising both deep vein thrombosis (DVT) and pulmonary embolism (PE), p. 1022

Virchow's triad Three important factors in the etiology of venous thrombosis: (1) venous stasis, (2) damage to the endothelium (inner lining of the vein), and (3) hypercoagulability of the blood, p. 1022

ELECTRONIC RESOURCES

Supplemental content related to Chapter 40 can be found ...

Evolve Web Site ⊖volve

http://evolve.elsevier.com/Canada/Lewis/medsurg
- Answer Guidelines for Case Study on p. 1034
- Clinical Reference: Laboratory Values
- Content Updates
- Customizable Nursing Care Plans:
  - Peripheral Arterial Disease of the Lower Extremities
- Electronic Calculators
- eNCP 40-1: After Surgical Repair of the Aorta

- eTables:
  - eTable 40-1: Drugs, Vitamins, and Minerals That Interact With Oral Anticoagulants
  - eTable 40-2: Nursing Interventions to Prevent Bleeding Complications in Patients Receiving Anticoagulants
- Examination Review Questions
- Glossary
- Interactive Case Studies:
  - Abdominal Aortic Aneurysm
  - Chronic Peripheral Arterial Disease
- Key Points (Printable and MP3 Download)
- Patient & Caregiver Teaching Guide: Anticoagulation Therapy

Problems of the vascular system include disorders of the arteries, veins, and lymphatic vessels. Arterial disorders are classified as aneurysmal, atherosclerotic, and nonatherosclerotic vascular diseases. Atherosclerotic vascular disease is divided into coronary, cerebral, peripheral, mesenteric, and renal artery disease (Hiatt et al., 2008). This chapter discusses peripheral artery disease (PAD), aortic aneurysm and dissection, and venous diseases, specifically venous thrombosis and chronic venous insufficiency.

Peripheral Arterial Disease

Peripheral artery disease (PAD) involves thickening of artery walls, which results in a progressive narrowing of the arteries of the upper and lower extremities. The risk for PAD increases with age, increasing substantially after age 70. In people with diabetes mellitus, PAD occurs much earlier. Aboriginal origin, gender, geographic location, and socioeconomic status are significant factors attributing to health discrepancies in Canada (Lovell et al., 2009). PAD is strongly related to other types of cardiovascular disease (CVD) and their risk factors. Patients with PAD have a significantly higher risk of mortality (in general), CVD mortality, and major coronary events (Ankle-Brachial Index Collaboration, 2008). Thus, PAD is a marker of advanced systemic atherosclerosis. Patients with PAD are more likely to have coronary artery disease (CAD) and/or cerebral artery disease. Many Canadians are unaware that PAD is a significant sign of atherosclerosis, with a high risk of morbidity and mortality (Lovell et al., 2009).

Etiology and Pathophysiology of Peripheral Artery Disease

The leading cause of PAD is *atherosclerosis*, a gradual thickening of the intima (the innermost layer of the arterial wall) and the media (middle layer of the arterial wall) that leads to progressive narrowing of the artery lumen. Although the exact cause(s) of atherosclerosis are unknown, inflammation and endothelial injury play a major role (see Chapter 36). The pathology of atherosclerosis includes migration and replication of smooth muscle cells, deposition of connective tissue, lymphocyte and macrophage infiltration, and accumulation of lipids.

Significant risk factors for PAD include tobacco use, hyperlipidemia, elevated high-sensitivity C-reactive protein, diabetes mellitus, and uncontrolled hypertension, with the most important being tobacco use (Ostchega et al., 2007). Other risk factors include family history, hypertriglyceridemia, hyperuricemia, increasing age, obesity, sedentary lifestyle, and stress (Lloyd-Jones et al., 2009) (Pradhan et al., 2008).

Atherosclerosis more commonly affects certain segments of the arterial tree. These include the coronary (see Chapter 36), carotid (see Chapter 60), common iliac, superficial femoral, popliteal, and tibial arteries (Figure 40-1). Clinical symptoms occur when vessels are 60 to 75% occluded.

Aortic Aneurysms

The aorta is the largest artery and supplies oxygen and blood to all vital organs. One of the most common problems affecting the aorta is an **aneurysm,** an outpouching or dilation of the vessel wall. Aneurysms occur in men more often than in women, and their incidence increases with age. Peripheral artery aneurysms also develop but are less common.

Etiology and Pathophysiology

Aortic aneurysms may involve the aortic arch, thoracic aorta, abdominal aorta, or a combination. Most aneurysms, however, are found in the abdominal aorta below the level of the renal arteries. The growth rate of aneurysms is unpredictable, but the

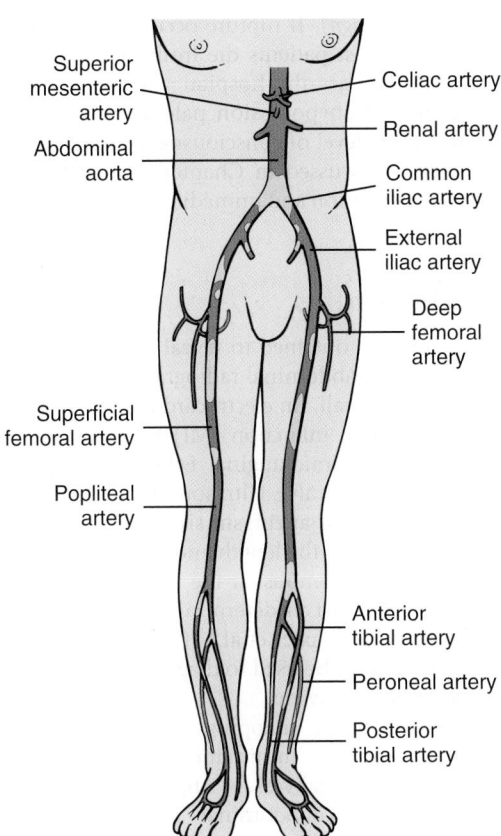

Figure 40-1 Common anatomical locations of atherosclerotic lesions (shown in *yellow*) of the abdominal aorta and lower extremities.

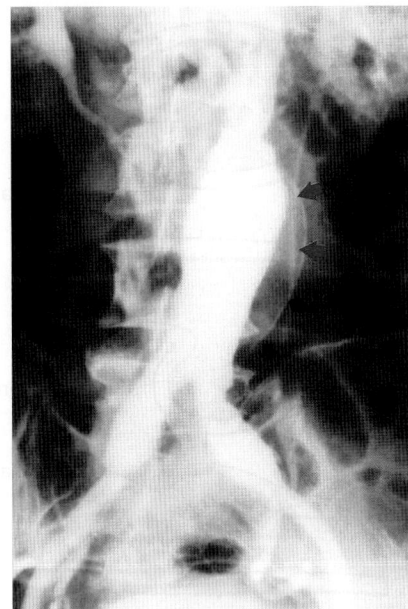

Figure 40-2 Angiography demonstrates a fusiform abdominal aortic aneurysm. Note calcification of the aortic wall *(arrows)* and extension of the aneurysm into the common iliac arteries.

Source: Courtesy Jo Menzoian, Boston.

larger the aneurysm, the greater the risk of rupture. The dilated aortic wall becomes lined with thrombi that can embolize, leading to acute ischemic symptoms to distal (downstream) branches. Three fourths of true aortic aneurysms occur in the abdomen (Figure 40-2) and one fourth in the thoracic aorta. Popliteal artery aneurysms rank third in frequency. Patients may have an aneurysm in more than one location.

Although various disorders are associated with aortic aneurysms, the primary cause may be classified as degenerative, congenital, mechanical, inflammatory, or infectious. The most common etiology of aneurysms of the aorta is atherosclerosis (Lloyd-Jones et al., 2009). It is known that atherosclerotic plaques deposit beneath the *intima* (the innermost layer of the arterial wall). This plaque formation is thought to cause degenerative changes in the *media* (middle layer of the arterial wall), leading to loss of elasticity, weakening, and eventual dilation of the aorta.

Male gender, age 65 years or older, and tobacco use are the major risk factors for abdominal aortic aneurysms (AAAs) of atherosclerotic origin. Other risk factors include the presence of CAD or PAD, high blood pressure (BP), and high cholesterol (Baxter, Terrin, & Dalman, 2008; Lederle et al., 2008). Studies have shown a strong genetic component to AAA development. The familial tendency is related to a number of congenital anomalies, including specific collagen defects (e.g., Ehlers-Danlos syndrome) and premature breakdown of vascular elastic tissue (Marfan syndrome) (Jagadesham, Scott, & Carding, 2008). Less

common causes of AAAs include penetrating or blunt trauma from motor vehicle collisions, inflammatory aortitis (e.g., Takayasu's or giant cell arteritis), and infectious aortitis (e.g., from syphilis or *Salmonella* or human immunodeficiency virus infection).

Classification

Aneurysms are classified as true or false (Figure 40-3). A *true aneurysm* is one in which the wall of the artery forms the aneurysm, with at least one vessel layer still intact. True aneurysms can be further subdivided into fusiform and saccular dilations. A *fusiform aneurysm* is circumferential and relatively uniform in shape. A *saccular aneurysm* is pouchlike with a narrow neck connecting the bulge to one side of the arterial wall.

A *false aneurysm*, or *pseudoaneurysm*, is not an aneurysm but a disruption of all layers of the arterial wall, resulting in bleeding that is contained by surrounding structures. False aneurysms may result from trauma or infection or occur after peripheral artery bypass graft surgery at the site of the graft–to–artery anastomosis. They may also result from arterial leakage after removal of cannulae such as lower extremity arterial catheters and intra-aortic balloon pump devices (Kalapatapu, Shelton, Ali, Moursi, & Eidt, 2008).

Clinical Manifestations

Thoracic aorta aneurysms are usually asymptomatic. When present, the most common symptom is deep, diffuse chest pain extending to the interscapular area. Aneurysms located in the ascending aorta and the aortic arch can produce hoarseness in the patient as a result of pressure on the recurrent laryngeal nerve. Pressure on the esophagus can cause dysphagia. If the aneurysm presses on the superior vena cava, it can cause decreased venous

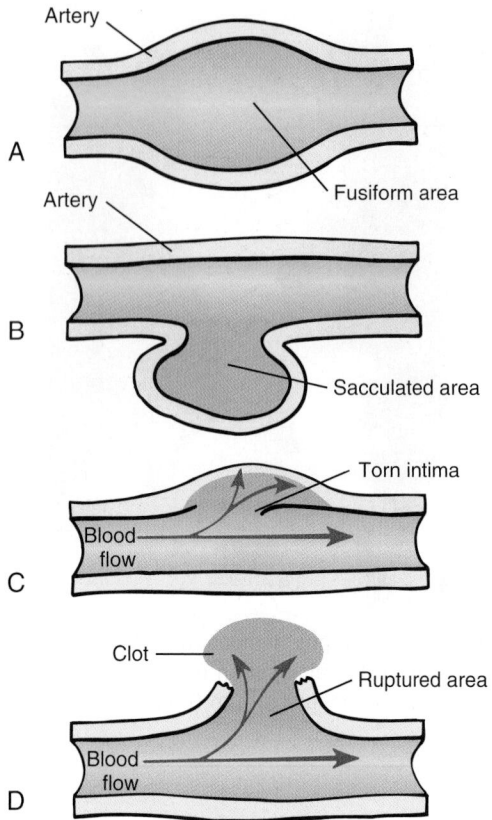

Figure 40-3 A, True fusiform abdominal aortic aneurysm. **B,** True saccular aortic aneurysm. **C,** Aortic dissection. **D,** False aneurysm or pseudoaneurysm.

drainage, resulting in distended neck veins and edema of the head and the arms.

AAAs are often asymptomatic and frequently detected on routine physical examination or when the patient is examined for an unrelated problem (e.g., abdominal radiographic examination, ultrasound, computed tomography [CT] scan, intravenous pyelogram, or abdominal surgery). On physical examination, a pulsatile mass in the periumbilical area slightly to the left of the midline may be detected. Bruits may be audible with a stethoscope placed over the aneurysm. These physical findings may be more difficult to detect in obese individuals.

Symptoms of an AAA may mimic pain associated with any abdominal or back disorder. Symptoms may result from compression of nearby anatomical structures. These include back pain caused by lumbar nerve compression and epigastric discomfort with or without alteration in bowel elimination resulting from compression on the bowel. Occasionally, aneurysms, even small ones, spontaneously embolize plaque. This can cause the "blue toe syndrome," in which patchy mottling of the feet and toes occurs in the presence of palpable pedal pulses.

Complications

The most serious complication is rupture of the aneurysm. If rupture occurs into the retroperitoneal space, bleeding may be tamponaded by surrounding anatomic structures, preventing exsanguination and death. In this case, the patient often has severe back pain and may or may not have back or flank ecchy-

mosis *(Grey Turner's sign).* If rupture occurs into the thoracic or abdominal cavity, most patients die from massive hemorrhage. The patient who reaches the hospital will be in hypovolemic shock with tachycardia, hypotension, pale clammy skin, decreased urine output, altered level of consciousness, and abdominal tenderness. (Shock is discussed in Chapter 69.) In this situation, simultaneous resuscitation and immediate surgical repair are necessary.

Diagnostic Studies

Chest radiographs are obtained to reveal abnormal widening of the thoracic aorta. An abdominal radiograph may show calcification within the aortic wall. An electrocardiogram (ECG) rules out evidence of myocardial infarction (MI) because thoracic aneurysm symptoms can mimic angina. Echocardiography assesses the function of the aortic valve. Ultrasound is useful for aneurysm screening and to monitor aneurysm size. A CT scan is the most accurate test to determine the length and cross-sectional diameter and the presence of thrombus in the aneurysm. Three dimensional CT scans can assist in determining what type of surgical repair should be done (Baxter et al., 2008). Magnetic resonance imaging (MRI) also may be used to diagnose and assess the location and severity of aneurysms.

Angiography, anatomic mapping of the aortic system by contrast imaging, provides information about the involvement of intestinal, renal, or distal vessels. Angiography is also useful if a suprarenal or thoracoabdominal aneurysm is suspected. (Chapter 34 and Table 34-5 discuss angiography.) A number of circulating biomarkers (e.g., fibrinogen, D-dimer, interleukin-6) are being investigated for use in determining the early diagnosis and prognosis of AAAs (Golledge, Tsao, Dalman, & Norman, 2008).

Collaborative Care

The goal of management is to prevent aneurysm rupture and extension of dissection. Therefore, early detection and prompt treatment are essential. A careful review of body systems is necessary to identify any co-morbidities, especially of the lungs, heart, or kidneys, because they may influence the patient's surgical risk. Correction of existing carotid and/or coronary artery obstructions may be needed before the aneurysm is repaired. Conservative therapy typically is initiated for small aneurysms (<5 cm). This consists of risk factor modification, decreasing BP, and annual monitoring of aneurysm size using ultrasound, CT, or MRI (Baxter et al., 2008). Surgical repair is done for aneurysms 5.5 cm or larger in men and 5 cm or larger in women (Ballard, Filardo, Fowkes, & Powell, 2008). Surgical intervention may occur sooner in younger, low-risk patients or if the aneurysm expands rapidly (i.e., >1-cm-diameter increase per year), if it becomes symptomatic, or if the risk of rupture is high (Criqui et al., 2008).

Surgical Therapy. For elective surgery, the patient is hydrated and any electrolyte, coagulation, and hematocrit abnormalities are corrected preoperatively. If the aneurysm has ruptured, emergent surgical intervention is required. Ruptured AAAs have up to a 90% mortality rate, with the lowest survival seen in women and older patients (Lloyd-Jones et al., 2009; McPhee, Hill, & Eslami, 2007). The open surgical technique involves a large abdominal incision through which the surgeon (1) incises the diseased aortic segment, (2) removes any thrombus or plaque, (3) sutures a

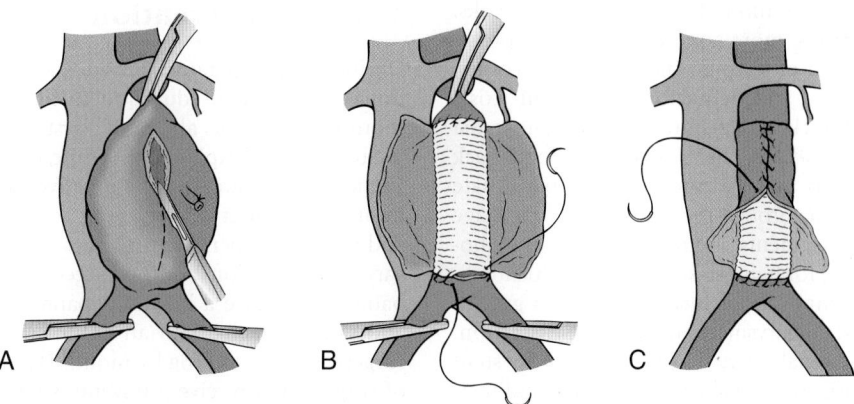

Figure 40-4 Surgical repair of an abdominal aortic aneurysm. **A,** Incising the aneurysmal sac. **B,** Insertion of synthetic graft. **C,** Suturing native aortic wall over synthetic graft.

synthetic graft (Dacron or polytetrafluoroethylene [PTFE]) to the normal aorta proximal and distal to the aneurysm, and (4) sutures the native aortic wall around the graft to act as a protective cover (Figure 40-4). If the iliac arteries are also aneurysmal, a bifurcated graft replaces the entire diseased segment. With saccular aneurysms, it may be possible to excise only the bulbous lesion, repairing the artery by primary closure (suturing the artery together) or by application of an autogenous or synthetic patch graft. *Autotransfusion*, which recycles the patient's own blood, reduces the need for blood transfusions during AAA surgery. (Chapter 33 discusses autotransfusion.)

All AAA resections require aortic cross-clamping proximal and distal to the aneurysm. Most resections are done in 30 to 45 minutes, after which time, the clamps are removed and blood flow is restored. If the cross clamp must be applied above the renal arteries, adequate renal perfusion after clamp removal should be determined before closure of the abdominal incision. The risk of postoperative renal complications such as acute renal failure increases significantly in patients who have surgical repair of AAAs above the level of the renal arteries.

Endovascular Graft Procedure. Minimally invasive endovascular aneurysm repair (EVAR) is an alternative to conventional surgical repair. EVAR involves the placement of a sutureless aortic graft into the abdominal aorta inside the aneurysm via femoral artery cutdowns. The graft, a Dacron cylinder consisting of several sections, is supported with multiple rings of flexible wire (Figure 40-5).

The main section of the graft is bifurcated and delivered through a femoral artery catheter. The second part of the graft is inserted through the opposite femoral artery. When all graft components are in place, they are released (deployed) against the vessel wall by balloon inflation (creating a circumferential seal). The blood then flows through the endovascular graft, thus preventing further expansion of the aneurysm (Tinkman, 2009). The aneurysmal wall will shrink over time because the blood is now being diverted through the endograft.

Patients must meet certain eligibility criteria to be candidates for EVAR. These include iliofemoral vessels that will allow for safe graft insertion and vessels of sufficient length and width to support the graft (Eliason & Upchurch, 2008). The benefits of EVAR include decreased anaesthesia and operative time,

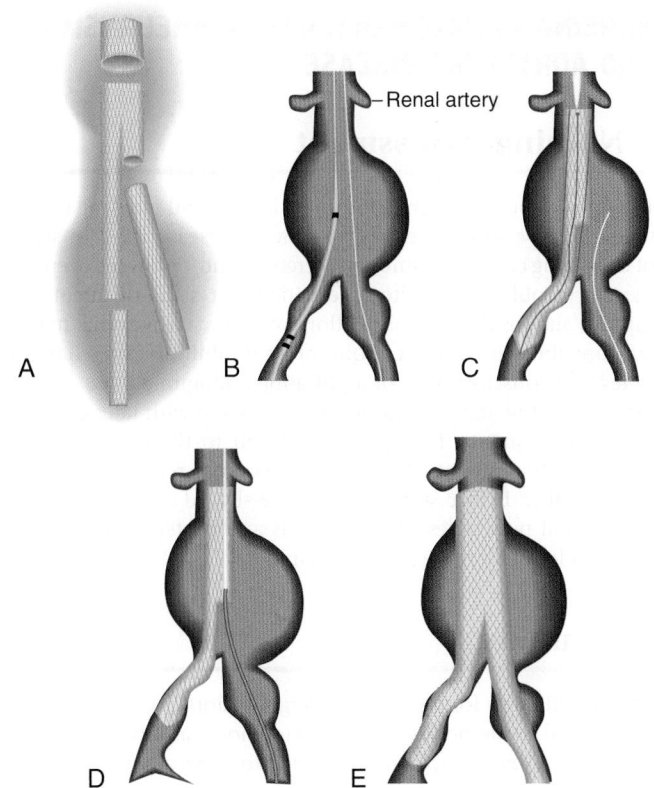

Figure 40-5 Bifurcated (two-branched) endovascular stent grafting of an aneurysm. **A,** The insertion of a woven polyester tube (graft) covered by a tubular metal web (stent). **B,** The stent graft is inserted through a large blood vessel (e.g., femoral artery) using a delivery catheter. The catheter is positioned below the renal arteries in the area of the aneurysm. **C,** The stent graft is slowly released (deployed) into the blood vessel. When the stent comes in contact with the blood vessel, it expands to a preset size. **D,** A second stent graft can be inserted in the contralateral (opposite) vessel if necessary. **E,** Fully deployed bifurcated stent graft.

Source: Medtronic, Minneapolis, MN.

limited blood loss, decreased morbidity and mortality risks, small bilateral groin incisions, more rapid resumption of physical activity, shortened length of hospital stays, quicker recovery, higher patient satisfaction, and reduction in overall costs (McPhee et al., 2007; Dimick & Upchurch, 2008). The most common complication is *endoleak*, the seepage of blood back into the old aneurysm. This may be caused by an inadequate seal at either graft end, a tear through the graft fabric, or leakage between overlapping graft segments and may require coil embolization (insertion of beads) for hemostasis (Eliason & Upchurch, 2008). Other potential complications include aneurysm growth above or below the graft aneurysm rupture, aortic dissection, bleeding, stent migration, renal artery occlusion caused by stent migration, graft thrombosis, incisional site hematoma, and incisional infection.

Graft dysfunction may require conversion to an open surgical repair. Patients must have regular follow-up visits with their health care provider and routine CT scans for the rest of their lives to monitor for complications (e.g., stent migration, aneurysm reoccurrence).

NURSING MANAGEMENT: AORTIC ANEURYSMS AND AORTOILIAC DISEASE

Nursing Assessment

The nurse should perform a thorough history and physical assessment. Because atherosclerosis is a systemic disease, look for signs of coexisting cardiac, pulmonary, cerebral, and/or lower extremity vascular problems. Monitor the patient for signs of aneurysm rupture, such as diaphoresis; pallor; weakness; tachycardia; hypotension; abdominal, back, groin, or periumbilical pain; changes in level of consciousness; or a pulsating abdominal mass. Establishing baseline data is critical for comparison with later postoperative assessments. Pay special attention to the character and quality of the patient's peripheral pulses and renal and neurological status. Before surgery, the nurse should mark and document pedal pulse sites (dorsalis pedis and posterior tibial) and any skin lesions on the lower extremities.

Planning

The overall goals for a patient undergoing aortic surgery include (1) normal tissue perfusion, (2) intact motor and sensory function, and (3) no complications related to surgical repair such as thrombosis or infection.

Nursing Implementation

Health Promotion

To promote overall health, encourage the patient to reduce CVD risk factors (see Table 35-3), including BP control, smoking cessation (see Chapter 36), increasing physical activity, and maintaining normal body weight and serum lipid levels. These measures also help ensure continued graft patency following surgical repair.

Acute Intervention

During the preoperative period, the nurse should provide emotional support and education to the patient and caregiver and thoroughly assess all body systems. Preoperative teaching includes a brief explanation of the disease process, the planned surgical procedure(s), preoperative routines, what to expect immediately after surgery (e.g., recovery room, tubes/drains), and usual postoperative timelines. Specific preoperative routines vary by institution and/or surgeon. In general, aortic surgery patients will have a bowel preparation (e.g., laxatives, enemas) and skin cleansing with an antimicrobial agent the day before surgery, receive nothing by mouth (NPO) after midnight the day of surgery, and receive intravenous (IV) antibiotics immediately before the incision is made. If appropriate, a preoperative visit to the critical care unit (CCU) may be helpful to the patient and caregiver. Patients with a history of CVD usually receive a β-blocker (e.g., metoprolol [Lopressor]) preoperatively (Smith et al., 2009).

Postoperatively, aortic surgery patients typically go to a CCU for 24 to 48 hours for close monitoring. When the patient arrives in the CCU, various devices are in place including an endotracheal tube for mechanical ventilation; an arterial line; a central venous pressure (CVP) or pulmonary artery (PA) catheter; peripheral IV lines; an indwelling urinary catheter; and depending on the approach and surgeon preference, a nasogastric (NG) tube. The patient will need continuous ECG and pulse oximetry monitoring. If the thorax is opened during surgery, chest tubes will be in place. Pain medication is administered via epidural catheter or patient-controlled analgesia (PCA). In addition to the usual goals of care for a postoperative patient (e.g., maintaining adequate respiratory function, fluid and electrolyte balance, and pain control [see Chapter 22]), the nurse should monitor graft patency and renal perfusion. The nurse should also monitor for and intervene to limit or treat dysrhythmias, infections, and neurological complications (Smith et al., 2009). See eNCP 40-1, available on the Evolve Web site for this chapter, for care of the patient with an aneurysm repair or other aortic surgery.

Graft Patency.
An adequate BP is important to maintain graft patency. Prolonged hypotension may result in graft thrombosis. Administration of IV fluids and blood components (as indicated) is essential for adequate blood flow. CVP readings or PA pressures and urinary output are monitored hourly in the immediate postoperative period to help assess the patient's hydration and perfusion status. Severe hypertension may cause undue stress on the arterial anastomoses, resulting in leakage of blood or rupture at the suture lines. Drug therapy with IV diuretics (e.g., furosemide [Lasix]) or IV antihypertensive agents (e.g., nitroprusside [Nipride], esmolol [Brevibloc], labetalol [Trandate]) may be indicated (Varon, 2008).

Cardiovascular Status.
In patients with CAD, myocardial ischemia or MI may occur in the perioperative period because of decreased myocardial oxygen supply or increased myocardial oxygen demands. Cardiac dysrhythmias may occur because of electrolyte imbalances, hypoxemia, hypothermia, or myocardial ischemia.

Nursing interventions include continuous ECG monitoring, frequent electrolyte and arterial blood gas determinations; administration of oxygen, IV antidysrhythmic and antihypertensive medications, and electrolytes as needed; adequate pain control; and resumption of cardiac medications.

Infection. A prosthetic vascular graft infection is a relatively rare but potentially life-threatening complication. Nursing interventions to prevent infection should include ensuring that the patient receives a broad-spectrum antibiotic as prescribed. Assess body temperature regularly, and promptly report elevations. Monitor laboratory data for an elevated white blood cell (WBC) count, which may be the first indication of an infection. The nurse should ensure adequate nutrition and assess the surgical incision for signs of infection (e.g., redness, swelling, drainage). All IV, arterial, and CVP or PA catheter insertion sites should be cared for using strict aseptic technique because they are ports of entry for bacteria. Meticulous perineal care for the patient with an in-dwelling urinary catheter is essential to minimize the risk of urinary tract infection. Keep surgical incisions clean and dry.

Gastrointestinal Status. After open abdominal aortic surgery, paralytic ileus may develop as a result of anaesthesia and the handling of the bowel during surgery. The intestines may become swollen and bruised, and peristalsis ceases for variable intervals. A retroperitoneal surgical approach can be used to decrease the risk of bowel complications. An NG tube may be placed during surgery and connected to low, intermittent suction to decompress the stomach, prevent aspiration of stomach contents, and decrease pressure on suture lines. Record the amount and character of the NG output. While the patient is NPO, provide oral care frequently. Ice chips or lozenges may be used to soothe a dry or irritated throat. Assess for bowel sounds. The passing of flatus signals returning bowel function and should be noted. Encourage early ambulation because this promotes the return of bowel functioning. A paralytic ileus rarely lasts beyond the fourth postoperative day.

If the blood supply to the bowel is disrupted during surgery, temporary ischemia or infarction (death) of intestinal tissue may result. Clinical manifestations of this rare but serious complication include absent bowel sounds, fever, abdominal distension, diarrhea, and bloody stools. If bowel infarction occurs, immediate reoperation is necessary to restore blood flow, with likely resection of the infarcted bowel.

Neurological Status. Neurological complications can occur after aortic surgery. When the ascending aorta and the aortic arch are involved, the nurse will assess the level of consciousness, pupil size and response to light, facial symmetry, tongue deviation, speech, ability to move upper extremities, and quality of hand grasps (see Chapter 59). When the descending aorta is involved, neurovascular assessment of the lower extremities is important. Record all assessments and report changes from baseline to the physician immediately.

Peripheral Perfusion Status. The aneurysm's anatomic location directs the areas of interest related to peripheral perfusion. The nurse should check and record all peripheral pulses hourly for several hours and then routinely, based on institutional policy. When the ascending aorta and aortic arch are involved, assess the carotid, radial, and temporal artery pulses. For surgery of the descending aorta, assess the femoral, popliteal, posterior tibial, and dorsalis pedis pulses (see Chapter 34, Figure 34-6).

When checking pulses, mark the locations with a felt-tip pen so that others can locate them easily. In some cases, a Doppler ultrasound may be needed to assess peripheral pulses. Check skin temperature and colour, capillary refill time, and sensation and movement of the extremities (see Chapter 34).

Occasionally, lower extremity pulses may be absent for a short time after surgery because of vasospasm and hypothermia. A decreased or absent pulse together with a cool, pale, mottled, or painful extremity may indicate embolization or graft occlusion. Report these findings to the physician immediately. Graft occlusion requires reoperation if identified early. Thrombolytic therapy may also be considered. In some patients, pulses may have been absent before surgery owing to coexistent PAD. It is essential to compare findings with the preoperative status to determine the cause of a decreased or absent pulse and the proper treatment.

Renal Perfusion Status. Postoperatively, the patient has an indwelling urinary catheter. In the immediate postoperative period, record hourly urine outputs. Maintain accurate fluid intake and output and record daily weights until the patient resumes a regular diet. CVP and PA pressures also provide important information about hydration status. Evaluate renal function by monitoring daily blood urea nitrogen (BUN) and serum creatinine levels. (For signs and symptoms of acute kidney injury, see Chapter 49.) Irreversible renal failure may occur after aortic surgery, particularly in high-risk individuals (e.g., patients with diabetes). Decreased renal perfusion can occur from embolization of the aortic thrombus/plaque to one or both renal arteries. This causes ischemia of one or both kidneys. Hypotension, dehydration, prolonged aortic clamping during surgery, or blood loss also can lead to decreased renal perfusion.

Ambulatory and Home Care

Instruct the patient and caregiver to increase activities gradually after they get home. Fatigue, poor appetite, and irregular bowel habits are common. The patient should avoid heavy lifting for 6 weeks after surgery. Any redness, swelling, increased pain, drainage from incisions, or fever greater than 37.8°C should be reported to a health care provider. Teach the patient and caregiver to look for changes in colour or warmth of the extremities. Patients and caregivers can learn to palpate peripheral pulses to assess changes in their quality. Sexual dysfunction in male patients is common after aortic surgery. Preoperatively, document baseline sexual function and recommend counselling as appropriate. A referral to an urologist may be useful if erectile dysfunction occurs.

Evaluation

Expected outcomes for the patient who undergoes aortic surgery are addressed in eNCP 40-1.

Aortic Dissection

Aortic dissection, often misnamed "dissecting aneurysm," is not a type of aneurysm. Rather, dissection results from the creation of a false lumen (between the intima and the media) through which blood flows (Figure 40-6; see also Figure 40-3).

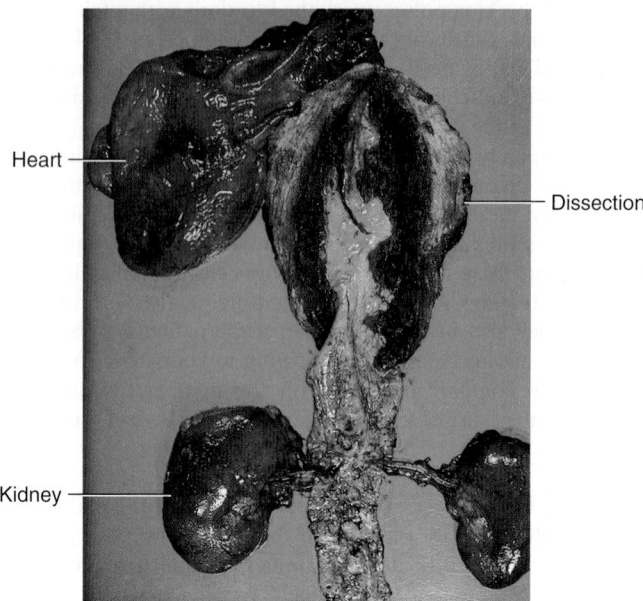

Figure 40-6 Aortic dissection of the thoracic aorta.

Source: Damjanov, I., & Linder, J. (1996). *Anderson's pathology* (10th ed.). St. Louis: Mosby.

Classification is based on anatomic location (ascending versus descending aorta) and duration of onset (acute versus chronic). Approximately 60 to 70% of dissections involve the ascending aorta and are acute in onset (Jonker, Schlösser, Moll, & Muhs, 2009; Tsai, Trimarchi, & Nienaber, 2009). Acute aortic dissections (i.e., diagnosed within 14 days of symptom onset) carry a mortality rate as high as 1% per hour (Patel & Arora, 2008). Chronic dissections almost exclusively involve the descending aorta.

Etiology and Pathophysiology

Most experts attribute nontraumatic aortic dissection to the degeneration of the elastic fibres in the medial layer. Chronic hypertension accelerates the degradation process. Aortic dissection is believed to arise from an intimal tear. Intimal tears typically occur in areas with the greatest rate of rise of BP, such as immediately above the aortic valve and just distal to the left subclavian artery. As the heart contracts, each systolic pulsation causes increased pressure on the damaged area, which further increases the dissection. Extension of the dissection may cut off blood supply to critical areas such as the brain, kidneys, spinal cord, and extremities. The false lumen may remain patent, become thrombosed (clotted), rejoin the true lumen by way of a distal tear, or rupture.

Aortic dissection affects men two to five times more often than women and occurs most frequently in their 50s to 70s. Approximately half of all dissections in women younger than 40 years occur during pregnancy (Patel & Arora, 2008). Predisposing factors include age, aortitis (e.g., syphilis, Takayasu arteritis), blunt or iatrogenic trauma, congenital heart disease (e.g., bicuspid aortic valve, coarctation of the aorta), connective tissue disorders (e.g., Marfan or Ehlers-Danlos syndrome), cocaine use, a history of cardiac surgery, atherosclerosis, male sex, pregnancy, hypertension, and Turner's syndrome (Tsai et al., 2009). Younger patients are more likely to have a bicuspid aortic valve, Marfan syndrome, prior aortic valve surgery, or recent trauma (Jonker et al., 2009).

Clinical Manifestations

The majority of patients with an acute ascending aortic dissection report sudden, severe onset of excruciating chest pain, back pain, or both, radiating to the neck or shoulders. The pain is frequently described as "sharp" and "worst ever" followed less frequently by "tearing" or "ripping." Patients with acute descending aortic dissection are more likely to report pain in their back, abdomen, or legs. Dissection pain can be differentiated from MI pain that is more gradual in onset and has increasing intensity. As the dissection progresses, pain may migrate. Older patients are less likely to have abrupt onset of chest or back pain and more likely to have hypotension and vague symptoms. Some patients have a painless aortic dissection, emphasizing the importance of the physical examination (Jonker et al., 2009; Tsai et al., 2009).

If the aortic arch is involved, the patient may exhibit neurological deficits, such as altered level of consciousness, weakened or absent carotid and temporal pulses, and dizziness or syncope. An ascending aortic dissection usually produces some degree of disruption in blood flow in the coronary arteries and aortic valvular insufficiency. The patient may develop angina, MI, and a new high-pitched, diastolic cardiac murmur. If severe enough, these complications can result in left ventricular failure with the development of dyspnea, orthopnea, and pulmonary edema. When either subclavian artery is involved, radial, ulnar, and brachial pulse quality and BP readings may be different between the left and the right arms. As the dissection progresses down the aorta, the abdominal organs and lower extremities demonstrate evidence of decreased tissue perfusion.

Complications

A severe and life-threatening complication of an acute ascending aortic dissection is cardiac tamponade, which occurs when blood from the dissection leaks into the pericardial sac. Clinical manifestations of tamponade include hypotension, narrowed pulse pressure, jugular venous distension, muffled heart sounds, and pulsus paradoxus (see Chapter 39). The aorta may rupture because it is weakened by the dissection. Hemorrhage may occur into the mediastinal, pleural, or abdominal cavities. Aortic rupture typically results in exsanguination and death. Dissection can lead to occlusion of the blood supply to vital organs. Symptoms of spinal cord ischemia range from weakness and decreased sensation to complete lower extremity paralysis. Renal ischemia can lead to renal failure. Manifestations of abdominal (mesenteric) ischemia include abdominal pain, decreased bowel sounds, altered bowel function, and bowel necrosis.

Diagnostic Studies

Diagnostic studies to detect aortic dissection are similar to those performed for suspected aneurysms (Table 40-1). A chest radiograph may show a widening of the mediastinal silhouette and left pleural effusion. Three-dimensional CT scanning and transesophageal echocardiography (TEE) have become the standard of care for the diagnosis of acute aortic dissection (Tsai et al., 2009). A CT scan can provide valuable information on the presence and severity of the dissection. Although an MRI has the highest accuracy for detecting aortic dissection, it is contraindicated in some patients (e.g., those with metallic implants, hemodynamically unstable patients) and may not be available on an emergency basis (Patel & Arora, 2008).

COLLABORATIVE CARE

Table 40-1 Aortic Dissection

Diagnostic	Collaborative Therapy
• Health history and physical examination	• Bed rest
• ECG	• Pain relief with opioids
• Chest radiograph	• Blood transfusion (if necessary)
• CT scan with three-dimensional reconstruction	• Control of blood pressure
	• Sodium nitroprusside (Nipride)
• TEE	• Calcium channel blockers (Table 35-8)
• MRI	• ACE inhibitors (Table 35-8)
	• Control of myocardial contractility
	• Metoprolol (Lopressor)
	• Labetalol (Trandate)
	• Surgical aortic resection and repair
	• Endovascular aortic dissection repair

ACE, angiotensin-converting enzyme; *CT,* computed tomography; *ECG,* electrocardiogram; *MRI,* magnetic resonance imaging; *TEE,* transesophageal echocardiogram.

Collaborative Care

Patients with acute aortic dissection are managed in the CCU. The initial goals of therapy for acute aortic dissection without complications are BP control and pain management. BP control reduces stress on the aortic wall by reducing systolic BP and myocardial contractility (see Table 40-1). An IV β-adrenergic blocker (e.g., esmolol) decreases BP and force of left ventricular contraction. Esmolol is particularly useful because it has a rapid onset and a short half-life. Other antihypertensive agents such as calcium channel blockers and angiotensin-converting enzyme (ACE) inhibitors are also used (Varon, 2008; Patel & Arora, 2008).

Conservative Therapy. The patient with an acute descending aortic dissection without complications can be treated conservatively (Tsai et al., 2009; Patel & Arora, 2008). Supportive treatment includes pain relief and BP control. Supportive treatment for an acute ascending aortic dissection serves as a bridge to surgery.

Endovascular Dissection Repair. Endovascular repair of chronic descending aortic dissection is an effective treatment option (Kim et al., 2009). Endovascular repair is the standard modality to treat acute descending aortic dissections with complications (e.g., hemodynamic instability, peripheral ischemia) (Tsai et al., 2009). Endovascular dissection repair is similar to EVAR. However, a temporary lumbar drain may be inserted for cerebrospinal fluid removal to reduce spinal cord edema and help prevent paralysis (Karmy-Jones, Simeone, Meissner, Granvall, & Nicholls, 2007).

Surgical Therapy. An acute ascending aortic dissection is considered a surgical emergency. Otherwise, surgery is indicated when drug therapy is ineffective or when complications (e.g., heart failure) occur. Because the aorta is fragile following dissection, surgery is delayed for as long as possible to allow time for edema to decrease and to permit clotting of the blood in the false lumen. Surgery involves resection of the aortic segment containing the intimal tear and replacement with a synthetic graft. Even with prompt surgical intervention, the in-hospital mortality rate of acute aortic dissection remains high. Women experience poorer surgical outcomes and higher mortality rates than men (Tsai et al, 2009). Causes of in-hospital mortality include aortic rupture, mesenteric ischemia, sepsis, and multiorgan failure (Patel & Arora, 2008).

NURSING MANAGEMENT: AORTIC DISSECTION

Preoperatively, nursing management includes keeping the patient in bed in a semi-Fowler's position and maintaining a quiet environment. These measures help to keep the systolic BP at the lowest possible level that maintains vital organ perfusion (typically between 110 and 120 mm Hg) (Patel & Arora, 2008). Opioids and sedatives are administered as ordered. The nurse must manage pain and anxiety for patient comfort and because these symptoms can cause elevations in the systolic BP.

Administration of IV antihypertensive agents requires careful supervision. This requires continuous ECG and intra-arterial BP monitoring (see Chapter 68). Monitor vital signs frequently, sometimes as often as every 2 to 3 minutes, until target BP is reached. The nurse should observe for changes in peripheral pulses and signs of increasing pain, restlessness, and anxiety. If the arteries branching off the aortic arch are involved, decreased cerebral blood flow may alter the level of consciousness. Postoperative care is similar to that after aortic aneurysm repair (see the section on nursing management of aortic aneurysms and aortoiliac disease earlier in this chapter, and eNCP 40-1).

In preparation for discharge, the nurse should focus on patient and caregiver teaching. All patients with a history of aortic dissection, regardless of anatomic location or treatment modality, require long-term medical therapy to control BP. Patients need to understand that antihypertensive drugs must be taken daily for the rest of their lives. β-Adrenergic blockers (e.g., metoprolol [Lopressor]) are used to control BP and decrease myocardial contractility. It is important that patients understand the drug regimen and potential adverse effects (e.g., dizziness, depression, fatigue, erectile dysfunction). Tell the patient to discuss any adverse effects with the health care provider before discontinuing the drug. Follow-up with regularly scheduled MRIs or CTs is essential (Patel & Arora, 2008). The most common cause of death in long-term survivors is aortic rupture from redissection or aneurysm formation. The nurse must instruct patients that, if the pain or other symptoms return, they should activate emergency medical services (EMS) for immediate care.

Peripheral Arterial Disease of the Lower Extremities

Lower extremity PAD may affect the aortoiliac, femoral, popliteal, tibial, or peroneal arteries, or any combination of these (see Figure 40-1). The femoral popliteal area is the site most commonly affected in nondiabetic patients. The patient with diabetes mellitus tends to develop PAD in the arteries below the knee, especially the anterior tibial, posterior tibial, and peroneal arteries. In advanced PAD, multiple levels of occlusions are found.

Clinical Manifestations

Generally, the severity of the clinical manifestations depends on the site and extent of the obstruction and the amount of collateral circulation. The classic symptom of lower extremity PAD is **intermittent claudication,** an ischemic muscle ache or pain that is precipitated by a consistent level of exercise, resolves within 10 minutes or less with rest, and is reproducible (Hirsch et al., 2006). The ischemic pain is a result of the accumulation of end products of anaerobic cellular metabolism, such as lactic acid. Once the patient stops exercising, the metabolites are cleared and the pain subsides. PAD of the aortoiliac arteries produces claudication in the buttocks and thighs, whereas calf claudication indicates femoral or popliteal artery involvement. Only about 10% of patients with PAD display the classic symptom of intermittent claudication (Hirsch et al., 2007).

If PAD involves the internal iliac (hypogastric) arteries, erectile dysfunction results. Some degree of sexual dysfunction occurs in a large portion of men with aortoiliac occlusion (Norgren et al., 2007).

Paresthesia, manifested as numbness or tingling in the toes or feet, may result from nerve tissue ischemia. True peripheral neuropathy occurs more commonly in patients with diabetes (see Chapter 52) and in those with longstanding ischemia. Neuropathy produces excruciating shooting or burning pain in the extremity, does not follow particular nerve roots, and may be present near ulcerated areas. Gradually diminishing perfusion to neurons produces loss of both pressure and deep pain sensations. Thus, patients may not notice lower extremity injuries.

The physical appearance of the limb provides important information about blood flow. The skin becomes thin, shiny, and taut and hair loss occurs on the lower legs. Diminished or absent pedal, popliteal, or femoral pulses are present. Pallor (blanching of the foot) develops in response to leg elevation (elevation pallor). Conversely, reactive hyperemia (redness of the foot) develops when the limb is in a dependent position (dependent rubour).

As PAD progresses and involves multiple arterial segments, continuous pain develops at rest. Rest pain most often occurs in the forefoot or toes and is aggravated by limb elevation. Rest pain occurs when there is insufficient blood flow to meet basic metabolic requirements of the distal tissues. Rest pain occurs more often at night because cardiac output tends to drop during sleep and the limbs are at the level of the heart. Patients often try to achieve partial pain relief by dangling the leg over the side of the bed or sleeping in a chair to allow gravity to maximize blood flow. The patient with chronic rest pain, ulceration, or gangrene has critical limb ischemia. Critical limb ischemia often leads to amputation within 6 months if untreated (Hirsch et al., 2006). Every attempt is made to save the limb, and surgical or endovascular revascularization is indicated. If a patient is not a candidate for revascularization and/or if revascularization is not technically possible, medical treatment is indicated (Norgren et al., 2007).

Complications

Lower extremity PAD progresses slowly. Prolonged ischemia leads to atrophy of the skin and underlying muscles. Because of the decreased arterial blood flow, even minor trauma to the feet (e.g., stubbing one's toe, blister from ill-fitting shoes) may result in delayed healing, wound infection, and tissue necrosis, especially in the diabetic patient. Arterial (ischemic) ulcers most commonly occur over bony prominences on the toes, feet, and lower leg

Table 40-2 Comparison of Peripheral Artery and Venous Disease

CHARACTERISTIC	ARTERIAL	VENOUS
Peripheral pulses	Decreased or absent	Present; may be difficult to palpate with edema
Capillary refill	>3 sec	<3 sec
Ankle–brachial index	<0.40	>0.91
Edema	Absent unless leg constantly in dependent position	Lower leg edema
Hair	Loss of hair on legs, feet, toes	Hair may be present or absent
Ulcer location	Tips of toes, foot, or lateral malleolus	Near medial malleolus
Ulcer margin	Rounded, smooth, looks "punched out"	Irregularly shaped
Ulcer drainage	Minimal	Moderate to large amount
Ulcer tissue	Black eschar or pale pink granulation	Yellow slough or dark red, "ruddy" granulation
Pain	Intermittent claudication or rest pain in foot; ulcer may or may not be painful	Dull ache or heaviness in calf or thigh; ulcer often painful
Nails	Thickened; brittle	Normal or thickened
Skin colour	Dependent rubour; elevation pallor	Bronze-brown pigmentation; varicose veins may be visible
Skin texture	Thin, shiny, taut	Skin thick, hardened, and indurated
Skin temperature	Cool, temperature gradient down the leg	Warm, no temperature gradient
Dermatitis	Rarely occurs	Frequently occurs
Pruritus	Rarely occurs	Frequently occurs

(Table 40-2). Nonhealing arterial ulcers and gangrene are the most serious complications. Amputation may be needed if blood flow is not restored adequately or if severe infection occurs. If PAD has been present for an extended period, collateral circulation may prevent gangrene of the extremity. Unmanageable pain or severe, spreading infection, or both, are indicators that an amputation is required in individuals who are not candidates for revascularization.

Diagnostic Studies

Various tests can assess blood flow and outline the vascular system (Table 40-3). Doppler ultrasound uses a probe that directs high-frequency sound waves toward the vessel being examined. Duplex imaging uses a colour Doppler system to systematically map blood flow throughout the entire region of an artery. When palpation of a peripheral pulse is difficult because of severe PAD, the Doppler can determine the degree of blood flow. A palpable pulse and a Doppler pulse are not equivalent, and the terms are

COLLABORATIVE CARE

Table 40-3 Peripheral Arterial Disease

Diagnostic

- Health history and physical examination, including palpation of peripheral pulses
- Doppler ultrasound studies
- Segmental blood pressures
- Ankle–brachial index (ABI)
- Duplex imaging
- Angiogram
- Magnetic resonance angiography (MRA)

Collaborative Therapy

Cardiovascular disease risk factor modification

- Smoking cessation
- Regular physical exercise
- Achieve/maintain ideal body weight
- Follow Dietary Approaches to Stop Hypertension (DASH) diet (see Table 35-7)
- Tight glucose control in diabetics
- Tight blood pressure control
- Treatment of hyperlipidemia and hypertriglyceridemia (see Table 36-7)
- Antiplatelet agent (aspirin or clopidogrel [Plavix])

- Angiotensin-converting enzyme inhibitors (see Table 35-8)
- Treatment of claudication symptoms
- Structured walking/exercise program
- Cilostazol (Pletal)
- Pentoxifylline (Trental)
- Nutritional therapy
- Proper foot care (see Chapter 52, Table 52-22)
- Percutaneous transluminal balloon angioplasty with or without stent
- Percutaneous transluminal atherectomy
- Percutaneous transluminal cryoplasty
- Peripheral arterial bypass surgery
- Patch graft angioplasty, often in conjunction with bypass surgery
- Endarterectomy (for localized stenosis but rarely done)
- Thrombolytic therapy (for acute ischemia only)
- Amputation

not interchangeable. Segmental blood pressures are obtained (using Doppler ultrasound and a sphygmomanometer) at the thigh, below the knee, and at ankle level while the patient is supine. A drop in segmental BP of greater than 30 mm Hg suggests PAD.

The *ankle–brachial index* (ABI) is performed using a handheld Doppler. The ABI is calculated by dividing the ankle systolic BPs by the higher of the left and right brachial systolic BP (Criqui et al., 2008). A normal ABI is 1.00 to 1.40 and indicates adequate BP in the extremities. An ABI between 0.91 and 0.99 is considered borderline, a value of 0.90 or less is abnormal, and values greater than 1.40 indicate noncompressible arteries (Rooke et al., 2011). The ABI also is used after revascularization to monitor bypass graft patency. An ABI has limited usefulness when arteries are calcified and noncompressible, as occurs in patients with diabetes mellitus. In these patients, the ABI frequently is falsely elevated.

Angiography and magnetic resonance angiography delineate the location and extent of PAD. They also provide information on inflow and outflow vessels to plan for surgery (see Table 34-5).

Collaborative Care

Table 40-3 summarizes the collaborative care for a patient with PAD.

Risk Factor Modification.
CVD is the leading cause of death in Canada (Goldenberg et al., 2011). Patients who have diabetes and atherosclerotic vascular disease such as CAD or PAD are at the highest risk for cardiovascular events such as MI, ischemic stroke, and CVD-related death. The Canadian Diabetes Association 2008 Clinical Practice Guidelines (Canadian Diabetes Association Clinical Practice Guidelines Expert Committee, 2008) stress the importance of lifestyle modifications such as achieving and maintaining a healthy body weight, regular physical activity, smoking cessation, optimal BP control, and optimal glycemic control to reduce CVD risk factors (Fitchett & Kraw, 2008). Risk factors may be modified with drug therapy and lifestyle changes on the part of the patient and caregiver (see Table 36-5). Nurse-led clinics have been effective for managing CVD risk factors with PAD (Hatfield, Gulati, Rahman, Coughlin, & Chetter, 2008). Smoking cessation is essential in the management of patients with PAD to reduce the risk of CVD events and mortality. Smoking cessation is a complex and difficult process with a high incidence of smoking relapse. All patients with PAD should have access to comprehensive smoking cessation interventions (see Chapter 11, eTables 11-1 and 11-2).

Canadian lipid guidelines recommend aggressive management with a low-density lipoprotein cholesterol (LDL-C) of 2.0 mmol/L or less, and a total cholesterol (TC) and high-density lipoprotein-cholesterol (HDL-C) ratio less than 4.0 mmol/L (Leiter et al., 2006). Although dietary change is also recommended, this alone is unlikely to achieve these goals. Research indicates that treatment of PAD patients with a statin (e.g., simvastatin [Zocor]) not only lowers cholesterol levels but also reduces CVD morbidity and mortality risks. Further, statin use by PAD patients is also associated with improved walking performance, increased bypass graft patency, and increased survival (Stalenhoef, 2009). (Table 36-6 discusses medications to lower cholesterol.)

Hypertension is a major risk factor for PAD progression as well as other CVD events (e.g., stroke, MI, heart failure). The Canadian Hypertension Education Program (CHEP) 2012 recommendations for the management of hypertension in patients with PAD and CVD include BP less than 140/90 mm Hg. In patients with diabetes mellitus, BP less than 130/80 mm Hg is recommended (CHEP, 2012). Initial antihypertensive drug therapy includes thiazides, ACE inhibitors, and angiotensin II receptor blocker (ARBs). Lifestyle changes are encouraged and include reducing dietary sodium and following the Dietary Approaches to Stop Hypertension (DASH) diet. (Chapter 35 discusses hypertension.)

Diabetes is a well-known risk factor for PAD and increases the risk of amputation in these patients (Norgren et al., 2007). It is recommended that diabetic patients maintain a glycosylated hemoglobin (A1C) below 7.0% and, optimally, as close as possible to 6.0%. (Chapter 52 discusses diabetes mellitus.)

Drug Therapy.
Antiplatelet agents are considered critically important for reducing the risks of CVD events and death in PAD patients. Guidelines for oral antiplatelet therapy recommend aspirin (75-325 mg/day). For patients who are aspirin intolerant, clopidogrel (Plavix) (75 mg/day) is indicated. Combination antiplatelet therapy with aspirin and clopidogrel is not recommended. Likewise, anticoagulants (e.g., warfarin [Coumadin]) are not recommended for the prevention of CVD events in PAD patients. The use of ACE inhibitors (e.g., ramipril [Altace]) decreases morbidity and mortality risks (Rooke et al., 2011).

Two drugs are used to treat intermittent claudication, cilostazol (Pletal) and pentoxifylline (Trental). Cilostazol is a phosphodiesterase inhibitor that promotes the effects of prostaglandin

I_2. This inhibits platelet aggregation and increases vasodilation. Cilostazol increases maximal walking distance and quality of life. It is recommended as first-line drug therapy for patients with intermittent claudication who do not respond to exercise therapy and are not candidates for surgical or radiological interventions (Norgren et al., 2007; Sobel & Verhaeghe, 2008). Although cilostazol improves symptoms, it does not reduce CVD morbidity and mortality risks and is contraindicated for patients with heart failure. Pentoxifylline increases red blood cell (RBC) flexibility and reduces blood viscosity. It is recommended as a second-line, alternative therapy to cilostazol. Anticoagulants, oral vasodilator prostaglandins (e.g., beraprost), and chelation are not recommended for the treatment of claudication symptoms (Hirsch et al., 2006). One promising approach to claudication treatment under investigation is carnitine, a naturally occurring derivative of the amino acid lysine. Carnitine improves initial and maximal treadmill walking distance and quality of life (Norgren et al., 2007).

Exercise Therapy.

The primary nondrug treatment for intermittent claudication is a formal, supervised exercise training program. Lack of exercise in PAD patients is related to low quality of life, particularly in men (Koivunen & Lukkarinen, 2006). Walking is the most effective exercise for PAD patients. A supervised, hospital-based PAD rehabilitation program is an effective means of improving exercise performance. Such programs typically include exercise for 30 to 60 min/day, three to five times a week, for 3 to 6 months. Supervised, treadmill exercise training improves walking performance and quality of life in PAD patients whether or not they have claudication (McDermott et al., 2009). A home exercise program is an alternative to a formal program. Encourage slow, progressive physical activity after a warm-up period. Instruct the patient to walk to the point of discomfort, stop and rest, and then resume walking until the discomfort recurs. Walking should be done for 30 to 40 min/day, three to five times a week for at least 6 months. An exercise therapy program should also be implemented in PAD patients after surgical interventions (discussed later in this chapter).

Nutritional Therapy.

PAD patients should be taught to adjust their dietary intake so that their body mass index is less than 25 kg/m^2 and their waist circumference is less than 101.6 cm (40 inches) for men and less than 89 cm (35 inches) for women (National Heart, Lung, and Blood Institute [NHLBI], 1998). A diet high in fruits, vegetables, and whole grains and low in cholesterol, saturated fat, and salt is recommended. Dietary cholesterol should be less than 200 mg/day, saturated fat intake should be substantially reduced, and dietary sodium should be 2 g/day or less (see Chapter 37, Tables 37-10 to 37-14).

Complementary and Alternative Therapies.

A number of vitamin, mineral, dietary, and herbal supplements have been investigated in the treatment of intermittent claudication. Currently, there are insufficient data to support the efficacy of supplemental fish oil, ginkgo biloba, L-arginine, or homocysteine-lowering vitamins (e.g., folate, vitamin B_6, cobalamin), in the treatment of claudication (Norgren et al., 2007; Sobel & Verhaeghe, 2008). Vitamin E is not recommended to treat claudication (Hirsch et al., 2006). Patients taking antiplatelet agents (e.g., aspirin), nonsteroidal anti-inflammatory agents (NSAIDs) (e.g., ibuprofen [Motrin]), and anticoagulants (e.g., warfarin) should consult with their health care provider before taking any dietary or herbal supplements owing to potential interactions and bleeding risks

(see the Complementary and Alternative Therapies box later in the chapter on p. 1017 (Frishman, Beroval, & Carosella, 2009).

Care of the Leg With Critical Limb Ischemia.

Critical limb ischemia is a condition characterized by pain at rest or at night and tissue loss such as ulcerations or gangrene of the leg attributed to PAD (Rooke et al., 2011). Optimal therapy is revascularization via surgery or endovascular procedure. Although palliative in nature, all patients with critical limb ischemia should have aggressive CVD risk factor modification and antiplatelet therapy to decrease the risk of a CVD event (Hirsch et al., 2006; Norgren et al., 2007; Gray et al., 2008).

Conservative management goals include protecting the extremity from trauma, decreasing ischemic pain, preventing and controlling infection, and maximizing perfusion. Carefully inspect, cleanse, and lubricate both feet to prevent cracking of the skin and infection. Avoid soaking feet to prevent skin maceration (or breakdown). If ulceration is present, keep the affected foot clean and dry. Cover any ulcers with a dry, sterile dressing to maintain cleanliness and protect the limb. Ulcers with significant depth may be treated with a variety of wound care products, but healing is unlikely without increased blood flow. Encourage the patient to select soft, roomy, and protective footwear and avoid extremes of heat and cold. Keep the patient's heels free of pressure. This may be accomplished by placing a pillow under the calves so that the heels are off the bed. Commercially available devices can also provide heel protection. Opioid analgesia and placing the bed in the reverse Trendelenburg position may control pain and facilitate perfusion to the lower extremities (Norgren et al., 2007). Some evidence indicates that spinal cord stimulation or hyperbaric oxygen therapy may be helpful in preventing amputation in patients with critical limb ischemia (Melamed et al., 2008). Another promising strategy under investigation is gene therapy to stimulate blood vessel growth (angiogenesis) (Nikol et al., 2008).

Interventional Radiology Catheter-Based Procedures.

Interventional radiology catheter-based procedures are alternatives to open surgical approaches for treatment of lower extremity PAD. These procedures take place in a catheterization laboratory rather than an operating room. Determining which intervention to use depends on stenosis location along with type and severity of the lesion. Most patients can ambulate the day of the procedure and return to normal activity within 24 to 48 hours (White & Gray, 2007). All of these procedures are similar to angiography in that they involve the insertion of a specialized catheter into the femoral artery. The percutaneous transluminal balloon angioplasty procedure uses a catheter that contains a cylindrical balloon at the tip. The end of the catheter is advanced to the narrowed (stenotic) area of the artery. When in position, the balloon is inflated, compressing the confining atherosclerotic intimal lining while also stretching the underlying media (White & Gray, 2007; Perera & Lyden, 2007).

Stents, expandable metallic devices, are positioned within the artery immediately after the balloon angioplasty is performed. The stent acts as a scaffold to keep the artery open and is used as a treatment for peripheral artery dissection (Nikol et al., 2008; White & Gray, 2007). Stents may be covered with Dacron or a drug-eluting agent (e.g., paclitaxel) to minimize re-stenosis by reducing the amount of new tissue growth in the stent.

Atherectomy is the removal of the obstructing plaque. A directional atherectomy device uses a high-speed cutting disc built into the catheter end that cuts long strips of the atheroma.

Laser atherectomy uses ultraviolet energy to break the molecular bonds of the atheroma to reduce the stenosis (White & Gray, 2007; Perera & Lyden, 2007; Shrikhande & McKinsey, 2008). Orbital or rotational atherectomy catheters have a diamond-coated tip that rotates at a high rate of speed (similar to a dentist drill) to pulverize the calcium within the atheroma into particles smaller than a blood cell. Cryoplasty combines two procedures: balloon angioplasty and cold therapy. The specialized balloon is inflated with liquid nitrous oxide that changes from liquid to gas as it enters the balloon. Expansion of the gas results in cooling to −10°C. The cold minimizes re-stenosis through reduction of smooth muscle cell activity (Wildgruber & Berger, 2008). Preprocedure and postprocedure nursing care is the same as for a diagnostic angiography. Antiplatelet agents are necessary after the procedure to reduce the risk of re-stenosis. Long-term, low-dose aspirin therapy is recommended postprocedure (Sobel & Verhaeghe, 2008). Re-stenosis rates depend on the procedure performed, lesion type and length, and target vessel characteristics. Immediate postprocedure success rates are high (>95%) for iliac and femoral interventions (White & Gray, 2007; Morgan, Belli, & Munneke, 2008).

Surgical Therapy. Surgery is indicated in patients with long areas of stenosis or severely calcified arteries (Gray et al., 2008). Various surgical approaches can be used to improve blood flow beyond a stenotic or occluded artery. The most common is a peripheral artery bypass operation with autogenous (native) vein or synthetic graft material to bypass or carry blood around the lesion (Figure 40-7).

Synthetic grafts (expanded PTFE or Dacron) typically are used for long bypasses such as an axillary–femoral or axillary–popliteal bypass. When a person's own vein is not available, human umbilical vein, cryopreserved vein, or a composite sequential bypass graft is an alternative (Ronayne, 2007). Balloon angioplasty with stenting also may be used in combination with bypass surgery. Other surgical options include *endarterectomy* (opening the artery and removing the obstructing plaque) and patch graft *angioplasty* (opening the artery, removing plaque, and sewing a patch to the opening to widen the lumen).

Not all patients with critical limb ischemia undergo revascularization. Amputation is the least desirable end-stage surgical option. Amputation may be required if tissue necrosis is extensive, infectious gangrene or osteomyelitis (infection in the bone) develops, or if all major arteries in the limb are occluded, precluding the possibility of successful surgery (Gray et al., 2008). Every effort is made to preserve as much of the limb as possible so that the potential for rehabilitation is optimized (see Chapter 64). Implementation of an amputee mobility protocol after surgery can increase functional mobility of patients with a lower limb amputation and maximize their rehabilitation potential (Marzen-Groller et al., 2008). (Amputation is discussed in Chapter 65.)

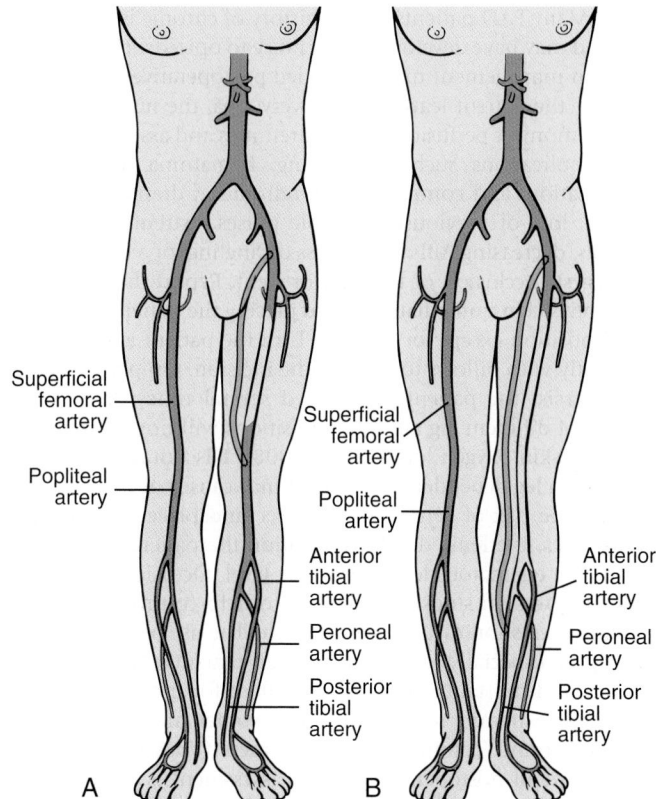

Figure 40-7 A, Femoral–popliteal bypass graft around an occluded superficial femoral artery. **B,** Femoral–posterior tibial bypass graft around occluded superficial femoral, popliteal, and proximal tibial arteries.

Source: Courtesy F. W. LoGerfo, Boston.

COMPLEMENTARY & ALTERNATIVE THERAPIES

Natural Health Products That May Affect Clotting

Effects

Increase Anticoagulant Effects
Angelica, anise, bilberry, bromelain, celery, chamomile, devil's claw, dong quai, fenugreek, feverfew, garlic, ginger, *Ginkgo biloba,* goldenseal, horse chestnut, licorice root, lovage root, meadowsweet, motherwort, parsley, passionflower, red clover, rue, turmeric, willow bark

Decrease Anticoagulant Effects
Coenzyme Q_{10}, ginseng, green tea, St. John's wort

Nursing Implications

- In general, these natural products should be used with caution or not at all in patients with bleeding or clotting disorders or those taking anticoagulant and antiplatelet drugs (e.g., warfarin [Coumadin], heparin, low–molecular weight heparin, aspirin, ticlopidine, or clopidogrel [Plavix]).
- Advise these patients to consult with a health care provider before using any of these natural products.
- These natural health products should be discontinued at least 2 to 3 wk before surgery to avoid potential complications. If this is not possible, the herbal product in its original container should be brought to the health care provider or the surgery site so the anaesthesia care provider knows exactly what the patient is taking.
- One common mechanism is to inhibit platelet aggregation.

NURSING MANAGEMENT: LOWER EXTREMITY PERIPHERAL ARTERIAL DISEASE

▪ Nursing Assessment

Table 40-4 presents subjective and objective data that the nurse should obtain from a patient with PAD.

▪ Nursing Diagnoses

Nursing care plan (NCP) 40-1 presents the priority nursing diagnoses for the patient with PAD of the lower extremities (who has not undergone surgery).

▪ Planning

The overall goals for the patient who has lower extremity PAD include (1) adequate tissue perfusion; (2) relief of pain;

NURSING ASSESSMENT

Table 40-4 Peripheral Arterial Disease

Subjective Data

Important Health Information

Past health history: Diabetes mellitus, tobacco use, hypertension, hyperlipidemia, hypertriglyceridemia, hyperuricemia, impaired renal function, obesity; ↑ high-sensitivity C-reactive protein, homocysteine or lipoprotein (a) [Lp(a)] levels; positive family history; exposure to environmental smoke; sedentary lifestyle; stress

High sodium, saturated fat and cholesterol intake; elevated hemoglobin (Hb) A1C

Exercise intolerance

Symptoms

- Buttock, thigh, or calf pain that is precipitated by exercise and that subsides with rest (intermittent claudication) or progresses to pain at rest; burning pain in forefeet and toes at rest; numbness, tingling, sensation of cold in legs or feet; progressive loss of sensation and deep pain in extremities
- Erectile dysfunction

Objective Data

Integumentary

Loss of hair on legs and feet; thick toenails; pallor with elevation; dependent rubour; thin, cool, shiny skin with muscle atrophy; skin breakdown and arterial ulcers, especially over bony areas; gangrene

Cardiovascular

Decreased or absent peripheral pulses; feet cool to touch; capillary refill >3 sec; bruits may be present at pulse sites

Neurological

Mobility or sensation impairment

Possible Diagnostic Findings

Arterial stenosis evident with duplex imaging, ↓ Doppler pressures, ↓ ankle–brachial index (ABI), angiography indicative of peripheral atherosclerosis

---

(3) increased exercise tolerance; and (4) intact, healthy skin on extremities.

▪ Nursing Implementation

▪ Health Promotion

Assess the patient for CVD risk factors and provide instructions on how to control them (see Chapter 36, Table 36-5). Also teach diet modification to reduce the intake of cholesterol, saturated fat, and refined sugars; proper care of the feet; and the avoidance of injury to the extremities. Encourage patients with positive family histories of cardiac, diabetic, or vascular disease to obtain regular follow-up care.

▪ Acute Intervention

After surgical or radiological intervention, the patient is moved to a recovery area for observation. Check the operative extremity every 15 minutes initially and then hourly for colour, temperature, capillary refill, presence of peripheral pulses, and sensation and movement. Loss of palpable pulses or a change in the Doppler sound over a pulse, or both, necessitates immediate notification of the physician or radiologist and prompt intervention. ABI measurements may be ordered, and the indexes should be higher than the patient's baseline and should remain stable if the bypass (or stent) remains patent. Compare all assessment findings with the patient's baseline and with findings in the opposite limb (Ronayne, 2007). Many PAD patients have a history of chronic ischemic rest pain and may have developed a tolerance to opioids. Thus, aggressive pain management may be needed postoperatively.

After the patient leaves the recovery area, the nurse will continue to monitor perfusion to the extremities and assess for potential complications such as bleeding, hematoma, thrombosis, embolization, and compartment syndrome. A dramatic increase in pain, loss of previously palpable pulses, extremity pallor or cyanosis, decreasing ABIs, numbness or tingling, or a cold extremity suggests occlusion of the graft or stent. Report these findings to the physician immediately. Avoid placing the patient in a knee-flexed position except for exercise. Turn the patient and position frequently with pillows to support the incision. On postoperative day 1, assist the patient out of bed several times daily. Short periods of different leg and body positions will not impair postoperative skin oxygen levels (Rich, 2008). Discourage prolonged sitting with leg dependency because it may cause pain and edema, increase the risk of venous thrombosis, and place stress on the suture lines. If edema develops, position the patient supine and elevate the edematous leg above heart level. Occasionally, graduated compression stockings are used to help control leg edema. Walking even short distances is desirable. The use of a walker may be helpful, especially in frail, older adult patients. Although graft patency and mortality rates are equivalent for men and women after lower extremity revascularization, women are more likely to develop wound complications than men (Vouyouka & Kent, 2007). Careful postoperative wound assessment is important. If no complications are present, discharge from the hospital can be anticipated 3 to 5 days postoperatively.

▪ Ambulatory and Home Care

Assess for CVD risk factors and be alert for opportunities to teach health promotion strategies to patients and their caregivers (see

NURSING CARE PLAN 40-1

Peripheral Arterial Disease of the Lower Extremities

NURSING DIAGNOSIS	**Ineffective tissue perfusion (peripheral)** *related to* decreased arterial blood flow *as evidenced by* intermittent claudication or rest pain; diminished or absent peripheral pulses; pallor or blanching on elevation of limb; or hyperemia when limb is dependent
Expected Patient Outcomes	**Nursing Interventions and *Rationales***
• Identifies activities that promote circulation • Identifies factors that impair circulation	• Assess for diminished or absent peripheral pulses in the extremities; colour or temperature changes in the extremities; altered sensation and movement of the extremities; increased pain level *because these are indicators of worsening peripheral perfusion.* • Compare extremities for warmth, capillary refill, and colour *because differences may indicate impaired blood flow.* • Encourage patient to participate in a structured walking program *to enhance O₂ utilization in the tissues.* • Teach the patient to reduce risk factors for peripheral arterial disease by stopping smoking (see Chapter 11), lowering serum cholesterol and triglyceride levels, and controlling hypertension and diabetes mellitus *to prevent worsening of the atherosclerosis.* • Teach patient to avoid tight girdles, garters, and socks, and avoid crossing legs, *because they impair peripheral circulation.*
NURSING DIAGNOSIS	**Impaired skin integrity** *related to* decreased peripheral circulation, altered sensation, and increased susceptibility to infection *as evidenced by* ulcerations, nonhealing wounds, or gangrenous areas on lower extremities
Expected Patient Outcomes	**Nursing Interventions and *Rationales***
• Maintains intact skin on lower extremities • Shows no evidence of wound or skin infection	• Teach patient to avoid trauma to lower extremities *because tissue is very fragile and wounds heal poorly as a result of poor circulation.* • Teach patient to check temperature of bath water with fingers rather than toes to avoid burns *because sensation in toes may be diminished.* • Teach patient and significant other proper care and daily inspection of feet; and the need to wear roomy, soft footwear and to obtain callus and toenail care by a health care provider *to avoid additional damage to the extremity.* • Teach patient to apply a mild lotion daily to the lower extremities *to keep the skin moist and avoid cracking.*
NURSING DIAGNOSIS	**Acute pain** *related to* tissue ischemia secondary to decreased peripheral circulation *as evidenced by* complaints of intermittent claudication or rest pain
Expected Patient Outcome	**Nursing Interventions and *Rationales***
• Experiences relief of pain	• Assess location, onset, degree, and duration of pain *so appropriate interventions are planned.* • Encourage the patient to rest when pain occurs so that tissue ischemia and pain are relieved or reduced, and explain rationale to patient *to increase cooperation.* • Teach patient relaxation techniques *because stress increases vasoconstriction and pain.* • Teach patient to report rest pain *because this is an indication of worsening of the arterial blockages.* • Teach patient the indications, the benefits, and the potential adverse effects of antiplatelet therapy (e.g., aspirin, ticlopidine [Ticlid]) to prevent thrombosis and cilostazol (Pletal) *because they help prevent pain and increase pain-free walking.*
NURSING DIAGNOSIS	**Activity intolerance** *related to* imbalance between oxygen supply and demand *as evidenced by* intermittent claudication
Expected Patient Outcome	**Nursing Interventions and *Rationales***
• Displays improved ability to ambulate without pain	• Assess the amount of exercise the patient can tolerate before the onset of pain *to provide a baseline for evaluation.* • Instruct the patient to develop a structured exercise program that includes warm-up exercises, progressive walking, and cool-down exercises *to prevent injury during exercise.* • Inform the patient that he or she should walk to point of pain, rest until pain subsides, and resume walking *so endurance can be increased and oxygen utilization in the tissues enhanced.*
NURSING DIAGNOSIS	**Ineffective self-health management** *related to* lack of knowledge of disease and self-care measures *as evidenced by* questions about disease process, wound, and treatment
Expected Patient Outcomes	**Nursing Interventions and *Rationales***
• Describes disease and treatment plan • Demonstrates how to care for leg ulcers • Identifies risk factors for PAD and how to manage them	• Identify factors that influence learning such as perception of severity, available support systems, cognitive ability, and physical ability *so that teaching plan can be individualized.* • Assess patient's knowledge of disease and its treatment *to determine extent of the problem and plan appropriate interventions.* • Teach patient about disease, treatment, activity restrictions, and ulcer care *so patient will be less anxious, be more cooperative with treatment plan, and make accurate adjustments in lifestyle.* • Explain the importance of smoking cessation *so patient understands the effects of nicotine.* • Emphasize the importance of meticulous foot care *to reduce the risk of infection and injury to feet.*

PAD, peripheral arterial disease.

Chapter 36). Tobacco use in any form (including environmental smoke) is contraindicated. Nicotine exerts vasoconstrictive effects and tobacco smoke impairs transport and cellular utilization of oxygen and increases blood viscosity and homocysteine levels. Continued tobacco use dramatically decreases the long-term patency rates of grafts and stents and increases the risk of an MI or stroke. Encourage physical activity and explain that it improves a number of CVD risk factors, including hypertension, hyperlipidemia, obesity, and glucose levels. Physical activity also improves peripheral circulation and increases walking distance (Badger, Soong, O'Donnell, Boreman, & McGuigan, 2007). Promoting self-efficacy when providing CVD risk factor education has shown to improve healthy food selections and exercise in PAD patients (Sol et al., 2008). (See Chapter 4 for discussion of patient and caregiver teaching.) Teach foot care to all patients with PAD. Meticulous foot care is especially important in the diabetic patient with PAD (see Table 52-21). Diabetic neuropathy increases the patient's susceptibility to traumatic injury and results in delay in seeking treatment. Instruct patients to inspect their legs and feet daily for mottling, changes in skin colour, skin texture, amount of subcutaneous fat, and reduction in hair growth. The nurse can also teach patients to check skin temperature and capillary refill and palpate pulses. Emphasize that they must report any changes in these findings or the development of any ulceration or inflammation to their health care provider. Thick or overgrown toenails and calluses are potentially serious and require regular attention by a skilled health care provider (e.g., podiatrist). Patients who have poor eyesight, back problems, obesity, or arthritis may need assistance with foot care. Encourage patients to wear clean, all-cotton or all-wool socks and comfortable shoes with rounded (not pointed) toes and soft insoles. Tell patients to lace shoes loosely and to break in new shoes gradually (Table 40-5).

Evaluation

NCP 40-1 addresses the expected outcomes for the patient with PAD of the lower extremities.

Acute Arterial Ischemic Disorders

Etiology and Pathophysiology

Acute arterial ischemia is a sudden interruption in the arterial blood supply to a tissue, organ, or extremity that, if left untreated, can result in tissue death. It is caused by embolism, thrombosis of a pre-existing atherosclerotic artery, or trauma. Embolization of a thrombus from the heart is the most frequent cause of acute arterial occlusion. Heart conditions in which thrombi can develop include infective endocarditis, MI, mitral valve disease, chronic atrial fibrillation, cardiomyopathies, and prosthetic heart valves. Noncardiac sources of emboli include aneurysms, ulcerated atherosclerotic plaque, recent endovascular procedures, venous thrombi, and rarely, arteritis. The thrombi become dislodged and may travel anywhere in the systemic circulation if they originate in the left side of the heart. The majority of emboli obstruct an artery of the lower extremity (e.g., iliofemoral, popliteal, tibial) (Sobel &

PATIENT & CAREGIVER TEACHING GUIDE

Table 40-5 Peripheral Artery Bypass Surgery

Include the following in a teaching plan:

1. Reduce risk factors by stopping the use of tobacco products, controlling blood pressure and blood glucose levels (if diabetic), and lowering cholesterol and triglyceride levels, achieving/maintaining ideal body weight, and exercising regularly.

2. Provide rationales for and basic mechanism of action of medications such as antiplatelets, antihypertensives, anticholesterol therapy, and pain medication and how long anticipated therapy will last.

3. Eat healthily—it is essential to recovery. Drink plenty of fluids, eat a well-balanced diet (e.g., foods high in protein, vitamins C and A, and zinc; high-fibre foods; fresh fruits and vegetables), and eat fewer high-fat foods and reduce salt intake.

4. Participate in a supervised exercise program and/or take a daily walk. In the beginning, take several short walks a day and rest between activities. Gradually increase your walking to 30 to 40 min/day 3 to 5 days/wk.

5. Care for your feet and legs. Inspect your feet and wash them daily. Wear clean cotton or wool socks and well-fitting shoes. File toenails straight across. Avoid sitting with your legs crossed, extreme hot and cold temperatures, and prolonged standing.

6. Follow routine postoperative wound care that includes keeping incision clean and dry; do not disturb Steri-Strips (if present).

7. Monitor for signs and symptoms of impaired healing and/or infection of the leg incision, and notify health care provider if any of the following occur:
   - Prolonged drainage or pus from the incision
   - Increased redness, warmth, pain, or hardness along incision
   - Separation of wound edges
   - Temperature greater than 37.8°C

8. Keep all follow-up appointments with your health care provider.

9. Notify health care provider if increased leg or foot pain or a change in the colour or temperature of foot and leg is experienced.

Verhaeghe, 2008). Thrombi that originate in the right side of the heart will travel to the lungs and cause a pulmonary embolus (see Chapter 29).

Arterial emboli tend to lodge at sites of arterial branching or in areas of atherosclerotic narrowing. An acute arterial occlusion causes the oxygen and blood supply distal to the embolus to decrease suddenly, producing ischemia. The amount of tissue and muscle at risk, degree of the ischemia, and extent of the symptoms depend on several factors, including (1) the location and size of the occlusion, (2) the occurrence of clot fragmentation with embolism to smaller vessels, (3) the degree of PAD already present, and (4) the presence of collaterals around the acute obstruction (Gray et al., 2008).

Sudden local thrombosis may occur at the site of an atherosclerotic plaque. Hypovolemia (e.g., shock), hyperviscosity (e.g., polycythemia), and hypercoagulability (e.g., chemotherapy) states predispose an individual to thrombotic arterial occlusion (Sobel & Verhaeghe, 2008). Traumatic injury to the extremity itself may cause partial or total occlusion. Acute arterial occlusion may also develop as a result of arterial dissection in the carotid artery or aorta or as a result of iatrogenic arterial injury (e.g., after angiography).

Clinical Manifestations

Clinical manifestations of acute arterial ischemia include the "six Ps": pain, pallor, paralysis, pulselessness, paresthesia, and poikilothermia (adaptation of the limb to the environmental temperature, most often cool). Without immediate intervention, ischemia may progress quickly to tissue necrosis and gangrene within a few hours. If the nurse detects these signs, the nurse should immediately notify the physician. Paralysis is a very late sign of acute arterial ischemia and signals the death of nerves supplying the extremity. Footdrop occurs as a result of nerve damage. Because nerve tissue is extremely sensitive to hypoxia, limb paralysis or ischemic neuropathy may be permanent even after revascularization.

Collaborative Care

Early treatment is essential to keep the affected limb viable during acute arterial ischemia. Anticoagulant therapy with continuous IV unfractionated heparin (UH) is started to prevent thrombus enlargement and inhibit further embolization (Norgren et al., 2007; Frishman et al., 2009). In patients undergoing embolectomy, UH should be followed by long-term anticoagulation with warfarin (see discussion of other anticoagulant options later in this chapter). To restore blood flow, the embolus/thrombus is removed as soon as possible. Options for embolus/thrombus removal consist of percutaneous catheter-directed thrombolytic therapy, percutaneous mechanical thrombectomy with or without thrombolytic therapy, surgical thrombectomy, or surgical bypass (Gray et al., 2008). Catheter-directed intra-arterial thrombolytic therapy (e.g., tissue plasminogen activator [tPA] [alteplase]) is recommended for patients with short-term (<14 days) thromboembolic disease (Sobel & Verhaeghe, 2008; Gray et al., 2008).

A percutaneous catheter is inserted into the femoral artery, threaded to the site of the clot, and the thrombolytic drug is infused. Thrombolytic agents work by directly dissolving the clot over a period of 24 to 48 hours. (Chapter 36 discusses thrombolytic therapy.) The catheter may act as a mechanical thrombectomy device, meaning it is also designed to remove or fragment the thrombus (Shrikhande & McKinsey, 2008).

Surgical intervention is recommended for some patients (e.g., those with ischemia for more than 14 days when catheter-based interventions are not possible such as an inability of the guidewire to transverse the thrombus) (Gray et al., 2008). Direct arteriotomy may be necessary to remove the clot. Surgical revascularization may be used in a patient with trauma (e.g., laceration of the artery) or with significant arterial occlusion. Amputation is reserved for patients with ischemic rest pain and tissue loss, for whom limb salvage is not possible. If the patient remains at risk for further embolization from a persistent source (e.g., chronic atrial fibrillation), long-term oral anticoagulation is recommended to prevent further acute arterial ischemic episodes (see Table 40-9 later in this chapter) (Sobel & Verhaeghe, 2008).

Thromboangiitis Obliterans

Thromboangiitis obliterans (Buerger's disease) is a nonatherosclerotic, segmental, recurrent inflammatory vaso-occlusive disorder of the small- and medium-sized arteries and veins of the upper and lower extremities. On very rare occasions, systemic manifestations of the disease may involve cerebral, mesenteric, or coronary arteries. The disorder occurs predominantly in young men (<40 yr) with a long history of tobacco use, but without other CVD risk factors (e.g., hypertension, hyperlipidemia, diabetes mellitus) (Chen et al., 2007).

In Buerger's disease, an inflammatory process damages the blood vessel wall. Lymphocytes and giant cells infiltrate the vessel wall accompanied by fibroblast proliferation (Paraskevas, Liapis, Briana, & Mikhailidis, 2007). Ultimately, thrombosis and fibrosis occur in the vessel, causing tissue ischemia. Patients with Buerger's disease have a high rate of periodontitis and the presence of *Porphyromonas gingivalis* (a periodontal pathogen) in the occluded blood vessels (Chen et al., 2007). This suggests a role for bacterial infection in the pathogenesis of Buerger's disease. Research is examining genetic factors in susceptible individuals (Chen et al., 2007; Paraskevas et al., 2007). The symptom complex of Buerger's disease often is confused with PAD and other inflammatory or autoimmune diseases (e.g., scleroderma). Patients may have intermittent claudication of the feet, hands, or arms. As the disease progresses, rest pain and ischemic ulcerations develop. Other signs and symptoms may include colour and temperature changes of the limbs, paresthesia, superficial vein thrombosis, and cold sensitivity. There are no laboratory or diagnostic tests specific to Buerger's disease. Diagnosis is made based on age of onset, history of tobacco use, clinical symptoms, involvement of distal vessels, presence of ischemic ulcerations, and exclusion of diabetes mellitus, autoimmune disease, thrombophilia (inherited tendency to clot), and proximal source of emboli (Chen et al., 2007).

Patients with Buerger's disease have RBC rigidity, elevated hematocrit, and increased blood viscosity (Paraskevas et al., 2007). The mainstay of treatment for Buerger's disease is the complete cessation of tobacco use in any form. Use of nicotine replacement products is contraindicated. Patients have a choice between their tobacco and their affected limbs, but not both. Conservative management includes the use of antibiotics to treat any infected ulcers and analgesics to manage the ischemic pain. Patients must avoid trauma to the extremities. A variety of novel drug therapies to treat Buerger's disease have been studied but the results have been marginal (Paraskevas et al., 2007). One therapy with modest effectiveness in Europe has been IV iloprost (a prostaglandin analogue). Another promising area of research is the intramuscular gene transfer of vascular growth factors (Nikol et al., 2008).

Surgical options include *sympathectomy* (transection of a nerve, ganglion, and/or plexus of the sympathetic nervous system), implantation of a spinal cord stimulator, and bypass surgery. Sympathectomy and implantation of a spinal cord stimulator are useful in improving distal blood flow and reducing pain, but neither alters the inflammatory process. Bypass surgery typically is not an option owing to the involvement of smaller, distal vessels but may be used in selected patients with severe ischemia (Paraskevas et al., 2007).

Painful ulcerations may require finger or toe amputations. Amputation below the knee may occur in severe cases. The amputation rate of patients who continue tobacco use is almost three times greater than for those who do not (Cooper et al., 2004).

Raynaud's Phenomenon

Raynaud's phenomenon is an episodic vasospastic disorder of small cutaneous arteries, most frequently involving the fingers and toes. It occurs primarily in young women (typically between

15 and 40 years of age) and it is more common in women than in men (Bakst, Merola, Franks, & Sanchez, 2008). The exact etiology of Raynaud's phenomenon remains unknown. One theory is that the vasospasm results from an exaggerated response to sympathetic nervous system stimulation. Other contributing factors include occupational-related trauma and pressure to the fingertips as noted in typists, pianists, and those who use handheld vibrating equipment. Exposure to heavy metals (e.g., lead) may also be a contributing factor. Primary Raynaud's phenomenon, the more common form of the disease, is associated with significantly lower physical and mental health–related quality of life (De Angelis, Salaffi, & Grassi, 2008). When symptoms occur in association with autoimmune diseases (e.g., rheumatoid arthritis, systemic lupus erythematosus), the disorder is called *secondary Raynaud's phenomenon*. Raynaud's phenomenon is characterized by vasospasm-induced colour changes of the fingers, toes, ears, and nose (white, blue, and red) (Figure 40-8). Decreased perfusion results in pallor (white). The digits then appear cyanotic (bluish-purple). These changes are followed by rubour (red), caused by the hyperemic response that occurs when perfusion is restored. The patient usually describes coldness and numbness in the vasoconstrictive phase followed by throbbing, aching pain; tingling; and swelling in the hyperemic phase. An episode usually lasts only minutes but, in severe cases, may persist for several hours. Exposure to cold, emotional upsets, tobacco use, and caffeine usually precipitate symptoms. After frequent, prolonged attacks, the skin may become thickened and the nails brittle. Occasionally, complications include *punctate* (small hole) lesions of the fingertips and superficial gangrenous ulcers in advanced stages. Diagnosis is based on persistent symptoms for at least 2 years. The primary focus of nursing management of Raynaud's phenomenon is patient teaching.

Instructions should focus on preventing recurrent episodes. Tell patients to wear loose, warm clothing as protection from the cold, including gloves when using the refrigerator or freezer or when handling cold objects. At all times, patients should avoid temperature extremes. Immersing hands in warm water often decreases the vasospasm. The patient should stop using all tobacco products and avoid caffeine and other drugs that have vasoconstrictive effects (e.g., amphetamines, cocaine, ergotamine, pseudoephedrine).

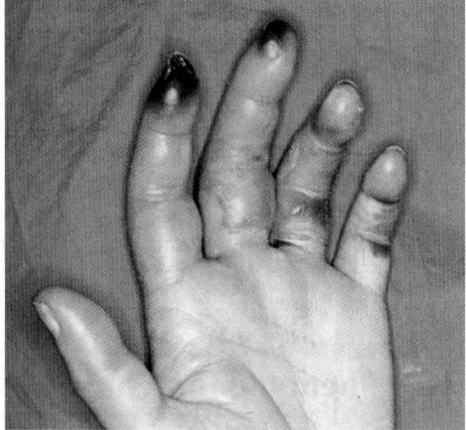

Figure 40-8 Raynaud's phenomenon.

Source: Kamal, A., & Brockelhurst, J. C. (1991). *Color atlas of geriatric medicine* (2nd ed.). St. Louis: Mosby–Year Book.

Patients with Raynaud's phenomenon often describe themselves as anxious or depressed, or both (De Angelis et al., 2008). Biofeedback, relaxation training, and stress management may be useful. If appropriate, encourage patients to explore these options. When a patient's episodes are severe and other therapies are ineffective, drug therapy is considered. Calcium channel blockers (e.g., diltiazem [Cardizem]) are the first-line drug therapy (Bakst et al., 2008). Calcium channel blockers relax smooth muscles of the arterioles by blocking the influx of calcium into the cells, thus reducing the frequency and severity of vasospastic attacks (Vinjar & Stewart, 2008).

Sympathectomy is considered only in advanced cases. Patients with Raynaud's phenomenon should receive routine follow-up to monitor for development of connective tissue or autoimmune diseases because Raynaud's phenomenon may be an early sign of scleroderma (Bakst et al., 2008).

Venous Disorders

Venous Thrombosis

Phlebitis is the inflammation (e.g., redness, tenderness, warmth, mild edema) of a superficial vein without the presence of a thrombus (clot) (Cesarone et al., 2007). It occurs in about 65% of all patients receiving IV therapy. It is rarely infectious and usually resolves quickly with removal of the IV catheter. *Venous thrombosis* involves the formation of a thrombus in association with inflammation of the vein. It is the most common disorder of the veins and is classified as either *superficial vein thrombosis* or *deep vein thrombosis*. **Superficial vein thrombosis (SVT)** is the formation of a thrombus in a superficial vein. **Deep vein thrombosis (DVT)** is a disorder involving a thrombus in a deep vein, most commonly the iliac and femoral veins (Milio et al., 2008). SVT is generally a benign disorder. However, there is a risk for extension of the clot to deeper veins if the thrombus involves the superficial femoral vein and/or is near the saphenofemoral junction (Cesarone et al., 2007). **Venous thromboembolism (VTE)** is the preferred terminology and represents the spectrum of pathology from DVT to pulmonary embolism (PE) (James, 2009) (Table 40-6). (PE is discussed in Chapter 30.)

Etiology

Three important factors (called **Virchow's triad**) in the etiology of venous thrombosis are (1) venous stasis, (2) damage of the endothelium (inner lining of the vein), and (3) hypercoagulability of the blood. The patient at risk for the development of venous thrombosis usually has predisposing conditions to these three disorders (Figure 40-9 and Table 40-7).

Venous Stasis. Normal blood flow in the venous system depends on the action of muscles in the extremities and the functional adequacy of venous valves, which allow unidirectional flow. *Venous stasis* occurs when the valves are dysfunctional or the muscles of the extremities are inactive. Venous stasis occurs more frequently in people who are obese or pregnant, have heart failure or atrial fibrillation, have been on long trips without regular exercise, have a prolonged surgical procedure, or are immobile for long periods (e.g., with spinal cord injury, fractured hip, limb paralysis).

Table 40-6 Comparison of Superficial Vein Thrombosis and Venous Thromboembolism

	SUPERFICIAL VEIN THROMBOSIS	VENOUS THROMBOEMBOLISM
Usual location	Superficial arm veins (e.g., IV catheters) and leg veins (e.g., varicosities)	Deep veins of arms (e.g., axillary, subclavian), legs (e.g., femoral), and pelvis (e.g., iliac or inferior or superior vena cava) and pulmonary system
Clinical findings	Tenderness, redness, warmth, pain, inflammation and induration along the course of the superficial vein; vein appears as a palpable cord; edema rarely occurs	Tenderness to pressure over involved vein, induration of overlying muscle, venous distension; edema; may have mild to moderate pain; deep reddish colour to area caused by venous congestion NOTE: Some patients may have no obvious physical changes in the affected extremity
Sequelae	Usually benign; if untreated, venous thromboembolism may occur if clot extends to deep veins.	Embolization to lungs (pulmonary embolism) may occur and may result in death*; pulmonary hypertension and chronic venous insufficiency with or without venous leg ulceration may develop

IV, intravenous.
*See Chapter 30 for clinical findings related to pulmonary embolism.

PATHOPHYSIOLOGY MAP

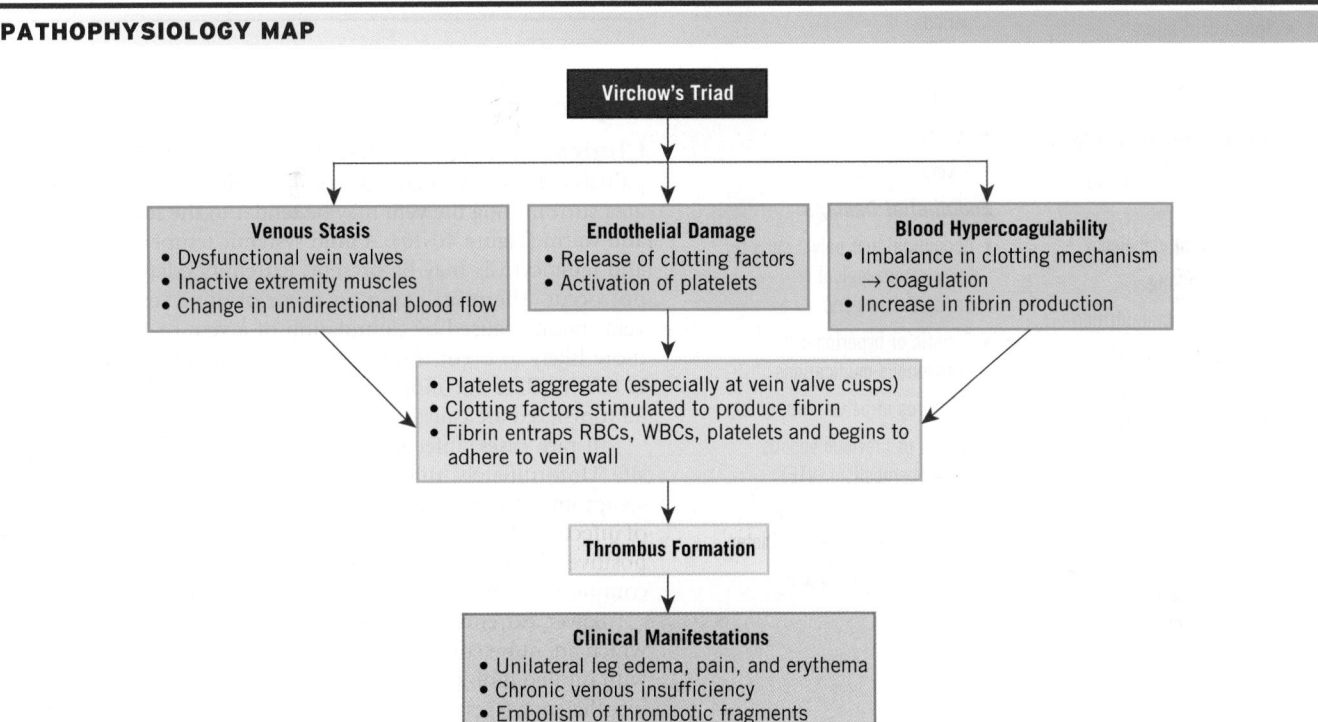

Figure 40-9 Pathophysiology of venous thromboembolism. *RBCs,* red blood cells; *WBCs,* white blood cells.

Endothelial Damage. Damage to the endothelium of the vein may be caused by direct (e.g., surgery, intravascular catheterization, trauma, fracture, burns) or indirect (chemotherapy, vasculitis, sepsis, hyperhomocysteinemia, diabetes) injury to the vessel (Merli, 2008). Damaged endothelium stimulates platelet activation and initiates the coagulation cascade. This results in decreased fibrinolytic capabilities and predisposes the patient to thrombus development.

Hypercoagulability of Blood. Hypercoagulability of blood occurs in many hematological disorders, particularly polycythemia, severe anemias, malignancies (e.g., cancers of the breast, brain, pancreas, and gastrointestinal tract), nephrotic syndrome, antithrombin III deficiency, elevated lipoprotein (a) [Lp(a)], elevated (clotting) Factor VIII, hyperhomocysteinemia, protein C deficiency, and protein S deficiency (James, 2009; Merli, 2008).

A patient with sepsis is predisposed to hypercoagulability owing to endotoxins that are released. Some medications (e.g., corticosteroids, estrogens) predispose a patient to thrombus formation.

Women of child-bearing age who take estrogen-based oral contraceptives or postmenopausal women who use oral hormone replacement therapy (HRT) are at increased risk for VTE (James, 2009; Hemelaar, van der Mooren, Rad, Kluft, & Kenemans, 2008). Women who use oral contraceptives and tobacco double their risk because of the vasoconstricting effects of nicotine. Smoking causes hypercoagulability by increasing plasma fibrinogen and homocysteine levels and activating the intrinsic coagulation pathway. Women who smoke, use oral contraceptives, are older than 35 years, and have a family history of VTE are at an extremely high risk for VTE. In women with a known thrombophilia, the benefits of HRT and raloxifene (Evista) must be weighed against

Table 40-7 Risk Factors for Venous Thromboembolism

Venous Stasis

- Advanced age
- Atrial fibrillation
- Heart failure
- Obesity
- Orthopedic surgery (especially lower extremity)
- Pregnancy and postpartum period
- Prolonged immobility
  - Bed rest
  - Fractured leg or hip
  - Long trips without adequate exercise
  - Spinal cord injury
- Stroke
- Varicose veins

Hypercoagulability of Blood

- Antiphospholipid antibody syndrome
- Antithrombin III deficiency
- Cigarette smoking
- Dehydration or malnutrition
- Elevated (clotting) factor VIII or lipoprotein (a) [Lp(a)]
- Factor V Leiden or prothrombin gene mutation

- High altitudes
- Oral hormone replacement therapy
- Hyperhomocysteinemia
- Malignancies (especially breast, brain, hepatic, pancreatic, and gastrointestinal)
- Nephrotic syndrome
- Oral contraceptives, especially in women >35 yr who smoke cigarettes
- Polycythemia vera
- Pregnancy and postpartum period
- Protein C deficiency
- Protein S deficiency
- Sepsis
- Severe anemias

Endothelial Damage

- Abdominal and pelvic surgery (e.g., gynecological or urological surgery)
- Caustic or hypertonic intravenous medications
- Fractures of pelvis, hip, or leg
- History of previous venous thromboembolism (VTE)
- In-dwelling, peripherally inserted, central vein catheter
- Intravenous drug abuse
- Trauma

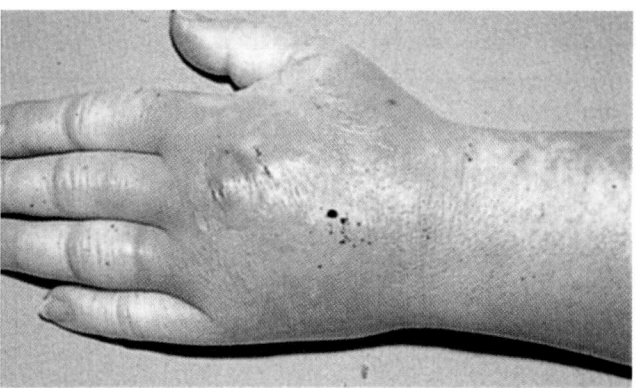

Figure 40-10 Superficial vein thrombosis of the hand following IV therapy.

Source: Grieg, J. D., & Garden, O. J. (1996). *Color atlas of surgical diagnosis*. London: Times Mirror International.

the risk for VTE (Merli, 2008). Transdermal or intranasal HRT may be safer than oral HRT with respect to risk for VTE (Hemelaar et al., 2008).

Pathophysiology

Localized platelet aggregation and fibrin entrap RBCs, WBCs, and more platelets to form a thrombus. A frequent site of thrombus formation is the valve cusps of veins, where venous stasis occurs. As the thrombus enlarges, increased numbers of blood cells and fibrin collect behind it, producing a larger clot with a "tail" that eventually occludes the lumen of the vein.

If a thrombus only partially occludes the vein, endothelial cells cover the thrombus and stop the thrombotic process. If the thrombus does not become detached, it undergoes lysis or becomes firmly organized and adherent within 5 to 7 days. The organized thrombi may detach and result in emboli. Turbulence of blood flow is a major contributing factor to embolization. The thrombus can become an embolus that flows through the venous circulation to the heart and lodges in the pulmonary circulation, becoming a PE (Figure 30-11).

Superficial Vein Thrombosis

Clinical Manifestations. The patient with SVT may have a palpable, firm, subcutaneous cordlike vein (see Table 40-6). The area surrounding the vein may be tender to the touch, reddened, and warm (Figure 40-10). A mild systemic temperature elevation and leukocytosis may be present. Extremity edema may or may not occur. The most common cause of upper extremity SVT is vein trauma caused by cannulation of a vein or IV therapy. It is more likely to occur if the catheter is located in a small vein, or is left in place for more than 48 hours, or if the IV solutions administered are caustic or hyperosmolar (Kearon et al., 2008).

In rare cases, infectious or suppurative SVT occurs at an IV site. Unfortunately, this type of SVT may have no local signs or symptoms. A high-grade fever or PE may be the first indication of infectious SVT (Cesarone et al., 2007). An elevated WBC count, positive blood cultures, or both, may also be found. The most common causative organism is *Staphylococcus aureus*.

Lower extremity SVT involves one or more varicose veins, which are more common in pregnant women and obese patients with limited mobility or older patients with longstanding venous insufficiency (Cesarone et al., 2007; Kearon et al., 2008). Other risk factors include thrombophilia, use of exogenous estrogens, recent sclerotherapy (e.g., treatment for varicose veins), and a history of VTE. SVT also can occur in people with endothelial alterations such as Buerger's disease, systemic lupus erythematosus, and other collagen disorders. The development of SVT in a healthy vein may be caused by a malignancy and may precede the cancer detection (Vinjar & Stewart, 2008). SVT typically is diagnosed based on physical examination alone. In the legs, a venous duplex ultrasound can be used to rule out extension of the clot to a deep vein (Milio et al., 2008).

Collaborative Care. The initial treatment of infusion-related SVT involves the immediate removal of the IV catheter. If edema is present, elevate the extremity to promote reabsorption of fluid from the interstitial space into the vasculature. The application of warm, moist heat may help relieve pain and inflammation. Oral NSAIDs (e.g., diclofenac [Voltaren]), topical NSAIDs (e.g., diclofenac gel), or topical heparin gels are used to treat symptoms for a maximum of 2 weeks (Cesarone et al., 2007). Suppurative infusion-related SVT typically requires drainage of the abscess, excision of the affected tissue, and systemic antibiotics (Cesarone et al., 2007). Systemic anticoagulants are not recommended for infusion-related SVT (Kearon et al., 2008).

For patients with an SVT involving the greater saphenous vein or the saphenofemoral junction, initial treatment consists of low-molecular-weight heparin (LMWH) or unfractionated heparin (UH) followed by warfarin (Kearon et al., 2008). Use of oral NSAIDs in combination with anticoagulants is not recommended. If the SVT affects a very short vein segment and is not near the saphenofemoral junction, anticoagulants are not necessary and oral or topical NSAIDs are appropriate. Additional interventions for SVT include educating the patient to wear graduated compression stockings and perform mild exercise such as walking.

Compression helps to reduce edema and walking increases endogenous fibrinolysis (Cesarone et al., 2007; Kearon et al., 2008).

Venous Thromboembolism

Clinical Manifestations. The patient with lower extremity VTE may or may not have unilateral leg edema, extremity pain, a sense of fullness in the thigh or calf, paresthesias, warm skin, erythema, and/or a systemic temperature greater than 38°C. If the calf is involved, it may be tender to palpation. A positive Homans sign (pain on forced dorsiflexion of the foot when the leg is raised) is a classic but very unreliable sign with frequent false positives (James, 2009) (see Table 40-6). If the inferior vena cava is involved, the legs may be edematous and cyanotic. If the superior vena cava is involved, symptoms may occur in the arms, neck, back, and face.

Complications. The most serious complications of VTE are PE, chronic venous insufficiency, and phlegmasia cerulea dolens (described later). PE is a potentially life-threatening complication of VTE (see Chapter 30).

Chronic venous insufficiency (CVI) results from valvular destruction, allowing retrograde flow of venous blood. Persistent edema, increased pigmentation, secondary varicosities, ulceration, and cyanosis of the limb when it is placed in a dependent position may occur in a person with CVI. Signs and symptoms of CVI typically do not develop until several years following VTE.

Phlegmasia cerulea dolens (swollen, blue, painful leg), a very rare complication, may develop in a patient in the advanced stages of cancer. It results from severe lower extremity VTE(s) that involve the major leg veins causing near-total occlusion of venous outflow. Patients typically experience sudden, massive swelling, deep pain, and intense cyanosis of the extremity. If untreated, the venous obstruction causes arterial occlusion and gangrene and requires amputation.

Diagnostic Studies. Table 40-8 presents the various diagnostic studies used to determine the site or location and extent of a VTE.

DIAGNOSTIC STUDIES

Table 40-8 Venous Thromboembolism*

STUDY	DESCRIPTION AND ABNORMAL FINDINGS
Blood Laboratory Studies	
ACT, aPTT, INR, bleeding time, Hb, Hct, platelet count	Alterations if patient has underlying blood dyscrasia (e.g., increased Hb and Hct in patient with polycythemia).
D-dimer	Fragment of fibrin formed as result of fibrin degradation and clot lysis. Elevated results suggest venous thromboembolism (VTE). *Normal results:* <250 mcg/L
Fibrin monomer complex	Forms when concentration of thrombin exceeds that of antithrombin. Presence is evidence of thrombus formation and suggests VTE. *Normal results:* <6.1 mg/L
Noninvasive Venous Studies	
Venous compression ultrasound	Evaluation of deep femoral, popliteal, and posterior tibial veins. *Normal finding:* Veins collapse with application of external pressure. *Abnormal finding:* Veins fail to collapse with application of external pressure; failure to collapse suggests a thrombus
Duplex ultrasound	Combination of compression ultrasound with spectral and colour flow Doppler. Veins examined for respiratory variation, compressibility, and intraluminal filling defects to help determine location and extent of thrombus (most widely used test to diagnose deep vein thrombosis).
Invasive Venous Studies	
Computed tomography venography (CTV)	Uses spiral CT to evaluate veins in the pelvis, thighs, and calves after injection of venous phase contrast material; uses less contrast material than traditional venography; may be performed simultaneously with CT angiography of pulmonary vessels for patients being evaluated for VTE.
Magnetic resonance venography	Uses MRI with specialized software to evaluate blood flow through veins; can be done with or without contrast; highly accurate for pelvic and proximal veins; less accurate for calf veins; can distinguish acute and chronic thrombus.
Contrast venography (phlebogram)	Radiographic determination of location and extent of clot using contrast media to outline filling defects; identifies the presence of collateral circulation; once the gold standard but currently rarely performed.

ACT, activated clotting time; *aPTT,* activated partial thromboplastin time; *CT,* computed tomography; *Hb,* hemoglobin; *Hct,* hematocrit; *INR,* international normalized ratio; *MRI,* magnetic resonance imaging.
*See Table 30-29 for diagnostic studies for pulmonary embolism.

Collaborative Care

Prevention and Prophylaxis. VTE prophylaxis in surgical patients is a core measure of quality health care in hospitalized surgical patients. In addition, it is recommended that hospitals have a formal, hospital-wide thromboprophylaxis policy that actively addresses VTE prevention on admission of all adult patients (Geerts et al., 2008).

In patients at risk for VTE, a variety of interventions are used. Early and aggressive mobilization based on the patient's condition is the easiest and most cost-effective method to decrease VTE risk (Crowther, 2007). Patients on bed rest need to change position every 2 hours. Unless contraindicated, teach patients to flex and extend their feet, knees, and hips every 2 to 4 hours while awake. Patients who are able to get out of bed need to be in a chair for meals and ambulate at least four to six times per day as tolerated. Reinforce the importance of these measures to the patient and caregiver. Research has shown that patients want additional information on VTE and prevention of VTE (Le Sage, McGee, & Emed, 2008). Early and frequent ambulation is sufficient prophylaxis for low-risk surgery patients who are undergoing minor procedures and have no additional VTE risk factors (Geerts et al., 2008).

Graduated compression (antiembolism) stockings (e.g., thromboembolic deterrent [TED] hose) are a part of VTE prevention. When fitted and worn properly, these stockings increase venous blood flow velocity, prevent venous wall dilation, improve venous valve function, and stimulate endothelial fibrinolytic activity (Walker & Lamond, 2008; Joanna Briggs Institute, 2008). It is critical to accurately measure the patient's legs, obtain the correct stocking size and length (thigh-high or knee-high), apply the stockings properly, and educate the patient and caregiver regarding proper use (Walker & Lamond, 2008; Winslow & Brosz, 2008). Correct use means the toe hole is under the toes, the heel patch is over the heel, the thigh gusset is on the inner thigh (thigh length only), and there are no wrinkles. The stockings are not to be rolled down, cut, or otherwise altered. Venous return is impeded by the stockings if the top elastic band is too tight or the stockings are rolled down. This actually increases the risk of VTE and skin damage (Joanna Briggs Institute, 2008). Monitor patients regularly to ensure the stockings are being worn properly, the size is still appropriate, and peripheral perfusion is adequate (Winslow & Brosz, 2008). If the patient's legs are swollen after surgery, remeasurement is necessary and a larger stocking size may be needed. Thoroughly assess the skin at least once a day with the stockings off or more frequently, depending on the patient's condition.

Sequential compression devices (SCDs) are inflatable garments wrapped around the legs that apply intermittent external pressure to the lower extremities. They are often used in combination with graduated compression stockings (Crowther, 2007; Joanna Briggs Institute, 2008). Benefits are similar to those provided by stockings. Like graduated compression stockings, the nurse must accurately measure the extremities to ensure correct fit. SCDs will not provide effective VTE prophylaxis if the device is not applied correctly, the fit is incorrect, or the patient does not wear the device continuously except during bathing, skin assessment, and ambulation (Crowther, 2007; Winslow & Brosz, 2008). SCDs are not to be worn when a patient has an active VTE owing to risk of PE. Preventive anticoagulation is recommended for many patients and depends on the patient's risk for VTE (Kakkos et al., 2008). This is determined by a number of factors including past medical history, current medications, medical diagnoses, and scheduled procedures (Geerts et al., 2008).

Drug Therapy. Anticoagulants are used routinely for VTE prevention and treatment. The goal of anticoagulation therapy for VTE prophylaxis is to prevent clot formation, whereas the goals in the treatment of confirmed VTE are to prevent propagation of the clot, development of any new thrombi, and embolization. Currently, four major classes of anticoagulants are available: (1) vitamin K antagonists, (2) indirect thrombin inhibitors, (3) direct thrombin inhibitors, and (4) Factor Xa inhibitors (Hirsh et al., 2008) (Table 40-9). The use of aspirin alone for VTE thromboprophylaxis is not recommended for any patient group (Geerts et al., 2008). Anticoagulant therapy does not dissolve the clot. Lysis of the clot begins spontaneously through the body's intrinsic fibrinolytic system (see Chapter 32).

Anticoagulant Therapy

Vitamin K Antagonists. The oral anticoagulant for long-term or extended anticoagulation is warfarin, a vitamin K antagonist. Warfarin inhibits activation of the vitamin K–dependent coagulation Factors II, VII, IX, and X, as well as the anticoagulant proteins C and S (Ansell et al., 2008). (Figure 32-4 displays the clotting pathways, and clotting factors are listed in Table 32-3.) Warfarin requires 48 to 72 hours to affect prothrombin time (PT) and takes several days to achieve a maximum effect. Thus, an overlap of a parenteral anticoagulant (e.g., UH or LMWH) and warfarin typically is required for 5 days (Hirsh et al., 2008). The level of anticoagulation is monitored daily using the international normalized ratio (INR). The INR is a standardized system of reporting PT (Table 40-10).

The nurse should take a careful history before starting warfarin. Antiplatelet agents (e.g., aspirin) generally are not given with warfarin owing to the increased bleeding risk (Schulman, Beyth, Kearon, Levine, & American College of Chest Physicians, 2008). Other drugs that interact with warfarin include NSAIDs; phenytoin (Dilantin); barbiturates; and many vitamin, mineral, dietary, and herbal supplements (Frishman et al., 2009) (see eTable 40-1, available on the Evolve Website for this chapter and the Complementary and Alternative Therapies box on p. 1017). A diet that frequently varies in vitamin K intake (e.g., green leafy vegetables) can make it difficult to achieve and maintain a therapeutic INR level. Variations in certain genes may influence how some people respond to warfarin. However, pharmacogenetic-based dosing is not recommended at this time (Dinwoodey & Ansell, 2008).

Indirect Thrombin Inhibitors. Indirect thrombin inhibitors are divided into two major classes: UH and LMWHs. UH (e.g., heparin) affects both the intrinsic and the common pathways of blood coagulation by way of the plasma antithrombin. Antithrombin inhibits thrombin-mediated conversion of fibrinogen to fibrin by affecting Factors II, IX, X, XI, and XII (see Figure 32-4).

Heparin can be given subcutaneously for VTE prophylaxis or by continuous IV for VTE treatment (Kearon et al., 2008; Hirsh et al, 2008). When given intravenously, heparin requires frequent laboratory monitoring of clotting status as measured by activated partial thromboplastin time (aPTT) (see Table 40-10). One serious adverse effect of heparin is *heparin-induced thrombocytopenia* (HIT). HIT is an immune reaction to heparin that causes a severe, sudden reduction in the platelet count along with a paradoxical increase in venous or arterial thrombosis (Dinwoodey & Ansell, 2008). HIT is diagnosed by measuring for the presence of heparin antibodies in the blood. Treatment requires immediately stopping heparin therapy and, if further anticoagulation is required, using a nonheparin anticoagulant (Dinwoodey & Ansell, 2008; Warkentin, Greinacher, Koster, Lincoff, & American

DRUG THERAPY

Table 40-9 Anticoagulant Therapy

ANTICOAGULANT	DRUG	ROUTE OF ADMINISTRATION	COMMENTS
Vitamin K antagonists	Warfarin (Coumadin)	PO	INR is used for monitoring therapeutic levels. Administer at the same time each day. Variations of certain genes (e.g., *CYP 2CP, VKO RC1*) may influence response to the drug. Antidote: vitamin K
Indirect Thrombin Inhibitors			
Unfractionated heparin (UH)	Heparin sodium (Heparin-Lock Flush)	Continuous IV Intermittent IV Subcut	Therapeutic effects measured at regular intervals by the aPTT or ACT. Monitor CBC at regular intervals. If administering subcutaneously, inject deep into subcutaneous tissue (preferably into the abdominal fatty tissue or above the iliac crest), inserting the entire length of the needle. Hold skinfold during injection but release before removing needle. Do not aspirate. Do not inject intramuscularly. Do not rub site after injection. Rotate sites. Antidote: protamine sulphate
Low-molecular-weight heparin (LMWH)	Enoxaparin (Lovenox) Tinzaparin (Innohep) Dalteparin (Fragmin) Nadroparin (Fraxiparine)	Subcut	Routine coagulation tests typically not required. Monitor CBC at regular intervals. Do not expel air bubble before administering subcutaneously. Follow remaining administration guidelines as described above for UH. Use extreme caution in patients with a history of HIT. Protamine partially reverses the effects of LMWH.
Direct Thrombin Inhibitors			
Hirudin derivatives	Lepirudin (Refludan) Bivalirudin (Angiomax)	IV or subcut IV IV or subcut	Therapeutic effect measured by ACT or aPTT. Used in patients with HIT when anticoagulation is still required. No antidote.
Synthetic thrombin inhibitors	Argatroban	IV	Therapeutic effect measured by aPTT. Used in patients at risk for or with HIT.
Factor Xa inhibitor	Fondaparinux (Arixtra)	Subcut	Routine coagulation tests not required. Monitor CBC and creatinine at regular intervals. Do not expel air bubble before administering. Follow remaining administration guidelines as described for UH. Approved for VTE prophylaxis and treatment. For surgical patients, initial dose should be given no earlier than 6 hr postoperatively. Use with caution in elderly patients and/or patients with impaired renal function. May cause thrombocytopenia. If uncontrollable bleeding occurs, treatment with recombinant factor VIIa may be effective.

ACT, activated clotting time; *aPTT,* activated partial thromboplastin time; *CBC,* complete blood count; *HIT,* heparin-induced thrombocytopenia; *INR,* international normalized ratio; *IV,* intravenous; *PO,* oral; *VTE,* venous thromboembolism.

College of Chest Physicians, 2008). Another adverse effect of long-term heparin therapy is osteoporosis (Hirsh et al, 2008). LMWHs (e.g., enoxaparin [Lovenox] and dalteparin [Fragmin]) are derived from heparin, but the molecule size is about one third that of UH (Geerts et al., 2008; Hirsh et al, 2008). LMWHs have a greater bioavailability, a more predictable dose response, a longer half-life, and a lower incidence of bleeding complications than UH. LMWHs also are less likely to cause HIT and osteoporosis (Hirsh et al, 2008; Schulman et al., 2008; Warkentin et al., 2008). LMWHs typically do not require anticoagulant monitoring and dose adjustment.

Direct Thrombin Inhibitors. Direct thrombin inhibitors are classified as hirudin derivatives or synthetic thrombin inhibitors. Hirudin is manufactured through recombinant DNA technology. It binds specifically with thrombin and directly inhibits its function without causing plasma protein and platelet interactions (Nutescu, Shapiro, & Chevalier, 2008). Hirudin derivatives (e.g., lepirudin [Refludan] and bivalirudin [Angiomax]) are administered by continuous IV infusion. Lepirudin is approved for prophylaxis or treatment of patients with HIT, whereas bivalirudin is approved for HIT patients undergoing percutaneous coronary angioplasty (Hirsh et al., 2008). Anticoagulant

Table 40-10 Tests of Blood Coagulation		
DRUGS MONITORED	**NORMAL VALUE**	**THERAPEUTIC VALUE**
International normalized ratio (INR)	0.75-1.25	2-3
• Vitamin K antagonists (e.g., warfarin [Coumadin])		
Activated partial thromboplastin time (aPTT)	25-35 sec	46-70 sec
• Unfractionated heparin (e.g., heparin [Heparin-Lock Flush])		
• Hirudin derivatives (e.g., bivalirudin [Angiomax])		
• Synthetic thrombin inhibitors (e.g., argatroban)		
Activated clotting time (ACT)	70-120 sec*	>300 sec
• Unfractionated heparin		
• Hirudin derivatives		
• Synthetic thrombin inhibitors		
Anti-factor Xa		
• Low-molecular-weight heparin (e.g., enoxaparin [Lovenox])	0 U/mL	0.6-1.0 U/mL
• Factor Xa inhibitors (e.g., fondaparinux [Arixtra])	0 U/mL	0.2-1.5 U/mL

*Varies based on type of system and test reagent or activator used.

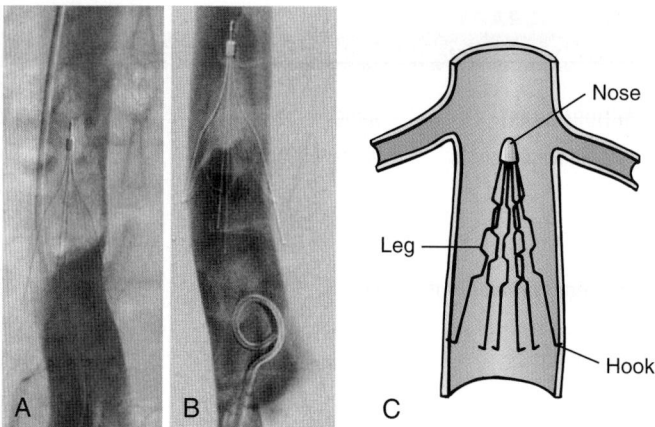

Figure 40-11 A, B, and **C,** Inferior vena caval interruption technique using a Greenfield stainless steel filter to prevent pulmonary embolism.

Source: **A** and **B,** Nicholson, D., & Botti, C. (2006). Case study: Successful prophylactic use of an inferior vena cava filter prevented a fatal pulmonary embolism. *Vascular Disease Management, 3*(5), 337-338.

activity for hirudin derivatives is monitored using aPTT or activated clotting time (ACT) (see Table 40-10). There is no antidote for hirudin derivatives if bleeding occurs (Schulman et al., 2008; Nutescu et al., 2008).

Argatroban, a synthetic direct thrombin inhibitor, inhibits thrombin. It is indicated for use in patients as an alternative to heparin for the prevention and treatment of HIT and for known HIT patients who require percutaneous coronary interventions (Hirsh et al, 2008; Warkentin et al., 2008). Anticoagulant activity is monitored for argatroban using aPTT or ACT. Similar to hirudin derivatives, the effects of argatroban are not reversible.

Factor Xa Inhibitors. Factor Xa inhibitors (e.g., fondaparinux [Arixtra]) inhibit Factor Xa directly or indirectly, producing rapid anticoagulation. Fondaparinux is recommended for both VTE treatment and prophylaxis (Crowther, 2007; Le Sage et al., 2008). It is given subcutaneously. Coagulation monitoring or dose adjustment is not needed, although its anticoagulant activity can be measured using anti-Xa assays (see Table 38-10). If uncontrollable bleeding occurs, recombinant Factor VIIa may be useful (Hirsh et al., 2008). Fondaparinux is contraindicated in patients with renal insufficiency.

Anticoagulation Therapy for Venous Thromboembolism Prophylaxis. For VTE prophylaxis, low-dose UH, LMWH, fondaparinux, or warfarin is prescribed. Patients with moderate VTE risk (e.g., general, gynecological, urological surgery; acute medical problem) should receive either UH, LMWH, or fondaparinux (Kearon et al., 2008). Patients with high VTE risk (e.g., major orthopedic surgery, trauma) should receive VTE prophylaxis with LMWH, fondaparinux, or warfarin until discharge (Geerts et al., 2008). It is recommended that high-risk gynecological (e.g., for cancer) and major orthopedic (e.g., total knee,

hip fracture) surgery patients be prescribed VTE prophylaxis up to 35 days after discharge. Similarly, all critically ill patients (e.g., trauma) should receive VTE prophylaxis while hospitalized (Geerts et al., 2008).

Anticoagulation Therapy for Venous Thromboembolism Treatment. Patients with confirmed VTE should receive initial treatment with LMWH, UH, or fondaparinux, and warfarin for at least 5 days or until the INR is 2.0 or higher for 24 hours (Kearon et al., 2008). Patients with one or more of multiple co-morbidities, complex medical issues, or a very large VTE usually are hospitalized for treatment and typically receive IV UH (Kearon et al., 2008). LMWH is recommended over UH for most patients with acute VTE. Depending on clinical presentation, these patients often can be safely and effectively managed as outpatients (Kearon et al., 2008). Fondaparinux may be particularly useful for VTE treatment in patients with a history of HIT.

Thrombolytic Therapy for Venous Thromboembolism Treatment. Another treatment option for patients with a thrombus is catheter-directed administration of a thrombolytic drug (e.g., urokinase, recombinant tissue plasminogen activator [r-tPA; alteplase]) (Kearon et al., 2008). Catheter-directed thrombolytics directly dissolve the clot(s), reduce the acute symptoms, and decrease the incidence of postphlebitic vein problems. Additional catheter-based interventions such as angioplasty, stents, or mechanical thrombectomy using a high-speed impeller to fragment the thrombus can be used in conjunction with the thrombolytic drug (Kearon et al., 2008). (Chapter 36 discusses thrombolytic therapy.)

Surgical Therapy. Although most patients are managed medically, a small number of patients undergo surgery. Surgical options include open venous thrombectomy and inferior vena cava interruption. Venous thrombectomy involves the removal of a thrombus through an incision in the vein (Kearon et al., 2008). Vena cava interruption devices (e.g., Greenfield, Vena Tech, or TrapEase filters) can be inserted percutaneously through the right femoral or right internal jugular veins. The filter device is opened and the spokes penetrate the vessel walls (Figure 40-11). These devices result in "sievetype" obstruction, permitting filtration of clots without interruption of blood flow. Complications after the insertion of the device are rare but include air embolism, improper placement, migration of the filter, and perforation of the vena cava with retroperitoneal bleeding (Kahn, Shrier, & Kearon, 2008). Over time, venous congestion can occur from accumulation of trapped clots. These can clog the filter and completely occlude the vena cava, requiring filter removal and replacement. A filter device is recommended if anticoagulant therapy is contraindicated owing to an increased risk of bleeding (Kearon et al., 2008; Kahn et al., 2008).

NURSING MANAGEMENT: VENOUS THROMBOEMBOLISM

Nursing Assessment

Table 40-11 presents the subjective and objective data to obtain from a patient with VTE.

Nursing Diagnoses

Nursing diagnoses and collaborative problems for the patient with VTE include, but are not limited to, the following:
- Acute pain *related to* venous congestion, impaired venous return, and inflammation
- Ineffective health maintenance *related to* lack of knowledge about disorder and its treatment
- Risk for impaired skin integrity *related to* altered peripheral tissue perfusion
- Potential complication: bleeding *related to* anticoagulant therapy
- Potential complication: PE *related to* embolization of thrombus, dehydration, and immobility

Planning

The overall goals for the patient with VTE include (1) pain relief, (2) decreased edema, (3) no skin ulceration, (4) no bleeding complications, and (5) no evidence of pulmonary emboli.

Nursing Implementation

Acute Intervention

Nursing care for the patient with VTE is directed toward the prevention of emboli formation and the reduction of inflammation. Because effective anticoagulation is essential, the nurse should review with the patient any medications, vitamins, minerals, and dietary and natural health products being taken that may interfere with anticoagulation therapy (Frishman et al., 2009) (see eTable 40-1, available on the Evolve Website for this chapter and the Complementary and Alternative Therapies box on p. 1017). Depending on the anticoagulant prescribed, the nurse will monitor INR, aPTT, ACT, anti–Factor Xa levels, complete blood count (CBC), creatinine, Factor X levels, hemoglo-

NURSING ASSESSMENT

Table 40-11 Venous Thromboembolism

Subjective Data

Important Health Information

Past health history: Trauma to vein, intravascular catheter (e.g., peripherally inserted central catheter) varicose veins, pregnancy or recent childbirth, bacteremia, obesity, prolonged bed rest, irregular heartbeat (e.g., atrial fibrillation), COPD, HF, cancer, coagulation disorders and hypercoagulable states, systemic lupus erythematosus, MI, spinal cord injury, stroke, prolonged air travel, recent bone fracture, dehydration, tobacco use

Medications: Use of estrogens (including oral contraceptives, hormone replacement therapy), tamoxifen (Istubol), raloxifene (Evistal), corticosteroids, excessive amounts of vitamin E, IV drug abuse

Surgery or other treatments: Any recent surgery, especially orthopedic, gynecological, gastric, or urological; previous surgery involving veins; central venous catheter

Symptoms
- Inactivity
- Pain in area on palpation or ambulation

Objective Data

General

Fever, anxiety, pain

Integumentary

Increased size of extremity when compared with extremity on other side; taut, shiny, warm skin, erythematous, tenderness to palpation. Some patients may have no physical changes in the affected extremity.

Cardiovascular

Distension and warmth of superficial veins in affected area; edema and cyanosis of extremities, neck, back, and face (if superior vena cava involvement)

Possible Findings

Leukocytosis, abnormal coagulation, anemia or ↑ hematocrit and RBC count, ↑ D-dimer level, positive venous compression Duplex ultrasound study, positive CTV, magnetic resonance venogram, or contrast venogram study.

COPD, chronic obstructive pulmonary disease; *CTV,* computed tomography venogram; *HF,* heart failure; *IV,* intravenous; *MI,* myocardial infarction; *RBC,* red blood cell.

bin, hematocrit, platelet levels, and/or liver enzymes (Hirsh et al., 2008; Dinwoodey & Ansell, 2008; Nutescu et al., 2008). Monitor platelet counts for patients receiving UH or LMWH to assess for HIT. Titrate doses of UH, warfarin, and direct thrombin inhibitors based on results of clotting studies and physician-established parameters. Direct thrombin inhibitors may need adjustment for patients with impaired renal and/or liver function (Nutescu et al., 2008). The nurse should always check the results of appropriate tests before initiating, administering, or adjusting anticoagulant therapy. While the patient is hospitalized, it is important to monitor for and reduce the risk of bleeding that may occur with anticoagulant administration (Table 40-12). The risk of bleeding is greater in people receiving UH who are elderly (>70 yr) and in patients receiving warfarin with a target INR greater than 3.0 (e.g., patients with mechanical heart valves) (Schulman et al., 2008). In the event

Table 40-12 Nursing Interventions for Patients Receiving Anticoagulants

Assessment

- Monitor vital signs as indicated.
- Examine urine and stool for overt signs of blood.
- Inspect skin frequently, especially under any splinting devices.
- Evaluate platelet count for signs of heparin-induced thrombocytopenia (HIT).
- Evaluate appropriate laboratory coagulation tests for target therapeutic levels.
- Evaluate lower extremity for ecchymosis/hematoma development if intermittent compression device used.
- Perform assessments frequently to observe for signs and symptoms of bleeding (e.g., hypotension, tachycardia) and/or clotting.
- Notify the health care provider of any abnormalities in assessments, vital signs, or laboratory values.

Injections

- Minimize venipunctures.
- Avoid intramuscular injections.
- Use small-gauge needles for venipunctures unless ordered therapy requires a larger gauge.
- Apply manual pressure for at least 10 min (or longer if needed) on venipuncture sites.

Patient Care

- Humidify O_2 source.
- Avoid restrictive clothing.
- Apply moisturizing lotion to skin.
- Use electric razors, not straight razors.
- Perform physical care in a gentle manner.
- Instruct patient not to forcefully blow nose.
- Avoid removing/disrupting established clots.
- Lubricate tubes (e.g., suction catheter) adequately before insertion.
- Use soft toothbrushes or foam swabs for oral care.
- Reposition the patient carefully at regular intervals.
- Limit tape application—use paper tape as appropriate.
- Administer stool softeners to avoid hard stools and straining.
- Avoid restraints if possible—use only soft, padded restraints if needed.
- Use support pads, mattresses, bed cradles, and therapeutic beds as indicated.
- Apply graduated compression stockings or sequential compression devices as ordered and with attention to proper size, application, and use.
- Perform fall assessment per institutional policy and implement safety measures as needed.

SAFETY ALERT

- Observe closely for any overt or occult bleeding.
  - Epistaxis and bleeding gingivae
  - Blood (visible or occult) in emesis, urine, stool, sputum
  - Oozing or visible bleeding from trauma site or surgical incision
  - Excessive menstrual bleeding
- Avoid intramuscular injections.
- Assess for mental status changes, especially in the older patient, because they may indicate cerebral bleeding.
- Monitor for signs of internal bleeding (e.g., decreased BP, increased heart rate).

Bed rest with limb elevation may be prescribed for patients with an acute VTE. Evidence indicates that early exercise when compared with bed rest does not increase the short-term risk of a PE in these patients (Young, Tang, Aukes, & Hughes, 2007). In addition, early exercise after VTE results in a more rapid decrease in edema and limb pain (Kearon et al., 2008). Emphasize to the patient and caregiver the importance of exercise and assist the patient to ambulate several times a day.

Ambulatory and Home Care

The nurse should focus discharge teaching on modification of VTE risk factors, use of graduated compression stockings, importance of monitoring laboratory values, medication instructions, and guidelines for follow-up. Once the edema is resolved, the patient should be measured for custom-fit, graduated compression stockings. Stocking use (or sleeves in the case of an upper extremity VTE) is recommended for at least 2 years after a VTE to support the vein walls and valves and decrease swelling and pain (Kearon et al., 2008). Regular use of graduated compression stockings reduces the occurrence of post-thrombotic syndrome (i.e., chronic venous insufficiency) (Giannakos, 2008).

If appropriate, the patient should be instructed to stop smoking and avoid all nicotine products, and to avoid constrictive clothing. If appropriate, women with a history of VTE should be instructed to stop using birth control pills or oral HRT (Hemelaar et al., 2008). Patients need to avoid standing or sitting in a motionless, leg-dependent position. Frequent knee flexion, ankle rotation, and active walking during long periods of sitting or standing, such as on car or airplane trips should be encouraged. For those at high risk for VTE who are planning a long trip, knee-high graduated compression stockings or one dose of LMWH before departure should be recommended (Geerts et al., 2008).

The patient and caregiver should be taught the signs and symptoms of PE such as sudden onset of dyspnea, tachypnea, and pleuritic chest pain. (Chapter 30 discusses PE.) They should contact EMS if these symptoms occur. However, adults older than 70 years are less likely to have calf or thigh swelling and/or pleuritic pain, two of the classic symptoms of VTE (Merli, 2008).

The patient and caregiver need thorough education regarding medication dosage, actions, and adverse effects, the need for routine blood tests, and what symptoms to report to the health care provider (Table 40-13). Devices are available for home monitoring of INR. Patients taking LMWH or fondaparinux or their caregivers should be taught how to administer the medication subcutaneously. Active or young patients need to avoid contact

of anticoagulation above therapeutic goals, protamine sulphate can be given to patients taking UH or LMWH, and vitamin K can be given to those taking warfarin. Fresh-frozen plasma can help to reverse the effects of direct thrombin inhibitors and Factor Xa inhibitors and is given for significant bleeding because it contains multiple clotting factors.

Table 40-13 Anticoagulant Therapy

Include the following information in the teaching plan for a patient receiving anticoagulant therapy and the patient's caregiver.

1. Reasons for and basic mechanism of action of anticoagulant therapy and how long anticipated therapy will last

2. Need to take medication at same time each day (preferably in afternoon or evening)

3. Depending on medication prescribed, need for frequent follow-up with blood tests to assess therapeutic effect of the drug and whether change in drug dosages is required

4. Adverse effects of drug therapy requiring medical attention:
   - Any bleeding that does not stop after a reasonable amount of time (usually 10-15 min)
   - Blood in urine or stool, or black, tarry stools
   - Unusual bleeding from gums, throat, skin, or nose, or heavy menstrual bleeding
   - Severe headaches or stomach pains
   - Weakness, dizziness, mental status changes
   - Vomiting blood
   - Cold, blue, or painful feet

5. Avoid any trauma or injury that might cause bleeding (e.g., vigorous brushing of teeth, contact sports, in-line rollerblading, use of straight razor).

6. Avoid all aspirin-containing drugs or nonsteroidal anti-inflammatory drugs.

7. Limit alcohol intake to small to moderate amount (12 oz beer, 4 oz wine, 1 oz hard liquor/day).

8. Wear a Medic Alert bracelet or necklace indicating what anticoagulant is being taken.

9. Avoid marked changes in eating habits, such as dramatically increasing foods high in vitamin K (e.g., broccoli, spinach, kale, greens). Do not take supplemental vitamin K.

10. Consult with health care provider before beginning or discontinuing any medication, vitamin, mineral, dietary, or herbal supplement (see Complementary and Alternative Therapies box on p. 1017).

11. Inform all health care providers, including dentist, of anticoagulant therapy.

12. Correct dosing is essential and supervision may be required (e.g., patients experiencing confusion or cognitive impairment) (Jagadesham, Scott, & Carding, 2008). Contact emergency medical services (EMS) immediately if chest pain, shortness of breath, palpitations (heart racing), or a feeling of passing out is experienced.

sports and high-risk (for trauma) activities (e.g., skiing). Older patients need to know to take safety precautions to prevent falls (e.g., not using throw rugs). Instruct the patient and caregiver to apply pressure for 10 to 15 minutes if bleeding occurs. If the bleeding persists, they should contact EMS.

A well-balanced diet including calcium and vitamin E is important because these affect coagulation. Patients taking warfarin should be taught to follow a consistent diet of foods containing vitamin K, to avoid taking any supplements containing vitamin K, and to avoid excessive amounts of vitamin E and alcohol. Proper hydration to prevent additional hypercoagulability of the blood, which may occur with dehydration, should be encouraged.

The overweight patient needs to not only limit caloric intake but also increase physical activity to achieve and maintain desired weight. A balanced program of rest and exercise also improves venous return. The nurse should assist the patient to develop an exercise program with an emphasis on walking and swimming. Water exercise is particularly beneficial because of the gentle, even pressure of the water. A 6-month exercise program of daily walking improves calf muscle flexibility, strength, and pump function and reduces post-thrombotic syndrome (Young et al., 2007).

■ Evaluation

The expected outcomes for the patient with VTE include:
- Minimal to no pain
- Intact skin
- No signs of hemorrhage or occult bleeding
- No signs of respiratory distress

Varicose Veins

Varicose veins, or *varicosities,* are dilated, tortuous subcutaneous veins most commonly found in the saphenous vein system. Varicosities may be small and innocuous or large and bulging. Primary varicose veins (idiopathic) are caused by a congenital weakness of the veins and are more common in women. Secondary varicose veins typically result from a previous VTE. Secondary varicose veins also may occur in the esophagus (esophageal varices), vulva, spermatic cords (varicoceles), and anorectal area (hemorrhoids), and as abnormal arteriovenous connections. Reticular veins are smaller varicose veins that appear flat, less tortuous, and bluish green. Telangiectasias (often referred to as *spider veins*) are very small visible vessels (generally <1 mm in diameter) that appear bluish-black, purple, or red.

Etiology and Pathophysiology

The etiology of varicose veins is multifactorial in nature. Superficial veins in the lower extremities become dilated and tortuous in response to increased venous pressure. Risk factors include chronic cough, constipation, family history of venous disease, congenital weakness of the vein structure, female gender, use of oral contraceptives or HRT, increasing age, obesity, pregnancy, venous obstruction resulting from thrombosis or extrinsic pressure by tumours, or occupations that require prolonged standing (Raju & Neglen, 2009). Although the exact etiology remains unknown, it is thought that the vein valve leaflets are stretched and become incompetent (do not fit together properly). Incompetent vein valves allow retrograde blood flow, particularly when the patient is standing, resulting in increased venous pressure and further venous distension.

Clinical Manifestations and Complications

Discomfort from varicose veins varies among people and tends to be worse after episodes of SVT. Many patients are concerned about cosmetic disfigurement. The most common varicose vein symptom is a heavy, achy feeling or pain after prolonged standing, which is relieved by walking or limb elevation. Some patients feel pressure or complain of an itchy, burning, or cramplike leg sensation. Swelling or nocturnal leg cramps also may occur. SVT is the most frequent complication of varicose veins and may occur spontaneously or after trauma, surgical procedures, or pregnancy. Rare complications include rupture of the varicose veins, resulting in external bleeding and skin ulcerations.

Diagnostic Studies and Collaborative Care

Superficial varicose veins can be diagnosed by appearance. A duplex ultrasound can detect obstruction and reflux in the venous system with considerable accuracy. It is the most widely used test to diagnose deep varicose veins.

Treatment usually is not indicated if varicose veins are only a cosmetic problem. If venous insufficiency develops, collaborative care involves rest with limb elevation, graduated compression stockings and exercise, such as walking. Two herbal therapies used for varicose vein treatment are horse chestnut seed extract (Aesculus hippocastanum) and butcher's broom (Ruscus aculeatus) (Frishman et al., 2009; Pittler & Ernst, 2006). (See discussion of chronic venous insufficiency later in this chapter.)

Sclerotherapy involves the injection of a substance that obliterates venous telangiectasias, reticular veins, and small, superficial varicose veins 5 mm or larger in diameter (Raju & Neglen, 2009) (Figure 40-12). Commonly used sclerosing agents include hypertonic saline, saline plus hypertonic dextrose, morrhuate sodium, glycerin, sodium tetradecyl sulphate, and polidocanol. Direct IV injection of a sclerosing agent induces inflammation and results in eventual thrombosis of the vein. This procedure is performed in an office setting and causes minimal discomfort. Potential complications include itching, pain, blistering, edema, hyperpigmentation, necrosis, recurrence of varicosities, SVT, visual disturbances, and VTE (Raju & Neglen, 2009). After injection, a thigh-high graduated compression stocking is worn or an elastic bandage is applied to the leg for several days to maintain pressure over the vein. Long-term compression therapy is advised to help prevent the development of further varicosities.

Newer, more costly, but noninvasive options for the treatment of venous telangiectasias include laser therapy and high-intensity pulsed-light therapy (Raju & Neglen, 2009). Laser or light therapy is indicated for isolated small telangiectasias or for patients in whom sclerotherapy is contraindicated or has been previously ineffective. Laser treatment typically requires more than one session, scheduled at 6- to 12-week intervals. Vascular lasers work by heating the hemoglobin in the vessels, which leads to thermocoagulation resulting in vessel sclerosis (Raju & Neglen, 2009). Pulsed-light therapy is similar to laser therapy, but uses a spectrum of light rather than a single wavelength. Potential complications of these therapies include pain, blistering, hyperpigmentation, and superficial erosions.

Surgical intervention is indicated for recurrent SVT or when chronic venous insufficiency cannot be controlled with conservative therapy. The traditional surgical intervention involves ligation of the entire vein (usually the greater saphenous vein) and dissection and removal of its incompetent tributaries. An alternative, but time-consuming, technique is ambulatory phlebectomy, which involves pulling the varicosity through a "stab" incision followed by excision of the vein. Potential complications include bleeding, bruising, and infection. In up to 30% of patients, a new vein forms to replace the one removed (Raju & Neglen, 2009).

A newer, less invasive procedure is endovenous ablation of the saphenous vein. Ablation involves the insertion of a catheter that emits energy. This causes collapse and sclerosis of the vein (Knipp et al., 2008). Potential complications include bruising, tightness along the vein, recanalization (reopening of the vein), and paresthesia (Knipp et al., 2008). Endovenous ablation also may be done in combination with saphenofemoral ligation or phlebectomy. Transilluminated powered phlebectomy involves the use of a powered tissue resector to destroy the varices and removes the pieces via aspiration.

NURSING MANAGEMENT: VARICOSE VEINS

Prevention is a key factor related to varicose veins. The patient should be instructed to avoid sitting or standing for long periods, maintain ideal body weight, take precautions against injury to the extremities, avoid wearing constrictive clothing, and walk daily.

After vein ligation surgery, the patient should be encouraged to deep breathe, which promotes venous return. It is important to check the extremities regularly for colour, movement, sensation, temperature, edema, and quality of pedal pulses. Bruising and discoloration are considered normal. Postoperatively, the legs should be elevated 15 degrees to limit edema. Graduated compression stockings should be applied, removed every 8 hours for short periods, and then reapplied. Long-term management of varicose veins is directed toward improving circulation and cosmetic appearance, relieving discomfort, and avoiding complications and ulceration. Varicose veins can recur in other veins after vein ligation. The patient needs to learn the proper use and care of custom-fitted graduated compression stockings. The patient should apply stockings in bed, before rising in the morning. In some instances, patients also will use SCDs at home to control edema (Giannakos, 2008). The importance of periodic positioning of the legs above the heart should be stressed. The overweight patient may need assistance with weight loss. The patient with a job that requires long periods of standing or sitting needs to frequently flex and extend her or his hips, legs, and ankles and change positions.

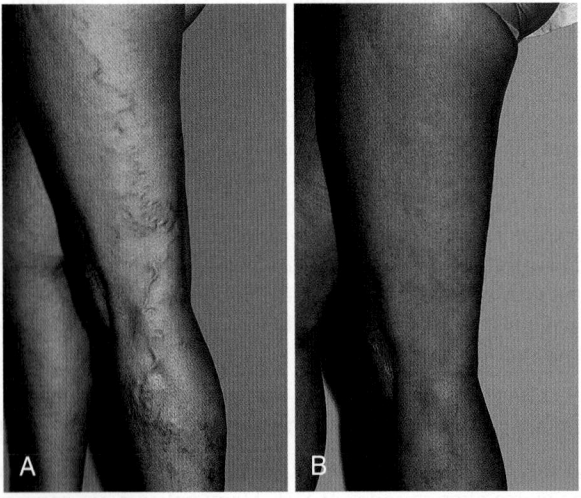

Figure 40-12 A, Lateral aspect of varicose veins before treatment. **B,** Lateral aspect of varicose veins 2 years after initial treatment with sclerotherapy.

Source: Goldman, M. P., Bergan, J. J., & Guex, J. J. (2007). *Sclerotherapy: Treatment of varicose and telangiectatic leg veins* (4th ed.). Philadelphia: Mosby.

Chronic Venous Insufficiency and Venous Leg Ulcers

Chronic venous insufficiency (CVI), a common medical problem in the elderly, is a condition in which the valves in the veins are damaged, which results in retrograde blood flow, pooling of blood in the legs, and swelling. CVI, which occurs as a result of previous episodes of VTE, can lead to venous leg ulcers (formerly called venous stasis ulcers or varicose ulcers). Although CVI and venous leg ulcers are not life-threatening diseases, they are painful, debilitating, and costly chronic conditions that adversely affect the quality of patients' lives (Koupidis, Paraskevas, Staphopoulos, & Mikhailidis, 2008).

Etiology and Pathophysiology

The causes of CVI include vein valve incompetence, deep vein obstruction, congenital venous malformation, and AV fistula (Raju & Neglen, 2009). The basic problem is incompetent valves of the deep veins. As a result, hydrostatic pressure in the veins increases and serous fluid and RBCs leak from the capillaries and venules into the tissue, resulting in edema. Enzymes in the tissue eventually break down RBCs, causing the release of *hemosiderin*, which causes a brownish skin discoloration. Over time, the skin and subcutaneous tissue around the ankle are replaced by fibrous tissue, resulting in thick, hardened, contracted skin.

Although the causes of CVI are known, the exact pathophysiology of venous ulcers is not known. It is known that increased cytokines, decreased fibrinolysis, inflammation, pericapillary fibrin cuffs, and WBC trapping occur in venous ulcers.

Clinical Manifestations and Complications

In individuals with CVI, the skin of the lower leg is leathery, with a characteristic brownish or "brawny" appearance from the hemosiderin deposition. Edema usually has been persistent for a prolonged period. Eczema, or "stasis dermatitis," is often present, and itching is a common complaint. Patients with CVI also have a higher skin temperature in the ankle area (Kelechi & Bonham, 2008).

Venous ulcers classically are located above the medial malleolus (Figure 40-13) (see Table 40-2). The ulcer is often quite painful, particularly when edema or infection is present (Koupidis et al., 2008). Pain may be worse when the leg is in a dependent position. If the venous ulcer is untreated, the wound becomes more extensive, eroding wider and deeper, and increasing the likelihood of wound infection and cellulitis. Recurrent episodes of cellulitis may lead to destruction of the superficial lymphatics, causing a secondary lymphedema to develop (Raju & Neglen, 2009). On very rare occasions, severe CVI with longstanding nonhealing venous ulcers may result in the need for amputation.

Collaborative Care

Compression is essential for CVI treatment, venous ulcer healing, and prevention of ulcer recurrence. A variety of options are available for compression therapy, including elastic wraps, custom-fitted graduated compression stockings, elastic tubular support bandages, a Velcro wrap (CircAid), SCDs, a paste bandage (Unna boot) with an elastic wrap, and multilayer (three or four) bandage systems (e.g., Profore) (Kelechi & Bonham, 2008). There are ben-

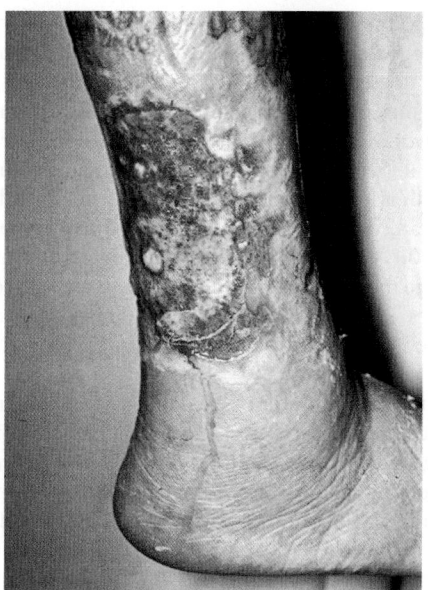

Figure 40-13 Venous leg ulcer.

Source: Kamal, A., & Brocklehurst, J. C. (1991). *Color atlas of geriatric medicine* (2nd ed.). St. Louis: Mosby–Year Book.

efits to each type of compression therapy. Evaluate each patient individually when choosing an extrinsic compression method. Before instituting compression therapy, assess the arterial status to make sure that coexistent PAD is not present. An ankle-brachial index (ABI) less than 0.9 suggests PAD and the patient should not have high levels of compression.

Moist environment dressings are the basis of wound care. A variety of these dressings are available and include transparent film dressings, hydrocolloids, hydrogels, foams, calcium alginates, impregnated gauze, gauze moistened with saline, and combination dressings. When used in conjunction with compression, moist environment dressings are more effective than dry dressings in hastening the healing of venous leg ulcers. (Chapter 14 and Table 14-10 discuss hydrocolloid and other dressings.) Evaluate the nutritional status of a patient with a venous ulcer. A balanced diet with adequate protein, calories, and micronutrients is essential for healing. Nutrients most important for healing include protein, vitamins A and C, and zinc. Foods high in protein (e.g., meat, beans, cheese, tofu), vitamin A (green leafy vegetables), vitamin C (citrus fruits, tomatoes, cantaloupe), and zinc (meat, seafood) must be provided.

For patients with diabetes mellitus, maintaining normal blood glucose levels assists the healing process. For overweight individuals with CVI and no active venous ulcer, a weight loss diet should be considered (Tobon, Whitney, & Jarrett, 2008). Routine antibiotic therapy is not indicated. Clinical signs of infection in a venous ulcer include change in quantity, colour, or odour of the drainage; presence of pus; erythema of the wound edges; change in sensation around the wound; warmth around the wound; increased local pain or edema, or both; dark-coloured granulation tissue; induration around the wound; delayed healing; and cellulitis. If signs of infection are present, obtain a wound culture before instituting antibiotic therapy. The usual treatment for infection is debridement, wound excision, and systemic antibiotics. A number of antimicrobial dressings (e.g., cadexomer iodine, silver, bacteriostatic polyvinyl alcohol foam) are available for use on contaminated or infected venous ulcers. If the ulcer does not heal with conservative therapy, alternative approaches may include drugs such as pentoxifylline, micronized purified flavonoid fraction (Daflon), and sulodexide (Sulonex) (Kearon et al., 2008). Alternative treatments also may include coverage with a split-thickness skin graft, cultured epithelial autograft, allograft, or bioengineered skin such as Dermagraft (Raju & Neglen, 2009). Before the graft is applied, the ulcer is debrided, varicosities in the area are removed, and veins are ligated. (Chapter 27 discusses skin grafting.) Although grafts may assist with healing, they do not replace the need for lifelong compression therapy.

A natural health product used for CVI treatment is horse chestnut seed extract (HCSE). Escins (the active ingredient) reduces leg pain, itching, and swelling (Pittler & Ernst, 2006). Minor adverse effects associated with HCSE include dizziness, gastrointestinal complaints, headache, and pruritus. The efficacy of HCSE in venous ulcer healing and recurrence has not been determined.

NURSING MANAGEMENT: CHRONIC VENOUS INSUFFICIENCY AND VENOUS LEG ULCERS

Long-term management of venous leg ulcers should focus on teaching the patient about self-care measures because the ulcers often recur (Kelechi & Bonham, 2008). The nurse should instruct the patient and caregiver to avoid trauma to the limbs and teach them proper skin care. The nurse should also demonstrate the correct application of graduated compression stockings and stress the importance of regular replacement.

It is important to discuss activity guidelines and proper limb positioning. Proper foot and leg care is essential to avoid additional skin trauma. Patients with CVI have dry, flaky, itchy skin caused by stasis dermatitis. Daily moisturizing decreases itching and prevents cracking of the skin. Venous dermatitis may result from contact with sensitizing products such as antibacterial agents (e.g., gentamicin, neomycin); additives in bandages or dressings (e.g., adhesives); ointments containing lanolin, alcohols, benzocaine, or balsam of Peru; and over-the-counter creams or lotions with fragrance or preservatives (Raju & Neglen, 2009; Kelechi & Bonham, 2008). With each dressing change, assess the wound for signs of infection.

Patients with CVI with or without a venous ulcer should be instructed to avoid standing or sitting for long periods. Standing or sitting with the legs in a dependent position decreases periulcer skin blood perfusion and oxygen levels. Venous ulcer patients should elevate their legs above the level of the heart to reduce edema. Patients should begin a daily walking program once an ulcer heals. Prescription graduated compression stockings should be worn daily and replaced every 4 to 6 months to reduce the occurrence of CVI (Kearon et al., 2008; Raju & Neglen, 2009).

CLINICAL DECISION-MAKING EXERCISE

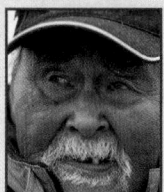

CASE STUDY:
Peripheral Arterial Disease

Source: © Picture Contact/Alamy.

Patient Profile

Mr. Assiniwe, a 76-year-old Aboriginal man, was admitted to the hospital with rest pain and a nonhealing ulcer of the big toe on the right foot.

Subjective Data

- History of a myocardial infarction, stroke, hypertension, arthritis, and diabetes mellitus
- Underwent a left femoral–popliteal bypass 5 years ago
- Has a smoking history of 45 pack-years
- Has been using insulin for 30 years
- Complains of intense right foot pain for past 6 weeks
- Sleeps in recliner with right leg in dependent position

Objective Data

Physical Examination

- Has a diminished right femoral pulse with no palpable pulses below that level
- Has a small necrotic ulcer on the tip of the right big toe
- Has thickened toenails; has shiny, thin skin on the legs; and hair is absent on both feet

Discussion Questions

1. What are Mr. Assiniwe's risk factors for peripheral arterial disease?
2. What additional information would the nurse like to know about Mr. Assiniwe?
3. Are Mr. Assiniwe's signs and symptoms evidence of an acute or a chronic peripheral arterial disease? Explain the answer.
4. What is the pathophysiology of rest pain?
5. What treatment modalities are possible for Mr. Assiniwe?
6. *Priority Decision:* What are the primary nursing responsibilities in caring for Mr. Assiniwe?
7. *Priority Decision:* Based on the assessment data presented, write one or more appropriate nursing diagnoses. Are there any collaborative problems?

℮volve *Answers are available at* **http://evolve.elsevier.com/ Canada/Lewis/medsurg**

REVIEW QUESTIONS

The number of the question corresponds to the same-numbered objective at the beginning of the chapter.

1. A 62-year-old woman weighs 92 kg and has a history of daily alcohol intake, smoking, high blood pressure, high sodium intake, and sedentary lifestyle. Which of the following risk factors are strongly related to peripheral arterial disease in this patient?
   a. Sex and age
   b. Weight and alcohol intake
   c. Cigarette smoking and hypertension
   d. Sedentary lifestyle and high sodium intake

2. The clinical manifestation of a pulsatile mass in the periumbilical area slightly to the left of the midline would be suggestive of which of the following?
   a. Thoracic aneurysm
   b. Aneurysm of the aortic arch
   c. Abdominal aortic aneurysm
   d. Thoracic and abdominal aortic aneurysm

3. Which if the following are important nursing measures after an abdominal aortic aneurysm repair?
   a. Elevate the legs.
   b. Assess cranial nerves and mental status.
   c. Administer IV heparin and monitor aPTT.
   d. Monitor urine output and creatinine.

4. Specific symptoms of aortic dissection may vary depending on which of the following?
   a. The medications that are administered
   b. How elevated the blood pressure becomes
   c. The aortic branches affected in the descent of the dissection
   d. The respiratory status of the patient before dissection occurs

5. Which of the following explains rest pain as a manifestation of peripheral arterial disease?
   a. The beginning of a venous leg ulcer
   b. Inadequate blood flow to the nerves of the feet
   c. Inadequate blood flow to the muscles during exercise
   d. Inadequate blood flow to the skin after application of the heat

6. A patient with infective endocarditis develops sudden left leg pain with pallor, paresthesia, and a loss of peripheral pulses. What should be the nurse's initial action?
   a. Notify the physician.
   b. Elevate the leg to promote venous return.
   c. Wrap the leg in a blanket to provide warmth.
   d. Perform passive range of motion exercises to stimulate circulation to the leg.

7. The medical treatment of Raynaud's phenomenon involves which of the following?
   a. Transluminal balloon angioplasty
   b. Amputation of the affected digits
   c. Peripheral arterial bypass surgery
   d. Administration of calcium channel blockers

8. Which of the following patients has the highest risk for venous thromboembolism?
   a. A 25-year-old obese woman who is 3 days postpartum
   b. A 40-year-old woman who smokes and uses oral contraceptives
   c. A 62-year-old man who has had a stroke with left-sided hemiparesis
   d. A 72-year-old man who had a suprapubic prostatectomy for cancer of the prostate

9. The nurse should suspect the presence of a venous thromboembolism when a patient demonstrates which of the following?
   a. Paresthesia and coolness of the leg
   b. Pain in the calf that occurs with exercise
   c. Generalized edema of the involved extremity
   d. Pallor and cyanosis of the involved extremity

10. Which of the following nursing interventions are indicated in the plan of care for the patient with superficial vein thrombosis and venous thromboembolism?
    a. Applying elastic compression stockings
    b. Administering anticoagulants as ordered
    c. Positioning the leg dependently to promote arterial circulation
    d. Encouraging walking and leg exercises to promote venous return

11. The nurse should include which of the following instructions for the patient discharged with an anticoagulant therapy regimen?
    a. Limit intake of vitamin C.
    b. Report symptoms of nausea to the physician.
    c. Have blood drawn routinely to check electrolytes.
    d. Be aware of and report signs or symptoms of bleeding.

12. The nurse should include which of the following interventions for healing venous leg ulcers when planning care and patient teaching?
    a. Application of antibiotic cream to the ulcers
    b. Debridement of the ulcers with skin grafting
    c. Elevation of the extremities to increase venous return
    d. Performance of leg exercises to increase collateral circulation

ANSWERS: 1. c; 2. c; 3. d; 4. c; 5. b; 6. a; 7. d; 8. b; 9. c; 10. b; 11. d; 12. c.

REFERENCES

Ankle-Brachial Index Collaboration. (2008). Ankle-brachial index combined with Framingham risk score to predict cardiovascular events and mortality, *Journal of the American Medical Association*, *300*, 197.

Ansell, J., Hirsh, J., Hylek, E., Jacobson, A., Crowther, M., & Palareti, G., & American College of Chest Physicians. (2008). Pharmacology and management of the vitamin K antagonists. American College of Chest Physicians evidence-based clinical practice guidelines (8th ed.). *Chest, 133*, 160S-198S. doi:10.1378/chest.08-0670

Badger, S., Soong, C., O'Donnell, M., Boreman, C., & McGuigan, K. (2007). Benefits of a supervised exercise program after lower limb bypass surgery. *Vascular Endovascular Surgery, 41*(1), 27-32. doi:10.1177/1538574406296209

Bakst, R., Merola, J. F., Franks, A. G., & Sanchez, M. (2008). Raynaud's phenomenon: Pathogenesis and management. *Journal of American Academic Dermatology, 59*(4), 633-653. doi:10.1016/j.jaad.2008.06.004

Ballard, D. J., Filardo, G., Fowkes, G., & Powell, J. T. (2008). Surgery for small asymptomatic abdominal aortic aneurysms. *Cochrane Database System Review, 8*(4), CD001835.

Baxter, B., Terrin, M., & Dalman, R. (2008). Medical management of small abdominal aortic aneurysms. *Circulation, 117*, 1883-1890. doi:10.1161/CIRCULATIONAHA.107.735274

Canadian Diabetes Association Clinical Practice Guidelines Expert Committee. (2008). Canadian Diabetes Association 2008 Clinical Practice Guidelines for the Prevention and Management of Diabetes in Canada (2008). *Canadian Journal of Diabetes, 32*(suppl 1), S1-S201. Available at *http://www.diabetes.ca/files/cpg2008/cpg-2008.pdf*

Canadian Hypertension Education Program (CHEP). (2012). 2012 Canadian recommendations for the management of hypertension: What's new? What's still really important? Retrieved from *http://toolkit.cfpc.ca/en/files/2012_CHEPRecsBooklet_EN_HCP1030.pdf*

Cesarone, M. R., Belcaro, G., Agus, G., Georgiev, M., Errichi, B. M., Marinucci, R., ..., Zukowski, A. (2007). Management of superficial vein thrombosis and thrombophlebitis: Status and expert opinion document. *Angiology, 58*(1S), 7S-14S. doi:10.1177/0003319706297643

Chen, Z., Takahashi, M., Naruse, T., Nakajima, T., Chen, Y.-W., Inoue, Y., ..., Kimura, A. (2007). Synergistic contribution of CD14 HLA loci in the susceptibility to Buerger's disease. *Human Genetics, 122*(3-4), 367-372. doi:10.1007/s00439-007-0408-1

Cooper, L. T., Tse, T. S., Mikhail, M. A., McBane, R. D., Stanson, A. W., & Ballman, K. V. (2004). Long-term survival and amputation risk in thromboangiitis obliterans (Buerger's disease). *Journal of the American College of Cardiology, 44*, 2410-2411. doi:10.1016/j.jacc.2004.09.029

Criqui, M., Alberts, M., Fowkes, G., Hirsh, A., O'Gara, P., & Olin, J. (2008). Atherosclerotic peripheral arterial disease symposium II screening for atherosclerotic vascular diseases: Should nationwide programs be instituted? *Circulation, 118*, 2830-2836. doi:10.1161/CIRCULATIONAHA.108.191172

Crowther, M. (2007). Deep vein thrombosis: Prevention. In B. Ackley, G. Ludwig, B. Swan, & S. Tucker (Eds.), *Evidence-based nursing care guidelines: Medical-surgical interventions*). St. Louis: Mosby.

De Angelis, R., Salaffi, F., & Grassi, W. (2008). Health-related quality of life in primary Raynaud phenomenon. *Journal of Clinical Rheumatology, 14*(4), 206-210. doi:10.1097/RHU.0b013e31817a2485

Dimick, J., & Upchurch, G. (2008). Endovascular technology, hospital volume and mortality with abdominal aortic aneurysm surgery. *Journal of Vascular Surgery, 47*(6), 1150-1154. doi:10.1016/j.jvs.2008.01.054

Dinwoodey, D., & Ansell, J. (2008). Heparins, low-molecular weight heparins, and pentasaccharides: Use in the older patient. *Cardiology Clinics, 26*(2), 145-155. doi:10.1016/j.ccl.2007.12.009

Eliason, J., & Upchurch, G. (2008). Endovascular abdominal aortic aneurysm repair. *Circulation, 117*, 1738-1744. doi:10.1161/CIRCULATIONAHA.107.747923

Fitchett, D., & Kraw, M. (2008). Vascular protection in people with diabetes. *Canadian Journal of Diabetes, 32*, S102-S106. Retrieved from *http://www.diabetes.ca/files/cpg2008/cpg-2008.pdf*

Frishman, W. H., Beravol, P., & Carosella, C. (2009). Alternative and complementary medicine for preventing and treating cardiovascular disease. *Disease-a-Month, 55*(3), 121-192. doi:10.1016/j.disamonth.2008.12.002

Geerts, W. H., Bergqvist, D., Pineo, G. F., Heit, J. L., Samama, C. M., Lassen, M. R., & Colwell, C. W. (2008). Prevention of venous thromboembolism. American College of Chest Physicians evidence-based clinical practice guidelines. *Chest, 133*(6 Suppl), 381S-453S. doi:10.1378/chest.08-0656

Giannakos, A. D. (2008). The role of compression in the prevention of post-thrombotic syndrome. *Phlebolymphology, 15*, 94.

Goldenberg I., Horr, S., Moss, A., Lopes, C., Barsheshet, A., McNitt, S., ..., Zhang, L. (2011). Risk for life-threatening cardiac events in patients with genotype-confirmed long-QT syndrome and normal-range corrected QT intervals. *Journal of the American College of Cardiology, 57*(1):51-9. doi:10.1016/j.jacc.2010.07.038

Golledge, J., Tsao, P. S., Dalman, R. L., & Norman, P. E. (2008). Circulating markers of abdominal aortic aneurysm presence and progression. *Circulation, 118*, 2382-2392. doi:10.1161/CIRCULATIONAHA.108.802074

Gray, B. H., Conte, M. S., Dake, M. D., Jaff, M. R., Kandarpa, K., Ramee, S. R., ..., Waksman, R. (2008). Atherosclerotic peripheral vascular disease symposium II: Lower extremity revascularization: State of the art. *Circulation, 118*, 2864-2872. doi:10.1161/CIRCULATIONAHA.108.191177

Hatfield, J., Gulati, S., Rahman, A., Coughlin, P., & Chetter, I. (2008). Nurse-led risk assessment/management clinics reduce predicted cardiac morbidity and mortality in claudicants. *Journal of Vascular Nursing, 26*(4), 118-122. doi:10.1016/j.jvn.2008.09.004

Hemelaar, M., van der Mooren, M. J., Rad, M., Kluft, C., & Kenemans, P. (2008). Effects of non-oral postmenopausal hormone therapy on markers of cardiovascular risk: A systematic review. *Fertility and Sterility, 90*(3), 642-672. doi:10.1016/j.fertnstert.2007.07.1298

Hiatt, W. R., Goldstone J., Smith, S. C., McDermott, M., Moneta, G., Oka, R., ..., Pearce, W. H. (2008). Atherosclerotic peripheral vascular disease symposium II: Nomenclature for vascular diseases. *Circulation, 118*(25), 2826-2829. doi:10.1161/CIRCULATIONAHA.108.191171

Hirsch, A. T., Haskal, Z. J., Hertzer, N. R., Bakal, C. W., Creager, M. A., Halperin, J. L., ..., White, R. A. (2006). ACC/AHA 2005 practice guidelines for the management of patients with peripheral arterial disease (lower extremity, renal, mesenteric, and abdominal aortic). *Circulation, 113*, e463-e654. doi:10.1161/CIRCULATIONAHA.106.174526

Hirsch, A. T., Murphy, T. P., Lovell, M. B., Twillman, G., Treat-Jacobson, D., Harwood, E. M., ..., Criqui, M. H. (2007). Gaps in public knowledge of peripheral arterial disease: The first national PAD public awareness survey. *Circulation, 116*, 2086-2094. doi:10.1161/CIRCULATIONAHA.107.725101

Hirsh, J., Bauer, K., Donati, M., Gould, M., Samama, M., & Wietz, J. (2008). Parenteral anticoagulants. American College of Chest Physicians evidence-based clinical practice guidelines (8th ed.). *Chest, 133*(6 Suppl), 141S-159S. doi:10.1378/chest.08-0689

Jagadesham, V. P., Scott, D. J., & Carding, S. R. (2008). Abdominal aortic aneurysms: An autoimmune disease? *Trends in Molecular Medicine, 14*(12), 522. doi:10.1016/j.molmed.2008.09.008

James, A. H. (2009). Venous thromboembolism in pregnancy. *Arteriosclerosis, Thrombosis and Vascular Biology, 29*(3), 326-331. doi:10.1161/ATVBAHA.109.184127

Joanna Briggs Institute. (2008). Graduated compression stockings for the prevention of post-operative venous thromboembolism. *Best Practice, 12*(4), 1-4. Retrieved from *http://connect.jbiconnectplus.org/ViewSourceFile.aspx?0=437*

Jonker, F. H. W., Schlösser, F. J. V., Moll, F. L., & Muhs, B. (2009). Dissection of the abdominal aorta: Current evidence and implications for treatment strategies: A review and meta-analysis of 92 patients. *Journal of Endovascular Therapy, 16*, 71. doi:10.1583/08-2601.1

Kahn, S. R., Shrier, I., & Kearon, C. (2008). Physical activity in patients with deep venous thrombosis: A systematic review. *Thrombosis Research, 122*, 763-773. doi:10.1016/j.thromres.2007.10.011

Kakkos, S. K., Caprini, J. A., Geroulakos, G., Nicolaides, A. N., Stansby, G., & Reddy, D. J. (2008). Combined intermittent pneumatic leg compression and pharmacologic prophylaxis for prevention of venous thromboembolism in high-risk patients. *Cochrane

Database System Review, 1, CD004174. doi:10.1002/14651858. CD005258.pub2

Kalapatapu, V. R., Shelton, K. R., Ali, A. T., Moursi, M. M., & Eidt, J. F. (2008). Pseudoaneurysm: A review. *Current Treatment Options in Cardiovascular Medicine, 10,* 173-183. doi:10.1007/s11936-008-0019-8

Karmy-Jones, R., Simeone, A., Meissner, M., Granvall, B., & Nicholls, S. (2007). Descending thoracic aortic dissections. *Surgical Clinics in North America, 87,* 1047. doi:10.1016/j.suc.2007.08.003

Kearon, C., Kahn, S. R., Agnelli, G., Goldhaber, S., Raskob, G. E., & Comerota, A. J. (2008). Antithrombotic therapy for venous thromboembolic disease: American College of Chest Physicians evidence-based clinical practice guidelines (8th ed.). *Chest, 133*(6 Suppl), 454S-545S. doi:10.1378/chest.08-0658

Kelechi, T. J., & Bonham, P. A. (2008). Lower extremity venous disorders: Implications for nursing practice. *Journal of Cardiovascular Nursing, 23*(2), 132-143. doi:10.1097/01.JCN.0000305070. 64860.87

Kim, U., Hong, S. J., Kim, J., Kim, J.-S., Young, G. K., Choi, D., ..., Shim, W. H. (2009). Intermediate to long-term outcomes of endoluminal stent-graft repair in patients with chronic type B aortic dissection. *Journal of Endovascular Therapy, 16,* 42-47. doi:10.1583/08-2563.1

Knipp, B. S., Blackburn, S. A., Bloom, J. R., Fellows, E., LaForge, W., Pfeifer, J. R., ..., Wakefield, T. W. (2008). Endovascular laser ablation: Venous outcomes and thrombotic complications are independent of the presence of deep venous insufficiency. *Journal of Vascular Surgery, 48*(6), 1538-1545. doi:10.1016/j.jvs.2008.07.052

Koivunen, K., & Lukkarinen, H. (2006). Lower limb atherosclerotic disease causes various deteriorations of patients' health-related quality of life. *Journal of Vascular Nursing, 24*(4), 102-115. doi:10.1016/j.jvn.2006.06.015

Koupidis, S. A., Paraskevas, K. I., Staphopoulos, V., & Mikhailidis, D. P. (2008). The impact of lower extremity venous ulcers due to chronic venous insufficiency on quality of life. *The Open Cardiovascular Medical Journal, 2,* 105-109. doi:10.2174/1874192400802010105

Lederle, F. A., Larson, J. C., Margolis, K. L., Allison, M. A., Freiberg, M. S., Cochrane, B. B., ..., Curb, J. D. (2008). Abdominal aortic aneurysm events in the Women's Health Initiative: Cohort study. *BMJ, 337,* a1724. doi:10.1136/bmj.a1724.

Leiter, L. A., Genest, J., Harris, S. B., Lewis, G., McPherson, R., Steiner, G., & Woo, V. (2006). Dyslipidemia in adults with diabetes. *Canadian Journal of Diabetes, 30*(3), 230-240.

Le Sage, S., McGee, M., & Emed, J. D. (2008). Knowledge of venous thromboembolism prevention among hospitalized patients. *Journal of Vascular Nursing, 26*(4), 109-117. doi:10.1016/j.jvn.2008.09.005

Lloyd-Jones, D., Adams, R., Carnethon, M., De Simone, G., Ferguson, T. B., Flegal, K., ..., Hong, Y. (2009). Heart disease and stroke statistics—2009 update: A report from the American Heart Association Statistics Committee and Stroke Statistics Subcommittee. *Circulation, 119*(3), e21-e181. doi:10.1161/CIRCULATIONAHA. 108.191261

Lovell, M., Harris, K., Forbes, T., Twillman, G., Abramson, B., Criqui, M. H., ..., Hirsch, A. T. (2009). Peripheral artery disease: Lack of awareness in Canada. *Canadian Journal of Cardiology, 25*(1): 39-45. doi:10.1016/S0828-282X(09)70021-2

Marzen-Groller, K. D., Tremblay, S. M., Kaszuba, J., Girodo, V., Swavely, D., Moyer, B., ..., Wilson, E. (2008). Testing the effectiveness of the Amputee Mobility Protocol: A pilot study. *Journal of Vascular Nursing, 26*(3), 74-81. doi:10.1016/j.jvn.2008.05.001

McDermott, M. M., Ades, P., Guralnik, J. M., Dyer, A., Ferrucci, L., Liu, K., ..., Criqui, M. H. (2009). Treadmill exercise and resistance training in patients with peripheral arterial disease with and without intermittent claudication: A randomized controlled trial. *JAMA, 301*(2), 165-174. doi:10.1001/jama.2008.962

McPhee, J., Hill, J., & Eslami, M. (2007). The impact of gender on presentation, therapy, and mortality of abdominal aortic aneu-

rysms in the US, 2001-2004. *Journal of Vascular Surgery, 45*(5), 891-899. doi:10.1016/j.jvs.2007.01.043

Melamed, M. L., Muntner, P., Michos, E., Uribarri, J., Weber, C., Sharma, J. & Raggi, P. (2008). Serum 25-hydroxyvitamin D levels and the prevalence of peripheral arterial disease: Results from the NHANES 2001-2004. *Arteriosclerosis, Thrombosis and Vascular Biology, 28,* 1179-1185. doi:10.1161/ATVBAHA.108. 165886

Merli, G. J. (2008). Pathophysiology of venous thrombosis and the diagnosis of deep vein thrombosis—Pulmonary embolism in the elderly. *Cardiology Clinics, 26*(2), 203-219. doi:10.1016/j. ccl.2007.12.013

Milio, G., Siragusa, S., Minà, C., Amato, C., Corrado, E., Grimaudo, S., & Novo, S. (2008). Superficial vein thrombosis: Prevalence of common genetic risk factors and their role on spreading to deep veins. *Thrombolytic Research, 123,* 194. doi:10.1016/j. thromres.2008.01.013

Morgan, R., Belli, A., & Munneke, G. (2008). *Peripheral vascular disease. Reference from A.D.A.M. Grainger and Allison's diagnostic radiology* (5th ed.). New York: Churchill Livingstone.

National Heart, Lung, and Blood Institute (NHLBI). (1998). *Clinical guidelines on the identification, evaluation, and treatment of overweight and obesity in adults: The evidence report (NIH pub no 98-4083).* Bethesda, MD: National Institutes of Health.

Nikol, S., Baumgartner, I., Van Belle, E., Diehm, C., Visonà, A., Capogrossi, M. C., ..., Meyer, F. (2008). Therapeutic angiogenesis with intramuscular NV1FGF improves amputation-free survival in patients with critical limb ischemia. *Molecular Therapy, 16*(5), 972-980. doi:10.1038/mt.2008.33

Norgren, L., Hiatt, W. R., Dormandy, J. A., Nehler, M. R., Harris, K. A., & Fowkes, F. G. R. (2007). Inter-Society consensus for the management of peripheral arterial disease. *Journal of Vascular Surgery, 45,* S5-S67. doi:10.1016/j.jvs.2006.12.037

Nutescu, E., Shapiro, N., & Chevalier, A. (2008). New anticoagulant agents: Direct thrombin inhibitors. *Cardiology Clinics, 26,* 169-187. doi:10.1016/j.ccl.2007.12.005

Ostchega, Y., Paulose-Ram, R., Dillon, C. F., Gu, Q., & Hughes, J. P. (2007). Prevalence of peripheral arterial disease and risk factors in persons aged 60 and older: Data from the National Health and Nutrition Examination Survey 1999-2004. *Journal of the American Geriatric Society, 55*(4), 583-589. doi:10.1111/j.1532-5415.2007.01123.x

Paraskevas, K. I., Liapis, C. D., Briana, D. D., & Mikhailidis, D. (2007). Thromboangiitis obliterans (Buerger's disease): Searching for a therapeutic strategy. *Angiology, 58,* 75-84. doi:10.1177/0003319706291169

Patel, P. D., & Arora, R. R. (2008). Pathophysiology, diagnosis, and management of aortic dissection. *Therapeutic Advances in Cardiovascular Disease, 2*(6), 439-468. doi:10.1177/1753944708090830

Perera, G., & Lyden, S. (2007). Current trends in lower extremity revascularization. *Surgical Clinics of North America, 87,* 1135-1147. doi:10.1016/j.suc.2007.07.004

Pittler, M. H., & Ernst, E. (2006). Horse chestnut seed extract for chronic venous insufficiency. *Cochrane Database System Review, 25*(1). CD003230.

Pradhan, A. D., Shrivastava, S., Cook, N. R., Rifai, N., Creager, M. A., & Ridker, P. M. (2008). Symptomatic peripheral arterial disease in women: Nontraditional biomarkers of elevated risk. *Circulation, 117,* 823-831. doi:10.1161/CIRCULATIONAHA.107.719369

Raju, S., & Neglen, P. (2009). Chronic venous insufficiency and varicose veins. *New England Journal of Medicine, 360,* 2319-2329. doi:10.1056/NEJMcp0802444

Rich, K. (2008). The effects of leg/body position on transcutaneous oxygen measurements after lower extremity arterial revascularization. *Journal of Vascular Nursing, 26,* 6. doi:10.1016/j. jvn.2007.09.002

Ronayne, R. (2007). Lower extremity peripheral arterial disease. In P. Lewis (Ed.), *Core curriculum for vascular nursing.* Salem, MA: Society for Vascular Nursing.

Rooke, T. W., Hirsch, A. T., Misra, S., Sdaway, A. N., Beckman, J. A., Findeiss, L. K., ..., Zierler, R. E. (2011). 2011 ACCF/AHA focused update of the guidelines for the management of patients with peripheral artery disease (updating the 2005 guideline): A report of the American College of Cardiology Foundation/American Heart Association task force on practice guidelines. *Circulation, 124*(18), 2020-2045. doi:10.1161/CIR.0b013e31822e80c3

Schulman, S., Beyth, R., Kearon, C., Levine, M. N., & American College of Chest Physicians. (2008). Hemorrhagic complications of anticoagulant and thrombolytic treatment. American College of Chest Physicians evidence-based clinical practice guidelines. *Chest, 133*(6), 257S-298S. doi:10.1378/chest.08-0673

Shrikhande, G., & McKinsey, J. (2008). Use and abuse of artherectomy: Where should it be used? *Seminars in Vascular Surgery, 21,* 204-209. doi:10.1053/j.semvascsurg.2008.11.007

Smith, D., DeVeaux, T., Dillard, C., Dinsmore, M., Fitzgerald, K., Flood, A., & Kohlman-Trigoboff, D. (2009). 2009 Clinical practice guideline for patients undergoing endovascular repair of abdominal aortic aneurysms. *Journal of Vascular Nursing, 27*(2), 48-63. doi:10.1016/j.jvn.2009.03.003

Sobel, M., & Verhaeghe, R. (2008). Antithrombotic therapy for peripheral artery occlusive disease. *Chest, 133*(6 Suppl), S815-S835. doi:10.1378/chest.08-0686

Sol, B., Graaf, Y., van der Bijl, J. J., Goessens, B. M. B., & Visseren, F. L. J. (2008). The role of self-efficacy in vascular risk factor management: A randomized control trial. *Patient Education and Counselling, 71*(2), 191-197. doi:10.1016/j.pec.2007.12.005

Stalenhoef, A. F. (2009). The benefit of statins in non-cardiac vascular surgery patients. *Journal of Vascular Surgery, 49,* 260-65. doi:10.1016/j.jvs.2008.11.070

Tinkman, M. (2009). The endovascular approach to abdominal aortic aneurysm repair. *AORN Journal, 89*(2), 289-306. doi:10.1016/j.aorn.2008.11.028

Tobon, J., Whitney, J. D., & Jarrett, M. (2008). Nutritional status and wound severity of overweight and obese patients with venous leg ulcers: A pilot study. *Journal of Vascular Nursing, 26*(2), 43-52. doi:10.1016/j.jvn.2007.12.002

Tsai, T. T., Trimarchi, S., & Nienaber, C. A. (2009). Acute aortic dissection: Perspectives from the International Registry of Acute Aortic Dissection. *European Journal of Endovascular Surgery, 37*(2), 149-159. doi:10.1016/j.ejvs.2008.11.032

Varon, J. (2008). Treatment of acute severe hypertension: Current and newer agents. *Drugs, 68*(3), 283-297. doi:10.2165/00003495-200868030-00003

Vinjar, B., & Stewart, M. (2008). Oral vasodilators for primary Raynaud's phenomenon. *Cochrane Database System Rev, 2,* CD00668. doi:10.1002/14651858.CD006687.pub2

Vouyouka, A., & Kent, K. (2007). Arterial vascular disease in women. *Journal of Vascular Surgery, 46*(6), 1295-1302. doi:10.1016/j.jvs.2007.07.057

Walker, L., & Lamond, S. (2008). Graduated compression stockings to prevent deep vein thrombosis. *Nursing Standard, 22*(40), 35-38.

Warkentin, T., Greinacher, A., Koster, A., Lincoff, A. M., & American College of Chest Physicians. (2008). Treatment and prevention of heparin-induced thrombocytopenia. American College of Chest Physicians evidence-based clinical practice guidelines (8th ed.). *Chest, 133*(6 Suppl), 340S-380S. doi:10.1378/chest.08-0677

White, C., & Gray, W. (2007). Endovascular therapies for peripheral arterial disease: An evidence-based review. *Circulation, 116,* 2203-2215. doi:10.1161/CIRCULATIONAHA.106.621391

Wildgruber, M., & Berger, H. (2008). Cryoplasty for the prevention of arterial stenosis. *Cardiovascular Interventional Radiology, 31,* 1050-1058. doi:10.1007/s00270-008-9364-y

Winslow, E. H., & Brosz, D. L. (2008). Graduated compression stockings in hospitalized postoperative patients: Correctness of usage and size. *American Journal of Nursing, 108*(9), 40. doi:10.1097/01.NAJ.0000334973.82359.11

Young, T., Tang, H., Aukes, J., & Hughes, R. (2007). Vena caval filters for the prevention of pulmonary embolism. *Cochrane Database System Review, 4,* CD006212. doi:10.1002/14651858.CD006212.pub3

CANADIAN RESOURCES

Canadian Cardiovascular Society
http://www.ccs.ca
Canadian Council of Cardiovascular Nurses
http://www.cccn.ca/index2.cfm
Canadian Society for Vascular Surgery
http://csvs.vascularweb.org
Heart and Stroke Foundation of Canada
http://ww2.heartandstroke.ca
Hypertension Canada
http://www.hypertension.ca/
Registered Nurses' Association of Ontario
Nursing Best Practice Guidelines: Assessment and Management of Venous Leg Ulcers. (2007).
http://www.rnao.org
Safer Healthcare Now—VTE
http://www.saferhealthcarenow.ca/en/interventions/vte/pages/default.aspx
Society of Vascular Nurses—Canadian Chapters
http://www.tigc.org

ⓔvolve *For additional Internet resources, see the Web site for this book at* **http://evolve.elsevier.com/Canada/Lewis/medsurg**

Problems of Ingestion, Digestion, Absorption, and Elimination

SECTION OUTLINE

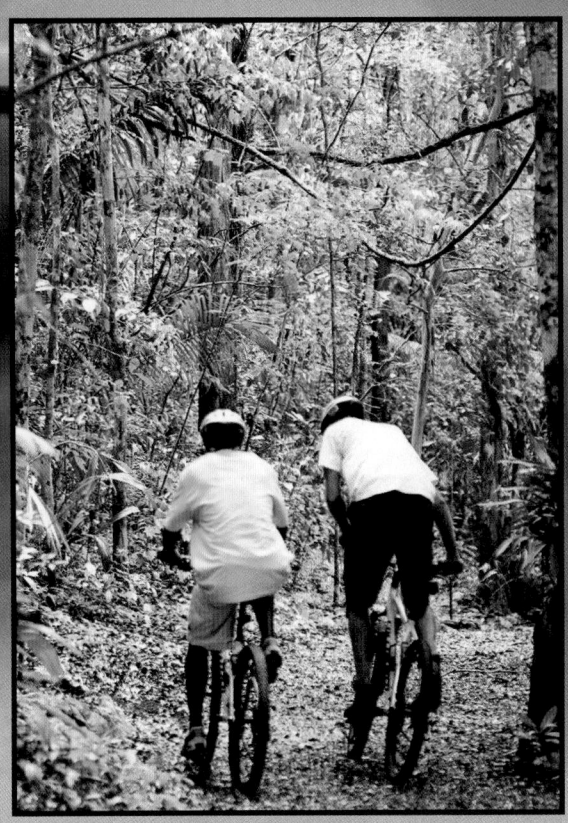

Nursing Assessment: Gastrointestinal System

Written by Juvann M. Wolff and Margaret McLean Heitkemper

Adapted by Donna Goodridge

LEARNING OBJECTIVES

1. Describe the structures and the functions of the organs of the gastrointestinal tract.
2. Describe the structures and functions of the liver, the gallbladder, the biliary tract, and the pancreas.
3. Differentiate between the processes of ingestion, digestion, absorption, and elimination.
4. Relate the age-related changes in the gastrointestinal system to differences in assessment findings.
5. Select the significant subjective and objective data related to the gastrointestinal system that should be obtained from a patient.

6. Describe the appropriate techniques used in the physical assessment of the gastrointestinal system.
7. Differentiate normal from abnormal findings of a physical assessment of the gastrointestinal system.
8. Describe the purpose, the significance of results, and nursing responsibilities related to diagnostic studies of the gastrointestinal system.

KEY TERMS

absorption Uptake of nutrients from the gut lumen to the bloodstream, p. 1045

bilirubin A pigment derived from the breakdown of aged red blood cells, p. 1047

borborygmi Audible abdominal sounds produced by hyperactive intestinal peristalsis; Table 41-11, p. 1054

cheilitis Inflammation of lips (usually lower) with fissuring, scaling, crusting; Table 41-11, p. 1054

cheilosis Softening, fissuring, and cracking of lips at angles of mouth; Table 41-11, p. 1054

defecation Discharge of feces from the rectum, p. 1046

deglutition Swallowing, p. 1043

digestion The process in the gastrointestinal tract by which food is broken down in order to convert food into a substance suitable for absorption and assimilation into the body; involves both mechanical digestion (mastication) and chemical digestion, p. 1044

endoscopy The direct visualization of a body structure through a lighted fibreoptic instrument (endoscope), p. 1060

hematemesis Vomiting of blood, which indicates bleeding in the upper gastrointestinal tract; Table 41-11, p. 1054

hepatocytes Specialized hepatic cells, p. 1046

ingestion The intake of food, p. 1041

Kupffer cells A type of macrophage found in the liver that removes bacteria and toxins from the blood, p. 1046

melena Abnormal, black, tarry stool containing digested blood; Table 41-11, p. 1055

pyrosis Heartburn; burning in epigastric or substernal area; Table 41-11, p. 1054

steatorrhea Passage of large amounts of fat as a fatty, frothy, foul-smelling stool as a result of failure to digest and absorb the fat; Table 41-11, p. 1055

tenesmus Spasmodic contraction of the anal sphincter with pain and persistent desire to empty the bowel; Table 41-11, p. 1055

Valsalva manoeuvre A manoeuvre that involves contraction of the chest muscles on a closed glottis with simultaneous contraction of the abdominal muscles, p. 1046

villi Minute, fingerlike projections in the mucous membrane of the small intestine, containing goblet cells that secrete mucus and epithelial cells that produce the intestinal digestive enzymes, p. 1043

ELECTRONIC RESOURCES

Supplemental content related to Chapter 41 can be found…

Evolve Web Site ⊖volve

http://evolve.elsevier.com/Canada/Lewis/medsurg
- Animation: Rectal Examination
- Assessment Case Study: Gastrointestinal System
- Clinical Reference: Laboratory Values
- Content Updates
- Electronic Calculators
- Examination Review Questions
- Glossary

- Key Points (Printable and MP3 Download)
- Video Clips:
  - Auscultation: Abdomen, Bowel Sounds
  - Percussion: Abdomen
  - Percussion: Liver
  - Percussion: Spleen
  - Palpation: Abdomen, Superficial and Deep
- Physical Examination Video Clips:
  - Abdomen: Inspection, Auscultation, and Percussion
  - Abdomen: Palpation

The main function of the gastrointestinal (GI) system is to supply nutrients to body cells. This is accomplished through the processes of *ingestion* (taking in food), *digestion* (breakdown of food), and *absorption* (transfer of food products into circulation). *Elimination* is the process of excreting the waste products of digestion.

The GI system (also called the *digestive system*) consists of the GI tract and its associated organs and glands. Included in the GI tract are the mouth, the esophagus, the stomach, the small intestine, the large intestine, the rectum, and the anus. The associated organs are the liver, the pancreas, and the gallbladder (Figure 41-1).

Factors outside the GI tract can influence its functioning. Both psychological and emotional factors, such as stress and anxiety, influence GI functioning in many people. Stress may be manifested as anorexia, nausea, epigastric and abdominal pain, or diarrhea. However, GI problems should never be attributed solely to psychological factors. Organic and psychologically based problems can exist independently or concurrently. Physical factors such as dietary intake, ingestion of alcohol and caffeine-containing products, cigarette smoking, and fatigue may also affect GI function. Some organic diseases of the GI system, such as peptic ulcer disease and ulcerative colitis, may be aggravated by stress.

Structures and Functions of the Gastrointestinal System

The GI tract is a tube approximately 9 m (30 ft) long, extending from the mouth to the anus. The entire tract is composed of four common layers. From the inside to the outside, these layers are (a) mucosa, (b) submucosa, (c) muscle, and (d) serosa (Figure 41-2). In the esophagus, the outer coat is fibrous tissue rather than serosa. The muscular coat consists of two layers: the circular (inner) and the longitudinal (outer).

The GI tract is innervated by the parasympathetic and the sympathetic branches of the autonomic nervous system. The parasympathetic system is mainly excitatory, and the sympathetic system is mainly inhibitory. For example, peristalsis is increased by parasympathetic stimulation and decreased by sympathetic stimulation. Sensory information is relayed via both sympathetic and parasympathetic afferent fibres.

The GI tract and accessory organs receive approximately 25 to 30% of the cardiac output. Circulation in the GI system is unique in that venous blood that drains from the GI tract organs empties into the portal vein, which then perfuses the liver. The upper portion of the GI tract receives its blood supply from the splanchnic artery. The small intestine receives its blood supply from branches of the hepatic and superior mesenteric arteries. The large intestine receives its blood supply mainly from the superior and inferior mesenteric arteries. Because such a large percentage of the cardiac output is used to perfuse these organs, the GI tract is a major source from which blood flow can be diverted during exercise or stress.

The two types of movement of the GI tract are *mixing* (segmentation) and *propulsion* (peristalsis). The secretions of the GI system consist of enzymes and hormones for digestion, mucus to provide protection and lubrication, and water and electrolytes.

The abdominal organs are almost completely covered by the peritoneum. The two layers of the peritoneum are the parietal, which lines the abdominal cavity wall, and the visceral, which covers the abdominal organs. The peritoneal cavity is the potential space between the parietal and visceral layers. The two folds of the peritoneum are the mesentery and the omentum. The mesentery is the attachment of the small intestine and part of the large intestine to the posterior abdominal wall and contains blood and lymph vessels. The lesser omentum extends from the lesser curvature of the stomach and the upper duodenum to the liver, and the greater omentum hangs from the stomach over the intestines like an apron. The omentum contains fat and lymph nodes.

The primary functions of the GI system are (a) ingestion and propulsion (movement) of food; (b) secretion of mucus, water, and enzymes; (c) digestion; (d) absorption; and (e) elimination. Each part of the GI system performs different activities to accomplish these functions.

Ingestion and Propulsion of Food

Ingestion is the intake of food. A person's appetite or desire to ingest food is a significant factor in how much food is eaten. Multiple factors are involved in the control of appetite. An

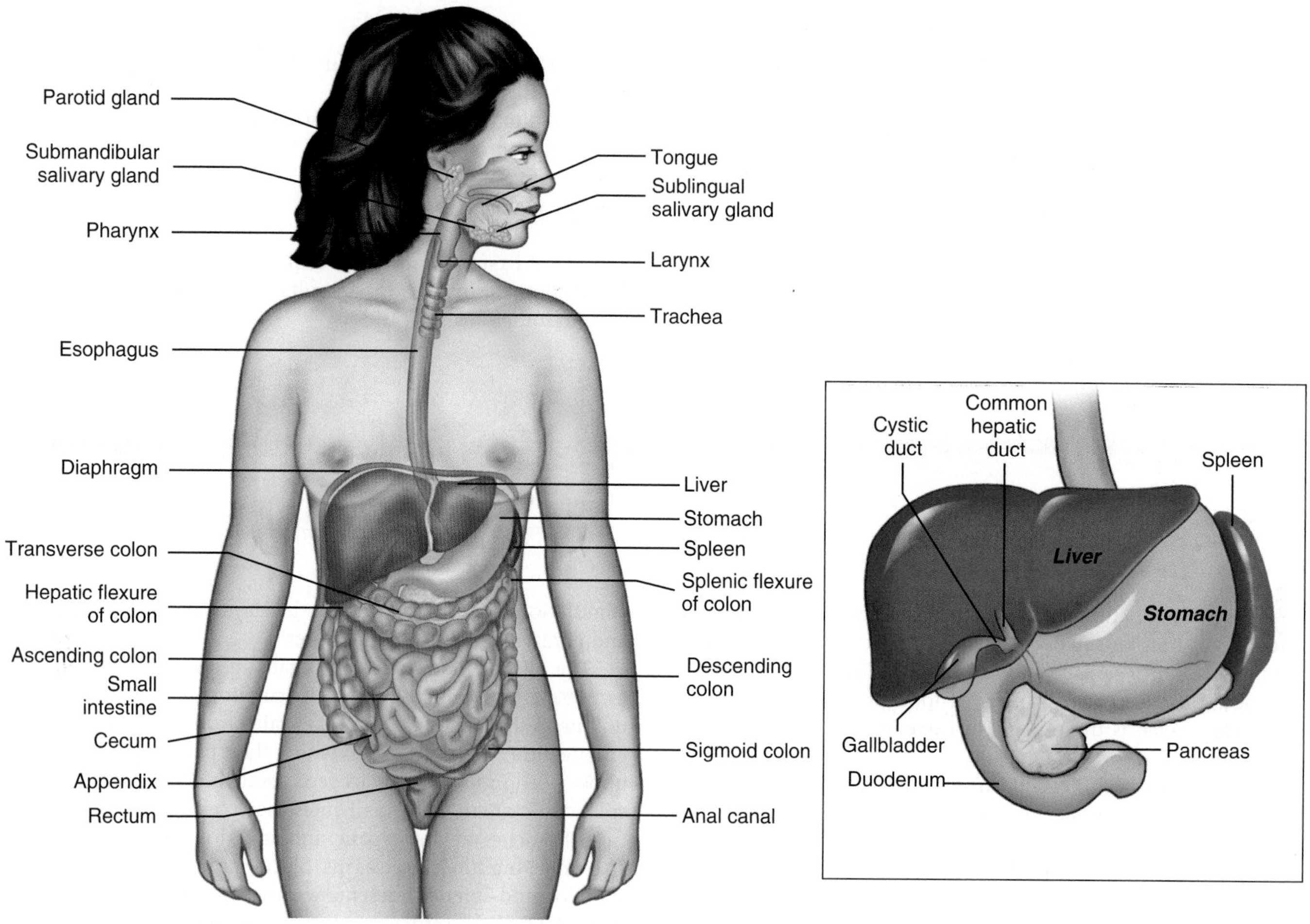

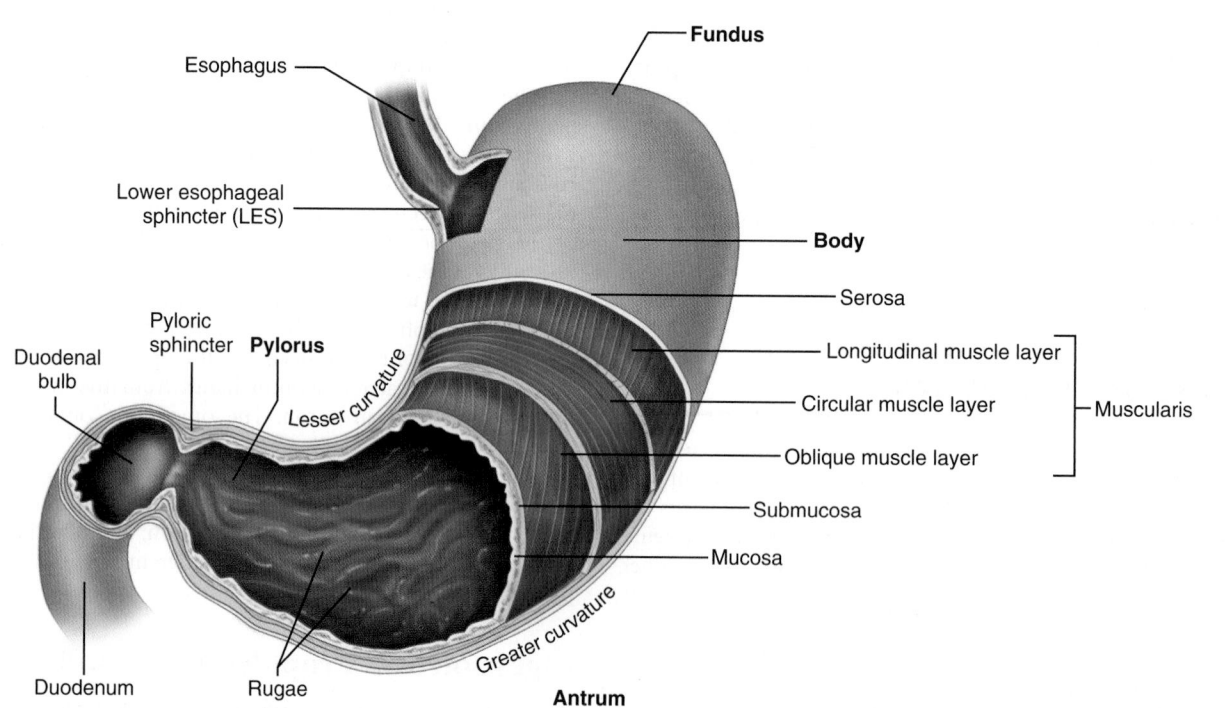

Figure 41-1 Location of organs of the gastrointestinal system.

Source: Patton, K. T., & Thibodeau, G. A. (2010). *Anatomy and physiology* (7th ed., p. 838, Figure 25-1). St. Louis: Mosby.

Figure 41-2 Parts of the stomach.

Source: Thibodeau G. A., & Patton, K. T. (2010). *The human body in health and disease* (5th ed., p. 499, Figure 17-15). St. Louis: Mosby.

appetite centre is located in the hypothalamus. It is directly or indirectly stimulated by hypoglycemia, an empty stomach, decrease in body temperature, and input from higher brain centres. The hormone *ghrelin* released from the stomach mucosa plays a role in appetite stimulation. Another hormone, *leptin*, is involved in appetite suppression. (Ghrelin and leptin are discussed further in Chapter 43). The sight, smell, and taste of food frequently stimulate appetite. Appetite may be inhibited by stomach distension, illness (especially accompanied by fever), hyperglycemia, nausea and vomiting, certain drugs (e.g., amphetamines), and psychological factors, such as depression.

Swallowing **(deglutition)** is the mechanical component of ingestion. The organs involved in the swallowing of food are the mouth, the pharynx, and the esophagus. Swallowed food is moved to the stomach by means of peristalsis, the coordinated, sequential contraction and relaxation of outer longitudinal and inner circular layers of muscles.

Mouth.

The mouth consists of the lips and the oral (buccal) cavity. The lips surround the orifice of the mouth and function in speech. The roof of the oral cavity is formed by the hard and soft palates. The oral cavity contains the teeth—used in mastication (chewing)—and the tongue. The tongue is a solid muscle mass and assists in chewing by keeping food between the teeth during chewing and moving the food to the back of the throat for swallowing. Taste receptors are found on the sides and the tip of the tongue. The tongue is also important in speech.

Within the oral cavity are three pairs of salivary glands: the parotid, the submaxillary, and the sublingual. These glands produce saliva, which consists of water, protein, mucin, inorganic salts, and salivary amylase. Approximately 1 L of saliva is produced each day. Saliva serves many roles, including the lubrication of food and prevention of bacterial overgrowth in the oral cavity.

Pharynx.

The pharynx is a musculomembranous tube that may be divided into the nasopharynx, the oropharynx, and the laryngeal pharynx. The mucous membrane of the pharynx is continuous with the nasal cavity, the mouth, the auditory tubes, and the larynx. The oropharynx secretes mucus, which aids in swallowing. The epiglottis is a lid of fibrocartilage that closes over the larynx during swallowing. During ingestion, the oropharynx provides a route for the food from the mouth to the esophagus. When receptors in the oropharynx are stimulated by food or liquid, the swallowing reflex is initiated.

Esophagus.

The esophagus is a hollow, muscular tube that receives food from the pharynx and moves it to the stomach by peristaltic contractions. It is 23 to 25 cm long and 2 cm in diameter. The esophagus is located in the thoracic cavity; it starts behind the trachea at the lower end of the pharynx and extends to the stomach. The upper one third of the esophagus is composed of striated skeletal muscle, and the distal two thirds are composed of smooth muscle.

With swallowing, the upper esophageal sphincter (cricopharyngeal muscle) relaxes, and a peristaltic wave moves the bolus into the esophagus. Between swallows, the esophagus is collapsed. It is structurally composed of four layers: the inner mucosa, submucosa, muscularis propria, and outermost adventitia. The muscular layers contract (peristalsis) and propel the food to the stomach. The lower esophageal sphincter (LES) at the distal end of the esophagus remains contracted except during swallowing, belching, or vomiting. The LES is an important

barrier that prevents reflux of acidic gastric contents into the esophagus.

Digestion and Absorption

Mouth.

Digestion begins in the mouth. *Digestion* involves both a mechanical process (mastication) and a chemical process. Saliva is the first secretion involved, and its main function is to lubricate and soften the food mass, thus facilitating swallowing. Saliva contains amylase (ptyalin), which hydrolyzes starches to maltose. However, salivary amylase is not necessary for the digestion of carbohydrates.

Stomach.

The functions of the stomach are to store food, secrete digestive juices, mix the food with gastric secretions, and empty the resulting content (called *chyme*) into the small intestine at a rate at which digestion can occur. The stomach absorbs only small amounts of water, alcohol, electrolytes, and certain drugs.

The stomach is usually J-shaped and lies obliquely in the epigastric, umbilical, and left hypochondriac regions of the abdomen (see Figure 41-7 later in the chapter). The shape and position of the stomach change according to the degree of gastric distension. It always contains gastric fluid and mucus. The three main parts of the stomach are the fundus, the body, and the antrum (see Figure 41-2). The pylorus is a small portion of the antrum that lies proximal to the pyloric sphincter. Food passes from the lower esophageal sphincter through the cardiac orifice into the stomach. The chyme is propelled through the pyloric sphincter into the duodenum.

The serous (outer) layer of the stomach is formed by the peritoneum. The muscular layer consists of the longitudinal (outer) layer, the circular (middle) layer, and the oblique (inner) layer. The mucosal layer forms folds called *rugae* that contain many small glands. In response to nutrient intake, these glands secrete most of the gastric juice. In the fundus, the glands contain chief cells, which secrete pepsinogen, and parietal cells, which secrete hydrochloric acid (HCl), water, and intrinsic factor. The secretion of HCl makes gastric juice acidic in comparison with other body fluids. This acidic pH aids in the protection against ingested organisms. Intrinsic factor promotes cobalamin (vitamin B_{12}) absorption in the small intestine. Mucus is secreted by glands in the cardiac and pyloric areas.

Small Intestine.

The two primary functions of the small intestine are digestion and *absorption* (uptake of nutrients from the gut lumen to the bloodstream). The small intestine is a coiled tube approximately 5 to 6 m in length and from 2.5 to 2.8 cm in diameter, diminishing in diameter at the lower end. It extends from the pylorus to the ileocecal valve. The small intestine is composed of the duodenum, the jejunum, and the ileum. The ileocecal valve, which separates the small intestine from the large intestine, prevents reflux of large intestine contents into the small intestine.

The serous coat of the small intestine is formed by the peritoneum. The mucosa is thick, vascular, and glandular. Folds in the mucosa slow the passage of food and provide a greater surface area for digestion and absorption.

Absorption occurs through the villi, which are functional units present throughout the entire small intestine. **Villi** are minute, finger-like projections in the mucous membrane. They contain goblet cells that secrete mucus and epithelial cells that produce the intestinal digestive enzymes. The epithelial cells on the villi also have *microvilli*, which compose the brush border. Thus the presence of villi and microvilli also greatly increases the surface area for absorption.

The digestive enzymes on the brush border of the microvilli chemically break down nutrients so that they can be absorbed. The villi are surrounded by the crypts of Lieberkühn, which contain the multipotent stem cells for the other epithelial cell types. (Stem cells are discussed in Chapter 16). Brunner's glands in the submucosa of the duodenum secrete mucus.

Physiology of Digestion.

Digestion is the physical and chemical breakdown of food into absorbable substances. Digestion in the GI tract is facilitated by the timely movement of food through the various organs and the secretion of specific enzymes. These enzymes break down foodstuffs to particles of appropriate size for absorption (Table 41-1).

The process of digestion begins in the mouth, where the food is chewed, mechanically broken down, and mixed with saliva.

The saliva lubricates the food. In addition, salivary amylase begins the breakdown of starch. Salivary gland secretion is stimulated by chewing movements and the sight, the smell, the thought, and the taste of food. The food is swallowed and passes into the esophagus, where peristaltic waves propel it to the stomach. No digestion or absorption occurs in the esophagus.

In the stomach, the digestion of proteins begins with the release of pepsinogen from chief cells. The acidic environment of the stomach results in the conversion of pepsinogen to its active form, pepsin. Pepsin begins the initial breakdown of proteins. In the stomach, digestion of starches and fats is minimal. The food is mixed with gastric secretions, which are under neural and hormonal control (Tables 41-2 and 41-3). The stomach also serves as a reservoir for food, which is slowly expelled into the small intestine. The length of time that food remains in the stomach depends on the composition of the food, but average meals remain from 3 to 4 hours.

Digestion is completed in the small intestine, where carbohydrates are hydrolyzed to monosaccharides, fats to glycerol and fatty acids, and proteins to amino acids. The physical presence of *chyme* (food mixed with gastric secretions), along with its chemical nature in the small intestine, stimulates motility and secretion. Secretions involved in digestion include enzymes from the pancreas, bile from the liver (see Table 41-1), and intestinal secretions from glands in the small intestine. Both secretion and motility are under neural and hormonal control.

When food enters the stomach and small intestine, hormones are released into the bloodstream (see Table 41-3). The hormone *secretin* stimulates the pancreas to secrete fluid with a high concentration of bicarbonate. This alkaline secretion enters the duodenum and neutralizes acid in the chyme. The duodenal mucosa also secrete mucus to protect against the HCl acid. In response

Table 41-1 Gastrointestinal Secretions Related to Digestion

DAILY AMOUNT (mL)	SECRETIONS OR ENZYMES	ACTION
Salivary Glands		
1000-1500	Salivary amylase (ptyalin)	Initiation of starch digestion
Stomach		
2500	Pepsinogen	Protein digestion
	HCl acid	Activation of pepsinogen to pepsin
	Lipase	Fat digestion
	Intrinsic factor	Essential for absorption of cobalamin in the ileum
Small Intestine		
3000	Enterokinase	Activation of trypsinogen to trypsin
	Amylase	Carbohydrate digestion
	Peptidases	Protein digestion
	Aminopeptidase	Protein digestion
	Maltase	Maltose to two glucose molecules
	Sucrase	Sucrose to glucose and fructose
	Lactase	Lactose to glucose and galactose
	Lipase	Fat digestion
Pancreas		
700	Trypsinogen	Protein digestion
	Chymotrypsin	Protein digestion
	Amylase	Starch to disaccharides and trisaccharides
	Lipase	Fat digestion
Liver and Gallbladder		
700-1200	Bile	Emulsification of fats and aid in absorption of fatty acids and fat-soluble vitamins (A, D, E, and K)

Table 41-2 Phases of Gastric Secretion

PHASE	STIMULUS TO SECRETION	SECRETION
Cephalic (nervous)	Sight, smell, taste of food (before food enters stomach); initiated in the CNS and mediated by the vagus nerve	HCl acid, pepsinogen, mucus
Gastric (hormonal and nervous)	Food in antrum of stomach, vagal stimulation	Release of gastrin from antrum into circulation to stimulate gastric secretions and motility
Intestinal (hormonal)	Presence of acidic chyme (pH <2) in small intestine stimulates release of secretin, gastric inhibitory polypeptide, and cholecystokinin into circulation to decrease acid secretion	Chyme (pH >3) stimulates release of duodenal gastrin to increase acid secretion

CNS, central nervous system; *HCl*, hydrochloric acid.

Table 41-3 Major Hormones Controlling Gastrointestinal Secretion and Motility

HORMONE	SOURCE	ACTIVATING STIMULI	FUNCTION
Gastrin	Gastric and duodenal mucosa	Stomach distension, partially digested proteins in pylorus	Stimulates gastric acid secretion and motility; maintains lower esophageal sphincter tone
Secretin	Duodenal mucosa	Acid entering small intestine	Inhibits gastric motility and acid secretion; stimulates pancreatic bicarbonate secretion
Cholecystokinin	Duodenal mucosa	Fatty acids and amino acids in small intestine	Causes contraction of gallbladder and relaxation of sphincter of Oddi, allowing increased flow of bile into duodenum; stimulates release of pancreatic digestive enzymes
Gastric inhibitory peptide	Duodenal mucosa	Fatty acids and lipids in small intestine	Inhibits gastric acid secretion and gastric motility

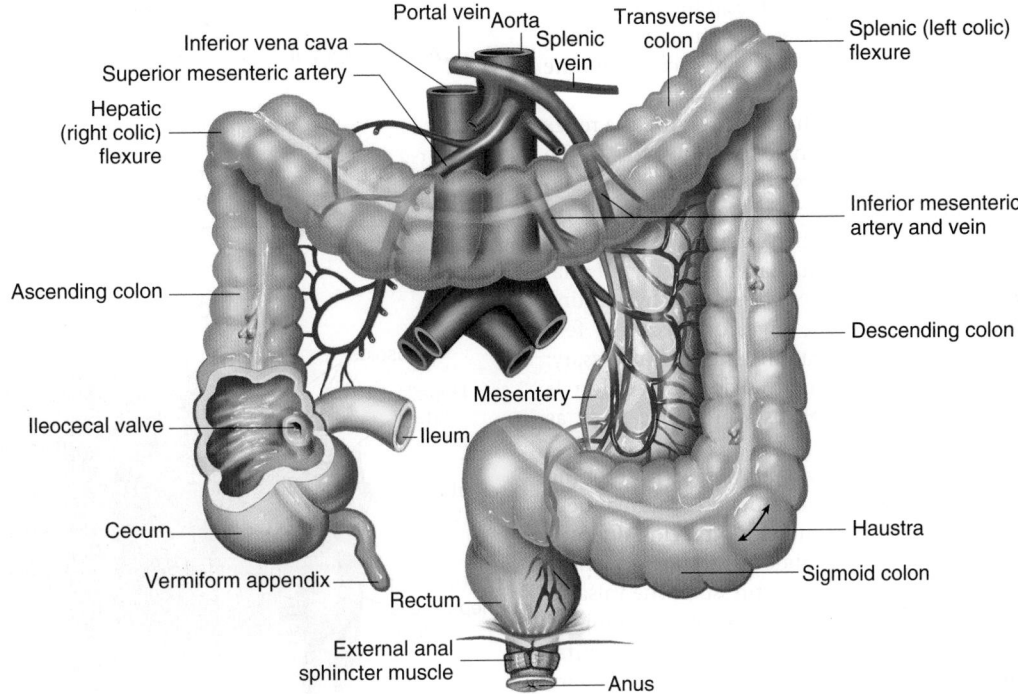

Figure 41-3 Anatomic locations of the large intestine.

Source: Patton, K. T., & Thibodeau, G. A. (2010). *Anatomy and physiology* (7th ed., p. 855, Figure 25-19A). St. Louis: Mosby.

to the presence of chyme, the hormone *cholecystokinin* (CCK), produced by the duodenal mucosa, enters the bloodstream and stimulates contraction of the gallbladder and relaxation of the sphincter of Oddi. These actions enable bile to flow from the common bile duct into the duodenum. Bile is necessary for the digestion of fats. CCK also stimulates the pancreas to synthesize and secrete enzymes for enzymatic digestion of carbohydrates, fats, and proteins.

Enzymes present on the brush border of the microvilli complete the digestion process. These enzymes hydrolyze disaccharides to monosaccharides and peptides to amino acids for absorption.

Absorption is the transfer of the end products of digestion across the intestinal wall to the circulation. Most absorption occurs in the small intestine. The surface area of the small intestine is greatly increased by its circular folds, villi, and microvilli. The movement of the villi enables the end products of digestion

to come in contact with the absorbing membrane. Monosaccharides (from carbohydrates), fatty acids (from fats), amino acids (from proteins), water, electrolytes, and vitamins are absorbed.

Elimination

Large Intestine. The large intestine is a hollow, muscular tube approximately 1.5 to 2 m long and 5 cm in diameter. The four parts of the large intestine are (a) the cecum and the appendix, a narrow tube at the end of the cecum; (b) the colon (ascending colon on the right side, transverse colon across the abdomen, descending colon on the left side, and the sigmoid colon); (c) the rectum; and (d) the anus, the terminal portion of the large intestine (Figure 41-3).

The most important function of the large intestine is the absorption of water and electrolytes. It also forms feces and serves as a reservoir for the fecal mass until defecation occurs. Feces are composed of water, bacteria, food residue, unabsorbed GI secretions, and desquamated epithelial cells. The large intestine secretes mucus, which acts as a lubricant and protects the mucosa.

Microorganisms in the colon play an important role in metabolism of bile salts, estrogens, androgens, lipids, carbohydrates, various nitrogenous substances, and drugs, as well as protecting against infection. Intestinal bacteria are responsible for the breakdown of proteins not digested or absorbed in the small intestine. These amino acids are deaminated by the bacteria, leaving ammonia, which is carried to the liver and converted to urea. Bacteria in the colon also synthesize vitamin K and some of the B vitamins. In addition, bacteria play a part in the production of flatus.

The movements of the large intestine are usually slow. When the circular muscles contract, they produce a kneading action termed *haustral churning*. Propulsive mass movement (peristalsis) also occurs. When food enters the stomach and the duodenum, the gastrocolic and duodenocolic reflexes are initiated, resulting in peristalsis in the colon. These reflexes are more active after the first daily meal and frequently result in bowel evacuation.

Defecation, the discharge of feces from the rectum, is a reflex action involving voluntary and involuntary control. Feces in the rectum stimulate sensory nerve endings that produce the urge to defecate. The reflex centre for defecation is in the sacral portion of the spinal cord (parasympathetic nerve fibres). These fibres produce contraction of the rectum and relaxation of the internal anal sphincter. Defecation is controlled voluntarily by relaxing the external anal sphincter when the urge to defecate is felt. An acceptable environment for defecation is usually necessary; otherwise the urge to defecate is suppressed. If defecation is suppressed over long periods, problems can occur, such as constipation or stool impaction.

Defecation can be facilitated by appropriate positioning (sitting or squatting) or by the **Valsalva manoeuvre.** This manoeuvre involves contraction of the chest muscles on a closed glottis with simultaneous contraction of the abdominal muscles. These actions result in increased intra-abdominal pressure. The Valsalva manoeuvre may be contraindicated in patients with head injury, cardiac problems, hemorrhoids, or liver cirrhosis with portal hypertension and in those who have undergone recent eye surgery or recent abdominal surgery.

Liver, Biliary Tract, and Pancreas

Liver. The liver is the largest internal organ in the body, weighing approximately 1200 to 1600 g in adults. It lies in the right hypochondriac and epigastric regions (see Figure 41-7 later in chapter) and is divided into right and left lobes (Figure 41-4). Glisson's capsule, which contains blood vessels, lymphatic vessels, and nerves, covers the liver. Liver disease or swelling may cause this capsule to become distended, leading to pain and oozing of lymphatic fluid into the peritoneal space.

The functional units of the liver are lobules (Figure 41-5). The lobule consists of plates of specialized hepatic cells (**hepatocytes**) arranged around a central vein. The capillaries (sinusoids) are located between the plates of hepatocytes and are lined with **Kupffer cells,** which carry out phagocytic activity (removal of bacteria and toxins from the blood). Kupffer cells also ingest aged red blood cells, breaking down hemoglobin into heme and globin. The heme is further broken down into iron and bilirubin, which is secreted into the bile. Interlobular bile ducts form from bile capillaries (*canaliculi*). The hepatic cells secrete bile into the canaliculi.

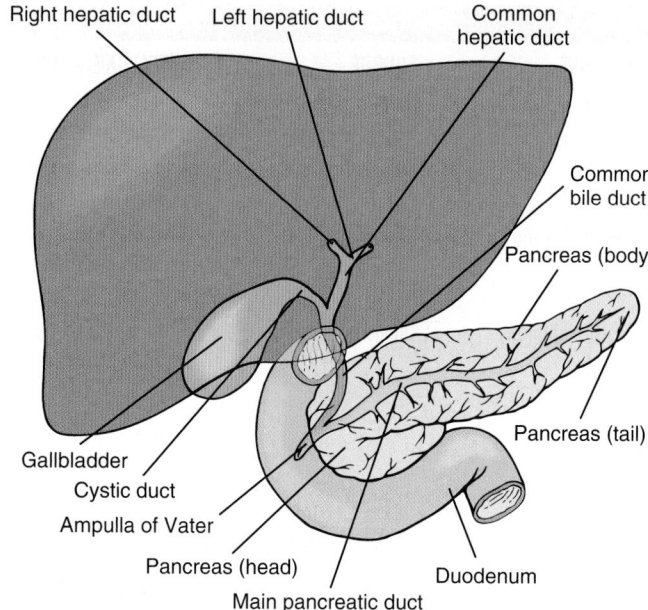

Figure 41-4 Gross structure of the liver, the gallbladder, and the pancreas and the duct system.

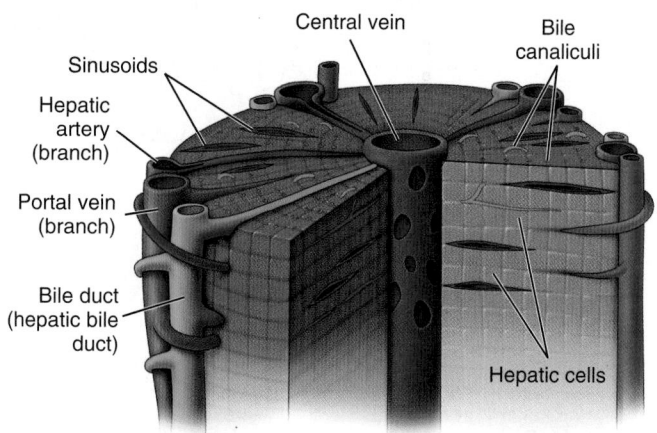

Figure 41-5 Microscopic structure of liver lobule.

Source: Herlihy, B. (2007). *The human body in health and illness* (3rd ed., p. 411, Figure 23-9B). St. Louis: W. B. Saunders.

The nerve supply to the liver is from the left vagus and the sympathetic celiac plexus. The liver receives both arterial and venous blood. About one third of the blood supply comes from the hepatic artery (branch of the celiac artery), and two thirds come from the portal vein.

A large amount of blood is required for the liver to fulfill its metabolic functions. The portal circulatory system (enterohepatic) brings blood to the liver from the stomach, intestines, spleen, and pancreas. This blood enters the liver through the portal vein. The portal vein carries absorbed products of digestion directly to the liver. In the liver, the portal vein branches and comes into contact with each lobule. The blood in the sinusoids is a mixture of arterial and venous blood.

The liver is essential for life. It functions in the manufacture, the storage, the transformation, and the excretion of a number of

Table 41-4 Major Functions of the Liver	
FUNCTION	DESCRIPTION
Metabolic Functions	
Carbohydrate metabolism	Glycogenesis (conversion of glucose to glycogen), glycogenolysis (process of breaking down glycogen to glucose), gluconeogenesis (formation of glucose from amino acids and fatty acids)
Protein metabolism	Synthesis of nonessential amino acids, synthesis of plasma proteins (except γ-globulin), urea formation from NH_3 (NH_3 formed from deamination of amino acids by action of bacteria on proteins in colon)
Fat metabolism	Synthesis of lipoproteins, breakdown of triglycerides into fatty acids and glycerol, formation of ketone bodies, synthesis of fatty acids from amino acids and glucose, synthesis and breakdown of cholesterol
Detoxification	Inactivation of drugs and harmful substances and excretion of their breakdown products
Steroid metabolism	Conjugation and excretion of gonadal and adrenal steroid hormones
Bile Synthesis	
Bile production	Formation of bile, containing bile salts, bile pigments (mainly bilirubin), and cholesterol
Bile excretion	Bile excretion by liver (≈1 L/day)
Storage	Glucose in form of glycogen; fat-soluble vitamins (A, D, E, and K) and water-soluble vitamins (B_1, B_2, cobalamin, folic acid); fatty acids; minerals (iron and copper); amino acids in form of albumin and β-globulins
Mononuclear Phagocyte System	
Kupffer cells	Breakdown of old RBCs, WBCs, bacteria, and other particles; breakdown of hemoglobin from old RBCs to bilirubin and biliverdin

NH_3, ammonia; *RBC,* red blood cell; *WBC,* white blood cell.

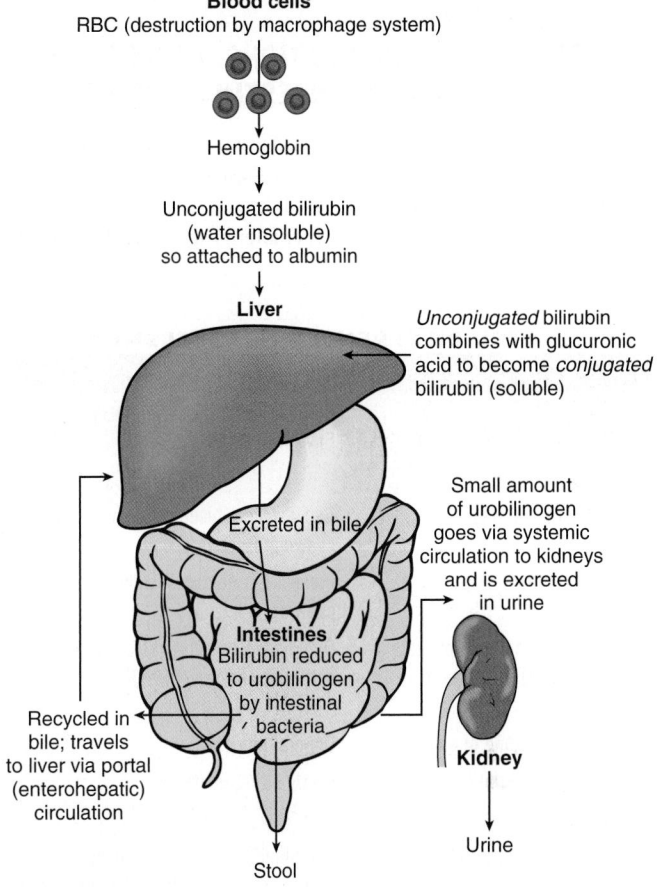

Figure 41-6 Bilirubin metabolism and conjugation. *RBC,* red blood cell.

substances involved in metabolism. The functions of the liver are numerous but can be classified into four main areas, as identified in Table 41-4.

Biliary Tract. The biliary tract consists of the gallbladder and the duct system. The gallbladder is a pear-shaped sac located below the liver. The function of the gallbladder is to concentrate and store bile. It can hold approximately 45 mL of bile.

Bile is produced by the hepatic cells and secreted into the biliary canaliculi of the lobules. Bile then drains into the interlobular bile ducts, which unite into the two main left and right hepatic ducts. The hepatic ducts merge with the cystic duct from the gallbladder to form the common bile duct (see Figure 41-4). Most bile is stored and concentrated in the gallbladder. It is then released into the cystic duct and moves down the common bile duct to enter the duodenum at the ampulla of Vater. In the intestines, most of the bilirubin is reduced to stercobilinogen and urobilinogen by bacterial action. Stercobilinogen accounts for the brown colour of stool. A small amount of conjugated bilirubin is reabsorbed by the blood. Some urobilinogen is reabsorbed by

the blood and returned to the liver through the portal circulation (enterohepatic) and excreted in the bile. An insignificant amount of urobilinogen is excreted in the urine.

Bilirubin Metabolism. **Bilirubin,** a pigment derived from the breakdown of aged red blood cells, is produced constantly (Figure 41-6). Because it is insoluble in water, it is bound to albumin for its transport to the liver. This form of bilirubin is referred to as *unconjugated.* In the liver, bilirubin is conjugated with glucuronic acid. Conjugated bilirubin is water soluble and is excreted in bile. Bile also consists of water, cholesterol, bile salts, electrolytes, and phospholipids. Bile salts are needed for fat emulsification and digestion.

Pancreas. The pancreas is a 20-cm long, slender gland lying behind the stomach and in front of the first and the second lumbar vertebrae. It consists of a head, a body, and a tail. The anterior surface is covered by peritoneum. The pancreas contains lobes and lobules. The pancreatic duct extends along the gland and enters the duodenum through the common bile duct (see Figure 41-4). The pancreas has both exocrine and endocrine functions. The exocrine function of the pancreas contributes to the process of digestion. Exocrine cells in the pancreas secrete pancreatic enzymes (see Table 41-1). The endocrine function occurs in the islets of Langerhans, whose beta cells secrete insulin; alpha cells secrete glucagon; delta cells secrete somatostatin; and F cells secrete pancreatic polypeptide.

AGE-RELATED CONSIDERATIONS: EFFECTS OF AGING ON THE GASTROINTESTINAL SYSTEM

The process of aging causes changes in the functional ability of the GI system, although to a lesser extent than in other organ systems (Table 41-5). Diet, alcohol intake, and obesity affect organs of the GI system, making it challenging to distinguish the effects of aging from lifestyle. Tooth enamel and dentin wear down, making the teeth susceptible to caries. Periodontal disease can lead to the loss of teeth. Xerostomia (decreased saliva production), or "dry mouth," affects many older adults and may be associated with difficulty swallowing (dysphagia). Dysphagia is much more common in this age group because of inadequate chewing or insufficient lubrication. The number of taste buds decreases, the sense of smell diminishes, and salivary secretions lessen, all of which can lead to a decrease in appetite and make eating less pleasurable.

Age-related changes in the esophagus include delayed emptying caused by smooth muscle weakness and an incompetent lower esophageal sphincter (Miller, 2012). Motility of the GI system decreases with age, but secretion and absorption are affected to a lesser extent. Many older adults experience a decrease in HCl secretion (hypochlorhydria), delayed gastric emptying, and constipation. With chronic atrophic gastritis, the number of parietal cells decreases, and the amount of acid and intrinsic factor secreted is subsequently reduced. Intestinal villi are shortened and become more convoluted. Intestinal absorption, motility, and blood flow decrease, thus hampering nutrient absorption.

Liver mass decreases after the age of 40 years, but results of liver function tests remain within normal ranges. Age-related enzyme changes in the liver decrease the liver's ability to metabolize drugs and hormones. Blood flow to the liver decreases, which affects the efficiency of drug metabolism. The size of the pancreas is unaffected by aging, but it does undergo structural changes such as fibrosis, fatty acid deposits, and atrophy. Secretion of digestive enzymes decreases. Aging does not cause changes in the structure and function of the gallbladder and bile ducts, although the incidence of gallstones increases (Heumann, 2011).

Rectal muscle mass is reduced, and the anal sphincter weakens. Changes in the enteric nervous system and a reduction in dietary fibre, along with reduced fluid intake and decreased physical activity, contribute to constipation in older adults.

Older adults, especially those older than 85, are at risk for decreased food intake, as a result of financial, environmental, and social circumstances (Miller, 2012). Financial constraints can affect both the quality and quantity of food available. Age-related changes in the GI system and differences in assessment findings are presented in Table 41-5.

AGE-RELATED DIFFERENCES IN ASSESSMENT

Table 41-5 Gastrointestinal System

POTENTIAL CHANGES	DIFFERENCES IN ASSESSMENT FINDINGS
Mouth	
Periodontal disease	Red, swollen, bleeding gums; painful chewing; loose or sensitive teeth
Loss of teeth	Presence of dentures, difficulty chewing
Decreased sensitivity of taste buds, decreased sense of smell	Diminished sense of taste (especially saltiness and sweetness)
Decreased volume of saliva	Dry oral mucosa
Atrophy of gingival tissue	Poorly fitting dentures
Esophagus	
Decreased tone and motility	Complaints of pyrosis (heartburn), dysphagia, eructation (belching), potential for hiatal hernia and aspiration
Stomach	
Atrophy of gastric mucosa, decreased blood flow	Food intolerances; signs of anemia as result of cobalamin malabsorption; slower gastric emptying
Small Intestine	
Slightly decreased secretion of most digestive enzymes, decreased motility	Complaints of indigestion; slowed intestinal transit; delayed absorption of fat-soluble vitamins
Liver, Gallbladder, Pancreas	
Decreased size and lowered in position	Easier palpation because lower border extends past costal margin
Decreased protein synthesis, decreased ability to regenerate cells	Decreased drug and hormone metabolism
Pancreatic ducts distension, lipase production decreased, pancreatic reserve impaired	Impaired fat absorption, decreased glucose tolerance
Large Intestine, Anus, Rectum	
Decreased anal sphincter tone and nerve supply to rectal area	Increased possibility of fecal incontinence
Decreased muscular tone, decreased motility	Flatulence, abdominal distension, relaxed perineal musculature
Increase in transit time, sensation to defecation decreased	Constipation, fecal impaction

Assessment of the Gastrointestinal System

Subjective Data

Important Health Information

Past Health History. Patients should be asked about changes in weight. Any unexplained or unplanned weight loss or weight gain within the past 12 months should be explored in detail. A history of chronic dieting and repeated weight loss and gain should also be documented. Usual patterns of elimination should be noted.

Information should be gathered about the history or existence of the following problems related to GI functioning: abdominal pain, nausea and vomiting, diarrhea, constipation, abdominal distension, jaundice, anemia, heartburn, dyspepsia, changes in appetite, hematemesis, food intolerance (including

Table 41-6 Potentially Hepatotoxic Drugs	
Dosage-Related	**Idiosyncratic/Rare**
• Acetaminophen	• Amiodarone
• D4T/DDI for HIV	• Alcohol
• Isoniazid (INH)	• Amoxicillin-clavulanic acid
• Methotrexate	• Carbamazepine
	• Ketoconazole
	• NSAIDs
	• Ramipril
	• Statins
	• Sulphonamides
	• Thiazolidinediones

D4T, stavudine; *DDI*, didanosine; *HIV*, human immunodeficiency virus; *NSAIDs*, nonsteroidal anti-inflammatory drugs.

Table 41-7 Surgical Procedures Involving the Gastrointestinal System	
SURGICAL PROCEDURE	**DESCRIPTION**
Antrectomy	Removal of antrum portion of stomach
Appendectomy	Removal of the appendix
Cecostomy	Opening into cecum
Cholecystectomy	Removal of gallbladder
Cholecystostomy	Opening into gallbladder
Choledochojejunostomy	Opening between common bile duct and jejunum
Choledocholithotomy	Opening into common bile duct for removal of stones
Colectomy	Removal of the colon
Colostomy	Opening into colon
Gastrectomy	Removal of stomach
Gastrostomy	Opening into stomach
Glossectomy	Removal of tongue
Hemiglossectomy	Removal of half of tongue
Ileostomy	Opening into ileum
Pyloroplasty	Enlargement and repair of pyloric sphincter area
Vagotomy	Resection of branch of vagus nerve

lactose) or allergies, dysphagia, indigestion, excessive gas, bloating, melena, hemorrhoids, and rectal bleeding. In addition, patients should be asked about the frequency of bowel movements, use of laxative and antacids, and history or existence of diseases such as gastritis, hepatitis, colitis, gallbladder disease, peptic ulcer, cancer, hernias (especially hiatal hernias), or infection with *Clostridium difficile*. (*C. difficile* is discussed in Chapter 45.)

Medications. The health history should include an assessment of the patient's past and current use of medications. The names of all drugs, their frequency of use, and their duration of use are important. This is a critical aspect of history taking because many medications not only may have an effect on the GI system but also may be affected by abnormalities of the GI system and surrounding organs. The medication assessment should include information about the use of over-the-counter (OTC) drugs, prescription drugs, and herbal products and nutritional supplements (see Chapter 12). Many chemicals and drugs are potentially hepatotoxic (Table 41-6) and can result in significant harm to the patient unless their use is monitored closely. For example, chronic high doses of acetaminophen may be hepatotoxic. NSAIDs (including aspirin) may predispose patients to upper GI bleeding if not taken cautiously with food or if a patient has severe liver disease. Antibiotics can cause changes in the normal bacterial composition in the GI tract that result in diarrhea. The nurse should ask patients about laxative or antacid use, including the type and the frequency.

Surgery or Other Treatments. Information should be obtained about hospitalizations for any problems related to the GI system, particularly any abdominal or rectal surgery, including the year, the reason for surgery, the postoperative course, and any blood transfusions. Terms related to surgery of the GI system are listed in Table 41-7.

Objective Data

In addition to collecting subjective data related to the patient's diet history and overall health (Table 41-8), objective data related to a nutritional assessment should be obtained. Examples of objective data include anthropometric measurements (height,

weight, skinfold thickness), results of blood studies such as serum protein, albumin, and hemoglobin levels, as well as a physical examination.

Physical Examination
Mouth

Inspection. The lips should be inspected for symmetry, colour, and size, and for abnormalities such as pallor or cyanosis, cracking, ulcers, or fissures. The dorsum (top) of the tongue should have a thin white coating; the undersurface should be smooth. The nurse should observe for any lesions. Using a tongue blade, the nurse should inspect the buccal mucosa and note the colour, any areas of pigmentation, and any lesions. Dark-skinned individuals normally have patchy areas of pigmentation. When assessing the teeth and gums, the nurse should look for caries; loose teeth; abnormal shape and position of teeth; and swelling, bleeding, discoloration, or inflammation of the gingivae. Any distinctive breath odour should be noted.

The pharynx is inspected by tilting the patient's head back and depressing the tongue with a tongue blade. The tonsils, the uvula, the soft palate, and the anterior and posterior pillars should be observed. The nurse should have the patient say, "Ah." The uvula and the soft palate should rise and remain in the midline.

Palpation. The nurse should palpate any suspect areas in the mouth such as ulcers, nodules, indurations, and areas of tenderness.

In older adults, the mouth must be assessed carefully. Particular attention should be given to the condition of the gums and the tongue, the fit and the condition of dentures (if present), ability to swallow, and the presence of lesions. A patient who has dentures must remove the dentures during an

HEALTH HISTORY

Table 41-8 Gastrointestinal System: Questions for Obtaining Subjective Data

Appetite

- Any change in appetite?* Are you more or less hungry?
- Any change in weight?* Do your clothes still fit the same as they used to? How much weight have you gained or lost? Over what time frame? Is the change in weight intentional?

Dysphagia

- Any problems swallowing?* How long have you had this problem?

Food Intolerance or Allergies

- Are there any foods you cannot eat?* What happens when you do eat them (e.g., heartburn, gas, bloating, indigestion, allergic reaction)?

Abdominal Pain

- Do you have any abdominal pain?* Please show me where it is.
- Is the pain in one spot, or does it move around?
- How long have you had this pain?
- Does it come and go, or is it constant? Does it get worse before or after meals? When is the pain worst (e.g., position, stress, activity)?
- Can you describe how it feels (e.g., cramping, burning, stabbing, aching)?
- What brings on the pain (e.g., menstruation, stress, overeating, fatigue)?
- Do any other symptoms occur when you have the pain (e.g., nausea and vomiting, gas, rectal bleeding, frequent urination, vaginal or penile discharge)?*
- What works to relieve the pain (e.g., rest, heat, walking, change of position, medication)?*

Nausea and Vomiting

- Any nausea or vomiting?* How much comes up?
- What colour is it? Is it bloody? Is there a particular odour?
- Do you have pain, diarrhea, fever, or chills at the same time as the nausea and vomiting?
- Does anyone else you have been in contact with over the past 24 hours have the same symptoms? Have you eaten any foods in the past 24 hours that you suspect may be the cause?

Bowel Habits

- How often do you have a bowel movement?*
- Any recent changes in colour, consistency, or frequency?
- Any problems with diarrhea or constipation?
- Do you use laxatives or stool softeners? Which ones? How often?

Past History

- Any past problems with your digestive system (e.g., ulcer, gallbladder problems, hepatitis, appendicitis, colitis, hernia)?*
- Any surgical procedures on your abdomen?*
- Do you know the results of any tests that were done relating to your abdomen?*

Medications

- What medications are you currently taking?
- How much alcohol do you drink each day? When was your last alcoholic drink?
- Do you smoke? How many packs a day?

Nutrition Assessment

- Describe your usual daily food and fluid intake.

Source: Based on Jarvis, C., Browne, A. J., MacDonald-Jenkins, J., & Luctkar-Flude, M. (Eds.). (2009). *Physical examination and health assessment* (1st Canadian ed., pp. 560-564). Toronto: W. B. Saunders.
*If yes, describe.

oral examination to allow for adequate visualization and palpation of the area.

Abdomen. Two anatomical systems are used to describe the surface of the abdomen. In one system, the abdomen is divided into four quadrants by a perpendicular line from the sternum to the pubic bone and by a horizontal line across the abdomen at the umbilicus (Figure 41-7, *A*; Table 41-9). In the other system, the abdomen is divided into nine regions (see Figure 41-7, *B*), but only the epigastric, umbilical, and suprapubic or hypogastric regions are commonly addressed.

Good lighting is required for the abdominal examination. The patient should be in the supine position and as relaxed as possible. To help relax the abdominal muscles, the patient should slightly flex the knees, and the head of the bed should be raised slightly. The patient should have an empty bladder. The nurse's hands should be warm when the abdominal examination is performed, to avoid eliciting muscle guarding. The patient should be instructed to breathe slowly through the mouth.

Inspection. The nurse should assess the abdomen for skin changes (colour, texture, scars, striae, dilated veins, rashes, and lesions), umbilicus (location and contour), symmetry, contour (flat, rounded [convex], concave, protuberant, distended), observable masses (hernias or other masses), and movement

(pulsations and peristalsis). A normal aortic pulsation may be visible in the epigastric area. The nurse should look across the abdomen tangentially (across the abdomen in a line) for peristalsis. Peristalsis is not normally visible in an adult but may be visible in a thin person.

Auscultation. During examination of the abdomen, the nurse should auscultate before percussion and palpation because these latter procedures may alter the bowel sounds. Auscultation of the abdomen includes listening for increased or decreased bowel sounds and vascular sounds. The diaphragm of the stethoscope is used to auscultate bowel sounds because they are relatively high pitched. The bell of the stethoscope is used to detect lower pitched sounds. Normal bowel sounds occur 5 to 35 times per minute and sound like high-pitched clicks or gurgles. Warming the stethoscope in the hands before auscultation helps prevent abdominal muscle contraction. The nurse should listen in the epigastrium and in all four quadrants (starting in the lower right quadrant) for bowel sounds for 2 to 5 minutes. A perfectly "silent abdomen" is uncommon (Jarvis, 2012). If the nurse listens for several minutes, he or she frequently finds that the sounds are not absent but hypoactive. If the nurse does not hear bowel sounds, the amount of time listened in each quadrant without hearing bowel sounds should be noted.

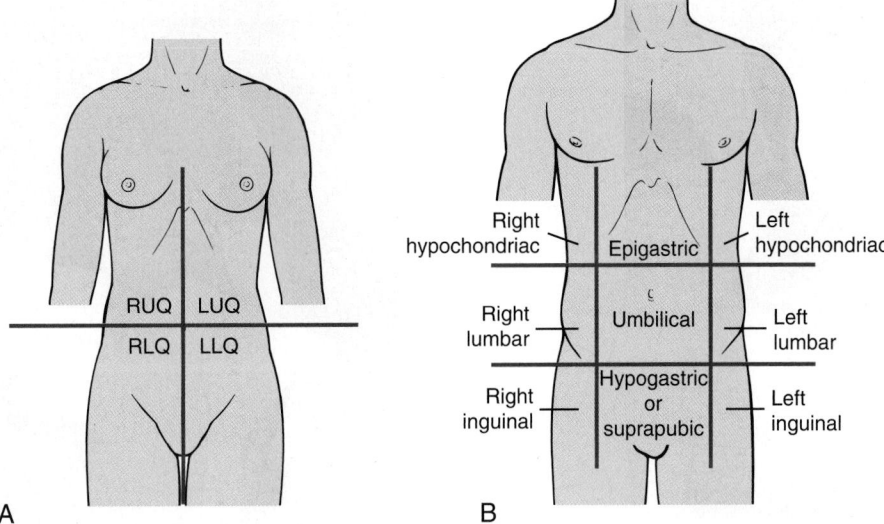

Figure 41-7 A, Abdominal quadrants. **B,** Abdominal regions. *LLQ,* left lower quadrant; *LUQ,* left upper quadrant; *RLQ,* right lower quadrant; *RUQ,* right upper quadrant.

Table 41-9 Abdominal Structures in Regions of Abdomen			
RIGHT UPPER QUADRANT	**LEFT UPPER QUADRANT**	**RIGHT LOWER QUADRANT**	**LEFT LOWER QUADRANT**
• Liver and gallbladder	• Left lobe of liver	• Lower pole of right kidney	• Lower pole of left kidney
• Pylorus	• Spleen	• Cecum and appendix	• Sigmoid flexure
• Duodenum	• Stomach	• Portion of ascending colon	• Portion of descending colon
• Head of pancreas	• Body of pancreas	• Bladder (can only be palpated if distended)	• Bladder (can only be palpated if distended)
• Right adrenal gland	• Left adrenal gland	• Right ovary and salpinx	• Left ovary and salpinx
• Portion of right kidney	• Portion of left kidney	• Uterus (can only be palpated if enlarged)	• Uterus (can only be palpated if enlarged)
• Hepatic flexure of colon	• Splenic flexure of colon	• Right spermatic cord	• Left spermatic cord
• Portion of ascending and transverse colon	• Portion of transverse and descending colon	• Right ureter	• Left ureter

The frequency and intensity of bowel sounds vary, depending on the phase of digestion. Normally, they sound relatively high pitched and gurgling. Loud gurgles indicate hyperperistalsis and are termed *borborygmi* (stomach growling). The bowel sounds are more high pitched (rushes and tinkling) when the intestines are under tension, such as in intestinal obstruction. The nurse should listen for decreased or absent bowel sounds. Terms used to describe bowel sounds include *present, absent, increased, decreased, high-pitched, tinkling, gurgling,* and *rushing.* Normally, no aortic bruits should be heard. A bruit, best heard with the bell of the stethoscope, is a swishing or buzzing sound and indicates turbulent blood flow.

Percussion. The purpose of percussion of the abdomen is to determine the presence of fluid, distension, and masses. Sound waves vary according to the density of underlying tissues. The presence of air produces a higher-pitched, hollow sound, termed *tympany,* and the presence of fluid or masses produces a short, high-pitched sound with little resonance, termed *dullness.* The nurse should lightly percuss all four quadrants of the abdomen and assess the distribution of tympany and dullness. Tympany is the predominant percussion sound of the abdomen.

To percuss the liver, the nurse should start below the umbilicus in the right midclavicular line and percuss lightly upward until dullness is heard, thus determining the lower border of liver dullness. After determining the lower border of the liver, the nurse should start at the nipple line in the right midclavicular line and percuss downward between ribs to the area of dullness, which indicates the upper border of the liver. The height or vertical space between the two areas should be measured to determine the size of the liver. The height of the person correlates directly with the span of the liver. The normal range of liver span is 6 to 12 cm.

Palpation. *Light palpation* is used to detect tenderness or cutaneous hypersensitivity, muscular resistance, masses, and swelling. It also helps patients to relax for deeper palpation. The nurse should keep fingers together and press gently with the pads of the fingertips, depressing the abdominal wall about 1 cm. Smooth movements should be used and all quadrants palpated (Figure 41-8, *A*). *Voluntary guarding* occurs when the person is ticklish, cold, or tense, and it occurs bilaterally. The nurse should help the person to relax because guarding interferes with deep palpation.

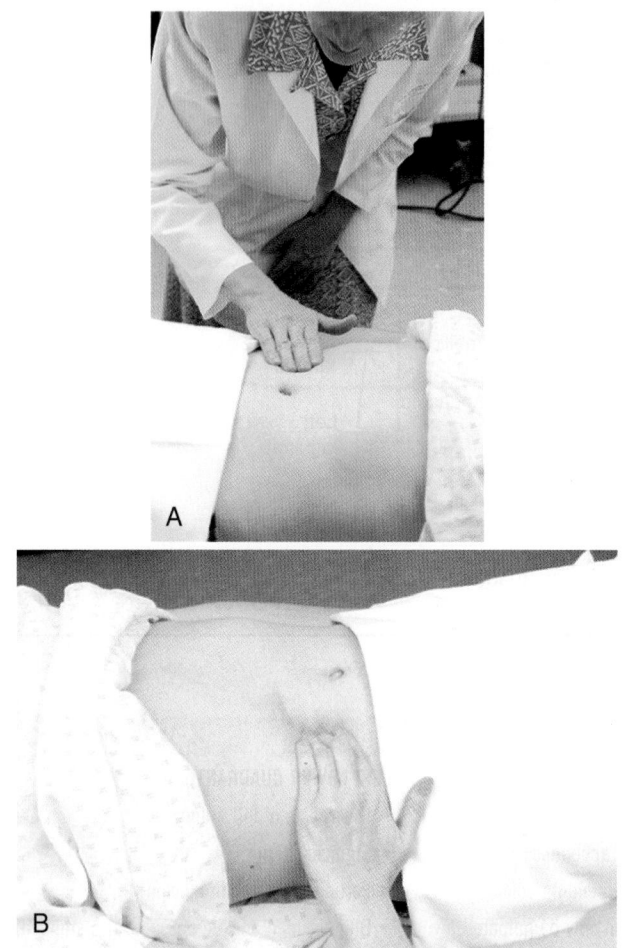

Figure 41-8 Palpation of the abdomen. **A,** Technique for light palpation. **B,** Technique for deep palpation.

Source: Doughty, D. B., & Jackson, D. B. (1993). *Mosby's clinical nursing series: Gastrointestinal disorders.* St. Louis: Mosby.

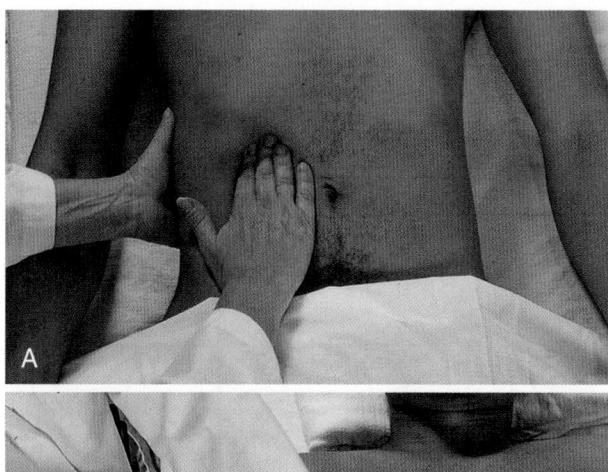

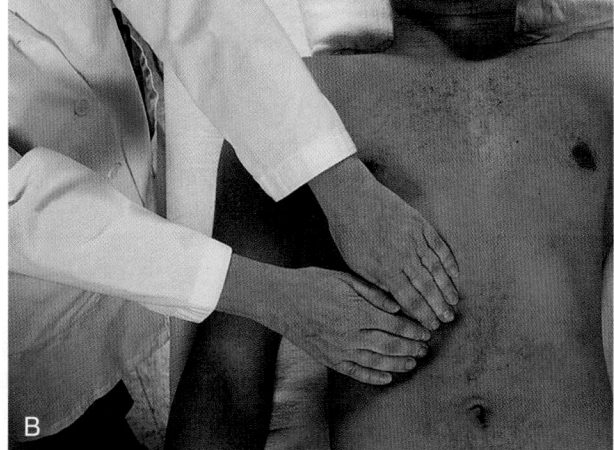

Figure 41-9 Liver palpation **A,** Technique with one hand under the patient. **B,** Alternative technique to palpate liver with fingers hooked over the coastal region.

Source: Jarvis, C. (2008). *Physical examination and health assessment* (5th ed., p. 578, Figures 21-26 and 21-27). St. Louis: Mosby.

Deep palpation is used to delineate abdominal organs and masses (see Figure 41-8, *B*). The palmar surfaces of the fingers should be used to press more deeply. Again, all quadrants should be palpated. When palpating masses, note the location, the size, the shape, and the presence of tenderness. The patient's facial expression should be observed during these manoeuvres because it will provide nonverbal cues of discomfort or pain.

An alternative method for deep abdominal palpation is the two-hand method. One hand is placed on top of the other. The fingers of the top hand apply pressure to the bottom hand. The fingers of the bottom hand feel for organs and masses. This method may be more effective with an obese abdomen. The nurse should practise both methods of deep palpation to determine which one is most effective.

Check any areas of concern for rebound tenderness by pressing in slowly and firmly over the painful site. The palpating fingers are withdrawn quickly. Pain on withdrawal of the fingers indicates peritoneal inflammation. Because assessing for rebound tenderness may produce pain and severe muscle spasm, it should be performed at the end of the examination and only by an experienced practitioner. The iliopsoas muscle test is performed when an acute or perforated appendix is suspected. With the patient in the supine position and the hip flexed, the right leg is

lifted up. As the patient tries to keep the leg up, push the leg down over the lower part of the right thigh. Pain is felt in the right lower quadrant when the iliopsoas muscle is inflamed, which occurs with appendix inflammation or perforation.

To palpate the liver, the nurse's left hand is placed beneath the supine patient to support the right eleventh and twelfth ribs (Figure 41-9). The patient may relax on the nurse's hand. The nurse should press the left hand forward and place the right hand on the patient's right abdomen lateral to the rectus muscle. The fingertips should be below the lower border of liver dullness and pointed toward the right costal margin. The nurse should gently press in and up. The patient should take a deep breath with the abdomen so that the liver drops and is in a better position to be palpated. The nurse should try to feel the liver edge as it comes down to the fingertips. During inspiration, the liver edge should feel firm, sharp, and smooth. The nurse should document the description of the surface, contour, and any tenderness.

To palpate the spleen, the nurse moves to the left side of the patient. The nurse places the right hand under the patient and supports and presses the patient's left lower rib cage forward. The left hand is placed below the left costal margin and presses it in toward the spleen. The nurse should ask the patient to breathe deeply. The nurse's fingertips can feel the tip or edge of an enlarged spleen. The spleen is not normally palpable. If it is palpable, the nurse should not continue because manual compression of an enlarged spleen may cause it to rupture.

Table 41-10 Normal Findings in Physical Assessment of the Gastrointestinal System

Mouth

- Moist, pink lips
- Moist, pink buccal mucosa and gingivae without plaques or lesions
- Teeth in good repair
- Protrusion of tongue in midline without deviation or fasciculations
- Pink uvula in midline, soft palate, tonsils, and posterior pharynx
- Smooth swallowing without coughing or gagging

Abdomen

- Flat without masses or scars
- No abdominal tenderness
- No bruises
- Bowel sounds in all quadrants
- Nonpalpable liver and spleen
- Liver 10 cm in right midclavicular line
- Generalized tympany

Anus

- Absence of lesions, fissures, and hemorrhoids
- Good sphincter tone
- Rectal walls smooth and soft
- No masses
- Stool soft, brown, and heme negative

The standard approach for examining the abdomen can be used on the older adult. Palpation is important because it may reveal a tumour. The abdominal musculature is thinner and more lax, unless the patient is obese, and so the organs may be easier to palpate. If the patient has chronic obstructive pulmonary disease, large lungs, or a low diaphragm, the liver may be palpated 1 to 2 cm below the right costal margin.

Rectum and Anus. The nurse should inspect the perianal and anal area for colour, texture, lumps, rashes, scars, erythema, fissures, and external hemorrhoids. Any lumps or unusual areas should be palpated with a gloved hand.

For the digital examination of the rectum, the gloved, lubricated index finger is placed against the anus while the patient strains (Valsalva manoeuvre). Then, as the sphincter relaxes, the nurse inserts the gloved, lubricated finger. The finger is pointed toward the umbilicus. The nurse should try to get the patient to relax. The finger is inserted into the rectum as far as possible, and all surfaces are palpated. Nodules, tenderness, or any irregularities should be assessed. A sample of stool can be removed with the gloved finger and checked for occult blood. However, a single guaiac-based fecal occult blood test has limited sensitivity in detecting colorectal cancer.

Documentation of a normal physical assessment of the GI system is described in Table 41-10. Age-related differences in the GI system and differences in assessment findings are described in Table 41-5. Common assessment abnormalities are listed in Table 41-11. A focused assessment is used to evaluate the status of previously identified GI problems and to monitor for signs of new problems (see Table 3-6). A focused assessment of the GI system is presented in the Focused Assessment box.

FOCUSED ASSESSMENT
Gastrointestinal (GI) System

Use this checklist to make sure the key assessment steps have been done.

Subjective

Ask the patient about any of the following and note responses.

Loss of appetite	Y	N
Abdominal pain	Y	N
Changes in stools; if so, check colour, consistency, frequency, for presence of blood and so forth	Y	N
Nausea, vomiting	Y	N
Painful swallowing	Y	N

Objective: Diagnostic

Check the following laboratory results for critical values.

Endoscopy: colonoscopy, sigmoidoscopy, esophagogastroduodenoscopy	✓
Radiology: upper GI series, lower GI series	✓
Stool for occult blood or ova and parasites	✓
Liver-function tests	✓

Objective: Physical Examination

Inspect

Skin for colour, lesions, scars, petechiae, and so forth	✓
Abdominal contour for symmetry and distension	✓
Anus and rectum for intact skin, presence or absence of hemorrhoids	✓

Auscultate*

Bowel sounds	✓

Palpate

Abdominal quadrants with light touch	✓
Abdominal quadrants with deep technique	✓

*Note: Perform auscultation before palpation.

Diagnostic Studies of the Gastrointestinal System

Diagnostic studies provide objective data for monitoring the patient's condition and planning appropriate interventions. Table 41-12 lists common diagnostic studies of the GI system. For most diagnostic studies, the nurse should make sure that a signed consent form for the procedure has been completed and is in the patient's health care record. It is the responsibility of the health care provider performing the procedure to explain the procedure and obtain the written consent. However, nurses play an important role in educating patients regarding the procedures. When preparing patients, the nurse must ask about any known allergies to drugs or contrast media.

Many of the diagnostic procedures of the GI system necessitate measures to cleanse the GI tract, as well as the ingestion or injection of a contrast medium or a radiopaque tracer. Often, the patient undergoes a series of GI diagnostic tests. Monitor the patient closely to ensure adequate hydration and nutrition during the testing period. Some diagnostic studies of the GI system are

Text continued on p. 1060

COMMON ASSESSMENT ABNORMALITIES

Table 41-11 Gastrointestinal System

FINDING	DESCRIPTION	POSSIBLE ETIOLOGY AND SIGNIFICANCE
Mouth		
Ulcer, plaque on lips or in mouth	Sore or lesion	Carcinoma, viral infections
Cheilosis	Softening, fissuring, and cracking of lips at angles of mouth	Riboflavin deficiency
Cheilitis	Inflammation of lips (usually lower) with fissuring, scaling, crusting	Often unknown
Geographic tongue	Scattered red, smooth (loss of papillae) areas on dorsum of tongue	Unknown
Smooth tongue	Red, slick appearance	Cobalamin deficiency
Leukoplakia	Thickened white patches	Premalignant lesion
Pyorrhea	Recessed gingivae, purulent pockets	Periodontitis
Herpes simplex	Benign vesicular lesion	Herpesvirus
Candidiasis	White, curdlike lesions surrounded by erythematous mucosa	*Candida albicans*
Glossitis	Reddened, ulcerated, swollen tongue	Exposure to streptococci, irritation, injury, vitamin B deficiencies, anemia
Acute marginal gingivitis	Friable, edematous, painful, bleeding gingivae	Irritation from ill-fitting dentures, calcium deposits on teeth, food impaction
Esophagus and Stomach		
Dysphagia	Difficulty in swallowing, sensation of food sticking in esophagus	Esophageal problems, cancer of esophagus
Hematemesis	Vomiting of blood	Esophageal varices, bleeding peptic ulcer (bleeding in upper GI tract)
Pyrosis	Heartburn, burning in epigastric or substernal area	Hiatal hernia, esophagitis, incompetent lower esophageal sphincter
Dyspepsia	Burning or indigestion	Peptic ulcer, gallbladder disease
Odynophagia	Painful swallowing	Cancer of esophagus, esophagitis
Eructation	Belching	Gallbladder disease
Nausea and vomiting	Feeling of impending vomiting, expulsion of gastric contents through mouth	GI infections, common manifestation of many GI diseases; stress, fear, and pathological conditions
Abdomen		
Distension	Excessive gas accumulation, enlarged abdomen; generalized tympany	Obstruction, paralytic ileus
Ascites	Accumulated fluid within abdominal cavity; eversion of umbilicus (usually)	Peritoneal inflammation, heart failure, metastatic carcinoma, cirrhosis
Bruit	Humming or swishing sound heard through stethoscope over vessel	Partial arterial obstruction (narrowing of vessel), turbulent flow (aneurysm)
Hyperresonance	Loud, tinkling rushes	Intestinal obstruction
Borborygmi	Audible waves of loud, gurgling abdominal sounds produced by hyperactive bowel	Hyperactive intestinal peristalsis; result of eating
Absent bowel sounds	No auscultation of bowel sounds	Peritonitis, paralytic ileus, obstruction
Absence of liver dullness	Tympany on percussion	Air from viscus (e.g., perforated ulcer)
Masses	Lump on palpation	Tumours, cysts
Rebound tenderness	Sudden pain when examiner's fingers are withdrawn quickly (Blumberg's sign)	Peritoneal inflammation, appendicitis
Inspiratory arrest	Sharp pain stops inspiration when the liver is palpated during a deep breath (Murphy's sign)	Cholecystitis
Nodular liver	Enlarged, hard liver with irregular edge or surface	Cirrhosis, carcinoma
Hepatomegaly	Enlargement of liver, liver edge >1-2 cm below costal margin	Metastatic carcinoma, hepatitis, venous congestion

COMMON ASSESSMENT ABNORMALITIES

Table 41-11 Gastrointestinal System—cont'd

FINDING	DESCRIPTION	POSSIBLE ETIOLOGY AND SIGNIFICANCE
Splenomegaly	Enlargement of spleen	Chronic leukemia, hemolytic states, portal hypertension, some infections
Hernia	Bulge or nodule in abdomen, usually appearing on straining	Inguinal (in inguinal canal), femoral (in femoral canal), umbilical (herniation of umbilicus), or incisional (defect in muscles after surgery)
Rectum and Anus		
Hemorrhoids	Thrombosed veins in rectum and anus (internal or external)	Portal hypertension, chronic constipation, prolonged sitting or standing, pregnancy
Mass	Firm, nodular edge	Tumour, carcinoma
Pilonidal cyst	Opening of sinus tract, cyst in midline just above coccyx	Probably congenital
Fissure	Ulceration in anal canal	Straining, irritation
Melena	Abnormal, black, tarry stool containing digested blood	Cancer, bleeding in upper GI tract from ulcers, varices
Tenesmus	Spasmodic contraction of the anal sphincter with pain and persistent desire to empty the bowel; painful and ineffective straining at stool	Ulcerative colitis, diarrhea secondary to GI infection such as food poisoning
Steatorrhea	Passage of large amounts of fat as a fatty, frothy, foul-smelling stool	Chronic pancreatitis, biliary obstruction, malabsorption problems (result of failure to digest and absorb fat)

GI, gastrointestinal.

DIAGNOSTIC STUDIES

Table 41-12 Gastrointestinal (GI) System

STUDY	DESCRIPTION AND PURPOSE	NURSING RESPONSIBILITY
Radiology		
Upper GI series or barium swallow study	Fluoroscopic radiographic study using contrast medium. Used to diagnose structural abnormalities of the esophagus, the stomach, and the duodenal bulb	Explain procedure to patient, including the need to drink contrast medium and to assume various positions on x-ray examination table. Keep patient NPO for 8-12 hr before procedure. Instruct patient to avoid smoking after midnight the night before the study. After radiograph, take measures to prevent contrast medium impaction (fluids, laxatives). Warn patient that stool may be white up to 72 hr after test.
Small bowel series	Fluoroscopic radiographic study using contrast medium. Images are obtained q30 min until medium reaches terminal ileum	Same as for upper GI series.
Lower GI series or barium enema study	Fluoroscopic radiographic examination of colon using contrast medium, which is administered rectally (enema). Double-contrast or air-contrast barium enema is test of choice. Air is infused after thick barium flows through transverse colon. Endoscopic procedures have made necessity for this test less common than in the past	The evening before the procedure, administer purgatives, laxatives, enemas, or a combination of these until colon is clear of stool. The patient is put on a clear liquid diet the evening before procedure. Keep patient NPO for 8 hr before test. Instruct patient about being given barium by enema. Explain that cramping and urge to defecate may occur during procedure and that patient may be placed in various positions on tilt table. After the procedure, administer fluids, laxatives, or suppositories to assist in expelling barium. Observe stool for passage of contrast medium.

GI, gasrointestinal; *NPO,* nothing by mouth.

Continued

DIAGNOSTIC STUDIES

Table 41-12 Gastrointestinal (GI) System—cont'd

STUDY	DESCRIPTION AND PURPOSE	NURSING RESPONSIBILITY
Cholangiography		
• Percutaneous transhepatic cholangiography (PTC)	Fluoroscopic radiographic study used to determine filling of hepatic and biliary ducts	Observe patient for signs of hemorrhage, bile leakage, and infection.
	After local anaesthesia is induced and with monitored anaesthesia care (formerly called *conscious sedation*), liver is entered with long needle (under fluoroscopy), bile duct is entered, bile withdrawn, and radiopaque contrast medium injected	Assess patient's medication for possible contraindications, precautions, or complications with use of contrast medium.
	IV antibiotics are administered prophylactically	
• Surgical cholangiography	Study performed during surgery on biliary structures, such as gallbladder	Explain to patient that anaesthetic and contrast medium will be used.
	Contrast medium is injected into common bile duct	Assess patient's medications for possible contraindications, precautions, or complications with the use of contrast medium.
• Magnetic resonance cholangiopancreatography (MRCP)	MRI technology used to obtain images of biliary and pancreatic ducts	Explain procedure to patient.
		Contraindicated in patient with metal implants (e.g., pacemaker) or who is pregnant.
Ultrasonography	Nonradiographic study used to show the size and configuration of organs	
	Noninvasive procedure in which high-frequency sound waves (ultrasound waves) are passed into body structures and recorded as they are reflected (bounded)	
• Abdominal ultrasonography	Ultrasound study used to detect abdominal masses (tumours and cysts), biliary and liver disease, gallstones (see Figure 41-10)	Keep patient NPO for 8-12 hr before procedure.
		Air or gas can reduce quality of images.
	A conductive gel (lubricant jelly) is applied to the skin and a transducer is placed on the area	Food intake can cause gallbladder contraction, resulting in suboptimal study results.
• Endoscopic ultrasonography (EUS)	Ultrasound study using a small transducer installed on tip of endoscope	Same as upper GI endoscopy.
	Because EUS transducer gets close to the organs being examined, images obtained are often more accurate and detailed than images provided by traditional ultrasonography	
	Detects and helps stage esophageal, gastric, rectal, biliary, and pancreatic tumours and abnormalities	
	Also used to guide fine-needle aspiration to diagnose cancer or dysplasia	
Nuclear imaging scans (scintigraphy)	Radionuclide studies used to show size, shape, and position of organ	Tell patient that substance to be ingested contains only traces of radioactivity and poses little to no danger.
	Functional disorders and structural defects may be identified	Schedule no more than one radionuclide test per day.
	Radionuclide (radioactive isotope) is injected IV, and a counter (scanning) device picks up radioactive emission, which is recorded on paper	Explain to patient the need to lie flat during the scan.
	Only tracer doses of radioactive isotopes are used	
• Gastric emptying studies	Radionuclide studies used to assess ability of stomach to empty solids or liquids in patients with emptying disorders resulting from peptic ulcer, ulcer surgery, diabetes, gastric malignancies, or functional disorders	Same as for nuclear imaging scans.
	• Solid-emptying study: cooked egg white containing ^{99m}Tc is eaten	
	• Liquid-emptying study: orange juice with ^{99m}Tc is swallowed	
	Sequential images from gamma camera are recorded q2min for up to 60 min	

DIAGNOSTIC STUDIES

Table 41-12 Gastrointestinal (GI) System—cont'd

STUDY	DESCRIPTION AND PURPOSE	NURSING RESPONSIBILITY
• Hepatobiliary scintigraphy (HIDA)	Radionuclide study used to identify obstructions of bile ducts (e.g., gallstones, tumours), diseases of gallbladder, and bile leaks Patient is given ^{99m}Tc IV and positioned under camera to record distribution of tracer in the liver, biliary tree, gallbladder, and proximal small bowel	Same as for nuclear imaging scans.
• Scintigraphy of GI bleeding	Radionuclide study used to reveal exact site of active GI blood loss Patient is given ^{99m}Tc-labelled sulphur colloid or patient's own red blood cells (RBCs) labelled with ^{99m}Tc, and images of the abdomen are obtained at intermittent intervals	Same as for nuclear imaging scans.
Computed tomography (CT)	Noninvasive radiological examination allows exposures at different depths Used to detect biliary tract, liver, and pancreatic disorders Use of oral and IV contrast media accentuates density differences	Explain procedures to patient. Determine sensitivity to iodine if contrast material is used.
Magnetic resonance imaging (MRI)	Noninvasive procedure using radiofrequency waves and a magnetic field Used to detect hepatobiliary disease, hepatic lesions, and sources of GI bleeding and to stage colorectal cancer IV contrast medium (gadolinium) may be used	Explain procedure to patient. Contraindicated in patients with metal implants (e.g., pacemaker) or who are pregnant.
Virtual colonoscopy	Combines CT scanning or MRI with computer virtual reality software to detect colon and bowel diseases, including polyps, colorectal cancer, diverticulosis, and lower GI bleeding Air is introduced via a tube placed in rectum to enlarge colon to enhance visualization Images obtained while patient is on back and stomach Computer combines images to form two- and three-dimensional images, which are viewed on monitor	Bowel preparation similar to that for colonoscopy (see below under "Endoscopy"). Unlike conventional colonoscopy, virtual colonoscopy necessitates no sedatives and no endoscope. Procedure takes about 15-20 min.
Endoscopy		
Esophagogastroduodenoscopy (EGD)	Enables direct visualization of mucosal lining of esophagus, stomach, and duodenum with flexible endoscope Video imaging may be used to visualize stomach motility Inflammations, ulcerations, tumours, varices, or Mallory-Weiss tear may be detected Biopsy samples may be obtained, and varices can be treated with band ligation or sclerotherapy	Before the procedure: Keep patient on NPO status for 8 hr. Make sure signed consent is obtained. Give preoperative medication if ordered. Explain to patient that local anaesthetic may be sprayed on throat before insertion of endoscope and that patient will be sedated during the procedure. After the procedure: Keep patient NPO until gag reflex returns (usually 2-4 hr). Gently tickle back of patient's throat to determine return of reflex. Instruct patient to use warm saline gargles for relief of sore throat. Check temperature q15-30min for 1-2 hr (sudden temperature spike is sign of perforation).

IV, intravenously; *NPO,* nothing by mouth; *RBCs,* red blood cells; *^{99m}Tc,* technetium-99m; *WBCs,* white blood cells. *Continued*

DIAGNOSTIC STUDIES

Table 41-12 Gastrointestinal (GI) System—cont'd

STUDY	DESCRIPTION AND PURPOSE	NURSING RESPONSIBILITY
Colonoscopy	Enables direct visualization of entire colon up to ileocecal valve with flexible fibreoptic endoscope Patient's position is changed frequently during procedure to assist with advancement of endoscope to cecum Used to detect/diagnose inflammatory bowel disease, polyps, tumours, and diverticulosis and to dilate strictures Procedure allows for removal of colonic polyps without laparotomy	Before the procedure: Bowel preparation is completed. Procedure varies with physician preference. For example, patient may be kept on clear fluids 1-2 days before procedure and cathartic, or enema, or both administered the night before. An alternative is to give 4.5 L (1 gal) of polyethylene glycol (GoLYTELY, Colyte) the evening before (8-oz glass q10min). Purgatives such as Pico-Salax may be administered. Explain to patient that a flexible endoscope will be inserted while patient is in side-lying position and that sedative will be given. After procedure: Be aware that patient may experience abdominal cramps caused by stimulation of peristalsis because bowel is constantly inflated with air during procedure. Observe for rectal bleeding and signs of perforation (e.g. malaise, abdominal distension, tenesmus). Check vital signs.
Capsule endoscopy	Study most commonly used to visualize small intestine and diagnose diseases such as Crohn's disease, small bowel tumours, celiac disease, and malabsorption syndrome and to identify sources of possible GI bleeding in areas not accessible by upper endoscopy or colonoscopy Patient swallows a capsule (approximately the size of a large vitamin) with a camera that provides endoscopic observation of GI tract (see Figure 41-12); camera takes >50,000 images during 8-hr examination Capsule relays images to monitoring device that patient wears on belt After examination, images are downloaded to a workstation Not used in patients with suspected intestinal strictures	Dietary preparation: similar to that for colonoscopy. The video capsule is swallowed, and patient is usually kept NPO until 4-6 hr later. Procedure is comfortable for most patients. Eight hours after swallowing the capsule, the patient returns to have the monitoring device removed. Peristalsis causes passage of the disposable capsule with a bowel movement.
Sigmoidoscopy	Enables direct visualization of rectum and sigmoid colon with lighted flexible endoscope Sometimes special table is used to tilt patient into knee-chest position Used to detect tumours, polyps, inflammatory and infectious diseases, fissures, hemorrhoids	Administer enemas evening before and morning of procedure. Make sure signed consent is obtained. Patient may have clear liquids day before or no dietary restrictions may be necessary. Explain to patient knee-chest position (unless patient is older or very ill), need to take deep breaths during insertion of scope, and possible urge to defecate as scope is passed. Encourage patient to relax and let abdomen go limp. Observe for rectal bleeding after polypectomy or biopsy.

IV, intravenously; *NPO,* nothing by mouth; *RBCs,* red blood cells; *^{99m}Tc,* technetium-99m; *WBCs,* white blood cells.

DIAGNOSTIC STUDIES

Table 41-12 Gastrointestinal (GI) System—cont'd

STUDY	DESCRIPTION AND PURPOSE	NURSING RESPONSIBILITY
Endoscopic retrograde cholangiopancreatography (ERCP)	Endoscopic technique enables direct visualization of structures Fiberoptic endoscope (using fluoroscopy) is inserted through the oral cavity into descending duodenum, and then common bile and pancreatic ducts are cannulated Contrast medium is then injected into ducts Technique can also be used to retrieve a gallstone from distal common bile duct, dilate strictures, obtain biopsy of tumours, or diagnose pseudocysts	Before the procedure, explain procedure to patient, including patient's role. Keep patient NPO for 8 hr before procedure. Make sure signed consent is obtained. Administer sedative immediately before and during procedure. Administer antibiotics if ordered. After the procedure, check vital signs. Check for signs of perforation or infection. Be aware that ERCP-induced pancreatitis is most common complication. This complication manifests as abdominal pain, nausea, and vomiting. Check for return of gag reflex.
Endoscopic ultrasonography	Combined use of endoscopy and ultrasonography with the use of an ultrasound transducer attached to an endoscope Enables visualization of esophagus, stomach, intestine, liver, pancreas and gallstones	Similar to that for upper GI endoscopy.
Laparoscopy (peritoneoscopy)	Enables visualization of peritoneal cavity and contents with laparoscope Biopsy specimen may be obtained Performed with patient under general anaesthesia in operating room Double-puncture peritoneoscopy enables better visualization of abdominal cavity, especially liver Can eliminate need for exploratory laparotomy in many patients	Keep patient on NPO status for 8 hr before study. Make sure signed consent is obtained. Administer preoperative sedative. Ensure that bladder and bowel are emptied. Inform patient that local anaesthetic is used before laparoscope insertion. Observe for possible complications of bleeding and bowel perforation after the procedure.
Blood Studies		
Amylase	Measures secretion of amylase by pancreas Is important in diagnosing acute pancreatitis Level peaks in 24 hr and then drops to normal in 48-72 hr Depending on method, reference range is 20-110 U/L	Obtain blood sample in acute attack of pancreatitis. Explain procedure to patient.
Lipase	Measures secretion of lipase by pancreas. Level stays elevated longer than that of serum amylase Reference range is <160 U/L	Explain procedure to patient.
Gastrin	Measures secretion of gastrin by the cells of the antrum of the stomach and by the pancreatic islets of Langerhans Reference interval: 25-100 pg/mL during fasting	Explain procedure to patient.
Liver biopsy	Percutaneous procedure uses needle inserted between sixth and seventh or between eighth and ninth intercostal spaces on the right side to obtain specimen of hepatic tissue Often performed under ultrasound or CT guidance	Before procedure, check patient's coagulation status (prothrombin time, clotting or bleeding time). Ensure that patient's blood is typed and crossmatched. Measure vital signs as baseline data. Explain holding of breath after expiration when needle is inserted. Make sure signed consent is obtained. After procedure, check vital signs to detect internal bleeding q15min × 2, q30min × 4, q1h × 4. Keep patient lying on right side for a minimum of 2 hr to splint puncture site. Keep patient in bed in flat position for 12-14 hr. Assess patient for complications such as bile peritonitis, shock, pneumothorax.

Continued

DIAGNOSTIC STUDIES

Table 41-12 Gastrointestinal (GI) System—cont'd		
STUDY	**DESCRIPTION AND PURPOSE**	**NURSING RESPONSIBILITY**
Miscellaneous Tests		
Fecal analysis	Form, consistency, and colour of fecal sample are noted	Observe patient's stools.
	Specimen examined for mucus, blood, pus, parasites, and fat content	Collect stool specimens.
		Check stools for blood.
	Tests for occult blood (guaiac test, Hemoccult, Hemoccult II, Hemoccult-SENSA, Hematest) are performed	Keep diet free of red meat for 24-48 hr before occult blood test.
	Single DNA test (Pre-Gen-Plus) is a panel of DNA markers used to detect and monitor colorectal cancer	
Stool culture	Tests for presence of bacteria, including *Clostridium difficile*	Collect stool specimen.

IV, intravenously; *NPO,* nothing by mouth; *RBCs,* red blood cells; *⁹⁹ᵐTc,* technetium-99m; *WBCs,* white blood cells.

especially difficult and uncomfortable for older adults. It may be necessary to individualize and make adjustments. Many radiological studies use either barium sulphate or diatrizoate meglumine and diatrizoate sodium (Gastrografin) as a contrast medium. Barium sulphate is more effective for visualizing mucosal detail. Gastrografin is water soluble and rapidly absorbed, so it is preferred when a perforation is suspected. If barium escapes into the peritoneal cavity, it can cause peritonitis. However, if the patient is at high risk for aspiration, use of water-soluble media is contraindicated and barium is preferred.

Radiological Studies

Upper Gastrointestinal Series. An upper GI series with small bowel follow-through enables visualization of the esophagus, the stomach, and the small intestine by means of fluoroscopy and radiographic examination. A barium swallow study is used to identify esophageal, stomach, and small intestine disorders such as esophageal strictures, varices, polyps, tumours, hiatal hernia, foreign bodies, and peptic ulcers in the stomach or duodenum. The barium swallow study begins with the patient swallowing a thick barium solution (contrast medium). The patient then assumes different positions on the x-ray examination table. The movement of the contrast medium through the upper GI tract is observed with fluoroscopy, and several radiographic images are obtained (see Table 41-12).

Lower Gastrointestinal Series. The purpose of a lower GI series (barium enema radiograph) is to observe by means of fluoroscopy the filling of the colon with contrast medium and to observe by radiograph the filled colon. This procedure helps identify polyps, tumours, and other lesions in the colon. The patient is administered an enema of contrast medium. The air-contrast barium enema provides better visualization of inflammatory bowel disease, polyps, tumours, and gallstones (Figure 41-10). Because the patient must retain the barium, this study is not tolerated well by older or immobile patients.

Abdominal Ultrasonography. Ultrasonography is a noninvasive, nonradiographic approach used to show the size and the configuration of organs. It is the diagnostic procedure of choice for detecting cholelithiasis (gallstones). Ultrasonography is also used for detecting appendicitis, acute cholecystitis, and other changes in abdominal organs (see Table 41-11).

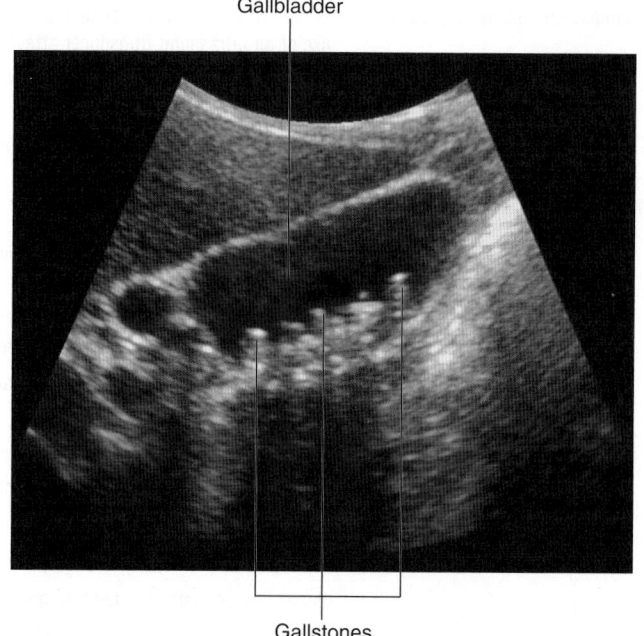

Figure 41-10 Ultrasound image of gallbladder, showing multiple gallstones.

Source: Drake, R. L., Vogl, W., & Mitchell, A. W. M. (2010). *Gray's anatomy for students* (2nd ed., p. 326, Figure 4.108). Edinburgh: Churchill Livingstone.

Endoscopy

Endoscopy is the direct visualization of a body structure through a lighted fibreoptic instrument (endoscope). The GI structures that can be examined through endoscopy include the esophagus, the stomach, the duodenum, the colon, and, with the aid of fluoroscopy and radiographs, the pancreas and the biliary tree. The pancreatic, hepatic, and common bile ducts can be visualized with side-viewing flexible endoscopes. This procedure is called *endoscopic retrograde cholangiopancreatography* (ERCP) and is illustrated in Figure 41-11.

The endoscope is an instrument channel through which biopsy forceps and cytology brushes may be passed. Cameras may be attached to take video recordings and still pictures. Endoscopy of the GI tract is often performed in combination with biopsy and cytological studies. The major complication of GI

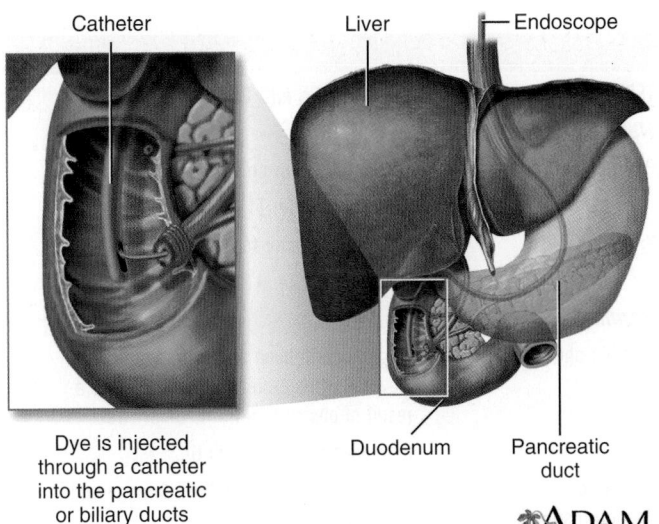

Figure 41-11 Endoscopic retrograde cholangiopancreatography.

Source: A.D.A.M. Inc., *http://www.adam.com.*

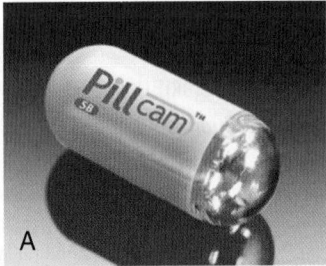

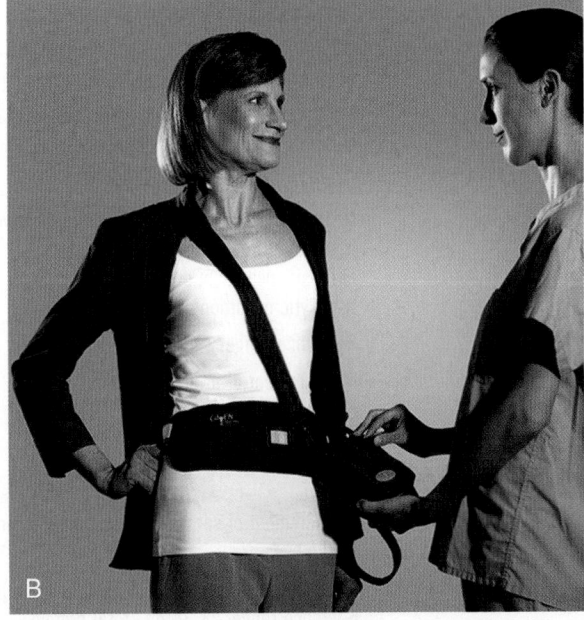

Figure 41-12 Capsule endoscopy. **A,** The video capsule has its own camera and light source. After it is swallowed, it travels through the GI tract and enables visualization of the small intestine. It sends messages to a monitoring device that is worn by the patient on a waist belt **(B).** During the 8-hour examination, the patient is free to move about. After the test, the images are viewed on a video monitor.

Source: Given Imaging, Inc., Norcross, Georgia.

endoscopy is perforation through the structure being viewed. The incidence of this complication is decreased with the use of the flexible fibreoptic endoscopes.

For all endoscopic procedures, informed written consent is required. Specific endoscopy procedures are discussed in Table 41-11. In addition to diagnostic procedures, many invasive and therapeutic procedures may be performed with endoscopes. These include procedures such as polypectomy, sclerosis of varices, laser treatment, cauterization of bleeding sites, papillotomy, removal of stones in the common bile duct, and balloon dilations. For many endoscopic procedures, patients require intravenous short-acting sedatives.

Endoscopic Ultrasonography. Endoscopic ultrasound (EUS) is a relatively new endoscopic technique that provides highly accurate images of the esophagus, GI tract, pancreas, and liver. EUS provides high-resolution imaging of the GI tract because of its unique ability to differentiate the histological layers of the GI tract wall. It is most often used for preoperative staging of esophageal, gastric, pancreatic, and colorectal cancers. It can also be used to detect gallstones.

Capsule Endoscopy. In capsule endoscopy, the patient swallows a capsule containing a disposable video camera (Figure 41-12). As the video camera passes through the intestine, images are transmitted by radiofrequency. This procedure is particularly useful in visualization of the portion of the small bowel that is not within reach of standard upper and lower endoscopy. It allows more access to the small bowel for patients with an obscure source of GI bleeding. This technology may be particularly helpful in discovering the cause of GI bleeding when results of standard upper endoscopy and colonoscopy are normal.

Liver Biopsy

A liver biopsy is performed when hepatic tissue is needed to establish a diagnosis such as fibrosis, cirrhosis, hepatitis, and

neoplasms. It may also be used for monitoring the progress of liver disease.

Liver biopsy may be performed as an open or closed procedure. The *open method* involves making an incision and removing a wedge of tissue. It is performed in the operating room, often concurrently with another surgical procedure, with the patient under general anaesthesia. The *closed,* or *needle, biopsy* is a percutaneous procedure in which the site is infiltrated with a local anaesthetic and a needle is inserted between the sixth and seventh or between the eighth and ninth intercostal spaces on the right side. The patient lies supine with the right arm over the head. The patient should be instructed to exhale fully and not breathe while the needle is inserted (see Table 41-11). It is important to perform a nursing assessment before and after a liver biopsy.

Liver Function Studies

Liver function tests are usually described separately from other GI diagnostic studies. Liver function tests are laboratory (blood) studies that reflect hepatic disease. Table 41-13 lists some common liver function tests.

DIAGNOSTIC STUDIES

Table 41-13 Liver Function Tests

TEST	DESCRIPTION AND PURPOSE	TEST	DESCRIPTION AND PURPOSE
Bile Formation and Excretion		**Hemostatic Functions**	
Serum bilirubin	Measurement of ability of liver to conjugate and excrete bilirubin; enables differentiation between unconjugated (indirect) and conjugated (direct) bilirubin in plasma	Prothrombin	Determination of prothrombin activity Reference range: 11-12.5 sec
		Vitamin K	Essential cofactor for many clotting factors Reference range: 0.22-4.88 nmol/L
• Total	Measurement of direct and indirect total bilirubin Reference range: 5.1-17 mcmol/L	**Serum Enzyme Tests**	
• Direct	Measurement of conjugated bilirubin; level is elevated in obstructive jaundice Reference range: 1.7-5.1 mcmol/L	Alkaline phosphatase (ALP)	Origination in bone and liver; serum level elevated when excretion is impaired as a result of obstruction in the biliary tract Reference range: 35-120 U/L
• Indirect	Measurement of unconjugated bilirubin; level is elevated in hepatocellular (hepatitis, cirrhosis, neoplasm or hepatic congestion) and hemolytic conditions Reference range: 3.4-12 mcmol/L	Aspartate aminotransferase (AST)	Serum level elevated in liver damage and inflammation Reference range: 0-35 U/L Women's values are slightly lower than men's
Urinary bilirubin	Measurement of urinary excretion of conjugated bilirubin Normal finding: 0 (negative)	Alanine aminotransferase (ALT)	Serum level elevated in liver damage and inflammation Reference range: 4-36 U/L
Protein Metabolism		γ-Glutamyl transpeptidase (GGT)	Present in biliary tract (not in skeletal muscle or cardiac tissue); serum level elevated in hepatitis and alcoholic liver disease; more sensitive for detecting biliary obstruction, cholangitis, or cholecystitis than ALP Reference ranges: 4-36 U/L
Serum protein levels	Measurement of serum proteins manufactured by the liver Albumin reference range: 35-50 g/L; globulin reference range: 23-34 g/L; total protein reference range: 64-83 g/L Normal A/G ratio: 1.5:1-2.5:1	**Lipid Metabolism**	
α-Fetoprotein	Tumour marker, especially for hepatic cancer Reference range: <40 mcg/L	Serum cholesterol	Synthesis and excretion by liver; serum level elevated in biliary obstruction, lowered in extensive liver disease and malnutrition Reference range: <5.2 mmol/L, age dependent LDL reference range: <3.37 mmol/L HDL reference ranges: LDL reference range: <2.59 mmol/L (optimal) HDL reference range: <1.036 mmol/L (low risk)
Ammonia	Conversion of ammonia to urea normally occurs in the liver; elevated ammonia level can result in hepatic encephalopathy secondary to liver cirrhosis Reference range: 6-47 mcmol/L		

HDL, high-density lipoprotein; *LDL*, low-density lipoprotein.

evolve *An assessment case study of the GI system is available at* **http://evolve.elsevier.com/Canada/Lewis/medsurg**

REVIEW QUESTIONS

The number of the question corresponds to the same-numbered objective at the beginning of the chapter.

1. A patient is admitted to the hospital with a diagnosis of diarrhea with dehydration. The nurse recognizes that increased peristalsis resulting in diarrhea can be related to which of the following mechanisms?
   a. Sympathetic inhibition
   b. Mixing and propulsion
   c. Sympathetic stimulation
   d. Parasympathetic stimulation

2. A patient has an elevated blood level of indirect (unconjugated) bilirubin. Which of the following might cause this finding?
   a. The gallbladder is unable to contract to release stored bile.
   b. Bilirubin is not being conjugated and excreted into the bile by the liver.
   c. The Kupffer cells in the liver are unable to remove bilirubin from the blood.
   d. There is an obstruction in the biliary tract preventing flow of bile into the small intestine.

3. Which of the following normally protects the bowel from the acidity of gastric contents as they move into the small intestine?
   a. Inhibition of secretin release
   b. Release of bicarbonate by the pancreas
   c. Release of pancreatic digestive enzymes
   d. Release of gastrin by the duodenal mucosa

4. An 80-year-old man states that although he adds a lot of salt to his food, it still does not have much flavour. Which of the following factors related to aging would account for this finding?
   a. Some disorder; he should not experience changes in the ability to taste
   b. Loss of taste buds, especially for sweetness and saltiness
   c. Some loss of taste sensation but no difficulty chewing food
   d. Loss of the sense of taste because the ability to smell is decreased

5. Which of the following questions is appropriate to initiate a GI assessment?
   a. "What is your usual bowel elimination pattern?"
   b. "What percentage of your income is spent on food?"
   c. "Have you travelled to a foreign country in the past year?"
   d. "Does stress give you diarrhea?"

6. Which of the following is appropriate for the nurse to undertake during an examination of the abdomen?
   a. Position the patient in the supine position with the bed flat and knees straight.
   b. Listen in the epigastrium and all four quadrants for 2 to 5 minutes for bowel sounds.
   c. Use the following order of techniques: inspection, palpation, percussion, auscultation.
   d. Describe bowel sounds as absent if no sound is heard in the lower right quadrant after 2 minutes.

7. Which of the following findings would be considered a normal physical assessment finding of the GI system? (More than one may be correct.)
   a. Nonpalpable liver and spleen
   b. Borborygmi in upper right quadrant
   c. Tympany on percussion of the abdomen
   d. Liver edge 2 to 4 cm below the costal margin
   e. Finding of a firm, nodular edge on the rectal examination

8. Which of the following is correct in preparing a patient for a colonoscopy?
   a. A signed consent form is not necessary.
   b. Sedation may be used during the procedure.
   c. Only one cleansing enema is necessary for preparation.
   d. A light meal should be eaten the day before the procedure.

ANSWERS: 1. d; 2. b; 3. b; 4. b; 5. a; 6. b; 7. a and c; 8. b.

REFERENCES

Heumann, D. M. (2011). *Cholelithiasis*. Retrieved from *http://emedicine.medscape.com/article/175667-overview*

Jarvis, C. (2012). *Physical examination and health assessment*. St. Louis: Elsevier Saunders.

Miller, C. A. (2012). Nursing for wellness in older adults (5th ed.). Philadelphia: Wolters Kluwer Health Lippincott, Williams & Wilkins.

RESOURCES

Resources for this chapter are listed in Chapter 42 on p. 1089, Chapter 44 on p. 1160, Chapter 45 on p. 1215, and Chapter 46 on p. 1263.

Nursing Management: Nutritional Problems

Written by Rose Ann DiMaria-Ghalili and Peggi Guenter
Adapted by Ellen Vogel, Christina Vaillancourt, Christine McCleary, and Andrea Miller

LEARNING OBJECTIVES

1. Relate the essential components of a nutritionally good diet to health.
2. Describe the common etiologic factors, clinical manifestations, and management of malnutrition.
3. Explain the indications, complications, and nursing management related to the use of enteral nutrition.
4. Describe the types of feeding tubes and related nursing management.
5. Explain the indications, complications, and nursing management related to the use of parenteral nutrition.
6. Compare the etiological factors, clinical manifestations, and nursing management of eating disorders.

KEY TERMS

anorexia nervosa A potentially life-threatening eating disorder characterized by self-imposed weight loss, endocrine dysfunction, and a distorted psychopathological attitude toward weight and eating, p. 1070

bulimia nervosa An eating disorder characterized by frequent binge eating, self-induced vomiting associated with loss of control over eating, and a persistent concern with body image, p. 1070

enteral nutrition (EN) Nutrition (e.g., a nutritionally balanced liquefied food or formula) provided through the gastrointestinal tract via a tube, catheter, or stoma that delivers nutrients distal to the oral cavity, p. 1076

food security Physical and economic access to sufficient, safe, and nutritious food that meets the food preferences and dietary needs for an active and healthy life, p. 1069

malabsorption syndrome A complex of symptoms defined as the impaired absorption of nutrients from the gastrointestinal tract and characterized by anorexia, weight loss, abdominal bloating, muscle cramps, bone pain, and steatorrhea; may result from decreased amounts of necessary enzymes or a reduced bowel surface area, p. 1070

malnutrition An excess, deficit, or imbalance in the essential components of a balanced diet, p. 1068

nutrition The process by which the body uses food for energy, growth, maintenance, and repair of body tissues, p. 1065

optimal nutritional status Achieved when nutrients are consumed in amounts that support daily requirements and metabolic demands resulting in overall good health, p. 1065

overnutrition Results from the consumption of nutrients—most frequently, calories, sodium, and fat—in excess of requirements, p. 1065

parenteral nutrition (PN) The administration of nutrients by a route other than the gastrointestinal tract (e.g., the bloodstream), p. 1082

protein–calorie malnutrition (PCM) The most common form of undernutrition, p. 1068

total parenteral nutrition (TPN) The delivery of a nutritionally adequate hypertonic solution consisting of glucose, protein hydrolysates, minerals, and vitamins, using an intravenous route, p. 1082

undernutrition Occurs when nutritional reserves become depleted or when nutrient intake is inadequate to meet daily requirements or metabolic demands p. 1065

ELECTRONIC RESOURCES

Supplemental content related to Chapter 42 can be found...

Evolve Web Site ⊖volve

http://evolve.elsevier.com/Canada/Lewis/medsurg
- Answer Guidelines for Case Study on p. 1087
- Clinical Reference: Laboratory Values
- Content Updates
- Customizable Nursing Care Plans:
  - Enteral Nutrition
  - Parenteral Nutrition
- Electronic Calculators
- eTables:
  - eTable 42-1: Recommended Dietary Reference Intakes and Manifestations of Imbalance

- eTable 42-2: Common Drug and Food–Nutrient Interactions
- eTable 42-3: Manifestations of Protein–Calorie Malnutrition
- eTable 42-4: Patient and Caregiver Teaching Guide: Good Nutrition
- eTable 42-5: Nutritional Therapy: High-Calorie, High-Protein Diet
- Examination Review Questions
- Glossary
- Key Points (Printable and MP3 Download)

As one of the fundamental requirements for sustaining life, eating is a highly symbolic and culturally meaningful act. It is unusual to hear a newscast that does not have several stories relating to the food we eat. Newspapers and bestseller lists frequently highlight nutrition- and food-related books, illustrating the importance of food and eating to Canadians. Nutrition is also inextricably linked to the development of and the recovery from illness. This chapter focuses on problems related to nutrition and the use of enteral and parenteral nutritional support.

Nurses, as the first point of contact for patients, frequently initiate patient referrals to dietitians. Thus, knowledge and skills in nutrition and nutritional screening are essential to ensure that patient's needs are met in an efficient and effective manner. Dietitians and nurses often collaborate in the development and implementation of nutritional care plans.

Dietitians, as part of the multidisciplinary team, provide expertise in the assessment of the nutritional status of individuals across the life cycle and in development of nutritional care plans for wide-ranging health concerns. Dietitians have extensive knowledge in the biochemical and nutritional components of foods and how these influence metabolic and physiological processes. In addition, dietitians understand the feeding environment and underlying psychosocial, economic, and health determinants that influence food intake at individual, family, and societal levels (Dietitians of Canada, 2011).

Nutritional Status

Nutritional status is the sum of processes by which one takes in and utilizes nutrients (Teitelbaum et al., 2005). Nutritional status can be viewed as a continuum from undernutrition to optimal nutrition to overnutrition. An alteration in the process of nutrient intake or utilization can potentially cause nutritional problems. Nutritional problems can occur in all age groups, cultures, ethnic groups, and socioeconomic classes and across all educational levels. Attitudes toward the importance of food and eating habits are established early. Cultural or religious preferences and requirements are frequently reflected in dietary intakes. The financial status of a family or an individual may influence the type and

amount of nutritionally sound food that can be purchased (Cook & Frank, 2008). Noncommunicable diseases or chronic diseases are a major health concern in Canada.

Numerous reports have shown that a significant portion of morbidity and mortality among Canadians is related to chronic diseases. It is estimated that three quarters of all deaths and 42% of total direct medical care expenditures in Canada are related to chronic diseases (Mirolla, 2004). Internationally, Canada's health care spending is among the highest in the world, representing 10% of the gross domestic product in 2002 (Canadian Institute for Health Information [CIHI], 2010). Poor nutrition is a key preventable risk factor for the major chronic diseases that take a huge toll in morbidity, disability, and premature death in Canada.

Undernutrition occurs when nutritional reserves become depleted or when nutrient intake is inadequate to meet daily requirements or metabolic demands. Undernutrition affects vulnerable groups including infants, children, pregnant women, new immigrants, individuals with low incomes, hospitalized people, and older adults. Undernutrition increases the risk of impaired growth and development, lowered resistance to infection and disease, delayed wound healing, longer hospital stays, and higher health-related expenses.

Optimal nutritional status is achieved when nutrients are consumed in amounts that support daily requirements and any increased metabolic demands related to growth, pregnancy, or illness. Individuals having optimal nutritional status are at lower risk of developing chronic diseases and, compared with those with a chronic illness, generally live longer.

Overnutrition results from the consumption of nutrients—most frequently, calories, sodium, and fat—in excess of requirements. A major nutritional problem today, overnutrition results in the development of chronic diseases such as obesity, some cancers, and Type 2 diabetes.

Nutritional Health

Nutrition is the process by which the body uses food for energy, growth, maintenance, and repair of body tissues. The nutrients required to optimize health over a lifetime are the same for all healthy individuals; however, the amount of each of those nutrients changes based on stages of the life cycle. Nutrition can be viewed as a continuum over the life cycle: a continuum that changes as individuals grow, age, and respond to variations in their environment, physical activity, and health. Optimal nutrition is essential for its contribution to overall health and well-being and in the prevention of chronic conditions.

Optimal nutrition in the absence of any underlying disease process results from the ingestion of a balanced diet. *Eating Well With Canada's Food Guide,* commonly referred to simply as Canada's Food Guide, provides Canadians with recommendations for healthy eating (Health Canada, 2011) (Figure 42-1). The guide is based on current nutritional science and defines four major foods groups. This standardization ensures that a diet based on the food guide will provide an adequate intake to support optimal nutritional status. It is important to note that Canada's Food Guide differs from the American "My Pyramid" in many ways, including the number of food groups and serving sizes and in graphic presentations.

Canada's Food Guide can be used by anyone in the planning of a healthy diet. The guide is flexible and can be adapted to include combination foods such as casseroles. In addition, the guide provides alternative choices to meat, milk, and other animal-based products.

Eating Well With Canada's Food Guide—First Nations, Inuit and Métis is a food guide tailored to reflect traditions and food choices of a specific population group (Health Canada, 2007a). This guide includes both traditional and store-bought foods that are generally available, affordable, and accessible to Aboriginal people across Canada.

Canada's Food Guide was developed in accordance with the daily Dietary Reference Intake (DRI) requirements, which represent a comprehensive set of nutrient reference values for healthy populations. The "rainbow" depicts the relative proportion of food intake from each of the four food groups in any given day. The broadest arc represents grain products, which is the food group consumed in the largest quantity; the smallest arc represents meat and alternatives that are to be consumed in smaller proportions. In addition to English, the guide is now available in 10 other languages: Arabic, Chinese, Farsi (Persian), Korean, Punjabi, Russian, Spanish, Tagalog, Tamil, and Urdu (Health Canada, 2012a).

There is a DRI set for each nutrient. These nutrient reference values are intended to help individuals optimize their health, prevent disease, and avoid overconsumption of any single nutrient. The reference values include the Estimated Average Requirement (EAR), the Recommended Dietary Allowance (RDA), the Adequate Intake (AI) and the Tolerable Upper Limit (UL) (Otten, Hellwig, & Meyers, 2006). The DRI values are designed to maintain health and prevent disease, not to restore health. Nutrient needs may exceed DRIs during times of acute stress or chronic illness.

In recent years, there has been considerable interest in vitamin, mineral, and herbal supplementation as a means of prevention and treatment of acute and chronic diseases. Although evidence does suggest that some nutrients, such as vitamin D, are beneficial to health, it is important to exercise caution when recommending daily supplementation. Exceeding the UL may place one at risk of deficiency or toxicity. Consumption of high levels of one vitamin or mineral may interfere with the absorption of another. For example, ingestion of high levels of zinc can interfere with the absorption of calcium; ingestion of high levels of vitamin C enhances the absorption of iron, which can lead to iron toxicity. Further, vitamin and mineral

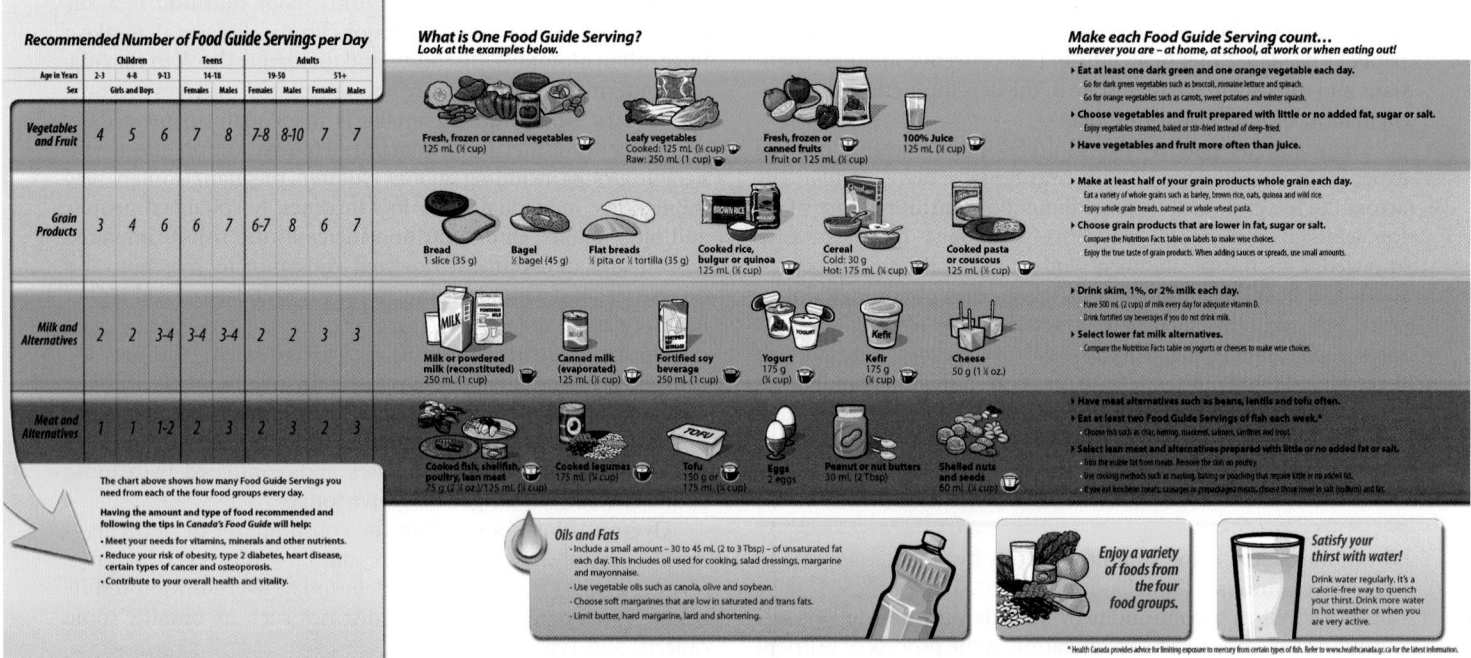

Figure 42-1 *Eating Well With Canada's Food Guide.* Visit *www.hc-sc.gc.ca/fn-an/food-guide-aliment/index_e.html* for additional information, plus interactive tools (My Food Guide) that allow nurses and their patients to personalize the information found in Canada's Food Guide.

Source: Extracted from Health Canada. (2011). *Eating Well With Canada's Food Guide.* Retrieved from *www.hc-sc.gc.ca/fn-an/alt_formats/hpfb-dgpsa/pdf/food-guide-aliment/view_eatwell_vue_bienmang-eng.pdf* © Her Majesty the Queen in Right of Canada, represented by the Minister of Health, 2007. This publication may be reproduced without permission. No changes permitted. HC Pub: 4651 Cat. H164-38/1-2007E.

supplements are not safe for everyone; daily β-carotene supplementation is associated with increased incidence of lung cancer in smokers and in people exposed to asbestos. In the case of herbal remedies, many herbal medicines contain natural drugs, such as willow bark, which contains salicin, a natural compound similar to acetylsalicylic acid (Aspirin), which may be harmful when consumed with other pharmaceuticals or by individuals with existing chronic diseases.

Patients should be encouraged to discuss vitamin, mineral, and herbal supplementation with their primary care physician or pharmacist, before using, to avoid harmful adverse effects.

Major Nutrients

The major nutritional constituents of foods are carbohydrates (and fibre), fats, proteins, vitamins, minerals, and water. Carbohydrates, fats, and proteins provide energy. Vitamins, minerals, and water do not provide energy; some serve as structure (calcium in bones); and all assist in body processes such as digestion of food, moving of muscles, disposing of wastes, growing of new tissues (wound healing), and obtaining energy from carbohydrates, proteins, and fats. The daily caloric requirements of a person are influenced by body build, age, sex, and physical activity. Adjustments in caloric intake are necessary depending on changes in health status and daily activity level. An average adult requires an estimated 20 to 35 cal/kg of body weight/day, leaning toward the higher end if the person is critically ill or very active and the lower end if the person is sedentary (Wooley & Frankenfield, 2007).

Carbohydrates, the body's primary source of energy, yield approximately 4 kcal/g. (*Kilocalorie* is the correct unit to designate caloric intake and expenditure; however, *calorie* is the term more commonly used.) Carbohydrates are either simple or complex. Simple carbohydrates are *monosaccharides* (e.g., glucose and fructose), which are found in fruits and honey, and *disaccharides* (e.g., sucrose, maltose, and lactose), which are found in such substances as table sugar, malted cereal, and milk. Complex carbohydrates or polysaccharides commonly appear in the diet as starches such as cereal grains, potatoes, and legumes. Carbohydrates are the chief protein-sparing ingredients in a nutritionally sound diet. Canada's Food Guide recommends that 55% of daily energy needs be supplied by carbohydrates, especially foods rich in complex carbohydrate and fibre. The rainbow design of the Food Guide places grain products, vegetables, and fruit in the outermost arcs to ensure that Canadians eat the recommended amount of carbohydrates.

Fibre is the indigestible parts of plant foods. Diets rich in fibre are associated with improved blood cholesterol and blood glucose levels, healthy bowel function, and body weights (Table 42-1).

Fats are stored in adipose tissue and in the abdominal cavity. Besides being a major source of energy, fats act as insulation, which reduces loss of body heat in cold environments and provides padding and protection for vital organs. Fats also act as carriers of essential fatty acids (linoleic and α-linolenic) and fat-soluble vitamins (A, D, E, and K). Fats provide a feeling of satiety after eating, partly from the flavour added and partly from their slow rate of digestion, which delays hunger.

Most Canadians eat far more fat than is recommended. Canada's Food Guide recommends that only about 30% of energy should come from fat and 10% from saturated fat (Health Canada, 2012b). One gram of fat yields 9 cal. A fat intake of 30% or less of a day's calories means an intake between 60 and 105 g of fat.

Fats in foods are made up of four different types of fatty acids—polyunsaturated, monounsaturated, saturated, and "*trans-*fats." Monounsaturated and polyunsaturated fats tend to lower the risk of heart disease. Polyunsaturated fats, made up of omega-3 and omega-6 essential fatty acids, are important to good health. These fatty acids are not synthesized by the body and so must be obtained from the diet. Omega-6 essential fatty acids are found in vegetable oils such as corn, sunflower, and soybean oils; omega-3 fatty acids are in some vegetable oils, such as canola and soybean oils, as well as in fish oils. Monounsaturated fats are found in vegetable oils, such as olive and canola.

Saturated fats are found naturally in both vegetable- and animal-based foods in forms such as coconut and palm oil and animal fats such as butter. *Trans-*fats are found naturally in some animal-based foods but are also formed when liquid oils are made into semisolid fats like shortening and hard margarine. Generally, saturated and *trans-*fats tend to increase the risk of heart disease because they raise the serum low-density lipoprotein (LDL) cholesterol levels (the so-called "bad" cholesterol) (Health Canada, 2007b). *Trans-*fats are particularly dangerous because they also reduce the blood levels of high-density lipoprotein (HDL) cholesterol (the so-called "good" cholesterol) (Health Canada, 2007b).

Proteins, another essential component of a well-balanced diet, are obtained from both animal and plant sources. Ideally, proteins provide 15 to 20% of daily caloric needs. The Recommended Daily Intake (RDI) for protein is 0.8 to 1 g/kg of body weight. One gram of protein yields 4 cal. Proteins are complex nitrogenous organic compounds, of which amino acids are the fundamental units of structure. The 22 amino acids can be classified as essential and nonessential. The body is capable of synthesizing nonessential amino acids if an adequate supply of protein is available. However, there are nine essential amino acids the body cannot synthesize, which are only available from dietary sources. Protein sources containing all the essential amino acids are considered to be high-quality proteins that are easier to digest. Generally, proteins that are of an animal source are easier to digest and are often referred to as *complete proteins* because they contain all of the essential amino acids (Table 42-2).

Grain products also contribute to protein intake. Plant-based proteins such as legumes and grains lack one or more of the essential amino acids and are more difficult to digest. These types of proteins are called *incomplete proteins.* This limitation can be overcome by combining high-protein plant-based foods. This concept is called *mutual supplementation.* Mutual supplementation is the strategy of combining two incomplete protein sources so that the amino acids in one food compensate for the missing ones in the other food. See Table 42-2 for a list of good sources of protein. Proteins are essential for tissue growth, repair, and maintenance; body regulatory functions; and energy production.

Table 42-1 Daily Recommended Intake (DRI) for Fibre	
	GRAMS OF FIBRE PER DAY
Men 19-50 years of age	38
Men ≥51 years of age	30
Women 19-50 years of age	25
Women ≥51 years of age	21

Table 42-2 Good Sources of Protein	
Complete Proteins	**Incomplete Proteins**
• Milk and milk products (e.g., cheese)	• Grains (e.g., corn)
• Eggs	• Legumes (e.g., navy beans, soybeans, peas)
• Fish	• Nuts (e.g., peanuts)
• Meats	• Seeds (e.g., sesame seeds, sunflower seeds)
• Poultry	

Vitamins are organic compounds required in small amounts by the body for normal metabolism. Vitamins function primarily in enzyme reactions that facilitate the metabolism of amino acids, fats, and carbohydrates. The body must rely on a dietary source to meet requirements for some vitamins, such as cobalamin (vitamin B_{12}). Vitamins are divided into two categories: water-soluble vitamins (vitamin C and the B-complex vitamins) and fat-soluble vitamins (vitamins A, D, E, and K). Vitamin D, in particular, has recently received widespread attention because of a growing body of evidence that suggests it may have a beneficial effect on some types of cancer, in particular colorectal cancer, and other immune-related diseases (Dietitians of Canada, 2012).

Mineral salts (e.g., magnesium, iron, calcium) make up approximately 4% of the total body weight. When minerals are present in minute amounts, they are referred to as *trace elements*. Minerals required in amounts greater than 100 mg/day are called *major minerals*. Minerals are necessary for the body to build tissues and regulate body fluids and assist in various body functions. Some minerals are stored in a manner similar to that of the fat-soluble vitamins and can be toxic if taken in excess amounts. The amount of minerals needed in the daily diet varies greatly from a few micrograms of trace minerals to 1 g or more of the major minerals, such as calcium, phosphorus, and sodium. A well-balanced diet usually meets the daily requirements of needed minerals without exceeding requirements.

CULTURALLY COMPETENT CARE

People have unique cultural heritages that may affect eating customs and nutritional status. Each culture has its own beliefs and behaviours related to food and the role that food plays in the etiology and treatment of disease. In addition, culture can dictate what food is considered edible as well as how it is prepared and when it is eaten. Both culture and religion may influence what foods are selected, when meals are eaten, how they are prepared, and who prepares them. It is important to consider cultural and ethnic influences when assessing the patient's nutritional status and suggesting interventions that require dietary changes. At the same time, the nurse should avoid *cultural stereotyping* by making assumptions or generalizations about diet based on the individual's cultural background. Dietary habits differ considerably within and among ethnic groups (Perez-Escamilla & Putnik, 2007). Acculturation, the extent to which immigrants adopt attributes of a new culture, can also affect dietary practices (Hoerr, Tsuei, Liu, Franklin, & Nicklas, 2008).

Special Diets

Vegetarian Diet

The common element among all vegetarians is the exclusion of meat, poultry, game, fish, shellfish or crustaceans, and meat by-products from the diet. Vegetarians base their diet on convictions founded in religious or cultural beliefs, respect for all living beings, ethical–ecological ideals, and economics. Many vegetarians are *vegans*, who are pure or total vegetarians and eat only plant-based food, whereas others are *lacto-ovo-vegetarians,* who eat plant-based foods and sometimes dairy products and eggs.

Vegetarians can be at risk for vitamin or protein deficiencies unless their diets are well planned. Plant protein, although of a lesser quality than that of animal origin, fulfills most of the protein requirements. Combinations of vegetable protein foods (e.g., rice and kidney beans) can increase the nutritional value. Lacto-ovo-vegetarians obtain additional protein sources from dairy products and eggs. Soy milk is an excellent protein source, and many palatable meat analogue products are now available.

The primary risk for deficiency in a strict vegan is lack of cobalamin (vitamin B_{12}), although many vegan foods are now supplemented with this vitamin. Vegans not using cobalamin supplements or foods fortified with cobalamin are susceptible to the development of megaloblastic anemia and the neurological signs of cobalamin deficiency. Strict vegetarians and lacto-ovo-vegetarians are also at risk for iron deficiency. The iron in plant foods such as legumes, dark green leafy vegetables, iron-fortified cereals, and whole grains and cereals is poorly absorbed.

Nutrition-Related Health Conditions

Malnutrition

Malnutrition is a deficit, excess, or imbalance of the essential components of a balanced diet (Soeters & Schols, 2009). Malnutrition can refer to alterations in macronutrients (carbohydrates, proteins, and fat) or micronutrients (electrolytes, minerals, and vitamins). Terms such as *undernutrition* and *overnutrition* are also used to describe malnutrition.

Undernutrition is often associated with developing countries in which adequate food sources do not exist and whose economic conditions often preclude a balanced diet (Norman, Prichard, Lochs, & Pirlich, 2008). Undernutrition, however, does exist in Canada, where income-related food insecurity is increasingly acknowledged as a key social determinant of health. The prevalence of household food insecurity is known to be higher in certain groups, including lone-parent families with one or more young children, those receiving social assistance, and Aboriginal people living off-reserve (Health Canada, 2007c). Malnutrition is common in hospitalized patients, within those that reside in long-term care facilities. It has been estimated that 37 to 55% of patients in hospitals and long-term care facilities are malnourished or at nutritional risk of malnourishment (Carrier, Ouellet, & West, 2007).

Types of Malnutrition

Protein–Calorie Malnutrition. Protein–calorie malnutrition (PCM) is the most common form of undernutrition and

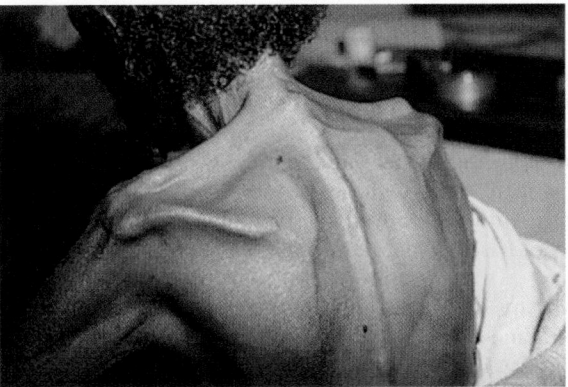

Figure 42-2 Patient with malnutrition.

Source: Morgan, S. L., & Weiniser, R. (1998). *Fundamental of clinical nutrition* (2nd ed.)
St. Louis: Mosby.

Table 42-3 Conditions That Increase the Risk for Malnutrition

- Dementia
- Depression
- Chronic alcoholism
- Eating disorders
- Swallowing disorders (e.g., neurological conditions, head and neck cancer, stroke)
- Decreased mobility that limits access to food or its preparation
- Nutrient losses from malabsorption, dialysis, fistulas, or wounds
- Drugs with antinutrient or catabolic properties, such as corticosteroids and oral antibiotics
- Extreme need for nutrients because of hypermetabolism or stresses such as infection, burns, trauma, or fever
- No oral intake, receiving standard intravenous solutions (e.g., 5% dextrose), or both for 5 days

results from either primary or secondary factors. Primary PCM occurs when nutritional needs are not met because of poor eating habits. Secondary PCM results when there is an alteration or defect in ingestion, digestion, absorption, or metabolism. In this type of malnutrition, tissue needs are not met even though the dietary intake would be satisfactory under normal conditions. Secondary malnutrition may occur as a result of gastrointestinal (GI) obstruction, surgical procedure, cancer, malabsorption syndromes, drugs, or infectious diseases. Secondary malnutrition is also referred to as *disease-related* malnutrition (Sorensen et al., 2008).

PCM may also be caused by the ingestion of foods deficient in protein. In addition to decreased quantities of protein, the diet is generally low in necessary vitamins and minerals. Most ill malnourished patients have combined (both primary and secondary) PCM (Figure 42-2).

Marasmus and Kwashiorkor. Marasmus and kwashiorkor are the most severe forms of PCM and are the most frequently seen in children of developing countries (Latham, 1997). *Marasmus* is characterized by generalized loss of body fat and muscle. Patients appear "wasted" or emaciated but may have normal serum protein levels. *Kwashiorkor* is caused by a deficiency of protein intake that is superimposed on a catabolic stress event, such as a GI obstruction, a surgical procedure, cancer, a malabsorption syndrome, or an infectious disease. Kwashiorkor is characterized by the presence of edema and low serum protein levels (Müller & Krawinkel, 2005). Marasmic-kwashiorkor is the combined form of marasmus and kwashiorkor. It is characterized by severe tissue wasting, loss of subcutaneous fat, and dehydration.

Etiology of Malnutrition

Many factors contribute to the development of malnutrition including socioeconomic factors, physical illnesses, incomplete diets, food–drug interactions, and psychological illness such as eating disorders. Table 42-3 lists conditions that increase the risk of malnutrition.

Socioeconomic Factors. At every stage of the life cycle, health is directly or indirectly influenced by key determinants of health such as education and literacy, income and social status, employment and working conditions, and social environments (Public Health Agency of Canada [PHAC], 2011). Increasingly,

evidence suggests that "the complex interaction between these determinants can influence health outcomes—both positively and negatively—and, depending on the individual, can result in the individual beginning and progressing through life stages at different times and rates" (p. 1).

The World Health Organization (WHO) defines **food security** as physical and economic access to sufficient, safe, and nutritious food that meets food preferences and dietary needs for an active and healthy life (Cook et al., 2008). Individuals or families with limited financial resources may have *food insecurity* (inadequate access). Food insecurity is problematic because it affects the overall quality of food that is available in both quantity and nutritional value. Families with food insecurity usually choose less expensive "filling" foods, which are more energy dense (high fat) and lack nutritional value. This type of diet increases the risk of nutrient deficiencies.

Individuals and families may utilize "safety net programs" including food assistance programs, housing and energy subsidies, and in-kind contributions from relatives, friends, food pantries, or charitable organizations to help them obtain food. The "heat or eat" phenomenon is problematic as families with limited economic resources struggle to pay household utility bills or put food on the table (DiMaria-Ghalili, 2008). Older adults on a fixed income have an added burden of deciding on whether to pay for medications or food. The nurse and the dietitian can assist patients in making food choices that meet nutritional requirements while staying within their limited resources.

Individual and families with lower social economic status are less likely to consume the nutrients needed for proper health and well-being than those living with higher incomes (PHAC, 2011). Studies have also linked food insecurity to the prevalence of unhealthy weights. Lower-income families consume more energy-dense, nutrient-poor diets whereas families with higher income consume more whole grains, lean meats, low-fat dairy products, and fresh vegetables and fruit.

Physical Illnesses. Regardless of the illness, an individual who is ill has increased nutritional needs. Pathological conditions are frequently aggravated by undernutrition and an existing deficiency is likely to become more severe during illness. Malnutrition is a common consequence of illness, surgery, injury, or hospitalization. The hospitalized patient, especially the older adult, is at risk of becoming malnourished. Prolonged illness, major surgery, sepsis, draining wounds, burns, hemorrhage, fractures, and immobilization can all contribute to malnutrition.

Anorexia, nausea, vomiting, diarrhea, abdominal distension, and cramping may accompany diseases of the GI system. Any combination of these symptoms interferes with usual food consumption and metabolism. Whereas *anorexia* is a loss of normal appetite and may occur as a result of physical or mental illness, *cachexia* refers to a wasting syndrome that causes weakness and loss of weight, fat, and muscle. Cachexia is a major cause of morbidity and mortality in cancer, human immunodeficiency virus (HIV), and other serious long-term illnesses such as chronic obstructive pulmonary disease (COPD).

Malabsorption syndrome is the impaired absorption of nutrients from the GI tract. It is characterized by anorexia, weight loss, abdominal bloating, muscle cramps, bone pain, and steatorrhea. It may result from decreased digestive enzymes or a reduced bowel surface area and can quickly lead to a deficiency state. Many drugs have undesirable GI adverse effects as well as alter normal digestive and absorptive processes. For example, antibiotics change the normal flora of the intestines, decreasing the body's ability to synthesize biotin.

Incomplete Diets.
Vitamin deficiencies are rare in most developed countries of the world. When present, vitamin deficiencies usually involve several vitamins. The recommended DRI for essential vitamins and minerals can be obtained by eating a diet consisting of foods from the four basic food groups outlined in Canada's Food Guide. When vitamin imbalances occur because of incomplete diets, they are usually found among people with a pattern of alcohol and drug abuse, people who are chronically ill, and individuals who follow poor dietary practices. People who have had surgery on the GI tract may be at risk for vitamin deficiencies. For example, resection of the terminal ileum poses a risk for deficiencies of fat-soluble vitamins. After a gastrectomy, patients require cobalamin supplementation. Followers of fad diets or poorly planned vegetarian diets are also at risk. Clinical manifestations of vitamin imbalances are most commonly exhibited as neurological manifestations. In the growing child, the central nervous system is primarily involved, whereas the peripheral nervous system is most affected in the adult. The recommended DRIs and manifestations of imbalance are presented in eTable 42-1, available on the Evolve Web site for this chapter.

Food–Drug Interactions.
When the patient's health conditions require drug therapy, drug and food interactions may not be explored before starting a prescription. Adverse interactions can include incompatibilities, altered drug effectiveness, and impaired nutritional status. Food–drug interactions can also occur with use of over-the-counter drugs and herbs and dietary supplements. The nurse's role is to monitor and prevent these potential interactions for patients while in the hospital and at home. Examples of common drug– and food–nutrient interactions are presented in eTable 42-2, available on the Evolve website for this chapter.

Eating Disorders.
Eating disorders are complex psychiatric disorders strongly associated with other mental illnesses, such as mood, personality, and anxiety disorders. Society's promotion of the thin body image has also been implicated. Although eating disorders are considered primarily psychiatric disorders, the mortality rate is significant. Eating disorders involve a serious disturbance in eating behaviour—eating either too much or too little—in addition to great concern over body size and shape. There is increasing evidence to suggest that up to 30% of all patients with an eating disorder are male. Male and female patients have similar psychological co-morbidities including depression and anxiety and similar behaviours and attitudes, except males tend to have less "drive for thinness" and more concern with the body shape or build compared with females (Practice Based Evidence in Nutrition [PEN], 2008).

Anorexia Nervosa. **Anorexia nervosa** is a serious, often chronic and life-threatening eating disorder characterized by self-imposed weight loss, endocrine dysfunction, and a distorted psychopathological attitude toward weight and eating (Gonzalez, Kohn, & Clarke, 2007). It manifests clinically as abnormal weight loss, deliberate self-starvation, intense fear of gaining weight or becoming fat, lanugo (soft, downy hair covering the body except the palms and soles), refusal to eat, continuous dieting, hair loss, sensitivity to cold, compulsive exercising, absent or irregular menstruation, dry skin, and constipation. Diagnostic studies often show iron-deficiency anemia and an elevated serum urea (nitrogen) level that is reflective of marked intravascular volume depletion and prerenal azotemia. Lack of potassium in the diet and loss of potassium in the urine lead to potassium deficiency that can cause muscle weakness, cardiac dysrhythmias, and renal failure. If the eating pattern continues for a prolonged time, body wasting and signs of severe malnutrition are evident, and death may become imminent.

Multidisciplinary treatment must involve a combination of nutritional support and psychiatric care. Although most of the treatment of an eating disorder is provided in the community, hospitalization may be necessary if there are severe physical complications that cannot be managed in an outpatient therapy program. Nutritional replenishment must be closely supervised to ensure consistent and ongoing weight gain. The use of tube or parenteral feedings may be necessary. Improved nutrition, however, is not a cure for anorexia nervosa. The underlying psychiatric problem must be identified and addressed.

Bulimia Nervosa. **Bulimia nervosa** is an eating disorder characterized by frequent binge eating, self-induced vomiting associated with loss of control over eating, and a persistent concern with body image (LeGrange, 2007). These individuals may have normal body mass index, but their weight may fluctuate with bingeing and purging. They may abuse diet drugs, laxatives, or diuretics. Signs of frequent vomiting—such as macerated knuckles, swollen salivary glands, broken blood vessels in the eyes, and dental problems—are common.

The patient with bulimia, similar to the one with anorexia nervosa, goes to great lengths to conceal abnormal eating habits. As the behaviour persists, many problems associated with the condition become increasingly hard to deal with effectively. As with anorexia, a treatment combination of psychological counselling and diet therapy is essential. Education and emotional support for the patient and the family are vital.

Starvation Process

Knowledge of the phases of the starvation process is useful in understanding the physiological changes that occur in PCM. Initially, the body selectively uses carbohydrates (glycogen) rather than fat and protein to meet metabolic needs. These carbohydrate stores, found in the liver and muscles, are minimal and may be depleted within 18 hours. During this early phase of starvation, the only use of protein is in its obligatory participation in cellular metabolism. However, once carbohydrate stores are depleted, protein begins to be converted to glucose for energy. Alanine and glutamine are the first amino acids to be used by the liver to form glucose in a process termed *gluconeogenesis*. The resulting available plasma glucose allows the metabolic processes to continue. With these amino acids being used as energy sources, the person may be in negative nitrogen balance (greater nitrogen excretion). However, within 5 to 9 days, body fat is fully mobilized to supply much of the needed energy.

In prolonged starvation, up to 97% of calories are provided by fat, and protein is conserved. Depletion of fat stores depends on the amount available; fat stores are generally used up in 4 to 6 weeks. Once fat stores are used, body proteins, including those in internal organs and plasma, can no longer be spared and rapidly decrease because they are the only remaining body source of energy available.

If the malnourished patient has surgery, experiences bodily trauma, or has an infection, the stress response with concomitant increase in energy expenditure is superimposed on the starvation response. These body insults cause an increase in the metabolic rate, with a subsequent increase in energy requirements. Protein stores are no longer spared and are used with increasing frequency for body energy because of the increased metabolic energy needs.

As protein depletion continues, liver function is impaired, and synthesis of proteins is diminished. The plasma oncotic pressure is decreased as a result of decreased protein synthesis. A major function of plasma proteins, primarily of albumin, is to maintain the osmotic pressure of the blood. Because of this decreased pressure, body fluids shift from the vascular space into the interstitial compartment. As protein ingestion decreases and body stores are depleted, albumin eventually leaks into the interstitial space along with the fluid. Edema becomes clinically observable. Often, the edema present in the face and the legs of the patient masks the muscle wasting that occurs.

As total blood volume is reduced, the skin appears dry and wrinkled. Ions also move with the shift of fluids to the interstitial space. Sodium (a predominant extracellular ion) is found in increased amounts within the cell, and potassium (a predominant intracellular ion) and magnesium shift to the extracellular space. The sodium–potassium exchange pump has high energy needs, using 20 to 50% of all calories ingested. When the diet is extremely deficient in calories and essential proteins, the pump will fail, leaving sodium inside the cell (along with water), and the cell will expand; this results in edema.

The liver is the body organ that loses the most mass during protein deprivation. It gradually becomes infiltrated with fat secondary to decreased synthesis of lipoproteins. Immediate intervention is required or death will rapidly ensue.

Clinical Manifestations

The clinical manifestations of malnutrition range from mild to emaciation and death. The most obvious clinical signs on physical examination are apparent in the skin (dry and scaly skin, brittle nails, rashes, and hair loss), mouth (crusting and ulceration, changes in tongue), muscles (decreased mass and weakness), and the central nervous system (cognitive changes such as confusion and irritability). The speed at which the malnutrition develops depends on the quantity and quality of the protein intake, caloric value, illness, and age of the person.

Clinical manifestations of malnutrition are the result of numerous interactions occurring at the cellular level. As protein intake is severely reduced, the muscles (the largest reservoir of body protein) become wasted and flabby, leading to weakness, fatigability, and decreased endurance. There is a decreased protein available for repair that can result in delayed wound healing. The person is more susceptible to all types of infections because humoral and cell-mediated immunity are deficient in PCM. There is a decrease in the number of leukocytes in the peripheral blood. Phagocytosis is altered as a result of the lack of energy (adenosine triphosphate) necessary to drive the process. Most malnourished people are anemic. Anemia resulting from PCM is usually caused by nutritional deficiencies in iron and folic acid, the necessary building blocks for red blood cells. A detailed listing of the clinical manifestations of malnutrition is available in eTable 42-3, available on the Evolve website for this chapter.

NURSING MANAGEMENT: HIGH-RISK NUTRITIONAL STATUS

Nursing Assessment

Regardless of setting, the nurse must be aware of the nutritional status of the patient. The nurse is often the first-line health care provider dealing with the patient. The patient's height, weight, and diet history are important components of any nursing assessment. Nutritional status may well be a major factor in the outcome of, and perhaps the underlying reason for, many illnesses.

In many institutions, the nurse is responsible for initial nutrition screening to identify individuals who are malnourished or at risk for malnutrition. Results of nutrition screening determine whether a more detailed nutrition assessment is necessary (Table 42-4).

Nutrition screening, the first step in assessing nutritional status, can be completed in any setting (e.g., clinic, home, hospital, long-term care facilities). Based on readily obtained data, nutrition screening is an efficient way to identify individuals at nutrition risk, including those who have experienced unintentional weight loss, inadequate food intake, or recent illness. Parameters used for nutrition screening include weight and weight history, diet information, medical history and routine laboratory data. A variety of valid tools are available for screening different populations, such as the Malnutrition Screening Tool (MST), which has been validated for use by nurses in hospitalized patients (Table 42-5).

The MST is a three-question screening tool that was developed and validated in 408 general medical–surgical adult hospital patients in Australia. This nutrition screening tool has a scoring potential of 7. A cut-off score of 2 has been determined to indicate risk of malnutrition. It is recommended that the MST be performed within 24 hours of hospitalization. This screen can be reliably completed by nurses and other members of the interprofessional health care team (Anthony, 2008).

Assessing Nutritional Intake

Individuals identified at nutritional risk during screening should be referred, where possible, to a dietitian to undergo a *comprehensive nutritional assessment*, which includes evaluation of

NURSING ASSESSMENT

Table 42-4 Malnutrition

Subjective Data	**Eyes**
Important Health Information	Pale or red conjunctivae, grey keratinized epithelium on conjunctiva (Bitot's spots); dryness and dull appearance of conjunctiva and cornea, soft cornea; blood vessel growth in cornea; redness and fissuring of eyelid corners
Past health history: Severe burns, major trauma, hemorrhage, draining wounds, bone fractures with prolonged immobility, chronic renal or liver disease, cancer, malabsorption syndrome, GI obstruction, infectious diseases (TB, AIDS)	
	Respiratory
	Decreased respiratory rate, ↓ vital capacity, crackles, weak cough
Medications: Corticosteroids, chemotherapeutic agents, diet pills	**Cardiovascular**
Surgery or other treatments: Recent surgery, radiation	Increase or decrease in heart rate, ↓ BP, dysrhythmias
Psychological factors: Alcohol or drug abuse; malaise, apathy	**Gastrointestinal**
Nutritional factors: Increase or decrease in weight, weight problems; increase or decrease in appetite, typical dietary intake; food preferences and aversions; food allergies or intolerance; ill-fitting or absent dentures; dry mouth, difficulty in chewing or swallowing; bloating or gas; sensitivity to cold; delayed wound healing	Swollen, smooth, raw, beefy red tongue (glossitis; see Fig. 33-2), hypertrophic or atrophic papillae; dental caries, absent or loose teeth, discoloured tooth enamel; spongy, pale, receded gums with a tendency to bleed easily, periodontal disease; ulcerations, white patches or plaques, redness, swelling of oral mucosa; distended, tympanic abdomen; ascites, hepatomegaly, decreased bowel sounds; steatorrhea
Elimination: Constipation, diarrhea, nocturia, decreased urinary output	**Neurological**
Activity: Increase or decrease in activity patterns; weakness, fatigue, decreased endurance	Decreased or loss of reflexes, tremor; inattention, irritability, confusion, syncope
Perception: Pain in mouth; paresthesias; loss of position and vibratory sense	
Objective Data	**Musculoskeletal**
General	Decreased muscle mass with poor tone, "wasted" appearance; bow legs, knock knees, beaded ribs, chest deformity, prominent bony structures
Listless, cachectic; underweight for height	**Possible Findings**
Integumentary	↓ Hemoglobin and hematocrit; ↓ MCV, MCH, or MCHC (iron deficiency); ↑ MCV or MHC (folic acid or cobalamin deficiency); altered serum electrolyte levels, especially hyperkalemia; ↓ BUN (serum urea [nitrogen]) and creatinine; ↓ serum albumin, transferrin, and prealbumin; ↓ lymphocytes; ↑ liver enzymes; ↓ serum vitamin levels
Dry, brittle, sparse hair with colour changes and lack of lustre, alopecia; dry, scaly lips, fever blisters, angular crusts and lesions at corners of mouth (cheilosis); brittle, ridged nails; decreased tone and elasticity of skin; cool, rough, dry, scaly skin with brown-grey pigment changes; reddened, scaly dermatitis, scrotal dermatitis; slight cyanosis; peripheral edema	

AIDS, acquired immune deficiency syndrome; *BP,* blood pressure; *BUN,* blood urea nitrogen; *GI,* gastrointestinal; *MCH,* mean corpuscular hemoglobin; *MCHC,* mean corpuscular hemoglobin concentration; *MCV,* mean corpuscular volume; *TB,* tuberculosis.

Table 42-5 Malnutrition Screening Tool (MST)

Have you lost weight recently without trying?	
No	0
Unsure	2
If yes, how much weight (kilograms) have you lost?	
1-5	1
6-10	2
11-15	3
>15	4
Unsure	2
Have you been eating poorly because of a decreased appetite?	
No	0
Yes	1
Total	

Source: Ferguson, M., Capra, S., Bauer, J., & Banks, M. (1999). Development of a valid and reliable malnutrition screening tool for adult acute hospital patients. *Nutrition, 15*(6), p. 461, Table IV. doi:10.1016/S0899-9007(99)00084-2

dietary history and clinical information, physical examination, and anthropometric measures.

Various methods for collecting current dietary intake information are available including the 24-hour recall, food frequency questionnaire, and food diary. Documentation of nutritional intake for hospitalized patients can best be achieved through calorie counts of nutrients consumed or infused.

■ **The 24-Hour Recall.** The most common method of obtaining information about dietary intake is the *24-hour recall.* The individual or family member is asked to recall everything eaten within the last 24 hours. It is important to be aware of potential information gaps when this method is used: (1) the individual or family member may not be able to recall type or amount of food eaten; (2) intake within the last 24 hours may be atypical of usual intake; (3) the individual or family member may alter the truth for a variety of reasons; and (4) snack items and use of gravies, sauces, and condiments may be under-reported.

■ **The Food Frequency Questionnaire.** To counter some of the challenges inherent in the 24-hour recall method, a *food frequency questionnaire* may also be completed. Information is collected related to how many times per day, week, or month an individual eats particular foods. The food frequency questionnaire does not quantify amount of food eaten, and similar to the 24-hour recall, it relies on the individual's or family member's memory.

■ **The Food Diary.** *Food diaries* require asking the individual or family member to write down everything consumed for a certain period of time. Three days—2 working and 1 nonworking day—are customarily used. A food diary is most accurate if the individual is instructed to record information immediately after eating. Potential challenges with the food diary include (1) non-adherence, (2) inaccurate recording, (3) atypical intake on the recording days, and (4) conscious alteration of diet during the recording period.

■ **Direct Observation.** *Direct observation* of the feeding and eating process can lead to detection of problems not readily identified through standard nutrition interviews. For example, observing the typical feeding techniques used by a parent or caregiver and the interaction between the individual and the caregiver can be of value when assessing failure to thrive in children or unintentional weight loss in older adults.

■ Anthropometric Measurements

Anthropometric measurements, which include gross measures of fat and muscle contents, are most beneficial in evaluating long-term effects of malnutrition or responses to nutritional interventions. They consist of measures of skinfold thickness at various sites, which is an indicator of subcutaneous fat stores, and midarm muscle circumference, an indicator of protein stores. Training and practice are required to perform these measurements accurately and reliably. To provide information on the patient's nutritional status in response to treatment, serial measurements are needed. These measurements may also be influenced by shifts in hydration status. The exact relationship of the midarm circumference measure to body composition of functional protein, both muscle and nonmuscle, remains to be established.

■ Laboratory Studies

The diagnosis of PCM can be determined by laboratory studies used in conjunction with the physical examination. Serum albumin has a half-life of approximately 20 to 22 days. In the absence of marked fluid loss, such as from hemorrhage or burns, the serum albumin value lags behind actual protein changes by more than 2 weeks and, therefore, is not a good indicator of acute changes in nutritional status. Prealbumin, a protein synthesized by liver, has a half-life of 2 days and is a better indicator of recent or current nutritional status. Serum transferrin level is another indicator of protein status. Transferrin, a protein synthesized by the liver, decreases during states of protein deficiency.

C-reactive protein (CRP) is a positive *acute-phase protein* and is typically elevated during inflammation. CRP levels should be obtained to help determine the extent to which low levels of visceral proteins are attributed to an inflammatory process or whether they are indeed an indicator of undernutrition (Jensen, 2008). However, it is still important to monitor albumin, preal-bumin, and transferrin levels in regard to nutrition assessment as indicators of disease severity, morbidity risk, and mortality risk (Russell & Mueller, 2007).

Serum electrolyte levels indicate changes in the intracellular and extracellular spaces. Serum potassium level is often elevated. The RBC count and the hemoglobin level indicate the presence

and degree of anemia. The total lymphocyte count decreases during malnutrition states. Liver enzyme levels, a reflection of liver function, may be elevated during malnutrition. Serum levels of fat- and water-soluble vitamins are usually diminished in a state of malnutrition. The lowered levels of the fat-soluble vita-mins correlate with the clinical signs of steatorrhea (fatty stools).

■ Nursing Diagnoses

The following are common causes/contributors to the development of malnutrition:
- Imbalanced nutrition: less than body requirements *related to* decreased access to or ingestion, digestion, or absorption of food or to anorexia.
- Self-care deficit (feeding) *related to* decreased strength and endurance, fatigue, and apathy.
- Constipation or diarrhea *related to* poor eating patterns, immo-bility, or medication effects.
- Deficient fluid volume *related to* factors affecting access to or absorption of fluids.
- Risk for impaired skin integrity *related to* poor nutritional state.
- Nonadherence *related to* alteration in perception, lack of moti-vation, or incompatibility of regimen with lifestyle or resources.
- Activity intolerance *related to* weakness, fatigue, and inadequate caloric intake or iron stores.

■ Planning

The overall goals are that the patient with malnutrition will (1) achieve weight gain, (2) consume a specified number of calories per day (with a diet individualized for the patient), and (3) have no adverse consequences related to malnutrition or nutrition therapies.

■ Nursing Implementation

High-calorie oral nutritional supplements may be used in the patient whose nutritional intake is deficient or impaired (dyspha-gia) or for patients in which their nutritional needs are increased (pressure ulcers). These supplements should not be used as meal substitutes but between meals as snacks as a means of increasing ingestion of calories and protein. In some long-term care facili-ties, these beverages are used instead of water with oral medica-tion administration to increase caloric intake (often referred to as *MedPass*).

■ Health Promotion

In the roles of caregiver, teacher, promoter of health, and resource person, the nurse can have a strong influence on the nutritional practices of patients and their families. The nurse is in an excel-lent position to collaborate with other health care providers (e.g., dietitians, social workers, physicians) in the nutritional assess-ment and health education of patients.

As part of a patient's health care team, the nurse can support a patient improving her or his health status by reinforcing healthy eating habits throughout the lifespan. Encouraging healthy eating by teaching Canada's Food Guide and encouraging patients to read food labels will support the patient in making positive changes. Nutrition labelling is mandatory on all prepared foods.

Nutrition Facts

Per 3/4 cup (175g)

Amount	% Daily Value
Calories 160	
Fat 2.5 g	**4** %
Saturated 1.5 g	**8** %
+ Trans 0 g	
Cholesterol 10 mg	
Sodium 75 mg	**3** %
Carbohydrate 25 g	**8** %
Fibre 0 g	**0** %
Sugars 24 g	
Protein 8 g	
Vitamin A 2 % Vitamin C	0 %
Calcium 20 % Iron	0 %

Figure 42-3 Nutrition facts table. An interactive version of this table with explanations of the components and other activities is available at the Health Canada Food and Nutrition Web site, *http://www.hc-sc.gc.ca/fn-an/label-etiquet/nutrition/cons/index-eng.php*

Source: Health Canada. (2012). Food and nutrition: Nutrition facts table. Retrieved from *http://www.hc-sc.gc.ca/fn-an/label-etiquet/nutrition/cons/index-eng.php* Reproduced with the permission of the Minister of Health, 2012.

The Nutrition Facts table (Figure 42-3) provides the information needed to make informed food choices and compare products by providing information on the amount of 13 core nutrients and calories in an amount of food. This information allows for the comparison of food products to facilitate healthier food purchases. The nurse can learn more about food labels on the Eat Right Ontario Web site and Health Canada's Web site (see the Resources at the end of this chapter). Recommendations for good nutrition are presented in eTable 42-4, available on the Evolve website for this chapter.

■ Ambulatory and Home Care

Patients may be discharged with instructions for a therapeutic diet regimen. Discharge preparation for the patient and the family is important. They must be aware of the cause of the undernourished state and ways to avoid the problem in the future. The patient must be made aware that undernourishment, whatever the cause, can recur and that a diet high in protein and calories for a few weeks cannot fully restore a normal nutritional state because many months are needed to reach this goal. Diet instruction is usually carried out by the dietitian, but it is important for the nurse to assess the patient's understanding and reinforce the information whenever possible. The ability to follow dietary instructions must be examined in light of past eating habits, religious and ethnic preferences, age, income, community or other resources, and state of health. Home visit follow-up may be required to ensure ongoing learning and determine whether the nutritional status of the patient is improving.

■ Acute Intervention

The patient's nutritional status is assessed at the same time that other physical problems are assessed (Kubrak & Jenson, 2007).

In states of increased stress, such as surgery, severe trauma, and sepsis, more calories and protein are needed. Wound healing requires increased protein synthesis. For patients undergoing major surgery or those with or at risk of malnutrition, several weeks of increased protein and calorie intake are needed preoperatively to promote healing and replenish body stores. When fever is present, the metabolic rate is increased and nitrogen loss is accelerated. Despite the return of body temperature to normal, the rate of protein breakdown and resynthesis may be accelerated for several weeks.

Daily weight measurement provides an ongoing record of weight gain or loss. Rapid gains and losses are usually the result of shifts in fluid balance. Body weight, in addition to accurate recording of food and fluid intake, provides a clearer picture of the patient's fluid and nutritional state. To ensure accuracy, weight should be measured at the same time each day, on the same scale, with the same type or amount of clothing, and with an empty bladder.

The protein and calorie intake required in the malnourished patient depends on the cause of the malnutrition, treatments, and stressors affecting the patient. If the patient is able to take food by mouth, a daily calorie count and food diary can provide an important record of food intake. The nurse and the dietitian working with the patient and the family can assist in the selection of high-calorie and high-protein foods (unless contraindicated). Preparation of foods preferred by the patient enhances the daily intake. Discussion with the patient and the family about foods that should be eaten to provide high-protein, high-calorie content is important. The family can be encouraged to bring the patient's favourite foods from home while the patient is still hospitalized. (See eTable 42-5 Nutritional Therapy: High-Calorie, High-Protein Diet, available on the Evolve Web site for this chapter.)

The undernourished patient requires additional calories, protein, fluids, and nutrients. This may be provided as either between-meal snacks or nutritional supplements. Nutritional supplements may be prepared in the dietary department, or they may be commercial products. Eating these items between meals increases the total daily intake by providing additional calories, protein, vitamins, and minerals. In addition, small frequent meals improve tolerance for food intake by distributing the amount of food more evenly throughout the day.

■ Evaluation

The following are expected outcomes for the patient who is malnourished:

• The patient will achieve and maintain optimal body weight.
• The patient will consume a well-balanced diet.
• The patient will experience no adverse outcomes related to malnutrition.

AGE-RELATED CONSIDERATIONS: MALNUTRITION

Older adults are particularly vulnerable to malnutrition. Older hospitalized adults with malnutrition are more likely to have poor wound healing, pressure ulcers, infections, decreased muscle

AGE-RELATED DIFFERENCES IN ASSESSMENT

Table 42-6 Factors Affecting Nutritional Intake in Older Adults

Physical Factors	Socioeconomic Factors
• Age	• Mental awareness
• Anorexia	• Social isolation
• Decreased number of taste buds	**Socioeconomic Factors**
• Dental problems	• Available time for food preparation and eating
• Food intolerances	• Availability of desired foods
• Health status	• Availability of transportation to food stores
• Physical disability	• Education level and nutritional knowledge
• Prescribed diets	• Food fads
• Prescribed or over-the-counter drugs	• Income level
Psychosocial Factors	• Lack of food preparation equipment
• Importance of food in the past	
• Loneliness or loss	

strength, postoperative complications, and increased morbidity and mortality risks (DiMaria-Ghalili & Amella, 2005; Amella, 2008). For a complete list of factors affecting nutritional intake of older adults, see Table 42-6. Older adults commonly report little or no appetite, problems with chewing or swallowing, inadequate servings of nutrients, and fewer than two meals per day. Limited incomes may cause them to restrict the number of meals eaten per day or the dietary quality of meals eaten. Social isolation is a problem in the older adult. Older adults who live alone may lose their desire to cook and report a decrease in their appetite. Older adults may have functional limitations that can affect their ability to purchase food as well as cook and prepare meals. Furthermore, older adults may lack access to transportation to buy food.

Chronic illnesses associated with aging can also potentially affect nutritional status. For example, depression and dysphagia (secondary to stroke) can affect intake (Palmer & Metheny, 2008). Poor oral health from cavities, gum disease, and missing teeth as well as xerostomia (dry mouth) can impair the older adult's ability to lubricate, masticate, and swallow food. Medications can cause dry mouth (e.g., antidepressants, antihypertensives, bronchodilators), can alter the taste of food, or can decrease appetite.

Lifestyle changes such as retirement or relocation to residence living can have a significant impact on the eating habits of the older adult. Other factors to assess include ethnic background, previous dietary practices, food preferences, knowledge of proper diet, availability and accessibility of food stores, transportation, and health status. Problems related to any or all of these areas can alert the nurse to the possibility of a nutritional problem. For older adult patients living in long-term care establishments, eating with others, having the freedom to choose the menu and one's table companions, having good help available, and enjoying a calm atmosphere contribute to residents' taking more pleasure and nutrition from their meals.

The nurse must be aware of common medical and psychosocial factors in the older adult and should incorporate interventions for overcoming these problems in the plan of care.

Some of the physiological changes associated with aging affect the nutritional status of older adults. The following changes are of particular interest:

1. Changes in the oral cavity (e.g., change in bite surfaces of the teeth, periodontal disease, drying of the mucous membranes of the mouth and tongue, poorly fitting dentures, decreased muscle strength for chewing, decreased number of taste buds, decreased saliva production)
2. Changes in digestion and motility (e.g., decreased absorption of cobalamin, vitamin A, and folic acid and decreased GI motility)
3. Changes in the endocrine system (e.g., decreased tolerance to glucose)
4. Changes in the musculoskeletal system (e.g., decreased bone density, degenerative joint changes)
5. Decrease in vision and hearing (e.g., procurement and preparation of food are more difficult)

Certain illnesses that are more prevalent in the older population are considered to be diet related. These include atherosclerosis, osteoporosis, diabetes mellitus, and diverticulosis. Multiple drugs are often required to treat these and other common chronic illnesses of the older patient. These drugs often have an adverse effect on the appetite of older adults, increasing the possibility of inadequate intake caused by anorexia.

To date, with the exception of calories, it has not been determined that older adults have different requirements for specific nutrients from those of middle-aged adults. Generally, caloric intake should decrease with age because of the progressive loss of lean body mass and a decrease in the basal metabolic rate. Unless caloric intake is decreased by reducing food intake or energy expenditure is increased through greater physical activity and exercise, obesity may result.

Malnutrition can occur in an older person even though the caloric requirements decrease with age. If malnutrition is present, few malnourished older people are able to ingest enough food to correct the malnourished state. Special strategies, such as adaptive devices (e.g., large-handled eating utensils), often are helpful in increasing dietary intake. Some older people may require nutritional support therapies until their strength and general health are improved. Before starting any nutritional support therapy (e.g., enteral nutrition [EN] or parenteral nutrition [PN]), review the older adult's advance directives regarding the use of artificial nutrition and hydration.

Some communities may have community nutritional programs that are available to the older person to make mealtime a pleasant, social event or home-delivered meal programs such as Meals on Wheels. However, these programs may not be able to fully support the older adult in accessing nutritious food for all three meals. It is not uncommon for older adults to also access food banks.

Pressure Ulcers

Pressure ulcers, as defined by the National Pressure Ulcer Advisory Panel (NPUAP), are "a localized injury to the skin and/or underlying tissue usually over a bony prominence, as a result of pressure, or pressure in combination with shear and/or friction," where pressure is the force per unit area, shear is mechanical stress, and friction is the force of two surfaces moving across one another (National Pressure Ulcer Advisory Panel [NPUAP], 2007).

Pressure ulcers develop in institutional and community settings and are often seen in the elderly, in debilitated and immobile patients (e.g., orthopedic patients), those with severe acute illness (e.g., in critical care units), and in individuals with neurological deficits (e.g., spinal cord injuries) (Registered Nurses' Association of Ontario [RNAO], 2005). Most pressure ulcers (95%) occur in the lower part of the body; the sacrum and heel are the most common cites (accounting for 36% and 30% of all pressure ulcers, respectively) (Thomas, 2006).

The nutritional care plans for pressure ulcers are designed to ensure that adequate calories, protein, fluids, vitamins, and minerals are provided to aid in wound healing. Referral to a dietitian and a wound management specialist is encouraged. (Pressure ulcers are discussed in Chapter 14.)

Dysphagia

Dysphagia is a symptom of disease or dysfunction and can be the result of a number of medical conditions. Among adults, the prevalence of dysphagia ranges from 10 to 50% in acute-care facilities and up to 66% in long-term care facilities (Dietitians of Canada, 2005). Defined as any impairment in eating, drinking, or swallowing, the consequences of unrecognized and untreated dysphagia can be life-threatening: protein–calorie malnutrition, dehydration, acute choking episodes that may lead to airway occlusion, chronic aspiration leading to frequent chest infections, and unnecessary long-term EN support (Dietitians of Canada, 2005).

Nurses must carefully assess all patients for the presence of signs of dysphagia (Table 42-7). A swallowing assessment, performed by a speech language pathologist can help identify patients at risk of aspiration, including the location of the swallowing problem and which food consistencies are safest. The speech language pathologist may also determine swallowing exercises, appropriate head positioning, and swallowing techniques.

The goal of nutrition intervention in dysphagia management should be to minimize weight loss (through adequate energy and protein intakes) and maintain hydration. Diet texture and fluid consistency modifications may be required for patient safety. Food texture may be modified with the addition of sauces or gravies and through mechanical alteration such as mincing or pureeing food. Fluid consistency may also be modified though the use of thickening agents added to beverages. Thickened fluids range in consistency from nectar-like to honey-like to pudding-like consistency.

Types of Specialized Nutrition Support

Oral Nutrition

High-calorie oral supplements may be used in the patient whose nutritional intake is deficient. This may include milkshakes, puddings, or commercially available products (e.g., Carnation Instant Breakfast Anytime, Ensure, Boost). Ingestion of these beverages may have a role in improving the nutritional status of elderly patients (Marian & McGinnis, 2007). It is important to note that these supplements should not be used as meal substitutes, but between meals as snacks. In some hospitals and long-term care facilities, these beverages are used instead of water with oral medication administration to increase caloric or protein intake (often referred to as *MedPass*). If patients are unable to maintain or achieve adequate nutritional status, nutrition support may be necessary.

Table 42-7 Indicators of Dysphagia
Obvious Indicators of Dysphagia
• Difficult, painful chewing or swallowing
• Regurgitation of undigested food
• Difficulty controlling food or liquid in the mouth
• Drooling
• Hoarse voice
• Coughing or choking before, during, or after swallowing
• Globus sensation (lump in the throat)
• Nasal regurgitation
• Feeling of obstruction
• Unintentional weight loss—for example, in people with dementia
Less Obvious Indicators of Dysphagia
• Change in respiration pattern
• Unexplained temperature spikes
• Wet voice quality
• Tongue fasciculation (may be indicative of motor neuron disease)
• Xerostomia
• Heartburn
• Change in eating—for example, eating slowly or avoiding social occasions
• Frequent throat clearing
• Recurrent chest infections
• Atypical chest pain

Source: National Institute for Health and Clinical Excellence. (2006). *Nutrition support in adults: Oral supplements, enteral and parenteral nutrition.* Retrieved from *www.nice.org.uk/guidance/index.jsp?action= download&o=29982*

If the patient is unable to consume enough nutrition orally, with a high-calorie, high-protein diet (food and supplements), nutrition support such as enteral feeds (tube feed) may be considered. If enteral feeds are not feasible, PN may be considered. For a decision-making plan related to nutrition support, see the algorithm in Figure 42-4.

Enteral Nutrition

Enteral nutrition (EN) is defined as nutrition (e.g., a nutritionally balanced liquefied food or formula) provided through the GI tract via a tube, catheter, or stoma that delivers nutrients distal to the oral cavity (Teitelbaum et al., 2005). EN may be ordered for the patient who has a functioning GI tract but is unable to take any or enough oral nourishment. Indications for EN may include those people with anorexia, orofacial fractures, head and neck cancer, or neurological or psychiatric conditions that prevent oral intake; extensive burns; critical illness; who are on mechanical ventilation; and those who are receiving chemotherapy or radiation therapy. EN is considered to be easily administered, safer, more physiologically efficient, and typically less expensive than PN. EN is used to provide nutrients by way of the GI tract either alone or as a supplement to oral nutrition or PN.

Common delivery options are continuous or cyclical infusion by pump, intermittent infusion by gravity, or by bolus by syringe. Continuous infusion is most often used with critically ill patients.

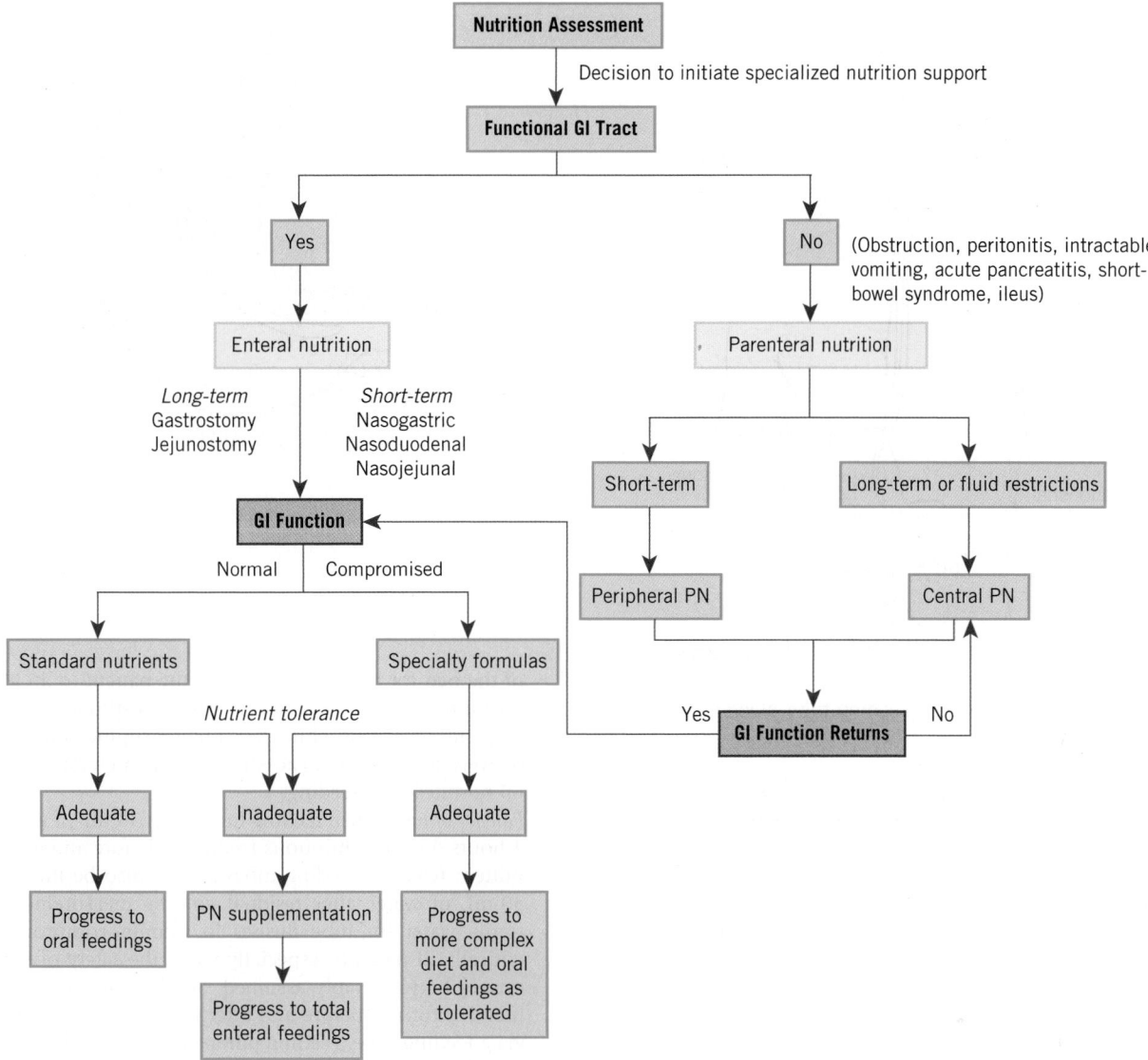

Figure 42-4 Nutrition support algorithm. *GI*, gastrointestinal, *PN*, parenteral nutrition.

Source: Adapted with permission of the American Society for Parenteral and Enteral Nutrition (ASPEN). ASPEN Board of Directors. (2002). Guidelines for the use of parenteral and enteral nutrition in adult and pediatric patients. *Journal of Parenteral and Enteral Nutrition, 26*(Suppl. 1), 8SA.

Intermittent feeding may be preferred as the patient improves or is receiving such feedings at home (Bankhead et al., 2009).

A nasogastric (NG) tube is commonly used for short-term feeding problems (<4 wk). If the feedings are necessary for an extended time, other means of feeding may be used, such as an esophagostomy tube, a gastrostomy tube, or a jejunostomy tube that delivers nutrients directly into the jejunum. Transpyloric (nasointestinal) tube placement or placement into the jejunum is used when physiological conditions warrant feeding the patient below the pyloric sphincter. Figure 42-5 shows the locations of commonly used enteral feeding tubes.

Nasogastric and Nasointestinal Tubes. Polyurethane or silicone feeding tubes are long, small in diameter, soft, and flexible, thereby decreasing the risk of mucosal damage from prolonged placement. Polyurethane and silicone tubes are radiopaque, making their position readily identified by radiograph. Placement into the small intestine theoretically decreases the likelihood of regurgitation of contents into the esophagus and subsequent aspiration. With the use of a stylet, these tubes can be placed in a comatose patient because the ability to swallow is not essential during insertion.

Although the smaller feeding tubes (12-8 French) have advantages over wider-lumen tubes (≥14 French), such as the standard decompression NG tube, there are some disadvantages. Because of the small diameter, these tubes are more easily occluded and it can be more problematic to check for gastric residual volumes. They are particularly prone to obstruction when oral drugs have not been thoroughly crushed and dissolved in water before administration. Failure to flush the tubing after both drug administration and residual volume determinations can result in tube clogging. When the tube becomes clogged, it may necessitate removal and insertion of a new tube, adding to cost and patient discomfort.

Gastrostomy and Jejunostomy. A gastrostomy tube may be used for a patient who requires EN over an extended time (>4-6 wk) (Figure 42-6). For the patient with chronic reflux, a

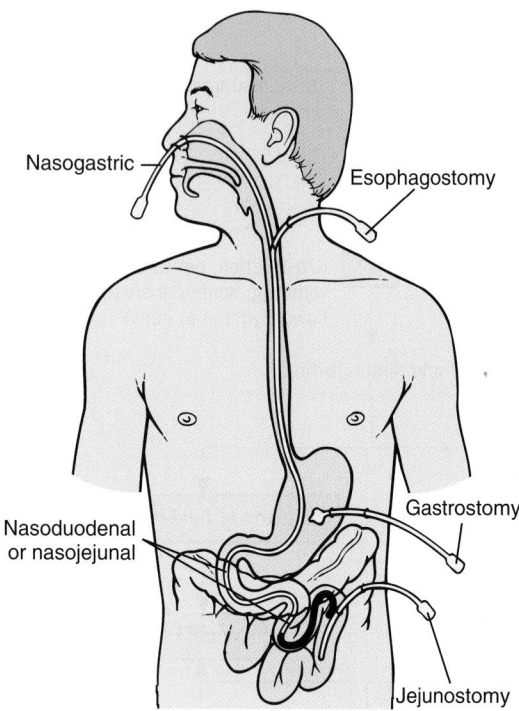

Figure 42-5 Common enteral feeding tube placement locations.

Source: Adapted from Mahan, L. K., Escott-Stump, S., & Raymond, J. L. (2012). *Krause's food and the nutrition care process* (13th ed., p. 309, Figure 14-2). Philadelphia: Saunders.

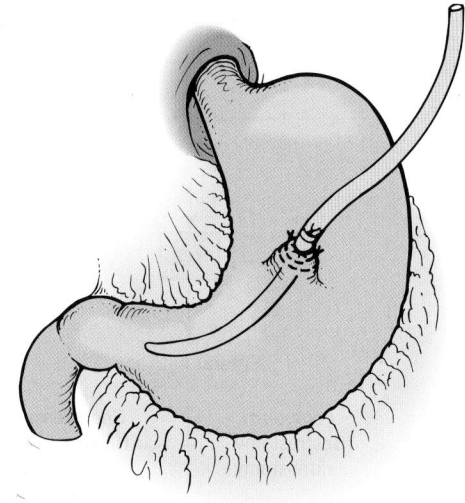

Figure 42-6 Placement of a gastrostomy tube.

Source: Redrawn from Mahan, L. K., & Arlin, M. (1992). *Krause's food, nutrition, and diet therapy* (8th ed.). Philadelphia: Saunders.

jejunostomy tube with continuous feedings may be appropriate to reduce the risk of aspiration (Bankhead et al., 2009).

Gastrostomy tubes can be placed surgically, fluoroscopically, laparoscopically, or endoscopically. The placement of a percutaneous endoscopic gastrostomy (PEG) tube is shown in Figure 42-7. The patient must have an intact, unobstructed GI tract, and the esophageal lumen must be wide enough to pass the endoscope for PEG tube placement. A PEG tube and a radiologically placed gastrostomy tube have several advantages. These procedures have fewer risks than surgical placement. Because they require no general anaesthesia and minimum sedation of the patient, these techniques can be done at a lower cost.

Enteral feedings can be started within 24 to 48 hours after a surgically placed gastrostomy or jejunostomy tube without waiting for flatus or a bowel movement and within 2 hours of insertion of a PEG tube, although this may be institution specific (Bankhead & Fang, 2007). The feeding tube is then marked at the skin insertion site, although many tubes are premarked. At regular intervals, the tube insertion length should be rechecked. The tube is most often connected to a pump for continuous feeding.

Procedures for Tube Feedings.
The following evidence-informed principles are based on the American Society for Parenteral and Enteral Nutrition's (ASPEN's) Enteral Nutrition Practice Recommendations (Bankhead et al., 2009).

1. *Patient position.* Elevate the head of bed to a minimum of 30 degrees, but preferably 45 degrees to prevent aspiration. A reverse Trendelenburg position can be used to elevate the head of the bed, unless contraindicated, when a back rest elevation is not tolerated. If it is necessary to lower the head

of the bed for a procedure, return the patient to an elevated position as soon as possible. Check institution policy for suspending feeding while the patient is supine. If intermittent delivery is used, the head should remain elevated for 30 to 60 minutes after feeding.

2. *Patency of tube.* Flush feeding tubes with 30 mL of water every 4 hours during continuous feeding or before and after intermittent feeding. Feeding tubes should also be flushed with 30 mL of water after residual volume measurements. Use sterile water for tube flushes in immunocompromised or critically ill patients, especially when the safety of tap water cannot be reasonably assumed. Sterile water is also recommended for use before and after medication administration via a feeding tube. Feeding pumps are equipped with alarms to indicate when the tube occluded. If no pump is available, monitor the drip rate frequently so that blockage does not occur from the patient lying on the tubing inadvertently or from too slow a drip rate.

3. *Tube position.* Obtain radiographic confirmation to determine whether a blindly placed NG or orogastric tube is properly positioned in the GI tract before administering feedings or medications. Smaller feeding tubes may be passed directly into the bronchus on insertion or may become dislodged and slip into the bronchus without any obvious respiratory manifestations. Do not rely on the auscultation method to differentiate between gastric and respiratory placement or to differentiate between gastric and small bowel placement. To determine whether a feeding tube has maintained the proper position, mark the exit site of the feeding tube at the time of the initial radiograph and observe for a change in the external tube length during feedings. If a significant increase in the external length is observed, use other bedside tests to help determine whether the tube has become dislocated. When in doubt, obtain a radiograph to determine tube location.

4. *Aspiration risk.* Evaluate enterally fed patients for risk of aspiration. Before starting feedings, ensure that the tube is in the proper position. Maintain head-of-bed elevation as described previously. Checking gastric residual volumes may be important when feedings are administered into the stomach

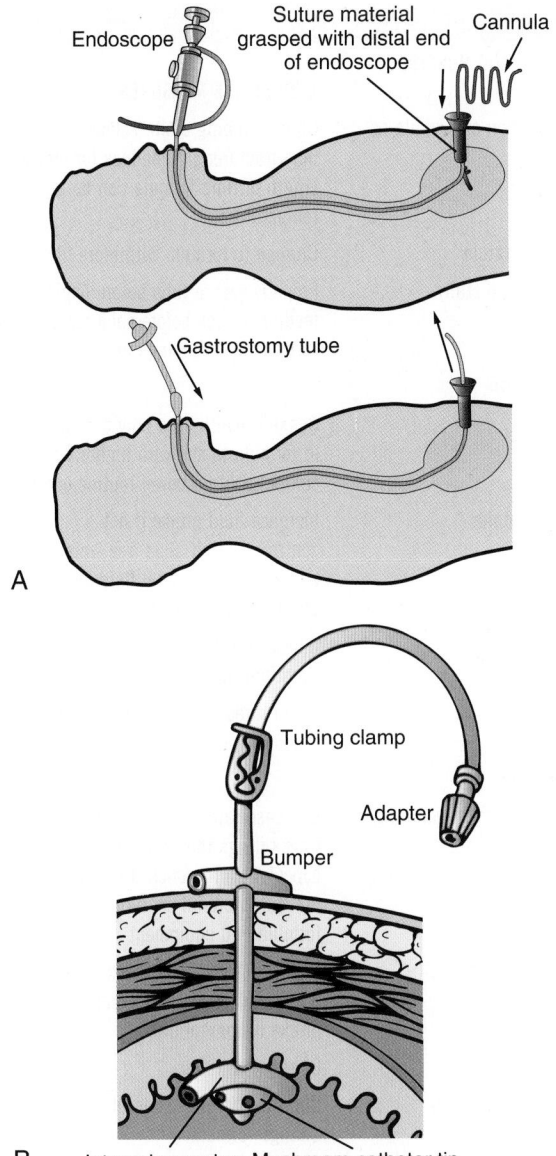

Figure 42-7 Percutaneous endoscopic gastrostomy.
A, Gastrostomy tube placement via percutaneous endoscopy. Using endoscopy, a gastrostomy tube is inserted through the esophagus into the stomach and then pulled through a stab wound made in the abdominal wall. **B,** A bumper secures the tube.

Source: Redrawn from Mahan, L. K., & Arlin, M. (1992). *Krause's food, nutrition, and diet therapy* (8th ed.). Philadelphia: Saunders.

(frequency of this assessment should be done per facility policy). To date, no adequately powered studies have demonstrated a relationship between aspiration pneumonia and gastric residual volumes. Current research suggests elevated gastric residue volumes "by themselves have little clinical meaning and that only when combined with vomiting, sepsis, sedation, or the need for pressor agents does the correlation with worsening patient outcome emerge" (Boullatta, Neimen, & Guenter, 2010, p. 279). Gastric residual volume can be affected by the type of tube inserted, tube bore (French) size, the position of the feeding tube's port in the gastric atrium, and the patient's position. Further, the presence of high

gastric residue volume may be a symptom of delayed gastric emptying (Boullatta et al., 2010).

Check gastric residual volumes every 4 hours during the first 48 hours for gastrically fed patients. After the enteral feeding goal rate is achieved, gastric residual monitoring may be decreased to every 6 to 8 hours in non–critically ill patients or continued every 4 hours in critically ill patients. (Corrective measures for residual volume are described in Table 42-8.)

Feeding tubes may need to be placed below the ligament of Treitz (jejunostomy) when gastric residual volumes consistently measure greater than 500 mL. Do not obtain residual volumes for EN delivered through a jejunostomy tube.

5. *Formula.* The use of a sterile, polymeric liquid EN formula is preferred to powdered or reconstituted formula. Formulas that are reconstituted in advance should be immediately refrigerated and discarded if unused within 24 hours of preparation. Powdered, reconstituted formulas should have a 4-hour hang time. Closed-system EN formulas can hang for 24 to 48 hours per manufacturer's guidelines. Sterile, decanted formula should have an 8-hour hang time. When starting a patient on EN, a full-strength isotonic commercial formula is preferred for initial feeding. Diluting the formula with water is not necessary and may increase the risk of diarrhea from microbial contamination. Ready-made, commercial formulas are preferable over blenderized foods for small-lumen tubes because of the lower risk of tube clogging, completeness of nutrition, and decreased risk of formula contamination.

Give the feeding at room or body temperature to decrease the likelihood of diarrhea and other GI complaints. The pleasurable aspects of eating, such as smelling, seeing, tasting, and chewing the food, are frequently denied the tube-fed patient. If the clinical condition permits, the patient may be allowed to smell, taste, and even chew small amounts of food before the feeding, and then the chewed food must be spit out.

6. *Administration of feeding.* The use of disposable gloves is recommended during setup and administration of EN. Feedings are administered either by the gravity drip method, by syringe, or by a feeding pump. The feeding rate or volume is increased gradually for 24 to 48 hours to minimize adverse effects, such as nausea or diarrhea. Gravity drip methods include bolus and intermittent feedings. Bolus feedings are typically delivered by gravity via a syringe over approximately 15 minutes when the feeding tube is placed in the stomach. A feeding container or bag is used for intermittent feedings and the volume is infused usually over 30 to 45 minutes either by gravity or with an enteral feeding pump. An enteral infusion pump is recommended for small bowel feedings and required for continuous feeding. Enteral feeding pumps should be routinely calibrated to ensure accuracy. It is important to remember that the patient still needs water (1 mL/cal formula received), and this may be administered with flush water or as additional boluses of water as tolerated.

7. *Medication administration.* Before giving medications, the enteral feeding formula should be stopped and the tube flushed with at least 15 mL of water. Dilute the medication as appropriate and administer via the feeding tube using a clean oral syringe (≥30 mL in size). Flush the tube again with at least 15 mL of water, taking into account the patient's volume status. Mixing medications with enteral feeding formula should be avoided. It may result in reduced drug absorption or increased risk of tube occlusion and is a

Table 42-8 Common Problems of Patients Receiving Tube Feedings

PROBLEMS AND POSSIBLE CAUSES	CORRECTIVE MEASURES	PROBLEMS AND POSSIBLE CAUSES	CORRECTIVE MEASURES
Vomiting and Aspiration		Contamination of formula or tubing	Change tubing q24h. Follow manufacturer's guidelines for maximum length of time formula can be at room temperature.
Improper tube placement	Replace tube in proper position. Check tube position before beginning feeding and q8h if feedings are continuous.	Low-fibre formula	Change to formula with more fibre.
Delayed gastric emptying, increased residual volume	Hold feeding 1 hr; then, if residual volume is less than before, resume feeding.	Tube moving distally	Properly secure tube before beginning feeding. Check before each feeding or at least q24h if feedings are continuous.
Aspiration risk	Keep head of bed elevated to 30- to 45-degree angle. Have patient sit up on side of bed or in chair. Encourage ambulation unless contraindicated.	**Constipation**	
		Low fibre	Consult health care provider for change in formula to one with higher fibre content. Obtain bowel routine order.
Contamination of formula	Refrigerate unused formula and record date opened. Discard outdated formula every 24 hr. Discard formula left standing for longer than manufacturer's guidelines: 8-12 hr for ready-to-feed formulas (cans) or 4 hr for reconstituted formula or closed system as per manufactures guidelines.	Poor fluid intake	Increase fluid intake if not contraindicated. Give free water, as well as formula. Give total fluid intake of 30 mL/kg body weight.
		Medications	Check for medications that may be constipating.
Diarrhea		Impaction	Perform rectal examinations to check and manually remove feces if present.
Feeding too fast, hypertonic formula, or medications	Evaluate number and volume of stools (if greater than three to five per day or >500 mL), consider patient's medical history, and assess abdomen for distension or pain. Contact physician, consider medications, and rule out infection (Clostridium difficile).	**Dehydration**	
		Excessive diarrhea, vomiting	Decrease rate or change formula. Check drugs that patient is receiving, especially antibiotics. Take care to prevent bacterial contamination of formula and equipment.
	Decrease rate of feeding. Change to continuous drip feedings. Check for drugs that may cause diarrhea (e.g., antibiotics).	Poor fluid intake	Increase intake and check amount and number of feedings. Increase amount of intake if appropriate.
		High-protein formula	Change formula.
		Hyperosmotic diuresis	Check blood glucose levels frequently. Change formula.

potential source of bacterial contamination. If giving more than one medication via an enteral feeding tube, separately dilute and administer each medication. Use liquid dosage forms when available and if appropriate. When liquid dosages are not available, only use immediate-release solid-dosage forms. Each tablet should be ground to a fine powder and mixed with sterile water before administration. Open hard gelatin capsules and mix the powder/liquid/beads with sterile water. Be aware that hyperosmolar medications delivered directly into the small intestine can increase the risk of GI distress and diarrhea.

8. *General nursing considerations.* Weigh the patient daily or several times a week, and maintain accurate intake and output records. Initially, blood glucose checks to assess glucose tolerance are performed at the bedside. An older patient who has baseline glucose intolerance is particularly at risk for hyperglycemia. Label feedings with the date and time that they are initially hung and clearly label "not for intravenous use." Enteral feeding sets (tubing and container) should be changed every 24 hours for open-system enteral feedings and per manufacturer's guidelines for closed-system feedings.

Complications Related to Tubes and Feedings.
The types of problems encountered in patients receiving tube feedings and corrective measures are presented in Table 42-8. When commercial products are used, the concentration, flavour, osmolarity, and amounts of protein, sodium, and fat vary according to the manufacturer. All commercial enteral formulas are lactose free. The concentrations range from 1 to 2 kcal/mL, with most between 1 and 1.5 kcal/mL.

The osmolality of the solution is determined by the number and size of particles in solution. The more hydrolyzed or broken down the nutrients, the greater the osmolality. Formulas are selected based on the individual patient's needs. The more calorically dense the formula, the less water it contains. Extra fluids may be provided through the feeding tube or, if permitted, by mouth. Tube feedings with high-sodium content maybe contraindicated in the patient with cardiovascular problems, such as heart failure. High-fat content is not advocated for a patient with short bowel syndrome or ileocecal resections because of impaired fat absorption.

With regard to EN (and nutrition in general), the dietitian is an important health care team member. Some institutions

Table 42-9 Nursing Management: Feeding Tubes

1. Check tube placement before feeding and before each drug administration.
2. Assess for bowel sounds before feeding.
3. Use liquid medications rather than pills, as appropriate.
   - Dilute viscous liquid medications.
   - Check to see if medications are intended to be taken with meals.
   - Avoid adding medications to enteral feeding formula.
4. If it is necessary to use tablets, be sure to crush drugs to a fine powder to prevent clogging feeding tubes.
5. Follow general principles of tube feeding (e.g., bed elevation, checking gastric residual volume, and flushing tube with water).
6. Assess regularly for complications (e.g., aspiration, diarrhea, abdominal distension, hyperglycemia, constipation, and fecal impaction).

EVIDENCE-INFORMED PRACTICE
Do Antibiotics Prevent Infection From Percutaneous Endoscopic Gastrostomy Tubes?

Clinical Question
For patients with PEG tubes (P), do prophylactic antibiotics (I) versus placebo or no intervention (C) reduce infections (O) after tube placement (T)?

Best Available Evidence
Systematic review of randomized controlled trials (RCTs)

Critical Appraisal and Synthesis of Evidence
- 10 RCTs (n = 1100) examining patients undergoing PEG placement and followed for 30 days.
- Risk of infection decreased by 19% when prophylactic antibiotics were used.

Conclusion
- Administration of systemic prophylactic antibiotics for PEG placement reduces risk of infection at the insertion site.

Implications for Nursing Practice
- Consult with endoscopist before PEG placement for antibiotic prophylaxis orders.
- Ensure that first dose of antibiotic is administered before skin incision.

Reference for Evidence
Lipp, A., & Lusardi, G. (2008). A systematic review of prophylactic antimicrobials in PEG placement, *Journal of Clinical Nursing*, 18(7), 938. doi:10.1111/j.1365-2702.2008.02585.x

PEG, percutaneous endoscopic gastrostomy; *PICO: P*, patient population of interest; *I*, intervention or area of interest; *C*, comparison of interest or comparison group; *O*, outcome(s) of interest; *RCTs*, randomized controlled trials; *T*, timing (see pp. 7-8).

have nutrition support teams composed of a physician, nurse, dietitian, and pharmacist whose function is to oversee the nutrition support of select inpatients and outpatients.

In patients receiving gastrostomy or jejunostomy feeding, be alert to two possible problems: (1) skin irritation and (2) pulling out of the tube. Skin care around the tube site is important because the action of the digestive juices is irritating to the skin. Assess the skin around the feeding tube daily for signs of redness and maceration. To keep the skin clean and dry, initially rinse it with sterile water and then dry it. Once the site has healed, it can be washed with mild soap and water. A protective ointment (zinc oxide, petroleum gauze) or a skin barrier (flange) may be used on the skin around the tube. Place a small dressing around the tube until the site is healed and change it promptly if it gets wet. Other types of drain or tube pouches may be used if there is a problem with skin irritation. An enterostomal therapist can provide great assistance if these issues arise. Teach the patient and caregiver how to care for the feeding tube. Accidental tube removal by the patient or caregiver can result in delayed feedings as well as potential discomfort with tube replacement. Teaching should include skin care, care of the tube, and complete information about feeding administration and potential complications. Nursing management of feeding tubes is summarized in Table 42-9.

An *enteral feeding misconnection* is an inadvertent connection between an enteral feeding system and a nonenteral system such as an intravascular line, a peritoneal dialysis catheter, or a tracheostomy tube cuff (Guenter et al., 2008). With an enteral feeding misconnection, nutritional formula intended for administration into the GI tract is administered via the wrong route, resulting in serious and potentially life-threatening patient complications. Nursing interventions aimed at decreasing the risk of enteral feeding misconnections are found in Table 42-10. (See also Nursing Care Plan [NCP] 42-1 for patients receiving EN.)

AGE-RELATED CONSIDERATIONS: ENTERAL FEEDS

EN strategies, including NG, nasointestinal, and gastrostomy feedings, are often used in the older patient to improve nutritional status. Because of physiological changes associated with aging, the older adult is more vulnerable to complications associated with nutrition interventions, especially fluid and electrolyte imbalances. Complications such as diarrhea can leave the patient dehydrated. Decreased thirst perception or impaired cognitive function decreases the ability of the patient to seek additional fluids.

With aging, there is decreased ability to handle glucose loads (glucose intolerance). As a result, the older patient may be susceptible to problems of hyperglycemia in response to the high-carbohydrate load of some enteral feeding formulas. If the older adult has compromised cardiovascular function (e.g., heart failure), there may be a decreased ability to handle large volumes of formula. In this situation, the use of more concentrated formulas (2.0 kcal/mL) may be warranted. The older adult also is at increased risk for aspiration caused by gastroesophageal reflux disease, delayed gastric emptying, hiatal hernia, or poor oral hygiene. Physical mobility, fine motor movement, and visual system changes associated with aging may contribute to difficulties in managing EN.

Table 42-10 Nursing Management: Decrease Risk of Enteral Feeding Misconnections

1. Teach visitors and nonclinical staff to notify nurse if an enteral feeding line becomes disconnected.

2. Teach visitors and nonclinical staff not to reconnect enteral feeding lines.

3. Do not modify or adapt IV or feeding devices, because this may compromise the safety features incorporated into their design.

4. When making a reconnection, the nurse should routinely trace lines back to their origins and then ensure that they are secure.

5. When patient arrives on a new unit or setting or during shift-to-shift handoff, nurses should recheck connections and trace all tubes.

6. Route tubes and catheters that have different purposes in unique and standardized directions (e.g., IV lines should be routed toward the patient's head, enteral lines should be routed toward the feet).

7. Package together all parts needed for enteral feeding and reduce the availability of additional adapters and connectors. This will minimize the availability of dissimilar tubes or catheters that could be improperly connected.

8. Label or colour-code feeding tubes and connectors, and educate staff about the labelling or colour-coding process in the institution's enteral feeding system.

9. Be sure to identify and confirm the solution's label, because a three-in-one parenteral nutrition solution can appear similar to an enteral nutrition formulation bag. Label the bags with large, bold statements such as "WARNING! For Enteral Use Only—NOT for IV Use."

10. Ensure that all connections are made under proper lighting conditions.

IV, intravenous.
Source: Adapted from Guenter, P., Hicks, R. W., Simmons, D., Crowley, J., Joseph, S., Croteau, R., ..., Vanderveen, T. W. (2008). Enteral feeding misconnections: A consortium position statement. *The Joint Commission Journal on Quality and Patient Safety, 34*(5), 289-290. Retrieved from *https://www.premierinc.com/safety/topics/tubing-misconnections/downloads/S5-JQPS-05-08-guenter.pdf*

Parenteral Nutrition

When the GI tract cannot be used for the ingestion, digestion, and absorption of essential nutrients, PN may be an alternative. **Parenteral nutrition (PN)** refers to the administration of nutrients by a route other than the GI tract (e.g., the bloodstream). PN has become a relatively safe and practical method of delivering nutritional needs. The goal of using PN is to meet the patient's nutritional needs. One form of PN is **total parenteral nutrition (TPN)**, the delivery of a nutritionally adequate hypertonic solution consisting of glucose, protein hydrolysates, minerals, and vitamins, using an intravenous route. *PN* is the correct term to use when a client is being fed via the vein any portion of their estimated nutrition needs or a component, e.g., carbohydrates and protein, but no lipids. *TPN* is the delivery of 100% of a patient's calculated nutritional requirements (carbohydrate, fat, protein, vitamins, minerals and often fluid). It is important to understand that a client receiving PN is not necessarily receiving 100% of his or her nutritional needs via that route.

Regular IV solutions of 5% dextrose (5 g dextrose/100 mL) in water (D5W) or 5% dextrose in lactated Ringer's solution contain no protein and have approximately 170 cal/L. The normal adult requires a minimum of 1200 to 1500 cal/day to carry out normal physiological functions. Patients who sustain severe injury, surgery, or burns and those who are malnourished as a result of medical treatment or disease processes have greatly increased nutritional needs. The volume of regular dextrose solutions needed to meet these high-caloric requirements could exceed the capacity of the cardiovascular system. Table 42-11 lists common indications for the use of PN.

Composition. Commercially prepared PN base solutions are available. These base solutions contain dextrose and protein in the form of amino acids. The pharmacy adds the prescribed electrolytes (e.g., sodium, potassium, chloride, calcium, magnesium, phosphate), vitamins, and trace elements (e.g., zinc, copper, chromium, manganese) to customize the solution for the needs of the patient. A three-in-one or total nutrient admixture containing an IV fat emulsion, dextrose, and amino acids is widely used.

Calories. Calories in PN are supplied primarily by carbohydrates in the form of dextrose and by fat in the form of fat emulsion. The administration of between 100 and 150 g of dextrose (1 g provides ~3.4 cal, as opposed to oral carbohydrates, which provide 4 cal) daily may have a protein-sparing effect. Adequate nonprotein calories in the form of glucose and fat must be provided to allow metabolism of amino acids for wound healing and not as energy. However, overfeeding can lead to metabolic complications. To minimize these problems, an energy intake of 25 to 35 cal/kg/day in a nonobese patient is often recommended.

The U.S. Food and Drug Administration (FDA) has approved the use of 10%, 20%, and 30% fat-emulsion solutions. Fat emulsions provide approximately 1.1 cal/mL (10% solution) or 2 cal/mL (20% solution). Thirty-percent fat-emulsion formulation is approved only for compounding of total nutrient admixture, not for direct IV administration (ASPEN, 2009). The contents of fat emulsion are primarily mixes of soybean or safflower oils with egg phospholipids added as an emulsifier. The maximum fat emulsion amount should not exceed a dose of 2.5 g/kg/day (Mirtallo, Dasta, Kleinschmidt, & Varon, 2010), and it should be administered slowly over 12 to 24 hours (Mirtallo et al., 2004). The preferred delivery method is a continuous low volume, such as 20% lipids delivered over 12 hours, depending on patient needs. Adverse reactions that can occur include allergic manifestations, dyspnea, cyanosis, fever, flushing, phlebitis, chest and back pain, and pain at the IV site. A major benefit derived from IV fat administration is that a large number of calories can be provided in a relatively small amount of fluid. This is especially beneficial when the patient is at risk for fluid overload.

Critically ill patients may not tolerate this dose, and close monitoring of triglyceride levels may be indicated. It is becoming more common to administer lipid-free PN for the first 3 to 5 days of critical illness (ASPEN, 2009). Nausea, vomiting, and elevated temperature have been reported, especially when lipids are infused quickly. The administration of fat emulsion is contraindicated in the patient with a disturbance in fat metabolism. It should also be used with caution in the patient who is in danger of fat embolism (e.g., fractured femur) and the patient with an allergy to eggs.

Protein. The normal healthy person of average body size needs approximately 45 to 65 g (0.8-1 g/kg/day) of protein daily. Protein should be provided at the rate of 1 to 1.5 g/kg/day

NURSING CARE PLAN 42-1

Enteral Nutrition

NURSING DIAGNOSIS	**Imbalanced nutrition: less than body requirements** *related to* inability to ingest food owing to physiological or psychological factors *as evidenced by* body weight at least 20% less than ideal, pale conjunctivae and mucous membranes, poor muscle tone
Expected Patient Outcomes	**Nursing Interventions and *Rationales***
• Achieves adequate nutritional status	**Nutrition therapy**
	• In collaboration with the dietitian, determine the number of calories and types of nutrients needed *to meet nutrition requirements.*
	• Determine need for enteral tube feedings.
	• Administer enteral feedings.
	• Discontinue use of tube feedings as oral intake is tolerated.
	Enteral tube feeding
	• Monitor weight three times a week initially, decreasing to once a month, *to make adjustments as needed in calorie intake.*
	• Monitor for presence of bowel regularity including for constipation and/or diarrhea.
	• Refrigerate open containers of enteral feed *to prevent bacterial growth.*
	• Discard enteral feeding containers and administration sets q24 hr *because they can become contaminated over time.*
NURSING DIAGNOSIS	**Risk for aspiration** *related to* enteral tube and tube feedings
Expected Patient Outcomes	**Nursing Interventions and *Rationales***
• Experiences no aspiration	**Enteral tube feeding**
	• Verify residuals q4-6h for the first 24 hr, then q8h during continuous feedings *to validate gastric emptying.*
	• Assess patient for abdominal distension, nausea, and vomiting *because these may be signs of gastric retention.*
	• Elevate head of the bed 30-45 degrees during feedings *to minimize the risk of aspiration.*
	• Complete oral care *to reduce the risk of aspiration of oropharyngeal secretions.*
	• Discontinue feedings 30-60 min before putting patient in a head-down position *to minimize risk of aspiration.*
NURSING DIAGNOSIS	**Risk for deficient fluid volume** *related to* diarrhea or inadequate water intake
Expected Patient Outcomes	**Nursing Interventions and *Rationales***
• Maintains adequate fluid volume	**Fluid/electrolyte management**
	• Assess patient's buccal membranes, sclerae, and skin for indications of altered fluid and electrolyte balance (e.g., dryness, cyanosis) *to identify signs of fluid volume deficit.*
	• Provide free water with tube feedings *to compensate for high-concentration enteral feedings.*
	Diarrhea management
	• Identify factors (e.g., medications, bacteria, tube feeding formula) that may cause or contribute to diarrhea.
	Enteral tube feeding
	• Check gravity drip rate or pump rate every hour *to maintain adequate fluid intake.*
	• Slow tube feeding rate and/or decrease strength *to control diarrhea.*
	• Irrigate the tube q4-6h during continuous feedings and after every intermittent feeding *to provide free water.*

Table 42-11 Common Indications for Parenteral Nutrition

- Chronic severe diarrhea and vomiting
- Complicated surgery or trauma
- Gastrointestinal obstruction
- Gastrointestinal tract anomalies and fistulas
- Intractable diarrhea
- Severe anorexia nervosa
- Severe malabsorption
- Short bowel syndrome

depending on the patient's needs. In a nutritionally depleted patient who is also under the stress of illness or surgery, protein requirements can exceed 150 g/day to ensure a positive nitrogen balance. In the most recent guidelines, protein intake levels of 1.5 to 2 g/kg/day are suggested for most patients who are experiencing moderate to severe stress (Bankhead et al., 2009).

Electrolytes. The assessment of individual requirements should take place daily at the beginning of therapy and then several times a week as the treatment progresses. The following are ranges for average daily electrolyte requirements for adult patients without renal or hepatic impairment (Mirtallo et al., 2004).

Sodium: 1 to 2 mEq/kg
Potassium: 1 to 2 mEq/kg
Chloride: as needed to maintain acid–base balance
Magnesium: 8 to 20 mEq
Calcium: 10 to 15 mEq
Phosphate: 20 to 40 mmol

The exact amount of electrolytes needed depends on the patient's health problem and on electrolyte levels as determined by blood testing.

Vitamins. Commercially available vitamin products for PN include single and mixtures of both fat and water-soluble vitamins. The daily addition of a multivitamin preparation to the PN generally meets the vitamin requirements.

Trace Elements. Zinc, copper, chromium, manganese, selenium, molybdenum, and iodine supplements may be added according to the patient's condition and needs. Levels of these elements are monitored in the patient receiving PN. The health care provider may order additional amounts of these elements to be added to the solutions according to the patient's requirements.

Methods of Administration.
PN may be administered as central parenteral nutrition (CPN) or peripheral parenteral nutrition (PPN). Both CPN and PPN are used in a patient who is not a candidate for EN.

Central Parenteral Nutrition. CPN is indicated when long-term support is necessary or when the patient has high protein and caloric requirements. CPN may be given through a central venous catheter that originates at the subclavian or jugular vein and whose tip lies in the superior vena cava (see Figure 42-8). It can also be given using peripherally inserted central catheters (PICCs) that are placed into the basilic or cephalic vein

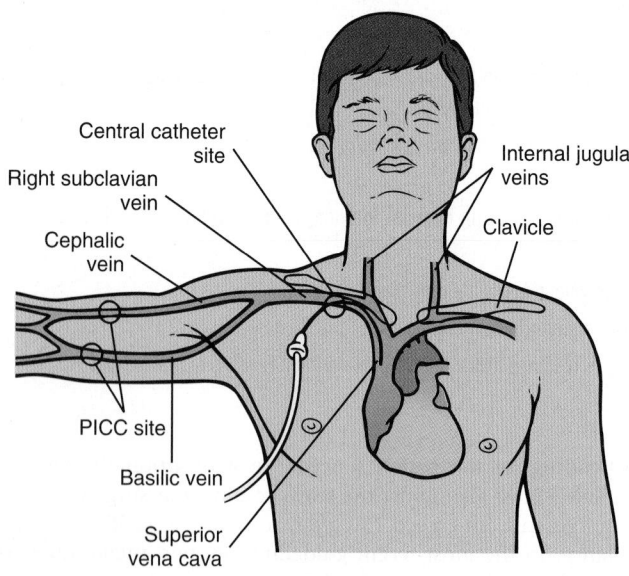

Figure 42-8 Placement of a catheter for central parenteral nutrition using the subclavian vein. Peripherally inserted central catheters (PICCs) are inserted using the basilic or the cephalic vein.

Source: Redrawn from Mahan, L. K., & Arlin, M. (1992). *Krause's food, nutrition, and diet therapy* (8th ed.). Philadelphia: Saunders.

and then advanced into the distal end of the superior vena cava (see Figure 42-8).

Peripheral Parenteral Nutrition. PPN is administered through a peripherally inserted catheter or vascular access device, which uses a large vein. PPN is used when (1) nutritional support is needed for only a short time, (2) protein and caloric requirements are not high, (3) the risk of a central catheter is too great, or (4) PN is used to supplement inadequate oral intake.

Comparison of Central and Peripheral Parenteral Nutrition. CPN and PPN differ in tonicity, which is measured in milliosmoles (mOsm; the concentration of particles in a fluid). Blood is isotonic and measures approximately 280 mOsm/L. The standard IV solutions of D5W and normal saline are essentially isotonic. CPN solutions are hypertonic, measuring at least 1600 mOsm/L. The high-glucose content ranges from 20 to 50%. CPN must be infused in a large central vein so that rapid dilution can occur. The use of a peripheral vein for CPN would cause irritation and thrombophlebitis. Nutrients can be infused using smaller volumes than PPN. PPN is hypertonic (typically using 10% glucose), but less so than CPN, and can be safely administered through a large peripheral vein, although phlebitis can occur. Another potential complication of PPN is fluid overload.

Catheter Placement. The central placement of the catheter into a large main vein for PN is performed by a physician. The vein most commonly used is the subclavian, although the innominate or jugular vein may be used. The procedure is the same as for the insertion of a central venous pressure line and is done under strict aseptic conditions.

A standard isotonic IV solution is infused through the central line until radiographic imaging confirms proper placement of the catheter tip in the superior vena cava and not in the jugular vein. The catheter insertion site is covered with a sterile dressing. The date is marked on the dressing.

Placement of a PICC is done under sterile conditions. A baseline measurement of the upper arm circumference is recommended. A tourniquet is then placed around the upper arm near the axilla to allow examination of the antecubital fossa and selection of a vein. If possible, the patient should be supine with the arm straight and at a 90-degree angle. Preparation of the insertion site should be done according to institutional policy. The sterile catheter is cut to the predetermined length, depending on the vein selected.

A local anaesthetic is usually used at the insertion site. This site should be cleaned, protected, and maintained according to institutional policy. As with the centrally placed line, a chest radiograph study is needed to verify proper tip placement before administering any PN solution. Proper placement of a catheter for CPN is illustrated in Figure 42-8. Complications frequently associated with catheter placement are hemorrhage, hydrothorax and pneumothorax, hemothorax, air embolus, and venous thrombosis. Once established for PN, a single-lumen central catheter should not be used for the administration of blood or antibiotics, the drawing of blood samples, or the monitoring of central venous pressure.

Administration of Solution. All PN solutions are prepared using strict aseptic techniques under a laminar flow hood. Nothing should be added to PN solutions after they are prepared in the pharmacy. The danger of drug incompatibilities and contamination is high. The fewer the personnel involved in the

Table 42-12 Complications of Parenteral Nutrition

Infection

- Fungal
- Gram-positive bacteria
- Gram-negative bacteria

Metabolic

- Hyperglycemia; hypoglycemia; and hyperosmolar, hyperglycemic state
- Prerenal azotemia
- Essential fatty acid deficiency
- Electrolyte and vitamin excesses and deficiencies
- Trace mineral deficiencies
- Dyslipidemia

Mechanical

- Insertion
- Air embolus
- Pneumothorax, hemothorax, and hydrothorax
- Hemorrhage
- Dislodgement
- Thrombosis of great vein
- Phlebitis

preparation and administration of PN, the lower the risk of infection. In most hospitals, PN solutions are ordered daily. In this way, the solution and additives can be adjusted to the patient's current needs. Each PN solution label indicates the nutrient content, all additives, the time mixed, and the date and time of expiration. In general, solutions are stable for 24 hours and must be refrigerated until a half hour before use.

Because PN solutions are excellent media for microbial growth, it is essential that proper aseptic techniques be followed. The FDA recommends that a 0.22-micron Millipore filter be placed on parenteral solutions not containing fat emulsion and a 1.2-micron filter be placed on solutions containing fat emulsion (Mirtallo et al., 2004). Filters and IV tubing are changed every 24 hours if PN with lipids is being administered and every 72 hours for PN with amino acids and dextrose (Gillies et al., 2005). The tubing and the filter should be clearly labelled with the date and the time they are put into use. Complications of PN can be divided into three categories: (1) infectious, (2) metabolic, and (3) mechanical. The major complications of each category are presented in Table 42-12.

To control the rate of infusion, PPN solutions should be administered with a volumetric controller and a pump is used for CPN solutions. If a PN formula bag should empty before the next solution is available, a 10 or 20% dextrose solution (based on the amount of dextrose in the CPN solution) or D5W solution (based on the amount of dextrose in the PPN solution) may be administered to prevent hypoglycemia.

NURSING MANAGEMENT: PARENTERAL NUTRITION

Monitor initial vital signs every 4 to 8 hours in the patient receiving PN. Daily weights provide an indication of the patient's hydration status as therapy progresses. Body weight is considered the sum of the changes in protein, fat, and water. On a daily basis, body water fluctuates more than protein or fat. Analysis must be made of whether gains or losses in weight are caused by fluid gained from edema, fluid lost through diuresis, or actual increase or decrease in tissue weight. Blood levels of glucose, electrolytes, and urea nitrogen; a complete blood count; and hepatic enzyme studies are followed a minimum of three times per week until stable and then weekly as the patient's condition warrants. Assessment of these important values assists the nurse in evaluating the patient's tolerance of PN.

Change dressings covering the catheter site according to institutional protocol, ranging from every other day to once a week. The procedure for changing the dressing is similar to that followed after catheter insertion. Carefully observe the catheter site for signs of inflammation and infection. Phlebitis can readily occur in the vein because of a hypertonic infusion, and the area can become infected. The patient receiving PN may be immunosuppressed and, thus, more susceptible to opportunistic infections. In this patient, signs of inflammation or infection can be subtle, if present at all. Some patients receiving PN may also be receiving chemotherapy, corticosteroids, or antibiotics, which can mask signs of infection. If an infection is suspected during a dressing change, a culture specimen of the site and drainage should be sent for analysis, and the health care provider should be notified immediately.

Hyperglycemia can be metabolic complication of PN in both those with and those without diabetes. Uncontrolled hyperglycemia may result in hyperglycemia hyperosmolar syndrome, coma and possible death owing to osmotic diuresis. An increase in blood glucose is expected on initiation of PN. To avoid hyperglycemia at initiation of PN, PN infusion rates are gradually increased in the first 24 hours. To assess for tolerance of PN initiation, blood glucose levels should be checked every 4 to 6 hours at the bedside with a blood glucose meter (see Chapter 46). Blood glucose targets will vary based on the patient's health status and co-morbid conditions. Tight glycemic control may be contraindicated owing to the risk for hypoglycemia. Regular or rapid-acting insulin or insulin as per an institutional algorithm (sliding scale) may be ordered to manage blood glucose levels (National Institute for Health and Clinical Excellence, 2006). (Care of the patient receiving PN is summarized in NCP 42-2.)

Re-feeding syndrome is characterized by fluid retention, electrolyte imbalances (hypophosphatemia, hypokalemia, hypomagnesemia), and hyperglycemia. Conditions that predispose patients to re-feeding syndrome include longstanding malnutrition states such as chronic alcoholism, vomiting and diarrhea, chemotherapy, and major surgery. Re-feeding syndrome can occur any time a malnourished patient is started on aggressive nutritional support. Hypophosphatemia is the hallmark of re-feeding syndrome and is associated with serious outcomes, including cardiac dysrhythmias, respiratory arrest, and neurological disturbances (e.g., paresthesias).

Before setting up and administering PN, check the label and ingredients in the solution to see that they match the PN order. Also examine the solution for leaks, colour changes, particulate matter, clarity, and fat emulsion cracking. If any of these abnormalities are suspected, promptly return it to the pharmacy for replacement. It is the nurse's responsibility to ensure that the PN solution is discontinued and replaced with a new solution if the bag is not empty at the end of 24 hours. At room temperature, the solution, especially when containing fat emulsion, is a medium for microorganism growth.

NURSING CARE PLAN 42-2

Parenteral Nutrition

NURSING DIAGNOSIS	***Risk for infection*** *related to* placement of a central venous access catheter, inadequate aseptic practices, and decreased defense mechanisms
Expected Patient Outcomes	**Nursing Interventions and *Rationales***
• Has no manifestations of infection • Has normal body temperature	• Use protocols for infusion of solution and tubing and filter changes; change occlusive dressing over catheter site according to institutional policy *to minimize the possibility of infection.* • Observe for signs of inflammation and infection; monitor vital signs q4h *to ensure early detection of infection.*
NURSING DIAGNOSIS	***Anxiety*** *related to* inability to ingest food and fluids; lack of knowledge regarding catheter position; benefits and management of PN as manifested by restlessness and apprehension; frequent questioning regarding care of catheter and PN line
Expected Patient Outcomes	**Nursing Interventions and *Rationales***
• Can state rationale for and demonstrate care of PN line	• Instruct patient on rationale and benefits of PN and care of line *because knowledge and facts may reduce anxiety.* • Illustrate catheter position by drawings and pictures *to increase patient understanding.*
Collaborative Problems	
Nursing Goals	**Nursing Interventions and *Rationales***
Potential complications of hyperglycemia, hypoglycemia, and electrolyte imbalances • Monitor blood glucose and serum electrolytes • Report deviations from acceptable parameters • Carry out medical and nursing interventions	• Monitor for signs of hyperglycemia such as thirst, polyuria, confusion, elevated blood glucose, blurred vision, dizziness, nausea and vomiting, and dehydration *to plan appropriate treatment.* • Monitor for signs of hypoglycemia such as sweating, hunger, weakness, and tremors *to ensure early intervention.* • Monitor serum electrolyte levels daily *to identify and treat complications early.* • Check for symptoms of hyperkalemia (e.g., muscle weakness, flaccid paralysis, cardiac dysrhythmias, abdominal cramps, diarrhea) and hypokalemia (e.g., general weakness, decreased muscle tone, weak or irregular pulse, low blood pressure, shallow respirations, abdominal distension, ileus).* • Maintain accurate infusion rate *to control the amount of glucose administered and prevent fluctuations in blood glucose levels.* • Never increase or decrease flow rate by more than 10% *to prevent fluctuations in blood glucose levels.†* • Never stop PN abruptly unless it is replaced by another glucose source *to prevent hypoglycemia.*

PN, parenteral nutrition.

*Other manifestations of electrolyte imbalances are discussed in Chapter 19.

†An infusion pump must be used during administration of PN so that the infusion rate can be maintained, and an alarm will sound if the tubing becomes obstructed. Even though an infusion pump is being used, the nurse should periodically check the volume infused because pump malfunctions can alter the rate.

Catheter-related infection and septicemia can occur in patients receiving PN. Local manifestations of infection include erythema, tenderness, and exudate at the catheter insertion site. Systemically, the patient may have fever, chills, nausea, vomiting, and malaise. If no other causes can be identified, a catheter-related infection is suspected. Because of the risk of infection, catheters with antibiotic or antiseptic surfaces may be used. To determine the causative organism, cultures are performed of the catheter tip if the catheter has been removed or if the blood in the catheter is still in place. Blood cultures are drawn simultaneously from the catheter and a peripheral vein. A chest radiograph is taken to detect changes in pulmonary status. When the catheter tip of a short-term catheter is the source of infection, antibiotic therapy may not be necessary because removal of the catheter can eliminate the problem (Zingg, Cartier-Fässler, & Walder, 2008). More permanent catheter-related infections may require antibiotics. A new central line may or may not be immediately placed depending on the patient's condition. When the PN therapy is completed and the catheter is removed, the dressing should be changed daily until the wound heals. Encourage oral nourishment and maintain a careful record of intake. A general rule is that 60% of caloric needs should be met orally before discontinuation of PN or EN.

▪ Home Nutrition Support

Home PN or EN is an accepted mode of nutritional therapy for the person who does not require hospitalization but who requires continued nutrition support. Some patients have been successfully treated at home for many months and even years. It is important for the nurse to educate the patient or caregiver about catheter or tube care, proper technique in mixing and handling of the solutions and tubing, and adverse effects and complications. The discharge planning team needs to be involved early in the admission to help plan for discharge. Home nutrition support may also be a burden on the patient and caregivers and may affect quality of life.

CLINICAL DECISION-MAKING EXERCISE

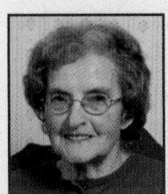

CASE STUDY:
Undernutrition

Source: © iStockphoto.com/Stan Rohrer.

Patient Profile

Mrs. Mary Smith is a 70-year-old White woman who is 162.5 cm tall and weighs 45.4 kg. She was recently admitted to the medical unit.

Subjective Data

- Reports 13.5-kg weight loss during past 2 months
- Has recently had a thrombotic stroke with hemiparesis and dysphagia
- Has had nothing by mouth for the past 24 hours and just started tube feedings
- Lives with her daughter, who is at her bedside

Objective Data
Physical Examination
- Has left-sided weakness
- Blood pressure is 150/90 mm Hg
- A percutaneous endoscopic gastrostomy (PEG) tube was recently placed

Laboratory Results
- Serum albumin 29 g/L
- Prealbumin 1.1 g/L

Discussion Questions

1. What are Mrs. Smith's risk factors for malnutrition?
2. What is her Malnutrition Screening Tool (MST) score?
3. What factors place her at risk for developing dysphagia?
4. What possible complications of tube feeding could Mrs. Smith be at risk for?
5. *Priority Decision:* What is the priority of the nursing care for Mrs. Smith?
6. *Priority Decision:* Based on the assessment data presented, what are the priority nutrition-related problems and the issues that the multidisciplinary team could collaborate on to improve Mrs. Smith's nutritional status?

evolve   *Answers are available at* **http://evolve.elsevier.com/ Canada/Lewis/medsurg**

REVIEW QUESTIONS

The number of the question corresponds to the same-numbered objective at the beginning of the chapter.

1. Which of the following reflects acceptable macronutrient ranges for adults (≥19 yr) as described in Canada's Food Guide?
   a. 10-20% carbohydrate, 30-45% protein, 10-25% fat
   b. 30-45% carbohydrate, 15-30% protein, 25-40% fat
   c. 5-15% carbohydrate, 35-55% protein, 5-20% fat
   d. 50% carbohydrate, 15-20% protein, 30% fat
2. During the first 24 hours of starvation, which of the following describes the order in which the body obtains substrate for energy?
   a. Glycogen, skeletal protein
   b. Visceral protein, fat stores, glycogen
   c. Fat stores, skeletal protein, visceral protein
   d. Liver protein, muscle protein, visceral protein
3. An older patient who recently had a stroke is exhibiting signs of severe dysphagia. What is the optimal form of nutrition support at this time?
   a. Parenteral nutrition
   b. Modified regular diet
   c. Nasoenteric tube feedings
   d. Nothing by mouth (NPO) until dysphagia resolves

4. What is one advantage of a percutaneous endoscopic gastrostomy tube placement relative to nasogastric (NG) feedings for the patient receiving long-term enteral nutrition?
   a. It increases patient comfort.
   b. It eliminates the risk of aspiration.
   c. Feedings can be initiated before bowel sounds are present.
   d. More calories can be delivered compared with NG feeding.
5. A patient is receiving peripheral parenteral nutrition. The parenteral nutrition solution is completed before the new solution arrives on the unit. The nurse administers
   a. 20% intralipids.
   b. 5% dextrose solution.
   c. 5% Ringer's lactate solution.
   d. 0.45% normal saline solution.
6. A patient with anorexia nervosa shows signs of malnutrition. During initial re-feeding, what does the nurse carefully assess the patient for?
   a. Hyperkalemia
   b. Hypoglycemia
   c. Hypercalcemia
   d. Hypophosphatemia

ANSWERS: 1. d; 2. a; 3. b; 4. a; 5. b; 6. a.

REFERENCES

Amella, E. J. (2008). Mealtime difficulties. In E. Capezuti, D. Zwicker, M. Mezey, T. Fulmer, D. Gray-Miceli, & M. Kluger (Eds.), *Evidence-based geriatric nursing protocols for best practice*, 3rd ed. (pp. 337-351). New York: Springer.

Anthony, P. (2008). Nutrition screening tools for hospitalized patients. *Nutrition in Clinical Practice*, 23(4):373382. doi:10.1177/0884533608321130

ASPEN. (2009). Clinical guidelines for the use of parenteral and enteral nutrition in adult and pediatric patients. *Journal of Enteral and Parenteral Nutrition*, 33(3), 255-259. doi:10.1177/0148607109333115

Bankhead, R., Boullatta, J., Brantley, S., Corkins, M., Guenter, P., Krenitsky, J., …, ASPEN Board of Directors. (2009). Enteral nutrition practice recommendations. *Journal of Enteral and Parenteral Nutrition*, 33(2), 122-167. doi:10.1177/0148607108330314

Bankhead, R. R., & Fang, J. C. (2007). Enteral access devices. In M. M. Gottschlich, M. H. DeLegge, T. Mattox, C. Mueller, P. Worthington, & P. Guenter (Eds.), *The A.S.P.E.N. nutrition support core curriculum: A case-based approach—The adult patient*. Silver Spring, MD: American Society of Parenteral and Enteral Nutrition (ASPEN).

Boullatta, J., Nieman, L., & Guenter, P. (Eds.). (2010). *ASPEN enteral nutrition handbook, 2010*. Silver Spring, MD: ASPEN.

Canadian Institute for Health Information (CIHI). (2010). *Health care in Canada, 2010* (White Paper). Retrieved from *www.CIHI.ca*

Carrier, N., Ouellet, D., & West, G. E. (2007). Nursing home food services linked with risk of malnutrition. *Canadian Journal of Dietetic Practice and Research*, 26(1), 14-20. doi:10.3148/68.1.2007.14

Cook, J. T., & Frank, D. A. (2008). Food security, poverty, and human development in the United States. *Annals of the New York Academy of Sciences*, 1136, 193. doi:10.1196/annals.1425.001

Cook, J. T., Frank, D. A., Casey, P. H., Rose-Jacobs, R., Black, M. M., Chilton, M., …, Cutts, D. B. (2008). A brief indicator of household energy security: Associations with food security, child health, and child development in US infants and toddlers. *Pediatrics*, 122, e867. doi:10.1542/peds.2008-0286

Dietitians of Canada. (2005). The role of the registered dietitian in dysphagia assessment and treatment—A discussion paper. Retrieved from *http://www.dietitians.ca/Downloadable-Content/Public/Role-DC-in-Dysphagia-Assessment-n-Treatment.aspx*

Dietitians of Canada. (2011). Career. Retrieved from *http://www.dietitians.ca/Career.aspx*

Dietitians of Canada. (2012). Vitamin D: What you need to know. Retrieved from *http://www.dietitians.ca/Nutrition-Resources-A-Z/Factsheets/Vitamins/Vitamin-D–What-you-need-to-know.aspx*

DiMaria-Ghalili, R. A. (2008). Nutrition risk factors in older coronary artery bypass graft patients. *Nutrition in Clinical Practice*, 23(5), 494. doi:10.1177/0884533608323428

DiMaria-Ghalili, R. A., & Amella, E. (2005). Nutrition in older adults. *American Journal of Nursing*, 105(3), 40. doi:10.1097/00000446-200503000-00020

Gillies, D., O'Riordan, L., Wallen, M., Morrison, A., Rankin, K., & Nagy, S. (2005). Optimal timing for intravenous administration set replacement. *Cochrane Database System Reviews* 4, CD003588.

Gonzalez, A., Kohn, M. R., & Clarke, S. D. (2007). Eating disorders in adolescents. *Australian Family Physician*, 36(8), 614-619.

Guenter, P., Hicks, R., Simmons, D., Crowley, J., Joseph, S., Croteau, R., …, Vanderveen, T. (2008). Enteral feeding misconnections: A consortium position statement. *The Joint Commission Journal on Quality and Patient Safety*, 34, 285-292. Retrieved from *https://www.premierinc.com/safety/topics/tubing-misconnections/downloads/S5-JQPS-05-08-guenter.pdf*

Health Canada. (2007a). *Eating well with Canada's food guide—First Nations, Inuit and Métis*. Ottawa: Author. Retrieved from *www.hc-sc.gc.ca/fn-an/pubs/fnim-pnim/index_e.html*

Health Canada. (2007b). *Trans fats: It's your health*. Ottawa: Author. Retrieved from *www.hc-sc.gc.ca/hl-vs/iyh-vsv/food-aliment/trans-eng.php*

Health Canada. (2007c). *Canadian community survey: Cycle 2.2 nutrition (2004): Income related household food insecurity in Canada*. Ottawa: Author. Retrieved from *http://www.hc-sc.gc.ca/fn-an/surveill/nutrition/commun/income_food_sec-sec_alim-eng.php*

Health Canada. (2011). *Eating well with Canada's food guide*. Ottawa: Author. Retrieved from *http://www.hc-sc.gc.ca/fn-an/alt_formats/hpfb-dgpsa/pdf/food-guide-aliment/view_eatwell_vue_bienmang-eng.pdf*

Health Canada. (2012a). *Canada's Food Guide: Translated versions of the guide*. Ottawa: Author. Retrieved from *http://www.hc-sc.gc.ca/fn-an/food-guide-aliment/order-commander/guide_trans-trad-eng.php*

Health Canada. (2012b). Do Canadian adults meet their nutrient requirements through food intake alone? Retrieved from *http://www.hc-sc.gc.ca/fn-an/alt_formats/pdf/surveill/nutrition/commun/art-nutr-adult-eng.pdf*

Hoerr, S. L., Tsuei, E., Liu, Y., Franklin, F., & Nicklas, T. (2008). Diet quality varies by race/ethnicity of head start mothers. *Journal of the American Dietetic Association*, 108(4), 651-659. doi:10.1016/j.jada.2008.01.010

Jensen, G. L. (2008). Nutrition assessment and requirements. In M. Marian, M. K. Russell, & S. A. Shikora (Eds.), *Clinical nutrition for surgical patients*. Boston: Jones & Bartlett.

Kubrak, C., & Jenson, L. (2007). Malnutrition in acute care patients: A narrative review. *International Journal of Nursing Studies*, 44, 1036-1054. doi:10.1016/j.ijnurstu.2006.07.015

Latham, M. C. (1997). *Human nutrition in the developing world*. Rome: Food and Agriculture Organizations of the United Nations.

LeGrange, D. (2007). *Treating bulimia in adolescents: A family-based approach*. New York: Guilford Press.

Marian, M., & McGinnis, C. (2007). Overview of enteral nutrition. In M. M. Gottschlich, M. H. DeLegge, T. Mattox, C. Mueller, P. Worthington, & P. Guenter (Eds.), *The A.S.P.E.N. nutrition support core curriculum: A case-based approach—The adult patient* (2nd ed., pp. 187-208). Silver Spring, MD: ASPEN.

Mirtallo, J., Canada, T., Johnson, D., Kumpf, V., Petersen, C., Sacks, G., …, Task Force for the Revision of Safe Practices for Parenteral Nutrition (TFPN). (2004). Safe practices for parenteral nutrition. *Journal of Parenteral and Enteral Nutrition*, 28(6), S39-S70.

Mirtallo, J. M., Dasta, J. K., Kleinschmidt, K. C., & Varon, J. (2010). State of the art: Intravenous fat emulsions—Current applications, safety profile and clinical manifestations. *Annals of Pharmacotherapy*, 44(4), 688-700.

Mirolla, M. (2004). *The cost of chronic disease in Canada* (White Paper). Retrieved from *www.gplatantic.org/pdf/health.chroniccanada.pdf*

Müller, O., & Krawinkel, M. (2005). Malnutrition and health in developing countries. *Canadian Medical Association Journal*, 173(3), 279-286. doi:10.1503/cmaj.050342

National Institute for Health and Clinical Excellence. (2006). *Nutrition support in adults: Oral supplements, enteral and parenteral nutrition*. Retrieved from *www.nice.org.uk/guidance/index.jsp?action=download&o=29982*

National Pressure Ulcer Advisory Panel (NPUAP). (2007). *Updated staging system*. Retrieved from *http://www.npuap.org/pr2.htm*

Norman, K., Prichard, C., Lochs, S., & Pirlich, M. (2008). Prognostic impact of disease-related malnutrition. *Clinical Nutrition*, 27(1), 5-15. doi:10.1016/j.clnu.2007.10.007

Otten, J. J., Hellwig, J. P., & Meyers, L. D. (Eds.) (2006). *Dietary reference intakes: The essential guide to nutrient requirements*. Washington, DC: The National Academies Press.

Palmer, J. L., & Metheny, N. A., (2008). Preventing aspiration in older adults with dysphagia. *American Journal of Nursing*, 108(2), 40-48. doi:10.1097/01.NAJ.0000308961.99857.33

Perez-Escamilla, R., & Putnik, P. (2007). The role of acculturation in nutrition, lifestyle, and incidence of type 2 diabetes among Latinos. *Journal of Nutrition*, 137, 860-870.

Practice Based Evidence in Nutrition. (2008). *Men's health: Key practice points.* Retrieved from *http://www.pennutrition.com/KnowledgePathway.aspx?kpid=9060&pqcatid=145&pqid=11301*

Public Health Agency of Canada (PHAC). (2011). *The Chief Public Health Officer's Report on the state of public health in Canada. 2011. Youth and young adults—Life in transition.* Retrieved from *http://publichealth.gc.ca/CPHOreport*

Registered Nurses' Association of Ontario (RNAO). (2005). *Risk assessment and prevention of pressure ulcers* (revised). Retrieved from *http://www.rnao.org/bestpractices*

Russell, M. K., & Mueller, C. (2007). Nutrition screening and assessment. In M. M. Gottschlich, M. H. DeLegge, T. Mattox, C. Mueller, P. Worthington, & P. Guenter (Eds.), *The A.S.P.E.N. nutrition support core curriculum: A case-based approach—The adult patient* (2nd ed., pp. 163-186.). Silver Spring, MD: ASPEN.

Soeters, P. B., & Schols, A. M. (2009). Advances in understanding and assessing malnutrition. *Current Opinion in Clinical Nutrition & Metabolic Care, 12*(5), 487-494. doi:10.1097/MCO.0b013e32832da243

Sorensen. J., Kondrup, J., Prokopowicz, J., Schiesser, M., Krähenbühl, L., Meier, R., & Liberda, M. (2008). EuroOOPS: An international, multicentre study to implement nutritional risk screening and evaluate clinical outcome. *Clinical Nutrition, 27*(3), 340-349. doi:10.1016/j.clnu.2008.03.012

Teitelbaum, D., Guenter, P., Howell, W., Kochevar, M., Roth, J., & Seidner, D. (2005). Definitions of terms, styles and conventions used in ASPEN guidelines and standards. *Nutrition in Clinical Practice, 20*(2), 281-285. doi:10.1177/0115426505020002281

Thomas, D. R. (2006). Prevention and treatment of pressure ulcers. *Journal of the American Medical Directors Association, 7*(1), 46-59. doi:10.1016/j.jamda.2005.10.004

Wooley, J. A., & Frankenfield, D. (2007). Energy. In M. M. Gottschlich, M. H. DeLegge, T. Mattox, C. Mueller, P. Worthington, & P. Guenter (Eds.), *The A.S.P.E.N. nutrition support core curriculum: A case-based approach—The adult patient* (2nd ed., pp. 20-21). Silver Spring, MD: ASPEN.

Zingg, W., Cartier-Fässler, V., & Walder, B. (2008). Central venous catheter-associated infections. *Best Practice & Research Clinical Anaesthesiology, 22*(3), 407-421. doi:10.1016/j.bpa.2008.05.007

CANADIAN RESOURCES

Canadian Diabetes Association
http://www.diabetes.ca
Canadian Intravenous Nurses Association
http://www.cina.ca

Canadian Mental Health Association
http://www.cmha.ca
Canadian Nutrition Society
http://www.cns-scn.ca/
Critical Care Nutrition
http://www.criticalcarenutrition.com
Dietitians of Canada
http://www.dietitians.ca
EatRight Ontario
http://www.eatrightOntario.ca
Health Canada: Eating Well With Canada's Food Guide
http://www.hc-sc.gc.ca/fn-an/food-guide-aliment/index-eng.php
Health Canada: Interactive Nutrition Facts Table
http://www.hc-sc.gc.ca/fn-an/label-etiquet/nutrition/cons/inl_main-eng.php
Health Canada, Therapeutic Products Directorate (TPD)
http://www.hc-sc.gc.ca/ahc-asc/branch-dirgen/hpfb-dgpsa/tpd-dpt/index-eng.php
Healthy Canadians (Government of Canada)
http://www.healthycanadians.gc.ca/index-eng.php
Heart and Stroke Foundation of Canada
http://www.heartandstroke.ca
National Eating Disorder Information Centre
http://www.nedic.ca
Oley Foundation
http://www.oley.org
Public Health Agency of Canada (PHAC)
http://www.phac-aspc.gc.ca
Registered Nurses' Association of Ontario (RNAO)
http://www.rnao.org

RELATED RESOURCES

Academy for Eating Disorders
http://www.aedweb.org
American Society for Parenteral and Enteral Nutrition (ASPEN)
http://www.nutritioncare.org
European Society for Parenteral and Enteral Nutrition (ESPEN)
http://www.espen.org/usefullinks.html
National Association of Anorexia Nervosa and Associated Disorders (ANAD)
http://www.anad.org

Ⓔvolve   *For additional Internet resources, see the Web site for this book at* **http://evolve.elsevier.com/Canada/Lewis/medsurg**

Nursing Management:
Obesity

Written by Judi Daniels
Adapted by J. Jacque E. Lovely

LEARNING OBJECTIVES

1. Discuss the epidemiology and etiology of obesity.
2. Describe the classification systems for determining a person's body size and associated health risks.
3. Explain the health risks associated with obesity.
4. Discuss nutritional, physical activity, and behaviour modification therapies for the obese patient.

5. Describe the different bariatric surgical procedures used to treat obesity.
6. Describe the nursing management related to conservative and surgical therapies for obesity.
7. Describe the etiology, the clinical manifestations, and the nursing and collaborative management of metabolic syndrome.

KEY TERMS

bariatric surgery A surgical procedure that is used to treat morbid obesity, p. 1102
body mass index (BMI) A ratio of weight to height; higher ranges are associated with increasing health risk, p. 1091
lipectomy Adipectomy; performed to remove unsightly skin folds and adipose tissue for cosmetic reasons, p. 1105
metabolic syndrome A collection of risk factors that increase an individual's chance of developing cardiovascular disease and diabetes mellitus, p. 1108
morbidly obese Classification describing individuals with a body mass index of greater than 40 kg/m², p. 1091

obese Classification used to describe individuals with body mass index values of 30 kg/m² or more, p. 1091
obesity A complex, chronic, multifactorial disease that develops from the interaction between genetics and the environment; manifests as an abnormal increase in the proportion of fat cells in the body, p. 1091
overweight Classification used to describe individuals with a body mass index value of 25.0 to 29.9 kg/m², p. 1091
waist-to-hip ratio (WHR) A method of describing the distribution of both subcutaneous and visceral adipose tissue by dividing the waist measurement by the hip measurement to calculate a ratio, p. 1091

ELECTRONIC RESOURCES

Supplemental content related to Chapter 43 can be found...

Evolve Web Site ⊖volve

http://evolve.elsevier.com/Canada/Lewis/medsurg
- Answer Guidelines for Case Study on p. 1109
- Content Updates
- Electronic Calculators

- eTable 43-1: Nutritional Therapy: Meal Plans for 1200-Calorie Weight Reduction Diet
- Examination Review Questions
- Glossary
- Interactive Case Study: Obese Patient
- Key Points (Printable and MP3 Download)

Obesity

Obesity is a complex, chronic, multifactorial disease that develops from the interaction between genetics and the environment. It manifests as an abnormal increase in the proportion of fat cells in the body. Weight gain in which the body is moving toward an overweight or obese state is characterized predominantly by adipocyte hypertrophy and hyperplasia (Halberg, Wernstedt-Asterholm, & Sherer, 2008). This is a process by which adipocytes can increase their volume several thousand times to accommodate large increases in lipid storage. In addition, preadipocytes are triggered to become adipocytes. This occurs primarily in the visceral (intra-abdominal) and subcutaneous tissues of the body (Figure 43-1).

Overweight and obesity result from a complex interaction of genetic, nutritional, physiological, psychological, behavioural, environmental, and social factors that create an imbalance between energy intake and energy expenditure (National Heart, Lung, and Blood Institute & National Institute of Diabetes and Digestive and Kidney Diseases, 1998; World Health Organization, 2000). There is increasing evidence that obesity is not a problem resulting from a lack of willpower and self-control but, instead, is a pervasive, progressive, and serious chronic condition that is strongly associated with a variety of comorbid conditions and has a major effect on the physical, mental, social, cultural, and economic health of those affected (World Health Organization, 2000). Interventions to address obesity must account for the complexity and progressive nature of the chronic condition and support appropriate lifelong management, which often necessitates sustained contact and support from trained health professionals (Kirk, Penney, McHugh, & Sharma, 2011).

Classifications of Body Weight and Obesity

The majority of obese people have *primary obesity,* which is calorie intake that exceeds the body's metabolic demands. Others have *secondary obesity,* which can result from various congenital anomalies, chromosomal anomalies, metabolic problems, or lesions and disorders of the central nervous system. The first step in the treatment of obesity is to determine whether the patient has any physical conditions that may be causing or contributing to the obesity. A thorough history and physical examination are necessary and will reveal the extent and duration of the obesity.

The degree to which a patient is classified as underweight, healthy (normal) weight, overweight, or obese is assessed with the use of a **body mass index (BMI)** chart (Figure 43-2). BMI is calculated by dividing weight (in kilograms) by height (in metres squared). Research studies in large groups of people have shown that the BMI can be classified into ranges associated with health risk (Table 43-1). Individuals with a BMI of 25 to 29.9 kg/m^2 are classified as being **overweight,** those with a BMI of 30 to 40 kg/m^2 are classified as **obese,** and those with a BMI of more than 40 kg/m^2 are classified as **morbidly obese.**

Waist circumference is another way to assess and classify weight (see Table 43-1) People who have visceral fat are especially at increased risk for cardiovascular disease and metabolic syndrome (discussed later in this chapter). The **waist-to-hip ratio (WHR)** can also be used to assess the health risks associated with obesity. This ratio reflects the distribution of both subcutaneous and visceral adipose tissue. To calculate the WHR, the waist measurement is divided by the hip measurement. A WHR of less than 0.80 is optimal; a WHR greater than 0.8 indicates that an individual is at greater risk for health complications. A simpler method for determining excess abdominal fat is measuring just the waist circumference. This is recommended for everyone with a BMI of 35 kg/m^2 and higher. Health risks increase if the waist circumference is greater than 101.6 cm (40 in) in men and greater than 88.9 cm (35 in) in women (Health Canada, 2003).

Obesity has also been classified by body shape or fat distribution. Individuals with fat located primarily in the abdominal area and the upper body (neck, arms, and shoulders; apple-shaped body) are at a greater risk for obesity-related complications than those whose fat is located primarily in the upper legs (pear-shaped body) (Table 43-2, Figure 43-3). Obese individuals with an apple-shaped body are classified as having *android obesity.* *Gynoid obesity* is a term used to classify obese people who are pear-shaped. Genetics play an important role in determining body fat distribution patterns.

Gynoid obesity carries a better prognosis but is more difficult to treat. It is believed that abdominal fat is more readily available and can be mobilized to maintain elevated triglyceride and lipid levels. Individuals with an apple shape carry more visceral fat than people with a pear shape and have increased amounts of fat around the organs. Pear-shaped individuals carry more subcutaneous fat, which causes more cellulite to appear. Abdominal and visceral fat have been linked to metabolic syndrome, a major

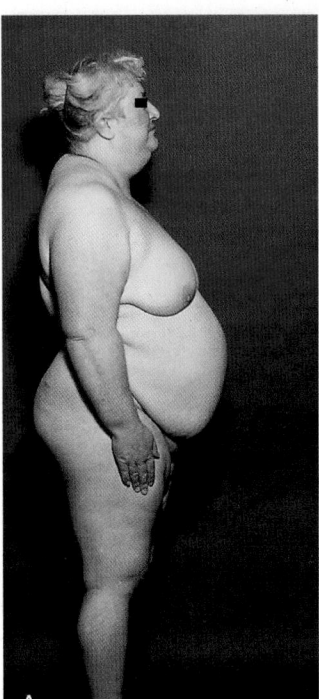
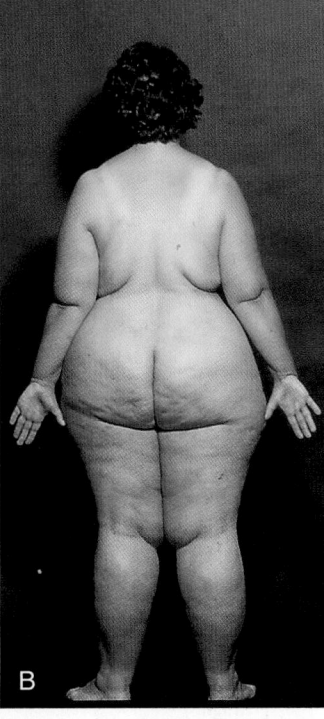

Figure 43-1 Obesity. **A,** This woman has excessive fat deposits in her abdominal area, upper arms, and breasts. **B,** This woman has excessive fat deposits in her upper arms, buttocks, and thighs. The fat distribution in both of these women is common in obese people.

Source: Forbes, C. D., & Jackson, W. F. (2003). *Color atlas and text of clinical medicine* (3rd ed., p. 327, Figures 7.115 and 7.116). London: Mosby.

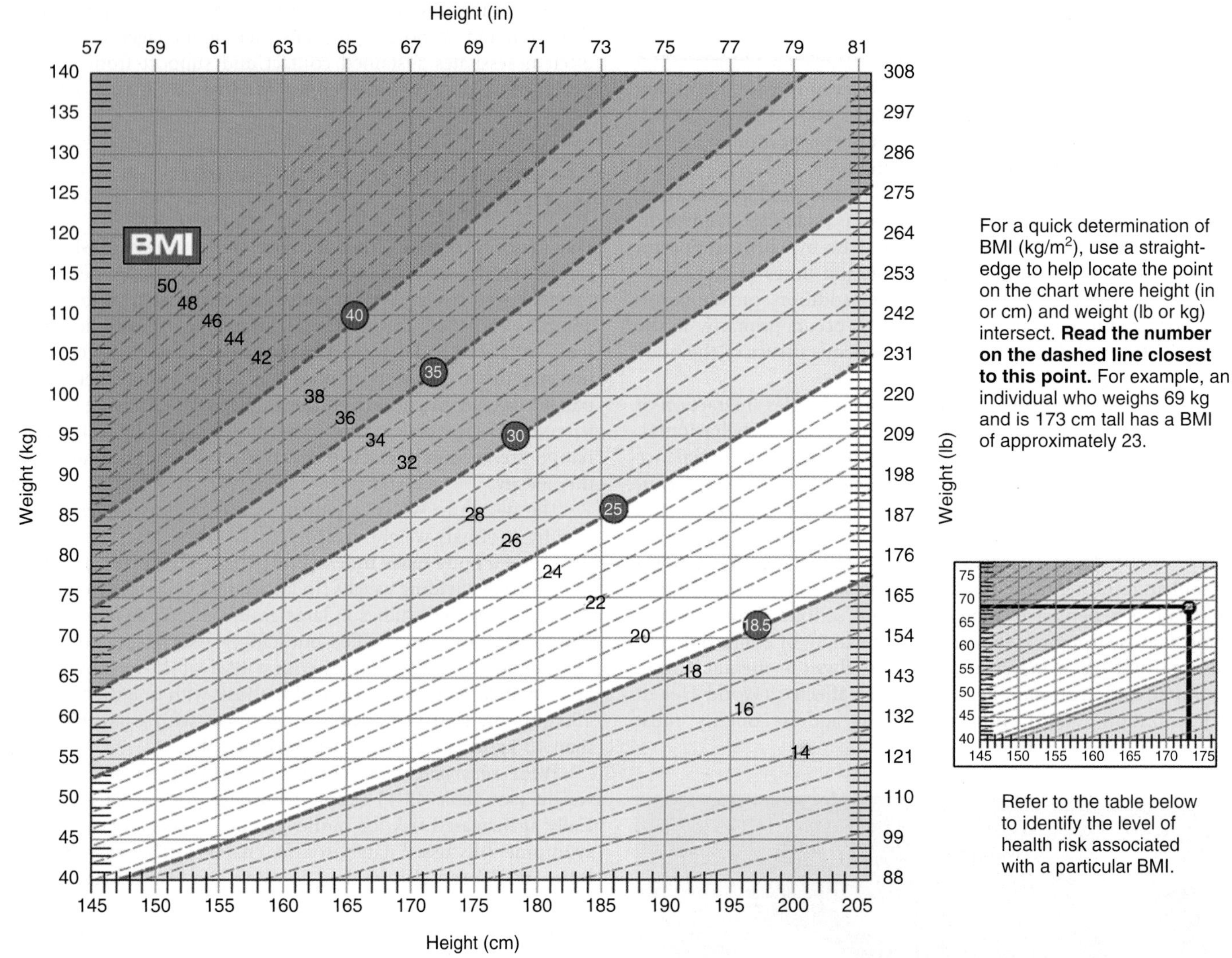
Height (in)
Weight (kg)
Weight (lb)
Height (cm)
BMI
For a quick determination of BMI (kg/m²), use a straight-edge to help locate the point on the chart where height (in or cm) and weight (lb or kg) intersect. **Read the number on the dashed line closest to this point.** For example, an individual who weighs 69 kg and is 173 cm tall has a BMI of approximately 23.
Refer to the table below to identify the level of health risk associated with a particular BMI.

Figure 43-2 Body mass index chart.

Source: Health Canada. (2003). *The 2003 Canadian guidelines for body weight classification in adults* (p. 37) (Cat. no. H49-179/2003E). Ottawa: Author. Retrieved from *http://www.hc-sc.gc.ca/fn-an/alt_formats/hpfb-dgpsa/pdf/nutrition/cg_quick_ref-ldc_rapide_ref-eng.pdf*

Table 43-1 Classification of Overweight and Obesity by BMI, Waist Circumference, and Associated Disease Risk*

			DISEASE RISK BASED ON WAIST CIRCUMFERENCE*	
CLASSIFICATION	**BMI (kg/m²)**	**OBESITY CLASS**	**MEN: ≤102 cm (40 in) WOMEN: ≤88 cm (35 in)**	**MEN: >102 cm (40 in) WOMEN: >88 cm (35 in)**
Underweight	<18.5	—	—	—
Normal†	18.5-24.9	—	—	—
Overweight	25.0-29.9	—	Increased	High
Obese	30.0-34.9	Class I	High	Very high
	35.0-39.9	Class II	Very high	Very high
Morbidly obese	≥40.0	Class III	Extremely high	Extremely high

Source: National Heart, Lung, and Blood Institute, North American Association for the Study of Obesity. (2000). *The practical guide: Identification, evaluation, and treatment of overweight and obesity in adults* (Pub. No. 00-4084). Washington, DC: U.S. Department of Health and Human Services.
BMI, body mass index.
*Disease risk for type 2 diabetes, hypertension, and cardiovascular disease in relation to that for a person of normal weight.
†Increased waist circumference can also be a marker for increased risk in people of normal weight.

Table 43-2 Relationship Between Body Shape and Health Risks

Gynoid (Pear)

Health Risks

- Osteoporosis
- Varicose veins
- Cellulite
- Subcutaneous fat, which traps and stores dietary fat
- Trapped fatty acids, which are stored as triglycerides

Android (Apple)

Health Risks

- Heart disease
- Diabetes mellitus
- Breast cancer
- Endometrial cancer

Results of Increased Visceral Fat (Which Is More Damaging)

- ↓ Insulin sensitivity
- ↑ Triglycerides
- ↓ HDL cholesterol
- ↑ Blood pressure
- ↑ Free fatty acid release into blood

HDL, high-density lipoprotein.

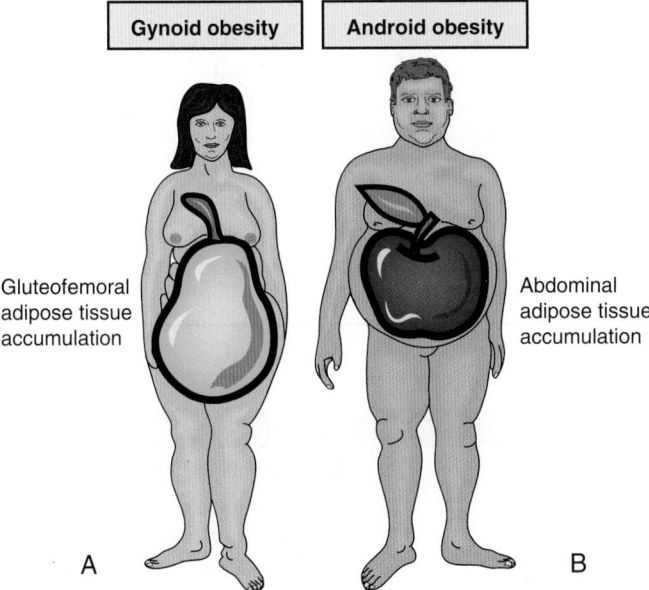

Figure 43-3 Two general classifications used to classify people by body fat distribution are **(A)** pear shape and **(B)** apple shape. Health risks are associated with each classification (see Table 43-2).

complication of obesity (Depres & Lemieux, 2006). Visceral fat actively harms the body by decreasing insulin sensitivity and levels of high-density lipoprotein (HDL) cholesterol and increasing blood pressure. Visceral fat also releases more free fatty acids into the bloodstream.

Epidemiology of Obesity

In developed and developing countries, obesity has reached epidemic proportions. Although adult obesity rates remain significantly lower in Canada (~25%) than in the United States (34%; Shields, Carroll, & Ogden, 2011), the prevalence of overweight and obesity among Canadians has approximately doubled since the early 1980s. According to measured height and weight data from 2007 to 2009, more than one in four Canadian adults (estimates range from 24.3 to 25.4%) 18 years of age or older are obese (Public Health Agency of Canada, 2011). The prevalence of obesity generally increases with each successive decade of life for both men and women up to age 65; the prevalence is highest between ages 55 and 64. Across all age groups, obesity prevalence is slightly higher among men except in the highest reported age category (75 years or older).

Perhaps most alarming is the marked shift in BMI and obesity classes over time. Between 1978/1979 and 2004, the prevalence of class I obesity increased from 10.5 to 15.2%; class II obesity increased from 2.3 to 5.1% (more than doubled); and class III obesity grew from 0.9 to 2.7% (a threefold increase). According to statistics that combine obesity with overweight, the prevalence among adults is 62.1%. The prevalence of obesity among Canadian children age 6 to 17 years is 8.6%. The prevalence of measured obesity among children and youth age 2 to 17 years has increased by 2.5 times since 2000, and the prevalence among youth age 12 to 17 has more than tripled from 3 to 9.4% (Shields, 2005). Although data for examining changes in obesity prevalence over time in Aboriginal populations are limited, obesity prevalence remains more prominent among adults and children in this population than among non-Aboriginal populations.

Lau (2007) warned that despite the major advances in medical knowledge and steady progress in the management of obesity, the health-related effects will continue. Obesity is a societal problem as much as a complex medical concern, because of the adverse health conditions related to weight gain and the associated expenses for health care. Anis and associates (2010) estimated that total costs of obesity to the Canadian health care system were $6.0 billion in 2006. This amount corresponds to 4.1% of the total health care expenditures in Canada for that year.

Etiology and Pathophysiology

In one sense, the etiology of obesity can be considered simplistically. It occurs because energy intake exceeds energy output. However, the processes leading to obesity are much more complex and still undergoing investigation. The causes of obesity involve significant genetic–biological susceptibility factors that are highly influenced by environmental and psychosocial factors.

Genetic–Biological Basis. Evidence from studies of twins, adoptees, and families indicate the existence of genetic factors in obesity (Bouchard, 2010). The heritability of obesity estimated from twin studies is high; values in twins raised apart are only slightly lower than in those raised together. Obesity is estimated to be an inherited problem in more than 50% of cases (Malis et al., 2005). Similarly, the BMI of adopted children correlated with that of their biological parents rather than that of their adoptive parents (Stunkard et al., 1986). The most common form of obesity is considered to be polygenic, arising from the interaction of multiple genetic and environmental factors (Li et al., 2010). Identifying the genes will contribute to a better understanding of the pathogenesis of obesity. Considerable research is being conducted on the genetic predisposition for obesity. A commonly occurring variant of the *FTO* gene has been discovered that may explain why some people become overweight and others do not: A strong link between the *FTO* variant and BMI has been found, and the strength of the genetic influence apparently depends on whether an individual has inherited one or two copies of the *FTO* gene variant (Frayling et al., 2007). Much more research is needed to better understand the role of genes related to obesity.

Regulation of eating behaviour, energy metabolism, and body fat metabolism are controlled by signals from the periphery that act on the hypothalamus (Figure 43-4). Appetite is influenced by many factors that are integrated by the brain, most importantly within the hypothalamus. Input to the hypothalamus is received from the periphery from many different hormones and peptides (Table 43-3). Obesity is associated with increased circulating plasma levels of leptin, insulin, and ghrelin and with decreased levels of peptide YY (Neary & Batterham, 2009; Sowers, 2008). Interaction of these hormones and peptides at the level of the hypothalamus may be an important determinant in factors contributing to obesity.

Adipocytes are not just a storage unit for triglycerides; they are also endocrine cells known to produce at least 100 different proteins. These proteins are secreted as enzymes, adipokines, growth factors, and hormones that contribute to the development of insulin resistance and atherosclerosis. Evidence now supports an association between the increased release of adipokines and certain cancers. Because visceral fat accumulation is associated

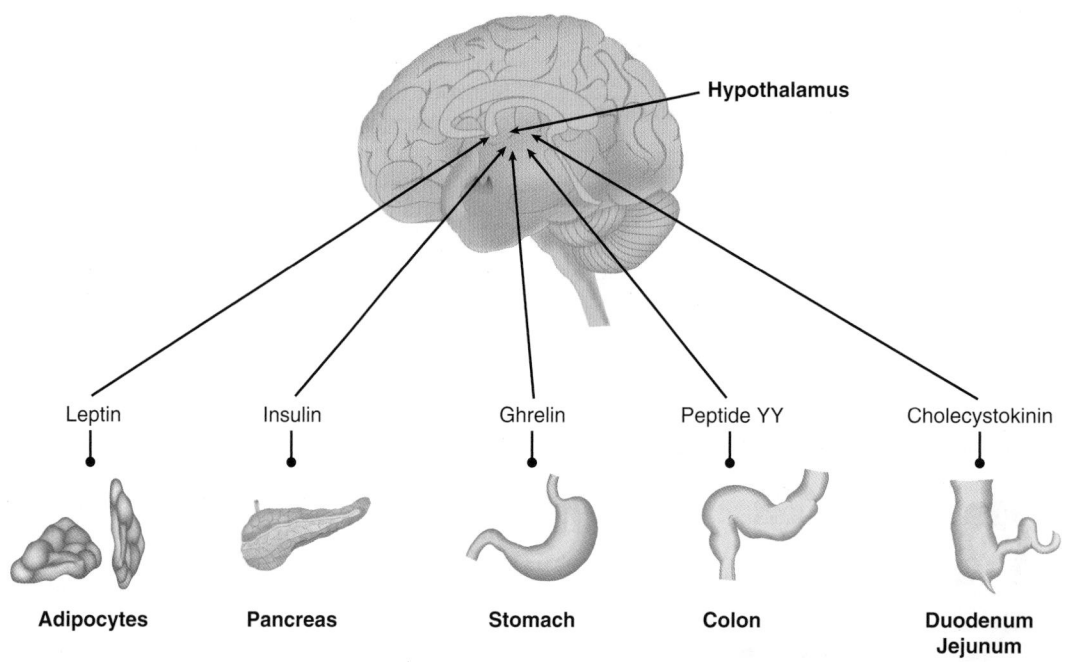

Figure 43-4 Some of the common hormones and peptides that interact with the hypothalamus to control and influence eating patterns, metabolic activities, and digestion. Obesity causes a disruption in this balance (see Table 43-3).

Table 43-3 Hormones and Peptides in Obesity			
HORMONE OR PEPTIDE	**WHERE PRODUCED**	**NORMAL FUNCTION**	**ALTERATION IN OBESITY**
Leptin	Adipocytes	Suppresses appetite and hunger Regulates eating behaviour	Obesity is associated with high leptin levels, and when leptin levels are high, leptin resistance develops; thus obese people may lose the effect of appetite suppression.
Insulin	Pancreas	Decreases appetite	Circulating levels are frequently high.
Ghrelin	Stomach (primarily)	Stimulates appetite ↑ After food deprivation ↓ In response to the presence of food in the stomach	Normal postprandial decline does not occur, which can lead to increased appetite and overeating.
Peptide YY	Descending colon and rectum	Inhibits appetite by slowing GI motility and gastric emptying	Circulating levels are decreased; release is decreased after eating.
Cholecystokinin	Duodenum Jejunum	Inhibits gastric emptying and sends satiety signals to hypothalamus	Role is unknown.

GI, gastrointestinal.

Table 43-4 Portion Sizes: Past Versus Present		
FOOD	**20 YEARS AGO**	**TODAY**
Turkey sandwich	320 cal	820 cal
Bagel	7.6 cm diameter: 140 cal	15.2 cm diameter: 350 cal
Cheeseburger	333 cal	590 cal
Soft drink	237 mL: 105 cal	591 mL: 250 cal

with more alterations of these adipokines, people with android obesity have more complications of obesity than those with gynoid obesity.

Environmental Factors. Environmental factors play an important role in obesity. In today's culture, there is greater access to food, particularly prepackaged and fast foods, as well as soft drinks, which have poor nutritional quality. Portion size of meals has also increased (Table 43-4). Obese individuals tend to underestimate food and caloric intake. Eating outside of the home impedes the ability to control the composition and the quality of food.

Lack of physical activity is another factor that contributes to weight gain and obesity (Swinburn & Shelly, 2008). The amount of physical activity has decreased, both in the workplace and at home. With increases in technology and labour-saving devices, Canadians are expending less energy in their everyday lives. Reduction of physical education programs in schools, along with increased time spent playing video games and watching TV, have increased sedentary habits among children. Numerous initiatives have been enacted in Canada to address inactivity and resultant obesity throughout the lifespan (Canadian Society for Exercise Physiology, 2011; Tremblay, 2007), but there is a need for further measures.

Socioeconomic status can affect obesity in a variety of indirect ways. People with low incomes may buy food that is less expensive but often has poorer nutritional quality and greater caloric content. For example, people with low incomes are more likely to purchase prepackaged foods than to buy fresh meats and produce. Low-income residents may be more likely to live in environments that do not accommodate outdoor activities, such as tennis and swimming (Davis, Forges, & Wylie-Rosett, 2009). Gyms tend to be attended by more affluent individuals.

Psychosocial Factors. People use food for many reasons beyond nutritional maintenance. Many food associations begin in childhood, such as using food for comfort and reward. Furthermore, when overeating begins in childhood and continues into adulthood, a person's ability to sense fullness, or *satiety*, is compromised. Whether the desire to eat is triggered by specific foods or by the availability of a wide variety, some people consume food beyond their body's needs. The social component of eating also develops early in life when food is associated with pleasure and fun at such events as birthday parties and religious holidays (Budge, Sebert, Sharkey, & Symonds, 2009). All these factors must be included when considering the etiology and treatment of obesity.

Health Risks Associated With Obesity

Hippocrates wrote that "corpulence is not only a disease itself, but the harbinger of others," thus recognizing that obesity has major adverse effects on health. Many health conditions occur at higher rates among obese people (Figure 43-5) than among people of normal weight (Guh et al., 2009). The mortality rate rises as the rate of obesity increases, especially when obesity is associated with visceral fat. Among people with a BMI of 30 kg/m² or higher, the mortality rates from all causes—especially from cardiovascular disease—are generally 50 to 100% higher than the rates for people with BMIs in the normal range. Being overweight was once thought to have fewer health consequences than being obese. However, evidence now shows a 20 to 40% increase in mortality rates among both men and women who are overweight in midlife (Adams et al., 2006). The number of years lived with obesity also has a direct link with the risk of mortality (Abdullah et al., 2011). In addition to these problems, obese patients have a reduced quality of life (Daniels, 2006). Fortunately, most of these conditions can improve if an individual loses weight. Loss of 5 to 10% of excess body weight can significantly improve obesity-related comorbid conditions (Lau, 2007).

Cardiovascular Problems. Obesity is a significant risk factor for predicting cardiovascular disease in both men and women. The WHR is the best predictor of these risks. Obesity, especially android obesity, is connected with increased levels of low-density lipoprotein (LDLs) and triglycerides and decreased levels of HDLs. Obesity is also associated with hypertension. Hypertension can occur because of increased circulating blood volume, abnormal vasoconstriction, decreased vascular relaxation, and increased cardiac output. Measurement of blood pressure in an obese patient requires the use of a larger cuff size to avoid artifactual increases.

Respiratory Problems. Severe obesity may be connected with sleep apnea and obesity hypoventilation syndrome. Affected patients also have reduced chest wall compliance, increased work of breathing, and decreased total lung capacity and functional residual capacity. Weight loss can bring substantial improvement in lung function.

Diabetes Mellitus. Hyperinsulinemia and insulin resistance are common features of obesity. Insulin resistance is more strongly related to visceral fat than to fat in other locations. Obesity is a major risk factor for type 2 diabetes (see Figure 43-9 later in this chapter). As many as 90% of cases of type 2 diabetes are associated with excess weight (Hossain, Kawar, & El Nahas, 2011). Weight loss and exercise are linked with improved glucose control in diabetes.

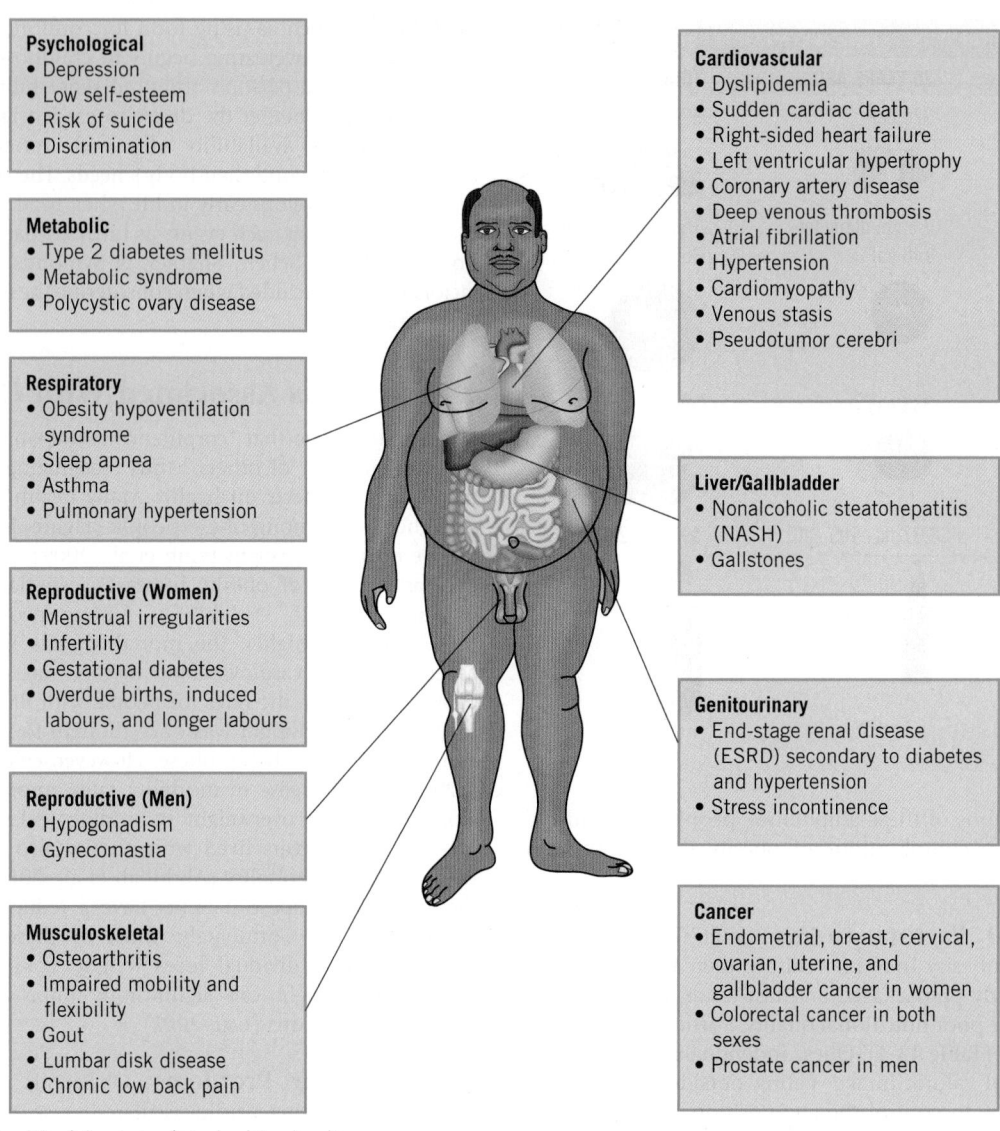

Psychological
- Depression
- Low self-esteem
- Risk of suicide
- Discrimination

Metabolic
- Type 2 diabetes mellitus
- Metabolic syndrome
- Polycystic ovary disease

Respiratory
- Obesity hypoventilation syndrome
- Sleep apnea
- Asthma
- Pulmonary hypertension

Reproductive (Women)
- Menstrual irregularities
- Infertility
- Gestational diabetes
- Overdue births, induced labours, and longer labours

Reproductive (Men)
- Hypogonadism
- Gynecomastia

Musculoskeletal
- Osteoarthritis
- Impaired mobility and flexibility
- Gout
- Lumbar disk disease
- Chronic low back pain

Cardiovascular
- Dyslipidemia
- Sudden cardiac death
- Right-sided heart failure
- Left ventricular hypertrophy
- Coronary artery disease
- Deep venous thrombosis
- Atrial fibrillation
- Hypertension
- Cardiomyopathy
- Venous stasis
- Pseudotumor cerebri

Liver/Gallbladder
- Nonalcoholic steatohepatitis (NASH)
- Gallstones

Genitourinary
- End-stage renal disease (ESRD) secondary to diabetes and hypertension
- Stress incontinence

Cancer
- Endometrial, breast, cervical, ovarian, uterine, and gallbladder cancer in women
- Colorectal cancer in both sexes
- Prostate cancer in men

Figure 43-5 Health risks associated with obesity.

Musculoskeletal Problems. Obesity is correlated with an increased incidence of osteoarthritis as a result of stress put on weight-bearing joints. Hyperuricemia and gout are often found in people who are obese and in those who have metabolic syndrome (discussed later in this chapter).

Gastrointestinal and Liver Problems. Gastroesophageal reflux disease and gallstones are more prevalent among obese people. Gallstones occur when bile becomes supersaturated with cholesterol. Nonalcoholic steatohepatitis (NASH) is more common in obese people. In NASH, lipids are deposited in the liver, resulting in a fatty liver. NASH is associated with increased production of hepatic glucose. NASH can eventually progress to cirrhosis and can be fatal. Weight loss can improve NASH.

Cancer. Obesity is one of the most important known preventable causes of cancer. Although the underlying mechanisms are difficult to determine, substantial evidence supports the link between obesity and many common cancers (Renehan, Tyson, Egger, Heller, & Zwalen, 2008). The risk of breast, endometrial, ovarian, and cervical cancer is increased in obese women, possibly because of the increased estrogen levels (estrogen is stored in fat cells) associated with obesity in postmenopausal women. Colorectal cancer has been linked to hyperinsulinemia. Increased waist circumference and WHR, indicators of abdominal obesity, are associated with increased risk of colon cancer in both men and women. Obese men have higher mortality rates with cancer of the prostate. Obesity often leads to acid reflux, also known as *gastroesophageal reflux disease* (GERD). Frequent or constant exposure of the esophageal lining to stomach acid and bile can lead to irritation and inflammation, which increases the risk of esophageal cancer.

Psychosocial Issues. The consequences of obesity extend beyond physical changes and often affect the individual's emotional well-being (Puhl & Heuer, 2009). Clear and consistent stigmatization of obese people and, in some cases, discrimination occur in three important areas of living: employment, education, and health care (Hramiak, Leiter, Paul, & Ur, 2007). In addition to the negative social impact, many obese people have low self-esteem, withdraw from social interaction, and experience major depression.

NURSING AND CONSERVATIVE COLLABORATIVE MANAGEMENT: OBESE PATIENTS

▪ Nursing Assessment

The nurse, working closely with the health care team, plays a major role in the planning and management of care for obese patients. Information that can assist the nurse in understanding an obese patient and provide a basis for intervention is presented in Table 43-5. Because many obese individuals have experienced weight bias in the past, the nurse should ensure that his or her approach and actions are free of any possible interpretation of continued insensitivity. By being sensitive when asking specific and leading questions, the nurse can often obtain information that the patient may otherwise withhold out of embarrassment or shyness (Table 43-6). The nurse must provide acceptable reasons for asking personally intrusive questions, respond to the patient's concerns about diagnostic tests, and interpret test outcomes. The patient's answers to questions must be treated with respect, understanding, and a nonjudgemental attitude. Knowledge regarding assessment and stepwise management for the treatment of obesity (Figure 43-6) can help the nurse, in conjunction with the interdisciplinary team, to guide patients and their families through weight loss interventions.

The health care provider should explore genetic and endocrine factors such as hypothyroidism, hypothalamic tumours, Cushing's syndrome, hypogonadism in men, and polycystic ovary disease in women. Laboratory tests of liver function, fasting glucose level, lipid panel (triglyceride level, and LDL and HDL cholesterol levels) assist in evaluating the cause and effects of obesity.

As part of the initial nursing history and physical examination, each body system should be examined, with particular attention to the organ system in which the patient has expressed a problem or concern. Measurements used with the obese person may include skinfold thickness, height, weight, and BMI. Specific documentation about these areas assists the health care provider with a more in-depth history and physical examination.

▪ Nursing Diagnoses

Nursing diagnoses for the patient with obesity include, but are not limited to, the following:

- Imbalanced nutrition: more than body requirements *related to* excessive intake in relation to metabolic needs
- Impaired skin integrity *related to* alterations in nutritional state (obesity), immobility, excess moisture, and multiple skinfolds
- Ineffective breathing pattern *related to* decreased lung expansion from obesity
- Chronic low self-esteem related to body size, inability to lose weight, and perceived unattractiveness
- Impaired physical mobility *related to* excess body weight
- Disturbed body image *related to* deviation from unusual or expected body size and inability to lose weight or retain weight loss

NURSING ASSESSMENT

Table 43-5 Obese Patient

Subjective Data

Important Health Information

Past health history: Time of obesity onset; diseases related to metabolism and obesity (e.g., hypertension, cardiovascular problems, stroke, cancer, chronic joint pain, respiratory problems, diabetes mellitus, cholelithiasis, metabolic syndrome); family history of obesity; history of weight gain and loss

Medications: Thyroid preparations, diet pills, herbal products

Surgery or other treatments: Prior bariatric surgery, other weight reduction procedures, or other major surgical procedures related to risk factors precipitated by obesity

Symptoms

- Irregularities in amount or frequency of eating, overeating in response to boredom, stress, specific times, or activities
- Constipation
- Drowsiness, somnolence; dyspnea on exertion, orthopnea, paroxysmal nocturnal dyspnea
- Sleep apnea
- Feelings of rejection, depression, isolation, guilt, or shame
- Change in financial status or family relationships; personal, social, and financial resources to support a reducing diet
- Menstrual irregularity, heavy menstrual flow in women, infertility
- Altered sexual activity and feelings of attractiveness

Objective Data

General

BMI ≥30 kg/m²; waist circumference: woman, >88 cm; man, >102 cm

Respiratory

Increased work of breathing; wheezing; rapid shallow breathing, sleep apnea

Cardiovascular

Hypertension, tachycardia, dysrhythmias

Musculoskeletal

Decreased joint mobility and flexibility; knee, hip, and low back pain

Reproductive

Menstrual irregularities and infertility in women; gynecomastia and hypogonadism in men

Possible Findings

Elevated levels of serum glucose, cholesterol, and triglycerides; chest radiograph demonstrating an enlarged heart; ECG tracing showing dysrhythmia; abnormal results of liver function tests

ECG, electrocardiogram.

▪ Planning

The overall goals are that the obese patient will (a) modify eating patterns, (b) participate in a program of regular physical activity, (c) achieve weight maintenance (stop historic pattern of continued weight gain over time) or achieve weight loss to a specified level, (d) maintain weight loss at a specified level, and (e) minimize or prevent health problems related to obesity.

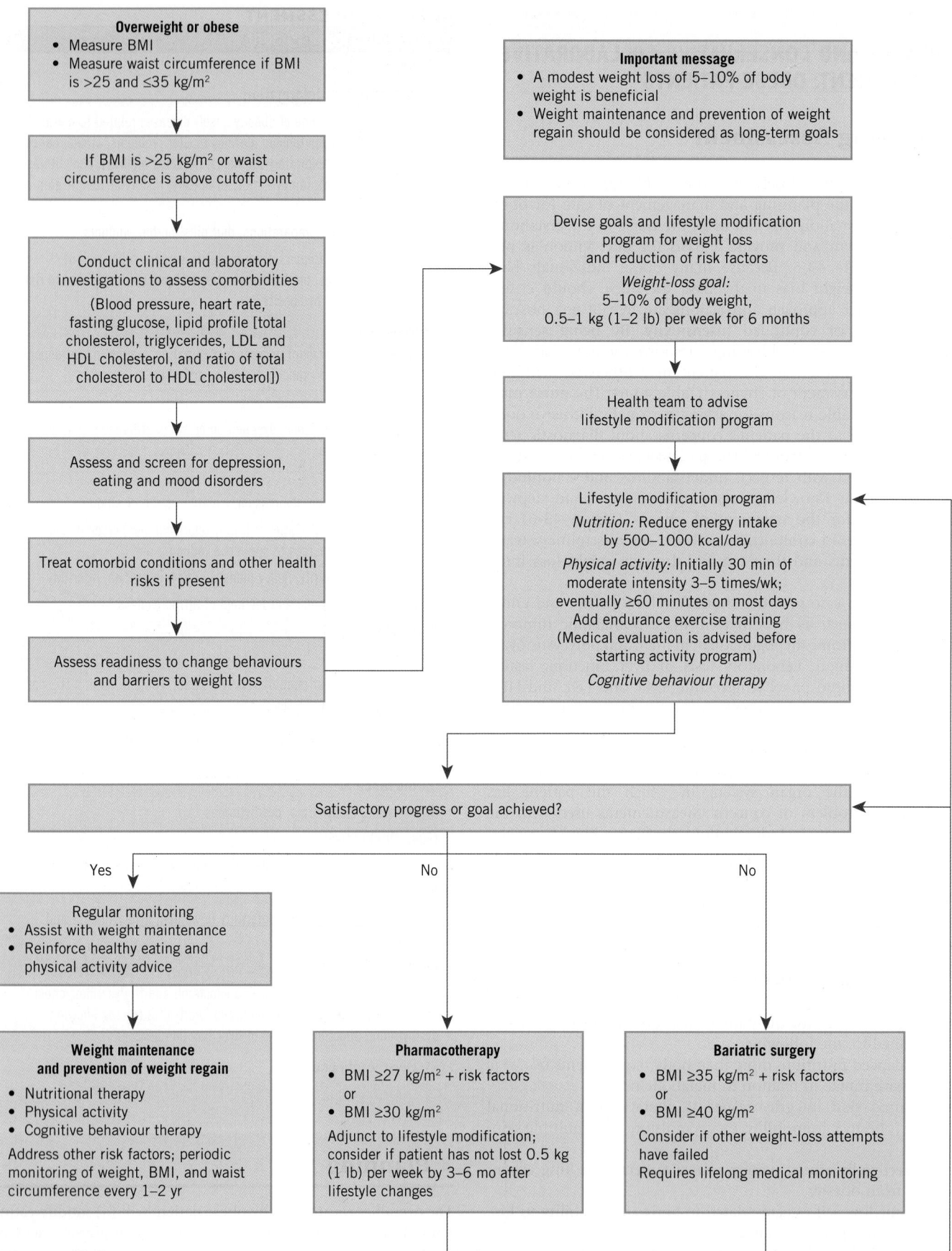

Figure 43-6 Algorithm for the assessment and stepwise management of overweight and obese adults. *BMI,* body mass index; *HDL,* high-density lipoprotein; *LDL,* low-density lipoprotein.

Source: Adapted from Lau, D. C. W. (2007). Synopsis of the 2006 Canadian clinical practice guidelines on the management and prevention of obesity in adults and children. *Canadian Medical Association Journal, 176*(8), 1103-1106.

When assessing a patient with obesity, the nurse should consider several different types of questions, such as the following:

- What is the patient's history with weight gain and weight loss?
- Is the patient interested in losing weight or managing weight differently?
- What does the patient think contributes to his or her weight?
- What sort of barriers does the patient feel impede weight loss efforts?
- What does food mean to the patient? How does the patient use food (e.g., to relieve stress, provide comfort)?
- Is the patient's food intake influenced by hunger?
- Are other family members overweight?
- Are there environmental or genetic factors influencing the weight gain?

Nursing Implementation

The nurse, working closely with the other members of the health care team, plays a major role in the planning and management of the care of an obese patient. To be effective, the nurse must be aware of his or her perceptions of and beliefs about obesity and obesity interventions. Although health care for obese patients has inherently greater demands, health care providers often fail to address these needs, and obese people underutilize health care opportunities available to them. In addition, health care providers are reluctant to counsel patients about obesity, often citing a lack of time during appointments, lack of professional reward for weight management, lack of reimbursement for weight management services, and a lack of knowledge of or faith in the effectiveness of weight management interventions. If a health care provider associates obesity with lack of willpower and with overindulgence, the patient can experience shame in a setting that claims to be a caring one. Nurses are in a pivotal position to help overweight and obese people deal with negative experiences and to educate other health care professionals to eliminate their bias against overweight patients.

Before selecting a weight-loss strategy with the patient, the following questions should be asked:

- What is the patient's motivation for losing weight?
- Is the patient experiencing any major stresses that will make it difficult to focus on weight control?
- Does the patient have any psychiatric illnesses—such as severe depression, substance abuse, or a binge-eating disorder—that will derail weight-loss efforts?
- Can the patient devote the minimal amount of time for physical activity (e.g., at least 15 to 30 minutes per day for the next 6 months) that is needed for a serious weight-loss effort?

Motivation should be assessed because it is essential for a favourable outcome. Lack of motivation is a huge barrier to change. However, the patient should be encouraged to focus on the reasons for wanting to lose weight as he or she faces the challenges in dealing with obesity.

When no organic cause (e.g., hypothyroidism) can be found for obesity, it should be considered a complex, chronic illness. Any supervised plan of care should be directed at (a) successful weight loss, which requires a short-term energy deficit, and (b) successful weight control, which requires long-term behaviour changes (Grief & Talamayan, 2008). A multipronged approach with attention to multiple factors—including nutrition therapy,

physical activity, cognitive–behavioural therapy, and perhaps pharmacotherapy and bariatric surgery—should be used (see Figure 43-6). Focusing on more than one aspect probably provides better balance to weight-loss and weight-control efforts. All opportunities for patient education should stress healthy eating habits and adequate physical activity as lifestyle patterns. A comprehensive, patient-centred, and collaborative approach should be the goal of the health care team (Lau et al., 2007).

Even with a comprehensive action plan, there is a high rate of weight regain among people in all age groups. This is discouraging when one considers the amount of time and effort expended in the process of attempting to lose weight. For successful management of obesity, it helps if obesity is viewed as a chronic condition that necessitates day-to-day attention to lose weight and maintain weight loss. It is essential that the nurse have a nonjudgemental approach in helping patients manage their problems related to obesity.

Nutritional Therapy

Restricted food intake is a cornerstone for any weight loss or maintenance program. A good weight-loss plan should promote healthy eating using Canada's Food Guide (Health Canada, 2011; see Chapter 42, Figure 42-1). Nutrition interventions should be developed with a qualified and experienced health professional, preferably a registered dietitian (Lau, 2007). To support a negative energy balance, it is recommended that energy intake be reduced by 500 to 1000 kcal/day below estimated energy needs to achieve a 0.5 to 1 kg (1 to 2 lb) weight loss per week (Academy of Nutrition and Dietetics, 2012). Diets may be classified as low-calorie (800 to 1200 cal/day) or very-low-calorie (less than 800 cal/day). Although an example of a low-calorie diet is presented in Table 43-7, it is important for the nurse to be aware that dietitians work with patients to develop diets that are based on the patients' current caloric consumption, with subsequent incremental reductions, because the diet must be sustainable over time for the resultant weight loss to be maintained. Once the patient has achieved one goal, subsequent progressive goals are set.

People on low-calorie and very–low-calorie diets need frequent professional monitoring because the severe energy restriction places them at risk for deficiency of multiple nutrients. A diet that includes adequate amounts of fruits and vegetables provides enough bulk to prevent constipation and meets daily vitamin A and vitamin C requirements. Lean meat, fish, and eggs provide sufficient protein, as well as B-complex vitamins. Restricting dietary intake so that it is below energy requirements is an effective way to reduce body weight.

Most overweight people have at some time attempted to lose weight. Some have had limited and temporary success, and others have met only with failure. Many individuals attempt weight loss by trying out a least one of the many fad diets that offer the enticement of quick weight loss with little effort. Often these fad diets advocate for the elimination of one or more categories of foods (e.g., carbohydrates) and should not be followed. Low-carbohydrate diets, for example, do produce a rapid weight loss, but they also may not allow for adequate amounts of fibre, vitamins, and minerals. These diets are difficult to maintain in the long term because of their restrictive nature. It is best to recommend a dietary approach in which caloric restriction includes all food groups. Patients find it easier to incorporate such changes into their lifestyles and do not become bored with their food options. The nurse must work to support patients' understanding

NUTRITIONAL THERAPY

Table 43-7 Sample 1200-Calorie Weight Reduction Diet*

GENERAL PRINCIPLES

1. Eat regularly. Do not skip meals.
2. Measure foods to determine the correct portion size.
3. Avoid concentrated sweets, such as sugar, candy, honey, pies, cakes, cookies, and regular soft drinks.
4. Reduce fat intake by baking, broiling, or steaming foods.
5. Maintain a regular physical activity program for successful weight loss.

MEAL	MENU PLAN†
Breakfast	30 g (¾ cup) dry cereal (unsweetened)
	1 small banana
	250 mL (1 cup) non-fat milk
	Coffee, black, unsweetened
Lunch	Beef & cheese enchiladas (made with 35 g cheese and 57 g lean, ground beef)
	2 corn tortillas with shredded lettuce
	2 tsp chile sauce
	1 cup sliced tomatoes and cucumbers
	30 mL (1 tbsp) low-fat salad dressing
	½ cup (approx 12) grapes
	2 cups water
Dinner	75 g baked chicken breast (no skin)
	5 mL (1 tsp) margarine
	2 cups tossed salad and 30 mL (1 tbsp) low-fat salad dressing
	½ cup strawberries
	½ cup whole grain rice
	250 mL (1 cup) non-fat milk

*For 1500 calories, add one meat and alternatives serving and two vegetable and fruit servings, and include one serving of the daily recommended oil and fats. For 1800 calories, add one grain product serving, one milk and alternative, two meat and alternative servings, two vegetable and fruit servings, and an additional serving of oil and fats.

†See eTable 43-1, available on the Evolve Web site for this chapter, for additional sample meal plans.

that following a well-balanced, low-calorie diet is an essential part of weight loss and is superior to fad diets in achieving and supporting weight loss and sustained weight maintenance. The degree of success of any reducing diet depends in part on the amount of weight to be lost. Moderately obese people attain the goal more easily than morbidly obese people. Perhaps because men have a higher percentage of lean body mass, men are able to lose weight more quickly than women. Women have a higher percentage of body fat, which is metabolically less active than muscle tissue. Postmenopausal women are particularly prone to weight gain, including increased abdominal fat.

Assessing and supporting readiness for change and patient motivation are essential steps in successful weight loss interventions. The obese patient must understand the need for weight loss and weight control and the advantages that will occur. The nurse can assist by helping the patient track eating patterns with a diet diary. A frank discussion of eating habits helps the patient realize that eating is often the result of bad habits picked up with time and not the result of hunger. The bad habits must be changed, or weight loss will be only temporary.

Setting a realistic and healthy goal, such as losing 0.5 to 1 kg (1 to 2 lb) per week, must be mutually agreed on at the outset. Trying to lose too much too fast usually results in a sense of frustration and failure for the patient. The nurse can help the patient understand that losing large amounts of weight in a short period causes skin and underlying tissue to lose elasticity and tone, resulting in loose folds of skin and tissue. Slower weight loss offers better cosmetic results. Inevitably, the patient reaches plateau periods during which no weight is lost. These plateaus may last from several days to several weeks. It is especially important for the patient to realize that these are normal occurrences during weight reduction, so that discouragement, frustration, and giving up of the prescribed dietary plan are prevented. A weekly check of body weight is a good method of monitoring progress. Daily weighing is not recommended because of the frequent fluctuations resulting from retained water (including urine) and elimination of feces. Instruct the patient to record his or her weight at the same time of the day, wearing the same type of clothing.

There is no firm agreement on the number of meals to be eaten when a person is on a diet; however, breakfast should not be missed. Some nutritionists advocate several small meals per day because the body's metabolic rate is temporarily increased immediately after eating. However, when several small meals are ingested per day, more calories may be consumed. The patient should be instructed to carefully adhere to portion sizes and stay within the total daily calorie allotment. There seems to be general agreement that consumption of most of the daily caloric intake at a large evening meal results in less weight loss than when the calories are evenly distributed throughout the day.

When a person first begins a weight reduction program, food portion sizes must be carefully determined to stay within the dietary guidelines. Portion sizes have increased considerably since the 1990s (Ello-Martin, Ledikwe, & Rolls, 2005; see Table 43-4). Food portions can be weighed on a scale, or everyday objects can be used as a visual cue to determine portion sizes; for example, the size of a woman's fist or a baseball is equivalent to one serving of vegetables or fruit. A serving of meat is about the size of an adult's palm or a deck of cards. A serving of cheese is about the size of a thumb or six dice (see the Alberta Health Services Web site listed in the Resources section at the end of this chapter for a sample patient teaching tool). A test on portion sizes is also available online (see the Resources at the end of this chapter).

As identified in Chapter 42, Canada's Food Guide provides a solid example of a balanced diet and instruction to assist individuals with making healthy choices, with appropriate portions from each of the food groups. The patients can be further assisted in understanding and exercising good portion control and choosing appropriate proportions from each of the food groups by describing a healthy meal by how portions fit on a plate (Figure 43-7). Half of a "healthy plate" consists of vegetables and fruit, one fourth consists of meat and meat alternatives, and one fourth consists of grain products.

A list of healthy, low-calorie foods serves as a good reference and enables the patient to eat an occasional meal at a restaurant. The patient who carefully follows the prescribed diet may not need to take vitamin supplements. Appropriate fluid intake should be encouraged. Alcoholic beverages are usually not permitted on a reducing diet because they increase the caloric intake and have low nutritional value.

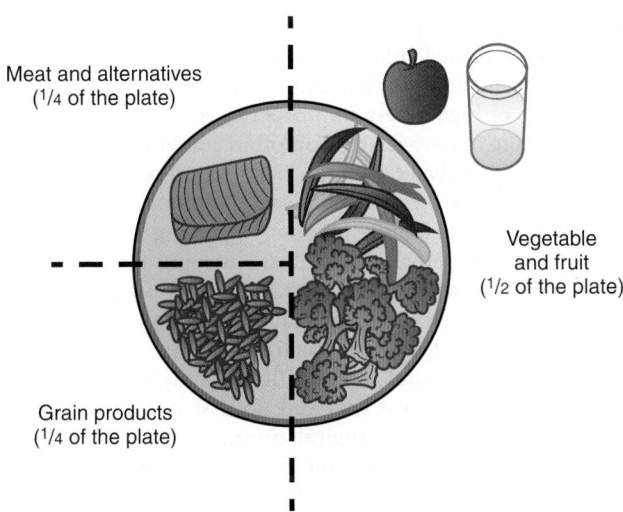

Meat and alternatives
(¹/₄ of the plate)

Vegetable
and fruit
(¹/₂ of the plate)

Grain products
(¹/₄ of the plate)

Figure 43-7 The sizes of healthy portions on a plate.

Source: Redrawn from Alberta Health Services. (2010). *What is a healthy plate?* Retrieved from *http://www.albertahealthservices.ca/SchoolsTeachers/if-sch-nfs-what-is-a-healthy-portion-size.pdf*

Physical Activity

Physical activity is an essential part of a weight-control program (Lau et al., 2007) and should be performed daily, preferably 30 minutes to an hour a day. There is no evidence that increased activity promotes an increase in appetite or leads to dietary excess. In fact, physical activity frequently has the opposite effect. The addition of physical activity produces more weight loss than does dieting alone. Increasing physical activity has a favourable effect on body fat distribution with a reduction in WHR. Physical activity is especially important in maintaining weight loss in overweight and obese people.

The nurse and the patient should explore possible ways to increase physical activity in daily routines. It may be as simple as parking farther from the place of employment or taking the stairs rather than an elevator. The patient should be encouraged to wear a pedometer to track daily activity. The goal is 10,000 steps a day. However, initial success may be in walking a third of the recommended steps, with incremental increases over time.

Joining a health club can be one mechanism of getting physical activity. Walking, swimming, and cycling are sensible forms of physical activity and have long-term benefits. Engaging in weekend exercise only or in spurts of strenuous activity is not advantageous and can actually be dangerous. When large muscles are involved in the physical activity program, a primary benefit is cardiovascular conditioning. Overweight men and women who are active and fit have lower rates of morbidity and mortality than overweight people who are sedentary and unfit. Therefore, physical activity is of benefit to overweight people even if it does not make them lean.

Many psychological benefits can be derived from an increased physical activity program. Reduction in tension and stress, better-quality sleep and rest, increased stamina and energy, improved self-concept and self-confidence, better attitudes toward work and play, and increased optimism about the future can be achieved.

Behaviour Modification

The assumption behind cognitive behaviour modification is twofold: (a) that obesity is a learned disorder caused by overeating and (b) that the critical difference between an obese person and a person of normal weight is in the cues that regulate eating behaviour. Therefore, most behaviour-modification programs de-emphasize the diet and focus on how and when the person eats. Participants often are taught to restrict their eating to designated meals and to increase the amount of physical activity in their lives. People who have undergone behaviour therapy are more successful in maintaining their losses over an extended time than are those who do not participate in such training.

Common behavioural techniques included in weight management interventions are (a) self-monitoring, (b) stimulus control, and (c) rewards. *Self-monitoring* may involve keeping a record of what and when foods are eaten, as well as how the person was feeling when the foods were consumed. *Stimulus control* is aimed at separating events that trigger eating from the act of eating. *Rewards* may be used as incentive for weight loss. Short- and long-term goals are useful benchmarks for earning rewards. It is important that the reward for a specified weight loss not be associated with food, such as dinner out or a favourite treat. Reward items do not have to have a monetary component. For example, time for a hot bath or an hour of pleasure reading would be an enjoyable reward for many people. People may participate in group or individual sessions, or both, as they work toward their goals.

Support Groups

The patient who is on any type of restrictive dietary program is often encouraged to join a group of other obese people who are receiving professional counselling to help them modify their eating habits. Many self-help groups are available to the person who wants to learn more about successful dieting and who likes the support of others who have the same problems and experiences. Take Off Pounds Sensibly (TOPS) is the oldest nonprofit organization of this type in the world. Behaviour modification is an integral part of the program, along with nutrition education. Weight Watchers International, Inc. is probably the most successful commercial weight-reduction enterprise. Weight Watchers offers a food plan that is nutritionally balanced and practical to follow, and its programs have included behaviour-modification techniques since 1974.

Commercial weight-reduction centres have proliferated across the nation. Many of these programs are staffed by nurses or dietitians, or both, and candidates must undergo an initial physical examination by a health care provider before being accepted for weight reduction. Although behaviour-modification training is often incorporated within these programs, they are often costly and the cost may be prohibitive for people with limited financial resources. In addition, many of these programs offer special prepackaged foods and supplements that must be purchased as part of the weight-reduction plan. Only these prescribed foods and drinks are to be consumed until an agreed-on amount of weight is lost. The patient is encouraged to buy the same type of foods for the maintenance phase of the program, which lasts from 6 months to 1 year. This is problematic for reasons beyond just the associated costs. Obesity, as with all chronic diseases, resumes its course when the intervention stops. Patients are often frustrated to find that the weight they lost is regained once they stop participating in the commercial program. Individuals who discontinue such programs must be supported to learn to adjust their diet appropriately to maintain their intervention and the resultant weight loss.

Many places of employment have started programs on health teaching and maintenance. The rationale for such programs is that better health repays the cost of the programs through improved work performance, decreased absenteeism, and eventually less hospitalization. Weight-reduction and hypertension-reduction programs have been instituted and are popular with employees.

Drug Therapy

Drugs have been used to treat obesity but only as adjuncts to nutrition, physical activity, and behavioural modification therapies. Pharmacotherapy should be reserved for patients with a BMI ≥27kg/m² who have existing comorbid conditions (e.g., hypertension, dyslipidemia, coronary artery disease, type 2 diabetes mellitus, and sleep apnea) and for those with a BMI ≥30 kg/m² (Lau, 2007). Currently, drugs approved for weight loss in Canada are the kind that decrease nutrient absorption. Drugs that decrease food intake by reducing appetite or increasing satiety (e.g., sibutramine [Meridia]) and drugs that increase energy expenditure (e.g., ephedrine) are not approved for weight loss in Canada at this time.

Nutrient Absorption–Blocking Drugs

Orlistat (Xenical), a drug that was developed for weight loss and maintenance, works by blocking fat breakdown and absorption in the intestine. It inhibits the action of intestinal lipases. The undigested fat is excreted in the feces. Although this drug has a high safety profile, levels of some fat-soluble vitamins may decrease, and those vitamins may have to be supplemented. Orlistat is associated with leakage of stool, flatulence, diarrhea, and abdominal bloating, which is accentuated if a high-fat diet is consumed. These adverse effects limit its acceptance as a weight-loss tool (Padwal, Rucker, Li, Curioni, & Lau, 2009). Drugs do not cure obesity, and the patient must understand that without substantial changes in food intake and increased physical activity, weight will be regained when short-term drug therapy is stopped. Supervised long-term drug therapy with safe compounds can contribute to weight management as well as weight loss. As with any pharmacological treatment, there are adverse effects. Careful evaluation for the presence of other medical conditions can help determine which drugs, if any, would be advisable for a given patient.

The role of the nurse in relation to drug therapy should centre on teaching the patient about proper administration and adverse events and the role of the drug fits into the larger weight-loss plan. Modifying the dosage without consulting a health care provider can have detrimental effects. The nurse should re-emphasize that the diet and physical activity regimens are the cornerstones of permanent weight loss. Drugs may be helpful, but they do not help the patient change eating behaviour. The purchase of over-the-counter diet aids should be discouraged.

Collaborative Surgical Therapy

Bariatric surgery is an invasive procedure used to treat morbid obesity. Bariatric surgery is currently the only treatment that has been found to help sustain weight loss in severely obese individuals. The majority of patients who undergo bariatric surgery have successfully improved their overall quality of life. A great deal of excess weight is lost, comorbid conditions resolve, and

patients' appearance, social opportunities, and economic opportunities are improved (Klarenbach et al., 2010).

Criteria guidelines for bariatric surgery include having a BMI of 40 kg/m² or higher, or a BMI of 35 kg/m² or higher plus one or more severe obesity-related comorbid conditions (e.g., hypertension, type 2 diabetes mellitus, heart failure, or sleep apnea). Many adults meet these criteria, and additional recommendations must be taken into account, including a documented history of conventional weight loss attempts that have been unsuccessful over time; a demonstrated history of accountability and responsibility marked by regular appointment attendance, practising self-monitoring, completing laboratory tests, regularly taking medications, and making time for healthy eating and activity. The patient must have full understanding of the benefits and limitations of a surgical procedure to assist with the management of obesity, and the risk of the surgical procedure must be lower than the risks of not providing the treatment (Karmali et al., 2010). Table 43-8 describes exclusion criteria for bariatric surgery (see also the Evidence-Informed Practice box "How Can Nurses Help Patients Who Are Considering Bariatric Surgery?").

Patients are not good candidates for bariatric surgery if they are (a) obese as a result of a treatable disorder (e.g., hypothyroidism); (b) have untreated depression or psychosis, binge eating disorder, or bulimia; (c) currently abuse drugs or alcohol; (d) have severe cardiac disease with prohibitive anaesthetic-related risks; (e) have severe coagulopathy; or (f) are unable to comply with nutritional requirements. Bariatric surgeries fall into one of three broad categories: restrictive, malabsorptive, or a combination of malabsorptive and restrictive (Table 43-9 and Figure 43-8). In restrictive procedures, the stomach is reduced in size (less food eaten), and in malabsorptive procedures, the length of the small intestine is decreased (less food absorbed).

Table 43-8 Exclusion Criteria for Bariatric Surgery

Patients *who are* or *who have* any of the following characteristics should not be offered bariatric surgery:

- BMI <35 kg/m²
- Age <18 yr or >65 yr
- A medical condition that makes surgery too risky
- Clinically significant or unstable mental health concerns
- An unrealistic postsurgical target weight
- Unrealistic expectations of a surgical procedure
- Not tried or optimized lifestyle or medical treatments
- A history of poor compliance with lifestyle, medical, or mental health interventions
- Pregnant, lactating, or plan for pregnancy within 2 yr of potential surgical treatment
- Lack of safe access to abdominal cavity or gastrointestinal tract
- Smokers (All smokers, regardless of their weight status, should quit smoking for at least 8 weeks before surgery as a goal of risk-factor management. All patients should be encouraged to remain nonsmokers or participate in smoking cessation programs.)

Source: Karmali, S., Johnson Stoklossa, C., Sharma, A., Stadnyk, J., Christiansen, S., Cottreau, D., & Birch, D. W. (2010). Bariatric surgery: A primer. *Canadian Family Physician, 56*, 874, Box 1.
BMI, body mass index.

How Can Nurses Help Patients Who Are Considering Bariatric Surgery?

Clinical (PICO) Question

For patients who are obese (P), what are the indications for recommending bariatric surgery (I) versus non-surgical weight-loss methods (C) to decrease the risk of conditions comorbid with obesity (O)?

Best Available Evidence

Clinical practice guidelines based on systematic review of randomized controlled trials

Critical Appraisal and Synthesis of Evidence

- Recommendations are based on high-quality evidence and benefits that exceed risk.
- Patients with BMI of ≥ 40 kg/m^2 are generally eligible for bariatric surgery when it is not associated with excessive risk.
- Patients with BMI of ≥ 35 kg/m^2 and severe comorbid conditions may also be eligible for bariatric surgery. These conditions include coronary artery disease, type 2 diabetes mellitus, obstructive sleep apnea, obesity-hypoventilation syndrome, pickwickian syndrome, hypertension, dyslipidemia, gastroesophageal reflux disease, asthma, venous stasis disease, severe urinary incontinence, debilitating arthritis, or considerably impaired quality of life.
- There is no strong evidence for preferred type of bariatric surgery for severely obese patients.
- Procedure of choice depends on surgical expertise, patient preference, and risk assessment specific to procedure.

Conclusion

- Bariatric surgery outcomes are generally positive for patients with a BMI of ≥ 40 kg/m^2 who do not have excessive risks and for patients with a BMI of ≥ 35 kg/m^2 who have one or more severe comorbid conditions.

Implications for Nursing Practice

- For patients with a BMI of <40 kg/m^2 who have no comorbid conditions, counsel and refer for weight loss management options.
- Collaborative care for types of bariatric surgery can vary widely.
- Obtain specific care and diet information related to surgical procedure to teach patient.

Reference for Evidence

Mechanick, J. I., Kushner, R. F., Sugerman, H. J., Gonzalez-Campoy, J. M., Collazo-Clavell, M. L., Guven, S., ..., Dixon, J. (2008). Medical guidelines for clinical practice for the perioperative nutritional, metabolic, and nonsurgical support of the bariatric surgery client. *Endocrine Practice*, 14(Suppl. 1), S1-S83.

BMI, body mass index.

Restrictive Surgeries

Restrictive bariatric surgery reduces the size of a stomach to a capacity for 30 mL or less, which causes the patient to feel full more quickly (Kaser & Kukla, 2009). The stomach and the intestine digest and absorb food normally when restrictive gastrointestinal surgery is performed. Because digestion is not altered, the risk for anemia or cobalamin deficiency is low. These procedures can be performed using a laparoscopic approach, which decreases the rate of wound infection and hernia formation. Weight loss is typically more gradual with these procedures. Several restrictive procedures are available. The most common are discussed as follows.

Vertical Banded Gastroplasty. *Vertical banded gastroplasty* involves partitioning the stomach into a small pouch in the upper portion along the lesser curvature of the stomach. This small pouch drastically limits capacity. In addition, the stoma opening to the rest of the stomach is banded to delay emptying of solid food from the proximal pouch. This procedure has been replaced by other procedures because of lack of sustained or desired weight loss and the high incidence of complications.

Adjustable Gastric Banding. With *adjustable gastric banding*, the stomach size is limited by an inflatable band placed around the fundus of the stomach. This restrictive procedure can be done using the Lap-Band system or the Realize Band system. The band is connected to a subcutaneous port and can be inflated or deflated (by fluid injection in the health care provider's office) to change the stoma size to meet the patient's needs as weight is lost. The procedure can be done laparoscopically and can be modified or reversed after the initial procedure. Adjustable gastric banding is the procedure most commonly performed, and it is the preferred option for patients who are at surgical risk because it is a less invasive approach.

Malabsorptive Surgery

In malabsorptive surgery to reduce weight, the surgeon bypasses various lengths of the small intestine so that less food is absorbed.

Biliopancreatic Diversion. Biliopancreatic diversion (BPD) involves removing approximately 75% of the stomach to produce both restriction of food intake and reduction of acid output. The remaining portion of the stomach is connected to the lower portion of the small intestine. Nutrients pass without being digested. The patient loses weight because most of the calories and nutrients are routed into the colon, where they are not absorbed.

This procedure can increase the risk of gallstone formation and may necessitate removal of the gallbladder. Patients should be aware of the possibilities of intestinal irritation and ulcers. Other risks from BPD include abdominal bloating and foul-smelling stool or gas. During the period when the intestines adjust, bowel movements can be very liquid and frequent. This condition may lessen over time, but it may be a lifelong condition. Patients should also monitor their protein, iron, and cobalamin intake to ensure that they do not develop malnutrition or anemia. Supplements and vitamins should be taken to offset these risks.

Biliopancreatic Diversion With Duodenal Switch. A variation of the BPD procedure involves a duodenal switch in which the surgeon leaves intact a larger portion of the stomach, as well as a small part of the duodenum. This procedure also enables sparing of the pyloric valve, which helps prevent dumping syndrome. (Dumping syndrome is discussed later in the chapter and in Chapter 44.)

Table 43-9 Surgical Interventions for Morbid Obesity*			
PROCEDURE	**ANATOMICAL CHANGES**	**ADVANTAGES**	**COMPLICATIONS**
Restrictive Surgery			
Vertical banded gastroplasty	Band is placed around stomach and staples used above band to create a small gastric pouch.	No surgical anastomosis More normal anatomy and physiology maintained Lower risk of infection	High complication rate Slow weight loss Rupture of staple line Dilated pouch Dumping syndrome (nausea, vomiting, and/or diarrhea related to ingestion of sweets, high-calorie liquids, or dairy products)
Adjustable gastric banding (Lap-Band, Realize Band)	Band encircles the stomach, creating a stoma and a gastric pouch with about 30 mL capacity	Low complication rate Food digestion occurs through normal process Adjustability of band to ↑ or ↓ restriction Procedure is reversible Absence of dumping syndrome Lack of malabsorption	Some nausea and vomiting initially Problems with adjustment device Slippage or erosion of band into stomach wall Gastric perforation
Vertical sleeve gastrectomy	Approximately 85% of stomach is removed leaving a sleeve-shaped stomach with 60-150 mL capacity	Preservation of stomach function No bypass of intestine Avoidance of complications of obstruction, anemia, vitamin deficiencies	Weight loss may be limited Leakage related to stapling
Malabsorptive Surgery			
Biliopancreatic diversion with or without duodenal switch	Approximately 70% of the stomach is removed horizontally Anastomosis between the stomach and the intestine decreases the amount of small intestine available for nutrient absorption Duodenal switch cuts the stomach vertically and is shaped like a tube	Increased amount of food intake Less food intolerance Greater long-term weight loss Rapid weight loss	Abdominal bloating, diarrhea, and foul-smelling gas (steatorrhea) Three or four loose bowel movements a day Malabsorption of fat-soluble vitamins Iron deficiency Protein-calorie malnutrition† Dumping syndrome†
Combination of Restrictive and Malabsorptive Surgery			
Roux-en-Y gastric bypass	Restrictive surgery on stomach creating pouch Small gastric pouch is connected to jejunum Remaining stomach and first segment of small intestine are bypassed	Better weight loss results than gastric restrictive procedures Lower incidences of malnutrition and diarrhea Rapid improvement of weight-related comorbid conditions	Leak at site of anastomosis Anemia: iron deficiency, cobalamin deficiency, folic acid deficiency Calcium deficiency Dumping syndrome

GI, gastrointestinal.
*See Figure 43-9.
†With duodenal switch, this problem is less common.

Combination of Restrictive and Malabsorptive Surgery

Roux-en-Y Surgical Procedure. The Roux-en-Y gastric bypass procedure is a combination of restrictive and malabsorptive surgery. Complication rates with this procedure are low, patient tolerance is excellent, and the procedure has proved to sustain long-term weight loss. Because of this, the Roux-en-Y gastric bypass procedure is the bariatric surgery most commonly performed. In this procedure, the stomach size is decreased with a gastric pouch anastomosis that empties directly into the jejunum. This surgery can be performed through an open abdominal incision or laparoscopically. Variations of this procedure include (a) stapling the stomach without transection to create a small gastric pouch (capacity, 20-30 mL); (b) creating an upper and a lower gastric pouch and totally disconnecting the pouches; and (c) creating an upper gastric pouch and completely removing the lower pouch. After the procedure, food bypasses 90% of the stomach, the duodenum, and a small segment of jejunum (Blackwood, 2005).

Weight loss is usually greatest during the first year after surgery. Weight tends to stabilize after 18 months. Outcomes include increased glucose tolerance, decreased BP, decreased levels of cholesterol and triglycerides, decreased incidence of

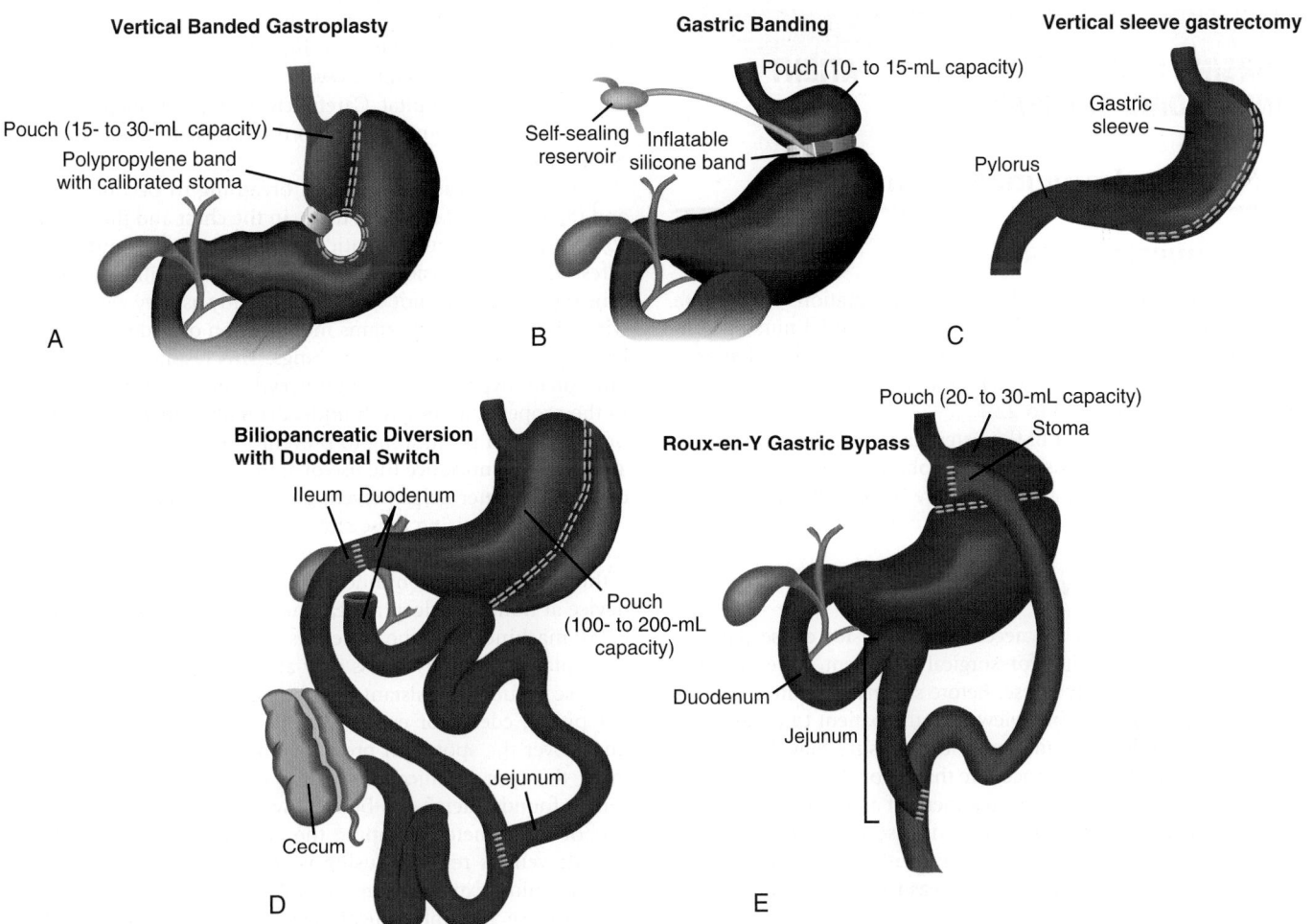

Figure 43-8 Bariatric surgical procedures. **A,** Vertical banded gastroplasty involves creating a small gastric pouch. **B,** Adjustable gastric banding involves the use of a band to create a gastric pouch. **C,** Vertical sleeve gastrectomy involves creating a sleeve-shaped stomach by removing approximately 85% of the stomach. **D,** Biliopancreatic diversion with duodenal switch procedure involves creating an anastomosis between the stomach and intestine. **E,** Roux-en-Y gastric bypass procedure involves constructing a gastric pouch whose outlet is a Y-shaped limb of small intestine.

gastroesophageal reflux disease (GERD), and decreased sleep apnea. A complication of this procedure is *dumping syndrome,* in which gastric contents empty too rapidly into the small intestine, overwhelming its ability to digest nutrients (see Chapter 44). Symptoms can include vomiting, nausea, weakness, sweating, faintness, and, on occasion, diarrhea. To avoid dumping syndrome, patients are discouraged from eating sugary foods after surgery. Because sections of the small intestine are bypassed, poor absorption of iron can cause iron-deficiency anemia. The patient needs to take a multivitamin with iron and calcium supplements. Chronic anemia caused by cobalamin deficiency may also occur. This problem usually can be managed with cobalamin injections or intranasal cobalamin preparations.

Cosmetic Surgeries to Reduce Fatty Tissue and Skinfolds

Lipectomy. Lipectomy (adipectomy) is performed to remove unsightly loose folds of adipose tissue and is performed for cosmetic reasons. In some patients, up to 15% of the total fat cells can be removed from the breasts, the abdomen, and the lumbar and femoral areas. There is no evidence that adipose tissue regenerates at the surgical sites. However, it must be emphasized to the patient that surgical removal does not prevent obesity from

recurring, especially if lifetime eating habits remain the same. Although body image and self-esteem may be enhanced by such procedures, these operations are not without complications. In obese patients, the effects of anaesthetics can be dangerous and wound healing has the potential to be poor. It is more useful for the majority of patients contemplating a lipectomy to be instructed in preventive health measures, such as slow weight reduction to maintain and preserve tissue integrity, the value of physical activity, and behaviour-modification techniques.

Liposuction. Another surgical procedure is *liposuction,* or suction-assisted lipectomy. The current use is for cosmetic purposes and not for weight reduction. This surgical intervention helps improve facial appearance and body contours. A good candidate for this type of surgery is a person who has achieved weight reduction but who has excess fat under the chin, along the jaw line, in the nasolabial folds, over the abdomen, or around the waist and upper thighs. A long, hollow, stainless steel cannula is inserted through a small incision over the fatty tissue to be suctioned. The purpose of this type of surgery is to improve body appearance, thereby enhancing body image and self-concept. It is not usually recommended for older patients because the skin is less elastic and does not accommodate the new underlying shape.

NURSING MANAGEMENT: OBESE PATIENT UNDERGOING SURGERY

Nursing Implementation

Perioperative Care

This section discusses general nursing considerations for the care of the obese patient who is having surgery. Special nursing considerations are described for the patient undergoing bariatric surgery. (Care of the patient before, during, and after surgery is discussed in Chapters 20 to 22.)

Many patients with a BMI greater than 30 kg/m² have several other medical conditions related to obesity that increase their surgical risk factors and affect their care before, during, and after surgery.

Preoperative Care

Special considerations are necessary to care for obese patients admitted to the hospital for surgical treatment, especially the ones who are morbidly obese. Before surgery, it is important to conduct a preoperative interview with the patient to obtain past and current health information and to ensure that the patient understands the surgical procedure that he or she is scheduled to undergo. A team approach to treatment of an obese patient may be necessary. If the patient has a disease other than obesity, it may be necessary to coordinate care with the patient's cardiologist, pulmonologist, gynecologist, gastroenterologist, or other specialist.

Every effort should be made to ensure the patient's dignity and privacy before admission. Most nursing units are not prepared to meet the needs of a patient who is often too large for a typical hospital bed or who does not fit into standard patient care gowns. To eliminate embarrassment for the patient and frustration for the staff, plans should be made to meet particular needs. Oversized BP cuffs should be ready for use when the patient arrives. A single-bed room may be necessary for the privacy of the patient and to accommodate the bed and sitting arrangements. A strongly reinforced trapeze bar should be placed over the bed to facilitate movement and positioning. In some cases, a specially constructed chair may have to be built and beds joined together to allow the patient to sit and sleep in comfort.

The nurse must consider how the patient will be weighed and transported within the hospital, and in what ways simple physical assessment strategies may have to be adjusted. Bariatric equipment such as an oversized wheelchair, bariatric bed, walker, and various lifting devices should be made available in the hospital and used.

Strategies for bathing, turning, and ambulating the patient may require extra staff, and a plan to meet this need should be in place before the patient's admission. Routine physical assessment strategies do not work well with morbidly obese patients, who have numerous layers of skinfolds covering areas that must be assessed. If alternative or unique methods of dealing with this problem are not identified, assessment of respiratory status and bowel sounds or even wound inspection could be awkward for the nurse and embarrassing for the patient. Wound infection is one of the most common complications after surgery (Baugh, Zeulzer, Meador, & Blankenship, 2007). Because of the many layers of excess skinfolds, especially in the abdominal area, preoperative skin preparation is important. Many patients are instructed to take several showers a day for a few days before admission to the hospital. Careful cleansing with soap and warm water of the abdominal area from the breasts to below the waist is emphasized.

Obesity can cause a patient's breathing to become shallow and rapid. The extra adipose tissue in the chest and the abdomen compresses the diaphragmatic, thoracic, and abdominal structures. This compression restricts the chest's ability to expand, causing the lungs to not work as efficiently as they would otherwise. Thus, the patient retains more carbon dioxide. In addition, less oxygen is delivered to the lungs. This results in hypoxemia, pulmonary hypertension, and polycythemia. Instruct the patient in the proper coughing technique, deep breathing, and methods of turning and positioning to prevent pulmonary complications after surgery. Introduce the use of spirometry before surgery. Use of the spirometer helps prevent and alleviate postoperative lung congestion. Practising these strategies preoperatively can aid the patient in performing them correctly after surgery. Furthermore, if the patient uses a continuous positive airway pressure (CPAP) device at home for sleep apnea, make arrangements for use of a CPAP machine while the patient is in the hospital.

Obtaining venous access may also be complicated by excess adipose tissue. An assistant may be needed to help. If a patient has pitting edema or excess fat, the nurse should hold a firm finger over the spot with pressure. The nurse may also want to mark the spot of injection with a sterile skin marker once a vein is found. Edema can become worse if the nurse chooses to anchor the catheter by taping the arm. This action can further impede venous return, causing venous stasis, pooling of intravenous fluids, extravasation, or infiltration. The nurse may also want to use multiple tourniquets to distend veins and hold back excess tissue. To avoid aggravating the edema, the tourniquet should be removed as soon as it is no longer needed. The nurse may also need a longer catheter (longer than 1 in.) to traverse overlying tissue. The cannula must reach far enough into the vein to ensure that it does not become dislodged or cause infiltration.

The use of anaesthetic agents during the surgery increases the patient's risk for failure to wean from mechanical ventilation. This risk is important for the patient to know to be aware of what to expect when he or she wakes up from the anaesthesia.

Special Considerations for Bariatric Surgery.
The hospital experience will depend on the type of procedure and surgical approach. The nurse should prepare the patient before surgery for the possibility of returning to the room with one or more of the following: urinary catheter, IV catheter, compression stockings, and a nasogastric tube. The nurse should emphasize that vital signs and general assessment will be conducted frequently to monitor for immediate complications. Furthermore, the patient must understand that he or she will be assisted with ambulation soon after surgery and encouraged to deep breathe to prevent pulmonary complications. Liquids will be started soon after surgery but only after the patient is fully awake and no anastomosis leaks are found.

Postoperative Care

The initial postoperative care focuses on careful assessment and immediate intervention for cardiopulmonary complications, thrombus formation, anastomosis leaks, and electrolyte imbalances. The transfer from surgery may require many trained staff members. During the transfer, the patient's airway should remain stabilized, and pain should be managed at a tolerable level. Maintain the head of the patient at a 35- to 40-degree angle to reduce abdominal pressure and increase tidal flow. If the patient is severely obese, the nursing team should closely monitor for rapid oxygen desaturation. The body stores anaesthetic agents in adipose tissue; thus the patient with excess adipose tissue is at risk for resedation. As adipose cells release anaesthetic back into the bloodstream, the patient may become sedated after surgery. If this happens, the nursing care team should be prepared to perform a head-tilt or jaw-thrust manoeuvre and keep the patient's oral and nasal airways opened. Early ambulation is essential for the postoperative bariatric patient. Preoperative teaching facilitates the patient's cooperation with what will be an uncomfortable activity. The patient should be informed that typically the evening after surgery, he or she will be assisted to walk and then be ambulated at least three or four times each day. The dangers of thrombophlebitis and measures to counteract its development are a routine part of preoperative teaching. The patient should know that sequential compression devices or elastic compression stockings will be applied to the legs and that active and passive range-of-motion exercises will be a frequent part of daily care. Low-dose heparin may be ordered. Depending on the size of the patient and the amount of pain he or she is experiencing, the patient may not be able to assist the nurse in turning. Extra nurses may be needed to help turn the patient safely.

The patient should also be informed that the nursing care team will also assess the patient's skin for delayed wound healing and the development of seromas, hematomas, wound dehiscence, wound evisceration, and wound infection. Skinfolds should be kept clean and dry to prevent dermatitis and secondary bacterial or fungal infections.

▪ Special Considerations for Bariatric Surgery.
The patient experiences considerable abdominal pain after bariatric surgery. Pain medications should be given as frequently as necessary during the immediate postoperative period (first 24 hours). The nurse must be diligent in assessing pain and be aware that pain could be caused by an anastomosis leak rather than typical surgical pain.

Abdominal wounds must be observed frequently for the amount and type of drainage, condition of the sutures, and signs of infection. The nurse must protect the incision against undue straining that accompanies turning and coughing. Wound dehiscence and wound healing are potential problems for all obese patients. Monitoring the vital signs assists in identifying problems such as infection.

If a nasogastric tube is inserted, the nurse must monitor it for the correct position. Vomiting with a nasogastric tube in place requires repositioning the tube, and the surgeon should be notified immediately. The upper gastric pouch is small, and irrigating the tube with too much solution or manipulating tube position can lead to disruption of the anastomosis or the staple line.

Skin care should be performed several times each shift. Perspiration may be excessive at times. The many layers of skin should be kept clean and dry so that this source of irritation is eliminated. For the patient who has an indwelling catheter, perineal care is important to prevent urinary tract infection.

During the immediate postoperative period (first 24 hours), water and sugar-free clear liquids are administered (30 mL every 2 hours while the patient is awake). Before discharge, the patient should be instructed about a measured amount of a high-protein liquid diet. The patient is taught to eat slowly and to stop when feeling full and not to consume liquids with solid food. Vomiting is a common complication during this time. A dietitian is typically a part of the bariatric team and assists with the transition to the new diet.

▪ Ambulatory and Home Care

▪ Special Considerations for Bariatric Surgery.
The patient who has undergone major surgical treatment for obesity has not, in the past, been successful in following or maintaining a prescribed diet. Now the patient is forced to reduce the oral intake as a result of the anatomical changes brought about by the operation. The patient finds that adherence to a regimen of reduced intake is necessary because of the concern for abdominal distension, cramping abdominal pain, and perhaps diarrhea.

Weight loss is considerable during the first 6 to 12 months. During this time, the patient must learn to adjust intake sufficiently to maintain a stable weight. Although behaviour modification was not an intended outcome when these surgical procedures were devised, it has become an unexpected and beneficial secondary benefit. The diet generally prescribed should be high in protein and low in carbohydrates, fat, and roughage, and consist of six small feedings daily. Fluids should not be ingested with the meal and, in some cases, fluids should be restricted to less than 1000 mL per day. Fluids and foods high in carbohydrate tend to promote diarrhea and symptoms of dumping syndrome. In general, calorically dense foods (foods high in fat) should be avoided to enable more nutritionally sound food to be consumed.

Proper diet must be clearly understood by the patient. Late complications can be anticipated after gastric bypass or gastroplasty, including anemia, vitamin deficiencies, diarrhea, and psychiatric problems. Failure to lose weight or loss of too much weight may be caused by the surgical formation of a stomach pouch that is too large or of an outlet that is much too small, respectively. Peptic ulcer formation, dumping syndrome, and small bowel obstruction may occur late in the recovery and rehabilitative stages.

Long-term follow-up care must be stressed, in part because of complications late in the recovery period. Encourage the patient to adhere strictly to the prescribed diet and to keep the health care provider informed of any changes in physical or emotional condition. Some patients have been known to overeat when they return home and gain rather than lose weight.

The nurse must anticipate and recognize several potential psychological problems after surgery. Some patients express guilt because the only way they could lose weight was by surgical means rather than by the "sheer willpower" of reduced dietary intake. The nurse should be ready to provide support so that such patients do not dwell on negative feelings.

Many morbidly obese patients who blamed their feelings of social inferiority or inadequacies on their appearance before bypass surgery may suffer from episodes of depression. By 6 to 8 months after surgery, considerable weight loss has occurred, and they are able to see clearly how much their appearance has changed. Massive weight loss often leaves the patient with large quantities of loose skin that can cause problems related to altered body image. Reconstructive surgery at least 1 full year after the initial surgery may alleviate this situation. Reduction of breasts, upper arms, thighs, and excess abdominal skinfolds are possible solutions. Discussion of this possible outcome with the patient before surgery and again during the rehabilitation phase of recovery helps facilitate the patient's adjustment to a new body image and social reintegration.

▪ Evaluation

The following outcomes are expected for obese patients after surgery:
• The patient will experience long-term weight loss.
• The patient will experience improvement in obesity-related comorbid conditions.
• The patient will integrate healthy practices into daily routines.
• The patient will monitor for adverse side effects of surgical therapy.
• The patient will have an improved self-image.

AGE-RELATED CONSIDERATIONS: OBESITY IN OLDER ADULTS

The prevalence of obesity is increasing in all age-groups, including older people (Public Health Agency of Canada, 2011). The number of obese older adults has risen markedly because of both an increase in the total number of older people and the percentage of older adults who are obese. Obesity is more common in older women than in older men. A decrease in energy expenditure is an important contributor to a gradual increase in body fat with increasing age.

Obesity in older adults can exacerbate age-related declines in physical function and lead to frailty and disability. Excess body weight places more demands on arthritic joints; mechanical strain on weight-bearing joints can lead to premature immobility. Older adults may find that excess intra-abdominal weight causes urinary incontinence. Excess weight may also contribute to hypoventilation and sleep apnea. Obesity is associated with shortened lifespan: individuals who are obese live 6 to 7 years less than do people of normal weight.

Obesity affects quality of life for older adults. Weight loss can improve quality of life and physical function and lessen obesity-related health complications. The same therapeutic approaches for obesity as discussed earlier also apply to older adults.

Metabolic Syndrome

Metabolic syndrome—also known as *syndrome X, insulin resistance syndrome,* and *dysmetabolic syndrome*—is a collection of risk factors that increase an individual's chance of developing cardiovascular disease and diabetes mellitus. The Canadian Heart Health Surveys, completed between 1986 and 1992, remain the most recent representative Canadian source of measured anthropometry and cardiovascular risk factors. Metabolic syndrome was noted at that time to be present in 17.5% of men and 11.2% of women, with an overall prevalence of 14.4% in Canadian adults from the 10 provinces (Brien & Katzmarzyk, 2006). Metabolic syndrome is diagnosed if an individual has three or more of the conditions listed in Table 43-10.

MEASUREMENT	CATEGORICAL CUTOFF POINT
Waist circumference	Men: ≥102 cm
	Women: ≥88 cm
Triglyceride levels	>1.7 mmol/L
	or
	Drug treatment for elevated triglyceride levels
HDL cholesterol level	Men: <0.9 mmol/L
	Women: <1.1 mmol/L
	or
	Drug treatment for reduced HDL cholesterol level
BP	≥130 mm Hg systolic
	or
	≥85 mm Hg diastolic
	or
	Drug treatment for hypertension
Fasting glucose level	≥10 mmol/L
	or
	Drug treatment for elevated glucose level

Table 43-10 Diagnostic Criteria for Metabolic Syndrome*

Source: Schneider, J. G., Tompkins, C., Blumenthal, R. S., & Mora, S. (2006). The metabolic syndrome in women. *Cardiology in Review, 14*(6), 286-291.
BP, blood pressure; *HDL,* high-density lipoprotein.
*At least three of the five measures must exceed the cutoff level for a diagnosis of metabolic syndrome.

PATHOPHYSIOLOGY MAP

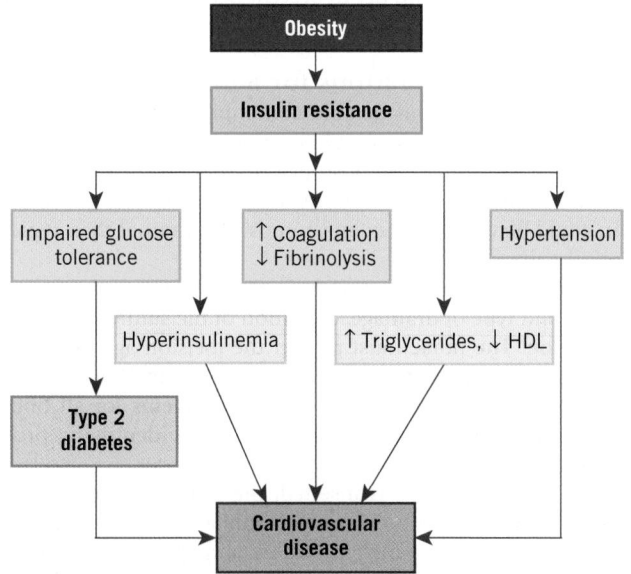

Figure 43-9 Relationships among insulin resistance, obesity, diabetes mellitus, and cardiovascular disease. *HDL,* high-density lipoprotein.

Etiology and Pathophysiology

The main underlying risk factors for metabolic syndrome are abdominal obesity and insulin resistance (Legro, 2009; Figure 43-9). In insulin resistance, the body's cells have a diminished ability to respond to the actions of insulin. To compensate, the pancreas secretes more insulin, which results in hyperinsulinemia. Most people with metabolic syndrome are overweight or obese.

Other characteristics associated with metabolic syndrome include hypertension, increased risk of clotting, and abnormalities in cholesterol levels. Genetics and environment have important roles in the development of metabolic syndrome.

Patients diagnosed with metabolic syndrome typically have diabetes and cannot maintain a proper level of glucose, have hypertension, and secrete a large amount of insulin, or they have survived a heart attack and have hyperinsulinemia.

NURSING AND COLLABORATIVE MANAGEMENT: METABOLIC SYNDROME

Lifestyle therapies are the first-line interventions to reduce the risk factors for metabolic syndrome. Management or reversal of metabolic syndrome can be achieved by reducing the major risk factors of cardiovascular disease: lowering LDL cholesterol level, smoking cessation, lowering BP, and reducing glucose levels. For long-term reduction of risk, weight should be decreased, physical activity increased, and healthy dietary habits established (Magkos, Yannakoulia, Chan, & Mantzoros, 2009).

No specific treatment for metabolic syndrome is available. Nurses can assist patients by providing information on healthy diets, physical activity, and positive lifestyle changes. The diet should be low in saturated fats and promote weight loss. Although low-carbohydrate diets may offer short-term weight loss, there is no strong evidence to support long-term weight loss with such diets. Weight reduction and maintenance of a lower weight should be the first priority in patients with abdominal obesity and metabolic syndrome.

Because sedentary lifestyles contribute to metabolic syndrome, increasing regular physical activity reduces a patient's risk factors. In addition to assisting in weight reduction, regular physical activity has been found to decrease the triglyceride level and increase the HDL cholesterol level in patients with metabolic syndrome.

Patients who are unable to reduce their risk factors with lifestyle therapies alone and those at high risk for a coronary event or diabetes may be considered for drug therapy. Although there is no medication for metabolic syndrome, cholesterol-lowering medication and antihypertensives can be used. Metformin (Glucophage) has also been used to prevent diabetes by lowering glucose levels and enhancing the cells' sensitivity to insulin.

CLINICAL DECISION-MAKING EXERCISE

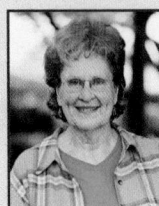

CASE STUDY
Obesity

Patient Profile

Mrs. Stella Roman is a 60-year-old White woman.

Subjective Data

- Reports gradual weight gain during past 40 years
- Spends most of her free time watching television
- Reports health problems related to type 2 diabetes mellitus, shortness of breath, hypertension, chest pressure, and osteoarthritis
- Underwent knee replacement surgery at age 56 for osteoarthritis

Objective Data

Physical Examination
- Height: 162.5 cm (5′4″); weight: 95 kg (210 lb)
- Has obese, nontender, soft abdomen
- Blood pressure: 160/100 mm Hg

Laboratory Results
- Fasting blood glucose level: 13.9 mmol/L
- Total cholesterol level: 5.3 mmol/L
- Triglyceride level: 3.36 mmol/L
- HDL cholesterol level: 0.8 mmol/L

Discussion Questions

1. What are Mrs. Roman's risk factors for obesity?
2. What is her estimated BMI?
3. Of the possible complications of obesity, which ones does Mrs. Roman have? Why did she develop them?
4. *Priority Decision:* How would the nurse assist Mrs. Roman in designing a successful program for weight loss and weight management?
5. What are Mrs. Roman's risk factors for metabolic syndrome?
6. Is Mrs. Roman a candidate for surgical intervention for obesity? If so, why? If not, why not?
7. *Priority Decision:* On the basis of the assessment data presented, what are the priority nursing diagnoses? Are there any collaborative problems?

evolve *Answers are available at* **http://evolve.elsevier.com/ Canada/Lewis/medsurg**

REVIEW QUESTIONS

The number of the question corresponds to the same-numbered objective at the beginning of the chapter.

1. Which of the following statements best describes the etiology of obesity?
   a. Obesity results primarily from a genetic predisposition.
   b. Psychosocial factors can override the effects of genetics in the etiology of obesity.
   c. Obesity is the result of complex interactions between genetic and environmental factors.
   d. Genetic factors are more important than environmental factors in the etiology of obesity.

2. Which obesity classification is *most* often associated with cardiovascular health problems?
   a. Primary obesity
   b. Secondary obesity
   c. Gynoid fat distribution
   d. Android fat distribution

3. Health risks associated with obesity include which of the following? *(Select all that apply.)*
   a. Colorectal cancer
   b. Rheumatoid arthritis
   c. Polycystic ovary disease.
   d. Nonalcoholic steatohepatitis.
   e. Systemic lupus erythematosus

4. What is the best nutritional therapy for a person who is obese?
   a. Low-carbohydrate diet
   b. High-protein diet
   c. Low-sugar diet
   d. Foods from the basic food groups

5. Which bariatric surgical procedure involves creating a stoma and gastric pouch that is reversible and does not involve malabsorption?
   a. Vertical gastric banding
   b. Biliopancreatic diversion
   c. Roux-en-Y gastric bypass
   d. Adjustable gastric banding

6. A morbidly obese patient has undergone Roux-en-Y gastric bypass surgery. In planning postoperative care, what should the nurse anticipate?
   a. The patient may have severe diarrhea early in the postoperative period.
   b. The patient will not be allowed to ambulate for 1 to 2 days postoperatively.
   c. The patient will require nasogastric suction until healing of the incision occurs.
   d. The patient may have only liquids orally, and in very limited amounts, during the early postoperative period.

7. Which of the following criteria must be met for a diagnosis of metabolic syndrome? *(Select all that apply.)*
   a. Hypertension
   b. Elevated triglyceride levels
   c. Elevated plasma glucose level
   d. Increased waist circumference
   e. Decreased LDL levels

ANSWERS: 1. c; 2. d; 3. a, c, d; 4. d; 5. d; 6. d; 7. a, b, c, d.

REFERENCES

Abdullah, A., Wolfe, R., Stoelwinder, J. U., de Courten, M., Stevenson, C., Walls, H. L., & Peeters, A. (2011). The number of years lived with obesity and the risk of all-cause and cause-specific mortality. *International Journal of Epidemiology, 40*(4), 985-986. doi:10.1093/ije/dyr018

Academy of Nutrition and Dietetics. (2012). Adult weight management evidence-based nutrition practice guideline. Retrieved from *http://www.adaevidencelibrary.com/topic.cfm?cat=3014*

Adams, K. F., Schatzkin, A., Harris, T. B., Kipnis, V., Mouw, T., Ballard-Barbash, R., ...Leitzmann, M. F. (2006). Overweight, obesity, and mortality in a large prospective cohort of persons 50 to 71 years old. *New England Journal of Medicine, 355,* 763-778. doi:10.1056/NEJMoa055643

Anis, A. H, Zhang, W., Bansback, N., Guh, D. P., Amarsi, Z., & Birmingham, C. L. (2010). Obesity and overweight in Canada: An updated cost-of-illness study. *Obesity Review, 11*(1), 31-40. doi:10.1111/j.1467-789X.2009.00579.x

Baugh, N., Zuelzer, H., Meador, J., & Blankenship J. (2007). Wounds in surgical patients who are obese. *American Journal of Nursing, 107*(6), 40-50. doi:10.1097/01.NAJ.0000271849.15344.71

Blackwood, H. S. (2005). Help your patient downsize with bariatric surgery. *Nursing2012, 35,* 4-9. Retrieved from *http://journals.lww.com/nursing/Fulltext/2005/09001/Help_your_patient_downsize_with_bariatric_surgery.2.aspx*

Bouchard, C. (2010). Defining the genetic architecture of the predisposition to obesity: A challenging but not insurmountable task. *American Journal of Clinical Nutrition, 91*(1), 5-6. doi:10.3945/ajcn.2009.28933

Brien, S. E., & Katzmarzyk, P. T. (2006). Physical activity and the metabolic syndrome in Canada. *Applied Physiology, Nutrition, and Metabolism, 31*(1), 40-47. doi:10.1139/h05-024

Budge, H., Sebert, S., Sharkey, D., & Symonds, M. E. (2009). Session on obesity: Adipose tissue development, nutrition in early life and its impact on later obesity. *The Proceedings of the Nutrition Society, 68*(3), 321-326. doi:10.1017/S0029665109001402

Canadian Society for Exercise Physiology. (2011). Canadian physical activity guidelines and Canadian sedentary behaviour guidelines. Retrieved from *http://www.csep.ca/english/view.asp?x=804*

Daniels, J. (2006). Obesity: America's epidemic. *American Journal of Nursing, 106*(1), 40-49. doi:10.1097/00000446-200601000-00028

Davis, N., Forges, B., & Wylie-Rosett, J. (2009). Role of obesity and lifestyle intervention in the prevention and management of type 2 diabetes. *Minerva Medica, 100*(3), 221-228.

Depres, J. P., & Lemieux, I. (2006). Abdominal obesity and the metabolic syndrome, *Nature, 444,* 881-887. doi:10.1038/nature05488

Ello-Martin, J. A., Ledikwe, J. H., & Rolls, B. J. (2005). The influence of food portion size and energy density on energy intake: Implications for weight management. *American Journal of Clinical Nutrition, 82*(Suppl.), 236S-241S.

Frayling, T. M., Timpson, N. J., Weedon, M. N., Zeggini, E., Freathy, R. M., Lindgren, C. M., …, McCarthy, M. I. (2007). A common variant in the *FTO* gene is associated with body mass index and predisposes to childhood and adult obesity. *Science, 316*(5826), 889-894. doi:10.1126/science.1141634

Grief, S., & Talamayan, K. (2008). Preventing obesity in the primary care setting. *Primary Care, 35,* 625-643. doi:10.1016/j.pop.2008.07.002

Guh, D. P., Zhang, W., Bansback, N., Amarsi, Z., Laird Birmingham, C., & Anis, A. H. (2009). The incidence of co-morbidities related to obesity and overweight: A systematic review and meta-analysis. *BMC Public Health, 9,* 88. doi:10.1186/1471-2458-9-88

Halberg, N., Wernstedt-Asterholm, I., & Sherer, P. (2008). The adipocyte as an endocrine cell. *Endocrinology and Metabolism Clinics of North America, 37*(3), 753-768. doi:10.1016/j.ecl.2008.07.002

Health Canada. (2003). *Canadian guidelines for body weight classification in adults.* Ottawa: Author. Retrieved from *http://www.hc-sc.gc.ca/fn-an/alt_formats/hpfb-dgpsa/pdf/nutrition/cg_quick_ref-ldc_rapide_ref-eng.pdf*

Health Canada. (2011). *Eating well with Canada's food guide.* Ottawa: Author. Retrieved from *http://www.hc-sc.gc.ca/fn-an/alt_formats/hpfb-dgpsa/pdf/food-guide-aliment/view_eatwell_vue_bienmang-eng.pdf*

Hossain, P., Kawar, B., & El Nahas, M. (2011). Obesity and diabetes in the developing world—A growing challenge. *New England Journal of Medicine, 356*(3), 213-215. doi:10.1056/NEJMp068177

Hramiak, I., Leiter, L., Paul, T. L., & Ur, E. (2007). 2006 Canadian clinical practice guidelines on the management and prevention of obesity in adults and children: Part 6. Assessment of obesity and its complications in adults. *Canadian Medical Association Journal, 176*(8), 36-39.

Karmali, S., Johnson Stoklossa, C., Sharma, A., Stadnyk, J., Christiansen, S., …, Birch, D. W. (2010). Bariatric surgery: A primer. *Canadian family physician, 56,* 873-879.

Kaser, N., & Kukla, A. (2009). Weight-loss surgery, *The Online Journal of Issues in Nursing, 14*(1). Retrieved from *http://nursingworld.org/MainMenuCategories/ANAMarketplace/ANAPeriodicals/OJIN/TableofContents/Vol142009/No1Jan09/Weight-Loss-Surgery.html*

Kirk, S. F. L., Penney, T. L., McHugh, T.-L. F., & Sharma, A. M. (2011). Effective weight management practice: A review of the lifestyle intervention evidence. *International Journal of Obesity, 36,* 178-185. doi:10.1038/ijo.2011.80

Klarenbach, S. Padwal, R., Wiebe, N., Hazel, M., Birch, D., Manns, B., …, Tonelli, M. (2010). *Bariatric surgery for severe obesity: Systematic review and economic evaluation (Technology report no. 129).* Ottawa: Canadian Agency for Drugs and Technologies in Health. Retrieved from *http://www.cadth.ca/index.php/en/hta/reports-publications/search?&type=16*

Lau, D. C. W. (2007). Synopsis of the 2006 Canadian clinical practice guidelines on the management and prevention of obesity in adults and children. *Canadian Medical Association Journal, 176*(8), 1103-1106. doi:10.1503/cmaj.070306

Lau, D. C. W., Douketis, J. D., Morrison, K. M., Hramiak, I. M., Sharma, A. M., Ur, E., & Obesity Canada Clinical Practice Guidelines Expert Panel. (2007). 2006 Canadian clinical practice guidelines on the management and prevention of obesity in in adults and children [summary]. *Canadian Medical Association Journal, 176*(8), S1-S13.

Legro, R. S. (2009). Insulin resistance in women's health: why it matters and how to identify it. *Current Opinion in Obstetrics and Gynecology, 21*(4), 301-305. doi:10.1097/GCO.0b013e32832e07d5

Li, S., Zhao, J. H., Luan, J., Luben, R. N., Rodwell, S. A., Kaw, K., …, Loos, R. J. F. (2010). Cumulative effects and predictive value of common obesity-susceptibility variants identified by genome-wide association studies. *American Journal of Clinical Nutrition, 91*(1), 184-190. doi:10.3945/ajcn.2009.28403

Magkos, F., Yannakoulia, M., Chan, J. L, & Mantzoros, C. S. (2009). Management of the metabolic syndrome and type 2 diabetes through lifestyle modification. *Annual Reviews of Nutrition, 29,* 223-256. doi:10.1146/annurev-nutr-080508-141200

Malis, C., Rasmussen, E. L., Poulsen, P., Petersen, I., Christensen, K., Beck-Nielsen, H., …, Vaag, A. A. (2005). Total and regional fat distribution is strongly influenced by genetic factors in young and elderly twins. *Obesity Research, 13,* 2139-2145. doi:10.1038/oby.2005.265

National Heart, Lung, and Blood Institute & National Institute of Diabetes and Digestive and Kidney Diseases. (1998). Clinical guidelines on the identification, evaluation, and treatment of overweight and obesity in adults. The evidence report. Retrieved from *http://www.ncbi.nlm.nih.gov/books/NBK2003*

Neary, M. T., & Batterham, R. L. (2009). Gut hormones: Implications for the treatment of obesity. *Pharmacology & Therapeutics, 124*(1), 44-56. doi:10.1016/j.pharmthera.2009.06.005

Padwal, R. S., Rucker, D., Li, S. K., Curioni, C., & Lau, D. C. W. (2009). Long-term pharmacotherapy for obesity and overweight. *Cochrane Metabolic and Endocrine Disorders Group.* doi:10.1002/14651858.CD004094.pub2

Public Health Agency of Canada. (2011). Obesity in Canada: A joint report from the Public Health Agency of Canada and the Canadian Institute for Health Information. Retrieved from *http://www.healthyenvironmentforkids.ca/sites/healthyenvironmentforkids.ca/files/Obesity_in_Canada.pdf*

Puhl, R., & Heuer, C. (2009). The stigma of obesity: A review and update. *Obesity, 17*(5), 941-964. doi:10.1038/oby/2008.636

Renehan, A. G., Tyson, M., Egger, M., Heller, R. F., Zwalen, M. (2008). Body-mass index and incidence of cancer: A systematic review and meta-analysis of prospective observational studies. *Lancet, 371,* 569-578. doi:10.1016/S0140-6736(08)60269-X

Shields, M. (2005). *Overweight Canadian children and adolescents. Nutrition: Findings from the Canadian Community Health Survey (Cat. No. 82-620-MWE).* Ottawa, ON: Statistics Canada.

Shields, M., Carroll, M. D. & Ogden, C. L. (2011). *Adult obesity prevalence in Canada and the United States (NCHS Data Brief No. 56).* Hyattsville, MD: National Center for Health Statistics. Retrieved from *http://www.cdc.gov/nchs/data/databriefs/db56.htm*

Sowers, J. R. (2008). Endocrine functions and adipose tissue: focus on adiponectin. *Clinical Cornerstone, 9*(1), 32-38. doi:10.1016/S1098-3597(08)60026-5

Stunkard, A., Sorensen, T. I., Hanis, C., Teasdale, T. W., Chakraborty, R., Schull, W. J., & Schulsinger, F. (1986). An adoption study of human obesity. *New England Journal of Medicine, 314*(4), 193-198. doi:10.1056/NEJM198601233140401

Swinburn, B., & Shelly, A. (2008). Effects of TV time and other sedentary pursuits. *International Journal of Obesity, 32*(Suppl. 7), 132-136. doi:10.1038/ijo.2008.249

Tremblay, M. S. (2007). Major initiatives related to childhood obesity and physical activity in Canada: The year in review. *Canadian Journal of Public Health, 98*(6), 457-459.

World Health Organization. (2000). *Obesity: Preventing and managing the global epidemic* (WHO Technical Report Series 894). Geneva, Switzerland: Author.

CANADIAN RESOURCES

Alberta Health Services: Choose Healthy Food Portions
http://www.albertahealthservices.ca/SchoolsTeachers/if-sch-nfs-what-is-a-healthy-portion-size.pdf

The Canadian Association of Bariatric Physicians and Surgeons
http://www.cabps.ca

Canadian Cancer Society Research Institute
http://www.cancer.ca/Research.aspx

Canadian Institute of Health Research Institute of Nutrition,
Metabolism & Diabetes (INMD)
http://www.cihr-irsc.gc.ca/e/13521.html
Canadian Obesity Network
http://www.obesitynetwork.ca
Canadian Physical Activity Guidelines
http://www.csep.ca/CMFiles/Guidelines/CSEP-Guidelines-
Handbook.pdf
Canadian Society for Exercise Physiology
http://www.csep.ca/english/view.asp?x=1
Dietitians of Canada
http://www.dietitians.ca
Health Canada
http://www.hc-sc.gc.ca
Health Canada BMI Nomogram
http://www.hc-sc.gc.ca/fn-an/alt_formats/hpfb-dgpsa/pdf/nutrition/
cg_quick_ref-ldc_rapide_ref-eng.pdf.
National Eating Disorder Information Centre
http://www.nedic.ca
Public Health Agency of Canada: Physical Activity
http://www.phac-aspc.gc.ca/pau-uap/paguide/index.html

RELATED RESOURCES

Academy for Eating Disorders
http://www.aedweb.org
National Eating Disorders Association
http://www.nationaleatingdisorders.org
National Heart, Lung, and Blood Institute: *Portion Distortion*
http://hp2010.nhlbihin.net/portion/index.htm
Overeaters Anonymous Headquarters
http://www.overeatersanonymous.org
Take Off Pounds Sensibly (TOPS)
http://www.tops.org
Weight Watchers, Inc.
http://www.weightwatchers.com

evolve *For additional Internet resources, see the Web site for this book*
at **http://evolve.elsevier.com/Canada/Lewis/medsurg**

Nursing Management: Upper Gastrointestinal Problems

Written by Margaret McLean Heitkemper

Adapted by Françoise Verville

LEARNING OBJECTIVES

1. Describe the etiology, complications, collaborative care, and nursing management of nausea and vomiting.
2. Describe the etiology, clinical manifestations, and treatment of common oral inflammations and infections.
3. Describe the etiology, clinical manifestations, complications, collaborative care, and nursing management of oral cancer.
4. Explain the types, pathophysiology, clinical manifestations, complications, and collaborative care including surgical therapy and nursing management of gastroesophageal reflux disease and hiatal hernia.
5. Describe the pathophysiology, clinical manifestations, complications, and collaborative care of esophageal cancer, diverticula, achalasia, and esophageal strictures.
6. Differentiate between acute and chronic gastritis, including the etiology, pathophysiology, collaborative care, and nursing management.
7. Explain the common etiology, clinical manifestations, collaborative care, and nursing management of upper gastrointestinal bleeding.
8. Compare and contrast gastric and duodenal ulcers, including the etiology and pathophysiology, clinical manifestations, complications, collaborative care, and nursing management.
9. Describe the clinical manifestations, collaborative care, and nursing management of gastric cancer.
10. Identify the common types of food poisoning and the nursing responsibilities related to food poisoning.

KEY TERMS

achalasia Cardiospasm, p. 1130

Barrett's esophagus A precancerous lesion that places the patient at risk for esophageal cancer, p. 1123

dysphagia Difficulty swallowing, p. 1120

esophageal cancer A rare malignant neoplasm of the esophagus, p. 1127

esophageal diverticula Saclike outpouchings of one or more layers of the esophagus, p. 1130

esophagitis Inflammation of the esophagus, p. 1123

gastric cancer An adenocarcinoma of the stomach wall, p. 1153

gastritis An inflammation of the gastric mucosa, p. 1131

gastroesophageal reflux disease (GERD) A syndrome denoting any clinically significant symptomatic condition or histopathological alteration presumed to be secondary to reflux of gastric contents into the lower esophagus, p. 1122

hiatal hernia Herniation of a portion of the stomach into the esophagus through an opening, or hiatus, in the diaphragm, p. 1126

leukoplakia A whitish precancerous lesion on the oral mucosa or tongue that results from chronic irritation, p. 1120

Mallory-Weiss tear A tear occurring in the esophageal mucosa at the junction of the esophagus and the stomach and resulting in severe bleeding; usually caused by severe retching and vomiting, p. 1134

nausea A feeling of discomfort in the epigastrium with a conscious desire to vomit, p. 1114

peptic ulcer disease (PUD) A condition characterized by erosion of the gastrointestinal mucosa resulting from the digestive action of HCl (hydrochloric acid) and pepsin, p. 1138

physiological stress ulcers Acute ulcers that develop following a major physiological insult such as trauma or surgery, p. 1141

vomiting The forceful ejection of partially digested food and secretions (emesis) from the upper gastrointestinal tract, p. 1114

ELECTRONIC RESOURCES

Supplemental content related to Chapter 44 can be found ...

Evolve Web Site ⊜volve

http://evolve.elsevier.com/Canada/Lewis/medsurg
- Answer Guidelines for Case Study on p. 1158
- Clinical Reference: Laboratory Values
- Content Updates
- Customizable Nursing Care Plans:
  - Nausea and Vomiting
  - Peptic Ulcer Disease

- Electronic Calculators
- Examination Review Questions
- Glossary
- Interactive Case Studies:
  - Oral Cancer
  - Peptic Ulcer Disease
- Key Points (Printable and MP3 Download)

Nausea and Vomiting

Nausea and vomiting are the most common manifestations of gastrointestinal (GI) diseases. **Nausea** is a feeling of discomfort in the epigastrium with a conscious desire to vomit. **Vomiting** is the forceful ejection of partially digested food and secretions *(emesis)* from the upper GI tract. Vomiting is a complex act that requires the coordinated activities of several structures: closure of the glottis, deep inspiration with contraction of the diaphragm in the inspiratory position, closure of the pylorus, relaxation of the stomach and lower esophageal sphincter (LES), and contraction of the abdominal muscles with increasing intra-abdominal pressure. These simultaneous activities force the stomach contents up through the esophagus, into the pharynx, and out the mouth. Although nausea and vomiting can occur independently, they are usually closely related and usually treated as one problem.

Etiology and Pathophysiology

Nausea and vomiting are found in a wide variety of GI disorders as well as in conditions that are unrelated to GI disease. These include pregnancy, infectious diseases, central nervous system (CNS) disorders (e.g., meningitis, CNS tumour), cardiovascular problems (e.g., myocardial infarction, heart failure), metabolic disorders (e.g., Addison's disease, uremia), adverse effects of drugs (e.g., narcotics, digitalis), and psychological factors (e.g., stress, fear).

Generally, nausea occurs before vomiting and is characterized by contraction of the duodenum and by slowing of gastric motility and emptying. A single episode of nausea accompanied by vomiting may not be significant. However, if vomiting occurs several times, it is important that the cause be identified.

A vomiting centre in the brainstem coordinates the multiple components involved in vomiting. This centre receives input from various stimuli. Neural impulses reach the vomiting centre via afferent pathways through branches of the autonomic nervous system. Visceral receptors for these afferent fibres are located in the GI tract, the kidneys, the heart, and the uterus. When stimulated, these receptors relay information to the vomiting centre, which then initiates the vomiting reflex (Figure 44-1).

In addition, the chemoreceptor trigger zone (CTZ), located on the floor of the fourth ventricle in the brain, responds to chemical stimuli of drugs and toxins. The CTZ also plays a role

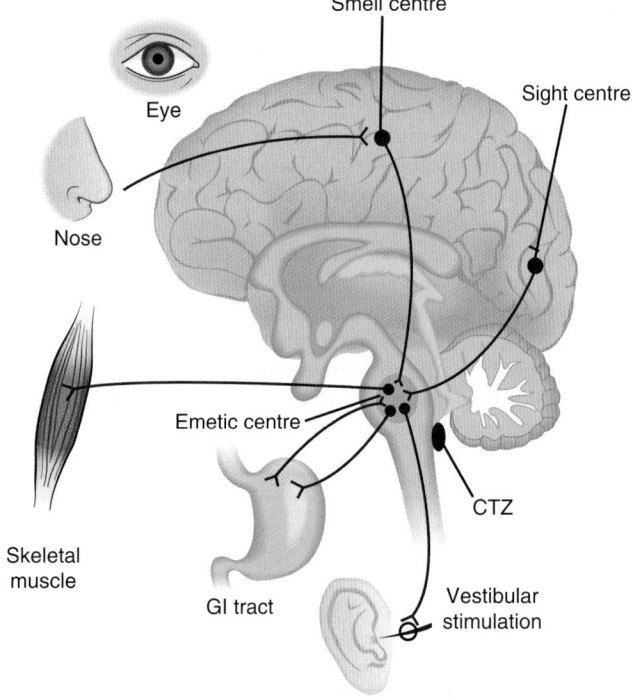

Figure 44-1 Stimuli involved in the act of vomiting. *CTZ*, chemoreceptor trigger zone; *GI*, gastrointestinal.

Source: McKenry, L., Tessier, E., & Hogan, M. (2006). *Mosby's pharmacology in nursing* (22nd ed.). St. Louis: Mosby.

in vomiting when it is caused by labyrinthine stimulation (e.g., motion sickness). Once stimulated, the CTZ transmits impulses directly to the vomiting centre.

Vomiting also can occur when the GI tract becomes overly irritated, excited, or distended. It can be a protective mechanism to rid the body of spoiled or irritating foods and liquids. Immediately before the act of vomiting, the person becomes aware of the need to vomit. The autonomic nervous system is activated, resulting in both parasympathetic and sympathetic nervous system stimulation. Sympathetic activation produces tachycardia, tachypnea, and diaphoresis. Parasympathetic stimulation causes relaxation of the lower esophageal (cardiac) sphincter, an increase in gastric motility, and a pronounced increase in salivation. These manifestations are experienced immediately before vomiting.

Clinical Manifestations

Nausea is a subjective complaint. *Anorexia* (lack of appetite) usually accompanies nausea and is brought on by unpleasant stimulation involving any of the five senses. When nausea and vomiting are prolonged, dehydration can rapidly occur. In addition to water, essential electrolytes (e.g., potassium, sodium, chloride, hydrogen) are also lost. As vomiting persists, there may be severe electrolyte imbalances, loss of extracellular fluid volume, decreased plasma volume, and eventually circulatory failure. Metabolic alkalosis can result from loss of gastric hydrochloric acid (HCl). (*Note:* The reader is advised to keep in mind throughout the chapter the word "acid" contained in the shorthand of the chemical formula, an important concept for an understanding of GI chemistry and function.) Metabolic acidosis can occur because of the loss of bicarbonate when contents from the small intestine are vomited. However, metabolic acidosis as a result of severe vomiting is less common than metabolic alkalosis. Weight loss resulting from fluid loss is evident in a short time when vomiting is severe.

The threat of pulmonary aspiration is a concern when vomiting occurs in the patient who is an older adult, is unconscious, or has other conditions that impair the gag reflex. The patient who cannot adequately manage self-care should be put in a semi-Fowler's or side-lying position to prevent aspiration.

Collaborative Care

The goals of collaborative care are to determine and treat the underlying cause of the nausea and vomiting and to provide symptomatic relief of nausea and vomiting. Determining the cause is often difficult because nausea and vomiting are manifestations of many conditions of the GI tract and of disorders of other body systems. An interprofessional approach to management of patients involving pharmacists, dieticians, and social workers should be considered.

A careful history must elicit important information regarding times when the vomiting occurs, precipitating factors, and a description of the contents of the vomitus or emesis. There are sex-related differences in risk for nausea and vomiting associated with both surgical procedures and motion sickness. Women are more likely than men to experience nausea and vomiting (Becker, 2010). In all patients, differentiation must be made between vomiting, regurgitation, and projectile vomiting. *Regurgitation* is a process in which partially digested food is slowly brought up from the stomach. Retching or vomiting seldom precedes it. *Projectile vomiting* is a very forceful expulsion of stomach contents without nausea and is a characteristic of CNS tumours.

The presence of fecal odour and bile after prolonged vomiting indicates intestinal obstruction below the level of the pylorus. The presence of bile in the emesis may suggest obstruction below the ampulla of Vater or bile reflux gastritis. The presence of partially digested food several hours after a meal is indicative of gastric outlet obstruction or delay in gastric emptying.

The colour of the emesis aids in determining the presence and the source of bleeding. Vomitus with a "coffee grounds" appearance is associated with bleeding in the stomach, where blood changes to dark brown as a result of its interaction with gastric acid. Bright red blood indicates active bleeding, which is suggestive of a tear in the mucosal lining of the lower esophagus

Table 44-1 Nausea and Vomiting

CLASSIFICATION	DRUG
Antiemetic and antipsychotic	Chlorpromazine
	Haloperidol
	Prochlorperazine
	Trifluoperazine
Antihistamine	Dimenhydrinate (Gravol)
	Diphenhydramine (Benadryl)
	Hydroxyzine (Atarax)
	Promethazine (Histantil)
Prokinetic	Domperidone
	Metoclopramide
Serotonin antagonist	Dolasetron (Anzemet)
	Granisetron (Kytril)
	Ondansetron (Zofran)
Antimuscarinic	Scopolamine
Others	Dexamethasone
	Corticosteroids
	Aprepitant (Emend)

or the fundus of stomach, bleeding gastric or duodenal ulcer or neoplasm, or bleeding esophageal varices.

Drug Therapy. The use of drugs in the treatment of nausea and vomiting depends on the cause of the problem. Many different drugs can be used (Table 44-1). Because the cause cannot always be readily determined, drugs must be used with caution. Antiemetics used before the cause of the vomiting is established can mask the underlying disease process and delay diagnosis and treatment. Many of the antiemetic drugs act on the CNS at the level of the CTZ. In general, they block the neurochemicals that appear to trigger nausea and vomiting.

Drugs that control nausea and vomiting include antimuscarinics (e.g., scopolamine), antihistamines (e.g., dimenhydrinate [Gravol]), and phenothiazines (e.g., chlorpromazine, prochlorperazine). Because many of these drugs have anticholinergic actions, their use is contraindicated for the patient with glaucoma, prostatic hyperplasia, pyloric or bladder neck obstruction, or biliary obstruction. They share many common adverse effects, which include dry mouth, hypotension, sedative effects, rashes, and GI disturbances such as constipation. Consultation with a pharmacist may be indicated before administering these drugs to the patient with multiple medical problems.

Other drugs with antiemetic properties include metoclopramide and domperidone. These drugs act both centrally and peripherally on dopamine receptors. Peripherally, they enhance the release of acetylcholine, resulting in increased gastric emptying. Because of this effect, these drugs are considered prokinetics. However, about 10 to 20% of patients taking metoclopramide experience CNS adverse effects ranging from anxiety to hallucinations. Extrapyramidal adverse effects including tremor and dyskinesias similar to Parkinson's disease may also occur. Domperidone does not cross the blood–brain barrier and thus produces fewer adverse effects than metoclopramide.

Antagonists to specific serotonin (5-HT) receptors have been found to act both centrally and peripherally to reduce nausea and vomiting. In particular, antagonists to the 5-HT3 receptors are effective in reducing cancer chemotherapy–induced vomiting, vomiting caused by total body radiation, GI motility disturbances, carcinoid syndrome, and nausea and vomiting related to migraine headache and anxiety. Serotonin antagonists, including ondansetron (Zofran), granisetron (Kytril), and dolasetron (Anzemet), act centrally in the vomiting centre as well as peripherally to enhance gastric emptying.

Dexamethasone is used in the management of cancer chemotherapy–induced emesis, usually in combination with other antiemetics. Dexamethasone alone or in combination with ondansetron reduces both acute and delayed chemotherapy-induced nausea and vomiting. Aprepitant (Emend), a substance P/neurokinin-1 receptor antagonist, is used for the prevention of chemotherapy-induced nausea and vomiting as well as prevention of postoperative nausea and vomiting. Co-administration with warfarin results in a decreased prothrombin time, the international normalized ratio (INR) must be closely monitored. The efficacy of hormonal contraceptives may also be reduced, necessitating an alternative method during treatment and for 1 month following the last dose.

Nutritional Therapy. The patient with severe vomiting requires intravenous (IV) fluid therapy with electrolyte and glucose replacement until able to tolerate oral intake. In some cases, a nasogastric (NG) tube and suction are used to decompress the stomach. Once the symptoms have subsided, oral nourishment beginning with clear liquids is started. Extremely hot or cold liquids are not usually well tolerated. Carbonated beverages, at room temperature and with the carbonation gone, and warm tea are more easily tolerated. The addition of dry toast or crackers may alleviate the feeling of nausea and help prevent vomiting. Water is the initial fluid of choice for rehydration by mouth.

As the patient's condition improves, a diet high in carbohydrates and low in fatty foods should be provided. Items such as a baked potato, plain gelatin, cereal with milk and sugar, and hard candy may be added. Foods that are known to be poorly tolerated include coffee, spicy foods, and highly acidic foods. Food should be eaten slowly and in small amounts to prevent overdistension of the stomach. When solid foods have been reintroduced, fluids should be taken between meals rather than with meals. It is advised that the patient avoid physical activity and sit upright for approximately 1 hour after meals. A dietitian may be consulted regarding appropriate foods that will maintain nutritional health and are well tolerated by the patient during the recovery process.

Some patients use herbs such as ginger and peppermint oil. Breathing exercises, massage, and changing body position or exercise may be helpful for some patients.

NURSING MANAGEMENT: NAUSEA AND VOMITING

▸ Nursing Assessment

Each patient with a history of prolonged and persistent nausea or vomiting requires a thorough nursing assessment before a specific plan of care is developed. Although the conditions asso-

ciated with nausea and vomiting are numerous, the nurse should have a basic understanding of the more common conditions and should be able to identify the patient who is at high risk. Knowledge of the physiological mechanisms involved in nausea and vomiting and the demonstration of a genuine regard for the patient are essential. Table 44-2 presents subjective and objective data that should be obtained from a patient with nausea and vomiting, regardless of the underlying cause.

▸ Nursing Diagnoses

Nursing diagnoses for the patient with nausea and vomiting may include, but are not limited to, those presented in Nursing Care Plan (NCP) 44-1.

▸ Planning

The overall goals are that the patient with nausea and vomiting will (1) experience minimal or no nausea and vomiting, (2) have normal electrolyte levels and hydration status, and (3) return to a normal pattern of fluid balance and nutrient intake.

▸ Nursing Implementation

▸ Acute Intervention

The majority of individuals with nausea and vomiting can be managed at home. However, when nausea and vomiting persist regardless of home treatment strategies, hospitalization may be necessary for diagnosis of the underlying problem. Until a diagnosis is confirmed, the patient is kept on nothing-by-mouth (NPO) status and given IV fluids. An NG tube connected to

NURSING ASSESSMENT

Table 44-2 Nausea and Vomiting

Subjective Data	Objective Data
Important Health Information	**General**
Past health history: GI disorders, chronic indigestion, food allergies, pregnancy, infection, CNS disorders, recent travel, bulimia, metabolic disorders, cancer, cardiovascular disease, renal disease	Lethargy, sunken eyeballs
	Integumentary
Medications: Use of antiemetics, digitalis, opioids, ferrous sulphate, aspirin, aminophylline, alcohol, antibiotics; general anaesthesia; chemotherapy	Pallor, dry mucous membranes, poor skin turgor
	Gastrointestinal
Surgery or other treatments: Recent surgery	Amount, frequency, character (e.g., projectile), content (undigested food, blood, bile, feces), and colour of vomitus (red, "coffee grounds," green-yellow)
Symptoms	**Urinary**
• Emesis, dry heaves, dry mouth, anorexia, weight loss	Decreased output, concentrated urine
• Weakness, fatigue	**Possible Findings**
• Abdominal tenderness or pain	Altered serum electrolytes (especially hypokalemia), metabolic alkalosis, abnormal upper GI findings on endoscopy or abdominal radiographs

CNS, central nervous system; *GI,* gastrointestinal.

NURSING CARE PLAN 44-1

Nausea and Vomiting

NURSING DIAGNOSIS	***Nausea*** *related to* multiple etiologies *as evidenced by* episodes of nausea and vomiting
Expected Patient Outcomes	**Nursing Interventions and *Rationales***
• Experiences minimal or no nausea • Reports satisfaction with care	• Assess duration, frequency, and nature of nausea and vomiting and aggravating and alleviating factors *to plan appropriate interventions.* • Remove visual stimuli and source of odours *to avoid precipitating triggers of nausea or vomiting.* • Provide mouth care; change soiled gown and linens *to ensure patient comfort.* • Maintain quiet environment and avoid unnecessary procedures or activities *to minimize triggers of vomiting.* • Administer antiemetic(s) as ordered. • Instruct patient to take several deep breaths; prevent sudden changes in position; keep head of bed elevated *to decrease stimulation of the vomiting centre.* • Instruct patient to avoid foods and beverages that stimulate nausea and vomiting.
NURSING DIAGNOSIS	***Deficient fluid volume*** *related to* prolonged vomiting and inability to ingest, digest, or absorb food and fluids *as evidenced by* decreased urine output and increased urine concentration, increased pulse rate, hypotension (postural), decreased intake, decreased skin turgor, and dry skin and mucous membranes
Expected Patient Outcomes	**Nursing Interventions and *Rationales***
• Shows no signs of dehydration	• Assess for signs of dehydration *to plan appropriate care.* • Administer and monitor amount and type of IV fluid *to maintain fluid and electrolyte balance.* • Provide small amounts of clear liquids when vomiting stops *to support hydration.* • Record amount and frequency of vomitus; maintain accurate intake and output records; weigh daily in acute phase *to monitor fluid balance accurately.* • Monitor laboratory results of serum sodium, potassium, chloride, and bicarbonate as indicators of electrolyte balance.
NURSING DIAGNOSIS	***Imbalanced nutrition: less than body requirements*** *related to* nausea and vomiting *as evidenced by* lack of interest in or aversion to food, perceived or actual inability to ingest food, and weight loss
Expected Patient Outcomes	**Nursing Interventions and Rationales**
• Shows gradual return to usual weight and eating habits	• Assess patient's interest in food, ability to ingest food, and weight *to determine if a problem is present.* • Maintain IV fluids or total parenteral nutrition until oral intake is possible *to provide necessary fluids, electrolytes, calories, and protein intake.* • Instruct patient to resume eating cautiously with bland, nonirritating foods in small amounts *to avoid irritating the stomach and initiating recurrence of nausea and vomiting.*

IV, intravenous.

suction may be necessary for the patient with persistent vomiting as well as for the patient in whom the possible diagnosis may be bowel obstruction or paralytic ileus. Keeping the stomach empty reduces the stimulus to vomit. The NG tube should be stabilized to eliminate its movement in the nose and back of the throat because this can stimulate nausea and vomiting.

With prolonged vomiting, there is a probability of dehydration and acid–base and electrolyte imbalances. The nurse plans care that includes accurate recording of intake and output, monitoring vital signs, assessing for signs of dehydration, proper positioning to prevent possible aspiration in the susceptible patient, and observing for changes in the patient's general physical comfort and mentation. The nurse takes responsibility for providing physical and emotional support; maintaining a quiet, odour-free environment; and giving explanations regarding any diagnostic tests or procedures performed.

Patients who are hospitalized for other health problems may be prone to episodes of nausea and vomiting. These individuals include the patient who is recovering immediately after surgery from the effects of the procedure, anaesthesia, and pain. Nausea and vomiting are common adverse effects in the patient with cancer receiving chemotherapeutic drugs. (Nursing care of the patient with cancer is found in Chapter 18.)

▪ Ambulatory and Home Care

The patient and caregiver may need instructions on (1) how to deal successfully with the unpleasant sensations of nausea, (2) methods of preventing nausea and vomiting, and (3) strategies to maintain fluid and nutritional intake. The occurrence of nausea or vomiting may be minimized if measures are taken to keep the immediate environment quiet, free of noxious odours, and well ventilated. The avoidance of sudden changes of position and unnecessary activity is also helpful. Use of relaxation techniques, acupressure, frequent rest periods, and diversional tactics help prevent nausea and vomiting and facilitate a more rapid recovery from their effects. Cleansing the face and the hands with a cool washcloth and mouth care between episodes increase the person's comfort level. When the symptoms occur, all foods and drugs should be stopped until the acute phase is past.

If a medication is suspected as the cause, the health care provider should be notified immediately so that either the dosage can be altered or a new drug can be prescribed. The patient should be reminded that stopping the drug without consulting the health care provider may eliminate the immediate cause of the nausea and vomiting but that omission of the prescribed drug may have detrimental effects on health or the disease state.

When food is identified as the precipitating cause of nausea and vomiting, the nurse should help the patient solve the problem. What food was it? When was it eaten? Has this food caused problems in the past? Is anyone else in the family sick?

When the patient believes some foods and fluids can be tolerated, the nurse might suggest that it would be helpful to begin with clear liquids or warm beverages, Gatorade, tea or broth, dry crackers or toast, and then plain gelatin. Bland foods, such as pasta, rice, and cooked chicken, are generally well tolerated in small amounts. An antiemetic drug should be taken only if prescribed by the health care provider. Taking over-the-counter (OTC) drugs for relief of symptoms may make the condition worse. Patients should be asked to describe any use of nontraditional preparations.

▪ Evaluation

The following are expected outcomes for the patient with nausea and vomiting:

- The patient will be comfortable with minimal or no nausea and vomiting.
- The patient will maintain body weight.
- The patient will have electrolyte levels within normal range.
- The patient will be able to maintain adequate intake of fluids and nutrients.
- The patient will maintain normal urine volume.

AGE-RELATED CONSIDERATIONS: NAUSEA AND VOMITING

The older adult patient experiencing nausea and vomiting requires careful assessment and monitoring, particularly during periods of fluid loss and subsequent rehydration therapy. Older adult patients are more likely to have cardiac or renal insufficiency that places them at greater risk for life-threatening fluid and electrolyte imbalances. In addition, excessive replacement of fluid and electrolytes may result in adverse consequences for the older adult person who has heart failure or renal disease. Finally, the older adult with a decreased level of consciousness may be at high risk for aspiration of vomitus. Close monitoring of the patient's physical status and level of consciousness during episodes of vomiting must be a primary concern for the nurse.

In addition, older adults are particularly susceptible to the CNS adverse effects of antiemetic drugs; these drugs may produce confusion. Dosages should be reduced and efficacy closely evaluated. Safety precautions also should be instituted for these patients.

Oral Inflammations and Infections

Oral infections and inflammations may be specific mouth diseases, or they may occur in the presence of some systemic diseases such as leukemia or vitamin deficiency. When oral inflammations and infections are present, they can severely impair the ingestion of food and fluids. Common inflammations and infections of the oral cavity are presented in Table 44-3. The patient who is immunosuppressed (e.g., patient with acquired immune deficiency syndrome [AIDS] or receiving chemotherapy) is most susceptible to oral infections. Patients receiving corticosteroid inhalant treatment for asthma are at risk for oral infections, especially candidiasis.

Oral infections may predispose to infections in other body organs. For example, the oral cavity can be considered a potential reservoir for respiratory pathogens. In addition, oral pathogens have also been associated with heart disease.

An important element in reducing oral infections and inflammation is good oral hygiene. Management of oral infections and inflammation is focused on identification of the cause, elimination of infection, provision of comfort measures, and maintenance of nutritional intake.

Table 44-3 Infections and Inflammation of the Mouth

CONDITION	ETIOLOGY	CLINICAL MANIFESTATIONS	TREATMENT
Gingivitis	Neglected oral hygiene, malocclusion, missing or irregular teeth, faulty dentistry, eating of soft rather than fibrous foods	Inflamed gingivae and interdental papillae; bleeding during toothbrushing; development of pus; formation of abscess with loosening of teeth (periodontitis)	Prevention through health teaching, dental care, gingival massage, professional cleaning of teeth, fibrous foods, conscientious brushing habits with flossing
Vincent's infection (acute necrotizing ulcerative gingivitis, trench mouth)	Fusiform bacteria; Vincent's spirochetes; predisposing factors of stress, excessive fatigue, poor oral hygiene, nutritional deficiencies (vitamins B and C)	Painful, bleeding gingivae; eroding necrotic lesions of interdental papillae; ulcerations that bleed; increased saliva with metallic taste; fetid mouth odour; anorexia, fever, and general malaise	Rest (physical and mental); avoidance of smoking and alcoholic beverages; soft, nutritious diet; correct oral hygiene habits; topical applications of antibiotics; mouth rinses with hydrogen peroxide and saline solutions
Oral candidiasis (moniliasis or thrush)	*Candida albicans* (a yeastlike fungus), debilitation, prolonged high-dose antibiotic or corticosteroid therapy	Pearly, bluish white "milk-curd" membranous lesions on mucosa of mouth and larynx; sore mouth; yeasty halitosis	Nystatin or amphotericin B as oral suspension or buccal tablets, good oral hygiene
Herpes simplex (cold sore, fever blister)	Herpes simplex virus type 1 or 2; predisposing factors of upper respiratory infections, excessive exposure to sunlight, food allergies, emotional tension, onset of menstruation	Lip lesions, mouth lesions, vesicle formation (single or clustered); shallow, painful ulcers	Spirits of camphor, corticosteroid cream, mild antiseptic mouthwash, viscous lidocaine; removal or control of predisposing factors, antiviral agents (e.g., acyclovir [Zovirax])
Aphthous stomatitis (canker sore)	Recurrent and chronic form of infection secondary to systemic disease, trauma, stress, or unknown causes	Ulcers of mouth and lips, causing extreme pain; ulcers surrounded by erythematous base	Corticosteroids (topical or systemic), tetracycline oral suspension
Parotitis (inflammation of parotid gland, surgical mumps)	Usually *Staphylococcus* species, *Streptococcus* species occasionally, debilitation and dehydration with poor oral hygiene, NPO status for an extended time	Pain and swelling in area of gland and ear, absence of salivation, purulent exudate from gland, erythema, ulcers	Antibiotics, mouthwashes, warm compresses; preventive measures such as chewing gum, sucking on hard candy, adequate fluid intake
Stomatitis (inflammation of mouth)	Trauma; pathogens; irritants (tobacco, alcohol); renal, liver, and hematological diseases; adverse effect of many cancer chemotherapy drugs and radiation	Excessive salivation, halitosis, sore mouth	Removal or treatment of cause, oral hygiene with soothing solutions, topical medications; soft, bland diet

NPO, nothing by mouth.

Oral Cancer

Oral (or oropharyngeal) cancer may occur on the lips or anywhere within the mouth (e.g., tongue, floor of the mouth, buccal mucosa, hard palate, soft palate, pharyngeal walls, tonsils). It was estimated that 4000 new cases of oral cancer would be diagnosed in Canada in 2012, and that 1150 persons would die from the disease (Canadian Cancer Society's Steering Committee on Cancer Statistics, 2012). It is more common after 50 years of age. Oral cancer occurs in all ethnic groups. It is more common in men (male-to-female ratio of 2 : 1). Squamous cell carcinoma is the most common oral malignant tumour (>90%). Mortality rates have been decreasing since the early 1980s. The 5-year survival for all stages of cancer of the oral cavity and pharynx combined is 63%.

Most of the oral malignant lesions occur on the lower lip. Other common sites are the lateral border and undersurface of the tongue, the labial commissure, and the buccal mucosa. Carcinoma of the lip has the most favourable prognosis of any of the oral tumours. This is probably because lip lesions are more apparent to the patient than other oral lesions and are usually diagnosed earlier.

Etiology and Pathophysiology

Although the definitive cause of oral cancer is unknown, there are a number of predisposing factors (Table 44-4). Factors that influence the development of oral cancer include tobacco use (e.g., cigar, cigarette, pipe, snuff), excessive alcohol intake, and chronic irritation such as from a jagged tooth or poor dental care. A positive history of tobacco and alcohol use, in the past or currently, is the most significant etiological factor in oral cancer. Constant overexposure to ultraviolet radiation from the sun is also a factor in the development of cancer of the lip. Irritation from the pipe stem resting on the lip is a factor in pipe smokers.

Table 44-4 Types and Characteristics of Oral Cancer

LOCATION	PREDISPOSING FACTORS	CLINICAL MANIFESTATIONS	TREATMENT
Lip	Constant overexposure to sun, ruddy and fair complexion, recurrent herpetic lesions, irritation from pipe stem, syphilis, immunosuppression	Indurated, painless ulcer	Surgical excision, radiation
Tongue	Tobacco, alcohol, chronic irritation, syphilis	Ulcer or area of thickening; soreness or pain; increased salivation, slurred speech, dysphagia, toothache, earache (later signs)	Surgery (hemiglossectomy or glossectomy), radiation
Oral cavity	Poor oral hygiene, tobacco usage (pipe and cigar smoking, snuff, chewing tobacco), chewing betel nut, chronic alcohol intake, chronic irritation (jagged tooth, ill-fitting prosthesis, chemical or mechanical irritants), exposure to HPV-16 and HPV-18	Leukoplakia; erythroplakia; ulcerations; sore spot; rough area; pain, dysphagia, difficulty in chewing and speaking (later signs)	Surgery (mandibulectomy, radical neck dissection, resections of buccal mucosa), internal and external radiation

HPV, human papillomavirus.

Clinical Manifestations

The common manifestations of oral cancer are leukoplakia, erythroplakia, ulcerations, a sore that bleeds easily and does not heal, and a rough area (felt with the tongue). **Leukoplakia,** called "white patch" or "smoker's patch," is often considered a precancerous lesion, although fewer than 5% of these lesions actually transform into malignant cells. It is a whitish patch on the mucosa of the mouth or the tongue that results from chronic irritation, especially from smoking. The patch becomes *keratinized* (hard and leathery) and is sometimes described as *hyperkeratosis. Erythroplasia* (erythroplakia), which is seen as a red velvety patch on the mouth or tongue, is also considered a precancerous lesion. Areas of erythroplakia have a 90% chance of becoming malignant. Later symptoms of oral cancer are pain, **dysphagia** (difficulty swallowing), and difficulty in moving the jaw (e.g., chewing and speaking).

Cancer of the lip usually appears as an indurated, painless ulcer on the lip. The first sign of carcinoma of the tongue is an ulcer or area of thickening. Soreness or pain of the tongue may occur, especially when eating hot or highly seasoned foods. Cancerous lesions are most likely to develop in the proximal half of the tongue. Some patients experience limitation of movement of the tongue. Later symptoms of cancer of the tongue include increased salivation, slurred speech, dysphagia, toothache, and earache. Approximately 30% of patients with oral cancer have an asymptomatic neck mass.

Diagnostic Studies

Biopsy of the suspected lesion with cytological examination is the best definitive diagnostic study for oral cancer. Oral exfoliative cytology involves scraping the suspicious lesion and spreading this scraping on a slide. Unlike biopsy, a negative cytological smear does not reliably rule out the possibility of a malignant condition, but it may be used as an initial screening test. The toluidine blue test may also be used as a screening test for oral cancer. Toluidine blue is applied topically to stain an area, and cancer cells preferentially take up the dye. However, the definitive diagnosis of cancer is based on biopsy and histology). Once cancer is diagnosed, computed tomography (CT) and magnetic

COLLABORATIVE CARE

Table 44-5 Oral Cancer

Diagnostic	*Collaborative Therapy**

• History and physical examination
• Biopsy
• Oral exfoliative cytology
• Toluidine blue test
• CT and MRI scans
	• Surgery
	  • Surgical excision of the tumour
	  • Radical neck dissection
	• Radiation (internal or external)
	• Combined surgical resection with radiation
	• Chemotherapy

CT, computed tomography; *MRI*, magnetic resonance imaging.
*Any of these approaches may be used, depending on the primary lesion and the extent of metastasis.

resonance imaging (MRI) are useful in the staging of oral cancer (Canadian Cancer Society, 2008).

Collaborative Care

Collaborative care of oral carcinoma usually consists of surgery, radiation, chemotherapy, or a combination of these (Table 44-5).

Surgical Therapy. Surgery remains the most effective treatment, especially for removing the central core of the tumour. Many of the operations are radical procedures involving extensive resections. Various surgical procedures may be performed, depending on the location and the extent of the tumour. Some examples are partial *mandibulectomy* (removal of the mandible), *hemiglossectomy* (removal of half of the tongue), *glossectomy* (removal of the tongue), resections of the buccal mucosa and the floor of the mouth, and radical neck dissection. Composite resections, which are combinations of the various surgical procedures, may be performed.

Because cancers of the oral cavity metastasize early to the cervical lymph nodes, a radical neck dissection is commonly performed. It includes wide excision of the involved primary lesion with removal of the regional lymph nodes, the deep cervical lymph nodes, and their lymphatic channels. In addition, the following structures may also be removed or transsected (depending on the extent of the primary lesion): sternocleidomastoid muscle and other closely associated muscles, internal jugular vein, mandible, submaxillary gland, part of the thyroid and parathyroid glands, and spinal accessory nerve. A tracheostomy is commonly performed along with the radical neck dissection. Drainage tubes are inserted into the surgical area and connected to suction to remove fluid and blood.

Nonsurgical Therapy. Chemotherapy and radiation therapy are used together when the lesions are more advanced or involve several structures of the oral cavity. Chemotherapy may also be used when surgery and radiation therapy fail or as the initial therapy for smaller tumours (see Chapter 18).

Palliative treatment may be the best management when the prognosis is poor, the cancer is inoperable, or the patient decides against surgery. Palliation aims to treat the symptoms and make the patient more comfortable. If it becomes difficult for the patient to swallow, a gastrostomy may be performed to allow for adequate nutritional intake. (Gastrostomy is discussed in Chapter 42.) Analgesic medication should be given freely to this patient. Frequent suctioning of the oral cavity becomes necessary when swallowing becomes difficult. (Other nursing measures for the terminally ill patient are discussed in Chapter 13.)

Nutritional Therapy. Because of depression, alcoholism, or presurgery radiation treatment, patients may be malnourished even before surgery. After radical neck surgery, the patient may be unable to take in nutrients through the normal route of ingestion because of swelling, location of sutures, or difficulty with swallowing. Parenteral fluids will be given for the first 24 to 48 hours. After this time, tube feedings are usually given via an NG or a nasointestinal tube that was placed during surgery. Sometimes, a temporary feeding gastrostomy may be used. (NG and gastrostomy feedings are described in Chapter 42.) Cervical esophagostomy and pharyngostomy have also been used. The nurse must observe for tolerance of the feedings and (in consultation with a dietitian) adjust the amount, the time, and the formula if nausea, vomiting, diarrhea, or distension occurs. The patient is instructed about the tube feedings. When the patient can swallow, small amounts of water are given. Close observation for choking is essential. Suctioning may be necessary to prevent aspiration.

NURSING MANAGEMENT: ORAL CANCER

▤ Nursing Assessment

Subjective and objective data that should be obtained from a patient with oral cancer are presented in Table 44-6.

▤ Nursing Diagnoses

Nursing diagnoses for the patient with oral cancer may include, but are not limited to, the following:

- Imbalanced nutrition: less than body requirements *related to* oral pain, difficulty chewing and swallowing, surgical resection, and radiation treatment

Table 44-6 Oral Cancer
Subjective Data
Important Health Information
Current health history: Use of alcohol or tobacco, pipe smoking, poor oral hygiene
Past health history: Recurrent oral herpetic lesions, syphilis, exposure to sunlight
Medications: Immunosuppressants
Surgery or other treatments: Removal of prior tumours or lesions
Symptoms
• Reduced oral intake, weight loss, difficulty in chewing or swallowing food; increased salivation; intolerance to certain foods or temperatures of food
• Mouth or tongue soreness or pain, toothache, earache, neck stiffness, difficulty speaking
Objective Data
Integumentary
Indurated, painless ulcer on lip; painless neck mass
Gastrointestinal
Areas of thickening or roughness, ulcers, leukoplakia, or erythroplakia on the tongue or the oral mucosa; limited movement of the tongue; increased salivation, drooling; slurred speech; poor oral hygiene, foul breath odour
Possible Findings
Positive exfoliative cytological smear (microscopic examination of cells removed by scraping); positive biopsy

- Chronic pain *related to* the tumour and surgical radiation
- Anxiety *related to* diagnosis of cancer, uncertain future, potential for disfiguring surgery, potential for recurrence, and prognosis
- Ineffective coping *related to* body image change
- Ineffective health maintenance *related to* lack of knowledge of disease process and therapeutic regimen and unavailability of a support system

▤ Planning

The overall goals are that the patient with carcinoma of the oral cavity will (1) have a patent airway, (2) be able to communicate, (3) have adequate nutritional intake to promote wound healing, and (4) have relief of pain and discomfort.

▤ Nursing Implementation

▤ Health Promotion

The nurse has a significant role in early detection and treatment of oral cancer. The nurse must provide the patient with information regarding predisposing factors, such as constant overexposure to the sun, tobacco, and other irritants like chewing betel nuts. Smoking and the long-term use of smokeless tobacco are the major risk factors for oral cancer. A patient identified as a smoker should be informed about smoking cessation programs available in the community. (Smoking cessation is discussed in Chapter 11. See also the link to the Registered Nurses' Association of Ontario's [RNAO's] *Integrating Smoking Cessation into Daily Nursing Practice* in the Resources at the end of this chapter.)

It is important that adolescents and teenagers be informed about the danger of using snuff and chewing tobacco. In addition, oral cancers have an increased chance of recurrence if risk factors are not reduced. The nurse should also teach correct oral hygiene and dental care and encourage the patient to seek preventive dental care. Risk factors should be identified. Because early detection of oral cancer is important, the patient should be taught to examine the mouth and to recognize danger signals of oral cancer. If any of these signals are present, the patient should be instructed to visit a health care provider. Danger signals include unexplained pain or soreness in the mouth, unusual bleeding from the oral cavity, dysphagia, and swelling or lump in the neck.

Any individual with an ulcerative lesion that does not heal within 2 to 3 weeks should be referred to a health care provider, and a biopsy of the lesion should probably be performed. The nurse should inspect the patient's oral cavity to detect suspicious lesions.

▪ Acute Intervention

Preoperative care for the patient who is to have a radical neck dissection involves consideration of the patient's physical and psychosocial needs. Physical preparation is the same as for any major surgery, with special emphasis on oral hygiene. Thorough assessment of alcohol intake should be done, and measures should be implemented early to assess and treat withdrawal if it is a problem. Explanations and emotional support are of special significance and should include postoperative measures relating to communication and feeding. The surgical procedure should be explained to the patient, and the nurse should make sure that the patient understands the information. Radical neck dissection and related nursing management are discussed in Chapter 29 and NCP 29-2.

▪ Evaluation

The following are expected outcomes for the patient with oral cancer:
- The patient will have no respiratory complications.
- The patient will be able to communicate.
- The patient will participate in regular follow-up examinations.
- The patient will maintain adequate nutritional intake to promote wound healing and overall health.
- The patient will experience minimal pain and discomfort with eating, drinking, and talking.

Esophageal Disorders

Gastroesophageal Reflux Disease

Etiology and Pathophysiology

Gastroesophageal reflux disease (GERD) is not a disease but a syndrome. The term *GERD* is defined as any clinically significant symptomatic condition or histopathological alteration presumed

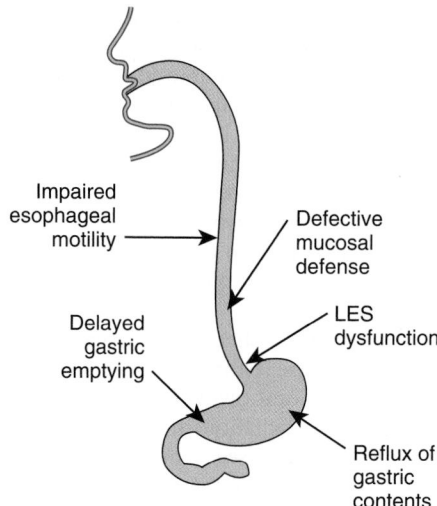

Figure 44-2 Factors involved in the pathogenesis of gastroesophageal reflux disease (GERD). *LES*, lower esophageal sphincter.

Source: Courtesy University of Washington, Division of Gastroenterology, St. Louis.

to be secondary to reflux of gastric contents into the lower esophagus. In Canada, GERD is the most prevalent acid-related disorder, with approximately 13% of Canadians suffering from GERD symptoms weekly (Canadian Society of Intestinal Research, 2011).

There is no one single cause of GERD. Several factors or a combination of factors can be involved (Figure 44-2). It results when the defences of the lower esophagus are overwhelmed by the reflux of stomach acidic contents into the esophagus. Predisposing conditions include hiatal hernia, incompetent lower esophageal sphincter (LES), decreased esophageal clearance (ability to clear liquids or food from the esophagus into the stomach) resulting from impaired esophageal motility, and decreased gastric emptying. The acidic gastric secretions that reflux up into the lower esophagus result in esophageal irritation and inflammation (esophagitis). In addition, the presence of the gastric enzyme pepsin and intestinal enzymes (e.g., trypsin) and bile salts are corrosive to the esophageal mucosa. The degree of inflammation depends on the amount and the composition of gastric reflux and on the ability of the esophagus to clear the acidic contents.

One of the primary factors in GERD is an incompetent LES. An incompetent LES results in a decrease in pressure in the distal portion of the esophagus. As a result, gastric contents are able to move from an area of higher pressure (stomach) to an area of lower pressure (esophagus) when the patient is in a supine position or has an increase in intra-abdominal pressure. Decreased LES pressure can be caused by certain foods (e.g., caffeine, chocolate) and drugs (e.g., anticholinergics). A common cause of GERD is a hiatal hernia, which is discussed in the next section.

Clinical Manifestations

The symptoms of GERD vary from individual to individual but the diagnosis can usually be made on the basis of history and physical examination. Heartburn *(pyrosis)* from gastroesophageal reflux is the most common clinical manifestation. It is caused by irritation of the esophagus by the gastric secretions. Heartburn is

Table 44-7 Factors Affecting Lower Esophageal Sphincter Pressure	
Increase Pressure	Peppermint, spearmint
Bethanechol (Duvoid)	Tea, coffee (caffeine)
Metoclopramide	β-Adrenergic blockers
Decrease Pressure	Calcium channel blockers
Alcohol	Diazepam (Valium)
Anticholinergics	Morphine sulphate
Chocolate (theobromine)	Nitrates
Fatty foods	Progesterone
Nicotine	Theophylline

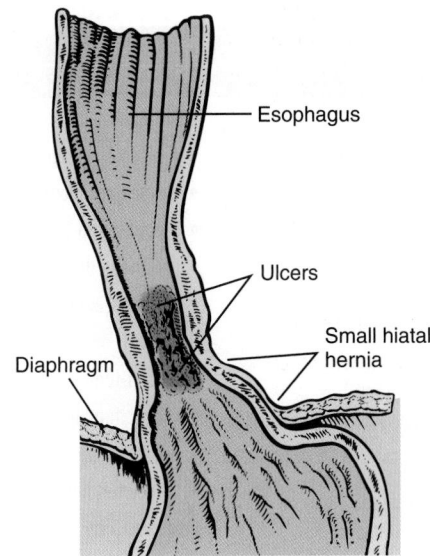

Figure 44-3 Esophagitis with esophageal ulcerations.

Source: Doughty, D. B., & Jackson, D. B. (1993). *Mosby's clinical nursing series: Gastrointestinal disorders.* St. Louis: Mosby.

described as a burning, tight sensation that is felt intermittently beneath the lower sternum and spreads upward to the throat or the jaw. The majority of individuals have mild symptoms including heartburn after a meal that occurs about once a week with no evidence of mucosal damage.

Heartburn may occur following ingestion of food or drugs that decrease the LES pressure or are directly irritating to the esophageal mucosa (Table 44-7). An individual with GERD may also report respiratory symptoms including wheezing, coughing, and dyspnea. Otolaryngological symptoms include hoarseness, sore throat, a globus sensation (sense of a lump in the throat), and choking. *Regurgitation* (effortless return of food or gastric contents from the stomach into the esophagus or mouth) is a fairly common manifestation of GERD. It is often described as hot, bitter, or sour liquid coming into the throat or mouth. Gastric symptoms including early satiety, bloating after a meal, nausea, and vomiting are related to delayed gastric emptying. Symptoms that would prompt endoscopic evaluation include dysphagia (solid food, progressive), odynophagia (painful swallowing), bleeding and subsequent anemia, weight loss, and persistent vomiting. Further investigation is indicated if suspected GERD symptoms are actually cardiac in origin, the patient has respiratory symptoms secondary to reflux, or for individuals who do not respond to medical therapy after 8 weeks (Flook, Jones, & Vakil, 2008; Toward Optimized Practice, 2009).

Complications

Complications of GERD are related to the direct local effects of gastric acid on the esophageal mucosa. **Esophagitis** (inflammation of the esophagus) is a frequent complication of GERD. Other risk factors for esophagitis include hiatal hernia, chemical irritation from lye, and physical irritants such as smoking, cold or hot liquids, and excessive alcoholic intake. Trauma to the esophagus may also produce inflammation. Esophagitis with esophageal ulcerations is shown in Figure 44-3.

Repeated exposure may cause scar tissue formation and decreased distensibility of the esophagus (*esophageal stricture*). This may result in dysphagia.

Another complication of GERD is **Barrett's esophagus** (esophageal metaplasia). Barrett's esophagus is considered a precancerous lesion and places the patient at risk for esophageal cancer. In Barrett's esophagus, there is replacement of the normal squamous epithelium of the esophagus with columnar epithelium. These cell changes are thought to be related to chronic reflux esophagitis. Signs and symptoms of Barrett's esophagus can range from none to mild to bleeding and perforation. Because

patients with Barrett's esophagus are at higher risk for adenocarcinoma, they may need to be monitored on a regular basis (every 3 yr) by endoscopy and biopsy.

Respiratory complications of GERD include bronchospasm, laryngospasm, and cricopharyngeal spasm. These complications are caused by irritation of the upper airway by gastric secretions. With GERD, there is also the potential for pneumonia as a result of aspiration of gastric contents into the respiratory system. Dental erosion, especially in the posterior teeth, may result from acid reflux into the mouth.

Diagnostic Studies

Diagnostic studies are performed to determine the cause of the GERD (e.g., hiatal hernia) (Table 44-8). Barium swallow may be done to determine whether there is protrusion of the upper part of the stomach (called the *gastric fundus*). Endoscopy is useful in assessing the competence of the LES and the extent of inflammation (if present), potential scarring, and strictures (Canadian Society of Intestinal Research, 2012). Biopsy and cytological specimens can be taken to differentiate carcinoma of the stomach or esophagus from Barrett's esophagus. Esophageal manometric studies can be performed to measure pressure in the esophagus as well as in the LES. The determination of pH using specially designed probes in the laboratory or using ambulatory monitoring systems may demonstrate the presence of acid in the normally alkaline esophagus. Radionuclide tests may also be performed to detect reflux of gastric contents and the rate of esophageal clearance.

Collaborative Care

Most patients with GERD can be successfully managed by lifestyle modifications and drug therapy. These are long-term approaches requiring patient teaching and adherence with therapies. When these therapies are ineffective, surgery is an option (see Table 44-8).

COLLABORATIVE CARE

Table 44-8 Gastroesophageal Reflux Disease (GERD) and Hiatal Hernia

Diagnostic

- History and physical examination
- Upper GI endoscopy with biopsy and cytological analysis
- Barium swallow
- Motility (manometry) studies
- pH monitoring (laboratory or 24-hr ambulatory)

Collaborative Therapy

Conservative

- Elevation of head of bed on 10- to 15-cm blocks
- High-protein, low-fat diet with avoidance of foods and fluids that decrease LES pressure or irritate acid-sensitive esophagus

- Antacids
- Antisecretory agents
- H₂-receptor blockers*
- Proton pump inhibitors*
- Prokinetic drug therapy*
- Cholinergic drugs

Surgical

- Nissen fundoplication
- Toupet fundoplication
- Hill gastropexy
- Belsey fundoplication

Endoscopic

- Stretta device

GI, gastrointestinal; *LES*, lower esophageal sphincter.
*See Table 44-9.

DRUG THERAPY

Table 44-9 Gastroesophageal Reflux Disease (GERD)

MECHANISM OF ACTION	EXAMPLES
Increase Lower Esophageal Sphincter Pressure	
Cholinergic	Bethanechol (Duvoid)
Promotility	
Prokinetic	Metoclopramide
Acid-Neutralizing	
Antacids	Maalox, Mylanta
Antisecretory	
H₂-receptor blockers	Famotidine (Pepcid)
	Nizatidine (Axid)
	Ranitidine (Zantac)
Proton pump inhibitors (PPIs)	Esomeprazole (Nexium)
	Dexlansoprazole (Dexilant)
	Lansoprazole (Prevacid)
	Omeprazole (Losec)
	Pantoprazole (Pantoloc)
	Rabeprazole (Pariet)
Cytoprotective	
Alginic acid-antacid	Gaviscon
Acid-protective	Sucralfate

Lifestyle Modifications. The patient with GERD is taught to avoid factors that aggravate symptoms. Particular attention is given to diet and drugs that may affect the LES, acid secretion, or gastric emptying. Patients who are overweight or obese are encouraged to lose weight.

Patients who smoke are encouraged to stop. Cigarette smoking has been associated with decreased acid clearance from the lower esophagus (Fock et al., 2008).

Nutritional Therapy. Diet does not cause GERD, but food can aggravate symptoms. No specific diet is necessary, but foods that cause reflux should be avoided. Fatty foods stimulate the release of cholecystokinin, a hormone from the duodenum that decreases LES pressure. High-fat foods also decrease the rate of gastric emptying. Foods that decrease LES pressure, such as chocolate, peppermint, coffee, and tea (see Table 44-7), should be avoided because they predispose to reflux. Milk products should be avoided, especially at bedtime, because milk increases gastric acid secretion. Small, frequent meals are advised to prevent overdistension of the stomach. The patient should avoid late-evening meals and nocturnal snacking. Fluids should be taken between rather than with meals to reduce gastric distension. Certain foods (e.g., tomato-based products, orange juice) may irritate the acid-sensitive esophagus and may have to be avoided. To reduce intraabdominal pressure, weight reduction is recommended if the patient is overweight.

Drug Therapy. Drug therapy for GERD is focused on improving LES function, increasing esophageal clearance, decreasing volume and acidity of reflux, and protecting the esophageal mucosa (Table 44-9). There are two approaches to drug therapy. The first is the "step-up" approach, which means starting with antacids and OTC histamine H₂-receptor (H₂R) blockers and progressing to prescription H₂R blockers and, finally, to proton pump inhibitors (PPIs). The "step-down" approach involves starting with a PPI and over time titrating down to prescription H₂R blockers and, finally, to OTC H₂R blockers and antacids.

Antacids produce quick but short-lived relief of heartburn. They act by neutralizing HCl. They should be taken 1 to 3 hours after meals and at bedtime. OTC antacids with or without alginic acid (e.g., Gaviscon) may be useful in patients with mild, intermittent heartburn. The alginic acid reacts with sodium bicarbonate and forms a viscous solution that floats to the surface of the gastric contents and coats the esophagus, acting as a mechanical barrier to reflux. However, in patients with moderate to severe or frequent symptoms or patients with documented esophagitis, these regimens are not effective in relieving symptoms or healing erosive lesions.

Antisecretory agents decrease the secretion of HCl by the stomach. H₂R blockers (e.g., ranitidine [Zantac], famotidine [Pepcid], nizatidine [Axid]) are available in OTC and prescription formulations. Some formulations include H₂R-plus-antacid combinations. For example, Pepcid Complete includes famotidine, calcium carbonate, and magnesium hydroxide. In prescription-strength doses, H₂R blockers reduce symptoms and promote esophageal healing in approximately 50% of patients. Patients frequently relapse (i.e., GERD symptoms return) with discontinuation of the drug.

PPIs such as omeprazole (Losec), esomeprazole (Nexium), pantoprazole (Pantoloc), lansoprazole (Prevacid), rabeprazole (Pariet), and dexlansoprazole (Dexilant) also decrease stomach HCl secretion. These agents act by inhibiting the proton pump mechanism responsible for the secretion of hydrogen ions (H⁺). PPIs promote esophageal healing in approximately 80 to 90% of patients but are more expensive than H₂R blockers. PPIs may also be beneficial in decreasing the incidence of esophageal strictures, a complication of chronic GERD.

Another drug that may be used to treat GERD is sucralfate, an antiulcer drug used for its cytoprotective properties. Cholinergic drugs, such as bethanechol (Duvoid), may be used to increase LES pressure, improve esophageal emptying in the supine position, and increase gastric emptying. However, the value of current cholinergic agents is limited because they also stimulate HCl secretion. Prokinetic (motility-enhancing) drugs such as metoclopramide promote gastric emptying and reduce the risk of gastric acid reflux (see Table 44-9).

Surgical Therapy.

Surgical therapy (antireflux surgery) may be necessary if long-term conservative therapy fails, if a hiatal hernia is present, or if complications exist, such as esophageal stricture and stenosis (narrowing), chronic esophagitis, and bleeding. Many surgical procedures are performed laparoscopically. The objective of surgical interventions for GERD is to reduce reflux of gastric contents by enhancing the integrity of the LES. Surgical interventions for GERD are called *antireflux procedures.* In these procedures, the fundus of the stomach is wrapped around the lower portion of the esophagus in varying positions.

The Nissen fundoplication is shown in Figure 44-4. Laparoscopically performed Nissen and Toupet fundoplications have become the standard antireflux surgeries. The use of laparoscopic antireflux surgery for GERD has reduced complications, overall morbidity, and the cost of hospitalization compared with a thoracic or open abdominal approach (Elakkary, Duffy, Roberts, & Bell, 2008).

NURSING MANAGEMENT: GASTROESOPHAGEAL REFLUX DISEASE

Patients with GERD must avoid factors that cause reflux. A patient teaching guide is provided in Table 44-10. The patient who is a smoker should stop. Smoking causes an almost immediate drop in LES pressure and decreases the ability to clear acid from the esophagus. The patient may need to be referred to other members of the health care team or to community resources for assistance in stopping smoking. (See Chapter 11 for additional information related to smoking cessation.) Substances that decrease LES pressure and tone should be avoided (see Table 44-7). If stress seems to cause symptoms, measures to cope with stress should be discussed. (See Chapter 8 for stress management techniques.) The patient should also be taught possible adverse effects of drugs.

Nursing care for the patient who is having acute symptoms consists mainly of encouraging the patient to follow the necessary regimen. The nurse should ensure that the head of the bed is elevated to approximately 30 degrees and that the patient does not lie down during the first 2 to 3 hours after eating. Teaching the patient to avoid food and activities that cause reflux is important (e.g., late-night eating should be avoided). The patient may be taking drugs to relieve heartburn, so the nurse must observe for adverse effects as well as evaluate the drugs' effectiveness. Even when symptoms are brought under control, the patient may need to continue drugs because the underlying problem is still present. Because of the link between GERD and metaplastic changes in

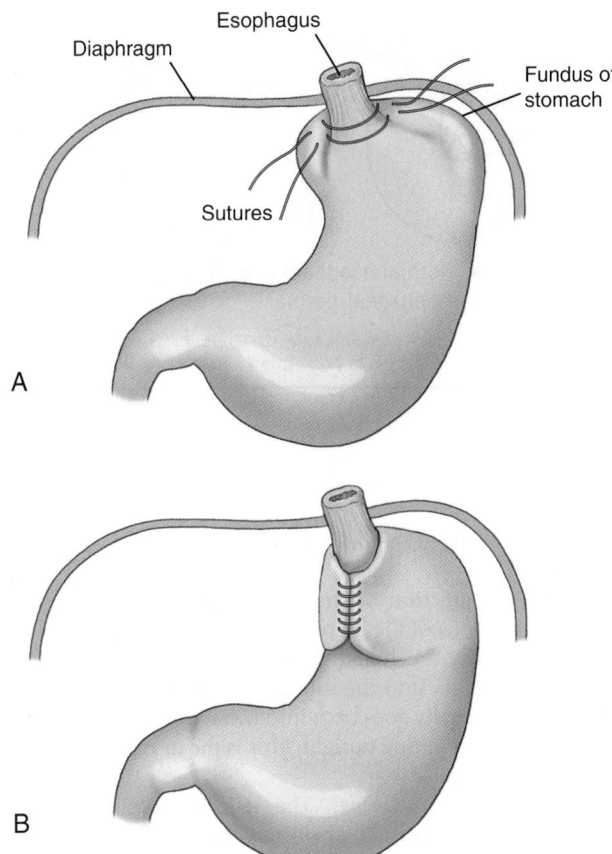

Figure 44-4 Nissen fundoplication for repair of hiatal hernia. **A,** The fundus of the stomach is wrapped around the distal esophagus. **B,** The fundus is then sutured to itself.

Source: Doughty, D. B., & Jackson, D. B. (1993). *Mosby's clinical nursing series: gastrointestinal disorders.* St. Louis: Mosby.

PATIENT & CAREGIVER TEACHING GUIDE

Table 44-10 Prevention of Gastroesophageal Reflux Disease (GERD)

The following are teaching guidelines for the patient and caregiver:

1. Explain the rationale for a high-protein, low-fat diet. If the patient is overweight or obese, discuss the need for weight loss.

2. Encourage the patient to eat small, frequent meals to prevent gastric distension.

3. Explain the rationale for avoiding alcohol, smoking (causes an almost immediate, marked decrease in LES pressure), and beverages that contain caffeine.

4. Teach the patient not to lie down for 2-3 hr after eating, wear tight clothing around the waist, or bend over (especially after eating).

5. Encourage the patient to sleep with head of bed elevated 30 degrees (gravity fosters esophageal emptying).

6. Teach information regarding drugs, including rationale for their use and common adverse effects.

7. Discuss strategies for weight reduction if appropriate.

8. Encourage patient and caregiver to share concerns about lifestyle changes and living with a chronic problem.

LES, lower esophageal sphincter.

the lower esophagus (Barrett's esophagus), patients are instructed to see their health care provider if symptoms persist.

The nurse must observe for and instruct the patient about adverse effects of the drugs being taken. Adverse effects with H_2R blockers and PPIs are rare. Antacids have minimal adverse effects. Antacids that contain aluminum tend to cause constipation, whereas those that contain magnesium tend to cause diarrhea. Several of the antacids are combinations of aluminum and magnesium designed to minimize these adverse effects. If the patient is taking bethanechol, adverse effects to observe for include urinary urgency, increased salivation, and abdominal cramping with diarrhea, nausea, vomiting, and hypotension. Such adverse effects often limit the effectiveness of cholinergic agents in the treatment of GERD. Adverse effects of metoclopramide include restlessness, anxiety, insomnia, and hallucinations. Adverse effects of sucralfate include drowsiness, dizziness, nausea, vomiting, constipation, urticaria, and rash.

Postoperative care focuses on concerns related to prevention of respiratory complications, maintenance of fluid and electrolyte balance, and prevention of infection. If a thoracic approach is used, a chest tube is inserted. Assessment and management related to closed chest drainage are important (see Chapter 30).

If an open abdominal incision is used, respiratory complications can occur in a patient because of the high abdominal incision. Respiratory assessment should include respiratory rate and rhythm, pulse rate and rhythm, and signs of pneumothorax (e.g., dyspnea, chest pain, cyanosis). Deep breathing is essential to fully expand the lungs.

The patient receives IV fluids and electrolytes until the return of peristalsis. Care should be taken to maintain patency of the NG tube (if present) to prevent the need to reinsert the tube. It is dangerous to attempt to replace the tube because of the possibility of perforation of the surgical repair. Immediately after the surgical procedure, the patient cannot voluntarily vomit or belch, and this may cause bloating and abdominal discomfort. When peristalsis returns, only fluids are given initially. Solids are added gradually so that the stomach is not overdistended. The nurse must maintain an accurate recording of intake and output and observe for fluid and electrolyte imbalances (see Chapter 19). (Care of the patient undergoing a laparotomy procedure is described in Chapter 42, NCP 42-1).

After surgical therapy, there should be no symptoms of gastric reflux. However, the recurrence rate may range from 10 to 30% over a 20-year period following surgery. The patient should be instructed to report symptoms such as heartburn and regurgitation. Such problems may be temporary and resolve with time. The patient should report persistent dysphagia, epigastric fullness, and bloating. A normal diet is gradually resumed. The patient should avoid foods that are gas forming and should try to prevent gastric distension. Food should be chewed thoroughly.

Hiatal Hernia

Hiatal hernia is herniation of a portion of the stomach into the esophagus through an opening, or hiatus, in the diaphragm. It is also referred to as *diaphragmatic hernia* and *esophageal hernia*. The incidence of hiatal hernia is difficult to determine. However, it is the most common abnormality found on radiographic examination of the upper GI tract. Hiatal hernias are common in older adults and occur more often in women than in men.

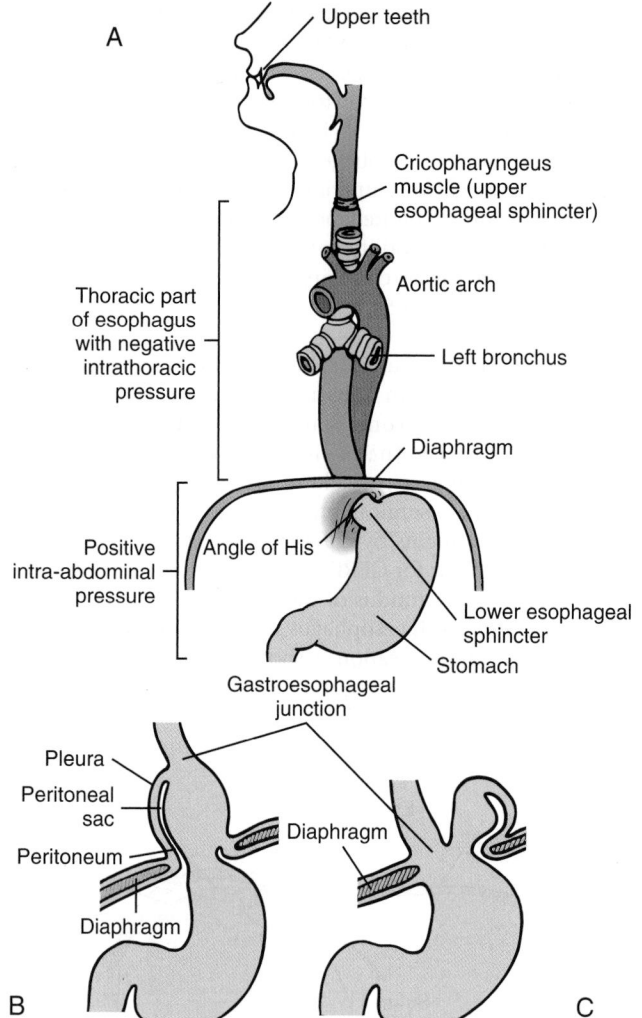

Figure 44-5 A, Normal esophagus. **B,** Sliding hiatal hernia. **C,** Rolling or paraesophageal hernia.

Source: Redrawn from Price, S. A., & Wilson, L. M. (2003). *Pathophysiology: Clinical concepts of disease processes* (6th ed., p. 322, Figure 23-6). St. Louis: Mosby.

Types

Hiatal hernias are classified into the following two types (Figure 44-5):

1. *Sliding:* The junction of the stomach and the esophagus is above the hiatus of the diaphragm, and a part of the stomach slides through the hiatal opening in the diaphragm. The stomach "slides" into the thoracic cavity when the patient is supine and usually goes back into the abdominal cavity when the patient is standing upright. This is the most common type of hiatal hernia.

2. *Paraesophageal* or *rolling:* The esophagogastric junction remains in the normal position, but the fundus and the greater curvature of the stomach roll up through the diaphragm, forming a pocket alongside the esophagus.

Etiology and Pathophysiology

The actual cause of hiatal hernia is unknown. Many factors contribute to the development of hiatal hernia. Structural changes, such as weakening of the muscles in the diaphragm around the esophagogastric opening, are usually contributing factors. Factors that increase intra-abdominal pressure, including obesity, pregnancy, ascites, tumours, tight corsets, intense physical exertion, and heavy lifting on a continual basis, may also predispose to development of a hiatal hernia. Other predisposing factors are increased age, trauma, poor nutrition, and a forced recumbent position, as when a prolonged illness confines the person to bed. In some cases, congenital weakness is a contributing factor.

Clinical Manifestations

Persons with hiatal hernia may be asymptomatic. When present, the signs and symptoms of hiatal hernia are similar to those described for GERD. Heartburn, especially after a meal or after lying supine, is a common symptom. Patients may complain of dysphagia. Frequently, the symptoms of hiatal hernia mimic gallbladder disease, peptic ulcer disease (PUD), and angina. However, some patients with hiatal hernia have no symptoms. Reflux and discomfort are also associated with position, occurring soon or several hours after lying down. Bending over may cause a severe burning pain, which is usually relieved by sitting or standing. Other common precipitating factors of pain include consumption of large meals and alcohol and smoking. Nocturnal symptoms of heartburn are common, especially if the person has eaten before going to sleep.

Complications

Complications that may occur with hiatal hernia include GERD, hemorrhage from erosion, stenosis (narrowing of the esophagus), ulcerations of the herniated portion of the stomach, strangulation of the hernia, and regurgitation with tracheal aspiration.

Diagnostic Studies

A barium swallow is an important diagnostic measure that may show the protrusion of gastric mucosa through the esophageal hiatus in the patient with hiatal hernia. Endoscopic visualization of the lower esophagus provides information on the degree of mucosal inflammation or other abnormalities. Other tests are similar to those described in Table 44-8.

NURSING AND COLLABORATIVE MANAGEMENT: HIATAL HERNIA

Conservative Therapy

Conservative therapy of hiatal hernia is similar to that described under GERD, including lifestyle modifications (e.g., reduction of intra-abdominal pressure by eliminating constricting garments, avoiding lifting and straining, eliminating alcohol and smoking, elevating the head of the bed) and the use of antacids and antisecretory agents (i.e., PPIs, H_2R blockers). Elevation of the bed on 10- to 15-cm blocks assists gravity in maintaining the stomach in the abdominal cavity and also helps prevent reflux and tracheal aspiration. If overweight, the patient should be encouraged to lose weight.

Surgical Therapy

The objective of surgical interventions for hiatal hernia is to reduce reflux by enhancing the integrity of the LES. There are four slightly varied procedures: the Nissen fundoplication, the Toupet fundoplication or technique, the Hill gastropexy, and the Belsey fundoplication. These surgical procedures are all variations of fundoplication, which involves "wrapping" the fundus of the stomach around the lower portion of the esophagus in varying positions. These procedures reduce the hernia, provide an acceptable LES pressure, and prevent movement of the gastroesophageal junction. The Nissen fundoplication is shown in Figure 44-4. Similar to GERD, laparoscopically performed Nissen and Toupet techniques have become the standard antireflux surgeries for hiatal hernia (Elakkary et al., 2008). A thoracic or open abdominal approach may also be used in selected cases.

AGE-RELATED CONSIDERATIONS: GASTROESOPHAGEAL REFLUX DISEASE AND HIATAL HERNIA

The incidence of both GERD and hiatal hernia increases with age. It is associated with weakening of the diaphragm, obesity, kyphosis, and use of corsets or other factors that increase intra-abdominal pressure. Some older adults with hiatal hernia are asymptomatic. The first indications may include esophageal bleeding secondary to esophagitis or respiratory complications (e.g., aspiration pneumonia) related to aspiration of gastric contents. The LES may become less competent with aging in some individuals.

The clinical course and the management of GERD and hiatal hernia in the older adult are similar to those for the younger adult. With the increased use of laparoscopic procedures, surgical risks have been reduced. However, an older adult with cardiovascular and pulmonary problems may not be a good candidate for surgical intervention. In addition, changes in lifestyle, including elimination of dietary factors such as caffeine-containing beverages and chocolate, and elevating the head of the bed on blocks, may be more difficult for the older adult.

Esophageal Cancer

Esophageal cancer, a rare malignant neoplasm of the esophagus, includes two main types, namely, squamous cell carcinoma and adenocarcinoma. The 5-year survival rate remains less than 15% despite multimodal treatment options. Cancer of the esophagus occurs three times more often in males than in females and the rate has remained relatively stable since the mid-1980s. Although still relatively rare in Canada, the incidence of one type of esophageal cancer (esophageal adenocarcinoma) doubled from 1986 to 2006 (Otterstatter et al., 2012). This may be because of the rising prevalence of obesity and GERD. It was estimated that 1850 new cases of esophageal cancer would be diagnosed in Canada during 2012 (Canadian Cancer Society's Steering Committee on Cancer Statistics, 2012). Adenocarcinomas arise from the glands lining the esophagus and resemble cancers of the stomach and the small intestine whereas squamous cell carcinoma starts in the squamous cells that line the esophagus. The incidence of esophageal cancer increases with age. One risk factor for esophageal adenocarcinoma is Barrett's esophagus. At this time, it is estimated that 1 in 200 cases of Barrett's esophagus will progress to esophageal cancer. (Barrett's esophagus is described earlier under the discussion of GERD.)

Etiology and Pathophysiology

The cause of esophageal cancer is unknown. Two important risk factors are smoking and excessive alcohol intake. Diets that are low in fruits and vegetables and certain minerals and vitamins may increase the risk of this cancer. Lye that is found in strong cleaners like drain cleaners can burn and destroy esophageal cells. As a result, a person who has swallowed lye has a higher risk of squamous cell cancer. A patient with a history of achalasia, a condition in which there is delayed emptying of the lower esophagus, is also at greater risk for squamous cell cancer. Other risk factors include exposure to asbestos and metal (Canadian Cancer Society, 2012).

The majority of esophageal tumours are located in the middle and lower portions of the esophagus. The malignant tumour usually appears as an ulcerated lesion and has often advanced by the time the patient experiences symptoms. The tumour may penetrate the muscular layer and even extend outside the wall of the esophagus. Obstruction of the esophagus occurs in the later stages.

Clinical Manifestations

The onset of symptoms is usually late in relation to the extent of the tumour. Progressive dysphagia is the most common symptom and may be expressed as a substernal feeling (globus sensation) as if food is not passing. Initially, the dysphagia occurs only with meat, then with soft foods, and eventually with liquids.

Pain develops late and is described as occurring in the substernal, epigastric, or back areas and usually increases with swallowing. The pain may radiate to the neck, the jaw, the ears, and the shoulders. If the tumour is in the upper third of the esophagus, symptoms such as sore throat, choking, and hoarseness may occur. Weight loss is fairly common. When esophageal stenosis is severe, regurgitation of blood-flecked esophageal contents is common.

Complications

Hemorrhage may occur if the cancer erodes through the esophagus and into the aorta. Esophageal perforation with fistula formation into the lung or the trachea sometimes develops. The tumour may enlarge enough to cause esophageal obstruction. There is spread via the lymph system, with the liver and the lung common sites of metastasis.

Diagnostic Studies

Barium swallow with fluoroscopy may demonstrate a narrowing of the esophagus at the site of the tumour (Table 44-11). Sometimes, a crater is visible. Endoscopy with biopsy is necessary to make a definitive diagnosis of carcinoma by identification of malignant cells. Endoscopic ultrasonography is an important tool used to stage esophageal cancer. A bronchoscopic examination may be performed to detect malignant involvement of the lung.

COLLABORATIVE CARE

Table 44-11 Esophageal Cancer

Diagnostic	Collaborative Therapy
• History and physical examination	• Surgical resection
• Endoscopy of esophagus with biopsy	• Esophagectomy
• Barium swallow	• Esophagogastrostomy
• Endoscopic ultrasonography	• Esophagoenterostomy
• Bronchoscopy	• Radiation
• CT and MRI	• Chemotherapy
	• Palliative therapy
	• Dilation
	• Stent or prosthesis
	• Laser therapy
	• Gastrostomy

CT, computed tomography; *MRI,* magnetic resonance imaging.

CT scanning and MRI are also used to assess the extent of the disease.

Collaborative Care

The treatment of esophageal cancer depends on the location of the tumour and whether invasion or metastasis has occurred (see Table 44-11). Esophageal cancer has a poor prognosis, mainly because it is not usually diagnosed until the disease is advanced. The best results may be obtained with a combination of surgery, chemotherapy, and radiation.

The types of surgical procedures that can be performed are (1) removal of part or all of the esophagus (*esophagectomy*) with use of a Dacron graft to replace the resected part, (2) resection of a portion of the esophagus and anastomosis of the remaining portion to the stomach (*esophagogastrostomy*), and (3) resection of a portion of the esophagus and anastomosis of a segment of colon to the remaining portion (*esophagoenterostomy*). The surgical approaches may be thoracic or both abdominal and thoracic. Minimally invasive esophagectomy (laparoscopic vagal nerve–sparing surgery) has the advantage of using smaller incisions, decreasing hospital stays, and fewer pulmonary complications. Overall outcomes appear to be similar to open resections of the esophagus. Chemotherapy in combination with radiation before surgery is currently used (Malthaner, Wong, Spithof, Rumble, & Zurow, 2008). Current treatment regimes can be found through the Canadian Cancer Society. If the tumour is in the cervical section (upper third) of the esophagus, radiation is usually indicated. A tumour in the lower third of the esophagus is usually resected surgically.

Palliative therapy consists of restoration of the swallowing function and maintenance of nutrition and hydration. Dilation, stent placement, or both can relieve obstruction. Dilation is done with various types of dilators (e.g., Celestin's tube). Dilation often relieves dysphagia and allows for improved nutrition. Placement of a stent or prosthesis may help when dilation is no longer effective. The prostheses are composed of silicone rubber or nylon-reinforced latex tubes with distal and proximal collars. The prosthesis is placed in the esophagus so that food and fluids can pass through the stenotic segment of the esophagus. The prosthesis can be placed endoscopically.

Endoscopic laser therapy or vaporization of the tumour may be used in combination with dilation. Obstruction recurs as the tumour grows, but laser therapy can be repeated. Sometimes, these procedures are combined with radiation therapy. Other measures for palliation include gastrostomy or esophagostomy tube placements for nutritional support and pain management.

Nutritional Therapy. After esophageal surgery, parenteral fluids are given. When fluids are allowed after bowel sounds have returned, 30 to 60 mL of water is given hourly, with gradual progression to small, frequent bland meals. The patient should be in an upright position to prevent regurgitation of the fluid. The patient is observed for signs of intolerance to the feeding or leakage of the feeding into the mediastinum. Symptoms that indicate leakage are pain, increased temperature, and dyspnea. Symptoms of food intolerance include vomiting and abdominal distension. A gastrostomy may be performed for the purpose of feeding the patient. (Gastrostomy and tube feedings are discussed in Chapter 42.)

NURSING MANAGEMENT: ESOPHAGEAL CANCER

Nursing Assessment

The patient should be asked about any history of GERD, hiatal hernia, achalasia, or Barrett's esophagus. The patient is also questioned regarding tobacco and alcohol use. The patient should be assessed for progressive dysphagia and *odynophagia* (burning, squeezing pain while swallowing). The nurse should question the patient regarding the type of substances ingested that cause dysphagia, such as meat, soft foods, and liquids. The patient is also assessed for pain (substernal, epigastric, or back areas), choking, heartburn, hoarseness, cough, anorexia, weight loss, and regurgitation (sometimes bloody).

Nursing Diagnoses

Nursing diagnoses for the patient with esophageal cancer include, but are not limited to, the following:
- Imbalanced nutrition: less than body requirements *related to* dysphagia, odynophagia, weakness, chemotherapy, and radiation therapy
- Chronic pain *related to* the tumour
- Deficient fluid volume *related to* inadequate intake
- Risk for aspiration *related to* impaired esophageal function
- Anxiety *related to* diagnosis of cancer, uncertain future, and poor prognosis
- Grieving *related to* diagnosis of life-threatening malignancy
- Ineffective health maintenance *related to* lack of knowledge of disease process and therapeutic regimen, unavailability of a support system, and chronic debilitating disease

Planning

The overall goals are that the patient with esophageal cancer will (1) have relief of symptoms including pain and dysphagia, (2) achieve optimal nutritional intake, (3) understand the prognosis of the disease, and (4) experience a quality of life appropriate to disease progression.

Nursing Implementation

Health Promotion

Patients with diagnosed GERD and hiatal hernia need to be counselled regarding regular follow-up evaluation. Health counselling should focus on elimination of smoking and excessive alcohol intake as well as other risk factors for GERD. Maintenance of good oral hygiene and dietary habits (intake of fresh fruits and vegetables) may also be helpful.

Patients diagnosed with Barrett's esophagus need to be monitored because this is considered a premalignant condition. Early diagnosis of esophageal tumours is important but difficult because the onset of symptoms is usually late. Patients are encouraged to seek medical attention for any esophageal problems, especially dysphagia. Patients who are at risk for esophageal adenocarcinoma, such as those with evidence of Barrett's esophagus and a diagnosis of achalasia (discussed later in the section on other esophageal disorders), may need regular endoscopic screening with biopsy and cytological study.

Acute Intervention

Preoperative Care. In addition to general preoperative teaching and preparation, particular attention to the patient's nutritional needs and oral care is important. Many patients are poorly nourished because of the inability to ingest adequate amounts of food and fluids before surgery. A high-calorie, high-protein diet is recommended. It may have to be in liquid form. Some patients may need IV fluid replacement or total parenteral nutrition. The patient, the family member, or both are instructed on how to keep an intake and output record and assess for signs of fluid and electrolyte imbalance. Some treatment protocols necessitate preoperative radiation and chemotherapy.

Meticulous oral care is essential. The mouth, including tongue, gingivae, and teeth or dentures, must be cleaned thoroughly. Milk of magnesia with mineral oil may be used to remove any crusting that has formed. A mixture of mouthwash (nonalcohol), ice, and water makes a refreshing rinse for the patient.

Teaching should include information about chest tubes (if a thoracic approach is used), IV lines, NG tube, gastrostomy feeding, turning, coughing, and deep breathing. (General preoperative care is presented in Chapter 20.)

Postoperative Care. The patient usually has an NG tube in place, and there may be bloody drainage for 8 to 12 hours. The drainage gradually changes to greenish yellow. Assessment of the drainage, maintenance of the tube, and oral and nasal care are nursing responsibilities. The NG tube should not be repositioned or reinserted without consulting with the surgeon.

Because of the location of the incision and the general condition of the patient, special emphasis must be placed on prevention of respiratory complications. Turning and deep breathing should be done every 2 hours. Use of an incentive spirometer helps to prevent respiratory complications.

The patient should be positioned in a semi-Fowler or Fowler position to prevent reflux and aspiration of gastric secretions. When the patient can drink fluids or eat, the upright position should be maintained for at least 2 hours after eating to assist the movement of food through the GI tract.

Ambulatory and Home Care

Many patients require long-term follow-up care after surgery for esophageal cancer. The patient may undergo chemotherapy and radiation treatment following surgery. The patient needs encouragement and assistance in maintaining adequate nutrition. The patient may need a permanent feeding gastrostomy. The patient usually has fears and anxieties about a diagnosis of cancer. The nurse should know what the health care provider has told the patient regarding the prognosis and then provide appropriate counselling.

Referral to a home health nurse may be necessary for continued care of the patient (e.g., gastrostomy teaching, follow-up wound care). (See Chapter 13 for management of the terminally ill patient and Chapter 18 for that of the patient with cancer.)

Evaluation

The following are expected outcomes for the patient with esophageal cancer:

- The patient will maintain a patent airway.
- The patient will have relief of pain.
- The patient will be able to swallow comfortably.
- The patient will consume adequate nutritional intake.
- The patient will understand the prognosis of the disease.
- The patient will experience quality of life appropriate to disease progression.

Other Esophageal Disorders

Esophageal Diverticula

Esophageal diverticula are saclike outpouchings of one or more layers of the esophagus. They occur in three main areas: (1) above the upper esophageal sphincter *(Zenker's diverticulum)*, which is the most common location; (2) near the esophageal midpoint *(traction diverticulum)*; and (3) above the LES *(epiphrenic diverticulum)* (Figure 44-6). Pharyngeal pouches (Zenker's diverticula) occur most commonly in older adults (>70 yr), and typical symptoms include dysphagia, regurgitation, chronic cough, aspiration, and weight loss. Traction diverticulum may not cause signs and symptoms. The patient frequently complains of tasting sour food and smelling a foul odour caused by the stagnant food. Complications include malnutrition, aspiration, and perforation. A diagnosis is easily established by barium studies.

There is no specific treatment for diverticula. Some patients find they can empty the pocket of food that collects by applying pressure at a point on the neck. The diet may have to be limited to foods that pass more readily (e.g., blenderized foods). Treatment of the diverticulum may be necessary if nutrition becomes disrupted. Treatment is surgical via an endoscopic or external cervical approach and should include a cricopharyngeal myotomy. Open approaches have been associated with significant morbidity because the majority of patients are older adults and often have general medical problems.

Esophageal Strictures

The most common cause of esophageal strictures (narrowings or constrictions of the esophagus) is chronic GERD. The ingestion

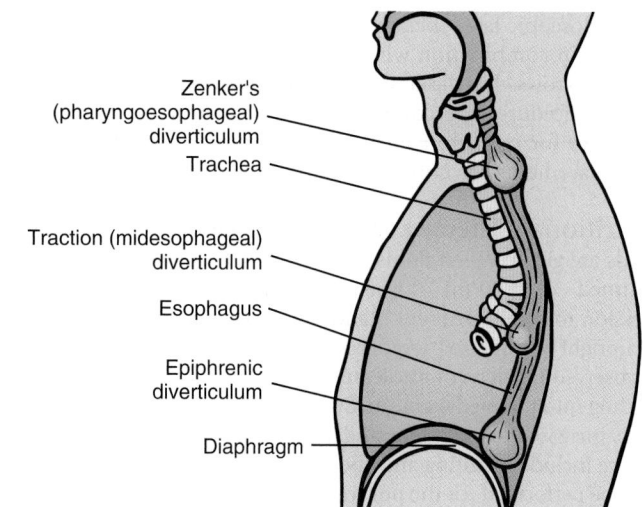

Figure 44-6 Possible sites for the occurrence of esophageal diverticula. These hollow outpouchings may occur just above the upper esophageal sphincter (Zenker's, the most common type of diverticulum), near the midpoint of the esophagus (traction), and just above the lower esophageal sphincter (epiphrenic).

Source: Redrawn from Price, S. A., & Wilson, L. M. (2003). *Pathophysiology: Clinical concepts of disease processes* (6th ed.). St. Louis: Mosby.

of strong acids or alkalis, external beam radiation, and surgical anastomosis can also create strictures. Trauma such as throat lacerations and gunshot wounds may also lead to strictures as a result of scar formation (collagen deposition) from healing. The strictures usually develop over a long time. Strictures can be dilated endoscopically using *bougies* (dilating instruments). Another technique is balloon dilation, which is done under endoscopy and does not require fluoroscopy. Surgical excision with anastomosis is sometimes necessary. The patient may have a temporary or permanent gastrostomy.

Achalasia

In **achalasia** (cardiospasm), peristalsis of the lower two thirds (smooth muscle) of the esophagus is absent. Pressure in the LES is increased, along with incomplete relaxation of the LES. Obstruction of the esophagus at or near the diaphragm occurs. Food and fluid accumulate in the lower esophagus. The result of this condition is dilation of the lower esophagus (Figure 44-7). The altered peristalsis is a result of impairment of the neurons that innervate the lower esophagus. There is a selective loss of inhibitory neurons, resulting in unopposed excitation of the LES. Achalasia affects all ages and both sexes. The course of the disease is chronic.

Dysphagia (difficulty swallowing) is the most common symptom and occurs with both liquids and solids. Patients may report a globus sensation (a lump in the throat). Substernal chest pain (similar to the pain of angina) occurs during or immediately after a meal. *Halitosis* (foul-smelling breath) and the inability to eructate (belch) are other symptoms. Another common symptom is regurgitation of sour-tasting food and liquids, especially when the patient is in a horizontal position. Patients with achalasia also report symptoms (e.g., heartburn) of GERD. Weight loss is typical.

Diagnosis usually involves obtaining radiographs and performing manometric studies of the lower esophagus, and endoscopy. The exact cause of achalasia is not known, so treatment is

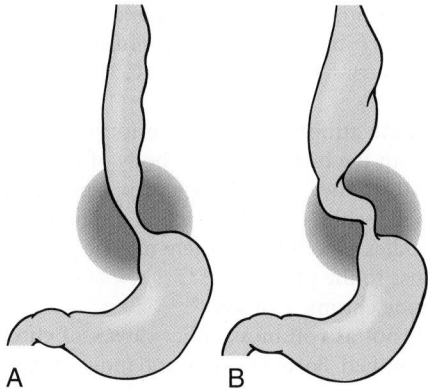

Figure 44-7 Esophageal achalasia. **A,** Early stage, showing tapering of lower esophagus. **B,** Advanced stage, showing dilated, tortuous esophagus.

Source: Redrawn from Price, S. A., & Wilson, L. M. (2003). *Pathophysiology: Clinical concepts of disease processes* (6th ed., p. 320, Figure 23-3). St. Louis: Mosby.

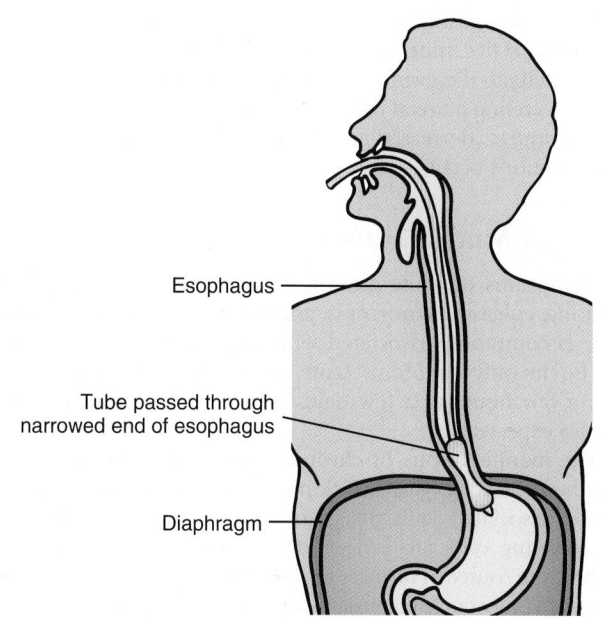

Esophagus

Tube passed through narrowed end of esophagus

Diaphragm

Figure 44-8 Pneumatic dilation attempts to treat achalasia by maintaining an adequate lumen and decreasing lower esophageal sphincter tone.

Source: Redrawn from Price, S. A., & Wilson, L. M. (2003). *Pathophysiology: Clinical concepts of disease processes* (6th ed.). St. Louis: Mosby.

focused on symptom management. Treatment consists of dilation, surgery, and use of drugs. All these therapies are directed at relieving the stasis caused by the increased LES pressure, the nonrelaxing LES, and the aperistaltic esophagus. Symptomatic treatment consists of a semisoft bland diet, eating slowly and drinking fluid with meals, and sleeping with the head elevated.

Esophageal dilation *(bougienage)* is an effective treatment measure for many patients. Pneumatic dilation of the LES with a balloon-tipped dilator passed orally is usually used. A variety of different dilators are available for this procedure. All depend on forcible expansion of a balloon in the LES (Figure 44-8). The forceful dilation does not restore normal esophageal motility, but it does provide for emptying of the esophagus into the stomach.

Surgical intervention may become necessary. An esophagomyotomy may be performed. In this procedure, the muscle fibres that enclose the narrowed area of the esophagus are divided. This allows the mucosa to pouch out through the division in the muscle layer so that food can be swallowed without obstruction.

A similar procedure is Heller's myotomy (cardiomyotomy), which disrupts the LES and reduces LES pressure. An antireflux procedure is often done with the myotomy. This procedure can be performed laparoscopically, reducing the potential for postoperative complications (Elakkary et al., 2008).

Drug therapy is used to manage early achalasia when there is no significant esophageal dilation. Drug therapy is used as a short-term measure and is considered as an alternative only in patients unfit to undergo pneumatic dilation or surgery. Endoscopic injection of botulinum toxin (Botox) into the LES can be offered for initial relief of symptoms, but the effects are short term, and symptoms will likely recur within 1 year. It works by inhibiting the release of acetylcholine from nerve endings, thereby promoting relaxation of the smooth muscle. This treatment does not carry the risk of perforation that can occur with pneumatic dilation. Repeated injections are required, or the patient must be switched to other therapy. However, there may be subsets of patients, such as older adult patients or those with multiple medical problems, who are poor candidates for more invasive procedures, for whom botulinum toxin injection is the preferred approach. Other classes of drugs used in the management of achalasia include anticholinergics, calcium channel blockers (e.g., nifedipine [Adalat]), and long-acting nitrates, which act by relaxing the smooth muscle.

Esophageal Varices

Esophageal varices are dilated, tortuous veins occurring in the lower portion of the esophagus as a result of portal hypertension. Esophageal varices are a common complication of liver cirrhosis and are discussed in Chapter 46.

Disorders of the Stomach and Upper Small Intestine

Gastritis

Types

Gastritis, an inflammation of the gastric mucosa, is one of the most common problems affecting the stomach. Gastritis may be acute or chronic and may be diffuse or localized. Chronic gastritis has been further divided into three subtypes including (1) autoimmune, which involves the body and the fundus of the stomach; (2) diffuse antral, which primarily affects the antrum; and (3) multifocal, which is diffuse throughout the stomach. At present, the causes of gastritis and its relationship to other gastric disorders, such as *Helicobacter pylori* infection and gastric cancer, are the focus of ongoing research.

Etiology and Pathophysiology

Gastritis occurs as the result of a breakdown in the normal gastric mucosal barrier. This mucosal barrier normally protects the stomach tissue from autodigestion by HCl and the proteolytic

Table 44-12 Causes of Gastritis	
Drugs	**Pathophysiological Conditions**
• Aspirin	• Burns
• Corticosteroid drugs	• Large hiatal hernia
• Nonsteroidal anti-inflammatory drugs	• Physiological stress
Diet	• Reflux of bile and pancreatic secretions
• Alcohol	• Renal failure (uremia)
• Spicy, irritating food	• Sepsis
Microorganisms	• Shock
• *Helicobacter pylori*	**Other Factors**
• *Salmonella*	• Endoscopic procedures
• *Staphylococcus* organisms	• Nasogastric suction
Environmental Factors	• Psychological stress
• Radiation	
• Smoking	

enzyme pepsin. When the barrier is broken, HCl can diffuse back into the mucosa. The acid back-diffusion results in tissue edema, disruption of capillary walls with loss of plasma into the gastric lumen, and possible hemorrhage.

Causes of gastritis are listed in Table 44-12. Drugs such as aspirin, nonsteroidal anti-inflammatory drugs (NSAIDs), and digitalis have direct irritating effects on the gastric mucosa. In addition, corticosteroids and NSAIDs are known to inhibit the synthesis of prostaglandins that are protective to the gastric mucosa. This leaves the gastric mucosa more susceptible to mucosal damage. NSAID-related gastritis is associated with many of the older drugs, including piroxicam (Pirox), naproxen (Naprosyn), sulindac (Sulin), indomethacin, diclofenac (Voltaren), and ibuprofen (Motrin, Advil). The use of cyclooxygenase-2 (COX-2) inhibitors has been associated with fewer GI adverse effects than nonselective NSAIDs. However, even these agents are associated with an increased risk of upper GI inflammation and bleeding.

Dietary indiscretions can also result in acute gastritis. After an alcoholic drinking binge, acute damage to the gastric mucosa can range from local destruction of superficial epithelial cells to desquamation and destruction of the mucosa, with mucosal congestion, edema, and hemorrhage. Prolonged damage induced by repeated alcohol abuse can result in chronic gastritis. Eating large quantities of spicy, irritating foods and metabolic conditions such as uremia can also cause acute gastritis.

An important causative factor in chronic gastritis, in particular in the diffuse antral and multifocal types, is *H. pylori* infection. *H. pylori*–associated gastritis is a common problem in adults, many of whom do not have symptoms of gastritis. It is currently thought that *H. pylori* infection is acquired in childhood and is able to persist in the hostile environment of the gastric lumen. For reasons not clearly understood, *H. pylori* is capable of promoting the breakdown of the gastric mucosal barrier, given certain "triggers" or conditions. Thus, given time, *H. pylori* will eventually have a destructive effect on its host environment. This is consistent with the finding that the incidence of chronic gastritis increases with age. However, studies also have shown that not all persons infected with *H. pylori* go on to develop chronic gastritis or PUD. Thus, a combination of factors may be at work to "turn

on" the virulent process by which *H. pylori* damages the gastric mucosal barrier. (The role of *H. pylori* in ulcer development is discussed in greater detail on pp. 1162-1163 in the context of drug therapy for PUD.)

Autoimmune atrophic gastritis is a form of chronic gastritis that affects both the fundus and the body of the stomach and is associated with an increased risk of gastric cancer. Approximately 30% of patients with *H. pylori* infection are found to have anti-gastric antibodies as well. Thus, there may be a link between the host's response to the presence of *H. pylori* and the development of autoimmune chronic gastritis.

Although not as common, other causes of chronic gastritis have been identified. Bacterial, viral, and fungal infections including *Mycobacterium*, cytomegalovirus, and syphilis are associated with chronic gastritis. Gastritis can occur from reflux of bile salts from the duodenum into the stomach as a result of anatomical changes following surgical procedures such as gastroduodenostomy and gastrojejunostomy. Prolonged vomiting may also cause reflux of bile salts. Intense emotional responses and CNS lesions may also produce inflammation of the mucosal lining as a result of hypersecretion of HCl or corticosteroids (Cushing's syndrome).

Progressive gastric mucosal atrophy from chronic alterations in the protective mucosal barrier causes the gastric chief and parietal cells to die eventually. With the decrease in the number of acid-secreting parietal cells and atrophy of the gastric mucosa, *hypochlorhydria* (decreased acid secretion) or *achlorhydria* (lack of acid secretion) occurs.

Clinical Manifestations

The symptoms of acute gastritis include anorexia, nausea and vomiting, epigastric tenderness, and a feeling of fullness. Hemorrhage is commonly associated with alcohol abuse and at times may be the only symptom. Acute gastritis is self-limiting, lasting from a few hours to a few days, with complete healing of the mucosa expected.

The manifestations of chronic gastritis are similar to those described for acute gastritis. Some patients have no symptoms directly associated with the gastric lesion. However, when the acid-secreting cells are lost or do not function as a result of atrophy, the source of *intrinsic factor* is also lost. The loss of intrinsic factor, a substance secreted by the gastric mucosa that is essential for the absorption of cobalamin (vitamin B_{12}) in the terminal ileum, ultimately results in cobalamin deficiency. With time, the body's storage of cobalamin in the liver is depleted, and a deficiency state exists. Lack of this important vitamin, which is essential for the growth and maturation of red blood cells (RBCs), results in the development of anemia and neurological complications. (Cobalamin deficiency anemia is discussed in Chapter 33.)

Diagnostic Studies

Diagnosis of acute gastritis is most often based on a history of drug and alcohol use. The diagnosis of chronic gastritis may be delayed or completely missed because the symptoms are nonspecific. Endoscopic examination with biopsy is necessary to obtain a definitive diagnosis. Breath, urine, serum, or gastric tissue biopsy tests are available for the determination of *H. pylori*. These tests are described later in this chapter in the discussion of PUD. Radiological studies are not helpful because the superficial mucosa is generally involved, and changes will not show clearly on radiograph. A complete blood count (CBC) may demonstrate the presence of anemia from blood loss or lack of intrinsic factor.

Stools are tested for the presence of occult blood. A gastric analysis, although currently not used as much, demonstrates the amount of HCl present, with achlorhydria being a common sign of severe atrophic gastritis. Serum tests for antibodies to parietal cells and intrinsic factor may be performed. Tissue biopsy with cytological examination is necessary to rule out gastric carcinoma.

NURSING AND COLLABORATIVE MANAGEMENT: GASTRITIS

▮ Acute Gastritis

Eliminating the cause and preventing or avoiding it in the future are generally all that is needed to treat acute gastritis. The plan of care is supportive and similar to that described for nausea and vomiting. If vomiting accompanies acute gastritis, bed rest, NPO status, and IV fluids may be prescribed. Dehydration can occur rapidly in acute gastritis with vomiting. Fluids and electrolytes lost through vomiting and occasionally diarrhea are replaced. Antiemetics are given for nausea and vomiting (see Table 44-1). In severe cases of acute gastritis, an NG tube may be used, either for lavage of the precipitating agent from the stomach or in conjunction with suction to keep the stomach empty and free of noxious stimuli. Clear liquids are resumed when acute symptoms have subsided, with gradual reintroduction of solid, bland foods.

If hemorrhage is considered likely, frequent checking of vital signs and testing the vomitus for blood are indicated. All of the management strategies discussed in the section on upper GI bleeding also apply to the patient with severe gastritis.

Drug therapy is focused on reducing irritation of the gastric mucosa and providing symptomatic relief. Antacids are beneficial in the relief of abdominal discomfort by raising intragastric pH to above 6. H_2R blockers (e.g., ranitidine [Zantac]) or PPIs (e.g., omeprazole [Losec], lansoprazole [Prevacid]) may be used to reduce gastric HCl secretion. It is essential that the nurse have knowledge of the action and the therapeutic effects of PPIs and H_2R blockers to teach the patient and to monitor the effects of the drugs.

▮ Chronic Gastritis

The treatment of chronic gastritis focuses on evaluating and eliminating the specific cause (e.g., cessation of alcohol intake, abstinence from drugs, *H. pylori* eradication). Currently, antibiotic and antisecretory agent combinations are used to eradicate infection with *H. pylori* (Table 44-13). For the patient with pernicious anemia, regular injections of cobalamin are needed (see Chapter 33). Discussion of the continued need for this essential vitamin must be included in the plan of care.

The patient undergoing treatment for chronic gastritis may have to adapt to many lifestyle changes and adhere strictly to a drug regimen. A nonirritating diet consisting of six small feedings a day and the use of an antacid after meals may help provide symptomatic relief. Smoking is contraindicated in the presence of all forms of gastritis. An interdisciplinary team approach in which the physician, the nurse, the dietitian, and the pharmacist provide consistent information and support may increase the patient's success in making these alterations. Because the inci-

DRUG THERAPY

Table 44-13 *Helicobacter pylori* Infection

TREATMENT	DURATION	ERADICATION RATE
Triple-Drug Therapy (Recommended as First-Line Therapy)		
Proton pump inhibitor*	7-14 days	>70-85%
Amoxicillin		
Clarithromycin (Biaxin)		
Dual Therapy		
Proton pump inhibitor	7-10 days	>45-50%
Clarithromycin (Biaxin)		
Quadruple Therapy		
Proton pump inhibitor*	10-14 days	85%
Bismuth		
Tetracycline		
Metronidazole (Flagyl)		
For penicillin-allergic patients		
Proton pump inhibitor, clarithromycin, and metronidazole (Chey & Wong, 2007)	10-14 days	70-85%

*See Table 44-9.

dence of gastric cancer is higher in the patient who has a history of chronic gastritis, especially atrophic gastritis, close medical follow-up should be stressed.

Upper Gastrointestinal Bleeding

Upper GI bleeding represents a significant clinical and societal burden because of the associated morbidity, mortality, and financial implications (Kovacs & Jensen, 2008). Despite advances in critical care, hemodynamic monitoring, and endoscopy, there has been little change in the mortality rate for upper GI bleeding, which has remained approximately 6 to 10% for the past 50 years. This is owing in part to the greater incidence of upper GI bleeding in older adults, especially women, related to the use of NSAIDs.

Etiology and Pathophysiology

Although the most serious loss of blood from the upper GI tract is characterized by a sudden onset, insidious occult bleeding can also be a major problem. The severity of bleeding depends on whether the origin is venous, capillary, or arterial. (Types of upper GI bleeding are presented in Table 44-14.) Bleeding from an arterial source is profuse, and the blood is bright red. The bright red colour indicates that the blood has not been in contact with the stomach's acid secretions. In contrast, "coffee grounds" vomitus reveals that the blood and other contents have been in the stomach for some time and have been changed by contact with gastric secretions. A massive upper GI hemorrhage is generally defined as a loss of more than 1500 mL of blood or a loss of 25% of intravascular blood volume. *Melena* (black, tarry stools) indicates slow bleeding from an upper GI source. The longer the passage of blood through the intestines, the darker the colour of the stool as a result of the degradation of hemoglobin and the release of iron.

Table 44-14 Types of Upper Gastrointestinal Bleeding

TYPE	CLINICAL MANIFESTATIONS
Obvious bleeding	
Hematemesis	Bloody vomitus appearing as fresh, bright red blood or "coffee grounds" appearance (dark, grainy digested blood)
Melena	Black, tarry stools (often foul smelling) caused by digestion of blood in the GI tract; the black appearance is caused by the presence of iron
Occult bleeding	Small amounts of blood in gastric secretions, vomitus, or stools not apparent by appearance; detectable by guaiac test

GI, gastrointestinal.

Table 44-15 Common Causes of Upper Gastrointestinal Bleeding

Drug-Induced	Stomach and Duodenum
• Corticosteroids	• Gastric cancer
• Nonsteroidal anti-inflammatory drugs	• Hemorrhagic gastritis
• Salicylates	• Peptic ulcer disease
Esophagus	• Polyps
• Esophageal varices	• Stress ulcer
• Esophagitis	**Systemic Diseases**
• Mallory-Weiss tear	• Blood dyscrasias (e.g., leukemia, aplastic anemia)
	• Renal failure (uremia)
	• Liver failure (cirrhosis)

Discovering the cause of the bleeding is not always an easy task. A variety of areas in the GI tract may be involved, and there may be many different reasons for the blood loss. Table 44-15 lists the common causes of bleeding. Although systemic diseases (e.g., leukemia, blood dyscrasias) that interfere with normal blood clotting must be considered whenever upper GI bleeding occurs, the most common sites are the esophagus, stomach, and duodenum.

Esophageal Origin. Bleeding from an esophageal source is most likely the result of chronic esophagitis, bleeding from a tear in the mucosa near the esophagogastric junction (Mallory-Weiss tear), or esophageal varices. Chronic esophagitis can be caused by the ingestion of chemicals, including drugs irritating to the mucosa. Alcohol and smoking are known irritants of the esophageal mucosa. GERD with or without a hiatal hernia can lead to chronic irritation and erosion. A **Mallory-Weiss tear** is usually caused by severe retching and vomiting. This tear occurs in the esophageal mucosa at the junction of the esophagus and the stomach and results in severe bleeding.

Esophageal varices usually occur secondary to cirrhosis of the liver. Branches of the vena cava and the azygos vein from the systemic circulation converge with the smaller vessels of the lower esophagus. These vessels are inelastic and become engorged and tortuous because of increased pressure exerted on them secondary to portal hypertension. Anything that may increase the pressure (e.g., coughing, sneezing, trauma) or cause mechanical irritation (e.g., vomiting, irritation, erosion) may result in sudden, massive bleeding. (Esophageal varices are discussed in Chapter 46.)

Stomach and Duodenal Origin. Bleeding ulcers account for 50% of the cases of upper GI bleeding (Kovacs & Jensen, 2008). Erosion of a blood vessel by an ulcer located in the stomach or duodenum must always be considered as a possible cause of upper GI bleeding. A gastric ulcer may penetrate the left gastric artery, and a duodenal ulcer may penetrate the superior pancreaticoduodenal artery.

Acute gastritis produced by ingestion of drugs or alcohol or the reflux of bile from the small intestine can result in bleeding. Drugs, either prescribed by the health care provider or OTC, are a major cause of upper GI bleeding. For example, the patient who regularly takes aspirin or aspirin-containing compounds may be at risk for bleeding episodes. Aspirin, NSAIDs (e.g., ibuprofen), and corticosteroids can cause irritation and disruption of the gastric mucosal barrier. Aspirin-containing products are sold without prescriptions as OTC drugs. It is not unusual for a patient to deny the use of aspirin because of lack of awareness, yet be self-medicating with aspirin-containing drugs such as Alka-Seltzer, Bufferin, and Excedrin. A careful history of all commonly used drugs is therefore necessary whenever upper GI bleeding is suspected.

Stress-related mucosal disease (SRMD), also called *physiological stress ulcers*, occurs in patients who have sustained severe burns or trauma or had major surgery. In SRMD, there is erosion of more superficial blood vessels than with PUD (Figure 44-9). Mucosal injury is found in approximately 70 to 90% of patients in the critical care unit (Singh, Houy, Singh, & Sekhon, 2008). Less-common causes of upper GI bleeding include tumours and vascular lesions. Gastric cancer causes steady blood loss as it grows and ulcerates through the mucosa and blood vessels located in its path.

Emergency Assessment and Management

Approximately 80 to 85% of patients who have massive upper GI hemorrhage spontaneously stop bleeding; however, the cause must be identified and treatment initiated immediately. Although a complete history of events leading to the bleeding episode is important in discovering the cause of the blood loss, it should be deferred until emergency care has been initiated. The immediate physical examination must include a systematic evaluation of the patient's condition with emphasis on blood pressure, rate and character of pulse, peripheral perfusion with capillary refill, and observation for the presence or absence of neck vein distension. Vital signs should be monitored every 15 to 30 minutes. Signs and symptoms of shock must be evaluated, and treatment should be started as soon as possible if it occurs (see Chapter 69). The patient's respiratory status is carefully assessed, along with a thorough abdominal examination. The presence or absence of bowel sounds should be assessed and noted. A tense, rigid, boardlike abdomen may indicate a perforation and peritonitis.

Once the immediate interventions have begun, the patient or the family should answer the following questions. Is there a history of previous bleeding episodes? Has weight loss been a recent problem? Has the patient received blood transfusions in the past, and were there any transfusion reactions? Is there a religious preference that prohibits the use of blood or blood products? Are there any other illnesses that may contribute to bleeding or interfere with treatment (e.g., heart failure, diabetes mellitus)?

Laboratory studies are ordered, including a CBC, blood urea nitrogen (BUN), serum electrolytes, blood glucose, prothrombin time, liver enzymes, arterial blood gases, and a type and cross-match for possible blood transfusions. Vomitus and stools can be tested for the presence of gross and occult blood. A urinalysis

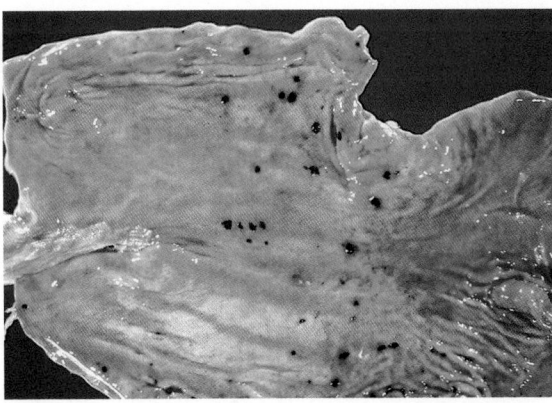

Figure 44-9 Multiple stress ulcers of the stomach, highlighted by dark digested blood on their surfaces.

Source: Kumar, V., Abbas, A. K., & Fausto, N. (2005). *Robbins and Cotran pathologic basis of disease* (7th ed.). Philadelphia: Saunders.

provides information on the presence of blood in the urine, and the specific gravity gives an immediate indication of the patient's hydration status.

Intravenous lines, preferably two, with a 16- or 18-gauge needle, should be established for fluid and blood replacement. The type and amount of fluids infused is dictated by physical and laboratory findings. It is generally best to begin with an isotonic crystalloid solution (e.g., lactated Ringer's solution). Whole blood, packed RBCs, and fresh-frozen plasma may be used for replacement of lost volume in massive hemorrhage. Because of the potential for fluid overload and immunological reactions, packed RBCs are often preferred over whole blood. (The use of blood transfusions and volume expanders is discussed in Chapter 33.) The hemoglobin and hematocrit values are not of immediate assistance in estimating the degree of blood loss, but they provide a baseline for guiding further treatment. The initial hematocrit may be normal and may not reflect the loss until 4 to 6 hours after fluid replacement has taken place because initially the loss of plasma and RBCs is equal. When upper GI bleeding is less profuse, infusion of isotonic saline solution followed by packed RBCs permits restoration of the hematocrit more quickly and does not create complications related to fluid volume overload. The use of supplemental oxygen may help increase blood oxygen saturation.

For most patients who are bleeding profusely, an indwelling urinary catheter is inserted so that urine volume can be accurately assessed every hour. A central venous pressure line may be inserted so that the patient's fluid volume status can be monitored easily. Empirical use of PPI therapy with high-dose bolus and subsequent infusion is often started before endoscopy.

Diagnostic Studies

Endoscopic procedures allow physicians to identify sources of GI bleeding through direct visualization. For example, a bleeding site from severe gastritis, an esophageal varix, a gastric or duodenal ulcer, or angiodysplasia can be easily determined and treated effectively. The endoscope is designed to facilitate the passing of various accessories, sclerosing drugs, and probes to control and stop GI bleeding. In addition to using endoscopic procedures to stop bleeding, these procedures also allow direct visualization of the bleeding site. Angiography is used in diagnosing upper GI bleeding only when endoscopy cannot be done. It is an invasive procedure requiring preparation and setup time and may not be appropriate for a patient at high risk whose condition is unstable. In this procedure, a catheter is placed into the left gastric or superior mesenteric artery and advanced until the site of bleeding is discovered.

Barium contrast studies are of little value in the identification of bleeding sites during the acute phase. After the acute bleeding phase, barium studies can document a lesion but cannot verify that it is the source of bleeding.

Collaborative Care

Endoscopic Therapy. The goal of endoscopic hemostasis is to identify and stop bleeding. This is done by removing clots that have formed to identify the bleeding site and to flush and prepare the area for treatment. Various methods based on physician preference and the types of GI bleeding are used to accomplish this. Endoscopy reduces the risk of surgical intervention.

Some causes of gastric bleeding are Mallory-Weiss tear, esophageal and gastric varices, bleeding ulcers and polyps, and angiodysplasia. Several methods are used to arrest the bleeding. Sclerosing needles are passed thought the endoscope, and medications, such as epinephrine (1 : 10,000 dilution) or Histoacryl (glue), are injected to stop bleeding. Endoclips are also passed through the endoscope. These clips can successfully clamp off the bleeding area. Multipolar and bipolar electrocoagulation probes can also be used endoscopically; the heat of the probe coagulates the tissue directly on the bleeding site. Overall, endoscopic therapy is more effective than medical management alone in reducing bleeding episodes.

Surgical Therapy. Surgical intervention is indicated when bleeding continues regardless of the therapy provided and when the site of the bleeding has been identified. A high percentage of patients are known to have another massive hemorrhage within 5 years after the first bleeding episode. The site of the hemorrhage determines the choice of operation. In addition, the surgeon must consider the age of the patient because mortality rates increase considerably when the patient is older than 60 years.

Drug Therapy. During the acute phase, drugs are used to decrease bleeding, decrease HCl secretion, and neutralize the HCl that is present. Drug therapy to decrease bleeding is administered during endoscopy. Injection therapy with absolute alcohol (ethanol) or epinephrine (1 : 10,000 dilution) is effective for acute hemostasis. These agents produce tissue edema and, ultimately, pressure on the source of bleeding. To prevent rebleeding, injection therapy is often combined with other therapies (e.g., thermocoagulation or laser treatment). A sclerosant (an agent that produces inflammation and results in fibrosis of the tissues) such as ethanolamine may be used, especially if the cause of bleeding is esophageal varices.

For variceal bleeding, vasopressin, which is posterior pituitary extract, can be used to produce vasoconstriction. It is used to treat upper GI bleeding in those patients who do not respond to other therapies and are poor surgical risks. It is administered systemically through a vein or intra-arterially at the local site of actual bleeding. Adverse effects of intravenously administered vasopressin include decreased myocardial contractility and decreased coronary blood flow. The patient undergoing vasopressin therapy must be closely monitored for its myocardial, visceral, and peripheral ischemic adverse effects. Vasopressin should be used with caution in the patient with a known history of vascular disease.

Efforts are made to reduce acid secretion because the acidic environment can alter platelet function as well as interfere with

DRUG THERAPY

Table 44-16 Gastrointestinal Bleeding

DRUG	SOURCE OF GI BLEEDING	MECHANISM OF ACTION
Antacids*	Duodenal ulcer, gastric ulcer, acute gastritis (corrosive, erosive, and hemorrhagic)	Neutralize acid and maintain gastric pH >5.5; elevated pH inhibits activation of pepsinogen
H$_2$-receptor blockers: cimetidine, famotidine (Pepcid), nizatidine (Axid), ranitidine (Zantac)	Duodenal ulcer, gastric ulcer, esophagitis, acute gastritis (especially hemorrhagic)	Inhibit action of histamine at H$_2$ receptors on parietal cells and decrease HCl secretion
Proton pump inhibitors: omeprazole (Losec), esomeprazole (Nexium), lansoprazole (Prevacid), pantoprazole (Pantoloc)		Inhibit the cellular pump, which is necessary for secretion of HCl
Vasopressin	Acute gastritis (corrosive, erosive, and hemorrhagic), esophageal varices	Causes vasoconstriction and increases smooth muscle activity of the GI tract; reduces pressure in the portal circulation and arrests bleeding
Octreotide (Sandostatin)	Upper gastrointestinal bleeding, esophageal varices	Somatostatin analogue that decreases splanchnic blood flow; decreases HCl secretion via decrease in release of gastrin

GI, gastrointestinal; *HCl*, hydrochloric acid.
*See Table 44-21.

clot stabilization. H$_2$R blockers (e.g., ranitidine [Zantac]) or PPIs (e.g., pantoprazole [Pantoloc]) are administered intravenously to decrease acid secretion. Table 44-16 reviews the mechanism of action of H$_2$R blockers and PPIs. Although these drugs have no proven ability to control active bleeding, they have become part of standard treatment protocols.

In patients with upper GI bleeding, early administration of the somatostatin analogue octreotide (Sandostatin) may be used. The drug reduces splanchnic blood flow as well as acid secretion. This drug is given in IV boluses up to 5 to 6 days after the initiation of bleeding.

Antacids have long been known to neutralize HCl and continue to be used as an adjunct therapy for PUD. Because antacids neutralize HCl and increase the pH of gastric contents to above 5, there is inhibition of the conversion of pepsinogen to its active form, pepsin. The most frequently used antacid preparations are magnesium hydroxide, magnesium trisilicate, aluminum hydroxide, calcium carbonate, and sodium bicarbonate (see Table 44-21 later in this chapter). Aluminum hydroxide and magnesium trisilicate are the most useful because they are nonabsorbable. Calcium carbonate and sodium bicarbonate are absorbable, and prolonged use can lead to systemic alkalosis.

Sedatives to control agitation and restlessness should be administered cautiously. They make accurate assessment of the patient's condition more difficult. Anticholinergic drugs are contraindicated for use in acute upper GI bleeding episodes.

NURSING MANAGEMENT: UPPER GASTROINTESTINAL BLEEDING

▪ Nursing Assessment

As the nurse begins care of the patient admitted with upper GI bleeding, a thorough and accurate nursing assessment is an essential first step. Subjective and objective data that should be obtained from the patient or significant others are presented in Table 44-17.

The patient experiencing upper GI bleeding may not be able to provide specific information about the cause of the bleeding

until the immediate physical needs are met. An immediate nursing assessment is performed while getting the patient ready for initial treatment. The assessment includes the patient's level of consciousness, vital signs, appearance of neck veins and skin colour, and capillary refill. The abdomen is checked for distension, guarding, and peristalsis. Immediate determination of vital signs indicates whether the patient is in shock from blood loss and also provides a baseline blood pressure and pulse by which to monitor the progress of treatment. Signs and symptoms of hypovolemic shock include low blood pressure; rapid, weak pulse; increased thirst; cold, clammy skin; and restlessness. Vital signs are monitored every 15 to 30 minutes, and the health care provider should be informed of any significant changes.

When obtaining vital signs, the nurse considers the patient's age and physical condition. Taking the blood pressure and pulse with the patient lying down and then sitting will indicate postural changes that occur after acute blood loss.

▪ Nursing Diagnoses

Nursing diagnoses for the patient with upper GI bleeding include, but are not limited to, the following:

- Deficient fluid volume *related to* acute loss of blood, as well as gastric secretions
- Ineffective peripheral tissue perfusion *related to* loss of circulatory volume
- Anxiety *related to* upper GI bleeding, hospitalization, uncertain outcome, source of bleeding
- Ineffective coping *related to* situational crisis and personal vulnerability
- Risk of aspiration *related to* active bleeding and altered level of consciousness
- Decreased cardiac output *related to* loss of blood

▪ Planning

The overall goals are that the patient with upper GI bleeding will (1) have no further GI bleeding, (2) have the cause of the bleeding identified and treated, (3) experience a return to a normal

NURSING ASSESSMENT

Table 44-17 Upper Gastrointestinal Bleeding

Subjective Data

Important Health Information

Past health history: Precipitating events before bleeding episode, previous bleeding episodes and treatment, peptic ulcer disease, esophageal varices, esophagitis, acute and chronic gastritis, stress-related mucosal disease; family history of bleeding; history of smoking or heavy alcohol use

Medications: Use of aspirin, nonsteroidal anti-inflammatory drugs, corticosteroids, anticoagulants

Symptoms

- Nausea, vomiting, weight loss; thirst
- Diarrhea; black, tarry stools; decreased urinary output; sweating
- Weakness, dizziness, fainting
- Epigastric pain, abdominal cramps

Objective Data

General

Fever

Integumentary

Clammy, cool, pale skin; pale mucous membranes, nail beds, and conjunctivae; spider angiomas; jaundice; peripheral edema

Respiratory

Rapid, shallow respirations

Cardiovascular

Tachycardia, weak pulse, orthostatic hypotension, slow capillary refill

Gastrointestinal

Red or "coffee grounds" vomitus; tense, rigid abdomen, ascites; hypoactive or hyperactive bowel sounds; black, tarry stools

Urinary

Decreased urinary output, concentrated urine

Neurological

Agitation, restlessness; decreasing level of consciousness

Possible Findings

↓ Hematocrit and hemoglobin; hematuria; guaiac-positive stools, emesis, or gastric aspirate; ↓ levels of clotting factors; ↑ liver enzymes; abnormal upper GI studies or endoscopy results

GI, gastrointestinal.

hemodynamic state, (4) experience minimal or no symptoms of pain or anxiety, and (5) be able to verbalize causative and preventive measures.

Nursing Implementation

Health Promotion

Although not all cases of upper GI bleeding can be anticipated and prevented, the nurse shares responsibility with the health care provider in trying to identify the patient who is at high risk. The patient with a history of chronic gastritis or PUD should always be considered in the high-risk category because of the increased incidence of bleeding associated with chronic irritation

or chronic ulcers. The patient who has had one major bleeding episode is more likely to have another. The patient is instructed to avoid gastric irritants such as alcohol and smoking, to prevent or decrease stress-inducing situations at home or at work, and to take only prescribed medications. OTC drugs can be harmful because they may contain ingredients (e.g., aspirin) that have potentially irritating effects on the mucosa.

The patient who requires regular administration of ulcerogenic drugs, such as aspirin, corticosteroids, or NSAIDs, needs instruction regarding the potential adverse effects that these agents may have on the GI mucosa. These drugs are avoided if at all possible. However, if aspirin must be prescribed, enteric-coated tablets can be substituted for regular tablets. Taking the drugs with meals or snacks lessens the potential irritating effects. For patients who must take NSAIDs, a change to a preparation with less GI toxicity may be considered. COX-2 inhibitors (e.g., celecoxib [Celebrex]) have less of an effect on the production of tissue prostaglandins and are associated with fewer GI adverse effects, although ongoing caution persists regarding cardiac risks associated with COX-2 inhibitors. The co-administration of an NSAID with a PPI can reduce bleeding risk. For the patient at risk for gastric ulcers because of NSAID use, misoprostol may also be prescribed. This prostaglandin analogue inhibits acid secretion and reduces upper GI bleeding episodes associated with NSAID use. However, the drug has several important adverse effects, including uterine cramping in women and diarrhea. Because of its effects on the uterus, its use is contraindicated in women of child-bearing age.

When the nurse is working with the patient who has a history of liver cirrhosis with esophageal varices, the instructions must be specific regarding the importance of avoiding known irritants, such as alcohol and smoking. The prompt treatment of an upper respiratory tract infection should be stressed. Severe coughing or sneezing can create increased pressure on the already fragile varices and may result in massive hemorrhage.

The patient who is known to have blood dyscrasias (e.g., aplastic anemia) or liver dysfunction or who is taking cancer chemotherapeutic drugs has a potential bleeding problem because of altered hemostasis caused by a decrease in clotting factors and platelets. When these patients also have a history of ulcer disease, gastritis, varices, or drug and alcohol abuse, they should be carefully instructed regarding their disease process and drugs, and they should be closely observed for bleeding.

Acute Intervention

The patient should be approached in a calm and assured manner to help decrease the level of anxiety. Caution should be used before administering sedatives for restlessness because it is one of the warning signs of shock and may be masked by the drugs.

Once an infusion has been started, the IV line must be maintained for fluid or blood replacement. An accurate intake and output record is essential so that the patient's hydration status can be assessed. Urine output should be measured hourly. A rate of at least 0.5 mL/kg/hr indicates adequate renal perfusion. Lesser amounts may indicate renal insufficiency secondary to loss of blood volume. Specific gravity readings consistently greater than 1.030 (normal is 1.005-1.030) indicate that the urine is extremely concentrated and that there is probably a low blood volume. The health care provider must be kept informed of these important parameters so that the IV solutions can be increased or decreased accordingly. If the patient has a central venous pressure line in place, readings should be recorded every 1 to 2 hours.

Hemodynamic monitoring provides an accurate and quick assessment of blood flow and pressure within the cardiovascular system (see Chapter 68).

The older adult or the patient with a history of cardiovascular problems should be observed closely for signs of fluid overload. However, the threat of volume overload and pulmonary edema must be a constant concern in all patients who are receiving large amounts of IV fluids within a short time. Therefore, auscultation of breath sounds and close observation of respiratory effort are important. Electrocardiographic monitoring can also be used to evaluate cardiac function.

Foods such as beets or even swallowed mouthwash can give vomitus a bloody appearance. Unless the contents of the vomitus are checked for occult blood, recorded observations gleaned from appearance alone may be false. Swallowed blood from a nosebleed must also be accurately noted to avoid misdiagnosis of an upper GI bleeding episode. When an NG tube is inserted, the nurse must pay special attention to keeping it in proper position and observing the aspirate for blood.

The nurse caring for a patient with upper GI bleeding should be well informed as to what constitutes blood in the stools. Black, tarry stools are not usually associated with a brisk hemorrhage but are indicative of the presence of bleeding of prolonged duration. Bright red blood in the stool is usually from a source in the lower bowel. (Lower GI bleeding is discussed in Chapter 45.) Menses and bleeding hemorrhoids should be ruled out as possible sources of blood in the stools. When vomitus contains blood but the stool contains no gross or occult blood, the hemorrhage is considered to have been of short duration.

Monitoring the patient's laboratory studies enables the nurse to estimate the effectiveness of therapy. The hemoglobin and hematocrit are usually evaluated about every 4 to 6 hours if the patient is actively bleeding. At first, the hematocrit level may not accurately reflect the amount of blood lost or the amount of blood replaced and will appear falsely high or low. The patient's BUN level is assessed. It is generally elevated with a significant hemorrhage because blood proteins are broken down by GI tract bacteria. However, renal disease may also result in an elevated BUN level. Many patients receive oxygen by mask or nasally to ensure that the circulating blood has an adequate oxygen content.

When oral nourishment is begun, the patient is observed for symptoms of nausea and vomiting and a recurrence of bleeding. Feedings initially consist of clear fluids or milk and are given hourly until tolerance is determined. These feedings help neutralize the gastric secretions and assist in the mucosal repair. Gradual introduction of foods follows if the patient exhibits no signs of discomfort. Consultation with a dietitian will ensure the introduction of appropriate foods and support the patient's nutrition.

The patient in whom hemorrhage was the result of chronic alcohol abuse requires close observation for the beginning of delirium tremens as withdrawal from alcohol takes place. Symptoms indicating the beginning of delirium tremens are agitation, uncontrolled shaking, sweating, and vivid hallucinations. (Alcohol withdrawal is discussed in Chapter 11.)

■ Ambulatory and Home Care

The patient and caregiver must be taught how to avoid future bleeding episodes. Ulcer disease, drug or alcohol abuse, and liver and respiratory diseases can all result in upper GI bleeding. The patient and caregiver must be made aware of the consequences of nonadherence to diet and drug therapy. It must be emphasized that no drugs (especially aspirin and NSAIDs) other than those prescribed by the health care provider should be taken. With the assistance of smoking or alcohol cessation or rehabilitation programs, smoking and alcohol should be eliminated because they are sources of irritation and interfere with tissue repair. The need for long-term follow-up care may be necessary because of the possibility of another bleeding episode. The patient and the family should be instructed on what to do if an acute hemorrhage occurs in the future.

■ Evaluation

The following are expected outcomes for the patient with upper GI bleeding:
- The patient will have no upper GI bleeding.
- The patient will maintain normal fluid volume.
- The patient will experience a return to a normal hemodynamic state.
- The patient will experience absence of or tolerable levels of pain and will be comfortable.
- The patient will understand potential etiological factors and make appropriate lifestyle modifications.

Peptic Ulcer Disease

Peptic ulcer disease is a condition characterized by erosion of the GI mucosa resulting from the digestive action of HCl and pepsin. Any portion of the GI tract that comes into contact with gastric secretions is susceptible to ulcer development, including the lower esophagus, stomach, duodenum, and margin of gastrojejunal anastomosis after surgical procedures.

Types

Peptic ulcers can be classified as acute or chronic, depending on the degree and duration of mucosal involvement (Figure 44-10), and gastric or duodenal, according to the location. The acute ulcer (see Figure 44-10) is associated with superficial erosion and minimal inflammation. It is of short duration and resolves

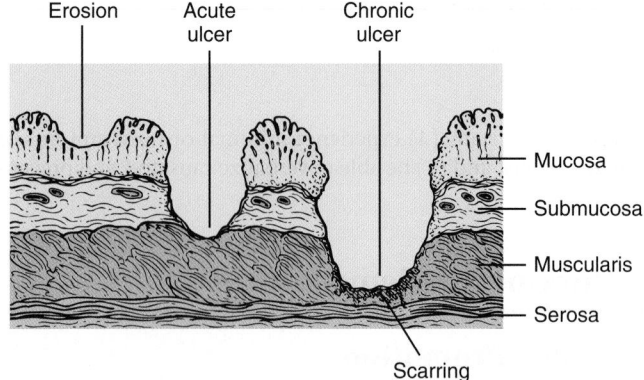

Figure 44-10 Peptic ulcers, including an erosion, an acute ulcer, and a chronic ulcer. Both the acute and the chronic ulcers may penetrate the entire wall of the stomach.

Source: Redrawn from Price, S. A., & Wilson, L. M. (2003). *Pathophysiology: Clinical concepts of disease processes* (6th ed., p. 331, Figure 24-4). St. Louis: Mosby.

quickly when the cause is identified and removed. A chronic ulcer (Figure 44-11) is one of long duration, eroding through the muscular wall with the formation of fibrous tissue. It is present continuously for many months or intermittently throughout the person's lifetime. A chronic ulcer is at least four times as common as acute erosion.

Gastric and duodenal ulcers, although defined as peptic ulcers, are different in their etiology and incidence (Table 44-18). Generally, the treatment of all types of ulcers is quite similar.

Etiology and Pathophysiology

Peptic ulcers develop only in the presence of an acid environment. The typical person with a gastric ulcer has normal to less-than-normal gastric acidity compared with the person with a

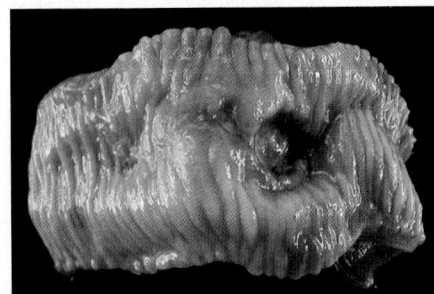

Figure 44-11 Peptic ulcer of the duodenum.

Source: Kumar, V., Abbas, A. K., & Fausto, N. (2005). *Robbins and Cotran pathologic basis of disease* (7th ed.). Philadelphia: Saunders.

duodenal ulcer. However, some intraluminal acid does seem to be essential for a gastric ulcer to occur.

Pepsinogen, the precursor of pepsin, is activated to pepsin in the presence of HCl and a pH of 2 to 3. The secretion of HCl by the parietal cells has a pH of 0.8. After mixing with the stomach contents, the pH reaches 2 to 3, a highly favourable range of acidity for pepsin activity. When the stomach acid level is neutralized by the presence of food or antacids, or acid secretion is blocked by drugs, the pH is increased to 3.5 or more. At a pH of 3.5 or more, pepsin has little or no proteolytic activity.

The stomach is normally protected from autodigestion by the gastric mucosal barrier. The GI tract has a high rate of cell turnover, and the surface mucosa of the stomach is renewed about every 3 days. As a result of this high turnover rate, the mucosa can continually repair itself except in extreme instances, when the cell breakdown surpasses the cell renewal rate. Normally, water, electrolytes, and water-soluble substances (e.g., glucose) can easily pass through the barrier. However, the mucosal barrier prevents the back-diffusion of acid from the gastric lumen through the mucosal layers to the underlying tissue.

Under specific circumstances, the mucosal barrier can be impaired, and back-diffusion of acid can occur (Figure 44-12). When the barrier is broken, HCl freely enters the mucosa and injury to the tissues occurs. This results in cellular destruction and inflammation. Histamine is released from the damaged mucosa, resulting in vasodilation and increased capillary permeability. The released histamine is then capable of stimulating further secretion of acid and pepsin.

As described in the section on gastritis, a variety of agents are known to destroy the mucosal barrier. By generating ammonia in the mucous layer, *H. pylori* may create a condition of chronic

Table 44-18 Comparison of Gastric and Duodenal Ulcers

	GASTRIC ULCERS	DUODENAL ULCERS
Lesion	Superficial; smooth margins; round, oval, or cone shaped	Penetrating (associated with deformity of duodenal bulb from healing of recurrent ulcers)
Location of lesion	Predominantly in the antrum, also in body and fundus of stomach	First 1-2 cm of duodenum
Gastric secretion	Normal to decreased	Increased
Incidence	• Greater in women • Peak age 50-60 yr • More common in persons of lower socioeconomic status and in unskilled labourers • Increased with smoking, drug, and alcohol use • Increased with incompetent pyloric sphincter and bile reflux • Increased with stress ulcers after severe burns, head trauma, and major surgery	• Greater in men, but increasing in women, especially postmenopausal • Peak age 35-45 yr • Associated with psychological stress • Increased with smoking, drug, and alcohol use • Associated with other diseases (e.g., chronic obstructive pulmonary disease, pancreatic disease, hyperparathyroidism, Zollinger-Ellison syndrome, chronic renal failure) • Burning, cramping, pressure-like pain across midepigastrium and upper abdomen; back pain with posterior ulcers
Clinical manifestations	• Burning or gaseous pressure in high left epigastrium and back and upper abdomen • Pain 1-2 hr after meals; if penetrating ulcer, aggravation of discomfort with food • Occasional nausea and vomiting, weight loss	• Pain 2-4 hr after meals and midmorning, midafternoon, middle of night; pain is periodic and episodic • Pain relief with antacids and food; occasional nausea and vomiting
Recurrence rate	High	High
Complications	Hemorrhage, perforation, outlet obstruction, intractability	Hemorrhage, perforation, obstruction

PATHOPHYSIOLOGY MAP

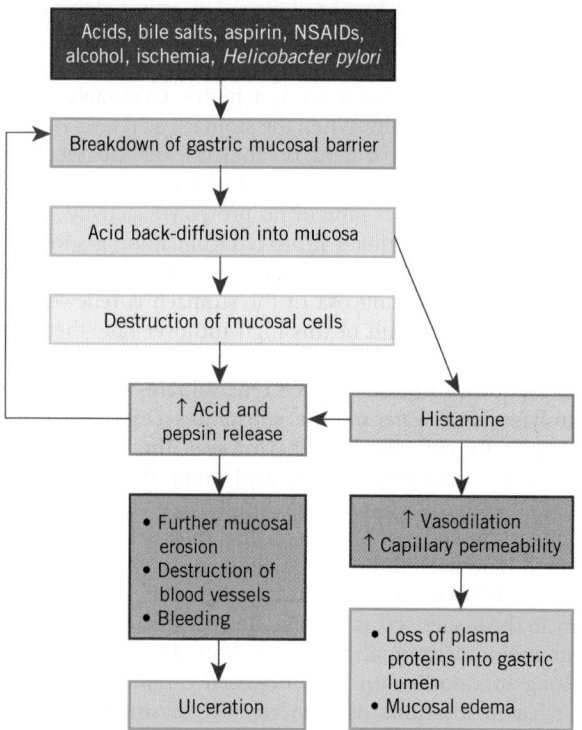

Figure 44-12 Disruption of gastric mucosa and pathophysiological consequences of back-diffusion of acids. *NSAIDs*, nonsteroidal anti-inflammatory drugs.

PATHOPHYSIOLOGY MAP

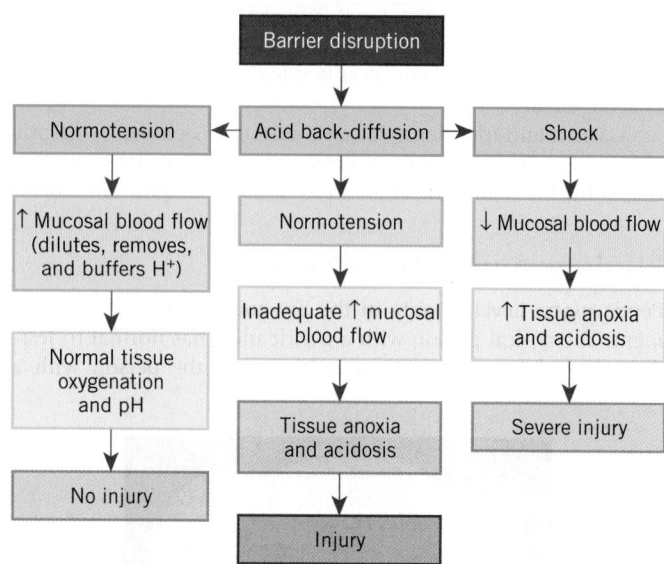

Figure 44-13 Relationship between mucosal blood flow and disruption of the gastric mucosal barrier.

inflammation, rendering the mucosa especially vulnerable to other noxious substances. Ulcerogenic drugs, such as aspirin and NSAIDs, inhibit synthesis of prostaglandins and cause abnormal permeability. Corticosteroids have the ability to decrease the rate of mucosal cell renewal and thereby decrease its protective effects. Lipid-soluble cytotoxic drugs can pass through the barrier and destroy it.

When the mucosal barrier is disrupted, there is a compensatory increase in blood flow (Figure 44-13). This phenomenon can occur in several ways. Prostaglandin-like substances and histamine act as vasodilators, thus increasing capillary blood flow. As blood flow increases within the affected mucosa, H^+ are rapidly removed from the area, buffers are delivered to help neutralize the H^+ present, nutrients necessary for cell function arrive, and the rate of mucosal cell replication increases. When the increase is sufficient to dilute, buffer, and remove the excess H^+, tissue damage may be minimal or may result in no injury at all. When blood flow is not sufficient to carry out these events, tissue injury results. Figure 44-13 shows a representation of the interrelationship between the mucosal blood flow and disruption of the gastric mucosal barrier.

Two mechanisms protect against damage. First, mucus is secreted by superficial mucous cells and forms a layer that can entrap or slow the diffusion of H^+ across the mucosal barrier in the stomach. Second, bicarbonate is secreted by the gastric and duodenal mucosa, and this helps neutralize HCl in the lumen of the GI tract.

Increased vagal nerve stimulation from a variety of causes (e.g., emotions) results in hypersecretion of HCl. Increased concentrations of HCl can alter the mucosal barrier. Duodenal ulcers

are associated with high acid content. It has been suggested that the continual response of the parietal cells to maximal stimulation results in hyperplasia of the cells.

Gastric Ulcers. Although gastric ulcers can occur in any portion of the stomach, they are most commonly found on the lesser curvature in close proximity to the antral junction. Gastric ulcers are less common than duodenal ulcers. Gastric ulcers are more prevalent in women and in older adults. The mortality rate from gastric ulcers is greater than that from duodenal ulcers because the peak incidence of gastric ulcers occurs in persons older than 50 years. Persons from the lower socioeconomic class and manual or unskilled workers are more prone to gastric ulcers.

Although gastric ulcers are characterized by a normal to low secretion of gastric acid, the back-diffusion of acid is greater with chronic gastric ulcers than with duodenal ulcers or in the healthy person. Therefore, the critical pathological process in gastric ulcer formation may not be the amount of acid that is secreted but the amount that is able to penetrate the mucosal barrier.

Gastric ulcers have also been attributed to various factors that can lead to acute episodes or to chronic involvement. The role of *H. pylori* in ulcer development is discussed under duodenal ulcers. It is thought that destruction of the gastric mucosa by noxious agents such as drugs or smoking may be enhanced by the presence of *H. pylori,* which further promotes gastric mucosal destruction.

Drugs can cause acute gastric ulcers and, in some cases, can lead to the development of chronic ulcers. The drugs most often implicated include aspirin, corticosteroids, NSAIDs (e.g., ibuprofen), and reserpine (Serpasil) (not commercially available in Canada). It is estimated that 1 to 3% of patients taking NSAIDs for 1 year experience serious GI complications, including gastritis, gastric ulcer, upper GI hemorrhage, or perforation. Other known causative factors of gastric ulcer formation are chronic alcohol abuse, chronic gastritis, and bile reflux gastritis from an incompetent pyloric sphincter. Cigarette smoking is positively linked with gastric ulcers. Nicotine seems to enhance reflux of duodenal contents into the antrum of the stomach. The ingestion of hot, rough, or spicy foods has been suggested as a causative factor, but there is no evidence to substantiate this claim.

Duodenal Ulcers. Duodenal ulcers account for about 80% of all peptic ulcers. Although duodenal ulcers still affect more men than women, the incidence of duodenal ulcers has followed a downward trend in men and a steady increase in women. The explanation for this change has not been clearly identified. Duodenal ulcers may occur at any age, but the incidence is especially high between the ages of 35 and 45 years. Duodenal ulcers can develop in anyone, regardless of occupation or socioeconomic group.

The development of duodenal ulcers is associated with a high HCl secretion. Several diseases have been identified with a high risk of duodenal ulcer development, including chronic obstructive pulmonary disease, cirrhosis of the liver, chronic pancreatitis, hyperparathyroidism, chronic renal failure, and Zollinger-Ellison syndrome. (*Zollinger-Ellison syndrome* is a rare condition characterized by severe peptic ulceration, gastric acid hypersecretion, elevated serum gastrin levels, and gastrinoma of the pancreas or the duodenum.) It is possible that the treatments used for these conditions may also promote ulcer development. Alcohol ingestion and heavy smoking habits are also associated with duodenal ulcer formation because both are known stimulants of acid secretion.

Although many factors are thought to contribute to the formation of duodenal ulcers, *H. pylori* has been identified as playing a key role. *H. pylori* is found in approximately 90 to 95% of patients with duodenal ulcers. However, a clear-cut direct causal relationship between *H. pylori* and duodenal ulcer formation has not yet been proved. Not all individuals with evidence of *H. pylori* go on to develop ulcers, suggesting that additional factors are needed to produce these conditions. *H. pylori* survives in the human upper GI tract for a long time as a result of its ability to move in mucus and attach to mucosal cells. In addition, it secretes a substance called urease, which buffers the area around the bacterium and protects it from destruction in an acidic environment.

Infection with *H. pylori* is highest in underdeveloped countries and in persons of low socioeconomic status. Although the routes of transmission are largely unknown, it is thought that infection occurs during childhood via transmission from family members to the child, possibly through a fecal–oral route, an oral–oral route, or both. In Canada and the United States, persons born before 1940 have a significantly higher risk of carrying *H. pylori* than those in younger age groups. This enhanced prevalence in older persons has been attributed to the presence of crowded living conditions and poor sanitation practices, which were more common in the first half of the last century.

Research into a genetic cause for ulcers has shown that some members of the same family are more prone to develop gastric or duodenal ulcers. Supporting a genetic etiology is the fact that persons with blood group O have an increased incidence of duodenal ulcers. Evidence is not complete, however, and the ulcer development could just as well be the result of sharing the same environment.

Physiological Stress Ulcers. Physiological stress ulcers are acute ulcers that develop following a major physiological insult such as trauma or surgery. A physiological stress ulcer is a form of erosive gastritis. It is believed that the gastric mucosa of the body of the stomach undergoes a period of transient ischemia in association with hypotension, severe injury, extensive burns, and complicated surgery. The ischemia is caused by decreased capillary blood flow or shunting of blood away from the GI tract so that blood flow bypasses the gastric mucosa. This occurs as a compensatory mechanism in hypotension or shock. The decrease in blood flow produces an imbalance between the destructive properties of HCl and pepsin and the protective factors of the stomach's mucosal barrier, especially in the fundic portion, resulting in ulceration. Multiple superficial erosions result, and these may bleed. Risk factors for development of stress ulcer bleeding are respiratory failure and coagulopathy. These patients should receive prophylaxis with antisecretory agents. The diagnosis of stress gastritis is made with endoscopy, and treatment is with aggressive reduction of gastric acid secretions using H_2R blockers or PPIs.

Clinical Manifestations

It is common for the person with gastric or duodenal ulcers to have no pain or other symptoms. The gastric and duodenal mucosas are not rich in sensory pain fibres, which may account for this phenomenon. When pain does occur with duodenal ulcer, it is described as "burning" or "cramplike." It is most often located in the midepigastric region beneath the xiphoid process. The pain associated with gastric ulcers is located high in the epigastrium and occurs spontaneously about 1 to 2 hours after meals. The pain is described as "burning" or "gaseous." The pain can occur when the stomach is empty or when food has been ingested. If the ulcer has eroded through the gastric mucosa, food tends to aggravate rather than alleviate the pain. Some persons do not experience any pain until the presence of the ulcer is demonstrated through a serious complication such as hemorrhage or perforation.

Ulcers located on the posterior aspect of the duodenum can be manifested by back pain. The pain usually occurs 2 to 4 hours after meals. It is relieved by antacids alone or in combination with an H_2R blocker or PPI and sometimes by foods that neutralize and dilute the HCl. A characteristic of duodenal ulcer is its tendency to occur continuously for a few weeks or months and then disappear for a time, only to recur some months later. Some patients claim their symptoms worsen in the spring and the fall of the year, thus strengthening the concept of a seasonal trend in occurrence.

Complications

The three major complications of chronic PUD are hemorrhage, perforation, and gastric outlet obstruction. All are considered emergency situations and are initially treated conservatively. However, surgery may become necessary at any time during the course of the therapy.

Hemorrhage. Hemorrhage is the most common complication of PUD. It develops from erosion of the granulation tissue found at the base of the ulcer during healing or from erosion of the ulcer through a major blood vessel. Duodenal ulcers account for a greater percentage of upper GI bleeding episodes than gastric ulcers.

Perforation. Perforation is considered the most lethal complication of peptic ulcer. Perforation is commonly seen in large penetrating duodenal ulcers that have not healed and are located on the posterior mucosal wall (Figure 44-14). Perforated gastric ulcers are most often located on the lesser curvature of the

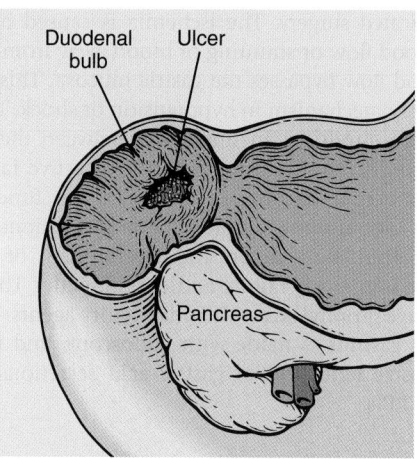

Figure 44-14 Duodenal ulcer of the posterior wall penetrating into the head of the pancreas, resulting in walled-off perforation.

Source: Redrawn from Price, S. A., & Wilson, L. M. (2003). *Pathophysiology: Clinical concepts of disease processes* (6th ed., p. 335, Figure 24-8). St. Louis: Mosby.

stomach. Even though duodenal ulcers are more prevalent and perforate more frequently, mortality rates associated with perforation of gastric ulcers are higher.

Perforation of a peptic ulcer occurs when the ulcer penetrates the serosal surface, with spillage of either gastric or duodenal contents into the peritoneal cavity. The size of the perforation is directly proportional to the length of time the patient has had the ulcer. The larger the perforation, the longer the history of the ulcer. Small perforations seal themselves and result in a cessation of symptoms; larger perforations require immediate surgical closure. Spontaneous sealing occurs as a result of large amounts of fibrin being produced in response to the perforation. This leads to fibrinous fusion of the duodenum or the gastric curvature to adjacent tissue, mainly the liver.

The clinical manifestations of perforation are characterized by their sudden and dramatic onset. The patient experiences sudden, severe upper abdominal pain that quickly spreads throughout the abdomen. The visceral and parietal layers of the peritoneum have an abundance of pain receptors, and this contributes to the abrupt, intense pain experienced. There may be shoulder pain if the spillage causes irritation to the phrenic nerve. The abdominal muscles contract, appearing rigid and boardlike as they attempt to protect the abdomen from further injury. The patient's respirations become shallow and rapid. Bowel sounds are usually absent. Nausea and vomiting may occur but are generally absent. Many patients report a history of ulcer disease or recent symptoms of indigestion.

The contents entering the peritoneal cavity from the stomach or the duodenum contain a variety of ingredients that include air, saliva, food particles, HCl, pepsin, bacteria, bile, and pancreatic fluid and enzymes. Bacterial peritonitis may occur within 6 to 12 hours. The intensity of the peritonitis is proportional to the amount and the duration of the spillage through the perforation. It is difficult to determine from the sudden onset of symptoms whether gastric or duodenal ulcer is the cause because the clinical characteristics of intestinal perforation are the same (see Chapter 45).

Gastric Outlet Obstruction. Ulcers located in the antrum and the prepyloric and pyloric areas of the stomach and the duodenum can predispose to gastric outlet obstruction. In the early phase of obstruction (often referred to as the *compensated phase*), gastric emptying is normal to near normal. Over time, increased contractile force needed to empty the stomach results in hypertrophy of the stomach wall. After longstanding obstruction, the stomach enters the decompensated phase, which results in dilation and atony. The obstruction is not totally the result of fibrous scar tissue because active ulcer formation is associated with edema, inflammation, and pylorospasm, all of which contribute to the narrowing of the pylorus.

The patient with gastric outlet obstruction generally has a long history of ulcer pain. Ulcer-like pain of short duration or complete absence of pain is more indicative of a malignant obstruction. The pain progresses to a more generalized upper abdominal discomfort that becomes worse toward the end of the day as the stomach fills and dilates. Relief may be obtained by belching or by self-induced vomiting. Vomiting is common and often projectile. The vomitus contains food particles that were ingested many hours or even a day or two before the vomiting episode. There is often an offensive odour if the contents have been dormant in the stomach for a time. The patient who vomits frequently will be anorectic, with evident weight loss, and will complain of thirst and an unpleasant taste in the mouth.

The patient with gastric outlet obstruction may show a swelling in the upper abdomen indicating dilation of the stomach. Loud peristalsis can be heard, and visible peristaltic waves are often observed passing across the abdomen from left to right. If the stomach is grossly dilated, it is possible to palpate it as well.

Diagnostic Studies

The diagnostic measures used to determine the presence and location of a peptic ulcer are similar to those used for acute upper GI bleeding. Endoscopy is the procedure most often used. It is more reliable than barium contrast studies because of the manoeuvrability of fibreoptic scopes for viewing the entire gastric and duodenal mucosa. This procedure can also be used to determine the degree of ulcer healing after treatment. During endoscopy, tissue specimens can be obtained for identification of *H. pylori* and to rule out gastric cancer.

Currently, several diagnostic tests are available to confirm *H. pylori* infection. These are classified as noninvasive and invasive. *Noninvasive tests* include serum or whole blood antibody tests, in particular, immunoglobulin G (IgG). This test is approximately 90 to 95% sensitive for *H. pylori* infection. However, because of the length of time that IgG levels remain elevated in the blood after the infection, the serological tests will not distinguish active from recently treated disease. The urea breath test can determine the presence of active infection. Urea is a by-product of the metabolism of *H. pylori* bacteria. *Invasive tests* involve biopsy of the stomach and include the rapid urease test as well as other histological markers of infection. These tests have greater sensitivity and specificity but involve an endoscopic procedure.

Barium contrast studies, although widely used, are not accurate in identifying shallow, superficial ulcers because of failure of the barium to properly fill the ulcer crater. Radiographic studies are also ineffective in differentiating a peptic ulcer from a malignant tumour. In addition, radiographs images do not as readily demonstrate the degree of healing that can be visually determined with the endoscope. Barium studies are of benefit in the diagnosis of gastric outlet obstruction. Barium normally should pass from the stomach within 2 hours, but with gastric outlet obstruction, 50% of the barium remains on follow-up films up to 6 hours later.

Gastric analysis has questionable value in the diagnosis of PUD because, in many patients, gastric secretions are normal in amount and composition. However, it can provide important data in (1) identifying a possible gastrinoma (Zollinger-Ellison syndrome), (2) determining the degree of gastric hyperacidity, and (3) evaluating the results of therapy such as vagotomy and antisecretory drug therapy. Gastric analysis procedure is described in Chapter 41.

Laboratory analyses, including a CBC, urinalysis, liver enzyme studies, serum amylase determination, and stool examination, should be performed. A CBC may indicate the presence of anemia secondary to bleeding from the ulcer. Liver enzyme studies help determine any liver problems, such as cirrhosis, that may complicate the treatment of the ulcer. Urine and stool are routinely tested for the presence of blood. A serum amylase determination is frequently ordered to provide information on pancreatic function in patients in whom posterior penetration of the pancreas is suspected.

Collaborative Care: Conservative Therapy

When the patient's clinical manifestations and health history suggest the diagnosis of PUD and diagnostic studies confirm it, a medical regimen is instituted (Table 44-19). The regimen consists of adequate rest, dietary modifications, drug therapy, elimination of smoking, and long-term follow-up care. The aim of the treatment program is to decrease the degree of gastric acidity, enhance mucosal defence mechanisms, and minimize the harmful effects on the mucosa.

Patients are generally treated in ambulatory care clinics. The healing of a peptic ulcer requires many weeks of therapy. Pain disappears after 3 to 6 days, but ulcer healing is much slower. Complete healing may take 3 to 9 weeks, depending on ulcer size and the treatment regimen employed. Healing of the ulcer should be assessed by means of radiographic or endoscopic examination. Barium contrast films provide a rough estimate of the degree of ulcer healing. However, it should be noted that endoscopic examination is the only accurate method by which to monitor ulcer healing.

Adequate rest, both physical and emotional, is important in the treatment process. A quiet, calm environment at home or on the job is not easy to achieve and may require some modifications in the patient's daily routine. The elimination or reduction of stressors helps decrease the stimulus for overproduction of HCl. Moderation in daily activity is essential.

When aspirin or nonselective NSAIDs must be continued, enteric-coated preparations or co-administration with a PPI or misoprostol should be considered.

Smoking has an irritating effect on the mucosa, increases gastric motility, and delays mucosal healing. It should be eliminated completely or severely reduced. The combination of adequate rest and abstinence from smoking accelerates ulcer healing.

Drug Therapy.
Drugs are a vital part of therapy. The patient must be well informed about each drug prescribed, why it is ordered, and the expected benefits. Strict adherence to the prescribed regimen of drugs is important. Drug therapy includes the use of antacids, H₂R blockers, PPIs, antibiotics, anticholinergics, and cytoprotective therapy (Tables 44-20 through 44-22).

Because recurrence of peptic ulcer is frequent, interruption or discontinuation of therapy can have detrimental results. The patient must be encouraged to comply with therapy and continue with follow-up care for at least 1 year. If changes in lifestyle are

COLLABORATIVE CARE

Table 44-19 Peptic Ulcer Disease

Diagnostic	Acute Exacerbation Without Complications
• History and physical examination	• NPO
• Upper GI endoscopy with biopsy	• Adequate rest
• *Helicobacter pylori* testing of breath, urine, blood, tissue	• Cessation of smoking
• Upper GI barium contrast study	• IV fluid replacement
• Complete blood count	• Drug therapy
• Urinalysis	• H₂-receptor blockers
• Liver enzymes	• Proton pump inhibitors
• Serum electrolytes	• Antacids
	• Anticholinergics
	• Sedatives

Collaborative Therapy Conservative Therapy	Acute Exacerbation With Complications (Hemorrhage, Perforation, Obstruction)
• Adequate rest	• NPO
• Bland diet (six small meals a day)	• NG suction
• Cessation of smoking	• Bed rest
• Drug therapy	• IV fluid replacement (lactated Ringer's solution)
• H₂-receptor blockers (see Table 44-20)	• Blood transfusions
• Proton pump inhibitors (see Table 44-20)	• Stomach lavage (possible)
• Antibiotics for *H. pylori* (see Table 44-13)	**Surgical Therapy**
• Antacids (see Table 44-21)	• Perforation—simple closure with omentum graft
• Anticholinergics	• Gastric outlet obstruction—pyloroplasty and vagotomy
• Cytoprotective drugs	• Ulcer removal or reduction
• Stress reduction	• Billroth I and II procedures
	• Vagotomy and pyloroplasty

GI, gastrointestinal; *IV*, intravenous; *NG*, nasogastric; *NPO*, nothing by mouth.

part of the prescribed therapy, they should be maintained. Antacids, H₂R blockers, and PPIs may be stopped after the ulcer has healed or may be prescribed in the form of low-dose maintenance therapy. No other drugs, unless prescribed by the health care provider, should be taken because they may have an ulcerogenic effect. Finally, the patient and the family should be told what to do in the event that pain and discomfort recur or blood is noted in the vomitus or stools.

Histamine-2 Receptor Blockers. H₂R blockers—ranitidine (Zantac), famotidine (Pepcid), and nizatidine (Axid)—are frequently used in the management of PUD. These drugs block the action of histamine on the H₂Rs and thus reduce HCl secretion. This decreases the conversion of pepsinogen to pepsin and accelerates ulcer healing. (Antihistamine drugs used to treat allergies are H₁R blockers and have no effect on gastric acid secretion.)

H₂R blocker drugs may be administered orally or intravenously; however, only ranitidine (Zantac) is available in an IV form. Depending on the specific drug, therapeutic effects last up to 12 hours. However, the onset of action (i.e., symptom relief)

DRUG THERAPY

Table 44-20 Peptic Ulcer Disease

Antisecretory	Cytoprotective
• H₂-receptor blockers	• Sucralfate bismuth subsalicylate (Pepto-Bismol)
• Ranitidine (Zantac)	**Neutralizing**
• Famotidine (Pepcid)	• Antacids*
• Nizatidine (Axid)	**Antibiotics for Helicobacter pylori**
• Proton pump inhibitors	• Amoxicillin
• Omeprazole (Losec)	• Metronidazole (Flagyl)
• Lansoprazole (Prevacid)	• Tetracycline
• Esomeprazole (Nexium)	• Clarithromycin (Biaxin)
• Pantoprazole (Pantoloc)	**Others**
• Dexlansoprazole (Dexilant)	• Tricyclic antidepressants
• Anticholinergics	• Imipramine
Antisecretory and Cytoprotective	• Doxepin (Sinequan)
• Misoprostol	

*See Table 44-21.

DRUG THERAPY

Table 44-21 Antacid Preparations

INGREDIENT	TRADE NAME
Single substance	
Aluminum carbonate	Basaljel
Aluminum hydroxide gel tablets	Amphojel
Aluminum phosphate	Phosphaljel
Calcium carbonate	Alka-2, Tums
Dihydroxyaluminum sodium carbonate	Rolaids
Magaldrate	Riopan
Magnesium hydroxide	Milk of magnesia
Sodium bicarbonate	Alka-Seltzer
Mixtures of aluminum hydroxide and magnesium salts	Gaviscon, Maalox/Diovol

DRUG THERAPY

Table 44-22 Adverse Effects of Antacid Therapy

ANTACID	REACTIONS
Aluminum hydroxide gels	Constipation, phosphorus depletion with chronic use
Calcium carbonate	Constipation or diarrhea, hypercalcemia, milk-alkali syndrome, renal calculi
Magnesium preparations	Diarrhea, hypermagnesemia
Sodium preparations	Milk–alkali syndrome if used with large amounts of calcium; used with caution in patients on sodium restrictions

is longer than that of antacids. H₂R blockers have demonstrated capabilities in the healing of gastric and duodenal ulcers. Famotidine, ranitidine, and nizatidine have longer half-lives than cimetidine, thus necessitating fewer doses and providing nocturnal HCl suppression. More adverse effects are associated with cimetidine. These include granulocytopenia, gynecomastia, diarrhea, fatigue, dizziness, rash, and in the older adult, mental confusion.

However, the rate of these adverse effects is low. Famotidine and nizatidine are considered more potent at reduced dosage levels than cimetidine, and adverse effects are minimal. OTC forms of H₂R blockers are currently available. H₂Rs are used in combination with antibiotics to treat ulcers related to *H. pylori*.

Proton Pump Inhibitors. PPIs, such as omeprazole (Losec), lansoprazole (Prevacid), pantoprazole (Pantoloc), esomeprazole (Nexium), and dexlanprazole (Dexilant), block the adenosine triphosphatase enzyme that is important for the secretion of HCl. These agents are more effective than H₂R blockers in reducing gastric acid secretion and promoting ulcer healing. PPIs are also used in combination with antibiotics to treat ulcers caused by *H. pylori*.

Antibiotic Therapy. Antibiotics are prescribed to eradicate *H. pylori* infection. The treatment of *H. pylori* is the most important element of treating ulcer disease in patients positive for *H. pylori*. When *H. pylori* is present, ulcer recurrence rates with H₂R blockers alone can be as high as 75 to 90%, whereas with antibiotic treatment, the recurrence rate may be less than 10%. Antibiotic therapy for *H. pylori* is shown in Table 44-13.

Once the presence of *H. pylori* has been determined, antibiotic treatment is instituted. The regimen of choice is based on the antibiotic susceptibility of the *H. pylori* organism, allergies, patient adherence, adverse effects, and costs. Most drug regimens involve treatment for 7 to 14 days (Bago et al., 2011). No single agents have been effective in eliminating *H. pylori* (see Table 44-13). Bismuth subsalicylate (Pepto-Bismol) is used as part of one therapy to facilitate healing. Bismuth is nonabsorbable and causes black stools.

Antacids. Antacids are used as adjunct therapy for PUD. They increase gastric pH by neutralizing the acid. As a result, the acid content of chyme reaching the duodenum is reduced. In addition, some antacids, such as aluminum hydroxide, can bind to bile salts, thus decreasing the detrimental effects of bile on the gastric mucosa. Patients who are vulnerable for physiological stress ulcer formation may be treated prophylactically with antacids along with an antisecretory agent.

Antacids consist of systemic and nonsystemic types. *Systemic antacids*, such as sodium bicarbonate, are extremely soluble and are absorbed into the circulation. Their long-term use can lead to systemic alkalosis; therefore, they are rarely used in ulcer treatment. The *nonsystemic antacids* are insoluble and poorly absorbed. The common commercial nonsystemic antacids consist of magnesium hydroxide or aluminum hydroxide as single preparations or in various combinations (see Table 44-21).

The antacid preparation may be in liquid or tablet form. A large number of tablets may be required to equal the same dose of a liquid preparation. Because the tablets are chewable, some of the drug is left coating the teeth and the gingivae instead of the stomach.

The neutralizing effects of antacids taken on an empty stomach last only 20 to 30 minutes because they are quickly evacuated. When antacids are taken after meals, the effects may last as long as 3 to 4 hours. Therapy regimens calling for frequent administration (e.g., hourly) often result in poor adherence.

The type and dosage of the antacid prescribed depends on adverse effects (see Table 44-22) as well as potential drug interactions. Preparations high in sodium should be used with caution in older adults and in the patient with liver cirrhosis, hypertension, heart failure, or renal disease. Magnesium preparations should not be prescribed for the patient with renal failure because of the risk of magnesium toxicity. The most frequent adverse effect experienced with magnesium antacids is diarrhea. Aluminum hydroxide causes constipation. An antacid combination of aluminum and magnesium salts seems to lessen the adverse effects of both.

Antacids have the capacity to interact unfavourably with some drugs. They can enhance the absorption of drugs such as dicumarol and amphetamines. The action of digitalis preparations can be potentiated when taken in combination with calcium or magnesium antacids. In some instances, antacids may decrease the absorption rates of prescribed drugs, such as tetracycline. Therefore, it is important to inform the health care provider of any drugs that are being taken before antacid therapy is begun.

Anticholinergic Drugs. Anticholinergic drugs are only occasionally ordered in the treatment of PUD. These drugs decrease cholinergic (vagal) stimulation of HCl secretion. Opinion is divided concerning their efficacy in preventing recurrences and their therapeutic effectiveness in alleviating symptoms and preventing complications. Because of their tendency to decrease gastric motility, they should not be used for gastric ulcers in which stasis of secretions increases the patient's pain and discomfort. Anticholinergics are associated with a number of adverse effects, such as dry mouth and skin, flushing, thirst, tachycardia, dilated pupils, blurred vision, and urine retention. Anticholinergics must be prescribed with caution in the patient with narrow-angle glaucoma, benign prostatic hyperplasia, and gastric outlet obstruction.

Cytoprotective Drug Therapy. Sucralfate is used for the short-term treatment of ulcers. It has proved to be cytoprotective of the esophagus, the stomach, and the duodenum. Its ability to accelerate ulcer healing is thought to be a result of the formation of an ulcer-adherent complex covering the ulcer and thereby protecting it from erosion caused by pepsin, acid, and bile salts. Sucralfate does not have acid-neutralizing capabilities. Its action is most effective at a low pH, and it should be given at least 30 minutes before or after an antacid. Adverse effects are minimal. However, it does bind with digoxin, warfarin (Coumadin), phenytoin (Dilantin), and tetracycline, causing reduced bioavailability of these drugs.

Misoprostol is a synthetic prostaglandin analogue. It has protective and some antisecretory effects on gastric mucosa. It is used for the prevention of gastric ulcers induced by NSAIDs and aspirin. A major advantage of misoprostol is that it does not interfere with the therapeutic effects of aspirin and NSAIDs. Persons who require chronic NSAID therapy, such as those with osteoarthritis, may benefit from the use of misoprostol. All NSAIDs, even COX-2 inhibitors, impair ulcer healing.

Other Drugs. Tricyclic antidepressants (e.g., imipramine, doxepin [Sinequan]) and serotonin reuptake inhibitors may be prescribed for patients with ulcer disease. Antidepressants may contribute to overall pain relief through their effects on afferent pain fibre transmission. In addition, tricyclic antidepressants have, to varying degrees, some anticholinergic properties, which result in reduced acid secretion.

Nutritional Therapy. Dietary modifications may be necessary so that foods and beverages irritating to the patient can be avoided or eliminated. A nonirritating or bland diet consisting of six small meals a day may be recommended for the patient during the symptomatic phase. However, there is considerable contro-

versy over the actual therapeutic benefits derived from a bland diet because the rationale is not supported by scientific evidence. Each patient should be instructed to eat and drink foods and fluids that do not cause any distressing symptoms. Alcohol and caffeine-containing products should be eliminated because of their irritating effects.

Dietary instructions should include a sample diet with a list of foods that usually cause distress and should, therefore, be eliminated from the diet. Foods known to irritate the gastric mucosa include hot, spicy foods and pepper, alcohol, carbonated beverages, tea, coffee, and broth (meat extract). These foods also have limited buffering ability in addition to stimulating gastric acid secretion. Foods high in roughage, such as raw fruit, salads, and vegetables, may irritate an inflamed mucosa. If these foods are well chewed, this seems to be less of a problem.

Protein is considered the best neutralizing food, but it also stimulates gastric secretions. Carbohydrates and fats are the least stimulating to HCl secretion, but they do not neutralize well. The patient must determine a suitable combination of these essential nutrients that does not cause undue distress.

Historically, milk was an essential part of ulcer therapy until it was learned that milk proteins and calcium stimulate gastric acid production. For this reason, milk as part of diet therapy for ulcers was out of favour for a time. However, milk is again used as part of the diet plan because it can neutralize gastric acidity and contains prostaglandins and growth factors, both of which may protect the GI mucosa from injury.

Therapy Related to Complications of Peptic Ulcer Disease

Acute Exacerbation. The patient with an acute exacerbation of peptic ulcer can usually be treated with the same regimen used for conservative therapy. However, the situation is considered more serious because of the possible complications of perforation, hemorrhage, and gastric outlet obstruction.

Bleeding, increased pain and discomfort, and nausea and vomiting frequently accompany an acute exacerbation. If the patient experiences recurrent vomiting or gastric outlet obstruction, an NG tube may be placed into the stomach with intermittent suction for about 24 to 48 hours.

If there is a history of an incompetent pyloric sphincter allowing reflux of duodenal contents into the stomach, an NG tube will remove intestinal contents from the stomach. This period of stomach rest eliminates any causative factors that may have precipitated the acute exacerbation and permits the resolution of edema and inflammation of the mucosa. Fluids and electrolytes are replaced by IV infusion until the patient is able to tolerate oral feedings without distress.

Management is similar to that described for upper GI bleeding. Blood or blood products may be administered. Careful monitoring of the vital signs, intake and output, laboratory studies, and signs of impending shock is important during this acute episode.

Endoscopic evaluation is performed to reveal the degree of inflammation or bleeding as well as the ulcer location. It is important to ascertain the presence of a prepyloric or pyloric ulcer that can cause gastric outlet obstruction. When endoscopic examination reveals no major problems and the patient's physical condition stabilizes, the plan of care for the patient should follow the same regimen of diet, activity, and drugs used in conservative therapy. A 5-year follow-up program is recommended after acute exacerbation. An increase in the healing rate is achieved after conservative treatment, but the treatment plan cannot prevent the scar formation that can result in gastric outlet obstruction.

Perforation. The immediate focus of management of a patient with a perforation is to stop the spillage of gastric or duodenal contents into the peritoneal cavity and restore blood volume. An NG tube is inserted into the stomach to provide continuous aspiration and gastric decompression to halt spillage through the perforation. Although duodenal aspiration is not achieved as promptly, placement of the tube as near to the perforation site as possible facilitates decompression.

Circulating blood volume must be replaced with lactated Ringer's and albumin solutions. These solutions substitute for the fluids lost from the vascular and interstitial space as the peritonitis develops. Blood replacement in the form of packed RBCs may be necessary. Unless contraindicated, a central venous pressure·line and an indwelling urinary catheter should be inserted and monitored hourly. Broad-spectrum antibiotic therapy should be started immediately to treat bacterial peritonitis. Administration of pain medications provides comfort.

The operative procedure involving the least risk to the patient is simple oversewing of the perforation and reinforcement of the area with a graft of omentum. The excess gastric contents are suctioned from the peritoneal cavity during the surgical procedure. There is controversy regarding the need for more definitive surgical treatment of a perforated ulcer than can be achieved with simple closure. Other types of surgical procedures depend on the location of the peptic ulcer and the surgeon's preference. If cure of the ulcer is the ultimate goal, the surgical procedures may include gastric resection or vagotomy and pyloroplasty.

Gastric Outlet Obstruction. The aim of therapy for obstruction is to decompress the stomach, correct any existing fluid and electrolyte imbalances, and improve the patient's general state of health. An NG tube is inserted into the stomach and attached to continuous suction to remove excess fluids and undigested food particles. With continuous decompression for several days, the stomach has the opportunity to regain its normal muscle tone, the ulcer can begin healing, and the inflammation and edema will subside.

The tube is clamped after several days of suction, and gastric residue is measured periodically. The frequency and amount of time the tube remains clamped are proportional to the amount of aspirate obtained and the comfort level of the patient. A method commonly followed is to clamp the tube overnight for approximately 8 to 12 hours and to measure the gastric residue in the morning. When the aspirate falls below 200 mL, it is considered to be within a normal range, and the patient can begin oral intake of clear liquids. Initially, oral fluids are begun at 30 mL/hr and then gradually increased in amount. The patient must be watched carefully for signs of distress or vomiting. As the amount of gastric residue decreases, solid foods are added and the tube is removed.

IV fluids and electrolytes are administered according to the degree of dehydration, vomiting, and electrolyte imbalance indicated by laboratory studies. Pain relief results from the decompression measures, and analgesics are usually not necessary. Antacids and antisecretory drug therapy (i.e., H_2R blockers, PPIs) are an integral part of treatment if the obstruction has been determined on endoscopic examination to be the result of an active ulcer. Pyloric obstruction may be treated nonsurgically by balloon dilations performed through the endoscope. Surgical intervention may be necessary to remove scar tissue.

NURSING MANAGEMENT: PEPTIC ULCER DISEASE

Nursing Assessment

Subjective and objective data that should be obtained from a patient with PUD are presented in Table 44-23.

Nursing Diagnoses

Nursing diagnoses related to PUD may include, but are not limited to, those presented in NCP 44-2.

Planning

Overall goals are that the patient with PUD will (1) comply with the prescribed therapeutic regimen, (2) experience a reduction or absence of discomfort related to PUD, (3) exhibit no signs of GI complications related to the ulcerative process, (4) have complete healing of the peptic ulcer, and (5) make appropriate lifestyle changes to prevent recurrence.

NURSING ASSESSMENT

Table 44-23 Peptic Ulcer Disease

Subjective Data

Important Health Information

Current health history: Chronic alcohol abuse, smoking, caffeine use

Past health history: Chronic kidney disease, pancreatic disease, chronic obstructive pulmonary disease, serious illness or trauma, hyperparathyroidism, cirrhosis of the liver, Zollinger-Ellison syndrome; family history of peptic ulcer disease

Medications: Use of aspirin, corticosteroids, nonsteroidal anti-inflammatory drugs

Surgery or other treatments: Complicated or prolonged surgery

Symptoms

- Weight loss, anorexia; nausea and vomiting, hematemesis; dyspepsia, heartburn, belching
- Black, tarry stools
- Burning, midepigastric or back pain occurring 2-4 hr after meals and relieved by food (duodenal ulcers), nocturnal pain common; high epigastric pain occurring 1-2 hr after meals (gastric ulcers), pain may be precipitated or aggravated by food

Objective Data

General

Anxiety, irritability

Gastrointestinal

Epigastric tenderness

Possible Findings

Anemia; guaiac-positive stools; positive blood, urine, breath, or stool tests for *Helicobacter pylori*; abnormalities revealed by upper gastrointestinal endoscopic and barium studies

Nursing Implementation

Health Promotion

Nurses must be involved in identifying patients at risk for ulcer development. Early detection and treatment of ulcers are important aspects of reducing morbidity associated with ulcers. Patients who are taking ulcerogenic drugs such as aspirin and NSAIDs are at risk for ulcer development. Patients need to be encouraged to take these drugs with food or milk. Patients should be taught to report symptoms related to gastric irritation, including epigastric pain, to their health care provider.

Acute Intervention

During the acute exacerbation of an ulcer, the patient generally complains of increased pain and nausea and vomiting, and some may have evidence of bleeding. Initially, many patients attempt to cope with the symptoms at home before seeking medical assistance.

During this acute phase, the patient may be maintained on NPO status for a few days, have an NG tube inserted and connected to intermittent suction, and have fluids replaced intravenously. The rationale for this therapy must be conveyed to the anxious patient and caregiver. They must understand that the

NURSING CARE PLAN 44-2

Peptic Ulcer Disease

Conservative Management

NURSING DIAGNOSIS	**Acute pain** related to increased gastric secretions, decreased mucosal protection, and ingestion of gastric irritants as evidenced by burning, cramplike pain in epigastrium and abdomen; pain onset 1-2 hr after meals with gastric ulcer; pain onset 2-4 hr after meals (midmorning, midafternoon) and middle of night with duodenal ulcer
Expected Patient Outcomes	**Nursing Interventions and Rationales**
• Verbalizes satisfaction with pain control	• Determine pain characteristics from verbal description and physical assessment data so that appropriate interventions can be planned.
	• Administer antacids, H$_2$-receptor blockers, proton pump inhibitors, anticholinergics, and cytoprotective agents as ordered to reduce pain.
	• Teach patient to avoid smoking and ingesting spicy, hot, or cold foods, coffee, tea, and cola drinks, and alcoholic beverages to prevent irritation and increasing acid production.
	• Teach patient stress reduction because relaxation results in decreased acid production and reduction in pain.
NURSING DIAGNOSIS	**Ineffective self-health management** related to lack of knowledge of long-term management of peptic ulcer disease and consequences of not following treatment plan and unwillingness to modify lifestyle as evidenced by frequent questions about home care, incorrect responses to questions about peptic ulcer disease, nonadherence with medical regimen
Expected Patient Outcomes	**Nursing Interventions and Rationales**
• Verbalizes plan to modify lifestyle and incorporate therapeutic regimen into lifestyle	• Explain peptic ulcer disease process at patient's level to foster understanding.
	• Help patient identify stressors and initiate modifications in daily routine because stress causes hypersecretion of HCl and pepsin, which can alter the mucosal barrier.
	• Discuss diet plan and assist with implementation at home and in work setting.
	• Explain rationale for the elimination of alcohol, spicy foods, coffee, tea, and colas from diet; explain the harmful effects of smoking because these agents increase acid production and directly irritate gastric mucosa.
	• Provide information on actions and adverse effects of drug therapy to ensure safe self-administration.
	• Inform patient what to do if symptoms related to ulcers recur to ensure early initiation of treatment.

Exacerbation Management

NURSING DIAGNOSIS	**Acute pain** related to exacerbation of disease process and inadequate comfort measures as evidenced by verbalization of increase in pain, nonverbal indicators of pain (e.g., moaning, crying, doubling up)
Expected Patient Outcomes	**Nursing Interventions and Rationales**
• Expresses satisfaction with pain management	• Encourage bed rest or light activity to conserve energy and promote comfort.
	• Provide quiet, relaxed environment and limit visitors to decrease stress and other factors that increase acid secretion.
	• Administer medications as ordered to relieve pain.

Continued

NURSING CARE PLAN 44-2

Peptic Ulcer Disease—cont'd

Collaborative Problem

POTENTIAL COMPLICATION	**Nausea** related to acute exacerbation of disease process as evidenced by episodes of nausea and/or vomiting (see NCP 44-1)
POTENTIAL COMPLICATION	**Hemorrhage** secondary to eroded mucosal tissue

Nursing Goals	Nursing Interventions and *Rationales*
• Monitor for signs of hemorrhage • Carry out medical and nursing interventions if hemorrhage occurs	• Assess for evidence of hematemesis, bright red or melena stool, abdominal pain or discomfort, symptoms of shock (e.g., decreased blood pressure; cool, clammy skin; dyspnea; tachycardia; decreased urine output) *to plan appropriate interventions.* • If ulcer is actively bleeding, observe NG tube aspirate or emesis for amount and colour *to assess degree of bleeding.* • Take vital signs q15-30min *to determine patient's hemodynamic status and as indicators of shock.* • Maintain IV infusion line *to provide ready access for blood and fluid replacement.* • If RBC transfusion is given, observe for transfusion reaction *so that appropriate actions can be taken immediately.* • Monitor hematocrit and hemoglobin as indicators of severity of hemorrhage and need for fluid and blood replacement. • Record intake and output *to monitor fluid balance.* • Reassure patient and caregiver *to decrease their anxiety.* • Remain calm and confident in plan of care *to foster calm and confidence in patient and caregiver.* • Prepare patient for possible endoscopy or surgery.

POTENTIAL COMPLICATION	**Perforation of GI mucosa** secondary to impaired mucosal tissue integrity

Nursing Goals	Nursing Interventions and *Rationales*
• Monitor for signs of perforation • Carry out appropriate medical and nursing interventions	• Observe for manifestations of perforation (e.g., sudden, severe abdominal pain; rigid, boardlike abdomen; radiating pain to shoulders; increasing distension; decreasing bowel sounds) *to ensure early recognition and intervention.* • Take vital signs q15-30 min *to determine patient's hemodynamic status and as indicators of shock.* • Maintain NG tube to suction to provide continuous aspiration and gastric decompression *to prevent further leakage of gastric fluid through the perforation.* • Administer pain medication *to promote comfort and reduce anxiety.* • Prepare patient for emergency diagnostic tests and possible surgery *to foster timely intervention.*

GI, gastrointestinal; *HCl,* hydrochloric acid; *IV,* intravenous; *NG,* nasogastric; *RBC,* red blood cell.

advantages far outweigh any temporary discomfort imposed by the presence of the tube. Regular mouth care alleviates the dry mouth. Cleansing and lubrication of the nares facilitates breathing and decreases soreness. When the stomach is kept empty of gastric secretions, the ulcer pain diminishes and ulcer healing begins. Usually, this form of intervention is effective.

Because the patient is on NPO status, IV fluids are ordered. The type and amount administered is directly related to the fluid lost, the manifestations exhibited by the patient, and the results of the hemoglobin, hematocrit, and electrolyte determinations. The nurse should be aware of any other current health problem that could be adversely affected by the type of fluid used or the rate of the infusion. Repeated monitoring of these parameters provides information on the hydration status and the effectiveness of treatment. Vital signs are initially taken at least hourly so that shock can be detected and treated.

Physical and emotional rest are conducive to ulcer healing. The patient's immediate environment should be quiet and restful. The use of a mild sedative or tranquilizer has beneficial effects when the patient is anxious and apprehensive. The nurse must use good judgement before sedating a person who is becoming increasingly restless. There is danger that the drug will mask the signs of shock secondary to upper GI bleeding.

If the patient's condition improves without progression of symptoms (e.g., increased pain, vomiting, and hemorrhage), the regimen outlined for conservative therapy is followed. However, complications such as hemorrhage, perforation, and obstruction can occur.

▮ **Hemorrhage.** Changes in the vital signs and an increase in the amount and redness of the aspirate often signal massive upper GI bleeding. When there is an increased amount of blood in the gastric contents, the patient's pain is often decreased because the blood helps to neutralize the acidic gastric contents. It is important to maintain the patency of the NG tube so that blood clots do not obstruct the tube. If the tube becomes blocked, the patient can develop abdominal distension. Similar interventions to those described for upper

GI bleeding in the section "Nursing Management: Upper Gastrointestinal Bleeding" on pp. 1136-1138 are used. The nurse must monitor the results of the hemoglobin and hematocrit determinations.

◼ **Perforation.** When there is sudden, severe abdominal pain unrelated in intensity and location to the pain that brought the patient to the hospital, the nurse must recognize the possibility of ulcer perforation. When any person with an ulcer, particularly a chronic duodenal ulcer, demonstrates these manifestations, perforation should be suspected and the health care provider notified immediately.

Perforation is indicated by a rigid, boardlike abdomen; severe generalized abdominal and shoulder pain; drawing up of the knees; and shallow, grunting respirations. The bowel sounds that may have been previously normal or hyperactive may diminish and become absent.

Vital signs are important parameters and should be promptly taken and recorded every 15 to 30 minutes. The nurse should temporarily stop all oral or NG drugs and feedings until the health care provider can be notified and a definitive diagnosis made. If perforation has taken place, anything taken internally can add to the spillage into the peritoneal cavity and increase discomfort. If IV fluids are being administered at the time of the perforation, the rate should be maintained or increased to replace the depleted plasma volume.

When perforation is confirmed, the nurse should ensure that any known patient allergies have been recorded on the chart. This is important because antibiotic therapy is usually started, and careful observation for allergic reactions must be made. When the perforation fails to seal spontaneously, surgical closure is necessary and is performed as soon as possible. There is often little time to prepare the patient and caregiver thoroughly for the surgical intervention, yet some instructions can be carried out while the immediate therapy is begun. If major reconstructive surgery is anticipated, the patient and caregiver may question the need when the problem is only a small hole.

◼ **Gastric Outlet Obstruction.** Gastric outlet obstruction can occur at any time and is most likely to occur in the patient whose ulcer is located close to the pylorus. Because the onset of symptoms is usually gradual, the condition is not generally as serious an emergency as hemorrhage or perforation. Relief of symptoms may be achieved by constant NG aspiration of stomach contents. This allows edema and inflammation to subside and then permits normal flow of gastric contents through the pylorus.

Obstruction can also occur during the treatment of an acute episode of peptic ulcer exacerbation. If these symptoms are experienced while the patient is still on NPO status, the patency of the NG tube should be questioned. Regular irrigation of the tube with a saline solution facilitates proper functioning. It may be helpful to reposition the patient from side to side so that the tube tip is not constantly lying against the mucosal surface.

When oral feedings have been resumed and symptoms of obstruction are observed, the health care provider should be promptly informed. Generally, all that is necessary to treat the problem is to resume gastric aspiration so that the edema and inflammation resulting from the acute episode have time to resolve. IV fluids with electrolyte replacement keep the patient hydrated during this period. The NG tube can be clamped, and gastric fluids can be aspirated to check for retention. It is important to maintain accurate intake and output records, especially of the gastric aspirate. The patient should be kept aware of why these

Table 44-24 Peptic Ulcer Disease

The following are teaching guidelines for the patient and caregiver:

1. Explain dietary modifications, including avoidance of foods that cause epigastric distress. This may include black pepper, spicy foods, and acidic foods. Small, frequent meals are better tolerated than large meals.

2. Explain the rationale for avoiding cigarettes. In addition to promoting ulcer development, smoking will delay ulcer healing.

3. Encourage the need to reduce or eliminate alcohol ingestion.

4. Explain the rationale for avoiding OTC drugs unless approved by the patient's health care provider. Many preparations contain ingredients, such as aspirin, that should not be taken unless approved by the health care provider. Check with the health care provider regarding the use of nonsteroidal anti-inflammatory drugs.

5. Explain the rationale for not interchanging brands of antacids and H$_2$-receptor blockers that can be purchased OTC without checking with the health care provider. Doing so can lead to harmful adverse effects.

6. Teach the need to take all medications as prescribed. This includes both antisecretory and antibiotic drugs. Failure to take medications as prescribed can result in relapse.

7. Explain the importance of reporting any of the following:
   • Increased nausea or vomiting
   • Increase in epigastric pain
   • Bloody emesis or tarry stools

8. Explain the relationship between symptoms and stress. Stress-reducing activities and relaxation strategies are encouraged.

9. Encourage patient and caregiver to share concerns about lifestyle changes and living with a chronic illness.

OTC, over-the-counter.

symptoms are being experienced. In some instances in which treatment is not successful, surgery may be performed after the acute phase has passed.

◼ **Ambulatory and Home Care.** The patient in whom PUD has been diagnosed has specific needs that must be met to prevent and avoid recurrence or complications. General instructions should cover aspects of the disease process itself, drugs, possible changes in lifestyle (including diet), and regular follow-up care. Table 44-24 provides a patient and caregiver teaching guide for the patient with PUD.

Knowing the cause of the ulcer and understanding the disease process may motivate the patient to become more involved in care and increase adherence with therapy. The patient must understand the dietary modifications and why they are important for recovery and health maintenance. The nurse and the dietitian should elicit a dietary history from the patient and plan for ways that dietary modifications can be easily incorporated into the patient's home and work setting. The patient who is following a diet prescribed for another illness needs to know how to balance the two so that neither condition is harmed by dietary interventions.

The patient does not always give the health care provider accurate information regarding habitual use of alcohol or cigarettes. The nurse should provide useful information about the detrimental effects of alcohol and cigarettes on ulcer disease and ulcer healing and provide resources on cessation and rehabilitation programs.

The nurse should teach the patient about prescribed drugs, including their actions, adverse effects, and inherent dangers if omitted for any reason. The patient should know why OTC drugs (e.g., aspirin) should not be taken unless approved by the health care provider. Because antacids and some H$_2$R blockers may be bought without a prescription, the patient must be informed that interchanging brands without checking with the health care provider or nurse can lead to harmful adverse effects.

Efforts should be made to obtain more information about the patient's psychosocial status. Knowledge of lifestyle, occupation, and coping behaviours can be helpful to the plan of care. The patient may be reluctant to talk about personal subjects, the stress experienced at home or on the job, the usual methods of coping, or dependence on drugs or alcohol. Unfortunately, the patient often does not see the relationship between lifestyle or occupation and ulcer disease. It is important to listen for subtle clues from the patient's statements and to observe for behaviours that broaden the database of what is known about the patient.

The need for long-term follow-up care must be stressed. Because successful treatment is frequently followed by a recurrence of the ulcer disease, the patient should be encouraged to seek immediate intervention if symptoms of the disease come back. The patient who has recurrence of ulcer disease following initial healing must learn to live with a disease that is chronic. The patient may be angry and frustrated, especially if the prescribed mode of therapy has been faithfully followed yet has failed to prevent the recurrence or extension of the disease process.

Unfortunately, many patients do not comply with the plan of care originally designed, and they experience repeated exacerbations. Patients quickly learn that they often experience no discomfort when they omit prescribed drugs or indulge in occasional dietary indiscretions. Consequently, they make no or little alteration in lifestyle. After an acute exacerbation, the patient is often more amenable to following the plan of care and open to suggestions for changes in lifestyle. Changes, such as smoking cessation and alcohol abstinence, are difficult for many people, and the idea of making them may be met with resistance. The patient may fare better from a reduction in his or her use of these substances rather than from total elimination. Although alcohol and smoking are known to interfere with ulcer healing, they frequently serve as coping mechanisms. From the patient's point of view, the distress caused by their total elimination may outweigh the benefits to be gained from abstention. The goal, however, should always be total cessation. A patient with chronic ulcers must be aware of the complications that may result from the disease, the clinical manifestations indicating their presence, and what to do until the health care provider can be seen.

■ Evaluation

Expected outcomes for the patient with PUD are addressed in NCP 44-2.

Collaborative Therapy: Surgical Therapy for Peptic Ulcer Disease

Fewer than 20% of patients with ulcers need surgical intervention. Because there is a high recurrence rate for both duodenal and gastric ulcers and complications increase with the duration of the ulcer, many health care providers believe that surgery is

necessary after therapy has been tried and has proved unsuccessful. The following criteria are used as general indications for surgical intervention:

- Intractability: failure of the ulcer to heal or recurrence of the ulcer after therapy
- History of hemorrhage or increased risk of bleeding during treatment
- Prepyloric or pyloric ulcers (both have high recurrence rates)
- Concurrent condition, such as severe burns, trauma, or sepsis
- Multiple ulcer sites
- Drug-induced ulcers, especially when withdrawal from the drug may put the person at risk
- Possible existence of a malignant ulcer
- Obstruction

A variety of surgical procedures are used to treat ulcer disease. They usually involve a partial gastrectomy, vagotomy, or pyloroplasty. Partial gastrectomy with removal of the distal two thirds of the stomach and anastomosis of the gastric stump to the duodenum is called a *gastroduodenostomy* or *Billroth I* operation (Figure 44-15). Partial gastrectomy with removal of the distal two thirds of the stomach and anastomosis of the gastric stump to the jejunum is called a *gastrojejunostomy* or *Billroth II* operation. In both procedures, the antrum and the pylorus are removed. Because the duodenum is bypassed, the Billroth II operation is the preferred surgical procedure to prevent recurrence of duodenal ulcers.

Vagotomy is the severing of the vagus nerve, either totally (truncal) or selectively at some point in its innervation to the stomach. In a truncal vagotomy, both the anterior and the posterior trunks are severed. *Selective vagotomy* consists of cutting the nerve at a particular branch of the vagus nerve, resulting in denervation of only a portion of the stomach, such as the antrum or the parietal cell mass.

Pyloroplasty consists of surgical enlargement of the pyloric sphincter to facilitate the easy passage of contents from the stomach. It is most commonly done after vagotomy or to enlarge an opening that has been constricted from scar tissue. A vagotomy decreases gastric motility and, subsequently, gastric emptying. A pyloroplasty accompanying vagotomy increases gastric emptying.

The combination of a Billroth I or II procedure with vagotomy has the advantage of eliminating the ulcer and the stimulus for acid secretion. Surgical removal of the antrum results in removal of the source of gastrin secretion. (Gastrin normally stimulates parietal and chief cells.) Vagotomy eliminates the stimulus of HCl and gastrin hormone secretion caused by vagal stimulation.

Postoperative Complications. The most common postoperative complications from peptic ulcer surgery are (1) dumping syndrome, (2) postprandial hypoglycemia, and (3) bile reflux gastritis.

Dumping Syndrome. *Dumping syndrome* is the direct result of surgical removal of a large portion of the stomach and the pyloric sphincter. These changes drastically reduce the reservoir capacity of the stomach. Although dumping syndrome is more commonly experienced after a Billroth II procedure, it can occur after any gastric reconstruction and vagotomy.

Dumping syndrome is associated with meals having a hyperosmolar composition. Normally, gastric chyme enters the small intestine in small amounts, and shifts in fluid from the extracellular space are minimal. After surgery, however, the stomach no longer has control over the amount of gastric chyme entering the small intestine. Consequently, a large bolus of hypertonic fluid enters the intestine and results in fluid being drawn into the bowel

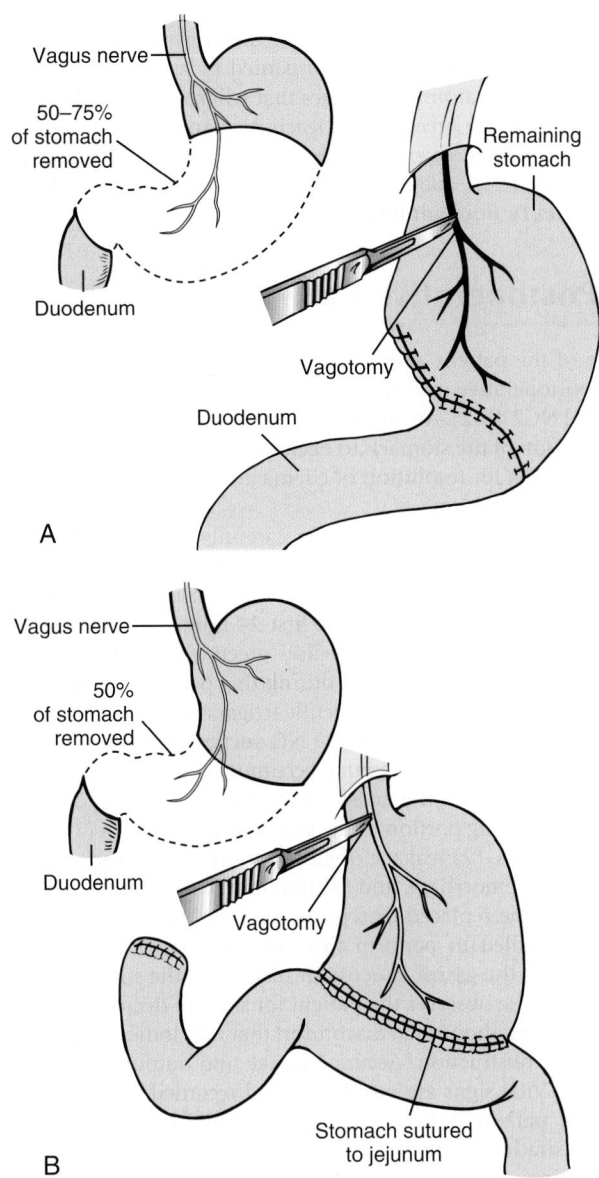

Figure 44-15 A, Billroth I procedure (subtotal gastric resection with gastroduodenostomy anastomosis). **B,** Billroth II procedure (subtotal gastric resection with gastrojejunostomy anastomosis).

lumen. This creates a decrease in plasma volume. A secondary consequence of this fluid shift is distension of the bowel lumen, which stimulates intestinal motility and the urge to defecate.

Approximately one third to one half of patients experience dumping syndrome after peptic ulcer surgery. The onset of symptoms occurs at the end of a meal or within 15 to 30 minutes after eating. The patient usually describes feelings of generalized weakness, sweating, palpitations, and dizziness. These symptoms are attributed to the sudden decrease in plasma volume. The patient complains of abdominal cramps, borborygmi (audible abdominal sounds produced by hyperactive intestinal peristalsis), and the urge to defecate. These manifestations usually last for no longer than an hour after meals.

Postprandial Hypoglycemia. Postprandial hypoglycemia is considered a variant of the dumping syndrome because it is the result of uncontrolled gastric emptying of a bolus of fluid high in carbohydrate into the small intestine. The bolus of concentrated carbohydrate results in hyperglycemia and the release of excessive amounts of insulin into the circulation. A secondary hypoglycemia then occurs, with symptoms appearing about 2 hours after meals. The symptoms experienced are the ones observed in any hypoglycemic reaction and include sweating, weakness, mental confusion, palpitations, tachycardia, and anxiety.

Bile Reflux Gastritis. Gastric surgery that involves the pylorus, either reconstruction or removal, can result in reflux alkaline gastritis. Prolonged contact of bile, especially bile salts, causes damage to the gastric mucosa. Chronic gastritis of this form may result in the back-diffusion of H⁺ through the gastric mucosa. Paradoxically, peptic ulcer may recur after surgical treatment that was intended as a cure.

The symptoms associated with reflux alkaline gastritis are continuous epigastric distress that increases after meals. Vomiting relieves the distress but only temporarily. The administration of cholestyramine, either before or with meals, has met with success. Cholestyramine binds with the bile salts that are the source of irritation in this condition. Aluminum hydroxide antacids have also been used in the treatment of this condition.

Nutritional Therapy. Discharge planning and instruction should be started as soon as the immediate postoperative period is successfully passed. Dietary instructions may be given by the dietitian and reinforced by the nursing staff. Because the stomach's reservoir has been greatly diminished after gastric resection, the meal size must be reduced accordingly. The patient should be advised to stop drinking fluids with meals. Dry foods with a low-carbohydrate content and moderate protein and fat content are better tolerated initially. These dietary changes, with the incorporation of a short rest period after each meal, reduce the likelihood of dumping syndrome. Reassurance that following these dietary measures will result in cessation of these symptoms within a few months is essential to long-term adherence.

Postprandial hypoglycemic reaction can be avoided if these dietary instructions are followed. The immediate ingestion of sugared fluids or candy relieves the hypoglycemic symptoms. The treatment of this type of hypoglycemia is similar to that of dumping syndrome. To avoid similar occurrences, the patient should be instructed to limit the amount of sugar consumed with each meal and to eat small, frequent meals with moderate amounts of protein and fat. Although only a small percentage of patients experience bile reflux gastritis, the patient must be cautioned to notify the health care provider of any continuous epigastric distress after meals that is similar to that felt before surgery.

With regard to dumping syndrome, the symptoms are self-limiting and often disappear within several months to a year after surgery. Interventions prescribed for the patient are diet instruction, rest, and reassurance. The diet should consist of small dry feedings daily that are low in carbohydrate, are restricted in refined sugars, and contain moderate amounts of protein and fat. Sample menu plans are presented in Table 44-25. Fluids should be taken between meals but not with the meal, and the patient should plan rest periods of at least 30 minutes after each meal. The recumbent position is the most beneficial if the patient can arrange it. Reassuring the patient that the unpleasant symptoms are usually of short duration is helpful in gaining cooperation. A small percentage of patients experience long-term problems and may require further reconstructive surgery.

NUTRITIONAL THERAPY

Table 44-25 Postgastrectomy Dumping Syndrome

Purpose

To slow the rapid passage of food into the intestine; to control symptoms of the dumping syndrome (dizziness, sense of fullness, diarrhea, tachycardia), which sometimes occur following a partial or total gastrectomy

Diet Principles

1. Meals are divided into six small feedings to avoid overloading intestines at mealtimes.

2. Fluids should not be taken with meals but at least 30-45 min before or after meals; this helps prevent distension or a feeling of fullness.

3. Concentrated sweets (e.g., honey, sugar, jelly, jam, candies, sweet pastries, sweetened fruit) are avoided because they sometimes cause dizziness, diarrhea, and a sense of fullness.

4. Protein and fats are increased to promote rebuilding of body tissues and to meet energy needs. Meat, cheese, eggs, and milk products are specific foods to increase in the diet.

5. The amount of time these restrictions should be followed varies. The health care provider decides the proper amount of time to remain on this prescribed diet according to the patient's clinical condition and progress.

Sample Menu

Breakfast	1 poached egg
	1 slice toast
	2 sausages
	Margarine
10 A.M. snack	180 g (0.75 cup) dry cereal
	120 mL (0.5 cup) milk
	Half a fresh banana
	Sugar substitute
Lunch	Grilled cheese sandwich with 55 g (2 oz) cheese, lettuce
	2 unsweetened pear halves
2 P.M. snack	120 mL (0.5 cup) plain yogurt
	2 graham crackers
Dinner	55 g (2 oz) tomato meat loaf
	120 mL (0.5 cup) mashed potatoes with gravy
	120 mL (0.5 cup) buttered green beans
	120 mL (0.5 cup) unsweetened apple sauce
8 P.M. snack	Half a sandwich with 1 slice bread, 30 g (1 oz) roast beef, lettuce, mayonnaise

NURSING MANAGEMENT: SURGICAL THERAPY FOR PEPTIC ULCER DISEASE

▪ Preoperative Care

When surgery is planned with the goal of curing the ulcer disease, the surgeon should provide necessary information about the procedure and the expected outcome so that the patient can make an informed decision. The nurse can help the patient and the family by clarifying and interpreting their questions. A discussion of the surgical procedure accompanied by a diagram or picture showing the anatomical changes that will result should be incorporated into the preoperative teaching plan. Instructions should be clear on what to expect after surgery, including comfort measures, pain relief, coughing and breathing exercises, use of an NG tube, and IV fluid administration (see Chapter 20).

▪ Postoperative Care

Care of the patient after major abdominal surgery is similar to the postoperative care after abdominal laparotomy (see Chapter 45 and NCP 45-2). An NG tube is used to decompress the remaining portion of the stomach to decrease pressure on the suture line and to allow for resolution of edema and inflammation resulting from surgical trauma.

The gastric aspirate must be carefully observed for colour, amount, and odour during the immediate postoperative period. The colour of the aspirate is expected to be bright red at first, with a gradual darkening within the first 24 hours after surgery. Normally, the colour changes to yellow-green within 36 to 48 hours. If the tube becomes clogged during this period, the health care provider may order periodic gentle irrigations with normal saline solution. It is essential that the NG suction is working and that the tube remains patent so that accumulated gastric secretions do not put a strain on the anastomosis. This can lead to distension of the remaining portion of the stomach and result in (1) rupture of the sutures, (2) leakage of gastric contents into the peritoneal cavity, (3) hemorrhage, and (4) possible abscess formation. If the tube must be replaced or repositioned, the health care provider must be called to perform this task because of the danger of perforating the gastric mucosa or disrupting the suture line.

The nurse observes the patient for signs of decreased peristalsis and lower abdominal discomfort that may indicate impending intestinal obstruction. Accurate intake and output records must be kept. Vital signs are monitored and recorded every 4 hours.

The patient is kept comfortable and free of pain by the administration of the prescribed drugs and by frequent changes in position. The incision is relatively high in the epigastrium and may interfere with deep-breathing and coughing measures. Splinting the area with a pillow while gently and persistently encouraging the patient to put forth the best efforts possible helps prevent pulmonary complications. Splinting also protects the abdominal suture line from rupturing during coughing. The dressing must be observed for signs of bleeding or odour and drainage indicative of an infection. Ambulation is encouraged and is increased daily.

While the NG tube is connected to suction, IV therapy is maintained. Potassium and vitamin supplements are added to the infusion until oral feedings are resumed. Before the NG tube is removed, the patient is started on oral feedings of clear liquids to determine the tolerance level. The stomach is aspirated within 1 or 2 hours to assess the amount remaining and its colour and consistency. When fluids are well tolerated, the tube is removed, and fluids are increased in frequency with a slow progression to regular foods. The regimen of six small meals a day is begun.

Pernicious anemia is a long-term complication of total gastrectomy and may occur after partial gastrectomy. Pernicious anemia is caused by the loss of intrinsic factor, which is produced by the parietal cells. Depending on the amount of parietal cell mass removed in surgery, the patient may eventually require regular injections of cobalamin (vitamin B_{12}). (Cobalamin deficiency and pernicious anemia are discussed in Chapter 33.)

PUD is a chronic problem, and ulcers can recur, especially at the site of the anastomosis. Adequate rest, nutrition, and avoidance of known irritants and stressors are keys to complete recovery. Avoiding the use of drugs not prescribed by the health care provider is re-emphasized, along with restrictions on smoking and alcohol use. If the patient is willing to make these kinds of adjustments in lifestyle, a successful rehabilitation is more likely.

AGE-RELATED CONSIDERATIONS: PEPTIC ULCER DISEASE

The incidence of peptic ulcers and, in particular, gastric ulcers in patients older than 60 years is increasing. This is related to the increased use of NSAIDs. In the older adult, pain may not be the first symptom associated with an ulcer. For some patients, the first manifestation may be frank gastric bleeding (e.g., hematemesis, melena) or a decrease in hematocrit. The morbidity and mortality rates associated with gastric ulcers in the older adult are higher than those for younger adults because of concomitant health problems (e.g., cardiovascular, pulmonary) and a decreased ability to withstand hypovolemia.

The treatment and management of ulcers in older adults are similar to that in younger adults. An emphasis is placed on prevention of both gastritis and peptic ulcers. This includes teaching the patient to take NSAIDs and other gastric-irritating drugs with food, milk, or antacids. The patient may be treated with antisecretory agents (i.e., PPIs or H_2R blockers). The patient should be instructed to avoid irritating substances, such as alcohol and smoking, and to report abdominal pain or discomfort to the health care provider.

Gastric Cancer

Gastric cancer is an adenocarcinoma of the stomach wall (Figure 44-16). It is the second most frequent cause of cancer death worldwide (Thomson & Young, 2011). Although less common in Canada, it was estimated that 3300 new gastric cancer cases would be diagnosed in 2012 (Canadian Cancer Society's Steering Committee on Cancer Statistics, 2012). Gastric cancer is more prevalent in men of the lower socioeconomic class, primarily those living in urban areas. Gastric or stomach cancer is typically at an advanced stage when diagnosed and is not usually amenable to surgical resection. Only 10 to 20% of patients develop disease confined to the stomach. The 5-year survival rate is 75% in patients with early stages of gastric cancer and less than 30% in those with advanced disease.

Etiology and Pathophysiology

Many factors have been implicated in the development of gastric cancer, yet no single causative agent has been identified. It is believed that a diet of smoked, highly salted, or spiced foods may have a carcinogenic effect. At the same time, there appears to be a negative association between fresh fruits and the development of gastric cancer. A genetic etiology has been postulated

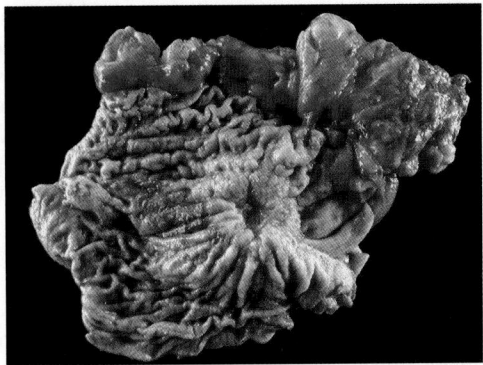

Figure 44-16 Stomach carcinoma. Gross photograph shows an ill-defined, excavated central ulcer surrounded by irregular, heaped-up borders.

Source: Kumar, V., Abbas, A. K., & Fausto, N. (2005). *Robbins and Cotran pathologic basis of disease* (7th ed.). Philadelphia: Saunders.

because of the greater than normal occurrence of stomach cancer in immediate family members. However, at the present time, there is no universally accepted genetic basis for gastric cancer.

Gastric carcinogenesis probably begins with a nonspecific mucosal injury as a result of aging, autoimmunity, or repeated exposure to irritants such as bile, anti-inflammatory agents, or alcohol. Nutritional or other undetermined genetic deficiencies may impede mucosal repair, resulting in chronic gastritis and subsequent proliferation of *H. pylori*. Infection with *H. pylori*, especially at an early age, is considered a definite risk factor for gastric cancer. It is possible that *H. pylori* and resulting metabolic changes can induce a sequence of transitions from dysplasia to carcinoma in situ.

Other predisposing factors associated with a high incidence of gastric cancer are atrophic gastritis, pernicious anemia, adenomatous polyps, hyperplastic polyps, and achlorhydria. The relationship between chronic gastric ulcers and the development of gastric cancer is still controversial. Malignant transformation of a benign chronic ulcer does occur but accounts for fewer than 5% of all gastric cancers. It is known that the person with achlorhydria or pernicious anemia is more likely to develop gastric cancer than is the person with normal gastric acid production.

Gastric cancers often spread to adjacent organs before any distressing symptoms occur. The tumour may grow to large dimensions without obstructing the lumen of the stomach simply because the lumen itself is so large. The interval from onset of symptoms to consultation with a health care provider may be as long as 6 months. This long delay is largely attributed to the vague, intermittent abdominal distress experienced by the patient. Unfortunately, most healthy persons at one time or another experience these symptoms as a result of dietary indiscretions, nervous tension, and anxiety.

Gastric cancer can occur in any portion of the stomach. Tumours located at the cardia and the fundus are associated with a poor prognosis. These tumours typically infiltrate rapidly to the surrounding tissue, regional lymph nodes, and liver. The patient with tumour growth along the lesser curvature has a better survival rate. Adenocarcinomas account for more than 95% of the cancers, and sarcomas (comprising lymphomas and leiomyomas) make up the rest.

The tumour growth is insidious and follows a pattern of continuous infiltration. Gastric cancer may spread by direct extension along the mucosal surface and infiltrate through the stomach wall. The rich lymphatic plexuses in the stomach facilitate distant metastasis. Seeding of tumour cells into the peritoneal cavity may occur late in the course of the disease. Evidence of spread to the peritoneal cavity is manifested by ascites and by spread to the ovaries.

Clinical Manifestations

The clinical manifestations exhibited by persons with gastric cancer can be categorized by signs and symptoms of anemia, PUD, or indigestion. Anemia is a common occurrence with stomach cancer. It is caused by chronic blood loss that occurs as the lesion erodes through the mucosa or as a direct result of pernicious anemia, which develops when intrinsic factor is lost. The person appears pale and weak and complains of fatigue, weakness, dizziness, and in extreme cases, shortness of breath. The stool may be positive for occult blood.

The symptoms of gastric cancer are sometimes identical to those of PUD. The pain and discomfort may be alleviated by belching and by the use of antacids, antisecretory agents, and diet modifications. Manifestations related to indigestion include vague epigastric fullness with feelings of early satiety after meals. Weight loss, dysphagia, and constipation frequently accompany epigastric distress. When nausea, vomiting, and hematemesis occur, they may indicate gastric outlet obstruction or may be a warning of impending hemorrhage.

With more advanced disease, the physical examination may reveal that the patient is pale and lethargic if anemia is present. When the appetite has been poor and weight loss has been considerable, the patient may appear cachectic. A mass may be detected beneath the abdominal wall and is seen to move with each inspiration. On palpation, the mass may be felt in the epigastrium. Masses that are predominantly in the antrum of the stomach are generally found to the left of the midline. Masses located to the right of midline usually tend to be metastases to the liver or indicate involvement of the perigastric lymph nodes. Supraclavicular lymph nodes that are hard and enlarged and located on the left side are suggestive of metastasis via the thoracic duct from the stomach lesion. The presence of ascites is a poor prognostic sign.

Diagnostic Studies

The diagnostic studies for gastric cancer are presented in Table 44-26. Upper GI barium studies may demonstrate alterations in gastric contractility and emptying. On radiographic examination, the malignant ulcer crater is more irregular around the edges and more elevated than the craters found with benign peptic ulcers. Barium studies do not always detect small lesions of the cardia and fundus.

Endoscopic examination of the stomach remains the best diagnostic tool. Lesions that go undetected on the radiograph can be more easily viewed and a biopsy performed when endoscopy is used. The stomach can be distended with air during the procedure so that the mucosal folds can be stretched. Fixation of the mucosa is indicative of malignancy.

Blood chemistry studies assist in the determination of anemia and its severity. Elevations in liver enzymes and serum amylase levels may indicate liver and pancreatic involvement. Stool examination provides evidence of occult or gross bleeding.

COLLABORATIVE CARE

Table 44-26 Gastric Cancer

Diagnostic	Collaborative Therapy
• History and physical examination	• Surgery
• Upper GI barium study	• Subtotal gastrectomy: Billroth I or II procedure
• Endoscopy and biopsy	• Total gastrectomy with esophagojejunostomy
• Exfoliative cytology	
• Endoscopic ultrasonography	• Adjuvant therapy
• Upper GI barium study	• Radiation therapy
• Complete blood count	• Chemotherapy
• Urinalysis	• Combination radiation therapy and chemotherapy
• Stool examination	
• Liver enzymes	
• Serum amylase	
• Tumour markers	
• Carcinoembryonic antigen (CEA)	
• Carbohydrate antigen (CA) 19-9	

GI, gastrointestinal.

Several tumour markers are often present in patients with gastric cancer including carbohydrate antigen (CA) 19-9 and carcinoembryonic antigen (CEA) (see Table 44-26). Serum tests for these markers are commonly performed before surgery for gastric cancer. Serum markers are not used as the only diagnostic tools for gastric cancer because elevations may be related to other factors such as smoking and the presence of benign lesions. (CEA and other tumour markers are discussed in Chapter 18.)

Collaborative Care

When the diagnosis of gastric cancer has been confirmed, the treatment of choice is surgical removal of the tumour. The preoperative management of the patient with gastric cancer focuses on the correction of nutritional deficits, treatment of anemia, and replacement of blood volume.

Transfusions of packed RBCs correct the anemia. If a gastric lesion has been located at or near the pylorus and is causing gastric outlet obstruction, gastric decompression may be necessary before surgery. When the tumour has extended into the transverse colon and partial colon resection is also required, special preparation of the bowel is necessary. This preparation may include a low-residue diet, enemas to cleanse the bowel, and the use of antibiotics to reduce the intestinal bacteria. Correction of malnutrition is important if surgery is planned. Malnutrition is associated with increased postoperative complications and mortality rates.

Surgical Therapy. The surgical intervention used in the treatment of gastric cancer may be the same surgical procedures used for PUD. The location and the extent of the lesion, the patient's physical condition, and the preference of the surgeon determine the specific surgery employed. When metastasis is widespread at the time of diagnosis, surgical intervention may be only palliative.

The surgical aim is to remove as much of the stomach as necessary to remove the tumour and a margin of normal tissue. When the lesion is located in the cardia or high in the fundus, a

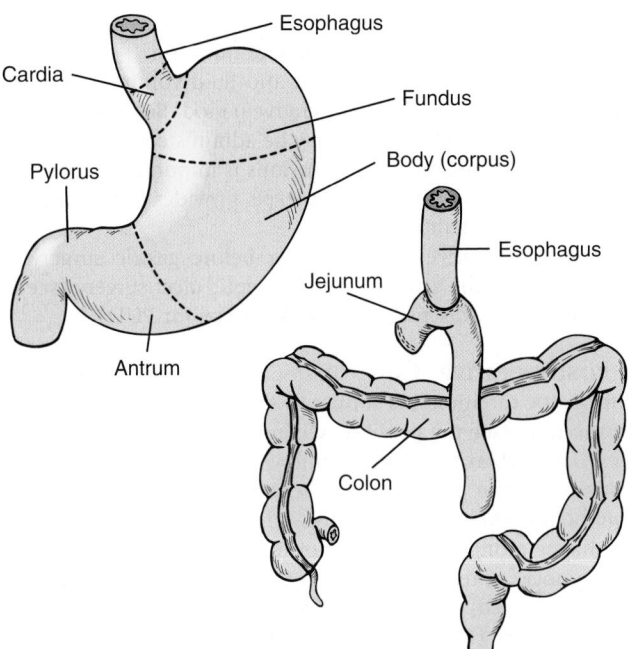

Figure 44-17 Total gastrectomy for gastric cancer (total gastrectomy with esophagojejunostomy).

total gastrectomy with esophagojejunostomy is performed. This procedure involves anastomosis of the lower end of the esophagus to the jejunum (Figure 44-17). Lesions located in the antrum or the pyloric region are generally treated by either a Billroth I or a Billroth II procedure. When metastasis has occurred to adjacent organs, such as the spleen, ovaries, or bowel, the surgical procedures must be modified and extended as necessary.

The chance of a complete cure by surgical means is decreased considerably when the lymph nodes are involved. Survival rates are considerably shortened when organs adjacent to the stomach show evidence of invasion at the time of surgery.

Adjuvant Therapy. Surgery is the only definitive means of achieving a cure. However, when the patient cannot physically withstand a surgical procedure or when surgical cure is not feasible, radiation or chemotherapy alone or in combination may be used. Neither radiation therapy nor chemotherapeutic agents have been very successful when used as the primary mode of treatment. Because the radiosensitivity of gastric cancers is low, radiation therapy has proved to be of little value. When radiation is used as a palliative measure, the tumour mass can be decreased, with temporary relief of the cardia or pyloric obstruction.

The combination of chemotherapy and radiation is now being used for patients who are at high risk for disease recurrence following surgery. Until recently, single-agent chemotherapy for gastric cancer has proved to be of little value. Agents that have been identified as having some effect on gastric cancer are a combination of 5-fluorouracil (5-FU), and cisplatin (BC Cancer Agency, 2012). Combination of radiation and chemotherapy involving 5-FU and leucovorin following surgical resection increases survival. Additional therapies including intraperitoneal administration of chemotherapeutic agents are undergoing evaluation. The role of biological therapy is still under investigation for use in gastric cancer. (These therapies are discussed in Chapter 18.)

NURSING MANAGEMENT: GASTRIC CANCER

▪ Nursing Assessment

The assessment of a person with possible gastric cancer is similar to that done for PUD (see Table 44-23). Important data that should be obtained from the patient and the family include a nutritional assessment, a psychosocial history, the patient's perceptions of the health problem and the need for hospitalization, and the physical examination of the patient.

The nutritional assessment must elicit information regarding appetite and changes in eating patterns over the previous 6 months. It is necessary to determine the patient's normal weight and any changes that may have occurred in the past few months. Unexplained weight loss is common in many types of cancer before diagnosis. A history of vague symptoms of dyspepsia, early satiety, feeling full after consuming even a small amount of food, or symptoms of gas pain should help the nurse differentiate these typical gastric cancer symptoms from those of peptic ulcer. The nurse should determine whether pain is present, where and when it occurs, and how it is relieved. When the pain has been controlled with ingestion of foods, fluids, or antacids for a time but now continues or worsens regardless of interventions, gastric cancer may be the underlying cause.

Psychosocial and demographic data include age, present or previous occupation, and financial status. Gastric cancer can occur at any age, but the risk increases with age. The majority of new cases occur in people over age 65. A family history of cancer, especially gastric cancer, puts a person at greater than normal risk.

It is important to determine the patient's personal perception of the health problem and method of coping with hospitalization, diagnostic tests, and procedures. The possibility of a diagnosis of cancer and a treatment regimen that may include surgery, chemotherapy, or radiation treatment forecast a prolonged stressful period and a possibly fatal outcome. Therefore, it is important for the nurse to support the patient and the family if tests result in an unfavourable diagnosis and complex treatment interventions are planned. If surgery is probable, the nurse should assess what the patient expects from surgery (cure or palliation) and how that patient has responded to any previous surgical procedures.

A complete physical examination reveals the patient's current functional abilities, the presence of other health problems, and an estimate of how well the patient may respond to therapy. Cachexia may be evident if the nutritional state has been compromised for an extended time. A malnourished patient does not respond well to chemotherapy or radiation therapy and is a poor surgical risk.

▪ Nursing Diagnoses

Nursing diagnoses for the patient with gastric cancer include, but are not limited to, the following:

- Imbalanced nutrition: less than body requirements *related to* inability to ingest, digest, or absorb nutrients
- Activity intolerance *related to* generalized weakness, abdominal discomfort, and nutritional deficits
- Anxiety *related to* lack of knowledge of diagnostic tests, unknown diagnostic outcome, disease process, and therapeutic regimen

- Acute pain *related to* underlying disease process and adverse effects of surgery, chemotherapy, or radiation therapy
- Grieving *related to* perceived unfavourable diagnosis and impending death

■ Planning

The overall goals are that the patient with gastric cancer will (1) experience minimal discomfort, (2) achieve optimal nutritional status, and (3) maintain a degree of spiritual and psychological well-being appropriate to the disease stage.

■ Nursing Implementation

■ Health Promotion

The nursing role in the early detection of cancer of the stomach is focused primarily on identification of the patient at risk because of specific disorders such as pernicious anemia and achlorhydria. The nurse should be aware of symptoms associated with gastric cancer, its method of spread, and the significant findings on physical examination. The nurse should understand that the cure rate is often quite dismal because symptoms arise late in the course of the disease process, are vague, and often mimic other conditions, such as PUD.

The nurse must be alert to problems suggesting gastric cancer, such as poor appetite, weight loss, fatigue, and persistent gastric distress. If any of these manifestations are present, medical attention should be obtained and the necessary diagnostic tests performed.

In addition, any patient with a positive family history of gastric cancer should be encouraged to undergo diagnostic evaluation if manifestations of anemia, peptic ulcer, or vague epigastric distress are present. It is important that the nurse recognize the possible existence of stomach cancer in a patient who is treated for peptic ulcer and who fails to have relief after 3 weeks of prescribed therapy.

■ Acute Intervention

■ Preoperative Care.
When the diagnostic tests confirm the presence of a malignancy, the patient and the family generally react with shock, disbelief, and depression, regardless of how thoroughly they may have been prepared for this possible outcome. Throughout this period, the nurse must give emotional and physical support, provide information, clarify test results, and maintain a positive attitude with respect to the patient's immediate recovery and long-term survival.

On admission to hospital, the patient may be in poor physical condition. Surgery may have to be delayed while the patient becomes more physically able to withstand the strain of major surgery. A positive nutritional state enhances wound healing as well as the ability to withstand infection and other possible postoperative complications. Often, the patient is better able to tolerate several small meals a day rather than three regular meals. The diet may be supplemented by a variety of commercial liquid supplements (see Chapter 42) and vitamins. The nurse is challenged to find innovative ways of persuading the patient to eat when lack of appetite and state of mind make eating difficult and unrewarding. Getting the patient's family to assist with meals and encourage intake may be beneficial. If the patient is unable to ingest oral feedings, it may be necessary to provide for nutritional needs with tube feedings or parenteral nutrition.

If needed, blood replacement and fluid volume restoration may be carried out in the preoperative period. Because anemia is usually present, packed RBCs may be administered. Close observation for reactions to the transfusions is important. Monitoring the hemoglobin and hematocrit levels provides information on the progress of therapy.

The preoperative teaching plan before gastric surgery for cancer is much the same as that for peptic ulcer surgery (see the previous section discussing surgical therapy for PUD).

■ Postoperative Care.
Postoperative care of the patient with gastric carcinoma is similar to that following a Billroth I or II procedure (see the previous section regarding surgical therapy for PUD). When the surgical intervention has involved a total gastrectomy, the plan of care is somewhat different. The operation performed usually requires some resecting of the lower esophagus along with the removal of the entire stomach and anastomosis of the esophagus to the jejunum. The chest cavity must be entered, and drainage is accomplished by the insertion of chest tubes. (Chest surgery and drainage tubes are discussed in Chapter 30.) After total gastrectomy, the NG tube does not drain a large quantity of secretions because removal of the stomach has eliminated the reservoir capacity. The NG tube is removed after several days, when intestinal peristalsis has resumed. Small amounts of clear fluid may then be started. The patient requires close observation for signs of leakage of the fluids at the anastomosis as evidenced by an elevation in the temperature and increasing dyspnea. When fluids are well tolerated without distress, the amount may be increased along with the addition of some solid foods.

As a consequence of a total gastrectomy, a patient experiences the symptoms of dumping syndrome. Unfortunately, weight loss is very common, and poor nutritional intake often contributes. Postoperative wound healing may be impaired because of inadequate dietary intake. This necessitates the IV or oral replacement of vitamins C, D, and K, the B-complex vitamins, and intramuscular administration of cobalamin. Because these vitamins (with the exception of cobalamin) are absorbed primarily in the upper part of the small intestine, they must be replaced because the duodenum has been bypassed in the surgical procedure.

A patient who has had a Billroth I or II operative procedure should receive the same postoperative care as someone who has had peptic ulcer surgery. This patient is also subject to the same type of postoperative complications such as dumping syndrome and postprandial hypoglycemia.

The patient with advanced malignant disease can be offered only palliative treatment. The chemotherapy agent found most useful for controlling symptoms of gastric cancer is 5-FU. When this drug or any of the combination drugs is prescribed, the nurse must have current information regarding the action and adverse effects of the drugs. The patient should be made aware of the potential benefits and hazards that can result from the chemotherapy. (The care of the patient receiving chemotherapy is discussed in detail in Chapter 18.)

Radiation therapy can be used as an adjuvant to surgery or for palliation. A patient is generally quite fearful of radiation and may develop many misconceptions regarding its value and dangers. To reassure the patient and ensure completion of the designated number of treatments, the nurse must provide detailed instruction. Because most therapy is completed on an outpatient basis, the nurse should assess the patient's knowledge of radiation, care of the skin, the need for good nutrition and fluid intake during therapy, and the appropriate use of antiemetic drugs. (Specific care of the patient receiving radiation therapy is discussed in Chapter 18.)

Ambulatory and Home Care

Before the patient is discharged, the need for teaching should be reviewed. Most dietary measures useful after peptic ulcer surgery are applicable after surgery for gastric carcinoma. Plans should be made for the relief of pain, including comfort measures and the judicious use of analgesics. Wound care, if needed, must be taught to the primary caregiver in the home situation. Dressings, special equipment, or special services may be required for the patient's continued care at home. A list of community agencies that are available for assistance can be provided before the patient goes home. The services of the Canadian Cancer Society are especially helpful.

When treatment in the form of chemotherapy or radiation therapy is to be continued after discharge, a referral to the home health nurse may be beneficial. The home health nurse can assist with recovery, determine the degree of patient adherence, and be a sympathetic health care provider with whom the patient can consult.

Long-term follow-up must be stressed. The patient must be encouraged to comply with the prescribed dietary and drug regimens, to keep appointments for chemotherapy administration or radiation treatments, and to keep the physician informed of changes in physical condition. (Long-term management of the patient with cancer is discussed in Chapter 18.)

Evaluation

Expected outcomes are the following for the patient with gastric cancer:

- The patient will experience no or minimal discomfort, pain, or nausea.
- The patient will achieve optimal nutritional status.
- The patient will maintain a degree of psychological well-being appropriate to the disease stage.

Food Poisoning

Food poisoning is a nonspecific term that describes acute GI symptoms such as nausea, vomiting, diarrhea, and colicky abdominal pain caused by the intake of contaminated food. Food most commonly causes illness if it is contaminated with microorganisms or their products. The GI tract is frequently the portal of entry for the microorganisms. The epidemiology of foodborne illness is changing. There are new organisms, and many have spread worldwide. The two main types of food poisoning are (1) acute gastroenteritis from bacteria and (2) neurological symptoms from botulism. The most common bacterial food poisonings are presented in Table 44-27.

Poisonous chemicals, such as mercury, arsenic, zinc, and potassium chlorate, may contaminate foods. Poisoning can also occur from ingestion of poisonous plants (e.g., certain mushroom species).

Prevention of occurrence is the focus of interventions. Teaching should include correct food preparation and cleanliness, adequate cooking, and refrigeration. If the patient is hospitalized, care focuses on correction of fluid and electrolyte imbalance from diarrhea and vomiting. With botulism, additional assessment and care relative to neurological symptoms are indicated (see Chapter 63).

Escherichia coli O157:H7 Poisoning

Of recent importance is the increase in number of cases of hemorrhagic colitis caused by the presence of the enterohemorrhagic

Table 44-27 Bacterial Food Poisoning					
CAUSATIVE AGENT	**SOURCES**	**ONSET OF SYMPTOMS**	**MANIFESTATIONS**	**TREATMENT**	**PREVENTION**
Staphylococcal					
Toxin from *Staphylococcus aureus*	Meat, bakery products, cream fillings, salad dressings, milk; skin and respiratory tract of food handlers	30 min-7 hr	Vomiting, nausea, abdominal cramping, diarrhea	Symptomatic, fluid and electrolyte replacement, antiemetics	Immediate refrigeration of foods, monitoring of food handlers
Clostridial					
Clostridium perfringens	Meat or poultry dishes cooked at lower temperature (stew or pot pie), rewarmed meat dishes, gravies, improperly canned vegetables	8-24 hr	Diarrhea, nausea, abdominal cramps, vomiting (rare); midepigastrium pain	Symptomatic, fluid replacement	Correct preparation of meat dishes, serving of food immediately after cooking or rapid cooling of food
Salmonella					
Salmonella typhimurium (grows in gut)	Improperly cooked poultry, pork, beef, lamb, and eggs	8 hr to several days	Nausea and vomiting, diarrhea, abdominal cramps, fever and chills	Symptomatic, fluid and electrolyte replacement	Correct preparation of food

Continued

Table 44-27 Bacterial Food Poisoning—cont'd

CAUSATIVE AGENT	SOURCES	ONSET OF SYMPTOMS	MANIFESTATIONS	TREATMENT	PREVENTION
Botulism					
Toxin from *Clostridium botulinum*; ingested toxin is absorbed from gut and blocks acetylcholine at neuromuscular junction	Improperly canned or preserved food, home-preserved vegetables, preserved fruits and fish, canned commercial products	12-36 hr	GI symptoms of nausea, vomiting, abdominal pain, constipation, distension Central nervous system symptoms of headache, dizziness, muscular incoordination, weakness, inability to talk or swallow, diplopia, breathing difficulties, paralysis, delirium, coma	Maintenance of ventilation, polyvalent antitoxin, guanidine HCl (enhances acetylcholine release)	Correct processing of canned foods, discard suspect canned goods
Escherichia coli					
E. coli serotype 0157:H7	Contaminated beef, pork, milk, cheese, fish	Varies by strain: 8 hr-1 wk	Bloody stools, hemolytic uremic syndrome, abdominal cramping, profuse diarrhea	Symptomatic, fluid and electrolyte replacement	Correct preparation of food
Listeria					
Gram-positive rod-shaped bacterium	Most cases associated with ingesting contaminated dairy products, poultry, and meat	1-90 days	In immunocompetent host: fever, diarrhea, fever Immunocompromised host (pregnant women, elderly, immunocompromised at greatest risk): meningitis ± septicemia	Ampicillin and trimethoprim-sulphamethoxazole or erythromycin	Pasteurization, proper washing, refrigeration, and cooking of foods potentially contaminated with animal manure or sewage

GI, gastrointestinal.

bacterial strain *Escherichia coli* 0157:H7. Widespread outbreaks have increased the public's awareness of this organism. Poisoning with *E. coli* 0157:H7 can be life threatening, particularly in the very young and the older adult. *E. coli* 0157:H7 is found primarily in undercooked meats, such as hamburger, roast beef, ham, and turkey. However, other sources include cheese sandwiches, apple cider, and unpasteurized milk. *E. coli* 0157:H7 can also be transmitted from person to person, particularly in settings such as long-term care facilities and day care centres. *E. coli* 0157:H7

may be responsible for 0.6 to 2.4% of all cases of nonbloody diarrhea and 15 to 36% of all cases of bloody diarrhea.

The clinical manifestations of *E. coli* 0157:H7 vary from mild diarrhea to bloody diarrhea and systemic complications, including hemolytic uremia and thrombocytopenic purpura and even death. The diarrhea may start out as watery but may progress to bloody. Treatment involves supportive care to maintain intravascular volume. Other therapies may include dialysis and plasmapheresis. The use of antibiotics remains controversial.

CLINICAL DECISION-MAKING EXERCISE

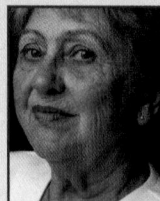

CASE STUDY
Hiatal Hernia

Source: © iStockphoto.com/Joseph Jean Rolland Dubé.

Patient Profile

Mrs. Blushke, a 63-year-old elementary school teacher, has had a sliding hiatal hernia for 10 years. Mrs. Blushke is admitted to the hospital for a hiatal hernia repair.

Subjective Data

- Reports increasing heartburn, especially at night
- Is currently on a bland diet and taking antacids
- Complains of substernal pain and heartburn
- Reports some problems with regurgitation

Objective Data

Physical Examination
- 157 cm tall and weighs 88 kg

Diagnostic Study
- Barium swallow and an endoscopy revealed a large sliding hiatal hernia.

Collaborative Care

Mrs. Blushke had a Nissen fundoplication through a laparoscopic approach.

Discussion Questions

1. Explain the pathophysiology of a hiatal hernia. What is the difference between a sliding and a paraesophageal hiatal hernia?
2. What are the characteristic symptoms of a hiatal hernia? Which of these did Mrs. Blushke have?

3. Describe a Nissen fundoplication procedure. What is the objective of this surgical procedure? Why was a laparoscopic approach used?
4. What are potential postoperative complications, and what nursing measures prevent them?
5. What should be included in a teaching plan for Mrs. Blushke?

6. *Priority Decision:* Based on the assessment data presented, what are the priority nursing diagnoses? Are there any collaborative problems?

evolve *Answers are available on* **http://evolve.elsevier.com/ Canada/Lewis/medsurg**

REVIEW QUESTIONS

The number of the question corresponds to the same-numbered objective at the beginning of the chapter.

1. Mrs. Mansour calls to tell the nurse that her elderly mother, who is 85 years of age, has been nauseated all day and has vomited twice. Before the nurse hangs up and telephones the health care provider to communicate her or his assessment data, what does the nurse instruct Mrs. Mansour to do?
   a. Administer antispasmodic drugs and observe skin turgor.
   b. Give her mother sips of water and elevate the head of her bed to prevent aspiration.
   c. Offer her mother a high-protein liquid supplement to drink to maintain her nutritional needs.
   d. Offer her mother large quantities of Gatorade to drink because older adults are at risk for sodium depletion.

2. The nurse explains to the patient with Vincent's infection that treatment will include which of the following?
   a. Smallpox vaccinations
   b. Viscous lidocaine rinses
   c. Amphotericin B suspension
   d. Topical application of antibiotics

3. The nurse is involved in health promotion related to oral cancer. Which behaviours are included in the teaching of adolescents regarding behaviours that put them at risk for oral cancer?
   a. Avoiding use of perfumed lip gloss
   b. Discouraging use of chewing gum
   c. Avoiding use of smokeless tobacco
   d. Discouraging drinking of carbonated beverages

4. What information is included when the nurse is explaining gastroesophageal reflux disease (GERD) to the patient with GERD?
   a. Results in acid erosion and ulceration of the esophagus caused by frequent vomiting
   b. Will require surgical wrapping or repair of the pyloric sphincter to control the symptoms
   c. Is the protrusion of a portion of the stomach into the esophagus through an opening in the diaphragm
   d. Often involves relaxation of the lower esophageal sphincter, allowing stomach contents to back up into the esophagus

5. A patient who has undergone an esophagectomy for esophageal cancer develops increasing pain, fever, and dyspnea when a full liquid diet is started postoperatively. What are these symptoms most indicative of?
   a. An intolerance to the feedings
   b. Extension of the tumour into the aorta
   c. Leakage of fluid or foods into the mediastinum
   d. Esophageal perforation with fistula formation into the lung

6. The pernicious anemia that may accompany gastritis is caused by which of the following?
   a. Chronic autoimmune destruction of cobalamin stores in the body
   b. Progressive gastric atrophy from chronic breakage in the mucosal barrier and blood loss
   c. A lack of intrinsic factor normally produced by acid-secreting cells of the gastric mucosa
   d. Hyperchlorhydria resulting from an increase in acid-secreting parietal cells and degradation of red blood cells

7. What information would the nurse's teaching plan for the patient being discharged following an acute episode of gastrointestinal (GI) bleeding include?
   a. Taking only drugs prescribed by the health care provider
   b. Avoiding taking aspirin with acidic beverages such as orange juice
   c. Taking all drugs 1 hour before mealtime to prevent further bleeding
   d. Reading all over-the-counter (OTC) drug labels to avoid those containing stearic acid and calcium

8. The nurse is teaching the patient and her family about possible causative factors for peptic ulcers. How does the nurse explain ulcer formation?
   a. Caused by a stressful lifestyle and other acid-producing factors such as *Helicobacter pylori*
   b. Inherited within families and reinforced by bacterial spread of *Staphylococcus aureus* in childhood
   c. Promoted by factors that tend to cause oversecretion of acid, such as excess dietary fats, smoking, and *H. pylori*
   d. Promoted by a combination of possible factors that may result in erosion of the gastric mucosa, including certain drugs and alcohol

9. What information should be included in an optimal teaching plan for an outpatient with gastric carcinoma receiving radiation therapy?
   a. Cancer support groups, alopecia, and stomatitis
   b. Avitaminosis, ostomy care, and community resources
   c. Prosthetic devices, skin conductance, and grief counselling
   d. Wound and skin care, nutrition, drugs, and community resources

10. Several patients are seen at an urgent care centre with symptoms of nausea, vomiting, and diarrhea that began 2 hours ago while attending a large family reunion potluck dinner. What kinds of foods that were ingested should the nurse question the patients specifically about?
    a. Beef
    b. Meat and milk
    c. Poultry and eggs
    d. Home-preserved vegetables

ANSWERS: 1. b, 2. d, 3. c, 4. d, 5. c, 6. c, 7. a, 8. d, 9. d, 10. b.

REFERENCES

Bago, I., Bago, J., Plecko, V., Aurer, A., Majstorovic, K., & Budimir, A. (2011). The effectiveness of systemic eradication therapy against oral *Helicobacter pylori*. *Journal of Oral Pathology & Medicine, 40*(5), 428-432. doi:10.1111/j.1600-0714.2010.00989.x

BC Cancer Agency. (2012). Chemotherapy protocols: Gastrointestinal. Retrieved from *http://www.bccancer.bc.ca/HPI/Chemo therapyProtocols/Gastrointestinal/default.htm#Esophagus,Stomach*

Becker, D. (2010). Nausea, vomiting, and hiccups: A review of mechanisms and treatment. *Anesthesia Progress, 57*(4), 150-157.

Billhult, A., Bergbom, I., & Stener-Victorin, E. (2007). Massage relieves nausea in women with breast cancer who are undergoing chemotherapy. *Journal of Alternative & Complementary Medicine, 13*(1), 53-57. doi:10.1089/acm.2006.6049

Canadian Cancer Society. (2008). Oral cancer: Understanding your diagnosis. Retrieved from *http://www.cancer.ca/~/media/CCS/ Canada%20wide/Files%20List/English%20files%20heading/ Library%20PDFs%20-%20English/Oral%20UYD%20-%20 complete%20PDF%20-%20English%202008_178729184.ashx*

Canadian Cancer Society. (2012). Overview on esophageal cancer. Retrieved from *http://info.cancer.ca/E/CCE/cceexplorer.asp?tocid=14*

Canadian Cancer Society's Steering Committee on Cancer Statistics. (2012). *Canadian cancer statistics 2012.* Toronto: Canadian Cancer Society. Retrieved from *https://www.cancer.ca/Canada-wide/ About%20cancer/~/media/CCS/Canada%20wide/Files%20List/ English%20files%20heading/PDF%20-%20Policy%20-%20 Canadian%20Cancer%20Statistics%20-%20English/Canadian%20 Cancer%20Statistics%202012%20-%20English.ashx*

Canadian Society of Intestinal Research. (2011). Report card: Acid Reflux and GERD. Retrieved from *http://www.badgut.org/ information-centre/gerd-report-card-1.html*

Canadian Society of Intestinal Research. (2012). Gastroesophageal reflux disease: Diagnosis. Retrieved from *http://www.badgut.org/ information-centre/gerd.html#diagnosis*

Chey, W., & Wong, B. (2007). American College of Gastroenterology guideline on the management of *Helicobacter pylori* infection. *American Journal of Gastroenterology, 102*(8), 1808-1825. doi:10.1111/j.1572-0241.2007.01393.x

Doran, K., & Halm, M. (2010). Integrating acupressure to alleviate postoperative nausea and vomiting. *American Journal of Critical Care, 19*(6), 553-556. doi:10.4037/ajcc2010900

Elakkary, E., Duffy, A., Roberts, K., & Bell, R. (2008). Recent advances in the surgical treatment of achalasia and gastroesophageal reflux disease. *Journal of Clinical Gastroenterology, 42*(5), 603-609. doi:10.1097/MCG.0b013e3181653a3b

Flook, N., Jones, R., & Vakil, N. (2008). Approach to gastroesophageal reflux disease in primary care: Putting the Montreal definition into practice. *Canadian Family Physician, 54*(5), 701-705.

Fock, K., Talley, N., Fass, R., Goh, K., Katelaris, P., Hunt, R., ..., Manatsathit, S. (2008). Asia-Pacific consensus on the management of gastroesophageal reflux disease. *Journal of Gastroenterology and Hepatology, 23*, 8-22.

Kovacs, T., & Jensen, D. (2008). The short-term medical management of non-variceal upper gastrointestinal bleeding. *Drugs, 68*(15), 2105-2111. doi:10.2165/00003495-200868150-00003

Malthaner, R., Wong, K., Spithof, K., Rumble, R., & Zurow, L. (2008). Pre-operative or post-operative therapy for respectable esophageal cancer: Guideline recommendations. *Cancer Care Ontario,* Series #2-11 V@.2008.

Nystrom, E., Ridderstrom, G., & Leffler, A. (2008). Manual acupuncture as an adjunctive treatment of nausea in patients with cancer in palliative care—A prospective, observational pilot study. *Acupuncture in Medicine, 26*(1), 27-32. doi:10.1136/aim.26.1.27

Otterstatter, M. C., Brierley, J. D., De, P., Ellison, L. F., Macintyre, M., Marret, L. D.,...Weir, H. K. (2012). Esophageal cancer in Canada: Trends according to morphology and anatomical location. *Canadian Journal of Gastroenterology, 26*(10), 723-727.

Singh, H., Houy, T., Singh, N., & Sekhon, S. (2008). Gastrointestinal prophylaxis in critically ill patients. *Critical Care Nursing Quarterly, 31*(4), 291-301. doi:10.1097/01.CNQ.0000336814.04548.ec

Thomson, G., & Young, K. (2011). Cancer in Canada: Framing the crisis and previewing the opportunity for donors. Retrieved from *http://www.charityintelligence.ca/cancer-in-canada*

Toward Optimized Practice. (2009). Guideline for the treatment of gastroesophageal disease in adults. Retrieved from *http://www.topalbertadoctors.org/cpgs.php?sid=14&cpg_cats=52*

CANADIAN RESOURCES

Canadian Association of Gastroenterology
   http://www.cag-acg.org
Canadian Cancer Society
   http://www.cancer.ca
Canadian Society of Gastroenterology Nurses and Associates
   http://www.csgna.com
Canadian Society of Intestinal Research
   http://www.badgut.org/
RNAO's Integrating Smoking Cessation into Daily Nursing Practice. Nursing Best Practice Guideline (Revised 2007)
   http://tobaccofreernao.ca/sites/tobaccofreernao.ca/files/BPG_ smokingcessation-rev-2007C.pdf

evolve   *For additional Internet resources, see the Web site for this book at* **http://evolve.elsevier.com/Canada/Lewis/medsurg**

Nursing Management: Lower Gastrointestinal Problems

Written by **Marilee Schmelzer**

Adapted by **Françoise Verville**

LEARNING OBJECTIVES

1. Explain the common etiologies, collaborative care, and nursing management of diarrhea, fecal incontinence, and constipation.
2. Describe the common causes of acute abdominal pain and nursing management of the patient following an exploratory laparotomy.
3. Describe the collaborative care and nursing management of acute appendicitis, peritonitis, and gastroenteritis.
4. Compare and contrast ulcerative colitis and Crohn's disease, including pathophysiology, clinical manifestations, complications, collaborative care, and nursing management.
5. Differentiate among mechanical, neurogenic, and vascular bowel obstructions, including causes, collaborative care, and nursing management.
6. Describe the clinical manifestations and collaborative management of colorectal cancer.
7. Explain the anatomical and physiological changes and nursing management of the patient with an ileostomy and the patient with a colostomy.
8. Differentiate between diverticulosis and diverticulitis, including clinical manifestations, collaborative care, and nursing management.
9. Compare and contrast the types of hernias, including etiology and surgical and nursing management.
10. Describe the types of malabsorption syndrome and collaborative care of tropical/nontropical syndrome, lactase deficiency, and short bowel syndrome.
11. Describe the types, clinical manifestations, collaborative care, and nursing management of anorectal conditions.

KEY TERMS

anal fissure A skin ulcer or a crack in the lining of the anal wall that is caused by trauma, local infection, or inflammation, p. 1212

anal fistula An abnormal tunnel leading out from the anus or the rectum, which may extend to the outside of the skin, the vagina, or the buttocks, p. 1212

appendicitis An inflammation of the appendix, p. 1177

celiac disease A chronic hereditary intestinal malabsorption disorder characterized by marked atrophy and flattening of the villi; the inability to absorb a portion of gluten results in the triggering of an immune response that damages the intestinal mucosa, p. 1190

colorectal cancer A malignant disease of the colon, the rectum, or both, p. 1196

constipation A decrease in frequency of bowel movements from what is "normal" for the individual; hard, difficult-to-pass stools; a decrease in stool volume; and retention of feces in the rectum, p. 1168

Crohn's disease A chronic, inflammatory bowel disorder of unknown origin that can affect any part of the gastrointestinal tract from the mouth to the anus, p. 1186

diarrhea The frequent passage of loose, watery stools, p. 1162

diverticulum A saccular dilation or outpouching of the mucosa through the circular smooth muscle of the intestinal wall, p. 1208

fecal impaction An accumulation of hardened feces in the rectum or the sigmoid colon that the individual is unable to move, p. 1166

fecal incontinence The involuntary passage of stool, p. 1165

gastroenteritis An inflammation of the mucosa of the stomach and the small intestine, p. 1179

hemorrhoids Varicosities in the lower rectum or the anus caused by congestion in the veins of the hemorrhoidal plexus, p. 1210

hernia A protrusion of a viscus through an abnormal opening or a weakened area in the wall of the cavity in which it is normally contained, p. 1209

inflammatory bowel disease (IBD) A term referring to two disorders of the gastrointestinal tract (Crohn's disease and ulcerative colitis [UC]) characterized by idiopathic inflammation and ulceration, p. 1179

intestinal obstruction Partial or complete obstruction of the intestine, preventing intestinal contents from passing through the gastrointestinal tract; may be classified as mechanical or nonmechanical, p. 1192

irritable bowel syndrome (IBS) A symptom complex characterized by intermittent and recurrent abdominal pain associated with an alteration in bowel function (diarrhea or constipation), p. 1176

lactase deficiency A condition in which the lactase enzyme is deficient or absent, p. 1191

ostomy A surgical procedure in which an opening is made to allow the passage of urine from the bladder or intestinal contents from the bowel to an incision or stoma surgically created in the wall of the abdomen, p. 1201

paralytic (adynamic) ileus Lack of intestinal peristalsis; the most common form of nonmechanical intestinal obstruction, p. 1193

peritonitis Results from a localized or generalized inflammatory process of the peritoneum, p. 1177

pilonidal sinus Refers to pilonidal cyst or abscess, a chronic infective skin disorder; pilonidal sinuses are narrow openings on the skin surface in the cleft of the buttocks; may be filled with hair, p. 1212

pseudo-obstruction An apparent mechanical obstruction of the intestine without demonstration of obstruction by radiological methods, p. 1193

short bowel syndrome (SBS) Syndrome resulting from extensive resection of the small intestine and characterized by rapid intestinal transit, impaired digestive and absorption processes, and fluid and electrolyte losses, p. 1192

steatorrhea Bulky, foul-smelling, yellow-grey, greasy stools with putty-like consistency, p. 1190

ulcerative colitis (UC) Chronic inflammatory bowel disease characterized by ulceration of the colon and the rectum, p. 1179

Valsalva manoeuvre A manoeuvre during straining: the patient takes a deep inspiration, the breath is held, and the glottis closes and traps the air; simultaneously with the contraction of the chest muscles against the closed airway, the abdominal muscles contract and try to push against the colon, p. 1168

ELECTRONIC RESOURCES

Supplemental content related to Chapter 45 can be found …

Evolve Web Site ⊝volve

http://evolve.elsevier.com/Canada/Lewis/medsurg
- Answer Guide to Case Study on p. 1213
- Audio Lectures:
  - Inflammatory Bowel Disease
  - Irritable Bowel Syndrome
- Clinical Reference: Laboratory Values
- Content Updates
- Customizable Nursing Care Plans:
  - Acute Infectious Diarrhea
  - Colostomy/Ileostomy
  - Inflammatory Bowel Disease
  - Laparotomy

- eFigures:
  - eFigure 45-1: Etiology of Acute Abdominal Pain and Pathophysiology Sequelae
  - eFigure 45-2: Acute Ulcerative Colitis
  - eFigure 45-3: Crohn's Disease
- eTable 45-1: Causes of Constipation
- Electronic Calculators
- Examination Review Questions
- Glossary
- Interactive Case Study: Ulcerative Colitis
- Key Points (Printable and MP3 Download)
- Patient & Caregiver Teaching Guides:
  - Colostomy Irrigation
  - Managing Constipation

Diarrhea

Diarrhea—the frequent passage of loose, watery stools—is not a disease but a symptom. The term *diarrhea* may mean different things to different patients. It is commonly used to denote an increase in stool frequency or volume and an increase in the looseness of stool.

Etiology and Pathophysiology

Causes of diarrhea can be divided into general classifications of decreased fluid absorption, increased fluid secretion, motility disturbances, or a combination of these (Table 45-1). Causes of acute infectious diarrhea are listed in Table 45-2.

Clinical Manifestations

Diarrhea may be acute or chronic. Acute diarrhea most commonly results from infection. Bacterial or viral infection of the intestine may result in explosive watery diarrhea, tenesmus (spasmodic contraction of anal sphincter with pain and persistent desire to defecate), and cramping abdominal pain. Perianal skin irritation may also develop. Systemic manifestations include fever, nausea, vomiting, and malaise. Leukocytes, blood, and mucus may be present in the stool, depending on the causative agent (see Table 45-2). Acute diarrhea is often self-limiting in the adult. Symptoms continue until the irritant or the causative agent is excreted. The mucous membrane lining of the gastrointestinal (GI) tract is composed of epithelial cells, which regenerate following the inflammatory response.

Table 45-1 Causes of Diarrhea

Decreased Fluid Absorption

- Oral intake of poorly absorbable solutes (e.g., laxatives)
- Maldigestion and malabsorption
- Mucosal damage: celiac disease, inflammatory bowel disease, radiation injury, ischemic bowel
- Pancreatic insufficiency (e.g., cystic fibrosis)
- Intestinal enzyme deficiencies (e.g., lactase)
- Bile salt deficiency
- Decreased surface area (e.g., intestinal resection, short gut syndrome)

Increased Fluid Secretion

- Infectious: bacterial endotoxins (e.g., cholera, *Escherichia coli*, *Shigella*, *Salmonella*, *Staphylococcus*, *Clostridium difficile*, viral agents [rotavirus], and parasitic agents [*Giardia lamblia*])
- Drugs: laxatives, antibiotics, suspensions, or elixirs containing sorbitol
- Foods: candy, gum, and mints containing sorbitol
- Hormonal: vasoactive intestinal polypeptide secretion from adenoma of the pancreas; gastrin secretion caused by Zollinger-Ellison syndrome; calcitonin secretion from carcinoma of the thyroid
- Tumour: villous adenoma

Motility Disturbances

- Irritable bowel syndrome: ↑ visceral sensitivity and transit
- Diabetic enteropathy: ↑ transit secondary to autonomic neuropathy
- Gastrectomy: ↑ transit as a result of dumping syndrome

Diarrhea is considered chronic when it persists for at least 2 weeks or when it subsides and returns more than 2 to 4 weeks after the initial episode. Severe diarrhea may be debilitating and life threatening. A patient may have severe dehydration (water and sodium loss) and electrolyte disturbances (e.g., hypokalemia). Malabsorption and malnutrition are also sequelae of chronic diarrhea. Throughout the world, diarrhea is one of the major causes of death.

Diagnostic Studies

Accurate diagnosis and management require a thorough history, physical examination, and when indicated, laboratory tests. A thorough history, including history of travel, medication use, diet and food allergies, previous surgery and adjunctive therapies, interpersonal contacts, and family history, should be obtained. Blood tests may identify anemia, elevated white blood cell (WBC) count, iron and folate deficiencies, elevated liver enzyme levels, and electrolyte disturbances. Stools may be examined for the presence of blood, mucus, WBCs, and ova and parasites. Stool cultures help to identify infectious organisms.

In a patient with chronic diarrhea, measurement of stool electrolytes, pH, and osmolality may help determine whether the diarrhea is related to decreased fluid absorption or increased fluid secretion (secretory diarrhea). Measurement of stool fat and undigested muscle fibre may indicate fat and protein malabsorption conditions, including pancreatic insufficiency. Elevated serum levels of GI hormones such as vasoactive intestinal polypeptide and gastrin may be present in some patients with secretory diarrhea. Endoscopy may be used to examine the

Table 45-2 Causes of Acute Infectious Diarrhea

	ONSET	DURATION	SYMPTOMS AND SIGNS
Viral			
Rotavirus	18–24 hr	3–8 days	Fever, vomiting, and profuse watery diarrhea
Norwalk virus	18–24 hr	24–48 hr	Nausea, vomiting, diarrhea, stomach cramping
Bacterial			
Escherichia coli	4–24 hr	3–4 days	Four or five loose stools per day, nausea, malaise, low-grade fever
Enterohemorrhagic *E. coli* (0157:H7)	4–24 hr	4–9 days	Bloody diarrhea, severe cramping, fever
Shigella	24 hr	7 days	Watery stools containing blood and mucus; tenesmus, urgency, severe cramping, fever
Salmonella	6–48 hr	2–5 days	Watery diarrhea, nausea, vomiting, abdominal cramps, fever
Campylobacter species	24 hr	<7 days	Profuse, watery diarrhea; malaise, nausea, abdominal cramps, low-grade fever
Clostridium perfringens	8–12 hr	24 hr	Watery diarrhea, abdominal cramps, vomiting
Clostridium difficile	4–9 days after start of antibiotics	24 hr	Associated with antibiotic treatment; symptoms range from mild, watery diarrhea to severe abdominal pain, fever, leukocytosis, leukocytes in stool
Parasitic			
Giardia lamblia	1–3 wk	Few days to 3 mo	Sudden onset; malodorous, explosive, watery diarrhea; flatulence, epigastric pain and cramping, nausea
Entamoeba histolytica	4 days	Weeks to months	Frequent soft stools with blood and mucus (in severe cases, watery stools), flatulence, distension, abdominal cramps, fever, leukocytes in stool
Cryptosporidium	2–10 days	1–6 mo	Watery diarrhea, nausea, vomiting, abdominal cramps, weight loss in AIDS

AIDS, acquired immune deficiency syndrome.

DRUG THERAPY
Table 45-3 Antidiarrheal Drugs

TYPE	MECHANISM OF ACTION	EXAMPLES
Demulcent	Soothes, coats, and protects mucous membranes	Bismuth subsalicylate* (Pepto-Bismol); calcium polycarbophil (Equalactin)
Anticholinergic (combination products)	Inhibits GI motility	Diphenoxylate with atropine sulphate (Lomotil), loperamide (Imodium)†‡
Antisecretory	Decreases intestinal secretion	Octreotide (Sandostatin), a synthetic analogue of somatostatin
Narcotic	Decreases CNS stimulation of GI tract motility and secretion; directly inhibits GI motility	Codeine
Probiotics	Alters balance of intestinal flora	*Saccharomyces, Lactobacillus*

CNS, central nervous system; *GI,* gastrointestinal.
*Also inhibits bacterial activity.
†Also absorbent, which contributes to the adhesiveness of the stool.
‡Has cholinergic and noncholinergic actions.

mucosa and to obtain specimens via biopsy for examination. Upper and lower radiographic studies with barium contrast may be helpful in detecting mucosal disease as well as structural abnormalities.

Collaborative Care

The treatment of diarrhea is based on the cause and aimed at replacing fluid and electrolytes and decreasing the number, volume, and frequency of stools. Oral solutions containing glucose and electrolytes (e.g., Gatorade, Pedialyte) may be sufficient to replace losses from mild diarrhea. In situations of severe diarrhea, parenteral administration of fluids, electrolytes, vitamins, and nutrition is warranted.

Once the cause of the diarrhea has been determined, pharmaceutical agents may be given to coat and protect mucous membranes, absorb irritating substances, inhibit GI motility, decrease intestinal secretions, and decrease central nervous system stimulation of the GI tract (Table 45-3). Antidiarrheal agents are not given to a patient who has infectious diarrhea because of the potential of prolonging exposure to the infectious agent. Regardless of the cause of diarrhea, antidiarrheal drugs should not be given for a prolonged time.

Antibiotics are reserved for treating specific bacterial organisms. Antibiotics can cause diarrhea by altering the normal bowel flora. Patients receiving antibiotics (e.g., clindamycin [Dalacin C]) are susceptible to *Clostridium difficile (C. difficile)* infection.

C. difficile is a Gram-positive, spore-forming bacterium that causes diarrhea and serious intestinal problems such as pseudomembranous colitis (Gould & McDonald, 2008). *C. difficile* is the most common cause of infectious diarrhea in the developed world and one of the most common infections in both hospitals and long-term care facilities in Canada. Health care workers should follow infection control precautions to prevent transmission of *C. difficile* from patient to patient

Table 45-4 Preventing Nosocomial Infections: The Four Moments for Hand Hygiene in Health Care

1. BEFORE initial patient–patient environment contact
2. BEFORE aseptic procedure
3. AFTER body fluid exposure risk
4. AFTER patient–patient environment contact

Source: Adapted from Public Health Ontario. (2011). *Just clean your hands—Your 4 moments for hand hygiene.* Retrieved from *http://www.oahpp.ca/services/jcyh/moments.html*

(Table 45-4). Symptoms of *C. difficile* include watery diarrhea with or without blood (at least three bowel movements per day for 2 or more days); fever; loss of appetite; nausea; and abdominal pain or tenderness.

This bacterium has been found to be present in normal bowel flora as well as in the genitourinary tract, in abdominal wounds, and on the skin of hospital workers. Patients entering hospitals may already be colonized with *C. difficile*, although healthy people are not usually vulnerable to the organism. Prolonged antibiotic therapy, cytotoxic chemotherapy, and advanced age are risk factors that may affect the bowel's resistance to colonization or its ability to suppress competing organisms, thus enhancing the growth of *C. difficile*. Laboratory confirmation may be made on the basis of a single, unpreserved stool sample. Metronidazole (Flagyl) is the first-line therapy for this infection followed by vancomycin. Fidaxomicin is currently being studied for its use in treating *C. difficile* (Grant, 2011).

NURSING MANAGEMENT: ACUTE INFECTIOUS DIARRHEA

Nursing Assessment

Nursing assessment should begin with a thorough history and physical examination (Table 45-5). The patient should be asked to describe the stool pattern and associated symptoms. Questions should focus on duration of diarrhea and frequency, character, and consistency of stool. A medication history should include use of antibiotics, laxatives, and other drugs known to cause diarrhea. Recent travel, stress, and health and family illnesses should be discussed. Dietary history should include questions about eating habits, appetite, and food intolerances, especially milk and dairy products, as well as food preparation practices.

Physical examination begins with obtaining vital signs, height, and weight. The patient's skin should be inspected for decreased turgor, dryness, and areas of breakdown. The abdomen should be inspected for distension, auscultated for bowel sounds, and palpated for tenderness.

Nursing Diagnoses

Nursing diagnoses for the patient with acute infectious diarrhea may include, but are not limited to, those presented in Nursing Care Plan (NCP) 45-1.

NURSING ASSESSMENT

Table 45-5 Diarrhea

Subjective Data

Important Health Information

Past health history: Recent travel, infections, stress; diverticulitis or malabsorption; metabolic disorders; inflammatory bowel disease; irritable bowel syndrome; chronic laxative abuse

Medications: Use of laxatives, magnesium-containing antacids, sorbitol-containing suspensions or elixirs, antibiotics, methyldopa, digitalis, colchicines; OTC antidiarrheal medications

Surgery or other treatments: Stomach or bowel surgery, radiation

Symptoms

- Malaise
- Food intolerances; anorexia, nausea, vomiting; weight loss; thirst
- Increased stool frequency, volume and looseness; change in colour and character of stools; steatorrhea, abdominal bloating; decreased urinary output
- Abdominal tenderness, abdominal pain and cramping; tenesmus

Objective Data

General

Lethargy, sunken eyeballs, fever, malnutrition

Integumentary

Pallor, dry mucous membranes, poor skin turgor, perianal irritation

Gastrointestinal

Frequent soft to liquid stools that may alternate with constipation; altered stool colour; abdominal distension, hyperactive bowel sounds; presence of pus, blood, mucus, or fat in stools; fecal impaction

Urinary Tract

Decreased output, concentrated urine

Possible Findings

Abnormal serum electrolyte levels; anemia; leukocytosis; eosinophilia, hypoalbuminemia; positive stool cultures; presence of ova, parasites, leukocytes, blood, or fat in stool; abnormal sigmoidoscopic or colonoscopic findings; abnormal lower GI series (barium enema study)

GI, gastrointestinal; *OTC,* over-the-counter.

◼ Planning

The overall goals are that the patient with diarrhea will (1) not transmit the microorganism causing the infectious diarrhea, (2) cease having diarrhea and resume normal bowel patterns, (3) have normal fluid and electrolyte and acid–base balance, (4) have normal nutritional intake, and (5) have no perianal skin breakdown.

◼ Nursing Implementation

Adherence to appropriate infection control practices and precautions (see Chapter 17, Table 17-8) is important and all cases of acute diarrhea should be considered infectious until the cause is determined. The use of precautions is effective in reducing the spread of infectious diarrhea.

Handwashing is the most important measure in preventing the transfer of microorganisms. Hands should be washed before and after contact with each patient and when body fluids of any kind are handled. The patient should be taught the principles of hygiene, infection control practices and precautions, and the potential dangers of an illness that is infectious to themselves and others. Family and visitors should also be advised of precautions. Proper handling, cooking, and storage of food should be discussed with the patient suspected of having infectious diarrhea.

Best practice guidelines for the management of *C. difficile* (see the Resources at the end of this chapter) state that all patients suspected of having *C. difficile* should be placed in a single room with dedicated toileting facilities such as a private bathroom or individual commode chair. When the number of patients with *C. difficile* exceeds the institution's single-room capacity, those patients with confirmed *C. difficile* may share a room. For patients in multibed rooms, the following precautions should be observed:

1. Signage indicating the precautions to be used should be visibly displayed.
2. A barrier supply cart should be easily accessible.
3. A laundry hamper should be placed as close to the patient's bed space as possible.
4. A commode chair should be dedicated for the patient's use.

Signage indicating that contact precautions are to be used should be posted on the door of any room of a patient with suspected or confirmed *C. difficile.* The nurse should ensure that appropriate environmental cleaning is taking place, including twice-daily cleaning with a hospital-grade disinfectant of all horizontal surfaces in the room and all items within reach of patients with suspected or confirmed *C. difficile.* Visitors should receive instruction from the nurse regarding the nature of *C. difficile* and the importance of hand hygiene and how to properly carry it out. If a visitor is providing care for the patient or having significant contact with the patient's immediate environment, gloves and gown should be worn. The visitor should also receive instruction from the nurse on the correct use of personal protective equipment and be instructed not to use the patient's toilet or go into other patients' rooms (Ontario Ministry of Health, 2009). Chapter 17 discusses contact precautions.

Fecal Incontinence

Etiology and Pathophysiology

Fecal incontinence, or the involuntary passage of stool, may result from multiple causes (Table 45-6). It is important to have an understanding of normal fecal continence to understand fecal incontinence. Normally, fecal contents pass from the sigmoid colon into the rectum, causing rectal distension. Sensory (stretch) receptors in the muscles surrounding the rectum provide the sensation of rectal filling. This causes a reflex relaxation of the internal anal sphincter and contraction of the external anal sphincter. Sensory receptors in the epithelium of the anal canal can usually distinguish among solid, liquid, and gas. The combination of contraction of the abdominal muscles, relaxation of the pelvic muscles, squatting (which straightens the anorectal angle), and voluntary relaxation of the external anal sphincter allows for elimination of feces. Therefore, motor (contraction of muscles) or sensory (ability to perceive presence of stool or to experience the urge to defecate)

NURSING CARE PLAN 45-1

Acute Infectious Diarrhea

NURSING DIAGNOSIS	*Diarrhea* related to acute infectious process *as evidenced by* frequent loose, watery stools
Expected Patient Outcomes	**Nursing Interventions and *Rationales***
• Maintains normal bowel elimination • Maintains afebrile condition	• Monitor frequency, amount, colour, and consistency of stools *to determine severity of diarrhea and need for intervention.* • Follow hospital procedure for infection control precautions; use strict medical asepsis when handling bedpans or commodes, linens, or patient *to prevent spread of infection.* • Administer anti-infective and antidiarrheal medications as ordered *to treat bacterial infection and relieve diarrhea.*
NURSING DIAGNOSIS	***Deficient fluid volume*** related to excessive fluid loss and decreased fluid intake secondary to diarrhea *as evidenced by* dry skin and mucous membranes, poor skin turgor, hypotension, tachycardia, decreased urine output, electrolyte imbalances
Expected Patient Outcomes	**Nursing Interventions and *Rationales***
• Has normal vital signs • Has normal skin turgor • Has moist mucous membranes • Has urine output >0.5 mL/kg/hr • Has normal serum electrolytes	• Assess for skin turgor changes, sunken eyes, rapid pulse, weakness, and anorexia *as indicators of fluid volume deficit.* • Monitor intake and output *to determine fluid balance.* • Monitor serum sodium and potassium levels *so that abnormalities can be reported to the health care provider.* • Monitor vital signs q4h *because changes can indicate hypovolemia.* • Weigh patient daily *to monitor fluid loss.* • Administer IV fluids as ordered, and increase intake of fluids as tolerated and medically indicated to at least 3000 mL/day, *to replace fluids and electrolytes lost in stools.* • Assess mouth for dryness and note patient's complaints of thirst *because these are indicators of dehydration.* • If patient is not vomiting, administer oral fluids as ordered and medically indicated *to replace fluids and electrolytes lost in stools.*
NURSING DIAGNOSIS	***Impaired skin integrity*** related to contact with diarrheal stools and inadequate perianal hygiene *as evidenced by* redness, irritation, swelling, possibly denuded skin, pain, and burning during defecation and urination
Expected Patient Outcome	**Nursing Interventions and *Rationales***
• Has no evidence of skin breakdown in perianal area	• Assess perianal skin area *to plan appropriate interventions.* • Cleanse area gently with warm water or perineal skin cleanser after each bowel movement, rinse well, and pat dry with a soft towel (do not rub) *to prevent skin breakdown and promote patient comfort.* • Apply barrier cream *to protect skin and promote healing.* • Monitor for skin rashes (e.g., yeast, fungal). • Administer warm sitz baths as needed *to relieve discomfort and cleanse skin.*

IV, intravenous.

problems or their combination can result in fecal incontinence. In addition, fecal incontinence can be secondary to **fecal impaction,** which is an accumulation of hardened feces in the rectum or the sigmoid colon that the individual is unable to move. Fecal incontinence caused by fecal impaction is a common problem in older adults.

Diagnostic Studies and Collaborative Care

The diagnosis and effective management of fecal incontinence require a thorough health history and physical examination with appropriate diagnostic studies. In all cases, a rectal examination should be performed, followed by examination with a flexible sigmoidoscope. Fecal impaction, internal prolapse, increased perineal descent, and rectocele may be identified by rectal examination. If the impaction is higher in the colon, an abdominal radiograph may be helpful. Flexible sigmoidoscopy may identify inflammation, tumours, fissures, and other sigmoid–rectal pathological conditions. Other studies may include barium enema, colonoscopy, endorectal ultrasound, and anorectal manometry.

Treatment of incontinence depends on the cause. If fecal incontinence is related to noninfectious diarrhea, dietary changes may be advised, and antidiarrheal agents may be prescribed. In contrast, the management of rectoceles (a defect of the rectovaginal septum) may include teaching the patient exercises to strengthen the muscles of the pelvic floor (Kegel exercises), insertion of a vaginal pessary, and in some cases, surgery (Serels, 2009).

Fecal impaction usually resolves after manual disimpaction and use of lubricants and cleansing enemas. To prevent recurrence, a high-fibre diet (see Table 45-9, later in this chapter),

Table 45-6 Causes of Fecal Incontinence

Traumatic
- Anorectal surgery
- Fistulectomy
- Hemorrhoidectomy
- Abdominal surgery (e.g., nerve injury)
- Traumatic injuries (e.g., gunshot wounds, impalements, foreign body insertion)
- Traumatic childbirth
- Sexual abuse
- Anal intercourse

Neurological
- Degenerative diseases
- Dementia
- Diabetes mellitus (secondary to neuropathic changes)
- Multiple sclerosis
- Spinal cord injuries
- Spinal cord tumour
- Stroke

Inflammatory
- Infection
- Radiation

Other
- Diarrhea
- Fecal impaction
- Loss of rectal elasticity

Pelvic Floor Dysfunction
- Medications
- Rectal prolapse

Functional
- Physical or mobility impairments affecting toileting ability

along with increased fluid intake, should be given unless contra-indicated. Dietary fibre supplements or bulk-forming laxatives (e.g., psyllium) can improve continence by increasing stool bulk, firming consistency, and promoting sensation of rectal filling. Protection of perianal skin and the use of appropriate fecal containment devices (e.g., perianal pouches or adult briefs) will help to protect skin and promote patient comfort and dignity.

Biofeedback therapy may be an option for the patient. This therapy is intended to (1) improve awareness of rectal sensation and coordination of the internal and external anal sphincters and (2) increase the strength of contraction of the external sphincter (Chiaroni & Whitehead, 2008). Biofeedback training requires adequate mental status and motivation to learn. It is a safe, pain-less, and inexpensive treatment for fecal incontinence. (Biofeedback is discussed further in Chapter 12.)

Surgery (e.g., sphincter repair procedures, diverting ostomy) should be considered only when conservative treatment fails.

NURSING MANAGEMENT: FECAL INCONTINENCE

Nursing Assessment

Fecal incontinence is not only an embarrassment to the patient but also a potential hazard to normal skin integrity. An assessment of the patient's general condition is necessary to identify the best alternative for managing the patient with fecal incontinence. The health care provider should identify normal bowel habits and current symptoms, including stool frequency and consistency. Information about the passage of blood or mucus, pain during defecation, and a feeling of incomplete evacuation is sought. The health care provider determines whether the patient has defecation urgency and is aware of leaking stool. The coexistence of urinary incontinence should be determined (Shmaliyan, Wyman, Bliss, Kane, & Wilt, 2007).

Assessment should also include history of multiple or traumatic childbirths, previous anorectal surgery, and injury. A neurological assessment that includes evaluation of mental status can be helpful in identifying the most effective treatment for the patient.

Nursing Diagnoses

Nursing diagnoses for the patient with fecal incontinence include, but are not limited to, the following:
- Bowel incontinence *related to* inability to control bowel function
- Risk for falls *related to* urgency and loss of voluntary control of bowel evacuation
- Toileting self-care deficit *related to* inability to manage bowel evacuation voluntarily
- Risk for situational low self-esteem *related to* inability to control bowel movements and hospital isolation protocols
- Risk for impaired skin integrity *related to* incontinence of stool
- Social isolation *related to* inability to control bowel functions

Planning

The overall goals are that the patient with fecal incontinence will (1) have normal bowel control, (2) maintain perianal skin integrity, and (3) not suffer any self-esteem problems related to problems with bowel control.

Nursing Implementation

If appropriate, prevention and treatment of fecal incontinence may be managed by implementing a bowel training program. Bowel training is effective in many patients because, once the bowel is empty, the rectum does not fill until the next day. The lack of stool in the rectum reduces the likelihood of incontinence. The patient should be assisted to a commode or bathroom at a regular time daily to assist with re-establishment of bowel regularity. A good time to establish this pattern is within 30 minutes after breakfast. Most individuals experience an urge to defecate following the first meal of the day because of the gastrocolic reflex. If the usual bowel habits differ from this pattern, efforts should be made to adhere to the patient's individual timing. Patients are at risk for injury owing to falls related to their inability to control bowel evacuation and attempting to reach a bathroom in time. Safety measures should be implemented to prevent this. Best practice guidelines on the prevention of falls are available from the Registered Nurses' Association of Ontario (RNAO) (2011).

If these techniques are ineffective in re-establishing bowel regularity, a bisacodyl (Dulcolax) or glycerin suppository or a small phosphate enema may be administered 15 to 30 minutes before the usual evacuation time. These preparations stimulate the anorectal reflex and often can be discontinued when a regular pattern is re-established.

Maintenance of skin integrity is important, especially in the bedridden or older adult patient. Nursing management may necessitate the use of fecal containment devices, incontinence briefs, and meticulous skin care. Rectal tubes and catheters are usually not recommended because their use for an extended period may decrease responsiveness of the rectal sphincter and cause ulceration or perforation of the rectal mucosa. Use of incontinence briefs may be helpful in maintaining skin integrity if changed frequently. Meticulous cleaning after each stool is required. Gentle washing, rinsing, thorough drying, and application of a protective barrier cream with each bowel movement are essential to the maintenance of skin integrity. Monitor the skin for the development of yeast or fungal infections.

Perianal pouching is an alternative in the management of fecal incontinence. These are pouches similar in appearance to one-piece ostomy pouches that are designed to be applied over the anus, allowing for the collection of stool. Pouching provides skin protection, odour control, fecal containment, comfort, and dignity. Because odour is often a problem, deodorant sprays and room deodorizers may be used. For the patient who is ambulatory, a regular chair or special tilt commode wheelchair may be used. Regardless of the patient's mobility, the nurse must make sure the skin is clean and intact and the odour is controlled.

Constipation

Constipation is a decrease in frequency of bowel movements from what is "normal" for the individual; hard, difficult-to-pass stools; a decrease in stool volume; retention of feces in the rectum; or some combination of these. Because individuals vary, it is important to compare current symptoms with the patient's normal pattern of elimination. It is important to remember that changes in bowel habits may also indicate bowel obstruction produced by an underlying disease process, such as a tumour.

Etiology and Pathophysiology

Constipation may be caused by insufficient dietary fibre, inadequate fluid intake, medications, and lack of exercise. If proper preventive measures are subsequently taken, constipation should not recur. Constipation may also occur as a result of behaviours related to sociocultural beliefs, environmental constraints, ignoring the urge to defecate, chronic laxative abuse, and multiple organic causes. Changes in diet, mealtime, or daily routines are a few environmental factors that may cause constipation. Depression and stress can also result in constipation. For many patients with constipation, however, it is not possible to identify the underlying cause (McCrea, Maiskowski, Stotts, Macera, & Varma, 2008). Causes of constipation are summarized in eTable 45-1, available on the Evolve Web site for this chapter.

Some patients believe that they are constipated if they do not have a daily bowel movement. This can result in chronic laxative use and subsequent cathartic colon syndrome. In this condition, the colon becomes dilated and *atonic* (lacking muscle tone).

Ignoring the urge to defecate for a time causes the muscles and mucosa in the rectal area to become insensitive to the presence of feces. In addition, the prolonged retention of feces in the

Table 45-7 Clinical Manifestations of Constipation	
• Abdominal distension or bloating	• Increased rectal pressure
• Abdominal pain	• Nausea
• Anorexia	• Palpable mass
• Decreased frequency of bowel movements	• Stone- or rock-shaped stool (fecalith)
• Hard, dry stool	• Stool with blood
• Headache	• Straining
• Increased flatulence	• Tenesmus

rectum results in drying of the stool because of the absorption of water. The harder and drier the feces, the more difficult they are to expel.

Clinical Manifestations

The clinical presentation of constipation may vary from a chronic discomfort to an acute event mimicking an "acute abdomen." Other clinical manifestations are presented in Table 45-7. Hemorrhoids, or dilated hemorrhoidal veins or varicosities, are the most common complication of chronic constipation. They result from venous engorgement caused by repeated executions of the Valsalva manoeuvre (straining) and venous compression from hard impacted stool. (Hemorrhoids are further discussed later in this chapter in the section on anorectal problems.)

The **Valsalva manoeuvre,** which occurs during straining to pass a hardened stool, may cause serious problems in patients with congestive heart failure, cerebral edema, hypertension, and coronary artery disease. During straining, the patient takes a deep inspiration, the breath is held, and the glottis closes and traps the air. Simultaneously with the contraction of the chest muscles against the closed airway, the abdominal muscles contract and try to push against the colon. Increases in intra-abdominal pressure and intrathoracic pressure occur, reducing venous return to the heart. The heart slows temporarily (bradycardia), the cardiac output is decreased, and there is a transient drop in arterial pressure. When the patient relaxes, there is decreased thoracic pressure and a sudden flow of blood into the heart, causing distension and an increase in heart rate. Immediately, the arterial pressure rises momentarily. These changes may be fatal for the patient who cannot compensate for sudden overload of blood flow returning to the heart.

Constipation may contribute to diverticulosis. Diverticula are thought to be caused by the increased intraluminal pressure and decreased intestinal compliance. Diverticulosis and diverticulitis are described later in this chapter.

In the presence of *obstipation*, or fecal impaction secondary to constipation, colonic perforation may occur. Perforation, which is life threatening, causes abdominal pain, nausea, vomiting, fever, and an elevated WBC count. An abdominal radiograph shows the presence of free air, which is diagnostic of perforation. Anal fissures and rectal mucosal ulcers may also occur as a result of stool stasis or straining.

Diagnostic Studies and Collaborative Care

A thorough history and physical examination should be performed to determine the underlying cause of constipation and

DRUG THERAPY

Table 45-8 Cathartic Agents

CATEGORY	MECHANISMS OF ACTION	EXAMPLE	ONSET OF ACTION	COMMENTS
Bulk-forming	Absorb water; increase bulk-stimulating peristalsis	Psyllium: Metamucil, Prodiem Plain, Mucillium	Usually within 24 hr	Must be taken with adequate fluids; can increase gas; contraindicated in patients with possible obstruction or known strictures
Stool softeners and lubricants	Lubricate intestinal tract and soften feces, making hard stools easier to pass; do not affect peristalsis	Mineral oil, docusate calcium (Soflax C), docusate sodium (Colace)	Softeners up to 72 hr, lubricants up to 8 hr	Can block absorption of fat-soluble vitamins A, D, E, and K
Saline and osmotic solutions	Cause retention of fluid in intestinal lumen due to osmotic effect	Magnesium salts: magnesium citrate, magnesium hydroxide (milk of magnesia) Sodium phosphates: Fleet enema, Fleet Phospho-Soda oral solution Lactulose Polyethylene glycol saline solutions: PegLyte, GoLYTELY, Colyte	15 min–3 hr	Magnesium-containing products may cause hypermagnesemia in patients with renal insufficiency; sodium phosphate products may cause electrolyte imbalances in patients with renal insufficiency (increased sodium, increased phosphate, decreased calcium)
Stimulants	Increase peristalsis by irritating colon wall and stimulating enteric nerves	Anthraquinone drugs: cascara sagrada, senna (Senokot) Bisacodyl (Dulcolax)	Usually within 12 hr	Can cause melanosis coli (brown or black pigmentation of colon); are most widely abused laxatives; should not be used in patients with impaction or obstipation

initiate treatment. Abdominal radiographs, barium enema, colonoscopy, sigmoidoscopy, and anorectal manometry may be helpful in the diagnosis. Many cases of constipation can be managed with diet therapy including increased intake of fibre and fluids and an exercise program. Consult a dietitian to review dietary influences. Laxatives (Table 45-8) should be used cautiously because with chronic overuse they may contribute to ongoing constipation. A stepwise approach for laxative use that progresses from bulk-forming fibre preparations to stimulants is recommended, depending on the acuteness of the constipation episode. Enemas are fast-acting and are beneficial in the immediate treatment of constipation, but their use for long-term treatment of constipation should be limited. Soapsuds enemas should be avoided because they may lead to inflammation of colonic mucosa. Excessive hypotonic enemas with tap water can cause water excess, and sodium phosphate enemas have been associated with electrolyte imbalances. Oil-retention enemas may be used to soften fecal impactions. Biofeedback therapy may benefit patients who are constipated as a result of *anismus* (uncoordinated contraction of the anal sphincter during straining) (Chiaroni & Whitehead, 2008).

Nurses must educate patients in whom the perception of constipation is related to beliefs and misinformation about bowel function. Appropriate information on normal bowel function must be given and discussed along with the adverse consequences of excessive use of laxatives and enemas. Best practice guidelines are available from professional organizations and may provide assistance in the assessment and management of individuals with constipation (World Gastroenterology Organization, 2010).

A patient with severe constipation related to bowel motility or mechanical disorders may require more intensive treatment. Diagnostic studies such as anorectal manometry, GI tract transit studies, and sigmoidoscopic rectal biopsies should be performed before treatment.

Nutritional Therapy. Diet is an important factor in the prevention of constipation. Many patients experience an improvement in their symptoms when they simply increase their intake of dietary fibre and fluids (Ghoshal, 2007). Dietary fibre is found in two forms: insoluble and soluble in water. Both are contained in most foods, but some foods are higher in soluble fibre (Table 45-9).

Insoluble fibre, which is found in higher concentrations in whole wheat and bran, remains essentially unchanged by the time it reaches the colon. Soluble fibres form gel-like substances that add viscosity to the digested contents, causing decreased gastric emptying and increased transit in the small intestine. When these fibres ferment and form gas, the gas increases stool bulk, promoting defecation and sequestering fluid, which softens stools. Soluble fibre is found in oat bran, fruits, vegetables, and psyllium. Patients should be told that fibre will increase gas production initially but that this effect decreases with time.

The diet should also include a fluid intake of at least 3000 mL/day, unless contraindicated by cardiac or renal disease. Increasing

NUTRITIONAL THERAPY

Table 45-9 High-Fibre Foods*

	FIBRE PER SERVING (G)	SIZE OF SERVING	CALORIES PER SERVING
Vegetables			
Asparagus	3.5	½ cup	18
Beans			
Navy	8.4	½ cup	80
Kidney	9.7	½ cup	94
Lima	8.3	½ cup	63
Pinto	8.9	½ cup	78
String	2.1	½ cup	18
Broccoli	3.5	½ cup	18
Carrots, raw	1.8	½ cup	15
Corn	2.6	½ medium ear	72
Peas, canned	6.7	½ cup	63
Potatoes			
Baked	1.9	½ medium	72
Sweet	2.1	½ medium	79
Squash, acorn	7.0	1 cup	82
Tomato, raw	1.5	1 small	18
Fruits			
Apple	2.0	½ large	42
Banana	1.5	½ medium	48
Blackberries	6.7	¾ cup	40
Orange	1.6	1 small	35
Peach	2.3	1 medium	38
Pear	2.0	½ medium	44
Raspberries	9.2	1 cup	42
Strawberries	3.1	1 cup	45
Grain Products			
Bread			
Rye	0.8	1 slice	62
White	0.7	1 slice	64
Whole wheat	1.3	1 slice	59
Cereal			
All-Bran (100%)	8.4	⅓ cup	70
Corn Flakes	2.6	¾ cup	70
Shredded Wheat	2.8	1 biscuit	70
Crackers, Graham	1.4	2 squares	53
Popcorn	3.0	3 cups	62
Rice			
Brown	1.6	⅓ cup	72
White	0.5	⅓ cup	76

*Recommended for patients with diverticulosis, irritable bowel syndrome, constipation, hemorrhoids, atherosclerosis, dyslipidemia, and diabetes mellitus.

fibre intake without increasing fluids may predispose the patient to worsening constipation, impaction, or obstruction. The nurse should consult a dietitian to help with patient food preferences and access. The patient's understanding of the diet and the importance of dietary fibre is important to ensuring compliance.

NURSING MANAGEMENT: CONSTIPATION

■ Nursing Assessment

Subjective and objective data that should be obtained from a patient with constipation are presented in Table 45-10.

■ Nursing Diagnoses

Nursing diagnoses for the patient with constipation can include, but are not limited to, the following:
- Constipation *related to* inadequate intake of dietary fibre and fluid and decreased physical activity

NURSING ASSESSMENT
Table 45-10 Constipation

Subjective Data

Important Health Information

*Current health history:** Chronic laxative or enema abuse; rigid beliefs regarding bowel routine; changes in diet or mealtime; inadequate fibre and fluid intake; immobility; change in daily activity routines; sedentary lifestyle

Past health history: Colorectal disease, neurological dysfunction, bowel obstruction, environmental changes, cancer, irritable bowel syndrome; history of chronic laxative or enema abuse

Medications: Use of aluminum and calcium antacids, anticholinergics, antidepressants, antihistamines, antipsychotics, diuretics, opioids, iron, laxatives, enemas

Symptoms

- Malaise
- Anorexia, nausea
- Hard, difficult-to-pass stool, decrease in frequency and amount of stools; flatus, abdominal distension; tenesmus, rectal pressure; fecal incontinence (if impacted)
- Dizziness, headache, anorectal pain; abdominal pain on defecation

Objective Data

General

Lethargy

Integumentary

Anorectal fissures, hemorrhoids

Gastrointestinal

Abdominal distension; hypoactive or absent bowel sounds; palpable abdominal mass, usually in LLQ; fecal impaction; small, hard, dry stool; stool streaked with blood

Possible Findings

Positive FOB; abdominal radiograph demonstrating stool in lower colon

FOB, fecal occult blood test; *LLQ*, left lower quadrant.
*See eTable 45-1 on the Evolve Web site for this chapter.

◾ Planning

The overall goals are that the patient with constipation will (1) increase dietary intake of fibre and fluids; (2) have the passage of soft, formed stools; and (3) not have any complications, such as bleeding hemorrhoids.

◾ Nursing Implementation

Nursing management should be based on the patient's symptoms (see Table 45-7) and the assessment of the patient (see Table 45-10). An important role of the nurse is teaching the patient the importance of dietary measures to prevent constipation. A patient and caregiver teaching guide for constipation is presented in Table 45-11. Emphasis should be placed on maintenance of a high-fibre diet, increasing fluid intake, and a regular exercise program. The patient should be taught to (1) establish a regular meal pattern, (2) maintain a regular time to defecate, and (3) avoid suppressing the urge to defecate. In many persons, the urge to defecate occurs after breakfast because of the stimulation of the gastrocolic reflex. The patient should be discouraged from using laxatives and enemas to achieve and maintain fecal elimination.

Proper position is important when defecating. For a patient in bed, the bedpan should be placed and the head of the bed should be elevated as high as the patient can tolerate. For the person who can sit on a toilet, a footstool may be placed in front of the toilet. Placing the feet on the footstool promotes flexion of the hips, which assists in defecation. For those requiring commodes, tilt commodes may provide proper positioning.

The patient with poor muscle tone should be assessed by a physiotherapist for abdominal muscle strength and taught to contract the abdominal muscles several times a day. Sit-ups and straight leg raises can also be used to improve abdominal muscle tone.

Acute Abdominal Pain

Etiology and Pathophysiology

The causes of an acute onset of abdominal pain are varied (Table 45-12).

Clinical Manifestations

Pain is the presenting symptom of greatest relevance. The patient may also complain of abdominal tenderness, nausea, vomiting, diarrhea, constipation, flatulence, fatigue, fever, and abdominal distension.

Diagnostic Studies and Collaborative Management

Many disorders must be ruled out before a diagnosis is confirmed. Diagnosis begins with a complete history and physical examination. Physical examination should include a rectal and pelvic examination. A complete blood count (CBC), urinalysis,

---

PATIENT & CAREGIVER TEACHING GUIDE

Table 45-11 Constipation

The following are teaching guidelines for the patient and caregiver(s):

1. **Eat dietary fibre.**
   Eat 20 to 30 g of fibre per day. Gradually, over 1 to 2 weeks, increase the amount of fibre eaten. Fibre softens hard stools and adds bulk to stool, promoting evacuation.
   - Foods high in fibre: raw vegetables and fruits, beans, breakfast cereals (All-Bran, oatmeal)
   - Fibre supplements: Metamucil, Citrucel, FiberCon

2. **Drink fluids.**
   Drink 3 L/day. Drink water or fruit juices; avoid large volumes of caffeinated coffee, tea, and cola. Fluids soften hard stools; caffeine promotes fluid loss through urination.

3. **Exercise regularly.**
   Walk, swim, or bike at least three times per week. Contract and relax abdominal muscles when standing or by doing sit-ups to strengthen muscles and prevent straining. Exercise stimulates bowel motility and moves stool through the intestine.

4. **Establish a regular time to defecate.**
   First thing in the morning or after the first meal of the day is a good time because people often have the urge to defecate at this time.

5. **Do not delay defecation.**
   Respond to the urge to have a bowel movement as soon as possible. Persistently delaying defecation results in hard stools and a decreased "urge" to defecate. More water is absorbed from stool by the intestine over time. The intestine becomes less sensitive to the presence of stool in the rectum.

6. **Record your bowel elimination pattern.**
   Record bowel movements on a calendar. Regular monitoring of bowel movement will assist in early identification of a problem.

7. **Avoid laxatives and enemas.**
   Do not overuse laxatives and enemas. They may actually promote constipation because the normal motility of the bowel is interrupted and bowel habituation cannot occur.

Table 45-12 Causes of Acute Abdominal Pain

• Abdominal penetrating trauma	• Mesenteric adenitis
• Acute ischemic bowel injury	• Pancreatitis
• Appendicitis	• Pelvic inflammatory disease
• Blunt abdominal trauma	• Peptic ulcer
• Bowel obstruction with perforation or necrosis	• Perforated gastrointestinal malignancy
• Cholecystitis	• Peritonitis
• Crohn's disease	• Postcolonoscopy bowel perforation
• Diverticulitis ± peritonitis	
• Foreign body perforation	• Ruptured abdominal aneurysm
• Gastritis	• Ruptured ectopic pregnancy
• Gastroenteritis	• Ruptured ovarian cyst
• Incarcerated or strangulated hernias	• Ulcerative colitis ± toxic megacolon
	• Uterine rupture
	• Volvulus

EMERGENCY MANAGEMENT

Table 45-13 Acute Abdominal Pain

ETIOLOGY	ASSESSMENT FINDINGS	INTERVENTIONS
Inflammation	**Abdominal and Gastrointestinal Findings**	**Initial**
• Appendicitis	• Diffuse, localized, dull, burning, or sharp abdominal pain or tenderness	• Ensure patent airway.
• Cholecystitis	• Rebound tenderness and guarding	• Administer oxygen via nasal cannula or nonrebreather mask if O_2 saturation <94%.
• Crohn's disease	• Abdominal distension	• Establish IV access with large-bore catheter and infuse warm normal saline or lactated Ringer's solution. Insert additional large-bore catheter if shock is present, as ordered.
• Diverticulitis	• Abdominal rigidity	
• Gastritis	• Nausea and vomiting	
• Pancreatitis	• Diarrhea	
• Ulcerative colitis	• Hematemesis	• Obtain blood for CBC and serum electrolytes assessment.
Vascular Problems	• Melena	• Consider ECG.
• Ruptured aortic aneurysm	**Hypovolemic Shock**	• Anticipate order for amylase level, pregnancy tests, clotting studies, and type and crossmatch as appropriate.
• Mesenteric vascular occlusion or ischemia	• ↓ Blood pressure	
Gynecological Problems	• ↓ Pulse pressure	• Insert indwelling urinary catheter.
• Pelvic inflammatory disease	• Tachycardia	• Obtain urine R&M, C&S.
• Ruptured ectopic pregnancy	• Cool, clammy skin	• Insert NG tube as needed.
• Ruptured ovarian cyst	• ↓ Level of consciousness	• Keep patient on NPO status.
Infectious Diseases		• Assess bowel sound characteristics.
• Giardiasis		**Ongoing Monitoring**
• Salmonellosis		• Monitor vital signs, level of consciousness, O_2 saturation, and intake–output.
Other		• Assess pain characteristics.
• Obstruction or perforation of abdominal organ		• Assess amount and character of emesis.
• Gastrointestinal bleeding		• Anticipate diagnostic tests.
• Trauma		• Anticipate surgical intervention.
		• Maintain NPO status.

CBC, complete blood count; *C&S*, culture and sensitivity; *ECG*, electrocardiogram; *IV*, intravenous; *NG*, nasogastric; *NPO*, nothing by mouth; *R&M*, routine and microscopic.

abdominal radiographic examination, and an electrocardiogram (ECG) are done initially. Pregnancy tests should be performed in women of child-bearing age who have acute abdominal pain to rule out ectopic pregnancy. The findings of these studies may provide some information about the cause of the acute abdomen.

Emergency management of the patient with acute abdominal pain is presented in Table 45-13. The goal of management is to stabilize the patient's condition and to identify and treat the cause. The health care provider attempts to make a differential diagnosis when the patient is seen with an acute condition in the abdomen because some causes of abdominal pain do not necessitate surgery (see Table 45-12). It was previously thought that pain medication should be withheld because analgesics might obscure progression of clinical manifestations and impede diagnosis. In fact, appropriate pain management that does not result in altered consciousness can decrease diffuse pain and abdominal rigidity and help localize the pain, leading to earlier diagnosis and treatment.

In addition to being a therapeutic measure, surgery can also be diagnostic. Operative exploration is usually done after a careful examination, a review of the patient status, and a review of diagnostic test results. Surgical exploration may be done lapa-roscopically or through an open midline abdominal wound (laparotomy). Direct examination may permit the cause to be identified and allow for completion of the definitive procedure.

NURSING MANAGEMENT: ACUTE ABDOMINAL PAIN

■ Nursing Assessment

Vital signs, including blood pressure and pulse rate, should be taken immediately to determine hypovolemic changes. An elevated temperature may indicate an inflammatory or infectious process. The abdomen should be inspected for distension, masses, abnormal pulsation, rashes, scars, and pigmentation changes. Bowel sounds should be auscultated. Bowel sounds that are diminished, absent, or hyperactive in a quadrant may indicate a complete bowel obstruction, acute peritonitis, or paralytic ileus. Palpation should be gentle.

A thorough assessment of the patient's symptoms should be made to determine onset, location, intensity, duration, frequency, and character of pain. The nurse should determine whether the pain has spread or moved to new locations (quadrants) as well as what makes the pain worse or better. It should also be determined whether the pain is associated with other symptoms, such as nausea, vomiting, changes in bowel and bladder habits, or vaginal discharge in women. Assessment of vomiting should include amount, colour, consistency, and odour of the vomitus. Bowel patterns and habits should also be assessed carefully.

Nursing Diagnoses

Nursing diagnoses for the patient with acute abdominal pain include, but are not limited to, the following:

- Acute pain *related to* inflammation of the peritoneum and abdominal distension
- Risk for deficient fluid volume *related to* anorexia, vomiting, intra-abdominal bleeding
- Imbalanced nutrition: less than body requirements *related to* anorexia, nausea, and vomiting
- Anxiety *related to* uncertainty of cause or outcome of condition and pain

Planning

The overall goals are that the patient with acute abdominal pain will have (1) resolution of the underlying process, (2) relief of abdominal pain, (3) freedom from complications (especially hypovolemic shock), and (4) normal nutritional status.

Nursing Implementation

Nursing interventions are based on the diagnosis and medical or surgical management of the patient. General care for the patient involves management of fluid and electrolyte imbalances, pain, and anxiety.

Acute Intervention

Preoperative Care. Emergency preparation of the patient with acute abdominal pain is usually limited to a CBC, typing and crossmatching of blood, and clotting studies. Catheterization, administration of medications (e.g., antibiotics), and the passage of a nasogastric (NG) tube may be done in the emergency department or operating room. (General care of the preoperative patient is discussed in Chapter 20.)

Postoperative Care. Postoperative care depends on the type of surgical procedure performed. The increased use of laparoscopic procedures has reduced the risk of potential postoperative complications related to wound care and altered GI motility. These newer procedures generally result in shorter hospital stays.

A general NCP for the postoperative patient is presented in Chapter 22. Nursing care for the patient following a laparotomy is presented in NCP 45-2.

An NG tube may or may not be present in the patient returning from surgery. If present, the NG tube is connected to suction as ordered. The purpose of the NG tube is to empty the stomach of secretions and gas to prevent gastric distension. GI peristaltic activity is often impaired because of the manipulative procedures of the surgery and anaesthesia.

If the upper GI tract has been entered, drainage from the NG tube may be dark brown to dark red for the first 12 hours. Later, it should be light yellowish brown, or it may have a greenish tinge because of the presence of bile. If a dark red colour continues or if bright red blood is observed, the health care provider should be notified at once of the possibility of hemorrhage. The "coffee grounds" appearance of the drainage is owing to the presence of small amounts of blood that have been chemically altered by gastric secretions.

The NG tube is checked regularly for patency. The tube may become obstructed with mucus, sediment, or blood clots. An order is usually written to irrigate the tube with 20 to 30 mL of tap water or normal saline solution if needed. An accurate record of intake and output, including emesis and gastric drainage, is essential. The nurse assesses serum electrolyte values and acid–base balance because prolonged gastric suctioning can result in loss of sodium, chloride, potassium, water, and hydrochloric acid.

The NG tube is removed when intestinal peristalsis returns, usually 24 to 72 hours after surgery. Motility of the stomach normally returns within 24 to 48 hours. Motility of the small intestine usually resumes within 12 to 24 hours, whereas return of large intestine motility may take as long as 3 to 5 days. Peristaltic activity can be assessed by auscultation for bowel sounds.

Mouth care and nasal care are essential. The patient tends to breathe through the mouth while the NG tube is in place. In addition, increased nasal secretions and crusting result from mechanical stimulation of the NG tube.

Parenteral fluids are administered to provide the patient with fluids and electrolytes until bowel sounds return. Ice chips may be ordered because they aid in the flow of saliva and prevent a dry mouth and sore throat. When bowel sounds return, fluids and food are increased gradually. Nausea and vomiting are not uncommon after abdominal surgery and are often self-limiting. Observation is important in determining the cause. Antiemetics such as dimenhydrinate (Gravol), ondansetron (Zofran), or metoclopramide may be ordered.

Abdominal distension and gas pains are also common after surgery; these are owing to swallowed air and impaired peristalsis resulting from immobility, manipulation of abdominal contents during surgery, and adverse effects of anaesthesia. The health care provider should be informed of abdominal distension and rigidity and worsening abdominal pain. Gradually, as intestinal activity increases, distension and gas pains decrease.

Ambulatory and Home Care

Preparation for discharge begins when the patient returns from the operating room. Instructions to the patient and family should include any modifications in activity, care of the incision, diet, and drug therapy. Small, frequent meals high in calories should be taken initially, with a gradually increased intake of food as tolerated.

Normal activities should be resumed gradually. Some activity restrictions may be required for 6 to 8 weeks. The patient should be aware of possible complications after surgery and should notify the health care provider immediately if vomiting, fever, pain, weight loss, incisional drainage, or changes in bowel function occur.

NURSING CARE PLAN 45-2

After Laparotomy

NURSING DIAGNOSIS	**Acute pain** *related to* surgical incision and inadequate pain control measures *as evidenced by* complaints of pain, body posturing, or unwillingness to move in bed or to ambulate
Expected Patient Outcome	**Nursing Interventions and *Rationales***
• Reports satisfactory level of pain control	• Provide patient-controlled analgesia.
	• Assess for pain and give pain medication every 3-4 hr as ordered for first 72 hr *to treat pain appropriately.*
	• Splint incision with pillows during coughing, deep breathing, and moving *to relieve pain while performing these activities.*
	• Position patient comfortably *to relieve pain.*
NURSING DIAGNOSIS	**Nausea** *related to* decreased GI motility, GI distension, and narcotics *as evidenced by* nausea, vomiting, lack of or diminished bowel sounds, or abdominal distension
Expected Patient Outcome	**Nursing Interventions and *Rationales***
• Reports relief of nausea and vomiting	• Administer antiemetic medications (as ordered) *to relieve nausea and vomiting.*
	• Assess response to pain medications to determine *if this is a possible cause of nausea and vomiting.*
	• Maintain patency of NG tube (if present) *to prevent accumulation of gastric secretions and subsequent vomiting.*
	• Assess for bowel sounds and abdominal distension *to determine return of peristalsis.*
	• Keep patient on NPO status until orders for postoperative diet are received.
	• Limit unpleasant sights, smells, and stimuli *to prevent initiating episodes of nausea and vomiting.*
NURSING DIAGNOSIS	**Constipation** *related to* immobility, pain, medication, and decreased GI motility *as evidenced by* decreased or absent bowel sounds, abdominal pain, abdominal distension, or inability to pass flatus or stool
Expected Patient Outcome	**Nursing Interventions and *Rationales***
• Will report bowel movement within 4-5 days	• Assess abdomen for distension and bowel sounds q8h *to determine need for intervention.*
	• Administer stool softener (if ordered) *to soften fecal mass or promote elimination.*
	• Encourage frequent position changes and ambulation as tolerated *to increase peristalsis.*
	• Encourage increased fluid intake as tolerated.

GI, gastrointestinal; *NG,* nasogastric; *NPO,* nothing by mouth.
NOTE: General nursing care for the postoperative patient is presented in NCP 22-1 in Chapter 22.

◾ Evaluation

The expected outcomes are that the patient with acute abdominal pain will have (1) resolution of the cause of the acute abdominal pain; (2) relief of abdominal pain and discomfort; (3) freedom from complications (especially hypovolemic shock and septicemia); and (4) normal fluid, electrolyte, and nutritional status.

Abdominal Trauma

Etiology and Pathophysiology

Injuries to the abdominal area most often occur as a result of blunt trauma (e.g., motor vehicle accident) or penetration injuries, primarily gunshot wounds or stab wounds to the abdomen. Blunt trauma is most common. Regardless of whether it is a blunt or penetration injury, the result is often the same: damage to or alteration of the internal organs.

Common injuries of the abdomen include lacerated liver, ruptured spleen, pancreatic trauma, mesenteric artery tears, diaphragmatic rupture, urinary bladder rupture, great vessel tears, renal injury, and stomach or intestinal rupture. These injuries may result in massive blood loss and hypovolemic shock. Surgery must be performed as early as possible to repair the damaged organs and to stop the bleeding. Common sequelae of intra-abdominal trauma are peritonitis and sepsis, particularly when the bowel is perforated.

Clinical Manifestations

Clinical manifestations of abdominal trauma are (1) guarding and splinting of the abdominal wall; (2) a hard, distended abdomen (may indicate intra-abdominal bleeding); (3) decreased or absent bowel sounds; (4) contusions, abrasions, or bruising over the flanks or the abdomen; (5) severe abdominal pain; (6) pain over the scapula caused by irritation of the phrenic nerve by free blood in the abdomen; (7) hematemesis or hematuria; and (8) signs of hypovolemic shock (Table 45-14). An ecchymotic

EVIDENCE-INFORMED PRACTICE

How Long After Gastrointestinal Surgery Should Patients Remain NPO?

Clinical Question

For patients undergoing GI surgery (P), does enteral feeding within 24 hours postoperative (I) versus maintaining NPO status (C) reduce postoperative mortality (O)?

Best Available Evidence

- Systematic review and meta-analysis of RCTs

Critical Appraisal and Synthesis of Evidence

- 13 RCTs (n = 1173); not all studies were blinded to intervention.
- Patients underwent upper or lower GI or hepatobiliary surgery.
- Wound infections, intra-abdominal abscesses, pneumonia, anastomotic leakage, mortality risk, length of hospital stay, and vomiting were assessed.

Conclusions

- Enteral feeding within 24 hr after GI surgery decreased patient mortality risk.
- Early postoperative feeding increased vomiting.

Implications for Nursing Practice

- Before surgery, patients are often malnourished owing to disease process, vomiting, and preparations for diagnostic testing or surgery. Severe malnourishment increases morbidity and mortality risks.
- Consult with surgeons and dietitians in advance for beginning enteral feeding in the first 24 hr postoperatively.
- Assess for nausea and vomiting with enteral feedings.

Reference for Evidence

Lewis, S. J., Andersen, H. K., & Thomas, S. (2009). Early enteral nutrition within 24 hr of intestinal surgery versus later commencement of feeding: A systematic review and meta-analysis, *Journal of Gastrointestinal Surgery, 3*, 569. doi:10.1007/s11605-008-0592-x

GI, gastrointestinal; *NPO*, nothing by mouth; *PICO:* patient population of interest *(P)*; intervention or area of interest *(I)*; comparison of interest or comparison group *(C)*; outcome(s) of interest *(O)*; *RCTs*, randomized controlled trials.

EMERGENCY MANAGEMENT

Table 45-14 Abdominal Trauma

ETIOLOGY	ASSESSMENT FINDINGS	INTERVENTIONS
Blunt	**Hypovolemic Shock**	**Initial**
• Falls	• ↓ Level of consciousness	• Ensure patent airway.
• Motor vehicle collisions	• Tachypnea	• Administer O_2 via face mask.
• Pedestrian accident	• Tachycardia	• Control external bleeding with direct pressure or sterile pressure dressing.
• Assault with blunt object	• ↓ Blood pressure	• Establish IV access with two large-bore catheters, and infuse warm normal saline or lactated Ringer's solution.
• Crush injuries	• ↓ Pulse pressure	
• Explosions	**Surface Findings**	• Obtain blood for type and crossmatch and CBC.
Penetrating	• Abrasions or ecchymoses on abdominal wall, flank, or perineum	• Remove clothing.
• Knife	• Open wounds: lacerations, eviscerations, puncture wounds, gunshot wounds	• Stabilize impaled objects with bulky dressing—do not remove.
• Gunshot wounds	• Impaled object	• Cover protruding organs or tissue with sterile, saline dressing.
• Other missiles	• Healed incisions or old scars	• Insert indwelling urinary catheter if there is no blood at the meatus, pelvic fracture, or boggy prostate.
	Abdominal and Gastrointestinal Findings	• Obtain urine for urinalysis.
	• Nausea and vomiting	• Insert NG tube if no evidence of facial neck trauma.
	• Bloody urine	• Anticipate diagnostic peritoneal lavage.
	• Abdominal pain	**Ongoing Monitoring**
	• Abdominal distension	• Monitor vital signs, level of consciousness, O_2 saturation, and urine output.
	• Abdominal rigidity	• Maintain patient warmth using blankets, warm IV fluids (40-45°C), or warm humidified oxygen.
	• Guarding	
	• Rebound tenderness	
	• Pain radiation to shoulder and back	

CBC, complete blood count; *IV,* intravenous; *NG,* nasogastric.

discoloration around the umbilicus (Cullen's sign) can indicate intra-abdominal or retroperitoneal hemorrhage.

Intra-abdominal injuries can also be associated with low rib fractures, fractured femur, fractured pelvis, and thoracic injury. If any of these injuries are present, the patient should be observed for abdominal trauma.

Diagnostic Studies

Specific diagnostic procedures include CBC, urinalysis, radiographs of the abdomen and the chest, high-resolution computed tomography (CT) scan, and abdominal ultrasound. With the availability of emergency department ultrasound and CT, peritoneal lavage is rarely performed as a diagnostic tool. If peritoneal lavage is performed (although contraindicated in pregnant women or those with pelvic fractures), the abdomen below the umbilicus is locally anaesthetized, and a large angiocatheter or peritoneal dialysis catheter is inserted into the abdomen. A syringe is attached to the catheter, and an attempt is made to gently aspirate any blood. If less than 10 mL of blood is aspirated, a litre of lactated Ringer's is then infused into the abdomen and drained. The fluid is observed for gross abnormalities, such as the presence of blood, bile, feces, or food fibres, and is sent to the laboratory for microscopic evaluation. In blunt abdominal trauma, positive findings may include (1) red blood cell (RBC) count greater than $100 \times 10^{12}/L$; (2) WBC count greater than $0.5 \times 10^9/L$; (3) high amylase level; and (4) presence of bacteria. In the case of stab wounds, the threshold for RBCs is lower ($1\text{-}5 \times 10^{12}/L$), allowing for detection of subtle diaphragmatic injuries. If the results are positive, immediate surgery is indicated. If the results are negative, continued observation of the patient is warranted. An impaled object should never be removed until skilled surgical care is available. Removal may cause further injury and bleeding.

NURSING AND COLLABORATIVE MANAGEMENT: ABDOMINAL TRAUMA

Emergency management of abdominal trauma focuses on establishing a patent airway and adequate breathing, fluid replacement, and prevention of hypovolemic shock (see Table 45-14). Intravenous (IV) lines are inserted, and volume expanders or blood is given if the patient is hypotensive. An NG tube is inserted to decompress the stomach and prevent the aspiration of vomitus.

Regardless of the mechanism of injury, physical evidence of abdominal trauma in a patient who is hemodynamically unstable mandates immediate laparotomy. In other cases, the indications for laparotomy must be correlated with the mechanism of injury. For example, if an individual has a gunshot wound or impaled object, surgery is usually indicated. If surgery is performed, the postoperative nursing care is similar to the care of the patient after laparotomy (see NCP 45-2).

Chronic Abdominal Pain

Chronic abdominal pain may originate from abdominal structures or may be referred from a site with the same or a similar nerve supply. Some common causes are irritable bowel syndrome (IBS), peptic ulcer disease, diverticulitis, chronic pancreatitis,

hepatitis, cholecystitis, pelvic inflammatory disease, and vascular insufficiency.

Diagnosis of chronic abdominal pain presents a challenge. Assessment should begin with a thorough history and identification of the specific pain pattern. Character and severity of pain, location, duration, and onset should be determined. The assessment should also include the relationship of pain to meals, defecation, and activity and factors that increase or decrease the pain. Chronic abdominal pain can be described as dull, aching, or diffuse.

Endoscopy, CT scans, magnetic resonance imaging (MRI), laparoscopy, and radiological barium studies have decreased the need for exploratory laparotomy. Treatment for chronic abdominal pain is comprehensive and directed toward palliation of symptoms using appropriate medications such as analgesics and antiemetics as well as psychological or behavioural therapies (e.g., relaxation therapies).

Irritable Bowel Syndrome

Irritable bowel syndrome (IBS) is a chronic functional disorder characterized by intermittent and recurrent abdominal pain associated with an alteration in bowel function (diarrhea or constipation or both). Other symptoms commonly found include abdominal distension, excessive flatulence, bloating, urge to defecate, urgency, and sensation of incomplete evacuation. IBS is a common problem affecting approximately 13 to 20% of the population in Canada (Canadian Society of Intestinal Research, 2011). Neurological hypersensitivity within the GI (enteric) nerves, physical and/or emotional stress, dietary issues such as food allergies or sensitivities, antibiotic use, GI infection, bile acid malabsorption, chronic alcohol abuse, abnormalities in GI secretions and/or digestive muscle contractions (peristalsis), acute infection or inflammation of the intestine (enteritis), such as traveller's diarrhea have been identified as factors that precipitate IBS symptoms (Canadian Society of Intestinal Research, 2011; Clarke & DeLegge, 2008). IBS is not a psychological disorder, even though stress, depression, panic, or anxiety may aggravate bowel symptoms.

The key to accurate diagnosis is a thorough history and physical examination. Emphasis should be on symptoms, past health history (including psychosocial aspects such as physical or sexual abuse), family history, and drug and dietary history. Diagnostic tests should be used to rule out more serious life-threatening disorders with symptoms similar to those of IBS, such as colorectal cancer, peptic ulcer disease, inflammatory bowel disease (IBD), and malabsorption disorders. Symptom-based criteria for IBS have been standardized and are referred to as the Rome III criteria (Talley, 2007). The Rome III criteria include abdominal discomfort or pain for at least 3 months, with onset at least 6 months before, that has at least two of the following characteristics: (1) relieved with defecation; (2) onset associated with a change in stool frequency; and (3) onset associated with a change in stool appearance (Heitkemper & Jarrett, 2008).

The health care provider should encourage the patient to verbalize concerns and anxiety. A diet containing at least 20 g/day of dietary fibre should be initiated (see Table 45-9). This may also include the addition of psyllium-containing products (e.g., Metamucil).

The patient whose primary symptoms are abdominal distension and increased flatulence should be advised to eliminate common gas-producing foods such as broccoli and cabbage from the diet and to use lactose-free products if there is lactose intolerance. Tegaserod (Zelnorm) has been recently used to treat women with IBS whose primary bowel symptom is constipation. It increases the movement of stools through the colon. Other therapies include relaxation and stress management techniques, antidepressants, acupuncture, and herbal therapy, although no single therapy has been found to be effective for all patients with IBS. Patients should be referred to a dietitian to review dietary practices. Maintaining a healthy diet according to Canada's Food Guide (see Chapter 42) should be encouraged.

Inflammatory Disorders

Appendicitis

Appendicitis is an inflammation of the appendix, a narrow blind tube that extends from the inferior part of the cecum. Appendicitis occurs in approximately 7% of the world's population. It can occur at any age but is most common in young adults (Pickhardt, Lawrence, Pooler, & Bruce, 2011).

Etiology and Pathophysiology

The most common causes of appendicitis are occlusion of the appendiceal lumen by a *fecalith* (accumulated feces) (Figure 45-1; see also eFigure 45-1, Etiology of Acute Abdominal pain and pathophysiological sequelae, available on the Evolve Web site for this chapter) and intramural thickening caused by hypergrowth of lymphoid tissue. Obstruction results in edema, venous engorgement, and the invasion by bacteria, which can lead to gangrene and perforation.

Clinical Manifestations

Appendicitis typically begins with periumbilical pain, followed by anorexia, nausea, and vomiting. The pain is persistent and continuous, eventually shifting to the right lower quadrant and localizing at the McBurney point (located halfway between the umbilicus and the right iliac crest). Further assessment of the

patient reveals localized tenderness, rebound tenderness, and muscle guarding. The patient usually prefers to lie still, often with the right leg flexed. Low-grade fever may or may not be present, and coughing aggravates pain. The Rovsing sign may be elicited by palpation of the left lower quadrant, causing pain to be felt in the right lower quadrant. Complications of acute appendicitis are perforation, peritonitis, and abscesses (Ng, Fleming, Drumm, Waldron, & Grace, 2008).

Diagnostic Studies and Collaborative Care

Examination of the patient includes a complete history and physical examination (particularly palpation of the abdomen) and a differential WBC count. A urinalysis may be done to rule out genitourinary conditions that mimic the manifestations of appendicitis.

The treatment of appendicitis may include surgical removal (appendectomy) if the inflammation is localized. If the appendix has ruptured and there is evidence of peritonitis or an abscess, conservative treatment consisting of antibiotic therapy and parenteral fluids may be used to prevent sepsis and dehydration for 6 to 8 hours before an appendectomy is performed.

NURSING MANAGEMENT: APPENDICITIS

The patient with abdominal pain is encouraged to see a health care provider and to avoid self-treatment, particularly the use of laxatives and enemas. The increased peristalsis from these may cause perforation of the appendix. Until the patient is seen by a health care provider, nothing should be taken by mouth (NPO) to ensure that the stomach is empty in the event that surgery is needed. Local application of heat is never used because it may cause the appendix to rupture. In addition, the patient should be observed for evidence of peritonitis. Surgery is usually performed as soon as a diagnosis is made.

Postoperative nursing management is similar to postoperative care of the patient after laparotomy (see NCP 45-2). Ambulation begins the day of surgery or the first postoperative day. The diet is advanced as tolerated. The patient is usually discharged on the first or second postoperative day, and normal activities are resumed 2 to 3 weeks after surgery.

Peritonitis

Etiology and Pathophysiology

Peritonitis results from a localized or generalized inflammatory process of the peritoneum. Causes of peritonitis are listed in Table 45-15. Peritonitis may appear in acute and chronic forms; trauma or rupture of an organ containing chemical irritants or bacteria (which are released into the peritoneal cavity) may cause it. Examples of a chemical peritonitis include peptic ulcer perforation and ruptured ectopic pregnancy. A chemical peritonitis is commonly followed by bacterial invasion. Bacterial peritonitis can be caused by a traumatic injury (e.g., gunshot wound, ruptured appendix), or it can be secondary to other diseases or conditions (e.g., pancreatitis, peritoneal dialysis).

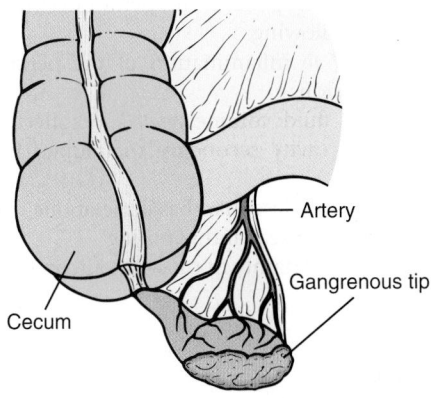

Figure 45-1 In appendicitis, the blood supply of the appendix is impaired by inflammation and bacterial infection in the wall of the appendix, which may result in gangrene.

Table 45-15 Causes of Peritonitis

Primary	
• Blood-borne organisms	• Diverticulitis with rupture
• Genital tract organisms	• Ischemic bowel disorders
• Cirrhosis with ascites	• Obstruction in the gastrointestinal tract
• GI tract organisms	• Pancreatitis
Secondary	• Perforated peptic ulcer
• Appendicitis with rupture	• Peritoneal dialysis
• Blunt or penetrating trauma to abdominal organs	• Postoperative anastomotic leak

GI, gastrointestinal.

The response of the peritoneum to the leakage of GI contents is to attempt to localize the offending agent by "walling it off" by exuding fibrin-containing fluids and swelling. Adhesions may form. These adhesions may reduce or disappear when the infection is eliminated. Normally, peritoneal injuries heal without formation of adhesions unless other factors, such as infection, ischemia, or foreign substances, are present.

Clinical Manifestations

Abdominal pain is the most common symptom of peritonitis. A universal sign of peritonitis is tenderness over the involved area. Rebound tenderness, muscular rigidity, and spasm are other major signs of irritation of the peritoneum. Abdominal distension or ascites, fever, tachycardia, tachypnea, nausea, vomiting, and altered bowel habits may also be present. These manifestations vary depending on severity and acuteness of the underlying cause. Complications of peritonitis include hypovolemic shock, septicemia, intra-abdominal abscess formation, paralytic ileus, and organ failure.

Diagnostic Studies

A CBC is done to determine elevations in WBC and hemoconcentration (Table 45-16). Peritoneal aspiration may be performed and the fluid analyzed for blood, bile, pus, bacteria, fungus, and amylase content. A radiograph of the abdomen may show dilated loops of bowel consistent with paralytic ileus, free air if perforation has occurred, or air–fluid levels if an obstruction is present. Ultrasound and CT scans may identify the presence of ascites and abscesses. *Peritoneoscopy* (an endoscope is placed through a stab wound in the abdomen to inspect the peritoneum) may be helpful in the patient without ascites. Direct examination of the peritoneum can be obtained along with biopsy specimens for diagnosis.

Collaborative Care

The goals of the management of peritonitis are to identify and eliminate the cause, combat infection, and prevent complications. Patients with milder cases of peritonitis or those who are poor surgical risks may be managed nonsurgically. Treatment consists of antibiotics, NG suction, analgesics, and IV fluid administration. Patients who require surgery need preoperative preparation as previously described. Those patients may be placed on total parenteral nutrition (TPN) because of increased nutritional requirements.

COLLABORATIVE CARE
Table 45-16 Peritonitis

Diagnostic	
• History and physical examination	• NG suction
• CBC	• Analgesics
• Serum electrolytes	• Preparation for surgery to include the above and nutritional support
• Abdominal radiographic examination	*Postoperative*
• Abdominal paracentesis and culture of fluid	• NPO status
• CT scan or ultrasound	• NG tube to suction
• Peritoneoscopy	• Semi-Fowler's position
Collaborative Therapy	• IV fluids with electrolyte replacement
Preoperative or Nonoperative	• Nutritional support as needed
• NPO status	• Antibiotic therapy
• Oxygen support	• Blood transfusions as needed
• Fluid replacement	• Sedatives and narcotics
• Antibiotic therapy	

CBC, complete blood count; *CT*, computed tomography; *IV*, intravenous; *NG*, nasogastric; *NPO*, nothing by mouth.

NURSING MANAGEMENT: PERITONITIS

Nursing Assessment

Assessment of the patient's pain, including the location, is important and may help in determining the cause of peritonitis. The patient should be assessed for the presence and the quality of bowel sounds, increasing abdominal distension, abdominal guarding, nausea, fever, and manifestations of hypovolemic and septic shock.

Nursing Diagnoses

Nursing diagnoses for the patient with peritonitis include, but are not limited to, the following:
• Acute pain *related to* inflammation of the peritoneum and abdominal distension
• Risk for deficient fluid volume *related to* collection of fluid in the peritoneal cavity secondary to trauma, infection, or ischemia
• Imbalanced nutrition: less than basal metabolic requirements *related to* anorexia, nausea, and vomiting
• Anxiety *related to* uncertainty of cause or outcome of condition and pain

Planning

The overall goals are that the patient with peritonitis will have (1) resolution of inflammation, (2) relief of abdominal pain, (3) freedom from complications, and (4) normal nutritional status.

Nursing Implementation

The patient with peritonitis is extremely ill and needs skilled supportive care. The patient is monitored for signs of sepsis, pain, and response to analgesic therapy. The patient may be positioned with knees flexed to increase comfort. The nurse should provide rest and a quiet environment. Sedatives may be given to allay anxiety.

Accurate monitoring of fluid intake and output and electrolyte status is necessary to determine replacement therapy. Vital signs are monitored frequently. Antiemetics may be administered to decrease nausea and vomiting and further fluid losses. The patient is on NPO status and may have an NG tube in place to decrease gastric distension.

If the patient has an open surgical procedure, drains are inserted to remove purulent drainage and excessive fluid. Postoperative care of the patient is similar to the care of the patient with an exploratory laparotomy (see NCP 45-2).

Gastroenteritis

Gastroenteritis is an inflammation of the mucosa of the stomach and the small intestine. Clinical manifestations include nausea, vomiting, diarrhea, abdominal cramping, and distension. Fever, increased WBCs, and blood or mucus in the stool may be present. Causative agents are varied (see Table 45-2). Most cases are self-limiting and do not necessitate hospitalization. However, older and chronically ill patients may be unable to consume sufficient fluids orally to compensate for fluid loss. Until vomiting has ceased, the patient should be on NPO status. If dehydration has occurred, IV replacement of fluids may be necessary. As soon as tolerated, oral fluids containing glucose and electrolytes should be given. If the causative agent is identified, appropriate pharmaceutical therapy is initiated.

NURSING MANAGEMENT: GASTROENTERITIS

Accurate monitoring of intake and output is important for successful replacement of lost fluid. Strict medical asepsis and infection control precautions should be instituted when indicated. The patient should be instructed in the importance of proper food handling and preparation of food to prevent infections such as salmonellosis and trichinosis (see Chapter 44, Table 44-27).

Symptomatic nursing care is given for nausea, vomiting, and diarrhea. The importance of rest and increased fluid intake should be stressed. The nurse should assess complaints of pain, vomiting, and diarrhea because gastroenteritis is often confused with appendicitis. To allay the patient's apprehension, the nurse should explain that gastroenteritis usually runs an acute course with no sequelae.

Inflammatory Bowel Disease

Inflammatory bowel disease (IBD) is an autoimmune disease that currently refers to two disorders of the GI tract (Crohn's disease and ulcerative colitis [UC]) characterized by idiopathic inflammation and ulceration. Although an antigen probably initiates the inflammation, the actual tissue damage is caused by an overactive, inappropriate, and sustained inflammatory response. Multiple factors are likely involved in the etiology of IBD (Noomen, Hommes, & Fidder, 2009). Both UC and Crohn's disease commonly occur during the teenage years and early adulthood, but both have a second peak in the fifties to seventies. Both are more prevalent in industrialized regions of the world. Epidemiological studies show a higher incidence of IBD in Whites (particularly those of Jewish descent) and in family members (especially monozygotic compared with dizygotic twins). Over 30 susceptibility genes have been linked to IBD (Cho, 2008). Some of the gene variations are associated with Crohn's disease only, whereas others are associated with both Crohn's disease and UC. The discovery of numerous gene variations suggests that IBD is a group of diseases (not just two) with multiple causes that produce similar types of mucosal destruction and thus manifest with similar symptoms (Achkar & Duerr, 2008). For both conditions, the clinical manifestations are varied, with unpredictable periods of remission interspersed with episodes of acute inflammation (Figure 45-2). Both diseases can be debilitating. In Canada, about 10,000 new cases of IBD are diagnosed annually. The incidence of newly diagnosed Crohn's disease appears to be increasing (Canadian Society of Intestinal Research, 2008).

Ulcerative Colitis

Ulcerative colitis (UC) is a chronic IBD characterized by inflammation and ulceration of the rectum and the colon. It may occur at any age but peaks between the ages of 15 and 25 years. There is a second, smaller peak onset between 60 and 80 years of age. UC equally affects both sexes (National Digestive Diseases Information Clearinghouse, 2006).

DETERMINANTS OF HEALTH
Colon Disorders

Physical Environment

- Inflammatory bowel disease (IBD) is more common in temperate regions of North America, South Africa, and Australia.
- Colorectal cancer is higher in Canada and the United States than in Japan, Finland, or Africa.

Biology and Genetic Endowment; Culture

- IBD is more common among Ashkenazi Jewish people and those of Scandinavian descent.

Etiology and Pathophysiology

The inflammation of UC is diffuse and involves the mucosa and the submucosa, with alternate periods of exacerbations and remissions (Table 45-17). The disease begins in the rectum and spreads proximally along the colon in a continuous fashion.

The mucosa of the rectum and the colon is hyperemic and edematous in the affected area (see eFigure 45-2, acute ulcerative colitis, available on the Evolve Web site for this chapter). Multiple abscesses develop in the crypts of Lieberkühn (intestinal glands).

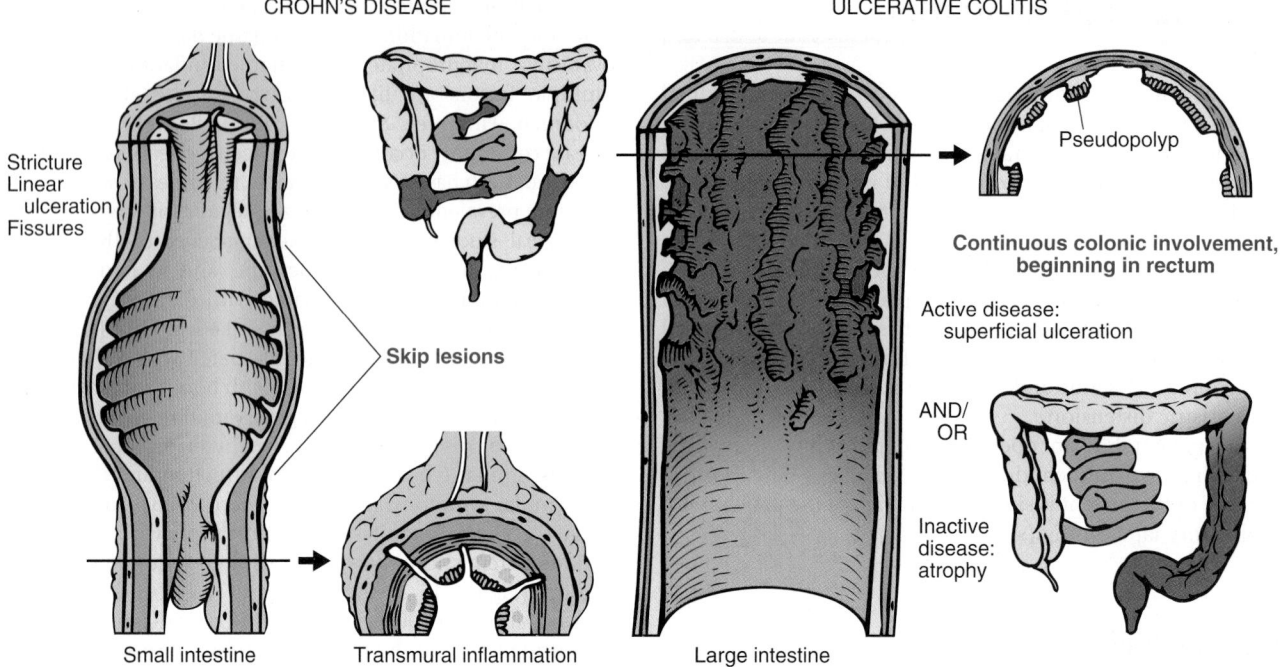

Figure 45-2 Comparison of distribution patterns of Crohn's disease and ulcerative colitis as well as different conformations of ulcers and wall thickenings.

Source: Kumar, V., Abbas, A. K., Fausto, N., & Mitchell, R. N. (2007). *Robbins basic pathology* (8th ed., p. 614, Figure 15-32). Philadelphia: Saunders.

EVIDENCE-INFORMED PRACTICE
Is Inflammatory Bowel Disease a Risk Factor for Osteoporosis?

Clinical Question
Do adults (P) with IBD (I) have a higher risk of osteoporosis (O) than adults without IBD (C)?

Best Available Evidence
Systematic review of research findings

Critical Appraisal and Synthesis of Evidence
- 40 studies (*n* = 48,000) with a majority being observations from IBD clinics.
- 50% of patients with Crohn's disease or ulcerative colitis had bone density levels within osteopenic or osteoporotic range.
- Hip fracture risk related to osteoporosis was greater in persons with IBD than in the general population.

Conclusion
- Patients with IBD are at higher risk for osteoporosis and related fractures.

Implications for Nursing Practice
- Counsel patients with IBD to modify osteoporosis risk factors where possible such as smoking cessation.
- Collaborate with health care providers to encourage osteoporosis treatment and prevention measures such as weight-bearing exercises and dietary or supplemental calcium and vitamin D.

Reference for Evidence
Lewis, N. R., & Scott, B. B. (2007). Guidelines for osteoporosis in inflammatory bowel disease and coeliac disease. London: British Society of Gastroenterology. Retrieved from *http://www.bsg.org.uk/images/stories/clinical/ost_coe_ibd.pdf*

IBD, inflammatory bowel disease.

As the disease advances, the abscesses break through the crypts into the submucosa, leaving ulcerations. These ulcerations also destroy the mucosal epithelium, causing bleeding and diarrhea. Losses of fluid and electrolytes occur because of the decreased mucosal surface area for absorption. Breakdown of cells results in protein loss through the stool. Areas of inflamed mucosa can form pseudopolyps, tonguelike projections into the bowel lumen.

Granulation tissue develops, and the mucosa musculature becomes thickened, shortening the colon.

Although the precipitating factors involved in UC are poorly understood, it is clear that the disease onset involves an inflammatory response. Specific proinflammatory cytokines such as tumour necrosis factor α (TNF-α) have been implicated in promoting this inflammatory response.

Table 45-17 Comparison of Ulcerative Colitis and Crohn's Disease

CHARACTERISTIC	ULCERATIVE COLITIS	CROHN'S DISEASE
Clinical		
Usual age at onset	Young to middle age	Young
Diarrhea	Common	Common
Abdominal cramping pain	Possible	Common
Fever (intermittent)	During acute episodes	Common
Weight loss	Common	Severe
Rectal bleeding	Common	Fairly common
Tenesmus	Severe	Rare
Malabsorption and nutritional deficiencies	Minimal incidence	Common
Pathological		
Location	Starts distally in the rectum and spreads proximally in a continuous fashion up the colon	Can occur anywhere along GI tract from mouth to anus, with characteristic skip lesions; most frequent site is terminal ileum
Distribution	Continuous	Segmental
Depth of involvement	Mucosa and submucosa	Entire thickness of bowel wall (transmural)
Granulomas	Absent	Common
Cobblestoning of mucosa	Rare	Common
Pseudopolyps	Common	Rare
Small bowel involvement	Minimal (backwash ileitis)	Common
Complications		
Fistulas	Rare	Common
Strictures	Rare	Common
Anal abscesses	Rare	Common
Perforation	Common	Common
Toxic megacolon	Common	Rare
Carcinoma	Increased incidence after 10 yr of disease	Slightly greater than general population
Recurrence after surgery	Cure with proctocolectomy	40-60% or more recurrence after segmental resections of small or large intestine

GI, gastrointestinal.

Table 45-18 Extraintestinal Manifestations of Inflammatory Bowel Disease

Musculoskeletal	***Metastatic Crohn's Disease***
• Peripheral arthritis (colitic)	**Mouth**
• Ankylosing spondylitis	• Aphthous ulcers (stomatitis)
• Sacroiliitis	**Ophthalmological**
• Osteoporosis	• Conjunctivitis
• Finger clubbing	• Uveitis
Dermatological	• Episcleritis
• Erythema nodosum	**Hepatobiliary**
• Pyoderma gangrenosum	• Gallstones
	• Primary sclerosing cholangitis
	• Portal vein thrombosis
	Genitourinary
	• Kidney stones

Pain may vary from the mild lower abdominal cramping associated with diarrhea to the severe, constant abdominal pain that may be associated with toxic megacolon and acute perforations. With mild disease, diarrhea may consist of one or two semi-formed stools containing small amounts of blood per day. The patient may have no other systemic manifestations. In moderate UC, there is increased stool output (four to five stools per day), increased bleeding, and systemic symptoms (fever, malaise, anorexia). In severe cases, diarrhea is bloody, contains mucus, and occurs 10 to 20 times a day. In addition, fever, weight loss greater than 10% of total body weight, anemia, tachycardia, and dehydration are present.

Complications

Complications of UC may be classified into those that are intestinal and those that are extraintestinal. Intestinal complications of UC include hemorrhage, perforation, toxic megacolon, and colonic dilation. Hemorrhage is a result of inflamed, ulcerated mucosa and is usually controlled with conservative medical therapy. Massive hemorrhage is unusual and requires emergency surgery. *Toxic megacolon* (extensive dilation and paralysis of the colon), bleeding, and fulminant colitis are the most common complications associated with UC. Colonic dilation, most often in the transverse colon, occurs as a result of severe acute inflammation of the entire colon wall. Perforation is most often associated with toxic megacolon but may occur alone. Most cases of perforation occur in the left side of the colon.

A patient who has had UC for more than 10 years is at greater risk of colorectal cancer. The risk of cancer depends on age at onset, duration, and extent of disease. The patient should be regularly screened with colonoscopy. Extraintestinal manifestations of the disease may be directly related to the colitis, or they may be nonspecific complications mediated by a disturbance in the immune system (Table 45-18). Colitis-related complications are associated with active inflammation and may respond to treatment of the underlying bowel disease. These manifestations can involve the joints, the skin, the mouth, and the eyes as well as disturbances of the hematological system including anemia, leukocytosis, and thrombocytosis. Skin lesions such as erythema

Clinical Manifestations

UC may appear as an acute fulminating crisis or, more commonly, as a chronic disorder with mild to severe acute exacerbations that occur at unpredictable intervals over many years. The major symptoms of UC are bloody diarrhea and abdominal pain.

COLLABORATIVE CARE

Table 45-19 Ulcerative Colitis

Diagnostic	Severe (Fulminant) Disease
• History and physical examination	• IV fluids with electrolytes
• Colonoscopy	• Blood transfusions
• Sigmoidoscopy	• NPO status
• Barium enema	• Nutritional support (parenteral therapy)
• CBC, electrolytes, BUN,* creatinine, albumin	• Antimicrobial therapy†
• Culture and sensitivity testing of stool (including *Clostridium difficile*)	• Immunosuppressants†
	• Immunomodulators†
Collaborative Therapy	• Corticosteroids†
Mild and Moderate Disease	• Surgery if no improvement
• Nutritional support (low-residue diet and no dairy products)	
• Antimicrobial therapy†	
• 5-Aminosalicylates†	
• Corticosteroids†	
• Antidiarrheal agents†	

BUN, blood urea nitrogen; *CBC,* complete blood count; *IV,* intravenous; *NPO,* nothing by mouth.
*Serum urea (nitrogen).
†See Table 45-20.

DRUG THERAPY

Table 45-20 Inflammatory Bowel Disease

CATEGORY	ACTION	EXAMPLES
Antimicrobial	Prevent or treat secondary infection	Metronidazole (Flagyl) Ciprofloxacin (Cipro)
5-Aminosalicylates (5-ASA)	Decrease GI inflammation*	*Systemic:* Sulphasalazine (Salazopyrin) Mesalazine (Asacol, Pentasa) Olsalazine (Dipentum) *Rectal suppository:* Mesalazine (Salofalk)
Corticosteroids	Decrease inflammation	*Systemic:* corticosteroids (cortisone, prednisone, budesonide) *Enemas:* hydrocortisone (Cortenema), budesonide (Entocort) *Rectal foam:* hydrocortisone (Cortifoam)
Antidiarrheal	Decrease GI motility†	Diphenoxylate (Lomotil)
Immunosuppressants	Suppress immune response	Azathioprine (Imuran), cyclosporine (Neoral)
Immunomodulators	Inhibit the cytokine tumour necrosis factor α (TNF-α)	Infliximab (Remicade), adalimumab (Humira)
Hematinics and vitamins	Correct iron deficiency anemia and promote healing	Oral iron: ferrous sulphate, ferrous gluconate Iron injection: iron dextran (Infufer), iron sucrose (Venofer)

GI, gastrointestinal.
*Mechanism of action unknown, possibly antimicrobial as well as anti-inflammatory.
†Used with caution during severe disease because of potential to produce toxic megacolon.

nodosum and pyoderma gangrenosum are among the most frequently seen extraintestinal manifestations (Agrawal, Rukkannagari, & Kethus, 2007). Uveitis is the most common eye problem. Hepatobiliary disease may accompany UC (Agrawal, et al., 2007).

Diagnostic Studies

Several studies are appropriate for diagnosis of UC (Table 45-19). Blood studies should include a CBC, serum electrolyte levels, and serum protein levels. A CBC typically shows iron-deficiency anemia from blood loss. An elevated WBC count may indicate toxic megacolon or perforation. Decreases in serum electrolytes, such as sodium, potassium, chloride, bicarbonate, and magnesium, are caused by fluid and electrolyte losses from diarrhea. Hypoalbuminemia is present with severe disease and results from protein loss from the bowel. The stool should be examined for blood, pus, and mucus. Stool cultures should be obtained to rule out infectious causes of inflammation.

Examinations with a sigmoidoscope and a colonoscope allow direct examination of the mucosa of the lower GI tract. Using a sigmoidoscope, the health care provider can view the rectum, the sigmoid colon, and the distal descending colon. The colonoscope allows for examination of the entire large intestine. The extent of inflammation, ulcerations, pseudopolyps, strictures, and lesions may be identified. Biopsy specimens should be taken for definitive diagnosis. Scopes should not be used when the rectum and the colon are severely inflamed because of the risk of perforation.

A double-contrast barium enema may show areas of granular inflammation with ulcerations. The colon may appear narrow and shortened, and pseudopolyps may be present. A double-contrast study (in which air is introduced into the bowel after the expulsion of barium) is effective in detecting mucosal abnormalities in UC.

Collaborative Care

The goals of treatment are to (1) rest the bowel, (2) control the inflammation, (3) manage fluids and nutrition, (4) manage patient stress, (5) provide education about the disease and treatment, and (6) provide symptomatic relief. The mainstays of drug therapy are sulphasalazine and corticosteroids. Hospitalization is indicated if the patient fails to respond to corticosteroid therapy or if complications are suspected.

Drug Therapy. Drug therapy is an extremely important aspect of treatment (Table 45-20) (Swaminath & Kornbluth, 2007).

The principal drug used is sulphasalazine, a combination of sulphapyridine and 5-aminosalicylic acid (5-ASA). It is effective in the maintenance of clinical remission and in the treatment of mild to moderately severe disease episodes. After remission is obtained, therapy is continued with a gradual reduction over several months. The maintenance dose is usually continued for at least 1 year.

During active disease, 5-ASA (the active form of sulphasalazine) and corticosteroid enemas are effective in the treatment of left-sided UC and proctitis. Topical salicylate therapy is the treatment of choice in patients with localized disease. 5-ASA (mesalazine) can also be administered orally. The acrylic-coated tablets provide delivery of the drug more distally in the intestine.

Corticosteroids are of proven benefit in the management of active UC. Oral prednisone or prednisolone is effective in treatment of mild to moderate disease without systemic manifestations. If remission is not achieved, the patient requires hospitalization and IV corticosteroid therapy. The patient is placed on a regimen of bowel rest. Fluids and electrolytes are administered intravenously. For *proctitis* (inflammation of the rectum and the anus), hydrocortisone enemas, rectal foams, or suppositories can be effective in the treatment of inflammation. Rectal foams are usually administered in 5-mL volumes, and patients can generally administer this themselves. Enemas are the preferred choice if the disease spreads beyond the rectum. Retention enemas have been shown to deliver drugs into the descending colon and beyond in patients with active disease. The patient taking corticosteroids needs to be monitored for common adverse effects such as Cushing's syndrome, hypertension, hirsutism, and mood swings.

Immunosuppressive drugs (e.g., cyclosporine) have been used in severe cases of UC when a patient has failed to respond to any of the usual drugs and before surgery is considered. Adverse effects of cyclosporine include renal dysfunction, hypertension, headache, and muscle cramps. Regular cyclosporine trough levels should be determined to ensure proper dosing of this medication. Therapeutic response to IV cyclosporine usually allows for conversion to an oral preparation for long-term therapy. Anti–TNF-α blocking agents (e.g., infliximab [Remicade]) were previously considered for use more with Crohn's disease; they are now considered more valuable in the management of moderate to severe refractory UC (Lawson, Thomas, & Akobeng, 2008).

Surgical Therapy.
Approximately 80 to 85% of patients with UC go into remission with conservative therapy and nursing management, but 15 to 20% require surgery. Surgery is indicated if (1) the patient fails to respond to treatment; (2) exacerbations are frequent and debilitating; (3) massive bleeding, perforation, strictures, or obstruction occur; (4) there are tissue changes that suggest that dysplasia is occurring; or (5) carcinoma develops.

Surgical procedures used to treat chronic UC include (1) total proctocolectomy with permanent ileostomy and (2) proctocolectomy with ileoanal reservoir.

Total Proctocolectomy with Permanent Ileostomy. Total proctocolectomy with a permanent ileostomy is a one-stage operation involving the removal of the colon, the rectum, and the anus, with closure of the anus. The end of the terminal ileum is brought out through the abdominal wall and forms a stoma, or ostomy. The stoma is usually placed in the right lower quadrant within the rectus muscle.

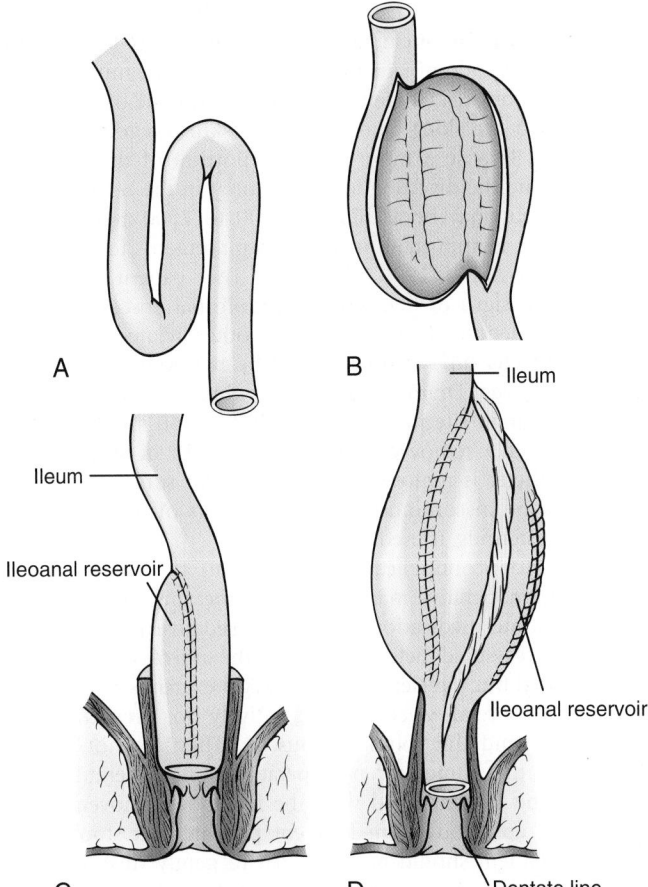

Figure 45-3 Ileoanal reservoir. **A,** Formation of a reservoir. **B,** Posterior suture lines completed. **C,** J-shaped configuration for an ileoanal reservoir. **D,** S-shaped configuration for an ileoanal reservoir.

Total Proctocolectomy with Ileoanal Reservoir. A more widely performed procedure involves total colectomy with the formation of an ileal reservoir and anal anastomosis (Figure 45-3). The ileoanal reservoir surgical procedure is usually a staged approach encompassing a combination of one to three procedures performed approximately 12 weeks apart. The initial procedure generally includes a colectomy with temporary end ileostomy and a possible mucous fistula. The second surgery involves takedown of the ileostomy and mucous fistula, resection of the rectal stump to just above the anal sphincters, and formation of the ileal reservoir and subsequent anastomosis to the anus, with a diverting temporary loop ileostomy (to protect the reservoir during healing). The final, third, surgery involves a takedown of the loop ileostomy, which functionalizes the reservoir. Depending upon the preoperative health of the patient, these staged surgeries may be combined into a two-stage procedure or a single operation. Adaptation to the reservoir occurs over the next 3 to 6 months, which usually results in a bowel movement frequency of four to eight pasty stools per day and good daytime continence.

Patient selection includes absence of colorectal cancer, small intestine free of disease (e.g., Crohn's disease), competent anorectal sphincter, and physical status adequate to permit lengthy surgery. In addition, the patient needs to be motivated and capable of understanding self-care instructions.

Postoperative Care. *Postoperative* care following surgical procedures to treat UC includes routine observations for patients who have had abdominal surgery. Stoma viability, mucocutaneous border (the area where the mucous membrane of the bowel is sutured to the skin), and peristomal skin integrity must be monitored. Because a more proximal portion of the bowel is used to create the diverting loop ileostomy in the second stage, stomal output may be as high as 1500 to 2000 mL/24 hr. IV fluid support is important, including replacements for excessive ileostomy losses (>1200 mL/24 hr). The patient must be observed for signs of hemorrhage, abdominal abscesses, small bowel obstruction, dehydration, and other related complications. If an NG tube is used, it will be removed when bowel function returns. Drainage of serosanguineous fluid from the abdominal drain site may vary from 100 to 150 mL/24 hr. The drain is usually removed within 3 to 4 days of surgery. The urinary catheter is removed 2 to 4 days after surgery. Systemic antibiotics are discontinued within 24 hours of the operation, and corticosteroids, if used, are tapered.

Transient incontinence of mucus from the reservoir is a result of intraoperative manipulation of the anal canal and the effects of some medications (narcotics, sedatives). The patient should be reassured before and after the operation regarding this potential but transient problem. Kegel exercises may be recommended several weeks postoperatively to strengthen the pelvic floor and the sphincter muscles. They are not recommended in the immediate postoperative period. Perianal skin care must be implemented with the first bowel movement to protect the epidermis from frequent pericare and stool irritation. The patient should be instructed to gently rinse the skin with water or a spray cleanser with a surfactant and dry thoroughly. A barrier cream should be used, and a perineal pad may be required.

The most frequent type of ileostomy that is constructed is a loop. This can present as a pouching challenge because the os (opening) may tilt down and drain inferiorly such that stool causes irritation to the surrounding skin. An enterostomal therapy (ET) nurse will help with these challenging problems. Self-care instructions should be taught and reviewed, and written information with discharge supplies should be provided before discharge. Stoma care is presented later in this chapter (see Nursing Management: Ostomy Surgery, p. 1222).

Nutritional Therapy. An important component in the treatment of UC is diet. The dietitian is an important member of the team and should be consulted regarding dietary recommendations. The goals of diet management are to provide adequate nutrition without exacerbating symptoms, to correct and prevent malnutrition, to replace fluid and electrolyte losses, and to prevent weight loss. The diet for each patient must be individualized.

Traditionally, during the acute phase, the patient may be on NPO status. When food is permitted, a high-calorie, high-protein, low-residue diet with vitamin and iron supplements is frequently prescribed. (A low-residue diet is presented in Table 45-21.) Special dietary restrictions are not usually necessary. Some health care providers allow the patient to eat anything that does not cause symptoms. Cold foods, high-residue foods (whole wheat bread, cereal with bran, nuts, raw fruit), and smoking increase GI motility and should be avoided. Fish oil preparations have been evaluated for their ability to reduce inflammation in active UC. However, their palatability has been low.

Often, enteral supplements and parenteral nutrition are necessary. Patients with systemic manifestations, significant fluid and electrolyte losses, or malabsorption may need parenteral nutrition or enteral feedings, such as elemental diets. Elemental diets are high in calories and nutrients, lactose free, and absorbed in the proximal small intestine.

Parenteral nutrition allows for a positive nitrogen balance. Vitamins, minerals, electrolytes, and other important nutrients (e.g., glucose, amino acids) can be administered to promote healing and correct nutritional deficiencies. (TPN is discussed in Chapter 42.)

Supplemental iron (ferrous sulphate or ferrous gluconate) may be necessary to prevent or treat iron-deficiency anemia resulting from chronic blood loss. Parenteral iron may be needed for patients who cannot tolerate oral iron. Iron dextran (DexIron, Infufer) administered intramuscularly by Z-track or intravenously may be necessary if anemia is severe. In patients receiving long-term sulphasalazine therapy, folic acid deficiency may develop, and supplementation may be necessary. Potassium supplements may be necessary if corticosteroid therapy is used because retention of sodium and loss of potassium can result in hypokalemia and subsequent toxic megacolon. Zinc deficiency can result from severe or chronic diarrhea, and supplementation may be necessary.

NURSING MANAGEMENT: ULCERATIVE COLITIS

Nursing Assessment

Subjective and objective data that should be obtained from a patient with UC are presented in Table 45-22.

Nursing Diagnoses

Nursing diagnoses for the patient with UC include, but are not limited to, those presented in NCP 45-3.

Planning

The overall goals are that the patient with UC will (1) respond to medical management, (2) maintain normal fluid and electrolyte balance, (3) be free from pain or discomfort, (4) participate in medical and surgical management, and (5) maintain nutritional balance.

Nursing Implementation

During the acute phase, attention is focused on hemodynamic stability, pain control, fluid and electrolyte balance, and nutritional support. Accurate intake and output records must be maintained. The number and characteristics of stools are monitored. Nursing care of the patient with UC is directed toward an intensive therapeutic and supportive program (see NCP 45-3). It is important that the nurse establishes a good working relationship and encourages the patient to talk about himself or herself and daily activities. An explanation of all

NUTRITIONAL THERAPY

Table 45-21 Low-Residue Diet

Purpose

Low-residue diet provides foods low in fibre, which will result in a reduced amount of fecal material in the lower intestinal tract.

General Principles

1. This diet eliminates foods that are indigestible or stimulating to the intestinal tract to reduce the amount of residue in the colon. Foods should be included or excluded according to the following list.

2. Hot and cold foods should be eaten slowly.

3. Milk products are limited to 2 cups daily. For a more restricted-residue diet, milk should be eliminated.

FOOD	FOODS INCLUDED	FOODS EXCLUDED
Beverages	Carbonated drinks, coffee, tea, cocoa, strained fruit juices	Alcohol, fruit juices with pulp
Bread	White bread, rolls, rusk, melba toast, crackers	Bread and crackers containing whole grain flour or bran; any hot breads such as biscuits, muffins, waffles, or pancakes
Cereals	Cooked, refined, or strained cereals: cream of wheat, cream of rice, farina, grits, dry cereals without bran; noodles; spaghetti; and macaroni	Whole grain cereals; cereals containing bran, nuts, and raisins; Shredded Wheat
Meat	Lean, tender ground beef, lamb, pork, veal or fish, broiled, stewed, or baked; canned tuna or salmon; shellfish; crisp bacon, chicken or turkey without skin, liver; creamy peanut butter	Fried, smoked, pickled, or cured meats; highly seasoned ham; fried fish; luncheon meats
Egg	All but fried	Fried or uncooked eggs
Cheese	Milk, cheese (aged cheddar), cottage cheese	All other cheeses
Milk	Limit to 1-2 cups (if tolerated), including that used in cooking; plain yogourt	Fruit yogourt
Fats	Butter, margarine, cream, oil, crisp bacon, mayonnaise, plain gravy	Any other; rich or spiced gravies
Soup	Cream and vegetable soups made from foods allowed and with quantity of milk allowed, bouillon, broth; strained vegetable juices	Cream and vegetable soups from foods not allowed (peas and dried beans)
Vegetables	Cooked or canned vegetables; strained vegetables; potatoes without skins; vegetable juices	Raw vegetables, all vegetables not strained, dried beans, peas, and legumes
Fruits	Strained fruit juices, cooked or canned fruits; ripe bananas, applesauce, pears, peaches, peeled apricots, Napoleon cherries, baked apple (no skin)	Raw fruits, fruits with skins, seeds
Desserts	Plain desserts (custards and puddings, plain ice cream for milk allowance), sherbet, plain gelatin desserts, angel food cake, sponge cake, plain butter cake, plain cookies	Nuts, coconut, raisins, rich desserts (pies, rich cakes, cobblers)
Condiments	Allspice, cinnamon, mace, paprika, salt, ground thyme, sugar, vinegar, lemon juice	All others

MENU PLAN	BREAKFAST	LUNCH		DINNER
MEAL	½ cup applesauce ½ cup Cream of Wheat 1 Scrambled egg White toast Butter or jelly 1 cup milk Coffee	Roast beef sandwich on 2 slices white bread (no lettuce or tomato) 1 tbsp mayonnaise 2 sugar cookies Canned peach halves Coffee		Baked chicken Mashed potato Cooked carrots White bread Butter Angel food cake 1 cup milk Coffee

procedures and treatment is necessary and may allay some apprehension.

Psychosocial support may be indicated if the patient is experiencing emotional problems, but the nurse must recognize that the patient's behaviour may result from factors other than emotional ones. Any person who has 10 to 20 bowel movements a day and has rectal discomfort may be anxious, frustrated, discouraged, and depressed. Along with other team members, the nurse can assist the patient to accept the chronic condition and to have an optimistic view with the possibility of cure after surgery. The nurse may find that inadequate coping mechanisms in the patient with UC are owing to early onset of the disease (often at 10-15 years of age), which may have interfered with usual growth, development, and maturation.

Restricted physical activity and possibly bed rest may be ordered if the patient has a severe exacerbation. Nursing interven-

NURSING ASSESSMENT

Table 45-22 Ulcerative Colitis

Subjective Data

Important Health Information

Past health history: Infection; autoimmune disorders; family history of inflammatory bowel disease

Medications: Use of antidiarrheal medications, steroids, other immunosuppressives; herbal, homeopathic, or naturopathic remedies

Symptoms

- Fatigue, malaise
- Nausea, vomiting, anorexia; weight loss; dietary intolerances
- Frequent bloody stools containing mucus and pus
- Lower abdominal pain (worse before defecating), cramping, tenesmus

Objective Data

General

Intermittent fever; emaciated appearance

Integumentary

Pale skin with poor turgor, dry mucous membranes; rash, nodules (on lower legs), or blisters; anorectal irritation

Gastrointestinal

Abdominal distension, hyperactive bowel sounds

Cardiovascular

Tachycardia, hypotension (including postural)

Possible Findings

Anemia; leukocytosis; electrolyte imbalance; hypoalbuminemia; vitamin and trace metal deficiencies; abnormal sigmoidoscopic, colonoscopic, and barium enema findings

tions to prevent complications of immobility should be instituted. Teaching related to treatment, drugs, diet, diagnostic tests, and the disease and its management is important.

Rest is important in the management of UC. Patients may lose much sleep because of frequent episodes of diarrhea and abdominal pain. Nutritional deficiencies and anemia leave the patient feeling weak and listless. Activities should be scheduled around rest periods. Nurses can provide physical and emotional support to the patient during acute exacerbations.

Until diarrhea is controlled, the patient must be kept clean, dry, and free of odour. Facilitating management of bowel movements, including close proximity to a bathroom or a bedside commode, is helpful. A deodorizer should be placed in the room. Antidiarrheal agents should be administered as ordered. If the patient has continuous diarrhea, the ET nurse may give helpful suggestions. Meticulous perianal skin care using plain water or a skin cleanser (no harsh soap) is necessary to treat and prevent skin breakdown. Use of skin barrier creams may help to protect perianal skin.

Evaluation

The expected outcomes for the patient with UC are presented in NCP 45-3.

Crohn's Disease

Crohn's disease is a chronic IBD of unknown origin that can affect any part of the GI tract from the mouth to the anus. Crohn's disease occurs most often between the ages of 15 and 30

NURSING CARE PLAN 45-3

Inflammatory Bowel Disease

NURSING DIAGNOSIS	*Diarrhea related to* irritated bowel and intestinal hyperactivity *as evidenced by* frequent diarrheal stools (>10/day)
Expected Patient Outcome	**Nursing Interventions and *Rationales***
• Reports fewer, firmer stools	• Monitor frequency and character of stools *to evaluate effectiveness of therapy and dietary restrictions.* • Maintain food and fluid restrictions *to rest bowel during exacerbations.* • Teach patient to avoid smoking, caffeine, and foods or fluids that are irritating to bowel or cause increased motility.
NURSING DIAGNOSIS	*Anxiety related to* diagnosis, possible social embarrassment, unfamiliar environment, diagnostic tests, and treatment *as evidenced by* expression of concerns about effect of disease on social relationships and questions about disease and treatment
Expected Patient Outcome	**Nursing Interventions and *Rationales***
• Experiences decreased anxiety	• Monitor for signs of anxiety *to plan appropriate interventions.* • Encourage open discussion of feelings about diagnosis *to demonstrate acceptance and concern for patient and allow verbalization of concerns.* • Explain disease treatments, diagnostic tests, and drugs *because understanding may reduce anxiety.* • Provide privacy *to reduce embarrassment and anxiety associated with frequent bowel movements.*

NURSING CARE PLAN 45-3

Inflammatory Bowel Disease—cont'd

NURSING DIAGNOSIS	*Imbalanced nutrition: less than body requirements* related to decreased intake, decreased absorption, and increased nutrient loss through diarrhea *as evidenced by* anorexia, weight loss, weakness, lethargy, or anemia.
Expected Patient Outcomes	**Nursing Interventions and *Rationales***
• Reports maintenance of body weight within normal range • Reports adequate nutritional intake • Reports increased strength and activity tolerance	• Assess for signs of malnutrition (e.g., hair loss, fatigue) *to direct plan for treating the problem.* • Record daily weights *to evaluate nutritional status and response to treatment.* • Perform ongoing calorie counts *to determine adequacy of caloric intake.* • Administer IV fluids and TPN as ordered *to allow for a positive nitrogen balance while resting the bowel.* • Give and instruct patient on high-calorie, nonspicy, caffeine-free, low-residue diet with small, frequent feedings *to reduce discomfort associated with eating.* • Administer nutritional supplements (as ordered) *to provide additional calories, protein, and fluid.* • Refer patient to a dietitian for assessment and management.
NURSING DIAGNOSIS	*Impaired skin integrity* related to diarrhea and altered nutritional status *as evidenced by* denuded perianal area and discomfort around perianal area during and after evacuation
Expected Patient Outcome	**Nursing Interventions and *Rationales***
• Has no evidence of skin breakdown in the perianal area	• Assess skin for signs of breakdown *to ensure early intervention.* • Cleanse perianal area after each bowel movement with warm water or perianal skin cleanser, and dry thoroughly *to remove stool, provide comfort, and prevent skin breakdown.* • Provide sitz baths for comfort and hygiene, and apply barrier cream. • Instruct patient and caregivers on proper skin care techniques *to enable them to participate fully in treatment plan.*
NURSING DIAGNOSIS	*Ineffective coping* related to chronic disease, lifestyle changes, stress, and pain *as evidenced by* inability to express feelings and concerns
Expected Patient Outcome	**Nursing Interventions and *Rationales***
• Expresses development of healthy coping behaviours	• Identify ineffective behaviours, and institute plan *to assist patient in learning more effective behaviours.* • Encourage patient's expression of feelings *to provide support as patient explores areas of concern and add to patient's feelings of self-worth.* • Offer reassurance and psychological support *to demonstrate caring and concern.* • Know limitations and refer to counselling when appropriate because more intensive treatment may be required *to deal with specific stress or problem areas.* • Refer patient to a social worker or spiritual services. • Identify community support groups.
NURSING DIAGNOSIS	*Ineffective self-health management* related to lack of knowledge of course of disease, appropriate lifestyle adjustments, and nutritional and drug therapy *as evidenced by* questioning about disease and treatment and poor decisions about activities of daily living
Expected Patient Outcome	**Nursing Interventions and *Rationales***
• Repeats correct information about disease and treatment	• Provide information about the disease *to ensure that patient has adequate knowledge about the disease and treatment.* • Teach about the relationships of stress to the disease *because stress may stimulate hyperreactivity of the colon in susceptible persons.* • Teach stress reduction techniques to assist patient in developing positive ways *to reduce stress.* • Recommend regular colorectal cancer screening *because of increased risk of cancer.*

IV, intravenous; *TPN,* total parenteral nutrition.

years. When it occurs in older adults, the morbidity and mortality rates are higher because of other chronic problems that may be present. Both sexes are affected, with a slightly higher incidence in women. Similar to UC, it occurs more often in Jewish and upper–middle-class urban populations. Canada may have one of the highest incidence rates of both Crohn's disease and UC in the world.

Etiology and Pathophysiology

Crohn's disease is characterized by inflammation of segments of the GI tract. It can affect any part of the GI tract but is most often seen in the terminal ileum and the colon. Approximately 5% of patients with Crohn's disease have ileojejunitis. Involvement of the esophagus, the stomach, or the duodenum is uncommon. The inflammation involves all layers of the bowel wall (i.e., transmural). Areas of involvement are usually discontinuous *skip lesions,* with segments of normal bowel occurring between diseased portions (see Table 45-17). Typically, ulcerations are deep and longitudinal and penetrate between islands of inflamed edematous mucosa, causing the classic cobblestone appearance (see eFigure 45-3, Crohn's Disease, on the Evolve Web site for this chapter). Thickening of the bowel wall occurs as well as narrowing of the lumen with stricture development. The areas of inflammation can extend through all layers of the bowel wall. Abscesses or fistula tracts that communicate with other loops of bowel, the skin, the bladder, the rectum, or the vagina may develop. Histologically, granulomas (chronic inflammatory lesions) are present in 50% of patients and may be located in any layer of the bowel wall.

TNF-α may be directly related to the pathogenesis of Crohn's disease. Levels of TNF-α are elevated in the stools of patients with Crohn's disease and correlate with disease activity. Treatment with the TNF-α blocker (discussed later in the section on drug therapy) decreases endoscopic and histological disease activity in Crohn's colitis (Swaminath & Kornbluth, 2007). Other proinflammatory cytokines may also be involved in the pathophysiology of Crohn's disease (e.g., interleukin-1 [IL-1], IL-6).

Clinical Manifestations

The manifestations depend largely on the anatomical site of involvement, the extent of the disease process, and the presence or absence of complications. The onset of Crohn's disease is usually insidious, with nonspecific complaints such as diarrhea, fatigue, abdominal pain, weight loss, and fever. Early diagnosis may be more difficult than for UC. The principal manifestations of Crohn's disease are diarrhea and abdominal pain. Diarrhea is usually nonbloody and is a result of the inflammatory process or malabsorption. Pain may be severe and intermittent or constant, depending on the cause. Other manifestations include abdominal cramping and tenderness, abdominal distension, fever, and fatigue. Similar to UC, extraintestinal complications may be directly related to the GI inflammation and small intestinal pathological conditions (malabsorption), or they may be nonspecific complications mediated by a disturbance in the immune system. Extraintestinal manifestations, such as arthritis and finger clubbing, may precede the onset of bowel disease. As the disease progresses, there is weight loss, malnutrition, dehydration, electrolyte imbalances, anemia, increased peristalsis, pain around the umbilicus and right lower quadrant, and possible perianal disease.

Crohn's disease is a chronic disorder with unpredictable periods of recurrence and remission. Attacks are intermittent, usually recurring over a period of several weeks to months.

Complications

Complications, both GI and extraintestinal, are common in Crohn's disease. Scar tissue from the inflammation and ulceration narrows the lumen of the intestine and may cause strictures and obstruction, a frequent complication. Fistulas are a cardinal feature and may develop between segments of bowel. Cutaneous fistulas, common in the perianal area, and rectovaginal fistulas also occur. Fistulas communicating with the urinary tract may cause urinary tract infections. Inflammation of the intestines may involve all layers, predisposing the patient to perforation and the formation of intra-abdominal abscesses and peritonitis (World Gastrointestinal Organization, 2009).

Impaired absorption causing various nutritional abnormalities may occur as a result of damage to areas of the intestinal mucosa. Fat malabsorption causes a deficiency in the fat-soluble vitamins (A, D, E, and K). The patient may have an intolerance to gluten (a protein found in barley, rye, and wheat).

Systemic complications are similar to those of UC and include arthritis, liver disease, cholelithiasis (especially with ileal involvement), ankylosing spondylitis, pyoderma gangrenosum, erythema nodosum, and uveitis. Renal disorders are common, especially nephrolithiasis (kidney stones) secondary to increased oxalate absorption.

Diagnostic Studies

Diagnosis of Crohn's disease can be made by means of a thorough history and physical examination, to establish clinical signs and symptoms; barium studies; and endoscopy with biopsy (Table 45-23). Laboratory studies may determine electrolyte disturbances and the presence of anemia. Barium studies are useful in determining location and extent of the disease and may reveal classic findings, such as stricture formations in the ileum (string sign), cobblestoning of the mucosa, fistulas, and areas of abnormal and normal mucosa. Endoscopic studies, such as

COLLABORATIVE CARE

Table 45-23 Crohn's Disease

Diagnostic	*Collaborative Therapy*
• History and physical examination	• High-calorie, high-vitamin, high-protein, low-residue, dairy-free diet
• CBC	• Antimicrobial agents*
• Serum chemistries	• Corticosteroid drugs*
• Testing of stool for occult blood	• Immunosuppressants*
• Radiological studies with barium contrast	• Immunomodulators*
• Sigmoidoscopy and colonoscopy with biopsy	• Supplementary parenteral nutrition
	• Elemental diet
	• Physical and emotional rest
	• Surgery†

CBC, complete blood count.
*See Table 45-20.
†See Table 45-24.

colonoscopy and sigmoidoscopy, are useful in detecting such early mucosal changes as patchy inflammation, small ulcerations, and skip areas that may not be seen radiologically. Biopsies may be performed to determine the presence of granulomas. Barium studies are performed to determine the degree of ileal involvement. Upper GI barium studies are done to diagnose upper gastroduodenal disease. Because an endoscope can enter only the distal ileum, capsule endoscopy may be used in the diagnosis of small intestine disease. Thus far, capsule endoscopy has been shown to have greater sensitivity than radiography when diagnosing Crohn's disease (Panaccione et al., 2008). However, biopsies cannot be obtained with either capsule endoscopy or barium enema.

Collaborative Care

The goal of collaborative care is to control the inflammatory process, relieve symptoms, correct metabolic and nutritional problems, and promote healing. Drug therapy and nutritional support are the mainstays of treatment.

Drug Therapy.
Drug therapy for Crohn's disease is presented in Table 45-20. Sulphasalazine is effective when the disease involves the large intestine but is much less effective when only the small intestine is involved. Corticosteroid therapy is effective in reducing inflammation and suppressing disease. The dosage and the route of administration depend on severity of the illness and the area involved. Once clinical symptoms subside, the dosage should be tapered (Swaminath & Kornbluth, 2007). Immunosuppressive agents (azathioprine) may be tried if repeated trials with corticosteroids fail. Patients require close monitoring because of the serious adverse effects of these drugs. Metronidazole (Flagyl) is useful in treating Crohn's disease of the perianal area. Marked exacerbations have been reported when the drug is stopped. In patients with Crohn's disease in remission, fish oil preparations have been evaluated for their ability to prevent recurrence of inflammation; however, their palatability has been low.

Biological drug therapies of Crohn's disease include monoclonal antibodies to TNF-α (infliximab [Remicade]), adalimumab [Humira]), and to a leukocyte adhesion molecule (natalizumab [Tysabri]). Infliximab has been shown to reduce the degree of inflammation in patients who are refractory to other drug therapies. However, not all patients with Crohn's disease respond to infliximab.

Nutritional Therapy.
Elemental diets and parenteral nutrition may be used in the patient with Crohn's disease (see Chapter 42). Parenteral nutrition may be given to patients with severe disease, small bowel fistulas, or short bowel syndrome (described later in this chapter). It is given before and after surgery to promote wound healing, reduce complications, and hasten recovery. The elemental diet provides a high-calorie, high-nitrogen, fat-free, no-residue substrate that is absorbed in the proximal small bowel. This diet can be given to most patients with Crohn's disease, even during acute exacerbations.

The diet should otherwise be low in residue, roughage, and fat but high in calories and protein. It may be difficult to maintain adequate absorption during periods of disease exacerbation and even during periods of remission. Milk and milk products may have to be excluded from the diet. Lactose, the primary disaccharide found in milk, may not be adequately digested because of the inability of the damaged intestinal mucosa to produce

Table 45-24 Indications for Surgical Therapy of Crohn's Disease

- Drainage of abdominal abscess
- Failure to respond to conservative therapy
- Fistulas
- Inability to decrease corticosteroids
- Intestinal obstruction
- Massive hemorrhage
- Perforation
- Secondary hydronephrosis
- Severe anorectal disease
- Suspicion of carcinoma

sufficient amounts of lactase. High-fat diets are poorly tolerated because of the loss of absorbing mucosa and altered bile salt metabolism and absorption.

Vitamin deficiencies may develop as a result of malabsorption. Cobalamin (vitamin B_{12}) injections every month may be needed because of the inability of the terminal ileum (if affected) to absorb this vitamin.

Surgical Therapy.
Surgery is used in patients with severe symptoms that are unresponsive to therapy and in those with life-threatening complications. The majority of patients with Crohn's disease eventually require surgery at least once in the course of their disease. Indications for surgery are outlined in Table 45-24. Unlike UC, Crohn's disease is not cured by surgery. The recurrence rate after surgery is high. The surgical procedure depends on the affected area and the condition of the patient. Conservative intestinal resection with anastomosis of healthy bowel is the procedure of choice.

NURSING MANAGEMENT: CROHN'S DISEASE

Care of the patient is similar to that of the patient with UC (see NCP 45-3). As the patient's condition improves, the nurse should allow for more self-care, provide frequent rest periods, and advise the patient of the importance of rest and avoidance or control of emotional stress. This may be difficult for the patient when told the nature of the disease and the limitations of the treatment. Patients who have perianal fistulas or abscesses may need special skin care. Postoperative care should be the same as for laparotomy.

In the majority of patients with Crohn's disease, the course is chronic and intermittent. The patient and significant others may need help in setting realistic short- and long-term goals. Teaching is important and should include (1) the importance of rest and diet management, (2) perianal care, (3) action and adverse effects of drugs, (4) symptoms of recurrence of disease, (5) when to seek medical care, and (6) use of stress management techniques.

AGE-RELATED CONSIDERATIONS: INFLAMMATORY BOWEL DISEASE

Although IBDs (i.e., UC and Crohn's disease) are considered diseases of young adults, a second peak in the distribution of these inflammatory conditions occurs around the age of 70 years. The pathogenesis, natural history, and clinical course of UC and Crohn's disease in older adults are similar to those observed in younger patients. However, the distribution of the inflammation appears to be somewhat different. In the older patient with UC, the distal colon is usually involved (proctitis). In the older patient with Crohn's disease, the colon rather than the small intestine tends to be involved. There is less recurrence of Crohn's disease in older patients treated with surgical resection. The degree of inflammation associated with both conditions tends to be less in the older adult than in the younger patient.

Collaborative care of the older patient with one of these conditions is similar to care of the younger patient. However, because of increased risk of cardiovascular and pulmonary complications, older adults tend to have increased morbidity associated with surgical procedures.

In addition to Crohn's disease and UC, older adults are also vulnerable to inflammation of the colon (colitis) from medication use and systemic vascular disease. Drugs such as nonsteroidal anti-inflammatory drugs (NSAIDs), digitalis, vasopressin, estrogen, and allopurinol (Zyloprim) have been associated with colitis development in the older adult patient. Colitis may also be secondary to ischemic bowel disease related to atherosclerosis and congestive heart failure.

Inflammation of the colon as a result of Crohn's disease or UC results in diarrhea, which may be bloody. The loss of fluid and electrolytes and possibly blood may leave the older adult more vulnerable to problems related to volume depletion and dehydration. This may be particularly problematic in the patient with diminished renal and cardiovascular function. Thus, nursing management is focused on careful assessment of fluid and electrolyte status and evaluation of the replacement therapies.

Malabsorption Syndrome

Malabsorption results from impaired absorption of fats, carbohydrates, proteins, minerals, and vitamins. The stomach, small intestine, liver, and pancreas regulate normal digestion and absorption. Digestive enzymes ordinarily break down nutrients so that absorption can take place through the intestinal mucosa and nutrients can get into the bloodstream. If there is an interruption in this process at any point, malabsorption may occur. Several problems can cause malabsorption (Table 45-25). They can be classified into malabsorptions caused by (1) biochemical or enzyme deficiencies, (2) bacterial proliferation, (3) disruption of small intestine mucosa, (4) disturbed lymphatic and vascular circulation, or (5) surface area loss. Lactose intolerance is the most common malabsorption disorder, followed by IBD, celiac disease, tropical sprue, and cystic fibrosis.

The most common clinical manifestation of malabsorption is **steatorrhea**, bulky, foul-smelling, yellow-grey, greasy stools with putty-like consistency that float in water and are difficult to flush (Table 45-26).

Tests used to determine the cause of malabsorption include qualitative examination of stool for fat (e.g., Sudan III stain), a 72-hour stool collection for quantitative measurement of fecal fat, serological testing for celiac disease, and fecal elastase testing to determine if there is pancreatic insufficiency. Other diagnostic studies include a CT scan and endoscopy to obtain a small bowel

Table 45-25 Common Causes of Malabsorption	
Biochemical or Enzyme Deficiencies	**Disturbed Lymphatic and Vascular Circulation**
Lactase deficiency	Lymphoma
Biliary tract obstruction	Ischemia
Pancreatic insufficiency	Lymphangiectasia
Cystic fibrosis	Heart failure
Chronic pancreatitis	**Surface Area Loss**
Zollinger-Ellison syndrome	Billroth II gastrectomy
Bacterial Proliferation	Gastrojejunal bypass surgery for obesity
Tropical sprue	Short bowel syndrome
Parasitic infection	Distal ileal resection, disease, or bypass
Small Intestinal Mucosal Disruption	
Celiac disease	
Whipple's disease	
Crohn's disease	

biopsy specimen for diagnosis. A small bowel barium enema is performed to identify abnormal mucosal patterns. Capsule endoscopy can be used to assess the small intestine for alterations in mucosal integrity and inflammation.

Tests for carbohydrate malabsorption include the D-xylose test and the lactose tolerance test. Laboratory studies that are frequently ordered include a CBC, measurement of prothrombin time (to see if vitamin K absorption is adequate), serum vitamin A and carotene levels, serum electrolytes, cholesterol, and calcium.

Celiac Disease

Celiac disease is an autoimmune disease characterized by damage to the small intestinal mucosa from the ingestion of wheat, barley, and rye in genetically susceptible individuals (Roos, Karner, & Hallert, 2009). It was previously considered a rare intestinal disease that began in childhood accompanied by symptoms of diarrhea, malabsorption, and malnutrition. We now know that it is relatively common, occurs at all ages, and has a wide variety of symptoms. *Celiac sprue* and *gluten-sensitive enteropathy* are other names for celiac disease. Celiac disease is not the same disease as *tropical sprue*, a chronic disorder acquired in tropical areas, that is characterized by progressive disruption of jejunal and ileal tissue resulting in nutritional difficulties. Tropical sprue is treated with folic acid and tetracycline. Celiac disease is most common in people of European ancestry, and it is estimated that approximately 1 in every 133 people in Canada is affected by celiac disease (Canadian Celiac Association, 2011).

Etiology and Pathophysiology

Three factors necessary for developing celiac disease are genetic predisposition, gluten ingestion, and an immune-mediated response. As with other autoimmune diseases, the tissue destruction that occurs with celiac disease is the result of chronic inflammation. Inflammation is activated by the ingestion of gluten found in wheat, rye, and barley. Gluten contains spe-

Table 45-26 Clinical Manifestations of Malabsorption

MANIFESTATIONS	PATHOPHYSIOLOGY
Gastrointestinal	
Weight loss	Malabsorption of fat, carbohydrates, and protein leading to loss of calories; marked reduction in caloric intake or increased use of calories
Diarrhea	Impaired absorption of water, sodium, fatty acids, bile, or carbohydrates
Flatulence	Bacterial fermentation of unabsorbed carbohydrates
Steatorrhea	Undigested and unabsorbed fat
Glossitis, cheilosis, stomatitis	Deficiency of iron, riboflavin, cobalamin, folic acid, and other vitamins
Hematological	
Anemia	Impaired absorption of iron, cobalamin, and folic acid
Hemorrhagic tendency	Vitamin C deficiency
	Vitamin K deficiency inhibiting production of clotting Factors II, VII, IX, and X
Musculoskeletal	
Bone pain	Osteoporosis from impaired calcium absorption
	Osteomalacia secondary to hypocalcemia, hypophosphatemia, inadequate vitamin D
Tetany	Hypocalcemia, hypomagnesemia
Weakness, muscle cramps	Anemia, electrolyte depletion (especially potassium)
Muscle wasting	Protein malabsorption
Neurological	
Altered mental status	Dehydration
Paresthesias	Cobalamin deficiency
Peripheral neuropathy	Cobalamin deficiency
Night blindness	Thiamine deficiency, vitamin A deficiency
Integumentary	
Bruising	Vitamin K deficiency
Dermatitis	Fatty acid deficiency, zinc deficiency, niacin and other vitamin deficiencies
Brittle nails	Iron deficiency
Hair thinning and loss	Protein deficiency
Cardiovascular	
Hypotension	Dehydration
Tachycardia	Hypovolemia, anemia
Peripheral edema	Protein malabsorption, protein loss in diarrhea

an inflammatory response. Inflammation damages the microvilli and brush border of the small intestine, decreasing the amount of surface area available for nutrient absorption (Martin, 2008). Damage is most severe in the duodenum, probably related to the greater exposure to gluten. The intestinal damage decreases distal to the duodenum. The inflammation continues until gluten ingestion ceases.

Clinical Manifestations

Classic signs of celiac disease include foul-smelling diarrhea, steatorrhea, flatulence, abdominal distension, and symptoms of malnutrition. Some people have no obvious GI symptoms, and may have atypical symptoms such as decreased bone density and osteoporosis, dental enamel hypoplasia, iron and folate deficiencies, peripheral neuropathy, and reproductive problems (Martin, 2008). A pruritic, vesicular skin lesion, called *dermatitis herpetiformis*, is sometimes present and occurs as a rash on the buttocks, scalp, face, elbows, and knees. Celiac disease is also associated with autoimmune diseases, particularly rheumatoid arthritis, type 1 diabetes mellitus, and thyroid disease. Protein, fat, and carbohydrate absorption is affected, leading to poor growth, weight loss, muscle wasting, and other signs of malnutrition. Abnormal folate, iron, and cobalamin levels can occur. Iron-deficiency anemia is one of the most common manifestations of celiac disease. Patients may exhibit lactose intolerance and eliminate lactose-containing products until the disease is under control. Inadequate calcium intake and vitamin D absorption can lead to decreased bone density and osteoporosis. Poor nutrition leads to reproductive problems.

Diagnostic Studies and Collaborative Care

Celiac disease is confirmed when (1) there is histological evidence of the disease following biopsy from the small intestine and (2) the symptoms and histological evidence disappear when the person eats a gluten-free diet (Martin, 2008). Diagnostic testing must be done before the person is placed on a gluten-free diet because the diet will alter the results. Biopsies show flattened mucosa and noticeable losses of villi. Celiac disease should be ruled out during a diagnostic workup of IBS because the symptoms are similar. Many people spend years seeking treatment for nonspecific complaints before celiac disease is diagnosed (thus the large number of people who are diagnosed in adulthood). Treatment with a gluten-free diet halts the process. Most patients recover completely within 3 to 6 months of treatment, but they need to maintain a gluten-free diet for life. Wheat, barley, oats, and rye products must be avoided. Although pure oats do not contain gluten, oat products can become contaminated with wheat, rye, and barley during the milling process. Gluten is also found in some medications and in many food additives, preservatives, and stabilizers. A combination of corticosteroids and a gluten-free diet is used to treat individuals who do not respond to the gluten-free diet alone.

Lactase Deficiency

Lactase deficiency is a condition in which the lactase enzyme is deficient or absent. *Lactase* is the enzyme that breaks down lactose into two simple sugars—glucose and galactose. Although primary lactase deficiency seems to be hereditary, milk intoler-

cific peptides called *prolamines*. In genetically susceptible individuals, partial digestion of gluten releases prolamine peptides, which are absorbed into the lamina propria in the intestinal submucosa.

Once in the lamina propria, peptides bind to human leukocyte antigen (HLA)-DQ2 and/or HLA-DQ8 antigens and activate

ance may not become clinically evident until late adolescence or early adulthood. About 5% of the adult population has primary lactase deficiency. The highest incidence in Canada is found in Blacks, Aboriginals, Hispanics, Asians, and persons of Jewish descent. Acquired lactase deficiency is often seen in conjunction with other GI diseases in which the mucosa has been damaged, including UC, Crohn's disease, gastroenteritis, and celiac disease.

Clinical Manifestations

The symptoms of lactose intolerance include bloating, flatulence, crampy abdominal pain, and diarrhea. They may occur within a half hour to several hours after drinking a glass of milk or ingesting a milk product. The diarrhea of lactose intolerance results from fluid secretion into the small intestine, a response to the osmotic action of undigested lactose.

NURSING AND COLLABORATIVE MANAGEMENT: LACTASE DEFICIENCY

Many lactose-intolerant persons are aware of their milk intolerance and avoid milk. A lactose intolerance test can be performed to rule out milk allergies. The patient is given 50 g of lactose orally. Blood samples are drawn before the consumption of lactose and at 15-, 30-, 60-, and 90-minute intervals. Failure of the blood glucose level to increase more than 20 mg/dL is suggestive of lactase deficiency. Results of the hydrogen breath test after ingestion of lactose are abnormal.

Treatment consists of eliminating lactose from the diet by avoiding milk and milk products. A lactose-free diet is given initially and is gradually advanced to a low-lactose diet as tolerated by the patient. Many lactose-intolerant persons may not exhibit symptoms if lactose is taken in small amounts. In some persons, lactose may be tolerated better if taken with meals.

The patient needs to be aware that milk, ice cream, cottage cheese, and cheese have a high lactose content. If the milk has been fermented (e.g., cultured buttermilk, yogourt, sour cream), the patient with low lactase levels may tolerate it better.

Lactase enzyme (Lactaid) is available commercially as an over-the-counter (OTC) product. It is mixed with milk and breaks down the lactose before the milk is ingested. Lactase tablets can also be taken with the ingestion of other dairy products.

Short-Bowel Syndrome

Short bowel syndrome (SBS) results from extensive resection of the small intestine. Rapid intestinal transit, impaired digestive and absorption processes, and fluid and electrolyte losses characterize the syndrome. In adults, extensive resection of the small intestine may be necessary for bowel infarction because of vascular thrombosis or insufficiency, abdominal trauma, cancer, radiation enteritis, or Crohn's disease.

The length and the portions of small bowel resected are associated with the number and severity of symptoms. Resections of up to 50% of the small intestine cause little disturbance of bowel

function, especially if the terminal ileum and the ileocecal valve remain intact. After large resections, the remaining intestine undergoes adaptive changes that are more pronounced in the ileum. The villi and the crypts increase in size, and absorptive capacity of the remaining intestine increases. Intestinal adaptation is enhanced by the presence of food, fibre, bile, and pancreatic secretions in the lumen and continues for up to 2 years. Resection of the ileum, the ileocecal valve, or the colon results in a rapid intestinal transit, decreasing absorption time. Ileal resection causes malabsorption of cobalamin, bile salts, and fat, resulting in steatorrhea.

Clinical Manifestations

The predominant manifestations of SBS are diarrhea, steatorrhea, and weight loss (Parekh & Steiger, 2007). There may be signs of malnutrition and multiple vitamin and mineral deficiencies (e.g., cobalamin and zinc deficiency, hypocalcemia). The patient may develop lactase deficiency and bacterial overgrowth. Oxalate kidney stones may form from increased colonic absorption of oxalate.

Collaborative Care

The overall goals are that the patient with SBS will have fluid and electrolyte balance, normal nutritional status, and control of diarrhea. In the period immediately following massive bowel resection, patients receive TPN to replace fluid, electrolyte, and nutrient losses. Hypersecretion of gastric acid, for which the cause is unknown, is reduced by proton pump inhibitors (e.g., omeprazole [Losec]).

A diet high in carbohydrate and low in fat is recommended. A high-carbohydrate, low-fat diet supplemented with soluble fibre and pectin may slow transit time and improve nutrient absorption, decrease stool output, and enable patients to wean off parenteral nutrition. The patient with SBS is encouraged to eat at least six to eight meals per day to increase the overall time food is present in and in contact with the intestine. Oral intake can be supplemented with elemental nutrient formulas and tube feeding during the night. For patients with severe malabsorption, TPN may be reinstituted. Oral supplements of calcium, zinc, and multivitamins are typically recommended.

Narcotic antidiarrheal drugs are the most effective in decreasing intestinal motility (see Table 45-3). For patients with limited ileal resections (<100 cm), cholestyramine reduces diarrhea resulting from unabsorbed bile acids and increases their excretion in feces. Bile acids stimulate intestinal fluid secretion and reduce colonic fluid absorption.

Intestinal Obstruction

Intestinal obstruction occurs when a partial or complete obstruction of the intestine prevents intestinal contents from passing through the GI tract; it requires prompt treatment. The causes of intestinal obstruction can be classified as mechanical or nonmechanical.

Types of Intestinal Obstruction

Mechanical. *Mechanical obstruction* may be caused by an occlusion of the lumen of the intestinal tract (Figure 45-4). Most

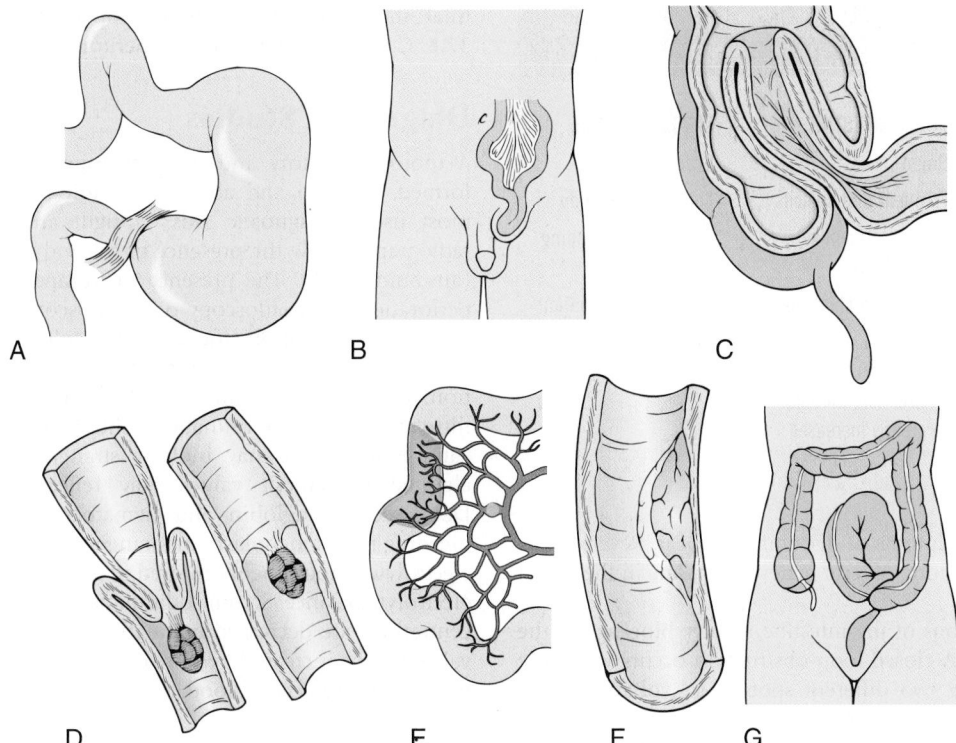

Figure 45-4 Bowel obstructions. **A,** Adhesions. **B,** Strangulated inguinal hernia. **C,** Ileocecal intussusception. **D,** Intussusception from polyps. **E,** Mesenteric occlusion. **F,** Neoplasm. **G,** Volvulus of the sigmoid colon.

intestinal obstructions occur in the small intestine, most often in the ileum. Adhesions account for 50%, hernias for 15%, and neoplasms for 15% of obstructions of the small intestine. Adhesions can develop after abdominal surgery. Obstruction can occur within days of surgery or years later. Carcinoma is the most common cause of large bowel obstruction, followed by volvulus and diverticular disease.

Nonmechanical. A *nonmechanical obstruction* may result from a neuromuscular or vascular disorder. **Paralytic (adynamic) ileus** (lack of intestinal peristalsis) is the most common form of nonmechanical obstruction. It can occur after any abdominal surgery. Other causes of paralytic ileus include inflammatory responses (e.g., acute pancreatitis, acute appendicitis), electrolyte abnormalities, and thoracic or lumbar spinal fractures.

Pseudo-obstruction is an apparent mechanical obstruction of the intestine without demonstration of obstruction by radiological methods. Collagen vascular diseases and neurological and endocrine disorders may cause pseudo-obstruction, but mostly, it is found to be idiopathic.

Vascular obstructions are rare and are due to an interference with the blood supply to a portion of the intestines. The most common causes are emboli and atherosclerosis of the mesenteric arteries. The celiac, inferior, and superior mesenteric arteries supply blood to the bowel. Emboli may originate from thrombi in patients with chronic atrial fibrillation, diseased heart valves, and prosthetic valves. Venous thrombosis may be seen in low–blood flow states, such as heart failure and shock.

Etiology and Pathophysiology

Normally, 6 to 8 L of fluid enters the small bowel daily. Most of the fluid is absorbed before it reaches the colon. Approximately 75% of intestinal gas is swallowed air. Bacterial metabolism produces methane and hydrogen gases. Fluid, gas, and intestinal contents accumulate proximal to the intestinal obstruction. This causes distension, and the distal bowel may collapse. The distension reduces the absorption of fluids and stimulates intestinal secretions. As the fluid increases, so does the pressure in the lumen of the bowel. The increased pressure leads to an increase in capillary permeability and extravasation of fluids and electrolytes into the peritoneal cavity. Edema, congestion, and necrosis from impaired blood supply as well as possible rupture of the bowel may occur. The retention of fluid in the intestine and the peritoneal cavity can lead to a severe reduction in circulating blood volume and result in hypotension and hypovolemic shock.

The electrolyte-rich fluids, which are normally absorbed in the bowel, are retained in the bowel and subsequently lost into the peritoneal cavity. The location of the obstruction determines the extent of fluid, electrolyte, and acid–base imbalances. If the obstruction is high, as in the pylorus, metabolic alkalosis may result from the loss of hydrochloric acid from the stomach through vomiting or NG intubation.

When the obstruction is located in the small bowel, dehydration occurs rapidly. Dehydration and electrolyte imbalances do not occur early in large bowel obstruction. If the obstruction is below the proximal colon, most GI fluids have been absorbed before reaching the point of the obstruction. Solid fecal material

Table 45-27 Clinical Manifestations of Small and Large Intestinal Obstructions

CLINICAL MANIFESTATION	SMALL INTESTINE	LARGE INTESTINE
Onset	Rapid	Gradual
Vomiting	Frequent and copious	Late manifestation
Pain	Colicky, cramplike, intermittent	Low-grade, cramping abdominal pain
Bowel movement	Feces for a short time	Absolute constipation
Abdominal distension	Dependent upon location of obstruction, minimal to greatly increased	Greatly increased

accumulates until symptoms of discomfort appear. Reverse peristalsis may cause vomiting of fecal material very late in the bowel obstruction.

Simple obstructions of the intestine involve blockage of the lumen in one spot. A closed-loop obstruction occurs when the lumen is blocked in two different spots (e.g., volvulus). This results in an isolated segment of bowel and obstruction proximal to that segment. Strangulation and gangrene are likely to develop if treatment is not immediate. A strangulated obstruction occurs when the circulation to the obstructed intestine is impaired. This is the most dangerous form of obstruction because it may lead to necrosis of the intestine (incarcerated). Volvulus, hernias, or adhesions are the most common causes.

Clinical Manifestations

The clinical manifestations of intestinal obstruction vary, depending on the location of the obstruction, and include nausea, vomiting, abdominal pain, distension, inability to pass flatus, and obstipation (Table 45-27). Obstruction located high in the small intestine produces rapid-onset, sometimes projectile vomiting with bile-containing vomitus. Vomiting from more distal obstructions of the small intestine is more gradual in onset. The vomitus may be orange-brown and foul smelling because of bacterial overgrowth. Vomiting may be entirely absent in large bowel obstruction if the ileocecal valve is competent; otherwise, the patient may eventually vomit fecal material.

Vomiting usually relieves abdominal pain in high intestinal obstructions. Persistent, colicky abdominal pain is seen with lower intestinal obstruction. A characteristic sign of mechanical obstruction is pain that comes and goes in waves. This is caused by intestinal peristalsis working to move bowel contents past the obstructed area. In contrast, paralytic ileus produces a more constant generalized discomfort. Strangulation causes severe, constant pain that is rapid in onset. Abdominal distension is a common manifestation of intestinal obstructions. It is usually absent or minimally noticeable in proximal obstructions of the small intestine and greatly increased in lower intestinal obstructions. Abdominal tenderness and rigidity are usually absent unless strangulation or peritonitis has occurred.

Auscultation of bowel sounds reveals high-pitched sounds above the area of obstruction. The patient often notes borborygmi (audible abdominal sounds produced by hyperactive intes-

tinal motility). The patient's temperature rarely rises above 37.8°C unless strangulation or peritonitis has occurred.

Diagnostic Studies

A thorough history and physical examination should be performed. CT scan and abdominal radiographic studies are the most useful diagnostic aids. Upright and lateral abdominal radiographs show the presence of gas and fluid in the intestines (air–fluid levels). The presence of intraperitoneal air indicates perforation. Sigmoidoscopy or colonoscopy may provide direct visualization of an obstruction in the colon.

Laboratory tests are important and provide essential information. A CBC and serum electrolyte, amylase, and blood urea nitrogen (BUN) determinations should be performed. An elevated WBC count may indicate strangulation or perforation; elevated hematocrit values may reflect hemoconcentration. Decreased hemoglobin and hematocrit values may indicate bleeding from a neoplasm or strangulation with necrosis. Serum electrolytes should be monitored to assess the patient's fluid and electrolyte balance. Serum sodium, potassium, and chloride concentrations are decreased in small-bowel obstruction. The BUN value may be increased because of dehydration. The stool should be checked for occult blood.

Collaborative Care

Treatment is directed toward decompression of the intestine by removal of gas and fluid, correction and maintenance of fluid and electrolyte balance, and relief or removal of the obstruction. NG tubes may be used to decompress the bowel. NG tubes may be inserted before surgery to empty the stomach and relieve distension. NG or venting percutaneous tubes are effective in the treatment of patients with neurogenic obstruction who do not require surgery.

Sigmoidoscopy may successfully reduce a sigmoid volvulus. Colon-decompression catheters may be passed through partially obstructed areas via a colonoscope to decompress the bowel before surgery.

IV infusions that contain normal saline solution and potassium should be given to maintain fluid and electrolyte balance. TPN may be necessary in some cases to correct nutritional deficiencies, improve the patient's nutritional status before surgery, and promote postoperative healing.

Most mechanical obstructions are treated surgically. Surgery may involve resecting the obstructed segment of bowel and anastomosing the remaining healthy bowel. Partial or total colectomy, colostomy, or ileostomy may be required when extensive obstruction or necrosis is present.

NURSING MANAGEMENT: INTESTINAL OBSTRUCTION

▪ Nursing Assessment

Intestinal obstruction is a potentially life-threatening condition. Nursing assessment must begin with a detailed patient history and physical examination. The type and the location of obstruction usually cause characteristic symptoms. The nurse should determine location, duration, intensity, and frequency of abdominal pain and whether abdominal tenderness or rigidity is present. Onset, frequency, colour, odour, and amount of vomitus should be recorded. Bowel function, including passage of flatus, should be determined. The nurse auscultates for bowel sounds and documents the character and the location; inspects the abdomen for scars, palpable masses, and distension; and observes for muscle guarding and tenderness.

Nursing Diagnoses

Nursing diagnoses for the patient with intestinal obstructions include, but are not limited to, the following:
- Acute pain *related to* abdominal distension and increased peristalsis
- Deficient fluid volume *related to* decrease in intestinal fluid absorption and loss of fluids secondary to vomiting
- Imbalanced nutrition: less than body requirements *related to* intestinal obstruction and vomiting

Planning

The overall goals are that the patient with an intestinal obstruction will have (1) relief of the obstruction and return to normal bowel function, (2) minimal to no discomfort, (3) normal fluid and electrolyte status, and (4) maintenance of adequate nutrition.

Nursing Implementation

The patient should be monitored closely for signs of dehydration and electrolyte imbalance. A strict intake and output record should be maintained. IV fluids should be administered as ordered. Serum electrolyte levels should be monitored. A patient with a high obstruction is more likely to have metabolic alkalosis; a patient with a low obstruction is at greater risk of metabolic acidosis. The patient is often restless and constantly changes position to relieve the pain. The nurse should provide comfort measures, promote a restful environment, and keep distractions and visitors to a minimum. Nursing care of the patient after surgery for an intestinal obstruction is similar to care of the patient after a laparotomy (see NCP 45-2, p. 1174).

Care of Nasogastric and Nasointestinal Tubes

Nurses may be instructed to insert NG tubes. Insertion is easier if the patient relaxes, takes deep breaths, and swallows when instructed. Once the tube is in place, it is extremely important to (1) confirm placement of the tube (e.g., by aspiration of gastric contents), (2) ensure the tube is properly secured to prevent dislodgement, and (3) provide appropriate nasal and mouth care. When an NG tube is in place, the patient breathes through the mouth, drying the mouth and lips. The nurse should encourage and assist the patient to brush the teeth frequently. Mouthwash and water for the patient to use in rinsing the mouth and petroleum jelly (if the patient is not on oxygen) or water-soluble lubricant for the lips should be provided at the bedside.

The patient's nose should be checked for signs of irritation from the NG tube. This area should be cleaned and dried daily with application of a water-soluble lubricant and retaping of the tube. NG tubes should be checked every 4 hours for patency. Characteristics of the NG losses may differ depending upon the underlying reason for the tube placement. Pale yellow to dark green bile drainage is more likely after abdominal surgery, whereas odoriferous thick drainage with food particles may be seen with bowel obstructions. Hemolyzed sanguineous drainage (often called "coffee grounds" owing to its dark brown, granular appearance) or fresh sanguineous drainage should be reported immediately to the physician or surgeon. The volume of NG losses should also be monitored. Excessive losses (>500-1000 mL/24 hr) may have to be replaced with IV fluids and electrolytes to maintain adequate hydration. Generally, NG tubes can be removed once normal bowel function returns (passing of gas and stool) and the patient is no longer vomiting.

Polyps of the Large Intestine

Colonic polyps arise from the mucosal surface of the colon and project into the lumen. They may be *sessile* (flat, broad based, and attached directly to the intestinal wall) or *pedunculated* (attached to the intestinal wall by a stalk). Polyps tend to be sessile when small and become pedunculated as they enlarge, especially if they are in the left or descending colon (Figure 45-5). They may be found anywhere in the large intestine but are most commonly found in the rectosigmoid area. Although most polyps are asymptomatic, rectal bleeding or occult blood in the stool are the most common manifestations.

Types of Polyps

The most common types of polyp are hyperplastic and adenomatous. *Hyperplastic polyps* originate from the epithelium and are non-neoplastic growths. They rarely grow larger than 5 mm and never cause clinical symptoms. Other benign (non-neoplastic) polyps include inflammatory polyps, lipomas, and juvenile polyps (Table 45-28) (Jass, 2008).

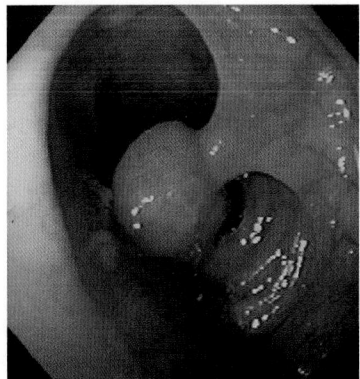

Figure 45-5 Endoscopic image of a pedunculated polyp in the descending colon.

Source: Courtesy David Bjorkman, MD, University of Utah School of Medicine, Department of Gastroenterology. In McCance, K. L., & Huether, S. E. (2010). *Pathophysiology: The biological basis for disease in adults and children* (6th ed., p. 1501, Figure 39-29A). St. Louis: Mosby.

Table 45-28 Types of Polyps of the Large Intestine

Neoplastic	Non-neoplastic
• Epithelial polyps (adenomatous)	• Epithelial polyps (hyperplastic)
• Tubular adenoma	• Hereditary polyposis syndromes
• Tubular villous adenoma	• Familial juvenile polyposis
• Villous adenoma	• Inflammatory polyps
• Hereditary polyposis syndromes (adenomatous polyposis syndrome)	• Pseudopolyps
• Familial adenomatous polyposis	• Benign lymphoid polyps
	• Submucosal
	• Lipomas
	• Leiomyomas
	• Fibromas

Adenomatous polyps are characterized by neoplastic changes in the epithelium. They are closely linked to colorectal adenocarcinoma. Structurally, there are three types, with tubular adenomas being the most prevalent. The risk of cancer in the polyp increases with polyp size and villous structure. Villous adenomas have a higher risk of turning cancerous than tubular adenomas. Removing adenomatous polyps decreases the occurrence of colorectal cancer.

Although there are several polyposis syndromes, they are relatively rare. Of these, *familial adenomatous polyposis* (FAP) is the most common (see the Genetics in Clinical Practice box on this page). This disorder is characterized by multiple polyps that at times number in the thousands and that are located in the large intestine and sometimes in other areas of the GI tract. Patients with a history of FAP have a lifetime risk of developing colorectal cancer that approaches 100%. They also develop cancer at an earlier age (i.e., <40 years of age) than patients with non-FAP colorectal cancer. For children of patients with FAP, screening must be initiated at puberty and then conducted annually. There is a 50% risk for these children to develop FAP. When there is indication of disease, total colectomy with ileostomy is the treatment of choice (Vasen et al., 2008).

Diagnostic Studies and Collaborative Care

Barium enema, sigmoidoscopy, colonoscopy and CT/MRI colonography (virtual colonoscopy) are used to diagnose polyps. All polyps are considered abnormal and should be removed. In patients whose polyps are identified through barium enema, removal (polypectomy) should be done through a colonoscope or a sigmoidoscope. If the polyp is not removable, a biopsy specimen should be taken for tissue examination. Surgery is not indicated unless carcinoma is present or certain cases of polyposis syndromes warrant it. The patient should be observed for rectal bleeding, fever, severe abdominal pain, and abdominal distension, which may indicate hemorrhage or perforation.

Colorectal Cancer

Colorectal cancer (a malignant disease of the colon, the rectum, or both) is the second most common cause of cancer death in

GENETICS IN CLINICAL PRACTICE

Familial Adenomatous Polyposis (FAP)

Genetic Basis
• Autosomal dominant disorder
• Mutation in *APC* gene located on chromosome 5

Incidence
• 1 in 5000-7500 people
• Men and women affected equally

Genetic Testing
• DNA testing available to detect *APC* gene mutation

Clinical Implications
• FAP is characterized by the presence of colorectal polyps (usually >1000).
• Polyps are not present at birth but appear during adolescence and early adulthood.
• FAP accounts for at least 1% of all colorectal cancers.
• If untreated, FAP almost always results in the development of colon cancer before the age of 40.
• With FAP, there is also increased incidence of gastric and small intestinal polyps.
• Many deaths related to FAP could be prevented with early and aggressive monitoring and treatment including frequent colonoscopies and total colectomy.
• Individuals with a family history of FAP could benefit from genetic counselling and teaching.

APC, adenomatous polyposis coli; *FAP*, familial adenomatous polyposis.

Canada. In 2012, it was estimated that there would be 23,300 new cases of colorectal cancer diagnosed in Canada, and that 9200 people would die from it (Canadian Cancer Society's Steering Committee on Cancer Statistics, 2012).

The incidence of colorectal cancer at specific sites varies (Figure 45-6). In both sexes, the incidence of right colon cancers has increased and cancers in the rectum have decreased. The highest percentages of colorectal cancers in Canada are currently located in the rectum, the ascending colon, and the sigmoid colon. Approximately 20% of colorectal cancers are within reach of the examining finger, and 50% are within reach of the sigmoidoscope.

Etiology and Pathophysiology

The causes of colorectal cancer remain unclear. Groups at high risk of colorectal cancer have been identified (Table 45-29). For at least 6% of patients who develop colorectal cancer, there is a clear genetic predisposition (see the Genetics in Clinical Practice boxes on this page and on p. 1197). Age is a risk factor in both men and women. The risk for development in the general population increases slightly after the age of 50 years and then rises rapidly in the following decades.

Adenocarcinoma is the most common type of colorectal cancer. Most colorectal cancers begin as adenomatous polyps that arise from the mucosa lining the lumen of the colon and the rectum. As it grows, the cancer progresses down from the tip of

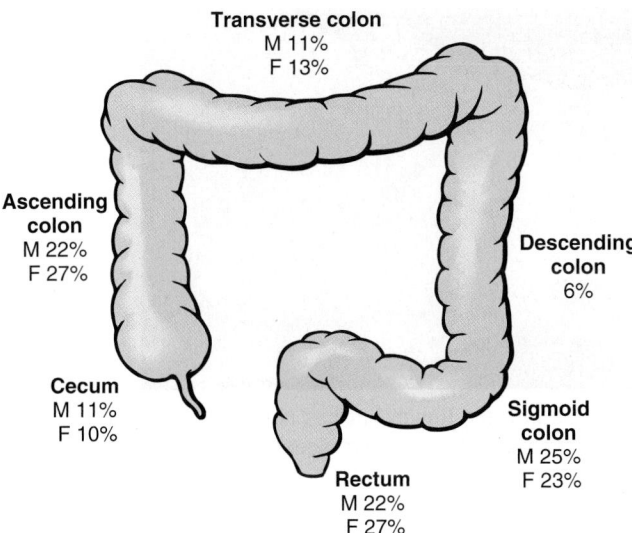

Figure 45-6 Incidence of colorectal cancer. Approximately one half of all colon cancers occur in the rectosigmoid area. Percentages are listed for males *(M)* and females *(F)*.

Table 45-29 Risk Factors for Colorectal Cancer

- Age >50 years
- Familial adenomatous polyposis (FAP)
- Colorectal polyps
- Chronic inflammatory bowel disease
- Family history of colorectal cancer or adenomas
- Previous history of colorectal cancer
- History of ovarian, endometrial, or breast cancer (women)
- High-fat or low-fibre diet (controversial)

GENETICS IN CLINICAL PRACTICE
Hereditary Nonpolyposis Colorectal Cancer

Genetic Basis
- Autosomal dominant disorder
- Mutations in genes that error-check DNA (repair genes)

Incidence
- 1 in 500-2000 people

Genetic Testing
- DNA testing available

Clinical Implications
- HNPCC accounts for 5% of all colorectal cancers.
- Individuals with gene mutation have 80-90% lifetime risk of developing colorectal cancer.
- Average age of diagnosis is in the mid-40s.
- Cancer arises from single colorectal lesion in absence of polyposis.
- Cancers tend to occur on right side of colon.
- HNPCC is less aggressive and survival rates are longer than colon cancers that develop without known risk factors.
- Persons with gene mutation are at high risk of developing other cancers, including uterine, ovarian, ureter, pancreas, stomach, and small intestinal cancer.
- Individuals with known gene mutations should be monitored with colonoscopy every year.
  Examination by pelvic ultrasound and endometrial biopsy should also be considered for women.

HNPCC, hereditary nonpolyposis colorectal cancer.

the polyp through the body and stalk. It becomes invasive and penetrates the muscularis mucosae. Once through the muscularis mucosae, tumour cells gain access to the regional lymph nodes and the vascular system and can spread to distant sites. (Carcinomas of the cecum and the colon are shown in Figure 45-7.) The most common sites of metastasis are the regional lymph nodes, liver, lungs, and peritoneum. Because venous blood leaving the colon and rectum flows through the portal vein and inferior rectal vein, the liver and lung are common sites of metastasis. The cancer spreads from the liver to other sites, including the lungs, bones, and brain. The cancer can also spread directly into adjacent structures. The growing tumour can obstruct the bowel. Other complications include bleeding, perforation, peritonitis, and fistula formation.

Clinical Manifestations

Clinical manifestations of colorectal cancer are usually nonspecific or do not appear until the disease is advanced. Cancer on the right side of the colon gives rise to clinical manifestations that are different from those on the left side of the colon (Colorectal Cancer Association of Canada, 2012). Rectal bleeding, the most common symptom of colorectal cancer, is most often seen with

left-sided lesions. Other commonly seen manifestations of left-sided lesions include alternating constipation and diarrhea, change in stool calibre (narrow, ribbon-like), and sensation of incomplete evacuation. Obstruction symptoms appear earlier with left-sided lesions because of the smaller lumen size (Figure 45-8).

Cancers of the right side of the colon are usually asymptomatic. Vague abdominal discomfort or crampy, colicky abdominal pain may be present. Iron-deficiency anemia and occult bleeding dictate further investigation. Weakness and fatigue result from anemia.

Diagnostic Studies

A thorough history with close attention to family history should be obtained, and a physical examination should be performed (Table 45-30). The digital rectal examination is the most important aspect of the physical examination because many rectal cancers are within reach of the finger. In the asymptomatic person who is 50 years or older with no risk factors (other than age), a *fecal occult blood test* (FOBT) or *fecal immunochemical test* (FIT) once a year and flexible sigmoidoscopy every 5 years beginning at age 50 are important aspects of the examination. Fecal occult blood tests have been used for more than 30 years to screen for colorectal cancer and continue to be widely used in North

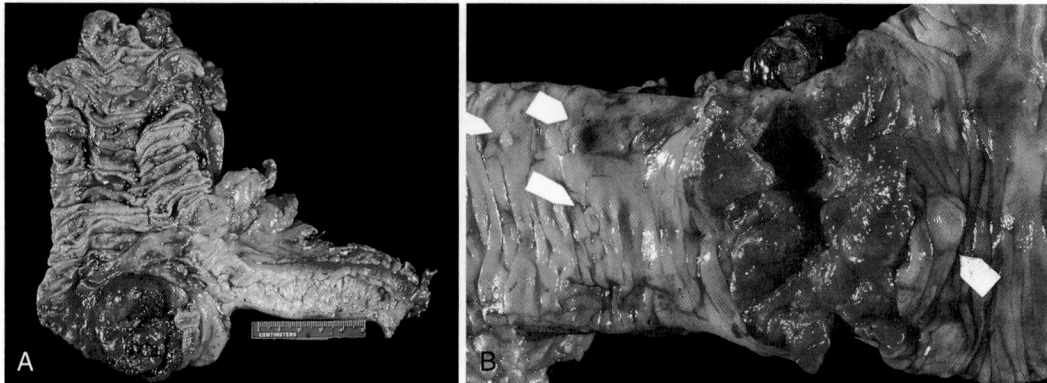

Figure 45-7 A, Carcinoma of the cecum. The fungating carcinoma projects into the lumen but has not caused obstruction. **B,** Carcinoma of the descending colon. This circumferential tumour has heaped-up edges and an ulcerated central portion. The *arrows* identify separate mucosal polyps.

Source: Kumar, V., Abbas, A. K., & Fausto, N. (2010). *Robbins and Cotran pathologic basis of disease* (8th ed.). Philadelphia: Saunders.

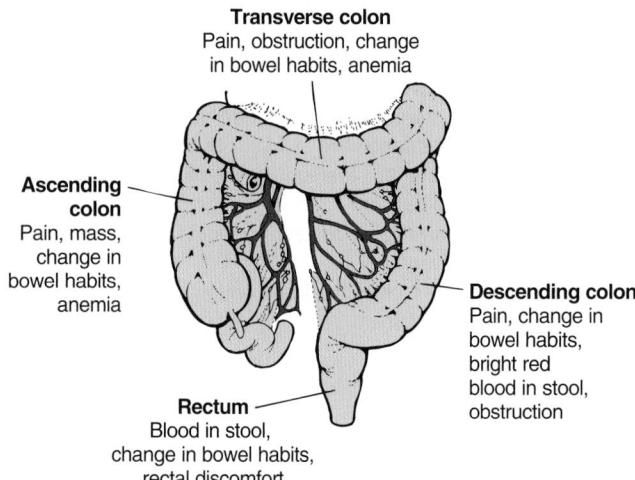

Transverse colon
Pain, obstruction, change
in bowel habits, anemia

Ascending colon
Pain, mass,
change in
bowel habits,
anemia

Descending colon
Pain, change in
bowel habits,
bright red
blood in stool,
obstruction

Rectum
Blood in stool,
change in bowel habits,
rectal discomfort

Figure 45-8 Signs and symptoms of colorectal cancer by location of primary lesion.

Source: McCance, K. L., & Huether, S. E. (2010). *Pathophysiology: The biologic basis for disease in adults and children* (6th ed., p. 1502, Figure 39-30A). St. Louis: Mosby.

COLLABORATIVE CARE

Table 45-30 Colorectal Cancer

Diagnostic	Collaborative Therapy
• History and physical examination	• Surgery
• Digital rectal examination	• Right hemicolectomy
• Sigmoidoscopy	• Left hemicolectomy
• Colonoscopy	• Abdominal–perineal resection
• Barium enema	• Laparoscopic colectomy
• CBC	• Radiation
• Liver function tests	• Chemotherapy
• Testing of stool for occult blood	
• Carcinoembryonic antigen test (CEA)	
• CT scan of abdomen	
• Ultrasound (including endorectal)	

CBC, complete blood count, *CT,* computed tomography.

America. Patients need to be taught to abstain from red meat, ASA and NSAIDs (if medically safe) before testing to avoid false positives. The FIT uses antibodies to detect human hemoglobin protein in stool. It is performed in much the same way as the FOBT, but there are no drug or dietary restrictions (Colorectal Cancer Association of Canada, 2011a).

Colonoscopy is the procedure of choice. Synchronous lesions may be present at other sites in the colon, and tissue diagnosis may be made by biopsy during the procedure. Other procedures include endorectal ultrasonography and *CT colonography (virtual colonoscopy)* to localize the lesion and determine its size or the presence of metastases.

Laboratory studies should include a CBC to check for anemia, clotting studies, and liver function tests. A CT scan of the abdomen may be helpful in detecting liver metastases, retroperitoneal and pelvic disease, and depth of penetration of tumour into the bowel wall. A CT scan should be done before surgery. Liver function tests are performed to determine liver metastases.

A carcinoembryonic antigen (CEA) test is often performed, although it is not specific for colorectal cancer. A normal level of CEA does not exclude the possibility of a malignant condition. This test is used most effectively in following the progress of a patient after surgery. Return to normal of a previously elevated CEA indicates successful removal of the tumour. In contrast, postoperative CEA levels that are persistently elevated or increase suggest the presence of residual tumour or tumour spread.

Collaborative Care

Prognosis and treatment correlate with pathological staging of the disease. Several methods of staging are available including Dukes Staging System and the TNM (tumour, nodes, metastasis) System (Table 45-31). The TNM system is widely used and describes a patient's cancer based on the degree of invasion of the primary tumour, lymph node involvement, and presence of

Table 45-31 Tumour–Node–Metastasis (TNM) Classification of Colorectal Cancer	
T	***Primary Tumour***
T_x	Primary tumour cannot be assessed because of incomplete information.
T_{is}	Carcinoma in situ. Cancer is in earliest stage and has not grown beyond mucosa layer.
T_1	Tumour has grown beyond mucosa into the submucosa.
T_2	Tumour has grown through submucosa into muscularis propria.
T_3	Tumour has grown through the muscularis propria into the subserosa but not to neighbouring organs or tissues.
T_4	Tumour has spread completely through the colon or rectal wall and into nearby tissues or organs.
N	***Lymph Node Involvement***
N_x	Lymph nodes cannot be assessed.
N_0	No regional lymph node involvement is found.
N_1	Cancer is found in one to three nearby lymph nodes.
N_2	Cancer is found in four or more nearby lymph nodes.
M	***Metastasis***
M_x	Presence of distant metastasis cannot be assessed.
M_0	No distant metastasis is seen.
M_1	Distant metastasis is present.

Stage	TNM		
0	T_{is}	N_0	M_0
IA	T_1	N_0	M_0
IB	T_2	N_0	M_0
II	T_1	N_2	M_0
	T_2	N_1	M_0
	T_3	N_0	M_0
IIIA	T_2	N_2	M_0
	T_3	N_{1-2}	M_0
IIIB	T_4	N_{0-1}	M_0
IV	T_4	N_2	M_0
	T_{1-4}	N_{0-2}	M_1

metastasis. The stage at diagnosis is key in determining prognosis and appropriate treatment (Nayak & Goel, 2011).

Several noninvasive procedures may be performed through a colonoscope to effectively treat certain types of colorectal cancer. Endoscopic polypectomy is a highly effective and safe procedure. Adequate treatment can be obtained if the resected margin of the polyp is free of cancer, the cancer is well differentiated, and there is no apparent lymphatic or blood vessel involvement. Laser therapy may be used to ablate nonresectable tumours. This is usually used only as palliative therapy in patients with obstructive symptoms.

Surgical Therapy. Surgery is the only curative treatment of colorectal cancer. The location and the extent of the cancer determine the type of surgery performed. Success of surgery depends on resection of the tumour with an adequate margin of healthy bowel and resection of the regional lymph nodes.

Right hemicolectomy is performed when the cancer is located in the cecum, the ascending colon, the hepatic flexure, or the transverse colon to the right of the middle colic artery. A portion of the terminal ileum, the ileocecal valve, and the appendix are removed, and an ileotransverse anastomosis is performed. A left hemicolectomy involves resection of the left transverse colon, the splenic flexure, the descending colon, the sigmoid colon, and the upper portion of the rectum.

Clear margins are most difficult to obtain with rectal carcinoma. Location of the rectal lesion determines the surgical procedure to be performed. There must be enough rectum left to ensure a secure anastomosis and preservation of anal sphincter function, or an abdominal–perineal resection is indicated. Abdominal–perineal resection is most often performed when the cancer is located within 5 cm of the anus, although ultra-low anterior resections can be performed (within 1-2 cm of the anus) by skilled surgeons.

In the abdominal–perineal resection, an abdominal incision is made, and the proximal sigmoid is brought through the abdominal wall as a permanent colostomy. The distal sigmoid, rectum, and anus are removed through a perineal incision. The perineal wound may be primarily closed with a drain or left open with appropriate dressings to allow healing by secondary intention. Complications that can occur are delayed wound healing, hemorrhage, persistent perineal sinus tracts, infections, and urinary tract and sexual dysfunctions.

Low anterior resection may be indicated for tumours of the rectosigmoid and the mid–to–upper rectum. The use of EEA (end-to-end anastomosis) staplers has allowed lower and more secure anastomoses. The stapler is passed through the anus, where the colon is stapled to the rectum. This technique has made it possible to resect lesions to a point as low as 1 to 2 cm from the anus.

Sphincter-sparing procedures are being performed on the patient who is a poor operative risk and on the patient with early disease. The number of these procedures may increase with continued early detection and surveillance. In these procedures, a local resection is performed, and the anal sphincters are left intact.

Laparoscopic colectomy is being evaluated for its effectiveness in eliminating cancer and improving survival. Potential benefits are faster return of bowel function, fewer incisional infections, shortened hospital stay, and improved cosmetic appearance (Chang, 2006).

Chemotherapy and Radiation Therapy. Chemotherapy is recommended when a patient has positive lymph nodes at the time of surgery or has metastatic disease. Chemotherapy is used both as an adjuvant therapy following colon resection and as primary treatment for nonresectable colorectal cancer. At present, the combination of 5-fluorouracil (5-FU) plus leucovorin and irinotecan (Camptosar) is approved as first-line chemotherapy for patients with metastatic colorectal cancer. Additional treatment protocols include the use of a variety of drugs in combination with 5-FU and leucovorin. For patients who are not considered appropriate candidates for this triple therapy, capecitabine (Xeloda) can be used as an acceptable alternative first-line treatment. Biological agents (bevacizumab [Avastin] and cetuximab [Erbitux]) may be used in combination with chemotherapeutic agent panitumumab (Vectibix). A human epidermal growth factor receptor (EGFR) monoclonal antibody is an option for patients with metastatic disease following standard chemotherapy regimens (Colorectal Cancer Association of

Canada, 2011b). Radiation may be used preoperatively as an adjuvant to colon resection and chemotherapy or as a palliative measure for patients with advanced lesions. As a palliative measure, its primary objective is to reduce tumour size and provide symptomatic relief. (For a discussion of radiation therapy, see Chapter 18.)

NURSING MANAGEMENT: COLORECTAL CANCER

▪ Nursing Assessment

Subjective and objective data that should be obtained from a patient with colorectal cancer are presented in Table 45-32.

▪ Nursing Diagnoses

Nursing diagnoses for the patient with cancer of the colon or the rectum include, but are not limited to, the following:

- Diarrhea or constipation *related to* altered bowel elimination patterns
- Acute pain *related to* difficulty in passing stools because of partial or complete obstruction from tumour

NURSING ASSESSMENT

Table 45-32 Colorectal Cancer

Subjective Data

Important Health Information

Past health history: Previous breast or ovarian cancer, familial adenomatous polyposis (FAP), callous adenoma, adenomatous polyps, inflammatory bowel disease; family history of colorectal, breast, or ovarian cancer

Medications: Use of any medication affecting bowel function (e.g., cathartics, antidiarrheal agents)

Symptoms

- Weakness, fatigue
- Anorexia, weight loss; nausea and vomiting
- Change in bowel habits; alternating diarrhea and constipation, defecation urgency; rectal bleeding; mucoid stools; black, tarry stools; increased flatus, decrease in stool calibre; feelings of incomplete evacuation
- Abdominal and low back pain, tenesmus

Objective Data

General

Pallor, cachexia, lymphadenopathy (later signs)

Gastrointestinal

Palpable abdominal mass (late sign), distension, ascites, and hepatomegaly (liver metastasis)

Possible Findings

Anemia; positive fecal occult blood; palpable mass on digital rectal examination; positive sigmoidoscopy, colonoscopy, barium enema, or CT scan; positive biopsy

CT, computed tomography.

- Fear *related to* diagnosis of colorectal cancer, surgical or therapeutic interventions, and possible terminal illness
- Ineffective coping *related to* diagnosis of cancer and adverse effects of treatment

▪ Planning

The overall goals are that the patient with colorectal cancer will have (1) appropriate treatment (removal of tumour, adjunctive therapy), (2) normal bowel elimination patterns, (3) quality of life appropriate to disease prognosis, (4) relief of pain, and (5) feelings of comfort and well-being.

▪ Nursing Implementation

▪ Health Promotion

The current recommendations from the Colorectal Cancer Association of Canada for colorectal cancer screening in patients who are not at high risk include FOBT or FIT performed every 1 to 2 years starting at the age of 50. Positive findings should be followed with flexible sigmoidoscopy, colonoscopy, or double-contrast barium enema (Colorectal Cancer Association of Canada, 2011a).

Screening for high-risk patients should begin before age 50, usually beginning with colonoscopy and continuing at more frequent intervals that vary according to risk factors (Colorectal Cancer Association of Canada, 2011a). Participation in early cancer screening is effective in decreasing mortality.

A number of epidemiology studies reported that use of NSAIDs (e.g., ibuprofen [Advil]) or long-term use of aspirin may reduce the development of adenomatous colorectal polyps and reduce the risk of colorectal cancer (Rostom et al., 2007).

▪ Acute Intervention

▪ **Preoperative Care.** Acute nursing care for the patient with a colon resection is similar to the care of the patient having a laparotomy (see NCP 45-2). In addition to general preoperative teaching and ostomy care instructions, the patient undergoing abdominal–perineal resection should be informed of the extent of the surgical procedure and the potential for sexual dysfunction after surgery. Comfortable positioning may be difficult with either an open or a closed perineal wound. Side-to-side positioning in bed and the use of pressure-reducing support surfaces for the bed and chair may be helpful. Doughnut cushions should not be used because these delay wound healing. The patient may experience phantom rectal sensation because the sympathetic nerves responsible for rectal control are not severed during the surgery. The nurse must be astute in distinguishing phantom sensations from perineal abscess pain.

▪ **Postoperative Care.** After an abdominal–perineal resection, there are two wounds, and a stoma is surgically constructed in the left lower quadrant. There is an abdominal incision through which the colon is resected, and an incision is made in the perineum. The management of a perineal incision differs according to the type of wound. Different approaches may be taken with the perineal wound: (1) packing of the entire open wound or (2) primary closure of the perineal wound with closed-suction drainage of the pelvic cavity. The type of management of the perineal wound is individualized. The open and packed method is used in patients with extensive bleeding in the perineal wound or when there are concerns about local wound infection. A Jackson-Pratt or a Hemovac suction device placed through the buttocks into the pelvic cavity is commonly used to provide drainage of the operative site during the early postoperative period. The drains usually remain until drainage is less than 50 mL/24 hr, which occurs after approximately 3 to 5 days.

A patient who has open and packed wounds requires meticulous postoperative care. During the immediate postoperative period, the perineal dressing may quickly become saturated with serosanguineous drainage. Proper containment of the drainage with appropriate topical dressings such as calcium alginates or hydrofibres will assist in the management of the wound. All drainage is carefully assessed for amount, colour, and consistency.

The nurse should examine the wound regularly and record bleeding, excessive drainage, and unusual odour. The perineal wound is usually irrigated with a normal saline solution when the dressings are changed. Topical dressing selection should be made applying wound care principles: reduce bacterial burden, facilitate moist wound healing, contain drainage, and protect periwound skin. Negative-pressure therapy may be an option to enhance wound healing. Aseptic technique is always used.

When the perineal wound is closed, the drains are left in place for approximately 3 to 5 days. During this time, the drainage is examined and observations recorded. The area around the drains is observed for signs of inflammation and is kept clean and dry. The nurse should observe for signs of induration, erythema, purulent drainage around the suture line, fever, and elevated WBC count. Perineal wound closure may be done with removable or dissolvable sutures. If removable sutures are used, these are generally left in place for 2 to 3 weeks.

If the patient complains of pain and itching in and around the wound, carefully inspect the wound for signs of local infection, maceration from wound drainage, or yeast. Use of a pressure-reducing chair cushion provides comfort when sitting, and side-to-side positioning in bed will help with comfort.

Sexual dysfunction is a possible complication of an abdominal–perineal resection and should be included in the plan of care. Although the effect of the procedure depends on the extent of pelvic dissection, the surgeon must inform the patient of the risk preoperatively. The nurse should understand that erection, ejaculation, and orgasm involve different nerve pathways and that a dysfunction of one does not mean total sexual dysfunction. The ET nurse is an important member of the team and can often provide factual information concerning sexual dysfunction and management options.

▪ Ambulatory and Home Care

Psychological support for the patient and family is important. The overall 5-year survival rate for all patients undergoing resection for colorectal cancer is less than 50%. This presents a problem for the patient and health care providers because of the often painful, debilitating, and demoralizing manifestations produced by the recurrent disease and the lack of any effective palliative therapy. Chemotherapy may be used as an adjuvant measure for the patient with evidence of local or distant metastasis. (The special needs of the patient with cancer are discussed in Chapter 18.)

The open perineal wound may not be completely healed before discharge. After discharge, the health care provider, home health nurse, and ET nurse usually see the patient. Regular reassessment of the wound to determine progress and ideal topical dressing management should be done. Clipping the buttock hair close to the perineal wound will aid dressing adherence and prevent wound bed irritation from long hairs. The nurse should report persistent drainage or prolonged wound healing because it may also indicate the presence of a foreign body, fistula, or rectal tissue not removed during surgery. The patient and significant others may be taught assessment and management of the wound. The patient and the family should be aware of all community services available for assistance.

▪ Evaluation

The following are expected outcomes for the patient with colorectal cancer:

- The patient will have regular bowel elimination patterns.
- The patient will have relief of pain.
- The patient will have balanced nutritional intake.
- The patient will have quality of life appropriate to disease prognosis.
- The patient will have feelings of comfort and well-being.

Ostomy Surgery

Types

The creation of an **ostomy** is a surgical procedure in which an opening is made to allow passage of urine from the bladder, or intestinal contents from the bowel, to an incision or stoma surgically created in the wall of the abdomen. In the context of intestinal reconstruction, the bowel is brought through an opening in the abdominal wall. The edges of the bowel are sutured to the surrounding skin, exposing the inner lining of the bowel (mucosa); this is the stoma. Bowel excretion will now occur through the stoma. The stoma may be permanent or temporary, depending upon the underlying reason for the surgery.

When the ileum is brought through the abdominal wall, it is called an *ileostomy*. It may also be called a *Brooke ileostomy* (Figure 45-9). It is commonly used in surgical treatment of UC, Crohn's disease, and FAP and may be used to temporarily protect distal anastomoses, such as in a low anterior resection.

A *cecostomy* describes the cecum being brought through the abdominal wall. Both cecostomies and ascending colostomies are rare. They are usually temporary and most often are used for fecal diversion and decompression before surgery or for palliation. An ileostomy is preferred over cecostomies or ascending colostomies.

A *colostomy* describes the colon being brought through the abdominal wall. *Colostomy* is a generic term and may be used to describe any part of the colon (large intestine) that is brought to the surface. Locations for colostomies are shown in Figure 45-10. A temporary colostomy may be created as an emergency measure following bowel obstruction (e.g., malignant tumour), abdominal trauma (e.g., gunshot wound), or a perforated diverticulum. Loop colostomy (see Figure 45-10) and double-barrelled colostomy (see Figure 45-9) may be created as temporary colostomies, but they may be permanent if the reason for surgery is palliation

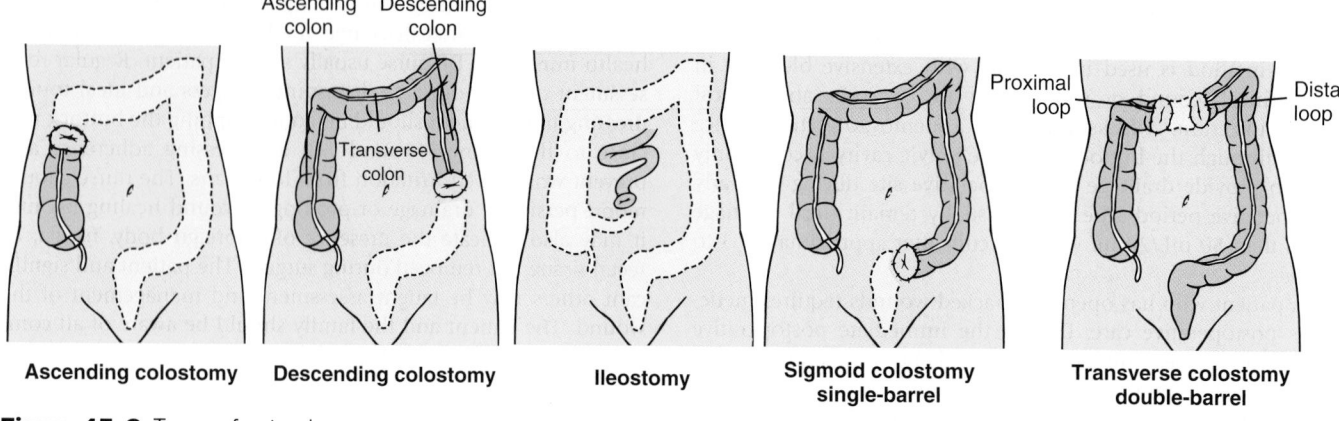

Figure 45-9 Types of ostomies.

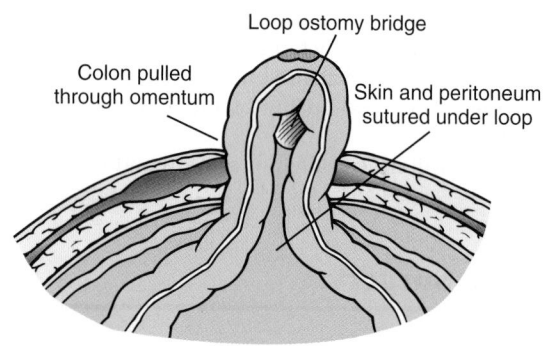

Figure 45-10 Loop colostomy.

Source: Redrawn from Meeker, M. H., & Rothrock, J. C. (1991). *Alexander's care of the patient in surgery* (9th ed.). St. Louis: Mosby.

for obstructing cancer. A comparison of colostomies and ileostomy is shown in Table 45-33.

Surgical Therapy

End Stoma. An *end stoma* is surgically constructed by dividing the bowel and bringing out the proximal end as a single stoma. The distal portion of the GI tract is either surgically removed or the distal segment is oversewn and left in the abdominal cavity with its mesentery intact. An end colostomy or ileostomy is then constructed. When the distal bowel is oversewn rather than removed, the result of the procedure is known as a *Hartmann's pouch* (Figure 45-11). If the distal bowel is removed, the stoma is permanent; if the distal bowel remains intact and oversewn, the potential exists for the bowel to be reanastomosed and the stoma to be closed (referred to as a *takedown*).

Loop Stoma. A *loop stoma* is constructed by bringing a loop of bowel to the abdominal surface and then opening the anterior wall of the bowel to provide fecal diversion. This results in one stoma with a proximal and distal opening as well as an intact posterior wall that separates the two openings. The loop of bowel may be supported by a plastic rod for 3 to 7 days after surgery to prevent it from slipping back into the abdominal cavity (see Figure 45-10). A loop stoma is usually temporary.

Table 45-33 Comparison of Colostomies and Ileostomy

	COLOSTOMY		ILEOSTOMY
	TRANSVERSE	**SIGMOID**	
Stool consistency	Semiliquid to semiformed	Formed	Liquid to pasty
Fluid requirement	Possibly increased	No change	Increased
Bowel regulation	No	Yes (if there is a history of a regular bowel pattern)	No
Pouch and skin barriers	Yes	Dependent on regulation	Yes
Irrigation	No	Possible every 24-48 hr (if patient meets criteria)	No
Indications for surgery	Palliation for distal, nonoperable obstructing cancers; trauma	Cancer of the rectum or rectosigmoid area; perforated diverticulitis; trauma; invading gynecological cancers	Ulcerative colitis, Crohn's disease, diseased or injured colon, birth defect, familial adenomatous polyposis; trauma; cancer; ischemic colitis

Double-Barrelled Stoma. When the bowel is divided, both the proximal and the distal ends are brought through the abdominal wall as two separate stomas (see Figure 45-9). The proximal one is the functioning stoma; the distal stoma is referred to as the mucus fistula. The double-barrelled stoma is usually temporary.

Ileoanal Reservoir. As described in the section on UC earlier in this chapter (pp. 1183-1186), this procedure involves total colectomy and ileoanal anastomosis with the formation of an ileal reservoir (see Figure 45-4).

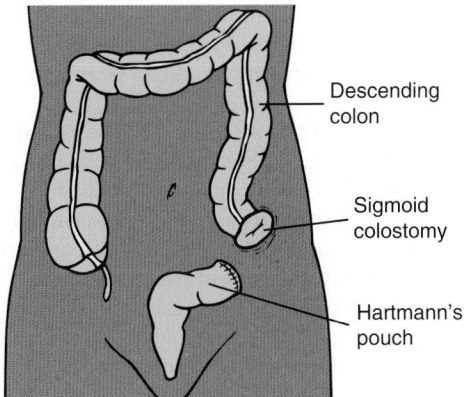

Figure 45-11 Sigmoid colostomy. Distal bowel is oversewn and left in place to create Hartmann's pouch.

Source: Redrawn from Hampton, B. G., & Bryant, R. A. (1992). *Ostomies and continent diversions*. St. Louis: Mosby.

NURSING MANAGEMENT: OSTOMY SURGERY

▪ Preoperative Care

It is important to review the information the patient has received from the health care provider. Psychological preparation and support are very important. The family and the patient usually have many questions concerning the procedures. If available, an ET nurse should visit with the patient and the family. An ET nurse is a nurse with additional education and training who specializes in the care and management of individuals with ostomies. The nurse or the ET nurse must determine the patient's ability to perform self-care, identify support systems, and determine potential adverse factors that could be modified to facilitate learning during rehabilitation. Preoperative assessment must be comprehensive and include physical, psychological, social, cultural, and educational components. Assessment is ongoing, including both the patient and the family. The ET nurse marks the stoma site before surgery. An improperly placed stoma complicates rehabilitation by increasing patient dependency on nursing support and increasing time, frequency, and expense of pouch change routine. It can also contribute to skin irritation and poor adaptation. Stomas should be placed within the rectus muscle, on the superior aspect of a skinfold, within the patient's visual field, above or below the belt line, and away from obvious creases and folds. The patient and the family should understand the extent of surgery, the type of stoma, and its care. Trained visitors from ostomy support groups may also provide reassurance and guidance for the patient and family. The patient and family have the opportunity to see a person who has adjusted well and who has experienced some of the same feelings and concerns. Bowel preparation before surgery may be required. Orally administered osmotic lavages (e.g., GoLYTELY) have shortened the classic 72-hour preparation with clear liquids, cathartics, and enemas. Preoperative IV antibiotics are given.

▪ Colostomy Care

Postoperative nursing care should focus on assessing the stoma, protecting the skin and the stoma, selecting the pouch, provid-

Table 45-34 Postoperative Characteristics of Stoma	
CHARACTERISTIC	**DESCRIPTION OR CAUSE**
Colour*	
Pink, rose to brick red	Viable stoma mucosa
Pale pink	May indicate anemia
Blanching, dark red to purple	May indicate inadequate blood supply to the stoma, low flow state, excessive tension on the bowel mesentery at the time of construction, or venous congestion; usually occurs in the first 72 hr after surgery
Edema†	
Mild to moderate edema	Normal in the initial postoperative period
	Trauma to the stoma
	Any medical condition that results in edema
Moderate to severe edema	Obstruction proximal to the stoma
Bleeding	
Small amount	Oozing from the stomal mucosa when touched or cleansed is normal because of its vascularity
Moderate to large amount‡	Moderate to large amount of bleeding from the stomal mucosa could indicate coagulation factor deficiency; trauma to the stoma
	Moderate to large amount from intestinal stoma opening could indicate lower gastrointestinal bleeding

*Sustained colour changes must be reported to surgeon.
†Closely observe, monitor, and report to the surgeon.
‡Report moderate to large amounts of bleeding to surgeon.

ing patient education on ostomy self-care, and assisting the patient to adapt psychologically to a changed body. Nursing care for the patient with a colostomy is presented in NCP 45-4 on pp. 1206-1207.

The stoma should be pink or red. A dusky purple stoma indicates ischemia, and a brown-black stoma indicates necrosis. The nurse should assess and document stoma colour every 8 to 12 hours for the first 72 hours after surgery, when necrosis is more likely to occur. There is initial mild to moderate swelling of the stoma, which will settle 4 to 6 weeks after surgery (Table 45-34). Application of an appropriate skin barrier is important to protect the peristomal skin. Several pouching options are available from ostomy supply companies, including ConvaTec, Coloplast, and Hollister. The peristomal skin should be cleansed with warm water and dried thoroughly before the new barrier is applied.

Principles of ostomy care and pouching selection include (1) protection of peristomal skin from effluent, trauma, or both; (2) protection of the stoma from trauma; (3) secured containment of odour and effluent; (4) preservation of patient dignity; and (5) cost containment of pouching system. Numerous pouching options are available. An ET nurse can assist with the education of the patient and selection of the most appropriate appliance. Openings to the traditional skin barrier should be cut 3 to 4 mm larger than the base of the stoma to allow for normal

NUTRITIONAL THERAPY

Table 45-35 Effects of Food on Stoma Output

Odour Producing*	Diarrhea Causing*
Eggs	Alcohol
Garlic	Beer
Onions	Cabbage family
Fish	Spinach
Asparagus	Green beans
Cabbage	Coffee
Broccoli	Spicy foods
Cauliflower	Fruits and vegetables (raw)
Alcohol	**Potential Obstruction in Ileostomy†**
Spicy foods	
Gas Forming*	Nuts
Beans and legumes	Raisins
Cabbage family	Popcorn
Onions	Seeds
Beer	Fruits and vegetables (raw)
Carbonated beverages	
Cheeses (strong)	
Asian vegetables	

*The effect of food on stoma output is individual. Patients are not discouraged from eating the above-listed foods and beverages.
†Patients are encouraged to chew high-roughage food well, or cook the foods and limit the amounts in the initial postoperative period (4-6 wk after surgery), and to drink increased amounts of fluids.

stomal peristalsis. Newer mouldable barriers eliminate the need for precise measuring and simplify the care for patients.

The volume, colour, and consistency of the drainage are recorded. Each time the pouch is changed, the condition of the skin and stoma are observed. If any abnormalities are noted (rash, blisters, ulcers), an ET nurse should be consulted for assessment and management.

A colostomy in the transverse colon has semiliquid to pasty stools and moderate to large volumes of flatus. A colostomy in the sigmoid or the descending colon has semiformed or formed stools and can sometimes be regulated by the irrigation method. Patients may choose to use drainable, closed-end pouches or pouch liners to manage the stool.

For most patients with colostomies, there are few, if any, dietary restrictions. A well-balanced diet and adequate fluid intake are important. The patient's medical and surgical history must be considered when individualizing dietary instructions. Table 45-35 lists foods and their effects on stoma output.

■ Colostomy Irrigations

Colostomy irrigations can be used to regulate bowel function, treat constipation, or prepare the bowel for surgery. When done to achieve a regular bowel pattern, the irrigations habituate the bowel to function at a specific time every day or every other day. If control is achieved, there should be little or no spillage between irrigations. The patient who establishes regularity may need to wear only a pad or small pouch over the stoma. Not all patients can be managed with irrigations. An ET nurse can help

to assess whether this is an appropriate management technique. The patient who is not eligible for irrigations or chooses not to establish regularity by irrigations must wear a pouch at all times.

All equipment should be assembled before irrigation. A commercially obtained irrigation set usually has all the equipment needed. The nurse should encourage the patient to watch the procedure and should explain each step to the patient. The cone tip on the tubing controls the depth of insertion and prevents the water from prematurely coming out from the stoma. If resistance is met, force should not be used because perforation of the intestine can result. However, this is unlikely when using a stoma cone. A hard plastic catheter is not recommended because of the risk of intestinal perforation. The procedure should not be rushed; the patient should feel relaxed. The patient or a family member must be instructed in the procedure and must be able to demonstrate the ability to irrigate before doing so independently. This can be done in the outpatient setting. Habituation of the bowel takes 3 to 6 weeks.

The patient should be able to perform a pouch change, care for skin and stoma, control odour, and identify signs and symptoms of complications. The patient should know the importance of fluids and food in the diet, have access to community resources, and know when to seek medical care. Home care and outpatient follow-up by an ET nurse are highly recommended. Patients should be discharged with written instructions for pouch change, teaching literature relevant to the type of stoma they have, a list and samples of products they use, a list of product retailers (including names and phone numbers), outpatient follow-up appointments with the surgeon and the ET nurse, and the phone numbers of the surgeon and the nurse. The patient and caregiver teaching guidelines are included in Table 45-36.

■ Ileostomy Care

Care of the ileostomy is presented in NCP 45-4. Ileostomy stomal protrusion of at least 2 cm makes care easier. When the stoma is flat, stool can undermine the seal and cause altered skin integrity. Stomal function is frequent, and the stool is extremely irritating to the skin. Regularity cannot be established, so a pouch must be worn at all times. An open-ended, drainable pouch is worn by the patient so that effluent can be emptied when the pouch is one-third full. The drainable pouch is usually worn for 4 to 7 days before being changed, as long as leakage does not occur under the pouching system. If pouch leakage occurs, the pouch should be promptly removed, the skin should be cleansed, and a new pouching system applied. Frequent leaks of the appliance warrant assessment by an ET nurse of appropriateness of the pouching. A transparent pouch may be used in the initial postoperative period to facilitate assessment of stoma viability and stoma function, but opaque pouches for discharge and home enhance aesthetics.

Immediately after surgery, intake and output must be accurately monitored. The patient should be observed for signs and symptoms of fluid and electrolyte imbalance, particularly potassium, sodium, and fluid deficits. In the first 24 to 48 hours after surgery, the amount of drainage from the stoma may be negligible. A person with an ileostomy has lost the absorptive functions provided by the colon as well as the delay feature provided by the ileocecal valve. Once peristalsis returns, the patient may experience a period of high-volume bilious output of 1200 to

Table 45-36 Ostomy Self-Care

The following are guidelines to include for patient and caregiver teaching.

1. Explain the following principles of ostomy care:
   - Routinely change appliances, cleanse skin, and inspect stoma and skin.
   - Empty pouch before it is one-third full.
   - Use deodorants as needed.
   - Explain how to contact the enterostomal therapy nurse.
   - Explain how to obtain additional supplies or accessories.
   - Ensure access to home health services.

2. Teach the following dietary and fluid intake guidelines:
   - Identify a well-balanced diet and dietary supplements if necessary to prevent nutritional deficiencies.
   - Identify foods to reduce diarrhea, gas, or obstruction (with ileostomy).
   - Identify foods to reduce constipation and gas (with colostomy).
   - Drink at least 1500-2000 mL/day of fluid to prevent dehydration (unless contraindicated).
   - Increase fluid intake during hot weather, excessive perspiration, or diarrhea to replace losses and prevent dehydration.
   - Get to know the signs and symptoms of dehydration and when to seek help from a health care provider.
   - Contact your registered dietitian with any questions.

3. Describe potential resources to assist with emotional and psychological adjustment.
   - Identify persons available to provide emotional support.
   - Identify community resources for psychosocial support.
   - Contact local ostomy support groups for information or peer support.

4. Explain the importance of follow-up care. Report signs and symptoms of the following:
   - Fluid and electrolyte deficits (dehydration)
   - Fever
   - Diarrhea
   - Constipation
   - Other stoma problems, including a change in appearance of the stoma or its function, a change in the peristomal skin, tenderness, erythema, or pain

1800 mL/day. Later on, the amount can average 800 mL daily because the proximal small bowel adapts and absorbs more fluid. If the small bowel has been shortened as a result of surgical resections, the drainage from the ileostomy may be greater. The patient must understand the importance of fluid and electrolyte balance. A dietitian is helpful in assessing and determining patient food and fluid requirements.

The patient should be instructed to drink at least 1.5 to 2 L of fluid daily; more may be necessary when diarrhea occurs and when perspiration is increased. Diarrhea from an ileostomy can produce dehydration and acidosis from the loss of bicarbonate. The patient may require brief hospitalization for IV fluid rehydration if large volumes of diarrhea occur.

Usually a low-residue diet is ordered initially. Insoluble fibre–containing foods are reintroduced gradually. Later, there are few dietary restrictions. It is important to limit the amount of high-roughage foods (e.g., popcorn), chew them well, and accompany them with fluids. The goal for the patient is a return to a normal, presurgical diet.

The stoma may bleed easily when it is touched or cleansed because it has a high vascular supply. The patient should be told that minimal oozing of blood is normal. If the terminal ileum has been removed, the patient may need cobalamin (vitamin B_{12}) injections or oral supplements.

Adaptation to an Ostomy

Adaptation to the ostomy is a gradual process. The patient experiences a grief reaction to the loss of a body part and an alteration in body image. Each person uses different coping mechanisms. The adjustment period for the person depends on the individual. Psychological support during the grieving process is needed. There are many concerns including body image, sexual activity, family responsibilities, and changes in lifestyle. The patient may become resentful and have fears of odour or leakage. Supportive measures by nurses include helping the patient acquire knowledge, providing or recommending support services, and identifying coping mechanisms that are effective. The nurse provides support by responding to the physiological needs of stoma care and psychosocial needs related to self-esteem.

Gradual involvement of the patient in self-care of the ostomy should be encouraged. Although initial visualization of the stoma and participation in care is distressing, supportive teaching from the nurse will enhance confidence and independence in care. Teaching at the appropriate time is an important part of the care and can contribute to a smooth adjustment process.

Gradual resumption of activities of daily living can occur within 2 to 3 weeks. Heavy lifting, physical exertion, and participation in sports should be avoided for 6 to 8 weeks. The patient's physical condition determines when sexual activity may be resumed. Bathing and swimming are not prohibited.

Sexual Dysfunction After Ostomy Surgery

Discussion of sexuality and sexual function must be incorporated in the plan of care. The nurse can help the patient understand that sexual function or sexual activity may be affected but that sexuality does not have to be altered.

Pelvic surgery can disrupt nerve and vascular supply to the genitals. Radiation, chemotherapy, and medications can also alter sexual function. Hormones and overall physical health of the patient influence desire. Certain pain medications and antiemetics can lower libido. Generalized fatigue caused by illness can also influence desire. By communicating this information to patients, they can plan sexual activity around a drug schedule and energy levels. Any pelvic surgery that removes the rectum has the potential of damaging the parasympathetic nerve plexus. Erection in men depends on the parasympathetic nerves that control blood flow and vascular supply to the pelvis and the pudendal nerves that transmit sensory responses from the genital area. Nerve-sparing surgical techniques are used when possible to preserve sexual function. Radiation therapy to the pelvis can reduce blood vascularity to the pelvis by causing scarring in the small blood vessels. Pelvic surgery usually does not affect a woman's arousal unless part of or the entire vagina is removed. Radiation therapy can affect vaginal expansion and lubrication.

NURSING CARE PLAN 45-4

Colostomy or an Ileostomy

NURSING DIAGNOSIS	**Risk for impaired skin integrity** *related to* fecal irritation, pouching product irritation, or lack of knowledge of skin care
Expected Patient Outcomes	**Nursing Interventions and *Rationales***
• Reports normal skin integrity • Has intact pouch seal	• Preoperative stoma site marking by the enterostomal therapy nurse *to ensure proper placement of the stoma site, avoiding body contours that may interfere with establishing a pouch seal.* • After surgery, monitor the pouch for leakage and change immediately if leakage noted *to prevent stool irritation.* • Assess the patient's reports of itching, burning, or pain to stomal area and remove pouch *to assess skin for stool irritation.* • During pouch change, assess skin for signs of skin irritation *to initiate treatment if indicated.* • Cleanse area with warm tap water, and dry thoroughly *to prevent irritation from intestinal contents and poor pouch adhesion.* • Apply skin barrier *to protect skin and prevent direct contact with stool.* • Teach patient stoma, skin, and appliance care *to ensure proper technique for long-term care.* • Plan for outpatient or home visit *for continued teaching and monitoring.* • Empty pouch when it is one-third full or inflated with gas *to prevent the pouch from leaking.*
NURSING DIAGNOSIS	**Disturbed body image** *related to* presence of ostomy *as evidenced by* verbalization of embarrassment or shame caused by presence of stoma
Expected Patient Outcomes	**Nursing Interventions and *Rationales***
• Expresses adjustment to altered body image • Reports control of odour	• Assess patient's attitude toward ostomy *to determine whether patient has concerns and, if indicated, plan appropriate education and intervention.* • Instruct patient on measures for odour control, including the use of pouch and room deodorants when pouch is emptied, and educate about foods that are known to increase odour *to minimize odours during pouch emptying.* • Discuss normal emotional response to stoma and encourage patient to express feelings *to assist patient in adjusting to change in body.* • Provide patient with information on local ostomy support groups *to offer patient and family an opportunity for additional education and support.* • Provide patient with education on self-care of ostomy, and ensure patient demonstrates skill before discharge *to increase independence and enhance self-esteem/image.*
NURSING DIAGNOSIS	**Imbalanced nutrition: less than body requirements** *related to* lack of knowledge of appropriate foods and decreased appetite *as evidenced by* weight loss, vitamin and mineral deficiencies, inability to tolerate certain foods
Expected Patient Outcome	**Nursing Interventions and *Rationales***
• Has adequate dietary intake to maintain weight at optimum level	• Assess volume of ostomy output to ensure losses are not in excess of 1200 mL/24 hr *because patient may require fluid replacements.* • Assess nutritional intake *to determine need for intervention.* • Initiate low-residue diet when patient progresses to solid foods *to minimize risk of bowel obstruction.* • Teach patient to chew food well *to facilitate digestion.* • Give list of foods (high-residue) that have potential for obstruction to ileostomy patients in the first 6-8 wk after surgery *so that patient has a ready source for reference.* • Arrange visit with dietitian if indicated *to ensure appropriate diet progression and adequate nutrition.*

NURSING CARE PLAN 45-4

Colostomy or an Ileostomy—cont'd

NURSING DIAGNOSIS	*Loss of sexuality* related to altered body image, perceived loss of sexual appeal, and concern about pouch leakage during sexual activity *as evidenced by* verbalization of concern about intimate relations with spouse or significant other
Expected Patient Outcome	**Nursing Interventions and *Rationales***
• Expresses confidence in ability to resume previous sexual activity	• Assess patient's attitude about impact of ostomy on sexual functioning *to determine if there are concerns and if there is a need to plan interventions.* • Encourage discussion of meaning of sexuality to patient and significant other *to allow patient opportunity to discuss sensitive topic in a supportive environment.* • Discuss ways to secure and conceal appliance during intimate relations *to decrease fear of embarrassment or withdrawal from intimate situations because of anxiety over appearance and leakage.* • If appropriate, arrange visit with person of same sex and condition *to discuss sexual concerns and share potential solutions; to provide an opportunity to ask questions; and to get practical, realistic answers from a supportive, understanding other.* • Provide information on intimate apparel that can be used during sexual activity, as well as use of smaller appliances such as stoma caps *to enhance body image during intimate activity.*
NURSING DIAGNOSIS	***Risk for deficient fluid volume*** related to excess fluid loss from ileostomy or diarrhea with a colostomy and inadequate oral intake
Expected Patient Outcomes	**Nursing Interventions and *Rationales***
• Has normal serum electrolytes • Has normal vital signs • Has good skin turgor • Has urine output >0.5 mL/kg/hr	• Assess for signs of weakness, poor skin turgor, sunken eyes, hypotension, tachycardia, hypokalemia, hyponatremia, decreased urine output *to determine presence of fluid volume deficit and, if present, plan appropriate interventions.* • Record intake and output including stoma drainage *to have an accurate record of fluid balance.* • Ensure fluid intake of at least 2000 mL/day in the initial postoperative period *to prevent dehydration.* • Administer additional IV fluid replacements, if initial ostomy outputs are excessive, *to prevent fluid and electrolyte imbalance.* • A patient with an ileostomy should ingest 1.5-2 L of fluid and increase it during hot weather, excessive perspiration, and during episodes of diarrhea *to ensure adequate fluid intake.* • Monitor serum electrolytes *to detect any imbalances.* • Instruct patient on signs and symptoms of sodium, potassium, and fluid deficits *to ensure early reporting and correction of underlying problem.*

IV, intravenous.

Muscular contraction and the genital pleasure that occur during orgasm are not disrupted by pelvic surgery. If the sympathetic nerves in the presacral area are damaged, the male mechanism of emission can be disrupted. This can occur with an abdominal–perineal resection. Orgasms can occur in both men and women who have had stoma surgery, although other aspects of the sexual response may be affected.

The psychological impact of the stoma and how it affects the patient's body image and self-esteem must be discussed. Emotional factors can contribute to sexual problems. A life-threatening illness can override concerns about sexual function. The nurse can assist a patient to identify ways of coping with depression and anxiety resulting from illness, surgery, or postoperative problems.

The social impact of the stoma is interrelated with its psychological, physical, and sexual aspects. Concerns of people

with stomas include the ability to resume sexual activity, altering clothing styles, the effect on daily activities, sleeping while wearing a pouch, passing gas, the presence of odour, cleanliness, and deciding when or whether to tell others about the stoma. The fear of rejection from a partner or the fear that others will not find them desirable as a sexual partner can be a concern. The nurse should encourage open communication about feelings and should realize that the patient needs time to adjust to the pouch and to body changes before feeling secure in her or his sexual functioning.

Pregnancy is possible with an ostomy. As the abdomen expands in the second and third trimesters, the stoma may retract and alternate pouching may be required. A woman with an ostomy who becomes pregnant should have regular medical care and assessment by an ET nurse.

Diverticulosis and Diverticulitis

A **diverticulum** is an outpouching of the mucosa through the circular smooth muscle of the intestinal wall. Diverticula may occur at any point within the GI tract but are most commonly found in the sigmoid colon. Clinically, diverticular disease occurs in two forms: diverticulosis and diverticulitis. Multiple noninflamed diverticula are present with *diverticulosis*. The patient is most often free of symptoms or may have alternating periods of constipation and diarrhea. In *diverticulitis*, inflammation of the diverticula occurs (Figures 45-12 and 45-13).

Etiology and Pathophysiology

Diverticular disease is a common GI disorder that affects 5% of the population by the age of 40 years and 60% by the age of 85 years. A diverticulum is a saccular dilation or outpouching of the

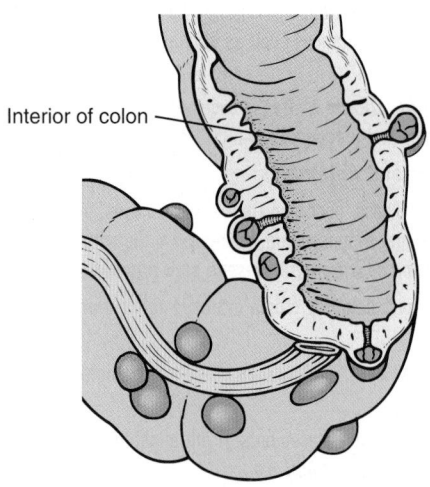

Figure 45-12 Diverticula are outpouchings of the colon. When they become inflamed, the condition is diverticulitis. The inflammatory process can spread to the surrounding area in the intestine.

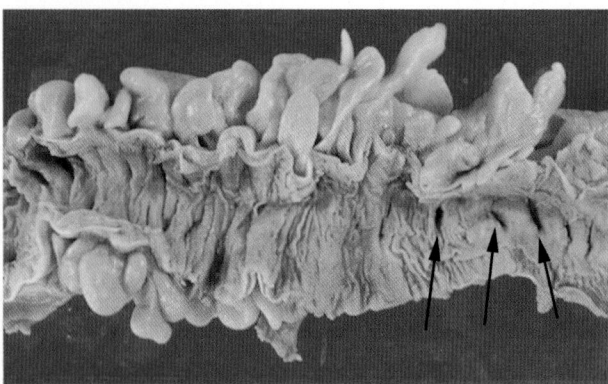

Figure 45-13 In diverticular disease, the outpouchings *(arrows)* of mucosa appear as slitlike openings from the mucosal surface of the open bowel.

Source: Stevens, A., & Lowe, J. (2000). *Pathology* (2nd ed.). London: Mosby.

mucosa through the circular smooth muscle of the intestinal wall. It affects men and women equally, but men seem to have a higher rate of complications. Most people are asymptomatic and are unaware that they have the disease.

There is no known cause of diverticular disease, but deficiency in dietary fibre has been associated with it. The disease is more prevalent in Western populations that consume diets low in fibre and high in refined carbohydrates; it is virtually unknown in other areas of the world, such as rural Africa, where high-fibre diets are consumed.

When diverticula form, the smooth muscle of the colon wall becomes thickened. Lack of dietary fibre slows transit time, and more water is absorbed from the stool, making its passage through the lumen more difficult. Decreased bulk of the stool, combined with a more acutely narrowed lumen in the sigmoid colon, causes high intraluminal pressures. These factors are believed to contribute to the formation of diverticula.

The cause of diverticulitis is related to the retention of stool and bacteria in the diverticulum, forming a hardened mass called a *fecalith*. This causes inflammation and usually small perforations. Inflammation of the diverticulum spreads to the surrounding tissues (Figure 45-14), causing it to become edematous. Abscesses may form, or complete perforation with peritonitis may occur.

Clinical Manifestations

The majority of patients with diverticulosis have no symptoms. Those with symptoms typically have crampy abdominal pain located in the left lower quadrant that is usually relieved by passage of flatus or bowel movement. Alternating constipation and diarrhea may be present.

Approximately 15% of patients with diverticulosis progress to acute diverticulitis. In patients with diverticulitis, abdominal pain is localized over the involved area of the colon. A tender left lower quadrant mass may be felt on palpation of the abdomen. Fever, chills, nausea, anorexia, and elevated WBC may be present.

PATHOPHYSIOLOGY MAP

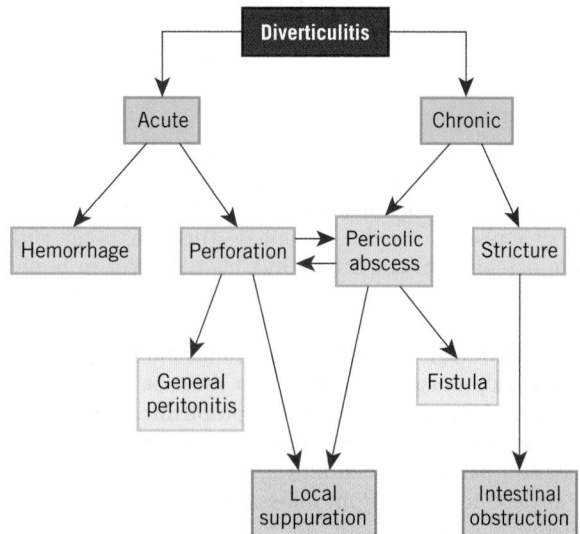

Figure 45-14 Complications of diverticulitis.

COLLABORATIVE CARE

Table 45-37 Diverticulosis and Diverticulitis

Diagnostic	Collaborative Therapy
• History and physical examination	**Ambulatory and Home Care**
• Testing of stool for occult blood	• High-fibre diet (during nonsymptomatic periods)
• Barium enema	• Dietary fibre supplements (during nonsymptomatic periods)
• Sigmoidoscopy	
• Colonoscopy	
• CBC	• Stool softeners
• CT scan with contrast	• Clear liquid diet
• Urinalysis	• Oral antibiotics
• Blood culture	**Acute Care: Diverticulitis**
	• IV antibiotics
	• NPO status
	• IV fluids
	• Possible colon resection for perforation, obstruction, or hemorrhage
	• Bed rest

CBC, complete blood count; *CT,* computed tomography; *IV,* intravenous; *NPO,* nothing by mouth.

Older adults with diverticulitis are frequently afebrile, with a normal WBC and little, if any, abdominal tenderness.

Complications of diverticulitis include perforation with peritonitis, abscess and fistula formation, bowel obstruction, ureteral obstruction, and bleeding. Diverticular bleeding is the most common cause of lower GI bleeding. Bleeding usually stops spontaneously.

Diagnostic Studies

A CT scan with oral contrast is the test of choice for diverticulitis. A CBC, urinalysis, and FOBT should be performed (Table 45-37). A barium enema is used to determine narrowing or obstruction of the colonic lumen. A colonoscopy may be performed to rule out possible hidden polyps or lesions. A patient with acute diverticulitis should not have a barium enema or colonoscopy because of the possibility of perforation and peritonitis.

NURSING AND COLLABORATIVE MANAGEMENT: DIVERTICULOSIS AND DIVERTICULITIS

Uncomplicated diverticular disease is treated with a high-fibre diet (see Table 45-9) and bulk laxatives, such as psyllium hydrophilic mucilloid (Metamucil). In acute diverticulitis, the goal of treatment is to allow the colon to rest and the inflammation to subside. The patient is kept on NPO status with parenteral fluids for hydration. The patient should be observed for signs of possible peritonitis. In acute diverticulitis, broad-spectrum antibiotic therapy is required. The temperature and the WBC count are monitored.

When the acute attack subsides, oral fluids are allowed, progressing to a semisolid diet. At this stage, the patient should be observed for a recurrent attack. If the patient has a bowel resection or colostomy, the nursing care is the same as for these procedures.

Approximately 30% of patients with acute diverticulitis require surgical intervention. Surgical intervention is necessary to drain abscesses and to resect an obstructing inflammatory mass or perforated segment. The usual surgical procedures involve resection of the involved colon with a temporary diverting colostomy. The bowel is reanastomosed after the colon has healed.

The patient should be provided with a full explanation of the condition. Consultation with a dietitian regarding high-fibre diets is recommended.

Hernias

A **hernia** is a protrusion of a viscus through an abnormal opening or a weakened area in the wall of the cavity in which it is normally contained. If the hernia can be placed back into the abdominal cavity, it is known as *reducible*. The hernia can be reduced by manipulation, or reduction can occur spontaneously when the person lies down. If the hernia cannot be placed back into the abdominal cavity, it is known as *irreducible*. In this situation (an incarcerated hernia), the intestinal flow may be obstructed. When the hernia is irreducible and the intestinal flow and blood supply are obstructed, the hernia is *strangulated*. The result is an acute intestinal obstruction and ischemia, necessitating surgery.

Types

The *inguinal hernia* is the most common type of hernia and occurs at the point of weakness in the abdominal wall where the spermatic cord emerges in men and the round ligament in women (Figure 45-15). When the protrusion escapes through the inguinal ring and follows the spermatic cord or the round ligament, it is termed an *indirect* hernia. When it escapes through the posterior inguinal wall, it is a *direct* hernia. An inguinal hernia is more common in men.

A *femoral hernia* occurs when there is a protrusion through the femoral ring into the femoral canal. It occurs below the inguinal (Poupart's) ligament as a bulge. It becomes strangulated easily and occurs more often in women. The umbilical hernia occurs when the rectus muscle is weak or the umbilical opening fails to close after birth.

Ventral, or incisional, hernia is caused by weakness of the abdominal wall at the site of a previous incision. It is found most commonly in patients who are obese, who have had multiple surgical procedures in the same area, and who have had inadequate wound healing because of poor nutrition or infection.

Clinical Manifestations

A hernia commonly occurs over the involved area when the patient stands or strains. Severe pain is caused if the hernia becomes strangulated. In this situation, the clinical manifestations of a bowel obstruction, such as vomiting, crampy abdominal pain, and distension, are found.

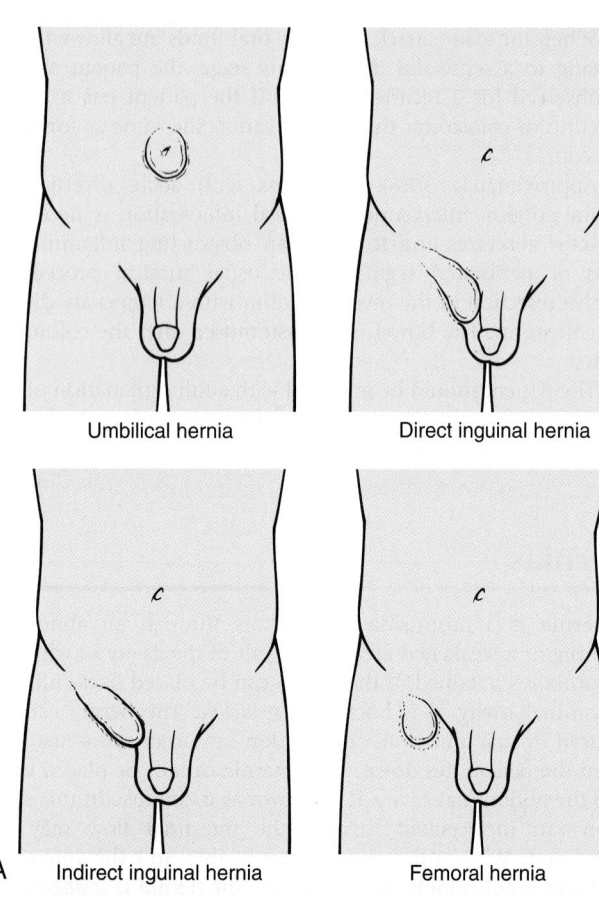

Umbilical hernia

Direct inguinal hernia

Indirect inguinal hernia

Femoral hernia

A

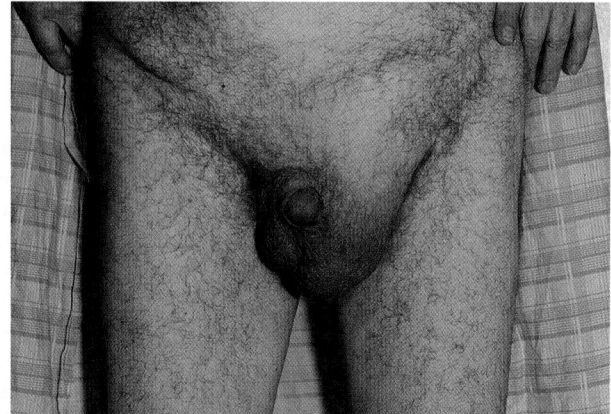

B

Figure 45-15 A, Types of hernias. **B,** Indirect inguinal hernia.

Source: **B** from Swartz, M. H. (2010). *Textbook of physical diagnosis: History and examination* (6th ed., p. 545, Figure 18-42). Philadelphia: Saunders.

NURSING AND COLLABORATIVE MANAGEMENT: HERNIAS

Diagnosis is based on history and physical examination findings. Surgery is the treatment of choice for hernias to prevent the possible complication of strangulation. The surgical repair of a hernia is known as a *herniorrhaphy*. The reinforcement of the weakened area with fascia or mesh is known as a *hernioplasty*. When there is strangulation, necrosis and gangrene may develop if immediate care is not given. A bowel resection of the involved area or a temporary ostomy may be needed to treat a strangulated hernia.

Some patients with inguinal hernias wear a truss, a firm pad placed over the hernia and held in place with a belt. The truss is worn to keep the hernia from protruding. The truss should be applied when the hernia is reduced. If the hernia cannot be reduced, the truss should not be used. If a patient wears a truss, the nurse should check for skin irritation caused by the continual rubbing and pressure of the truss.

After an inguinal hernia repair, the patient may have difficulty voiding; thus, the nurse should observe for a distended bladder. An accurate intake and output record is important. Scrotal edema is a painful complication after an inguinal hernia repair. A scrotal support may help relieve discomfort. Coughing is not encouraged, but deep breathing and turning should be done. If the patient needs to cough or sneeze, the incision should be splinted during coughing or sneezing. After discharge, the patient may be restricted from heavy lifting or activities for 6 to 8 weeks. Some surgeons do not put any limitations on physical activities.

Anorectal Problems

Hemorrhoids

Hemorrhoids are varicosities in the lower rectum or the anus caused by congestion in the veins of the hemorrhoidal plexus. They may be *internal* (occurring above the internal sphincter) or *external* (occurring outside the external sphincter) (Figures 45-16 and 45-17). Symptoms of hemorrhoids, including bleeding, pruritus, prolapse, and pain, are common in all age groups. In affected persons, hemorrhoids appear periodically, depending on the amount of anorectal pressure.

Etiology and Pathophysiology

Hemorrhoids are thought to develop as a result of shearing forces during defecation. This force damages supporting muscles. When supporting tissues in the anal canal weaken, usually as a result of straining at defecation, venules become dilated. In addition, blood flow through the veins of the hemorrhoidal plexus is impaired. An intravascular clot in the venule results in a thrombosed external hemorrhoid. They are the most common cause of bleeding with defecation. The amount of blood lost at one time may be small but may lead to iron-deficiency anemia over time.

Hemorrhoids may be precipitated by many factors, including pregnancy, prolonged constipation, straining in an effort to defecate, heavy lifting, prolonged standing and sitting, and portal hypertension (as found in cirrhosis).

Clinical Manifestations

The patient with internal hemorrhoids may be asymptomatic. However, when internal hemorrhoids become constricted, the patient will report pain. Internal hemorrhoids can bleed, resulting in blood on toilet paper after defecation or blood on the outside of stool. The patient may report a chronic, dull, aching discomfort, particularly when the hemorrhoids have prolapsed.

External hemorrhoids are reddish blue and seldom bleed or cause pain unless a vein ruptures. If the blood clots in external

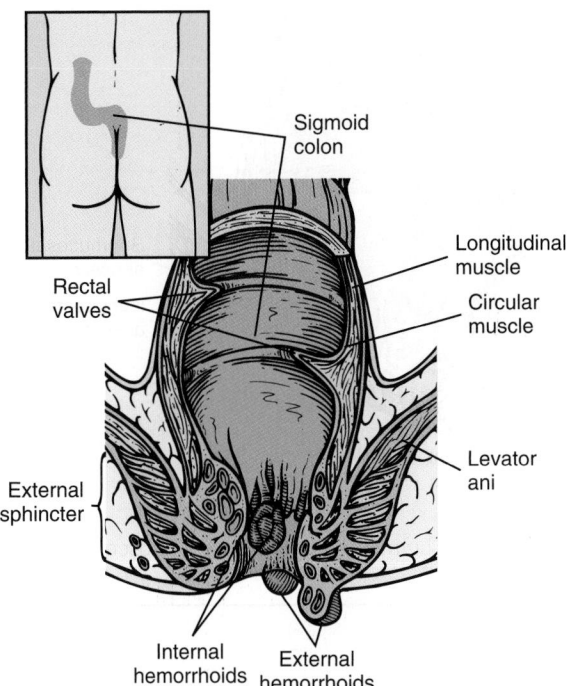

Figure 45-16 Anatomical structures of the rectum and the anus with external and internal hemorrhoids.

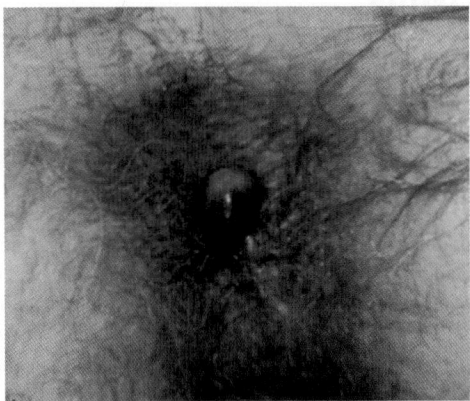

Figure 45-17 Thrombosed external hemorrhoids.

Source: Townsend, C. M., Beauchamp, R. D., Evers, B. M., & Mattox, K. L (Eds.). (2009). *Sabiston textbook of surgery: The biological basis of modern surgical practice* (18th ed.). Saunders: Philadelphia.

hemorrhoids, they become inflamed and painful and are said to be thrombosed. External hemorrhoids cause intermittent pain, pain on palpation, itching, and burning. Patients also report bleeding associated with defecation. Constipation or diarrhea can aggravate these symptoms.

Diagnostic Studies and Collaborative Care

Internal hemorrhoids are diagnosed by digital examination, anoscopy, or sigmoidoscopy. External hemorrhoids can be diagnosed by visual inspection and digital examination. Therapy should be directed toward the causes and the patient's symptoms. A high-fibre diet and increased fluid intake prevent constipation

and reduce straining, which allows engorgement of the veins to subside. Ointments, creams, suppositories, and impregnated pads that contain anti-inflammatory agents (e.g., hydrocortisone), or astringents and anaesthetics (e.g., witch hazel, benzocaine) may be used to shrink the mucous membranes and relieve discomfort. Stool softeners may be ordered to keep the stools soft; sitz baths may be ordered to relieve pain.

Surgical excision and clot removal are generally recommended for thrombosed external hemorrhoids. For internal hemorrhoids, one of four nonsurgical approaches can be used. The first is *band ligation*. Through an anoscope, the hemorrhoid is identified and then ligated with a rubber band. The constrictive effect impairs circulation, and the tissue becomes necrotic, separates, and sloughs off. There is some local discomfort with this procedure, but no anaesthetic is required. *Infrared coagulation* can be used to treat bleeding internal hemorrhoids. In this procedure, either infrared or electrical current reduces local inflammation. *Cryotherapy* involves rapid freezing of the hemorrhoid. Because this method can result in acute pain, it is used less often. Finally, *laser treatment* can be used to treat internal hemorrhoids. This procedure involves expensive equipment and tends to be more costly than band ligation and coagulation therapies.

A *hemorrhoidectomy* is the surgical excision of hemorrhoids. Surgery is indicated when there is prolapse, excessive pain or bleeding, or large hemorrhoids. In general, hemorrhoidectomy is reserved for patients with severe symptoms related to multiple thrombosed hemorrhoids or marked protrusion. Surgical removal may be done by cautery, clamp, or excision. One surgical approach is to leave the area open so that healing takes place by secondary intention. In another approach, the hemorrhoids are removed, the tissue is sutured, and healing takes place by primary intention wound healing.

NURSING MANAGEMENT: HEMORRHOIDS

Conservative nursing management for the patient with hemorrhoids includes teaching measures regarding prevention of constipation, avoidance of prolonged standing or sitting, proper use of OTC drugs available for hemorrhoidal symptoms, and the need to seek medical care for severe symptoms of hemorrhoids (e.g., excessive pain and bleeding, prolapsed hemorrhoids) when necessary. Sitz baths (15-20 minutes) two to three times each day for 7 to 10 days may be helpful to reduce the discomfort and swelling associated with hemorrhoids.

Pain caused by sphincter spasm is a common problem after a hemorrhoidectomy. The nurse must be aware that, although the procedure is minor, the pain is severe. Narcotics are usually given initially. Sitz baths are started 1 to 2 days after surgery. A warm sitz bath provides comfort and keeps the anal area clean. Initially, the patient should not be left alone because of the possibility of weakness or fainting.

Packing may be inserted into the rectum to absorb drainage. A T-binder may hold the dressing in place. If packing is inserted, it usually is removed on the first or second postoperative day. The nurse should assess for rectal bleeding. The patient may be embarrassed when the dressing is changed, and privacy should be provided. The patient usually dreads the first bowel movement and often resists the urge to defecate. Pain medication may be given before the bowel movement to reduce discomfort.

A stool softener such as docusate (Colace) is usually ordered for the first few postoperative days. If the patient does not have a bowel movement within 2 to 3 days, other oral laxatives may be given.

Patients are taught the importance of diet, care of the anal area, symptoms of complications (especially bleeding), and avoidance of constipation and straining. Sitz baths are recommended for 1 to 2 weeks. The health care provider may order a stool softener to be taken for a time. Hemorrhoids may recur. Occasionally, anal strictures develop and dilation is necessary. Regular checkups are important in the prevention of any further problems.

Anal Fissure

An **anal fissure** is a skin ulcer or a crack in the lining of the anal wall that is caused by trauma, local infection, or inflammation. Fissures are considered either primary or secondary based on their etiology. *Primary fissures* usually occur as a result of local trauma associated with defecation or anal intercourse. When there is high pressure in the internal anal sphincter, it can result in ischemia, which can lead to fissuring. Thus, sexual practices and conditions that promote constipation are likely to be associated with fissure development. *Secondary fissures* are caused by a variety of conditions, including IBD, prior anal surgery, infection (syphilis, tuberculosis, chlamydia, gonorrhea, herpes simplex virus), and human immunodeficiency virus (HIV) infection.

The most common clinical manifestations are painful spasms of the anal sphincter and severe, burning pain during defecation. Some bleeding may occur, and constipation results because of fear of pain associated with bowel movements.

Anal fissures are diagnosed through physical examination. Treatment of anal fissures is directed at correcting the underlying conditions, such as hard stools. Most acute fissures require 2 to 4 weeks to heal. Conservative treatment consists of bowel regulation with mineral oil and stool softeners. Warm sitz baths (15-20 minutes, three times a day) and anal anaesthetic suppositories (Anusol) are also ordered.

For chronic fissures, other invasive procedures may be needed. These include coagulation therapy or surgical treatment (sphincterotomy). Surgical treatment involves excision of the fissure. Postoperative nursing care is the same as the care for the patient who has had a hemorrhoidectomy.

Anorectal Abscess

Anorectal abscesses are undrained collections of perianal pus (Figure 45-18). They are the result of obstruction of the anal glands, leading to infection and subsequent abscess formation. Abscess formation can occur secondary to anal fissures, trauma, or IBD.

The most common causative organisms are *Escherichia coli*, staphylococci, and streptococci. Clinical manifestations include local pain and swelling, foul-smelling drainage, tenderness, and elevated temperature. Sepsis can occur as a complication. Anorectal abscesses are diagnosed by rectal examination.

Surgical therapy consists of drainage of abscesses. The wound will be left open and allowed to heal by secondary intention. Topical dressing selection is determined based on wound care principles (maintain moist wound environment, manage bacterial burden, protect from further trauma). Care must be taken to avoid soiling the dressing during urination or defecation. A low-

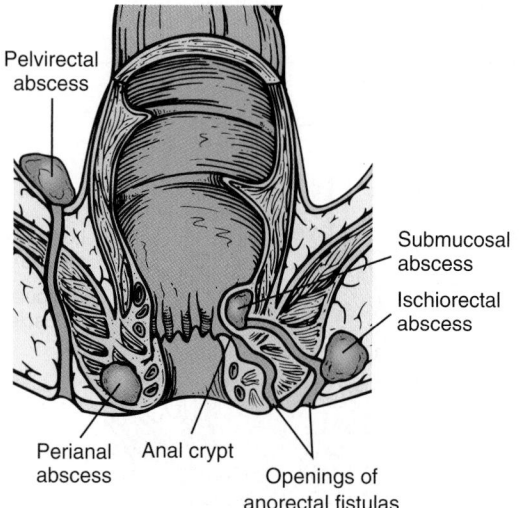

Figure 45-18 Common sites of anorectal abscesses and fistula formation.

residue diet is given. Discharge teaching should include access to home health care, wound care, and the importance of sitz baths; thorough cleaning after bowel movements, and follow-up visits to a health care provider.

Anal Fistula

An **anal fistula** is an abnormal tunnel leading out from the anus or the rectum. It may extend to the outside of the skin, the vagina, or the buttocks. Anal fistulas are a complication of Crohn's disease (occurring in the perianal area). This condition often precedes an anorectal abscess.

Feces enter the fistula and may cause a localized infection. There may be persistent, blood-stained, purulent discharge or stool leakage from the fistula. The patient may need to use dressings to contain the drainage and protect perifistular skin.

Surgical therapy may involve a fistulotomy or a fistulectomy. In a *fistulotomy*, the fistula is opened and healthy tissue is allowed to granulate. A *fistulectomy* is an excision of the entire fistulous tract. Appropriate topical therapy is used, and the wound is allowed to heal by secondary intention. In severe cases of perianal disease caused by Crohn's disease, a diverting loop ileostomy may be required to manage the fistulas. Care is the same as that given after a hemorrhoidectomy.

Pilonidal Sinus

A **pilonidal sinus** is a small tract under the skin between the buttocks in the sacrococcygeal area. It is thought to be of congenital origin. It may have several openings and is lined with epithelium and hair, thus given the name *pilonidal* ("a nest of hair").

The skin in the sacrococcygeal region is moist, and the movement of the buttocks causes the short, wiry hair to penetrate the skin. The irritated skin becomes infected and forms a pilonidal cyst or abscess. There are no symptoms unless there is an infection. If it becomes infected, the patient complains of pain and swelling at the base of the spine, and there may be spontaneous drainage of pus.

The formed abscess requires incision and drainage. The wound may be primarily closed or left open to heal by secondary intention. The wound is packed with appropriate topical therapeutic material. The wounds are often very painful, and the patient may require premedication before dressing changes. The patient is usually more comfortable lying on the abdomen or side. Sitting for prolonged periods of time may be difficult.

Activities that contribute to shear in the area (running, sports, long walks) should be avoided until the wound heals. Because the area is poorly vascularized, healing of open pilonidal wounds may be prolonged. Ensuring that surrounding hair is clipped and kept out of the wound bed is imperative. Unfortunately, despite excision of the tract, pilonidal cysts or abscesses may reoccur.

CLINICAL DECISION-MAKING EXERCISE

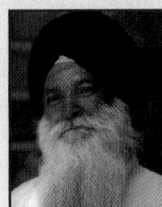

CASE STUDY:
Colorectal Cancer

Source: © Corbis/Lindsay Hebberd.

Patient Profile
Parminder Singh is a 58-year-old South Asian man living in southern Ontario. His family has brought him to the hospital for evaluation because of a recent deterioration in his health.

Subjective Data
- Complains of bright red bleeding during a bowel movement
- Family states that he has become thinner over the past several months and has little appetite
- Describes feeling weak and being easily fatigued; he appears ill
- Complains of abdominal pain and a feeling of fullness
- He has noticed a change in the size of his stools (more thin, pencil-like)
- No prior screening for colorectal cancer; family history of colorectal cancer is unknown

Objective Data
Physical Examination
- Temperature: 38°C
- Heart rate is 100 beats per minute; blood pressure is 120/74 mm Hg

- Weight, 63.6 kg; height, 172.5 cm
- Mild palpation of descending colon elicits discomfort
- Digital rectal examination reveals a mass
Diagnostic Tests
- Colonoscopy reveals distal rectal cancer
- Hematocrit, 0.26
- Hemoglobin, 5.6 mmol/L

Discussion Questions
1. What are the signs and symptoms of colorectal cancer that Mr. Singh manifests?
2. What is the significance of Mr. Singh's tachycardia?
3. What types of diagnostic information are available from a colonoscopy versus a double-contrast barium enema?
4. *Priority Decision:* What priority nursing interventions are indicated for Mr. Singh at this stage of his illness?
5. What does the nurse need to do to support Mr. Singh and his family in making decisions about his continued health care?
6. *Priority Decision:* Based on the assessment data, what are the priority nursing diagnoses? Are there any collaborative problems?

Evolve *Answers are available on* **http://evolve.elsevier.com/ Canada/Lewis/medsurg**

REVIEW QUESTIONS

The number of the question corresponds to the same-numbered objective at the beginning of the chapter.

1. What is included in the collaborative therapy for the patient with acute diarrhea caused by rotavirus?
   a. Increase fluid intake.
   b. Administer an antibiotic.
   c. Administer antimotility drugs.
   d. Quarantine the patient to prevent spread of the virus.
2. What procedures should be included during the nursing assessment of a patient with acute abdominal pain?
   a. Perform deep palpation before auscultation.
   b. Obtain blood pressure and pulse rate to determine hypovolemic changes.
   c. Auscultate bowel sounds because hyperactive bowel sounds suggest paralytic ileus.
   d. Measure body temperature because an elevated temperature may indicate an inflammatory or infectious process.

3. How can a nurse increase the comfort of the patient with appendicitis?
   a. Have the patient lie prone.
   b. Flex the patient's right knee.
   c. Sit the patient upright in a chair.
   d. Turn the patient onto his or her left side.
4. In planning care for the patient with Crohn's disease, the nurse recognizes that there are major differences between ulcerative colitis (UC) and Crohn's disease. Which feature below is more indicative of Crohn's disease?
   a. Frequently results in toxic megacolon
   b. Causes fewer nutritional deficiencies than does UC
   c. Often recurs after surgery, whereas UC is curable with a proctocolectomy
   d. Is manifested by rectal bleeding and anemia more frequently than is UC

5. The nurse performs a detailed assessment of the abdomen of a patient with a possible bowel obstruction. What is a manifestation of an obstruction in the large intestine?
   a. A largely distended abdomen
   b. Diarrhea that is loose or liquid
   c. Persistent, colicky abdominal pain
   d. Profuse vomiting that relieves abdominal pain

6. A patient with metastatic colorectal cancer is scheduled for both chemotherapy and radiation therapy. What information would be included in patient teaching regarding these therapies?
   a. Chemotherapy can be used to cure colorectal cancer.
   b. Radiation is routinely used as adjuvant therapy following surgery.
   c. Both chemotherapy and radiation can be used as palliative treatments.
   d. The patient should expect few if any adverse effects from chemotherapeutic agents.

7. Which ostomy surgery maintains the most normal functioning of the bowel?
   a. A sigmoid colostomy
   b. A transverse colostomy
   c. A descending colostomy
   d. An ascending colostomy

8. In contrast to diverticulitis, what manifestations does the patient with diverticulosis have?
   a. Has rectal bleeding
   b. Often has no symptoms
   c. Has localized crampy pain
   d. Frequently develops peritonitis

9. Which nursing intervention is most appropriate to decrease postoperative scrotal edema and pain following an inguinal herniorrhaphy?
   a. Applying a truss to the hernia site
   b. Allowing the patient to stand to void
   c. Supporting the incision during routine coughing
   d. Elevating the scrotum with a support

10. After dietary teaching for the patient with celiac disease, the selection of which menu items by the patient would demonstrate that the goals of teaching have been met?
    a. Scrambled eggs and sausage
    b. Whole grain pancakes with syrup
    c. Oatmeal, skim milk, and orange juice
    d. Yogourt, strawberries, and rye toast with butter

11. Which of the following should a patient be taught after a hemorrhoidectomy?
    a. Do not use the Valsalva manoeuvre.
    b. Eat a low-fibre diet to rest the colon.
    c. Administer an oil-retention enema to empty the colon.
    d. Use prescribed pain medication before a bowel movement.

ANSWERS: 1. a; 2. d; 3. b; 4. c; 5. a; 6. c; 7. a; 8. b; 9. d; 10. a; 11. d.

REFERENCES

Achkar, J., & Duerr, R. (2008). The expanding universe of inflammatory bowel disease genetics. *Current Opinion in Gastroenterology, 24*(4), 429. doi:10.1097/MOG.0b013e3283009c92

Agrawal, D., Rukkannagari, S., & Kethus, S. (2007). Pathogenesis and clinical approach to extraintestinal manifestations of inflammatory bowel disease. *Minerva Gastroenterologica, 53,* 233-248.

Canadian Cancer Society's Steering Committee on Cancer Statistics. (2012). *Canadian cancer statistics 2012.* Toronto: Canadian Cancer Society.

Canadian Celiac Association. (2011). About celiac disease. Retrieved from *http://www.celiac.ca/index.php/about-celiac-disease-2/symptoms-treatment-cd*

Canadian Society of Intestinal Research. (2008). Frequently asked questions about IBD. Retrieved from *http://www.badgut.com/index.php?contentFile=ibd_faq&title=Inflammatory%20Bowel%20Disease%20FAQ*

Canadian Society of Intestinal Research. (2011). Irritable bowel syndrome. Retrieved from *http://www.badgut.org/information-centre/irritable-bowel-syndrome.html*

Chang, G. (2006). Laparoscopic treatment of colorectal neoplasms. *Current Treatment Options in Gastroenterology, 9,* 256-264. doi:10.1007/s11938-006-0044-1

Chiaroni, G., & Whitehead, W. (2008). The role of biofeedback in the treatment of gastrointestinal disorders. *Nature Clinical Practice Gastroenterology & Hepatology, 5,* 371-382. doi:10.1038/ncpgasthep1150

Cho, J. (2008). The genetics and immunopathogenesis of inflammatory bowel disease. *Nature Review, 8,* 458-466. doi:10.1038/nri2340

Clarke, C., & DeLegge, M. (2008). Irritable bowel syndrome: A practical approach. *Nutrition in Clinical Practice, 23,* 263-267. doi:10.1177/0884533608318107

Colorectal Cancer Association of Canada. (2011a). Screening. Retrieved from *http://www.colorectal-cancer.ca/en/screening/screening-tests/*

Colorectal Cancer Association of Canada. (2011b). Treatments and side effects. Retrieved from *http://www.colorectal-cancer.ca/en/treating-cancer/treatment-cancer/#STDRUGS*

Colorectal Cancer Association of Canada. (2012). Symptoms. Retrieved from *http://www.colorectal-cancer.ca/en/just-the-facts/symptoms/*

Ghoshal, U. (2007). Review of pathogenesis and management of constipation. *Tropical Gastroenterology, 28,* 91-95.

Gould, C., & McDonald, L. (2008). Bench to bedside review: *Clostridium difficile* colitis. *Critical Care, 12,* 203. doi:10.1186/cc6207

Grant, E. M. (2011). Fidaxomicin: New therapy for *Clostridium difficile*–associated diarrhea. *Formulary, 46*(8), 297-308.

Heitkemper, M. M., & Jarrett, M. E. (2008). Update on irritable bowel syndrome and gender differences. *Nutrition in Clinical Practice, 23*(3), 275-283. doi:10.1177/0884533608318672

Jass, J. (2008). Colorectal polyposes: From phenotype to diagnosis. *Pathology, Research & Practice, 204,* 431-447. doi:10.1016/j.prp.2008.03.008

Lawson, M., Thomas, A., & Akobeng, A. (2008). Tumor necrosis factor alpha blocking agents for induction of remission in ulcerative colitis. *Cochrane Database of Systemic Reviews, 2,* CD005112.

Martin, S. (2008). Against the grain: An overview of celiac disease. *Journal of the American Academy of Nurse Practitioners, 20,* 243. doi:10.1111/j.1745-7599.2008.00314.x

McCrea, G., Miaskowski, C., Stotts, N., Macera, L., & Varma, M. (2008). Pathophysiology of constipation in the older adult. *World Journal of Gastroenterology, 14,* 2631-2638. doi:10.3748/wjg.14.2631

National Digestive Diseases Information Clearinghouse. (2006). Statistics on IBD. Retrieved from *http://digestive.niddk.nih.gov/ddiseases/pubs/colitis/*

Nayak, J., & Goel, S. (2011). Revised TNM staging for colorectal cancer: Did we miss the golden opportunity to do right by the staging? *Clinical Colorectal Cancer, 10*(3), 207-209. doi:10.1016/j.clcc.2011.03.016

Ng, S., Fleming, F., Drumm, J., Waldron, P., & Grace, P. A. (2008). Current trends in the management of acute appendicitis. *Irish Journal of Medical Science, 177*, 121-125. doi:10.1007/s11845-008-0116-4

Noomen, C. G., Hommes, D. W., & Fidder, H. H. (2009). Update on genetics in inflammatory disease. *Best Practices and Research: Clinical Gastroenterology, 23*, 233. doi:10.1016/j.bpg.2009.02.005

Ontario Ministry of Health. (2009). *Control of Clostridium difficile infection (CDI) outbreaks in hospitals: A guide for health and hospital unit staff.* Retrieved from *http://www.health.gov.on.ca/patient_safety/pro/cdad/pro_resource/guide_cdi_infect_control.pdf*

Panaccione, R., Rutgeerts, P., Sandborn, W. J., Feagan, B., Schreiber, S. & Ghosh, S. (2008). Review article: Treatment algorithms to maximize remission and minimize corticosteroid dependence in patients with inflammatory bowel disease. *Alimentary Pharmacology & Therapeutics, 28*, 674. doi:10.1111/j.1365-2036.2008.03753.x

Parekh, N., & Steiger, E. (2007). Short bowel syndrome. *Current Treatment Options in Gastroenterology, 101*, 10-23. doi:10.1007/s11938-007-0052-9

Pickhardt, P., Lawrence, E., Pooler, B., & Bruce, R. (2011). Diagnostic performance of multidetector computed tomography for suspected acute appendicitis. *Annals of Internal Medicine, 154*(12), 789-796.

Registered Nurses' Association of Ontario (RNAO). (2011). Prevention of falls and fall injuries in the older adult. Retrieved from *http://www.rnao.org/Storage/80/7444_BPG_Falls-and_SUPP.pdf*

Roos, S., Karner, A., & Hallert, C. (2009). Gastrointestinal symptoms and well-being of adults living on a gluten-free diet: A case for nursing in celiac disease. *Gastroenterology Nursing, 32*, 196. doi:10.1097/SGA.0b013e3181a85e7b

Rostom, A., Dube, C., Lewin, G., Tsertsvadze, A., Barrowman, N., Code, C., ..., Moher, D. (2007). Clinical guidelines. Nonsteroidal anti-inflammatory drugs and cyclooxygenase-2 inhibitors for primary prevention of colorectal cancer: A systematic review prepared for the U.S. Preventive Services Task Force. *Annals of Internal Medicine, 146*(5), 376-389.

Serels, S. (2009). Surgical correction of vaginal vault prolapse. *Urology Times—Clinical Edition,* June, S12. Retrieved from *http://digital.healthcaregroup.advanstar.com/nxtbooks/advanstar/ut_200906/index.php?startid=s12#/74*

Shmaliyan, T., Wyman, J., Bliss, D., Kane, R., & Wilt, T. (2007). Prevention of urinary and fecal incontinence in adults. *Evidence Report/Technology Assessment, 161*, 1-379.

Swaminath, A., & Kornbluth, A. (2007). Optimizing drug therapy in inflammatory bowel disease. *Current Gastroenterology Reports, 9*, 513-520. doi:10.1007/s11894-007-0068-2

Talley, N. (2007). Functional gastrointestinal disorders in 2007 and Rome III: Something new, something borrowed, something objective. *Reviews in Gastroenterological Disorders, 7*, 97-105.

Vasen, H., Möslein, G., Alonso, A., Aretz, S., Bernstein, I., Bertario, L., ..., Wijnen, J. (2008). Guidelines for the clinical management of familial adenomatous polyposis. *Gut, 57*, 704-713. doi:10.1136/gut.2007.136127

World Gastrointestinal Organization. (2009). Inflammatory bowel disease: a global perspective. Retrieved from *http://www.worldgastroenterology.org/assets/downloads/en/pdf/guidelines/21_inflammatory_bowel_disease.pdf*

World Gastroenterology Organization. (2010). Constipation: A global perspective. Retrieved from *http://www.worldgastroenterology.org/assets/export/userfiles/05_constipation.pdf*

CANADIAN RESOURCES

Canadian Association of Gastroenterology
http://www.cag-acg.org
Canadian Cancer Society
http://www.cancer.ca
Canadian Celiac Association
http://www.celiac.ca/
Canadian Society for Enterostomal Therapy
http://www.caet.com
Canadian Society of Gastroenterology and Associates
http://www.csgna.com
The Canadian Society of Intestinal Research
http://www.badgut.com
Colorectal Cancer Association of Canada
http://www.ccac-accc.ca
Crohn's & Colitis Foundation of Canada (CCFC)
http://www.ccfc.ca
United Ostomy Association (UOA)
http://www.ostomycanada.com

evolve *For additional Internet resources, see the Web site for this book* at **http://evolve.elsevier.com/Canada/Lewis/medsurg**

Written by Anne Croghan and Margaret McLean Heitkemper
Adapted by Colina Yim

LEARNING OBJECTIVES

1. Define jaundice, and describe signs and symptoms that may occur with the different types of jaundice.
2. Differentiate among the types of viral hepatitis, including etiology, pathophysiology, clinical manifestations, complications, and collaborative care.
3. Describe the nursing management of patients with viral hepatitis.
4. Explain the etiology, pathophysiology, clinical manifestations, complications, and collaborative care of patients with cirrhosis.
5. Describe the nursing management of patients with cirrhosis.
6. Describe the clinical manifestations and management of hepatocellular carcinoma.
7. Describe the pathophysiology, clinical manifestations, complications, and collaborative care of patients with acute and chronic pancreatitis.
8. Describe the nursing management of patients with pancreatitis.
9. Explain the clinical manifestations and collaborative care of patients with pancreatic cancer.
10. Explain the pathophysiology, clinical manifestations, complications, and collaborative care, including surgical therapy, of patients with gallbladder disorders.
11. Describe the nursing management of patients undergoing conservative or surgical treatment of cholecystitis and cholelithiasis.

KEY TERMS

acute pancreatitis An acute inflammatory process of the pancreas, p. 1248

ascites The accumulation of serous fluid in the peritoneal or the abdominal cavity, p. 1235

asterixis Flapping tremors (liver flap) commonly affecting the arms and hands, that are a manifestation of hepatic encephalopathy, p. 1236

cholecystitis Inflammation of the gallbladder, p. 1255

cholelithiasis Stones in the gallbladder, p. 1255

chronic pancreatitis Progressive destruction of the pancreas with fibrotic replacement of pancreatic tissue, p. 1252

cirrhosis A chronic progressive disease of the liver characterized by extensive degeneration and destruction of the liver parenchymal cells, p. 1233

esophageal varices A complex of tortuous veins at the lower end of the esophagus, enlarged and swollen as a result of portal hypertension, p. 1234

fetor hepaticus A musty, sweet odour of the patient's breath caused by accumulation of digestive by-products that the liver is unable to degrade, p. 1236

fulminant hepatic failure An acute clinical syndrome characterized by severe impairment of liver function associated with hepatic encephalopathy, p. 1245

fulminant hepatitis An acute clinical syndrome that results in severe impairment or necrosis of liver cells and potential liver failure, p. 1220

hepatic encephalopathy Changes in neurological and mental function, ranging from lethargy to deep coma, resulting when liver damage causes ammonia to enter the systemic circulation without liver detoxification, p. 1236

hepatitis An inflammation of the liver, p. 1218

hepatorenal syndrome (HRS) A serious complication of cirrhosis characterized by functional kidney failure with advancing azotemia, oliguria, and intractable ascites, p. 1236

jaundice A yellowish discoloration of body tissues resulting from an alteration in normal bilirubin metabolism or flow of bile into the hepatic or biliary duct systems, p. 1217

nonalcoholic fatty liver disease (NAFLD) A spectrum of disease that ranges from simple fatty liver that causes no hepatic inflammation to severe liver scarring; characterized by hepatic steatosis not associated with other causes, p. 1230 nonalcoholic steatohepatitis (NASH) A condition characterized by the accumulation of fat in the liver cells, causing inflammation and liver cell injury; occurs in people who drink little or no alcohol, p. 1231

paracentesis A needle puncture of the abdominal cavity, performed to remove ascitic fluid, p. 1237

portal hypertension Hypertension characterized by increased venous pressure in the portal circulation, as well as splenomegaly, large collateral veins, ascites, systemic hypertension, and esophageal varices, p. 1234

pseudocyst A cavity continuous with or surrounding the outside of the pancreas, p. 1249

spider angiomas Small, dilated blood vessels of the skin with a bright red centre and spiderlike branches, p. 1233

ELECTRONIC RESOURCES

Supplemental content related to Chapter 46 can be found...

Evolve Web Site ⊝volve

http://evolve.elsevier.com/Canada/Lewis/medsurg
- Answer Guidelines for Case Study on p. 1260
- Clinical Reference: Laboratory Values
- Concept Map for Case Study on p. 1260
- Content Updates
- Customizable Nursing Care Plans:
  - Acute Pancreatitis
  - Acute Viral Hepatitis
  - Cirrhosis

- Electronic Calculators
- eNCP 46-1: Acute Pancreatitis
- eTable 46-1: Diagnostic Findings in Jaundice
- Examination Review Questions
- Glossary
- Interactive Case Studies:
  - Acute Pancreatitis
  - Cholelithiasis and Cholecystitis
  - Hepatitis
  - Postnecrotic Cirrhosis
- Key Points (Printable and MP3 Download)

The liver, the pancreas, and the biliary tract are critical organs that are responsible for many functions vital to life. In addition to playing a central role of metabolizing carbohydrates, lipids, and proteins, the liver produces bile and detoxifies endogenous and exogenous substances such as hormones and drugs. The gallbladder stores and concentrates the bile transported through the biliary tract. Bile is essential for digestion of dietary fats and absorption of fats and fat-soluble vitamins from the digestive tract. The pancreas regulates blood glucose levels by secreting insulin and glucagon, as well as contributing enzymes that aid in food digestion.

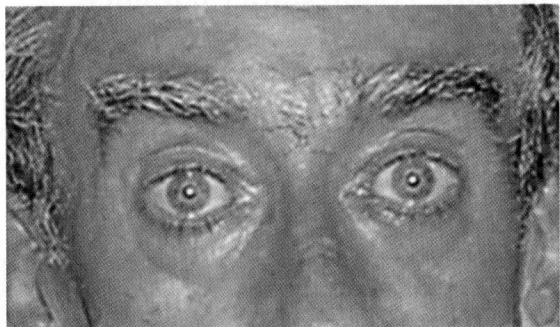

Figure 46-1 Patient with jaundice.

Source: From Butcher, G. P. (2004). *Gastroenterology: An illustrated colour text*. London: Churchill Livingstone.

Jaundice

Jaundice, a yellowish discoloration of body tissues, results when the concentration of bilirubin in the blood becomes abnormally increased. It is a symptom rather than a disease. The term *jaundice* is often used interchangeably with *hyperbilirubinemia*. However, a careful clinical examination cannot detect jaundice until the serum bilirubin level is higher than 34 mcmol/L, twice the normal upper limit. Jaundice is usually first observed in the sclera and later in the skin (Figure 46-1).

Most of the body's bilirubin is formed from the breakdown of hemoglobin (from red blood cells) by macrophages (see Chapter 41, Figure 41-6). This unconjugated (indirect) bilirubin is released into the blood circulation tightly bound to albumin and is not water soluble. Because the unconjugated bilirubin is not water soluble, it cannot be filtered in the kidneys and is not excreted in the urine. In the liver, the unconjugated bilirubin is conjugated with glucuronic acid to form conjugated (direct) bilirubin, which is water soluble. Conjugated bilirubin is secreted into bile, which flows through the hepatic and the biliary duct system into the small intestine. In the large intestine, bilirubin is converted to stercobilinogen and urobilinogen by bacterial action. Stercobilinogen is responsible for the characteristic brown colour of feces. Some urobilinogen is reabsorbed into the portal circulation and returned to the liver. Normally, a very small amount of urobilinogen is excreted in urine.

Jaundice can be classified as prehepatic, hepatic, and posthepatic (or cholestatic). There is, however, much overlap, particularly between the hepatic and posthepatic varieties. Diagnostic findings associated with these types of jaundice may be found in eTable 46-1, available on the Evolve website for this chapter.

Prehepatic Jaundice

Prehepatic jaundice results from an increase in the load of bilirubin before the bile arrives at the liver. The most common cause of this increased load is overproduction of unconjugated bilirubin, as in hemolysis (excessive breakdown of red blood cells). Hemolysis can be related to blood transfusion reactions, sickle cell crisis, and hemolytic anemia. In benign hereditary conditions, such as Gilbert's syndrome, the amount of unconjugated bilirubin in the blood is increased. The liver is unable to handle this increased bilirubin load. Bilirubin cannot be detected in the urine (see eTable 46-1).

Hepatic Jaundice

Hepatic jaundice results from an alteration in the liver's ability to take up bilirubin from the blood or to conjugate or excrete it into bile. In hepatocellular disease, the hepatocytes are damaged and leak bilirubin; thus levels of conjugated bilirubin are increased (see eTable 46-1). In severe liver injuries, levels of both unconjugated and conjugated bilirubin are elevated as a result of both the inability of hepatocytes to conjugate bilirubin and continued leaking of conjugated bilirubin from cells. Through reflux, conjugated bilirubin returns to the circulation and is excreted in urine because it is water soluble. The most common causes of hepatic jaundice are hepatitis, cirrhosis, and hepatocellularcarcinoma (HCC).

Posthepatic (Cholestatic) Jaundice

Posthepatic jaundice is caused by failure of bile to reach the duodenum, mostly because of obstruction of bile flow through the liver or biliary duct system. The obstruction may be intrahepatic or extrahepatic. Intrahepatic obstructions result from swelling or fibrosis of the liver's canaliculi and bile ducts. This can be caused by damage from liver tumours, hepatitis, or cirrhosis.

Causes of extrahepatic obstruction include obstruction of the common bile duct by a stone, sclerosing cholangitis, and pancreatic cancer. Laboratory findings show an elevation of levels of both unconjugated and conjugated bilirubin and urine bilirubin (see eTable 46-1). Because bilirubin does not enter the intestines, the level of fecal or urinary urobilinogen is decreased or nonexistent. When obstruction is complete, the stools are clay coloured.

Disorders of the Liver

Viral Hepatitis

Hepatitis is defined as inflammation of the liver. The most common cause of hepatitis is a viral infection. The types of infectious viruses that are the primary causes of viral hepatitis are *A, B, C, D, E,* and *G.* Other viruses—such as cytomegalovirus, Epstein-Barr virus, herpesvirus, coxsackievirus, and rubella virus—may cause hepatitis, but the liver is usually not the primary infected organ. Hepatitis may also be caused by chemicals and drugs (including alcohol; see Chapter 41, Table 41-6) autoimmune diseases, metabolic disorders, and genetic abnormalities. In rare cases, hepatitis is caused by bacteria, such as streptococci, *Salmonella* organisms, and *Escherichia coli.*

Viral hepatitis is a major public health concern. The most common types in Canada are those caused by hepatitis A, B, and C viruses. Surveillance of these three viruses is carried out by the National Notifiable Disease Reporting System of Health Canada, and confirmed cases must therefore be reported. The only definitive way to distinguish among the various forms of viral hepatitis is by the presence of the antigens and the subsequent development of antibodies to them. However, the person who is immune to one virus can still develop another type of viral hepatitis. The major characteristics of the hepatitis viruses are presented in Table 46-1. Each type of viral hepatitis is discussed in detail later in this chapter. See also the Determinants of Health box, "Disorders of the Liver, Pancreas, and Gallbladder."

Table 46-1 Characteristics of Hepatitis Viruses

CHARACTERISTIC	HEPATITIS A VIRUS (HAV)	HEPATITIS B VIRUS (HBV)	HEPATITIS C VIRUS (HCV)	HEPATITIS D VIRUS (HDV)	HEPATITIS E VIRUS (HEV)
Virus type	RNA	DNA	RNA	RNA	RNA
Incubation (days)	15–45	30–180	15–60	21–140	15–65
Transmission	Fecal–oral	Percutaneous, sexual, perinatal	Percutaneous, perinatal (uncommon)	HBV infection must precede HDV infection; percutaneous, sexual, perinatal	Fecal–oral
Acute hepatitis progressing to chronic disease	None	Adults: <5%; preschoolers: 25%; neonates: 90%	70–80%	Usual in superinfection; rare in co-infection	None
Prevention	Immunization before and after exposure	Immunization before and after exposure	Blood donor screening, risk behaviour modification	Immunization for HBV prevents HDV infection	Ensure safe drinking water

Source: Adapted from Peltekian, K. M., & Hirsh, G. (2007). Viral hepatitis. In Gray, J. (Ed.), *Therapeutic choices* (5th ed., Chapter 52). Ottawa: Canadian Pharmacists Association. Adapted with permission from Canadian Pharmacists Association.
DNA, deoxyribonucleic acid; *RNA,* ribonucleic acid.

Table 46-2 Clinical Manifestations of Hepatitis	
Acute	• Splenomegaly
• Anorexia	• Weight loss
• Nausea, vomiting	• Jaundice
• Right upper quadrant discomfort	• Pruritus
• Constipation or diarrhea	• Dark urine
• Altered taste and smell	• Light stools
• Fever	• Fatigue
• Malaise	**Chronic**
• Headache	• Malaise
• Arthralgias	• Easy fatigability
• Urticaria	• Myalgia and arthralgia
• Hepatomegaly	• Hepatomegaly

Pathophysiological Features

Liver. The pathophysiological changes in the various types of viral hepatitis are similar. Hepatitis involves widespread inflammation of liver tissue. During acute infection, liver damage is mediated by cytotoxic cytokines and natural killer cells that cause lysis of infected hepatocytes (liver cells). Liver cell damage results in liver cell necrosis (death). Inflammation of the periportal areas may interrupt bile flow, causing cholestasis (impaired flow of bile). Liver cells can normally regenerate through cellular replication, and if no complications occur, they should resume their normal function. If liver cell loss is massive, cellular replication may not be possible.

Systemic Effects. The antigen–antibody complexes between the virus and its corresponding antibody form a circulating immune complex in the early phases of hepatitis. The circulating immune complexes activate the complement system (see Chapter 16). The clinical manifestations of this activation are rash, angioedema, arthritis, fever, and malaise. *Cryoglobulinemia* (presence of abnormal proteins in the blood), glomerulonephritis, and vasculitis have also been found secondary to immune complex activation.

Clinical Manifestations

The clinical manifestations of viral hepatitis can be classified into acute and chronic hepatitis (Table 46-2). The acute phase is the time of initial exposure to that particular virus. Many individuals with acute hepatitis have no symptoms—(i.e., 30% with acute hepatitis B, 80% with acute hepatitis C). Individuals who are immunosuppressed may also have no symptoms. For those with no symptoms during the acute phase, infections are often not known to be present and therefore not diagnosed.

The clinical symptoms, if present, in acute infections are similar across all types of hepatitis viruses. However, the course of infections varies between the types of hepatitis (discussed in detail in individual sections on viral hepatitis). In general, hepatitis A and E have a similar clinical course. Almost all cases of acute hepatitis A resolve, whereas many cases of acute hepatitis B and C result in lifelong infections.

Acute Phase. The acute phase of a viral hepatitis infection usually lasts 1 to 4 months. During the incubation period, symptoms are mostly gastrointestinal, which may include anorexia, nausea, occasional vomiting, right upper quadrant discomfort, constipation, or diarrhea. The infected person may find food or alcohol repugnant and, if a smoker, may develop a distaste for cigarettes. Other symptoms that may also occur during this phase are malaise, fatigue, headache, low-grade fever, arthralgias, and skin rashes. Physical examination may reveal hepatomegaly, lymphadenopathy, and sometimes splenomegaly. The acute phase is the period of maximal infectivity.

The acute phase may be icteric (jaundice) or anicteric (no jaundice). Jaundice results when bilirubin diffuses into the tissues. The urine may darken because of excretion of excess bilirubin by the kidneys. If conjugated bilirubin cannot flow out of the liver because of obstruction or inflammation of the bile ducts, the stools are light or clay coloured. Pruritus sometimes accompanies the jaundice and occurs as a result of the accumulation of bile salts beneath the skin. When jaundice occurs, other symptoms decrease in severity.

The convalescent period of the acute phase begins as jaundice is disappearing and lasts from weeks to months; the average is 2 to 4 months. During this period, the patient's major complaint is malaise and easy fatigability. Hepatomegaly remains for several weeks, but splenomegaly usually subsides.

Chronic Phase. Almost all cases of acute hepatitis A resolve with no progression to a chronic state. In a few patients, relapse occurs a few months after the infection. The disappearance of jaundice does not mean resolution of the virus infection. Many hepatitis B and C infections result in chronic (lifelong) disease.

Most patients with chronic viral hepatitis have no symptoms. Others may have nonspecific symptoms, including malaise, fatigue, myalgias, arthralgias, and hepatomegaly (see Table 46-2). Chronic hepatitis B and C can progress to severe scarring of the liver (cirrhosis) and liver failure if left untreated.

Complications

The overall mortality rate for acute viral hepatitis is less than 1%. The risk of death is higher in older adults and those with underlying debilitating illnesses, including chronic liver disease. Fulminant hepatitis can develop as a complication.

Fulminant hepatitis is an acute clinical syndrome that results in severe impairment or necrosis of liver cells and potential liver failure. It occurs only in a small percentage of patients. It may develop in co-infection with HBV and HDV. It is less frequent with acute HCV infection and rarely occurs with acute HAV. Toxic reactions to drugs and congenital metabolic disorders may also cause fulminant hepatitis and liver failure. Liver failure usually causes death unless liver transplantation is performed. (Fulminant hepatitis is further discussed later in this chapter)

Diagnostic Studies

Viral Serological Tests. The viral antigens and antibodies are serological markers used to diagnose the different types of viral hepatitis. The specific markers and their interpretations for each type of viral hepatitis are explained under the headings of the particular viruses.

Serum Liver Enzymes. These tests cannot differentiate one type of hepatitis from another, but they are helpful in determining the type of liver injury, whether it is related to liver cell injury or bile duct abnormalities.

Aspartate aminotransferase (AST) and alanine aminotransferase (ALT) are liver enzymes whose levels can indicate liver cell injury. In severe acute viral hepatitis, the levels can be markedly increased to more than 1000 U/L. Elevated levels of alkaline phosphatase (ALP) and γ-glutamyl transpeptidase (GGT) are usually associated with bile duct injuries, but these levels can rise to a lesser extent in viral hepatitis infections.

Liver Function Tests. The term *liver function tests* (LFTs) was often used broadly to include liver enzyme measurements, and that is misleading. The LFTs that more accurately reflect liver function are serum albumin, serum bilirubin, and prothrombin time, which is standardized to the international normalized ratio (INR). In mild acute viral hepatitis, serum albumin, serum bilirubin, and INR remain normal. When jaundice is detectable on physical examination, the serum bilirubin level is usually at least twice the normal upper limit (>34 mcmol/L). Deteriorating liver function is demonstrated by increased INR and serum bilirubin, and decreased serum albumin.

Hepatitis A

Canada has a relatively low incidence of hepatitis A (World Health Organization [WHO], 2010), and it has been slowly decreasing since the introduction of hepatitis A vaccine in 1996. The World Health Organization estimates an annual total of 1.5 million cases of hepatitis A worldwide (WHO, 2011), but seroprevalence data suggest that tens of millions of HAV infec-

tions occur each year (Public Health Agency of Canada, 2011). In developing countries, hepatitis A infection is nearly universal during childhood.

Hepatitis A Virus (HAV). HAV is an RNA virus transmitted predominantly through the fecal–oral route. The virus is found in feces 2 weeks or more before the onset of symptoms and up to 1 week after the onset of jaundice (Figure 46-2). It is present in blood only briefly. Anti-HAV immunoglobulin M (IgM) appears in the serum as the stool becomes negative for the virus. The presence of anti-HAV IgM indicates acute hepatitis, and the presence of anti-HAV IgG is an indicator of past infection. The presence of IgG antibody provides lifelong immunity (Table 46-3).

The mode of transmission of HAV is usually fecal–oral (mainly by ingesting food or liquid infected with the virus) and rarely parenteral. Poor hygiene, improper handling of food, crowded situations, and poor sanitary conditions are related factors. Foodborne hepatitis A outbreaks usually result from

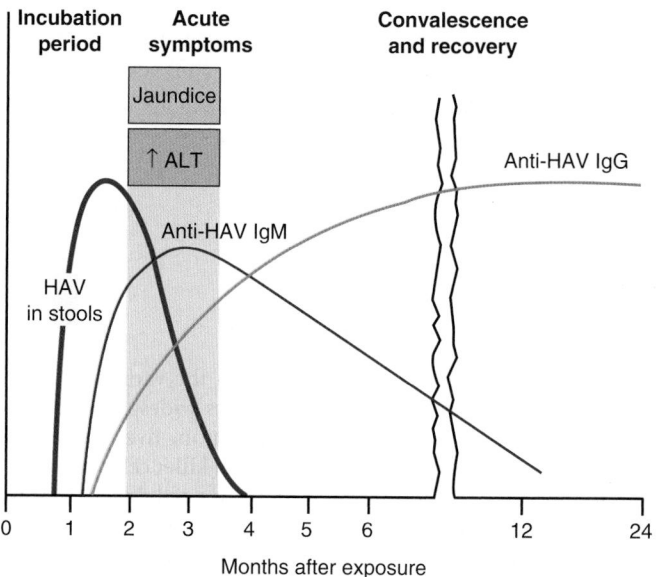

Figure 46-2 Course of infection with hepatitis A virus (HAV). *ALT,* alanine aminotransferase; *anti-HAV IgG,* immunoglobulin G class antibody to hepatitis A virus; *anti-HAV IgM,* immunoglobulin M class antibody to hepatitis A virus.

Source: From McCance, K. L., & Huether, S. E. (2010). *Pathophysiology: The biologic basis for disease in adults and children* (6th ed., p. 1488, Figure 39-20). St. Louis: Mosby.

Table 46-3 Serological Markers of HAV Infection

MARKER	DESCRIPTION
Anti-HAV IgM (Antibody to HAV, immunoglobulin M)	Antibody produced in response to infection; positive finding indicates acute infection
Anti-HAV IgG (Antibody to HAV, immunoglobulin G)	Antibody produced from previous infection or vaccination; positive finding indicates long-term immunity

HAV, hepatitis A virus.

contamination of food during preparation by an infected food handler. The virus is present in feces during the incubation period, and so it can be carried and transmitted by people who have undetectable, subclinical infections. The risk of transmission is highest before clinical symptoms are apparent. The virus can also be transmitted by patients with anicteric (asymptomatic) hepatitis A.

Clinical Manifestations. Hepatitis A usually causes acute symptoms in adults but not in younger children. Typical symptoms include anorexia, nausea, fatigue, fever and jaundice (see Table 46-2). The symptom severity increases with age. Only fewer than 10% of affected children younger than 6 years develop jaundice. Recovery usually takes 4 to 6 weeks, but it may take months. Although relapse occurs in about 15% of the cases, hepatitis A does not lead to chronicity. Recovery from HAV infection confers lifelong immunity against the virus.

Hepatitis A rarely causes fulminant hepatic failure. The overall estimated rate of mortality associated with hepatitis A is 0.1 to 0.3%, but it increases to 12.5% in patients older than 60 who are hospitalized (Public Health Agency of Canada, 2007a). There is no specific treatment for hepatitis A. Infected people generally recover in 4 to 6 weeks. Hospitalization is normally unnecessary unless the patient is severely dehydrated. Management is focused on relief of symptoms.

Prevention. HAV is usually the cause of outbreaks of viral hepatitis. Preventive measures include personal and environmental hygiene and health education to promote good sanitation. Careful handwashing, especially after bowel movements and before eating, is essential and is probably the most important precaution. Both hepatitis A vaccine and immune globulin (IG) are administered for prevention.

From a public health perspective, vaccination, or active immunization, is an important and effective means of controlling hepatitis A. Canada currently does not have a universal HAV immunization program. People at risk are advised to receive the vaccine as pre-exposure prophylaxis. People at risk include those who travel to HAV-endemic regions, those who use illicit drugs, men who have sex with men, those with chronic liver disease, those with clotting factor disorders (e.g. hemophilia), and residents of communities where hepatitis A is highly endemic (Public Health Agency of Canada, 2007a).

The HAV vaccine is inactivated hepatitis A virus and is currently available in several forms, including Havrix, Vaqta, and Avaxim. Primary immunization consists of a single dose administered intramuscularly in the deltoid muscle. A booster is recommended between 6 and 12 months after the initial primary dose to ensure adequate antibody titres and long-term protection. Primary immunization provides immunity within 30 days after a single dose in more than 95% of those vaccinated. Postvaccination testing is therefore not necessary. The adverse effects of the vaccine are mild and are usually limited to soreness and redness at the injection site. Twinrix, a combined HAV and HBV vaccine, is available for children and adults. The primary immunization consists of three doses, given on a 0-, 1-, and 6-month schedule, the same schedule used for the single HBV vaccine. Booster doses are not needed in people who completed the primary three doses. Twinrix may be given to individuals at high risk for hepatitis infection, as previously mentioned.

Hepatitis A immune globulin can be administered either before or after exposure. IG provides temporary (6 to 8 weeks) passive immunity and is effective for preventing hepatitis A if given within 1 to 2 weeks after exposure. IG is recommended for those without anti-HAV antibodies who are exposed to hepatitis A by close contact (e.g., household, day care centre) with people who have HAV or through food-borne exposure. Although IG may not prevent infection in all people, it may modify the illness to a subclinical infection. It may also be administered as a prophylactic measure for travellers to countries that have a high incidence of hepatitis A.

Hepatitis B

Hepatitis B is an important vaccine-preventable infectious disease in Canada. It is the most prevalent viral hepatitis strain in the globe. Worldwide, nearly 2 billion people are infected with HBV and, of these, 350 million have been unable to clear the infection and have become chronically infected. In Canada, the incidence of HBV was approximately 2.0 cases per 100,000 people, and the prevalence was estimated at 250,000 or 0.7 to 0.9% of the Canadian population (Public Health Agency of Canada, 2012). Because of the heterogeneity of the Canadian population, immigrants—particularly those from regions highly endemic for hepatitis B—constitute the largest group of carriers of chronic hepatitis B.

Hepatitis B Virus (HBV).
HBV is a DNA virus that is much more infectious than the human immunodeficiency virus (HIV). Nine hepatitis B genotypes (genotype A to I) have been identified thus far. The genotype distribution varies among different parts of the world. Genotype A is common in North America and Europe, whereas genotype D is found predominantly in Southern Europe, the Middle East, and South Asia. Most Asians who are infected have genotype C or D. Genotypes have implications for treatment responses and disease outcomes.

HBV has a complex structure. It expresses a few viral proteins or antigens that can be measured in blood. Each antigen has a corresponding antibody that may develop in response to the HBV infection. Hepatitis B surface antigen (HBsAg) represents the outer protein coat of the virus. The persistence of HBsAg in the blood for 6 to 12 months or longer indicates a chronic hepatitis B state. Development of antibody toward HBsAg (anti-HBs) signifies immunity. The core HBV antigen (HBcAg) can be observed only in the liver and not in blood, but its antibody (anti-HBc) can be measured, and its presence in blood indicates infection. Hepatitis B e antigen (HBeAg) is a third viral protein excreted by the virus. Its presence is associated with an active viral replication state and high infectivity. The absence of HBeAg, however, does not always rule out active disease because some people can have mutant viruses that cannot express e-antigen and hence they have active e-antigen negative c hepatitis B. The different serological markers of hepatitis B are explained in Table 46-4.

The diagnosis of an acute versus chronic hepatitis B infection is based on accurate interpretation of the serological markers (Table 46-5).

HBV is highly infectious and can live outside a human body for up to 7 days. It is transmitted perinatally by mothers with the viral infection; percutaneously (e.g., IV drug use, accidental needle-stick punctures, tattoos); sexually; or horizontally by permucosal exposure to infectious blood, blood products, or other body fluids (e.g., semen, vaginal secretions). Transmission occurs when infected blood or other body fluids enter the body of a person who is not immune to the virus.

In people who have HBV, HBsAg has been detected in almost every body fluid. Infected semen and saliva contain much lower concentrations of HBV than does blood, and the risk of virus transmission via these secretions is very low. There is no evidence that urine, feces, tears, and sweat are infective.

Breastfeeding is safe and does not contribute to mother-to-child transmission when the newborn receives both vaccination and IGs at birth (Shi et al., 2011). Kissing, hugging, sharing food items, and casual contacts with infected individuals does not transmit HBV infection.

Table 46-4 Serological Markers of HBV Infection

MARKER	DESCRIPTION
HBsAg (hepatitis B surface antigen)	Virus surface protein; positive result indicates infection; persistence of positive result >6 months indicates chronic infection
HBeAg (hepatitis B e antigen)	Virus protein secreted during active viral replication; positive finding indicates high virus activity and high degree of infectiousness; negative result is usually associated with lower virus replication and less infectious state
Anti-HBe (antibody to hepatitis B e antigen)	Antibody produced in response to HBeAg; positive result is usually associated with lower rate of virus replication and less infectious state; in cases of mutant viruses, positive result can be associated with active virus replication and high infectivity
Anti-HBc total (total antibody to hepatitis B core antigen)	Antibody to viral core protein; positive result indicates past or ongoing infection; seropositivity persists for life
Anti-HBc IgM (IgM class antibody to hepatitis B core antigen)	Early-phase IgM class antibody to viral core protein; positive result indicates acute infection; is sometimes observed in acute flares of chronic infection
Anti-HBs (antibody to hepatitis B surface antigen)	Protective antibody produced with recovery from infection or in response to vaccination

HBV, hepatitis B virus; *IgM,* immunoglobulin M.

The Public Health Agency of Canada (2007b) identified people who use IV drugs and those have unprotected sex with multiple sexual partners as the populations at highest risk for acquiring hepatitis B. People at moderate risk are those who have spent time in prison, homosexual men, and individuals from areas of the world where the virus is common (i.e., Africa, Southeast Asia, the Middle East, southern and western Pacific Islands, the Amazon basin, Haiti, the Dominican Republic). At low risk are people with hemophilia, those who undergo hemodialysis, and health care workers.

Acute Hepatitis B. Most acutely infected individuals, especially neonates and young children born to mothers with hepatitis B, have no symptoms. Fulminant hepatitis is uncommon but can be life-threatening. Those most at risk are individuals with chronic liver disease of any etiology. Symptoms of fulminant hepatitis include jaundice, encephalopathy (manifested by altered mental state), and ascites (abdominal swelling).

The course of an acute HBV infection that spontaneously resolves is shown in Figure 46-3. After an acute infection, the percentage of infected people in whom the infection does not resolve and becomes chronic varies with age. Up to 90% of neonates who contract HBV at birth become chronically infected. In contrast, more than 95% of adults can clear the HBV infection except for those who are immunocompromised, such as those with HIV co-infection. Children with HBV have a 20% risk for chronic infection (WHO, 2012).

Acute hepatitis B normally does not necessitate antiviral treatment. Management focuses on relief of symptoms and counselling to prevent virus transmission, including contacts tracing. If HBsAg is detected in the blood 6 months after the initial confirmation test, HBV infection has progressed to a chronic state. People with chronic HBV may have a normal liver, low-grade disease, or severe liver disease. Severe liver fibrosis or cirrhosis occurs in up to 25% of cases of chronic hepatitis B. All adults infected with chronic HBV are at risk for developing hepatocellular carcinoma.

Chronic Hepatitis B. The course of chronic hepatitis B is highly variable and rather complex. Some infected individuals may have exacerbations and remissions of inflammatory activity in the liver, some have continuous active inflammation, and others have no inflammation whatsoever for life. The course of chronic hepatitis B infection (Figure 46-4) can be divided into four phases.

The first phase, the so-called immune-tolerant phase, is characterized by a high level of virus replication (HBV DNA or viral

Table 46-5 Interpretation of HBV Serological Profile

HEPATITIS B SURFACE ANTIGEN (HBSAG)	ANTIBODY TO HEPATITIS B CORE ANTIGEN (ANTI-HBC)	IGM CLASS ANTIBODY TO HEPATITIS B CORE ANTIGEN (IGM ANTI-HBC)	ANTIBODY TO HEPATITIS B SURFACE ANTIGEN (ANTI-HBS)	INTERPRETATION
−	−	−	−	No exposure
+	−	±	−	Acute infection
+	+	−	−	Chronic infection
−	−	−	+	Immunity from vaccination
−	+	−	+	Immunity from past exposure
−	+	−	−	Past exposure/occult HBV infection

HBV, hepatitis B virus; *IgM,* immunoglobulin M.

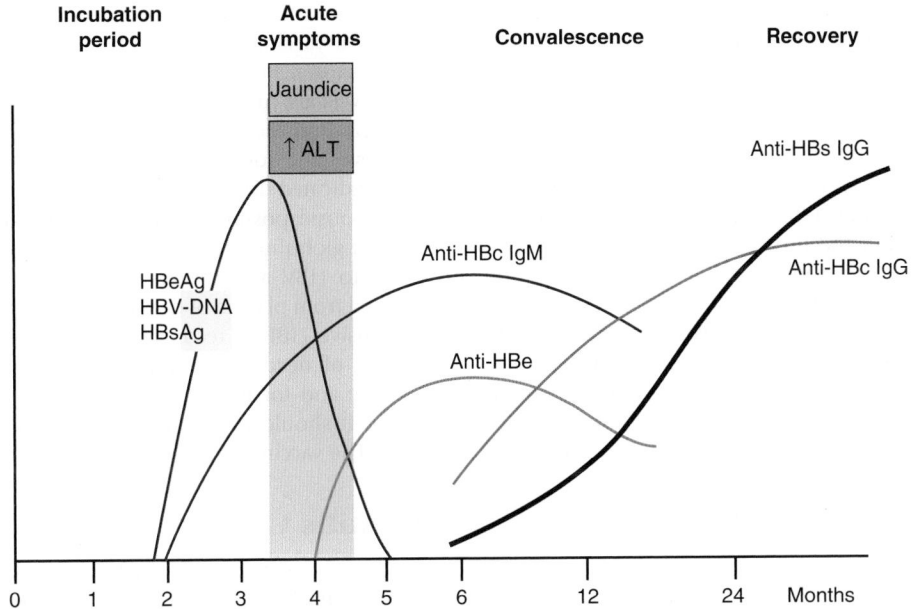

Figure 46-3 Course of a resolved hepatitis B (HBV) infection. *ALT,* alanine aminotransferase; *anti-HBc,* antibody to hepatitis B core antigen; *anti-HBe,* antibody to *HBeAg; anti-HBs,* antibody to HBsAg; *HBeAg,* hepatitis B e antigen; *HBsAg,* hepatitis B surface antigen; *HBV,* hepatitis B virus; *IgG,* immunoglobulin G; *IgM,* immunoglobulin M.

Source: From McCance, K. L., & Huether, S. E. (2010). *Pathophysiology: The biologic basis for disease in adults and children* (6th ed., p. 1489, Figure 39-21). St. Louis: Mosby.

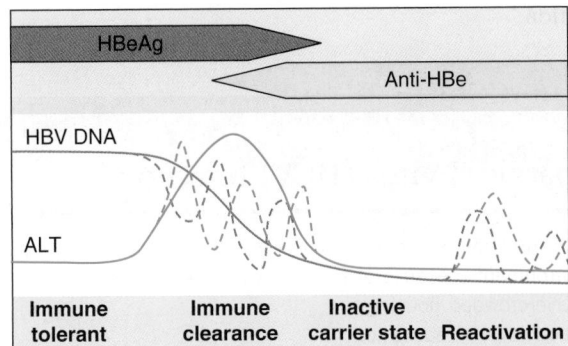

Figure 46-4 Phases of chronic hepatitis B infection. *ALT,* alanine aminotransferase; *Anti-HBe,* antibody to hepatitis B e antigen (HBeAg).

Source: From Dooley, J. S., Lok, A .S. F., Burroughs, A., & Heathcote, E. J. (2011). *Sherlock's diseases of the liver and biliary system* (12th ed., p. 378). Chichester, UK: Wiley-Blackwell.

load) in the blood but no or minimal hepatic inflammation. Affected individuals are HBeAg seropositive but have normal ALT levels (<40 IU/mL) because of the lack of immune response to the virus. In the second phase, the immune clearance phase, hepatitis is intermittent, with varying degrees of inflammatory activity. HBV DNA load in this phase is also high, and liver enzyme levels are abnormal because the immune response against the virus has begun. Seroconversion from HBeAg positivity to anti-HBe positivity may occur during this phase. The third phase is an inactive stage during which the viral load is low and there is no inflammatory activity in the liver, so liver enzyme levels are normal and HBV DNA is low or undetectable. Some individuals remain in this phase and have inactive hepatitis B throughout life. Others develop a high viral load and abnor-

mal liver enzyme levels, signalling the reactivation of HBV infection.

In general, patients in whom the HBeAg infection clears have a better prognosis than patients who remain HBeAg-positive for a prolonged time. Every year, about 1% of patients become cleared of HBsAg. Patients with chronic hepatitis B are at risk for the development of hepatocellular carcinoma.

Drug Therapy.   Drug therapy for chronic HBV usually includes interferon (IFN) and oral antiviral agents, with the aim is to decrease (a) the viral load, (b) liver enzyme levels, and (c) the rate of disease progression. The ultimate goals are to prevent cirrhosis, liver failure, and hepatocellular carcinoma. Current drug therapies for chronic HBV suppress but do not eradicate the virus (Lok & McMahon, 2009).

Interferon.   IFN has both antiviral and immunomodulatory activity and was the first approved treatment for hepatitis B. IFN is available in two forms: conventional (Intron A) and pegylated. Conventional IFN has a short half-life, which necessitates frequent subcutaneous administrations (three times per week). In contrast, pegylated IFN is long-acting, and subcutaneous administration is needed only once per week. The long-acting preparations are made by conjugating a conventional IFN with polyethylene glycol (PEG), in a process known as *pegylation.* Because of their convenience, these products are preferred to conventional IFN and are used to treat both hepatitis C and hepatitis B.

In patients with HBV who are receiving IFN, one third exhibit a significant reduction of serum HBV DNA levels, normalization of ALT levels, and loss of HBeAg. The response to treatment may vary on the basis of viral genotype. IFN treatment is associated with a number of adverse drug events (see Table 46-7 on p. 1226). These adverse events are dosage related and tend to decrease in severity with continued treatment. For patients receiving IFN, blood cell counts and liver enzyme levels should be measured at least every 4 weeks, or more often as needed. Duration of therapy ranges from 24 to 48 weeks (Myers, Ramji, Bilodeau, Wong, & Feld, 2012).

Nucleoside and Nucleotide Analogues. The oral nucleoside analogue class of antiviral agents used to treat HBV infection include lamivudine (Heptovir), telbivudine (Sebivo), and entecavir (Baraclude); the nucleotide analogues are adefovir (Hepsera) and tenofovir (Viread). They are given during active viral replication to inhibit viral DNA synthesis and to reduce viral load and liver enzymes. Most patients with HBV infection require long-term treatment with these medications, unless *"e" seroconversion* (loss of HBeAg and development of anti-HBe) occurs. Seroconversion occurs in 5 to 20% of patients with HBV infection treated with nucleoside and nucleotide analogues.

Development of drug resistance is an issue with oral antiviral drugs. Of patients who take lamivudine for more than 3 years, up to 70% develop resistance. Patients with lamivudine-resistant HBV infection can be treated with another class of drugs (i.e., adefovir or tenofovir). Because adefovir is considerably less potent and associated with an increasing rate of resistance, it is no longer commonly prescribed. Adefovir and entecavir should not be taken by women who are pregnant. Tenofovir demonstrated no drug resistance development in a 5-year follow-up study (Marcellin et al., 2011). Lactic acidosis has been reported with the use of nucleoside and nucleotide analogues. Acute, severe exacerbations of hepatitis B have been reported after discontinuation of these drugs. If these drugs are discontinued, liver function should be monitored closely for several months.

SAFETY ALERT

Adefovir (Hepsera) and Tenofovir (Viread)

- These drugs are nephrotoxic.
- Serum creatinine levels should be monitored, especially in patients at risk, including those with pre-existing renal disease and those taking nephrotoxic drugs (e.g. cyclosporine, aminoglycoside, vancomycin).

Adefovir (Hepsera) and Entecavir (Baraclude)

- These drug should not be taken by women who are pregnant.

Prevention. Immunization with hepatitis B vaccine is the most effective means of preventing HBV infection. Since the late 1990s, universal immunization against HBV is part of the vaccine programs offered by all provinces and territories in Canada. Although different jurisdictions offer the vaccines for people of different ages, the HBV vaccine programs ensure that every child is vaccinated by the end of high school. It is also important to vaccinate adults in the major risk groups, such as people who use injection drugs, household members living with a hepatitis B carrier, and health care providers. It is hoped that universal vaccination will lead to eventual prevention and control of hepatitis B.

Hepatitis B vaccine is produced through recombinant DNA technology (see Chapter 16, Figure 16-15). The vaccines are Recombivax HB and Engerix-B. The vaccine is given in a series of three injections in the deltoid muscle. The second dose is administered within 1 month of the first one, and the third one within 6 months of the first. The vaccine is more than 95% effective. Successful vaccination should result in anti-HBs titres of 10 IU/mL or greater. Boosters (additional doses) to increase the antibody levels are currently not recommended. Only minor adverse reactions have been reported with vaccination, including transient fever and soreness at the injection site. The vaccine is not contraindicated during pregnancy.

For postexposure prophylaxis, the vaccine and hepatitis B immune globulin (HBIG) are administered. HBIG contains antibodies to HBV and confers temporary passive immunity. It is prepared from plasma of donors with a high titre of anti-HBs and is expensive. HBIG is recommended for postexposure prophylaxis in cases of needlestick, mucous membrane contact, or sexual exposure and for infants born to mothers who are positive for HBsAg. It should be given after exposure, preferably within 24 hours. The vaccine series should also be started.

Hepatitis C

Worldwide, approximately 170 million people are chronically infected with hepatitis C virus (HCV). In Canada, the estimated prevalence is 0.8% of the total population, which is approximately 245,000 Canadians (Myers et al., 2012). The highest rate of acute HCV infection in Canada among men is in the 25- to 34-year age group, and that among women is in the 15- to 24-year age group. This phenomenon is probably related to the engagement of high-risk behaviours including injection drug use. See the Determinants of Health box "Hepatitis C Virus (HCV) Infection."

DETERMINANTS OF HEALTH
Hepatitis C Virus (HCV) Infection

- HCV infection occurs in people who are vulnerable in the social environment, because of the following risk factors:
  - Overcrowded housing
  - Low level of education
  - Low income and social status
  - Social isolation
- These create barriers to seeking testing and treatment for HCV infection.
- A comprehensive approach is the best strategy to address the broader context of HCV infection in people who are vulnerable.

Of all the forms of hepatitis, hepatitis C is the most likely to cause long-term liver damage: Up to 80% of people with HCV infection develop a chronic infection. Chronic hepatitis C is a significant medical and economic burden in Canada and is the most common indication for liver transplantation in Canada. Modelling data suggest that the number of patients with hepatitis C–related sequelae—including decompensated liver disease, hepatocellular carcinoma, and liver transplantation—is expected to rise through 2025 (Myers et al., 2012).

Co-infection with HCV and HIV is increasing. The modelled estimate of the number of HCV–HIV co-infected individuals as of 2008 is 13,000, which corresponds to 20% of the HIV-positive population (Remis, 2010). People who use injection drugs and men who have sex with men are the two populations with the highest rates of dual infection. The presence of both HIV and HCV infection increases the risk for end-stage liver disease.

Hepatitis C Virus (HCV).
HCV is an RNA virus that is primarily transmitted percutaneously. HCV is 10 times more likely than HIV to be transmitted by infected blood (Hoffman, Rockstroh, & Kamps, 2007). In Canada, the most common mode of HCV transmission is the sharing of contaminated needles and equipment among people who use injection drugs. Transmission during blood transfusion has been eliminated. The proportion of cases related to high-risk sexual behaviour (unprotected sex, multiple partners) has increased in recent years. However, sexual transmission among monogamous heterosexual partners remains rare. The risk of perinatal transmission is approximately 5% but is higher in women with HIV–HCV co-infection. People who were born in regions where HCV is common are also at risk because of the lack of universal precautions and medical practices in which contaminated equipment is used (e.g., during childhood immunization). Other transmission risks are related to needlestick injuries and hemodialysis.

In the 1980s, up to 20,000 Canadians were infected with HCV after receiving tainted blood transfusions. After the Commission of Inquiry on the Blood System in Canada (the Krever Inquiry), the Canadian Blood Services Agency and Hema Quebec were established in 1998 to monitor the blood system and prevent such occurrences in the future. A reliable antibody test for HCV was not widely available before 1992, and so people who received blood or blood products before then are at risk for chronic HCV infection and should be tested.

Diagnostic Tests.
Unlike antibodies to HAV and HBV, antibodies to HCV are not protective and their presence in the blood does not indicate immunity. A positive result of an anti-HCV test can be related to either a past or current exposure (Table 46-6). To confirm if disease is active or not, HCV RNA (the presence of replicating HCV) should be tested through polymerase chain reaction. In those whose HCV infection has resolved, anti-HCV results are positive but HCV RNA are negative.

After initial exposure to the virus, HCV RNA (replicating virus) appears in blood earlier than anti-HCV, and patients can test positive at approximately 2 weeks after exposure. Therefore, HCV RNA helps identify the presence of the virus in exposed individuals (e.g., health care workers) before antibodies develop. HCV RNA detection is particularly useful in the immunocompromised patient (e.g., patient with HIV) who has active disease but whose anti-HCV is negative because antibody production is very low (below the detection level of the antibody tests).

Six genotypes and more than 50 subtypes of HCV have been identified. In Canada, 75% of HCV infections are caused by HCV genotype 1. Genotyping currently plays an important role in the management of patients receiving treatment. Patients with genotypes 2 and 3 in general have better treatment response and require shorter treatment duration than those with genotype 1. The role of genotyping may change with future development of drugs that are effective for all genotypes.

Drug Therapy

Acute Hepatitis C. The rate of spontaneous clearance of acute hepatitis C (AHC) has been reported as more than 50% in some studies. Therefore, treatment for patients with AHC can be delayed for at least 12 weeks, allowing time for spontaneous clearing of the virus infection. The younger the patient is when infected, the higher the likelihood of spontaneous clearance. Patients with symptoms also have higher chance of eliminating the infection. Studies thus far have shown that treatment with IFN alone is successful in eradicating the virus in AHC (Sherman et al., 2007).

Chronic Hepatitis C. Unlike hepatitis B, chronic hepatitis C can be cured with drug treatment. Drug therapy (Table 46-7) for chronic hepatitis C is directed at completely eradicating the virus thus slowing progression of the disease. Treatment for HCV is a combination of pegylated IFN α-2a (Pegasys) plus ribavirin (combination is Pegasys RBV), or IFN α-2b (PEG-Intron) plus ribavirin (combination is Pegetron) for all HCV genotypes. Relapse after treatment, usually within 3 to 6 months, can occur. The overall cure rate with combination drug therapy for genotype non2/3 is 40 to 50%, whereas for genotypes 2 and 3 it is better, at more than 80%.

In 2011, the addition of protease inhibitors (PIs) was approved in Canada as triple therapy for HCV genotype 1. PIs inhibit the protease enzymes necessary for HCV to replicate. The two approved PIs are boceprevir (Victrelis) and telaprevir (Incivek). Triple therapy can improve the cure rate for HCV genotype 1 up to 75% (Myers et al., 2012). Another benefit of triple therapy is a potentially shorter treatment duration.

Pegylated IFN is injected once weekly and ribavirin is taken orally twice daily. Ribavirin, given in combination with IFN, has a synergistic effect and reduces the rate of relapse. PIs for genotype 1 are also taken orally every 8 hours. Telaprevir is to be taken with pegylated IFN and ribavirin during the first 12 weeks of treatment. However, boceprevir is given after 4 weeks of pegylated IFN and ribavirin combination. Detailed treatment regimens, dosing schedule, duration and monitoring can be found in the 2012 Canadian consensus guidelines on the management of chronic hepatitis C (Myers et al., 2012).

Patients with advanced fibrosis or cirrhosis can be treated with drug therapy as long as liver decompensation (e.g., ascites, esophageal hemorrhage, jaundice, wasting, encephalopathy) is not present. These drugs have many adverse events (see Table 46-7), and some may not be tolerable by all patients receiving therapy. Patients receiving treatment require intense monitoring for adverse events and drug–drug interactions, especially those receiving triple therapy.

Table 46-6 Serological Tests for HCV Infection	
MARKER	**DESCRIPTION**
Anti-HCV (antibody to hepatitis C virus)	Positive result indicates either past exposure or current infection
	An initial screening test for HCV
HCV RNA by PCR assay	Positive result indicates active ongoing viral replication
	Reported result is either qualitative (positive or negative) or quantitative (provides the viral replication amount, also referred as viral load)

HCV, hepatitis C virus; *PCR,* polymerase chain reaction.

Table 46-7 HCV Drug Therapy: Most Common Adverse Effects

Interferon	Ribavirin
Influenza-Like Symptoms	• Anemia
• Arthralgia	• Anorexia
• Asthenia	• Cough
• Chills	• Dyspnea
• Fatigue	• Insomnia
• Headache	• Pruritus
• Low grade fever	• Rash
• Nausea	• Teratogenicity (interferes with normal fetal development)
Other Effects	**Boceprevir**
• Depression	• Anemia
• Hair thinning	• Dysgeusia (bad taste in mouth)
• Insomnia	• Fatigue
• Irritability	• Headache
• Itching/dry skin	• Nausea
• Mood swings	**Telaprevir**
• Thyroid dysfunction	• Anemia
• Weight loss	• Anorectal itch
	• Fatigue
	• Pruritus
	• Nausea
	• Rash

HCV, hepatitis C virus.

SAFETY ALERT

Ribavirin

• During treatment, pregnancy must be avoided, both by women taking the drug and by women whose male partners are taking the drug.

Boceprevir (Victrelis), Telaprevir (Incivek)

• To avoid development of drug resistance, drug dosage must not be reduced.

• These drugs must not be taken alone; they must be taken with pegylated IFN and ribavirin.

• Telaprevir must be taken with high-fat food for absorption.

• A detailed medication history from the patient is essential to avoid potential drug–drug interactions with these two drugs.

IFN, interferon.

Many patients with HIV infection also have HCV infection. Patients who have stable HIV infection and relatively intact immune systems (CD4$^+$ counts >200/microlitre) are treated for hepatitis C with the goal of eradicating HCV infection and reducing the risk of progression to cirrhosis. As of December 2012, triple therapy had not yet been approved for HIV–HCV co-infection. HCV treatment with combination of IFN and ribavirin may reduce CD4$^+$ counts, worsen leukopenia, and increase the patient's risk for anemia. HIV medications may need to be altered because of the potential for drug interactions between some HIV medications and ribavirin.

Prevention. No vaccine for the prevention of HCV infection is currently available. The Public Health Agency of Canada does not recommend globulin (IG) for postexposure prophylaxis (e.g., needlestick exposure from an infected person) for HCV infection. After an acute exposure (e.g., through needlestick), baseline anti-HCV and ALT levels should be measured in both the person already infected (i.e., the source) and the person exposed to HCV. Follow-up testing for anti-HCV and ALT activity should be performed 4 to 6 months later. If the source is someone with known HCV infection, HCV RNA should be measured 2 weeks later to confirm viral transmission. Whether antiviral therapy initiated immediately after exposure has any positive effect is not yet known (Sherman, et al., 2007).

Hepatitis D

Hepatitis D virus (HDV), also called *delta virus,* is a defective single-stranded RNA virus that cannot survive on its own. Of the 350 million people infected with HBV worldwide, 15 million are co-infected with HDV. Eight genotypes of HDV have been reported, with variations in their geographical distribution (Hughes, Wedemeyer, & Harrison, 2011). HDV prevalence is generally highest in regions where hepatitis B is endemic. Although the prevalence of HDV in Canada is extremely low, people who are at risk for HBV infection (e.g., people who use injection drugs) should also be screened for HDV.

HDV requires the helper function of HBV to replicate. People infected with HDV can be co-infected (acquired HBV and HDV at the same time) or super-infected (existing HBV infection, then infected with HDV at a later time). HBV–HDV co-infection can cause fulminant hepatitis and more severe acute disease than HBV infection alone. A positive anti-HDV (hepatitis D antibody) test indicates exposure to HDV. To confirm whether the infection is current and active, HDV RNA must be measured. Currently in Canada, HDV RNA testing is not available in commercial laboratories and can be performed only in government-approved laboratories.

HDV, like HBV, is transmitted percutaneously. HDV is rarely acquired through sexual transmission. The symptoms of acute infection are the same as those of other viral hepatitis infection. People at risk for HDV infection are only those at risk for HBV, including people from highly HBV-endemic regions, those with multiple sexual partners, and those who use injection drugs. No vaccine for HDV is available; however, vaccination against HBV reduces risk of HDV co-infection. Treatment of HDV infection is with interferon alfa. However, response rates are poor (<30%), and relapse is common.

Hepatitis E

Hepatitis E virus (HEV) is an RNA virus and has four genotypes. Genotypes 1 and 2 infect humans exclusively, whereas genotypes 3 and 4 also infect other mammalian species, including pigs. HEV is transmitted via the fecal–oral route, most commonly through drinking contaminated water. Infection with HEV, initially thought to occur primarily in developing countries, has been reported in increasing numbers in many developed countries, including the United States (Aggarwal & Jameel, 2011). Current prevalence of hepatitis E in Canada remains unknown and has not been reported as a public health threat. In areas with poor sanitation, outbreaks or sporadic cases of HEV are common. HEV infection causes acute self-limiting hepatitis. Pregnant women, however, are at risk for more severe disease. In immunosuppressed people, hepatitis E may progress to a chronic infection and even cirrhosis. The diagnosis is confirmed through detection of IgM anti-HEV antibodies. Two vaccines have undergone successful human trials but were not yet commercially available at time of writing.

Hepatitis G

Hepatitis G virus (HGV) and GB virus-C (GBV-C) were once thought to be the same entity but are now considered different strains of the same virus. HGV is transmitted parenterally and sexually. People at risk include those who use injection drugs, those with hemophilia and patients receiving hemodialysis (because of frequent exposure to blood products), and sexually promiscuous individuals. HGV–GBV-C co-infection is found in 1 to 4% of Canadian blood donors. HGV–GBV-C co-infection is often found along with other viruses, such as HBV, HCV, and HIV.

Acute HGV–GBV-C co-infection rarely becomes chronic. A positive anti-GBV E2 antibody test result indicates previous infection and immunity. In immunocompromised individuals, such as those with HIV, HGV is less likely to be cleared but it does not appear to cause liver damage by itself. No association between GBV-C and liver cancer has ever been reported. Collaborative care for the patient with viral hepatitis is described in Table 46-8.

NURSING MANAGEMENT: VIRAL HEPATITIS

▪ Nursing Assessment

Subjective and objective data that should be obtained from a person with hepatitis are presented in Table 46-9.

▪ Nursing Diagnoses

Nursing diagnoses for the patient with hepatitis may include, but are not limited to, those presented in Nursing Care Plan 46-1.

▪ Planning

The overall goals are that the patient with viral hepatitis will (a) have relief of discomfort, (b) be able to resume normal activities, and (c) experience a return to normal liver function without complications.

▪ Nursing Implementation

▪ Health Promotion

Viral hepatitis is a public health problem. The nurse has a significant role in the control and prevention of this infectious disease. The nurse must first understand the epidemiology of the

COLLABORATIVE CARE

Table 46-8 Viral Hepatitis

Diagnostic

- History and physical examination
- Liver enzyme measurements
  - Alanine aminotransferase (ALT)
  - Aspartate aminotransferase (AST)
- Liver function tests
  - Albumin, bilirubin, INR
- Hepatitis serological profiles
  - Anti-HAV: IgM or IgG
  - HBsAg (HBeAg in suspected chronic cases)
  - Anti-HBs
  - Anti-HBc: IgM or total (IgM + IgG)
  - HBV DNA
  - Anti-HCV
  - HCV RNA
  - Anti-HDV

Collaborative Therapy

Acute and Chronic

- Well-balanced diet
- Vitamin supplements if needed
- Rest if fatigue is present
- Avoidance of alcohol and hepatotoxic drugs

Chronic HBV

- Interferon therapy
  - Conventional IFN (Intron A), pegylated IFN α-2a (Pegasys), pegylated IFN α-2b (PegIntron)
- Oral antiviral agents
  - Lamivudine (Heptovir), adefovir (Hepsera), telbivudine (Sebivo), entecavir (Baraclude), tenofovir (Viread)

Chronic HCV

- Pegylated IFN α-2a (Pegasys) + ribavirin (combination is Pegasys RBV), pegylated IFN α-2b (PegIntron) + ribavirin (combination is Pegetron)
- Boceprevir (Victrelis), Telaprevir (Incivek): must be administered with the combination pegylated IFN drugs

Anti-HBc, antibody to hepatitis B core antigen; *anti-HBs*, antibody to surface antigen; *HAV*, hepatitis A virus; *HbeAg*, hepatitis B e antigen; *HBsAg*, hepatitis B surface antigen; *HBV*, hepatitis B virus; *HCV*, hepatitis C virus; *HDV*, hepatitis D virus; *IgG*, immunoglobulin G; *IgM*, immunoglobulin M; *IFN*, interferon; *INR*, international normalized ratio.

different types of viral hepatitis, including risk factors for acquisition, before considering appropriate control measures.

▪ **Hepatitis A.** Vaccination is the best protection against HAV infection. Vaccination is recommended for people 2 years of age and older who travel to areas with increased rates of hepatitis A, for men who have sex with men, for people who use injection and noninjection drugs, for people with clotting factor disorders (e.g., hemophilia), and for people with chronic liver disease.

Preventive measures include personal and environmental hygiene and health education to promote good sanitation (Table 46-10). Handwashing before and after bowel movements

NURSING ASSESSMENT

Table 46-9 Hepatitis

Subjective Data

Important Health Information

Past health history: Family history of or exposure to person infected with viral hepatitis; exposure to benzene, carbon tetrachloride or other hepatotoxic agents, including herbal preparations; recent travel; exposure to contaminated medical or dental equipment; hemodialysis; blood or blood product transfusions; organ transplantation; misuse of alcohol; previous injection drug use; previous cocaine use; smoking history; high-risk sexual behaviour; exposure as health care worker; chronic care institution resident; incarceration

Medications: Exposure to new drug therapies; use and misuse of acetaminophen, phenytoin, halothane, methyldopa

Symptoms

- Weight loss, anorexia, vomiting, feeling of fullness in right upper quadrant
- Malaise; taste change
- Skin rashes or hives, pruritus
- Right upper quadrant pain and tenderness
- Jaundice, dark urine; light-coloured stools
- Fatigue, arthralgias, myalgias

Objective Data

General

Low-grade fever, lethargy, lymphadenopathy

Integumentary

Rash, other skin changes, jaundice, icteric sclera, interferon injection sites

Gastrointestinal

Hepatomegaly, splenomegaly

Possible Diagnostic Findings

Abnormal results of liver enzyme studies: ↑ serum total bilirubin level, hypoalbuminemia, anemia, bilirubin in urine, and ↑ urobilinogen; prolonged prothrombin time (INR); positive test results for hepatitis, including anti-HAV IgM, anti-HAV IgG, HBsAg, HBeAg, anti-HBc IgM, HBV DNA, anti-HCV, HCV RNA, and anti-HDV; abnormal findings on radiological imaging

HAV, hepatitis A virus; *HBc,* hepatitis B core antigen; *HBeAg,* hepatitis B e antigen; *HBsAg,* hepatitis B surface antigen; *HBV,* hepatitis B virus; *HCV,* hepatitis C virus; *HDV,* hepatitis D virus; *IgG,* immunoglobulin G; *IgM,* immunoglobulin M; *INR,* international normalized ratio.

and before eating is essential and is probably the most important precaution. When hepatitis A infection occurs in a food handler, IG should be administered to all other food handlers at the establishment. Patrons should also be offered IG.

The patient with acute hepatitis A is hospitalized only when symptoms are severe. Isolation is generally not required for hepatitis A; however, infection control precautions must be used (see Chapter 17, Table 17-8). A private room is indicated if the patient is incontinent of stool or has poor personal hygiene.

■ **Hepatitis B.** The use of the hepatitis B vaccine is the best means of protection. Control and prevention of hepatitis B also focus on identification of possible exposure via percutaneous and sexual transmission (see Table 46-10). The nurse must be aware

Table 46-10 Viral Hepatitis: Health Promotion and Preventative Measures

Hepatitis A

General Measures

- Good handwashing
- Proper personal hygiene
- Environmental sanitation
- Control and screening (signs, symptoms) of food handlers
- Serological screening
- Active immunization for people in at-risk groups

Use of Immune Globulin

- Early administration (1-2 wk after exposure) to those exposed
- Prophylaxis for travellers to areas where hepatitis A is common if they have not previously received HAV vaccine

Special Considerations for Health Care Providers

- Washing hands after contact with an affected patient or after removal of gloves
- Use of infection control precautions

Hepatitis B and C Percutaneous Transmission

- Screening of donated blood
  - Hepatitis B: HBsAg
  - Hepatitis C: anti-HCV antibody
- Use of disposable needles and syringes

Sexual Transmission

- Acute exposure: HBIG administration to sexual partner of HBsAg-positive person
- Administration of HBV vaccine series to uninfected sexual partners
- Use of condoms for sexual intercourse

General Measures

- Good handwashing
- Avoidance of sharing toothbrushes and razors
- HBIG administration for one-time exposure (needlestick, contact of mucous membranes with infectious material)
- Active immunization: HBV vaccine

Special Consideration for Health Care Providers

- Use of infection control precautions
- Handling the blood of all patients as potentially infectious
- Proper disposal of needles
- Use of needleless IV access devices when possible

HBIG, hepatitis B immunoglobulin; *HBsAg,* hepatitis B surface antigen; *IV,* intravenous.

of which individuals are at risk for contracting hepatitis B and teach ways to reduce risks of transmission.

Good hygienic practices, including handwashing and the use of gloves when expecting contact with blood, are important. A condom is advised for sexual intercourse before the partner undergoes vaccination. Razors, toothbrushes, and other personal items should not be shared. Close contacts of the person with hepatitis B should all be screened and vaccinated when necessary.

According to the Public Health Agency of Canada guidelines (PHAC, 1997), infection control precautions for people with

NURSING CARE PLAN 46-1

Acute Viral Hepatitis

NURSING DIAGNOSIS	*Imbalanced nutrition: less than body requirements* related to anorexia, nausea, and reduced metabolism of nutrients by liver *as evidenced by* inadequate food intake, perceived inability to ingest food, and weight loss
Expected Patient Outcomes	**Nursing Interventions and *Rationales***
• Maintains adequate nutritional intake • Progresses toward or maintains normal body weight	• Collaborate with health care provider, dietitian, and family to provide appropriate diet *so that the proper nutritional requirements can be provided.* • Assess patient's appetite and adequacy of intake *so that appropriate interventions can be planned.* • Offer frequent small meals and provide oral care before meals *to enhance patient's dietary intake.* • Allow patient to choose food items; serve high-carbohydrate and high-protein foods at time of day when the patient feels most like eating *to increase likelihood of adequate intake.* • Provide attractively served meals in pleasant surroundings *to stimulate patient's appetite.* • Measure weight daily on same scale, at same time, with same clothing *to monitor weight loss secondary to poor appetite.*
NURSING DIAGNOSIS	*Activity intolerance* related to fatigue and weakness *as evidenced by* verbal report of fatigue or weakness and altered response to activity
Expected Patient Outcome	**Nursing Interventions and *Rationales***
• Shows increased tolerance for activity	• Assist patient in scheduling rest periods *to maximize the benefits of rest and relaxation.* • Increase patient's activity gradually, as tolerated, *to allow previous activity pattern to be resumed.* • Conserve patient's strength by carefully monitoring activity *to prevent increasing weakness and fatigue.* • Teach patient to monitor and control activities that provoke fatigue *to prevent setback of activity progression.* • Limit environmental stimuli (e.g., light and noise) *to facilitate relaxation.*
NURSING DIAGNOSIS	*Ineffective therapeutic regimen management* related to lack of knowledge of follow-up care *as evidenced by* frequent questions about the disease, transmission risks, activities allowed, and general follow-up care
Expected Patient Outcomes	**Nursing Interventions and *Rationales***
• Verbalizes understanding of follow-up care • Explains methods of transmission and methods of preventing transmission to others	• Educate patient on the basic facts about illness, modes of transmission, diet, activities allowed, avoidance of alcohol, and need for follow-up care *to ensure patient's complete adherence to follow-up plan.* • Teach patient to watch for and report signs of disease complications, such as bleeding gums, black stools, and worsening of symptoms, *to enable prompt intervention.* • Teach use of infection control precautions *to reduce risk of cross-contamination.*

bloodborne pathogens (HBV, HBC, and HIV) include the use of disposable needles and syringes, which should be disposed of in puncture-resistant disposal units without recapping, bending, or breaking. (See Chapter 17, Table 17-8, for various types of infection control precautions.)

■ **Hepatitis C.** No vaccine is currently available. The primary measures to prevent HCV transmission are screening of blood, organ, and tissue donors; use of infection control precautions; and modification of high-risk behaviour. As with HBV prevention, the nurse should identify individuals at high risk for contracting HCV and teach different ways to reduce risks. Individuals at risk include those who use injection drugs (or have ever used them, even once or many years ago), people who received blood or blood products before 1992,

patients who are or have been undergoing hemodialysis, workers in hemodialysis units and laboratories in which blood is handled, people with multiple sexual partners, prisoners, and sexual partners of individuals with HCV infection. As with hepatitis B prevention, the use of universal precautions is important. A condom is advised for sexual intercourse with an individual with HCV. Razors, toothbrushes, and other personal items should not be shared. Health promotion and preventive measures for hepatitis A, B, and C are summarized in Table 46-10.

■ **Acute Intervention**

■ **Jaundice.** In light-skinned people, jaundice is usually observed first in the sclera of the eyes and later in the skin. In dark-skinned people, jaundice is observed in the hard palate of the mouth and the inner canthus of the eyes. The urine may be dark brown or brownish red because of the presence of bilirubin. Comfort measures should be used to relieve pruritus (if present), headache, and arthralgias (see Nursing Care Plan 46-1).

Ensuring that the patient receives adequate nutrition can be a challenge. Anorexia and a distaste for food can cause nutritional problems. Dietary assessment should be performed. Small, frequent meals may be preferable to three large ones and may help prevent nausea. Measures to stimulate the appetite—such as mouth care, antiemetics, and attractively served meals in pleasant surroundings—should be included in the nursing care plan. Carbonated beverages, ginger, and avoidance of very hot or very cold foods may help counteract the symptom of nausea. Adequate hydration is important.

■ **Rest.** Patients with symptomatic acute viral hepatitis have fatigue and decreased energy. Rest is important to help conserve energy. The nurse should help the patient space activities both to conserve energy and to avoid overexertion. The nurse must assess the patient's response to the rest and activity plan and modify it accordingly. Assessment of symptoms and the liver function tests should continue as a guide to activity.

■ **Ambulatory and Home Care**

Most individuals with acute viral hepatitis are cared for at home, and so the nurse must assess patients' knowledge of nutrition and provide the necessary dietary teaching. Rest and adequate nutrition are important for those with impaired liver synthetic functions. Patients should be cautioned about overexertion and the need to follow the health care provider's advice about when to return to work. The patient and family should be taught how to prevent transmission among household members and what symptoms should be reported to the health care provider. Symptoms of worsening liver function include bleeding tendencies (caused by increased INR), abdominal swelling (from ascites), and confusion (caused by encephalopathy). Patients should be instructed to have regular follow-up for at least 1 year after the diagnosis of acute viral hepatitis. Those who are unable to resolve the acute infection and become chronic HBV and HCV carriers should be assessed for the need of a referral for a hepatologist, if it is not already done. All patients with chronic HBV or HCV infection should avoid excessive use of alcohol, to prevent acceleration of disease progression.

Patients who remain seropositive for HBsAg should not donate blood, semen, or organs. Patients who receive interferon for the treatment of hepatitis B or C require education regarding this drug and its adverse effects. Patients and caregivers need to be taught how to administer a subcutaneous injection. They must also be informed about the numerous adverse effects with the therapy, including influenza-like symptoms (e.g., fever, malaise, fatigue, chills; see Table 46-7). (Additional information on interferon is presented in Chapters 16 and 18.)

■ **Evaluation**

Expected outcomes for the patient with viral hepatitis are addressed in Nursing Care Plan 46-1.

Control of Viral Hepatitis in Health Care Personnel

Hepatitis A. Hepatitis A is rarely transmitted from patients to health care personnel. When transmission does occur, it is associated with undiagnosed hepatitis A in patients who are being treated for other problems. If the patient is incontinent of stool, infection control precautions must be strictly enforced to prevent transmission.

Hepatitis B. Health care workers may be exposed to HBV from needlesticks, blood contamination, or transmission through mucous membranes or nonintact skin. After a needlestick injury, the chance that the health care worker will become infected with HBV is 6 to 30% (Centers for Disease Control and Prevention, 2011). Vaccination is the most effective method of preventing HBV. All health care workers in Canada are strongly advised to be immunized against HBV. Many health care organizations provide free hepatitis B vaccinations through the occupational health department to their at-risk employees.

Hepatitis C. Transmission usually results from percutaneous needle exposure or other blood exposure and undetected parenteral transmission. Measures to prevent transmission of the viruses from patients to health care personnel are presented in Table 46-11. Of particular concern to the public has been the issue of health care workers infected with bloodborne agents such as hepatitis virus and HIV. Many Canadian hospitals have committees that advise on the practice modifications needed for infected workers.

Nonalcoholic Fatty Liver Disease and Nonalcoholic Steatohepatitis

Nonalcoholic fatty liver disease (NAFLD) is a spectrum of disease that ranges from simple fatty liver that causes no hepatic

Table 46-11 Measures to Prevent Transmission of Hepatitis Viruses From Patients to Health Care Personnel*	
HAV	**HBV AND HCV**
Maintain good personal hygiene.	Use infection control precautions.†
Wash hands after contact with a patient or after removal of gloves.	Wash hands frequently and after each patient contact.
Use infection control precautions.†	Avoid direct contact with blood or blood-containing secretions.
	Handle the blood of all patients as potentially infective.
	Dispose of needles properly.
	Receive HBV vaccine.
	Use needleless IV access devices when they are available.

HAV, hepatitis A virus; *HBV*, hepatitis B virus; *HCV*, hepatitis C virus; *IV*, intravenous.

*To prevent the nurse from contracting viral hepatitis from patients with diagnosed and undiagnosed hepatitis, one suggested guideline for general practice is for the nurse to wear disposable gloves, goggles, and gown (sometimes) when fecal or blood contamination is likely in handling (a) soiled bedpans, urinals, and catheters and (b) patient's bed linens soiled by body excreta or secretions.

†See Chapter 17, Table 17-8.

inflammation to severe liver scarring. It is characterized by hepatic *steatosis* (accumulation of fat in the liver) not associated with other causes such as viral hepatitis, autoimmune disease, or alcohol.

Histologically, liver cells exhibit fatty changes. This accumulation of fat causes inflammation and scarring that is called **nonalcoholic steatohepatitis (NASH)**. NASH is diagnosed histologically by evidence of liver cell ballooning and presence of Mallory bodies. People with NASH can develop advanced scarring *(cirrhosis)*, and the risk for developing liver cancer and liver failure is increased. When the liver fails, liver transplantation is the only treatment alternative.

Causes

NAFLD is emerging as the most common chronic liver disease in the Western world (Kopec & Burns, 2011). The most common cause of fatty liver disease is obesity. According to the *Obesity in Canada* report (Public Health Agency of Canada & Canadian Institute for Health Information, 2011), one in four Canadians is obese. Obesity rates almost doubled among both sexes in most age groups in the adults and youth categories. Obesity is linked to many chronic diseases, and fatty liver disease is one of them. About 75% of obese people are at risk of developing simple fatty liver, and of those, up to 25% are at risk of developing fatty liver with inflammation (i.e., NASH).

NAFLD also occurs in patients with other risk factors such as diabetes, hyperlipidemia, severe weight loss (especially in those whose weight loss was recent), and metabolic syndrome. Poor diet, tuberculosis, intestinal bypass, and medications (e.g., corticosteroids) can also lead to NAFLD. Environmental exposure to certain chemicals, such as organic solvents and dimethylformamide, has also been associated with NAFLD.

Clinical Manifestations and Diagnostic Studies

Most patients with NAFLD have no symptoms. NAFLD is usually diagnosed during the routine medical checkup or during evaluation of other health problems such as hypertension, diabetes, or obesity. Elevations in liver enzyme levels (ALT, AST) are often the first signs of NAFLD. However, such elevations may be associated with other liver disorders. Symptoms, if present, are nonspecific and may include fatigue, malaise, and vague pain in the right upper abdominal quadrant. Enlarged liver (hepatomegaly) and enlarged spleen (splenomegaly) may be detected on first examination of the patient. Only a small number of patients exhibit signs of serious liver disease (e.g., ascites, anasarca, variceal hemorrhage). Jaundice occurs late in NASH and indicates advanced liver disease. As the disease progresses, serum albumin level is reduced and serum bilirubin level and prothrombin time are increased.

Definitive diagnosis is made through liver biopsy and histological examination of hepatocytes. Ultrasonography and computed tomography (CT) are also used to diagnose NAFLD.

Collaborative Care

NAFLD can progress to liver cirrhosis, liver failure, and hepatocellular carcinoma. Patients with NAFLD who are older, are obese, or have diabetes are at risk for advanced liver disease. No definitive treatment is available, and therapy is directed at reduction of risk factors, including treatment of diabetes, reduction in body weight, and elimination of harmful medications.

For patients with NAFLD who are overweight, weight reduction is important. Weight loss improves insulin sensitivity and reduces liver enzyme levels. No specific dietary therapy is recommended; however, a heart-healthy diet is appropriate. Lifestyle counselling interventions that focused on physical activities and eating behaviours have enabled significant improvement in liver function test results. Patients should have liver function monitored during weight loss because too rapid loss of weight is associated with liver failure.

Health promotion and patient education are important in preventing the development of NAFLD. Ways to prevent fatty liver include maintaining a healthy body mass index (≤25), avoiding increased abdominal fat (for men, keeping waist circumference <102 cm; for women, <88 cm), eating a heart-healthy diet, exercising at least three times weekly, limiting alcohol to no more than two drinks at a time, taking only medications that are needed, and following physicians' recommendations.

Toxic and Drug-Induced Hepatitis

Liver injury and death may occur after the inhalation, parenteral injection, or ingestion of certain chemical substances (see Chapter 41, Table 41-6). The two major types of chemical hepatotoxicity are toxic and drug-induced hepatitis. Agents producing toxic hepatitis are generally systemic poisons (e.g., carbon tetrachloride, gold compounds) or are those converted in the liver to toxic metabolites (e.g., acetaminophen). Liver necrosis generally occurs within 2 to 3 days of acute exposure to a toxic substance.

SAFETY ALERT

Acetaminophen (Tylenol)

- Drug is safe if taken at recommended levels and not combined with alcohol. However, it is also present in a variety of pain relievers, fever reducers, and cough medicines as a somewhat "hidden" ingredient; thus patients taking several drugs may not realize that they are taking a higher amount of acetaminophen.

- Its toxic effects are dose related. Ingestion of more than 10 g/day leads to acute liver failure.

- Idiosyncratic drug reactions produce drug-induced hepatitis. Such agents as isoniazid (INH), sulphasalazine, amiodarone, and methyldopa may produce idiosyncratic reactions because of patient susceptibility (metabolic reactivity) to these agents or immunologically mediated hypersensitivity responses. Most liver injuries occur within the first 6 months after drug initiation. Certain herbal preparations, weight loss agents, and other nutritional supplements have been found to cause liver injury.

The pathophysiological changes in the liver and the clinical manifestations of toxic and drug-induced hepatitis are similar to those of viral hepatitis. The usual presenting clinical findings are anorexia, nausea, vomiting, hepatomegaly, splenomegaly, and abnormal results of liver function studies. Treatment is largely supportive, as in acute viral hepatitis. Recovery may be rapid if the hepatotoxin is identified and removed. Liver transplantation may be necessary in cases with severe liver injuries.

Autoimmune and Genetic Liver Diseases

Autoimmune Hepatitis

Autoimmune hepatitis (AIH) is a chronic inflammatory disorder of the liver that occurs when the body's immune system attack its own liver cells. The cause is unknown, but its occurrence may be related to genetic and environmental factors or to drug, virus, or toxin exposure that triggers the activation of the immune system. However, the immune system remains activated after the trigger is removed. AIH is classified as type 1 or type 2. Type 1 is more common and affects people of all ages, whereas type 2 affects mainly children. The majority (70 to 80%) of patients with type 2 AIH are women, and many affected patients have other autoimmune diseases such as celiac disease or hypothyroidism.

The course of AIH is variable. Some patients have no symptoms, whereas others have an acute presentation with symptoms similar to those of acute viral hepatitis. Symptoms include fatigue, arthralgia, abdominal pain, and occasionally jaundice. Viral hepatitis must therefore be ruled out. Diagnosis is usually based on the presence of autoantibodies (i.e., antinuclear antibodies and anti–smooth muscle antibodies), high levels of serum immunoglobulins, and elevated liver enzymes. Liver cancer develops in approximately 6% of patients with AIH.

Daily treatment with prednisone alone or in combination with azathioprine (Imuran) induces remission in approximately 80% of patients. If these drugs are not effective, other immunosuppressive therapies (e.g., cyclosporine, tacrolimus [Prograf], or mycophenolate mofetil [CellCept]) are administered. Many patients who stop treatment experience relapse; therefore, treatment is usually lifelong to maintain remission. The most common cause of relapse is failure to adhere to the treatment regimen. Patients who do adhere and respond do not have a shortened life expectancy. However, liver transplantation is indicated for those with liver failure.

Wilson's Disease

Wilson's disease is a genetic disorder of copper metabolism that affects mainly the liver but also the brain, eyes, and kidneys. It is associated with increased storage of copper. The pattern of inheritance is autosomal recessive. The affected gene, *ATP7B*, codes for a protein expressed mainly in hepatocytes and affects the transmembrane transport of copper. Mutations in the *ATP7B* gene lead to decreased hepatocellular excretion of copper into bile. This results in copper accumulation in the liver, which causes liver cell injury. Wilson's disease has an average worldwide prevalence of 1 per 30,000.

Wilson's disease can manifest as liver disease or as neuropsychiatric disease. The hallmark of the disease is corneal Kayser-Fleischer rings, which are brownish red rings seen in the cornea near the limbus. In addition to liver disease, many affected patients also have neurological dysfunction, including movement disorders (tremor, involuntary movements), drooling, dysarthria, rigid dystonia, seizures, migraine headaches, and insomnia.

Diagnosis is based on clinical findings, including the corneal findings and presence of neurological symptoms. Serum ALT and AST levels are elevated, serum ceruloplasmin levels are low, serum uric acid levels are decreased, and urinary copper excretion levels are increased. Measurable copper concentrations from liver biopsy samples can also be present.

The mainstay initial treatment of symptomatic patients or those with active disease is with chelating agents such as D-penicillamine or trientine (not commercially available in Canada) that promote the excretion. Treatment is lifelong. Liver transplantation is reserved for acute liver failures or for treatment failures.

Hereditary Hemochromatosis

Hereditary hemochromatosis (HH) is a genetic disorder that affects the liver, heart, pancreas, and endocrine system. It is an inherited condition that is related to the mutation in the *HFE* gene, causing an increase and inappropriate absorption of dietary iron. Prolonged increased iron absorption can lead to complications such as cirrhosis, hepatocellular carcinoma, diabetes, and heart disease.

The clinical condition begins at approximately 20 to 40 years of age with clinically insignificant iron accumulation that progresses to a stage of iron overload without disease. If left untreated, it may progress to a stage of iron overload with organ damage (usually at ~40 years of age). The degree of iron overload has a direct impact on life expectancy of the individual with hemochromatosis. The major causes of death are cirrhosis, hepatocellular carcinoma, diabetes mellitus, and cardiomyopathy. (Hemochromatosis is discussed further in Chapter 32.)

Primary Biliary Cirrhosis

Primary biliary cirrhosis (PBC) is a chronic and slowly progressive disease caused by inflammation and destruction of small bile ducts in the liver. A T cell–mediated attack on the small bile duct epithelial cells results in loss of bile ducts and ultimately *cholestasis* (blockage of bile flow). Over time, this leads to liver fibrosis and cirrhosis. Although the etiology of PBC is not completely understood, it appears that both genetic and environmental factors such as chemical exposure and infection may play a role.

Patients with PBC present with generalized pruritus, hepatomegaly, hyperpigmentation of the skin, and fatigue. Patients with PBC are at increased risk for hepatocellular cancer. Most patients (95%) diagnosed with PBC are women, usually 30 to 60 years of age. The disease is associated with other autoimmune disorders such as rheumatoid arthritis, Sjögren's syndrome, and scleroderma.

In the early stages, patients may have no symptoms and may seek treatment for symptoms of fatigue and pruritus. Jaundice is a sign of late-stage disease. Osteoporosis is also found in a significant number of patients with PBC, and they may also have signs of fat malabsorption, including low levels of fat-soluble vitamins, which occur because of decreased bile secretion. Levels of serum alkaline phosphatase, antimitochondrial antibodies, antinuclear antibodies, and serum lipid levels are also elevated in patients with PBC. Histological evidence of disease is found on liver biopsy.

The goals of treatment are suppression of ongoing liver damage, prevention of complications, and symptom management. The only drug approved for treatment of PBC in Canada is ursodeoxycholic acid. This drug increases the rate of bile acid secretion and appears to have a cytoprotective effect. Management includes a focus on malabsorption, skin disorders such as pruritus and xanthomas (cholesterol deposits in the skin), hyperlipidemia, vitamin deficiencies, anemia, and fatigue. Cholestyramine is administered to treat pruritus. Patients are monitored for progression to cirrhosis. Liver transplantation is a treatment option for end-stage liver disease in patients with PBC.

Cirrhosis of the Liver

Cirrhosis is a diffuse pathological process, characterized by fibrosis (scar tissue) and conversion of normal liver architecture to abnormal nodules (Figure 46-5). Fibrosis occurs when the liver cells attempt to regenerate after liver injuries but the regenerative process is disorganized. The overgrowth of new and fibrous connective tissue distorts the normal lobular structure, resulting in lobules of irregular size and shape with impeded blood flow. Eventually, irregular and disorganized regeneration, poor cellular nutrition, and hypoxia caused by inadequate blood flow and scar tissue result in decreased functioning of the liver. Cirrhosis is the final stage of chronic liver disease; however, it is now known that cirrhosis is reversible because of fibrosis regression.

Cirrhosis is an important cause of morbidity and mortality. It is ranked as the thirteenth leading cause of death in Canadians (Statistics Canada, 2008); the incidence is highest between ages 40 and 60. It is twice as common in men as in women.

Etiology

Any chronic liver disease—including chronic viral hepatitis, NAFLD, and autoimmune hepatitis—as well as excessive alcohol intake can cause cirrhosis. The specific cause of cirrhosis may not be determined in all patients. However, excessive alcohol ingestion remains one of the most common causes of cirrhosis. Alcohol has a direct hepatotoxic effect, and it causes cell necrosis and fatty infiltration in the liver. Some controversy continues as to whether the cause of cirrhosis is alcohol or the malnutrition that frequently coexists with chronic ingestion of alcohol. A common problem in people with alcoholism is protein malnutrition. Cases of nutrition-related cirrhosis have resulted from extreme dieting, malabsorption, and obesity. Environmental factors, as well as a genetic predisposition, may also lead to the development of cirrhosis, regardless of dietary or alcohol intake. Approximately 20% of patients with chronic hepatitis C and 25% of those with chronic hepatitis B develop cirrhosis. Chronic inflammation and cell necrosis result in fibrosis and, ultimately,

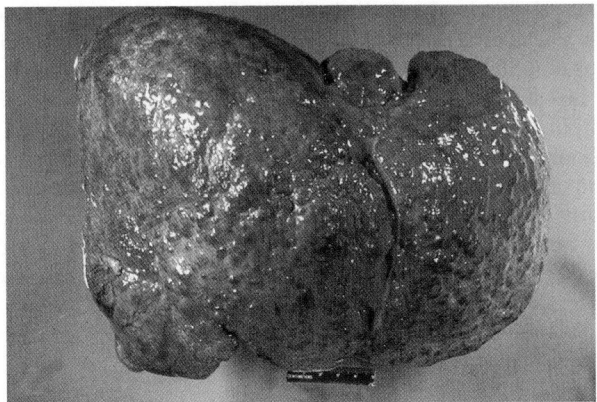

Figure 46-5 Cirrhosis that developed secondary to alcoholism. The characteristic diffuse nodularity of the surface is caused by the combination of regeneration and scarring of the liver.

Source: From Kumar, V., Abbas, A. K., Fausto, J. N., & Aster, J. (2010). *Robbins and Cotran pathologic basis of disease* (8th ed., p. 858, Figure 18-24,A). Philadelphia: W. B. Saunders.

cirrhosis. The combination of chronic hepatitis and excessive alcohol use accelerates the degree of liver damage.

Biliary causes of cirrhosis include primary biliary cirrhosis (described earlier in this chapter) and primary sclerosing cholangitis. *Primary sclerosing cholangitis* is a chronic inflammatory condition affecting the liver and bile ducts. It occurs most frequently in men. The cause of primary sclerosing cholangitis is unknown; however, it is strongly associated with ulcerative colitis. The chronic inflammation can ultimately progress to cirrhosis and end-stage liver disease.

Cardiac cirrhosis includes a spectrum of hepatic derangements that result from longstanding, severe right-sided heart failure. The treatment is aimed at managing the underlying heart failure.

Clinical Manifestations

Cirrhosis can be classified as compensated or decompensated. In well-compensated cirrhosis, the liver is able to continue to function normally despite severe hepatic cell injury. Results of liver function tests—including albumin level, bilirubin level, and prothrombin time—are normal. In decompensated cirrhosis, one or more of the complications from cirrhosis (discussed in the following section) occurs.

The onset of cirrhosis is usually insidious. Most patients with early compensated cirrhosis have no specific physical symptoms. Some patients may complain of abdominal pain, described as a dull, heavy feeling in the right upper quadrant or epigastrium. The pain may be caused by swelling and stretching of the liver capsule, spasm of the biliary ducts, intermittent vascular spasm, or a combination of these. Other early manifestations are nonspecific, and they include lassitude, fatigue, slight weight loss, and enlargement of the liver and the spleen.

Early symptoms of decompensated cirrhosis that leads to liver failure can be abrupt. Symptoms may include anorexia, dyspepsia, nausea and vomiting, weakness, muscle loss, and diarrhea or constipation. These symptoms occur as a result of the liver's altered metabolism of carbohydrates, fats, and proteins.

Manifestations of Advanced Cirrhosis.
When cirrhosis progresses, more symptoms start to develop. They may be severe and result from the complications of portal hypertension and liver failure. Jaundice, peripheral edema, and ascites develop gradually as the liver's synthesis function further deteriorates. Other late symptoms include skin lesions, hematological disorders, endocrine disturbances, and peripheral neuropathies (Figure 46-6). In the advanced stages, the liver becomes small and nodular and feels firm on palpation.

Jaundice. The appearance of jaundice is suggestive of disease decompensation. Jaundice occurs as a result of the liver's decreased ability to excrete conjugated bilirubin (hepatic jaundice). The jaundice may be minimal or severe, depending on the degree of liver damage. If obstruction of the biliary tract occurs, obstructive jaundice may also occur and is usually accompanied by pruritus. The pruritus is caused by an accumulation of bile salts underneath the skin.

Skin Lesions. Various skin manifestations are commonly seen in cirrhosis. **Spider angiomas** (*telangiectasia* or *spider nevi*) are small, dilated blood vessels with a bright red centre and spider-like branches. They occur on nose, cheeks, upper trunk, neck, and shoulders. *Palmar erythema* (a red area that blanches with pressure) appears on the palms of the hands. Both of these

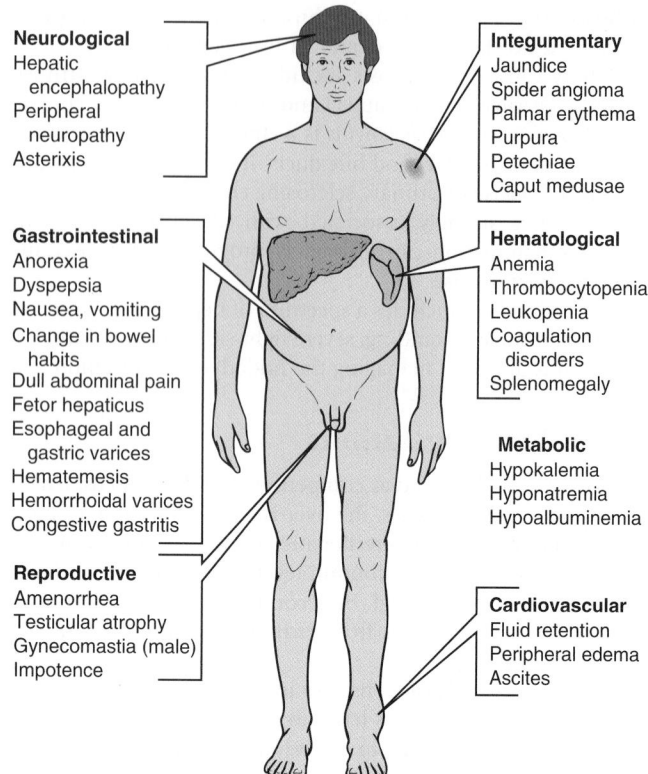

Neurological
Hepatic
  encephalopathy
Peripheral
  neuropathy
Asterixis

Gastrointestinal
Anorexia
Dyspepsia
Nausea, vomiting
Change in bowel
  habits
Dull abdominal pain
Fetor hepaticus
Esophageal and
  gastric varices
Hematemesis
Hemorrhoidal varices
Congestive gastritis

Reproductive
Amenorrhea
Testicular atrophy
Gynecomastia (male)
Impotence

Integumentary
Jaundice
Spider angioma
Palmar erythema
Purpura
Petechiae
Caput medusae

Hematological
Anemia
Thrombocytopenia
Leukopenia
Coagulation
  disorders
Splenomegaly

Metabolic
Hypokalemia
Hyponatremia
Hypoalbuminemia

Cardiovascular
Fluid retention
Peripheral edema
Ascites

Figure 46-6 Systemic clinical manifestations of advanced liver cirrhosis.

lesions are attributed to an increase in circulating estrogen as a result of the damaged liver's inability to metabolize steroid hormones.

Hematological Problems. Hematological problems include thrombocytopenia, leukopenia, anemia, and coagulation disorders. Thrombocytopenia is the strongest indicator of cirrhosis. Thrombocytopenia, leukopenia, and anemia are probably caused by splenomegaly, which results from backup of blood from the portal vein into the spleen. Overactivity of the enlarged spleen results in increased removal of blood cells, particularly the platelets, from circulation. The anemia also results from inadequate red blood cell production and survival. Other factors involved in the anemia are related to poor diet, poor absorption of folic acid, and bleeding from varices.

The coagulation problems result from the liver's inability to produce prothrombin and other factors essential for blood clotting. Coagulation problems are manifested by hemorrhagic phenomena or bleeding tendencies, such as epistaxis, purpura, petechiae, easy bruising, gingival bleeding, and heavy menstrual bleeding.

Endocrine Disturbances. Several signs and symptoms that occur in cirrhosis are related to the metabolism and inactivation of adrenocortical hormones, estrogen, and testosterone. Normally, the liver metabolizes these hormones. When the damaged liver is unable to do so, various manifestations occur. In men, gynecomastia, loss of axillary and pubic hair, testicular atrophy, and impotence with loss of libido may occur as a result of estrogen accumulation. In younger women, amenorrhea may occur, and older women may have vaginal bleeding. The liver fails to

metabolize aldosterone adequately, which results in hyperaldosteronism with subsequent sodium retention, water retention, and potassium loss.

Peripheral Neuropathy. Peripheral neuropathy is a common finding in alcoholic cirrhosis and is probably caused by a dietary deficiency of thiamine, folic acid, and cobalamin (vitamin B_{12}). The neuropathy usually results in mixed neurological symptoms, but sensory symptoms may predominate. (See Figure 46-6.)

Complications

Major complications of cirrhosis are portal hypertension with resultant esophageal or gastric varices (or both), peripheral edema and ascites, hepatic encephalopathy (manifested as coma), and hepatorenal syndrome. One or more of these complications are suggestive of disease decompensation.

Portal Hypertension and Esophageal and Gastric Varices.

Because of the structural changes in the liver as a result of the cirrhotic process, the portal and hepatic veins and sinusoids are compressed and damaged. These changes result in obstruction to the normal flow of blood through the portal system, which causes portal hypertension.

Portal hypertension is characterized by increased venous pressure in the portal circulation, as well as by splenomegaly, large collateral veins, ascites, systemic hypertension, and esophageal varices. Many pathophysiological changes result from portal hypertension. Collateral circulation develops in an attempt both to reduce this high portal pressure and to reduce the increased plasma volume and lymphatic flow. The common areas where the collateral channels form are in the lower esophagus (the anastomosis of the left gastric vein and the azygos veins), the anterior abdominal wall, the parietal peritoneum, and the rectum. Varicosities may develop in areas where the collateral and systemic circulations communicate, resulting in esophageal and gastric varices, *caput medusae* (ring of varices around the umbilicus), and hemorrhoids.

Varices are complexes of tortuous veins, enlarged and swollen as a result of portal hypertension. **Esophageal varices** are located at the lower end of the esophagus, and gastric varices are located in the upper portion (fundus) of the stomach. These collateral vessels contain little elastic tissue and are quite fragile. They tolerate the high pressure poorly, and the result is distended veins that bleed easily. Large varices are more likely to bleed.

Bleeding esophageal varices are the most life-threatening complication of cirrhosis. The varices rupture and bleed in response to ulceration and irritation. Factors producing ulceration and irritation include alcohol ingestion, swallowing of poorly masticated food, ingestion of coarse food, acid regurgitation from the stomach, and increased intra-abdominal pressure caused by nausea, vomiting, straining at stool, coughing, sneezing, or lifting heavy objects. The patient may have melena or hematemesis. Hemorrhage may be slow and oozing or massive. Massive hemorrhage is a medical emergency.

Peripheral Edema and Ascites.

Peripheral edema sometimes precedes ascites, but in some patients, its development coincides with or occurs after ascites. Edema is caused by decreased colloidal oncotic pressure as a result of impaired liver synthesis of albumin and by increased portocaval pressure from portal hypertension. Peripheral edema manifests as ankle and presacral edema.

PATHOPHYSIOLOGY MAP

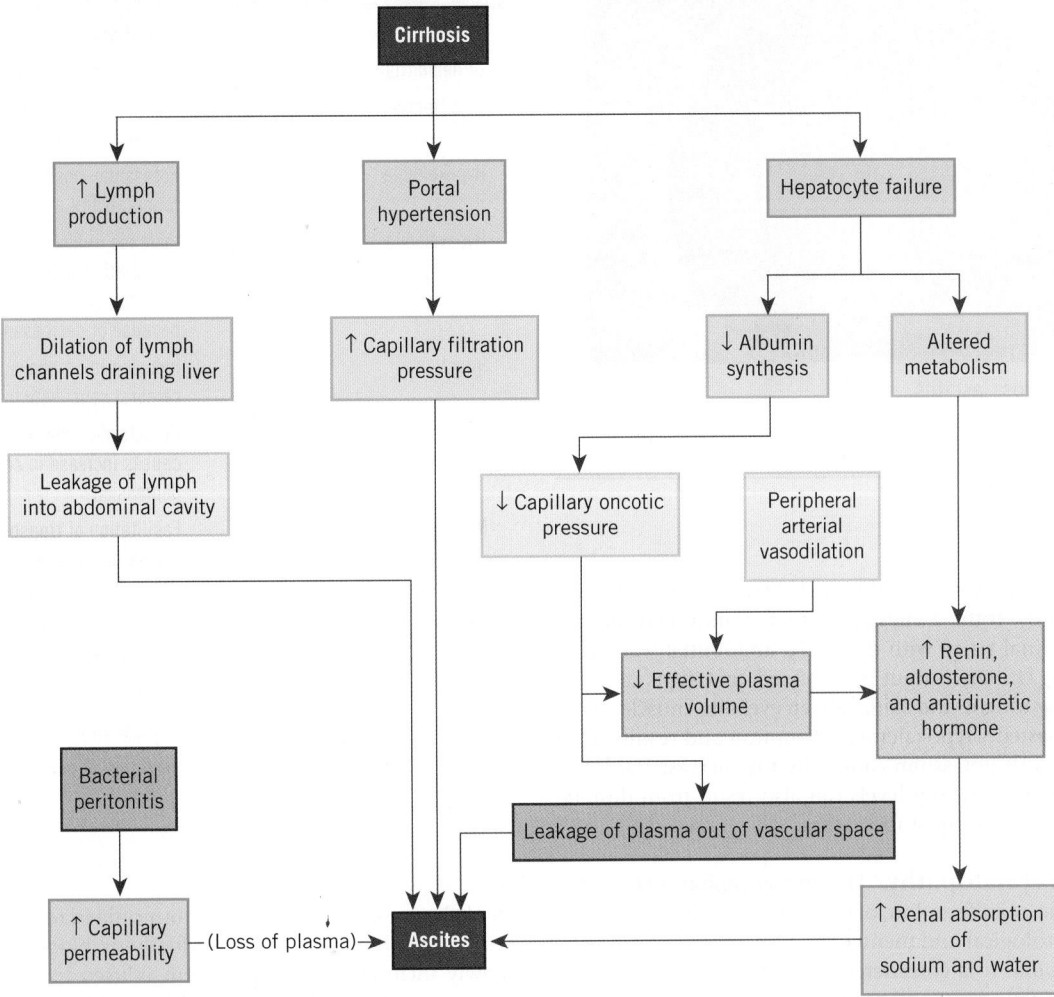

Figure 46-7 Mechanisms for development of ascites.

Source: Adapted from McCance, K. L., & Huether, S. E. (2010). *Pathophysiology: The biologic basis for disease in adults and children* (6th ed., p. 1484, Figure 39-17). St. Louis: Mosby.

Ascites is the accumulation of serous fluid in the peritoneal or the abdominal cavity. When the portal pressure is elevated in the liver, as occurs in cirrhosis, proteins shift from the blood vessels via the larger pores of the sinusoids (capillaries) into the lymph space (Figure 46-7). When the lymphatic system is unable to carry off the excess proteins and water, they leak through the liver capsule into the peritoneal cavity. The osmotic pressure of the proteins pulls additional fluid into the peritoneal cavity (Table 46-12).

A second mechanism of ascites formation is hypoalbuminemia, which results from the inability of the liver to synthesize albumin. The hypoalbuminemia results in decreased colloidal oncotic pressure. A third mechanism of ascites, hyperaldosteronism, results when aldosterone is not metabolized by damaged hepatocytes. The increased level of aldosterone causes an increase in sodium reabsorption by the renal tubules. This retention of sodium, as well as an increase in antidiuretic hormone, causes additional water retention in affected patients. Because of edema formation, intravascular volume and, subsequently, renal blood flow and glomerular filtration are decreased.

Table 46-12 Factors Involved in the Development of Ascites	
FACTOR	**MECHANISM**
Portal hypertension	Increase in resistance of blood flow through liver
Increased flow of hepatic lymph	Leaking of protein-rich lymph from surface of cirrhotic liver; intrahepatic blockage of lymph channels
Decreased serum colloidal oncotic pressure	Impairment of liver synthesis of albumin; loss of albumin into peritoneal cavity
Hyperaldosteronism	Increase in aldosterone secretion, stimulated by decreased renal blood flow; decreased liver metabolism of aldosterone
Impaired water excretion	Reduction in renal vascular flow and excessive serum levels of antidiuretic hormone

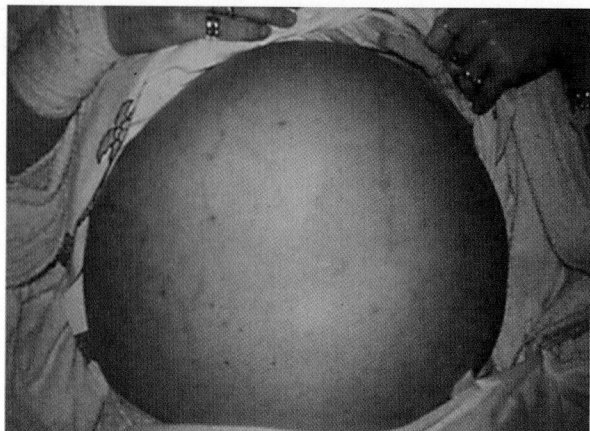

Figure 46-8 Gross ascites.

Source: From Butcher, G. P. (2004). *Gastroenterology: An illustrated colour text*, London: Churchill Livingstone.

Table 46-13 Factors Precipitating Hepatic Encephalopathy

FACTOR	MECHANISM
GI hemorrhage	Increase in ammonia in GI tract
Constipation	Increase in ammonia from bacterial action on feces
Hypokalemia	Potassium ions are needed by brain to metabolize ammonia
Hypovolemia	Increase in blood ammonia, caused by hepatic hypoxia; impairment of cerebral, hepatic, and renal function because of decreased blood flow
Infection	Increase in catabolism; increase in cerebral sensitivity to toxins
Cerebral depressants (e.g., narcotics)	No detoxification by liver, which causes increase in cerebral depression
Metabolic alkalosis	Facilitation of transport of ammonia across blood–brain barrier; increase in renal production of ammonia
Paracentesis	Loss of sodium and potassium ions; decrease in blood volume
Dehydration	Potentiation of ammonia toxicity
Increased metabolism	Increase in workload of liver
Uremia (kidney failure)	Retention of nitrogenous metabolites

GI, gastrointestinal.

Ascites is manifested by abdominal distension with weight gain (Figure 46-8). If the ascites is severe, the umbilicus may be everted. Abdominal striae with distended abdominal wall veins may be present. Urinary output is decreased, and signs of dehydration (e.g., dry tongue and skin, sunken eyeballs, muscle weakness) are manifested. Hypokalemia is common and results from an excessive loss of potassium caused by the increased aldosterone. Lowering of potassium levels can also result from diuretic therapy administered to treat the ascites.

Hepatic Encephalopathy. **Hepatic encephalopathy** is a neuropsychiatric manifestation of liver damage, manifested as changes in neurological and mental function, ranging from lethargy to deep coma. It is considered a terminal complication in liver disease. Hepatic encephalopathy can occur in any condition in which ammonia enters the systemic circulation without detoxification by the damaged liver.

The pathogenesis of hepatic encephalopathy is multifactorial and includes the neurotoxic effects of ammonia, abnormal neurotransmission, astrocyte swelling, and inflammatory cytokines. Hepatic encephalopathy is associated with rising levels of ammonia. However, the exact mechanism of action of ammonia remains to be determined. A major source of ammonia is the bacterial and enzymatic deamination of amino acids in the intestines. The ammonia that results from this deamination process normally goes to the liver via the portal circulation and is converted to urea, which is then excreted by the kidneys. When the blood is shunted past the liver via the collateral anastomoses, or when the liver is unable to convert ammonia to urea, ammonia levels in the systemic circulation rise. The ammonia crosses the blood–brain barrier and produces neurotoxic manifestations. A number of factors may precipitate hepatic encephalopathy, mostly because they increase the amount of circulating ammonia (Table 46-13). Hepatic encephalopathy is also an outcome of surgical shunt procedures and creation of transjugular intrahepatic portosystemic shunt (TIPS), which are used to reduce portal hypertension (Haussinger & Schliess, 2008).

Clinical manifestations of encephalopathy are changes in neurological and mental responsiveness, ranging from sleep disturbances to lethargy to deep coma. Changes may occur suddenly because of an increase in ammonia in response to bleeding varices, or they may occur gradually as blood ammonia levels slowly increase. A grading system is used to classify the stages of hepatic encephalopathy (Table 46-14). In the early stages (grades 0 and 1), manifestations include euphoria, depression, apathy, irritability, memory loss, confusion, yawning, drowsiness, insomnia, and agitation. Grades 2 and 3 are characterized by slow and slurred speech, impaired judgement, hiccups, slow and deep respirations, hyperactive reflexes, and a positive Babinski reflex.

Clinical manifestations of impending coma (grade 4) include disorientation as to time, place, or person. A characteristic symptom of hepatic encephalopathy is **asterixis** (flapping tremors) involving the arms and hands. When asked to hold the arms and hands stretched out, the patient is unable to hold this position, and the hands exhibit a series of rapid flexion and extension movements. Other signs of asterixis are rhythmic movements of the legs with dorsiflexion of the foot and rhythmic movements in the face with strong closure of the eyelids. Impairments in writing involve difficulty in moving the pen or pencil from left to right and *constructional apraxia* (the inability to construct simple figures). Other signs include hyperventilation, hypothermia, and grimacing and grasping reflexes.

Fetor hepaticus—a musty, sweet odour of the patient's breath—occurs in some patients with encephalopathy. This odour results from the accumulation of digestive by-products that the liver is unable to degrade.

Hepatorenal Syndrome. **Hepatorenal syndrome (HRS)** is a serious complication of cirrhosis. It is characterized by

	Table 46-14 Grading Scale for Hepatic Encephalopathy		
GRADE	**LEVEL OF CONSCIOUSNESS**	**INTELLECTUAL FUNCTION**	**NEUROLOGICAL FINDINGS**
0	Insomnia, sleep disturbances	Subtle change in computational skills	Impaired handwriting, tremor
1	Lack of awareness, personality change	Short attention span, mild confusion, depression	Incoordination, asterixis
2	Lethargy, drowsiness, inappropriate behaviour	Disorientation	Asterixis, abnormal reflexes
3	Sleep, ability to be roused	Loss of meaningful conversation, marked confusion, incomprehensible speech	Asterixis, abnormal reflexes
4	Not rousable, inability to be roused	Absent	Decerebrate posturing; possible responsiveness to painful stimuli

functional kidney failure with advancing azotemia, oliguria, and intractable ascites. It is not characterized by structural abnormality of the kidneys. The etiology is complex, but the final common pathway is likely to be that portal hypertension, along with liver decompensation, results in splanchnic and systemic vasodilation and decreased arterial blood volume. As a result, renal vasoconstriction occurs, leading to kidney failure. This kidney failure can be reversed by liver transplantation. In patients with cirrhosis, HRS frequently follows diuretic therapy, GI hemorrhage, or paracentesis (Mukherjee, 2008).

Diagnostic Studies

In well-compensated cirrhosis, liver function test results (bilirubin, albumin, and INR) remain normal although AST and ALT levels may or may not be elevated (see Table 46-6 for tests). When the liver starts to deteriorate and fail, most of the liver tests yield abnormal results.

Levels of liver enzymes—including AST, ALT, alkaline phosphatase, and γ-glutamyl transpeptidase—are elevated because of the release of these enzymes from damaged liver cells and bile ducts. Total protein and albumin levels in the blood are decreased because they are synthesized by the liver. γ-Globulins (antibodies), produced by B lymphocytes, often increase in number in cirrhosis, which indicates increased synthesis or decreased removal. Abnormalities in fat metabolism are reflected by decreased cholesterol levels. The prothrombin time or INR is prolonged, and bilirubin level is increased.

Liver Biopsy. Liver biopsy is a procedure in which a small amount of liver tissue is removed for histological examination. The degree of inflammatory activity and the amount of fibrosis (scar tissue) can be characterized. Liver biopsy is unnecessary to confirm cirrhosis if cirrhosis is clinically evident (e.g., nodular appearance of the liver on ultrasonography, presence of thrombocytopenia). However, biopsy may be needed to confirm the underlying causes of the liver disease.

Liver biopsy is normally performed percutaneously. In patients with advanced cirrhosis who have abnormal coagulation, biopsy must be performed via the transjugular vein. The most common risk of liver biopsy is bleeding.

Noninvasive Fibrosis Markers. Transient elastography (FibroScan) is a noninvasive imaging technique by which the degree of hepatic fibrosis is measured. Its use in Canada was approved in 2010. It is an ultrasonography-based imaging technique for detecting liver stiffness without the need for liver biopsy. Meta-analyses have revealed transient elastography to have excellent diagnostic accuracy for the diagnosis of cirrhosis, regardless of the underlying causes of the liver disease (Stebbing et al., 2010).

Models of serum markers (e.g., FibroTest) are also noninvasive tests that can be performed with blood samples. FibroTest is most commonly used in Canada. In this model, five parameters are used (levels of bilirubin, γ-glutamyl transpeptidase, haptoglobin, apolipoprotein, and α2-macroglobulin), in addition to patient's age and sex, to calculate a fibrosis score for predicting the degree of liver fibrosis.

Collaborative Care in Advanced Cirrhosis of the Liver

Rest. Although there is no specific therapy for advanced cirrhosis, certain measures can be taken to prevent or treat complications (Table 46-15). Rest may be required for patients with decompensated cirrhosis and constitutional symptoms, including fatigue and lassitude. It has long been thought that rest may reduce metabolic demands of the liver.

Ascites. Management of ascites is focused on sodium restriction, diuretics, and fluid removal. Affected patients are encouraged to limit sodium intake to 2 g (88 mmol) per day. More stringent sodium restriction is no longer recommended because it can result in reduced nutritional intake and subsequent malnutrition problems. Fluid restriction is usually not necessary unless severe ascites develops. Fluid and electrolyte balance should be accurately assessed and controlled. Salt-poor albumin may be administered to help maintain intravascular volume and adequate urinary output by increasing plasma colloid osmotic pressure.

Diuretic therapy is an important part of management. A combination of drugs that work at multiple sites in the nephron is often more effective than just one. Spironolactone (Aldactone) is an effective diuretic. It is an antagonist of aldosterone and is potassium sparing. Other potassium-sparing diuretics include amiloride (Apo-Amilzide) and triamterene (Teva-Triamzide). A high-potency loop diuretic, such as furosemide (Lasix), is frequently administered in combination with a potassium-sparing drug. Hydrochlorothiazide is rarely administered because it is not as potent as the loop diuretics.

Paracentesis (needle puncture of the abdominal cavity) may be performed to remove ascitic fluid. However, it is indicated only when the diuretic therapy fails and for relief of symptoms such

COLLABORATIVE CARE

Table 46-15 Advanced Cirrhosis of the Liver

Diagnostic	Ascites
• History and physical examination	• Diuretics
• Liver function studies (albumin, bilirubin, INR)	• Low-sodium diet
• Liver enzyme measurements (AST, ALT, ALP, GGT)	• Paracentesis (if indicated)
• Liver biopsy (if indicated)	• TIPS
• Endoscopy (esophagogastroduodenoscopy)	**Esophageal and Gastric Varices**
• Liver ultrasonography	• Drugs
• Computed tomography (CT)	• β-Adrenergic blockers (e.g., nadolol)
• Magnetic resonance imaging (MRI)	• Vasopressin
• Serum electrolyte measurements	• Octreotide (Sandostatin)
• CBC	• Endoscopic sclerotherapy or band ligation
• Testing of stool for occult blood	• Balloon tamponade
	• Surgical shunting procedure
Collaborative Therapy	• TIPS
Conservative Therapy	**Hepatic Encephalopathy**
• Rest (in decompensated cirrhosis)	• Antibiotics
• Avoidance of alcohol, aspirin, and nonsteroidal anti-inflammatory drugs (NSAIDs)	• Lactulose

ALP, alkaline phosphatase; *ALT,* alanine aminotransferase; *AST,* aspartate aminotransferase; *CBC,* complete blood count; *GGT,* γ-glutamyl transpeptidase; *INR,* international normalized ratio; *TIPS,* transjugular intrahepatic portosystemic shunt.

as abdominal pain or difficulty breathing. The relief provided by paracentesis is only temporary because the fluid reaccumulates.

TIPS (discussed later in this section) is being used increasingly to alleviate ascites.

Esophageal Varices. The main therapeutic goal related to esophageal and gastric varices is prevention of bleeding. Risk factors for esophageal bleeding include variceal size, decreased wall thickness, and degree of liver dysfunction. Patients who have esophageal varices should avoid ingesting alcohol, aspirin, nonsteroidal inflammatory drugs (NSAIDs), and irritating foods. Upper respiratory infections should be treated promptly, and coughing should be controlled. For patients who have esophageal varices that have not bled, prophylactic treatment with nonselective β-adrenergic blockers (e.g., propranolol or nadolol) has been shown to reduce the risk of bleeding, as well as the number of bleeding-related deaths (Garcia-Tsao, Sanyal, Grace, Carey, & Practice Guidelines Committee of the American Association for the Study of Liver Diseases, 2007.)

Management of bleeding varices includes emergency, therapeutic, and prophylactic interventions. The combination of drug and endoscopic therapy is more successful than either approach alone (Garcia-Tsao et al., 2007). Drug therapy may include octreotide (Sandostatin), vasopressin, nitroglycerin, and

β-adrenergic blockers. Endoscopic therapies include sclerotherapy, ligation of varices, and shunt therapy.

When esophageal variceal bleeding does occur, the first step is to stabilize the patient and manage the airway. IV therapy is initiated and may include administration of blood products. Variceal bleeding is diagnosed on endoscopic examination. At the time of endoscopy, sclerotherapy or banding of the varices may be performed. The main goal of drug therapy is to stop the bleeding. Gastric varices are more difficult to manage than esophageal varices. The initial measures to stop the bleeding include IV administration of vasopressin to produce vasoconstriction of the splanchnic arterial bed, to decrease portal blood flow, and to decrease portal hypertension. Because vasopressin has adverse effects (including decreased coronary blood flow and heart rate and increased blood pressure), nitroglycerin is often administered in combination with vasopressin for reducing the detrimental effects of the vasopressin while enhancing its beneficial effect. Vasopressin should be avoided or administered cautiously in older adults because of the risk of cardiac ischemia (Garcia-Tsao et al., 2007).

Endoscopic sclerotherapy is a treatment method for both acute and chronic bleeding varices. The sclerosing agent, introduced via endoscopy, thromboses and obliterates the distended veins.

Another procedure for managing acute variceal bleeding is endoscopic ligation or banding of the varices. A small rubber band (elastic O-ring) is slipped around the base of the varix. Endoscopic variceal ligation can be achieved with clips instead of the O-rings (endoscopic clipping). Endoscopic ligation is as effective as endoscopic sclerotherapy with fewer complications. A combination of endoscopic sclerotherapy and ligation may be used and seems to be more effective than either treatment alone.

Balloon tamponade may be used in patients with brisk esophageal or gastric variceal hemorrhage that cannot be controlled on initial endoscopy. Balloon tamponade controls the hemorrhage by mechanical compression of the varices. Either the Minnesota or Sengstaken-Blakemore tube (Figure 46-9) is used for this purpose. These tubes have two balloons, one gastric and one esophageal. The Sengstaken-Blakemore tube has three lumens: one for the gastric balloon, one for the esophageal balloon, and one for gastric aspiration. The Minnesota tube has an esophageal aspiration port. When inflated, the gastric and esophageal balloons put mechanical compression on the varices. The gastric balloon anchors the tube in position and also applies pressure to any bleeding gastric varices.

Supportive measures during an acute variceal bleed include administration of fresh-frozen plasma and packed red blood cells, vitamin K, proton pump inhibitors, and histamine H$_2$-receptor blockers. Lactulose and neomycin administration may be started to prevent hepatic encephalopathy from breakdown of blood and the release of ammonia in the intestine.

Long-Term Management. The incidence of recurrent bleeding is high, as is the mortality risk with each bleeding episode, and so continued therapy is necessary. Long-term management of patients who have had an episode of bleeding includes the use of β-adrenergic blockers, repeated sclerotherapy, endoscopic ligation, and portosystemic shunts.

A nonselective β-adrenergic blocker (e.g., propranolol, nadolol) can be administered orally to prevent recurrent GI

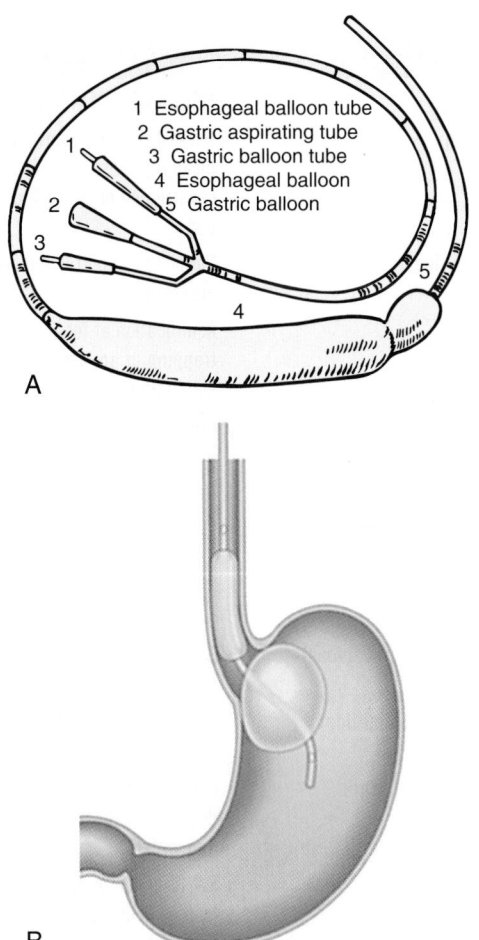

Figure 46-9 A, Diagram of Sengstaken-Blakemore tube.
B, Diagram of tube inserted into esophagus and stomach.

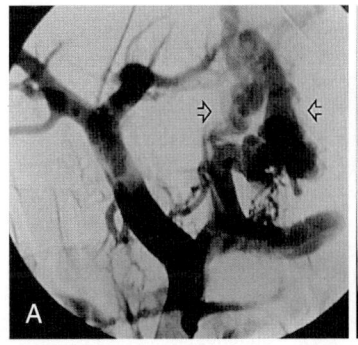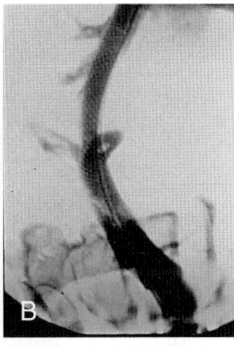

Figure 46-10 Total portal diversion after insertion of a transjugular intrahepatic portosystemic shunt (TIPS). **A,** Portal venogram before TIPS insertion shows filling of large esophageal varices *(arrows)*. **B,** After TIPS insertion, flow to varices is eliminated. The direction of intrahepatic portal vein flow is now reversed, toward the TIPS.

Source: From LaBerge, J. M., Ring, E. J., Lake, J. R., Ferrell, L. D., Doherty, M. M., Gordon, R. L., …, Ascher, N. L. (1992). Transjugular intrahepatic portosystemic shunts: Preliminary results in 25 patients. *Journal of Vascular Surgery, 16,* 258. doi:10.1016/0741-5214(92)90116-P

bleeding. Such medication reduces portal venous pressure. This effect is caused by reduced cardiac output and, possibly, constriction of splanchnic vessels.

Shunting Procedures. Surgical and nonsurgical methods of shunting blood away from the esophageal varices are available. Shunting procedures tend to be used more commonly after a second major bleeding episode than after an initial bleeding episode. In TIPS, a tract (shunt) between the systemic and portal venous systems is nonsurgically created to redirect portal blood flow (Figure 46-10).

Under radiological guidance, the catheter is placed in the jugular vein and then threaded through the superior and inferior venae cavae to the hepatic vein. The wall of the hepatic vein is punctured, and the catheter is directed to the portal vein. Stents are positioned along the passageway, overlapping in the liver tissue and extending into both veins.

This procedure reduces portal venous pressure and decompresses the varices, thus controlling bleeding. This procedure does not interfere with future liver transplantation. Limitations of the TIPS procedure include the increased risk of hepatic encephalopathy and stenosis of the stent.

Various surgical shunting procedures are no longer in common use but may be used to decrease portal hypertension by diverting some of the portal blood flow and simultaneously allow adequate liver perfusion. The surgical shunts still in use are the portacaval shunt and the distal splenorenal shunt (see Figure 46-10). Surgical shunts are more likely to be used in emergency situations. Although a prophylactic portacaval shunt decreases bleeding episodes, it does not prolong life. Patients can develop hepatic encephalopathy as a result of the diversion of the ammonia past the liver and into the systemic circulation. The distal splenorenal shunt (Warren shunt) leaves portal venous flow intact (Figure 46-11), and so the incidence of associated hepatic encephalopathy is lower. However, with time the flow of blood through the liver decreases. Like the TIPS, surgical stents are also prone to occlusion, which necessitates angiography and stent dilation.

Hepatic Encephalopathy. The goal of the management of hepatic encephalopathy is the reduction of ammonia formation. Several measures are used to reduce ammonia formation in the intestines. Lactulose is a synthetic keto analogue of lactose. In the colon, it is split into lactic acid and acetic acid, which decreases the pH from 7.0 to 5.0. The acidic environment discourages bacterial growth. The lactulose traps the ammonia in the gut, and the laxative effect of the drug expels the ammonia from the colon. It is usually administered orally to prevent encephalopathy but can be given as a retention enema or via a nasogastric (NG) tube if a patient is in the later stage of encephalopathy.

Antibiotics that are poorly absorbed from the GI tract, such as neomycin sulphate, are given orally or rectally. Because neomycin may cause renal toxicity and hearing impairments, other antibiotics such as metronidazole (Flagyl) are administered. They reduce the bacterial flora of the colon. Bacterial action on protein in the feces results in ammonia production. Cathartics and enemas are also administered to decrease bacterial action. Constipation should be prevented.

Control of hepatic encephalopathy also involves treatment of precipitating causes (see Table 46-13). One strategy involves controlling GI hemorrhage and removing the blood from the GI tract to decrease the protein in the intestine. Electrolyte disorders, acid–base imbalances, and infections should also be treated.

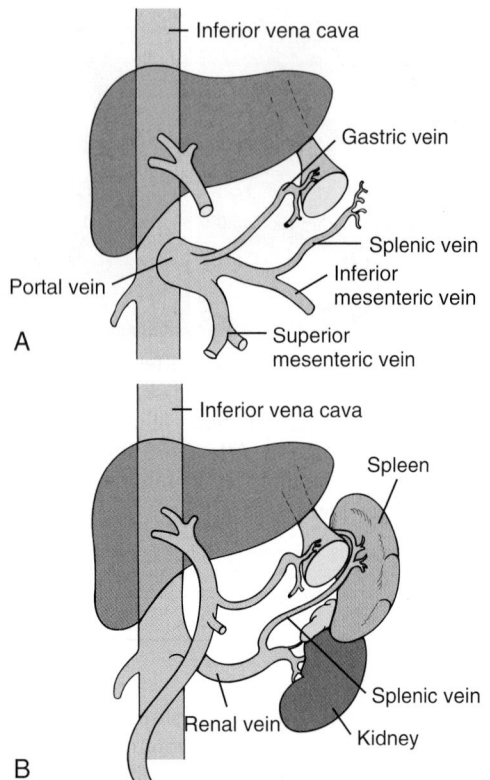

Figure 46-11 Portosystemic shunts. **A,** Portacaval shunt. The portal vein is anastomosed to the inferior vena cava, diverting blood from the portal vein to the systemic circulation. **B,** Distal splenorenal shunt. The splenic vein is anastomosed to the renal vein. The portal venous flow remains intact, and esophageal varices are selectively decompressed (by decompression of the short gastric veins). The spleen conducts blood from the high pressure of the esophageal and gastric varices to the low-pressure renal vein.

DRUG THERAPY

Table 46-16 Advanced Cirrhosis

DRUG	MECHANISM OF ACTION
Vasopressin	Hemostasis and control of bleeding in esophageal varices; constriction of splanchnic arterial bed
Propranolol (Inderal) or nadolol	Reduction of portal venous pressure
Lactulose	Acidification of feces in bowel and trapping of ammonia, causing its elimination in feces
Neomycin sulphate	Decrease in bacterial flora, decrease formation of ammonia
Histamine (H_2) blocker (e.g., ranitidine [Zantac]) or proton pump inhibitors (e.g., pantoprazole [Pantoloc])	Decrease in gastric acidity
Diuretics	
Spironolactone (Aldactone)	Blocking action of aldosterone; potassium sparing
Amiloride (Apo-Amilzide)	Inhibiting reabsorption of sodium and secretion of potassium
Chlorothiazide (Diuril)	Action on proximal tubule to decrease reabsorption of sodium and water
Furosemide (Lasix)	Rapid action on distal tubule and loop of Henle to prevent reabsorption of sodium and water
Triamterene (Teva-Triamzide)	Inhibiting reabsorption of sodium and secretion of potassium
Magnesium sulphate	Magnesium replacement*
Vitamin K	Correction of clotting abnormalities

*Hypomagnesemia occurs with liver dysfunction.

Liver transplantation may be considered in patients with recurring hepatic encephalopathy and end-stage liver disease. The decision to perform liver transplantation depends on a number of factors, including the cause of the cirrhosis and other systemic medical problems.

Drug Therapy. No drug therapy specifically for cirrhosis is available. However, a number of drugs are administered to treat symptoms and complications of advanced liver disease (Table 46-16).

Nutritional Therapy. The diet for the patient with cirrhosis without complications is high in calories (3000 kcal/day) with high carbohydrate content and moderate to low fat levels. Protein restriction may be appropriate in some patients immediately after a severe flare of symptoms (i.e., episodic hepatic encephalopathy). However, protein restriction is rarely justified in patients with cirrhosis and persistent hepatic encephalopathy. Indeed, malnutrition is a more serious clinical problem than hepatic encephalopathy for many of these patients.

Sufficient carbohydrate intake must be provided to maintain an intake of 1500 to 2000 calories to prevent hypoglycemia and catabolism. Glucose polymer (Polycose) is protein free and can be used as a source of calories. It can be administered orally or via NG tube. Many patients with alcoholic cirrhosis have protein–calorie malnutrition and may benefit from receiving enteral formulas containing protein from branched-chain amino acids that are metabolized by the muscles. They provide protein that is more easily metabolized by the liver. Total parenteral nutrition or tube feedings may be required.

In patients with ascites and edema, diet must be low in sodium. The degree of sodium restriction varies depending on a patient's condition. Table salt is the most common source of sodium. Patients must avoid foods that are high in sodium content. These include canned soups and vegetables, salted snacks such as potato chips, nuts, smoked meats and fish, crackers, breads, olives, pickles, ketchup, and beer.

Sodium is also present in many OTC drugs (e.g., antacids); however, most antacids now have a lower sodium content than previously. Carbonated beverages tend to be high in sodium, but low-sodium and sodium-free carbonated drinks are also available. Patients should be advised to read food labels; foods high in protein usually have large amounts of sodium. Alternative protein supplements that are low in sodium may have to be administered. Food can be made more palatable by the use of seasonings such as garlic, parsley, onion, lemon juice, and spices.

NURSING MANAGEMENT: CIRRHOSIS

Nursing Assessment

Subjective and objective data that should be obtained from an individual with cirrhosis are presented in Table 46-17.

NURSING ASSESSMENT
Table 46-17 Cirrhosis

Subjective Data

Important Health Information

Past health history: Previous viral, toxic, or idiopathic hepatitis; chronic biliary obstruction and infection; severe right-sided heart failure; chronic alcoholism

Medications: Adverse reaction to any medication; use of anticoagulants, aspirin, nonsteroidal anti-inflammatory drugs, acetaminophen

Symptoms

- Weakness, fatigue, difficulty with concentration
- Change in sleep–wake pattern
- Anorexia, muscle loss
- Gum bleeding
- Yellow sclera or skin; pruritus; easy bruising
- Dull pain in right upper quadrant or epigastric region
- Erectile dysfunction; amenorrhea

Objective Data

General

Fever, cachexia, muscle wasting

Integumentary

Icteric sclera, jaundice, petechiae, ecchymoses, spider angiomas, palmar erythema, alopecia, clubbing, peripheral edema

Respiratory

Shallow, rapid respirations, epistaxis

Gastrointestinal

Abdominal distension, ascites, distended abdominal wall veins, palpable liver and spleen, foul breath; hematemesis; black, tarry stools; hemorrhoids, fetor hepaticus

Neurological

Confusion, asterixis

Reproductive

Gynecomastia and testicular atrophy (men), erectile dysfunction (men), loss of libido (men and women), amenorrhea or heavy menstrual bleeding (women)

Possible Findings

Anemia, thrombocytopenia; leukopenia; ↓ serum albumin and potassium levels; abnormal liver function studies; ↑ INR and bilirubin levels; abnormal abdominal ultrasonographic appearance

INR, international normalized ratio.

Nursing Diagnoses

Nursing diagnoses for the patient with advanced cirrhosis include, but are not limited to, those presented in Nursing Care Plan 46-2.

Planning

The overall goals are that the patient with advanced cirrhosis will (a) have relief of discomfort, (b) have minimal to no complications (ascites, esophageal varices, hepatic encephalopathy), and (c) maintain as normal a lifestyle as possible.

Nursing Implementation

Health Promotion

The common causes of cirrhosis are alcohol, viral hepatitis, biliary obstruction, and right-sided heart failure. Prevention and early treatment of cirrhosis must focus on eliminating the primary cause. Alcoholism must be treated. Patients should be urged to avoid alcohol ingestion, and their efforts should be supported. Adequate nutrition, especially for those at risk for cirrhosis, is essential to prevent muscle loss. Chronic viral hepatitis must be identified and treated early so that it does not progress to cirrhosis or liver failure. Biliary disease should be treated to avoid biliary obstruction and infection. The underlying cause (e.g., chronic lung disease) of right-sided heart failure must be treated so that the heart failure does not lead to cirrhosis.

Acute Intervention. The focus of nursing care for the patient with advanced cirrhosis is on conserving the patient's energy (see Nursing Care Plan 46-2). Provide rest periods for patients for recovery. Allow patients to engage in activities as tolerated. Modify the activity and rest schedule according to signs of clinical improvement (e.g., decreasing jaundice, improvement in results of liver function studies).

Anorexia, nausea, and vomiting, pressure from ascites, and poor eating habits create problems in maintaining adequate nutrition. Oral hygiene before meals may improve the patient's taste sensation. Between-meal nourishments should be available at times when the patient can best tolerate them. Food preferences should also be available whenever possible. The nurse should explain to the patient and caregivers the reason for any dietary restrictions.

Nursing assessment and care should include the patient's physiological response to cirrhosis. If jaundice is present, where it is observed—sclera, skin, hard palate—should be documented. If the jaundice is accompanied by pruritus, cholestyramine may be ordered to help relieve the pruritus. Other measures to help alleviate pruritus include baking soda baths, lotions containing antihistamines, and calamine. The patient's nails should be kept short and clean.

The colour of the urine and stools should be noted. With jaundice, the urine is often dark brown and foamy when shaken. The stool is grey or tan.

Edema and ascites are frequent manifestations of cirrhosis and necessitate nursing assessment and interventions. Accurate calculation and recordings of intake and output, as well as daily body weight measurements, help in the ongoing assessment of the location and the extent of the edema.

NURSING CARE PLAN 46-2

Advanced Cirrhosis

NURSING DIAGNOSIS	***Imbalanced nutrition: less than body requirements*** *related to* anorexia, impaired use and storage of nutrients, and nausea, *as evidenced by* lack of interest in food, weight loss, and reported inadequate food intake
Expected Patient Outcomes	**Nursing Interventions and *Rationales***
• Maintains adequate intake of nutrients • Maintains normal body weight	• Monitor weight *to evaluate nitrogen balance.* • Provide oral care before meals *to remove foul tastes and improve taste of food.* • Administer antiemetics as ordered *to relieve nausea and prevent vomiting.* • Provide small, frequent meals with nourishing content *to prevent feeling of fullness and to maintain nutritional status.* • Determine patient's food preferences *to increase nutritional appeal because a low-sodium diet may be unpalatable.*
NURSING DIAGNOSIS	***Impaired skin integrity*** *related to* edema, ascites, and pruritus *as evidenced by* complaints of itching; areas of excoriation caused by scratching; taut, shiny skin over edematous areas; and areas of skin breakdown
Expected Patient Outcomes	**Nursing Interventions and *Rationales***
• Maintains of skin integrity • Reports relief of pruritus	• Restrict sodium intake as ordered *to prevent additional fluid retention.* • Restrict fluids, if such restriction is ordered, *to reduce fluid retention.* • Administer prescribed diuretics *to prevent fluid retention and promote diuresis.* • Monitor intake and output *to maintain necessary fluid restrictions and assess kidney function.* • Assess location and extent of edema by weighing patient at the same time each day and taking daily measurements of extremities and of abdominal girth (same location each time) *to determine patient's response to treatment.* • Provide meticulous skin care *to prevent breakdown of edematous tissues.* • Reposition patient at least q2h *to relieve pressure over bony prominences.* • Elevate edematous areas *to promote venous drainage.* • Assess the patient regularly with the Braden Scale *to evaluate the level of risk for pressure ulcer development.* • Provide nail care *to prevent skin excoriation caused by pruritus secondary to deposit of bile salts on skin.* • Administer antipruritic medication as ordered *to relieve itching.* • Provide diversions and distractions *to assist patient in coping with the discomfort of itching and edema.*
NURSING DIAGNOSIS	***Ineffective breathing pattern*** *related to* pressure on diaphragm and reduced lung volume secondary to ascites *as evidenced by* dyspnea, cyanosis, cough, and changes in pulse or respiratory rate, depth, or pattern
Expected Patient Outcomes	**Nursing Interventions and *Rationales***
• Breathes with minimal difficulty • Demonstrates effective breathing pattern • Experiences absence of cyanosis and other signs and symptoms of hypoxia	• Place patient in semi-Fowler's or Fowler's position and support the arms and chest with pillows *to facilitate breathing by relieving pressure on diaphragm.* • Auscultate chest for crackles *to identify collection of fluid in lungs.* • Assess respiratory rate and rhythm *to identify increasing dyspnea.*
NURSING DIAGNOSIS	***Risk for injury*** *related to* diminished sensory perception secondary to peripheral neuropathy
Expected Patient Outcome	**Nursing Interventions and *Rationales***
• Has no injury caused by decreased sensory perception	• Assess for numbness and tingling and decreased sensation in lower extremities *to determine risk for injury.* • Prevent excess stimulation or trauma to extremities *because patient may not be able to detect harmful stimuli.* • Do not use restrictive bed linens *to avoid pressure placed on edematous tissue.* • Instruct patient to avoid tight clothing *to avoid interfering with blood circulation.* • Use heat and cold applications with care *to avoid skin injury because patient's ability to perceive temperature is impaired.* • Assist with ambulation *to assess patient's ability to safely ambulate and to prevent injury.*

NURSING CARE PLAN 46-2

Advanced Cirrhosis—cont'd

NURSING DIAGNOSIS	*Risk for infection related to* increased susceptibility to environmental pathogens *as evidenced by* leukopenia
Expected Patient Outcome	**Nursing Interventions and *Rationales***
• Shows no signs or symptoms of infections	• Use appropriate infection control measures *to avoid infection.*
	• Assess patient for risk factors, including leukopenia, altered immune response, and altered circulation *to ensure early identification of infection.*
	• Monitor patient's temperature every 4 hours *to rule out sepsis.*
	• Observe for any local and systemic manifestations of infection *to enable early diagnosis and treatment.*
	• Protect patient from other people with infections *to reduce the risk of infection secondary to decreased resistance.*
	• Monitor white blood cell count *to assess patient's response to treatment.*

Collaborative Problems

POTENTIAL COMPLICATION	*Hepatic encephalopathy related to* inability of liver to detoxify toxin *as evidenced by* episodes of drowsiness
Nursing Goals	**Nursing Interventions and *Rationales***
• Monitor for signs of hepatic encephalopathy • Report deviation from acceptable parameters • Carry out appropriate medical and nursing interventions	• Monitor for encephalopathy by assessing patient's general behaviour, orientation to time and place, and speech *to detect encephalopathy early and provide prompt treatment.* • Provide laxatives and enemas as ordered *to move toxins out of the body system.* • Watch for signs of infection *to reduce risk of encephalopathy.*
POTENTIAL COMPLICATION	*Hemorrhage related to* bleeding tendency secondary to altered clotting factors and rupture of esophageal or gastric varices
Nursing Goals	**Nursing Interventions and *Rationales***
• Monitor for signs of hemorrhage • Initiate appropriate medical and nursing interventions	• Monitor for hemorrhage by assessing for epistaxis, purpura, petechiae, easy bruising, gingival bleeding, hematuria, and melena *to provide early intervention if any of these are present.* • Provide gentle nursing care *to minimize the risk of tissue trauma.* • Watch for bleeding episodes, including hematuria and melena, *to enable prompt intervention.* • Use smallest-gauge needle possible when giving injections and apply gentle but prolonged pressure after injection *to minimize risk of bleeding into tissue.* • Advise use of soft-bristle toothbrush and avoidance of irritating food *to reduce trauma because mucous membranes have increased risk of injury as a result of high vascularity.* • Teach patient to avoid straining at stool, vigorous blowing of nose, and coughing *to reduce risk of hemorrhage.* • Observe for bruising on the skin *to detect bleeding early and enable prompt intervention or modification of care protocol.* • Monitor laboratory results (hematocrit, hemoglobin, and prothrombin time) *as indicators of anemia, active bleeding, or impending complications.*

When paracentesis is required, the patient should void immediately before the procedure to prevent puncture of the bladder. After the procedure, the nurse should monitor vital signs for hypovolemia and check the dressing for bleeding and leakage from the puncture site.

Dyspnea is a frequent problem for the patient with ascites. A semi-Fowler's or Fowler's position allows for maximal respiratory efficiency. Pillows can be used to support the arms and the chest and may increase the patient's comfort and ability to breathe.

Meticulous skin care is essential because the edematous tissues are prone to breakdown. An alternating–air pressure mattress or other special mattress should be used, if possible. A turning schedule (minimum of every 2 hours) must be adhered to rigidly. The patient's abdomen should be supported with pillows. If the abdomen is taut, cleansing must be done very gently. Patients with ascites tends to move very little because of the abdominal discomfort and dyspnea, so range-of-motion exercises, deep breathing, and coughing exercises are helpful in preventing respiratory problems. The lower extremities may be elevated. If scrotal edema is present, a scrotal support provides some comfort.

When the patient is taking diuretics, the nurse should monitor levels of serum electrolytes, including sodium, potassium, chloride, and bicarbonate. The nurse should observe for signs of fluid and electrolyte imbalance, especially hypokalemia. Hypokalemia may be manifested by cardiac dysrhythmias, hypotension, tachycardia, and generalized muscle weakness. Water excess is manifested by muscle cramping, weakness, lethargy, and confusion.

Observations and nursing care in relation to hematological disorders (bleeding tendencies, anemia, increased susceptibility to infection) are the same as for patients with advanced liver disease (see Nursing Care Plan 46-2).

The nurse must assess the patient's response to altered body image as a result of jaundice, spider angiomas, palmar erythema, ascites, and gynecomastia. The patient may experience a great deal of anxiety regarding these changes. The nurse should explain these phenomena and be a supportive listener. Nursing care with concern and warmth regardless of physical changes helps the patient maintain self-esteem.

Bleeding Esophageal Varices.

If the patient has esophageal or gastric varices, the nurse should observe for signs of bleeding from the varices, such as hematemesis and melena. If hematemesis occurs, the nurse must call the physician and be ready to assist with whatever treatment is used to control the bleeding. The patient may be admitted to the critical care unit. The patient's airway must be maintained.

To stop the bleeding, the physician may perform sclerotherapy or ligation procedures. Balloon tamponade is not used as first-line therapy for bleeding varices. However, it is used in cases of refractory bleeding that is unresponsive to sclerotherapy or ligation. When balloon tamponade is used, the initial nursing task is to explain the use of the tube and how it will be inserted. The balloons should be checked for patency. It is usually the physician's responsibility to insert the tube. It may be inserted via the nose or the mouth (see Figure 46-9). Then the gastric balloon is inflated with approximately 250 mL of air, and the tube is retracted until resistance (gastroesophageal junction) is felt. The tube is secured by placement of a piece of sponge or foam rubber at the nostrils (nasal cuff). For continued bleeding, the esophageal balloon is then inflated. A sphygmomanometer is used to measure and maintain the desired pressure at 20 to 40 mm Hg. The positions of the balloons are verified radiologically.

Nursing care includes monitoring for complications of rupture or erosion of the esophagus, regurgitation and aspiration of gastric contents, and occlusion of the airway by the balloon. If the gastric balloon breaks or is deflated, the esophageal balloon will slip upward, obstructing the airway and causing asphyxiation. If this happens, the nurse must cut the tube or deflate the esophageal balloon; thus scissors should be kept at the patient's bedside. Regurgitation is minimized by oral and pharyngeal suctioning and by keeping the patient in a semi-Fowler's position.

The patient is unable to swallow saliva because the esophagus is occluded by the inflated esophageal balloon. With the Minnesota tube, which has an esophageal aspiration lumen, this problem can be alleviated. The patient should be encouraged to expectorate, and an emesis basin and tissues should be provided. Frequent oral and nasal care provides relief from the taste of blood and irritation from mouth breathing.

Hepatic Encephalopathy.

The focus of nursing care of the patient with hepatic encephalopathy is on maintaining a safe environment, sustaining life, and assisting with measures to reduce episodes of drowsiness. The nurse should assess (a) the patient's level of responsiveness (e.g., reflexes, pupillary reactions, orientation), (b) sensory and motor abnormalities (e.g., hyperreflexia, asterixis, motor coordination), (c) fluid and electrolyte imbalances, (d) acid–base imbalances, and (e) the effect of treatment measures.

Assessment of the neurological status should include an exact description of the patient's behaviour and should be performed at least every 2 hours. The care of the patient with neurological problems is based on the severity of the encephalopathy.

Constipation, which is a common precipitating factor for encephalopathy, should be prevented. Drugs, laxatives, and enemas should be given as ordered. Patients must be instructed to not strain while moving their bowels because this may cause bleeding of hemorrhoidal varices. Any GI bleeding may worsen encephalopathy. Patients who are taking lactulose for diarrhea and excessive fluid and electrolyte losses must be evaluated. It is desirable to have two to three loose bowel movements per day to promote elimination of toxins.

Ambulatory and Home Care

The patient with cirrhosis may be faced with a prolonged course and the possibility of serious, life-threatening problems and complications. The patient and the caregivers need to understand the importance of continuous health care and medical supervision and ways to reduce mortality risk (Table 46-18).

Patients with cirrhosis should receive vaccination for hepatitis A and B, if they are not already immune. Infection with these viruses in patients with cirrhosis can lead to fulminant hepatitis. Patients should avoid aspirin, NSAIDs, and aminoglycosides, which can cause bleeding, edema, and renal complications. Patients should also avoid sleeping pills or sedatives that contain codeine because they can lead to encephalopathy. Total abstinence from alcohol is mandatory. A low-sodium diet should be followed at home. Patients with cirrhosis have higher risks for

---

PATIENT & CAREGIVER TEACHING GUIDE

Table 46-18 Cirrhosis in Ambulatory and Home Care Setting

1. Explain the importance of continuous medical care with the goal to prolong survival and to avoid disease complications.

2. Teach patients and caregivers the symptoms of complications (e.g., black stools, confusion) and when to seek medical attention to enable prompt treatment of complications.

3. Teach about the importance of a low-sodium diet and how to make food more palatable by using herbs and spices.

4. Teach patients to avoid certain drugs:
   - Aspirin: increases risk of bleeding
   - NSAIDs: increase risk of bleeding, edema
   - Aspirin, NSAIDs, aminoglycoside: increase risk of renal impairment
   - ACE inhibitors: cause fluid retention
   - Sleeping pills/sedatives/cough syrups that contain narcotics: may cause confusion

5. Encourage complete abstinence from alcohol because alcohol can further injure the liver.

6. Teach patients to seek medical attention promptly for any type of infections to avoid complications.

7. Teach patients to avoid heavy lifting (e.g., Valsalva manoeuvre), which increases portal pressure and heightens risk of hemorrhage.

8. Encourage patients to receive hepatitis A and B vaccine, if the patient is not immune, to prevent risk of fulminant hepatitis when exposed to these viruses.

9. Ensure that patients undergo ultrasound surveillance every 6 months for early detection of liver cancer.

ACE, angiotensin-converting enzyme; *NSAID,* nonsteroidal anti-inflammatory drug.

infection and surgical complications, and so any infections must be promptly treated, and surgical procedures that necessitate general anaesthesia must first be discussed with the liver specialist. Patients with cirrhosis are at high risk for hepatocellular carcinoma. The current recommendation is hepatoma surveillance with abdominal ultrasonography every 6 months. Hepatocellular carcinoma, when small, is curable.

Cirrhosis is a chronic disorder. The patient is affected not only physically but also psychologically, socially, and economically. Major lifestyle changes may be required, especially if alcohol abuse is the primary cause. The nurse should provide information regarding community support programs, such as Alcoholics Anonymous, for help with alcohol abuse. Other health teaching should include information about early signs of disease decompensation such as black stools and abdominal swelling. Counselling information regarding sexual problems may be needed. The emphasis of home care for patients with cirrhosis should focus on helping patients maintain the highest level of wellness possible and initiate and maintain necessary lifestyle changes.

▪ Evaluation

Expected outcomes for the patient with advanced cirrhosis are addressed in Nursing Care Plan 46-2.

Fulminant Hepatic Failure

Fulminant hepatic failure, or *acute liver failure,* is a clinical syndrome characterized by severe impairment of liver function in association with hepatic encephalopathy. The most common cause is drugs, usually acetaminophen in combination with alcohol. People who abuse alcohol are particularly susceptible to detrimental effects of acetaminophen on the liver. Other drugs that can cause fulminant hepatitis include isoniazid, halothane, sulpha-containing drugs, and NSAIDs. Drugs can cause liver cell failure by disrupting essential intracellular processes or causing an accumulation of toxic metabolic products.

Hepatitis viruses, particularly HBV, are the second most common cause of fulminant hepatic failure. Hepatic failure may also occur with HAV infection and less frequently with HCV infection. Mushroom poisoning is also associated with fulminant liver failure. The majority of mushroom poisonings occur with *Amanita phalloides* (also known as "death cap").

Fulminant hepatic failure is characterized by the rapid onset of severe liver dysfunction in someone with no history of liver disease. In general, the disease runs its course over 8 weeks, but it can last as long as 26 weeks. Depending on the cause, survival rates range from 10 to 40% with intensive support.

Clinical Manifestations and Diagnostic Studies

Manifestations include jaundice, coagulation abnormalities, and encephalopathy. In acute liver failure, changes in mentation are the first clinical sign. Patients with acute liver failure are susceptible to a wide variety of complications. These include cerebral edema, renal failure, hypoglycemia, metabolic acidosis, sepsis, and multiorgan failure.

Fulminant hepatic failure is identified in most patients by abnormalities in laboratory values and clinical manifestations

resulting from hepatic necrosis and fibrosis. Most often, serum bilirubin levels are elevated and the prothrombin time is prolonged. Liver enzyme levels (AST, ALT) are often markedly elevated. Additional laboratory tests include blood chemistry evaluation (especially glucose because hypoglycemia may be present and require correction); complete blood cell counts; screening for acetaminophen and other drugs and toxins; viral hepatitis serological testing (especially for HAV and HBV); and measurements of serum ceruloplasmin (enzyme synthesized in liver) levels, α_1-antitrypsin levels, iron levels, and autoantibodies (antinuclear and anti–smooth muscle antibodies). Plasma ammonia levels may also be measured.

Liver biopsy, most often performed via the transjugular route because of coagulopathy, may be indicated when conditions such as autoimmune hepatitis, metastatic liver disease, and lymphoma are suspected. In addition, ultrasonography, CT, or magnetic resonance imaging (MRI) is helpful in providing information about the liver size and contour, presence of ascites, presence of tumours, and patency of the blood vessels.

Collaborative Care

Because fulminant hepatic failure may progress rapidly, with hour-by-hour changes in consciousness, early transfer to the critical care unit is preferred once the diagnosis is made. Planning for transfer to a transplantation centre should begin in patients with grade 1 or 2 encephalopathy because the condition may worsen rapidly. Early transfer is important because the risks involved with patient transport may increase or even preclude transfer once stage 3 or 4 encephalopathy develops (see Table 46-14).

Acute and chronic renal failure is a frequent complication in patients with liver failure and may be caused by dehydration, hepatorenal syndrome, or acute tubular necrosis. The frequency of renal failure may be even greater with acetaminophen overdose or other toxins, in which direct renal toxicity occurs. Although few patients die of renal failure alone, it often contributes to mortality risk and may imply a poorer prognosis.

The nurse should protect a patient's renal function by maintaining adequate hemodynamics, withholding nephrotoxic agents (e.g., aminoglycosides, NSAIDs), and promptly identifying and treating infection. Liver transplantation is the treatment of choice for fulminant liver failure. Liver transplantation increases length of survival in 50 to 85% of patients with acute liver failure. Cerebral edema, cerebellar herniation, and brainstem compression are the most common causes of death. Treatment of cerebral edema is described in Chapter 59.

NURSING MANAGEMENT: FULMINANT HEPATIC FAILURE

The nurse checks a patient's mental status frequently if the level of consciousness declines. To minimize agitation, the patient's environment should be kept quiet. Additional measures include padding bedrails to avoid injury from possible seizures, close observation to avoid injuries, monitoring of intake and output for renal function, and providing good skin and oral care to avoid breakdown and infection.

Monitoring and management of hemodynamic and renal parameters, glucose levels, electrolyte levels, and acid–base status are critical. The nurse should conduct frequent neurological evaluations for signs of elevated intracranial pressure. The patient should be positioned with the head elevated at 30 degrees. Stimulation of the patient should be avoided. Manoeuvres that cause straining, or Valsalva-like movements, may increase intracranial pressure. It may be advisable to use endotracheal lidocaine before endotracheal suctioning. The use of any sedatives should be avoided because of their effects on mental status. Only minimal doses of benzodiazepines should be administered because of their delayed metabolism by the failing liver. Intracranial pressure should be maintained below 20 to 25 mm Hg if possible; cerebral perfusion pressure should be maintained above 50 to 60 mm Hg. Support of systemic blood pressure may be necessary to maintain adequate cerebral perfusion pressure.

Liver Cancer

Hepatocellular carcinoma (HCC), the primary liver cancer, is the third most common cancer in the world. It is also the fifth most common cause of cancer-related death in men and the seventh in women (Sherman, Burak, et al., 2011). The Multidisciplinary Canadian Consensus for the Management and Treatment of Hepatocellular Carcinoma reported the incidence rate among men 40 to 84 years old was 15.4 per 100,000 in the years 2006 to 2010 (Sherman, Burak, et al., 2011). The incidence rate for women is lower but has also shown an increasing trend (Sherman, Burak, et al., 2011). HCC is four to eight times more common in men than in women.

Unlike other cancers, risk factors for HCC have been identified and well described. About 80 to 90% of people with hepatocellular carcinoma have cirrhosis of the liver. Cirrhosis is therefore a major risk factor regardless of the cause of cirrhosis. In North America, chronic HCV infection is the major underlying cause. Among those with chronic HBV infection, the risk of HCC is further increased if they are male, are older, have a family history of HCC, or are infected with HBV genotype C. Alcoholic cirrhosis and nonalcoholic fatty liver disease are also well established risk factors for HCC although to a lesser extent than HBV and HCV infections.

In liver cancer, hemorrhage and necrosis in the liver are common. Single or multiple tumours can occur; they can be well defined or diffusely spread over the entire liver. Some tumours infiltrate other organs, such as the gallbladder, or other structures, such as the peritoneum or the diaphragm. (Primary liver tumours commonly metastasize to the lungs). The liver is a common site of metastatic growth because of its high rate of blood flow and extensive capillary network. Cancer cells in other parts of the body are commonly carried to the liver via the portal circulation (Figure 46-12).

Clinical Manifestations and Diagnostic Studies

Liver cancers usually produce no symptoms until they become very large. Diagnosing small liver cancers in the presence of cirrhosis is sometimes a challenge when the liver is nodular and severely scarred. Clinical manifestations in later stages of cancer include weight loss, epigastric or right upper quadrant pain, anorexia, nausea and vomiting, weakness, and jaundice. More severe clinical symptoms such as ascites, peripheral edema, encephalopathy, and variceal bleeding occur in the setting of decompensated liver disease. A hemorrhagic tumour can

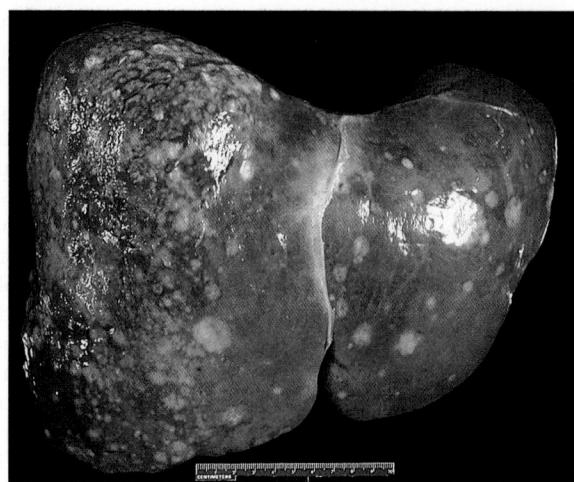

Figure 46-12 Multiple hepatic metastases from a primary colon cancer.

Source: From Kumar, V., Abbas, A. K., & Fausto, N. (2005). *Robbins and Cotran pathologic basis of disease* (7th ed.). Philadelphia: W. B. Saunders.

cause blood clots to form, leading to pulmonary emboli as a complication.

Liver cancer is diagnosed increasingly with the use of imaging tests that include ultrasonography, CT, and MRI. The test for α-fetoprotein may yield positive results in hepatocellular carcinoma. α-Fetoprotein levels are elevated in approximately 60% of patients with hepatocellular carcinoma (Sherman, Burak, et al., 2011), and this finding helps distinguish primary cancer from metastatic cancer. (α-Fetoprotein is discussed in Chapter 18.)

NURSING AND COLLABORATIVE MANAGEMENT: LIVER CANCER

Treatment of liver cancer depends on the size and number of tumours, presence of spread beyond of the liver, and the age and overall health of the patient. Surgical resection (partial hepatectomy) is performed when there is no evidence of portal hypertension, when liver function is normal, and in the absence of invasion of hepatic blood vessels. Hepatectomy offers the best chance for cure of liver cancer. Liver transplantation is performed when the tumour is localized with underlying liver disease.

Other treatment options commonly used are radiofrequency ablation, chemoembolization, and chemotherapies (El-Serag, Marrero, & Rudolph, 2008). *Radiofrequency ablation* has become the most frequently used modality for treating tumours that are less than 2 to 3 cm in diameter. The overall survival rates are 100% and 98% at 1 and 2 years, but the 5-year recurrence rates are as high as 70% (El-Serag, 2011). In radiofrequency ablation, a thin needle is inserted into the core of the tumour. Electrical energy is then used to create heat in a specific location for a limited amount of time. The end result is destruction of tumour cells. Complications can include infection, bleeding, dysrhythmias, and skin burn; however, they are not common.

Chemoembolization (sometimes called *transarterial chemoembolization*) is a minimally invasive procedure performed in the interventional radiology department. A catheter is placed in the arteries to the tumour, and an embolic agent is administered, often mixed with one or more chemotherapeutic agents. The embolic agent reduces the blood supply to the tumour, thus allowing greater exposure of liver cells to the chemotherapy drugs. A postembolization syndrome of fever and abdominal pain related to liver ischemia occurs in up to 50% of patients receiving chemoembolization.

Chemotherapy is used for patients with liver cancer who are not likely to benefit from other procedures; it is mostly palliative. Sorafenib (Nexavar) is a targeted therapy, approved in Canada in 2006 for treating HCC. Sorafenib is administered orally and works by inhibiting cancer cell growth. It has many adverse effects (including rash on the hands and feet, diarrhea, and fatigue) and is often not well tolerated by patients. It can prolong survival by only 2 to 3 months.

Nursing intervention for patients with liver cancer focuses on keeping patients as comfortable as possible. (See Chapter 18 for care of patients with cancer.) The prognosis for patients with liver cancer depends on how early the tumour is detected. Therefore, nurses play a very important role in health promotion and health teaching for prevention of HCC. HBV vaccination for people at high risk for HBV infection can drastically reduce the occurrence of liver cancer. Treatment for chronic hepatitis B and C disease, if given early before the establishment of cirrhosis, helps decrease risk for liver cancer. For patients with established cirrhosis, cancer surveillance with ultrasonography every 6 months is beneficial, inasmuch as small cancers are potentially curable.

Liver Transplantation

The first human liver transplantation was performed in 1963 at the University of Colorado by Thomas Starzl. Canada's first liver transplantation was performed in Montreal in 1970. In 2010, 2153 organ transplantations were performed in Canada; of those, 443 were liver transplantations (Canadian Institute for Health Information, 2010), half of which were for hepatitis C–related liver disease. Canada has one of the lowest organ donation rates among industrialized nations: only 14 donors per 1 million people, in comparison with 34 per 1 million in Spain (London Health Sciences Centre, 2012).

Liver transplantation has become a therapeutic option and an accepted treatment modality for many people with end-stage liver disease. It improves overall health and affects quality of life. Among recipients, 1-year survival rates are 85 to 95%, and 5-year survival rates are 75% (Haque et al., 2010). Indications for liver transplantation include end-stage liver disease from many different underlying causes, HCC, and fulminant hepatic failure. On occasion, other disease conditions that do not result in liver failure but may be cured by liver transplantation (e.g., familial amyloidosis polyneuropathy) are treated this way.

Liver transplantation is contraindicated in patients with widespread malignant disease. Potential candidates for transplantation undergo numerous diagnostic tests and a thorough assessment by a multidisciplinary team to evaluate the extent of other comorbid conditions. This review ensures that recipients have adequate social supports and are healthy enough to withstand the process of transplantation.

The major postoperative complications are rejection and infection. Rejection is the most feared but the most easily treated complication. It often necessitates only adjustment of immunosuppressive drug dosages. Cyclosporine, the initial immunosuppressant drug, improved the rates of success of liver transplantation. Tacrolimus is currently the first-line immuno-suppressive drug in most programs. Both these drugs are calcineurin inhibitors. The mechanism of action and adverse effects of cyclosporine are discussed in Chapter 16 and Table 16-15. Other immunosuppressants used include mycophenolate mofetil (Cellcept, Myfortic), azathioprine (Imuran), corticosteroids, and sirolimus (Rapamune; see Chapter 16, Table 16-15). The interleukin-2 receptor antagonist basiliximab (Simulect) and polyclonal antilymphocyte antibodies, such as thymoglobulin, may be administered to patients at high risk for complications.

Immunosuppressive drugs have allowed for great success in transplantation; however, they produce a host of adverse effects, including hypertension, hyperlipidemia, renal impairment, and diabetes. (See the Interdisciplinary Research box "Adverse Effects of Immunosuppressive Drugs.") Other factors in the improved success rate are advances in surgical techniques, including options such as living donor liver transplantation, and improved management of the underlying liver disease and complications of cirrhosis before surgery.

INTERDISCIPLINARY RESEARCH
Adverse Effects of Immunosuppressive Drugs

Citation
Doebbel, F., Moons, P., Abraham, I., Larsen, C. P., Du Pont, L., & de Geest, S. (2008). Measuring symptom experience of side-effects of immunosuppressive drugs: The Modified Transplant Symptom Occurrence and Distress Scale. *Transplant International*. doi: 10.1111/j.1432-2277.2008.00674.x

Purpose
This study was conducted to update and validate the Modified Transplant Symptom Occurrence and Symptom Distress Scale (MTSOSD) for novel immunosuppressive regimens.

Methods
This study comprised four steps: (a) literature review to identify immunosuppressant-related symptoms; (b) screening of adverse event forms; (c) international experts' evaluation of the appropriateness of each symptom; and (d) a pilot study in 24 renal transplant recipients to test the clarity of instructions and items and a pilot study in 84 lung transplant recipients to determine content and discriminant validity. The instrument was modified and adapted to create a new version of the scale, the MTSOSD-59R.

Results and Conclusions
This study established the content and discriminant validity of the new instrument, the MTSOSD-59R. The revised instrument proved easy to complete, had understandable items and instructions, and demonstrated good discrimination between male and female patients and between depressed and nondepressed patients.

Implications for Nursing Practice
Measurement of patients' subjective experience of the adverse effects of immunosuppressants is a critical post-transplantation outcome. Measuring the patient's symptom experience allows nurses to identify patients with high levels of symptom distress and those at risk for nonadherence to the treatment regimen, so that appropriate interventions can be instituted.

Almost all liver diseases may recur. Because of the development of effective antiviral agents for the management of HBV infection and the concurrent use of hepatitis B immune globulin, HBV reinfection is rare. Hepatitis C recurrence, as evidenced by histological damage, is almost universal after transplantation in HCV-viremic patients. Approximately 20 to 30% of such patients develop cirrhosis in the transplanted liver by the fifth year after transplantation (Burton, Sonnenberg, & Rosen, 2004). Antiviral therapy for HCV initiated after transplantation—even before the development of histological evidence of recurrence—is aimed at altering this trend (Berenguer et al., 2006). Overall, liver transplantation provides good long-term survival.

The patient who has undergone liver transplantation requires competent and highly skilled nursing care, either in an ICU or in a dedicated transplantation unit. Postoperative nursing care includes assessing neurological status; monitoring for signs of hemorrhage; preventing pulmonary complications; monitoring for drainage, electrolyte levels, and urinary output; and monitoring for signs and symptoms of infection and rejection. Common respiratory problems are pneumonia, atelectasis, and pleural effusions.

Measures such as coughing, deep breathing, incentive spirometry, and repositioning are needed to prevent complications. Drainage from the Jackson-Pratt drain, the nasogastric tube, and the T-tube should be measured, and the colour and the consistency of drainage noted.

A critical aspect of nursing care after liver transplantation is monitoring for infection because this is the most common cause of mortality and morbidity. Infections can be viral, fungal, or bacterial. Nutrition, physiotherapy, and patient education focused on medication regimens, signs and symptoms of infection, and lifestyle practices are all key to lifelong success in transplant recipients. Emotional support for the patient and family is also essential for successful transplantation outcomes.

AGE-RELATED CONSIDERATIONS: LIVER DISEASE IN OLDER PATIENTS

The incidence of liver disease increases with age. With aging, liver volume decreases, drug metabolism slows, and hepatobiliary function is altered. The ability of the liver to respond to injury, particularly to regenerate after injury, is also decreased (Premoli et al., 2009). Transplanted livers take longer to regenerate in older adults than in younger adults.

Older patients are particularly vulnerable to drug-induced hepatitis. This is a result of several factors, including decline in body weight, and increased use of prescription and over-the-counter drugs, which can lead to drug interactions and potential drug toxicity. Age-related decreases in liver function caused by decreased liver blood flow and enzyme activity result in decreased drug metabolism. In addition, with aging, the liver's ability to recover from drug-induced injury is reduced.

A growing number of older adults have chronic hepatitis C and subsequent cirrhosis. The presence of HCV and elevated liver enzyme levels are often found during a routine health assessment. Drug therapy for HCV has been shown to be less effective in older adults. Because older adults have more comorbid conditions, liver transplantation for liver failure may not be an option. The older adult undergoing hemodialysis is at risk for exposure to both HCV and HBV.

Lifetime health behaviours may also influence the development of chronic liver disease in the older adult. Chronic alcohol abuse and obesity can contribute to alcoholic cirrhosis, NASH, and subsequent liver failure. Because of comorbid cardiovascular and pulmonary diseases, older adults are less able to tolerate variceal bleeding. In older adults with liver disease, hepatic encephalopathy may be misdiagnosed as dementia.

Disorders of the Pancreas

Acute Pancreatitis

Acute pancreatitis is an acute inflammatory process of the pancreas. The degree of inflammation varies from mild edema to severe hemorrhagic necrosis. Acute pancreatitis is most common in middle-aged men and women. The severity of the disease varies according to the extent of pancreatic destruction. Some patients recover completely, others have recurring attacks, and chronic pancreatitis develops in others. Acute pancreatitis can be life-threatening.

Etiology and Pathophysiology

Many factors can cause injury to the pancreas. In Canada, the most common cause is alcoholism, followed by gallbladder disease (gallstones). Acute pancreatitis attacks are also associated with hypertriglyceridemia (serum triglyceride level >11 mmol/L). Less common causes include trauma (postsurgical, abdominal), viral infections (mumps, coxsackievirus), penetrating duodenal ulcer, cysts, abscesses, cystic fibrosis, certain drugs (azathioprine, corticosteroids, thiazides, estrogens, sulphonamides, HIV medications, anti-inflammatory drugs), metabolic disorders (hyperparathyroidism, renal failure), and vascular disease. Pancreatitis may occur after surgical procedures on the pancreas, the stomach, the duodenum, or the biliary tract. Pancreatitis can also occur after endoscopic retrograde cholangiopancreatography (ERCP). In some cases, the cause is unknown (idiopathic).

The most common pathogenic mechanism is believed to be autodigestion of the pancreas (Figure 46-13). Injury to pancreatic cells or activation of the pancreatic enzymes is caused in the pancreas rather than in the intestine. It is not clear how the activation of pancreatic enzymes occurs. One possible cause is believed to be the reflux of bile acids into the pancreatic ducts through an open or distended sphincter of Oddi. This reflux may result from blockage created by gallstones. Obstruction of a pancreatic duct results in pancreatic ischemia.

Trypsinogen is an inactive proteolytic enzyme produced by the pancreas. Normally, it is released into the small intestine via the pancreatic duct. In the intestine, it is activated to trypsin by enterokinase. Normally, trypsin inhibitors in the pancreas and the plasma bind and inactivate any trypsin that is inadvertently produced. In pancreatitis, activated trypsin is present in the pancreas. This enzyme can digest the pancreas and can activate other proteolytic enzymes such as elastase and phospholipase A.

Elastase and phospholipase A play a major role in autodigestion of the pancreas. Elastase causes hemorrhage by producing dissolution of the elastic fibres of blood vessels. Phospholipase A is probably activated by trypsin and bile acids and causes fat necrosis.

PATHOPHYSIOLOGY MAP

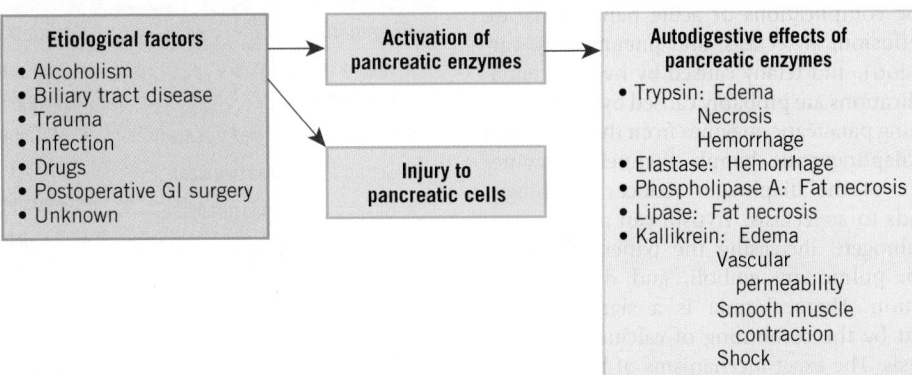

Figure 46-13 Pathogenic process of acute pancreatitis. *GI*, gastrointestinal.

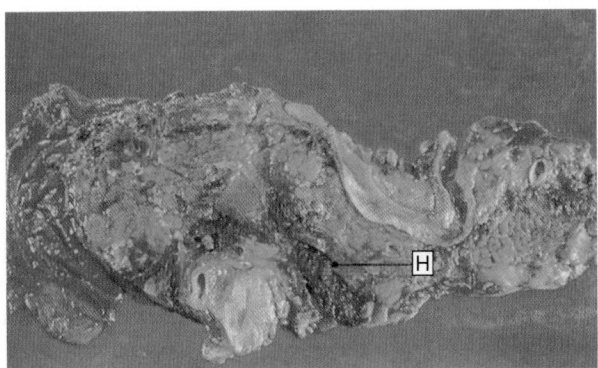

Figure 46-14 In acute pancreatitis, the pancreas appears edematous and is commonly hemorrhagic *(H)*.

Source: From Stevens, A., & Lowe, J. (2000). *Pathology: Illustrated review in colour* (2nd ed.). London: Mosby.

It is not entirely clear how chronic alcohol use causes acute pancreatitis. It is thought that alcohol increases the production of digestive enzymes in the pancreas. However, because only 5 to 10% of people who abuse alcohol develop pancreatitis, other factors such as environment (high-fat diet, smoking) and genetics may also contribute to the cause.

The pathophysiological involvement of acute pancreatitis ranges from mild (*edematous* or *interstitial pancreatitis*) to severe (*necrotizing pancreatitis;* Figure 46-14). In patients with mild pancreatitis, the functions of the gland return to normal upon recovery. In approximately half of the patients with severe pancreatitis, endocrine and exocrine function decrease permanently. Such patients are also at risk of developing pancreatic necrosis, organ failure, and septic complications, which results in a 25% mortality rate (Lindberg, 2009).

Clinical Manifestations

Abdominal pain is the predominant symptom of acute pancreatitis. The pain is usually located in the left upper quadrant, but it may be in the midepigastrium. It commonly radiates to the back because of the retroperitoneal location of the pancreas. The pain has a sudden onset and is described as severe, deep, piercing, and continuous or steady. It is aggravated by eating, and it frequently occurs when the patient is recumbent; it is not relieved by vomiting. The pain may be accompanied by flushing, cyanosis, and dyspnea. The patient may assume various positions involving flexion of the spine in an attempt to relieve the severe pain. The pain is caused by distension of the pancreas, peritoneal irritation, and obstruction of the biliary tract.

Other manifestations of acute pancreatitis include nausea and vomiting, low-grade fever, leukocytosis, hypotension, tachycardia, and jaundice. Abdominal tenderness with muscle guarding is common. Bowel sounds may be decreased or absent. Ileus may occur and causes marked abdominal distension. The lungs are frequently involved, with crackles present. Intravascular damage from circulating trypsin may cause areas of cyanosis or greenish to yellow-brown discoloration of the abdominal wall. Other areas of ecchymoses are the flanks (*Grey Turner's spots* or *sign,* a bluish flank discoloration) and the periumbilical area (*Cullen's sign,* a bluish periumbilical discoloration). These ecchymoses result from seepage of blood-stained exudate from the pancreas and may occur in severe cases.

Shock may occur as a result of hemorrhage into the pancreas, toxemia from the activated pancreatic enzymes, or hypovolemia as a result of massive shift of exudates of blood and plasma proteins into the retroperitoneal space.

Complications

Two significant local complications of acute pancreatitis are pseudocyst and abscess. A pancreatic **pseudocyst** is a cavity continuous with or surrounding the outside of the pancreas. The pseudocyst is filled with necrotic products and liquid secretions, such as plasma, pancreatic enzymes, and inflammatory exudates. As pancreatic enzymes escape from the pseudocyst, the serosal surfaces next to the pancreas become inflamed; granulation tissue subsequently forms, encapsulating the exudate. Manifestations of pseudocyst are abdominal pain, palpable epigastric mass, nausea, vomiting, and anorexia. The serum amylase level frequently remains elevated. These cysts usually resolve spontaneously within a few weeks, but they may perforate, causing peritonitis, or they may rupture into the stomach or duodenum. Treatment consists of an internal drainage procedure with an anastomosis between the pancreatic duct and the jejunum.

A pancreatic abscess is a large fluid-containing cavity within the pancreas. It results from extensive necrosis in the pancreas. It may become infected or perforate into adjacent organs. Manifestations of an abscess include upper abdominal pain, abdominal mass, high fever, and leukocytosis. Pancreatic abscesses must be surgically drained promptly to prevent sepsis.

The main systemic complications of acute pancreatitis are pulmonary (pleural effusion, atelectasis, and pneumonia), cardiovascular (hypotension), and tetany caused by hypocalcemia. The pulmonary complications are probably caused by the passage of the exudate containing pancreatic enzymes from the peritoneal cavity through transdiaphragmatic lymph channels. Enzyme-induced inflammation of the diaphragm reduces diaphragm movement, which leads to atelectasis. Trypsin can activate prothrombin and plasminogen, increasing the patient's risk for intravascular thrombi, pulmonary emboli, and disseminated intravascular coagulation. Hypocalcemia is a sign of severe disease, caused in part by the combining of calcium and fatty acids during fat necrosis. The exact mechanisms of how or why hypocalcemia occurs are not well understood.

Diagnostic Studies

The primary diagnostic tests for acute pancreatitis are measurements of serum amylase and lipase. The serum amylase level is usually elevated early and remains so for 24 to 72 hours. The serum lipase level is also elevated and is important for differentiating acute pancreatitis from other disorders such as mumps and cerebral trauma. Other abnormal findings include an increase in liver enzyme, triglyceride, glucose, and bilirubin levels and a decrease in calcium level.

The urinary amylase level from a 24-hour collection may be increased to more than 5000 IU. Urinary trypsinogen-2 measurement is a better screening test than amylase.

Abdominal ultrasonography, radiography, or CT can be used to identify pancreatic problems. CT with IV contrast material is the best imaging for confirming a diagnosis of pancreatitis. Magnetic resonance cholangiopancreatography (MRCP) is superior to CT for detecting complications and related complications such as pseudocysts and abscesses and does not require the use of IV contrast material. It often replaces the use of ERCP, which itself can cause acute pancreatitis.

Collaborative Care

Objectives of collaborative care for acute pancreatitis include (a) relief of pain; (b) prevention or alleviation of shock; (c) reduction of pancreatic secretions; (d) control of fluid and electrolyte imbalance; (e) prevention or treatment of infections; and (f) removal of the precipitating cause, if possible (Table 46-19).

Conservative Therapy. Treatment is focused principally on supportive care, including aggressive hydration, pain management, management of metabolic complications, and minimization of pancreatic stimulation. A primary consideration in the treatment of acute pancreatitis is the relief and control of pain. IV morphine may be administered. Pain medications may be combined with an antispasmodic. However, atropine-like drugs should be avoided when paralytic ileus is present because they may contribute to the problem. Other medications that relax smooth muscles (spasmolytics), such as nitroglycerin or papaverine, may be administered.

If shock is present, plasma or plasma volume expanders such as dextran or albumin may be given. Fluid and electrolyte imbalances are corrected with lactated Ringer's solution. Central venous pressure readings may be used to assist in determining requirements for fluid replacement. Vasoactive drugs such as dopamine

COLLABORATIVE CARE

Table 46-19 Acute Pancreatitis

Diagnostic	Collaborative Therapy
• History and physical examination	• Pain medication (e.g., morphine)
• Serum amylase measurement	• NPO status with NG tube to suction
• Serum lipase measurement	• Albumin (if shock is present)
• Blood glucose measurement	• IV calcium gluconate, 10% (if tetany is present)
• Serum calcium measurement	
• Triglyceride measurement	• Lactated Ringer's solution
• Flat-plate radiography of the abdomen	• Histamine blockers, proton pump inhibitors
• Abdominal ultrasonography	• Antibiotics (if necrotizing pancreatitis is present)
• Endoscopic ultrasonography	
• Contrast medium–enhanced CT	
• MRCP	
• ERCP	
• Chest radiography	

CT, computed tomography; *ERCP*, endoscopic retrograde cholangiopancreatography; *IV*, intravenous; *MRCP*, magnetic resonance cholangiopancreatography; *NG*, nasogastric; *NPO*, nothing by mouth.

may be administered to increase systemic vascular resistance in patients with ongoing hypotension.

Pancreatic enzyme secretion must be reduced or suppressed in order to decrease stimulation of the pancreas and allow it to rest. Suppression of pancreatic secretion is accomplished by keeping the patient on nothing-by-mouth (NPO) status and by using NG suction to reduce vomiting and gastric distension and to prevent gastric acidic contents from entering the duodenum. Certain drugs may also be administered for this purpose (Table 46-20). The inflamed and necrotic pancreatic tissue is a good medium for bacterial growth; therefore, it is important to prevent infections. The prophylactic use of antibiotics is somewhat controversial. The patient should be monitored closely so that antibiotic therapy can be instituted early if infection occurs.

Surgical Therapy. When the acute pancreatitis is related to the presence of gallstones, urgent ERCP and endoscopic sphincterotomy may be performed and followed by laparoscopic cholecystectomy to reduce the potential for recurrence. Surgical intervention may also be indicated when the diagnosis is uncertain and in patients who do not respond to conservative therapy. Patients with severe acute pancreatitis may require drainage of necrotic fluid collections. This can be accomplished either surgically, under guidance by CT, or endoscopically. A pseudocyst can be drained percutaneously, and a drainage tube is left in place.

Drug Therapy. Several different drugs may be used in the treatment of both acute and chronic pancreatitis (see Table 46-20). A number of drugs are administered in an effort to suppress pancreatic secretion, but these drugs have not proved effective in the management of pancreatitis.

Nutritional Therapy. Initially, patients with acute pancreatitis are kept on NPO status to reduce pancreatic secretion. When food is allowed, small, frequent feedings are given. The diet is usually high in carbohydrate content because that is the least

DRUG THERAPY

Table 46-20 Acute and Chronic Pancreatitis

DRUG	MECHANISM OF ACTION OR RATIONALE
Acute Pancreatitis	
Morphine, meperidine (Demerol)	Relief of pain
Nitroglycerin or papaverine	Relaxation of smooth-muscles and relief of pain
Antispasmodics (e.g., dicyclomine [Bentylol]*	Decrease of vagal stimulation, motility, and pancreatic outflow (through inhibition of volume and concentration of bicarbonate and enzymatic secretion)
Carbonic anhydrase inhibitor (acetazolamide [Diamox])	Reduction in volume and bicarbonate concentration of pancreatic secretion
Antacids	Neutralization of gastric HCl secretion and subsequent decrease in secretin, which stimulates production and secretion of pancreatic secretions
Histamine H$_2$-receptor antagonists (cimetidine [Tagamet], ranitidine [Zantac]); proton pump inhibitors (omeprazole [Prevacid])	Decrease in HCl secretion (HCl stimulates pancreatic activity)
Chronic Pancreatitis	
Pancreatin (Viokase), pancrelipase (Cotazym)	Replacement therapy for pancreatic enzymes
Insulin	Treatment for diabetes mellitus, if it occurs, or for hyperglycemia

*Contraindicated in patients with paralytic ileus.
HCl, hydrochloric acid.

stimulating to the exocrine portion of the pancreas. Intolerance to oral foods should be suspected if a patient reports pain, has increasing abdominal girth, or has elevated amylase and lipase levels. The patient needs to abstain from alcohol. Supplemental fat-soluble vitamins may be administered. Depending on the severity of the pancreatitis, the patient may require enteral feeding via nasojejunal tube. Because of infection risk, parenteral nutrition is reserved for patients who cannot tolerate enteral nutrition (see Chapter 42).

NURSING MANAGEMENT: ACUTE PANCREATITIS

▮ Nursing Assessment

Subjective and objective data that should be obtained from a person with acute pancreatitis are presented in Table 46-21.

▮ Nursing Diagnoses

Nursing diagnoses for patients with acute pancreatitis may include, but are not limited to, those presented in eNCP 46-1, available on the Evolve Web site for this chapter.

NURSING ASSESSMENT

Table 46-21 Acute Pancreatitis

Subjective Data

Important Health Information

Past health history: Biliary tract disease, alcohol use, abdominal trauma, duodenal ulcers, infection, metabolic disorders

Medications: Thiazides, immunosuppressive agents, anti-inflammatory drugs

Surgery or other treatments: Surgical procedures on the pancreas, stomach, duodenum, or biliary tract; ERCP

Symptoms

- Weakness or lassitude
- Nausea, vomiting, or both; anorexia
- Dyspnea
- Severe abdominal pain that may radiate to the back and is aggravated by food and or alcohol

Objective Data

General

Restlessness, anxiety, low-grade fever

Integumentary

Flushing, diaphoresis, discoloration of abdomen and flanks, cyanosis, jaundice; decreased skin turgor; dry mucous membranes

Respiratory

Tachypnea, basilar crackles

Cardiovascular

Tachycardia, hypotension

Gastrointestinal

Abdominal distension, tenderness, and muscle guarding; diminished bowel sounds

Possible Findings

↑ Serum amylase and lipase levels, leukocytosis, hyperglycemia, ↑ urine amylase level, dyslipidemia, hypocalcemia, abnormal findings on ultrasonography and CT of pancreas, abnormal findings on ERCP

CT, computed tomography; *ERCP,* endoscopic retrograde cholangiopancreatography.

▮ Planning

The overall goals are that patients with acute pancreatitis will have (a) relief of pain, (b) normal fluid and electrolyte balance, (c) minimal to no complications, and (d) no recurrent attacks.

▮ Nursing Implementation

▮ Health Promotion

Health promotion is focused on the assessment of the predisposing and etiological factors of pancreatitis and on encouragement of early intervention to prevent occurrence of acute pancreatitis. The nurse should promote the early diagnosis and treatment of biliary tract disease, such as cholelithiasis. The patient should be advised to eliminate alcohol intake, especially if there have been any previous episodes of pancreatitis. Attacks of pancreatitis become milder or disappear when alcohol use is discontinued.

■ Acute Intervention

During the acute phase, it is important to monitor vital signs. Hemodynamic stability may be compromised by hypotension, fever, and tachypnea, which may result in fluid volume deficit. IV fluids are ordered, and the response to therapy is monitored. A vital part of the nursing care plan for this patient is monitoring for electrolyte imbalances. Frequent vomiting, along with gastric suction, may cause electrolyte levels to decrease. Respiratory failure may develop in patients with severe acute pancreatitis. It is important that respiratory function be assessed (e.g., breath sounds, oxygen saturation levels). If acute respiratory distress syndrome develops, the patient may require intubation and mechanical ventilatory support. Because hypocalcemia can also occur, the nurse must observe for symptoms of tetany, such as jerking, irritability, and muscular twitching. Numbness or tingling around the lips and in the fingers is an early indicator of hypocalcemia. The patient should be assessed for a positive Chvostek or Trousseau sign (see Chapter 19). Calcium gluconate (as ordered) should be given to treat symptomatic hypocalcemia. In addition, hypomagnesemia may develop, necessitating the observation of serum magnesium levels.

Because abdominal pain is a prominent symptom of pancreatitis, a major focus of nursing care is the relief of pain (see eNCP 46-3). Pain and restlessness can increase body metabolism and subsequent stimulation of pancreatic secretions. Morphine or meperidine may be administered for pain relief. The nurse should assess and document the duration of pain relief. Measures such as comfortable positioning, frequent changes in position, and relief of nausea and vomiting assist in reducing the restlessness that usually accompanies the pain. Assuming positions that flex the trunk and draw the knees up to the abdomen may decrease pain. A side-lying position with the head elevated 45 degrees decreases tension on the abdomen and may also help ease the pain. Nursing measures for the patient who is kept NPO or has an NG tube should include frequent oral and nasal care to relieve the dryness of the mouth and nose.

Oral care is essential to prevent parotitis. If the patient is taking anticholinergics to decrease GI secretions, dryness of the mouth is exacerbated. If antacids are taken to neutralize gastric acid secretions, they should be sipped slowly or administered through the NG tube.

The patient with acute pancreatitis is susceptible to infections. The nurse should monitor for fever and other manifestations of infection. Respiratory infections are common because the retroperitoneal fluid raises the diaphragm, which causes the patient to take shallow, guarded abdominal breaths. Measures to prevent respiratory infections include frequent turning, coughing, deep breathing, and assuming a semi-Fowler's position. Other important assessments are for signs of paralytic ileus, renal failure, and mental changes. The blood glucose level should be monitored to assess damage to the β cells of the islets of Langerhans in the pancreas.

After pancreatic surgery, the patient may require special wound care for an anastomotic leak or a fistula. To prevent skin irritation, measures such as skin barriers (Stomahesive or Karaya paste), pouching, and drains should be used. In addition to protecting the skin, pouching also provides a more accurate determination of fluid and electrolyte losses and increases patient comfort.

■ Ambulatory and Home Care

After acute pancreatitis, most patients need home care follow-up to prevent infection, monitor pain, and detect complications. Physiotherapy may be needed if the patient has lost physical reserve and muscle strength. Patient counselling should include alcohol abstinence and cigarette smoking cessation. Abstinence from alcohol prevents future pancreatitis attacks. Because tobacco can stimulate the pancreatic enzymes secretions, smoking should be avoided. Counselling recommendations and strategies for smoking cessation, including resources, can be referenced from the *Integrating Smoking Cessation into Daily Nursing Practice* best practice guideline by the Registered Nurses' Association of Ontario (2007).

Dietary teaching should include restriction of fats because they stimulate the secretion of cholecystokinin, which then stimulates the pancreas. Carbohydrates are less stimulating to the pancreas. The patient should be advised to avoid crash dieting and bingeing because they can precipitate attacks. The patient and the caregivers should be taught the symptoms of infection, diabetes mellitus, or steatorrhea (foul-smelling, frothy stools). These changes indicate possible ongoing destruction of pancreatic tissue, so they must be recognized and reported promptly. The patient and the caregivers should also be educated about the prescribed regimen, including the importance of taking the required medications and following the recommended diet.

■ Evaluation

Expected outcomes for patients with acute pancreatitis are presented in eNursing Care Plan 46-3.

Chronic Pancreatitis

Chronic pancreatitis is a continuous, prolonged inflammatory and fibrosing process of the pancreas. The pancreas becomes progressively destroyed as it is replaced with fibrotic tissues. Strictures and calcifications may also occur in the pancreas.

Etiology and Pathophysiology

Chronic pancreatitis may follow acute pancreatitis, but it may also occur in the absence of any history of acute episodes. In some patients, an identifiable cause may not be found (*idiopathic pancreatitis*). In the Western countries, 70% of cases of chronic pancreatitis are associated with alcohol abuse. However, not all people who abuse alcohol develop chronic pancreatitis, which suggests that affected people have cofactors that predispose them to the direct toxic effect of the alcohol on the pancreas.

Chronic pancreatitis can be classified into different types according to the causes. The two major types are *chronic obstructive pancreatitis* and *chronic calcifying pancreatitis*. Chronic calcifying pancreatitis is characterized by inflammation and sclerosis, mainly in the head of the pancreas and around the pancreatic duct. In chronic calcifying pancreatitis, the ducts are obstructed with protein precipitates. These precipitates block the pancreatic duct and eventually calcify. This is followed by fibrosis and glandular atrophy. Pseudocysts and abscesses commonly develop. Alcohol abuse is the most common cause of calcifying pancreatitis.

Obstructive pancreatitis is associated with biliary disease. The most common cause is inflammation of the sphincter of Oddi associated with cholelithiasis. Cancer of the ampulla of Vater, the duodenum, or the pancreas can also cause this type of chronic pancreatitis.

Clinical Manifestations

As with acute pancreatitis, a major manifestation of chronic pancreatitis is abdominal pain. The patient may have episodes of acute pain, but it usually is chronic (recurrent attacks at intervals of months or years). The attacks may become more and more frequent until they are almost constant, or they may diminish as the pancreatic fibrosis develops. The pain is located in the same areas as in acute pancreatitis but is usually described as a heavy, gnawing feeling or sometimes as burning and cramplike. The pain is not relieved with food or antacids. Other clinical manifestations are symptoms of pancreatic insufficiency, including malabsorption with weight loss, constipation, mild jaundice with dark urine, steatorrhea, and diabetes mellitus. The steatorrhea may become severe, with voluminous, foul, fatty stools. Urine and stool may be frothy. Some abdominal tenderness may be present. Chronic pancreatitis is also associated with a variety of complications. These include pancreatic pseudocyst formation, bile duct or duodenal obstruction, diabetes mellitus, pancreatic ascites or pleural effusion, splenic vein thrombosis, pseudoaneurysms, and pancreatic cancer.

Diagnostic Studies

The diagnosis is based on the patient's signs and symptoms, results of laboratory studies, and findings on imaging. In chronic pancreatitis, the levels of serum amylase and lipase may be elevated slightly or not at all, depending on the degree of pancreatic fibrosis. Serum bilirubin and alkaline phosphatase levels may be increased. Mild leukocytosis is usually present, and the sedimentation rate is usually elevated.

The secretin stimulation test is used to assess pancreatic function. In the normal pancreas, secretin stimulates secretion of pancreatic carbonate (HCO_3^-). In the stimulation test, secretin is given intravenously, and gastric–duodenal secretions are collected with a double-lumen tube for separate gastric and duodenal aspiration. In chronic pancreatitis, the volume of secretions and the bicarbonate concentration are reduced. Normally, secretin stimulates the production of pancreatic fluid high in bicarbonate content. The stimulation test is not widely available.

Stool samples are examined for fecal fat content. Deficiencies of fat-soluble vitamins and cobalamin, glucose intolerance, and possibly diabetes may also be found in patients with chronic pancreatitis. Arteriographic and radiographic studies may demonstrate fibrosis and calcification. ERCP is used to visualize the pancreatic and common bile ducts. Changes in the pancreatic ductal system, such as gross dilation and microcysts, can be visualized. Imaging studies, such as CT, MRI, MRCP, transabdominal ultrasonography, and endoscopic ultrasonography, are useful in patients with chronic pancreatitis. These tests show a variety of changes, including calcifications, ductal dilation, pseudocysts, and pancreatic enlargement.

Collaborative Care

When a patient with chronic pancreatitis is experiencing an acute attack, the therapy is identical to that for acute pancreatitis. At other times, the focus is on prevention of further attacks, relief of pain, and control of pancreatic exocrine and endocrine insufficiency. Sometimes, doses of analgesics must be large and frequent to relieve the pain.

Diet, pancreatic enzyme replacement, and control of the diabetes are measures used to control the pancreatic insufficiency. The diet should be bland and low in fat. Small, frequent meals should be encouraged. Fatty, rich, and stimulating foods should be avoided in order to decrease pancreatic secretions. Alcohol must be totally eliminated from the diet.

Pancreatic enzyme products (e.g., pancreatin [Viokase] and pancrelipase [Cotazym]) contain amylase, lipase, and trypsin and are administered to replace the deficient pancreatic enzymes. They are usually enteric coated to prevent their breakdown or inactivation by gastric hydrochloric acid. Bile salts are sometimes administered to facilitate the absorption of the fat-soluble vitamins (A, D, E, and K) and to prevent further fat loss. If diabetes develops, it is controlled with insulin or oral hypoglycemic agents. Acid-neutralizing (e.g., antacids) and acid-inhibiting drugs (e.g., histamine H_2-receptor blockers, proton pump inhibitors, anticholinergics) may be administered to decrease hydrochloric acid levels, but they have little overall effect on the outcome of the disease.

When biliary disease is present or if obstruction or pseudocyst develops, surgery may be indicated. Surgical procedures can divert bile flow or relieve ductal obstruction. A choledochojejunostomy diverts bile around the ampulla of Vater, where spasm or hypertrophy of the sphincter may be present. In this procedure, the common bile duct is anastomosed into the jejunum. One type is the Roux-en-Y pancreatojejunostomy, in which the pancreatic duct is opened and an anastomosis is made with the jejunum. Pancreatic drainage procedures relieve ductal obstruction. Some patients may undergo ERCP with either sphincterotomy or stent placement at the site of obstruction, or both. These patients require follow-up ERCP to either exchange or remove the stent.

NURSING MANAGEMENT: CHRONIC PANCREATITIS

Except during an acute episode, the focus of nursing management is on chronic care and health promotion. Patients must be instructed to take measures to prevent further attacks. Dietary control, along with adherence to pancreatic enzyme treatment regimens, is essential. The pancreatic extracts are taken with meals or snacks. Patients' stools should be examined for steatorrhea to help determine the effectiveness of the enzyme treatment. Patient and caregivers must be given clear instructions on stool assessment.

If diabetes has developed, patients need instruction about testing of blood glucose levels and medications (see Chapter 52). Ensure that patients who are taking antisecretory agents take them as ordered to control gastric acidity. Antacids should be taken after meals and at bedtime.

Alcohol must be avoided, and patients may need assistance with this problem. If a patient has developed a dependence on alcohol, referral to other agencies or resources may be necessary (see Chapter 11).

Pancreatic Cancer

Pancreatic cancer is a disease with a dismal outcome. In Canada, it was estimated that 4100 new cases of pancreatic cancer would be diagnosed in 2011. It has one of the lowest rates of survival of all cancers (Canadian Cancer Encyclopedia, 2011). Pancreatic cancer affects older people; the incidence peaks among those 65 to 75 years of age. The prognosis of pancreatic cancer is poor. The majority of patients die within 5 to 12 months of the initial diagnosis, and the overall 5-year survival rate is less than 5% (Maitra & Hruban, 2008).

Etiology and Pathophysiology

Cigarette smoking is the most consistently reported risk factor for pancreatic cancer (Lynch et al., 2009). People who smoke are twice as likely to develop pancreatic cancers than are people who do not smoke. The risk is related to both duration and amount of cigarettes smoked.

Other risk factors are obesity, diabetes, genetic dispositions and long-term exposure to chemicals such as certain types of pesticides and dyes.

Most pancreatic tumours are adenocarcinomas originating from the epithelium of the ductal system. More than half the tumours occur in the head of the pancreas. As such a tumour grows, the common bile duct becomes obstructed, and obstructive jaundice develops. Tumours starting in the body or the tail often do not produce symptoms until their growth is advanced. Metastases to the lymph nodes are common. Molecular and histopathological analyses have identified precursor lesions. These are microscopic lesions (<5 mm), defined as neoplastic epithelial proliferations in the small pancreatic ducts; they progress from normal tissue to invasive cancer and are associated with genetic alterations.

Clinical Manifestations

Common manifestations of pancreatic cancer include abdominal pain (dull, aching), anorexia, nausea, and rapid and progressive weight loss. Jaundice occurs when the cancer is in the head of the pancreas because of the ductal obstruction. Pruritus may accompany obstructive jaundice.

Pain is common and is related to the location of malignancy. Extreme, unrelenting pain is related to extension of the cancer into the retroperitoneal tissues and nerve plexuses. The pain is frequently located in the upper abdomen or the left hypochondrium and often radiates to the back. Its onset is commonly related to eating, and it also occurs at night. Weight loss results from poor digestion and absorption caused by lack of digestive enzymes from the pancreas.

Diagnostic Studies

Endoscopic ultrasonography, CT, ERCP, MRI, and MRCP are the imaging techniques most commonly used for diagnosing pancreatic diseases, including cancer. Endoscopic ultrasonography involves imaging the pancreas with the use of an endoscope positioned in the stomach and duodenum. It also allows for fine-needle aspiration of the tumour. CT is often the initial study and provides information on metastasis and vascular involvement. When ERCP is used, pancreatic secretions, as well as tissue, can be collected for analysis of different tumour markers. MRI and MRCP are used for diagnosing and staging the cancer.

Tumour markers are used both for establishing the diagnosis of pancreatic adenocarcinoma and for monitoring the response to treatment. Cancer-associated antigen (CA-19-9) is elevated in pancreatic cancer and is the most commonly used tumour marker.

Collaborative Care

Surgery is the most effective treatment for cancer of the pancreas. Only 15 to 20% of affected patients have resectable tumours. The classic surgical procedure is a *radical pancreaticoduodenectomy,* or *Whipple's procedure* (Figure 46-15). This entails resection of the proximal pancreas (proximal pancreatectomy), the adjoining duodenum (duodenectomy), the distal portion of the stomach (partial gastrectomy), and the distal segment of the common bile duct, and the removal of the gallbladder. An anastomosis of

Before surgery

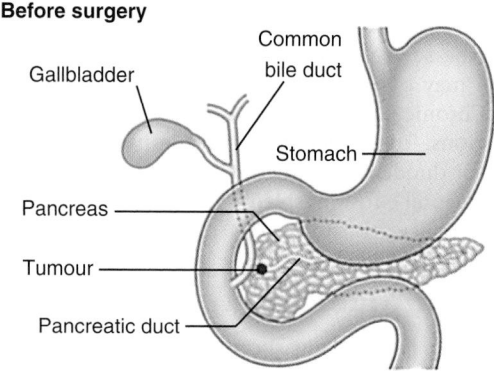

Whipple's operation

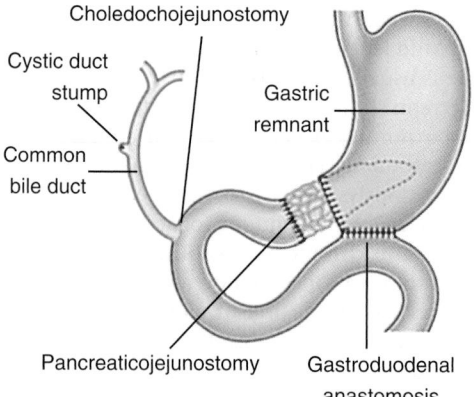

Figure 46-15 Whipple's procedure, or radical pancreaticoduodenectomy. This surgical procedure involves resection of the proximal pancreas, adjoining duodenum, distal portion of the stomach, and distal segment of the common bile duct, and the removal of the gallbladder. An anastomosis of the pancreatic duct, common bile duct, and stomach to the jejunum is created.

Source: Modified from Butcher, G. P. (2004). *Gastroenterology: An illustrated colour text.* London: Churchill Livingstone.

the pancreatic duct, the common bile duct, and the stomach to the jejunum is created. A total pancreatectomy is performed in some institutions. Sometimes, a simple bypass procedure, such as a cholecystojejunostomy to relieve biliary obstruction, may be used as a palliative measure. Some surgeons suggest a more radical resection, such as a total pancreaticoduodenectomy with splenectomy. Biliary stents (e.g., Cotton-Leung stent) can be used as a palliative measure when tumours compress the bile duct.

Radiation therapy has little effect on survival, but it is effective for pain relief. External radiation is usually used, but internal radiation seeds have also been implanted into the tumour. The current role of chemotherapy in pancreatic cancer is limited. Chemotherapy usually consists of 5-fluorouracil (5-FU) and gemcitabine (Gemzar), either alone or in combination with agents such as capecitabine (Xeloda) or erlotinib (Tarceva). Erlotinib is a targeted therapy. Because of the aggressive nature of pancreatic cancer, experimental chemotherapy is focused on subjective clinical benefits, including reductions in pain.

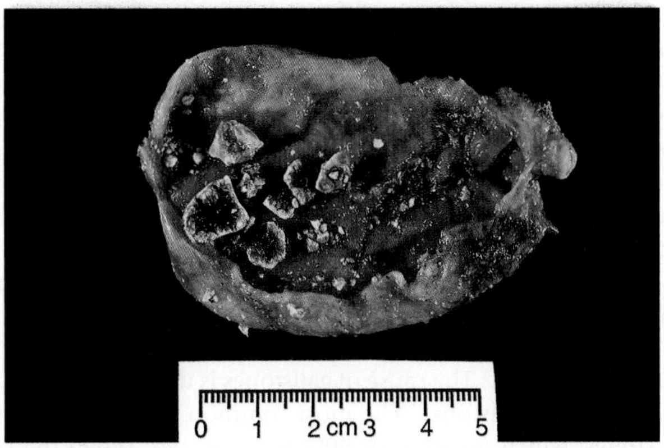

Figure 46-16 Cholesterol gallstones in a gallbladder that was removed.

Source: From Kumar, V., Abbas, A. K., & Fausto, N. (2005). *Robbins and Cotran pathologic basis of disease* (7th ed.). Philadelphia: W. B. Saunders.

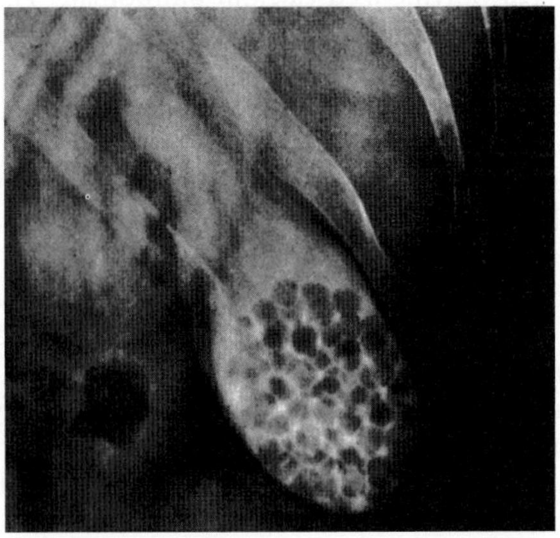

NURSING MANAGEMENT: PANCREATIC CANCER

Because the patient with pancreatic cancer has many of the same problems as the patient with pancreatitis, nursing care includes the same measures (see eNCP 46-1, Patient with Acute Pancreatisis, available on the Evolve Web site for this chapter.). The nurse should provide symptomatic and supportive nursing care. The nurse should administer analgesics and comfort measures to relieve pain. Psychological support to both the patient and the family is essential, especially during times of anxiety or depression.

Adequate nutrition is an important part of the nursing care plan. Frequent and supplemental feedings may be necessary. Measures to stimulate the appetite and to overcome anorexia, nausea, and vomiting should be included in the nursing care. Because bleeding can result from impaired vitamin K production, the nurse should assess for bleeding from body orifices and mucous membranes. If a patient is undergoing radiation therapy, the nurse should observe for adverse reactions, such as anorexia, nausea, vomiting, and skin irritation. The prognosis for patients with pancreatic cancer is not good. A significant component of the nursing care is helping the patient and the family or significant others through the grieving process.

Figure 46-17 Radiograph of a gallbladder with gallstones.

Disorders of the Biliary Tract

Cholelithiasis and Cholecystitis

The most common disorder of the biliary system is **cholelithiasis** (stones in the gallbladder) (Figures 46-16 and 46-17). **Cholecystitis** (inflammation of the gallbladder) is usually associated with cholelithiasis. The stones may be lodged in the neck of the gallbladder or in the cystic duct. Cholecystitis may be acute or chronic.

Cholelithiasis occurs in 10 to 15% of adults in North America and in Europe. The prevalence is lower in Africa and Asia. *Cholecystectomy* (removal of the gallbladder) ranks among the most common surgical procedures. Although gallstones are common,

more than 80% of affected patients have no symptoms. The incidence of cholelithiasis is higher in women, particularly multiparous women, and in people older than 40 years. Postmenopausal women receiving estrogen therapy are at somewhat greater risk than are women who are taking birth control pills. Oral contraceptives alter the character of bile, resulting in increased cholesterol saturation. Other factors that increase the occurrence of gallbladder disease are a sedentary lifestyle, a familial tendency, and obesity. Obesity causes increased secretion of cholesterol in bile. The incidence of gallstones in industrialized and developing societies will probably escalate because of the increase in dietary fat and carbohydrate intake coupled with reductions in dietary fibre intake.

Etiology and Pathophysiology

Cholecystitis. Cholecystitis is most commonly associated with obstruction caused by gallstones or biliary sludge. Cholecystitis that occurs in the absence of obstruction (acalculous cholecystitis) is most common in older adults and in patients who have trauma, have extensive burns, or have recently undergone surgery. Acalculous cholecystitis can also occur as a result of prolonged immobility and fasting, prolonged total parenteral nutrition, and diabetes mellitus. Bacteria (reaching the gallbladder via the vascular or the lymphatic route) or chemical irritants in the bile can also produce cholecystitis.

Inflammation is the major pathophysiological process in cholecystitis; it may be confined to the mucous lining, or it may involve the entire wall of the gallbladder. During an acute attack of cholecystitis, the gallbladder is edematous and hyperemic. It may be distended with bile or pus. The cystic duct is also involved and may become occluded. The wall of the gallbladder becomes scarred after an acute attack. Functioning is decreased if large amounts of tissue undergo fibrosis.

Cholelithiasis.

The cause of gallstones is unknown. There are three types of gallstones. The most common type is cholesterol gallstones, which account for 90% of gallstones. When the bile secreted by the liver is supersaturated with cholesterol (lithogenic bile), the bile in the gallbladder also becomes supersaturated with cholesterol. When that happens, precipitation of cholesterol occurs. Risk factors for developing cholesterol gallstones can be genetic, dietary, and medication related.

Black pigment gallstones account for 2% of gallstones, and they consist of polymerized calcium bilirubinate. Patients with hemolytic anemia, cirrhosis, and ileal diseases are at highest risk for developing black pigment stones.

Brown pigment gallstones are infrequent and usually formed in the bile ducts as a result of stasis of bile and infection. These stones consist of unconjugated bilirubin and calcium salts. People at risk include those with duodenal diverticula, bile duct strictures, or parasitic diseases.

The stones may remain in the gallbladder or migrate to the cystic duct or to the common bile duct. They cause pain as they pass through the ducts, and they may lodge in the ducts and produce an obstruction. Small stones are more likely to move into a duct and cause obstruction. Table 46-22 lists the changes and the manifestations that occur when the stones obstruct the common bile duct. If the blockage occurs in the cystic duct, the bile can continue to flow into the duodenum directly from the liver. However, when the bile in the gallbladder cannot escape, this stasis of bile may lead to cholecystitis.

Clinical Manifestations

Manifestations of cholecystitis vary from indigestion to moderate to severe pain, fever, and jaundice. Initial symptoms of acute cholecystitis include pain and tenderness in the right upper quadrant (which may be referred to the right shoulder and scapula) and indigestion. The pain may be acute and be accompanied by nausea and vomiting, restlessness, and diaphoresis. Manifestations of inflammation include leukocytosis and fever. Physical findings include tenderness in the right upper quadrant and abdominal rigidity. Affected patients may have a history of fat intolerance. Symptoms of chronic cholecystitis include dyspepsia, heartburn, and flatulence.

Cholelithiasis may produce severe symptoms or none at all (*silent cholelithiasis*). The severity of symptoms depends on whether the stones are stationary or mobile and whether obstruction is present. When a stone is lodged in the ducts or when stones are moving through the ducts, spasms may result. The gallbladder spasms occur in response to the stone. This sometimes produces severe pain, which is termed *biliary colic* even though the pain is rarely colicky; it is more often steady. The pain can be excruciating and accompanied by tachycardia, diaphoresis, and prostration. The severe pain may last up to an hour, and when it subsides, there is residual tenderness in the right upper quadrant. The attacks of pain frequently occur 3 to 6 hours after a high-fat meal or when the patient lies down. When total obstruction occurs, symptoms related to bile blockage are manifested (see Table 46-22).

Complications

Complications of cholecystitis include subphrenic abscess, acute pancreatitis, *cholangitis* (inflammation of bile ducts), biliary cirrhosis, fistulas, and rupture of the gallbladder, which can cause bile peritonitis. Many of the same complications can result from cholelithiasis, including cholangitis, biliary cirrhosis, carcinoma, and peritonitis. *Choledocholithiasis* (stone in the common bile duct) may occur, producing symptoms of obstruction.

Diagnostic Studies

Ultrasonography is 90 to 95% accurate in detecting stones. It is especially useful for patients who are allergic to contrast medium. ERCP allows for visualization of the gallbladder, the cystic duct, the common hepatic duct, and the common bile duct. Bile samples taken during ERCP are sent for culture to identify possibly infecting organisms. Laboratory tests may demonstrate elevations in levels of some liver enzymes, such as alkaline phosphatase, ALT, and AST. The white blood cell count is increased as a result of inflammation. Both the direct and indirect bilirubin levels are elevated, as is the urinary bilirubin level if an obstructive process is present. If the common bile duct is obstructed, no bilirubin reaches the small intestine to be converted to urobilinogen. The serum amylase level is increased if the pancreas is involved.

Collaborative Care

Conservative Therapy

Cholecystitis. During an acute episode of cholecystitis, the focus of treatment is on control of pain, control of possible

Table 46-22 Clinical Manifestations Caused by Obstructed Bile Flow

CLINICAL MANIFESTATION	ETIOLOGY
Obstructive jaundice	No bile flow into duodenum
Dark amber urine, which foams when shaken	Soluble bilirubin in urine
No urobilinogen in urine	No bilirubin reaching small intestine to be converted to urobilinogen
Clay-coloured stools	Blockage of flow of bile salts out of the liver
Pruritus	Deposition of bile salts in skin tissues
Intolerance of fatty foods (nausea, sensation of fullness, anorexia)	No bile in small intestine for fat digestion
Bleeding tendencies	Lack of or decreased absorption of vitamin K, resulting in decreased production of prothrombin
Steatorrhea	No bile salts in duodenum, preventing fat emulsion and digestion

COLLABORATIVE CARE

Table 46-23 Cholelithiasis and Acute Cholecystitis

Diagnostic

- History and physical examination
- Liver enzyme measurements
- WBC count
- Serum bilirubin measurement
- Ultrasonography
- ERCP

Collaborative Therapy

Conservative Therapy

- IV fluids
- NPO status with NG tube, later progressing to low-fat diet
- Antiemetics
- Analgesics

- Fat-soluble vitamins (A, D, E, and K)
- Anticholinergics (antispasmodics)
- Antibiotics (for secondary infection)
- ERCP with sphincterotomy (papillotomy)
- Extracorporeal shock-wave lithotripsy

Dissolution Therapy

- Ursodeoxycholic acid
- Ursodiol
- Chenodeoxycholic acid

Surgical Therapy*

- Laparoscopic cholecystectomy
- Incisional cholecystectomy

*See Table 46-24.
ERCP, endoscopic retrograde cholangiopancreatography; *IV*, intravenous; *NG*, nasogastric; *NPO*, nothing by mouth; *WBC*, white blood cell.

Table 46-24 Gallbladder Surgery Procedures

NAME	DESCRIPTION
Cholecystectomy	Removal of gallbladder
Cholecystostomy (usually an emergency procedure)	Incision into gallbladder (usually for removal of stones)
Choledocholithotomy	Incision into common bile duct for removal of stones
Cholecystogastrostomy	Anastomosis between stomach and gallbladder
Cholecystoduodenostomy	Anastomosis between gallbladder and duodenum to relieve obstruction at distal end of common bile duct
Laparoscopic cholecystectomy	Removal of gallbladder via laparoscopy through the use of a dissecting laser

infection with antibiotics, and maintenance of fluid and electrolyte balance (Table 46-23). If nausea and vomiting are severe, an NG tube may be inserted and gastric decompression may be used to prevent further gallbladder stimulation. Anticholinergics are administered to decrease secretion and counteract smooth muscle spasms. Analgesics are given for pain relief.

Cholelithiasis. The treatment of gallstones depends on the stage of the disease. Bile acids (cholesterol solvents) such as ursodeoxycholic acid and chenodeoxycholic acid (chenodiol) are administered to dissolve stones. However, the gallstones may recur. Gallstones are not usually treated with drugs because of the high use and success of laparoscopic cholecystectomy.

Standard ERCP clears stones from the common bile duct in approximately 90% of patients (Figure 46-18). This procedure allows for visualization of the biliary system, placement of stents, and sphincterotomy (papillotomy) if warranted. In this procedure, the endoscope is passed to the duodenum. With an electrodiathermy knife attached to the endoscope, the sphincter of Oddi is widened (sphincterotomy). A basket is used to retrieve the stone. The stone may be removed in the basket, but more commonly it is left in the duodenum and will be passed naturally in the stool.

Extracorporeal shock-wave lithotripsy (ESWL) is another nonsurgical treatment for gallstones. In ESWL, high-energy shock waves are used to disintegrate gallstones. Ultrasonography is first performed to locate the stones and to determine where to direct the shock waves. The shock waves are directed with a lithotriptor through the abdomen as a water-filled cushion is pressed against the area. It usually takes 1 to 2 hours to disintegrate the stones. After they are broken up, the fragments pass through the common bile duct and into the small intestine. Usually ESWL and oral dissolution therapy are used together.

Surgical Therapy. Surgical interventions for cholelithiasis are listed in Table 46-24. Laparoscopic cholecystectomy is the

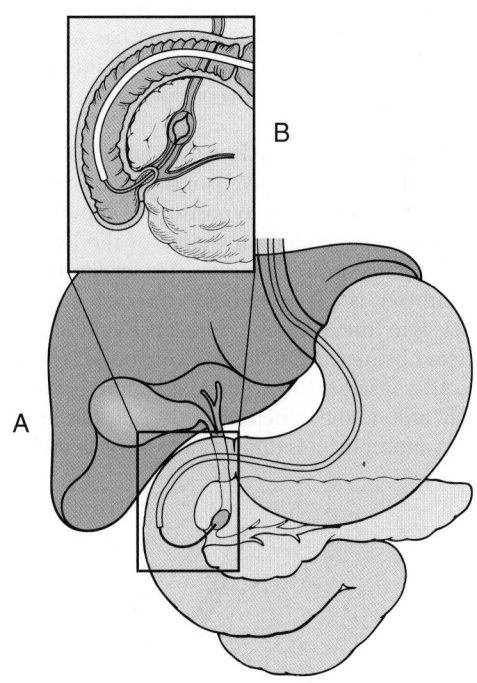

Figure 46-18 Standard endoscopic retrograde cholangiopancreatography (ERCP). **A,** During endoscopic sphincterotomy, an endoscope is advanced through the mouth and stomach until its tip sits in the duodenum opposite the common bile duct. **B,** After widening the duct mouth by incising the sphincter muscle, the physician advances a basket attachment into the duct and snags the stone.

treatment of choice for symptomatic cholelithiasis. Approximately 92% of all cholecystectomies are performed laparoscopically. In this procedure, the gallbladder is removed through one of four small punctures in the abdomen. A 1-cm puncture is made slightly above the umbilicus, and the surgeon inflates the abdominal cavity with 3 to 4 L of CO_2 to improve visibility. A laparoscope that has a camera attached is inserted into the abdomen. Two additional punctures made just below the ribs are used for insertion of grasping forceps. A dissection laser is inserted into the fourth puncture. (The incision sites may vary.) Using closed-circuit monitors to view the abdominal cavity, the surgeon retracts and dissects the gallbladder and removes it with grasping forceps.

This procedure is relatively minor and entails few complications. Most patients experience minimal postoperative pain and are discharged the day of or the day after surgery. In most cases, they are able to resume normal activities and return to work within 1 week. Advantages of the laparoscopic cholecystectomy include decreased postoperative pain, shorter hospital stay, and earlier return to work and full activity. The main complication is injury to the common bile duct.

There are few contraindications to laparoscopic cholecystectomy. The primary ones are peritonitis, cholangitis, gangrene or perforation of the gallbladder, portal hypertension, and serious bleeding disorders.

On selected patients, an incisional (open) cholecystectomy may be performed. This involves removal of the gallbladder through a right subcostal incision. A T-tube is inserted into the common bile duct during surgery when a common bile duct exploration is part of the surgical procedure (Figure 46-19). This ensures patency of the duct until the edema produced by the trauma of exploring and probing the duct has subsided. It also allows the excess bile to drain while the small intestine is adjusting to receiving a continuous flow of bile.

Transhepatic Biliary Catheter.
The transhepatic biliary catheter can be used preoperatively in biliary obstruction and in hepatic dysfunction secondary to obstructive jaundice. It can also be inserted when inoperable carcinoma of the liver, pancreatic duct, or bile duct obstructs bile flow. Under fluoroscopic guidance, the catheter is percutaneously inserted across the liver parenchyma into the common bile duct and duodenum. It decompresses obstructed extrahepatic bile ducts so that bile can flow freely. After insertion, the catheter is connected to a drainage bag. The skin around the catheter insertion site has to be cleansed daily with an antiseptic. It is important to observe for bile leakage at the insertion site. Depending on the reason the catheter was inserted, the patient may be discharged with it in place.

Drug Therapy.
The drugs most commonly administered in the treatment of gallbladder disease are analgesics, anticholinergics (antispasmodics), fat-soluble vitamins, and bile salts. Morphine or meperidine (Demerol) may be administered for pain management. Anticholinergics such as atropine and other antispasmodics may be administered to relax the smooth muscle and decrease ductal tone. If a patient has chronic gallbladder disease or any biliary tract obstruction, fat-soluble vitamins (A, D, E, and K) will probably be given. Bile salts may be administered to facilitate digestion and vitamin absorption. For treatment of pruritus, cholestyramine may provide relief. This is a resin that binds bile salts in the intestine, increasing their excretion in the feces. Cholestyramine is administered in powder form and should be mixed with milk or juice. Adverse effects include nausea, vomiting, diarrhea or constipation, and skin reactions.

Nutritional Therapy.
Many patients have fewer problems if they eat smaller, more frequent meals, with some fat at each meal to promote gallbladder emptying. If obesity is a problem, a reduced-calorie diet is indicated. The diet should be low in saturated fats (e.g. butter, shortening) and high in fibre and calcium. Rapid weight loss should be avoided because it can promote gallstone formation. After a laparoscopic cholecystectomy, the patient should have liquids for the rest of the day and eat light meals for a few days. If an incisional cholecystectomy is performed, the patient may progress from liquids to a bland diet once bowel sounds have returned. The amount of fat in the postoperative diet depends on the patient's tolerance of fat. A low-fat diet may be helpful if the flow of bile is reduced (usually only in the early postoperative period) or if the patient is overweight. Some patients need to restrict fats for 4 to 6 weeks. Otherwise, no special dietary instructions are needed other than to eat nutritious meals and avoid excessive fat intake.

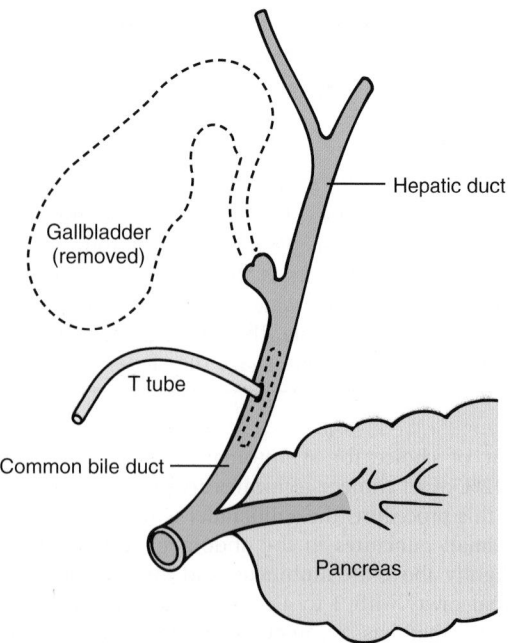

Figure 46-19 Placement of T-tube during cholecystectomy. *Dotted lines* indicate parts removed.

NURSING MANAGEMENT: GALLBLADDER DISEASE

▪ Nursing Assessment

Subjective and objective data that should be obtained from a person with gallbladder disease are presented in Table 46-25.

▪ Nursing Diagnoses

Nursing diagnoses for patients with gallbladder disease treated surgically include, but are not limited to, the following:
• Acute pain *related to* surgical procedure
• Ineffective self-health management *related to* lack of knowledge of diet and postoperative management

▪ Planning

The overall goals are that the patient with gallbladder disease will have (a) relief of pain and discomfort, (b) no complications

NURSING ASSESSMENT

Table 46-25 Cholecystitis or Cholelithiasis

Subjective Data

Important Health Information

Past health history: Obesity, multiparity, infection, cancer, extensive fasting, pregnancy; positive family history; sedentary lifestyle

Medications: Use of estrogen or oral contraceptives

Surgery or other treatments: Previous abdominal surgery

Symptoms

- Weight loss, anorexia; indigestion, fat intolerance, nausea and vomiting, dyspepsia; chills
- Clay-coloured stools, steatorrhea, flatulence; dark urine
- Moderate to severe pain in right upper quadrant that may radiate to the back or scapula; pruritus

Objective Data

General

Fever, restlessness

Integumentary

Jaundice, icteric sclera; diaphoresis

Respiratory

Tachypnea, splinting during respirations

Cardiovascular

Tachycardia

Gastrointestinal

Palpable gallbladder, abdominal guarding and distension

Possible Findings

↑ Levels of serum liver enzymes and bilirubin; absence of urobilinogen in urine; ↑ level of urinary bilirubin; leukocytosis; abnormal findings on ultrasonography

postoperatively, and (c) no recurrent attacks of cholecystitis or cholelithiasis.

Nursing Implementation

Health Promotion

In general health screening, the nurse should recognize the predisposing factors of gallbladder disease. Patients at risk should be taught initial clinical manifestations and be instructed to seek medical care if these manifestations occur. Patients with chronic cholecystitis do not have acute symptoms and may not seek help until jaundice and biliary obstruction occur. Earlier detection in these patients is beneficial so that the condition can be managed with lifestyle modifications (e.g., a low-fat diet).

Acute Intervention

Nursing objectives for the patient undergoing conservative therapy include managing pain, relieving nausea and vomiting, providing comfort and emotional support, maintaining fluid and electrolyte balance, maintaining nutrition, making accurate assessments of effectiveness of treatment, and observing for complications.

Many patients with acute cholecystitis or cholelithiasis experience severe pain. The medications ordered to relieve the pain should be administered as required by patients and before the pain becomes more severe. The nurse should determine what medications relieve the pain and how much medication is required. The nurse must also observe for adverse effects of the medications. Nursing comfort measures, such as a clean bed, comfortable positioning, and oral care, are appropriate.

For patients who have severe nausea and vomiting, insertion of a nasogastric tube and gastric decompression may be necessary. The elimination of food intake also prevents further stimulation of the gallbladder. Oral hygiene, care of nares, accurate intake and output measurements, and maintenance of suction should be a part of the nursing care plan for such patients. For patients with less severe nausea and vomiting, antiemetics are usually adequate. When a patient is vomiting, comfort measures such as frequent mouth rinses should be provided. Any vomitus must be removed immediately from the patient's view.

If pruritus occurs with jaundice, measures to relieve itching include baking soda or oatmeal baths; lotions, such as those containing calamine; antihistamines; soft, old linen; and control of the temperature (not too hot and not too cold). The patient's nails should be kept short and clean. Patients should be taught to rub with their knuckles rather than scratch with their nails when they cannot resist scratching.

The nursing care plan for such patients also includes assessment of progression of the symptoms and development of complications. The nurse should observe for signs of bile duct obstructions: jaundice; clay-coloured stools; dark, foamy urine; steatorrhea; fever; and increased WBC count.

When symptoms of obstruction are present (see Table 46-22), the nurse must be aware of the possibility of bleeding as a result of decreased prothrombin production. Common sites to observe for bleeding are the mucous membranes of the mouth, the nose, the gingivae, and injection sites. If injections are given, a small-gauge needle should be used and gentle pressure applied after the injection. The nurse should know the patient's prothrombin time and use this as a guide in the assessment process.

Assessment for infections includes monitoring of vital signs. Fever with chills and jaundice may indicate choledocholithiasis. Nursing care of the patient after ERCP with papillotomy includes assessment to detect complications such as pancreatitis, perforation, infection, and bleeding. The patient's vital signs should be monitored. Abdominal pain and fever may indicate pancreatitis. The patient should be rested for several hours and ingest nothing by mouth until the gag reflex returns.

Postoperative Care

Postoperative nursing care after a laparoscopic cholecystectomy includes monitoring for complications such as bleeding, making the patient comfortable, and preparing the patient for discharge. A common postoperative problem is referred pain to the shoulder because of the CO_2 that was not released or was absorbed by the body. The CO_2 can irritate the phrenic nerve and the diaphragm, causing some difficulty breathing. Placing the patient in Sims's position (left side with right knee flexed) helps move the gas pocket away from the diaphragm. Deep breathing and early ambulation should be encouraged. Severe pain can be relieved by narcotic analgesics such as oxycodone (OxyContin) or codeine. The patient is allowed clear liquids and can walk to the bathroom to void. Many patients go home the same day as the procedure, but some stay overnight.

Postoperative nursing care for incisional cholecystectomy is the same as general postoperative nursing care (see Chapter 22).

Table 46-26 Laparoscopic Cholecystectomy: Postoperative Care

1. Remove the bandages on the puncture site the day after surgery, and bathe or shower.

2. Notify the surgeon of any of the following signs and symptoms:
   - Redness; swelling; bile-coloured drainage or pus from any incision
   - Severe abdominal pain, nausea, vomiting, fever, chills

3. Resume normal activities gradually.

4. Return to work within 1 week of surgery if no complications ensue.

5. Resume normal diet; a low-fat diet, however, is usually better tolerated for several weeks after surgery.

The goal is to prevent postoperative complications. If the patient has a T-tube (see Figure 46-19), nursing care plan should focus on maintaining bile drainage and observing for the T-tube functioning and drainage. The T-tube is connected to a closed-gravity drainage system. If the Penrose or Jackson-Pratt drain or the T-tube is draining large amounts, a sterile pouching system should be used to protect the skin.

▪ Ambulatory and Home Care

When a patient has conservative therapy, long-term nursing management depends on symptoms and on whether surgical intervention is being planned. Dietary teaching is usually necessary. The food should be low in fat. If the patient is obese, a weight-reduction program should be recommended. The patient may need to take fat-soluble vitamin supplements. The patient should be provided instructions about symptoms that indicate obstruction (stool and urine changes, jaundice, and pruritus). The nurse should explain the importance of continued health care. Patients who undergo a laparoscopic cholecystectomy are discharged soon after the surgery; therefore, home care is important. Teaching is essential; a teaching guide is presented in Table 46-26.

After an incisional cholecystectomy, the patient may be discharged in 2 to 3 days. The patient must avoid heavy lifting for 4 to 6 weeks. Usual sexual activities, including intercourse, can be resumed as soon as the patient feels ready, unless the physician instructs otherwise. If the patient is required to remain on a low-fat diet for 4 to 6 weeks, a dietary teaching plan is necessary. A weight-reduction program may be helpful if the patient is overweight. Most patients tolerate a regular diet with no difficulties but should avoid excessive fats.

▪ Evaluation

The overall expected outcomes are that the patient with gallbladder disease will (a) be comfortable and free of pain and (b) will verbalize understanding of activity level and dietary restrictions.

Gallbladder Cancer

Primary cancer of the gallbladder is uncommon. The majority of gallbladder carcinomas are adenocarcinomas and arise in the inner lining of the gallbladder. There seems to be a definite relationship between cancer of the gallbladder and chronic cholecystitis and cholelithiasis. The early symptoms of carcinoma of the gallbladder are insidious and are similar to those of chronic cholecystitis and cholelithiasis, which makes diagnosis difficult. Later symptoms are usually those of biliary obstruction.

Diagnosis and staging of gallbladder cancer is done using endoscopic ultrasonography, transabdominal ultrasonography, CT, MRI, MRCP, or a combination of these methodologies. Unfortunately, gallbladder cancer often is not detected until the advanced stage. When it is found early, surgery can be curative. Several factors influence successful surgical outcomes, including the depth of cancer invasion, extent of liver involvement, presence of venous or lymphatic invasion, and lymph node metastasis. Extended cholecystectomy with lymph node dissection has improved the outcomes for patients with gallbladder cancer. When surgery is not an option, endoscopic implantation of stents in the biliary tree to reduce obstructive jaundice may be warranted. Adjuvant therapies, including radiation therapy and chemotherapy, may be used, depending on the disease state. Overall, cancer of the gallbladder has a poor prognosis. Nursing management involves supportive care with special attention to nutrition, hydration, skin care, and pain relief. Many of the nursing care measures used for patients with cholecystitis and cholelithiasis are frequently applied, as are nursing care measures for patients with cancer (see Chapter 18).

CLINICAL DECISION-MAKING EXERCISES

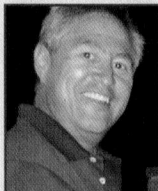

CASE STUDY:
Cirrhosis of the Liver

Courtesy Sharon L. Lewis.

Patient Profile

Mr. Begay is a 55-year-old man admitted with a diagnosis of decompensating cirrhosis of the liver.

Subjective Data

- Was informed 10 years ago that he had cirrhosis
- Had a blood transfusion 25 years ago after a car accident
- Acknowledges that he has been drinking heavily for more than 30 years
- Complains of anorexia, nausea, and abdominal discomfort

Objective Data

Physical Examination
- Is thin and malnourished
- Has moderate ascites
- Has jaundice of sclera and skin
- Has 4+ pitting edema of the lower extremities
- Has palpable liver and spleen

Laboratory Values
- Total bilirubin: 150 mcmol/L
- Albumin: 26 U/L
- AST: 210 U/L

- ALT: 190 U/L
- Platelet count: 75,000
- INR: 1.3
- Anti-HCV (antibody to hepatitis C) positive and HCV RNA negative
- HBsAg (hepatitis B surface antigen) negative and anti-HBs (antibody to hepatitis B surface antigen) positive

Discussion Questions

1. What are the possible causes of cirrhosis? What is the most likely etiology responsible for Mr. Begay's cirrhosis?
2. Describe the pathophysiological changes that occur in the liver as cirrhosis develops.
3. List Mr. Begay's clinical manifestations of liver failure. For each manifestation, explain the pathophysiological basis.
4. Explain the significance of the results of his laboratory values.
5. If Mr. Begay begins to manifest signs and symptoms of hepatic encephalopathy, what would the nurse monitor? What measures should be instituted to control or decrease encephalopathy?
6. Mr. Begay was being closely observed for the possibility of gastrointestinal bleeding. Why is this considered a possible complication?
7. *Priority Decision:* On the basis of the assessment data presented, what are the nursing diagnoses? Are there any collaborative problems?
8. *Priority Decision:* What are the priority nursing interventions for the patient at this stage of his illness?

evolve *Answers are available on* **http://evolve.elsevier.com/ Canada/Lewis/medsurg**

REVIEW QUESTIONS

The number of the question corresponds to the same-numbered objective at the beginning of the chapter.

1. During assessment of a patient with cholestatic (obstructive) jaundice, which of the following would the nurse expect to find?
   a. Clay-coloured stools
   b. Dark urine and stools
   c. Pyrexia and severe pruritus
   d. Elevated urinary urobilinogen level
2. A patient with hepatitis A is in the acute phase. Which of the following should the nurse's plan of care consider?
   a. Pruritus is a common problem with jaundice in this phase.
   b. The patient is most likely to transmit the disease during this phase.
   c. Gastrointestinal symptoms are not as severe in hepatitis A as they are in hepatitis B.
   d. Extrahepatic manifestations of glomerulonephritis and polyarteritis are common in this phase.
3. A patient with acute hepatitis B is being discharged in 2 days. Which of the following instructions should the nurse include in the discharge teaching plan?
   a. Resume alcohol as soon as he is symptom free.
   b. Use a condom during sexual intercourse.
   c. Have family members get an injection of immune globulin.
   d. Follow a low-protein, moderate-carbohydrate, moderate-fat diet.
4. The patient with advanced cirrhosis asks the nurse why his abdomen is so swollen. The nurse's response is based on the knowledge of which of the following?
   a. A lack of clotting factors promotes the collection of blood in the abdominal cavity.
   b. Portal hypertension and hypoalbuminemia cause a fluid shift into the peritoneal space.
   c. Decreased peristalsis in the gastrointestinal tract contributes to gas formation and distension of the bowel.
   d. Bile salts in the blood irritate the peritoneal membranes, causing edema and pocketing of fluid.
5. A patient has been told that her liver enzyme levels are elevated as a result of NAFLD. Which of the following instructions should the nurse's teaching plan include?
   a. Have genetic testing performed.
   b. Follow a heart-healthy diet and regular exercise program.
   c. Join Weight Watchers to lose weight quickly.
   d. Avoid alcohol until the liver enzyme levels return to normal.
6. In caring for a patient with metastatic liver cancer, which of the following should the nurse perform?
   a. Focus primarily on symptomatic and comfort measures.
   b. Reassure the patient that chemotherapy offers a good prognosis for recovery.
   c. Promote the patient's confidence that surgical excision of the tumour will be successful.
   d. Provide information necessary for the patient to make decisions regarding liver transplantation.
7. The nurse explains to the patient that the most common pathogenic mechanisms of acute pancreatitis is which of the following?
   a. Cellular disorganization
   b. Overproduction of enzymes
   c. Lack of secretion of enzymes
   d. Autodigestion of the pancreas
8. Which of the following would be included in nursing management of a patient with acute pancreatitis?
   a. Checking for signs of hypercalcemia
   b. Observing stools for signs of steatorrhea
   c. Providing a diet low in carbohydrates with moderate fat
   d. Monitoring for infection, particularly respiratory infection

9. A patient with pancreatic cancer is admitted to the hospital for evaluation for treatment. The patient asks the nurse to describe Whipple's procedure, which the surgeon has planned. Which of the following would the nurse include in her explanation?
   a. Creating a bypass around the obstruction caused by the tumour by joining the gallbladder to the jejunum
   b. Resection of the entire pancreas and the distal portion of the stomach, with anastomosis of the common bile duct and the stomach into the duodenum
   c. Removal of part of the pancreas, part of the stomach, the duodenum, and the gallbladder, with joining of the pancreatic duct, the common bile duct, and the stomach to the jejunum
   d. Radical removal of pancreas, duodenum, and spleen, and attaching the stomach to the jejunum, which requires oral supplementation of pancreatic digestive enzymes and insulin replacement therapy

10. The nursing management of a patient with cholecystitis in association with cholelithiasis should include which of the following?
    a. Recommendation of a low-fat diet
    b. Information that gallstones once removed tend not to recur
    c. Avoidance of morphine in the management of pain
    d. Treatment with oral bile salts that dissolve gallstones

11. What information should be included in teaching about home management after a laparoscopic cholecystectomy?
    a. Keeping the bandages on the puncture sites for 48 hours
    b. Reporting any bile-coloured drainage or pus from any incision
    c. Using over-the-counter antiemetics if nausea and vomiting occur
    d. Emptying and measuring the contents of the bile bag from the T-tube every day

ANSWERS: 1. a; 2. b; 3. b; 4. b; 5. b; 6. a; 7. d; 8. d; 9. c; 10. a; 11. b.

REFERENCES

Aggarwal, R., & Jameel S. (2011). Hepatitis E. *Hepatology, 54*(6), 2218-2226. doi:10.1002/hep.24674

Berenguer, M., Palau, A., Fernandez, A., Benllock, S., Aguilera, V., Prieto, M., …, Berenguer, J. (2006). Efficacy, predictors or response and potential risks associated with antiviral therapy in liver transplant recipients with recurrent hepatitis C. *Liver Transplantation, 12*, 1067-1076. doi:10.1002/lt.20737

Burton, J. R., Sonnenberg, A., & Rosen, H. R. (2004). Retransplantation for recurrent hepatitis C in the MELD era: Maximizing utility. *Liver Transplantation, 10*(Suppl. 2), S59-S64. doi:10.1002/lt.20259

Canadian Cancer Encyclopedia. (2011). Statistics for pancreatic cancer. Retrieved from *http://info.cancer.ca/cce-ecc/default.aspx?Lang=E&toc=36&cceid=1215*

Canadian Institute for Health Information. (2010). e-Statistics Report on Transplant, Waiting List, and Donor Statistics. Table 1A. Retrieved from *http://www.cihi.ca/CIHI-ext-portal/pdf/internet/REPORT_STATS2010_PDF_EN*

Centers for Disease Control and Prevention. (2011). Bloodborne pathogens—Occupational exposure. Retrieved from *http://www.cdc.gov/oralhealth/infectioncontrol/faq/bloodborne_exposures.htm*

El-Serag, H. B. (2011). Hepatocellular carcinoma. *New England Journal of Medicine, 365*, 1118-1127. doi:10.1056/NEJMra1001683

El-Serag, H., Marrero, J., & Rudolph, L. (2008). Diagnosis and treatment of hepatocellular carcinoma. *Gastroenterology, 134*, 1752. doi:10.1053/j.gastro.2008.02.090

Garcia-Tsao, G., Sanyal, A. J., Grace, N. D., Carey, W., & Practice Guidelines Committee of the American Association for the Study of Liver Diseases. (2007). Prevention and management of gastroesophageal varices and variceal hemorrhage in cirrhosis. *Hepatology, 46*, 922-938. doi:10.1002/hep.21907

Haque, M., Scudamore, C. H., Steinbrecher, U. P., Chung, S. W., Buczkowski, A. K., Erb, S. R., & Yoshida, E. M. (2010). Liver transplantation: Current status in British Columbia. *British Columbia Medical Journal, 52*(4), 203-210. Retrieved from *http://www.bcmj.org/article/liver-transplantation-current-status-british-columbia*

Haussinger, D., & Schliess, F. (2008). Pathogenetic mechanisms of hepatic encephalopathy. *Gut, 57*, 1156. doi:10.1136/gut.2007.122176

Hoffman, C., Rockstroh, J. K., & Kamps, B. S. (Eds.) (2007). *HIV medicine 2007*. Paris: Flying Publisher. Retrieved from *http://www.hivmedicine.com/hivmedicine2007.pdf*

Hughes, S., Wedemeyer, H., & Harrison, P. M. (2011). Hepatitis delta virus. *The Lancet, 378*, 73-85. doi:10.1016/S0140-6736(10)61931-9

Kopec, K. L., & Burns, D. (2011). Nonalcoholic fatty liver disease: A review of the spectrum of disease, diagnosis and therapy. *Nutrition in Clinical Practice, 26*(5), 565-576. doi:10.1177/0884533611419668

Lindberg, D. A. (2009). Acute pancreatitis and hypertriglyceridemia. *Gastroenterology Nursing, 32*(2), 75-82. doi:10.1097/SGA.0b013e31819de3e0

Lok, A. S. F., & McMahon, B. J. (2009). Chronic hepatitis B: Update 2009. *Hepatology, 50*(3), 661-662. doi:10.1002/hep.23190

London Health Sciences Centre. (2012). Statistics. Retrieved from *http://www.lhsc.on.ca/About_Us/MOTP/Statistics/index.htm*

Lynch, S. M., Vrieling, A., Lubin, J. H., Kraft, P., Mendelsohn, J. B., Hartge, P., …, Stolzenberg-Solomon, R. Z. (2009). Cigarette smoking and pancreatic cancer: A pooled analysis from the Pancreatic Cancer Cohort Consortium. *American Journal of Epidemiology, 170*, 403-413. doi:10.1093/aje/kwp134

Maitra, A., & Hruban, R. H. (2008). Pancreatic cancer. *Annual Review of Pathology, 3*, 157-188. doi:10.1146/annurev.pathmechdis.3.121806.154305

Marcellin, P., Heathcote, J., Corsa, A., Liu, Y., Miller, M. D., & Kitrinos, K. M. (2011). No detectable resistance to Tenofovir Disoproxil Fumarate (TDF) following up to 240 weeks of treatment in patients with HBeAg+ and HbeAg- chronic hepatitis B virus infection. *Hepatology, 54*(238):480A.

Mukherjee, S. (2008). Hepatorenal syndrome. Retrieved from *http://www.emedicine.com/med/topic1001.htm*

Myers, R. P., Ramji, A., Bilodeau, M., Wong, S., & Feld, J. J. (2012). An update on the management of hepatitis C: Consensus guidelines from the Canadian Association for the Study of the Liver. *Canadian Journal of Gastroenterology, 26*(6), 359-375. Retrieved from *http://www.buksa.com/CASL/2012HepCGuidelines_CJG.pdf*

Premoli, A., Paschetta, E., Hvalryq, M., Spandre, M., Bo, S., & Durazzo, M. (2009). Characteristics of liver diseases in the elderly: A review. *Minerva Gastrointestinologica e Dietologica, 55*(1), 71-78.

Public Health Agency of Canada. (1997). Preventing the transmission of bloodborne pathogens in health care and public service settings. Retrieved from *http://www.collectionscanada.gc.ca/webarchives/20071124030210/http://www.phac-aspc.gc.ca/publicat/ccdr-rmtc/97vol23/23s3/index.html*

Public Health Agency of Canada. (2007a). Canadian immunization guide: Seventh Edition–2006: Hepatitis A. Retrieved from *http://www.phac-aspc.gc.ca/publicat/cig-gci/p04-hepa-eng.php*

Public Health Agency of Canada. (2007b). Canadian immunization guide: Seventh Edition–2006: Hepatitis B. Retrieved from *http://www.phac-aspc.gc.ca/publicat/cig-gci/p04-hepb-eng.php*

Public Health Agency of Canada. (2011). Hepatitis A virus: Pathogen safety data sheet—Infectious substances. Retrieved from *http://www.phac-aspc.gc.ca/lab-bio/res/psds-ftss/hepa-eng.php*

Public Health Agency of Canada. (2012). Hepatitis C fact sheet. Retrieved from *http://www.phac-aspc.gc.ca/hcai-iamss/bbp-pts/hepatitis/hep_c_e.html*

Public Health Agency of Canada & Canadian Institute for Health Information. (2011). Obesity in Canada report. Retrieved from *http://www.phac-aspc.gc.ca/hp-ps/hl-mvs/oic-oac/index-eng.php*

Registered Nurses' Association of Ontario. (2007). Integrating smoking cessation into daily nursing practice. Retrieved from *http://rnao.ca/bpg/guidelines/integrating-smoking-cessation-daily-nursing-practice*

Remis, R. S. (2010). Reaching for the STARHS. *Sexually Transmitted Infections, 86*(7):486-7. doi:10.1136/sti.2010.046771

Sherman, M., Burak, K., Maroun, J., Metrakos, P., Knox, J. J., Myers, R. P., ..., Wong, R. (2011). Multidisciplinary Canadian consensus recommendations for the management and treatment of hepatocellular carcinoma. *Current Oncology, 18*, 228-240. doi:10.3747/co.v18i5.952

Sherman, M., Shafran, S., Burak, K., Doucette, K., Wong, W., Girgrah, N., ..., Deschênes, M. (2007). Management of chronic hepatitis C: Consensus guidelines. *Canadian Journal of Gastroenterology, 21*(Suppl. C), 25C-34C.

Shi, Z., Yang, Y., Wang, H., Ma, L., Schreiber, A., Li, X., & An, Y. (2011). Breastfeeding of newborns by mothers carrying hepatitis B virus: A meta-analysis and systematic review. *Archives of Pediatric & Adolescent Medicine, 165*(9), 837-846. doi:10.1001/archpediatrics.2011.72

Statistics Canada. (2008). Selected leading causes of death, by sex. Retrieved from *http://www5.statcan.gc.ca/bsolc/olc-cel/olc-cel?catno=84-215-x&lang=eng&lang=eng*

Stebbing, J., Farouk, L., Panos, G., Anderson, M., Jiao, L., Mandalia, S., ..., Nelson, M. (2010). A meta-analysis of transient elastography for the detection of hepatic fibrosis. *Journal of Clinical Gastroenterology, 44*(3):214-219. doi:10.1097/MCG.0b013e3181b4af1f

World Health Organization. (2010). The global prevalence of hepatitis A virus infection and susceptibility: A systematic review. Retrieved from *http://whqlibdoc.who.int/hq/2010/WHO_IVB_10.01_eng.pdf*

World Health Organization. (2011). Hepatitis A. Retrieved from *http://www.who.int/biologicals/vaccines/hepatitis_A/en/index.html*

World Health Organization. (2012). Global alert and response: Hepatitis B. Retrieved from *http://www.who.int/csr/disease/hepatitis/whocdscsrlyo20022/en/index3.html*

CANADIAN RESOURCES

BC Centre for Disease Control
http://www.bccdc.ca
Canadian Association for the Study of the Liver
http://www.hepatology.ca/
Canadian Hemophilia Society
http://www.hemophilia.ca
Canadian Liver Foundation
http://www.liver.ca
Canadian Nurses Association: *Hepatitis C—A Nursing Guide*
http://www2.cna-aiic.ca/cna/documents/pdf/publications/Hep_C_2002_e.pdf
CATIE Canada's Source for HIV and Hepatitis C Information
http://www.hepcinfo.ca
Hepatitis Central: Hepatitis C Support Groups
http://www.hepatitis-central.com/hcv/support/canada/toc.html

⊙volve *For additional Internet resources, see the Web site for this book at* **http://evolve.elsevier.com/Canada/Lewis/medsurg**

Problems of Urinary Function

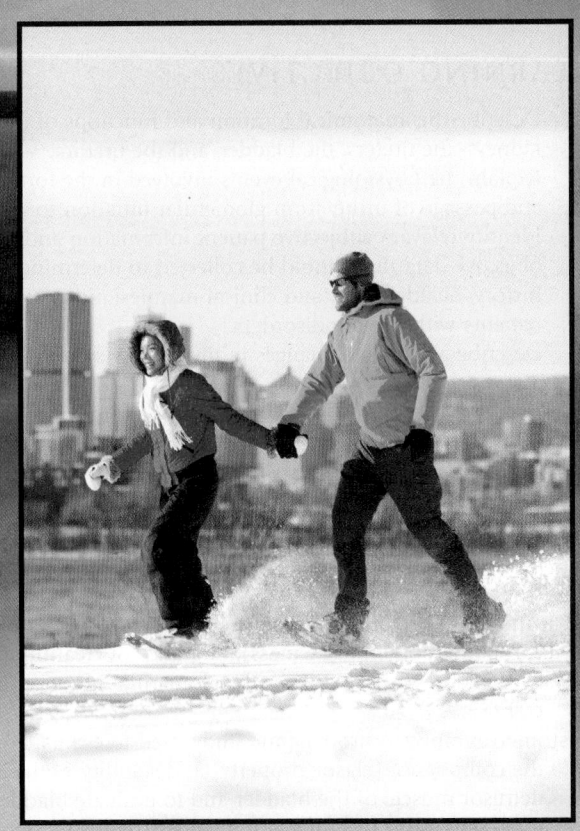

Nursing Assessment: Urinary System

Written by Vicki Y. Johnson

Adapted by Lynn Jansen

LEARNING OBJECTIVES

1. Describe the anatomical location and functions of the kidneys, the ureters, the bladder, and the urethra.
2. Explain the physiological events involved in the formation and passage of urine, from glomerular filtration to voiding.
3. Identify relevant subjective patient information and objective data that should be collected to determine health history, health status, and clinical manifestations of patients with urinary disorders.
4. Describe age-related changes in the urinary system.
5. Describe the appropriate techniques used in the physical assessment of the urinary system.
6. Differentiate normal from common abnormal findings of a physical assessment of the urinary system.
7. Describe the range of tests performed in the analysis of urine.
8. Describe the normal physical and chemical characteristics of urine.

KEY TERMS

costovertebral angle A physical examination landmark used to locate the kidneys, formed by the rib cage and the vertebral column, p. 1276

creatinine A waste product produced by protein breakdown (primarily body muscle mass); clearance of creatinine by the kidney approximates the glomerular filtration rate, p. 1283

cystometrography A urodynamic study used to evaluate the compliance (elastic property) and stability of the detrusor muscle of the bladder and to evaluate bladder tone, sensations of filling, and bladder (detrusor) stability, p. 1285

cystoscopy A radiological bladder procedure in which contrast material is instilled into the bladder to inspect the interior of the bladder and evaluate the vesicoureteral reflux with a tubular lighted instrument called a cystoscope, p. 1285

glomerular filtration rate (GFR) The amount of blood filtered by the glomeruli in a given time, p. 1270

glomerulus A capillary network within the kidneys that comprises up to 50 capillaries, p. 1269

intravenous pyelography (IVP) A diagnostic study in which an intravenous contrast medium circulates in the blood and is excreted through the urinary system; used to evaluate the presence, position, size, and shape of the kidneys, ureters, and bladder, p. 1283

nephron The functional unit of the kidney; each kidney has 800,000 to 1.2 million nephrons, p. 1268

renal arteriography A radiological study performed by injecting contrast material into the renal artery via a catheter inserted into the femoral artery; the purpose is to visualize renal blood vessels, p. 1283

renal biopsy Procedure to obtain renal tissue for examination to establish a diagnosis or to follow progress of renal disease; may be open biopsy or, more commonly, a skin (percutaneous) biopsy conducted through needle insertion into the lower lobe of the kidney, p. 1284

retrograde pyelography Radiographic visualization of the kidneys, the ureter, and the bladder after direct injection of a contrast material into the kidney, p. 1283

urinalysis A general examination of urine for routine and microscopic findings; may establish baseline information, provide information about possible abnormalities, indicate what further studies need to be done, and supply information on the progression of a diagnosed disorder, p. 1278

urodynamics testing A set of studies designed to measure urinary tract function: the storage of urine within the bladder and the flow of urine through the urinary tract to the outside of the body, p. 1285

ELECTRONIC RESOURCES

Supplemental content related to Chapter 47 can be found...

Evolve Web Site ⓔvolve

http://evolve.elsevier.com/Canada/Lewis/medsurg
- Assessment Case Study
- Clinical Reference: Laboratory Values
- Content Updates

- Electronic Calculators
- Examination Review Questions
- Glossary
- Key Points (Printable and MP3 Download)
- Physical Examination Video Clips:
  - Abdomen: Inspection, Auscultation, and Percussion
  - Abdomen: Palpation

"**B**ones can break, muscles can atrophy, glands can loaf, even the brain can go to sleep without immediate danger to survival. But should the kidneys fail...neither bone, muscle, gland, nor brain could carry on" (Smith, 1953). This statement underlines the importance of kidneys to our lives. Adequate functioning of the kidneys is essential to the maintenance of a healthy body. If the kidneys fail completely and treatment is not given, death is inevitable.

The primary functions of the kidneys are (a) to filter waste products from the bloodstream, (b) to maintain fluid and electrolyte and acid–base balance in the body, and (c) to excrete metabolic waste products. The two kidneys perform the primary physiological functions. Secondary functions of the kidneys are to regulate (a) blood pressure, (b) bone density, and (c) erythropoiesis. The kidneys are connected to two narrow tubules, the ureters, which reabsorb 99% of filtered products and transport urine from the kidney to the bladder. Urine flows from the bladder and from the body through the urethra (Figure 47-1).

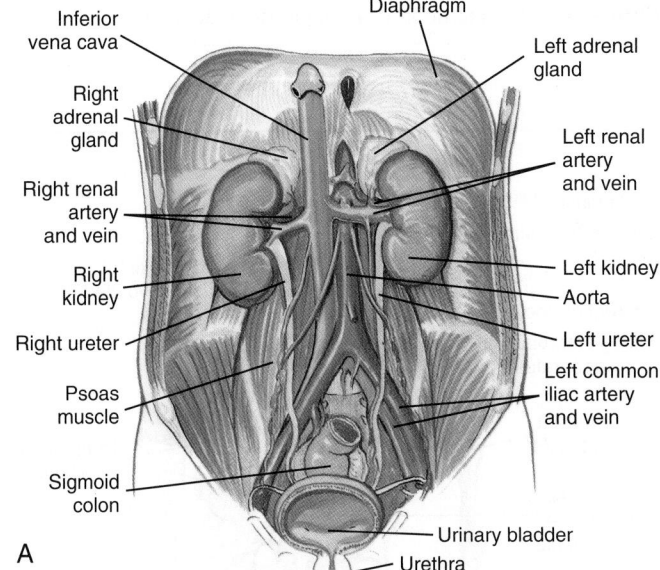

A

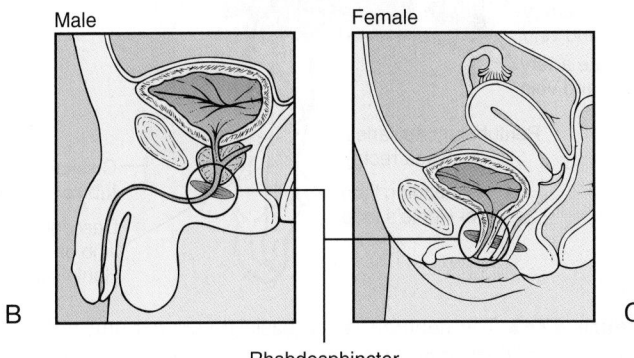

B   C

Rhabdosphincter

Figure 47-1 Illustrations of organs of the urinary system. **A,** Upper urinary tract in relation to other anatomical structures. **B,** Male urethra in relation to other pelvic structures. **C,** Female urethra in relation to other pelvic structures.

Source: A, From Thibodeau, G. A., & Patton, K. T. (2007). *Anatomy and physiology* (6th ed.). St. Louis: Mosby.

Structures and Functions of the Urinary System

Kidneys

Macrostructure. The paired kidneys are bean-shaped organs that are retroperitoneal (behind the peritoneum) on either side of the vertebral column at about the level of the twelfth thoracic (T12) vertebra to the third lumbar (L3) vertebra. Each kidney weighs 115 to 175 g and is about 12 cm long. With the liver above it, the right kidney is at the level of the twelfth rib, lower than the left kidney. An adrenal gland lies on top of each kidney.

Each kidney is surrounded by a considerable amount of fat and connective tissue that serve to support and maintain its position. The surface of the kidney is covered by a thin, smooth layer of fibrous membrane called the *capsule*. These structures protect the kidney and serve as a shock absorber should the kidney be subjected to a sudden force from a blunt object striking the abdomen or back. The *hilus* on the medial side of the kidney serves as the entry site for the renal artery and nerves, as well as the exit site for the renal vein and the ureter.

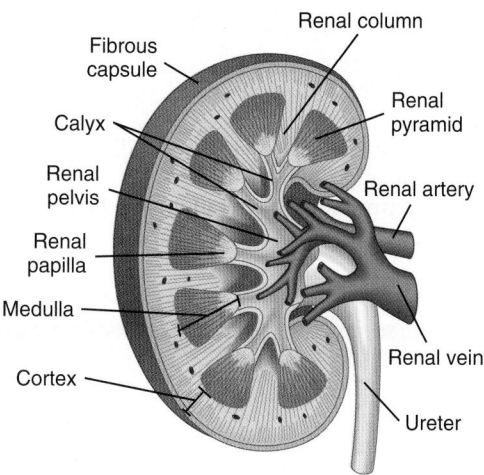

Figure 47-2 Illustration of a longitudinal section of the kidney.

Source: Adapted from Patton, K. T., & Thibodeau, G. A. (2010). *Anatomy and physiology* (7th ed., p. 949, Figure 28-3,*A*). St. Louis: Mosby.

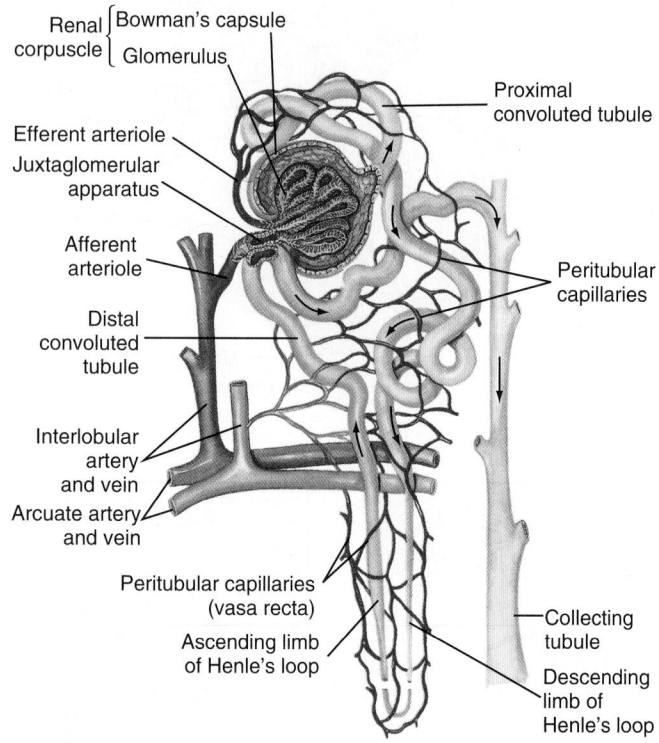

Figure 47-3 The nephron is the basic functional unit of the kidney. This illustration of a single nephron unit also shows the surrounding blood vessels.

Source: From Thibodeau, G. A., & Patton, K. T. (2005). *Anatomy and physiology* (4th ed.). St. Louis: Mosby.

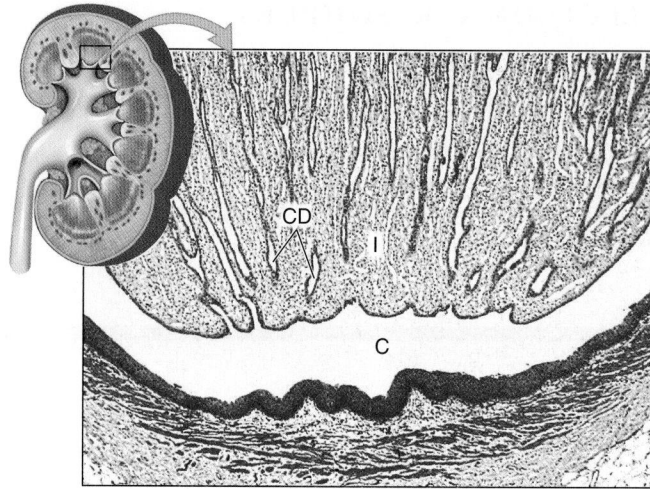

Figure 47-4 Illustration of collecting ducts *(CD)* seen opening into a calyx *(C)* at the papillary tip. The interstitial tissue *(I)* includes some loops of Henle.

Source: From Patton, K. T. & Thibodeau, G. A. (2010). *Anatomy and physiology* (7th ed., p. 957, Figure 28-16). St. Louis: Mosby.

On a longitudinal section of the kidney (Figure 47-2), the parenchyma (actual tissue) of the kidney can be visualized. The outer layer is termed the *cortex*, and the inner layer is called the *medulla*. The medulla consists of a number of pyramids. The apices of these pyramids are called *papillae*, and urine passes through the papillae to enter the calyces. The minor calyces widen and merge to form major calyces, which form a funnel-shaped

sac called the *renal pelvis*. The minor and major calyces transport urine to the renal pelvis in preparation for transportation to the bladder via the ureter. The renal pelvis can store a small volume of urine (3 to 5 mL).

Microstructure. The functional unit of the kidney is the **nephron.** Each kidney has about 1 million nephrons (Quaggin & Kreidberg, 2008). A nephron is composed of a glomerulus, Bowman's capsule, and the tubular system. The tubular system consists of the proximal convoluted tubule, the loop of Henle, and the distal convoluted tubule (Figure 47-3). The glomeruli, Bowman's capsule, the proximal tubule, and the distal tubule are located in the cortex of the kidney. The loop of Henle and the collecting ducts are located in the medulla (Figure 47-4; see also Figure 47-2). Several nephrons converge into a collecting duct, which eventually merges into a pyramid and empties via the papilla into a minor calyx (see Figures 47-2 and 47-4).

Blood Supply. A blood supply of about 1200 mL/min, which is 20 to 25% of total cardiac output, flows to the two kidneys (Tortora & Derrickson, 2006). Blood reaches the kidneys via the renal artery, which arises from the aorta and enters the kidney through the hilus. The renal artery divides into secondary branches and then into still smaller branches, each of which eventually forms an afferent arteriole. The afferent arteriole divides into a capillary network termed the *glomerulus,* which is a tuft of up to 50 capillaries. The capillaries of the glomerulus eventually unite in the efferent arteriole (Figure 47-5). This arteriole splits to form a capillary network called the *peritubular capillaries,* which, as the name suggests, surround the tubular system. All peritubular capillaries eventually drain into the venous system. The renal vein empties into the inferior vena cava.

Physiology of Urine Formation. The process of urine formation is extremely complex. It represents the outcome of a multistep process of filtration, reabsorption, secretion, and excretion of water, electrolytes, and metabolic waste products. Although urine formation is the result of this process, the primary

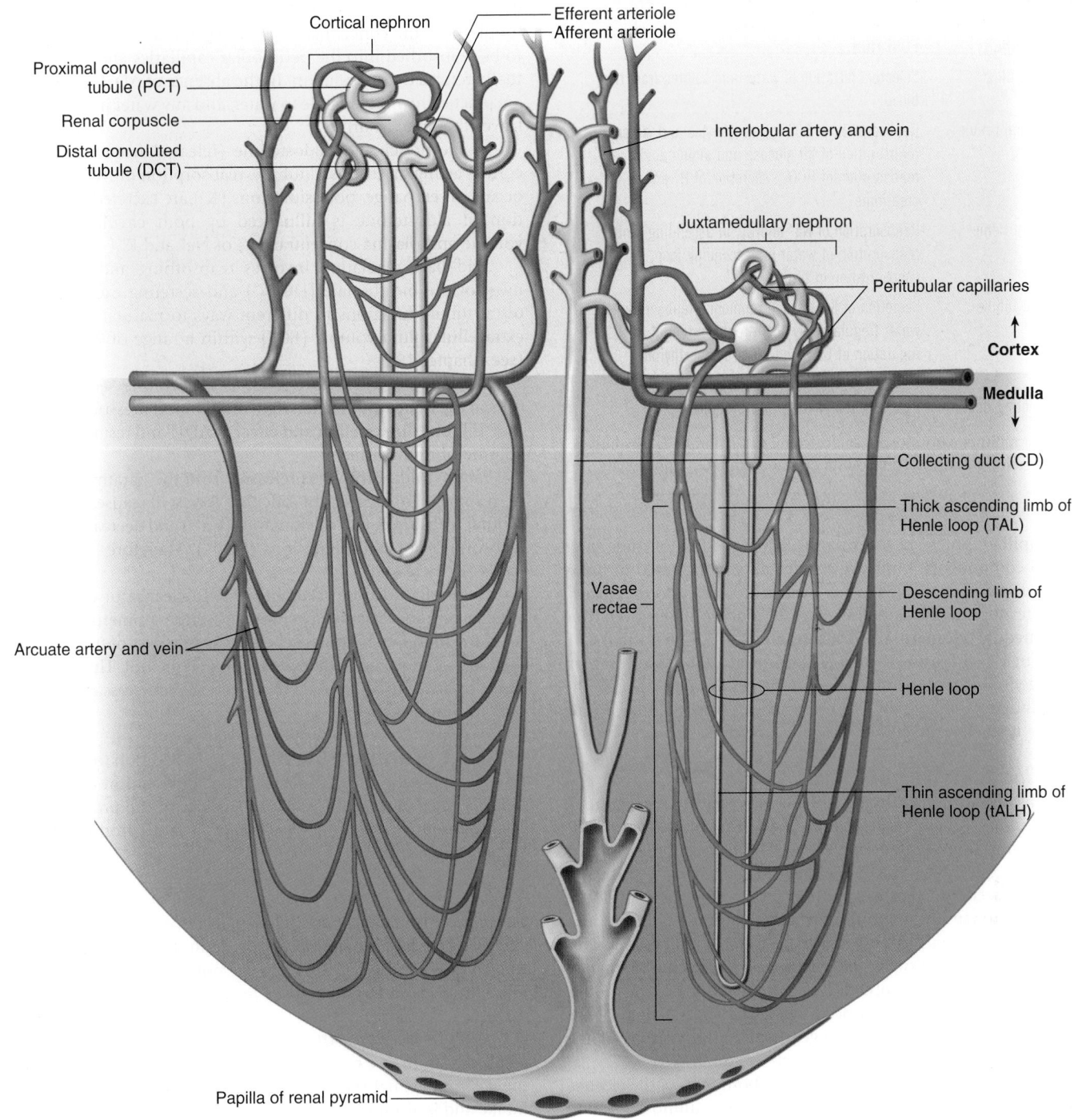

Figure 47-5 Blood supply of nephrons. In this illustration, two types of nephrons (cortical and juxtaglomerular) are shown surrounded by the peritubular blood supply.

Source: From Patton, K. T. & Thibodeau, G. A. (2010). *Anatomy and physiology* (7th ed., p. 957, Figure 28-17). St. Louis: Mosby.

function of the kidneys is to filter the blood and maintain the body's internal homeostasis.

Glomerular Function. Urine formation starts at the glomerulus, where blood is filtered. The **glomerulus,** a capillary network within the kidneys that comprises up to 50 capillaries, is a semipermeable membrane and so allows for filtration (see Figure 47-3). The hydrostatic pressure of the blood within the

glomerular capillaries causes a portion of blood to be filtered across the semipermeable membrane into Bowman's capsule, where the filtered portion of the blood, called the *glomerular filtrate*, begins to pass down to the tubule. Filtration is more rapid in the glomerulus than in ordinary tissue capillaries because of the porosity of the glomerular membrane. The ultrafiltrate is similar in composition to blood except that it lacks blood cells, platelets, and large plasma proteins. Under normal conditions,

Table 47-1 Functions of the Segments of the Nephron	
COMPONENT	**FUNCTION**
Glomerulus	Selective filtration of water and solutes from the blood
Proximal tubule	Reabsorption of 80% of electrolytes and water; reabsorption of all glucose and amino acids; reabsorption of HCO_3^-; secretion of H^+ and creatinine
Loop of Henle	Reabsorption of Na^+ and Cl^- in ascending limb; reabsorption of water in descending loop; concentration of filtrate
Distal tubule	Secretion of K^+, H^+, and ammonia; reabsorption of water (regulated by ADH); reabsorption of HCO_3^-; regulation of Ca^{2+} and PO_4^{2-} by parathyroid hormone, regulation of Na^+ and K^+ by aldosterone
Collecting duct	Reabsorption of water (ADH required)

ADH, antidiuretic hormone; Ca^{2+}, calcium; Cl^-, chloride; H^+, hydrogen; HCO_3^-, bicarbonate; K^+, potassium; Na^+, sodium; PO_4^{2-}, phosphate.

the capillary pores are too small to allow the loss of these large blood components. Capillary permeability is increased in many renal diseases, enabling plasma proteins to pass into the urine.

The amount of blood filtered by the glomeruli in a given time is termed the **glomerular filtration rate (GFR)**. The normal GFR is about 125 mL/min (Tortora & Derrickson, 2006). However, on average, only 1 mL is excreted as urine per minute because the peritubular capillary network reabsorbs most glomerular filtrate before it reaches the end of the collecting duct.

Tubular Function. Because the glomerular membrane is a selective filtration membrane that filters primarily by size, provision is made for the reabsorption of essential materials and the excretion of nonessential ones (Table 47-1). The tubules and the collecting ducts carry out these functions by means of reabsorption and secretion. Reabsorption is the passage of a substance from the lumen of the tubules through the tubule cells and into the capillaries. This process involves both active and passive transport. Tubular secretion is the passage of a substance from the capillaries through the tubular cells into the lumen of the tubule. Reabsorption and secretion occur along the entire length of the tubule, causing numerous changes in the composition of the glomerular filtrate as it moves through the tubules.

In the proximal convoluted tubule, about 80% of the electrolytes are reabsorbed. Normally, all the glucose, amino acids, and small proteins are reabsorbed. For the most part, reabsorption occurs by active transport. Hydrogen ions (H^+) and creatinine are secreted into the filtrate (McCance & Huether, 2010).

The loop of Henle is important in conserving water and thus concentrating the filtrate. Reabsorption continues in the loop of Henle. The descending loop is permeable to water and moderately permeable to sodium, urea, and other solutes. In the ascending limb, chloride ions (Cl^-) are actively reabsorbed, followed passively by sodium ions (Na^+). About 25% of the filtered sodium is reabsorbed in the ascending limb.

Two important functions of the distal convoluted tubules are final regulation of water balance and acid–base balance (Miller, 2009). Antidiuretic hormone (ADH), released by the posterior portion of the pituitary gland, is required for water reabsorption. The stimuli for ADH release are increased serum osmolality and

decreased blood volume. ADH makes the distal convoluted tubules and the collecting ducts permeable to water, allowing it to be reabsorbed into the peritubular capillaries and to be eventually returned to circulation. In the absence of ADH, the tubules are practically impermeable to water, and any water in the tubules leaves the body as urine.

In the presence of aldosterone (released from the adrenal cortex) acting on the distal tubule, reabsorption of Na^+ and water occurs. In exchange, potassium ions (K^+) are excreted. The secretion of aldosterone is influenced by both circulating blood volume and plasma concentrations of Na^+ and K^+.

Acid–base regulation involves reabsorbing and conserving most of the bicarbonate (HCO_3^-) and secreting excess H^+. The distal tubule functions in different ways to maintain the pH of extracellular fluid volume (ECF) within a range of 7.35 to 7.45 (see Chapter 19).

Atrial natriuretic factor (ANF) is a hormone secreted from cells in the right atrium when right atrial blood pressure increases. ANF inhibits the secretion and effect of ADH and results in a large volume of dilute urine.

Parathyroid hormone is released from the parathyroid gland in response to low serum calcium levels. It causes increased tubular reabsorption of calcium ions (Ca^{2+}) and decreased tubular reabsorption of phosphate ions (PO_4^{2-}). Therefore, serum Ca^{2+} levels are increased.

The basic function of nephrons is to cleanse or clear blood plasma of unnecessary substances. After the glomerulus has filtered the blood, the tubules separate the portions of tubular fluid that are useful to the body from those that are not. The necessary portions are returned to the blood, and the unnecessary portions pass into urine as waste.

Other Functions of the Kidney. In addition to their function of regulating the volume and the composition of ECF, the kidneys have other vital functions, including the production of erythropoietin, activation of vitamin D, and production and secretion of renin.

Production of Erythropoietin. Erythropoietin is a hormone produced by the kidney and released in response to hypoxia and decreased renal blood flow. Erythropoietin stimulates the production of red blood cells (RBCs) in the bone marrow. A deficiency of erythropoietin in renal failure leads to anemia.

Activation of Vitamin D. Metabolites of vitamin D, a fat-soluble vitamin, are essential for the absorption of calcium from the gastrointestinal (GI) tract. Vitamin D is obtained from food intake and is also produced in interaction with cholesterol in the skin after exposure to sunlight or ultraviolet radiation. The raw forms of vitamin D are inactive, and two more reactions are needed for those forms to become active metabolites or steroid hormones. The first step in activation occurs in the liver. The second step occurs in the kidneys. Patients with renal failure have a deficiency of an active metabolite of vitamin D and manifest problems related to altered calcium and phosphate balance (see Chapter 49).

Production and Secretion of Renin. Renin, an enzyme, is important in the regulation of blood pressure. Renin is released from the *juxtaglomerular apparatus* of the nephron (Figure 47-6) in response to decreased arterial blood pressure, renal ischemia, ECF depletion, increased norepinephrine, and increased urinary Na^+ concentration. Renin catalyzes the splitting of the plasma

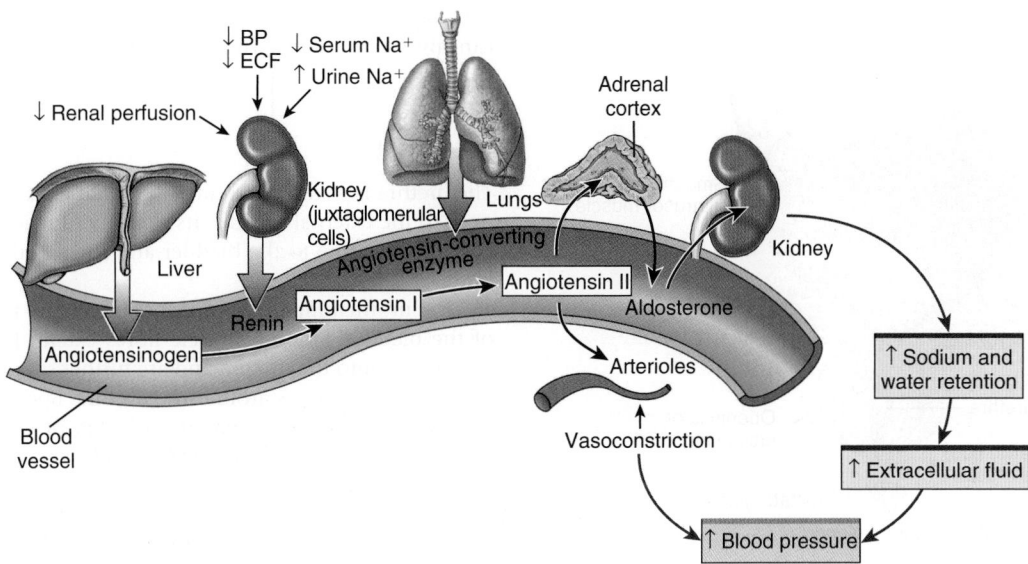

Figure 47-6 Renin-angiotensin-aldosterone system.

BP, blood pressure; *ECF*, extracellular fluid; *Na⁺*, sodium ion.
Source: Adapted from Herlihy, B. (2007). *The human body in health and illness* (3rd ed., p. 432, Figure 24-3). Philadelphia: W. B. Saunders.

protein angiotensinogen (from the liver) into angiotensin I, which is subsequently converted to angiotensin II by a converting enzyme made in the lungs. Angiotensin II stimulates the release of aldosterone from the adrenal cortex, which causes retention of Na⁺ and water, leading to an increase in ECF. Angiotensin II also causes increases in peripheral vasoconstriction. The increases in ECF and vasoconstriction cause an elevation in blood pressure, which inhibits renin release. Excessive renin production caused by impaired renal perfusion may be a contributing factor in hypertension (see Chapters 35 and 49). ANF acts directly on the medullary collecting ducts and indirectly on other tubular segments (by inhibiting several steps in the renin-angiotensin-aldosterone pathway) to inhibit sodium reabsorption. It inhibits secretion of renin and aldosterone and causes an increase in GFR (through its effects on the renal arterioles), all of which increase excretion of sodium and water.

Prostaglandins (PGs) are synthesized by most body tissues from the precursor, arachidonic acid. PGs, which are involved in the regulation of cell function, exert their influence primarily on cells or tissues that are close to the site where they are synthesized. (See Chapter 14 for a more detailed discussion of PGs.)

In the kidney, PG synthesis (primarily PGE₂ and PGI₂) occurs primarily in the medulla. These PGs have a vasodilating action in addition to increasing renal blood flow and promoting Na⁺ excretion. They also counteract the vasoconstrictor effect of substances such as angiotensin and norepinephrine. Renal PGs may have a systemic effect in lowering blood pressure by decreasing systemic vascular resistance (Kiela & Ghishan, 2009). In addition, they are associated with hypertension that develops in renal failure. With a loss of functioning tissue, these renal vasodilators are also lost (see Chapter 49).

Ureters

The ureters are tubes approximately 25 to 35 cm long and 2 to 8 mm in diameter that carry urine from the renal pelvis to the bladder (see Figure 47-1). The narrow area where the ureter joins the renal pelvis is termed the *ureteropelvic junction*. After coursing down along the psoas muscle, the ureter crosses over the pelvic brim and the iliac artery and inserts into the base of the bladder at the *ureterovesical junction* (UVJ). The ureteral lumen is narrowest at these junctions; consequently, they are often the sites of urinary stone (calculi) obstruction. Because the lumen of the ureter is narrow, it can be easily occluded internally (e.g., by calculi) or externally (e.g., by tumours, adhesions, or inflammation).

Sympathetic and parasympathetic nerves, along with the vascular supply, surround the mucosal lining of the ureter. Circular and longitudinal smooth muscle fibres are arranged in a meshlike outer layer and contract to promote the peristaltic one-way flow of urine. These muscle contractions can be affected by distension, as well as by neurological, endocrine, and pharmacological factors. Stimulation of these nerves during passage of a stone or clot may cause acute, severe pain termed *renal colic*.

Because the renal pelvis holds only 3 to 5 mL of urine, kidney damage can result from a backflow of more than that amount of urine. The UVJ relies on the ureter's angle of bladder penetration and muscle fibre attachments with the bladder to prevent the backflow of urine (reflux) and ascending infection. The distal ureter entering the bladder has more longitudinal muscle fibres than the upper ureter. This segment enters the bladder laterally at its base, courses along obliquely through the bladder wall for about 1.5 cm, and intermingles with muscle fibres of the bladder base. Circular and longitudinal bladder muscle fibres adjacent to the embedded ureter help secure it. When bladder pressure rises (e.g., during voiding or coughing), muscle fibres that the ureter shares with the bladder base contract first to help promote urethral lumen closure. The bladder then contracts against its base to further close the UVJ and prevent urine from moving back through the junction.

Bladder

The urinary bladder is a distensible organ positioned behind the symphysis pubis and is anterior to the vagina and the rectum. (Figure 47-7 shows the male urinary bladder.) Its primary

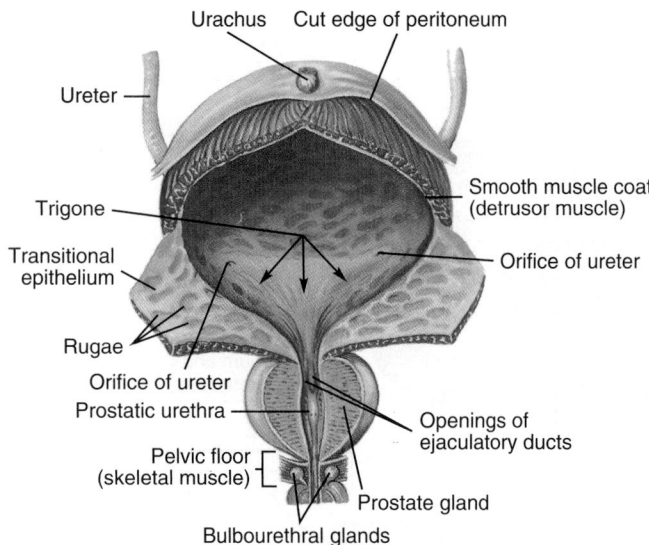

Figure 47-7 Illustration of the male urinary bladder.

Source: Adapted from Patton, K. T., & Thibodeau, G. A. (2010). *Anatomy and physiology* (7th ed., p. 950, Figure 28-5). St. Louis: Mosby.

functions are to serve as a reservoir for urine and to help the body eliminate waste products. Normal adult urine output is approximately 1500 mL/day, which varies with food and fluid intake. The volume of urine produced at night is less than half of that formed during the day because of hormonal influences (e.g., ADH). This diurnal pattern of urination is normal. Most people urinate five to six times during the day and only occasionally at night.

The triangular area formed by the two ureteral openings and the bladder neck at the base of the bladder is the *trigone*. It is affixed to the pelvis by many ligaments, and it does not change its shape during bladder filling or emptying. The bladder muscle, the *detrusor*, is composed of layers of intertwined smooth muscle fibres and is capable of considerable distension during bladder filling and contraction during emptying. It is affixed to the abdominal wall by an umbilical ligament. As the bladder fills, it rises toward the umbilicus. The dome, anterior, and lateral aspects of the bladder expand and contract. When the bladder is empty, it appears as multiple folds within the pelvis.

On average, 200 to 250 mL of urine in the bladder causes moderate distension and the urge to urinate. When the quantity of urine reaches about 400 to 600 mL, the person feels uncomfortable. Bladder capacity varies with the individual, usually ranging from 600 to 1000 mL. Evacuation of urine is termed *urination, micturition,* or *voiding*.

The lining of the bladder is identical to that of the renal pelvis, the ureter, and the bladder neck. It is called *transitional cell epithelium* or *urothelium* and is unique to the urinary tract. Transitional cell epithelium is resistant to absorption of urine. Therefore, urinary wastes produced by the kidneys do not leak out of the urinary system after they leave the kidneys. Microscopically, transitional cell epithelium is several cells deep. These cells stretch out in the bladder so that the epithelium is only a few cells deep as it accommodates filling. As the bladder empties, the epithelium resumes its multicellular layer formation.

Because the linings of these organs are similar, transitional cell tumours that occur in one section of the urinary tract can easily metastasize to other urinary tract areas. Malignant cells may move down from upper urinary tract tumours and

become established in the bladder, or large bladder tumours can invade the ureter. Tumour recurrence within the bladder is common.

Urethra

The urethra is a small muscular tube that leads from the bladder neck to the external meatus. Its primary function is to serve as a conduit for urine to the bladder and then to the outside of the body.

The urothelium and submucosal layers are the same as those of the bladder. Smooth muscle fibres extend from the bladder neck down into the urethra and are further supported by circular smooth muscle fibres around the urethra. Special C-shaped striated muscle fibres (the rhabdosphincter, or external sphincter) surround a portion of the urethra and, when bladder pressure increases, voluntarily contract and prevent leaking.

The female urethra is 3 to 5 cm long and lies behind the symphysis pubis but anterior to the vagina (see Figure 47-1, *C*). The rhabdosphincter encircles the middle third of the urethra. The shortness of the urethra is a contributing factor to the increased incidence of urinary tract infections in women.

The male urethra, which is about 20 to 25 cm long, originates at the bladder neck and extends the length of the penis (see Figure 47-1, *B*). It is often viewed as consisting of three parts. The prostatic urethra extends from the bladder neck through the prostate to the urogenital diaphragm. The membranous urethra passes through the urogenital diaphragm. The rhabdosphincter encircles this portion. Because of the concentrated muscular support, this short portion is not very expandable. As a consequence, stricture formation in this area after instrumentation is common. The penile urethra continues through the corpus spongiosum, a cavernous penile body, through the urogenital diaphragm to a distal dilated area, the fossa navicularis, before terminating at the meatus.

Urethrovesical Unit Function

Together, the bladder, the urethra, and the pelvic floor muscles form the *urethrovesical unit*. Normal voluntary control of this unit is defined as *continence*. Various areas of the brain send stimulating and inhibiting impulses to the thoracolumbar (T11 to L2) and sacral (S2-4) areas of the spinal cord to control voiding. Distension of the bladder stimulates stretch receptors within the bladder wall. Impulses are transmitted to the sacral spinal cord and then to the brain, causing a desire to urinate. If the time is not appropriate for voiding, inhibitor impulses in the brain are stimulated and transmitted back to the thoracolumbar and sacral nerves innervating the bladder. In a coordinated manner, the detrusor accommodates to the pressure (does not contract) while the sphincter and pelvic floor muscles tighten to resist bladder pressure. If the time is appropriate for voiding, cerebral inhibition is voluntarily suppressed, and impulses are transmitted via the spinal cord for the bladder neck, the sphincter, and the pelvic floor muscles to relax and for the bladder to contract. The sphincter closes, and the detrusor muscle relaxes when the bladder is empty.

Any disease or trauma that affects function of the brain, the spinal cord, or the nerves that directly innervate the bladder, the bladder neck, the external sphincter, or the pelvic floor can affect bladder function. These conditions include diabetes mellitus, paraplegia, and tetraplegia (quadriplegia). Drugs affecting nerve transmission also can affect bladder function.

AGE-RELATED CONSIDERATIONS: EFFECTS OF AGING ON THE URINARY SYSTEM

Anatomical changes in the aging kidney include a 20 to 30% decrease in size and weight between the ages of 30 and 90 years. This loss in renal mass is predominantly in the cortex. The aging nephron fails as a unit because glomerular and tubular function appears to decrease at the same rate. By the seventh decade of life, 30 to 50% of glomeruli have lost their function. Despite losing this original kidney volume, older individuals maintain body fluid homeostasis unless they encounter diseases or other physiological stressors (Cheung, Ponnusamy, & Anderton, 2008).

Blood flow to and within the kidneys also decreases with age. There is no evidence, however, that atherosclerotic vascular disease is primarily responsible for the age-related changes in the kidneys.

Physiological changes in the aging kidney include a decrease in renal blood flow; a decrease in GFR; and decreases in the abilities to conserve Na^+, dilute or concentrate urine, and excrete an acid load. Under normal conditions, the aging kidney is able to maintain homeostasis, but after abrupt changes in blood volume, acid load, or other insults, the kidney may not be able to function effectively because much of its renal reserve has been lost (Liamis, Milionis, & Elisaf, 2008).

Physiological changes also occur in the aging bladder and urethra. Estrogen receptors exist in the female urethra, bladder, vagina, and pelvic floor. As estrogen levels decrease with age, tissues become less elastic, thin, and less vascular. Estrogen replacement may be prescribed to minimize these changes. Periurethral striated muscle fibres and muscles supporting the bladder relax. Consequently, older women are more prone to urethral irritation, urinary incontinence, and urethral and bladder infections (Baum, 2006). Although urinary incontinence in older women has long been associated with diminished estrogen levels, the incidence of incontinence has been found to be higher in menopausal women who use hormone replacement therapy (Palmer & Newman, 2007). These findings may promote changes in therapy for postmenopausal urinary incontinence. Men's prostates enlarge as they age, and because the prostate surrounds the proximal urethra, increasing prostate size may affect urinary patterns in men, causing hesitancy, retention, slow stream, and bladder infections. Constipation, a complaint often expressed by older adults, can also affect urination. Partial urethral obstruction may occur because of the rectum's close proximity to the urethra. (See the guidelines of the Registered Nurses' Association of Ontario [2011] for management of urinary incontinence.)

A summary of age-related changes in the urinary system and differences in assessment findings is presented in Table 47-2.

Assessment of the Urinary System

Subjective Data

Important Health Information

Past Health History. The patient should be questioned about the presence or history of diseases that are known to be related to renal or other urological problems. Some of these diseases are hypertension, diabetes mellitus, gout and other metabolic problems, connective tissue disorders (e.g., systemic lupus erythema-

AGE-RELATED DIFFERENCES IN ASSESSMENT

Table 47-2 Urinary System

CHANGES	DIFFERENCES IN ASSESSMENT FINDINGS
Kidney	
↓ Amount of renal tissue	Less palpable
↓ Number of nephrons and renal blood vessels; thickened basement membrane of Bowman's capsule and glomeruli	↓ Creatinine clearance, ↑ BUN level
↓ Function of loop of Henle and tubules	Alterations in drug excretion; nocturia; loss of normal diurnal excretory pattern because of ↓ ability to concentrate urine; less concentrated urine
Ureter, Bladder, and Urethra	
↓ Elasticity and muscle tone	Palpable bladder after urination because of retention
Weakening of urinary sphincter	Stress incontinence (especially during Valsalva's manoeuvre), dribbling of urine after urination
↓ Bladder capacity and sensory receptors	Frequency, urgency, nocturia, overflow incontinence
Estrogen deficiency, leading to thinning and dryness of vaginal tissue	Stress or overactive bladder, dysuria
↑ Prevalence of unstable bladder contractions	Overactive bladder
Prostatic enlargement	Hesitancy, frequency, urgency, nocturia, straining to urinate, retention, dribbling

BUN, blood urea nitrogen.

tosus, systemic sclerosis [scleroderma]), skin or upper respiratory infections of streptococcal origin, tuberculosis, viral hepatitis, congenital disorders, neurological conditions (e.g., stroke, back injury), and trauma. Specific urinary problems such as cancer, infections, benign prostatic hyperplasia, and calculi should be noted.

Medications. An assessment of the patient's current and past use of medications is important. This list should include over-the-counter drugs, prescription medications, and herbs. Drugs affect the urinary tract in several ways. Many drugs are known to be nephrotoxic (Table 47-3). Certain drugs may alter the quantity and the character of urine output (e.g., diuretics). Numerous drugs such as phenazopyridine (Pyridium) and nitrofurantoin change urine colour. Anticoagulants may cause hematuria. Many antidepressants, calcium channel blockers, antihistamines, and drugs used to treat neurological and musculoskeletal disorders affect the ability of the bladder or the sphincter to contract or relax normally.

Surgery and Other Treatments. The patient should also be questioned about any previous hospitalizations related to renal or urological diseases and about all urinary problems during past

Table 47-3 Potentially Nephrotoxic Agents	
Antibiotics	**Other Agents**
• Amikacin	• Anaesthetics
• Amphotericin B	• Captopril
• Bacitracin	• Cimetidine
• Cephalosporins	• Cisplatin
• Gentamicin	• Cocaine
• Kanamycin	• Contrast medium
• Neomycin	• Cyclosporine (Neoral, Sandimmune)
• Polymyxin B	• Ethylene glycol
• Streptomycin	• Gold
• Sulphonamides	• Heavy metals
• Tobramycin	• Heroin
• Vancomycin	• Lithium
	• Methotrexate
	• Nitrosoureas (e.g., carmustine)
	• Nonsteroidal anti-inflammatory drugs (e.g., ibuprofen, indomethacin)
	• Phenacetin
	• Quinine
	• Rifampin
	• Salicylate (large quantities)

pregnancies. The duration, the severity, and the patient's perception of any problem and its treatment should be sought. Past surgical procedures, particularly pelvic surgery, and urinary tract instrumentation should be documented. Information should be obtained from the patient about any radiation or chemotherapy treatment for cancer.

Key Questions. Nurses must convey sensitivity and understanding while asking urinary health assessment questions to maintain the patient's physical and emotional comfort. Key questions to ask a patient with problems related to the urinary system are listed in Table 47-4.

Health History. The nurse should ask about the patient's general health, particularly when disease affecting the kidneys is suspected. Sometimes responses such as "feeling tired all the time," changes in weight or appetite, excess thirst, fluid retention, and complaints of headache, pruritus, or blurred vision may be related to abnormal kidney function. Similarly, in older patients, malaise and nonlocalized abdominal discomfort may be the only symptoms of a urinary tract infection (Liang & Mackowiak, 2007).

An occupational history should be taken. Exposure to certain chemicals can affect the kidneys and the urinary tract system. Phenol and ethylene glycol are examples of nephrotoxic chemicals. Aromatic amines and certain organic chemicals may increase the risk of bladder cancers. Textile workers, painters, hairdressers, and industrial workers have a high incidence of bladder tumours.

A smoking history should be obtained. Cigarette smoking is a major factor in the risk for bladder cancer. Bladder tumours occur four times more frequently in cigarette smokers than in nonsmokers.

Places where a patient has lived may affect the incidence and prevalence of renal disease. Higher mineral content of the soil and water may be a contributing factor. People living in Middle Eastern countries or Africa can acquire certain parasites that can cause cystitis or bladder cancer.

A family history of certain renal or urological problems increases the likelihood that similar problems will occur in the patient. The nurse should ask about family members who have had any of the diseases referred to in the past health history, as well as polycystic renal disease and congenital urinary tract abnormalities, such as Alport's syndrome (congenital nephritis).

Nutritional Assessment. The usual quantity and types of fluid that a patient drinks are important information in relation to urinary tract disease. Dehydration may contribute to urinary infections, calculi formation, and renal failure. Large intake of particular foods, such as dairy products or foods high in proteins, may also lead to calculi formation. Asparagus may cause the urine to smell musty, and redness of urine caused by beet ingestion may be mistaken for blood. Coffee, alcohol, carbonated beverages, or spicy foods often aggravate urinary inflammatory diseases. An unexplained weight gain may be the result of fluid retention secondary to a renal problem. Anorexia, nausea, and vomiting can dramatically affect fluid status and require careful assessment. Information on vitamin and mineral supplements and herbal therapies should be obtained. The patient may not think of these supplements and therapies when listing over-the-counter drugs; supplements are often considered part of nutritional intake.

Elimination Assessment. Questions about urine elimination patterns are the cornerstone of the health history in patients with a lower urinary tract disorder. This line of inquiry begins with a question of how patients manage urine elimination. The majority of patients eliminate urine by spontaneous voiding, and they should be asked about daytime (diurnal) voiding frequency and the frequency of nocturia. Patients should also be queried about additional bothersome lower urinary tract symptoms, including urgency, incontinence, or urinary retention. Table 47-5 lists some of the common clinical manifestations of urinary tract disorders. Changes in the colour and the appearance of urine are often significant and should be evaluated. If blood is visible in the urine, it should be determined whether it occurs at the beginning, throughout, or at the end of urination.

Bowel function should also be investigated. Problems with fecal incontinence may signal neurological causes of bladder problems because of shared nerve pathways. Constipation and fecal impaction can partially obstruct the urethra, causing inadequate bladder emptying, overflow incontinence, and infection.

The nurse should find out patients' methods of handling a urinary problem. A patient may already be using a catheter or collection device. Sometimes a patient has to assume a particular position to urinate or must perform such manoeuvres as pressing on the lower abdomen (Credé method), straining (Valsalva manoeuvre), or stretching the rectum to empty the bladder.

Activity Assessment. The patient's level of activity should be assessed. A sedentary person is more likely than an active individual to have stasis of urine, which can predispose to infection and calculi. Demineralization of bones in a person with limited physical activity causes increased urine calcium precipitation.

An active person may find that increasing activity aggravates a urinary problem. A patient who has had prostate surgery or who

HEALTH HISTORY

Table 47-4 Urinary System: Questions for Obtaining Subjective Data

Health History

- How is your energy level in comparison with that of a year ago?
- Have you ever smoked? If yes, how many packs per day?
- What occupations or work positions have you held?
- Do you have any history of kidney disease, kidney stones, urinary tract infections?*
- Have you had any tests or surgical procedures on your kidney, bladder, or [in men] prostate?*
- Do certain activities aggravate any urinary problems you might have?*
- Have urinary problems caused you to alter or stop any activity or exercise?*
- How do you move or get to the bathroom?*
- What medications are you currently taking?*
- Do you take vitamin or mineral supplements?*

Nutritional Assessment

- How much and what kinds of fluids do you drink daily? Describe when fluid intake occurs over a day.
- Do you drink coffee? Colas? Alcohol? How often? How much?
- Do you eat chocolate? How often? How much?
- Do you spice your food heavily?*

Elimination Assessment

- Do you ever have difficulty holding your urine (water) long enough to get to the toilet? [Or] How long can you hold your urine after you first feel the need to go to the bathroom?
- Do you ever leak urine? If so, what causes urine leakage? Do you leak when you cough or sneeze, laugh, walk, run, or lift a heavy object? Do you leak when you touch a doorknob or attempt to open the bathroom door or if you are unable to reach a toilet right away? When did the leaking begin?
- What have you done to manage the problem of leaking? (Have you cut down on the amount of fluids that you drink? Do you empty your bladder as a precautionary measure?)
- Are there certain things that make the problem worse or better?
- Does it happen all of the time, or just at certain times?
- Are you able to sit through a 2-hour meeting or ride in a car for 2 hours without urinating?
- Do you ever leak urine at night? If so, how often and how much do you leak? [If the response is affirmative, the nurse should try to differentiate between this symptom and the habit of going to the bathroom after waking up for some other reason.]
- Do you ever find that you have leaked without awareness of doing so?

- Do you use special devices or supplies for urine elimination or control? If so, (a) What types of devices or supplies do you use? (b) How often do you use these devices or supplies? (c) How many of these devices or supplies do you use on a daily basis?
- Immediately after urinating (passing your water), does it feel as if you have not emptied your bladder completely? Do you experience any hesitancy and straining? A weakened force of stream? Any dribbling?
- Do you have to exert pressure during urination to feel as if your bladder is being completely emptied?
- [Men] When you urinate (pass water), do you have any difficulty starting the stream or keeping the stream going?
- Do you ever notice blood in your urine?* If so, at what point in the urination does it occur?
- How often do you move your bowels? Do you ever experience constipation (hardened stools that are difficult to pass or a sensation that you are unable to completely evacuate your bowels)?

Activity Assessment

- Have you changed any of your activities because you need to stay near a toilet?
- Do you avoid going to certain places because of difficulty holding your urine (water)?

Pain Assessment

- Do you ever have pain when you urinate?* If so, where is the pain?
- [Women] Do you feel any pressure in your pelvic area?

Self-Concept Assessment

- How does the urinary problem make you feel about yourself?
- Have you been perceiving your body differently since the urinary problem developed?
- Does the urinary problem interfere with your relationships with family or friends?*
- Has the urinary problem caused a change in your job status or affected your ability to carry out job-related responsibilities?*

Sexuality Assessment

- Has the urinary problem caused any change in your sexual pleasure or performance?*
- Do you ever notice any blood or red-tinged urine when you urinate after intercourse?

Coping Assessment

- Have you ever sought help or talked to a primary care provider or other health care professional about this problem?
- Do you feel able to manage the problems associated with your urinary problem? If not, explain.
- What strategies are you using to cope with your urinary problem?

*Describe.

Source: Adapted from Jarvis, C., Browne, A. J., MacDonald-Jenkins, J., & Luctkar-Flude, M. (Eds.). (2008). *Physical examination and health assessment* (1st Canadian ed., pp. 759-763). Toronto: Elsevier Canada; and Miller, C. A. (2009). Urinary function. In C. A. Miller (Ed.), *Nursing for wellness in older adults* (5th ed., pp. 390-416). Philadelphia: Lippincott Williams & Wilkins.

Table 47-5 Clinical Manifestations of Disorders of the Urinary System

General Manifestations

- Anorexia
- Blurred vision
- Chills
- Change in body weight
- Change in mentation
- Excess thirst
- Fatigue
- Headaches
- Hypertension
- Itching
- Nausea and vomiting

Urinary System Symptoms

Pain

- Dysuria
- Flank or costovertebral angle
- Groin
- Suprapubic

Changes in Patterns of Urination

- Change in stream
- Dribbling
- Dysuria
- Frequency
- Hesitancy of stream
- Incontinence
- Nocturia
- Overactive bladder
- Retention
- Stress incontinence
- Urgency

Changes in Urine Output

- Anuria
- Oliguria
- Polyuria

Changes in Urine Composition

- Colour (red, brown, yellowish green)
- Increased concentration
- Dilution
- Hematuria
- Pyuria

Edema

- Anasarca
- Ankle
- Ascites
- Facial (periorbital)
- Sacral

has weakened pelvic floor muscles may leak urine when attempting particular activities such as running. Some men may develop chronic inflammatory prostatitis or epididymitis after heavy lifting or long-distance driving.

Nocturia is a common and a particularly bothersome lower urinary tract symptom that often leads to sleep deprivation, daytime sleepiness, and fatigue. It occurs in multiple disorders affecting the lower urinary tract, including urinary incontinence, urinary retention, and interstitial cystitis. Nocturia also may be attributable to polyuria from renal disease, poorly controlled diabetes mellitus, alcoholism, excessive fluid intake, or obstructive sleep apnea. When the nurse asks the patient about nocturia, it is helpful to determine whether the desire to urinate is what causes the patient to arise from sleep or whether pain or some other symptom interrupts sleep and the person urinates as a matter of habit before returning to bed. Up to one episode of nocturia is considered normal in younger adults, and up to two episodes are considered acceptable among adults age 65 years or older. Sleep problems associated with a urinary disorder should be documented. Older adults may awaken many times during the night to urinate and may need to be assured that this may be normal. However, a complete assessment should be made to rule out any problem.

Pain Assessment. Pain is a frequent symptom of urinary tract disease. Types of pain associated with renal and urological problems include dysuria, groin pain, costovertebral pain, and suprapubic pain. If pain is present, the location, the character, and the duration should be assessed. The absence of pain when other urinary symptoms exist is also significant. Many urinary tract tumours are painless in the early stages.

Self-Concept Assessment. Problems associated with the urinary system—such as incontinence, urinary diversion procedures, and chronic fatigue—can result in loss of self-esteem and a negative body image. Sensitive questioning may elicit cues to problems in this area.

Relationship and Sexuality Assessment. Urinary problems can affect many aspects of a person's life, including the ability to work and relationships with others. These factors have important implications for future treatment and management. The nurse must be alert to cues from the patient.

Urinary system problems may be serious enough to cause problems in job-related and social situations. Chronic dialysis therapy often makes regular employment or full-time homemaking difficult. Also, concurrent poor health and negative body image can seriously alter existing roles. The nurse should assess this area to plan appropriate interventions.

The nurse should ask about the effect of a renal or urological problem on the patient's sexual patterns and satisfaction. Problems related to personal hygiene and fatigue can seriously affect a sexual relationship. Although urinary incontinence is not directly associated with sexual dysfunction, it often has a devastating effect on self-esteem and on social and intimate relationships. Counselling of both the patient and the partner may be indicated.

Objective Data

Physical Examination

Inspection. The nurse should assess for changes in the following:

Skin: Pallor, yellow-grey cast, excoriations, changes in turgor, bruises, texture (e.g., rough, dry skin)

Mouth: Stomatitis, ammonia breath odour

Face and extremities: Generalized edema, peripheral edema, bladder distension, masses, enlarged kidneys

Abdomen: Skin changes described earlier, as well as striae, abdominal contour for midline mass in lower abdomen (may indicate urinary retention) or unilateral mass (occasionally observed in adults, indicating enlargement of one or both kidneys from large tumour or polycystic kidney)

Weight: Weight gain secondary to edema; weight loss and muscle wasting in renal failure.

General state of health: Fatigue, lethargy, and diminished alertness

Palpation. The kidneys are posterior organs protected by the abdominal organs, the ribs, and the heavy back muscles. A landmark useful in locating the kidneys is the **costovertebral angle** (CVA) formed by the rib cage and the vertebral column. The normal-sized left kidney is rarely palpable because the spleen lies directly on top of it. On occasion, the lower pole of the right kidney is palpable.

To palpate the right kidney, the examiner's left hand is placed behind and supports the patient's right side between the rib cage and the iliac crest (Figure 47-8). The patient's right flank is elevated with the examiner's left hand, and the examiner's right hand is used to palpate deeply for the patient's right kidney. The lower pole of the right kidney may feel like a smooth, rounded mass that descends on inspiration. If the kidney is palpable, its

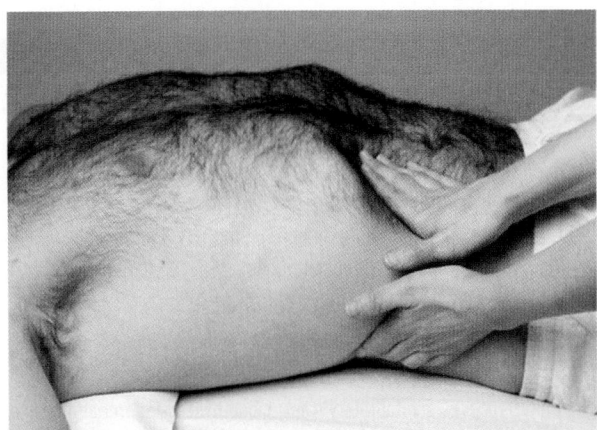

Figure 47-8 Palpating the right kidney.

Source: From Brundage, D. J. (1992). *Renal disorders*. St. Louis: Mosby.

Table 47-6 Evidence of Normal Physical Findings

- No costovertebral angle tenderness
- Nonpalpable kidney and bladder
- No palpable masses

size, contour, and tenderness should be noted. Kidney enlargement is suggestive of neoplasm or other serious renal pathological conditions.

The urinary bladder is normally not palpable unless it is distended with urine. If the bladder is full, it may feel like a smooth, round, firm organ and is sensitive to palpation.

Percussion. Tenderness in the flank area may be detected by fist percussion. This technique is performed by striking the fist (kidney punch) of one hand against the dorsal surface of the other hand, which is placed flat on the patient along the posterior CVA margin. Normally a firm blow in the flank area should not elicit pain. Tenderness and pain at the CVA may indicate a kidney infection or polycystic kidney disease.

Normally, a bladder is not percussible until it contains 150 mL of urine. If the bladder is full, dullness is heard above the symphysis pubis. A distended bladder may be percussed as high as the umbilicus.

Auscultation. The diaphragm of the stethoscope may be used to auscultate over both CVAs and in the upper abdominal quadrants. With this technique, the abdominal aorta and the renal arteries are auscultated for a bruit (an abnormal murmur), which indicates impaired blood flow to the kidneys.

Table 47-6 lists the normal physical assessment findings in the urinary system. Table 47-7 lists common assessment abnormalities of the urinary system. Variations in assessment findings may be normal in older adults. Table 47-2 shows the age-related changes in the urinary system and differences in assessment findings. The nurse should use a focused assessment to evaluate the status of previously identified urinary system problems and to monitor for signs of new problems). A focused assessment of the urinary system is presented in the Focused Assessment: Urinary System box.

FOCUSED ASSESSMENT
Urinary System

Use this checklist to ensure that the key assessment steps have been performed.

Subjective
Ask the patient about any of the following, and note responses

Painful urination	Y	N
Changes in colour of urine (blood, cloudy)	Y	N
Change in characteristics of urination (diminished, excessive)	Y	N
Problems with frequent nighttime urination (nocturia)	Y	N

Objective: Diagnostic
Check the following laboratory results for critical values

Blood urea nitrogen	✓
Serum creatinine	✓
Urinalysis	✓
Urine culture and sensitivity	✓

Objective: Physical Examination
Inspect

Abdomen	✓
Urinary meatus for inflammation or discharge	✓

Palpate

Abdomen for bladder distention, masses, or tenderness	✓

Percuss

Costovertebral angle for tenderness	✓

Auscultate

Renal arteries for bruits	✓

Diagnostic Studies

Table 47-8 lists and describes diagnostic tests common to the urinary system. It is important to conduct appropriate diagnostic tests to locate, understand, and manage urinary problems. The accuracy of the results is influenced by (a) adherence to the proper procedures related to the study and (b) cooperation of the patient in restricting fluids, collecting urine specimens, lying quietly on the examination table, and following other instructions.

For many radiological investigations, a bowel preparation must be used the evening before the study to clear the lower GI tract of feces and flatus. Because the kidneys lie in a retroperitoneal location, the contents of the colon may obstruct visualization of the urinary tract. If a bowel preparation is not properly performed, a test may be unsuccessful and must be rescheduled. Commonly used bowel preparations include enemas, castor oil, magnesium citrate, and bisacodyl (Dulcolax) tablets or suppositories. Some bowel preparations, such as magnesium citrate and Fleet enema, are contraindicated for use in patients with renal failure: Magnesium cannot be excreted by patients with renal failure (see Chapter 49).

When a patient has repeated diagnostic studies on consecutive days, it is important to prevent dehydration. It is not uncommon for a patient to take nothing by mouth (NPO) after

COMMON ASSESSMENT ABNORMALITIES

Table 47-7 Urinary System

FINDING	DESCRIPTION	POSSIBLE ETIOLOGY AND SIGNIFICANCE
Anuria	Technically no urination (24-hr urine output of <100 mL)	Acute renal failure, end-stage renal disease, bilateral ureteral obstruction
Burning on urination	Stinging pain in urethral area	Urethral irritation, urinary tract infection
Dysuria	Painful or difficult urination	Sign of urinary tract infection, interstitial cystitis, and a wide variety of pathological conditions
Enuresis	Involuntary nocturnal urinating	Symptom of lower urinary tract disorder
Frequency	Increased incidence of urinating	Acutely inflamed bladder, retention with overflow, excess fluid intake
Hematuria	Blood in the urine	Cancer of genitourinary tract, blood dyscrasias, renal disease, urinary tract infection, stones in kidney or ureter, medications (anticoagulants)
Hesitancy	Delay or difficulty in initiating urination	Partial urethral obstruction
Incontinence	Inability to voluntarily control discharge of urine	Neurogenic bladder, bladder infection, injury to external sphincter
Nocturia	Frequency of urination at night	Renal disease with impaired concentrating ability, bladder obstruction, heart failure, diabetes mellitus. May occur after renal transplantation
Oliguria	Diminished amount of urine in a given time (24-hr urine output of 100-400 mL)	Severe dehydration, shock, transfusion reaction, kidney disease, end-stage renal disease
Pain	Presence over suprapubic area (related to bladder), urethral pain (irritation of bladder neck), flank (CVA) pain	Infection, urinary retention, foreign body in urinary tract, urethritis, pyelonephritis, renal colic or stones
Pneumaturia	Passage of urine containing gas	Fistula connections between bowel and bladder, gas-forming urinary tract infections
Polyuria	Large volume of urine in a given time	Diabetes mellitus, diabetes insipidus, chronic renal failure, diuretics, excess fluid intake
Retention	Inability to urinate, even though bladder contains excessive amount of urine	Urethral stricture or obstruction; neurogenic bladder; postanaesthesia status. May occur after pelvic surgery, childbirth, catheter removal
Stress incontinence	Involuntary urination with increased pressure (sneezing or coughing)	Weakness of sphincter control
Urgency	Strong desire to urinate	Inflammatory lesions in bladder or urethra, acute bacterial infections

CVA, costovertebral angle.

midnight, spend all morning in the radiology department, be too tired to eat, sleep all afternoon, and be on NPO status after midnight again because of studies scheduled for the next day. Severe dehydration, especially in a diabetic, debilitated, or older patient, may lead to acute renal failure. The nurse is responsible for ensuring that a patient undergoing diagnostic studies is properly hydrated and given adequate nourishment between studies. The nurse should also check with the health care provider regarding the insulin dose for diabetic patients who are NPO.

Analysis of Urine

Urinalysis. In evaluating disorders of the urinary tract, one of the first studies performed is a **urinalysis** (Table 47-9; see Table 47-8). This test is a general examination of urine for routine and microscopic findings and may establish baseline information, provide information about possible abnormalities, indicate what further studies need to be done, and supply information on the progression of a diagnosed disorder.

For a routine urinalysis, a specimen may be collected at any time of the day. However, it is best to obtain the first specimen urinated in the morning. This concentrated specimen is more likely to contain abnormal constituents if they are present in the urine. The specimen should be examined within 1 hour of urination. If it is not, bacteria multiply rapidly, RBCs hemolyze, casts (moulds of renal tubules) disintegrate, and the urine becomes alkaline as a result of urea-splitting bacteria. If it is not possible to send the specimen to the laboratory immediately, it should be refrigerated. However, to obtain the best results, the nurse should coordinate specimen collection with routine laboratory hours.

Multiple reagent strips (also called *urine dipsticks*) are commonly used by laboratories and in outpatient settings to provide

Text continued on p. 1282

DIAGNOSTIC STUDIES

Table 47-8 Urinary System

STUDY	DESCRIPTION AND PURPOSE	NURSING RESPONSIBILITY
Urine Tests		
Urinalysis	This is a general examination of urine for routine and microscopic evaluation, to establish baseline information or provide data to establish a tentative diagnosis and determine whether further tests are to be ordered (see Table 47-9).	Usually the first urinated morning specimen is required, but it may not be appropriate for all diagnostic purposes. Ensure that the specimen is examined within 1 hr of urinating. Wash patient's perineal area if soiled with menses or fecal material.
Creatinine clearance	Creatinine is a waste product of protein breakdown (primarily body muscle mass). Clearance of creatinine by the kidney approximates the GFR. Normal creatinine clearance varies with age and is approximately 20% higher in men. Normal finding is 1.42-2.25 mL/sec (85-135 mL/min).	Collect 24-hr urine specimen. Discard sample from first urination when test is started. Save urine from all subsequent urinations for 24 hr. Instruct patient to urinate at end of 24 hr and add that specimen to collection. Ensure that serum creatinine clearance is determined during 24-hr period.
Urine for culture and sensitivity (C&S) ("clean catch," "midstream")	Test is performed to confirm suspected urinary tract infection and identify causative organisms. Normally, the bladder is sterile, but the urethra contains bacteria and a few WBCs. If specimen is properly collected, stored, and handled: <10,000 organisms/mL usually indicates no infection; 10,000-100,000/mL is usually not diagnostic, and test may have to be repeated; >100,000/mL indicates infection.	Use sterile container for collection of urine. Touch only outside of container. For women, separate labia with one hand and clean meatus with other hand, using at least three sponges (saturated with cleansing solution) in a front-to-back motion. For men, retract foreskin (if present) and cleanse glans with at least three cleansing sponges. After cleaning, instruct patient to start urinating and then continue voiding in sterile container. (The initial voided urine flushes out most contaminants in the urethra and the perineal area.) Catheterization may be needed if patient is unable to cooperate with this procedure.
Concentration test	Study is an evaluation of renal concentration ability. Concentration is measured from specific gravity readings. Normal finding is 1.020-1.035.	Instruct patient to fast after a given time in evening (in usual procedure). Collect three urine specimens at hourly intervals in morning.
Residual urine	Test is a determination of amount of urine left in bladder after urination. Finding may be abnormal in patients who have problems with bladder enervation, sphincter impairment, BPH, equine syndrome (nerve compression), or urethral strictures. Normal finding is ≤50 mL urine (increases with age).	If residual urine test is ordered, catheterize patient immediately after patient urinates, or use bladder ultrasonography equipment, including portable scanner. If a large amount of residual urine is obtained, health care provider may order catheter to be left in bladder.
Protein dipstick determination (Albustix, Combistix)	Test detects protein (primarily albumin) in urine. Normal finding is grade 0 to trace amounts.	Dip end of stick in urine, and read result by comparison with colour chart on label as directed. Grading is from 0 to 4+. Interpret with caution. A positive result may not indicate significant proteinuria; some medications may produce false-positive readings.
Quantitative test for protein	A 12- or 24-hr collection yields a more accurate indication of the amount of protein in urine. Persistent proteinuria usually indicates glomerular renal disease. Normal finding is <0.15 g/24 hr (<150 mg/24 hr), and protein consists mainly of albumin.	Perform 12- or 24-hr urine collection.
Urine cytology	Test is used to identify changes in cellular structure indicative of malignancy, especially bladder cancer.	Obtain urine and send immediately to laboratory. The first morning specimen should not be used.
Blood Tests		
Bicarbonate (HCO_3^-)	Most patients in renal failure have metabolic acidosis and low serum HCO_3^- levels. Normal finding is 21-28 mmol/L.	Explain test, and watch for postpuncture bleeding.
BUN	Test is most commonly used to identify presence of renal problems. Concentration of urea in blood is regulated by rate at which kidney excretes urea. Normal finding is 3.6-7.1 mmol/L.	Nonrenal factors (e.g., rapid cell destruction from infections, fever, GI bleeding, trauma, athletic activity and excessive muscle breakdown, corticosteroid therapy) may cause increase in BUN level. A low BUN level could result from overhydration or advanced liver disease.
Creatinine	Study is more reliable than BUN as a determinant of renal function. Creatinine is end product of muscle and protein metabolism and is liberated at a constant rate. Normal values: 53-106 mcmol/L for men, 44-97 mcmol/L for women. Normal finding is 44-133 mcmol/L.	Explain test, and watch for postpuncture bleeding.
Urea/creatinine ratio	Normal finding is 10:1.	—

Continued

Table 47-8 Urinary System—cont'd

STUDY	DESCRIPTION AND PURPOSE	NURSING RESPONSIBILITY
Blood Tests—cont'd		
Calcium (Ca^{2+})	Calcium is main mineral in bone and aids in muscle contraction, neurotransmission, and clotting. In renal disease, decreased reabsorption of Ca^{2+} leads to renal osteodystrophy. Normal calcium levels in adults range from 2.25 to 2.75 mmol/L.	Explain test, and watch for postpuncture bleeding.
Potassium (K^+)	Kidneys are responsible for excreting majority of body's potassium. In renal disease, K^+ determinations are critical because K^+ is one of the first electrolytes whose levels become abnormal. Highly elevated K^+ levels (>6 mmol/L) can lead to muscle weakness and cardiac dysrhythmias. Normal values are 3.5-5 mmol/L.	Explain test, and watch for postpuncture bleeding.
Phosphorus	Phosphorus balance is inversely related to Ca^{2+} balance. In renal disease, phosphorus levels are elevated because the kidney is the primary excretory organ. Normal values are 0.97-1.45 mmol/L.	Explain test, and watch for postpuncture bleeding.
Sodium (Na^+)	Sodium is the main extracellular electrolyte determining blood volume. Values usually stay within normal range until late stages of renal failure. Normal finding is 135-145 mmol/L.	Explain test, and watch for postpuncture bleeding.
Uric acid	Study is used as a screening test primarily for disorders of purine metabolism but can indicate kidney disease as well. Values depend on renal function and rate of purine metabolism and dietary intake of food rich in purines. Normal findings are 0.16-0.43 mmol/L for women and 0.24-0.51 mmol/L for men.	Explain test, and watch for postpuncture bleeding.
Radiological Procedures		
Kidneys, ureters, bladder (KUB)	Study involves radiographic examination of abdomen and pelvis and delineates size, shape, and position of kidneys.	Perform bowel preparation (if ordered).
Intravenous pyelography (IVP)	Radiographic examination visualizes urinary tract after IV injection of contrast material.	Assess renal function. If BUN and creatinine levels are elevated, use of contrast dye in diagnostic procedure may not be safe. Evening before procedure, administer cathartic or enema to empty colon of feces and gas. Keep patient on NPO status 8 hr before procedure. Before procedure, assess patient for iodine sensitivity to avoid anaphylactic reaction. Inform patient that procedure involves lying on table and having serial radiographs taken. After procedure, encourage fluids (if permitted) to flush out contrast material.
Nephrotomography	Radiograph is performed with rotating tubes. Test delineates segments of the kidney at different levels. Multiple exposures are obtained to visualize specific sections of the kidney after IV injection of contrast material.	Explain procedure, and prepare patient as for IVP.
Retrograde pyelography	Radiograph of urinary tract is performed after injection of contrast material into kidneys. Cystoscope is inserted, and ureteral catheters are inserted through it into renal pelvis. Contrast material is injected through catheters.	Prepare patient as for IVP. Inform patient that pain may be experienced from distension of pelvis and discomfort from cystoscope. Inform patient that anaesthetic may be administered for procedure.
Renal arteriography (angiography)	Study helps visualize renal blood vessels. Contrast material is injected into renal artery via catheter inserted into femoral artery.	Prepare patient evening before procedure by administering cathartic or enema. Before injection of contrast material, test for iodine sensitivity. After procedure, check insertion site for bleeding, and measure peripheral pulses in involved leg every 30-60 min to detect occluded blood flow, if any.
Renal ultrasonography	Small external ultrasound probe is placed on patient's skin. Conductive gel is applied to the skin. Noninvasive procedure involves passing sound waves into body structures and recording images as the waves are reflected back. Computer interprets tissue density on the basis of sound waves and displays it in picture form. Study is most valuable in detection of renal or perirenal masses, differential diagnosis of renal cysts, solid masses, and identification of obstructions. It can be used safely in patients with renal failure.	Explain procedure to patient.

DIAGNOSTIC STUDIES

Table 47-8 Urinary System—cont'd

STUDY	DESCRIPTION AND PURPOSE	NURSING RESPONSIBILITY
Radiological Procedures—cont'd		
CT	Study provides excellent visualization of kidneys. Kidney size can be evaluated; tumours, abscesses, suprarenal masses (e.g., adrenal tumours, pheochromocytomas), and obstructions can be detected. Advantage of CT over ultrasonography is its ability to distinguish subtle differences in density. Use of IV-administered contrast media during CT accentuates density of renal tissue and helps differentiate masses.	Explain procedure to patient. Before injection of contrast material, ask patient about iodine sensitivity.
MRI	Computer-generated images rely on radiofrequency waves and alteration in magnetic field. Useful for visualization of kidneys. Not proven useful for detecting urinary calculi or calcified tumours.	Explain procedure to patient. Have patient remove all metal objects. Patients with a history of claustrophobia may need to be sedated.
Cystography	Purpose of study is to visualize bladder and evaluate vesicoureteral reflux. Contrast material is instilled into bladder via cystoscope or catheter.	Explain procedure to patient. If procedure is performed via cystoscope, follow nursing care related to cystoscopy.
Renal Radionuclide Imaging		
Renal scan	Purpose of scan is to show blood flow, glomerular filtration, tubular function, and excretion. Radioactive isotopes are injected by IV route. Radiation detector probes are placed over kidney, and scintillation counter monitors radioactive material in kidney. Radioisotope distribution in kidney is scanned and mapped. Test is useful in showing location, size, and shape of kidney and, in general, assessing blood perfusion and kidney's ability to secrete urine. Abscesses, cysts, and tumours may appear as cold spots because of presence of nonfunctioning tissue.	Requires no dietary or activity restriction. Inform patient that no pain or discomfort should be felt during test.
Surgical Study		
Renal biopsy	Purpose is to obtain renal tissue for examination to determine type of renal disease or to monitor progress of renal disease. This technique is usually performed percutaneously (skin biopsy) through needle insertion into lower lobe of kidney. Can be guided by CT or ultrasonography.	Before procedure, ascertain coagulation status through patient's history, medication history, CBC, hematocrit, prothrombin time, and bleeding and clotting times. Type and crossmatch for blood. Ensure consent form is signed. After procedure, apply pressure dressing to biopsy site and check frequently for bleeding. Measure vital signs frequently. Observe urine for gross bleeding. Determine microscopic bleeding by use of dipstick. Assess patient for flank pain. Monitor hematocrit levels.
Endoscopy		
Cystoscopy	Study involves use of tubular lighted cystoscope to inspect bladder. Lithotomy position is used. It may be performed while patient receives local or general anaesthesia, depending on needs and condition of patient.	Before procedure, force fluids or administer IV fluids if general anaesthesia is to be used. Ensure that consent form is signed. Explain procedure to patient. Administer preoperative medication. After procedure, explain that burning on urination, pink-tinged urine, and urinary frequency are expected effects after cystoscopy. Do not let patient walk alone immediately after procedure because orthostatic hypotension may occur. Offer warm sitz baths, heat, and mild analgesics to relieve discomfort.
Urodynamics Testing		
Cystometrography	Purpose of study is to evaluate bladder tone, sensations of filling, and bladder (detrusor) stability. Study involves insertion of catheter and instillation of water or saline solution into bladder. Measurements of pressure exerted against bladder wall are recorded.	Explain procedure to patient. Observe patient for manifestations of urinary infection after procedure.

BPH, benign prostatic hyperplasia; *BUN*, blood urea nitrogen; *CBC*, complete blood cell count; *CT*, computed tomography; *GFR*, glomerular filtration rate; *GI*, gastrointestinal; *IV*, intravenous; *MRI*, magnetic resonance imaging; *NPO*, nothing by mouth; *WBC*, white blood cell.

Table 47-9 Urinalysis Findings

EVALUATION	NORMAL FINDING	ABNORMAL FINDINGS AND SIGNIFICANCE
Colour	Amber yellow	Dark, smoky colour suggests hematuria. Yellow-brown to olive green indicates excessive bilirubin. Orange-red or orange-brown colour is caused by phenazopyridine (Pyridium). Cloudiness of freshly voided urine indicates infection. Colourless urine indicates excessive fluid intake, renal disease, or diabetes insipidus.
Smell	Aromatic	After standing, smell becomes more ammonia-like. In urinary tract infections, urine smells unpleasant.
Protein	<0.15 g/day	Persistent proteinuria is characteristic of acute and chronic renal disease, especially involving glomeruli. In absence of disease, positive reading may be caused by high-protein diet, strenuous exercise, dehydration, fever, or emotional stress. Vaginal secretions may contaminate urine specimen and produce positive reading.
Glucose	None	Glycosuria indicates diabetes mellitus or low renal threshold for glucose reabsorption (if blood glucose level is normal). Small amounts may be found after glucose loading (e.g., glucose tolerance test).
Ketones	None	Altered carbohydrate and fat metabolism indicates diabetes mellitus and starvation. Findings can also occur in dehydration, vomiting, and severe diarrhea.
Bilirubin	None	Bilirubinuria is as significant as jaundice in detection of liver disorders. Bilirubin may appear in urine before jaundice becomes visible or may be present in persons with hepatic disorders who do not have recognizable jaundice.*
Specific gravity	1.005-1.030 Maximum concentrating ability of kidney (1.025-1.030)	*Low*: dilute urine and possibly excessive diuresis. *High*: dehydration. *Fixed at about 1.010*: kidneys are unable to concentrate urine, which suggests that kidneys are progressing to end-stage renal disease.
Osmolality (random specimen)	50-1200 mmol/kg	Measurement is a more accurate method than specific gravity for determining diluting and concentrating ability of kidneys. Deviations from normal indicate tubular dysfunction. Findings indicate whether kidney has lost ability to concentrate or dilute urine. (Not part of routine urinalysis.)
pH	4.6-8.0 (average, 6.0)	A pH of >8.0 may be the result of standing of urine or urinary tract infections because bacteria decompose urea to form ammonia. A pH of <4.0 may indicate respiratory or metabolic acidosis.
RBC	0-4/hpf	Bleeding in urinary tract is caused by calculi, cystitis, neoplasm, glomerulonephritis, tuberculosis, kidney biopsy, or trauma.
WBC	0-5/hpf	Increased number of WBCs in urine (pyuria) indicates urinary tract infection or inflammation.
Casts	None; occasional hyaline casts	Casts are moulds of the renal tubules and may contain protein, WBCs, RBCs, or bacteria. Noncellular casts are hyaline in appearance, and a few may be found in normal urine. Casts indicate renal dysfunction or upper urinary tract infections.
Culture for organisms	No organisms in bladder; count of <104 organisms/mL is result of normal urethral flora	Bacteria counts >105/mL indicate urinary tract infection. Organisms most commonly found in urinary tract infections are *Escherichia coli*, enterococci, *Klebsiella* species, *Proteus* species, and streptococci.

*See Chapter 46 for further discussion.

hpf, high-powered field (or what can be seen in one view of the slide through the microscope); *RBC*, red blood cells; *WBC*, white blood cells.

chemical analysis of urine, along with a microscopic interpretation. The results of a urinalysis usually include a description of the appearance, specific gravity (mass and density), pH, glucose, ketones, and protein in the urine and a microscopic examination of urine sediment for white blood cells (WBCs), RBCs, crystals, and casts (see Table 47-9).

Composite Urine Collections.
Composite urine specimens are collected over a period that may range from 2 to 24 hours. The purpose of a composite specimen is to examine or measure specific components, such as electrolytes, glucose, protein, 17-ketosteroids, catecholamines, creatinine, and minerals. These specimens may have to be refrigerated, or preservatives may have to be added to the container used for collecting urine.

For collection of a composite urine specimen, the patient is instructed to urinate and discard this first urine specimen. This time is noted as the start of the test. All urine from subsequent urinations is saved in a container for the designated period. Finally, at the end of the period, the patient is asked to urinate, and this urine sample is added to the container. Incomplete collections do not provide valid results. Reminding the patient to save all urine during the study period is critical.

Creatinine Clearance.
One of the most common composite indicators used to analyze urinary system disorders is creati-

nine clearance. **Creatinine** is a waste product produced by protein breakdown (primarily body muscle mass). Urinary excretion of creatinine is a measure of the amount of active muscle tissue in the body, not of body weight; therefore, people with larger muscle mass have higher values. Because almost all creatinine in the blood is normally excreted by the kidneys, creatinine clearance is the most accurate indicator of renal function. The result of a creatinine clearance test closely approximates that of the GFR (National Kidney Foundation, 2011). A blood specimen for serum creatinine determination should be obtained during the period of urine collection.

Creatinine levels remain remarkably constant for each person because they are not significantly affected by protein ingestion, muscular exercise, water intake, or rate of urine production. Normal creatinine clearance values range from 1.42 to 2.25 mL/sec (85-135 mL/min). After age 40, the creatinine clearance rate decreases at a rate of about 1 mL/min/yr.

Urine Cytology. Urine can be checked for abnormal cellular structures that occur with bladder cancer. Specimens may be obtained from voiding, catheterization, or bladder irrigation (bladder washing). The first morning's voided specimen should not be used because epithelial cells may change in appearance in urine held in the bladder overnight. As with urinalysis, the specimen should be fresh or brought to the laboratory within the hour. An alcohol-based fixative is then added to preserve the cellular structure. Urine cytological study is used for detection and monitoring the prognosis of bladder cancer.

Radiological Studies

Diagnostic urine studies are summarized in Table 47-8.

Kidney, Ureter, and Bladder Radiography. The kidney, ureter, and bladder (KUB) radiograph is an abdominal view obtained without use of a contrast medium to show the renal outline, the psoas shadow, and the full bladder. Radiopaque stones and foreign bodies can be seen on this radiograph. The form, the size, and the position of the kidneys can also be seen. Abscesses, tumours, and cysts may distort anatomical relationships on the KUB image. Sometimes nephrotomography (sectional views that focus on a single plane of the kidney) is ordered at the same time as the KUB study to maximize visualization of the kidneys.

Intravenous Pyelography. Intravenous pyelography (IVP), or excretory urography, enables visualization of the urinary tract. The presence, the position, the size, and the shape of the kidneys, the ureters, and the bladder can be evaluated. Cysts, tumours, lesions, and obstructions cause a distortion in the normal appearance of these structures.

The procedure consists of injecting an IV dose of contrast material, which circulates in the blood and is excreted by the kidneys into the urine. As with all contrast studies, possible iodine and shellfish allergies should be determined before the study. During injection, the patient may experience sensations of warmth, facial flushing, and a salty taste. After injection, radiographs are taken sequentially. The sequencing of images is planned so that contrast excretion can be followed from the cortex of the kidney to the bladder. The presence of bladder atony or outlet obstruction also can be detected by an image obtained after urination, which shows the residual volume of urine in the bladder.

Patients with significantly decreased renal function should not undergo IVP because the contrast material is not properly excreted by the kidneys. Contrast medium can also be nephrotoxic and can worsen renal function.

Retrograde Pyelography. **Retrograde pyelography** is the radiographic visualization of the kidneys, the ureter, and the bladder after direct injection of contrast material into the kidney via a ureteral catheter introduced through a cystoscope. It may be performed if IVP does not visualize the urinary tract or if the patient is allergic to IV contrast material or has decreased renal function. The risks associated with retrograde pyelography are similar to those related to cystoscopy, including the risk of infection and the use of anaesthetics.

Antegrade Pyelography. Antegrade pyelography is performed to evaluate the upper urinary tract when the patient has an allergy to contrast media, when renal function is decreased, or when abnormalities prevent passage of a ureteral catheter. Contrast media may be injected percutaneously into the renal pelvis or via a nephrostomy tube that is already in place (this method is also called *nephrostography*) when tube function or ureteral integrity must be determined after trauma or surgery. Complications of antegrade pyelography include hematuria, infection, and hematoma.

Renal Ultrasonography. Renal ultrasonography uses high-frequency sound waves to image the kidneys, the ureter, and the bladder. Because radiation exposure is avoided, a number of images can be obtained, and studies can be repeated over a brief period. Images can be obtained with the patient in both the prone and the supine positions. A bowel preparation is not required for renal ultrasonography.

Computed Tomography. Computed tomography (CT) of the abdomen and the pelvis may be performed to detect tumours and possible metastases. CT can differentiate these from cysts or abscesses. Contrast material may be used to help visualize urinary structures more clearly in the computer-generated images. The patient is instructed to lie very still during the procedure while the machine takes precise transaxial images. Sedation may be required if the patient is unable to cooperate.

Renal Arteriography. The purpose of **renal arteriography** (angiography) is to visualize the renal blood vessels. In this radiological study, contrast material is injected into the renal artery via a catheter inserted into the femoral artery. The findings in arteriography can assist in diagnosing renal artery stenosis (Figure 47-9), additional or missing renal blood vessels, and renovascular hypertension and can assist in differentiating between a renal cyst and a renal tumour. Renal arteriography is also included in the workup of a potential renal transplant donor.

The patient is given a local anaesthetic at the site of catheter insertion. A catheter is usually inserted into the femoral artery and passed up the aorta to the level of the renal arteries (Figure 47-10). Contrast media is then injected to outline the renal blood supply, and x-ray images are taken.

The patient may experience a transient warm feeling along the course of the blood vessel when the contrast material is injected. After the catheter is removed, a pressure dressing is placed over the femoral injection site. It is important to observe the site for bleeding. Bed rest with the affected leg kept straight

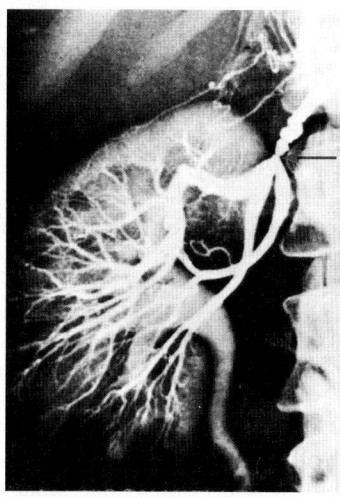

Figure 47-9 Renal arteriogram showing stenosis *(arrow)* of the right renal artery.

Source: From Brundage, D. J. (1992). *Renal disorders.* St. Louis: Mosby.

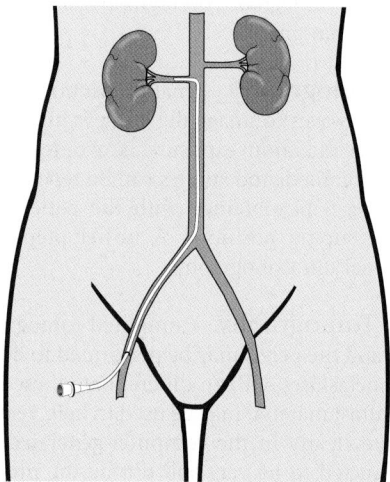

Figure 47-10 Diagram of catheter insertion for renal arteriography.

is usually prescribed. Peripheral pulses in the involved leg should be measured at least every 30 to 60 minutes to detect occlusion of blood flow caused by a thrombus, if any. Complications that may result from renal arteriography include thrombus, embolus, local inflammation, and hematoma. Patients with baseline renal insufficiency may experience a decrease in renal function secondary to the nephrotoxic contrast material.

Cystography. The purpose of cystography is to outline and visualize the bladder and evaluate the UVJ for reflux. In addition to suspected vesicoureteral reflux, indications for cystography include a neurogenic bladder and recurrent urinary tract infections. Cystography can also delineate abnormalities of the bladder, such as diverticula, calculi, and tumours. In this procedure, a contrast material is instilled via a cystoscope or catheter into the bladder.

Voiding cystourethrography (VCUG) is a voiding study of the bladder opening (bladder neck) and urethra. The bladder is filled

with contrast material. During urination, images are obtained to visualize the bladder and the urethra. After urination, another image is obtained to assess for residual urine. VCUG can detect abnormalities of the lower urinary tract, urethral stenosis, bladder neck obstruction, and prostatic enlargement (Digesu et al., 2006).

Urethrography. Urethrography is similar to cystography. Contrast material is injected in a retrograde manner into the urethra to identify strictures, diverticula, or other urethral pathological conditions. When urethral trauma is suspected, urethrography is performed before catheterization.

Loopography. Loopography is used to detect obstructions, anastomotic leaks, stones, reflux, and other uropathological features when a patient has a urinary pouch or ileal conduit. Because urinary diversions are created with sections of bowel, contrast absorption is a risk. The patient should be closely monitored for reactions to the contrast media.

Renal Radionuclide Imaging. Renal scans involving the use of radionuclides are useful in evaluating the anatomical structures, perfusion, and function of the kidneys. The results reveal the difference between the two kidneys with regard to blood flow, tubular function, and excretion. A normal scan shows symmetrical functioning of both kidneys. Normally, the distribution of activity is recorded throughout the kidneys. A lesion (e.g., a tumour) is indicated by the absence of radioactivity in the involved area and the appearance of the resultant defect on the scan. This study is particularly useful in detecting renal vascular disease, acute renal failure, and upper urinary tract obstruction. It is also useful in monitoring the function of a transplanted kidney.

Renal Biopsy. The purpose of **renal biopsy** is to obtain renal tissue for examination to establish a diagnosis or to monitor progress of renal disease. Biopsy material can be obtained through open biopsy or closed percutaneous needle biopsy. Open biopsy is rarely performed because it is a surgical procedure that necessitates general anaesthesia. Percutaneous needle biopsy, conducted through needle insertion into the lower lobe of the kidney, is more common.

Absolute contraindications to a percutaneous renal biopsy are bleeding disorders, the presence of a single kidney, and uncontrolled hypertension. Relative contraindications include suspected renal infection, hydronephrosis, and possible vascular lesions. Patients about to undergo biopsy should stop taking aspirin or warfarin (Coumadin) before the procedure as advised by their physicians.

In this procedure, the patient lies prone with a pillow or sandbag to elevate the abdomen and the kidneys. The position of the kidney is marked on the body under guidance with CT, IVP, or ultrasonography. Local anaesthetic is used, and a biopsy needle is inserted into the kidney just below the twelfth rib. The patient is instructed to hold his or her breath while the biopsy specimen is being taken.

After the procedure, a pressure dressing is applied, and the patient is kept prone for 30 to 60 minutes. Usually bed rest is prescribed for 24 hours. Vital signs should be measured every 5 to 10 minutes during the first hour and then, if no problems are noted, with decreasing frequency. The biopsy site should be inspected frequently for bleeding. Serial urine specimens should be assessed for gross and microscopic hematuria. A dipstick can be used to test for bleeding, even when hematuria is not obvious. The physician may order all urine sent for laboratory analysis to detect possible hematuria. The patient should be assessed for flank pain, hypotension, decreasing hematocrit, and temperature elevation and should also be observed for chills, urinary frequency, and dysuria.

Complications of a renal biopsy include renal hemorrhage, hematoma, and infection. Even if no complications occur, the patient should be instructed to avoid lifting heavy objects for 5 to 7 days. The patient should be instructed not to take any anticoagulant drugs until permission is given by the physician who performed the biopsy.

Endoscopy

Cystoscopy. **Cystoscopy** is a radiological bladder procedure in which contrast material is instilled into the bladder. The main purpose is to inspect the interior of the bladder and evaluate the vesicoureteral reflux with a tubular lighted endoscope called a *cystoscope* (Figure 47-11).

Cystoscopes can be used to insert ureteral catheters, remove calculi, obtain biopsy specimens of bladder lesions, and treat bleeding lesions. In most cases, bladder disorders can be determined by cystoscopic examination.

Cystoscopy is usually performed in a cystoscopy room in the radiology department, in a urology clinic, or in the operating room. Most of the pain associated with cystoscopy results from spasms and contractions of bladder and sphincter. Relaxation and deep breathing by the patient may alleviate some of the bladder and sphincter spasms. A local anaesthetic is instilled into the urethra before cystoscope insertion. During the examination, saline solution is instilled slowly to distend the bladder. This improves visualization but causes an urge to urinate.

After the procedure, the patient can expect to have some burning on urination, blood-tinged urine, and urinary frequency from the irritation of cystoscope insertion and manipulation. The nurse should observe for bright red bleeding, which is not normal. After the procedure, the nurse is responsible for keeping the patient well hydrated, administering mild analgesics, providing sitz baths, and applying heat to decrease the patient's discomfort. Complications that may result from cystoscopy include urinary retention, urinary tract hemorrhage, bladder infection, and perforation of the bladder.

Urodynamics Testing

Urodynamics testing is a set of studies designed to measure urinary tract function. Urodynamic tests entail study of the storage of urine within the bladder and the flow of urine through the urinary tract to the outside of the body. A combination of techniques may be used to provide a detailed assessment of urinary incontinence.

Urinary Flow Study. The urinary flow study (uroflow) entails measurement of urine volume in a single voiding, expelled in a specified time and expressed in millilitres per second. As the patient voids, the stream pattern is depicted graphically on a printout.

The patient is asked to start the test with a reasonably full bladder, urinate into a special container, and try to empty the bladder completely. The container generates a graph in which flow rate is compared to time. This test is used to (a) assess the degree of outflow obstruction caused by such conditions as benign prostatic hyperplasia or stricture; (b) assess bladder or sphincter dysfunction effects on voiding such as occurs with neuropathological conditions; and (c) evaluate the effects of treatment for lower urinary tract problems. Residual urine volume should be measured immediately after a urinary flow study to help identify the degree of chronic urinary retention that is often associated with abnormal flow patterns.

A normal maximum flow rate is about 20 to 25 mL/sec for men and about 25 to 30 mL/sec for women. However, the volume voided and the patient's age can affect the flow rate; thus variations are normal and common. Graphic displays can illustrate straining and intermittent flow patterns or other abnormal voiding disorders.

Cystometrography. **Cystometrography** is an evaluation of the compliance (elastic property) and stability of the detrusor muscle of the bladder, as well as bladder tone, sensations of filling, and bladder (detrusor) stability. It is a measurement of intravesical pressure during the course of bladder filling. It is usually ordered if a patient has incontinence or neurogenic bladder. The procedure consists of insertion of a specially designed catheter while the patient is in a supine position. If abdominal pressure is also to be measured, a second tube is inserted into the rectum or the vagina. This tube is typically attached to a small fluid-filled balloon to allow pressure recording. Saline or sterile water for

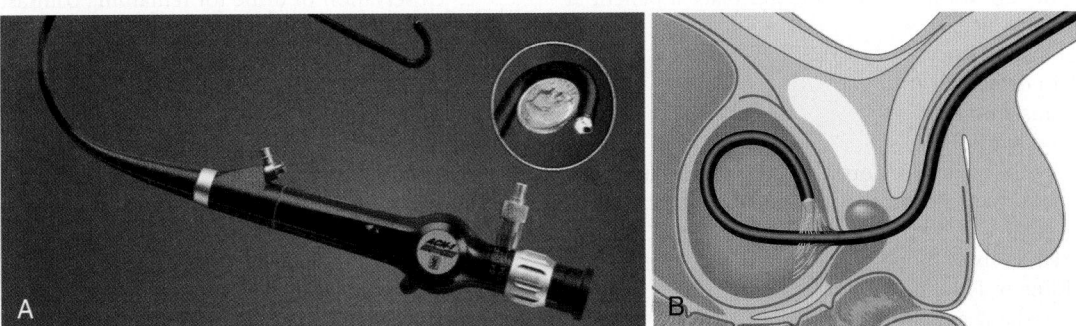

Figure 47-11 Cystoscopic examination of the bladder. **A,** Flexible Cysto nephroscope. **B,** Illustration of nephroscope inserted into male bladder.

irrigation or contrast used for cystography is infused into the bladder, and pressures are measured. During the infusion, the patient is asked about sensations of bladder filling, usually including the first urge to urinate, a strong urge to urinate, and perception of bladder fullness.

Sphincter Electromyography.

In electromyography (EMG), the electrical activity created when the nervous system stimulates motor units within a muscle is recorded. Through the placement of needles, percutaneous wires, or patches near the urethra, the pelvic floor muscle activity can be assessed. During filling cystometrography, sphincter EMG is used to identify voluntary pelvic floor muscle contractions and the response of these muscles to bladder filling, coughing, and other provocative manoeuvres.

Voiding Pressure Flow Study.

The voiding pressure flow study combines a urinary flow rate, cystometric pressures (intravesical, abdominal, and detrusor pressures), and a sphincter EMG for detailed evaluation of micturition. It is completed by assisting the patient to a specialized toilet and allowing him or her to urinate while the various pressure tubes and EMG apparatus remain in place.

Videourodynamics Testing.

Videourodynamics testing is a combination of the filling cystometrography, sphincter EMG, and/or urinary flow study with anatomical imaging of the lower urinary tract, typically via fluoroscopy. This combination is used in selected cases to identify an obstructive lesion and characterize anatomical changes in the bladder and lower urinary tract.

Radionuclide Cystography.

Radionuclide cystography is used to detect and grade vesicoureteral reflux. Similar to VCUG, a small dose of radioisotope tracer is instilled into the bladder via urethral catheter. The procedure is more sensitive than VCUG, and the radiation dose is one-thousandth that used in VCUG.

Whitaker's Study.

Whitaker's study is used to measure the pressure differential between the renal pelvis and the bladder. The presence of a ureteral obstruction can be assessed. Percutaneous access to the renal pelvis is achieved by placement of a catheter in the renal pelvis. A catheter is also placed in the bladder. Fluid is perfused through the percutaneous tube or needle at a rate of 10 mL/min. Pressure data are then collected. These pressure measurements are studied in combination with fluoroscopic imaging to identify the level of obstruction.

⊘volve   *An assessment case study of the urinary system is available at* **http://evolve.elsevier.com/Canada/Lewis/medsurg**

REVIEW QUESTIONS

The number of the question corresponds to the same-numbered objective at the beginning of the chapter.

1. Which of the following is affected by a renal stone in the pelvis of the kidney?
   a. The structural support of the kidney
   b. Regulation of the concentration of urine
   c. The entry and exit of blood vessels at the kidney
   d. Collection and drainage of urine from the kidney
2. A patient with renal disease has oliguria and a creatinine clearance rate of 40 mL/min. Which of the following functions of the kidney is most directly implicated in these abnormal findings?
   a. Tubular secretion
   b. Glomerular filtration
   c. Capillary permeability
   d. Concentration of filtrate
3. Which of the following conditions might place a patient at risk for urinary calculi?
   a. Adrenal insufficiency
   b. Serotonin deficiency
   c. Hyperaldosteronism
   d. Hyperparathyroidism
4. Which of the following are normal changes associated with aging of the urinary system that the nurse might expect to find?
   a. Decreased levels of blood urea nitrogen
   b. Postvoiding residual urine
   c. Increased bladder capacity
   d. More easily palpable kidneys

5. Which of the following does the nurse undertake during physical assessment of the urinary system?
   a. Percussion of the flank area with a firm blow
   b. Palpation of an empty bladder as a small nodule
   c. Prone positioning of the patient to palpate the kidneys
   d. Auscultation to determine the level of urine in the bladder
6. Which of the following are normal findings expected by the nurse on physical assessment of the urinary system?
   a. Nonpalpable left kidney
   b. Auscultation of renal artery bruit
   c. CVA tenderness elicited by a kidney punch
   d. Palpable bladder to the level of the pubic symphysis
7. Which of the following is an important nursing responsibility after IVP?
   a. Assessment of the patient for flank pain
   b. Encouragement of extra oral fluid intake
   c. Observation of urine for remaining contrast material
   d. Encouragement of ambulation 2 to 3 hours after the study
8. Which of the following would the nurse expect to find on reading the urinalysis results of a dehydrated patient?
   a. A pH of 8.4
   b. RBC measurement of 4/high-powered field
   c. Colour and appearance: yellow, cloudy
   d. Specific gravity of 1.035

ANSWERS: 1. d; 2. b; 3. d; 4. b; 5. a; 6. a; 7. b; 8. d.

REFERENCES

Baum, N. (2006). Urinary incontinence in the geriatric patient, *Clinical Geriatrics, 14*(4), 35-38.

Cheung, C. M., Ponnusamy, A., & Anderton, J. G. (2008). Management of acute renal failure in the elderly patient: A clinician's guide. *Drugs & Aging, 25,* 455-476. doi:10.2165/00002512-200825060-00002

Digesu, G. A., Athanasiou, S., Chaliha, C., Michalas, S., Salvatore, S., Selvaggi, L., & Khullar, V. (2006). Urethral retro-resistance pressure and urodynamic diagnoses in women with lower urinary tract symptoms. *British Journal of Obstetrics and Gynecology, 113*(1), 34-38. doi:10.1111/j.1471-0528.2005.00787.x

Kiela, P. R., & Ghishan, F. K. (2009). Recent advances in the renal-skeletal-gut axis that controls phosphate homeostasis. *Laboratory Investigation, 89,* 7-14. doi:10.1038/labinvest.2008.114

Liamis, G., Milionis, M. E., & Elisaf, M. (2008). Blood pressure therapy and electrolyte disturbances. *International Journal of Clinical Practice, 62*(10), 1572-1580. doi:10.1111/j.1742-1241.2008.01860.x

Liang, S. Y., & Mackowiak, P. A. (2007). Infections in the elderly patient. *Clinics in Geriatric Medicine, 23,* 441-456. doi:10.1016/j.cger.2007.01.010

McCance, K. L., & Huether, S. E. (2010). *Pathophysiology: The biologic basis for disease in adults and children* (6th ed.). St. Louis: Mosby.

Miller, C. A. (2009). Urinary function. In C. A. Miller (Ed.), *Nursing for wellness in older adults* (5th ed., pp. 390-416). Philadelphia: Lippincott Williams & Wilkins.

National Kidney Foundation. (2011). Frequently asked questions about GFR estimates. Retrieved from *http://www.kidney.org/professionals/kls/pdf/12-10-4004_KBB_FAQs_AboutGFR-1.pdf*

Palmer, M. H., & Newman, D. K. (2007). Urinary incontinence and estrogen: Is hormone replacement therapy an effective treatment? *American Journal of Nursing, 107*(3), 35-37. Retrieved from *http://www.nursingcenter.com/pdf.asp?AID=698029*

Quaggin, S. E., & Kreidberg, J. A. (2008). Development of the renal glomerulus: Good neighbors and good fences. *Development, 135*(4), 609-20. doi:10.1242/dev.001081

Registered Nurses' Association of Ontario. (2011). Nursing best practice guidelines: Promoting continence using prompted voiding. Retrieved from *http://rnao.ca/bpg/guidelines/promoting-continence-using-prompted-voiding*

Smith, H. W. (1953). *Fish to philosopher.* Boston: Little, Brown.

Tortora, G. J., & Derrickson, B. H. (2006). Principles of anatomy and physiology (11th ed.). Hoboken, NJ: Wiley.

RESOURCES

Resources for this chapter are listed in Chapter 48, p. 1331 and Chapter 49, p. 1367.

Nursing Management: Renal and Urological Problems

Written by Vicki Y. Johnson
Adapted by Lynn Jansen

LEARNING OBJECTIVES

1. Describe the pathophysiology, clinical manifestations, collaborative care, and drug therapy of cystitis, urethritis, and pyelonephritis.
2. Explain the nursing management of urinary tract infections.
3. Describe the immunological mechanisms involved in glomerulonephritis.
4. Explain the clinical manifestations and the nursing and collaborative management of acute poststreptococcal glomerulonephritis, Goodpasture's syndrome, and chronic glomerulonephritis.
5. Describe the common causes, clinical manifestations, collaborative care, and nursing management of nephrotic syndrome.
6. Compare and contrast the etiology, clinical manifestations, collaborative care, and nursing management of various types of urinary calculi.
7. Explain the common causes and management of renal trauma, renal vascular problems, and hereditary renal problems.
8. Describe the mechanisms of renal involvement in metabolic and connective tissue disorders.
9. Describe the clinical manifestations and collaborative care of kidney and bladder cancer.
10. Describe the common causes and management of bladder dysfunctions.
11. Differentiate among ureteral, suprapubic, nephrostomy, and urethral catheters with regard to indications for use and nursing responsibilities.
12. Explain the nursing and collaborative management of the patient undergoing nephrectomy or urinary diversion surgery.

KEY TERMS

calculus An abnormal stone formed in body tissues by an accumulation of mineral salts, p. 1304

cystitis An inflammatory condition of the urinary bladder, characterized by pain, urgency and frequency of urination, and hematuria, p. 1290

glomerulonephritis An immune-related inflammation of the glomeruli characterized by proteinuria, hematuria, decreased urine production, and edema, p. 1299

Goodpasture's syndrome An example of cytotoxic autoimmune disease, characterized by the presence of circulating antibodies against the glomerular basement membrane and the alveolar basement membrane, p. 1301

hydronephrosis Dilation or enlargement of the renal pelvis and the calyces resulting from increased bladder pressure and backflow of urine to the kidney caused by obstruction in the lower urinary tract, p. 1303

hydroureter Dilation of the renal pelvis caused by backflow of urine, p. 1303

ileal conduit Urinary diversion procedure; ureters are anastomosed into a segment of ileum that is converted into a conduit for urinary drainage; the other end of the bowel is brought out through the abdominal wall to form a stoma, p. 1326

interstitial cystitis (IC) Chronic, painful inflammatory disease of the bladder, believed to be associated with an autoimmune or allergic response, p. 1298

lithotripsy The use of sound waves to break renal stones into small particles that can be eliminated from the urinary tract, p. 1307

nephrolithiasis The formation of stones in the urinary tract, p. 1304

nephrosclerosis A vascular disease of the kidney characterized by sclerosis of the small arteries and arterioles of the kidney resulting in renal tissue destruction, p. 1310 nephrotic syndrome An abnormal condition of the kidney characterized by peripheral edema, massive proteinuria, p. 1301

polycystic kidney disease (PKD) A genetic kidney disorder in which the cortex and the medulla are filled with thin-walled cysts that enlarge and destroy surrounding tissue, p. 1311

pyelonephritis Inflammation (usually caused by infection) of the renal parenchyma and collecting system, p. 1295

renal artery stenosis A partial occlusion of one or both renal arteries and their major branches; a major cause of abrupt onset hypertension, p. 1310

renal vein thrombosis An embolus occurring in the renal vein, p. 1311

stricture An abnormal temporary or permanent narrowing of the lumen of a hollow organ such as the ureter or the urethra, p. 1308

urethritis Inflammation of the urethra, p. 1297

urinary incontinence (UI) An uncontrolled leakage loss of urine that is of sufficient magnitude to be a problem, p. 1315

urinary retention The inability to empty the bladder despite micturition or the accumulation of urine in the bladder because of an inability to urinate, p. 1315

ELECTRONIC RESOURCES

Supplemental content related to Chapter 48 can be found…

Evolve Web Site ⏀volve

http://evolve.elsevier.com/Canada/Lewis/medsurg
- Answer Guidelines for Case Study on p. 1328
- Clinical Reference: Laboratory Values
- Content Updates
- Customizable Nursing Care Plans:
  - Acute Renal Lithiasis
  - Ileal Conduit
  - Urinary Tract Infection

- Electronic Calculators
- Examination Review Questions
- Glossary
- Interactive Case Studies:
  - Bladder Cancer With Urinary Diversion
  - Glomerulonephritis and Chronic Kidney Disease
- Key Points (Printable and MP3 Download)
- Patient & Caregiver Teaching Guides:
  - Changing Your Ileal Conduit Appliances
  - Urinary Tract Infection

Renal and urological disorders encompass a wide spectrum of clinical problems. The diverse causes of these disorders may involve infectious, immunological, obstructive, metabolic, collagen-related and vascular, traumatic, congenital, neoplastic, and neurological mechanisms. This chapter discusses specific disorders of the kidneys, ureters, bladder, and urethra. Acute kidney injury and chronic kidney disease are discussed in Chapter 49. Female reproductive problems are discussed in Chapter 56. Male genitourinary problems are discussed in Chapter 57.

Infectious and Inflammatory Disorders of the Urinary System

Urinary Tract Infection

Urinary tract infections (UTIs) are the second most common bacterial disease the human body is subject to, and they affect all age groups. Women are the most susceptible to UTIs and account for more than 500,000 visits to a physician per year in Canada (Kidney Foundation of Canada, 2007). During their lifetime, more than half of women will have a UTI, and up to 50% of these will have another infection within a year (Griebling, 2007). In the older adult population, the prevalence of UTI varies from 30 to 50% in women and 25 to 40% in men. In some cases, patients who develop Gram-negative bacteremia die, and one third of these cases are caused by bacterial infections originating in the

urinary tract (Griebling, 2007; Lin, Fajardo, & U.S. Preventive Services Task Force, 2008).

Inflammation of the urinary tract may be attributable to a variety of disorders, but bacterial infection is by far the most common (Griebling, 2007; Nicolle et al., 2006). In the majority of healthy persons, the bladder and its contents are free from bacteria. Nevertheless, minorities of otherwise healthy individuals, including many young adult women and older women and men, have some bacteria colonizing the bladder. This condition is called *asymptomatic bacteriuria* and does not warrant treatment. In contrast, an infection of the urinary system is diagnosed when bacterial invasion of the urinary tract occurs. Bacterial counts of 10^5 colony-forming units per millilitre (CFU/mL) or higher typically indicate a clinically significant UTI. However, counts as low as 10^2 to 10^3 CFU/mL in a person with signs and symptoms are indicative of UTI.

Escherichia coli (E. coli) (Table 48-1) is the most common pathogen leading to a UTI. Although fungal and parasitic infections may also cause UTIs, they are uncommon. UTIs from these causes are sometimes observed in patients who are immunosuppressed, have diabetes mellitus, or have undergone multiple courses of antibiotic therapy. They also may be seen in persons living in or having travelled to certain developing countries.

Classification

Several classification systems can be used for UTIs (Griebling, 2007; Lin et al., 2008). For example, a UTI can be broadly classified as an upper or a lower UTI according to its location within

Table 48-1 Common Micro-organisms Causing Urinary Tract Infections	
Escherichia coli*	Proteus
Enterococcus	Pseudomonas
Klebsiella	Staphylococcus
Enterobacter	Candida
Serratia	

*Causes about 80% of infections in persons who do not have urinary tract structural abnormalities or calculi.

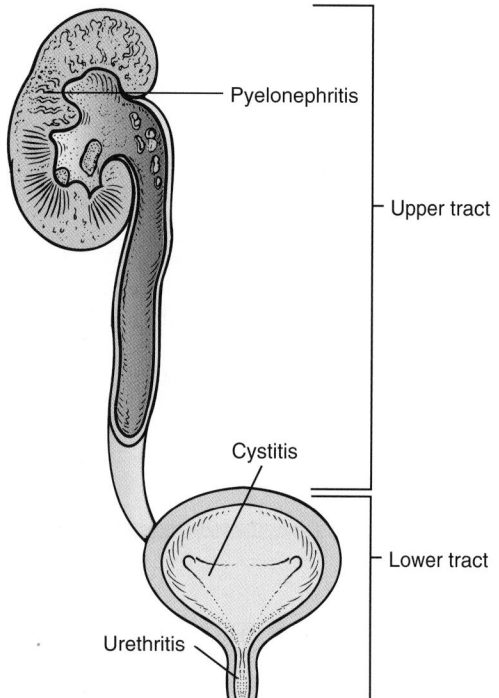

Figure 48-1 Sites of infectious processes in the urinary tract.

Table 48-2 Predisposing Factors to Urinary Tract Infections
Factors Increasing Urinary Stasis
• Intrinsic obstruction (stone, tumour of urinary tract)
• Extrinsic obstruction (tumour, fibrosis compressing urinary tract)
• Urinary retention (including neurogenic bladder and low bladder-wall compliance)
Foreign Bodies
• Urinary calculi
• Indwelling catheter
• Ureteral stent (close proximity of urethral and anal orifices)
Anatomical Factors
• Congenital defects leading to obstruction or urinary stasis
• Fistula (abnormal opening) exposing urinary stream to skin, vagina, or fecal stream
• Shorter female urethra (close proximity of urethral and anal orifices)
Factors Compromising Immune Response
• Human immunodeficiency virus infection
• Diabetes mellitus
Functional Disorders
• Constipation
• Voiding dysfunction with detrusor sphincter dyssynergia

the urinary system (Figure 48-1). Infection of the upper urinary tract (involving the renal parenchyma, renal pelvis, and ureters) typically causes fever, chills, and flank pain, whereas a UTI confined to the lower urinary tract does not usually have systemic manifestations. Specific terms are used to further delineate the location of a UTI or inflammation. For example, **pyelonephritis** implies inflammation (usually caused by infection) of the renal parenchyma and the collecting system. **Cystitis** indicates an inflammatory condition of the urinary bladder, characterized by pain, urgency and frequency of urination, and hematuria. **Urethritis** means inflammation of the urethra.

Classifying a UTI as complicated or uncomplicated is also useful. *Uncomplicated infections* are those that occur in an otherwise normal urinary tract (Norrby, 2007). *Complicated infections* include those that occur concurrently with the presence of obstruction, stones, or catheters; existing diabetes or neurological diseases; or an infection that is recurrent. The individual with a complicated infection is at risk for renal damage.

UTIs can also be classified according to their natural history. An *initial infection* (sometimes called a first or an isolated infection) refers to an uncomplicated UTI in a person who has never had an infection or experiences one that is remote from any previous UTI (usually separated by a period of years). In contrast, a *recurrent UTI* is a reinfection in a person who experienced a previous infection that was successfully eradicated. If a recurrent UTI occurs because the original infection is not adequately eradicated, it is classified as unresolved bacteriuria or bacterial persistence. *Unresolved bacteriuria* occurs when bacteria are initially resistant to the antibiotic used to treat an infection, when the antibiotic agent fails to achieve adequate concentrations in the urine or the bloodstream to kill bacteria, or when the drug is discontinued before the underlying bacteriuria is completely eradicated. *Bacterial persistence* also may occur when bacteria develop resistance to the antibiotic agent selected for treatment or when a foreign body in the urinary system serves as a harbour or anchor allowing bacteria to survive despite appropriate therapy.

Etiology and Pathophysiology

The urinary tract above the urethra is normally sterile. Several physiological and mechanical defence mechanisms assist in maintaining sterility and preventing UTIs. These defences include normal voiding with complete emptying of the bladder, normal antibacterial capability of the bladder mucosa and urine, uretero-vesical junction competence, and peristaltic activity that propels urine toward the bladder. An alteration in any of these defence mechanisms increases the risk of contracting a UTI. Table 48-2 lists predisposing factors to UTIs.

The organisms that usually cause UTIs are introduced via the ascending route from the urethra. Other, less common routes are via the bloodstream or the lymphatic system. Most infections are caused by Gram-negative bacilli normally found in the gastro-intestinal (GI) tract, although Gram-positive organisms such as streptococci, enterococci, and *Staphylococcus saprophyticus* can also

Table 48-3 Lower Urinary Tract Symptoms

Emptying Symptoms

Weak urinary stream.

Hesitancy—difficulty starting the urine stream resulting in a delay between initiation of urination by relaxation of the urethral sphincter and when urine stream actually begins.

Intermittency—interruption of the urinary stream while voiding.

Postvoid dribbling—urine loss after completion of voiding.

Urinary retention or incomplete emptying—inability to empty urine from the bladder, which can be caused by atonic bladder or obstruction of the urethra. Can be acute or chronic.

Dysuria—difficulty voiding.

Pain on urination.

Storage Symptoms

Urinary frequency—an abnormally frequent (usually eight times in a 24-hr period) desire to void, often of only small quantities (e.g., <200 mL).

Urgency—a sudden, strong or intense desire to void immediately, usually accompanied by frequency.

Incontinence—involuntary or unwanted loss or leakage of urine.

Nocturia—waking up two or more times at night because of the need or the urge to void.

Nocturnal enuresis—complaint of loss of urine during sleep. In children, it is called *bedwetting*.

---

cause urinary infections. A common factor contributing to ascending infection is urological instrumentation (e.g., catheterization, cystoscopic examinations). Instrumentation allows bacteria that are normally present at the opening of the urethra to enter the urethra or the bladder. Sexual intercourse promotes "milking" of bacteria from the vagina and the perineum and may cause minor urethral trauma that predisposes women to UTIs.

Rarely do UTIs result from a hematogenous route, where bloodborne bacteria secondarily invade the kidneys, the ureters, or the bladder from elsewhere in the body. For a kidney infection to occur from hematogenous transmission, there must be prior injury to the urinary tract, such as obstruction of the ureter, damage caused by stones, or renal scars.

An important source of UTIs is hospital-acquired, or hospital-associated, infection. The cause of hospital-associated infection is often *E. coli* and, less frequently, *Pseudomonas* organisms. Urological instrumentation, particularly with an indwelling urinary catheter, is the most common predisposing factor.

Clinical Manifestations

Bothersome lower urinary tract symptoms (LUTS) are seen in UTIs of the upper urinary tracts as well as those confined to the lower tract. These symptoms are related to either bladder storage or bladder emptying. These symptoms are defined in Table 48-3.

These symptoms include dysuria, frequency of urination (>q2h), urgency, and suprapubic discomfort or pressure. The urine may contain grossly visible blood (hematuria) or sediment, giving it a cloudy appearance. Flank pain, chills, and the presence of a fever indicate an infection involving the upper urinary tract (pyelonephritis). It is important to remember that these symptoms, considered characteristic of a UTI, are often absent in older adults. Older adults tend to experience nonlocalized abdominal discomfort rather than dysuria and suprapubic pain (Krause, Mowassee, & Auerhahn, 2008). In addition, they may have cognitive impairment. Older adults are also less likely to experience a fever with infection of the upper urinary tract. Patients older than age 80 may experience a slight decline in temperature. People with significant bacteriuria may have no symptoms or may have nonspecific symptoms such as fatigue or anorexia.

Multiple factors may produce bothersome LUTS like those that can accompany a UTI. For example, patients with bladder tumours or those receiving intravesical chemotherapy or pelvic radiation usually experience urinary frequency, urgency, and dysuria. Interstitial cystitis, discussed later in this chapter, is a chronic inflammatory condition of unknown etiology, also producing bothersome urinary symptoms that sometimes cause it to be confused with a UTI.

Diagnostic Studies

Dipstick urinalysis should be obtained initially to identify the presence of nitrites (indicating bacteriuria), white blood cells (WBCs), and leukocyte esterase (an enzyme present in WBCs). These findings can be confirmed by microscopic urinalysis. Following confirmation of bacteriuria and pyuria, a urine culture may be obtained. A urine culture is indicated in complicated or hospital-associated UTIs, persistent bacteria, or frequently recurring UTIs (more than two to three episodes per year). Urine also may be cultured when the infection is unresponsive to empirical therapy or the diagnosis is questionable. A voided midstream technique yielding a clean-catch urine sample is preferred for obtaining a urine culture in most circumstances. (See Chapter 47, Table 47-8 for a description of this technique). However, a specimen obtained by catheterization or suprapubic needle aspiration provides more accurate results and may be necessary when an adequate clean-catch specimen cannot be readily obtained.

A urine culture is accompanied by *sensitivity testing* to determine the bacteria's susceptibility to a variety of antibiotic drugs. The results of this test allow the health care provider to select an antibiotic known to be capable of destroying the bacterial strain producing a UTI in a specific patient.

Imaging studies of the urinary tract are indicated in selected cases. For example, an intravenous pyelogram (IVP) or abdominal computed tomography (CT) scan may be obtained when obstruction of the urinary system is suspected of causing a UTI.

Collaborative Care and Drug Therapy

Once a UTI has been diagnosed, appropriate antimicrobial therapy is initiated. An antibiotic may be selected based on the health care provider's best judgement (empirical therapy) or the results of sensitivity testing. The collaborative care and drug therapy of cystitis are summarized in Table 48-4. Uncomplicated cystitis can be treated by a short-term course of antibiotics, typically for 1 to 3 days. In contrast, complicated UTIs require longer-term treatment, lasting 7 to 14 days or even longer (Norrby, 2007).

Trimethoprim–sulphamethoxazole (TMP–SMX) or nitrofurantoin is often used to empirically treat uncomplicated or initial UTIs. TMP–SMX has the advantages of being relatively inexpensive and is taken twice daily. Nitrofurantoin is normally given three to four times daily, but a long-acting preparation (Macro-BID) is available that is taken twice daily. Ampicillin or amoxicil-

COLLABORATIVE CARE

Table 48-4 Urinary Tract Infection

Diagnostic

- History and physical examination
- Urinalysis
- Urine for culture and sensitivity (if indicated)
- Imaging studies of urinary tract (e.g., IVP, cystoscopy) (if indicated)

Collaborative Therapy

Uncomplicated UTI

- Antibiotic: 1- to 3-day treatment regimen
  - Trimethoprim–sulphamethoxazole (Bactrim, Septra)
  - Nitrofurantoin (Macrodantin, Macrobid)
- Adequate fluid intake
- Urinary analgesic such as phenazopyridine (Pyridium) or combination agent
- Counselling about risk of recurrence and reduction of risk factors

Recurrent, Uncomplicated UTI

- Repeat urinalysis and consideration of need for urine culture and sensitivity testing
- Antibiotic: 3- to 5-day treatment regimen
  - Trimethoprim–sulphamethoxazole (Septra)
  - Nitrofurantoin
  - Sensitivity-guided antibiotic (ampicillin, amoxicillin, first-generation cephalosporin, fluoroquinolone)
- Consideration of 3- to 6-mo trial of suppressive antibiotics
- Adequate fluid intake
- Urinary analgesic such as phenazopyridine (Pyridium) or combination agent
- Counselling about risk of recurrence and reduction of risk factors
- Imaging study of urinary tract in selected cases

IVP, intravenous pyelogram; *UTI*, urinary tract infection.

lin is not frequently selected when empirically treating an uncomplicated UTI because they must be administered three to four times daily. In addition to these agents, the fluoroquinolones (including ciprofloxacin [Cipro], levofloxacin [Levaquin], and norfloxacin) may be used to treat complicated UTIs (Nicolle et al., 2006).

A number of prescription drugs may be used in combination with antibiotic agents to relieve the discomfort associated with a UTI. Phenazopyridine (Pyridium) is a drug that provides a soothing effect on the urinary tract mucosa. It also stains the urine a reddish orange that may be mistaken for blood in the urine, and it may permanently stain underclothing. Although this drug is typically effective in relieving the transient acute discomfort associated with a UTI, patients should be advised to avoid long-term use of phenazopyridine because it can produce hemolytic anemia.

Prophylactic or *suppressive antibiotics* are sometimes administered to patients who experience repeated UTIs (see the Evidence-Informed Practice box). A low dose of TMP–SMX, nitrofurantoin, or another antibiotic, such as ciprofloxacin, may be administered on a daily basis in an attempt to prevent recurring UTIs, or a single dose may be taken before an event likely to provoke a UTI, such as intercourse. However, although suppres-

EVIDENCE-INFORMED PRACTICE

Are Prophylactic Antibiotics Effective for Recurrent Urinary Tract Infection?

Clinical Question

In women (P), is long-term prophylactic antibiotic use (I) more effective than placebo (C) in preventing recurrent urinary tract infections (O)?

Best Available Evidence

Systematic review of randomized controlled trials (RCTs)

Critical Appraisal and Synthesis of Evidence

- 10 RCTs (*n* = 430 women) comparing antibiotic use for 6-12 mo against a placebo for recurrent urinary tract infections (UTI).
- Recurrence is defined as three or more UTI episodes during a 12-mo period.
- Antibiotics reduced the number of UTI recurrences in premenopausal and postmenopausal women with recurrent UTI.
- Antibiotic group had higher incidence of adverse effects, including vaginal itching, skin rash, and nausea.

Conclusions

- Prophylactic antibiotic administration in women who experience recurrent UTIs reduces recurrence.

Implications for Nursing Practice

- Patient treatment preference should be considered when weighing the discomfort of recurrent UTIs and the adverse effects of prophylactic antibiotics.
- UTI prophylaxis for longer than 12 mo has not been studied.

Reference for Evidence

Albert, X., Huertas, I., Pereiro, I., Sanfélix, J., Gosalbes, V., Perrotta, C. (2004 [assessed as up to date 2007]). Antibiotics for preventing recurrent urinary tract infection in non-pregnant women. *Cochrane Database of Systematic Reviews*, 3, CD001209. doi:10.1002/14651858.CD001209.pub2

PICO: P, patient population of interest; *I*, intervention or area of interest; *C*, comparison of interest or comparison group; *O*, outcome(s) of interest.

sive therapy is often effective on a short-term basis, this strategy is limited because of the risk of antibiotic resistance ultimately leading to breakthrough infections with increasingly virulent pathogens (Griebling, 2007; Lin et al., 2008).

NURSING MANAGEMENT: URINARY TRACT INFECTION

Nursing Assessment

Subjective and objective data that should be obtained from a patient with a UTI are presented in Table 48-5.

NURSING ASSESSMENT
Table 48-5 Urinary Tract Infection

Subjective Data

Important Health Information

Past health history: Previous urinary tract infections; urinary calculi, stasis, reflux, strictures, or retention; neurogenic bladder; pregnancy; prostatic hyperplasia; sexually transmitted infection; bladder cancer

Medications: Use of antibiotics, anticholinergics, antispasmodics

Surgery or other treatments: Recent urological instrumentation (catheterization, cystoscopy, surgery)

Symptoms

- Nausea, vomiting, and anorexia; chills
- Lassitude, malaise
- Urinary frequency, urgency, hesitancy; nocturia
- Suprapubic or low back pain, pressure in bladder area, costovertebral tenderness; bladder spasms, dysuria, burning on urination, sense of incomplete emptying

Objective Data

General

Fever

Urinary

Hematuria; cloudy, foul-smelling urine; tender, enlarged kidney

Possible Findings

Leukocytosis; urinalysis positive for bacteria, pyuria, RBCs, and WBCs; positive urine culture; IVP, CT scan, ultrasound, voiding cystourethrogram and cystoscopy demonstrating abnormalities of urinary tract

CT, computed tomography; *IVP,* intravenous pyelogram; *RBCs,* red blood cells; *WBCs,* white blood cells.

Nursing Diagnoses

Nursing diagnoses for the patient with a UTI may include, but are not limited to, those presented in Nursing Care Plan (NCP) 48-1.

Planning

The overall goals are (1) that the patient with a UTI will have relief from bothersome LUTS, (2) prevention of upper urinary tract involvement, and (3) prevention of recurrence.

Nursing Implementation

Health Promotion

Health promotion measures include recognizing individuals who are at risk for a UTI. Debilitated persons, older adults, patients with underlying diseases (e.g., cancer, human immunodeficiency virus [HIV], or diabetes mellitus) that compromise host immune responses, and patients treated with immunosuppressive drugs or corticosteroids are at high risk for UTIs. Especially for these individuals, health promotion activities can help decrease the frequency of infections and promote early detection of infection. Health promotion activities include

working with the patient to promote knowledge about preventive measures, such as (1) emptying the bladder regularly and completely, (2) evacuating the bowel regularly, (3) wiping the perineal area from front to back after urination and defecation, and (4) drinking an adequate amount of liquid each day. The recommended daily liquid intake for the ambulatory adult is approximately 33 mL/kg of body weight per day. Thus, a 70-kg person would require 2310 mL each day. Because the person will obtain approximately 20% of this fluid from food, this leaves 1848 mL obtained by drinking, or nearly eight 236-mL glasses of fluid. Although suppressive antibiotics are not generally recommended, daily intake of cranberry juice (consumed as pure juice, 236 mL twice daily) or cranberry essence tablets may reduce the risk of certain UTIs (Jepson & Craig, 2008). In addition, it is important to advise the patient to seek early treatment once symptoms are identified.

The nurse can play a major role in the prevention of hospital-associated infections. Avoidance of unnecessary catheterization and early removal of indwelling catheters are the most effective means for reducing hospital-associated UTIs. All patients undergoing instrumentation of the urinary tract are at risk for developing a hospital-associated UTI. Aseptic technique must always be followed during these procedures. Washing hands before and after contact with each patient and wearing gloves for care involving the urinary system are especially important. When a catheter has been inserted, special measures must be employed as explained in the section on urethral catheterization later in this chapter.

Routine and thorough perineal hygiene is important for all hospitalized patients, especially when a bedpan is used. Answering the call light quickly or offering the bedpan or urinal at frequent intervals to the bedridden patient should reduce the number of incontinent episodes.

Acute Intervention

Acute intervention for a patient with a UTI includes ensuring adequate fluid intake if it is not contraindicated. It is sometimes difficult to get the patient to maintain an adequate fluid intake because the person may think it will worsen the discomfort and frequency associated with a UTI. The patient needs to be told that fluids will increase frequency of urination at first but will also dilute the urine, making the bladder less irritable. Fluids will help flush out bacteria before they have a chance to colonize in the bladder. Caffeine, alcohol, citrus juices, chocolate, and highly spiced foods or beverages should be avoided because they are potential bladder irritants.

Application of local heat to the suprapubic area or lower back may relieve the discomfort associated with a UTI. The patient can be advised to apply a heating pad (turned to its lowest setting) against the back or suprapubic area. A warm shower can also be effective in providing temporary relief. The patient should be instructed about the prescribed drug therapy, including adverse effects. The nurse should emphasize the importance of taking the full course of antibiotics. Often patients stop antibiotic therapy once symptoms disappear. This practice can lead to inadequate treatment and recurrence of infection or to bacterial resistance to antibiotics. Sometimes a second drug or a reduced dose of drug is ordered after the initial course to suppress bacterial growth in certain patients susceptible to recurrent UTI. The patient should be advised to watch for any changes in the colour or the consistency of the urine and a decrease in or cessation of symptoms as a sign of the effectiveness

NURSING CARE PLAN 48-1

Urinary Tract Infection

NURSING DIAGNOSIS	**Impaired urinary elimination** related to effects of urinary tract infection (UTI) as evidenced by pain and burning on urination and flank, suprapubic, and/or lower back pain

Expected Patient Outcomes	Nursing Interventions and *Rationales*
Pain control	**Pain management**
• Uses nonanalgesic relief measures • Uses analgesics appropriately	• Perform a comprehensive assessment of pain to include location, characteristics, onset and duration, frequency, quality, intensity or severity, and precipitating factors *to establish history and baseline pain level.* • Share information about the use of nonpharmacological techniques (e.g., heating pad to suprapubic area or lower back, warm showers) along with other relief measures *to supplement pain medication and increase pain relief.* • Provide the patient optimal pain relief with prescribed analgesics (such as phenazopyridine [Pyridium]) or combination agents *to promote comfort.*

NURSING DIAGNOSIS	**Impaired urinary elimination** related to UTI as evidenced by bothersome urgency, daytime voiding frequency, nocturia, or hematuria and verbalization of concern over altered elimination pattern

Expected Patient Outcomes	Nursing Interventions and *Rationales*
Urinary elimination	**Urinary elimination management**
Reports relief of bothersome urinary tract symptoms: • Experiences normal urinary elimination patterns • Experiences nocturia not more than two times at night • Urine passes without urgency and frequency • Urine passes without burning sensation • Urine free of visible blood • Has adequate fluid intake	• Monitor urinary elimination including frequency, consistency, odour, volume, and colour (as appropriate) *to assess elimination status.* • Obtain midstream voided specimen for urinalysis (as appropriate) *to determine pathogen causing UTI or to monitor effectiveness of treatment.* • Administer antimicrobial drugs as ordered *to eliminate symptoms by inhibiting bacterial growth.* • Advise patient and monitor for signs and symptoms of UTI *to monitor effectiveness of treatment and recognize symptoms of recurrence.* • Encourage patient to drink 236 mL (8 oz.) of liquid with meals, between meals, and in early evening *to help prevent infection and dehydration.*

NURSING DIAGNOSIS	**Ineffective self-health management** related to lack of knowledge regarding treatment regimen and prevention of recurrent infections as evidenced by response to questions regarding therapeutic management and verbalization of desire to manage treatment of illness and prevent infections.

Expected Patient Outcomes	Nursing Interventions and *Rationales*
• Verbalizes knowledge of treatment regimen • Expresses intent to carry out treatment regimen	**Teaching: disease process** • Appraise patient's current level of knowledge related to specific disease process *to plan how to teach and manage symptom management with the patient.* • Explain pathophysiology of the disease and how it relates to anatomy and physiology *to promote patient understanding.* • Describe rationale behind disease management, *to promote patient's knowledge application of therapy and/or treatment recommendations.* • Describe possible chronic complications *to emphasize the need for completion of treatment.* **Teaching: prescribed medication** • Present purpose and action of each medication and ask the patient if he or she has any questions *to promote patient understanding.* • Describe possible adverse effects of each medication *so patient can identify problems.* • Identify appropriate actions to take if adverse effects occur *to prevent serious problems.*

Table 48-6 Urinary Tract Infection

The following are important to assist the patient with a UTI to prevent recurrence:

1. Explain the importance of taking all antibiotics as prescribed. Symptoms may improve after 1-2 days of therapy, but organisms may still be present.

2. Instruct the patient on appropriate hygiene, including the following:
   a. Careful cleansing of perineal region
   b. Wiping from front to back after urinating
   c. Cleansing with soap and water after each bowel movement

3. Explain the importance of emptying the bladder before and after intercourse and temporarily discontinuing the use of a diaphragm (if used).

4. Advise the patient to urinate regularly, approximately q2-4hr during the day.

5. Discuss information with the patient about how to maintain adequate fluid intake (33 mL [1 oz.] per kilogram of body weight per day).

6. Explain why harsh soaps, bubble baths, powders, and sprays should not be applied in the perineal area.

7. Advise the patient to report symptoms or signs of recurrent UTI (e.g., cloudy urine, pain on urination, urgency, frequency).

UTI, urinary tract infection.

of therapy. The patient should be counselled that persistence of bothersome LUTS beyond the antibiotic treatment course or the onset of flank pain or fever should be reported promptly to a health care provider.

▪ Ambulatory and Home Care

The nurse's responsibility in ambulatory and home care settings is to work with the patient to promote understanding about the need for ongoing care (Table 48-6).

The patient must understand the need for follow-up care with urine culture to determine if the infection has been adequately treated. Recurrent symptoms caused by bacterial persistence or inadequate treatment typically occur within 1 to 2 weeks after completion of therapy. If the patient has been adherent, a relapse indicates the need for further evaluation.

▪ Evaluation

The expected outcomes for the patient with a UTI are presented in NCP 48-1.

Acute Pyelonephritis

Etiology and Pathophysiology

Pyelonephritis is an inflammation of the renal parenchyma (Figure 48-2) and collecting system (including the renal pelvis). The most common cause is bacterial infection, but fungi, protozoa, or viruses sometimes infect the kidney (Czaja, Scholes, Hooton, & Stam, 2007; Schaefer, 2007).

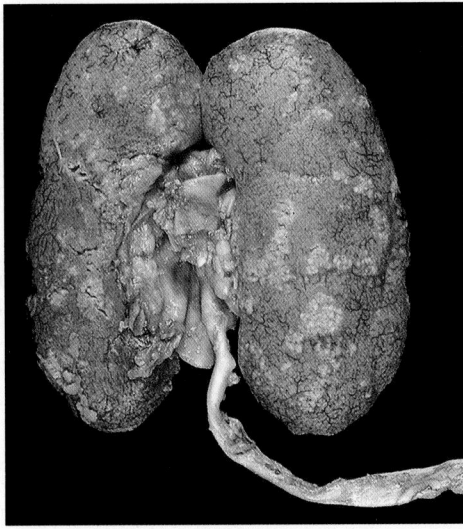

Figure 48-2 Acute pyelonephritis. Cortical surface shows greyish white areas of inflammation and abscess formation.

Source: Kumar, V., Abbas, A. K., Fausto, N., & Aster, J. (2010). *Robbins and Cotran pathologic basis of disease* (8th ed., p. 941, Figure 20-28). Philadelphia: Saunders.

Urosepsis is a systemic infection arising from a urological source. Its prompt diagnosis and effective treatment are critical because, unless promptly eradicated, it typically leads to septic shock and death in 15% of cases. Septic shock is the outcome of unresolved bacteremia involving a Gram-negative organism. (Septic shock is discussed in Chapter 69.)

Pyelonephritis usually begins with colonization and infection of the lower urinary tract via the ascending urethral route. Bacteria normally found in the intestinal tract, such as *E. coli, Proteus, Klebsiella,* or *Enterobacter* species, frequently cause pyelonephritis. A pre-existing factor is often present, such as *vesicoureteral reflux* (retrograde or backward movement of urine from lower to upper urinary tract) or dysfunction of lower urinary tract function such as obstruction from benign prostatic hyperplasia (BPH), a stricture, or a urinary stone.

Acute pyelonephritis commonly starts in the renal medulla and spreads to the adjacent cortex. Recurring episodes of pyelonephritis, especially in the presence of obstructive abnormalities, can lead to a scarred, poorly functioning kidney and a condition called *chronic pyelonephritis.*

Clinical Manifestations and Diagnostic Studies

The clinical manifestations of acute pyelonephritis vary from mild fatigue to the sudden onset of chills, fever, vomiting, malaise, flank pain, and the bothersome LUTS characteristic of cystitis. *Costovertebral tenderness* is typically present on the affected side. The clinical manifestations usually subside within a few days, even without specific therapy, but bacteriuria and pyuria usually persist.

Urinalysis shows pyuria, bacteriuria, and varying degrees of hematuria. WBC casts may be found in the urine, indicating involvement of the renal parenchyma. A complete blood count (CBC) will show leukocytosis and a shift to the left with an increase in immature neutrophils (bands). Urine cultures must be obtained when pyelonephritis is suspected. In patients with more severe illness who are hospitalized, blood cultures are also obtained.

Imaging studies, such as an IVP or CT scan, requiring intravenous injection of contrast materials are usually not obtained in the early stages of pyelonephritis to prevent the possible spread of infection. Alternatively, ultrasonography of the urinary system may be obtained to identify anatomical abnormalities or the presence of an obstructing stone and reduce the need for catheterization. Imaging studies are also used to assess for complications of pyelonephritis such as impaired renal function, scarring, chronic pyelonephritis, or abscesses.

Urosepsis is characterized by bacteriuria and bacteremia (presence of bacteria in blood). If bacteremia is a possibility, close observation and monitoring of vital signs is essential. Prompt recognition and treatment of septic shock may prevent irreversible damage or death.

Collaborative Care and Drug Therapy

The diagnostic tests and the collaborative therapy of acute pyelonephritis are summarized in Table 48-7. Patients with severe infections or complicating factors, such as nausea and vomiting with dehydration, require hospital admission.

The patient with mild symptoms may be treated as an outpatient with antibiotics for 14 to 21 days (see Table 48-7). Parenteral antibiotics are often given initially in the hospital to rapidly establish high serum and urinary drug levels. When initial treatment resolves acute symptoms and the patient is able to tolerate oral fluids and drugs, the person may be discharged on a regimen of oral antibiotics for an additional 14 to 21 days. Symptoms and signs typically improve or resolve within 48 to 72 hours after starting therapy (Schaefer, 2007).

Relapses may be treated with a 6-week course of antibiotics. Reinfections may be treated as individual episodes of disease or managed with long-term antibiotic therapy. Antibiotic prophylaxis may also be used for recurrent infections. The effectiveness of therapy is evaluated in accordance with the presence or absence of bacterial growth on urine culture.

NURSING MANAGEMENT: ACUTE PYELONEPHRITIS

■ Nursing Assessment

Subjective and objective data that should be obtained from a patient with pyelonephritis are presented in Table 48-5.

■ Nursing Diagnoses

Nursing diagnoses for the patient with pyelonephritis include, but are not limited to, those for the patient with a UTI (see NCP 48-1).

■ Planning

The overall goals are that the patient with pyelonephritis will have (1) relief of pain, (2) normal body temperature, (3) no complications, (4) normal renal function, and (5) no recurrence of symptoms.

COLLABORATIVE CARE

Table 48-7 Acute Pyelonephritis

Diagnostic

- History and physical examination
- Urinalysis
- Urine for culture and sensitivity
- Ultrasound (initially), IVP, VCUG, radionuclide imaging, CT scan
- CBC count with WBC differential
- Blood culture (if bacteremia is suspected)
- Palpation for flank pain

Collaborative Therapy

Mild Symptoms

- Outpatient management or short hospitalization for IV antibiotics:
  - Empirically selected broad-spectrum antibiotics (ampicillin, vancomycin) combined with an aminoglycoside (e.g., tobramycin, gentamicin [Garamycin])
  - Switch to sensitivity-guided therapy (when results available) for 14-21 days
  - Trimethoprim–sulphamethoxazole (Septra)
  - Fluoroquinolones (e.g., ciprofloxacin [Cipro], norfloxacin)
- Adequate fluid intake
- Nonsteroidal anti-inflammatory drugs or antipyretic drugs
- Urinary analgesics (e.g., phenazopyridine [Pyridium])
- Follow-up urine culture and imaging studies

Severe Symptoms

- Hospitalization
- Parenteral antibiotics:
  - Empirically selected broad-spectrum antibiotics (e.g., ampicillin, vancomycin) combined with an aminoglycoside (e.g., tobramycin, gentamicin)
  - Switch to sensitivity-guided antibiotic therapy when results of urine and blood culture are available
  - Oral antibiotics when patient tolerates oral intake; administer for 7-21 days
- Adequate fluid intake (initially parenteral; switched to oral fluids as nausea, vomiting, and dehydration subside)
- Nonsteroidal anti-inflammatory or antipyretic drugs to reverse fever and relieve discomfort
- Urinary analgesics (e.g., to relieve bothersome lower urinary tract symptoms)
- Follow-up urine culture and imaging studies

CBC, complete blood count; *CT*, computed tomography; *IV*, intravenous; *IVP*, intravenous pyelogram; *VCUG*, voiding cystourethrogram; *WBC*, white blood cell.

■ Nursing Implementation

■ Health Promotion

Health promotion and maintenance measures are similar to those for cystitis (see p. 1317). In addition, it is important that the patient receive early treatment for cystitis to prevent ascending infections. Because the patient with structural abnormalities of the urinary tract is at high risk for infection, the need for regular medical care should be stressed to these patients.

Acute Intervention and Home Care

Nursing interventions vary depending on the severity of symptoms. These interventions include teaching and working with the patient to promote understanding about the disease process with emphasis on (1) the need to continue drugs as prescribed, (2) the need for a follow-up urine culture to ensure proper management, and (3) identification of risk for recurrence or relapse (see Table 48-5 and NCP 48-1). In addition to antibiotic therapy, the patient should be encouraged to drink at least eight glasses of fluid every day, even after the infection has been treated. Rest is often indicated to increase patient comfort. The patient with frequent relapses or reinfections may be treated with long-term, low-dose antibiotics. Understanding the rationale for therapy is important to enhance patient application of knowledge for disease management.

Evaluation

The expected outcomes for the patient with pyelonephritis are presented in NCP 48-1.

Chronic Pyelonephritis

Chronic pyelonephritis is a term used to describe a kidney that has become shrunken and has lost function owing to scarring or fibrosis (Tolkoff-Rubin, Cotran, & Rubin, 2008). It usually occurs as the outcome of recurring infections involving the upper urinary tract. However, it also may occur in the absence of an existing infection and a recent or remote history of UTIs. Alternative terms used to describe this condition include *interstitial nephritis*, *chronic atrophic pyelonephritis*, or *reflux nephropathy* (when scarring occurs in the presence of vesicoureteral reflux).

Chronic pyelonephritis is diagnosed by radiological imaging and histological testing rather than clinical features. Imaging studies reveal a small, contracted kidney with a thinned parenchyma. The collecting system may be small or hydronephrotic. Pathological analysis reveals loss of functioning nephrons, infiltration of the parenchyma with inflammatory cells, and fibrosis.

The level of renal function in chronic pyelonephritis varies, depending on whether one or both kidneys are affected, the magnitude of scarring, and the presence of coexisting infection. Chronic pyelonephritis often progresses to end-stage renal disease when both kidneys are involved, even if the underlying infection is successfully eradicated. (Nursing and collaborative management of the patient with chronic kidney disease is discussed in Chapter 49.)

Urethritis

Urethritis is an inflammation of the urethra. Causes of urethritis include a bacterial or viral infection, *Trichomonas* and monilial infection (especially in women), chlamydia, and gonorrhea (especially in men). In men, urethritis usually arises from sexual transmission; purulent discharge usually indicates a gonococcal urethritis, whereas a clear discharge typically signifies a nongonococcal urethritis. (Sexually transmitted infections are discussed in Chapter 55.) Urethritis also produces bothersome LUTS, including dysuria and frequent urination, similar to those seen with cystitis.

Urethritis is difficult to diagnose in women. It frequently produces bothersome LUTS as described previously, but urethral discharge may not be present. Cultures on split urine collections (taken at beginning of urine flow and then midstream) or any urethral discharge may confirm a diagnosis of urethral infection.

Treatment is based on identifying and treating the cause and providing symptomatic relief. Sulphamethoxazole with trimethoprim or nitrofurantoin are examples of drugs used for bacterial infections. Metronidazole (Flagyl) and clotrimazole (Mycelex) may be used for treating *Trichomonas*. Drugs such as nystatin (Mycostatin) or fluconazole (Diflucan) may be prescribed for monilial infections. In chlamydial infections, doxycycline (Vibramycin) may be used. Women with negative urine cultures and no pyuria do not usually respond to antibiotics. Hot sitz baths may temporarily relieve bothersome symptoms. The patient should be instructed to avoid the use of vaginal deodorant sprays, properly cleanse the perineal area after bowel movements and urination, and avoid intercourse until symptoms subside. Patients with sexually transmitted urethritis should be instructed to refer their sex partners for evaluation and testing if they had sexual contact in the 60 days preceding onset of symptoms or diagnosis.

Urethral Diverticula

Urethral diverticula are the result of obstruction and subsequent rupture of the periurethral glands into the urethral lumen with epithelialization (regrowth of tissue) over the opening of the resulting periurethral cavity (Dmochowski, 2007). Urethral diverticula are much more common in females than in males, with an incidence in women of 1 to 5%. The rare cases reported in males generally have been associated with lower urinary tract congenital anomalies or surgical trauma. Urethral diverticula occur mostly in the area of the periurethral glands. These glands are found along the entire length of the urethra, with the majority draining into the distal third of the urethra; Skene's glands are the largest and most distal. In many cases, a person may have more than one diverticulum. Causes include urethral trauma from childbearing, urethral instrumentation, dilation or infection with gonococcal organisms, and normal vaginal flora. Urethral diverticula present some of the more challenging diagnostic and reconstructive cases in urology.

Symptoms include dysuria, postvoid dribbling, frequent urination (>q2h), urgency, suprapubic discomfort or pressure, dyspareunia, and a feeling of incomplete bladder emptying. Urinary incontinence is frequently seen. However, one of four women may have no symptoms. The urine may contain gross hematuria or sediment, giving it a cloudy appearance. An anterior vaginal wall mass may be noted on physical examination, which, upon palpation, may be quite tender and express purulent discharge through the urethra. Radiographic studies such as voiding cystourethrography (VCUG) should be used to confirm the diagnosis. Additional studies include ultrasound and magnetic resonance imaging (MRI) to determine the size of the diverticulum in relation to the urethral lumen.

Surgical options include transurethral incision of the diverticular neck, marsupialization (creation of a permanent opening) of the diverticular sac into the vagina (often referred to as a *Spence procedure*), and surgical excision. Surgical excision of a urethral diverticulum should be performed with caution because the diverticular sac may be adherent to the adjacent urethral lumen, and careless excision of the sac may result in a large urethral defect requiring construction of a neourethra (new urethra).

Other important considerations during surgery include identification and closure of the diverticular neck, complete removal of the mucosal lining of the diverticular sac to prevent recurrence, and a multiple-layered closure to prevent postoperative urethrovaginal fistula formation. A complication of the surgery may be stress urinary incontinence.

Interstitial Cystitis

Interstitial cystitis (IC) is a chronic, painful inflammatory disease of the bladder believed to be associated with an autoimmune or allergic response. It is thought to affect as many 101,228 Canadians (3%). The average age at onset is 40 years (Hanno, 2007). The ratio of women to men with IC is 10 to 12 : 1 (Clemens, Joyce, Wise, & Payne, 2007). Although the etiology of IC remains unknown, probable contributing factors include chronic inflammation with mast cell invasion of the bladder wall (possibly provoked by an infection or an autoimmune disorder), defects of the glycosaminoglycan layer that protects the bladder mucosa from the irritating effects of urine exposure, abnormal constituents in the urine, and neurological dysfunction (Hanno, 2007).

The two primary clinical manifestations that characterize IC are pain and bothersome LUTS (e.g., frequency, urgency). The pain associated with IC is usually located in the suprapubic area but may involve the vagina, labia, or entire perineal region. It varies from moderate to severe in intensity and is exacerbated by bladder filling, postponing urination, physical exertion, pressure against the suprapubic area, dietary intake of certain foods, and emotional distress. The pain is transiently relieved by urination. Bothersome LUTS are very similar to those with a UTI, and the condition is often misdiagnosed as a recurring or chronic UTI. The pain and bothersome voiding symptoms produced by IC remit and exacerbate over time. Some patients experience an onset of symptoms that disappear altogether after a period of weeks to months, whereas others have persistent symptoms over a period of months to years.

IC is a diagnosis of exclusion. The condition is suspected whenever a patient experiences symptoms of a UTI despite the absence of bacteriuria, pyuria, or a positive urine culture. A careful history and physical examination are necessary to exclude a variety of disorders that may produce somewhat similar symptoms, such as UTI or endometriosis. This evaluation must include at least one negative urine culture during a period of active symptoms. Cystoscopic examination may reveal a small bladder capacity and superficial ulcerations with bladder filling called *glomerulations*, but these findings are frequently absent and are not unique to IC. Criteria for diagnosing IC are presented in Table 48-8.

Collaborative Care and Drug Therapy

Because the etiology of IC is unknown, no single treatment has been identified that consistently reverses or relieves symptoms. Various therapies have been effective in alleviating or relieving bothersome symptoms in most patients (Chuang & Chancellor, 2009). Dietary and lifestyle alterations are used to relieve pain and diminish voiding frequency and nocturia. Dietary alterations include elimination of foods and beverages likely to exacerbate the symptoms. A diet low in acidic foods and avoiding consumption of beverages such as coffee, tea, and carbonated and alcoholic drinks can be helpful in reducing IC symptoms. Patients may be advised that an over-the-counter dietary supplement

Table 48-8 Clinical Criteria for the Diagnosis of Interstitial Cystitis
Inclusion Criteria
• Pain with bladder filling or postponing urination
• Bothersome urinary urgency
• Small bladder capacity on urodynamic testing
• Cystoscopic evidence of ulcerations or glomerulations (not specific to interstitial cystitis)
Exclusion Criteria
• Bladder capacity >350 mL on urodynamic testing
• Overactive bladder contractions on urodynamic testing
• Daytime voiding frequency (eight or more times per day)
• Active genital herpes
• History of chemotherapy, particularly if treated with cyclophosphamide (Procytox)
• Tubercular cystitis
• History of pelvic radiation
• Bladder tumour

called calcium glycerophosphate (Prelief) alkalinizes the urine and can provide relief from the irritating effects of certain foods. This agent may be particularly helpful when dining away from home where the patient has less control over the preparation of foods.

A number of tricyclic antidepressants, including amitriptyline (Elavil) and doxepin, are used to reduce the burning pain and urinary frequency. Pentosan (Elmiron) is a drug used to enhance the protective effects of the glycosaminoglycan layer of the bladder. It is thought to relieve pain associated with IC by reducing the irritating effects of urine on the bladder wall. Drugs that provide modest relief from IC symptoms in certain cases include nifedipine, which is a calcium channel blocker. These drugs are effective over time (weeks to months), but they do not provide the immediate relief that may be needed when a patient experiences an acute exacerbation of symptoms. In this case, a short course of opioid analgesics may be given.

Several agents may be instilled directly into the bladder through a small catheter. Dimethyl sulphoxide probably acts by desensitizing pain receptors in the bladder wall. Heparin and hyaluronic acid also may be instilled into the bladder to relieve IC symptoms. Like pentosan, they are thought to enhance the protective properties of the glycosaminoglycan layer of the bladder. These drugs are often administered with lidocaine, which rapidly desensitizes the bladder wall, rendering the patient better able to tolerate instillation of additional heparin or hyaluronic acid and providing transient relief from pain. Bacille Calmette-Guérin (BCG), an attenuated form of *Mycobacterium bovis* administered intravesically, is now in clinical trials. The mechanism of action of BCG is unclear, but it may alleviate a possible autoimmune disorder provoking the chronic inflammation characteristic of the disorder.

Distension of the bladder during endoscopic examination relieves IC-related pain and voiding frequency, probably by temporarily disrupting sensory nerve endings in the bladder wall. Several surgical procedures have been used in an attempt to relieve severe, debilitating pain. Urinary diversion, the surgical removal of the bladder and rerouting flow of urine to an ostomy on the abdomen, is an approach that can be used when other measures fail. Unfortunately, some patients have reported pain within the urinary diversion, possibly indicating that components of the urine may contribute to IC in certain cases.

NURSING MANAGEMENT: INTERSTITIAL CYSTITIS

Assessment focuses on characterization of the pain associated with IC. The patient is asked about specific dietary or lifestyle factors known to exacerbate or alleviate pain and about the intensity of the pain. Objective data collection includes a bladder log or voiding diary kept over a period of at least 3 days to determine diurnal voiding frequency and patterns of nocturia. A simultaneous pain record may be useful.

Reassurance that IC is a real condition experienced by others and that it can be effectively treated may relieve the anxiety, anger, guilt, and frustration related to experiences of chronic pain and voiding dysfunction in the absence of a clear-cut diagnosis and treatment strategy. A UTI may occur during the course of IC management. A UTI is likely to produce an acute exacerbation of bothersome LUTS and urinary frequency as well as dysuria (not typically associated with IC) and odorous urine, possibly with hematuria.

The patient also must be given instruction about the need to maintain good nutrition, particularly in light of the broad dietary restrictions often necessary to control IC-related pain. Specifically, the patient may be advised to take a multivitamin containing no more than the recommended dietary allowance for essential vitamins and to avoid high-potency vitamins, because these formulations may irritate the bladder. The patient is also advised to obtain information from support organizations such as the Sunnybrook Women's Health Network in Canada and the Interstitial Cystitis Association in the United States, which includes recipes and menus for a well-balanced diet that is specifically designed to avoid bladder-irritating foods and beverages.

Elimination of a variety of foods and beverages from the diet that are likely to irritate the bladder typically provides modest to profound relief from symptoms. Typical bladder irritants include caffeine, alcohol, citrus products, aged cheeses, nuts, foods containing vinegar, curries or hot peppers, and foods or beverages likely to lower urinary pH. In addition, the patient should be taught to self-manage the use of Prelief. The patient is advised to avoid clothing that creates suprapubic pressure, including pants with tight belts or restrictive waistlines.

Written educational materials concerning diet, coping with the need for frequent urination, and strategies for coping with the emotional burden of IC are available from the Interstitial Cystitis Association. Providing such materials affords an excellent opportunity for the nurse to introduce the patient to the existence of this patient advocacy group and to participate in local support groups when desired.

Renal Tuberculosis

Renal tuberculosis (TB) is rarely a primary lesion. It is usually secondary to TB of the lung. In a small percentage of patients with pulmonary TB, the tubercle bacilli reach the kidneys via the bloodstream. Onset occurs 5 to 8 years after the primary infection. The patient is often asymptomatic when the kidney is initially infiltrated with bacilli. Sometimes, the patient complains of fatigue and develops a low-grade fever. As the lesions ulcerate, infection descends to the bladder, and the patient experiences frequent urination, burning on voiding, and epididymitis (in men). Symptoms of a UTI are the first sign in the majority of patients with renal TB. Renal lesions may calcify as they heal. Infrequently, renal colic, lumbar and iliac pain, and hematuria may be present. A diagnosis is based on localization of tubercle bacilli in the urine and on IVP findings.

Long-term complications of renal TB depend on the duration of the disease before treatment. Scarring of the renal parenchyma and the development of ureteral strictures occur. The earlier treatment is initiated, the less likely renal failure is to develop. Reduced bladder volume may be irreversible in advanced disease. The patient may require long-term urological follow-up. (Nursing and collaborative management for the patient with TB is discussed in Chapter 30.)

Immunological Disorders of the Kidney

Glomerulonephritis

Immunological processes involving the urinary tract predominantly affect the renal glomerulus. The disease process results in **glomerulonephritis,** an immune-related inflammation of the glomeruli characterized by proteinuria, hematuria, decreased urine production, and edema. The condition affects both kidneys equally. Although the glomerulus is the primary site of inflammation, tubular, interstitial, and vascular changes also occur. Glomerulonephritis is divided into a number of classifications, which may describe (1) the extent of damage (diffuse or focal), (2) the initial cause of the disorder (systemic lupus erythematosus, systemic sclerosis [scleroderma], streptococcal infection), or (3) the extent of changes (minimal or widespread).

Etiology and Pathophysiology

Two types of antibody-induced injury can initiate glomerular damage. In the first type, the antibodies have specificity for antigens within the glomerular basement membrane (GBM). These are termed anti-GBM antibodies. Immunoglobulins and complement are deposited along the basement membrane. The mechanism that causes development of antibodies against a person's own GBM is not known. Production of autoantibodies (antibodies to one's own tissue) may be stimulated by a structural alteration in the GBM or by an interaction between the basement membrane and an exogenous agent (e.g., hydrocarbon, viruses).

In the second type of immune process, the antibodies react with circulating nonglomerular antigens and are randomly deposited as immune complexes along the GBM. On electron microscopy of renal tissue sections, the deposits appear uneven. In this immune complex process, the antigens do not come from the glomeruli but from either endogenous circulating native DNA or exogenous sources (e.g., bacteria, viruses, chemicals, drugs). Bacterial products appear to be important in poststreptococcal glomerulonephritis. Viral agents have been recognized in certain cases of glomerulonephritis that develop after hepatitis B or C and rubella (measles).

All forms of immune-complex disease are characterized by an accumulation of antigen, antibody, and complement in the glomeruli, which can result in tissue injury. The immune complexes activate complement (see Chapters 14 and 16). Complement activation results in the release of chemotactic factors that attract polymorphonuclear leukocytes and cause the release of histamine and other inflammatory mediators. These processes cause inflammation, whose end result is glomerular injury.

Clinical Manifestations

Clinical manifestations of glomerulonephritis include varying degrees of hematuria (ranging from microscopic to gross) and urinary excretion of various formed elements, including red blood cells (RBCs), WBCs, and casts. Proteinuria and elevated serum urea (blood urea nitrogen [BUN]) and serum creatinine levels are other manifestations. In most cases, recovery from the acute illness is complete. However, if progressive involvement occurs, the result is destruction of renal tissue and marked renal insufficiency.

The patient's history provides important information related to glomerulonephritis. It is necessary to assess exposure to drugs, immunizations, microbial infections, and viral infections such as hepatitis. It is also important to evaluate the patient for more generalized conditions involving immune disorders, such as systemic lupus erythematosus and systemic sclerosis.

Acute Post-streptococcal Glomerulonephritis

Acute post-streptococcal glomerulonephritis (APSGN) is most common in children and young adults, but all age groups can be affected. APSGN develops 5 to 21 days after an infection of the pharynx or the skin (e.g., streptococcal sore throat, impetigo) by certain nephrotoxic strains of group A β-hemolytic streptococci. The person produces antibodies to the streptococcal antigen. Although the specific mechanism is not known, the antigen–antibody complexes are deposited in the glomeruli and activate complement (Zhang & Rothenbacher, 2008). Complement activation causes an inflammatory reaction to the injury. The response to the injury is also a decrease in the filtration of metabolic waste products from the blood and an increase in the permeability of the glomerulus to larger protein molecules.

Clinical Manifestations and Complications

The clinical manifestations of APSGN appear as a variety of signs and symptoms, which may include generalized body edema, hypertension, oliguria, hematuria with a smoky or rusty appearance, and proteinuria. Fluid retention occurs as a result of decreased glomerular filtration. The edema appears initially in low-pressure tissues, such as around the eyes (periorbital edema), but later progresses to involve the total body as ascites or peripheral edema in the legs. Smoky urine indicates bleeding in the upper urinary tract. The degree of proteinuria varies with the severity of the glomerulonephropathy. Hypertension primarily results from increased extracellular fluid volume. The patient with APSGN may have abdominal or flank pain. At times, the patient has no symptoms, and the problem is found on routine urinalysis.

Table 48-9 Acute Glomerulonephritis

Diagnostic	Collaborative Therapy
• History and physical examination • Urinalysis • CBC • BUN, serum creatinine, and albumin • Complement levels and ASO titre • Renal biopsy (if indicated)	• Rest • Sodium and fluid restriction • Diuretics • Antihypertensive therapy • Adjustment of dietary protein intake to level of proteinuria and uremia

ASO, antistreptolysin O; *BUN,* blood urea nitrogen; *CBC,* complete blood count.

More than 95% of patients with APSGN recover completely or improve rapidly with conservative management. Chronic glomerulonephritis develops in 5 to 15% of the affected persons, and irreversible renal failure occurs in less than 1% of patients (Zhang & Rothenbacher, 2008).

Diagnostic Studies

The diagnosis of APSGN is based on a complete history and physical examination and laboratory studies (Table 48-9) to determine the presence or history of a group A β-hemolytic streptococcus in a throat or skin lesion. An immune response to the streptococcus is often demonstrated by assessment of antistreptolysin O (ASO) titres. The finding of decreased complement components (especially C3 and CH50) indicates an immune-mediated response. A renal biopsy may be performed to confirm the presence of the disease.

Dipstick and urine sediment microscopy will reveal the presence of erythrocytes in significant numbers. Erythrocyte casts are highly suggestive of acute glomerulonephritis. Proteinuria may range from mild to severe. Screening blood tests include BUN and serum creatinine to assess the extent of renal impairment.

NURSING AND COLLABORATIVE MANAGEMENT: ACUTE POST-STREPTOCOCCAL GLOMERULONEPHRITIS

The management of APSGN focuses on symptomatic relief (see Table 48-9). Rest is recommended until the signs of glomerular inflammation (proteinuria, hematuria) and hypertension subside. Edema is treated by restricting sodium and fluid intake and by administrating diuretics. Severe hypertension is treated with antihypertensive drugs. Dietary protein intake may be restricted if there is evidence of an increase in nitrogenous wastes (e.g., elevated BUN). The restriction varies with the degree of proteinuria. (Low-protein, low-sodium, fluid-restricted diets are discussed in Chapter 49.) Antibiotics should be given only if the streptococcal infection is still present. Corticosteroids and cytotoxic drugs have not been shown to be of value.

One of the most important ways to prevent the development of APSGN is to encourage early diagnosis and treatment of sore throats and skin lesions. If streptococci are found in the culture, treatment with appropriate antibiotic therapy (usually penicillin) is essential. The patient must be encouraged to take the full course of antibiotics to ensure that the bacteria have been eradicated. Good personal hygiene is an important factor in preventing the spread of cutaneous streptococcal infections. (The Kidney Foundation of Canada Web site provides information on the management of kidney disease and support groups.)

Goodpasture's Syndrome

Goodpasture's syndrome, an example of cytotoxic (type II) autoimmune disease, is characterized by the presence of circulating antibodies against the GBM and the alveolar basement membrane (Goligher & Detsky, 2009). Although the primary target organ is the kidney, the lungs are also involved. In the course of this pathological syndrome, the binding of the antibody causes an inflammatory reaction mediated by complement fixation and activation (see Chapters 14 and 16). The causative factors for development of autoantibody production are unknown, although type A influenza viruses, hydrocarbons, penicillamine, and unknown genetic factors may be involved.

Goodpasture's syndrome is a rare disease that is seen mostly in young male smokers. The clinical manifestations include hemoptysis, pulmonary insufficiency, crackles, wheezes, renal involvement with hematuria and renal failure, weakness, pallor, and anemia. Pulmonary hemorrhage usually occurs and may precede glomerular abnormalities by weeks or months. Abnormal diagnostic findings include low hematocrit and hemoglobin levels, elevated BUN and serum creatinine levels, hematuria, and proteinuria. Circulating serum anti-GBM antibodies parallel the activity of the renal disease and are diagnostic of this syndrome.

NURSING AND COLLABORATIVE MANAGEMENT: GOODPASTURE'S SYNDROME

Until recently, the prognosis for the patient with Goodpasture's syndrome was poor (Goligher & Detsky, 2009). However, with the development of immunosuppressive therapy and advances in transplantation techniques, the outlook has improved. Management consists of corticosteroids, immunosuppressive drugs (e.g., cyclophosphamide [Procytox], azathioprine [Imuran]), plasmapheresis (see Chapter 16), and dialysis. Plasmapheresis removes the circulating anti-GBM antibodies, and immunosuppressive therapy inhibits further antibody production. Renal transplantation can be attempted after the circulating anti-GBM antibody titre decreases. Although recurrences may develop, the disease is not a contraindication to transplantation. In selected patients with severe pulmonary hemorrhage, bilateral nephrectomy has been helpful. The exact mechanism for improvement has not been determined.

Nursing management appropriate for a critically ill patient who is experiencing symptoms of acute kidney failure and respiratory distress is instituted. Death is often secondary to hemorrhage in the lungs and respiratory failure. (Nursing interventions for a patient in acute renal failure are discussed in Chapter 49, and nursing interventions for a patient with respiratory failure are discussed in Chapter 70.) Because this syndrome is rare and primarily affects previously healthy young adults, support and understanding of the patient and family are of major importance. The patient and family need instructions concerning current therapy, drugs, and complications of the disease process.

Rapidly Progressive Glomerulonephritis

Rapidly progressive glomerulonephritis (RPGN) is glomerular disease associated with rapid, progressive loss of renal function over days to weeks. Renal failure may occur within weeks to months, in contrast to chronic glomerulonephritis, in which it develops insidiously and progresses over many years. The manifestations of RPGN are hypertension, edema, proteinuria, hematuria, and RBC casts.

RPGN can occur in a variety of situations: (1) as a complication of inflammatory or infectious disease (e.g., APSGN), (2) as a complication of a multisystemic disease (e.g., systemic lupus erythematosus, Goodpasture's syndrome), (3) as an idiopathic disease, or (4) in association with the use of certain drugs (e.g., penicillamine).

Treatment is directed toward correction of fluid overload, hypertension, uremia, and inflammatory injury to the kidney. Treatment includes corticosteroids, cytotoxic agents, and plasmapheresis. Dialysis therapy and transplantation are used as maintenance therapy for the patient with RPGN. Following renal transplantation, RPGN may recur.

Chronic Glomerulonephritis

Chronic glomerulonephritis is a syndrome that reflects the end stage of glomerular inflammatory disease. Most types of glomerulonephritis and nephrotic syndrome can eventually lead to chronic glomerulonephritis.

The syndrome is characterized by proteinuria, hematuria, and the slow development of uremic syndrome (see Chapter 49) as a result of decreasing renal function. Chronic glomerulonephritis does not usually follow an acute course. It progresses insidiously toward renal failure over a few to as many as 30 years.

Chronic glomerulonephritis is often found coincidentally as an abnormality on a urinalysis or when elevated blood pressure is detected. It is common to find that the patient has no recollection or history of acute nephritis or any renal problems. A renal biopsy may be performed to determine the exact cause and nature of the glomerulonephritis. However, ultrasound and CT scanning are generally preferred as diagnostic measures.

Treatment is supportive and symptomatic. Hypertension and UTIs should be treated vigorously. Protein and phosphate restrictions may slow the rate of progression of kidney disease. (Management of chronic kidney disease is discussed in Chapter 49.)

Nephrotic Syndrome

Etiology and Clinical Manifestations

Nephrotic syndrome describes a clinical course that can be associated with a number of disease conditions. Some of the more common causes of nephrotic syndrome are listed in Table 48-10.

Table 48-10 Causes of Nephrotic Syndrome

Primary Glomerular Disease

- Primary nephrotic syndrome
- Focal glomerulonephritis
- Inherited nephrotic disease

Extrarenal Causes

Multisystem Disease

- Systemic lupus erythematosus
- Diabetes mellitus
- Amyloidosis

Infections

- Bacterial (streptococcal, syphilis)
- Viral (hepatitis, human immunodeficiency virus infection)
- Protozoal (malaria)

Neoplasms

- Hodgkin's disease
- Solid tumours of lungs, colon, stomach, breast
- Leukemias

Allergens (e.g., bee sting, pollen)

Drugs

- Penicillamine
- Nonsteroidal anti-inflammatory drugs
- Captopril
- Heroin

In adults, about one third of patients with nephrotic syndrome will have a systemic disease such as diabetes or systemic lupus erythematosus. The remainder will be categorized as having idiopathic nephrotic syndrome.

The characteristic manifestations include peripheral edema, massive proteinuria, dyslipidemia, and hypoalbuminemia. Characteristic blood chemistries include decreased serum albumin, decreased total serum protein, and elevated serum cholesterol. The increased glomerular membrane permeability found in nephrotic syndrome is responsible for the massive excretion of protein in the urine. This results in decreased serum protein and subsequent edema formation. Ascites and anasarca develop if there is severe hypoalbuminemia.

The diminished plasma oncotic pressure from the decreased serum proteins stimulates hepatic lipoprotein synthesis, which results in dyslipidemia. Initially, cholesterol and low-density lipoproteins are elevated. Later, the triglyceride level is also increased. Fat bodies (fatty casts) commonly appear in the urine.

Immune responses, both humoral and cellular, are altered in nephrotic syndrome. As a result, infection is an important cause of morbidity and mortality. Calcium and skeletal abnormalities may occur, including hypocalcemia, blunted calcemic response to parathyroid hormone, hyperparathyroidism, and osteomalacia.

With nephrotic proteinuria, loss of clotting factors can result in a relative hypercoagulable state. Hypercoagulability with thromboembolism is potentially the most serious complication of nephrotic syndrome. The renal vein is the site most commonly involved for thrombus formation. Pulmonary emboli occur in about 40% of nephrotic patients with thrombosis.

Collaborative Care

Treatment of nephrotic syndrome is symptomatic (Mayo Clinic Staff, 2012). The goals are to relieve edema and cure or control the primary disease. Management of the edema includes the cautious use of angiotensin-converting enzyme inhibitors, nonsteroidal anti-inflammatory drugs, and a low-sodium (2-3 g/day), low- to moderate-protein diet (0.5-0.6 g/kg of body weight per day). Dietary salt restrictions are a key to managing edema. In some individuals, thiazide or loop diuretics may be needed. If urine protein loss exceeds 10 g/24 hr, additional dietary protein may be needed.

The treatment of dyslipidemia is often unsuccessful. However, treatment with lipid-lowering agents, such as colestipol (Colestid) and lovastatin (Mevacor), may result in moderate decreases in serum cholesterol levels. If thrombosis is detected, anticoagulant therapy may be necessary for up to 6 months.

Corticosteroids and cyclophosphamide (Procytox) may be used for the treatment of severe cases of nephrotic syndrome. Management of diabetes and treatment of edema are the only measures used for nephrotic syndrome related to diabetes.

NURSING MANAGEMENT: NEPHROTIC SYNDROME

A major nursing intervention for a patient with nephrotic syndrome is related to edema. It is important to assess the edema by weighing the patient daily, accurately recording intake and output, and measuring abdominal girth or extremity size. Comparing this information daily provides the nurse with a tool for assessing the effectiveness of treatment. The edematous skin must be cleaned carefully. Trauma should be avoided, and the effectiveness of diuretic therapy must be monitored.

The patient with nephrotic syndrome has the potential to become malnourished from the excessive loss of protein in the urine. Maintaining a low- to moderate-protein diet that is also low in sodium is not always easy. The patient is usually anorexic. Serving small, frequent meals in a pleasant setting may encourage better dietary intake.

Because the patient is susceptible to infection, measures should be taken to avoid exposure to persons with known infections. The person with nephrotic syndrome is often ashamed of an edematous appearance and needs support in dealing with an altered body image.

Obstructive Uropathies

Urinary obstruction refers to any anatomical or functional condition that blocks or impedes the flow of urine (Figure 48-3). It may be congenital or acquired. Obstruction may be the result of (1) intrinsic causes such as anomalies, diverticula, tumours, or benign growth within the urinary tract; (2) extrinsic causes such as tumours, adhesions, retroperitoneal fibrosis, or prolapsed adjacent organs; or (3) functional causes as a result of neurological or psychogenic factors. Some common intrinsic obstructions are narrowing of the ureteropelvic junction (UPJ), bladder neck contracture, BPH, urethral stricture, and urethral meatal stenosis. Common extrinsic causes include pelvic and abdominal tumours or a prolapsed uterus. Examples of functional causes are

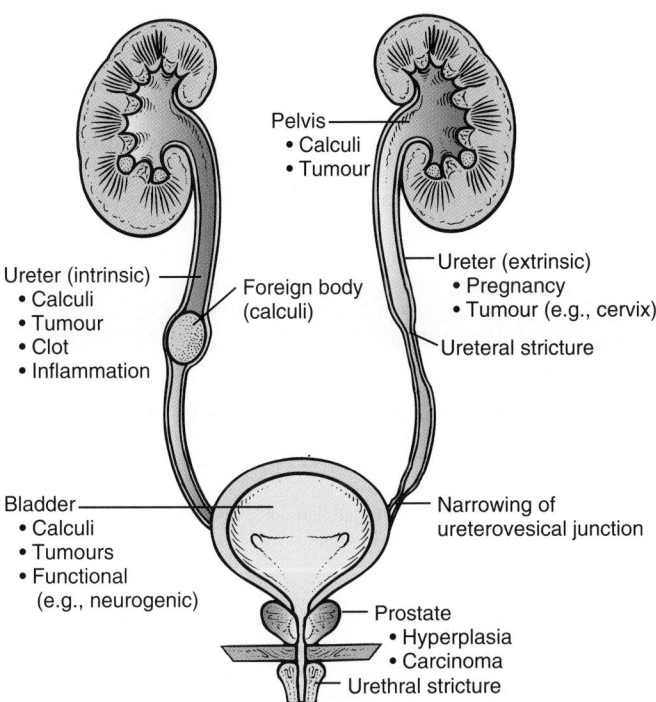

Figure 48-3 Common causes of urinary tract obstruction.

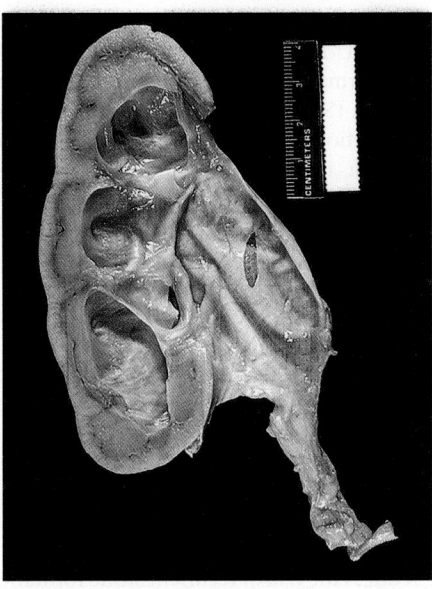

Figure 48-4 Hydronephrosis of the kidney with marked dilation of the pelvis and the calyces and thinning of the renal parenchyma.

Source: Kumar, V., Abbas, A. K., Fausto, N., & Aster, J. (2010). *Robbins and Cotran pathologic basis of disease* (8th ed., p. 961, Figure 20-50). Philadelphia: Saunders.

neurogenic bladder and vesicosphincter dyssynergia (disturbance in muscle coordination) after spinal cord injury.

Damaging effects from urinary tract obstruction affect the system above the level of the obstruction. The severity of these effects depends on location, duration of obstruction, amount of pressure or dilation, presence of urinary stasis, and whether infection is present. Infection increases the risk of irreversible damage.

Although obstruction distal to the prostate in men or the bladder neck in women causes mucosal scarring and a slower stream, it rarely results in major obstructive uropathy because the urethral wall pressure is less than that of the bladder neck and bladder. Urethral obstruction may contribute to outlet resistance and cause lower or upper urinary tract damage when other obstructive or dysfunctional factors are also present. For example, there is an increased risk of compromised renal function in the patient with a spinal cord injury with vesicosphincter dyssynergia.

When obstruction occurs at the level of the bladder neck or the prostate, significant bladder changes can occur. Detrusor muscle fibres *hypertrophy* (increase in size) to contract harder-to-push urine out a narrower pathway. Over a long period, the detrusor loses its ability to compensate for this resistance. Muscle bundles separate and become less compliant. This separation is called *trabeculation*. Trabeculation is caused by the deposition of collagen in the bladder wall that separates the smooth muscle fascicles. Trabeculation may hasten the decompensation of the detrusor. The areas between these muscle bundles are called *cellules*. Because these areas have no muscle support, the bladder mucosa can herniate between detrusor muscle bundles, forming sacs that drain poorly, called *diverticula*. Residual urine can be very high in a noncompensating bladder.

Pressure increases during bladder filling or storage and can be transmitted to the ureter when *bladder outlet obstruction* is present. This pressure overcomes the normal peristaltic pressure and leads to *reflux* (a backflow of urine), which in turn causes

ureteral dilation, kinking, and tortuosity; **hydroureter** (dilation of the renal pelvis); vesicoureteral reflux (backflow or backward movement of urine from the lower to upper urinary tracts); and **hydronephrosis** (dilation or enlargement of the renal pelvis and the calyces) (Figure 48-4) and consequent chronic pyelonephritis and renal atrophy. If only one kidney is obstructed, the other kidney may try to compensate by hypertrophy, but the ureter will not be dilated on this contralateral side.

Partial obstruction may occur in the ureter or at the UPJ. If the pressure remains low or moderate, the kidney may continue to dilate with no noticeable loss of function. There is an increased risk of pyelonephritis because of urinary stasis and reflux. If only one kidney is involved and the other kidney is functioning, the patient may be free of symptoms. If both kidneys or only one functioning kidney is involved (e.g., if the patient has only one kidney), alterations in renal function (e.g., increased BUN or serum creatinine levels) are found. If the obstruction progresses, oliguria or anuria develops. Often, episodes of oliguria are followed by polyuria if the obstruction is a stone that becomes dislodged. Treatment calls for location and relief of the blockage. This can include insertion of a tube (e.g., urethral or ureteral), surgical correction of the disease process, or diversion of the urinary stream above the level of blockage.

Urinary Tract Calculi

One out of 10 Canadians will have a kidney stone at some point in life (Kidney Foundation of Canada, 2003). Many of these people require hospitalization. In Canada, the incidence of kidney stones is highest in the East and decreases to the West. Except for struvite (magnesium–ammonium phosphate) stones associated with UTI, stone disorders are more common in men than in women (National Kidney and Urologic Diseases Information Clearinghouse [NKUDIC], 2007).

The majority of patients with stones are between 20 and 55 years of age. The incidence is also higher in persons with a family history of stone formation. Recurrence of stones can occur in up to 50% of patients (Sakhaee, 2009). There is seasonal variation, with stone formation occurring more often in the summer months in Canada, thus supporting the role of dehydration in this process. Stone formation in the kidney also seems to increase in incidence as countries become more industrialized whereas the incidence of bladder stones decreases.

Etiology and Pathophysiology

Many factors are involved in the incidence and the type of stone formation, including metabolic, dietary, genetic, climatic, lifestyle, and occupational influences (Table 48-11). Many theories have been proposed to explain the formation of stones in the urinary tract. No single theory can account for stone formation in all cases. Crystals, when in a supersaturated concentration, can precipitate and unite to form a stone. Keeping urine dilute and free flowing reduces the risk of recurrent stone formation in many individuals. It is known that a *mucoprotein* is formed (the matrix for the stone) in the kidneys that forms stones. Urinary pH, solute load, and inhibitors in the urine affect the formation of stones. The lower the pH is, the less soluble uric acid and cystine are. The higher the pH, the less soluble calcium and phosphate.

Other important factors in the development of stones include obstruction with urinary stasis and urinary infection with urea-splitting bacteria (e.g., *Proteus, Klebsiella, Pseudomonas,* and some species of staphylococci). These bacteria cause the urine to become alkaline and contribute to the formation of struvite (magnesium–ammonium phosphate) stones (Carpentier et al., 2009). Infected stones, when they are entrapped in the kidney, may assume a staghorn configuration as they enlarge (Figure 48-5). Infected stones are frequent in the patient with an external urinary diversion, long-term indwelling catheter, neurogenic bladder, or urinary retention. Genetic factors may also contribute to urine stone formation. Cystinuria is an autosomal recessive disorder. In this disorder, there is a marked increased excretion of cystine.

Types

A **calculus** is an abnormal stone formed in body tissues by an accumulation of mineral salts. The term *calculus* refers to the stone, and *lithiasis* refers to stone formation (**nephrolithiasis** thus indicating the formation of stones in the urinary tract). The five major categories of stones are (1) calcium phosphate, (2) calcium

Table 48-11 Risk Factors for the Development of Urinary Tract Calculi
Metabolic
Abnormalities that result in increased urine levels of calcium, oxaluric acid, uric acid, or citric acid
Climate
Warm climates that cause increased fluid loss, low urine volume, and increased solute concentration in urine
Diet
Large intake of dietary proteins that increases uric acid excretion
Excessive amounts of tea or fruit juices that elevate urinary oxalate level
Large intake of calcium* and oxalate
Low fluid intake that increases urinary concentration
Genetic
Family history of stone formation, cystinuria, gout, or renal acidosis
Lifestyle
Sedentary occupation, immobility

*Recent research suggests that a high dietary calcium intake, which was previously thought to contribute to kidney stones, may actually lower the risk by reducing the urinary excretion of oxalate, a common factor in many stones (National Kidney and Urologic Diseases Information Clearinghouse, 2009).
Source: National Kidney and Urologic Information and Clearing House. (2009). Diet for Kidney Stone Prevention. Retrieved from *http://kidney. niddk.nih.gov/KUDiseases/pubs/kidneystonediet/index.aspx#calcium/*

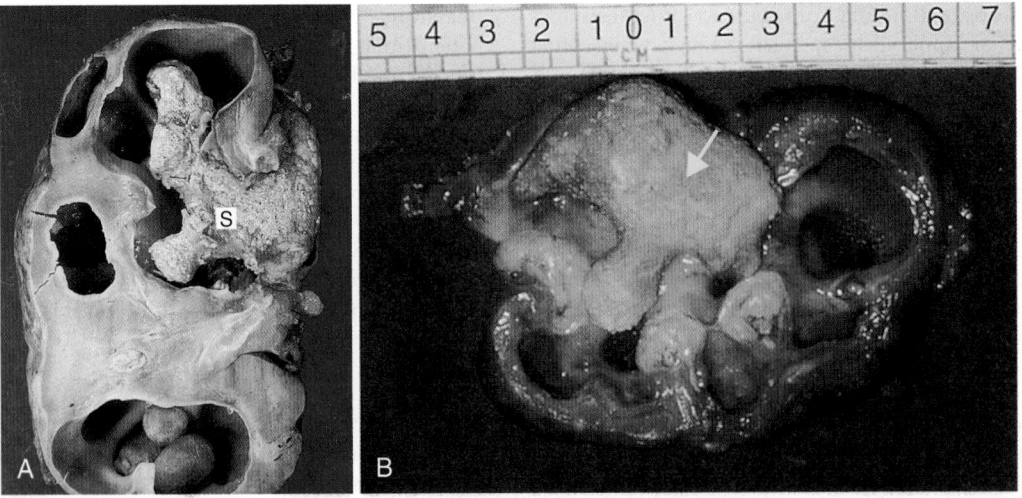

Figure 48-5 A, Renal staghorn calculus. The renal pelvis is filled with a large calculus that is shaped to its contours, resembling the horn of a stag *(S).* **B,** Embedded staghorn calculus *(yellow arrow)* in a hydronephrotic, infected, nonfunctioning kidney.

Source: **A** from Stevens, A., & Lowe, J. (2000). *Pathology: Illustrated review in color* (2nd ed.). London: Mosby; **B** from Bullock, N., Doble, A., Turner, W., & Cuckow, P. (2008). *Urology: An illustrated colour text.* London: Churchill Livingstone.

Table 48-12 Types of Urinary Tract Calculi

URINARY STONE	INCIDENCE (%)	CHARACTERISTICS	PREDISPOSING FACTORS	THERAPEUTIC MEASURES
Calcium oxalate*	35-40	Small, often possible to get trapped in ureter; more frequent in men than in women	Idiopathic hypercalciuria; hyperoxaluria, family history; independent of urinary pH	Increase hydration. Reduce dietary oxalate.† Give thiazide diuretics. Give cellulose phosphate to chelate calcium and prevent GI absorption. Give potassium citrate to maintain alkaline urine. Give cholestyramine to bind oxalate. Give calcium lactate to precipitate oxalate in GI tract.
Calcium phosphate	8-10	Mixed stones (typically), occur with struvite or oxalate stones	Alkaline urine, primary hyperparathyroidism	Treat underlying causes and other stones.
Struvite ($MgNH_4PO_4$)	10-15	Three to four times more common in women than men, always in association with urinary tract infections, large staghorn type (usually)‡	Urinary tract infections (usually *Proteus* organisms)	Administer antimicrobial agents, acetohydroxamic acid. Use surgical intervention to remove stone. Take measures to acidify urine.
Uric acid	5-8	Predominant in men, high incidence in Jewish men	Gout, acid urine, inherited condition	Reduce urinary concentration of uric acid. Alkalinize urine with potassium citrate. Administer allopurinol. Reduce dietary purines.†
Cystine	1-2	Genetic autosomal recessive defect, defective absorption of cystine in GI tract and kidney, excess concentrations causing stone formation	Acid urine	Increase hydration. Give α-penicillamine and tiopronin to prevent cystine crystallization. Give potassium citrate to maintain alkaline urine.

GI, gastrointestinal.

*Calcium stones can exist as calcium oxalate, calcium phosphate, or a mixture of both. Calcium stones account for the majority of all stones.
†See Table 48-13.
‡See Figs. 48-5 and 48-6.

oxalate, (3) uric acid, (4) cystine, and (5) struvite (magnesium–ammonium phosphate) (Table 48-12). Stone composition may be mixed, although calcium stones are the most common. Calculi can be found in various locations in the urinary tract.

Clinical Manifestations

Urinary stones cause clinical manifestations when they obstruct urinary flow. Common sites of complete obstruction are at the UPJ (the point where the ureter crosses the iliac vessels) and the ureterovesical junction (UVJ). Symptoms include abdominal or flank pain (usually severe), hematuria, and renal colic. The pain may be associated with nausea and vomiting. The type of pain is determined by the location of the stone. If the stone is nonobstructing, pain may be absent. If the obstruction is in a calyx or at the UPJ, the patient may experience dull costovertebral flank pain or even colic. Pain resulting from the passage of a calculus down the ureter is intense and colicky. The patient may be in mild shock with cool, moist skin. As a stone nears the UVJ, pain will be felt in the lateral flank and sometimes down into the testicles, the labia, or the groin. Other clinical manifestations include the presence of urinary infection accompanied by fever, vomiting, nausea, and chills.

Diagnostic Studies

Diagnostic studies useful in the evaluation and management of renal lithiasis include urinalysis, urine culture, IVP, retrograde pyelogram, ultrasound, and cystoscopy. A plain film of the abdomen and renal ultrasound will identify larger, radiopaque stones. An IVP or retrograde pyelogram is used to localize the degree and the site of obstruction or to confirm the presence of a radiolucent stone, such as a uric acid or cystine calculus (see Figure 48-5,*B*). Ultrasonography can be used to identify a radiopaque or radiolucent calculus in the renal pelvis, the calyx, or the proximal ureter. It is less useful when attempting to locate stones trapped in the midureter. A CT scan may be used to differentiate a nonopaque stone from a tumour.

Retrieval and analysis of the stones is important in the diagnosis of the underlying problem contributing to stone formation. The patient's BUN and serum creatinine levels are also measured to assess renal function. A careful history, including previous stone formation, prescribed and over-the-counter medications and dietary supplements, and family history of urinary calculi is useful. Measurement of urine pH is useful in the diagnosis of struvite stones and renal tubular acidosis (tendency to alkaline pH) and uric acid stones (tendency to acidic pH).

Collaborative Care

Evaluation and management of a patient with renal lithiasis consists of two concurrent approaches. The first approach is directed toward management of the acute attack. This involves treating the symptoms of pain, infection, or obstruction as indicated for the individual patient. Narcotics are typically required at frequent intervals for relief of renal colic pain. Many stones pass spontaneously. However, stones larger than 4 mm are unlikely to pass through the ureter.

The second approach is directed toward evaluation of the cause of the stone formation and the prevention of further development of stones. Information to be obtained from the patient includes family history of stone formation, geographic residence, nutritional assessment including the intake of vitamins A and D, activity pattern (active or sedentary), history of periods of prolonged illness with immobilization or dehydration, and any history of disease or surgery involving the GI or genitourinary tract.

Therapy for people who are active stone formers requires a concerted management approach, with primary emphasis on teaching and on developing a therapeutic regimen with which the patient can manage. Adequate hydration, dietary sodium restrictions, dietary changes (Table 48-13), and the use of drugs

NUTRITIONAL THERAPY

Table 48-13 Urinary Tract Calculi

The following is a list of foods high in purine, calcium, or oxalate content. Initial nutritional management should include limiting oxalate- and purine-rich foods. Recommendations for intake of calcium are changing, however; whereas high dietary calcium has traditionally been viewed as a risk factor for stone formation (see Table 48-11), recent research suggests that calcium may actually lower the risk of stone formation by reducing the urinary excretion of oxalate (Traver, Passman, Leroy, Passmore, & Assimos, 2009).

Purine

High: Sardines, herring, mussels, liver, kidney, goose, venison, meat soups, sweetbreads

Moderate: Chicken, salmon, crab, veal, mutton, bacon, pork, beef, ham

Calcium

Milk, cheese, ice cream, yogourt, sauces containing milk; all beans (except green beans), lentils; fish with fine bones (e.g., sardines, kippers, herring, salmon); dried fruits, nuts; chocolate, cocoa, Ovaltine

Oxalate

Spinach, rhubarb, asparagus, cabbage, tomatoes, beets, nuts, celery, parsley, runner beans; chocolate, cocoa, instant coffee, Ovaltine, tea; Worcestershire sauce

keep urinary stone formation to a minimum. Various drugs are prescribed, depending on the specific problem underlying stone formation. These drugs prevent stone formation in various ways, including altering urine pH, preventing excessive urinary excretion of a substance, or correcting a primary disease (e.g., hyperparathyroidism).

Treatment of struvite stones calls for control of infection. This may be difficult if the stone remains in place. In addition to antibiotics, acetohydroxamic acid may be used in the treatment of kidney infections that result in the continual formation of struvite stones. Acetohydroxamic acid, an inhibitor of the chemical action caused by the persistent bacteria, can be used effectively to retard struvite stone formation (Pietrow & Karellas, 2006). If the infection cannot be controlled, the stone may have to be removed surgically.

Indications for endourological, lithotripsy, or open surgical stone removal include the following:
1. Stones too large for spontaneous passage.
2. Stones associated with bacteriuria or symptomatic infection.
3. Stones causing impaired renal function.
4. Stones causing persistent pain, nausea, or ileus.
5. Inability of patient to be treated medically.
6. Patient with one kidney.

Endourological Procedures. If the stone is located in the bladder, a cystoscopy is done to remove small stones. For large stones (Figure 48-6), a *cystolitholapaxy* is done. In this procedure, large stones can be broken up with an instrument called a *lithotrite* (stone crusher). The bladder is then irrigated and the crushed stones washed out. A *cystoscopic lithotripsy* uses an ultrasonic lithotrite to pulverize stones. Complications associated with these cystoscopic procedures include hemorrhage, retained stone fragments, and infection.

Flexible *ureteroscopes,* inserted via a cystoscope, can be used to remove stones from the renal pelvis and the upper urinary tract. Ultrasonic, laser, or electrohydraulic lithotripsy can be used in conjunction with the ureteroscope to pulverize and break the stone into fragments.

In *percutaneous nephrolithotomy,* a nephroscope is inserted through a sinus tract from the skin into the kidney pelvis. Stones can be fragmented using ultrasound, electrohydraulic, or laser lithotripsy. The stone fragments are removed and the pelvis irri-

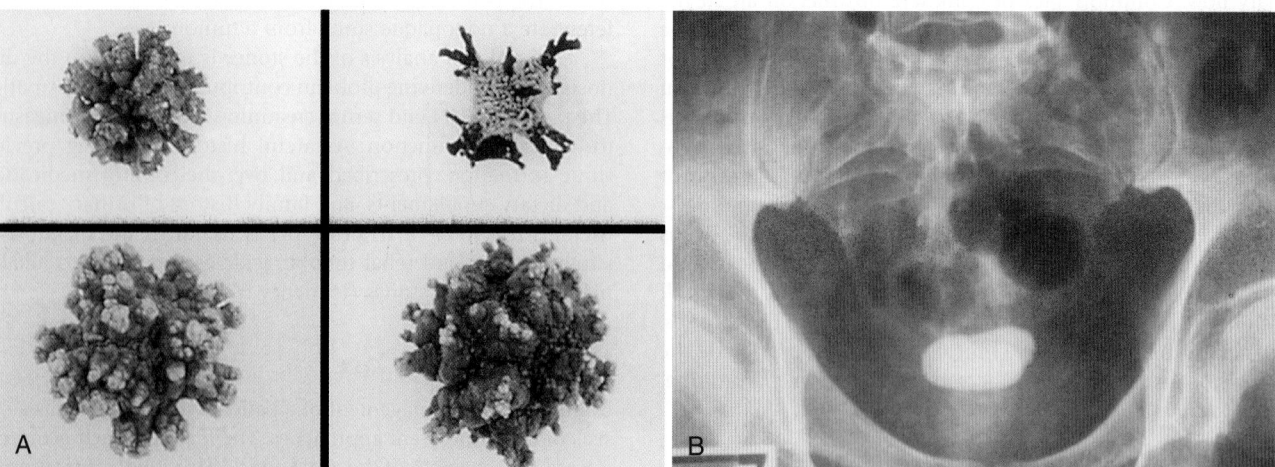

Figure 48-6 A, Calcium oxalate stones. **B,** Plain abdominal radiograph shows a large bladder calculus.

gated. A percutaneous nephrostomy tube is usually left in place to ensure that the ureter is not obstructed. Complications include bleeding, injury to adjacent structures, and infection.

Lithotripsy.

Lithotripsy involves the use of sound waves to break renal stones into small particles that can be eliminated from the urinary tract. Lithotripsy techniques include percutaneous ultrasonic lithotripsy, electrohydraulic lithotripsy, laser lithotripsy, and extracorporeal shock-wave lithotripsy (Perlmutter et al., 2008).

Extracorporeal shock-wave lithotripsy and laser lithotripsy are the most common. In *percutaneous ultrasonic lithotripsy,* an ultrasonic probe is placed in the renal pelvis via a percutaneous nephroscope (inserted through a small incision in the flank) and is positioned against the stone. (The patient is given general or spinal anaesthesia for this procedure.) The probe produces ultrasonic waves, which break the stone into sandlike particles. Percutaneous lithotripsy is not used as much as a primary approach to renal or upper ureteral stones unless the stone is large and other lithotripsy procedures have failed.

The *electrohydraulic lithotripsy* probe is also placed directly on a stone, but it breaks the stone into small fragments that are removed by forceps or suction. A continuous saline irrigation flushes out the stone particles, and all outflow drainage is strained so that the particles can be analyzed. Forceps or basket extraction can also be used to remove the calculi. Complications are rare but include hemorrhage, sepsis, and abscess formation. Postoperatively, the patient usually complains of moderate to severe colicky pain. The first few voids are bright red; as the bleeding subsides, the urine becomes dark red or turns a smoky colour. Antibiotics are usually given for 2 weeks to reduce the risk of infection.

Laser lithotripsy probes are used to fragment lower ureteral and large bladder stones. A holmium laser medium is preferred; it fragments stones but does not injure the surrounding tissue.

In *extracorporeal shock-wave lithotripsy,* a noninvasive procedure, the patient is anaesthetized (spinal or general) and placed in a water bath. Anaesthesia is necessary to keep the patient very still during the procedure. Some of the newer-generation lithotripters do not require submersion and use other means of initiating shock waves. The lithotripters are categorized as electrohydraulic, electromagnetic, and piezoelectric. The second-generation lithotripters use less power to fragment stones. Lower power reduces a patient's pain, but usually some sedation or analgesia is necessary.

Fluoroscopy or ultrasound is used to focus the lithotripter on the affected kidney, and a high-voltage spark generator produces high-energy acoustic shock waves that shatter the stone without damaging the surrounding tissues. The stone is broken into fine sand, which is excreted into the patient's urine within a few days after the procedure.

Hematuria is common after lithotripsy procedures. A self-retaining ureteral stent is often placed after the procedure to promote passage of sand from the fragmented stone and to prevent obstruction caused by its buildup in the ureter. The stent is removed 1 to 2 weeks after lithotripsy. A primary advantage of these techniques compared with open surgery is the decrease in the length of hospitalization and the patient's earlier return to normal activities. Additional treatment may be necessary, especially if a stone is large and in the midureter or the distal ureter.

Surgical Therapy.

A small group of select patients need open surgical procedures, such as the very obese patient or the individual with complex abnormalities in the calyces or at the UPJ. The type of open surgery performed depends on the location of the stone. A *nephrolithotomy* is an incision into the kidney to remove a stone. A *pyelolithotomy* is an incision into the renal pelvis to remove a stone. If the stone is located in the ureter, a *ureterolithotomy* is performed. A *cystotomy* may be indicated for bladder calculi. For open surgery on the kidney or ureter, a flank incision directly below the diaphragm and across the side is usually the preferred surgical approach. Complications related to hemorrhage are the most common following these surgical procedures.

Nutritional Therapy.

When managing an obstructing stone, the patient is advised to drink adequate fluids to avoid dehydration. Forcing fluids is avoided, because this strategy has not proved effective in assisting the patient to spontaneously "pass" (excrete) the stone via the urine. In addition, forcing fluids may exacerbate the colic associated with this episode.

After an episode of urolithiasis, however, a high fluid intake (~3000 mL/day) is recommended to produce a urine output of at least 2 L/day. High urine output prevents supersaturation of minerals (i.e., dilutes the concentration) and flushes them out before the minerals have a chance to precipitate and form a stone. Increasing the fluid intake is especially important for the patient who is active in sports, lives in a dry climate, performs physical exercise, has a family history of stone formation, or works in an occupation that requires outdoor work or a great deal of physical activity that can lead to dehydration. Water is the preferred fluid, and consumption of colas, coffee, and tea should be limited because high intake of these beverages tends to increase rather than diminish the risk of recurring urinary calculi (Traver, Passman, LeRoy, Passmore, & Assimos, 2009).

Dietary intervention may be important in the management of urolithiasis. In the past, calcium restriction was routinely implemented for the patient with kidney stones. However, more recent research suggests that a high dietary calcium intake, which was previously thought to contribute to kidney stones, may actually lower the risk by reducing the urinary excretion of oxalate, a common factor in many stones (Traver et al., 2009). Initial nutritional management should include limiting oxalate-rich foods and thereby reducing oxalate excretion. Foods high in calcium, oxalate, and purines are presented in Table 48-13.

NURSING MANAGEMENT: RENAL CALCULI

Nursing Assessment

Subjective and objective data that should be obtained from a patient with urinary tract lithiasis are presented in Table 48-14.

Nursing Diagnoses

Nursing diagnoses for the patient with urinary tract lithiasis include, but are not limited to, those presented in NCP 48-2.

Planning

The overall goals are that the patient with urinary tract calculi will have (1) relief of pain, (2) no urinary tract obstruction, and (3)

NURSING ASSESSMENT

Table 48-14 Urinary Tract Calculi

Subjective Data

Important Health Information

Current health history: Dietary intake of purines, calcium, oxalates, phosphates; low fluid intake

Past health history: Recent or chronic UTI; bed rest or sedentary lifestyle; immobilization; previous urinary tract stones, obstruction, or kidney disease with urinary stasis; gout; prostatic hyperplasia; hyperparathyroidism; family history of renal calculi

Medications: Prior use of medication for prevention of stones or treatment of UTI; allopurinol, analgesics

Surgery or other treatments: External urinary diversion, long-term indwelling urinary catheter

Symptoms

- Nausea, vomiting; chills
- Decreased urinary output, urinary urgency, frequency, feeling of bladder fullness
- Acute, severe, colicky pain in flank, back, abdomen, groin, or genitalia; burning on urination, dysuria, anxiety

Objective Data

General

Guarding, fever

Integumentary

Warm, flushed skin or pallor with cool, moist skin (mild shock)

Gastrointestinal

Abdominal distension, absence of bowel sounds

Urinary

Oliguria, hematuria, tenderness on palpation of renal areas, passage of stone or stones

Possible Findings

↑ Serum urea (BUN) and serum creatinine levels; RBCs, WBCs, pyuria, crystals, casts, minerals, bacteria on urinalysis; ↑ uric acid, calcium, phosphorus, oxalate, or cystine values on 24-hr urine sample; calculi or anatomical changes on IVP or KUB radiographic study; direct visualization of obstruction on cystoureteroscopy

BUN, blood urea nitrogen; *IVP,* intravenous pyelogram; *KUB,* kidneys, ureters, bladder; *RBCs,* red blood cells; *UTI,* urinary tract infection; *WBCs,* white blood cells.

an understanding of measures to prevent further recurrence of stones.

■ Nursing Implementation

A program to prevent stone recurrence always includes adequate fluid intake to produce a urine output of approximately 2 L/day, and it may include measures to alleviate metabolic or secondary risk factors. The nurse should consult with the health care provider concerning recommendations for fluid intake in a given patient. In the modestly active, ambulatory person, this requires the patient to drink about 2000 to 2200 mL/day with the residual 20 to 30% of fluids gained through consumption of foods. The volume of necessary fluids will be higher in the highly active patient who works outdoors or who regularly engages in demand-

ing athletic activities. In contrast, fluid intake will be less for the very sedentary or immobile person. Preventive measures related to the person who is on bed rest or is relatively immobile for a prolonged time include maintaining an adequate fluid intake, turning the patient every 2 hours, and helping the patient to sit or stand, if possible, to maximize urinary flow.

Additional preventive measures focus on reducing metabolic or secondary risk factors. For example, dietary restriction of purines may be helpful to the patient at risk for developing uric acid stones. Reduced intake of oxalates may be indicated in the person with recurring calcium oxalate calculi. The patient is taught about dosage, scheduling, and potential adverse effects of drugs used to reduce the risk of stone formation. Selected patients may be taught to self-monitor urinary pH, or they may be asked to measure urinary output.

Pain management and patient comfort are primary nursing responsibilities when managing an obstructing stone and renal colic (see NCP 48-2). It is important to ensure that the patient retrieves any spontaneously passed stones. All urine voided by the patient should be strained through gauze or a special urine strainer in an effort to detect the stone. The high fluid intake necessary for stone prevention is suspended, but consumption should be adequate to meet daily needs and prevent dehydration. Ambulation is generally encouraged to promote the movement of the stone from the upper to the lower urinary tract, but the patient should not walk unattended when experiencing acute colic, particularly if opioid analgesics are being used.

■ Evaluation

The expected outcomes for the patient with urinary calculi are presented in NCP 48-2.

Strictures

A **stricture** is an abnormal temporary or permanent narrowing of the lumen of a hollow organ, in this context of the ureter or the urethra.

Ureteral Strictures

Ureteral strictures can affect the entire length of the ureter, from the UPJ to UVJ. These strictures are usually an unintended result of surgical intervention, usually secondary to adhesions or scar formation. Depending on its severity, ureteral obstruction can threaten the function of the kidney. Clinical manifestations of a ureteral stricture include mild to moderate colic; this pain may be of moderate to severe intensity if the patient consumes a large volume of fluids (alcohol, in particular) over a brief period. Infection is unusual unless a calculus or foreign object such as a stent or nephrostomy tube is present.

The discomfort and obstruction of a ureteral stricture may be temporarily bypassed by placing a stent under endoscopic control or by diverting urinary flow via a nephrostomy tube inserted into the renal pelvis of the affected kidney. Definitive correction requires dilation with a balloon or catheter. If the stricture is severe or recurs after initial balloon or catheter dilation, it may be incised under endoscopic control *(endoureterotomy).* In selected cases, an open surgical approach may be required to excise the stenotic area and reanastomose the ureter to the contralateral

NURSING CARE PLAN 48-2

Acute Renal Lithiasis

NURSING DIAGNOSIS	**Acute pain** related to irritation of stone and inadequate pain control or comfort measures as evidenced by complaints of pain, facial grimacing, and restlessness
Expected Patient Outcomes	**Nursing Interventions and Rationales**
• Reports minimal or no pain • Reports decrease in pain and satisfaction with pain control	• Assess for pain location and severity to plan appropriate interventions. • Administer pain medication as ordered to promote comfort. • Apply heat to flank area as needed because heat reduces reflex muscle spasm and promotes comfort.
NURSING DIAGNOSIS	**Anxiety** related to uncertain outcome and lack of knowledge regarding possible surgery as evidenced by expressions of concern about future treatments
Expected Patient Outcomes	**Nursing Interventions and Rationales**
• Reports relief of anxiety • Expresses confidence in treatment plan	• Assess cause and level of anxiety to plan appropriate interventions. • Explain surgical or nonsurgical procedure (include insertion of urethral catheters) because accurate information often decreases anxiety and fosters control. • Encourage patient to express feelings of anxiety and fear of surgery to validate feelings and provide support.
NURSING DIAGNOSIS	**Ineffective self-health management** related to lack of knowledge about prevention of recurrence, diet, fluid requirements, and symptoms of recurrence as evidenced by questions that indicate inadequate knowledge of disorder
Expected Patient Outcomes	**Nursing Interventions and Rationales**
• Verbalizes correct self-care measures • Identifies symptoms of recurrence	• Advise patient during initial hospital stay regarding increasing fluids unless contraindicated and diet restrictions and rationale to prepare for home self-care. • Inform patient about rationale, dosage, and adverse effects of medication to foster adherence to medication regimen. • Involve patient with teaching about how to strain all urine through a urine strainer or piece of gauze (if necessary) to determine if stones are passed and to bring stone to physician for analysis. • Teach patient about symptoms of recurrence (e.g., hematuria, flank pain) to ensure early reporting and initiation of treatment. • Encourage resumption of high fluid intake after acute episode has passed unless contraindicated because stones form more readily in concentrated urine. Provide opportunities for patient to reflect on and ask questions about self-care.
NURSING DIAGNOSIS	**Impaired urinary elimination** related to trauma or blockage of ureters or urethra as evidenced by decrease in urinary output or bloody urine
Expected Patient Outcomes	**Nursing Intervention and Rationale**
• Maintains free flow of urine • Has minimal to no hematuria • Maintains balanced intake and output	• Monitor urine amount and character to ensure patency in urinary system and that hematuria is not excessive.
NURSING DIAGNOSIS	**Risk for infection** related to introduction of bacteria following manipulations of the urinary tract and obstructed urinary flow
Expected Patient Outcome	**Nursing Interventions and Rationales**
• Reports no urinary tract infections	• Assess for elevation in temperature; chills; cloudy, foul-smelling urine as indicators of potential infection. • Monitor vital signs and observe for fever because abnormalities may indicate infection.

ureter (*ureteroureterostomy*) or to the renal pelvis. Alternatively, distal ureteral strictures may be managed by a *ureteroneocystostomy* (reimplantation of the ureter into the bladder wall).

Urethral Stricture

A *urethral stricture* is the result of fibrosis or inflammation of the urethral lumen (Bernier & Sims, 2009). Causes of urethral stric-

tures include trauma, urethritis (particularly following gonococcal infection), and a congenital defect in the canalization of the urethra; causes can also be iatrogenic (following surgical intervention). Once the process of inflammation and fibrosis begins, the lumen of the urethra narrows, and its compliance (ability to close or open in response to bladder filling or micturition) is compromised. Meatal stenosis, a narrowing of the urethral opening, is also common. A urethral stricture creates symptoms when it causes voiding dysfunction or bladder outlet obstruction (Bernier & Sims, 2009).

Clinical manifestations associated with a urethral stricture include a diminished force of the urinary stream, spraying, or a split urine stream. The patient may report feelings of incomplete bladder emptying with urinary frequency and nocturia. Moderate to severe obstruction of the bladder outlet may lead to acute urinary retention. The patient may report a history of urethritis, difficulty with placement of a urinary catheter, or trauma involving the penis or the perineum. However, many patients are unable to recall any such events, thus leading to a diagnosis of an idiopathic stricture. A history of a UTI is not uncommon, particularly if the stricture involves the distal urethra.

Initial management of a stricture may be based on dilation. A metal instrument (urethral sound) may be placed, or a series of progressively enlarging stents can be placed into the urethra (filiforms and followers) to expand its lumen in a stepwise fashion. Although initially successful, recurring stenosis is frequent. Recurrences may be managed by teaching the patient to repeatedly dilate the urethra by self-catheterization every few days. Alternatively, an endoscopic or open surgical procedure may be completed to provide a more durable solution to an obstructive urethral stricture. Shorter strictures may be managed by resection of the fibrotic area with primary reanastomosis. Longer strictures may require autotransplantation of a substitute segment such as a skin flap.

Renal Trauma

A rise in the incidence of traumatic renal injuries is related to an increase in the mechanization and speed of transportation and to the increase in violent crimes and injuries (Geehan & Santucci, 2006). The majority of incidents occur in men younger than 30 years. Blunt trauma is the most common cause. Injury to the kidney should be considered in multiple or sports injuries, traffic accidents, and falls. It is especially likely when the patient injures the abdomen, the flank, or the back. Penetrating injuries may result from violent encounters (e.g., gunshot or stabbing incidents) or may be of iatrogenic origin.

Clinical findings include a history of trauma to the area of the kidneys. Gross or microscopic hematuria may be present. Diagnostic studies include urinalysis, IVP with cystography, ultrasound, CT, or MRI evaluation. Renal arteriography may also be used. Both the injured kidney and the uninvolved kidney should be evaluated to provide information for further management.

The severity of renal trauma depends on the extent of the injury. Treatments range from bed rest, fluids, and analgesia to surgical exploration and repair or nephrectomy.

Nursing interventions vary with the type and the extent of associated injuries. Specific interventions related to renal trauma include ensuring increased fluid intake, providing comfort measures, monitoring for shock (e.g., penetrating injury), monitoring intake and output, observing for hematuria, determining the presence of myoglobinuria, assessing the cardiovascular status, and monitoring the use of potentially nephrotoxic antibiotics.

Renal Vascular Problems

Vascular problems involving the kidney include (1) nephrosclerosis, (2) renal artery stenosis, and (3) renal vein thrombosis.

Nephrosclerosis

Nephrosclerosis is a vascular disease of the kidney characterized by sclerosis of the small arteries and arterioles of the kidney, resulting in renal tissue destruction. There is decreased blood flow, which results in patchy necrosis of the renal parenchyma. Ischemic necrosis and destruction of glomeruli with subsequent fibrosis also occur.

Benign nephrosclerosis usually occurs in adults 30 to 50 years of age. It is caused by vascular changes resulting from hypertension and from the process of atherosclerosis. Atherosclerotic vascular changes account for most of the loss of renal function associated with aging. There is a direct relation between the degree of nephrosclerosis and the severity of hypertension. The patient with benign nephrosclerosis may have normal renal function in the early stages. The only detectable abnormality may be hypertension.

Accelerated nephrosclerosis, or *malignant nephrosclerosis,* is associated with malignant hypertension, a complication of hypertension characterized by a sharp increase in blood pressure with a diastolic pressure greater than 130 mm Hg (Schrier, 2007). The patient is usually a young adult, with a male–to–female predominance of 2:1. Renal insufficiency progresses rapidly.

Treatment for benign nephrosclerosis is the same as that for essential hypertension (see Chapter 35). Malignant nephrosclerosis is treated with aggressive antihypertensive therapy (see Chapter 35). The availability and use of antihypertensives have improved the prognosis for the patient with benign and malignant nephrosclerosis. Renal dysfunction and renal failure (in some persons) constitute two of the major complications of hypertension. The prognosis for the patient with malignant hypertension is poor, with the major cause of death related to renal failure.

Renal Artery Stenosis

Renal artery stenosis, a partial occlusion of one or both renal arteries and their major branches, is a major cause of abrupt-onset hypertension. It can be caused by atherosclerotic narrowing or fibromuscular hyperplasia. Renal artery stenosis accounts for 1 to 2% of all cases of hypertension (Schrier, 2007).

When hypertension develops rather abruptly, renal artery stenosis should be considered as a possible cause, especially in the patient younger than 30 or older than 50 years and in the patient with no familial history of hypertension. This contrasts with the age distribution for essential hypertension, which peaks between 30 and 50 years of age. A renal arteriogram is the best diagnostic tool for identifying renal artery stenosis.

The goals of therapy are control of blood pressure and restoration of perfusion to the kidney. Percutaneous transluminal renal angioplasty is the procedure of first choice, especially in older patients who are poor surgical risks. Surgical revascularization of the kidney is indicated when blood flow is decreased enough to cause renal ischemia or when evidence indicates that renovascular hypertension is present that might be resolved by surgical intervention. The surgical procedure usually involves anastomoses between the kidney and another major artery, usually the splenic artery or the aorta. In selected cases of unilateral renal involvement with high renin production, unilateral nephrectomy may be indicated.

Renal Vein Thrombosis

Renal vein thrombosis, an embolus occurring in the renal vein, may occur unilaterally or bilaterally. Trauma, extrinsic compression (e.g., tumour, aortic aneurysm), renal cell carcinoma, pregnancy, contraceptive use, and nephrotic syndrome are associated with renal vein thrombosis.

The patient has symptoms of flank pain, hematuria, or fever or has nephrotic syndrome. Anticoagulation is important in treatment because there is a high incidence of pulmonary emboli. Corticosteroids may be used for the patient with nephrosis. Surgical thrombectomy may be performed instead of or along with anticoagulation (Schrier, 2007).

Hereditary Renal Diseases

Hereditary renal diseases involve developmental abnormalities of the renal parenchyma. These abnormalities are either isolated or part of more complex malformation syndromes. The majority of inherited structural abnormalities are cystic. However, cysts may also develop as a result of obstructive uropathies, metabolic derangements, or neurological diseases. Cysts may be evaluated to rule out any tumour content.

Polycystic Kidney Disease

Polycystic kidney disease (PKD) is one of the most common genetic diseases in Canada. It may first become apparent in either childhood or adulthood. It involves both kidneys and occurs in both men and women. The cortex and the medulla are filled with thin-walled cysts that are several millimetres to several centimetres in diameter (Figure 48-7). The cysts enlarge and destroy surrounding tissue by compression. They are filled with fluid and may contain blood or pus.

There are two forms of hereditary polycystic renal disease. The adult form of PKD is an autosomal dominant disorder. It is latent for many years and is usually evidenced between 30 and 40 years of age. However, PKD has also been found in newborns. The childhood form of PKD is a rare autosomal recessive disorder that is often rapidly progressive (see the Genetics in Clinical Practice box).

Clinical Manifestations

In the patient with PKD (Figure 48-8), symptoms appear when the cysts begin to enlarge. A common early symptom of adult PKD is abdominal or flank pain, which is steady and dull or abrupt in onset as well as episodic and colicky. This pain is often caused by bleeding into the cysts. On physical examination, pal-

GENETICS IN CLINICAL PRACTICE
Polycystic Kidney Disease

	Adult	Child
Genetic basis	• Autosomal dominant	• Autosomal recessive
Incidence	• 1 in 500 to 1000	• 1 in 6000 to 40,000
Gene location	• Chromosomes 4 and 16	• Chromosome 6
Genetic testing	• DNA testing available	• DNA testing available
Age of onset	• Usually between the ages of 30 and 40 yr, but can begin earlier	• Infancy or childhood
Clinical implications	• Multisystem involvement • Systemic hypertension occurs in 60-80% of patients • Families at risk should be screened	• 30-50% of affected newborns die shortly after birth

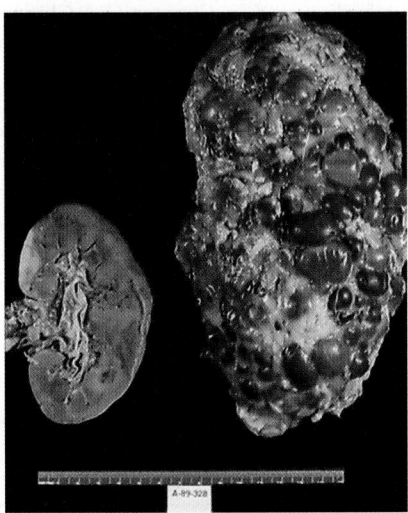

Figure 48-7 Comparison of polycystic kidney with normal kidney.

Source: Brundage, D. J. (1992). *Renal disorders.* St. Louis: Mosby.

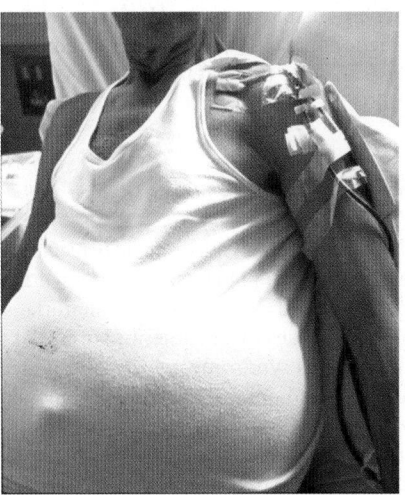

Figure 48-8 Man with an 11-kg polycystic kidney.

Source: Lemmi, F. O., & Lemmi, C. A. E. (2000). *Physical assessment findings* (CD-ROM). Philadelphia: Saunders.

pable bilateral enlarged kidneys are often found. Other clinical manifestations include hematuria (from rupture of cysts), UTI, and hypertension.

Diagnosis is based on clinical manifestations, family history, IVP, ultrasound, or CT scan. Usually, the disease progresses to end-stage renal failure, although some individuals have relatively mild disease and die from unrelated problems. Loss of kidney function to the point of end-stage renal disease occurs by age 60 in 50% of patients (Chapman, 2009).

Collaborative Care

There is no specific treatment for PKD. A major aim of treatment is to prevent infections of the urinary tract or to treat them with appropriate antibiotics if they occur. Nephrectomy may be necessary if pain, bleeding, or infection becomes a chronic, serious problem.

When the patient begins to experience progressive renal failure, the interventions are determined by the remaining renal function. Nursing measures are those used for management of end-stage renal disease (see Chapter 49). They include diet modification, fluid restriction, drugs (e.g., antihypertensives), assisting the patient to accept the chronic disease process, and assisting the patient and family to deal with physical, socioeconomic, and emotional reactions to the disease.

The patient who has adult polycystic disease often has children by the time the disease is diagnosed. Each child of a parent with PKD has a 50% chance of having the disease. The patient will need appropriate counselling regarding plans for having more children. In addition, genetic counselling resources should be provided for the children.

Medullary Cystic Disease

Medullary cystic disease is a hereditary disorder that occurs in two forms. The *autosomal recessive form* is associated with renal failure before age 20; the *autosomal dominant form* is associated with renal failure after age 20. Most cysts are located in the medulla. The kidneys are asymmetrical and are significantly scarred. There are defects in the concentration ability of the kidneys. Polyuria, progressive renal failure, severe anemia, metabolic acidosis, and poor sodium conservation are common. Hypertension can be a terminal event. Genetic counselling may be helpful in family planning. Treatment measures are those related to end-stage renal disease (see Chapter 49).

Alport's Syndrome

Alport's syndrome is also known as *chronic hereditary nephritis.* Two forms of the disease exist: (1) classic Alport's syndrome, which is inherited as a sex-linked disorder with hematuria, sensorineural deafness, and deformities of the anterior surface of the lens, and (2) nonclassic Alport's syndrome, which is inherited as an autosomal trait that causes hematuria but not deafness or lens deformities (Devarajan, 2008). Men are affected earlier and more severely than women. The disease is often diagnosed in the first decade of life. The basic defect is altered synthesis of the GBM. The patient most commonly has hematuria and progressive uremia. Treatment is supportive. Corticosteroids and cytotoxic drugs are not effective. The disease does not recur after kidney transplantation.

Renal Involvement in Metabolic and Connective Tissue Diseases

Various metabolic and connective tissue disease processes may have an effect on renal function. The pathophysiological effects on the renal parenchyma are not always specific to each process. The clinical course of renal involvement is that of chronic progressive nephropathy, which can result in uremia and death. Management includes treatment of the primary disorder along with symptomatic relief of renal involvement. If renal involvement progresses to end-stage renal disease, management includes dialysis or transplantation (see Chapter 49). Nursing interventions include teaching the patient about the primary disease process, the renal involvement, and the resulting need to comply with dietary and fluid restrictions and drug regimens.

Diabetic nephropathy is the primary cause of end-stage renal failure in Canada (Canadian Diabetes Association Clinical Practice Guidelines Expert Committee, 2008). Diabetes mellitus may affect the kidneys in several ways. Microangiopathic changes in diabetes consist of diffuse glomerulosclerosis, involving thickening of the GBM, and nodular glomerulosclerosis (Kimmelstiel–Wilson syndrome), which is characterized by nodular lesions. Nodular glomerulosclerosis is reasonably specific for type 1 diabetes mellitus. The diabetic patient prone to glomerulonephropathy (e.g., the presence of trace proteinuria or retinopathy) requires careful monitoring of glucose levels and insulin requirements. (Diabetes mellitus is discussed in Chapter 52.)

Gout is a syndrome of acute attacks of arthritis caused by hyperuricemia (see Chapter 67). Monosodium urate crystals deposited in joints are responsible for the syndrome. Renal disease may develop as a result of damage caused by deposition of uric acid crystals in the renal interstitium and the tubules.

Amyloidosis is a group of disorders evidenced by impaired organ function from the infiltration of tissues with a hyaline substance (amyloid). The hyaline consists largely of protein. Kidney involvement is common in amyloidosis. Proteinuria is often the first clinical manifestation.

Systemic lupus erythematosus is a connective tissue disorder characterized by the involvement of several tissues and organs, particularly the joints, the skin, and the kidneys. (Systemic lupus erythematosus is discussed in Chapter 67.) Clinical manifestations of lupus nephritis are similar to those of other forms of glomerulonephritis. Renal failure frequently occurs in systemic lupus erythematosus and has a poor prognosis.

Systemic sclerosis (scleroderma) is a disease of unknown etiology characterized by widespread alterations of connective tissue and vascular lesions in many organs (see Chapter 67). In the kidney, vascular lesions are associated with fibrosis. An immune complex mechanism has been postulated as a possible etiological factor. The severity of renal involvement varies. The patient who develops severe renal lesions has a poor prognosis.

Urinary Tract Tumours

Kidney Cancer

The incidence of kidney cancer in Canada is rising. From 2003 to 2007, kidney cancer rates increased among males by 2.6% per year. From 1998 to 2007, the incidence in kidney cancer in women increased by 1.9% per year. In the same time period, mortality rates decreased slightly (0.8% for men and 0.9% for women) (Canadian Cancer Society's Steering Committee on Cancer Statistics, 2012). In 2012 it was estimated that 5600 new cases would be diagnosed in Canada that year, and that 1700 would die from it. Kidney cancers arise from the cortex or the pelvis (and the calyces). Tumours arising from both areas may be benign or malignant. However, malignant tumours are more frequent. Renal cell carcinoma (adenocarcinoma) is the most common type. Adenocarcinoma occurs twice as often in men as in women and is typically discovered when the person is 50 to 70 years old. Cigarette smoking is the most significant risk factor for the development of renal cell carcinoma. Other risk factors are obesity and the use of phenacetin-containing analgesics and exposure to asbestos, cadmium, and gasoline (Moldawer & Figlin, 2008).

There are no characteristic early symptoms. Generalized symptoms of weight loss, weakness, and anemia are the earliest manifestations. The classic manifestations of gross hematuria, flank pain, and a palpable mass are those of advanced disease. The most common sites of metastases include the lungs, liver, and long bones. Local extension of kidney cancer into the renal vein and the vena cava is common (Figure 48-9). Renal cystic disease and renal-associated carcinomas may develop in the patient with end-stage renal disease who is receiving maintenance renal dialysis (see Chapter 49).

Several studies are used to diagnose kidney cancer. IVP with nephrotomography is the primary examination by which most masses are detected and evaluated. Ultrasounds have improved the ability to differentiate between a tumour and a cyst. Angiography, percutaneous needle aspiration, CT, and MRI are also used in the diagnosis of renal tumours. Small renal tumours are found earlier because of the increased use of CT scans and MRI. Radionuclide isotope scanning is used to detect metastases.

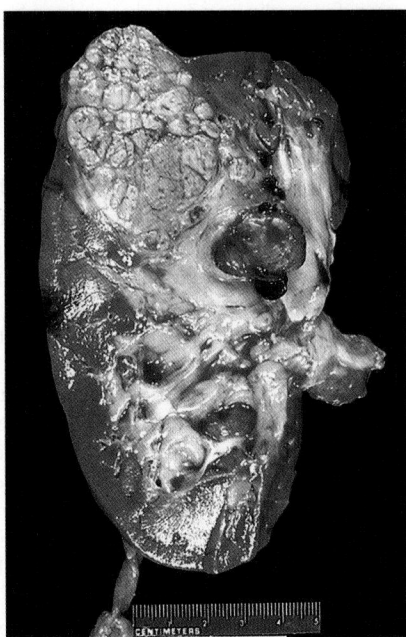

Figure 48-9 Renal cell carcinoma. Cross-section shows yellowish cancer in one pole of the kidney. The tumour also involves the dilated thrombosed renal vein.

Source: Kumar, V., Abbas, A. K., Fausto, N., & Aster, J. (2010). *Robbins and Cotran pathologic basis of disease* (8th ed., p. 965, Figure 20-53). Philadelphia: Saunders.

Robson's system of staging renal carcinoma is presented in Table 48-15. The treatment of choice is a radical nephrectomy. Radical nephrectomy is the removal of the kidney, the adrenal gland, the surrounding fascia, part of the ureter, and the draining lymph nodes. Radiation therapy is used palliatively in inoperable cases and when there are metastases to bone or lungs.

Chemotherapy using 5-fluorouracil (5-FU), floxuridine (FUDR), and gemcitabine (Gemzar) is used to treat metastatic disease. However, renal cell carcinoma is refractory to most chemotherapy drugs. Biological therapy, including interferon α and interleukin-2 (IL-2), is most promising in the treatment of metastatic disease (Gollob et al., 2007). Adverse effects of IL-2 include capillary leakage syndrome, fever, chills, fatigue, and hypotension.

Patients with early-stage kidney cancer can expect a 60 to 70% 5-year survival after undergoing radical nephrectomy. The 5-year survival rate for patients with metastatic disease is only 3 to 10%. However, patients with metastatic disease often remain stable for a prolonged period (Greenberg, 2007).

Bladder Cancer

It was estimated that 7800 Canadians would be diagnosed with bladder cancer in 2012 and that 2100 Canadians would die from this disease (Canadian Cancer Society's Steering Committee on Cancer Statistics, 2012). Bladder cancer is the sixth most common type of cancer diagnosed in Canadians. The most frequent malignant tumour of the urinary tract is transitional cell carcinoma of the bladder. Most bladder tumours are papillomatous growths within the bladder (Figure 48-10). Cancer of the bladder is most common between the ages of 60 and 70 years and is at least three times as common in men as in women. Risk factors for bladder cancer include cigarette smoking, exposure to dyes used in the rubber and cable industries, and chronic abuse of phenacetin-containing analgesics. Women treated with radiation for cervical cancer and patients receiving cyclophosphamide (Procytox) also have increased risk, but the reason is unknown.

Individuals with chronic, recurrent stones (often bladder) and chronic lower urinary infections have an increased risk of squamous cell cancer of the bladder. Patients who have indwelling catheters for long periods can develop these chronic conditions.

Clinical Manifestations and Diagnostic Studies

Gross, painless hematuria (chronic or intermittent) is the most common clinical finding. Bladder irritability with dysuria, fre-

Table 48-15 Robson's System of Staging Renal Carcinoma	
STAGE	**DESCRIPTION**
I	Limitation to renal capsule
II	Spreading to perirenal fat but confined within fascia; includes metastasis to adrenal gland
III	Regional lymph node involvement, tumour thrombus in renal vein or vena cava, involvement of renal vein or vena cava
IV	Presence of distant metastases

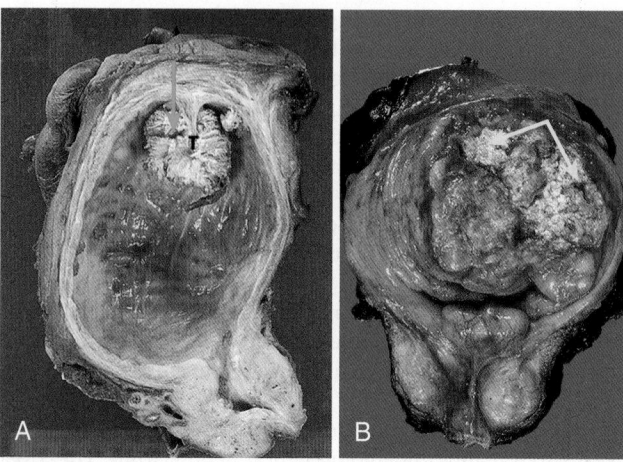

Figure 48-10 A, A papillary transitional cell carcinoma is seen arising from the dome of the bladder as a cauliflower-like lesion. **B,** Opened bladder shows a bladder cancer at an advanced stage. The yellow areas represent ulcerations and necrosis.

Source: **A** from Stevens, A., & Lowe, J. (2000). *Pathology: Illustrated review in color* (2nd ed.). London: Mosby; **B** from Kumar, V., Abbas, A. K., Fausto, N., & Aster, J. (2010). *Robbins and Cotran pathologic basis of disease* (8th ed., p. 979, Figure 21-12). Philadelphia: Saunders.

COLLABORATIVE CARE

Table 48-16 Bladder Cancer

Diagnostic
- History and physical examination
- Urinalysis
- Intravenous pyelogram (IVP)
- Cystoscopy with biopsy
- Cytology studies
- Ultrasound
- CT scan

Collaborative Therapy
- Surgical treatment
  - Transurethral resection with fulguration
  - Laser photocoagulation
  - Open loop resection or fulguration
  - Segmental cystectomy
  - Radical cystectomy

- Radiation
- Intravesical immunotherapy
  - Bacille Calmette-Guérin (BCG)
  - α-Interferon
- Intravesical chemotherapy
  - Thiotepa
  - Mitomycin
  - Doxorubicin (Adriamycin)
  - Valrubicin (Valtaxin)
- Systemic chemotherapy

CT, computed tomography.

quency, and urgency may also occur. When cancer is suspected, urine specimens for cytology can be obtained to determine the presence of neoplastic or atypical cells. Exfoliated cells from the epithelial surface of the bladder can readily be detected in voided specimens. Other recent urine tests assess for specific factors associated with bladder cancer, such as bladder tumour antigens. Bladder cancers can be detected using IVP, ultrasound, CT, or MRI. However, the presence of cancer is confirmed by cystoscopy and biopsy.

The depth of invasion of the bladder wall and surrounding tissue determines the clinical staging of carcinoma of the bladder. The Jewett–Strong–Marshall classification system broadly classifies bladder cancer as superficial (carcinoma in situ, O, A), invasive (B_1, B_2, C), or metastatic (D_1-D_4) disease. Pathological grading systems are also used to classify the malignant potential of tumour cells, indicating a scale from well-differentiated to anaplastic categories. Low-stage, low-grade bladder cancers are the most responsive to treatment and are more easily cured.

NURSING AND COLLABORATIVE MANAGEMENT: BLADDER CANCER

Collaborative care of the patient with bladder cancer is outlined in Table 48-16.

Surgical Therapy

Surgical therapies include a variety of procedures. *Transurethral resection with fulguration* (electrocautery) is used for the diagnosis and treatment of superficial lesions with a low recurrence rate. This procedure is also used to control bleeding in the patient who is a poor operative risk or who has advanced tumours. With this technique, the tumour mass is excised by means of a blade inserted through the cystoscope. The remaining portions of the tumour are cauterized.

A second technique, *laser photocoagulation,* is also used to treat superficial bladder cancers. This procedure can be repeated a number of times to manage recurrences. The advantages of laser include bloodless destruction of the lesion, minimal risk of perforation, and lack of need for a urinary catheter. The primary disadvantage is that, owing to destruction of the tumour, pathological evaluation for grading and staging cannot be completed.

A third technique used is *open loop resection* (snaring of polyp types of lesion) *with fulguration.* It is used for the control of bleeding, for large superficial tumours, and for multiple lesions. Treatment of large lesions entails a segmental resection of the bladder (*segmental cystectomy*).

Postoperative management of the patient who has had any of these surgical procedures includes instructions to drink a large volume of fluid each day for the first week following the procedure and to avoid intake of alcoholic beverages. The patient is taught to self-monitor the urine. It is anticipated to be pink during the first several days after the procedure, but it should not be bright red or contain blood clots. Approximately 7 to 10 days following tumour resection or ablation, the patient may observe dark red or rust-coloured flecks in the urine. These are anticipated and represent scabs from the healing tumour resection sites. Opioid analgesics may be required for a brief period after the procedure, along with stool softeners. The patient can be encouraged to take a 15- to 20-minute sitz bath two to three times a day to promote muscle relaxation and to reduce the risk of urinary retention. The nurse should also help the patient and family cope with fears about cancer, surgery, and sexuality and should emphasize the importance of regular follow-up care. Frequent routine cystoscopies are required.

When the tumour is invasive or when it involves the trigone (the area where the ureters insert into the bladder) and the patient is free from metastasis beyond the pelvic area, a partial or radical cystectomy with urinary diversion is the treatment of choice (see the section on urinary diversion later in the chapter). A *partial cystectomy* includes resection of that portion of the bladder wall containing the tumour, along with a margin of normal tissue. A *radical cystectomy* involves removal of the bladder, the prostate, and the seminal vesicles in men and the bladder, the uterus, the cervix, the urethra, and the ovaries in women (Eggener, 2008).

Radiation Therapy and Chemotherapy

Radiation therapy is used with cystectomy or as the primary therapy when the cancer is inoperable or when surgery is refused. Increasingly, radiation therapy is being combined with systemic chemotherapy. Sometimes, combination systemic chemotherapy is used for bladder cancer, usually preoperatively or before radiation therapy, or is used to treat distant metastases. Chemotherapy drugs used in treating invasive bladder cancer include cisplatin, vinblastine, and methotrexate.

Intravesical Therapy

Chemotherapy with local instillation of chemotherapeutic or immune-stimulating agents can be delivered directly into the bladder by a urethral catheter. Protocols vary, but intravesical therapy is usually initiated at weekly intervals for 6 to 12 weeks. The chemotherapeutic agents are instilled directly into the patient's bladder and retained for about 2 hours. The patient's position may be changed every 15 minutes for maximum contact in all areas of the bladder, especially if the tumour occurred on the bladder dome. The use of maintenance therapy after the initial induction regimen may be beneficial.

BCG, a weakened strain of *Mycobacterium bovis,* is the treatment of choice for carcinoma in situ. BCG stimulates the immune system rather than acting directly on cancer cells in the bladder. When BCG alone fails, interferon α may be used in addition to BCG. Other treatments that can be used when BCG fails include thiotepa, an alkylating agent, and valrubicin (Valtaxin), an antineoplastic antibiotic.

Most patients have irritation upon voiding and hemorrhagic cystitis following intravesical therapy. Thiotepa (when absorbed into circulation from the bladder wall) can significantly reduce WBC and platelet counts in some individuals. BCG may cause flulike symptoms, hematuria, or systemic infection. Other adverse effects usually associated with chemotherapy, such as nausea, vomiting, and hair loss, are not experienced with intravesical chemotherapy.

Nursing responsibilities include encouraging the patient to increase the daily fluid intake and to quit smoking, assessing the patient for secondary UTI, and stressing the need for routine urological follow-up. The patient may have fears or concerns about sexual activity or bladder function that will have to be addressed.

Urinary Incontinence and Retention

Urinary incontinence (UI) is defined as an uncontrolled loss of urine that is of sufficient magnitude to be a problem. Approximately 3.3 million Canadians experience incontinence across the age spectrum, including 10% of children 6 years of age and up, 25% of women middle-aged and older, and 15% of all men aged 60 years and older (Canadian Continence Foundation, 2010). Among younger adults, UI affects far more women than men. Although the prevalence of incontinence is higher among older women and older men, it is not a natural consequence of aging. Although UI has traditionally been viewed as a social or hygienic problem, it is now known to affect quality of life as well as contribute to serious health problems in older adults).

Anything that interferes with bladder or urethral sphincter control can result in UI. Causes may be transient (e.g., caused by confusion or depression, infection, drugs, restricted mobility, or stool impaction). Congenital disorders that produce incontinence include exstrophy of the bladder, epispadias, spina bifida with myelomeningocele, and ectopic ureteral orifice. Acquired disorders are described in Table 48-17. Patients may have more than one type of incontinence. Patients may not disclose symptoms of UI because of the stigma associated with this condition. Nurses' relational care approaches through listening to patients' questions and valuing patients' knowledge about UI are required to promote patients' understanding and application of UI management techniques.

Urinary retention is the inability to empty the bladder despite micturition or the accumulation of urine in the bladder because of an inability to urinate. In certain cases, it is associated with dribbling urinary leakage called *overflow UI. Acute urinary retention* is the total inability to pass urine via micturition; it is a medical emergency. *Chronic urinary retention* is defined as incomplete bladder emptying despite urination. The postvoid residual volumes in patients with chronic urinary retention vary widely; values of 150 to 200 mL or higher generally necessitate further evaluation. Even smaller volumes may justify evaluation when they produce bothersome LUTS or occur in a context of recurring UTIs. Urinary retention is caused by two different dysfunctions of the urinary system: bladder outlet obstruction and deficient detrusor contraction strength. Obstruction leads to urinary retention when the blockage is sufficiently severe that the bladder can no longer evacuate its contents despite a detrusor contraction. A common cause of obstruction in men is an enlarged prostate. Urinary retention also results when the detrusor muscle no longer has the strength to contract with enough force or for long enough to completely empty the bladder.

Common causes of deficient detrusor muscle contraction strength are neurological diseases affecting sacral segments 2, 3, and 4; longstanding diabetes mellitus; overdistension; chronic alcoholism; and drugs (e.g., anticholinergic drugs).

Diagnostic Studies

The basic evaluation for UI and urinary retention includes a focused history, physical assessment, and a bladder log or voiding record whenever possible. Information should be obtained regarding the onset of UI, factors that provoke urinary leakage, and associated conditions. The nurse should pay special attention to factors known to produce transient UI, particularly when a relatively sudden onset of urine loss is reported. The physical examination begins with an assessment of general health and functional issues associated with urinary function, including mobility, dexterity, and cognitive function. A pelvic examination includes careful inspection of the perineal skin for signs of erosion or rashes related to UI. Local innervation and pelvic muscle strength should also be evaluated. Whenever possible, the patient is asked to keep a bladder log or voiding diary documenting the timing of urinations, episodes of urinary leakage, and frequency of nocturia for a period of 1 to 7 days. This record can be kept by nursing staff if the person is in an inpatient facility.

The urinalysis is used to identify possible factors contributing to transient UI or urinary retention (e.g., urinary infection, diabetes mellitus). A postvoid residual urine must be measured in the patient undergoing evaluation for urinary retention and UI. The postvoid residual volume is obtained by asking the patient to urinate, followed by catheterization within a relatively brief period (preferably 5-10 min). Alternatively, a bladder scan device can be used to estimate the residual volume. Although less accurate than the catheterized residual measurement, this technique avoids catheterization with its associated discomfort and risk of UTI. Urodynamic testing is indicated in selected cases of UI and urinary retention (Fung, Spencer, Eslami, & Crandall, 2009). Imaging studies of the upper urinary tract (e.g., ultrasound, IVP) are obtained when retention or UI is associated with UTIs or when there is evidence of upper urinary tract involvement.

DETERMINANTS OF HEALTH
Urinary Incontinence

Gender

Men
- Urinary incontinence is a common manifestation of benign and malignant prostate enlargement in men.
- Urinary incontinence in men most often is overflow incontinence caused by urinary retention.

Women
- Prevalence of urinary incontinence is higher in women than in men.
- Women more frequently experience stress and urge incontinence than men.

Collaborative Care: Urinary Incontinence

An estimated 80% of incontinence can be cured or significantly improved. Transient, reversible factors are corrected initially, followed by management of established UI (see Table 48-17). In general, less invasive treatments are attempted before more invasive methods (e.g., surgery) are used. Nevertheless, the choice of initial treatment is highly individualized and based on patient preference, the type and severity of UI, and associated anatomical defects.

Several therapies may be employed to improve urinary continence (Fader, Bliss, Cottenden, Moore, & Norton, 2010). These interventions are outlined in Table 48-18. Pelvic muscle training (Kegel exercises) is used to manage stress, urge, or mixed UI (Table 48-19). Biofeedback is used to assist the patient to identify, isolate, contract, and relax the pelvic muscles (see the Complementary and Alternative Therapies box). Strength training is used to improve the efficiency of the sphincter. Neuromuscular education is used to teach patients how and when to contract the pelvic floor muscles to maximize continence. Bladder training or habit training involves rigidly scheduled toileting intervals designed to enhance bladder capacity and reduce the frequency and volume of urine loss. *Prompted toileting* is a behavioural technique used in patients with functional UI. In this case, the patient with impaired cognitive function is regularly reminded

to urinate, assisted to the toilet, and offered praise for successful toileting.

COMPLEMENTARY AND ALTERNATIVE THERAPIES
Biofeedback for Urinary Incontinence in Women

Clinical Uses
Kegel exercises help to strengthen the pelvic floor muscles. Biofeedback helps to isolate muscle groups in the pelvis.

Effects
Sensors for biofeedback are placed in the vagina or on the skin outside of the vagina. These sensors measure electrical signals produced when muscles contract. Biofeedback training develops an awareness of and control of the pelvic floor muscles.

Nursing Implications
If done correctly, pelvic floor exercise is effective treatment for mild to moderate urinary incontinence and other conditions related to pelvic floor weakness. Unfortunately, many women do not do these exercises correctly. Biofeedback is a tool to make sure that these exercises are done correctly. Most insurance companies cover the cost of biofeedback.

Electrical stimulation of the pelvic floor muscles relies on very-low-voltage and low-frequency pulses to stimulate muscle contraction and diminish overactive bladder contractions. It can be used as monotherapy for the treatment of urge or mixed UI or in conjunction with pelvic muscle training in the management of stress UI. Minimally invasive electrical stimulation uses a transvaginal or transrectal probe, or a device can be surgically implanted near the pelvic nerve roots.

Drug Therapy. Drug therapy varies according to the UI type (Table 48-20). Drugs have a very limited role in the management of stress UI. α-Adrenergic agonists can be used to increase urethral resistance at the level of the sphincter mechanism. Unfortunately, they exert a limited beneficial effect, and they are associated with adverse effects including exacerbation of hypertension and tachycardia. Drugs play a more central role in the management of urge or reflex UI. Antimuscarinic (also called anticholinergic or antispasmodic) drugs relax the bladder muscle and inhibit overactive detrusor contractions. Two preparations, long-acting tolterodine (Detrol LA) and oxybutynin in a releasing capsule (Ditropan XL), are preferred because of their efficacy and the modest incidence of their adverse effects compared with older antimuscarinic agents.

Surgical Therapy. Surgical techniques also vary according to the type of UI (Hinoul, Roovers, Ombelet, & Vanspauwen, 2009). The Marshall–Marchetti procedure involves suspending the urethra and the bladder neck by suturing the anterior vaginal wall on each side to the periosteum of the pubic bones and the lower rectum through an abdominal incision. The Pereyra procedure and subsequent modifications involve suspending the tissues adjacent to the bladder neck to the abdominal fascia, mainly through a transvaginal approach. Placement of a suburethral sling, using autologous fascia, cadaveric fascia, or a synthetic

Table 48-17 Acquired Disorders Causing Urinary Incontinence

TYPE AND DESCRIPTION	CAUSES	TREATMENT
Stress Incontinence*		
Sudden increase in intra-abdominal pressure causes involuntary passage of urine. It can occur during coughing, heavy lifting, straining, or laughing.	*Females:* Condition is found most commonly in women with relaxed pelvic musculature (frequently from obstetrical complications or multiple pregnancies). Structures of the female urethra atrophy when estrogen decreases. *Males:* Prostate surgery for benign prostatic hyperplasia or prostatic carcinoma.	Perineal muscle exercises (e.g., Kegel exercises), weight loss if patient is obese, insertion of vaginal pessary, estrogen (vaginal creams, tablets, or vaginal ring) Condom catheters or penile clamp, surgery Urethral inserts, patches, or bladder neck support devices to correct underlying problem
Urge Incontinence*		
Condition occurs randomly when involuntary urination is preceded by warning a few seconds to a few minutes in advance. Leakage is periodic but frequent. Nocturnal frequency and incontinence are common. Condition may appear with varying severity during psychological stress.	Condition is caused by uncontrolled contraction or overactivity of detrusor muscle. Bladder escapes central inhibition and contracts reflexively. Conditions include central nervous system disorders (e.g., cerebrovascular disease, Alzheimer's disease, brain tumour, Parkinson's disease), bladder disorders (e.g., carcinoma in situ, radiation effects, interstitial cystitis), interference with spinal inhibitory pathways (e.g., malignant growth in spinal cord, spondylosis), and bladder outlet obstruction, as well as conditions of unknown etiology.	Treatment of underlying cause, instruction to have patient urinate more frequently or on time schedule, anticholinergic drugs (e.g., imipramine) at bedtime, calcium channel blockers, condom catheters, vaginal estrogen
Overflow Incontinence		
Pressure of urine in overfull bladder overcomes sphincter control. Urination may also occur frequently in small amounts during the night. Bladder remains distended and is usually palpable.	Disorder is caused by outlet obstruction (prostatic hyperplasia, bladder neck obstruction, urethral stricture) or by underactive detrusor muscle caused by myogenic or neurogenic factors (e.g., herniated disk, diabetic neuropathy). It may also occur after anaesthesia and surgery (especially procedures such as hemorrhoidectomy, herniorrhaphy, cystoscopy). Neurogenic bladder (flaccid type) is another cause.	Urinary catheterization to decompress bladder, implementation of Credé's or Valsalva's manoeuvre, α-adrenergic blocker (e.g., prazosin [Minipress]) to decrease outlet resistance, bethanechol (Duvoid) to enhance bladder contractions, intermittent catheterization, surgery to correct underlying problem
Reflex Incontinence		
No warning or stress precedes periodic involuntary urination. Urination is frequent, is moderate in volume, and occurs equally during the day and night.	Spinal cord lesion above S2 interferes with central nervous system inhibition. Disorder results in detrusor hyperreflexia and interferes with pathways coordinating detrusor contraction and sphincter relaxation.	Treatment of underlying cause, bladder decompression to prevent ureteral reflux and hydronephrosis, intermittent self-catheterization, α-adrenergic blocker (e.g., prazosin) to relax internal sphincter, diazepam or baclofen to relax external sphincter, prophylactic antibiotics, surgical sphincterotomy
Incontinence After Trauma or Surgery		
Vesicovaginal or urethrovaginal fistula may occur in women. Alteration in continence control in men involves proximal urethral sphincter (bladder neck and prostatic urethra) and distal urethral sphincter (external striated muscle).	Fistulas may occur during pregnancy, after delivery of baby, as a result of hysterectomy or invasive cancer of cervix, or after radiation therapy. Incontinence is found as postoperative complication after transurethral, perineal, or retropubic prostatectomy.	Surgery to correct fistula, urinary diversion surgery to bypass urethra and bladder, external condom catheter, penile clamp, placement of artificial implantable sphincter
Functional incontinence		
Loss of urine resulting from problems of patient mobility or environmental factors.	Older adults often have problems that affect balance and mobility.	Modifications of environment or care plan that facilitate regular, easy access to toilet and promote patient safety (e.g., better lighting, ambulatory assistance equipment, clothing alterations, timed voiding, different toileting equipment)

*Patients can have a combination of stress and urge incontinence that is referred to as *mixed incontinence.*

Table 48-18 Interventions for Urinary Incontinence

INTERVENTION	DESCRIPTION
Lifestyle Modifications	

	• Self-management strategies to reduce or eliminate risk factors, including the following:
	  • Smoking cessation
	  • Weight reduction
	  • Good bowel regimen
	  • Reduction of bladder irritants such as caffeine
	  • Fluid modifications for those with urge incontinence

Scheduling Voiding Regimens	
• Timed voiding	Toileting on a fixed schedule (typically q2-3h during waking hours).
• Habit retraining	Scheduled toileting with adjustments of voiding intervals (longer or shorter) based on the individual's voiding pattern.
• Prompted voiding	Scheduled toileting that requires prompts to void from a caregiver (typically q3 h). Used in conjunction with operant conditioning techniques for rewarding individuals for maintaining continence and appropriate toileting.
• Bladder retraining and urge-suppression strategies	Scheduled toileting with progressive voiding intervals. Includes teaching of urge-control strategies using relaxation and distraction techniques, self-monitoring, use of reinforcement techniques, and other strategies such as conscious contraction of pelvic floor muscles.
Pelvic Floor Muscle Rehabilitation	
• Pelvic floor muscle (Kegel) exercises or training	See Table 48-19.
• Vaginal weight training	Active retention of increasing vaginal weights at least twice a day. Typically used in combination with pelvic floor muscle exercises.
• Biofeedback	See Complementary and Alternative Therapies box.
• Electrical stimulation	Application of low-voltage electric current to sacral and pudendal afferent fibres through vaginal, anal, or surface electrodes. Used to inhibit bladder overactivity and improve awareness, contractility, and efficiency of pelvic muscle contraction.
Anti-incontinence Devices	
• Intravaginal support devices (pessaries and bladder neck support prostheses)	Devices support bladder neck, relieve minor pelvic organ prolapse, and change pressure transmission to the urethra.
• Transvaginal sling device	Prevents involuntary release of urine through urethral support.
• Intraurethral occlusive device (urethral plug)	Single-use device that is worn in the urethra to provide mechanical obstruction to prevent urine leakage. Removed for voiding.
• Penile compression device	Mechanical fixed compression applied to the penis to prevent any flow or leakage via the urethra. Must be released hourly to void.
Containment Devices	
• External collection devices	External catheter (condom) systems (i.e., penile sheaths) direct urine into a drainage bag. Most commonly used by men.
• Absorbent products	Variety of reusable and disposable pads and pant systems.

material, is also used to correct stress UI in women. An artificial urethral sphincter can be used in women or men with intrinsic sphincter deficiency and severe stress UI. Bolsters can also be implanted in men with stress UI to increase urethral resistance. This procedure is technically similar to the suburethral sling surgery often performed in women. A tension-free synthetic vaginal tape also can be used to treat stress UI. This transvaginal slinglike material is placed under the midurethra through incisions in the abdominal and vaginal wall (Kociszewski et al., 2012). Alternatively, one of several bulking agents can be injected underneath the mucosa of the urethra to correct stress UI in women or men (Keegan, Atiemo, Cody, McClinton, & Pickard, 2007). Bulking agents include glutaraldehyde cross-linked bovine collagen (GAX collagen), small silicone beads (Durasphere), or polytetrafluoroethylene (Teflon). Because of the risk of migration

of Teflon particles, GAX collagen or Durasphere injections are most commonly used today.

NURSING MANAGEMENT: URINARY INCONTINENCE

The nurse must recognize both the physical and the emotional problems associated with UI. The patient's dignity, privacy, and feelings of self-worth must be maintained or enhanced. This often includes a two-step approach comprising containment devices to manage existing urinary leakage and a definitive plan of management designed to reduce or resolve the factors leading to UI.

PATIENT & CAREGIVER TEACHING GUIDE

Table 48-19 Pelvic Floor Muscle or Kegel Exercises

What Is the Pelvic Floor Muscle?

Your pelvic floor muscle provides support for your bladder and rectum and, in women, the vagina and the uterus. If it weakens or is damaged, it cannot support these organs and their position can change. This causes problems with the normal bladder and rectal function. If you have a weak pelvic floor muscle, you might want to do special exercises to make the muscle stronger, prevent unwanted urine leakage, and lessen urinary urgency.

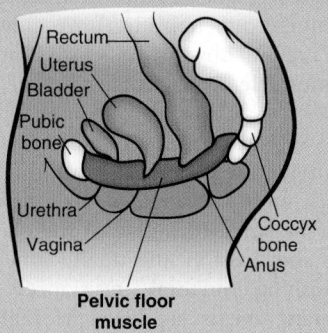 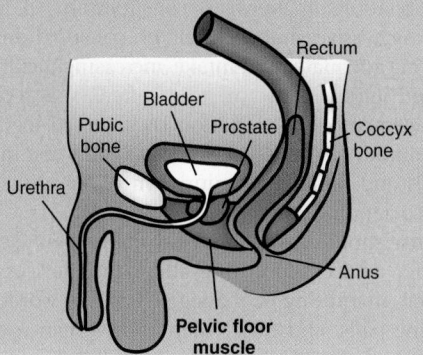

Finding the Pelvic Floor Muscle

Without tensing the muscles of your leg, buttocks, or abdomen, imagine that you are trying to control the passing of gas or pinching off a stool. Or imagine you are in an elevator full of people and you feel the urge to pass gas. What do you do? You tighten or pull in the ring of muscle around your rectum—your pelvic floor muscle. You should feel a lifting sensation in the area around the vagina or a pulling in of your rectum.

How to Do the Exercises

There are two different kinds of exercises—short squeezes and long squeezes.

1. To do the *short squeezes,* tighten your pelvic floor muscle quickly, squeeze hard for 2 sec, and then relax the muscle. Also, when you have strong urinary urges, try to tighten your pelvic floor muscle quickly and hard several times in a row until the urge passes.

2. To do the *long squeezes,* tighten the muscle for 5-10 sec before you relax. Do both of these exercises 40-50 times each day.

When to Do These Exercises

You can do these exercises anytime and anywhere. You can do these exercises in any position, but sitting or lying down may be the easiest.

How Long Does It Take Before You Notice a Change?

After 4-6 wk of doing these exercises, you should start to see less urine leakage and urinary urgency.

Source: Courtesy of Diane Newman. *Kegel exercises.* Retrieved from *http://www.seekwellness.com/incontinence/tip-sheets.htm*

DRUG THERAPY

Table 48-20 Voiding Dysfunction*

DRUG CLASS AND MECHANISM OF ACTION	DRUG	DRUG CLASS AND MECHANISM OF ACTION	DRUG
Muscarinic Receptor Antagonists and Anticholinergics		**Tricyclic Antidepressants**	
Reduce overactive bladder contractions in urge urinary incontinence and overactive bladder	Oxybutynin (Ditropan XL, Oxytrol transdermal system)	Reduce sensory urgency and burning pain of interstitial cystitis	Imipramine
	Tolterodine (Detrol, Detrol LA)	Reduce overactive bladder contractions	Amitriptyline (Elavil)
	Dicyclomine (Bentylol)	**Calcium Channel Blockers**	
	Flavoxate (Urispas)	Reduce smooth muscle contraction strength	Nifedipine (Adalat)
α-Adrenergic Antagonists			Diltiazem (Cardizem)
Reduce urethral sphincter resistance to urinary outflow	Doxazosin (Cardura)	May reduce burning pain of interstitial cystitis	Verapamil (Isoptin)
	Terazosin (Hytrin)	**Hormone Replacement Therapy**	
	Tamsulosin (Flomax)	Local application reduces urethral irritation and increases host defences against UTI	Estrogen cream (Premarin, Estrace)
5α-Reductase Inhibitors			Estrogen vaginal ring (Estring)
Androgen suppression that results in epithelial atrophy and a decrease in total prostate size	Finasteride (Proscar)		Estrogen vaginal tablets (Vagifem)

*The type of drug therapy depends on the type of incontinence.
UTI, urinary tract infection.

Management includes working with the patient to promote adequate fluid intake and reduction or elimination of bladder irritants (particularly caffeine and alcohol) from the diet. The patient is advised to maintain a regular, flexible schedule of urination (usually q2-3h while awake). In addition, patients are strongly advised to quit smoking because this habit increases the risk of stress incontinence. Patients should also be counselled about the relationship between constipation, UI, and urinary retention. Aggressive management of constipation, beginning with ensuring adequate fluid intake, increasing dietary fibre, light exercise, and judicious use of stool softeners, is recommended. (The management of constipation is discussed in Chapter 45.) As well, promoting continence strategies can assist in the prevention of falls and fall-related injuries in older adults (Registered Nurses' Association of Ontario [RNAO], 2011).

The nurse should assess strategies the patient uses to contain UI and offer advice concerning alternative devices when indicated. When attempting to manage UI, many women use feminine hygiene pads, and many men and women use household products such as rags, paper towels, or folded toilet tissue. Unfortunately, none of these products is adequately designed to wick urine away from the skin, prevent soiling of clothing, and reduce or eliminate odour. Instead, the nurse should share information on products specifically designed to contain urine. For example, patients with mild to moderate UI often benefit from incontinent pads containing Superabsorbent, a material specifically designed to absorb many times its weight in water. Patients with higher volume urine loss or those with double urinary and fecal incontinence may benefit from disposable or reusable incontinence briefs or pad–pant systems designed for more severe cases.

Several behavioural interventions are used in the management of UI. Habit training or prompted toileting are useful for patients with urge, mixed, and functional UI, respectively. Habit training uses the results of a voiding diary or bladder log to determine patterns of daytime voiding frequency. The patient and nurse then negotiate a goal for voiding frequency, usually ranging from 2 to 3 hours. The patient is taught to schedule rigidly during waking hours according to the baseline urinary frequency identified on the bladder log. At night, the person is advised to urinate as normal if awakened from sleep with the desire to void. This interval is increased in a stepwise fashion to the goal negotiated with the nurse, usually over a period of 2 to 6 weeks. Habit training may be combined with pelvic muscle training, focusing on techniques such as urge suppression. Prompted toileting is indicated for patients with altered cognitive function and functional UI (usually coexisting with urge UI). In this case, caregivers are taught to remind the patient to toilet on a regular basis (usually q2-3h), and the patient is assisted to the toilet and given praise for successful toileting. A trial of prompted toileting, in conjunction with a urological evaluation, is used to predict the ultimate success of such a program.

In the hospital, nursing management includes maximizing toilet access. This assistance may take the form of offering the urinal or bedpan or assisting the patient to the bathroom every 2 to 3 hours or at scheduled times. The nurse ensures that toilets are accessible to patients and that adequate privacy occurs to allow effective urine elimination.

Collaborative Care: Urinary Retention

Behavioural therapies also may be used in the management of urinary retention (Fader et al., 2010). Scheduled toileting and double voiding may be effective in chronic urinary retention with moderate postvoid residual volumes. However, for acute or chronic urinary retention, catheterization may be required. Ideally, intermittent catheterization is used to manage urinary retention. It allows the patient to remain free of an indwelling catheter with its associated risk of UTI and urethral irritation. Despite these potential advantages, an indwelling catheter is preferred in certain cases (e.g., the patient who is unwilling or unable to perform intermittent catheterization). An indwelling catheter is also used when urethral obstruction renders intermittent catheterization uncomfortable or unfeasible.

Drug Therapy. Several drugs may be administered to promote bladder evacuation. For the patient with obstruction at the level of the bladder neck, an α-adrenergic blocker may be prescribed. These drugs relax the smooth muscle of the bladder neck, the prostatic urethra, and possibly the dually innervated rhabdosphincter, diminishing urethral resistance. Examples of α-adrenergic blocking agents are listed in Table 48-20. They are indicated for use in patients with BPH, bladder neck dyssynergia, or detrusor sphincter dyssynergia. Finasteride (Proscar) is a 5α-reductase enzyme inhibitor that reduces prostate size by inhibiting the conversion of testosterone to dihydrotestosterone. Finasteride is also useful for the hematuria that occasionally complicates symptomatic BPH in older men. Bethanechol chloride (Duvoid) is sometimes prescribed to promote contractility in the weakened detrusor muscle (Skidmore-Roth, 2008).

Surgical Therapy. Surgical interventions are often useful when managing urinary retention caused by obstruction. Transurethral or open surgical techniques are used to treat benign or malignant prostatic enlargement, bladder neck contracture, urethral strictures, or dyssynergia of the bladder neck in selected patients. Pelvic reconstruction using an abdominal or transvaginal approach can be used to correct bladder outlet obstruction in women with severe pelvic organ prolapse.

Unfortunately, surgery plays little role in the management of urinary retention caused by deficient detrusor contraction strength. Attempts to create a bladder stimulator (implanted device capable of stimulating micturition) have proved largely unsuccessful because of the difficulty in achieving a coordinated detrusor contraction associated with pelvic muscle and striated sphincter relaxation.

NURSING MANAGEMENT: URINARY RETENTION

Acute urinary retention is a medical emergency that requires prompt recognition and bladder drainage. The nurse should insert a catheter (as prescribed) unless otherwise directed. A catheter with a retention balloon is used in anticipation of the need for an indwelling catheter.

The patient with acute urinary retention (as well as the patient predisposed to these episodes) should be taught strategies to minimize risk, including avoiding intake of large volumes of fluid over a brief period. Instead, the patient is advised to drink small volumes throughout the day. The patient is advised to warm up before attempting urination when chilled and to avoid large volumes of alcohol intake because it leads to polyuria and a diminished awareness of the need to urinate until the bladder is distended. A patient who is unable to urinate is advised to drink

Table 48-21 Indications for Urinary Catheterization

Indwelling Catheter

- Relief of urinary retention caused by lower urinary tract obstruction, paralysis, or inability to void
- Bladder decompression preoperatively and operatively for lower abdominal or pelvic surgery
- Facilitation of surgical repair of urethra and surrounding structures
- Splinting of ureters or urethra to facilitate healing after surgery or other trauma in area
- Accurate measurement of urinary output in critically ill patient
- Measurement of residual urine after urination (referred to as postvoid residual [PVR]) if portable ultrasound not available
- Contamination of stage III or IV pressure ulcers with urine that has impeded healing, despite appropriate personal care for the incontinence
- Terminal illness or severe impairment, which makes positioning or clothing changes uncomfortable, or which is associated with intractable pain

Straight (In-and-Out) Catheter

- Study of anatomical structures of urinary system
- Urodynamic testing
- Collection of sterile urine sample in selected situations
- Instillation of medications into bladder

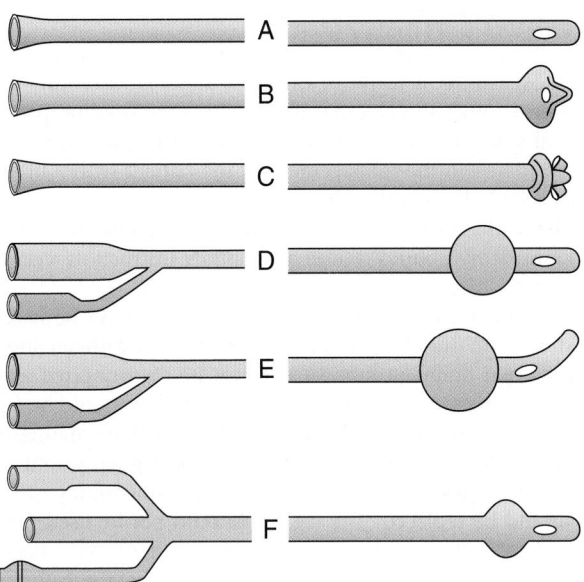

Figure 48-11 Different types of commonly used catheters. **A,** Simple urethral catheter. **B,** Mushroom or Pezzar (can be used for suprapubic catheterization). **C,** Winged-tip or Malecot. **D,** Indwelling with inflated balloon. **E,** Indwelling with Coudé tip or Tiemann. **F,** Three-way indwelling (the third lumen is used for irrigation of the bladder).

a cup of coffee or brewed tea containing caffeine to create or maximize urinary urgency and to take a warm shower and attempt to urinate while in the bath tub or shower. The patient can be reassured that he or she can easily bathe immediately following bladder evacuation. If this does not lead to successful urination, the patient is advised to seek immediate care.

Patients with chronic urinary retention may be managed by behavioural methods, indwelling or intermittent catheterization (Table 48-21), surgery, or drugs (Pellatt, 2007). Scheduled toileting and double voiding are the primary behavioural interventions used for chronic retention. Scheduled toileting is used to reduce rather than expand bladder capacity. In this case, patients are asked to void every 3 to 4 hours regardless of the desire to urinate. This intervention is particularly useful in the patient with chronic overdistension, diabetes mellitus, or chronic alcoholism characterized by a large bladder capacity and diminished or delayed sensations of bladder filling and urgency. Double voiding is an attempt to maximize bladder evacuation. The patient is asked to urinate, sit on the toilet for 3 to 4 minutes, and urinate again before exiting the bathroom.

Instrumentation

Reasons for short-term urinary catheterization are listed in Table 48-21. Two reasons that are not valid indications for catheterization are (1) routine acquisition of a urine specimen for laboratory analysis and (2) convenience of the nursing staff or the patient's family. The risks of hospital-associated infection are too high to allow catheterization of a patient for the convenience of hospital personnel or family members. Catheterization to obtain sterile urine specimens may occasionally be indicated when patients

have a history of complicated urinary infection. These specimens have to be as free of contaminants as possible. A catheter should be the final means of providing the patient with a dry environment for prevention of skin breakdown and protection of dressings or skin lesions.

Urinary catheterization is used when indicated in the management of the hospitalized patient. However, it is not without serious risks. The urinary tract is the most common site of hospital-associated infections. Urinary catheterization is a major cause of UTIs. Strict aseptic technique is mandatory when a urinary catheter is inserted. After insertion, maintenance and protection of the closed drainage system are major nursing responsibilities. Irrigation of the catheter should not be routinely performed.

While the patient has a catheter in place, nursing actions should include maintaining patency of the catheter, managing fluid intake, providing for the comfort and safety of the patient, and preventing infection. Attention should be given to the psychological implications of urinary drainage. Concerns of the patient can include embarrassment related to exposure of the body, an altered body image, and fear concerning the care of the catheter that results in increased dependency.

Catheters vary in construction materials, tip shape (Figure 48-11), and size of the lumen. Catheters are sized according to the French scale. Each French unit equals 0.33 mm of diameter. The diameter measured is the internal diameter of the catheter. The size used varies with the size of the individual and the purpose for catheterization. In women, urethral catheter sizes 12 to 14F are the most common; in men, sizes 14 to 16F are used. The primary problem resulting from too large a catheter is tissue erosion secondary to excessive pressure on the meatus or the urethra. Four routes are used for urinary tract catheterization: urethral, ureteral, suprapubic, and via a nephrostomy tube.

Urethral Catheterization

The most common route of catheterization is insertion of the catheter through the external meatus into the urethra, past the internal sphincter, and into the bladder. Principles that should be considered in the management of the patient with a urethral catheter include the following:

1. The catheterized patient, particularly the person who is ambulatory, should receive appropriate instruction regarding catheter care.
2. A sterile, closed drainage system should always be used in short-term catheterization. The distal urinary catheter and the proximal drainage tube should not be disconnected except for necessary catheter irrigation. The catheter should be taped to the leg. Unobstructed downhill flow must be maintained. The collecting bag should be emptied regularly and kept below the level of the bladder. A poorly functioning catheter should be replaced. The leg bag should not be used for the patient in the hospital setting on a short-term basis because the risk of bacterial infection is great when the catheter is disconnected and the drainage bags are exchanged.
3. Perineal care (one to two times per day and when necessary) should include cleaning of the meatus–catheter junction with soap and water. Following this, an antimicrobial ointment may be applied. Lotion or powder should not be used near the catheter. The catheter should be properly secured to the leg to prevent movement and urethral traction.
4. Sterile technique must be used whenever the collecting system is opened. Catheter irrigation is performed only when obstruction or blood clots are suspected or, in the case of long-term catheterization, to reduce sediment buildup. If frequent irrigations are necessary in short-term catheterization for catheter patency, a triple-lumen catheter may be preferable, permitting continuous irrigations within a closed system. Small volumes of urine for culture can be aspirated from the distal catheter by means of a sterile syringe and a 21-gauge needle after the drainage tubing is clamped. The puncture site must first be prepared with a tincture of iodine or alcohol solution. Many drainage systems are now equipped with a sampling port. Silicone or plastic catheters do not self-seal. Urine for chemical analysis (e.g., electrolytes) can be obtained from the drainage bag.
5. When the patient is catheterized for less than 2 weeks, routine catheter change is not necessary. For long-term use of an indwelling catheter, regular replacement is necessary. With long-term use of a catheter, a leg bag may be used. If the collection bag is reused, it should be washed in soap and water and rinsed thoroughly. When not reused immediately, it should be filled with 0.5 cup of vinegar and drained. The vinegar is effective against *Pseudomonas* and other organisms and eliminates odours.

Ureteral Catheters

The ureteral catheter is placed through the ureters into the renal pelvis. The catheter is inserted either (1) by being threaded up the urethra and bladder to the ureters under cystoscopic observation or (2) by surgical insertion through the abdominal wall into the ureters. The ureteral catheter is used after surgery to splint the ureters and to prevent them from being obstructed by edema. The urine volume from the ureteral catheter should be recorded separately from other urinary catheters. The patient is usually kept on bed rest while a ureteral catheter is in place until specific orders indicate that ambulation is permissible. The self-retaining ureteral catheter is often inserted after a lithotripsy procedure or when ureteral obstruction from adjacent tumours or fibrosis threatens renal function. The double-J ureteral catheter is often used and allows the patient to ambulate. One end coils up in the kidney pelvis, and the other coils in the bladder.

The placement of the ureteral catheter should be checked frequently, and tension on the catheter should be prevented. The catheter drains urine from the renal pelvis, which has a capacity of 3 to 5 mL. If the volume of urine in the renal pelvis increases, the additional pressure will cause tissue damage to the pelvis. Therefore, the ureteral catheter should not be clamped. If the physician orders irrigation of the ureteral catheter, strict aseptic technique is required. If output is decreased, the physician should be notified immediately. Drainage should be checked often (at least q1-2h). It is normal for some urine to drain around the ureteral catheter into the bladder. Accurate recording of urine output from both the ureters and the urethral catheter is essential. Sometimes, a ureteral catheter may be used as a stent and is not expected to drain. It is important to check with the physician as to the type of catheter and what to expect.

Suprapubic Catheters

Suprapubic catheterization is the simplest and oldest method of urinary diversion. The two methods of insertion of a suprapubic catheter into the bladder are (1) through a small incision in the abdominal wall and (2) by the use of a trocar. A suprapubic catheter is placed while the patient is under general anaesthesia for another surgical procedure or at the bedside with a local anaesthetic. The catheter may be sutured into place. The nursing responsibility includes taping the catheter to prevent dislodgement. The care of the tube and catheter is similar to that of the urethral catheter. A pectin-base skin barrier (e.g., Stomahesive) is effective around the insertion site in protecting the skin from breakdown.

The suprapubic catheter is used in temporary situations such as bladder, prostate, and urethral surgery. The suprapubic catheter is also used long-term in selected patients (e.g., male tetraplegic [quadriplegic] patient who tends to form penoscrotal fistulas).

A suprapubic catheter is prone to poor drainage because of mechanical obstruction of the catheter tip by the bladder wall, sediment, and clots. Nursing interventions to ensure patency of the tube include (1) preventing tube kinking by coiling the excess tubing and maintaining gravity drainage, (2) having the patient turn from side to side, and (3) milking the tube. If these measures are not effective, the catheter is irrigated with sterile technique after a physician's order has been obtained.

If the patient experiences bladder spasms that are difficult to control, urinary leakage may result. Oxybutynin (Ditropan) or other oral antispasmodics or belladonna and opium (B&O) suppositories may be prescribed to decrease bladder spasms.

Nephrostomy Tubes

The nephrostomy tube (catheter) is inserted on a temporary basis to preserve renal function when a complete obstruction of the ureter is present. It is inserted directly into the pelvis of the kidney and attached to connecting tubing for closed drainage. The principle is the same as with the ureteral catheter; that is, the catheter should never be kinked, laid or leaned on, or clamped. If the patient complains of excessive pain in the area or if there is excessive drainage around the tube, the catheter should be checked for patency. If irrigation is ordered, strict aseptic technique is required. No more than 5 mL of sterile saline solution is gently instilled at one time to prevent overdistension of the kidney pelvis and renal damage. Infection and secondary stone formation are complications associated with the insertion of a nephrostomy tube.

Intermittent Catheterization

An alternative approach to a long-term in-dwelling catheter is intermittent catheterization (Gotteli et al., 2008). It is being used with increasing frequency in conditions characterized by neurogenic bladder (e.g., spinal cord injuries, chronic neurological diseases) or bladder outlet obstruction in men and can be self-managed. This type of catheterization may also be used in the oliguric and anuric phases of acute kidney injury to reduce the possibility of infection from an indwelling catheter. Intermittent catheterization is also used postoperatively, often after a surgical procedure for female incontinence or radioactive seed implantation into the prostate for cancer. The main goal of intermittent catheterization is to prevent urinary retention, stasis, and compromised blood supply to the bladder caused by prolonged pressure.

The technique consists of inserting a urethral catheter into the bladder every 3 to 5 hours. Some patients do intermittent catheterization only once or twice a day to measure residual urine and to ensure an empty bladder. Patients should be instructed to wash and rinse the catheter and their hands with soap and water before and after catheterization. Lubricant is necessary for men and may make catheterization more comfortable for women. The catheter may be inserted by the patient or the care provider. The bladder is emptied, and the catheter is removed. The catheter can be dried and placed in a carrying pouch or purse or folded in a paper towel until it is next needed. The same catheter can be used for weeks at a time. In general, patients should change the catheter every 2 to 4 weeks.

In the hospital, sterile technique is used. For home care, a clean technique that includes good handwashing with soap and water is used. There has been no significant increase in infection with the use of an appropriate clean technique as compared with sterile technique. The patient is taught to observe for signs of UTI so that treatment can be instituted early. If indicated, some patients are placed on a regimen of prophylactic antibiotics.

Surgery of the Urinary Tract

Renal and Ureteral Surgery

The most common indications for nephrectomy are a renal tumour, polycystic kidneys that are bleeding or severely infected, massive traumatic injury to the kidney, and the elective removal of a kidney from a donor. Surgery involving the ureters and the kidneys is most commonly performed to remove calculi that become obstructive, correct congenital anomalies, and divert urine when necessary.

Preoperative Management

The basic needs of the patient undergoing renal and ureteral surgery are similar to those of any patient who experiences surgery (see Chapters 20 through 22). In addition, it is especially important preoperatively to ensure adequate fluid intake and a normal electrolyte balance. The patient should be told that there will probably be a flank incision on the affected side and that surgery will require a hyperextended, side-lying position. This position frequently causes the patient to experience muscle aches after surgery. If a nephrectomy is planned, the patient must be assured that one working kidney is sufficient to maintain normal renal function.

Postoperative Management

Specific postoperative needs of a patient are related to urine output, respiratory status, and abdominal distension.

Urine Output. In the immediate postoperative period, urine output should be determined at least every 1 to 2 hours. Drainage from various catheters should be recorded separately. The catheter or tube should not be clamped or irrigated without a specific order. The total urine output should be at least 0.5 mL/kg/hr. Peak flow rates can be measured with a urometer. It is also important to assess for urine drainage on the dressing and to estimate the amount. Daily weighing of the patient is important. The same scale should be used and properly balanced, and the patient should wear similar clothing and dressings each time.

It is important to observe and monitor the colour and the consistency of urine. Urine with increased amounts of mucus, blood, or sediment may occlude the drainage tubing or catheter.

Respiratory Status. Renal surgery is often performed through a flank incision just below the diaphragm and often involves removal of the twelfth rib. Postoperatively, it is important to ensure adequate ventilation. The patient is often reluctant to turn, cough, and deep breathe because of the incisional pain. Adequate pain medication should be given to ensure the patient's comfort and ability to perform coughing and deep-breathing exercises. Frequently, additional respiratory devices such as an incentive spirometer are used every 2 hours while the patient is awake. In addition, early and frequent ambulation assists in maintaining adequate respiratory function.

Abdominal Distension. Abdominal distension is present to some degree in most patients who have had surgery on their kidneys or ureters. It is most commonly the result of paralytic ileus caused by manipulation and compression of the bowel during surgery. Oral intake is restricted until bowel sounds are present (usually 24-48 hr after surgery). Intravenous fluids are given until the patient can take oral fluids. Progression to a regular diet follows.

Laparoscopic Nephrectomy

Laparoscopic nephrectomy can be performed in select situations to remove a diseased kidney. Laparoscopic nephrectomy can also be used to obtain a kidney from a living donor to be transplanted into a person with end-stage renal disease. In contrast to the open incision of about 18 cm required in a conventional nephrectomy, a laparoscopic nephrectomy is performed using five puncture sites. One incision is to view the kidney and another is to dissect it. The laparoscope contains a miniature camera so that the surgeons can watch what they are doing on a video monitor. Once dissected, the kidney is manoeuvred into a nylon impermeable sack, and its contents can then be safely removed from the patient. Compared with conventional nephrectomy, the laparoscopic approach is less painful and requires no sutures or staples, involves a shorter hospital stay, and has a much faster recovery. NCP 48-3 for care of patients with an ileal conduit identifies key

NURSING CARE PLAN 48-3

Ileal Conduit

NURSING DIAGNOSIS	**Anxiety** *related to* effects of ileal conduit on lifestyle and relationships; lack of knowledge regarding surgical procedure, appliance, and its use *as evidenced by* frequent questions about surgical procedure, restlessness, and inability to sleep
Expected Patient Outcome	**Nursing Interventions and *Rationales***
• Is knowledgeable about preoperative, operative, and postoperative procedures, including both stoma and appliance	• Support patient in preoperative, operative, and postoperative procedures including diet, drugs, nasogastric tube, IVs, NPO status, pain management, turning, deep breathing, and leg exercises *to reduce anxiety and facilitate patient's progress through postoperative recovery.* • Demonstrate how to apply appliance and use equipment *because knowledge before surgery reduces patient's postoperative concerns.* • Answer questions honestly and provide emotional support *to reduce fear of the unknown and to convey a caring attitude.* • Arrange for visit by person with an ileal conduit or by an enterostomal therapy nurse *to provide patient with significant information related to ostomy care.*
NURSING DIAGNOSIS	**Risk for infection** *related to* surgical procedure, ureteral obstruction, chronic use of external appliance, and incorrect or inadequate stoma care
Expected Patient Outcome	**Nursing Interventions and *Rationales***
• Has no urinary tract infection	• Assess patient for elevation in body temperature, pain in back or abdomen, bloody or cloudy urine, or decrease in urinary output *to ensure early detection of UTI.* • Empty appliance q2-3h or when one-third to one-half full of urine *to reduce risk of urinary reflux.* • Use bedside drainage bag at night *to prevent reflux of urine into conduit.* • Advise patient about symptoms to be reported *as indicators of possible infection.*
NURSING DIAGNOSIS	**Deficient fluid volume** *related to* active fluid volume loss or failure of regulatory mechanisms
Expected Patient Outcomes	**Nursing Interventions and *Rationales***
• Excretes >800-1500 mL of urine in 24 hr (30-52 mL/hr) • Maintains normal blood pressure, pulse, and body temperature	• Monitor urine output and quality, maintain total fluid intake and output q8h or every hour for unstable patients, treat postoperative nausea, and regulate oral and IV fluid intake *to maintain fluid and electrolyte balance.* • Monitor vital signs q15min for unstable patient *to ensure that they remain within acceptable limits.* • Observe for decreased pulse pressure, hypotension, tachycardia, and pulse volume and for changes in body temperature *to detect subtle changes that might be early indicators of complications.*
NURSING DIAGNOSIS	**Disturbed body image** *related to* effects of change in body function on lifestyle or relationships *as evidenced by* negative feelings about self, refusal to look at or touch stoma or participate in self-care, and expression of concern about effect on family and lifestyle
Expected Patient Outcome	**Nursing Interventions and *Rationales***
• Accepts changes in body image and function	• Encourage patient to share feelings *to provide opportunity to assist with issues and misconceptions and plan appropriate interventions.* • Demonstrate willingness to listen and answer questions *to convey interest in the patient's concerns and to provide needed information.* • Determine the need for additional support (e.g., psychiatric support, visit by an ostomate) *because these persons may provide new information and suggestions of ways to modify lifestyle.* • Encourage gradual involvement in self-care *because independence in self-care helps to improve self-esteem.*
NURSING DIAGNOSIS	**Ineffective self-health management** *related to* lack of knowledge regarding stoma and appliance care *as evidenced by* expression of concern about how to manage ileal conduit, or frequent questions or inaccurate responses regarding stoma care
Expected Patient Outcomes	**Nursing Interventions and *Rationales***
• Demonstrates ability to change stoma bag and clean stoma • Demonstrates ability to maintain permanent appliance	• Demonstrate proper method of changing stoma bag and have patient give return demonstration *to teach correct care and evaluate learning.* • Teach measures such as high fluid intake, regular activity, and urine acidification *to prevent urinary calculi and infection.* • Teach practices such as proper stoma and pouch care; empty or change pouch when one-third to one-half full; avoid odour-producing foods such as onions, fish, eggs, cheese; drink cranberry juice or use a liquid appliance deodorant *to enable satisfactory self-care.*

NURSING CARE PLAN 48-3

Ileal Conduit—cont'd

NURSING DIAGNOSIS	**Risk for impaired skin integrity** *related to* ill-fitting appliance, inadequate hygiene, and lack of knowledge regarding stoma care
Expected Patient Outcomes	**Nursing Interventions and *Rationales***
• Has intact, viable stoma • Maintains clean and intact skin surrounding stoma	• Assess skin for improperly fitted appliance, reddened and irritated skin around stoma *to ensure prompt identification of the problem.* • Check appliance position *to prevent leakage of caustic drainage onto skin.* • Observe stoma for any bleeding or eroded areas *for early identification and treatment of complications.* • Cleanse stoma as ordered *to reduce encrustations and bacterial contact with the stoma and surrounding skin.* • Allow no tight clothing or binders over stoma *to enable unobstructed circulation of blood and flow of urine.*
NURSING DIAGNOSIS	**Ineffective sexuality pattern** *related to* perceived or actual effects of surgery on sexual activity *as evidenced by* verbalizing concerns about sexuality and unwillingness to discuss sexual issues with partner
Expected Patient Outcome	**Nursing Interventions and *Rationales***
• Expresses satisfaction with sexual practices	• Assess patient's concerns related to sexuality such as future sexual functioning and lack of understanding by significant other *to determine presence and extent of problem.* • Provide accurate information related to sexual activity *so that patient will know the effect of this surgery on sexual activities and practices.*

IVs, intravenous lines; *NPO,* nothing by mouth; *UTI,* urinary tract infection.

Table 48-22 Types of Urinary Diversion Surgery Requiring Collection Devices

TYPE	DESCRIPTION	ADVANTAGES	DISADVANTAGES	SPECIAL CONSIDERATIONS
Ileal	Conduit ureters are implanted into part of ileum or colon that has been resected from intestinal tract. Abdominal stoma is created.	Relatively good urine flow with few physiological alterations	External appliance necessary to continually collect urine	Surgical procedure is more complex. Postoperative complications may be increased. Reabsorption of urea by ileum occurs. Meticulous attention is necessary to care for stoma and collecting device.
Cutaneous ureterostomy	Ureters are excised from bladder and brought through abdominal wall, and stoma is created. Ureteral stomas may be created from both ureters, or ureters may be brought together and one stoma created.	No need for major surgery as required with ileal conduit	External appliance necessary because of continuous urine drainage; possibility of stricture or stenosis of small stoma	Periodic catheterizations may be required to dilate stomas to maintain patency.
Nephrostomy	Catheter is inserted into pelvis of kidney. Procedure may be done to one or both kidneys and may be temporary or permanent. It is most frequently done in advanced disease as palliative procedure.	No need for major surgery	High risk of renal infection; predisposition to calculus formation from catheter	Nephrostomy tube may have to be changed every month. Catheter must never be clamped.

nursing diagnoses that apply to the care of a patient with a nephrectomy pertaining to (1) management of anxiety related to lack of knowledge regarding a major surgical procedure, (2) knowledge deficits about preoperative, operative, and postoperative procedures, (3) risks for infection related to the surgical procedure, and (4) deficient fluid volume.

Urinary Diversion

Urinary diversion may be performed with and without cystectomy. Urinary diversion procedures are performed to treat cancer of the bladder, neurogenic bladder, congenital anomalies, stric-

tures, trauma to the bladder, and chronic infections with deterioration of renal function. Numerous urinary diversion techniques and bladder substitutes are possible, including an incontinent urinary diversion, continent urinary diversion catheterized by patient, or an orthotopic bladder so that the patient voids urethrally. Types of these surgical procedures are presented in Table 48-22 and Figure 48-12.

Incontinent Urinary Diversion

Incontinent urinary diversion is diversion to the skin, requiring an appliance. The simplest form is the cutaneous ureterostomy, but scarring and strictures of the ureter have led to the use of ileal or

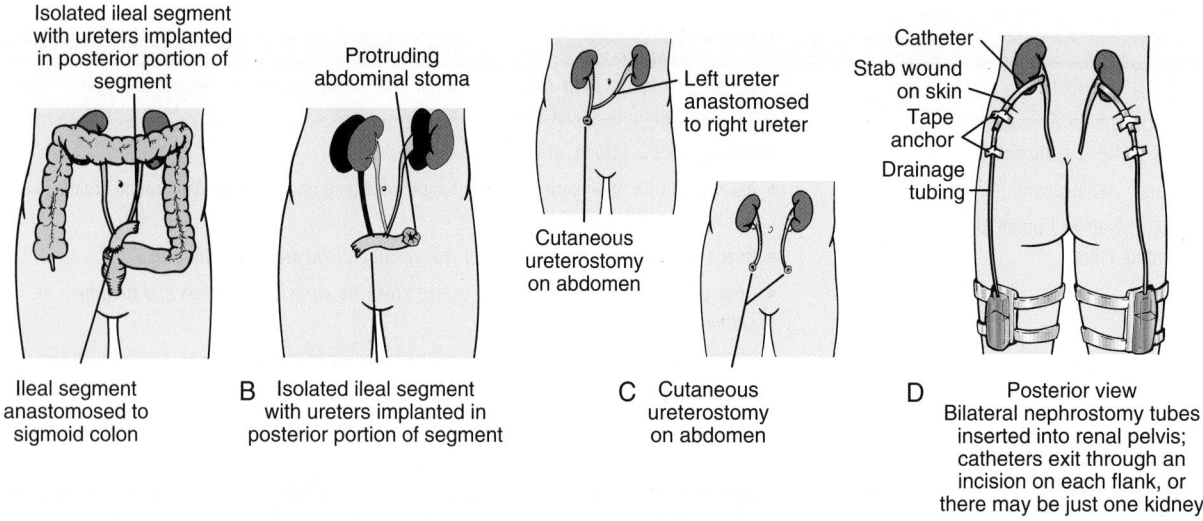

Figure 48-12 Methods of urinary diversion. **A,** Ureteroileosigmoidostomy. **B,** Ileal loop (or ileal conduit). **C,** Ureterostomy (transcutaneous ureterostomy and bilateral cutaneous ureterostomies). **D,** Nephrostomy.

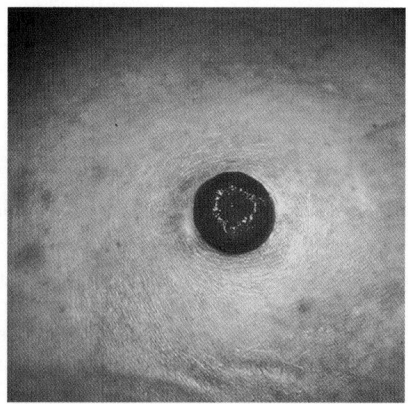

Figure 48-13 Ideal urinary stoma. It is symmetrical, has no skin breakdown, and protrudes about 1.5 cm. The mucosa is a healthy red, and the configuration is flat when the patient is upright and supine.

Source: Courtesy Lynda Brubacher, Virginia Mason Hospital, Seattle, WA.

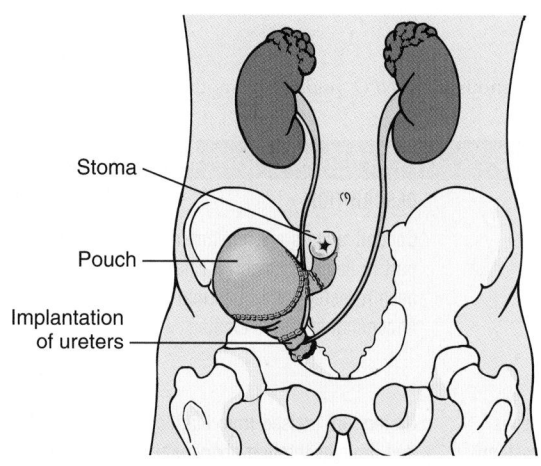

Figure 48-14 Creation of a Kock pouch with implantation of ureters into one intussuscepted portion of the pouch and creation of a stoma with the other intussuscepted portion.

colonic conduits. The most commonly performed incontinent urinary diversion procedure is the **ileal conduit** (ileal loop). In this procedure, a 15- to 20-cm segment of the ileum is converted into a conduit for urinary drainage. The colon (colon conduit) can be used instead of the ileum. The ureters are anastomosed into one end of the conduit, and the other end of the bowel is brought out through the abdominal wall to form a stoma (Figure 48-13). Although the segment of bowel remains supported by the mesentery, it is completely isolated from the intestinal tract. The bowel is anastomosed and continues to function normally. Because there is no valve and no voluntary control over the stoma, drops of urine flow from the stoma every few seconds, requiring the use of a permanent external collecting device. The visible stoma and the need for external collection devices are obvious disadvantages of this procedure. The lifelong care and dealing with the stoma and collection devices may be psychologically difficult. These problems have stimulated the increasing use of continent diversions and orthotopic bladder substitutes.

Continent Urinary Diversions

A *continent urinary diversion* is an intra-abdominal urinary reservoir that is catheterizable or has an outlet controlled by the anal sphincter. Continent diversions are internal pouches created similarly to the ileal conduit. Reservoirs have been constructed from the ileum, ileocecal segment, or colon. Large segments of bowel are altered to prevent peristaltic action. A continence mechanism is formed between this large, low-pressure reservoir and the stoma by intussuscepting a portion of bowel. In this way, a patient does not leak involuntarily. The patient with a continent reservoir needs to self-catheterize every 4 to 6 hours but does not need to wear external attachments. Examples of continent diversions are the Kock (Figure 48-14), Mainz, Indiana, and Florida pouches. A main difference among the various diversions is the segment of bowel used. For example, the Indiana pouch uses the right colon as a reservoir and has become a popular form of continent urinary diversion.

Orthotopic Bladder Substitution

Orthotopic bladder substitutes can be derived from various segments of the intestines. An isolated segment of the distal ileum is often preferred. Various procedures include the hemi-Kock pouch, Studer pouch, and the ileal W-neobladder. In these procedures, the bowel is surgically reshaped to become a neobladder. The ureters and urethra are sutured into the neobladder. Orthotopic bladder reconstruction has become a more viable option for both men and women if cancer does not involve the bladder neck or urethra (Swearingen, 2007). The advantage of orthotopic bladder substitution is that it allows for natural micturition. Incontinence is a possible problem with this technique, and intermittent catheterization may be required.

NURSING MANAGEMENT: URINARY DIVERSION

▪ Preoperative Management

The patient awaiting cystectomy and urinary diversion must be given a great deal of information. The nurse must assess ability and readiness to learn before initiating a teaching program. If the patient is not ready to learn, the teaching plan should be adjusted. The patient's anxiety and fear may be decreased by the information. However, the anxiety and fear may also interfere with learning. The patient's family and caregivers should be involved in the teaching process. A discussion of the social aspects of living with a stoma (including clothing, changes in body image and sexuality, exercise, and odour) provides the patient with facts that may allay some fears. The patient who will have a continent diversion must be taught to catheterize and irrigate the pouch and be able to adhere to a strict catheterization schedule. The patient with an orthotopic neobladder may have problems with incontinence. Concerns about the effect on sexual activities should be discussed. The enterostomal therapy nurse should be involved in the preoperative phase of the patient's care. A visit from an ostomate or enterostomal therapy nurse can be helpful. Additional interventions are presented in NCP 48-3.

▪ Postoperative Management

Nursing interventions during the postoperative period (see NCP 48-3 for care after an ileal conduit) should be planned to prevent surgical complications such as postoperative atelectasis and shock (see Chapter 22). After pelvic surgery, there is an increased incidence of thrombophlebitis. With removal of part of the bowel, the incidence of paralytic ileus and small bowel obstruction is increased, the patient is kept on nothing by mouth status, and a nasogastric tube is necessary for 3 to 5 days.

Specific attention should be given to preventing injury to the stoma and maintaining urine output. Mucus is present in the urine because it is secreted by the intestines as a result of the irritating effect of the urine. The patient should be told that this is a normal occurrence. A high fluid intake is encouraged to "flush" the ileal conduit or continent diversion.

When an ileal conduit is created, the skin around the stoma requires meticulous care. Alkaline encrustations with dermatitis may occur when alkaline urine comes in contact with exposed skin (Figure 48-15). Other common peristomal skin problems

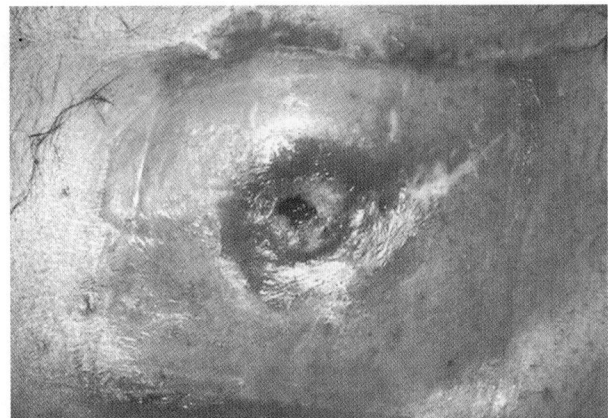

Figure 48-15 Ammonia salt encrustation secondary to alkaline urine.

Source: Courtesy Lynda Brubacher, Virginia Mason Hospital, Seattle, WA.

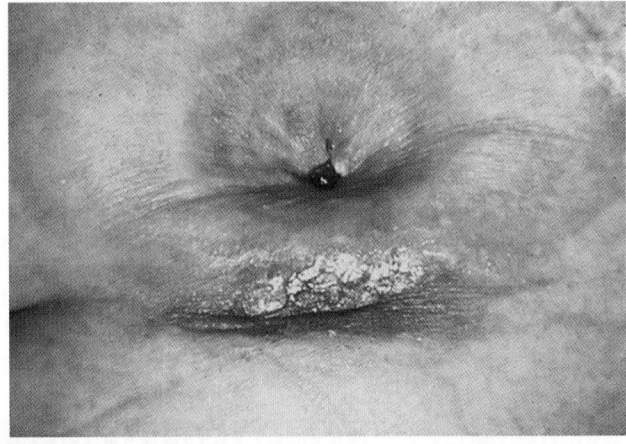

Figure 48-16 Retracted urinary stoma with pressure sore from faceplate above stoma.

Source: Courtesy Lynda Brubacher, Virginia Mason Hospital, Seattle, WA.

include yeast infections, product allergies, and shearing-effect excoriations. Changing appliances (pouches) is described in Table 48-23. A properly fitting appliance is essential to prevent skin problems. The appliance should be about 0.2 cm larger than the stoma. It is normal for the stoma to shrink within the first few weeks after surgery. The urine is kept acidic to prevent alkaline encrustations.

Acceptance of the surgery and of alterations in body image is needed to ensure the patient's best adjustment. Concerns of the patient include fear that the stoma will be offensive to others and will interfere with sexual, personal, professional, and recreational activities. The patient should know that few activities, if any, will be restricted as a result of the urinary diversion.

Discharge planning after an ileal conduit includes teaching the patient symptoms of obstruction or infection and care of the ostomy. The patient with an ileal conduit is fitted for a permanent appliance 7 to 10 days after surgery and may need to be refitted at a later time, depending on the degree of stoma shrinkage. Appliances are made of a variety of products, including natural and synthetic rubbers, plastics, and metals. Most appliances have a faceplate that adheres to the skin, a collecting pouch, and an opening to drain the pouch. The faceplate may

PATIENT & CAREGIVER TEACHING GUIDE

Table 48-23 Changing Ileal Conduit Appliances

Temporary Appliance	Permanent Appliance*
1. Cut hole in pouch to fit over stoma (pouch 3.2 mm [one-eighth inch] larger than stoma).	1. Keep appliance in place for 2-14 days.
2. Remove old pouch.	2. Change appliance when fluid intake has been restricted for several hours.
3. Clean area gently, and remove old adhesive.	3. Have patient sit or stand in front of mirror.
4. Wash area with warm water.	4. Moisten edge of faceplate with adhesive solvent and gently remove.
5. Place wick (rolled-up 4 × 4–inch) over stoma to keep area dry during rest of procedure.	5. Clean skin with adhesive solvent.
6. Dry skin around stoma.	6. Wash skin with warm water. (Patient may shower.)
7. Apply a prescribed skin protectant around stoma to area where pouch will be placed.	7. Dry skin and inspect.
8. Apply pouch by first smoothing its edges toward side and lower portion of body.	8. Place wick (rolled-up 4 × 4–inch) over stoma to keep skin free of urine.
9. Remove wick and complete application of bag.	9. Apply skin cement to faceplate and skin.
10. If patient is usually in bed, apply bag so that it lies toward side of body.	10. Place appliance over stoma.
11. If patient is ambulatory, apply bag so that it lies vertically.	11. Wash removed appliance with soap and lukewarm water; soak in distilled vinegar; rinse with lukewarm water and air dry.
12. Connect drainage tubing to pouch.	
13. Keep drainage pouch on same side of bed as stoma.	

*Many disposable appliances with self-adhesive backing are used as permanent appliances.

be secured to the skin with glues, adhesives, or adhering synthetic wafers. Some appliances do not require adhesives, but their design relies on pressure to keep the pouch in place. If improperly fitted or applied, the faceplate may cause skin problems (Figure 48-16). A bag may be used for night drainage. The patient needs information on where to purchase supplies, emergency telephone numbers, location of ostomy clubs, and follow-up visits with an enterostomal therapist. Physician follow-up is imperative to monitor and correct homeostatic abnormalities and to prevent complications and renal function deterioration.

CLINICAL DECISION-MAKING EXERCISE

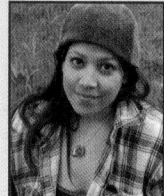

CASE STUDY:
Urinary Tract Infection

Source: blackie/iStockphoto.

Patient Profile

Ms. Guinto, a 28-year-old woman with diabetes, was seen in the nurse practitioner's office for a history of painful, frequent urination.

Subjective Data

- Has had history of painful, frequent urination with passage of small volumes of urine for 3 days
- Has had intermittent fever, chills, and back pain during these 3 days
- Was frightened when she saw blood in her urine
- Is anxious because her father died of kidney cancer

Objective Data

Physical Examination

- Complains of bilateral flank pain and abdominal tenderness to palpation
- Temperature is 38°C

Diagnostic Study

- Urinalysis: pyuria and hematuria

Discussion Questions

1. What are the most common organisms that cause urinary tract infections (UTIs)?
2. What factors predispose a patient to a UTI?
3. What is the difference between upper and lower UTIs?
4. *Priority Decision:* What are the priority nursing interventions that will help Ms. Guinto cope with her symptoms?
5. What can the nurse do to help Ms. Guinto prevent another UTI?
6. Why might she be having recurrent bouts of UTIs? What other diagnostic tests may be indicated?
7. *Priority Decision:* Based on the data presented, write one or more appropriate nursing diagnoses. Are there any collaborative problems?

evolve   *Answers are available on* **http://evolve.elsevier.com/
Canada/Lewis/medsurg**

REVIEW QUESTIONS

The number of the question corresponds to the same-numbered objective at the beginning of the chapter.

1. In teaching a patient with pyelonephritis about the disorder, the nurse will explain that organisms that cause pyelonephritis most commonly reach the kidneys through which means?
   a. The bloodstream
   b. The lymphatic system
   c. A descending infection
   d. An ascending infection

2. What should the nurse teach the female patient who has frequent urinary tract infections (UTIs)?
   a. Urinate after sexual intercourse.
   b. Take tub baths with bubble bath.
   c. Take prophylactic sulphonamides for the rest of her life.
   d. Restrict fluid intake to prevent the need for frequent voiding.

3. Which of the following immunological mechanisms are involved in glomerulonephritis?
   a. Tubular blocking by precipitates of bacteria and antibody reactions
   b. Deposition of immune complexes and complement along the glomerular basement membrane (GBM)
   c. Thickening of the GBM from autoimmune microangiopathic changes
   d. Destruction of glomeruli by proteolytic enzymes contained in the GBM

4. What is one of the most important roles of the nurse in relation to acute poststreptococcal glomerulonephritis?
   a. Promote early diagnosis and treatment of sore throats and skin lesions.
   b. Encourage patients to request antibiotic therapy for all upper respiratory infections.
   c. Teach patients with acute post-streptococcal glomerulonephritis (APSGN) that long-term prophylactic antibiotic therapy is necessary to prevent recurrence.
   d. Monitor patients for respiratory symptoms that indicate that the disease is affecting the alveolar basement membrane.

5. Why does edema occur in nephrotic syndrome?
   a. Decreased aldosterone secretion from adrenal insufficiency
   b. Increased hydrostatic pressure caused by sodium retention
   c. Increased fluid retention caused by decreased glomerular filtration
   d. Decreased colloidal osmotic pressure caused by loss of serum albumin

6. A patient is admitted to the hospital with severe renal colic caused by renal lithiasis. What is the nurse's first priority in management of the patient?
   a. Administer narcotics as prescribed.
   b. Obtain supplies for straining all urine.
   c. Encourage fluid intake of 3 to 4 L/day.
   d. Keep the patient on nothing by mouth status in preparation for surgery.

7. In which of the following conditions should the nurse recommend genetic counselling for the patient's children?
   a. Nephrotic syndrome
   b. Chronic pyelonephritis
   c. Malignant nephrosclerosis
   d. Adult-onset polycystic renal disease

8. Which of the following complications would represent the primary reason a nurse would recommend strict diabetic control in a patient prone to diabetic nephropathy?
   a. Uric acid calculi and nephrolithiasis
   b. Renal sugar-crystal calculi and cysts
   c. Lipid deposits in the glomeruli and the nephrons
   d. Thickening of the GBM and glomerulosclerosis

9. Which of the following conditions in a patient's history would the nurse identify as a risk factor for kidney and bladder cancer?
   a. Aspirin use
   b. Tobacco use
   c. Chronic alcohol abuse
   d. Use of artificial sweeteners

10. Which of the following are important in planning nursing interventions to increase bladder control in the patient with urinary incontinence?
    a. Restricting fluids to diminish the risk of urinary leakage
    b. Counselling the patient concerning choice of incontinence containment device
    c. Clamping and releasing a catheter to increase bladder tone
    d. Teaching the patient biofeedback mechanisms to suppress the urge to void

11. A patient with a ureterolithotomy returns from surgery with a nephrostomy tube in place. What would postoperative nursing care of the patient include?
    a. Encouraging the patient to drink fruit juices and milk
    b. Forcing fluids of at least 2 to 3 L/day after nausea has subsided
    c. Notifying the physician if nephrostomy tube drainage is more than 30 mL/hr
    d. Irrigating the nephrostomy tube with 10 mL of normal saline solution as needed

12. A patient has had a cystectomy and ileal conduit diversion performed. Four days postoperatively, mucous shreds are seen in the drainage bag. Which action should the nurse undertake?
    a. Notify the physician.
    b. Notify the charge nurse.
    c. Irrigate the drainage tube.
    d. Chart it as a normal observation.

ANSWERS: 1. d; 2. a; 3. b; 4. a; 5. d; 6. a; 7. d; 8. d; 9. b; 10. d; 11. b; 12. d.

REFERENCES

Bernier, F., & Sims, T. W. (2009). Management of clients with urinary disorders. In J. M. Black & J. H. Hawks (Eds.), *Medical-surgical nursing: Clinical management for positive outcomes* (8th ed., pp. 727-778). St. Louis: Elsevier Saunders.

Canadian Cancer Society's Steering Committee on Cancer Statistics. (2012). *Canadian cancer statistics 2012.* Toronto: Canadian Cancer Society. Retrieved from *http://www.cancer.ca/~/media/CCS/Canada%20wide/Files%20List/English%20files%20heading/PDF%20-%20Policy%20-%20Canadian%20Cancer%20Statistics%20-%20English/Canadian%20Cancer%20Statistics%202012%20-%20English.ashx*

Canadian Continence Foundation. (2010). Facts on incontinence. Retrieved from *http://www.canadiancontinence.ca/english/consumers/facts.html*

Canadian Diabetes Association Clinical Practice Guidelines Expert Committee. (2008). Canadian Diabetes Association clinical practice guidelines for the prevention and management of diabetes in Canada. *Canadian Journal of Diabetes, 32*(Suppl 1): S1-S201.

Carpentier, X., Daudon, M., Traxer, O., Jungers, P., Mazouyes, A., Matzen, G., ..., Bazin, D. (2009). Relationships between carbonation rate of carbapatite and morphologic characteristics of calcium phosphate stones and etiology. *Urology, 73*(5), 968-975. doi:10.1016/j.urology.2008.12.049

Chapman, A. (2009). Polycystic kidney disease: The cadence of kidney growth in ADPKD. *Nature Reviews Nephrology, 5,* 311-312. doi:10.1038/nrneph.2009.75

Chuang, Y. C. & Chancellor, M. (2009). Treatment of painful bladder syndrome and pelvic organ prolapse. *Reviews of Urology, 11*(1), 28-32.

Clemens J. Q., Joyce, G. F., Wise, M., & Payne, C. K. (2007). Interstitial cystitis and painful bladder syndrome. In M. S. Litwin, & C. S. Saigal (Eds.), *Urologic diseases in America* (NIH Publication No. 07-5512:125-154). US Department of Health and Human Services, Public Health Service, National Institutes of Health, National Institute of Diabetes and Digestive and Kidney Diseases. Washington, DC: US Government Printing Office.

Czaja, C. A., Scholes, D., Hooton, T. M., & Stam, W. E. (2007). Population-based epidemiologic analysis of acute pyelonephritis. *Clinical Infectious Diseases, 45*(3), 273-280. doi:10.1086/519268

Devarajan, P. (2008). Alport syndrome. Retrieved from *http://emedicine.medscape.com/article/981126-overview*

Dmochowski, R. (2007). Urethral diverticula. In A. J. Wein, L. R. Kavoussi, A. C. Novick, et al. (Eds.). *Campbell-Walsh urology* (9th ed.). Philadelphia: Saunders.

Eggener, S. E. (2008). Radical cystectomy. Retrieved from *http://www.emedicine.com/MED/topic3061.htm*

Fader, M., Bliss, D., Cottenden, A., Moore, K., & Norton, C. (2010). Continence products: Research priorities to improve the lives of people with urinary and/or fecal leakage. *Neurourology and Urodynamics, 29*(4), 640-4. doi:10.1002/nau.20918

Fung, C. H., Spencer, B., Eslami, M., & Crandall, C. (2009). Quality indicators for the screening and care of urinary incontinence in vulnerable elders. *Journal of the American Geriatric Society, 55* (Suppl 2), S443-S449.

Geehan, D. M., & Santucci, R. A. (2006). Renal trauma. Retrieved from *http://www.emedicine.com/MED/topic2853.htm*

Goligher, E. C., & Detsky, A. S. (2009). Migratory pulmonary infiltrates: Goodpasture syndrome. *Canadian Medical Association Journal, 180*(1), 75-77. doi:10.1503/cmaj.081117

Gollob, J. A., Rathmell, W. K., Richmond, T. M., Marino, C. B., Miller, E. K., Grigson, G., ..., Wright, J. J. (2007). Phase II trial of Sorafenib plus interferon alfa-2β as first- or second-line therapy in patients with metastatic renal cell cancer. *Journal of Clinical Oncology, 25,* 3288-3295. doi:10.1200/JCO.2007.10.8613

Gotteli, J. M., Merryman, P., Carr, C., McElveen, L., Epperson, C., & Bynum, D. (2008). A quality improvement approach to reduce the complications associated with indwelling catheters. *Urological Nursing, 28*(6), 465-473.

Greenberg, D. (2007). Incidence, mortality and survival in kidney cancer in East Anglia. Retrieved from *info.cancerresearchuk.org/cancerstats/types/kidney/survival/#stage*

Griebling, T. L. (2007). Urinary tract infection in women. In M. S. Litwin, C. S. Saigal (Eds.), *Urologic Diseases in America.* DHHS, PHS, NIH, NIDDK (NIH pub. no. 07-5512; pp. 3-7). Washington, DC: Government Printing Office.

Hanno, P. M. (2007). Painful bladder syndrome/interstitial cystitis and related disorders. In A. J. Wein (Ed.), *Campbell-Walsh, urology* (9th ed., pp. 330-370). Philadelphia: Saunders.

Hinoul, P., Roovers, J. P., Ombelet, W., & Vanspauwen, R. (2009). Surgical management of urinary stress incontinence in women: A historical and clinical overview. *European Journal of Obstetrics Gynecology and Reproductive Biology, 145*(2), 219-225. doi:10.1016/j.ejogrb.2009.04.020

Jepson, R. G., & Craig, J. C. (2008). Cranberries for preventing urinary tract infections. *Cochrane Database Systematic Reviews, 1,* CD001321. doi:10.1002/14651858.CD001321.pub4

Keegan, P. E., Atiemo, K., Cody, J., McClinton, S., & Pickard, R. (2007). Periurethral injection therapy for urinary incontinence in women. *Cochrane Database for Systematic Reviews, 3,* CD003881.

Kidney Foundation of Canada. (2003). Kidney stones. Retrieved from *http://www.kidney.ca/page.aspx?pid=328*

Kidney Foundation of Canada. (2007). Urinary tract infections. Retrieved from *http://www.kidney.ca/document.doc?id=316*

Kociszewski, J., Rautenberg, O., Kuszka, A., Eberhard, J., Hilgers, R., & Viereck, V. (2012). Can we place tension-free vaginal tape where it should be? The one-third rule. *Ultrasound in Obstetrics and Gynecology, 39,* 210-214. doi:10.1002/uog.10050

Krause K., Mowassee M., & Auerhahn, C. (2008). Urinary tract infections in the elderly: Symptomatology and prevention. *American Journal for Nurse Practitioners, 12*(9), 57-63.

Lin K., Fajardo, K., & U. S. Preventive Services Task Force. (2008). Screening for asymptomatic bacteriuria in adults: Evidence for the US Preventive Services Task Force reaffirmation recommendation statement, *Annuls of Internal Medicine, 149*(1), W20.

Mayo Clinic Staff. (2012). Nephrotic syndrome. Retrieved from *http://www.mayoclinic.com/health/nephrotic-syndrome/DS01047*

Moldawer, N. P., & Figlin, R. (2008). Renal cell carcinoma: The translation of molecular biology into new treatments, new patient outcomes, and nursing implications, *Oncology Nursing Forum, 35*(4), 699-708. doi:10.1188/08.ONF.699-708

National Kidney and Urologic Diseases Information Clearinghouse (NKUDIC). (2007). Kidney Stones in Adults. Retrieved from *http://kidney.niddk.nih.gov/KUDiseases/pubs/stonesadults/index.aspx#who*

National Kidney and Urologic Diseases Information and Clearinghouse. (2009). Diet for Kidney Stone Prevention. Retrieved from *http://kidney.niddk.nih.gov/KUDiseases/pubs/kidneystonediet/index.aspx#calcium/*

Nicolle, L., Anderson, P. A. M., Conly, J., Mainprize, T. C., Meuser, J., Nickel, J. C., ..., Zhanel, G. (2006). Uncomplicated urinary tract infection in women: Current practice and the effect of antibiotic resistance on empiric treatment. *Canadian Family Physician, 52,* 612-618.

Norrby, S. R. (2007). Approach to the patient with urinary tract infection. In L. Goldman & D. Ausiello (Eds.), *Cecil textbook of medicine* (23rd ed.). Philadelphia: Saunders.

Pellatt, G., (2007). Urinary elimination: Part 2—Retention, incontinence and catheterization. *British Journal of Nursing, 16*(8), 480-485.

Perlmutter, A. E., Talug, C., Tarry, W. F., Zaslau, S., Mohseni, H., & Kandzari, S. J. (2008). Impact of stone location on success rates of endoscopic lithotripsy for nephrolithiasis, *Urology, 71*(2), 214-217. doi:10.1016/j.urology.2007.09.023

Pietrow, P. K., & Karellas, M. E. (2006). Medical management of common urinary calculi, *American Family Physician, 74*(1), 86-94.

Registered Nurses' Association of Ontario (RNAO). (2011). Prevention of falls and fall injuries in the older adult. Registered Nurses'

Association of Ontario Best Practice Guideline Supplement. Retrieved from *http://rnao.ca/bpg/guidelines/prevention-falls-and-fall-injuries-older-adult*

Sakhaee, K. (2009). Recent advances in the pathophysiology of nephrolithiasis. *Kidney International Review, 75*(6), 585-595. doi:10.1038/ki.2008.626

Schaefer, A. J. (2007). Infections of the urinary tract. In: A. J. Wein, L. R. Kavoussi, A. C. Novick, et al. (Eds.), *Campbell-Walsh urology* (9th ed.). Philadelphia: Elsevier.

Schrier, R. (2007). *Disease of the kidney and urinary tract* (8th ed., vol. 2). St. Louis: Lippincott, Williams & Wilkins.

Skidmore-Roth, L. (2008). *2008 Mosby's nursing drug reference*. St. Louis: Mosby.

Swearingen, P. L. (2007). *Manual of medical-surgical nursing care* (6th ed.). St. Louis: Mosby, Elsevier.

Tolkoff–Rubin, N. E., Cotran, R. S., & Rubin, R. H. (2008). Urinary tract infection, pyelonephritis, and reflux nephropathy. In B. M. Brenner (Ed.). *Brenner and Rector's The Kidney* (8th ed., Chapter 34). Philadelphia: Saunders.

Traver, M. A., Passman, C., LeRoy, T., Passmore, L., & Assimos, D. G. (2009). Is the Internet a reliable source for dietary recommendations for stone formers? *Journal of Endourology, 23*(4), 715-717. doi:10.1089/end.2008.0490

Zhang, Q., & Rothenbacher, D. (2008). Prevalence of chronic kidney disease in population-based studies: Systematic review. *BMC Public Health, 8*, 117. doi:10.1186/1471-2458-8-117.

CANADIAN RESOURCES

Canadian Interstitial Cystitis Resource Centre
http://www.canadaic.com
Canadian Kidney Foundation Educational Resources
http://www.kidney.ca/page.asp?intNodeID=20234

Canadian Association of Nephrology Nurses and Technologists
http://cannt.ca
Canadian Urological Association
http://www.cua.org
Cancer Care Ontario Toolbox: Evidence-Based Guidelines
https://www.cancercare.on.ca/toolbox/qualityguidelines/
Kidney Foundation of Canada
http://www.kidney.ca/
Registered Nurses' Association of Ontario Best Practice Guidelines
http://www.rnao.org/Page.asp?PageID=924&ContentID=1274
Sunnybrook and Women's College Health Sciences Centre
http://www.womenshealthmatters.ca
United Ostomy Association of Canada
http://www.ostomycanada.ca/

RELATED RESOURCES

American Cancer Society
http://www.cancer.org
Bladder Health Council
http://www.afud.org/education/bladder.html
International Continence Foundation (ICF)
http://www.icsoffice.org
Interstitial Cystitis Association
http://www.ichelp.com
Wound, Ostomy and Continence Nurses Society
http://www.wocn.org

evolve *For additional Internet resources, see the Web site for this book at* **http://evolve.elsevier.com/Canada/Lewis/medsurg**

Written by Carol M. Headley
Adapted by Marsha Wood

LEARNING OBJECTIVES

1. Differentiate between acute kidney injury and chronic kidney disease.
2. Identify criteria used in the classification of acute kidney injury using the acronym RIFLE (risk, injury, failure, loss, end-stage kidney disease).
3. Describe the clinical course of acute kidney injury.
4. Explain the collaborative care and nursing management of a patient with acute renal failure.
5. Define chronic kidney disease and delineate the five stages of chronic kidney disease based on the glomerular filtration rate.

6. Select risk factors that contribute to the development of chronic kidney disease.
7. Summarize the significance of cardiovascular disease in individuals with chronic kidney disease.
8. Explain the collaborative care and related nursing management of the patient with chronic kidney disease.
9. Differentiate among renal replacement therapies for individuals with chronic kidney disease.
10. Discuss the role of the nurse in the management of individuals who receive a renal transplant.

KEY TERMS

acute kidney injury (AKI) Renal impairment that ranges from mild, calling for little intervention, to severe, necessitating renal replacement therapy; the changes in renal function are acute in nature and usually occur over a 48-hr period, p. 1333

acute renal failure (ARF) The advanced stages of acute kidney injury that call for aggressive management and often necessitate renal replacement therapy, p. 1333

acute tubular necrosis (ATN) Necrosis of the renal tubular cells caused by nephrotoxic substances or ischemia, p. 1335

arteriovenous fistula (AVF) The preferred hemodialysis access created by the surgical connection of a vein and an artery, usually in the forearm, p. 1354

arteriovenous graft (AVG) A hemodialysis access created with a synthetic graft that is attached to an artery and vein; used for people who do not have suitable vessels for an AVF, p. 1355

automated peritoneal dialysis (APD) Also called *continuous cycling peritoneal dialysis*, it involves the use of a machine to perform, or automate, the dialysis exchanges, p. 1353

chronic kidney disease (CKD) The presence of kidney damage or renal insufficiency that is unlikely to be reversed that is present for a period of 3 months or more and can be classified at one of five stages, depending on level of severity based on glomerular filtration rate, p. 1339

chronic kidney disease–mineral and bone disorder (CKD–MBD) A clinical syndrome involving characteristic bone abnormalities and changes in mineral balance and vascular and other soft tissue calcification, p. 1343

continuous ambulatory peritoneal dialysis (CAPD) A type of peritoneal dialysis that consists of a minimum of four exchanges of dialysis fluid over a 24-hr period, p. 1353

continuous renal replacement therapy (CRRT) A 12- to 24-hr continuous dialysis type of therapy (hemofiltration) for patients who are hemodynamically unstable or require large amounts of fluid removal, p. 1358

dialysis A clinical technique, used to correct fluid and electrolyte imbalances and to remove waste products in renal failure, in which substances move from the blood through a semipermeable membrane (dialyzer/ peritoneal membrane) and into a dialysis solution (dialysate), p. 1350

end-stage renal disease (ESRD) Also known as *CKD stage 5* or advanced kidney disease with glomerular filtration rate <15 mL/min when most patients with CKD require some form of renal replacement therapy, p. 1340

hemodialysis (HD) A type of dialysis that uses a machine to remove waste products and excess fluid from the blood by pumping the blood through an artificial semipermeable membrane, p. 1350

oliguria A urine output of less than 400 mL in 24 hours, p. 1335

paired organ donation An option that allows a living donor to donate a kidney to a different compatible recipient, with the intent that another donor will donate to the first donor's designated recipient, p. 1360

peritoneal dialysis (PD) A type of dialysis that uses a natural semipermeable membrane, the peritoneum; dialysis fluid is infused into the peritoneal cavity, and excess fluid and waste products pass across the membrane into the fluid, which is then drained and discarded, p. 1350

renal osteodystrophy A disorder of the bones associated with CKD that results in bone demineralization from derangements of calcium, phosphorous, vitamin D, and parathyroid hormone metabolism, p. 1343

renal replacement therapy (RRT) All forms of life-supporting therapies for renal failure including hemodialysis, peritoneal dialysis, hemofiltration, and renal transplantation, p. 1333

uremia A constellation of signs and symptoms resulting from the buildup of waste products and excess fluid associated with kidney failure; these may include, but are not limited to, elevated serum creatinine and blood urea nitrogen, abnormal electrolytes, acidosis, anemia, fluid volume excess, nausea, loss of appetite, fatigue, decreased cognition, pruritus, and neuropathy, p. 1340

ELECTRONIC RESOURCES

Supplemental content related to Chapter 49 can be found...

Evolve Web Site ⊝volve

http://evolve.elsevier.com/Canada/Lewis/medsurg
- Answer Guidelines for Case Study on p. 1364
- Clinical Reference: Laboratory Values
- Content Updates
- Customizable Nursing Care Plan: Chronic Kidney Disease
- Electronic Calculators

- eTables:
  - eTable 49-1: Manifestations of Acute Kidney Injury
  - eTable 49-2: Intrarenal Cause of Acute Kidney Injury Following Surgery
- Examination Review Questions
- Glossary
- Interactive Case Studies:
  - Glomerulonephritis and Chronic Kidney Disease
  - Kidney Transplant
- Key Points (Printable and MP3 Download)

---

*K*idney disease may result in the partial or complete impairment of kidney function. It results in an inability to excrete metabolic waste products and water as well as functional disturbances of all body systems. This impairment may be acute or chronic in nature (Table 49-1). Acute kidney injury (AKI) has a rapid onset. Chronic kidney disease (CKD) usually develops slowly over months to years. If CKD progresses to stage 5 (worst functioning), **renal replacement therapy (RRT)** (dialysis or transplantation) is necessary for long-term survival. Early CKD care focuses on prevention and delaying progression of disease and educating patients about the treatment options for RRTs so an informed decision can be made when the time comes. As with other chronic illnesses in Canada, CKD is much more common in the older population. Over half of the people starting dialysis in 2009 were ages 65 years or older (Canadian Institute for Health Information [CIHI], 2011a). At the end of 2009, 37,744 Canadians had stage 5 CKD, with 22,310 people receiving some form of dialysis and 15,434 people living with a functioning kidney transplant (CIHI, 2011a).

Acute Kidney Injury

Acute kidney injury (AKI), previously known as **acute renal failure (ARF)**, is a more inclusive term encompassing a broader subset of patients with varying degrees of kidney injury (Dirkes, 2011; Murphy & Byrne, 2010). AKI is characterized by an abrupt decline in kidney function leading to a rise in serum creatinine or a reduction in urine output, or both (Murphy & Byrne, 2010; Yaklin, 2011). The severity of dysfunction may be mild, calling for little intervention, to severe, necessitating renal replacement therapy.

Although AKI is potentially reversible, despite advances in its treatment, the mortality rate is high (Cheung, Ponnusamy, & Anderton, 2008; Dirkes, 2011; Murphy & Byrne, 2010; Yaklin, 2011). AKI usually affects people with other life-threatening conditions. Most commonly, AKI follows severe, prolonged hypotension or hypovolemia or exposure to a nephrotoxic agent.

The ARF associated with AKI usually develops over hours or days with progressive elevations of blood urea nitrogen (BUN), creatinine, and potassium with or without oliguria. Severe AKI develops in over 60% of critical care unit (CCU) patients, with mortality rates of 70 to 80%.

One of the most commonly used classification systems uses serum creatinine, glomerular filtration rate (GFR), and urine output to identify *risk, injury, failure, loss,* and *end-*stage kidney disease (the RIFLE Criteria) (Figure 49-1) (Yaklin, 2011). The criteria for evaluating AKI have been found to correlate with outcome and are a good predictor of mortality in hospitalized patients (Dirkes, 2011; Murphy & Byrne, 2010; Yaklin, 2011).

Etiology and Pathophysiology

AKI is a complex disorder with many etiological factors and varied clinical manifestations that range from minimal elevation in serum creatinine to anuric renal failure (Murphy & Byrne,

Table 49-1 Comparison of Acute Kidney Injury and Chronic Kidney Disease

	ACUTE KIDNEY INJURY	CHRONIC KIDNEY DISEASE
Onset	Sudden	Gradual, often over many years
Most common cause	Acute tubular necrosis	Diabetic nephropathy
Diagnostic criteria	Acute reduction in urine output and/or elevation in serum creatinine	GFR <60 mL/min/1.73m² for >3 mo and/or kidney damage >3 mo
Reversibility	Potentially	Progressive and irreversible
Mortality	High (~60%)	19-24% (patients on dialysis)
Primary cause of death	Infection	Cardiovascular disease

GFR, glomerular filtration rate.
Source: Kellum, J., Bellomo, R., & Ronco, C. (2008). Definition and classification of acute kidney injury. *Nephron Clinical Practice, 109*(4), 182-187. doi:10.1159/000142926; and U.S. Renal Data System. (2008). USRDS 2008 annual data report: Atlas of end-stage renal disease. Bethesda, MD: National Institute of Diabetes and Digestive and Kidney Diseases.

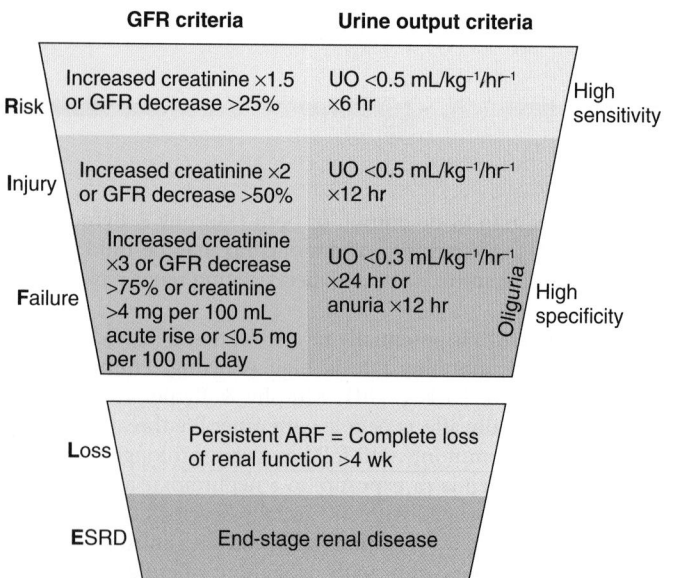

Figure 49-1 RIFLE (risk, injury, failure, loss, end-stage kidney disease) Criteria. *ARF,* acute renal failure; *ESRD,* end-stage renal disease; *GFR,* glomerular filtration rate; *UO,* urine output.

Source: Ricci, Z., Cruz, D., & Ronco, C. (2008). The RIFLE criteria and mortality in acute kidney injury: A systematic review. *Kidney International, 73*(5), 538-546. doi:10.1038/sj.ki.5002743

Table 49-2 Common Causes of Acute Kidney Injury

Prerenal

- Hypovolemia
- Dehydration
- Hemorrhage
- GI losses (diarrhea, vomiting)
- Excessive diuresis
- Hypoalbuminemia
- Burns
- Decreased cardiac output
- Cardiac dysrhythmias
- Cardiogenic shock
- Heart failure
- Myocardial infarction
- Pericardial tamponade
- Pulmonary edema
- Valvular heart disease
- Decreased peripheral vascular resistance
- Anaphylaxis
- Antihypertensive drugs
- Neurological injury
- Septic shock
- Decreased renovascular blood flow
- Bilateral renal vein thrombosis
- Embolism
- Hepatorenal syndrome
- Renal artery thrombosis

Intrarenal

- Prolonged prerenal ischemia
- Nephrotoxic injury
- Drugs (aminoglycosides [gentamicin, amikacin], amphotericin B)
- Radiocontrast agents
- Hemolytic blood transfusion reaction
- Severe crush injury
- Chemical exposure (ethylene glycol, lead, arsenic, carbon tetrachloride)
- Acute glomerulonephritis
- Thrombotic disorders
- Toxemia of pregnancy
- Malignant hypertension
- Systemic lupus erythematosus
- Interstitial nephritis
- Allergies (antibiotics [sulphonamides, rifampin], nonsteroidal anti-inflammatory drugs, ACE inhibitors)
- Infections (bacterial [acute pyelonephritis], viral [CMV], fungal [candidiasis])

Postrenal

- Benign prostatic hyperplasia
- Cancer (bladder, prostate, cervical, colorectal)
- Calculi formation
- Neuromuscular disorders
- Spinal cord disease
- Strictures
- Trauma (back, pelvis, perineum)

ACE, angiotensin-converting enzyme; CMV, cytomegalovirus; GI, gastrointestinal.

Although renal tubular and glomerular function is preserved, glomerular filtration is reduced as a result of decreased perfusion. Hypovolemia, decreased cardiac output, decreased peripheral vascular resistance, and vascular obstruction can all decrease the effective circulating volume of the blood. With a decrease in circulating blood volume, autoregulatory mechanisms that increase angiotensin II, aldosterone, norepinephrine, and antidiuretic hormone attempt to preserve blood flow to essential organs. Prerenal azotemia results in a reduction in the excretion of sodium (<20 mmol/L), increased salt and water retention, and decreased urine output.

Prerenal AKI can also be caused by vasoactive medications such as angiotensin-converting enzymes (ACE) inhibitors, angiotensin receptor blockers (ARBs), epinephrine, and large doses of dopamine that cause intrarenal vasoconstriction leading to hypo-

2010; Yaklin, 2011). The causes leading to AKI with renal failure are divided into prerenal, intrarenal (or intrinsic), and postrenal categories (Table 49-2).

Prerenal causes of AKI are those that reduce renal blood flow and lead to decreased glomerular perfusion and filtration.

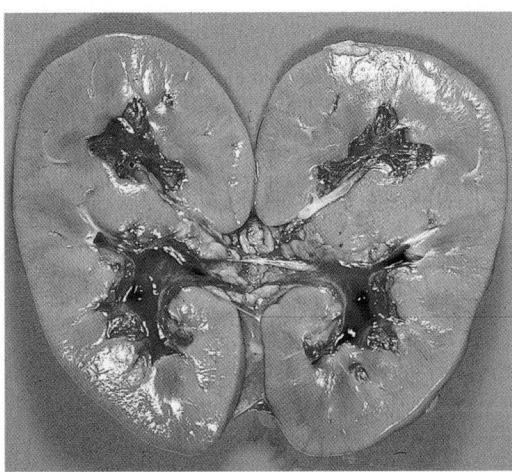

Figure 49-2 Acute tubular necrosis. In acute tubular necrosis, the kidneys are swollen and pale.

Source: Stevens, A., & Lowe, J. (2000). *Pathology: Illustrated review in color* (2nd ed.). London: Mosby.

perfusion of the glomeruli (Yaklin, 2011). AKI associated with prerenal causes is usually reversible. If the course of prerenal failure is prolonged, intrarenal damage may ensue, usually resulting in acute tubular necrosis.

Intrarenal causes include conditions that cause direct damage to the renal tissue (parenchyma), resulting in impaired nephron function. Intrarenal causes of AKI are usually owing to prolonged ischemia or the presence of nephrotoxins, hemoglobin released from hemolyzed red blood cells (RBCs), or myoglobin released from necrotic muscle cells. Nephrotoxins can cause obstruction of intrarenal structures by crystallization or by actually damaging the epithelial cells of the tubules. Hemoglobin and myoglobin block the tubules and cause renal vasoconstriction. Primary renal diseases such as acute glomerulonephritis and systemic lupus erythematosus may also cause AKI.

Acute tubular necrosis (ATN) is the most common intrarenal cause of AKI and is primarily the result of ischemia, nephrotoxins, or sepsis (Figure 49-2). Severe renal ischemia causes a disruption in the basement membrane and patchy destruction of the tubular epithelium. Nephrotoxic agents cause necrosis of tubular epithelial cells, which slough off and plug the tubules. ATN is potentially reversible if the basement membrane is not destroyed and the tubular epithelium regenerates.

Possible pathological processes involved in ATN include the following:

1. Hypovolemia and decreased renal blood flow stimulate renin release, which activates the renin–angiotensin–aldosterone system (see Chapter 47, Figure 47-4) and results in constriction of the peripheral arteries and the renal afferent arterioles. With decreased renal blood flow, there is decreased glomerular capillary pressure and GFR as well as tubular dysfunction and, ultimately, oliguria.
2. Ischemia alters glomerular epithelial cells and decreases glomerular capillary permeability. This reduces the GFR, which significantly reduces blood flow and leads to tubular dysfunction.
3. When tubules are damaged, interstitial edema occurs, and necrotic epithelial cells accumulate in the tubules. The debris lowers the GFR by obstructing the tubules and increasing intratubular pressure.

4. Glomerular filtrate leaks back into plasma through holes in the damaged tubular membranes, which decreases intratubular fluid flow.

Postrenal causes of AKI involve mechanical obstruction of urinary outflow. As the flow of urine is obstructed, urine refluxes into the renal pelvis, impairing kidney function. The most common causes are benign prostatic hyperplasia, prostate cancer, calculi, trauma, and extrarenal tumours. Postrenal causes of AKI account for less than 5% of the cases (Price-Rabetoy, 2006). Postrenal AKI is almost always treatable if identified before permanent kidney damage occurs.

Clinical Manifestations

Prerenal and postrenal AKI that has not caused intrarenal damage usually resolves quickly with correction of the cause. However, if parenchymal damage has occurred from either prerenal or postrenal causes, or intrarenal causes, ATN results and the course of AKI is prolonged. Clinically, ATN progresses through three phases: initiation, maintenance, and recovery (Murphy & Byrne, 2010; Yaklin, 2011). In some situations, the patient does not recover from AKI and CKD results.

Initiation Phase. This is characterized by an increase in serum creatinine and BUN and a decrease in urine output (Murphy & Byrne, 2010).

Maintenance Phase. This phase may last from days to weeks. During this phase, patients may be anuric, oliguric, or nonoliguric. In this case, a dilute urine (low specific gravity) is being made but uremic toxins are not being removed. The oliguric phase usually lasts 10 to 14 days, but it can last months in some cases. The longer the oliguric phase lasts, the poorer the prognosis for recovery of complete renal function. (Manifestations of AKI are presented in eTable 49-1 available on the Evolve Web site for this chapter.)

The manifestations of the oliguric phase are changes in urinary output, fluid and electrolyte abnormalities, and uremia (for a definition of uremia, see the discussion of the clinical manifestations of CKD later in this chapter). The nurse must be alert for the signs and symptoms of these changes.

Urinary Changes. The most common initial manifestation of ATN is **oliguria**, in which urine output generally decreases to less than 400 mL/24 hr. If ATN is caused by ischemia, oliguria will occur within 24 hours. If ATN is caused by nephrotoxic drugs, the onset may be delayed for as long as a week. The duration of the oliguric phase is generally 10 to 14 days, but it can last months in some cases.

Oliguria associated with ATN is characterized by urine with a normal specific gravity (1.010) and a high sodium concentration (>40 mmol/L), and urine osmolality at about 300 mmol/kg, indicating that the injured tubules cannot respond to autoregulatory mechanisms. The urine sediment may show RBCs and white blood cells (WBCs), casts, and proteinuria. The casts are formed from mucoprotein impressions of the necrotic renal tubular epithelial cells, which detach or slough into the tubules.

Fluid Volume Excess. When urinary output decreases, fluid retention occurs. The severity of the symptoms depends on the extent of the fluid overload. The neck veins may become distended with a bounding pulse. Edema and hypertension may develop. Fluid overload can eventually lead to congestive heart failure (CHF), pulmonary edema, and pericardial and pleural effusions.

Metabolic Acidosis. In renal failure, the kidneys cannot synthesize ammonia, which is needed for hydrogen ion excretion, or to excrete acid products of metabolism. The serum bicarbonate level decreases because bicarbonate is used up in buffering hydrogen ions. In addition, defective reabsorption and regeneration of bicarbonate occurs. The patient may develop Kussmaul's respirations (rapid, deep respirations) to increase the excretion of carbon dioxide. Lethargy and stupor will occur if treatment is not started.

Sodium Balance. Damaged tubules cannot conserve sodium. Consequently, the urinary excretion of sodium may increase, resulting in normal or below-normal levels of serum sodium. Excessive intake of sodium should be avoided because it can lead to volume expansion, hypertension, and CHF. Uncontrolled hyponatremia or water excess can lead to cerebral edema.

Potassium Excess. Hyperkalemia is a common life-threatening complication seen in the patient with oliguria. Serum potassium levels increase because the normal ability of the kidneys to regulate and excrete potassium is impaired. Hyperkalemia associated with ARF may be precipitated by a number of causes. Massive tissue trauma may result in the release of additional potassium into the extracellular fluid by the damaged cells. Bleeding and blood transfusions may cause cellular destruction, releasing more potassium into the extracellular fluid. Acidosis worsens hyperkalemia as hydrogen ions enter the cells and potassium is driven out of the cells into the extracellular fluid.

Most of the time patients with hyperkalemia are asymptomatic. Some patients may complain of weakness with severe hyperkalemia. Severe hyperkalemia requires immediate treatment. Before clinical signs of hyperkalemia are apparent, the electrocardiogram (ECG) will show tall, peaked T waves; widening of the QRS complex; and ST depression. Progressive changes in the ECG that are related to increasing potassium levels are depicted in Chapter 19, Figure 19-14. Because cardiac muscle is very intolerant of acute increases in potassium, treatment is essential when hyperkalemia develops.

Hematological Disorders. Several hematological disorders are seen in connection with ARF. Anemia occurs because renal failure results in impaired erythropoietin production. Uremia decreases platelet adhesiveness and can lead to bleeding from multiple sources (e.g., intestines, brain). WBCs are also altered, causing immunodeficiency. This leaves the patient susceptible to numerous systemic and local infections. Infection (sepsis) in combination with AKI is associated with a mortality rate of over 80% (Akcay, Turkman, Lee, & Edelstein, 2010, p. 133).

Calcium Deficit and Phosphate Excess. Activated vitamin D must be present for calcium absorption from the gastrointestinal (GI) tract to occur. Only functioning kidneys can activate vitamin D. Thus, in the presence of kidney failure, GI absorption of calcium decreases and a low serum calcium level results. When hypocalcemia occurs, the parathyroid gland secretes parathyroid hormone (PTH), which stimulates bone demineralization and causes calcium to be released from the bones. Phosphate is released as well, leading to hyperphosphatemia, which is worsened by the decreased excretion of phosphate by the kidneys. Normally, plasma calcium is found ionized or free (physiologi-

cally active form) or bound to protein. In the acidotic state associated with renal failure, more calcium is in the ionized form. Although it is unusual for hypocalcemia to be symptomatic in renal failure, an ionized calcium level that does decrease significantly can lead to tetany.

Waste Product Accumulation. The kidneys are the primary excretory organs for urea, an end product of protein metabolism, and creatinine, an end product of endogenous muscle metabolism. The BUN and creatinine levels are elevated in kidney failure. An elevated BUN level must be interpreted with caution because dehydration, corticosteroids, catabolism resulting from infections, fever, severe injury, and GI bleeding can also elevate BUN. The best serum indicator of renal failure is creatinine because it is not significantly altered by other factors. Measuring creatinine clearance by using radioactive tracer (inulin) is the most accurate method for assessing renal function, but it is expensive and impractical. Clinically, the recommended method to evaluate the kidney function is with an estimated glomerular filtration rate (eGFR) (Kinzner & Hain, 2007).

Neurological Disorders. Neurological changes can occur as nitrogenous waste products accumulate in the brain and other nervous tissue. The symptoms can be as mild as fatigue and difficulty concentrating or can escalate to seizures, stupor, and coma.

Eventually, all body systems become involved in the acute uremic syndrome. The extrarenal manifestations are generally similar to those found in the patient with chronic uremia (see the discussion of CKD later in this chapter).

Recovery Phase. The recovery phase is marked by a return of BUN and creatinine and GFR toward normal ranges (Murphy & Byrne, 2010). During this phase, patients may experience a diuretic phase that can result in fluid and electrolyte abnormalities. The diuretic phase begins with a gradual increase in daily urine output to 1 to 3 L/day, but it may reach 3 to 5 L or more per day. Although urine output is increasing, the nephrons are still not fully functional. The high urine volume is caused by osmotic diuresis from the high urea concentration in the glomerular filtrate and the inability of the tubules to concentrate the urine. In this phase, the kidneys have recovered their ability to excrete wastes but not to concentrate the urine. Hypovolemia and hypotension can occur from massive fluid losses. Because of the large losses of fluid and electrolytes, the patient must be monitored for hyponatremia, hypokalemia, and dehydration. The diuretic phase may last 1 to 3 weeks. Near the end of this phase, the patient's acid–base, electrolyte, and waste product (BUN, creatinine) values begin to normalize. Although the major improvements occur in the first 1 to 2 weeks of this phase, renal function may take up to 12 months to stabilize.

The outcome of AKI is influenced by the patient's overall health, the severity of renal failure, and the number and type of complications. Some individuals do not recover and progress to CKD. The older adult patient is less likely to recover full kidney function than the younger patient. Among the individuals who recover, the majority achieve clinically normal kidney function with no complications (e.g., hypertension).

Diagnostic Studies. Urinalysis is an important diagnostic test. Urine sediment containing abundant cells, casts, or proteins suggests intrarenal disorders. The urine osmolality, sodium content, and specific gravity help to differentiate the types of

AKI. Urine sediment may be normal in both prerenal and postrenal AKI. Hematuria, pyuria, and crystals may be seen with postrenal AKI.

To establish a diagnosis of AKI, other testing may be required. A renal ultrasound is often the first test done and provides information about anatomy and function. Ultrasound does not require the use of nephrotoxic contrast agents. A renal scan can assess renal blood flow and the integrity of the collecting system. A computed tomography (CT) scan can identify lesions and masses as well as well as obstruction; but exposure to radiation is higher and it may involve contrast that can be nephrotoxic. Magnetic resonance imaging (MRI) and magnetic resonance angiography (MRA) are not recommended. Gadolinium, a contrast medium used with MRI and MRA, has been associated with the development of *nephrogenic systemic fibrosis* in patients with compromised renal function.

Collaborative Care

Because AKI is potentially reversible, the primary goals of treatment are to eliminate the cause, manage the signs and symptoms, and prevent complications while the kidneys recover (Table 49-3). The first step is to determine whether there is sufficient intravascular volume and cardiac output to ensure adequate perfusion of the kidneys. Diuretic therapy is often administered along with volume expanders to prevent fluid overload. Diuretic therapy usually includes loop diuretics (e.g., furosemide [Lasix]) or an osmotic diuretic (e.g., mannitol). If AKI is already established, forcing fluids and diuretics will not be effective and may, in fact, be harmful. Medical management without RRT may be all that is necessary until renal function improves. The general trend is to initiate early and frequent RRT to minimize symptoms and prevent complications.

Fluid intake must be closely monitored during the oliguric phase. The general rule for calculating the permitted fluid intake is to add all losses for the previous 24 hours (e.g., urine, diarrhea, emesis, blood) plus 600 mL for insensible losses (e.g., respiration, diaphoresis). For example, if a patient excreted 300 mL of urine on Tuesday with no other losses, the fluid intake on Wednesday would be restricted to 900 mL.

Hyperkalemia is one of the most serious complications in AKI because it can cause life-threatening cardiac dysrhythmias. The various therapies used to treat elevated potassium levels are listed in Table 49-4. Both insulin and salbutamol temporarily shift potassium into the cells, but it will eventually shift back out. Calcium gluconate raises the threshold at which dysrhythmias will occur, serving to temporarily stabilize the myocardium. Only cation exchange resins, such as sodium polystyrene sulphonate (Kayexalate) or calcium resonium, and dialysis actually remove potassium from the body. Sodium polystyrene sulphonate should not be given to patients who do not have normal bowel function or mixed with sorbitol because of associated bowel necrosis (U.S. Food and Drug Administration [FDA], 2011).

The most common indications for RRT in AKI include (1) volume overload resulting in compromised cardiac or pulmonary status, or both; (2) elevated potassium levels; (3) metabolic acidosis (serum bicarbonate level <15 mmol/L); (4)BUN level

COLLABORATIVE CARE

Table 49-3 Acute Kidney Injury

Diagnostic	Collaborative Therapy
• History and physical examination	• Treatment of precipitating cause
• Identification of precipitating cause	• Fluid restriction (allowance = 600 mL + previous 24-hr fluid loss)
• Serum creatinine and BUN levels	• Nutritional therapy
• Serum electrolytes	• Adequate protein intake (0.6-2 g/kg/day) depending on degree of catabolism
• Urinalysis	• Potassium restriction
• Renal ultrasound	• Phosphate restriction
• Renal scan (as indicated)	• Sodium restriction
• CT scan (as indicated and without contrast if possible)	• Measures to lower potassium (if elevated)*
• Retrograde pyelogram (as indicated)	• Calcium supplements or phosphate-binding agents
	• Total parenteral nutrition (if indicated)†
	• Enteral nutrition (if indicated)†
	• Initiation of renal replacement therapy (if necessary)

BUN, blood urea nitrogen; *CT,* computed tomography.
*See Table 49-4.
†Renal formulations of these two forms of nutrition are available.

Table 49-4 Treatment of Hyperkalemia

Stabilize Myocardium

• If the ECG shows hyperkalemia-related abnormalities, *calcium gluconate IV* is given. Calcium raises the threshold potential, thus counteracting the toxic effect of potassium on the myocardium, which can induce life-threatening dysrhythmias.

Shift Potassium Into Cells

• *Regular IV insulin administration* causes potassium to move into cells. Glucose is given concurrently to prevent hypoglycemia. When effects of insulin diminish, potassium shifts back out of cells.
• *Salbutamol* will also temporarily shift potassium back into cells.
• *Sodium bicarbonate* can correct acidosis and causes shift of potassium into cells.

Enhance Potassium Removal

• *Cation exchange resins* such as *sodium polystyrene sulphonate (Kayexalate)* are administered by mouth or retention enema. When resin is in the bowel, potassium is exchanged for sodium. Therapy removes 1 mmol of potassium/g of drug. *Calcium resonium* is another such resin.
• Loop diuretics such as *furosemide* can increase potassium excretion in the urine if the patient has any urine output.
• *Dialysis,* particularly *hemodialysis,* can bring potassium levels to normal within 30 min to 2 hr.

Long-term Treatment

• *Restrict intake of dietary potassium* to 40 mmol/day and avoid potassium-containing salt substitutes.
• Limit or discontinue medications that can precipitate or exacerbate hyperkalemia such as ACE inhibitors, ARBs, and potassium-sparing diuretics.

ACE, angiotensin-converting enzyme; *ARBs,* angiotensin receptor blockers; *ECG,* electrocardiogram; *IV,* intravenous.

greater than 43 mmol/L; (5) significant change in mental status; and (6) pericarditis, pericardial effusion, or cardiac tamponade. Although laboratory values provide rough parameters, the best guide to treatment is good clinical assessment.

If RRT is required, many options are available, but there is no consensus regarding the best approach. Even though peritoneal dialysis (PD) is considered a viable option for RRT, it is rarely used. Intermittent hemodialysis (HD) (e.g., at intervals of 4 hr either daily or every other day, or three to four times per week) and continuous renal replacement therapy (CRRT) have both been used effectively. CRRT is provided continuously over approximately 24 hours and has much slower blood flow rates than intermittent HD.

HD is the method of choice when rapid changes are required in a short time. It is technically more complicated because specialized staff and equipment are required. It also requires anticoagulation to prevent the patient's blood from clotting when it contacts the foreign material in the dialysis circuit. Rapid fluid shifts during HD may cause hypotension.

RRT, PD, HD, and CRRT are discussed later in this chapter.

Nutritional Therapy. The challenge of nutritional management in AKI is to provide adequate calories to prevent catabolism despite the restrictions required to prevent electrolyte and fluid disorders and azotemia. Adequate energy should be provided from carbohydrate and fat sources to prevent ketosis from endogenous fat breakdown and gluconeogenesis from muscle-protein breakdown. The daily caloric intake for patients with AKI should be about 25 to 35 kcal/kg based on estimated metabolic stress and protein energy requirements (Gervasio, Garmon & Holowatyj, 2011). Protein dosage varies from 1.5 to 2.5 g/kg/day depending on the stage of AKI and whether or not RRT is required (Gervasio, Garmon & Holowatyj, 2011; Maursetter, Kight, Mennig, & Hofmann, 2011).

Potassium and sodium are regulated in accordance with plasma levels. Sodium is restricted as needed to prevent edema, hypertension, and CHF. Hyperphosphatemia, hypocalcemia, and hypermagnesemia are common and must be monitored and regulated (Gervasio et al., 2011). Dietary fat intake is increased so that the patient receives at least 30 to 40% of total calories from fat. Fat-emulsion intravenous (IV) infusions can also be given as a nutritional supplement and provide a good source of nonprotein calories (see Chapter 42). If a patient cannot maintain adequate oral intake, enteral nutrition is the preferred route for nutritional support (see Chapter 42). When the GI tract is not functional, total parenteral nutrition (TPN) is necessary for the provision of adequate nutrition. The patient treated with TPN may need daily HD or CRRT to remove the excess fluid. Concentrated TPN formulas are available to minimize fluid volume (Kinzner & Hain, 2007).

NURSING MANAGEMENT: ACUTE KIDNEY INJURY

▪ Nursing Assessment

An assessment of the patient with AKI includes the specific areas presented in eTable 49-1 (see the Evolve Web site for this chapter). It is important to monitor the vital signs and intake and output.

The urine should be examined for colour, specific gravity, glucose, protein, blood, and sediment. The patient's general appearance should be assessed, including skin colour, peripheral edema, neck vein distension, and bruises.

If the patient is receiving RRT, the access site should be observed for signs of inflammation. Evaluate the patient's mental status and level of consciousness. Examine the oral mucosa for dryness and inflammation. Auscultate the lung fields for crackles and wheezes or diminished breath sounds. Monitor the heart for the presence of a third heart sound (S3 or gallop), murmurs, or a pericardial friction rub. Assess ECG readings for the presence of dysrhythmias. Review laboratory values and diagnostic test results. All of the previous data are essential for developing a collaborative plan of care.

▪ Nursing Diagnoses

Nursing diagnoses and potential complications for the patient with AKI include, but are not limited to, the following:

- Excess fluid volume *related to* renal failure and fluid retention
- Risk for infection *related to* invasive lines, uremic toxins, and altered immune responses secondary to kidney failure
- Imbalanced nutrition: less than body requirements *related to* altered metabolic state and dietary restrictions
- Disturbed thought processes *related to* effects of uremic toxins on central nervous system (CNS)
- Fatigue *related to* anemia, metabolic acidosis, and uremic toxins
- Anxiety *related to* disease process, therapeutic interventions, and uncertainty of prognosis
- Potential complication: dysrhythmias *related to* electrolyte imbalances
- Potential complication: metabolic acidosis *related to* inability to excrete H^+, impaired HCO_3^- reabsorption, and decreased synthesis of ammonia

▪ Planning

The overall goals are that the patient with AKI will (1) completely recover without any loss of kidney function, (2) maintain normal fluid and electrolyte balance, (3) have decreased anxiety, and (4) understand and adhere to the treatment plan and follow-up care.

▪ Nursing Implementation

▪ Health Promotion

Prevention of AKI is essential because of the high mortality rate associated with it and is primarily directed toward identifying and monitoring high-risk populations, controlling nephrotoxic drugs and industrial chemicals, and preventing prolonged episodes of hypotension and hypovolemia. In the hospital, the factors that increase the risk for developing AKI are advanced age, massive trauma, major surgical procedures, extensive burns, cardiac failure, sepsis, obstetrical complications, and baseline renal insufficiency caused by hypertension or diabetes mellitus. Careful monitoring of intake and output and of fluid and electrolyte balance is essential. Assess and record extrarenal losses of fluid from vomiting, diarrhea, hemorrhage, and increased insensible losses. Prompt replacement of significant fluid losses will help prevent ischemic tubular damage associated with trauma, burns, and extensive surgery. Intake and output records and the patient's weight provide valuable indicators of fluid volume status. Aggressive diuretic therapy for the patient with fluid overload resulting from any cause can lead to decreased renal blood flow.

For patients with any level of renal insufficiency, and particularly the older adult or diabetic patient with renal insufficiency who is undergoing diagnostic studies requiring IV contrast media, special attention must be given to prevent a nephrotoxic injury secondary to the dye. Adequate hydration before and after the test is critical. The use of acetylcysteine (Mucomyst) may be helpful in providing added protection to the kidneys (Venkataraman, 2008). Patients with urinary tract infections need prompt treatment and careful follow-up care. Chemotherapeutic drugs that cause hyperuricemia also can put a patient at risk for renal injury.

The individual who is taking drugs that are potentially nephrotoxic (see Chapter 47, Table 47-3) must have renal function monitored. Nephrotoxic drugs should be used sparingly in high-risk patients. When these drugs must be used, they should be given in the smallest effective doses for the shortest possible periods. The patient should be cautioned about the abuse of over-the-counter analgesics (especially nonsteroidal anti-inflammatory drugs [NSAIDs]) because some of these may worsen renal function in the patient with borderline renal insufficiency by decreasing glomerular pressure or causing interstitial nephritis. ACE inhibitors can also decrease perfusion pressure and cause hyperkalemia, and their use may be contraindicated in renal insufficiency. Industrial and agricultural chemicals and products (e.g., organic solvents, insecticides, cleaning agents) must be monitored regularly to assess their safety for employees and the general population.

Acute Intervention

The patient with AKI is most often critically ill and often has a high burden of co-morbid illness (e.g., diabetes, cardiovascular disease) that also affects renal function. The nurse needs to focus on the patient holistically because there are many physical and emotional needs. Usually, the changes caused by AKI arise suddenly. Both the patient and the family need assistance in understanding that the functioning of the whole body can be disrupted by renal failure.

The nurse has an important role in managing fluid and electrolyte balance during the oliguric and diuretic phases. Observing and recording accurate intake and output are essential. Measure weights daily with the same scale at the same time each day to allow for the evaluation and detection of excessive gains or losses of body fluid (1 kg is equivalent to 1000 mL of fluid). The nurse needs to be knowledgeable about the common signs and symptoms of hypervolemia (in the oliguric phase) or hypovolemia (in the diuretic phase), potassium and sodium disturbances, and other electrolyte imbalances that may occur in AKI (see Chapter 19).

Because infection is the leading cause of death in AKI, meticulous aseptic technique is critical. Protect the patient from other individuals with infectious diseases. Be alert for local manifestations of infection (e.g., swelling, redness, pain) as well as systemic manifestations (e.g., malaise, leukocytosis), but realize that an elevated temperature may not be present. Patients with renal failure have a blunted febrile response to an infection (e.g., pneumonia). If antibiotics are used to treat an infection, the type, frequency, and dosage must be carefully considered because the kidneys are the primary route of excretion for many antibiotics.

Dosages and dosing intervals need to be considered in relation to the patient's level of kidney function if the drug is primarily eliminated by the kidneys. Nephrotoxic drugs (see Chapter 47, Table 47-3) should be avoided.

Skin care and measures to prevent pressure ulcers should be performed because the patient usually develops edema as well as decreased muscle tone. Mouth care is important to prevent stomatitis, which develops when ammonia (produced by bacterial breakdown of urea) in saliva irritates the mucous membranes.

Ambulatory and Home Care

Recovery from AKI is highly variable and depends on the underlying illness, the general condition and the age of the patient, the length of the oliguric phase, and the severity of nephron damage. Good nutrition, rest, and activity are necessary. Dietary restrictions should be regulated in accordance with kidney function. Follow-up care and regular evaluation of renal function are necessary. Teach the patient the signs and symptoms of recurrent kidney disease. Emphasize measures to prevent the recurrence of AKI.

The long-term convalescence of 3 to 12 months may cause psychosocial and financial hardships for the family. Make referrals for counselling as appropriate. If the kidneys do not recover, the patient will need to transition to life on chronic dialysis or possible future transplantation.

Evaluation

The following are expected outcomes for the patient with AKI:
- Regain and maintain normal fluid and electrolyte balance.
- Comply with treatment regimen.
- Experience no infectious complications.
- Have complete recovery.

AGE-RELATED CONSIDERATIONS: ACUTE KIDNEY INJURY

The older adult is more susceptible than the younger adult to AKI because the number of functioning nephrons decreases with age. Impaired function of other organ systems (e.g., cardiovascular disease, impaired pancreas function) can increase the risk of developing AKI. The aging kidney is less able to compensate for changes in fluid volume, solute load, and cardiac output. Common causes of AKI in the older adult include dehydration, hypotension, diuretic therapy, aminoglycoside therapy, obstructive disorders (e.g., prostatic hyperplasia), surgery, infection, and radiocontrast agents.

Chronic Kidney Disease

Chronic kidney disease (CKD), involves the progressive, irreversible loss of kidney function. The Kidney Disease Outcomes Quality Initiative (KDOQI) defines CKD as either kidney damage or GFR <60 mL/min/1.73 m² for 3 months or longer. CKD is classified as one of five stages, depending on the level of severity based on GFR (Table 49-5). CKD involves progressive, irreversible

Table 49-5 Stages* and Descriptions of Chronic Kidney Disease†

	DESCRIPTION	GFR (ml/min/1.73 m²)	ACTION‡
Stage 1	Kidney damage with normal or ↑ GFR	≥90	Diagnosis and treatment of co-morbid conditions CVD risk reduction
Stage 2	Kidney damage with mild ↓ GFR	60-89	Estimation of progression
Stage 3	Moderate ↓ GFR	30-59	Evaluation and treatment of complications
Stage 4	Severe ↓ GFR	15-29	Preparation for renal replacement therapy
Stage 5	Kidney failure	<15 (or dialysis)	Renal replacement therapy (if uremia present and patient desires treatment)

CVD, cardiovascular disease; *GFR*, glomerular filtration rate.
*Stages 1 to 5 identify patients who have chronic kidney disease.
†Chronic kidney disease is defined as either kidney damage or GFR <60 mL/min/1.73 m² for 3 mo. Kidney damage is defined as pathological abnormalities or markers of damage, including abnormalities in blood or urine tests or imaging studies.
‡Includes actions from preceding stages.
Source: National Kidney Foundation. 2002 Kidney Disease Outcomes Quality Initiative clinical practice guidelines for chronic kidney disease: Evaluation, classification, and stratification (Table 3). Retrieved from *http://www.kidney.org/Professionals/Kdoqi/guidelines_ckd/toc.htm*

destruction of the nephrons in both kidneys. Not all people with CKD will progress to stage 5, in which RRT would be necessary; however, all those affected will require ongoing monitoring.

Identifying the stage of CKD allows for early intervention to reduce cardiovascular risk, delay progression, and prevent the need for RRT (Dinwiddie, Burrows-Hudson, & Peacock, 2006). RRTs include PD, HD, and renal transplantation. Stage 5 CKD, often referred to as **end-stage renal disease (ESRD)**, is advanced kidney disease with GFR less than 15 mL/min, when most patients with CKD require some form of RRT. At this point, RRT (dialysis or transplantation) is usually required. In 2009, there were 5375 new dialysis patients in Canada. Of these, over half (54%) were older than 65 years (CIHI, 2011a). Although there are many causes of CKD, the leading causes of CKD in Canada are diabetes mellitus (34%) and renal vascular disease (19%) (CIHI, 2011a).

The kidneys have remarkable functional reserve. Up to 80% of the GFR (reflected in creatinine clearance measurements) may be lost with few overt changes in the functioning of the body. A person is born with about 2 million nephrons and can survive without RRT until almost 90% of the nephrons are lost. In the majority of cases, the individual passes through the early stages of CKD without recognizing the disease state because the remaining nephrons hypertrophy to compensate. The prognosis and the course of CKD are highly variable depending on the etiology, the individual's condition and age, and the adequacy of medical follow-up. Some individuals live normal, active lives with

compensated renal failure, whereas others may rapidly progress to ESRD.

Since 1973, many deaths have been prevented through the use of RRTs. Dialysis modalities remain the most common RRT for people with stage 5 CKD because of (1) a lack of donated organs, (2) medical conditions that preclude transplantation, or (3) personal reasons in which an individual may decline transplantation as a treatment option. With the advances made in medical science, an increasing number of individuals are receiving RRTs, including older adults and those with complex medical problems. All people with advanced CKD, regardless of age, should be offered RRT unless it is medically contraindicated.

Clinical Manifestations

As renal function progressively deteriorates, excretory, regulatory, and endocrine function are lost, and these effects are manifested in every body system, no matter what the underlying cause of CKD. These excretory, regulatory, and endocrine functional impairments are manifested in retained substances, including urea, creatinine, phenols, hormones, electrolytes, water, and many other substances. **Uremia** is a constellation of signs and symptoms resulting from the buildup of waste products and excess fluid associated with kidney failure. These may include, but are not limited to, elevated serum creatinine and BUN, abnormal electrolytes, acidosis, anemia, fluid volume excess, nausea, loss of appetite, fatigue, decreased cognition, pruritus, and neuropathy (Figure 49-3). It is important to recognize that the manifestations of uremia vary among patients, according to the cause of the kidney disease, co-morbid conditions, age, and degree of adherence to the prescribed medical regimen. Many patients are very tolerant of the changes that occur because they develop gradually. Uremia often occurs when the GFR is 10 mL/min/1.73m² or lower.

Urinary System. In the early stage of CKD, polyuria results from the inability of the kidneys to concentrate urine. This happens most often at night, and the patient must arise several times to urinate (nocturia). Because of the decrease in renal

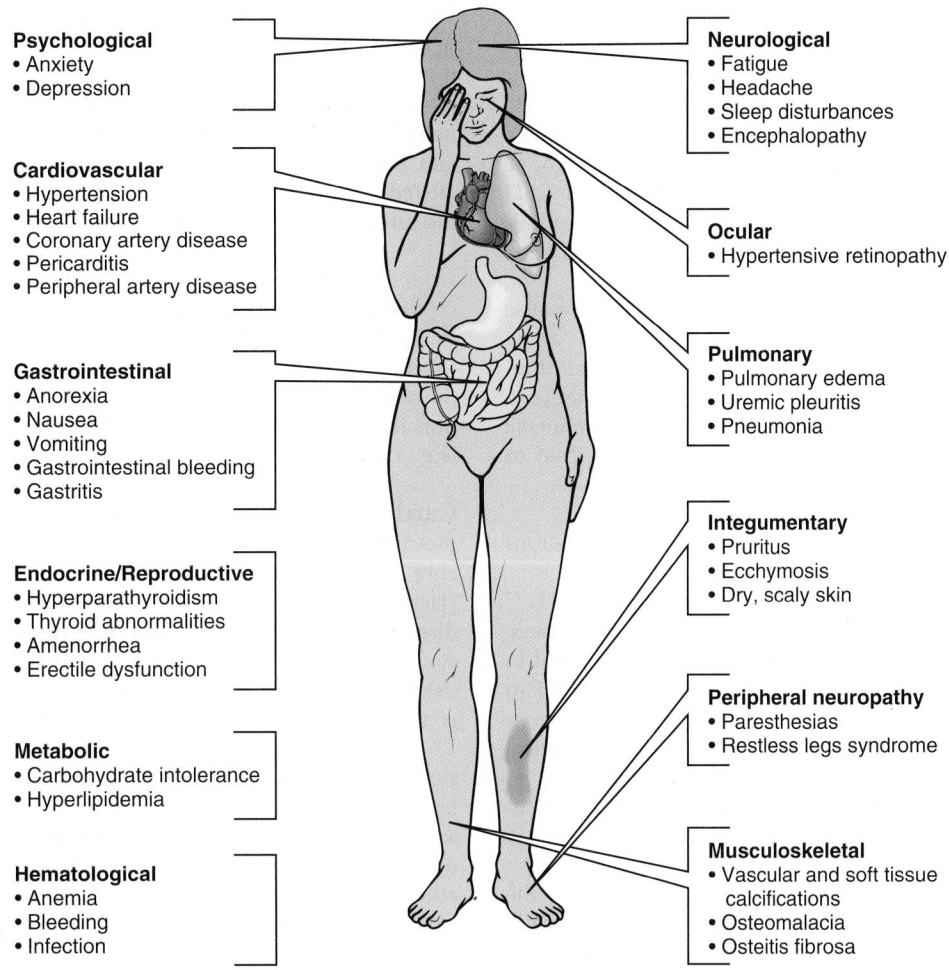

Psychological
• Anxiety
• Depression

Cardiovascular
• Hypertension
• Heart failure
• Coronary artery disease
• Pericarditis
• Peripheral artery disease

Gastrointestinal
• Anorexia
• Nausea
• Vomiting
• Gastrointestinal bleeding
• Gastritis

Endocrine/Reproductive
• Hyperparathyroidism
• Thyroid abnormalities
• Amenorrhea
• Erectile dysfunction

Metabolic
• Carbohydrate intolerance
• Hyperlipidemia

Hematological
• Anemia
• Bleeding
• Infection

Neurological
• Fatigue
• Headache
• Sleep disturbances
• Encephalopathy

Ocular
• Hypertensive retinopathy

Pulmonary
• Pulmonary edema
• Uremic pleuritis
• Pneumonia

Integumentary
• Pruritus
• Ecchymosis
• Dry, scaly skin

Peripheral neuropathy
• Paresthesias
• Restless legs syndrome

Musculoskeletal
• Vascular and soft tissue calcifications
• Osteomalacia
• Osteitis fibrosa

Figure 49-3 Clinical manifestations of chronic uremia.

concentrating ability, the specific gravity of urine gradually becomes fixed at around 1.010 (the osmolar concentration of plasma). As CKD worsens, oliguria develops, and eventually anuria (urine output 40 mL/24 hr) develops. If the patient is still producing urine, proteinuria, casts, pyuria, and hematuria could be present depending on the cause of the kidney disease.

Metabolic Disturbances

Waste Product Accumulation. As GFR declines, the serum creatinine and BUN levels increase. Accumulation of nitrogenous waste products in advanced stages of CKD often manifest with symptoms of nausea, vomiting, lethargy, fatigue, impaired thought processes, and headaches as a result of the multisystemic involvement of CKD.

Serum creatinine continues to be the most common biochemical parameter to estimate the GFR, but it alone is not an accurate measure of GFR (Kinzner & Hain, 2007). Serum creatinine tends to be an ineffective marker of early as well as advanced kidney disease. eGFR is a better measure of overall kidney function than creatinine or BUN. The eGFR may be calculated by the laboratory using mathematical formulas. If this method is not available, GFR calculators and tables can be used (see link to the MDRD calculator in the Resources at the end of this chapter.). The serum creatinine level in an older adult patient with ESRD will be lower than in a younger person with the same degree of renal dysfunction. Decreased muscle mass and decreased muscle

activity from aging account for this finding because creatinine is an end product of muscle metabolism.

Altered Carbohydrate Metabolism. Defective carbohydrate metabolism is caused by impaired glucose use resulting from cellular insensitivity to the normal action of insulin. The exact nature of this insulin resistance is unclear, but it may be related to circulating insulin antagonists, alterations in hormone receptors, or abnormalities of transport mechanisms. Moderate hyperglycemia, hyperinsulinemia, and abnormal glucose tolerance tests may be seen. Insulin and glucose metabolism may improve (but not to normal values) after the initiation of dialysis.

Patients with diabetes who become uremic may require less insulin than before the onset of CKD. This is because insulin, which is dependent on the kidneys for excretion, remains in circulation longer. The insulin regimen must be individualized and glucose levels monitored carefully.

Elevated Triglycerides. Hyperinsulinemia stimulates hepatic production of triglycerides. Almost all patients with uremia develop dyslipidemia, with elevated very low density lipoproteins, normal or decreased low-density lipoproteins, and lowered high-density lipoproteins. The altered lipid metabolism is related to decreased levels of the enzyme lipoprotein lipase, which is important in the breakdown of lipoproteins.

Electrolyte and Acid–Base Imbalances

Potassium. Hyperkalemia is a serious electrolyte disorder associated with kidney disease. Fatal dysrhythmias can occur when the serum potassium level reaches 7 to 8 mmol/L. Hyperkalemia results from the decreased excretion by the kidneys, the breakdown of cellular protein, bleeding, and metabolic acidosis. The most common causes of hyperkalemia in CKD are associated with diet, dietary supplements, drugs, and IV infusions.

Sodium. Sodium may be normal or low in renal failure. Because of impaired sodium excretion, sodium is retained along with water. If large quantities of body water are retained, dilutional hyponatremia occurs. Sodium retention can contribute to edema, hypertension, and congestive heart failure. Sodium intake must be individually determined but is generally restricted to 2 g/24 hr.

Calcium and Phosphate. Calcium and phosphate alterations are in the section on the musculoskeletal system (p. 1343).

Magnesium. Magnesium is excreted primarily by the kidneys. Magnesium is sometimes used as a phosphate-binding agent in patients with CKD. Hypermagnesemia is generally not a problem unless the patient is ingesting magnesium (e.g., milk of magnesia, magnesium citrate, antacids containing magnesium). Clinical manifestations of hypermagnesemia can include absence of reflexes, decreased mental status, cardiac dysrhythmias, hypotension, and respiratory failure.

Metabolic Acidosis. Metabolic acidosis results from the impaired ability of the kidneys to excrete the acid load (primarily ammonia) and from defective reabsorption and regeneration of bicarbonate. The average adult produces 80 to 90 mmol/day of acid. In renal failure, plasma bicarbonate, which is an indirect measure of acidosis, usually falls to a new steady state at around 16 to 20 mmol/L. It generally does not progress below this level because hydrogen ion production is usually balanced by buffering from demineralization of the bone (the phosphate buffering system). Although Kussmaul's respiration is uncommon in CKD, this breathing pattern reduces the severity of acidosis by increasing carbon dioxide excretion.

Hematological System

Anemia. Anemia is very common in CKD. A normocytic, normochromic anemia is associated with CKD and is a result of decreased production of the hormone erythropoietin by the kidneys, resulting in decreased erythropoiesis by the bone marrow (Nguyen & Wells, 2011). Erythropoietin stimulates precursor cells in the bone marrow to produce RBCs. Other factors contributing to anemia are nutritional deficiencies, decreased RBC lifespan, increased hemolysis of RBCs, frequent blood samplings, and bleeding from the GI tract. For patients receiving maintenance HD, blood loss in the dialyzer may also contribute to the anemic state. Elevated levels of PTH (produced to compensate for low serum calcium levels) can inhibit erythropoiesis, shorten survival of RBCs, and cause bone marrow fibrosis, which can result in decreased numbers of hematopoietic cells.

Sufficient iron stores are needed for erythropoiesis. Many patients with renal failure are iron deficient and require iron replacement. Folic acid, which is water soluble and essential for RBC maturation, is removed with dialysis and needs to be replaced in the diet with supplementation (1 mg/day).

Bleeding Tendencies. The most common cause of bleeding in uremia is a qualitative defect in platelet function. This dysfunction is caused by impaired platelet aggregation and impaired release of platelet Factor III. In addition, alterations in the coagulation system with increased concentrations of both Factor VIII and fibrinogen are found in the serum of these patients. The altered platelet function, hemorrhagic tendencies, and GI bleeding can usually be corrected with regular HD or PD.

Infection. Patients with advanced CKD have an increased susceptibility to infection. Infectious complications are caused by changes in leukocyte function and altered immune response and function. Both cellular and humoral immune responses are suppressed. Other factors contributing to the increased risk of infection include malnutrition, hyperglycemia, and external trauma (e.g., catheters, needle insertions into vascular access sites).

Cardiovascular System. Morbidity and mortality from cardiovascular disease are high in patients with CKD, and the presence of CKD worsens the outcomes of cardiovascular disease (Herzog et al., 2011). Many patients will die from cardiovascular disease before CKD stage 5 requiring dialysis develops (Herzog et al., 2011; Levin et al., 2008). Management of cardiovascular risk factors in patients with CKD should be a focus of care (Levin et al., 2008).

The most common cardiovascular abnormality is hypertension, which usually exists before ESRD sets in and is worsened by sodium retention and increased extracellular fluid volume. In some individuals, increased renin production contributes to the problem (see Chapter 47, Figure 47-6). Hypertension accelerates atherosclerotic vascular disease, produces intrarenal arterial spasm, and eventually leads to left ventricular hypertrophy and congestive heart failure (Herzog et al., 2011, p. 574). Hypertension also causes retinopathy, encephalopathy, and nephropathy.

The vascular changes from longstanding hypertension and the accelerated atherosclerosis from elevated triglyceride levels are responsible for many cardiovascular complications (e.g., myocardial infarction, stroke). Diabetes mellitus is a major risk factor for the development of vascular problems.

CHF from left ventricular hypertrophy can lead to pulmonary edema. Peripheral edema is often present. Cardiac dysrhythmias may result from hyperkalemia, hypocalcemia, and decreased coronary artery perfusion.

Uremic pericarditis can develop and occasionally progresses to pericardial effusion and cardiac tamponade. Pericarditis is manifested by a friction rub, chest pain, and low-grade fever.

Respiratory System. Respiratory changes include dyspnea from fluid overload, pulmonary edema, uremic pleuritis (pleurisy), pleural effusion, a predisposition to respiratory infections, and in very advanced CKD, Kussmaul's respirations. "Uremic lung," or uremic pneumonitis, is typically found in CKD and shows up as interstitial edema on chest radiograph. This condition usually responds to vigorous fluid removal during dialysis treatments.

Gastrointestinal System. Every part of the GI system is affected as a result of inflammation of the mucosa caused by excessive urea. Stomatitis with exudates and ulcerations, a metallic taste in the mouth, and *uremic fetor* (a urinous odour of the breath) are commonly found. As CKD progresses, anorexia, nausea, and vomiting caused by irritation of the GI tract by waste products may be present. Patients are also at risk for weight loss and malnutrition. Diabetic gastroparesis (delayed gastric emptying) can compound these problems for patients with diabetes. GI bleeding is also a risk because of irritation of the mucosa by waste products coupled with the platelet defect. Constipation may be caused by the ingestion of iron salts or calcium-containing phosphate binders, or both. Constipation can be made worse by the limited fluid intake and inactivity.

Neurological System.
Neurological changes are expected as renal failure progresses. They are attributed to increased nitrogenous waste products, electrolyte imbalances, metabolic acidosis, and axonal atrophy and demyelination of nerve fibres (Burrows & Muller, 2007). High levels of uremic toxins have been implicated in axonal damage.

The CNS becomes depressed, resulting in lethargy, apathy, decreased ability to concentrate, fatigue, irritability, and altered mental ability. Although uncommon, seizures and coma may result from a rapidly increasing BUN and hypertensive encephalopathy.

Peripheral neuropathy is initially manifested by a slowing of nerve conduction to the extremities. The patient complains of restless legs syndrome and may describe it as "bugs crawling inside the leg." Paresthesias occur most often in the feet and legs and may be described by the patient as a burning sensation. Eventually, motor involvement may lead to bilateral foot drop, muscular weakness and atrophy, and loss of deep tendon reflexes. Muscle twitching, jerking, asterixis (hand-flapping tremor), and nocturnal leg cramps also occur. In patients with diabetes, uremic neuropathy is compounded by the neuropathy associated with diabetes mellitus.

The treatment for neurological problems is dialysis or transplantation. Dialysis should improve the general CNS symptoms and may slow or halt the progression of neuropathies. However, motor neuropathy may not be reversible.

Musculoskeletal System.
CKD–mineral and bone disorder (CKD–MBD) is a term used to describe the systemic components of this clinical syndrome that include characteristic bone abnormalities, changes in mineral balance (calcium, phosphorus, PTH, and vitamin D), and vascular and other soft tissue calcification (Smith & Smelt, 2009, p. 49). These manifestations develop owing to progressive deterioration in kidney function (Figure 49-4). As kidney function declines, phosphorus elimination decreases and less vitamin D is converted to its active form, resulting in decreased serum levels (Smith & Smelt, 2009; Soroka, Thomas, & Girvan, 2010). To absorb calcium from the GI tract, activated vitamin D is necessary. Thus, decreased active vitamin D levels result in less calcium absorption from the intestine and, therefore, decreased serum calcium levels (Hudson, 2006). When hypocalcemia occurs, the parathyroid gland secretes PTH, which stimulates bone demineralization with the release of calcium from the bones. Phosphate is released as well, leading to elevated serum phosphate levels. Hyperphosphatemia has been shown to directly decrease serum calcium levels and further reduce the ability of the kidneys to activate vitamin D (Smith & Smelt, 2009).

Hyperphosphatemia, decreased vitamin D level, and hypocalcemia lead to overstimulation of the parathyroid glands, resulting in excess secretion of PTH (Soroka et al., 2010). PTH that remains elevated for long periods of time leads to hypertrophy of the parathyroid gland and bone disease (Smith & Smelt, 2009).

CKD–MBD is a common complication of CKD and results in both skeletal (renal osteodystrophy) and extraskeletal complica-

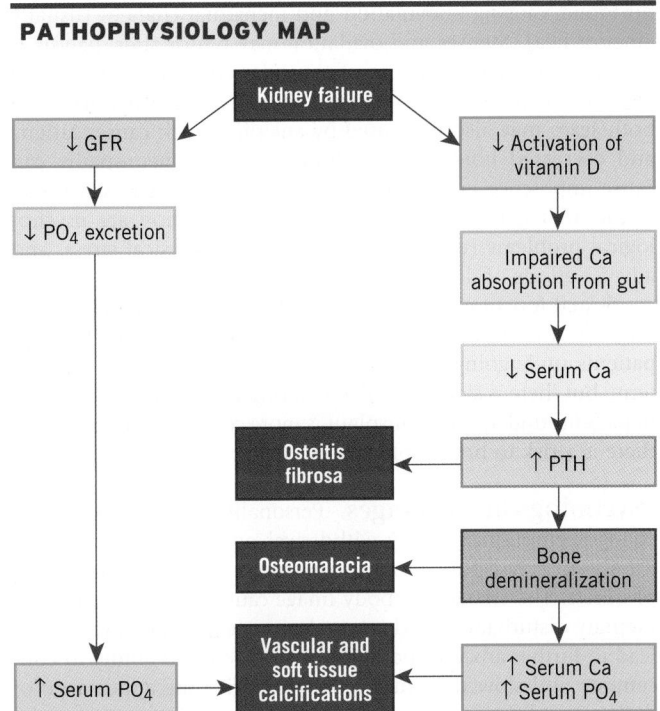

PATHOPHYSIOLOGY MAP

Figure 49-4 Mechanisms of chronic kidney disease–mineral and bone disorder (CKD–MBD).

Ca, calcium; *GFR*, glomerular filtration rate; *PO₄*, phosphate; *PTH*, parathyroid hormone.

tions (vascular and soft tissue complications). **Renal osteodystrophy** includes a number of skeletal disorders: (1) *osteitis fibrosa*, in which there is an increased number of osteoclasts and osteoblasts, high bone turnover, and fibrosis of the marrow; (2) *osteomalacia* with low bone turnover and abnormal mineralized bone; (3) *adynamic bone disorder*, in which there is low bone turnover with normal mineralization; and (4) *mixed osteodystrophy* with high bone turnover and abnormal mineralization (Raymond, Wazny, & Sood, 2010; Soroka et al., 2010).

Extraskeletal complications include vascular and soft tissue calcification (Smith & Smelt, 2009). The excess phosphate binds with calcium, leading to the formation of insoluble calcifications that are deposited in the vascular walls and soft tissue. Common sites are blood vessels, GI tract, lungs, muscles, skin, subcutaneous tissues, myocardium, and eyes (McCarley & Arjomand, 2008). Cardiovascular calcification is an important contributor to cardiovascular disease in this population (Benavente et al., 2008), and vascular calcification is the likely cause of high cardiovascular morbidity and mortality in patients with CKD (Soroka et al., 2010).

Integumentary System.
Pruritus is highly prevalent in patients with CKD. It most commonly results from a combination of the dry skin, calcium–phosphate deposition in the skin, and sensory neuropathy. The itching may be so intense that it can lead to bleeding or infection secondary to scratching. Uremic frost is a rare condition in which urea crystallizes on the skin and is usually seen only when BUN levels are extremely high.

Reproductive System.
Both men and women can experience infertility and a decreased libido. Women usually have decreased levels of estrogen, progesterone, and luteinizing

hormone, causing anovulation and menstrual changes (usually amenorrhea). Menses and ovulation may return after dialysis is started. Men experience loss of testicular consistency, decreased testosterone levels, and low sperm counts. Sexual dysfunction in both sexes may also be caused by anemia, which causes fatigue and decreased libido. In addition, peripheral neuropathy can cause impotence in men and anorgasmy in women. Additional factors that may cause changes in sexual function are psychological problems (e.g., anxiety, depression), physical stress, and adverse effects of drugs.

Sexual function may improve with maintenance dialysis and may become normal with successful transplantation. Pregnant patients undergoing dialysis have been able to carry a fetus to term, but there is significant risk to mother and infant. Pregnancy in patients undergoing transplant is more common, but here, too, there is a risk to both mother and fetus.

Psychological Changes. Personality and behavioural changes, emotional lability, withdrawal, and depression are commonly observed. Fatigue and lethargy contribute to the feeling of illness. The changes in body image caused by edema, integumentary disturbances, and access devices (e.g., fistulas, catheters) lead to further anxiety and depression. Decreased ability to concentrate and slowed mental activity can give the appearance of dullness and disinterest in the environment. There are also significant changes in lifestyle, occupation, family responsibilities, and financial status that must be dealt with by the patient. Long-term survival depends on drugs, dietary restrictions, dialysis, and possibly transplantation. The patient will also grieve the loss of renal function. This can be a prolonged process for some individuals.

Diagnostic Studies

Adverse outcomes of CKD can often be prevented or delayed through early detection and treatment. Early stages of CKD can be detected through routine laboratory measurements (Table 49-6). Proteinuria is one of the most important risk factors for the progression of chronic kidney disease leading to dialysis and is the earliest marker of kidney damage (Levin et al., 2008). Patients at high risk for kidney disease such as those with diabetes, hypertension, vascular disease, autoimmune disease, GFR less than 60 mL/min, and edema should be screened for proteinuria (Levin et al., 2008). The preferred method for screening for proteinuria is the measurement of urine protein to creatinine or of albumin to creatinine (Levin et al., 2008). A dipstick evaluation for protein in the urine may be done but is not as accurate. Patients with diabetes need to have examination of their urine for microalbuminuria if none is detected on routine urinalysis. The presence of proteinuria in two or three consecutive urine samples is needed to determine persistent proteinuria (Levin et al., 2008) A person with persistent proteinuria (1+ protein on standard dipstick testing two or more times over a 3-mo period) should have further assessment of risk factors and a diagnostic workup with blood and urine tests. A urine test for albumin-to-creatinine ratio provides an accurate estimate of the protein and albumin excretion rate. A ratio greater than 300 mg albumin/1 g creatinine signals CKD (Snyder & Collins, 2009).

A urinalysis can detect RBCs, WBCs, protein, casts, and glucose. Imaging of the kidneys to exclude obstruction and note the size of the kidneys is usually done by ultrasound. Other diagnostic studies (see Table 49-6) help establish the diagnosis and cause of CKD.

COLLABORATIVE CARE

Table 49-6 Management of Chronic Kidney Disease

Diagnostic

- History and physical examination
- Identification of reversible renal disease
- Renal ultrasound
- Renal scan
- CT scan
- Renal biopsy
- BUN, serum creatinine, and eGFR
- Serum electrolytes
- Serum calcium, phosphorous, albumin, and parathyroid hormone levels
- Protein/creatinine ratio in first, morning-voided specimen
- Urinalysis and urine culture
- Serum hemoglobin level and iron indices

Collaborative Therapy

- Correction of extracellular fluid volume overload or deficit
- Nutritional therapy*
- Erythropoietin therapy
- Calcium supplementation, phosphate binders, or both
- Antihypertensive therapy
- Measures to lower potassium†
- Adjustment of drug dosages according to degree of renal function
- Renal replacement therapy (dialysis, kidney transplant)

BUN, blood urea nitrogen; *CT*, computed tomography; *eGFR*, estimated glomerular filtration rate.
*See Tables 49-8 and 49-9.
†See Table 49-4.

Serum creatinine alone poorly reflects kidney function, and a rise in blood creatinine is observed only after significant loss of functioning nephrons (National Kidney Foundation, 2011). GFR is the preferred measure used to determine kidney function. Several GFR calculators are available. The two equations used most frequently to estimate GFR are the Cockcroft-Gault formula and the Modification of Diet in Renal Disease (MDRD) Study equation (Table 49-7). The National Kidney Foundation KDOQI guidelines recommend the MDRD Study equation to estimate GFR (Komaba, Tanaka, & Fukagawa, 2008).

Collaborative Management of Chronic Kidney Disease

The focus in CKD is on prevention and early identification to deter the progression of kidney disease. When a patient is diagnosed as having CKD, every effort is made to detect and treat potentially reversible causes (e.g., cardiac failure, dehydration, infections, nephrotoxins, urinary tract obstruction, renal artery stenosis). A renal biopsy may be necessary to provide a definitive diagnosis. The goals of CKD care are to preserve existing renal function, delay progression of renal disease, treat clinical manifestations, prevent complications, educate patients and families regarding kidney disease and options for care, and prepare patients for RRT (Kopyt, 2007; McCarley, 2006; McCarley &

Table 49-7 Serum Creatinine Is a Poor Indicator of Kidney Function

Calculation of GFR is considered the best index to estimate kidney function as indicated by the following example.

	TYPE OF PATIENT	
ESTIMATION OF GFR	**76-YEAR-OLD WHITE WOMAN (WEIGHT 56 kg)**	**28-YEAR-OLD WHITE MAN (WEIGHT 74 kg)**
SCr	155 mmol/L	155 mmol/L
GFR—estimated by the Cockcroft-Gault formula*	28.4 mL/min	65.7 mL/min
GFR—estimated by MDRD equation†	30 mL/min/1.73 m²	49 mL/min/1.73 m²

GFR, glomerular filtration rate; *MDRD,* modification of diet in renal disease; *SCr,* serum creatinine.

*Cockcroft-Gault GFR = [(140 − age) × (weight in kg) × 1.2]/(SCr (mmol/L). For women, multiply the result by 0.85 (Dersch & McCormack, 2008).

†GFR as estimated by MDRD and Cockcroft-Gault equation calculator can be accessed at *http://www.mdrd.com.*

Burrows-Hudson, 2006). The care of the patient with CKD must be tailored to the stage of CKD. Early CKD care can lead to effective planning and appropriate timing of dialysis start and creation of the dialysis access. In the early stages of CKD, pharmacological and nutritional therapy and supportive care are essential components of the CKD care plan.

Drug Therapy

Hyperkalemia. There are multiple strategies for managing hyperkalemia (see Table 49-4). Every effort is made to control hyperkalemia with the restriction of high-potassium foods and drugs. Acute hyperkalemia may require urgent intervention. The level of potassium that should be treated has not been firmly established; however, based on a systematic review (Elliott, Ronksley, Clase, Ahmed, & Hemmelgarn, 2010), it is suggested that nonpharmacological steps be instituted for management of potassium levels above 5.5 mmol/L and pharmacological intervention at potassium levels of 6.0 mmol/L or greater. An ECG should be considered to assess for cardiac dysrhythmias that may require treatment. Common ECG changes associated with hyperkalemia include peaked T waves and widened QRS complexes. Patients with ECG changes consistent with severe hyperkalemia should be treated with IV calcium-based salts such as calcium gluconate or calcium chloride (Elliott et al., 2010). Acute hyperkalemia may require treatment with IV glucose and insulin and/or β2-adrenergic agonists such as salbutamol to shift potassium into the cells. Rebound after potassium-shifting therapy occurs within 2 hours if steps have not been taken to reduce potassium either through urine excretion or HD (Elliott et al., 2010). A cation exchange resin, such as sodium polystyrene sulphonate (Kayexalate), is commonly used to lower potassium levels and can be administered on an outpatient basis. Cation exchange resins take hours to days to reduce potassium. Sodium polystyrene sulphonate should not be given to patients who do not have normal bowel function or mixed with sorbitol because of associated bowel necrosis (U.S. FDA, 2011).

Because sodium polystyrene sulphonate exchanges sodium ions for potassium ions, the patient should be observed for

sodium and water retention. If life-threatening dysrhythmias are present, dialysis may be required.

Hypertension. The progression of CKD can be delayed by controlling hypertension (McCarley & Arjomand, 2008). Treatment of hypertension consists of lifestyle modifications (e.g., exercise, weight reduction, avoidance of alcohol, stress management), dietary sodium and fluid restriction, and the administration of antihypertensive drugs. The Canadian Hypertension Education Program (CHEP, 2012) recommends a target blood pressure for patients with nondiabetic CKD and patients with diabetes less than 140/90 mm Hg; for those with diabetes mellitus, it is less than 130/80 mm Hg.

For patients with nondiabetic CKD and proteinuria, ACE inhibitors (e.g., ramapril [Altace], enalapril [Vasotec]) or ARBs (e.g., irbesartan [Avapro], losartan [Cozaar]) are recommended as initial therapy (CHEP, 2012). ACE inhibitors and ARBs decrease proteinuria and delay the progression of renal failure. For additional therapy, the use of thiazide diuretics (e.g., hydrochlorothiazide) or loop diuretics (e.g., furosemide [Lasix]) for volume overload is suggested (CHEP, 2012).

For patients with renovascular disease, CHEP suggests cautious use of ACE inhibitors and ARBs as patients with bilateral disease or a solitary kidney are at increased risk for AKI (CHEP, 2012).

For patients with diabetes, CHEP (2012) suggests use of ACE inhibitors or ARBs as initial therapy. Other antihypertensive drugs commonly used include dihydropyridine calcium channel blockers (nifedipine [Adalat], amlodipine [Norvasc] and thiazide or thiazide-like diuretics.

ACE inhibitors and ARBs must be used cautiously in CKD because they can further decrease the GFR and increase serum potassium levels. Most people require a number of antihypertensives to achieve target blood pressure, and regimens must be individualized based on other existing co-morbidities.

Blood pressure (BP) should periodically be measured in supine, sitting, and standing positions to effectively monitor the effect of antihypertensive drugs. The patient should be taught how to monitor the BP at home and what BP readings require immediate intervention. BP control is essential to slow atherosclerotic changes that could further impair renal function.

Chronic Kidney Disease–Mineral and Bone Disorder. Interventions for CKD–MBD include limiting dietary phosphorus, administering phosphate binders, and supplementing vitamin D. Phosphate intake is generally restricted to less than 1000 mg/day, but usually dietary control is not adequate. Calcium-based phosphate binders such as calcium carbonate (e.g., Tums, Caltrate) and calcium acetate (e.g., PhosLo) are used to bind the phosphate, which is then excreted in the stool. Giving a calcium-based binder when the phosphate levels are still high (1.98 mmol/L) may cause the formation of calcium–phosphate deposits. Sevelamer (Renagel) is a phosphate binder that contains neither calcium nor aluminum.

Because dementia (aluminum toxicity) and bone disease (osteomalacia) are associated with excessive absorption of aluminum, aluminum preparations (e.g., Basaljel) should be avoided if possible and used with caution in patients with renal failure. Magnesium-containing antacids (Maalox, Mylanta) are used in moderation because magnesium is dependent on the kidneys for excretion. Phosphate binders should be administered with each meal to be effective because most phosphate is absorbed within 1 hour after eating. Hypercalcemia may occur with calcium supplementation and is associated with increased cardiac calcifications and mortality in ESRD patients. Calcium binders are generally limited to a maximum of 1500 mg/day with the total daily calcium intake including diet not exceeding 2 g. Constipation is a frequent adverse effect of phosphate binders and may necessitate the use of stool softeners.

Hypocalcemia is often a problem because of the inability of the GI tract to absorb calcium in the absence of vitamin D. If hypocalcemia persists even when serum phosphate levels are controlled and supplemental calcium is given, the active form of vitamin D should be given. It is commercially available in oral preparations such as calcitriol (Rocaltrol) and in IV form as calcitriol (Calcijex). It is important to lower the phosphate level before administering calcium or vitamin D because these drugs may contribute to soft tissue calcification if both calcium and phosphate levels are elevated. Calcimimetics such as cinacalcet (Sensipar) may be prescribed to lower PTH and may also cause hypocalcemia (Sloand, 2007).

If renal osteodystrophy remains severe despite medical management, a subtotal parathyroidectomy may be performed to decrease the synthesis and secretion of PTH. In some situations, a total parathyroidectomy is performed, and some parathyroid tissue is transplanted into the forearm. The transplanted cells produce PTH as needed. If production of PTH becomes excessive, some of the cells can be removed from the forearm under local anaesthesia.

The most common methods for evaluating the status of the bone disease are skeletal radiographs, bone scans, bone biopsy, and bone densitometry. PTH and alkaline phosphatase levels should also be measured. Alkaline phosphatase is elevated when there is demineralization of the bone but can also be increased by liver disease.

Anemia. The most important cause of anemia in CKD is a decreased production of erythropoietin. With the use of recombinant DNA technology (see Chapter 16, Figure 16-15), erythropoiesis-stimulating agents (ESAs) are available for the treatment of anemia. ESAs can be administered intravenously or subcutaneously. They have been very effective in treating anemia. A significant increase in hemoglobin is usually not seen for 2 to 3 weeks. The patient who is receiving erythropoietin has improved exercise tolerance and an enhanced quality of life.

Significant morbidity and mortality have been associated with trying to normalize hemoglobin levels (Levin et al., 2008, p. 1158). The Canadian Society of Nephrology (CSN) *Guidelines for the Management of Chronic Kidney Disease* recommend a target hemoglobin of 110 g/L, with an acceptable range between 100 and 120 g/L (Levin et al., 2008, p. 1158). A common adverse effect of ESAs is the development or acceleration of hypertension. The underlying mechanism is related to the hemodynamic changes (e.g., increased whole blood viscosity) that occur as the anemia is corrected. Patients with significantly elevated BP should not receive ESAs.

Another adverse effect of ESA therapy is the development of functional iron deficiency resulting from the increased demand for iron to support erythropoiesis. The CSN *Guidelines for the Management of Chronic Kidney Disease* recommend a target ferritin greater than 100 ng/mL and a transferring saturation level greater than 20% (Levin et al., 2008, p. 1159). Most patients receive iron supplements. The GI adverse effects of oral iron, including gastric irritation and constipation, may lead to nonadherence to therapy. Orally administered iron should not be taken at the same time as phosphate binders because calcium binds the iron, preventing

absorption. The patient should be advised that iron may make the stool dark in colour.

Most patients on HD receive IV iron. Supplemental folic acid is usually given because it is needed for RBC formation and is removed by dialysis.

Blood transfusions should be avoided in treating anemia unless the patient experiences an acute blood loss or has symptomatic anemia (i.e., dyspnea, excess fatigue, tachycardia, palpitations, chest pain). Undesirable effects of transfusions are the suppression of erythropoiesis as a result of a decrease in the hypoxic stimulus, the possible transmission of hepatitis B or C or human immunodeficiency virus (HIV), the possibility of developing antibodies that may affect transplantation, and the possibility of iron overload because each unit of blood contains about 250 mg of iron.

Dyslipidemia. There is a high prevalence of dyslipidemia for patients with CKD (Levin et al., 2008). Currently, good evidence-informed research is lacking to guide the management of dyslipidemia in CKD. The CSN *Guidelines for the Management of Chronic Kidney Disease* support the use of statins in patients with stages 1 to 3 CKD, as per guidelines for the general population (Levin et al., 2008, p. 1157).

Complications of Drug Therapy. Because the kidneys play a large role in absorption, distribution, metabolism, and elimination of drugs, the CKD population is at risk for medication-related problems that can lead to increased morbidity and mortality (Liles, 2011). Many drugs are partially or totally excreted by the kidneys. Delayed and decreased elimination lead to an accumulation of drugs in the body and potential for drug toxicity. Dialysis may remove or lower drug levels. Drug doses and frequency of administration must be adjusted based on the level of kidney function and whether or not the patient is receiving dialysis. Drugs of particular concern include digoxin, oral glycemic agents (e.g., metformin, glyburide), antibiotics, and opioid medication (e.g., hydromorphone [Dilaudid], morphine).

Patients should be advised to avoid NSAIDs. These drugs block the synthesis of the renal prostaglandins that promote vasodilation. This can worsen renal hypoperfusion and cause interstitial nephritis. Many NSAIDs are available over the counter, so it is essential that the patient be cautioned. Acetaminophen can be substituted.

Nutritional Therapy

Protein Restriction. The diet is designed to be as normal as possible to maintain good nutrition (Table 49-8). All patients with CKD should be seen by a dietitian. Protein energy wasting in CKD is a strong predictor of mortality (Kovesdy & Kalantar-Zadeh, 2012). Protein is moderately restricted because BUN is an end product of protein metabolism. For the patient who is not undergoing dialysis, one guide is to restrict protein intake to 0.6 to 0.75 g/kg of ideal body weight (IBW)/day when the creatinine clearance is less than 25 mL/min (Atkins et al., 2008; Goldstein-Fuch, 2006). This moderate restriction may slow progression of CKD for these patients. For patients with more severe renal insufficiency, low-protein diets should be used with caution because these patients are at risk for developing malnutrition.

Once the patient starts dialysis, protein intake can be increased to 1.2 to 1.3 g/kg of IBW/day. Dietary protein guidelines for PD differ from those for HD because excessive amounts of protein

NUTRITIONAL THERAPY

Table 49-8 Daily Requirements for the Patient With Chronic Kidney Disease

	CKD STAGES 3-4 MANAGEMENT	HEMODIALYSIS	PERITONEAL DIALYSIS
Fluid allowance	Urine output + 600 mL	Urine output + 600 mL	Often no restriction
Protein*	0.6-0.75 g/kg body weight	1.2-1.3 g/kg IBW	≥1.2-1.3 g/kg IBW
Calories	30-35 kcal/kg EDW	30-35 kcal/kg EDW†	30-35 kcal/kg IBW†
Fat	Determined by caloric requirement	Determined by caloric requirement	Determined by caloric requirement
Carbohydrate	Unlimited intake of sugars, starches; bread and cereal products limited owing to protein restriction	Same as for conservative management	Dependent on individual patient needs
Iron	Variable	Variable	Variable
Potassium	2-3 g	2-3 g	3-4 g, no restrictions
Sodium	2-3 g	2-3 g	2-4 g
Phosphorus	800-1000 mg	1000 mg	1000 mg
Calcium	Variable	1000-1500 mg	1000-1500 mg
Folic acid	1-mg supplement	1-mg supplement	1-mg supplement

CKD, chronic kidney disease; *EDW*, estimated dry weight; *IBW*, ideal body weight.
*At least 50% of protein intake should be of high biological value (e.g., coming from eggs, milk, meat).
†Includes dialysate calories.

are lost in the dialysate. The protein intake must be high enough to compensate for the losses so that the nitrogen balance is maintained. The recommended protein intake is at least 1.2 g/kg of IBW/day and can be increased depending on the individual needs of the patient. At least 50% of protein intake should have high biological value containing all of the essential amino acids (e.g., eggs, milk, meat, poultry).

Sufficient calories from carbohydrates and fat are needed to minimize catabolism of body protein and to maintain body weight. Therefore, 100 g of carbohydrates and an appropriate amount of fat are prescribed to maintain an intake of 30 to 35 kcal/kg body weight/day. See Table 49-8 for specific guidelines.

For patients with malnutrition or inadequate caloric intake, commercially prepared products that are high in calories and low in protein, sodium, and potassium are available.

Because the diet for CKD is deficient in vitamins, and water-soluble vitamins are lost through dialysis, multivitamins are prescribed.

Sodium and Fluid Restriction. Fluid intake for patients with CKD depends on the daily urine output and overall fluid balance. For patients not yet on dialysis, fluids are generally not restricted and diuretics and a low-sodium diet help to manage fluid retention. For patients receiving HD, fluids are generally restricted as urine output begins to decline. Generally, 600 mL (from insensible loss) plus an amount equal to the previous day's urine output is allowed for a patient receiving dialysis. Foods that are liquid at room temperature (e.g., gelatin, ice cream) should be counted as fluid intake. The fluid allotment should be spaced throughout the day so that the patient does not become thirsty. For the patient receiving long-term HD, fluid intake is adjusted so that weight gains are no more than 1 to 3 kg between dialyses.

To achieve the optimal fluid balance, the sodium must also be restricted. Sodium-restricted diet allowances may vary from 2 to 4 g depending on the degree of edema and hypertension. Sodium and salt should not be equated because the sodium

NUTRITIONAL THERAPY

Table 49-9 High-Potassium Foods

Fruits and Fruit Juices	*Vegetables*	*Cereal*
• Apple juice	• Beans, white and pinto*	• All-Bran*
• Grapefruit juice	• Broccoli	• Raisin bran*
• Orange juice*	• Carrots	*Meat and Poultry*
• Prune juice*	• Lima beans, cooked*	• Beef,* pork, cooked
• Tomato juice*	• Mushrooms, fresh*	• Chicken
• Oranges	• Potato, baked*	• Turkey
• Tomatoes	• Squash, baked*	*Miscellaneous*
• Honeydew melons*	• Spinach, cooked*	• Chocolate
• Raisins*	*Dairy*	• Molasses
• Avocados*	• Milk*	• Sunflower seeds*
• Bananas*	• Yogourt*	
• Prunes*		

*>10 mmol of potassium per serving.

content in 1 g of sodium chloride is equivalent to 400 mg of sodium. The patient should be instructed to avoid high-sodium foods such as cured meats, pickled foods, canned soups and stews, frankfurters, cold cuts, soy sauce, and salad dressings (see Chapter 37, Tables 37-11 through 37-14). Most salt substitutes should not be used because they contain potassium chloride.

Potassium Restriction. The potassium restriction depends on the ability of the kidneys to excrete this electrolyte. Dietary allowances for potassium range from about 2 to 4 g. Some PD patients do not need potassium restrictions. Some foods with high potassium content that should be avoided are oranges, bananas, melons, tomatoes, prunes, raisins, deep green and yellow vegetables, beans, and legumes (Table 49-9).

Phosphate Restriction. CKD alters the homeostasis of calcium, phosphorus, and vitamin D (Goldstein-Fuch, 2006). As CKD progresses, phosphorus excretion diminishes, resulting in hyperphosphatemia. Phosphate should be limited to approximately 1000 mg/day. Foods that are high in phosphate include dairy products (e.g., milk, ice cream, cheese, yogourt) and foods containing dairy products (pudding). Most foods that are high in phosphate are also high in calcium. Restricting phosphate will restrict calcium intake.

NURSING MANAGEMENT: CHRONIC KIDNEY DISEASE

▪ Nursing Assessment

The nurse should obtain a complete history of any existing renal disease or family history of renal disease because some renal disorders have a hereditary basis (e.g., polycystic kidney disease, Alport's syndrome). Information on long-term health problems such as hypertension, diabetes, recurrent urinary tract infections, and systemic lupus erythematosus should be obtained because these conditions can lead to CKD. Because the kidneys play a large role in absorption, distribution, metabolism, and elimination of drugs and the fact that many drugs are potentially nephrotoxic, both current and past use of prescription and over-the-counter drugs must be reviewed.

The nurse should assess the patient's dietary habits and discuss any problems. The height and weight should be measured, and any recent weight changes must be evaluated.

Clinical manifestations of CKD are apparent in multiple body systems (see Figure 49-3). Fatigue, lethargy, and pruritus are often the early symptoms of CKD. Hypertension and changes in urine characteristics are often the first signs.

CKD is a lifelong and life-limiting illness. The chronicity of renal disease and the long-term nature of treatment modalities affect every area of a person's life, including family relationships, social and work activities, and self-image and emotional state. Support systems should be assessed. The choice of treatment modality may be related to support systems available to the patient.

It is important to respect the patient's choice not to receive treatment. Many times, patients will initiate the conversation about palliative care themselves. The discussion needs to focus on moving from the curative approach to promotion of comfort care and consideration for end-of-life care. Listen to the patient and caregiver, allowing them to do most of the talking, and pay special attention to their hopes and fears (Haras, 2008) (Table 49-10). (Palliative and end of-life care is discussed in Chapter 13.)

▪ Nursing Diagnoses

Nursing diagnoses for the patient with CKD in stage 4 may include, but are not limited to, those presented in Nursing Care Plan (NCP) 49-1.

Table 49-10 Summary of Recommendations for Decision Support for Adults Living With Chronic Kidney Disease

PRACTICE RECOMMENDATIONS

Patient Decision-Making Needs

1.0 Nurses know the common decisions faced by an adult with CKD.
Nursing Actions:
- Nurses identify the decision the patient is facing at a particular point in time.

2.0 Nurses screen the patient for decisional conflict at initial contact and as the patient's situation and condition changes.
Nursing Actions:
- Nurses screen for decisional conflict.

3.0 Nurses determine the source of patient's decisional conflict.
Nursing Actions:
- Nurses assess the patient's knowledge and expectations about the options.
- Nurses assess and discuss the availability of resources.
- Nurses objectively measure the patient's confidence and ability for making decisions and self-managing their CKD.
- Nurses assist the patient to clarify his or her values.
- Nurses clarify the patient's preferred role in decision making and who else the patient wants to involve in the decision-making process.

Decision Support Interventions

4.0 Nurses understand the difference between providing patient education and decision support.
Nursing Actions:
- Nurses describe patient education.
- Nurses describe the additional elements involved with decision support.

5.0 Nurses use patient decision aids and other tools to provide decision support.
Nursing Actions:
- Nurses remain neutral when supporting the patient in decision-making process.
- Nurses use validated tools to provide decision support.
- Nurses help the patient to build confidence in participation in decision making.
- Nurses meet the patient's knowledge needs.
- Nurses help the patient clarify his or her values.
- Nurses help the patient mobilize resources.
- Nurses help the patient to communicate with others during the decision-making process.
- Nurses obtain commitment from the patient for the next decision-making step(s).

CKD, chronic kidney disease.
Source: Excerpted from Registered Nurses' Association of Ontario (RNAO) (2009). Decision support for adults living with chronic kidney disease. RNAO Clinical Best Practice Guideline (p. 8). Retrieved from *http://rnao.ca/sites/rnao-ca/files/Decision_Support_for_Adults_Living_with_Chronic_Kidney_Disease_1.pdf*

▪ Planning

The majority of CKD care occurs in the ambulatory care setting. The overall goals are that a patient with CKD will (1) demonstrate knowledge and ability to comply with the therapeutic regimen, (2) participate in decision making for the plan of care and future

NURSING CARE PLAN 49-1

Chronic Kidney Disease in Stage 4

NURSING DIAGNOSIS	*Excess fluid volume* related to inability of kidneys to excrete excess fluid *as evidenced by* edema, hypertension, bounding pulse, weight gain, shortness of breath, and pulmonary edema
Expected Patient Outcomes	**Nursing Interventions and *Rationales***
• Maintains an acceptable body weight and fluid balance with dietary modifications or with peritoneal dialysis or hemodialysis treatments	• Monitor BP, periorbital, sacral and peripheral edema, and dyspnea, *which are indicators of fluid excess.* • Monitor weight, intake and output *to determine effect of treatment on volume status.* • Provide appropriate diet instruction *to help control edema and hypertension.* • Instruct patient and/or caregivers on measures instituted to treat the hypervolemia (e.g., daily weights, fluid restrictions) *to help monitor and control fluid overload and related hypertension.*
NURSING DIAGNOSIS	*Decreased functional ability* related to anemia resulting from iron deficiency and kidneys' inability to produce erythropoietin *as evidenced by* fatigue, decreased exercise tolerance, and reported impaired quality of life
Expected Patient Outcomes	**Nursing Interventions and *Rationales***
• Reports decreased fatigue and improved exercise tolerance and improved quality of life • Has hemoglobin, transferrin percent saturation, and ferritin levels within acceptable ranges • Demonstrates appropriate technique for ESA administration	• Assess patient for dyspnea, excess fatigue, tachycardia, palpitations, chest pain, *which are indicators of anemia.* • Monitor trends in hemoglobin and iron stores (e.g., ferritin, total iron-binding capacity and transferring saturation *to determine effect of treatment on anemia.* ***Teaching Anemia Management:*** Provide information about causes of CKD anemia, symptoms, treatment, benefits of treatment and potential adverse effects *to increase patient knowledge and promote self-management of adherence to treatment plan.* • Instruct patient to administer subcutaneous ESA *to promote self confidence and skill mastery.* • Discuss importance of adhering to medication regimen (iron and ESA) *because a major reason of poor response to ESA therapy is nonadherence.*

Other nursing diagnoses related to the patient with CKD stage 4:

Risk for impaired skin integrity *related to* pruritus *resulting from* elevated phosphorus and fluid volume excess *as evidenced by* dry skin, scratching, and peripheral edema

Imbalanced nutrition: less than body requirements *related to* restricted intake of nutrients (especially protein), nausea, vomiting, anorexia, and stomatitis *as evidenced by* loss of appetite and weight

Grieving *related to* loss of kidney function *as evidenced by* expression of feelings of sadness, anger, inadequacy, hopelessness

BP, blood pressure; *CKD*, chronic kidney disease; *ESA*, erythropoiesis-stimulating agent.

treatment modality, (3) demonstrate effective coping strategies, and (4) continue with activities of daily living within physiological limitations.

Nursing Implementation

Health Promotion

Identify individuals at risk for CKD. These include people with a history (or a family history) of renal disease, hypertension, diabetes mellitus, and repeated urinary tract infection. These individuals should have regular checkups including assessments of serum creatinine and BUN and urinalysis. People with diabetes should have their urine checked for microalbuminuria if routine urinalysis is negative for protein. They should be advised that any changes in urine appearance (colour, odour), frequency, or volume must be reported to the health care provider. If a patient must be prescribed a potentially nephrotoxic drug, it is important to monitor renal function with serum creatinine and BUN.

Individuals identified as at risk need to take measures to prevent or delay the progression of CKD and reduce the risk for cardiovascular disease. These include glycemic control for patients with diabetes (see Chapter 52), optimizing BP control, and lifestyle modifications including smoking cessation.

Care Considerations for Chronic Kidney Disease in Stages 4 to 5

The specific nursing management of the patient with CKD in stages 4 to 5 is detailed in NCP 49-1. It is important to teach the patient and the family because diet, drugs, and follow-up medical care are the responsibilities of the patient (Table 49-11). The patient should check weight daily, learn to take daily BPs, and be able to identify signs and symptoms of fluid overload, hyperkalemia, and other electrolyte imbalances. The patient and the family must understand the importance of strict dietary adherence. A registered dietitian should meet with the patient and the family on a regular basis for diet planning. A diet history and consideration of cultural variations will facilitate diet planning and adherence.

The patient needs a complete understanding of prescribed drugs, the dosages, and the common adverse effects. It may be helpful to make a list of the drugs and the times of administration that can be posted in the home. The patient must be instructed to avoid certain over-the-counter drugs such as NSAIDs and natural and herbal preparations. ACE inhibitors may have to be discontinued if they are contributing to hyperkalemia or decreased GFR.

Motivation on the part of the patient to assume the primary role in the management of the disease is essential. The period of

Table 49-11 Chronic Kidney Disease in Stages 4 and 5

1. Explain dietary (protein, sodium, potassium, phosphate) and fluid restrictions incorporating the patient's own cultural dietary patterns.

2. Encourage discussion of difficulties in modifying diet and fluid intake.

3. Explain signs and symptoms of electrolyte imbalance, especially high potassium.

4. Teach alternative ways of reducing thirst, such as sucking on ice cubes, lemon, or hard candy.

5. Explain the rationale for prescribed drugs and common adverse effects. Examples:
   - Phosphate binders should be taken with meals.
   - Iron supplements should be taken between meals.

6. Explain the importance of reporting any of the following:
   - Weight gain >2 kg
   - Increasing blood pressure
   - Shortness of breath
   - Edema
   - Increasing fatigue or weakness
   - Confusion or lethargy

7. Encourage patient and caregiver(s) to share concerns about lifestyle changes, living with a chronic illness, and decisions about type of dialysis or transplantation.

predialysis care provides an opportunity to evaluate each patient's ability to manage the disease. This knowledge will be helpful when determining the treatment modality.

Ambulatory and Home Care

The length of time that a patient with CKD can be managed without RRT is highly variable and depends on the progression of renal failure and the presence of other co-morbid conditions. When RRT is required, HD, PD, and transplantation are the available treatment options.

Extensive and ongoing teaching and discussion about RRTs should occur early (CKD in stage 3) in order for the patient to make an informed decision about future therapies including RRT and advanced directives.

The patient and the family need a clear explanation of what is involved in dialysis and transplantation. The patient should be informed that, if dialysis is chosen, the option of transplantation still remains, if the patient is medically suitable. It should be emphasized that, if a transplanted organ fails, the patient can return to dialysis. The patient should also be counselled that retransplantation may also be an option.

Evaluation

The expected outcomes for the patient with CKD are presented in NCP 49-1.

Dialysis

Dialysis is the movement of fluid and molecules across a semipermeable membrane from one compartment to another. Clini-

NURSING RESEARCH

Self-Management in Chronic Kidney Disease

Citation

Costantini, L., Beanlands, H., McCay, E., Cattran, D., Hladunewich, M., & Francis, D. (2008). The self-management experience of people with mild to moderate chronic kidney disease. *Nephrology Nursing Journal, 35*(2), 147-155.

Purpose

To explore, describe, and stimulate interest in the self-management experiences of patients with mild to moderate chronic kidney disease (CKD).

Methods

A qualitative exploratory study that was part of a larger descriptive–cross-sectional–quantitative design examined psychosocial variables and health behaviours in people with mild to moderate CKD. The 60 participants from the larger study in central Canada completed standardized questionnaires and, from these, 14 participants were selected using an approach that ensured representation of men and women of varying ages. A qualitative semistructured interview was conducted to elicit perceptions of health, kidney disease, illness management, and supports needed for self-management. Open-ended questions were used in audiotaped sessions. Thematic analysis was used to analyze the interviews.

Results and Conclusions

Patients with CKD use a process for renegotiating life with their chronic illness. This process encompasses discovering and learning to live with kidney disease. Themes identified include searching for evidence, realizing kidney disease is forever, managing the illness, taking care of the self, and the need for disease-specific information. Findings indicate that patients with early CKD want to self-manage their illness in collaboration with health care providers and need guidance and support from health providers to do this successfully.

Implications for Nursing Practice

Nurses caring for people with CKD are uniquely positioned to provide the needed guidance and support to assist patients with CKD to self-manage their illness and to collaborate with other health care providers to facilitate self-management.

cally, dialysis is a technique in which substances move from the blood through a semipermeable membrane (dialyzer) and into a dialysis solution (dialysate). It is used to correct fluid and electrolyte imbalances and to remove waste products in renal failure. It can also be used to treat drug overdoses. The two methods of dialysis available are PD and HD (Table 49-12). **Peritoneal dialysis (PD)** is a method of removing waste products and excess fluid from the blood using a natural semipermeable membrane, the peritoneum. Dialysis fluid is infused into the peritoneal cavity, and excess fluid and waste products pass across the membrane into the fluid, which is then drained and discarded. In **hemodialysis (HD)**, waste products and excess fluid are removed from the blood using a machine to pump the blood through an

Table 49-12 Comparison of Peritoneal Dialysis and Hemodialysis

Peritoneal Dialysis	Hemodialysis
Advantages	**Advantages**
• Less complicated than hemodialysis	• Rapid fluid removal
• Portable system with CAPD	• Rapid removal of urea and creatinine
• Fewer dietary restrictions	• Effective potassium removal
• Relatively short training time	• Less protein loss
• Usable in the patient with vascular access problems	• Lowering of serum triglycerides
• Less cardiovascular stress	• Home dialysis possible
• Home dialysis possible	• Temporary access can be placed at bedside
• Preferable for the diabetic patient	**Disadvantages**
Disadvantages	• Vascular access problems
• Bacterial or chemical peritonitis	• Dietary and fluid restrictions
• Protein loss into dialysate	• Heparinization may be necessary
• Exit-site and tunnel infections	• Extensive equipment necessary
• Self-image problems with catheter placement	• Hypotension during dialysis
• Hyperglycemia	• Added blood loss that contributes to anemia
• Aggravated dyslipidemia	• Specially trained personnel necessary (if in-centre option chosen)
• Surgery for catheter placement	• Longer training time for home hemodialysis vs peritoneal
• Contraindication in the patient with multiple abdominal surgeries, trauma, unrepaired hernia	• Surgery for permanent access placement
• Catheter can migrate	• Self-image problems with permanent access

CAPD, continuous ambulatory peritoneal dialysis.

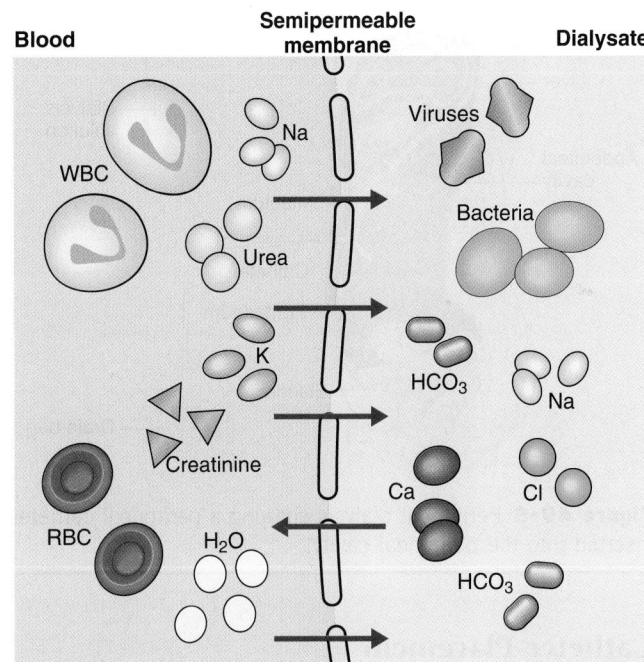

Figure 49-5 Osmosis and diffusion across a semipermeable membrane.

Ca, calcium; *Cl*, chlorine; *HCO₃*, bicarbonate; *H₂O*, water; *K*, potassium; *Na*, sodium; *RBC*, red blood cell; *WBC*, white blood cell.

artificial semipermeable membrane (usually made of cellulose-based or synthetic materials).

When CKD progresses to the point that the patient's symptoms, fluid volume status, or both can no longer be managed without dialysis, dialysis therapy is initiated. Generally, dialysis is initiated when the GFR (or creatinine clearance) is less than 15 mL/min/1.73 m². This criterion can vary widely in different clinical situations. Certain uremic complications, including encephalopathy, neuropathies, uncontrolled hyperkalemia, pericarditis, and accelerated hypertension, indicate a need for immediate dialysis.

General Principles of Dialysis

Solutes and water move across the semipermeable membrane from the blood to the dialysate or from the dialysate to the blood in accordance with concentration gradients. The principles of diffusion, osmosis, and ultrafiltration are involved in dialysis (Figure 49-5). *Diffusion* is the movement of solutes from an area of greater concentration to an area of lesser concentration. In

renal failure, urea, creatinine, uric acid, and electrolytes (potassium, phosphate) move from the blood to the dialysate with the net effect of lowering their concentration in the blood. RBCs, WBCs, and plasma proteins are too large to diffuse through the pores of the membrane. Bacteria and viruses that may be present in the dialysate are too large to migrate through the pores into the blood.

Osmosis is the movement of fluid from an area of lesser to an area of greater concentration of solutes. Glucose is added to the dialysate and creates an osmotic gradient across the membrane, pulling excess fluid from the blood.

Ultrafiltration (water and fluid removal) results when there is an osmotic gradient or pressure gradient across the membrane. In PD, excess fluid is removed by increasing the osmolality of the dialysate (osmotic gradient) with the addition of glucose. In HD, the gradient is created by increasing pressure in the blood compartment (positive pressure) or decreasing pressure in the dialysate compartment (negative pressure). Extracellular fluid moves into the dialysate because of the pressure gradient. The excess fluid is removed by creating a pressure differential between the blood and the dialysate solution with a combination of positive pressure in the blood compartment and negative pressure in the dialysate compartment.

Peritoneal Dialysis

Although PD was first used in 1923, it did not come into widespread use for chronic treatment until the 1970s with the development of soft, pliable peritoneal solution bags and the introduction of the concept of continuous PD. In Canada, 18.8% of patients were receiving peritoneal dialysis compared with 77.8% who were receiving HD in 2009 (CIHI, 2011a).

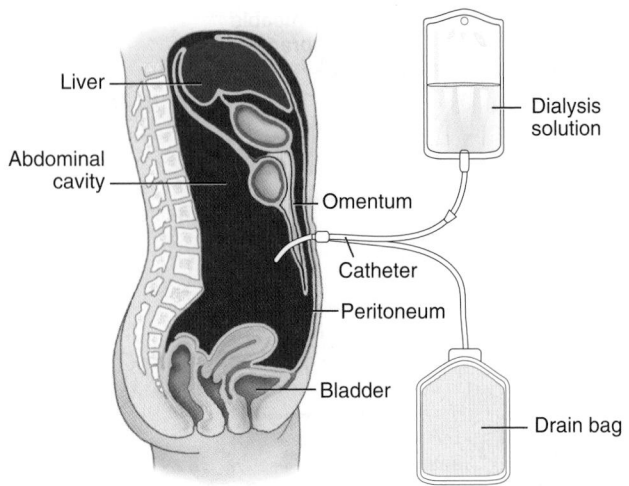

Figure 49-6 Peritoneal dialysis showing a peritoneal catheter inserted into the peritoneal cavity.

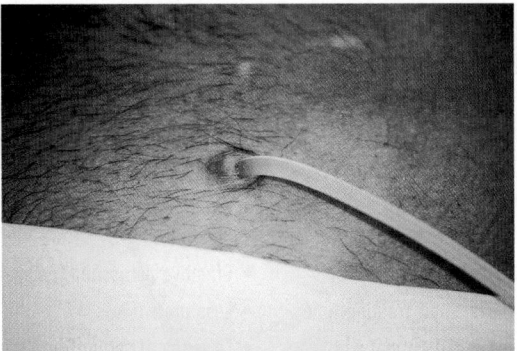

Figure 49-7 Peritoneal catheter exit site.

Source: Courtesy of Mary Jo Holechek, Baltimore, Maryland.

Catheter Placement

Peritoneal access is obtained by inserting a catheter through the anterior abdominal wall (Figure 49-6). Most catheter exit sites are in the abdomen; however, some catheters are inserted using a presternal technique where the catheter exits on the chest (Ponferrada, Prowant, & Satalowich, 2008; Prowant, 2006). The catheters vary in length and have one or two Dacron cuffs on the subcutaneous and peritoneal portions of the catheter that act as anchors and prevent the migration of microorganisms down the shaft from the skin. Within a few weeks of insertion, fibrous tissue grows into the Dacron cuff, holding the catheter in place and preventing bacterial penetration into the peritoneal cavity. The tip of the catheter rests in the peritoneal cavity and has many perforations spaced along the distal end of the tubing to allow fluid to flow in and out of the catheter. There are numerous types of PD catheters.

The technique for catheter placement varies. Although it is possible to place a permanent catheter in the peritoneal cavity at the bedside with a trocar, it is usually done via surgery so that its placement can be directly visualized, minimizing potential complications. Preparation of the patient for catheter insertion includes emptying the bladder and the bowel, weighing the patient, and obtaining a signed consent form.

In the nonsurgical (bedside) approach, an area approximately 2 cm below the umbilicus is numbed with a local anaesthetic, and a small stab wound is made. A stylet is inserted, and the abdomen is distended with dialysis solution. The catheter is then placed into the peritoneal cavity. When the patient feels pressure in the rectal area and has the urge to defecate, the catheter is in place.

In the surgical approach, a midline umbilical incision is made, and a small puncture is made to one side and below this incision. The distal end of the catheter is placed in the peritoneum, and it is tunnelled under the skin to the puncture site. The tunnel helps prevent peritonitis. After the catheter is inserted, the skin is cleaned with an antiseptic solution, and a sterile dressing is applied. Complications of catheter insertion include perforation of the bladder, the bowel, or a blood vessel and the introduction of bacteria.

The catheter is connected to a sterile tubing system and secured to the abdomen with tape. The catheter is irrigated immediately with heparinized dialysate (usually 500 mL) to clear blood and fibrin from it. Prophylactic antibiotics may also be given. Catheter placement is usually same-day surgery, and the patient is discharged home with a sterile dressing covering the PD catheter. The patient needs instructions on keeping the dressing dry, avoiding accidentally pulling the catheter, and receiving follow-up care.

Before starting PD, it is preferable to allow a waiting period of 7 to 14 days for proper sealing of the catheter and for tissue to grow into the cuffs. Postoperative exit-site care should be restricted to trained staff (Prowant, 2006). About 2 to 4 weeks after catheter implantation, the exit site should be clean, dry, and free of redness and tenderness (Figure 49-7). Once the catheter incision site is healed, routine care should be done daily or every other day. This care includes the use of antibacterial soap or mild medical-grade disinfectants as well as examination of the catheter site for signs of infection. Each centre will have a policy about exit-site care and patients are taught how to examine and care for their PD catheter and exit site by the PD nursing staff.

Dialysis Solutions and Cycles

PD is accomplished by putting dialysis solution into the peritoneal space. The three phases of the PD cycle are *inflow* (fill), *dwell* (equilibration), and *drain*. The three phases are called an *exchange*. The dialysis prescription is tailored to the patient's needs. During inflow, a prescribed amount of solution, usually 2 L, is infused through an established catheter over about 10 minutes. After the solution has been infused, the inflow clamp is closed before air enters the tubing.

The next part of the cycle is the dwell phase, or equilibration, during which diffusion and osmosis occur between the patient's blood and the peritoneal cavity. The duration of the dwell time can last 20 to 30 minutes to 8 or more hours, depending on the goals of PD.

Drain time takes 15 to 30 minutes. The cycle starts again with the infusion of another 2 L of solution. For manual PD, a period of about 30 to 50 minutes is required to complete an exchange.

Dialysis solutions vary, and the choice of exchange volume is primarily determined by the size of the peritoneal cavity. A larger person may tolerate a 3-L volume without any difficulty whereas an average-size person usually tolerates a 2-L exchange.

Ultrafiltration (fluid removal) during PD depends on osmotic forces, with glucose being the most effective agent available. Dextrose remains the most commonly used osmotic agent available in PD solutions. It is relatively safe but has been associated with high rates of peritoneal glucose absorption leading to

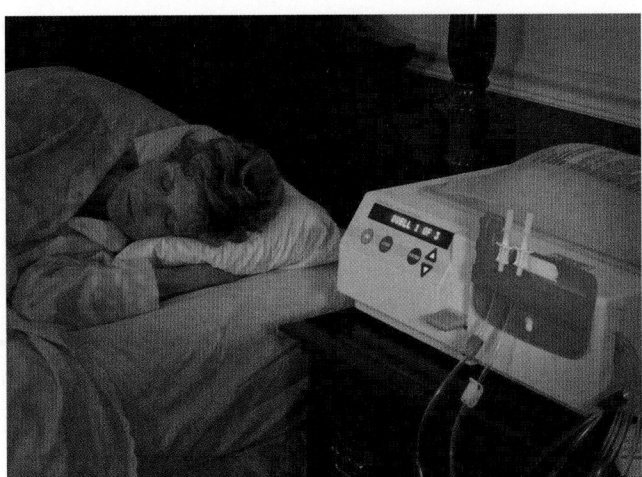

Figure 49-8 Automated peritoneal dialysis cycler, which can be used while the patient is sleeping at night or for hospitalized patients who require frequent exchanges.

Source: Courtesy Baxter Healthcare Corporation, McGaw Park, Illinois.

hypertriglyceridemia, hyperglycemia, and long-term peritoneal membrane dysfunction. The amount of dextrose in the solution varies among 0.5%, 1.5%, 2.5%, and 4.25% depending on the fluid volume goal. Alternate osmotic agents include icodextrin and amino acid solutions.

Peritoneal Dialysis Systems

Two types of PD currently being used are automated peritoneal dialysis (APD) and continuous ambulatory peritoneal dialysis (CAPD).

Automated Peritoneal Dialysis. Automated peritoneal dialysis (APD), also called *continuous cycling peritoneal dialysis,* is a popular form of PD that is done while the patient sleeps. An automated device called a *cycler* is used to perform the dialysis exchanges (Figure 49-8). The automated cycler times and controls the fill, dwell, and drain phases. The machine cycles four or more exchanges per night with 1 to 2 hours per exchange. Alarms and monitors are built into the system to make it safe for the patient to dialyze while sleeping. The patient disconnects from the machine in the morning and usually leaves fluid in the abdomen during the day. One to two daytime manual exchanges may also be prescribed to ensure adequate dialysis.

Continuous Ambulatory Peritoneal Dialysis. Continuous ambulatory peritoneal dialysis (CAPD) is a type of PD that is done during the day and consists of a minimum of four exchanges of dialysis fluid per day. CAPD exchanges are carried out manually by exchanging 1.5 to 3 L of peritoneal dialysate at least four times daily, with dwell times averaging 4 hours. For example, one schedule starts the exchanges at 7 A.M., 12 noon, 5 P.M., and 10 P.M.

Dialysis fluid is instilled into the peritoneal cavity and remains (dwells) there for a specified period, allowing for the removal of waste products and excess fluid; it is then drained and fresh fluid is instilled. It is continuous in that dialysis fluid is always in the peritoneal cavity so dialysis is continuously going on. After the equilibration period, the dialysate (effluent) is drained from the peritoneal cavity, and a new 2-L bag of

dialysate solution is infused. It is critical in PD to maintain aseptic technique to avoid peritonitis. Several tubing connections and devices are commercially available to help maintain an aseptic system.

Potential contraindications for PD include the following:
1. History of multiple abdominal surgical procedures or severe abdominal pathological condition (e.g., severe pancreatitis, diverticulitis).
2. Recurrent abdominal wall or inguinal hernias.
3. Excessive obesity with large abdominal wall and fat deposits.
4. Pre-existing vertebral disease (e.g., chronic back problems).
5. Severe obstructive pulmonary disease.

Complications of Peritoneal Dialysis

Exit-Site Infection. Infection of the peritoneal catheter exit site is most commonly caused by *Staphylococcus aureus* or *Staphylococcus epidermidis* (from skin flora). Superficial exit-site infections caused by these organisms are generally resolved with antibiotic therapy. Clinical manifestations of an exit-site infection include redness at the site, tenderness, and drainage. If not treated immediately, subcutaneous tunnel infections usually result in abscess formation and may cause peritonitis, necessitating catheter removal.

Peritonitis. Peritonitis results from contamination or from progression of an exit-site or tunnel infection. Most frequently peritonitis occurs because of improper technique in making or breaking connections for exchanges. Less commonly, peritonitis results from bacteria in the intestine crossing over into the peritoneal cavity. Peritonitis is usually caused by *S. aureus* or *S. epidermidis.*

The primary clinical manifestation of peritonitis is a cloudy peritoneal effluent that has a WBC count of over $0.1 \times 10^9/L$ (particularly neutrophils) or demonstration of bacteria in the peritoneal effluent by Gram stain or culture. GI manifestations may also be present, including diffuse abdominal pain, diarrhea, vomiting, abdominal distension, and hyperactive bowel sounds. Fever may or may not be present. Cultures, Gram stain, and a cell count with WBC differential of the peritoneal effluent are used to confirm the diagnosis of peritonitis. Antibiotics can be given by mouth or by IV or intraperitoneal route. The patient is usually treated on an outpatient basis. Repeated infections may necessitate the removal of the peritoneal catheter and termination of PD. The formation of adhesions in the peritoneum can result from repeated infections and interferes with the peritoneal membrane's ability to act as a dialyzing surface.

Abdominal Pain. Although not severe, pain is a common complication caused by the low pH of the dialysate solution, peritonitis, intraperitoneal irritation (which usually subsides in 1 to 2 weeks), and placement of the catheter. Pain can also occur when the tip of the catheter touches the bladder, the bowel, or the peritoneum. A change in the position of the catheter should correct this problem. Accidental infusion of air or infusing the dialysate too rapidly may cause referred pain in the shoulder. If the infusion rate is decreased, the pain usually subsides.

Outflow Problems. It is expected that at least 80% of the volume instilled in the peritoneal cavity is returned when draining the cavity after an exchange. Causes of poor outflow include constipation, a kink in the catheter or transfer set, omentum wrapped around the catheter, and migration of the catheter out of the pelvic region. Laxatives and stool softeners can be used to relieve constipation and promote regular bowel movements. Outflow problems related to omental entrapment or migration may necessitate radiological intervention, surgical manipulation of the catheter, or both.

Hernias. Because of increased intra-abdominal pressure secondary to the dialysate infusion, umbilical or inguinal hernias or diastasis recti can develop in predisposed individuals such as multiparous women and older men. However, in most situations after hernia repair, PD can be resumed after several days using small dialysate volumes and keeping the patient supine.

Lower Back Problems. Increased intra-abdominal pressure can cause or aggravate lower back pain. The lumbosacral curvature is increased by intraperitoneal infusion of dialysate. Orthopedic binders and a regular exercise program for strengthening the back muscles have been beneficial for some patients.

Bleeding. Effluent drained after the first few exchanges may be pink or slightly bloody because of the trauma of catheter insertion. Bloody effluent over several days or the new appearance of blood in the effluent can indicate active intraperitoneal bleeding. If this occurs, BP and hemoglobin should be checked. Blood may also be present in the effluent of women who are menstruating or ovulating; this necessitates no intervention.

Pulmonary Complications. Atelectasis, pneumonia, and bronchitis may occur from repeated upward displacement of the diaphragm, resulting in decreased lung expansion. The longer the dwell time, the greater the likelihood of pulmonary problems. Frequent repositioning and deep-breathing exercises can help. When the patient is lying in bed, elevation of the head of the bed may prevent these problems.

Protein Loss. The peritoneal membrane is permeable to plasma proteins, amino acids, and polypeptides. These substances are lost in the dialysate fluid. The amount of loss may be as much as 5 to 15 g/day. This loss may increase to up to 40 g/day during episodes of peritonitis as the membrane becomes more permeable. Positive nitrogen balance can be maintained with adequate protein intake.

Carbohydrate and Lipid Abnormalities. Dialysate glucose is absorbed via the peritoneum in quantities that may be as high as 100 to 150 g/day. Continuous absorption of glucose results in increased insulin secretion and increased plasma insulin levels. The hyperinsulinemia stimulates hepatic production of triglycerides.

Effectiveness of and Adaptation to Chronic Peritoneal Dialysis

Learning the self-management skills required to do PD involves a relatively short training program. PD provides independence and flexibility with treatment, and travelling is easier. A major advantage of PD is its simplicity and that it is a home-based treatment that allows the patient to be in control.

Clinically, the patient receiving PD does as well as the patient receiving HD and sometimes better. There are fewer dietary restrictions, and greater mobility is possible than with conventional HD. The major disadvantage is the possibility of developing peritonitis.

PD is especially indicated for the individual who has vascular access problems or responds poorly to the hemodynamic stresses of HD (e.g., the older adult patient with diabetes and cardiovascular disease). The diabetic patient with ESRD does better with PD than with HD. The advantages of PD for the diabetic patient include better BP control, less hemodynamic instability because fluid shifts are gradual, and prevention of retinal hemorrhage because heparin is not required as it is in HD.

Hemodialysis

HD is a method of removing waste products and excess fluid from the blood using a machine to pump the blood through an artificial semipermeable membrane (dialyzer).

Vascular Access Sites for Hemodialysis

Obtaining vascular access is one of the greatest challenges associated with HD. To carry out HD, a very rapid blood flow is required, and access to a large blood vessel is essential. The types of vascular access in current use include arteriovenous fistulas (AVFs) and grafts (AVGs), and tunnelled and nontunnelled central venous catheters (CVCs). AVFs are superior to synthetic AVGs and CVCs and are associated with better long-term survival, lower infection and complication rates, and lower health care expenditure (Gilpin & Nichols, 2010; Jindal et al., 2006).

Arteriovenous Fistulas and Grafts. A native **arteriovenous fistula (AVF)** is the preferred HD access created by surgically connecting a vein and an artery, usually in the forearm (Gilpin & Nichols, 2010; Jindal et al., 2006) (Figures 49-9, *A* and 49-10). The preferred sites for creating an AVF are the wrist (radiocephalic) and the elbow (brachiocephalic) (Gilpin & Nichols, 2010). The fistula provides for arterial blood flow through the vein. The increased pressure of the arterial blood flow through the vein causes the vein to dilate and become tough, making it amenable to repeated venipuncture. The vein is accessed using two large-gauge needles.

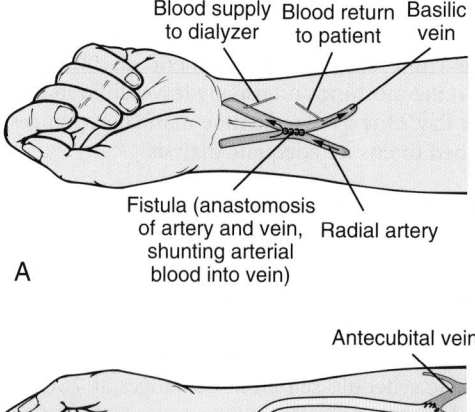

Figure 49-9 Vascular access for hemodialysis. **A,** Arteriovenous fistula. **B,** Arteriovenous graft.

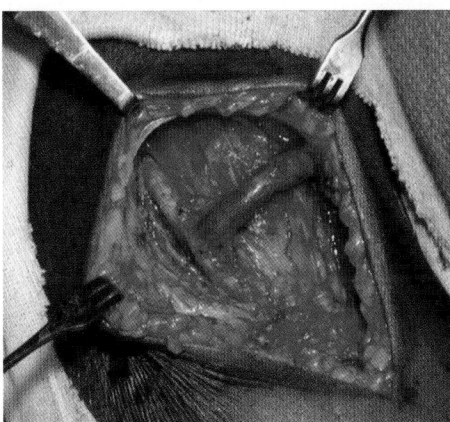

Figure 49-10 Arteriovenous fistula created by anastomosing an artery and a vein.

Source: Courtesy Dr. Stephen Van Voorst, MD.

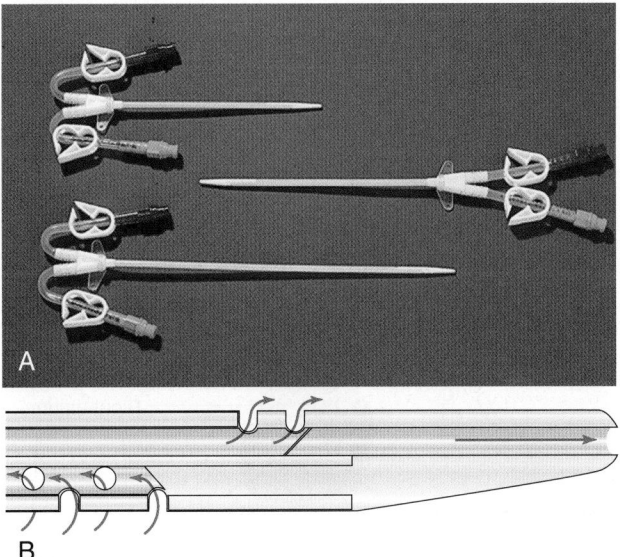

Figure 49-11 Temporary double-lumen vascular access catheter for acute hemodialysis. **A,** Soft, flexible dual-lumen tube is attached to a Y hub. **B,** Blood is withdrawn continuously through the red lumen (upstream) and returned through the blue lumen (downstream), thus reducing recirculation.

Source: **A,** Courtesy Quinton Instrument Co., Seattle, Washington.

AVFs have the best overall patency rates and the least number of complications (e.g., thrombosis, infection) of all vascular accesses. The CSN *Clinical Practice Guidelines for Vascular Access* suggest that the AVF should be created at least 3 to 4 months before starting dialysis (Jindal et al., 2006). The AVF requires 4 to 6 weeks, and preferably 3 months, to mature (dilate and toughen) sufficiently for use. AVFs are more difficult to create in people with severe peripheral vascular disease, diabetes, prolonged IV drug use, or previous multiple IV procedures in the forearm. For these individuals, a synthetic graft may be required.

An **arteriovenous graft (AVG)** is an HD access created with a synthetic graft that is attached to an artery and a vein. It is used for people who do not have suitable vessels for an AVF. The preferred site for a synthetic graft is a forearm, using a curved loop radiocephalic graft. The graft is a surgically created anastomosis between an artery (usually radial) and a vein (usually cephalic) (see Figure 49-9, *B*). An interval of 3 to 6 weeks is usually necessary to allow the graft to heal, but some centres may use it earlier (Jindal et al., 2006). The graft, like the fistula, is under the skin and is accessed using two large-gauge needles. The graft material is self-healing, meaning it should close over any puncture site after the needle is removed. Infections in other parts of the body can result in infection and damage to the graft and have a tendency to be thrombogenic (Gilpin & Nichols, 2010, p. 82).

Normally, a *thrill* can be felt by palpating the area of anastomosis, and a bruit can be heard with a stethoscope. The bruit and the thrill are created by the turbulence of arterial blood rushing into the vein. BPs, IV insertion, and venipuncture should not be performed on an extremity with an AVF or AVG. This is to prevent thrombosis and infection in the vascular access. Protection of the vascular access site is of paramount importance.

The AVF is much less likely to clot and become infected than a graft. Thrombosis in AVGs is common but can often be corrected using interventional radiology techniques or a surgical procedure. AVFs and AVGs can cause the development of distal ischemia (steal syndrome) because too much of the arterial blood is being shunted or "stolen" from the distal extremity. This is usually seen soon after surgery and may require surgical correction. Aneurysms can also develop at the fistula site and can rupture if left untreated. AVG infections are not uncommon, and immediate treatment is essential to salvage the graft and prevent bacteremia. Severe AVG infections may necessitate graft removal.

Central Venous Catheters. In some situations when immediate vascular access is required, a temporary CVC is placed by percutaneous cannulation of the internal jugular or the femoral vein. Internal jugular vein cannulation is associated with a low incidence of thrombosis, which is the primary reason this method is preferred over subclavian cannulation. In addition to vessel thrombosis and stenosis, subclavian vein cannulation has been associated with pneumothorax and brachial plexus; therefore, this site should be used as a last resort. A flexible Teflon, silicone rubber, or polyurethane catheter can be inserted at the bedside into the internal jugular vein and provides access to circulation without surgery (Figure 49-11, *A*). The catheters usually have a double external lumen with an internal septum separating the two internal segments (see Figure 49-11, *B*). One lumen is used for blood removal and the other for blood return. Femoral catheters should be sutured into place and can be left in place as long as there are no complications (Jindal et al., 2006).

Disadvantages of femoral vessel cannulation include the following: (1) the location encourages catheter kinking and (2) the groin is not a clean site. Potential complications of femoral catheterization are femoral vein thrombosis with pulmonary emboli (especially if the treatment is prolonged), infections, immobility, and inadvertent blood vessel punctures with hematoma formation. Temporary catheters are generally stiff and inflexible. They can cause trauma to the vessel, so bed rest is recommended. Temporary catheters in the internal jugular vein should be sutured in place and should be replaced as soon as possible by a tunnelled catheter that can be left in place for several weeks. Proper catheter position should be confirmed using radiography before use (Jindal et al., 2006). Temporary catheters are generally left in place only for short periods or until a tunnelled catheter can be inserted.

Tunnelled catheters, which are soft and flexible, may be an option for patients who have exhausted all other vascular access

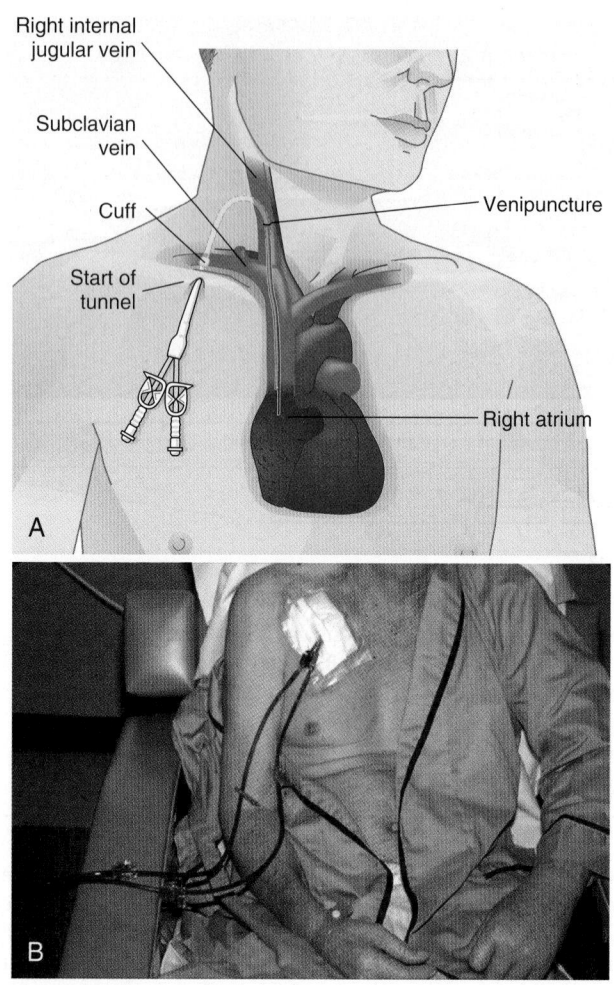

Figure 49-12 A, Right internal jugular placement for a tunnelled, cuffed semipermanent catheter. **B,** Long-term cuffed hemodialysis catheter.

Source: **B,** Courtesy Dr. Stephen Van Voorst, MD.

sites. These catheters can be used as temporary access while awaiting fistula placement and development or as long-term access when other forms of access have failed. This type of catheter exits on the upper chest wall and is tunnelled subcutaneously to the internal jugular vein (Figure 49-12). The catheter tip rests in the right atrium. It has one or two subcutaneous Dacron cuffs that prevent infection from tracking along the catheter and anchor the catheter, eliminating the need for sutures.

For CVCs, no drugs should be administered or blood withdrawn via the catheter by nondialysis staff. This is to minimize the risk of infection, catheter loss, and accidental injection of heparin. Trained dialysis staff will instill heparin into the lumens of the catheter at the end of each treatment to ensure patency and withdraw it before the next treatment.

Dialyzers

The dialyzer is a long plastic cartridge that contains thousands of parallel hollow tubes or fibres (Figure 49-13). The fibres are the semipermeable membrane made of cellulose-based or other synthetic materials. The blood is pumped into the top of the cartridge and is dispersed into all of the fibres. Dialysis fluid

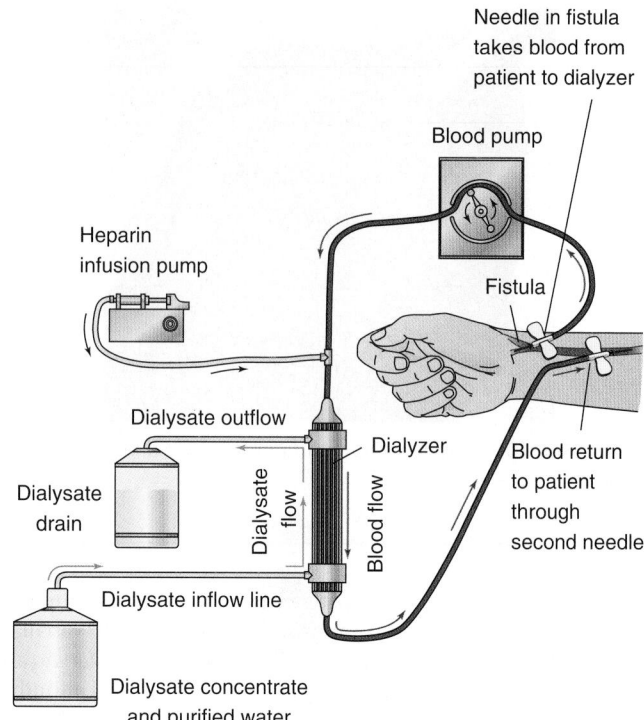

Figure 49-13 Components of a hemodialysis system. Blood is removed via a needle inserted in a fistula or via catheter lumen. It is propelled to the dialyzer by a blood pump. Heparin is infused to prevent clotting. Dialysate is pumped in and flows in the opposite direction of the blood. The dialyzed blood is returned to the patient through a second needle or catheter lumen. Old dialysate and ultrafiltrate are drained and discarded.

(dialysate) is pumped into the bottom of the cartridge and bathes the outside of the fibres with dialysis fluid. Ultrafiltration, diffusion, and osmosis occur across the pores of this semipermeable membrane. When the dialyzed blood reaches the end of the semipermeable fibres, it converges into a single tube that returns it to the patient. Dialyzers available differ in regard to surface area, membrane composition and thickness, clearance of waste products, and removal of fluid.

Procedure

To initiate chronic dialysis in a patient with an AVG or AVF, two needles are placed in the fistula or graft. One needle is used to draw blood from the patient and circulate it through the extracorporeal circuit and dialyzer, and the other needle is used to return the blood. If the patient has a catheter, the two blood lines are attached to the two catheter lumens and blood is circulated through the dialysis blood circuit similar to that of the AVF and is sent to the dialyzer with the assistance of a blood pump. Heparin is added to the blood as it flows into the dialyzer because any time blood contacts a foreign substance it has a tendency to clot. When the blood enters the extracorporeal circuit, it is propelled through the top of the dialyzer by a blood pump at a flow rate of 200 to 500 mL/min, while the dialysate circulates in the opposite direction at a rate of 300 to 900 mL/min. Blood is returned from the dialyzer to the patient through the second needle or the blue (venous) catheter lumen.

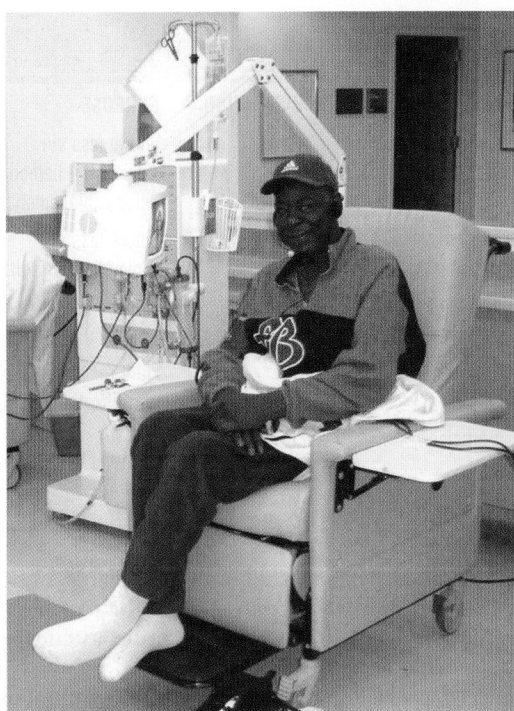

Figure 49-14 Patient receiving in-centre hemodialysis.

Source: Courtesy Vascular Access Services, LLC, St. Louis, Missouri.

In addition to the dialyzer, there is a dialysate delivery and monitoring system (Figure 49-14). This system pumps the dialysate through the dialyzer in the direction opposite the blood flow.

Before beginning treatment, the nurse must complete an assessment of the patient that includes fluid status (weight, BP, peripheral edema, lung and heart sounds), condition of vascular access, temperature, and general skin condition. The difference between the last postdialysis weight and the present predialysis weight represents the amount of fluid weight gained since the last treatment. This information is used to determine the ultrafiltration or the amount of fluid to be removed. Each kilogram represents approximately 1 L of fluid. Ideally, no more than 1 to 1.5 kg should be gained between treatments to prevent the hypotension associated with the removal of larger volumes of fluid. Many patients gain 2 to 3 kg between treatments, and this volume usually can be removed if their BP is not labile. While the patient is on dialysis, vital signs should be taken at least every 30 to 60 minutes because rapid changes may occur in the BP.

Most maintenance dialysis units use reclining chairs that allow for elevation of the feet if hypotension develops. Most people sleep, read, talk, or watch television during dialysis. Treatments usually last 3 to 5 hours and are done a minimum of three times per week to achieve adequate clearance and maintain fluid balance.

Settings for Hemodialysis.

HD units and treatments are performed in a variety of settings. Acutely ill patients may require dialysis in the CCU setting. Most large teaching hospitals in Canada have dialysis units that accommodate patients who are in hospital as well as a chronic outpatient population. Many satellite and outpatient clinics provide chronic HD treatments. The patient may choose to do self-care with backup support from trained personnel if needed. Self-care patients generally put in their dialysis needles, set up the machine, and

monitor the course of their treatment. Patients receiving HD are able to travel if dialysis treatments can be arranged at another dialysis unit.

Dialysis done at home is an optimal option for patients requiring RRT. Treatments are more cost effective and have many benefits for the patient (Harwood & Leitch, 2006). HD can also be done at home. Today, almost 1.3% of patients receiving HD use it at home (Harwood & Leitch, 2006). One of the main advantages of home HD is that it allows greater freedom in choosing dialysis times. Some modifications for a special electrical outlet, plumbing, and water treatment are necessary to accommodate the HD machine in the home setting.

Complications of Hemodialysis

Hypotension. Hypotension that occurs during HD primarily results from rapid removal of vascular volume (hypovolemia), decreased cardiac output, and decreased systemic intravascular resistance. The drop in BP during dialysis may precipitate light-headedness, nausea, vomiting, seizures, vision changes, and chest pain from cardiac ischemia. The usual treatment for hypotension includes decreasing the volume of fluid being removed and infusion of 0.9% saline solution (100-300 mL). If a patient experiences recurrent hypotensive episodes, a reassessment may have to be done of dry weight and BP drugs. BP drugs should be held before dialysis if there are frequent episodes of hypotension during dialysis.

Muscle Cramps. Painful muscle cramps are a common problem. They result from rapid removal of sodium and water or from neuromuscular hypersensitivity. Treatment includes reducing the ultrafiltration rate and infusing hypertonic saline or a normal saline bolus. The nurse should also educate the patient about restricting salt and fluid in the diet to reduce weight gains between dialysis treatments.

Loss of Blood. Blood loss may result from blood not being completely rinsed from the dialyzer, accidental separation of blood tubing, dialysis membrane rupture, or bleeding after the removal of needles at the end of dialysis. If a patient has received too much heparin or has clotting problems, there can be significant postdialysis bleeding. It is essential to rinse back all blood, to closely monitor heparinization to prevent excess anticoagulation, and to hold firm but nonocclusive pressure on access sites until the risk of bleeding has passed.

Hepatitis. The causes of hepatitis B and C in dialysis patients include blood transfusions or the lack of adherence to precautions used to prevent the spread of infection. Because blood is now screened for hepatitis B and C, blood is an unlikely source of infection. IV drug use and unprotected sex can also contribute to the incidence of hepatitis in the dialysis population. The incidence of hepatitis B has decreased with frequent testing for hepatitis B surface antigen in patients, isolation of dialysis patients who are positive for hepatitis B, and the use of disposable equipment, the hepatitis B vaccine, and infection control precautions. All patients and personnel in dialysis units should receive hepatitis B vaccine.

Currently, hepatitis C is responsible for the majority of cases of hepatitis in dialysis patients. (Hepatitis is discussed in more detail in Chapter 46.) The CSN recommendations for the *Prevention of Transmission of Blood-Borne Pathogens in Hemodialysis Patients* suggests that isolation of the HD patient who has hepatitis C is not required; however, strict adherence to good infection practice is required to prevent transmission in HD units (Burns et al., 2005). (Infection control precautions are discussed in Chapter 17.) Currently, no vaccine is available for hepatitis C.

Sepsis. Sepsis is most often related to infections of vascular access sites. Bacteria can also be introduced during the dialysis treatment as a result of poor technique or interruption of blood tubing or dialyzer membranes. Bacterial endocarditis can occur because of the frequent and prolonged access to the vascular system. Aseptic technique is essential to prevent this problem. Nurses must monitor patients for signs and symptoms of sepsis such as fever, hypotension, and an elevated WBC count.

Disequilibrium Syndrome. *Disequilibrium syndrome* is a rare complication of modern HD and develops as a result of very rapid changes in the composition of the extracellular fluid. Urea, sodium, and other solutes are removed more rapidly from the blood than from the cerebrospinal fluid and the brain. This creates a high osmotic gradient in the brain resulting in the shift of fluid into the brain, causing cerebral edema. Manifestations include nausea, vomiting, confusion, restlessness, headaches, twitching and jerking, and seizures. The rapid changes in osmolality may cause muscle cramps and worsen hypotension. Treatment consists of slowing or stopping dialysis and infusing hypertonic saline solution, albumin, or mannitol to draw fluid from the brain cells back into the systemic circulation. It is more commonly observed in the initial treatment of the patient when the BUN level is high. First dialysis treatment sessions are purposely short with limited total solute removal to prevent this rare syndrome.

Effectiveness of and Adaptation to Hemodialysis

HD is still an imperfect technique to treat stage 5 CKD. It cannot fully replace the metabolic and hormonal functions of the kidneys. It can ease many of the symptoms of CKD and, if started early, can prevent certain complications. It does not alter the accelerated atherosclerosis.

The 5-year survival rate for patients receiving maintenance HD is 41.4% (CIHI, 2011a). Age and primary diagnosis are associated with survival of dialysis patients. The 5-year survival rate is 24% for those age 75 and older, whereas patients with renal vascular disease and diabetes have a 5-year survival rate of 35% and 38%, respectively (CIHI, 2011a).

Individual adaptation to maintenance HD varies considerably. Initially, many patients feel positive about the dialysis because it makes them feel better and keeps them alive, but there is often great ambivalence about whether it is worthwhile. Dependence on a machine is a reality, and some have dreams about being tied to the machine. In response to their illness, patients undergoing dialysis may demonstrate nonadherence to medical therapy, depression, and suicidal tendencies. The primary nursing goals are to help the patient regain or maintain positive self-esteem and control of her or his life and continue to be productive in society.

Continuous Renal Replacement Therapy

Continuous renal replacement therapy (CRRT) is an alternative or adjunctive method for treating AKI. It provides a means by which uremic toxins and fluids are removed from a hemody-

Table 49-13 Types of Continuous Renal Replacement Therapies

THERAPIES	ABBREVIATION	PURPOSE
Continuous venovenous hemofiltration*	CVVH	Solute loss via convection; hemodilution using replacement fluid
Continuous venovenous hemodialysis*	CVVHD	Solute loss via convection and diffusion
Continuous venovenous hemodiafiltration	CVVHDF	—
Slow continuous ultrafiltration	SCUF	Fluid removal via ultrafiltration
Slow low-efficiency dialysis	SLED	—

*Most commonly used therapies.

namically unstable patient, while acid–base status and electrolytes are adjusted slowly and continuously. The patients selected are usually those who do not respond to dietary interventions and pharmacological agents.

Various types of CRRT are available such as continuous venovenous hemofiltration (CVVH), continuous venovenous hemodialysis (CVVHD), and continuous venovenous hemodiafiltration (CVVHDF) (Claure-Del Grando, Macedo, & Mehta, 2012) (Table 49-13). Various hybrid modalities that combine aspects of conventional HD and CRRT can be used and are determined based on the needs of the patient. Some common hybrid modalities include slow low-efficiency dialysis (SLED) and slow continuous ultrafiltration (SCUF) (Claure-Del Grando et al., 2012).

Vascular access for CRRT is achieved through the use of a double-lumen catheter (as used in HD, noted in Figure 49-13, *A* on p. 1356) placed in the femoral or the jugular vein. The subclavian vein should be used only if no other access site is available, owing to the increased complication rates of pneumothorax, hemorrhage, and stenosis (Claure-Del Grando et al., 2012). Under the influence of hydrostatic pressure and osmotic pressure, water and nonprotein solutes pass out of the filter into the extracapillary space and drain through the ultrafiltrate port into a collection device (Foley bag) (Figure 49-15). The remaining fluid continues through the filter and returns to the patient via the return port of the double-lumen catheter. While the ultrafiltrate drains out of the hemofilter, fluid and electrolyte replacements can be infused into the infusion port located after the filter as the blood returns to the patient. This fluid is designed to replace volume and solutes such as sodium, chloride, bicarbonate, and glucose. It will also further dilute intravascular fluid, decreasing the concentration of unwanted solutes such as BUN, creatinine, and potassium. The infusion rate of replacement fluid is determined by the degree of the fluid and electrolyte imbalance. Replacement fluid may also be infused into the infusion port before the hemofilter. This method allows for greater clearance of urea and can decrease filter clotting.

Anticoagulation (e.g., heparin) is needed to prevent blood clotting during CRRT. Heparin dosage is based on the patient's activated clotting time (ACT), partial prothrombin time (PPT), or prothrombin time (PT).

Several features of CRRT differ from those of HD:
1. It is continuous rather than intermittent. Large volumes of fluid can be removed over days (24 hr to >2 wk) versus hours (3 to 4 hr).

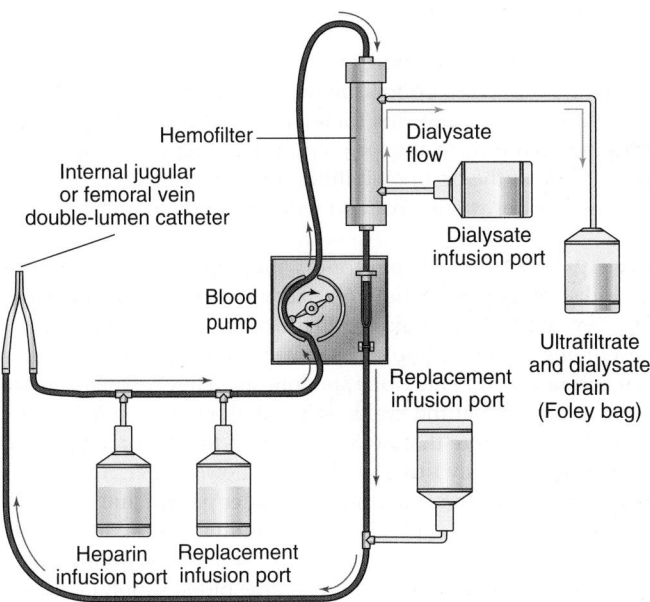

Figure 49-15 Basic schematic of continuous venovenous therapies. Blood pump is required to pump blood through the circuit. Replacement ports are used for continuous venovenous hemofiltration (CVVH) and continuous venovenous hemodialysis (CVVHD) only; replacements can be given prefilter or postfilter. Dialysate port is used for CVVHD only. Regardless of modality, ultrafiltrate is drained via the ultrafiltration drain port.

2. Solute removal can occur by convection (no dialysate required) in addition to osmosis and diffusion.
3. It causes less hemodynamic instability (e.g., hypotension).
4. It does not require constant monitoring by a specialized HD nurse but does require a trained CCU nurse.
5. It does not require complicated HD equipment, but a blood pump is needed for venovenous therapies.

The type of CRRT is customized to the needs of the patient. Some types involve the use of replacement fluids. Large volumes of fluid may be removed hourly (200-800 mL), and then a portion of this fluid is replaced. The type of fluid replacement is dependent on the stability of the patient's condition and the patient's individualized needs. Ultrafiltration and convective losses occur, and solute concentrations in the blood are diluted with the replacement fluid.

CRRT can be continued as long as 30 to 40 days, but the hemofilter should be changed every 24 to 48 hours because of loss of filtration efficiency and the potential for clotting.

The nurse responsible for the care of the patient with AKI who is receiving CRRT may be a critical care nurse or a nephrology nurse specialist, working in collaboration with other health care providers. Specific nursing interventions include obtaining weights and monitoring and documenting laboratory values daily to ensure adequate fluid and electrolyte balance. Hourly intake–output measurements and monitoring of vital signs and hemodynamic status are essential. Although reductions in central venous pressure and pulmonary artery pressure are expected, there should be little change in mean arterial pressure or cardiac output. Patency of the CRRT system is assessed and maintained, and the patient's vascular access site is cared for to prevent infection. Treatment is discontinued and the vascular access is removed once the patient's ARF is

resolved or there is a decision to withdraw treatment owing to patient deterioration.

Kidney Transplantation

Major progress has been made in organ transplantation since the first kidney transplant was performed in 1954 in Boston between identical twins. The advances made in organ procurement and preservation, surgical techniques, tissue typing and matching, understanding the immune system, immunosuppressant therapy, and preventing and treating rejection have dramatically increased the success of organ transplantation.

The disparity between the supply and the demand for organs is significant. In Canada, over 22,000 patients received dialysis in 2010, representing an increase of 189% since 1991. Over 16,000 patients were living with a kidney transplant, more than double the number in 1991 (CIHI, 2011b). According to CIHI data, 10,641 adult patients received renal transplants between 2000 and 2009. Transplantation from a deceased donor usually requires a prolonged waiting period, with median waiting times between 2007 and 2009 of 3.6 years (CIHI, 2011a). By province, the longest median wait time was British Columbia (5.8 years) and the shortest median wait time was in Nova Scotia, at just more than 2 years (CIHI, 2011a).

Kidney transplantation is extremely successful, with 1-year graft survival rates of about 90% for deceased donor transplants and greater than 95% for live donor transplants (CIHI, 2011a). An advantage of kidney transplantation when compared with dialysis is that when normal kidney function is restored, many of the pathophysiological changes associated with renal failure are reversed. It also eliminates the dependence on dialysis and the accompanying dietary and lifestyle restrictions. Transplantation is also less expensive than dialysis after the first year.

Ethical Issues

Transplant health care in Canada is governed by laws and statutes. It is complex and involves many people, professionals, services, functions, and levels of government. Voluntary consent must be given by the donor (Giles, 2005); in some provinces, one can provide advance written consent on a driver's licence or in a will (although permission from the donor's legal next of kin is still required after brain death is determined). In the absence of formal written consent at death, family or significant others can donate organs of the deceased if they had prior knowledge of the donor's intent. Kidneys may be obtained from deceased or live donors. It is illegal to buy or sell organs in Canada. Ethical issues in transplantation are also discussed in Chapter 16 and in the Ethical Dilemmas box.

Recipient Selection

Appropriate recipient selection is important for a successful outcome. Candidacy is determined by a variety of medical and psychosocial factors that vary among transplant centres. A careful evaluation is completed in an attempt to identify and minimize potential complications after transplantation. Certain patients, particularly those with cardiovascular disease and diabetes mellitus, are considered high risk. With careful evaluation and monitoring, high-risk patients can achieve the same success rates as other patients. Some patients who are approaching ESRD can receive a transplant before dialysis is required if they have a living

ETHICAL DILEMMAS
Allocation of Resources

Situation

A transplant nurse coordinator is considering her feelings about two patients who are being evaluated for placement on the deceased donor kidney transplant waiting list. One patient is a 40-year-old school teacher. She is married and has two children. The other patient is a 22-year-old unemployed man who is actively using cocaine. He misses three to four dialysis treatments per month and does not take his phosphate binders or antihypertensive drugs consistently.

Important Points for Consideration

- Psychological, physiological, and adherence factors are included in the assessment process for eligibility for organ transplantation.
- In kidney transplantation, the organ is transplanted into the patient who has received the most points based on a scoring system, regardless of the health care provider's opinion of the patient's worth. If a patient is denied transplant candidacy on this basis, he or she must be given a chance to change or improve the problem or condition in a specified period.
- The national organ procurement system is designed to be unbiased about the patient in all respects. Once a patient is placed on the list for transplantation, that patient is deemed of no greater or lesser worth than any other patient.
- Because organ donation is voluntary in Canada, any concerns that the system of procurement and transplantation is not fair may negatively affect the pool of available organs.

Clinical Decision-Making Questions

1. What guidance is provided by the Canadian Nurses Association (CNA) *Code of Ethics for Registered Nurses* (2008) to help nurses address kidney transplant issues?
2. What are the nurse's feelings about which of the patients should receive the next available organ?

donor. This approach is most advantageous for patients with diabetes, who have a much higher mortality rate on dialysis than people who do not have diabetes.

Contraindications to transplantation include disseminated malignancies, refractory or untreated cardiac disease, chronic respiratory failure, extensive vascular disease, chronic infection, and unresolved psychosocial disorders (e.g., nonadherence to medical regimens, alcoholism, drug addiction). The presence of hepatitis B or C is not a contraindication to transplantation.

Surgical procedures may be required before transplantation based on the results of the recipient evaluation. Coronary artery bypass may be indicated for advanced coronary artery disease. Cholecystectomy may be necessary for patients with a history of gallstones, biliary obstruction, or cholecystitis. On rare occasions, bilateral nephrectomies may be done for patients with refractory hypertension, recurrent urinary tract infections, or grossly enlarged kidneys resulting from polycystic kidney disease.

Histocompatibility Studies

Histocompatibility testing is discussed in Chapter 16.

Donor Sources

Kidneys for transplantation may be obtained from compatible blood–type deceased donors, blood relatives, emotionally related living donors (e.g., spouses, friends), and altruistic living donors who are unknown to the recipient. Expanding the living donor pool is one of the best possibilities for decreasing the size of the deceased donor waiting list and reducing waiting times.

Living Donors. Living donors must undergo an extensive multidisciplinary evaluation to be certain they are in good health and have no history of disease that would place them at risk for developing kidney failure or operative complications. Psychosocial and financial evaluations are done as well. Crossmatches are done at the time of the evaluation and about a week before the transplant to ensure that no antibodies to the donor are present or that the antibody titre is below the allowed level. Advantages of a living donor transplant include better patient and graft survival rates regardless of histocompatibility match, immediate organ availability, immediate function because of minimal cold time (kidney out of body and not getting blood supply), and the opportunity to have the recipient in the best possible medical condition because the surgery is elective.

The potential donor will see a nephrologist for a complete history and physical and laboratory and diagnostic studies. Laboratory studies include a 24-hour urine study for creatinine clearance and total protein, complete blood count, and chemistry and electrolyte profiles. Hepatitis B and C, HIV, and cytomegalovirus (CMV) testing are done to assess for the presence of any transmissible diseases. An ECG and chest radiography are also obtained. A renal ultrasound and a renal arteriogram or three-dimensional CT are performed to ensure that the blood vessels supplying each kidney are adequate and that there are no anomalies and to determine which kidney will be removed.

A transplant psychologist or social worker will determine whether the individual is emotionally stable and able to deal with the issues related to organ donation. All donors must be informed about the risks and benefits of donation, the potential short- and long-term complications, and what can be expected during the hospitalization and recovery phases. Although the cost of the evaluation and surgery are covered by the recipient's insurance, there is no compensation available for lost wages during the posthospitalization recovery period. This period can last 6 weeks or longer.

Incompatibility between a potential transplant recipient and a prospective donor is a major barrier to living donor transplants. **Paired organ donation** is another option that allows a living donor to donate a kidney to a different compatible recipient, with the intent that another donor will donate to the first donor's designated recipient (Gentry, Montgomery, & Segev, 2011, p. 144; Veys & Bramstedt, 2010). In 2009, the Canadian Blood Services launched a pilot project for a living donor paired exchange (LDPE) registry that is now available to every province (The Organ Registry Team [ORT] [Ottawa] & The Organ and Tissue Donation and Transplantation [OTDT] Team [Ottawa and Edmonton], 2011). The registry is designed to facilitate transplants between recipients and living donors who have an incompatible match with other recipient donor pairs in the same situation (ORT & OTDT, 2011). The recipient–donor pairs in the LDPE registry are entered in a complex computer algorithm that identifies opportunities for transplants between them (ORT & OTDT, 2011).

Deceased Donors. Deceased (cadaver) kidney donors are relatively healthy individuals who have suffered an irreversible brain injury with a declaration of brain death. The most common causes of injury are cerebral trauma from motor vehicle accidents or gunshot wounds, intracerebral or subarachnoid hemorrhage, and anoxic brain damage caused by cardiac arrest. The donor must have effective cardiovascular function and be supported on a ventilator to preserve the organs. The age range of most suitable kidney donors is from 2 to 70 years. The age of the donor is less important than the quality of kidney function. The donor must be free of active IV drug use; severe hypertension; longstanding diabetes mellitus; malignancies; sepsis; and communicable diseases, including HIV, hepatitis B and C, syphilis, and tuberculosis. Permission from the donor's legal next of kin is required after brain death is determined, even if the donor carried a signed donor card.

The kidneys are removed and preserved. They can be preserved for up to 72 hours, but most transplant surgeons prefer to transplant kidneys before the cold time reaches 24 hours. Experience has shown that prolonged cold time increases the likelihood that the kidney will not function immediately and the transplant recipient will require dialysis until the ATN from the extended cold time resolves.

In Canada, patients who receive a kidney from deceased donors are selected from provincial waiting lists that use an objective computerized point system. ABO group, human lymphocyte antigen (HLA) typing, age, antibody level, and length of time waiting are entered into the computer matching program for each candidate when they are listed. When a donor becomes available, the donor's HLA data, ABO type, and other key information are compared with the data of all patients awaiting transplantation locally. Donors and recipients must have the same blood type. The kidney is offered to the recipient with the most points. If there are no patients in the local area who are suitable, the organ is then offered in the region, and then to the nation. When a kidney arrives at the recipient's transplant centre, a final crossmatch is done. The final crossmatch must be negative for the deceased donor transplant to proceed. (Crossmatching is discussed in Chapter 16.)

Surgical Procedure

Live Donor. The donor nephrectomy is performed by a urologist or transplant surgeon. The donor's surgery begins an hour or 2 before the recipient's surgery is started. The recipient is surgically prepared for the kidney transplant in a nearby operating room.

Laparoscopic donor nephrectomy is the most common approach to removing a kidney from a living donor. (Laparoscopic nephrectomy is discussed in Chapter 48.) The laparoscopic approach significantly decreases the hospital stay, pain, operative blood loss, debilitation, and length of time off work.

For a conventional nephrectomy, the donor is placed in the lateral decubitus position on the operating table so that the flank is presented laterally. An incision is made at the level of the eleventh rib. The rib may have to be removed to provide adequate visualization of the kidney.

Kidney Transplant Recipient. The transplanted kidney is usually placed extraperitoneally in the iliac fossa. The right iliac fossa is preferred to facilitate anastomoses and minimize the occurrence of ileus.

Before any incisions are made, a urinary catheter is placed into the bladder. An antibiotic solution is instilled to distend the bladder and decrease the risk of infection. A crescent-shaped incision is made, extending from the iliac crest to the symphysis pubis (Figure 49-16). The peritoneum is left intact. The iliac and the hypogastric vessels are dissected free.

Rapid revascularization is critical to prevent ischemic injury to the kidney. The donor artery is anastomosed to the recipient's internal iliac (hypogastric) or external iliac artery. The donor vein is anastomosed to the recipient's external iliac vein. Kidney transplants with living donors can be technically more difficult because the blood vessel lengths can be shorter than in cadaveric transplants.

When the anastomoses are complete, the clamps are released, and blood flow to the kidney is re-established. The kidney should

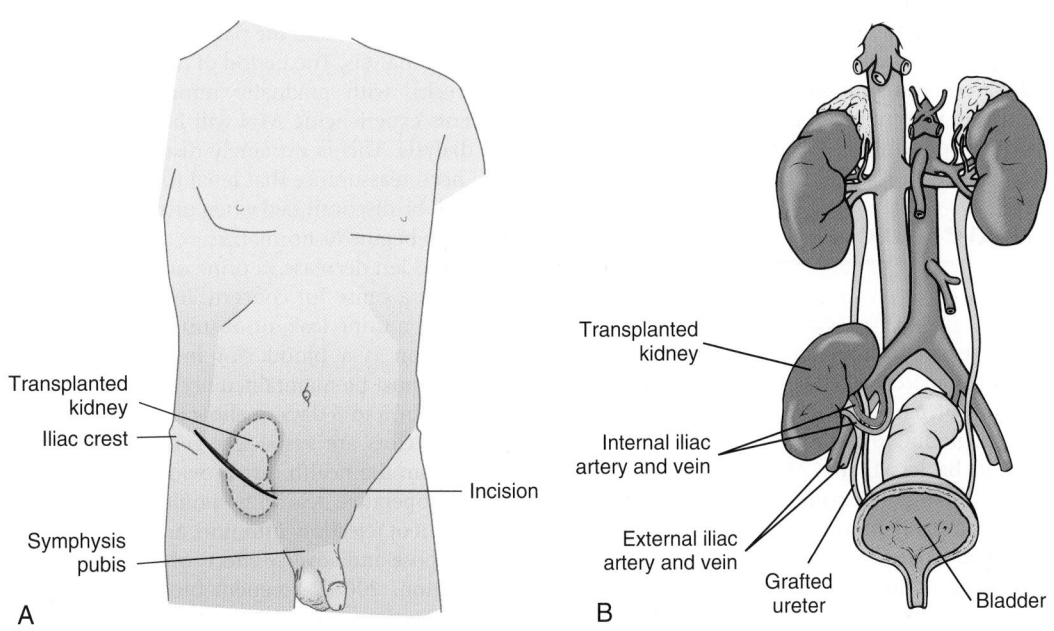

Figure 49-16 A, Surgical incision for a renal transplant. **B,** Surgical placement of a transplanted kidney.

become firm and pink. Urine may begin to flow from the ureter immediately. Mannitol or furosemide (Lasix) may be administered to promote diuresis.

The donor ureter in most cases is then tunnelled through the bladder submucosa before entering the bladder cavity and being sutured in place. This approach is called *ureteroneocystostomy*. This allows the bladder wall to compress the ureter as it contracts for micturition, thereby preventing reflux of urine up the ureter into the transplanted kidney. The transplant surgery takes approximately 3 to 4 hours.

NURSING MANAGEMENT: KIDNEY TRANSPLANT RECIPIENT

The successful recovery and rehabilitation of the recipient are made possible with careful nursing assessment, diagnosis, intervention, and evaluation of all body systems. With a length of hospital stay averaging 4 to 5 days, discharge planning and teaching needs must be identified and addressed early in the hospital course.

▪ Preoperative Care

Nursing care of the patient in the preoperative phase includes emotional and physical preparation for surgery. Because the patient and the family may have been waiting years for the kidney transplant, a review of the operative procedure and what can be expected in the immediate postoperative recovery period is necessary. It is important to stress that there is a chance the kidney may not function immediately and that dialysis may be required for days to weeks. The need for immunosuppressive drugs and measures to prevent infection must be reviewed.

To ensure the patient is in optimal physical condition for surgery, an ECG, chest radiograph, and laboratory studies are ordered. Dialysis may be required before surgery for any significant abnormality such as fluid overload or hyperkalemia. A patient on PD must empty the peritoneal cavity of all dialysate solution before going to surgery. Because dialysis may be required after transplant, the patency of the vascular access must be maintained. The vascular access extremity should be labelled "dialysis access, no procedures" to prevent use of the affected extremity for BP measurement, blood drawing, or IV infusions.

▪ Postoperative Care

▪ Living Donor

The usual postoperative care for the donor is similar to that following conventional or laparoscopic nephrectomy (see Chapter 48). Close monitoring of renal function, to assess for impairment, and of the hemoglobin, to assess for bleeding, is essential. The creatinine should be less than 124 micromol/L, and the hemoglobin should be stable. The pain experienced by a donor who has had a conventional nephrectomy is greater than that of the donor who had a laparoscopic procedure. Generally, all donors have more pain than the recipients. Conventional donors are ready to be discharged from the hospital in 4 to 7 days and can usually return to work in 6 to 8 weeks. Laparoscopic donors are able to be discharged from the hospital in 2 to 4 days and

can return to work in 4 to 6 weeks. The donor is seen by the surgeon 1 to 2 weeks after discharge.

Nurses caring for the living donor need to acknowledge the precious gift that this person has given. The donor has taken physical, emotional, and financial risks to assist the recipient. It is vital that this individual not be forgotten after surgery. The donor will need even greater support if the donated organ does not work immediately or, for some reason, fails.

▪ Kidney Transplant Recipient

The first priority during this period is maintenance of fluid and electrolyte balance. In some centres, kidney transplant recipients spend the first 12 to 24 hours in the CCU because of the close monitoring required. Very large volumes of urine may be produced soon after the blood supply to the transplanted kidney is re-established. This diuresis is owing to (1) the new kidney's ability to filter BUN, which acts as an osmotic diuretic; (2) the abundance of fluids administered during the operation; and (3) initial renal tubular dysfunction, which inhibits the kidney from concentrating urine normally. Urine output during this phase may be as high as 1 L/hr and gradually decreases as the BUN and creatinine levels become more normal. Urine output is replaced millilitre for millilitre hourly for the first 12 to 24 hours. Central venous pressure readings are essential for monitoring postoperative fluid status. Dehydration must be prevented to prevent subsequent renal hypoperfusion and renal tubular damage. Electrolyte monitoring is critical to assess for the hyponatremia and hypokalemia often associated with rapid diuresis. Treatment with potassium supplements or 0.9% normal saline solution infusion may be indicated. IV sodium bicarbonate may also be required if the patient becomes acidotic.

ATN is becoming more common because of prolonged cold times and the use of marginal deceased donors (those who are medically suboptimal). The ischemic damage from extended cold times causes ATN. While ATN is present, dialysis may be required to maintain fluid and electrolyte balance. If high-output ATN is present, the ability to excrete fluid is intact, but not the ability to regulate metabolic wastes or electrolytes. If oliguric or anuric ATN is present, there is risk of fluid overload in the immediate postoperative period, and the patient must be assessed closely for the need for dialysis. The period of ATN can last anywhere from days to weeks, with gradually improving kidney function. Most patients experiencing ATN will be discharged from the hospital on dialysis. This is extremely discouraging for the patient, who will need reassurance that renal function usually improves. Dialysis will be discontinued when urine output increases and kidney function begins to normalize.

A sudden decrease in urine output in the early postoperative period is a cause for concern. It may be owing to dehydration, rejection, a urine leak, or obstruction. A common cause of early obstruction is a blood clot in the urinary catheter. Catheter patency must be maintained because the catheter remains in the bladder for 3 to 5 days to allow the bladder anastomosis to heal. If blood clots are suspected, gentle catheter irrigation with an order from the health care provider can re-establish patency.

Postoperative teaching should include the prevention and treatment of rejection, infection, and complications of surgery and the purpose and adverse effects of immunosuppression (Alleman & Longton, 2008). Frequent blood tests and clinic visits help detect rejection early. Patient education to ensure a smooth transition from hospital to home is an integral part of the nursing care.

Immunosuppressive Therapy

The goal of immunosuppression is to adequately suppress the immune response to prevent rejection of the transplanted kidney while maintaining sufficient immunity to prevent overwhelming infection. Immunosuppressive therapy is discussed in Chapter 16 and in Table 16-15.

Complications of Transplantation

Rejection. Rejection is one of the major problems following kidney transplantation. Rejection can be hyperacute or acute or chronic. These types of rejection are discussed in Chapter 16 on p. 306. Prevention and early diagnosis of rejection is essential for long-term graft function.

Infection. Infection remains a significant cause of morbidity and mortality after transplantation (Ding, 2010). The transplant recipient is at risk for infection because of suppression of the body's normal defence mechanisms by surgery, immunosuppressive drugs, and the effects of ESRD. Underlying systemic illness such as diabetes mellitus or systemic lupus erythematosus, malnutrition, and older age can further compound the negative effects on the immune response. At times, the signs and symptoms of infection can be subtle. Nurses caring for transplant recipients must be astute in their observation and assessment because prompt diagnosis and treatment of infections will improve patient outcomes.

The most common infections observed in the first month after transplantation are similar to those acquired by any postoperative patient, such as pneumonia, wound infections, IV line and drain infections, and urinary tract infections. Fungal and viral infections are not uncommon because of the patient's immunosuppressed state. Fungal infections can include *Candida, Cryptococcus, Aspergillus,* and *Pneumocystis jiroveci*. Fungal infections are difficult to treat, require prolonged treatment periods, and often involve the administration of nephrotoxic drugs. Transplant recipients usually receive prophylactic antifungal drugs to prevent these infections, such as nystatin (Mycostatin), fluconazole (Diflucan), and sulphamethoxazole-trimethoprim (Septra DS).

Viral infections including CMV, Epstein-Barr virus, herpes simplex virus (HSV), varicella-zoster virus, and polyomavirus (e.g., BK virus) can be primary or reactivation of existing disease (Ding, 2010). Primary infections occur as new infections after transplantation from an exogenous source such as the donated organ or blood transfusion. Reactivation occurs when a virus exists in a patient and becomes reactivated after transplantation because of immunosuppression.

CMV is one of the most common viral infections. If a recipient has never had CMV and receives an organ from a donor with a history of CMV, antiviral prophylaxis will be administered (IV ganciclovir, valganciclovir [Valcyte]). If a primary active CMV infection is diagnosed or there is symptomatic reactivation of CMV, IV ganciclovir will be given along with an immune globulin that contains CMV antibodies. To prevent HSV infections, oral acyclovir is given for several months after the transplant.

Cardiovascular Disease. Transplant recipients have an increased incidence of atherosclerotic vascular disease. Cardiovascular disease is the leading cause of death after renal transplantation (Murphy, 2011). Hypertension, dyslipidemia, diabetes mellitus, smoking, rejection, infections, and increased homocysteine levels can all contribute to cardiovascular disease. Immunosuppressants can worsen hypertension and dyslipidemia. It is important that the patient be taught to control risk factors such as elevated cholesterol, triglycerides, and blood glucose and weight gain. Adherence to the prescribed antihypertensive and dyslipidemia regimen is essential not only to prevent cardiovascular events but also to prevent damage to the new kidney. (Hypertension is discussed in Chapter 35.)

Malignancies. The overall incidence of malignancies in kidney transplant recipients is about 6%, which is 100 times greater than in the general population. The primary cause of this increased incidence is the immunosuppressive therapy. Not only do immunosuppressants suppress the immune system, but they also suppress the ability to fight infection and the production of abnormal cells such as cancer cells. The malignancies include cancers of the skin, lips, kidney, hepatobiliary system, vulva, and perineum; lymphomas; and Kaposi's sarcoma and other sarcomas. Regular screening for cancer is an important part of the transplant recipient's preventive care. The patient must also be advised to avoid sun exposure by using protective clothing and sunscreens to minimize the incidence of skin cancers and to check the skin regularly and report any suspicious lesions.

Recurrence of Original Renal Disease. Recurrence of the original disease that destroyed the native kidneys occurs in some kidney transplant recipients. It is most common with certain types of glomerulonephritis, immunoglobulin A nephropathy, diabetes mellitus, and focal segmental sclerosis. Disease recurrence can result in the loss of a functioning kidney transplant. Patients must be advised before transplant if they have a disease known to recur.

Corticosteroid-Related Complications. Aseptic necrosis of the hips, the knees, and other joints can result from chronic corticosteroid therapy and renal osteodystrophy. Most transplant recipients receive calcium supplements, vitamin D, and bisphosphonates in an effort to prevent or minimize the bone disorders associated with corticosteroid use. Patient teaching should include the importance of regular bone mineral density testing, weight-bearing exercise, smoking cessation, and limiting alcohol consumption. Other significant problems related to corticosteroids include peptic ulcer disease, glucose intolerance and diabetes, cataracts, dyslipidemia, and an increased incidence of infections and malignancies. In the first year after transplant, corticosteroid doses are usually decreased to 5 to 10 mg a day. The use of tacrolimus and cyclosporine has allowed for the corticosteroid doses to be much lower than they were in the past. Some patients have been successfully withdrawn from corticosteroids 1.5 to 2 years after transplantation, thus eliminating these problems. Vigilant monitoring for adverse effects of corticosteroids and early treatment are essential.

AGE-RELATED CONSIDERATIONS: CHRONIC KIDNEY DISEASE

The incidence of stage 5 CKD in Canada is increasing most rapidly in older patients. The incidence of stage 5 CKD increased nearly 20% in 5 years, from 13/100,000 people in 1997 to 16/100,000 in 2001. Of all new patients in 2009, 54% were 65 years of age or older as compared to 33% in 1990 (CIHI, 2011a).

This rate has been relatively stable since 2001 (CIHI, 2011a). The most common diseases leading to renal failure in the older adult are diabetes and hypertension. HD is the predominant RRT for older patients starting dialysis. In 2009, 81% of those ages 64 to 75, and 86% of those 75 or older, started with HD as compared to other RRTs (CIHI, 2011a). Expenditures can be expected to increase as the CKD-affected population ages and has a correspondingly greater number of co-morbid conditions.

The care of the older adult with CKD is particularly challenging, not only because of the normal physiological changes of aging that occur but also because of the number of co-morbid conditions that develop (Mathers, 2006). Physiological changes of clinical importance in the older patient with CKD include diminished cardiopulmonary function, bone loss, immunodeficiency, altered protein synthesis, impaired cognition, and altered drug metabolism. Malnutrition is common in the older CKD patient for a variety of reasons, including lack of mobility, lack of understanding of basic nutritional requirements, social isolation, physical disability, impaired cognitive function, and malabsorption problems (Mathers, 2006).

The older patient needs to consider what is the best treatment modality based on his or her health, personal preferences, and the support available. Home PD allows the patient to be more mobile and to enjoy an increased sense of control over the illness. PD causes less hemodynamic instability than HD but does require self-care or assistance from another person. The older adult may not have adequate help in the home to provide assistance. Establishing vascular access for HD may be difficult in an older patient because of atherosclerotic changes. Travel to and from the HD unit may also be problematic if the patient does not drive or have access to reliable public transportation. Although transplantation is an option, older adult patients must be carefully screened to ensure that the benefits outweigh the risks. A living donor is preferable so that there is not a prolonged waiting time.

The most common cause of death in the elderly CKD patient is cardiovascular disease (myocardial infarction, stroke) followed by withdrawal from dialysis. If a competent patient decides to withdraw from dialysis, it is essential to support the patient and the family. Ethical issues (see the Ethical Dilemmas box) to be considered in this situation include patient competency, benefit versus burden of treatment, and futility of treatment. Withdrawal from treatment is not a failure if the patient is well informed and comfortable with the decision.

The increasing number of older, debilitated patients with CKD receiving dialysis has raised a number of ethical concerns about the use of scarce resources in a population with a limited life expectancy. Substantial evidence exists showing success of dialysis (especially PD) in older adults. Quality of life has also been reported to be good to excellent in many older patients with CKD. There appears to be no justification for excluding the older adult from dialysis programs. Rationing dialysis on the basis of age alone is not supported based on current outcome and quality-of-life data.

ETHICAL DILEMMAS
Withdrawing Treatment

Situation

A 70-year-old patient with diabetes mellitus and chronic renal failure who has been receiving dialysis for 10 years tells the nurse that he wants to discontinue his dialysis. His quality of life has diminished during the past 2 years since his wife died. He is not a prospective transplant patient.

Important Points for Consideration

- Quality of life is an important consideration for patients when evaluating whether to begin or discontinue treatment.
- Quality-of-life decisions often weigh the benefit of treatment against the burden of treatment. When a treatment becomes too burdensome, the patient (if competent) may request to withdraw the treatment.
- A determination must be made whether there is some other treatable problem such as depression that may be clouding the patient's judgement.
- Patient autonomy, or the patient's right to self-determination regarding treatment decisions, applies to both initiating and discontinuing treatment.
- If a decision is made to withdraw treatment, the health care team, the patient, and the family should develop an appropriate follow-up plan that includes palliative care and hospice support.

Clinical Decision-Making Questions

1. How should the nurse respond to the patient's request?
2. What is the position of the Canadian Nurses Association (CNA) on withdrawing or withholding treatment that no longer benefits the patient or causes suffering?

CLINICAL DECISION-MAKING EXERCISE

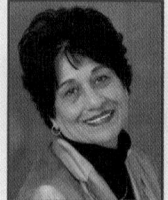

CASE STUDY:
Chronic Kidney Disease

Source: © iStockphoto.com/Michael Blackburn.

Patient Profile

Mrs. Crowe, a 46-year-old Aboriginal schoolteacher, has been treated for type 2 diabetes mellitus since the age of 25. Her nephrologist has observed her for the past several years for manifestations of progressive chronic kidney disease. Eight weeks ago, she had an arteriovenous fistula created in preparation for starting hemodialysis. Over the past week, she has experienced anorexia, nausea, vomiting, problems with concentration, and pruritus.

Subjective Data

- Complains of swelling in her feet and hands
- Has gained 4.5 kg in the past 2 weeks
- Complains of dyspnea and weakness when walking

Objective Data

Laboratory Data

- Estimated glomerular filtration rate (eGFR): 8.0 mL/min/1.73 m^2
- Serum creatinine: 560 mmol/L
- Blood urea nitrogen (BUN): 32 mmol/L
- Potassium: 6 mmol/L
- Hemoglobin: 95 g/dL

Chest Radiograph

- Pulmonary edema

Discussion Questions

1. Explain the basic pathophysiological changes that resulted in the development of Mrs. Crowe's diabetic nephropathy.

2. What are the indications for dialysis in this patient?
3. Identify the abnormal diagnostic study results, and explain why each would occur.
4. Explain why Mrs. Crowe developed each of the clinical manifestations she shows.
5. *Priority Decision:* What are the priority nursing interventions for Mrs. Crowe and her family?
6. *Priority Decision:* Based on the assessment data provided, what are the priority nursing diagnoses? Are there any collaborative problems?

evolve *Answers are available at* **http://evolve.elsevier.com/ Canada/Lewis/medsurg**

REVIEW QUESTIONS

The number of the question corresponds to the same-numbered objective at the beginning of the chapter.

1. Which of the following characterizes acute kidney injury? *(Select all that apply.)*
   a. Most always reversible with low mortality rates.
   b. An abrupt decline in kidney function with a rise in serum creatinine.
   c. Mechanical obstruction of urinary outflow is the most common cause.
   d. Cardiovascular disease is the most common cause of death.

2. The RIFLE Criteria define three stages of AKI based on changes in which of the following?
   a. Blood pressure (BP) and urine osmolality
   b. Urine output and urinary creatinine
   c. Fractional excretion of urinary sodium and glomerular filtration rate (GFR)
   d. Baseline serum creatinine and urine output

3. In the oliguric phase of acute kidney injury (AKI), for which symptoms does the nurse monitor the patient?
   a. Hypotension
   b. Pulmonary edema
   c. Hypernatremia
   d. Hypokalemia

4. The nurse monitors the patient in the diuretic phase of AKI for which serum electrolyte imbalances?
   a. Hyperkalemia and hyponatremia
   b. Hyperkalemia and hypernatremia
   c. Hypokalemia and hyponatremia
   d. Hypokalemia and hypernatremia

5. Which systemic effect best characterizes chronic kidney disease (CKD)?
   a. Progressive irreversible damage of the kidneys
   b. Rapid decrease in urinary output with an elevated blood urea nitrogen (BUN)
   c. Progressive increase in creatinine clearance
   d. Rapid rise in serum creatinine from baseline

6. Nurses need to educate patients at risk for developing CKD. Which of the following individuals are considered to be at increased risk? *(Select all that apply.)*
   a. Older Black Canadians
   b. Older than 60 years
   c. History of pancreatitis
   d. Obesity

7. Patients with CKD experience an increased incidence of cardiovascular disease related to which of the following? *(Select all that apply.)*
   a. Vascular calcification
   b. Genetic predisposition
   c. Hypertension
   d. Increased high-density lipoproteins

8. Patients with CKD stages 3-4 require a collaborative approach to care that focuses on delaying the progression of CKD by which of the following?
   a. Educating patients and caregivers about BP control
   b. Instructing patients to significantly restrict protein in their diet
   c. Instructing patients that radiocontrast agents are not harmful at this stage of CKD
   d. Educating patients to restrict their sodium intake to 3.5 g/day

9. Which of the following interventions should the nurse undertake to assess the patency of a newly placed arteriovenous graft for dialysis?
   a. Irrigate the graft daily with low-dose heparin.
   b. Monitor for any increase in blood pressure in the affected arm.
   c. Listen with a stethoscope over the graft for the presence of a bruit.
   d. Frequently monitor the pulses and the neurovascular status distal to the graft.

10. Following a kidney transplant, which signs of rejection would the nurse include in her or his patient education?
    a. Fever, weight loss, increased urinary output, increased BP
    b. Fever, weight gain, increased urinary output, increased BP
    c. Fever, weight loss, decreased urinary output, decreased BP
    d. Fever, weight gain, decreased urinary output, increased BP

REFERENCES

Akcay, A., Turkman, K., Lee, D., & Edelstein, C. (2010). Update on the diagnosis and management of acute kidney injury. *International Journal of Nephrology and Renal Disease, 3*, 129-140. doi:10.2147/IJNRD.S8641

Alleman, K., & Longton, S. (2008). Transplantation. In C. S. Counts (Ed.), *Core curriculum for nephrology nursing* (5th ed.). Pitman, NJ: Anthony J. Jannetti.

Atkins, K., Clement, L., Cotton, A. B., Karalis, M., Patel, C., Stover, J., & Terrill, C. J. (2008). Nutrition in kidney disease, dialysis, and transplantation. In C. S. Counts (Ed.), *Core curriculum for nephrology nursing* (5th ed., pp. 519-563). Pitman, NJ: Anthony J. Jannetti.

Benavente, G. S., Counts, C. S., McCarley, P. B., Pelfrey, N. J., Petroff, S., & Stackiewicz, L. (2008). Chronic kidney disease. In C. S. Counts (Ed.), *Core curriculum for nephrology nursing* (5th ed.). Pitman, NJ: Anthony J. Jannetti.

Burns, K., Toffelmire, T., Barre, P., Dorval, M., Jastrzebski, J., Jindal, K., ..., Taylor, G. (2005). The prevention of transmission of blood-borne pathogens in hemodialysis patients. The Canadian Society of Nephrology Recommendations. Retrieved from *https:// www.csnscn.ca/images/Docs_Misc/VAWG/The_Prevention_of_ Transmission_of_Blood-_Borne_Pathogens_in_Hemodialysis_ Patients.pdf*

Burrows, L., & Muller, R. (2007). Chronic kidney disease and cardiovascular disease: Pathophysiologic links. *Nephrology Nursing Journal, 34*(1), 55-63.

Canadian Hypertension Education Program (CHEP). (2012). Recommendations for management of hypertension. Retrieved from *http://www.hypertension.ca/images/2012_CHEPFullRecommendations_ EN_HCP1009.pdf*

Canadian Institute for Health Information (CIHI). (2011a). 2009 Annual report—Treatment of end-stage organ failure in Canada, 2000-2009. Retrieved from *http://secure.cihi.ca/cihiweb/products/ 2011_CORR_Annual_Report_final_e.pdf*

Canadian Institute for Health Information. (2011b). *Canadian Organ Replacement Register Annual Report: Treatment of End-Stage Organ Failure in Canada, 2001 to 2010.* Ottawa: CIHI. Retrieved from *https://secure.cihi.ca/free_products/2011_CORR_Annua_Report_ EN.pdf*

Canadian Nurses Association. (2008). Code of ethics for registered nurses. Retrieved from *http://www.cna-aiic.ca/CNA/practice/ethics/ code/default_e.aspx*

Cheung, C., Ponnusamy, A., & Anderton, J. (2008). Management of acute renal failure in the elderly patient: A clinician's guide. *Drugs and Aging, 25*(6), 455-476. Retrieved from *http://adisonline.com/ aging/toc/2008/25060*

Claure-Del Grando, R., Macedo, E., & Mehta, R. (2012). Management options: Continuous renal replacement therapy. In E. Lerma & A. Nissenson, *Nephrology secrets* (3rd ed.). Philadelphia: Mosby.

Dersch, D., & McCormack, J. (2008). Estimating renal function for drug dosing: Rewriting the gospel? *The Canadian Journal of Hospital Pharmacy, 61*(2), 138-143. Retrieved from *http://www.cjhp-online.ca/index.php/cjhp/article/view/31/30*

Ding, D. (2010). Post-kidney transplant rejection and infection complications. *Nephrology Nursing, 37*(4), 419-426.

Dinwiddie, L. C., Burrows-Hudson, S., & Peacock, E. J. (2006). Stage 4 chronic kidney disease: Preserving kidney function and preparing patients for stage 5 kidney disease. *American Journal of Nursing, 106*(9), 40-51. doi:10.1097/00000446-200609000-00024

Dirkes, S. (2011). Acute kidney injury: Not just acute renal failure anymore? *Critical Care Nurse, 31*(1), 37-49. doi:10.4037/ ccn2011946

Elliott, M., Ronksley, P., Clase, C., Ahmed, S., & Hemmelgarn, B. (2010). Management of patients with acute hyperkalemia. *CMAJ, 182*(15), 1631-1635. doi:10.1503/cmaj.100461

Gentry, S., Montgomery, R., & Segev, D. (2011). Kidney paired donation: Fundamentals, limitations, and expansions. *American Journal of Kidney Diseases, 57*(1), 144-151. doi:10.1053/j. ajkd.2010.10.005

Gervasio, J., Garmon, W., & Holowatyj, M. (2011). Nutrition support in acute kidney injury. *Nutrition in Clinical Practice, 26*(4), 374-381. doi:10.1177/0884533611414029

Giles, S. (2005). An antidote to the emerging two tier organ donation policy in Canada: The Public Cadaveric Organ Donation Program. *Journal of Medical Ethics, 31*(4), 188-191. doi:10.1136/jme. 2003.002931

Gilpin, V., & Nichols, W. (2010). Vascular access for hemodialysis: Thrills and thrombosis. *Journal of Vascular Nursing, 28*(2), 78-83. doi:10.1016/j.jvn.2010.03.001

Goldstein-Fuch, J. (2006). Nutrition in chronic kidney disease. In A. Molzahn & E. Butera (Eds.), *Contemporary nephrology nursing: Principles and practices* (2nd ed.). Pitman, NJ: Anthony J. Jannetti.

Haras, M. S. (2008). Planning for a good death: A neglected but essential part of ESRD care. *Nephrology Nursing Journal, 35*(5), 541.

Harwood, L., & Leitch, R. (2006). Home dialysis therapies. In A. Molzahn & E. Butera (Eds.), *Contemporary nephrology nursing: Principles and practices* (2nd ed.). Pitman, NJ: Anthony J. Jannetti.

Herzog, C., Asinger, R., Berger, A., Charytan, D., Diez, J., Hart, R., ..., Ritz, E. (2011). Cardiovascular disease in chronic kidney disease. A clinical update from Kidney Disease: Improving Global Outcomes (KDIGO). *Kidney International, 80*(6), 572-586. doi:10.1038/ki.2011.223

Hudson, J. (2006). Secondary hyperparathyroidism in chronic kidney disease: Focus on clinical consequences and vitamin D therapies. *Annals of Pharmacotherapy, 40*(9), 1584-1593. doi:10.1345/ aph.1G724

Jindal, K., Chan, C. T., Deziel, C., Hirsch, D., Soroka, S. D., Tonelli, M., ..., Canadian Society of Nephrology Committee for Clinical Practice Guidelines. (2006). Chapter 4: Vascular access. In *Hemodialysis clinical practice guidelines for the Canadian Society of Nephrology. Journal of the American Society of Nephrology, 17*(3 Suppl 1), S1-S27.

Kinzner, C. L., & Hain, D. J. (2007). Understanding the eGFR. *Nephrology Nursing Journal, 34*(6), 655-657.

Komaba, H., Tanaka, M., & Fukagawa, M. (2008). Treatment of chronic kidney disease–mineral and bone disorder (CKD-MBD). *Internal Medicine, 47*(11), 989. doi:10.2169/internalmedicine. 47.1051

Kopyt, N. (2007). Management and treatment of chronic kidney disease. *The Nurse Practitioner, 32*(11), 14-23. doi:10.1097/01. NPR.0000298267.70526.b8

Kovesdy, C. & Kalantar-Zadeh, K. (2012) Nutrition and malnutrition. In E. Lerma, & A. Nissenson, *Nephrology secrets* (3rd ed.). Philadelphia: Mosby Elsevier.

Levin, A., Hemmelgarn, B., Culleton, B., Tobe, S., MacFarlane, P., Ruzicka, M., ..., Tonelli, M. (2008). Guidelines for the management of chronic kidney disease. *Canadian Medical Association Journal, 179*(11), 1154-1162. doi:10.1503/cmaj.080351

Liles, A. M. (2011). Medication considerations for patients with chronic kidney disease who are not yet on dialysis. *Nephrology Nursing Journal, 38*(3), 263-270.

Mathers, T. (2006). The older adult with chronic kidney disease. In A. Molzahn & E. Butera (Eds.), *Contemporary nephrology nursing: Principles and practices* (2nd ed.). Pitman, NJ: Anthony J. Jannetti.

Maursetter, L., Kight, C., Mennig, J., & Hofmann, R. (2011). Review of the mechanism and nutrition recommendations for patients undergoing continuous renal replacement therapy. *Nutrition in Clinical Practice, 26*(4), 382-390. doi:10.1177/0884533611413899

McCarley, P. (2006). Diagnosis, classification and management of chronic kidney disease. In A. Molzahn & E. Butera (Eds.), *Contemporary nephrology nursing: Principles and practices* (2nd ed.). Pitman, NJ: Anthony J. Jannetti.

McCarley, P., & Arjomand, M. (2008). Mineral and bone disorders in patients on dialysis: Physiology and clinical consequences. *Nephrology Nursing Journal, 35*(1), 59-64.

McCarley, P., & Burrows-Hudson, S. (2006). Chronic kidney disease and cardiovascular disease: Using the ANNA standards and practice guidelines to improve care. *Nephrology Nursing Journal, 33*(6), 666-674.

Murphy, F. (2011). Managing post-transplant patients in primary care. *Practice Nursing, 22*(6), 292, 294-297.

Murphy, F., & Byrne, G. (2010). The role of the nurse in the management of acute kidney injury. *British Journal of Nursing, 19*(3), 146-152.

National Kidney Foundation. (2011). Frequently asked questions about GFR estimates. Retrieved from *http://www.kidney.org/ professionals/kls/pdf/12-10-4004_KBB_FAQs_AboutGFR-1.pdf*

Nguyen, T., & Wells, D. (2011) Establishing maintenance doses of IV iron in anemia management to improve patient outcomes. *Nephrology Nursing Journal, 38*(1), 55-59.

Organ Registry Team (ORT) (Ottawa) & the Organ and Tissue Donation and Transplantation (OTDT) Team (Ottawa and Edmonton). (2011). Living donor paired exchange registry helps kidney patients get the transplants they need. *CANNT, 21*(1), 12.

Ponferrada, L., Prowant, B., & Satalowich, R. J. (2008). Peritoneal dialysis. In C. S. Counts (Ed.), *Core curriculum for nephrology nursing* (5th ed.). Pitman, NJ: Anthony J. Jannetti.

Price-Rabetoy, C. (2006). Acute renal failure. In A. Molzahn & E. Butera (Eds.), *Contemporary nephrology nursing: Principles and practices* (2nd ed.). Pitman, NJ: Anthony J. Jannetti.

Prowant, B. (2006). Peritoneal dialysis access. In A. Molzahn & E. Butera (Eds.), *Contemporary nephrology nursing: Principles and practices* (2nd ed.). Pitman, NJ: Anthony J. Jannetti.

Raymond, C., Wazny, L., & Sood, A. (2010). Update on the new Kidney Disease: Improving Global Outcomes (KDIGO) guidelines for mineral and bone disorders (MBD)—A focus on medications. *CANNT, 20*(1), 42-46.

Sloand, J. (2007). Treating hyperparathyroidism with cinacalcet HCl (sensipar). *Nephrology Nursing Journal, 34*(3), 341-342.

Smith, K., & Smelt, S. (2009). Consequences of chronic kidney disease–mineral and bone disorder: A progressive disease. *Nephrology Nursing Journal, 36*(1), 49-55.

Snyder, J. J., & Collins, A. J. (2009). KDOQI hypertension, dyslipidemia and diabetes care guidelines and current care patterns in the United States CKD population: National Health and Nutrition Examination Survey 1999-2004. *American Journal of Nephrology, 30*(1), 44.

Soroka, S., Thomas, A., & Girvan, C. (2010). *Module 5: Chronic kidney disease–mineral and bone disorder in Essential Concepts in Chronic Renal Failure.* Mississauga, ON: Amgen Canada Inc.

U.S. Food and Drug Administration. (2011). U.S. Food and Drug Administration safety information: Kayexalate (sodium polystyrene sulfonate) powder. Retrieved from *http://www.fda.gov/Safety/ MedWatch/SafetyInformation/ucm186845.htm*

Venkataraman, R. (2008). Can we prevent acute kidney injury? *Critical Care Medicine, 36*(4 Suppl), S166-S171. doi:10.1097/ CCM.0b013e318168c74a

Veys, C., & Bramstedt, K. (2010). Stranger donors: A key link in transplant chains. *Progress in Transplantation, 20*(4), 366-371. Retrieved from *http://search.proquest.com/docview/818750578/ fulltextPDF/13340F1DFDE15FF8CA1/12?accountid=26764*

Yaklin, K. M. (2011), Acute kidney injury: An overview of pathophysiology and treatments. *Nephrology Nursing Journal, 38*(1), 13-18, 30.

CANADIAN RESOURCES

Canadian Association of Nephrology Nurses and Technologists (CANNT)
http://www.cannt.ca/

Canadian Institute for Health Information
http://www.cihi.ca

Canadian Organ Replacement Register (CORR)
http://www.cihi.ca/CIHI-ext-portal/internet/en/document/ types+of+care/specialized+services/organ+replacements/ services_corr

Canadian Society of Nephrology (CSN)
https://www.csnscn.ca/en/

Hypertension Canada
http://www.hypertension.ca/

The Kidney Foundation of Canada
http://www.kidney.ca/

RELATED RESOURCES

International Society of Nephrology (ISN)
http://www.isn-online.org

International Transplant Nurses Society
http://www.itns.org

National Kidney Foundation
http://www.kidney.org

National Kidney Foundation: Calculators for Health Care Professionals
http://www.kidney.org/professionals/kdoqi/gfr_calculator.cfm

RenalWEB Patient Education
http://www.renalweb.com/topics/patiented/patiented.htm

United Network for Organ Sharing (UNOS)
http://www.unos.org

ⓔvolve *For additional Internet resources, see the Web site for this book at* **http://evolve.elsevier.com/Canada/Lewis/medsurg**

Problems Related to Regulatory and Reproductive Mechanisms

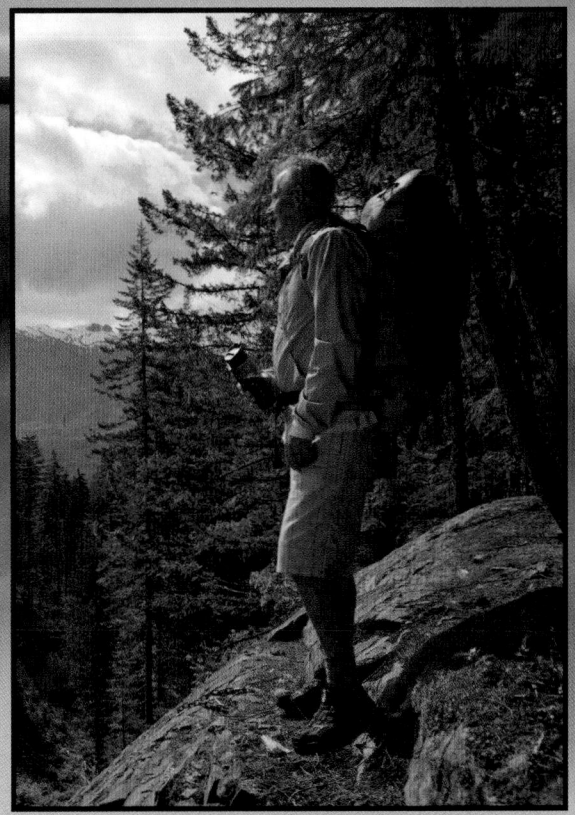

Noel Hendrickson/Digital Vision/Thinkstock

SECTION OUTLINE

Nursing Assessment: Endocrine System

Written by Ian M. Camera

Adapted by Daphne Connolly

LEARNING OBJECTIVES

1. Describe the common characteristics and the functions of hormones.
2. Identify the locations of the endocrine glands.
3. Describe the functions of hormones secreted by the pituitary, thyroid, parathyroid, and adrenal glands and the pancreas.
4. Describe the locations and the roles of hormone receptors.
5. Identify the significant subjective and objective assessment data related to the endocrine system that should be obtained from a patient.
6. Identify the appropriate technique to use in the physical assessment of the thyroid gland.
7. Relate age-related changes in the endocrine system to differences in assessment findings.
8. Differentiate normal from common abnormal findings in the physical assessment of the endocrine system.
9. Describe the purpose, significance of results, and nursing responsibilities related to diagnostic studies of the endocrine system.

KEY TERMS

aldosterone A potent mineralocorticoid that maintains extracellular fluid volume, p. 1378

antidiuretic hormone (ADH) Also called *vasopressin*; a potent vasoconstrictor, its major physiological role is regulation of fluid volume, p. 1377

catecholamines Usually considered neurotransmitters but are hormones when secreted by the adrenal medulla; an essential part of the body's response to stress, p. 1378

corticosteroid Any of the hormones synthesized by the adrenal cortex (excluding androgens), p. 1378

cortisol The most abundant and potent glucocorticoid; one major function is the regulation of blood glucose concentration, p. 1378

glucagon A hormone synthesized and released from pancreatic α cells in response to low levels of blood glucose, to protein ingestion, and to exercise; increases blood glucose level by stimulating glycogenolysis, gluconeogenesis, and ketogenesis, p. 1379

growth hormone A hormone that affects the growth and development of skeletal muscles and long bones, thereby affecting a person's size and height, p. 1376

hormone A chemical substance synthesized and secreted by a specific organ or tissue; hormones control a number of physiological activities, p. 1371

insulin The principal regulator of the metabolism and storage of ingested carbohydrates, fats, and proteins, p. 1379

islets of Langerhans The hormone-secreting portion of the pancreas, p. 1379

negative feedback The most common type of feedback system; increases or decreases the secretion of a hormone on the basis of feedback from various factors, p. 1373

positive feedback A second feedback system; increases the target organ action beyond normal, p. 1373

thyroxine (T$_4$) The most abundant hormone produced by the thyroid gland and the precursor to triiodothyronine, p. 1377

triiodothyronine (T$_3$) Thyroid hormone that regulates metabolic rate of all cells and processes of cell growth and tissue differentiation, p. 1377

tropic hormones Hormones that control the secretion of hormones by other glands, p. 1377

ELECTRONIC RESOURCES

The endocrine system and the nervous system are two of the primary communicating and coordinating systems in the body. The nervous system communicates through nerve impulses; the endocrine system communicates through chemical substances known as *hormones*, and it plays a role in reproduction, growth and development, and regulation of energy. The endocrine glands include the hypothalamus, pituitary gland, thyroid, parathyroids, adrenal glands, pancreas, ovaries, testes, and pineal gland (Figure 50-1). The pineal gland secretes melatonin and is involved in regulation of gonadal function and development, as well as chronobiological rhythms (Stehle et al., 2011). In addition to the endocrine glands, other body organs secrete hormones. For example, the kidneys secrete erythropoietin, the heart secretes atrial natriuretic peptide, and the gastrointestinal tract secretes numerous peptide hormones (e.g., gastrin). These hormones are discussed in their respective assessment chapters.

Structures and Functions of the Endocrine System

Glands

The organs of the endocrine system are referred to as *glands*. Endocrine glands produce chemical substances called *hormones* and secrete them into blood, by which they eventually affect specific target tissues. A *target tissue* is the body tissue or organ on which the hormone has its effect. For example, the thyroid (the gland) synthesizes thyroxine (the hormone), which influences all body tissues (target tissue). It is important to note that not all glands in the body belong to the endocrine system. There are two types of glands: *Exocrine glands* secrete their substances into ducts that then empty into a body cavity or onto a surface (e.g., skin). For example, salivary glands produce saliva, which is secreted through salivary ducts into the mouth. *Endocrine glands*, in contrast, secrete their substances directly into the blood, not into ducts.

Hormones

Classifications and Functions. A **hormone** is a chemical substance synthesized and secreted by a specific organ or tissue. Most hormones have common characteristics, including (a) secretion in small amounts at variable but predictable rates,

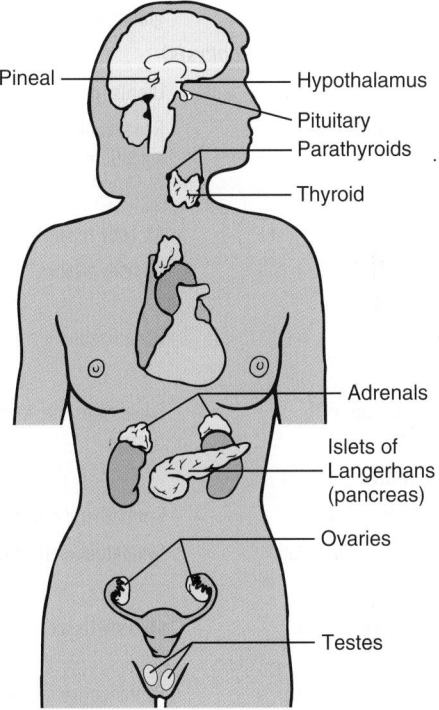

Figure 50-1 Location of the major endocrine glands. The parathyroid glands lie on the posterior surface of the thyroid.

(b) circulation through the blood, and (c) binding to specific cellular receptors either in the cell membrane or within the cell.

Hormones are classified by their chemical structure: *lipid-soluble hormones* and *water-soluble* (protein-based) *hormones*. Lipid-soluble hormones include steroid hormones (all hormones produced by the adrenal cortex and the sex glands) and thyroid hormones. All other hormones are water soluble (Low, 2011). The differences in solubility are important for understanding how the hormone interacts with the target cell.

Hormones control a number of physiological activities. Important hormonal functions are related to reproduction, response to stress and injury, electrolyte balance, energy metabolism, growth, maturation, and aging. Hormones also play a role in the function of the nervous system. Some hormones have a

Table 50-1 Major Endocrine Glands and Hormones

HORMONES	TARGET TISSUE	FUNCTIONS
Anterior pituitary (Adenohypophysis)		
Growth hormone or somatotropin	All body cells	Promotes protein anabolism (growth, tissue repair) and lipid mobilization and catabolism
Thyroid-stimulating hormone (TSH) or thyrotropin	Thyroid gland	Stimulates synthesis and release of thyroid hormones, growth and function of thyroid gland
Adrenocorticotropic hormone (ACTH)	Adrenal cortex	Fosters growth of adrenal cortex; stimulates secretion of corticosteroids
Gonadotropic hormones	Reproductive organs	Stimulates sex hormone secretion, reproductive organ growth, reproductive processes
• Follicle-stimulating hormone (FSH)		
• Luteinizing hormone (LH)		
Melanocyte-stimulating hormone (MSH)	Melanocytes in skin	Increases melanin production in melanocytes to make skin darker in colour
Prolactin	Ovary and mammary glands in girls and women	Stimulates milk production in lactating women; increases response of follicles to LH and FSH; has unclear function in men
Posterior pituitary (Neurohypophysis)		
Oxytocin	Uterus; mammary glands	Stimulates milk secretion, uterine contractility
Antidiuretic hormone (ADH; vasopressin)	Renal tubules, vascular smooth muscle	Promotes reabsorption of water, vasoconstriction
Thyroid		
Thyroxine (T_4)	All body tissues	Precursor to T_3
Triiodothyronine (T_3)	All body tissues	Regulates metabolic rate of all cells and processes of cell growth and tissue differentiation
Calcitonin	Bone tissue	Regulates calcium and phosphorus blood levels; decreases serum Ca^{2+} levels
Parathyroids		
Parathyroid hormone (PTH; parathormone)	Bone, intestine, kidney tissues	Regulates calcium and phosphorus blood levels; promotes bone demineralization and increases intestinal absorption of Ca^{2+}; increases serum Ca^{2+} levels
Adrenal Medulla		
Epinephrine (adrenaline)	Sympathetic effectors	Response to stress; enhances and prolongs effects of sympathetic nervous system
Norepinephrine (noradrenaline)	Sympathetic effectors	Response to stress; enhances and prolongs effects of sympathetic nervous system
Adrenal Cortex		
Corticosteroids (e.g., cortisol, hydrocortisone)	All body tissues	Promotes metabolism, response to stress; anti-inflammatory
Androgens (e.g., testosterone, androsterone) and estrogen	Reproductive organs	Promotes masculinization in men, growth and sexual activity in women
Mineralocorticoids (e.g., aldosterone)	Kidney	Regulates sodium and potassium balance and thus water balance
Pancreas (Islets of Langerhans)		
Insulin (from β cells)	General	Promotes movement of glucose out of blood and into cells
Amylin (from β cells)	Liver, stomach	↓ Gastric motility, ↓ glucagon secretion, ↓ endogenous glucose release from liver, ↑ satiety
Glucagon (from α cells)	General	Stimulates glycogenolysis and gluconeogenesis
Somatostatin	Pancreas	Inhibits insulin and glucagon secretion
Pancreatic polypeptide	General	Influences regulation of pancreatic exocrine function and metabolism of absorbed nutrients
Gonads		
Women: Ovaries		
Estrogen	Reproductive system, breasts	Stimulates development of secondary sex characteristics, preparation of uterus for fertilization, and fetal development; stimulates bone growth
Progesterone	Reproductive system	Maintains lining of uterus necessary for successful pregnancy
Men: Testes		
Testosterone	Reproductive system	Stimulates development of secondary sex characteristics, spermatogenesis

regulatory effect on nervous tissue. For example, catecholamines are hormones when they are secreted by the adrenal medulla, but they act as neurotransmitters when secreted by nerve cells in the brain and the peripheral nervous system. When epinephrine travels through the blood, it is a hormone and affects target tissues. When it travels across synaptic junctions, it acts as a neurotransmitter (Low, 2011). Hormones can also influence behaviour. For example, excess growth hormone, cortisol, and parathyroid hormone can cause mood swings. Depression has been associated with adrenal insufficiency and hypothyroidism. Table 50-1 summarizes the major hormones, glands or tissues from which they are synthesized, target organs or tissues, and functions.

Hormone Transport. Hormones are carried by the blood to other sites in the body where their actions are exerted. Some hormones (e.g., steroid and thyroid hormones) are not water soluble. Therefore, these types of hormones are bound to plasma proteins for transport in the blood. Although hormones are inactive when bound to plasma proteins, they can be released when appropriate and immediately exert their action at the target tissue. Water-soluble hormones (e.g., protein hormones, catecholamines) circulate freely in the blood and are not dependent on proteins for transport.

Targets and Receptors. As mentioned, hormones exert their effects on target tissue. The hormone recognizes the target tissue by attaching to receptors (the site that interacts with the hormone) in the cell membrane (e.g., protein-type hormone receptors) or within cells of the target tissue (e.g., thyroid and steroid hormone receptors). The specificity of hormone–target cell interaction is determined by receptors in a "lock-and-key" type of mechanism. Thus, a hormone acts only on cells that have a receptor specific for that hormone (Figure 50-2). The location of the receptor sites affects the mechanism of action for the hormone.

Protein Hormone Receptors. Protein hormone action is a two-step process. The receptor is located in the target cell membrane; thus the hormone itself acts as a "first messenger." The hormone–receptor interaction stimulates the production of a "second messenger" such as cyclic adenosine monophosphate (cAMP). cAMP works by activating enzymes to regulate intracellular activity (Figure 50-3).

Steroid Hormone Receptors. Steroid and thyroid hormone receptors are located inside the cell. Because these hormones are lipid soluble, they pass through the target cell membrane by passive diffusion and bind to receptor sites located in the cytoplasm or nucleus of the target cell (Cooper & Ladenson, 2011). Intracellular hormone–receptor complexes, such as those observed in steroid hormone action, bind to specific sites on DNA to stimulate or inhibit the synthesis of messenger RNA. When new messenger RNA is synthesized, it migrates to the cytoplasm, where it stimulates the synthesis of new protein. These new proteins produce specific effects in the target cell (see Figure 50-3).

Regulation of Hormonal Secretion. Endocrine activity is regulated by specific mechanisms of varying levels of complexity. These mechanisms stimulate or inhibit hormone synthesis and secretion and include simple feedback, complex feedback, nervous system control, and physiological rhythms.

Simple Feedback. The regulation of hormone levels in the blood depends on a highly specialized mechanism called *feedback.* Feedback is based on the blood level of a particular substance. The substance may be a hormone or another chemical compound regulated by, or responsive to, a hormone. In **negative feedback,** the most common type of feedback system, the gland responds by increasing or decreasing the secretion of a hormone on the basis of feedback from various factors (Cooper & Ladenson, 2011). Negative feedback is similar to the functioning of a thermostat in which cold air in a room activates the thermostat to release heat and hot air turns off the thermostat to prevent more warm air from entering the room.

The pattern of insulin secretion is a physiological example of negative feedback between glucose and insulin. Elevated blood glucose levels stimulate the secretion of insulin from the pancreas. As blood glucose levels decrease, the stimulus for insulin secretion also decreases (Figure 50-4). The homeostatic mechanism is considered negative feedback because it reverses the change in blood glucose level. Another example of negative feedback is the relationship between calcium and parathyroid hormone (PTH). Low blood levels of calcium stimulate the parathyroid gland to release PTH, which acts on bone, the intestine, and the kidneys to increase blood calcium levels. The increased blood calcium levels then inhibit further PTH release (Figure 50-5).

Positive feedback is a second method of regulation of hormone secretion. The positive feedback mechanism increases the target organ action beyond normal. The action of oxytocin during childbirth is an example. The hormone oxytocin from the posterior pituitary gland stimulates and increases uterine contractions. The release of oxytocin is stimulated by pressure receptors in the vagina. As the fetus enters the vagina during childbirth, the pressure receptors sense increased pressure and signal the brain

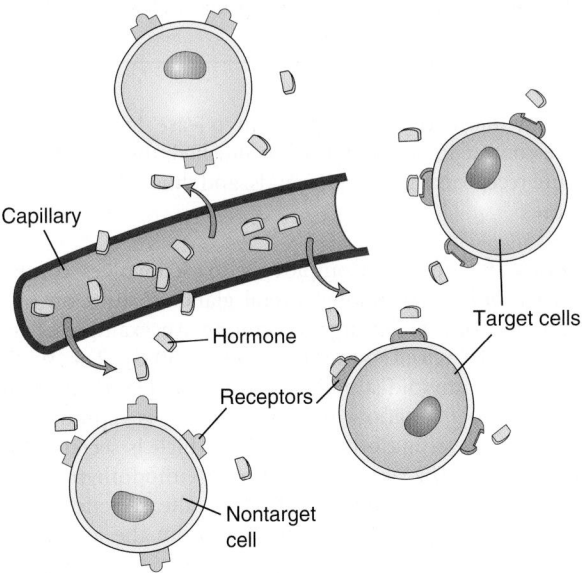

Figure 50-2 The target cell concept. Hormones act only on cells that have receptors specific to that hormone because the shape of the receptor determines which hormone can react with it. This is an example of the lock-and-key model of biochemical reactions.

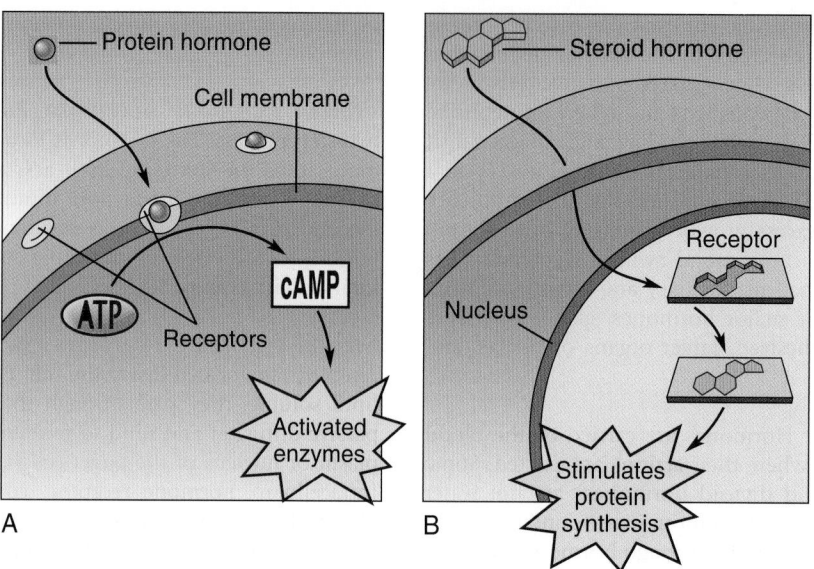

Figure 50-3 Actions of protein and steroid hormones. **A,** Protein hormones bind to receptors located on the surface of the cell membrane. The hormone–receptor interaction stimulates the formation of cyclic adenosine monophosphate (cAMP), thereby activating various cell processes. **B,** Steroid hormones penetrate the cell membrane and interact with intracellular receptors. The hormone–receptor complex activates the cell by stimulating protein synthesis. *ATP,* adenosine triphosphate.

Source: From Herlihy, B. (2011). *The human body in health and illness* (4th ed., p. 253, Figure 14-2). Philadelphia: W. B. Saunders.

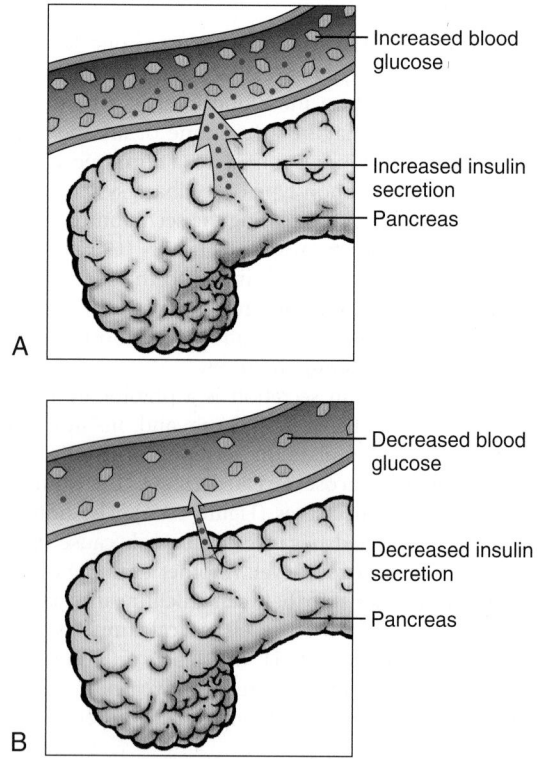

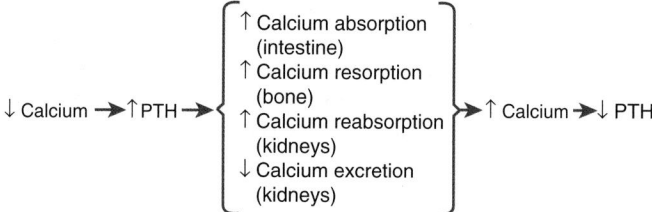

Figure 50-5 Feedback mechanism between parathyroid hormone (PTH) and calcium.

Figure 50-4 Feedback mechanism between blood glucose and insulin. **A,** Increased blood glucose stimulates increased insulin secretion from the pancreas. **B,** As blood glucose levels decline, insulin secretion decreases.

Source: Adapted from Herlihy, B. (2007). *The human body in health and illness* (3rd ed., p. 242, Figure 14-3). Philadelphia: W. B. Saunders.

to release more oxytocin. Oxytocin release leads to stronger uterine contractions. When birth is finished, the stimulus to the pressure receptors in the vagina ends, and thus oxytocin secretion decreases.

Complex Feedback. Complex feedback involves communication via hormones among several glands to turn on or turn off secretion of a target organ hormone. An example of this is regulation of thyroid hormones (Figure 50-6). The synthesis and release of thyroid-stimulating hormone (TSH) or thyrotropin from the anterior pituitary gland is stimulated by thyrotropin-releasing hormone (TRH), which is secreted by the hypothalamus. The thyroid hormones, triiodothyronine and thyroxine, have an inhibitory effect on the secretion of both TRH from the hypothalamus and TSH from the anterior pituitary gland.

Nervous System Control. In addition to chemical regulation, some endocrine glands are directly affected by the activity of the nervous system. Pain, emotion, sexual excitement, and stress can stimulate the nervous system to modulate hormone secretion.

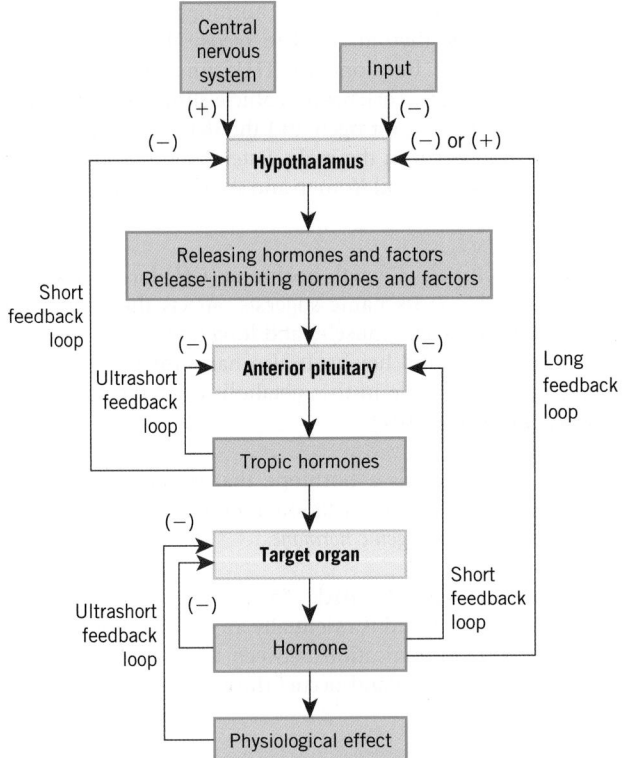

Figure 50-6 General model for control and negative feedback to hypothalamus–pituitary target organ systems. Negative feedback regulation is possible at three levels: target organ (ultrashort feedback), anterior pituitary gland (short feedback), and hypothalamus (long feedback).

Source: Redrawn from McCance, K. L., & Huether, S. E. (2010). *Pathophysiology: The biologic basis for disease in adults and children* (6th ed., p. 699, Figure 20-2). St. Louis: Mosby.

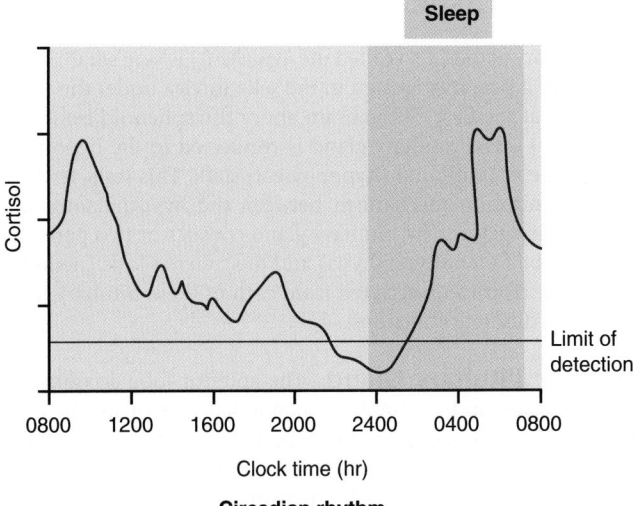

Figure 50-7 Circadian rhythm of cortisol secretion.

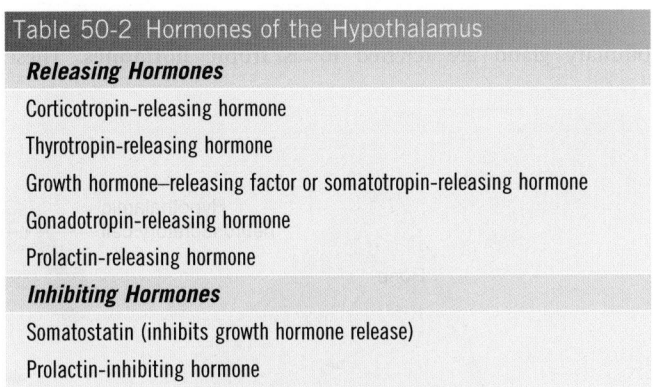

Table 50-2 Hormones of the Hypothalamus
Releasing Hormones
Corticotropin-releasing hormone
Thyrotropin-releasing hormone
Growth hormone–releasing factor or somatotropin-releasing hormone
Gonadotropin-releasing hormone
Prolactin-releasing hormone
Inhibiting Hormones
Somatostatin (inhibits growth hormone release)
Prolactin-inhibiting hormone

Neural involvement is initiated by the central nervous system and implemented by the sympathetic nervous system. For example, stress is sensed by the central nervous system, and the sympathetic nervous system secretes catecholamines that increase heart rate and blood pressure to deal with stress more effectively. (Effects of stress are discussed further in Chapter 8.)

Rhythms. Another regulatory mechanism affecting many hormonal secretions involves the rhythms of secretions. These rhythms originate in brain structures. A common physiological rhythm is the *circadian rhythm,* in which a hormone level fluctuates predictably during a 24-hour period (Stehle et al., 2011). These rhythms may be related to sleep–wake or dark–light cycles. For example, in a person who sleeps at night, the cortisol level rises early in the day, declines toward evening, and rises again toward the end of sleep to peak by morning (Figure 50-7). Secretion of growth hormone and prolactin peaks during sleep. TSH secretion is also maximal during sleep and ebbs 3 hours after a person awakens in the morning. The menstrual cycle is an example of a body rhythm that is longer than 24 hours *(ultradian).* These rhythms must be considered when hormone levels on laboratory results are interpreted. (See the Diagnostic Studies of the Endocrine System section in this chapter and Chapter 51.)

Hypothalamus

The relationship between the hypothalamus and the pituitary gland is one of the most important aspects of the endocrine system. Although the pituitary gland has been referred to as the "master gland," most of its functions rely on an interrelationship with the hypothalamus. The hypothalamus and the pituitary gland integrate communication between nervous and endocrine systems. Thus neuroendocrinology is the study of interactions between these two systems (Low, 2011).

The hypothalamus is located in the most central part of the diencephalon area of the brain (see Figure 50-1). Although it is part of the brain, the hypothalamus secretes many hormones. Two important groups of hormones from the hypothalamus are releasing hormones and inhibiting hormones (Radu, 2011). The function of these hormones is to either stimulate (release) or inhibit the secretion of hormones from the anterior pituitary (Table 50-2).

The hypothalamus also contains neurons, which receive input from the brainstem and limbic system. These neurons influence the limbic system, brainstem, and spinal cord. This creates a circuit to facilitate the coordination of the endocrine system, the autonomic nervous system, and the expression of complex behavioural responses, such as anger and feelings of fear and pleasure.

Pituitary Gland

The pituitary gland (also called the *hypophysis*) is very small: about the size of a pea. It is located in the sella turcica under the hypothalamus at the base of the brain above the sphenoid bone (see Figure 50-1). The pituitary gland is connected to the hypothalamus by the infundibular (hypophyseal) stalk. This stalk serves as a communication mechanism between the hypothalamus and the pituitary gland. The pituitary gland consists of two parts, the *anterior* lobe (adenohypophysis) and the *posterior* lobe (neurohypophysis). Hormones secreted from each of these pituitary lobes serve very different functions.

Anterior Pituitary Gland.
The anterior lobe accounts for 80% of the gland by weight. As mentioned previously, the anterior pituitary is regulated by the hypothalamus through releasing and inhibiting hormones. These hypothalamic hormones reach the anterior pituitary through a network of capillaries known as the *hypothalamus–hypophyseal portal system*. The releasing and inhibiting hormones in turn affect the secretion of six hormones from the anterior pituitary gland (Figure 50-8; see Table 50-2).

Tropic Hormones. Several hormones secreted by the anterior pituitary gland are referred to as **tropic hormones**. These hormones control the secretion of hormones by other glands. TSH stimulates the thyroid gland to secrete thyroid hormones. Adrenocorticotropic hormone (ACTH) stimulates the adrenal cortex to secrete corticosteroids. Follicle-stimulating hormone stimulates secretion of estrogen and the development of ova in the female and sperm in the male. Luteinizing hormone stimulates ovulation in girls and women and secretion of sex hormones in both sexes.

Growth Hormone. **Growth hormone (GH)** has effects on all body tissue. GH, as its name suggests, affects the growth and development of skeletal muscles and long bones, thereby affecting a person's size and height. It also has numerous biological actions, including a role in the metabolism of protein, fat, and carbohydrate (Radu, 2011).

Prolactin. Prolactin is a hormone that stimulates the breast development necessary for lactation after childbirth. Prolactin is also referred to as *lactogenic hormone*.

Posterior Pituitary Gland.
The posterior pituitary is composed of nerve tissue and is essentially an extension of the hypothalamus. The communication between the hypothalamus and the posterior pituitary gland occurs through nerve tracts known

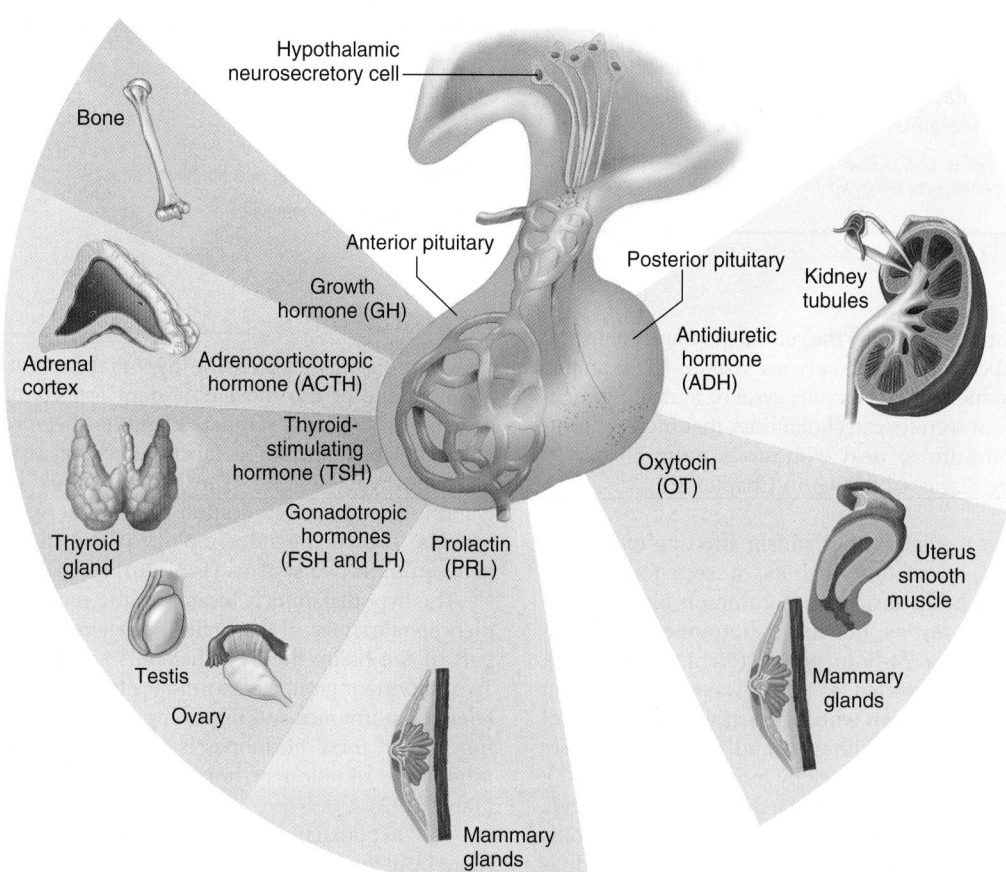

Figure 50-8 Relationship among the hypothalamus, the pituitary gland, and the target organs. The hypothalamus communicates with the anterior pituitary gland via a capillary system and with the posterior pituitary via nerve tracts. The anterior and posterior pituitary hormones are shown with their target tissues. *FSH,* follicle-stimulating hormone; *LH,* luteinizing hormone.

as the *median eminence*. The hormones secreted by the posterior pituitary gland—antidiuretic hormone and oxytocin—are actually produced in the hypothalamus. These hormones travel down the nerve tracts from the hypothalamus to the posterior pituitary gland and are stored until their release is triggered by the appropriate stimuli (see Figure 50-8).

Antidiuretic Hormone. The major physiological role of **antidiuretic hormone (ADH)**—also called *vasopressin*—is regulation of fluid volume by stimulating reabsorption of water in the renal tubules. ADH is also a potent vasoconstrictor.

The most important stimulus of ADH secretion is *plasma osmolality*, a measure of solute concentration of circulating blood (Figure 50-9). Plasma osmolality increases when there is a decrease in extracellular fluid or an increase in solute concentration. The increased plasma osmolality activates osmoreceptors, which are extremely sensitive, specialized neurons in the hypothalamus. These activated osmoreceptors stimulate ADH release (Radu, 2011). Table 50-3 lists factors that affect ADH release. When ADH is released, the renal tubules reabsorb water, causing urine to be more concentrated. When ADH release is inhibited, renal tubules do not reabsorb water, causing urine to be more dilute.

Oxytocin. Oxytocin stimulates both ejection of milk into mammary ducts and contraction of uterine smooth muscle. Oxytocin secretion is increased by stimulation of touch receptors in the nipples of lactating women and of vaginal pressure receptors.

Thyroid Gland

The thyroid gland is located in the anterior portion of the neck, in front of the trachea. It consists of two encapsulated lateral lobes connected by a narrow isthmus (Figure 50-10). The thyroid is a highly vascular organ and is regulated by TSH from the anterior pituitary. The three hormones produced and secreted by the thyroid gland are thyroxine, triiodothyronine, and calcitonin.

Thyroxine and Triiodothyronine.
The major function of the thyroid gland is the production, storage, and release of the thyroid hormones: **thyroxine (T_4)** and **triiodothyronine (T_3)**. T_4 is by far the most abundant thyroid hormone, accounting for 90% of thyroid hormone produced by the thyroid gland. T_3, however, is much more potent and has greater metabolic effects. About 20% of circulating T_3 is secreted directly by the thyroid gland, and the remainder is obtained by peripheral conversion of T_4 (Radu, 2011). Iodine is necessary for the synthesis of thyroid hormones. T_4 and T_3 affect metabolic rate, caloric requirements, oxygen consumption, carbohydrate and lipid metabolism, growth and development, brain function, and nervous system activity. More than 99% of thyroid hormones are bound to plasma proteins, especially T_4-binding globulin synthesized by the liver. Only the unbound "free" hormones are biologically active.

Thyroid hormone production and release is stimulated by TSH from the anterior pituitary gland. When circulating levels of thyroid hormone are low, the hypothalamus releases TRH, which in turn causes the anterior pituitary gland to release TSH. High levels of circulating thyroid hormone have an inhibitory effect on the secretion of both TRH from the hypothalamus and TSH from the anterior pituitary gland (Radu, 2011).

Calcitonin.
Calcitonin is a hormone produced by C cells (parafollicular cells) of the thyroid gland in response to high circulating calcium levels. Calcitonin inhibits calcium resorption (loss of substance) from bone, increases calcium storage in bone,

Table 50-3 Factors Affecting Release of Antidiuretic Hormone	
Stimulate Release	**Inhibit Release**
Increased plasma osmolality	Decreased plasma osmolality
Decreased fluid volume	Increased fluid volume
Hypotension	β-Adrenergic agonists
Nausea and vomiting	Alcohol
Pain	

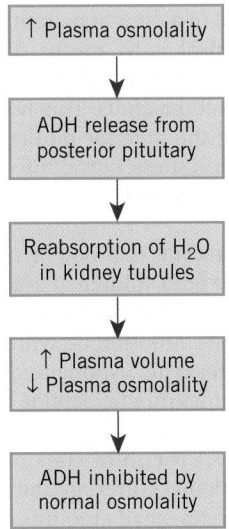

Figure 50-9 Relationship of plasma osmolality to antidiuretic hormone (ADH) release and action.

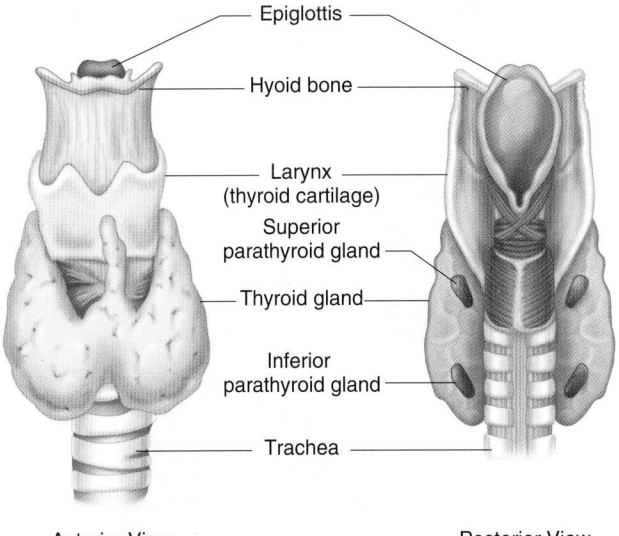

Anterior View   Posterior View

Figure 50-10 Thyroid and parathyroid glands. Note the surrounding structures.

Source: From Thibodeau, G. A., & Patton, K. T. (2010). *The human body in health and disease* (5th ed., p. 321, Figure 11-7). St. Louis: Mosby.

and increases renal excretion of calcium and phosphorus, thereby lowering serum calcium levels. Although it provides a counter-mechanism to PTH, calcitonin does not play a critical role in calcium balance (Goodman, 2009).

Parathyroid Glands

The parathyroid glands are small, oval structures usually arranged in pairs behind each thyroid lobe (see Figure 50-10). Most people have four such glands. The major cell type of the glands is epithelial, and the glands are richly supplied with blood from the inferior and superior thyroid arteries.

Parathyroid Hormone.
The parathyroids secrete PTH (also called *parathormone*). Its major role is to regulate the blood level of calcium. PTH acts on bone, the kidneys, and, indirectly, the gastrointestinal tract. In bone, PTH stimulates bone resorption and inhibits bone formation, which results in the release of calcium and phosphate into the blood. In the kidneys, PTH increases calcium reabsorption and phosphate excretion. In addition, PTH stimulates the renal conversion of vitamin D to its most active form ($1,25$-dihydroxyvitamin D_3). This active form then enhances the intestinal absorption of calcium.

The secretion of PTH is directly regulated by a feedback system (see Figure 50-5) and is not under pituitary and hypothalamic control. When the serum calcium level is low, PTH secretion increases; when the serum calcium level rises, PTH secretion falls. In addition, high levels of active vitamin D inhibit PTH secretion, and low levels of magnesium stimulate PTH secretion.

Adrenal Glands

The adrenal glands are small, paired, highly vascularized glands located on the upper portion of each kidney. Each gland consists of two parts: the medulla and the cortex (Figure 50-11). Each part has distinct functions, and the glands act independently of one another.

Adrenal Medulla.
The adrenal medulla is the inner part of the gland and consists of sympathetic postganglionic neurons. The medulla secretes the catecholamines epinephrine (the major

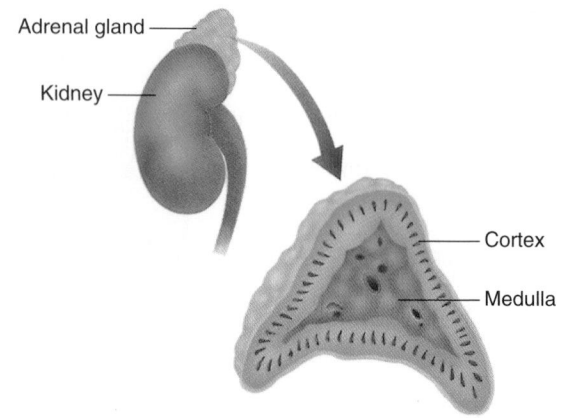

Figure 50-11 The adrenal gland is composed of the adrenal cortex and the adrenal medulla.

Source: From Solomon, E. P. (2009). *Introduction to human anatomy and physiology* (3rd ed., p. 167, Figure 9-8). St. Louis: W. B. Saunders.

hormone), norepinephrine, and dopamine. **Catecholamines,** usually considered neurotransmitters, are hormones when secreted by the adrenal medulla because they are released into the circulation and transported to their target organs. Catecholamines exert their effects after binding to adrenergic receptors on cells, and they have widespread effects on all body systems. Catecholamines are an essential part of the body's response to stress (see Chapter 8).

Adrenal Cortex.
The adrenal cortex is the outer part of the adrenal gland. It secretes more than 50 steroid hormones, which are classified as glucocorticoids, mineralocorticoids, and androgens. Cholesterol is the precursor for steroid hormone synthesis. Glucocorticoids (e.g., cortisol) are named for their effects on glucose metabolism. Mineralocorticoids (e.g., aldosterone) are essential for the maintenance of fluid and electrolyte balance. Adrenal androgens are produced and secreted in small but significant amounts. The term *corticosteroid* refers to any of the hormones synthesized by the adrenal cortex (excluding androgens).

Cortisol. **Cortisol,** the most abundant and potent glucocorticoid, is necessary to maintain life. One major function of cortisol is the regulation of blood glucose concentration. Cortisol increases blood glucose through stimulation of hepatic gluconeogenesis (conversion of amino acids to glucose) and inhibiting protein synthesis (Carroll, Aron, Findling, & Tyrrell, 2011). Cortisol also decreases peripheral glucose use in the fasting state.

Another major effect of glucocorticoids is their anti-inflammatory action and supportive actions in response to stress. A marked increase in the rate of cortisol secretion by the adrenal cortex aids the body in coping more effectively with stressful situations (see Chapter 8). Cortisol decreases the inflammatory response by stabilizing the membranes of cellular lysosomes and preventing increased capillary permeability. The lysosomal stabilization reduces the release of proteolytic enzymes and thereby limits their destructive effect on surrounding tissue. Cortisol can also inhibit production of prostaglandins, thromboxanes, and leukotrienes and alter the cell-mediated immune response.

Cortisol helps maintain vascular integrity and fluid volume. It has a mineralocorticoid effect because it can bind to mineralocorticoid receptors.

Cortisol is secreted in a diurnal pattern (see Figure 50-7). The major control of cortisol is by means of a negative feedback mechanism that involves the secretion of corticotropin-releasing hormone from the hypothalamus. This hormone stimulates the secretion of ACTH by the anterior pituitary. Cortisol levels are also increased by surgical stress, burns, infection, fever, psychoses, acute anxiety, and hypoglycemia.

Aldosterone. **Aldosterone** is a potent mineralocorticoid that maintains extracellular fluid volume. It acts at the renal tubule to promote renal reabsorption of sodium and excretion of potassium and hydrogen ions. Aldosterone synthesis and secretion are stimulated by angiotensin II, hyponatremia, and hyperkalemia and inhibited by atrial natriuretic peptide and hypokalemia.

Adrenal Androgens. The third class of steroids synthesized and secreted by the adrenal cortex are the androgens. Normally, the adrenal cortex secretes small amounts of androgens. Adrenal androgens stimulate pubic and axillary hair growth and sex drive in women. In girls and women, androgens are converted to estrogen in the peripheral tissues. In postmenopausal women, the major source of estrogen is from the peripheral conversion of adrenal androgen to estrogen. The effects of adrenal androgen in men are negligible in comparison with testosterone secreted by the testes.

Pancreas

The pancreas is a long, tapered, lobular, soft gland located behind the stomach and anterior to the first and second lumbar vertebrae. The pancreas has both exocrine and endocrine functions. The hormone-secreting portion of the pancreas is referred to as the **islets of Langerhans.** The islets account for less than 2% of the gland and consist of four types of hormone-secreting cells: α, β, δ, and F (or PP) cells. α Cells produce and secrete the hormone glucagon. Insulin and amylin are produced and secreted by β cells. Somatostatin is produced and secreted by the δ cells. Pancreatic polypeptide is secreted by the F cells.

Glucagon. Glucagon is synthesized and released from pancreatic α cells in response to low levels of blood glucose, to protein ingestion, and to exercise. Glucagon increases blood glucose levels by stimulating glycogenolysis, gluconeogenesis, and ketogenesis. Usually, glucagon and insulin function in a reciprocal manner to maintain normal blood glucose levels. The exception is after ingestion of a high-protein, carbohydrate-free diet, in which case both hormones are secreted. In this instance, glucagon counteracts the inhibitory effect of insulin on gluconeogenesis, and normal blood glucose levels are maintained.

Insulin. Insulin is the principal regulator of the metabolism and storage of ingested carbohydrates, fats, and proteins. Insulin facilitates glucose transport across cell membranes in most tissues. However, the brain, nerves, lens of the eye, hepatocytes, erythrocytes, and cells in the intestinal mucosa and kidney tubules are not dependent on insulin for glucose uptake. An increased blood glucose level is the major stimulus for insulin synthesis and secretion. Other stimuli to insulin secretion are increased amino acid levels and vagal stimulation. Insulin secretion is usually inhibited by low blood glucose levels and by glucagon, somatostatin, hypokalemia, and catecholamines (Table 50-4).

A major effect of insulin on glucose metabolism occurs in the liver, where the hormone enhances glucose incorporation into glycogen and triglycerides by altering enzymatic activity and inhibiting gluconeogenesis. Another major effect occurs in peripheral tissues, where insulin facilitates glucose transport into cells, transport of amino acids across muscle membranes and

their synthesis into protein, and transport of triglycerides into adipose tissue. Thus, insulin is a storage, or *anabolic*, hormone.

The endocrine system functions to regulate body processes and maintain internal homeostasis despite vastly changing substrates, as is observed in glucose homeostasis after food ingestion. After a meal, insulin is responsible for the storage of nutrients (anabolism). In the fasting state (during which ingested glucose is not readily available), hormones such as catecholamines, cortisol, and glucagon break down stored complex fuels (*catabolism*) to provide simple glucose as fuel for energy.

AGE-RELATED CONSIDERATIONS: THE ENDOCRINE SYSTEM

Normal aging has many effects on the endocrine system (Table 50-5). These include (a) decreased hormone production and secretion, (b) altered hormone metabolism and biological activity, (c) decreased responsiveness of target tissues to hormones, and (d) alterations in circadian rhythms.

Assessment of the effects of aging on the endocrine system is difficult because the subtle changes of aging often mimic manifestations of endocrine disorders. Some endocrine changes associated with aging are obvious; others are subtle. The nurse must be aware that endocrine problems may manifest differently in an older adult than in a younger person. Older adults may have multiple comorbid conditions and take multiple medications that alter the body's usual response to endocrine dysfunction. Symptoms of endocrine dysfunction such as fatigue, constipation, or mental impairment in older adults are often missed because they are attributed solely to aging. It is important that the nurse consider age-related endocrine changes when assessing an older adult (Eliopoulos, 2010).

Assessment of the Endocrine System

Hormones affect every body tissue and system, causing great diversity in the signs and symptoms of endocrine dysfunction. Therefore, assessment of the endocrine system is often difficult, and keen clinical skills are required to detect manifestations of disorders. Endocrine dysfunction may result from deficient or excessive hormone secretion, transport abnormalities, an inability of the target tissue to respond to a hormone, or inappropriate stimulation of the target-tissue receptor.

Endocrine disorders may have specific or nonspecific (vague) clinical manifestations. When signs and symptoms are specific, such as the classic "polys" (polyuria, polydipsia, and polyphagia) in diabetes mellitus, the assessment is easier; nonspecific signs and symptoms, such as tachycardia, palpitations, fatigue, or altered mood, are more problematic. Nonspecific changes should alert the health care provider to the possibility of an endocrine disorder. The most common nonspecific symptoms, fatigue and depression, often are accompanied by other manifestations such as changes in energy level, alertness, sleep patterns, mood, affect, weight, skin, hair, personal appearance, and sexual function.

Subjective Data

The lack of clear-cut manifestations of endocrine problems necessitates a conscientious and detailed health history. A thorough

Table 50-4 Factors Influencing Secretion of Insulin	
Stimulate Secretion	**Inhibit Secretion**
↑ Glucose levels	↓ Glucose levels
↑ Amino acid levels	↓ Amino acid levels
↑ Gastrointestinal hormone levels	↓ Potassium levels
↑ Vagal stimulation	↑ Corticosteroid hormone levels
↑ Fats	↑ Catecholamine levels
	↑ Somatostatin levels
	↑ Glucagon levels (usually)
	↑ Insulin levels

AGE-RELATED DIFFERENCES IN ASSESSMENT

Table 50-5 Endocrine System

CHANGES	CLINICAL SIGNIFICANCE
Thyroid	
Atrophy of thyroid gland; decrease in TSH and T$_3$ secretion	Increased incidence of hypothyroidism with aging; however, most older adults maintain adequate thyroid function
Parathyroid	
Increased basal level of PTH and increased secretion	Increased calcium resorption from bone (demineralization); hypercalcemia, hypercalciuria
Adrenal Cortex	
Adrenal cortex: more fibrotic and slightly smaller	Unknown; possibly contributes to a decreased response to sodium restriction and to upright posture
Higher plasma levels of cortisol	
Decreased plasma levels of adrenal androgens and aldosterone	
Adrenal Medulla	
Increased secretion and basal level of norepinephrine	Decreased responsiveness to β-adrenergic agonists and receptor blockers
No change in plasma epinephrine levels	
Decreased β-adrenergic receptor response to norepinephrine	May partly explain increased incidence of hypertension with aging
Pancreas	
Increase in fibrosis and fatty deposits in pancreas	May partly contribute to increased incidence of diabetes mellitus with advanced aging
Increased glucose intolerance and decreased sensitivity to insulin	
Gonads	
Female: decline in estrogen secretion	Women experience symptoms associated with menopause and have increased risk for atherosclerosis and osteoporosis
Male: decline in testosterone secretion	Men may or may not experience symptoms

PTH, parathyroid hormone; *TSH*, thyroid-stimulating hormone; *T$_3$*, triiodothyronine.

health history yields data to help sort out possible causes and the effect of the problem on the person's life (Table 50-6).

Important Health Information

Past Health History. During an assessment, the patient should be questioned about the general state of health and whether any changes in it have occurred. In addition, the patient or significant other should be specifically questioned about previous or current endocrine abnormalities and abnormal patterns of growth and development.

Family History. Heredity can play a major role in the occurrence of endocrine problems. The patient should be questioned about the following conditions in family members: diabetes mellitus or insipidus; hyperthyroidism or hypothyroidism; goitre; hypertension or hypotension; obesity; infertility; growth problems; pheochromocytoma (neoplastic tumour of the adrenal medulla or sympathetic ganglia); autoimmune diseases (e.g., Addison's disease); and adrenal hyperplasia. Such questioning frequently elicits information about a familial tendency.

Medications. The patient should be questioned about the use of all medications (both prescription and over-the-counter drugs) and the use of herbs and dietary supplements. The patient should be asked the reason for taking the drug, the dosage, and the length of time taken. The patient should specifically be asked about the use of hormone replacements. Information that the patient is currently taking hormone replacements such as insulin, thyroid hormone, or corticosteroids (e.g., prednisone) helps direct the nurse with regard to possible problems associated with the use of these agents. For example, corticosteroids may cause glucose intolerance in susceptible patients by increasing glycogenolysis and insulin resistance. The adverse effects of many nonhormone medications can contribute to problems affecting endocrine function. For example, many drugs can affect blood glucose levels.

Surgery and Other Treatments. The nurse should inquire about previous hospitalizations, surgery, chemotherapy, and radiation therapy (especially irradiation of the neck). Surgery of the brain or a severe blow to the head could have resulted in pituitary or hypothalamic alterations.

Objective Data

Most endocrine glands are inaccessible for direct examination. With the exception of the thyroid and the male gonads, the glands are deeply encased in the body, protected against injury and trauma. However, assessment can be accomplished with a variety of objective data. The nurse must understand the actions of hormones so that by monitoring the target tissue, he or she can assess the function of a gland.

Physical Examination. The nurse must remember that the endocrine system affects every body system. Clinical manifestations of endocrine function vary significantly, depending on the gland involved. Specific clinical findings for the various endocrine problems are discussed in Chapters 51 and 52. Regardless of the type of endocrine dysfunction, the following general examination procedure should be followed.

Vital Signs. All vital signs are measured at the beginning of the examination. Variations in temperature may be associated with thyroid dysfunction. Cardiovascular changes such as tachycardia, bradycardia, hypotension, or hypertension may occur with a variety of endocrine-related problems.

Height and Weight. Assessment of the endocrine system includes a history of growth and development patterns, weight distribution and changes, and comparisons of these factors with normal findings. Growth pattern abnormalities are suggestive of problems associated with growth hormone. Changes in weight also may be associated with endocrine dysfunction. Thyroid disorders and diabetes mellitus are examples of endocrine disorders that can affect body weight. Body mass index is a height-to-weight ratio used to assess nutritional status (see Chapter 43, Figure 43-2).

HEALTH HISTORY

Table 50-6 Endocrine System: Questions for Obtaining Subjective Data

Assess the patient's general health and health care behaviours. This might result in the identification of vague, nonspecific symptoms that could suggest an endocrine problem.

Past History

- Do you have any previous or current problems with your endocrine system (e.g., problems with thyroid, diabetes, changes in facial or body hair)?
- Have you had any previous hospitalizations, surgical procedures, or treatments for endocrine problems?
- Are you currently taking or have you ever taken medications for an endocrine problem such as a thyroid disorder or diabetes?

Family History

- Is there any family history of diabetes mellitus or insipidus; hyperthyroidism or hypothyroidism; goitre; hypertension or hypotension; obesity; infertility; growth problems; pheochromocytoma (neoplastic tumour of the adrenal medulla or sympathetic ganglia); autoimmune diseases (e.g., Addison's disease); or adrenal hyperplasia?
- Have any other members of your family ever had a problem similar to your problem today?

Social and Occupational History

- Are you married? Do you have any children? Do you think you are able to take care of your family and your home? If not, why not?
- Where do you work? What kind of work do you do? Are you able to do what is expected of you and what you expect of yourself?
- If you are retired, what do you do with your time? What did you do before you retired?
- If you are unemployed, are you looking for work?
- Is your income adequate for your needs?

Self-Care History

- Do you have a planned exercise program? If yes, what is it, and have you had to make any changes in this routine lately? If so, why and what kinds of changes?
- Women: Have you had a mammogram or Pap smear recently? Men: Have you had a prostate examination recently? Both: If so, what were the results and dates of these tests? How often do you have these tests?

General

- What is your usual day like?
- What is your usual activity pattern during a typical day? Have you been more or less active than usual?*
- Have you noticed any changes in your ability to perform your usual activities in comparison with last year? Five years ago?*
- Do you experience fatigue with or without activity?*

Nutrition History

- What is your weight and height?
- How much do you want to weigh?
- Have there been any changes in your appetite or weight?*

Eyes, Ears, Nose, and Throat

- Have you experienced any blurring or double vision?*
- When was your last eye examination?
- Have you noticed any difficulty swallowing, or are your shirts harder to button at the neck?*

Cardiovascular

- Do you experience heart palpitations?*

Musculoskeletal

- Do you have difficulty holding things because of shakiness of your hands?*

Gastrointestinal

- Describe your usual bowel pattern. Have you noted any bowel changes?*
- Do you use anything, such as laxatives, to help you move your bowels?*

Genitourinary

- Do you have to get up at night to urinate? If so, how many times? Do you keep water by your bed at night?
- Have you ever had a kidney stone?*

Neurological–Psychological

- Do you feel more nervous than you used to? Do you notice your heart pounding or that you sweat when you do not think you should be sweating?
- How is your memory? Have you noticed any changes?
- How long can you concentrate on any one thing? Has this changed lately?
- What kind of stressors do you have?
- How do you deal with stress or problems?
- What is your support system? To whom do you turn when you have a problem?
- Do you feel sad or uninterested in life?*

Integumentary

- Have you noticed any changes in the distribution of the hair anywhere on your body?*
- Have you noticed any changes in the colour of your skin, particularly on your face, neck, hands, or body creases?*
- Has the texture of your skin changed? For example, does it seem thicker and drier than it used to?*

Sleep History

- How many hours do you sleep at night? Do you feel rested on awakening?
- Are you ever awakened by sweating during the night?*
- Do you have nightmares?*
- Does anyone in your family complain about your snoring?*

Sexual and Reproductive History

Women

- When did you start to menstruate? Was this earlier or later than other women in your family? Do you have scant, heavy, or irregular menstrual flows?
- How many children have you had? How much did they weigh at birth? Were you told you had diabetes during any pregnancy?*
- Were you able to nurse your children if you wanted to?
- Are you attempting to get pregnant but cannot?*

Men

- Have you noticed any changes in your ability to have an erection?*
- Are you trying to have children but cannot?*

Other Health Information

- Do you feel that most rooms are too hot or too cold? Do you frequently have to put on a sweater, or do you feel as though you need to open windows when others in the room seem comfortable?*

*If yes, describe.

It may also be helpful to compare the patient's current body weight to the usual body weight in order to assess changes. Weight change (percentage) is calculated by subtracting the current body weight from the usual weight, dividing by usual body weight, and multiplying by 100.

Mental–Emotional Status. Throughout the examination, the patient's orientation, alertness, memory, affect, personality, anxiety, appropriateness of dress, and speech pattern should be assessed objectively. Endocrine disorders can commonly cause changes in mental and emotional status.

Integument. The nurse should note the colour and the texture of skin, hair, and nails. The overall skin colour should be noted, as should pigmentation, and any ecchymosis should be documented. Hyperpigmentation, or "bronzing," of the skin (particularly on knuckles, elbows, knees, genitalia, and palmar creases) is a classic finding in Addison's disease but also is present with ACTH-producing tumours and acromegaly (Jarvis, Browne, MacDonald-Jenkins, & Luctkar-Flude, 2009). The nurse should palpate the skin for texture and presence of moisture. The nurse should also examine the hair distribution, not only on the head but also on the face, the trunk, and the extremities. The appearance and texture of the hair should be examined. Dull, brittle hair; excessive hair growth; or hair loss may indicate endocrine dysfunction.

Head. The size and contour of the head are inspected. Facial features should be symmetrical. Inspect the eyes for position, symmetry, shape, movement, opacity over the lens, eyelid lag, and edema. Visual acuity should also be checked because changes may be associated with a pituitary tumour or diabetic retinopathy. In the mouth, the buccal mucosa, the condition of the teeth (malocclusion and mottling), and tongue size should be inspected, and fasciculations (localized, uncoordinated, uncontrollable twitching of a single muscle group) documented.

Neck. When inspecting the thyroid gland, the nurse should make observations first in the normal position (preferably with side lighting), then with the patient's neck in slight extension, and then as the patient swallows some water. The trachea should be midline, and the neck should appear symmetrical. Any unusual bulging over the thyroid area should be noted. If enlargement of the thyroid gland is not noticeable, palpation can be performed. (Because palpation can trigger the release of thyroid hormones, palpation should be deferred in patients with a visibly enlarged thyroid gland.) When the thyroid is enlarged, the lateral lobes should be auscultated with the stethoscope bell to determine the presence of a bruit.

The thyroid gland is difficult to palpate. Thyroid palpation requires considerable practice, as well as validation by a more experienced examiner. Water should always be available for the patient to swallow as part of this examination. There are two acceptable approaches to thyroid palpation: anterior and posterior. For anterior palpation, the nurse stands in front of the patient, with the patient's neck flexed. The nurse places a thumb horizontally with the upper edge along the lower border of the patient's cricoid cartilage. The thumb is then moved over the isthmus as the patient swallows water. The fingers are then placed laterally to the anterior border of the sternocleidomastoid muscle, and each lateral lobe is palpated before and while the patient swallows water.

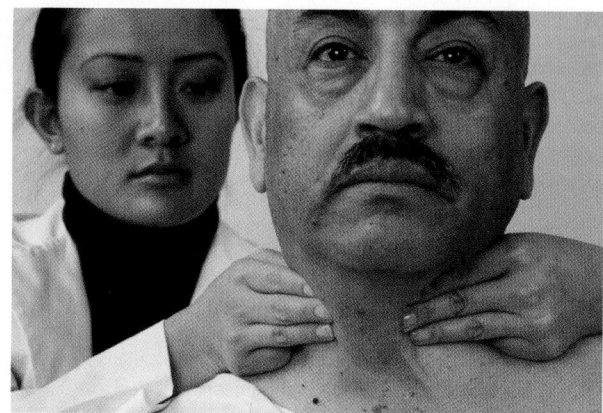

Figure 50-12 Posterior palpation of the thyroid gland.

Source: From Wilson, S., & Giddens, J. F. (2009). *Health assessment for nursing practice* (4th ed., p. 193, Figure 11-48, *A*). St. Louis: Mosby Elsevier.

For posterior palpation, the nurse stands behind the patient. With the thumbs of both hands resting on the nape of the patient's neck, the nurse uses the index and middle fingers of both hands to feel for the thyroid isthmus and for the anterior surfaces of the lateral lobes. To facilitate the examination of each lobe and to relax the neck muscles, the nurse asks the patient to flex the neck slightly forward and to the right. The thyroid cartilage is displaced to the right by the nurse's left hand and fingers. The nurse palpates with the right hand after placing the thumb deep and behind the sternocleidomastoid muscle with the index and middle fingers in front of it; the area is palpated with the right hand (Figure 50-12). While this is done, the patient is asked to swallow water. This procedure is repeated on the left side. The thyroid is palpated for its size, shape, symmetry, and tenderness and for any nodules.

The thyroid is often not palpable. If palpable, it usually feels smooth, with a firm consistency, and is not tender with gentle pressure. Nodules, enlargement, asymmetry, or hardness is abnormal, and the patient should be referred for further evaluation.

Thorax. The thorax should be inspected for shape and characteristics of the skin. The presence of gynecomastia in men should be noted. The nurse auscultates lung sounds and heart sounds, noting the presence of adventitious lung sounds or extra heart sounds.

Abdomen. No abdominal examination findings are specific for endocrine dysfunction other than skin characteristics and hyperactive or hypoactive bowel sounds.

Extremities. The nurse assesses the size, shape, symmetry, and general proportion of hands and feet. The skin is inspected for changes in pigmentation and presence of lesions and edema. Muscle strength is evaluated, as are deep tendon reflexes. In the upper extremities, the nurse assesses for the presence of tremors by placing a piece of paper in the patient's outstretched fingers, palm down.

Genitalia. The nurse inspects the hair distribution pattern. A diamond pubic hair distribution pattern in women or a triangular pattern in men are abnormal findings and might indicate endocrine dysfunction. For men, the testes should be palpated; for women, any clitoral enlargement should be noted.

Common assessment abnormalities related to the endocrine system are presented in Table 50-7. A focused assessment is used to evaluate the status of previously identified endocrine problems and to monitor for signs of new problems (see Table 3-6). A focused assessment of the endocrine system is described in the Focused Assessment box, "Endocrine System."

Diagnostic Studies of the Endocrine System

Accurately performed laboratory tests and radiological examinations contribute to the diagnosis of an endocrine problem. Laboratory tests usually involve blood and urine testing. Ultrasonography may be used as a screening tool to localize endocrine

COMMON ASSESSMENT ABNORMALITIES

Table 50-7 Endocrine System

FINDING	DESCRIPTION	POSSIBLE ETIOLOGY AND SIGNIFICANCE
Integument		
Hyperpigmentation	Darkening of the skin, particularly in creases and skinfolds caused by increased secretion of melanocyte-stimulating hormone	Addison's disease
Striae	Purplish-red marks below the skin surface, usually observed on abdomen, breasts, and buttocks	Cushing's syndrome
Changes in skin texture	Thick, cold, dry skin	Hypothyroidism
	Thick, leathery, oily skin	Growth hormone excess (acromegaly)
	Warm, smooth, moist skin	Hyperthyroidism
Changes in hair distribution	Hair loss	Hypothyroidism, hyperthyroidism, decreased pituitary secretion
	Diminished axillary and pubic hair	Cortisol deficiency
	Hirsutism (excessive facial hair on women)	Cushing's syndrome, prolactinoma (a pituitary tumour)
Skin ulceration	Areas of ulcerated skin, most commonly observed on legs and feet	Peripheral neuropathy and peripheral vascular disease, which are contributory factors in the development of diabetic foot ulcers
Edema	Generalized edema	Mucopolysaccharide accumulation in tissue in hypothyroidism
Head and Neck		
Visual changes	Decreased visual acuity or decreased peripheral vision	Pituitary gland enlargement or tumour, which leads to pressure on optic nerve
Exophthalmos	Protrusion of eyeballs from orbits	Hyperthyroidism; results from fluid accumulation in eye and retro-orbital tissue
Moon facies	Periorbital edema and facial fullness	Increased cortisol secretion as a result of Cushing's syndrome
Myxedema	Puffiness, periorbital edema, masklike affect	Infiltration of dermis by hydrophilic mucopolysaccharides in hypothyroidism
Goitre	Generalized enlargement of thyroid gland	Hyperthyroidism, hypothyroidism, iodine deficiency
Thyroid nodule (one or more)	Localized enlargement of thyroid gland	May be benign or malignant
Cardiovascular		
Chest pain	Angina caused by increased metabolic demands	Hyperthyroidism
Dysrhythmias	Tachycardia, atrial fibrillation	Hypothyroidism, hyperthyroidism, pheochromocytoma
Hypertension	Elevation in blood pressure caused by increased metabolic demands and catecholamines	Hyperthyroidism, pheochromocytoma, Cushing's syndrome
Musculoskeletal		
Changes in muscular strength or muscle mass	Generalized weakness, fatigue, or both	Common symptoms associated with many endocrine problems, including pituitary, thyroid, parathyroid, and adrenal dysfunction; diabetes mellitus; diabetes insipidus
	Decreased muscle mass	Specifically observed in growth hormone deficiency and in Cushing's syndrome secondary to protein wasting
Enlargement of bones and cartilage	Coarsening of facial features; increases in size of hands and feet over a period of several years	Growth hormone excess in adults, as in acromegaly

Continued

Table 50-7 Endocrine System—cont'd

FINDING	DESCRIPTION	POSSIBLE ETIOLOGY AND SIGNIFICANCE
Nutrition		
Changes in weight Altered glucose levels	Weight loss	Hyperthyroidism; caused by increases in metabolism, diabetic ketoacidosis
	Weight gain	Hypothyroidism, Cushing's syndrome
	Increased serum glucose level	Diabetes mellitus, Cushing's syndrome, growth hormone excess
Neurological		
Lethargy	State of mental sluggishness or somnolence	Hypothyroidism
Tetany	Intermittent involuntary muscle spasms usually involving the extremities	Severe calcium deficiency that can occur with hypoparathyroidism
Seizure	Sudden involuntary contraction of muscles	Consequence of a pituitary tumour; fluid and electrolyte imbalance associated with excessive ADH secretion; complications of diabetes mellitus; severe hypothyroidism
Increased deep tendon reflexes	Hyperreflexia	Hyperthyroidism, hypoparathyroidism
Gastrointestinal		
Constipation	Infrequent defecation characterized by passage of hard stools	Hyperthyroidism, hypothyroidism; hyperparathyroidism caused by calcium imbalances
Reproductive		
Changes in reproductive function	Menstrual irregularities, decreased libido, decreased fertility, erectile dysfunction	Various endocrine abnormalities, including pituitary hypofunction, growth hormone excess, thyroid dysfunction, and adrenocortical dysfunction
Other		
Polyuria	Excessive urinary output	Diabetes mellitus (secondary to hyperglycemia) or diabetes insipidus (associated with decreased ADH secretion)
Polydipsia	Excessive thirst	Extreme water losses in diabetes mellitus (with severe hyperglycemia) and diabetes insipidus
Decreased urine output	Reabsorption of water from kidney tubules	Syndrome of inappropriate antidiuretic hormone (SIADH)
Thermoregulation	Cold sensitivity	Hypothyroidism caused by a slowing of metabolic processes
	Heat intolerance	Hyperthyroidism caused by excessive metabolism

ADH, antidiuretic hormone.

growths such as thyroid nodules. Radiological tests include regular radiography, computed tomography, and magnetic resonance imaging. For all diagnostic testing, the nurse is responsible for explaining the procedure to the patient and family. Diagnostic studies common to the endocrine system are described in Table 50-8.

Laboratory Studies

Laboratory studies used to diagnose endocrine problems may include direct measurement of the hormone level or an indirect indication of gland function by evaluation of blood or urine components affected by the hormone (e.g., electrolytes).

Hormones with fairly constant basal levels (e.g., T_4) need be measured only once. Notation of sample time on the laboratory slip and sample is important for hormones with circadian or sleep-related secretion (e.g., cortisol). Evaluation of other hormones may require multiple blood sampling, as in suppression tests (e.g., dexamethasone) and stimulation tests (e.g., glucose tolerance). In these situations, it is often necessary to obtain intravenous access to administer medications and fluids and to collect multiple blood samples.

Pituitary Studies. Disorders associated with the pituitary gland can manifest in a wide variety of ways because of the number of hormones produced. Many diagnostic studies are available to evaluate these hormones either directly or indirectly (see Table 50-8).

Thyroid Studies. There are a number of tests available to evaluate thyroid function. The most sensitive and accurate laboratory test is measurement of TSH; thus it is often recommended as a first diagnostic test for evaluation of thyroid function (Toward Optimized Practice Clinical Practice Guideline Working Group, 2008). Common additional tests ordered in the presence of abnormal TSH levels include measurements of total serum T_4, free T_4, and total serum T_3. Free T_4 is the unbound T_4, and its level is a more accurate reflection of thyroid function than that of total T_4. Less common tests that help in the differentiation of various types of thyroid disease include measurement of T_3, assessment of free T_3 resin uptake, measurement of thyroid autoantibodies, thyroid scanning, ultrasonography, and biopsy. These tests are performed to help differentiate various types of thyroid disorders.

Text continued on p. 1391

FOCUSED ASSESSMENT

Endocrine System

Use this checklist to ensure the key assessment steps have been done.

Subjective

Ask the patient about the following, and note responses

Excessive or increased thirst	Y	N
Excessive or decreased urination	Y	N
Excessive hunger	Y	N
Intolerance of heat or cold	Y	N
Excessive sweating	Y	N
Recent weight gain or loss	Y	N

Objective: Diagnostic

Check the following laboratory results for critical values

Potassium level	✓
Glucose level	✓
Sodium level	✓
Glycosylated hemoglobin (HbA$_{1c}$) level	✓
Thyroid studies: TSH, T$_3$, and T$_4$ levels	✓

TSH, Thyroid-stimulating hormone; T$_3$, triiodothyronine; T$_4$, thyroxine.

Objective: Physical Examination

Inspect/Measure

Body temperature	✓
Height and weight	✓
Alertness and emotional state	✓
Skin, for changes in colour and texture	✓
Hair, for changes in colour, texture, and distribution	✓

Auscultate

Heart rate, blood pressure	✓

Palpate

Extremities, for edema	✓
Skin, for texture and temperature	✓
Neck, for thyroid size, shape	✓

DIAGNOSTIC STUDIES

Table 50-8 Endocrine System

STUDY	PURPOSE AND DESCRIPTION	NORMAL VALUES	NURSING RESPONSIBILITY
Pituitary Studies			
Serum Studies			
Growth hormone (GH; somatotropin)	Evaluation of GH secretion Used to identify GH deficiency or excess GH levels are affected by time of day, food intake, and stress.	Men: <5 mcg/L; women: <10 mcg/L Values >50 mcg/L suggest acromegaly	Make sure that patient has been fasting and has not recently been emotionally or physically stressed. Indicate patient fasting status and recent activity level on the laboratory slip. Send blood sample to laboratory immediately.
Insulin-like growth factor (IGF-1; somatomedin C)	Evaluation of GH secretion Provides a more accurate reflection of mean plasma concentration of GH because it is not subject to circadian rhythm and fluctuations	5-14.4 nmol/L Low levels indicate GH deficiency; high levels indicate GH excess	Overnight fasting is preferred.
GH stimulation test	Needed to adequately diagnose GH deficiency Measurement of GH secretion in response to stimulation (insulin, arginine) For insulin, baseline blood levels for GH, glucose, and cortisol are obtained; insulin is then administered IV; blood samples for GH are obtained 0, 60, and 90 min after insulin is administered; blood glucose levels are monitored at 15- to 30-min intervals; blood glucose should drop to less than 2.2 mmol/L for effective test results, and GH level should rise twofold to threefold over baseline levels Response is subnormal or absent in GH deficiency	Growth hormone levels >10 mcg/L	Ensure that patient or family understands this procedure. Patient must be on NPO status after midnight. Water is permitted on morning of the test. IV access is established for administration of medications and frequent blood sampling. Continually assess for hypoglycemia and hypotension. A 50% dextrose and a 5% dextrose IV solution should be kept at patient's bedside in case severe hypoglycemia occurs.

Continued

DIAGNOSTIC STUDIES

Table 50-8 Endocrine System—cont'd

STUDY	PURPOSE AND DESCRIPTION	NORMAL VALUES	NURSING RESPONSIBILITY
Pituitary Studies—cont'd			
Serum Studies			
Measurement of gonadotropin levels • Follicle-stimulating hormone (FSH) • Luteinizing hormone (LH)	Useful in distinguishing primary gonadal problems from pituitary insufficiency Normal levels vary according to age and sex Levels are low in pituitary insufficiency and high in primary gonadal failure	**FSH** Female patients • Follicular phase: 1.37-9.9 IU/L • Ovulatory peak: 6.7-17.2 IU/L • Luteal phase: 1.09-9.2 IU/L • Postmenopause levels: 19.3-100.6 IU/L Male patients • 1.42-15.4 IU/L **LH** Female patients • Follicular phase: 1.68-15 IU/L • Ovulatory peak: 21.9-56.6 IU/L • Luteal phase: 0.61-16.3 IU/L • Postmenopause levels: 14.2-52.3 IU/L Male patients • 1.24-7.8 IU/L	There is no special preparation of the patient. Note on the laboratory slip time of menstrual cycle or whether female patient is postmenopausal.
Water deprivation test	Used to differentiate causes of polyuria, including central (neurogenic) DI or nephrogenic DI ADH or vasopressin is administered IV or subcutaneously	In patients with central DI, urine osmolality increases after ADH administration In patients with nephrogenic DI, there is little or no response to ADH	Caution: Severe dehydration may occur with central or nephrogenic DI during this test. Test should be performed only if serum sodium level is normal and urine osmolality is <300 mOsm/kg. Test lasts 6 hr, usually from 6 A.M. to 12 noon. Obtain baseline weight and urine and plasma osmolality. Assess urine hourly for volume and specific gravity. Send hourly samples for measuring urine osmolality. Discontinue test and rehydrate if patient's weight drops more than 2 kg at any time. Rehydrate with oral fluids. Check orthostatic BP and pulse after rehydration to ensure adequate fluid volume.
Prolactin level	Evaluation of prolactin level	Male patients • <20 mcg/L Female patients • Nonlactating: <25 mcg/L • Levels above normal reflect potential pituitary tumour	Draw blood within 3-4 hours after patient awakens. Specimen must be sent to the laboratory immediately. If there is a delay, the specimen is placed on ice.

ADH, antidiuretic hormone; *BP*, blood pressure; *DI*, diabetes insipidus; *IV*, intravenous; *NPO*, nothing by mouth; *PO*, by mouth.

DIAGNOSTIC STUDIES

Table 50-8 Endocrine System—cont'd

STUDY	PURPOSE AND DESCRIPTION	NORMAL VALUES	NURSING RESPONSIBILITY
Pituitary Studies—cont'd			
Radiology			
Magnetic resonance imaging (MRI)	Examination of choice for radiological evaluation of the pituitary gland and hypothalamus Useful in identification of tumours involving the hypothalamus or pituitary gland	—	Inform patient of the need to lie as still as possible during the test; explain that tests are painless and noninvasive.
Computed tomography with contrast media	Used to detect presence and size of tumour Oral and/or IV contrast medium may be used	—	Inform patient of the need to lie still during the procedure. If IV contrast medium is to be used, check for iodine allergy before test.
Thyroid Studies			
Serum Studies			
Thyroid-stimulating hormone (TSH)	Measurement of TSH levels Considered the most sensitive method for evaluating thyroid disease Generally recommended as first diagnostic test for thyroid dysfunction	2-10 mU/L	Explain blood collection procedure to patient. No specific preparations are necessary.
Thyroxine (T_4), total	Measurement of total serum level of T_4 Useful in evaluating thyroid function and monitoring thyroid therapy	Male patients: 51-154 nmol/L Female patients: 64-154 nmol/L	Same as for TSH measurement.
Triiodothyronine (T_3)	Measurement of serum levels of T_3 Helpful in diagnosing hyperthyroidism if T_4 levels are normal	Ages 20-50: 1.2-3.4 nmol/L Ages >50: 0.6-2.8 nmol/L	Same as for TSH measurement.
Free T_4	Measurement of active component of total T_4 Because level remains constant, this is considered better indication of thyroid function than T_4	10-36 pmol/L	Same as for TSH measurement.
T_3 resin uptake (T_3RU)	Indirect measurement of binding capacity of thyroid-binding globulin	24-34 AU	Same as for TSH measurement.
Thyroid antibodies (Ab) • Thyroid peroxidase (TPO) Ab • Thyroglobulin Ab • Thyroid-stimulating Ab	Measurements of levels of thyroid antibodies Assist in the diagnosis of an autoimmune thyroid disease and distinguishes it from thyroiditis One or more antibody tests may be ordered, depending on symptoms	—	Same as for TSH measurement.
Thyroglobulin	Test to identify the presence of functioning thyroid tissue or thyroid cancer cells; result used primarily as a tumour marker for patients being treated for thyroid cancer	Male patients: 0.5-53 mcg/L Female patients: 0.5-43 mcg/L	Same as for TSH measurement.
Radiology			
Ultrasonography	Evaluation of thyroid nodule or nodules to determine whether they are fluid filled (cystic) or solid tumour	—	Explain that gel and a transducer will be used over the neck. The test will last 15 min. Neither fasting nor sedation is required.

AU, arbitrary units (T_3RU).

Continued

DIAGNOSTIC STUDIES

Table 50-8 Endocrine System—cont'd

STUDY	PURPOSE AND DESCRIPTION	NORMAL VALUES	NURSING RESPONSIBILITY
Thyroid Studies—cont'd			
Radiology			
Thyroid scan and uptake	Scan: Used to evaluate nodules of the thyroid. Radioactive isotopes are given PO or IV. Scanner passes over thyroid and makes graphic record of radiation emitted. Normal thyroid scan reveals homogeneous pattern with symmetrical lobes. Benign nodules appear as warm spots because they take up the radionuclide; malignant tumours appear as cold spots because they tend not to take up the radionuclide. Radioactive iodine uptake (RAIU): Provides direct measurement of thyroid activity. Useful for evaluation of functional activity of solitary thyroid nodules. Patient is given radioactive iodine either PO or IV. The uptake by the thyroid gland is measured with a scanner at several time intervals such as 2- to 4-hr intervals and at 24 hr. The values of RAIU are expressed in percentage of uptake.	—	Explain procedure to the patient. Check for iodine and shellfish allergy before test. Be sure patient understands that radioactive iodine taken orally is harmless. No special preparation is required. Patient should not have supplemental iodine for several weeks before the test. Thyroid medications interfere with test results.
Parathyroid Studies			
Serum Studies			
Parathyroid hormone (PTH)	Measurement of PTH level in serum. Results must be interpreted in terms of concomitantly measured serum calcium level	Intact (whole): 10-65 ng/L	Fasting specimen preferred. Inform patient that blood sample will be collected. Sample must be kept on ice. Apply pressure to venipuncture site.
Total serum calcium	Measurement of total serum calcium to help detect bone and parathyroid disorders. Hypercalcemia can indicate primary hyperparathyroidism, and hypocalcemia can indicate hypoparathyroidism	2.25-2.75 mmol/L	Inform patient that blood sample will be collected. Avoid prolonged tourniquet application. Apply pressure to venipuncture site.
Ionized calcium	Measurement of free form of calcium unaffected by variable serum albumin levels	1.05-1.3 mmol/L	Same as for total serum calcium.
Serum phosphate	Measurement of inorganic phosphorus. Hyperphosphatemia indicates primary hypoparathyroidism or secondary causes (e.g., renal failure); hypophosphatemia indicates hyperparathyroidism. Phosphorus and calcium levels are inversely related	0.97-1.45 mmol/L	Fasting preferred. Inform patient that blood sample will be collected. Take specimen to laboratory immediately. Apply pressure to venipuncture site.
Adrenal Studies			
Serum Studies			
Cortisol	Measures amount of total cortisol in serum and evaluation of status of adrenal cortex function	138-635 nmol/L at 8 A.M.; 83-359 nmol/L at 4 P.M.	Cortisol has diurnal variation: levels are higher in the morning than in evening. Sample should be collected in morning; evening samples may also be ordered. Mark time of blood collection on laboratory slip. Patient's anxiety should be minimized.
Aldosterone	Measurement of aldosterone levels to evaluate for hyperaldosteronism	Upright posture: 0.14-0.8 nmol/L Supine position: 0.08-0.3 nmol/L	Usually, morning blood sample is preferred. On laboratory slip, indicate patient position (supine, sitting, standing) during venipuncture.

DIAGNOSTIC STUDIES

Table 50-8 Endocrine System—cont'd

STUDY	PURPOSE AND DESCRIPTION	NORMAL VALUES	NURSING RESPONSIBILITY
Adrenal Studies—cont'd			
Serum Studies			
Adrenocorticotropic hormone (ACTH, corticotropin)	Measurement of the plasma level of ACTH Although ACTH is a pituitary hormone, it controls adrenal cortex secretion; this value helps determine whether underproduction or overproduction of cortisol is caused by dysfunction of the adrenal gland or pituitary gland	Morning: <18 pmol/L Evening: <11 pmol/L	Patient should be on NPO status after midnight before morning blood collection. Minimize patient's stress. Diurnal levels correspond with variation of cortisol levels; that is, levels are higher in morning, lower in evening. ACTH is very unstable; blood tube must be placed on ice and sent to laboratory immediately.
ACTH stimulation with cosyntropin	Used to evaluate adrenal function Baseline plasma cortisol levels are measured; IV cosyntropin (synthetic ACTH) is administered; samples are collected 30 and 60 min after bolus	For the rapid stimulation test, cortisol levels increase more than 193 nmol/L above baseline	Inject cosyntropin with a plastic syringe, and collect blood samples in plastic heparinized tubes. Ensure sample collection at appropriate times.
ACTH suppression (dexamethasone suppression)	Assessment of adrenal function; especially helpful if hyperactivity is suspected Useful in evaluation of Cushing's syndrome Dexamethasone is administered at 11 P.M. to suppress secretion of corticotropin-releasing hormone; plasma cortisol sample is collected at 8 A.M.	Cortisol level <138 nmol/L indicates normal adrenal response (50% decrease in cortisol production)	Ensure that patient has fasted. Inform patient that blood sample will be collected. Observe venipuncture site for bleeding and hematoma formation. Do not test acutely ill patients; those under stress are not tested. ACTH may override suppression. Screen patient for drugs such as estrogen and glucocorticoids, which may produce false-positive results. Ensure accurate timing of medication and sample collection.
Metanephrine	Screening for pheochromocytoma; more accurate than urinary vanillylmandelic acid (VMA) and catecholamine measurements	—	Ask about recent history of vigorous exercise, high levels of stress, or starvation (may artificially ↑ levels). Ingestion of caffeine, alcohol, levodopa, lithium, nitroglycerin, acetaminophen, and medications containing epinephrine or norepinephrine can alter test results.
Urine Studies			
17-Ketosteroids	Measurement of androgen metabolites in urine and evaluation of adrenocortical and gonadal function	Male patients: 20-70 mcmol/day Female patients: 20-60 mcmol/day	Instruct patient regarding 24-hr urine collection. Tell patient that specimen must be kept refrigerated or on ice during collection. Determine whether preservative is required for method used.
Aldosterone	Measurement of urinary aldosterone level to evaluate adrenal function Useful in determining therapy for hypertension	6-72 nmol/24 hr	Ensure that patient is on unrestricted diet with normal salt intake and no medication for 3 wk before collection. Instruct patient regarding 24-hr urine collection.
Free cortisol	Measurement of free (unbound) cortisol Preferred test for evaluating hypercortisolism	<276 nmol/day	Instruct patient about 24-hr urine collection and avoidance of stressful situations and excessive physical exercise. Some drugs (e.g., reserpine, diuretics, phenothiazines, amphetamines) may elevate levels. Ensure that patient is on low-sodium diet.

Continued

DIAGNOSTIC STUDIES

Table 50-8 Endocrine System—cont'd

STUDY	PURPOSE AND DESCRIPTION	NORMAL VALUES	NURSING RESPONSIBILITY
Adrenal Studies—cont'd			
Urine Studies			
Vanillylmandelic acid (VMA)	Measurement of urinary excretion of catecholamine metabolite; helpful in diagnosing pheochromocytoma	Normal values are <35 mcmol/24 hr; elevated values indicate pheochromocytoma	Collect specimen with a preservative. Keep on ice. Consult with laboratory or physician about whether patient should discontinue any drugs 3 days before urine collection and a VMA-restricted diet.
Radiology			
Abdominal computed tomography (CT)	The radiological examination of choice for the adrenal gland Used to detect tumour and size of tumour mass or metastatic spread Oral or IV contrast medium, or both, may be used	—	Inform patient of the need to lie still during the procedure. If IV contrast medium is to be used, check for iodine and shellfish allergy before test.
Pancreatic Studies			
Serum Studies			
Fasting blood glucose (FBS) level	Measurement of circulating glucose level	4-6 mmol/L	Patient should fast for at least 4-8 hr; water intake is permitted. If patient has an IV infusion containing dextrose, test result is not considered valid.
Oral glucose tolerance test (OBTT)	**2-Hour Test** Used to diagnose diabetes mellitus if FBS result is equivocal Patient drinks 75 g of glucose; samples for glucose are collected immediately at 30, 60, and 120 min. **5-Hour Test** Used to evaluate hypoglycemia Patient drinks 100 g of glucose; samples of glucose are collected immediately and at 30, 60, 90, 120, 180, 240, and 300 min Baseline cortisol level test is performed if patient becomes symptomatic Patients with reactive hypoglycemia have adrenergic symptoms and glucose level <3.3 mmol/L between 30 min and 5 hr after glucose ingestion	<11.1 mmol/L at 30 and 60 min; <7.8 mmol/L at 120 min	Ensure that tests are not performed on patients who are malnourished, confined to bed for >3 days, or severely stressed. Instruct patient to refrain from smoking and ingesting caffeine and to fast for 12 hr before test. Ensure that patient's diet 3 days before test included 150-300 g of carbohydrate with intake of at least 1500 cal/day. Screen for estrogens, phenytoin (Dilantin), and corticosteroids, and check for hypokalemia, which may impair glucose tolerance. Simultaneously monitor glucose levels with capillary glucose monitoring.
Capillary glucose monitoring	Provides immediate glucose values with glucose oxidase or electrochemical methods	Capillary values (whole blood): 10-15% less than serum values Most capillary blood glucose meters automatically accommodate for this discrepancy	Obtain large drop of blood from clean finger, touch strip to drop of blood (not finger), time accurately, and compare colours in good lighting if visual method is used. Use digital readout if it is available. Use automatic finger-puncture device if it is available. Be sure to change section of device that touches patient's fingers between uses.

DIAGNOSTIC STUDIES

Table 50-8 Endocrine System—cont'd

STUDY	PURPOSE AND DESCRIPTION	NORMAL VALUES	NURSING RESPONSIBILITY
Pancreatic Studies—cont'd			
Serum Studies			
Glycosylated or glycated hemoglobin (hemoglobin A$_{1c}$)	Measurement of degree of glucose control during previous 3 mo (lifespan of hemoglobin molecule).	Less than 6% for nondiabetic patients Less than 7% for patients with good diabetic control (values vary; check with laboratory)	Inform patient that fasting is not necessary and that blood sample will be collected. Observe venipuncture site for bleeding or hematoma formation.
Urine Studies			
Glucose	Estimation of amount of glucose in urine through use of an enzymatic method Dipstick is dipped into the urine and read for colour changes after 1 min.	No glucose in the urine	Use freshly voided urine specimen collected at appropriate time. Know that many different drugs alter glucose readings and that errors are great if directions for timing are not followed exactly. Follow package directions.
Ketones	Measurement of amount of acetone excreted in urine as result of incomplete fat metabolism Tested with a dipstick as described for glucose study.	Negative or trace amount of ketone is normal Positive result can indicate lack of insulin and diabetic ketoacidosis	Use freshly voided urine specimen. Test is often performed with glucose test. Directions must be followed exactly. Certain drugs can produce false-positive and false-negative results.
Radiology			
Abdominal computed tomography (CT)	The radiological examination of choice for pancreas Used to identify tumours or cysts. Oral or IV (or both) contrast medium may be ordered.	—	Inform patient of the need to lie still during the procedure. If IV contrast is to be used, check for iodine allergy before test.

Parathyroid Studies. The only hormone secreted by the parathyroid glands is PTH. Because the function of PTH is to regulate serum calcium and phosphate levels, abnormalities in PTH secretion are reflected in the calcium and phosphate levels. For this reason, diagnostic tests for the parathyroid gland typically include measurements of PTH, serum calcium, and serum phosphate.

Adrenal Studies. Diagnostic tests associated with the adrenal glands focus on the three types of hormones secreted: glucocorticoids, mineralocorticoids, and androgens. These hormone levels can be measured both in blood plasma and in urine. Urine studies are usually performed as 24-hour urine collections. The major advantage of a 24-hour urine sample is that the short-term fluctuations in hormone levels seen in plasma samples are eliminated (Pagana & Pagana, 2011).

Pancreatic Studies. The tests found in Table 50-8 are geared toward evaluating the metabolism of glucose. They are important in the diagnosis and management of diabetes. (Diagnostic studies for diabetes are discussed in Chapter 52.)

evolve   *An assessment case study of the endocrine system is available at* **http://evolve.elsevier.com/Canada/Lewis/medsurg**

REVIEW QUESTIONS

The number of the question corresponds to the same-numbered objective at the beginning of the chapter.

1. What is a characteristic of all hormones?
   a. They circulate in the blood bound to plasma proteins.
   b. They influence cellular activity of specific target tissues.
   c. They accelerate the metabolic processes of all body cells.
   d. They enter cells to alter the cell's metabolism or gene expression.

2. A patient is receiving radiation therapy for cancer of the kidney. The nurse monitors the patient for signs and symptoms of damage to which gland?
   a. Pancreas
   b. Thyroid
   c. Adrenal
   d. Posterior pituitary gland

3. A patient has a serum sodium level of 152 mmol/L. What is a normal hormonal response to this situation?
   a. Release of ADH
   b. Release of renin
   c. Secretion of aldosterone
   d. Secretion of corticotropin-releasing hormone

4. All cells in the body are believed to have intracellular receptors for which of the following?
   a. Insulin
   b. Glucagon
   c. Growth hormone
   d. Thyroid hormone

5. The nurse asks specifically about which of the following when obtaining subjective data from a patient during assessment of the endocrine system?
   a. Energy level
   b. Intake of vitamin C
   c. Employment history
   d. Frequency of sexual intercourse

6. What is an appropriate technique to use during physical assessment of the thyroid gland?
   a. Asking the patient to hyperextend the neck during palpation
   b. Percussing the neck for dullness to define the size of the thyroid
   c. Having the patient swallow water during inspection and palpation of the gland
   d. Using deep palpation to determine the extent of a visibly enlarged thyroid gland

7. Why do endocrine disorders often go unrecognized in older adults?
   a. Symptoms are often attributed to aging.
   b. They rarely have identifiable symptoms.
   c. Endocrine disorders are relatively rare.
   d. They usually have subclinical endocrine disorders.

8. Which of the following would the nurse consider an abnormal finding during an endocrine assessment?
   a. A blood pressure of 100/70
   b. Soft, formed stool every other day
   c. Excessive facial hair on a woman
   d. A 2.2-kg weight gain over the last 6 months

9. A patient has a total serum calcium level of 0.75 mmol/L. If this finding reflects hypoparathyroidism, what would the nurse expect further diagnostic testing to reveal?
   a. Decreased serum PTH
   b. Increased serum ACTH
   c. Increased serum glucose
   d. Decreased serum cortisol levels

ANSWERS: 1. b; 2. c; 3. a; 4. d; 5. a; 6. c; 7. a; 8. c; 9. a.

REFERENCES

Carroll, T. B., Aron, D. C., Findling, J. W., & Tyrell, J. B. (2011). Glucocorticoids and adrenal androgens. In D. Gardner, D. Shoback, & F. S. Greenspan (Eds.), *Greenspan's basic and clinical endocrinology* (9th ed., pp. 346-395). New York: McGraw-Hill.

Cooper, D. S., & Ladenson, P. W. (2011). The thyroid gland. In D. Gardner, D. Shoback, & F. S. Greenspan (Eds.), *Greenspan's basic and clinical endocrinology* (9th ed., pp. 163-225). New York: McGraw-Hill.

Eliopoulos, C. (2010). *Gerontological nursing* (7th ed.). Philadelphia: Lippincott, Williams & Wilkins.

Goodman, H. (2009). *Basic medical endocrinology* (4th ed.). Philadelphia: W. B. Saunders.

Jarvis, C., Browne, A. J., MacDonald-Jenkins, J., & Luctkar-Flude, M. (Eds.). (2009). *Physical examination and health assessment* (1st Canadian ed.). Toronto: Elsevier Canada.

Low, M. J. (2011). Neuroendocrinology. In S. Melmed, K. S. Polonsky, P. R. Larsen, & H. M. Kronenberg (Eds.), *Williams textbook of endocrinology* (12th ed., pp.103-175). Philadelphia: W. B. Saunders.

Pagana, K. D., & Pagana, T. J. (2011). *Mosby's diagnostic and laboratory test reference* (10th ed.). St. Louis: Mosby.

Radu, M. (2011). Physiology of the pituitary, thyroid and adrenal glands. *Surgery (Oxford)*, *29*(9), 419-427. doi:10.1016/j.mpsur.2011.06.017

Stehle, J. H., Saade, A., Rawashdeh, O., Ackermann, K., Jilg, A., Sebesteny, T., & Maronde, E. (2011). A survey of molecular details in the human pineal gland in the light of phylogeny, structure, function, and chronobiological diseases. *Journal of Pineal Research*, *51*(1), 17-43. doi:10.1111/j.1600-079X.2011.00856.x

Toward Optimized Practice Clinical Practice Guideline Working Group. (2008). Clinical practice guideline: Investigation and management of primary thyroid dysfunction. Retrieved from *http://www.topalbertadoctors.org/download/350/thyroid_guideline.pdf*

RESOURCES

Resources for this chapter are listed in Chapter 51, p. 1427 and Chapter 52, p. 1469.

Nursing Management:
Endocrine Problems

Written by Ian M. Camera

Adapted by Daphne Connolly

LEARNING OBJECTIVES

1. Describe the pathophysiology, clinical manifestations, collaborative care, and nursing management of the patient with an imbalance of hormones produced by the anterior pituitary gland.
2. Describe the pathophysiology, clinical manifestations, collaborative care, and nursing management of the patient with an imbalance of hormones produced by the posterior pituitary gland.
3. Describe the pathophysiology, clinical manifestations, collaborative care, and nursing management of the patient with thyroid dysfunction.
4. Describe the pathophysiology, clinical manifestations, collaborative care, and nursing management of the patient with an imbalance of the hormone produced by the parathyroid glands.

5. Describe the pathophysiology, clinical manifestations, collaborative care, and nursing management of the patient with an imbalance of hormones produced by the adrenal cortex.
6. Describe the pathophysiology, clinical manifestations, collaborative care, and nursing management of the patient with an excess of hormones produced by the adrenal medulla.
7. Explain the adverse effects of corticosteroid therapy.
8. Describe common nursing assessments, interventions, rationales, and expected outcomes related to patient teaching for management of chronic endocrine problems.

KEY TERMS

acromegaly A condition caused by excessive secretion of growth hormone and characterized by an overgrowth of the bones and soft tissues, p. 1394

Addison's disease Hypofunction of the adrenal cortex, in which the supply of all three classes of adrenal corticosteroids is reduced, p. 1420

cretinism Hypothyroidism that develops in infancy, p. 1409

Cushing's syndrome A metabolic disorder caused by excess corticosteroids, particularly glucocorticoids; most common causes are iatrogenic administration of exogenous corticosteroids (e.g., prednisone) in large doses for several weeks or longer and the chronic and excessive production of cortisol by the adrenal cortex, p. 1416

diabetes insipidus (DI) A group of conditions associated with deficient production or secretion of antidiuretic hormone (ADH) or with a decreased renal response to ADH; caused by injury to the neurohypophyseal system, p. 1399

exophthalmos Protrusion of the eyeballs from the orbits; caused by increased fat deposits and fluid in the retro-orbital tissues, p. 1404

goitre Enlargement of the thyroid gland that may be associated with hyperthyroidism, hypothyroidism, or normal thyroid function, p. 1401

Graves' disease An autoimmune disease of unknown origin that is marked by diffuse thyroid enlargement and excessive thyroid hormone secretion, p. 1403

hyperthyroidism A clinical syndrome characterized by a sustained increase in synthesis and release of thyroid hormones by the thyroid gland, p. 1403

hypopituitarism A rare disorder that involves a decrease in one or more of the pituitary hormones, p. 1397

hypothyroidism Insufficient circulation of thyroid hormones, resulting in a hypometabolic state, p. 1409

myxedema The characteristic facies of severe longstanding hypothyroidism (i.e., puffiness, periorbital edema, and masklike affect) caused by an accumulation of hydrophilic mucopolysaccharides in the dermis and other tissues, p. 1410

myxedema coma The progression of the mental sluggishness, drowsiness, and lethargy of hypothyroidism to a notable impairment of consciousness or coma that is a medical emergency, p. 1410

pheochromocytoma A rare condition characterized by a tumour of the adrenal medulla that produces excessive catecholamines, causing severe hypertension, p. 1424

syndrome of inappropriate antidiuretic hormone (SIADH) A condition characterized by fluid retention, serum hypo-osmolality, dilutional hyponatremia, hypochloremia, and concentrated urine in the presence of normal or increased intravascular volume; results from an abnormal production or sustained secretion of antidiuretic hormone despite normal or low plasma osmolarity, p. 1398

thyroiditis An inflammation of the thyroid gland that may cause hyperthyroid or hypothyroid manifestations, p. 1403

thyrotoxicosis A hypermetabolic state caused by excessive circulating levels of thyroxine, triiodothyronine, or both, p. 1403

ELECTRONIC RESOURCES

Supplemental content related to Chapter 51 can be found…

Evolve Web Site ⊖volve

http://evolve.elsevier.com/Canada/Lewis/medsurg

- Answer Guidelines for Case Study on p. 1425
- Clinical Reference: Laboratory Values
- Content Updates
- Customizable Nursing Care Plans:
  - Cushing's Syndrome
  - Hyperthyroidism
  - Hypothyroidism

- Electronic Calculators
- eTable 51-1: Comparison of SIADH and DI
- Examination Review Questions
- Glossary
- Interactive Case Studies:
  - Addison's Disease
  - Cushing's Syndrome
  - Hyperthyroidism
- Key Points (Printable and MP3 Download)
- Patient & Caregiver Teaching Guide: Corticosteroid Therapy

Disorders of the Anterior Pituitary Gland

Acromegaly

Etiology and Pathophysiology

Growth hormone (GH), an anabolic hormone, promotes protein synthesis and mobilizes glucose and free fatty acids. GH is produced by the anterior pituitary and stimulates the liver to produce insulin-like growth factor 1 (IGF-1), also known as *somatomedin C*. IGF-1 stimulates growth of bones and soft tissues. Normally, IGF-1 also signals the anterior pituitary gland to reduce GH production. Overproduction of GH is usually caused by a benign pituitary tumour (adenoma). The pituitary tumour secretes GH despite elevated IGF-1 levels, which leads to inordinate growth of bones and other soft tissue. Overproduction of GH also causes elevation of blood glucose levels through insulin antagonism. Prolonged elevation of glucose levels in association with elevation in GH leads to glucose intolerance. In affected children, excessive secretion of GH results in *gigantism*. When the onset of GH excess occurs before closure of the epiphyses, the long bones are still capable of longitudinal growth. The excessive growth is usually proportional. These children may grow as tall as 240 cm and weigh more than 136 kg.

In adults, excessive secretion of GH results in **acromegaly,** a condition characterized by a thickening of bones and soft tissues. Because the problem develops after epiphyseal closure in adults, the bones are unable to grow longer. Acromegaly is relatively rare.

The estimated annual incidence is up to 10 cases per 1 million population (Melmed, 2011). Both genders are affected in equal numbers.

Clinical Manifestations

Manifestations of acromegaly begin gradually, usually in the third and fourth decades of life. Typically, the time between the initial onset of symptoms and the final diagnosis is an average of 7 to 10 years (Miller, Learned-Miller, Trainer, Paisley, & Blanz, 2011). Individuals experience enlargement of the hands and feet. The enlargement of the bones and cartilage may cause symptoms that range from mild joint pain to deforming, crippling arthritis. Changes in physical appearance occur, with thickening and enlargement of bony and soft tissue on the face and head (Figure 51-1). Enlargement of the mandible causes the jaw to jut forward. The paranasal and the frontal sinuses enlarge, as does the bony tissue of the forehead. Enlargement of soft tissue around eyes, nose, and mouth results in a coarsening of facial features. Enlargement of the tongue results in speech difficulties, and the voice deepens as a result of hypertrophy of the vocal cords.

Sleep apnea may also occur and is thought to be related to upper airway narrowing that results from changes in pharyngeal soft tissues (Melmed, 2011). The skin becomes thick, leathery, and oily. People with acromegaly may also experience peripheral neuropathy and proximal muscle weakness. Women may develop menstrual disturbances. Individuals with acromegaly are more likely to develop polyps in the colon and colon cancer.

The enlarged pituitary gland can exert pressure on surrounding structures within the brain, leading to visual disturbances and headaches. Because GH mobilizes stored fat for energy, it increases free fatty acid levels in the blood, which predisposes patients to

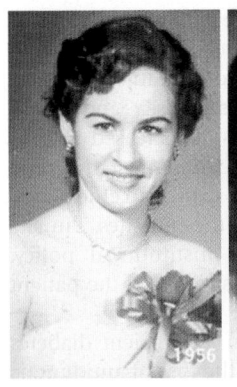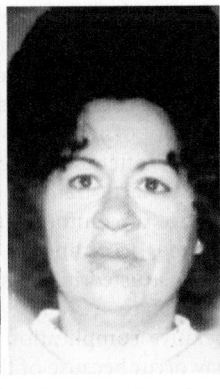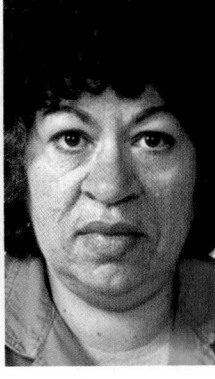

Figure 51-1 Example of progressive changes in facial features in acromegaly.

Source: Courtesy Linda Haas, Seattle, Washington.

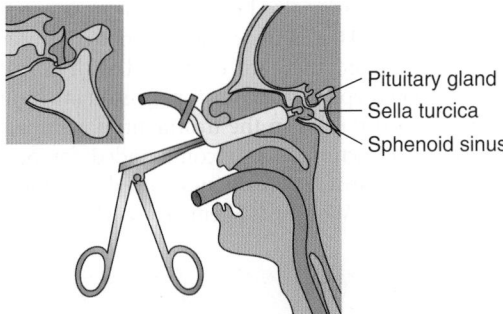

Figure 51-2 Surgery on the pituitary gland is most commonly performed with the trans-sphenoidal approach. An incision is made in the inner aspect of the upper lip and gingiva. The sella turcica is entered through the floor of the nose and the sphenoid sinuses.

atherosclerosis. The hormone also antagonizes the action of insulin and causes hyperglycemia. Manifestations of diabetes mellitus may occur, including polydipsia and polyuria. Prolonged secretion of GH leads to glucose intolerance.

Untreated acromegaly leads to a number of changes in the body. Effects on the cardiovascular system include cardiomegaly, left ventricular hypertrophy, angina pectoris, and hypertension. For this reason, disease of the cardiovascular system is associated with increased mortality rates among these individuals. Other systems that undergo changes include the gastrointestinal (GI), genitourinary, musculoskeletal, and nervous systems.

Diagnostic Studies

In addition to the history and physical examination, diagnosis of GH excess requires evaluation of plasma IGF-1 levels and GH response to an oral glucose tolerance test (OGTT). A single measurement of serum GH is of limited value in the diagnosis of acromegaly because GH levels normally fluctuate. IGF-1 levels are more constant and thus provide a more reliable measure. The definitive test for acromegaly is the OGTT. Normally, GH concentration falls during an OGTT. In acromegaly, these levels do not fall (Verrua et al., 2010).

Magnetic resonance imaging (MRI) is indicated for the identification and the localization of the pituitary tumour and the determination of its extension into surrounding tissue. High-resolution computed tomography (CT) with contrast media may also be used to localize the tumour. A complete ophthalmological examination, including evaluation of visual fields, is typically performed because the tumour (especially a macroadenoma larger than 10 mm in diameter) can cause pressure on the optic chiasm or the optic nerves.

Collaborative Care

The therapeutic goal in acromegaly is to return GH levels to normal. This is accomplished by surgery, radiation therapy, drug therapy, or a combination of these therapies. The prognosis depends on age at onset, age when treatment is initiated, and tumour size. Usually, bone growth can be arrested and soft tissue hypertrophy can be reversed. However, sleep apnea and diabetic and cardiac complications may persist in spite of treatment.

Surgical Therapy. Surgery is the treatment of choice and offers the best hope for a cure, especially for smaller tumours.

More than 90% of pituitary surgical procedures to remove tumours associated with acromegaly are accomplished with the transsphenoidal approach (Buchfelder & Schlaffer, 2009; Figure 51-2). Surgery produces an immediate reduction in GH levels that is followed by a drop in IGF-1 levels within a few weeks. Patients with larger tumours or those with GH levels higher than 50 mcg/L may require adjunctive drug or radiation therapy (Buchfelder & Schlaffer, 2009).

When the entire pituitary gland is removed during surgery *(hypophysectomy)*, the loss of pituitary hormones is permanent. Rather than replacing the pituitary (tropic) hormones, which requires parenteral administration, the essential hormones produced by target organs (glucocorticoids, thyroid hormone, and sex hormones) can be replaced orally. Hormone replacement must be continued throughout life.

Radiation Therapy. Radiation therapy is considered when surgery has failed to produce complete remission and for patients considered to be at high risk for surgical complications. External irradiation can successfully reduce GH levels in 30 to 70% of patients, but the primary disadvantage is the long delay (10 to 20 years) before GH levels normalize (Melmed, 2011). Radiation therapy is usually offered in combination with drugs that reduce GH levels. Radiation therapy has also been used to reduce the size of a tumour before surgery. Hypopituitarism commonly results from radiation therapy and necessitates hormone replacement therapy.

Stereotactic radiosurgery (gamma-knife surgery) may be used for small, surgically inaccessible pituitary tumours (see Chapter 59). This procedure consists of a single dose of radiation delivered to one site from multiple angles. It is used to occlude the blood vessels that supply the tumour and results in cell death.

Drug Therapy. Three groups of drugs are used in the treatment of acromegaly: somatostatin analogues, dopamine agonists, and GH-receptor antagonists. These drugs reduce GH levels and can be used as initial treatment or as adjunct therapy with surgery or radiation. The most common drug used for acromegaly is octreotide (Sandostatin), a somatostatin analogue that reduces GH levels to within the normal range in many patients. Octreotide is given by subcutaneous injection three times a day. Two long-acting analogues, octreotide (Sandostatin LAR), and lanreotide (Somatuline Autogel), are available as intramuscular (IM) injections every 2 to 4 weeks. Dopamine agonists, such as cabergoline (Dostinex) and bromocriptine mesylate

(Apo-bromocriptine), may also be used in the treatment of acromegaly to suppress GH secretion. They are not commonly used as sole therapy; rather, they are combined with somatostatin analogues. A GH receptor antagonist, pegvisomant (Somavert), has been developed for use in the treatment of acromegaly and directly blocks GH action. It is recommended for patients in whom surgery, somatostatin analogues, and dopamine agonists have failed (Sherlock, Woods, & Sheppard, 2011).

NURSING MANAGEMENT: ACROMEGALY

■ Nursing Assessment

The nurse must assess for signs and symptoms of abnormal tissue growth and evaluate changes in the physical size of each patient. Patients should be questioned about increases in hat, ring, glove, and shoe sizes and about changes in appearance. Photographs are helpful for evaluating any changes. Because physical changes occur slowly and over a long time, it is possible that the individual is not even aware of them.

■ Nursing Implementation

Patients typically have many questions and concerns regarding surgery. It is important for the nurse to offer reassurance and to provide accurate information regarding this process. The individual treated surgically needs skilled neurosurgical nursing care and must be prepared before surgery for postoperative care. After surgery in which a transsphenoidal approach has been used, the head of the patient's bed should be elevated at a 30-degree angle at all times. This elevation prevents pressure on the sella turcica and decreases the incidence of headaches, a frequent postoperative problem. Neurological status, including pupillary response, should be monitored in order to detect neurological complications. Patients should be instructed to avoid vigorous coughing, sneezing, and straining at stool (Valsalva's manoeuvre) to prevent leakage of cerebrospinal fluid from the point at which the sella turcica was entered.

Any clear nasal drainage should be sent to the laboratory to be tested for glucose. A glucose level higher than 1.67 mmol/L indicates leakage of cerebrospinal fluid from an open connection to the brain. If this happens, the patient is at an increased risk for meningitis. Complaints of persistent and severe generalized or supraorbital headache may indicate leakage of cerebrospinal fluid into the sinuses. A cerebrospinal fluid leak usually resolves within 72 hours when treated with head elevation and bed rest. If the leak persists, daily spinal taps may be performed to reduce pressure to below-normal levels and allow the fossa to heal. When a patient has a cerebrospinal fluid leak, IV antibiotics should be administered as ordered to prevent meningitis. If the leak does not respond to treatment within 72 hours, surgical intervention may be required.

Mild analgesics are given for headaches. The nurse should perform mouth care every 4 hours to keep the surgical area clean and free of debris and to promote patient comfort. Tooth brushing should be avoided for at least 10 days to prevent disrupting the suture line and to avoid discomfort.

If stereotactic radiosurgery is performed, the patient is usually moved from the specialized radiation centre to the neurosurgical nursing unit for overnight observation. The patient is in a stereotactic head frame. Vital signs, neurological status, and fluid volume status must be carefully monitored. Possible complications include increased headaches, seizures, nausea, and vomiting. A patient with a history of seizures is at increased risk for seizures for at least 24 hours after the procedure. All staff should know how to remove a stereotactic frame in case of an emergency. The patient may experience discomfort at the pin sites. Pin site care should be performed according to institutional policy. Family members can be instructed in pin site care if the patient is discharged with pins in place.

A possible postoperative complication is transient diabetes insipidus (DI). This may occur because of the loss of antidiuretic hormone (ADH), which is stored in the posterior lobe of the pituitary gland, or because of cerebral edema related to manipulation of the pituitary gland during surgery. To assess for DI, urine output and serum and urine osmolarity must be closely monitored. Clinical manifestations and treatment of DI are discussed in more detail later in this chapter.

If a hypophysectomy is performed or the pituitary gland is damaged, replacement of ADH, cortisol, and thyroid hormone is necessary. These medications must be taken for life; therefore, careful patient teaching is essential.

Surgery may result in permanent loss or deficiencies in follicle-stimulating hormone (FSH) and luteinizing hormone (LH). This can lead to decreased fertility. The nurse should assist patients in working through the grieving process associated with these losses.

The need for continued drug therapy reduces the patient's perception of independence and requires considerable emotional adjustment. The teaching plan should include self-administration of subcutaneous injections if prescribed. Cost issues related to the expense of ongoing medication, as well as other therapies, may be another area for nursing intervention.

The nurse must consider the emotional impact of a hypophysectomy when counselling patients and planning the educational program related to hormone replacement. Serial photographs to show improvement may be helpful. Psychological support from the nurse and from the patient's family and friends is needed to promote positive mental health outcomes for a patient with acromegaly. Patients with acromegaly are at higher risk for colon polyps and colorectal cancer and should undergo screening colonoscopy every 3 to 4 years (Melmed, 2011).

Excesses of Other Tropic Hormones

Excesses of tropic hormones and overproduction of a single anterior pituitary hormone usually cause syndromes related to hormone excess from the target organ. If the adrenocorticotropic hormone (ACTH) level is increased, Cushing's disease results; if the thyroid-stimulating hormone (TSH) level is excessive, hyperthyroidism develops.

Prolactinomas (prolactin-secreting adenomas) are the most frequently occurring pituitary tumours. Common manifestations experienced by women with prolactinomas include galactorrhea, ovulatory dysfunction (anovulation, infertility), menstrual dysfunction (oligomenorrhea or amenorrhea), decreased libido, and hirsutism. In men, erectile dysfunction and decreased libido and sperm density may result. Headaches and visual problems may also occur. The visual problems are secondary to pressure on the optic chiasm. Because prolactinomas do not typically enlarge, drug therapy is usually the first-line treatment (Yang, Hong, Lee, Lee, & Kim, 2011). Dopamine agonists such as cabergoline (Dostinex) and bromocriptine have been used successfully to treat this disorder. Surgery with the transsphenoidal approach discussed previously may be considered, depending on the size and extent of the tumour. Radiation therapy for treatment of prolactinomas has been used to a somewhat limited degree, mainly in patients in whom the tumour has failed to respond to medical or surgical therapy.

Hypofunction of the Pituitary Gland

Hypopituitarism is a rare disorder that involves a decrease in one or more of the pituitary hormones; signs and symptoms relate to the underlying disorder and to the specific pituitary hormones that are deficient or absent. The anterior pituitary gland secretes ACTH, TSH, FSH, LH, GH, and prolactin; the posterior pituitary gland secretes ADH and oxytocin. A deficiency of only one pituitary hormone is referred to as *selective hypopituitarism*. Total failure of the pituitary gland results in deficiency of all pituitary hormones; this condition is referred to as *panhypopituitarism*. The hormone deficiencies most commonly associated with hypopituitarism involve GH and the gonadotropins (e.g., LH, FSH).

Etiology and Pathophysiology

The most common cause of pituitary hypofunction is a pituitary tumour. Autoimmune disorders, infections, pituitary infarction (Sheehan's syndrome), or destruction of the pituitary gland (as a result of trauma, irradiation, or surgical procedures) can also cause hypopituitarism. *Sheehan's syndrome* is a postpartum condition of pituitary necrosis and hypopituitarism after circulatory collapse resulting from uterine hemorrhaging.

Hormone deficiencies involving anterior pituitary hormones lead to end-organ failure; thus the effects of hypopituitarism depend on the specific pituitary hormone or hormones that are lacking. For example, infertility may be the first indication of pituitary hypofunction associated with a pituitary tumour. Deficiencies of TSH and ACTH are life-threatening. ACTH deficiency causes a tendency toward shock and may result in an episode of acute adrenal insufficiency (refractory and life-threatening shock from sodium and water depletion). (Adrenal shock is discussed later in this chapter.)

Clinical Manifestations

The signs and symptoms associated with pituitary hypofunction vary with the degree and the speed of onset of pituitary dysfunction and are related to hyposecretion of the target glands, a growing pituitary tumour, or both. Common symptoms associated with a space-occupying lesion include headaches, visual changes (decreased peripheral vision or decreased visual acuity), *anosmia* (loss of the sense of smell), and seizures.

Many adults with GH deficiency have subtle, nonspecific clinical findings. They have truncal obesity and decreased muscle mass causing reduced strength, decreased energy, and reduced exercise capability. They may have a flat affect or appear depressed. Impaired psychological well-being is a common finding associated with GH deficiency in adults.

Deficiencies of FSH and LH in women are first manifested as menstrual irregularities, diminished libido, and changes in secondary sex characteristics (e.g., decreased breast size). Men with deficiencies of FSH and LH experience testicular atrophy, diminished spermatogenesis, loss of libido, erectile dysfunction, and decreased facial hair and muscle mass.

Deficiencies of ACTH and cortisol often produce a nonspecific clinical picture. Signs and symptoms may include weakness, fatigue, headache, dry and pale skin, and diminished amounts of axillary and pubic hair. Affected individuals may have postural hypotension, fasting hypoglycemia, diminished tolerance for stress, and poor resistance to infection.

The clinical presentations of individuals with thyroid hormone deficiency associated with hypopituitarism are similar (although usually milder) to those of patients with primary hypothyroidism. Common symptoms include cold intolerance, constipation, fatigue, lethargy, and weight gain. (Hypothyroidism is discussed in greater detail later in this chapter.)

Diagnostic Studies

In addition to a history and physical examination, diagnostic studies are useful in the diagnosis and treatment of hypopituitarism. Radiological tests such as MRI and CT are indicated to determine the presence of a pituitary tumour. The laboratory tests indicated for hypopituitarism vary widely but generally involve the direct measurement of pituitary hormones or an indirect determination of the hormone level. Diagnostic tests are also used to evaluate the effectiveness of therapy. See Chapter 50 for more information regarding diagnostic studies.

Nursing and Collaborative Management

Treatment of hypopituitarism consists of surgery or radiation therapy for tumour removal, followed by permanent hormone replacement. Surgery and radiation therapy for pituitary tumours are discussed earlier in this chapter. Hormone replacement therapy is carried out with the appropriate pituitary hormone (e.g., GH, corticosteroids, thyroid hormone, and sex hormones). Hormone replacement therapies for thyroid hormone and corticosteroids are discussed later in this chapter.

A primary nursing role in anterior pituitary insufficiency is assessment and recognition of signs and symptoms associated with hypopituitarism. Nursing management is directed at problems that result from hormone deficiency. The nurse also plays a pivotal role in teaching patients about diagnostic procedures, the disease process, and collaborative care options. Because the need for hormone therapy is lifelong, patient teaching must cover hormonal administration, adverse drug effects, and follow-up therapy.

Somatropin (Humatrope) is used for GH replacement therapy. Adults with GH deficiency respond well to GH replacement and experience increased energy, increased lean body mass, a feeling of well-being, and improved body image. The adverse drug effects most commonly reported by adults include swelling in the feet and the hands, pain in the joints, and headache. Somatropin is given as a subcutaneous injection. The dosage and administration is variable because it is adjusted according to the degree of relief from symptoms, IGF-1 levels, and the development of adverse effects.

Although gonadal deficiency is not life-threatening, replacement therapy is offered to improve sexual function and general well-being. This therapy, however, is contraindicated in individuals with certain medical conditions, such as breast cancer, phlebitis, pulmonary embolism in women, and prostate cancer in men. Estrogen and progesterone replacement therapy may be indicated for hypogonadal women to treat hot flashes, vaginal dryness, and decreased libido. Hormone replacement for women is discussed in greater detail in Chapter 56. Testosterone is used to treat men with gonadotropin deficiency. The benefits achieved with testosterone therapy include a return of male secondary sex characteristics, improvement in libido, and increased muscle mass, bone mass, and bone density. Hormone replacement for men is discussed in greater detail in Chapter 57.

Disorders of the Posterior Pituitary Gland

The hormones secreted by the posterior pituitary—ADH and oxytocin—are actually produced in the hypothalamus and then transported to and stored in the posterior pituitary gland. ADH, also referred to as *arginine vasopressin* (AVP) or *vasopressin*, plays a major role in the regulation of water balance and osmolarity (see Chapter 50).

The two primary conditions associated with ADH secretion are a result of either overproduction or underproduction of ADH. Overproduction or oversecretion of ADH results in the **syndrome of inappropriate antidiuretic hormone (SIADH)**. Underproduction or undersecretion of ADH results in a condition referred to as *diabetes insipidus*.

Syndrome of Inappropriate Antidiuretic Hormone

Etiology and Pathophysiology

SIADH occurs when ADH is released despite normal or low plasma osmolarity (Figure 51-3). SIADH results from an abnormal production or sustained secretion of ADH and is characterized by fluid retention, serum hypo-osmolality, dilutional hyponatremia, hypochloremia, concentrated urine in the presence of normal or increased intravascular volume, and normal renal function. This syndrome occurs more commonly in older adults (Soiza & Talbot, 2011).

The abnormal production or sustained secretion of ADH that leads to SIADH has various causes (Table 51-1). The most common cause is malignancy, especially small cell lung cancer. This relationship is strong enough that an evaluation for the presence of such a tumour is recommended when SIADH is otherwise unexplained (Robinson & Verbalis, 2011). SIADH tends to be self-limiting when caused by head trauma or drugs but is chronic in nature when associated with tumours or metabolic diseases.

Clinical Manifestations

Excess ADH increases both permeability of the distal tubules and collecting ducts and reabsorption of water into the circulation. Consequently, extracellular fluid volume expands, plasma osmolality declines, the glomerular filtration rate increases, and sodium levels decline (dilutional hyponatremia). Hyponatremia causes muscle cramps and weakness. Patients with SIADH experience low urinary output and increased body weight (Robinson & Verbalis, 2011). As the serum sodium level falls

PATHOPHYSIOLOGY MAP

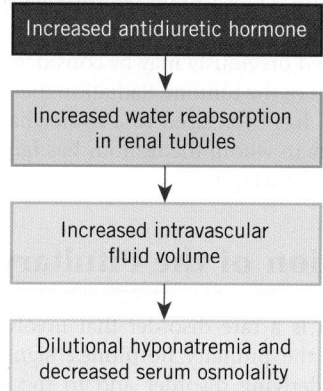

Figure 51-3 Pathophysiological development of the syndrome of inappropriate antidiuretic hormone (SIADH).

Source: Redrawn from Urden, L. D., Stacy, K. M., & Lough, M. E. (2010). *Critical care nursing: Diagnosis and management* (6th ed., p. 926, Figure 37-7). St. Louis: Mosby.

Table 51-1 Causes of Syndrome of Inappropriate Antidiuretic Hormone

Malignant Tumours	*Drug Therapy*
• Small cell carcinoma of the lung	• Carbamazepine (Tegretol)
• Pancreatic cancer	• Chlorpropamide
• Lymphoid cancers (Hodgkin's disease, non-Hodgkin's lymphoma, lymphocytic leukemia)	• General anaesthetic agents
	• Opioids
	• Oxytocin
• Thymus cancer	• Thiazide diuretics
• Prostate cancer	• SSRI antidepressants
• Colorectal cancer	• Tricyclic antidepressants
Central Nervous System Disorders	• Antineoplastic agents (vincristine, vinblastine, cyclophosphamide [Procytox])
• Head injury (skull fracture, subdural hematoma, subarachnoid hemorrhage)	*Miscellaneous Conditions*
	• Hypothyroidism
• Cerebrovascular injury	• Lung infection (pneumonia, tuberculosis, lung abscess)
• Brain tumours	
• Infection (encephalitis, meningitis)	• Chronic obstructive pulmonary disease
• Cerebral atrophy	• Positive pressure mechanical ventilation
• Guillain-Barré syndrome	• HIV infection
• Systemic lupus erythematosus	• Adrenal insufficiency

HIV, human immunodeficiency virus; *SSRI,* selective serotonin reuptake inhibitor.

(usually to less than 120 mmol/L), manifestations become more severe and include vomiting, abdominal cramps, muscle twitching, and seizures. As plasma osmolality and serum sodium levels continue to decline, cerebral edema may occur, leading to lethargy, anorexia, confusion, headache, seizures, and coma.

Diagnostic Studies

SIADH is diagnosed from simultaneous measurements of urine and serum osmolality. The dilutional hyponatremia is indicated by a serum sodium level of less than 134 mmol/L, serum osmolality of less than 280 mmol/kg, and a urine specific gravity greater than 1.005. A serum osmolality much lower than the urine osmolality indicates the inappropriate excretion of concentrated urine in the presence of dilute serum.

Collaborative Care

Once SIADH is identified, treatment is directed at the underlying cause of the disorder. Medications that stimulate the release of ADH should be avoided or discontinued (see Table 51-1). The immediate treatment goal is to restore normal fluid volume and osmolality. If symptoms are mild and the serum sodium level exceeds 125 mmol/L, the only treatment may be restriction of fluids to between 800 and 1000 mL/day. This restriction should result in gradual, daily reductions in weight, a progressive rise in serum sodium concentration and osmolality, and improvement in symptoms.

In cases of severe hyponatremia (serum sodium level < 120 mmol/L), especially in the presence of neurological symptoms such as seizures, IV hypertonic saline solution (3 to 5%) may be administered. Hypertonic saline must be administered very slowly on an infusion pump to avoid too rapid a rise in sodium. A diuretic such as furosemide (Lasix) may be used to promote diuresis, but only if the serum sodium level is at least 125 mmol/L because it may promote further loss of sodium. Because furosemide increases potassium, calcium, and magnesium losses, supplements may be needed. A fluid restriction of 500 mL/day is also indicated for patients with severe hyponatremia.

In chronic SIADH, water restriction of between 800 and 1000 mL/day is recommended. Because this degree of restriction may not be tolerated, agents that block the effect of ADH on the renal tubules may be prescribed, thereby allowing more dilution of urine. Tolvaptan (Samsca), a vasopressin receptor antagonist, is used to treat euvolemia-hyponatremia in hospitalized patients. This medication should be initiated in a closely monitored setting to prevent rapid correction of the serum sodium level.

Table 51-2 Nursing Assessment and Management: Syndrome of Inappropriate Antidiuretic Hormone

Assessment

- Frequent measurement of vital signs
- Frequent measurement of intake (oral and parenteral) and output
- Frequent measurement of urine specific gravity
- Daily weight measurement
- Monitoring of level of consciousness
- Observation for signs of hyponatremia (e.g., decreased neurological function, seizures, nausea and vomiting, muscle cramping)
- Monitoring of heart and lung sounds

Management

- Restricting total fluid intake to no more than 1000 mL/day (including that taken with medications)
- Positioning of head of bed flat or with no more than 10 degrees of elevation to enhance venous return to heart and increase left atrial filling pressure, thereby reducing ADH release
- Protection from injury (i.e., assist with ambulation, bed alarm) because of potential alterations in mental status
- Seizure precautions
- Frequent turning, positioning, and range of motion exercise (if patient is bedridden)
- Frequent oral hygiene
- Provision of distractions to decrease the discomfort of thirst related to fluid restrictions
- Provision of support for patient and significant others regarding diagnosis and any mental status changes

ADH, antidiuretic hormone.

NURSING MANAGEMENT: SYNDROME OF INAPPROPRIATE ANTIDIURETIC HORMONE

The nurse can be instrumental in the early detection and treatment of SIADH. An appropriate nursing assessment (Table 51-2) should be conducted for patients at risk for SIADH and those who have confirmed SIADH. Specifically, the nurse should be alert for low urinary output with a high specific gravity, a sudden weight gain, or a decline in serum sodium level. Nursing management of acute onset of SIADH is presented in Table 51-2.

When SIADH is chronic, patients must learn to self-manage treatment regimens. Fluids are restricted to between 800 and 1000 mL/day. Ice chips or sugarless chewing gum can help decrease thirst. If drinking liquids is an aspect of socialization, patients should be assisted in planning fluid intake so that liquid allowances are saved for social occasions. Patients may be treated with a diuretic to remove excess fluid volume. The diet should be supplemented with sodium and potassium, especially if diuretics are prescribed. Solutions of these electrolytes must be well diluted to prevent gastrointestinal irritation or damage. They are best taken at mealtime to allow mixing with and dilution by food. Patients should be taught the symptoms of fluid and electrolyte imbalances, especially those involving sodium and potassium, so that responses to treatment can be monitored (see Chapter 19).

Diabetes Insipidus

Etiology and Pathophysiology

Diabetes insipidus (DI) is a group of conditions associated with a deficiency of production or secretion of ADH or with a decreased renal response to ADH caused by injury to the neurohypophyseal system. The decrease in ADH results in fluid and electrolyte imbalances caused by increased urinary output and increased plasma osmolality (Figure 51-4). Depending on the cause, DI may be transient or a chronic lifelong condition.

Diabetes insipidus has several classifications (Table 51-3). *Central DI* (also known as *neurogenic DI*) occurs when any organic lesion of the hypothalamus, the infundibular stem, or the posterior pituitary gland interferes with ADH synthesis, transport, or release.

PATHOPHYSIOLOGY MAP

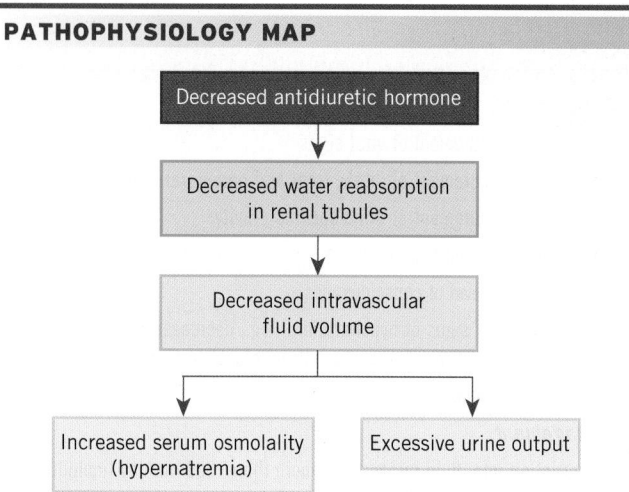

Figure 51-4 Pathophysiological development of diabetes insipidus.

Source: Redrawn from Urden, L. D., Stacy, K. M., & Lough, M. E. (2010). *Critical care nursing: Diagnosis and management* (6th ed., p. 922, Figure 37-6). St. Louis: Mosby.

Table 51-3 Types and Causes of Diabetes Insipidus

TYPES	CAUSES
Central diabetes insipidus (neurogenic)	Problem stems from an interference with ADH synthesis or release. Multiple causes include brain tumour, head injury, brain surgery, CNS infections.
Nephrogenic diabetes insipidus	Problem stems from inadequate renal response to ADH despite presence of adequate levels of ADH. Causes include drug therapy (especially lithium), renal damage, or hereditary renal disease.
Primary diabetes insipidus	Problem stems from excessive water intake. Causes are structural lesion in thirst centre and psychological disorder.

ADH, antidiuretic hormone; *CNS,* central nervous system.

Nephrogenic DI is a term for conditions in which the ADH level is adequate but the response to ADH is decreased in the kidneys. Lithium is one of the most common causes of drug-induced nephrogenic DI. Hypokalemia and hypercalcemia may also lead to nephrogenic DI.

Primary (also called *psychogenic*) *DI,* a less common condition, is associated with excessive water intake. This can be caused by a structural lesion in the thirst centre, or it may be caused by psychological disorders.

Clinical Manifestations

DI is characterized by increased thirst (polydipsia) and increased urination (polyuria; see Figure 51-4). The primary characteristic of DI is the excretion of large quantities of urine (5-20 L per day) with a very low specific gravity (<1.005) and urine osmolality of less than 100 mmol/kg. Serum osmolality is elevated (usually >295 mmol/kg) as a result of hypernatremia caused by pure water loss in the kidneys. Most affected patients compensate for fluid loss by drinking great amounts of water so that serum osmolality is normal or only moderately elevated. Patients may be fatigued from nocturia and may experience generalized weakness.

Central DI usually occurs suddenly with excessive fluid loss. After intracranial surgery, DI usually has a triphasic pattern: the acute phase, with abrupt onset of polyuria; an interphase, in which urine volume apparently normalizes; and a third phase, in which central DI is permanent. The third phase is usually apparent within 10 to 14 days postoperatively. Central DI that results from head trauma is usually self-limiting and improves with treatment of the underlying problem. DI following cranial surgery is more likely to be permanent. Although the clinical manifestations of nephrogenic DI are similar, the onset and the amount of fluid losses are less dramatic.

If oral fluid intake cannot keep up with urinary losses, severe fluid volume deficit results. This deficit is manifested by weight loss, constipation, poor tissue turgor, hypotension, tachycardia, and shock. In addition, affected patients shows central nervous system (CNS) manifestations, ranging from irritability and mental dullness to coma. These manifestations are related to increasing serum osmolality and hypernatremia. Because of the polyuria, severe dehydration and hypovolemic shock may occur.

Diagnostic Studies

Because DI may be central, nephrogenic, or psychogenic in origin, identification of the cause is the initial step. A complete history is documented, and a thorough physical examination is performed. Primary or psychogenic DI is associated with overhydration and hypervolemia rather than with the dehydration and hypovolemia seen in other forms of DI. A water deprivation test is usually performed to confirm the diagnosis of central DI. Before the water deprivation test, the patient's baseline weight, pulse, urine and plasma osmolalities, specific gravity of urine, and blood pressure (BP) are measured. All fluids are withheld for 8 to 16 hours. Patients may be anxious and should be reassured that the test will be stopped if fluid volume deficit becomes severe. Patients should be observed throughout the test because of the craving to drink. During the test, the patient's BP, weight, and urine osmolality are assessed hourly. The test continues until urine osmolality stabilizes (hourly increase of <30 mmol/kg in 3 consecutive hours), body weight declines by 3%, or orthostatic hypotension develops. ADH is then given, and urine osmolality is measured 1 hour later. In central DI, the rise in urinary osmolality after vasopressin administration exceeds 9%. Individuals with nephrogenic DI will have no response (Pagana & Pagana, 2011).

Collaborative Care

Determining and treating the primary cause is central in the collaborative management of DI. The therapeutic goal is maintenance of fluid and electrolyte balance.

For central DI, fluid and hormonal replacement is the cornerstone of treatment. In acute DI, hypotonic saline is administered IV and titrated to replace urinary output (Gardner, 2011). Hormone replacement is necessary because of the lack of ADH production or secretion. Desmopressin acetate (DDAVP), an analogue of ADH, is the hormone replacement of choice for central DI. DDAVP can be administered orally, IV, or as a nasal spray. Another drug available for ADH replacement is vasopressin. Several drugs can be used for the treatment of partial central DI, including carbamazepine (Tegretol).

Hormone replacement has little effect in the treatment of nephrogenic DI because the kidney is unable to respond to ADH. Instead, the treatment for nephrogenic DI revolves around dietary measures (low-sodium diet) and thiazide diuretics. Limiting sodium intake to no more than 3 g per day is thought to help decrease urine output. Thiazide diuretics (e.g., hydrochlorothiazide) are able to slow the glomerular filtration rate and allow the kidneys to reabsorb more water in the loop of Henle and the distal tubules. When low-sodium diet and thiazides are not effective, indomethacin (Indocin) may be prescribed. Indomethacin, a nonsteroidal anti-inflammatory agent, helps increase renal responsiveness to ADH.

NURSING MANAGEMENT: DIABETES INSIPIDUS

Nursing management of patients with DI revolves around early detection, maintenance of adequate hydration, and patient teaching for long-term management.

Acute DI is treated with fluids and hormone replacement. Fluids are replaced orally or IV, depending on the patient's condition and ability to drink copious amounts of fluids. Adequate amounts of fluids should be kept at the patient's bedside. If IV glucose solutions are used, the serum glucose level should be monitored because hyperglycemia and glucosuria can lead to osmotic diuresis, which increases the fluid volume deficit. Accurate records of intake and output, urine specific gravity, and daily weights are mandatory in the assessment of fluid volume status.

Nursing interventions also include the administration of DDAVP. Patients should be assessed for weight gain, headache, restlessness, and signs of hyponatremia and water intoxication. By monitoring fluid intake and output and the urine specific gravity, the nurse can assess the adequacy of treatment. The health care provider should be notified immediately if the patient with DI develops increased urine volume with a low specific gravity because this indicates need for increasing the dosage of DDAVP.

The patient with chronic DI requiring long-term ADH replacement needs instruction in self-management. DDAVP can be taken orally or intranasally. Nasal irritation may result from nasal administration. Headache, nausea, and other signs of hyponatremia may indicate overdosage, whereas failure to improve may indicate underdosage. The patient should be instructed to report any of these symptoms. Patients taking DDAVP should be instructed to monitor their weight daily; increases in weight may indicate fluid retention. The need for close follow-up, including laboratory studies, is an essential part of the teaching plan.

Table 51-4 compares diabetes insipidus and SIADH. (See eTable 51-1, available on the Evolve Web site for this chapter, for a more detailed comparison.)

Disorders of the Thyroid Gland

The thyroid hormones, thyroxine (T_4) and triiodothyronine (T_3), regulate energy metabolism, growth, and development. Disorders of the thyroid gland include enlargement, benign and malignant nodules, inflammation, and hyperfunctioning and hypofunctioning states (Figure 51-5).

Thyroid Enlargement: Goitre

A **goitre** is an enlarged thyroid gland. In a person with a goitre, the thyroid cells are stimulated to grow, which may result in an

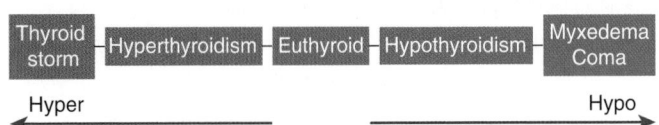

Figure 51-5 Continuum of thyroid dysfunction.

Table 51-4 Comparison of Diabetes Insipidus and SIADH		
FEATURE	**DIABETES INSIPIDUS**	**SIADH**
Definition	Deficiency of antidiuretic hormone (ADH) results in inability to conserve water.	Excessive amounts of ADH are secreted from posterior pituitary and other ectopic sources.
Pathophysiological features	With ADH deficiency, permeability of water is diminished, which results in excretion of large volumes of hypotonic fluid. Three patterns may develop: (a) transient diabetes insipidus—abrupt onset within first few days after neurosurgery, resolves; (b) permanent diabetes insipidus—abrupt and early onset, persists for several weeks or for life; (c) triphasic diabetes insipidus—an acute phase with abrupt onset of polyuria; an interphase, in which urine volume apparently normalizes; and a third phase, in which central diabetes insipidus is permanent.	Key features of ADH excess are (a) water retention, (b) hyponatremia, and (c) hypo-osmolality. Continual release of ADH causes water retention from renal tubules and collecting ducts; extracellular fluid volume increases with dilutional hyponatremia; and hyponatremia suppresses renin and aldosterone secretions, which causes decrease in proximal tubule reabsorption of Na^+.
Clinical manifestations	Genitourinary: polyuria: a few liters to 18 L/day; clear urine; urinary frequency; nocturia Gastrointestinal: weight loss; polydipsia (if thirst mechanism intact) Integumentary: dry skin and mucous membranes Neurological: mentation changes as electrolyte imbalance and hypotension worsen	Related to degree of hyponatremia: confusion, lethargy, irritability, seizures, coma Gastrointestinal: decreased motility with anorexia, nausea, vomiting; abrupt weight gain *without edema* in 5-10% of affected patients

Source: Adapted from Black, J. M., & Hawks, J. H. (2009). *Medical-surgical nursing: Clinical management for positive outcomes* (8th ed., pp. 1058-1059). St. Louis: Saunders Elsevier.
Note: a more detailed version of this table is available on the Evolve Web site for this chapter.
SIADH, syndrome of inappropriate antidiuretic hormone.

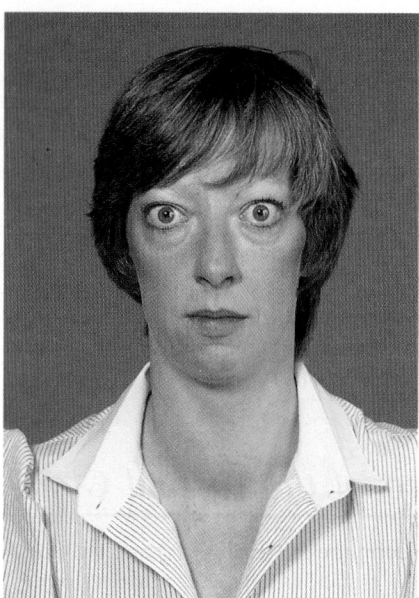

Figure 51-6 Exophthalmos and goitre of Graves' disease.

Source: Forbes, C. D., & Jackson, W. F. (2003). *Color atlas and text of clinical medicine* (3rd ed., p. 309, Figure 7.55). London: Mosby.

Table 51-5 Drugs That Are Goitrogens	
Thyroid Inhibitors	*Others*
• Propylthiouracil	• Sulphonamides
• Methimazole (Tapazole)	• Salicylates
• Iodine in large doses	• Para-aminosalicylic acid
	• Lithium
	• Amiodarone (Cordarone)

overactive thyroid (hyperthyroidism) or an underactive one (hypothyroidism). Goitres are common in patients with Graves' disease (Figure 51-6). A goitre that produces excess thyroid hormone is called a *toxic goitre.* A nontoxic goitre produces normal levels of thyroid hormone. Goitre as a clinical manifestation of thyroid disorders is further discussed in the following sections.

The most common cause of goitre worldwide is a lack of iodine in the diet. In Canada, where most people use iodized salt, goitre is more often caused by the overproduction or underproduction of thyroid hormones or by nodules that develop in the gland itself. Foods or drugs that contain thyroid-inhibiting substances (goitrogens) can cause goitre (Table 51-5).

In a person with a goitre, TSH and T_4 levels are measured to determine whether a goitre is associated with hyperthyroidism, hypothyroidism, or normal thyroid function. Thyroid antibodies are measured to assess for thyroiditis (inflammation of the thyroid). Treatment with thyroid hormone may prevent further thyroid enlargement. Large goiters are removed surgically.

Thyroid Nodules and Cancer

A *thyroid nodule,* a palpable deformity of the thyroid gland, may be benign or malignant. More than 95% of all thyroid nodules are benign. The incidence of thyroid nodules increases with age.

Benign nodules are usually not dangerous, but they can cause tracheal compression if they become too large. Nodules should be assessed and evaluated (discussed in the section Diagnostic Studies).

Thyroid cancer is the most common endocrine-related carcinoma. It was estimated that 5600 new cases of thyroid cancer would be diagnosed in Canada in 2012 (Canadian Cancer Society's Steering Committee on Cancer Statistics, 2012), the majority of these in women. The primary sign of thyroid cancer is the presence of a painless, palpable nodule or nodules in an enlarged thyroid gland. Patients or health care providers discover most of these nodules during routine palpation of the neck.

Types of Thyroid Cancer

The four main types of thyroid cancer include papillary, follicular, medullary, and anaplastic. *Papillary* thyroid cancer is the most common type, accounting for about 70 to 80% of all thyroid cancers. Papillary cancer tends to grow slowly and spreads initially to lymph nodes in the neck (Elaraj & Sturgeon, 2009).

Follicular thyroid cancer, which accounts for approximately 10 to 15% of all thyroid cancers, tends to occur in older adults. Follicular cancer first grows into the cervical lymph nodes. Follicular cancer is more likely than papillary cancer to grow into blood vessels and, from there, to spread to the lungs and bones.

Medullary thyroid cancer, which accounts for 5 to 10% of all thyroid cancers, is more likely to occur in families and to be associated with other endocrine problems. It can be diagnosed through genetic testing. In family members of a person with medullary thyroid cancer, a positive finding of the *RET* proto-oncogene can enable early diagnosis and treatment of medullary thyroid cancer.

Anaplastic thyroid cancer, which accounts for less than 5% of all thyroid cancers, is the most advanced and aggressive thyroid cancer. It is the least likely to respond to treatment.

Diagnostic Studies

Nodular enlargement of the thyroid gland or palpation of a mass usually necessitates radiological evaluation. Ultrasonography is often the first radiological test used in the diagnostic workup of a thyroid nodule. CT, MRI, and ultrasonography-guided fine-needle aspiration (FNA) are other diagnostic options. FNA is indicated when a tissue sample is necessary for pathological examination.

FNA is considered one of the most effective methods of identifying malignancy (Coorough et al., 2011). A thyroid scan may also be performed to evaluate for possible malignancy. The scan shows whether nodules on the thyroid are "hot" or "cold." Thyroid tumours may or may not take up radioactive iodine. Tumours that take up the radioactive iodine are called "hot" nodules and are nearly always benign. If the nodule does not take up the radioactive iodine, it appears as "cold" and has a higher risk of being malignant (Figure 51-7). Measurement of serum calcitonin is also helpful in diagnosis because increased levels are associated with medullary thyroid carcinoma.

Nursing and Collaborative Care

Surgical removal of the tumour is usually indicated in the treatment of thyroid cancer. Surgical procedures may range from unilateral total lobectomy with removal of the isthmus to total thyroidectomy with bilateral lobectomy. The latter choice is

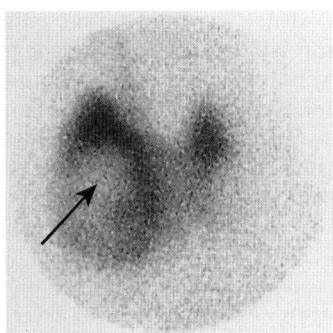

Figure 51-7 A large "cold" nodule *(arrow)* on the thyroid gland, detected on a scan.

Source: Forbes, C. D., & Jackson, W. F. (2003). *Color atlas and text of clinical medicine* (3rd ed., p. 313, Figure 7.72). London: Mosby.

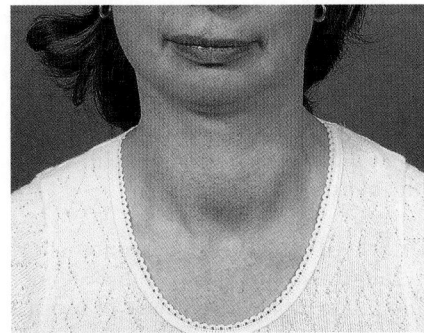

Figure 51-8 Appearance of the neck in Hashimoto's thyroiditis.

Source: Belchetz, P. E., & Hammond, P. (2003). *Mosby's color atlas and text of diabetes and endocrinology.* London: Mosby.

desirable because it is more likely to preserve the function of the parathyroid gland (Fitzgibbons, Brams, & Wei, 2008). In addition, many thyroid cancers are TSH dependent, and thyroid hormone in hyperphysiological doses is often prescribed to inhibit pituitary secretion of TSH. Radiation therapy may be used as the primary treatment or as palliative treatment for patients with metastatic thyroid cancer. Nursing care for patients with thyroid tumours is similar to care for patients who have undergone thyroidectomy and should also include general nursing measures for patients with cancer (see Chapter 18).

Thyroiditis

Thyroiditis is an inflammation of the thyroid gland that can have several causes. *Subacute granulomatous thyroiditis* is thought to be caused by a viral infection. *Acute thyroiditis* is caused by a bacterial or fungal infection. Subacute and acute forms of thyroiditis have abrupt onsets, and the thyroid gland is painful. *Chronic autoimmune thyroiditis* (Hashimoto's thyroiditis) can lead to hypothyroidism. *Hashimoto's thyroiditis* is a chronic autoimmune disease in which thyroid tissue is replaced by lymphocytes and fibrous tissue (Figure 51-8). It is the most common cause of goitrous hypothyroidism. *Silent thyroiditis,* a form of lymphocytic thyroiditis, has a variable onset and no apparent symptoms. *Postpartum thyroiditis* occurs frequently in women with a history of thyroid disease who have recently given birth. In most respects, silent and postpartum thyroiditis resemble Hashimoto's thyroiditis, except that the gland tends to recover and thyroid hormone treatment needs to be administered for only a few weeks (Thyroid Foundation of Canada, 2011).

T_4 and T_3 levels are initially elevated in subacute, acute, and silent thyroiditis but may become depressed over time. TSH levels are initially low and then elevated. Thyroid hormone levels are usually low in chronic Hashimoto's thyroiditis, but the TSH level is high. Radioactive iodine uptake (RAIU) is suppressed in subacute and silent thyroiditis. Antithyroid antibodies are present in patients with Hashimoto's thyroiditis.

Recovery from thyroiditis may be complete in weeks or months without treatment. If the condition is bacterial in origin, treatment may include specific antibiotics or surgical drainage. In subacute and acute forms, salicylates and nonsteroidal anti-inflammatory drugs are administered. If patients do not respond to these drugs in 48 hours, corticosteroids are administered.

Propranolol (Inderal) or atenolol (Tenormin) may be used for the cardiovascular symptoms of a hyperthyroid condition. Thyroid hormone replacement is indicated if a patient is hypothyroid.

Nursing care of patients with thyroiditis involves teaching about treatment and encouraging adherence to the treatment regimen. Patients are instructed to remain under close health care supervision so that progress can be monitored and any change in symptoms can be reported immediately to the health care provider.

Patients with thyroiditis of autoimmune origin may be susceptible to other autoimmune disorders such as Addison's disease, pernicious anemia, premature gonadal failure, or Graves' disease (Hubbard, 2011). Patients should be taught the signs and symptoms of these disorders, particularly Addison's disease. A patient receiving thyroid hormone replacement must be taught the expected adverse effects of these drugs and how to manage them. Patients treated surgically need care similar to that given to patients undergoing thyroidectomy.

Hyperthyroidism

Hyperthyroidism is hyperactivity of the thyroid gland with sustained increase in synthesis and release of thyroid hormones. **Thyrotoxicosis** is the clinical syndrome of hypermetabolism caused by excess circulating levels of T_4, T_3, or both. Hyperthyroidism and thyrotoxicosis usually occur together, as in Graves' disease. However, in some forms of thyroiditis, thyrotoxicosis may occur without hyperthyroidism (Hubbard, 2011).

Hyperthyroidism is more prevalent among women than among men; the frequency is highest among people 20 to 40 years old. The most common form of hyperthyroidism is Graves' disease. Other causes include toxic nodular goitre, thyroiditis, exogenous iodine excess, pituitary tumours, and thyroid cancer.

Etiology and Pathophysiology

Graves' Disease. **Graves' disease** is an autoimmune disease of unknown etiology marked by diffuse thyroid enlargement and excessive thyroid hormone secretion. Precipitating factors such as insufficient iodine supply, infections, and stressful life events may interact with genetic factors to cause Graves' disease. In Canada, Graves' disease accounts for 90% of the cases of hyperthyroidism (Thyroid Foundation of Canada, 2011). Patients with this disease develop antibodies to the TSH receptor. These antibodies attach to the receptors and stimulate the thyroid gland to release T_3, T_4, or both. The excessive release of thyroid hormones leads to the clinical manifestations associated with thyrotoxicosis. The disease is characterized by remissions and exacerbations, with or without treatment. It may progress to destruction of thyroid tissue, which causes hypothyroidism.

Toxic Nodular Goitres. Nodular goitres are characterized by thyroid hormone–secreting nodules that are independent of TSH stimulation. If associated with signs of hyperthyroidism, a nodule is termed *toxic*. A goitre may have multiple nodules (multinodular goitre) or a single nodule (solitary autonomous nodule). The nodules are usually benign follicular adenomas. Toxic nodular goitres occur equally in men and women. Although they can appear at any age, the frequency of toxic multinodular goitre is highest among people older than 40 years.

Clinical Manifestations

The clinical manifestations of hyperthyroidism are related to the effects of excess amounts of thyroid hormones. Excess amounts of circulating thyroid hormone directly increase metabolism. They also increase tissue sensitivity to stimulation by the sympathetic nervous system.

Palpation of the thyroid gland may reveal a goitre. When the thyroid gland is excessively large, a goitre may be visible. Auscultation of the thyroid gland may reveal bruits, a reflection of increased blood supply. Another common finding associated with hyperthyroidism is *ophthalmopathy,* a term used to describe abnormal eye appearance or function. A classic finding in Graves' disease is **exophthalmos,** a protrusion of the eyeballs from the orbits (see Figure 51-6). Exophthalmos is a type of infiltrative ophthalmopathy that results from impairment of venous drainage from the orbit, which causes increased fat deposits and fluid (edema) in the retro-orbital tissues. Because of increased pressure, the eyeballs are forced outward and protrude. This sign is seen in 20 to 50% of patients with Graves' disease. It is usually bilateral but can be unilateral or asymmetrical. In ophthalmopathy, the upper eyelids are usually retracted and elevated, with the sclera visible above the iris. When the eyelids do not close completely, the exposed corneal surfaces become dry and irritated. Serious consequences, such as corneal ulcers and eventual loss of vision, can occur.

Other common manifestations of thyroid hyperfunction are summarized in Table 51-6. A patient with advanced disease may exhibit many of the manifestations, whereas a patient in the early stages of hyperthyroidism may exhibit only weight loss and increased nervousness. Manifestations of hyperthyroidism (e.g., palpitations, tremors, weight loss) in older adults do not differ significantly from those in younger adults (Jett, 2008). In some instances in which confusion and agitation are reported, dementia may be suspected, and this suspicion may delay the diagnosis. In Table 51-7, features of hyperthyroidism in younger and older adult patients are compared.

Complications

Thyrotoxic crisis (also called *thyroid storm*) is an acute, rare condition in which all hyperthyroid manifestations are intensified. Although thyrotoxic crisis is considered a life-threatening emergency, death is rare when treatment is initiated early. The cause is thought to be stressors (e.g., infection, trauma, surgery) in a patient with pre-existing hyperthyroidism, either diagnosed or undiagnosed. Heart and nerve tissues become more sensitive to sympathetic nervous system activation because more binding sites for epinephrine and norepinephrine are present.

Manifestations include severe tachycardia, heart failure, shock, hyperthermia (temperature up to 40.7°C), restlessness, agitation, seizures, abdominal pain, nausea, vomiting, diarrhea, delirium, and coma. Treatment is aimed at reducing circulating thyroid hormone levels and the clinical manifestations of this disorder by appropriate drug therapy. Supportive therapy is directed at managing respiratory distress, fever reduction, fluid replacement, and elimination or management of the initiating stressor or stressors.

Diagnostic Studies

The two primary laboratory findings used to confirm the diagnosis of hyperthyroidism are decreased TSH levels and elevated free T_4 levels (Simmons, 2010). Total T_3 and T_4 levels may also be assessed, but these are not as definitive. Measurements of total T_3 and T_4 include both free and bound (to protein) hormone levels. The free hormone is the only form of the hormone that is biologically active.

The radioactive iodine uptake test is indicated to differentiate Graves' disease from other forms of thyroiditis. The 24-hour test of radioiodine uptake in patients with Graves' disease reveals a diffuse, homogeneous uptake of 35 to 90%, whereas in patients with thyroiditis, the amount of uptake is less than 20%. Patients with nodular goitre demonstrate uptake in the high-normal range (see Table 51-7).

Collaborative Care

The overall goal in the treatment of hyperthyroidism is to block the adverse effects of thyroid hormones and stop their oversecretion. The three primary treatment options for patients with hyperthyroidism are antithyroid medications, radioactive iodine therapy, and subtotal thyroidectomy (Table 51-8). In general, the treatment of choice in nonpregnant adults is radioactive iodine therapy. However, the choice of treatment is influenced by the patient's age, severity of the disorder, complicating features (including pregnancy), and the patient's preferences. If surgery is to be performed, antithyroid drugs and iodine are usually administered to produce a euthyroid state and possibly β-adrenergic blockers to relieve symptoms preoperatively.

Drug Therapy. Drugs used in the treatment of hyperthyroidism include antithyroid drugs, iodine, and β-adrenergic blockers. It is important to note that although these drugs are useful in the treatment of thyrotoxic states, they are not considered curative. Radiation therapy or surgery may ultimately be required.

Antithyroid Drugs. The first-line antithyroid drugs used in the treatment of hyperthyroidism are thioamides, such as propylthiouracil (Propyl-Thyracil) and methimazole (Tapazole). These drugs inhibit the synthesis of thyroid hormones. Propyl-Thyracil also blocks peripheral conversion of T_4 to T_3. Individual response is considerably varied; however, improvement usually begins 1 to 2 weeks after the initiation of therapy, and good results are seen within 4 to 8 weeks. Therapy is usually continued for 6 months to 2 years to allow for spontaneous remission. The major disadvantages of these drugs are possible patients' nonadherence to the regimen and a high rate of recurrence of hyperthyroidism

Table 51-6 Clinical Manifestations: Thyroid Hormone Dysfunction

HYPOFUNCTION	HYPERFUNCTION	HYPOFUNCTION	HYPERFUNCTION
Cardiovascular system		**Musculoskeletal System**	
• Increased capillary fragility	• Systolic hypertension	• Fatigue	• Fatigue
• Decreased rate and force of cardiac contractions	• Increased rate and force of cardiac contractions	• Weakness	• Muscle weakness
• Varied changes in blood pressure	• Bounding, rapid pulse	• Muscular aches and pains	• Proximal muscle wasting
• Cardiac hypertrophy	• Increased cardiac output	• Slow movements	• Dependent edema
• Distant heart sounds	• Cardiac hypertrophy	• Arthralgia	• Osteoporosis
• Anemia	• Systolic murmurs	**Nervous System**	
• Tendency to develop heart failure, angina, myocardial infarction	• Dysrhythmias	• Apathy	• Difficulty in focusing eyes
	• Palpitations	• Lethargy	• Nervousness
	• Atrial fibrillation (more common in older adults)	• Fatigue	• Fine tremor (of fingers and tongue)
	• Angina	• Forgetfulness	• Insomnia
Respiratory System		• Slowed mental processes	• Lability of mood, delirium
• Dyspnea	• Increased respiratory rate	• Hoarseness	• Restlessness
• Decreased breathing capacity	• Dyspnea on mild exertion	• Slow, slurred speech	• Personality changes: irritability, agitation
Gastrointestinal System		• Delayed relaxation of deep tendon reflexes	• Exhaustion
• Decreased appetite	• Increased appetite, thirst	• Stupor, coma	• Hyperreflexia of tendon reflexes
• Nausea and vomiting	• Weight loss	• Paresthesias	• Depression, fatigue, apathy (in older adults)
• Weight gain	• Increased peristalsis	• Anxiety, depression	• Inability to concentrate
• Constipation	• Diarrhea, frequent defecation	• Polyneuropathy	• Stupor, coma
• Distended abdomen	• Increased bowel sounds	**Reproductive System**	
• Enlarged, scaly tongue	• Splenomegaly	• Prolonged menstrual periods or amenorrhea	• Menstrual irregularities
	• Hepatomegaly	• Decreased libido	• Amenorrhea
Integumentary System		• Infertility	• Decreased libido
• Dry, thick, inelastic, cold skin	• Warm, smooth, moist skin		• Erectile dysfunction in men
• Thick, brittle nails	• Thin, brittle nails detached from nail bed (onycholysis)		• Gynecomastia in men
• Dry, sparse, coarse hair	• Hair loss (may be patchy)		• Decreased fertility
• Poor turgor of mucosa	• Clubbing of fingers (thyroid acropachy)	**Other**	
• Generalized interstitial edema	• Palmar erythema	• Increased susceptibility to infection	• Intolerance of heat
• Puffy face	• Fine, silky hair	• Increased sensitivity to narcotics, barbiturates, anaesthetics	• Increased sensitivity to stimulant drugs
• Decreased sweating	• Premature greying (in men)	• Intolerance of cold	• Elevated basal temperature
• Pallor	• Diaphoresis	• Decreased hearing	• Eyelid lag, stare
	• Pretibial myxedema (infiltrative dermopathy)	• Sleepiness	• Eyelid retraction
		• Goitre	• Exophthalmos
			• Goitre
			• Rapid speech

when the drugs are discontinued. Indications for use of antithyroid drugs include Graves' disease in young patients, hyperthyroidism during pregnancy, and the need to attain a euthyroid state before surgery or radiation therapy.

Iodine. Iodine is used with other antithyroid drugs in the preparation of a patient for thyroidectomy or for treatment of thyrotoxic crisis. The administration of iodine in large doses rapidly inhibits synthesis of T_3 and T_4 and blocks the release of these hormones into the circulation. It also decreases the vascularity of the thyroid gland, which makes surgery safer and easier. The effect of iodine is usually maximal within 1 to 2 weeks. Because the therapeutic effect lessens, long-term iodine therapy is not effective in controlling hyperthyroidism. Iodine is available in the form of Lugol's solution (Health Canada, 2011).

β-Adrenergic Blockers. β-Adrenergic blockers are used for symptomatic relief of thyrotoxicosis that results from increased β-adrenergic receptor stimulation caused by excess thyroid hormones. Propranolol (Inderal) is usually administered with

Table 51-7 Comparison of Hyperthyroidism in Younger and Older Adults

FEATURES	YOUNGER ADULTS	OLDER ADULTS
Common causes	Graves' disease in >90% of cases	Graves' disease or toxic nodular goitre
Common symptoms	Nervousness; irritability; weight loss; heat intolerance; warm, moist skin	Anorexia, weight loss, apathy, lassitude, depression, confusion
Goitre	Present in >90% of cases	Present in ~50% of cases
Ophthalmopathy	Exophthalmos present in 20-50% of cases	Occasional exophthalmos
Cardiac features	Tachycardia and palpitations common, but without heart failure	Angina, dysrhythmias (especially atrial fibrillation), or heart failure may occur

COLLABORATIVE CARE

Table 51-8 Hyperthyroidism

Diagnostic
- History and physical examination
- Ophthalmological examination
- Electrocardiography
- Laboratory tests
  - Serum free T_4, TSH levels
  - TRH stimulation test
- Radioactive iodine uptake

Collaborative Therapy

Drug Therapy
- Antithyroid drugs
  - Propylthiouracil (Propyl-Thyracil)
  - Methimazole (Tapazole)
- Iodine
- β-Adrenergic blockers (e.g., propranolol [Inderal])

Radiation Therapy
- Radioactive iodine

Surgical Therapy
- Subtotal thyroidectomy

Nutritional Therapy
- High-calorie diet
- High-protein diet
- Frequent meals

T_4, thyroxine; *TRH*, thyrotropin-releasing hormone; *TSH*, thyroid-stimulating hormone.

other antithyroid agents and rapidly provides symptomatic relief. Atenolol (Tenormin) is the preferred β-adrenergic blocker for use in hyperthyroid patients with asthma or heart disease.

Radioactive Iodine Therapy.
Radioactive iodine (RAI) therapy is the treatment of choice for most nonpregnant adults. (Before initiation of therapy, a pregnancy test is performed on all women who menstruate.) RAI damages or destroys thyroid tissue, thus limiting thyroid hormone secretion. Patients should be instructed that radiation-related thyroiditis and parotiditis are possible and may cause dryness and irritation of the mouth and throat. Relief may be obtained with frequent sips of water, ice chips, or the use of normal saline or a baking soda solution (e.g., 10 mL of baking soda in 250 mL of water) to gargle three or four times per day. The discomfort should subside in 3 to 4 days. If dryness and irritation persist, patients should contact the health care provider. The response to radioactive iodine is delayed, and the effect may not be maximal for 2 to 3 months. For this reason, patients are usually treated with antithyroid drugs and propranolol before and during the first 3 months after the initiation of RAI until the effects of irradiation become apparent. Although this method of treatment is usually effective, the biggest disadvantage is the high incidence of post-treatment hypothyroidism, which results in the need for lifelong thyroid hormone replacement (Simmons, 2010). Patients and the family or caregiver should be taught about the symptoms of hypothyroidism and instructed to seek medical help if these symptoms occur.

Surgical Therapy.
Thyroidectomy is indicated when a large goitre causes tracheal compression, when patients do not respond to antithyroid therapy, and in patients with thyroid cancer. In addition, surgery may be performed when an individual is not a candidate for RAI. One advantage of thyroidectomy over RAI is a more rapid reduction in T_3 and T_4 levels. A *subtotal thyroidectomy* is the preferred surgical procedure and involves the removal of a significant portion (90%) of the thyroid gland. If too much tissue is taken, the gland does not regenerate after surgery, and hypothyroidism results.

Endoscopic thyroidectomy is a minimally invasive procedure. In this procedure, several small incisions are made through which an endoscope and other instruments can be passed to remove thyroid tissue or nodules. It is an appropriate procedure for patients with small nodules (<3 cm in diameter) in whom there is no evidence of malignancy. Advantages of endoscopic thyroidectomy over the traditional approach are less scarring, less pain, and a faster return to normal activity.

Before surgery, antithyroid drugs, iodine, and β-adrenergic blockers may be administered to achieve a euthyroid state and to control symptoms. Iodine reduces vascularization of the gland, thereby reducing the risk of hemorrhage. Postoperative complications include hypothyroidism, damage to or inadvertent removal of parathyroid glands (causing hypoparathyroidism and hypocalcemia), hemorrhage, injury to the recurrent or the superior laryngeal nerve, thyrotoxic crisis, and infection.

Nutritional Therapy.
The potential for nutritional deficits is high when the metabolic rate is increased. A high-calorie diet (4000 to 5000 kcal/day) may be ordered to satisfy hunger and prevent tissue breakdown. This is accomplished with six full meals a day and snacks high in protein, carbohydrates, minerals, and vitamins, particularly vitamin A, thiamine, vitamin B_6, and vitamin C. The protein allowance should be 1 to 2 g/kg of ideal body weight. Increased carbohydrates should compensate for disturbed metabolism, provide energy, and spare body protein stores. Highly seasoned and high-fibre foods should be avoided because they can further stimulate the already hyperactive GI tract. Substitutes should be provided for caffeine-containing beverages such as coffee, tea, and cola because their stimulating effects increase restlessness and sleep disturbances. The nurse should consult a dietitian for guidance in meeting the nutritional needs of a patient with hyperthyroidism.

NURSING MANAGEMENT: HYPERTHYROIDISM

Nursing Assessment

Subjective and objective data that should be obtained from an individual with hyperthyroidism are presented in Table 51-9.

NURSING ASSESSMENT
Table 51-9 Hyperthyroidism

Subjective Data

Important Health Information

Past health history: Pre-existing goitre; recent infection or trauma; immigration from iodine-deficient area; autoimmune disease; positive family history of thyroid or autoimmune disorders

Medications: Use of thyroid hormones or herbal therapies that may contain thyroid hormone

Symptoms

- Insufficient iodine intake; weight loss; increased appetite or thirst; nausea
- Diarrhea; polyuria
- Chest pain; dyspnea on exertion; palpitations
- Insomnia
- Muscle weakness, fatigue
- Heat intolerance; pruritus; sweating
- Decreased libido; erectile dysfunction, gynecomastia (in men); amenorrhea (in women)
- Emotional lability, irritability, restlessness, personality changes, delirium, nervousness

Objective Data

General Observation

Agitation, rapid speech and body movements; hyperthermia, enlarged or nodular thyroid gland

Eyes

Exophthalmos, eyelid retraction; infrequent blinking

Integumentary

Warm, diaphoretic, velvety skin; thin, loose nails; fine, silky hair and hair loss; palmar erythema; digital clubbing; white pigmentation of skin (vitiligo); diffuse edema of legs and feet

Respiratory

Tachypnea

Cardiovascular

Tachycardia, bounding pulse, systolic murmurs, dysrhythmias, hypertension

Gastrointestinal

Increased bowel sounds; hepatosplenomegaly

Neurological

Hyper-reflexia; diplopia; fine tremors of hands, tongue, eyelids; stupor; coma

Musculoskeletal

Muscle wasting

Reproductive

Menstrual irregularities, infertility in women; erectile dysfunction, gynecomastia in men

Possible Findings

↑ T_3 level, ↑ T_4 level; ↑ T_3 resin uptake; ↓ serum TSH level; chest radiograph showing enlarged heart, findings of tachycardia, atrial fibrillation on ECG

ECG, electrocardiogram; T_3, triiodothyronine; T_4, thyroxine; *TSH,* thyroid-stimulating hormone.

Nursing Diagnoses

Nursing diagnoses for patients with hyperthyroidism include, but are not limited to, those presented in Nursing Care Plan 51-1.

Planning

The overall goals are that patients with hyperthyroidism will (a) experience relief from symptoms, (b) have no serious complications related to the disease or treatment, (c) maintain nutritional balance, and (d) adhere to the therapeutic plan.

Nursing Implementation

Acute Intervention

Individuals who have hyperthyroidism are usually treated in an out-patient setting. However, patients who develop acute thyrotoxicosis and those who undergo thyroidectomy require hospitalization and acute care.

Acute Thyrotoxicosis.
Acute thyrotoxicosis is a systemic syndrome that necessitates aggressive treatment, often in a critical care unit. Medications that block thyroid hormone production and the sympathetic nervous system (see previous discussion) should be administered. Supportive therapy includes monitoring for cardiac dysrhythmias and decompensation, ensuring adequate oxygenation, and administering IV fluids to replace fluid and electrolyte losses. This is especially important in patients who develop vomiting and diarrhea.

The patient's room should be kept calm and quiet because increased metabolism causes sleep disturbances. Provision of adequate rest may be a challenge because of the patient's irritability and restlessness. Specific interventions may include (a) placing the patient in a cool room, away from very ill patients and noisy, high-traffic areas; (b) using light-weight bed coverings and changing the linen frequently if the patient is diaphoretic; (c) encouraging and assisting with exercise involving large muscle groups (tremors can interfere with small-muscle coordination) to allow the release of nervous tension and restlessness; and (d) establishing a supportive, trusting relationship to help the patient cope with aggravating events and lessen anxiety.

Exophthalmos, when present, incurs a potential for corneal injury related to irritation and dryness. Affected patients may also have orbital pain. Nursing interventions to relieve eye discomfort and prevent corneal ulceration include applying artificial tears to soothe and moisten conjunctival membranes. Salt restriction may help reduce periorbital edema. Elevation of the patient's head promotes fluid drainage from the periorbital area; the patient should sit upright as much as possible. Dark glasses reduce glare and prevent irritation from air currents, dust, and dirt. If the eyelids cannot be closed, they should be lightly taped shut for sleep. To maintain flexibility, the patient should be taught to exercise the intraocular muscles several times a day by turning the eyes in the complete range of motion. Good grooming can be helpful in reducing the loss of self-esteem that can result from an altered body image. If the exophthalmos is severe, corticosteroids, radiation of retro-orbital tissues, orbital decompression, or corrective eyelid or muscle surgery may be helpful.

NURSING CARE PLAN 51-1

Hyperthyroidism

NURSING DIAGNOSIS	*Activity intolerance* related to fatigue, exhaustion, and heat intolerance secondary to hypermetabolism *as evidenced by* complaints of weakness, inability to perform usual activities, dyspnea, tachycardia, irritability
Expected Patient Outcomes	**Nursing Interventions and *Rationales***
• Achieves a program of activity that balances physical activity with energy-conserving activities • Reports increased tolerance of activity with less weakness and fatigue	**Energy management** • Assess for evidence of excess physical and emotional fatigue *because hyperthyroidism results in protein catabolism, overactivity, and increased metabolism, all leading to exhaustion.* • Monitor cardiorespiratory response to activity (e.g., tachycardia, other dysrhythmias, dyspnea, diaphoresis, pallor, BP, and respiratory rate) *because tachycardia and BP elevations can indicate excessive thyroid hormone activity.* • Assist with regular physical activities (e.g., ambulation, transfers, turning, and personal care) *to ensure that patient's daily needs are met.* • Assist the patient to understand energy conservation principles (e.g., the requirement for restricted activity or bedrest) *to avoid fatiguing patient.* • Assist the patient in scheduling rest periods *to avoid fatigue.* • Avoid performing care activities during scheduled rest periods *to promote adequate rest.*
NURSING DIAGNOSIS	***Imbalanced nutrition: less than body requirements*** related to hypermetabolism and inadequate diet *as evidenced by* complaints of weight loss and suboptimal body weight
Expected Patient Outcomes	**Nursing Interventions and *Rationales***
• Maintains weight appropriate for height • Consumes food and fluid in adequate amounts to meet nutritional needs • Corrects nutritional deficiencies	**Nutritional management** • Assess patient's food preferences *to determine extent of the problem and to plan appropriate interventions.* • Consult dietitian to determine the number of calories and type of nutrients needed *to meet nutrition requirements.* • Provide patient with high-protein, high-calorie, nutritious finger foods and drinks that can be readily consumed *to prevent muscle breakdown and weight loss caused by increased metabolic rate as a result of hyperthyroidism.* • Offer snacks (e.g., frequent drinks, fresh fruits/juice) *to maintain adequate caloric intake.* • Monitor recorded intake for nutritional content and calories *to evaluate nutritional status.* • Weigh patient at appropriate intervals *to evaluate effectiveness of nutritional plan.* • Provide patient with appropriate information about nutritional needs and how to meet them *to promote self-care.* • Assist patient in receiving help from appropriate community nutritional programs *to ensure that support is ongoing.*

BP, blood pressure.

■ **Thyroid Surgery.** When subtotal thyroidectomy is the treatment of choice, patients must be adequately prepared in order to avoid postoperative complications. To alleviate thyrotoxicosis, iodine treatment or propylthiouracil may be given before surgery. Iodine is mixed with water or juice and sipped through a straw after meals. The nurse assesses patients for signs of iodine toxicity, such as swelling of buccal mucosa and other mucous membranes, excessive salivation, nausea and vomiting, and skin reactions. If toxicity occurs, iodine administration should be discontinued and the physician notified.

Preoperative teaching should include comfort and safety measures in which patients can participate. Coughing, deep breathing, and leg exercises should be practised and their importance explained. Patients should be taught how to support the head manually while turning in bed because this manoeuvre minimizes stress on the suture line after surgery. Range-of-motion exercises of the neck should be practised. The nurse should

explain routine postoperative care such as IV infusions. Patients should be told that talking is likely to be difficult for a short time after surgery.

SAFETY ALERT

• Airway obstruction, although not common, may occur postoperatively.

• Airway obstruction is an emergency situation.

• Oxygen, suction equipment, and a tracheostomy tray should be readily available in the patient's room.

Recurrent laryngeal nerve damage leads to vocal cord paralysis. If both cords are paralyzed, spastic airway obstruction may occur, necessitating an immediate tracheostomy.

Respiration may also become difficult because of excess swelling of the neck tissues, hemorrhage, hematoma formation, and laryngeal stridor. *Laryngeal stridor* (harsh, vibratory sound) may occur during inspiration and expiration as a result of edema of the laryngeal nerve. Laryngeal stridor may also be related to tetany, which occurs if the parathyroid glands are removed or damaged during surgery, which leads to hypocalcemia. To treat tetany, calcium salts such as calcium gluconate and calcium chloride should be readily available for IV administration. After a thyroidectomy, the patient should be cared for as follows:

1. Assessment every 2 hours for 24 hours for signs of hemorrhage or tracheal compression, such as irregular breathing, neck swelling, frequent swallowing, sensations of fullness at the incision site, choking, and blood on the dressings.
2. Placement in a semi-Fowler's position, and support of the patient's head with pillows, with care to avoid flexion of the neck and any tension on the suture lines.
3. Monitoring of vital signs. The nurse completes the initial assessment by checking for signs of hypocalcemia and tetany secondary to hypoparathyroidism (e.g., tingling sensation in toes, in fingers, or around the mouth; muscular twitching; apprehension) and by evaluating difficulty in speaking and hoarseness. The nurse should also check for the presence of Trousseau's and Chvostek's signs for 72 hours (see Chapter 19, Figure 19-15). Some hoarseness is to be expected for 3 to 4 days after surgery because of edema.
4. Control of postoperative pain with medication.

If postoperative recovery is uneventful, patients are ambulated within hours after surgery, are permitted to take fluid as soon as tolerated, and eat soft foods the day after surgery.

The appearance of the incision may be distressing to patients. They can be reassured that the scar will fade and eventually look like a normal neck wrinkle. A scarf, jewellery, a high collar, or other covering can effectively camouflage a fresh scar.

◾ Ambulatory and Home Care

◾ Postoperative Care.
Patients and family need to be aware that thyroid hormone balance should be monitored periodically to ensure that normal function has returned. Most patients experience a period of relative hypothyroidism soon after surgery because of the substantial reduction in the size of the thyroid. The remaining tissue usually hypertrophies, recovering the capacity to produce the hormone needed by the body, but this takes time. Thyroid hormone is not administered because exogenous hormone inhibits pituitary production of TSH and delays or prevents the restoration of normal gland function and thyroid tissue regeneration.

To prevent weight gain, caloric intake must be reduced substantially below the amount that was required before surgery. Adequate iodine is necessary to promote thyroid function, but excesses inhibit the thyroid. Seafood once or twice a week or normal use of iodized salt should provide sufficient iodine intake. Regular exercise stimulates the thyroid gland and should be encouraged. High environmental temperature should be avoided because it inhibits thyroid regeneration.

Regular follow-up care is necessary. Patients should be seen biweekly for a month and then at least semiannually to assess for the development of hypothyroidism. If a complete thyroidectomy has been performed, patients need instruction in lifelong thyroid replacement. Patients should be taught the signs and symptoms of progressive thyroid failure and instructed to seek medical care if these develop. Hypothyroidism is relatively easy to manage with oral administration of thyroid replacement.

◾ Evaluation

The following are expected outcomes for patients with hyperthyroidism:

- Relief from symptoms
- No serious complications related to the disease or the treatment
- Adherence to the therapeutic plan

Hypothyroidism

Etiology and Pathophysiology

Hypothyroidism affects approximately 2 per 100 people (Thyroid Foundation of Canada, 2011). Hypothyroidism results from insufficient circulating thyroid hormone as a result of various abnormalities. Hypothyroidism can be primary (related to destruction of thyroid tissue or defective hormone synthesis) or secondary (related to pituitary disease with decreased secretion of TSH or hypothalamic dysfunction with decreased secretion of thyrotropin-releasing hormone [TRH]). It may also be transient, related to thyroiditis or discontinuation of thyroid hormone therapy.

Iodine deficiency is the most common cause of hypothyroidism worldwide. In Canada, the most common cause of primary hypothyroidism in the adult is atrophy of the thyroid gland. This atrophy is the end result of Hashimoto's thyroiditis and Graves' disease. These autoimmune diseases destroy the thyroid gland. Hypothyroidism also may develop as a result of treatment for hyperthyroidism, specifically the surgical removal of the thyroid gland or radioactive iodine therapy. Drugs such as amiodarone (which contains iodine) and lithium (which blocks hormone production) are known to produce hypothyroidism.

Hypothyroidism that develops in infancy (**cretinism**) is caused by thyroid hormone deficiencies during fetal or early neonatal life. All infants in Canada are screened for decreased thyroid function at birth.

Clinical Manifestations

All hypothyroid states have certain features in common, regardless of the cause. Manifestations vary, depending on the severity and the duration of thyroid deficiency, as well as the patient's age at onset of the deficiency.

Hypothyroidism has systemic effects characterized by an insidious and nonspecific slowing of body processes. The clinical presentation can range from no symptoms to classic symptoms and physical changes easily detected on examination. Unless hypothyroidism occurs after thyroidectomy or thyroid ablation or during treatment with antithyroid drugs, the onset of symptoms may occur unnoticed over months to years. The severity of symptoms experienced depends on the degree of thyroid hormone deficiency and the long-term physiological effects of thyroid hormone deficiency. Long-term effects may involve any body system but are more pronounced in neurological, cardiovascular, GI, reproductive, and hematological systems.

Many affected patients are fatigued and lethargic and experience personality and mental changes. The mental changes observed in hypothyroidism include impaired memory, slowed speech, decreased initiative, and somnolence. Many individuals with hypothyroidism appear depressed. Although patients with hypothyroidism sleep for long periods, the stages of sleep are altered (Dursunoglu, Ozkurt, & SarÄłkaya, 2009).

Hypothyroidism is associated with decreased cardiac output and decreased cardiac contractility. The patient may experience low exercise tolerance and shortness of breath on exertion. In patients with a pre-existing cardiovascular condition, hypothyroidism may cause significant hemodynamic compromise (Simmons, 2010).

Anemia is a common feature of hypothyroidism. Erythropoietin levels may be low or normal. Oxygen demand is decreased, and the bone marrow is hypocellular; the result is a low hematocrit. Other hematological problems are related to cobalamin, iron, and folate deficiencies. The patient may bruise easily. Increased serum cholesterol and triglyceride levels and the accumulation of mucopolysaccharides in the intima of small blood vessels can result in coronary atherosclerosis. This accumulation is seldom symptomatic (i.e., characterized by angina) because of the decreased myocardial oxygen consumption that has been observed in hypothyroidism.

GI motility is decreased in hypothyroidism, and achlorhydria (absence or decrease of hydrochloric acid) is common. Constipation, which is a common complaint, may progress to obstipation and, in rare cases, to intestinal obstruction. Other physical changes include cold intolerance, hair loss, dry and coarse skin, brittle nails, hoarseness, muscle weakness and swelling, and weight gain. Weight gain is probably a result of decreased metabolic rate.

Patients with severe long-standing hypothyroidism may display **myxedema,** the accumulation of hydrophilic mucopolysaccharides in the dermis and other tissues (Figure 51-9). This mucinous edema causes the characteristic facies of hypothyroidism (i.e., puffiness, periorbital edema, and masklike affect). Individuals with hypothyroidism may describe impaired self-image in regard to their disabilities and altered appearance.

Women with hypothyroidism frequently complain of menorrhagia. In addition, cycles may be anovulatory, and subsequent infertility may occur (Dittrich et al., 2011).

In older adults, the typical manifestations of hypothyroidism (including fatigue, cold and dry skin, hoarseness, hair loss, constipation, and cold intolerance) may be attributed to normal aging. For this reason, these symptoms may not raise suspicion about an underlying condition. Older adults who have confusion, lethargy, and depression should be evaluated for thyroid disease.

Complications

The mental sluggishness, drowsiness, and lethargy of hypothyroidism may progress gradually or suddenly to a notable impairment of consciousness or coma. This situation, **myxedema coma,** constitutes a medical emergency. Myxedema coma can be precipitated by infection, drugs (especially narcotics, tranquilizers, and barbiturates), exposure to cold, and trauma. It is characterized by subnormal temperature, hypotension, and hypoventilation. For patients to survive, vital functions must be supported and IV thyroid hormone replacement must be administered.

Diagnostic Studies

The most common and reliable laboratory tests used to evaluate thyroid function are measurements of TSH and free T_4 (Simmons, 2010). These values, when correlated with symptoms evident in the history and physical examination, confirm the diagnosis. Serum TSH levels help determine the cause of hypothyroidism: They are high when the defect is in the thyroid and low when it is in the pituitary or hypothalamus. An increase in TSH level after injection of TRH suggests hypothalamic dysfunction, whereas no change suggests anterior pituitary dysfunction (Table 51-10). The presence of thyroid peroxidase antibodies suggests an autoimmune origin of the problem (Zelaya, Stotts, Nader, & Moreno, 2010). Other abnormal laboratory findings are elevated cholesterol and triglyceride levels, anemia, and increased creatine kinase level.

Collaborative Care

The overall goal for treatment in a patient with hypothyroidism is restoration of a euthyroid state as safely and rapidly as possible

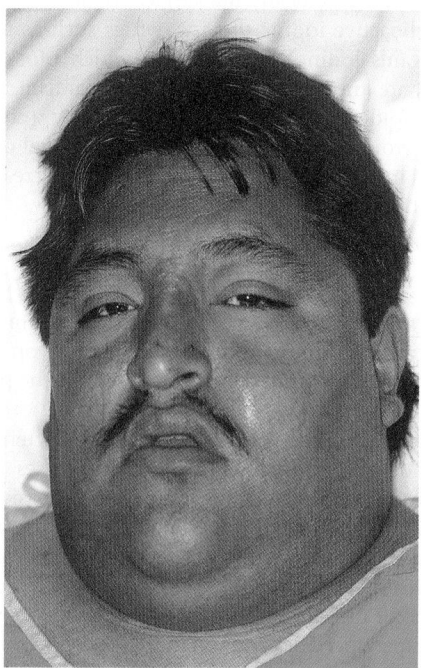

Figure 51-9 Patient with myxedema, displaying the characteristic facies of hypothyroidism (i.e., puffiness, periorbital edema, and masklike affect).

Source: Seidel, H. M., Ball, J., Dains, J., Flynn, J. A., Solomon, B. S., & Stewart, R. W. (2011). *Mosby's guide to physical examination* (7th ed., p. 247, Figure 10-10). St. Louis: Mosby. (Originally from Lemmi, F. O., Lemmi, C. A. E. [2000]. Physical assessment findings CD-ROM. 2000, Saunders, Philadelphia.)

COLLABORATIVE CARE

Table 51-10 Hypothyroidism	
Diagnostic	**Collaborative Therapy**
• History and physical examination	• Thyroid hormone replacement (e.g., levothyroxine)
• Serum TSH and free T_4 levels	• Monitoring thyroid hormone levels and adjusting dosage (if needed)
• Serum T_3 and serum T_4 levels	• Nutritional therapy to promote weight loss
• TRH stimulation test	
• Thyroid peroxidase antibodies	• Patient and caregiver teaching (see Table 51-11)

T_3, triiodothyronine; T_4, thyroxine; *TRH*, thyrotropin-releasing hormone; *TSH*, thyroid-stimulating hormone.

with hormone replacement therapy. A low-calorie diet is indicated to promote weight loss.

Levothyroxine (Synthroid, Eltroxin) is the drug of choice to treat hypothyroidism. In young and otherwise healthy patients, the maintenance replacement dose is adjusted according to patients' response and laboratory findings. In older adult patients and in patients with compromised cardiac status, a lower initial dosage is recommended because the usual dosage may increase myocardial oxygen demand. The increased oxygen demand may cause angina and cardiac dysrhythmias. Any chest pain experienced by a patient starting thyroid replacement should be reported immediately; electrocardiography (ECG) must be performed and serum cardiac enzymes measured. In patients without adverse effects, the dose is increased at 4- to 6-week intervals. It is important that patients take replacement medication regularly. Lifelong thyroid replacement therapy is usually required.

Multiple levothyroxine preparations are currently available. Patients taking levothyroxine must have serum TSH levels checked 4 to 6 weeks after changing levothyroxine preparation.

NURSING MANAGEMENT: HYPOTHYROIDISM

Nursing Assessment

Careful assessment may reveal the early and subtle changes that indicate dysfunction. Assessment of a patient who is suspected of having hypothyroidism should include questions about weight gain, mental changes, fatigue, slowed and slurred speech, cold intolerance, skin changes such as increased dryness or thickening, constipation, and dyspnea. The patient should be questioned about recent introduction of iodine-containing medications. The patient should be assessed for bradycardia; distended abdomen; dry, thick, cold skin; thick, brittle nails; paresthesias; and muscular aches and pains.

Nursing Diagnoses

Nursing diagnoses for patients with hypothyroidism may include, but are not limited to, those presented in Nursing Care Plan 51-2.

Planning

The overall goals are that patients with hypothyroidism will (a) experience relief from symptoms, (b) maintain a euthyroid state, (c) maintain a positive self-image, and (d) adhere to a lifelong regimen of thyroid replacement therapy.

Nursing Implementation

Health Promotion

There is currently no consensus regarding thyroid function screening. Although hypothyroidism is relatively common, particularly among women older than 50, screening of the general population is not strongly justified (Zelaya et al., 2010). Research

suggests that populations at high risk for thyroid dysfunction should be screened for subclinical (asymptomatic) thyroid disease. Individuals at risk include those with a family history of thyroid disease, those with a history of neck irradiation, women older than 50, and women who have just given birth.

Acute Intervention

Most individuals with hypothyroidism do not require acute nursing care. However, a patient who develops myxedema coma does require acute nursing care, often in a critical care setting. Mechanical respiratory support and cardiac monitoring are frequently necessary. Thyroid hormone replacement therapy and all other medications should be administered IV because paralytic ileus may be present with myxedema coma. If the patient is hyponatremic, hypertonic saline may be administered until the serum sodium level reaches at least 130 mmol/L. Core temperature should be monitored because many patients with myxedema coma are hypothermic.

The nurse monitors a patient's progress by assessing vital signs, body weight, fluid intake and output, and visible edema. Cardiac assessment is especially important because the cardiovascular response to the hormone determines the medication regimen. Energy level and mental alertness should be noted. These should increase within 2 to 14 days and continue to rise steadily to normal levels.

Ambulatory and Home Care

Patient and caregiver teaching is essential for patients with hypothyroidism (Table 51-11). Initially, patients with hypothyroidism need more time than usual to comprehend all the necessary information. It is important to provide written instructions, repeat the information often, and assess the patient's comprehension level regularly.

The need for lifelong drug therapy must be stressed. Patients should be taught expected and unexpected adverse drug effects.

PATIENT & CAREGIVER TEACHING GUIDE

Table 51-11 Hypothyroidism

1. Explain the nature of thyroid hormone deficiency and self-care practices necessary to prevent complications. Patient and family caregivers must understand thyroid replacement therapy. It is especially important to emphasize the need for lifelong replacement, the need to take the medication continually, and the need for regular follow-up care.

2. Emphasize the need for a comfortable, warm environment because of intolerance of cold.

3. Teach measures to prevent skin breakdown. Soap should be used sparingly and lotion applied to skin.

4. Caution patients, especially older adults, to avoid sedatives. If they must be used, suggest that the lowest dose be used. Caregivers should closely monitor patient's mental status, level of consciousness, and respiration.

5. Discuss with patients measures to minimize constipation. Suggestions should include a gradual increase in activity and exercise, increased fibre in diet, use of stool softeners, and maintenance of a regular bowel elimination time. Enemas should not be used because they produce vagal stimulation, which can be hazardous if cardiac disease is present.

NURSING CARE PLAN 51-2

Hypothyroidism

NURSING DIAGNOSIS	*Imbalanced nutrition: more than body requirements* related to calorie intake in excess of metabolic rate secondary to hypometabolism *as evidenced by* weight gain
Expected Patient Outcomes	**Nursing Interventions and *Rationales***
• Attains weight appropriate for height • Maintains caloric intake that meets nutritional needs	**Weight management** • Discuss the medical conditions that may affect weight *to reassure patient that optimal weight can be maintained with treatment of hypothyroidism.* • Discuss the relationship between food intake, exercise, weight gain, and weight loss *to promote understanding of weight management.* • Determine ideal body weight *to plan weekly weight loss goals.* • Assist in developing well-balanced meal plans consistent with level of energy expenditure *to promote weight loss progress.* • Develop with the patient a method of keeping a daily record of intake, exercise sessions, and changes in body weight *to promote progress toward final goal.* **Nutrition management** • Determine, in collaboration with dietitian, number of calories and type of nutrients needed to meet nutrition requirements *to plan meals.* • Provide appropriate information about nutritional needs and how to meet them *to encourage patient to be more amenable to dietary restrictions.* • Monitor recorded intake for nutritional content and calories *to evaluate patient's management of nutrition.* • Weigh patient at appropriate intervals *to monitor progress toward target weight.*
NURSING DIAGNOSIS	*Constipation* related to gastrointestinal hypomotility *as evidenced by* irregular, hard stools
Expected Patient Outcome	**Nursing Interventions and *Rationales***
• Reports stools are regular, soft, and easy to pass	• Assess bowel pattern and characteristics, including frequency, consistency, shape, volume, and colour, *to plan appropriate interventions.* • Encourage increased fluid intake (e.g., 2-3 L/day) *to maintain softness of stool.* • Instruct patient and caregivers about high-fibre diet *to increase their knowledge of how to increase fecal mass.* • Suggest use of laxatives or stool softeners, if necessary, *to stimulate bowel evacuation.*
NURSING DIAGNOSIS	*Impaired memory* related to hypometabolism *as evidenced by* forgetfulness, memory loss, somnolence, and personality changes
Expected Patient Outcome	**Nursing Interventions and *Rationales***
• Demonstrates cognitive orientation with correction of hormone deficiency	• Monitor for changes in orientation, cognitive and behavioural functioning, and quality of life *to determine appropriate interventions.* • Inform patient of person, place, and time *to decrease confusion.* • Provide a low-stimulation environment for patient in whom disorientation is increased by overstimulation *to limit disorientation.* • Speak to patient slowly and distinctly with appropriate volume *to enable patient to understand.* • Use environmental cues (e.g., signs, pictures, clocks, calendars) *to maintain patient's orientation to time and day.* • Explain all procedures, including sensations likely to be experienced during the procedure, *to reduce patient's anxiety and frustration.*

Specifically, the signs and symptoms of hypothyroidism or hyperthyroidism that indicate hormone imbalance should be included in the teaching plan. Toxic symptoms should be clearly defined. Table 51-6 lists signs of hyperthyroidism that are the same as toxic symptoms of thyroid hormone replacement.

Patients must be taught to contact a health care professional immediately if signs of overdose such as orthopnea, dyspnea, rapid pulse, palpitations, nervousness, or insomnia appear. A patient with diabetes mellitus should test his or her capillary blood glucose level at least daily because return to the euthyroid state frequently increases insulin requirements. In addition, thyroid preparations potentiate the effects of anticoagulants and decrease the effect of digitalis compounds. Thus the patient should be taught the toxic signs and symptoms of these medications and should remain under close medical observation until his or her condition is stable.

It is sometimes difficult for patients to recognize signs of overdosage or underdosage of drug therapy; therefore, a family member or friend should also receive instructions. Handouts for patients should be written in understandable language and should accompany verbal instruction. The handouts should be reviewed with patients and the family to assess understanding, and information should be clarified when necessary.

With treatment, striking transformations occur in both appearance and mental function. In most adults, both return to normal. Cardiovascular conditions and (occasionally) psychosis may persist despite corrections of the hormonal imbalance. Relapses occur if treatment is interrupted.

■ Evaluation

The following are expected outcomes for patients with hypothyroidism:
- Relief from symptoms
- Maintenance of a euthyroid state as evidenced by normal thyroid hormone and TSH levels
- Adherence to lifelong therapy

Disorders of the Parathyroid Glands

Hyperparathyroidism

Etiology and Pathophysiology

Hyperparathyroidism is a condition involving increased secretion of parathyroid hormone (PTH). PTH helps regulate calcium and phosphate levels by stimulating bone resorption of calcium, renal tubular reabsorption of calcium, and activation of vitamin D. Thus oversecretion of PTH is associated with increased serum calcium levels. Hyperparathyroidism affects approximately 0.1 to 0.4% of the general population, it occurs more frequently among women, and the incidence increases with age (Pallan & Khan, 2011).

Hyperparathyroidism is classified as primary, secondary, or tertiary. *Primary hyperparathyroidism* results from an increased secretion of PTH, which leads to disorders of calcium, phosphate, and bone metabolism. The most common cause is a benign neoplasm or a single adenoma in the parathyroid gland. Primary hyperparathyroidism usually occurs between the ages of 30 and 70 years. The incidence peaks in the fifth and sixth decades of life. Patients who have previously undergone head and neck irradiation may have an increased risk of developing a parathyroid adenoma.

Secondary hyperparathyroidism appears to be a compensatory response to states that induce or cause hypocalcemia, the main stimulus of PTH secretion. Disease conditions associated with secondary hyperparathyroidism include vitamin D deficiencies, malabsorption, chronic renal failure, and hyperphosphatemia.

Tertiary hyperparathyroidism occurs when the parathyroid glands become hyperplastic and negative feedback is lost from circulating calcium levels; thus, PTH is secreted autonomously, even with normal calcium levels. This condition is observed in patients who have undergone kidney transplantation after a long period of dialysis treatment for chronic renal failure (see Chapter 49).

Excessive levels of circulating PTH usually lead to hypercalcemia and hypophosphatemia, creating a multisystem effect (Table 51-12). In the skeleton, decreased bone density, cyst formation, and general weakness can occur as a result of the effect of PTH on osteoclastic activity (bone resorption) and osteoblastic activity (bone formation). In the kidneys, the excess calcium cannot be reabsorbed; as a result, levels of calcium in the urine increase (hypercalciuria). This urinary calcium level, along with a large amount of urinary phosphate, can lead to calculi formation (Pallan & Khan, 2011). In addition, PTH stimulates the synthesis of a biologically active form of vitamin D, a potent stimulator of calcium transport in the intestine. In this way, PTH indirectly increases GI absorption of calcium, contributing further to the high serum calcium levels.

Clinical Manifestations and Complications

Clinical manifestations of hyperparathyroidism range from no symptoms (the condition is diagnosed through testing for unrelated problems) to overt symptoms. Clinical manifestations are associated with hypercalcemia and are summarized in Table 51-12. The major manifestations include muscle weakness, loss of appetite, constipation, fatigue, emotional disorders, and shortened attention span. Major signs include loss of calcium from bones (osteoporosis), fractures, and kidney stones (nephrolithiasis). Neuromuscular abnormalities are characterized by muscle weakness, particularly in the proximal muscles of the lower extremities. Asymptomatic cases are often identified through routine calcium screening. Serious complications of hyperparathyroidism are renal failure; pancreatitis; cardiac changes; and fractures of long bones, ribs, and vertebrae.

Diagnostic Studies

PTH levels are elevated in hyperparathyroidism. Serum calcium levels usually exceed 2.5 mmol/L. Because of its inverse relation

Table 51-12 Clinical Manifestations: Parathyroid Dysfunction

HYPOFUNCTION	HYPERFUNCTION	HYPOFUNCTION	HYPERFUNCTION
Cardiovascular		**Neurological**	
Decreased contractility of heart muscle	Dysrhythmias	Personality changes	Personality disturbances
Decreased cardiac output	Shortened Q-T interval on ECG	Psychiatric manifestations of depression, anxiety, psychosis	Emotional irritability
Prolongation of QT and ST intervals on ECG	Hypertension	Irritability	Memory impairment
Dysrhythmias		Memory impairment	Psychosis, depression
Gastrointestinal		Headache	Delirium, confusion, coma
Abdominal cramps	Vague abdominal pain	Seizures	Poor coordination
Fecal incontinence (in older adults)	Anorexia	Positive Chvostek's or Trousseau's sign	Hyperactive deep tendon reflexes
Malabsorption	Nausea and vomiting	Tremor	Abnormalities of gait
	Constipation	Paresthesias of perioral area, hands, and feet	Psychomotor retardation
	Pancreatitis	Hyperactive deep tendon reflexes	Headache
	Peptic ulcer disease	Disorientation, confusion (in older adults)	Paraesthesias
	Cholelithiasis	**Renal**	
	Weight loss	Urinary frequency	Hypercalciuria
Integumentary		Urinary incontinence	Kidney stones (nephrolithiasis)
Dry, scaly skin	Skin necrosis		Urinary tract infections
Hair loss on scalp and body	Moist skin		Polyuria
Brittle nails, transverse ridging		**Other**	
Changes in developing teeth, lack of tooth enamel		Eye changes, including lenticular opacities, cataracts, papilledema	Corneal calcification on slit-lamp examination
Musculoskeletal			
Fatigue	Skeletal pain		
Weakness	Backache		
Painful muscle cramps	Weakness, fatigue		
Skeletal radiograph changes, osteosclerosis	Pain on weight bearing		
Soft tissue calcification	Osteoporosis		
Difficulty in walking	Pathological fractures of long bones		
	Compression fractures of spine		
	Decreased muscle tone, muscle atrophy		

ECG, electrocardiogram.

with the calcium level, the serum phosphorus level is usually below 0.1 mmol/L. Elevations occur in other laboratory values: urine calcium, serum chloride, uric acid, creatinine, amylase (if pancreatitis is present), and alkaline phosphatase (if bone disease is present). Bone density measurements may also be used to detect bone loss. Imaging studies, such as MRI, CT, and ultrasonography, may help localize the adenoma.

Collaborative Care

The treatment objectives are to relieve the manifestations and prevent complications caused by excess PTH. The choice of therapy depends on the urgency of the clinical situation, the degree of hypercalcemia, and the underlying cause of the disorder.

Surgical Therapy. The most effective treatment of primary and secondary hyperparathyroidism is surgical intervention. Parathyroidectomy leads to rapid reduction of chronically high calcium levels. Criteria for surgery include serum calcium levels higher than 0.25 mmol/L above normal level; creatinine clearance rate of less than 60 mL/min; *T*-score lower than −2.5 at any site on bone mineral density testing, previous fracture fragility, or both; and age younger than 50 (Pallan & Khan, 2011; Pyram, Mahajan, & Gliwa, 2011). The surgical procedure involves partial or complete removal of the parathyroid glands. The most common procedure involves use of an endoscope and is performed on an outpatient basis. Successful removal of the parathyroid glands is facilitated by preoperative nuclear scanning with sestamibi. (Pata et al., 2011).

Autotransplantation of normal parathyroid tissue in the forearm or near the sternocleidomastoid muscle may be performed, which allows PTH secretion to continue with normalization of calcium levels. If autotransplantation is not possible, or if it fails, patients need to take calcium supplements for the rest of their lives.

Nonsurgical Therapy. A conservative management approach is used if a patient does not meet the criteria for surgical intervention, is an older adult, or is at increased surgical risk from other health problems. This approach includes an annual examination with tests for serum calcium and creatinine clearance and evaluation of bone density every 1 to 2 years (three sites). Continued ambulation and the avoidance of immobility are critical aspects of management. Dietary measures also include maintenance of a high fluid intake and a moderate calcium intake.

Phosphorus intake is usually supplemented unless this is contraindicated by an increased risk for urinary calculi formation. Several drugs currently used in the treatment of hyperparathyroidism are helpful in lowering calcium levels but do not treat the underlying problem. Bisphosphonates (e.g., alendronate [Fosamax]) inhibit osteoclastic bone resorption and rapidly normalize serum calcium levels. Estrogen or progestin therapy can reduce serum and urinary calcium levels in postmenopausal women and may slow the demineralization of the skeleton. Oral phosphate may be used to inhibit the calcium-absorbing effects of vitamin D in the intestine. Phosphates should be used only if a patient has normal renal function and low serum phosphate levels. Calcimimetic agents (e.g., cinacalcet [Sensipar]) are a class of drugs that increase the sensitivity of the calcium receptor on the parathyroid gland, resulting in decreased PTH secretion and calcium blood levels and thus sparing calcium stores in the bone. Drugs in this class are currently indicated for secondary hyperparathyroidism in individuals with chronic kidney disease who are undergoing dialysis, for patients with parathyroid cancer, and for patients with symptomatic hypercalcemia in primary hyperparathyroidism (Pallan & Khan, 2011).

NURSING MANAGEMENT: HYPERPARATHYROIDISM

Nursing care for patients after a parathyroidectomy is similar to that for patients after thyroidectomy. The major postoperative complications are associated with hemorrhage and fluid and electrolyte disturbances. *Tetany*, a condition of neuromuscular hyperexcitability associated with a sudden decrease in calcium levels, is another concern. It is usually apparent early in the postoperative period but may develop over several days. Mild tetany, characterized by an unpleasant tingling sensation of the hands and around the mouth, may be present but should abate without problems. If tetany becomes more severe (e.g., muscular spasms or laryngospasms develop), IV calcium may be given. IV calcium gluconate should be readily available for patients after parathyroidectomy in case acute tetany occurs.

The nurse monitors intake and output to evaluate fluid status. Calcium, potassium, phosphate, and magnesium levels are assessed frequently, as are Chvostek's and Trousseau's signs (see Chapter 19, Figure 19-15). The nurse also encourages mobility to promote bone calcification.

If surgery is not performed, treatment to relieve symptoms and prevent complications is initiated. The nurse can assist patients with hyperparathyroidism adapt the meal plan to their lifestyle. A referral to a dietitian may be useful. Because immobility can aggravate the bone loss, the nurse must stress to patients the importance of an exercise program. Patients should be encouraged to keep the regular appointments, and the tests being performed should be explained. Patients should also be instructed in the symptoms of hypocalcemia or hypercalcemia and to report them, should they occur. Hypocalcemia and hypercalcemia are discussed in Chapter 19.

Hypoparathyroidism

Etiology and Pathophysiology

Hypoparathyroidism, a condition associated with inadequate levels of circulating PTH, is uncommon. It is characterized by hypocalcemia that results from a lack of PTH to maintain serum calcium levels. PTH resistance at the cellular level may also occur (pseudohypoparathyroidism). This is caused by a genetic defect that results in hypocalcemia in spite of normal or high PTH levels and is often associated with hypothyroidism and hypogonadism.

The most common cause of hypoparathyroidism is iatrogenic. This may include accidental removal of the parathyroids or damage to the vascular supply of the glands during neck surgery (e.g., thyroidectomy, radical neck surgery). Idiopathic hypoparathyroidism resulting from the absence, fatty replacement, or atrophy of the glands is a rare disease that usually occurs early in life and may be associated with other endocrine disorders. Affected patients may have antiparathyroid antibodies. Severe hypomagnesemia also leads to a suppression of PTH secretion (Bringhurst, Demay, & Kronenberg, 2011).

Clinical Manifestations

The clinical features of acute hypoparathyroidism result from a low serum calcium level (see Table 51-12). Sudden decreases in calcium concentration cause tetany. This state is characterized by tingling sensations in the lips, the fingertips, and occasionally the feet and by increased muscle tension, which escalates to paresthesias and stiffness. Painful tonic spasms of smooth and skeletal muscles can cause dysphagia, a constricted feeling in the throat, and laryngospasms that can compromise breathing. Patients are usually anxious and apprehensive. Abnormal laboratory findings include decreased serum calcium and PTH levels and increased serum phosphate levels. Other causes of chronic hypocalcemia include chronic renal failure, vitamin D deficiency, and hypomagnesemia.

NURSING AND COLLABORATIVE MANAGEMENT: HYPOPARATHYROIDISM

The primary management objectives for a patient with hypoparathyroidism are to treat acute complications such as tetany, maintain normal serum calcium levels, and prevent long-term complications. Emergency treatment of tetany requires the administration of IV calcium. IV calcium chloride or calcium gluconate should be infused slowly because high blood levels of calcium can cause hypotension, serious cardiac dysrhythmias, or cardiac arrest; thus ECG monitoring is indicated when calcium is administered. Patients who take digoxin are particularly vulnerable. IV calcium can cause venous irritation and inflammation. Extravasation may cause cellulitis, necrosis, and tissue sloughing. IV patency should be assessed before administration.

Rebreathing may partially alleviate acute neuromuscular symptoms associated with hypocalcemia, such as generalized muscle cramps or mild tetany. Patients who can cooperate should be instructed to breathe in and out of a paper bag or breathing mask. This reduces carbon dioxide excretion from the lungs, increases carbonic acid levels in the blood, and lowers the pH.

A lower pH (acidic environment) enhances the degree of ionization of calcium, causing an increase in the proportion of total body calcium available in the active form. This then temporarily alleviates the manifestations of hypocalcemia.

Patients with hypoparathyroidism need instruction in the management of long-term drug therapy and nutrition. Oral calcium supplements of at least 1.5 to 3 g/day in divided doses are usually prescribed. PTH replacement is not a recommended drug therapy because of the expense and the need for parenteral administration. Vitamin D is administered to patients with chronic and resistant hypocalcemia to enhance intestinal calcium absorption and bone resorption. The primary preparation is calcitriol (Rocaltrol). This drug raises calcium levels rapidly and is quickly metabolized. Rapid metabolism is desired because vitamin D is a fat-soluble vitamin, and toxicity can cause irreversible renal impairment.

A high-calcium meal plan includes foods such as dark green vegetables, soybeans, and tofu. Patients should be told to avoid foods containing oxalic acid (e.g., spinach, rhubarb), phytic acid (e.g., bran, whole grains), and phosphorus because they reduce calcium absorption.

Patients should be instructed about the need for lifelong treatment and follow-up care, including the monitoring of calcium levels three to four times a year.

Disorders of the Adrenal Cortex

There are three main classifications of adrenal steroid hormones. *Glucocorticoids* regulate metabolism, increase blood glucose levels, and are critical in the physiological stress response. In humans, the primary glucocorticoid is cortisol. *Mineralocorticoids* regulate sodium and potassium balance. The primary mineralocorticoid is aldosterone. *Androgens* contribute to growth and development in both genders and to sexual desire and satisfaction in women. The term *corticosteroid* refers to any one of these three types of hormones produced by the adrenal cortex.

Cushing's Syndrome

Etiology and Pathophysiology

Cushing's syndrome is a spectrum of clinical abnormalities caused by excess levels of corticosteroids, particularly glucocorticoids. Several conditions can cause this metabolic disorder (Table 51-13). The most common causes are iatrogenic administration of exogenous corticosteroids (e.g., prednisone) in large doses for several weeks or longer and the chronic and excessive production of cortisol by the adrenal cortex. Approximately 85% of cases of endogenous Cushing's syndrome result from an ACTH-secreting pituitary tumour (Cushing's disease). Other causes of Cushing's

---

Table 51-13 Causes of Cushing's Syndrome

- Prolonged administration of high doses of corticosteroids
- ACTH-secreting pituitary tumour (Cushing's disease)
- Cortisol-secreting neoplasm within the adrenal cortex that can be either carcinoma or adenoma
- Excess secretion of ACTH from carcinoma of the lung or other malignant growth outside the pituitary or the adrenal glands

ACTH, adrenocorticotropic hormone.

---

syndrome include adrenal tumours and ectopic ACTH production by tumours outside the hypothalamic-pituitary-adrenal axis (usually of the lung or the pancreas). Cushing's disease and primary adrenal tumours are most common in women age 20 to 40 years; ectopic ACTH production is more common in men.

Clinical Manifestations

The clinical manifestations of Cushing's syndrome can occur in most body systems and are related to excess levels of corticosteroids (Table 51-14). Although manifestations of glucocorticoid excess usually predominate, symptoms of mineralocorticoid and androgen excess may also appear.

Corticosteroid excess causes pronounced changes in physical appearance (Figure 51-10). Weight gain, the most common feature, results from the accumulation of adipose tissue in the trunk, the face, and the cervical area (see Figure 51-10). Transient weight gain from sodium and water retention may be present because of the mineralocorticoid effects of cortisol. Hyperglycemia occurs because of glucose intolerance (associated with cortisol-induced insulin resistance) and increased gluconeogenesis by the liver.

The catabolic effects of cortisol on peripheral tissue cause protein wasting. Muscle wasting leads to muscle weakness, especially in the extremities. Loss of protein matrix in bone leads to osteoporosis with subsequent pathological fractures (e.g., vertebral compression fractures) and bone and back pain. Loss of collagen makes the skin weaker and thinner; therefore, the skin bruises more easily. Catabolic processes predominate, and wound healing is delayed. Mood disturbances (e.g., irritability, anxiety, euphoria), insomnia, irrationality, and occasionally psychosis may occur.

Mineralocorticoid excess may cause hypertension (secondary to fluid retention), whereas adrenal androgen excess may cause pronounced acne, virilization in women, and feminization in men. Menstrual disorders and hirsutism in women and gynecomastia and erectile dysfunction in men occur more commonly with adrenal carcinomas.

The clinical presentation is the first indication of Cushing's syndrome (Figure 51-11). Of particular importance are (a) centripetal (truncal) obesity or generalized obesity; (b) so-called moon facies (fullness of the face) with facial plethora; (c) purplish red striae, which are usually depressed below the skin surface, on the abdomen, the breast, or the buttocks (Figure 51-12); (d) hirsutism in women; (e) menstrual disorders in women; (f) hypertension; and (g) unexplained hypokalemia.

Diagnostic Studies

When Cushing's syndrome is suspected, a 24-hour urine sample is collected to measure free cortisol (see Chapter 50). If the free cortisol results are borderline, a low-dose dexamethasone suppression test is performed. Plasma cortisol (the primary glucocorticoid) levels may be elevated, with loss of diurnal variation. Elevation in the midnight serum cortisol level confirms the diagnosis of Cushing's syndrome with 100% sensitivity (Liubinas, Porto, & Kaye, 2011). False-positive results can occur in patients with depression, those under acute stress, and those who are actively alcoholic. CT and MRI of the pituitary and adrenal glands may be used.

Plasma ACTH levels may be low, normal, or elevated, depending on the underlying problem. High or normal levels indicate ACTH-dependent Cushing's disease, whereas low or undetectable

Table 51-14 Clinical Manifestations: Adrenocortical Hormone Dysfunction

CATEGORY	HYPOFUNCTION (ADDISON'S DISEASE)	HYPERFUNCTION (CUSHING'S SYNDROME)
Glucocorticoids		
General appearance	Weight loss	Centripetal (truncal) obesity, thin extremities, rounding of face (moon facies), fat deposits on back of neck and on shoulders (buffalo hump)
Integumentary system	Bronzed or smoky hyperpigmentation of face, neck, hands (especially creases), buccal membranes, nipples, genitalia, and scars (if pituitary function is normal); vitiligo, alopecia	Thin, fragile skin; purplish red striae; petechial hemorrhages; bruises; florid cheeks (facial plethora); acne; poor wound healing
Cardiovascular system	Hypotension, tendency to develop refractory shock, vasodilation	Hypervolemia, hypertension, edema of lower extremities
Gastrointestinal system	Anorexia, nausea and vomiting, cramping abdominal pain, diarrhea	Increase in secretion of pepsin and hydrochloric acid; anorexia
Urinary system	—	Glycosuria, hypercalciuria, kidney stones
Musculoskeletal system	Fatigability	Muscle wasting in extremities, proximal muscle weakness, fatigue, osteoporosis, awkward gait, back and joint pain, weakness
Immune system	Propensity for coexisting autoimmune diseases	Inhibition of immune response, suppression of allergic response, inhibition of inflammation
Hematological system	Anemia, lymphocytosis	Leukocytosis, lymphopenia, polycythemia, increased coagulability
Fluids and electrolytes	Hyponatremia, hypovolemia, dehydration, hyperkalemia	Sodium and water retention, edema, hypokalemia
Metabolism	Hypoglycemia, insulin sensitivity, fever	Hyperglycemia, negative nitrogen balance, dyslipidemia
Emotional state	Neurasthenia, depression, exhaustion or irritability, confusion, delusions	Euphoria, irritability, hypomania to depression, emotional lability
Mineralocorticoids		
Fluid and electrolytes	Sodium loss, decreased volume of extracellular fluid, hyperkalemia, salt craving	Marked sodium and water retention, tendency toward edema, marked hypokalemia, alkalosis
Cardiovascular system	Hypovolemia, tendency toward shock, decreased cardiac output, decrease in heart size	Hypertension, hypervolemia
Androgen		
Integumentary system	Decreased axillary and pubic hair (in women)	Hirsutism, acne, hyperpigmentation
Reproductive system	No effect in men; decreased libido in women	Menstrual irregularities and enlargement of clitoris in women; gynecomastia and testicular atrophy in men
Musculoskeletal system	Decrease in muscle size and tone	Muscle wasting and weakness

levels indicate an adrenal or exogenous etiology. Other findings on diagnostic tests associated with, but not diagnostic of, Cushing's syndrome include granulocytosis, lymphopenia, eosinopenia, hyperglycemia, glycosuria, hypercalciuria, and osteoporosis. Hypokalemia and alkalosis occur in ectopic ACTH syndrome and adrenal carcinoma.

Collaborative Care

The primary goal of treatment for Cushing's disease is to normalize hormone secretion. The specific treatment is dependent on the underlying cause (Table 51-15). If the underlying cause is a pituitary adenoma, the standard treatment is surgical removal of the tumour through the trans-sphenoidal approach (Liubinas et al., 2011). (The trans-sphenoidal approach is discussed earlier in this chapter.) Irradiation of the pituitary adenoma may be necessary if surgical outcomes are not optimal or if a patient is at high risk for surgical complications. Adrenalectomy is indicated for Cushing's syndrome caused by

adrenal tumours or hyperplasia. On occasion, bilateral adrenalectomy is necessary.

Laparoscopic adrenalectomy is considered an appropriate surgical approach except for patients with known or suspected malignant adrenal tumours. An open surgical adrenalectomy is the treatment of choice for adrenal cancer. Patients with ectopic ACTH-secreting tumours are managed by treating the primary neoplasm.

Drug therapy is used when surgery is contraindicated or as an adjunct to surgery. The goal of drug therapy is the inhibition of adrenal function (medical adrenalectomy). Mitotane (Lysodren) suppresses cortisol production, alters peripheral metabolism of cortisol, and decreases plasma and urine corticosteroid levels. Ketoconazole can be used to inhibit cortisol synthesis. These drugs are used cautiously because they are often toxic at doses needed to reduce corticosteroid synthesis.

If Cushing's syndrome has developed during the course of prolonged administration of corticosteroids (e.g., prednisone), one or more of the following alternatives may be tried: (a) gradual

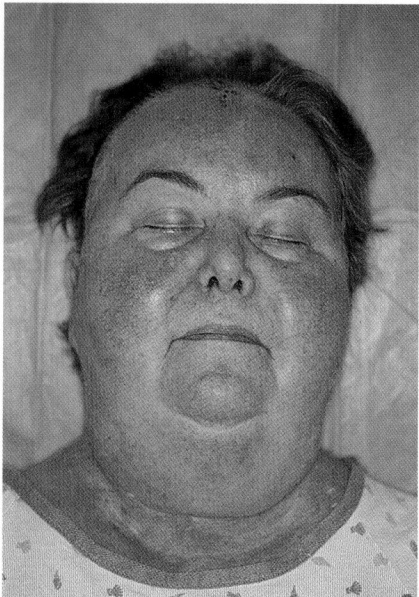

Figure 51-10 Cushing's syndrome. Facies include a rounded face (moon facies) with thin, reddened skin. Hirsutism may also be present.

Source: Seidel, H. M., Ball, J., Dains, J., & Benedict, G. W. (2006). *Mosby's guide to physical examination* (6th ed., p. 272, Figure 10-17). St. Louis: Mosby.

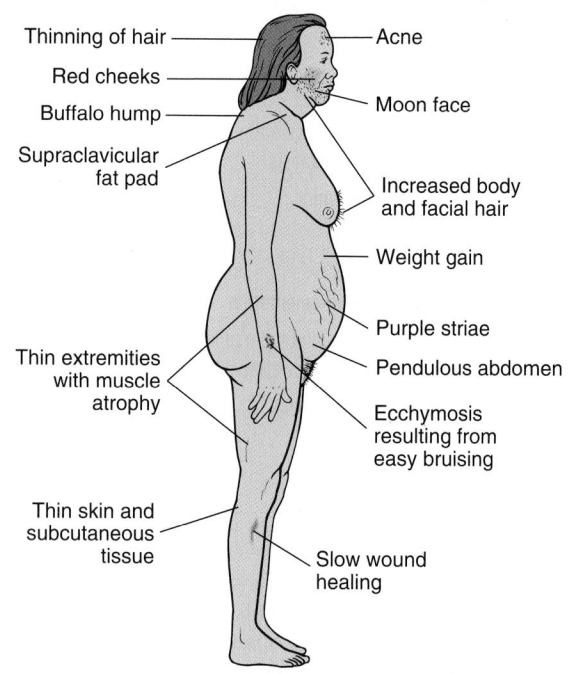

Figure 51-11 Common characteristics of Cushing's syndrome.

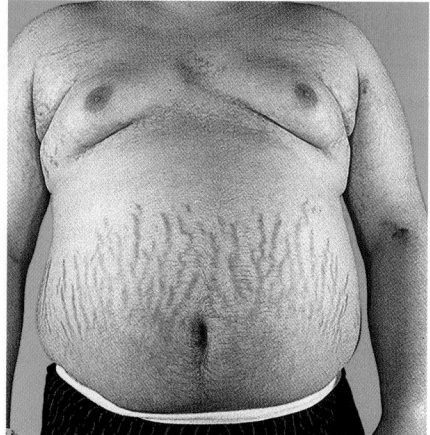

Figure 51-12 Appearance of torso in Cushing's syndrome. Truncal obesity; broad, purple striae; and easy bruising (left antecubital fossa).

Source: Chew, S. L., & Leslie, D. (2006). *Clinical endocrinology and diabetes: An illustrated colour text.* Edinburgh: Churchill Livingstone.

COLLABORATIVE CARE

Table 51-15 Cushing's Syndrome

Diagnostic	Collaborative Therapy*
• History and physical examination	**Adrenocortical Adenoma, Carcinoma, or Hyperplasia**
• Mental status examination	• Adrenalectomy (open or laparoscopic)
• Measurement of plasma cortisol levels for diurnal variations	• Drug therapy
	• Mitotane (Lysodren)
• Measurement of plasma ACTH level	• Ketoconazole (Nizoral)
• Complete blood cell count	**Pituitary Adenoma**
• Blood chemistry evaluation for sodium, potassium, and glucose	• Trans-sphenoidal resection
	• Radiation therapy
	Ectopic ACTH-Secreting Tumour
• Dexamethasone suppression test	• Treatment of the tumour responsible (surgical removal or radiation therapy)
• 24-hour urine collection for free cortisol measurement	**Exogenous Corticosteroid Therapy**
• Examination of visual field	• Discontinuance of or alteration in administration of exogenous corticosteroids
• CT, MRI	

ACTH, adrenocorticotropic hormone; *CT*, computed tomography; *MRI*, magnetic resonance imaging.
*Treatment is based on underlying cause.

discontinuance of corticosteroid therapy, (b) reduction of the corticosteroid dose, and (c) conversion to an alternate-day regimen. Gradual tapering of the corticosteroids is necessary to avoid potentially life-threatening adrenal insufficiency. An alternate-day regimen is one in which twice the daily dosage of a shorter-acting corticosteroid is given every other morning to minimize hypothalamic-pituitary-adrenal suppression, growth suppression, and altered appearance. This regimen is not used when the corticosteroids are given as endocrine replacement therapy (Stewart & Krone, 2011).

NURSING MANAGEMENT: CUSHING'S SYNDROME

Nursing Assessment

Subjective and objective data that should be obtained from a patient with Cushing's syndrome are presented in Table 51-16.

Figure 51-11 labels:
Thinning of hair — Acne
Red cheeks
Buffalo hump — Moon face
Supraclavicular fat pad
Increased body and facial hair
Weight gain
Thin extremities with muscle atrophy
Purple striae
Pendulous abdomen
Ecchymosis resulting from easy bruising
Thin skin and subcutaneous tissue
Slow wound healing

NURSING ASSESSMENT

Table 51-16 Cushing's Syndrome

Subjective Data

Important Health Information

Past health history: Pituitary tumour (Cushing's disease); adrenal, pancreatic, or pulmonary neoplasms; GI bleeding; frequent infections

Medications: Use of corticosteroids

Symptoms

- Malaise, weakness, fatigue
- Weight gain, anorexia
- Polyuria
- Prolonged wound healing, easy bruising
- Insomnia, poor sleep quality
- Headache; back, joint, bone, and rib pain; poor concentration and memory
- Negative feelings regarding changes in personal appearance
- Amenorrhea, erectile dysfunction, decreased libido
- Anxiety, mood disturbances, emotional lability, psychosis

Objective Data

General

Centripetal (truncal) obesity, supraclavicular fat pads, buffalo hump, moon facies

Integumentary

Facial plethora; hirsutism of body and face, thinning of head hair; thin, friable skin; acne; petechiae; purpura; hyperpigmentation; purplish red striae on breasts, buttocks, and abdomen; edema of lower extremities

Cardiovascular

Hypertension

Musculoskeletal

Muscle wasting, thin extremities, awkward gait

Reproductive

Gynecomastia, testicular atrophy (in men); enlarged clitoris (in women)

Possible Findings

Hypokalemia, hyperglycemia, dyslipidemia; polycythemia, granulocytosis, lymphocytopenia, eosinopenia; ↑ plasma cortisol level; high, low, or normal ACTH levels; abnormal result of dexamethasone suppression test; ↑ levels of urine free cortisol and 17-ketosteroids; glycosuria, hypercalciuria; osteoporosis on radiograph

ACTH, adrenocorticotropic hormone; *GI,* gastrointestinal.

Nursing Diagnoses

Nursing diagnoses for patients with Cushing's syndrome may include, but are not limited to, the following:

- Risk for infection *related to* lowered resistance to stress and suppression of immune system
- Imbalanced nutrition: more than body requirements *related to* increased appetite, high caloric content of foods, and inactivity
- Disturbed body image *related to* altered body appearance and emotional lability
- Impaired skin integrity *related to* excess corticosteroids, immobility, and altered skin fragility

Planning

The overall goals for patients with Cushing's syndrome are as follows:

- Relief from symptoms.
- No serious complications.
- Maintenance of a positive self-image.
- Active participation in the therapeutic plan.

Nursing Implementation

Health Promotion

Health promotion is focused on identifying patients at risk for Cushing's syndrome. Patients receiving long-term, exogenous cortisol for a variety of diseases are at risk. Teaching patients about the medication use and monitoring of adverse drug effects are important preventive measures.

Acute Intervention

Patients with Cushing's syndrome are seriously ill. Because the therapeutic interventions produce many adverse drug effects, the focus of daily assessment is on signs and symptoms of hormone and drug toxicity and complicating conditions such as cardiovascular disease, diabetes mellitus, and infection. Nursing assessment should include monitoring of vital signs, daily weighing, and measuring glucose levels. Because signs and symptoms of inflammation, such as fever and redness, may be minimal or absent, the nurse must assess for pain, loss of function, and purulent drainage as signs of possible infection. The nurse also monitors for signs and symptoms of thromboembolic events, such as sudden chest pain, dyspnea, or tachypnea.

Another important focus of nursing care is emotional support. Changes in appearance such as centripetal obesity, multiple bruises, hirsutism in women, and gynecomastia in men can be distressing. Patients may feel unattractive or unwanted. The nurse can help by remaining sensitive to patients' feelings and offering respect and unconditional acceptance. Patients can be reassured that the physical changes and much of the emotional lability will resolve when hormone levels return to normal.

If treatment involves surgical removal of a pituitary adenoma, an adrenal tumour, or one or both adrenal glands, nursing care has an additional focus on preoperative and postoperative care.

Preoperative Care. Before surgery, the patient should be brought to optimal physical condition. Hypertension and hyperglycemia must be controlled, and hypokalemia is corrected with diet and potassium supplements. A high-protein meal plan helps correct the protein depletion. Preoperative teaching depends on the type of surgical approach planned (hypophysectomy or adrenalectomy), but should include information regarding the postoperative care that patients should anticipate. Patients should be told that in the postoperative period (for both open and laparoscopic adrenalectomy), they will probably have a nasogastric tube, urinary catheter, IV therapy, central venous pressure monitoring, and leg sequential compression devices to prevent emboli. Preoperative management for patients undergoing a hypophysectomy is discussed earlier in this chapter.

■ **Postoperative Care.** Surgery on the adrenal glands poses risks beyond those of other types of operations. Because the glands are highly vascular, the risk of hemorrhage is increased. Manipulation of glandular tissue during surgery may cause the release of large amounts of hormone into the circulation, which produce marked fluctuations in the metabolic processes affected by these hormones. After surgery, BP, fluid balance, and electrolyte levels tend to be unstable because of these hormone fluctuations.

High doses of corticosteroids (e.g., hydrocortisone [Solu-Cortef]) are administered IV during surgery and for several days afterward to ensure adequate responses to the stress of the procedure. If large amounts of endogenous hormone have been released into the systemic circulation during surgery, hypertension is likely to develop, increasing the risk of hemorrhage. High levels of corticosteroids also increase susceptibility to infection and delay wound healing.

Any significant changes in BP, respirations, or heart rate should be reported to the physician. Fluid intake and output should be monitored carefully and assessed for potential imbalances. The critical period for circulatory instability ranges from 24 to 48 hours after surgery. IV corticosteroids are given, and the dosage and the rate of flow are adjusted to the patient's clinical manifestations and fluid and electrolyte balances. Oral doses are given as tolerated. The IV line may be kept in place after IV corticosteroids are withdrawn to maintain access for quick administration of corticosteroids or vasopressors. Morning urine levels of cortisol (assessed at the same time each morning) are measured to evaluate the effectiveness of the surgery.

If the corticosteroid dosage is tapered too rapidly after surgery, acute adrenal insufficiency may develop. Vomiting, increased weakness, dehydration, and hypotension may indicate hypocortisolism. In addition, patients may complain of painful joints, pruritus, or peeling skin and may experience severe emotional disturbances. These signs and symptoms should be reported so that drug doses can be adjusted. The nurse must constantly be alert for signs of corticosteroid imbalance. After surgery, the patient is usually maintained on bed rest until the BP stabilizes. Because the usual inflammatory responses are suppressed, the nurse must be alert for subtle signs of postoperative infections. The nurse must use meticulous care when changing the dressing and during any other procedures that necessitate access to body cavities, circulation, or areas under the skin, so that infection is prevented. A nursing care plan for patients with Cushing's syndrome is available on the Evolve Web site for this chapter.

■ Ambulatory and Home Care

Discharge instructions are based on the patient's lack of endogenous corticosteroids and resulting inability to react to stressors physiologically. The nurse should consider a referral for a visiting nurse, especially for older adults, because of the need for ongoing evaluation and educational needs. Patients should wear medical alert bracelets at all times and carry medical identification and instructions in a wallet or purse. Exposure to extremes of temperature, infections, and emotional disturbances should be avoided as much as possible. Stress may produce or precipitate acute adrenal insufficiency because the remaining adrenal tissue cannot meet an increased hormonal demand. Many patients can be taught to adjust their corticosteroid replacement therapy in accordance with their stress levels. The nurse should consult with each patient's health care provider to determine the param-

eters for dosage changes if this plan is feasible. If a patient cannot adjust his or her own medication or if weakness, fainting, fever, or nausea and vomiting occur, the patient should contact the health care provider for a possible adjustment in corticosteroid dosage. Many patients require lifetime replacement therapy; however, it may take several months to adjust the hormone dose satisfactorily, and patients should be prepared for this.

■ Evaluation

The expected outcomes for patients with Cushing's syndrome are as follows:
- No signs or symptoms of infection
- Appropriate weight for height
- Increased acceptance of appearance
- Healing and maintenance of intact skin

Adrenocortical Insufficiency

Causes and Pathophysiological Features

Adrenocortical insufficiency (hypofunction of the adrenal cortex) may have a primary cause (known as *Addison's disease*) or a secondary cause (lack of pituitary ACTH secretion). In **Addison's disease**, the supply of all three classes of adrenal corticosteroids (glucocorticoids, mineralocorticoids, and androgens) is reduced. In secondary adrenocortical insufficiency, levels of corticosteroids and androgens are deficient, but those of mineralocorticoids rarely are. ACTH deficiency may be caused by pituitary disease or suppression of the hypothalamic-pituitary-adrenal axis as a result of the administration of exogenous corticosteroids.

The most common cause of Addison's disease in industrialized nations is an autoimmune response. Adrenal tissue is destroyed by antibodies against the patient's own adrenal cortex. Susceptibility genes for Addison's disease are beginning to be identified (Husebye & Løvås, 2009). Often, other endocrine conditions are present, and Addison's disease is considered a component of polyglandular autoimmune syndrome (Reddy, 2011). Tuberculosis causes Addison's disease worldwide, but tuberculosis is now rare in North American and industrialized nations (Yokoyama, Toda, Kimura, Mikagi, & Aizawa, 2009). Other causes include infarction, fungal infections (e.g., histoplasmosis), acquired immune deficiency syndrome (AIDS), and metastatic cancer. Iatrogenic Addison's disease may be caused by adrenal hemorrhage, often related to anticoagulant therapy, antineoplastic chemotherapy, ketoconazole therapy for AIDS, or bilateral adrenalectomy. Adrenal insufficiency most often occurs in adults younger than 60 years and affects both genders equally. Addison's disease, if caused by an autoimmune response, is most common in White women.

Clinical Manifestations

Because manifestations do not tend to become evident until 90% of the adrenal cortex is destroyed, the disease is often advanced before it is diagnosed. The manifestations have a very slow (insidious) onset and include progressive weakness, fatigue, weight loss, and anorexia as primary features. Skin hyperpigmentation, a striking feature, is observed primarily in sun-exposed areas of the body, at pressure points, over joints, and in creases (Figure 51-13). It is most likely caused by increased secretion of β-lipotropin

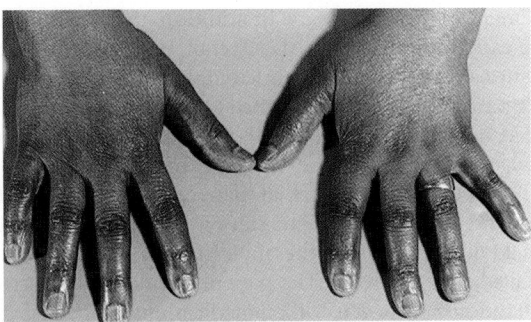

Figure 51-13 Hyperpigmentation typically observed in Addison's disease.

Source: Chew, S. L., & Leslie, D. (2006). *Clinical endocrinology and diabetes: An illustrated colour text*. Edinburgh: Churchill Livingstone.

COLLABORATIVE CARE

Table 51-17 Addison's Disease

Diagnostic	*Collaborative Therapy*
• History and physical examination	• Daily glucocorticoid (e.g., hydrocortisone) replacement (two thirds on awakening in morning, one third in late afternoon)*
• Measurement of plasma cortisol levels	
• Measurement of urine cortisol and aldosterone levels	• Daily mineralocorticoid (fludrocortisone [Florinef]) replacement in morning*
• Measurement of serum electrolytes	• Salt additives for excess heat or humidity
• ACTH stimulation test	• Increased dose of cortisol for stress situations (e.g., surgery, hospitalization)
• CT, MRI	

*For conditions of normal daily stress in individuals with usual daytime activity.
ACTH, adrenocorticotropic hormone; *CT,* computed tomography; *MRI,* magnetic resonance imaging.

(which contains melanocyte-stimulating hormone [MSH]). Secretion of this tropic hormone is increased because of decreased negative feedback and subsequent low corticosteroid levels. Other frequent manifestations are hypotension, hyponatremia, hyperkalemia, nausea and vomiting, and diarrhea. Irritability and depression may also occur in primary adrenal hypofunction.

Secondary adrenocortical hypofunction shares many signs and symptoms in common with Addison's disease, but hyperpigmentation is not characteristic because ACTH and related peptide levels are low.

Complications

Patients with adrenocortical insufficiency are at risk for an acute adrenal insufficiency *(addisonian crisis)*, a life-threatening emergency caused by insufficient adrenocortical hormones or a sudden sharp decrease in these hormones. Addisonian crisis is triggered by stress (e.g., from infection, surgery, trauma, hemorrhage, or psychological distress); by sudden withdrawal of corticosteroid hormone replacement therapy (which often occurs when a patient who lacks knowledge of the importance of replacement therapy stops following the regimen); by adrenal surgery; or by sudden pituitary gland destruction.

During acute adrenal insufficiency, manifestations of glucocorticoid and mineralocorticoid deficiencies are severe and include hypotension (particularly postural), tachycardia, dehydration, hyponatremia, hyperkalemia, hypoglycemia, fever, weakness, and confusion. Hypotension may lead to shock. Circulatory collapse associated with adrenal insufficiency is often unresponsive to the usual treatment (vasopressors and fluid replacement). GI manifestations include nausea, vomiting, diarrhea, and pain in the abdomen. Pain may also occur in the lower back or the legs.

Diagnostic Studies

In addition to clinical features, cortisol levels that are subnormal or fail to rise over basal levels with an ACTH stimulation test can be diagnostic for Addison's disease. A failure of cortisol levels to rise in response to ACTH stimulation indicates primary adrenal disease. A positive response to ACTH stimulation indicates that the adrenal gland is functioning and that the probable cause is pituitary disease (see Chapter 50).

Other abnormal laboratory findings include hyperkalemia, hypochloremia, hyponatremia, hypoglycemia, anemia, and increased blood urea nitrogen levels. Urine levels of free cortisol are low, as is the urine level of aldosterone (Pagana & Pagana, 2011). An ECG may show low voltage and a vertical QRS axis. In addition, peaked T-waves caused by hyperkalemia may be evident. CT and MRI are used to localize tumours or identify adrenal calcifications or enlargement (Table 51-17).

Collaborative Care

Treatment of adrenocortical insufficiency is focused on management of the underlying cause when possible. The mainstay of treatment for adrenocortical insufficiency is replacement therapy (see Table 51-17). Hydrocortisone, the most commonly used form of replacement therapy, has both glucocorticoid and mineralocorticoid properties. During situations associated with physiological stress, glucocorticoid dosage must be increased to prevent addisonian crisis. Mineralocorticoid replacement with fludrocortisone acetate (Florinef) is administered daily with increased salt in the diet.

Addisonian crisis is a life-threatening emergency requiring aggressive management. Treatment must be directed toward shock management and high-dose hydrocortisone replacement. Large volumes of 0.9% saline solution and 5% dextrose are administered to reverse hypotension and electrolyte imbalances until BP returns to normal.

NURSING MANAGEMENT: ADDISON'S DISEASE

Nursing Implementation

Acute Intervention

When the patient with Addison's disease is hospitalized—whether for diagnosis, an acute crisis, or some other health problem—frequent nursing assessment is necessary. Vital signs and signs of fluid volume deficit and electrolyte imbalance should be assessed for the first 24 hours every 30 minutes to 4 hours, depending on how unstable the patient's condition is. Daily weighings, diligent corticosteroid administration, protection against exposure to

Table 51-18 Addison's Disease

The following should be included in a teaching plan for the patient and caregiver:

1. Names, dosages, and actions of drugs

2. Symptoms of overdosage and underdosage

3. Conditions necessitating increased medication (e.g., trauma, infection, surgery, emotional crisis)

4. Course of action to take with regard to changes in medication
   - Increase in dose of corticosteroid
   - Administration of large dose of corticosteroid intramuscularly, including demonstration and return demonstration
   - Consultation with health care provider

5. Prevention of infection and need for prompt and vigorous treatment of existing infections

6. Need for lifelong replacement therapy

7. Need for lifelong medical supervision

8. Need for medical identification device

infection, and complete assistance with hygiene are also needed. The patients should be protected from noise, light, and environmental temperature extremes. The patients cannot cope with these stresses because of the inability to produce corticosteroids.

The patient who is hospitalized because of adrenal crisis usually responds by the second day and can start oral corticosteroid replacement. Instruct the patient about the importance of keeping scheduled follow-up appointments.

◾ Ambulatory and Home Care

The nurse has an important role in the long-term management of Addison's disease. The serious nature of the disease and the need for lifelong replacement therapy necessitate a well-organized and carefully presented teaching plan. Table 51-18 outlines the major areas that must be included in the teaching plan.

Glucocorticoids are usually given in divided doses, two thirds in the morning and one third in the afternoon. Mineralocorticoids are given once daily, preferably in the morning. This dosage schedule reflects normal circadian rhythm in endogenous hormone secretion and decreases the intensity of adverse effects associated with corticosteroid replacement therapy. Because the aim of replacement therapy is to return hormone levels to normal, nursing care is designed to help patients maintain hormone balance and manage the medication regimen.

Because the patient with Addison's disease is unable to tolerate physical or emotional stress without additional exogenous corticosteroids, long-term care revolves around recognizing the need for extra medication and techniques for stress management. The need for corticosteroid hormone is proportional to stress levels. A patient who cannot produce endogenous hormone must adjust the dose of exogenous hormone to the stress level. Examples of situations requiring corticosteroid adjustment are fever, influenza, extraction of teeth, and rigorous physical activity, such as playing tennis on a hot day or running a marathon. Doses are usually doubled in situations of minor stress (e.g., a respiratory infection, dental work) and tripled in situations of major stress (e.g., divorce, loss of parent). When the stress level is in doubt, it is better to err on the side of over-replacement. If vomiting or diarrhea occurs, as may happen with influenza, the health care provider must be notified immediately because electrolyte

replacement may be necessary. In addition, these manifestations may be early indicators of crisis. Overall, patients who take their medications consistently can anticipate a normal life expectancy.

The patient must be taught the signs and symptoms of corticosteroid deficiency and excess and to report these signs to the health care provider so the dosage can be adjusted to each patient's need. It is critical that patients wear a medical alert bracelet and carry a wallet card stating that they have Addison's disease so that appropriate therapy can be initiated in case of an unexpected stressful event. The patient should be instructed and given handouts related to other medications that cause a need to increase glucocorticoid dosage (e.g., phenytoin [Dilantin], barbiturates, rifampin [Rifadin], and antacids). Estrogen inhibits steroid metabolism. The nurse should instruct patients receiving mineralocorticoid therapy (fludrocortisone [Florinef]) how to measure their BP, to increase salt intake, and to report significant changes to their health care provider. Changes may indicate a need for dosage adjustment.

Patients should carry an emergency kit at all times. The kit should consist of 100 mg of intramuscular (IM) hydrocortisone, syringes, and instructions for use. The patient and significant others should be instructed in how to administer an IM injection in case the replacement therapy cannot be taken orally. The patient should verbalize instructions, practise IM injections with saline, and receive written instructions about when to alter the dose (National Institute of Diabetes and Digestive and Kidney Diseases, 2009).

Corticosteroid Therapy

Cortisol and related glucocorticoids are used to relieve the signs and symptoms associated with many diseases (Table 51-19). The long-term administration of corticosteroids in therapeutic dosages often leads to serious complications and adverse drug effects (Table 51-20). For this reason, corticosteroid therapy is not recommended for minor chronic conditions. Therapy should be reserved for diseases in which there is a risk of death or permanent loss of function and conditions in which short-term therapy is likely to produce remission or recovery. The potential benefits of treatment must always be weighed against the risks.

Effects of Corticosteroid Therapy

Corticosteroid therapy has multiple effects. Although these actions can prove to be beneficial and therapeutic in some situations, they can contribute to adverse effects as well. The expected effects of corticosteroid therapy include the following:

1. *Anti-inflammatory action.* Corticosteroids decrease the number of circulating lymphocytes, monocytes, and eosinophils. They enhance the release of polymorphonuclear leukocytes from bone marrow, inhibit the accumulation of leukocytes at the site of inflammation, and inhibit the release of substances involved in the inflammatory response (e.g., kinins, prostaglandins, histamine) from the leukocytes. As a result, manifestations of inflammation, including redness, tenderness, heat, swelling, and local edema, are suppressed.

2. *Immunosuppression.* Corticosteroids cause atrophy of lymphoid tissue, suppress the cell-mediated immune responses, and decrease the production of antibodies.

3. *Maintenance of normal blood pressure.* Corticosteroids potentiate the vasoconstrictor effect of norepinephrine and act on the renal tubules to increase sodium reabsorption and enhance potassium and hydrogen excretion. Retention of

DRUG THERAPY

Table 51-19 Diseases and Disorders Treated With Corticosteroids

For Hormone Replacement	Endocrine Diseases
• Adrenal insufficiency	• Hypercalcemia
• Congenital adrenal hyperplasia	• Hashimoto's thyroiditis
For Therapeutic Effect	• Thyrotoxic crisis (thyroid storm)
Allergic Reactions	**Liver Diseases**
• Anaphylaxis	• Alcohol-related hepatitis
• Bee stings	• Autoimmune hepatitis
• Contact dermatitis	**Neurological Diseases**
• Drug reactions	• Prevention of cerebral edema and increase in intracranial pressure
• Serum sickness	
• Urticaria	• Head trauma
Collagen Diseases	**Pulmonary Diseases**
• Giant cell arteritis	• Aspiration pneumonia
• Mixed connective tissue disorders	• Asthma
• Polymyositis	• Chronic obstructive pulmonary disease
• Polyarteritis nodosa	
• Rheumatoid arthritis	**Other Diseases/Disorders**
• Systemic lupus erythematosus	• Skin diseases
Gastrointestinal Diseases	• Malignancies, leukemia, lymphoma
• Inflammatory bowel disease	• Immunosuppression (after organ transplantation)
• Celiac disease	
	• Inflammation
	• Nephrotic syndrome

DRUG THERAPY

Table 51-20 Adverse Effects of Corticosteroids

- Hypokalemia may develop.
- Patient is predisposed to peptic ulcer disease.
- Skeletal muscle atrophy and weakness occur.
- Mood and behaviour changes may be observed.
- Glucose intolerance predisposes to diabetes mellitus.
- Fat from extremities is redistributed to trunk and face.
- Hypocalcemia related to anti–vitamin D effect may occur.
- Healing is delayed, and patient is at increased risk for wound dehiscence.
- Susceptibility to infection is increased. Infection develops more rapidly and spreads more widely.
- Suppression of pituitary ACTH synthesis occurs. Corticosteroid deficiency is likely if hormone treatment is withdrawn abruptly. Corticosteroid doses should be tapered.
- BP increases because of excess blood volume and potentiation of vasoconstrictor effects. Hypertension predisposes to heart failure.
- Protein depletion decreases bone formation, density, and strength; patient is thus predisposed to pathological fractures, especially compression fractures of the vertebrae (osteoporosis).

ACTH, adrenocorticotropic hormone; *BP,* blood pressure.

SAFETY ALERT

Corticosteroids

- Instruct patients not to discontinue therapy abruptly.
- Instruct patients to monitor for signs of infection.
- Instruct patients with diabetes to closely monitor blood glucose levels.

sodium (and subsequently water) increases blood volume and helps maintain BP. Mineralocorticoids have a direct effect on sodium reabsorption in the distal tubules of the kidneys; as a result, sodium retention and water retention are increased.

4. *Carbohydrate and protein metabolism.* Corticosteroids antagonize the effects of insulin and can induce glucose intolerance by increasing hepatic glycogenolysis and insulin resistance. They also stimulate the breakdown of protein for gluconeogenesis, which can lead to skeletal muscle wasting. Although corticosteroids mobilize free fatty acids and cause redistribution of fat in cushingoid patterns, the mechanism underlying this process is unknown.

Complications Associated With Corticosteroid Therapy

A beneficial effect in one situation may be a harmful one in another. For example, the vasopressive effect of a hormone is critical in enabling the organism to function in stressful situations, but it can produce hypertension when used for drug therapy. Suppression of inflammation and the immune response may help save the lives of the victim of anaphylaxis and the transplant recipient, but it causes reactivation of latent tuberculosis and greatly reduces resistance to other infections and cancers. In addition, corticosteroids inhibit the antibody response to vaccines. Specific adverse effects related to corticosteroid therapy are listed in Table 51-20.

NURSING AND COLLABORATIVE MANAGEMENT: CORTICOSTEROID THERAPY

Many patients receive corticosteroid therapy, particularly glucocorticoid therapy, for nonendocrine reasons (see Table 51-19). Thorough instruction is necessary to ensure patient adherence to the regimen. When corticosteroids are used as nonreplacement therapy, they are taken once daily or once every other day. They should be taken early in the morning with food to decrease gastric irritation. Because exogenous corticosteroid administration may suppress endogenous ACTH and therefore endogenous cortisol (suppression is time and dose dependent), the danger of abrupt cessation of corticosteroid therapy must be emphasized to patients and significant others. When taken for longer than 1 week, corticosteroids suppress adrenal production, and oral steroids should be tapered. Nurses must ensure that increased doses of steroid are prescribed in acute care or home care situations with increased physical or emotional stress.

Because patients often receive corticosteroid treatment for prolonged periods (>3 months), corticosteroid-induced osteoporosis is an important concern (Furukawa et al., 2011). Therapies to reduce the resorption of bone may include increased calcium intake, vitamin D supplementation, administration of bisphosphonates (e.g., alendronate [Fosamax]), and institution of a low-impact exercise program. Further instruction and interventions to minimize the adverse effects and complications of corticosteroid therapy are listed in Table 51-21.

Table 51-21 Corticosteroid Therapy

The nurse must teach patients and caregivers the following:

1. Plan a diet high in protein, calcium, and potassium but low in fat and concentrated simple carbohydrates such as sugar, honey, syrups, and candy.

2. Identify measures to ensure adequate rest and sleep, such as daily naps and avoidance of caffeine late in the day.

3. Develop and maintain an exercise program to help maintain bone integrity.

4. Recognize edema and ways to restrict sodium intake to less than 2000 mg/day if edema occurs.

5. Monitor glucose levels and recognize symptoms and signs of hyperglycemia (e.g., polydipsia, polyuria, blurred vision) and glycosuria (glucose in the urine). Patients should be instructed to report hyperglycemic symptoms or capillary glucose levels higher than 10 mmol/L or urine findings that are positive for glucose.

6. Notify health care provider if patients are experiencing postprandial heartburn or epigastric pain that is not relieved by antacids.

7. See an eye specialist yearly to assess development of possible cataracts.

8. Use safety measures such as getting up slowly from a bed or a chair, and use good lighting to prevent accidental injury.

9. Maintain good hygiene practices and avoid contact with people with colds or other contagious illnesses to prevent infection.

10. Inform all health care providers about long-term corticosteroid use.

11. Realize that doses of corticosteroids may need to be increased in times of physical and emotional stress.

12. Never abruptly stop taking the corticosteroids because this could lead to addisonian crisis and possibly death.

Hyperaldosteronism

Etiology and Pathophysiology

Hyperaldosteronism is characterized by excessive aldosterone secretion. The main effects of aldosterone are retention of sodium and excretion of potassium and hydrogen ion. Thus the hallmark of this disease is hypertension with hypokalemic alkalosis. *Primary hyperaldosteronism* (PA) is most commonly caused by a small, solitary adrenocortical adenoma. On occasion, multiple lesions are involved and are associated with bilateral adrenal hyperplasia. PA affects both sexes equally and occurs most frequently between the ages of 30 and 50 years. It is estimated that approximately 1% of cases of hypertension are caused by PA. *Secondary hyperaldosteronism* occurs in response to a nonadrenal cause of elevated aldosterone levels such as renal artery stenosis, renin-secreting tumours, or chronic renal disease.

Clinical Manifestations

Elevations in aldosterone levels are associated with retention of sodium and elimination of potassium. Sodium retention leads to hypernatremia, hypertension, and headache. Edema does not usually occur because the rate of sodium excretion increases, which prevents more severe sodium retention. The potassium wasting leads to hypokalemia, which causes generalized muscle weakness, fatigue, cardiac dysrhythmias, glucose intolerance, and metabolic alkalosis that may lead to tetany.

Diagnostic Studies

The diagnosis of hyperaldosteronism should be suspected in all hypertensive patients with hypokalemia that is not being treated with diuretics. PA is associated with elevations in plasma aldosterone levels and decreased plasma renin activity, elevated sodium levels, and decreased serum potassium levels. Adenomas are localized by means of CT or MRI. If a tumour is not found, plasma 18-hydroxycorticosterone is measured after overnight bed rest. A level higher than 1.38 nmol/L indicates the presence of an adenoma.

NURSING AND COLLABORATIVE MANAGEMENT: PRIMARY HYPERALDOSTERONISM

The preferred treatment for PA is surgical removal of the adrenal gland that has the adenoma (adrenalectomy). Although this surgery can be performed as an open procedure, laparoscopic adrenalectomy is increasingly performed because of the benefits offered by this minimally invasive surgery (Phitayakorn & McHenry, 2008). Before surgery, patients should be treated with a low-sodium diet, potassium-sparing diuretics (spironolactone [Aldactone] or eplerenone [Inspra]), and antihypertensive agents to normalize serum potassium levels and BP. Spironolactone and eplerenone block the binding of aldosterone to the mineralocorticoid receptor in the terminal distal tubules and collecting ducts of the kidneys, thus increasing the excretion of sodium and water and the retention of potassium. Oral potassium supplements and sodium restrictions may also be necessary. Potassium supplementation and a potassium-sparing diuretic should not be started simultaneously because of the danger of hyperkalemia. Patients taking eplerenone should be instructed to avoid grapefruit juice.

Patients with bilateral adrenal hyperplasia are treated with a potassium-sparing diuretic. Calcium channel blockers may also be used to control BP. Dexamethasone may be used to decrease the hyperplasia.

Nursing care includes careful assessment for signs of fluid and electrolyte imbalance (especially potassium imbalance) and cardiovascular status. BP should be monitored frequently before and after surgery because unilateral adrenalectomy is successful in controlling hypertension in only 80% of patients with adenoma. Patients receiving maintenance therapy with spironolactone need instruction about the possible adverse effects (gynecomastia, erectile dysfunction, and menstrual disorders), as well as knowledge about the signs and symptoms of hypokalemia and hyperkalemia. Patients should be taught how to monitor their own BP and the need for frequent monitoring. The need for continued health supervision should be stressed.

Disorders of the Adrenal Medulla

Pheochromocytoma

Etiology and Pathophysiology

Pheochromocytoma is a rare condition characterized by a tumour of the adrenal medulla that produces excessive amounts of catecholamines (epinephrine, norepinephrine). The secretion of excessive catecholamines results in severe hypertension. If undiagnosed and untreated, pheochromocytoma may lead to diabetes mellitus, cardiomyopathy, and death. It occurs most commonly in young to middle-aged adults. In most cases affecting adults, the tumour is benign, encapsulated, unilateral, and solitary. On occasionally, tumours are bilateral.

Clinical Manifestations

The most striking clinical features of pheochromocytoma include severe, episodic hypertension accompanied by the classic manifestations of severe, pounding headache, tachycardia with palpitations, profuse sweating, and unexplained abdominal or chest pain. Such "attacks" may be provoked by many medications, including antihypertensives, opioids, radiological contrast media, and tricyclic antidepressants. The duration of the episodes varies from a few minutes to several hours.

Diagnostic Studies

Although pheochromocytoma is associated with a number of symptoms, the correct diagnosis is often missed. Pheochromocytoma is an uncommon cause of hypertension, accounting for only 0.1% of all cases. This condition should be considered in patients who do not respond to traditional hypertensive treatments.

The diagnosis is confirmed by demonstrating elevated blood and urine levels of catecholamines and their metabolites (Cook, 2009; Pagana & Pagana, 2011). Measurement of serum catecholamines is preferable during an attack. CT and MRI are used for tumour localization.

NURSING AND COLLABORATIVE MANAGEMENT: PHEOCHROMOCYTOMA

The primary treatment consists of surgical removal of the tumour. Preoperatively, calcium channel blockers are used to control BP and other excess catecholamine symptoms. Sympathetic blocking agents such as prazosin (Minipress) may be administered to reduce BP and alleviate other symptoms of catecholamine excess along with the calcium channel blockers. Sympathetic blocking agents may result in orthostatic hypotension. Patients must be advised to make postural changes cautiously. β-Adrenergic blockers (e.g., propranolol [Inderal]) are also used to decrease tachycardia and other dysrhythmias.

Surgery is more commonly performed via laparoscopic adrenalectomy than via open abdominal incision. Complete removal of the adrenal tumour cures the hypertension in the majority of affected individuals, but hypertension persists in approximately 10 to 30% of patients. For these individuals, BP management involves standard antihypertensive drug therapy. If surgery is not an option, medication is used to diminish catecholamine production by the tumour and simplify chronic management.

Case finding is an important nursing function. Any patient with hypertension accompanied by symptoms of sympathoadrenal discharge should be referred to a health care provider for definitive diagnosis. An important part of the nursing assessment is observation of patients for the classic triad of symptoms of pheochromocytoma (severe pounding headache, tachycardia, and profuse sweating). BP should be monitored immediately if a patient is experiencing an attack. The nurse should be prepared to check BP when any of the drugs that might precipitate an attack are administered.

The nurse should attempt to make patients with pheochromocytoma as comfortable as possible. All diagnostic samples should be collected appropriately. Capillary blood glucose levels should be monitored to assess for diabetes mellitus. Patients need rest, nourishing food, and emotional support during this period.

Preoperative and postoperative care is similar to that for any patient undergoing adrenalectomy except that BP fluctuations from catecholamine excesses tend to be severe and must be carefully monitored. Because hypertension may persist even when the tumour is removed, the nurse should stress the importance of follow-up care and routine BP monitoring. If a patient is taking catecholamine synthesis inhibitors, he or she should be instructed to rise slowly while holding on to a secure object because this medication can cause orthostatic hypotension.

CLINICAL DECISION-MAKING EXERCISE

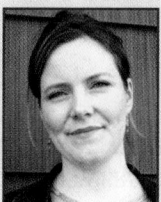

CASE STUDY:
Graves' Disease

Source: © iStockphoto.com/Lancia Klein.

Patient Profile

Elizabeth Minton, a 43-year-old woman, was admitted to the hospital with a high fever. After an endocrine workup, she received a diagnosis of Graves' disease.

Subjective Data

- Reports recent job loss because of inability to cope with job stress
- Reports symptoms including fatigue, unintentional weight loss, insomnia, palpitations, and heat intolerance

Objective Data

Physical Examination

- Has a fever of 40°C
- Has BP of 150/78, pulse of 118, and respiratory rate of 24
- Has hot, moist skin
- Has fine tremors of the hands
- Has grade 4+ deep tendon reflexes and muscle strength of grades 1 to 2

Collaborative Care

- Subtotal thyroidectomy planned for 2 months later
- Therapy with propylthiouracil and propranolol (Inderal) started

Discussion Questions

1. What is the cause of Ms. Minton's symptoms?
2. What diagnostic studies were probably ordered? What results have established the diagnosis of Graves' disease?

3. Why was surgery delayed?
4. What was the purpose of the drug therapy?
5. *Priority Decision:* What are Ms. Minton's priority learning needs? What teaching strategies would the nurse use if Ms. Minton could not read?
6. What are the nursing interventions for successful long-term management of Ms. Minton after the subtotal thyroidectomy? How would nursing interventions differ if she were 70 years old?

7. *Priority Decision:* On the basis of the assessment data presented, what are the priority nursing diagnoses pertinent to Ms. Minton while she is hospitalized? Are there any collaborative problems?

ℯvolve *Answers are available at* **http://evolve.elsevier.com/ Canada/Lewis/medsurg**

REVIEW QUESTIONS

The number of the question corresponds to the same-numbered objective at the beginning of the chapter.

1. What would the nurse include in teaching a patient who develops hypopituitarism after a hypophysectomy for treatment of acromegaly?
   a. Hormone replacement with ACTH, TSH, FSH, and luteinizing hormone is necessary.
   b. Permanent ADH replacement therapy is needed if the diabetes insipidus does not reverse.
   c. Frequent monitoring of blood and urine glucose is needed to identify the development of diabetes mellitus.
   d. The elimination of the source of excess growth hormone reverses the physiological effects of acromegaly.

2. What symptom would the nurse expect to find in a patient who develops SIADH after a head injury?
   a. Edema
   b. Weight gain
   c. Urine specific gravity of 1.004
   d. Serum sodium of 140 mmol/L

3. The health care provider prescribes levothyroxine (Synthroid) for a patient with myxedema. In accordance with teaching regarding this therapy, which of the following indicates that further instruction by the nurse is needed?
   a. The patient expects to return to normal function with the use of the drug.
   b. The patient expects the medication dose to be increased every several weeks.
   c. The patient expects to only need to take this medication until the symptoms improve.
   d. The patient will report any chest pain or difficulty breathing to the doctor right away.

4. After a patient undergoes thyroid surgery, the nurse suspects damage or removal of the parathyroid glands when the patient develops which of the following?
   a. Laryngeal stridor
   b. Muscle weakness
   c. Hoarseness and difficulty swallowing
   d. Hyperthermia and severe tachycardia

5. What is an important nursing intervention in caring for a patient with Cushing's syndrome?
   a. Restrict protein intake.
   b. Observe for signs of hypotension.
   c. Administer medication in equal doses.
   d. Protect the patient from exposure to infection.

6. After an adrenalectomy for pheochromocytoma, which of the following is the patient most likely to experience?
   a. Hypokalemia
   b. Hyperglycemia
   c. Marked sodium and water retention
   d. Marked fluctuations in blood pressure

7. Which of the following does the nurse teach the patient to control the adverse effects of pharmacological corticosteroid therapy?
   a. Increase calcium intake to 1500 mg per day.
   b. Perform glucose monitoring for hypoglycemia.
   c. Carry an emergency kit of hydrocortisone in case of severe stress.
   d. Avoid abrupt position changes because of orthostatic hypotension.

8. What does the nurse teach the patient about the best time to take corticosteroids for replacement purposes?
   a. Once a day at bedtime
   b. Every other day on awakening
   c. On arising and in the late afternoon
   d. At consistent intervals every 6 to 8 hours

ANSWERS: 1. b; 2. b; 3. c; 4. b; 5. d; 6. d; 7. a; 8. c.

REFERENCES

Bringhurst, F., Demay, M., & Kronenberg, H. (2011) Hormones and disorders of mineral metabolism. In S. Melmed, K. S. Polonsky, P. R. Larsen, & H. M. Kronenberg (Eds.), *Williams textbook of endocrinology* (12th ed., pp.1237-1304). Philadelphia: W. B. Saunders.

Buchfelder, M., & Schlaffer, S. (2009). Surgical treatment of pituitary tumours. *Best Practice & Research Clinical Endocrinology & Metabolism, 23*(5), 677-692. doi:10.1016/j.beem.2009.05.002

Canadian Cancer Society's Steering Committee on Cancer Statistics. (2012). *Canadian Cancer Statistics 2012*. Toronto, ON: Canadian

Cancer Society. Retrieved from *http://www.cancer.ca/Canada-wide/ About%20cancer/~/media/CCS/Canada%20wide/Files%20List/ English%20files%20heading/PDF%20-%20Policy%20-%20 Canadian%20Cancer%20Statistics%20-%20English/Canadian%20 Cancer%20Statistics%202012%20-%20English.ashx*

Cook, L. K. (2009). Pheochromocytoma. *The American Journal of Nursing, 109*(2), 50-3. doi:10.1097/01.NAJ.0000345437.83475.48

Coorough, N., Hudak, K., Buehler, D., Selvaggi, S., Sippel, R., & Chen, H. (2011). Fine needle aspiration of the thyroid: A contemporary experience of 3981 cases. *Journal of Surgical Research, 170*(1), 48-51. doi:10.1016/j.jss.2011.02.048

Dittrich, R., Beckmann, M. W., Oppelt, P. G., Hoffmann, I., Lotz, L., Kuwert, T., & Mueller, A. (2011). Thyroid hormone receptors and reproduction. *Journal of Reproductive Immunology, 90*(1), 58-66. doi:10.1016/j.jri.2011.02.009

Dursunoglu, N., Ozkurt, S., & SarÄłkaya, S. (2009). Is the clinical presentation different between men and women admitting to the sleep laboratory? *Sleep and Breathing, 13,* 295-298. doi:10.1007/s11325-008-0243-1

Elaraj, D. M., & Sturgeon, C. (2009). Adequate surgery for papillary thyroid cancer. *The Surgeon, 7*(5), 286-289. doi:10.1016/S1479-666X(09)80006-1

Fitzgibbons, S. C., Brams, D. M., & Wei, J. P. (2008). Invited commentary: The treatment of thyroid cancer. *American Surgeon, 74*(5), 389-399.

Furukawa, F., Kaminaka, C., Ikeda, T., Kanazawa, N., Yamamoto, Y., Ohta, C., ..., Hata, M. (2011). Preliminary study of etidronate for prevention of corticosteroid-induced osteoporosis caused by oral glucocorticoid therapy. *Clinical and Experimental Dermatology, 36*(2), 165-168. doi:10.1111/j.1365-2230.2010.03856.x

Gardner, D. G. (2011). Endocrine emergencies. In D. Gardner & D. Shoback (Eds.), *Greenspan's basic and clinical endocrinology* (9th ed., pp. 763-787). New York: McGraw Hill.

Health Canada. (2011). Drug product database. Retrieved from *http://www.hc-sc.gc.ca/dhp-mps/prodpharma/databasdon/index-eng.php*

Hubbard, J. G. H. (2011). Thyrotoxicosis and thyroiditis. *Surgery (Oxford), 29*(9), 440-445. doi:10.1016/j.mpsur.2011.06.003

Husebye, E., Løvås, K. (2009). Pathogenesis of primary adrenal insufficiency. *Best Practice & Research Clinical Endocrinology & Metabolism, 23*(2), 147-157. doi:10.1016/j.beem.2008.09.004

Jett, K. F. (2008). Chronic diseases in late life. In P. Ebersole, T. A. Touhy, P. Hess, K. Jett, & A. Schmidt Luggen (Eds.), *Toward healthy aging: human needs and nursing responses* (7th ed.). Philadelphia: Mosby.

Liubinas, S. V., Porto, L. D., & Kaye, A. H. (2011). Management of recurrent Cushing's disease. *Journal of Clinical Neuroscience, 18*(1), 7-12. doi:10.1016/j.jocn.2010.05.001

Melmed, S. (2011). *The pituitary* (3rd ed.). St. Louis: Academic Press.

Miller, R. E., Learned-Miller, E. G., Trainer, P., Paisley, A., & Blanz, V. (2011). Early diagnosis of acromegaly: Computers vs clinicians. *Clinical Endocrinology, 75,* 226-231. doi:10.1111/j.1365-2265.2011.04020.x

National Institute of Diabetes and Digestive and Kidney Diseases. (2009). Adrenal insufficiency and Addison's disease. Retrieved from *http://endocrine.niddk.nih.gov/pubs/addison/addison.aspx#emergency*

Pagana, K. D., & Pagana, T. J. (2011). *Mosby's diagnostic and laboratory test reference* (10th ed.). St. Louis: Mosby.

Pallan, S., & Khan, A. (2011). Primary hyperparathyroidism: Update on presentation, diagnosis, and management in primary care. *Canadian Family Physician, 57*(2), 184-189. Retrieved from *http://www.cfp.ca/content/57/2/184.full*

Pata, G., Casella, C., Magri, G. C., Lucchini, S., Panarotto, M. B., Crea, N., ..., Salerni, B. (2011). Financial and clinical implications of low-energy CT combined with 99m technetium–sestamibi SPECT for primary hyperparathyroidism. *Annals of Surgical Oncology, 18*(9), 2555-2563. doi:10.1245/s10434-011-1641-3

Phitayakorn, R., & McHenry, C. R. (2008). Laparoscopic and selective open resection for adrenal and extraadrenal neuroendocrine tumors. *American Surgeon, 74*(1), 37-42.

Pyram, R., Mahajan, G., & Gliwa, A. (2011). Primary hyperparathyroidism: Skeletal and non-skeletal effects, diagnosis and management. *Maturitas, 70*(3), 246-255. doi:10.1016/j.maturitas.2011.07.021

Reddy, P. (2011). Clinical approach to adrenal insufficiency in hospitalised patients. *International Journal of Clinical Practice, 65,* 1059-1066. doi:10.1111/j.1742-1241.2011.02718.x

Robinson, A. G., & Verbalis, J. G. (2011). Posterior pituitary. In S. Melmed, K. S. Polonsky, P. R. Larsen, & H. M. Kronenberg (Eds.), *Williams textbook of endocrinology* (12th ed., pp. 291-327). Philadelphia: W. B. Saunders.

Sherlock, M., Woods, C., & Sheppard, M.C. (2011). Medical therapy in acromegaly. *Nature Reviews Endocrinology, 7*(5), 291-300. doi:10.1038/nrendo.2011.42

Simmons, S. (2010). A delicate balance: Detecting thyroid disease. *Nursing, 40*(7), 22-29. doi:10.1097/01.NURSE.0000383445.23626.82

Soiza, R., & Talbot, H. (2011). Management of hyponatraemia in older people: Old threats and new opportunities. *Therapeutic Advances in Drug Safety, 2*(1), 9-17. doi:10.1177/2042098610394233

Stewart, P. M. & Krone, N. P. (2011). The adrenal cortex. In S. Melmed, K. S. Polonsky, P. R. Larsen, & H. M. Kronenberg (Eds.), *Williams textbook of endocrinology* (12th ed., pp. 479-544). Philadelphia: W. B. Saunders.

Thyroid Foundation of Canada. (2011). Health guides on thyroid disease. Retrieved from *http://www.thyroid.ca/educational_material.php*

Verrua, E., Filopanti, M., Ronchi, C. L., Olgiati, L., Ferrante, E., Giavoli, C., ..., Spada, A. (2010). GH response to oral glucose tolerance test: A comparison between patients with acromegaly and other pituitary disorders. *Journal of Clinical Endocrinology, 96*(1), E83-E88. doi:10.1210/jc.2010-1115

Yang, M. S., Hong, J. W., Lee, S. K., Lee, E. J., & Kim, S. H. (2011). Clinical management and outcome of 36 invasive prolactinomas treated with dopamine agonist. *Journal of Neuro-Oncology, 104*(1), 195-204. doi:10.1007/s11060-010-0459-3

Yokoyama, T., Toda, R., Kimura, Y., Mikagi, M., & Aizawa, H. (2009). Addison's disease induced by miliary tuberculosis and the administration of rifampicin. *Internal Medicine, 48*(15), 1297-1300. doi:10.2169/internalmedicine.48.1974

Zelaya, A. S., Stotts, A., Nader, S., & Moreno, C. A. (2010). Antithyroid peroxidase antibodies in patients with high normal range thyroid stimulating hormone. *Family Medicine, 42*(2), 111-115. Retrieved from *http://www.stfm.org/fmhub/toc.cfm?xmlFileName=fm2010/fammedvol42issue2.xml*

CANADIAN RESOURCES

Canadian Addison Society
http://www.addisonsociety.ca
The Canadian Society of Endocrinology and Metabolism
http://www.endo-metab.ca/
Thyroid Foundation of Canada
http://www.thyroid.ca

RELATED RESOURCES

American Association of Clinical Endocrinologists (AACE)
https://www.aace.com
American Society for Bone and Mineral Research
http://www.asbmr.org
Endocrine Nurses Society (ENS)
http://www.endo-nurses.org
Endocrine Society
http://www.endo-society.org
EndocrineWeb.com
http://www.endocrineweb.com/
National Endocrine and Metabolic Diseases Information Service
http://endocrine.niddk.nih.gov
Pituitary Network Association
https://www.pituitary.org
Society for Endocrinology
http://www.endocrinology.org/

evolve *For additional Internet resources, see the Web site for this book at* **http://evolve.elsevier.com/Canada/Lewis/medsurg**

52

Nursing Management: Diabetes Mellitus

Written by Brenda Michel

Adapted by Tess Montada-Atin

LEARNING OBJECTIVES

1. Describe the pathophysiology and clinical manifestations of diabetes mellitus.
2. Describe the differences between type 1 and type 2 diabetes mellitus.
3. Describe the collaborative care of the patient with diabetes mellitus.
4. Describe the role of nutrition and exercise in the management of diabetes mellitus.
5. Describe the nursing management of a patient with newly diagnosed diabetes mellitus.
6. Describe the nursing management of the patient with diabetes mellitus in the ambulatory and home care settings.
7. Identify the pathophysiology and clinical manifestations of acute and chronic complications of diabetes mellitus.
8. Explain the collaborative care and nursing management of the patient with acute and chronic complications of diabetes mellitus.

KEY TERMS

diabetes mellitus (DM) A multisystem disease related to abnormal insulin secretion, impaired insulin action, or both, p. 1429

diabetic ketoacidosis (DKA) An acute metabolic complication of diabetes occurring when fats are metabolized in the absence of insulin; characterized by hyperglycemia, ketosis, acidosis, and dehydration, p. 1455

diabetic nephropathy A microvascular complication of diabetes mellitus associated with damage to the small blood vessels that supply the glomeruli of the kidney, p. 1463

diabetic neuropathy Nerve damage that occurs because of the metabolic derangements associated with diabetes mellitus, p. 1463

glycemic index (GI) Term used to describe the rise in blood glucose levels after a person has consumed carbohydrate-containing food, p. 1444

hyperosmolar hyperglycemic state (HHS) A life-threatening syndrome that can occur in the patient with diabetes who is able to produce enough insulin to prevent diabetic

ketoacidosis but not enough to prevent severe hyperglycemia, osmotic diuresis, and extracellular fluid depletion, p. 1458

insulin resistance A condition in which body tissues do not respond to the action of insulin, p. 1433

lipodystrophy Hypertrophy or atrophy of subcutaneous tissue, p. 1441

prediabetes Also known as impaired glucose tolerance (IGT) or impaired fasting glucose (IFG); is noted when fasting or a 2-hour plasma glucose level is higher than normal but lower than that considered diagnostic for diabetes; places the individual at risk for developing diabetes and its complications, p. 1431

Somogyi effect Produces a decline in blood glucose level in response to too much insulin; counter-regulatory hormones are released that cause rebound hyperglycemia and ketosis resulting in high blood glucose levels at morning testing; treatment is reduction of insulin dosage, p. 1441

ELECTRONIC RESOURCES

Supplemental content related to Chapter 52 can be found...

Evolve Web Site ⓔvolve

http://evolve.elsevier.com/Canada/Lewis/medsurg
- Answer Guidelines for Case Study on p. 1466
- Patient & Caregiver Teaching Guides:
  - Exercise Guidelines for Patients With Diabetes Mellitus
  - Foot Care for Patients With Diabetes or Peripheral Vascular Problems
  - Insulin Administration
  - Management of Diabetes Mellitus
  - Self-Monitoring of Blood Glucose (SMBG)

- Clinical Reference: Laboratory Values
- Concept Map for Case Study on p. 1466
- Content Updates
- Customizable Nursing Care Plan: Diabetes Mellitus
- Electronic Calculators
- Examination Review Questions
- Glossary
- Interactive Case Studies:
  - Diabetic Ketoacidosis
  - Type 2 Diabetes Mellitus
- Key Points (Printable and MP3 Download)

Diabetes Mellitus

Diabetes mellitus (DM) is a multisystem disease related to abnormal insulin production, impaired insulin utilization, or both. DM is a serious health problem throughout the world. According to the World Health Organization (WHO), 346 million people have DM (WHO, 2011). By 2030, this figure is expected to top 366 million. Canadian data indicate that the prevalence of diagnosed DM in adults is 6.2% (~2 million people) (Health Canada, 2009).

Approximately 80% of people with DM will die as a result of heart disease or stroke (Cheng, 2009, p. 1). DM is a contributing factor in the deaths of approximately 41,500 Canadians each year. Canadian adults with DM are twice as likely to die prematurely as people without DM. For example, a Canadian with DM is four times more likely to die at age 35 than a 35-year-old without DM. Life expectancy for people with type 2 DM may be shortened by 5 to 10 years (Canadian Diabetes Association [CDA], 2009, p.1). The financial burden of DM and its complications on people with the disease and on the Canadian health care system is enormous. A person with DM incurs medical costs that are two to three times higher than those of a person without DM. A person with DM can face direct costs for medication and supplies ranging from $1000 to $15,000 a year. DM and its complications cost the Canadian health care system an estimated $11.7 billion in 2010 and will rise to $16 billion by 2020 (CDA and Diabetes Quebec [DQ], 2011, p. 20).

Approximately 10% of people with DM have type 1 DM. However, the number of people with type 2 DM is increasing dramatically owing to a number of factors. In the Western world, people are living longer, obesity rates are rising, and lifestyles are becoming increasingly sedentary. There is increased immigration from high-risk populations, with 77% of Canadians coming from populations that are at higher risk for type 2 DM. These populations include people of Hispanic, Asian, South Asian, and African descent (CDA and DQ, 2011, p. 17) (see Determinants of Health box). Risk levels for these groups are between two and six times higher than for White Canadians.

There are three recognized groups of Aboriginal people in Canada: First Nations, Inuit, and Métis. These populations are three to five times more likely than the general population to

DETERMINANTS OF HEALTH
Diabetes

Income and Social Status
- Low income appears to be associated with a higher prevalence of diabetes and diabetes-related complications.*
- Diabetes may be up to two times more prevalent in low-income populations than in wealthy populations.†

Biology and Genetics
- Aboriginal people are three to five times more likely to have type 2 diabetes than the general Canadian population.‡
- Almost 80% of new Canadians come from populations that are at higher risk for type 2 diabetes (e.g., people of Hispanic, Asian, South Asian, or African descent).‡

Personal Health Practices and Coping Skills
- Progression to type 2 diabetes can be prevented or delayed through lifestyle modifications such as weight loss and control, eating a healthy diet, and exercising.‡

Sex
- Type 2 diabetes increases the risk of coronary heart disease (CHD) more markedly in women than in men.

*Rabi, D., Edwards, L., Southern, D., et al. (2006). Association of socio-economic status with diabetes prevalence and utilization of diabetes care services. *BMC Health Services Research, 6*, 124.
†Dasgupta, K., Khan, S., & Ross, N. (2010). Type 2 diabetes in Canada: Concentration of risk among most disadvantaged men but inverse social gradient across groups in women. *Diabetic Medicine, 27*(5), 522-531.
‡Canadian Diabetes Association (CDA). (2009). *The prevalence and costs of diabetes facts.* Retrieved from *http://www.diabetes.ca/documents/about-diabetes/PrevalanceandCost_09.pdf*
Source: Boucher, J., & Hurrell, D. (2008). Cardiovascular disease and diabetes. *Diabetes Spectrum, 21*, 154. doi:10.2337/diaspect.21.3.154

develop type 2 DM (CDA, 2008, p. 187). An estimated 25% of individuals in First Nations communities on reserves who are over age 45 have DM. According to the CDA Clinical Practice Guidelines Expert Committee (CDA, 2008), the prevalence of type 2 DM in Canadian Aboriginal children 5 to 18 years of age

Table 52-1 Characteristics of Type 1 and Type 2 Diabetes Mellitus

FACTOR	TYPE 1 DIABETES MELLITUS	TYPE 2 DIABETES MELLITUS	FACTOR	TYPE 1 DIABETES MELLITUS	TYPE 2 DIABETES MELLITUS
Age at onset	More common in young people but can occur at any age	Usually ≥35 yr but can occur at any age Incidence is increasing in children	Endogenous insulin	Minimal or absent	Possibly excessive; adequate but delayed secretion or reduced utilization; secretions diminish over time
Type of onset	Signs and symptoms abrupt, but disease process may be present for several years	Insidious, may go undiagnosed for years	Nutritional status	Thin, normal or obese	Obese or normal
			Symptoms	Thirst, polyuria, polyphagia, fatigue, weight loss	Frequently none, fatigue, recurrent infections
Prevalence	Accounts for 5-10% of all types of diabetes	Accounts for 90% of all types of diabetes	Ketosis	Prone at onset or during insulin deficiency	Resistant except during infection or stress
Environmental factors	Virus, toxins	Obesity, lack of exercise	Nutritional therapy	Essential	Essential
Primary defect	Absent or minimal insulin production	Insulin resistance, decreased insulin production over time, and alterations in production of adipokines	Insulin	Required for all	Required for some
			Oral antihyperglycemic agents	Not indicated	Usually beneficial
Islet-cell antibodies	Often present at onset	Absent	Vascular and neurological complications	Frequent	Frequent

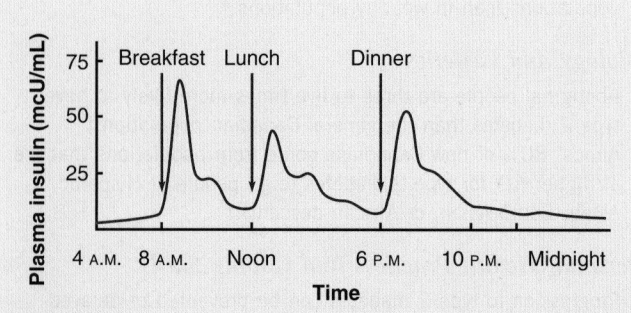

Figure 52-1 Normal endogenous insulin secretion. In the first hour or 2 after meals, insulin concentrations rise rapidly in blood and peak at about 1 hour. After meals, insulin concentrations promptly decline toward preprandial values as carbohydrate absorption from the gastrointestinal tract declines. After carbohydrate absorption from the gastrointestinal tract is complete and during the night, insulin concentrations are low and fairly constant, with a slight increase at dawn.

is noted to be as high as 1%, with the highest in the Plains Cree people of central Canada. Screening every 2 years should also be considered from age 10 or established puberty in Aboriginal children with more than one additional risk factor (CDA, 2008, p. 187).

DM is a serious problem for the Métis, more frequently affecting women, the older adult, the obese, and the less educated. The disease has a negative impact on quality of life and is associated with significant co-morbidities in this population (Shah, Cauch-

Dudek, & Pigeau, 2011, p. 2555; Martens et al., 2011, p. 814). It has been documented that Aboriginal communities in Canada experience prevalence rates of DM that are among the highest in the world (CDA and DQ, 2011, p. 16). Comparing First Nations with non–First Nations in Manitoba, it was found that rates of DM and amputation were higher (Martens et al., 2011, p. 814).

Etiology and Pathophysiology

Current theories link the causes of DM, singly or in combination, to genetic, autoimmune, viral, and environmental factors (e.g., obesity, sedentary lifestyle, stress). Regardless of its cause, DM is primarily a disorder of glucose metabolism related to absent or insufficient insulin supply or poor utilization of the insulin that is available.

Although the CDA *2008 Clinical Practice Guidelines* recognize 11 different classifications of the disease, most of these types are rarely encountered in routine nursing practice (CDA, 2008, p. S194). The two most common types of DM are classified as type 1 and type 2 DM (Table 52-1). Gestational diabetes mellitus (GDM), prediabetes, and secondary DM (discussed later in this chapter) are other classifications of DM commonly seen in clinical practice.

Normal Insulin Metabolism. Insulin is a hormone produced by the β cells in the islets of Langerhans of the pancreas. Under normal conditions, insulin is continuously released into the bloodstream in small pulsatile increments (a basal rate), with increased release (bolus) when food is ingested (Figure 52-1). The activity of released insulin lowers blood glucose and facilitates a stable, normal glucose range of approximately 4 to 6 mmol/L. The average amount of insulin secreted daily by an adult is approximately 40 to 50 units, or 0.6 units/kg of body weight.

Other hormones (glucagon, epinephrine, growth hormone, and cortisol) work to oppose the effects of insulin and are often referred to as *counter-regulatory hormones*. These hormones work to increase blood glucose levels by stimulating glucose production and output by the liver and by decreasing the movement of glucose into the cells. Insulin and these counter-regulatory hormones provide a sustained but regulated release of glucose for energy during food intake and periods of fasting and usually maintain blood glucose levels within the normal range. An abnormal production of any or all of these hormones may be present in DM.

Insulin is released from the pancreatic β cells as its precursor, proinsulin, and is then routed through the liver. Proinsulin is composed of two polypeptide chains, chain A and chain B, which are linked by the C-peptide chain. Insulin is formed when enzymes cleave C off, leaving the A and B chains. The presence of C peptide in serum is a useful indicator of β-cell function.

Insulin facilitates glucose transport from the bloodstream across the cell membrane to the cytoplasm of the cell. The rise in plasma insulin after a meal stimulates storage of glucose as glycogen in liver and muscle, inhibits gluconeogenesis, enhances fat deposition in adipose tissue, and increases protein synthesis. The fall in insulin level during normal overnight fasting facilitates the release of stored glucose from the liver, protein from muscle, and fat from adipose tissue. For this reason, insulin is known as the *anabolic* or storage hormone.

Skeletal muscle and adipose tissue have specific receptors for insulin and are considered insulin-dependent tissues. Other tissues (e.g., brain, liver, blood cells) do not directly depend on insulin for glucose transport but require an adequate glucose supply for normal function. Although liver cells are not considered insulin-dependent tissue, insulin receptor sites on the liver facilitate the hepatic uptake of glucose and its conversion to glycogen.

Type 1 Diabetes Mellitus.
Formerly known as "juvenile-onset" or "insulin-dependent" DM, *type 1 DM* most often occurs in people who are younger than 30 years, with a peak onset between ages 11 and 13. The rate of type 1 DM in children is highest in Europe (United Kingdom, Russian Federation, and Germany) (International Diabetes Federation [IDF], 2011). Most cases of type 1 DM are sporadic; only 10 to 15% of affected individuals have a first-degree relative with type 1 DM at the time of diagnosis. Typically, it is seen in people with a lean body type, although it can occur in people who are overweight. This form includes *latent autoimmune diabetes mellitus in adults* (LADA), the term is used to describe the small number of people with apparent type 2 DM who appear to have immune-mediated loss of pancreatic β cells (CDA, 2008, p. S10).

Etiology and Pathophysiology. Type 1 DM results from progressive destruction of pancreatic β cells owing to an autoimmune process in susceptible individuals. Autoantibodies to the islet cells cause a reduction of 80 to 90% of normal β-cell function before hyperglycemia and other manifestations occur (Figure 52-2). A genetic predisposition and exposure to a virus are factors that may contribute to the pathogenesis of type 1 DM. Occasionally, type 1 DM may be caused by nonimmune factors of unknown (idiopathic) etiologies. This type of DM is known as *type 1B DM*. When type 1 DM is caused by an immune mechanism, the disease is known as *type 1A*.

Predisposition to type 1 DM is believed to be related to human leukocyte antigens (HLAs). (See Chapter 14 for a discussion of HLAs and disease associations.) Theoretically, when an individual with certain HLA types is exposed to viral infections, the β cells of the pancreas are destroyed, either directly or through an autoimmune process. The HLA types associated with an increased risk for type 1 DM include HLA-DR3 and HLA-DR4 (see Genetics in Clinical Practice box on p. 1433).

Onset of Disease. Type 1 DM is associated with a long preclinical period. The islet-cell autoantibodies responsible for β-cell destruction are present for months to years before the onset of symptoms. Manifestations of type 1 DM develop when the person's pancreas can no longer produce insulin. Once this occurs, the onset of symptoms is usually rapid, and the patient comes to the emergency department with impending or actual ketoacidosis. The patient usually has a history of recent and sudden weight loss as well as the classic symptoms of *polydipsia* (excessive thirst), *polyuria* (frequent urination), and *polyphagia* (excessive hunger).

The individual with type 1 DM requires a supply of insulin from an outside source *(exogenous insulin)*, such as an injection, in order to sustain life. Without insulin, the patient will develop **diabetic ketoacidosis (DKA)**, a life-threatening condition resulting in metabolic acidosis that, if untreated, could be fatal. Newly diagnosed patients with type 1 DM may experience a remission, or "honeymoon period," soon after treatment is initiated. During this time, the patient requires very little injected insulin because β-cell mass remains sufficient for glucose control as the progressive destruction continues to occur. Eventually, as more β cells are destroyed, blood glucose levels increase, more insulin is needed, and the honeymoon period ends. It is critical for the patient to monitor blood glucose very closely during this period. The honeymoon period usually lasts 3 to 12 months, after which the person will require insulin on a permanent basis.

Prediabetes.
Prediabetes, also known as *impaired glucose tolerance* (IGT) or *impaired fasting glucose* (IFG), is noted when a fasting or a 2-hour plasma glucose level is higher than normal (6.1-6.9 mmol/L for IFG and 7.1-11 mmol/L for IGT) but lower than that considered diagnostic for DM. Up to 6 million Canadians have prediabetes, putting them at risk for developing DM and its complications, particularly cardiovascular disease. About 50% of Canadians with prediabetes develop type 2 DM in their lifetime (CDA and DC, 2011, p. 8).

Long-term damage to the body, especially the heart and blood vessels, may already be occurring in patients with prediabetes. People with prediabetes usually do not have symptoms. Individuals with prediabetes should test their blood glucose regularly and watch for the symptoms of DM, such as polyuria, polyphagia, or polydipsia. If action is taken to manage blood glucose, patients with prediabetes can delay or prevent the development of type 2 DM. Maintaining a healthy weight, exercising regularly, eating a healthy diet, and using medication when required are measures found to reduce the risk of developing DM in people with prediabetes by up to 58% (CDA, 2008, p. S17; Gillies et al., 2007, p. 1).

Type 2 Diabetes Mellitus.
Type 2 DM is, by far, the most prevalent type of DM, accounting for over 90% of patients with DM. Type 2 DM usually occurs in people older than 35 years, and 80 to 90% of patients are overweight at the time of diagnosis.

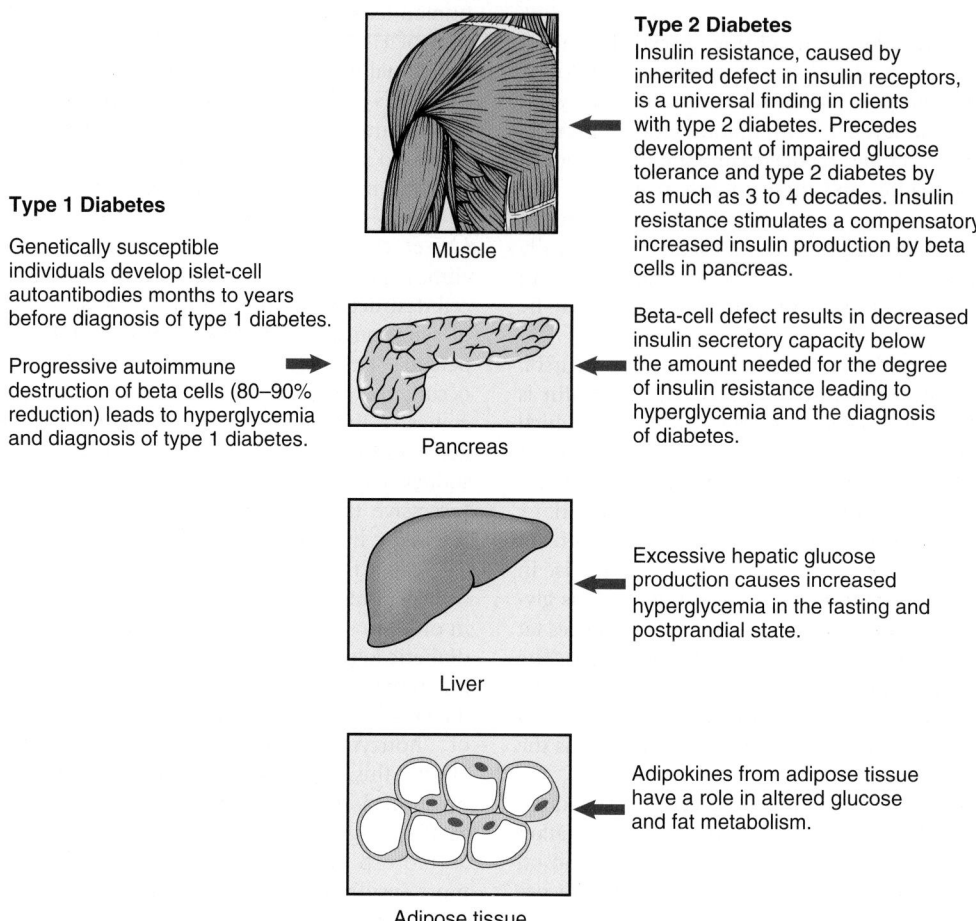

Type 1 Diabetes

Genetically susceptible individuals develop islet-cell autoantibodies months to years before diagnosis of type 1 diabetes.

Progressive autoimmune destruction of beta cells (80–90% reduction) leads to hyperglycemia and diagnosis of type 1 diabetes.

Muscle

Pancreas

Liver

Adipose tissue

Type 2 Diabetes

Insulin resistance, caused by inherited defect in insulin receptors, is a universal finding in clients with type 2 diabetes. Precedes development of impaired glucose tolerance and type 2 diabetes by as much as 3 to 4 decades. Insulin resistance stimulates a compensatory increased insulin production by beta cells in pancreas.

Beta-cell defect results in decreased insulin secretory capacity below the amount needed for the degree of insulin resistance leading to hyperglycemia and the diagnosis of diabetes.

Excessive hepatic glucose production causes increased hyperglycemia in the fasting and postprandial state.

Adipokines from adipose tissue have a role in altered glucose and fat metabolism.

Figure 52-2 Altered mechanisms in type 1 and type 2 diabetes mellitus.

The most powerful risk factor is believed to be obesity, specifically abdominal and visceral adiposity. Visceral adipocytes release an excess amount of free fatty acids, which are associated with insulin resistance at the level of the liver, as well as several adipocytokines, which cause insulin resistance in the muscle (Gastaldelli, 2008, p. 1118). Obesity has a tendency to run in families and probably has a genetic basis (see Genetics in Clinical Practice box later).

Other risk factors for type 2 DM are membership in a high-risk population (e.g., people of Aboriginal, Hispanic, South Asian, Asian, or African descent), history of IGT or IFG, presence of complications associated with DM, vascular disease, history of GDM, and history of delivery of a macrosomic infant. Hypertension, dyslipidemia, being overweight, abdominal obesity, polycystic ovary syndrome (PCOS), and acanthosis nigricans are associated with insulin resistance and are also risk factors for type 2 DM. Insulin resistance with compensatory hyperinsulinemia is a common feature of PCOS, in both lean and obese women. The exact mechanisms for abnormalities of insulin action in PCOS are not fully understood (Nestler, 2008, p. 47). Acanthosis nigricans is a cutaneous sign of an underlying condition and is characterized by a velvety, light brown to black hyperpigmented thickening of the skin, usually on the back, the sides of the neck, the axillae, and flexural surfaces (Kong et al., 2010, p. 477). The pathways that lead to acanthosis nigricans are not well known. However, the association of acanthosis nigricans with disorders such as DM characterized by insulin resistance suggests that hyperinsulinemia plays a key role in the development of acanthosis nigricans (Torley, Bellus, & Munro, 2002, p. 1096). The incidence of type 2 DM is at least three times higher in people with schizophrenia than in the general population and is thought to be related to antipsychotic medications (Llorente, & Urrutia, 2006, p. 18; CDA, 2008, p. S14). These medications have contributed to the prevalence of obesity in patients with schizophrenia, which is a known risk factor for insulin resistance and type 2 DM.

Prevalence of type 2 DM increases with age, with about half of the people diagnosed being older than 55. In the past, type 2 DM was known as "adult-onset" DM. This term is no longer considered appropriate because the disease is now being seen in a rapidly growing number of children and adolescents, particularly in the Aboriginal population. In a large study, people at risk for type 2 DM were able to cut that risk by 58% by exercising moderately for 30 minutes a day and by losing 5 to 7% of their body weight. In people older than 60, the risk was cut by almost 71% (CDA, 2009, p. 2). Other large studies have shown similar results in reducing risk.

Etiology and Pathophysiology. In type 2 DM, the pancreas usually continues to produce some *endogenous* (self-made) insulin. However, the insulin that is produced is either insufficient for the needs of the body, is poorly utilized by the tissues, or both. In contrast, there is a virtual absence of endogenous insulin in type 1 DM. The presence of endogenous insulin is the major pathophysiological distinction between type 1 and type 2 DM.

Genetic mutations that lead to insulin resistance and a higher risk for obesity have been found in many people with type 2 DM. It is likely that multiple genes are involved in this complex, multifactorial disorder (see Genetics in Clinical Practice box).

GENETICS IN CLINICAL PRACTICE
Types 1 and 2 Diabetes Mellitus

	Type 1 Diabetes Mellitus	Type 2 Diabetes Mellitus
Genetic basis	Associations between specific human leukocyte antigens (HLA-DR3, HLA-DR4)	Majority of cases are polygenic.
	As many as 20 genes (and maybe more) influence susceptibility.	Genetic defects of β-cell function referred to as maturity-onset diabetes of the young (MODY) types 1-6.*
Incidence	Accounts for about 5-10% of cases in Canada.	Accounts for about 90% of cases in Canada.
Risk to offspring and twins	Risk to offspring of mothers with diabetes is only 1-4%.	Risk to offspring is 8-14%.
	Risk to offspring of diabetic fathers is 5-6%.	
	Identical twin concordance is 30-40%.	Identical twin concordance often exceeds 60-75%.
Clinical implications	Disease is a result of complex interaction of genetic, autoimmune, and environmental factors.	Disease is a result of complex genetic interactions, which are modified by environmental factors such as body weight and exercise.

*MODY is often considered a subtype of type 2 diabetes that accounts for 1-5% of people with diabetes and is a result of a defect in a single gene.

Four major metabolic abnormalities have a role in the development of type 2 DM. The first factor is **insulin resistance** in glucose and lipid metabolism, which is a condition in which body tissues do not respond to the action of insulin. This is owing to insulin receptors that are unresponsive to the action of insulin, insufficient in number, or both. Most insulin receptors are located on skeletal muscle, fat, and liver cells. Insulin mediates glucose uptake into fat tissue and skeletal muscle through GLUT4 glucose transporters. Insulin resistance in fat cells is associated with a

decrease in the number of GLUT4 transporters and its activity in those with type 2 DM (Shepherd & Kahn, 1999, p. 251; Ismail-Beigi, 2012, p. 1319). When insulin is not properly used, the entry of glucose into the cell is impeded, resulting in hyperglycemia. In the early stages of insulin resistance, the pancreas responds to high blood glucose by producing greater amounts of insulin (if β-cell function is normal). This creates a temporary state of hyperinsulinemia that coexists with the hyperglycemia.

A second factor in the development of type 2 DM is a marked decrease in the ability of the pancreas to produce insulin, as the β cells become fatigued from the compensatory overproduction of insulin or when β-cell mass is lost. The resulting IFG and IGT place the individual at risk for developing DM and its complications. This does not necessarily mean that all people with prediabetes will progress to DM. A significant proportion will revert to normal blood glucose levels (CDA, 2008, p. S11). The underlying basis for the failure of β cells to adapt is unknown. However, it may be linked to the adverse effects of chronic hyperglycemia or high circulating free fatty acids.

A third factor is inappropriate glucose production by the liver. Instead of properly regulating the release of glucose in response to blood levels, the liver does so in a haphazard way that does not correspond to the body's needs at the time. Furthermore, there is in increased secretion of glucagon from the α cells of the pancreas that stimulates glucose production by the liver, adding to the increase in blood sugar. However, this is not considered a primary factor in the development of type 2 DM.

A fourth factor is alteration in the production of hormones and cytokines by adipose tissue *(adipocytokines)*. Adipocytokines appear to play a role in glucose and fat metabolism and are likely to contribute to the pathophysiology of type 2 DM. The two main adipocytokines believed to affect insulin sensitivity are adiponectin and leptin. Others include tumour necrosis factor α (TNF-α), interlukin-6 (IL-6), and resistin. The role of resistin in the pathogenesis of obesity-mediated insulin resistance and type 2 DM, however, remains controversial (Kuminski, McTernan, & Kumar, 2005, p. 243). Figure 52-2 depicts the altered mechanisms in type 1 and type 2 DM.

Metabolic syndrome (also known as insulin resistance syndrome) is a cluster of abnormalities that act synergistically to greatly increase the risk for cardiovascular disease. Metabolic syndrome is characterized by abdominal obesity, hypertension, dyslipidemia, insulin resistance, and dysglycemia. Patients with metabolic syndrome are at significant risk for developing DM and cardiovascular disease (CDA, 2008, p. S11). Lifestyle interventions have been shown to be highly effective in delaying or preventing the onset of DM in people with IGT. Risk factors for metabolic syndrome include, but are not limited to, abdominal obesity, sedentary lifestyle, urbanization and Westernization, and certain ethnicities (First Nations, Hispanics, and African Canadians). Overweight individuals with metabolic syndrome can prevent or delay the onset of DM through a program of weight loss and regular physical activity. (Metabolic syndrome is discussed in further detail in Chapter 43.)

Onset of Disease. Disease onset in type 2 DM is usually gradual. The person may go for many years with undetected hyperglycemia that might produce few, if any, symptoms. Many people are diagnosed on routine laboratory testing. If the patient with type 2 DM has marked hyperglycemia (e.g., 28 to 55 mmol/L), a sufficient endogenous insulin supply may prevent DKA from occurring. However, osmotic fluid and electrolyte loss related to hyperglycemia may become severe and lead to hyperosmolar hyperglycemic state. (Complications of DM are discussed later in this chapter.)

Gestational Diabetes.

Gestational diabetes mellitus (GDM) develops during pregnancy. It occurs in about 4% of pregnancies in the non-Aboriginal population and in about 8 to 18% of pregnancies in Aboriginal populations in Canada (CDA, 2008, p. S171). It is detected between 24 and 28 weeks of gestation, usually following a gestational diabetes screen (GDS)—50 g glucose load, with a 1-hr postplasma glucose. Women with multiple risk factors should be screened during the first trimester (CDA, 2008, p. S172). Treatment of GDM reduces perinatal death and neonatal complications such as birth trauma, hypoglycemia, hyperbilirubinemia, and respiratory distress syndrome (CDA, 2008, p. S173). Nutritional counselling is considered to be the first-line therapy. Physical activity should be encouraged as tolerated. If nutritional counselling alone does not achieve target fasting, or postprandial blood glucose levels, or both, insulin therapy is usually indicated. Approximately 10% of patients progress to DM soon after pregnancy. Although most women with GDM will have normal glucose levels within 6 weeks' postpartum, their risk for developing type 2 DM in 5 to 10 years is increased. Women should be screened postpartum to determine their glucose status. The 2008 CDA guidelines recommend a 75-g oral glucose tolerance test (OGTT) be done between 6 weeks and 6 months postpartum. Education on lifestyle modifications to prevent DM should continue postpartum. GDM and management of the pregnant patient with DM is a specialized area not covered in detail in this chapter. The reader is advised to consult a DM and obstetrics text for information about this subject.

Secondary Diabetes.

In some people, DM occurs because of another medical condition or as a result of the treatment of a medical condition that causes abnormal blood glucose levels. Conditions that may cause secondary DM include schizophrenia, cystic fibrosis, Cushing's syndrome, hyperthyroidism, immunosuppressive therapy, and the use of parenteral nutrition. Commonly used medications that can induce DM in some people include corticosteroids (prednisone), phenytoin (Dilantin), and atypical antipsychotics (e.g., clozapine [Clozaril]). Secondary DM may resolve when the underlying condition is treated.

Clinical Manifestations

Type 1 Diabetes Mellitus.

Because the onset of type 1 DM is rapid, the initial manifestations are usually acute. The classic symptoms are *polyuria* (frequent urination), *polydipsia* (excessive thirst), and *polyphagia* (excessive hunger). The osmotic effect of glucose produces the manifestations of polydipsia and polyuria. Polyphagia is a consequence of cellular malnourishment when insulin deficiency prevents utilization of glucose for energy. Weight loss may occur because the body cannot get glucose and turns to other energy sources, such as fat and protein. Weakness and fatigue may also be experienced, because body cells lack needed energy from glucose. There may be pronounced changes in visual acuity owing to changes in the lens with hyperglycemia and fluid retention. Women may have vaginal yeast infections. Ketoacidosis, a complication associated with untreated type 1 DM, is associated with additional clinical manifestations that are discussed later in this chapter.

Type 2 Diabetes Mellitus.

The clinical manifestations of type 2 DM are often nonspecific, although it is possible that an individual with type 2 DM will experience some of the classic symptoms associated with type 1. Some of the more common manifestations associated with type 2 DM include fatigue, recurrent infections, prolonged wound healing, visual acuity changes, and painful peripheral neuropathy in the feet. Unfortunately, the clinical manifestations appear so gradually that, before the person knows it, he or she may have complications.

Complications

Complications of DM are discussed in detail later in this chapter.

Diagnostic Studies.

Regardless of the type, the diagnosis of DM can be made through one of four methods. Whichever method is used, diagnosis of DM must be confirmed on a subsequent day by any of the four methods (CDA, 2008, p. S10; Goldenberg, Cheng, Punthakee, & Clement, 2011, p. 247). These methods and their criteria for diagnosis are as follows:

1. Hemoglobin A1C (A1C) ≥6.5%, using a standardized, validated assay, in the absence of conditions that affect the accuracy of the A1C.
2. Fasting plasma glucose (FPG) level ≥7 mmol/L. *Fasting* is defined as no caloric intake for at least 8 hours.
3. Random, or casual, plasma glucose measurement ≥11.1 mmol/L, plus classic symptoms of DM, such as polyuria, polydipsia, and unexplained weight loss. *Casual* is defined as any time of day without regard to the interval since the last meal.
4. Two-hour OGTT level ≥11.1 mmol/L, using a glucose load of 75 g.

For many years, A1C has been used to monitor glucose control in people diagnosed with DM. In July 2011, the CDA recommended the use of A1C for diagnosing DM. The A1C has several advantages over the FPG, including greater convenience because fasting is not required and there are fewer day-to-day alterations during periods of stress and illness (Goldenberg et al., 2011, p. 247). The FPG test, confirmed by repeat testing on another day, is another method of diagnosis. When overt symptoms of hyperglycemia (polyuria, polydipsia, and polyphagia) coexist with FPG levels of 7 mmol/L or greater, further testing using the OGTT may not be necessary to make a diagnosis (CDA, 2008, p. S11).

IFG and IGT each represent an intermediate stage between normal glucose homeostasis and DM. The stage is called *prediabetes* (see discussion on prediabetes earlier in this chapter). When the fasting blood glucose level is 6.1 to 6.9 mmol/L, the individual is considered to have IFG. IGT is classified as a 2-hour OGTT level that is greater than or equal to normal (≥7.8 mmol/L) but lower than that considered diagnostic for DM (11.1 mmol/L) (CDA, 2008, p. S11).

Measurement of glycosylated hemoglobin, also known as the *hemoglobin A1C (A1C) test*, is useful in determining glycemic control over time. The test works by showing the amount of glucose that has been attached to hemoglobin molecules, which are attached to the red blood cell (RBC) for the life of the cell (~120 days). Therefore, an A1C test indicates the overall glucose control for the previous 90 to 120 days. All patients with DM should have regular assessments of A1C every 3 to 6 months. Major studies have demonstrated that people with DM who can maintain near-normal A1C levels over time have a greatly reduced risk for the development of retinopathy, nephropathy, and neuropathy. For most people with DM, the ideal A1C goal is 7% or less. Normal range is 6% or less. A target A1C of less than 6.5%

can be considered in some patients with type 2 DM to further lower the risk of nephropathy but must be balanced against the risk of hypoglycemia and increased mortality in those at an elevated risk for cardiovascular disease (CDA, 2008, p. S31). Diseases affecting RBCs (e.g., sickle cell anemia, thalassemia trait) or recent blood transfusions can affect the A1C results and should be taken into consideration in the interpretation of this test result.

Collaborative Care

The goals of DM management are to promote well-being, reduce symptoms, prevent acute complications of hyperglycemia and hypoglycemia, and delay the onset and progression of long-term complications. These goals are most likely to be met when the patient is able to maintain blood glucose levels as near to normal as possible. Patient teaching, which enables the patient to become the most active participant in her or his own care, is essential for a successful treatment plan. Nutritional therapy, exercise, self-monitoring of blood glucose, and drug therapy are the tools used in the management of DM (Table 52-2). All individuals with type 1 DM require insulin from the time of diagnosis. For some people with type 2 DM, lifestyle modifications including healthy eating, regular physical activity, and maintenance of desirable body weight will be sufficient to attain an optimal level of blood glucose control. For the majority, however, drug therapy with oral antihyperglycemic agents (OHAs), insulin, or both will be necessary.

Drug Therapy: Insulin

Exogenous (injected) insulin is needed when a patient has inadequate insulin to meet specific metabolic needs and the combination of nutritional therapy, exercise, and OHAs cannot maintain a satisfactory blood glucose level. Exogenous insulin is always required for the management of type 1 DM. Individuals with type 2 DM may be treated with insulin alone or with insulin in combination with OHAs (CDA, 2008, p. S56). Insulin requirement may increase significantly during periods of severe stress, such as illness or surgery.

Types of Insulin. In Canada, beef insulin was withdrawn in 1999 but can be bought from international sources. Human biosynthetic insulin is now the most widely used insulin. Human insulin is derived from common bacteria (e.g., *Escherichia coli*) or yeast cells using recombinant DNA technology (see Chapter 16). Insulin analogues are made by modifying the amino acid sequence of the insulin molecule (Cheng, 2011, p. 4). Insulins differ in regard to onset, peak action, and duration (Figure 52-3). The specific properties and different combinations of these insulins can be used to tailor treatment to the patient's specific patterns of blood glucose levels, lifestyle, eating, and activity. Different types of insulin are listed in Table 52-3. Most insulin preparations start with regular insulin as a base. By adding zinc, acetate buffers, and protamine to insulin in various ways, the onset of activity, peak, and duration times can be manipulated. Zinc and protamine are added to make NPH (neutral protamine Hagedorn). In rare instances, these additives may cause an allergic reaction at the injection site. Switching the brand or the type of insulin may alleviate this localized reaction.

Insulin Regimens. Examples of insulin regimens ranging from one to four injections per day are presented in Table 52-4.

COLLABORATIVE CARE

Table 52-2 Diabetes Mellitus

Diagnostic

- History and physical examination
- Blood tests: including fasting blood glucose, postprandial blood glucose, glycosylated hemoglobin (A1C), fasting lipid profile, serum creatinine, electrolytes, calculation of creatinine clearance, TSH
- Fundoscopic examination—dilated eye examination
- Neurological examination, including monofilament test for sensation to lower extremities
- ECG (if indicated)
- Blood pressure
- Monitoring of weight
- Doppler scan—ankle-brachial index (if indicated)
- Dental examination
- Foot (podiatric) examination
- Random urine for microalbuminuria (MAU), complete urinalysis, and acetone if indicated

Collaborative Therapy

- Nutritional therapy (see Table 52-8)
- Exercise therapy (see Tables 52-9 and 52-10)
- Drug therapy
  - Insulin (see Figure 52-3 and Tables 52-3 and 52-4)
  - Oral antihyperglycemic agents (see Table 52-7)
- Vascular protection
  - Enteric-coated aspirin (80 mg or 325 mg)
  - Angiotensin-converting enzyme (ACE) inhibitors or angiotensin II receptor antagonists (ARBs) (high risk of a cardiovascular event) (see Chapter 35, Table 35-8)
  - Lipid-lowering therapy (high risk of a cardiovascular event) (see Chapter 35, Table 35-8)
- Self-monitoring of blood glucose (SMBG)
- Blood pressure control
  - Target <130/80 mm Hg
- Patient and caregiver teaching and follow-up programs

ECG, electrocardiogram; *TSH,* thyroid-stimulating hormone.
Source: Canadian Diabetes Association (CDA) Clinical Practice Guidelines Expert Committee. (2008). Clinical practice guidelines for the prevention and management of diabetes in Canada. *Canadian Journal of Diabetes, 32*(Suppl 1), S195.

The exogenous insulin regimen that most closely mimics endogenous insulin production is the basal–bolus regimen, which uses rapid- or short-acting (bolus) insulin before meals and intermediate- or long-acting (basal) background insulin once or twice a day. The basal–bolus regimen is *intensive insulin therapy,* which consists of multiple daily insulin (MDI). The goal is to achieve a near-normal glucose level of 4 to 7 mmol/L before meals, or 4 to 6 mmol/L if this can be reached safely without severe hypoglycemia. The Diabetes Control and Complications Trial (DCCT) Research Group demonstrated that people with type 1 DM who have tight glucose control through intensive management develop fewer and less severe complications (DCCT, 1993, p. 977). Ideally, regimens should be collaboratively selected by the patient and the health care provider (CDA, 2008, p. S46). The criteria for selection are based on the type of DM and the required, desired,

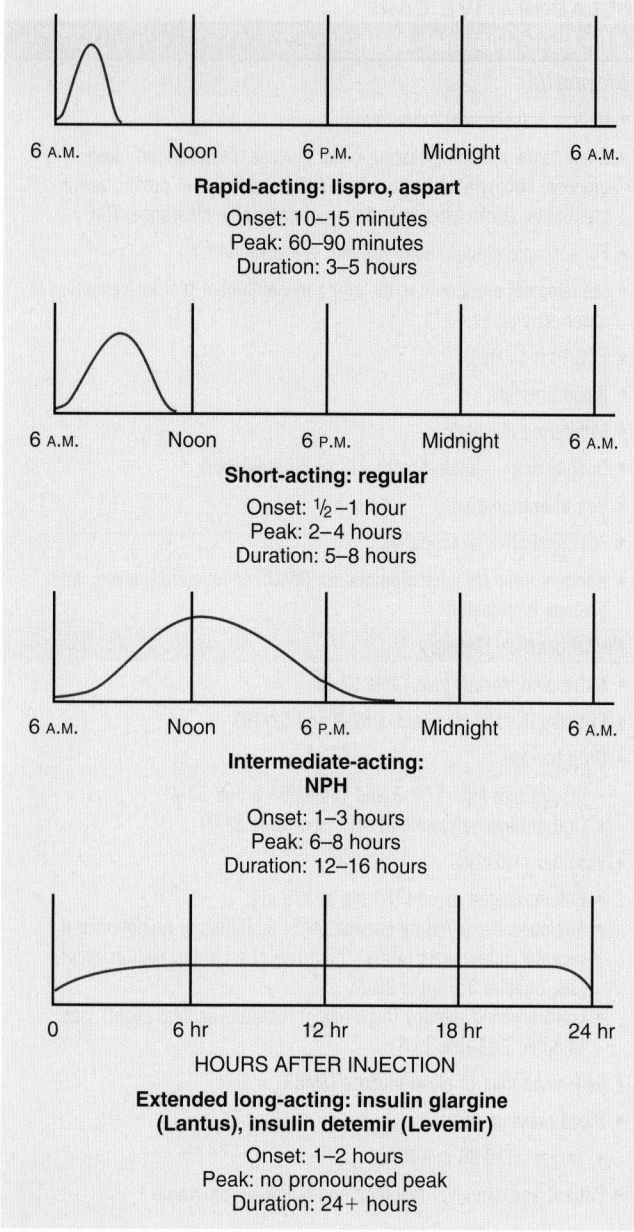

Figure 52-3 Commercially available insulin preparations showing onset, peak, and duration of action of relative plasma insulin level. *NPH*, neutral protamine Hagedorn.

Table 52-3 Types of Insulin*

CLASSIFICATION	EXAMPLES
Rapid-acting analogue (clear)	Lispro (Humalog)
	Aspart (NovoRapid)
	Glulisine (Apidra)
Short-acting (clear)	Regular (Novolin ge Toronto, Humulin R)
Intermediate-acting (cloudy)	NPH (Humulin N, Novolin ge NPH)
Extended long-acting analogue (clear)	Glargine (Lantus)
	Detemir (Levemir)
Premixed (cloudy)	Regular/NPH 30/70† (Humulin 30/70, Novolin ge 30/70)
	Regular/NPH 50/50 and 40/60
	Lispro/lispro protamine 25/75 (Humalog Mix 25); 50/50 (Humalog Mix 50)
	Aspart/aspart protamine 30/70 (NovoMix 30)

NPH, neutral protamine Hagedorn.
*The intermediate-acting insulin (lente) and long-acting (ultralente) were discontinued in Canada at the end of 2005, and 10/90 and 20/80 in July 2007, owing to underutilization and the introduction of the new long-acting basal insulin analogues and premixes.
†These numbers refer to percentages of each type of insulin.

acting insulin is so short. Other benefits of rapid-acting insulin include decreased postmeal hyperglycemia, decreased hypoglycemic episodes, and increased flexibility compared to regular insulin (Fowler, 2008, p. 35; Shlafer, 2009, p. 658). Regular insulin is also a mealtime insulin and has an onset of action of 30 to 60 minutes and should be injected 30 to 45 minutes before a meal to ensure that the onset of action coincides with meal absorption. Because timing an injection 30 to 45 minutes before a meal is difficult for people to incorporate into their lifestyles, the rapid-acting insulins are often preferred by people who take insulin with meals (Shlafer, 2009, p. 658).

Long- or Intermediate-Acting (Basal) Background Insulin. Insulin glargine (Lantus) and detemir (Levemir) are extended long-acting basal insulins that are released steadily and continuously over 24 hours. They do not have a peak of action (see Figure 52-3). Both may be used for once-daily subcutaneous administration at bedtime in patients with type 1 and type 2 DM who require basal (long-acting) insulin for the control of hyperglycemia. Because they lack a peak action time, the risk for hypoglycemia is greatly reduced. They are both clear, colourless insulins. The nurse should be aware of the potential danger of confusing glargine and detemir with other clear insulins (rapid- or short-acting) (Registered Nurses' Association of Ontario [RNAO], 2009, p. 73). Glargine and detemir must not be diluted or mixed with any other insulin or solution (Shlafer, 2009, p. 658).

Intermediate-acting insulin NPH is also used as a basal insulin that has a duration of 10 to 16 hours. The disadvantage is that it has a peak at 4 to 10 hours, which can result in hypoglycemia. It is the only basal insulin that can be mixed with the short- and rapid-acting insulins. NPH is a cloudy insulin that must be gently agitated before administration (Fowler, 2008, p. 36).

and feasible levels of glycemic control in addition to economic factors and flexibility.

Mealtime Insulin (Bolus). Synthetic rapid-acting insulins include lispro (Humalog), aspart insulin (NovoRapid), and glulisine (Apidra). They have an onset of action of approximately 10 to 15 minutes (as compared with 30 to 60 min for regular insulin). Rapid-acting insulin is considered to be the type that best mimics natural insulin secretion in response to a meal. It should be administered 0 to 15 minutes before meals and can be given up to 15 minutes after meals. However, preprandial administration achieves better postprandial glycemic control. When rapid-acting insulin is used as mealtime coverage in people with type 1 DM, an additional and longer-acting insulin must also be used as basal background insulin because the duration of rapid-

DRUG THERAPY

Table 52-4 Common Insulin Regimens

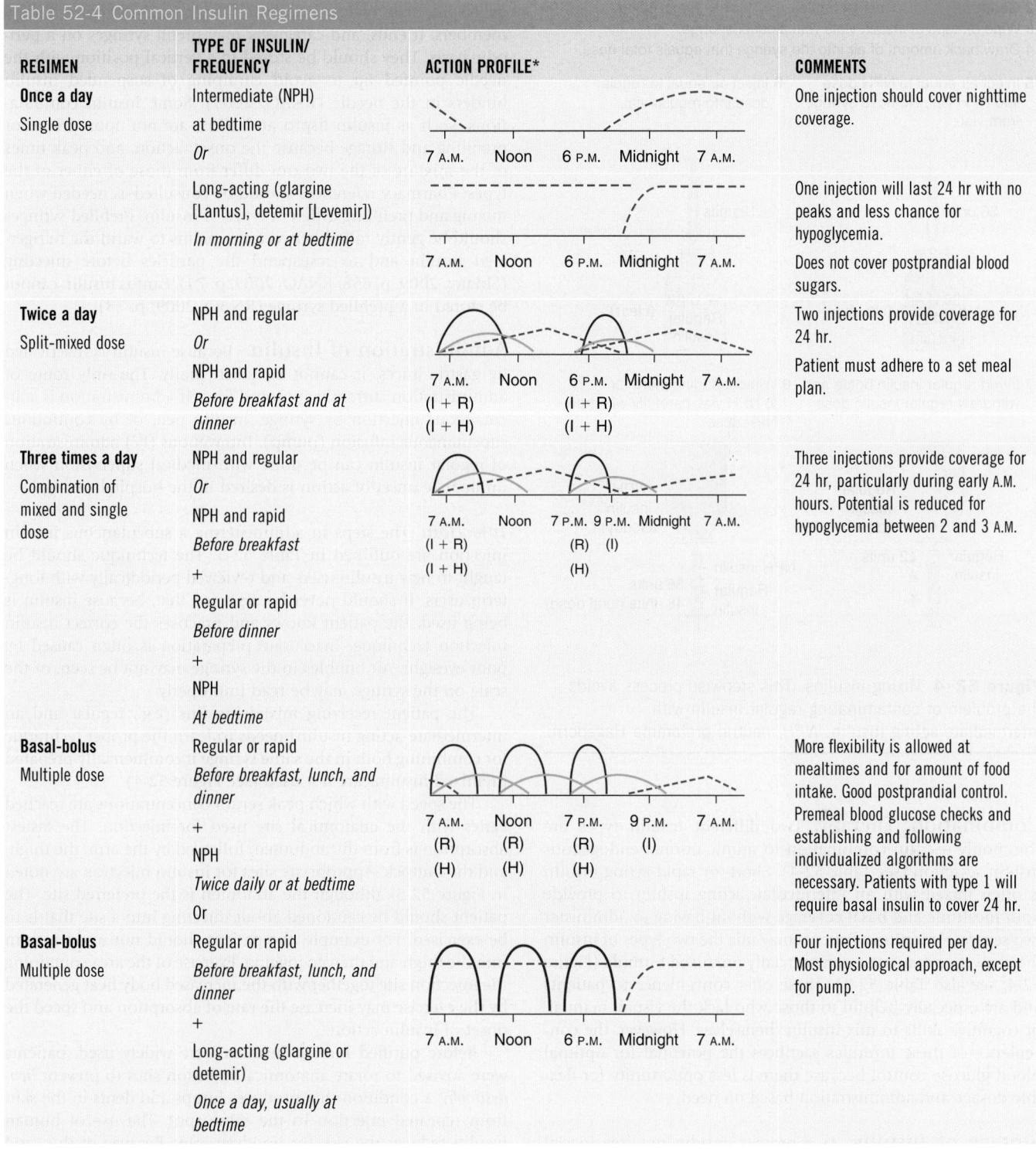

REGIMEN	TYPE OF INSULIN/ FREQUENCY	ACTION PROFILE*	COMMENTS
Once a day Single dose	Intermediate (NPH) at bedtime *Or*		One injection should cover nighttime coverage.
	Long-acting (glargine [Lantus], detemir [Levemir]) *In morning or at bedtime*		One injection will last 24 hr with no peaks and less chance for hypoglycemia. Does not cover postprandial blood sugars.
Twice a day Split-mixed dose	NPH and regular *Or* NPH and rapid *Before breakfast and at dinner*	(I + R) (I + R) (I + H) (I + H)	Two injections provide coverage for 24 hr. Patient must adhere to a set meal plan.
Three times a day Combination of mixed and single dose	NPH and regular *Or* NPH and rapid *Before breakfast* + Regular or rapid *Before dinner* + NPH *At bedtime*	(I + R) (R) (I) (I + H) (H)	Three injections provide coverage for 24 hr, particularly during early A.M. hours. Potential is reduced for hypoglycemia between 2 and 3 A.M.
Basal-bolus Multiple dose	Regular or rapid *Before breakfast, lunch, and dinner* + NPH *Twice daily or at bedtime* *Or*	(R) (R) (R) (I) (H) (H) (H)	More flexibility is allowed at mealtimes and for amount of food intake. Good postprandial control. Premeal blood glucose checks and establishing and following individualized algorithms are necessary. Patients with type 1 will require basal insulin to cover 24 hr.
Basal-bolus Multiple dose	Regular or rapid *Before breakfast, lunch, and dinner* + Long-acting (glargine or detemir) *Once a day, usually at bedtime*		Four injections required per day. Most physiological approach, except for pump.

NPH, neutral protamine Hagedorn.

*Key:

————————Rapid-acting (lispro, aspart, glulisine) insulin.

————————Short-acting (regular) insulin.

- - - - - - - - - -Intermediate-acting (NPH) or long-acting (glargine, detemir) insulin.

1 Wash hands.
2 Gently rotate NPH insulin bottle.
3 Wipe off tops of insulin vials with alcohol sponge.
4 Draw back amount of air into the syringe that equals total dose.

5 Inject air equal to NPH dose into NPH vial. Remove syringe from vial.

6 Inject air equal to regular dose into regular vial.

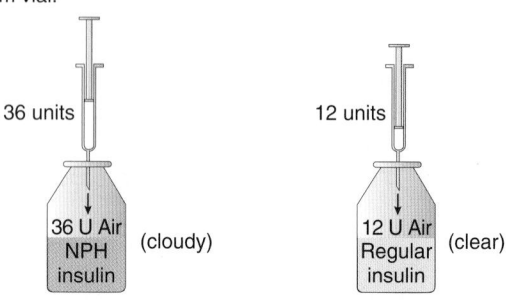

7 Invert regular insulin bottle and withdraw regular insulin dose.

8 Without adding more air to NPH vial, carefully withdraw NPH dose.

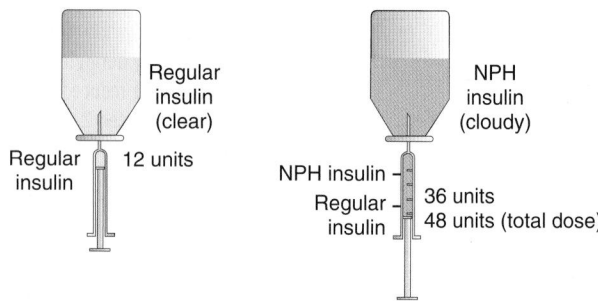

Figure 52-4 Mixing insulins. This stepwise process avoids the problem of contaminating regular insulin with intermediate-acting insulin. *NPH,* neutral protamine Hagedorn.

Combination Therapy. Two different insulin types are commonly used in combination to mimic normal endogenous insulin secretion (see Table 52-4). Short- or rapid-acting insulin is often mixed with an intermediate-acting insulin to provide both mealtime and basal coverage without having to administer two separate injections. Patients may mix the two types of insulin themselves or may use a commercially premixed formula (Figure 52-4; see also Table 52-3). These offer convenience to patients and are especially helpful to those who lack the visual, manual, or cognitive skills to mix insulin themselves. However, the convenience of these formulas sacrifices the potential for optimal blood glucose control because there is less opportunity for flexible dosage and administration based on need.

Storage of Insulin. As a protein, insulin requires special storage considerations. Heat and freezing alter the insulin molecule. The insulin vial or cartridge that the patient is currently using may be left at room temperature for up to 4 weeks, unless the room temperature is higher than 30°C or below freezing (<2°C). Unopened vials and cartridges must be refrigerated. Prolonged exposure to direct sunlight should be avoided. Insulin pens should not be stored in the refrigerator. The same principles apply for a patient who is travelling. Insulin can be stored in a thermos or cooler to keep it cool (not frozen) if the patient is travelling in hot climates (RNAO, 2009, p. 74).

Prefilled syringes, including mixed insulins, are stable for up to 30 days when stored in the refrigerator. This may be beneficial to patients who are sight impaired or who lack the manual dexterity to fill their own syringes at home. In these cases, family members, friends, and caregivers may prefill syringes on a periodic basis. They should be stored in a vertical position with the needle pointed up to avoid clumping of suspended insulin binders in the needle (RNAO, 2009). Some insulin combinations, such as insulin lispro and NPH, are not appropriate for prefilling and storage because the onset, action, and peak times of the mixture of the two can differ from those of either of the types. Pharmacy references should be consulted as needed when mixing and prefilling different types of insulin. Prefilled syringes should be gently rolled between the palms to warm the refrigerated insulin and to resuspend the particles before injecting (Shlafer, 2009, p. 658; RNAO, 2009, p. 74). Lantus insulin cannot be stored in a prefilled syringe (RNAO, 2009, p. 73).

Administration of Insulin. Because insulin is inactivated by gastric juices, it cannot be taken orally. The only route of administration currently approved for self-administration is subcutaneous injection by syringe, insulin pen, or by continuous subcutaneous infusion (pump). Intravenous (IV) administration of regular insulin can be done with medical supervision when immediate onset of action is desired in the hospital setting.

Injection. The steps in administering a subcutaneous insulin injection are outlined in Table 52-5. The technique should be taught to new insulin users and reviewed periodically with long-term users. It should never be assumed that, because insulin is being used, the patient knows and practises the correct insulin injection technique. Inaccurate preparation is often caused by poor eyesight. Air bubbles in the syringe may not be seen, or the scale on the syringe may be read improperly.

The patient receiving mixed insulins (e.g., regular and an intermediate-acting insulin) needs to learn the proper technique for combining both in the same syringe if commercially prepared premixed insulins are not used (see Figure 52-4).

The speed with which peak serum concentrations are reached varies with the anatomical site used for injection. The fastest absorption is from the abdomen, followed by the arm, the thigh, and the buttock. Appropriate sites for insulin injection are noted in Figure 52-5, although the abdomen is the preferred site. The patient should be cautioned about injecting into a site that is to be exercised. For example, the patient should not inject insulin into the thigh and then go jogging. Exercise of the area containing the injection site together with the increased body heat generated by the exercise may increase the rate of absorption and speed the onset of insulin action.

Before purified human insulins were widely used, patients were advised to rotate anatomical injection sites to prevent *lipodystrophy,* a condition that produces lumps and dents in the skin from repeated injection in the same spot. The use of human insulin reduces the risk for lipodystrophy. Because of this, and because rotating sites causes variability in insulin absorption, rotation of injection sites to different anatomical sites is no longer the recommended practice. Instead, patients are advised to rotate the injection within one particular site, such as the abdomen. Sometimes, it is helpful to think of the entire abdomen as a checkerboard, with each square representing an injection site as the patient rotates sites systematically across the board.

Most commercial insulin is available as U100, indicating that 1 mL contains 100 units of insulin. U100 insulin must be used with a U100-marked syringe. Disposable plastic insulin syringes are available in a variety of sizes, including 1, 0.5, and 0.3 mL. The 0.5-mL size may be used for doses of 50 units or less, and

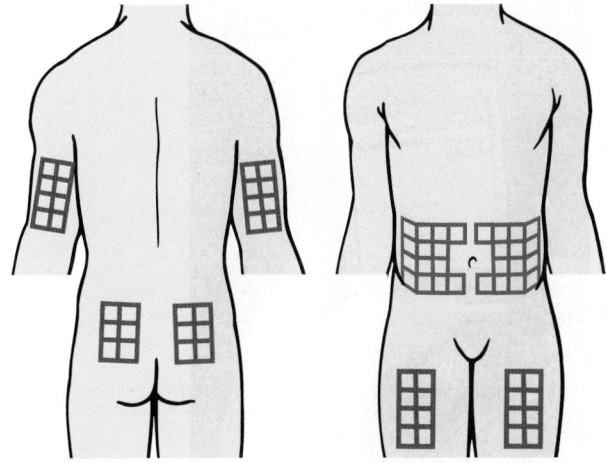

Figure 52-5 Injection sites for insulin. The abdomen is the preferred site.

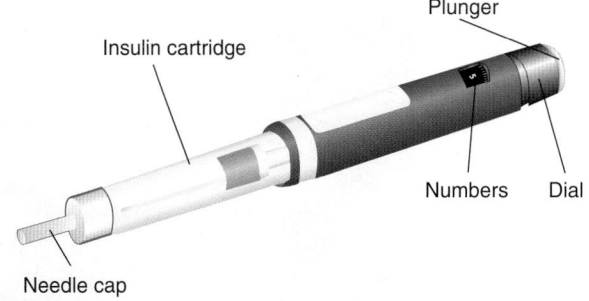

Figure 52-6 Parts of an insulin pen.

PATIENT & CAREGIVER TEACHING GUIDE

Table 52-5 Insulin Therapy

1. Wash hands thoroughly.
2. Check insulin type and expiration date.
3. If a cloudy insulin is used, gently roll container to resuspend insulin. It should look uniformly milky.
4. Remove the cover from the needle.
5. Pull the plunger down until the tip of the plunger is at the line for the number of units required. Put the needle into the vial and push the air into the vial.
6. Turn the vial upside down and slowly push plunger up and down to get rid of air bubbles and then pull plunger down until it is at the line for the correct dose of insulin.
7. Check that the amount of insulin is correct and that there are no large air bubbles in the syringe. Remove the syringe.
8. Select proper injection site and inject following the procedure for any subcutaneous injection (see Figure 52-5). In sites where subcutaneous tissue is adequate, inject commercial insulin needles at 45- (slim individuals) to 90-degree angle. (The use of 8-mm needles is recommended.)
9. After injecting insulin, leave needle in place for 10 sec to ensure that all insulin has been injected and to prevent leakage of the insulin. Apply a dry cotton ball at site when withdrawing needle.
10. Dispose of single-use syringe safely. *Note:* When instructing patient to self-inject insulin, use the following guidelines (if appropriate):
    - Inspect insulin for any changes before each use (i.e., clumping, precipitation, change in clarity or colour).
    - Aspiration does not need to be done before injection.
    - The injection site does not need to be cleansed with alcohol.

the 0.3-mL syringe can be used for doses of 30 units or less. Smaller syringes offer a number of advantages. The major benefit is increased accuracy and reliability when delivering smaller doses because wider line markings are easier to see. Patients should be cautioned to check dosage lines carefully when changing syringe types because some use a scale of 1-unit increments and others use 2-unit increments.

Recapping should be done only by the person using the syringe. The nurse must never recap a needle that has been used by a patient. The use of an alcohol swab on the site before self-injection is no longer recommended. Routine hygiene such as washing with soap and rinsing with water is adequate. This applies primarily to patient self-injection technique. When injection occurs in a health care facility, policy may dictate site preparation with alcohol to prevent hospital-acquired infection. Injection should be performed at a 45- to 90-degree angle, depending on the thickness of the patient's fat pad.

An insulin pen is a compact portable device that serves the same function as a needle and syringe but is handier to use (Figure 52-6). The insulin pen uses 300-unit cartridges, which are packaged in a box of five, for a total of 1500 units. One of the advantages of insulin pens is that they are less "medical" looking. The insulin pen has a numerical dial-up device that clicks for each unit being dialled. The pen can dial up to a maximum of 60 to 70 units depending on the device. This is a safer and more convenient option for most patients, especially those with visual impairment, dexterity problems, and peripheral neuropathy. Pen-needle tips are finer than syringe tips and must be changed with every injection. They are manufactured in a variety of sizes—4, 5, 6 , 8, and 12 to 12.7 mm—for a variety of body-fat types (Forum for Injection Technique [FIT] Canada, 2011, p. 8).

Alternate Delivery Methods. Continuous subcutaneous insulin infusion can be administered using an insulin pump, a small battery-operated device that resembles a standard paging device in size and appearance (Figure 52-7). Usually worn on the belt or under clothing, the pump is connected via a small plastic tube to a catheter inserted into the subcutaneous tissue in the abdominal wall. Every 2 to 3 days, the insertion site is changed and the pump is refilled with insulin and reprogrammed. The device is programmed to deliver a continuous infusion of rapid-acting insulin 24 hours a day, known as the *basal rate.* Basal insulin can be temporarily increased or decreased based on activity level changes or illness. At mealtime, the user programs the pump to deliver a bolus infusion of insulin appropriate to the amount of carbohydrate ingested and to bring down high premeal blood glucose, if necessary. A major advantage of the insulin pump is the reduction of hypoglycemia episodes. Pumps also offer the benefit of a more normal lifestyle, allowing users more flexibility with meal and activity patterns as insulin delivery becomes very similar to the normal physiological pattern. The insertion site should be checked daily for redness and swelling (White, 2007, p. 845; American Association of Diabetes Educators [AADE], 2009, p. 6).

Problems With Insulin Therapy. Hypoglycemia, allergic reactions, lipodystrophy, and Somogyi effect are the problems associated with insulin therapy. Hypoglycemia is discussed in detail later in this chapter. (Guidelines for assessing patients treated with insulin are presented in Table 52-6.)

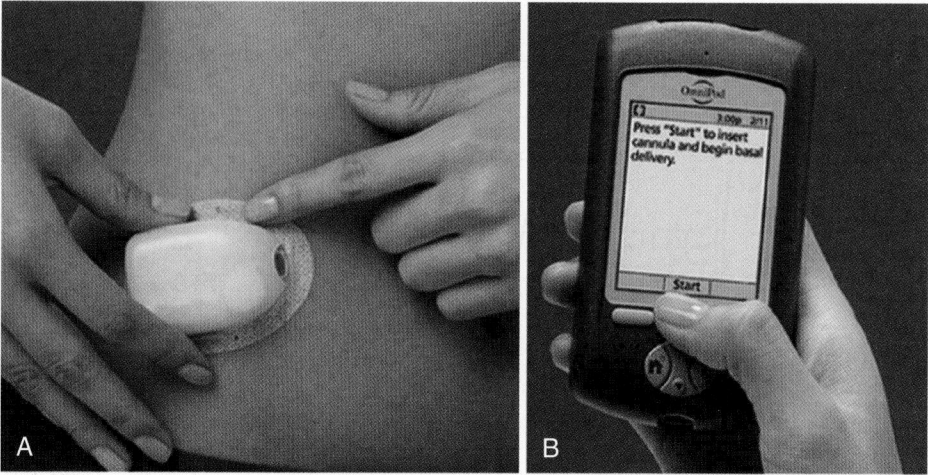

Figure 52-7 A, OmniPod Insulin Management System. The Pod holds and delivers insulin. **B,** The Personal Diabetes Manager (PDM) wirelessly programs insulin delivery via the Pod. The PDM has a built-in glucose meter.

Source: Courtesy Insulet Corporation.

Table 52-6 Assessing the Patient Treated With Oral Antihyperglycemic Agents and Insulin	
FOR PATIENT WITH NEWLY DIAGNOSED DIABETES OR RE-EVALUATION OF MEDICATION REGIMEN	
Cognitive	Is patient or responsible other able to understand why insulin or OHAs are being used as part of diabetes management?
	Is patient or responsible other able to understand concepts of asepsis, combining insulins, insulin–OHA actions, and adverse effects?
	Is patient able to remember to take >1 dose/day?
	Does patient take medications at right times in relation to meals?
Psychomotor	Is patient or responsible other physically able to prepare and administer accurate doses of the medication?
Affective	What emotions and attitudes are patient and responsible others displaying in regard to diagnosis of diabetes and insulin or OHA treatment?
FOR FOLLOW-UP OF PATIENT TREATED WITH ORAL ANTIHYPERGLYCEMIC AGENTS AND INSULIN	
Effectiveness of therapy	Is patient having symptoms of hyperglycemia or hypoglycemia?
	Does blood glucose record show good or poor control?
	Is glycosylated hemoglobin (A1C) consistent with glucose records?
Adverse effects of therapy	Has patient had hypoglycemic episodes? If so, how often? What time of day? What was the precipitating event? Inconsistent meal timing, meal carbohydrate content, alcohol, or exercise?
	Are there complaints of nightmares, night sweats, or early-morning headaches?
	Has patient had skin rash, GI upset, ankle edema, or weight gain since taking the oral antihyperglycemic agent?
	Is atrophy or hypertrophy present at injection sites?
Self-management behaviours	If patient is having hypoglycemic episodes, how are those episodes managed? Has the patient analyzed episodes to determine reason?
	How much insulin or OHA is the patient taking and at what time of day? Is patient adjusting insulin or OHA dose? Under what circumstances and by how much?
	Has exercise pattern changed?
	Is patient adhering to healthy eating recommendations? Are meals taken at times corresponding to peak insulin action? Is patient performing SMBG?

GI, gastrointestinal; *OHA,* oral antihyperglycemic agent; *SMBG,* self-monitoring of blood glucose.

Allergic Reactions. Local inflammatory reactions to insulin, such as itching, erythema, and burning around the injection site, may occur. Local reactions may be self-limiting within 1 to 3 months or may improve with a low dose of antihistamine. A true insulin allergy is a systemic response with urticaria and possibly anaphylactic shock generally resulting from the use of animal insulins. Fortunately, this type of allergy is rare, particularly since human insulin has become available. Zinc or protamine used as preservatives in the insulin and the latex rubber stoppers on the vials have been implicated in insulin reactions.

Lipodystrophy. **Lipodystrophy** (hypertrophy or atrophy of subcutaneous tissue) may occur if the same injection sites are used frequently. Hypertrophy, a thickening of the subcutaneous tissue, eventually regresses if the patient does not use the site for at least 6 months. The use of hypertrophied sites may result in erratic insulin absorption. Lipodystrophies have been most commonly associated with beef or beef and pork insulin and rarely with human insulin.

Somogyi Effect and Dawn Phenomenon. Wide differences in early-morning (low) and fasting (high) glucose levels characterize the Somogyi effect. Usually occurring during the hours of sleep, the **Somogyi effect** produces a decline in blood glucose level in response to too much insulin. Counter-regulatory hormones are released, stimulating lipolysis, gluconeogenesis, and glycogenolysis, which in turn produce rebound hyperglycemia and ketosis. The danger of this effect is that, when blood glucose levels are measured in the morning, hyperglycemia is apparent, and the patient (or the health care provider) may, therefore, increase the insulin dose. The Somogyi effect is associated with the occurrence of undetected hypoglycemia during sleep, although it can happen at any time.

The patient may report headaches on awakening and may recall night sweats or nightmares. If the Somogyi effect is suspected as a cause for early-morning high blood glucose, the patient may be advised to check blood glucose levels between 2 and 4 A.M. to determine whether hypoglycemia is present at that time. If it is, the insulin dosage of administration affecting the early-morning blood glucose is reduced.

The *dawn phenomenon* is characterized by hyperglycemia that is present on awakening in the morning owing to the release of counter-regulatory hormones in the predawn hours. It has been suggested that growth hormone and cortisol are possible factors in this occurrence. The dawn phenomenon affects the majority of people with DM and tends to be most severe when growth hormone is at its peak in adolescence and young adulthood.

Careful assessment is required to document each phenomenon because the treatment for each differs. The treatment for Somogyi effect is reduction of insulin dosage. The treatment for dawn phenomenon is an adjustment in the timing of insulin administration or an increase in insulin. The assessment must include insulin dose, injection sites, and variability in the time of meals or insulin administration. In addition, the patient is asked to measure and document bedtime, nighttime (between 2 and 4 A.M.), and morning fasting blood glucose levels on several occasions. If the predawn levels are below 3.3 mmol/L and signs and symptoms of hypoglycemia are present, the insulin dosage should be reduced. If the 2- to 4-A.M. blood glucose is high, the insulin dosage should be increased. In addition, the patient should be counselled on appropriate bedtime snacks.

Drug Therapy: Oral Antihyperglycemic Agents

OHAs are not insulin, but they work to improve the mechanisms by which insulin and glucose are produced and used by the body. The term *oral antihyperglycemic agents* is used by the CDA *2008 Clinical Practice Guidelines* and encompasses all oral medications for the management of blood glucose control. For any of the OHAs to be effective, the patient must have some circulating endogenous insulin. There are currently no OHAs for the treatment of type 1 DM. OHAs may be used in combination with agents from several classes or with insulin to achieve blood glucose targets. Guidelines for assessing patients receiving OHAs are shown in Table 52-6.

Currently, many classes of oral medications are available to improve DM control for patients with type 2 DM (Fowler, 2007, p. 131). These agents are listed in Table 52-7.

Insulin Secretagogues. *Sulphonylureas* have been widely used to treat type 2 DM since the 1950s. The primary action of the sulphonylureas is to increase β-cell insulin production from the pancreas. Caution must be exercised in dosage determination in older adults and patients with renal impairment owing to the increased risk of hypoglycemia. Therapy with sulphonylureas is generally more effective early in the course of type 2 DM. According to one study, up to a third of patients on monotherapy with a sulfonylurea will require a second agent within 5 years (Kahn et al. 2006, p. 2427).

Nonsulphonylureas (Meglitinides). Like the sulphonylureas, repaglinide (GlucoNorm) and nateglinide (Starlix) increase insulin production from the pancreas. But because they are more rapidly absorbed and eliminated, they offer a reduced potential for hypoglycemia. When taken just before meals, pancreatic insulin production increases during and after the meal, mimicking the normal blood glucose response to eating. Patients should be instructed to take meglitinides anytime from 30 minutes before each meal right up to the time of the meal, and not to take a dose if they are not eating. They are safer to use in patients with irregular mealtimes.

Biguanides. Metformin (Glucophage) is the only biguanide glucose-lowering agent available worldwide. It can be used alone or with sulphonylureas, other OHAs, or insulin to treat type 2 DM. The primary action of Glucophage is to reduce glucose production by the liver. It also enhances insulin sensitivity at the tissue level and improves glucose transport into the cells. Glucophage is recommended as the first-line medication for most people with type 2 DM (CDA, 2008, p. S53). Besides being an effective blood glucose–lowering agent, metformin has other advantages. Unlike insulin secretagogues and insulin, Glucophage does not promote weight gain. It also has beneficial effects on plasma lipids. Glucophage is also used to treat prediabetes, especially in individuals who are obese and have impaired fasting glucose.

α-Glucosidase Inhibitors. Also known as *starch blockers*, glucosidase inhibitors work by slowing down the absorption of carbohydrate in the small intestine. Acarbose (Glucobay) is the available drug in this class. Taken with the first bite of each main meal, they are most effective in lowering postprandial blood glucose. Effectiveness of these medications is measured by checking 2-hour postprandial glucose levels. Medications from this

DRUG THERAPY

Table 52-7 Antihyperglycemic Agents for Diabetes Mellitus

TYPE	MECHANISM OF ACTION	ADVERSE EFFECTS
Insulin Secretagogues: Sulphonylureas		
Gliclazide (Diamicron, Diamicron MR) Glimepiride (Amaryl) Glyburide (Diabeta) (chlorpropamide and tolbutamide are available in Canada but rarely used)	Stimulate release of insulin from β cells; decrease glycogenolysis and gluconeogenesis; glimepiride may improve insensitivity in tissues	Weight gain, hypoglycemia
Nonsulphonylureas		
Nateglinide (Starlix) Repaglinide (GlucoNorm)	Stimulate a rapid and short-lived release of insulin from the pancreas	Less weight gain, decreased incidence of hypoglycemia compared to glyburide
Biguanide		
Metformin (Glucophage, Glumetza)	Inhibits hepatic glucose production; increases peripheral sensitivity to insulin and inhibits GI absorption of glucose	Nausea, upset stomach, diarrhea; less weight gain than sulphonylureas and does not cause hypoglycemia; potential lactic acidosis in renal or hepatic impairment; has to be held at the time of or before procedure and held for 48 hr after administration of IV contrast media
α-Glucosidase Inhibitors		
Acarbose (Glucobay)	Delay absorption of glucose and digestion of CHO in small intestine, lowering after-meal blood glucose levels	Flatulence, abdominal pain, diarrhea
Thiazolidinediones		
Pioglitazone (Actos) Rosiglitazone (Avandia)	↑ Glucose uptake in muscle and fat; inhibit hepatic glucose production	Edema, weight gain, CHF, causes ovulation in premenopausal women with PCOS; not recommended for patients with heart failure
Dipeptidyl Peptidase-4 Inhibitors		
Sitagliptin (Januvia) Saxagliptin (Onglyza) Linagliptin (Tradjenta)	Enhances the incretin system, stimulates release of insulin from pancreatic beta cells, and inhibits hepatic glucose production	Upper respiratory tract infection, sore throat, headache, diarrhea
Incretin Mimetic (Injectable)		
Liraglutide (Victoza) Exenatide (Byetta)	Stimulates release of insulin; decreases glucagon secretion, increases satiety, decreases gastric emptying	Nausea, vomiting, hypoglycemia, diarrhea, headache
Combination Therapy		
Avandamet (rosiglitazone [Avandia] and metformin [Glucophage]) Janumet (sitagliptin [Januvia] and metformin [Glucophage])	See mechanism of action for individual drugs above	See adverse effects for individual drugs above

CHF, congestive heart failure; *CHO,* carbohydrates; *GI,* gastrointestinal; *IV,* intravenous; *PCOS,* polycystic ovarian syndrome.

class are not effective against fasting hyperglycemia (Banting and Best Diabetes Centre [BBDC], 2009, p. 29).

Thiazolidinediones.
Sometimes referred to as *insulin sensitizers,* thiazolidinediones include pioglitazone (Actos) and rosiglitazone (Avandia). They are most effective for people who have insulin resistance. They improve insulin sensitivity, transport, and utilization at target tissues.

Because they do not increase insulin production, thiazolidinediones will not cause hypoglycemia when used alone, but the risk is still present when a thiazolidinedione is used in combination with an insulin secretagogue or insulin. Patients taking

these medications may experience a secondary benefit of improved triglyceride, high-density lipoprotein (HDL), and blood pressure levels (CDA, 2008, p. 55; BBDC, 2009, p. 29). Use with insulin is not approved in Canada because the combination potentiates the adverse effect of edema and subsequent weight gain.

Dipeptidyl Peptidase-4 Inhibitors.
A newer class of glucose-lowering drugs available in Canada include the dipeptidyl peptidase-4 (DPP-4) inhibitors. This class of drugs includes sitagliptin (Januvia) and saxagliptin (Onglyza). The incretin hormones, which are part of the physiological process that regulates

glucose homeostasis, are normally inactivated by DPP-4. By inhibiting DDP-4, these medications slow the inactivation of incretin hormones. Incretin hormones are released by the intestines throughout the day, but levels increase in response to a meal. When glucose levels are normal or elevated, incretins increase insulin synthesis and release from the pancreas as well as decrease hepatic glucose production. DPP-4 inhibitors manage type 2 DM by increasing and prolonging increased incretin levels. These drugs are glucose-dependent (i.e., they respond to the presence of elevated glucose and result in insulin release only when needed), and therefore, they lower the potential for hypoglycemia. The main benefit of these drugs over other medications for DM with similar effects is the absence of weight gain as a adverse effect. These drugs may be taken alone or in combination with other OHAs (Ross & Ekoe, 2010, p. 641; Bristol-Myers Squibb [BMS] Canada, 2011).

Combination Therapy. A few combination drugs are currently available. These drugs combine two different classes of medications to treat DM. These agents are listed in Table 52-6. One advantage of combined therapy is improved patient compliance.

Incretin Mimetic. Liraglutide (Victoza) and exenatide (Byetta) are the incretin mimetics available in Canada. These drugs stimulate one of the incretin hormones (glucagon-like peptide-1 [GLP-1]) found to be decreased in people with type 2 DM. The mechanisms of action of these drugs are similar to those performed by the incretin hormone it mimics. They stimulate the release of insulin from the pancreatic β cells. Other mechanisms of actions are (1) suppression of glucagon secretion from the pancreatic β cells, which reduces glucose output from the liver; (2) reduction of food intake by increasing satiety, thereby reducing caloric intake; and (3) slowing gastric emptying. It is not indicated for use with insulin. Liraglutide and exenatide are administered using a subcutaneous injection in a prefilled pen. (NovoNordisk, 2011; Eli Lilly Canada, 2011)

Other Drugs Affecting Blood Glucose Levels.
Both the patient and the health care provider must be aware of drug interactions that can potentiate hypoglycemic and hyperglycemic effects. For example, β-adrenergic blockers can mask symptoms of hypoglycemia and prolong the hypoglycemic effects of insulin. Thiazide and loop diuretics can potentiate hyperglycemia by inducing potassium loss, although low-dose therapy with a thiazide is usually considered safe.

Nutritional Therapy

Although nutritional therapy is the cornerstone of care for the person with DM, it is also its most challenging aspect. Nutritional therapy can reduce A1C by an absolute 1 to 2% with the greatest impact at the initial stages of DM. The effects of nutritional therapy are apparent anywhere between 6 weeks and 3 months from initiation (Franz, Boucher, Green-Pastors, & Powers, 2008, p. 52; BBDC, 2009, p. 10). Achieving nutritional goals requires a coordinated team effort that takes into account the behavioural, cognitive, socioeconomic, cultural, and spiritual aspects of the person. Because of these complexities, it is recommended that a DM nurse educator and a registered dietitian, with expertise in DM management, be members of the team.

Nutritional therapy for the management of DM is based on a plan of healthy eating that is appropriate and beneficial for all members of the general population, whether they have DM or not. In an institutional setting, the prescribed diet is often labelled "diabetic diet" or "no added sugar," indicating that the meal plan follows the CDA's current nutritional recommendations.

Eating Well with Canada's Food Guide (see Chapter 42, Figure 42-1) summarizes and illustrates nutritional guidelines and nutrient needs. These are appropriate in guiding the food choices of people with DM. Nutritional therapy and meal planning should be individualized to accommodate the person's preferences, age, needs, culture, lifestyle, and readiness to change. Tools used to measure the effectiveness of nutritional therapy include blood glucose, A1C, and lipid values; tests of renal status; and clinical measurements such as body weight, body mass index, waist circumference, and blood pressure (CDA, 2008, p. S40). Table 52-8 describes nutritional therapy for type 1 and type 2 DM.

NUTRITIONAL THERAPY

Table 52-8 Diabetes Mellitus

FACTOR	TYPE 1 DIABETES MELLITUS	TYPE 2 DIABETES MELLITUS
Total calories	Increase in caloric intake possibly necessary to achieve desirable body weight and restore body tissues	Reduction in caloric intake desirable for overweight or obese patient
Effect of diet	Diet and insulin necessary for glucose control	Diet alone possibly sufficient for glucose control
Distribution of calories	Equal distribution of carbohydrates through meals or adjustment of carbohydrates for insulin activity	Equal distribution recommended; low-fat diet desirable; consistency of carbohydrate at meals desirable
Consistency in daily intake	Necessary for glucose control	Desirable for weight reduction and moderation of blood glucose levels
Uniform timing of meals	Crucial for NPH insulin programs; flexibility with multidose rapid-acting insulin	Desirable but not essential, unless using insulin or sulphonylureas
Intermeal and bedtime snacks	Frequently necessary	Is based on patient's eating habits and preferences; may be necessary if using insulin or sulphonylurea
Nutritional supplement for exercise programs	Carbohydrates 20 g/hr for moderate physical activities	May be necessary if patient's blood glucose levels are controlled on sulphonylurea or insulin

NPH, neutral protamine Hagedorn.

The CDA provides a variety of nutrition teaching tools to assist health care providers. These are accessible online at the CDA's Web site or through the CDA office. The CDA resource *Just the Basics: Healthy Eating for Diabetes Management and Prevention* is an example of such a tool. It provides tips for healthy eating, DM prevention, and management for support until the person can see a dietitian. This tool highlights the need for the following:

1. Eating three meals per day at regular times and eating at intervals no more than 6 hours apart
2. Limiting sugars and sweets such as sugar, regular pop, desserts, candies, jam, and honey
3. Limiting the amount of high-fat food such as fried foods, chips, and pastries
4. Eating more high-fibre foods (whole-grain breads and cereals, lentils, dried beans and peas, brown rice, fruits, and vegetables)
5. Drinking water if thirsty
6. Adding physical activity to the lifestyle (CDA, 2008, p. S40)

Type 1 Diabetes Mellitus. Meal planning should be based on the individual's usual food intake and balanced with insulin and exercise patterns. The insulin regimen should be developed with the patient's eating habits and activity pattern in mind. Patients using rapid-acting insulin can make adjustments in dosage before the meal, based on the current blood glucose level and the carbohydrate content of the meal or snack. Intensified insulin therapy, such as multiple daily injections or the use of an insulin pump, allows considerable flexibility in food selection and can be adjusted for deviations from usual eating and exercise habits. All people with type 1 DM should be seen by a registered dietitian to learn about carbohydrate-counting strategies.

Type 2 Diabetes Mellitus. The emphasis for nutritional therapy in type 2 DM should be placed on achieving glucose, lipid, and blood pressure goals. Because 80 to 90% of people with type 2 DM are overweight, calorie and fat reduction is a goal. Weight loss has been shown to improve glycemic control by increasing insulin sensitivity and glucose uptake and decreasing hepatic glucose output (CDA, 2008, p. S77).

There is no one proven strategy or method that can be uniformly recommended. A nutritionally adequate meal plan with a reduction of total fat (especially saturated fats), an increase of fibre, and a decrease in simple sugars can bring about decreased calorie and carbohydrate consumption. Eating many small meals is another strategy that can be adopted to spread nutrient intake throughout the day. A weight loss of 5 to 7% of body weight often improves glycemic control, even if desirable body weight is not achieved. Weight loss is best attempted by a moderate decrease in calories and an increase in caloric expenditure. Regular exercise and learning new behaviours and attitudes can help facilitate long-term lifestyle changes. Monitoring of blood glucose levels, A1C, lipids, and blood pressure provides feedback on how well the goals of nutritional therapy are being met.

Food Composition. DM has been called a disease of carbohydrate metabolism, but it is actually a general metabolic disorder involving three categories of energy-providing nutrients: carbohydrates, fats, and proteins. Therefore, the nutrient balance of a diabetic diet is essential to maintenance of blood glucose levels. The nutritional energy intake should be constantly balanced with the energy output of the individual, taking into account exercise and metabolic work of the body. The following

are general recommendations for nutrient balance; each patient's individual meal plan should be developed with a dietitian and with her or his lifestyle and health goals in mind and is based on Canada's food guide (Health Canada, 2007; CDA, 2008, p. S40; American Diabetes Association [ADA], 2008, p. S61):

- *Protein:* 15 to 20% of energy. There is no evidence that usual protein intake (15-20% of energy) should be modified. Those with diabetic nephropathy should limit protein intake to 15% of energy and be monitored closely by a registered dietitian.
- *Fat:* less than 35% of energy. Reduce combined saturated fats and *trans*-fatty acids to less than 7% of energy intake. Limit polyunsaturated fat to less than 10% of energy intake. Include foods rich in polyunsaturated omega-3 fatty acids and plant oils.
- *Fibre:* approximately 25 to 50 g/day from a variety of food sources, including soluble and cereal fibres.
- *Carbohydrate:* 45 to 60% of energy. Carbohydrates should include whole grains, fruits, vegetables, and low-fat milk. Patients should try to consume higher-fibre sources of carbohydrate. Less than 10% of daily energy should come from sucrose (sugar). Low-carbohydrate diets are not recommended for DM management.

Glycemic index (GI) is the term used to describe the rise in blood glucose levels after a person has consumed carbohydrate-containing food. The GI of foods was developed to compare the postprandial responses of the body to carbohydrate-containing foods. A GI of 100 refers to the response to 50 g of glucose or white bread in a normal person without DM. All other food with an equivalent carbohydrate value is measured against this standard. For example, the GI of an apple is 52, regular milk 27, baked potato 93, cornflake cereal 119, and baked beans 69 (ADA, 2008, p. S63) (see the Resources at the end of this chapter for an online calculator for GI).

The GI of carbohydrates should be considered when choosing them in a meal plan. Foods with a high GI (e.g., potatoes, white bread) will cause a sharp rise in blood glucose, whereas those with a low GI (e.g., brown rice) steadily increase blood glucose over a longer period. Although the GI affects blood glucose, the total amount of carbohydrates is more important than the source (CDA, 2008, p. S40).

Nutritive and nonnutritive sweeteners may be included in a healthy meal plan in moderation. Nonnutritive sweeteners include the sugar substitutes saccharin, aspartame, sucralose, acesulphame-K and cyclamate (CDA, 2008, p. S41).

Alcohol. Alcohol is high in calories, has no nutritive value, and can be a partner in contributing to hypertriglyceridemia. In addition, it has detrimental effects on the liver (see Chapter 46). The inhibitory effect of alcohol on glucose production by the liver can cause severe hypoglycemia in patients taking insulin or OHAs that increase insulin secretion. Hypoglycemia may occur up to 24 hours after alcohol consumption in those with type 1 DM. Because alcohol consumption can make blood glucose more difficult to control, patients should be encouraged to discuss the use of alcohol honestly with their health care providers (CDA, 2008, p. S42).

Alcohol can also cause other serious adverse effects when used in conjunction with certain OHAs used to treat DM. For example, there is a risk of lactic acidosis in patients who have alcohol dependency and use Glucophage. Alcohol consumption should be limited to 1 to 2 standard drinks per day (e.g., 1 glass or 142 mL wine) or fewer than 14 standard drinks per week for men and fewer than 9 for women (CDA, 2008, p. S42). Alcohol can sometimes be incorporated into healthy eating if blood glucose is well controlled and if the patient is not on medications that will cause adverse effects. A patient can reduce the risk for alcohol-induced hyperglycemia or hypoglycemia by consuming alcohol with food, using sugar-free mixes, and drinking dry, light wines (CDA, 2008, p. S42).

Healthy Eating Education. Dietitians are the primary source of nutrition education. However, all members of the interdisciplinary team should be prepared to answer basic questions about healthy eating and DM. Access to a dietitian may not be possible for patients who live in remote areas, and nurses often assume responsibility for teaching basic dietary management. *Eating Well with Canada's Food Guide* (see Chapter 42, Figure 42-1) is a simple, accessible, and appropriate tool for health care team members to use to educate people with DM about nutrition.

An effective method of presenting the basics of meal planning is the *plate method*. This simple method helps the patient visualize the amount of vegetables, starch, and protein that should fill a dinner plate (RNAO, 2009, p. 79). For lunch and dinner, one half of the plate is filled with vegetables, one fourth is filled with a starch, and one fourth is filled with 60 to 90 g (2 to 3 oz) of lean meat or other protein source. A glass of low-fat milk and a small piece of fresh fruit complete the meal. The breakfast plate is filled halfway with starch, and one fourth of the plate contains an optional protein. Low-fat milk and fresh fruit complete the breakfast. Assuming low-fat and nonfat foods are selected, following the plate method will provide a well-balanced diet.

Nutrition education should include the patient's family and significant others, and it is most effective to teach the person who will be cooking. However, it is important that the responsibility for making healthy food choices not fall to someone other than the patient with DM. A support network of family and friends is the key to making successful and sustainable nutritional and lifestyle changes.

In an acute health care facility, the nutritional needs of the patient with DM vary slightly from the normal meal plans. Previously, standardized calorie-level meal patterns were used, but new alternatives are now being used, such as the consistent-carbohydrate DM meal plan. Under this system, meal plans are not created according to calorie levels, but instead are created with consistent carbohydrate content. For example, every day, each breakfast contains the same amount of carbohydrates as the previous day; the same method is used for lunch and dinner (ADA, 2008, p. S73).

Exercise

Regular, consistent exercise is considered an essential part of DM and prediabetes management. Exercise increases insulin sensitivity and can have a direct effect on lowering the blood glucose levels. It also contributes to weight loss, which also decreases insulin resistance. The therapeutic benefits of regular physical activity may result in a decreased need for DM medicines in order to reach target blood glucose goals. Regular exercise may also help reduce triglyceride and low-density lipoprotein (LDL) cholesterol levels, reduce blood pressure, and improve circulation (Levene & Donnelly, 2008, p. 29; CDA, 2008, p. S37). Any new exercise program in the person with DM should be started only after medical clearance and should be started slowly with gradual progression toward the desired goal. People with type 2 DM should accumulate at least 150

minutes of moderate-intensity aerobic activity—such as brisk walking, cycling, or dancing—each week, spread over at least 3 separate days. Performance of resistance exercises three times per week should also be encouraged in addition to aerobic exercise (CDA, 2008, p. S38).

Before starting an exercise program, all patients with DM should undergo a pre-exercise assessment by a medical doctor and should be started slowly with gradual progression toward the desired goal (CDA, 2008, p. S37). Patients who use insulin and insulin secretagogues, such as sulphonylureas or meglitinides, are at increased risk for hypoglycemia when there is an increase in physical activity, especially if the patient exercises at the time of peak drug action or if food intake has not been sufficient to maintain adequate blood glucose levels. This can also occur if a normally sedentary patient with DM has an unusually active day. The glucose-lowering effects of exercise can last up to 48 hours after the activity, so it is possible for hypoglycemia to occur during that time. It is recommended that patients who use medications that can cause hypoglycemia schedule exercise about 1 hour after a meal or have a 10- to 15-g carbohydrate snack before exercising. Several small carbohydrate snacks can be taken every 30 minutes during exercise to prevent hypoglycemia. Patients using medications that place them at risk for hypoglycemia should always carry a fast-acting source of carbohydrate, such as juice, glucose tablets, or hard candies, when exercising. Table 52-9 gives guidelines on the number of calories burned per hour for different activities.

Although exercise is generally beneficial to blood glucose levels, strenuous activity can be perceived by the body as a stress, causing a release of counter-regulatory hormones that results in a temporary elevation of blood glucose. As a result, hyperglycemia may occur in cases of poorly controlled type 2 DM or in patients with type 1 DM who exercise at a time of day when insulin action is waning. Some patients may have to inject a small bolus of rapid-acting or regular insulin if the blood glucose level is elevated before exercising to prevent progressive hyperglycemia. Furthermore, patients should exercise with caution if the blood glucose is elevated and there are no ketones. However, exercise should be avoided when the blood sugar is elevated and urine ketones are present (ADA, 2011, p. S24). Additional information about exercise and DM that is important for both the patient and the health care provider is provided in the Patient and Caregiver Teaching Guide (Table 52-10).

Table 52-9 Activities That Affect Caloric Expenditure		
LIGHT ACTIVITY (100–200 kcal/hr)	**MODERATE ACTIVITY (200–350 kcal/hr)**	**VIGOROUS ACTIVITY (400–900 kcal/hr)**
• Driving a car	• Active housework	• Aerobic exercise
• Fishing	• Bicycling (light)	• Bicycling (vigorous)
• Light housework	• Bowling	• Hard labour
• Secretarial work	• Dancing	• Ice skating
• Teaching	• Gardening	• Outdoor sports
• Walking casually	• Golfing	• Running
	• Roller skating	• Soccer
	• Walking briskly	• Tennis
		• Wood chopping

Table 52-10 Exercise for Patients With Diabetes Mellitus

1. Exercise does not have to be vigorous to be effective. The blood glucose–reducing effects of exercise can be attained with exercise such as brisk walking. The exercises selected should be enjoyable to foster regularity.

2. It is important to have properly fitting footwear.

3. The exercise session should have a warm-up period and a cool-down period. The program should be started gradually and increased slowly.

4. Exercise plans should be individualized for each patient and monitored by the health care provider.

5. Exercise is best done after meals, when the blood glucose level is rising.

6. It is important to self-monitor blood glucose levels before, during, and after exercise to determine the effect exercise has on blood glucose level at particular times of the day.
   - Before exercise, if blood glucose <5.5 mmol/L, eat a 10- to 15-g carbohydrate snack (one small apple or four to six crackers). After 15-30 min, retest blood glucose levels. Do not exercise if <5.5 mmol/L.
   - If blood glucose >14 mmol/L before exercise in a person with type 1 diabetes and ketones are present, vigorous activity should be avoided.
   - Recheck blood glucose at the end of the exercise program.

7. Take sources of carbohydrate with you during exercise at all times. Liquid sources may be the best tolerated and quickest to take effect in case of hypoglycemia.

8. Be alert to the possibility of delayed exercise-induced hypoglycemia, which may occur several hours after the completion of exercise.

9. Taking a glucose-lowering medication does not mean that planned or spontaneous exercise cannot occur.

10. It is important to compensate for extensive planned and spontaneous activity by monitoring blood glucose level to make adjustments in the insulin dose (if taken) and food intake.

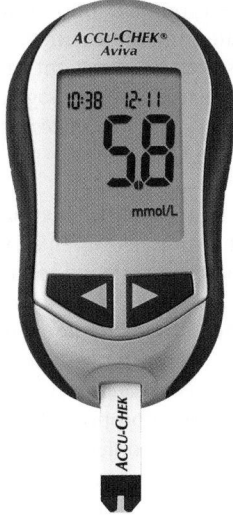

Figure 52-8 A blood glucose monitor (Accu-Chek Aviva) is used to measure blood glucose levels.

Source: Courtesy Roche Diagnostics Canada, Laval, QC.

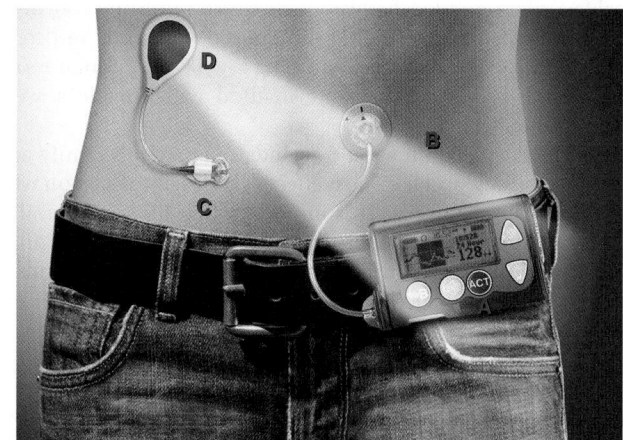

Figure 52-9 The MiniMed Paradigm insulin pump **(A)** delivers insulin into a cannula **(B)** that sits under the skin. Continuous glucose monitoring occurs through a tiny sensor **(C)** inserted under the skin. Sensor data are sent continuously to the transmitter **(D).** The transmitter sends data to the insulin pump through wireless technology.

Source: Courtesy Medtronic Diabetes.

Monitoring Blood Glucose

Self-monitoring of blood glucose (SMBG) is a cornerstone of DM management. By providing a "real-time" blood glucose reading, SMBG enables the patient to make self-management decisions regarding diet, exercise, and medication. SMBG is also important for detecting episodic hyperglycemia and hypoglycemia.

Portable blood glucose meters are used at the hospital bedside and by patients who perform SMBG independently. A wide variety of blood glucose meters are available (Figure 52-8). Disposable lancets are usually used to obtain a small drop of capillary blood (usually from a finger stick) that is placed onto a glucose testing strip. After a specified time, the meter displays a digital reading of the blood glucose. The technology of SMBG is a rapidly changing field, with more convenient systems being introduced every year. Newer systems allow the user to collect blood from alternative sites such as the forearm or the palm but will not register rapidly changing blood glucose readings. Therefore, finger sticks are still recommended if symptoms of low blood glucose are present. The most advanced systems require 4 seconds to provide results with only 0.3 µL of capillary blood.

The only invasive glucose monitor available in Canada is the Medtronic MiniMed Paradigm REAL-Time System (Figure 52-9). Using a sensor inserted under the skin, it displays glucose values continuously with updated values occurring every 5 minutes. The sensor is inserted by the patient using an automatic insertion device. Data are sent from the sensor to a transmitter, which displays the glucose value on an insulin pump. This system assists the patient and health care provider to identify trends and track patterns. These data are particularly useful for the management of insulin therapy. The patient is alerted during episodes of hypoglycemia and hyperglycemia, allowing corrective action to be taken quickly. Both systems still require finger-stick measurements using a blood glucose monitor to calibrate the sensor and to make treatment decisions.

The blood glucose level reported by a laboratory is sometimes higher than the patient's home glucose monitor or the hospital's portable meter. This is because some meters give capillary blood glucose values from whole blood (via finger stick), whereas venous samples taken in the laboratory provide plasma readings. Plasma samples, or venous samples, are approximately 10 to 12% higher. Most meters are automatically calibrated to give a "plasma" test result (although whole blood was used for the sample) so that the home readings can be more readily compared with laboratory values. The literature accompanying a meter will identify whether that particular meter is calibrated to give plasma or whole blood readings.

Instructions for using a blood glucose meter accompany each product. Because errors in monitoring technique can cause errors in management strategies, thorough patient education is crucial. Initial education should be followed up at regular intervals with reassessment. In addition, patients must be taught to calibrate and use control solutions that are a part of each blood glucose monitoring kit (AADE, 2010, p. 1). Table 52-11 lists the steps that should be taught to the patient learning to perform SMBG.

The primary advantage of SMBG is that it supplies immediate information about blood glucose levels that can be used to make adjustments in food intake, activity patterns, and medication dosages. It also produces accurate records of daily glucose fluctuations and trends as well as alerting the patient to acute episodes of hyperglycemia and hypoglycemia. Furthermore, it provides patients with a tool for achieving and maintaining specific glycemic goals. SMBG is recommended as an essential part of daily DM management for all people using insulin or OHAs. The frequency of monitoring depends on several factors, including the patient's glycemic goals, the type of DM that the patient has, the patient's ability and willingness to perform the test independently, and the treatment regimen. It is recommended that patients with type 1 DM test at least three times per day and include both preprandial and postprandial testing. Those using an insulin pump may test more frequently. People with type 2 DM treated with OHAs or lifestyle alone will have more variable and individualized testing regimens. For patients with type 2 DM treated with once-daily insulin and OHAs, monitoring at least once daily is recommended (CDA, 2008, p. S32).

Blood glucose testing should also be performed whenever hypoglycemia is suspected so that immediate action can be taken if necessary. When the person with DM is ill, the blood glucose should be tested at 4-hour intervals to determine the effects of this stressor on the blood glucose level (BBDC, 2009, p. 76).

SMBG is an empowering tool that allows the patient to be an active partner in the treatment of DM. Achieving the desired level of patient participation does require time and effort from the health care provider. The nurse involved in this aspect of management should anticipate a close working relationship with patients as they refine their techniques and learn appropriate decision making about managing their DM. A patient who is visually impaired, cognitively impaired, or limited in manual dexterity needs careful evaluation of the degree to which SMBG can be performed independently. Nurses working in home health and outpatient settings may need to identify caregivers who can assume this responsibility. Adaptive devices are available to help patients with certain limitations. These include "talking meters" and other equipment for the visually impaired as well as devices to stabilize insulin vials and syringes for those with limitations affecting dexterity.

PATIENT & CAREGIVER TEACHING GUIDE

Table 52-11 Obtaining a Capillary Sample for Blood Glucose Testing

1. Wash hands with soap and warm water. It is not necessary to clean the site with alcohol, and it may interfere with test results by artificially lowering them.

2. If it is difficult to obtain an adequate drop of blood for testing, do any or all of the following: warm the hands in warm water, let the arm hang down for a few minutes before the finger puncture is made, use a new lancet with every puncture, or use a higher setting on the lancing device.

3. If the puncture is made on the finger, use the side of the finger pad rather than near the centre. There are fewer nerve endings along the side of the finger pad. If an alternative site is used (e.g., forearm), special equipment may be needed. Alternative-site testing is not recommended after a meal or for people with erratic blood glucose control experiencing hypoglycemia. Refer to manufacturer's instructions for alternative-site use.

4. The puncture should be only deep enough to obtain a sufficiently large drop of blood. Unnecessarily deep punctures may cause pain and bruising.

5. Lancets should be disposed of in designated "sharps" containers obtained from drug stores. Lancets and needles should not be placed in garbage cans, recycling bins, toilets, or glass jars.

CULTURALLY COMPETENT CARE: DIABETES MELLITUS

Because culture can have a strong influence on dietary preferences and meal preparation practices, culturally competent care has special relevance for the patient with diabetes. This is especially pertinent when considering the prevalence of diabetes in diverse Canadian cultural groups such as people of Aboriginal, Hispanic, and South Asian, Asian, or African descent. The influence of culture on food choices and meal planning should be explored with the patient as part of the health history. When giving diet instructions, efforts should be made to consider the food preferences of the cultural group. Nutritional resources specifically designed for members of different cultural groups are available from the Canadian Diabetes Association.

NURSING MANAGEMENT: DIABETES MELLITUS

Nursing Assessment

Table 52-12 provides initial subjective and objective data that might be obtained from a person with DM. After the initial assessment, periodic patient assessments should be done on a regular basis.

NURSING ASSESSMENT

Table 52-12 Diabetes Mellitus

Subjective Data

Important Health Information

Past health history: Mumps, rubella, coxsackievirus, or other viral infections; recent trauma, infection, or stress; pregnancy, gave birth to infant >4 kg; chronic pancreatitis; Cushing's syndrome, acromegaly; family history of type 1 or type 2 diabetes mellitus; obesity

Date of last eye and dental examination, compliance with diet in patients with previously diagnosed diabetes

Medications: Use of and compliance with insulin or OHAs; use of corticosteroids, diuretics, phenytoin (Dilantin)

Surgery or other treatments: Any recent surgery

Symptoms

- Malaise
- Weight loss (type 1), weight gain (type 2)
- Thirst, hunger, nausea and vomiting
- Poor healing, especially involving the feet
- Constipation or diarrhea; frequent urination, nocturia, urinary incontinence
- Skin infections, pruritus
- Muscle weakness, fatigue
- Abdominal pain, headache; blurred vision; numbness or tingling of extremities
- Erectile dysfunction; frequent vaginal infections; decreased libido
- Depression, irritability, apathy

Objective Data

Eyes

Vitreal hemorrhages; cataracts; soft, sunken eyeballs*

Integumentary

Dry, warm, inelastic skin; pigmented lesions (on legs); ulcers (especially on feet), loss of hair on toes

Respiratory

Rapid, deep respirations (Kussmaul's respirations)

Cardiovascular

Hypotension; weak, rapid pulse, peripheral pulses diminished, feet pale and cool to touch

Gastrointestinal

Dry mouth, vomiting, fruity breath

Neurological

Altered reflexes, restlessness, confusion, stupor, coma, reduced sensation and/or vibration sense in feet

Musculoskeletal

Muscle wasting

Possible Findings

- Glucose level ≥7.0 mmol/L; glucose tolerance test ≥11.1 mmol/L; glycosylated hemoglobin (≥6%)
- Urinalysis: glycosuria, ketonuria, microalbuminuria, or proteinuria
- Other: serum electrolyte abnormalities; acidosis; ↑ creatinine, ↑ total cholesterol, LDL, VLDL and triglycerides; ↓ HDL; leukocytosis

HDL, high-density lipoprotein; *LDL,* low-density lipoprotein; *OHA,* oral antihyperglycemic agent; *VLDL,* very low density lipoprotein.
*Indicates manifestations of ketoacidosis.

Nursing Diagnoses

Nursing diagnoses related to DM may include, but are not limited to, those found in Nursing Care Plan (NCP) 52-1.

Planning

The overall goals for the patient with DM include the following: (1) to be an active participant in the management of the DM regimen; (2) to experience few or no episodes of hypoglycemia or acute hyperglycemic emergencies; (3) to maintain blood glucose levels at normal or near-normal levels; (4) to prevent, minimize, or delay the occurrence of chronic complications of DM; and (5) to adjust lifestyle to accommodate DM regimen with a minimum of stress.

Nursing Implementation

Health Promotion

The role of the nurse in health promotion and maintenance relates to the identification, the monitoring, and the education of the patient at risk for the development of DM. Obesity is the number one predictor of type 2 DM. The Diabetes Prevention Program (DPP) found that a modest weight loss of 5 to 10% of body weight and regular exercise of 30 minutes five times a week lowered the risk of developing type 2 DM up to 58% (DPP, 2002, p. 2165).

The CDA recommends screening every 3 years in individuals 40 years of age or older with no other risk factors and more frequently in individuals younger than 40 years with risk factors. The FPG is the preferred method for screening in clinical settings, although the OGTT is also suitable in those with IFG plus risk factors. Testing should be considered at a younger age or be carried out more frequently in individuals who meet the criteria listed in Table 52-13 (CDA, 2008, p. S15). It is important to know where an individual is on the glucose continuum (Figure 52-10).

Acute Intervention

Acute situations involving the patient with DM include hypoglycemia, DKA, and HHS. Nursing management for these situations is discussed in more detail later in this chapter. Other areas of acute intervention relate to management during stress, such as during acute illness and surgery.

Stress of Acute Illness and Surgery.
Both emotional and physical stress can increase the blood glucose level and result in hyperglycemia. Because it is impossible to totally avoid stress in life, certain situations may require more intense management, such as extra insulin, to maintain glycemic goals and prevent hyperglycemia.

Acute illness, injury, and surgery are situations that may evoke a counter-regulatory hormone response resulting in hyperglycemia. Even minor illnesses such as a viral upper respiratory infection or the flu can cause this. When patients with DM are ill, they should continue with the regular meal plan while increasing the intake of noncarbohydrate-containing fluids, such as broth, water, and other decaffeinated beverages. They should also continue taking OHAs and insulin as prescribed and check blood

NURSING CARE PLAN 52-1

Diabetes Mellitus

NURSING DIAGNOSIS	*Ineffective self-health management* related to insufficient knowledge as evidenced by continued hyperglycemia, inaccurate statements regarding diabetes and its management, and stated confusion regarding the pathophysiology of diabetes and its treatment
Expected Patient Outcomes	**Nursing Interventions and *Rationales***

Expected Patient Outcomes

- Verbalizes key elements of the therapeutic regimen, including knowledge of disease and treatment plan
- Describes self-care measures that may prevent or decrease progression of chronic complications

Nursing Interventions and *Rationales*

Teaching: disease process

- Appraise the patient's current level of knowledge related to specific disease process *to determine the scope and extent of required teaching.*
- Describe the disease process and therapy or treatment recommendations *to enable patient to better understand rationale behind treatment regimen and lifestyle changes.*
- Instruct patient on measures to prevent or minimize symptoms *to promote management of the disease.*
- Discuss lifestyle changes that may be required *to prevent future complications and control the disease process to encourage patient to actively participate in determining changes that will be acceptable.*
- Describe possible chronic complications as appropriate *to increase awareness of the long-term effects of inadequate control of disease process.*
- Plan individualized exercise program with patient *because exercise is an integral part of diabetes management.*
- Review steps to prevent hyperglycemia and hypoglycemia *because activity changes can cause changes in insulin needs.*
- Instruct patient on which signs and symptoms to report to health care provider *to ensure prompt treatment.*
- Review insulin administration (if used); have patient give return demonstration of insulin injection *to ensure proper technique.*
- Review OHA regimen; have patient explain timing and purpose of medication *to ensure understanding.*
- Refer patient to local community agencies or support groups *to provide continuing support and education.*

NURSING DIAGNOSIS	*Imbalanced nutrition: more than body requirements* related to intake in excess of activity expenditure or medication coverage as evidenced by hyperglycemia, weight gain
Expected Patient Outcome	**Nursing Interventions and *Rationales***

Expected Patient Outcome

- Maintains a balance of nutrition, activity, and insulin availability that results in normal blood glucose levels and optimum weight

Nursing Interventions and *Rationales*

Teaching: prescribed diet

- Determine patient's/caregiver's feelings and attitude toward prescribed diet and expected degree of dietary compliance *to determine readiness to learn.*
- Assist the patient to accommodate food preferences in the prescribed diet *to improve adherence.*
- Refer patient and significant other to dietitian or nutritionist *to provide continuing diet education and evaluation.*

Teaching: prescribed activity and exercise

- Inform the patient of the purpose for, and the benefits of, the prescribed activity and exercise *to improve commitment to activity.*
- Instruct the patient how to monitor tolerance of the activity and exercise *to prevent injury.*
- Assist the patient to incorporate activity and exercise regimen into daily routine or lifestyle *because it is an integral part of diabetes control.*

Hyperglycemia management

- Monitor for signs and symptoms of hyperglycemia: polyuria, polydipsia, polyphagia, weakness, lethargy, malaise, blurring of vision, or headache *to alert patient to glucose–insulin imbalance and need for treatment.*
- Anticipate situations in which insulin requirements will increase (e.g., illness) *to allow patient to adjust insulin dosage appropriately and avoid undue fatigue.*
- Facilitate adherence to diet and exercise regimen *to promote diabetes control.*
- Restrict exercise when blood glucose levels are >14 mmol/L, especially when ketones are present, *to decrease the body's requirement for already unavailable glucose.*

NURSING CARE PLAN 52-1

Diabetes Mellitus—cont'd

NURSING DIAGNOSIS	*Risk for injury* related to decreased tactile sensation, episodes of hypoglycemia
Expected Patient Outcomes	**Nursing Interventions and *Rationales***

- Experiences no injury resulting from decreased sensation in feet
- Experiences no injury resulting from hypoglycemia

Teaching: foot care

- Perform a comprehensive foot assessment for neuropathy using a 10-g monofilament or 128-Hz tuning fork *to establish baseline findings.*
- Provide information regarding the relationship between neuropathy, injury, and vascular disease and the risk for ulceration and lower extremity amputation in people with diabetes *to promote commitment to care.*
- Caution about potential sources of injury to the feet (e.g., heat, cold, cutting corns or calluses, chemicals, use of strong antiseptics or astringents, use of adhesive tape, and going barefoot or wearing thongs, open-toe shoes, or ill-fitting shoes) *to prevent injury to feet.*
- Instruct individual to inspect inside of shoes daily for foreign objects, nail points, torn linings, and rough areas *to avoid injury by factors that are not felt.*
- Recommend specialist care for thick fungal or ingrown toenails, corns, calluses *to ensure safe treatment of feet.*

Hypoglycemia management

- Monitor for signs and symptoms of hypoglycemia *to alert patient to glucose–insulin imbalance and need for treatment.*
- Determine patient's recognition of hypoglycemia signs and symptoms *to assess learning needs.*
- Instruct patient to have simple carbohydrate available at all times *to treat hypoglycemia.*
- Instruct patient to obtain and carry or wear appropriate emergency identification *to facilitate treatment by others.*

NURSING DIAGNOSIS	*Risk for peripheral neurovascular dysfunction* related to vascular effects of diabetes
Expected Patient Outcomes	**Nursing Interventions and *Rationales***

- Verbalizes effects of diabetes on peripheral artery circulation
- Implements measures to increase peripheral circulatory status
- Experiences no injury to feet from impaired circulation

Circulatory care: arterial insufficiency

- Perform a comprehensive appraisal of peripheral circulation (e.g., check peripheral pulses, edema, capillary refill, colour, and temperature) *to establish baseline findings.*
- Inspect skin for arterial ulcers or tissue breakdown *to provide treatment and to prevent infection and additional necrosis.*
- Protect the extremity from injury (e.g., sheepskin under feet and lower legs, footboard or bed cradle at foot of bed; well-fitted shoes) *to prevent conditions that favour skin breakdown.*
- Maintain adequate hydration *to decrease blood viscosity.*
- Encourage the patient to obtain exercise as tolerated *to increase peripheral circulation.*
- Instruct the patient on factors that interfere with circulation (e.g., smoking, restrictive clothing, exposure to cold temperatures, crossing of legs and feet) *to prevent impairment of circulation.*
- Instruct the patient on proper foot care, including footwear, *to prevent injury and infection* (see Table 52-21).

OHA, oral antihyperglycemic agent.

---

glucose at least every 4 hours around the clock. With type 1 DM, if the glucose is greater than 14 mmol/L, urine should be tested for ketones every 3 to 4 hours. Patients should report moderate to large ketone levels to the health care provider.

When the illness causes the patient to eat less than normal, the patient should continue to take OHAs, insulin, or both as prescribed while supplementing food intake with carbohydrate-containing fluids. Examples include soups, juices, and regular decaffeinated soft drinks (BBDC, 2009, p. 76). The health care provider should be notified promptly if the patient is unable to keep anything down, and the patient should go to the emergency department if vomiting occurs more than twice in 12 hours. The patient should understand that medication for DM, including

insulin, should not be withheld during times of illness because counter-regulatory mechanisms often increase the blood glucose level dramatically. Food intake is also important during this time because the body requires extra energy to deal with the stress of the illness. Extra insulin may be necessary to meet this demand and to prevent the onset of DKA in the patient with type 1 DM (Wesorick, O'Malley, & Rushakoff, 2008, p. S20).

During the perioperative period, adjustments in the DM regimen can be planned to ensure glycemic control. For patients undergoing major surgery who require insulin (type 1 or type 2 DM), IV fluids with dextrose and insulin are administered immediately before, during, and after surgery. For patients undergoing minor or moderate surgery who require insulin (type 1 or type 2

Table 52-13 Criteria for Testing in Asymptomatic, Undiagnosed Individuals

Type 1 Diabetes Mellitus

Testing presumably healthy individuals for the presence of any immune markers (e.g., HLA), outside of a clinical trial setting, is not recommended.

Type 2 Diabetes Mellitus

In asymptomatic, undiagnosed individuals, testing for diabetes should be considered in all individuals at ≥40 yr and, if normal, should be repeated at 3-yr intervals.

Testing* should be considered at a younger age, or be carried out more frequently, in individuals who

- Have a first-degree relative with type 2 diabetes
- Are members of a high-risk ethnic population (Aboriginal, Hispanic, South Asian, Asian, or African descent)
- Have a history of impaired fasting glucose or impaired glucose tolerance
- Have complications associated with diabetes
- Have vascular disease
- Have a history of gestational diabetes mellitus
- Have delivered a macrosomic infant (>4.4 kg)
- Have hypertension
- Have dyslipidemia
- Are overweight, particularly with abdominal obesity
- Have polycystic ovary syndrome
- Have acanthosis nigricans
- Have schizophrenia

HLA, human lymphocyte antigen.
*Testing may include fasting plasma glucose (FPG) or oral glucose tolerance test (OGTT). The FPG is the recommended diagnostic test because of its ease of administration, convenience, acceptability to patients, and lower cost.
Source: Adapted from Canadian Diabetes Association (CDA) Clinical Practice Guidelines Expert Committee. (2008). Clinical practice guidelines for the prevention and management of diabetes in Canada. *Canadian Journal of Diabetes Care, 32*(Suppl 1), S14.

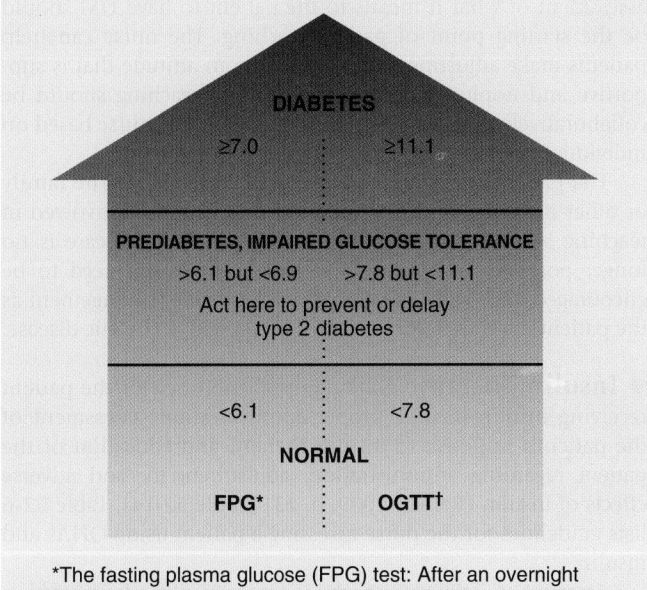

*The fasting plasma glucose (FPG) test: After an overnight fast, blood glucose is measured in the morning.

†The 2-hour oral glucose tolerance test (OGTT): Includes a fasting blood glucose test and glucose measurements 2 hours after drinking a glucose-containing solution.

Note: The Canadian Diabetes Association believes that either test is appropriate to measure prediabetes (impaired glucose tolerance) and diabetes.

Figure 52-10 The glucose continuum. Numbers represent blood glucose levels in millimoles per litre (mmol/L).

▮ Ambulatory and Home Care

Successful management of DM requires ongoing interaction among the patient, the family, and the health care team. It is important that a DM nurse educator be involved in the care of the patient and the family. This person provides expertise in many areas of specialized care needs.

Because DM is a complex, chronic condition, a great deal of patient contact takes place in outpatient and home settings. The major goal of patient care in these settings is to enable the patient or caregiver to reach an optimal level of independence in self-care activities. Unfortunately, many patients with DM face challenges in reaching these goals. DM increases the risk for other chronic conditions that can affect self-care activities. These include visual impairment, lower extremity problems that affect mobility, and other functional limitations related to cardiovascular disease. Therefore, important nursing functions are to assess the ability of patients and caregivers in such activities as meal preparation, SMBG, safe administration of OHAs, and insulin injection techniques. Assistive devices for self-administration of insulin include syringe magnifiers, vial stabilizers, and dose-preparation aids for the visually impaired as well as pill organizers for those taking OHAs. In some cases, the nurse will make referrals to others who can help the patient achieve the self-care goals. These may include a community health nurse, pharmacist, dietitian, occupational therapist, or social worker.

A diagnosis of DM affects the patient in many profound ways. Patients with DM must continually contend with lifestyle choices that affect the food they eat, the activities they engage in, and the demands on their time and energy. In addition, they face the prospect of the devastating complications of this disease. Careful

DM), recommendations will be provided by the physician to reduce the insulin dosage the night before and day of surgery. For patients taking OHAs who are undergoing major, moderate, or minor surgery, DM medications may be put on hold for as long as 24 hours before the day of surgery, and IV fluids with dextrose and insulin may be administered. The patient should understand that this is a temporary measure and is not to be interpreted as a worsening of DM. Patients who are undergoing surgery or any radiological procedures that involve the use of a contrast medium are instructed to hold their Glucophage at the time of or before surgery or the procedure. They will also be instructed not to resume the Glucophage until 48 hours after the surgery or the procedure and after their serum creatinine has been checked and is normal (Bristol-Meyers Squibb [BMS] Company, 2008).

The nurse caring for an unconscious surgical patient receiving insulin must be alert for signs of hypoglycemia, such as sweating, tachycardia, and tremors. Frequent monitoring of blood glucose will prevent episodes of severe hypoglycemia in such a patient (BBDC, 2009, p. 66).

assessment of what it means to the patient to have DM should be the starting point of patient teaching. The nurse can help patients make adjustments by displaying an attitude that is supportive and nonjudgemental. The goals of teaching should be collaboratively determined by the patient and the nurse based on individual needs as well as therapeutic requirements.

The patient's support system must be identified. The family or other members of the support system need to be involved in teaching so they can care for the patient when self-care is no longer possible. The family and significant others need to be encouraged to provide emotional support and encouragement as the patient deals with the reality of living with a chronic disease.

▮ Insulin Therapy.

Nursing responsibilities for the patient receiving insulin include proper administration, assessment of the patient's response to insulin therapy, and education of the patient regarding administration, adjustment to, and adverse effects of insulin (RNAO, 2009, p. 23) (Table 52-14). Table 52-6 lists guidelines for the nurse assessing a patient using OHAs and insulin.

Assessment of the patient who is new to insulin administration must include an evaluation of the patient's ability to manage this therapy safely. This includes the ability to understand the interaction of insulin, diet, and activity and to be able to recognize and treat the symptoms of hypoglycemia appropriately. If the patient does not have the cognitive skills to do these things, another responsible person must be identified and educated. The patient or caregiver must also have the cognitive and the manual skills needed to prepare and inject the insulin. If the patient or family lacks these, additional resources will be needed to assist the patient.

Many patients are fearful when they first begin using insulin. Some patients find it difficult to self-inject because they are afraid of needles or the pain associated with an injection. Some are afraid they will hurt themselves by giving too much or too little insulin. And in some cases, the patient believes that using insulin is a "last ditch" effort and that he or she is now in the final stages of the disease process. Therefore, it is important to explore the patient's underlying fears before beginning the teaching (Shaefer, 2007, p. S41; RNAO, 2009, p. 20).

Follow-up assessment of the patient who has been using insulin therapy includes an inspection of injection sites for signs of lipodystrophy and other reactions; review of insulin preparation, storage, timing, and injection technique; a history of hypoglycemic episodes; and review of the patient's method for handling hypoglycemic episodes. A review of the patient's recorded blood glucose tests is also important in assessing overall glycemic control.

▮ Oral Agents.

Nursing responsibilities for the patient taking OHAs are similar to those for the patient taking insulin. Proper administration, assessment of the patient's use of and response to the OHA, and education of the patient and the family about OHAs are all part of the nurse's function.

The nurse's assessment can be extremely valuable in determining the most appropriate OHA for a patient. Factors such as the patient's financial situation, cognitive status, eating habits, home environment, attitude toward DM, and medication history all play a significant role in determining the most appropriate OHA for the individual patient. For example, frail older adults who live alone are at high risk for severe hypoglycemia because low blood glucose is frequently undetected and untreated in this population. This is especially true if the patient has a short-term memory deficit. In these cases, an OHA that

PATIENT & CAREGIVER TEACHING GUIDE

Table 52-14 General Guidelines for the Management of Diabetes Mellitus

Disease Process
- Include an introduction about the pancreas and the islets of Langerhans.
- Describe how insulin is made and what affects its production.
- Discuss the relationship between insulin and glucose.

Physical Activity
- Discuss the importance of regular exercise on the management of blood glucose, improvement of cardiovascular function, and general health.

Menu Planning
- Educate the patient on the importance of a well-balanced diet as part of a diabetes management plan.
- Explain the impact of carbohydrates on the glycemic index and blood glucose levels.

Medication Adherence
- Ensure that the patient is well educated on the proper use of insulin (see Table 52-5) and oral agents.
- Account for any physical limitations or inabilities for self-medication on the patient's part. If necessary, involve the family or caregiver in proper use of medication.
- Discuss all adverse effects and safety issues regarding medication.

Monitoring Blood Glucose
- Teach how to correctly monitor blood glucose levels.
- Include when blood glucose levels should be checked, how to record them, and if necessary, how to adjust insulin levels accordingly.

Risk Reduction
- Ensure that the patient understands and appropriately responds to the signs and symptoms of hypoglycemia and hyperglycemia (see Table 52-16).
- Stress the importance of proper foot care (see Table 52-21), regular eye examinations, and consistent glucose monitoring.
- Inform the patient about the effect that stress can have on blood glucose.

Psychosocial
- Advise the patient of resources that are available to facilitate the adjustment and answer questions about living with a chronic condition such as diabetes (see Resources at end of chapter).

does not cause hypoglycemia, or a shorter-acting OHA, would be most appropriate.

Patient education is an essential nursing function when caring for the patient who uses OHAs for blood glucose control. Some patients may assume that their DM is not a serious condition if they are taking "only a pill" for glycemic control. Therefore, the patient should be instructed that these agents will help keep blood glucose controlled and will help prevent serious long- and short-term complications of DM. Patients should be instructed that OHAs are used in addition to healthy eating and activity as therapy for DM and that they should continue with their meal and activity plans. Patients should not take extra pills if overeating has occurred unless specifically instructed to do so by their health care provider. If the patient uses insulin secretagogues, instructions should be given with regard to prevention, symptom recognition, and management of hypoglycemia.

The patient should also be instructed to contact a health care provider if periods of illness or extreme stress occur. During such a period, insulin therapy may be required to prevent or treat hyperglycemic symptoms and avoid an acute hyperglycemic emergency.

■ **Personal Hygiene.** The potential for microvascular complications and infections necessitates diligent skin and dental hygiene practices on the part of the patient. Because of the susceptibility to periodontal disease, daily brushing and flossing should be encouraged in addition to regular visits to the dentist. When dental work must be done, the dentist should be informed that the patient has DM.

Routine care should include an emphasis on foot care, including daily assessment of feet (RNAO, 2007, p. 31). Problems associated with the feet and the lower extremities are presented later in this chapter. If cuts, scrapes, or burns occur, they should be treated promptly and monitored carefully. The area should be washed, and a nonabrasive or nonirritating antiseptic ointment may be applied. The area should be covered with a dry, sterile pad. If the injury does not begin to heal within 24 hours, or if signs of infection develop, the health care provider should be notified immediately.

■ **Medical Identification and Travel.** The patient should be instructed to carry medical identification at all times indicating that he or she has DM (Figure 52-11). Police, paramedics, and many private citizens are aware of the need to look for this identification when working with sick or unconscious people. Every person with DM should wear a medical alert bracelet or necklace. An identification card can supply valuable information, such as the name of the health care provider and the type and dose of insulin or OHA.

Travel for a patient with DM requires advance planning. The patient should have a full set of DM care supplies in the carry-on luggage when travelling by plane, train, or bus. This includes blood glucose monitoring equipment, insulin, and pen needles or syringes. When pen needles, syringes, and lancing devices are carried onto a commercial airliner, a letter from the prescribing health care provider indicating medical necessity may prevent delays at security checkpoints. Screeners should be notified if an insulin pump is used so they can inspect it while it is on the body, rather than remove it.

For patients who use insulin or an OHA that can cause hypoglycemia, snack items and a fast-acting carbohydrate source for treating hypoglycemia should be included in the carry-on luggage and on the person at all times. Extra insulin should be available in case a vial or cartridge breaks or gets lost. In addition, the patient should carry a full day's supply of food to be prepared for possibly cancelled flights, delayed meals, and closed restaurants. If the patient is planning a trip out of the country, it is wise to have a letter from the health care provider explaining that the patient has DM and requires all the materials being transported, particularly pen needles and syringes, for ongoing health care.

Some travel involves significant time changes such as travelling coast to coast or across the International Date Line. The patient should contact the DM health care provider to plan an appropriate meal and insulin schedule. During travel, most patients find it helpful to keep watches set to the time of the city of origin until they reach their destination, and then switch to travel destination time as soon as possible. The key to travel when taking insulin is to know the type of insulin being taken, its onset of action, the anticipated peak time, and mealtimes.

■ **Patient and Caregiver Teaching.** The goals of DM self-management education are to enable the patient to become the most active participant in her or his care, while matching level of self-management to the ability of the individual patient. Patients who actively manage their DM care have better outcomes than those who do not. For this reason, an educational approach that facilitates informed decision making on the part of the patient is widely advocated. Sometimes, this is referred to as the *empowerment approach* to education.

Unfortunately, patients can encounter a variety of physical, psychological, emotional, and socioeconomic barriers when it comes to effectively managing their DM. These barriers may include feelings of inadequacy about one's own abilities, unwillingness to make the necessary behavioural changes, ineffective coping strategies, lack of resources, and cognitive deficits. If the patient is not able to manage the disease, a family member may be able to assume part of this role. If the patient or the family cannot make decisions related to DM management, the nurse may refer the patient to a social worker or other resources within the community. These resources can assist the patient and the family in outlining a feasible treatment program that meets their capabilities. Patient and health care provider resources are listed at the end of this chapter.

An assessment of the patient's knowledge of DM and lifestyle preferences is useful in planning a teaching program. Tables 52-14 and 52-15 present guidelines to use for patient and caregiver teaching. The nurse should assess the patient's knowledge base frequently so that gaps in knowledge or incorrect or inaccurate ideas can be quickly corrected.

The CDA offers pamphlets, booklets, and a bimonthly magazine called *Diabetes Dialogue*. Chapters of the CDA are located in all major Canadian cities, and most can be reached by accessing CDA online. The CDA also publishes research and education materials and sponsors conferences for health care providers concerned with DM education, research, and management of patients. The 2008 *Clinical Practice Guidelines for the Prevention and Management of Diabetes in Canada* published by the CDA were released in the fall of 2008. Prepared under the leadership of the Clinical and Scientific Section of the Canadian Diabetes Association, the guidelines represent the contributions of more than 99 experts from a broad range of health care disciplines. These experts have evaluated and graded the international literature on the best evidence to

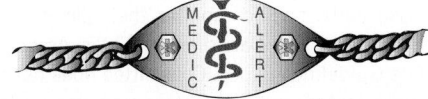

Figure 52-11 Medical Alerts. A patient with diabetes should carry a card and wear a bracelet or necklace that indicates diabetes. If the patient with diabetes is unconscious, these measures will ensure prompt and appropriate attention.

PATIENT & CAREGIVER TEACHING GUIDE

Table 52-15 Instructions for Patients With Diabetes Mellitus

DO	DO NOT	DO	DO NOT
Blood Glucose		**Nutrition**	
• Monitor your blood glucose at home and record results in a log. • Take your insulin or OHA as prescribed. • Rotate injection site areas weekly. • Obtain an A1C blood test every 3-6 mo as an indicator of your long-term blood glucose control. • Know signs and symptoms of hypoglycemia and hyperglycemia. • Carry some form of glucose at all times so you can treat hypoglycemia quickly. • Instruct family members in the use of glucagon administration in the case of emergencies owing to severe hypoglycemia.	• Skip doses of your insulin, especially when you are sick. • Run out of insulin. • Ignore the symptoms of hypoglycemia and hyperglycemia.	• Follow a healthy eating plan, and eat regular meals at regular times. • Choose foods low in saturated and *trans*-fats and high in fibre. • Limit the amount of alcohol you drink. • Know your cholesterol level.	• Drink excessive amounts of alcohol because this may lead to unpredictable low blood glucose reactions and high triglycerides. • Enroll in a fad diet. • Drink regular pop or lots of fruit juices.
		Other Guidelines	
		• Obtain an annual eye examination by an ophthalmologist. • Obtain annual urine testing for protein. • Examine your feet at home daily. • Change socks daily. • Trim nails straight across. • Wear well-fitting shoes to help prevent foot injury. Break in new shoes gradually. • Always carry identification that says you have diabetes. • Have other medical problems treated, especially high blood pressure and high cholesterol. • Quit smoking.	• Smoke cigarettes. • Go barefoot. • Put baby oil or lotion between your toes. • Ignore the signs of infection. • Apply hot or cold directly to your feet. • Wear tight socks, garters, or elastics or knee-highs.
Exercise			
• Learn how exercise and food affect your blood glucose levels. • Begin an exercise program after approval from a health care provider.	• Forget that exercise will lower your blood glucose level. • Exercise if your blood glucose levels are very elevated. This may lead to a temporary worsening of your blood glucose levels.		

OHA, oral antihyperglycemic agent.

guide screening, prevention, diagnosis, care, management, and education for Canadians living with type 1, type 2, and GDM. The CDA also gives recognition to education programs that meet the international standards of DM education and can provide a list of these programs. Pharmaceutical and diagnostic companies specializing in DM-related products also have promotions and free educational materials for patients and health care providers.

▮ Evaluation

The expected outcomes for the patient with DM are addressed in NCP 52-1.

Acute Complications of Diabetes Mellitus

Acute complications of DM arise from events associated with *hyperglycemia* or *hypoglycemia* (also referred to as *insulin reaction* or *low blood glucose*). It is important for the health care provider to be able to distinguish between hyperglycemia and

COMPLEMENTARY AND ALTERNATIVE THERAPIES

Herbs and Supplements That May Affect Glucose Levels

Possible Hypoglycemic Herbs and Supplements*
  Aloe, fish oils, goldenseal, bilberry eleuthero, ginseng, milk thistle, Chinese cinnamom (Cinnamomum cassia) and sage.
Possible Hyperglycemic Herbs and Supplements*
  St. John's wort, celery seed, rosemary, and melatonin

Nursing Implications

It is very important that patients with diabetes consult with their health care provider before using herbs or nutritional supplements. Patients who use herbs should monitor their blood glucose levels carefully and regularly. The Canadian Diabetes Association (CDA) Clinical Practice Guidelines Expert Committee does not recommend the use of complementary and alternative medicine for the management of diabetes as there is insufficient evidence regarding its safety and efficacy (CDA, 2008, p. S91).

*www.naturalstandard.com.

Table 52-16 Comparison of Hyperglycemia and Hypoglycemia

HYPERGLYCEMIA	HYPOGLYCEMIA	HYPERGLYCEMIA	HYPOGLYCEMIA
Manifestations*		**Treatment**	
Elevated blood glucose†	Blood glucose <4.0 mmol/L	Get medical care.	Immediate ingestion of 15-20 g of simple carbohydrates
Increase in urination	Cold, clammy skin	Continuance of OHA or insulin as ordered; may need increase in dose	
Increase in appetite followed by lack of appetite	Numbness of fingers, toes, mouth		Ingestion of another 15-20 g of simple carbohydrates in 15 min if no relief obtained
Weakness, fatigue	Rapid heartbeat	Check blood glucose frequently. Check urine for ketones. Record results.	
Blurred vision	Emotional changes		Follow-up with snack if regular meal more than 1 hr away, and contact health care provider if no effect.
Headache	Headache	Hourly drinking of fluids	
Glycosuria	Nervousness, tremors	IV fluids may be necessary.	Discussion with health care provider about insulin or OHA dosage
Nausea and vomiting	Faintness, dizziness		
Abdominal cramps	Unsteady gait, slurred speech	**Preventive Measures**	
Progression to DKA or HHS	Hunger	Taking prescribed dose of medication at proper time	Taking prescribed dose of medication at proper time
	Changes in vision	Accurate administration of insulin and OHA	Accurate administration of insulin and OHA
	Seizures, coma		Ingestion of all recommended foods at proper time
Causes		Maintenance of diet	
Illness, infection	Alcohol intake without food	Maintenance of good personal hygiene	Provision of compensation for exercise
Corticosteroids	Too little food—delayed, omitted, inadequate intake		Ability to recognize and know symptoms and treat them immediately
Too much food		Adherence to sick-day rules when ill	
Too little or no diabetes medication	Too much diabetic medication		Carrying of simple carbohydrates
	Too much exercise without compensation	Checking of blood for glucose as ordered	Education of friends, family, fellow employees about symptoms and treatment
Inactivity	Diabetes medication or food taken at wrong time		
Emotional, physical stress		Contacting of health care provider regarding ketonuria	Checking blood glucose as ordered
Poor absorption or lack of insulin	Loss of weight without change in medication		
	Use of β-adrenergic blockers interfering with recognition of symptoms	Wearing of diabetic identification	Wearing medical alert (diabetic) identification

DKA, diabetic ketoacidosis; *HHS*, hyperosmolar hyperglycemic state; *IV*, intravenous; *OHA*, oral antihyperglycemic agent.
*There is usually a gradual onset of symptoms in hyperglycemia and a rapid onset in hypoglycemia.
†Specific clinical manifestations related to elevated levels of blood glucose vary according to the patient.

hypoglycemia because hypoglycemia worsens rapidly and constitutes a serious threat if action is not immediately taken. Table 52-16 compares manifestations, causes, treatment, and prevention of hyperglycemia and hypoglycemia.

Diabetic Ketoacidosis

Etiology and Pathophysiology

Diabetic ketoacidosis (DKA), also referred to as *diabetic acidosis* and *diabetic coma,* is an acute metabolic complication of DM occurring when fats are metabolized in the absence of insulin. It is caused by a profound deficiency of insulin and is characterized by hyperglycemia, ketosis, metabolic acidosis, and dehydration (volume depletion). It is most likely to occur in people with type 1 DM but may be seen in type 2 in conditions of severe illness or stress when the pancreas cannot meet the extra demand for insulin. Precipitating factors include illness, infection, inadequate insulin dosage, insulin omission, undiagnosed type 1 DM, and poor self-management.

When the circulating supply of insulin is insufficient, glucose cannot be properly used for energy, so the body breaks down fat stores as a secondary source of fuel (Figure 52-12). Ketones

are acidic by-products of fat metabolism that can cause serious problems when they become excessive in the blood. Ketosis alters the pH balance, causing metabolic acidosis to develop. Ketonuria is a process that begins when ketone bodies are excreted in the urine. During this process, electrolytes become depleted as cations (sodium, potassium, and ammonium salts) are eliminated along with the anionic ketones in an attempt to maintain electrical neutrality.

Insulin deficiency impairs protein synthesis and causes excessive protein degradation. This results in nitrogen losses from the tissues. Insulin deficiency also stimulates the production of glucose from amino acids (from proteins) in the liver and leads to further hyperglycemia. But because there is a deficiency of insulin, the additional glucose cannot be used and the blood glucose level rises further, adding to the osmotic diuresis. Untreated, this leads to severe depletion of sodium, potassium, chloride, magnesium, and phosphate. Potassium is most affected in DKA. Acidosis causes hydrogen ions to move from the extracellular fluid to the intracellular space. Hydrogen movement into the cell promotes potassium movement out of the cell into the extracellular compartment, resulting in severe potassium depletion in the intracellular space. Most of the shifted extracellular potassium is lost in the urine because of osmotic diuresis. The serum potassium can be normal or even high, but this is misleading because there is an intracellular and total body loss of potassium (Kitabchi, Umpierrez, Miles, & Fisher, 2009, p. 1340).

Vomiting caused by the acidosis results in more fluid and electrolyte losses. Eventually, hypovolemia, followed by shock, will ensue.

Renal failure may eventually occur from hypovolemic shock. This causes the retention of ketones and glucose, and the metabolic acidosis progresses. Untreated, the patient becomes comatose as a result of dehydration, electrolyte imbalance, and acidosis. If the condition is not treated, death is inevitable.

Clinical Manifestations

Signs and symptoms of DKA include polyuria and polydipsia leading to dehydration. Dehydration is manifested by poor skin turgor, dry mucous membranes, tachycardia, and orthostatic hypotension. Early symptoms may include lethargy and weakness. As the patient becomes severely dehydrated, the skin becomes dry and loose, and the eye sockets become sunken. Nausea and vomiting are common symptoms. Abdominal pain is occasionally seen. This may be owing to dehydration of muscle tissue, delayed gastric emptying, and ileus induced by electrolyte disturbance and metabolic acidosis (DeBeer et al., 2008, p. 6). Finally, Kussmaul's respirations (rapid, deep breathing associated with dyspnea) are the body's attempt to reverse metabolic acidosis through the exhalation of excess carbon dioxide. Acetone is noted on the breath as a sweet, fruity odour. (See Chapter 19 for a discussion of respiratory compensation of metabolic acidosis.) Laboratory findings include a blood glucose level above 14 mmol/L, arterial blood pH below 7.35, serum bicarbonate level less than 15 mmol/L, and ketones in the blood and urine (DeBeer et al., 2008, p. 7).

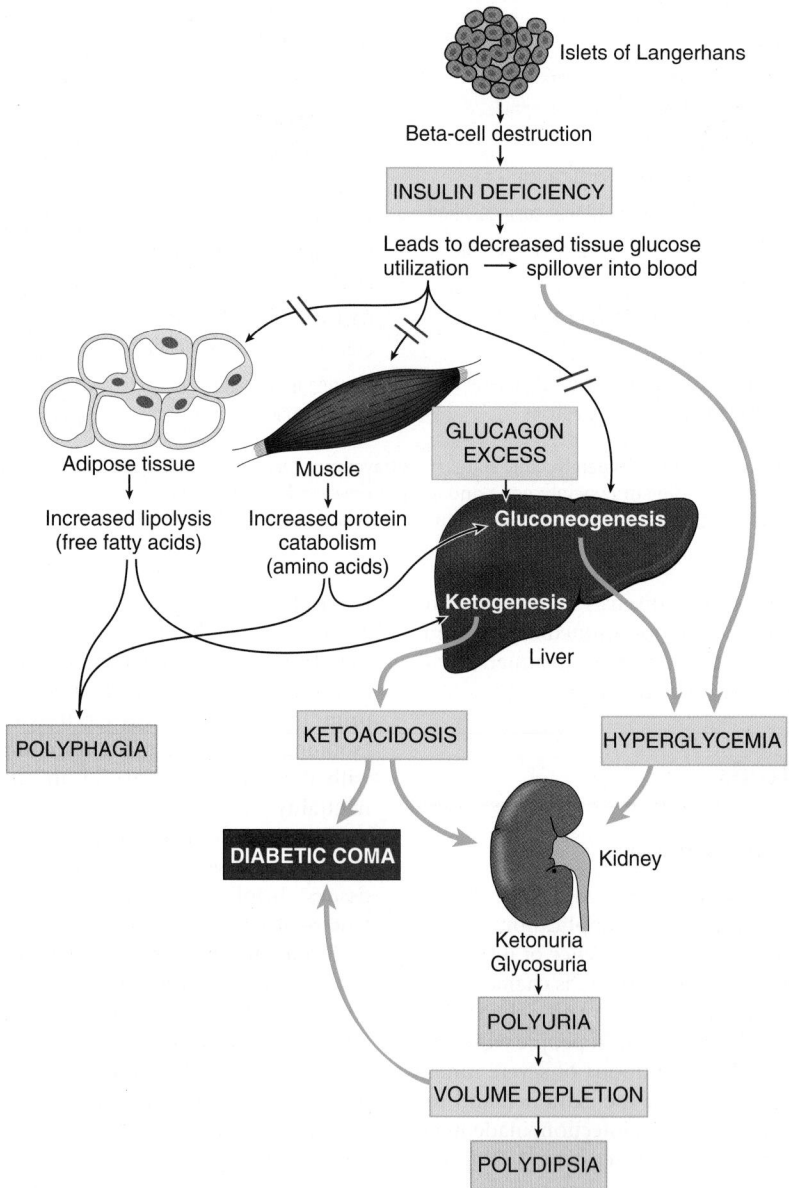

Figure 52-12 Metabolic events leading to diabetic ketoacidosis and diabetic coma.

Source: Kumar, V., Abbas, A. K., Fausto, N., & Aster, J. (2010). *Robbins and Cotran pathologic basis of disease* (8th ed., p. 1144, Figure 24-39). Philadelphia: Saunders.

Collaborative Care

Before the advent of self-monitoring of blood glucose and β-hydroxybutyrate (capillary blood ketones), all patients with DKA required hospitalization for treatment. Today, hospitalization may not be required. In instances in which fluid and electrolyte imbalances are not severe and blood glucose levels can be safely monitored at home, early stages of DKA may be managed on an outpatient basis (Table 52-17). However, the decision as to the location where the patient is managed must also take other factors into consideration. These include the presence of fever, nausea, vomiting, and diarrhea; altered mental status; nature of the cause of the ketoacidosis; and availability of frequent communication with the health care provider (every few hours).

Regardless of the setting in which it occurs, DKA is a serious condition that proceeds rapidly and must be treated promptly. (Table 52-18 describes the emergency management of a patient with DKA.) Because fluid imbalance is potentially life threatening, the initial goal of therapy is to establish IV access and begin fluid and electrolyte replacement. Typically, the initial fluid therapy regimen comprises an infusion of 0.45% or 0.9% NaCl IV solution at a rate to restore urine output to 30 to 60 mL/hr and to raise blood pressure. When blood glucose levels approach 14 mmol/L, 5% dextrose is added to the fluid regimen to prevent hypoglycemia (DeBeer et al., 2008, p. 9; CDA, 2008, p. S66).

The aim of fluid and electrolyte therapy is to replace extracellular and intracellular water and to correct deficits of sodium, chloride, bicarbonate, potassium, phosphate, magnesium, and nitrogen. Early potassium replacement is essential because hypokalemia is a significant cause of preventable death during treatment of DKA. Although initial serum potassium may be normal or high, levels can rapidly decrease once therapy starts because insulin drives potassium into the cells, leading to life-threatening hypokalemia.

IV insulin administration is therapy directed toward correcting hyperglycemia and hyperketonemia. Insulin therapy is withheld until fluid resuscitation is under way and serum potassium is greater than 3.3 mmol/L because insulin allows water and potassium to enter the cell along with glucose and can lead to a depletion of vascular volume and hypokalemia. Initially, a bolus of insulin is delivered, followed by a continuous infusion (CDA, 2008, p. 67).

COLLABORATIVE CARE

Table 52-17 Diabetic Ketoacidosis (DKA) and Hyperosmolar Hyperglycemic State (HHS)

Diagnostic

- History and physical examination
- Blood studies, including immediate blood glucose, complete blood count, ketones, pH, electrolytes, blood urea nitrogen, arterial blood gases
- Urinalysis, including specific gravity, pH, glucose, ketones

Collaborative Therapy

- Administration of IV fluids
- IV administration of rapid- or short-acting insulin
- Electrolyte replacement
- Assessment of mental status
- Recording of intake and output
- Central venous pressure monitoring (if indicated)
- Assessment of blood glucose levels
- Assessment of blood and urine for ketones
- ECG monitoring
- Assessment of cardiovascular and respiratory status

ECG, electrocardiogram; *IV,* intravenous.

EMERGENCY MANAGEMENT

Table 52-18 Diabetic Ketoacidosis

ETIOLOGY	ASSESSMENT FINDINGS	INTERVENTIONS
- Undiagnosed diabetes mellitus - Inadequate treatment of existing diabetes mellitus - Insulin not taken as prescribed, or omitted - Infection - Dehydration owing to illness with vomiting or diarrhea - Change in diet, insulin, or exercise regimen	- Dry mouth - Thirst - Abdominal pain - Nausea and vomiting - Gradually increasing restlessness, confusion, lethargy - Flushed, dry skin - Eyes appear sunken - Breath odour of acetone - Rapid, weak pulse, orthostatic hypotension - Laboured breathing (Kussmaul's respirations) - Fever - Urinary frequency - Serum glucose >14 mmol/L - Glucosuria and ketonuria - Oral or vaginal *Candida albicans* (yeast infection)	**Initial** - Ensure patent airway. - Administer oxygen as per physician's order. - Establish IV access with large-bore catheter. - Begin fluid resuscitation with 0.9% NaCl solution until BP stabilized and urine output 30-60 mL/hr. - Begin continuous regular insulin drip 0.1 units/kg/hr as needed. - Administer potassium IV to correct hypokalemia. - Administer IV sodium bicarbonate if severe acidosis (pH <7.0). - Identify history of diabetes, time of last food, and time and amount of last insulin injection. **Ongoing Monitoring** - Monitor vital signs, level of consciousness, cardiac rhythm, oxygen saturation, and urine output. - Assess breath sounds for fluid overload. - Monitor serum glucose, pH, and serum potassium.

BP, blood pressure; *IV,* intravenous.

SAFETY ALERT

Too rapid administration of IV fluid and a rapid lowering of serum glucose can lead to cerebral edema.

Hyperosmolar Hyperglycemic State

Hyperosmolar hyperglycemic state (HHS) is a life-threatening syndrome that can occur in the patient with DM who is able to produce enough insulin to prevent DKA but not enough to prevent severe hyperglycemia, osmotic diuresis, and extracellular fluid depletion (Figure 52-13). HHS is less common than DKA. The main difference between HHS and DKA is that the patient with HHS usually has enough circulating insulin so that ketoacidosis does not occur. Because HHS produces fewer symptoms in the earlier stages, blood glucose levels can climb quite high before the problem is recognized. The higher blood glucose levels increase serum osmolality and produce more-severe neurological manifestations, such as somnolence, coma, seizures, hemiparesis, and aphasia. HHS often occurs in the older adult patient with type 2 DM and is often related to impaired thirst sensation, a functional inability to replace fluids, or both. There is usually a history of inadequate fluid intake, increasing mental depression, and polyuria. Laboratory values in HHS include blood glucose greater than 34 mmol/L and a marked increase in serum osmolality. Ketone bodies are absent or minimal in both blood and urine.

Collaborative Care

HHS constitutes a medical emergency and has a high mortality rate. Therapy is similar to that for the treatment of DKA and includes immediate IV administration of either 0.9% or 0.45% NaCl at a rate that is dependent on cardiac status and the degree of fluid volume deficit. Regular insulin is given by IV bolus, followed by an infusion after fluid replacement therapy is instituted to aid in reducing the hyperglycemia. When blood glucose levels fall to approximately 14 mmol/L, IV fluids containing glucose are administered to prevent hypoglycemia. Electrolytes are monitored and replaced as needed. Hypokalemia is not as significant in HHS as it is in DKA, although fluid losses may result in milder potassium deficits that necessitate replacement. Vital signs, intake and output, tissue turgor, laboratory values, and cardiac monitoring are assessed to monitor the efficacy of fluid and electrolyte replacement. Patients with renal or cardiac compromise require special monitoring to avoid fluid overload during fluid replacement. This includes monitoring of serum osmolality and frequent assessment of cardiac, renal, and neurological status (DeBeer et al., 2008, p. 9; CDA, 2008, p. S68).

The management for both DKA and HHS is similar, except that HHS necessitates greater fluid replacement (see Table 52-17). Once the patient is stabilized, attempts to detect and correct the underlying precipitating cause should be initiated.

NURSING MANAGEMENT: DIABETIC KETOACIDOSIS AND HYPEROSMOLAR HYPERGLYCEMIC STATE

When hospitalized, the patient is closely monitored with appropriate blood and urine tests. The nurse is responsible for monitor-

PATHOPHYSIOLOGY MAP

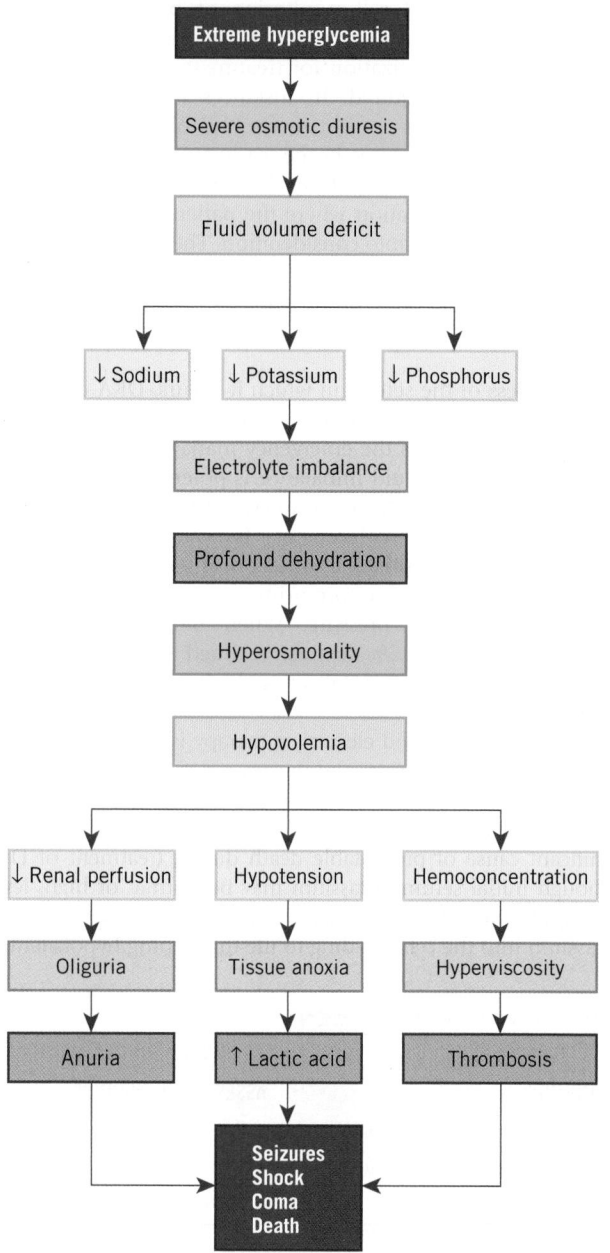

Figure 52-13 Pathophysiology of hyperosmolar hyperglycemic state (HHS).

Source: Redrawn from Urden, L. D., Stacy, K. M., & Lough, M. E. (2010). *Critical care nursing: Diagnosis and management* (6th ed., p. 917, Figure 37-4). St. Louis: Mosby.

ing blood glucose and urine for output and ketones as well as using laboratory data to support care.

Nursing responsibilities include monitoring the administration of IV fluids to correct dehydration, insulin therapy to reduce blood glucose and serum ketones, and electrolytes to correct electrolyte imbalance; assessment of renal status; assessment of the cardiopulmonary status related to hydration and electrolyte levels; and monitoring of the level of consciousness.

The nurse must also monitor the signs of potassium imbalance resulting from hypoinsulinemia and osmotic diuresis (see Chapter 19). When treatment for hyperglycemia is begun with insulin, serum potassium levels may decrease rapidly because potassium moves into the cells once insulin becomes available. This movement of potassium into and out of extracellular fluid influences cardiac functioning. Cardiac monitoring is a useful aid in detecting hyperkalemia and hypokalemia because characteristic changes indicating potassium excess or deficit are observable on electrocardiogram (ECG) tracings (see Chapter 19, Figure 19-14). Vital signs should be assessed often to determine the presence of fever, hypovolemic shock, tachycardia, and Kussmaul's breathing (Brenner, 2006, p. 55).

Hypoglycemia

Hypoglycemia, or low blood glucose, occurs when there is too much insulin in proportion to available glucose in the blood. This causes the blood glucose level to drop to less than 4 mmol/L. Once plasma glucose drops below 4 mmol/L, neuroendocrine hormones are released and the autonomic nervous system is activated. Suppression of insulin secretion and production of glucagon and epinephrine provide defense against hypoglycemia. Epinephrine release causes manifestations that include diaphoresis, tremors, hunger, nervousness, anxiety, pallor and palpitations. Because the brain requires as a primary energy source a constant supply of glucose in sufficient quantities to function properly, hypoglycemia can eventually affect cognitive functioning. These manifestations are referred to as *neuroglycopenic signs* and may include irritability, visual disturbances, difficulty speaking, stupor, confusion and coma. Manifestations of hypoglycemia can mimic alcohol intoxication. Untreated hypoglycemia can progress to loss of consciousness, seizures, coma, and death.

Hypoglycemic unawareness (or *asymptomatic hypoglycemia*) is a condition in which a person does not experience the usual autonomic warning signs and symptoms of hypoglycemia, increasing his or her risk for dangerously low blood glucose levels. This is often related to autonomic neuropathy of DM that interferes with the secretion of counter-regulatory hormones that produce these symptoms. Older adult patients and patients who use β-adrenergic blockers are also at risk for hypoglycemic unawareness. It is usually not safe for patients with risk factors for hypoglycemic unawareness to aim for tight blood glucose control owing to the increased potential of hypoglycemia. They are usually managed with blood glucose goals that are somewhat higher than patients who are able to detect and manage the onset of hypoglycemia.

Hypoglycemic symptoms may occur when a very high blood glucose level falls too rapidly, for example, a blood glucose level of 16 mmol/L falling quickly to 8 mmol/L. Although the blood glucose level is above normal by definition and measurement, the sudden metabolic shift can evoke hypoglycemic symptoms. Too vigorous management of hyperglycemia with insulin can induce this type of situation.

Causes of hypoglycemia are often related to a mismatch in the timing of food intake and the peak action of insulin or OHAs that increase endogenous insulin secretion. The balance between blood glucose and insulin can be disrupted by the administration of too much insulin or medication, the ingestion of insufficient carbohydrates, delaying the time of eating, and performing unusual amounts of exercise. Insulin reactions can occur at any time, but most reactions occur when the OHA or insulin is at its peak of action. Although hypoglycemia is more common with insulin therapy, it can occur with OHAs and may be severe and

persist for an extended time because of the longer duration of action.

NURSING AND COLLABORATIVE MANAGEMENT: HYPOGLYCEMIA

Hypoglycemia can usually be quickly reversed with effective and rapid treatment. At the first sign of hypoglycemia, the blood glucose should be checked if possible (Table 52-19). If it is below 4 mmol/L, the patient should begin treatment immediately. If the blood glucose is above 4 mmol/L, other causes of the signs and symptoms should be investigated. If the patient has manifestations of hypoglycemia and monitoring equipment is not available, hypoglycemia should be assumed and treatment should be initiated.

Hypoglycemia is treated by ingesting 15 to 20 g of a simple (fast-acting) carbohydrate, such as three or four glucose tablets, 175 mL of fruit juice or regular soft drink, or six Life Savers candies. Commercial products such as gels or tablets containing specific amounts of glucose are convenient for carrying in a purse or pocket to be used in such situations.

Treatment with sweet foods containing fat, such as chocolate bars, cookies, and ice cream, should be avoided because fat will slow down the absorption of the sugar and delay the response to treatment. Overtreatment with large quantities of simple carbohydrates should be avoided to prevent a rapid fluctuation to

COLLABORATIVE CARE

Table 52-19 Hypoglycemia

Diagnostic

- Capillary blood glucose (evaluated and reported on an emergency basis)
- History (if possible) and physical examination

Collaborative Therapy

Determination of cause of hypoglycemia (after correction of condition)

Conscious Patient With Mild to Moderate Hypoglycemia

- Administration of 15-20 g of fast-acting (simple) carbohydrate (e.g., commercial dextrose products [per label instructions]; 175 mL of fruit juice or regular soft drink; 6-8 Life Savers; for patient taking acarbose: 15 mL (1 Tbsp) syrup or honey, or 125-150 mL low-fat milk, or dextrose tabs (because the absorption of glucose itself is not affected)*
- Repetition of treatment in 15 min (if no improvement)
- Administration of additional food or longer-acting combination such as carbohydrate plus protein or fat (e.g., crackers with peanut butter or cheese) after symptoms subside, if meal is longer than 1 hr away
- Immediate notification of health care provider or emergency service (if patient is outside hospital) if symptoms do not subside after two or three administrations of fast-acting carbohydrate

Severe Hypoglycemia or Unconscious Patient

- Subcutaneous or intramuscular injection of 1 mg glucagon
- Intravenous administration of 20-50 mL of dextrose 50% in water (D50W) given over 1-3 min

*Canadian Diabetes Association (CDA) Clinical Practice Guidelines Expert Committee. (2008). 2008 Clinical practice guidelines for the prevention and management of diabetes in Canada. *Canadian Journal of Diabetes Care, 32*(Suppl), S62.

hyperglycemia. A prompt but moderate approach is best. Blood glucose should be checked 15 minutes after the initial treatment and repeated if blood glucose remains lower than 4 mmol/L. Once the blood glucose is greater than 4 mmol/L, the patient should eat a snack if the next regularly scheduled meal is more than an hour away in order to prevent hypoglycemia from recurring. Good snacks include one protein and one starch choice such as a peanut butter sandwich, cheese and crackers, or cereal and milk. Blood glucose should also be checked again about 45 minutes after treatment to ensure that hypoglycemia is not recurring (CDA, 2008, p. S63; BBDC, 2009, p. 65).

If there is no significant improvement in the patient's condition after two to three doses of 15 to 20 g of simple carbohydrate or if the patient is not alert enough to swallow, 1 mg of glucagon may be administered by intramuscular or subcutaneous injection. Glucagon stimulates a strong hepatic response to convert glycogen to glucose, making glucose rapidly available. Rebound hypoglycemia is a potential adverse effect of glucagon. Having the patient ingest a starch snack after recovery may prevent this from happening. Patients with minimal glycogen stores will not respond to glucagon. These include patients with alcohol-related hepatic disease, starvation, and adrenal insufficiency. In an acute care setting, patients with hypoglycemia are treated with 20 to 50 mL of 50% dextrose by IV push.

Once the hypoglycemic episode has resolved, the nurse should explore with the patient the reasons why the situation developed. This assessment may indicate the need for additional education of the patient and the family to prevent future episodes of hypoglycemia. The danger of hypoglycemic episodes must be stressed; safety concerns include risks such as driving a motorized vehicle or bicycle, operating heavy machinery, and falls; and they also have a long-term impact upon memory.

Chronic Complications of Diabetes Mellitus

Chronic complications of DM are primarily those of end-organ disease that result from damage to the large and small blood vessels (angiopathy) secondary to chronic hyperglycemia (Figure 52-14). Angiopathy, or blood vessel disease, is estimated to account for the majority of deaths among patients with DM. These chronic blood vessel dysfunctions are divided into two categories: *macrovascular complications* and *microvascular complications*.

Several theories exist as to how and why chronic hyperglycemia damages cells and tissues. Possible causes include (1) the accumulation of damaging by-products of glucose metabolism, such as sorbitol, which is associated with damage to nerve cells; (2) the formation of abnormal glucose molecules in the basement membrane of small blood vessels such as those that circulate to the eye and the kidney; and (3) a derangement called *oxidative stress* in RBC function that leads to a decrease in oxygenation to the tissues.

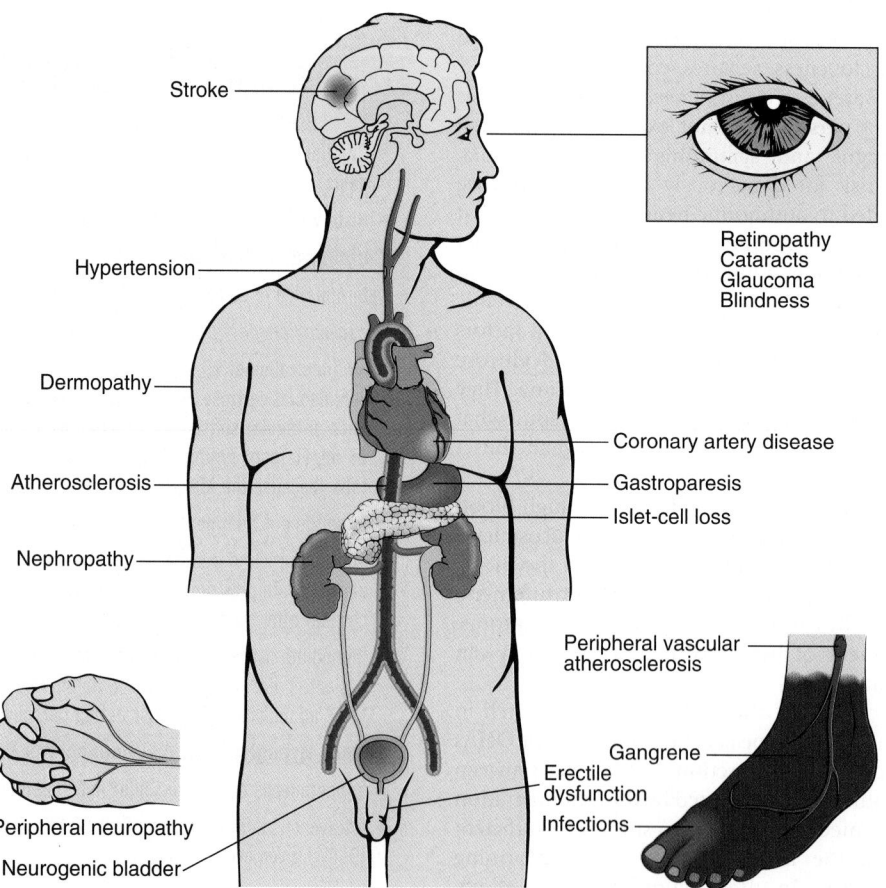

Figure 52-14 Long-term complications of diabetes mellitus.

Source: Kumar, V., Abbas, A. K., Fausto, N., & Aster, J. (2010). *Robbins and Cotran pathologic basis of disease* (8th ed., p. 1139, Figure 24-32). Philadelphia: Saunders.

The Diabetes Control and Complication Trial (DCCT) was a landmark study that has greatly influenced DM management since its results were announced in 1993 (DCCT, 1993, p. 977). This study demonstrated that, in patients with type 1 DM, the risk for microvascular complications could be significantly reduced by keeping blood glucose levels as near to normal as possible for as much of the time as possible (intensive insulin therapy). In this study, patients were randomly assigned to one of two groups: intensive or standard treatment. The intensive treatment group took three or more insulin injections a day or used an insulin pump and tested their blood glucose four to five times a day. The patients in the standard treatment group took one to two injections a day and tested their blood glucose once or twice a day. The average A1C in the intensive treatment group was 7.2%; in the standard treatment group, it was 9%. (The normal range for A1C in a person without DM is 4 to 6%.) The results showed that the subjects in the intensive therapy group reduced their risk for the development of retinopathy, nephropathy, and peripheral neuropathy. The adverse effects associated with intensive therapy were an increase in frequency of hypoglycemic episodes and weight gain.

Based on the findings of the DCCT, the CDA (2008) *Clinical Practice Guidelines* included recommendations for treatment goals to maintain blood glucose levels as near to normal as possible (see the Evidence-Informed Practice box "What Level of Hemoglobin A1C Is Associated With Fewer Diabetes Mellitus Complications?"). Specific targets for individual patients must take into account the risk for severe or undetected hypoglycemia as an adverse effect of tight glucose control.

The United Kingdom Prospective Diabetes Study (UKPDS) demonstrated that intensive treatment of type 2 DM with OHAs alone, in combination with insulin, or using insulin alone, can also significantly lower the risk for developing DM-related microvascular complications such as retinopathy, nephropathy, and neuropathy. The findings from this study showed a 25% reduction of microvascular disease in subjects who maintained long-term glycemic control, including a 1% reduction in A1C, regardless of the initial value (UKPDS, 1998, p. 837).

Because of the devastating effects of long-term complications, patients with DM require scheduled and ongoing monitoring for the detection and prevention of chronic complications. The recommendations for ongoing evaluation are listed in Table 52-20. It is imperative that patients understand the importance of regular follow-up examinations (CDA, 2008, p. 196; BBDC, 2009, p. 82).

Macrovascular Complications

Macrovascular complications are diseases of the large and medium-sized blood vessels that occur with greater frequency and with an earlier onset in people with DM. Although atherosclerotic plaque formation is believed to have a genetic origin, its development seems to be promoted by the altered lipid metabolism common to DM. Tight glucose control may help delay the atherosclerotic process (DCCT, 1993, p. 977; UKPDS, 1998, p. 837). Macrovascular diseases include cerebrovascular, cardiovascular, and peripheral vascular disease. Adults with DM have two to three times the risk of heart and cerebrovascular disease of those without DM (CDA, 2008, p. S95). Although genetic makeup cannot be altered, vascular protection may be addressed by the addition of an angiotensin-converting enzyme (ACE) inhibitor, antiplatelet therapy such as acetylsalicylic acid, blood pressure control, glycemic control, lifestyle modifications, healthy weight, lipid control, and smoking cessation. Optimizing blood pressure

---

EVIDENCE-INFORMED PRACTICE

What Level of Hemoglobin A1C Is Associated With Fewer Diabetes Mellitus Complications?

Clinical Question

For patients with diabetes mellitus (P), does maintaining a hemoglobin A1C level <7% (I) compared with maintaining a level >7% (C) decrease microvascular and neuropathic complications (O)?

Best Available Evidence

- Clinical practice guidelines based on systematic review of clinical trials

Critical Appraisal and Synthesis of Evidence

- Studies included adults, older adults, and children with type 1 and type 2 diabetes.
- Assessed were blood glucose, hemoglobin A1C, blood lipids, blood pressure, vascular disease, obesity, dyslipidemia, hypertension, nephropathy, and quality of life.
- Lowering hemoglobin A1C (to average of 7%) reduced microvascular and neuropathic complications.
- Tighter glycemic control (a normal A1C <6%) may further reduce complications but increases hypoglycemia risk.

Conclusion

- Lowering A1C to an average of 7% decreases diabetes complications.

Implications for Nursing Practice

- Counsel patient that recommendations are to maintain A1C at <7%.
- Individualize goals based on the patient's health status.
- Urge patients to actively manage their blood glucose and A1C levels.

Reference for Evidence

Canadian Diabetes Association (CDA) Clinical Practice Guidelines Expert Committee. (2008). 2008 Clinical practice guidelines for the prevention and management of diabetes in Canada. *Canadian Journal of Diabetes Care, 32*(Suppl), S29.

PICO: P, patient population of interest; *I*, intervention or area of interest; *C*, comparison of interest or comparison group; *O*, outcome(s) of interest.

---

control in patients with DM is significant for the prevention of cardiovascular and renal disease. The target blood pressure for people with DM is 130/80 mm Hg. Control of lifestyle risk factors, hyperglycemia, hypertension, and dyslipidemia will reduce mortality risk by 50% in patients with DM (Gaede, Lund-Anderson, Parving, & Pedersen, 2008, p. 580).

Insulin resistance seems to play an important role in the development of cardiovascular disease and is implicated in the pathogenesis of essential hypertension and dyslipidemia. The term *metabolic syndrome* is applied to the clinical association of insulin resistance, hypertension, and increased very low density lipoprotein (VLDL) and decreased HDL cholesterol concentrations. The role of insulin resistance in the pathogenesis of cardiovascular disease is not well understood, but it seems to combine

Table 52-20 Prevention, Detection, and Monitoring of Long-Term Complications of Diabetes Mellitus*

COMPLICATION	TYPE OF EXAMINATION	FREQUENCY
Retinopathy	Fundoscopic–dilated-eye examination by experienced professional	Type 1: annually starting 5 yr after onset of diabetes Type 2: at diagnosis; then every 1-2 yr if normal
Nephropathy	Random urinalysis for albumin/creatinine ratio (ACR), serum creatinine converted to eGFR.	Type 1 annually, if no CKD, starting 5 yr after onset of diabetes Type 2 at diagnosis and then annually if normal; if CKD present ACR and eGFR at least every 6 mo.
Neuropathy (foot and lower extremities)	Visual examination of foot Comprehensive foot examination: Assessment of structural abnormalities, neuropathy (monofilament, tuning fork), vascular disease (peripheral pulses), ulcerations, and evidence of infection	Daily by patient Every visit by health care provider Type 1: annually starting 5 yr after onset of diabetes Type 2: at diagnosis and annually
Cardiovascular disease	Blood pressure Lipid panel	Every visit At the time of diagnosis, and then every 1-3 yr
	Exercise stress testing (may include stress ECG, stress echocardiogram, perfusion imaging)	As needed based on risk factors

CKD, chronic kidney disease; *ECG*, electrocardiogram; *eGFR*, estimated glomerular filtration rate.

*Based on the recommendations of the Canadian Diabetes Association (CDA) Clinical Practice Guidelines Expert Committee. (2008). 2008 Clinical practice guidelines for the prevention and management of diabetes in Canada. *Canadian Journal of Diabetes Care, 32*(Suppl), S196.

with dyslipidemia in contributing to greater risk of cardiovascular disease in patients with DM. All patients with DM should be screened for dyslipidemia at the time DM is diagnosed. Most people with DM are considered at high risk for a vascular event (Dokken, 2008, p. 160).

Lifestyle changes such as healthy eating and exercise are first-line interventions to achieve an optimal lipid profile. If unsuccessful, lipid-lowering therapy such as statins, fibrates, or both may be added to optimize lipid levels, thereby reducing risk of a vascular event.

Microvascular Complications

Microvascular complications result from thickening of the vessel membranes in the capillaries and arterioles in response to conditions of chronic hyperglycemia. They differ from the macrovascular complications in that they are specific to DM. Although microangiopathy can be found throughout the body, the areas most noticeably affected are the eyes (retinopathy), the kidneys (nephropathy), the nerves (neuropathy), and the skin (dermopathy). Thickening of the basement membrane has been found in some people with DM before or at the time of diagnosis or before the onset of symptoms of DM. However, clinical manifestations may not appear until 10 to 20 years after the onset of DM, depending on the glycemic control over that period of time as measured by A1C.

Diabetic Retinopathy

Etiology and Pathophysiology

Diabetic retinopathy refers to the process of microvascular damage to the blood vessels in the retina as a result of chronic hyperglycemia, presence of nephropathy, and hypertension in patients with DM. After 15 years with DM, nearly all patients with type 1 DM and 80% with type 2 DM will have some degree of retinal disease. Diabetic retinopathy is estimated to be the most common cause of new cases of blindness in people of working age (CDA, 2008, p. S134; ADA, 2011, p. S40).

Retinopathy can be classified as nonproliferative or proliferative. In *nonproliferative retinopathy*, the most common form, partial occlusion of the small blood vessels in the retina causes the development of microaneurysms in the capillary walls. The walls of these microaneurysms are so weak that capillary fluid leaks out, causing retinal edema and eventually hard exudates or intraretinal hemorrhages. Vision may be affected if the macula is involved.

Proliferative retinopathy, the most severe form, involves the retina and the vitreous. When retinal capillaries become occluded, the body compensates by forming new blood vessels to supply the retina with blood, a pathological process known as *neovascularization*. These new vessels are extremely fragile and hemorrhage easily, producing vitreous contraction. Eventually, light is prevented from reaching the retina as the vessels become torn and bleed into the vitreous cavity. The patient sees black or red spots or lines. If these new blood vessels pull the retina while the vitreous contracts, causing a tear, partial or complete retinal detachment will occur. If the macula is involved, vision is lost. Without treatment, more than half of patients with proliferative diabetic retinopathy will be blind.

Collaborative Care

The earliest and most treatable stages of diabetic retinopathy often produce no changes in the vision. Because of this, the patient with DM must have regular dilated-eye examinations by an ophthalmologist or a specially trained optometrist for early detection and treatment.

The most common forms of treatment for diabetic retinopathy are early laser photocoagulation therapy of the retina, and vitrectomy. Photocoagulation by laser destroys the ischemic areas of the retina that produce growth factors that encourage neovascularization, thereby preventing further vision loss, and reduces legal blindness up to 90% in people with severe nonproliferative retinopathy and proliferative retinopathy (CDA, 2008, p. 135). (Photocoagulation is discussed in Chapter 24.)

Vitrectomy is the aspiration of blood, membrane, and fibres from the inside of the eye through a small incision just behind the cornea. Vitrectomy is indicated in patients with advanced proliferative retinopathy with vitreous hemorrhage or retinal detachment of the macula. (Vitrectomy is discussed in Chapter 24.)

People with DM are also prone to other visual problems. Glaucoma occurs as a result of the occlusion of the outflow channels secondary to neovascularization. This type of glaucoma is difficult to treat and often results in blindness. Cataracts develop at an earlier age and progress more rapidly in people with DM.

Nephropathy

Diabetic nephropathy is a microvascular complication associated with damage to the small blood vessels that supply the glomeruli of the kidney. It is the leading cause of end-stage renal disease (ESRD) in Canada. The risk of nephropathy is similar in patients with either type 1 or type 2 DM. Risk factors for the development of diabetic nephropathy include hypertension, genetic predisposition, smoking, and chronic hyperglycemia. Results of the DCCT and UKPDS studies have demonstrated that kidney disease can be significantly reduced when near-normal blood glucose control is achieved and maintained (DCCT, 1993, p. 977; UKPDS, 1998, p. 837).

Hypertension significantly accelerates the progression of diabetic nephropathy, retinopathy, and risk of stroke. Therefore, aggressive blood pressure management is indicated for all patients with DM. ACE-inhibitor drugs (e.g., ramipril [Altace]) are commonly prescribed to patients with DM because they are effective blood pressure–lowering agents with few adverse effects. In addition, ACE inhibitors are often prescribed to patients with DM even when they are not hypertensive because drugs in this class have a protective effect on the kidney that prevents the progression of diabetic nephropathy independent of hypertension control (CDA, 2008, p. S129; Strippoli, Bonifati, Craig, Navaneethan, & Craig, 2006, p. 2). Angiotensin II receptor blockers (e.g., losartan [Cozaar]) may also be used for their kidney-protective benefits. (See Chapter 35 for a discussion of hypertension and Chapter 49 for a discussion of renal failure.)

Standards for the prevention and detection of nephropathy in patients with DM include yearly screening for the presence of microalbuminuria (MAU). This test detects kidney damage at an earlier stage than the standard dipstick test for macroprotein in the urine. Screening for MAU should be performed using a random urine for albumin/creatinine ratio (ACR) and serum creatinine for estimated glomerular filtration rate (eGFR). A 24-hour urine collection for determination of creatinine clearance and serum creatinine may be performed when there is doubt about the accuracy of an eGFR (Basi & Lewis, 2007, p. 439; CDA, 2008, p. S128).

Neuropathy

Diabetic neuropathy is nerve damage that occurs because of the metabolic derangements associated with DM. About 40 to 50% of patients with DM have some degree of neuropathy, with neurological complications occurring equally in type 1 and type 2 DM (CDA, 2008, p. S140). The most common type of neuropathy affecting people with DM is peripheral sensory neuropathy.

This can lead to the loss of protective sensation in the lower extremities, and, coupled with other factors, this significantly increases the risk for complications that can result in a lower limb amputation. Seven out of 10 nontraumatic lower extremity amputations in Canada occur in people with DM (CDA, 2008, p. S143; Canadian Association of Wound Care [CAWC], 2011).

Etiology and Pathophysiology

The pathophysiological processes of diabetic neuropathy are not well understood. Several theories exist, including metabolic, vascular, and autoimmune elements. The prevailing theory suggests that persistent hyperglycemia leads to an accumulation of sorbitol and fructose in the nerves that causes damage by an unknown mechanism. The result is reduced nerve conduction and demyelinization. Ischemia in blood vessels damaged by chronic hyperglycemia that supply the peripheral nerves is also implicated in the development of diabetic neuropathy. Neuropathy can precede, accompany, or follow the diagnosis of DM.

Classification

The two major categories of diabetic neuropathy are sensory neuropathy, which affects the peripheral nervous system, and autonomic neuropathy, which affects the central nervous system. Each of these types can take on several forms.

Sensory Neuropathy. The most common form of sensory polyneuropathy is distal symmetrical neuropathy, which affects the hands, the feet, or both bilaterally. This is sometimes referred to as *stocking-glove neuropathy*. Characteristics of distal symmetrical neuropathy include paresthesias, abnormal sensations, pain, and loss of sensation. The paresthesias may be associated with tingling, burning, and itching sensations. The patient may report a feeling of walking on pillows or numb feet. At times, the skin becomes so sensitive (hyperesthesia) that even light pressure from bed sheets cannot be tolerated. Complete or partial loss of sensitivity to touch and temperature is common. The pain, which is often described as burning, cramping, crushing, or tearing, is usually worse at night and may occur only at that time. Foot injury and ulcerations can occur without the patient ever having pain (Figure 52-15). Neuropathy can also cause atrophy of the small muscles of the hands and feet, causing deformity and limiting fine movement.

Control of blood glucose is the only treatment for diabetic neuropathy. It is effective in many, but not all, cases. Drug therapy may be used to treat neuropathic symptoms, particularly pain. Medications commonly used include topical creams (e.g., capsaicin), tricyclic antidepressants (e.g., amitriptyline [Elavil]), selective serotonin and norepinephrine reuptake inhibitors (e.g., duloxetine [Cymbalta]), and antiseizure medications (e.g., gabapentin [Neurontin]; pregablin [Lyrica]). Capsaicin is a moderately effective topical cream made from chili peppers. It depletes the accumulation of pain-mediating chemicals in the peripheral sensory neurons. The cream is applied with gloves three to four times a day. There is usually an increase in symptoms at the start of therapy, which is followed by relief of pain in 2 to 3 weeks. Tricyclic antidepressants are also moderately effective in treating the symptoms of diabetic neuropathy. They work by inhibiting the reuptake of norepinephrine and serotonin, which are neurotransmitters that are believed to play a role in the transmission of pain through the spinal cord (Unger & Cole, 2007, p. 900). Duloxetine is thought to relieve pain by increasing the levels of

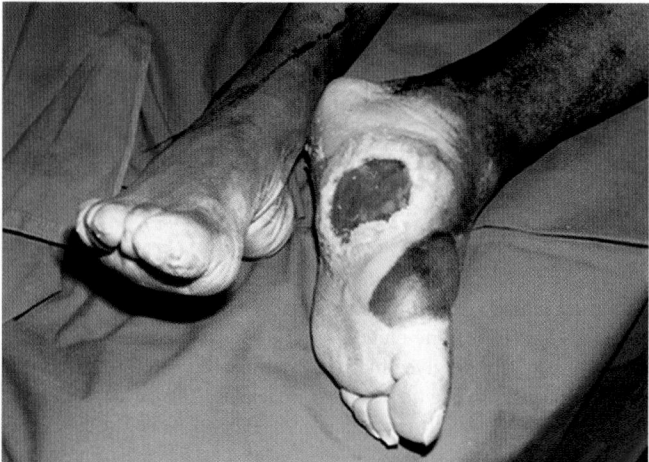

Figure 52-15 Neuropathy: neurotrophic ulceration.

Source: Urden, L. D., Stacy, K. M., & Lough, M. E. (2009). *Thelan's critical care nursing: Diagnosis and management* (6th ed.). St. Louis: Mosby.

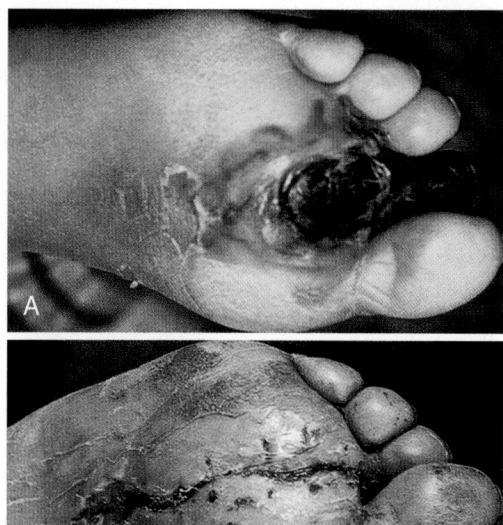

Figure 52-16 The necrotic toe developed as a complication of diabetes. **A,** Before amputation. **B,** After amputation.

Source: Chew, S. L., & Leslie, D. (2006). *Clinical endocrinology and diabetes: An illustrated colour text.* Edinburgh: Churchill Livingstone.

serotonin and norepinephrine, which improves the body's ability to regulate pain. Although gabapentin has been found to be effective in treating the pain of diabetic neuropathy, its mechanism of action is not well understood.

Autonomic Neuropathy. Autonomic neuropathy can affect nearly all body systems and lead to hypoglycemic unawareness, bowel incontinence and diarrhea, and urinary retention. Delayed gastric emptying (gastroparesis) is a complication of autonomic neuropathy that can produce anorexia, nausea, vomiting, gastroesophageal reflux, and persistent feelings of fullness. Gastroparesis can trigger hypoglycemia by delaying food absorption. Cardiovascular abnormalities associated with autonomic neuropathy are postural hypotension, resting tachycardia, and "silent" or painless myocardial infarction. A patient with postural hypotension should be instructed to change slowly from a lying or sitting position to a standing position.

DM can affect sexual function in men and women. Erectile dysfunction in diabetic men is well recognized and common, often being the first manifestation of autonomic failure. Erectile dysfunction associated with DM is believed to result from damage to the sacral parasympathetic nerves. Determining whether this problem is of organic or psychological origin is an important part of the assessment. Decreased libido is a problem for some women with DM. Monilial and nonspecific vaginitis are also common. Organic erectile dysfunction or sexual dysfunction in either the male or the female patient requires sensitive therapeutic counselling for both the patient and the patient's partner (Unger & Cole, 2007, p. 902). (See Chapter 57 for a further discussion of erectile dysfunction.)

A neurogenic bladder may develop as sensation in the inner bladder wall decreases, causing urinary retention. A patient with retention has infrequent voiding, difficulty in voiding, and a weak stream of urine. Emptying the bladder every 3 hours in a sitting position helps prevent stasis and subsequent infection. Tightening the abdominal muscles during voiding and using Credé's manoeuvre (mild massage downward over the lower abdomen and bladder) may also help with complete bladder emptying. Cholinergic agonist drugs such as bethanechol (Urecholine) may be used. The patient may also have to learn self-catheterization (see Chapter 48).

Complications of the Foot and the Lower Extremity

Foot complications are the most common cause of hospitalization in the person with DM (CAWC, 2011). The development of diabetic foot complications is a multifactorial process (Crawford, Inkster, Kleijnen, & Fahey, 2007, p. 65). They result from a combination of microvascular and macrovascular diseases that place the patient at risk for injury and serious infection that may lead to amputation (Figure 52-16). Sensory neuropathy and peripheral vascular disease (PVD) are risk factors, and clotting abnormalities, impaired immune function, and autonomic neuropathy also play important roles. Smoking is deleterious to the health of lower extremity blood vessels and increases the risk for amputation.

Sensory neuropathy is a major risk factor for lower extremity amputation in the person with DM. Loss of protective sensation (LOPS) often prevents the patient from becoming aware that a foot injury has occurred. Improper footwear and injury from stepping on foreign objects while barefoot are common causes of undetected foot injury in the person with LOPS. Because the primary risk factor for lower extremity amputation is LOPS, annual screening using a *monofilament* is an extremely important preventive measure. This is done by applying a thin, flexible filament to several spots on the plantar surface of the foot and toes and asking the patient to report if it is felt. Insensitivity to a 10-g Semmes-Weinstein monofilament has been shown to greatly increase the risk for diabetic foot ulcers that can lead to amputation. If the patient has LOPS, aggressive measures must be taken to teach the patient how to prevent foot ulceration. These measures include the selection of proper footwear, including prescription shoes. Other measures are to carefully avoid injury to the foot, to practise diligent skin and nail care, to inspect the foot thoroughly each day, and to treat small problems promptly (CDA, 2008, p. 200; Edwards, 2008, p. 21).

PVD increases the risk for amputation by causing a reduction in blood flow to the lower extremities. When blood flow is decreased, oxygen, white blood cells, and vital nutrients are not available to the tissues. Therefore, wounds take longer to heal and the risk for infection increases. Signs of PVD include intermittent claudication, pain at rest, cold feet, loss of hair, delayed capillary filling, and dependent rubor (redness of the skin that occurs when the extremity is in a dependent position). The disease is diagnosed by history, ankle–brachial index (ABI), and angiography. Management includes control or reduction of risk factors, particularly smoking, high saturated fat intake, and hypertension. Femoral bypass or graft surgery is indicated in some patients. Proper care of the feet is essential for the patient with PVD. Guidelines for patient teaching are listed in Table 52-21.

The Doppler instrument is used to perform the ABI to diagnose the presence or degree of PVD. Similar to an electronic stethoscope, this device amplifies sound. The procedure is noninvasive and can measure blood pressure and blood flow velocity in the lower extremities. It can indicate areas of stenosis or

occlusion and is useful as an indicator of the need for additional vascular tests. To determine location and extent of PVD, an angiography can be completed. Angiography is an invasive procedure and it provides information on the actual blood vessel condition.

Proper care of a diabetic foot ulcer is critical to prevention of infections. Management requires an interdisciplinary approach that addresses glycemic control, infection, lower extremity vascular status, and local wound care (CDA, 2008, p. S144). The fundamentals of good wound care involve an optimal wound environment, off-loading of the ulcer site, and in nonischemic wounds, regular debridement of nonviable tissue.

Neuropathic arthropathy, or *Charcot foot*, results in ligament softening and bony deformities that ultimately lead to joint dysfunction and foot drop. The pathogenesis of Charcot foot is not clear but it is likely owing to a combination of mechanical and vascular factors resulting from peripheral neuropathy and is mediated through an uncontrolled inflammation in the foot (Hordon, 2011, p. 1; Rogers et al., 2011, p. 2123). Changes that occur with Charcot foot happen gradually and create an abnormal distribution of weight over the foot, further increasing the chances of developing an ulcer on the plantar aspect of the foot as new pressure points emerge. Neuropathic ulcers resemble a "BB-shot" or "punched-out" wound and are usually painless. This high-risk foot complication requires immediate attention such as foot radiographic studies and referral to a high-risk foot team of chiropody, orthopedic surgery, and plastic surgery specialists. Infection and subsequent amputation is a danger and necessitates the long-term use of antibiotics and weeks of avoidance of weight bearing on the affected limb (Edmonds, 2008, p. S20; Bentley & Foster, 2008, p. S18).

Integumentary Complications

The skin is often affected in patients with DM. *Acanthosis nigricans* is a dark, coarse, thickened skin predominantly seen in flexures and on the neck. Acanthosis nigricans is a risk factor for type 2 DM and is associated with hyperinsulinemia and insulin resistance (CDA, 2008, p. S14; Kong et al., 2007, p. 203). Skin disorders such as diabetic dermopathy and necrobiosis lipoidica diabeticorum are attributed to microangiopathy. Shin spots are brown spots located on the anterior surfaces of the lower extremities. They are harmless and painless and initially measure less than 1 cm in diameter. *Necrobiosis lipoidica diabeticorum* (Figure 52-17) is believed to be the result of the breakdown of collagen in the skin. It usually appears as red-yellow lesions, with atrophic skin that becomes shiny and transparent, revealing tiny blood vessels under the surface. Because the thin skin is prone to injury, special care must be taken to protect affected areas from injury and ulceration. This condition is not common, but it may appear before other clinical signs or symptoms of DM. It is more frequently seen in young women. *Granuloma annulare*, associated mainly with type 1 DM, is probably autoimmune in nature and forms partial rings of papules, often on the dorsal surface of hands and feet.

Infection

A patient with DM is more susceptible to infections than other patients. The mechanisms for this phenomenon include a defect in the mobilization of inflammatory cells and an impairment of phagocytosis by neutrophils and monocytes. Organisms such as

PATIENT & CAREGIVER TEACHING GUIDE

Table 52-21 Foot Care

1. Wash feet daily with a mild soap and warm water. Test water temperature with a thermometer or hands first.

2. Pat feet dry gently, especially between toes.

3. Examine feet daily for cuts, blisters, swelling, and red, tender areas. Do not depend on feeling sores. If eyesight is poor, have others inspect feet.

4. Use lanolin on feet to prevent skin from drying and cracking. Do not apply between toes.

5. Do not use commercial remedies or sharp blades to remove calluses or corns.

6. Cleanse cuts with warm water and mild soap, covering with clean dressing. Do not use iodine, rubbing alcohol, or strong adhesives.

7. Report skin infections or nonhealing sores to health care provider immediately.

8. Cut and file toenails even with rounded contour of toes. Do not cut down corners. The best time to trim nails is after a shower or bath. See a foot care specialist if advice or treatment is needed.

9. Separate overlapping toes with cotton or lamb's wool.

10. Avoid open-toe, open-heel, and high-heel shoes. Leather shoes are preferred to synthetic ones. Wear slippers at home and shoes on the beach. Do not go barefoot. Shake out shoes before putting on.

11. Wear clean, absorbent (cotton or wool) socks or stockings that have not been mended. Coloured socks must be colourfast.

12. Do not wear socks or stockings that leave impressions, hindering circulation.

13. Do not use hot water bottles or heating pads to warm feet. Wear socks for warmth.

14. Guard against frostbite.

15. Exercise feet daily either by walking or by flexing and extending feet in suspended position. Avoid prolonged sitting, standing, and crossing of legs.*

*Registered Nurses Association of Ontario (RNAO). (2007). *Reducing foot complications for people with diabetes.* In RNAO, Nursing Best Practice Guidelines. Toronto: Author.

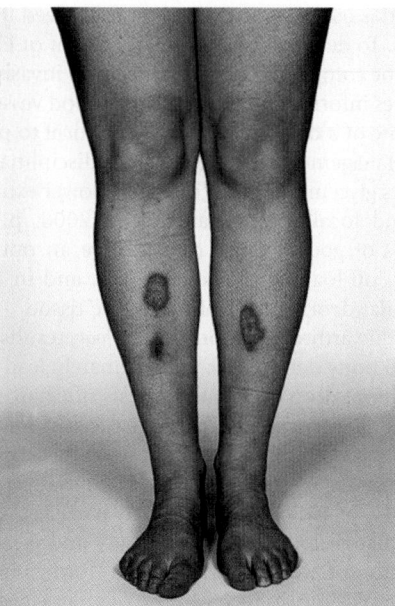

Figure 52-17 Necrobiosis lipoidica diabeticorum.

Source: Chew, S. L., & Leslie, D. (2006). *Clinical endocrinology and diabetes: An illustrated colour text.* Edinburgh: Churchill Livingstone.

yeast thrive in a high–blood glucose environment. Thus, recurring or persistent infections such as *Candida albicans,* as well as boils and furuncles, in the undiagnosed patient often lead the health care provider to suspect DM. Loss of sensation (peripheral neuropathy) may delay the detection of an infection in the feet.

Persistent glycosuria may predispose to bladder infections, especially in patients with a neurogenic bladder. Decreased circulation resulting from angiopathy can prevent or delay the immune response. Antibiotic therapy has prevented infection from being a major cause of death in patients with DM. The treatment of infections must be prompt and vigorous.

AGE-RELATED CONSIDERATIONS: DIABETES MELLITUS

The prevalence of DM increases with age. A major reason for this is that the process of aging is associated with a reduction in β-cell function, decreased insulin sensitivity, and altered carbohydrate metabolism (BBDC, 2009, p. 42). Aging is also associated with a number of conditions that are more likely to be treated with medications that impair insulin action (e.g., corticosteroids, anti-hypertensives, phenothiazines). Undiagnosed and untreated DM is more common in the older adult, partly because many of the normal physiological changes of aging, such as visual changes and decreased glomerular filtration, resemble those of DM.

Although good glycemic control is important to people of all ages with DM, several factors are taken into account when determining glycemic goals for an older adult. One is that hypoglycemic unawareness is more common in this age group, making these patients more likely to suffer adverse consequences from blood glucose–lowering therapy. They may also have delayed psychomotor function that could interfere with the ability to treat hypoglycemia. Other factors to consider in establishing glycemic goals for the older adult patient include the patient's own desire for treatment and other coexisting medical problems such as cognitive impairment. Compounding the challenge, DM has been found to contribute to a greater rate of decline of cognitive function. Although it is generally agreed that treatment is indicated for older adults with DM to prevent acute complications and avoid unpleasant symptoms, strict glycemic control may be difficult to achieve (Meneilly, 2011, p. 14).

As with any group, healthy eating and exercise are recommended as therapy for older adult patients with DM. This should take into account functional limitations that may interfere with physical activity and the ability to prepare meals. Because of the physiological changes that occur with aging, the therapeutic outcome for the older adult with DM who receives OHAs may be altered. The short-acting insulin secretagogues (e.g., repaglinide [GlucoNorm]) are usually well tolerated and appear to have fewer adverse effects and fewer drug interaction problems than longer-acting insulin secretagogues (glyburide [Diabeta]). Other OHAs described earlier in this chapter may also be used in older adult patients with DM. Insulin therapy may be instituted if OHAs are not effective. However, it is important to recognize that older adult patients are more likely to have limitations in manual dexterity and visual acuity, both of which are necessary for accurate insulin administration (CDA, 2008, p. S182).

Patient teaching should be based on the individual's needs, using a slower pace with simple printed materials. It is important to include family or a support person in the teaching. The patient education issues for the older adult patient include those related to vision, mobility, cognitive status, memory, functional ability, financial and social situation, the effect of multiple medications, eating habits, the potential for undetected hypoglycemia, and quality-of-life issues.

CLINICAL DECISION-MAKING EXERCISE

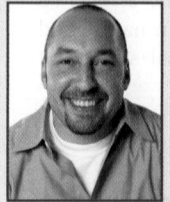

CASE STUDY:
Diabetic Ketoacidosis

Source: © iStockphoto.com/Justin Horracks.

Patient Profile

Hector LeBlanc, a 34-year-old White man, was admitted to the emergency department after he was found unconscious in his apartment by his wife.

Subjective Data (Provided by Wife)

- Was diagnosed with type 1 diabetes mellitus 12 months ago
- Was taking 48 units of insulin daily: 12 units of regular insulin plus 20 units of neutral protamine Hagedorn (NPH) insulin before breakfast, 8 units of regular insulin before dinner, and 8 units of NPH at bedtime
- Has history of flu for 1 week with vomiting and anorexia
- Stopped taking insulin 2 days ago when he was unable to eat

Objective Data

Physical Examination
- Breathing is deep and rapid
- Acetone smell on breath
- Skin flushed and dry

Diagnostic Studies
- Blood glucose level of 40.5 mmol/L
- Blood pH of 7.26

Discussion Questions

1. Briefly explain the pathophysiology of the development of diabetic ketoacidosis (DKA) in this patient.
2. What clinical manifestations of DKA does Mr. LeBlanc exhibit?

3. What factors precipitated Mr. LeBlanc's DKA?
4. *Priority Decision:* What is the priority nursing intervention for Mr. LeBlanc?
5. What distinguishes this case history from one of hyperosmolar hyperglycemic state (HHS) or hypoglycemia?
6. What teaching should be done with Mr. LeBlanc and his family?
7. What role should Mr. LeBlanc's wife have in the management of his diabetes?
8. *Priority Decision:* Based on the assessment data presented, what are the priority nursing diagnoses? Are there any collaborative problems?

Evolve *Answers are available on* **http://evolve.elsevier.com/ Canada/Lewis/medsurg**

REVIEW QUESTIONS

The number of the question corresponds to the same-numbered objective at the beginning of the chapter.

1. What are polydipsia and polyuria related to diabetes mellitus primarily caused by?
   a. The release of ketones from cells during fat metabolism
   b. Fluid shifts resulting from the osmotic effect of hyperglycemia
   c. Damage to the kidneys from exposure to high levels of glucose
   d. Changes in red blood cells resulting from attachment of excessive glucose to hemoglobin
2. What should the nurse recognize when a patient with type 2 diabetes mellitus is admitted to the hospital with pneumonia?
   a. The patient must receive insulin therapy to prevent the development of ketoacidosis.
   b. The patient has islet-cell antibodies that have destroyed the ability of the pancreas to produce insulin.
   c. The patient has minimal or absent endogenous insulin secretion and requires daily insulin injections.
   d. The patient may have sufficient endogenous insulin to prevent ketosis but is at risk for development of hyperosmolar hyperglycemic state.
3. What does effective collaborative management of diabetes include?
   a. Using insulin with all patients to achieve glycemic goals
   b. Relying on the health care provider as the central figure in the program for good control
   c. Relying solely on nutritional therapy as the initial treatment modality for all patients with diabetes
   d. Aiming for a balance of nutrition, activity, and medications together with appropriate monitoring and patient and caregiver teaching

4. The nurse is responsible for counselling the person with diabetes regarding lifestyle changes. Which of the following would be appropriate for the nurse to discuss?
   a. The use of the same diabetes diet for all people with diabetes
   b. The importance of calorie restriction to control blood sugars
   c. The use of Canada's Food Guide to support a well-balanced nutrition plan
   d. The importance of carbohydrate counting and insulin adjustment for all people with diabetes
5. What information should the nurse include when teaching a person with newly diagnosed type 1 diabetes "survival skills"?
   a. Weight-loss measures
   b. Elimination of sugar from diet
   c. The need to reduce physical activity
   d. Self-monitoring of blood glucose
6. What is an appropriate teaching measure for the patient with diabetes mellitus related to foot care?
   a. Use heat to increase blood supply.
   b. Avoid softening lotions and creams.
   c. Inspect all surfaces of the feet daily.
   d. Use iodine to disinfect cuts and abrasions.
7. A patient with diabetes has a serum glucose level of 36 mmol/L and is unresponsive. Following assessment of the patient, the nurse suspects diabetic ketoacidosis (DKA) rather than hyperosmolar hyperglycemic state. Which of the following is characteristic of DKA?
   a. Polyuria
   b. Severe dehydration
   c. Rapid, deep respirations
   d. Decreased serum potassium
8. Which of the following is an appropriate therapy for patients with diabetes mellitus?
   a. Use of diuretics to prevent and treat renal problems
   b. Use of angiotensin-converting enzyme inhibitors to prevent and treat renal problems
   c. Use of commercial remedies or sharp blades to remove calluses or corns
   d. Use of sugar-free drinks to treat hypoglycemia

REFERENCES

American Association of Diabetes Educators (AADE). (2009). *Insulin pump therapy: Guidelines for successful outcomes.* AADE 2008 Consensus Summit. Retrieved from *http://www.diabeteseducator.org/export/sites/aade/_resources/pdf/Insulin_Pump_White_Paper.pdf*

American Association of Diabetes Educators (AADE) (2010). *Position statement: Self-monitoring of blood glucose, 1-9.* Chicago: Author. Retrieved from *http://www.diabeteseducator.org/export/sites/aade/_resources/pdf/research/Self-Monitoring_of_Blood_Glucose.pdf*

American Diabetes Association (ADA). (2008) Nutrition recommendations and interventions for diabetes. *Diabetes Care, 31*(Suppl 1), S61-S78, doi:10.2337/dc08-S061

American Diabetes Association (ADA). (2011). Position statement: Standards of medical care in diabetes. *Diabetes Care, 34*(Suppl 1), S11-S61: doi:10.2337/dc11-S011

Banting and Best Diabetes Centre (BBDC). Diabetes Care and Education Committee. (2009). *Approach to the management of diabetes mellitus* (7th ed.). Retrieved from *http://www.bbdc.org/diabetesmanagement/*

Basi, S., & Lewis, J. (2007). Microalbuminuria as a target to improve cardiovascular and renal outcomes in diabetic patients. *Current Diabetes Reports, 7*(6), 439-442. doi:10.1007/s11892-007-0074-7

Bentley, J., & Foster, A. (2008). Management of the diabetic foot ulcer: Exercising control. *British Journal of Community Nursing, 13*(3), S16, S18.

Brenner, Z. (2006). Management of hyperglycaemic emergencies. *AACN Clinical Issues, 17*(1), 56-65. doi:10.1097/00044067-200601000-00008

Bristol-Myers Squibb (BMS) Canada. (2011). *Product monograph: Onglyza.* Montreal: Author.

Bristol-Myers Squibb (BMS) Company. (2008). *Glucophage (metformin hydrochloride tablets) prescribing information—Revised 2008.* New York: Author.

Canadian Association of Wound Care (CAWC). (2011). Diabetes foot ulcers. Retrieved from *http://cawc.net/index.php/public/facts-stats-and-tools/statistics/*

Canadian Diabetes Association (CDA). (2009). *The prevalence and costs of diabetes facts.* Toronto: Author. Retrieved from *http://www.diabetes.ca/documents/about-diabetes/PrevalanceandCost_09.pdf*

Canadian Diabetes Association (CDA) Clinical Practice Guidelines Expert Committee. (2008). 2008 Clinical practice guidelines for the prevention and management of diabetes in Canada. *Canadian Journal of Diabetes, 32*(Suppl.1), S1-S201. Retrieved from *http://www.diabetes.ca/files/cpg2008/cpg-2008.pdf*

Canadian Diabetes Association (CDA) and Diabetes Quebec (DC). (2011). *Diabetes: Canada at the tipping point charting a new path.* Toronto: Author. Retrieved from *http://www.diabetes.ca/documents/get-involved/WEB_Eng.CDA_Report_.pdf*

Cheng, A. (2009). Cardiovascular disease and diabetes: Key elements from the CDA 2008 Clinical Practice Guidelines. Retrieved from *http://www.diabetes.ca/documents/about-diabetes/Synopsis_Final.pdf*

Cheng, A. (2011). The rule of 3's: Insulin use in type 2 diabetes. *Canadian Diabetes, 24*(1), 3-9.

Crawford, F., Inkster, M., Kleijnen, J., & Fahey, T. (2007). Predicting foot ulcers in patients with diabetes: A systematic review and meta-analysis. *Quality Journal of Medicine, 100,* 65-86. doi:10.1093/qjmed/hcl140

DeBeer, K., Michael, S., Thacker, M., Wynne, E., Pattni, C., Gomm, M., …, Ullah, K. (2008). Diabetic ketoacidosis and hyperglycemic hyperosmolar syndrome—Clinical guidelines. *Nursing in Critical Care, 13*(1), 5-11. doi:10.1111/j.1478-5153.2007.00259.x

Diabetes Control and Complications Trial (DCCT) Research Group. (1993). The effect of intensive treatment of diabetes on the development and progression of long-term complications in insulin-dependent diabetes mellitus. *New England Journal of Medicine, 329*(14), 977-986.

Diabetes Prevention Program (DPP) Research Group. (2002). Reduction in the incidence of type 2 diabetes with lifestyle intervention or metformin. *New England Journal of Medicine, 346,* 393. doi:10.2337/diacare.25.12.2165

Dokken, B. (2008). The pathophysiology of cardiovascular disease and diabetes: Beyond blood pressure and lipids. *Diabetes Spectrum, 21*(3), 160-65. doi:10.2337/diaspect.21.3.160

Edmonds, M. (2008). A natural history and framework for managing diabetic foot ulcers. *British Journal of Nursing, 17*(11, Suppl), S20-S29.

Edwards, M. (2008). Risk reduction and care for the diabetic foot. *Practice Nurse, 36*(4) 21-26.

Eli Lilly Canada. (2011). *Product monograph: Byetta.* Toronto: Author.

Forum for Injection Technique (FIT) Canada. FIT Board (2011). *Recommendations for best practice in injection technique, 1-26.* Retrieved from *http://www.bd.com/resource.aspx?IDX=25063*

Fowler, M. (2007). Diabetes treatment. Part 2: Oral agents for glycemic management. *Clinical Diabetes, 25,* 131-134. doi:10.2337/diaclin.25.4.131

Fowler, M. (2008). Diabetes treatment. Part 3: Insulin and incretins. *Clinical Diabetes, 26,* 35-39. doi:10.2337/diaclin.26.1.35

Franz, M. J., Boucher, J. L., Green-Pastors J., & Powers, M. A. (2008). Evidence-based nutrition practice guidelines for diabetes and scope and standards of practice. *Journal of the American Dietetic Association, 108*(4 Suppl 1), S52-S58. doi:10.1016/j.jada.2008.01.021

Gaede, P., Lund-Anderson, H., Parving, H., & Pedersen, O. (2008). Effects of multifactorial intervention on mortality in type 2 diabetes. *New England Journal of Medicine, 358,* 580-591. doi:10.1056/NEJMoa0706245

Gastaldelli, A. (2008). Abdominal fat: Does it predict the development of type 2 diabetes? *American Journal of Clinical Nutrition, 87*(5), 1118-1119. Retrieved from *http://www.ajcn.org/content/87/5/1118.full.pdf+html*

Gillies, C., Abrams, K., Lambert, P., Cooper, N. J., Sutton, A. J., Hsu, R. T., & Khunti, K. (2007). Pharmacological and lifestyle interventions to prevent or delay type 2 diabetes in people with impaired glucose tolerance: Systematic review and meta-analysis. *British Medical Journal, 334,* 1-9. doi:10.1136/bmj.39063.689375.55

Goldenberg, R., Cheng, A., Punthakee, Z., & Clement, M. (2011). Position Statement: Use of glycated hemoglobin (A1C) in the diagnosis of type 2 diabetes mellitus in adults. *Canadian Journal of Diabetes, 35*(3), 247-253.

Health Canada. (2007). *Eating well with Canada's food guide.* Ottawa: Author. Retrieved from *http://www.hc-sc.gc.ca/fn-an/food-guide-aliment/index-eng.php*

Health Canada. (2009). *Report from the national diabetes surveillance system: Diabetes in Canada 2009.* Ottawa: Author. Retrieved from *http://www.phac-aspc.gc.ca/publicat/2009/ndssdic-snsddac-09/1-eng.php#intro*

Hordon, L. (2011). *Diabetic neuropathic arthropathy. 2012 UpToDate.* Philadelphia: Wolters-Kluwer Health. Retrieved from *http://www.uptodate.com/contents/diabetic-neuropathic-arthropathy#H24803269*

International Diabetes Federation (IDF). (2011). *Diabetes Atlas* (5th ed.). Retrieved from *http://www.idf.org/diabetesatlas*

Ismail-Beigi, F. (2012). Glycemic management of type 2 diabetes mellitus. *New England Journal of Medicine, 366*(14), 1319-27. doi:10.1056/NEJMcp1013127

Kahn, S., Haffner, S., Heise, M., Herman, W. H., Holman, R. R., Jones, N. P., …, Viberti, G. (2006). Glycemic durability of rosiglitazone, metformin or glyburide monotherapy. *New England Journal of Medicine, 355*(23), 2427-2443. doi:10.1056/NEJMoa066224

Kitabchi, A., Umpierrez, G., Miles, J., & Fisher, J. (2009) Hyperglycemic crises in adult patients with diabetes. *Diabetes Care, 32,* 1335-1343. doi:10.2337/dc09-9032

Kong, A., Williams, R., Rhyne, R., Urias-Sandoval, V., Cardinali, G., Weller, N. F., …, PRIME Net Clinicians. (2010). Acanthosis nigricans: High prevalence and association with diabetes in a practice-based research network consortium—A PRImary care Multi-Ethnic network (PRIME Net) study. *Journal of the American Board of Family Medicine, 23*(4), 476-485. doi:10.3122/jabfm.2010.04.090221

Kong, A., Williams, R., Smith, M., Sussman, A. L., Skipper, B., Hsi, A. C., & Rhyne, R. L. (2007). Acanthosis nigricans and diabetes risk factors: Prevalence in young people seen in southwestern U.S. primary care practices. *Annals of Family Medicine, 5*(3), 202-208. doi:10.1370/afm.678

Kuminski, C., McTernan, P., & Kumar, S. (2005). Role of resistin in obesity, insulin resistance and type II diabetes. *Clinical Science, 109*, 243-256. doi:10.1042/CS20050078

Levene, S., & Donnelly, R. (2008). *Management of type 2 diabetes mellitus* (2nd ed.). St. Louis: Mosby.

Llorente, M., & Urrutia, V. (2006). Diabetes, psychiatric disorders and the metabolic effects of antipsychotic medications. *Clinical Diabetes, 24*(1), 18-24. doi:10.2337/diaclin.24.1.18

Martens, P., Barlett, J., Prior, H., Sanguins, J., Burchill, C. A., Burland, E. M. J., & Carter, S. (2011). What is the comparative health status and associated risk factors for the Métis? A population-based study in Manitoba, Canada. *BMC Public Health, 11*(1), 814. doi:10.1186/1471-2458-11-814

Meneilly, G. (2011). Diabetes in the elderly. *Canadian Journal of Diabetes, 35*(1), 13-16.

Nestler, J. E. (2008). Metformin for the treatment of polycystic ovarian syndrome. *New England Journal of Medicine, 358*(1), 47-54. doi:10.1056/NEJMct0707092

NovoNordisk. (2011). *Product monograph: Victoza.* Mississauga, ON: Novo-Nordisk Canada Inc. Retrieved from *http://www.novonordisk.ca/PDF_Files/VictozaProductMonographEnglish_22-Mar-11.pdf*

Registered Nurses' Association of Ontario (RNAO). (2007). Assessment and management of foot ulcers for people with diabetes. In *RNAO, Nursing Best Practice Guidelines.* Toronto: Author.

Registered Nurses' Association of Ontario (RNAO). (2009). Subcutaneous administration of insulin in adults with type 2 diabetes—Revision. In *RNAO, Nursing Best Practice Guidelines.* Toronto: Author.

Rogers, L., Frykberg, R., Armstrong, D., Boulton, A. J., Edmonds, M., Van, G. H., ..., Uccioli, L. (2011). The Charcot foot in diabetes. *Diabetes Care, 34*, 2123-2129. doi:10.2337/dc11-0844

Ross, S., & Ekoe, J. M. (2010). Incretin agents in type 2 diabetes. *Canadian Family Physician, 56*, 639-648.

Shaefer, C. (2007). Patient and physician barriers to instituting insulin therapy: A case-based overview. *Insulin, 2*(Suppl B), S41-S46. doi:10.1016/S1557-0843(07)80070-4

Shah, B. R., Cauch-Dudek, K., & Pigeau, L. (2011). Diabetes prevalence and care in the Métis population of Ontario, Canada. *Diabetes Care, 34*(12), 2555-2556. doi:10.2337/dc11-0945

Shepherd, P., & Kahn, B. (1999). Glucose transporters and insulin action—Implications for insulin resistance and diabetes mellitus. *New England Journal of Medicine, 341*(4), 248-257. doi:10.1056/NEJM199907223410406

Shlafer, M. (2009). Drugs for diabetes mellitus. In R. S. Lehne (Ed.), *Pharmacology for nursing care* (7th ed., pp. 658-717). St. Louis: Saunders.

Strippoli, G., Bonifati, C., Craig, M., Navaneethan, S., & Craig, J. (2006). Angiotensin-converting enzyme inhibitors and angiotensin II receptor antagonists for preventing the progression of diabetic kidney disease. *Cochrane Database of Systematic Reviews, 4*, CD006257, 1-93. doi:10.1002/14651858.CD006257

Torley, D., Bellus, G. A., & Munro, C. S. (2002). Genes, growth factors and acanthosis nigricans. *British Journal of Dermatology, 147*(6), 1096. doi:10.1046/j.1365-2133.2002.05150.x

Unger, J., & Cole, E. (2007). Recognition and management of diabetic neuropathy. *Primary Care, 34*, 887. doi:10.1016/j.pop.2007.07.003

United Kingdom Prospective Diabetes Study (UKPDS). (1998). Intensive blood glucose control with sulphonylureas or insulin compared with conventional treatment and risk of complications in patients with type 2 diabetes. *Lancet, 352*, 837-853.

Wesorick, D., O'Malley, C., & Rushakoff, R. (2008). Management of diabetes and hyperglycemia in hospital: A practical guide to subcutaneous insulin use in the non-critically ill, adult patient. *Journal of Hospital Medicine, 3*(5), S17. doi:10.1002/jhm.353

White, R. (2007). Insulin pump therapy (continuous subcutaneous insulin infusion). *Primary Care: Clinics in Office Practice, 34*(4), 845-71. doi:10.1016/j.pop.2007.07.005

World Health Organization (WHO). (2011). Diabetes. Geneva: Author. Retrieved from *http://www.who.int/mediacentre/factsheets/fs312/en/*

CANADIAN RESOURCES

Canadian Diabetes Association
http://www.diabetes.ca
Dietitians of Canada
http://www.dietitians.ca
Heart and Stroke Foundation
http://ww2.heartandstroke.ca
Registered Nurses' Association of Ontario (RNAO) Nursing Best Practice Guidelines
http://www.rnao.org/bestpractices/index.asp

RELATED RESOURCES

American Diabetes Association (ADA)
http://www.diabetes.org
Diabetes 123
http://www.parknicollet.com/Diabetes
Glycemic Index Calculator (University of Sydney)
http://www.glycemicindex.com
International Diabetes Federation (IDF)
http://www.idf.org
Joslin Diabetes Center
http://www.joslin.harvard.edu
National Diabetes Information Clearinghouse
http://www.niddk.nih.gov

evolve *For additional Internet resources, see the Web site for this book at* **http://evolve.elsevier.com/Canada/Lewis/medsurg**

Written by Shannon Ruff Dirksen
Adapted by Maureen A. Barry

LEARNING OBJECTIVES

1. Describe the structures and functions of the male and female reproductive systems.
2. Summarize the functions of the major hormones essential for functioning of the male and female reproductive systems.
3. Explain the physiological changes that occur in a man and in a woman during the stages of sexual response.
4. Relate the age-related changes of the male and female reproductive systems to the differences in assessment findings.
5. Identify significant subjective and objective data related to the male and female reproductive systems and information

about sexual function that should be obtained from a patient.
6. Describe appropriate techniques to use in the physical assessment of the male and female reproductive systems.
7. Differentiate normal from common abnormal findings of a physical assessment of the male and female reproductive systems.
8. Describe the purpose, significance of results, and nursing responsibilities related to diagnostic studies of the male and female reproductive systems.

KEY TERMS

amenorrhea Absence of menstruation, p. 1478

clitoris Erectile tissue that lies anterior to the urethral meatus and the vaginal orifice and becomes engorged during sexual excitation, p. 1474

ductus deferens (or vas deferens) Long, thick tube through which sperm exit the epididymis, p. 1472

dyspareunia Abnormal pain during sexual intercourse, p. 1482

epididymis A very long, tightly coiled, comma-shaped tubular structure located on the top and behind each testis inside the scrotum; transports the sperm as they mature, p. 1472

gonads The primary reproductive organs (i.e., ovaries in the female and testes in the male), p. 1471

menarche The first episode of menstrual bleeding; indicates that a female has reached puberty, p. 1478

menopause The physiological cessation of menses associated with declining ovarian function, p. 1478

menstrual cycle The monthly process mediated by hormonal activity from the beginning of one menstrual period to the beginning of the next; repeats during each month between puberty and menopause in which an egg is not fertilized, p. 1478

mons pubis A fatty layer lying over the pubic bone that is covered in coarse hair after puberty, p. 1474

spermatogenesis Process of sperm production, p. 1472

ELECTRONIC RESOURCES

Supplemental content related to Chapter 53 can be found...

Evolve Web Site ⊖volve

http://evolve.elsevier.com/Canada/Lewis/medsurg

- Animations:
  - Lymphatic Drainage of the Breast
  - The Menstrual Cycle
- Assessment Case Study
- Clinical Reference: Laboratory Values
- Content Updates
- Electronic Calculators
- Examination Review Questions
- Glossary
- Key Points (Printable and MP3 Download)
- Physical Examination Video Clips:
  - Breasts
  - Breasts and Heart

- Abdominal Reflexes, Abdominal Muscles, and Inguinal Area
- Genitalia and Rectum (Female)
- Rectum and Prostate Gland (Male)
- Video Clips:
  - Inspection and Palpation: External Genitalia—Standing Position (Male)—1
  - Inspection and Palpation: External Genitalia—Standing Position (Male)—2
  - Inspection: Female Breasts—Sitting Position
  - Inspection: External Genitalia (Female)
  - Inspection: Speculum Examination (Female)
  - Palpation: Bimanual Examination (Female)
  - Palpation: Female Breasts—Supine Position
  - Palpation: Inguinal Hernia Evaluation (Male)

Structures and Functions of the Male and Female Reproductive Systems

The reproductive system of both males and females consists of primary (or essential) organs and secondary (or accessory) organs. The primary reproductive organs are referred to as **gonads**. The female gonads are the ovaries; the male gonads are the testes. The primary responsibility of the gonads is secretion of hormones and production of gametes (ova and sperm). Secondary or accessory organs are responsible for transporting and nourishing the ova and sperm as well as preserving and protecting the fertilized eggs.

Male Reproductive System

The three primary roles of the male reproductive system are (1) production and transportation of sperm, (2) deposit of sperm in the female reproductive tract, and (3) secretion of hormones. The primary reproductive organs in the male are the testes. Secondary reproductive organs include ducts (epididymis, ductus deferens, ejaculatory duct, and urethra), sex glands (prostate gland, Cowper's glands, and seminal vesicles), and the external genitalia (scrotum and penis) (Figure 53-1).

Testes. The paired testes are ovoid, smooth, firm organs measuring 3.5 to 5.5 cm long and 2 to 3 cm wide. They are within

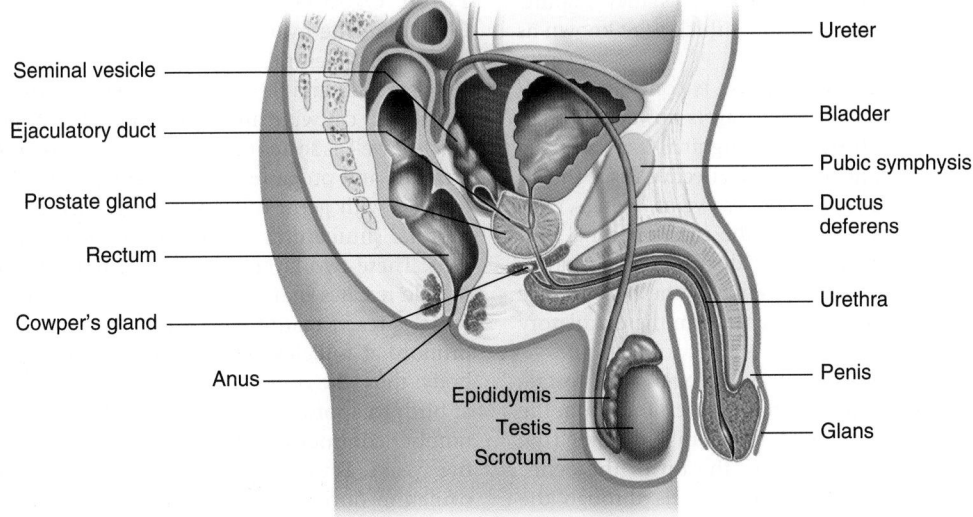

Figure 53-1 External and internal male sex organs.

Source: Patton, K. T., & Thibodeau, G. A. (2010). *Anatomy and physiology* (7th ed., p. 1021, Figure 31-1). St. Louis: Mosby.

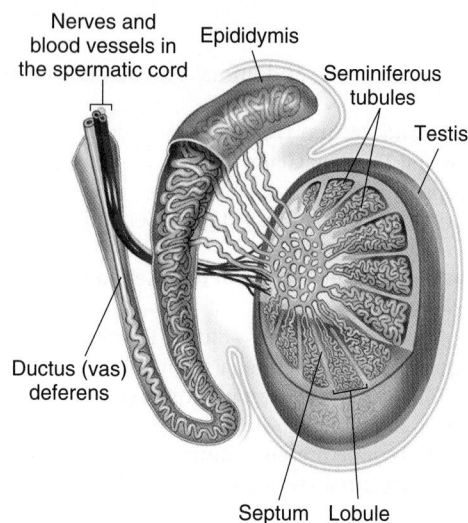

Figure 53-2 Seminiferous tubules, testis, epididymis, and ductus (vas) deferens in the male.

Source: Adapted from Patton, K. T., & Thibodeau, G. A. (2010). *Anatomy and physiology* (7th ed., p. 1023, Figure 31-3). St. Louis: Mosby.

the scrotum, which is a loose protective sac composed of a thin, loose outer layer of skin over a tough connective tissue layer. Within the testes, coiled structures known as seminiferous tubules form *spermatozoa* (immature sperm). The process of sperm production is called **spermatogenesis.** Interstitial cells of the testes lie between the seminiferous tubules and produce the male sex hormone testosterone.

Ducts. Sperm formed in the seminiferous tubules move through a series of ducts. These ducts transport the sperm from the testes to the outside of the body. As sperm exit the testes, they enter and pass through the epididymis, the ductus deferens, the ejaculatory duct, and the urethra.

The **epididymis** is a comma-shaped structure located on the posterior-superior aspect of each testis within the scrotum (Figure 53-2; see also Figure 53-1). It is a very long, tightly coiled tubular structure that measures about 6 m in length (Thibodeau & Patton, 2008). The epididymis transports the sperm as they mature. Sperm exit the epididymis through a long, thick tube known as the ductus deferens.

The **ductus deferens (or vas deferens)** is continuous with the epididymis within the scrotal sac. It travels upward through the scrotum and continues through the inguinal ring into the abdominal cavity. The spermatic cord is a connective tissue sheath that encloses the ductus deferens, arteries, veins, nerves, and lymph vessels as it ascends up through the inguinal canal (see Figure 53-2). In the abdominal cavity, the ductus deferens travels up, over, and behind the bladder. Posterior to the bladder, the ductus deferens joins the seminal vesicle to form the ejaculatory duct (see Figure 53-1).

The ejaculatory duct passes downward through the prostate gland, connecting with the urethra. The urethra extends from the bladder, through the prostate, and ends in a slitlike opening (the meatus) on the ventral side of the *glans,* the tip of the penis. During the process of ejaculation, sperm travels through the urethra and out of the penis.

Glands. The seminal vesicles, prostate gland, and Cowper's (bulbourethral) glands are the accessory glands of the male reproductive system. These glands produce and secrete seminal fluid (semen), which surrounds the sperm and forms the *ejaculate.*

The seminal vesicles lie just behind the bladder and between the rectum and the bladder. The ducts of the seminal vesicles fuse with the ductus deferens to form the ejaculatory ducts that enter the prostate gland. The prostate gland lies underneath the bladder. Its posterior surface is in contact with the rectal wall. The prostate normally measures 2 cm wide and 3 cm long and is divided into right and left lateral lobes and an anteroposterior median lobe. Cowper's glands lie on each side of the urethra and slightly posterior to it, just below the prostate. The ducts of these glands enter directly into the urethra.

Secretions from the seminal vesicles, prostate, and Cowper's glands make up most of the fluid in the ejaculate. These various secretions serve as a medium for the transport of sperm and create an alkaline, nutritious environment that promotes sperm motility and survival.

External Genitalia. The external genitalia consist of the penis and the scrotum. The penis consists of a shaft, and the tip is known as the glans. The glans is covered by a fold of skin, the prepuce (or foreskin), that forms at the junction of the glans and the shaft of the penis. In circumcised males, the prepuce has been removed. The broadened segment of the glans at the junction is the corona. The shaft of the penis consists of erectile tissue composed of the corpus cavernosum, the corpus spongiosum, the fibrous sheath that encases the erectile tissue, and the urethra. The skin covering the penis is thin, loose, and essentially hairless.

Female Reproductive System

The three primary roles of the female reproductive system are (1) production of ova (eggs), (2) secretion of hormones, and (3) protection and facilitation of the development of the fetus in a pregnant female. Like the male, the female has primary and secondary reproductive organs. The primary reproductive organs in the female are the paired ovaries. Secondary reproductive organs include ducts (fallopian tubes), the uterus, the vagina, sex glands (Bartholin's glands and breasts), and the external genitalia (vulva).

Pelvic Organs

Ovaries. The ovaries are usually located on either side of the uterus, just behind and below the fallopian (uterine) tubes (Figures 53-3 and 53-4). The ovaries are firm and solid, approximately 1.5 cm wide and 3 cm long. Their functions include *ovulation* as well as secretion of the two major reproductive hormones, estrogen and progesterone. The outer zone of the ovary contains follicles with germ cells, or *oocytes.* Each follicle contains a primordial (immature) oocyte surrounded by granulosa and theca cells. These two layers protect and nourish the oocyte until the follicle reaches maturity and ovulation occurs. However, not all follicles reach maturity. In a process termed *atresia,* most of the primordial follicles become smaller and are reabsorbed by the body; thus, the number of follicles declines from 2 to 4 million at birth to approximately 300,000 to 400,000 at menarche. This number continues to decrease throughout a woman's reproductive years. Fewer than 500 oocytes are actually released by ovulation during the reproductive years of the normal healthy woman.

Fallopian Tubes. Normally, each month during a woman's reproductive years, one ovarian follicle reaches maturity, and the

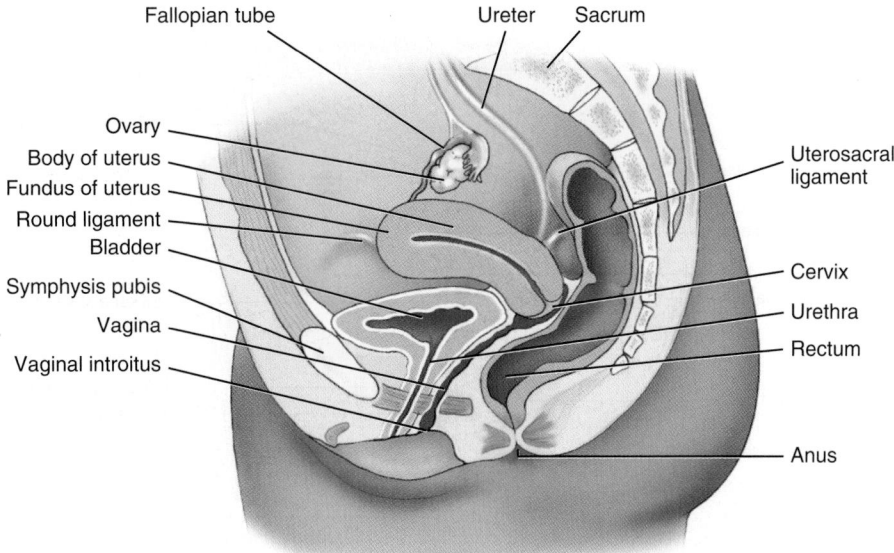

Figure 53-3 Female reproductive tract and related organs.

Source: Adapted from McKenry, L., Tessier, E., & Hogan, M. (2006). *Mosby's pharmacology in nursing* (22nd ed., p. 889, Figure 50-1). St. Louis: Mosby.

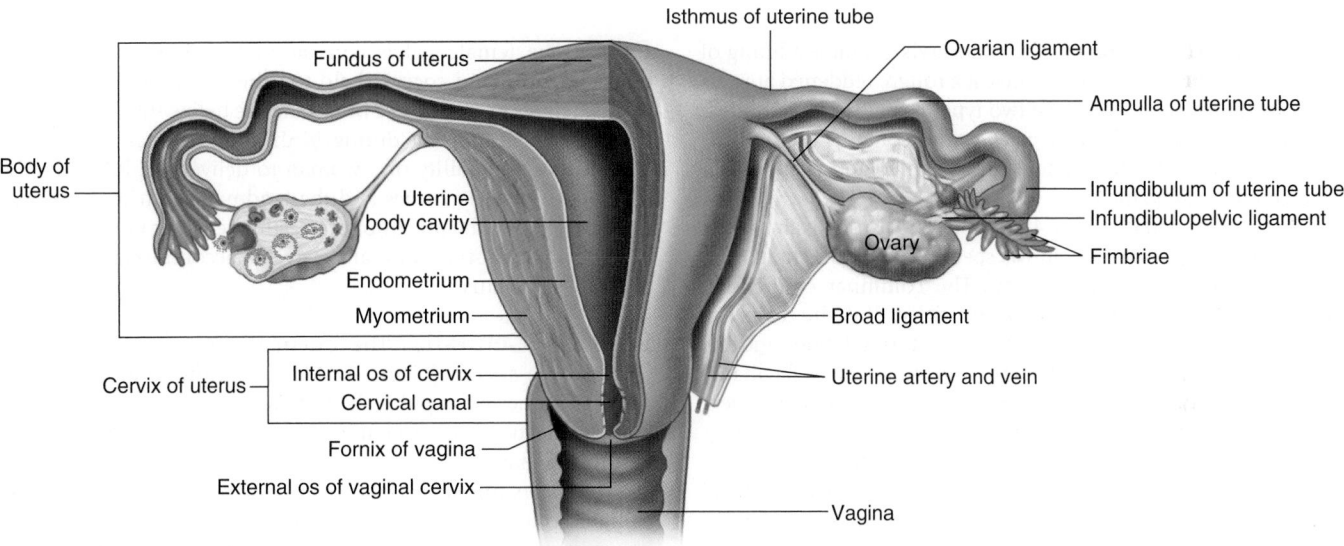

Figure 53-4 Female reproductive tract.

Source: Patton, K. T., & Thibodeau, G. A. (2010). *Anatomy and physiology* (7th ed., p. 1042, Figure 32-3A). St. Louis: Mosby.

ovum is ovulated, or expelled, from the ovary through the stimulus of the gonadotropic hormones, follicle-stimulating hormone (FSH) and luteinizing hormone (LH). The ovum then travels up a fallopian tube, where fertilization by sperm may occur. An ovum can be fertilized up to 72 hours after its release.

The distal ends of the fallopian tubes consist of finger-like projections called *fimbriae* that "massage" the ovaries at ovulation to help extract the mature ovum. The tubes, which average 12 cm in length, extend from the fimbriae to the superior lateral borders of the uterus. Fertilization usually takes place within the outer one third of the fallopian tubes.

Uterus. The uterus is a pear-shaped, hollow, muscular organ (see Figures 53-3 and 53-4). It is located between the bladder and

the rectum. In the mature *nulliparous* (never pregnant) female, the uterus is approximately 6 to 8 cm long and 4 cm wide. The uterine walls consist of an outer serosal layer, the perimetrium; a middle muscular layer, the myometrium; and an inner mucosal layer, the endometrium.

The uterus consists of the fundus, the body (or corpus), and the cervix (see Figure 53-4). The body makes up about 80% of the uterus and connects with the cervix at the isthmus, or neck. The cervix is the lower portion of the uterus that projects into the anterior wall of the vaginal canal. It makes up about 15 to 20% of the uterus in the nulliparous female. The cervix consists of the *ectocervix*, the outer portion that protrudes into the vagina, and the *endocervix*, the canal in the opening of the cervix. The ectocervix is covered with squamous epithelial cells, which give it a

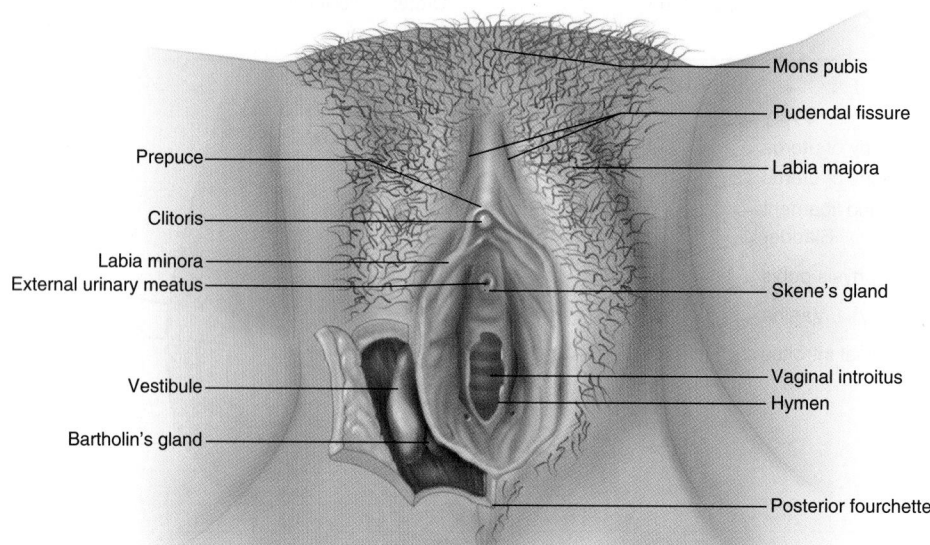

Figure 53-5 External female genitalia.

Source: Modified from Thibodeau, G. A., & Patton, K. T. (2010). *Anatomy and physiology* (7th ed., p. 1049, Figure 32-9A). St. Louis: Mosby.

smooth, pinkish appearance. The endocervix contains a lining of columnar epithelial cells, which give it a rough, reddened appearance. The junction at which the two types of epithelial cells meet is termed the *squamocolumnar junction* and contains the optimal types of cells needed for an accurate Papanicolaou (Pap) smear to screen for malignancies.

The cervical canal is 2 to 4 cm long and is relatively tightly closed. The cervix, however, allows sperm to enter the uterus and also allows menstruation to occur. The columnar epithelium, under hormonal influence, provides elasticity; thus, the cervix can stretch to allow for the passage of a fetus during labour and the birth process. The entrance of sperm into the uterus is facilitated by mucus produced by the cervix under the influence of estrogen. Under normal conditions, the cervical mucus becomes watery, stretchy, and more abundant at ovulation. This mucus facilitates the passage of sperm into the uterus. The postovulatory cervical mucus, under the influence of progesterone, is thick and inhibits sperm passage.

The anterior and posterior peritoneal covering of the uterus is called the *broad ligament.* It separates the uterus from the bladder and the rectum but does not provide support for the uterus or the *adnexa* (ovaries and tubes). The round ligament, which extends anteriorly to the labia majora, provides some support but is easily weakened by pregnancy. The firmest support for the uterus is provided by the uterosacral ligaments, which pull the uterus back and away from the vaginal orifice.

Vagina. The vagina is a tubular structure 8 to 10 cm long that is lined with squamous epithelium. The secretions of the vagina consist of cervical mucus, desquamated epithelium, and during sexual stimulation, a direct transudate secretion. These fluids protect against vaginal infection. The muscular and erectile tissue of the vaginal walls allows enough dilation and contraction to accommodate the passage of the fetus during labour as well as penetration of the penis during intercourse. The anterior vaginal wall lies along the urethra and the bladder. The posterior vaginal wall is adjacent to the rectum.

Pelvis. The female pelvis consists of four bones (two pelvic bones, sacrum, and coccyx) held together by several strong ligaments. The sections of these bones that lie below the iliopectineal line are very important during birth and are often a factor in determining the ability of a woman to deliver a child vaginally. Knowledge of these bones and the landmarks that they form in the pelvis allows the practitioner to estimate pelvic measurements and the potential for a woman's pelvis to accommodate the birth of a full-term fetus.

External Genitalia. The external portion of the female reproductive system (Figure 53-5), commonly called the *vulva,* consists of the mons pubis, labia majora, labia minora, clitoris, urethral meatus, Skene's glands, vaginal introitus (opening), and Bartholin's glands.

The **mons pubis** is a fatty layer lying over the pubic bone. It contains coarse hair that lies in a triangular pattern. (The male hair pattern is diamond shaped.) The labia majora are folds of adipose tissue that form the outer borders of the vulva. These hair-covered folds contain sweat glands and sebaceous glands. The hairless labia minora form the borders of the vaginal orifice and extend anteriorly to enclose the clitoris (Gibbs, Karlan, Haney, & Nygaard, 2008).

The *vestibule* is a boat-shaped fossa between the labia minora, extending from the clitoris at the anterior end to the vaginal opening at the posterior end. The perineum is the area between the vagina and the anus. The vaginal introitus is surrounded by thin membranous tissue called the *hymen.* In the adult female, the hymen usually appears as folds or hymenal tags and separates the external genitalia from the vagina. Although all females have this structure, there is wide anatomical variation in its morphology. At the posterior aspect of the vagina, a tense band of mucous membrane connecting the posterior ends of the labia minora is referred to as the *posterior fourchette.*

The **clitoris** is erectile tissue that becomes engorged during sexual excitation. It lies anterior to the urethral meatus and the vaginal orifice and is usually covered by the prepuce (Gibbs et al.,

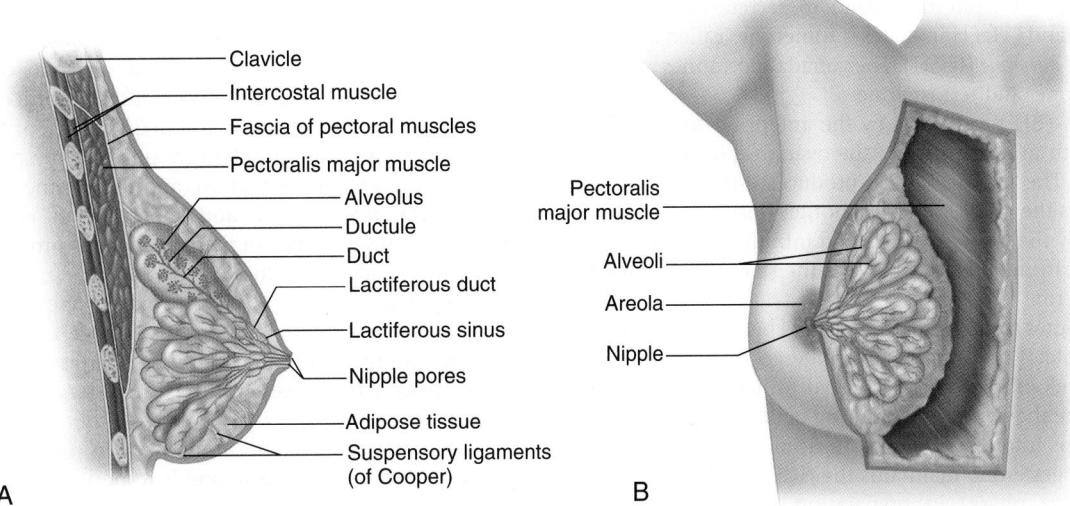

Figure 53-6 The lactating female breast. **A,** Sagittal section of a lactating breast. Glandular structures are anchored to the overlying skin and to the pectoral muscle by suspensory ligaments of Cooper. Each lobule of glandular tissues is drained by a lactiferous duct that eventually opens through the nipple. **B,** Anterior view of a lactating breast. In nonlactating breasts, the glandular tissue is much less evident, with adipose tissue making up most of each breast.

Source: Thibodeau, G. A., & Patton, K. T. (2010). *Anatomy and physiology* (7th ed., p. 1059, Figure 32-16). St. Louis: Mosby.

2008). Clitoral stimulation is an important part of sexual activity for many women.

Ducts of the Skene's glands lie alongside the urinary meatus and are thought to help lubricate the urinary meatus (McCance, Huether, Brashers, & Rote, 2010). Bartholin's glands, located at the posterior and lateral aspects of the vaginal orifice, secrete a thin, mucoid material believed to contribute slightly to lubrication during sexual intercourse. These glands are not usually palpable unless sebaceous-like cysts form or an infection is present, such as a sexually transmitted infection (STI).

Breasts. The breasts are a secondary sex characteristic; they develop during puberty in response to estrogen and progesterone. Cyclical hormonal changes lead to regular changes in breast tissue to prepare it for lactation when fertilization and pregnancy occur. The breasts are also considered a major organ of sexual stimulation.

The breasts extend from the second to the sixth ribs, with an area called the *tail of Spence* reaching the axilla. The fully mature breast is dome shaped and contains a pigmented centre termed the *areola*. The areolar region contains Montgomery's tubercles, which are similar to sebaceous glands and assist in lubricating the nipple. During lactation, the alveoli secrete milk (Figure 53-6). The milk then flows into a ductal system and is transported to the lactiferous sinuses. The nipple contains 15 to 20 tiny openings through which the milk flows during breastfeeding. The fibrous and fatty tissue that supports and separates the channels of the mammary duct system is primarily responsible for the varying sizes and shapes of the breasts in different individuals.

The breast has a rich lymphatic network that drains into the axillary and clavicular channels (Figure 53-7). Superficial lymph nodes are located in the axilla and are accessible to examination. This system is often responsible for the metastasis of a malignant tumour from the breast to other parts of the body.

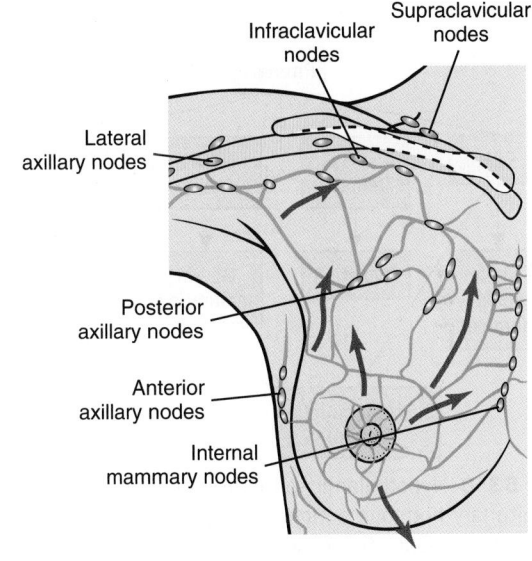

Figure 53-7 Lymphatic drainage of the breast. *Arrows* indicate direction of drainage.

Neuroendocrine Regulation of the Reproductive System

The hypothalamus, the pituitary gland, and the gonads secrete numerous hormones (Figure 53-8). (Endocrine hormones are discussed in Chapter 50.) These hormones regulate the processes of ovulation, spermatogenesis (formation of sperm), and fertilization and the formation and function of the secondary sex characteristics. In women, the hormones secreted by the anterior pituitary gland cause cyclical changes in the ovaries. The hypothalamus secretes gonadotropin-releasing hormone (GnRH), which stimulates the pituitary gland to secrete its hormones, including FSH and LH. LH in males is sometimes called *interstitial cell–stimulating hormone* (ICSH). The gonadal hormones are estrogen, progesterone, and testosterone.

In women, FSH production by the anterior pituitary stimulates the growth and maturity of the ovarian follicles necessary for ovulation. The mature follicle produces estrogen, which in turn suppresses the release of FSH. Another hormone, inhibin, is also secreted by the ovarian follicle and inhibits both GnRH and FSH secretion. In men, FSH stimulates the seminiferous tubules to produce sperm.

LH contributes to the ovulatory process because it causes follicles to complete maturation and undergo ovulation. It also causes the development of the ruptured follicle, or the area on the ovary where the ovum exited during ovulation. The ruptured follicle develops into a corpus luteum from which progesterone is secreted. Progesterone maintains the rich vascular state of the uterus (secretory phase) in preparation for fertilization and implantation. In men, LH or ICSH triggers testosterone production by the interstitial cells of the testes and, thus, is essential for the full maturation of sperm. Prolactin has no known function in men. In women, prolactin stimulates the development and

growth of the mammary glands. During lactation, it initiates and maintains milk production.

The gonadal hormones, estrogen and progesterone, are produced by the ovaries in women. Small amounts of an estrogen precursor are also produced in the adrenal cortices. Estrogen is essential to the development and maintenance of the secondary sex characteristics, the proliferative phase of the menstrual cycle immediately after menstruation, and the uterine changes essential to pregnancy. The role and importance of estrogen in men are not well understood. In men, estrogen is produced predominantly in the adrenal cortex.

Progesterone plays a major role in the menstrual cycle but most specifically in the secretory phase. Like estrogen, progesterone is involved in the bodily changes associated with pregnancy. Adequate progesterone is necessary to maintain an implanted egg.

The major gonadal hormone of men, testosterone, is produced by the testes. Testosterone is responsible for the development and maintenance of secondary sex characteristics as well as for adequate spermatogenesis. Androgens are produced in females by the adrenal glands and the ovaries in small amounts.

The circulating levels of gonadal hormones are controlled primarily by a negative feedback process. Receptors within the hypothalamus and the pituitary are sensitive to the circulating blood levels of the hormones (Table 53-1). Increased levels of hormones stimulate a hypothalamic response that decreases the high circulating levels. Likewise, low circulating levels provoke a hypothalamic response that increases the low circulating levels. For example, if the circulating level of testosterone in men is low, the hypothalamus is stimulated to secrete GnRH. This triggers the anterior pituitary to secrete greater amounts of FSH and ICSH, which in turn set off an increase in the production of testosterone. The high levels of testosterone then stimulate a decrease in the production of GnRH and thus of FSH and ICSH.

In women, however, there is a slight variation. The circulating levels are controlled through a combination of both a negative and a positive feedback system. A negative feedback control mechanism exists similar to that described previously. When circulating estrogen levels are low at the beginning of the follicular phase (see the later discussion of the menstrual cycle), the hypothalamus is stimulated to increase its production of GnRH. GnRH stimulates the pituitary to secrete greater amounts of FSH and LH, resulting in higher levels of estrogen production by the ovaries. Reciprocally, higher levels of circulating estrogen result in a decreasing secretion of GnRH and, thus, bring about a decrease in the secretion of FSH by the pituitary.

There is also a positive feedback control mechanism in women. Thus, with the increased levels of circulating estrogen, a greater level of GnRH is produced, resulting in an increased

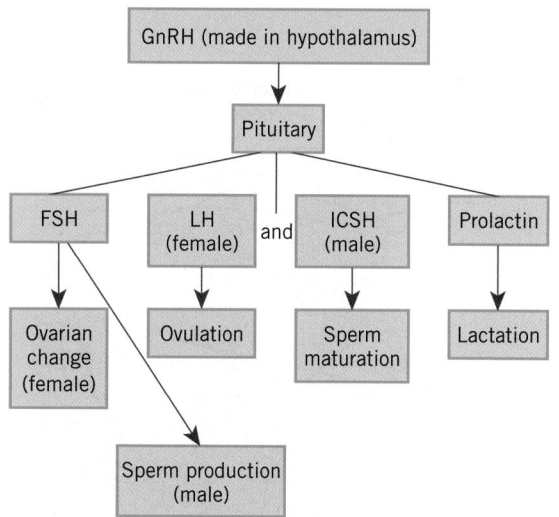

Figure 53-8 Hypothalamic–pituitary–gonadal axis. Only the major pituitary hormone actions are depicted. *FSH*, follicle-stimulating hormone; *GnRH*, gonadotropin-releasing hormone; *ICSH*, interstitial cell–stimulating hormone; *LH*, luteinizing hormone.

Table 53-1 Gonadal Feedback Mechanisms						
Negative Feedback						
↓ Estrogen	→	↑ GnRH (hypothalamus)	→	↑ FSH (pituitary)	→	↑ Estrogen (ovaries)
Positive feedback						
↑ Estrogen	→	↑ GnRH (hypothalamus)	→	↑ LH (pituitary)		
Testes (negative feedback)						
↓ Testosterone	→	↑ GnRH (hypothalamus)	→	↑ FSH and ICSH (pituitary)	→	↑ Testosterone (testes)

FSH, follicle-stimulating hormone; *GnRH*, gonadotropin-releasing hormone; *ICSH*, interstitial cell–stimulating hormone; *LH*, luteinizing hormone.

level of LH from the pituitary, which instigates ovulation. Likewise, lowered levels of estrogen result in a lowered level of LH.

Menarche

Menarche is the first episode of menstrual bleeding and indicates that a female has reached puberty. Menarche usually occurs at approximately 12 to 13 years of age but can occur as early as 10 years of age in some individuals (Styne & Grumbach, 2008). As puberty approaches, there are changes associated with the elevated rate of estrogen and progesterone secretion by the ovaries. These changes include the development of breast buds and pubic hair, and later, the development of axillary hair. During this time, there is a decrease in the sensitivity of the hypothalamic–pituitary axis that allows for increased secretion of FSH and LH and a resultant increase in estrogen. It is during this time that the adult pattern of gonadotropin secretion sets in, resulting in the menstrual cycle. Menstrual cycles are often irregular for the first 1 to 2 years following menarche because of *anovulatory* cycles (cycles without ovulation).

Menstrual Cycle

The major functions of the ovaries are ovulation and the secretion of hormones. These functions are accomplished during the normal **menstrual cycle,** a monthly process mediated by the hormonal activity of the hypothalamus, the pituitary gland, and the ovaries. Menstruation occurs during each month in which an egg is not fertilized (Figure 53-9). The endometrial cycle is divided into three phases labelled in relation to uterine and ovarian changes: (1) the *proliferative* or *follicular phase,* (2) the *secretory* or *luteal phase,* and (3) the *menstrual* or *ischemic phase.* The length of the menstrual cycle ranges from 20 to 40 days, the average being 28 days.

The menstrual cycle begins on the first day of one menstrual period, which usually lasts 4 to 6 days, and ends on the first day of the next (Farage, Neill, & MacLean, 2009). Table 53-2 includes characteristics of the menstrual cycle and related patient teaching. During this time, estrogen and progesterone levels are low, but FSH levels begin to increase. During the follicular phase, a single follicle matures fully under the stimulation of FSH. (The mechanism that ensures that usually only one follicle reaches maturity is not known.) The mature follicle stimulates estrogen production, causing the negative feedback that results in decreased FSH secretion.

Although the initial stage of follicular maturation is stimulated by FSH, complete maturation and ovulation occur only with the presence of LH. When estrogen levels peak on about the twelfth day of the cycle, there is a surge of LH, which triggers ovulation a day or two later. After ovulation (maturation and release of an ovum), LH promotes the development of the corpus luteum.

The fully developed corpus luteum continues to secrete estrogen and initiates progesterone secretion. If fertilization occurs, high levels of estrogen and progesterone continue to be secreted owing to the continued activity of the corpus luteum from stimulation by human chorionic gonadotropin (hCG). If fertilization does not take place, menstruation occurs because of a decrease in estrogen production and progesterone withdrawal.

During the follicular phase, the endometrial lining of the uterus also undergoes change. As larger amounts of estrogen are produced, the endometrial lining undergoes proliferative changes,

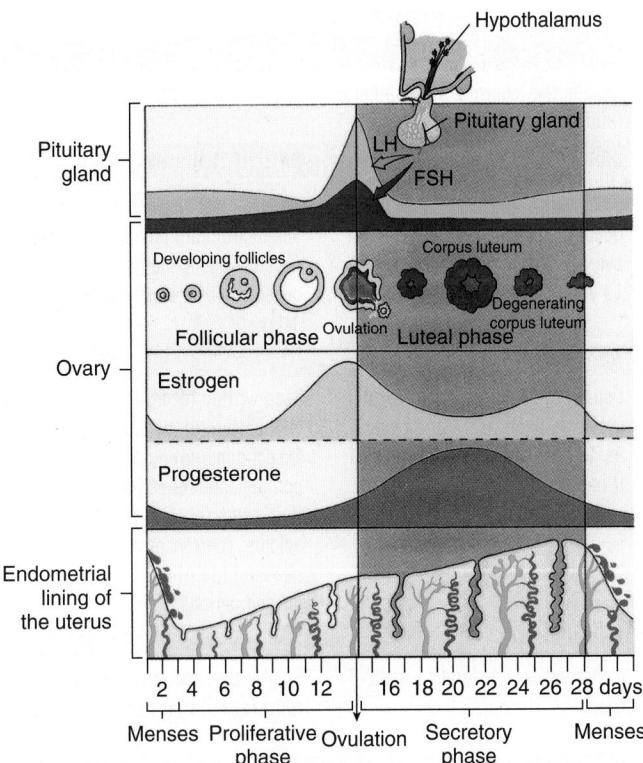

Figure 53-9 Events of the menstrual cycle. The various lines depict the changes in blood hormone levels, the development of the follicles, and the changes in the endometrium during the cycle. *FSH,* follicle-stimulating hormone; *LH,* luteinizing hormone.

Source: Thibodeau, G. A., & Patton, K. T. (2010). *Anatomy and physiology* (7th ed., p. 1055, Figure 32-14). St. Louis: Mosby.

and there is an increase in cellular growth, including an increase in the length of blood vessels and glandular tissue.

With ovulation and the resulting increased levels of progesterone, the luteal (or secretory) phase begins. In this phase, the blood vessels begin to coil, increasing the surface area of the vascular supply. The glandular tissues mature and secrete a glycogen-rich substance, and the glandular ducts dilate. If the corpus luteum regresses (i.e., fertilization does not occur) and estrogen and progesterone levels fall, the endometrial lining can no longer be supported. As a result, the blood vessels contract, and tissue begins to slough (fall away). This sloughing results in the menses and the start of the menstrual phase (Farage et al., 2009).

Menopause

Menopause is the physiological cessation of menses associated with declining ovarian function. It is usually considered complete after 1 year of **amenorrhea** (absence of menstruation) (Grady & Barrett-Connor, 2008). (Menopause is discussed in Chapter 56.)

Phases of the Sexual Response

The sexual response is a complex interplay of psychological and physiological phenomena and is influenced by a number of variables, including daily stress, illness, and crisis. The changes that

PATIENT & CAREGIVER TEACHING GUIDE

Table 53-2 Characteristics of Menstruation

Include the following information when teaching the patient and their family about menstruation

CHARACTERISTIC	PATIENT TEACHING
Menarche	
Occurs between ages 9 and 16 yr; average age at onset is 12 or 13 yr.	See health care provider regarding possible endocrine or developmental abnormality when delayed.
Interval	
Usually is 21-35 days, but regular cycles as short as 17 or as long as 45 days are considered normal if pattern is consistent for individual.	Keep written record to identify own pattern of menstrual cycle. Expect some irregularity in perimenopausal period. Be aware that drugs (phenothiazines, opioids, contraceptives) and stressful life events can result in missed periods.
Duration	
Menstrual flow generally lasts 2-8 days.	Realize that pattern is fairly constant but that wide variations do exist.
Amount	
Menstrual flow varies from 20 to 80 mL per menses; average is 30 mL; amount varies among women and in the same woman at different times; it is usually heaviest first 2 days.	Count pads or tampons used per day. The average tampon or pad, when completely saturated, absorbs 20-30 mL. Very heavy flow is indicated by complete soaking of two pads in 1-2 hr. Flow increases and then gradually decreases in perimenopausal period. IUD or drugs such as anticoagulants and thiazides can produce heavy menses.
Composition	
Menstrual discharge is a mixture of endometrium, blood, mucus, and vaginal cells; it is dark red and less viscous than blood and usually does not clot.	Clots indicate heavy flow or vaginal pooling.

IUD, intrauterine device.

occur during sexual excitement are similar for men and women. Masters and Johnson (1966) described the sexual response in terms of excitement, plateau, orgasmic, and resolution phases.

Male Sexual Response. The penis and the urethra are essential to the transport of sperm into the vagina and the cervix during intercourse. This transport is facilitated by penile erection in response to sexual stimulation during the *excitement phase.* Erection results from the filling of the large venous sinuses within the erectile tissue of the penis. In the flaccid state, the sinuses hold only a small amount of blood, but during the erection stage, they are congested with blood. Because the penis is richly endowed with sympathetic, parasympathetic, and pudendal nerve endings, it is readily stimulated to erection. The loose skin

of the penis becomes taut as a result of the intense venous congestion. This erectile tautness allows for easy insertion during intercourse.

As the man reaches the *plateau phase,* the erection is maintained, and a small increase in diameter occurs as a result of a slight increase in vasocongestion. There is also an increase in testicle size. Sometimes, a change in colour occurs in the glans penis, which becomes more reddish purple.

The subsequent contraction of the penile and urethral musculature during the *orgasmic phase* propels the sperm outward through the meatus. In this process, termed *ejaculation,* sperm are released into the ductus deferens during contractions. Sperm advance through the urethra, where fluids from the prostate and the seminal vesicles are added to the ejaculate. The sperm continue their path through the urethra, receiving a small amount of fluid from Cowper's glands, and are finally ejaculated through the urinary meatus. Orgasm is characterized by the rapid release of the vasocongestion and muscular tension (myotonia) that have developed. The rapid release of muscular tension (through rhythmic contractions) occurs primarily in the penis, the prostate gland, and the seminal vesicles. After ejaculation, a man enters the *resolution phase.* During this phase, the penis undergoes involution, gradually returning to its unstimulated, flaccid state.

Female Sexual Response. The changes that occur in a woman during sexual excitation are similar to those in a man. In response to stimulation, the clitoris becomes congested and vaginal lubrication increases as a result of secretions from the cervix, Bartholin's glands, and vaginal walls. This initial response is the *excitation phase.*

As excitation is maintained in the *plateau phase,* the vagina expands and the uterus is elevated. In the *orgasmic phase,* contractions occur in the uterus from the fundus to the lower uterine segment. There is a slight relaxation of the cervical os, which helps the entrance of the sperm, and rhythmic contractions of the vagina. Muscular tension is rapidly released through rhythmic contractions in the clitoris, the vagina, and the uterus. This phase is followed by a *resolution phase* in which these organs return to their pre-excitation state. However, women do not have to go through the resolution (refractory) recovery state before they can be orgasmic again. They can be multiorgasmic without resolution between orgasms.

AGE-RELATED CONSIDERATIONS: THE REPRODUCTIVE SYSTEM AND SEXUAL RESPONSE

With advancing age, changes occur in the male and female reproductive systems. In women, many of these changes are related to the altered estrogen production that is associated with menopause. A reduction in circulating estrogen along with an increase in androgens in postmenopausal women is associated with breast and genital atrophy, reduction in bone mass, and increased rate of atherosclerosis. Vaginal dryness may occur, which can lead to urogenital atrophy and changes in the quantity and composition of vaginal secretions (Weismiller, 2009). A gradual hormonal decline in elderly men also occurs (Gooren, 2008). Manifestations of hormonal decline in men can be physical, psychological, or sexual. Some of the changes include an increase in prostate size, decreased testosterone level, decreased sperm production, decreased muscle tone of the scrotum, and a decrease in the size and firmness of the testicles. Erectile dysfunction and sexual dysfunction occur in some men as a result of these changes. Age-related changes in the reproductive systems and differences in assessment findings are presented in Table 53-3.

Gradual changes resulting from advancing age occur in the sexual responses of men and women (Table 53-4). These changes occur at different rates and to varying degrees. The cumulative effects of these changes, as well as the negative social attitude toward sexuality in older adults, can affect the sexual practices of people in this age-group. Nurses have an important role in providing accurate and unbiased information about sexuality and age. Nurses should emphasize the normalcy of sexual activity in older adults. Counselling may be necessary to help older patients accommodate to these normal physiological changes.

Table 53-3 Age-Related Differences in Assessment of the Reproductive System

CHANGES	DIFFERENCES IN ASSESSMENT FINDINGS
Male	
Penis: decreased subcutaneous fat, decreased skin turgor	Easily retractable foreskin (if uncircumcised); decrease in size; fewer sustained erections
Testes: decreased testosterone production	Decrease in size; change in position (lower); increase in firmness
Prostate: benign hyperplasia	Enlargement
Breasts: enlargement	Gynecomastia (abnormal enlargement)
Female	
Breasts: decreased subcutaneous fat, increased fibrous tissue, decreased skin turgor	Less resilient, looser, more pendulous tissue; decreased size; duct around nipple may feel like stringy strand
Vulva: decreased skin turgor	Atrophy; decreased amount of pubic hair; decreased size of clitoris and labia
Vagina: atrophy of tissue, decreased muscle tone; pH becomes alkaline	Pale and dry mucosa; relaxation of outlet; mucosa thins; vagina narrower and shorter; increased potential for infection
Urethra: decreased muscle tone	Cystocele (protrusion of bladder through vaginal wall)
Uterus: decreased thickness of myometrium	Decrease in size; uterine prolapse
Ovaries: decreased ovarian function	Nonpalpable ovaries; decreased size

Table 53-4 Age-Related Changes in Sexual Functioning

Male
- Increased stimulation necessary for erection
- Force of ejaculation decreased
- Decreased ability to attain erection
- Decreased size and rigidity of the penis at full erection
- Decreased libido and interest in sex

Female
- Decreased vaginal lubrication
- Decreased sensitivity with labia shrinking and more clitoris exposed
- Difficulty in maintaining arousal
- Difficulty in achieving orgasm after stimulation
- Decreased libido and interest in sex

Assessment of the Male and Female Reproductive Systems

Subjective Data

Important Health Information. In addition to general health information, the nurse must elicit information specifically relating to the reproductive system. Reproduction and sexual issues are often considered extremely personal and private. The nurse must develop trust to elicit such information. A professional demeanour is important when taking a reproductive or sexual history. The nurse must be sensitive, ask gender-neutral questions, and maintain an awareness of a patient's culture and beliefs. It is helpful if the nurse begins with the least sensitive information (e.g., menstrual history) before asking questions about more sensitive issues, such as sexual practices or STIs.

Past Health History. The past health history should include information about major illnesses, hospitalizations, and surgeries. The nurse should also inquire about any infections involving the reproductive system, including STIs. Women should also have a complete obstetrical and gynecological history taken.

Common pediatric illnesses that affect reproductive function are mumps and rubella. The occurrence of mumps in young men has been associated with an increase in sterility. Bilateral testicular atrophy can occur secondary to mumps-related orchitis. In the health history, the nurse should ask if male patients have had mumps, have been immunized with mumps vaccine, or have any indications of sterility.

Rubella is of primary concern to women of childbearing age. If rubella occurs during the first 3 months of pregnancy, the possibility of congenital anomalies is increased. For this reason, nurses should encourage immunization for all women of childbearing age who have not been immunized for rubella or have not already had the disease. However, women should not be immunized if they are already pregnant (Coonrod et al., 2008). Women are also advised not to conceive for at least 3 months after immunization. Rubella immunity can be determined by antibody titres.

The nurse should also question the patient regarding the patient's current health status and the presence of any acute or chronic health problems. Problems in other body systems are often related to problems with the reproductive system. Questions relating to possible endocrine disorders, particularly diabetes mellitus (DM), hypothyroidism, and hyperthyroidism, must be asked because these disorders directly interfere with women's menstrual cycles and with sexual performance. Men who have DM may experience erectile dysfunction (ED) and retrograde ejaculation. In women with uncontrolled DM, pregnancy and the use of oral contraceptives may constitute significant risks to health. Many other chronic illnesses such as cardiovascular disease, respiratory disorders, anemia, cancer, and kidney and urinary tract disorders may affect the reproductive system and sexual functioning.

A history of a stroke should be determined. In men, strokes may cause physiological or psychological ED. Men who have suffered a myocardial infarction (MI) may experience ED because of the fear of precipitating another heart attack resulting from sexual activity. This same concern is shared by the woman both as a partner of someone who has had an MI and as the person recovering from an MI. Although most patients have concerns about sexual activity following an MI, many are not comfortable expressing these concerns to the nurse. The nurse must be sensitive to this concern. In women, a history of cardiovascular disease (e.g., hypertension, thrombophlebitis, angina) causes a higher incidence of morbidity and mortality with pregnancy or oral contraceptive use.

Family History. The nurse should inquire about a history of cancer, particularly cancer of the reproductive organs. Having a first-degree relative who has cancer of the breast, the ovaries, the uterus, or the prostate significantly increases the risk of cancer for the patient.

Medications. A list of all prescription and over-the-counter medications that the patient is taking should be documented, including the reason for using the medication, the dosage, and the length of time that the medication has been taken. All drugs taken by female patients should be evaluated for possible teratogenic effects in women of childbearing age. The patient should be asked about the use of herbal products and dietary supplements.

Particularly relevant in the assessment of the reproductive system is the use of diuretics (sometimes prescribed for premenstrual edema), psychotropic agents (which may interfere with sexual performance), and antihypertensives (some of which may cause ED). Thus, patients who use calcium channel blockers such as amlodipine (Norvasc), nonselective β-blockers such as propranolol (Inderal), angiotensin II antagonists such as losartan (Cozaar), and certain diuretics such as spironolactone (Aldactone) must be closely assessed for these problems (Shiri et al., 2007). The nurse must also note the use of drugs such as alcohol, marijuana, barbiturates, amphetamines, and phencyclidine (PCP; also called *angel dust*), which can have serious behavioural and physiological effects on the functioning of the reproductive system.

In women, the use of oral contraceptives or other hormones should be noted. The long-term use of both estrogen and progesterone in hormone replacement therapy (HRT) appears to increase the risk of cardiovascular disease, stroke, and breast cancer in postmenopausal women (National Institutes of Health [NIH], 2008). The short-term use of HRT appears to be appropriate for women experiencing moderate to severe menopausal symptoms. (HRT is discussed in Chapter 56.)

A history of cholecystitis and hepatitis is important information because these conditions may be contraindications for oral contraceptive use; cholecystitis is often aggravated by oral contraceptives, and chronic active inflammation of the liver generally precludes the use of estrogen products because they are metabolized by the liver. Chronic obstructive pulmonary disease may be a contraindication to oral contraceptive use because progesterone thickens respiratory secretions.

Surgery or Other Treatments. Any surgical procedures should be noted in the health history. Surgical procedures involving the reproductive system are listed in Table 53-5. Therapeutic or spontaneous abortions should also be documented.

Taking a Health History Related to a Reproductive Problem.

When collecting information related to reproductive health, the nurse should start with questions of lesser sensitivity, proceeding to more sensitive issues after rapport has been established. The nurse is also in a unique position to discuss general health issues related to women or men and to emphasize health promotion and self-care activities. The key questions to ask a patient with a reproductive problem are presented in Table 53-6 and discussed in more detail in the paragraphs below.

Menstrual History. The menstrual history includes the date of the last menstrual period, description of menstrual flow, age

Table 53-5 Surgeries of the Reproductive Systems	
SURGERY	**DESCRIPTION**
Male	
Herniorrhaphy	Repair of hernia
Orchiectomy	Removal of one or both testes
Prostatectomy	Removal of prostate gland
Repair of testicular torsion	Correction of axial rotation of spermatic cord, which cuts off blood supply to the testicle, epididymis, and other structures
Transurethral resection of prostate (TURP)	Removal of prostate tissue via the urethra (e.g., obstructive benign prostatic hyperplasia)
Varicocelectomy	Repair of varicose vein of scrotum
Vasectomy	Removal of part of ductus (vas) deferens; can be an elective procedure for sterilization or contraception
Female	
Cryosurgery	Use of subfreezing temperature to destroy tissue, especially for treatment of abnormal cells in the cervix
Dilation and curettage (D & C)	Dilation of uterus and scraping of endometrium, performed to diagnose disease of uterus, correct heavy or prolonged vaginal bleeding, or empty uterus of products of conception; also used in the treatment of infertility to correlate state of endometrium and time of cycle
Hysterectomy	Removal of uterus
Mastectomy	Removal of one or both breasts
Oophorectomy	Removal of one or both ovaries
Repair of cystocele	Correction of protrusion of urinary bladder into vagina
Repair of rectocele	Correction of protrusion of rectum into vagina
Salpingectomy	Removal of one or both fallopian tubes
Tubal ligation or sterilization	Ligation of fallopian tubes

HEALTH HISTORY

Table 53-6 Reproductive System

Menstrual History (Women)

Tell the nurse about your menstrual periods—date of last menstruation, description of menstrual flow, problems with menstruation, age of menarche, age of menopause.

Obstetrical History (Women)

Tell the nurse about your pregnancy history—number of times pregnant, number of living children, number of miscarriages or abortions. Do you think you could be pregnant now?

Menopause (Women)

Have your periods changed or stopped? Are you experiencing any of the symptoms of menopause—hot flashes, headaches, heavy sweats, vaginal dryness? Are you taking or have you taken HRT? How are you feeling about menopause?

Nutritional History (Women)

- Have you had any problems with anemia?*
- Have you had problems with eating disorders?*

Self-Care History

Women: Explain how you examine your breasts. Have you had a Pap test or mammogram recently? If so, what were the results and dates of these tests? How often do you have these checks?

Men: Explain how you examine your testes. Have you had a prostate examination recently? If so, what were the results and dates of these tests?

Elimination

- Do you experience problems with urination (e.g., pain; burning; dribbling; inability to control urine; frequency; small amounts; urinating at night; blood in the urine; urine that is dark, cloudy, or foul smelling)? Do you urinate when you sneeze or laugh or cough?
- Do you have any discharge from your vagina or penis?*
- Do you experience problems with bowel movements?*

General and Past History

- Are you having any problems in the area of your genitals?*
- Have you had treatment for problems in the past, and how were those treated?
- Have you had any surgery on your uterus, ovaries, vagina, or prostate?*
- Any history of kidney disease, kidney stones, prostate problems?*
- Have you had bladder infections? If so, when? How often?

Family History

Describe the health of your family members. Any history of breast, uterine, ovarian, or prostate cancer?

Sexual History

See Table 53-7.

HRT, hormone replacement therapy; *Pap,* Papanicolaou.
*If yes, describe.

of menarche, and if applicable, age at menopause. Menstrual history data are used in the detection of pregnancy, infertility, and numerous other gynecological concerns. Changes in the usual menstrual pattern must be explicitly described to determine whether the change is transient and unimportant or connected with a more serious gynecological problem. *Metrorrhagia* (spotting or bleeding between menstruations), *menorrhagia* (excessive menstrual bleeding), *amenorrhea* (lack of menstrua-

tion), and *postcoital bleeding* are examples of such problems. Changes in menstrual patterns associated with the use of contraceptive pills, intrauterine devices (IUDs), subdermal estrogen-only implant (Norplant), or medroxyprogesterone (Depo-Provera) injections must be identified. Contraceptive pills usually decrease the amount and duration of flow, and some IUDs may cause an increase in the amount and duration. Some IUDs also increase the severity of dysmenorrhea. However, newer IUDs contain progestin and may be therapeutic.

Obstetrical History. The obstetrical history includes the number of pregnancies, full-term births, preterm births, and live births. Other obstetrical information should include information about any ectopic pregnancies or abortions, either spontaneous or therapeutic. Any problems that occurred with pregnancy should be documented.

Menopause. Taking a menopause history includes asking the date of the last menstrual period and asking about any other symptoms of menopause such as hot flashes, heavy sweats, vaginal dryness, headaches, sleeping problems, mood changes, decreased libido, and urinary problems. Women should be asked if they are using or have ever used HRT. It is also important to explore how the woman feels about menopause because the drop in estrogen levels during perimenopause and menopause can lead to depression in some individuals. Women are also more prone to osteoporosis and heart disease after menopause owing to the lower levels of estrogen, and there has to be some discussion of ways to prevent and reduce the risk of these diseases.

Nutritional History. Anemia is a common problem in women in their reproductive years, particularly during pregnancy and the postpartum period. The adequacy of the diet should be evaluated with this condition in mind.

A thorough nutritional and psychological history should be taken to assess for the presence of an eating disorder. Anorexia can cause amenorrhea and the subsequent problems, such as osteoporosis, that are related to estrogen cessation. From early adolescence, women can be counselled regarding adequate calcium intake and the role of calcium in the prevention of osteoporosis. The patient's daily calcium intake should be estimated to determine whether there is a need for supplementation. Folic acid intake for women in their reproductive years should be evaluated because a deficiency can result in spina bifida and other neural tube defects in the fetus (Kelly, 2008).

Self-Care History. It is important to establish the patient's perception of his or her own health and measures that the patient takes to maintain health. Specifically, it is important to ask about self-examination practices and screenings. Breast self-examination (BSE), mammography according to age-specific guidelines (see Chapter 54), and Papanicolaou (Pap) tests are integral to a woman's health. Testicular self-examination (TSE) should be practised by all men, starting from age 15 years (Canadian Cancer Society, 2011a). Men older than 50 years are advised to talk to their physician about their personal risk for prostate cancer and the advisability of them having screening tests for early detection of prostate cancer such as a digital rectal examination (DRE) and a prostate-specific antigen (PSA) test (Canadian Cancer Society, 2011b). Prostate Cancer Canada (2011) and the Canadian Urological Association (2011) do, however, still endorse baseline screening for all men aged 40 to 49, as well as PSA and DRE every 2 to 4 years for men aged 50 and those older than 40 of African or Caribbean descent or having a close relative with prostate cancer.

Assessment of the reproductive system is incomplete without knowledge of the patient's lifestyle choices. The nurse should know whether a woman uses cigarettes, alcohol, caffeine, or other drugs because these substances can be detrimental to both mother and fetus. Cigarette smoking may delay conception and can also increase the risk of morbidity in women using oral contraceptives. Early menopause is also associated with smoking in women. These substances may also adversely affect the sperm count in men and cause ED or decreased libido.

Elimination. Stress and urge incontinence are common in older women because of relaxation of the pelvic musculature caused by multiple births or advancing age. Vaginal infections predispose patients to chronic or recurrent urinary tract infections. Metastasis of malignant tumours of the reproductive system to the genitourinary system is possible because of their proximity. Benign prostatic hyperplasia is a common problem of older men. It can alter normal urination, causing retention and difficulty in initiating the urinary stream.

Sexual History. The extent and the depth of the interview about a patient's sexuality depend primarily on the expertise of the interviewer and on the needs and the willingness of the patient. Before taking a sexual history, interviewers should assess their comfort with their own sexuality because any discomfort in questioning becomes obvious to the patient. Interviews must be carried out in an environment that provides reassurance, confidentiality, and a nonjudgemental attitude (Wallace, 2008).

Table 53-7 outlines specific questions for a sexual history. A sexual history should include information regarding sexual activity, beliefs, and practices. Sexual preference (heterosexual, homosexual, bisexual), the frequency and type of sexual activity (penile–vaginal, penile–rectal, recipient rectal, oral), and the number of partners and protective measures against STIs and pregnancy should be explored. The patient's knowledge of safe sexual practices should be determined. A history of multiple sex partners and unprotected sex increases the risk of contracting an STI. For a woman, this can increase the risk of pelvic inflammatory disease, which can compromise her ability to become pregnant.

Both men and women should be asked about their general satisfaction with sexuality. The patient should be questioned about sexual beliefs and practices and whether orgasm is achieved. Any unexplained change in sexual practices or performance should be explored. Problems of the reproductive system can cause physiological or psychological problems that can lead to **dyspareunia** (painful intercourse), ED, sexual dysfunction, or infertility. Both the cause and the effect of such problems should be determined.

Inclusive and Appropriate Health Care for Sexual and Gender Minority Communities. People who identify themselves as LGBTTTIQQ (lesbian, gay, bisexual, transsexual, transgender, two-spirit, intersex, queer, or questioning) account for as much as 5 to 10% of the population (Registered Nurses Association of Ontario [RNAO], 2007; The Centre, 2006). Members of sexual and gender minority communities experience barriers to inclusive and appropriate health care (Tjepkema, 2008). LGBTTTIQQ Canadians are in fact "dying younger and experiencing poorer health than heterosexual and non-trans people" (The Centre, 2006). Because prevailing attitudes in

Table 53-7 Sexual History Format
• Are you currently in a relationship that involves sexual intercourse? If yes, do you have one or multiple partners?
• How frequently do you engage in sexual activities? Are you and your partner(s) satisfied with the sexual relationship?
• Do you have a significant other? If yes, is this relationship satisfying? If no, explain.
• How many sexual partners have you had in the past 6 mo?
• Do you prefer relationships with men, women, or both? (If the patient is gay or lesbian, inquire whether he or she is in a significant relationship.)
• Has your sex life changed during the past year? If yes, how?
• What kind of sex do you engage in (e.g., oral, vaginal, rectal)?
• Are you experiencing any problems that are affecting your sexuality? If yes, describe.
• Have you ever had a sexually transmitted infection? If yes, what?
• What are you doing to protect yourself from sexually transmitted infections? If protection is used, what type? Do you use protection every time you have intercourse?
• Are you currently using any birth control measures? If yes, what type?
• How long have you been using this product? How effective do you feel this has been?
• Have you ever been in a relationship with anyone who hurt you? Have you ever been forced into sexual acts as a child or an adult?
• How often have you experienced erectile dysfunction (male) or difficulty with vaginal lubrication (female) or pain with intercourse?

Source: Adapted from Wilson, S. F., & Giddens, J. F. (2009). *Health assessment for nursing practice* (4th ed.). St. Louis: Mosby.

society discourage self-disclosure, LGBTTTIQQ people often seek help later in the disease process (Canadian Research Network for Care in the Community [CRNCC], 2007). They underutilize the health care system because they often encounter insensitivity or homophobic attitudes as well as discrimination in some health care settings. A growing body of international research indicates that, after excluding illnesses related to human immunodeficiency virus (HIV) and acquired immune deficiency syndrome (AIDS), sexual- and gender-minority communities experience higher rates of cervical, breast, and anal cancer; eating disorders; depression and other mental health issues; as well as a higher incidence of smoking- and alcoholism-related health problems (CRNCC, 2007).

Nurses must understand the unique needs of the LGBTTTIQQ community and provide inclusive and appropriate health care. Members of sexual- and gender-minority communities need "to *see, hear,* and *feel* that they are welcome, have rights, and are safe" (Stonewall Scotland and National Health Services [NHS], 2006).

See. The physical environment must acknowledge that LGBTTTIQQ people exist and are welcome (e.g., signage, posters, brochures, agency literature).

Hear. Language and agency forms and assessment tools should not assume heterosexuality as the norm but should allow individuals "to disclose their sexual identity, same sex partnerships and sexual behaviour without fear of discrimination" (Stonewall Scotland & NHS, 2006). Some examples of inclusive care are the use of the following language and concepts: "partner" instead of "husband" or "wife," "significant relationships" instead of "next of kin," and a broad definition of family that goes beyond traditional concepts to recognize as family whomever the patient considers that family to be.

Feel. LGBTTTIQQ patients and their families need "affirmation that their identity is acknowledged and respected" (CRNCC, 2007). As well, the behaviour of the health care provider must demonstrate "understanding of any implications of sexual orientation for the service user" (Stonewall Scotland & NHS, 2006).

Objective Data

Physical Examination: Male.
The examination of the male external genitalia includes inspection and palpation. An examination may be performed with the patient lying or standing. The standing position is generally preferred. The examiner should be seated in front of the standing patient. Gloves should be used during examination of the male genitalia.

Pubis. Observe the distribution and general characteristics of the pubic hair and the skin. Normally, the hair is in a diamond-shaped pattern. The hair is usually coarser than scalp hair. The absence of hair is not a normal finding.

Penis. Note the size and the skin texture of the penis and any lesions, scars, or swelling. Also note the location of the urethral meatus as well as the presence or absence of a foreskin. If present, the foreskin should be retracted to note cleanliness and then replaced over the glans after observation. The glans is compressed to note any discharge and its amount, colour, and odour if present. Palpate the penile shaft for tenderness or masses and observes the ventral and dorsal aspects.

Scrotum and Testes. This part of the examination is performed by a nurse with advanced skills. The nurse would start by performing a complete skin examination by lifting each testis to inspect all sides of the scrotal sac. Palpation of the scrotum is done to note changes in consistency or the presence of masses. It is important to note if the testes are descended. The left testis usually hangs lower than the right. Undescended testis is a major risk factor for testicular cancer as well as a potential cause of male infertility.

Inguinal Region and Spermatic Cord. This part of the examination is performed by a nurse with advanced skills. The nurse would first inspect the skin overlying the inguinal regions for rashes or lesions. The patient should be asked to bear down or cough. While he is straining, the inguinal area should be inspected for the presence of a bulge. No bulging should be seen.

Examination of the inguinal area continues with palpation. The right and left inguinal rings should be palpated using the index or the middle finger. The finger should be inserted into the lower aspect of the scrotum and should follow the spermatic cord upward through the triangular, slitlike opening of the inguinal ring. At this point, the patient should be asked to bear down and cough. The nurse determines whether the strain produces a bulging of the intestines through the ring, indicating the presence of a hernia, a condition that necessitates follow up. The inguinal lymph nodes should also be palpated. Enlargement of the lymph nodes (termed *lymphadenopathy*) could suggest a pelvic organ infection or malignancy.

Anus and Prostate. Inspect the anal sphincter and the perineal region for lesions, masses, and hemorrhoids. A DRE is required for all men who have symptoms of prostate trouble, such as difficulty in initiating the flow and the urge to void frequently. This examination should be performed annually for all men 50 years of age or older.

Physical Examination: Female.
Physical examination of women often begins with inspection and palpation of the breasts and then proceeds to the abdomen and the genitalia. Examination of the abdomen provides an opportunity to detect pain or any masses that may involve the genitourinary system. Abdominal examination is discussed in Chapter 41.

Breasts. First examine the breasts by visual inspection. With the patient seated, observe the breasts for symmetry, size, shape, skin colour and texture, vascular patterns, dimpling, and the presence of unusual lesions. Ask the patient to put her arms at her sides, arms overhead, lean forward, and press hands on hips. Observe for any abnormalities during these manoeuvres. Palpate the axillae and the clavicular areas for enlarged lymph nodes.

After the patient assumes a supine position, place a pillow under her back on the side to be examined. Ask the patient to put her arm above and behind her head. These manoeuvres flatten breast tissue and make palpation easier. Then palpate the breast in a systematic fashion. Use the distal finger pads for palpation. Include the tail of Spence (the upper outer tail of breast tissue that extends into the axilla) in the examination because this area and the upper outer quadrant are the areas where most breast malignancies develop. Finally, palpate the area around the areolae for masses. Compress the nipple to determine the presence of discharge or any masses. Document the colour, consistency, and odour of any discharge.

External Genitalia. Use gloves for examination of the external genitalia. Inspect the mons pubis, labia majora, labia minora, posterior fourchette, perineum, and anal region for characteristics of skin, hair distribution, and contour. Note any lesions, inflammation, swelling, and discharge. Separate the labia to fully inspect the clitoris, the urethral meatus, and the vaginal orifice.

Internal Pelvic Examination. This part of the examination is performed by a nurse with advanced skills. During the speculum examination, the examiner observes the walls of the vagina and the cervix for inflammation, discharge, polyps, and suspicious growths. During this examination, it is possible to obtain a Pap test and collect secretions for culture and microscopic examination. After the speculum examination, a bimanual examination is performed to allow assessment of the size, the shape, and the consistency of the uterus, the ovaries, and the tubes. The tubes are not normally palpable.

Parts of the pelvic and bimanual examinations are not included in this text because they are considered advanced skills and are not usually within the scope of the nurse generalist.

Table 53-8 provides an example of a recording format for the physical assessment findings for the male and female reproductive systems. Tables 53-9 through 53-11 summarize common assessment abnormalities of the breasts, the female reproductive system, and the male reproductive system, respectively.

A *focused assessment* is used to evaluate the status of previously identified reproductive problems and to monitor for signs of new problems (see Table 3-7). A focused assessment of the reproductive system is presented in the box on p. 1486.

Table 53-8 Normal Physical Assessment of the Reproductive System

MALE	FEMALE
Breasts	
Symmetrical. No masses or tenderness behind nipple. No drainage, retraction, or lesions noted. No lymphadenopathy.	Symmetrical without dimpling. No masses or tenderness behind nipple. Nipples soft; no drainage, retraction, or lesions noted. No lymphadenopathy.
External Genitalia	
Diamond-shaped hair distribution. No lesions or discharge noted. Scrotum symmetrical, testes descended; no masses. No inguinal hernia.	Triangular hair distribution. Genitalia dark pink; no lesions, redness, swelling, or inflammation in perineal region. No vaginal discharge noted. No tenderness with palpation of Skene's ducts and Bartholin's glands.
Anus	
No hemorrhoids, fissures, or lesions noted.	No hemorrhoids, fissures, or lesions noted.

Diagnostic Studies of the Reproductive Systems

Numerous diagnostic studies are available to assess the reproductive system. Table 53-12 summarizes the most commonly used diagnostic studies in the assessment of the reproductive systems and select studies are described in more detail later in the chapter.

Urine Studies

Pregnancy Testing. Occurrence of pregnancy is generally validated by measuring human chorionic gonadotropin (hCG) in the urine. A solution containing monoclonal antibodies specific for hCG is mixed with a small amount of urine. The presence of hCG causes a change in colour of the tested urine.

Home pregnancy test kits use the same assay principle described in the preceding paragraph. Positive results are based on the presence of hCG in urine. Some tests can detect pregnancy as early as the first day following a missed menstrual period. These tests are 98% accurate if the test is performed exactly per

COMMON ASSESSMENT ABNORMALITIES

Table 53-9 Breast

FINDING	DESCRIPTION	POSSIBLE ETIOLOGY AND SIGNIFICANCE
Nipple inversion or retraction	Recent onset, erythematous, pain, unilateral	Abscess, inflammation, cancer
	Recent onset (usually within past year), unilateral, lack of tenderness	Neoplasm
Nipple secretions		
• Galactorrhea (female)	Milky, no relationship to lactation, unilateral or bilateral or intermittent or consistent presentation	Drug therapy, particularly phenothiazines, tricyclic antidepressants, methyldopa; hypofunction or hyperfunction of thyroid or adrenal glands; tumours of hypothalamus or pituitary gland; excessive estrogen; prolonged suckling or breast foreplay
• Galactorrhea (male)	Milky, bilateral presentation	Chorioepithelioma of testes, manifestation of pituitary tumour
• Purulent	Grey-green or yellow colour; frequent unilateral presentation; association with pain, erythema, induration, nipple inversion	Puerperal (after birth) mastitis (inflammatory condition of breast) or abscess
	Same description as mastitis or abscess but usually without nipple inversion	Infected sebaceous cyst
• Serous discharge	Clear appearance, unilateral or bilateral or intermittent or consistent presentation	Intraductal papilloma
• Dark green or multicoloured discharge	Thick, sticky, and frequently bilateral	Ductal ectasia (dilation of mammary ducts)
• Serosanguineous or bloody drainage	Unilateral presentation	Papillomatosis (widespread development of nipple-like growths), intraductal papilloma, carcinoma
Scaling or irritation of nipple	Unilateral or bilateral presentation, crusting, possible ulceration	Paget's disease, eczema, infection
Nodules, lumps, or masses	Multiple, bilateral, well-delineated, soft or firm, mobile cysts; pain; premenstrual occurrence	Fibrocystic changes
	Rubbery consistency, fluid-filled interior, pain	Ductal ectasia
	Soft, mobile, well-delineated cyst; absence of pain	Lipoma, fibroadenoma
	Erythema, tenderness, induration	Infected sebaceous cysts, abscesses
	Usually singular, hard, irregularly shaped, poorly delineated, nonmobile	Neoplasm
Dimpling of breast	Unilateral, recent onset, no pain	Neoplasm

COMMON ASSESSMENT ABNORMALITIES

Table 53-10 Female Reproductive System

FINDING/DESCRIPTION	POSSIBLE ETIOLOGY AND SIGNIFICANCE	FINDING/DESCRIPTION	POSSIBLE ETIOLOGY AND SIGNIFICANCE
Vulvar Discharge		**Vulvar Growths**	
Plaquelike consistency; frequent itching and inflammation; lack of odour; yeastlike smell	Candidiasis (*Candida* or yeast infection), vaginitis	Soft, fleshy growth; nontender	Condyloma acuminatum
		Flat and warty appearance, nontender	Condyloma latum
Greyish colour, copious flow, frothy appearance, vulvar irritation	Bacterial vaginosis infection	Same as either of preceding descriptions, possible pain	Neoplasm
Greyish green or yellow colour; malodorous or "fishy" odour	*Trichomonas vaginalis*	Reddened base, vesicles, and small erosions; pain	Lymphogranuloma venereum, genital herpes, chancroid
Bloody colour	*Chlamydia trachomatis* or *Neisseria gonorrhoeae* infection, menstruation, trauma, cancer	Indurated, firm ulcers; lack of pain	Chancre (painless ulcer associated with syphilis), granuloma inguinale
Vulvar Erythema		**Abdominal Pain or Tenderness**	
Bright or beefy red colour, itching	*Candida albicans,* allergy, chemical vaginitis	Intermittent or consistent tenderness in right or left lower quadrant	Salpingitis (infection of fallopian tube), ectopic pregnancy, ruptured ovarian cyst, PID, tubal or ovarian abscess
Reddened base, painful vesicles or ulcerations	Genital herpes	Periumbilical location, consistent occurrence	Cystitis, endometritis (inflammation of endometrium), ectopic pregnancy
Macules or papules, itching	Chancroid (STI), contact dermatitis, scabies, pediculosis		

PID, pelvic inflammatory disease; *STI,* sexually transmitted infection.

COMMON ASSESSMENT ABNORMALITIES

Table 53-11 Male Reproductive System

FINDING/ DESCRIPTION	POSSIBLE ETIOLOGY AND SIGNIFICANCE	FINDING/ DESCRIPTION	POSSIBLE ETIOLOGY AND SIGNIFICANCE
Penile Growths or Masses		**Scrotal Masses**	
Indurated, smooth, disclike appearance; absence of pain; singular presentation	Chancre	Localized swelling with tenderness, unilateral or bilateral presentation	Epididymitis (inflammation of epididymis), testicular torsion, orchitis (mumps)
Papular to irregularly shaped ulceration with pus, lack of induration	Chancroid	Swelling, tenderness	Incarcerated hernia
Ulceration with induration and nodularity	Cancer	Unilateral or bilateral presentation; swelling without pain; translucent, cordlike or wormlike appearance	Hydrocele (accumulation of fluid in outer covering of testes), spermatocele (firm, sperm-containing cyst of epididymis), varicocele (dilation of veins that drain testes), hematocele (accumulation of blood within scrotum)
Flat, wartlike nodule	Condyloma latum		
Elevated, fleshy, moist, elongated projections with single or multiple projections	Condyloma acuminatum		
Localized swelling with retracted, tight foreskin	Paraphimosis (inability to replace foreskin to its normal position after retraction), trauma	Firm, nodular testes or epididymis; frequent unilateral presentation	Tuberculosis, cancer
		Penile Discharge	
Vesicles, Erosions, or Ulcers		Clear to purulent colour, minimal to copious flow	Urethritis or gonorrhea, *Chlamydia trachomatis* infection, trauma
Painful, erythematous base; vesicular or small erosions	Genital herpes, balanitis (inflammation of glans penis), chancroid	**Penile or Scrotal Erythema**	
		Macules and papules	Scabies, pediculosis
Painless, singular, small erosion with eventual lymphadenopathy	Lymphogranuloma venereum, cancer	**Inguinal Masses**	
		Bulging, unilateral presentation during straining	Inguinal hernia
		Shotty (hard, round, and small), 1- to 3-cm nodules	Lymphadenopathy

Reproductive System

Use this checklist to ensure the key assessment steps have been done.

Subjective

Ask the patient about any of the following and note responses

Vaginal discharge/itching, unusual bleeding	Y	N
Penile pain, lesions, discharge	Y	N
Medications: oral contraceptives, antihypertensives, psychotropics, hormones	Y	N
Self-examinations (breast or testicular examination) and results	Y	N
Clinical examinations of reproductive systems (breast, pelvis, testicular, prostate) and results	Y	N
Pain in the abdomen, pelvis, or genitalia	Y	N

Objective: Diagnostic

Check the following for results and critical values

Serum hCG	✓
Serum PSA	✓
Culture and sensitivity test results	✓
Hormone levels (testosterone, progesterone, estrogen) if done	✓
Screen for STIs (e.g., *Chlamydia*, gonorrhea)	✓
Laboratory reports: wet mounts, dark-field microscopy	✓
Radiograph of pelvis or breasts	✓
Ultrasound of prostate	✓

Objective: Physical Examination

Inspect

External genitalia for redness, swelling, drainage	✓
Breasts for swelling, dimpling, retraction, drainage	✓

Palpate

Breast tissue for masses or inflammation	✓

hCG, human chorionic gonadotropin; PSA, prostate-specific antigen; STIs, sexually transmitted infections.

---

instructions. A second test is recommended within a week if the first test is negative (assuming menses have not yet occurred) (Scolaro, Braxton-Lloyd, & Helms, 2008).

Hormone Studies. Although estrogen studies are performed on urine, the results are frequently inaccurate because of variable estrogen levels during the normal cycle and the difficulty in estimating the day of the cycle in women with irregular menses. Adrenal androgens are precursors of estrogens and can be measured in the urine of both men and women. FSH can be measured in a 24-hour urine specimen. Increased and decreased FSH levels can indicate gonadal failure due to pituitary dysfunction. For more information regarding hormone studies, see Chapter 50.

Blood Studies

Hormone Studies. Serum assays for hCG can detect pregnancy before a woman misses her menstrual period, as early as 10 days after conception (Pagana & Pagana, 2009). The prolactin assay is used primarily in the workup of a patient with amenorrhea. High levels of prolactin are normally associated with low levels of estrogen, such as those that occur during lactation. However, the same finding can occur with pituitary adenomas, especially with otherwise unexplained *galactorrhea* (excessive secretion of breast milk). Serum progesterone and estradiol are sometimes measured in ovarian function assessment, particularly for amenorrhea. In addition, hormonal blood studies are essential components of a thorough fertility workup.

Tumour Markers. Biological tumour markers are substances associated with malignant disease. Measurement of these markers is useful in monitoring therapy (marker levels rise as disease progresses and fall with disease regression) because marker levels may rise months before new disease or metastasis is evident. α-Fetoprotein (AFP), hCG, and CA-125 are tumour markers for reproductive system malignancies. A specific tumour antigen such as prostate-specific antigen (PSA) is another type of tumour marker frequently used for prostate cancer.

Serology Tests for Syphilis. The Venereal Disease Research Laboratory (VDRL) test and the rapid plasma reagin (RPR) test detect the presence of antibodies in the serum of patients infected with syphilis. These tests are inexpensive and reliable but have high levels of false-positive results because they test for a nonspecific antibody. The fluorescent treponemal antibody absorption (FTA-Abs) test is highly reliable and should be used after a positive VDRL or RPR, even if it is weakly positive or questionable.

Cultures and Smears

Cultures and smears are most frequently employed in the diagnosis of STI. Specimens for cultures and smears are most commonly taken from the vagina, the endocervix, and the rectum for females and the urethra and the rectum for males. For a culture, the specimen is placed on a special culture medium; a smear involves rubbing the specimen on a slide for direct examination. Gram stain smears have been shown to be effective in the diagnosis of *Chlamydia* infection. A nucleic acid amplification test (NAAT) can screen for both gonorrhea and *Chlamydia* from a wide variety of samples, including vaginal, endocervical, urine, and urethral specimens. Dark-field microscopy involves the direct examination of a specimen obtained from a syphilitic chancre for the diagnosis of syphilis.

Cytological Studies

Cytology involves the study of cells under microscopic examination. The Pap smear is a screening test to detect abnormal cells obtained from the cervix or vagina. It is performed by obtaining cells from the cervical canal, preferably the endocervix, as well as from the vagina. The cells are placed in a fixative for examination by a cytologist for cellular abnormalities. Screening guidelines for the Pap test (also called a *smear*) are discussed in Chapter 56.

Cytological study is also indicated for nipple discharge. Cytological examination can detect the presence of malignant cells and distinguish the discharge from one associated with infection.

Radiological Studies

Mammography. Mammography has become one of the most frequently used diagnostic tools in reproductive system assessment. It is used to detect breast masses and can do so before they are palpable. Mammography and screening guidelines for mammography are discussed in Chapter 54.

Text continued on p. 1490

DIAGNOSTIC STUDIES

Table 53-12 Male and Female Reproductive Systems

STUDY	DESCRIPTION AND PURPOSE	NURSING RESPONSIBILITY
Urine Studies		
Human chorionic gonadotropin (hCG)	Used to detect pregnancy. Also used to detect hydatidiform moles and chorioepithelioma (in men and women). *Males and nonpregnant females*: negative	Obtain menstrual history from patient, including birth control methods. Determine presence or absence of presumptive signs of pregnancy (e.g., breast changes, increased whitish vaginal discharge).
Testosterone levels	Tumours and developmental anomalies of the testes can be detected. *Female*: 6.9-41.6 nmol/24 hr *Male*: 139-469 nmol/24 hr	Instruct patient to collect 24-hr urine specimen and to keep refrigerated.
Follicle-stimulating hormone (FSH)	Indicates gonadal failure because of pituitary dysfunction. *Female*: Follicular phase: 1.37-9.9 IU/L/24 hr Midcycle: 6.17-17.2 IU/L/24 hr Luteal phase: 1.09-9.2 IU/L/24 hr Postmenopause: 19.3-100.6 IU/L/24 hr *Male*: 1.42-15.4 IU/L/24 hr	Instruct patient to collect 24-hr urine specimen. Indicate phase of menstrual cycle, if menopausal, and if taking oral contraceptives or hormones.
Blood Studies		
Prolactin	Detects pituitary dysfunction that can cause amenorrhea. *Female*: <25 mcg/L *Male*: <20 mcg/L	Observe venipuncture site for bleeding or hematoma.
Prostate-specific antigen (PSA)	Used to detect prostate cancer. Also a sensitive test for monitoring response to therapy. Reference interval: (<4 mcg/L)	No food or fluid restrictions. Collect 5 mL blood. Observe venipuncture site for bleeding.
hCG	Used to detect pregnancy; can also be used as a tumour marker for testicular malignancy. Also used to detect hydatidiform moles. *Males and nonpregnant females*: <5 mLU/mL	Elicit where she is in her menstrual cycle and whether she has missed menses and, if so, how late she is.
Testosterone	Determine whether elevated androgens are owing to adrenal or ovarian dysfunction or pituitary tumours. Serum testosterone is also drawn to assess male infertility and tumours of the testicle or the ovary. *Male*: 9.75-38 nmol/L *Female*: <2.43 nmol/L	Collect health history to eliminate potential sources of interference with accuracy of results (e.g., use of corticosteroids or barbiturates, presence of hypothyroidism or hyperthyroidism).
Progesterone	Frequently used to detect functioning corpus luteum cyst *Female*: Follicular phase: <1.6 nmol/L Luteal phase: 9.54-79.5 nmol/L Postmenopause: <1.27 nmol/L *Male*: 0.32-1.6 nmol/L	Observe venipuncture site for bleeding or hematoma. Include last menstrual period and trimester of pregnancy because progesterone levels vary with gestation.
Estradiol	Measures ovarian function. Particularly useful in assessing estrogen-secreting tumours and states of precocious female puberty. May be used to confirm perimenopausal status. Increased serum estradiol levels in men may be indicative of testicular tumours. *Female*: Follicular phase: 73-1285 pmol/L Luteal phase: 110-1652 pmol/L Postmenopause: ≤73 pmol/L *Male*: 37-184 pmol/L	Observe venipuncture site for bleeding or hematoma.

hCG, human chorionic gonadotropin.

Continued

DIAGNOSTIC STUDIES

Table 53-12 Male and Female Reproductive Systems—cont'd

STUDY	DESCRIPTION AND PURPOSE	NURSING RESPONSIBILITY
Blood Studies—cont'd		
FSH	Indicates gonadal failure owing to pituitary dysfunction; used to validate menopausal status. *Female:* Follicular phase: 1.37-9.9 IU/L Ovulatory peak: 6.7-17.2 IU/L Luteal phase: 1.09-9.2 IU/L Postmenopause: 19.3-100.6 IU/L *Male:* 1.42-15.4 IU/L	No food or fluid restrictions required. State phase of menstrual cycle, if menopausal, and if taking oral contraceptive or hormones.
Venereal Disease Research Laboratory (VDRL) (flocculation)	Nonspecific antibody tests used to screen for syphilis. Positive readings can be made within 1-2 wk after appearance of primary lesion (chancre) or 4-15 wk after initial infection. *Reference interval:* Negative or nonreactive	Observe venipuncture site for bleeding or hematoma.
Rapid plasma regain (RPR) (agglutination)	Nonspecific antibody tests used to screen for syphilis. *Reference interval:* Negative or nonreactive	Obtain data to determine presence or absence of problems such as hepatitis, pregnancy, and autoimmune diseases that may interfere with the accuracy of results.
Fluorescent treponemal antibody absorption (FTA-Abs)	Detects syphilis antibodies. Also detects early syphilis with great accuracy. Usually performed if results of above nonspecific tests are questionable. *Reference interval:* Negative or nonreactive	Observe venipuncture site for bleeding or hematoma formation.
Cultures and Smears		
Dark-field microscopy	Direct examination of specimen obtained from potential syphilitic lesion (chancre) is performed to detect *Treponema pallidum.*	Avoid direct skin contact with open lesion.
Wet mounts	Direct microscopic examination of specimen of vaginal discharge is performed immediately after collection. Determines presence or absence and number of *Trichomonas* organisms, bacteria, white and red blood cells, and candidal buds or hyphae. Other clues or causes of inflammation or infection may be determined.	Explain procedure and purpose to patient. Instruct patient not to douche before examination. Prepare for collection of specimens (glass slide, 10-20% potassium hydroxide [KOH] solution, sodium chloride [NaCl] solution, and cotton-tipped applicators).
Cultures	Specimens of vaginal, urethral, or cervical discharge are cultured and used to assess presence of gonorrhea or *Chlamydia.* Rectal and throat cultures may also be taken, depending on data obtained from sexual history.	Obtain specific contact and sexual history inclusive of oral and rectal intercourse. Instruct against douching before examination. Obtain urethral specimen from men before they void. Instruct women who are sexually active with multiple partners to have at least a yearly culture for gonorrhea and *Chlamydia.* Instruct sexually active men to have any discharge evaluated immediately to rule out gonorrhea strains that do not cause classic symptoms of dysuria.
Nucleic acid amplification test (NAAT)	A wide variety of samples, including vaginal, endocervical, urine, and urethral specimens, can be used to screen for both gonorrhea and *Chlamydia.*	Same as above.
Gram stain	Used for rapid detection of gonorrhea. Presence of gram-negative intracellular diplococci generally warrants initiation of treatment. Not highly accurate for women. Has also been shown as accurate alternative for *Chlamydia* testing.	Same as above.

FSH, follicle-stimulating hormone.

DIAGNOSTIC STUDIES

Table 53-12 Male and Female Reproductive Systems—cont'd

STUDY	DESCRIPTION AND PURPOSE	NURSING RESPONSIBILITY
Cytological Studies		
Papanicolaou (Pap) smear	Microscopic study of exfoliated cells via special staining and fixation technique detects abnormal cells. Cells most commonly studied are those obtained directly from endocervix and ectocervix.	Instruct women who are sexually active and who are between the ages of 21 and 69 to have Pap smears according to Canadian Cancer Society guidelines (q1-3 yr, depending on provincial and territorial screening guidelines).* Instruct patients not to douche for at least 24 hr before examination. Collect careful menstrual and gynecological history.
Nipple discharge test	Cytological study of nipple discharge is performed.	Indicate if breastfeeding, or history of amenorrhea, or whether hormonal preparations or other drugs are being taken. Instruct that nipple discharge should always be evaluated.
Radiological Studies		
Mammography • Screening • Diagnostic	Low-dose radiographic image of breast tissue is used to assess breast tissue. Used to detect benign and malignant masses. Performed when patient has suspicious clinical symptoms or abnormalities found on screening mammogram. Additional views of affected breast are taken.	Instruct patient about advantages of the examination. The Canadian Cancer Society recommends screening with mammography q2yr for women who are 50-69 yr of age (see Chapter 54 for more information).†
Ultrasound mammography (abdominal and transvaginal)	Measures and records high-frequency sound waves as they pass through tissues of variable density. It is very useful in detecting masses >3 cm, such as ectopic pregnancies, IUDs, ovarian cysts, uterine fibroids, and hydatidiform moles. In men, is used to detect testicular torsion or masses.	Instruct patient that a full bladder may be required, depending on the reason for the study.
Computed tomography (CT) of pelvis	Pelvic CT is used to detect tumour within the pelvis.	Inform patient of procedure. Patient must lie still during the procedure. If IV contrast medium is used, check for iodine allergy.
Magnetic resonance imaging (MRI)	Radio waves and magnetic field are used to view soft tissue. Useful if there is an abnormal mammogram or breast dysplasia. Also used to diagnose abnormalities in the female and male reproductive systems.	Screen patient for metal parts and pacemaker. Inform patient that the procedure is painless. Patient must lie still during the procedure.
Invasive Procedures		
Breast biopsy	Histological examination of excised breast tissue is performed, either by needle aspiration or excisional biopsy.	Before surgery, instruct patient about operative procedures and sedation. After surgery, perform wound care and instruct patient about breast self-examination.
Hysteroscopy	Allows visualization of uterine lining through insertion of scope through cervix. Used mainly to diagnose and treat abnormal bleeding such as fibroids or polyps. Biopsy may be taken during the procedure.	Explain purpose and method of procedure and that it might be done in the physician's office. Inform patient that mild cramping and slight bloody discharge after procedure is normal.
Hysterosalpingogram	Involves instillation of contrast media through cervix into uterine cavity and subsequently through and out fallopian tubes. Radiographs are taken to detect abnormalities of uterus and its adnexa (ovaries and tubes) as contrast progresses through them. Test may be most useful in diagnostic assessment of fertility (e.g., to detect adhesions near ovary, an abnormal uterine shape, blockage of tubal pathways).	Inform patient about procedure and that it may be fairly uncomfortable. Determine possibility of iodine allergy.
Colposcopy	Direct visualization of cervix with binocular microscope that allows magnification and study of cellular dysplasia and cervix abnormalities. Used as follow-up study for abnormal Pap test and for examination of women exposed to DES in utero. Biopsy of cervix may be taken during examination. Valuable in decreasing number of false-negative cervical biopsies.	Inform patient about this outpatient procedure. Inform patient that this examination is similar to speculum examination.

DES, diethylstilbestrol; *IUDs*, intrauterine devices.

Continued

DIAGNOSTIC STUDIES

Table 53-12 Male and Female Reproductive Systems—cont'd

STUDY	DESCRIPTION AND PURPOSE	NURSING RESPONSIBILITY
Invasive Procedures—cont'd		
Conization	Cone-shaped sample of squamocolumnar tissue of cervix is removed for direct study.	Explain purpose and method of procedure and that it requires use of surgical facilities and anaesthesia. Instruct patient to rest for at least 3 days after procedure and to have 3-wk follow-up appointment.
Loop electrosurgical excision of transformation zone (LEETZ)	Excision of cervical tissue via an electrosurgical instrument.	Explain purpose and method of procedure and that it may be done in the physician's office.
Loop electrosurgical excision procedure (LEEP)	Same as above.	Same as above.
Culdotomy, culdoscopy, and culdocentesis	Culdotomy is an incision made through posterior fornix of cul-de-sac and allows visualization of peritoneal cavity (i.e., uterus, tubes, and ovaries). Culdoscope can then be used to study these structures closely. This technique is valuable in fertility evaluations. Withdrawal of fluid (culdocentesis) allows examination of fluid characteristics.	Explain purpose and method of procedure. Prepare patient for vaginal operation with preoperative instruction and sedation. Perform assessment of bleeding and discomfort after surgery.
Laparoscopy (peritoneoscopy)	Allows visualization of pelvic structures via fibreoptic scopes inserted through small abdominal incisions. Instillation of carbon dioxide into cavity improves visualization. Used in diagnostic assessment of uterus, tubes, and ovaries (Figure 53-10). Can be used in conjunction with tubal sterilization.	Before surgery, instruct patient about procedure, prepare abdomen, and reassure patient about sedation. Tell patient to rest for 1-3 days after surgery. Inform patient of probability of shoulder pain owing to air in the abdomen.
Dilatation and curettage (D & C)	Operative procedure dilates cervix and allows curetting of endometrial lining. Used in assessment of abnormal bleeding and cytological evaluation of lining.	Before surgery, instruct patient about procedure and sedation. Perform postoperative assessment of degree of bleeding (frequent perineal pad check during first 24 hr).
Fertility Studies		
Semen analysis	Semen is assessed for volume (2-5 mL), viscosity, sperm count (>20 million/mL), sperm motility (60% motile), and percent of abnormal sperm (60% with normal structure).	Instruct patient to bring in fresh specimen within 2 hr of ejaculation.
Basal body temperature assessment	Measurement indicates indirectly whether ovulation has occurred. (Temperature rises at ovulation and remains elevated during secretory phase of normal menstrual cycle.)	Instruct woman to take her temperature using special basal temperature thermometer (calibrated in tenths of degrees) every morning before getting out of bed. Tell woman to record temperature on graph.
Huhner test or Sims-Huhner	Mucus sample of cervix is examined within 2-8 hr after intercourse. Total number of sperm is assessed in relation to number of live sperm. Used to determine whether cervical mucus is "hostile" to passage of sperm from vagina into uterus.	Instruct couples to have intercourse at estimated time of ovulation and be present for test within 2-8 hr after intercourse.
Endometrial biopsy	Small curette is used to obtain piece of endometrial lining to assess endometrial changes common to progesterone secretion after ovulation.	Tell patient that test must be performed post ovulation. Explain that procedure should cause only short period of uterine cramping.
Hysterosalpingogram	Same as operative procedures.	Same as operative procedures.
Serum progesterone	Same as blood studies.	Same as blood studies.

*Canadian Cancer Society. (2011). *Canadian cancer encyclopedia: Screening for cervical cancer.* Retrieved from *http://info.cancer.ca/cce-ecc/default.aspx?cceid=809&toc=12&Lang=E*
†Canadian Cancer Society. (2011). *Canadian cancer encyclopedia: Breast cancer overview.* Retrieved from *http://info.cancer.ca/cce-ecc/default.aspx?Lang=E&toc=10*

Ultrasonography. Ultrasonography has many applications for diagnostic study. Pelvic ultrasonography is used to obtain images of the pelvic organs. Transvaginal ultrasonography can be used to aid in diagnosing abnormalities of the ovaries or the uterus. These types of ultrasound are also used to detect pregnancy in the uterus, ectopic pregnancy, ovarian cysts, and other pelvic masses. Breast ultrasonography is useful in the detection of fluid-filled masses. In men, ultrasonography is used to detect testicular masses and testicular torsion. Transrectal ultrasonography is useful in locating prostate tumours.

Pelvic Computed Tomography and Magnetic Resonance Imaging. Pelvic computed tomography or magnetic resonance imaging (MRI) is used to detect primary or metastatic tumours of the reproductive organs. Contrast medium may be used in conjunction with the CT procedure.

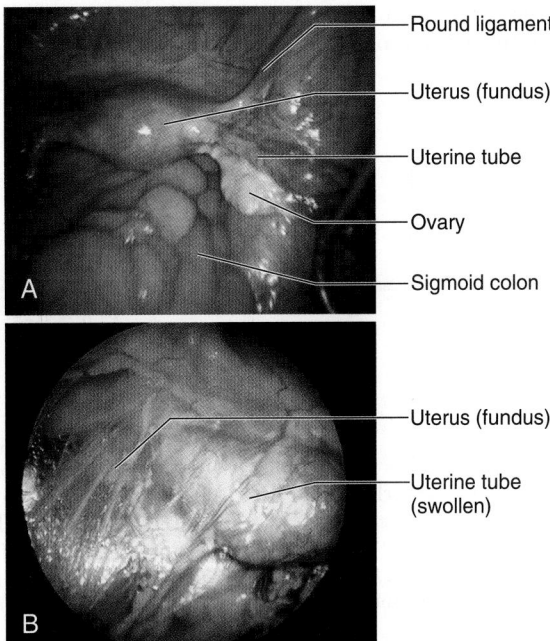

Figure 53-10 Laparoscopic views of the female pelvis. **A,** Normal image. **B,** Pelvic inflammatory disease. Note the reddish inflammatory membrane covering and fixing the ovary and uterus to the surrounding structures.

Source: Thibodeau, G. A., & Patton, K. T. (2010). *Anatomy and physiology* (7th ed., p. 1064, Figure 32-20). St. Louis: Mosby.

ⓔvolve   *An assessment case study of the reproductive system is available at* **http://evolve.elsevier.com/Canada/Lewis/medsurg**

REVIEW QUESTIONS

The number of the question corresponds to the same-numbered objective at the beginning of the chapter.

1. Which of the following is a normal reproductive function that may be altered in a patient who undergoes a prostatectomy?
   a. Sperm production
   b. Production of testosterone
   c. Production of seminal fluid
   d. Release of sperm from the epididymis

2. What does estrogen production by the mature ovarian follicle cause?
   a. Decreased secretion of follicle-stimulating hormone (FSH) and luteinizing hormone (LH)
   b. Increased production of gonadotropin-releasing hormone (GnRH) and FSH
   c. Release of GnRH and increased secretion of LH
   d. Decreased release of FSH and decreased progesterone production

3. Female orgasm is the result of which of the following?
   a. Uterine and vaginal contractions and rapid release of muscular tension
   b. Vaginal enlargement and secretion with penile insertion
   c. Clitoral swelling, vaginal lubrication, and uterine elevation
   d. Clitoral swelling and increased vaginal lubrication

4. Which of the following is an age-related finding noted by the nurse during assessment of the older woman's reproductive system?
   a. Gynecomastia
   b. Vaginal dryness
   c. Nipple retraction
   d. Increased sensitivity of labia

5. Which of the following should be included as significant information about a patient's past medical history related to the reproductive system?
   a. Extent of sexual activity
   b. General satisfaction with sexuality
   c. Previous sexually transmitted infections
   d. Self-image and relationships with others

6. Which of the following examination techniques is used to evaluate the prostate?
   a. Palpation
   b. Percussion
   c. Inspection
   d. Auscultation

7. Which of the following would be considered an abnormal finding during physical assessment of the male reproductive system?
   a. Slight clear urethral discharge
   b. The glans covered with prepuce
   c. Symmetrical scrotum
   d. Descended testes

8. Which of the following is a screening criterion for assessing prostate cancer?
   a. Baseline ultrasonography of the prostate at age 40
   b. Baseline ultrasonography of the prostate at age 50
   c. Yearly digital rectal examination for men older than age 30
   d. Yearly digital rectal examination for men older than age 50

ANSWERS: 1. c; 2. c; 3. a; 4. b; 5. c; 6. a; 7. a; 8. d.

REFERENCES

Canadian Cancer Society. (2011a). Canadian cancer encyclopedia: Testicular cancer overview. Retrieved from *http://info.cancer.ca/cce-ecc/SearchDetails.aspx?Lang=E&lf=testicular%2520self%2520examination&cceid=4339&rk=60302525&fp=file%253a%252f%252fcispublicweb%252fe_html%252f50_4339.html&sqg=9eb83606-2dff-4acf-978c-8abacd6ec281*

Canadian Cancer Society. (2011b). Canadian cancer encyclopedia: Early detection of prostate cancer. Retrieved from *http://info.cancer.ca/cce-ecc/default.aspx?cceid=6567&toc=41&Lang=E*

Canadian Research Network for Care in the Community (CRNCC). (2007). Diversity: Sexual orientation in home and community care. Retrieved from *http://www.ryerson.ca/crncc/knowledge/factsheets/pdf/InFocus-Diversity-SexualOrientationinHomecommunityCareJuly2011.pdf*

Canadian Urological Association. (2011). PSA testing still essential—CUA position contrasts the US position. Retrieved from *http://www.cua.org/userfiles/files/CUA-PSA-position-statement-ENG-Nov-15-2011-FINAL(3).pdf*

The Centre: A Community Centre Serving and Supporting Lesbian, Gay, Transgender, Bisexual Persons and Their Allies. (2006). LGTB health matters: An educational and training resource for health and social services sectors. Retrieved from *http://www.sexualhealthcentresaskatoon.ca/pdfs/p_lgbt.pdf*

Coonrod, D. V., Jack, B. W., Boggess, K. A., Long, R., Conry, J. A., Cox, S. N., …, Dunlop, A. L. (2008). The clinical content of preconception care: Immunizations as part of preconception care. *American Journal of Obstetrics and Gynecology, 199*(6 Suppl 2), S290-S295. doi:10.1016/j.ajog.2008.08.062

Farage, M., Neill, S., & MacLean, A. B. (2009). Physiological changes associated with the menstrual cycle: A review. *Obstetrical and Gynecological Survey, 64*(1), 58-72. doi:10.1097/OGX.0b013e3181932a37

Gibbs, R., Karlan, B., Haney, A., & Nygaard, I. (2008). *Danforth's obstetrics and gynecology* (10th ed.). Philadelphia: Lippincott Williams & Wilkins.

Gooren, L. (2008). Recent perspectives on the age-related decline of testosterone. *Journal of Men's Health, 5*(1), 86-93. doi:10.1016/j.jomh.2007.12.003

Grady, D., & Barrrett-Connor, E. (2008). Menopause. In L. Goldman & D. Ausiello (Eds.), *Cecil's medicine* (23rd ed.). Philadelphia: Saunders Elsevier.

Kelly, B. (2008). Possible indicators of fetal abnormalities. In S. Ratliffe (Ed.), *Family medicine obstetrics* (3rd ed.). St. Louis: Mosby.

Masters, W. H., & Johnson, E. (1966). *Human sexual response.* Boston: Little Brown.

McCance, K. L., Huether, S. E., Brashers, V. L., & Rote, N. S. (2010). *Pathophysiology: The biologic basis for disease in adults and children* (6th ed.). St. Louis: Mosby.

National Institutes of Health (NIH). (2008). WHI follow-up study confirms health risks of long-term combination hormone therapy outweigh benefits for postmenopausal women. Retrieved from *http://public.nhlbi.nih.gov/newsroom/home/GetPressRelease.aspx?id=2554*

Pagana, K. D., & Pagana, T. J. (2009). *Mosby's manual of diagnostic and laboratory tests* (4th ed.). St. Louis: Mosby.

Prostate Cancer Canada. (2011). Early detection guidelines update. Retrieved from *http://www.prostatecancer.ca/In-The-News/Prostate-Cancer-News/Early-Detection-Guidelines-Update*

Registered Nurses Association of Ontario (RNAO). (2007). Position statement: Respecting sexual orientation and gender identity. Retrieved from *http://www.rnao.org/Storage/30/2486_Respecting_Sexual_Orientation_and_Gender_Identity.pdf*

Scolaro, K., Braxton-Lloyd, K., & Helms, K. (2008). Devices for home evaluation of women's health concerns. *American Journal of Health-System Pharmacy, 65,* 299-314. doi:10.2146/ajhp060565

Shiri, R., Koskimäki, J., Häkkinen, J., Auvinen, A., Tammela, T., & Hakama, M. (2007). Cardiovascular drug use and the incidence of erectile dysfunction. *International Journal of Impotence Research, 19*(2), 208-212. doi:10.1038/sj.ijir.3901516

Stonewall Scotland and National Health Services (NHS). (2006). Fair for all—The wider challenge: Good LGBT practice in the NHS. Retrieved from *http://www.healthscotland.com/uploads/documents/6307-Fair%20For%20All%20-%20Good_LGBT_Practice_NHS.pdf*

Styne, D., & Grumbach, M. (2008). Puberty: Ontogeny, endocrinology, physiology and disorders. In H. M. Kronenberg, S. Melmed, K. S. Polonsky & P. R. Larsen (Eds.), *Williams textbook of endocrinology* (11th ed.). Philadelphia: Mosby.

Thibodeau, G. A., & Patton, K. T. (2008). *Structure and function of the body* (13th ed.). St. Louis: Mosby.

Tjepkema, M. (March, 2008). Health care use among gay, lesbian and bisexual Canadians. *Health Reports—Statistics Canada, 19*(1). Retrieved from *http://www.statcan.gc.ca/pub/82-003-x/2008001/article/10532-eng.pdf*

Wallace, M. (2008). Assessment of sexual health in older adults. *American Journal of Nursing, 108*(9), 47-53. doi:10.1097/01.NAJ.0000336417.50193.90

Weismiller, D. G. (2009). Menopause. *Primary Care: Clinics in office practice, 36*(1), 199-226. doi:10.1016/j.pop.2008.10.007

RESOURCES

Resources for this chapter are listed in Chapter 56, p. 1574, and Chapter 57, p. 1603.

Written by Deborah Hamolsky
Adapted by Jackie Hartigan-Rogers

LEARNING OBJECTIVES

1. Summarize screening guidelines for the early detection of breast cancer.
2. Describe the technique of breast self-awareness, including rationale and reasons for referral.
3. Explain the types, causes, clinical manifestations, collaborative care, and the nursing management of common benign breast disorders.
4. Assess the risk factors for breast cancer.
5. Describe the pathophysiology and clinical manifestations of breast cancer.
6. Describe the collaborative care and the nursing management of breast cancer.
7. Specify the physical and psychological preoperative and postoperative aspects of nursing management for patients undergoing a mastectomy.
8. Explain the indications for reconstructive breast surgery; types, potential risks, and complications of reconstructive breast surgery; and nursing management after reconstructive breast surgery.

KEY TERMS

fibroadenoma A common cause of discrete benign breast lumps in young women; painless, round, well-delineated, and very mobile, p. 1497

fibrocystic changes A benign condition of the breasts characterized by development of excess fibrous tissue, hyperplasia of the epithelial lining of the mammary ducts, proliferation of mammary ducts, and cyst formation, p. 1496

galactorrhea A milky secretion from the nipple caused by inappropriate lactation, p. 1498

gynecomastia A transient, noninflammatory enlargement of one or both breasts in men, p. 1498

lumpectomy Breast-conserving surgery that involves the removal of the entire tumour along with a margin of normal surrounding tissue, p. 1503

lymphedema Accumulation of lymph in soft tissue that results from the excision or irradiation of lymph nodes, p. 1503

mammoplasty Surgical change in the size or shape of the breast, p. 1513

mastalgia Breast pain; most common breast-related complaint in women, p. 1496

mastectomy Surgical removal of the breast, the pectoral muscles, the axillary lymph nodes, and all fat and adjacent tissue, p. 1502

mastitis An inflammatory condition of the breast that occurs most frequently in lactating women; usually caused by staphylococcal infection, p. 1496

Paget's disease A rare breast malignancy characterized by a persistent lesion of the nipple and areola with or without a palpable mass, p. 1501

ELECTRONIC RESOURCES

Supplemental content related to Chapter 54 can be found ...

Evolve Web Site ⊖volve

http://evolve.elsevier.com/Canada/Lewis/medsurg
- Answer Guidelines for Case Study on p. 1515
- Clinical Reference: Laboratory Values
- Content Updates

- Customizable Nursing Care Plan: Mastectomy or Lumpectomy
- Electronic Calculators
- Examination Review Questions
- Glossary
- Interactive Case Study: Breast Cancer
- Key Points (Printable and MP3 Download)

Breast disorders are a significant health concern for women. Most breast pain is of a benign nature; however, in a Canadian woman's lifetime, she has a chance of one in nine that she will receive a diagnosis of breast cancer (Canadian Cancer Society, 2011a). Whether the actual diagnosis is one of a benign condition or a malignancy, the initial discovery of a lump or change in the breast often triggers intense feelings of anxiety, fear, and denial. These feelings can be associated with both the fear of death and the possible loss of a breast. Throughout history, the female breast has been regarded as a symbol of beauty, femininity, sexuality, and motherhood. The potential loss of a breast, or part of a breast, may be devastating for many women because of the significant psychological, social, sexual, and body image implications associated with it.

The most frequently encountered breast disorders in women are fibrocystic changes, breast cancer, fibroadenoma, intraductal papilloma, and duct ectasia. In men, gynecomastia is the most common breast disorder.

Assessment of Breast Disorders

It is critical that breast disorders be detected early, diagnosed accurately, and treated promptly. The frequency of these examinations is determined by the woman's age, the presence of significant risk factors, and her medical history. Guidelines established in Canada regarding breast surveillance practices include the following:
- Women of all ages should be familiar with their breasts and report any changes to their health care providers.
- Women ages 40 to 49 should discuss individual risk for breast cancer, along with the risks and benefits of mammography, with a health care provider.
- Women ages 50 to 69 should undergo mammography every 2 years.
- Women ages 70 or older should talk to a health care provider about an individualized screening program.
- A health care provider may also perform a physical examination of the breasts (clinical breast examination).
- Women who are at high risk for developing breast cancer should talk to their health care providers about a personal plan of testing (Canadian Cancer Society, 2011b).

It is recommended that all women discuss the risks and benefits of mammography with their health care providers (Canadian Cancer Society, 2010a). The benefits of early detection of breast cancer are well established. The use of screening mammography has significantly improved early and accurate detection of breast malignancies. Mammography can identify breast abnormalities that may be cancer before physical symptoms appear. In Canada, national guidelines have been established on the basis of research that women aged 50 to 69 benefit most from regular breast screening (Canadian Cancer Society, 2012a).

There has been some confusion with regard to the value of breast self-examination (BSE) and screening mammography for younger women and its role in reducing rates of mortality from breast cancer (Canadian Task Force on Preventive Health Care, 2011; Rosolowich, 2006). The emphasis now is on helping women become aware of how their breasts normally look and feel and to understand that there is no right or wrong way for women to check their breasts (Figure 54-1). Nurses should teach women that it is important to get to know the whole area of breast tissue including up to the collarbone and under armpits

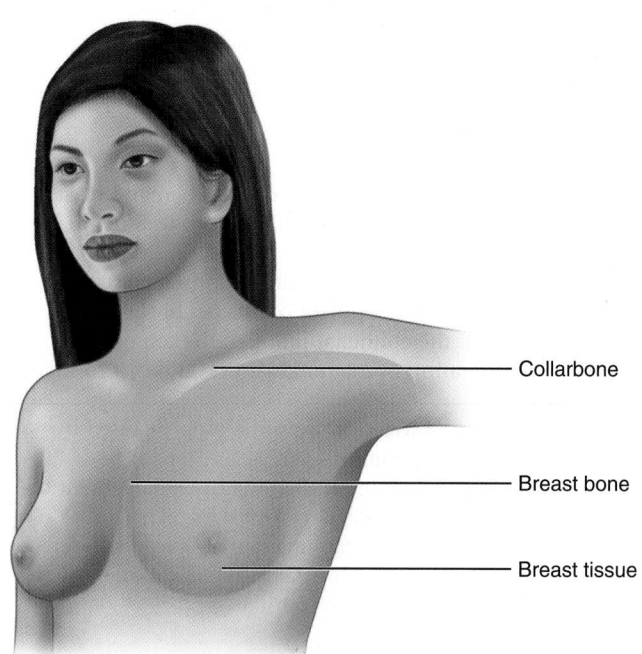

Figure 54-1 Every women should know her breasts. She should be aware of what is normal by looking at and feeling her breasts any way that works best for her. She should get to know the whole area of her breast tissue: up to the collarbone, under the armpits, and including the nipples. Every woman should get to know her breasts well enough to notice changes.

Source: Canadian Cancer Society. (2010). *Know your breasts.* Retrieved July 7, 2012, from *http://www.cancer.ca/Canada-wide/Prevention/Knowing%20your%20body/Know%20your%20breasts.aspx?sc_lang=en*

and nipples (Canadian Cancer Society, 2010b). Women should be encouraged to report any new breast changes (e.g., nipple discharge, finding a lump) to their health care providers (Canadian Cancer Society, 2010c).

If a woman decides she wants to practise BSE and undergo mammography screening, health care providers must ensure that the benefits and risks, as well as the woman's values and preferences, be discussed fully (Canadian Task Force on Preventive Health Care, 2011; Rosolowich, 2006).

It is also important that nurses ensure patients' awareness of Canada's clinical practice guidelines for the care and treatment of breast cancer. The guidelines developed in 1998 provide important information for health care providers and patients and make a significant contribution toward ensuring quality care for patients with breast cancer (Latosinsky, Fradette, Lix, Hildebrand, & Turner, 2007). A primary goal of the development of these guidelines was to decrease the variation in breast cancer care across Canada (Folkes, Urquhart, Zitzelsberger, & Grunfeld, 2008). All patients who have completed primary treatment for breast cancer should have regular follow-up surveillance that comprises a medical history, physical examination, and annual mammography. The frequency of visits must be adjusted according to the individual patient's needs. Special topics of concern that have to be addressed with patients who have breast cancer include cognitive functioning, fatigue, weight management, osteoporosis, sexual functioning, and pregnancy (Grunfeld, Dhesy-Thind, & Levine, 2005).

Diagnostic Studies

Several techniques can be used to screen for breast disorders or provide a diagnosis of a suspect physical finding. *Mammography* is a method used to visualize the internal structure of the breast with the use of radiography (Figure 54-2). This generally well-tolerated procedure can detect suspect findings that cannot be felt by palpation. Mammography has significantly improved the early and accurate detection of breast malignancies. Improved imaging technology has also reduced the amount of radiation used in mammography.

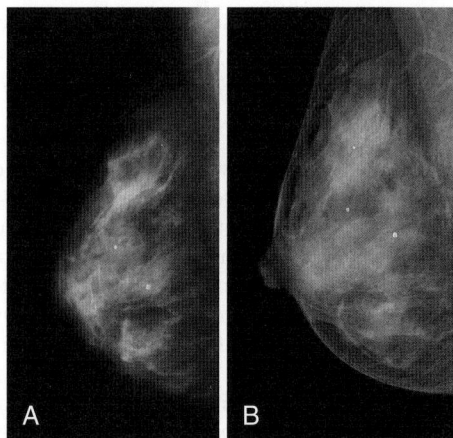

Figure 54-2 Screening mammograms showing dense breast tissue and benign, scattered microcalcifications of a 57-year-old. **A,** Image obtained with conventional radiography. **B,** Image obtained with digital radiography.

Source: Adam, A. (2008). *Grainger and Allison's diagnostic radiology* (5th ed.). St. Louis: Churchill Livingstone.

Digital mammography is a newer technique in which x-ray images are digitally coded into a computer. This allows for a clearer and more accurate image than conventional mammography (Costaridou, Skiadopoulos, Karahaliou, Arikidis, & Panayiotakis, 2009; see Figure 54-2).

Calcifications are the abnormality most easily recognized on mammograms (see Figure 54-2). These deposits of calcium crystals form in the breast for many reasons, such as inflammation, trauma, and aging. Although most calcifications are benign, they also may be associated with preinvasive cancer.

A comparison of current and prior mammograms may reveal early cancerous tissue changes. Because some tumours metastasize late, early detection by mammography allows for earlier treatment and the prevention of metastasis of lesions that are smaller or less aggressive. In younger women, mammography is less sensitive because of the breast tissue is more dense and because developing breast tissue is radiosensitive (Miltenburg & Speights, 2008). About 10 to 15% of all breast cancers cannot be seen on mammograms and are detected only by palpation. If the clinical findings are suspect, a biopsy may be recommended with normal mammography.

Ultrasonography is used in conjunction with mammography. It may be used to differentiate a solid mass from a cystic mass, to evaluate a mass in a pregnant or lactating woman, or to locate and guide biopsy for a suspect lesion on breast magnetic resonance imaging (MRI). Palpable masses should be investigated with both mammography and ultrasonography (Miltenburg & Speights, 2008).

MRI is recommended as a sensitive screening tool for women at high risk for breast cancer, for women whose findings on mammography or ultrasonography are suspect for malignancy, and for women in whom breast cancer was previously detected by mammography. Limitations of MRI include its high cost, which may result in less frequent use of this method of screening (Palacio, 2010).

A definitive diagnosis of a suspect area is made by means of histological examination of a biopsy sample of tissue. Biopsy techniques include *fine-needle aspiration* (FNA) biopsy, stereotactic or ultrasonography-guided core biopsy, and surgical biopsy (also called *open biopsy*).

In FNA biopsy, a needle is inserted into the lesion and cellular fluid aspirated into a syringe. Three or four passes are usually made. FNA and cytological evaluation may be helpful in making a diagnosis and planning treatment. The procedure should be performed by an experienced cytologist. If the results are negative but the lesion is suspect, an additional biopsy may be necessary. Biopsy results are usually available within 24 to 48 hours.

Stereotactic core biopsy is a reliable diagnostic technique for obtaining a biopsy sample of an abnormality seen on a mammogram. The patient is positioned lying face down on a table with an opening in the table for the breast and should be informed that the procedure is uncomfortable. Mammography is then used to locate the lesion. The skin is anaesthetized, and a small skin incision is made to allow the entrance of a biopsy gun device. The gun is fired and removes a core sample of the lesion. This is repeated several times, and the core samples are sent for pathological analysis.

In *ultrasonography-guided core biopsy*, ultrasound waves are used to locate the lesion with the patient lying on her back. To obtain the tissue sample, the same technique as described for stereotactic core biopsy is used. These outpatient techniques have several advantages over an open surgical biopsy, including minimal scarring, local anaesthesia, reduced cost, and shorter recovery time. An open surgical biopsy involves removal of part or all of a suspect lesion through an incision into the breast. If the lesion is small, deep, and difficult to locate, a wire localization technique may be used during surgery. A special wire is placed into the lesion under radiographic guidance, and then the surgeon follows this wire to help locate the lesion.

Benign Breast Disorders

Mastalgia

Mastalgia (breast pain) is the most common breast-related complaint in women. The most common form is *cyclic mastalgia*, which coincides with the menstrual cycle (Rodden, 2009). It is described as diffuse breast tenderness or heaviness. Breast pain may last 2 to 3 days or most of the month. The pain is related to hormonal sensitivity. The symptoms often decrease with menopause. *Noncyclic mastalgia* has no relationship to the menstrual cycle and can continue into menopause. It may be constant or intermittent throughout the month and last for several years. Symptoms include a burning sensation, aching, or soreness in the breast. The cause of the pain of noncyclic mastalgia is not known (Rodden, 2009).

Mammography is not usually necessary for mastalgia unless the woman is older than 40 years and did not undergo mammography in the previous year. Cyclic pain may be relieved somewhat by reductions in caffeine and dietary fat intake; by vitamins E, A, and B complex and γ-linolenic acid (evening primrose oil); and by continual wearing of a support bra. Massage with ice or heat, analgesics, and anti-inflammatory medications may also help (Rodden, 2009). Medications that might be recommended include oral contraceptives and danazol (Danocrine). Because of the androgenic adverse effects of danazol (acne, edema, hirsutism), this therapy is unacceptable for many women.

Breast Infections

Mastitis. **Mastitis** is an inflammatory condition of the breast that occurs most frequently in lactating women (Table 54-1). *Lactational mastitis* manifests as a localized area that is erythematous, painful, and tender on palpation. Fever is often present. The infection develops when organisms, usually staphylococci, gain access to the breast through a cracked nipple. In its early stages, mastitis can be cured with antibiotics. Breastfeeding should continue unless an abscess is forming or a purulent drainage is noted. The mother may wish to use a nipple shield or to hand-express milk from the involved breast until the pain subsides. She should see her health care provider promptly to begin a course of antibiotic therapy. Any breast that remains red, tender, and not responsive to antibiotics necessitates follow-up care and evaluation for inflammatory breast cancer.

Lactational Breast Abscess. If lactational mastitis persists after several days of antibiotic therapy, a lactational breast abscess may have developed. In this condition, the skin may become red and edematous over the involved breast, often with a corresponding palpable mass, and the patient may have a fever. Antibiotics alone constitute insufficient treatment for a breast abscess. Ultrasonography-guided drainage of the abscess or surgical incision and drainage are necessary (Spencer, 2008). The drainage is cultured, sensitivities are measured, and therapy with an appro-

Table 54-1 Selected Benign Breast Disorders		
DISORDER	**INCIDENCE**	**CLINICAL MANIFESTATIONS**
Lactational mastitis	Occurs in up to 10% of postpartum lactating mothers (both primipara and multipara), usually 2-4 wk after parturition	Warm to touch, indurated, painful, often unilateral; most commonly caused by *Staphylococcus aureus*
Fibrocystic changes	Most common between ages 35 and 50	Not usually discrete masses but nodularity instead (movable, soft); usually accompanied by cyclic pain and tenderness; mass(es) often cyclic in occurrence
Cysts	Most common after age 35, incidence decreases after menopause; develop in 1 per 14 women	Palpable fluid-filled mass (movable, soft); multiple cysts can occur and recur; rarely associated with breast cancer
Fibroadenoma	Occurs in 10% of all women aged 15-40	Palpable mass (movable, firm), usually 2-3 cm in size; rarely associated with breast cancer
Fat necrosis	Many women report previous history of trauma to breast	Usually a hard, very tender, mobile, indurated mass with irregular borders
Duct ectasia	Perimenopausal woman: most common in women in their 50s; previous lactation; inverted nipples	Fixation of nipple, usually accompanied by nipple discharge of thick, grey material; often associated with breast pain

priate antibiotic is begun. Breastfeeding can continue in most cases with ongoing treatment of the abscess (Spencer, 2008).

Fibrocystic Changes

Fibrocystic changes in the breast constitute a benign condition characterized by changes in breast tissue (Figure 54-3). The changes include the development of excess fibrous tissue, hyperplasia of the epithelial lining of the mammary ducts, proliferation of mammary ducts, and cyst formation. As a result of these changes, pain is caused by nerve irritation from edema in the connective tissue and by fibrosis from pinching of the nerve. The term *fibrocystic disease* is incorrect because the cluster of problems is actually an exaggerated response to hormonal influence; the terms *fibrocystic condition* and *fibrocystic complex* are more accurate. Fibrocystic changes are not associated with increased risk for breast cancer. Masses or nodularities can appear in both breasts. They are often found in the upper, outer quadrants and usually occur bilaterally.

Fibrocystic changes are the most frequently occurring breast disorder. They occur most frequently in women between 35 and 50 years of age but often begin as early as 20 years of age. Pain

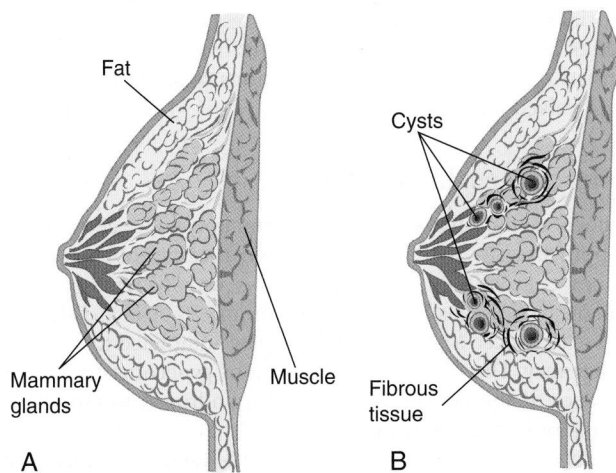

Figure 54-3 Diagrams of types of breast tissue. **A,** Normal breast tissue. **B,** Fibrocystic breast tissue.

and nodularity often increase over time but tend to subside after menopause unless high doses of estrogen replacement are used. Fibrocystic changes are thought to result from a heightened responsiveness of breast tissue to circulating estrogen and progesterone (Morgan & McCance, 2008).

Fibrocystic changes most commonly occur in women with premenstrual abnormalities, nulliparous women, women with a history of spontaneous abortion, nonusers of oral contraceptives, and women with early menarche and late menopause. Symptoms related to fibrocystic changes often worsen in the premenstrual phase and subside after menstruation.

Manifestations of fibrocystic breast changes include one or more palpable lumps that are often round, well delineated, and freely movable within the breast (see Table 54-1). Discomfort ranging from tenderness to pain may also occur. The lump is usually observed to increase in size and perhaps in tenderness before menstruation. Cysts may enlarge or shrink rapidly, becoming larger before menstruation and shrinking afterward. Nipple discharge associated with fibrocystic breasts is often milky, watery-milky, yellow, or green.

Mammography may be helpful in distinguishing fibrocystic changes from breast cancer. However, in some women the breast tissue is so dense that it is difficult to obtain a mammographic study. In these situations, ultrasonography may be more useful in differentiating a cystic mass from a solid mass.

NURSING AND COLLABORATIVE MANAGEMENT: FIBROCYSTIC CHANGES

With the initial discovery of a discrete mass in the breast by a woman or her health care provider, aspiration or surgical biopsy may be indicated. A wait of 7 to 10 days may be planned in order to note any changes that may be related to the menstrual cycle. For large or frequent cysts, surgical removal may be favoured over repeated aspiration. An excisional biopsy would be recommended (a) if no fluid is found on aspiration, (b) if the fluid that is found is hemorrhagic, or (c) if, after fluid aspiration, a residual mass remains. Excisional biopsy is performed in an outpatient surgery unit.

Biopsy may be indicated for women with fibrocystic disorders who are at increased risk for breast cancer. Atypical hyperplasia, which is discovered on breast biopsy, increases a woman's risk for developing breast cancer later in life.

The woman with cystic changes should be encouraged to return regularly for follow-up examinations throughout her life. She may also be taught BSE to self-monitor changes. Severe fibrocystic changes may make palpation of the breast more difficult. Any changes in symptoms or changes found during the BSE should be reported and evaluated.

Treatment for a fibrocystic condition is similar to that described earlier for mastalgia. The nurse's role in the care of patients with fibrocystic breast changes is primarily one of teaching. Patients should be taught that the cysts may recur in one or both breasts until menopause and that the cysts may enlarge or become painful just before menstruation. In addition, patients should be reassured that the cysts do not "turn into" cancer. Patients should be advised that any new lump that does not respond in a cyclic manner over 1 to 2 weeks should be examined by a health care provider promptly.

Fibroadenoma

Fibroadenoma is a common cause of discrete benign breast lumps in young women, generally between 15 and 40 years of age. It is the most frequent cause of breast masses in women younger than 25 years. The possible cause of fibroadenoma may be increased estrogen sensitivity in a localized area of the breast. Fibroadenomas are usually small but can be large (2 to 3 cm) and are typically painless, round, well delineated, and very mobile. They may be soft but are usually solid, firm, and rubbery in consistency. Retraction and nipple discharge are not associated with them. Such lumps are often painless. Fibroadenomas may appear as a single unilateral mass, although multiple bilateral fibroadenomas have been reported. Growth is slow and often ceases when the size reaches 2 to 3 cm. Size is not affected by menstruation. However, pregnancy can stimulate dramatic growth.

NURSING AND COLLABORATIVE MANAGEMENT: FIBROADENOMA

Fibroadenomas are easily detected on physical examination and may be visible on mammography and ultrasonography. Definitive diagnosis, however, requires an image-guided core needle biopsy or excisional biopsy and tissue examination by a pathologist. Treatment of fibroadenomas can include observation with regular monitoring, after a malignancy has been ruled out, or surgical excision (Figure 54-4). In women older than 35 years, all new lesions should be evaluated with breast ultrasonography and, possibly, biopsy.

In some clinical settings as an alternative to surgery, tumours can be removed with cryoablation after an established diagnosis of a fibroadenoma. In *cryoablation*, a cryoprobe is inserted into the tumour under ultrasound guidance. Extremely cold gas is piped into the tumour. The frozen tumour dies and is either reduced in size or completely eliminated. Benefits include minimal scarring and quick recovery time.

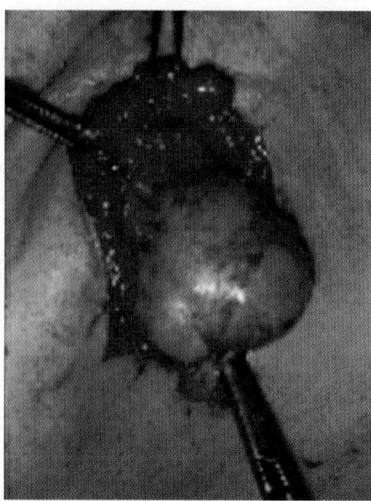

Figure 54-4 Well-defined encapsulated fibroadenoma.

Source: Mansell, R. E., Webster, D., & Sweetland, H. (2009). *Hughes, Mansell & Webster's benign disorders and diseases of the breast* (3rd ed., Figure 7-4). Philadelphia: W. B. Saunders.

The nurse needs to emphasize to the woman with a fibroadenoma the benign nature of the lesion and encourage her to have follow-up examinations.

Nipple Discharge

Nipple discharge may occur spontaneously or as a result of nipple manipulation. A milky secretion constitutes inappropriate lactation (**galactorrhea**) and may be a result of problems such as drug therapy, endocrine problems, and neurological disorders. Nipple discharge may also be idiopathic.

Secretions can also be serous, grossly bloody, or brown to green (Rodden, 2009). These secretions may be caused by either benign or malignant disease. Cytological study of the secretion may help determine the specific disease. Diseases associated with nipple discharge include malignancies, cystic disease, intraductal papilloma, and duct ectasia. Treatment depends on identification of the cause (Rodden, 2009). In most cases, nipple discharge is not related to malignancy.

Intraductal Papilloma. An *intraductal papilloma* is a benign, soft, wartlike growth found in the mammary ducts. It is usually unilateral. It is typically accompanied by a bloody discharge from the nipple that can be intermittent or spontaneous. Most intraductal papillomas are beneath the areola and cannot be palpated. They are usually found in women aged 40 to 60 years. A single duct or several ducts may be involved. Treatment includes excision of the papilloma and the involved duct or duct system. Papillomas may be associated with an increased risk of cancer.

Duct Ectasia. *Duct ectasia* (duct dilation) is a benign breast disorder of perimenopausal and postmenopausal women that involves the ducts in the subareolar area. Several bilateral ducts are usually involved. Multicoloured, sticky discharge is the primary symptom. Duct ectasia is initially painless but may progress to burning sensation, itching, and pain around the nipple, as well as swelling in the areolar area. Inflammatory signs are often present, the nipple may retract, and the discharge may become bloody in more advanced disease. Duct ectasia is not associated with malignancy. If an abscess develops, warm compresses and antibiotics are usually effective treatments. Therapy consists of close follow-up examinations or surgical excision of the involved ducts.

Gynecomastia in Men

Gynecomastia, a transient, noninflammatory enlargement of one or both breasts, is the most common breast problem in men (Hines et al., 2008). The condition is usually temporary and benign. Gynecomastia by itself is not an established risk factor for breast cancer. Mammography may be completed to screen for malignancy. The most common cause of gynecomastia is a disturbance of the normal ratio of active androgen to estrogen in plasma or within the breast itself.

Gynecomastia may also be a manifestation of other problems. It may accompany developmental abnormalities of the male reproductive organs. It may also accompany organic diseases, including testicular tumours, cancer of the adrenal cortex, pituitary adenomas, hyperthyroidism, and liver disease (Jarvis, Browne, MacDonald-Jenkins, & Luctkar-Flude, 2009). Gynecomastia may occur as an adverse effect of drug therapy, particularly with administration of estrogens and androgens, digitalis, isoniazid (Isotamine), ranitidine (Zantac), and spironolactone (Aldactone). Use of heroin and marijuana can also cause gynecomastia.

Senescent Gynecomastia. *Senescent gynecomastia* occurs in up to 57% of older men (Hines et al.). A probable cause is the elevation in plasma estrogen in older adult men as the result of increased conversion of androgens to estrogens in peripheral circulation. Although initially unilateral, the tender, firm, centrally located enlargement may become bilateral. When gynecomastia is characterized by a discrete, circumscribed mass, it must be differentiated from the rarer breast cancer in men. Senescent hyperplasia necessitates no treatment and generally regresses within 6 to 12 months.

AGE-RELATED CONSIDERATIONS: BREAST CHANGES

The loss of subcutaneous fat and structural support and the atrophy of mammary glands often cause breasts to become pendulous in postmenopausal women. The nurse should encourage older women to wear a well-fitting bra. Adequate support can improve physical appearance and reduce pain in the back, shoulders, and neck. It can also prevent *intertrigo* (dermatitis caused by friction between opposing surfaces of skin). Surgical lifting of sagging breasts is possible and may be desirable when reconstruction after a mastectomy is performed.

The decrease in glandular tissue in older women makes a breast mass easier to palpate. This decreased density is probably age related and occurs to a lesser degree with women receiving hormone replacement therapy. Rib margins may be palpable in older women and can be confused with a mass. As a woman becomes more familiar with her own breasts and is reassured about her findings, the anxiety about this finding should decrease. The nurse should encourage older women to continue examining their breasts and to talk to their health care providers about an individualized screening program because the incidence of breast cancer increases with age.

Breast Cancer

Breast cancer is the most common cancer in Canadian women, excluding nonmelanoma skin cancer. It is second only to lung cancer as the leading cause of death from cancer in women. In 2011, an estimated 23,400 new cases of breast cancer were diagnosed in women in Canada, and approximately 190 new cases were diagnosed in men. Each year in Canada, approximately 5155 deaths (5100 women and 55 men) occur in relation to breast cancer. The number of deaths of women from breast cancer in every age group have declined partly as a result of increased mammography screening (Canadian Cancer Society, 2010a, 2010c). The decline in breast cancer incidence among Canadian women may also be the result of the decreased use of hormone replacement therapy (De, Neutel, Olivotto, & Morrison, 2010).

Etiology and Risk Factors

Although the etiology is not completely understood, a number of factors are thought to relate to the cause of breast cancer. Heredity or genetically related susceptibility plays a role. Hormonal regulation of the breast is related to the development of breast cancer, but the mechanisms are poorly understood. Sex hormones (estrogen and progesterone) may act as tumour promoters to stimulate breast cancer growth if malignant changes in the cells have already occurred. Modifiable risk factors include weight gain during adulthood, sedentary lifestyle, dietary fat intake, obesity, and alcohol intake (Canadian Cancer Society, 2012b). Environmental factors such as radiation exposure may also play a role.

Some factors that increase the risk for breast cancer have been identified (Table 54-2). Women are at far greater risk than men because 99% of breast cancers occur in women. Increasing age also increases the risk of developing breast cancer. The incidence of breast cancer in women is very low before 25 years of age and increases gradually until age 60. After age 60, the incidence increases dramatically. Family history is an important risk factor, especially if the involved family member also had ovarian cancer, was premenopausal, had bilateral breast cancer, and is a first-degree relative (e.g., mother, sister, daughter). Having any first-degree relative with breast cancer increases a woman's risk of breast cancer 1.5 to 3 times, depending on age. Data from the Women's Health Initiative study have shown that the use of combined hormone replacement therapy (estrogen plus progesterone) increases the risk of breast cancer and also the risk that the breast cancer will be larger and more advanced at diagnosis (De et al., 2010). The use of estrogen replacement therapy alone (for women who have had a prior hysterectomy) does not currently appear to increase breast cancer risk. Oral contraceptives that contain both estrogen and progesterone cause a slight increase in the risk of breast cancer, particularly for women who have used them for 10 years or longer (Canadian Cancer Society, 2012a). (The Determinants of Health box discusses other factors contributing to breast cancer.)

Risk factors appear to be cumulative and interacting. Therefore, the presence of other risk factors may greatly increase the overall risk, especially for people with a positive family history. Identification of risk factors increases the need for careful clinical surveillance of a patient and for participation in cancer screening measures. However, the identifiable risk factors most associated with breast cancer include female gender and advancing age.

Table 54-2 Risk Factors for Breast Cancer

INCREASED RISK	COMMENTS
Female gender	Women account for 99% of breast cancer cases.
Age 50 or older	Majority of breast cancers are found in postmenopausal women. After age 60, the incidence is greatly elevated.
Family history	Breast cancer in a first-degree relative—particularly when the person is premenopausal or the tumour is bilateral—increases risk. Gene mutations (*BRCA1* or *BRCA2*) play a role in 5-10% of breast cancer cases.
Personal history of breast cancer, colon cancer, endometrial cancer, ovarian cancer	Personal history significantly increases risk of breast cancer, risk of cancer in the other breast, and recurrence.
Early menarche (<age 12); late menopause (>age 55)	A long menstrual history increases the risk of breast cancer.
First full-term pregnancy after age 30; nulliparity	Prolonged exposure to unopposed estrogen increases risk for breast cancer.
Benign breast disorder with atypical epithelial hyperplasia, LCIS	Atypical changes in breast biopsy increase the risk of breast cancer.
Weight gain and obesity after menopause	Fat cells store estrogen.
Exposure to ionizing radiation	Radiation (e.g., prior treatment for Hodgkin's lymphoma) damages DNA.
Alcohol consumption	Women who drink ≥1 alcoholic beverage per day have an increased risk of breast cancer.
Physical inactivity	Breast cancer risk is decreased in physically active women by 33% in comparison with sedentary women.

DNA, deoxyribonucleic acid; *LCIS,* lobular carcinoma in situ.

As many as 5 to 10% of all patients with breast cancer may have inherited a specific genetic abnormality contributing to the development of their breast cancer (Canadian Cancer Society, 2010a). The first genetic alteration to be identified was in the tumour suppressor gene *p53*. The *BRCA1* gene, located on chromosome 17, and the *BRCA2* gene, located on chromosome 11, are tumour suppressor genes that, when functioning normally, inhibit tumour development. Women with inherited *BRCA1* or *BRCA2* mutations have up to an 80% lifetime chance of developing breast cancer (Canadian Cancer Society, 2010a). These women are also at high risk for developing ovarian cancer (Canadian Cancer Society, 2010a). Routine screening for genetic abnormalities in women without evidence of a strong family history of breast cancer is not warranted (see the Genetics in Clinical Practice box "Breast Cancer").

In women with *BRCA1* or *BRCA2* mutations, prophylactic bilateral oophorectomy can decrease the risk of breast cancer and ovarian cancer (Metcalfe & Narod, 2007). In deciding whether and when to undergo this surgical procedure, women should

DETERMINANTS OF HEALTH
Breast Cancer

Personal Health Practices and Coping Skills

- Moderate diets or lifestyles that produce a normal body mass index may be associated with better breast cancer outcomes.*
- Physical exercise can assist overall improvement in quality of life, cardiorespiratory fitness, and physical functioning and can alleviate fatigue.†

Gender

Breast cancer is more common in women; it can also occur in men, although it is rare.‡

Income

Women with higher incomes have a slightly higher incidence of breast cancer, which may be related to having children later in life or having fewer children.‡

Physical Environment

Women living in rural and urban areas receive different primary treatments for breast cancer. Rural women experience more difficulties accessing treatment facilities because of geographic location, which may play a role in determining the type of treatment they receive; they have more problems negotiating traditional gender roles during and after treatment; they have less health information about their breast cancer available to them; and they have less access to mental health therapy.§

*Weihofen, D. L. (2010). Fighting cancer with food and nutrition. *Journal of Gynecologic Oncology Nursing, 20*(1), 22–35.

†Alfano, C. M., Day. J. M., Katz, M. L., Herndon, J. E. 2nd, Bittoni, M. A., Oliveri J. M., ..., Paskett, E. D. (2009). Exercise and dietary change after diagnosis and cancer-related symptoms in long-term survivors of breast cancer: CALGB 79804. *Psycho-Oncology, 18*, 128–133. doi:10.1002/pon.1378

‡Canadian Cancer Society. (2012). *Canadian cancer encyclopedia: Risk factors for breast cancer.* Retrieved from http://info.cancer.ca/cce-ecc/default.aspx?cceid=185&toc=10&lf=stomach&Lang=E

§Bettencourt, B. A., Schlegel, R. J., Talley, A. E., & Molix, L. A. (2007). The breast cancer experience of rural women: A literature review. *Psycho-Oncology, 16*, 875–887. doi:10.1002/pon.1235

GENETICS IN CLINICAL PRACTICE
Breast Cancer

Genetic Basis

- Mutations in genes *BRCA1* and *BRCA2*
- Autosomal dominant transmission

Incidence

- Approximately 5–10% of breast cancers are related to *BRCA1* and *BRCA2* gene mutations.
- Women with *BRCA1* and *BRCA2* gene mutations have a 40 to 80% lifetime risk of developing breast cancer.
- *BRCA1* and *BRCA2* gene mutations are associated with early-onset breast cancer.
- Family history of both breast and ovarian cancer increases the risk of having a *BRCA1* mutation (Morgan & McCance, 2008).

Genetic Testing

- DNA testing is available for *BRCA1* and *BRCA2* gene mutations.

Clinical Implications

- Bilateral oophorectomy, bilateral mastectomy, or both reduce the risk of breast cancer in women with *BRCA1* and *BRCA2* mutations.
- Genetic counselling and testing for *BRCA* mutations should be considered for women whose personal or family history puts them at high risk for a genetic predisposition to breast cancer.

Table 54-3 Types of Breast Cancer

TYPE	FREQUENCY OF OCCURRENCE
Infiltrating ductal carcinoma	63–68%
• Colloid (mucinous)	
• Inflammatory	
• Paget's disease	
• Medullary	
• Papillary	
• Tubular	
Infiltrating lobular carcinoma	10–15%
Noninvasive	22%
• Ductal carcinoma in situ	

receive counselling about the risks and benefits of prophylactic oophorectomy, including fertility issues.

A woman who has a high risk of developing breast cancer (i.e., related to factors such as family history and prior tissue biopsy findings) may, in consultation with her physician, choose to undergo prophylactic bilateral mastectomy. Research has shown that contralateral prophylactic mastectomy can decrease the risk of contralateral breast cancer, but survival rates have not been determined (R. Nelson, 2008).

Women with hereditary (non-*BRCA*) breast cancer have a higher risk of developing a secondary primary breast cancer in the unaffected (contralateral) breast. These women may also choose to have the unaffected breast removed prophylactically at the time of initial surgery for breast cancer or at a later time. The rate of contralateral prophylactic mastectomies in women has been steadily increasing (R. Nelson, 2008).

Predisposing risk factors for breast cancer in men include states of hyperestrogenism, a family history of breast cancer, and radiation exposure. A thorough examination of the male breast should be a routine part of a physical examination for all men.

Pathophysiology

Various types of breast cancer have been identified on the basis of their histological characteristics and growth patterns (Table 54-3). The main components of the breast are lobules (milk-producing glands) and ducts (milk passages that connect the lobules and the nipple). In general, breast cancer arises from the epithelial lining of the ducts (ductal carcinoma) or from the epithelium of the lobules (lobular carcinoma). Breast cancers may be in situ (within the duct or lobule) or invasive (arising from the duct or lobule and invading through the wall of the duct or lobule).

Metastatic breast cancer is breast cancer that has spread to bone, the liver, the lungs, or the brain. Cancer growth rate can range from slow to rapid. Factors that affect cancer prognosis are tumour size, axillary node involvement (the more nodes involved, the worse the prognosis), tumour differentiation, estrogen and progesterone receptor status, and human epidermal growth factor receptor 2 (HER-2) status. HER-2 is a transmembrane receptor that helps regulate cell growth. In many patients with breast cancer, it is overexpressed (Buzdar, 2009).

Noninvasive Breast Cancer. An estimated 22% of all breast cancers are noninvasive. These intraductal cancers include ductal carcinoma in situ (DCIS) and lobular carcinoma in situ (LCIS). DCIS tends to be unilateral and would probably progress to invasive breast cancer if left untreated.

Although the management of DCIS can be controversial, patients should discuss all treatment options with their physician, including local excision, mastectomy with breast reconstruction, breast-conserving surgery (lumpectomy), radiation therapy, and tamoxifen (Nolvadex) therapy.

The term *lobular carcinoma in situ* is somewhat misleading. Although LCIS is a risk factor for developing breast cancer, it is not known to be a premalignant lesion. Although no treatment is necessary, patients with LCIS should increase their surveillance for breast cancer. Tamoxifen may be given as a chemopreventive agent in some patients.

Paget's Disease. *Paget's disease* is a rare breast malignancy characterized by a persistent lesion of the nipple and areola with or without a palpable mass. (This is different from Paget's disease of the bone, which is discussed in Chapter 66.) Itching, burning sensation, bloody nipple discharge with superficial erosion, and ulceration may be present. Diagnosis of Paget's disease is confirmed by pathological examination of the erosion. Nipple changes are often diagnosed as an infection or dermatitis, which can lead to delays in proper treatment. The treatment of Paget's disease may include lumpectomy and radiation therapy or a simple or modified radical mastectomy. The prognosis is good when the cancer is confined to the nipple. The nursing care for patients with Paget's disease is the same as the care for patients with breast cancer.

Inflammatory Breast Cancer. *Inflammatory breast cancer,* the most malignant form of all breast cancers, is rare. It is an aggressive and fast-growing cancer with a high risk for metastasis. The skin of the breast looks red, feels warm, and has a thickened appearance that is often described as resembling an orange peel *(peau d'orange)*. Sometimes, the breast develops ridges and small bumps that look like hives. The inflammatory changes, often mistaken for an infection, are caused by blockage of lymph channels by cancer cells. Neoadjuvant chemotherapy, which is chemotherapy given before surgery, is usually the first course of treatment. It is often followed by radiation. Surgery and hormone therapy may also be indicated. Biological therapy (e.g., trastuzumab [Herceptin]) may be effective in cancers in which HER-2 is overexpressed (Buzdar, 2009).

Clinical Manifestations

Breast cancer is detected as a lump or mammographic abnormality in the breast. It occurs most often in the upper outer quadrant of the breast because it is the location of most of the glandular tissue (Figure 54-5). Breast cancers vary in growth rate. If palpable, breast cancer is characteristically hard and may be irregularly shaped, poorly delineated, nonmobile, and nontender.

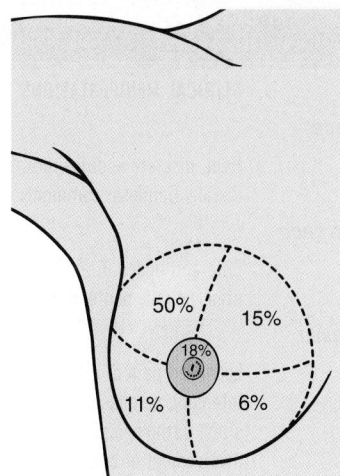

Figure 54-5 Distribution of where breast cancer occurs.

A small percentage of breast cancers cause nipple discharge. The discharge is usually unilateral and may be clear or bloody. Nipple retraction may occur. Peau d'orange may result from the plugging of the dermal lymphatic vessels. With large cancers, infiltration, induration, and dimpling (pulling in) of the overlying skin may also be noted.

Complications

The main complication of breast cancer is recurrence (Table 54-4). Recurrence may be local or regional (skin or soft tissue near the mastectomy site, axillary or internal mammary lymph nodes) or distant (most commonly involving bone, lung, brain, and liver). However, metastatic disease can be found in any distant site.

Widely disseminated or metastatic disease involves the growth of colonies of cancerous breast cells in parts of the body distant from the breast. Metastases primarily occur through the lymphatic vessels, principally those of the axilla (see Chapter 53, Figure 53-7). However, the cancer can spread to other parts of the body without invading the axillary nodes even when the primary breast tumour is small. Even with node-negative breast cancer, there is a possibility of distant metastasis.

Diagnostic Studies

In addition to studies used to diagnose breast cancer (see discussion earlier in this chapter), other tests are useful in predicting the risk of local or systemic recurrence. These tests include axillary lymph node status, tumour size, estrogen and progesterone receptor status, and cell proliferative indices. Results of many of these diagnostic studies are useful prognostic indicators of the disease.

Axillary lymph node involvement is one of the most important prognostic factors in breast cancer. An *axillary lymph node dissection (ALND)* is often performed to determine whether cancer has spread to the axilla on the side of the breast cancer (Swenson, Nissen, Leach, & Post-White, 2009). The more nodes involved, the higher the risk of recurrence. Patients with four or more positive nodes have the highest risk of recurrence.

Lymphatic mapping and *sentinel lymph node dissection (SLND)* helps the surgeon identify the lymph node or nodes that drain first from the tumour site *(sentinel node)*. SLND is less invasive

Table 54-4 Common Sites of Breast Cancer Recurrence and Metastasis

SITE	CLINICAL MANIFESTATIONS
Local Recurrence	
Skin, chest wall	Firm, discrete nodules; occasionally pruritic, usually painless; commonly in or near a scar
Regional Recurrence	
Lymph nodes	Enlarged nodes in axilla or supraclavicular area, usually nontender
Distant Metastases	
Skeletal	Localized pain of gradually increasing intensity; percussion tenderness at involved sites; pathological fracture caused by involvement of bone cortex
Spinal cord	Progressive back pain, localized and radiating; change in bladder or bowel function; loss of sensation in lower extremities
Brain	Headache described as "different"; unilateral sensory loss; focal muscular weakness, hemiparesis, incoordination (ataxia); nausea or vomiting unrelated to medication; cognitive changes
Pulmonary (including lung nodules and pleural effusions)	Shortness of breath, tachypnea, nonproductive cough (not present in all patients)
Liver	Abdominal distension; right lower quadrant abdominal pain, sometimes with radiation to scapular area; nausea and vomiting, anorexia, weight loss; weakness and fatigue; hepatomegaly, ascites, jaundice; peripheral edema; elevated liver enzyme levels
Bone marrow	Anemia; infection; increased bleeding, bruising, petechiae; weakness and fatigue; mild confusion, light-headedness; dyspnea

than ALND (Swenson et al., 2009). A radioisotope or blue dye is injected into the tumour site, and intraoperatively it is determined in which sentinel lymph nodes the radioisotope or blue dye is located. A local incision is made in the axilla, and the surgeon dissects the blue-stained sentinel node or the radioactive lymph node. In general, in SLND, one to four axillary lymph nodes are removed. The nodes are then sent for a frozen-section pathological analysis. If the results are negative, no further axillary surgery is required. If the results are positive, the surgeon may choose to remove additional lymph nodes during the same procedure or during a follow-up surgical procedure in consultation with the patient. SLND has been associated with lower rates of lymphedema and other arm symptoms (Swenson et al., 2009).

Tumour size is a valuable prognostic variable: the larger the tumour, the poorer the prognosis. The wide variety of histological types of breast cancer explains the heterogeneity of the disease. In general, the more well differentiated the tumour is, the less aggressive it is. Poorly differentiated tumours appear morphologically disorganized and are more aggressive.

Another diagnostic test useful for both treatment decisions and prediction of prognosis is measurement of estrogen and progesterone receptor status. Receptor-positive tumours (a) commonly show histological evidence of being well differentiated, (b) frequently have a diploid (more normal) deoxyribonucleic acid (DNA) content and low proliferative indices, (c) have a lower chance for recurrence, and (d) are frequently hormone dependent and responsive to hormone therapy. Receptor-negative tumours (a) are often poorly differentiated histologically, (b) have a high incidence of aneuploidy (abnormally high or low DNA content) and higher proliferative indices, (c) frequently recur, and (d) are usually unresponsive to hormonal therapy.

Ploidy status correlates with tumour aggressiveness. Diploid tumours have been shown to have a significantly lower risk of recurrence than do aneuploid tumours.

Cell-proliferative indices indirectly measure the rate of tumour cell proliferation. The percentage of tumour cells in the synthesis (S) phase of the cell cycle (see Chapter 18, Figure 18-1) is another important prognostic indicator. Patients with cells that have high S-phase fractions have a higher risk for recurrence and a higher probability of earlier death from cancer (Mackey et al., 2009).

Another prognostic indicator is the marker HER-2, which is a protein that can be measured in breast tissue. Overexpression of this receptor has been associated with a greater risk for recurrence and a poorer prognosis in breast cancer. Between 25 and 30% of metastatic breast cancers produce excessive HER-2. High numbers of HER-2 receptors are associated with unusually aggressive tumour growth. The presence of this marker assists in the selection and sequence of chemotherapy and the prediction of a patient's response to treatment (Buzdar, 2009).

Collaborative Care

Historically, a **mastectomy** (removal of breast, pectoral muscles, axillary lymph nodes, and all fat and adjacent tissue) was the standard of care. Currently, a wide range of treatment options is available (Tables 54-5 and 54-6). Prognostic factors are considered when treatment decisions are made about a specific breast cancer. Some of these factors also enter into the staging of breast cancer. The most widely accepted staging method for breast cancer is the American Joint Committee on Cancer's TNM system (Canadian Cancer Society, 2012c). In this system, tumour size (T), nodal involvement (N), and presence of metastasis (M) are used to determine the stage of disease. The stage of a breast cancer describes its size and the extent to which it has spread (Table 54-7).

The stages range from I to IV, with stage I being very small tumours (≤2 cm) with no lymph node involvement and no metastasis. Further classification within these stages depends on the size of the tumour and the number of lymph nodes involved. Stage IV indicates the presence of metastatic spread, regardless of tumour size or lymph node involvement.

The therapeutic regimen is often dictated by the clinical stage and biology of the cancer. (Adverse drug effects and appropriate nursing management of general treatment modalities for cancer are discussed in Chapter 18.)

In spite of the advent of new prognostic indicators such as determination of DNA content and analysis of cell-cycle phases, the presence or absence of malignant cells in lymph nodes remains a powerful prognostic factor related to local recurrence or metastasis after primary therapy.

Surgical Therapy. Breast-conserving surgery with radiation therapy and modified radical mastectomy with or without reconstruction are currently the most common options for resectable

COLLABORATIVE CARE

Table 54-5 Breast Cancer

Diagnostic	Collaborative Therapy

• Health history, including risk factors
• Physical examination, including breast and lymph nodes
• Mammography
• Ultrasonography
• Biopsy
• Breast MRI (if indicated)
	• Surgery
	  • Breast-conserving (lumpectomy) with sentinel lymph node biopsy and dissection, axillary lymph node dissection, or both
	  • Modified radical mastectomy (may include reconstruction)
	• Radiation therapy
	  • Primary radiotherapy
	  • Adjuvant radiotherapy
	  • High-dose brachytherapy
	  • Palliative radiotherapy
	• Drug therapy
	  • Chemotherapy
	  • Neoadjuvant or adjuvant chemotherapy
	  • Chemotherapy for recurrent or metastatic disease
	• Hormonal therapy (see Table 54-6)
	• Biological and targeted therapy

Staging Workup	
• Complete blood cell count, platelet count • Calcium and phosphate levels • Liver function tests • Chest radiograph • Bone scan (if indicated) • CT of chest, abdomen, pelvis (if indicated) • MRI (if indicated) • PET (if indicated)	

CT, computed tomography; *MRI,* magnetic resonance imaging; *PET,* positron emission tomography.

DRUG THERAPY

Table 54-6 Hormonal Therapy for Breast Cancer

MECHANISM OF ACTION	EXAMPLES	INDICATIONS FOR USE
Blocking estrogen receptors	Tamoxifen (Nolvadex)	Prevention, adjuvant and metastatic disease
Destroying estrogen receptors	Fulvestrant (Faslodex)	Metastatic disease
Preventing production of estrogen by inhibiting aromatase	Anastrozole (Arimidex) Letrozole (Femara) Exemestane (Aromasin)	Neoadjuvant, adjuvant, and metastatic disease

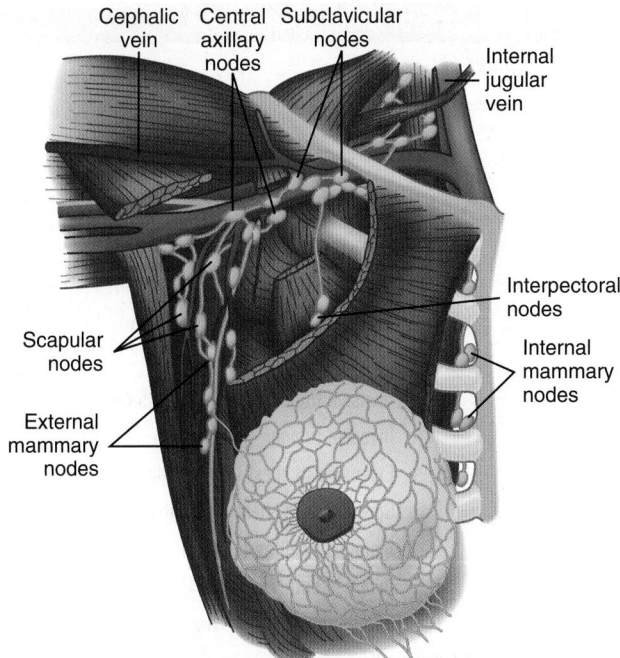

Figure 54-6 Illustration of lymph nodes and drainage in the axilla. The sentinel lymph node is usually found in the external mammary nodes. In a complete axillary dissection, all nodes would be removed.

Source: Townsend, C. M., Beauchamp, R. D., Evers, B. M., & Mattox, K. L. (2009). *Sabiston textbook of surgery* (18th ed.). St. Louis: Mosby.

breast cancer. Most women with a diagnosis of early-stage breast cancer (≤4 to 5 cm in size) are candidates for either treatment choice. The overall survival rate with lumpectomy and radiation is about the same as that with modified radical mastectomy (M. C. Nelson, Norton, & Greene, 2011).

Axillary Node Dissection. ALND on the same side as the breast cancer is often performed and until the early 2000s was the standard of care for invasive breast cancer. In general, ALND typically involves the removal of 12 to 20 nodes. SLND has replaced ALND for patients in whom malignant cells are not identified in the sentinel nodes (Figure 54-6). If one or more sentinel lymph nodes contain malignant cells, ALND is generally recommended. Examination of the lymph nodes provides prognostic information and helps determine further treatment (chemotherapy, hormone therapy, or both).

Lymphedema (accumulation of lymph in soft tissue) can occur as a result of the excision or irradiation of lymph nodes (Swenson et al., 2009; see Figure 54-6). When the axillary nodes cannot return lymph fluid to the central circulation, the fluid accumulates in the arm, causing obstructive pressure on the veins and venous return (Figure 54-7). Patients may experience heaviness, pain, impaired motor function in the arm, and numbness and paraesthesia in the fingers as a result of lymphedema. Cellulitis and progressive fibrosis can result from lymphedema. Although lymphedema is not always preventable, it can be controlled somewhat after surgery or radiation therapy (see discussion later in this chapter).

Breast-Conserving Surgery. Breast-conserving surgery (also called **lumpectomy**) involves the removal of the entire tumour along with a margin of normal surrounding tissue. After surgery, radiation therapy is delivered to the entire breast, ending with a boost to the tumour bed. Depending on the staging of the disease, chemotherapy may be administered before radiation therapy. Contraindications to breast-conserving surgery include the following: breast size too small in relation to the tumour size to yield an acceptable cosmetic result, masses and calcifications that are multifocal (within the same breast quadrant), masses that are multicentric (in more than one quadrant), diffuse calcifications in more than one quadrant, or central location of tumour near the nipple. Contraindications to radiation therapy (e.g. active lupus or prior radiation therapy in the radiation field may make mastectomy a better surgical option.

Table 54-7 Staging of Breast Cancer

Primary Tumour (T)

TX	Primary tumour cannot be assessed
T0	No evidence of primary tumour
Tis	Carcinoma in situ (noninvasive cancer)
T1	Invasive tumour, ≤2 cm
T1mic	Microinvasion, ≤0.1 cm
T1a	Tumour, >0.1 cm but not >0.5 cm
T1b	Tumour, >0.5 cm but not >1 cm
T1c	Tumour, >1 cm but not >2 cm
T2	Invasive tumour, >2 cm but ≤5 cm
T3	Invasive tumour, >5 cm
T4	Extension to chest wall or skin
T4a	Spread to the chest wall but not to pectoral muscle
T4b	Includes swelling (edema), including peau d'orange, ulceration of skin of the breast, or skin nodules in breast
T4c	Includes both T4a and T4b
T4d	Inflammatory breast cancer

Regional Lymph Nodes (N)

NX	Regional lymph nodes cannot be assessed
N0	No regional lymph node metastasis (lymph node–negative breast cancer)
N1	Regional lymph node metastasis (lymph node–positive breast cancer); cancer has spread to axillary lymph nodes, internal mammary lymph nodes, or both
N2	Regional lymph node metastasis (lymph node–positive breast cancer); cancer has spread to axillary lymph nodes, internal mammary lymph nodes, or both
N3	Regional lymph node metastasis (lymph node–positive breast cancer); cancer has spread to axillary lymph nodes (with or without spread to internal mammary nodes) or to infraclavicular or supraclavicular lymph nodes

Distant Metastasis (M)

M0	No distant metastasis
M1	Distant metastasis (includes spread to cervical or internal mammary lymph nodes on the side opposite the breast cancer)

STAGE GROUPING FOR BREAST CANCER

UICC/AJCC STAGE	TNM DESIGNATION			EXPLANATION
Stage 0	Tis	N0	M0	In situ cancer: not spread to nearby breast tissue, nodes, or distant sites
Stage I	T1	N0	M0	Tumour, ≤2 cm ; not spread to lymph nodes or distant sites
Stage IIA	T0	N1	M0	No breast tumour; cancer in 1-3 axillary nodes; not spread to distant sites
	T1	N1	M0	Tumour ≤2 cm ; cancer in 1-3 axillary or internal mammary lymph nodes, or both; not spread to distant sites
	T2	N0	M0	Tumour >2 cm but not >5 cm; not spread to lymph nodes or distant sites
Stage IIB	T2	N1	M0	Tumour >2 cm but not >5 cm; cancer in 1-3 axillary or internal mammary lymph nodes, or both; not spread to distant sites
	T3	N0	M0	Tumour >5 cm; not spread to lymph nodes or distant sites
Stage IIIA	T0	N2	M0	No breast tumour; cancer in 4-9 axillary nodes or internal mammary lymph nodes; not spread to distant sites
	T1	N2	M0	Tumour ≤2 cm ; cancer in 4-9 axillary nodes or has spread to internal mammary lymph nodes; not spread to distant sites
	T2	N2	M0	Tumour >2 cm but not >5 cm; cancer in 4-9 axillary nodes or has spread to internal mammary lymph nodes; not spread to distant sites
	T3	N1, N2	M0	Tumour >5 cm; cancer has spread to 1-9 axillary nodes or to internal mammary lymph nodes; not spread to distant sites
Stage IIIB	T4	N0, N1, N2	M0	Extension to chest wall or skin. One of the following applies: cancer has not spread to any lymph nodes, or has spread to 1-9 axillary nodes; may or may not have spread to internal mammary lymph nodes; not spread to distant sites

AJCC, American Joint Committee on Cancer; *UICC*, International Union Against Cancer.

	STAGE GROUPING FOR BREAST CANCER—cont'd			
UICC/AJCC STAGE	**TNM DESIGNATION**			**EXPLANATION**
Stage IIIC	Any T	N3	M0	Tumour of any size. One of the following applies: cancer has spread to 10 or more axillary nodes, to 1 or more infraclavicular or supraclavicular nodes, or to >3 axillary nodes and to internal mammary lymph nodes, or cancer has not spread to distant sites
	T4d			Inflammatory breast cancer
Stage IV	Any T	Any N	M1	Tumour of any size with any degree of lymph node involvement; cancer has spread to distant sites such as bone, liver, brain, lung, or lymph nodes far from the breast

Table 54-7 Staging of Breast Cancer—cont'd

Source: Adapted from Canadian Cancer Society. (2012). *Canadian cancer encyclopedia: Common staging system.* Retrieved from *http://info.cancer.ca/ cce-ecc/default.aspx?cceid=185&toc=10&lf=stomach&Lang=E.*

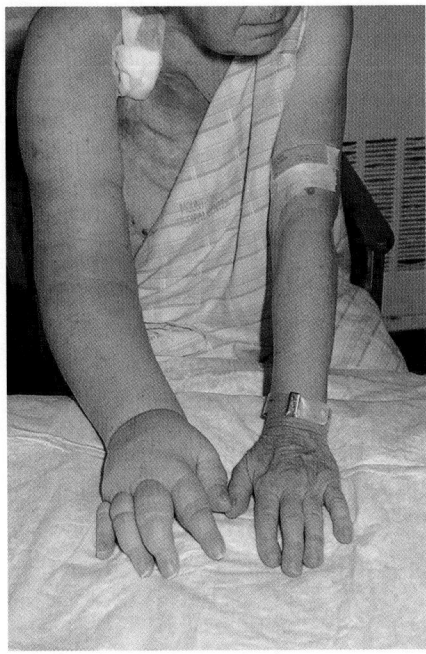

Figure 54-7 Lymphedema. Accumulation of fluid in the tissue after excision of lymph nodes.

Source: Swartz, M. H. (2010). *Textbook of physical diagnosis: History and examination* (6th ed., p. 443, Figure 15-3). Philadelphia: W. B. Saunders.

One of the main advantages of breast-conserving surgery and radiation therapy is that the breast, including the nipple, is preserved. The goal of the combined surgery and radiation is to both maximize the benefits of both cancer treatment and cosmetic outcome and minimize risks. Disadvantages of this approach include the increased cost of the surgery plus radiation therapy over surgery alone and the possible adverse effects of irradiation. Table 54-8 lists treatment options, adverse effects, complications, and patient issues related to the most common surgical procedures currently used to treat breast cancer.

Modified Radical Mastectomy. A modified radical mastectomy includes removal of the breast and the axillary lymph nodes, but it spares the pectoralis major muscle. This surgery is preferred over breast-conserving surgery if the tumour is too large

to excise with adequate margins, and if it is so large that excision would produce a poor cosmetic result. . Some patients may select this surgical procedure over lumpectomy when presented with a choice.

When a modified radical mastectomy is performed, patients have the option of breast reconstruction. If a patient chooses to have reconstructive surgery, it can be performed immediately after the mastectomy, or it can be delayed until postoperative recovery is complete (Weaver, 2009).

Follow-up and Survivorship Care. After surgery, the woman must be monitored for the rest of her life at regular intervals. Most women have professional examinations every 6 months for 2 years and then annually thereafter. In addition, it is recommended that the woman perform monthly BSE on both breasts or on the remaining breast and the surgical site. The most common site of local recurrence of breast cancer is at the surgical site. The woman should undergo appropriate breast imaging at regular intervals (usually 6 months to 1 year), as determined by her risk of recurrence and breast cancer history.

Postmastectomy Pain Syndrome. Postmastectomy pain syndrome can occur after a mastectomy or an axillary node dissection. Common symptoms include chest and upper arm pain, tingling sensations down the arm, numbness, shooting or pricking pain, and unbearable itching that persist beyond the normal 3-month healing time. The cause most commonly theorized about the onset of this syndrome is injury to intercostobrachial nerves, which are sensory nerves that exit chest wall muscles and provide sensation to the shoulder and the upper arm.

Treatments include nonsteroidal anti-inflammatory drugs (NSAIDs), antidepressants, topical lidocaine patches, eutectic mixture of local anaesthetics (EMLA: lidocaine and prilocaine), and antiseizure drugs (e.g., gabapentin [Neurontin]). Other possible treatment modalities include imagery, biofeedback, physical therapy to prevent "frozen shoulder" syndrome as a result of inadequate movement, and psychological counselling with a person trained in the management of chronic pain syndromes.

Adjuvant Therapy. The decision to recommend adjuvant (additional) therapy after surgery depends on the stage of the disease (number of involved nodes and tumour size); the menstrual status, health, and age of the patient; cancer cell characteristics; and presence or absence of estrogen, progesterone, and HER-2 receptors. Adjuvant therapies include local radiation

Table 54-8 Surgical Procedures for Breast Cancer

PROCEDURES	DESCRIPTION	ADVERSE EFFECTS	POTENTIAL COMPLICATIONS	PATIENT ISSUES
Modified radical mastectomy	Removal of breast, preservation of pectoralis muscle, SLND or ALND	Chest wall tightens, scar Phantom breast sensations Lymphedema Sensory changes Impaired range of motion	Short-term: skin flap necrosis, seroma, hematoma, infection Long-term: sensory loss, muscle weakness, lymphedema	Loss of breast Incision Body image Need for prosthesis Impaired arm mobility
Breast-conserving surgery (lumpectomy) with radiation therapy	Wide excision of tumour, SLND or ALND, radiation therapy	Breast soreness Breast edema Skin reactions Arm swelling Sensory changes in breast and arm	Short-term: moist desquamation,* hematoma, seroma, infection Long-term: fibrosis, lymphedema,† myositis, pneumonitis,* rib fractures*	Prolonged treatment* Impaired arm mobility† Change in texture and sensitivity of breast
Tissue expansion and breast implants	Expander used to slowly stretch tissue; saline gradually injected into reservoir over weeks to months Insertion of implant under musculofascial layer of chest wall	Discomfort Sensation of chest wall tightness	Short-term: skin flap necrosis, wound separation, seroma, hematoma, infection Long-term: capsular contractions, displacement of implant	Body image Prolonged physician visits to expand implants Potential additional surgical procedures for nipple construction, symmetry
Breast reconstruction flap procedures	Most common is TRAM flap procedure‡ A musculocutaneous flap (muscle, skin, fat, blood supply) is transposed from abdomen to the mastectomy site	Pain related to two surgical sites and extensive surgery	Short-term: delayed wound healing, infection, skin flap necrosis, abdominal hernia, hematoma	Prolonged postoperative recovery

ALND, axillary lymph node dissection; *SLND,* sentinel lymph node dissection; *TRAM,* transverse rectus abdominis musculocutaneous.
*Specific to radiation therapy.
†If ALND is performed (less likely with SLND).
‡May be performed concurrently with mastectomy.

therapy and systemic therapies such as chemotherapy and hormone therapy (Buzdar, 2009; Mackey et al., 2009).

Radiation Therapy. Radiation therapy may be used as (a) primary treatment to prevent local breast recurrences after breast-conserving surgery (see the Evidence-Informed Practice box), (b) adjuvant treatment after mastectomy to prevent local and nodal recurrences, and (c) palliative treatment for pain caused by local, regional. or distant recurrence.

Primary Radiation Therapy. When radiation therapy is the primary treatment, it is usually performed after local excision of the breast mass. The breast (and the regional lymph nodes in some cases) is irradiated 5 days per week over the course of approximately 5 to 6 weeks. An external beam of radiation is used to deliver an approximate total dose of 4500 to 5000 cGy (4500 to 5000 rads). A "boost" is a dose of radiation delivered to the area in which the original tumour was located. It can be delivered by external beam and represents eight additional treatments in the total number given. Fatigue, skin changes, and breast edema may be temporary adverse effects of external beam radiation therapy. To decrease the risk of axillary recurrence, irradiation of the axilla or supraclavicular nodes, or both, may be indicated when lymph nodes are involved. Chemotherapy may be used systemically before radia-

tion therapy to enhance the local effects of radiation. (Nursing management of patients receiving radiation therapy is discussed in Chapter 18.)

The decision to use radiation therapy after mastectomy is based on the probability that local residual cancer cells are present (related to tumour size and biology and number of involved lymph nodes). Irradiating the area does not prevent the appearance of distant metastasis at a later date. The site of the radiation therapy field (lymph nodes, chest wall, or both) depends on the risk of recurrence.

High-Dose Brachytherapy. *Brachytherapy* (internal radiation) is an alternative to traditional radiation treatment for early-stage breast cancer. For many years, internal radiation therapy has been delivered primarily through a multicatheter implant method that requires many catheters to be placed in the breast. After placement, a radioactive seed is delivered into each catheter to treat the target area.

A developing technology in the treatment of breast cancer is partial breast radiation. Currently, the most widely practised method is balloon brachytherapy. Traditional radiation treatments can take 5 to 6 weeks; in contrast, high-dose brachytherapy with the balloon catheter may require only 5 days.

The MammoSite Radiation Therapy System (MammoSite RTS) is a minimally invasive method of delivering internal radia-

EVIDENCE-INFORMED PRACTICE

Does Radiotherapy After Breast Cancer Surgery Reduce Recurrence?

Clinical Question

For women with ductal carcinoma in situ (DCIS) who undergo breast-conserving surgery (P), does the addition of radiotherapy (I) versus no radiotherapy (C) decrease the risk of cancer recurrence in the treated breast (O) in the first 5 years (T)?

Best Available Evidence

Systematic review of randomized controlled trials (RCTs)

Critical Appraisal and Synthesis of Evidence

- Four RCTs (N = 3295) with average follow-up time of 4.4 to 10.5 years.
- Radiotherapy reduced recurrence risk for DCIS and invasive cancer in treated breast.
- Long-term harm from radiotherapy was not found.
- Information on short-term toxicity or quality of life was not available.

Conclusion

- Benefit of adding radiotherapy to breast-conserving surgery for all women treated for DCIS was confirmed.

Implications for Nursing

- Advise women with DCIS considering treatment options to discuss benefits of radiotherapy with health care providers.
- Counsel women on well-known short-term adverse effects of radiotherapy.

Reference for Evidence

Goodwin, A., Parker, S., Ghersi, D., & Wilcken, N. (2009). Postoperative radiotherapy for ductal carcinoma in situ of the breast. *Cochrane Database System Review*, (4), CD000563. doi:10.1002/14651858.CD000563.pub6

P, patient population of interest; *I*, intervention or area of interest; *C*, comparison of interest or comparison group; *O*, outcome(s) of interest; *T*, timing.

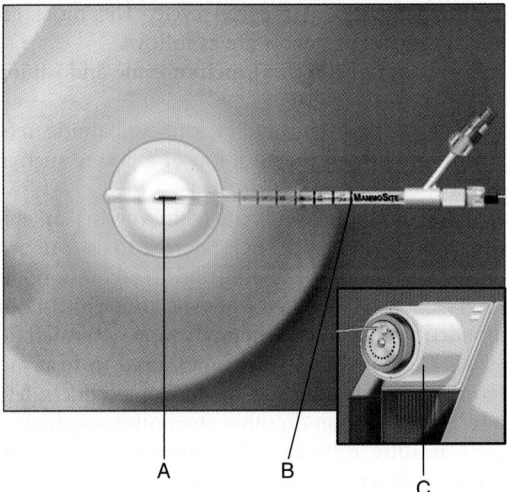

Figure 54-8 High-dose brachytherapy for breast cancer. The MammoSite Radiation Therapy System involves the insertion of a single small balloon catheter *(B)* at the time of the lumpectomy or shortly thereafter into the tumour resection cavity (the space that is left after the surgeon removes the tumour). A tiny radioactive seed *(A)* is inserted into the balloon, connected to a machine called an *afterloader (C)*, and delivers the radiation therapy.

Source: Courtesy Cytyc Corporation and Affiliates, Marlborough, Massachusetts.

tion therapy. In this technique, a balloon catheter is used to insert radioactive seeds into the breast after the tumour is removed (Figure 54-8). Radiation is emitted by a tiny radioactive seed attached by a wire on the way to an afterloader, a computer-controlled machine. The seed travels through the MammoSite RTS applicator into the inflated balloon. The radiation dose is focused on the area of the breast at highest risk for tumour recurrence.

Radiation therapy with the MammoSite RTS is performed over a 1- to 5-day period on an outpatient basis. Patients typically receive treatments twice a day for 5 days.

The MammoSite RTS may also be used as boost therapy in conjunction with external irradiation.

The source of radiation does not remain in the body between treatments or after the final treatment is over. The tiny radioactive seed is inserted only during treatment and then removed. Once the final session is completed, the balloon is deflated, and the system is removed.

Palliative Radiation Therapy. In addition to reducing the primary tumour mass with a resultant decrease in pain, radiation therapy is used to stabilize symptomatic metastatic lesions in such sites as bone, soft tissue organs, the brain, and the chest. Radiation therapy often relieves pain and is successful in controlling recurrent or metastatic disease.

Systemic Therapy. The goal of systemic therapy is to destroy tumour cells that may have spread to distant sites. Systemic therapy as an adjuvant to primary local treatment (in the absence of demonstrable metastases) can decrease the rate of recurrence and increase the length of survival. Because of the high risk for recurrent disease, nearly all women with evidence of node involvement, particularly those whose hormone receptor status is negative, have some type of systemic therapy. Some women, particularly those with a larger tumour or a more aggressive type of tumour, are at higher risk for recurrent or metastatic disease. Systemic therapy is often recommended for such women even when no evidence of node involvement is found. Weighing the risk and benefits of adjuvant therapy is a complex process.

Chemotherapy. *Chemotherapy* is the use of cytotoxic drugs to destroy cancer cells. Many breast cancers are responsive to chemotherapy. In some patients, chemotherapy is administered preoperatively. Preoperative (neoadjuvant) chemotherapy can decrease the size of the primary tumour, possibly enabling surgery to be less extensive. Breast cancer survival rates with preoperative chemotherapy are no different from those with postoperative chemotherapy (Kong, Moran, Zhang, Haffty, & Yang, 2011).

Combinations of drugs yield results superior to those of a single drug. The benefits of combination treatment result from the use of drugs that have different mechanisms of action and work at different parts of the cell cycle. The more common combination-therapy protocols are as follows:

- Cyclophosphamide (Procytox), methotrexate, and 5-fluorouracil (5-FU), referred to as *CMF*
- Doxorubicin (Adriamycin) and cyclophosphamide, referred to as AC, with or without the addition of a taxane such as paclitaxel (Taxol) or docetaxel (Taxotere)
- Cyclophosphamide, doxorubicin (Adriamycin) or epirubicin (Pharmorubicin PFS), and 5-FU, referred to as *CAF* or *CEF*

Docetaxel, capecitabine (Xeloda), and an albumin-bound form of paclitaxel (Abraxane) are used when metastatic breast cancer has not responded to standard chemotherapy (Palmieri, Frye, & Mahon, 2009). Vinorelbine (Navelbine), used to treat metastatic breast cancer, is better tolerated because it produces fewer and milder adverse effects than do other chemotherapy drugs.

Because healthy cells are also affected by chemotherapy, various adverse effects accompany this treatment modality. The incidence and severity of predictable and commonly observed adverse effects are influenced by the specific drug combination, drug schedule, and doses of the drug or drugs. Usually, body organs with rapidly dividing cells are the most strongly affected. The most common adverse effects involve the gastrointestinal tract, bone marrow, and hair follicles, resulting in nausea, anorexia, weight loss, bone marrow suppression and subsequent fatigue, and alopecia (hair loss). Weight gain is common with breast cancer treatment (Ligibel et al., 2010).

Cognitive changes during and after treatment, especially with chemotherapy, have been reported in patients with cancer. These changes include difficulties in concentration, memory, and maintaining focus and attention (Simmons, 2009). This phenomenon, called *chemobrain*, may affect 17 to 75% of cancer survivors (Mayfield, 2009). Ongoing research is focusing on why the cognitive impairment occurs.

Hormonal Therapy. Estrogen can promote the growth of breast cancer cells if the cells are estrogen receptor positive. Hormonal therapy blocks the source of estrogen, thus promoting tumour regression (Rugo, 2008).

Two advances have increased the use of hormone therapy in breast cancer. First, hormone receptor assays, which are reliable diagnostic tests, have been developed to identify women who are likely to respond to hormone therapy. Both the estrogen- and progesterone-receptor status of the tumour can be determined. The importance of these assays is their ability to predict whether hormonal therapy is a treatment option for women with breast cancer, either at the time of initial therapy or if the cancer recurs. Second, drugs have been developed that can inactivate the hormone-secreting glands as effectively as surgery or radiation. Chances of tumour regression are significantly greater in women whose tumours contain estrogen and progesterone receptors (Rugo, 2008).

Estrogen deprivation can occur when ovarian function is damaged by surgery, radiation therapy, or drug therapy (see Table 54-6). Hormonal therapy can (a) block or destroy the estrogen receptors or (b) suppress estrogen synthesis through inhibiting aromatase, an enzyme needed for endogenous estrogen synthesis. Hormone therapy may be used as an adjuvant to primary treatment or in patients with recurrent or metastatic cancer.

Tamoxifen (Nolvadex) has for many years been the hormonal agent of choice in estrogen receptor–positive women with breast cancer of all stages (Litsas, 2008). Tamoxifen, an antiestrogen drug, blocks the estrogen-receptor sites of malignant cells and thus inhibits the growth-stimulating effects of estrogen. It is commonly used in early-stage and advanced breast cancer and to treat recur-

rent disease. Tamoxifen may also be used to prevent breast cancer in individuals at high risk for its development. Adverse effects of tamoxifen may include hot flashes, mood swings, vaginal discharge and dryness, and other effects commonly associated with decreased estrogen levels. It also increases the risk of blood clots, cataracts, stroke and endometrial cancer in postmenopausal women. Treatment with tamoxifen generally lasts 5 years (Litsas, 2008).

Fulvestrant (Faslodex) may be administered when advanced breast cancer no longer responds to tamoxifen. This drug slows cancer progression by destroying estrogen receptors in the breast cancer cells. Fulvestrant is given intramuscularly on a monthly basis. Common adverse effects include fatigue, hot flashes, and nausea.

Aromatase inhibitor drugs interfere with the enzyme that synthesizes endogenous estrogen and are used in the treatment of breast cancer in postmenopausal women. These drugs include anastrozole (Arimidex), letrozole (Femara), and exemestane (Aromasin). Aromatase inhibitors do not block the production of estrogen by the ovaries; thus they are of little benefit and may be harmful in premenopausal women.

Clinical trials have demonstrated improved disease-free survival when these drugs are given after tamoxifen treatment has ended (Rugo, 2008). They also appear to be more effective than tamoxifen in preventing breast cancer recurrence and possibly more effective in preventing contralateral disease (disease in the other breast). The adverse effects of aromatase inhibitors are different from those of tamoxifen. Aromatase inhibitors only rarely cause blood clots, and they do not cause endometrial cancer. Because they block the production of estrogen in postmenopausal women, osteoporosis and bone fractures may occur. These drugs have also been associated with night sweats, nausea, arthralgias, and myalgias.

Raloxifene (Evista), a drug used to prevent bone loss, is now being used to reduce the risk of breast cancer in postmenopausal women without stimulating endometrial growth. Raloxifene may act by blocking estrogen receptors in the breast, which is similar to its action in the bone. (Raloxifene is discussed in the section on osteoporosis in Chapter 66.)

Less common hormone-deprivation strategies include bilateral oophorectomy, adrenalectomy, and hypophysectomy.

Biological and Targeted Therapy. Some breast cancers make excessive amounts of the HER-2 protein. For patients who are HER-2 positive, trastuzumab (Herceptin) is a monoclonal antibody to HER-2. After the antibody attaches to the antigen, it is taken into the cancer cells and eventually kills them. It can be used alone or in combination with other chemotherapy such as docetaxel (Taxotere) or paclitaxel (Taxol) to treat patients whose tumours overexpress the *HER-2* gene. Additional genetic testing may offer information on which patients are good candidates for treatment with trastuzumab. (The use of biological and targeted therapies is discussed further in Chapter 18.)

Lapatinib (Tykerb) may be used in combination with capecitabine (Xeloda) for patients with advanced, metastatic disease whose tumours produce excessive HER-2. The combination treatment is indicated for women in whom disease has become resistant to other cancer drugs (Litsas, 2008). Lapatinib works inside the cell by blocking the function of the HER-2 protein. Adverse effects can include diarrhea, nausea, vomiting, rash, and a syndrome of numbness, tingling, swelling, and pain in the hands and feet. Cardiotoxicity has also been reported.

Angiogenesis inhibitors prevent the formation of blood vessels into newly developing cancerous tumours. Bevacizumab

(Avastin), an angiogenesis inhibitor, is now being given in combination with chemotherapy to extend the survival of women with newly diagnosed advanced breast cancer. However, clinical trials are re-evaluating the safety of this drug.

Cultural Safety: Breast Cancer. Among diverse ethnic groups, differences exist in the incidence, mortality rates, and relevant care issues related to breast cancer. In addition, cultural differences may involve gender roles, health beliefs, religion, and family structure. Other differences may be related to dietary factors and disparities in the access to and use of clinical breast examinations and screening mammography. Cultural values strongly influence how women respond to and cope with breast cancer and treatment. Nurses need to consider how health behaviours are influenced by cultural norms and, in particular, the cultural value of breasts and the cultural factors related to the disease of breast cancer. Women may delay screening or treatment for varying reasons, including an acceptance of disease as inevitable fate or "God's will," a mistrust of Western medicine, lack of health care access, or the stigma of a cancer diagnosis.

NURSING MANAGEMENT: BREAST CANCER

▪ Nursing Assessment

Many factors need to be considered when a nurse is assessing a patient with a breast problem. The history of the breast disorder assists in establishing the diagnosis. The presence of nipple discharge, pain, rate of growth of the lump, breast asymmetry, and correlation with the menstrual cycle should all be investigated.

The size and location of the lump or lumps should be carefully documented. The physical characteristics of the lesion, such as consistency, mobility, and shape, should be assessed. If nipple discharge is present, the colour and consistency should be noted, as well as whether it occurs from one or both breasts.

Subjective and objective data that should be obtained from an individual with suspected or diagnosed breast cancer are presented in Table 54-9.

▪ Nursing Diagnoses

Nursing diagnoses related to the care of a patient with diagnosed breast cancer vary. After diagnosis and before a treatment plan has been selected, the following diagnoses apply:
- Decisional conflict *related to* lack of knowledge about treatment options and their effects
- Fear, anxiety, or both *related to* diagnosis of breast cancer
- Disturbed body image *related to* anticipated physical and emotional effects of treatment modalities

If a mastectomy or lumpectomy is planned, the nursing diagnoses may include, but are not limited to, those presented in Nursing Care Plan 54-1.

▪ Planning

The overall goals are that patients with breast cancer will (a) actively participate in the decision-making process related to treatment options, (b) adhere to the therapeutic plan, (c) manage

NURSING ASSESSMENT

Table 54-9 Breast Cancer

Subjective Data

Important Health Information

Past health history:
- Family history of breast cancer (especially mother or sister, young age at diagnosis)
- History of abnormal mammogram findings or atypical findings in prior biopsy
- Benign breast disorders with atypical changes
- Previous unilateral breast cancer
- Menstrual history (early menarche with late menopause)
- Pregnancy history (nulliparity or first full-term pregnancy after age 30)
- Previous endometrial, ovarian, or colon cancer
- Hyperestrogenism and testicular atrophy (in men)
- Dietary habits and history of history of alcohol use
- Level of usual physical activity, weight, and BMI

Medications: Use of hormones, especially as postmenopausal hormone replacement therapy and in oral contraceptives; infertility treatments

Surgeries or other treatments: Exposure to therapeutic radiation (e.g., for Hodgkin's lymphoma or thyroid cancer)

Symptoms
- Palpable change found on self-examination
- Obesity; unexplained severe weight loss (possible indicator of metastasis)
- Changes in cognition, headache; bone pain (possible indicators of metastasis)
- Unilateral nipple discharge (clear, milky, or bloody)
- Change in breast contour, size, or symmetry
- Psychological stress
- Anxiety regarding threat to self-esteem

Objective Data

General

Axillary and supraclavicular lymphadenopathy

Integumentary

Firm, discrete nodules at mastectomy site (possible indicator of local recurrence); peripheral edema (possible indicator of metastasis)

Respiratory

Pleural effusions (possible indicator of metastasis)

Gastrointestinal

Hepatomegaly, jaundice; ascites (possible indicators of liver metastasis)

Reproductive

Hard, irregular, nonmobile breast lump, most often in upper outer sector, possibly fixated to fascia or chest wall; nipple inversion or retraction, erosion; edema (peau d'orange appearance), erythema, induration, infiltration, or dimpling (in later stages)

Possible Findings

Finding of mass or change in tissue on breast examination; abnormal findings on mammography, ultrasonography, or breast MRI; positive results of FNA or surgical biopsy or similar results with needle biopsy

BMI, body mass index; *FNA,* fine-needle aspiration; *MRI,* magnetic resonance imaging.

the adverse effects of adjuvant therapy, and (d) access and benefit from the support provided by significant others and health care providers.

Nursing Implementation

Acute Intervention

The time between the diagnosis of breast cancer and the selection of a treatment plan is a difficult period for the woman and her family. Although the primary care provider has discussed treatment options, the woman often relies on the nurse to clarify and expand on these options. During this often stressful time, the woman may not be coping effectively. Appropriate nursing interventions are to explore the woman's usual decision-making patterns, to help the woman accurately evaluate the advantages and disadvantages of the options, to provide information relevant to the decision, and to support the patient and family once the decision is made.

During this period, the woman may exhibit signs of distress or tension—such as tachycardia, increased muscle tension, sleep disturbances, and restlessness—whenever she focuses on the decision to be made. The nurse should assess the woman's body language, motor activity, and affect during periods of high stress and indecision so that appropriate interventions can be used.

Regardless of the surgery planned, patients must be provided with sufficient information to ensure informed consent. Some patients seek extensive, detailed information, whereas others avoid information. Sensitivity to the individual's need for and type of information is essential. The information includes (a) preoperative instructions on turning, coughing, and deep breathing; (b) a review of postoperative exercises; and (c) explanation of the recovery period from the time of surgery until discharge.

Many women who undergo breast-conserving surgery have an uncomplicated postoperative course with variable pain intensity. Pain is most affected by the extent of the lymph node dissection performed. If an ALND or a mastectomy has been performed, drains are generally left in place, and patients are discharged home with them. Patients and their families need to be taught, with a return demonstration, how to manage the drains at home.

Restoring arm function on the affected side after mastectomy and axillary lymph node dissection is a key nursing goal. The woman should be placed in a semi-Fowler's position with the arm on the affected side elevated on a pillow. Flexing and extending the fingers should begin in the recovery room, with progressive increases in activity encouraged.

Postoperative arm and shoulder exercises are instituted gradually with a surgeon's direction (Figure 54-9). These exercises are designed to prevent contractures and muscle shortening, maintain muscle tone, and improve lymph and blood circulation. The difficulty and pain encountered by the woman in performing the previously simple tasks included in the exercise program may cause frustration and depression. The goal of all exercise is a gradual return to full range of motion within 4 to 6 weeks.

The nurse can minimize postoperative discomfort by administering analgesics about 30 minutes before the patient initiates exercises. When the patient is able to shower, the warm water on the involved shoulder often has a muscle-relaxing effect and reduces joint stiffness. Whenever possible, the same nurse should work with the woman so that progress can be monitored and problems can be identified.

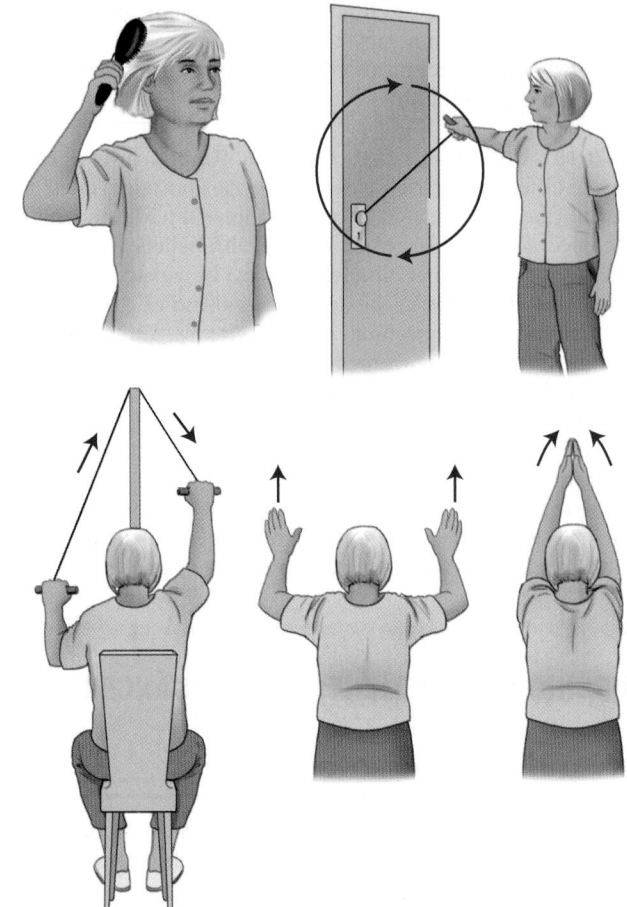

Figure 54-9 Postoperative exercises for patient with a mastectomy or lumpectomy with axillary lymph node dissection.

Measures to prevent or reduce lymphedema after ALND must be used by the nurse and taught to the woman. The affected arm should not be dependent, even during sleep. Blood pressure readings, venipunctures, and injections should not be performed on the affected arm. Elastic bandages should not be used in the early postoperative period because they inhibit collateral lymph drainage. The woman must be instructed to protect the arm on the operative side from even minor trauma such as a pinprick or sunburn. If trauma to the arm occurs, the area should be washed thoroughly with soap and water, and a topical antibiotic ointment and a bandage or other sterile dressing should be applied. The woman must be taught to advise the surgeon of the trauma, and the site of injury must be observed closely for evidence of inflammation. The patient must understand that for the rest of her life, she is at risk for developing lymphedema (Singer, 2009).

When lymphedema is acute (see Figure 54-7), complete decongestive therapy may be recommended (Singer, 2009). This therapy consists of a massage-like technique to mobilize the subcutaneous accumulation of fluid. This is then followed by compression bandaging and the wearing of a pneumatic compression sleeve. This sleeve intermittently applies mechanical massage to the arm and facilitates lymph drainage up toward the heart. Diuretics, isometric exercises, and elevation of the arm so that it is level with the heart may be recommended to reduce the fluid volume in the arm. The patient may need to wear a fitted elastic pressure-gradient sleeve (a) during waking hours to maintain maximum volume reduction and (b) preventively during air travel.

Psychological Care

Throughout interactions with a woman with breast cancer, the nurse should be aware of the extensive psychological effect of the disease. Effective care includes sensitivity to the woman's efforts to cope with a life-threatening disease. A relationship in which the woman can express her authentic feelings is therapeutic. The nurse can help to meet the woman's psychological needs in the following ways:

1. Providing a safe environment for the expression of the full range of feelings

NURSING CARE PLAN 54-1

After Mastectomy or Lumpectomy*

NURSING DIAGNOSIS	**Acute pain** *related to* tissue trauma and manipulation *as evidenced by* (a) verbalization of pain at operative area and (b) nonverbal behaviours indicating pain
Expected Patient Outcomes	**Nursing Interventions and *Rationales***
• Verbalizes progressive reduction in pain • Uses pain control measures appropriately	• Assess verbal and nonverbal indicators of pain *to identify degree of discomfort and need for and effectiveness of analgesia.* • Perform a comprehensive pain assessment (i.e., location, characteristics, intensity [0-10 scale] *to plan individualized pain management.* • Encourage use of nonpharmacological techniques (e.g., distraction, imagery, and relaxation) *to complement analgesia.* • Provide appropriate analgesics on a regular schedule (i.e., before ROM exercises and ADLs) *to maintain comfort level and mobility in affected arm.* • Support the arm and limit its activity *to prevent tension on suture line.*
NURSING DIAGNOSIS	**Anxiety** *related to* a situational crisis and unpredictable outcome secondary to a diagnosis of cancer *as evidenced by* insomnia, crying, and questioning of prognosis
Expected Patient Outcomes	**Nursing Interventions and *Rationales***
• Acknowledges and discusses concerns • Reports anxiety is reduced to a manageable level • Demonstrates effective use of coping strategies that provide reduction of anxiety	• Encourage verbalization of feelings, perceptions, and fears *to promote successful resolution of fear and establish effective coping mechanisms.* • Encourage the family to verbalize feelings *to help increase their overall effectiveness as a support system.* • Provide factual information concerning diagnosis, treatment, and prognosis *to help decrease fear of the unknown.*
NURSING DIAGNOSIS	**Disturbed body image** *related to* perceived effects of mastectomy *as evidenced by* (a) verbalization of concern about appearance and feelings of loss of femininity and (b) refusal to view incision
Expected Patient Outcomes	**Nursing Interventions and *Rationales***
• Discusses feelings about and the meaning of changes in physical appearance • Identifies community resources and self-help groups available for support	• Identify support groups available to patient *so that social support will be available.* • Help patient separate physical appearance from feelings of personal worth *to increase self-esteem.* • Facilitate contact with individuals with similar change in body image (e.g., Reach to Recovery) *to serve as a peer support and provide hope for recovery and a normal future.* • Help patient discuss changes caused by illness and surgery *to promote grief work and maintain support from family/friends.* • Help patient identify actions that will enhance appearance (e.g., prosthesis, breast reconstruction) *to assist with coping and adaptation to changed body image.*
NURSING DIAGNOSIS	**Impaired physical mobility** *related to* weakness and muscle loss *as evidenced by* limitation in movement of upper extremity on surgical side
Expected Patient Outcomes	**Nursing Interventions and *Rationales***
• Identifies activities that can reduce postoperative edema and mobility • Demonstrates appropriate hand and arm exercises	• Instruct patient and caregivers how to systematically perform passive, assisted, or active ROM exercises *to prevent contractures and muscle shortening, maintain muscle tone, and improve lymph and blood circulation.* • Incorporate ADLs into exercise protocol *to reduce dependent behaviours, raise self-esteem, and maintain mobility of affected arm.* • Encourage use of motor activities that require attention to and use of both sides of the body *to prevent guarding of operative side and loss of function.*

ADLs, activities of daily living; *ROM,* range of motion.

*Many of the specific interventions in this care plan also relate to the patient who has also had an axillary node dissection.　　　　*Continued*

NURSING CARE PLAN 54-1

After Mastectomy or Lumpectomy—cont'd

Collaborative Problem

POTENTIAL COMPLICATION	*Lymphedema* *related to* impaired lymphatic drainage and lack of knowledge of preventive measures
Nursing Goals	**Nursing Interventions and *Rationales***
• Monitor for signs of lymphedema, and report deviations • Carry out appropriate medical and nursing interventions	• Assess for signs of lymphedema (such as edema in hand or arm, or both on operative side; heaviness; and localized pain) *to enable early diagnosis and intervention to prevent and treat the complication.* • Instruct patient about self-care strategies and precautions to reduce risk of lymphedema *so that patient will be an active, informed participant of care.* • Teach patient to protect affected arm from injury, ensuring that no procedures are performed (blood pressure, venipuncture, injections), *to reduce risk of injury and infection in affected arm.* • Avoid dependent position of affected arm *to allow proper wound healing and decrease stress on incision site.* • Encourage ROM exercises in affected arm *to promote circulation.* • Explain that elastic compression bandage or sleeve may help control swelling, if necessary, *to reduce edema and promote venous return.*

2. Helping her identify sources of support and strength, such as her partner, family, and spiritual or religious practices
3. Encouraging her to identify and learn individual coping strengths
4. Promoting communication between the patient and her family, friends, or both
5. Providing accurate and complete answers to her questions about the disease, treatment options, and reproductive, fertility, or lactation issues (if appropriate)
6. Offering information about community resources, such as Reach to Recovery, Cancer Connection, CanSurmount, Living with Cancer, Look Good Feel Better, and local support organizations and groups

The nurse can promote the woman's recovery by referring her to peer support resources, such as a Reach to Recovery volunteer, if the service is available. The Reach to Recovery program of the Canadian Cancer Society is a rehabilitation program for women who have undergone breast surgery. It is designed to help them meet their psychological, physical, and cosmetic needs.

The volunteers, who have had breast cancer, can answer questions about expectations, surgery, and recovery. The Canadian Cancer Society and the Canadian Cancer Society Research Institute can provide excellent materials to assist the nurse in meeting the special needs of women with breast cancer.

It is important for health care providers to remain sensitive to the complex psychological effect that a diagnosis of cancer and subsequent breast surgery can have on a woman and her family (Weaver, 2009). Diverse emotional responses are common. The nurse's accepting attitude and the offering of resources can greatly alleviate the common feelings of fear, anger, anxiety, and depression experienced by many patients.

■ Ambulatory and Home Care

The nurse should explain the specific follow-up routine to patients and emphasize the importance of ongoing monitoring and breast self-awareness. To address needs for individual and family support in addition to coping needs, referral to a mental health care provider may be indicated. Immediately after surgery, symptoms that should be reported to the clinician include fever, inflammation at the surgical site, erythema, postoperative constipation, and unusual swelling. Other changes to report in the future are new back pain, weakness, shortness of breath, and confusion. For women who have undergone mastectomy without breast reconstruction, a variety of products are available to meet specific individual needs. These include garments ranging from camisoles with soft breast prosthetic inserts to a fitted prosthesis with bra. Should the woman choose a breast prosthesis, a certified fitter can help the woman select a comfortable, more permanent weighted prosthesis and bra, generally at 4 to 8 weeks postoperatively. The role of the nurse is to present the choices and resources without judgement.

The implications of the loss of a breast for the sexual identity and relationships of the woman vary. The nurse can initiate a discussion of sexuality by inviting questions about relationships or intimacy concerns within the recovery framework (Fobair & Spiegel, 2009). To be effective sources of support for the patient, the husband, sexual partner, or family members often need help in dealing with their emotional reactions to the diagnosis and surgery. There are no physical reasons for a mastectomy to prevent sexual satisfaction. The woman taking hormonal therapy may have a decreased sexual drive or vaginal dryness. She may need to use lubrication to prevent discomfort during intercourse. Concerns about sexuality are not well addressed by many health care providers (Fobair & Spiegel, 2009). If difficulty in adjustment or other problems develop, counselling may be necessary to deal with the emotional component of a mastectomy and the diagnosis of cancer.

Depression and anxiety may occur with the continued stress and uncertainty of a cancer diagnosis. A woman's self-esteem and identity may also be threatened. Psychological support and self-care teaching are indicated interventions with a breast cancer recurrence. The support of family and friends and participation in a cancer support group are important aspects of care that are often helpful in improving quality of life and have been found to have a clinically significant effect on survival.

▪ Evaluation

The expected outcomes for patients after a mastectomy or lumpectomy are presented in Nursing Care Plan 54-1.

Mammoplasty

Mammoplasty is the surgical change in the size or shape of the breast. It may be performed electively for cosmetic purposes to either enlarge or reduce the size of the breasts. It may also be performed to reconstruct the breast after a mastectomy.

A professional, nonjudgemental attitude and clear information about surgical breast options are most useful for women engaged in decision making about mammoplasty. The desire to alter the appearance of the breasts has special significance for each woman as she attempts to alter or re-create her body image. It is important for the nurse to be aware of the cultural value placed on the breast by the woman. It is important that the woman set realistic expectations about what mammoplasty can accomplish and about possible complications, such as hematoma formation, hemorrhage, and infection. If an implant is involved, the woman must understand that capsular contracture and loss of the implant are possible (Health Canada, 2007).

Breast Augmentation

In augmentation mammoplasty (the procedure to enlarge the breasts), an implant is placed in a surgically created pocket between the capsule of the breast and the pectoral fascia or, ideally, under the pectoral muscle. Most implants are silicone envelopes filled with a fluid such as dextran, saline, or silicone. Because of their resemblance to the human breast, implants filled with silicone were the most widely used. In 1992, Health Canada asked manufacturers to stop the sale of silicone implants in Canada in response to potential health hazards related to silicone leakage. Currently in Canada, two types of breast implants (saline-filled and silicone gel–filled) have the required licensing from Health Canada. All implants contain an insert that identifies all potential risks related to breast implant surgery (Health Canada, 2007).

Breast Reduction

For some women, large breasts can be a source of physical and psychological discomfort. They can interfere with normal daily activities such as walking, typing, and driving a car. The weight of large breasts can lead to back, shoulder, and neck problems, including degenerative nerve changes. Overly large breasts can interfere with self-esteem and self-image, and the comfort in wearing some clothing may be affected. Reduction in the size of the breasts can have positive effects on both the psychological and the physical health of the patient. Reduction mammoplasty is performed by resecting wedges of tissue from the upper and lower quadrants of the breast. The excess skin is removed, and the areola and nipple are relocated on the breast. Lactation can usually be accomplished if massive amounts of tissue are not removed and the nipples are left connected during surgery.

NURSING MANAGEMENT: BREAST AUGMENTATION AND REDUCTION

Breast augmentation and breast reduction may be performed in the outpatient surgical area, or they may involve overnight hospitalization. General anaesthesia is used. Drains are generally placed in the surgical site to prevent hematoma formation and then removed 2 to 3 days after surgery or when drainage is less than 20 to 30 mL per day. The drainage must be examined for colour and odour to detect postoperative infection or hemorrhage. The woman's temperature should also be monitored. Dressings should be changed as necessary, with sterile technique, and prescribed. After surgery, the woman should be assured that the appearance of the breast will improve when healing is completed. Depending on physician instructions, patients may be instructed to wear a bra that provides good support continuously for 2 to 3 days after breast reduction or augmentation. Depending on the extent of the operation, most women can resume normal activities within 2 to 3 weeks. Strenuous exercise may not be appropriate until several weeks later.

Breast Reconstruction

Breast reconstructive surgery may be performed simultaneously with a mastectomy or some time afterward to achieve symmetry and to restore or preserve body image. The timing of reconstruction surgery should be based on the psychological needs of individual patients. Immediate breast reconstruction after mastectomy is commonly performed. The advantages of immediate reconstruction are the fact that only one surgical procedure is needed, anaesthesia induction is needed only once, and only one recovery period is needed. Also, reconstructive surgery takes place before the development of scar tissue or adhesions. Early reconstruction does not delay or influence further treatment or adversely affect predicted survival.

Indications. The main indication for breast reconstruction is to improve a woman's self-image, help her regain a sense of normality, and assist in coping with the loss of the breast. Patient-reported outcomes are similar, however, between women who choose breast reconstruction after a mastectomy for breast cancer and those who do not choose reconstruction (Lee, Sunu, & Pignone, 2009). Current techniques cannot restore lactation, nipple sensation, or nipple erectility. Therefore, the erotic functions of the breast are not present. Although the breast will not fully resemble its premastectomy appearance, the reconstructed appearance usually represents an improvement over the mastectomy scar (Figure 54-10). The contour of the breast is restored without the use of an external prosthesis.

Types of Reconstruction

Breast Implants and Tissue Expansion. Breast implants are placed in a pocket under the pectoralis muscle, which protects the implant and provides soft tissue coverage over the implant. Implants can be placed either at the time of mastectomy or later. A small magnet is embedded in most expanders. Therefore, a woman with a magnet in place should not undergo MRI. Because many patients who have undergone mastectomy have insufficient tissue, simple placement of an implant may lead to small breast

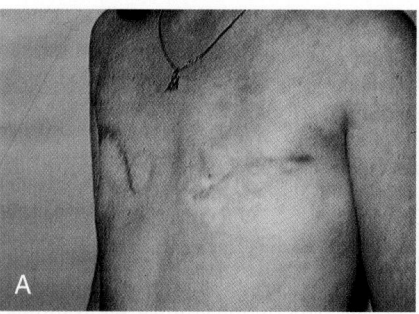
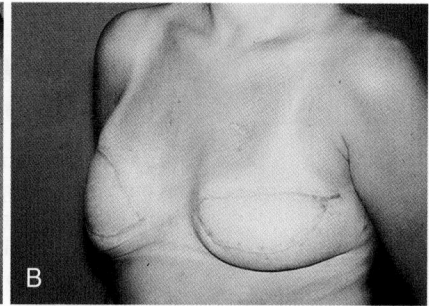
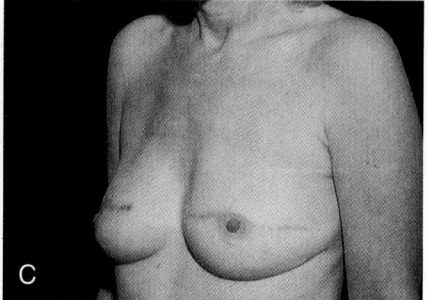

Figure 54-10 Appearances after breast surgery. **A,** Appearance of chest after bilateral mastectomy. **B,** Postoperative breast reconstruction before nipple-areolar reconstruction. **C,** Postoperative breast reconstruction after nipple-areolar reconstruction.

Source: Fortunato, N., & McCullough, S. M. (1998). *Plastic and reconstructive surgery.* St. Louis: Mosby. Courtesy Brian Davies, MD.

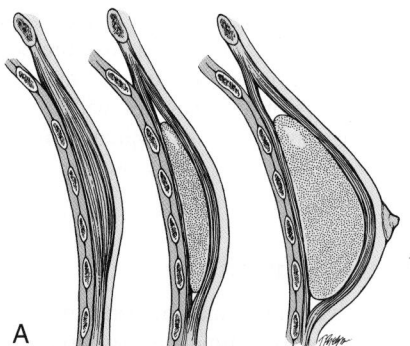

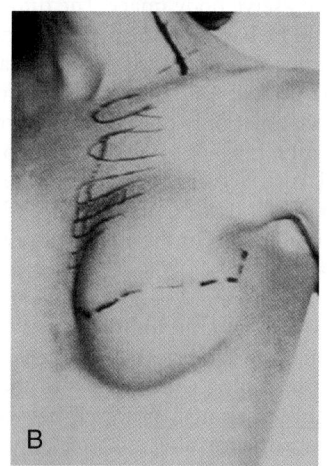

Figure 54-11 Tissue expansion. **A,** Diagram of tissue expander with gradual expansion. **B,** Tissue expander in place after mastectomy.

Sources: **A,** From Cameron, J. (1995). *Current surgical therapy* (5th ed.). St. Louis: Mosby. **B,** From Fortunato, N., & McCullough, S. M. (1998). *Plastic and reconstructive surgery.* St. Louis: Mosby. Courtesy Brian Davies, MD.

reconstruction that is tight or firm. Autologous (one's own) tissue reconstruction may then be recommended.

A tissue expander can be used to stretch the skin and muscle at the mastectomy site before implants are inserted (Figure 54-11). The use of tissue expanders and breast implants is the most common breast reconstruction technique currently used. Placement of the expander can be performed at the time of mastectomy or at a later date. The tissue expander, which is minimally inflated at the time of surgery, is gradually filled by weekly injec-

tions of sterile water or saline solution, which stretch the skin and muscle. Once the tissue is adequately stretched and the anticipated breast size is reached, the expander is surgically removed and a permanent implant is inserted. Some expanders are designed to remain in place and become the implant, eliminating the need for a second surgical procedure. Tissue expansion does not work well in individuals with extensive scar tissue from surgery or radiation therapy.

The body's natural response to the presence of a foreign substance is the formation of a fibrous capsule around the implant (Health Canada, 2007). If excessive capsular formation occurs as a result of infection, hematoma, trauma, or reaction to a foreign body, a contracture can develop, resulting in deformation of the breast. Surgeons differ in their approaches to the prevention of contracture formation, although gentle manual massage around the implant is routine. Prevention of the problems that cause excessive capsule formation is critical. Other postoperative complications include skin ulceration, hypertrophic scar formation, intercostal neuralgia, and wound infection.

Musculocutaneous Flap Procedure. An additional choice for breast reconstruction is the use of autologous tissue to re-create a breast mound. If insufficient muscle is left after mastectomy or if the chest wall has been irradiated, the person's own tissue may be used to repair the soft tissue defects. Musculocutaneous flaps are most often taken from the back (latissimus dorsi muscle) or the abdomen (transverse rectus abdominis muscle). In the latissimus dorsi musculocutaneous flap, a block of skin and muscle from the patient's back is used to replace tissue removed during mastectomy. A small implant may be needed beneath the flap to obtain reasonable breast shape and size. A disadvantage of this technique is an additional scar on the back.

The *transverse rectus abdominis musculocutaneous (TRAM)* flap is the most frequently used flap operation (Dell, Weaver, Kozempel, & Barsevick, 2008). The rectus abdominis muscles are paired flat muscles running from the rib cage down to the pubic bone. Arteries running inside the muscles provide branches at many levels, and these branches supply the fat and skin across a large expanse of the abdomen. In this technique, the surgeon elevates a large block of tissue from the lower abdominal area but leaves it attached to the rectus muscle (Figure 54-12). This tissue is then tunnelled or placed as "free flaps" under the skin up to the area where the breast will be reconstructed. Then it is moulded and fashioned to form a breast. The abdominal incision is closed, which results in an appearance similar to that of an abdominoplasty. This surgical procedure can last 2 to 8 hours, and recovery

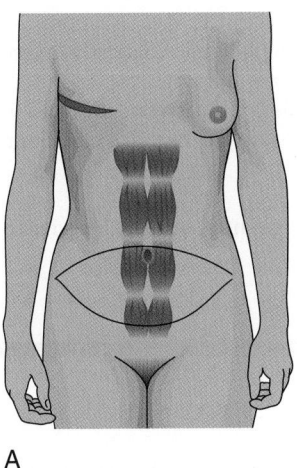 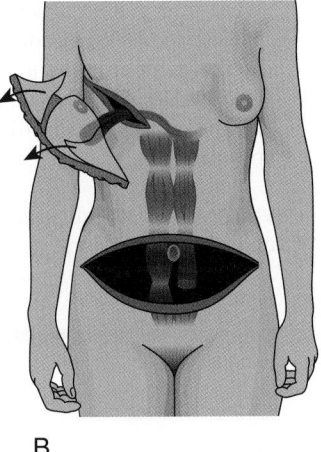 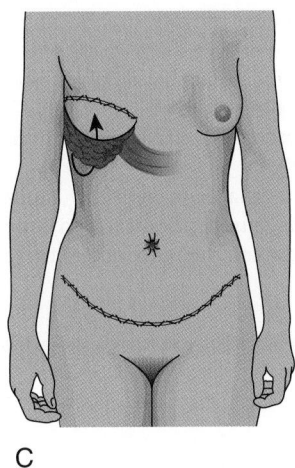 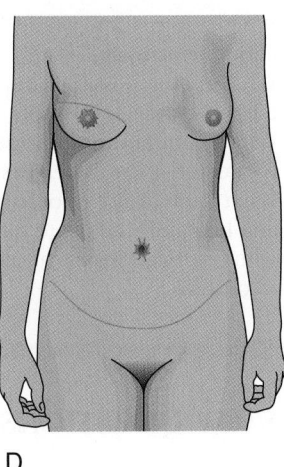

A   B   C   D

Figure 54-12 Diagrams of the transverse rectus abdominis musculocutaneous (TRAM) flap procedure. **A,** TRAM flap is planned. **B,** The abdominal tissue, while attached to the rectus muscle, nerve, and blood supply, is tunnelled through the abdomen to the chest. **C,** The flap is trimmed to shape the breast. The lower abdominal incision is closed. **D,** Nipple and areola are reconstructed after the breast is healed.

Sources: Adapted from Beare, P. G., & Myers, J. L. (1998). *Adult health nursing* (3rd ed.). St. Louis: Mosby; and from Fortunato, N., & McCullough, S. M. (1998). *Plastic and reconstructive surgery*. St. Louis: Mosby.

takes 6 to 8 weeks. Some patients have reported pain and fatigue for up to 3 months (Dell et al., 2008). Complications include bleeding, seroma, hernia, infection, and low back pain. An implant may be used in addition to the flap if the flap does not provide the desired cosmetic result alone. Patients who smoke, are too thin, or are overweight are not good candidates for this type of procedure.

Nipple-Areolar Reconstruction. The majority of patients who undergo breast reconstruction also receive nipple-areolar reconstruction. Nipple reconstruction gives the reconstructed breast a much more natural appearance. Nipple-areolar reconstruction is usually done a few months after breast reconstruction. Tissue to construct a nipple may be taken from the opposite breast or from a small flap of tissue on the reconstructed breast mound. The areola may be grafted from the labia, skin in area of the groin, or lower abdominal skin, or it may be tattooed with a permanent pigmented dye. In some patients, a small implant may be placed under the completed nipple-areolar reconstruction to add additional projection.

CLINICAL DECISION-MAKING EXERCISE

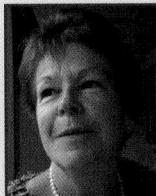

CASE STUDY:
Breast Cancer

Source: © iStockphoto.com/Jessica Jones.

Patient Profile

Ms. Maria Yanez, a 67-year-old married Hispanic woman, found a large lump in the upper outer quadrant of her left breast while showering. She states, "My breasts are lumpy, but this feels different."

Subjective Data

- Has family history of breast cancer: mother's diagnosed at age 60, and sister's diagnosed at age 40; grandmother had "some kind of female cancer"
- Had onset of menarche at age 11
- Has two daughters (34 and 32) and a son (30)
- Has no prior history of breast cancer
- Has taken combined hormone replacement therapy for 14 years

- Last mammogram and clinical breast examination 2 years ago
- States she is afraid she has cancer

Objective Data

- A palpable, firm, fixed, 1.5-cm mass is in upper outer quadrant of left breast.
- Left breast density is evident on mammogram.
- Both MRI and ultrasonography show a mass.
- No skin or nipple changes or lymphadenopathy is present.
- Results of ultrasonography-guided FNA indicate diagnosis of breast cancer; laboratory findings indicate estrogen and progesterone receptor positivity, HER-2 positivity.

Collaborative Care

- Scheduled for lumpectomy and sentinel lymph node dissection with possible axillary dissection

Discussion Questions

1. What characteristics of malignancy could be determined by palpation of Ms. Yanez's breast mass?
2. What in Ms. Yanez's breast cancer experience with her family members might influence her coping response?

3. What information would the nurse provide to Ms. Yanez about her surgery?
4. What are the possible complications that she may face after a lumpectomy and lymph node dissection?
5. Which common postoperative exercises will Ms. Yanez need to practise if she undergoes ALND?
6. What community resources are available to help Ms. Yanez and her family adjust to the change in her body and to cope with the diagnosis of cancer? How can the nurse access these resources?

7. What information about breast cancer risks is important to provide to Ms. Yanez and her daughters? What early-detection measures are important for them to know?
8. *Priority Decision:* On the basis of the assessment data, what are the priority nursing diagnoses? Are there any collaborative problems?

evolve *Answers are available at* **http://evolve.elsevier.com/ Canada/Lewis/medsurg**

REVIEW QUESTIONS

The number of the question corresponds to the same-numbered objective at the beginning of the chapter.

1. An occupational health nurse is planning a program on breast screening practices for women in the company. Which method should the nurse use to promote learning and adherence among participants?
   a. A movie that demonstrates the procedure of breast self-awareness
   b. Distribution of detailed written instructions for use at home
   c. Explanations emphasizing the value of early detection of breast cancer
   d. An opportunity to practise breast self-awareness on themselves with individual guidance from the nurse

2. Which of the following techniques is the most appropriate way to teach a patient how to know her breasts?
   a. Teach her palpation of cervical lymph nodes.
   b. Teach her to practise hard squeezing of the breast tissue.
   c. Teach her the importance of a mammogram to evaluate breast tissue.
   d. Teach her inspection of the whole area of breast tissue for any changes.

3. What explanation should the nurse provide when teaching a patient with painful fibrocystic breast changes about the condition?
   a. All discrete breast lumps must be subjected to biopsy to rule out malignant changes.
   b. The symptoms will probably subside after menopause unless hormone replacement is used.
   c. The lumps will become progressively larger and more painful, eventually necessitating surgical removal.
   d. Restrictions of coffee and chocolate and supplements of vitamin E may relieve the discomfort for many patients.

4. While the nurse discusses risk factors for breast cancer with a group of women, which of the following should the nurse stress as the greatest known risk factor for breast cancer?
   a. Being a woman older than 60 years
   b. Experiencing menstruation for 40 years or more
   c. Using estrogen replacement therapy during menopause
   d. Having a paternal grandmother with postmenopausal breast cancer

5. A patient has a lumpectomy with sentinel lymph node biopsy that yields results positive for cancer. Which of the following results supports the most favourable prognosis?
   a. Well-differentiated tumour
   b. Receptor-negative tumour
   c. Involvement of two to four axillary nodes
   d. Overexpression of *HER-2* cell marker

6. A patient with breast cancer has been scheduled for a modified radical mastectomy with an axillary node dissection. Which of the following should the nurse perform postoperatively to restore arm function on the affected side?
   a. Apply heating pads or blankets to increase circulation.
   b. Place daily ice packs to minimize the risk of lymphedema.
   c. Teach passive exercises with the affected arm in a dependent position.
   d. Emphasize regular exercises for the affected shoulder to increase range of motion.

7. Which of the following should the nurse implement preoperatively to meet the psychological needs of a woman scheduled for a modified radical mastectomy?
   a. Discuss the limitations of breast reconstruction.
   b. Include her significant other in all conversations.
   c. Promote an environment for expression of feelings.
   d. Explain the importance of regular follow-up screening.

8. Which of the following statements is the correct way to teach patients how to prevent capsular formation after breast reconstruction with implants?
   a. Gently massage the area around the implant.
   b. Bind the breasts tightly with elastic bandages.
   c. Exercise the arm on the affected side to promote drainage.
   d. Avoid strenuous exercise until implant healing has occurred.

ANSWERS: 1. d; 2. d; 3. d; 4. a; 5. a; 6. d; 7. c; 8. a.

REFERENCES

Buzdar, A. U. (2009). Role of biologic therapy and chemotherapy in hormone receptor- and HER2-positive breast cancer. *Annals of Oncology, 20*(6), 993-999. doi:10.1093/annonc/mdn739

Canadian Cancer Society. (2010a). *Benefits and risks of screening for breast cancer.* Retrieved from *http://www.cancer.ca/Canada-wide/ Prevention/Getting%20checked/Benefits%20and%20risks%20of%20 screening%20for%20breast%20cancer.aspx?sc_lang=en*

Canadian Cancer Society. (2010b). *Know your breasts.* Retrieved from *http://www.cancer.ca/Canada-wide/Prevention/Knowing%20 your%20body/Know%20your%20breasts.aspx?sc_lang=en*

Canadian Cancer Society. (2010c). *Signs and symptoms of breast cancer.* Retrieved from *http://www.cancer.ca/Canada-wide/About%20cancer/ Types%20of%20cancer/Signs%20and%20symptoms%20of%20 breast%20cancer.aspx?sc_lang=en*

Canadian Cancer Society. (2011a). *Breast cancer statistics at a glance.* Retrieved from *http://www.cancer.ca/Canada-wide/About%20cancer/ Cancer%20statistics/Stats%20at%20a%20glance/Breast%20 cancer.aspx?sc_lang=en*

Canadian Cancer Society. (2011b). *Breast cancer.* Retrieved from *http://www.cancer.ca/Canada-wide/Prevention/Getting%20checked/ Breast%20cancer%20NEW.aspx?sc_lang=en*

Canadian Cancer Society. (2012a). *Breast cancer screening in your 40s.* Retrieved from *http://www.cancer.ca/Canada-wide/Prevention/ Getting%20checked/Breast%20cancer%20screening%20in%20 your%2040s.aspx?sc_lang=en*

Canadian Cancer Society. (2012b). *Canadian Cancer Encyclopedia: Risk factors for breast cancer.* Retrieved from *http://info.cancer.ca/cce-ecc/ default.aspx?cceid=185&toc=10&lf=stomach&Lang=E*

Canadian Cancer Society. (2012c). *Canadian Cancer Encyclopedia: Stages of breast cancer.* Retrieved from *http://info.cancer.ca/cce-ecc/ default.aspx?cceid=185&toc=10&lf=stomach&Lang=E*

Canadian Task Force on Preventive Health Care. (2011). Recommendations on screening for breast cancer in average-risk women aged 40-74 years. *Canadian Medical Association Journal, 183,* 1991-2001. doi:10.1503/cmaj.110334

Costaridou, L., Skiadopoulos, S., Karahaliou, A., Arikidis, N., & Panayiotakis, G. (2009). Computer-aided diagnosis in breast imaging: Trends and challenges. In T. P. Exarchos, A. Papadopoulos, & D. I. Fotiadis (Eds.), *Handbook of research on advanced techniques in diagnostic imaging and biomedical applications* (pp. 142-159). Hershey, PA: IGI Global. doi:10.4018/978-1-60566-314-2.ch010

De, P., C., Neutel, C. I., Olivotto, I., & Morrison, H. (2010). Breast cancer incidence and hormone replacement therapy in Canada. *Journal of the National Cancer Institute, 102,* 1489-1495. doi:10.1093/jnci/djq345

Dell, D. D., Weaver, C., Kozempel, J., & Barsevick, A. (2008). Recovery after transverse rectus abdominis myocutaneous flap breast reconstruction surgery. *Oncology Nursing Forum, 35*(2), 189-196. doi:10.1188/08.ONF.189-196

Fobair, P., & Spiegel, D. (2009). Concerns about sexuality after breast cancer. *The Cancer Journal, 15*(1), 19-26. doi:10.10971PP0.0b013 e31819587bb

Folkes, A., Urquhart, R., Zitzelsberger, L., & Grunfeld, E. (2008). Breast cancer guidelines in Canada: A review of development and implementation. *Breast Care (Basel), 3*(2), 108-113. doi:10. 1159/ 000121732

Grunfeld, E., Dhesy-Thind, S., & Levine, M. (2005). Clinical practice guidelines for the care and treatment of breast cancer: Follow-up after treatment for breast cancer (summary of the 2005 update). *Canadian Medical Association Journal, 172*(10), 1319-1320. doi: 10.1503/cmaj.045062

Health Canada. (2007). *It's your health: Breast implants.* Retrieved from *http://www.hc-sc.gc.ca/hl-vs/alt_formats/pacrb-dgapcr/pdf/iyh-vsv/ med/implants-eng.pdf*

Hines, S. L., Tan, W., Larson, J. M., Thompson, K. M., Keels, H., Jorn, S., & Files, J. A. (2008). Evaluation of breast masses in older men. *Geriatrics, 63*(6), 19-24.

Jarvis, C., Browne, A., MacDonald-Jenkins, J., & Luctkar-Flude, M. (Eds.). (2009). *Physical examination and health assessment* (1st Canadian ed.). Toronto: Elsevier Canada.

Kong, X., Moran, M. S., Zhang, N., Haffty, B., & Yang, Q. (2011). Meta-analysis confirms achieving pathological complete response after neoadjuvant chemotherapy predicts favourable prognosis for breast cancer patients. *European Journal of Cancer, 47*(14), 2084-2091. doi:10.1016/j.ejca.2011.06.014

Ligibel, J. A., Partridge, A., Giobbie-Hurder, A., Campbell, N., Shockro, L., Salinadri, T., & Winer, E. P. (2010). Physical and psychological outcomes among women in a telephone-based exercise intervention during adjuvant therapy for early stage breast cancer. *Journal of Women's Health, 19*(8), 1553-1559. doi:10.1089/jwh.2009. 1760

Latosinsky, S., Fradette, K., Lix, L., Hildebrand, K., & Turner, D. (2007). Canadian breast cancer guidelines: Have they made a difference? *Canadian Medical Association Journal, 176,* (6), 771-776. doi:10.1503/cmaj.060854

Lee, C., Sunu, C., & Pignone, M. (2009). Patient-reported outcomes of breast reconstruction after mastectomy: A systematic review. *Journal of the American College of Surgeons, 209*(1), 123-133. doi:10.1016/j.jamcollsurg.2009.02.061

Litsas, G. (2008). Sequential therapy with tamoxifen and aromatase inhibitors in early-stage postmenopausal breast cancer: A review of the evidence. *Oncology Nursing Forum, 35*(4), 714-721. doi:10.1188/08.ONF.714-721

Mackey, J., McLeod, D., Ragaz, J., Gelmon, K., Verma, S., Pritchard, K., …, Charbonneau, L. F. (2009). Adjuvant targeted therapy in early breast cancer. *Cancer, 115,* 1154-1168. doi:10.1002/ cncr.24112

Mayfield, E. (2009). Delving into possible mechanisms for chemobrain. *National Cancer Institute Cancer Bulletin, 6*(6). Retrieved from *http://www.cancer.gov/aboutnci/ncicancerbulletin/archive/2009/ 032409/page8/print*

Metcalfe, K. A., & Narod, S. A. (2007). Breast cancer prevention in women with a *BRCA1* or *BRCA2* mutation. *Open Medicine, 1*(3). Retrieved from *http://www.openmedicine.ca/article/view/11/100*

Miltenburg, D., & Speights, V. O. (2008). Benign breast disease. *Obstetrics and Gynecology Clinics of North America, 35*(2), 285-300. doi:10.1016/j.ogc.2008.03.008

Morgan, K., & McCance, K. L. (2008). Alterations of the reproductive systems, including sexually transmitted infections. In S. E. Huether & K. L. McCance (Eds.), *Understanding pathophysiology* (4th ed., pp. 848-903). St. Louis: Mosby.

Nelson, M. C., Norton, H. J., & Greene, F. L. (2011). Breast conservation therapy versus mastectomy in the community-based setting: Can this rate be used as a benchmark for cancer care? *Surgical Oncology Clinics of North America, 20*(3), 427-437. doi:10.10161j. soc.2011.01.005

Nelson, R. (2008). Contralateral prophylactic mastectomy. *American Journal of Nursing, 108*(2), 26-27. doi:10.1097/01.NAJ. 0000310326.63056.22

Palacio, M. (2010). Breast imaging alternatives. *Applied Radiology, 39*(3), 34-36.

Palmieri, F. M., Frye, D. K., & Mahon, S. M. (2009). Current clinical issues in systemic therapy for metastatic breast cancer. *Clinical Journal of Oncology Nursing, 131*(1), 4-10. doi:10.1188/09.CJON. 51.4-10

Rodden, A. (2009). Common breast concerns. *Primary Care Clinical Office Practice, 36,* 103-113. doi:10.1016/j.pop.2008.10.006

Rosolowich, V. (2006). Breast self-examination. *Journal of Obstetrics and Gynaecology Canada, 28*(8), 728-730.

Rugo, H. S. (2008). The breast cancer continuum in hormone-receptor–positive breast cancer in postmenopausal women: Evolving management options focusing on aromatase inhibitors. *Annals of Oncology, 19*(1), 16-27. doi:10.1093/annonc/mdm282

Simmons, C. (2009). Chemo brain, antiestrogens, and me. *Clinical Journal of Oncology Nursing, 13*(3), 253-254. doi:10.1188/09. CJON.253-254

Singer, M. (2009). Lymphedema in breast cancer: Dilemmas and challenges. *Clinical Journal of Oncology Nursing, 13*(3), 350-352. doi:10.1188/09.CJON.350-352

Spencer, J. P. (2008). Management of mastitis in breastfeeding women. *American Family Physician, 78*(6), 727-732.

Swenson, K. K., Nissen, M. J., Leach, J. W., & Post-White, J. (2009). Case-control study to evaluate predictors of lymphedema after breast cancer surgery. *Oncology Nursing Forum, 36*(2), 185-193. doi:10.1188/09.ONF.185-193

Weaver, C. (2009). Caring for a patient after mastectomy. *Nursing, 39*(5), 44-48. doi:10.1097/01.NURSE.0000350757.93924.b5

CANADIAN RESOURCES

Breast Cancer Society of Canada
http://www.bcsc.ca

Canadian Association of Provincial Cancer Agencies (CAPCA)
http://www.capca.ca

Canadian Breast Cancer Foundation (CBCF)
http://www.cbcf.org

Canadian Breast Cancer Network (CBCN)
http://www.cbcn.ca

Canadian Cancer Society
http://www.cancer.ca

Canadian Cancer Society Research Institute
http://www.cancer.ca/Research.aspx

Canadian Oncology Societies (COS)
http://www.cos.ca

Canadian Partnership Against Cancer
http://www.partnershipagainstcancer.ca

Canadian Society of Plastic Surgeons
http://www.plasticsurgery.ca

Society of Obstetricians and Gynaecologists of Canada
http://www.sogc.org

Willow Breast Cancer Support Canada
http://www.willow.org

RELATED RESOURCES

American Cancer Society: Reach to Recovery
http://www.cancer.org/treatment/supportprogramsservices/reach-to-recovery

American Society of Plastic Surgeons: Plastic Surgery Education Foundation
http://www.plasticsurgery.org

Living Beyond Breast Cancer
http://www.lbbc.org

NABCO (National Alliance of Breast Cancer Organizations)
http://www.nabco.org

National Breast Cancer Coalition
http://www.natlbcc.org

National Cancer Institute
http://www.nci.nih.gov

National Coalition for Cancer Survivorship (NCS)
http://www.canceradvocacy.org

National Lymphedema Network (NLN)
http://www.lymphnet.org

OncoLink (cancer information site of the Abramson Cancer Center, University of Pennsylvania)
http://www.oncolink.upenn.edu

Oncology Nursing Society (ONS)
http://www.ons.org

Susan G. Komen for the Cure (formerly Susan G. Komen Breast Cancer Foundation)
http://www.komen.org

evolve *For additional Internet resources, see the Web site for this book at* **http://evolve.elsevier.com/Canada/Lewis/medsurg**

Nursing Management: Sexually Transmitted Infections

Written by JoAnn Grove
Adapted by Shelley L. Cobbett

LEARNING OBJECTIVES

1. Identify the factors contributing to the high incidence of sexually transmitted infections.
2. Explain the etiology, the clinical manifestations, the complications, and the diagnostic abnormalities of gonorrhea, syphilis, chlamydial infections, genital herpes, and genital warts.
3. Compare primary genital herpes with recurrent genital herpes.
4. Explain the collaborative care and the drug therapy for gonorrhea, syphilis, chlamydial infections, genital herpes, and genital warts.
5. Identify the nursing assessment and the nursing diagnoses for patients who have a sexually transmitted infection.
6. Describe the nursing role in the prevention and control of sexually transmitted infections.
7. Describe the nursing management of patients with sexually transmitted infections.

KEY TERMS

chancre Painless indurated lesion found on the penis, the vulva, the lips, the mouth, the vagina, and the rectum; characteristic of syphilis, Table 55-3, p. 1525

chlamydial infections Superficial mucosal infections caused by *Chlamydia trachomatis*, p. 1526

genital herpes A sexually transmitted infection caused by the herpes simplex virus (HSV), usually type 2, resulting in painful genital or anal vesicular lesions, p. 1527

gonorrhea Infection of the genitalia, the rectum, or the oropharynx by *Neisseria gonorrhoeae*; elicits an inflammatory response that, if left untreated, leads to the formation of fibrous tissue and adhesions, p. 1521

gummas Chronic, destructive nodular lesions associated with late syphilis and affecting any organ of the body, especially the skin, bones, the liver, and mucous membranes, Table 55-3, p. 1525

sexually transmitted infections (STIs) Infectious diseases transmitted most commonly through sexual intercourse or genital contact, p. 1520

syphilis Infection of organs and tissues of the body by *Treponema pallidum*, p. 1522

tabes dorsalis Neurological degeneration caused by inflammatory damage to the dorsal roots of sensory nerves in neurosyphilis; also called *progressive locomotor ataxia*, p. 1523

venereal infections A term used historically to describe any illness transmitted by intimate sexual contact, or sexually transmitted infections, p. 1520

ELECTRONIC RESOURCES

Supplemental content related to Chapter 55 can be found …

Evolve Web Site ⊖volve

http://evolve.elsevier.com/Canada/Lewis/medsurg
• Answer Guidelines for Case Study on p. 1535
• Clinical Reference: Laboratory Values

• Content Updates
• Electronic Calculators
• Examination Review Questions
• Glossary
• Key Points (Printable and MP3 Download)

Sexually Transmitted Infections

Sexually transmitted infections (STIs) are infectious diseases transmitted most commonly through sexual contact (Table 55-1). Historically, they have been referred to as **venereal infections,** a term used to describe any illness transmitted by intimate sexual contact. Many of the agents causing STIs are easily inactivated by drying, heating, and washing. These infections can be bacterial (gonorrhea, chlamydial infection, syphilis), viral (genital herpes, genital warts), or both. Most infections start as lesions on the genitalia and other sexually exposed mucous membranes. The infections can then be widely disseminated to other areas of the body. A latent or subclinical phase occurs with all STIs. This can lead to a long-term persistent infection and the transmission of disease from a person who has no symptoms (but is infected) to another contact. Different STIs can coexist within one person. For example, if a person has gonorrhea, chlamydial infection may also be present.

In Canada, three nationally reportable STIs—gonorrhea, syphilis, and chlamydial infection—must be reported to the Communicable Disease Division in each province and territory (Public Health Agency of Canada [PHAC], 2010b). Since 1997, there has been a steady increase in the rates of all three of these infections (PHAC, 2010b). Infections that are associated with sexual transmission can also be contracted by other routes, such as contact with blood and blood products and autoinoculation.

The more commonly diagnosed STIs are discussed in this chapter. Human immunodeficiency virus (HIV) infection and related problems are discussed in Chapter 17. Hepatitis B infection and related problems are discussed in Chapter 46.

Factors Affecting Incidence of Sexually Transmitted Infection

Many factors contribute to the current dramatic increase in STI rates. Earlier reproductive maturity and increased longevity have resulted in a longer sexual lifespan. The increase in the total population has resulted in an increase in the number of susceptible hosts. Other factors include greater sexual freedom, failure to use barrier methods (e.g., condom, dental dam) during sexual activity, and an increased emphasis in the media on sexuality. In addition, increased leisure time, more national and international travel, expansion of anonymous partnering venues, and urbanization have brought together people with varying social behaviours

and value systems. Use of illicit drugs (e.g., 3-4-methylenedioxy-methamphetamine [ecstasy], crystal methamphetamine) is being increasingly linked to unsafe sexual practices (Fang, Oliver, Jayaraman, & Wong, 2010).

Changes in the methods of contraception that are typically used are also reflected in the incidence of STIs. The condom is considered the only contraceptive device that is prophylactic with regard to STIs (Sarkar, 2008). Although condom use is increasing in selected populations, condoms are not used frequently in the general population. Commonly used oral contraceptives cause the secretions of the cervix and the vagina to become more alkaline. This change produces a more favourable environment for the growth of organisms that cause STIs at these sites. Women who take oral contraceptives have a lower risk of pelvic inflammatory disease (PID) as a result of the ability of the cervical mucus to act as a barrier against bacteria. However, the proliferation of *Chlamydia* organisms, the leading cause of nongonococcal PID, may be enhanced by oral contraceptive use. Whether users of intrauterine devices (IUDs) are at increased risk of PID is controversial, but IUDs do not confer protection from STIs. Long-acting contraceptives such as levonorgestrel (Norplant) and medroxyprogesterone (Depo-Provera) also confer no protection from STIs. Lack of awareness of this fact may be a factor leading to STIs in people who use these products.

Nurses need to strive to attend to the physiological and psychological needs of the large number of people living with incurable STIs in Canada. Chronic viral STI can have long-standing negative effects on a patient's psychosocial well-being, which highlights the need for strengthened prevention efforts. There are also some noteworthy trends related to populations at high risk for STIs, such as injection-drug users, men who have sex with men, survival sex workers, street youth, and Aboriginals (PHAC, 2010b).

Bacterial Infections

Gonococcal Infection

Gonorrhea is the second most frequently occurring STI. After years of constant decline in Canada, the rates of infection for gonorrhea rose from 17.6 cases per 100,000 in 1999 to 33.1 cases per 100,000 in 2009 (PHAC, 2010a). Most affected are men from 20 to 24 years of age and girls and women from 15 to 19 years of age (PHAC, 2010b). Continued monitoring for

Table 55-1 Microorganisms Responsible for Sexually Transmitted Infections

MICROORGANISM	INFECTION
Bacteria	
Chlamydia trachomatis	Nongonococcal urethritis; cervicitis; lymphogranuloma venereum
Neisseria gonorrhoeae	Gonorrhea
Treponema pallidum	Syphilis
Viruses	
Cytomegalovirus	Encephalitis, esophagitis, retinitis, pneumonitis in immunocompromised patients
Hepatitis B virus	Hepatitis B
Herpes simplex virus (HSV)	Genital herpes
Human immunodeficiency virus (HIV)	HIV infection, acquired immune deficiency syndrome (AIDS)
Human papillomavirus (HPV)	Genital warts
Poxvirus	Molluscum contagiosum
Trichomonas vaginalis	Trichomoniasis

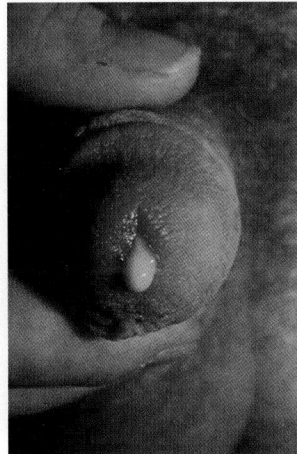

Figure 55-1 Profuse, purulent drainage in a patient with gonorrhea.

Source: Marx, K., Walls, R., & Hockberger, R. (2010). *Rosen's emergency medicine: Concepts and clinical practice* (7th ed.). St Louis: Mosby.

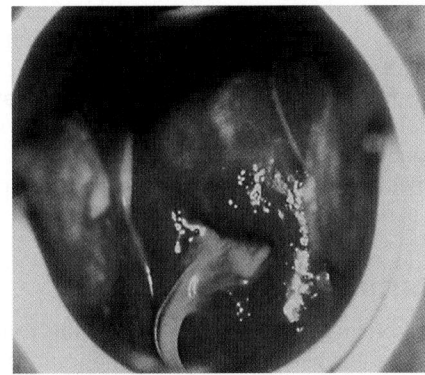

Figure 55-2 Endocervical gonorrhea. Cervical redness and edema with discharge.

Source: Morse, S., Moreland, A., & Holmes, K. (Eds.). (1996). *Atlas of sexually transmitted diseases and AIDS*. London: Mosby-Wolfe.

antimicrobial resistance is important to prevent the spread of drug-resistant gonorrhea and to ensure successful cure rates for this treatable infection. Most provinces have enacted laws that permit examination and treatment of minors without parental consent.

Etiology and Pathophysiology

Gonorrhea is an infection of the genitalia, the rectum, the oropharynx, or a combination of the three caused by *Neisseria gonorrhoeae*, a Gram-negative diplococcus. The disease is spread by direct physical contact with an infected host, usually during sexual activity (vaginal, oral, or anal). Mucosa with columnar epithelium is susceptible to gonococcal infection. This tissue is present in the genitalia (urethra in men, cervix in women), the rectum, and the oropharynx. Neonates can develop gonorrhea during delivery from an infected mother. The delicate gonococcus is easily killed by drying, heating, or washing with an antiseptic solution. As a consequence, indirect transmission by instruments or linens is rare.

The incubation period is 3 to 8 days. The disease confers no immunity to subsequent reinfection. Gonorrhea elicits an inflammatory response that, if left untreated, leads to the formation of fibrous tissue and adhesions. This fibrous scarring is subsequently responsible for many complications in women such as strictures and tubal abnormalities, which can lead to tubal pregnancy, chronic pelvic pain, and infertility (Trigg, 2008).

Clinical Manifestations

The initial site of infection in men is usually the urethra. Symptoms of urethritis consist of dysuria and profuse, purulent urethral discharge that develops 2 to 5 days after infection (Figure 55-1). The testicles may also become painful or swollen. Men generally seek medical evaluation early in the disease course because their symptoms are usually obvious and distressing. It is unusual for men with gonorrhea to be asymptomatic.

Most women who contract gonorrhea, in contrast, have no symptoms or have minor symptoms that are often overlooked, which makes it possible for them to remain a source of infection. A few affected women may complain of vaginal discharge, dysuria, or frequency of urination. Changes in menstruation may be a symptom, but many affected women disregard these changes. After the incubation period, redness and swelling occur at the site of contact, which is usually the cervix or the urethra (Figure 55-2). A greenish-yellow purulent exudate often develops, with a potential for abscess formation. The disease may remain local or can spread by direct tissue extension to the uterus, the fallopian tubes, and the ovaries. Although the vulva and the vagina are uncommon sites for a gonorrheal infection, they may become involved when little or no estrogen is present, as is the case in prepubertal girls and postmenopausal women. Because the vagina acts as a natural reservoir for infectious secretions, transmission is often more efficient from men to women than it is from women to men.

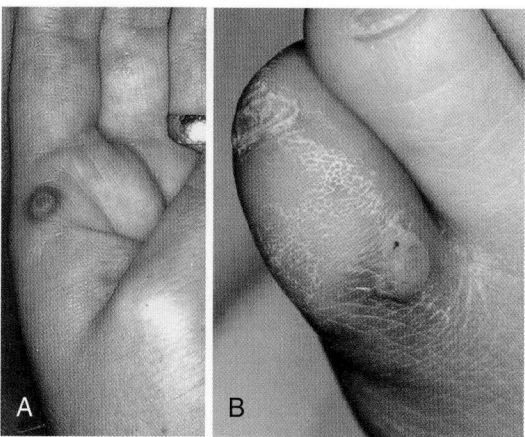

Figure 55-3 Skin lesions from disseminated gonococcal infection. **A,** On hand. **B,** On the fifth toe.

Sources: **A,** Cohen, J., & Powderly, W. G. (2004). *Infectious diseases* (2nd ed.). St. Louis: Mosby. **B,** Mandell, G. L., Bennett, J. E., & Dolin, R. (2010). *Mandell, Douglas, and Bennett's principles and practice of infectious diseases* (7th ed.). Philadelphia: Churchill Livingstone.

Anorectal gonorrhea may be present and is usually caused by anal intercourse. Symptoms may include soreness, itching, and discharge. In a small percentage of individuals, gonococcal pharyngitis results from orogenital sexual contact. Most patients with rectal infections and infections in the throat have few symptoms. When the gonococcus can be demonstrated by a laboratory culture, individuals of either sex can transmit the infection to their sexual partners.

Complications

Because men often seek treatment early in the course of the disease, they are less likely to develop complications. The complications that do occur in men are prostatitis, urethral strictures, and sterility from orchitis or epididymitis. Because women without symptoms seldom seek treatment, complications are more common and usually constitute the reason for seeking medical attention. PID, Bartholin's abscess, ectopic pregnancy, and infertility are the main complications of gonorrhea in women. A small percentage of infected people, mainly women, may develop disseminated gonorrhea. In this condition, the appearance of skin lesions, fever, arthralgia, or arthritis usually causes the patient to seek medical help (Figure 55-3).

Eye Infections in Newborns. Most provinces and territories require the instillation of a prophylactic drug such as erythromycin or tetracycline into the eyes of all newborns as a precaution. (Perry et al., 2013). Gonorrheal eye infections in newborns (ophthalmia neonatorum) are therefore relatively rare today. Infants with untreated infection develop permanent blindness.

Diagnostic Studies

For men, a diagnosis of gonorrhea is presumed if a man has a history of sexual contact with a new or infected partner, followed within a few days by a urethral discharge. Typical clinical manifestations, combined with a positive finding in a Gram-stained smear of the purulent discharge from the penis, render the diag-nosis almost certain. A culture of the discharge is indicated for men whose smears are negative in the presence of strong clinical evidence.

The immediate identification of *N. gonorrhoeae* is usually made with a Gram stain of smears made from the exudate. A reliable way to confirm gonorrhea is to isolate the organism in culture. Cultures of the discharge or secretion can provide a definitive diagnosis after incubation for 24 to 48 hours. Although culture is the recommended diagnostic test because it allows for antibiotic resistance testing, the nucleic acid amplification test (NAAT) can be used when transportation or storage conditions are not ideal for culture. NAATs are the only available diagnostic method in some areas of Canada and may be useful when patients resist pelvic examination or urethral swabbing (Fang et al., 2010). NAAT can also be used to detect reinfection 3 weeks after completion of therapy (PHAC, 2010b).

Diagnosing gonorrhea in women on the basis of symptoms is difficult because most infected women are symptom free or have complaints that may be confused with other conditions. Smears and purulent discharge do not establish a diagnosis of gonorrhea because the female genitourinary tract normally harbours a large number of organisms that resemble *N. gonorrhoeae*. A culture must be performed to confirm the diagnosis.

Collaborative Care

Collaborative care for the patient with a gonorrheal infection is presented in Table 55-2.

Drug Therapy. Because of a short incubation period and high infectivity, treatment is generally instituted before culture results are available, even in the absence of any signs or symptoms (PHAC, 2010b). As a result of penicillin-resistant strains, the first choice of treatment in Canada is cefixime (Suprax). Azithromycin (Zithromax) or spectinomycin (Trobicin) should be reserved for patients who are allergic to cephalosporin or who have anaphylactic reactions to penicillin (PHAC, 2010b). Quinolones such as ciprofloxacin and ofloxacin are no longer preferred drugs for the treatment of gonorrhea in Canada because of the rapid increase in quinolone-resistant strains of *N. gonorrhoeae* (PHAC, 2010b). Patients with coexisting syphilis are likely to be treated with the same drugs used for gonorrhea.

All sexual contacts of patients with gonorrhea must be examined and treated to prevent reinfection after resumption of sexual relations. The "ping-pong" effect of re-exposure, treatment, and reinfection can cease only when infected partners are treated simultaneously. In addition, the patient should be counselled to abstain from sexual intercourse and alcohol during treatment. Sexual intercourse allows the infection to spread and can delay complete healing, and alcohol has an irritant effect on the healing urethral walls. Men should be cautioned against squeezing the penis to look for further discharge. Follow-up examination and repeated culture may be performed at least once after treatment, usually in 4 to 7 days. Reinfection, rather than treatment failure, is the main cause for infections identified after treatment has ended.

Syphilis

The incidence of **syphilis** has steadily increased in Canada, from 191 cases in 1999 to 1683 cases in 2009 (PHAC, 2010b). In Canada, infectious syphilis rates are highest among men having

COLLABORATIVE CARE

Table 55-2 Gonorrhea

Diagnostic

- History and physical examination
- Gram-stained smears of urethral or endocervical exudate
- Cultures for *Neisseria gonorrhoeae*
- NAAT to detect *N. gonorrhoeae*
- Testing for other STIs (syphilis, HIV, *Chlamydia*)

Collaborative Therapy

Drug Therapy

- Urethral, endocervical, rectal, pharyngeal gonorrheal infections: cefixime (Suprax) 400 mg PO in a single dose (preferred); or alternatives such as ceftriaxone 125 mg IM in a single dose; or azithromycin (Zithromax) 2 g PO in a single dose; or Spectinomycin 2 g IM in a single dose; or ciprofloxacin 500 mg PO in a single dose; or ofloxacin 400 mg PO in a single dose
- Also treated for chlamydial infection, unless a *Chlamydia* test result is available and negative
- All regimens followed by empirical treatment for chlamydial and nongonococcal infections
- Gonococcal infections reportable to the public health department in all provinces and territories
- Treatment of sexual contacts
- Instruction on abstinence from sexual intercourse and alcohol
- Re-examination if symptoms persist or recur after completion of treatment

HIV, human immunodeficiency virus; *IM,* intramuscularly; *PO,* by mouth (per os); *NAAT,* nucleic acid amplification test; *STI,* sexually transmitted infection.
Source: Modified from Centers for Disease Control and Prevention. (2010). Sexually transmitted diseases: Treatment guidelines, 2010. *Morbidity and Mortality Weekly Report, 59*(RR-12), 1-126. Retrieved from *http://www.cdc.gov/STD/treatment;* and from Public Health Agency of Canada. (2010). *Canadian guidelines on sexually transmitted infections (Updated 2006 Edition)*. Ottawa: Author.

sex with men and among sex trade workers and in situations in which sex is exchanged for food, shelter, or protection (survival sex; PHAC, 2010b). Syphilis remains an important health problem.

Etiology and Pathophysiology

The causative organism of syphilis is *Treponema pallidum*, a spirochete. This bacterium is thought to enter the body through very small breaks in the skin or mucous membranes. Its entry is facilitated by the minor abrasions that often occur during sexual intercourse. Syphilis is a complex disease in which many organs and tissues of the body can become infected with *T. pallidum*. The infection causes the production of antibodies that also react with normal tissues. Not all people who are exposed to syphilis acquire the disease; in about one third of cases, infection is acquired after intercourse with an infected person. In addition to sexual contact, syphilis may be spread through contact with infectious lesions and sharing of needles among people who use intravenous (IV) drugs. *T. pallidum* is extremely fragile and easily destroyed by drying, heating, or washing. The incubation period for syphilis

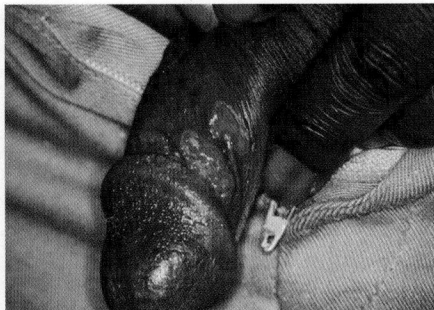

Figure 55-4 Primary syphilis chancre.

Source: Rakel, R. (2007). *Textbook of family medicine* (7th ed.). Philadelphia: W. B. Saunders.

ranges from 10 to 90 days (average, 21 days; Frenkel & Potts, 2008). In congenital syphilis, the infection is transmitted from an infected mother to the fetus in utero after the tenth week of gestation. Universal screening of pregnant women has remained the standard of care in Canada (PHAC, 2010b).

Patients with syphilis are often also infected with HIV (Tucker et al., 2011). The presence of syphilitic lesions on the genitals enhances HIV transmission. HIV-infected patients with syphilis appear to be at greatest risk for clinically significant central nervous system (CNS) involvement and may require more intensive treatment with penicillin than do other patients with syphilis. The treatment failure rate is higher in HIV-positive patients with syphilis than in HIV-negative patients who acquire syphilis (Lin et al., 2011). Therefore, the assessment of all patients with syphilis should also include testing for HIV (with the patient's consent).

Clinical Manifestations

Syphilis produces a variety of signs and symptoms that mimic those of a number of other diseases (Domantay-Apostol, Handog & Gabriel, 2008; Figures 55-4, 55-5, and 55-6); thus in comparison with other STIs, it is more difficult to recognize syphilis. If it is not treated, specific clinical stages are characteristic of the progression of the disease (Table 55-3).

Complications

Complications of the disease occur mostly in the late stage of syphilis. The gummas of benign late syphilis may produce irreparable damage to bone, liver, or skin but seldom result in death. In cardiovascular syphilis, the resulting aneurysm may press on structures such as the intercostal nerves, causing pain. The possibility of a rupture rises as the aneurysm increases in size. Scarring of the aortic valve results in aortic valve insufficiency and, eventually, heart failure.

Neurosyphilis is responsible for degeneration of the brain with mental deterioration (Ferrando & Freyberg, 2008). Other neurological deficits may be evident. Inflammatory damage to the dorsal roots of sensory nerves causes **tabes dorsalis** (progressive locomotor ataxia), characterized by sudden attacks of pain anywhere in the body, which can confuse the diagnosis with other conditions. Loss of vision and sense of position in the feet and legs can also occur with tabes dorsalis. Walking may become even more difficult as joint stability is lost. (Late syphilis is also discussed in Chapter 63.)

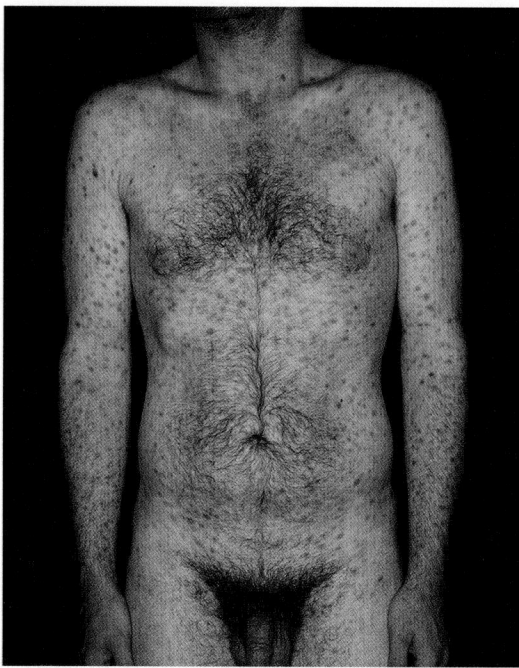

Figure 55-5 Secondary syphilis. Bilateral, symmetrical cutaneous lesions.

Source: Habif, T. (2004). *Clinical dermatology: A color guide to diagnosis and therapy* (4th ed., p. 319, Figure 10-9). St. Louis: Mosby.

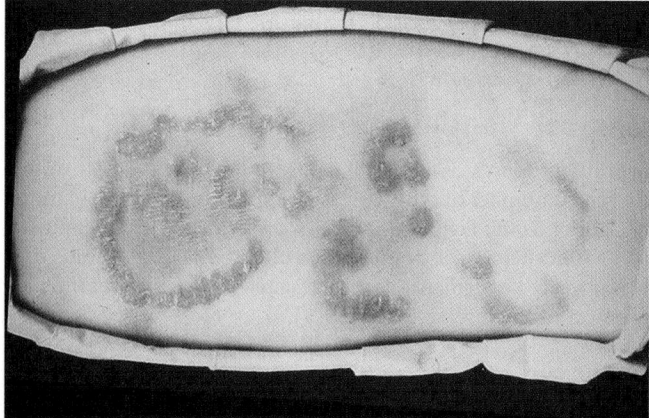

Figure 55-6 Destructive skin gummas associated with tertiary syphilis.

Source: Cohen, J., & Powderly, W. G. (2004). *Infectious diseases* (2nd ed.). St. Louis: Mosby.

Diagnostic Studies

The first step in diagnosis is to obtain a detailed and accurate sexual history. Instead of asking whether a patient is homosexual or asking only about sexual preference, it is often useful to be more specific and ask whether the patient has sex with men or women or both. Some men who have sex with men do not identify themselves as homosexual or bisexual. In addition, the examiner should inquire whether the patient has vaginal, oral, or anal sex. A physical examination should be performed to identify any suspicious lesions, as well as to note other significant signs and symptoms. Because syphilis is "the great imitator" of other conditions, it is easily missed, and oral sex is an important transmission route that necessitates attention.

The presence of spirochetes on dark-field microscopic examination and direct fluorescent antibody tests of lesion exudate or tissue can confirm a clinical diagnosis of syphilis. However, syphilis is more commonly diagnosed through a serological test. Tests for syphilis may be classified as those performed for screening and those performed for confirmation of a positive screening result. Nonspecific antitreponemal antibodies can be detected by tests such as the Venereal Disease Research Laboratory (VDRL) test and the rapid plasma reagin (RPR) test. These nontreponemal tests are suitable for screening purposes and usually yield positive results 10 to 14 days after the appearance of a chancre. The fluorescent treponemal antibody absorption (FTA-ABS) test and the *T. pallidum* particle agglutination (TP-PA) test detect specific antitreponemal antibodies and are suitable for confirming the diagnosis.

False-negative and false-positive results do occur with the nontreponemal tests (VDRL, rapid plasma reagin [RPR]). A false-negative result may be obtained during primary syphilis if the test is performed before the individual has had time to produce antibodies. A false-positive finding may occur after smallpox vaccination or with other diseases or conditions such as hepatitis, infectious mononucleosis, collagen diseases (e.g., systemic lupus erythematosus), pregnancy, or aging. Positive nontreponemal test results should be confirmed by more specific treponemal tests to rule out other causes. In the CSF, changes such as increased white blood cell count, increased total protein levels, and a positive result of the treponemal antibody test are diagnostic of asymptomatic neurosyphilis.

If a patient is treated with antibiotics early in the course of the disease on the basis of the history and the symptoms, the results of serological testing may not indicate the presence of syphilis. Once a person has positive serological findings for syphilis, indicating the presence of antibodies, these findings may remain positive for an indefinite period in spite of successful treatment.

Collaborative Care

Drug Therapy. Management of syphilis is aimed at eradication of all syphilitic organisms (Table 55-4). However, treatment cannot reverse damage that is already present in the late stage of the disease. Penicillin G benzathine remains the treatment of choice for all stages of syphilis (Frenkel & Potts, 2008). To date, since confirmation of its effectiveness in 1943, there is no evidence to suggest a decrease in the effectiveness of penicillin against *T. pallidum*. Therapy for the various stages of syphilis that is in accordance with national STI guidelines provided by the PHAC is described in Table 55-5. All stages of syphilis should be treated. When symptoms are chronic or recur after drug therapy has ended, the patient should undergo repeated treatment. All patients with neurosyphilis must be carefully monitored, with periodic serological testing, clinical evaluation at 6-month intervals, and repeat CSF examinations for at least 3 years. Specific management is based on the symptoms. It is also very important that all sexual contacts in the previous 90 days be treated.

In pregnant women with syphilis, penicillin G benzathine, 2.4 million U by intramuscular route weekly for 1 to 3 doses is administered, depending on the stage of syphilis. Treatment administered in the second half of pregnancy may pose a risk of

Table 55-3 Stages of Syphilis

CLINICAL STAGE	CHARACTERISTIC FINDINGS	COMMUNICABILITY	DURATION OF STAGE
Primary	**Chancre** (painless indurated lesion [see Figure 55-4]; appears 10 to 90 days after inoculation) Regional lymphadenopathy Genital ulcers	Exudate from chancre is highly infectious; blood is infectious Most infectious stage	3-8 wk
Secondary	Occurs a few weeks after chancre appears Systematic manifestations: flu-like symptoms Cutaneous lesions: bilateral, symmetrical rash that begins on truck and involves the palms and soles (see Figure 55-5); mucous patches in the mouth, tongue or cervix; condylomata lata in the anal and genital area Weight loss, alopecia	Exudate from skin and mucous membrane lesions is highly infectious	1-2 yr
Latent	Absence of signs or symptoms Diagnosis based on positive specific treponemal antibody test together with normal CSF and absence of clinical manifestations	Noninfectious after 4 yr; possible placental transmission Almost 25% of people with latent syphilis; in some cases occurring many years later	Throughout life or progression to late stage
Late (tertiary)*	Appearance 3-20 yr after initial infection	Noninfectious	Chronic (without treatment), possibly fatal
• Benign	**Gummas** (chronic, destructive lesions affecting any organ of body, especially skin, bone, liver, mucous membranes) (see Figure 55-6)	CSF possibly containing organism	—
• Cardiovascular	Aortic valve insufficiency or saccular aneurysm of thoracic aorta, aortitis	—	—
• Neurosyphilis	General paresis (personality changes from minor to extreme [psychosis], tremors, physical and mental deterioration) Tabes dorsalis (ataxia, areflexia, paresthesias, lightning pains, damaged joints [Charcot's joints]) Speech disturbances	—	—

CSF, cerebrospinal fluid.
*Several forms, such as cardiovascular and neurosyphilis, occur together in approximately 25% of untreated cases.

COLLABORATIVE CARE

Table 55-4 Syphilis

Diagnostic	*Collaborative Therapy*

• History and physical examination
• Dark-field microscopy
• Nontreponemal or treponemal serological testing
• Testing for other STIs (HIV infection, gonorrhea, chlamydial infection)
	• Appropriate drug therapy (see Table 55-5)
	• Confidential counselling and testing for HIV infection
	• Case finding
	• Surveillance
	  • Repeat of quantitative nontreponemal tests at 6 and 12 months
	  • Examination of cerebrospinal fluid at 1 year if treatment involves alternative antibiotics or treatment failure has occurred

HIV, human immunodeficiency virus; *STI,* sexually transmitted infections.

SAFETY ALERT

• Reports from some jurisdictions have indicated inappropriate use of short-acting benzylpenicillin (Penicillin G) intramuscularly for the treatment of infectious syphilis rather than long-acting benzathine penicillin G (Bicillin-LA; PHAC, 2010b).

• Nurses need to be aware of the similar names of these two products to prevent and avoid inappropriate and inadequate treatment.

premature labour and fetal distress. Pregnant women receiving treatment should be advised to seek medical care if fetal movements decrease.

Chlamydial Infections

Chlamydial infections are the most prevalent bacterial STIs in Canada today. More than 87,000 cases are reported annually, and approximately 1 of every 2 cases reported occurs in women (PHAC, 2010b). Underreporting is substantial because most

DRUG THERAPY

Table 55-5 Syphilis

STAGE	PREFERRED TREATMENT	ALTERNATIVE TREATMENT*
All non-pregnant adults: • primary syphilis • secondary syphilis • early latent syphilis (<1 year duration)	Benzathine penicillin G (Bicillin L-A) 2.4 million units IM in a single dose	• Doxycycline (Vibramycin) 100 mg PO twice a day for 2 wk • Alternate agent (to be used in exceptional circumstances)—ceftriaxone 1 g IV or IM daily for 10 days
All non-pregnant adults • Late latent syphilis • Latent syphilis of unknown duration • Cardiovascular syphilis and other tertiary syphilis not involving central nervous system	Benzathine penicillin G (Bicillin L-A) three doses of 2.4 million units each, IM, at 1-wk intervals (total dose, 7.2 million units)	• Consider penicillin desensitization • Doxycycline (Vibramycin) 100 mg PO twice a day for 28 days • Alternate agent (to be used in exceptional circumstances)—ceftriaxone 1 g IV or IM daily for 10 days
All adults • Neurosyphilis	Penicillin G 3-4 million units every 4 hr IV for 10-14 days (total dose, 16-24 million units)	• Strongly consider penicillin desensitization followed by treatment with penicillin • Ceftriaxone 2 g IV or IM daily for 10-14 days

IM, intramuscularly; *IV*, intravenously; *PO*, by mouth (per os).
*Given when penicillin is contraindicated.
Source: Modified from Public Health Agency of Canada. (2010). *Canadian guidelines on sexually transmitted infections* (p. 15). Ottawa: Author.

infected people have no symptoms and therefore do not seek testing. Chlamydial infections are a major contributor to PID, ectopic pregnancy, and infertility among women and to non-gonococcal urethritis in men (Bender et al., 2011).

Etiology and Pathophysiology

Chlamydial infections are superficial mucosal infections caused by *Chlamydia trachomatis*, a Gram-negative bacterium. *Chlamydia* can be transmitted during vaginal, anal, or oral sex. Numerous different serotypes, or strains, of *C. trachomatis* cause urogenital infections (e.g., nongonococcal urethritis in men and cervicitis in women), ocular trachoma, and lymphogranuloma venereum. Pregnant women with chlamydial infections are more likely to have premature rupture of fetal membranes and a preterm birth (Blas, Canchihuaman, Alva, & Hawes, 2007).

Women younger than 25 years are five times more likely to have a chlamydial infection than are women older than 30 (Lin & Ramsey, 2008). Women with chlamydial infection may also be at high risk for acquiring HIV from an infected partner.

Because chlamydial infections are closely associated with gonorrhea, clinical differentiation may be difficult. Therefore, both infections are usually treated concurrently even without diagnostic evidence that both are present. The incubation period of 1 to 3 weeks for chlamydial infection is longer than that for gonorrhea. The incidence of recurrence may be high because of failure to treat the sexual partners of infected people. Table 55-6 lists the risk factors for chlamydial infection. Because of the high prevalence of asymptomatic infections, screening of populations at high risk is needed to identify those infected.

Clinical Manifestations and Complications

Chlamydial infection is known as a silent disease because symptoms may be absent or minor in most infected women and in many men; symptoms that do manifest in men are often milder than those of gonorrhea. Like gonorrhea, chlamydial infections result in a superficial mucosal infection that can become more invasive. Signs and symptoms in men include urethritis (dysuria,

Table 55-6 Risk Factors for Chlamydial Infection

• Female sex and age in teens
• New or multiple sex partners
• History of STIs, coexisting and cervical ectopy
• Early age at first sexual intercourse
• Inconsistent or incorrect use of barrier contraception (condoms, dental dams)
• Membership in a vulnerable populations (people who use injection drugs, incarcerated individuals, sex trade workers, street youth)
• Use of alcohol and drugs (indirect risk factors)

STIs, sexually transmitted infections.
Source: Faber, M., Nielsen, A., Nygard, M., Sparen, P., Tryggvadottie, L., Hansen, B., …, Kjaer, S. (2011). Genital chlamydia, genital herpes, trichomonas vaginalis and gonorrhea prevalence, and risk factors among nearly 70,000 randomly selected women in 4 Nordic countries. *Sexually Transmitted Diseases, 38*(8), 727-734. doi:10.1097/OLQ.0b013e318214bb9b

urethral discharge), epididymitis (unilateral scrotal pain, swelling, tenderness, fever), and proctitis (rectal discharge and pain during defecation). Signs and symptoms in women include cervicitis (mucopurulent discharge and hypertrophic ectopy [area that is edematous and bleeds easily]), urethritis (dysuria, frequent urination, and pyuria), bartholinitis (purulent exudate), PID (abdominal pain, nausea, vomiting, fever, malaise, abnormal vaginal bleeding, and menstrual abnormalities), and perihepatitis (fever, nausea, vomiting, and right upper quadrant pain).

Complications often develop when chlamydial infections are poorly managed, inaccurately diagnosed, or undiagnosed. The infection is often not diagnosed until complications appear. Rare complications for men generally result from epididymitis, with possible infertility and Reiter's disease (a systemic condition characterized by urethritis, conjunctivitis, arthritis, and mucocutaneous lesions; Trojian, Lishnak, & Heiman, 2009). Complications from chlamydial infections in women may result in PID, which can lead to chronic pelvic pain and infertility. For this reason, the PHAC's (2010) publication *Canadian Guidelines on Sexually Transmitted Infections* emphasizes the importance of screening all sexually active women younger than 25 years and all people (either sex, any age) who have risk factors for chlamydial infection (see Table 55-6). The guidelines also stress the value of repeat screening 6 months after treatment for chlamydial infection in view of the risk of reinfection.

Diagnostic Studies and Collaborative Care

Chlamydial infections in men can be diagnosed by ruling out gonorrhea. The cervical or urethral discharge appears to be less purulent, less watery, and less painful in chlamydial infections than in gonorrhea. Culture is the preferred method for medicolegal purposes, and culture is recommended for throat specimens (PHAC, 2010b). NAATs are more sensitive and specific than culture, enzyme immunoassay, and direct fluorescent antibody assay. For nonmedicolegal purposes, NAATs should be used whenever possible for urine and for urethral or cervical specimens.

Drug Therapy. When diagnosed, chlamydial infection can be easily treated and cured. Chlamydial infections respond to treatment with doxycycline (Vibramycin) or azithromycin (Zithromax; Toro, 2008). Alternative regimens include erythromycin. Follow-up care should include advising the patient to return if the symptoms persist or recur, treatment of sex partners, and encouraging the use of condoms during all sexual contacts.

Viral Infections

Genital Herpes

Genital herpes is not required to be reported in most provinces and territories (only in the Atlantic provinces); therefore, its true incidence is difficult to determine, and the PHAC must use U.S. statistics when stating the incidence of herpes. Genital herpes is considered one of the most common STIs in North America.

Approximately 1.6 million Americans are infected with genital herpesvirus each year (PHAC, 2010b), which indicates how widespread this infection is. Between 1976 and 1994, the prevalence of herpes simplex virus type 2 (HSV-2) infection has risen by 30% (PHAC, 2010b).

Etiology and Pathophysiology

Genital herpes is a sexually transmitted infection caused by the herpes simplex virus (HSV), usually type 2. The virus enters through the mucous membranes or breaks in the skin during contact with an infected person (Figure 55-7). HSV then reproduces inside the cell and spreads to the surrounding cells. The virus next enters the peripheral or autonomic nerve endings and ascends to the sensory or autonomic nerve ganglion, where it often becomes dormant. Viral reactivation (recurrence) may occur when the virus descends to the initial site of infection, either the mucous membranes or the skin. When a person is infected with HSV, the infection is usually chronic within the individual for life. Transmission occurs through direct contact with skin or mucous membrane or through asymptomatic viral shedding (Nikolic & Piguet, 2010).

Two different strains of HSV cause infection. In general, HSV type 1 (HSV-1) causes infection above the waist, involving the gingivae, the dermis, the upper respiratory tract, and the CNS. HSV-2 most frequently infects the genital tract and the perineum (i.e., locations below the waist). However, either strain can cause disease on the mouth or the genitals. The incidence and prevalence of HSV-1 genital infection are increasing globally, particularly among college students. The majority of genital herpes cases, however, are caused by HSV-2 infection (Anzivino et al., 2009).

Clinical Manifestations

In the primary (initial) episode of genital herpes, the patient may complain of a burning or tingling sensation at the site of inoculation. The painful vesicular lesions—which may appear on the penis, the scrotum, the vulva, the perineum, the perianal region, the vagina, or the cervix—contain large quantities of infectious viral particles (Figure 55-8). The lesions rupture and form shallow, moist ulcerations. Finally, crusting and epithelialization of the

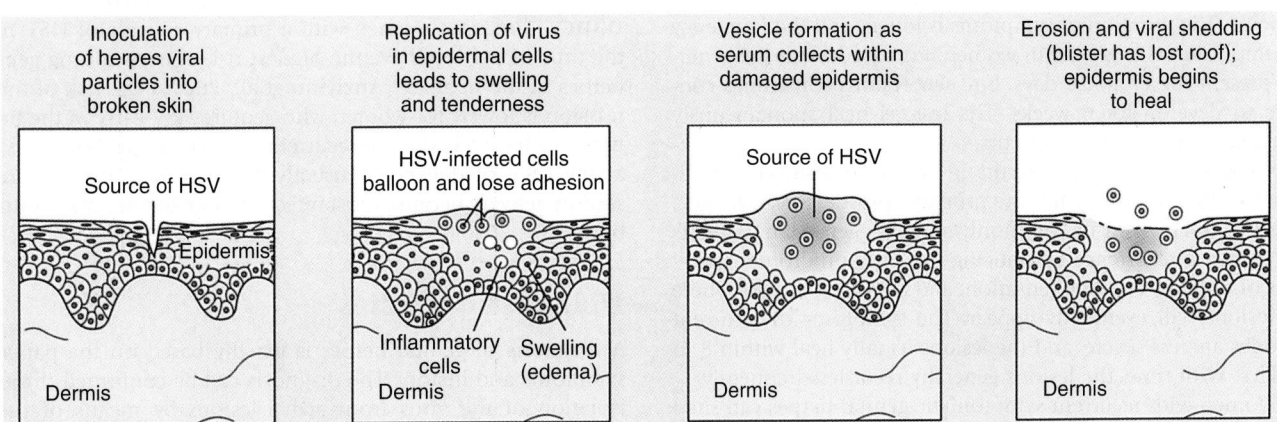

Figure 55-7 Stages of infection with herpes simplex virus (HSV).

Source: Morse, S., Moreland, A., & Holmes, K. (Eds.). (1996). *Atlas of sexually transmitted diseases and AIDS*. London: Mosby-Wolfe.

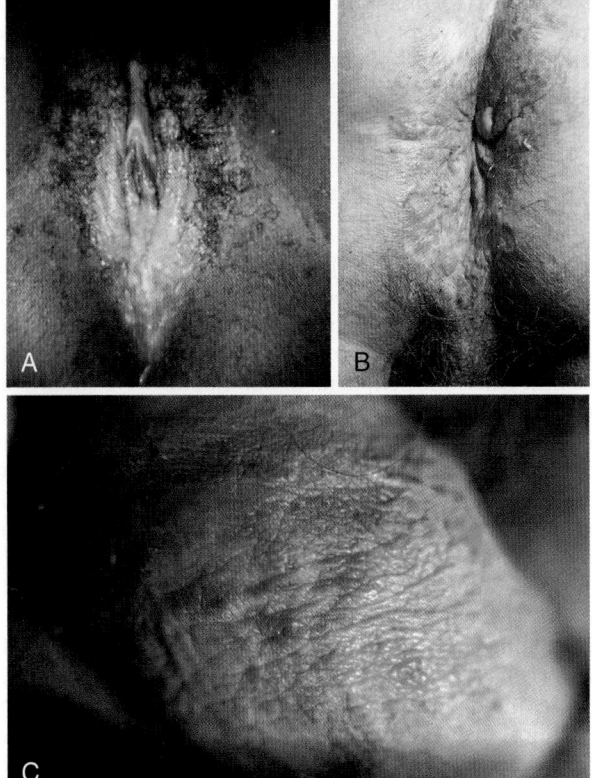

Figure 55-8 Unruptured vesicles of herpes simplex virus type 2 (HSV-2). **A,** Vulvar area. **B,** Perianal area. **C,** Penile herpes simplex, ulcerative stage.

Sources: **A** and **C,** From the Centers for Disease Control and Prevention; courtesy Susan Lindsley. **B,** From Morse, S., Moreland, A., & Holmes, K. (Eds.). (1996). *Atlas of sexually transmitted diseases and AIDS*, London: Mosby-Wolfe.

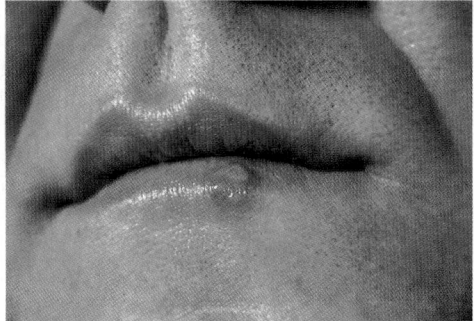

Figure 55-9 Autoinoculation of herpes simplex virus (HSV) to the lips.

Source: Centers for Disease Control and Prevention public image library. Retrieved from *http://phil.cdc.gov/phil/quicksearch.asp* (image #5434).

erosions occur. Primary infections tend to be associated with local inflammation and pain, accompanied by systemic manifestations such as fever, headache, malaise, myalgia, and regional lymphadenopathy.

Urination may be painful because the urine touches active lesions. Urinary retention may occur as a result of HSV urethritis or cystitis. A purulent vaginal discharge may develop with HSV cervicitis. The duration of symptoms is longer and the frequency of complications is greater in women. Primary lesions are generally present for 17 to 20 days, but new lesions sometimes continue to develop for 6 weeks. The lesions heal spontaneously unless secondary infection occurs.

Recurrent genital herpes occurs in about 50 to 80% of individuals during the year after the primary episode. Stress, fatigue, sunburn, and menses are commonly noted triggers. Many patients can predict a recurrence by noticing the early prodromal symptoms of tingling, burning sensation, and itching at the site where the lesions will eventually appear. The symptoms of recurrent episodes are less severe, and the lesions usually heal within 8 to 12 days. With time, the lesions generally recur less frequently.

Women with recurrent symptomatic genital herpes can shed the virus up to 1% of the time even when no visible lesions are present. Suppressive therapy with antiviral drugs has been shown to reduce the rate of transmission by 48% (PHAC, 2010b). Barrier forms of contraception, especially condoms, used during asymp-

tomatic periods may decrease transmission of the virus. When lesions are present, the patient should avoid sexual activity altogether because even barrier protection is not satisfactory in preventing disease transmission.

Complications

Although most infections are of a relatively benign nature, complications of genital herpes may involve the CNS, causing aseptic meningitis and lower motor neuron damage. Neuron damage may result in atonic bladder, erectile dysfunction, and constipation. Another complication is *autoinoculation* of the virus to extragenital sites such as the lips (Figure 55-9), the breasts, and, most commonly, the fingers (herpetic whitlow).

Herpes Simplex Virus–Related Keratitis. HSV infection of the eye usually resolves within 1 to 2 weeks, but it can progress, resulting in the development of ulcers. Symptoms include blurred vision, acute pain, and conjunctivitis with the possibility that recurrent attacks could result in scarring of the cornea and blindness (Toma et al., 2008). Primary treatment is topical antiviral agents, and the ulcer may need debridement. Corneal transplantation may be needed to replace an opacified cornea.

Herpes Simplex Virus Infection During Pregnancy. Pregnant women with a primary episode of HSV near the time of delivery have the highest risk of transmitting genital herpes to the neonate (Anzivino et al., 2009). The risk of transmission is lowest for women who acquire HSV early in the pregnancy or have a history of recurrent HSV. An active genital lesion at the time of delivery is usually an indication for Caesarean section delivery because most infections in neonates occur during birth.

Diagnostic Studies

A diagnosis of genital herpes is usually based on the patient's symptoms and history. The diagnosis can be confirmed through isolation of the virus from active lesions by means of tissue culture, and this is the most common method currently used in Canada (PHAC, 2010b). Polymerase chain reaction assay is four times more sensitive than HSV culture and is 100% specific; however, it has not yet replaced the culture for routine screening in Canada (PHAC, 2010b). Other techniques to detect HSV include direct immunofluorescence, enzyme immunoassay, and DNA amplification. These tests enable more rapid identification of HSV than does a culture. Highly accurate serological methods for detecting the HSV type are available. The Tzanck smear, because of its low specificity, is no longer considered a reliable test for the confirmation of diagnosis (PHAC, 2010b).

Collaborative Care

Drug Therapy. Three antiviral agents are available for the treatment of HSV: acyclovir (Zovirax), valacyclovir (Valtrex), and famciclovir (Famvir). These drugs inhibit herpetic viral replication and are prescribed for primary and recurrent infections (Table 55-7). Acyclovir, valacyclovir, and famciclovir are also used to suppress frequent recurrences (more than six episodes per year). Although not a cure, these drugs shorten the duration of viral shedding and the healing time of genital lesions and reduce

COLLABORATIVE CARE

Table 55-7 Genital Herpes

Diagnostic

- History and physical examination
- Viral isolation by tissue culture
- Antibody assay for specific HSV viral type

Collaborative Therapy

Treatment for First Episode

- For severe primary disease, IV acyclovir 5 mg/per kg over 60 min every 8 hours with later conversion to oral drug therapy
- Acyclovir (Zovirax) 200 mg PO five times daily for 5–10 days; or famciclovir (Famvir) 250 mg PO three times daily for 5 days; or valacyclovir (Valtrex) 1000 mg PO twice daily for 10 days; or acyclovir 400 mg PO three times daily for 7–10 days (recommended by Centers for Disease Control).

Treatment for Recurrent Episodes

- Valacyclovir 500 mg PO twice daily or 1 g daily for 3 days; or famciclovir 125 mg PO twice daily for 5 days; acyclovir 200 mg PO five times daily for 5 days or 800 mg PO three times daily for 2 days

Suppressive Therapy for Frequent Recurrence in Non-pregnant Patients

- Acyclovir 200 mg PO 3–5 times daily or 400 mg PO twice daily; or famciclovir 250 mg PO twice daily; or valacyclovir 500 mg PO daily (patients with ≤9 recurrences per year) or 1000 mg PO daily (patients with >9 recurrences per year)

Other Considerations

- Attempt to identify trigger mechanisms
- Yearly Pap smear
- Abstinence from sexual contact while lesions are present; however, virus may be shed without lesions
- Symptomatic care
- Confidential counselling and testing for HIV

Source: Modified from Public Health Agency of Canada. (2010). *Canadian guidelines on sexually transmitted infections.* Ottawa: Author. *HIV,* human immunodeficiency virus; *HSV,* herpes simplex virus; *IV,* intravenously; *Pap,* Papanicolaou; *PO,* by mouth (per os).

outbreaks by 75% (Centers for Disease Control and Prevention, 2010). Continued use of oral acyclovir as suppressive therapy for up to 6 years is safe and effective. Adverse reactions are mild and include headache, occasional nausea and vomiting, and diarrhea. The safety of these drugs for treatment of pregnant women has not been established. Acyclovir ointment appears to have no clinical benefit in the treatment of recurrent lesions, either in speed of healing or in resolution of pain, and is not commonly recommended. IV acyclovir is reserved for severe or life-threatening infections in which hospitalization is required for the treatment of disseminated infections, CNS infections (meningitis), or pneumonitis. Nephrotoxicity has been observed with high-dose IV administration.

Symptomatic Care. Symptomatic treatment such as good genital hygiene and the wearing of loose-fitting cotton undergarments should be encouraged. The lesions should be kept clean and dry. To ensure complete drying of the perineal area, women may use a hair dryer set at a cool setting. Frequent sitz baths may soothe the area and reduce inflammation. Drying agents such as colloidal oatmeal (Aveeno) and aluminum salts (Burow's solution) may provide some relief from the burning sensation and itching. Techniques to reduce pain on urination include pouring a pitcher of water onto the perineal area while voiding to dilute the urine, and voiding in a warm tub of water or shower. Pain may require a local anaesthetic such as lidocaine (Xylocaine) or systemic analgesics such as codeine and aspirin. Sexual transmission of HSV has been documented during asymptomatic periods, and the use of barrier methods, especially condoms, should be encouraged.

Genital Human Papillomavirus Infections

Human papillomavirus (HPV) causes skin and mucosal infections and has a strong affinity for the moist mucosa of the anal, genital, and aerodigestive tracts. There are more than 130 types of the virus; 13 high-risk HPV types were confirmed in the International Agency for Research on Cancer monograph on human papillomaviruses (IARC, 2007) as necessary factors in the etiology of cervical cancer, whereas other HPV types have been implicated in skin and oral-pharyngeal cancers, as well as with cancers of the anus and penis (PHAC, 2010b). Most types do not cause any symptoms and go away on their own. The most common low-risk genotypes are 6 and 11, which cause condylomata acuminata (genital warts), and the most common high-risk genotypes are 16 and 18, predisposing to precancerous or cancerous lesions (PHAC, 2010b). HPV infection is a highly contagious STI frequently observed in young, sexually active adults and is the most common viral STI. Risk factors include young age, less education, less vegetable consumption, more sexual partners, young age at first sexual experience, more pregnancies, and high alcohol consumption (Bell et al., 2011). Of the adult population in Canada, 70% have at least one genital HPV infection over their lifetime (PHAC, 2010b).

Minor trauma during intercourse can cause abrasions that allow HPV to enter the body. The incubation period of the virus is generally 3 to 4 months but may be longer. Prevention is hampered by a high proportion of asymptomatic infections and lack of curative treatment. In Canada, the reporting of HPV infection is not required.

Clinical Manifestations and Complications

The discussion of clinical manifestations, complications, and care focuses on the low-risk HPV genotypes resulting in genital warts; cervical cancer is discussed in Chapter 56. Genital warts are discrete single or multiple papillary growths that are white to grey and flesh-pink. They may grow and coalesce to form large, cauliflower-like masses. Most affected patients have from 1 to 10 genital warts. In men, the warts may occur on the penis and the scrotum, around the anus, or in the urethra. In women, the warts may be located on the vulva, the vagina, or the cervix and in the perianal area (Figure 55-10). There are usually no other signs or symptoms. Itching may occur with anogenital warts. Bleeding on defecation may occur with anal warts.

During pregnancy, genital warts tend to grow rapidly and increase in size (Hollier & Workowski, 2008). An infected mother may transmit the condition to her newborn (Nigam & Mishra, 2011). Caesarean delivery is not routinely indicated unless the birth canal becomes blocked by massive warts.

Diagnostic Studies and Collaborative Care

Genital warts can be diagnosed on the basis of the gross appearance of the lesions. However, the warts may be confused with condylomata lata of secondary syphilis, carcinoma, or benign neoplasms. The HPV DNA test is recommended with women who have abnormal Papanicolaou (Pap) test results (PHAC, 2010b). The HPV DNA test can identify women who are infected with the high-risk HPV strains (types 16 and 18) associated with cervical cancer. At present, access to HPV DNA tests in Canada is limited to a small number of jurisdictions, and HPV cannot be confirmed by culture (PHAC, 2010b).

The primary goal in treating visible genital warts is the removal of symptomatic warts. The removal may or may not decrease infectivity. Genital warts are difficult to treat and often necessitate multiple office visits with a variety of treatment modalities. The therapy should be modified if a patient has not experienced improvement after three treatments or if after six treatments the warts have not completely disappeared. Treatment consists of chemical or ablative (removal with laser or electrocautery) methods. One common treatment is the use of 50 to 80% trichloroacetic acid (TCA) or bichloroacetic acid (BCA) solutions

in 70% alcohol, applied directly to the wart surface. Petroleum jelly is applied to the surrounding normal skin to minimize irritation before a small amount of TCA is applied to the wart with a cotton swab. A sharp stinging pain is often felt with initial acid contact, but this quickly subsides. TCA is not washed off after treatment and is safe for use during pregnancy.

Podophyllin resin (10 to 25%), a cytotoxic agent, is recommended therapy for small external genital warts (Hollier & Workowski, 2008). When podophyllin is used, it is applied carefully to each wart, with normal tissue being avoided, and is then thoroughly washed off in 1 to 4 hours. This substance encourages the sloughing off of skin containing viral particles. Podophyllin produces toxic symptoms that can be local (e.g., pain, burning sensation) or systemic (e.g., nausea, dizziness, leukopenia, respiratory distress). Its use is contraindicated in pregnant women. In general, warts located on moist surfaces respond better to topical treatment (e.g., TCA, podophyllin) than do warts on drier surfaces.

Patient-managed treatment is also an option. Podofilox gel is available by prescription (Condylox and Condylox Gel). The patient applies the gel every 12 hours for 3 successive days, followed by 4 days of no treatment. Treatment can be repeated for up to 6 weeks or until the lesions resolve. Imiquimod cream (Aldara) is an immune-response modifier that is applied three times a week (usually at bedtime) for up to 16 weeks; it should be washed off after 6 to 8 hours. None of these treatments is recommended for use during pregnancy or lactation.

If the warts do not regress with any of these therapies, treatments such as cryotherapy, electrocautery, laser therapy, and surgical excision may be indicated (PHAC, 2010b). Because treatment does not destroy the virus, merely the infected tissue, recurrences and reinfection are possible, and careful long-term follow-up is advised.

Human Papillomavirus Immunization

HPV infection has been linked to cervical and vulvar cancer in women and to anorectal and squamous cell carcinoma of the penis in men. HPV types 16 and 18 cause approximately 70% of cervical cancers, and types 6 and 11 cause approximately 90% of anogenital warts (PHAC, 2010b). Vaccines available to protect against HPV types 6, 11, 16, and 18 (Gardasil) and HPV types 16

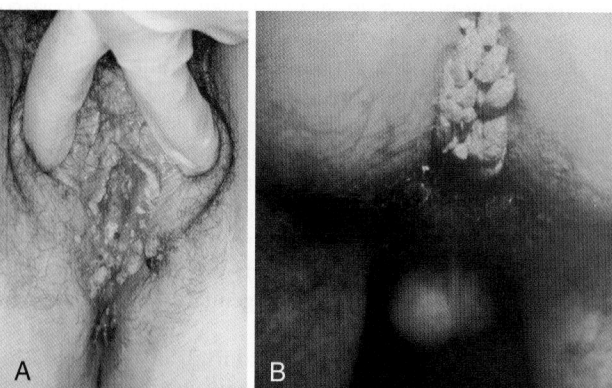
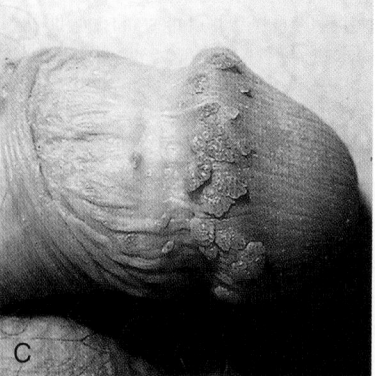

Figure 55-10 Genital warts. **A,** Severe vulvular warts. **B,** Perineal wart. **C,** Multiple genital warts of the glans penis.

and 18 (Cervarix) have been approved for use in Canada in female patients aged 9 to 26 years. Gardasil is also recommended for male patients aged 9 to 26 years. HPV vaccination of male patients helps prevent future genital warts or anal cancer and potentially reduce the spread of HPV from men to women (Centers for Disease Control and Prevention, 2010). Giuliano and colleagues (2011) studied the efficacy of the HPV vaccine in men and suggest that the vaccine's rates of efficacy may be similar for both sexes. They concluded that quadrivalent HPV vaccine prevents infection with HPV types 6, 11, 16, and 18 and the development of related external genital lesions in boys and men 16 to 26 years of age. Because of reported cases of syncope during vaccine administration, the patient should remain seated or lying down and be closely observed for 15 minutes after vaccination. These vaccines do not treat active HPV infections. Ideally, they should be administered before the start of sexual activity, but people who are sexually active, as well as those infected, would still obtain protection from the HPV types not already acquired.

NURSING MANAGEMENT: SEXUALLY TRANSMITTED INFECTIONS

▪ Nursing Assessment

Subjective and objective data that should be obtained from a person with an STI are presented in Table 55-8.

▪ Nursing Diagnoses

Nursing diagnoses for the patient with an STI include, but are not limited to, the following:
- Risk for infection *related to* lack of knowledge about mode of transmission, inadequate personal and genital hygiene, and failure to practise precautionary measures
- Anxiety *related to* effect of condition on relationships, disease outcome, and lack of knowledge of disease
- Ineffective health maintenance *related to* lack of knowledge about disease process, appropriate follow-up measures, and possibility of reinfection

▪ Planning

The overall goals are that the patient with an STI will (a) demonstrate understanding of the mode of transmission of STIs and the risk posed by STIs, (b) complete treatment and return for appropriate follow-up, (c) notify or assist in notification of sexual contacts about their need for testing and treatment, (d) abstain from intercourse until infection is resolved, and (e) demonstrate knowledge of safer sex practices.

▪ Nursing Implementation

▪ Health Promotion

Many approaches to curtailing the spread of STIs have been advocated and have met with varying degrees of success. Nurses should

NURSING ASSESSMENT

Table 55-8 Sexually Transmitted Infections

Subjective Data

Important Health Information

Past health history: Contact with individuals with STIs, multiple sexual partners, pregnancy, shared needles during IV drug use, previous vaccination against HPV.

Medications: Use of oral contraceptives; allergy to any antibiotics, especially penicillin

Symptoms
- Malaise; chills
- Nausea, vomiting, anorexia, pharyngitis, oral lesions
- Itching at infected site; lesions that cause pain or burning sensation
- Dysuria, urinary frequency, retention; urethral discharge; tenesmus, proctitis
- Arthralgia, headache
- Dyspareunia; vaginal discharge, menstrual abnormalities; presence of genital or perianal lesions
- Alopecia

Objective Data

General

Fever, lymphadenopathy (generalized or inguinal)

Integumentary
- Syphilis:
  - Primary: painless, indurated genital, oral, or perianal lesions
  - Secondary: bilateral, symmetrical rash on palms, soles, or entire body; mucous patches on mouth or tongue; alopecia
- Genital herpes: Painful genital or anal vesicular lesions
- Genital warts: Single or multiple grey or white genital or anal warts (possibly becoming massive)

Gastrointestinal

Purulent rectal discharge (indicator of gonorrhea), rectal lesions, proctitis

Urinary

Urethral discharge, erythema

Reproductive

Cervical discharge, lesions, inflamed Bartholin's glands

Possible Findings
- *Gonorrhea:* Positive Gram stain, smears, cultures, and DNA amplification for *Neisseria gonorrhoeae*
- *Syphilis:* Positive findings on VDRL and RPR tests, spirochetes observed on dark-field microscopic examination
- *Chlamydial infection:* Positive culture or DNA amplification for *Chlamydia* organisms
- *Genital herpes:* Positive tissue culture for HSV-2; positive anti–HSV-2 antibody titre

HPV, human papillomavirus; *HSV-2,* herpes simplex virus type 2; *IV,* intravenous; *RPR,* rapid plasma reagin; *STI,* sexually transmitted infection; *VDRL,* Venereal Disease Research Laboratory.

Table 55-9 Sexually Transmitted Infections

1. Instruct patient in hygienic measures, such as washing and urinating after intercourse to flush out some of the causative organisms.

2. Explain the importance of taking all antibiotics as prescribed. Symptoms improve after 1 to 2 days of therapy, but organisms may still be present.

3. Teach patient about the need for treatment of sexual partners with antibiotics to prevent transmission of disease.

4. Instruct patient to abstain from sexual intercourse during treatment and to use condoms when sexual activity is resumed, to prevent spread of infection and prevent reinfection.

5. Explain the importance of follow-up examination and repeated culture at least once after treatment if appropriate, to confirm complete cure and prevent relapse.

6. Allow patient and partner to verbalize concerns to clarify areas that need explanation.

7. Instruct patient about symptoms of complications and need to report problems to ensure proper follow-up and early treatment of reinfection.

8. Explain precautions to take, such as being monogamous; asking potential partners about sexual history; avoiding sex with partners who use intravenous drugs or who have visible oral, inguinal, genital, perineal, or anal lesions; using male or female condoms or dental dams; and voiding and washing genitalia after intercourse to reduce the occurrence of reinfection.

9. Inform patient regarding state of infectivity to prevent a false sense of security, which might result in careless sexual practices and poor personal hygiene.

10. Provide information related to HPV vaccination.

be prepared to discuss practices with all patients, not only those who are perceived to be at risk. These practices include abstinence, monogamy with an uninfected partner, avoidance of certain high-risk sexual practices, and use of barriers (e.g., dental dams, condoms) to limit contact with potentially infectious body fluids or lesions. Sexual abstinence is a certain method of avoiding all STIs, but few adults consider this a feasible alternative to sexual expression. Limiting sexual intimacies outside of a well-established monogamous relationship can reduce the risk of contracting an STI. A patient and caregiver teaching guide related to the patient with an STI is presented in Table 55-9.

All sexually active women should be screened for cervical cancer. Women with a history of STIs are at greater risk for cervical cancer than are women without this history. Pap smears are discussed in Chapter 56.

■ **Measures to Prevent Infection.** An inspection of the sexual partner's genitals before coitus is recommended. The presence of discharge, sores, blisters, or rash should be viewed with concern. A patient who is aware of specific signs and symptoms of infection can intelligently make the decision to continue the sexual interaction with modifications or elect not to have sexual relations. The patient should remember that, when engaging in sex, there is exposure to the infections of everyone with whom the partner has ever had sex. Men should be told that some protection is provided if they void immediately after intercourse and wash their genitalia and the adjacent areas with soap and water.

Women may also benefit from postcoital voiding and washing. However, emphasize that this does not provide adequate protection against STIs after exposure to infection.

Spermicidal jellies and creams have a mild detergent effect that may reduce the risk of contracting STIs, but this has not been proved. These same barriers can serve as supplementary lubrication, thereby decreasing irritation and friction and chances for development of a minor laceration that could serve as an entry point for the organism. A latex condom, when used properly, is a highly effective mechanical barrier to infection (see Evidence-Informed Practice box, "What Is the Effectiveness of Condom Promotion Interventions?"). The condom should be undamaged and correctly in place throughout all phases of sexual activity. A deterrent to condom usage is alcohol and drug use (Gerbi, Habtemariam, Tameru, Nganwa, & Robnett, 2009). Use of barrier contraceptives requires planning and motivation, both of which are impaired with alcohol or drug ingestion. The patient should be given specific verbal and written instructions on the proper use of condoms (see Chapter 17, eFigure 17-1 and Table 17-19). The objections to condom usage, such as interference with spontaneity and the presence of a barrier, should be discussed by the partners. Information about the mechanics of sexual arousal and incorporating the use of a condom into lovemaking can help in overcoming patient or partner resistance to its use. Female condoms are lubricated polyurethane sheaths with a ring at each end designed for vaginal use (see Chapter 17, eFigure 17-2 and Table 17-20).

Sexual contact with people known or suspected to have HIV infection should be avoided (see Chapter 17). Among couples with one infected partner, consistent and scrupulous barrier use can reduce transmission to the uninfected partner. Sexually active individuals can reduce risk by minimizing the number of sexual contacts. Unprotected anal intercourse and other high-risk behaviours should be eliminated, and condoms should be used if sexual contact continues.

Initiate a discussion to assess the patient's risk for contracting an STI. Questions to ask include number of partners, type of birth control used, use of condoms and dental dams, use of intravenous drugs, history of STIs, and sexual preference. Patient education can be planned on the basis of the response to these questions. Interpersonal skills necessary for this interview include respect, compassion, and a nonjudgemental attitude. Counselling should be tailored to the individual patient. The nurse should not assume that older people are not at risk, inasmuch as an increasing number of older people are acquiring STIs.

■ **Screening Programs.** Screening programs that are used to identify infected patients can also help prevent certain STIs. For many years, there have been various screening programs to find cases of syphilis. With the increase of infection rates across Canada, more stringent screening and follow-up treatment are required. Many institutions offer voluntary prenatal HIV and syphilis testing and counselling for pregnant women.

Screening programs have also been developed and implemented for detection of gonorrhea and chlamydial infection. These programs are targeted to women because women are more likely to have asymptomatic gonorrhea and thereby serve as sources of infection. Gonorrheal and chlamydial testing during pelvic examinations and prenatal visits is becoming a major routine part of these programs. Mass application of screening programs for genital chlamydial infections, genital herpes, and HPV infections may also be possible with the advent of rapid, cost-effective tests.

What Is the Effectiveness of Condom Promotion Interventions?

Clinical Question

In sexually active men and women (P), are condom promotion interventions (I) as opposed to no promotion interventions (C) effective in reducing the number of unwanted pregnancies and STIs (O)?

Best Available Evidence

Systematic review of randomized controlled trials (RCTs)

Critical Appraisal and Synthesis of Evidence

- In 139 RCTs (n = 143,000), 181 different interventions were evaluated.
- Of the interventions, 156 involved sexual behaviour change, 19 involved sexual and intravenous drug behavioural change, and 6 involved condom design.
- Despite the public health importance of increasing condom use, there is little reliable evidence for the effectiveness of condom promotion interventions.
- Because of the low proportion of trials using the same outcome, the potential for bias from selective reporting of outcomes is considerable.

Conclusions

Reported results in the trials in this review are generally consistent with modest benefits. However, reporting for trials promoting effective condom use must be agreed upon, and consensus regarding which outcomes should be reported must be reached.

Implications for Nursing Practice

- Educate patients about proper condom use.
- Explore innovative alternative means of distributing condoms because condom distribution proximal to the time of sex has been shown to increase condom use.
- Conduct RCTs of the female reality condom for anal sex because results from a low-quality trial suggested that the female reality condom may be less likely to slip than a standard condom.

Reference for Evidence

Free, C., Roberts, I., Abramsky, T., Fitzgerald, M., & Wensley, F. (2011). A systematic review of randomised controlled trials of interventions promoting effective condom use. *Journal of Epidemiology in Community Health*, *65*, 100-110. doi:10.1136/jech.2008.085456

P, patient population of interest; *I*, intervention or area of interest; *C*, comparison of interest or comparison group; *O*, outcome of interest.

Confidentiality

Situation

A nurse in a clinic gives the positive results of a test for *Chlamydia* infection to a patient and advises her to tell her sexual partners that she has this infection. The patient refuses to tell her boyfriend because he will then know that she has had sex with another partner. Should the nurse contact the boyfriend?

Important Points for Consideration

- Nurses and other health care providers have both a legal and an ethical obligation to maintain confidentiality of patient information. If confidentiality is violated, trust is eroded and patients may not share privileged information that is essential to plan effective care.
- Health care providers have an obligation to maintain confidentiality unless there is a risk to the health or life of innocent third parties. Each province and territory has requirements for reporting communicable infections and other health-related data.
- The nurse's primary obligation is to the patient seeking care. However, there are long-term health consequences for this patient, as well as the public in general.
- Patient teaching is one way to establish a partnership with this woman. Information should be shared about the effects of the infection being untreated, the risks and consequences of re-infection, and the results that the infection may have on others who may not know they are infected. The patient can then be encouraged to inform her partners of the diagnosis for the good of everyone.

Clinical Decision-Making Questions

1. What are your provincial or territorial requirements for reportable conditions?
2. What information would you share with this patient regarding the transmission of chlamydial infection so that she may be more willing to discuss the results with her boyfriend?
3. In your opinion, what is the best way to balance the needs of an individual patient with those of the general public?

contacts are often not informed about the origin of the information naming them as a contact, so that greater cooperation and privacy is ensured. (See the Ethical Dilemmas box on patient confidentiality.)

▌ **Educational and Research Programs.** Nurses can actively encourage their communities to provide better education about STIs for their citizens. Teenagers, who are known to have a high incidence of infection, should be a prime target for such educational programs. STI rates are on the rise among older adults; they are less likely to use condoms and, in general, have a more difficult time engaging in a discussion of sexual health issues (Bodley-Tickell et al., 2008). Hotline services, reliable Internet sites, school nurses, nurse practitioners, nurse midwives, and outreach programs sponsored by Canada's Health Protection Branch are effective. The PHAC (2010b) has published the *Canadian Guidelines for Sexual Health Education* to provide education and support. These guidelines are available online (see the

▌ **Case Finding.** Interviewing and case finding are other processes used to control STIs. These activities are directed toward locating and examining all contacts of each known patient with an STI as soon after sexual exposure as possible so that effective treatment can be initiated. Trained interviewers may often find cases even if they are supplied with only limited information. The caseworkers, who are often nurses, are aware of the social implications of these diseases and the need for discretion. Sexual

Resources at the end of this chapter). Obtaining a highly effective HPV vaccine that protects against cervical cancer and genital warts should be encouraged before the start of sexual activity.

Knowledge and understanding can decrease the STI epidemic. Efforts are being made to develop vaccines for syphilis, gonorrhea, genital herpes, and HIV. The development of effective vaccines is viewed by many clinicians as a prerequisite for eradication of STIs.

Harm Reduction.
Behavioural interventions to promote condom use, to modify HIV sexual risk behaviours, or both include individual counselling, skills training, coping strategies, peer education, and social and educational support (Carvalho et al., 2011). For these interventions to achieve a reduction in STIs in the population, they must reach a broad sector of the community, be of sufficient intensity, and occur in supportive social environments and contexts (Wohlfeiler & Ellen, 2010). For individuals identified as being at ongoing risk for STIs, screening is recommended at 3-month intervals for HIV, gonorrhea, syphilis, and chlamydial infection. Ongoing contact with a health care provider is an opportunity for reinforcement of safer sex practices. Interventions to promote safer sex, testing, counselling, and education, as well as health care workers' awareness, should be integrated in harm-reduction programs and health care settings to prevent STIs and reduce HIV transmission (Coffin et al., 2010). Canada has an annual Sexual and Reproductive Health Day, which occurs in February (see the Resources at the end of this chapter).

Acute Intervention

Psychological Support.
The diagnosis of an STI may be met with a variety of emotions, such as shame, guilt, anger, and a desire for vengeance. The nurse should provide counselling and try to help the patient verbalize feelings. Couples in marital or committed relationships are confronted with an added problem when an STI is diagnosed. The implication of sexual activity by one of the partners with a person outside the relationship might have to be faced; however, because some of the STIs have long latency periods, this may not be an issue. Support and counselling for the couple are needed.

A patient who has genital herpes is faced with the fact that infections can recur and that no cure is available. This can be frustrating and disruptive to the patient's physical, emotional, social, and sexual life. Helping the patient identify and avoid any factors that may precipitate the condition is indicated. Inform the patient that the incidence and severity of recurrences will decrease over time.

HPV infections involve a prolonged course of treatment. The patient can become frustrated and distressed because of frequent office visits, associated costs, potential for unpleasant adverse effects as a result of treatment, and effects of the infection on future health and sexual relationships. Tremendous support and a willingness to listen to the patient's concerns are needed. Support groups are also available.

Follow-Up.
A nurse working in public health facilities, clinics, or other outpatient settings may care for patients with STIs more often than a nurse in a hospital. This nurse is in a position to explain and interpret treatment measures such as the purpose and possible adverse effects of prescribed drugs and the need for follow-up care.

Single-dose treatment for gonococcal, chlamydial, and syphilitic infections frequently helps prevent the problems associated with nonadherence to drug therapy. Patients who require multiple-dose therapy should be given special instructions in completing the prescribed regimen and should be informed about problems resulting from nonadherence. All patients should return to the treatment centre for a repeat culture from the infected sites or for serological testing at designated times to determine the effectiveness of the treatment. Explaining to the patient that cures are not always obtained on the first treatment can reinforce the need for a follow-up visit. The patient should also be advised to inform sexual partners of the need for testing and treatment, regardless of whether they are free of symptoms or are experiencing symptoms.

Hygiene Measures.
The nurse must emphasize certain hygiene measures to patients with an STI. An important measure is frequent handwashing and bathing. Bathing and cleaning of the involved areas can provide local comfort and prevent secondary infection. Douching may spread the infection or undermine local immune responses and is therefore contraindicated. The synthetic materials used in most undergarments frequently increase or exacerbate local irritations by trapping moisture. Cotton undergarments provide better absorption and are cooler and more comfortable for the patient with an STI.

Sexual Activity.
Sexual abstinence is indicated during the communicable phase of the disease. If sexual activity occurs before treatment of the patient has been completed, the use of condoms may prevent the spread of infection and reinfection. Condom usage after treatment should be encouraged to prevent future exposure to infection. The patient can also choose to relate to a partner in an intimate way that avoids both coitus and oral–genital contact. It is important to note that even single-dose treatments can take up to 1 week to be effective and that the patient's condition is thus infectious during this period.

Ambulatory and Home Care

Because many STIs are cured with a single dose or short course of antibiotic therapy, many people are casual about the outcome of these diseases. The consequences of this attitude can include delays in treatment, nonadherence to instructions, and subsequent development of complications. The complications are serious and costly; they can result in disfigurement and destruction of important tissues and organs.

Surgery and prolonged therapy are indicated for many patients with disease-related complications. Major surgical procedures such as resection of an aneurysm or aortic valve replacement may be necessary to treat cardiovascular problems caused by syphilis. Pelvic surgery and procedures to correct fertility problems secondary to an STI may include lysis of adhesions, dilation of strictures, reconstructive tuboplasty, and in vitro fertilization.

Evaluation

The following are expected outcomes for a patient with an STI:
- The patient will describe modes of transmission.
- The patient will use appropriate hygienic measures.
- The patient will experience no reinfection.
- The patient will demonstrate adherence to a follow-up protocol.

CLINICAL DECISION-MAKING EXERCISE

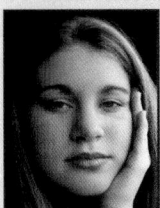

CASE STUDY:
Chlamydial Infection and Gonorrhea

Source: © iStockphoto.com/Roberta Osborne.

Patient Profile

Jade Krycek is a 17-year-old girl who visits the outpatient Teen Clinic seeking birth control pills. She had sexual intercourse for the first time 8 weeks ago.

Subjective Data

- Did not use condom or spermicide
- Has not asked boyfriend about his sexual practices
- Last menstrual period was 2 weeks ago
- Denies any symptoms
- Interested in using birth control
- Very nervous

Objective Data

- Cervical ectopy noted during Pap test
- Mucopurulent cervical discharge
- Tests for *Chlamydia* and gonococci: positive results
- Urine pregnancy test: negative result
- Patient crying and very upset when informed of positive test results

Collaborative Care

- Doxycycline, 100 mg PO twice a day for 7 days
- Ceftriaxone, 250 mg intramuscularly once

Discussion Questions

1. What were Ms. Krycek's risk factors for acquiring chlamydial and gonococcal infections?
2. What complications could have occurred if Ms. Krycek's infection had not been detected?
3. What effect is the diagnosis likely to have on Ms. Krycek's self-image? On her relationship with her sexual partner?
4. What instructions should Ms. Krycek receive to ensure successful treatment? To prevent reinfection? To prevent further transmission of the infection?
5. *Priority Decision:* What are the priority nursing interventions for Ms. Krycek?
6. *Priority Decision:* On the basis of the assessment data presented, what are the priority nursing diagnoses? Are there any collaborative problems?

evolve *Answers are available at* **http://evolve.elsevier.com/ Canada/Lewis/medsurg**

REVIEW QUESTIONS

The number of the question corresponds to the same-numbered objective at the beginning of the chapter.

1. Which of the following women has the lowest risk for sexually transmitted pelvic inflammatory disease?
   a. Woman who uses oral contraceptives
   b. Woman who uses barrier methods of contraception
   c. Woman who uses an intrauterine device for contraception
   d. Woman who uses a Norplant implant or injectable Depo-Provera for contraception

2. To help in obtaining subjective assessment data from a woman reported as a sexual contact of a man with chlamydial infection, which of the following does the nurse keep in mind about the symptoms of chlamydial infections in women?
   a. They are frequently absent.
   b. They mimic those of genital herpes.
   c. They include a macular palmar rash in later stages.
   d. They may involve chancres hidden inside the vagina.

3. What is the difference between a primary HSV infection and recurrent episodes?
   a. Primary infection is of shorter duration than recurrent episodes.
   b. Only primary infections are sexually transmissible.
   c. In primary infections, systemic manifestations such as fever and myalgia are more common.
   d. Transmission of the virus to a fetus is less likely during primary infection.

4. Why should the nurse explain to a patient with gonorrhea that treatment will include both ceftriaxone and doxycycline?
   a. Most patients do not respond to ceftriaxone alone.
   b. Coverage with more than one antibiotic prevents reinfection.
   c. No single agent successfully eradicates all strains of gonorrhea.
   d. The high rate of coexisting chlamydial infection and gonorrhea indicates dual coverage.

5. Which STI is most likely to include a nursing diagnosis of disturbed body image that hinders future sexual relationships?
   a. Syphilis
   b. Gonorrhea
   c. Genital warts
   d. Chlamydial infection
6. Teaching by the nurse to prevent infection and transmission of STIs includes explanations of which of the following?
   a. The appropriate use of birth control pills
   b. Sexual positions that can be used to avoid infection
   c. Sexual practices that are considered high-risk behaviours
   d. The necessity of annual Pap smears for patients with HPV

7. Which of the following is an appropriate nursing intervention to provide emotional support to a patient with an STI?
   a. Use concerned listening when the patient expresses negative feelings.
   b. Reassure the patient that the disease is curable with appropriate treatment.
   c. Offer information on how safe sexual practices can prevent STIs.
   d. Help the patient who received the STI from his or her sexual partner in forgiving the partner.

ANSWERS: 1. b; 2. a; 3. c; 4. d; 5. c; 6. c; 7. a.

REFERENCES

Anzivino, E., Fioriti, D., Mischetelli, M., Bellizzi, A., Barucca, V., Chiarini, F., & Pietropaolo, V. (2009). Herpes simplex virus infection in pregnancy and in neonate: Status of art epidemiology, diagnosis, therapy and prevention. *Virology Journal, 6*, 40. doi:10.1186/1743-422X-6-40

Bell, M., Schmidt-Grimminger, D., Jacobsen, C., Chauhan, S., Maher, D., & Buchwald, D. (2011). Risk factors for HPV infection among American Indian and white women in the Northern Plains. *Gynecologic Oncology, 121*(3), 532-536. doi:10.1016/j.ygyno.2011.02.032

Bender, N., Hermann, B., Anderson, B., Hocking, J. S., vanBergen, J., Morgan, J., ..., & Low, N. (2011). *Chlamydia* infection, pelvic inflammatory disease, ectopic pregnancy and infertility: A cross national study. *Sexually Transmitted Infections, 87*(7), 601-608. doi:10.1136/sextrans-2011-050205

Blas, M. M., Canchihuaman, F. A., Alva, I. E., & Hawes, S. E. (2007). Pregnancy outcomes in women infected with *Chlamydia trachomatis*: A population-based cohort study in Washington State. *Sexually Transmitted Infections, 83*(4):314-318. doi:10.1136/sti.2006.022665

Bodley-Tickell, A. T., Olowokure, B., Bhaduri, S., White, D. J., Ward, D., Ross, J., ..., Goold, P. (2008). Trends in sexually transmitted infections (other than HIV) in older people: Analysis of data from an enhanced surveillance system. *Sexually Transmitted Infections, 84*, 312-317. doi:10.1136/sti.2007.027847

Carvalho, F., Goncalves, T., Faria, E., Shoveller, J., Piccinini, C., Ramos, M., & Medeiros, L. (2011). Behavioural interventions to promote condom use among women living with HIV. *Cochrane Database of Systematic Reviews 2011, 9*, CD007844. doi:10.1002é14651858.CD007844.pub2

Centers for Disease Control and Prevention. (2010). Sexually transmitted diseases treatment guidelines. *Morbidity and Mortality Weekly Report (MMWR), 59*(RR-12), 1-126. Retrieved from http://www.cdc.gov/STD/treatment/2010/STD-Treatment-2010-RR5912.pdf

Coffin, L., Newberry, A., Hagan, H., Cleland, C., Des Jarlais, D., & Perlman, D. (2010). Syphilis in drug users in low and middle income countries. *International Journal of Drug Policy, 21*(1), 20-27. doi:10.1016/j.drugpo.2009.02.008

Domantay-Apostol, G., Handog, E., & Gabriel, T. (2008). Syphilis: The international challenge of the great imitator. *Dermatology Clinics, 24*, 889-905. doi:10.1016/j.det.2007.12.001

Fang, L., Oliver, A., Jayaraman, G., & Wong, T. (2010). Trends in age disparities between younger and middle-age adults among reported rates of chlamydia, gonorrhoea and infectious syphilis infections in Canada: Findings from 1997 to 2007. *Sexually Transmitted Diseases, 37*(1), 18-25. doi:10.1097/OLQ.0b013e3181b617dc

Ferrando, S., & Freyberg, Z. (2008). Neuropsychiatric aspects of infectious diseases. *Critical Care Clinics, 24*(4), 889-919. doi:10.1016/j.ccc.2008.05.007

Frenkel, T., & Potts, J. (2008). Sexually transmitted infections. *Urologic Clinics of North America, 35*, 33-41. doi:10.1016/j.ucl.2007.09.003

Gerbi, G., Habtemariam, T., Tameru, B., Nganwa, D., & Robnett, V. (2009). The correlation between alcohol consumption and risky sexual behaviours among people living with HIV/AIDS. *Journal of Substance Use, 14*(2), 90-100. doi:10.1080/14659890802624261

Giuliano, A. R., Palefsky, J. M., Goldstone, S., Moreira, E. D., Penny, M. E., Aranda, C., ..., Guris, D. (2011). Efficacy of quadrivalent HPV vaccine against HPV infection and disease in males. *New England Journal of Medicine, 364*(5), 401-411. doi:10.1056/NEJMoa0909537

Hollier, L. M., & Workowski, K. (2008). Treatment of sexually transmitted infections in women. *Infectious Diseases Clinics of North America, 22*, 665-691. doi:10.1016/j.idc.2008.05.009

International Agency of Research on Cancer. (2007). IARC Monographs on the Evaluation of Carcinogenic Risks to Humans, Volume 90: *Human Papillomaviruses*. Retrieved from http://monographs.iarc.fr/ENG/Monographs/vol90/index.php

Lin, K. W., & Ramsey, L. (2008). Screening for chlamydial infection. *American Family Physician, 78*, 1349-1354.

Lin, L., Zheng, W., Tong, M., Fu, Z., Liu, G., Fu, J., ..., Yang, T. (2011). Further evaluation of the characteristics of *Treponema pallidum*–specific IgM antibody in syphilis serofast reaction patients. *Diagnostic Microbiology and Infectious Disease, 71*(3), 201-207. doi:10.1016/j.diagmicrobio.2011.07.005

Nigam, A., & Mishra, A. (2011). Condyloma acuminatum: Atypical presentation during pregnancy. *International Journal of STD & AIDS, 22*(9), 534-535. doi:10.1258/ijsa.2009.009114

Nikolic, D., & Piguet, V. (2010). Vaccines and microbicides preventing HIV-1, HSV-2 and HPV mucosal transmission. *Journal of Investigative Dermatology, 130*, 352-361. doi:10.1038/jid.2009.227

Perry, S. E., Hockenberry, M. J., Lowdermilk, D. L., Wilson, D., Sams, C., & Keenan-Lindsay, L. (2013). *Maternal child nursing care in Canada*. Toronto: Mosby Canada.

Public Health Agency of Canada. (2010a). *Reported cases and rates of gonorrhea by province/territory and sex, 1980 to 2009*. Community Acquired Infections Division. Centre for Communicable Diseases and Infection Control. Retrieved from http://www.phac-aspc.gc.ca/std-mts/sti-its_tab/gonorrhea_pts-eng.php

Public Health Agency of Canada. (2010b). *Canadian guidelines on sexually transmitted infections (Updated 2006 Edition)*. Ottawa: Author.

Sarkar, N. (2008). Barriers to condom use. *European Journal of Contraceptive & Reproductive Health Care, 13,* 114-123. doi:10.1080/13625180802011302

Toma, H. S., Murina, A. T., Areaux, R. G., Neumann, D. M., Bhattacharjee, P. S., Foster, T. P., ..., Hill, J. M. (2008). Ocular HSV-1 latency, reactivation and recurrent disease. *Seminars in Ophthalmology, 23*(4), 249-273. doi:10.1080/08820530802111085

Toro, M. (2008). Combating infection: Closing in on *Chlamydia. Nursing, 38,* 61-69.

Trigg, B. (2008). Sexually transmitted disease and pelvic inflammatory disease in women. *Medical Clinics of North America, 92,* 1083-1102.

Trojian, T. H., Lishnak, T., & Heiman, D. (2009). Epididymitis and orchitis: An overview. *American Family Physician, 79,* 583-592.

Tucker, J. D., Li, J. Z., Robbins, G. K., Davis, B. T., Lobo, A. M., Kunkel, J., & Felsenstein, D. (2011). Ocular syphilis among HIV-infected patients: A systematic analysis of the literature. *Sexually Transmitted Infections, 87,* 4-8. doi:10.1136/sti.2010.043042

Wohlfeiler, D., & Ellen, J. (2010). The limits of behavioral interventions for HIV prevention. In L. Cohen, V. Chavez, & S. Chehimi (Eds.), *Prevention is primary: Strategies for community well being* (2nd ed.). San Francisco: Jossey-Bass.

CANADIAN RESOURCES

Canadian Federation for Sexual Health
http://www.cfsh.ca
CATIE: Canada's Source for HIV and Hepatitis C Information
http://www.catie.ca/en/home

Health Canada: Sexually Transmitted Infections
http://www.hc-sc.gc.ca/hc-ps/dc-ma/sti-its-eng.php
International Herpes Resource Center
http://www.herpesresourcecenter.com/
Phoenix Association—Toronto Help
http://www.torontoherpes.com/
Public Health Agency of Canada
   Sexual and Reproductive Health Day
      http://www.phac-aspc.gc.ca/cpho-acsp/statements/20120213-eng.php
   Sexual Health Promotion/Education: FAQs on Emergency Contraception
      http://www.phac-aspc.gc.ca/std-mts/ec_cu-eng.php
   Sexual Health and Sexually Transmitted Infections
      http://www.phac-aspc.gc.ca/std-mts
   Canadian Guidelines for Sexual Health Education
      http://www.phac-aspc.gc.ca/std-mts/sti-its/pdf/sti-its-eng.pdf
Sex Information and Education Council of Canada
   http://www.sieccan.org
SexualityandU.ca
   http://www.sexualityandu.ca/

℮volve   *For additional Internet resources, see the Web site for this book at* **http://evolve.elsevier.com/Canada/Lewis/medsurg**

Nursing Management: Female Reproductive Problems

Written by Nancy J. MacMullen and Laura Dulski
Adapted by Maureen A. Barry

LEARNING OBJECTIVES

1. Identify causes of infertility and the strategies for diagnosis and treatment of infertility.
2. Describe the etiology, clinical manifestations, and nursing and collaborative management of menstrual problems and abnormal vaginal bleeding.
3. Identify the risk factors, clinical manifestations, and collaborative care of ectopic pregnancy.
4. Discuss the changes related to menopause and the nursing and collaborative management of the patient with menopausal symptoms.
5. Differentiate among the common problems that affect the vulva, vagina, and cervix and related nursing and collaborative management.
6. Describe the assessment, collaborative care, and nursing management of women with pelvic inflammatory disease and endometriosis.
7. Explain the clinical manifestations, diagnostic studies, collaborative care, and surgical therapy for cervical, endometrial, ovarian, and vulvar cancers.
8. Summarize the preoperative and the postoperative nursing management for the patient requiring surgery of the female reproductive system.
9. Differentiate among the common problems that occur with cystoceles, rectoceles, and fistulas and the related nursing and collaborative management.
10. Summarize the clinical manifestations of sexual assault and the appropriate nursing and collaborative management of the patient who has been sexually assaulted.

KEY TERMS

abortion The loss or termination of a pregnancy before the fetus has developed to a state of viability, p. 1541

amenorrhea Absence of menstruation, p. 1545

cystocele Herniation or protrusion of the urinary bladder through the wall of the vagina; occurs when connective tissue support between the vagina and the bladder is weakened; also known as anterior wall prolapse, p. 1567

dysmenorrhea Abdominal cramping pain or discomfort associated with menstrual flow, p. 1544

ectopic pregnancy The implantation of the fertilized ovum anywhere outside the uterine cavity, p. 1547

endometriosis The presence of normal endometrial tissue in sites outside the endometrial cavity, p. 1554

hysterectomy Surgical removal of the uterus, p. 1546

infertility The inability to achieve a pregnancy after at least 1 year of frequent intercourse without contraception, p. 1539

leiomyomas Benign smooth muscle tumours that occur most commonly within the uterus, the stomach, the esophagus,

or the small intestine; uterine leiomyoma is also called a *uterine fibroid*, p. 1557

menopause The physiological cessation of menses associated with declining ovarian function, p. 1548

menorrhagia Excessive or prolonged menstrual bleeding, p. 1545

metrorrhagia Irregular uterine bleeding or bleeding between menses, p. 1545

oligomenorrhea Long intervals between menses, generally longer than 35 days, p. 1545

pelvic inflammatory disease (PID) An infectious condition of the pelvic cavity that may involve infection of the fallopian tubes, the ovaries, and the pelvic peritoneum, p. 1553

perimenopause A normal life transition that begins with the first signs of change in menstrual cycles and ends after cessation of menses, p. 1548

postmenopause The time in a woman's life after menopause, p. 1548

premenstrual syndrome (PMS) A common disorder in women in which a group of physical and psychological symptoms occur during the last few days of the menstrual cycle and before the onset of menstruation, p. 1542

rectocele Herniation or protrusion of the rectum through the wall of the vagina resulting from weakening of the connective tissue support between the vagina and the rectum; also known as posterior wall prolapse, p. 1567

sexual assault The legal term used to refer to any form of sexual contact imposed on another person without that person's voluntary consent, p. 1568

uterine prolapse The downward displacement of the uterus into the vaginal canal as a result of impaired pelvic support, p. 1566

ELECTRONIC RESOURCES

Supplemental content related to Chapter 56 can be found ...

Evolve Web Site ⊖volve

http://evolve.elsevier.com/Canada/Lewis/medsurg
- Answer Guidelines to Case Study on p. 1571
- Assessment Case Study
- Clinical Reference: Laboratory Values

- Content Updates
- Customizable Nursing Care Plan: Abdominal Hysterectomy
- Electronic Calculators
- Examination Review Questions
- Glossary
- Interactive Case Study: Endometrial Cancer
- Key Points (Printable and MP3 Download)

Infertility

Infertility is the inability to achieve a pregnancy after at least 1 year of regular unprotected intercourse (Quaas & Dokras, 2008). Current evidence indicates a 9% prevalence of infertility (over 12 months) with 56% of couples seeking medical care for infertility (Boivin, Bunting, Collins, & Nygren, 2007). Approximately 10 to 15% of couples in North America are infertile (Lowdermilk, Perry, Cashion, & Rhodes Alden, 2012). Assessment and therapy measures can be invasive, expensive, and lengthy. Understandably, infertility can constitute a physical and emotional crisis.

Etiology and Pathophysiology

Infertility may be caused by either female, male, or combined factors. Conditions that cause male infertility are discussed in Chapter 57. In 10 to 20% of the couples evaluated, the cause of infertility may not be identified (Quaas & Dokras, 2008). The most frequent female causes of infertility include factors associated with ovulation (anovulation or inadequate corpus luteum), tubal obstruction or dysfunction (endometriosis or damage from pelvic infection), and uterine or cervical factors (fibroid tumours or structural anomalies). Risk factors for infertility include tobacco and illicit drug use and an abnormal body mass index (BMI) indicating obesity or low body weight. In women, the risk for infertility increases with age. In particular, the probability of becoming pregnant begins decreasing at age 35 and decreases even further after age 40.

Diagnostic Studies

A detailed history and general physical examination of the woman and her partner provide the basis for selecting diagnostic studies (Table 56-1). The possibility of medical, genetic, or gynecological diseases is explored before tests are performed to determine problems affecting general health as well as fertility. These tests include hormonal levels, ovulatory studies, tubal patency studies, and postcoital studies.

Ovulatory Studies. A basal body temperature record is kept to determine whether there is regular ovulation (Figure 56-1). The woman is instructed to take and graph her temperature, referred to as *basal body temperature*, on awakening, before any activity. The same site (e.g., oral, rectal) for taking the temperature should be used each time. Any cause for variation, such as sleeplessness or illness, should be noted. As ovulation approaches, the production of estrogen increases. This may cause a drop in temperature. When ovulation occurs, progesterone is produced, causing a rise in temperature. The temperature graph thus helps detect ovulation and suggests the optimal timing of intercourse if pregnancy is desired. Rigid adherence to a schedule for intercourse can produce psychological stress sufficient to inhibit sexual relations.

Ovulation prediction kits are now available for use by women at home. These kits are generally used daily to measure luteinizing hormone (LH) levels in urine samples. Ovulation occurs about 28 to 36 hours after the first rise of LH, so intercourse can be timed accordingly. Other tests for ovulation include cervical and vaginal smears, endometrial biopsy, and plasma progesterone levels.

Tubal Patency Studies. Tubal factors (occlusion or deformity) are assessed most commonly by means of hysterosalpingogram. This procedure consists of the radiographic visualization of the uterus and tubes by injecting a radiopaque dye through the cervix. Tubal patency, shape, and position and any distortions of the endometrial cavity can be determined. Laparoscopy may be used when a hysterosalpingogram is contraindicated or other pathological pelvic conditions appear likely.

Postcoital Studies. Examination of the cervical mucus can reveal whether it undergoes favourable changes at ovulation,

COLLABORATIVE CARE

Table 56-1 Infertility

Diagnostic

- History and physical examination of both partners, including psychosocial functioning
- Counselling
- Review of menstrual and gynaecological history
- Assessment of possible sexually transmitted infections
- Hormone levels
  - Serum hormone levels (e.g., FSH, LH, prolactin)
  - Urinary LH
- Ovulatory study
  - Basal body temperature record
  - Ovulation predication tests
  - Endometrial biopsy
- Tubal patency study
  - Hysterosalpingogram
- Postcoital test
  - Cervical mucus
  - Sperm penetration assay
  - Semen analysis
- Pelvic ultrasonography
- Genetic screening

Collaborative Therapy

- Hormone supplement therapy
- Drug therapy (see Table 56-2)
- Intrauterine insemination
- Assisted reproductive technologies (ARTs)

FSH, follicle-stimulating hormone; *LH,* luteinizing hormone.

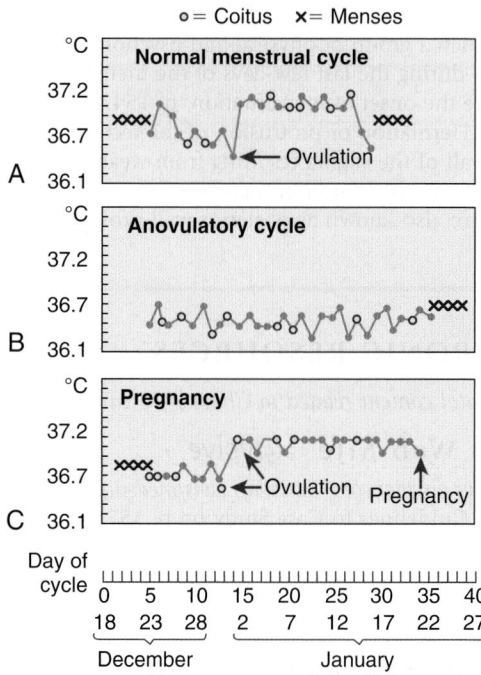

Figure 56-1 Basal body temperature chart. **A,** Typical biphasic temperature curve indicative of ovulation and normal progesterone effect. **B,** Irregular monophasic curve characteristic of anovulatory cycles. **C,** Ovulatory curve with sustained temperature elevation following conception and the first missed period.

enabling penetration, survival, and normal motility of the sperm. A postcoital test can determine whether the cervical environment is favourable for the sperm. The couple is asked to have intercourse about the time ovulation is expected and 2 to 12 hours before the office visit. Douching or bathing should be avoided before the test. The cervical and vaginal secretions are aspirated and examined for the number and the motility of sperm present.

NURSING AND COLLABORATIVE MANAGEMENT: INFERTILITY

The management of infertility problems depends on the cause. If infertility is secondary to an alteration in ovarian function, supplemental hormone therapy to restore and maintain ovulation may be attempted (Kendall, 2008). Drug therapy used to treat infertility is presented in Table 56-2. Chronic cervicitis and inadequate estrogenic stimulation are cervical factors causing infertility. Antibiotic therapy is indicated for cervicitis. Inadequate estrogenic stimulation is treated by the administration of estrogen.

When a couple has not succeeded in conceiving while under infertility management, an option is intrauterine insemination (IUI) with sperm from the partner or a donor. If this technique does not succeed, assisted reproductive technologies (ARTs) may be used. ARTs include in vitro fertilization (IVF), gamete intrafallopian transfer (GIFT), zygote intrafallopian transfer (ZIFT), donor gametes, and embryo cryopreservation. IVF is the removal of mature oocytes from the woman's ovarian follicle via laparoscopy, followed by IVF of the ova with the partner's sperm. When fertilization and cleavage have occurred, the resulting embryos are transferred into the woman's uterus. The procedure requires 2 to 3 days to complete and is used in cases of fallopian tube obstruction, diminished sperm count, and unexplained infertility. Frequently, multiple attempts are needed for successful implantation. IVF is costly and emotionally stressful. However, it has become a recognized and accepted method of therapy for infertile couples.

With the increasing sophistication of ARTs, couples have an increased potential for pregnancy. However, the use of ART often poses many ethical, legal, and social concerns.

Nurses can assist women experiencing infertility by providing information about the physiology of reproduction and infertility evaluation and addressing the psychological and social distress that can accompany infertility. Reducing psychological stress can improve the emotional climate, making it more conducive to achieving a pregnancy.

The nurse has a major responsibility for teaching and providing emotional support throughout infertility testing and treatment. Feelings of anger, frustration, grief, and helplessness may heighten as additional diagnostic tests are performed. Infertility can generate great tension in a marriage as the couple exhausts financial and emotional resources. Few insurance carriers cover the high cost of infertility testing or expensive infertility

DRUG THERAPY
Table 56-2 Infertility

DRUG	MECHANISM OF ACTION
Selective Estrogen Receptor Modulator	
Clomiphene (Clomid, Serophene)	Stimulate hypothalamus to ↑ production of GnRH, which ↑ release of LH and FSH; end result is stimulation of ovulation.
Menotropin (Human Menopausal Gonadotropin)	
Repronex	Product made of equal amounts of FSH and LH that promote the development and maturation of follicles in the ovaries.
Follicle-Stimulating Hormone Agonists	
Urofollitropin (Bravelle) Follitropin alpha (Gonal-F & Gonal-F pen)	Stimulate follicle growth and maturation by mimicking the actions of the body's natural FSH.
GnRH Antagonists	
Cetrorelix (Cetrotide) Ganirelix (Orgalutran)	Prevent premature LH surges and premature ovulation in women undergoing ovarian stimulation.
GnRH Agonists	
Leuprolide (Lupron, Eligard) Nafarelin (Synarel)	Suppress release of LH and FSH with continuous use. May also be used in the treatment of endometriosis.
Human chorionic gonadotropin (hCG) Pregnyl	Induce ovulation by stimulating the release of eggs from follicles.

FSH, follicle-stimulating hormone; *GnRH,* gonadotropin-releasing hormone; *hCG,* human chorionic gonadotropin; *LH,* luteinizing hormone.

treatment. Recognizing and taking steps to deal with the psychological and financial factors that surface can assist the couple to better cope with the situation. Couples should be encouraged to participate in a support group for infertile couples as well as individual therapy.

Abortion

An **abortion** is the loss or termination of a pregnancy before the fetus has developed to a state of viability. Abortions are classified as *spontaneous* (those occurring naturally) or *induced* (those occurring as a result of mechanical or medical intervention). *Miscarriage* is the common term for the unintended loss of a pregnancy. *Habitual recurrent abortion* is defined as a history of three or more aborted pregnancies or miscarriages in succession.

Spontaneous Abortion

Spontaneous abortion is the natural loss of pregnancy before 20 weeks of gestation. Fetal chromosomal anomalies account for 50% of miscarriages before 8 weeks of gestation. Other causes of spontaneous abortions include endocrine abnormalities, maternal infection, acquired anatomical abnormalities (e.g., uterine fibroids, endometriosis), immunological factors, and environmental factors. About 10 to 15% of all clinically recognized pregnancies end as a result of spontaneous abortion (Davidson, London, & Ladewig, 2012).

Uterine cramping coupled with vaginal bleeding often indicates a spontaneous abortion. Cramping is usually absent if the vaginal bleeding is caused by other conditions, such as polyps. Serial measurements of serum β-human chorionic gonadotropin hormone (β-hCG) and vaginal ultrasonography examination of the pelvis are the most reliable indicators of early pregnancy viability. The gestational sac can be visualized using ultrasonography as early as 6 weeks of gestation.

Treatment for a possible spontaneous abortion is limited. Although bed rest and avoiding vaginal intercourse are often recommended, there is no evidence that these measures improve the outcome. The woman is advised to report any bleeding to her health care provider. Most women proceed to abortion regardless of treatment. If the products of conception do not pass completely or bleeding becomes excessive, a *dilation and curettage* (D & C) procedure is generally performed. The D & C involves dilating the uterine cervix and scraping the endometrium of the uterus to empty the contents of the uterus. A medical abortion may also be performed.

Women who are experiencing bleeding and cramping during pregnancy may be admitted to the hospital. Vital signs and estimated blood loss are monitored. Any tissue or blood clots that might contain tissue are examined for products of conception. Women are very distressed and experience both physical and emotional pain. Nurses should use comfort measures to provide the needed physical and mental rest. Arranging for someone to stay with the patient provides important emotional support. The nurse should be aware of the grieving process that results from pregnancy loss (Gerber-Epstein, Leichtentritt, & Benyamini, 2009). Support of the patient and her family is essential.

Induced Abortion

Induced abortion is an intentional or elective termination of a pregnancy. Induced abortion is done at the request of the woman (elective) or for medical reasons (therapeutic). The number of induced abortions for every 100 live births in Canada was 31.7 in 2004 (excluding Ontario) (Public Health Agency of Canada [PHAC], 2008a). The number of induced abortions performed in Canada in 2009 was approximately 93,755 (Canadian Institute for Health Information [CIHI], 2009). Induced abortions continue to be most common among women in their early 20s. Women aged 20 to 24 years had the highest induced abortion rate in 2004, followed by the 25- to 29-year-age group (PHAC, 2008a).

Several techniques are used to induce abortion surgically, including manual vacuum aspiration (MVA), suction curettage, dilation and evacuation (D & E), and drug therapy. Deciding which technique to use to terminate a pregnancy depends on the gestational age (length of the pregnancy) and the woman's condition and preference. Suction curettage may be performed at up to 14 weeks of gestation and accounts for more than 90% of abortion procedures (Burkman, 2007). D & E is conducted in the second semester. Table 56-3 lists current methods for induced abortion available in Canada.

Table 56-3 Methods for Inducing Abortion

METHOD	LENGTH OF PREGNANCY	PROCEDURE	ADVANTAGES	DISADVANTAGES
Early Abortion				
Methotrexate with misoprostol	≤7 wk	Methotrexate is administered intramuscularly. Misoprostol is given intravaginally 5-7 days later.	Safe, effective; avoids surgery and the risk of damage to the uterus with surgical instruments. May feel less invasive than surgery. May seem more private to some women because much of the procedure can occur at home.	Prolonged bleeding possible. Takes place over a week or more and involves several trips to the health care provider. Risk of incomplete abortion; surgical abortion may be necessary. Drugs may have unpleasant adverse effects.
Manual vacuum aspiration (MVA)	Usually ≤6 wk after first missed period	Cervix is dilated and a catheter is inserted through cervix into uterus, and manual suction is applied. Endometrium and contents of uterus are aspirated.	Low cost, simple, done at outpatient facility with or without anaesthesia or cervical dilation, minimally traumatic.	Continuation of pregnancy possible; potential for uterine injury and bleeding.
Suction curettage	≤14 wk	Cervix is usually dilated, uterine aspirator is introduced, and vacuum suction is applied, removing endometrial tissue and implanted pregnancy.	Outpatient procedure, involving local or general anaesthesia, 1- to 2-day recovery period.	Infection, uterine perforation possible.
Dilation and evacuation (D & E)	10-16 wk (approximate)	Cervix is dilated, and products of conception are removed by vacuum cannula and the use of other instruments as needed.	Safe and effective procedure for more advanced pregnancy, outpatient procedure with general anaesthesia, 2-day recovery period.	Potentially more psychological trauma, more expensive, greater risk with general anaesthesia, more invasive procedure.
Late Abortion				
After 22 weeks, late abortion is available in Canada only under special circumstances such as risk to the health of the mother or a nonviable fetus.				

Once the decision is made to have an abortion, the woman and her significant others need support and acceptance. The patient should be prepared for what to expect both emotionally and physically. Grief and sadness are normal emotions after an abortion. The patient needs to understand the procedure, including instructions for preprocedure and postprocedure care. The nurse's caring, nonjudgemental attitude can be a positive factor in the patient's experience.

Follow-up care includes instructions on signs and symptoms of possible complications, including abnormal vaginal bleeding, severe abdominal cramping, fever, and foul drainage. The need to avoid intercourse, tampons, and douching until re-examination in 2 weeks should be stressed. The patient needs to return for re-examination in 2 weeks. Contraception can be started the day of the procedure or during the patient's return visit in accordance with her needs and desires.

Problems Related to Menstruation

The normal menstrual cycle is discussed in Chapter 53. The hormonal influences related to the menstrual cycle are shown in Figure 53-9. Menstruation may be irregular during the first few years after menarche and the years preceding menopause. Once established, a woman's menstrual cycles usually have a predictable pattern. However, considerable normal variation exists among women in cycle length as well as in the duration, amount, and character of the menstrual flow (see Table 53-2).

Premenstrual Syndrome

Premenstrual syndrome (PMS) is a symptom complex related to the luteal phase of the menstrual cycle that resolves with menstruation (Davidson et al., 2012). The symptoms can be severe enough to impair interpersonal relationships or interfere with usual activities. Because many symptoms are associated with PMS, it is difficult to concisely define it. However, PMS symptoms always occur cyclically during the luteal phase before the onset of menstruation and are not present at other times of the month.

Etiology and Pathophysiology

The etiology and pathophysiology are not well understood. It may have a biologic trigger with compounding psychosocial factors. Neurotransmitters, such as serotonin, could also be involved. Some women may have a genetic predisposition to

Abortion

Situation

A recently married, 39-year-old woman is informed that the results of her amniocentesis indicate that her fetus has major chromosomal abnormalities and is expected to have severe physical and mental disabilities. The patient has no children, but her husband has three children from a previous marriage. She asks the nurse what she should do. How would the nurse respond?

Important Points for Consideration

- Decisions about whether to continue a pregnancy with a child who has severe disabilities are extremely personal and emotional. The woman and her husband will need support and information to explore their options and their values.
- Pregnancy counselling is warranted about the woman's choices, her feelings about the pregnancy, her desire to have a child with her husband, her concerns about raising a child with severe disabilities, her feelings about abortion, and concerns about possible future pregnancies.
- Patient autonomy ensures that a woman decide for herself whether or not to continue a pregnancy.
- Abortion is legal in Canada. Canada is one of a small number of countries without a law restricting abortion. Abortion is governed by provincial and medical regulations and treated like any other medical procedure. In the first trimester, abortion is a private matter between a woman and her physician. An abortion can be obtained in a clinic or hospital in many, but not all, provinces and territories.
- The role of the health care provider in these difficult situations is to provide education and support in order to facilitate a decision consistent with the patient's values.

Clinical Decision-Making Questions

1. How would the nurse's feelings about abortion affect her or his ability to care for this patient?
2. What counselling and genetic testing are available to the patient regarding genetic abnormalities?

COLLABORATIVE CARE

Table 56-4 Premenstrual Syndrome

Diagnostic
- History and physical examination
- Symptom diary

Collaborative Therapy
- Stress management and relaxation therapy
- Nutritional therapy
- Aerobic exercise
- Drug therapy
  - Diuretics
  - Prostaglandin inhibitors (e.g., ibuprofen [Advil])
  - Selective serotonin reuptake inhibitors (e.g., sertraline [Zoloft])
  - Combined oral contraceptives

---

palpitations, dizziness) have been reported by women with PMS. Anxiety, depression, irritability, and mood swings are some of the emotional symptoms that women may experience.

Diagnostic Studies and Collaborative Care

PMS can be diagnosed only when other possible causes for the symptoms have been eliminated. A focused health history and physical examination are done to identify any underlying conditions, such as thyroid dysfunction, uterine fibroids, or depression, that may account for the symptoms. No definitive diagnostic test is available for PMS. When PMS or PMDD is a possible diagnosis, a woman is given a symptom diary to record her symptoms prospectively for two or three menstrual cycles (Raines, 2010). Diagnosis is based on an evaluation of the woman's symptoms.

Nonpharmacological and pharmacological strategies can relieve some PMS symptoms (Table 56-4). However, no single treatment is available. The goal of treatment is to reduce the severity of symptoms and enhance the woman's sense of control and quality of life.

Several conservative approaches to managing PMS symptoms are considered helpful, including stress management, diet changes, exercise, education, and counseling. Techniques for stress reduction include yoga, meditation, imagery, and biofeedback (see Chapter 12). To decrease autonomic nervous system arousal, women should avoid caffeine, reduce dietary intake of refined carbohydrates, exercise on a regular basis, and practise relaxation techniques. Eating complex carbohydrates with high fibre, foods rich in vitamin B_6, and sources of tryptophan (dairy and poultry) are thought to promote serotonin production, which improves the symptoms. Vitamin B_6 may be found in such foods as pork, milk, egg yolk, and legumes. Although no strongly supportive data exist, limiting salt intake before menstruation and increasing calcium intake have been proposed to alleviate fluid retention, weight gain, bloating, breast swelling, and tenderness.

Exercise results in a release of endorphins, leading to mood elevation. Aerobic exercise can also have a relaxing effect. Because fatigue tends to exaggerate the symptoms of PMS, adequate rest in the premenstrual period is a priority.

Explanations about PMS help the woman understand the complexity of the disorder and ways that she can regain a better

---

PMS. Other proposed causes of PMS include hormone imbalance and nutritional deficiencies. It occurs in 20 to 30% of premenopausal women. *Premenstrual dysphoric disorder* (PMDD) is the term applied to a type of PMS that affects 3 to 8% of premenopausal women (Biggs & Demuth, 2011). Women with PMDD have a severe mood disorder (marked depression and anxiety) in addition to PMS (Raines, 2010).

Clinical Manifestations

PMS is extremely variable in its clinical manifestation. Variation is common, both among women and for an individual woman, from one cycle to another. Commonly occurring physical symptoms include breast discomfort, peripheral edema, abdominal bloating, sensation of weight gain, episodes of binge eating, and headache. Abdominal bloating and breast swelling are caused by fluid shifts because total body weight does not generally change. Symptoms of autonomic nervous system arousal (e.g., heart

sense of control. The patient needs to be assured that her symptoms are real, PMS exists, and she is not "crazy." Acknowledgement of having PMS can itself be therapeutic. Teaching the woman's partner about the nature of PMS assists the partner to better understand PMS and to provide support to the woman in making lifestyle changes to reduce the symptoms of PMS.

Drug Therapy. Drug therapy is considered when symptoms persist or interfere with daily functioning. At present, no single drug can treat all the symptoms associated with PMS. One therapy may be tried for a time, and if no improvement is observed, another approach is tried. Many treatments are symptom specific. For fluid retention, diuretics such as spironolactone (Aldactone) are used. For reducing cramps, backache, and headache, prostaglandin inhibitors such as ibuprofen (Advil) are used. To improve negative mood, vitamin B_6 supplementation (50 mg daily) may be used. Calcium and magnesium supplementation may also be effective in alleviating psychological and physiological symptoms. For anxiety, buspirone taken during the luteal phase has helped some women. Women with PMDD may benefit from antidepressants, including fluoxetine HCl (Prozac) and tricyclic antidepressants (e.g., amitriptyline).

Other pharmacological treatments are directed at PMS in general. Selective serotonin reuptake inhibitors (SSRIs) (e.g., sertraline [Zoloft]) have provided significant relief to women with severe PMS (Brown, O'Brien, Marjoribanks, & Wyatt, 2009). Other general treatments include oral contraceptives containing estrogen and progesterone. Evening primrose oil may help some women.

Dysmenorrhea

Dysmenorrhea is abdominal cramping pain or discomfort associated with menstrual flow. The degree of pain and discomfort varies with the individual. The two types of dysmenorrhea are primary (no pathology exists) and secondary (pelvic disease is the underlying cause). Dysmenorrhea is one of the most common gynecological problems, affecting approximately 50% of all women (Rapkin & Gambone, 2010).

Etiology and Pathophysiology

Primary dysmenorrhea is not a disease. It is caused by an excess of prostaglandin $F_{2\alpha}$ ($PGF_{2\alpha}$), an increased sensitivity to it, or both. Stimulation of the endometrium by estrogen, and then followed by progesterone, results in a dramatic increase in prostaglandin production by the endometrium. With the onset of menses, degeneration of the endometrium releases prostaglandin. Locally, prostaglandins increase myometrial contractions and constriction of small endometrial blood vessels. This causes tissue ischemia and increased sensitization of the pain receptors, resulting in menstrual pain. Primary dysmenorrhea begins in the first few years after menarche, typically with the onset of regular ovulatory cycles.

Secondary dysmenorrhea is usually acquired after adolescence, occurring most commonly at 30 to 40 years of age. Common pelvic conditions that cause secondary dysmenorrhea include endometriosis, chronic pelvic inflammatory disease (PID), and uterine fibroids. Because secondary dysmenorrhea is caused by multiple conditions, symptoms vary. However, painful menses are present in all situations.

Clinical Manifestations

Primary dysmenorrhea starts 12 to 24 hours before the onset of menses. The pain is most severe the first day of menses and rarely lasts more than 2 days. Characteristic manifestations include lower abdominal pain that is colicky in nature, frequently radiating to the lower back and the upper thighs. The abdominal pain is often accompanied by nausea, diarrhea, loose stools, fatigue, headache, and lightheadedness.

Secondary dysmenorrhea usually occurs after the woman has experienced problem-free periods for some time. The pain may be unilateral and it is generally more constant and continues longer than in primary dysmenorrhea. Depending on the cause, symptoms such as *dyspareunia* (painful intercourse), painful defecation, or irregular bleeding may occur at times other than menstruation.

Collaborative Care

Evaluation begins with distinguishing primary from secondary dysmenorrhea. A complete health history with special attention to menstrual and gynecological history should be obtained. A pelvic examination is also performed. If the history reveals an onset shortly after menarche and symptoms associated only with menses in addition to normal pelvic examination findings, the probable diagnosis is primary dysmenorrhea. If any specific cause of dysmenorrheal is evident, the diagnosis is secondary dysmenorrhea.

Treatment for primary dysmenorrhea includes heat, exercise, and drug therapy. Heat is applied to the lower abdomen or back. Regular exercise is thought to be beneficial because it may reduce endometrial hyperplasia and subsequently reduce prostaglandin production. The primary drug therapy is nonsteroidal anti-inflammatory drugs (NSAIDs) such as naproxen (Naprosyn), which has antiprostaglandin activity. NSAIDs should be started at the first sign of menses and continued every 4 to 8 hours to maintain a sufficient level of the drug to inhibit prostaglandin synthesis for the usual duration of discomfort. Oral contraceptives may also be used. They decrease dysmenorrhea by reducing endometrial hyperplasia.

Acupuncture and transcutaneous nerve stimulation (TENS) also provide varying degrees of relief. (See Chapter 12 for a discussion of acupuncture.) These methods may be used for women who obtain inadequate relief from medications or who prefer not to take medications. Patients who are unresponsive to these treatments should be evaluated for chronic pelvic pain.

Treatment of secondary dysmenorrhea depends on the cause. Some individuals with secondary dysmenorrhea will be helped by the approaches used for primary dysmenorrhea. Depending on the underlying causes of dysmenorrhea, additional drug or surgical interventions are used.

NURSING MANAGEMENT: DYSMENORRHEA

One of the primary roles of the nurse is teaching. Women should be taught why dysmenorrhea occurs as well as how to treat it. Teaching and supportive therapy can provide women with a foundation for coping with this common occurrence and increase feelings of control and self-reliance.

Women often ask the nurse what can be done for minor discomforts associated with menstrual cycles. Women should be advised that, during acute pain, relief may be obtained by lying down for short periods, drinking hot beverages such as herbal teas, applying heat to the abdomen or the back, taking warm baths, and taking NSAIDs for analgesia (Smith, 2008). The nurse can also suggest noninvasive pain-relieving practices such as distraction and guided imagery.

Other health care measures to reduce the discomfort of dysmenorrhea include regular exercise and proper nutritional habits. Avoiding constipation, maintaining good body mechanics, and eliminating stress and fatigue, particularly during the time preceding menstrual periods, can also decrease discomfort.

Abnormal Vaginal Bleeding

Abnormal vaginal or uterine bleeding is a common gynecological concern. Irregularities include **oligomenorrhea** (long intervals between menses, generally longer than 35 days), **amenorrhea** (absence of menstruation), **menorrhagia** (excessive or prolonged menstrual bleeding), and **metrorrhagia** (irregular uterine bleeding or bleeding between menses). The cause of abnormal bleeding may vary from anovulatory menstrual cycles to more serious causes such as ectopic pregnancy or endometrial cancer. The age of the woman provides direction for identifying the cause of bleeding. For example, a postmenopausal woman with abnormal bleeding must always be evaluated for endometrial cancer but does not need to be evaluated for possible pregnancy. For a 20-year-old woman with abnormal bleeding, the possibility of pregnancy must always be considered, and the possibility of endometrial cancer would be unlikely. When bleeding is caused by a disruption in the menstrual cycle (e.g., anovulation), it is called *dysfunctional uterine bleeding.*

Abnormal bleeding may be caused by dysfunction of the hypothalamic–pituitary–ovarian axis such as a pituitary adenoma. Another cause may be infection. Changes in lifestyle such as marriage, recent moves, a death in the family, financial stress, and other emotional crises can also cause irregular bleeding. Because psychological factors can influence endocrine function, they should be considered when the patient is evaluated.

Types of Irregular Bleeding

Oligomenorrhea and Secondary Amenorrhea.

Anovulation is the most common cause for missing menses once pregnancy has been ruled out. Additional causes of amenorrhea are listed in Table 56-5. *Primary amenorrhea* refers to the failure of menstrual cycles to begin by age 16 years or by age 14 years if secondary sex characteristics are present. *Secondary amenorrhea* refers to cessation of menstrual cycles once established.

Ovulation is often erratic for several years following menarche and before menopause. Thus, oligomenorrhea owing to anovulation is common for women at the beginning and end of menstruation (Ayers & Montgomery, 2009). In anovulatory cycles, the corpus luteum that produces progesterone does not form. This may result in a situation referred to as *unopposed estrogen.* When unopposed by progesterone, estrogen can cause excessive buildup of the endometrium. Persistent overgrowth of the endometrium increases a woman's risk for endometrial cancer. To reduce this risk, progesterone or oral contraceptives are prescribed to ensure that the patient's endometrial lining will be shed at least four to six times per year.

Table 56-5 Causes of Amenorrhea
Hypothalamic–Pituitary Axis
• Reversible CNS-mediated causes (e.g., emotional stress, anorexia nervosa or severe dieting, strenuous exercise, chronic or acute illness)
• Prolactinoma or other causes of hyperprolactinemia (e.g., drugs)
• Brainstem or pituitary tumours
• Vascular disease (e.g., hypothalamic vasculitis)
• Pituitary tumours
Ovaries
• Autoimmune disease (often involving thyroid, adrenal, and islet cells)
• Premature menopause
• Polycystic ovary disease
• Congenital or genetic conditions (e.g., Turner's syndrome)*
• Infection (e.g., mumps oophoritis)
• Toxins (especially alkylating chemotherapeutic agents)
• Radiation
• Tumours
Hormonal Synthesis and Action
Male pseudohermaphroditism (e.g., testicular feminization)*

CNS, central nervous system.
*Usually manifests as primary amenorrhea.

Menorrhagia. The excessive bleeding associated with menorrhagia can be characterized as an increased duration (>7 days), increased amount (>80 mL), or both. Anovulatory uterine bleeding is the most common cause of menorrhagia. An unopposed estrogen state continues to build up the endometrium until it becomes unstable, resulting in menorrhagia. For young women with excessive bleeding, clotting disorders must be considered. Uterine fibroids (also called *leiomyomas*) and endometrial polyps are a common cause of menorrhagia for women in their 30s and 40s.

Metrorrhagia. Metrorrhagia, also referred to as *spotting* or *breakthrough bleeding,* is bleeding between menstrual periods. For all women of reproductive age, pregnancy complications such as spontaneous abortion or ectopic pregnancy must be considered as a possible cause. Other causes include cervical or endometrial polyps, infection, and carcinoma. Spotting is common during the first three cycles of oral contraceptives. If spotting continues past the woman's third cycle using oral contraceptives and if other causes of metrorrhagia have been ruled out, a different pill formulation can be prescribed when other causes of metrorrhagia have been ruled out. Spotting with long-acting progestin therapy, (e.g., Mirena IUD) or progestin-only pills (Depo-Provera) is also common. For postmenopausal women, endometrial cancer must be considered whenever spotting is experienced. In postmenopausal women, exogenous estrogen administration during hormone replacement therapy (HRT) is a common cause of metrorrhagia. *Menometrorrhagia* is excessive bleeding that occurs at irregular intervals. It may be caused by endometrial cancer or uterine fibroids.

Diagnostic Studies and Collaborative Care

Because abnormal vaginal bleeding has multiple causes, the diagnostic and collaborative care varies. A health history and physical examination directed at the most likely causes of vaginal bleeding for the woman's age group is the first step. These findings will provide the basis for selecting the necessary laboratory tests and diagnostic procedures. Treatment depends on the nature of the problem (e.g., menorrhagia, amenorrhea), the degree of threat to the patient's health, and whether children are desired in the future.

Combined oral contraceptives may be prescribed for a woman with amenorrhea to ensure regular shedding of endometrium if she also wants contraception. If she wants to become pregnant, a fertility drug may be prescribed. If she does not need birth control, progesterone may be prescribed to ensure a shedding of the endometrial lining four to six times per year. Tranexamic acid (Cyklokapron), a nonhormonal product, may be used to treat heavy menstrual bleeding. This drug stabilizes a protein that helps blood to clot. Adverse effects may include headache, sinus and nasal symptoms, back pain, abdominal pain, muscle and joint pain, muscle cramps, anemia, and fatigue. Use of tranexamic acid while taking hormonal contraceptives may increase risk of blood clots, stroke, or heart attack. Women using hormonal contraception should take tranexamic acid only if there is a strong medical need.

The treatment goal for women with menorrhagia is to minimize further blood loss. If menorrhagia is the result of anovulatory cycles, the endometrium must be stabilized by a combination of oral estrogen and progesterone.

Balloon thermotherapy is a technique for menorrhagia that involves the introduction of a soft, flexible balloon into the uterus; the balloon is then inflated with sterile fluid (Figure 56-2). The fluid in the balloon is heated and maintained for 8 minutes, then causing ablation (removal) of the uterine lining. When the treatment is completed, the fluid is withdrawn from the balloon and the catheter is removed from the uterus. The uterine lining sloughs off in the following 7 to 10 days. Uterine balloon thermotherapy is contraindicated for women desiring to maintain their fertility and for women with

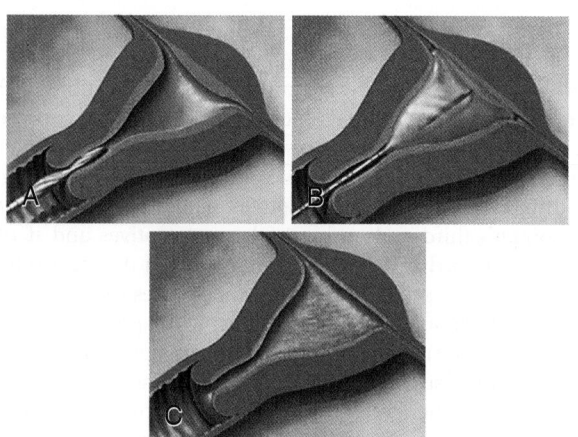

Figure 56-2 Balloon thermotherapy for treatment of menorrhagia. **A,** Balloon-tipped catheter is inserted into the uterus through the vagina and cervix. **B,** The balloon is inflated with a sterile fluid that expands to fit the size and shape of the uterus. The fluid is heated to 87°C and maintained for 8 minutes while the uterine lining is treated. **C,** Fluid is withdrawn from the balloon and the catheter is removed.

Source: Courtesy Ethicon, Inc., Cornelia, GA.

any suspected uterine abnormalities such as fibroids, suspected endometrial cancer, prior Caesarean section or myomectomy. With severe bleeding, hospitalization is indicated. All patients with menorrhagia should be evaluated for anemia and treated as indicated.

Surgical Therapy. Surgery may be indicated, depending on the underlying cause of the abnormal vaginal bleeding. D & C was once a common therapy for excessive bleeding or for spotting in perimenopausal women. Now D & C is used only in extreme cases of bleeding or for older women when endometrial biopsy and ultrasonography have not provided the necessary diagnostic information. Endometrial ablation for menorrhagia may be done by laser, thermal balloon, cryotherapy, microwave energy, or electrosurgical technique for patients who do not want to have children (Ayers & Montgomery, 2009). If menorrhagia is caused by uterine fibroids, a **hysterectomy** (surgical removal of the uterus) may be performed. A *myomectomy* (removal of fibroids without removal of the uterus) may be performed if the patient wants to preserve her uterus. The myomectomy is done via laparotomy, laparoscopy, or hysteroscopy. Hormonal regimens and embolization of blood vessels supplying the fibroid are other treatment options.

NURSING MANAGEMENT: ABNORMAL VAGINAL BLEEDING

Infrequent or no menses might seem a desirable state by the woman. Teaching women about the characteristics of the menstrual cycle will assist them to identify normal variations.

Table 53-2 in Chapter 53 includes characteristics of the menstrual cycle and related patient teaching. This knowledge can diminish apprehension and dispel misconceptions about the menstrual cycle. If the patient's menstrual cycle pattern does not fall within the normal range, the nurse should urge her to visit her health care provider. Myths concerning activities allowed during menstruation are common. The nurse should be prepared to clarify the facts. The patient should be assured that bathing and hair washing are safe. A daily warm tub bath may actually relieve some of the associated pelvic discomfort. Women can swim, exercise, have intercourse, and basically continue their usual daily activities.

Frequent changing of tampons or pads meets comfort and hygiene needs during menstruation. The selection of internal or external sanitary protection is a matter of personal preference. Tampons are convenient and make menstrual hygiene easier, whereas pads may provide better protection. Using a combination of tampons and pads and avoiding prolonged use of superabsorbent tampons may decrease the risk of *toxic shock syndrome* (TSS). TSS is an acute condition caused by a toxin from *Staphylococcus aureus*. Symptoms of TSS may initially include flulike symptoms such as high fever, nausea, vomiting, diarrhea, dizziness, fainting and confusion. Other symptoms may include low blood pressure, shock, dehydration, myalgia, and a sunburn-like rash (Health Canada, 2011).

Whenever excessive, the amount of the patient's vaginal bleeding should be assessed as accurately as possible. The number and size of pads or tampons used and the degree of saturation should be reported and recorded. The patient's fatigue level, along with variations in blood pressure and pulse, should be monitored because anemia and hypovolemia may be present. If a surgical procedure is indicated, the nurse should provide appropriate preoperative and postoperative care.

Ectopic Pregnancy

An **ectopic pregnancy** is the implantation of the fertilized ovum anywhere outside the uterine cavity (Figure 56-3). In 2004 to 2005, the rate of ectopic pregnancies was 11.9 per 1000 reported pregnancies in Canada (PHAC, 2008a). The incidence of ectopic pregnancy increases with maternal age (Best Start Resource Centre and Halton Region Health Department, 2007).

Ectopic pregnancy is a life-threatening condition. Earlier identification has contributed to a decrease in mortality rates. Ectopic pregnancy accounts for about 6.5% of the maternal deaths reported by Statistics Canada for the years 1993 to 2004 (PHAC, 2008a). Approximately 98% of ectopic pregnancies occur in the fallopian tube (see Figure 56-3). The remaining 2 to 3% may be ovarian, abdominal, or cervical (McQueen, 2011).

Etiology and Pathophysiology

Any blockage of the tube or reduction of tubal peristalsis that impedes or delays the zygote passing to the uterine cavity can result in tubal implantation. After implantation, the growth of the gestational sac expands the tubal wall. Eventually, the tube ruptures, causing acute peritoneal symptoms. Less acute symptoms usually begin within 6 to 8 weeks after the last normal menstrual period and weeks before rupture would occur.

Risk factors for ectopic pregnancy include a history of PID, prior ectopic pregnancy, current progestin-releasing intrauterine device (IUD), progestin-only birth control failure, and prior pelvic or tubal surgery. Additional risk factors for ectopic pregnancy comprise procedures used in infertility treatment, including in vitro fertilization procedures, embryo transfer, and ovulation induction.

Clinical Manifestations

The classic symptoms of ectopic pregnancy are abdominal or pelvic pain, missed menses, and irregular vaginal bleeding. Other symptoms include amenorrhea, morning sickness, breast tenderness, gastrointestinal disturbance, malaise, and syncope. Pain is almost always present and is caused by distension of the fallopian tube. It may start unilaterally and then spread to become bilateral. The character of the pain varies among women and can be colicky or vague. If tubal rupture occurs, the pain is intense and may be referred to the shoulder as a result of irritation of the diaphragm by blood released into the abdominal cavity. Symptom severity does not necessarily correlate with the extent of external bleeding present. With rupture, the risk of hemorrhage and hypovolemic shock is present. Suspected rupture is treated as an emergency.

The vaginal bleeding that may accompany ectopic pregnancy is usually described as "spotting." However, it is also possible that bleeding may be heavier and can be confused with menses. The woman may also experience abnormal bleeding.

Diagnostic Studies

Because of the life-threatening nature of ectopic pregnancy, it should be considered whenever pregnancy is even remotely possible. Ectopic pregnancy can be a diagnostic challenge because of its similarity to other pelvic and abdominal disorders, such as salpingitis, spontaneous abortion, ruptured ovarian cyst, appendicitis, and peritonitis. A serum (radioimmunoassay) pregnancy test should be performed. If the test is negative, an ectopic pregnancy is not likely. If ectopic pregnancy cannot be excluded by the pregnancy test, further evaluation is warranted. If the patient is in a stable condition, a combination of serial β-hCG assessment and vaginal ultrasonography is used. β-hCG is expected to double about every 48 hours in a normal pregnancy. If the β-hCG level fails to double, the patient may have an ectopic pregnancy. Transvaginal ultrasonography can be used to confirm the presence of an intrauterine pregnancy once the β-hCG level has reached 1500 to 2000 mIU/mL (Shamonki, Nelson, & Gambone, 2010).

Absence of a normal intrauterine pregnancy means that the diagnosis is probably spontaneous abortion or ectopic pregnancy. With a spontaneous abortion, serial β-hCG levels will decrease over time. A complete blood count is obtained when there is any concern regarding the amount of blood loss or if surgery is contemplated. A gradually decreasing hematocrit may indicate internal bleeding.

NURSING AND COLLABORATIVE MANAGEMENT: ECTOPIC PREGNANCY

Surgery remains the primary approach for treating ectopic pregnancies and should be performed immediately. However, medical management with intramuscular injection of methotrexate is being used with increasing success and safety in patients who are hemodynamically stable and have a mass smaller than 3.5 to 4 cm (Barnhart, 2009). A conservative surgical approach limits damage to the reproductive system as much as possible. Removal of the pregnancy from the tube is preferred to removing the tube. Laparoscopy is preferable to laparotomy because it decreases blood loss and the length of the hospital stay. If the tube ruptures, conservative surgical approaches may not be possible. The patient may need a blood transfusion and supplemental intravenous (IV) fluid therapy to relieve shock and restore a satisfactory blood volume for safe anaesthesia and surgery. The use of microsurgery techniques has resulted in fewer repeated ectopic pregnancies and a higher rate of future successful pregnancies.

Nursing care depends on the condition of the patient. Before the diagnosis has been confirmed, the nurse should be alert to

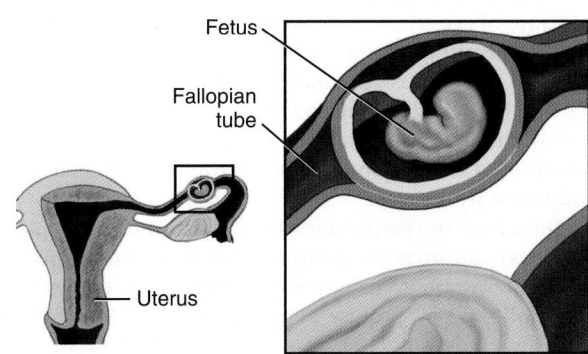

Figure 56-3 Ectopic pregnancy occurring in the fallopian tube.

Fetus
Fallopian tube
Uterus

signs of increasing pain and vaginal bleeding, which may indicate that rupture of the tube has occurred. Vital signs are monitored closely, along with observation for signs of shock. Explanations and preparation for diagnostic procedures are given when appropriate. Preparation of the patient for abdominal surgery may follow rapidly. The patient's emotional status should be assessed. Reassurance and support for the surgery should be given to the patient and her family. Postoperatively, the patient may express a fear of future ectopic pregnancies and have many questions about the impact of this experience on her future fertility.

Perimenopause and Postmenopause

The **perimenopause** is a normal life transition that begins with the first signs of change in menstrual cycles and ends after cessation of menses. **Menopause** is the physiological cessation of menses associated with declining ovarian function. It is made retrospectively after 1 year of *amenorrhea* (absence of menstruation). Menopause starts gradually and is usually associated with changes in menstruation, including menstrual flows that are increased, decreased, irregular, or some combination of these. Cessation of menses finally occurs. **Postmenopause** is a term that refers to the time in a woman's life after menopause.

The age at which menopause occurs ranges from 44 to 55 years, with the average being 51 years (Lund, 2008). Menopause may occur earlier as a result of illness, surgical removal of the uterus or both ovaries, adverse effects of radiation therapy or chemotherapy, or drugs. The age at which menopause occurs is not affected by age at menarche, physical characteristics, number of pregnancies, date of last pregnancy, or oral contraceptive use. However, genetic factors, autoimmune conditions, cigarette smoking, and racial or ethnic factors, have been linked to earlier age at menopause (Cooper, 2009).

Changes within the ovary start the cascade of events that finally result in menopause. The regression of the follicles within each ovary begins with puberty and accelerates after age 35. With age, fewer and fewer follicles remain that are responsive to follicle-stimulating hormone (FSH). FSH normally stimulates the dominant follicle to secrete estrogen. When the follicles can no longer respond to FSH, ovarian production of estrogen and progesterone declines. However, perimenopausal women can get pregnant until menopause has occurred. This is because many women have long anovulatory cycles interspersed with shorter, ovulatory cycles.

With decreased ovarian function, there are decreased levels of estrogen that cause a gradual increase in FSH and LH as a result of the negative feedback process. By the time menopause occurs, there is a ten- to twenty-fold increase in FSH. The elevated FSH level may take several years to return to the premenopausal level. The reduced estrogen level also causes a decrease in the frequency of ovulation and results in changes in the reproductive organs and tissues (e.g., atrophy of vaginal tissue).

Clinical Manifestations

Clinical manifestations of perimenopause and postmenopause are presented in Table 56-6. The perimenopause is a time of erratic hormonal fluctuation. Irregular vaginal bleeding is common. With decreasing estrogen, hot flashes and other symptoms begin. The signs and symptoms of diminished estrogen are

Table 56-6 Clinical Manifestations of Perimenopause and Postmenopause

PERIMENOPAUSE	POSTMENOPAUSE
Irregular menses	Cessation of menses
Occasional vasomotor symptoms (hot flashes and night sweats)	Vasomotor instability (hot flashes and night sweats)
Atrophy of genitourinary tissue with decreased support	Atrophy of genitourinary tissue (e.g., vaginal epithelium)
Stress and urge incontinence	Stress and urge incontinence
Osteoporosis	Breast tenderness
Mood changes	

Table 56-7 Signs and Symptoms of Estrogen Deficiency

Vasomotor
- Hot flashes
- Night sweats

Genitourinary
- Atrophic vaginitis
- Dyspareunia secondary to poor lubrication
- Incontinence

Psychological
- Emotional lability
- Change in sleep pattern
- Decreased REM sleep

Skeletal
- Increased fracture rate, especially of vertebral bodies but also of humerus, distal radius, and upper femur

Cardiovascular
- Decreased high-density lipoproteins (HDLs)
- Increased low-density lipoproteins (LDLs)

Dermatological
- Diminished collagen content of skin
- Breast tissue changes

REM, rapid eye movement.

listed in Table 56-7. The loss of estrogen plays a significant role in the cause of age-related alterations. Changes most critical to a woman's well-being are the increased risks for coronary artery disease and osteoporosis secondary to bone density loss. Other changes include a redistribution of fat, a tendency to gain weight more easily, muscle and joint pain, loss of skin elasticity, changes in hair amount and distribution, and atrophy of external genitalia and breast tissue.

Hallmarks of the perimenopause include *vasomotor instability* (hot flashes) and irregular menses. A hot flash is described as a sensation of warmth in the upper part of the chest, the neck, and the face followed by profuse perspiration (Alraek & Malterud, 2009). These sensations last from several seconds to 5 minutes and occur most often at night, thereby disturbing sleep. The cause of hot flashes, or vasomotor instability, is not clearly understood. It has been theorized that temperature regulators in the brain are in proximity to the area where gonadotropin-releasing hormone (GnRH) is released. The lowered estrogen levels are correlated with dilation of cutaneous blood vessels, resulting in hot flashes and increased sweating. The more sudden the withdrawal of estrogen (e.g., surgical removal of the ovaries), the more likely the symptoms will be severe if no hormone replacement is provided. These symptoms subside over time with or without HRT. Hot flashes can be triggered by situations that affect body temperature, such as eating a hot meal, hot weather, drinking an alcoholic beverage, stress, or warm clothing.

Atrophic vaginal changes secondary to decreased estrogen include thinning of the vaginal mucosa and disappearance of rugae. Vaginal secretions also decrease and become more alkaline. As a result of these changes, the vagina is easily traumatized and more susceptible to infection, including a higher risk for human immunodeficiency virus (HIV) transmission if exposed. *Dyspareunia* (painful intercourse) may also occur. This can lead to unnecessary and premature cessation of sexual activity. Dryness is a problem that can be easily corrected with water-soluble lubricants or, if needed, with hormonal creams or systemic HRT. In general, the extent and the severity of the symptoms of menopause vary and are not easily predicted.

Atrophic changes in the lower urinary tract also occur with a decrease in estrogen. Bladder capacity decreases, and the bladder and urethral tissue lose tone. These changes can cause symptoms that mimic a bladder infection (e.g., dysuria, urgency, frequency) when no infection is present.

Whether decreasing estrogen is responsible for the psychological changes associated with perimenopause is unclear. The attributed depression, irritability, and cognitive problems could result from life stressors or sleep deprivation from hot flashes. Depressive symptoms appear to improve when hormone levels stabilize (Accortt, Freeman, & Allen, 2008).

Collaborative Care

The diagnosis of perimenopause should be made only after careful consideration of other possible causes for the woman's symptoms. Depression, thyroid dysfunction, anemia, or anxiety could be responsible for the same symptoms. An accurate history of menstrual patterns should be reviewed as part of establishing the diagnosis (Currie, 2008). Because of the hormonal fluctuations that occur before menopause, routine testing of the serum FSH level is not indicated.

Drug Therapy. HRT was once standard therapy in Canada for treating menopausal symptoms. HRT includes estrogen for women without ovaries or estrogen and progesterone for women with a uterus.

Beginning in 2002, findings from the Women's Health Initiative (WHI) clinical trials have changed this practice. The data showed that women who had taken estrogen plus progestin had an increased risk of breast cancer, stroke, heart disease, and emboli. However, these women had fewer hip fractures and a lower risk of developing colorectal cancer. In women who took only estrogen (Premarin), there was an increased risk for stroke and emboli. However, these women had decreased risk for fractures with no increased risk for heart disease or breast or colorectal cancer. Neither estrogen plus progestin nor estrogen alone affected the risk of death (Department of Health and Human Services/National Institute of Health/National Heart, Lung, and Blood Institute, 2011). (See also the Evidence-Informed Practice box regarding HRT and cognitive function.)

EVIDENCE-INFORMED PRACTICE

Can Hormone Replacement Therapy (HRT) Improve Cognitive Function?

Clinical Question

For postmenopausal women (P), does HRT (I) versus no replacement (C) improve or maintain cognitive function (O) over a 5-yr period (T)?

Best Available Evidence

- Systematic review of randomized controlled trials (RCTs)

Critical Appraisal and Synthesis of Evidence

- 16 double-blind RCTs ($n = 10,114$) of postmenopausal healthy women 29 to >75 yr old.
- Women without dementia on HRT (estrogen alone or estrogen and progesterone) for 2 wk (short term) up to 5 yr (long term).
- Cognitive function measured through global and specific tests including verbal and visual memory, attention, and reasoning.

Conclusion

- Neither type of HRT maintained or improved cognitive function on a short- or long-term basis.

Implications for Nursing Practice

- Advise patients that HRT may be given as short-term therapy for menopausal symptoms such as intolerable hot flashes or night sweats.
- Counsel patients that current evidence does not support taking HRT to maintain cognitive function, and that HRT increases the risk of stroke and breast cancer.

Reference for Evidence

Lethaby, A., Hogervorst, E., Richards, M., Yesufu, A., & Yaffe, K. (2008). Hormone replacement therapy for cognitive function in postmenopausal women. *Cochrane Database of Systematic Reviews*, 1, CD003122. doi:10.1002/14651858.CD003122. pub2

If women wish to consider taking HRT for the short-term treatment (4 to 5 years) of menopausal symptoms, the risks and benefits of therapy (e.g., minimizes bone loss, hot flashes, vaginal atrophic changes) should be considered carefully. The decision to take HRT, and which ones to take, should be thoroughly discussed between the woman and her health care provider. If a woman chooses to use HRT, the lowest effective dose should be used (North American Menopause Society, 2010; Birkhauser et al., 2008). The age that a woman starts HRT may determine her risk of heart disease. The risk appears to increase the further a woman moves away from menopause (Society of Obstetricians and Gynaecologists of Canada [SOGC], 2009).

The adverse effects of estrogen include nausea, fluid retention, headache, and breast enlargement. Adverse effects of progesterone include increased appetite, weight gain, irritability, depression, spotting, and breast tenderness. A commonly used estrogen preparation is 0.625 mg of conjugated estrogen (Premarin) daily. For symptom relief, a higher dose may be needed. To receive the protective benefit of progesterone, 5 to 10 mg of medroxyprogesterone (Provera) is indicated for 12 days of each month on a cyclical regimen or 2.5 mg if on a continuous regimen. If the estrogen is to be increased for symptom relief, the progesterone should also be increased. Other forms of progesterone include norethindrone (Brevicon, Synphasic) and micronized progesterone creams, dermal patches, gels, and lotions; rings placed around the cervix; and subcutaneous pellets. Vaginal creams are especially useful for urogenital symptoms (e.g., dryness). Transdermal (skin patch) estrogen has the advantage of bypassing the liver but has the disadvantage of causing skin irritation.

Antidepressants known as selective serotonin reuptake inhibitors (SSRIs), including paroxetine (Paxil), fluoxetine (Prozac), and venlafaxine (Effexor XR), are an effective alternative to HRT in reducing hot flashes. This effect is noted even if the user is not depressed (Birkhauser et al., 2008). The mechanism of action is unknown. Clonidine (Catapres), an antihypertensive drug, and gabapentin (Neurontin), an antiseizure drug, have also been shown to relieve hot flashes.

Selective estrogen receptor modulators (SERMs), such as raloxifene (Evista), are also used in treating menopausal problems. These drugs have some of the positive benefits of estrogen, such as preventing bone loss, without the negative effects, such as endometrial hyperplasia. Raloxifene competes with estrogen for estrogen receptor sites. It decreases bone loss and serum cholesterol but has minimal effects on breast and uterine tissue.

Bisphosphonates including alendronate (Fosamax, Fosavance) and risedronate (Actonel/Actonel DR) are also used to decrease the risk for osteoporosis in postmenopausal women. These drugs enhance bone mineral density by suppressing resorption. SERMs and bisphosphonates are discussed further in Chapter 66 with respect to their role in the management of osteoporosis.

Nonhormone Therapy.

Because of the risks associated with HRT, alternative therapies are often tried by many women to relieve menopausal symptoms. Hot flash frequency and severity can be reduced by promoting measures that would lead to a decrease in heat production and an increase in heat loss. Keeping a cool environment and limiting caffeine and alcohol intake lowers heat production. Behavioural changes, such as relaxation techniques, also help. To promote heat loss at night when hot flashes can disrupt sleep, increasing air circulation in the room and avoiding bedding that traps the heat (e.g., heavy quilts) may help. Loose-fitting clothes do not retain body heat, unlike clothes with tight necks and wrists. Cool cloths applied to flushed areas also aid heat loss. Daily intake of vitamin E in doses up to 800 IU may help reduce hot flashes in some women.

A focus on improving behaviours related to good nutrition with adequate amounts of exercise and sleep can help decrease anxiety and depression. Changing sleep patterns may be helped by avoiding alcohol and controlling hot flashes. Stress reduction techniques can promote a better night's sleep by decreasing anxiety. A regular, moderate program (three to four times per week) of aerobic and weight-bearing exercises can slow the process of bone loss and a tendency toward weight gain. Exercise is important at menopause in modifying coronary artery disease risk factors, including stress, obesity, physical inactivity, and hypertension.

Nutritional Therapy.

Good nutrition can decrease the risk of cardiovascular disease and osteoporosis in addition to assisting with vasomotor symptoms. A daily intake of about 30 kcal/kg of body weight with maintenance of sound nutrition is recommended. A decrease in metabolic rate and careless eating habits can cause the weight gain and fatigue often attributed to menopause. An adequate intake of calcium and vitamin D helps maintain healthy bones and counteracts loss of bone density. Postmenopausal women who are not receiving supplemental estrogen should have a daily calcium intake of at least 1500 mg. Those who are taking estrogen replacement need at least 1000 mg/ day. Calcium supplements are best absorbed when taken with meals. Either dietary calcium or calcium supplements may be used (see Chapter 66, Tables 66-14 and 66-15).

The diet should be high in complex carbohydrates and vitamin B complex, especially B_6. Phytoestrogens from plant sources may reduce menopausal symptoms. Foods containing phytoestrogens include soy, tofu, chickpeas, and sunflower seeds. Herbal remedies, such as black cohosh, have become popular in treating menopausal symptoms (see the Complementary and Alternative Therapies box on this page). Consultation with an experienced herbal practitioner is recommended before initiating therapy. Many herbs can cause serious adverse effects.

COMPLEMENTARY AND ALTERNATIVE THERAPIES
Herbs and Supplements for Menopause

Herb	Scientific Evidence	Nursing Implications
Black cohosh	Good evidence for treatment of menopausal symptoms*; further research is needed	• Generally well tolerated in recommended doses for ≤6 mo. • May lower blood pressure.
Soy	Good evidence for treatment of menopausal symptoms*; further research is needed	Women with a history of breast, ovarian, or uterine cancer or endometriosis should consult with their health care provider before using soy or soy products. • Soy may interact with warfarin. Patients taking warfarin should consult their health care provider before using soy or soy products.

*Based on a systematic review of scientific literature. Available at *http://www.naturalstandard.com*

CULTURALLY COMPETENT CARE: MENOPAUSE

Menopause is a universal phase in a woman's life, but the perception of this change varies by culture. Nurses must be aware of the differences in attitudes and beliefs regarding menopause among women from various ethnic backgrounds. In many cultures, menopause is considered a normal part of aging, and little emphasis is placed on the physical and emotional symptoms that accompany the loss of fertility. A study of Hindu women found that these women looked forward to menopause (Rani, 2009). In cultures in which the elderly are revered, menopause is seen as a liberating transition to a state of being a "wise woman" (Brockie, 2008). North American culture is generally negative toward aging and places a high value on youth. Menopause is often considered a disorder that requires treatment. Menopausal symptoms may be viewed as troublesome, with a strong need to treat hot flashes and mood swings. Numerous substances, from HRT to herbal preparations, are often used to treat menopausal symptoms.

Although menopause is experienced by all women, its meaning and symptoms vary. Menopause is a milestone in a woman's life that is embedded in her own personality and culture. Approaching the menopausal woman with this understanding is important to provide culturally competent care.

NURSING MANAGEMENT: PERIMENOPAUSE AND POSTMENOPAUSE

Nurses can play a key role in helping women to understand perimenopausal changes and options to minimize unwanted symptoms that are bothersome (see Table 56-7). Nurses can foster a positive image of perimenopause as a time of vitality and attractiveness. Perimenopause can provide women with a renewed incentive to enhance self-care and well-being.

Nurses must provide teaching and reassurance to perimenopausal women who experience difficulty in managing their symptoms. They should be informed that the symptoms are normal and only temporary. Nonpharmacological approaches to managing symptoms should be discussed. The nurse must address misconceptions about menopause to reduce unnecessary anxiety.

Dry skin can be improved by the use of moisturizing soaps and body lotions. Kegel exercises may help decrease stress incontinence (see Table 48-19). Sexual function can continue with little change in the vast majority of postmenopausal women. Cessation of menstruation and ability to bear children should not be equated with cessation of sexual capability; in fact, it may be liberating. Femininity and libido do not disappear with menopause. Atrophic changes in vaginal epithelium associated with decreased estrogen may lead to dyspareunia. A water-soluble lubricant (e.g., Replens, K-Y jelly) is often effective in managing this problem. An active sex life helps increase lubrication and maintains the pliability of vaginal tissues. The patient should be given an opportunity to candidly discuss concerns related to sexual functioning.

Conditions of the Vulva, the Vagina, and the Cervix

Etiology and Pathophysiology

Infection and inflammation of the vagina, the cervix, and the vulva tend to occur when the natural defences of the acid vaginal secretions (maintained by sufficient estrogen levels) and the presence of *Lactobacillus* are disrupted. The woman's resistance may also be decreased as a result of aging, poor nutrition, and the use of drugs (e.g., antibiotics, hormones) that alter the bacterial flora or mucosa. Organisms gain entrance to the areas through contaminated hands, clothing, and douche tips and during intercourse, surgery, and childbirth. Table 56-8 relates the specific etiological factors, clinical manifestations and diagnostic methods, and collaborative care of common inflammations and infections.

Most lower genital tract infections are related to sexual intercourse. Intercourse can transmit organisms, injure tissues, and alter the acid–base balance of the vagina. Vulvar infections caused by viruses such as herpes and genital warts can be sexually transmitted when no lesions are apparent. Oral contraceptives, antibiotics, and corticosteroids may produce changes in the vaginal pH and trigger an overgrowth of the organisms present. For example, *Candida albicans* may be present in small numbers in the vagina. An overgrowth of this organism causes vulvovaginitis.

Clinical Manifestations

Abnormal vaginal discharge and reddened vulvar lesions are common clinical manifestations. In addition to a thick, white, curdlike discharge, women with vulvovaginal candidiasis (VVC) often experience intense itching and dysuria, which is the result of urine coming into contact with fissures and irritated areas on the vulva. The hallmark of bacterial vaginosis is the fishy odour of the discharge. Women with cervicitis may notice spotting after intercourse.

Common vulvar lesions include herpes infection and genital warts. Initial or primary herpes infections may be extremely painful. Herpes begins as a small vesicle followed by a superficial red ulcer. Most herpes lesions are painful. Dysuria is common when urine touches the lesion. Genital warts, caused by the human papillomavirus (HPV), vary in appearance. Irregularly shaped "cauliflower" lesions are common. Genital warts are painless unless traumatized. (Herpes infection and genital warts are discussed in Chapter 55.)

Postmenopausal women may develop gynecological problems such as *lichen sclerosis* (Valdivielso-Ramos, Bueno, & Hernanz, 2008). This chronic inflammatory condition is associated with intense itching in the genital skin area (e.g., labia minora, clitoris). The lesions are white with a "tissue paper" appearance initially, although scratching produces changes in the appearance. The cause is unknown. High-potency topical corticosteroid ointment such as clobetasol (Clobex) helps relieve itching.

Collaborative Care

Genital problems are evaluated by taking a history, performing a physical examination, and obtaining the appropriate laboratory and diagnostic studies. Because many problems relate to sexual activity, a sexual history is essential. The nature of the problem directs specific aspects of the evaluation. Ulcerative lesions should be cultured for herpes. A blood test for syphilis may be done when ulcerative lesions are present. Genital warts are usually identified by their clinical appearance. Vulvar dystrophies may be examined via colposcopy, and a biopsy is taken for diagnosis.

Problems involving vaginal discharge are evaluated by microscopy and cultures. The most common vaginal conditions (i.e., bacterial vaginosis, VVC, and trichomoniasis) are diagnosed by a procedure called a *wet mount*. The findings that are characteristic of each condition are shown in Table 56-8. To assess for cervicitis, endocervical cultures are obtained for *Chlamydia* and gonorrhea. If purulent discharge is observed coming from the cervix, a

Table 56-8 Infections of the Lower Genital Tract

INFECTION/ETIOLOGY	CLINICAL MANIFESTATIONS AND DIAGNOSTIC METHODS	DRUG THERAPY
Vulvovaginal Candidiasis (VVC) (Monilial Vaginitis)		
Candida albicans (fungus)	Commonly found in mouth, gastrointestinal tract, and vagina; pruritus, thick white, curdlike discharge; KOH microscopic examination—pseudohyphae; pH 4-4.7	Intravaginal, over-the-counter azole ovules and creams (e.g., clotrimazole, miconazole) Fluconazole 150 mg PO as single dose (contraindicated in pregnancy)
Trichomoniasis Vaginitis		
Trichomonas vaginalis (protozoa)	Sexually transmitted; pruritus; frothy greenish or grey discharge; hemorrhagic spots on cervix or vaginal walls; saline microscopic examination—swimming trichomonads; pH >4.5	Metronidazole (Flagyl) 2 g PO in single dose or 500 mg PO BID for 7 days for patient and partner
Bacterial Vaginosis		
Gardnerella vaginalis Corynebacterium vaginale	Mode of transmission unclear; watery discharge with fishy odour; may or may not have symptoms; saline microscopic examination—epithelial cells; pH >4.5	Metronidazole (Flagyl) 500 mg PO BID for 7 days Metronidazole (Flagyl) gel 0.75%, on applicator (5 g) once a day intravaginally for 5 days Clindamycin cream 2%, one applicator (5 g) intravaginally for 7 days Examine and treat partner Alternatives: Metronidazole 2 g PO in a single dose Clindamycin (Dalacin C) 300 mg PO BID for 7 days
Cervicitis		
Chlamydia trachomatis	Sexually transmitted; mucopurulent discharge with postcoital spotting from cervical inflammation; culture for C. trachomatis and Neisseria gonorrhoeae	Azithromycin (Zithromax) 1 g PO as a single dose or doxycycline (Doxycin) 100 mg PO BID for 7 days; treat partners with same drugs
Severe Recurrent Vaginitis		
C. albicans (most often)	May be indicative of HIV infection; all women who are unresponsive to first-line treatment should be offered HIV testing	Drug appropriate to opportunistic organism

HIV, human immunodeficiency virus; KOH, potassium hydroxide.
Source: Adapted from Public Health Agency of Canada [PHAC]. (2008 edition). *Canadian guidelines on sexually transmitted infections*. Ottawa: Author. Retrieved from *http://www.phac-aspc.gc.ca/std-mts/sti-its/guide-lignesdir-eng.php*

sample of endocervical cells may be taken to be evaluated by Gram's staining. The Gram-stained slide is examined with a microscope to identify white blood cells and Gram-negative diplococci (indicative of gonorrhea). (Sexually transmitted infections [STIs] are discussed in Chapter 55.)

Drug therapy is based on the diagnosis and is shown in Table 56-8. Antibiotics taken as directed will cure bacterial infections. Antifungal preparations (in oral and cream preparations) are indicated for VVC. Women with vaginal conditions or cervical infection should abstain from intercourse for at least 1 week. Douching has been adversely linked to pelvic inflammatory disease (PID), sexually transmitted infection (STIs), and ectopic pregnancy and, thus, should be avoided (Cotrell Hansen & Close, 2008). Sexual partners must be examined and treated if the patient is diagnosed with trichomoniasis, chlamydial infection, gonorrhea, syphilis, or HIV.

Treatment of vulvar dystrophies is symptomatic because no cures are available. Treatment involves controlling the itching and, hence, the scratching. Interrupting the "itch–scratch cycle" prevents further secondary damage to the skin.

NURSING MANAGEMENT: CONDITIONS OF THE VULVA, THE VAGINA, AND THE CERVIX

Nurses have the opportunity to teach women about common genital conditions and how to reduce their risks. Recognizing symptoms that indicate a problem helps women seek care in a timely manner. Discussing problems concerning one's genitals or sexual intercourse is frequently difficult. The nurse's nonjudgemental attitude makes women feel more comfortable and empowers them to ask questions and seek accurate information.

When a woman is diagnosed with a pathological genital condition, the nurse should ensure that she fully understands the directions for treatment. Taking the full course of medication is especially important to decrease the chance of relapse. Because genitalia are such a private area, use of graphs and models is especially helpful for patient teaching. When a woman will be using a vaginal medication for the first time, showing her the applicator and how to fill it is important. The woman should be taught where and how the applicator should be inserted, using visual aids or models. Vaginal creams should be inserted before going to bed so that the medication will remain in the vagina for a long time. Women using vaginal creams or suppositories may wish to use panty liners during the day, when the residual medication may drain out.

Pelvic Inflammatory Disease

Pelvic inflammatory disease (PID) is an infectious condition of the pelvic cavity that may involve infection of the cervix (endocervicitis), fallopian tubes (salpingitis), and pelvic peritoneum (peritonitis) (Soper, 2010). A tubo-ovarian abscess may also form (Figure 56-4). There are about 100,000 cases of symptomatic PID annually in Canada (PHAC, 2008b). PID is referred to as "silent" when women do not perceive any symptoms. Other women with PID will be in acute distress. Pelvic pain may also be chronic in nature.

Etiology and Pathophysiology

PID is often the result of untreated cervicitis. The organism infecting the cervix ascends higher into the uterus, fallopian tubes, ovaries, and peritoneal cavity. *Chlamydia trachomatis* and *Neisseria gonorrhoeae* are the most common causative organisms of PID. These organisms, as well as anaerobes, mycoplasma, streptococci, and enteric Gram-negative rods, gain entrance during sexual intercourse or after pregnancy termination, pelvic surgery, or childbirth. It is important to remember that not all cases of PID are the result of an STI.

Women at increased risk for chlamydial infections (younger than 24 years of age, who have multiple sex partners, or who have a new sex partner) should be routinely tested for *Chlamydia*. Chlamydial infections can be asymptomatic and unknowingly transmitted during intercourse. Silent PID can cause damage that cannot be reversed. PID remains a major cause of female infertility.

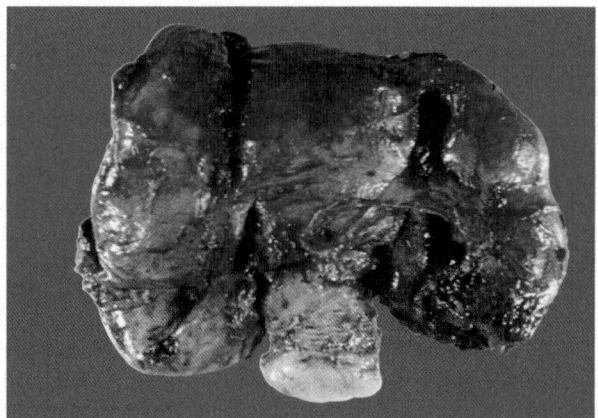

Figure 56-4 Pelvic inflammatory disease. Acute infection of the fallopian tubes and ovaries. The tubes and ovaries have become an inflamed mass attached to the uterus. A tubo-ovarian abscess is also present.

Source: Kumar, V., Abbas, A. K., Fausto, N., & Aster, J. (2010). *Robbins and Cotran pathologic basis of disease* (8th ed., p. 1010, Figure 22-4A). Philadelphia: Saunders.

Chronic pelvic pain is pain 6 months or longer in duration and is located below the umbilicus and between the hips (Mayo Clinic, 2011). Up to one third of women have chronic pelvic pain after PID. Additional factors also associated with chronic pelvic pain include interstitial cystitis, irritable bowel syndrome, adhesions, endometriosis, and dysmenorrhea (Ortiz, 2008).

Clinical Manifestations

Women with PID usually go to a health care provider because they are experiencing lower abdominal pain. The pain typically starts gradually and then becomes constant. The intensity may vary from mild to severe. Movement such as walking can increase the pain; pain is also frequently associated with intercourse. Spotting after intercourse and purulent cervical or vaginal discharge may also be noted. Fever and chills may also be present. Women with less acute symptoms notice increased cramping pain with menses, irregular bleeding, and some pain with intercourse. Women who have mild symptoms may go untreated either because they did not seek care or the health care provider misdiagnosed their complaints.

PID is a clinical diagnosis based on the patient's signs and symptoms. The diagnosis of PID is obtained during the bimanual portion of the pelvic examination. Women with PID have lower abdominal tenderness, adnexal tenderness (tenderness of uterine appendages such as fallopian tubes, ovaries, and ligaments that hold the uterus in place), and positive cervical motion tenderness. Additional criteria useful for diagnosis include fever and abnormal discharge (vaginal or cervical). Cultures for *N. gonorrhoeae* and *Chlamydia* are also obtained, and a pregnancy test should be done to rule out ectopic pregnancy. Drug therapy begins when minimal diagnostic criteria are met; thus, treatment is not delayed for culture results. If the patient's pain or obesity compromises the pelvic examination and a tubo-ovarian abscess is considered a possibility, a vaginal ultrasonography is indicated.

Complications

Immediate complications of PID include septic shock and *Fitz–Hugh–Curtis syndrome,* which occurs when PID spreads to the liver and causes acute perihepatitis. The patient will have symptoms of right upper quadrant pain, but liver function tests will be normal. Tubo-ovarian abscesses may "leak" or rupture, resulting in pelvic or generalized peritonitis. As the general circulation is flooded with bacterial endotoxins from the infected areas, septic shock may result. Embolisms may occur as the result of thrombophlebitis of the pelvic veins.

PID can cause adhesions and strictures to develop in the fallopian tubes. Ectopic pregnancy may result when a tube is partially obstructed because the sperm can pass through the stricture but the fertilized ovum cannot reach the uterus. After one episode of PID, the risk of having an ectopic pregnancy increases ten-fold. Women with PID are also at increased risk of recurrent infection (Soper, 2010). Further damage can obstruct the fallopian tubes and cause infertility.

Collaborative Care

PID is usually treated on an outpatient basis. The patient is given a combination of antibiotics such as cefoxitin and doxycycline (Vibramycin) to provide broad coverage against the causative organisms. With effective antibiotic therapy, the pain should subside. The patient must have no intercourse for 3 weeks. Her partner(s) must be examined and treated. An important part of care is physical rest and oral fluids. Re-evaluation in 48 to 72 hours, even if symptoms are improving, is an essential part of outpatient care.

If outpatient treatment is unsuccessful or if the patient is acutely ill or in severe pain, admission to hospital is indicated. If a tubo-ovarian abscess is present, hospitalization is necessary. Maximum doses of parenteral antibiotics are given in hospital. Corticosteroids may be added to the antibiotic regimen to reduce inflammation, allowing for faster recovery and improvement in subsequent fertility. Application of heat to the lower abdomen or sitz baths may be used to improve circulation and decrease pain. Bed rest in the semi-Fowler position promotes drainage of the pelvic cavity by gravity and may prevent the development of abscesses high in the abdomen. Analgesics to relieve pain and IV fluids to prevent dehydration are also used.

An indication for surgery is the presence of abscesses that fail to resolve with IV antibiotics. The abscess may be drained by laparoscopy or laparotomy. In extreme cases, a hysterectomy may be performed. When surgery is necessary, the capacity for childbearing is preserved whenever possible.

Treatment for chronic pelvic pain should focus on the underlying disorder (Ortiz, 2008). If the source of the pain is unknown, treatment is directed at managing the symptoms.

NURSING MANAGEMENT: PELVIC INFLAMMATORY DISEASE

Subjective and objective data that should be obtained from the woman with PID are presented in Table 56-9. Prevention, early recognition, and prompt treatment of vaginal and cervical infections can help prevent PID and its serious complications. Nurses should urge women to seek medical attention for any unusual vaginal discharge or possible infection of their reproductive organs. Women should be helped to understand that not all discharge is indicative of infection, but that early diagnosis and treatment of an infection, if present, can prevent serious complications. Women should be informed of the methods to decrease the risk of getting STIs and to recognize the signs of infection in their partner(s).

The patient may have guilt feelings about having PID, especially if it was associated with an STI. She may also be concerned about the complications associated with PID, such as adhesions and strictures of the fallopian tubes, infertility, and the increased incidence of ectopic pregnancy. Discussion with the patient regarding her feelings and concerns can assist her to cope more effectively with them.

For patients requiring hospitalization, nurses have an important role in implementing drug therapy, monitoring the patient's health status, and providing symptom relief and patient teaching. Vital signs and character, amount, colour, and odour of the vaginal discharge should be recorded. Explanations about the need for limited activity, maintaining a semi-Fowler position, and increased fluid intake should increase patient cooperation. Assessing the degree of abdominal pain will provide information about the effectiveness of drug therapy.

NURSING ASSESSMENT

Table 56-9 Pelvic Inflammatory Disease

Subjective Data

Important Health Information

Past health history:

Use of IUD; previous PID, gonorrhea, or chlamydial infection; multiple sexual partners; exposure to partner with urethritis; infertility

Medications: Use of and allergy to any antibiotics

Surgery or other treatments: Recent abortion or pelvic surgery

Symptoms

- Malaise
- Nausea, vomiting; chills
- Urinary frequency, urgency
- Lower abdominal and pelvic pain; low back pain; pain on fundal palpation and cervical motion; onset of pain just after a menstrual cycle; dysmenorrhea, dyspareunia, dysuria, vulvar pruritus
- Abnormal vaginal bleeding and menstrual irregularity; vaginal discharge

Objective Data

General

Fever

Reproductive

Mucopurulent cervicitis, vulvar maceration, vaginal discharge (heavy and purulent to thin and mucoid), tenderness on motion of cervix and uterus; presence of inflammatory masses on palpation

Possible Findings

Leukocytosis; ↑ erythrocyte sedimentation rate; positive culture of secretions or endocervical fluid; pelvic inflammation and positive endometrial biopsy on laparoscopic examination; abscess or inflammation on ultrasonography

IUD, intrauterine device; *PID,* pelvic inflammatory disease.

Endometriosis

Endometriosis is the presence of endometrial epithelial and/or stromal cells in sites outside the uterine cavity (Holoch & Lessey, 2010). The most frequent sites are in or near the ovaries, the uterosacral ligaments, and the uterovesical peritoneum (Figure 56-5). However, endometrial tissues can be in many other locations such as the stomach, the lungs, the intestines, and the spleen. The tissue responds to the hormones of the ovarian cycle and undergoes a "mini-menstrual cycle" similar to the uterine endometrium.

The typical patient with endometriosis is in her late 20s or early 30s, is White, and has never had a full-term pregnancy. Although it is not a life-threatening condition, endometriosis can cause considerable pain. It also increases the risk of ovarian cancer. Endometriosis is one of the most common gynaecologic problems affecting over 5.5 million females in North America (Cleveland Clinic, 2010).

Etiology and Pathophysiology

The etiology is poorly understood, and many theories about the cause of endometriosis have been proposed. The most widely

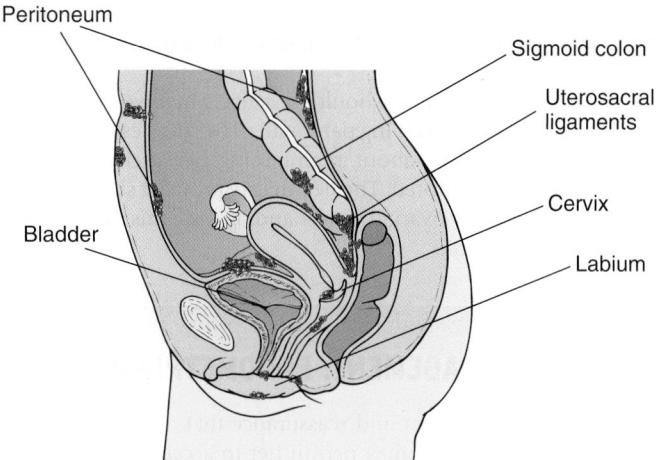

Figure 56-5 Common sites of endometriosis.

Source: Adapted from Stenchever, M. A., Droegemueller, W., Herbst, A. L., & Mishell, D. R. (2001). *Comprehensive gynecology* (4th ed.). St. Louis: Mosby.

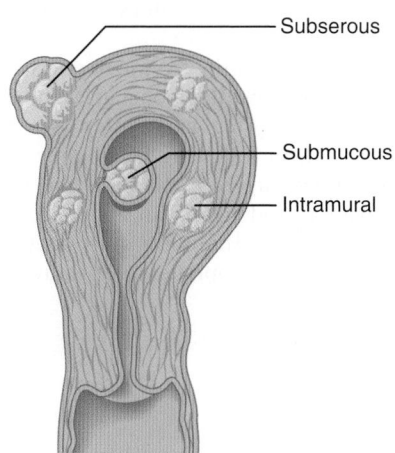

Figure 56-6 Leiomyomas. Uterine section shows the whorl-like appearance and locations of leiomyomas, which are also called *uterine fibroids*.

Source: McCance, K. L., & Huether, S. E. (2010). *Pathophysiology: The biologic basis for disease in adults and children* (6th ed., p. 838, Figure 23-14A). St. Louis: Mosby.

accepted view is that retrograde menstrual flow passes through the fallopian tubes carrying viable endometrial tissues into the pelvis (Holoch & Lessey, 2010). The tissue attaches to various sites shown in Figure 56-6. Another theory suggests that undifferentiated embryonic peritoneal cavity cells remain dormant in the pelvic tissue until the ovaries produce sufficient hormones to stimulate their growth. Other proposed causes are a genetic predisposition and altered immune function.

Clinical Manifestations

In patients with endometriosis, a wide range of clinical manifestations and severity exists. The magnitude of a woman's symptoms does not necessarily correlate with the clinical extent of her endometriosis. Dysmenorrhea after years of relatively pain-free menses and infertility may serve as clues to the presence of endometriosis. The most common manifestations are secondary dys-

COLLABORATIVE CARE

Table 56-10 Endometriosis

Diagnostic

- History and physical examination
- Pelvic examination
- Laparoscopy
- Pelvic ultrasonography
- MRI

Collaborative Therapy

- Conservative therapy (watch and wait)

Drug Therapy

- Nonsteroidal anti-inflammatory agents
- Oral contraceptives
- Danazol (Cyclomen)
- GnRH agonists (e.g., leuprolide [Lupron])

Surgical Therapy

- Laparotomy to remove implants and adhesions
- Total abdominal hysterectomy and bilateral salpingo-oophorectomy (TAH-BSO)

GnRH, gonadotropin-releasing hormone; *MRI*, magnetic resonance imaging.

menorrhea, infertility, pelvic pain, dyspareunia, and irregular bleeding. Less common manifestations include backache, painful bowel movements, and dysuria. These symptoms may or may not correspond to the woman's menstrual cycles. With menopause, estrogen is no longer produced in the ovaries. This may lead to the disappearance of the symptoms.

When the ectopic endometrial tissues "menstruate," the blood collects in cystlike nodules that have a characteristic bluish black colour. Nodules in the ovaries are sometimes called *chocolate cysts* because of the thick, chocolate-coloured material they contain. When a cyst ruptures, the pain may be acute, and the resulting irritation promotes the formation of adhesions, which fix the affected area to another pelvic structure. Endometrial adhesions may become severe enough to cause a bowel obstruction or painful micturition.

Collaborative Care

Endometriosis may be suspected from a woman's history of the characteristic symptoms and the health care provider's palpation of firm nodular lumps in the adnexa on bimanual examination. However, laparoscopy is necessary for a definitive diagnosis. The treatment of endometriosis is influenced by the patient's age, desire for pregnancy, symptom severity, and the extent and the location of the disease. When symptoms are not disruptive, a "watch-and-wait" approach is used (Table 56-10). When endometriosis is identified as a probable cause of infertility, therapy proceeds more rapidly.

Drug Therapy. Drug therapy is used to reduce symptoms. Pain may be relieved with NSAIDs such as ibuprofen (Advil) and diclofenac (Voltaren). Drugs to inhibit estrogen production by the ovary are often given to shrink the endometrial tissue. These drugs imitate a state of pregnancy or menopause. Continuous use (for 9 months) of combined oral contraceptives causes regression of endometrial tissue. Ovulation is suppressed, and *pseudopregnancy* (hyperhormonal amenorrhea) is produced by progestin agents such as medroxyprogesterone (Depo-Provera). Another approach to hormonal treatment is danazol (Cyclomen), a synthetic androgen that inhibits the anterior pituitary. This drug produces a *pseudomenopause* (ovarian suppression) with atrophy of ectopic endometrial tissue. Subjective relief of symptoms is noted within 6 weeks of danazol use. Adverse effects include weight gain, acne, hot flashes, and hirsutism. These adverse effects and the expense of this drug restrict its use.

Another class of drugs used is gonadotropin-releasing hormone (GnRH) agonists (e.g., leuprolide [Lupron, Eligard], nafarelin [Synarel]). These drugs cause a hypoestrogenic state resulting in amenorrhea. The adverse effects reported by patients are usually the same as menopause (hot flashes, vaginal dryness, and emotional lability). Loss of bone density has also been reported in women who remain on the therapy longer than 6 months. Endometriosis is controlled but not cured by hormone therapy. Persistent lesions give rise to subsequent recurrences once the menstrual cycle is re-established.

Surgical Therapy. The only cure for endometriosis is surgical removal of all the endometrial implants. Surgical therapy may be conservative or definitive. Conservative surgery is done to confirm the diagnosis or to remove implants. It involves removal or destruction of endometrial implants and lysing or excision of adhesions by means of laparoscopic laser surgery or laparotomy. GnRH agonist therapy (e.g., leuprolide) can be administered for 4 to 6 months to reduce the size of the lesions before surgery. By reducing the extent of the surgery, this preoperative drug treatment helps reduce the development of adhesions that may further threaten fertility.

For women wishing to get pregnant, conservative surgical therapy is used to remove implants blocking the fallopian tube.

Adhesions are removed from the tubes, the ovaries, and the pelvic structures. Efforts are made to conserve all tissues necessary to maintain fertility.

The individual woman should be actively involved in making the decision about preserving part or all of her ovaries if surgically possible. Her feelings about maintaining her cyclical ovarian function must be explored. The health care provider should assess the woman's risk for ovarian cancer and provide this information for her consideration.

NURSING MANAGEMENT: ENDOMETRIOSIS

Education of the patient and reassurance that a life-threatening situation does not exist may permit her to accept a conservative and progressive treatment. When the symptoms are less severe, teaching about nondrug comfort measures may be helpful. Nurses must assist patients to understand the drugs that have been ordered to treat their condition. The action of the prescribed drug should be explained as well as the possible adverse effects. Psychological support may be needed for women experiencing severe disabling pain, sexual difficulties secondary to dyspareunia, and infertility.

If conservative surgery is the treatment selected, the nursing care is similar to the general preoperative and postoperative care of a patient undergoing laparotomy (see Nursing Care Plan 45-2 for the patient following laparotomy in Chapter 45, p. 1174). If definitive surgery is planned, the nursing care is similar to the patient undergoing an abdominal hysterectomy (Nursing Care Plan 56-1). The nurse must know the extent of the procedure so that appropriate preoperative teaching can be done.

NURSING CARE PLAN 56-1
Abdominal Hysterectomy

NURSING DIAGNOSIS	***Disturbed body image*** *related to* perceived loss of femininity and future inability to conceive *as evidenced by* crying, weeping, or depression; verbalization of perceived loss of femininity and/or ability to conceive
Expected Patient Outcomes	**Nursing Interventions and *Rationales***
• Verbalizes confidence in ability to adjust to postsurgical state • States acceptance of self and changes resulting from surgery	• Determine patient's body image expectations *to establish need and plan for interventions.* • Determine patient's and family's perceptions of the alteration in body image versus reality *to provide accurate facts and decrease fear of consequences of hysterectomy.* • Determine if a change in body image has contributed to increased social isolation *to identify need for intervention.* • Identify support groups available to the patient *to minimize emotional impact of hysterectomy through open discussion.* • Assist the patient to discuss stressors affecting body image owing to surgery (e.g., surgical menopause) *so patient is informed about possible treatment* (e.g., hormone replacement therapy).
NURSING DIAGNOSIS	***Acute pain*; ineffective breathing pattern*; nausea*; risk for imbalanced fluid volume*; risk for infection****
Collaborative Problems*	Hemorrhage*; urinary retention*; paralytic ileus*

*Postoperative care of the patient with an abdominal hysterectomy includes nursing diagnoses for the postoperative patient found in eNCP 22-1: Postoperative Patient, available on the Evolve Web site for that chapter.

Benign Tumours of the Female Reproductive System

Leiomyomas

Etiology and Pathophysiology

Leiomyomas (uterine fibroids) are benign smooth muscle tumours that occur most commonly within the uterus. Leiomyomas are the most common benign tumours of the female genital tract (Ellenson & Pirog, 2010) (see Figure 56-6). Estimates of the prevalence of fibroids in women range from 20 to 77%, but the literature provides weak evidence of the overall burden of disease posed by uterine fibroids (Viswanathan et al., 2007). The cause of leiomyomas is unknown. They appear to depend on ovarian hormones because they grow slowly during the reproductive years and undergo atrophy after menopause.

Clinical Manifestations

The majority of women with leiomyomas do not have any symptoms. Of the women who develop symptoms, the most common include abnormal uterine bleeding, pain, and symptoms associated with pelvic pressure. Increased bleeding is thought to be associated with the increased endometrial surface area that is associated with leiomyomas. Pain is associated with infection or twisting of the pedicle from which the tumour is growing. Devascularization and blood vessel compression are also thought to contribute to pain. Pressure on surrounding organs may result in rectal, bladder, and lower abdominal discomfort. Large tumours may cause a general enlargement of the lower abdomen. These tumours are sometimes associated with miscarriage and infertility.

Collaborative Care

Clinical diagnosis is based on the characteristic pelvic findings of an enlarged uterus distorted by nodular masses. Treatment depends on the symptoms, the age of the patient, her desire to bear children, and the location and size of the tumour or tumours. If the symptoms are minor, the health care provider may elect to follow the patient closely for a time.

Persistent heavy menstrual bleeding causing anemia and large or rapidly growing tumours are indications for surgery. The leiomyomas are removed by hysterectomy or myomectomy. A myomectomy is performed for women who wish to have children. In this case, only the fibroids are removed to preserve the uterus. Small tumours may be removed using a hysteroscope and laser resection instruments.

Uterine artery embolization is an increasingly used alternative treatment for uterine fibroids. In the short term, it involves less blood loss, shorter hospital stays, and a quicker return to work but there is evidence of a higher reintervention rate in the longer term (van der Kooij, Bipat, Henekamp, Ankum, & Reekers, 2011). In the procedure, embolic material (small plastic or gelatin beads) is injected into the uterine artery and carried to the fibroid branches.

Cryosurgery is another option. In cases of large leiomyomas, a GnRH agonist (e.g., leuprolide [Lupron]) may be used preoperatively to shrink the size of the tumour. However, the risks and benefits of this drug should be fully discussed, including the

potential for irreversible loss of bone mass. The treatment should not be used on women planning to have children.

Another treatment option uses magnetic resonance imaging (MRI)–guided focused ultrasonography to target and destroy uterine fibroids. Treatment requires repeated targeting and heating of the fibroid tissue while the patient lies inside the MRI machine. The procedure can last as long as 3 to 4 hours and the patient must lie in a prone position. Long-term studies are needed to provide reliable evidence of its clinical effectiveness and safety as well as its cost-effectiveness (Stovall, 2011).

Cervical Polyps

Cervical polyps are benign pedunculated lesions that generally arise from the endocervical mucosa and are seen protruding through the cervical os during a speculum examination. Polyps are a characteristic bright cherry red and are soft and fragile in consistency. They are generally small, measuring less than 3 cm in length, and may be single or multiple. Their cause is unknown. Symptoms are usually not present, but metrorrhagia and bleeding after straining and coitus can occur. Polyps are prone to infection. When the polyp is small, it can be excised in an outpatient procedure. If the point of attachment of the polyp cannot be identified and is not accessible to cautery, a polypectomy is performed in an operating room. All tissue removed is sent for pathological review because polyps occasionally undergo malignant changes.

Benign Ovarian Tumours

There are many different types of benign tumours. The cause of most of them is unknown. They can be divided into cysts and neoplasms. *Cysts* are usually soft, are surrounded by a thin capsule, and may be detected during the reproductive years. Follicle and corpus luteum cysts are common ovarian cysts (Figure 56-7). Multiple small ovarian follicles may occur in a condition called *polycystic ovary syndrome* (PCOS) (discussed in the next section). Epithelial ovarian neoplasms may be cystic or solid, small or extremely large. Cystic teratomas, or dermoid cysts,

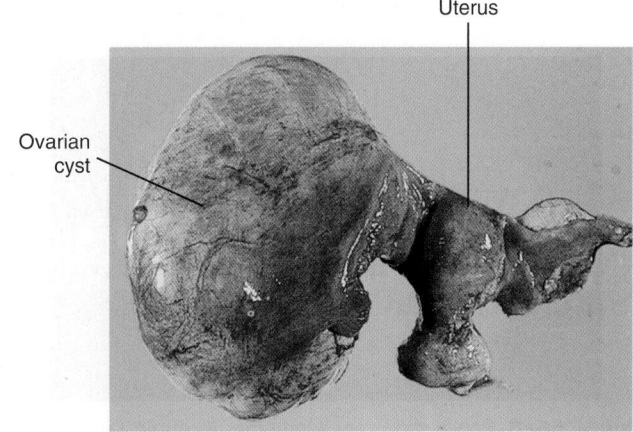

Figure 56-7 Large ovarian cyst.

Source: Symonds, E. M., & MacPherson, M. B. A. (1994). *Colour atlas of obstetrics and gynecology.* London: Mosby.

originate from germ cells and can contain bits of any type of body tissue, such as hair or teeth.

Ovarian masses are often asymptomatic until they are large enough to cause pressure in the pelvis. Constipation, menstrual irregularities, urinary frequency, a full feeling in the abdomen, anorexia, and peripheral edema may occur, depending on the size and the location of the tumour. There may be an increase in abdominal girth. Pelvic pain may be present if the tumour is growing rapidly. Severe pain results when the cyst twists on its pedicle (ovarian torsion).

Pelvic examination reveals a mass or an enlarged ovary that demands further investigation. If the mass is cystic and smaller than 8 cm, the patient is asked to return for re-examination in 4 to 6 weeks. If the mass is cystic and greater than 8 cm or is solid, laparoscopic surgery or laparotomy is performed. Immediate surgery is necessary if ovarian torsion occurs, causing the ovary to rotate and cutting off circulation. Surgical techniques are used to save as much of the ovary as possible.

Polycystic Ovary Syndrome

PCOS is a chronic disorder in which many benign cysts form on the ovaries. It most commonly occurs in women younger than 30 years and is a cause of infertility. It affects about 5 to 10% of women of reproductive age (Radosh, 2009). PCOS is caused by hormonal abnormalities in which the ovaries produce estrogen and excess testosterone but not progesterone. Fluid-filled cysts develop from mature ovarian follicles that fail to rupture (thereby releasing an egg) each month (Figure 56-8). This problem affects both ovaries.

Clinical manifestations include irregular menstrual periods (particularly long cycles), amenorrhea or oligomenorrhea, dysfunctional uterine bleeding, infertility, hirsutism, obesity, and acne. Many women start with normal menstrual periods, and then, after 1 to 2 years, the periods become irregular and then infrequent. If left untreated, cardiovascular disease, metabolic syndrome with type 2 diabetes mellitus, infertility, and ovarian and endometrial cancers may develop (Ahonen, 2010; Buckworth & Hsu, 2010).

Pelvic ultrasonography will reveal enlarged ovaries with multiple small cysts. Successful management includes early diagnosis and treatment to improve quality of life and decrease the risk of complications. Oral contraceptives are useful in regulating

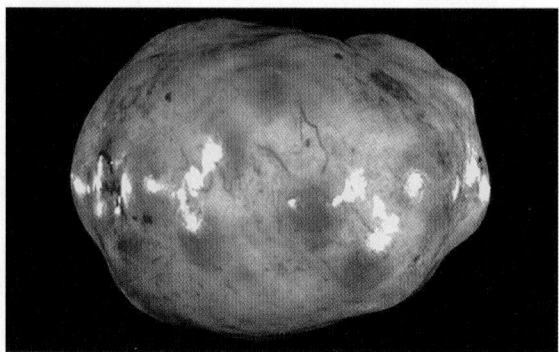

Figure 56-8 Polycystic ovary syndrome. Multiple fluid-filled cysts in the ovary.

Source: Patton, K. T., & Thibodeau, G. (2010). *Anatomy and physiology* (7th ed., p. 1065, Figure 32-22). St Louis: Mosby.

menstrual cycles. Hyperandrogenism can be treated with flutamide (Euflex) and a GnRH agonist such as leuprolide (Lupron). Metformin (Glucophage) reduces hyperinsulinemia and has been shown to improve hyperandrogenism and restore ovulation. For women desiring to become pregnant, fertility drugs (e.g., clomiphene [Clomid, Serophene]) may be used to induce ovulation. If all other treatments are unsuccessful, a hysterectomy with bilateral salpingo-oophorectomy may be performed.

Patient teaching for the patient with PCOS includes the importance of weight management and exercise to decrease insulin resistance. Obesity exacerbates the problems related to PCOS. Lipid profile and fasting glucose levels should be monitored. Regular follow-up care is important to monitor the effectiveness of therapy and to detect any complications.

Cancer of the Female Reproductive System

Cervical Cancer

Cervical cancer is the second most common female cancer in the world, with 83% of these cases occurring in under-resourced countries (Gakidou, Nordhagen, & Obermeyer, 2008). Noninvasive cervical cancer is about four times more common than invasive cervical cancer. In 2012, it was estimated that 1350 Canadian women would be diagnosed with cervical cancer and 390 women would die of the disease. The lifetime probability of a woman developing cervical cancer in Canada is 1 in 153 (Canadian Cancer Society's Steering Committee on Cancer Statistics, 2012).

The most important risk factor for developing cervical cancer is infection with HPV. An increased risk of cervical cancer is also associated with low socioeconomic status, early sexual activity, multiple sexual partners, weakened immune system, long term use of oral contraceptives (>10 years), high parity (seven or more children), smoking, and being the daughter of a mother who took diethylstilbestrol (DES) (Canadian Cancer Society [CCS], 2011a).

The number of deaths from cervical cancer in women who undergo regular screening and follow-up has fallen steadily since the 1950s. This is attributable to better and earlier diagnosis with the widespread use of the Papanicolaou (Pap) test. In addition to cancer, the Pap test detects precancerous changes. By treating precancerous lesions, progression to cervical cancer can be prevented.

Etiology and Pathophysiology

The progression from normal cervical cells to dysplasia and then to cervical cancer appears to be related to repeated injuries to the cervix. The progression occurs slowly over years rather than months. There is a strong relationship between dysplasia and HPV.

Clinical Manifestations

Precancerous changes are asymptomatic. This highlights the importance of routine screening. The peak incidence of noninvasive cervical cancer is in women in their early 30s. The average age for women with invasive cervical cancer is 50 (Figure 56-9). Early cervical cancer is generally asymptomatic, but leucorrhea

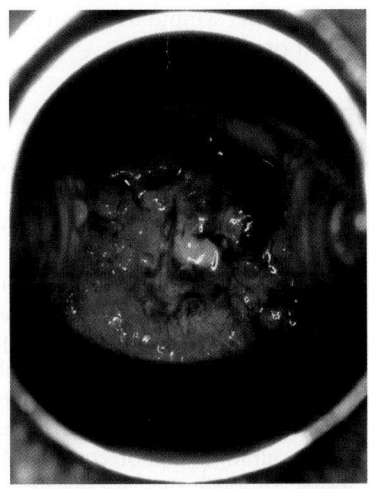

Figure 56-9 Cervical cancer. View through a speculum inserted into the vagina.

Source: Drake, R. L., Vogl, W., & Mitchell, A. W. M. (2010). *Gray's anatomy for students* (2nd ed., p. 457, Figure 5.55). Edinburgh: Churchill Livingstone.

Table 56-11	Staging and Treatment of Cervical Cancer	
STAGE	**EXTENT**	**TREATMENT**
Stage I	Confinement to cervix	Radiation, radical hysterectomy
Stage II	Extension to nearby tissues such as the upper part of the vagina or tissues next to the cervix	Radiation, cisplatin-based chemotherapy, radical hysterectomy
Stage III	Extension to the lower part of the vagina and/or the pelvic wall, and/or causes hydronephrosis or nonfunctioning kidney	Radiation, cisplatin-based chemotherapy
Stage IV	Extension beyond true pelvis or clinical involvement (biopsy proven) of the mucosa of bladder or rectum	Radiation, surgery (e.g., pelvic exenteration), cisplatin-based chemotherapy

Source: Adapted from FIGO Committee on Gynecologic Oncology. (2009). Revised FIGO staging for carcinoma of the vulva, cervix, and endometrium. *International Journal of Gynecology and Obstetrics, 105*(2), 103-104.

and intermenstrual bleeding eventually occur. The discharge is usually thin and watery but becomes dark and foul smelling as the disease advances, suggesting the presence of an infection. The vaginal bleeding is initially only spotting. As the tumour enlarges, the bleeding becomes heavier and more frequent. Pain is a late symptom and is followed by weight loss, anemia, and cachexia.

Diagnostic Studies

Cervical cancer screening is recommended in Canada for sexually active women between the ages of 21 and 69. Some provinces or territories may offer screening at earlier or later ages. The CCS (2011b) recommends that women have a Pap test every 1 to 3 years, depending on the screening guidelines in their province or territory and depending on their previous test results. After age 69, women should talk to their health care provider about the possibility of stopping the Pap test following two or three previously normal (negative) Pap results. Women who have sex with women should follow the same cervical screening guidelines. Women with previous abnormal Pap tests may be screened more often (CCS, 2011b). Women who have had a total hysterectomy (uterus and cervix removed) do not need to be screened for cervical cancer, unless the surgery was done for cervical precancer or cancer.

Pap tests are less than 100% accurate. There are problems with both false-positive and false-negative reports. ThinPrep, a newer liquid-based technique for Pap tests, has reduced the number of inaccurate Pap test results.

The finding of an abnormal Pap smear indicates the need for follow-up. The type of follow-up depends on the findings. Women with minor changes may be followed with a repeated Pap test in 4 to 6 months for 2 years. Up to 80% may revert to normal spontaneously. Women with more prominent changes will receive additional procedures, such as colposcopy and biopsy, before a definitive diagnosis can be made. Colposcopy involves examination of the cervix with a binocular microscope with low levels of magnification (10× to 40×). The procedure helps in the identification of possible epithelial abnormalities and suggests areas for biopsy. The LUMA Cervical Imaging System may be used

with colposcopy to identify these sites. Biopsies are sent to pathology for evaluation. Colposcopy and biopsy have improved diagnosis and allow more focused treatments to be selected.

The type and the extent of the biopsy vary with the abnormality seen. A punch biopsy may be done on an outpatient basis with special punch biopsy forceps. The excision of a cone-shaped section of the cervix may be used for both diagnosis and treatment. Conization is accomplished using one of several techniques. The choice of procedure is determined by the health care provider's experience and the availability of equipment. *Cryotherapy* (freezing) and laser cone vaporization destroy the tissue. Laser cone excision and *loop electrosurgery excision procedure* (LEEP) remove the identified tissue and allow for histological examination to ensure that all microinvasive tissue has been removed. These procedures can be performed as outpatient procedures with mild analgesics or sedation. Complications of these procedures include excessive bleeding and possible cervical stenosis after healing.

Collaborative Care

Vaccines against HPV (e.g., Gardasil, Cervarix) reduce the incidence of both cervical-related neoplasia and cervical cancer caused by infection from HPV types 16 and 18. HPV types 16 and 18 together cause 70% of cervical cancers (Maine, Hurlburt, & Greeson, 2011). The other 30% of cervical cancers are from HPV types not covered by the vaccine (CCS, 2011a). Vaccination is recommended for females aged 9 to 26. (Vaccines are discussed further in Chapter 55, pp. 1530-1531.)

The treatment of cancer of the cervix is guided by the stage of the tumour and the patient's age and general state of health (Table 56-11). There are four procedures in which fertility can be preserved. Conization may be the only type of therapy needed for noninvasive cervical cancer if analysis of removed tissue demonstrates that a wide area of normal tissue surrounds the excised tissue. Laser treatments can be used in which a directed infrared beam is employed to destroy abnormal tissue. Cautery and cryo-surgery may also be used.

Invasive cancer of the cervix is treated with surgery, irradiation, and chemotherapy as single treatments or in combination. Surgical procedures include hysterectomy, radical hysterectomy (involving adjacent structures), and rarely, pelvic exenterations. (Surgical therapy is discussed on p. 1546.) Irradiation may be external (e.g., cobalt) or internal implants (e.g., cesium, radium). Standard radiation treatment is 4 to 6 weeks of external irradiation followed with one or two treatments with internal implants (brachytherapy). (Radiation therapy is discussed in Chapter 18.) Cisplatin-based chemotherapy regimens have benefit for patients with cancer spread beyond the cervix.

Endometrial or Uterine Cancer

Cancer of the endometrium is the most common gynecological malignancy, accounting for nearly 50% of female genital tract neoplasms. The probability of a Canadian woman developing uterine cancer in her lifetime is 1 in 40. In 2012, it was estimated that there would be 5300 new cases of endometrial cancer in Canada and that 900 women would die from the disease (Canadian Cancer Society's Steering Committee on Cancer Statistics, 2012). Endometrial cancer has a relatively low mortality rate because most cases are diagnosed early. The survival rate is 95% if the cancer has not spread at the time of diagnosis.

Etiology and Pathophysiology

The major risk factor for endometrial cancer is estrogen, especially unopposed estrogen. Additional risk factors include increasing age, nulliparity, late menopause, obesity, smoking, diabetes mellitus, and having a personal or family history of hereditary nonpolyposis colorectal cancer (HNPCC) (see the Genetics in Clinical Practice box for HNPCC in Chapter 45, p. 1197). Obesity is a risk factor because adipose cells store estrogen. This increases endogenous estrogen. Pregnancy and oral contraceptives are protective factors.

Endometrial cancer arises from the lining of the endometrium. Most tumours are adenocarcinomas. The precursor may be a hyperplasic state that progresses to invasive carcinoma. Hyperplasia occurs when estrogen is not counteracted by progesterone. The cancer extends directly into the cervix and through the uterine serosa. As invasion of the myometrium occurs, regional lymph nodes, including the paravaginal and para-aortic, become involved. Hematogenous metastases develop concurrently. The usual sites of metastases are the lung, bone, the liver, and eventually, the brain. Malignant cells can be found in the peritoneal cavity, probably having arrived by transport through the fallopian tubes.

Prognostic factors include histological differentiation, myometrial invasion, peritoneal cytology, lymph node and adnexal metastases, and tumour size. Endometrial cancer grows slowly, metastasizes late, and is amenable to therapy if diagnosed early.

Clinical Manifestations

The first sign of endometrial cancer is abnormal uterine bleeding, usually in postmenopausal women. Because perimenopausal women have sporadic periods for a time, it is important that this sign not be ignored or attributed to menopause. Pain occurs late in the disease process. Other symptoms that may arise are related to metastasis to other organs.

Collaborative Care

Endometrial biopsy is the primary diagnostic procedure for endometrial cancer. Endometrial biopsy, which is done on an outpatient basis, involves obtaining endometrial tissue from the uterus. Any occurrence of abnormal or unexpected bleeding in a postmenopausal woman mandates obtaining a tissue sample to exclude endometrial cancer. It is recommended that an endometrial biopsy be performed at menopause and then periodically in women who are at risk. The Pap test is not a reliable diagnostic tool for endometrial cancer, but it can rule out cervical cancer.

Treatment of endometrial cancer is a total abdominal hysterectomy and bilateral salpingo-oophorectomy (TAH-BSO) with lymph node biopsies. Although they are not in widespread use, molecular markers help identify high-risk groups that could benefit from postoperative adjuvant therapy. These markers include p53 and p16 overexpression (tumour markers of high proliferative activity) and the expression of estrogen or progesterone receptors, or both, by the tumour cells. The absence of estrogen and progesterone receptors is a poor prognostic indicator.

Most cases of endometrial cancer are diagnosed at an early stage when surgery alone may result in cure. Surgery may be followed by irradiation, to either the pelvis or the abdomen externally or intravaginally, to decrease local recurrence.

Treatment of advanced or recurrent disease is difficult. Progesterone hormone therapy (e.g., megestrol [Megace]) is the treatment of choice when the progesterone receptor status is positive and the tumour is well differentiated. Tamoxifen (Nolvadex-D), either alone or in combination with progesterone therapy, is also effective in women with advanced or recurrent endometrial cancer. Chemotherapy is considered when progesterone therapy is unsuccessful. The most common agents used are doxorubicin (Adriamycin), cisplatin (Cisplatin), 5-fluorouracil (5-FU), carboplatin, and paclitaxel (Taxol).

Ovarian Cancer

Ovarian cancer is a malignant neoplasm of the ovaries. In 2012, it was estimated that there would be 2600 new cases of ovarian cancer in Canada and that 1750 women would die from the disease (Canadian Cancer Society's Steering Committee on Cancer Statistics, 2012). Ovarian cancer has the highest mortality rate of all gynecological cancers because most women have advanced disease at diagnosis. In Canada, the lifetime probability of a woman dying from ovarian cancer in is 1 in 92 (Canadian Cancer Society's Steering Committee on Cancer Statistics, 2012). It occurs most frequently in women between 55 and 65 years of age.

Etiology and Pathophysiology

The cause of ovarian cancer is not known. Women who have mutations of the *BRCA* genes have increased susceptibility for ovarian and breast cancer (Jelovac & Armstrong, 2011; Lanceley et al., 2011). The *BRCA* genes are tumour suppressor genes that inhibit tumour growth when functioning normally. When they mutate, they lose their tumour suppressor ability. This results in an increased risk for women to develop ovarian or breast cancer (see the Genetics in Clinical Practice box on ovarian cancer).

GENETICS IN CLINICAL PRACTICE

Ovarian Cancer

Genetic Basis

- Mutations in genes *BRCA1* and *BRCA2*.
- Autosomal dominant transmission.
- Mutations can be passed down from either mother or father.

Incidence

- About 10% of cases of ovarian cancer are related to hereditary factors.
- Women with *BRCA1* mutations have a 25-40% lifetime risk of developing ovarian cancer.
- Women with *BRCA2* mutations have a 10-20% lifetime risk of developing ovarian cancer.
- Family history of both breast and ovarian cancer increases the risk of having a *BRCA* mutation.
- *BRCA* mutations occur in 10-20% of patients with ovarian cancer who have no family history of breast or ovarian cancer.
- Family of genes associated with hereditary nonpolyposis colorectal cancer accounts for 10% of ovarian cancers.

Genetic Testing

- DNA testing is available for *BRCA1* and *BRCA2* genetic mutations.

Clinical Implications

- Bilateral oophorectomy reduces the risk of ovarian cancer in women with *BRCA1* and *BRCA2* mutations.
- Genetic counselling and testing for *BRCA* mutations should be considered for women whose personal or family history puts them at high risk for a genetic predisposition to ovarian cancer.

COLLABORATIVE CARE

Table 56-12 Ovarian Cancer

Diagnostic

- History and physical examination
- Pelvic examination
- Abdominal and transvaginal ultrasonography
- CA 125 levels
- Laparotomy for diagnostic staging

Collaborative Therapy

- Surgery
  - Abdominal hysterectomy and bilateral salpingo-oophorectomy with pelvic lymph node biopsies
  - Debulking for advanced disease
- Chemotherapy
  - Adjuvant and palliative
- Radiation therapy
  - Adjuvant and palliative

CA, carbohydrate antigen.

differentiated (grade II), and *poorly differentiated* (grade III). Grade III lesions carry a poorer prognosis than the other grades.

Ovarian cancer can metastasize directly by shedding malignant cells, which frequently implant on the uterus, bladder, bowel, and omentum. Ovarian cancer can metastasize by lymphatic spread.

Clinical Manifestations

Clinical manifestations are vague in the early stages. An accumulation of fluid initially causes abdominal enlargement. Nonspecific persistent symptoms have been identified as warranting further evaluation if they occur on an almost daily basis for at least 3 weeks including (1) pelvic or abdominal pain, (2) bloating, (3) urinary urgency or frequency, and (4) difficulty in eating or feeling full quickly (American Cancer Society, 2011, p. 17). Women who have one or more of these symptoms, especially if they are new, persistent, or worsening, are advised to see their health care provider. Vaginal bleeding rarely occurs and pain is not an early symptom. Later signs are increased abdominal girth, unexplained weight loss or gain, and menstrual irregularities.

Diagnostic Studies

No screening test exists for ovarian cancer. Because early ovarian cancer has vague symptoms, yearly bimanual pelvic examinations should be performed to identify the presence of an ovarian mass (Table 56-12). Postmenopausal women should not have palpable ovaries, so a mass of any size should be suspected as possible ovarian cancer. An abdominal or transvaginal ultrasonography can be used to detect ovarian masses. An exploratory laparotomy may be used to establish the diagnosis and stage the disease.

A test called OVA1 can help detect whether a pelvic mass is benign or malignant. OVA1 uses a blood sample to test for levels of five proteins that change owing to ovarian cancer. It is not intended for ovarian cancer screening or for a definitive diagnosis of ovarian cancer.

The major risk factor for ovarian cancer is family history (one or more first-degree relatives with ovarian cancer). Having a family history of breast or colon cancer is also a risk factor. Other risk factors include a personal history of breast or colon cancer and HNPCC (see the Genetics in Clinical Practice box on HNPCC in Chapter 45 on p. 1197). Women who have never been pregnant (nulliparity) are also at higher risk. Other risk factors include increasing age, high-fat diet, increased number of ovulatory cycles (usually associated with early menarche and late menopause), HRT, and possibly the use of infertility drugs. The use of oral contraceptives is associated with lower ovarian cancer risk.

Breastfeeding, multiple pregnancies, oral contraceptive use (>5 years), and early age at first birth seem to reduce the risk of ovarian cancer. It is thought that these factors have a protective effect because they reduce the number of ovulatory cycles and, thus, reduce the exposure to estrogen.

About 90% of ovarian cancers are epithelial carcinomas that arise from malignant transformation of the surface epithelial cells. Epithelial ovarian cancer is primarily a disease of postmenopausal women in the sixth or seventh decade of life (Jelovac & Armstrong, 2011). Germ cell tumours account for another 10%. Histological grading is an important prognostic determinant. Tumours are graded according to the level of differentiation. These include *well differentiated* (grade I), *moderately well*

For women with a high risk for ovarian cancer, screening using a combination of the tumour marker (carbohydrate antigen-125 [CA-125]) and ultrasonography is recommended in addition to a yearly pelvic examination. CA-125 is positive in 80% of women with epithelial ovarian cancer and is used to monitor the course of the disease. However, levels of CA-125 may be elevated with other nonovarian malignancies or with benign conditions such as fibroids or endometriosis. Clinical trials are actively investigating serum biomarkers that may detect ovarian cancer at an early stage (Visintin et al., 2008). Currently, only 20% of ovarian cancers are diagnosed at an early stage.

Collaborative Care

Women identified as being at high risk based on family and health history may require counselling regarding options such as prophylactic oophorectomy and oral contraceptives. It is important to note that, although oophorectomy will significantly reduce the risk of ovarian cancer, it will not completely eliminate the possibility of disease.

Ovarian cancer staging is critical for guiding treatment decisions. Stage I describes disease limited to the ovaries; stage II, disease limited to the true pelvis; stage III, disease limited to the abdominal cavity; and stage IV, distant metastatic disease. The overall survival rate is 89% with early disease, 36% with local spread, and 17% with distant metastases.

The treatment for stage I ovarian cancer is usually a TAH-BSO with removal of as much of the tumour as possible (i.e., tumour debulking). The addition of chemotherapy or the instillation of intraperitoneal radioisotopes is usually suggested for stage I disease that is poorly differentiated. The patient with stage II disease may receive external abdominal and pelvic irradiation, intraperitoneal irradiation, or systemic combined chemotherapy after tumour-reducing surgery. After completion of systemic chemotherapy in the patient who is clinically free of symptoms, a "second-look" surgical procedure is often performed to determine whether there is any evidence of disease. This option does not necessarily improve the outcome. If no disease is found, the patient is monitored for recurrent disease.

Chemotherapy (e.g., cisplatin, carboplatin) is used for the treatment of stage III and stage IV diseases. Paclitaxel (Taxol) and topotecan (Hycamtin) are used to treat metastatic ovarian cancer. Surgical debulking is often done in conjunction with chemotherapy for advanced disease. Intraperitoneal chemotherapy is being used for the patient who has minimum residual disease after surgery for advanced ovarian cancer (Anderson & Hacker, 2008). Gemcitabine (Gemzar) in combination with carboplatin is used to treat recurrent ovarian cancer.

With metastasis, recurrent pleural effusion often causes shortness of breath requiring frequent paracentesis. Palliative radiation may be used to shrink the tumour to relieve pressure and pain.

Vaginal Cancer

Primary vaginal cancers are rare. The peak incidence is between 50 and 70 years of age. Vaginal tumours are usually secondary sites or metastases of other cancers such as cervical or endometrial carcinomas. The most common type of vaginal cancer is squamous cell carcinoma. Intrauterine exposure to DES places a woman at risk for clear cell adenocarcinoma of the vagina.

Treatment of vaginal cancer depends on the type of cells involved and the stage of the disease, the size of the tumour, and the location of the tumour. Squamous cell carcinomas can be treated with both surgery and radiation.

Vulvar Cancer

Cancer of the vulva is relatively rare. Similar to cervical cancer, preinvasive lesions referred to as *vulvar intraepithelial neoplasia* (VIN) precede invasive vulvar cancer. The invasive form occurs mainly in women older than 60 years, with the highest incidence being in women in their 70s. Patients with vulvar neoplasia may have symptoms of vulvar itching or burning, pain, bleeding, or discharge. Women who are immunosuppressed or have diabetes mellitus, hypertension, or chronic vulvar dystrophies are at a higher risk for developing vulvar cancers. Several subtypes of HPV have been identified in some but not all vulvar cancers. Vaccines (Gardasil, Cervarix) are now available to protect against some vaginal and vulvar cancers that are caused by these HPV subtypes. (Vaccines are discussed further in Chapter 55, p. 1530.)

Diagnosis of vulvar cancer is determined by the pathology report on the biopsy of the suspicious lesion. VIN is managed by eradicating the lesion medically with 5-FU or by surgical excision. Larger lesions may necessitate more extensive surgery and skin graft. The traditional treatment for vulvar cancer has been radical vulvectomy. However, the procedure results in extensive morbidity related to scarring and wound breakdown. For this reason, more conservative surgical techniques such as radical hemivulvectomy are being used. The cure rates are comparable between the radical vulvectomy and the hemivulvectomy. However, the morbidity and loss of function have been significantly decreased with the hemivulvectomy procedure.

Surgical Procedures: Female Reproductive System

A variety of surgical procedures are performed when benign or malignant tumours of the genital tract are found (Table 56-13). A *hysterectomy* (removal of the uterus) is the type of surgery performed for excision of cancerous tumours of the female reproductive system. A hysterectomy may be done either vaginally or abdominally. A vaginal route is often used when vaginal repair is to be done in addition to removal of the uterus. The abdominal route is used when large tumours are present and the pelvic cavity is to be explored or when the tubes and ovaries are to be removed at the same time (Figure 56-10). The abdominal route can present more postoperative problems because it involves an incision and the opening of the abdominal cavity.

In both vaginal and abdominal hysterectomies, the ligaments that support the uterus are attached to the vaginal cuff so that normal depth of the vagina is maintained. The cervix may or may not be removed depending on the findings.

Laparoscopic-assisted vaginal hysterectomy (LAVH) is a modified approach to a vaginal hysterectomy. LAVH utilizes a laparoscope to assist with the removal of the uterus. Another alternative is laparoscopic subtotal hysterectomy, which allows the cervix to remain in place. The advantage of these newer procedures is quicker recovery time and fewer complications (Candiani et al., 2009).

Table 56-13 Surgical Procedures Involving the Female Reproductive System	
TYPE OF SURGERY	**DESCRIPTION**
Hysterectomy	
• Subtotal hysterectomy	Removal of uterus without cervix (rarely done today)
• Total hysterectomy	Removal of uterus and cervix
• Total abdominal hysterectomy and bilateral salpingo-oophorectomy (TAH-BSO)	Removal of uterus, cervix, fallopian tubes, and ovaries
• Radical hysterectomy	TAH-BSO, partial vaginectomy, and dissection of lymph nodes in pelvis
• Laparoscopic-assisted vaginal hysterectomy (LAVH)	Vaginal removal of the uterus with laparoscopic assistance
Vulvectomy	
• Simple vulvectomy	Excision of vulva and wide margin of skin
• Radical vulvectomy	Excision of tissue from anus to few centimetres above symphysis pubis (skin, labia majora and minora, and clitoris) with superficial and deep lymph node dissection
Vaginectomy	Removal of vagina
Pelvic Exenteration	Radical hysterectomy, total vaginectomy, removal of bladder with diversion of urinary system, and resection of bowel with colostomy
• Anterior pelvic exenteration	Pelvic exenteration without bowel resection
• Posterior pelvic exenteration	Pelvic exenteration without bladder removal

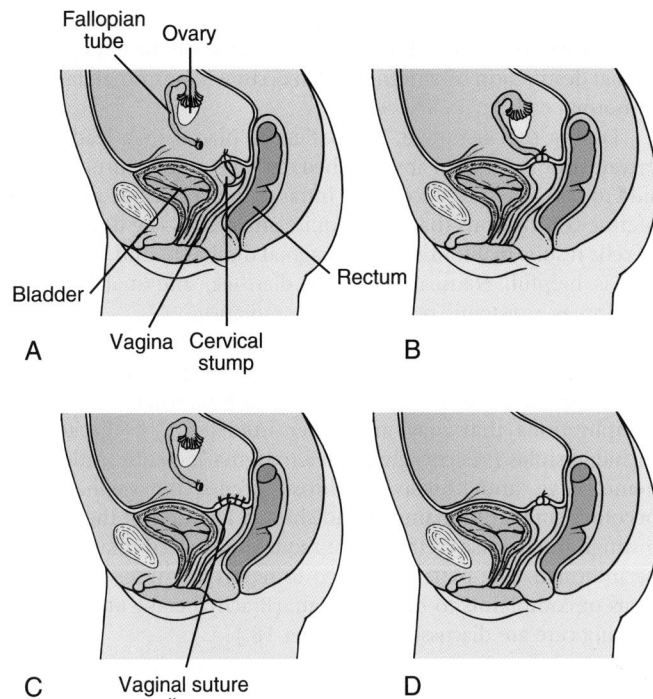

Figure 56-10 A, Cross-section of subtotal hysterectomy. Note that the cervical stump, fallopian tubes, and ovaries remain. **B,** Cross-section of total hysterectomy. Note that the fallopian tubes and ovaries remain. **C,** Cross-section of vaginal hysterectomy. Note that the fallopian tubes and ovaries remain. **D,** Total hysterectomy, salpingectomy, and oophorectomy. Note that the uterus, fallopian tubes, and ovaries are completely removed.

Source: Phipps, W. J., Sands, J. K., & Marek, J. F. (1999). *Medical-surgical nursing: Concepts and clinical practice* (6th ed.). St. Louis: Mosby.

Radiation Therapy: Cancers of the Female Reproductive System

Radiation is used to cure, control, or act as a palliative measure for cancers of the female reproductive system, either alone or in combination with other treatments. The goal of radiation therapy is to deliver a specific amount of high-energy (or ionizing) radiation to the cancer and with minimal damage to the normal surrounding tissue. Radiation therapy may be external or internal (brachytherapy).

External Radiation Therapy

With external radiation therapy, a source outside of the body delivers electromagnetic radiation in the form of waves. (External radiation therapy and related nursing care is discussed in Chapter 18.)

Internal Radiation Therapy (Brachytherapy)

Brachytherapy allows the radiation to be placed near or into the tumour. This method can deliver a high dose of radiation directly to the tumour. The dose decreases sharply as distance from the source increases, causing less damage to the surrounding normal tissue. A variety of forms are used to deliver internal radiation therapy, including wires, capsules, needles, tubes, and seeds. Brachytherapy is used in the management of cervical and endometrial cancer because of the accessibility of these body parts and the favourable results obtained. Radium and cesium are two commonly used isotopes. In preparation of the patient for the treatment, a cleansing enema is given to prevent straining at stool, which could cause displacement of the isotope. An indwelling catheter is inserted to prevent a distended bladder from coming into contact with the radioactive source.

A variety of applicators have been developed for intrauterine treatment. Applicators are inserted into the endometrial cavity and the vagina of an anaesthetized patient in the operating room. When the applicator contains the radioactive material, this is known as *preloading.* In *afterloading,* the applicator is implanted in the operating room but is not loaded with the radioactive material until its correct placement is verified and the patient has been returned to her room. Radiation exposure to the patient is precisely controlled. The radiation exposure to the physician and other personnel involved in the implantation is reduced when the afterload technique is used. The applicator is secured with vaginal packing and is left in place for 24 to 72 hours. The radiation oncologist determines the exact amount of radioactive substance to be used and the length of time it will be left in place so that destruction of cancer cells can occur with minimal damage to normal cells.

During the treatment, the patient is placed in a lead-lined private room and is on absolute bed rest. She may be turned from side to side. The presence of an intrauterine applicator produces uterine contractions that may require analgesics. The destruction of cells results in a foul-smelling vaginal discharge, and a deodorizer is helpful. Nausea, vomiting, diarrhea, and malaise may develop as a systemic reaction to the radiation.

At the end of the prescribed period of radiation, the radioactive material and the catheter are removed. The patient is allowed off bed rest and is discharged from the hospital when stable. Late complications that may arise after irradiation of the uterus include fistulas (vesicovaginal, ureterovaginal), cystitis, phlebitis, hemorrhage, and fibrosis. If fibrosis occurs, the vaginal wall becomes smaller in diameter and shorter. Dilation of the vagina through intercourse or the use of sequentially sized dilators may be indicated. The patient is urged to report any unusual symptoms or complaints to her physician. (Brachytherapy and related nursing care are discussed in Chapter 18.)

NURSING MANAGEMENT: CANCERS OF THE FEMALE REPRODUCTIVE SYSTEM

Nursing Assessment

Malignant tumours of the female reproductive system can be found in the cervix, endometrium, ovaries, vagina, and vulva. The patient with any of these malignant tumours may experience a variety of clinical manifestations, including leucorrhea, irregular vaginal bleeding, vaginal discharge, increase in abdominal pain and pressure, bowel and bladder dysfunction, and vulvar itching and burning. Assessment for these signs and symptoms is an important nursing responsibility.

Nursing Diagnoses

Nursing diagnoses for the female patient with cancer of the reproductive system include, but are not limited to, the following:

- Anxiety *related to* threat of a malignancy and lack of knowledge about the disease process and prognosis
- Acute pain *related to* pressure secondary to enlarging tumour
- Disturbed body image *related to* loss of body part and loss of good health
- Ineffective sexuality patterns *related to* physiological limitations and fatigue
- Ineffective breathing pattern *related to* presence of ascites and effusions
- Grieving *related to* poor prognosis of advanced disease

Planning

The overall goals are that the patient with a malignant tumour of the female reproductive system will (1) actively participate in treatment decisions, (2) achieve satisfactory pain and symptom management, (3) recognize and report problems promptly, (4) maintain preferred lifestyle as long as possible, and (5) continue to practise cancer detection strategies.

Nursing Implementation

Health Promotion

Through their contact with women in a variety of settings, nurses can teach women the importance of routine screening for cancers of the reproductive system. Cancer may be prevented when screening reveals precancerous conditions of the vulva, cervix, endometrium, and rarely, the ovaries. Also, routine screening increases the chance that a cancer will be identified in its early stage. When cancer is identified earlier, treatment can be more conservative and the woman's prognosis improves. Regular pelvic examinations and Pap tests will allow the health care provider to detect lesions on the vulva or any uterine or ovarian irregularities and screen for cervical cancer. Nurses can assist women to view routine cancer screening as an important self-care activity and can recommend vaccination against cervical cancer for those women at high risk.

Educating women about risk factors for cancers of the reproductive system is also important. Limiting sexual activity during adolescence, using condoms, having fewer sexual partners, and not smoking reduce the risk of cervical cancer. A high-fat diet increases risk for ovarian cancer. When high-risk behaviours are identified, nurses should assist women to identify lifestyle changes to decrease risk.

Acute Intervention Related to Surgery

All patients experience a degree of anxiety when surgery is contemplated, but the prospect of major gynecological surgery may heighten these concerns. Some women may fear a loss of femininity and worry about possible changes in their secondary sex characteristics. Others may experience feelings of guilt, anger, or embarrassment. Still others may focus on the effect the surgery will have on their reproductive and sexual functions. Some women view the whole process as annoying, whereas others are relieved by the thought of no longer having menstrual periods or becoming pregnant. Each patient must be understood in light of her fears and concerns and must be approached and evaluated individually. The nurse who exhibits interest and a willingness to listen can provide considerable psychological support.

Preoperatively, the patient is prepared physically for surgery with the standard perineal or abdominal preparation. A vaginal douche and enemas may be given, according to the preference of the surgeon. The bladder should be emptied before the patient is sent to the operating room. An indwelling catheter is commonly inserted preoperatively (see Chapter 20 for discussion of general preoperative patient care).

Hysterectomy. Postoperatively, the patient who has had a hysterectomy will have an abdominal dressing (abdominal hysterectomy) or a sterile perineal pad (vaginal hysterectomy). (See NCP 56-1 for care of the patient after a total abdominal hysterectomy. See Chapter 22 for potential surgical complications, wound care, and other postoperative care.) The dressing should be observed frequently for any sign of bleeding during the first 8 hours after surgery. A moderate amount of serosanguineous drainage on the perineal pad is expected following a vaginal hysterectomy. The patient with an abdominal hysterectomy often has only a small amount of serosanguineous vaginal drainage.

The patient may experience urinary retention postoperatively because of temporary bladder atony resulting from edema or nerve trauma. This problem is more acute when a radical hysterectomy has been performed. At times, an indwelling catheter is used for 1 to 2 days postoperatively to maintain constant drainage of the bladder and prevent strain on the suture line. If an indwelling catheter is not used, catheterization may be necessary if the patient has not urinated for 8 hours postoperatively. If residual urine is suspected after the removal of an indwelling catheter, catheterization is done to prevent bladder infection caused by pooling of urine. Accidental ligation of a ureter is a serious surgical complication. Any complaint of backache or decreased urine output should be reported to the surgeon.

Abdominal distension may develop from the sudden release of pressure on the intestines when a large tumour is removed or from paralytic ileus secondary to anaesthesia and manipulation of the bowel. Food and fluids may be restricted if the patient is nauseated. A rectal tube may be prescribed to relieve abdominal flatus. Early ambulation is encouraged to relieve abdominal pain related to flatus and to prevent abdominal distension.

Special care must be taken to prevent the development of deep venous thrombosis (DVT). Frequent changes of position, avoidance of the high Fowler position, and avoidance of pressure under the knees minimize stasis and pooling of blood. Leg exercises should be encouraged to promote circulation.

The loss of the uterus may bring about grief responses similar to any great personal loss. The ability to bear children is central to society's image of being a woman. Although not experienced by all women, grief over this loss is normal. Eliciting the woman's feelings and concerns about her surgery will provide the needed information to give understanding care. When surgery removes the ovaries as well, women experience surgical menopause. Estrogen is no longer available from the ovaries, so symptoms of estrogen deficiency will arise. To counter this, HRT may be initiated in the early postoperative period.

Discharge teaching should prepare the patient for what to expect following surgery (e.g., she will not menstruate). Teaching should include specific activity restrictions. Intercourse should be avoided until the wound is healed (~4 to 6 weeks). If a vaginal hysterectomy is performed, the woman needs to know that there may be a temporary loss of vaginal sensation. She should be reassured that sensation will return in several months.

Physical restrictions are limited for a short time. Heavy lifting should be avoided for 2 months. Activities that may increase pelvic congestion, such as dancing and walking swiftly, should be avoided for several months, whereas activities such as swimming may be both physically and mentally helpful. Wearing a girdle is allowed and may provide comfort. Assure the patient that once healing is complete, all previous activity can be resumed.

Salpingectomy and Oophorectomy.
Postoperative care of the woman who has undergone removal of a fallopian tube (salpingectomy) or an ovary (oophorectomy) is similar to that for any patient having abdominal surgery. However, if a large ovarian cyst is removed, there may be abdominal distension caused by the sudden release of pressure in the intestines. An abdominal binder may provide relief until the distension subsides.

When both ovaries are removed (bilateral oophorectomy), surgical menopause results. The symptoms are similar to those of regular menopause but may be more severe because of the sudden withdrawal of hormones. Attempts may be made to leave at least a portion of an ovary.

Vulvectomy.
Although cancer of the vulva is relatively uncommon, it is important that the nurse recognize the extent of the vulvectomy and the significant effect it is likely to have on the patient's life. An honest, open attitude with the patient and her partner preoperatively can be most helpful in the postoperative period.

After a vulvectomy (see Table 56-13), the patient returns to the unit with a wound in the perineal area extending to the groin. The wound may be covered or left exposed and frequently has drains attached to portable suction (e.g., Hemovac). A heavy pressure dressing is often in place for the first 24 to 48 hours. The wound is cleaned with normal saline solution or an antiseptic twice daily. Solutions can be applied with an aseptic bulb syringe or a Water Pik machine. A heat lamp or a hair dryer is then used to dry the area. Wound care must be meticulous to prevent infection, which results in delayed healing.

Special attention to bowel and bladder care is needed. A low-residue diet and stool softeners prevent straining and wound contamination. An indwelling catheter is used to provide urinary drainage. Great care is taken not to dislodge the catheter because extensive edema makes its reinsertion difficult. Heavy, taut sutures are often used to close the wounds, resulting in severe discomfort for the patient. In other instances, the wound may be allowed to heal by granulation. Analgesics may be required frequently to control pain. Careful positioning of the patient through the use of strategically placed pillows provides comfort. Ambulation is usually begun on the second postoperative day, but this varies with the preference of the surgeon. Anticoagulant therapy to prevent DVT is common.

Because the surgery causes mutilation of the perineal area and the healing process is slow, the patient is likely to become discouraged. Opportunities for the patient to express her feelings and concerns about the operation should be provided. The patient needs specific instructions in self-care before she is discharged. She should be told to report any unusual odour, fresh bleeding, breakdown of incision, or perineal pain. Home care nursing can benefit the patient during her adjustment period. Sexual function is often retained. Whether clitoral sensation is retained may be critical to some women, particularly if it was a primary source of orgasmic satisfaction. A discussion of alternative methods of achieving sexual satisfaction may also be indicated.

Pelvic Exenteration.
When other forms of therapy fail to control the spread of cancer and no metastases have been found outside of the pelvis, pelvic exenteration may be performed. Although different types are done, this radical surgery usually involves removal of the uterus, ovaries, fallopian tubes, vagina, bladder, urethra, and pelvic lymph nodes. In some situations, the descending colon, rectum, and anal canal may also be removed. Candidates for this procedure are selected on the basis of their likelihood of surviving the surgery and their ability to adjust to and accept the resulting limitations.

Postoperative care is similar to that of a patient who has had a radical hysterectomy, an abdominal perineal resection, and an ileostomy or colostomy. The physical, emotional, and social adjustments to life on the part of the woman and her family are great. There are urinary or fecal diversions in the abdominal wall, a reconstructed vagina, and the onset of menopausal symptoms.

The patient's rehabilitative process should keep pace with her acceptance of the situation. Much understanding and support is needed from the nursing staff during a long recovery period. The patient should be gently encouraged to regain her independence. She needs to verbalize her feelings about her altered body structure. Inclusion of the family in the plan of care is important.

The patient will need to return to her health care provider at specified intervals. Early recurrence of the cancer may be identified and treated. At this time, the patient's physical and emotional adjustment to the changes in body image produced by the surgery and her ability to carry our any treatment measures can also be assessed. Additional teaching and counselling can then be provided.

Acute Intervention With Radiation Therapy

Nursing management of the patient receiving brachytherapy requires special considerations. The nurse should not stay in the immediate area any longer than is necessary to give proper care and attention. No individual nurse should attend the patient for more than 30 minutes per day. The nurse should stay at the foot of the bed or at the entrance to the room to minimize radiation exposure. Visitors need to be told to stay about 2 m away from the bed and limit visits to less than 3 hours a day. Efficient organization of nursing care is essential so that the nurse does not stay in the immediate area of the patient any longer than is necessary. The reasons for these precautions must be explained fully to the patient and her visitors. (A more detailed discussion of nursing care of the patient receiving brachytherapy is given in Chapter 18.)

When the patient is to receive external radiation, she should be told to urinate immediately before the treatment to minimize radiation exposure to the bladder. She should be advised about radiation adverse effects, including enteritis and cystitis. These are natural reactions to radiotherapy and do not indicate an overdose. The patient should be fully informed of the possible adverse effects and measures to use to reduce their impact.

Evaluation

The expected outcomes are that the patient with cancer of the female reproductive system will:

- Actively participate in treatment decisions.
- Achieve satisfactory pain and symptom management.
- Recognize and report problems promptly.
- Maintain preferred lifestyle as long as possible.
- Continue to practise cancer-detection strategies.

Problems With Pelvic Support

The most commonly occurring problems with pelvic support are uterine prolapse, cystocele, and rectocele. Female pelvic organ prolapse (also called *genital* or *genitourinary prolapse*) is a common condition referring to the loss of fibromuscular support of the pelvic viscera causing the descent or herniation of the pelvic organs into the vagina (Tinelli et al., 2010). Although vaginal birth increases the risk for these problems, these conditions can occur in women who have never experienced childbirth. Obesity,

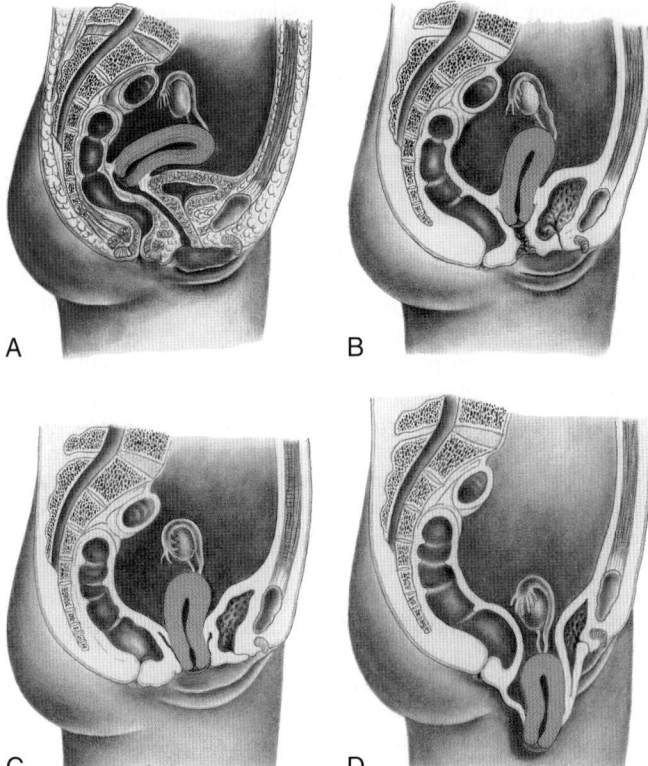

Figure 56-11 Uterine prolapse. **A,** Expected uterine position. **B,** First-degree prolapse of the uterus. **C,** Second-degree prolapse of the uterus. **D,** Complete prolapse of the uterus.

Source: Seidel, H. M., Ball, J., Dains, J., & Benedict, G. W. (2011). *Mosby's guide to physical examination* (7th ed., p. 592, Figure 18-58). St. Louis: Mosby.

chronic coughing, and straining during bowel movements can increase the likelihood of these problems. The decreased estrogen that normally accompanies the perimenopause also reduces some connective tissue support.

Uterine Prolapse

Uterine prolapse is the downward displacement of the uterus into the vaginal canal as a result of impaired pelvic support (Prasad & Alvero, 2011) (Figure 56-11). Prolapse is rated by degrees. In first-degree prolapse, the cervix rests in the lower part of the vagina. Second-degree prolapse means the cervix is at the vaginal opening. A third-degree prolapse means the uterus protrudes through the introitus. Symptoms vary with the degree of prolapse. The patient may describe a feeling of "something coming down." She may have dyspareunia, a dragging or heavy feeling in the pelvis, backache, and bowel or bladder problems if cystocele or rectocele is also present. Stress incontinence is a common and troubling problem. When third-degree uterine prolapse occurs, the protruding cervix and vaginal walls are subjected to constant irritation, and tissue changes may occur.

Therapy depends on the degree of prolapse and how much the woman's daily activities have been affected. Pelvic floor muscle exercises (PFMEs) or Kegel exercises may be effective for some women (Hagen & Stark, 2011) (see Chapter 48, Table 48-19). Women need proper training to perform PFMEs and there is some evidence that proper training and consistent interpersonal support from health care providers increases the effectiveness of PFMEs (Tsai & Liu, 2009). If PFMEs do not provide improvement, a pessary may be used. A *pessary* is a device that is placed in the vagina to help support the uterus (Herbruck, 2008). A wide variety of shapes exist, including rings, arches, and balls. Most are made of plastic or wire coated with plastic. When a woman first receives a pessary, she needs instructions for its cleaning and for follow-up. Pessaries that are left in place for long periods are associated with erosion, fistulas, and an increased incidence of vaginal carcinoma. If more conservative measures are not successful, surgery is indicated. Surgery generally involves a vaginal hysterectomy with anterior and posterior repair of the vagina and the underlying fascia.

Cystocele and Rectocele

Cystocele or anterior wall prolapse occurs when support between the vagina and the bladder is weakened (Figure 56-12). Similarly, a **rectocele** or posterior wall prolapse results from weakening

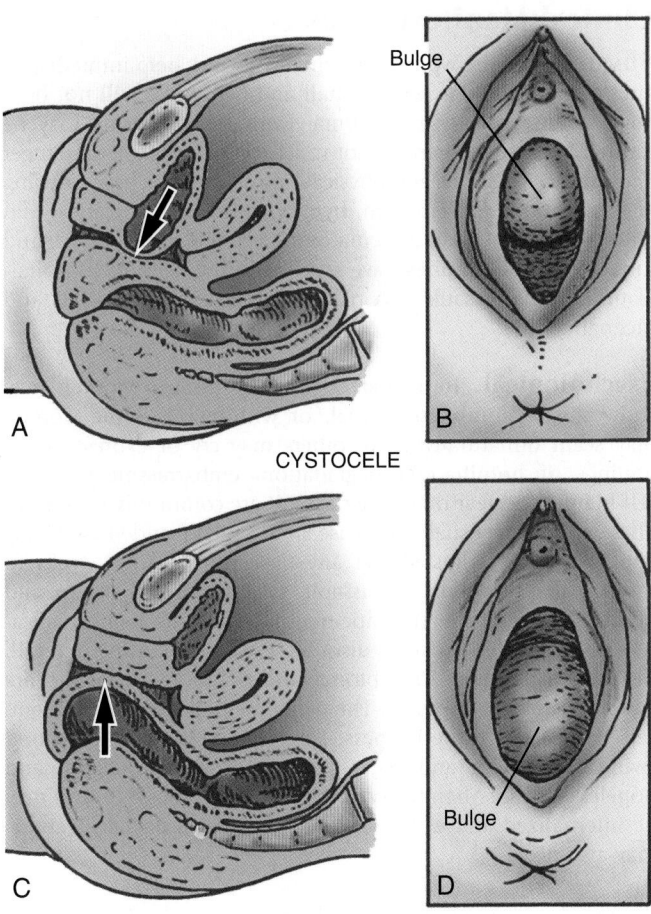

Figure 56-12 A, Cystocele. Note the bulging of the anterior vaginal wall. The urinary bladder is displaced downward. **B,** The cystocele pushes the anterior vaginal wall downward into the vagina. **C,** Rectocele. Note the bulging of the posterior vaginal wall. **D,** The rectocele pushes the posterior vaginal wall into the vagina.

Source: Black, J. M., & Hawks, J. H. (2009). *Medical-surgical nursing: Clinical management for positive outcomes* (8th ed., p. 930, Figure 39-7). St. Louis: Saunders.

between the vagina and the rectum (see Figure 56-12). These problems are common and asymptomatic in many women. With large cystoceles, complete emptying of the bladder can be difficult, predisposing women to bladder infections. A woman with a large rectocele may not be able to completely empty her rectum when defecating unless she helps push the stool out by putting her fingers in her vagina.

As with uterine prolapse, Kegel exercises (see Chapter 48, Table 48-19) may be used to strengthen the weakened perineal muscles if the cystocele or rectocele is not too problematic. A pessary may be helpful for cystoceles. Surgery designed to tighten the vaginal wall is generally the method of treatment. A cystocele is corrected with a procedure called an *anterior colporrhaphy,* whereas a *posterior colporrhaphy* is done for a rectocele. If further surgery is needed to relieve stress incontinence, procedures to support the urethra and restore the proper angle between the urethra and the posterior bladder wall are used.

NURSING MANAGEMENT: PROBLEMS WITH PELVIC SUPPORT

Nurses can assist women to avoid or decrease problems with pelvic support by teaching them how to do Kegel exercises. Women of all ages can benefit from these exercises. However, Kegel exercises are especially important following childbirth or whenever women begin to have incontinence. To instruct a patient in this exercise, she should be told to pull in or contract her muscles as if she were trying to stop the flow of urine. She should hold the contraction for several seconds and then relax. Sets of 5 to 10 contractions each should be done several times daily.

If vaginal surgery is necessary, the preoperative preparation may include a cleansing douche the morning of surgery. A cathartic and a cleansing enema are usually given when a rectocele repair is scheduled. A perineal shave may be done.

In the postoperative period, the goals of care are to prevent wound infection and pressure on the vaginal suture line. This necessitates perineal care at least twice a day and after each urination or defecation. An ice pack applied locally may relieve the initial perineal discomfort and swelling. A disposable glove filled with ice and covered with a cloth works well for this purpose. Later, sitz baths may be used.

After an anterior colporrhaphy, an indwelling catheter is usually left in the bladder for 2 to 3 days to allow the local edema to subside. The catheter keeps the bladder empty, preventing strain on the sutures. Catheter care with an antiseptic is generally done twice daily. The amount of urine left in the bladder after voiding is checked for the first few voidings to make sure it is less than 150 mL. This is checked by intermittent catheterization after the patient has voided (postresidual) or by using a bladder scanner. After posterior colporrhaphy, straining at stool is avoided by means of a low-residue diet and the prevention of constipation. A stool softener is usually given each night.

Discharge instructions should be reviewed before the patient leaves the hospital. They include the use of douches or a mild laxative as needed; restriction of heavy lifting and prolonged standing, walking, or sitting; and avoidance of intercourse until the physician gives permission. There may be a loss of vaginal sensation, which can last for several months. The patient needs to be reassured that this situation is temporary.

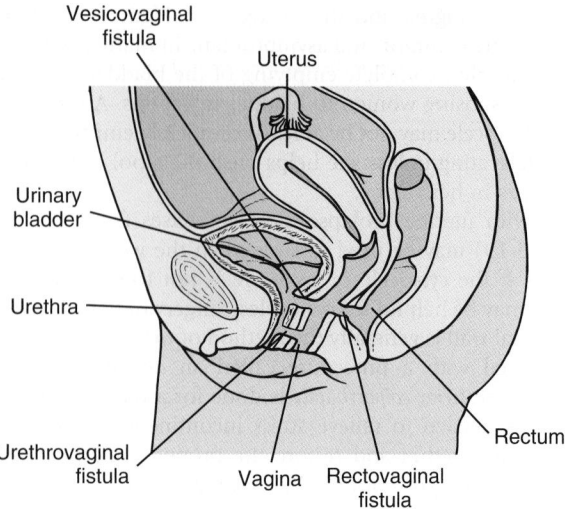

Figure 56-13 Common fistulas involving the vagina.

Fistula

A *fistula* is an abnormal opening between internal organs or between an organ and the exterior of the body (Figure 56-13). Gynecological procedures cause the majority of urinary tract fistulas. Other causes include injury during childbirth and disease processes, such as carcinoma. They may develop between the vagina and the bladder, the urethra, the ureter, or the rectum. When *vesicovaginal* fistulas (between the bladder and the vagina) develop, some urine leaks into the vagina, whereas with recto-vaginal fistulas (between the rectum and the vagina), flatus and feces escape into the vagina. In both instances, excoriation and irritation of the vaginal and vulvar tissues occur and may lead to severe infections. In addition to wetness, offensive odours may develop, causing embarrassment and severely limiting socialization.

Because small fistulas may heal spontaneously within a matter of months, treatment may not be needed (McGee & Delaney, 2009). If the fistula does not heal, surgical excision is required. Inflammation and tissue edema must be eliminated before surgery is attempted. This may involve a wait of up to 6 months for the surgery. The fistulectomy may result in the patient's having an ileal conduit or temporary colostomy.

NURSING MANAGEMENT: FISTULAS

Perineal hygiene is of great importance, both preoperatively and postoperatively. The perineum should be cleansed every 4 hours. Warm sitz baths should be taken three times daily if possible. Perineal pads should be changed frequently. The patient should be encouraged to maintain an adequate fluid intake. Encouragement and reassurance are needed to help the patient cope with her problems.

Postoperatively, nursing care emphasis is on avoidance of stress on the repaired areas and prevention of infection. Care should be taken so that the indwelling catheter, usually in place for 7 to 10 days, is draining at all times. Oral fluids should be urged to provide for internal catheter irrigation. Minimal pres-

sure and strict asepsis are used if catheter irrigation becomes necessary. The first stool after bowel surgery may be purposely delayed to prevent contamination of the wound. Later, stool softeners or mild laxatives may be given. (See Chapter 48 for care of a patient with an ileal conduit and Chapter 45 for care of a patient with a colostomy.) Surgical repair of fistulas is not always effective, even in the best conditions. Therefore, support-ive nursing care for the patient and her significant others is especially important.

Sexual Assault

In Canada, **sexual assault** is the legal term used to refer to any form of sexual contact imposed on another person without that person's voluntary consent. Kissing, fondling, vaginal and oral or anal intercourse, penetration, or both are all examples of sexual assault if they are done without voluntary consent. People of either gender can be victims of sexual assault but this section is dealing with sexual assault of women in particular.

Clinical Manifestations

Physical. Of the women and men who seek help immediately after the assault, between one half and two thirds will not have any evidence of physical trauma. Evidence of trauma may be limited because women do not resist for fear of physical danger and injury. When present, physical injuries may include bruising and lacerations to perineum, hymen, vulva, vagina, cervix, and anus. Fractures, subdural hematomas, cerebral concussions, and intra-abdominal injuries have resulted in the need for hospital-ization. Sexual assault also places women at risk for STIs and pregnancy.

Psychological. Immediately after the assault, women may show shock, numbness, denial, or withdrawal. Some women may seem unnaturally calm; others may cry or express anger. Feelings of humiliation, degradation, embarrassment, anger, self-blame, and fear of another assault are commonly expressed. These symptoms usually decrease after 2 weeks, and victims may appear to have adjusted. Yet any time from 2 to 3 weeks to months to years after the assault, symptoms may return and become more severe. The rape-trauma syndrome is a classifica-tion of post-traumatic stress disorder. Flashbacks, intrusive recall, sleep disturbances, GI symptoms, and numbing of feelings are common initial symptoms. The person will feel embarrassment, self-blame, and powerlessness. Later symptoms include mood swings, irritability, and anger. Feelings of despair, shame, and hopelessness are often the cause of the anger. These feelings may be internalized and expressed as depression. Suicidal ideations may also occur.

Collaborative Care

In the acute care of an assault survivor, ensuring emotional and physical safety has the highest priority. Table 56-14 outlines the emergency management of the patient who has been sexually assaulted. Most emergency departments (EDs) have identified personnel who have received special training in order to work with women who have been assaulted. Each province and terri-tory has created the position of sexual assault nurse examiner (SANE). The SANE is a registered nurse who is certified to provide

EMERGENCY MANAGEMENT

Table 56-14 Sexual Assault

ETIOLOGY	ASSESSMENT FINDINGS	INTERVENTIONS
• Sexual molestation • Sodomy • Assault involving genitalia (male or female) without consent	• Emotional or physical manifestations of shock • Agitation • Hysteria • Crying • Anger • Silence • Decreased level of consciousness • Hyperventilation • Oral, vaginal, and rectal injuries • Extragenital injuries • Pain in genital area or extragenital area	**Initial** • Treat shock and other urgent medical problems (e.g., head injury, hemorrhage, wounds, fractures). • Assess emotional state. • Contact support person (i.e., social worker, rape advocate, sexual assault nurse examiner). • Do *not* clean the patient until all evidence is collected. Make sure the patient does not wash, douche, urinate, brush teeth, or gargle. • Place sheet on floor. Then have patient stand on sheet to remove clothing. Place sheet with clothing in paper bag. • SANE will collect forensic evidence per local protocol (i.e., body hair, nail scrapings, tissue, dried semen, vaginal washing, blood samples). • Maintain chain of evidence for all legal specimens. Clearly label evidence and keep in locked cabinet until given to law enforcement agency. • Obtain baseline HIV, syphilis, and other STI screening. • Obtain toxicology sample to evaluate drug-facilitated sexual assault. • Determine method of contraception, date of last menstrual period, and date of last tetanus immunization. • Consider tetanus prophylaxis if lacerations contain soil or dirt. • Vaccinate with hepatitis B if not already done. **Ongoing Monitoring** • Monitor vital signs and emotional status. • Provide clothing as needed. • Counsel patient regarding confidential HIV and STI testing.

HIV, human immunodeficiency virus; *SANE,* sexual assault nurse examiner; *STI,* sexually transmitted infection.

care to victims of sexual assault, while ensuring evidence is safeguarded. Special procedures are followed in taking the history and conducting the examination in order to preserve all evidence in case of future prosecution.

When the survivor of an assault is admitted to the ED or clinic, a specific chain of events occurs (Table 56-15). A signed informed consent is obtained before any data are collected. All materials gathered are well documented, labelled, and given to the appropriate person, such as the pathologist or a police officer. The materials are handled by as few people as possible, and signatures of all responsible for keeping and handling the data are obtained. Many items can be used as evidence if the victim chooses to pursue a police investigation. Consequently, the integrity of the material must be maintained. The nurse's involvement in the medicolegal process depends on the policies of the individual institution and provincial or territorial law.

A gynecological and sexual history and an account of the assault (who, what, when, and where) as well as a general physical and pelvic examination add further information about the sexual assault. Laboratory tests are done primarily to gather forensic evidence, determine the presence of sperm in the vagina, and identify any existing STIs or pregnancy.

Follow-up physical and psychological care is essential. Victims of assault should return weekly for the first month following the assault. This includes the time period when psychological reactions may be the most severe. Health care providers should have the telephone numbers and names of contact people for local resources for sexual assault survivors, including rape crisis centres, legal and law enforcement authorities, and human services.

NURSING MANAGEMENT: SEXUAL ASSAULT

Nurses can assist people to become aware of prevention tactics (Table 56-16). They should also be encouraged to learn some basic techniques of self-defence. Local high schools and the YWCA usually have self-defence classes in which formal instruction is given. Practising the various techniques with a friend builds up a person's confidence in his or her ability to fight back. Learning self-defence can make a person less vulnerable and more self-reliant.

When a sexual assault survivor is brought to the clinic or ED, a quiet, private area should be used for the initial assessment and the examinations that follow. The patient should not be left alone. Whenever possible, the same nurse should remain with the person throughout the hospital stay and provide needed emotional support. The patient's actions and words in relation to the incident may be inconsistent, confused, and inappropriate. The nurse should maintain a nonjudgemental attitude.

The patient usually has many feelings and thoughts about the assault and generally wants to talk about them to an interested

Table 56-15 Evaluation of Alleged Sexual Assault

1. Medicolegal

- Valid written consent for examination, photographs, laboratory tests, release of information, and laboratory samples
- Appropriate "chain of evidence" documentation

2. History

- History of assault (who, what, when, where)
- Penetration, ejaculation, extragenital acts
- Activities since assault (e.g., changed clothes, bathed, douched)
- Inquire about safety
- Menstrual and contraceptive history
- Medical history
- Emotional status
- Current symptoms

3. General Physical Examination

- Vital signs and general appearance
- Extragenital trauma—mouth, breasts, neck
- Cuts, bruises, scratches (photograph taken)

4. Pelvic Examination

- Vulvar trauma, erythema; hymen, anal, and rectal status
- Matted hairs or free hairs
- Vaginal examination with unlubricated speculum for discharge, blood, lacerations
- Uterine size
- Adnexa, especially hematomas

5. Laboratory Samples

- Vaginal vault content sampling
- Vaginal smears—microscope evaluation for trichomonads and semen
- Oral or rectal swabs and smears, if indicated
- Blood samples—VDRL serology, pregnancy test; serological testing for HIV and hepatitis B infection, toxicology
- Freeze serum sample for later HIV testing
- Cultures—cervix and other areas (if indicated) for gonorrhea and chlamydial infection
- Fingernail scrapings
- Pubic hair scrapings
- Clipping of matted pubic hairs

6. Treatment

- Care of injuries and emotional trauma
- Prophylaxis for STIs, tetanus, and hepatitis B (see appropriate chapters)
- Follow-up for pregnancy test in 2-3 wk (if appropriate)
- Testing for HIV, syphilis, and hepatitis B may be done at 6-8 wk
- Protection of legal rights
- Recommendation of continued follow-up and services of rape crisis centre

HIV, human immunodeficiency virus; *STIs,* sexually transmitted infections; *VDRL,* Venereal Disease Research Laboratory.

PATIENT AND CAREGIVER TEACHING GUIDE

Table 56-16 Sexual Assault Prevention

1. Place and maintain lights at all entrances to your home.
2. Keep your doors locked, and do not open them to a stranger; ask for identification if a service person comes to the door.
3. Do not advertise that you live alone; list only your initials with your last name in the telephone directory or on the mailbox; never reveal to a caller that you are home alone.
4. Avoid walking alone in deserted areas; walk to the parking lot with a friend; be sure you see each other leave.
5. Have your keys ready as you approach your car or home.
6. Keep all doors locked and windows up when driving.
7. Never get on an elevator with a suspicious person; pretend you have forgotten something and get off.
8. Say what you mean in social situations; be sure your voice and body language reflect your response.
9. Carry a loud whistle and use it when you think you are in danger.
10. Yell "fire" if you are attacked, and run toward a lighted area.
11. Proceed with caution in online correspondence.
12. Do not leave your beverage unattended or accept a drink from an open container.
13. Consume alcohol in moderation if you drink. Many sexual assaults involve the use of alcohol by the offender, the victim, or both.

listener. Talking may help the patient feel better and gain understanding of her or his reactions to the incident. When the nurse listens carefully, the patient feels less alone and is better able to gain control over the situation.

The nurse should assess the patient's stress level in preparation for the various procedures that will follow. The patient's coping mechanisms are supported when he or she knows what to expect and what is expected as well as why the particular procedure must be done. Because the pelvic examination may trigger a flashback of the attack, the nurse should answer all related questions before the examination and be a supportive presence during the examination.

Following the examinations, the patient's physical comfort needs should be considered. The patient needs a change of clothing because her or his original garments may be torn or soiled or kept as evidence. Most people who have been sexually assaulted feel dirty and would appreciate a place to wash as well as use a mouthwash, especially if oral sex was involved. Food and drink may also provide comfort to the victim. The possibility of pregnancy should be discussed and the patient can be offered emergency contraception (sold as "Plan B" in Canada) to prevent an unintended pregnancy. It is similar to birth control pills but taken in different doses and can be used up to 72 hours after unprotected sex, reducing the risk of getting pregnant to approximately 75% (PHAC, 2009).

Many sexual assault survivors are unaware of the availability of compensation or financial assistance programs and appreciate information about the application process. All provinces except Newfoundland and Labrador and the territories have financial compensation programs for victims and survivors of violent crime such as sexual assault (Canadian Resource Centre for Victims of Crime, 2011). The programs were created to recognize the harm done to innocent people and to ease the financial burden that often accompanies victimization. All other coverage must be exhausted before claims for compensation are considered (Canadian Resource Centre for Victims of Crime, 2011).

When the patient is discharged, the nurse should make certain the patient has transportation home. If friends or family members are not available, the hospital or clinic should make arrangements with an appropriate community resource. The patient should not be sent home alone. The victim's partner and family have a tremendous potential for both negative and positive influence.

Many communities today have crisis centres. These public service organizations have trained professional and nonprofessional volunteers who provide an emotional support system for survivors on request. Their programs provide advocacy to ensure dignified treatment throughout the medical and police procedures, short-term counselling for the woman and her family, and court assistance and public education on rape-related issues.

CLINICAL DECISION-MAKING EXERCISE

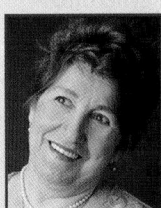

CASE STUDY:
Uterine Prolapse and Vaginal Hysterectomy

Source: © 2011 JupiterImages Corporation.

Patient Profile

Thérèse Pelletier is a 62-year-old French-Canadian woman who has developed lower pelvic discomfort and stress incontinence. She has type 2 diabetes and hypertension. She is the mother of four children. A second-degree uterine prolapse is diagnosed. She was treated conservatively with a pessary, but her symptoms did not improve. She comes to the hospital for a vaginal hysterectomy and anterior and posterior repair.

Subjective Data

- Was initially reluctant about surgery
- Concerned about her dyspareunia and her husband's reaction to the surgery
- Concerned she may have uterine cancer

Objective Data

Physical Examination

- Second-degree uterine prolapse on vaginal examination
- Blood pressure (BP) is 150/100 mm Hg, pulse 110 beats per minute, respirations 20 breaths per minute
- Stress incontinence and pelvic discomfort

Laboratory Studies

- Hemoglobin 100 g/L
- Hemoglobin A_{1c} 9%

Postoperative Status

- Returned to room with indwelling urinary catheter in place
- Vaginal packing in place
- Sequential compression devices are present on lower extremities
- Patient-controlled analgesia pump for pain management

Discussion Questions

1. What are the common causes of uterine prolapse?
2. Ms. Pelletier asks about the effect of the surgery on her sexuality. How would the nurse respond?
3. *Priority Decision:* What are the priorities of care for Ms. Pelletier?
4. What possible complications (including their basis for development) can arise after vaginal hysterectomy?
5. What does Ms. Pelletier need to be taught before discharge related to her diabetes and hypertension?
6. *Priority Decision:* Based on the assessment data presented, what are the priority nursing diagnoses? Are there any collaborative problems?

evolve *Answers are available at* **http://evolve.elsevier.com/Canada/Lewis/medsurg**

REVIEW QUESTIONS

The number of the question corresponds to the same-numbered objective at the beginning of the chapter.

1. What should the nurse explain to a patient with infertility about what she and her partner should expect during the infertility assessment?
   a. Ovulatory studies can help determine tube patency.
   b. A hysterosalpingogram is a common diagnostic study.
   c. The cause will remain unexplained for 40% of couples.
   d. If postcoital studies are normal, tests for infection will be done.

2. Which of the following is the most appropriate question to ask the patient with painful menstruation to differentiate primary from secondary dysmenorrhea?
   a. "Does your pain become worse with activity or overexertion?"
   b. "Have you had a recent personal crisis or change in your lifestyle?"
   c. "Is your pain relieved by nonsteroidal anti-inflammatory medications?"
   d. "When in your menstrual history did the pain with your period begin?"

3. The nurse is caring for a patient after an ectopic pregnancy was surgically removed. What should the nurse advise the recovering patient?
   a. She has an increased risk for salpingitis.
   b. Bed rest must be maintained for 12 hours to assist healing.
   c. Having one ectopic pregnancy increases her risk for another.
   d. Intrauterine devices and infertility treatments should be avoided.

4. The nurse is teaching a patient who chooses not to take hormone therapy how to prevent or decrease age-related changes that occur after menopause. Which of the following is the most important self-care measure that the nurse should teach?
   a. Maintaining usual sexual activity
   b. Increasing the intake of dairy products
   c. Performing regular aerobic, weight-bearing exercise
   d. Taking vitamin E and B-complex vitamin supplements

5. The patient has a history indicating thick, white, and curdlike vaginal discharge and vulvar pruritus. What are these symptoms most consistent with?
   a. Trichomoniasis
   b. Monilial vaginitis
   c. Bacterial vaginosis
   d. Chlamydial cervicitis

6. Why does the nurse caring for a patient with pelvic inflammatory disease place her in a semi-Fowler position?
   a. To relieve severe pain
   b. To promote drainage to prevent abscesses
   c. To improve circulation and promote healing
   d. To prevent complication of bowel obstruction

7. Which of the following is a nursing responsibility related to the care of the patient receiving brachytherapy for endometrial cancer?
   a. Maintaining absolute bed rest
   b. Keeping the patient in high Fowler's position
   c. Allowing visitors to stay if they remain 1 m (3 ft) from the bed
   d. Limiting direct nurse-to-patient contact to 30 minutes per shift

8. Why should the nurse plan early and frequent ambulation for the patient who has undergone an abdominal hysterectomy?
   a. To prevent urinary retention
   b. To promote pelvic circulation
   c. To promote intestinal peristalsis
   d. To maintain a sense of normalcy

9. Which of the following postoperative interventions are included in the nursing care of a woman with a gynecological fistula?
   a. Ambulation and bladder training
   b. Bladder training and warm sitz baths
   c. Warm sitz baths and perineal hygiene
   d. Perineal hygiene and bladder training

10. What is the first nursing intervention for the patient who has been sexually assaulted?
    a. Treat urgent medical problems.
    b. Contact a support person for the patient.
    c. Provide supplies for the patient to cleanse himself or herself.
    d. Document bruises and lacerations of the perineum and the cervix.

ANSWERS: 1. b; 2. d; 3. c; 4. c; 5. b; 6. b; 7. a; 8. c; 9. c; 10. a.

REFERENCES

Accortt, E. E., Freeman, M. P., & Allen, J. B. (2008). Women and major depressive disorder: Clinical perspectives on causal pathways. *Journal of Women's Health, 17*(10), 1583-1590.

Ahonen, K. A. (2010). Polycystic ovary syndrome: Recognize and intervene early. *The Nurse Practitioner, 35*(9), 49-52. doi:10.1097/01.NPR.0000387144.87541.c4

Alraek, T., & Malterud, K. (2009). Acupuncture for menopausal hot flashes: A qualitative study about patient experiences. *Journal of Alternative Complementary Medicine, 15*(2), 153-158. doi:10.1089/acm.2008.0310

American Cancer Society. (2011). *Cancer facts and figures 2011.* Retrieved from *http://www.cancer.org/acs/groups/content/@epidemiologysurveilance/documents/document/acspc-029771.pdf*

Anderson N., & Hacker E. (2008). Fatigue in women receiving intraperitoneal chemotherapy for ovarian cancer. *Clinical Journal of Oncology Nursing, 12*(3), 445-454. doi:10.1188/08.CJON.445-454

Ayers, D., & Montgomery, M. (2009). Putting a stop to dysfunctional bleeding. *Nursing, 39*(1), 44-50. doi:10.1097/01.NURSE.0000343457.81247.df

Barnhart, K. T. (2009). Ectopic pregnancy. *New England Journal of Medicine, 361*(4), 379-387. doi:10.1056/NEJMcp0810384

Best Start Resource Centre and Halton Region Health Department. (2007). *Reflecting on the trend: Pregnancy after age 35.* Retrieved from *http://www.beststart.org/resources/rep_health/pdf/bs_pregnancy_age35.pdf*

Biggs, W. S., & Demuth, R. H. (2011). Premenstrual syndrome and premenstrual dysphoric disorder. *American Family Physician, 84*(8), 918-924.

Birkhauser, M. H., Panay, N., Archer, D. F., Barlow, D., Burger, H., Gambacciani, M., …, Sturdee, D. W. (2008). Updated practical recommendations for hormone replacement therapy in the peri- and postmenopause. *Climacteric, 11*(2), 108-123. doi:10.1080/13697130801983921

Boivin, J., Bunting, L., Collins, J. A., & Nygren, K. G. (2007). International estimates of infertility prevalence and treatment-seeking: Potential need and demand for infertility medical care. *Human Reproduction, 22*(6), 1506-1512. doi:10.1093/humrep/dem046

Brockie, J. (2008). Physiology and effects of the menopause. *Nurse Prescribing, 6*(5), 202-207.

Brown, J., O'Brien, P. M., Marjoribanks, J., & Wyatt, K. (2009). Selective serotonin reuptake inhibitors for premenstrual syndrome. *Cochrane Database of Systematic Reviews, 2*, CD001396. doi:10.1002/14651858.CD001396.pub2

Buckworth, J., & Hsu, Y. (2010). Polycystic ovary syndrome: Challenges for practitioners and clients. *ACSM's Health & Fitness Journal, 14*(3), 15-20. doi:10.1249/FIT.0b013e3181daa6c5

Burkman, R. T. (2007). Contraception and family planning. In A. H. De Cheney, L. Nathan, T. Murphy Goodman, & N. Laufer (Eds.), *Current diagnosis and treatment obstetrics and gynecology* (10th ed.). New York: McGraw-Hill.

Canadian Cancer Society. (2011a). Canadian cancer encyclopedia: Risk factors for cervical cancer. Retrieved from *http://info.cancer.ca/cce-ecc/default.aspx?cceid=801&toc=12&Lang=E*

Canadian Cancer Society. (2011b). *Canadian cancer encyclopedia: Screening for cervical cancer*. Retrieved from *http://info.cancer.ca/cce-ecc/default.aspx?Lang=E&toc=12*

Canadian Cancer Society's Steering Committee on Cancer Statistics. (2012, May). *Canadian Cancer Statistics 2012*. Toronto, ON: Canadian Cancer Society.

Canadian Institute for Health Information [CIHI]. (2009). *Induced Abortions Performed in Canada in 2009: Table 1—Number of Induced Abortions Performed in Canada in 2009, by Province/Territory of Hospital or Clinic*. Retrieved from *http://www.cihi.ca/CIHI-ext-portal/pdf/internet/TA_09_ALLDATATABLES20111028_EN*

Canadian Resource Centre for Victims of Crime. (2011). *Crimes compensation*. Retrieved from *http://www.crcvc.ca/en/compensation.php*

Candiani, M., Izzo, S., Bulfoni, A., Riparini, J., Ronzoni, S., & Marconi, A. (2009). Laparoscopic vs. vaginal hysterectomy for benign pathology. *American Journal of Obstetrics and Gynecology, 200*(3), 368.e1-368.e7. doi:10.1016/j.ajog.2008.09.016

Cleveland Clinic. (2010). *Facts about endometriosis*. Retrieved from *http://my.clevelandclinic.org/disorders/endometriosis/hic_facts_about_endometriosis.aspx*

Cooper, M. (2009). How modern women can manage the menopause. *Primary Health Care, 19*(1), 24-29.

Cottrell Hansen, B., & Close, F. T. (2008). Vaginal douching among university women in the southeastern United States. *Journal of American College Health, 56*(4), 177-182.

Currie, H. (2008). Prescribing HRT. *Practice Nurse, 35*(4), 31-32, 35, 38.

Davidson, M. R., London, M. L., & Ladewig, P. A. (2012). *Maternal-newborn nursing and women's health across the lifespan* (9th ed.). Upper Saddle River, NJ: Pearson Prentice Hall.

Department of Health and Human Services/National Institutes of Health/National Heart, Lung, and Blood Institute. (2011). *Women's Health Initiative: Findings from the WHI postmenopausal hormone therapy trials*. Retrieved from *http://www.nhlbi.nih.gov/whi*

Ellenson, L., & Pirog, E. (2010). The female genital tract. In V. Kumar, A. Abbas, & N. Fausto (Eds.). *Robbins and Cotran pathologic basis of disease* (8th ed.). Philadelphia: Saunders.

Gakidou, E., Nordhagen, S., & Obermeyer, Z. (2008). Coverage of cervical cancer screening in 57 countries: Low average levels and large inequalities. *PloS (Public Library of Science) Medicine 5*(6), e132. doi:10.1371/journal.pmed.0050132

Gerber-Epstein, P., Leichtentritt, R. D., & Benyamini, Y. (2009). The experience of miscarriage in first pregnancy: The women's voices. *Death Studies, 33*(1), 1-29. doi:10.1080/07481180802494032

Hagen, S., & Stark, D. (2011). Conservative prevention and management of pelvic organ prolapse in women. *Cochrane Database of Systematic Reviews 2011*, 12, CD003882. doi:10.1002/14651858.CD003882.pub4

Health Canada. (2011). *Toxic shock syndrome (TSS)*. Retrieved from *http://www.hc-sc.gc.ca/hl-vs/iyh-vsv/prod/tampons-eng.php*

Herbruck, L. (2008). Urinary incontinence in the childbearing woman. *Urologic Nursing, 28*(3), 163-171.

Holoch, K., & Lessey, B. (2010). Endometriosis and Infertility. *Clinical Obstetrics and Gynecology, 53*(2), 429-438. doi:10.1097/GRF.0b013e3181db7d71

Jelovac, D., & Armstrong, D. K. (2011). Recent progress in the diagnosis and treatment of ovarian cancer. *CA: A Cancer Journal for Clinicians, 61*(3), 183-203. doi:10.3322/caac.20113

Kendall, J. (2008). Women's health. Female infertility 2: Treatments. *Practice Nursing, 19*(1), 35-38.

Lanceley, A., Fitzgerald, D., Jones, V., Miles, T., Elliott, E., Darragh, L., & Peck, L. (2011). Ovarian cancer: Symptoms, treatment and long-term patient management. *Primary Health Care, 21*(7), 31-37.

Lowdermilk, D. L., Perry, C. S., Cashion, K., & Rhodes Alden, K. (2012). *Maternity and women's health care* (10th ed.). St Louis: Mosby.

Lund, K. (2008). Menopause and the menopausal transition. *Medical Clinics of North America, 92*(5), 1253-1271. doi:10.1016/j.mcna.2008.04.009

Maine, D., Hurlburt, S., & Greeson, D. (2011). Cervical cancer prevention in the 21st century: Cost is not the only issue. *American Journal of Public Health, 101*(9), 1549-1555. doi:10.2105/AJPH.2011.300204

Mayo Clinic. (2011). *Chronic pelvic pain*. Retrieved from *http://www.mayoclinic.com/health/chronic-pelvic-pain/DS00571*

McGee, M., & Delaney, C. (2009). Stomas and fistulas. In D. Walsh, A. Caraceni, R. Fainsinger, K. M. Foley, P. Glare, C. Goh, …, L. Radbruch (Eds.), *Palliative medicine (Chapter 89)*. Philadelphia: Saunders.

McQueen, A. (2011). Ectopic pregnancy: Risk factors, diagnostic procedures and treatment. *Nursing Standard, 25*(37), 49-56.

North American Menopause Society. (2010). *Position statement: Estrogen and progesterone use in menopausal women*. Retrieved from *http://www.menopause.org/PSht10.pdf*

Ortiz, D. (2008). Chronic pelvic pain in women. *American Family Physician, 77*(11), 1535-1542.

Prasad, A. G., & Alvero, R. (2011). Uterine prolapse. In F. Ferri (Ed.), *Ferri's clinical advisor 2011: Instant diagnosis and treatment*. Philadelphia: Mosby.

Public Health Agency of Canada [PHAC]. (2008a). *Canadian perinatal health report*. Retrieved from *http://www.phac-aspc.gc.ca/publicat/2008/cphr-rspc/pdf/cphr-rspc08-eng.pdf*

Public Health Agency of Canada [PHAC]. (2008b). *Pelvic inflammatory disease (PID)*. Updated: January 2010. *Canadian Guidelines on Sexually Transmitted Infections*. Available at *http://www.phac-aspc.gc.ca/std-mts/sti-its/pdf/404pelviinfla-eng.pdf*

Public Health Agency of Canada [PHAC]. (2009). *Frequently asked questions on emergency contraception*. Retrieved from *http://www.phac-aspc.gc.ca/std-mts/ec_cu-eng.php*

Quaas, A., & Dokras, A. (2008). Diagnosis and treatment of unexplained infertility. *Reviews in Obstetrics and Gynecology, 1*(2), 69-76.

Radosh, L. (2009). Drug treatments for polycystic ovary syndrome. *American Family Physician, 79*(8), 671-676. Retrieved from *http://www.aafp.org/afp/2009/0415/p671.html*

Raines, K. (2010). Diagnosing premenstrual syndrome. *Journal for Nurse Practitioners, 6*(3), 224-225. doi:10.1016/J.Nupra.2009.12.013

Rani, S. (2009). The psychosexual implications of menopause. *British Journal of Nursing, 18*(6), 370-373.

Rapkin, A. J., & Gambone, J. C. (2010). Pelvic pain. In N. F. Hacker, J. C. Gambone, & C. J. Hobel (Eds.), *Hacker and Moore's essentials of obstetrics and gynecology* (5th ed.). Philadelphia: Saunders.

Shamonki, M., Nelson, A. L., & Gambone, J. C. (2010). Ectopic pregnancy. In N. F. Hacker, J. C. Gambone, & C. J. Hobel (Eds.), *Hacker and Moore's essentials of obstetrics and gynecology* (5th ed.). Philadelphia: Saunders.

Smith, R. P. (Ed.). (2008). *Netter's obstetrics and gynecology* (2nd ed.). Philadelphia: Saunders.

Society of Obstetricians and Gynaecologists of Canada (SOGC). (2009). *Media backgrounder: Menopause and osteoporosis update 2009*. Retrieved from *http://www.sogc.org/media/pdf/advisories/MenoOsteoBackgrounder-090122.pdf*

Soper, D. (2010). Pelvic inflammatory disease. *Obstetrics & Gynecology, 116*(2), 419-428. doi:10.1097/AOG.0b013e3181e92c54

Stovall, D. (2011). Alternatives to hysterectomy: Focus on global endometrial ablation, uterine fibroid embolization, and magnetic resonance-guided focused ultrasound. *Menopause, 18*(4), 443-450. doi:10.1097/gme.0b013e318207fe15

Tinelli, A., Malvasi, A., Rahimi, S., Negro, R., Vergara, D., Martignago, R., …, Cavallotti, C. (2010). Age-related pelvic floor modifications and prolapse risk factors in postmenopausal women. *Menopause, 17*(1), 204-212. doi:10.1097/gme.0b013e3181b0c2ae

Tsai, Y.-C., & Liu, C.-H. (2009). The effectiveness of pelvic floor exercises, digital vaginal palpation and interpersonal support on stress urinary incontinence: An experimental study. *International Journal of Nursing Studies, 46*(9), 1181-1186. doi:10.1016/j.ijnurstu.2009.03.003

Valdivielso-Ramos, M., Bueno, C., & Hernanz, J. M. (2008). Significant improvement in extensive lichen sclerosus with tacrolimus ointment and PUVA. *American Journal of Clinical Dermatology, 9*(3), 175-179. doi:10.2165/00128071-200809030-00006

van der Kooij, S. M., Bipat, S., Henekamp, W. J. K., Ankum, W. M., & Reekers, J. A. (2011). Uterine artery embolization versus surgery in the treatment of symptomatic fibroids: A systematic review and metaanalysis. *American Journal of Obstetrics and Gynecology, 205*(317), e1-18. doi:10.1016/j.ajog.2011.03.016

Visintin, I., Feng, Z., Longton, G., Ward, D. C., Alvero, A. B., Lai, Y., ..., Mor, G. (2008). Diagnostic markers for early detection of ovarian cancer. *Clinical Cancer Research, 14*(4), 1065-1072. doi:10.1158/1078-0432.CCR-07-1569

Viswanathan, M., Hartmann, K., McKoy, N., Stuart, G., Rankins, N., Thieda, P., ..., Lohr, K. N. (2007). *Management for uterine fibroids: An update of the evidence.* Evidence Report/Technology Assessment No. 154 (Prepared by RTI International—University of North Carolina Evidence-based Practice Center under Contract No. 290-02-0016). AHRQ Publication No. 07-E011. Rockville, MD: Agency for Healthcare Research and Quality. Retrieved from *http://www.ncbi.nlm.nih.gov/books/bv.fcgi?rid=hstat1b.section.55718*

CANADIAN RESOURCES

Canadian Cancer Society
http://www.cancer.ca
Canadian Fertility and Andrology Society
http://www.cfas.ca/
Centre for Chronic Prevention and Control (Public Health Agency of Canada)
http://www.phac-aspc.gc.ca/ccdpc-cpcmc/cc-ccu/index_e.html
Cervical Cancer Control in Canada (CCCiC)
http://www.cancerview.ca/cv/portal/Home/PreventionAndScreening/ PSProfessionals/PSScreeningAndEarlyDiagnosis/CervicalCancer- ControlInCanada?_afrLoop=1782622997038000&_afrWindow- Mode=0&_adf.ctrl-state=pyzb01eh7_4

endometriosisinfo.ca: The facts of endometriosis
http://endometriosisinfo.ca/index_e.aspx
myfertility.ca
http://www.myfertility.ca/index.asp?C=28633409132596180556
National Ovarian Cancer Coalition (NOCC)
http://www.ovarian.org/about_us.php
Ovarian Cancer Canada
http://www.ovariancanada.org
SexualityandU.ca
http://www.sexualityandu.ca/
Society of Obstetricians and Gynaecologists of Canada
http://www.sogc.org/index_e.asp
Women's Health Matters
http://www.womenshealthmatters.ca/

RELATED RESOURCES

American Cancer Society
http://www.cancer.org
American College of Obstetricians and Gynecologists
http://www.acog.org
American Urological Association
http://www.auanet.org
Hysterectomy Educational Resources and Services (HERS) Foundation
http://www.hersfoundation.com/
North American Menopause Society
http://www.menopause.org
Sexuality Information and Education Council of the United States (SIECUS)
http://www.siecus.org

evolve *For additional Internet resources, see the Web site for this book at* **http://evolve.elsevier.com/Canada/Lewis/medsurg**

Nursing Management: Male Reproductive Problems

Written by Shannon Ruff Dirksen

Adapted by Shelley L. Cobbett

LEARNING OBJECTIVES

1. Describe the pathophysiology, clinical manifestations, and collaborative care of benign prostatic hyperplasia.
2. Discuss the nursing management of benign prostatic hyperplasia.
3. Describe the pathophysiology, clinical manifestations, and collaborative care of prostate cancer.
4. Discuss the nursing management of prostate cancer.
5. Describe the pathophysiology, clinical manifestations, and collaborative and nursing management of

6. problems of the penis, problems of the scrotum, and prostatitis.
7. Explain the clinical manifestations and collaborative care of testicular cancer.
8. Discuss the nursing management of problems related to male sexual functioning.
9. Identify the psychological and emotional implications related to male reproductive problems.

KEY TERMS

benign prostatic hyperplasia (BPH) A nonmalignant, noninflammatory enlargement of the prostate gland caused by an increase in the number of epithelial cells and the amount of stromal tissue, p. 1576

epididymitis Inflammation of the epididymis, usually as a result of infection and rarely as a result of trauma or urinary reflux down the vas deferens from the urethra, p. 1593

epispadias A congenital opening of the penis on the dorsum of the penis, p. 1592

erectile dysfunction (ED) The inability to attain or maintain an erect penis that allows satisfactory sexual performance, p. 1597

hydrocele A nontender, fluid-filled mass that results from interference with lymphatic drainage of the scrotum and swelling of the tunica vaginalis that surrounds the testis, p. 1594

hypospadias An abnormal congenital opening of the male urethra upon the undersurface of the penis, p. 1592

orchitis An acute inflammation of the testis, p. 1593

paraphimosis Narrowing or edema of the retracted uncircumcised foreskin, preventing normal return over the glans and causing strangulation, p. 1592

phimosis Constriction of the uncircumcised foreskin around the head of the penis, making retraction over the glans penis difficult, p. 1592

prostate-specific antigen (PSA) A glycoprotein found only in the epithelial cells of the prostate that, when elevated, indicates a pathological condition of the prostate, although not necessarily prostate cancer, p. 1585

prostatitis Acute or chronic inflammatory conditions affecting the prostate gland, usually as a result of infection, p. 1591

radical prostatectomy Surgical removal of the entire prostate gland, the seminal vesicles, and part of the bladder neck (ampulla), p. 1586

spermatocele A firm, sperm-containing, painless cyst of the epididymis, p. 1594

testicular torsion Involves a twisting of the spermatic cord that supplies blood to the testes and epididymis, causing an interruption to the blood supply, p. 1594

transurethral resection of the prostate (TURP) A surgical procedure involving the removal of prostate tissue with the use of a resectoscope inserted through the urethra, p. 1579

varicocele A dilation of the veins that drain the testes, p. 1594

vasectomy Bilateral surgical ligation or resection of the vas deferens performed for the purpose of sterilization, p. 1596

ELECTRONIC RESOURCES

Supplemental content related to Chapter 57 can be found...

Evolve Web Site

http://evolve.elsevier.com/Canada/Lewis/medsurg

- Answer Guidelines for Case Study on p. 1600
- Clinical Reference: Laboratory Values
- Content Updates
- Customizable Nursing Care Plan: Prostate Surgery
- eFigure 57-1: Vacuum Constriction Device
- Electronic Calculators
- Examination Review Questions
- Glossary
- Interactive Case Study: Benign Prostatic Hyperplasia
- Key Points (Printable and MP3 Download)
- Patient & Caregiver Teaching Guide: Testicular Self-Examination

Problems of the male reproductive system can involve a variety of structures, including the prostate, the penis, the urethra, the ejaculatory duct, the scrotum, the testes, the epididymis, the vas deferens, and the rectum (Figure 57-1).

Problems of the Prostate Gland

Benign Prostatic Hyperplasia

Benign prostatic hyperplasia (BPH) is an enlargement of the prostate gland resulting from an increase in the number of epithelial cells and the amount of stromal tissue. It is the most common urological problem in male adults (Rawson & Saad, 2010). BPH occurs in about 50% of men older than 50 years and in over 80% of men older than 80 years. Approximately 25% of men require some form of treatment by the time they reach age 80. Prostate hyperplasia does not predispose to the development of prostate cancer (Andriole, 2009).

Etiology and Pathophysiology

Although the cause of BPH is not completely understood, it is thought that BPH results from endocrine changes associated with the aging process. Possible causes include excessive accumulation of dihydroxytestosterone (the principal intraprostatic androgen), stimulation by estrogen, and local growth hormone action. Typically, BPH develops in the inner part of the prostate. (Prostate cancer is most likely to develop in the outer part.) This enlargement gradually compresses the urethra, eventually leading to partial or complete obstruction (Figure 57-2). It is the compression of the urethra that ultimately leads to the development of clinical symptoms. There is no direct relationship between the size of the prostate and the degree of obstruction. It is the location of the enlargement that is most significant in the development of obstructive symptoms. For example, it is possible for mild hyperplasia to cause severe obstruction; likewise, it is possible for extreme hyperplasia to cause few obstructive symptoms.

Risk factors for BPH include a family history (particularly involving first-degree relatives), environment, and diet. Although men from both Western and Eastern cultures develop BPH disease

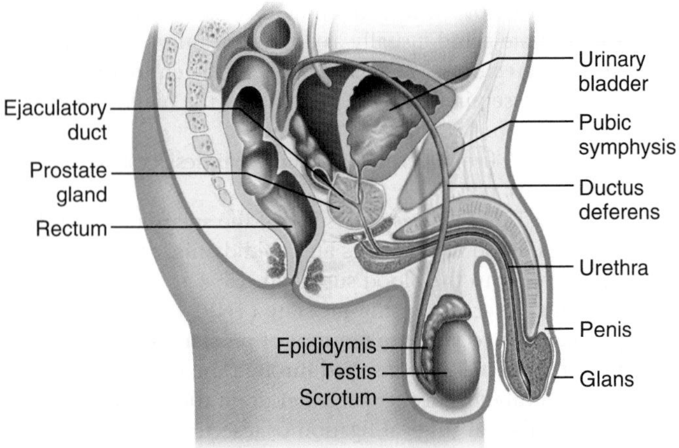

Figure 57-1 Areas of the male reproductive system in which problems are likely to develop.

Source: Adapted from Patton, K. T., & Thibodeau, G. A. (2010) *Anatomy and physiology* (7th ed., p. 1021, Figure 31-1). St Louis: Mosby.

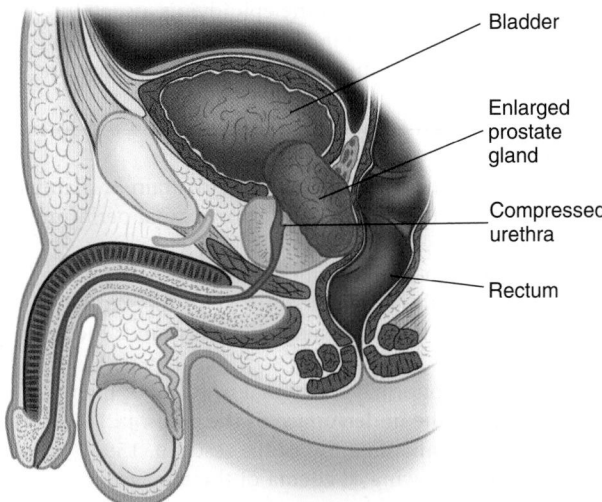

Figure 57-2 Benign prostatic hyperplasia. The enlarged prostate compresses the urethra.

Source: Adapted from Seidel, H. M., Ball, J. W., Dains, J. E., Flynn, J. A., Solomon, B. S., & Stewart, R. W. (2011). *Mosby's guide to physical examination* (6th ed., p. 645, Figure 20-14). St. Louis: Mosby.

at about the same rates, men from Western cultures are much more likely to develop obstructive problems. Higher risk for BPH has been found in association with obesity and a diet high in zinc, butter, and margarine, whereas individuals who eat lots of fruits and vegetables are thought to have a lower risk for BPH. Physical activity and moderate alcohol consumption also have been found to decrease the risk of BPH (Tanguay et al., 2009).

Clinical Manifestations

The symptoms of BPH experienced by the patient result from urinary obstruction. Symptoms are usually gradual in onset and may not be noticed until prostatic enlargement has been present for some time. Early symptoms are usually minimal because the bladder can compensate for a small amount of resistance to urine flow. The symptoms gradually worsen as the degree of urethral obstruction increases.

Symptoms fall into one of two groups: obstructive symptoms and irritative symptoms. *Obstructive symptoms* include a decrease in the calibre and force of the urinary stream, difficulty in initiating voiding, intermittency (stopping and starting stream several times while voiding), and dribbling at the end of urination. *Irritative symptoms,* which include urinary frequency, urgency, dysuria, bladder pain, nocturia, and incontinence, are associated with inflammation or infection. The American Urological Association (AUA) Symptom Index for BPH (Table 57-1) is a tool used in both Canada and the United States as well as other countries to assess voiding symptoms associated with obstruction (Barry et al., 1992). Although this tool is not diagnostic, it is useful in determining the degree of symptoms.

Complications

The majority of complications that develop in BPH are related to urinary obstruction. Acute urinary retention is a common complication and is an indication for surgical intervention in about 25 to 30% of patients (Tanguay et al., 2009). Another common complication is urinary tract infection (UTI) and, potentially, sepsis secondary to UTI. Incomplete bladder emptying (associated with partial obstruction) results in residual urine, providing a favourable environment for bacterial growth. Calculi may develop in the bladder because of the alkalinization of the residual urine. Although bladder stones are eight times more common in men with BPH, risk of renal calculi is not significantly increased. Other less common but potential complications include renal failure caused by *hydronephrosis* (distension of the pelvis and the calyces of the kidney by urine that cannot flow through the ureter to the bladder), pyelonephritis, and bladder damage if treatment for acute urinary retention is delayed.

Diagnostic Studies

The primary methods used to diagnose BPH include a history and physical examination. The prostate can be palpated by digital rectal examination (DRE). Using DRE, the health care provider can estimate the size, the symmetry, and the consistency of the prostate gland. In BPH, the prostate is symmetrically enlarged, firm, and smooth.

Additional diagnostic tests may be indicated, depending on the type and the severity of symptoms and clinical findings.

Table 57-1 American Urological Association Symptom Index to Determine Severity of Prostatic Problems

AMERICAN UROLOGICAL ASSOCIATION (AUA) SYMPTOM SCORE*

(CIRCLE ONE NUMBER ON EACH LINE)

QUESTIONS TO BE ANSWERED	NOT AT ALL	LESS THAN 1 TIME IN 5	LESS THAN HALF THE TIME	ABOUT HALF THE TIME	MORE THAN HALF THE TIME	ALMOST ALWAYS
Over the past month:	0	1	2	3	4	5
1. How often have you had a sensation of not emptying your bladder completely after you finished urinating?						
2. How often have you had to urinate again, <2 hr after you finished urinating?	0	1	2	3	4	5
3. How often have you found you stopped and started again several times when you urinated?	0	1	2	3	4	5
4. How often have you found it difficult to postpone urination?	0	1	2	3	4	5
5. How often have you had a weak urinary stream?	0	1	2	3	4	5
6. How often have you had to push or strain to begin urination?	0	1	2	3	4	5
7. How many times did you most typically get up to urinate from the time you went to bed at night until the time you got up in the morning?	0 (None)	1 (1 time)	2 (2 times)	3 (3 times)	4 (4 times)	5 (≥5 times)
Sum of circled numbers (AUA Symptom Score):* _____						

*Score is interpreted as 0-7, mild; 8-19, moderate; 20-35, severe.
Source: Barry, M. J., Fowler, F. J., Jr., O'Leary, M. P., Bruskowitz, R. C., Holtgrewe, H. L., Mebust, W. K., & Cockett, A. T. (1992). The American Urological Association symptom index for benign prostatic hyperplasia. *Journal of Urology, 148*(5), 1549-1557. Used with permission.

A urinalysis with culture is routinely done to determine the presence of infection. The presence of bacteria, white blood cells, or microscopic hematuria is an indication of infection or inflammation. The prostate-specific antigen (PSA) blood level is usually measured to rule out prostate cancer (Ferri, 2009). However, PSA levels may be slightly elevated in patients with BPH. Serum creatinine may be ordered to rule out renal insufficiency.

In patients with an abnormal DRE and elevated PSA, a *transrectal ultrasonography* (TRUS) scan is typically indicated. This examination allows for accurate assessment of prostate size and is helpful in differentiating BPH from prostate cancer. Biopsies can be taken during the ultrasonography procedure. *Uroflowmetry*, a study that measures the volume of urine expelled from the bladder per second, is helpful in determining the extent of urethral blockage and thus the type of treatment needed. Postvoid residual urine volume is often measured to determine the degree of urine flow obstruction. *Cystourethroscopy*, a procedure allowing internal visualization of the urethra and the bladder, is performed if the diagnosis is uncertain and in patients who are scheduled for prostatectomy. Diagnostic studies are outlined in Table 57-2.

Collaborative Care

The goals of collaborative care are to restore bladder drainage, relieve the patient's symptoms, and prevent or treat the complications of BPH. Treatment is generally based on the degree to which the symptoms bother the patient or the presence of complications rather than the size of the prostate. Alternatives to surgical intervention for some patients now include drug therapy and minimally invasive procedures, for example, holmium laser enucleation (Lingeman, 2011).

COLLABORATIVE CARE

Table 57-2 Benign Prostatic Hyperplasia

Diagnostic	Invasive Therapy*
• History and physical examination	• Transurethral resection of the prostate (TURP)
• Digital rectal examination (DRE)	• Open prostatectomy
• Urinalysis with culture	• Transurethral incision of the prostate (TUIP)
• Serum creatinine	**Minimally Invasive Therapy***
• Prostate-specific antigen (PSA)	• Transurethral microwave thermotherapy (TUMT)
• Postvoid residual	• Transurethral needle ablation (TUNA)
• Uroflowmetry	
• Transrectal ultrasonography (TRUS)	• Laser prostatectomy
• Cystourethroscopy	• Transurethral electrovaporization of the prostate (TUVP)
Collaborative Therapy	
Conservative Therapy ("Watchful Waiting")	• Intraprostatic urethral stents
Drug Therapy	
• 5α-Reductase inhibitors	
• α-Adrenergic receptor blockers	
• Saw palmetto	

*See Table 57-3.

The most conservative initial treatment for BPH is referred to as *watchful waiting*. When there are no symptoms or only mild ones (AUA symptom scores <7), a wait-and-see approach is taken (Rakel & Bope, 2008). Because symptoms may come and go, a conservative approach has value. Dietary changes (decreasing intake of caffeine and artificial sweeteners, limiting spicy or acidic foods), avoiding medication such as decongestants and anticholinergics, and restricting evening fluid intake may result in improvement of symptoms. A timed voiding schedule may reduce or eliminate symptoms, thus negating the need for further intervention. If the patient begins to have signs or symptoms that indicate an increase in obstruction, further treatment is indicated.

Drug Therapy. Drugs that have been used to treat BPH with variable degrees of success include 5α-reductase inhibitors and α-adrenergic receptor blockers. Combination therapy has been shown to be more effective in reducing symptoms than using one drug alone (Barry & McNaughton-Collins, 2008).

5α-Reductase Inhibitors. These drugs work by reducing the size of the prostate gland. Finasteride (Proscar) blocks the enzyme 5α-reductase, which is necessary for the conversion of testosterone to dihydroxytestosterone, the principal intraprostatic androgen. This drug causes regression of hyperplastic tissue through suppression of androgens and may also lower the risk of low-grade early-stage prostate cancer. Finasteride is an appropriate treatment option for individuals who score between 12 and 26 on the AUA Symptom Index for BPH (see Table 57-1). Although 40 to 50% of those treated show improvement, it takes between 3 and 6 months to be effective, and the medication must be taken on a continuous basis to maintain therapeutic results. Dutasteride (Duragen) is a dual inhibitor of 5α-reductase types 1 and 2 isoenzymes. (Finasteride inhibits only the type 2 isoenzyme.) Adverse effects of 5α-reductase inhibitors include decreased libido, decreased volume of ejaculate, and erectile dysfunction (ED).

α-Adrenergic Receptor Blockers. Another drug treatment option for BPH is agents that block α₁-adrenergic receptors. Although this group of drugs is more commonly used for treatment of hypertension, these drugs promote smooth muscle relaxation in the prostate. $α_1$-Adrenergic receptors are abundant in the prostate and are increased in hyperplastic prostate tissue. Relaxation of the smooth muscle ultimately facilitates urinary flow through the urethra. Currently, the α-adrenergic blockers are the most widely prescribed drug for the patient with BPH who is experiencing moderate symptoms without the presence of other complications. These agents demonstrate a 50 to 60% efficacy in improvement of symptoms. Improvement of symptoms occurs within 2 to 3 weeks.

Several α-adrenergic blockers, including silodosin (Rapaflo), alfuzosin (Uroxatral), prazosin (Minipress), doxazosin (Cardura), terazosin (Hytrin), and tamsulosin (Flomax), are currently being used. Adverse effects include postural hypotension, dizziness, fatigue, retrograde ejaculation, and nasal congestion. It must be pointed out that, although these drugs offer symptomatic relief of BPH, they do not treat hyperplasia.

Herbal Therapy. Herbs extracted from plants have been used in the management of BPH. In particular, plant extracts, such as saw palmetto *(Serenoa repens)*, have been used. However, current evidence indicates that saw palmetto has no benefit over a placebo (Tacklind, MacDonald, Rutks, & Wilt, 2009). Pygeum, an extract from the African prune tree, provides moderate relief of the urinary symptoms associated with BPH but more research is required (Edgar, Levin, Constantinou, & Denis, 2007) (see the Complementary and Alternative Therapies box on pygeum).

COMPLEMENTARY & ALTERNATIVE THERAPIES

Pygeum

Clinical Uses

Benign prostatic hyperplasia (BPH); treatment of lower urinary tract symptoms

Effects

Appears to be effective in managing specific parameters of bladder function associated with BPH

Nursing Implications

Generally well tolerated. Minimal adverse effects such as nausea and abdominal pain. No known drug interactions. Advise patient to consult a physician for the correct diagnosis of BPH.

Source: Edgar, A. D., Levin, R., Constantinou, C. C., & Denis, L. (2007). A critical review of the pharmacology of the plant extract of *Pygeum africanum* in the treatment of LUTS. *Neurourology and Urodynamics, 26*(4), 458-463. doi:10.1002/nau.20136

Invasive Therapy. Invasive treatment of symptomatic BPH primarily involves resection or ablation of the prostate. The choice of the treatment approach depends on the size and the location of the prostatic enlargement as well as patient factors such as age and surgical risk. Various invasive treatments are summarized in Table 57-3.

Invasive therapy is indicated when there is a decrease in urine flow sufficient to cause discomfort, persistent residual urine, acute urinary retention because of obstruction with no reversible precipitating cause, or hydronephrosis. Intermittent catheterization or insertion of an indwelling catheter can temporarily reduce symptoms and bypass the obstruction. However, long-term catheter use should be avoided because of the increased risk of infection.

Transurethral Resection of the Prostate. **Transurethral resection of the prostate (TURP)** is a surgical procedure involving the removal of prostate tissue using a resectoscope inserted through the urethra. TURP has long been considered the "gold standard" surgical treatment for obstructing BPH. Although this procedure remains by far the most common operation performed, there has been a decrease in the number of TURP procedures done in recent years owing to the development of less invasive technologies (Steels, 2008).

TURP is performed under a spinal or general anaesthetic. No external surgical incision is made. A resectoscope is inserted through the urethra to excise and cauterize obstructing prostatic tissue (Figure 57-3). A large three-way indwelling catheter with a 30-mL balloon is inserted into the bladder after the procedure to provide hemostasis and to facilitate urinary drainage. Usually for the first 24 hours, the bladder is irrigated, either continuously or intermittently, to prevent obstruction from mucus and blood clots.

The outcome for 80 to 90% of patients is excellent, with marked improvements in symptoms and urinary flow rates. TURP is a surgical procedure with relatively low risk. Some of the postoperative complications include bleeding, clot retention, bladder spasms, and dilutional hyponatremia associated with irrigation. Because bleeding is a common complication, patients taking aspirin or warfarin (Coumadin) must discontinue these medications several days before surgery.

Transurethral Incision of the Prostate. Transurethral incision of the prostate (TUIP) is a surgical procedure that is indicated for men with moderate to severe symptoms and small prostates who are poor surgical candidates. It is done under local anaesthesia and is as effective as TURP in symptom relief.

Prostatectomy. This is the surgery of choice for large prostates and is discussed later in this chapter on pp. 1586-1587.

Minimally Invasive Therapy. Minimally invasive nonsurgical therapies are an alternative to watchful waiting and surgical treatment. They generally do not necessitate hospitalization or catheterization and are associated with few adverse events. When compared with invasive techniques, many minimally invasive therapies are less effective in improving urine flow and symptoms (Lourenco et al., 2008).

Transurethral Microwave Thermotherapy. Transurethral microwave thermotherapy (TUMT) is an outpatient procedure that involves the delivery of microwaves directly to the prostate through a transurethral probe in order to raise the temperature of the prostate tissue to about 45°C (Bankhead, 2010). The heat causes death of tissue, thus relieving the obstruction. A rectal temperature probe is used during the procedure to ensure that the rectal temperature is kept below 43.5°C to prevent rectal tissue damage.

Postoperative urinary retention is a common complication. Thus, the patient is generally sent home with an indwelling catheter for 2 to 7 days to maintain urinary flow and to facilitate the passing of small clots or necrotic tissue. Antibiotics, pain medication, and bladder antispasmodic medications are used to treat and prevent postprocedure problems. The procedure is not appropriate for men with rectal problems. Anticoagulant therapy should be stopped 10 days before treatment. Mild adverse effects include occasional problems of bladder spasm, hematuria, dysuria, and retention.

Transurethral Needle Ablation. Transurethral needle ablation (TUNA) is another procedure that increases the temperature of prostate tissue, thus causing localized necrosis. TUNA differs from TUMT in that low-wave radiofrequency is used to heat the prostate, and only prostate tissue in direct contact with the needle is affected, allowing greater precision in removal of the target tissue. The extent of tissue removed by this process is determined by the amount of tissue contact (needle length), amount of energy delivered, and duration of treatment. Seventy percent of patients undergoing TUNA report an improvement in symptoms, making this an attractive treatment option for men with BPH.

This procedure is performed in an outpatient unit or physician's office using local anaesthesia and intravenous or oral

Table 57-3 Treatment Options for Benign Prostatic Hyperplasia

TREATMENT	DESCRIPTION	ADVANTAGES	DISADVANTAGES
Invasive			
Transurethral resection of the prostate (TURP)	Use of excision and cauterization to remove prostate tissue cystoscopically. Considered the most effective treatment of BPH.	Best long-term relief of prostatic obstruction. Erectile dysfunction unlikely.	Bleeding. Retrograde ejaculation.
Transurethral incision of the prostate (TUIP)	Involves making transurethral slits or incisions into prostatic tissue to relieve obstruction. Effective for men with relatively little prostatic enlargement.	Outpatient procedure. Minimal complications. Good for high-risk patients. Low occurrence of erectile dysfunction or retrograde ejaculation.	Urinary catheter needed after procedure. Retreatment may be needed.
Open prostatectomy	Surgery of choice for men with large prostates or complicating factors. Involves external incision with three possible approaches (see Figure 57-4).	Complete visualization of prostate and surrounding tissue. Usually indicated only if prostate gland is very large.	Erectile dysfunction, retrograde ejaculation. Bleeding. Postoperative pain. Risk of infection.
Minimally Invasive			
Transurethral microwave thermotherapy (TUMT)	Use of microwave-radiating heat to produce coagulative necrosis of the prostate.	Short, outpatient procedure. Erectile dysfunction and retrograde ejaculation are rare.	Potential for damage to surrounding tissue. Urinary catheter needed after procedure. May need retreatment.
Transurethral needle ablation of the prostate (TUNA)	Low-wave radiofrequency used to heat the prostate and cause necrosis.	Short outpatient procedure. Erectile dysfunction and retrograde ejaculation are rare. Precise delivery of heat to desired area. Very little pain experienced.	Urinary retention common. Irritative voiding symptoms. Hematuria. May need retreatment.
Laser prostatectomy	Procedure uses a laser beam to cut or destroy part of the prostate. Different techniques are available: Visual laser ablation of the prostate (VLAP). Contact laser technique. Interstitial laser coagulation (ILC). Photovaporization of the prostate (PVP).	Short procedure. Comparable results with TURP. Minimal bleeding. Fast recovery time. Rapid symptom improvement.	Postprocedure catheterization (≤7 days) needed because of edema and urinary retention. Delayed sloughing of tissue. Takes several weeks to reach optimal effect. Retrograde ejaculation.
Transurethral electrovaporization of prostate (TUVP)	Electrosurgical vaporization and desiccation are used together to destroy prostatic tissue.	Minimal risks. Minimal bleeding and sloughing.	Retrograde ejaculation. Intermittent hematuria.
Intraprostatic urethral stents	Insertion of self-expandable metallic stent into the urethra where enlarged area of prostate occurs.	Safe and effective. Low risk.	Stent may move. Long-term effect is unknown.

sedation. The TUNA procedure typically lasts only 30 minutes. The patient normally experiences little pain and an early return to regular activities. Complications include urinary retention, UTI, and irritative voiding symptoms (e.g., frequency, urgency, dysuria). Some patients require a urinary catheter for a short duration. Patients typically have hematuria for up to a week.

Laser Prostatectomy. The use of laser therapy through visual or ultrasonography guidance is an effective alternative to TURP in treating BPH (Chung et al., 2011). The laser beam is delivered transurethrally through a fibre instrument and is used for cutting, coagulation, and vaporization of prostatic tissue. There are a variety of laser procedures using different sources, wavelengths,

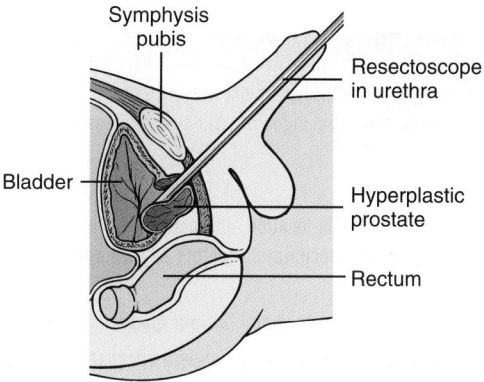

Figure 57-3 Transurethral resection of the prostate.

and delivery systems. A common laser procedure is laser coagulation of the prostate, often referred to as *visual laser ablation of the prostate* (VLAP). VLAP uses the laser beam to produce deep coagulation necrosis of the prostate. The affected prostate tissue gradually sloughs in the urinary stream. It takes several weeks before the patient reaches optimal results following this type of laser therapy. At the completion of VLAP, a urinary catheter is inserted to allow for drainage.

Contact laser techniques involve the direct contact of the laser to the prostate tissue. This produces an immediate vaporization of the prostate tissue. Blood vessels near the laser tip are immediately cauterized; thus, bleeding during the procedure is rare. A three-way catheter with slow-drip irrigation is placed immediately after the procedure for a short time. Typically, the catheter is removed within 6 to 8 hours after the procedure. Advantages of this procedure over TURP include minimal bleeding both during and after the procedure, faster recovery time, and ability to perform the surgery on patients taking anticoagulants.

Another approach to laser prostatectomy is *interstitial laser coagulation* (ILC) (Woods, 2010). The prostate is viewed through a cystoscope. A laser is used to quickly treat precise areas of the enlarged prostate by placement of interstitial light guides directly into the prostate tissue.

Intraprostatic Urethral Stents. For patients seeking care who have contraindications to surgery or anaesthesia, prostatic stenting can serve as a temporary or permanent solution for bladder outlet obstruction caused by BPH (see Table 57-3).

NURSING MANAGEMENT: BENIGN PROSTATIC HYPERPLASIA

Because the nurse is most directly involved with care of patients with BPH having invasive procedures, the focus of nursing management in this section is on preoperative and postoperative care.

◾ Nursing Assessment

Subjective and objective data that should be obtained from a patient with BPH are presented in Table 57-4.

Table 57-4 Benign Prostatic Hyperplasia
Subjective Data
Important Health Information
Past health history: Family history of BPH; obesity; diet high in fat or zinc
Medications: Estrogen or testosterone supplementation
Surgeries or other treatments: Previous treatment for BPH
Symptoms
Voluntary fluid restriction; urinary urgency; urinary dysuria; diminution in calibre and force of urinary stream; hesitancy in initiating voiding; postvoiding dribbling; urinary retention; incontinence; nocturia; bladder discomfort; anxiety about sexual functioning
Objective Data
General
Older adult male
Urinary
Distended bladder on palpation; smooth, firm, elastic enlargement of prostate on rectal examination
Possible Findings
Enlarged prostate on ultrasonography; vesicle neck obstruction on cystourethroscopy; residual urine with postvoiding catheterization; presence of white blood cells, bacteria, or microscopic hematuria with infection; ↑ serum creatinine levels with renal involvement

BPH, benign prostatic hyperplasia.

◾ Nursing Diagnoses

Nursing diagnoses for the patient with BPH preoperatively may include, but are not limited to, the following:
- Acute pain *related to* bladder distension secondary to enlarged prostate
- Risk for infection *related to* an indwelling catheter, urinary stasis, or environmental pathogens

Nursing diagnoses for the patient with BPH who has surgery may include, but are not limited to, those presented in Nursing Care Plan (NCP) 57-1.

◾ Planning

The overall preoperative goals for the patient with BPH having invasive procedures are to have (1) restoration of urinary drainage, (2) treatment of any UTI, and (3) understanding on the patient's part of the upcoming procedure, the implications for sexual functioning, and urinary control. The overall postoperative goals are to have (1) no complications, (2) restoration of urinary control, (3) complete bladder emptying, and (4) satisfying sexual expression.

◾ Nursing Implementation

Health Promotion

The cause of BPH is largely attributed to the aging process. The focus of health promotion is on early detection and treatment.

NURSING CARE PLAN 57-1

Prostate Surgery*

NURSING DIAGNOSIS	**Acute pain** *related to* bladder irritability, irrigations, and distension; presence of catheter; and surgical trauma *as evidenced by* reports of pain; nonverbal signs of pain such as moaning, crying, and legs drawn to abdomen
Expected Patient Outcome	**Nursing Interventions and *Rationales***
• Reports satisfactory pain control	• Perform a comprehensive assessment of pain to include location, characteristics, onset and duration, frequency, quality, intensity, or severity of pain, and precipitating factors *to plan appropriate interventions*.† • Monitor intake and output carefully *to evaluate fluid balance and prevent bladder distension*. • Percuss bladder or use bladder scanner to check for distension *to validate adequate emptying of the bladder*. • Maintain patency of catheter *to ensure continuous flow of urine from the bladder and no clots because they may cause obstruction of urine flow, resulting in bladder spasms*. • Increase continuous bladder irrigation rate if there is increased hematuria postoperatively; irrigate manually if occluded *to prevent clots and possible occlusion of catheter*. • Instruct patient to try not to urinate around catheter *because this increases the occurrence of spasm*. • Give belladonna and opium suppository as needed; instruct patient in relaxation techniques such as deep-breathing exercises, distraction therapy, and visual imagery *to relieve pain and decrease spasms*. • Assess comfort status *to continue or revise plan as necessary*.
NURSING DIAGNOSIS	**Ineffective self-health management** *related to* lack of knowledge regarding need for follow-up care and activity restriction postoperatively *as evidenced by* questioning or inaccurate comments about postoperative activity
Expected Patient Outcome	**Nursing Interventions and *Rationales***
• Describes follow-up care and activity restrictions	• Teach patient to avoid heavy lifting (not more than 4.5 kg), straining during defecation, prolonged periods of travel, stair climbing, driving, and sexual activity until surgeon approves such activity *to prevent increases in intra-abdominal pressure and the possibility of bleeding*. • Teach patient about the need for follow-up care *to evaluate prostate (if present) and overall health*.
NURSING DIAGNOSIS	**Urge urinary incontinence** *related to* poor sphincter control *as evidenced by* involuntary leakage of urine
Expected Patient Outcome	**Nursing Interventions and *Rationales***
• Reports decrease in urine leakage between voidings	• Identify factors that contribute to incontinence episodes *to plan appropriate interventions*. • Instruct patient to respond immediately to urge to void *to prevent involuntary leakage*. • Explain etiology of problem and rationale for actions *to help patient plan appropriate interventions*. • Limit ingestion of bladder irritants (e.g., colas, coffee, tea, chocolate) *to decrease urinary urgency*. • Limit fluids for 2-3 hr before bedtime *to avoid nighttime urgency*. • Advise patient about devices for short-term management of dribbling (e.g., incontinence garment or pad, condom catheter, penile clamp) *so patient is aware of various devices and can make an informed decision among alternatives*. • Teach patient Kegel exercises *to strengthen sphincter tone*.

*The specific nursing management will vary depending on the type of surgical intervention for benign prostatic hyperplasia (BPH) or prostate cancer.
†See eNCP 22-1, Postoperative Patient, on the Evolve Web site for that chapter for further nursing interventions and rationales for the nursing diagnosis of acute pain.

The Canadian Cancer Society (2011) recommends that if men are older than 50 years, are in good health, and have no symptoms of prostate cancer (or older than 40 if a man is at high risk), they should talk with their health care provider about PSA testing for prostate cancer. Early prostate cancer screening may reduce the mortality rate by as much as 35%, and men with prostate cancer who engaged in vigorous activity have a lower mortality rate (Kenfield, Stampfer, Giovannuncci, & Chan, 2011). Men in high-risk groups should consider testing at a younger age. When symptoms of prostatic hyperplasia become evident, further diagnostic screening may be necessary (see Table 57-2).

Some men find that the ingestion of alcohol and caffeine tends to increase prostatic symptoms because the diuretic effect of these substances increases bladder distension. Compounds found in common cough and cold remedies such as pseudoephedrine (e.g., Sudafed) and phenylephrine (e.g., Dimetapp) often worsen the symptoms of BPH. These drugs are α-adrenergic agonists that cause smooth muscle contraction. If this happens, the patient should avoid these drugs.

The patient with obstructive symptoms should be advised to urinate every 2 to 3 hours and when first feeling the urge. This will minimize urinary stasis and acute urinary retention. Fluid intake should be maintained at a normal level to prevent dehydration or fluid overload. The patient may believe that, if he restricts his fluid intake, symptoms will be less severe, but this only increases the chances of an infection. However, if the patient increases his intake too rapidly, bladder distension can develop because of the prostatic obstruction.

▪ Acute Intervention

The following discussion focuses on preoperative and postoperative care for the patient undergoing a TURP.

▪ Preoperative Care.
Urinary drainage must be restored before surgery. Prostatic obstruction may result in acute retention or inability to void. A urethral catheter such as a coudé (curvedtip) catheter may be needed to restore drainage. In many health care settings, 10 mL of sterile 2% lidocaine gel is injected into the urethra before insertion of the catheter. The lidocaine gel not only acts as a lubricant but also provides local anaesthesia and helps open the urethral lumen. If a sizable obstruction of the urethra exists, a urologist may insert a filiform catheter with sufficient rigidity to pass the obstruction. Aseptic technique is important at all times to avoid introducing bacteria into the bladder. (Urinary catheters are discussed in Chapter 48.)

Antibiotics are usually administered before any invasive procedure. Any infection of the urinary tract must be treated before surgery. Restoring urine drainage and encouraging a high fluid intake (2 to 3 L/day unless contraindicated) are also helpful in managing the infection.

Patients are often concerned about the impact of the impending surgery on sexual functioning. Data gathered from the health history relating to sexual activities will identify possible problem areas. Provide an opportunity for the patient and partner to express their concerns. Inform the patient that surgery may affect sexual functioning. Most types of prostatic surgery result in some degree of retrograde ejaculation. Inform the patient that the ejaculate may be decreased in amount or totally absent. This may decrease orgasmic sensations felt during ejaculation. Retrograde ejaculation is not harmful because the semen is eliminated during the next urination.

▪ Postoperative Care.
The main complications following surgery are hemorrhage, bladder spasms, urinary incontinence, and infection. The plan of care should be adjusted to the type of surgery, the reasons for surgery, and the patient's response to surgery.

After surgery, the patient will have a standard catheter or a triple-lumen catheter. Bladder irrigation is typically done to remove clotted blood from the bladder and ensure drainage of urine. The bladder is irrigated either manually on an intermittent basis or, more commonly, as continuous bladder irrigation with sterile normal saline solution or another prescribed solution. If manual irrigation of the bladder is ordered, instill 50 mL of irrigating solution (commonly normal saline) and then withdraw with a syringe to remove clots that may be in the bladder and catheter. Painful bladder spasms often occur as a result of manual irrigation. With continuous bladder irrigation, irrigating solution is continuously infused and drained from the bladder. The rate of infusion is based on the colour of drainage. Ideally, the urine drainage should be light pink without clots. The

inflow and outflow of irrigant must be continuously monitored. If outflow is less than inflow, the bladder should be assessed immediately and the catheter patency checked. If the outflow is blocked and patency cannot be re-established by manual irrigation, continuous bladder irrigation is stopped and the physician notified.

Use careful aseptic technique when irrigating the bladder because bacteria can easily be introduced into the urinary tract. Proper care of the catheter is important. To prevent urethral irritation and minimize the risk of bladder infection, the catheter must be secured to the leg or the abdomen with tape or catheter strap. The catheter should be connected to a closed-drainage system and should not be disconnected unless it is being removed, changed, or irrigated. The secretions that accumulate around the meatus can be cleansed daily with soap and water.

Blood clots are expected after prostate surgery for the first 24 to 36 hours. However, large amounts of bright red blood in the urine can indicate hemorrhage. Postoperative hemorrhage may occur from displacement of the catheter, dislodgement of a large clot, or increases in abdominal pressure. Release or displacement of the catheter dislodges the balloon that provides counterpressure on the operative site. Traction on the catheter may be applied to provide counterpressure (tamponade) on the bleeding site in the prostate, thereby decreasing bleeding. Such traction can result in local necrosis if pressure is applied for too long. Pressure should, therefore, be relieved on a scheduled basis by qualified personnel. Activities that increase abdominal pressure, such as sitting or walking for prolonged periods and straining to have a bowel movement (Valsalva's manoeuvre), should be avoided in the postoperative recovery period.

Bladder spasms are a distressing complication for the patient after transurethral procedures. They occur as a result of irritation of the bladder mucosa from the insertion of the resectoscope, presence of a catheter, or clots leading to obstruction of the catheter. The patient should be instructed not to urinate around the catheter because this increases the likelihood of spasm. If bladder spasms develop, the catheter should be checked for clots. If present, the clots should be removed by irrigation so that urine can flow freely. Antispasmodics (e.g., belladonna and opium suppositories, oxybutynin [Oxytrol]), along with relaxation techniques, are used to relieve the pain and decrease spasm. The catheter is often removed 2 to 4 days after surgery. The patient should urinate within 6 hours after catheter removal. If he cannot, a catheter is reinserted for a day or two. If the problem continues, the nurse may need to instruct the patient in clean intermittent self-catheterization (see Chapter 48).

Sphincter tone may be poor immediately after catheter removal, resulting in urinary incontinence or dribbling. This is a common but distressing situation for the patient. Sphincter tone can be strengthened by having the patient practise Kegel exercises (pelvic floor muscle technique) 10 to 20 times per hour while awake. The patient should be encouraged to practise starting and stopping the stream several times during urination. This facilitates learning of the pelvic floor exercises. It usually takes several weeks to achieve urinary continence. In some instances, control of urine may never be fully regained. Continence can improve for up to 12 months. If continence has not been achieved by that time, the patient may be referred to a continence clinic. A variety of methods, including biofeedback, have been used to achieve positive results. The patient can also be instructed to use a penile clamp, condom catheter, or incontinence pads or briefs to avoid embarrassment from dribbling. In severe cases, an occlusive cuff that serves as an artificial sphincter can be surgically implanted to restore continence. Assist the patient in finding ways to manage the problem that will allow him to continue socializing and interacting with others.

Observe the patient for signs of postoperative infection. If an external wound is present (from an open prostatectomy), assess the area for redness, heat, swelling, and purulent drainage. Special care must be taken if a perineal incision is present because of the proximity of the anus. Rectal procedures, such as taking rectal temperatures and administering enemas, should be avoided. The insertion of well-lubricated belladonna and opium suppositories is acceptable.

Dietary intervention and stool softeners are important in the postoperative period to prevent the patient from straining while having bowel movements. Straining increases the intra-abdominal pressure, which can lead to bleeding at the operative site. Adequate fluid intake and a diet high in fibre facilitate the passage of stool.

▣ Ambulatory and Home Care

Discharge planning and home care issues are important aspects of care after prostate surgery. Instructions include (1) caring for an indwelling catheter (if one is left in place); (2) managing urinary incontinence; (3) maintaining oral fluids between 2000 and 3000 mL/day; (4) observing for signs and symptoms of UTI and wound infection; (5) preventing constipation; (6) avoiding heavy lifting (>4.5 kg); and (7) refraining from driving or intercourse after surgery as directed by the physician.

The patient may experience a change in sexual functioning following surgery, for example, retrograde ejaculation or physiological erectile dysfunction (if the nerves are cut or damaged during surgery). The patient may experience anxiety over the change owing to a perceived loss of his sex role, self-esteem, or quality of sexual interaction with his partner. Discuss these changes with the patient and his partner and allow them to ask questions and express their concerns. Sexual counselling and treatment options may be necessary if ED becomes a chronic or permanent problem. ED is discussed later in the chapter. It should be pointed out that, although some patients experience concerns regarding change in sexual functioning, this is not a universal concern. It may take up to 1 year for complete sexual functioning to return.

The bladder may take up to 2 months to return to its normal capacity. The patient should be instructed to drink at least 2 L of fluid per day and urinate every 2 to 3 hours to flush the urinary tract. Bladder irritants such as caffeine products, citrus juices, and alcohol should be avoided or limited to small amounts. Because the patient may be experiencing incontinence or dribbling, he may incorrectly believe that decreasing fluid intake will relieve this problem. Urethral strictures may result from instrumentation or catheterization. Treatment may include teaching the patient intermittent clean catheterization or having a urethral dilation.

Advise the patient to continue having a yearly DRE and discussion with his physician about a PSA if he has had any procedure other than complete removal of the prostate. Hyperplasia or cancer can occur in the remaining prostatic tissue.

▣ Evaluation

Expected outcomes for the patient with BPH are presented in NCP 57-1.

Prostate Cancer

Prostate cancer is a malignant tumour of the prostate gland. In 2012 it was estimated that 26,500 new cases of prostate cancer would be diagnosed in Canada that year, and that 4000 men would die of it (Canadian Cancer Society's Steering Committee on Cancer Statistics, 2012), meaning that on average, 72 Canadian are diagnosed with prostate cancer each day and 11 men die from it. Prostate cancer is the most common cancer among men, excluding skin cancer. The majority (>75%) of cases occur in men older than age 65. However, many cases occur in younger men, who sometimes have a more aggressive type of cancer. There was a large increase in the incidence of newly diagnosed cases of prostate cancer between 1988 and 1993. This increase in number was attributed to the widespread use of PSA as a screening procedure, allowing early detection of prostate cancer. The incidence of prostate cancer has increased because of reporting differences, with most provinces opting to use projections based upon modelling rather than averaging (Canadian Cancer Society Steering Committee on Cancer Statistics, 2011).

Etiology and Pathophysiology

Prostate cancer is an androgen-dependent adenocarcinoma. The majority of tumours occur in the outer aspect of the prostate gland. Prostate cancer is usually slow growing. It can spread by three routes: direct extension, through the lymph system, or through the bloodstream. Spread by direct extension involves the seminal vesicles, the urethral mucosa, the bladder wall, and the external sphincter. The cancer later spreads through the lymphatic system to the regional lymph nodes. The veins from the prostate seem to be the mode of spread to the pelvic bones, the head of the femur, the lower lumbar spine, the liver, and the lungs.

Age, ethnicity, and family history are three nonmodifiable risk factors for prostate cancer. Most men diagnosed with prostate cancer are older than 65 years. Rates of prostate cancer for men of African ancestry are higher than those for White men at all ages. Men of African ancestry are also diagnosed with tumours that are more aggressive and advanced, whereas men of Asian ancestry have lower rates of prostate cancer (Turner & Drudge-Coates, 2010). These racial differences may, of course, be based on environmental rather than genetic factors. Factors such as a family history of prostate cancer, especially first-degree relatives (fathers, brothers), long-term exposure to testosterone, diet high in fats, and occupational exposure are also associated with an increased risk (Turner & Drudge-Coates, 2010) whereas recent research suggests that consumption of tomatoes, tomato-based products, and garlic may protect patients against prostate cancer (Salem et al., 2011).

Clinical Manifestations and Complications

Prostate cancer is usually asymptomatic in the early stages. Eventually, the patient may have symptoms similar to those of BPH, including dysuria, hesitancy, dribbling, frequency, urgency, hematuria, nocturia, retention, interruption of urinary stream, and inability to urinate. Pain in the lumbosacral area that radiates down to the hips or the legs, when coupled with urinary symptoms, may indicate metastasis.

Early recognition and treatment are required to control growth, prevent metastasis, and preserve quality of life. The tumour can spread to pelvic lymph nodes, bones, bladder, lungs,

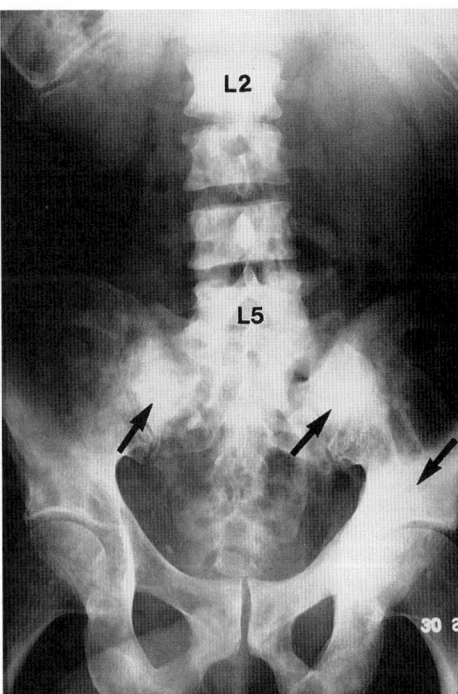

Figure 57-4 Metastasis *(arrows)* of prostate cancer to the pelvis and lumbar spine.

Source: Mettler, F. (2004). *Essentials of radiology* (2nd ed.). Philadelphia: Saunders.

and liver. Once the tumour has spread to distant sites, the major problem becomes the management of pain. As the cancer spreads to the bones (a common site of metastasis), pain can become severe, especially in the back and the legs because of compression of the spinal cord and destruction of bone (Figure 57-4).

Diagnostic Studies

Improved diagnostic techniques have greatly enhanced the detection of prostate cancer. The two primary screening tools are a digital rectal examination (DRE) and a blood test for **prostate-specific antigen (PSA),** a glycoprotein produced by the prostate. On DRE, an abnormal prostate may feel hard, nodular, and asymmetrical.

Elevated levels of PSA (normal level 0-4 mcg/L) indicate a pathological condition of the prostate, although not necessarily prostate cancer. Mild elevations in PSA may occur with aging, BPH, recent ejaculation, drugs (e.g., finasteride [Proscar]), acute or chronic prostatitis, urinary retention, or after long bike rides. In addition, cystoscopy, indwelling urethral catheters, and prostate biopsies may produce an elevation. When prostate cancer exists, serum PSA levels are a useful marker of tumour volume (i.e., the higher the PSA level, the greater the tumour mass).

At the core of the controversy as to whether routine screening should be recommended is that many people live and die *with* prostate cancer but not *from* it. As screening has become more widespread, smaller cancers are being found in older men. Early detection of aggressive cancers by PSA testing has saved lives; however, PSA is not solely specific to prostate cancer and the search for a better prostate cancer biomarker continues (Fiorentino, Capizzi, & Loda, 2010). Men are now being advised to discuss individually with their health care provider the potential benefits and harm of PSA testing (Canadian Cancer Society, 2010).

PSA is used not only to detect prostate cancer but also to monitor the success of treatment. When the treatment has been successful in removing prostate cancer, PSA levels should fall to undetectable levels. Regular measurement of PSA levels following treatment is important to evaluate the effectiveness of treatment and the possible recurrence of prostate cancer.

Elevated levels of prostatic isoenzyme of serum acid phosphatase (prostatic acid phosphatase [PAP]) is another indication of prostate cancer, especially if there is extracapsular spread. With advanced prostate cancer, serum alkaline phosphatase is increased as a result of bone metastasis. Investigation is now under way to locate a serum marker for prostate cancer similar to carbohydrate antigen (CA)-125, which is a useful marker in ovarian cancer. (Ovarian cancer is discussed in Chapter 56.)

Neither PSA nor DRE is a definitive diagnostic test for prostate cancer. If PSA levels are elevated or if the DRE is abnormal, biopsy of the prostate tissue is indicated and necessary to confirm the diagnosis of prostate cancer. The biopsy is typically done using TRUS because it allows the physician to visualize the prostate and pinpoint abnormalities. When a suspicious area is

Table 57-5 Whitmore-Jewett Staging Classification of Prostate Cancer

Stage A: Clinically Unrecognized	
A1	<5% of prostatic tissue neoplastic
A2	>5% of prostatic tissue neoplastic, all high-grade tumours
Stage B: Clinically Intracapsular	
B1	Nodule <2 cm and surrounded by palpably normal tissue
B2	Nodule >2 cm or multiple nodules
Stage C: Clinically Extracapsular	
C1	Minimal extracapsular extension
C2	Large tumours involving seminal vesicles, adjacent structures, or both
Stage D: Metastatic Disease	
D1	Pelvic lymph node metastases or ureteral obstruction causing hydronephrosis
D2	Distant metastases to bone, viscera, or other soft tissue structures

COLLABORATIVE CARE

Table 57-6 Prostate Cancer

Diagnostic	*Collaborative Therapy*
• History and physical examination	**Stage A**
• Digital rectal examination (DRE)	• Watchful waiting with annual PSA and DRE
• Prostate-specific antigen (PSA)	• Radical prostatectomy
	• Radiation therapy
• Prostatic acid phosphatase (PAP)	• External beam
	• Brachytherapy
• Transrectal ultrasonography (TRUS)	**Stage B**
	• Radical prostatectomy
• Biopsy of prostate and lymph nodes	• Radiation therapy
	Stage C
• Computed tomography (CT), magnetic resonance imaging (MRI), bone scan (to evaluate for metastatic disease)	• Radical prostatectomy
	• Radiation therapy
	• Hormone therapy
	• Orchiectomy
	Stage D
	• Hormone therapy
	• Orchiectomy
	• Chemotherapy
	• Radiation therapy to metastatic bone areas

located, a special biopsy needle is inserted into the prostate to obtain a tissue sample. A pathological examination of the specimen is done to assess for malignant changes. Other tests used to determine the location and the extent of the spread of the cancer may include bone scan, computed tomography (CT), and magnetic resonance imaging (MRI) using an endorectal probe.

Collaborative Care

Early-stage prostate cancer is a curable disease in most men. Based on findings from diagnostic studies, the prostate cancer is staged and graded. Two common classification systems for staging prostate cancer, the Whitmore-Jewett and tumour–node–metastasis (TNM) systems, are both based on the size (volume) of the tumour and spread (Table 57-5). Both classification systems are used in Canada, with description and treatment based upon the Whitmore-Jewett classification (i.e., stage A, B, C, or D) and description of the extent of the cancer based upon the TNM system. Approximately 80% of patients with prostate cancer are initially diagnosed when the cancer is in either a local or a regional stage. The lifetime probability of a man dying from prostate cancer in Canada is 1 in 28 (Canadian Cancer Society, 2011).

Grading of the tumour is done based on tumour histology using the Gleason scale. With this scale, tumours are graded from 1 to 5 based on the degree of glandular differentiation. Grade 1 represents the most well differentiated (most like the original cells), and grade 5 represents the most poorly differentiated (undifferentiated). Gleason grades are given to the two most commonly occurring patterns of cells and added together. The Gleason score is a number from 2 to 10. This scale is used to predict how quickly the cancer will progress.

The collaborative care of the patient with prostate cancer depends on the stage of the cancer and the overall health of the patient. At all stages, there is more than one possible treatment option. The decision of which treatment course to pursue is made jointly by the patient and the health care team based on a careful analysis of the facts and the patient's preference (Saca-Hazboun, 2008). Table 57-6 summarizes the various treatment options available.

Conservative Therapy. Prostate cancer is relatively slow growing, and a conservative approach to the management of prostate cancer is "watchful waiting." The decision to adopt a strategy of watchful waiting is appropriate when there is (1) a life expectancy of less than 10 years, (2) presence of significant co-morbid disease, and (3) presence of a low-grade, low-stage tumour. These patients are typically followed with frequent PSA measurements, along with DRE, to monitor the progress of the disease. Significant changes in either PSA, DRE, or development of symptoms warrant a re-evaluation of treatment options.

Surgical Therapy

Radical Prostatectomy. With **radical prostatectomy**, the entire prostate gland, the seminal vesicles, and part of the bladder neck (ampulla) are surgically removed. The entire prostate is removed because the cancer tends to be in many different locations within the gland. In addition, a retroperitoneal lymph node dissection is usually done (Streif, 2008). A radical prostatectomy is the surgical procedure considered the most effective treatment for long-term survival. Thus, it is the preferred treatment for men younger than 70 years who are in good health and with the cancer confined to the prostate (stages A and B). Surgery is usually not considered an option for stage D cancer (except to relieve symptoms associated with obstruction) because metastasis has already occurred. The two most common approaches for radical prostatectomy are retropubic and perineal resection (Figure 57-5). With the *retropubic* approach, a low midline abdominal incision is made to access the prostate gland, and the pelvic lymph nodes can be dissected. With the *perineal* resection, an incision is made between the scrotum and the anus. This procedure does not permit the removal of lymph nodes. More recent approaches to treatment, laparoscopic or robotic-assisted prostatectomy, have similar surgical outcomes to traditional approaches with improved recovery times (Parsons & Bennett, 2008).

After surgery, the patient has a large indwelling catheter with a 30-mL balloon placed in the bladder via the urethra. This catheter is typically left in place for 1 to 2 weeks. A drain is left in the surgical site to aid in the removal of drainage from the area. This drain is typically removed after a couple of days. Because the perineal approach has a higher risk of postoperative infection (owing to the location of the incision related to the anus), careful dressing changes and perineal care after each bowel movement are important for comfort and to prevent infection. The typical length of hospital stay postoperatively is 3 days.

The two major complications following a radical prostatectomy are ED and incontinence. The incidence of ED is dependent on the patient's age and preoperative sexual functioning, whether nerve-sparing surgery was performed, and the expertise of the surgeon. Problems with urinary control occur in nearly all men for the first few months following surgery because the bladder must be reattached to the urethra after the prostate is removed. Over time, the bladder adjusts and most men regain control (YuKo & Sawatzky, 2008). Kegel exercises strengthen the urinary sphincter and may help improve incontinence (see the Evidence-Informed Practice box). Other common complications associated with surgery include hemorrhage, urinary retention, infection, wound dehiscence, deep vein thrombosis, and pulmonary emboli.

Nerve-Sparing Procedure. In close proximity to the prostate gland are neurovascular bundles that maintain erectile functioning. The preservation of these bundles during a prostatectomy is possible while still removing all of the cancer. This procedure is not indicated for patients with cancer outside of the prostate gland. Although the risk of ED is significantly reduced with this procedure, there is no guarantee that potency will be maintained. However, most men younger than 50 years with good preoperative erectile function and low-stage prostate cancer can expect a return of potency after nerve-sparing prostatectomy.

Cryosurgery. *Prostatic cryosurgery* is a surgical technique that destroys cancer cells by freezing the tissue. It has been used both as an initial treatment and as a second-line treatment after radiation treatment failures. A TRUS probe is inserted to visualize the prostate gland. Probes containing liquid nitrogen are then inserted into the prostate. Liquid nitrogen delivers freezing temperatures, destroying the tissue. The treatment takes about 2 hours under general or spinal anaesthesia and does not involve an abdominal incision. Possible complications of prostatic cryosurgery include damage to the urethra and, in rare cases, a urethrorectal fistula (an opening between the urethra and the rectum) or a urethrocutaneous fistula (an opening between the urethra and the skin). Tissue sloughing, ED, urinary incontinence, prostatitis, and hemorrhage have also been reported.

Radiation Therapy. Radiation therapy is a common treatment option for prostate cancer, especially for men older than 70, patients who are poor surgical risks, or those who wish to avoid surgery. Radiation therapy may be offered as the only treatment, or it may be offered in combination with surgery or with hormonal therapy. Salvage radiation therapy given for cancer recurrence after a radical prostatectomy has shown promise in improving survival in some men (Trock et al., 2008).

External Beam Irradiation. External beam is the most widely used method of delivering radiation treatments for those with prostate cancer. This therapy can be used to treat patients with prostate cancer confined to the prostate, the surrounding tissue, or both (stages A, B, and C). Patients are treated on an outpatient basis 5 days a week for 6 to 8 weeks. Each treatment lasts only a few minutes. Adverse effects from irradiation can be acute (occurring during treatment or within 90 days that follow) or delayed (occurring months or years after treatment). Common adverse effects involve the skin (dryness, redness, irritation, pain), GI tract (diarrhea, abdominal cramping, bleeding), urinary tract (dysuria, frequency, hesitancy, urgency, nocturia), sexual functioning (ED), fatigue, and bone marrow suppression. These problems usually resolve 2 to 3 weeks after the completion of radiation therapy. In patients with clinically localized disease, cure rates

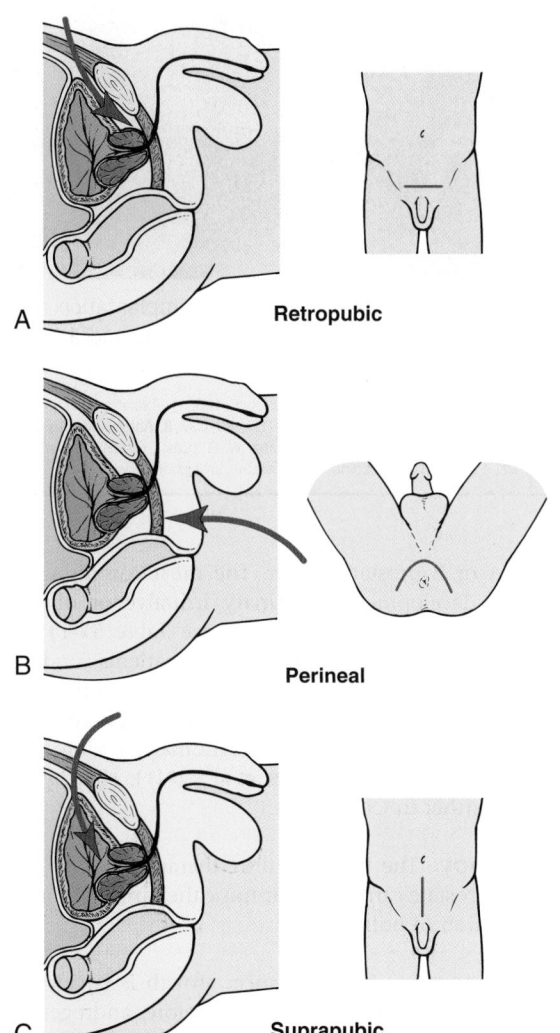

Figure 57-5 Three approaches used to perform a prostatectomy. **A,** Retropubic approach involves a midline abdominal incision. **B,** Perineal approach involves an incision between the scrotum and the anus. **C,** Suprapubic approach involves an abdominal incision.

What Therapy Works Best for Urinary Incontinence Following Radical Prostatectomy?

Clinical Question

In men who have undergone radical prostatectomy (P), does the combination of pelvic floor muscle training plus biofeedback (I) as compared with no treatment (C) reduce the frequency and duration of urinary incontinence (O)?

Best Available Evidence

Systematic review of randomized controlled trials (RCTs)

Critical Appraisal and Synthesis of Evidence

- 17 RCTs (n = 402) of men after radical prostatectomy.
- Quality of trials included in review was reported as moderate.
- Outcome measures were self-reports of incontinence and leakage symptoms by pad counts, diary, interview, or questionnaire.

Conclusions

- The evidence was inconclusive regarding the role of conservative management in treating incontinence in patients after prostatectomy.
- The frequency and amount of urinary incontinence generally decreased with time, irrespective of treatment modality.

Implications for Nursing Practice

- Use biofeedback with pelvic floor muscle training exercises when urinary catheter is removed postoperatively to promote a return to continence.
- Research is needed on effects of conservative management for long-term incontinence.

Reference for Evidence

Hunter, K. F., Moore, K. N., & Glazener, C. M. A. (2007). Conservative management for postprostatectomy urinary incontinence. *Cochrane Database of Systematic Reviews* 2007, 2, CD001843. doi:10.1002/14651858.CD001843.pub3

P, patient population of interest; *I*, intervention or area of interest; *C*, comparison of interest or comparison group; *O*, outcome(s) of interest.

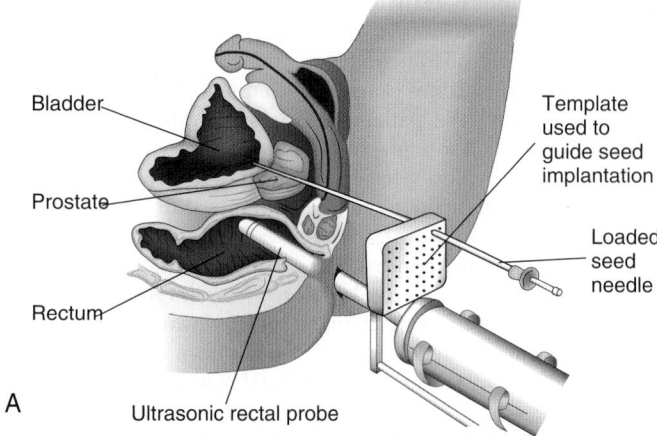

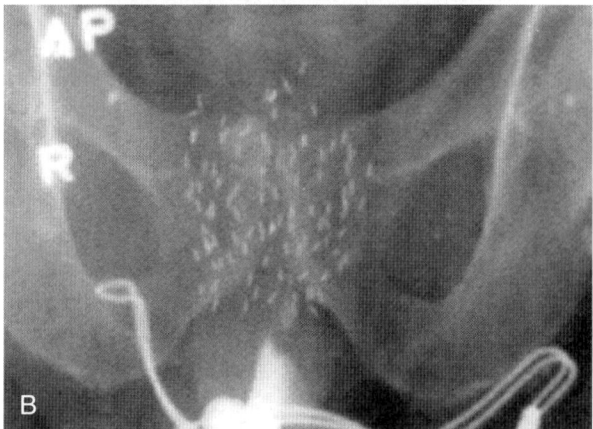

Figure 57-6 A, Prostate brachytherapy. Implantation of seeds with a needle guided by ultrasonography and a template grid. **B,** Radioactive seeds.

Source: **A,** Adapted from Iwamoto, R. R., & Maher, K. E. (2001). Radiation therapy for prostate cancer. *Seminars in Oncology Nursing, 17*(2), 90-100. **B,** Abeloff, M., Armitage, J. O., Niederhuber, J. D., Kastan, M. B., & McKenna, W. G. (Eds.). (2008). *Abeloff's clinical oncology* (4th ed., Figure 88-12A). Edinburgh: Churchill Livingstone.

with external beam radiation are comparable with those with radical prostatectomy.

Brachytherapy. Brachytherapy involves the implantation of radioactive seed implants into the prostate gland, allowing higher radiation doses directly in the tissue while sparing the surrounding tissue (rectum and bladder). The radioactive seeds are placed in the prostate gland with a needle through a grid template guided by TRUS (Figure 57-6). The grid template and ultrasonography ensure accurate placement of the seeds. Because brachytherapy is a one-time outpatient procedure, many patients find this more convenient than external beam radiation treatment. Brachytherapy is best suited for patients

with stage A or B prostate cancer. The most common adverse effect is the development of urinary irritative or obstructive problems. The AUA Symptom Index (see Table 57-1) can be used to measure urinary function for patients undergoing brachytherapy and can be incorporated into postoperative nursing management. For those with more advanced tumours, brachytherapy may be offered in combination with external beam radiation treatment (Pieters et al., 2011). (Brachytherapy is discussed further in Chapter 18.)

Drug Therapy. The forms of drug therapy available for the treatment of prostate cancer are hormone therapy, chemotherapy, or a combination of both.

Hormone Therapy. Prostate cancer growth is largely dependent on the presence of androgens. Therefore, androgen deprivation is the primary therapeutic approach for men with prostatic cancer. Hormone therapy, also known as *androgen deprivation therapy,* is focused on reducing the levels of circulating androgens in order to reduce the tumour growth. Androgen deprivation therapy can also be used as adjunct therapy before surgery or radiation therapy to reduce tumour size and in men with locally advanced disease (stage C). One of the biggest chal-

DRUG THERAPY

Table 57-7 Hormone Therapy for Prostate Cancer

THERAPY	MECHANISM OF ACTION
Luteinizing Hormone–Releasing Hormone (LH-RH) Agonists	
Goserelin (Zoladex)	Prevents release of LH
	Decreases testosterone production
Leuprolide (Lupron, Eligard)	Suppress release of LH-RH
Buserelin (Suprefact)	Decrease testosterone production
Triptorelin (Trelstar)	
Androgen Receptor Blockers	
Bicalutamide (Casodex)	Block the action of testosterone by competing with receptor sites
Flutamide (Euflex)	
Nilutamide (Anandron)	
Orchiectomy	
Surgical removal of testicles	Removes 95% of testosterone source

LH, luteinizing hormone; *LH-RH,* luteinizing hormone–releasing hormone.

lenges with androgen deprivation therapy is that almost all tumours will become resistant to this therapy (hormone-refractory) within a few years. An elevated PSA level is often the first sign that hormone therapy is no longer effective. Androgen ablation can be produced by interference with androgen production (e.g., luteinizing hormone–releasing hormone [LH-RH] agonists, orchiectomy) or androgen receptor blockers (Table 57-7). Bisphosphonate drugs are the currently recommended treatment to reduce bone mineral loss in these patients (Greenspan, 2008).

Luteinizing Hormone–Releasing Hormone Agonists. LH-RH is released from the hypothalamus to stimulate the anterior pituitary to produce luteinizing hormone (LH) and follicle-stimulating hormone (FSH). LH stimulates the testicular Leydig cells to produce testosterone. The LH-RH agonists superstimulate the pituitary. This ultimately results in down-regulation of the LH-RH receptors, leading to a refractory condition in which the anterior pituitary is unresponsive to LH-RH. These drugs cause an initial transient increase in LH and testosterone called a "flare," and a worsening of symptoms may occur during this time. However, with continued administration, LH and testosterone levels are decreased. Current antiandrogen therapy includes leuprolide (Lupron, Eligard), goserelin (Zoladex), and triptorelin (Trelstar). This therapy essentially produces a chemical castration similar to the effects of an orchiectomy. Antiandrogen medications are given by subcutaneous or intramuscular injections on a regular basis, and they must be taken indefinitely. Viadur (leuprolide acetate implant) is an implant that is placed subcutaneously and delivers leuprolide continuously for 1 year (Therigy Drug Reference Series, 2008).

Androgen Receptor Blockers. Another classification of antiandrogens is drugs that compete with circulating androgens at the receptor sites. Flutamide (Euflex), nilutamide (Anandron), and bicalutamide (Casodex) are nonsteroidal androgen receptor blockers. They can be used in combination with goserelin or leuprolide. The combination has been found to be safe and well tolerated as a potency-sparing, androgen-ablative therapy. Adverse effects of androgen receptor blockers include loss of libido, ED,

and hot flashes. Breast pain and gynecomastia may also occur in men treated with androgen receptor blockers. Combining an androgen receptor blocker with an LH-RH agonist is an often-used treatment and results in combined androgen blockade (Turner & Drudge-Coates, 2010).

Orchiectomy. Testosterone, produced by the testes, stimulates growth of the prostate cancer. A bilateral orchiectomy is the surgical removal of the testes that may be done alone or in combination with prostatectomy. For advanced stages of prostate cancer (stage D), an orchiectomy is one treatment option for cancer control. Another possible benefit of this procedure is the rapid relief of bone pain associated with advanced tumours. Orchiectomy may also induce sufficient shrinkage of the prostate to relieve urinary obstruction in later stages of disease when surgery is not an option.

Adverse effects of orchiectomy include hot flashes, ED, loss of sex drive, and irritability. Weight gain and loss of muscle mass, which are also common, can alter a man's physical appearance. Osteoporosis has also been reported as a consequence of orchiectomy. These physical changes can affect self-esteem, leading to grief and depression. Although this procedure is permanent and cost effective (compared with chemical hormone manipulation using LH-RH agonists), many men prefer drug therapy to orchiectomy.

Chemotherapy. The use of chemotherapeutic agents has primarily been limited to treatment for those with hormone-resistant prostate cancer in late-stage disease. In hormone-resistant prostate cancer, the cancer is progressing despite treatment. This occurs in patients who have taken an antiandrogen for a certain period of time. Historically, prostate cancer has been poorly responsive to chemotherapy, which has not been shown to improve survival. Thus, the goal of chemotherapy is palliation. Some of the more commonly used chemotherapy drugs include docetaxel (Taxotere), mitoxantrone, cyclophosphamide (Procytox), idarubicin (Idamycin), epirubicin (Pharmorubicin), and estramustine (Emcyt). Docetaxel, when administered with prednisone, estramustine, or mitoxantrone, is now the standard of care (Armstrong et al., 2010). Adverse effects include nausea, alopecia, reduced left ventricular ejection, and bone marrow suppression.

CULTURALLY COMPETENT CARE: PROSTATE CANCER

Demographic characteristics should be considered when providing information about the risk for prostate cancer and screening recommendations. It is important to be aware of the epidemiological differences that occur with prostate cancer as well as the differences that exist in health promotion practice.

Despite the availability of early screening measures (PSA and DRE), individuals in lower socioeconomic groups frequently do not use such services. Although exposure to electronic and print media is successful in informing some men about prostate cancer, significant differences of effectiveness exist based on demographic variables such as ethnicity, age, education level, and socioeconomic level. Canadian men of African or Caribbean descent are at the highest risk for development of prostate cancer (Prostate Cancer Canada, 2011). Consider the best method to communicate this information to men of all cultures and ethnicities that will result in the greatest degree of understanding and participation in prostate cancer screening.

NURSING MANAGEMENT: PROSTATE CANCER

▮ Nursing Assessment

Subjective and objective data that should be obtained from a patient with prostate cancer are presented in Table 57-8.

▮ Nursing Diagnoses

Nursing diagnoses for the patient with prostate cancer depend on the stage of the cancer. General nursing diagnoses, which may or may not apply to every patient with cancer of the prostate, may include, but are not limited to, the following.

- Decisional conflict *related to* numerous alternative treatment options
- Acute pain *related to* surgery, prostatic enlargement, bone metastasis, and bladder spasms

NURSING ASSESSMENT

Table 57-8 Prostate Cancer

Subjective Data

Important Health Information

Past health history: Family history of prostate cancer; diet high in fat

Medications: Use of testosterone supplements or any other medications affecting urinary tract such as morphine, anticholinergics, monoamine oxidase inhibitors, and tricyclic antidepressants

Surgeries or other treatments: History of urinary tract infections or prostate problems

Symptoms

- *Urinary:* Hesitancy or straining to start stream; weak stream; urinary urgency or frequency; retention with dribbling; hematuria; nocturia
- *Other:* Low back pain radiating to legs or pelvis; bone pain (possible indicators of metastasis); anorexia, weight loss (possible indicators of metastasis); increasing fatigue and malaise; anxiety related to self-concept or sexuality

Objective Data

General

Older adult male; pelvic lymphadenopathy (late sign)

Urinary

Distended bladder on palpation; unilaterally hard, enlarged, fixed prostate on rectal examination

Musculoskeletal

Pathological fractures (metastasis)

Possible Findings

↑ Serum PSA; ↑ serum PAP (metastasis); nodular and irregular prostate on ultrasonography, positive biopsy results; anemia

PAP, prostatic acid phosphatase; *PSA,* prostate-specific antigen.

- Urinary retention *related to* obstruction of urethra or bladder neck by the prostate, blood clots, and loss of bladder tone
- Impaired urinary elimination *related to* bladder neck sphincter damage
- Constipation or diarrhea *related to* treatment interventions
- Sexual dysfunction *related to* effects of treatment
- Anxiety *related to* uncertain outcome of disease process on life and lifestyle and effect of treatment on sexual functioning

▮ Planning

The overall goals are that the patient with prostate cancer will (1) be an active participant in the treatment plan, (2) have satisfactory pain control, (3) follow the therapeutic plan, (4) accept the effect of the therapeutic plan on sexual function, and (5) find a satisfactory way to manage the impact on bladder or bowel function.

▮ Nursing Implementation

▮ Health Promotion

Prostate Cancer Canada (2011) strongly believes in the merits of screening and endorses the Canadian Urological Association screening guidelines that include baseline screening for men aged 40 to 49; PSA and DRE every 2 to 4 years for men aged 50; and those between 40 and 50 with a family history of prostate cancer.

▮ Acute Intervention

Preoperative and postoperative phases of radical prostatectomy are similar to surgical procedures for BPH (see pp. 1579-1584). Nursing interventions for the patient who undergoes radiation therapy and chemotherapy are discussed in Chapter 18. An additional consideration is the psychological response of the patient to a diagnosis of cancer. The nurse should provide sensitive, caring support for the patient and his family to help them cope with the diagnosis of cancer. Prostate support groups are available for men and their families to encourage them to be active, informed participants in their own care.

▮ Ambulatory and Home Care

Teach appropriate catheter care if the patient is discharged with an indwelling catheter. Instruct the patient to clean the urethral meatus with soap and water once a day; maintain a high fluid intake; keep the collecting bag lower than the bladder at all times; keep the catheter securely anchored to the inner thigh or the abdomen; and report any signs of bladder infection, such as bladder spasms, fever, or hematuria. If urinary incontinence is a problem, patients should be encouraged to practise pelvic floor muscle exercises (Kegel exercises) at every urination and throughout the day. Continuous practice during the 4- to 6-week healing process improves the success rate. Products used for incontinence specifically designed for men are available through home care product catalogues and many retail stores.

Although prostate cancer has a high cure rate if detected and treated early, prognosis for stage D prostate cancer is poor. Palliative and end-of-life care is often appropriate and beneficial to the patient and family (see Chapter 13.) Common problems experienced by the patient with advanced prostate cancer include fatigue, bladder outlet obstruction and ureteral obstruction (caused by compression of the urethra, ureters, or both from tumour mass or lymph node metastasis), severe bone pain and fractures (caused by bone metastasis), spinal cord compression (from spinal metastasis), and leg edema (caused by lymphedema, deep vein thrombosis, and other medical conditions). Nursing interventions must focus on all of these problems. However, management of pain is one of the most important aspects of nursing care for these patients. Pain control is managed through ongoing pain assessment, administration of prescribed medications (both opioid and nonopioid agents), and the use of non-pharmacological methods of pain relief. (Pain management is discussed further in Chapter 10.)

▪ Evaluation

Evaluation is based on expected outcomes. The outcomes are that the patient with prostate cancer will:

- Be an active participant in the treatment plan.
- Have satisfactory pain control.
- Follow the therapeutic plan.
- Understand the effect of the treatment on sexual function.
- Find a satisfactory way to manage the impact on bladder or bowel function.

Prostatitis

Etiology and Pathophysiology

Prostatitis is a broad term that describes a group of acute or chronic inflammatory conditions affecting the prostate gland, usually as a result of infection. It is the most common urological problem in men younger than 50 years. Prostatitis is a common health care issue and affects 10 to 14% of men of all ages, demographic groups, and ethnicities (Naber, 2008). Classifications for prostatitis include four categories: (1) acute bacterial prostatitis, (2) chronic bacterial prostatitis, (3) chronic prostatitis–chronic pelvic pain syndrome, and (4) asymptomatic inflammatory prostatitis (Anothaisintawee et al., 2011).

Both acute and chronic bacterial prostatitis generally result from organisms reaching the prostate gland by one of the following routes: ascending from the urethra, descending from the bladder, and invasion via the bloodstream or the lymphatic channels. Common causative organisms are *Escherichia coli, Klebsiella, Pseudomonas, Enterobacter, Proteus, Chlamydia trachomatis, Neisseria gonorrhoeae,* and group D streptococci. Chronic bacterial prostatitis differs from acute prostatitis in that it involves recurrent episodes of infection.

Chronic prostatitis–chronic pelvic pain syndrome describes a syndrome with prostate and urinary pain in the absence of an obvious infectious process. The etiology of chronic prostatitis–chronic pelvic pain syndrome is unclear. It may occur after a viral illness, or it may be associated with sexually transmitted infections, particularly in a younger adult. The etiology is not known, and a culture reveals no causative organisms. However, leukocytes may be found in prostatic secretions.

Asymptomatic inflammatory prostatitis is usually diagnosed in individuals who have no symptoms but are found to have an inflammatory process in the prostate. These patients are usually diagnosed during the evaluation of other genitourinary tract problems. Leukocytes are present in the seminal fluid from the prostate, but the cause of this process is unclear.

Clinical Manifestations and Complications

Common clinical manifestations of acute bacterial prostatitis include fever, chills, back pain, and perineal pain, along with acute urinary symptoms such as dysuria, urinary frequency, urgency, and cloudy urine (Anothaisintawee et al., 2011). The patient may also have acute urinary retention caused by prostatic swelling. With DRE, the prostate is extremely swollen, very tender, and firm. The complications of prostatitis are epididymitis and cystitis. Sexual functioning may be affected as evidenced by post-ejaculation pain, libido problems, and ED. Prostatic abscess is also a potential but uncommon complication.

Chronic bacterial prostatitis and chronic prostatitis–pelvic pain syndrome manifest with similar symptoms that are generally milder than those associated with acute bacterial prostatitis. These include irritative voiding symptoms (frequency, urgency, dysuria), backache, perineal or pelvic pain, and ejaculatory pain. Obstructive symptoms are uncommon unless the patient has coexisting BPH. With DRE, the prostate feels enlarged and firm (often described as boggy) and is slightly tender with palpation. Chronic prostatitis can predispose the patient to recurrent UTIs.

The clinical features of prostatitis can be mimicked by UTI. However, acute cystitis is not common in men.

Diagnostic Studies

Because patients with prostatitis have urinary symptoms, a urinalysis and urine culture are indicated; often white blood cells and bacteria are present. If the patient has a fever, white blood cell count and blood cultures are also indicated. The PSA test may be done to rule out prostate cancer. However, PSA levels are often elevated with prostatic inflammation (Benway & Moon, 2008). Thus, it is not considered diagnostic in itself.

Microscopic evaluation and culture of expressed prostate secretion is considered useful in the diagnosis of prostatitis. Expressed prostate secretion is obtained using a premassage and postmassage test. The patient is asked to void into a specimen cup just before and just after a vigorous prostate massage. Prostatic massage (for expressed prostate secretion) should be avoided if acute bacterial prostatitis is suspected because compression is extremely painful and can increase the risk of bacteria spread (Latendresse & McCance, 2011). TRUS has not been particularly useful in the diagnosis of prostatitis. However, transabdominal ultrasonography or MRI may be done to rule out an abscess on the prostate.

NURSING AND COLLABORATIVE MANAGEMENT: PROSTATITIS

Antibiotics commonly used for acute and chronic bacterial prostatitis include trimethoprim–sulfamethoxazole and cipro-floxacin (Cipro). Doxycycline (Vibramycin) or tetracycline may be prescribed for those patients with multiple sex partners. Antibiotics are usually given orally for up to 4 weeks for acute bacterial prostatitis. However, if the patient has high fever or other signs of impending sepsis, hospitalization and intravenous antibiotics are prescribed. Patients with chronic bacterial prostatitis are given oral antibiotic therapy for 4 to 12 weeks. A short course of oral antibiotics is usually prescribed for those with chronic prostatitis–chronic pelvic pain syndrome. However, antibiotic therapy often is ineffective for patients whose prostatitis is not caused by bacteria.

Although patients with acute and chronic bacterial prostatitis tend to experience a great amount of discomfort, the pain resolves as the infection is treated. Pain management for patients with chronic prostatitis–chronic pelvic pain syndrome is more difficult because the pain persists for weeks to months. Anti-inflammatory agents are the most common agents used for pain control in prostatitis, but these provide only moderate pain relief. Opioid pain medications can be used, but if the pain is chronic in nature, multimodal therapies should be considered. Relaxation of muscle tissue in the prostate using α-adrenergic blockers has been shown to be effective in reducing discomfort for some men (Pontari, 2008).

Acute urinary retention can develop in acute prostatitis, necessitating bladder drainage with suprapubic catheterization. Passage of a catheter through the inflamed urethra in acute prostatitis is contraindicated. Repetitive prostatic massage is thought to be therapeutic for most types of prostatitis, but it is not an appropriate measure for acute bacterial prostatitis. This measure relieves congestion within the prostate by squeezing out excess prostatic secretions, thus providing pain relief. Prostatic massage is performed by using the index finger of a gloved hand and pressing down on the prostate, covering the entire gland's surface in longitudinal strokes. This is done two to three times a week for 6 to 12 weeks (Mishra, Browne, & Emberton, 2008). Measures to stimulate ejaculation (masturbation and intercourse) help drain the prostate as well and are encouraged.

Because the prostate can serve as a source of bacteria, fluid intake should be kept at a high level for all patients experiencing prostatitis. Nursing interventions are aimed at encouraging the patient to drink plenty of fluids. This is especially important for those with acute bacterial prostatitis because of the increased fluid needs associated with fever and infection. Management of fever is also an important nursing intervention.

Problems of the Penis

Health problems of the penis are rare if sexually transmitted infections are excluded (see Chapter 55). Problems of the penis may be classified as congenital, problems of the prepuce, problems with the erectile mechanism, and cancer.

Congenital Problems

Hypospadias is a urological abnormality in which the urethral meatus is located on the ventral surface of the penis anywhere from the corona to the perineum. Hormonal influences in utero, environmental factors, and genetic factors are possible causes. Surgical repair of hypospadias may be necessary if it is associated with *chordee* (a painful downward curvature of the penis during erection) or if it prevents intercourse or normal

urination. Surgery may also be done for cosmetic reasons or emotional well-being.

Epispadias, an opening of the urethra on the dorsal surface of the penis, is a complex birth defect that is usually associated with other genitourinary tract defects. Corrective surgery to place the urethra in a normal position in the penis is usually done in early childhood.

Problems of the Prepuce

Problems of the prepuce are rare in Canada because, up until the 1990s, circumcision was a routine procedure for most male infants. Circumcision, the surgical removal of the foreskin of the penis, is a procedure done to male infants for religious or cultural reasons. It is believed to prevent problems such as *phimosis, paraphimosis,* and cancer of the penis.

Phimosis is a constriction of the uncircumcised foreskin around the head of the penis, making retraction over the glans penis difficult. It is caused by edema or inflammation of the foreskin, usually associated with poor hygiene techniques that allow bacterial and yeast organisms to become trapped under the foreskin (Figure 57-7, *A*).

Paraphimosis is narrowing or edema of the retracted uncircumcised foreskin, preventing normal return over the glans and causing strangulation. This can occur when the foreskin is pulled back during bathing, use of urinary catheters, or intercourse and is not placed back in the forward position. Antibiotics, warm soaks, and sometimes circumcision or dorsal slitting of the prepuce may be required. Careful cleaning followed by replacement of the foreskin generally prevents these problems (see Figure 57-7, *B*).

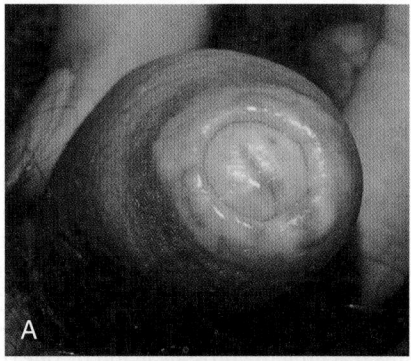
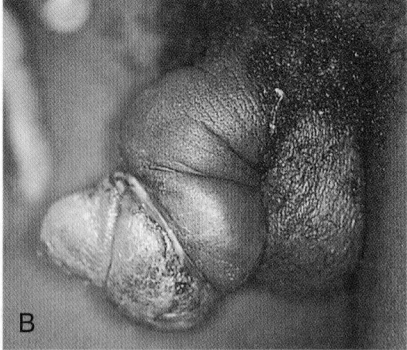

Figure 57-7 A, Phimosis. Unable to retract the foreskin owing to secondary lesions on the prepuce. **B,** Paraphimosis. Ulcer with edema from the foreskin remaining contracted over the prepuce.

Problems of the Erectile Mechanism

Priapism is a painful erection lasting longer than 4 hours and may constitute a medical emergency (Burnett & Bivalacqua, 2011). Causes of priapism include thrombosis of the corpus cavernosal veins, leukemia, sickle cell anemia, diabetes mellitus, degenerative lesions of the spine, neoplasms of the brain or spinal cord, prolonged foreplay, injection of vasoactive medications into the corpus cavernosa, and use of certain medications and cocaine. Treatment may include sedatives, injection of smooth muscle relaxants directly into the penis, aspiration and irrigation of the corpora cavernosa with a large-bore needle, and the surgical creation of a shunt to drain the corpora. Complications may include penile tissue necrosis caused by lack of blood flow or hydronephrosis from bladder distension. After an episode of priapism, the patient may be unable to achieve a normal erection.

Peyronie's disease, sometimes referred to as curved or crooked penis, is caused by plaque formation in one of the corpora cavernosa of the penis. The palpable, nontender, hard plaque formation is usually found on the posterior surface. It may result from trauma to the penile shaft or may occur spontaneously. The plaque prevents adequate blood flow into the spongy tissue, which results in a curvature during erection. The condition is not dangerous but can result in painful erections, ED, or embarrassment. If conservative measures do not correct the problem, surgery may be necessary.

Cancer of the Penis

Cancer of the penis is rare. Major risk factors include human papillomavirus infection, smoking, and psoriasis (Latendresse & McCance, 2011). The tumour may appear as a superficial ulceration or a pimple-like nodule. The nontender warty lesion may be mistaken for a venereal wart. The majority of malignancies (95%) are well-differentiated squamous cell carcinomas. Treatment in the early stages is laser removal of the growth. A radical resection of the penis may be done if the cancer has spread. Surgery, radiation, or chemotherapy may be tried, depending on the extent of the disease, lymph node involvement, or metastasis.

Problems of the Scrotum and Testes

Inflammatory and Infectious Problems

Skin Problems

The skin of the scrotum is susceptible to a number of common skin diseases. The most common conditions of the scrotal skin are fungal infections, dermatitis (neurodermatitis, contact dermatitis, seborrheic dermatitis), and parasitic infections (scabies, lice). These conditions involve discomfort for the patient but are associated with few, if any, severe complications (see Chapter 26).

Epididymitis

Epididymitis is an inflammatory process of the epididymis (Figure 57-8), usually secondary to an infectious process (sexually or nonsexually transmitted) and rarely as a result of trauma or urinary reflux down the vas deferens from the urethra. Swelling

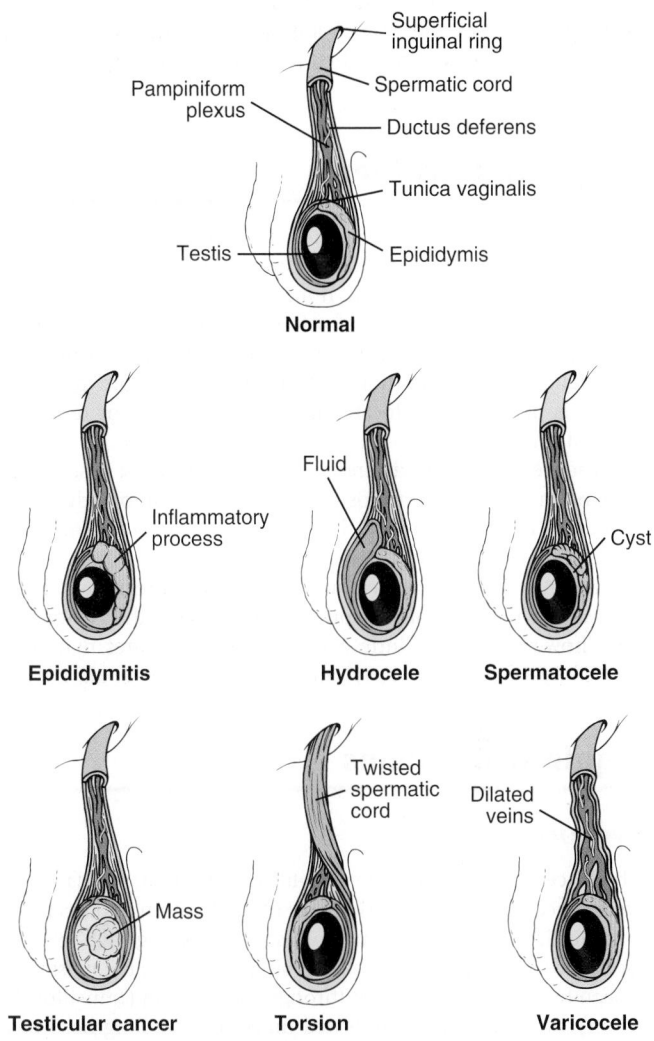

Figure 57-8 Scrotal masses.

may progress to the point that the epididymis and the testis are indistinguishable. In men younger than 35 years, the most common cause is through sexual transmission of either gonorrhea or *Chlamydia* (Trojian, Lishnak, & Heiman, 2009). The use of antibiotics is important for both partners if the transmission is through sexual contact. Patients should be encouraged to refrain from sexual intercourse during the acute phase. If they do engage in intercourse, a condom should be used. Conservative treatment consists of bed rest with elevation of the scrotum, use of ice packs, and analgesics. Ambulation places the scrotum in a dependent position and increases pain. Most tenderness subsides within 1 week, although swelling may last for weeks or months.

Orchitis

Orchitis refers to an acute inflammation of the testis. In orchitis, the testis is painful, tender, and swollen. It generally occurs after an episode of bacterial or viral infections such as mumps, pneumonia, tuberculosis, or syphilis. It can also be an adverse effect of epididymitis, prostatectomy, trauma, infectious mononucleosis, influenza, catheterization, or complicated UTI. Mumps orchitis is a condition contributing to infertility, and its incidence could easily be decreased by childhood vaccination against mumps. Treatment involves the use of antibiotics (if the organism is known), pain medications, or bed rest with the scrotum elevated on an ice pack.

Congenital Problems

Cryptorchidism (undescended testes) is failure of the testes to descend into the scrotal sac before birth. It is the most common congenital testicular condition. It may occur bilaterally or unilaterally and may be the cause of infertility if corrective surgery is not done by 2 years of age. The incidence of testicular cancer is also higher if the condition is not corrected before puberty. Surgery is performed to locate and suture the testis or testes to the scrotum.

Absence of the vas deferens is a rare condition associated most often with cystic fibrosis. With the advent of advanced techniques to treat infertility, this defect can be circumvented by aspirating the sperm directly from the testis.

Maternal use of acetaminophen during pregnancy may increase the risk of male offspring being born with cryptorchidism; however, there is little evidence that implicates maternal use of ibuprofen and/or acetylsalicylic acid (Jensen et al., 2011).

Acquired Problems

Hydrocele

A **hydrocele** is a nontender, fluid-filled mass that results from interference with lymphatic drainage of the scrotum and swelling of the tunica vaginalis that surrounds the testis (Figure 57-9; see also Figure 57-8). Diagnosis is fairly simple because the mass can be seen by shining a flashlight through the scrotum (transillumination). No treatment is indicated unless the swelling becomes very large and uncomfortable, in which case aspiration or surgical drainage of the mass is performed.

Spermatocele

A **spermatocele** is a firm, sperm-containing, painless cyst of the epididymis that may be visible with transillumination (see Figure 57-8). The cause is unknown, and surgical removal is the treatment. It is important for the patient to see his doctor if he feels any scrotal lumps. The patient would be unable to distinguish this cyst from cancer when performing self-examination.

Varicocele

A **varicocele** is a dilation of the veins that drain the testes (Figure 57-10; see Figure 57-8). The scrotum feels wormlike when palpated. The cause of the problem is unknown. The varicocele is usually located on the left side of the scrotum as a consequence of retrograde blood flow from the left renal vein. Surgery is indicated if the patient is infertile because persistent varicoceles are associated with 40 to 50% of cases of infertility. Repair of the varicocele may be through injection of a sclerosing agent or by surgical ligation of the spermatic vein.

Testicular Torsion

Testicular torsion is the result of the testis rotating on its vascular pedicle. It involves a twisting of the spermatic cord that supplies blood to the testes and epididymis, causing an interruption to the blood supply (see Figure 57-8). It is most commonly seen in males younger than age 20. The patient experiences severe scrotal pain, tenderness, swelling, nausea, and vomiting. Urinary symptoms, fever, and white blood cells or bacteria in the urine are absent. The pain does not usually subside with rest or elevation of the scrotum. Nuclear technetium scan of the testes or Doppler ultrasonography is typically performed to assess blood flow within the testicle. The cremasteric reflex is absent on the side of the swelling, and a decrease or absence in blood flow confirms the diagnosis. Unless the torsion resolves spontaneously, surgery to untwist the cord and restore the blood supply must be performed immediately. Torsion constitutes a surgical emergency because, if the blood supply to the affected testicle is not restored within 4 to 6 hours, ischemia to

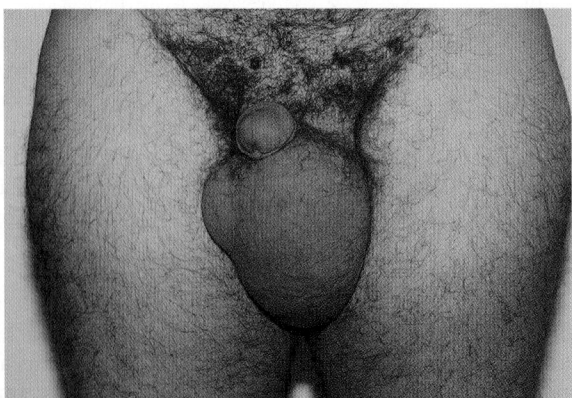

Figure 57-9 Hydrocele.

Source: Swartz, M. H. (2010). *Textbook of physical diagnosis: History and examination* (6th ed., p. 537, Figure 18-28). Philadelphia: Saunders.

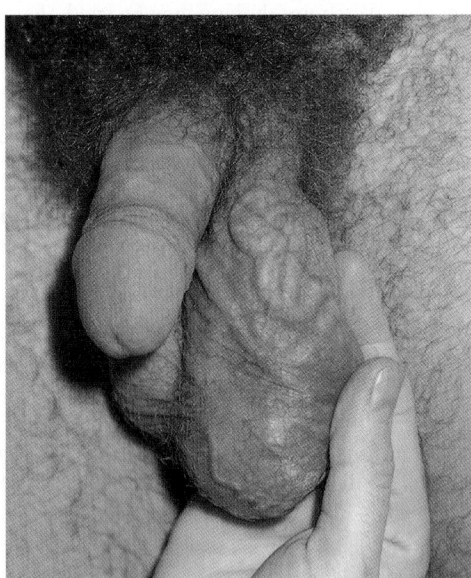

Figure 57-10 A large varicocele.

Source: Swartz, M. H. (2010). *Textbook of physical diagnosis: History and examination* (6th ed., p. 537, Figure 18-27). Philadelphia: Saunders.

the testis will occur, leading to necrosis and the possible need for removal.

Testicular Cancer

Etiology and Pathophysiology

Testicular cancer is relatively rare, accounting for less than 1% of all cancers found in males. However, testicular cancer is the most common type of cancer in young men between 15 and 35 years of age (Zoltick, 2011). The incidence of testicular cancer continues to increase in Canada at a rate that continues to be statistically significant (1.5%/yr between 1998 and 2007) for reasons that are not well understood (Canadian Cancer Society Steering Committee on Cancer Statistics, 2011). In Canada in 2011, it was estimated there would be 970 new cases of testicular cancer with a 5-year survival rate of 95% (Canadian Cancer Society Steering Committee on Cancer Statistics, 2011). White males are four times more likely to contract testicular cancer than non-Whites (Jarvis, Browne, MacDonald-Jenkins, & Luctkar-Flude, 2009). Testicular cancer occurs more commonly in the right testicle than the left (Latendresse & McCance, 2011). Testicular tumours are also more common in males who have had undescended testes (cryptorchidism) or a family history of testicular cancer or anomalies. Other predisposing factors include orchitis, human immunodeficiency virus infection, maternal exposure to diethylstilbestrol, and testicular cancer in the contralateral testis.

Most testicular cancers develop from embryonic germ cells. The two types of germ cell cancers are seminomas and nonseminomas. Although seminoma germ cell cancers are the most common, they are the least aggressive. Nonseminoma testicular germ cell tumours are rare but are very aggressive. Non–germ cell tumours arise from other testicular tissue and include Leydig cell and Sertoli cell tumours. These account for less than 10% of testicular cancers.

Clinical Manifestations and Complications

Testicular cancer may have a slow or rapid onset depending on the type of tumour. The patient may notice a painless lump in his scrotum as well as scrotal swelling and a feeling of heaviness. The scrotal mass usually is nontender and very firm. Some patients complain of a dull ache or heavy sensation in the lower abdomen, the perianal area, or the scrotum. Acute pain is the presenting symptom in about 10% of patients. Manifestations associated with metastasis to other systems are varied and include back pain, cough, dyspnea, hemoptysis, dysphagia (difficulty swallowing), alterations in vision or mental status, papilledema, and seizures.

Diagnostic Studies

Palpation of the scrotal contents is the first step in diagnosing testicular cancer. A cancerous mass is firm and does not transilluminate. Ultrasonography of the testes is indicated whenever testicular cancer is suspected (e.g., palpable mass) or when persistent or painful testicular swelling is present. If a testicular neoplasm is suspected, blood is obtained to determine the serum levels of α-fetoprotein, lactate dehydrogenase, and human chorionic gonadotropin. (These tumour markers are discussed in Chapter 18.) A chest radiographic examination and CT scan of the abdomen and pelvis are done to detect metastasis. Anemia

may be present and liver function may be elevated in metastatic disease.

NURSING AND COLLABORATIVE MANAGEMENT: TESTICULAR CANCER

▥ Testicular Self-Examination

As with many forms of cancer, the survival of the patient is closely associated with early recognition of the tumour. The scrotum is easily examined, and beginning tumours are usually palpable. Every male from the age of 15 years of age should be taught and encouraged to perform a monthly testicular self-examination (TSE) to check what is normal for his testicles so that he can notice any changes. The nurse should teach the patient how to perform TSE with a particular emphasis on males with a history of an undescended testis or a previous testicular tumour.

The procedure for TSE is not difficult. The man may indicate some reluctance to examine his own genitals, but with encouragement, he can learn this simple procedure. He should be encouraged to perform TSEs frequently until he is comfortable with the procedure. The scrotum should then be examined once a month. Videotapes and illustrations on shower hangers are available as teaching aids and ideally should be introduced during high school or college physical education classes. Free information is available through the Canadian Cancer Society and on various medical Web sites.

Guidelines for TSE of the scrotum are presented in Table 57-9 and Figure 57-11. The nurse should make this procedure as simple and uncomplicated for the man as possible. The man should choose a technique that is comfortable and consistent for him.

▥ Collaborative Care

Collaborative care of testicular cancer generally involves an orchiectomy or a radical orchiectomy (surgical removal of the affected

PATIENT & CAREGIVER TEACHING GUIDE

Table 57-9   Testicular Self-Examination
1. Just after a shower or bath is the best time to examine the testes. Warm temperatures make the testes hang lower in the scrotum.
2. Stand in front of a mirror. Look for any swelling on the skin of the scrotum.
3. Hold your scrotum in the palms of your hands so that you can feel the size and weight of each testicle. It is normal for one testicle to be larger and hang lower than the other.
4. Gently roll each testicle between your thumb and your fingers (see Figure 57-9, *A*). Feel for lumps or bumps. If you feel a soft, tender tube cord leading upward from the back of each testicle, that is normal (see Figure 57-10, *B*).
5. Notify the health care provider at once if any abnormalities are found.

Source: Adapted from Canadian Cancer Society. (2008). *Testicular self-examination (TSE).* Retrieved from https://129.33.170.43/Canada-wide/About%20cancer/Types%20of%20cancer/Testicular%20self-examination%20TSE.aspx?sc_lang=en

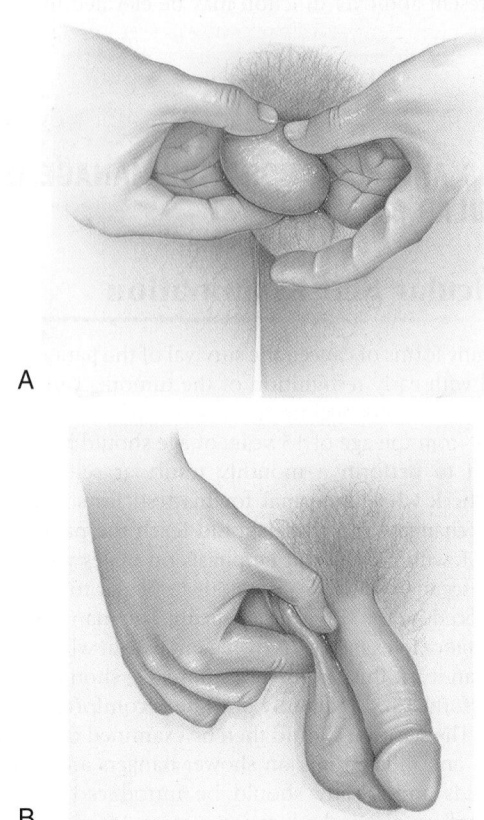

Figure 57-11 Testicular self-examination. **A,** The testicle is checked for smoothness by rolling it between the thumb and the fingers. **B,** The spermatic cord or vas deferens can be felt toward the back of the testicle and should feel soft and tender.

Source: *The wellness way: Testicular examination.* Copyright 1987, 1994, 2000, 2001, 2002. The StayWell Company.

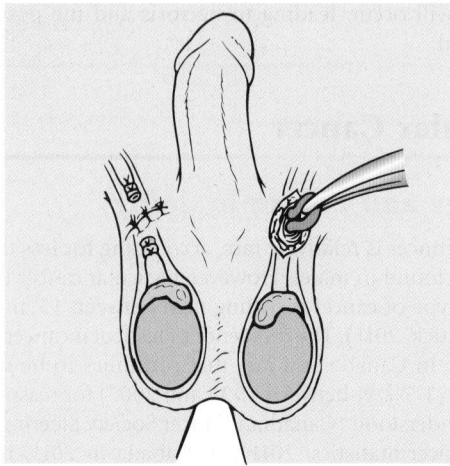

Figure 57-12 Vasectomy procedure. The vas deferens is ligated or resected for the purpose of sterilization.

testis, the spermatic cord, and regional lymph nodes). Postorchiectomy treatment involves surveillance, radiation therapy, or chemotherapy, depending on the stage of the cancer. Chemotherapy protocols use combination therapy: bleomycin, etoposide (VePesid), and cisplatin; or etoposide (VePesid), ifosfamide (Ifex), and cisplatin. (Testicular germ cell tumours are more sensitive to systemic chemotherapy than any other adult solid tumour.)

Of patients with testicular cancer, 95% obtain complete remission if the disease is detected in the early stages. As a result of treatment successes, the majority of men with testicular cancer are long-term survivors, and treatment-related toxicity is a significant issue (Gospodarowicz, 2008). All patients with testicular cancer, regardless of pathological condition or stage, require meticulous follow-up and regular physical examinations, chest radiographic examinations, CT scans, and assessment of human chorionic gonadotropin and α-fetoprotein. The goal is to detect relapse when the tumour burden is minimal. Secondary malignancies that occur as a result of chemotherapy and radiation are described in Chapter 18.

The man with testicular cancer should have the opportunity to discuss fertility and sperm banking before any treatment. The nurse should be sensitive to any psychosocial problems this type of cancer can have on a man's feelings of self-worth or sexual performance (Carpentier, Fortenberry, Ott, Brames, & Einhorn, 2011). Treatment has the potential to interfere with both erections and fertility.

Sexual Functioning

Vasectomy

Vasectomy is the bilateral surgical ligation or resection of the vas deferens performed for the purpose of sterilization (Figure 57-12). The procedure requires only 15 to 30 minutes and is usually performed on an outpatient basis with the patient under local anaesthesia. Vasectomy is considered a permanent form of sterilization, although some successful reversals *(vasovasotomy)* have been reported.

After vasectomy, the patient should not notice any difference in the look or feel of the ejaculate because its major component is seminal and prostatic fluid. The patient will need to use an alternative form of contraception until semen examination reveals no sperm. This usually requires at least 10 ejaculations or 6 weeks, until sperm distal to the surgical site are evacuated. Sperm cells continue to be produced by the testes but are absorbed by the body rather than being passed through the vas deferens. Occasionally, postoperative hematoma and swelling of the scrotum occur.

Vasectomy does not affect the production of hormones, the ability to ejaculate, or the physiological mechanisms related to erection or orgasm. Psychological adjustment may be a problem after surgery. It may be difficult for the patient to separate vasectomy from castration at a subconscious level. Some men may develop ED or may feel the need to become much more sexually active than they were in the past to prove their masculinity. Careful discussion of the procedure and its outcome before the surgery can be helpful in detecting patients who may have problems with psychological adjustment. Surgery should be delayed for these patients. (The Ethical Dilemmas box discusses sterilization.)

Sterilization

Situation

A 43-year-old male patient is requesting a vasectomy and informs the nurse that he does not wish to discuss this with his wife. The physician's policy is to have the spouse or partner sign a form acknowledging the patient's desire to be sterilized. This patient explains that, although his wife wants to have more children, the one they already have is all he wants.

Important Points for Consideration

- Patient autonomy suggests that matters of reproduction are left to the privacy and discretion of the individual. Competent adults may legally choose to be sterilized for medical reasons or convenience.
- To prevent possible future harm, this man should include his wife in the decision to permanently eliminate his ability to procreate.
- In most provinces and territories, women can terminate a pregnancy without proof that their husbands are aware of their intentions. Sterilization, conversely, is a more permanent decision that has consequences for both parties in the relationship.
- This physician's standard is to have evidence of the spouse's or significant other's knowledge of the intent for sterilization. The nurse should inform the man of the standard in this particular physician's practice and the benefits to the integrity of his marriage.
- If the patient is still unwilling to discuss the matter with his wife, either the nurse or the physician should inform the man that they will not participate in deception and he is free to select another physician to perform the procedure.

Clinical Decision-Making Questions

1. How would the nurse approach this situation?
2. Should the nurse tell the wife of her husband's plans?
3. Are there ever circumstances in which deception of a patient or family would be justified?

Erectile Dysfunction

Erectile dysfunction (ED) is the inability to attain or maintain an erect penis that allows satisfactory sexual performance (Ellsworth & Kirshenbaum, 2008). Although sexual function is a topic that many individuals are uncomfortable discussing, health care providers must be able and willing to address ED. Treatment may include phosphodiesterase type 5 inhibitors, a class of medications used to treat ED, including tadalafil (Cialis), vardenafil (Levitra), and sildenafil (Viagra).

The effects of ED potentially interfere with a man's self-esteem, confidence, relationships, and overall sense of well-being. ED is a condition that is significant because of its prevalence; it is estimated that 34% of men in Canada experience ED (College of Family Physicians of Canada, 2007). ED can occur at any age, but it is a more common disorder in men aged 40 and older. The prevalence increases to 25% of men aged 65 years and 55% of men aged 75, with 65% of men in their 80s experiencing ED

(Wong, Lawen, Kiberd, & Alkhudair, 2007). The problem is increasing in all segments of the sexually active male population and affects both the man and his partner. In younger men, the increase is attributed to substance use, such as recreational drugs and alcohol. Middle-aged men are affected by medical conditions such as diabetes, hypertension, renal disease, organ transplants, coronary artery bypass surgeries, and cancer or the therapy for these problems. Men are living longer and expect to remain sexually active, regardless of any existing medical conditions.

Etiology and Pathophysiology

ED can result from a number of factors in two general categories: physiological (organic) and psychological. *Physiological ED* can result from a number of etiological factors (Table 57-10). Common causes include vascular disease (most common cause), diabetes mellitus, adverse effects from medications, result of surgery (such as prostatectomy), trauma, chronic illness, and decreased gonadal hormone secretion (Rakel & Bope, 2008). *Psychological ED* can be caused by a number of issues but is most often associated with stress, difficulty in a relationship, depression, or low self-esteem.

Normal physiological age-related changes are associated with changes in erectile function and may be an underlying cause of ED for some men (LeRoy & Broderick, 2011). Table 57-11 lists age-related changes in sexual functioning. Explanation of these age-related changes may be necessary to reassure an anxious older man regarding normal changes in his sexual abilities.

Clinical Manifestations and Complications

A patient's self-report of problems associated with sexual performance is the typical symptom of ED. The patient usually describes an inability to attain or maintain an erection. The symptoms may occur only occasionally, may be continual and have a gradual onset, or may occur with a sudden onset. A gradual onset of symptoms usually is associated with physiological ED, whereas sudden or rapid onset of symptoms is typically associated with ED caused by psychological issues.

Although the patient may specifically seek help to alleviate the problem, many men have misconceptions about ED that make them less likely to present this as their chief complaint. More often, ED is identified from the history-taking process. This underscores the need for nurses to conduct interviews that address sexuality with men of all ages.

The major complication of ED is that the man's inability to perform sexually can cause great distress in his interpersonal relationships and may interfere with his concept of himself as a man. Our society promotes images of a man being strong, capable, and sexually responsive. Problems with ED can lead to a number of personal issues, including anger or depression.

Diagnostic Studies

The first step in diagnosis and management of ED begins with a thorough sexual, health, and psychosocial history. Self-administered assessment and treatment-related questionnaires have been developed and may prove useful as primary screening tools, for example, the Erection Quality Scale (Rosen et al., 2007). Second, a physical examination should be performed that focuses on secondary sexual characteristics, including pubic hair distribution, size and appearance of the penis and scrotum, and

Table 57-10 Risk Factors for Erectile Dysfunction

Anatomical Genitourinary

Congenital deformities of the penis (e.g., hypospadias)

Peyronie's disease

Cystectomy

Hydrocele

Perineal or suprapubic prostatectomy

Phimosis

After kidney transplant

Postpriapism

Prostatitis

Renal failure

Varicocele

Cardiorespiratory

Angina pectoris

Atherosclerosis

Emphysema

Hypertension

Myocardial infarction

Postcardiac surgery

Drug-Induced Neurological and Nerve Conduction

5α-Reductase inhibitors (finasteride [Proscar])

Alcohol

Antiandrogens

Antilipidemic agents

Antihypertensives

Caffeine

Diuretics (chlorothiazide [Diuril], spironolactone [Aldactone])

Drugs for Parkinson's disease (carbidopa–levodopa [Sinemet])

Estrogens

Major tranquilizers (diazepam [Valium], alprazolam [Xanax])

Marijuana, cocaine, LSD

Opioids

Nicotine

Tricyclic antidepressants (amitriptyline [Elavil])

Central nervous system disorders

Electroshock therapy

Multiple sclerosis

Parkinson's disease

Peripheral neuropathic conditions

Spina bifida

Stroke

Sympathectomy

Trauma to the spinal cord

Tumours or transection of spinal cord

Psychogenic

Depression

Excessive stress in family, work, or interpersonal relationships

Fatigue

Fear of failure to perform

Endocrine

Addison's disease

Diabetes mellitus

Prolactin (high levels)

Obesity

Pituitary tumour

Testosterone deficiency

Thyrotoxicosis

Vascular

Aortic aneurysm

Aortofemoral bypass surgery

Atherosclerosis of pelvic blood vessels

LSD, lysergic acid diethylamide.

Table 57-11 Age-Related Changes in Sexual Functioning

- Time lag between perceiving sexual opportunity and full erection
- Diminished size and rigidity of the penis at full erection
- Increased time interval to ejaculation
- Changed nature of ejaculation (e.g., less intensity)
- Shortened period between ejaculation and flaccidity
- Increase in time to next reaction to sexual stimulation

COLLABORATIVE CARE

Table 57-12 Erectile Dysfunction

Diagnostic	Collaborative Therapy
<ul><li>History and physical examination</li><li>Sexual history</li><li>Serum glucose and lipid profile</li><li>Testosterone, prolactin, and thyroid hormone levels</li><li>Nocturnal penile tumescence and rigidity testing</li><li>Vascular studies</li></ul>	<ul><li>Modify reversible causes</li><li>Drug therapy [sildenafil (Viagra), vardenafil (Levitra), tadalafil (Cialis)]</li><li>Vacuum constriction device (VCD)</li><li>Intraurethral medication pellet</li><li>Intracavernosal self-injection</li><li>Topical gels</li><li>Penile implants</li><li>Sexual counselling</li></ul>

method that involves the continuous measurement of penile circumference and axial rigidity during sleep. Such measurements are used to differentiate between physiological and psychological causes of ED as well as to evaluate the effectiveness of drug therapy. Vascular studies, including penile arteriography, penile blood flow study, and duplex Doppler ultrasonography studies, are used to assess penile blood inflow and outflow. Such studies help assess vascular problems interfering with erection.

Collaborative Care

The goal of ED therapy is for the patient and his partner to achieve a satisfactory sexual relationship. The treatment for ED is based on the underlying cause. A variety of treatment options are available (LeRoy & Broderick, 2011) (Table 57-12). The results of these interventions are usually most satisfactory when both partners are involved in the decision-making process and have realistic expectations of the treatment.

It is important to determine whether ED is reversible before treatment is started. For example, if ED appears to be an adverse effect of prescribed drugs, alternative agents or treatments should be explored. When there is an established diagnosis of testicular failure (hypogonadism), androgen replacement therapy may sometimes be effective in improving erectile function. For individuals who have ED that is psychological in nature, counselling by a qualified therapist for the patient (and possibly his partner) is recommended (Dean et al., 2008).

Oral Drug Therapy. Sildenafil (Viagra), tadalafil (Cialis), and vardenafil (Levitra) are erectogenic drugs. These drugs cause smooth muscle relaxation and increased arterial inflow with corporal veno-occlusion resulting in an erection. They are taken

rectal examination. Assessment of blood pressure, palpation of peripheral pulses, and sensation of the genitalia should also be included.

Further examination or diagnostic testing is typically based on findings from the history and physical examination. A serum glucose and lipid profile is recommended to rule out diabetes mellitus. Hormonal levels for testosterone, prolactin, LH, and thyroid may help identify endocrine-related problems, and other blood chemistries (e.g., PSA level) and a complete blood count may be helpful in identifying unrecognized systemic diseases.

Other diagnostic tests may be conducted to diagnose ED. Nocturnal penile tumescence and rigidity testing is a noninvasive

orally about 1 hour before sexual activity, but not more than once a day. Although rare, these drugs have been shown to cause vision and hearing loss (Nehra, 2009). Patients who experience a temporary decrease or permanent loss of vision or hearing should stop taking the medication and be examined promptly. Because they potentiate the hypotensive effect of nitrates, their use is contraindicated for individuals taking nitrates (such as nitroglycerin).

Vacuum Constriction Devices. Vacuum constriction devices are suction devices that can be applied to the flaccid penis to produce an erection by pulling blood up into the corporeal bodies (see eFigure 57-1, available on the Evolve Web site for this chapter). A penile ring or constrictive band is placed around the base of the penis to retain venous blood, thereby preventing the erection from subsiding. Special care must be taken in using these devices to prevent tissue bruising.

Intraurethral Devices. These interventions include the use of vasoactive drugs administered as topical gel, an injection into the penis (intracavernosal self-injection), or insertion of a medication pellet (alprostadil) into the urethra (intraurethral) using a medicated urethral system for erection device. These vasoactive drugs enhance blood flow into the penile arteries. Current vasoactive medications include papaverine (topical gel or injection), alprostadil (Caverject) (topical gel, transurethral pellet, or injection), and phentolamine (Rogitine).

The vasoactive medication dose is regulated on an individual basis to prevent adverse effects. Adverse effects may include penile pain, priapism, corporal fibrosis, fibrotic nodules, and hypotension. It is important to instruct patients carefully on the specific administration techniques and precautions for any of the vasoactive medications.

Home injection therapy instruction is given to those men who are suitable candidates for the therapy. The injection is nearly painless and generally begins to work in 20 to 30 minutes. Success rates have been high when there is adequate patient teaching and follow-up. This treatment is not suitable for men with severe vascular problems, intolerance for transient hypotension, severe psychiatric disease, poor manual dexterity, or poor vision or those receiving anticoagulant therapy. The man may discontinue treatment if he perceives a lack of spontaneity, has a needle phobia, or wants a more permanent treatment option.

Penile Implants. Surgical implantation of semirigid or inflatable penile prostheses is shown in Figure 57-13. These surgical procedures are highly invasive and associated with potential complications. Thus, they are usually indicated for men with severe ED for which other interventions are ineffective.

The devices are implanted into the corporeal bodies to provide an erection firm enough for penetration. The semirigid malleable implant is displayed in Figure 57-13, A. The inflatable implant consists of cylinders in the penis, a small pump in the scrotum, and a reservoir in the lower abdomen (Figure 57-13, B). The main problems associated with penile prostheses are mechanical failure, infection, and erosions.

Sexual Counselling. Sexual counselling is often recommended before and after treatment. The ability to please both partners enhances satisfaction levels. Counselling should address psychological or interpersonal factors that may enhance sexual expression as well as other factors that are of concern. Counselling can be effective for the individual patient, but it is typically preferred to include his partner, particularly if he is involved in

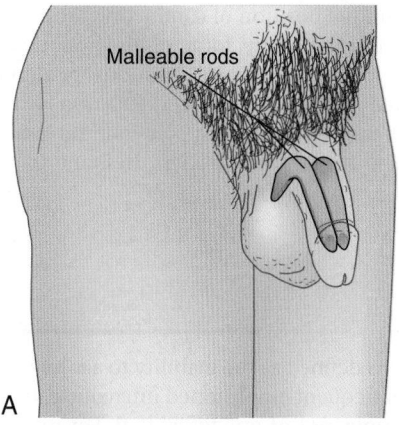

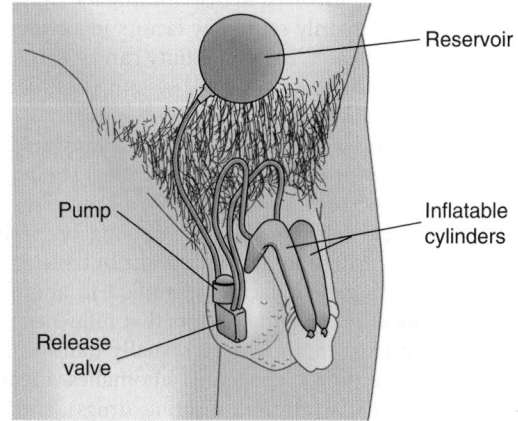

Figure 57-13 Penile implants. **A,** Malleable implant is always erect but can be bent close to the body for concealment. **B,** Inflatable implant consists of cylinders in the penis, a small pump in the scrotum, and a reservoir in the lower abdomen. When activated, the pump fills the cylinders with fluid from the reservoir. A small release valve permits the fluid to drain back into the reservoir after intercourse.

a long-term relationship (Dean et al., 2008). Counselling should begin after the start of medical treatment for ED.

NURSING MANAGEMENT: ERECTILE DYSFUNCTION

The man experiencing ED requires a great deal of emotional support for both himself and his partner. Men often do not feel comfortable discussing their problems with others because of society's expectations of a man's sexual abilities. The man may experience and demonstrate isolation from support systems, and he may also lose self-esteem.

The patient needs reassurance that confidentiality will be maintained. In conjunction with medical treatment, it often becomes necessary to provide counselling and therapy for the couple to establish realistic expectations and develop meaningful communication patterns. The majority of men delay seeking medical assistance. They are often highly motivated and expect immediate solutions to their problems. The health care team should provide a support system and accurate information as soon as possible.

Nurses are in a unique position of conducting routine health assessments on men seeking any form of medical treatment. This provides an opportunity to ask questions pertaining to general health as well as sexual health and function. Given the opportunity and when they know that someone cares and can provide them with answers, men are less hesitant to answer these questions.

Infertility

Infertility in a couple is defined as the inability to achieve conception despite 1 year of frequent, unprotected intercourse. Infertility is a disorder of a couple, not of one individual. For this reason, both partners must be involved in determining the cause of infertility. Infertility is primarily caused by factors involving the man in about 33% of the cases. Male infertility can be caused by disorders of the hypothalamic–pituitary system, disorders of the testes, and abnormalities of the ejaculatory system.

The physical causes are generally divided into three categories: pretesticular, testicular, and post-testicular. The *pretesticular or endocrine causes* occur in only about 3% of the cases and can generally be treated with medication or surgery. Seventy-five percent of all male infertility factors are attributable to primary *testicular causes* with genetic factors identified in about 15% of these cases (Krausz, 2011). Other factors that influence the testes include infection (e.g., mumps virus, sexually transmitted infections, bacterial infections), congenital anomalies, medications, radiation, substance use (alcohol, nicotine, drugs), and environmental hazards. *Post-testicular causes* account for approximately 5 to 7% of the cases, with obstruction, infection, or the result of a surgical procedure being the primary causes. The remaining 40% are classified as *idiopathic,* or of unknown cause.

A careful health history and examination may reveal the cause of a patient's infertility. Thus, the history is a starting point for determining cause and treatment. The history should include age; occupation; past injury, surgery, or infections to the genital tract; lifestyle issues such as use of hot tubs, weight training, or wearing tight undergarments; sexual practices; frequency of intercourse; and emotional factors such as stress levels and the desire for children. The use of drugs, such as chemotherapeutic agents, anabolic steroids (testosterone), sulphasalazine, cimetidine, and recreational drugs, should be documented because these can reduce sperm count. A physical examination can disclose a varicocele, Peyronie's disease, or other physical abnormalities.

The first test in an infertility study is a semen analysis. The test determines the sperm concentration (count >20 million/mL), forward progressive motility (at least 60% with a grade >2), and morphology (at least 60% have a normal oval head and long tail). Additional tests that may be helpful in determining the etiology include plasma testosterone and serum LH and FSH measurements. A test for sperm penetration abilities may also be done. The specific cause of infertility is often not determined.

The nurse should be concerned and tactful in dealing with the male patient undergoing infertility studies. For many men, fertility and masculinity are equated. The nurse must be sensitive to the problem of gender identity in the infertile man.

Treatment options for the man include medications, conservative lifestyle changes (e.g., avoidance of scrotal heat, substance abuse, high stress), in vitro fertilization techniques, and corrective surgery. Infertility can seriously strain a marriage, and the couple may require counselling and discussion of alternatives if conception is not achieved. (Female infertility is discussed in Chapter 56.)

CLINICAL DECISION-MAKING EXERCISE

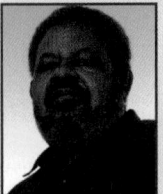

CASE STUDY:
Benign Prostatic Hyperplasia

Source: © iStockphoto.com/drbimages.

Patient Profile
Reggie Keller, a 71-year-old married man, comes to the emergency department because of an inability to void for the past 12 hours.

Subjective Data
- Complains of severe bladder pain and pressure
- Is very restless and agitated
- Relates history of three cans of beer the previous evening; has not voided since then

Objective Data
- Has prostate enlargement on digital rectal examination
- Has hematuria and white blood cells in urine
- Has palpable bladder above umbilicus
- Prostate-specific antigen (PSA) test: 6 mcg/L (normal: <4 mcg/L)

Collaborative Care
- Indwelling catheter inserted by a urology resident
- Admitted to hospital

Discussion Questions
1. What risk factors for acute urinary retention and benign prostatic hyperplasia (BPH) are present in Mr. Keller?
2. Explain the etiology of the objective symptoms Mr. Keller exhibited.
3. Discuss the drug options available to Mr. Keller.
4. Discuss the invasive options available to Mr. Keller.
5. Mr. Keller asks about the effect of the various treatment options on his ability to have sex. How would the nurse respond?
6. *Priority Decision:* What is the priority nursing intervention for Mr. Keller?
7. *Priority Decision:* What are the priority nursing diagnoses based on the assessment data presented? Are there any collaborative problems?
8. On further assessment, the nurse notes that Mr. Keller has a nursing diagnosis of decisional conflict. How would the nurse help him resolve this conflict related to treatment options?

evolve *Answers are available at* **http://evolve.elsevier.com/ Canada/Lewis/medsurg**

REVIEW QUESTIONS

The number of the question corresponds to the same-numbered objective at the beginning of the chapter.

1. A patient with benign prostatic hyperplasia (BPH) experiences hesitancy in initiating voiding and a feeling of incomplete bladder emptying. In assessing for complications related to these symptoms, the nurse would specifically ask about the presence of which of the following symptoms?
   a. Constipation
   b. Dysuria and urgency
   c. Gross blood in the urine
   d. Decreased force of the urinary stream

2. Postoperatively, a patient who has had a transurethral prostatectomy has continuous bladder irrigation with a three-way Foley with a 30-mL balloon and traction applied. Which nursing intervention is most appropriate when the patient complains that he feels the urge to void even with the catheter in place?
   a. Hand-irrigate the catheter to ensure that it is patent.
   b. Deflate the catheter balloon to 10 mL to decrease bulk in the bladder.
   c. Encourage the patient to try to have a bowel movement to relieve colon pressure.
   d. Explain that this feeling is normal and that he should not try to urinate around the catheter.

3. In teaching health promotion related to early detection of prostate cancer for men older than 50 years, what should the nurse advise?
   a. Screening should be based on your risk factors and discussion with your primary care provider.
   b. Annual urinalysis and prostatic ultrasonography are recommended.
   c. Annual PSA (prostate-specific antigen) and DRE (digital rectal examination) are recommended.
   d. Prostatic acid phosphatase (PAP) and PSA are recommended when urinary symptoms are present.

4. A patient scheduled for a prostatectomy for prostate cancer expresses the fear that he will have erectile dysfunction (ED). Which of the following should the nurse keep in mind when responding to the patient?
   a. ED is a possibility even with a nerve-sparing procedure.
   b. The most common complication of this surgery is postoperative urinary retention.
   c. Pain control will be a more important factor than sexual function or the long-term consideration of his condition.
   d. A penile implant is the best method to treat ED and should be considered after he has recovered from his surgery.

5. Which of the following is a component of the management of chronic prostatitis?
   a. A permanent indwelling catheter
   b. Regular injection of sclerosing agents
   c. Sexual activities that result in ejaculation
   d. Aspiration or surgical drainage of abscesses

6. While assessing a patient for testicular cancer, the nurse should know that manifestations of this disease include which of the following?
   a. Acute back spasms and testicular pain
   b. Rapid onset of scrotal swelling and fever
   c. Fertility problems and bilateral scrotal tenderness
   d. Painless mass and heaviness sensation in the scrotal area

7. What information should the nurse include in discharge teaching for the patient who has had a vasectomy?
   a. The procedure blocks the production of sperm.
   b. The ejaculate will be about half the volume it was before the procedure.
   c. An alternative form of contraception will be necessary for 6 to 8 weeks.
   d. ED is temporary and will return with continued sexual activity.

8. Which of the following is a nursing measure that can decrease the patient's discomfort over care involving his reproductive organs?
   a. Relating his sexual concerns to his sexual partner
   b. Arranging to have only male nurses care for the patient
   c. Maintaining a nonjudgemental attitude toward his sexual practices
   d. Using only technical terminology when discussing reproductive function

ANSWERS: 1. b; 2. d; 3. a; 4. a; 5. c; 6. d; 7. c; 8. c.

REFERENCES

Andriole, G. L. (2009). Overview of pivotal studies for prostate cancer risk reduction, past and present. *Urology, 73*(5), S36-S43. doi:10.1016/j.urology.2009.02.017

Anothaisintawee, T., Attia, J., Nickel, J., Thammakraisorn, S., Numthavaj, P., McEvoy, M., & Thakkinstian, A. (2011). Management of chronic prostatitis/chronic pelvic pain syndrome: A systematic review and network meta-analysis. *JAMA, 305*(1), 78-86. doi:10.1001/jama.2010.1913

Armstrong, A., Tannock, I., de Wit, R., George, D., Eisenberger, M., & Halabi, S. (2010). The development of risk groups in men with metastatic castration-resistant prostate cancer based on risk factors for PSA decline and survival. *European Journal of Cancer, 46*(3), 517-525. doi:10.1016/j.ejca.2009.11.007

Bankhead, C. (2010). Nanoparticle-enhanced TUMT shows promise for BPH. *Urology Times, 38*(13), 20.

Barry, M., Fowler, F., O'Leary, M., Bruskewitz, R., Holtgrewe, L., Mebust, W., & Cockett, A. T. (1992). The American Urologic Association symptom index for benign prostatic hyperplasia. *Journal of Urology, 148*(5),1549-1557.

Barry, M., & McNaughton-Collins, M. (2008). Benign prostate disease and prostatitis. In L. Goldman & D. Ausiello (Eds.), *Cecil textbook of medicine* (23rd ed., pp. 916-921). St. Louis: Saunders.

Benway, B. M., & Moon, T. (2008). Bacterial prostatitis. *Urologic Clinics North America, 35*(1), 81-92. doi:10.1016/j.ucl.2007.09.008

Burnett, A., & Bivalacqua, T. (2011). Priapism: New concepts in medical and surgical management. *Urologic Clinics of North America, 38*(2), 185-194. doi:10.1016/j.ucl.2011.02.005

Canadian Cancer Society. (2010). *Prostate cancer.* Retrieved from *http://www.cancer.ca/Canada-wide/Prevention/Getting%20checked/Prostate%20cancer%20NEW.aspx?sc_lang=en*

Canadian Cancer Society. (2011). *Prostate cancer statistics at a glance.* Retrieved from *http://www.cancer.ca/canada-wide/about%20cancer/cancer%20statistics/stats%20at%20a%20glance/prostate%20cancer.aspx*

Canadian Cancer Society's Steering Committee on Cancer Statistics. (2012). *Canadian Cancer Statistics 2012.* Toronto, ON: Canadian Cancer Society.

Canadian Cancer Society's Steering Committee on Cancer Statistics. (2011). *Canadian Cancer Statistics 2011.* Toronto, ON: Canadian Cancer Society. Retrieved from *http://www.cancer.ca/~/media/CCS/Canada%20wide/Files%20List/English%20files%20heading/PDF%20-%20Policy%20-%20Canadian%20Cancer%20Statistics%20-%20English/Canadian%20Cancer%20Statistics%202011%20-%20English.ashx*

Prostate Cancer Canada. (2011). *Prostate cancer and Black history month.* Retrieved from *http://www.prostatecancer.ca/Special-Pages/Prostate-Cancer-Canada-s-Blog-(1)/Prostate-Cancer-Canada-s-Blog/Prostate-Cancer-and-Black-History-Month*

Carpentier, M., Fortenberry, J., Ott, M., Brames, M., & Einhorn, L. (2011). Perceptions of masculinity and self-image in adolescent and young adult testicular cancer survivors: Implications for romantic and sexual relationships. *Psycho-Oncology, 20*(7), 738-745. doi:10.1002/pon.1772

Chung, D., Wysock, J., Lee, R., Melamed, S., Kaplan, S., & Te, A. (2011). Outcomes and complications after 532 nm laser prostatectomy in anticoagulated patients with benign prostatic hyperplasia. *Journal of Urology, 186*(3), 977-981. doi:10.1016/j.juro.2011.04.068

College of Family Physicians of Canada. (2007). *Erectile dysfunction—Learning the causes and what you can do.* Retrieved from *http://www.cfpc.ca/english/cfpc/programs/patient%20education/erectile%20dysfunction/default.asp?s=1*

Dean, J., Ruoio-Aurioles, E., McCabe, M., Eardly, I., Speakman, M., Buvat, J., …, & Fisher, W. (2008). Integrating partners into erectile dysfunction treatment: Improving the sexual experience for the couple. *International Journal of Clinical Practice, 62*(1), 127-133. doi:10.1111/j.1742-1241.2007.01636.x

Edgar, A. D., Levin, R., Constantinou, C. C., & Denis, L. (2007). A critical review of the pharmacology of the plant extract of *Pygeum africanum* in the treatment of LUTS. *Neurourology and Urodynamics, 26*(4), 458-456. doi:10.1002/nau.20136

Ellsworth, P., & Kirshenbaum, E. (2008). Current concepts in the evaluation and management of erectile dysfunction. *Urologic Nursing, 28*(5), 357-369.

Ferri, F. (Ed.). (2009). *Ferri's clinical advisor 2009.* St. Louis: Mosby.

Fiorentino, M., Capizzi, E., & Loda, M. (2010). Blood and tissue biomarkers in prostate cancer: State of the art. *Urologic Clinics of North America, 37*(1), 131. doi:10.1016/j.ucl.2009.11.006

Gospodarowicz, M. (2008). Testicular cancer patients: Considerations in long-term follow-up. *Hematologic Oncology Clinics of North America, 22*(2), 245-254. doi:10.1016/j.hoc.2008.01.003

Greenspan, S. (2008). Approach to the prostate cancer patient with bone disease. *Journal of Clinical Endocrinology and Metabolism, 93*(1), 2-7. doi:10.1210/jc.2007-1402

Jarvis, C., Browne, A. J., MacDonald-Jenkins, J., & Luctkar-Flude, M. (Eds.). (2009). *Physical examination and health assessment* (1st Canadian ed.). Toronto: Elsevier Canada.

Jensen, M. S., Henriksen, T. B., Rebordosa, C., Thulstrup, A. M., Toft, G., Sørensen, H. T., …, Olsen, J. (2011). Analgesics during pregnancy and cryptorchidism: Additional analyses. *Epidemiology, 22*(4), 610-612. doi:10.1097/EDE.0b013e31821eca69

Kenfield, S. A., Stampfer, M. J., Giovannuncci, E., & Chan, J. M. (2011). Physical activity and survival after prostate cancer diagnosis in the Health Professionals Follow-Up Study. *Journal of Clinical Oncology, 29*(6), 726-732. doi:10.1200/JCO.2010.31.5226

Krausz, C. (2011). Male infertility: Pathogenesis and clinical diagnosis. *Best Practice & Research Clinical Endocrinology & Metabolism, 25*(2), 271-285. doi:10.1016/j.beem.2010.08.006

Latendresse, G., & McCance, K. L. (2011). Alterations of the reproductive systems, including sexually transmitted infections. In S. E. Huether & K. L. McCance (Eds.), *Understanding pathophysiology* (5th ed., pp. 799-870). St. Louis: Mosby.

LeRoy, T., & Broderick, G. (2011). Doppler blood flow analysis of erectile function: Who, when and how. *Urologic Clinics of North America, 38*(2), 147-154. doi:10.1016/j.ucl.2011.03.003

Lingeman, J. (2011). Holmium laser enucleation of the prostate—If not now, when? *Journal of Urology, 186*(5), 1762-1763. doi:10.1016/j.juro.2011.08.020

Lourenco, T., Pickard, R., Vale, L., Grant, A., Fraser, C., MacLennan, G., …, N'Dow, J. (2008). Minimally invasive treatments for benign prostatic enlargement: Systematic review of randomised controlled trials. *BMJ, 337*, a1662. doi:10.1136/bmj.a1662

Mishra, V., Browne, J., & Emberton, M. (2008). Role of repeated prostatic massage in chronic prostatitis: A systematic review of the literature. *Urology, 72*(4), 731-735. doi:10.1016/j.urology.2008.04.030

Naber, K. (2008). Management of bacterial prostatitis: What's new? *BJU International, 101*(Suppl 3), 7-10. doi:10.1111/j.1464-410X.2008.07495.x

Nehra, A. (2009). Can Viagra really cause hearing and vision loss? If so, is this a reason to avoid using it? *Mayo Clinic Health Letter, 26*(7), 8.

Parsons, J., & Bennett, J. (2008). Outcomes of retropubic, laparoscopic and robotic-assisted prostatectomy. *Urology, 72*(2), 412-416. doi:10.1016/j.urology.2007.11.026

Pieters, B., Rezaie, E., Geusen, E., Koedooder, K., van der Grient, J., Blank, L., …, Koning, C. (2011). Development of late toxicity and international prostate symptom score resolution after external-beam radiotherapy combined with pulse dose rate brachytherapy for prostate cancer. *International Journal of Radiation Oncology, Biology, Physics, 81*(3), 758-764. doi:10.1016/j.ijrobp.2010.05.044

Pontari, M. A. (2008). Chronic prostatitis/chronic pelvic pain syndrome. *Urologic Clinics of North America, 35*(1), 81-88. doi:10.1016/j.ucl.2007.09.005

Prostate Cancer Canada. (2011). Early detection guidelines update. Retrieved from *http://www.Prostatecancer.ca/In-The-News*

Rakel, R., & Bope, E. (2008). *Conn's current therapy 2008* (60th ed.). Philadelphia: Saunders.

Rawson, N., & Saad, F. (2010). The aging male population and medical care for benign prostatic hyperplasia in Canada. *Canadian Urologic Association Journal, 4*(2), 123-127.

Rosen, R., Wincze, J., Mollen, M., Gondek, K., McLeod, L., & Fisher, W. (2007). Responsiveness and minimum important differences for the erection quality scale. *Journal of Urology, 178*(5), 2076-2081. doi:10.1016/j.juro.2007.07.019

Saca-Hazboun, H. (2008). Advances in prostate cancer treatment: How do providers help patients choose appropriate treatments? *Oncology Nursing Society Connect, 23*(9), 8-12.

Salem, S., Salahi, M., Mohseni, M., Ahmadi, H., Mehrsai, A., Jahani, Y., & Pourmand, G. (2011). Major dietary factors and prostate cancer risk: A prospective multicenter case-control study. *Nutrition and Cancer, 63*(1), 21-27. doi:10.1080/01635581.2010.516875

Steels, E. (2008). Probing the prostate—Safe and effective treatments for BPH. *Total Health, 30*(2), 34. Retrieved from *http://totalhealthmagazine.com/features/mens-health/probing-the-prostate-safe-and-effective-treatments-for-bph.html*

Streif, D. (2008). An overview of prostate cancer: Diagnosis and treatment. *Medsurg Nursing, 17*(4), 258.

Tacklind, J., MacDonald, R., Rutks, I., & Wilt, T. J. (2009). Serenoa repens for benign prostatic hyperplasia. *Cochrane Database of*

Systematic Reviews 2009, 2, CD001423. doi:10.1002/14651858. CD001423.pub2

Tanguay, S., Awde, M., Brock, G., Casey, R., Kozak, J., Lee, J., ..., Saad, F. (2009). Diagnosis and management of benign prostatic hyperplasia in primary care. *Canadian Urological Association Journal*, 3(3), S92-S100.

Therigy Drug Reference Series. (2008). VIADUR Drug fact sheet for professionals. Retrieved from *https://resources.therigy.com/news/view_article.html?article_id=89105820fef1814daeb42669a4758131&dir_cat_id=9c1e8fc1e6ee8f86e14aafd399b500f8*

Trock, B., Han, M., Freedland, S. J., Humphreys, E., DeWeese, T., Partin, A., & Walsh, P. (2008). Prostate cancer-specific survival following salvage radiotherapy vs observation in men with biochemical recurrence after radical prostectomy. *Journal of the American Medical Association*, 299(23), 2760-2769. doi:10.1001/jama.299.23.2760

Trojian, T., Lishnak, T., & Heiman, D. (2009). Epididymitis and orchitis: An overview. *American Family Physician*, 79(7), 583-587. doi:1668359621

Turner, B., & Drudge-Coates, L. (2010). Prostate cancer: Risk factors, diagnosis and management. *Cancer Nursing Practice*, 9(10), 29-35.

Wong, J., Lawen, J., Kiberd, B., & Alkhudair, W. (2007). Prevalence and prognostic factors for erectile dysfunction in renal transplant recipients. *Canadian Urological Association Journal*, 1(4), 383-387.

Woods, E. (2010). Laser ablation of the prostate: A safe effective treatment of obstructive benign prostatic disease. *Canadian Urological Association Journal*, 4(5), 344-346. doi:10.5489/cuaj.10073

YuKo, W., & Sawatzky, J. (2008). Understanding urinary incontinence after radical prostatectomy: A nursing framework. *Clinical Journal of Oncology Nursing*, 12(4), 647-658. doi:10.1188/08.CJON.647-654

Zoltick, B. (2011). Shedding light on testicular cancer. *The Nurse Practitioner*, 36(7), 32-39. doi:10.1097/01.NPR.0000398870.16580.86

CANADIAN RESOURCES

Canadian Cancer Society
http://www.cancer.ca
Canadian Urological Association
http://www.cua.org
EDHELP: Canadian Erectile Difficulties Help Centre
http://www.edhelp.ca
Prostate Cancer Canada
http://www.prostatecancer.ca
Prostate Cancer Center
http://www.prostatecancercentre.ca
The Prostate Centre: Princess Margaret Hospital—Toronto
http://www.prostatecanada.net/index.html
The Prostate Centre at Vancouver General Hospital
http://www.prostatecentre.com

RELATED RESOURCES

Men's Health Center, Mayo Clinic
http://www.mayoclinic.com
Prostate Calculator: Forecasting the Course of Disease (Artificial Neural Networks in Prostate Cancer Project)
http://prostatecalculator.org

evolve For additional Internet resources, see the Web site for this book at **http://evolve.elsevier.com/Canada/Lewis/medsurg**

Problems Related to Movement and Coordination

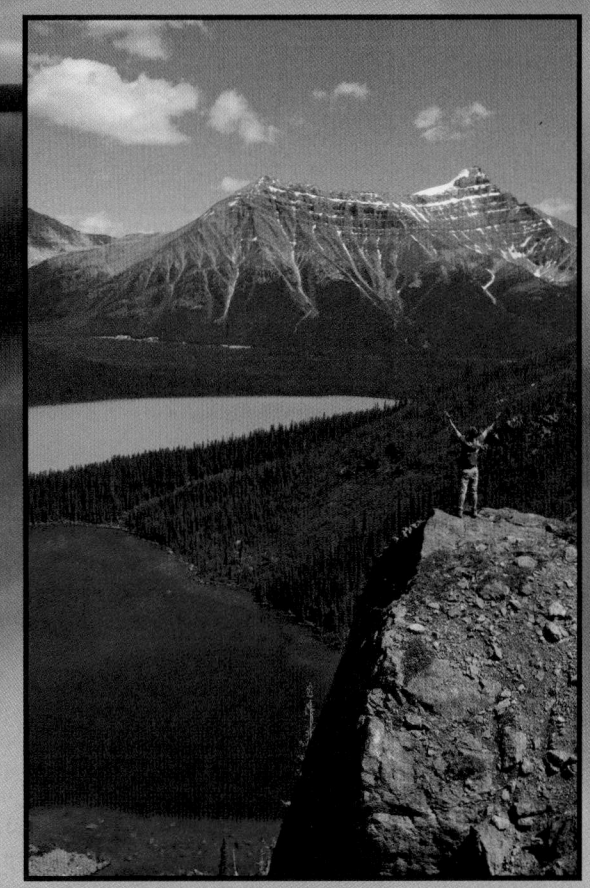

© Mountainpz/Dreamstime.com

Nursing Assessment: Nervous System

Written by DaiWai M. Olson

Adapted by Donna Goodridge

LEARNING OBJECTIVES

1. Describe the functions of neurons and glial cells.
2. Explain the electrochemical aspects of nerve impulse transmission.
3. Explain the anatomical location and functions of the cerebrum, brainstem, cerebellum, spinal cord, peripheral nerves, and cerebrospinal fluid.
4. Identify the major arteries supplying the brain.
5. Describe the functions of the 12 cranial nerves.
6. Compare the functions of the two divisions of the autonomic nervous system.
7. Describe age-related changes in the neurological system and differences in assessment findings.
8. Identify the significant subjective and objective data related to the nervous system that should be obtained from a patient.
9. Select appropriate techniques in physical assessment of the nervous system.
10. Differentiate normal from common abnormal findings of a physical assessment of the nervous system.
11. Describe the purpose, the significance of results, and the nursing responsibilities related to diagnostic studies of the nervous system.

KEY TERMS

autonomic nervous system (ANS) The division of the nervous system that governs involuntary functions of cardiac muscle, smooth (involuntary) muscle, and glands, p. 1615

blood–brain barrier A physiological barrier between blood capillaries and brain tissue that protects the brain from certain potentially harmful agents while allowing nutrients and gases to enter, p. 1616

central nervous system (CNS) The division of the nervous system that consists of the brain, the spinal cord, and cranial nerves I and II, p. 1607

cerebrospinal fluid (CSF) Fluid that provides cushioning for the brain and the spinal cord, allows fluid shifts from the cranial cavity to the spinal cavity, and carries nutrients, p. 1614

cranial nerves (CN) The 12 paired nerves composed of cell bodies with fibres that exit from the cranial cavity, p. 1615

dermatome The area of skin innervated by the sensory fibres of a single dorsal root of a spinal nerve, p. 1614

glial cells The cells in the nervous system that provide support, nourishment, and protection to neurons, p. 1607

lower motor neurons (LMNs) The final common pathway through which descending motor tracts influence skeletal muscle, the effector organ for movement, p. 1611

meninges Three layers of protective membranes that surround the brain and the spinal cord, p. 1616

neurons The primary functional units of the nervous system, p. 1607

neurotransmitter A chemical agent involved in the transmission of an impulse across the synaptic cleft, p. 1609

peripheral nervous system (PNS) The division of the nervous system that consists of cranial nerves III to XII, the spinal nerves, and the peripheral components of the autonomic nervous system, p. 1607

reflex An involuntary response to a stimulus, p. 1612

synapse The structural and functional junction between two neurons, p. 1609

upper motor neurons (UMNs) The classification of motor pathways contained completely within the central nervous system, p. 1611

ELECTRONIC RESOURCES

Supplemental content related to Chapter 58 can be found...

Evolve Web Site ⊖volve

http://evolve.elsevier.com/Canada/Lewis/medsurg
- Animations:
  - Motor Pathways and Clinical Evaluation of the Central Nervous System
  - Reflex Arc
  - Sensory Pathways and Clinical Evaluation of the Central Nervous System
- Assessment Case Study
- Clinical Reference: Laboratory Values
- Content Updates
- Electronic Calculators
- Examination Review Questions
- Glossary
- Key Points (Printable and MP3 Download)
- Physical Examination Video Clips:
  - Head and Face; Eyes; Ears
  - Nose, Mouth, and Pharynx

- Neck
- Abdominal Reflexes, Abdominal Muscles, and Inguinal Area
- Neurological System: Sensory Function; Motor Function and Coordination; Gait and Balance
- Video Clips:
  - Evaluation: Smell, Cranial Nerve I: Olfactory Nerve
  - Evaluation: Central Vision and Visual Acuity, Cranial Nerve II: Optic Nerve
  - Evaluation: Pupil Responses, Direct and Accommodation, Cranial Nerves III, IV, and VI: Oculomotor, Trochlear, and Abducens Nerves
  - Evaluation: Sensory and Light Touch, Face and Upper and Lower Extremities, Cranial Nerve V: Trigeminal Nerve
  - Inspection: Fine Motor Coordination, Upper Extremities
  - Inspection: Fine Motor Coordination, Lower Extremities
  - Evaluation: Sensory, Face, and Upper Extremities
  - Evaluation: Deep Tendon Reflex, Patellar Tendon

Structures and Functions of the Nervous System

The human nervous system is a highly specialized system responsible for the control and integration of the body's many activities. The nervous system has two main divisions: the **central nervous system (CNS)** and the **peripheral nervous system (PNS)**. The CNS consists of the brain, the spinal cord, and cranial nerves I and II. The PNS consists of cranial nerves III to XII, the spinal nerves, and the peripheral components of the autonomic nervous system (ANS). Components of the ANS are found in both the CNS and the PNS, although the ANS is considered part of the PNS (McCance & Huether, 2010).

Cells of the Nervous System

The nervous system is made up of two types of cells: neurons and glial cells. Glial cells provide structural support and are more numerous than neurons. **Neurons**—the primary functional unit of the nervous system—were long thought to be nonmitotic and therefore after being damaged could not be replaced. However, discovery of neuronal stem cells demonstrated that neurogenesis may occur in adult brains after cerebral injury (Colucci-D'Amato & di Porzio, 2008). Glial cells are mitotic and can replicate.

Neurons. The neurons of the nervous system come in many different shapes and sizes, but they share three characteristics: (a) *excitability*, or the ability to generate a nerve impulse; (b) *conductivity*, or the ability to transmit the impulse to other portions of the cell; and (c) the ability to *influence* other neurons, muscle cells, and glandular cells by transmitting nerve impulses to them.

A typical neuron consists of a cell body, an axon, and several dendrites (Figure 58-1). The cell body, which contains the nucleus and the cytoplasm, is the metabolic centre of the neuron. Dendrites are short processes extending from the cell body. They receive nerve impulses from the axons of other neurons and conduct impulses toward the cell body. The nerve axon projects varying distances from the cell body, ranging from several micrometres to more than a metre. Its function is to carry nerve impulses to other neurons or to end organs. The end organs are smooth and striated muscles and glands. Axons may be myelinated or unmyelinated. Many axons present in the CNS and the PNS are covered by a segmentally interrupted myelin sheath composed of a white, lipid substance that acts as an insulator for the conduction of impulses. In general, the smaller fibres are unmyelinated.

Glial Cells. **Glial cells** provide support, nourishment, and protection to neurons. They constitute almost half the brain and spinal cord mass and are 5 to 10 times more numerous than neurons. Different types of glial cells, including oligodendrocytes, astrocytes, ependymal cells, and microglia, have specific functions. *Oligodendrocytes* are specialized cells that produce the myelin sheath of nerve fibres in the CNS (Schwann cells myelinate the nerve fibres in the periphery) and are found primarily in the white matter of the CNS.

Astrocytes provide structural support to neurons and their delicate processes, form the blood–brain barrier with the endothelium of the blood vessels, and play a role in synaptic transmission (conduction of impulses between neurons). They are found primarily in grey matter. When the brain is injured, astrocytes act as phagocytes for neuronal debris. They help restore the neurochemical milieu and provide support for repair. Proliferation of

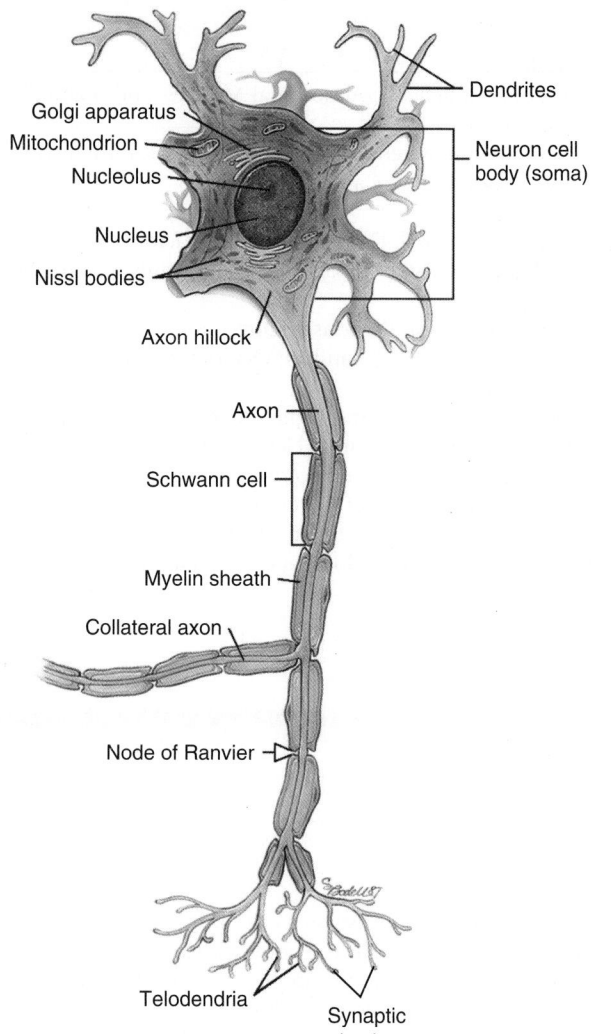

Figure 58-1 Structural features of neurons: dendrites, cell body, and axons.

Source: Adapted from Patton, K. T., & Thibodeau, G. A. (2010). *Anatomy and physiology* (7th ed., p. 379, Figure 12-5). St. Louis: Mosby.

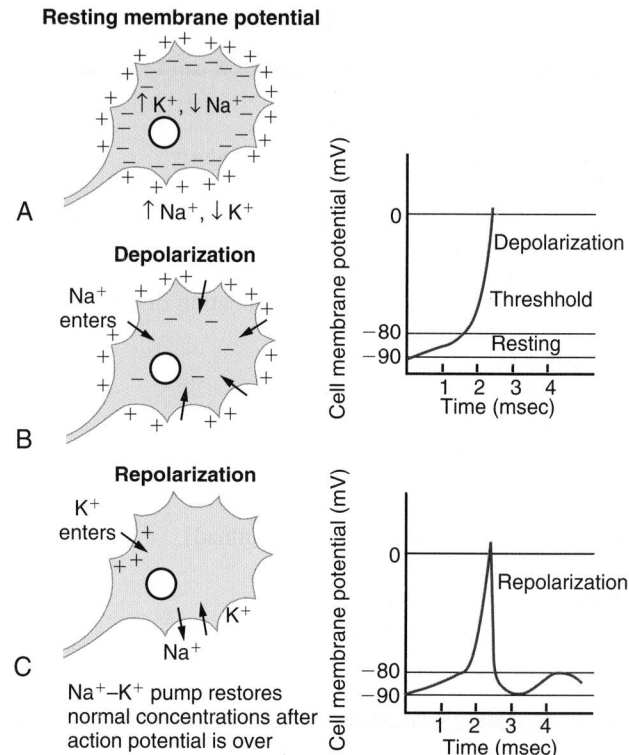

Figure 58-2 The events occurring in a cell for an action potential. **A,** Resting membrane potential. **B,** Depolarization. **C,** Repolarizarion. K^+, potassium ions; Na^+, sodium ions.

astrocytes contributes to the formation of scar tissue (gliosis) in the CNS.

Ependymal cells line the brain ventricles and aid in the secretion of cerebrospinal fluid. *Microglia*, a type of macrophage, are relatively rare in normal CNS tissue. They are phagocytes and are important in host defence.

Most primary CNS tumours involve glial cells. Primary malignancies involving neurons are rare.

Neurogenesis

If the axon of a nerve cell is damaged, the cell attempts to repair itself. When damaged, all nerve cells attempt to grow back to their origins by sprouting many branches from the damaged ends of their axons. Unfortunately, axons in the CNS are less successful than peripheral axons in regenerating. Endogenous inhibitors (e.g., neurite outgrowth inhibitor, myelin-associated glycoprotein) decrease axon regeneration.

In the PNS (outside the brain and the spinal cord), injured nerve fibres can successfully regenerate by growing within the protective myelin sheath of the supporting Schwann cells if the cell body is intact. The final result of nerve regeneration depends on the number of axon sprouts that join with the appropriate Schwann cell columns and re-innervate appropriate end organs.

Nerve Impulse

The function of a neuron is to initiate, receive, and process messages about events both within and outside the body. The initiation of a neuronal message (nerve impulse) involves the generation of an action potential. Once an action potential is initiated, a series of action potentials travel along the axon. When the impulse reaches the end of the nerve fibre, it is transmitted across the junction between nerve cells (synapse) by a chemical interaction involving neurotransmitters. This chemical interaction generates another set of action potentials in the next neuron. These events are repeated until the nerve impulse reaches its destination.

Action Potential. When nerve cells are in a resting (nonactive) state, the inside of the cell carries an electrical charge that is negative in relation to the outside of the cell. Sodium ions (Na^+) are in high concentration outside the cell, and potassium ions (K^+) are in high concentration inside the cell. The difference in electrical charge across the cell membrane is termed the *resting membrane potential* (Figure 58-2). An action potential occurs when a stimulus is of sufficient magnitude to alter the membrane potential.

During the action potential, the cell membrane becomes more permeable to Na^+, allowing the Na^+ to move readily into the cell. The resulting change in the voltage across the cell membrane is called *depolarization*. The inside of the cell temporarily becomes positive in relation to the outside. After rapid depolarization, *repolarization* (in which the inside of the cell becomes negative in relation to the outside) is facilitated by a slower increase in K^+ permeability, which in turn is caused by the depolarization associated with entry of Na^+ into the cell. The whole process of depolarization and repolarization of the nerve cell membrane takes only 1 to 2 msec. With repeated action potentials, the cells accumulate Na^+. An active metabolic process within the cell is required to move Na^+ out of the cell and K^+ back in. This metabolic process is accomplished by the sodium–potassium pump, which requires energy from the breakdown of adenosine triphosphate.

Once the cell depolarizes enough to cause an action potential, the size of the action potential is independent of the strength of the stimulus. When an action potential is initiated at one point of a neuron, it is transmitted along the axon without losing its intensity.

Because of its insulating capacity, myelination of nerve axons facilitates the conduction of an action potential. Many peripheral nerve axons have gaps, termed *nodes of Ranvier*, at regular intervals in the myelin sheath surrounding them. An action potential travelling down one of these axons hops from node to node without traversing the insulated membrane segment between nodes, which makes the action potential travel much faster than it would otherwise. This is called *saltatory* (hopping) conduction. In an unmyelinated fibre, the wave of depolarization traverses the entire length of the axon, and each portion of the membrane becomes depolarized in turn. Figure 58-3 depicts a comparison of nerve impulse transmission of myelinated and unmyelinated fibres.

Synapse. A **synapse** is the structural and functional junction between two neurons. It is the point at which the nerve impulse is transmitted from one neuron to another or from a neuron to glands or muscles. The essential structures of synaptic transmission are a presynaptic terminal, a synaptic cleft, and a receptor site on the postsynaptic cell (Figure 58-4). There are two types of synapses: electrical and chemical. In an electrical synapse, an action potential moves from neuron to neuron directly by allowing electrical current to flow between neurons. In a chemical synapse, an action potential reaches the end of the axon (presynaptic terminal); then it causes release of a chemical substance (neurotransmitter) from tiny vesicles within the axon terminal. This release depends on influx of calcium, initiated by depolarization of the nerve terminal. The neurotransmitter then crosses the microscopic space (synaptic cleft) between the two neurons and attaches to receptor sites of the receiving (postsynaptic) neuron. This causes a change in the permeability of the postsynaptic cell membrane to specific ions, such as Na^+ and K^+, and a change in the electric potential of the membrane. Parts of the synapse include the neurotransmitters, the inactivators, and the receptors (see Figure 58-4).

Neurotransmitters. A **neurotransmitter** is a chemical agent that affects the transmission of an impulse across the synaptic

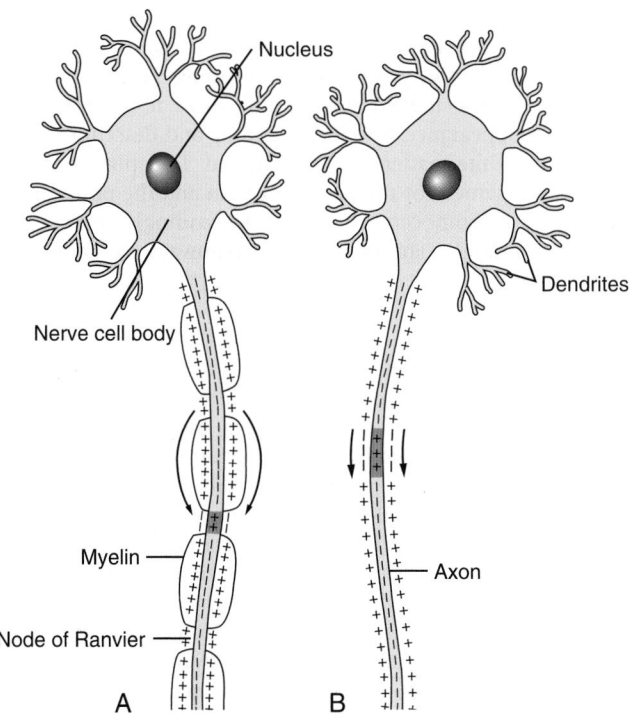

Figure 58-3 Nerve impulse transmission. **A,** Saltatory conduction in a myelinated nerve. **B,** Depolarization in an unmyelinated fibre.

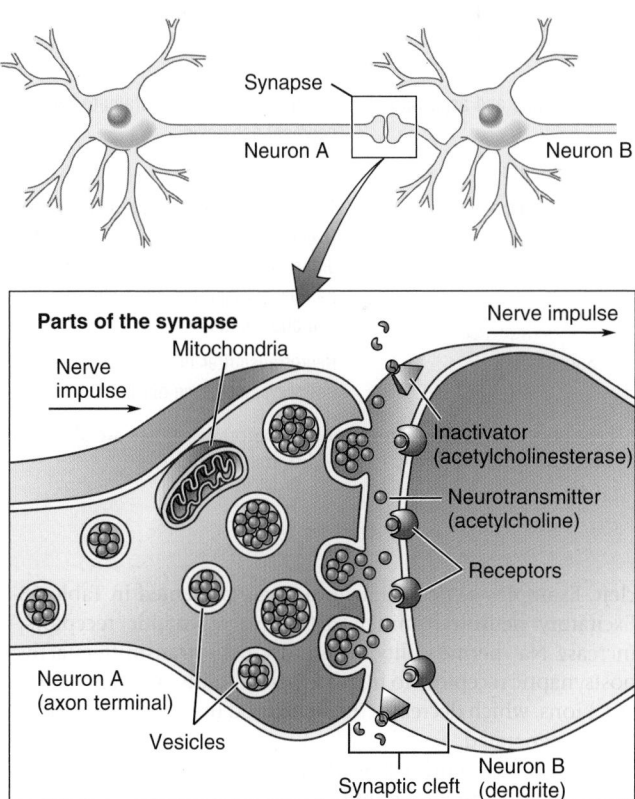

Figure 58-4 The synapse is located in the space between neuron A and neuron B. Parts of the synapse include the neurotransmitters, the inactivators, and the receptors. The neurotransmitters are located in the vesicles of neuron A. The inactivators are located on the membrane of neuron B. The receptors are located on the membrane of neuron B.

Source: Adapted from Herlihy, B. (2007). *The human body in health and illness* (3rd ed., p. 170, Figure 10-9). Philadelphia: W. B. Saunders.

Table 58-1 Examples of Neurotransmitters

SUBSTANCE	CLINICAL RELEVANCE*
Acetylcholine	The number of acetylcholine-secreting neurons decreases in Alzheimer's disease; myasthenia gravis results from a reduction in acetylcholine receptors.
Amines	
• Epinephrine	Acts as a hormone when secreted by the neurosecretory cells of the adrenal medulla.
• Norepinephrine	Cocaine and amphetamines increase the release and block the reuptake of norepinephrine, resulting in overstimulation of postsynaptic neurons.
• Serotonin	Involved in moods, emotions, and sleep.
• Dopamine	Involved in emotions and moods and regulating motor control. Parkinson's disease results from destruction of dopamine-secreting neurons.
Amino Acids	
• γ-Aminobutyric acid (GABA)	Drugs that increase GABA function have been used to treat seizure disorders.
• Glutamate and aspartate	Sustained release of glutamate triggers neuronal apoptosis.
Neuropeptides	
• Endorphins and enkephalins	The opiates morphine and heroin bind to endorphin and enkephalin receptors on presynaptic neurons and reduce pain by blocking the release of neurotransmitter.
• Substance P	Neurotransmitter in pain transmission pathways; morphine blocks its release.

*These are examples only; most of the neurotransmitters are also found in other locations and may have additional functions.

cleft. Examples of neurotransmitters are presented in Table 58-1. Excitatory neurotransmitters activate postsynaptic receptors to increase Na^+ permeability. Inhibitory neurotransmitters activate postsynaptic receptors to increase permeability of K^+ and chloride (Cl^-) ions, which decreases the likelihood that an action potential will be generated.

Each of the hundreds to thousands of synaptic connections of a single neuron has an influence on that neuron. The net effect of the input is sometimes excitatory and sometimes inhibitory. In general, the net effect depends on the number of presynaptic neurons that are releasing neurotransmitters on the postsynaptic cell. A presynaptic cell that releases an excitatory neurotransmitter does not always cause the postsynaptic cell to depolarize enough to generate an action potential. However, when many presynaptic cells release excitatory neurotransmitters on a single neuron, the sum of their input is enough to generate an action potential.

The presynaptic input can be summed by the number of presynaptic cells firing *(spatial summation)* or by the frequency of firing of a single presynaptic cell *(temporal summation)*. Both types of summation usually occur simultaneously.

Neurotransmitters continue to combine with the receptor sites at the postsynaptic membrane until they are inactivated by enzymes, are taken up by the presynaptic endings, or diffuse away from the synaptic region. In addition, the action of neurotransmitters can be affected by drugs and toxins, which can modify their function or block their attachment to receptor sites on the postsynaptic membrane.

γ-Aminobutyric acid (GABA) is the main inhibitory neurotransmitter in the nervous system, acting to dampen neural transmissions within the system. Decreased amounts of GABA in the spinal cord have been shown to contribute to the development of neuropathic pain (Porter & Kaplan, 2011). Enkephalins and endorphins are also considered neurotransmitters. These substances have opiate-like properties. They are found in multiple areas of the CNS and the PNS and act to inhibit pain perception (see Chapter 10).

Central Nervous System

Major structural components of the CNS are the cerebrum (cerebral hemispheres), telencephalon and diencephalon, brainstem, cerebellum, and spinal cord.

Spinal Cord. The spinal cord is continuous with the brainstem and exits from the cranial cavity through the foramen magnum. A cross-section of the spinal cord reveals grey matter that is centrally located in an H shape and is surrounded by white matter (Figure 58-5). The grey matter contains the cell bodies of voluntary motor neurons and preganglionic autonomic motor neurons, as well as cell bodies of association neurons (interneurons). The white matter contains the axons of the ascending sensory and the descending (suprasegmental) motor fibres. The myelin surrounding these fibres gives them their white appearance. Specific ascending and descending pathways in the white matter can be identified. The spinal pathways or tracts are named for the point of origin and the point of destination (e.g., spinocerebellar tract [ascending], corticospinal tract [descending]). The major spinal pathways are depicted in Figure 58-6.

Ascending Tracts. In general, the ascending tracts carry specific sensory information to higher levels of the CNS. This information comes from special sensory endings (receptors) in the skin, the muscles and joints, the viscera, and the blood vessels and enters the spinal cord by way of the dorsal roots of the spinal nerves. The fasciculus gracilis and the fasciculus cuneatus (together, commonly called the *dorsal* or *posterior column*) carry information and transmit impulses concerned with touch, deep pressure, vibration, position sense, and kinaesthesia (appreciation of movement, weight, and body parts). The *spinocerebellar tracts* carry information about muscle tension and body position to the cerebellum for coordination of movement. The *spinothalamic tracts* carry pain and temperature sensations. Thus the ascending tracts are organized by sensory modality, as well as by anatomy.

Other ascending tracts may also participate in transmission of sensory information. The symptoms of various neurological diseases suggest the existence of alternative pathways for touch, position sense, and vibration.

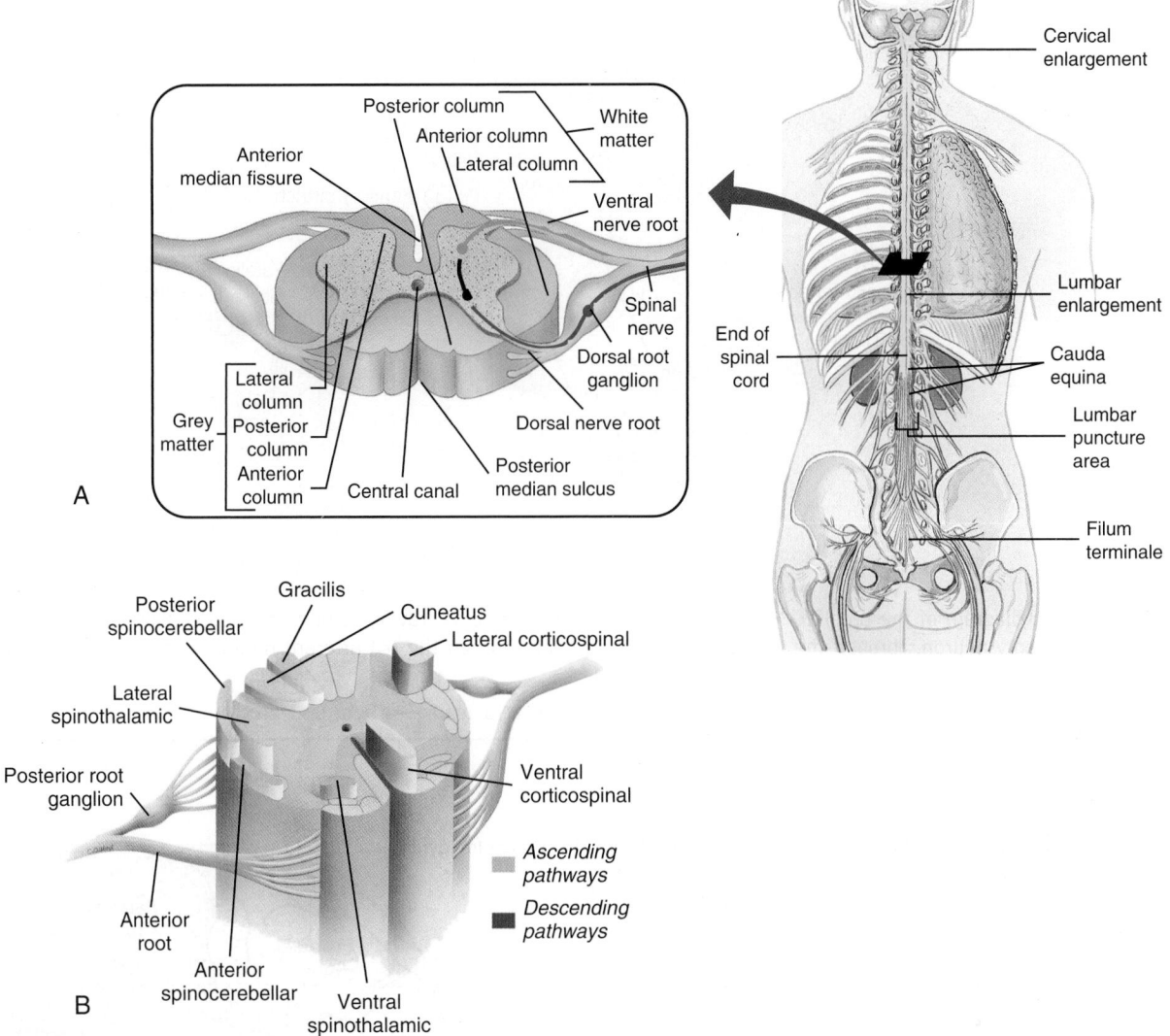

Figure 58-5 Spinal cord. **A,** Broad view of the spinal cord; *inset,* a transverse cross-section. **B,** Another cross-section of the spinal cord, showing the horns, the pathways (nerve tracts), and the roots.

Source: Adapted from Patton, K. T., & Thibodeau, G. A. (2010). *Anatomy and physiology* (7th ed., pp. 418-419, Figures 13-6 and 13-7). St. Louis: Mosby.

Descending Tracts. Descending tracts carry impulses that are responsible for muscle movement. Among the most important descending tracts are the corticobulbar and corticospinal tracts, collectively termed the *pyramidal tract.* These tracts carry volitional (voluntary) impulses from the cortex to the cranial and the peripheral nerves. Another group of descending motor tracts carries impulses from the extrapyramidal system, which includes all motor systems (except the pyramidal system) concerned with voluntary movement. It includes descending pathways originating in the brainstem, basal ganglia, and cerebellum. The motor output exits the spinal cord by way of the ventral roots of the spinal nerves.

Lower Motor Neurons. **Lower motor neurons (LMNs)** are the final common pathway through which descending motor tracts influence skeletal muscle, the effector organ for movement. The cell bodies of LMNs, which send axons to innervate the skeletal muscles of arms, trunk, and legs, are located in the anterior horn of the corresponding segments of the spinal cord (e.g.,

cervical segments contain LMNs for the arms). LMNs for skeletal muscles of eyes, face, mouth, and throat are located in the corresponding segments of the brainstem. These cell bodies and their axons make up the somatic motor components of the cranial nerves. LMN lesions generally cause weakness or paralysis, denervation atrophy, hyperreflexia or areflexia, and decreased muscle tone (flaccidity).

Upper Motor Neurons. **Upper motor neurons (UMNs)** are the classification of motor pathways contained completely within the CNS. They originate in the cerebral cortex and project downward. The corticobulbar tract ends in the brainstem, and the corticospinal tract descends into the spinal cord. The primary functions of UMNs include directing, influencing, and modifying reflex arcs, lower-level control centres, and motor (and some sensory) neurons (McCance & Huether, 2010). UMN lesions generally cause weakness or paralysis, disuse atrophy, hyperreflexia, and increased muscle tone (spasticity).

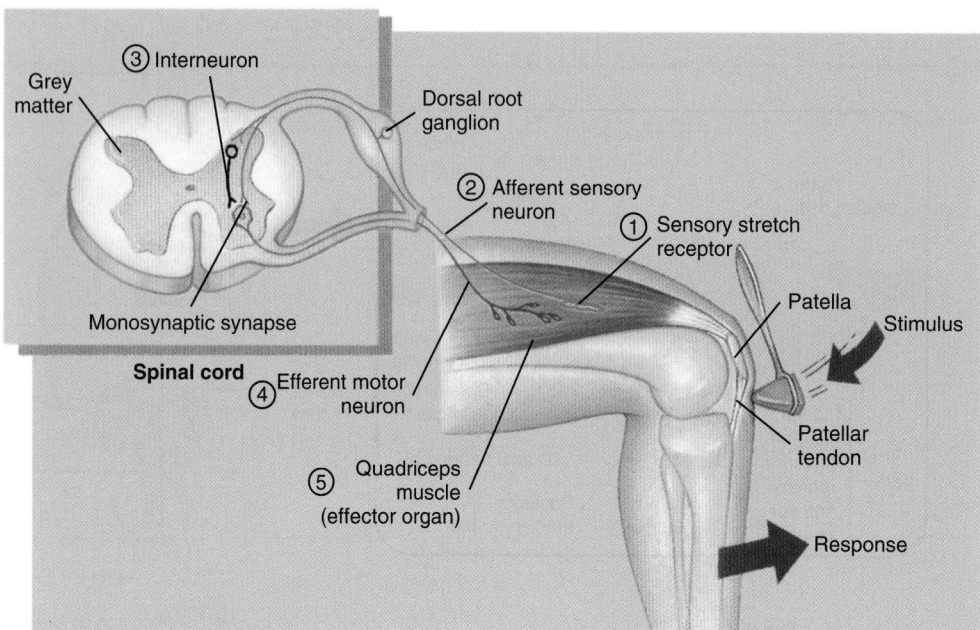

Figure 58-6 Basic diagram of the patellar "knee-jerk" reflex arc. The impulse travels through the (1) sensory stretch receptor and (2) afferent sensory neuron, through the (3) interneuron, and back through the (4) efferent motor neuron and to the (5) quadriceps muscle (effector organ).

Source: Adapted from Thibodeau, G. A., & Patton, K. T. (2008). *Structure and function of the body* (13th ed., p. 192, Figure 8-5). St. Louis: Mosby.

Reflex Arc. A **reflex** is defined as an involuntary response to a stimulus. The components of a monosynaptic reflex arc (the simplest kind of reflex arc) are a receptor organ, an afferent neuron, an effector neuron, and an effector organ (e.g., skeletal muscle). The afferent neuron synapses with the efferent neuron in the grey matter of the spinal cord. A reflex arc is shown in Figure 58-6. In more complex reflex arcs, the effector neuron is influenced by other neurons (interneurons) in addition to the afferent neuron. In the spinal cord, reflex arcs play an important role in maintaining muscle tone, which is essential for body posture.

Brain. The brain can be divided into three major components: cerebrum, brainstem, and cerebellum.

Cerebrum. The *cerebrum* is composed of the right and left cerebral hemispheres. Both hemispheres can be further divided into four major lobes: frontal, temporal, parietal, and occipital (Figure 58-7). These divisions are useful for delineating portions of the neocortex (grey matter), which makes up the outer layer of the cerebral hemispheres. Neurons in specific parts of the neocortex are essential for various highly complex and sophisticated aspects of mental functioning, such as language, memory, and appreciation of visual–spatial relationships. The frontal lobe controls higher cognitive function, memory, voluntary eye movements, voluntary motor movements, and expressive speech in Broca's area. The temporal lobe contains Wernicke's area, which is responsible for receptive speech and for integration of somatic, visual, and auditory data. The parietal lobe is composed of the sensory cortex, controlling and interpreting spatial information. Processing of visual data takes place in the occipital lobe.

The functions of the cerebrum are multiple and complex. Specific areas of the cerebral cortex are associated with specific functions. Table 58-2 summarizes the location and function of the parts of the cerebrum.

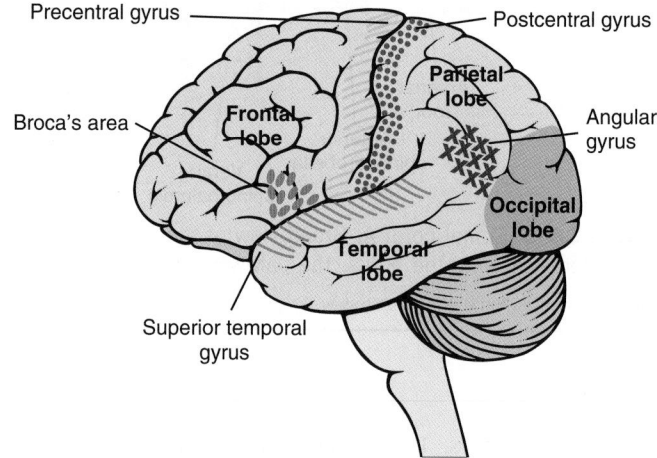

Figure 58-7 Left hemisphere of cerebrum, lateral surface, showing major lobes and areas of the brain.

The basal ganglia, the thalamus, the hypothalamus, and the limbic system are also located in the cerebrum. The basal ganglia are a group of paired structures located centrally in the cerebrum and the midbrain; most of them are on both sides of the thalamus. The function of the basal ganglia is to modulate initiation, execution, and completion of voluntary movements and automatic movements associated with skeletal muscle activity, such as swinging of the arms during walking, swallowing saliva, and blinking.

The thalamus (part of the diencephalon) lies directly above the brainstem (Figure 58-8) and is the major relay centre for sensory and other afferent (i.e., cerebellar) inputs to the cerebral cortex. The hypothalamus is located just inferior to the thalamus

Table 58-2 Location and Function of the Parts of the Cerebrum

PART	LOCATION	FUNCTION	PART	LOCATION	FUNCTION
Cortical Areas			**Language**		
Motor			• Comprehension	Wernicke's area	Integrates auditory language (understanding of spoken words)
• Primary	Precentral gyrus	Facilitates motor control and movement on the opposite side of the body	• Expression	Broca's area	Regulates verbal expression
• Supplemental	Anterior to precentral gyrus	Facilitates proximal muscle activity, including activity for stance and gait, spontaneous movement, and coordination	**Other Functions**		
			• Basal ganglia	Near lateral ventricles of both cerebral hemispheres	Control and facilitate learned and automatic movements
Sensory					
• Somatic	Postcentral gyrus	Processes sensory response from the opposite side of body	• Thalamus	Below basal ganglia	Relays sensory and motor inputs to cortex and other parts of cerebrum
• Visual	Occipital lobe	Registers visual images			
• Auditory	Superior temporal gyrus	Registers auditory inputs	• Hypothalamus	Below thalamus	Regulates endocrine and autonomic functions (e.g., feeding, sleeping, emotional and sexual responses)
• Association areas	Parietal lobe	Integrates somatic and sensory inputs			
	Posterior temporal lobe	Integrates visual and auditory inputs for language comprehension	• Limbic system	Lateral to hypothalamus	Influences affective (emotional) behaviour and basic drives such as feeding and sexual behaviour
	Anterior temporal lobe	Integrates past experiences			
	Anterior frontal lobe	Controls higher-order processes (e.g., judgement, insight, reasoning, problem solving, planning)			

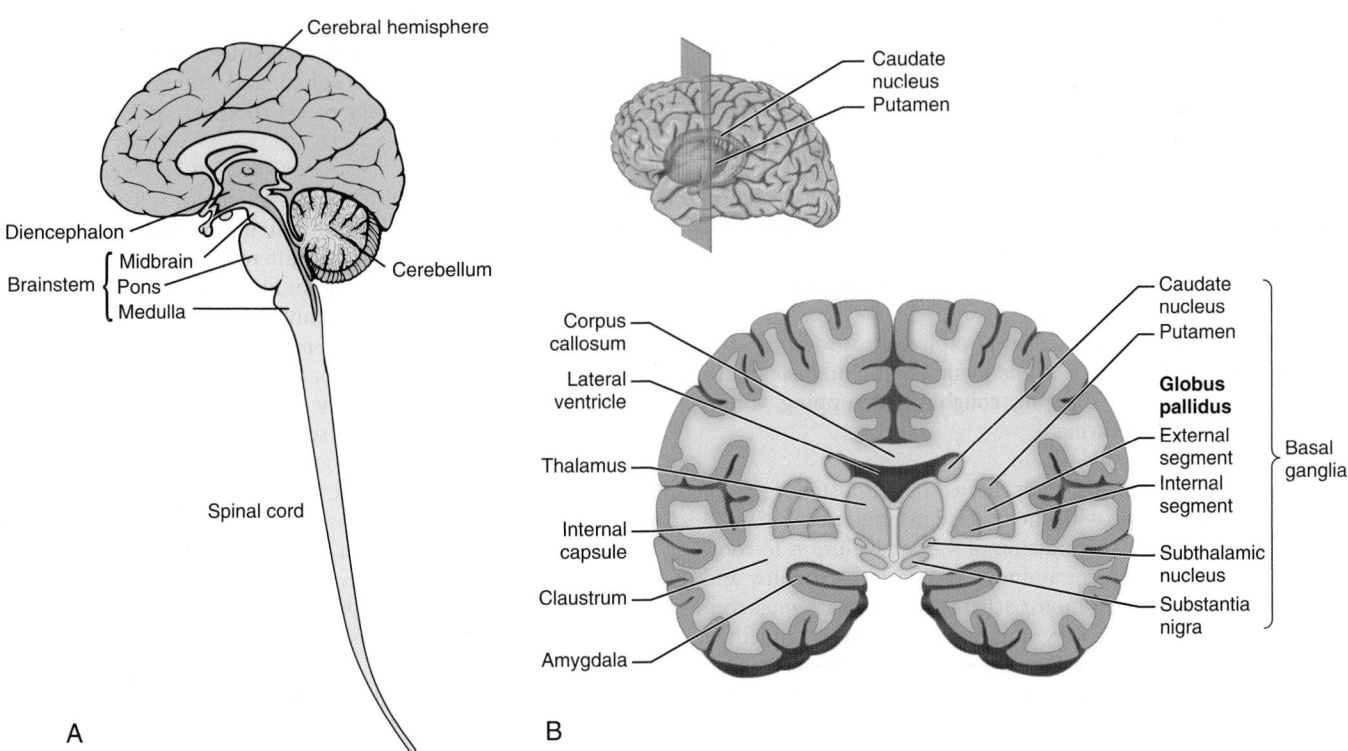

Figure 58-8 The central nervous system. **A,** Side view of major divisions. **B,** Coronal overview of the components of the basal ganglia.

Source: **B,** Redrawn from Ropper, A. H., & Brown, R. H. (2005). *Adams and Victor's principles of neurology* (8th ed.). New York: McGraw-Hill.

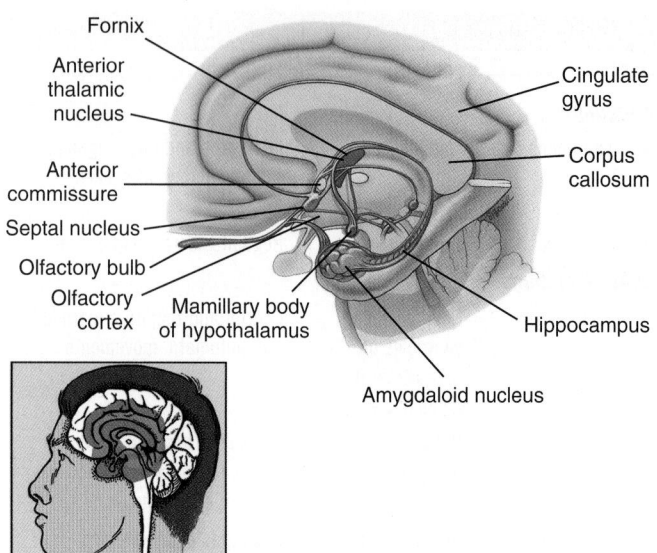

Figure 58-9 Structures of the limbic system.

Source: Adapted from Patton, K. T., & Thibodeau, G. A. (2010). *Anatomy and physiology* (7th ed., p. 436, Figure 13-22). St. Louis: Mosby.

and slightly in front of the midbrain. It regulates the ANS and the endocrine system. The limbic system is, phylogenetically, an old part of the human cerebrum. It is located near the inner surfaces of the cerebral hemispheres (Figure 58-9) and is concerned with emotion, aggression, feeding behaviour, and sexual response.

Brainstem. The *brainstem* includes the midbrain, the pons, and the medulla (see Figure 58-8). Ascending and descending fibres pass through the brainstem between the cerebrum and the cerebellum. The cell bodies, or nuclei, of cranial nerves III through XII are in the brainstem. Also located in the brainstem is the *reticular formation*, a diffusely arranged group of neurons and their axons that extends from the medulla to the thalamus and the hypothalamus. The functions of the reticular formation include relaying sensory information, influencing excitatory and inhibitory control of spinal motor neurons, and controlling vasomotor and respiratory activity. The reticular activating system is part of the reticular formation and is the regulatory system for arousal, a component of consciousness.

The vital centres concerned with respiratory, vasomotor, and cardiac function are located in the medulla. The brainstem also contains the centres for sneezing, coughing, hiccupping, vomiting, sucking, and swallowing.

Cerebellum. The cerebellum is located in the posterior part of the cranial fossa, along with the brainstem, under the occipital lobe of the cerebrum. The function of the cerebellum is to coordinate voluntary movement and to maintain trunk stability and equilibrium. It influences motor activity through its axonal connections to the motor cortex, the brainstem nuclei, and their descending pathways. To perform these functions, the cerebellum receives information from the cerebral cortex, the muscles, the joints, and the inner ear.

Ventricles and Cerebrospinal Fluid. Several supporting structures located within the CNS are important in regulating neuronal function and physical support of the brain. The ven-

tricles are four fluid-filled cavities within the brain that connect with one another and with the spinal canal. The lower portion of the fourth ventricle becomes the central canal in the lower part of the brainstem. The spinal canal is located in the centre and extends the full length of the spinal cord. Figure 58-10 depicts the ventricles and the flow of CSF in the CNS.

Cerebrospinal Fluid. **Cerebrospinal fluid (CSF)** is a clear, colourless fluid similar to blood plasma and interstitial fluid (McCance & Huether, 2010). CSF circulates within the subarachnoid space that surrounds the brain, the brainstem, and the spinal cord; provides cushioning for the brain and the spinal cord; allows fluid shifts from the cranial cavity to the spinal cavity; and carries nutrients. The formation of CSF in the choroid plexus in the ventricles involves both passive diffusion and active transport of substances. Although CSF is continually being formed, many physiological factors influence its rate of absorption and formation. The ventricles and the central canal are normally filled with an average of 135 mL of CSF.

The CSF circulates throughout the ventricles and seeps into the subarachnoid space surrounding the brain and the spinal cord. It is absorbed primarily through the *arachnoid villi* (tiny projections into the subarachnoid space), into the intradural venous sinuses, and eventually into the venous system. The analysis of CSF composition provides useful diagnostic information relating to certain nervous system diseases. CSF pressure is often measured in patients with actual or suspected intracranial diseases. Increases in intracranial pressure, indicated by increased CSF pressure, can lead to herniation of the brain and compression of vital brainstem structures. The signs marking this event are part of the herniation syndrome (see Chapter 59).

Peripheral Nervous System

The PNS includes all of the neuronal structures that lie outside the CNS. It consists of the spinal and cranial nerves, their associated ganglia (groupings of cell bodies), and portions of the ANS.

Spinal Nerves. The spinal cord is a series of spinal segments, one on top of another. In addition to the cell bodies, each segment contains a pair of dorsal (afferent) sensory nerve fibres or roots and ventral (efferent) motor fibres or roots, which innervate a specific region of neck, trunk, or limbs. This combined motor–sensory nerve is called a *spinal nerve* (Figure 58-11). The cell bodies of the voluntary motor system are located in the anterior horn of the spinal cord grey matter. The cell bodies of the autonomic (involuntary) motor system are located in the anterolateral portion of spinal cord grey matter. The cell bodies of sensory fibres are located in the dorsal root ganglia just outside the spinal cord. On exiting the spinal column, each spinal nerve divides into ventral and dorsal rami, a collection of motor and sensory fibres that eventually extend to peripheral structures (e.g., skin, muscles, viscera). The sympathetic ganglia are attached to the ventral rami of the spinal nerves by grey and white rami communicantes.

A **dermatome** is the area of skin innervated by the sensory fibres of a single dorsal root of a spinal nerve. The locations of dermatomes indicate the general pattern of somatic sensory innervation by spinal segments. A *myotome* is a muscle group innervated by the primary motor neurons of a single ventral root. The dermatomes and myotomes of a given spinal segment

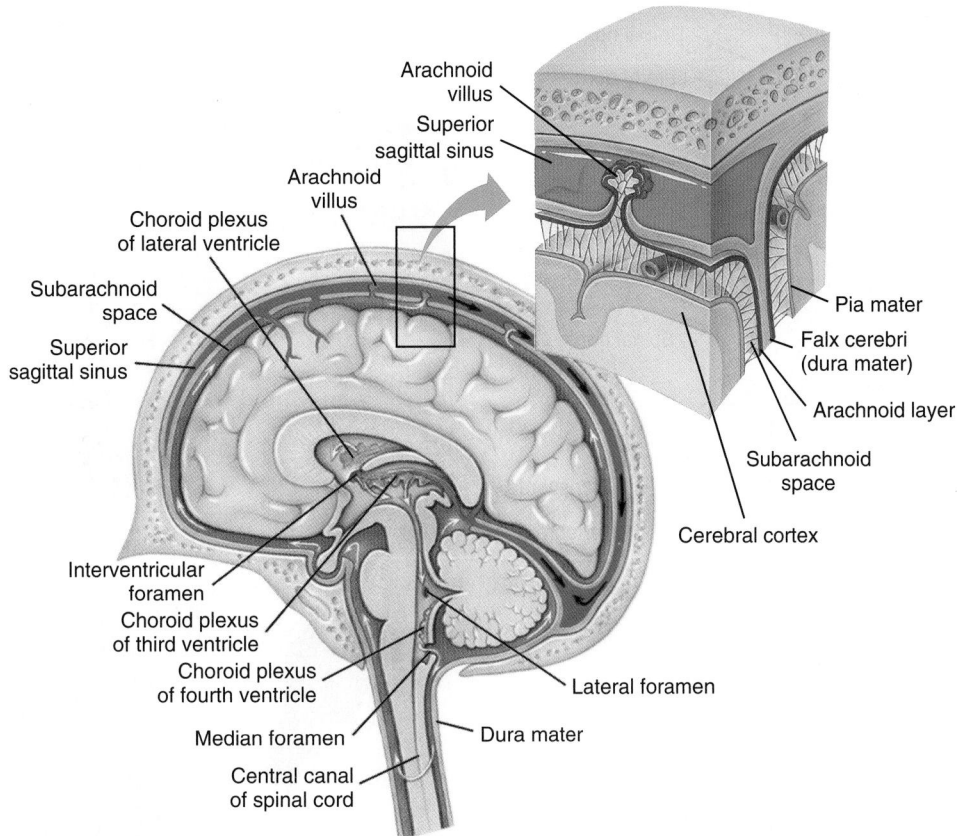

Figure 58-10 Flow of cerebrospinal fluid (CSF). The fluid produced by filtration of blood by the choroid plexus of each ventricle flows inferiorly through the lateral ventricles, the interventricular foramen, the third ventricle, the cerebral aqueduct, the fourth ventricle, and the subarachnoid space and to the blood.

Source: Adapted from Patton, K. T., & Thibodeau, G. A. (2010). *Anatomy and physiology* (7th ed., p. 417, Figure 13-5). St. Louis: Mosby.

overlap with those of adjacent segments because of the development of ascending and descending collateral branches of nerve fibres.

Cranial Nerves. The **cranial nerves (CNs)** are the 12 paired nerves composed of cell bodies with fibres that exit from the cranial cavity. Unlike the spinal nerves, which always have both afferent sensory and efferent motor fibres, some cranial nerves have only afferent and some only efferent fibres; others have both. Table 58-3 summarizes the motor and sensory components of the cranial nerves. Figure 58-12 shows the position of the cranial nerves in relation to the brain and the spinal cord. Just as the cell bodies of the spinal nerves are located in specific segments of the spinal cord, the cell bodies (nuclei) of the cranial nerves are located in specific segments of the brain. Exceptions are the nuclei of the olfactory and optic nerves. The primary cell bodies of the olfactory nerve are located in the nasal epithelium, and those of the optic nerve are in the retina.

Autonomic Nervous System. The **autonomic nervous system (ANS)** governs involuntary functions of cardiac muscle, smooth (involuntary) muscle, and glands.

The ANS is divided into two components, sympathetic and parasympathetic, that are anatomically and functionally different. These two systems function together to maintain a relatively balanced internal environment. The ANS is both an efferent and an afferent system. It consists of preganglionic nerves and postganglionic nerves.

The preganglionic cell bodies of the *sympathetic nervous system* (SNS) are located in spinal segments T1 through L2. The sympathetic ganglia, which contain the cell bodies of the postganglionic neurons, lie close to the spinal column, along the vertebral bodies in the rami communicantes. These ganglia and the connecting nerves are called the *paravertebral chain*. The major neurotransmitter released by the postganglionic fibres of the SNS is norepinephrine, and the neurotransmitter released by the preganglionic fibres is acetylcholine.

In contrast, the preganglionic cell bodies of the *parasympathetic nervous system* (PSNS) are located in the brainstem and in the sacral spinal segments (S2 through S4). The parasympathetic ganglia are located in or near the structures that they innervate. Acetylcholine is the neurotransmitter released at both preganglionic and postganglionic nerve endings.

The ANS provides dual and often reciprocal innervation to many structures. For example, the SNS increases the rate and force of the heart contraction, and the PSNS decreases the rate and force. The SNS dilates bronchi and bronchioles of the lungs, and the PSNS constricts them. Some structures are innervated by only one system (e.g., the hair follicles and the sweat glands are innervated only by the SNS). Table 58-4 lists the effects of the SNS and PSNS.

The result of SNS stimulation is activation of mechanisms required for the "fight or flight" response that occurs throughout

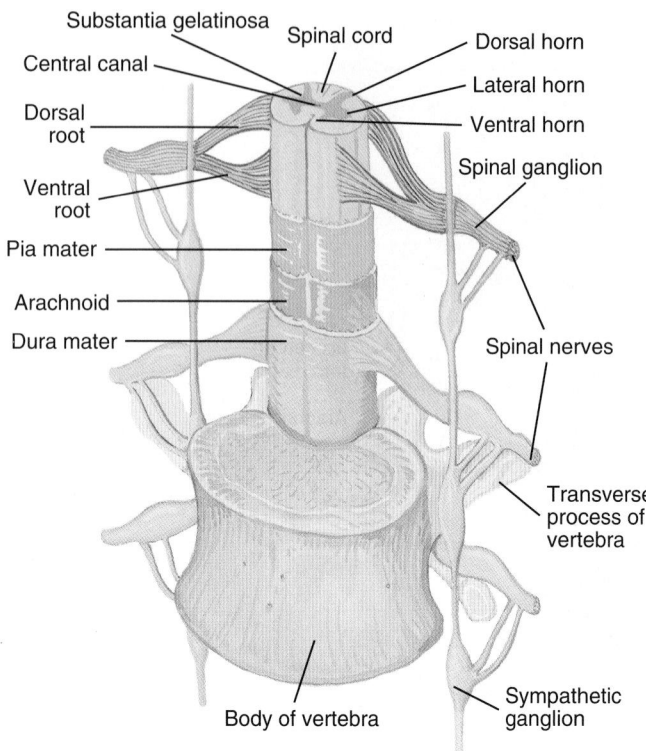

Figure 58-11 Illustration of a cross-section of spinal cord, showing attachments of spinal nerves and coverings of the spinal cord.

Source: Adapted from Thibodeau, G. A., & Patton, K. T. (2008). *Structure and function of the body* (13th ed., p. 205, Figure 8-13). St. Louis: Mosby.

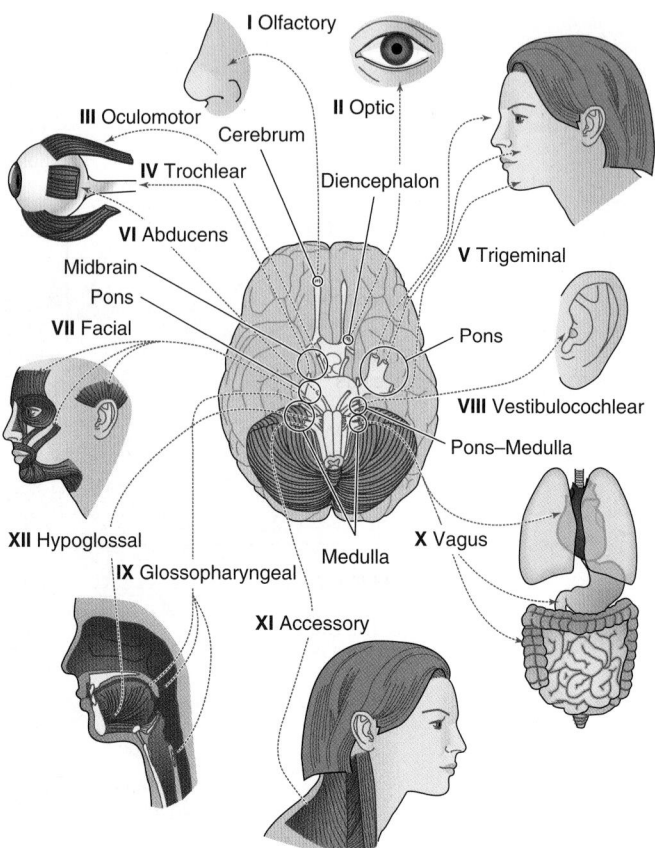

Figure 58-12 The cranial nerves are numbered from anterior to posterior, according to the order in which they leave the brain.

Source: Redrawn from McCance, K. L., & Huether, S. E. (2010). *Pathophysiology: The biologic basis for disease in adults and children* (6th ed., p. 466, Figure 14-23). St. Louis: Mosby.

the body. In contrast, the PSNS is geared to act in localized and discrete regions. It serves to conserve and restore the energy stores of the body.

Cerebral Circulation

Knowledge of the distribution of the major arteries of the brain and the area supplied is essential for understanding and evaluating the signs and symptoms of cerebrovascular disease and trauma. The blood supply of the brain arises from the internal carotid arteries (anterior circulation) and the vertebral arteries (posterior circulation), which are depicted in Figure 58-13.

Each internal carotid artery supplies the ipsilateral hemisphere, whereas the basilar artery, formed by the junction of the two vertebral arteries, supplies structures within the posterior fossa (cerebellum and brainstem). The *circle of Willis* arises from the basilar artery and the two internal carotid arteries (Figure 58-14). This vascular circle may act as a safety valve when differential pressures are present in these arteries. It also may function as an anastomotic pathway when a major artery on one side of the brain becomes occluded. In general, the two anterior cerebral arteries supply the medial portion of the frontal lobes. The two middle cerebral arteries supply the outer portions of the frontal, parietal, and superior temporal lobes. The two posterior cerebral arteries supply the medial portions of the occipital and inferior temporal lobes. Figure 58-13 shows the major cerebral arteries. Venous blood drains from the brain through the dural sinuses, which form channels that drain into the two jugular veins.

Blood–Brain Barrier. The **blood–brain barrier** is a physiological barrier between blood capillaries and brain tissue. It is composed of cellular structures that selectively inhibit certain substances in the blood from entering the interstitial spaces of the brain or the CSF (McCance & Huether, 2010). Some substances that normally pass readily into most tissues are prevented from entering brain tissue. This barrier protects the brain from certain potentially harmful agents, while allowing nutrients and gases to enter. Because the blood–brain barrier affects the penetration of drugs, only certain ones can enter the CNS from the bloodstream. Lipid-soluble compounds enter the brain easily, whereas water-soluble and ionized drugs enter the brain and spinal cord slowly. Damage to the blood–brain barrier results in the penetration of drugs and other substances into brain tissue.

Protective Structures

Meninges. The **meninges** are three layers of protective membranes that surround the brain and the spinal cord. The thick *dura mater* forms the outermost layer, and the *arachnoid layer* and *pia mater* are the next two layers. The *falx cerebri* is a fold of the dura that separates the two cerebral hemispheres and prevents expansion of brain tissue in situations such as the presence of a rapidly growing tumour or acute hemorrhage. The expanding brain must

Table 58-3 Cranial Nerves

NERVE	NAME	CONNECTION WITH BRAIN	PATH OF INTERVENTION
I	Olfactory nerves and tract	Anterior ventral cerebrum	*Sensory:* from olfactory epithelium of superior nasal cavity
II	Optic nerve	Lateral geniculate body of the thalamus	*Sensory:* from retina of eyes
III	Oculomotor nerve	Midbrain	*Motor:* to four eye-movement muscles and levator palpebrae *Parasympathetic:* smooth muscle in eyeball
IV	Trochlear nerve	Midbrain	*Motor:* to one eye-movement muscle, the superior oblique
V	Trigeminal nerve		
	• Ophthalmic branch	Pons	*Sensory:* from forehead, eye, superior nasal cavity
	• Maxillary branch	Pons	*Sensory:* from inferior nasal cavity, face, upper teeth, mucosa of superior mouth
	• Mandibular branch	Pons	*Sensory:* from surfaces of jaw, lower teeth, mucosa of lower mouth, and anterior tongue *Motor:* to muscles of mastication
VI	Abducens nerve	Pons	*Motor:* to one eye-movement muscle, the lateral rectus
VII	Facial nerve	Junction of pons and medulla	*Motor:* to facial muscles of expression and cheek muscle, the buccinator *Sensory:* taste from anterior two thirds of tongue
VIII	Vestibulocochlear nerve		
	• Vestibular branch	Junction of pons and medulla	*Sensory:* from equilibrium sensory organ, the vestibular apparatus
	• Cochlear branch	Junction of pons and medulla	*Sensory:* from auditory sensory organ, the cochlea
IX	Glossopharyngeal nerve	Medulla	*Sensory:* from pharynx and posterior tongue, including taste *Motor:* superior pharyngeal muscles
X	Vagus nerve	Medulla	*Sensory:* much of viscera of thorax and abdomen *Motor:* larynx and middle and inferior pharyngeal muscles *Parasympathetic:* heart, lungs, most of digestive system
XI	Accessory nerve	Medulla and superior spinal segments	*Motor:* to several neck muscles, sternocleidomastoid and trapezius
XII	Hypoglossal nerve	Medulla	*Motor:* to intrinsic and extrinsic muscles of tongue

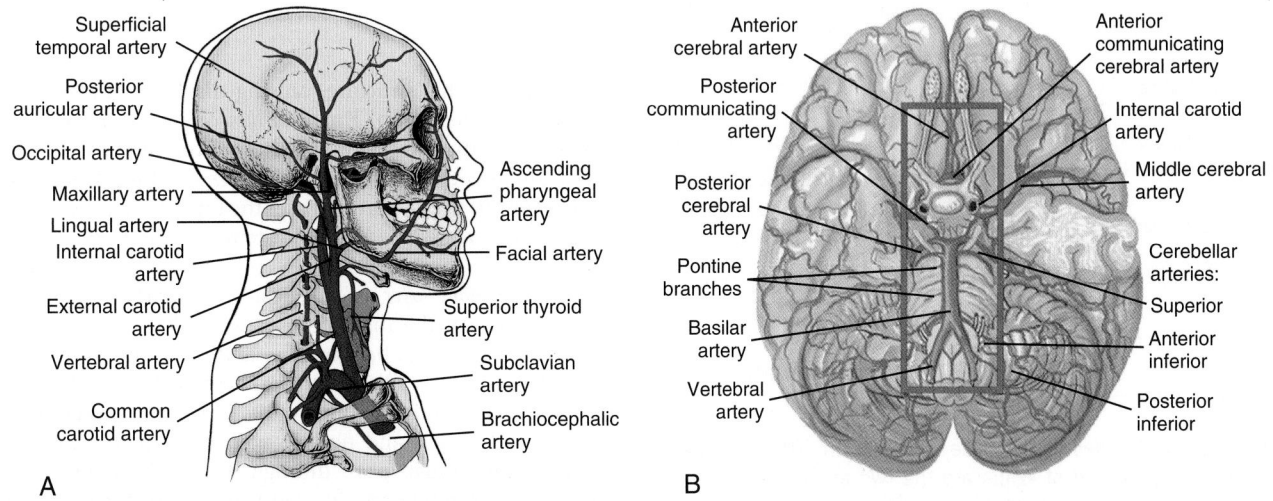

Figure 58-13 Arteries of the head and neck. **A,** Right lateral view: brachiocephalic artery, right common carotid artery, right subclavian artery, and their branches. The major arteries to the head are the common carotid and vertebral arteries. **B,** Inferior view of the brain, showing the vertebral, basilar, and internal carotid arteries and their branches.

Source: Adapted from Patton, K. T., & Thibodeau, G. A. (2010). *Anatomy and physiology* (7th ed., p. 633, Figure 18-19). St. Louis: Mosby.

Table 58-4 Effect of Sympathetic and Parasympathetic Nervous Systems

VISCERAL EFFECTOR	EFFECT OF SYMPATHETIC NERVOUS SYSTEM*	EFFECT OF PARASYMPATHETIC NERVOUS SYSTEM†
Heart	Increase in rate and strength of heartbeat (β-receptors)	Decrease in rate and strength of heartbeat
Smooth muscle of blood vessels		
• Skin blood vessels	Constriction (α-receptors)	No effect
• Skeletal muscle blood vessels	Dilation (β-receptors)	No effect
• Coronary blood vessels	Dilation (β-receptors), constriction (α-receptors)	Dilation (β-receptors)
• Abdominal blood vessels	Constriction (α-receptors)	No effect
• Blood vessels of external genitals	Ejaculation (contraction of smooth muscle in male ducts [e.g., epididymis, ductus deferens])	Dilation of blood vessels, causing penile erection
Smooth muscle of hollow organs and sphincters		
• Bronchi	Dilation (β-receptors)	Constriction (α-receptors)
• Digestive tract, except sphincters	Decrease in rate of peristalsis (β-receptors)	Increase in rate of peristalsis
• Sphincters of digestive tract	Contraction (α-receptors)	Relaxation
• Urinary bladder	Relaxation (β-receptors)	Contraction
• Urinary sphincters	Contraction (α-receptors)	Relaxation
Eye		
• Iris	Contraction of radial muscle, dilation of pupil	Contraction of circular muscle, constriction of pupil
• Ciliary	Relaxation, accommodation for far vision	Contraction, accommodation for near vision
Hairs (pilomotor muscles)	Contraction producing goose pimples or piloerection (α-receptors)	No effect
Glands		
• Sweat	Increase in sweat (neurotransmitter, acetylcholine)	No effect
• Digestive (e.g., salivary, gastric)	Decrease in secretion of saliva; not known for others	Increase in secretion of saliva and gastric HCl acid
• Pancreas, including islets	Decrease in secretion	Increase in secretion of pancreatic juice and insulin
• Liver	Increase in glycogenolysis (β-receptors), increase in blood glucose level	No effect
Adrenal medulla‡	Increase in epinephrine secretion	No effect

Source: Adapted from Patton, K. T., & Thibodeau, G. A. (2010). *Anatomy and physiology* (7th ed., p. 483, Table 14-6). St. Louis: Mosby.

*Neurotransmitter is norepinephrine unless otherwise stated.

†Neurotransmitter is acetylcholine unless otherwise stated.

‡Sympathetic preganglionic axons terminate in contact with secreting cells of the adrenal medulla. Thus the adrenal medulla functions as what is sometimes called a *giant sympathetic postganglionic neuron.*

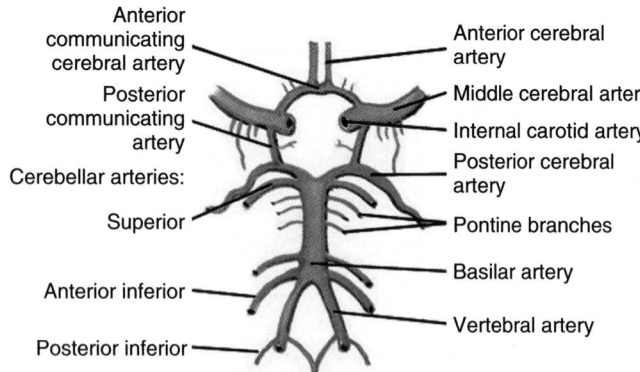

Figure 58-14 Arteries at the base of the brain. The arteries that compose the circle of Willis are the two anterior cerebral arteries, joined to each other by the anterior communicating cerebral artery and to the posterior cerebral arteries by the posterior communicating arteries.

Source: Adapted from Patton, K. T., & Thibodeau, G. A. (2010). *Anatomy and physiology* (7th ed., p. 634, Figure 18-20). St. Louis: Mosby.

squeeze under this structure, causing displacement toward the side opposite the lesion. The *tentorium cerebelli* is a fold of dura that separates the cerebral hemispheres from the posterior fossa, which contains the brainstem and the cerebellum. Expansion of mass lesions in the cerebrum forces the brain to herniate through the opening created by the brainstem. This is termed *tentorial herniation* (see Chapter 59).

The *arachnoid layer* is a delicate, impermeable membrane that lies between the thick dura mater and the pia mater. The *subarachnoid space* lies between the arachnoid layer and the pia mater. This space is filled with CSF. Structures passing to and from the brain and the skull or its foramina (holes through which blood vessels and nerves enter and exit the intracranial compartment) must pass through the subarachnoid space. Therefore, all cerebral arteries and veins lie in this space, as do the cranial nerves. A larger subarachnoid space is present in the region of the third and fourth lumbar vertebrae, which is the area penetrated to obtain CSF during a lumbar puncture. (The spinal cord itself ends between the first and second lumbar vertebrae.)

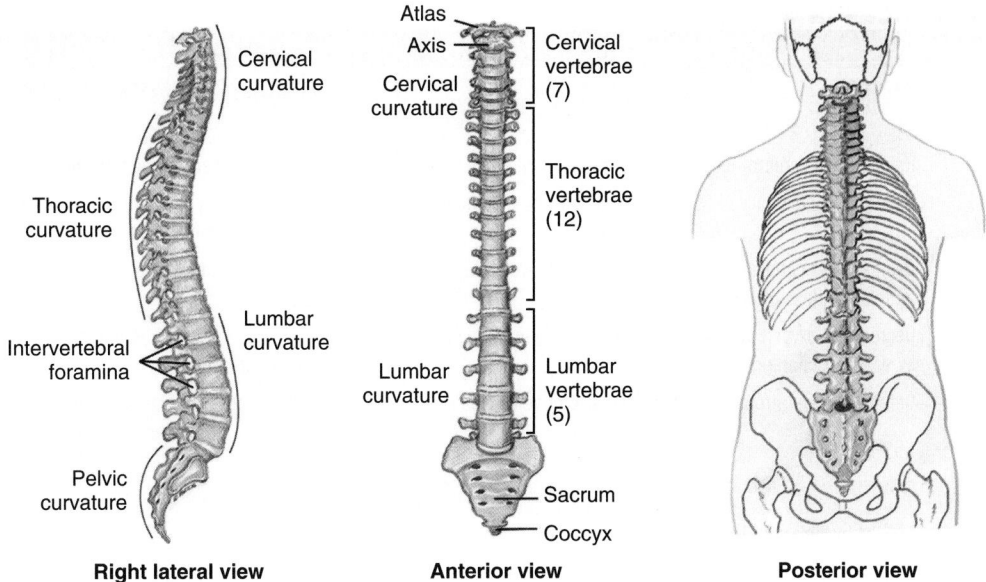

Figure 58-15 Vertebral column (three views).

Source: Adapted from Patton, K. T., & Thibodeau, G. A. (2010). *Anatomy and physiology* (7th ed., p. 237, Figure 8-13). St. Louis: Mosby.

Skull. The bony skull protects the brain from external trauma. It is composed of 8 cranial bones and 14 facial bones. The structure of the skull cavity accounts for the physiology of head injuries (see Chapter 59). Although the top and the sides of the inside of the skull are relatively smooth, the bottom surface is uneven; it has many ridges, prominences, and foramina (holes through which blood vessels and nerves enter the intracranial vault). The largest hole is the foramen magnum, through which the brainstem extends to the spinal cord. This foramen is the only major space for the expansion of brain contents when increased intracranial pressure occurs.

Vertebral Column. The vertebral column protects the spinal cord, supports the head, and provides flexibility. The vertebral column is made up of 33 individual vertebrae: 7 cervical, 12 thoracic, 5 lumbar, 5 sacral (fused into one, the sacrum), and 4 coccygeal (fused into one, the coccyx). Each vertebra has a central opening through which the spinal cord passes. The vertebrae are held together by a series of ligaments. Intervertebral discs occupy the spaces between vertebrae. Figure 58-15 depicts the vertebral column in relation to the trunk.

AGE-RELATED CONSIDERATIONS: EFFECTS OF AGING ON THE NERVOUS SYSTEM

Several parts of the nervous system are affected by aging. In the CNS, neurons are lost in certain areas of the brainstem, the cerebellum, and the cerebral cortex. This loss is a gradual process that begins in early adulthood. With loss of neurons, the ventricles widen. Brain weight also decreases by 10 to 15% between the second and ninth decades of life (Porter & Kaplan, 2011). There is compensatory lengthening and an increase in the number of dendrites of the remaining nerve cells as nerve cells deteriorate and die.

Cerebral blood flow decreases, and CSF production declines. Changes in neurotransmitters of the dopaminergic and cholinergic systems result in decreasing amounts of acetylcholine, serotonin, and catecholamines.

In the PNS, degenerative changes in myelin cause a decrease in nerve conduction. Coordinated neuromuscular activity, such as the maintenance of blood pressure in response to changing from a lying to a standing position, is altered with aging. As a result, older adults are more vulnerable to problems with orthostatic hypotension. Similarly, coordination of neuromuscular activity to maintain body temperature is also less efficient with aging. Older adults are less able to adapt to extremes in environmental temperature and are more vulnerable to both hypothermia and hyperthermia.

In general, the intellectual performance of older adults who do not have brain dysfunction remains fairly consistent. A slowdown in central processing may result in needing longer to perform certain tasks. Sensory changes, including decreases in taste and smell perception, may result in decreased dietary intake in older adults. Changes in pain perception may occur. Decline in visual and auditory acuity can result in perceptual challenges. Problems with balance and coordination can increase older adults' risk for falls and subsequent fractures.

Changes in assessment findings result from age-related alterations in the various components of the nervous system. Age-related changes in the nervous system and differences in assessment findings are presented in Table 58-5.

Assessment of the Nervous System

Because of the complexity of the nervous system, neurological assessment is challenging and lengthy. Involving family members in the assessment is critical because patients with neurological problems often experience cognitive, emotional, and

AGE-RELATED DIFFERENCES IN ASSESSMENT

Table 58-5 Nervous System

COMPONENT	CHANGES	DIFFERENCES IN ASSESSMENT FINDINGS
Central Nervous System		
Brain	Reduction in cerebral blood flow and metabolism	Alterations in certain mental functions
	Decrease in efficiency of temperature-regulating mechanism	Decrease in body temperature, impairment of ability to adapt to environmental temperature
	Decrease in neurotransmitter volume, disruption in integration as result of loss of neurons	Conduction of nerve impulses slowed, response time slowed
	Decrease in oxygen supply, changes in basal ganglia caused by vascular changes	Changes in gait and ambulation; diminished kinaesthetic sense
	Cerebral tissue atrophy and increased size of ventricles	Altered balance, vertigo, syncope; increased postural hypotension; decreased proprioception; decreased sensation
Peripheral Nervous System		
Cranial and spinal nerves	Loss of myelin and increase in conduction time in some nerves	Decrease in reaction time in specific nerves
	Cellular degeneration, death of neurons	Decrease in speed and intensity of neuronal reflexes
Functional Divisions		
Motor	Decrease in muscle bulk	Diminished strength and agility
	Decrease in electrical activity	Increased reaction and movement time
Sensory*	Decrease in sensory receptors caused by degenerative changes and involution of fine corpuscles of nerve endings	Diminished sense of touch; inability to localize stimuli; decrease in appreciation of touch, temperature, and peripheral vibrations
	Decrease in electrical activity	Slowing of or alteration in sensory reception
	Atrophy of taste buds	Signs of malnutrition, weight loss
	Degeneration and loss of fibres in olfactory bulb	Diminished sense of smell
	Degenerative changes in nerve cells in vestibular system of inner ear, cerebellum, and proprioceptive pathways in nervous system	Poor ability to maintain balance, widened gait
Reflexes	Possible decrease in deep tendon reflexes	Below-average reflex score
	Decrease in sensory conduction velocity as result of myelin sheath degeneration	Sluggish reflexes, lengthened reaction time
Reticular Formation		
Reticular activating system	Modification of hypothalamic function, reduction in stage IV sleep	Increase in frequency of spontaneous awakening, together with tiredness, interrupted sleep, insomnia
Autonomic Nervous System		
SNS and PSNS	Morphological changes in features of ganglia, slowing of ANS responses	Orthostatic hypotension, systolic hypertension

*Specific changes related to the eye and the ear are in Chapter 24.
ANS, autonomic nervous system; *PSNS*, parasympathetic nervous system; *SNS*, sympathetic nervous system.

motivational deficits. Careful observation is an especially important nursing skill because many neurological changes are subtle.

Subjective Data

The history should begin with an open-ended and indirect inquiry that allows the patient to describe his or her chief complaint and current health (Black & Hawks, 2009). Three points should be considered in documenting the history of a patient with neurological problems. First, questions about symptoms should be open-ended. It is better to ask "What is your headache like?" or "Is there anything about your right side that bothers you?" rather than to ask leading questions such as "Is your headache throbbing?" or "Are you weak on the right side?" Second, the mode of onset and the course of the illness are especially important aspects of the history. The nature of a neurological disease process can often be described by these facts alone, and the nurse should obtain all pertinent data in the history of the present illness, especially data related to the characteristics and progression of the symptoms. Third, because many neurological diseases affect a patient's mental functioning, mental status must be assessed accurately before the nurse assumes that the history is factual. If the patient is not considered a reliable historian, the history should be obtained from a person who has first-hand knowledge of the patient's problems and complaints.

In many cases, a health history cannot be obtained, and the nurse must proceed with only objective data.

Important Health Information

Past Health History. The health history helps guide the approach for the neurological examination; that is, it can direct the nurse toward the parts of the nervous system that must be closely assessed. If the patient's primary complaint is dizziness, the examination may be focused on visual, vestibular, and cerebellar functions rather than on somatic motor and sensory functions.

Medications. Special attention should be given to obtaining a careful medication history, especially the use of sedatives, narcotics, tranquilizers, mood-elevating drugs, over-the-counter medications, and herbal remedies. Many drugs can cause adverse neurological effects.

Surgery or Other Treatments. The nurse should inquire about any surgery involving any part of the nervous system, such as the head, the spine, or the sensory organs. If a patient has had surgery, the date, the cause, the procedure, the recovery, and the current status should be investigated.

The perinatal history may reveal exposure to toxic agents such as viruses, alcohol, tobacco, drugs, and radiation, which are known to adversely influence the development of the nervous system. The history may reveal a difficult labour and delivery, which can cause brain damage as a result of hypoxia, forceps delivery, or Rh incompatibility.

Growth and developmental history can be important in ascertaining whether nervous system dysfunction was present at an early age. The nurse should specifically inquire about major developmental tasks such as walking and talking. Successes at school or identified problems in an educational setting are other important developmental data to gather. Often, this information is not available when an older patient is interviewed.

Health Status. Key questions to ask a patient with a neurological problem are presented in Table 58-6.

General Health Practices. The nurse should ask about the patient's general health practices that may affect the nervous system, such as substance use and smoking, nutrition, participation in physical and recreational activities, use of seat belts and helmets, and control of hypertension. The nurse should ask about previous hospitalizations for neurological problems. A careful family history may determine whether the neurological problem has a hereditary or congenital background.

If the patient has an existing neurological problem, the nurse should ask about how it affects daily living and the ability to carry out self-care. After a careful review of information, and with the patient's permission, the nurse may find it helpful to ask someone who knows the patient well whether any mental or physical changes have been noticed in the patient. The patient with a neurological problem may not be aware of it or may be unable to provide enough specific data to aid in the diagnosis.

Nutritional Problems. Neurological problems can result in inadequate nutrition. Problems related to chewing, swallowing, facial nerve paralysis, and muscle coordination could make it difficult for affected patients to ingest adequate nutrients. Also, certain vitamins such as thiamine (B_1), niacin, and pyridoxine (B_6) are essential for the maintenance and health of the CNS.

Deficiencies in one or more of these vitamins could result in such nonspecific complaints as depression, apathy, neuritis, weakness, mental confusion, and irritability. Risk for cobalamin (vitamin B_{12}) deficiency is higher in older adults because they may have problems with vitamin absorption. Untreated, this deficiency may cause a decline in mental function (Werder, 2010).

Bowel and Bladder Problems. Bowel and bladder problems are often associated with neurological problems, such as stroke, head injury, spinal cord injury, multiple sclerosis, and dementia. To plan appropriate interventions, it is important to determine whether the bowel or bladder problem was present before or after the neurological event. Incontinence of urine and feces and urinary retention are the most common elimination problems associated with a neurological problem. For example, nerve root compression leads to a sudden onset of incontinence. The details of the problem—such as number of episodes, accompanying sensations or lack of sensations, and measures taken to control the problem—must be documented carefully.

Motor Problems. Many neurological disorders can cause problems in the patient's mobility, strength, and coordination. These problems can result in changes in the patient's usual activity and exercise patterns. Falls can also result from such problems. Many aspects of daily living, such as getting out of a bed or chair, ambulating, preparing meals, and performing personal hygiene, can be affected and should be assessed. The ability to perform fine motor tasks may be affected, which increases the possibility of personal injury.

Sleep Problems. Sleep pattern disruptions can be both a cause of and a response to many neurologically related concerns. Discomfort from pain and inability to move and change to a position of comfort because of muscle weakness and paralysis could interfere with sound sleep. Hallucinations resulting from dementia or drugs can also interrupt sleep. The nurse should carefully document the sleep problem and the patient's methods of dealing with the problem.

Cognition and Sensory Problems. Because the nervous system controls cognition and sensory integration, many neurological disorders affect these functions. The nurse should assess orientation, memory, language, calculation ability, problem-solving ability, insight, and judgement. A structured mental status questionnaire is often used to evaluate these functions and provide baseline data.

Information about sensory changes related to hearing, sight, and touch should be sought. The patient should be questioned about problems with vertigo and sensitivity to heat and cold.

Ability to both use and understand language is a cognitive function that the nurse should assess. Appropriateness of responses is a useful indicator of cognitive and perceptual ability, but it is culturally determined.

Pain is a common event associated with many health problems. Pain is often the reason why patients seek health care. A patient's pain should be assessed carefully (see Chapter 10).

Emotional Problems. Neurological disease can drastically alter control over one's life and create dependency on others for daily needs. A patient's physical appearance and emotional control can be affected. The nurse should ask about the patient's evaluation of self-worth, perception of abilities, body image, and

HEALTH HISTORY

Table 58-6 Nervous System: Questions for Obtaining Subjective Data

Headaches

- Any unusually frequent or severe headaches?
- When did this start? How often does this happen?
- Show me where you feel the pain in your head.
- What do you think the headaches are caused by?

Head Injury

- Please describe any head injuries you have had.
- Which part of your head was injured?
- Did you lose consciousness? For how long?

Dizziness or Vertigo

- Have you ever felt light-headed or faint?
- When does this feeling occur? Do activity or change in position bring this on?
- Do you ever feel something called *vertigo* (a spinning sensation)? Does the room spin (objective vertigo)? Do you feel you are spinning (subjective vertigo)?

Seizures

- Have you ever had seizures or convulsions? When did they start? How often did they occur?
- When a seizure starts, do you have any warning? What do you experience?
- Where in your body do the seizures begin? On one side or both? Do they travel through your body? Are your muscles tense or limp?
- Are there other signs that go along with the seizures (loss of consciousness, colour change in face or lips, eyelid fluttering, eye-rolling, lip smacking, or incontinence)?
- After the seizure, are you told that you fall asleep or experience confusion, weakness, headache, or muscle ache?
- What seems to bring on the seizures (activity, discontinuing medications, fatigue, stress)?
- Are you taking medication for the seizures?
- How have the seizures affected your daily life?

Tremors

- Have you experienced any shaking or tremors in the hands or the face? When did these start?
- Are the tremors worse with anxiety? With deliberate movement? With rest?
- Are the tremors better with rest? With activity? With alcohol?
- Do the tremors affect your daily activity?

Weakness

- Do you have any weakness or problem moving any body part? Is this generalized or local?
- Does this occur with any particular movement? (Example: Difficulty getting out of a chair may signal proximal or large muscle weakness, whereas distal or small muscle weakness makes it difficult to open a jar or write.)

Coordination

- Do you have any problems with coordination or balance when walking?
- Do you list to one side? Do you have any problems with falling? Which way? Do your legs give out from under you? Do you have any clumsy movement?

Numbness or Tingling

- Have you experienced any numbness or tingling? Does it feel like pins and needles? When did this start? Is it worse with activity?
- Show me where you feel this.

Difficulty Swallowing

- Any difficulty swallowing? Does this occur with solids or liquids?
- Have you experienced excessive saliva or drooling?

Difficulty Speaking

- Have you had any problems with forming words or with saying what you meant to say?
- When did this start? How long did it last?

Significant Past History

- Have you ever had a stroke, a spinal cord or head injury, or meningitis or encephalitis? Do you have any congenital defects? Have you had past problems with alcohol or drug use?

Environmental and Occupational Hazards

- Are you exposed to any environmental or occupational hazards such as insecticides, lead, or organic solvents?
- Are you taking any medications now, including pain medications?
- How much alcohol do you drink? Each day? Each week?
- Do you use any mood-altering drugs: marijuana, barbiturates, tranquilizers?

Source: Adapted from Jarvis, C., Browne, A. J., MacDonald-Jenkins, J., & Luctkar-Flude, M. (Eds.). (2009). *Physical examination and health assessment* (1st Canadian ed., pp. 661-663). Toronto: W. B. Saunders.

general emotional pattern in a sensitive manner. The physical sequelae of a neurological problem can seriously strain the patient's coping abilities. The nurse should determine whether coping abilities are sufficient to meet the challenges faced by the patient.

Relationship Problems. The patient should be asked whether changes resulting from a neurological problem have occurred in such roles as spouse, parent, or breadwinner. Physical impairments such as weakness and paralysis can alter or limit participation in usual roles and activities. Cognitive changes, however, can

permanently change a person's ability to maintain previous roles. These changes can dramatically affect both the patient and significant others. Dependent relationships can develop.

Sexual Problems. Because many nervous system disorders can affect sexual functioning, sexual health may be an important part of the assessment for some patients. Cerebral lesions may inhibit the desire phase or the reflex responses of the excitement phase. Brainstem and spinal cord lesions may partially or completely interrupt the connections between the brain and the effector systems necessary for intercourse.

Neuropathies and spinal cord lesions that affect sensation, especially in the erotic zones, may decrease desire. Autonomic neuropathies and lesions of the sacral cord and the cauda equina may prevent reflex activities of the sexual response. The nurse should determine whether the patient and the spouse or significant other are satisfied with their sexual activity. The use or need for alternative methods of achieving sexual satisfaction should be explored. Despite neurologically related changes in sexual functioning, many people can achieve satisfying expression of intimacy and affection.

Objective Data

Physical Examination. The standard neurological examination helps determine the presence, the location, and the nature of disease of the nervous system. In this examination, six categories of functions are assessed: mental status, function of cranial nerves, motor function, cerebellar function, sensory function, and reflex function. The choice of particular parts of the examination depends on what information is needed. If a comprehensive baseline assessment of neurological functioning is desired, all components of the examination are performed. However, if a specific problem is to be evaluated, only certain components may be assessed. For example, if a patient's primary complaint is lack of feeling in the feet, the examination may be focused only on movement and sensation of the lower limbs. Similarly, if a patient comes into the emergency department after a head injury and is unconscious, a limited examination is conducted because the patient is not able to respond to verbal instructions. The nurse should develop a systematic and consistent approach to assessment.

Mental Status. Assessment of mental status (cerebral functioning) gives an indication of how the patient is functioning. It involves determination of complex and high-level cerebral functions that are governed by many areas of the cerebral cortex. Much of the mental status examination can be conducted during the routine history and may not need to be evaluated further. For example, language and memory can be assessed when the patient is asked for details of the illness and significant past events. The patient's cultural and educational background should be taken into account when mental status is evaluated.

The components of the mental status examination are as follows:

- *General appearance and behaviour:* This component includes motor activity, body posture, dress and hygiene, facial expression, and speech.
- *Level of consciousness (LOC):* This is the most sensitive indicator of changes in neurological status (Black & Hawks, 2009). LOC concerns arousal and wakefulness and the ability to respond to the environment. The Glasgow Coma Scale is often used to assess a patient's response to stimuli (see Chapter 59).
- *Cognition:* The nurse should note the patient's orientation to time, place, person, and situation. Further assessment of memory, intellectual ability, insight, judgement, problem solving, and calculation may be warranted (see Chapter 62). The nurse should consider whether the patient's plans and goals match the patient's physical ·and mental capabilities. Problems with memory may have implications for retention of new information, and impaired judgement and insight may jeopardize the patient's safety.
- *Mood and affect:* The nurse should note restlessness, agitation, anger, depression, or euphoria and the appropriateness of these states. The nurse should also note whether the affect is appropriate for the situation.
- *Thought content:* The nurse should note the presence of illusions, hallucinations, delusions, or paranoia.

Cranial Nerves. Testing of each cranial nerve (CN) is an essential component of the neurological examination (see Table 58-3).

Olfactory Nerve. After determining that both nostrils are patent, the olfactory nerve (CN I) is tested by asking the patient to close one nostril, close both eyes, and sniff from a bottle containing coffee, spice, soap, or some other readily recognized odour. The same procedure is done for the other nostril. In general, olfaction is not tested unless the patient has some disturbance with smell. Chronic rhinitis, sinusitis, and heavy smoking can often decrease the sense of smell. Disturbance in ability to smell may be associated with a tumour involving the olfactory bulb, or it may be the result of a basilar skull fracture that has damaged the olfactory fibres as they pass through the delicate cribriform plate of the skull.

Optic Nerve. Visual fields and visual acuity are assessed to test the function of the optic nerve (CN II). Visual fields are assessed by gross confrontation. The examiner, positioned directly opposite the patient, asks the patient to close one eye, look directly at the bridge of the examiner's nose, and indicate when an object (finger, pencil tip, head of pin) presented from the periphery of each of the four visual field quadrants becomes visible (Figure 58-16). The same test is repeated for the other eye. The examiner is used as a control because both examiner and patient are sharing the same visual field. It is important to remember that the nasal side of the visual field is narrower because of the nasal bridge. Visual field defects may arise from lesions of the optic nerve, the optic chiasm, or the tracts that extend through the temporal, parietal, and occipital lobes. Visual field changes resulting from brain lesions are usually either a *hemianopsia* (one half of the visual field is affected), a *quadrantanopsia* (one fourth of the visual field is affected), or monocular.

To test visual acuity, the patient reads a Snellen chart from 6 metres away. The nurse records the number of the lowest line that the patient can read with 50% accuracy. The patient who wears glasses should wear them during testing, unless they are used only for reading. The eyes should be tested individually and together. If a Snellen chart is not available, the patient should be asked to read newsprint for a gross assessment of acuity. The distance from the patient to the newsprint required for accurate reading should be recorded. Acuity may not be testable by these means if the patient does not read English or is aphasic.

Funduscopy reveals the physical condition of the optic disc (head of the optic nerve), as well as that of the retina and the blood vessels. This procedure is routinely performed when the optic nerve is tested. Optic nerve atrophy and papilledema can be detected by this method.

Oculomotor, Trochlear, and Abducens Nerves. Because the oculomotor (CN III), trochlear (CN IV), and abducens (CN VI) nerves all help move the eye, they are tested together for what are termed *extraocular movements* (EOM). The patient is asked to follow the examiner's finger as it moves horizontally and vertically (making a cross) and diagonally (making an X; Figure 58-17). If weakness or paralysis is present in one of the eye muscles, the eyes do not move together, and the patient has a *disconjugate gaze*. The presence and direction of *nystagmus* (fine,

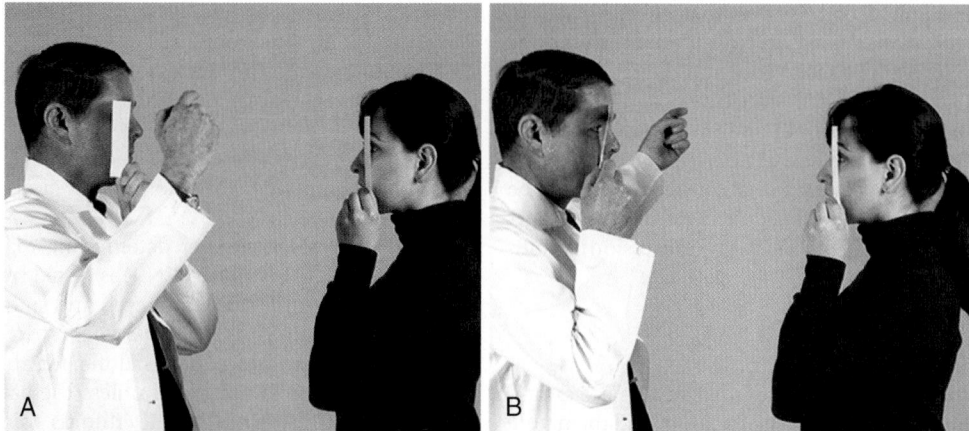

Figure 58-16 Assessment of visual fields by gross confrontation. In gross confrontation, the target is moved in a flat plane between the nurse and the patient. The nurse compares his monocular field with that of that patient.

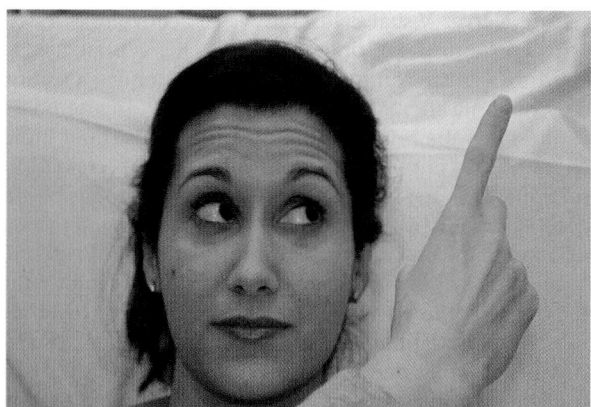

Figure 58-17 Nurse checking extraocular movement. Normally, both eyes move together. Eye movements should be smooth and coordinated.

rapid jerking movements of the eyes) are observed at this time, even though this condition most often indicates vestibulocerebellar problems.

Other functions of the oculomotor nerve are tested by checking for pupillary constriction and for *convergence* (eyes turning inward) and *accommodation* (pupils constricting with near vision). To test pupillary constriction, the examiner shines a light into the pupil of one eye and looks for ipsilateral constriction of the same pupil and contralateral (consensual) constriction of the opposite eye. The size and shape of the pupils are also noted. For this reflex to occur, the optic nerve must be intact. Testing for papillary constriction is an important component of the neurological assessment of patients at risk for herniation syndrome (see Chapter 59). Because the oculomotor nerve exits at the top of the brainstem at the tentorial notch, it can be easily compressed by expanding mass lesions in the cerebral hemispheres. The result is that the pupil does not constrict in response to light; it may become dilated because the sympathetic input to the pupil acts unopposed. To test convergence and accommodation, the patient focuses on the examiner's finger as it moves toward the patient's nose. Another function of the oculomotor nerve is to keep the eyelid open. Damage to the nerve can cause *ptosis* (drooping eyelid), pupillary abnormalities, and eye muscle weakness.

Trigeminal Nerve. To test the sensory component of the trigeminal nerve (CN V), the patient is asked to identify light touch (cotton) and pinprick in each of the three divisions (ophthalmic, maxillary, and mandibular) of the nerve on both sides of the face. The patient's eyes should be closed during this part of the examination. To test the motor component, the patient clenches the teeth, and the masseter muscles, just above the mandibular angle, are palpated. The corneal reflex test, in which CN V and CN VII are evaluated simultaneously, involves applying a cotton wisp strand to the cornea. The sensory component of this reflex (corneal sensation) is innervated by the ophthalmic division of CN V. The motor component (eye blink) is innervated by the facial nerve (CN VII). This reflex is not normally tested in patients who are awake and alert because other tests are used to evaluate these two nerves. However, for patients with a decreased level of consciousness, the corneal reflex test provides an opportunity to evaluate the integrity of the brainstem at the level of the pons because the fibres of CN V and CN VII have connections in this area.

Facial Nerve. The facial nerve (CN VII) innervates the muscles of facial expression. To test its function, the patient raises the eyebrows, closes the eyes tightly, purses the lips, draws back the corners of the mouth in an exaggerated smile, and frowns. The examiner should note any asymmetry in the facial movements because they can indicate damage to the facial nerve. Although taste discrimination of salt and sugar in the anterior two thirds of the tongue is a function of this nerve, it is not routinely tested unless a peripheral nerve lesion is suspected.

Vestibulocochlear Nerve. To test the cochlear portion of the acoustic (vestibulocochlear) nerve (CN VIII), the patient closes the eyes and indicates when a ticking watch or the rustling of the examiner's fingertips is heard as the stimulus is brought closer to the patient's ear. Each ear is tested individually, and the distance from the patient's ear to the sound source when first heard is recorded. This test identifies only gross deficits in hearing. For more precise assessment of hearing, an audiometer is used (see Chapter 23). The vestibular portion of this nerve is not routinely tested unless the patient complains of dizziness, vertigo, or unsteadiness or has auditory dysfunction. In an unconscious patient, the oculocephalic reflex (movement of the eyes when the head is briskly turned to the side) may be assessed.

Glossopharyngeal and Vagus Nerves. The glossopharyngeal and vagus nerves are tested together because both innervate the pharynx. The glossopharyngeal nerve (CN IX) is primarily sensory. In the gag reflex (bilateral contraction of the palatal muscles initiated by stroking or touching either side of the posterior pharynx or soft palate with a tongue blade), the sensory component is mediated by CN IX and the major motor component by the vagus nerve (CN X). It is important to assess the gag reflex in patients who have a decreased level of consciousness, a brainstem lesion, or a disease involving the throat musculature. If the reflex is weak or absent, the patient is in danger of aspirating food or secretions. The strength and efficiency of swallowing are important to test in these patients for the same reason. In another test for an awake, cooperative patient, the patient phonates by saying "ah" and the examiner notes the bilateral symmetry of elevation of the soft palate. Any asymmetry can indicate weakness or paralysis. To assess swallowing, the examiner's hands are held lightly on either side of the patient's throat while the patient swallows. Any asymmetry is noted. If the patient is endotracheally intubated, the cough reflex (elicited when the suction catheter contacts the carina of the respiratory tree) is a method of assessing cranial nerve X).

Spinal Accessory Nerve. To test the spinal accessory nerve (CN XI), the patient shrugs the shoulders against resistance and turns the head to either side against resistance. The contraction of the sternomastoid and trapezius muscles should be smooth. Symmetry, atrophy, or fasciculation of the muscle should also be noted.

Hypoglossal Nerve. To test the hypoglossal nerve (CN XII), the patient sticks out the tongue. It should protrude in the midline. The patient should also be able to push the tongue to either side against the resistance of a tongue blade. Again, any asymmetry, atrophy, or fasciculation should be noted.

Motor System. The motor system examination includes assessment of bulk, tone, and power of the major muscle groups of the body, as well as assessment of balance and coordination. To test strength, the patient pushes and pulls against the resistance of the examiner's arm as it opposes flexion and extension of the patient's muscle. The patient should be asked to offer resistance at the shoulders, elbows, wrists, hips, knees, and ankles. The patient's grip strength can also be tested. To test for mild weakness of the upper extremities, the patient extends both arms forward at shoulder height with palms up while the eyes are closed. Mild weakness of the arm is demonstrated by downward drifting of the arm or pronation of the palm *(pronator drift)*. Any weakness or asymmetry of strength between the same muscle groups of the right and left side should be noted.

To test tone, the limbs are passively moved through their range of motion; there should be a slight resistance to these movements. Abnormal tone is described as *hypotonia* (flaccidity) or *hypertonia* (spasticity). Involuntary movements—such as tics, tremor, myoclonus (spasm of muscles), athetosis (slow, writhing, involuntary movements of extremities), chorea (involuntary, purposeless, rapid motions), and dystonia (impairment of muscle tone)—should be noted.

To test cerebellar function, balance and coordination are assessed. A good screening test for both balance and muscle strength is to observe the patient's stance (posture while standing) and gait. The examiner should note the pace and rhythm of the gait and observe the arm swing. (The arms should move symmetrically and in the opposite direction of the leg on the same side.) The patient's ability to ambulate is a key factor in determining the amount of nursing care that is needed and the risk of injury from falling. A patient with cerebellar disease may have an ataxic or staggering gait, in which the feet are placed wide apart and the steps are unsteady.

Coordination can be easily tested in several ways. In the finger-to-nose test, the patient alternately touches the nose with the index finger and then touches the examiner's finger. The examiner repositions the finger while the patient is touching the nose so that the patient must adjust to a new distance each time the examiner's finger is touched. These movements should be performed smoothly and accurately. Other tests include asking the patient to pronate and supinate both hands rapidly and to perform a shallow knee bend, first on one leg and then on the other. Dysarthria or slurred speech should be noted because it is a sign of incoordination of the speech muscles.

In the heel-to-shin test, the patient places one heel on the opposite shin below the knee and moves the heel down the shin to the ankle. This procedure is repeated for the other leg. These movements should flow smoothly without jerking or hesitation.

Sensory System. Several modalities are tested in the somatic sensory examination. Each modality is carried by a specific ascending pathway in the spinal cord before it reaches the sensory cortex.

There are some general guidelines for performing the sensory examination. The patient should always have the eyes closed to avoid visual clues. The examiner should avoid giving verbal cues such as "Is this sharp?" The sensory stimulus should be applied in such a way that the patient does not expect it; that is, the examiner should avoid rhythmic application of the stimulus. In the routine neurological examination, sensory testing of the four extremities is sufficient. However, if a disturbance in sensory function of the skin is identified, the boundaries of that dysfunction should be carefully delineated.

Light Touch. The sensation of light touch is usually tested first. The examiner gently strokes each of the four extremities with a cotton wisp and asks the patient to indicate when the stimulus is felt by saying "touch." (The sensory examination of the trigeminal nerve may be delayed until this time because the same material for testing sensation is used.)

Pain and Temperature. Pain is tested by touching the skin with the sharp end of a safety pin. This stimulus is irregularly alternated with a simple touch stimulus with the dull end of the pin to determine whether the patient can distinguish the two stimuli.

The sensation of temperature is tested by applying tubes of warm and cold water to the skin and asking the patient to identify the stimuli with the eyes closed. If pain sensation is intact, assessment of temperature sensation may be omitted because both sensations are carried by the same ascending pathways.

Vibration Sense. To assess vibration sense, a vibrating C128 tuning fork is applied to the patient's fingernails and the bony prominences of the hands, the legs, and the feet while the patient's eyes are closed. The examiner asks the patient whether the vibration or "buzz" is felt. The examiner then asks the patient to indicate when the vibration ceases. The examiner stops the vibration with the hand as desired.

Position Sense. To assess position sense, the examiner's thumb and forefinger are placed on either side of the patient's forefinger or great toe and gently move the patient's digit up or down. The patient is asked to indicate the direction in which the digit is moved.

Another test of position sense of the lower extremities is Romberg's test. The patient is asked to stand with the feet together and then to close his or her eyes. If the patient is able to maintain balance with the eyes open but sways or falls with the eyes closed (i.e., a positive result of Romberg's test), disease may be present in the posterior columns of the spinal cord or the cerebellum. It is important that the nurse ensure the patient's safety during this test.

Cortical Sensory Functions. Several tests are used to evaluate cortical integration of sensory perceptions (which occurs in the parietal lobes). To assess two-point discrimination, the two points of a calibrated compass are placed on the tips of the patient's fingers and toes. The minimum recognizable separation is 4 to 5 mm in the fingertips and a greater degree of separation elsewhere. This test is important in diagnosing diseases of the sensory cortex and the PNS.

To test *graphaesthesia* (ability to feel writing on skin), the patient is asked to identify numbers traced on the palm of the hands. To test *stereognosis* (ability to perceive the form and nature of objects), the patient is asked to identify the size and shape of easily recognized objects (e.g., coins, keys, a safety pin) placed in the hands. To evaluate sensory extinction or inattention, the examiner touches both sides of the patient's body simultaneously. An abnormal response occurs when the patient perceives the stimulus only on one side. The other stimulus is "extinguished."

Reflexes. Tendons attached to skeletal muscles have receptors that are sensitive to stretch. A reflex contraction of the skeletal muscle occurs when the tendon is stretched. A simple muscle stretch reflex is initiated by briskly tapping the tendon of a stretched muscle, usually with a reflex hammer (Figure 58-18). The response (muscle contraction of the corresponding muscle) is measured as follows: 0 represents absence of response—always abnormal; 1+, slight but definitely present response—may or may not be normal; 2+, brisk response—normal; 3+, a very brisk response—may or may not be normal; and 4+, tap elicits repeating reflex (clonus)—always abnormal. *Clonus,* an abnormal response, is a continued rhythmic contraction of the muscle with continuous application of the stimulus.

In general, the biceps, triceps, brachioradialis, and patellar and Achilles tendon reflexes are tested. The examiner elicits the biceps reflex by placing his or her thumb over the patient's biceps tendon in the antecubital space and striking the thumb with a hammer. The patient should have the arms partially flexed at the elbow with the palms up. The normal response is flexion of the arm at the elbow or contraction of the biceps muscle that can be felt by the examiner's thumb.

To elicit the triceps reflex, the examiner strikes the patient's triceps tendon above the elbow while the patient's arm is flexed. The normal response is extension of the arm or visible contraction of the triceps.

To elicit the brachioradialis reflex, the examiner strikes the patient's radius 3 to 5 cm above the wrist while the patient's arm is relaxed. The normal response is flexion and supination at the elbow or visible contraction of the brachioradialis muscle.

To elicit the patellar reflex, the examiner strikes the patient's patellar tendon just below the patella. The patient can be

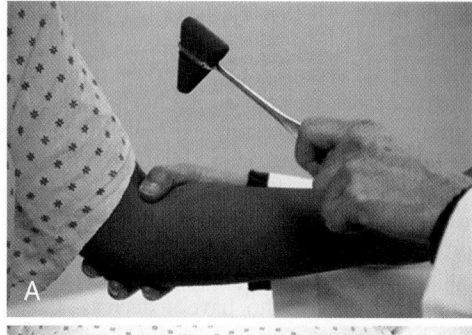
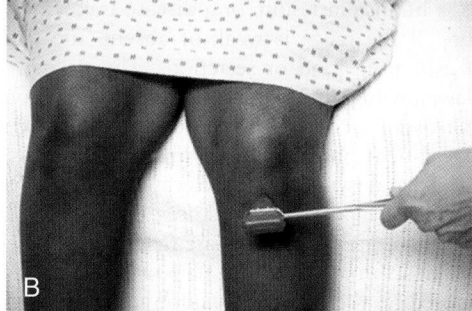

Figure 58-18 The examiner strikes a swift blow over a stretched tendon to elicit a stretch reflex. **A,** Biceps reflex. **B,** Patellar reflex.

sitting or lying as long as the leg being tested hangs freely. The normal response is extension of the leg with contraction of the quadriceps.

To elicit the Achilles tendon reflex, the examiner strikes the patient's Achilles tendon while the patient's leg is flexed at the knee and the foot is dorsiflexed at the ankle. The normal response is plantar flexion at the ankle.

A focused assessment is used to evaluate the status or previously identified neurological problems and to monitor for signs of new problems (see Table 3-6). A focused assessment of the neurological system is presented in the Focused Assessment box.

Table 58-7 is a listing of normal findings in a neurological assessment. Common abnormal assessment findings of the neurological system are presented in Table 58-8.

Diagnostic Studies of the Nervous System

Numerous diagnostic studies are available to assess the nervous system. Table 58-9 presents the most commonly encountered studies.

Cerebrospinal Fluid Analysis.
CSF analysis provides information about a variety of CNS diseases. Normal CSF fluid is clear, colourless, and free of red blood cells and contains little protein. Normal CSF values are listed in Table 58-10.

Lumbar Puncture.
Lumbar puncture is the most common method of obtaining CSF for analysis. It is contraindicated in the presence of increased intracranial pressure or infection at the site of puncture.

Nurses often assist in this procedure because it is usually performed in the patient's room. Before the procedure, the patient should empty the bladder. The patient should lie in the lateral recumbent position, with the back as near as possible to the edge of the bed. The nurse should assist the patient in drawing up the

FOCUSED ASSESSMENT
Neurological System

Use this checklist to make sure the key assessment steps have been performed.

Subjective

Ask the patient about any of the following, and note responses

Blackouts/loss of memory	Y	N
Weakness, numbness, tingling sensation in arms or legs	Y	N
Headaches, especially of new onset	Y	N
Loss of balance/coordination	Y	N
Orientation to person, place, and time	Y	N

Objective: Diagnostic

Check the following laboratory results for critical values

Lumbar puncture	✓
CT or MRI of brain	✓
EEG	✓

Objective: Physical Examination

Inspect/Observe

General level of consciousness/orientation	✓
Oropharynx for gag reflex and soft palate movement	✓
Peripheral sensation of light touch and pinprick (face, hands, feet)	✓
Sense of smell with an alcohol wipe	✓
Eyes for extraocular movements, PERRLA, peripheral vision, nystagmus	✓
Gait for smoothness and coordination	✓

Palpate

Strength of neck, shoulders, arms, and legs, full and symmetrical	✓

Percuss

Reflexes	✓

CT, computed tomography; EEG, electroencephalogram; MRI, magnetic resonance imaging; PERRLA, pupils equal, round, and reactive to light and accommodation.

Table 58-7 Normal Physical Assessment of the Nervous System*

Mental Status

Alert and oriented, orderly thought processes, appropriate mood and affect

Cranial Nerves†

Sense of smell intact for soap and coffee; visual fields full to confrontation; visual acuity 20/20 in both eyes; intact extraocular movements; no nystagmus; pupils equal, round, reactive to light and accommodation; intact facial sensation for touch and pinprick; facial movements full; intact gag and swallow reflexes; symmetrical elevation of soft palate; full strength with head turning and shrugging of shoulders against resistance; midline protrusion of tongue

Motor System

Normal gait and station; normal tandem walk; negative result of Romberg's test; normal and symmetrical muscle bulk, tone, strength; smooth performance of finger–nose, heel–shin movements

Sensory System

Intact sensation to light touch, position sense, vibration, pinprick, heat and cold, two-point discrimination; intact stereognosis and graphaesthesia

Reflexes‡

Biceps, triceps, brachioradialis, patellar, and Achilles tendon reflexes 2+ bilaterally; downward-pointing toes with plantar stimulation

*If some portion of the neurological examination was not performed, this should be indicated (e.g., "Smell not tested").
†May also be recorded as "CNs [cranial nerves] I to XII intact."
‡May also be recorded as drawing of stick figure indicating reflex strength at appropriate sites.

withdrawn in a series of tubes and sent for analysis. Some examiners believe that the patient should be kept lying flat for at least a few hours after the procedure to avoid a spinal headache, which is presumably caused by loss of the cushioning effect of CSF as a result of leakage of CSF at the puncture site. The prone position may be effective in preventing CSF leakage. Other examiners do not believe that the lying position is necessary because headache seems to develop in some patients despite precautions. Meningeal irritation (nuchal rigidity) or signs and symptoms of local trauma (e.g., hematoma, pain) may develop in some patients.

Radiological Studies

Cerebral Angiography. Cerebral angiography is indicated when vascular lesions or tumours are suspected. A catheter is inserted into the femoral (sometimes brachial) artery. It is then passed up the artery to the aortic arch and into the base of a carotid or a vertebral artery for injection of radiopaque contrast medium. Radiographs are taken in a timed sequence so that pictures of the arteries, smaller vessels, and veins can be obtained (Figure 58-19). This study can help localize and determine the presence of abscesses, aneurysms, hematomas, arteriovenous malformations, arterial spasm, and certain tumours.

Because this is an invasive procedure, adverse reactions may occur. The patient may have an allergic (anaphylactic) reaction to the contrast medium. This reaction usually occurs immediately after injection of the contrast medium and may necessitate

knees to the abdomen and flexing the head to the chest. This helps separate the vertebrae so that the needle can be inserted more easily.

Using strict sterile technique, the physician inserts a long needle below the third lumbar vertebra. This may cause some local discomfort. There is no danger of injuring the spinal cord because the cord terminates between the first and second lumbar vertebrae. However, the patient may experience some pain radiating down the leg or muscle twitching if the needle irritates the spinal root. The nurse can assure the patient that this is temporary and that the patient is not in danger of being paralyzed.

A manometer is attached to the needle, and CSF pressure is determined after the patient is asked to relax and extend the legs. If the patient does not relax and extend the legs, the pressure reading is abnormally high. Normal CSF pressure is approximately 9 to 14 mm Hg (Black & Hawks, 2009). CSF is

Text continued on p. 1631

Table 58-8 Nervous System

FINDING	DESCRIPTION	POSSIBLE ETIOLOGY AND SIGNIFICANCE
Altered consciousness	Inability to speak, obey commands, open eyes appropriately with verbal or painful stimulus	Intracranial lesions, metabolic disorder, psychiatric disorders
Anisocoria	Inequality of pupil size	Lesion, injury, or intracranial pressure in area of midbrain
Agnosia	Inability to determine meaning or significance of sensory stimulus	Cerebral cortex lesion
Apraxia	Inability to perform learned movements; defect in motor planning	Cerebral cortex lesion
Aphasia	Loss of language faculty (language comprehension, language expression, or both)	Cerebral cortex lesion
Analgesia	Loss of pain sensation	Lesion in spinothalamic tract or thalamus, lack of or damage to sensory nerve endings
Anaesthesia	Absence of sensation	Lesions in spinal cord, thalamus, sensory cortex, or peripheral sensory nerve
Hyperaesthesia	Increase in sensation	Shingles, nerve compression, stress, or chronic pain
Hypoaesthesia	Decrease in sensation	Impingement or damage of a nerve (e.g., peripheral neuropathy in diabetes)
Anosognosia	Inability to recognize bodily defect or disease	Lesions in right parietal cortex, common in right-sided brain stroke
Astereognosis	Inability to recognize form of object by touch	Lesions in parietal cortex
Ataxia	Lack of coordination of movement	Lesions of sensory or motor pathways, cerebellum; anticonvulsant drug, sedative, or hypnotic drug toxicity (including alcohol)
Muscle atrophy (disuse or denervation atrophy)	Wasting away or diminution in size of muscle	Suprasegmental (upper motor neuron) lesions, segmental (lower motor neuron) lesions
Bladder dysfunction		
• Atonic (autonomous)	Absence of muscle tone and contractility, enlarged capacity, no discomfort, overflow with large residual, inability to voluntarily empty or empty by reflex	Early stage of spinal cord injury
• Hypotonic	More ability to empty by reflex than with atonic bladder but less than normal	Interruption of afferent pathways from bladder
• Hypertonic	Increase in muscle tone, diminished capacity, reflex emptying, dribbling, incontinence	Lesions in pyramidal tracts (efferent pathways)
Diplopia	Double vision	Lesions affecting nerves of extraocular muscles, cerebellar damage
Dysarthria	Lack of coordination in articulating speech	Lesions in cerebellum or pathway of cranial nerves (including brainstem); anticonvulsant drug, sedative, or hypnotic drug toxicity (including alcohol)
Dyskinesia	Impaired power of voluntary movement, resulting in fragmentary or incomplete movements	Disorders of basal ganglia, idiosyncratic reaction to psychotropic drugs
Dysphagia	Difficulty in swallowing	Lesions involving motor pathways of cranial nerves IX and X (including lower brainstem)
Extensor plantar response (Babinski's sign)	Upward-pointing toes with plantar stimulation	Suprasegmental or upper motor neuron lesion
Homonymous hemianopsia	Loss of vision in one side of visual field	Injury or lesions in area of optic tract or its radiations to occipital cortex
Hemiplegia	Paralysis on one side	Stroke and other lesions involving motor cortex
Nystagmus	Jerking or bobbing of eyes as they track moving object	Lesions in cerebellum, brainstem, vestibular system; toxic effects of anticonvulsants, sedatives, hypnotics (including alcohol)
Ophthalmoplegia	Paralysis of eye muscles	Lesions in brainstem or cranial nerves III, IV, and VI
Opisthotonus	Extreme arching of back with retraction of head	Meningitis, tonic phase of grand mal seizure
Papilledema	Swelling of optic disk	Increase in intracranial pressure
Paraplegia	Paralysis of lower extremities	Spinal cord transection or mass lesion (thoracolumbar region)
Tetraplegia (quadriplegia)	Paralysis of all extremities	Spinal cord transection or mass lesion (cervical region or brainstem)

DIAGNOSTIC STUDIES

Table 58-9 Nervous System

STUDY	DESCRIPTION AND PURPOSE	NURSING RESPONSIBILITY
Cerebrospinal Fluid Analysis		
Lumbar puncture	CSF is aspirated by needle insertion in L3-4 or L4-5 interspace to assess many CNS diseases. (See Table 58-10.)	Help patient assume and maintain lateral recumbent position with knees flexed. Ensure maintenance of strict aseptic technique. Ensure labelling of CSF specimens in proper sequence. Encourage patient to drink fluids. Monitor neurological and VS. Administer analgesia as needed.
Radiological		
Skull and spine radiographs	Simple radiographs of skull and spinal column can help detect fractures, spinal misalignment, bone erosion, calcifications, or abnormal vascularity.	Explain that procedure is noninvasive. Explain positions to be assumed.
Cerebral angiography	Serial radiographic visualization of intracranial and extracranial blood vessels can help detect vascular lesions and tumours of brain. Contrast medium is used.	Assess for risk of stoke because thrombi may be dislodged during procedure. Withhold preceding meal. Explain that patient will experience hot flush of head and neck when contrast medium is injected. Explain need to be absolutely still during procedure. Monitor neurological and VS every 15-30 min for first 2 hr, every hour for next 6 hr, then every 2 hr for 24 hr. Maintain pressure dressing and ice on injection site. Maintain bed rest until patient is alert and VS are stable. Report any signs of change in neurological status.
Computed tomography (CT)	Computer-assisted radiographic views of several levels or thin cross-sections of body parts can help detect problems such as hemorrhage, space-occupying lesions, cerebral edema, brain atrophy, and other abnormalities.	Explain that procedure is noninvasive (if no contrast medium is used). Observe for allergic reaction, and note puncture site (if contrast medium is used). Explain appearance of scanner. Instruct patient to remain absolutely still during procedure.
Magnetic resonance imaging (MRI)	Imaging of brain, spinal cord, and spinal canal by means of magnetic energy helps detect infarctions, multiple sclerosis, tumours, trauma, herniation, and seizures. No invasive procedures are required.	Screen patient for joint replacements and pacemaker in body. Instruct patient to lie very still for up to 1 hr. Sedation may be necessary if patient is claustrophobic.
Magnetic resonance angiography (MRA)	Differential signal characteristics of flowing blood are studied to evaluate extracranial and intracranial blood vessels. Test provides both anatomical and hemodynamic information. MRA can be used in conjunction with contrast media (contrast-enhanced MRA [cMRA]). MRA is rapidly replacing cerebral angiography for use in diagnosing cerebrovascular diseases.	Nursing responsibilities are similar to those for MRI.
Positron emission tomography (PET)	Metabolic activity of brain regions is measured to assess cell death or damage. Test involves the use of radioactive material that shows up as a bright spot on the image.	Explain procedure to patient. Explain that two IV lines will be inserted. Instruct patient not to take sedatives or tranquilizers and to empty bladder before procedure. Patient may be asked to perform different activities during test.
Single-photon emission computed tomography (SPECT)	This method of scanning is similar to PET, but more stable substances and different detectors are used. Radiolabelled compounds are injected, and their photon emissions can be detected. Images made are accumulation of labelled compound. SPECT is used to visualize blood flow or oxygen or glucose metabolism in the brain. It is useful in diagnosing strokes, brain tumours, and seizure disorders.	Nursing responsibilities are similar to those for PET.

CNS, central nervous system; *CSF*, cerebrospinal fluid; *IV*, intravenous; *VS*, vital signs.

Continued

DIAGNOSTIC STUDIES

Table 58-9 Nervous System—cont'd

STUDY	DESCRIPTION AND PURPOSE	NURSING RESPONSIBILITY
Electrographic		
Electroencephalography (EEG)	Electrical activity of brain is recorded by scalp electrodes to evaluate cerebral disease, CNS effects of systemic diseases, and brain death.	Inform patient that procedure is painless and without danger of electric shock. Withhold stimulants. Inform patient that he or she may be asked to perform various activities such as hyperventilation during test. Determine whether any medications (e.g., tranquilizers, anticonvulsant drugs) should be withheld. Resume medications after test. Assist patient in washing electrode paste out of hair.
Magnetoencephalography (MEG)	A sensitivity machine called a *biomagnetometer* is used to detect very small magnetic fields generated by neural activity. It can accurately pinpoint the part of the brain involved in a stroke, seizure, or other disorder or injury. Extracranial magnetic fields, as well as scalp electrical field (EEG), are measured.	MEG, a passive sensor, does not make physical contact with patient. Explain procedure to patient.
Electromyography (EMG) and nerve conduction	Electrical activity associated with nerve and skeletal muscle is recorded by insertion of needle electrodes to detect muscle and peripheral nerve disease.	Inform patient of slight discomfort associated with insertion of needles.
Evoked potentials	Electrical activity associated with nerve conduction along sensory pathways is recorded by electrodes placed on skin and scalp. Stimulus generates the impulse. Procedure is used to diagnose disease, locate nerve damage, and monitor function intraoperatively.	Explain procedure to patient. Avoid hair spray, gel or other hair care products and sedative drugs such as benzodiazepines and barbiturates.
Ultrasonography		
Carotid duplex studies	Sound waves are used to determine blood flow velocity, which may indicate presence of occlusive vascular disease.	Explain procedure to patient.
Transcranial Doppler ultrasonography	Technology is the same as that for carotid duplex studies, but intracranial vessels are evaluated.	Explain procedure to patient.

Table 58-10 Normal Cerebrospinal Fluid Values

PARAMETER	NORMAL VALUE
Specific gravity	1.007
pH	7.35
Appearance	Clear, colourless
RBCs	None
WBCs	Adult: $0-5 \times 10^6$/L
Protein	
• Lumbar	0.15-0.45 g/L
• Cisternal	0.15-0.25 g/L
• Ventricular	0.05-0.15 g/L
Glucose	2.2-3.9 mmol/L
Microorganisms	None
Pressure	60-150 mm H_2O

RBCs, red blood cells; *WBCs*, white blood cells.

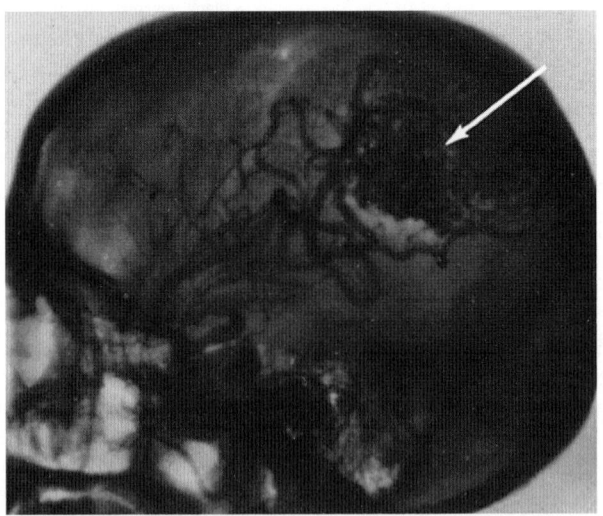

Figure 58-19 Cerebral angiogram illustrating an arteriovenous malformation *(arrow)*.

Source: From Chipps, E., Clanin, N., & Campbell, V. (1992). *Neurologic disorders*. St. Louis: Mosby.

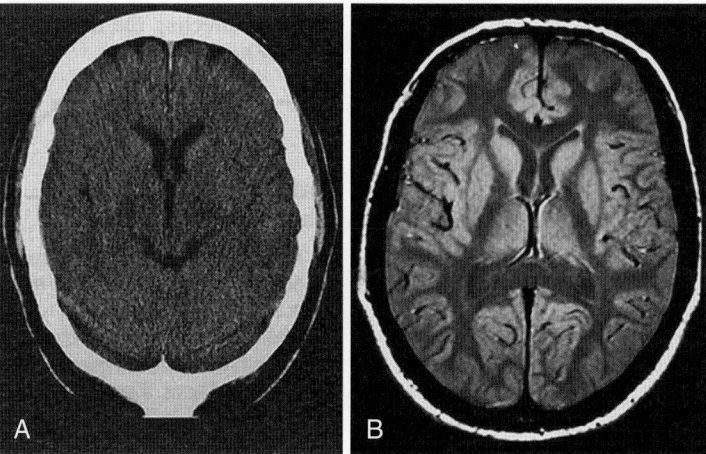

Figure 58-20 Normal images of the brain. **A,** Computed tomography. **B,** Magnetic resonance imaging.

Source: From Fuller, G., & Manford, M. (2006). *Neurology: An illustrated colour text.* Edinburgh: Churchill Livingstone.

emergency resuscitation measures in the procedure room. The most common precaution for nurses to take in caring for the patient after the return to the room is observation for bleeding at the catheter puncture site (usually the groin). A pressure dressing and ice are usually placed on the site to promote hemostasis and prevent swelling.

Computed Tomography.

Computed tomography (CT) is a noninvasive procedure, although intravenous injection of contrast medium may be used to enhance visualization of the blood vessels and identify disruptions in the blood–brain barrier. CT can be performed on an outpatient basis. A number of radiographic scans of different levels of the brain are compiled with computer assistance and presented in a series of black-and-white pictures. These pictures, which illustrate "slices" of the brain (Figure 58-20, *A*), can show hemorrhages, tumours, cysts, edema, infarction, brain atrophy, and hydrocephalus. CT does not illustrate structures in the posterior fossa and the base of the brain as clearly as does magnetic resonance imaging (MRI).

Magnetic Resonance Imaging.

Rather than using x rays, MRI involves two kinds of magnetism. The patient is placed within a giant magnetic field that aligns the protons of the hydrogen ions in the cells of the body. Bursts of radiofrequency magnetism are introduced to flip the protons out of alignment. When the radiofrequency magnetism is turned off, the protons realign. The resulting magnetic field change is picked up by the machine and processed by a computer. Vivid black-and-white pictures (see Figure 58-20, *B*) are then produced.

MRI is useful in evaluating brain and spinal cord edema, hemorrhage, infarction, blood vessels, tumours, herniation, and bone lesions. It is used in the detection of early strokes and multiple sclerosis. Intravenous injection of gadolinium can enhance the images obtained with MRI. Because the images of soft tissue structures have greater contrast with MRI than with CT, MRI is the diagnostic test of choice for many neurological diseases.

Positron Emission Tomography.

Positron emission tomography (PET) is used to determine regional metabolism in the brain. PET provides a noninvasive means of determining biochemical processes that occur in the brain. PET is increasingly used to monitor patients with stroke, Alzheimer's disease, seizure disorders, epilepsy, tumours, and Parkinson's disease.

Electrographic Studies

Electroencephalography.

Electroencephalography (EEG) is the recording of the electrical activity of the surface cortical neurons of the brain using 8 to 16 electrodes placed on specific areas of the scalp. This test is done to evaluate not only cerebral disease but also the CNS effects of many metabolic and systemic diseases and to determine brain death. Among the cerebral diseases and other conditions assessed with EEG are epilepsy, mass lesions (e.g., tumour, abscess, hematoma), cerebrovascular lesions, and brain injury. The procedure is noninvasive. Patients sometimes have the misconception that the recording electrodes will give them an electric shock. They should be assured that this is not true and that the procedure is similar to electrocardiography.

Electromyography and Nerve Conduction Studies.

Electromyography (EMG) is the recording of electrical activity associated with innervation of skeletal muscle. The recording is displayed on a computer screen and may be played on a loudspeaker for simultaneous analysis. Needle electrodes are inserted into the muscle to record specific motor units because recording from the skin is not sufficient. Normal muscle at rest shows no electrical activity. Typical electrical activity occurs when the muscle contracts. This activity may be altered in diseases of muscle itself (e.g., myopathic conditions) or in disorders of muscle innervation (e.g., segmental or LMN lesions, peripheral neuropathic conditions). *Fibrillations* are spontaneous, independent contractions of individual muscle fibres that can be detected only by EMG. They appear on EMG 1 to 3 weeks after a muscle has lost its nerve supply.

In *nerve conduction studies,* a brief electrical stimulus is applied to a distal portion of a sensory or mixed nerve, and the resulting wave of depolarization is recorded at some point proximal to the stimulation. For example, a stimulus can be applied to the forefinger and a recording electrode placed over the median nerve at the wrist. The time between the onset of the stimulus and the initial wave of depolarization at the recording electrode is measured. The speed of this response is termed *nerve conduction velocity.* Damaged nerves have slower conduction velocities.

Evoked Potentials.

Evoked potentials are recordings of electrical activity associated with nerve conduction along sensory pathways. The activity is generated by a specific sensory stimulus related to the type of study (e.g., checkerboard patterns for visual evoked potentials, clicking sounds for auditory evoked potentials, mild electrical pulses for somatosensory evoked potentials). Electrodes placed on specific areas of the skin and scalp record the electrical activity, and these data are stored and averaged by a computerized instrument. A wave pattern appears on a screen and is printed on paper. Peaks in the wave pattern correspond to conduction of the stimulus through certain points along the sensory pathway (e.g., peripheral nerve, brainstem, cortical areas). Increases in the time from stimulus onset to a given peak (latency) indicate slowed nerve conduction or nerve damage. This technique is useful in diagnosing abnormalities of the visual or auditory systems because it reveals whether a sensory impulse is reaching the appropriate part of the brain. Purposes for these tests include evaluation of the optic nerve in conditions such as multiple sclerosis (optic neuritis) and the vestibulocochlear nerve in acoustic neuroma.

Combined Doppler and Ultrasound (Duplex) Studies

Carotid Duplex.

In a duplex study, ultrasonography and pulsed Doppler technology are combined. A technician places a probe on the patient's skin over the carotid artery and slowly moves the probe along the course of the common carotid artery to the bifurcation of the external and internal carotid arteries. The ultrasound signal emitted from the probe reflects off the moving blood cells within the vessel. The frequency of the reflected signal corresponds to the blood flow velocity. This response is amplified and is registered on a graphic record and also as sound. The graphic record registers blood flow velocity. Increases in blood flow velocity can indicate stenosis of a vessel. Duplex scanning is a noninvasive study in which the degree of stenosis of the carotid and vertebral arteries is evaluated.

Transcranial Doppler Sonography.

The same technology used in duplex studies is used in transcranial Doppler sonography, except that blood flow velocities of the intracranial blood vessels are recorded. The probe is placed on the patient's skin at various "windows" in the skull (areas in the skull that have only a thin bony covering) to register velocities of the middle cerebral artery, anterior cerebral artery, posterior cerebral artery, terminal carotid artery, and occasionally the anterior and posterior communicating arteries. The temporal, orbital, and suboccipital sites are used. The ultrasound signal received is recorded graphically as a waveform. Peak blood flow velocities and systolic–diastolic ratios can be calculated from this information. Transcranial Doppler sonography is a noninvasive technique that is useful in assessing vasospasm associated with subarachnoid hemorrhage, altered intracranial blood flow dynamics associated with occlusive vascular disease, presence of emboli, and cerebral autoregulation.

ⓔvolve　*An assessment case study of the nervous system is available at* **http://evolve.elsevier.com/Canada/Lewis/medsurg**

REVIEW QUESTIONS

The number of the question corresponds to the same-numbered objective at the beginning of the chapter.

1. In a patient with a disease that affects the myelin sheath of nerves, such as multiple sclerosis, which glial cells are affected?
   a. Microglia
   b. Astrocytes
   c. Oligodendrocytes
   d. Ependymal cells
2. A state of hypoxia alters the repeated action potentials necessary for transmission of nerve impulses. Which of the following requires energy?
   a. Repolarization of the cell membrane
   b. Creation of cell membrane permeability
   c. Movement of sodium into the nerve cell
   d. Maintenance of the resting membrane potential
3. Drugs or diseases that impair the function of the extrapyramidal system may cause the loss of which of the following?
   a. Sensations of pain and temperature
   b. Regulation of the ANS
   c. Integration of somatic and special sensory inputs
   d. Automatic movements associated with skeletal muscle activity

4. Which of the following will be affected by an obstruction of the anterior cerebral arteries?
   a. Visual imaging
   b. Balance and coordination
   c. Judgement, insight, and reasoning
   d. Visual and auditory integration for language comprehension
5. Data regarding mobility, strength, coordination, and activity tolerance are important for the nurse to obtain for which of the following reasons?
   a. Many neurological diseases affect one or more of these abilities.
   b. Patients are less able to identify other neurological impairments.
   c. These are the first functions to be lost in neurological disease.
   d. Aspects of movement are the most important function of the nervous system.
6. What is a result of stimulation of the parasympathetic nervous system?
   a. Dilation of skin blood vessels
   b. Increased secretion of insulin
   c. Increased blood glucose levels
   d. Relaxation of the urinary sphincters

7. Why can the muscle strength of older adults not be compared with that of younger adults?
   a. Stroke is more common in older adults.
   b. Nutritional status is better in young adults.
   c. Most young people exercise more than older people.
   d. Aging leads to a decrease in muscle bulk and strength.

8. A lesion of which cranial nerve would cause paralysis of the lateral gaze?
   a. Cranial nerve II
   b. Cranial nerve III
   c. Cranial nerve IV
   d. Cranial nerve VI

9. During neurological testing, the patient is able to perceive pain elicited by pinprick. On the basis of this finding, which of the following tests may the nurse omit?
   a. Position sense
   b. Patellar reflexes
   c. Temperature perception
   d. Heel-to-shin movements

10. A patient's eyes jerk as they follow the nurse's moving finger. How would the nurse record this finding?
    a. Nystagmus
    b. Normal tracking
    c. Ophthalmoplegia
    d. Ophthalmic dyskinesia

11. Which of the following are nursing responsibilities for lumbar puncture?
    a. Ensuring the patient has a full bladder
    b. Placing the patient in the lateral recumbent position
    c. Straightening the patient's legs just before the puncture
    d. Having the patient cough when the needle has been inserted

ANSWERS: 1. c; 2. d; 3. d; 4. c; 5. a; 6. b; 7. d; 8. d; 9. c; 10. a; 11. b.

REFERENCES

Black, J. M., & Hawks, J. H. (2009). *Medical-surgical nursing: Clinical management for positive outcomes* (8th ed.). St. Louis: Saunders.

Colucci-D'Amato, L., & di Porzio, U. (2008). Neurogenesis in the adult CNS: From denial to opportunities and challenges for therapy. *Bioessays, 30,* 135. doi:10.1002/bies.20703

McCance, K. L., & Huether, S. E. (2010). *Pathophysiology: The biologic basis for disease in adults and children* (6th ed.) St. Louis: Mosby.

Porter, R. S., & Kaplan, J. L. (2011). *Merck manual of diagnosis and therapy* (19th ed.). West Point, PA: Merck & Co.

Werder, S. F. (2010). Cobalamin deficiency, hyperhomocysteinemia, and dementia. *Neuropsychiatric Disease and Treatment, 6,* 159-195. doi:10.2147/NDT.S6564

RESOURCES

Resources for this chapter are listed in Chapter 59, p. 1671; Chapter 60, p. 1699; Chapter 61, p. 1735; Chapter 62, p. 1758; and Chapter 63, p. 1795.

Nursing Management:
Acute Intracranial Problems

Written by Meg Zomorodi

Adapted by Sarah L. Johnston

LEARNING OBJECTIVES

1. Identify the physiological mechanisms that maintain normal intracranial pressure.
2. Describe the common etiologies, clinical manifestations, and collaborative care of the patient with increased intracranial pressure.
3. Describe the collaborative care and nursing management of the patient with increased intracranial pressure.
4. Differentiate between the types of head injury by mechanism of injury and clinical manifestations.
5. Describe the collaborative care and nursing management of the patient with a head injury.

6. Explain the types, clinical manifestations, and collaborative care of brain tumours.
7. Discuss the nursing management of the patient with a brain tumour.
8. Discuss the nursing management of the patient undergoing cranial surgery.
9. Compare the primary causes, collaborative care, and nursing management of meningitis, encephalitis, and brain abscess.

KEY TERMS

brain abscess Accumulation of pus within the brain tissue that can result from a local or systemic infection, p. 1668

cerebral edema Increased accumulation of fluid in the extravascular spaces of brain tissue, p. 1637

coma Profound state of unconsciousness, p. 1638

concussion Sudden transient mechanical head injury with disruption of neural activity and a change in the level of consciousness, p. 1650

contusion Bruising of the brain tissue within a focal area, p. 1651

diffuse axonal injury (DAI) Widespread axonal damage occurring after a mild, moderate, or severe traumatic brain injury, p. 1651

encephalitis Acute inflammation of the brain, p. 1666

epidural hematoma Collection of blood that results from bleeding between the dura and the inner surface of the skull; produces compression of the dura mater and thus of the brain, p. 1652

Glasgow Coma Scale (GCS) Quick, practical, and standardized system for assessing the degree to which consciousness is impaired, p. 1644

head injury Any trauma to the scalp, the skull, or the brain, p. 1649

intracranial pressure (ICP) Pressure exerted because of the combined total volume of the three components within the skull: brain tissue, blood, and cerebrospinal fluid, p. 1635

intraparenchymal or intracerebral hematoma Collection of blood within the parenchyma of the brain, possibly from the rupture of an intracerebral vessel at the time of a head injury, p. 1653

meningitis Acute inflammation of meningeal tissues (the pia mater and the arachnoid membrane) surrounding the brain and the spinal cord, p. 1663

nuchal rigidity Resistance to flexion of the neck, p. 1664

subdural hematoma Collection of blood between the dura mater and the arachnoid layer of the meninges of the brain that is usually of venous origin, usually caused by injury, p. 1653

unconsciousness Abnormal state of complete or partial unawareness of self or environment, p. 1638

ELECTRONIC RESOURCES

Supplemental content related to Chapter 59 can be found...

Evolve Web Site ⊖volve

http://evolve.elsevier.com/Canada/Lewis/medsurg
- Animation: Functional Areas of the Brain
- Answer Guidelines for Case Study on p. 1669
- Clinical Reference: Laboratory Values
- Content Updates
- Customizable Nursing Care Plans:
  - Bacterial Meningitis
  - Increased Intracranial Pressure

- eFigure 59-1: Systematic Approach to Nursing Assessment of Unconscious Patient
- eTable 59-1: Patient & Caregiver Teaching Guide: Head Injury
- Electronic Calculators
- Examination Review Questions
- Glossary
- Interactive Case Studies:
  - Head Injury
  - Meningitis
- Key Points (Printable and MP3 Download)

Acute intracranial problems include diseases and disorders that can increase intracranial pressure (ICP). This chapter discusses the mechanisms that maintain normal ICP, increased ICP, head injury, brain tumours, and cerebral inflammatory disorders.

Intracranial Pressure

Understanding the mechanisms associated with ICP is important in caring for patients with many different neurological problems. The skull is like a closed box with three essential components constituting its volume: brain tissue, blood, and cerebrospinal fluid (CSF) (Figure 59-1). The brain compartment, made up of neurons, neuroglial cells, and intracellular and extracellular fluids of brain tissue, makes up approximately 78% of this volume. Blood in the arterial, the venous, and the capillary networks makes up 12% of the volume, and the remaining 10% is the volume of the CSF. Under normal conditions, the volume of these three compartments is relatively stable, maintaining ICP within normal limits. Factors that influence ICP under normal circumstances are changes in (1) blood pressure (BP), (2) cardiac function, (3) intra-abdominal and intrathoracic pressure, (4) body position, (5) temperature, and (6) blood gases, particularly CO_2 levels. The degree to which these factors increase or decrease the ICP depends on the ability of the brain to accommodate to the changes.

Regulation and Maintenance of Intracranial Pressure

Normal Intracranial Pressure. Intracranial pressure (ICP) is the pressure exerted because of the combined total volume of the three components within the skull: brain tissue, blood, and CSF. The modified Monro-Kellie doctrine describes how a state of dynamic equilibrium is maintained by the volume relationship of these three components within the rigid skull structure. If the volume in any one of the three components increases within the cranial vault and the volume from another component is displaced, the total intracranial volume will not change (Cushing, 1925). If the volume of any one of these three components increases without a corresponding

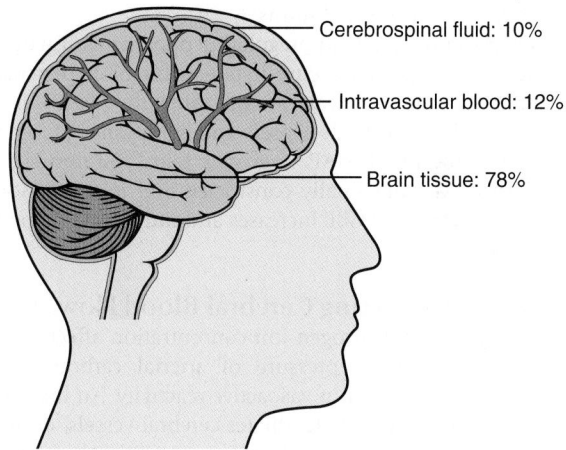

Cerebrospinal fluid: 10%

Intravascular blood: 12%

Brain tissue: 78%

Figure 59-1 Components of the brain.

---

decrease in another component, the result is an elevated ICP. This hypothesis is not applicable in situations in which the skull is not rigid (e.g., in neonates, in adults with unfused skull fractures).

Normal Compensatory Adaptations. Intrinsic compensatory mechanisms exist to resist increases in ICP. A major compensatory mechanism involves changes in the CSF volume. These are achieved primarily by the displacement of CSF into the spinal subarachnoid space or to the basal subarachnoid cisterns and to a lesser degree by altering CSF production and absorption rates. Alterations in intracranial blood volume occur through the compression of cerebral veins and dural sinuses, regional cerebral vasoconstriction or dilation, and changes in venous outflow. Brain tissue volume compensates through distension of the dura or compression of brain tissue. Initially, an increase in volume produces no increase in ICP as a result of these compensatory mechanisms. However, compensatory adaptations are finite, and progressive increases in volume eventually exhaust compensatory mechanisms (Cushing, 1925). The result is increased ICP, neuronal compression, and ischemia. The indications for and methods of monitoring ICP are discussed later in the chapter.

Cerebral Blood Flow

Cerebral blood flow (CBF) is the amount of blood in millilitres (mL) passing through 100 grams (g) of brain tissue per minute. In adults, this equates to approximately 50 mL of blood/min/100 g of brain tissue or approximately 750 mL/min. Unlike other organs, the brain lacks the ability to store oxygen or glucose, and therefore the maintenance of adequate blood flow to the brain is critical for neuronal functioning and survival. Although the brain accounts for only about 2% of body weight, it uses 20% of the body's oxygen and 25% of its glucose.

Autoregulation of Cerebral Blood Flow. The brain's intrinsic ability to regulate its own blood flow in response to its metabolic needs in spite of wide fluctuations in systemic arterial pressure is termed *autoregulation*. Autoregulation is the automatic alteration in the diameter of the cerebral blood vessels to maintain a constant blood flow to the brain during changes in BP. The purpose of autoregulation is to ensure adequate CBF to meet the metabolic needs of brain tissue and to maintain cerebral perfusion pressure within normal limits.

In healthy individuals, autoregulation operates within limited parameters. In cases of extreme hypotension or hypertension, autoregulation fails. If mean arterial pressure (MAP) is less than 50 mm Hg, CBF is decreased and symptoms of cerebral ischemia may occur. If MAP is greater than 150 mm Hg, the cerebral vessels are maximally constricted and further vasoconstrictor response is lost; CBF increases and intracranial hypertension may occur.

Other Factors Affecting Cerebral Blood Flow. Carbon dioxide, oxygen, and hydrogen ion concentration affect cerebral vessel tone. The partial pressure of arterial carbon dioxide ($PaCO_2$) is a potent factor in vasoactive reactivity. An increase in $PaCO_2$ relaxes smooth muscle, dilates cerebral vessels, decreases cerebrovascular resistance, and increases CBF. Alternately, a decrease in $PaCO_2$ reverses this process and decreases CBF. Cerebral oxygen tension (PaO_2) below 50 mm Hg results in cerebral vascular dilation. This dilation decreases cerebral vascular resistance and increases CBF. If PaO_2 is not raised, anaerobic metabolism begins, resulting in an accumulation of lactic acid. As lactic acid increases and hydrogen ions accumulate, the cerebral environment becomes more acidic. Within this acidic environment, further vasodilation occurs in a continued attempt to increase blood flow. The combination of a severely low arterial oxygen pressure (PaO_2) and an elevated hydrogen ion concentration (acidosis), which are both potent cerebral vasodilators, may produce a state wherein autoregulation is lost and compensatory mechanisms fail to meet tissue metabolic demands (Cushing, 1925).

CBF can be globally affected by cardiac or respiratory arrest, systemic hemorrhage, and other pathophysiological states (e.g., diabetic coma, encephalopathies, infections, toxicities). Regional CBF can also be affected by trauma, tumours, cerebral hemorrhage, or stroke. When regional or global autoregulation is lost, CBF is no longer maintained at a constant level but is directly influenced by changes in systemic BP, $PaCO_2$, or catecholamines. CBF can be indirectly reflected by calculating *cerebral perfusion pressure* (CPP). CPP is the pressure needed to ensure adequate brain tissue perfusion. CPP is equal to the MAP minus the ICP (CPP = MAP − ICP) (see example in Table 59-1). If CPP is inadequate, brain perfusion can be improved by either decreasing ICP or increasing mean arterial pressure (MAP).

As the CPP decreases, autoregulation fails and CBF decreases. Normal CPP is 70 to 100 mm Hg, and a minimum of 50 to 60 mm Hg is necessary for adequate cerebral perfusion. CPP less than 50 mm Hg is associated with cerebral ischemia. A CPP below 30 mm Hg results in cellular ischemia and is incompatible with life. Under normal circumstances, autoregulation maintains an adequate CBF and perfusion pressure primarily by cerebral vasoreactivity and metabolic adjustments that affect ICP. It is of paramount importance to maintain MAP when ICP is elevated. It should be remembered that CPP does not reflect perfusion pressure in all parts of the brain. There may be local areas of swelling and compression limiting regional perfusion pressure. Thus, a higher CPP may be needed for these patients to prevent localized tissue damage.

Pressure Changes. The relationship of pressure to volume is depicted in the pressure–volume curve (Figure 59-2). The curve is affected by the brain's compliance.

Compliance is the expandability of the brain. It is represented as the volume increase for each unit increase in pressure. With low compliance, small increases in volume result in greater increases in pressure.

$$\text{Compliance} = \text{Volume/Pressure}$$

The pressure–volume curve can be used to represent the stages of increased ICP (see Figure 59-2). At stage 1 on the curve,

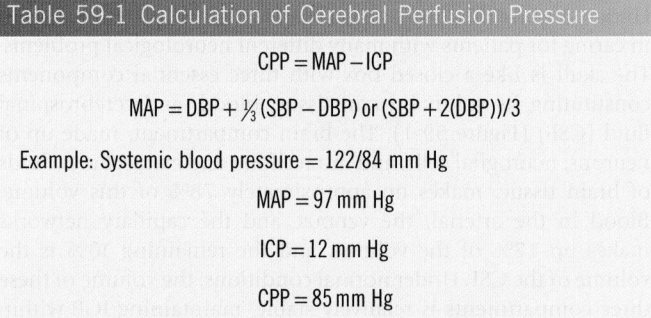

Table 59-1 Calculation of Cerebral Perfusion Pressure
CPP = MAP − ICP
MAP = DBP + ⅓(SBP − DBP) or (SBP + 2(DBP))/3
Example: Systemic blood pressure = 122/84 mm Hg
MAP = 97 mm Hg
ICP = 12 mm Hg
CPP = 85 mm Hg

CPP, cerebral perfusion pressure; *DBP*, diastolic blood pressure; *ICP*, intracranial pressure; *MAP*, mean arterial pressure; *SBP*, systolic blood pressure.

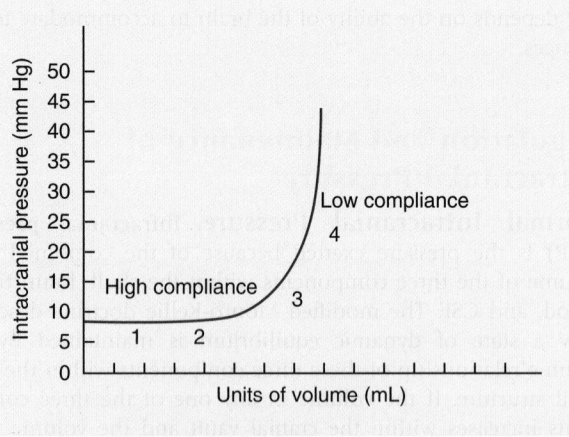

Figure 59-2 Intracranial pressure–volume curve. (See text for descriptions of *1*, *2*, *3*, and *4*.)

there is high compliance. The brain is in total compensation, with accommodation and autoregulation intact. An increase in volume (in brain tissue, blood, or CSF) does not increase the ICP. At stage 2, the compliance is lessening, and an increase in volume places the patient at risk of increased ICP. At stage 3, there is low compliance as compensatory mechanisms are becoming exhausted. Any small addition of volume causes a great increase in ICP. As compensatory mechanisms fail, there is a loss of autoregulation, and the patient may exhibit symptoms indicating increased ICP, such as headache, changes in level of consciousness (LOC), or pupil responsiveness.

As the patient enters stage 4, the ICP rises to lethal levels with even slight increases in volume. Here the patient is at significant risk of hypoperfusion and brain herniation and death.

Increased Intracranial Pressure

Increased ICP is a life-threatening situation resulting from an increase in any or all of the three components (brain tissue, blood, CSF) of the skull. Elevated ICP (above the threshold of 20 mm Hg) is clinically significant because it diminishes CPP, increasing risk of brain ischemia and infarction, and is associated with a poor prognosis (Brain Trauma Foundation [BTF], 2007).

Mechanisms of Increased Intracranial Pressure

The brain component of ICP can be increased by cerebral neoplasm, contusion, abscess, or cerebral edema. Conditions that increase the cerebral blood volume include intracranial hematomas or hemorrhages, metabolic and physiological factors (e.g., CO_2, O_2, fever, pain), and vascular anomalies. Increases in the CSF volume can result from CSF-secreting tumours or hydrocephalus. These cerebral insults may result in hypercapnia, cerebral acidosis, impaired autoregulation, and systemic hypertension, which promote the formation and spread of cerebral edema. This edema distorts brain tissue, further increasing the ICP, which leads to even more tissue hypoxia and acidosis. Figure 59-3 illustrates the progression of increased ICP.

Crucial to preservation of tissue is maintenance of CBF. Elevations in pressure that are more evenly distributed throughout the brain or slow increases in ICP (e.g., an enlarging brain lesion) preserve blood flow better than a rapid increase, as in primary brain injury. Sustained increases in ICP result in brainstem compression and herniation of the brain from one compartment to another.

Displacement and herniation of brain tissue cause a potentially reversible pathophysiological process to become irreversible. Ischemia and edema are further increased, compounding the pre-existing problem. Herniations force the cerebellum and the brainstem downward through the foramen magnum. If compression of the brainstem is unrelieved, respiratory arrest may occur. Compression of brain tissue, brainstem structures, cranial nerves, and vessels may be fatal. Figure 59-4 illustrates herniation. (Herniation is further described in the later section on complications of ICP.)

Cerebral Edema

As shown in Table 59-2, there are a variety of causes of **cerebral edema** (increased accumulation of fluid in the extravascular spaces of brain tissue). Regardless of the cause, cerebral edema

PATHOPHYSIOLOGY MAP

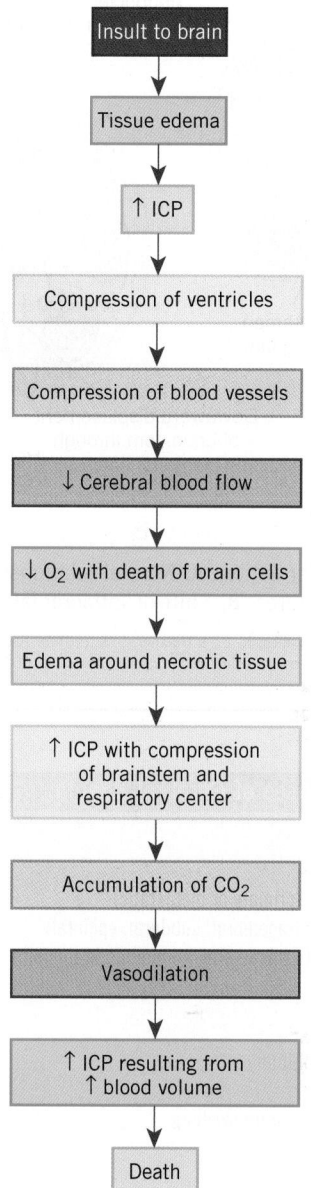

Figure 59-3 Progression of increased intracranial pressure (ICP).

results in an increase in tissue volume that carries the potential for increased ICP. Factors that contribute to the degree of cerebral edema are the extent and the severity of the original insult as well as the cascade of secondary cellular events that occur in the hours and days following insult or injury.

Three types of cerebral edema have been distinguished: vasogenic, cytotoxic, and interstitial. More than one type may result from a single insult in the same patient.

Vasogenic Cerebral Edema. *Vasogenic cerebral edema,* the most common type of edema, occurs mainly in the white matter and is attributed to changes in the endothelial lining of cerebral capillaries. These changes allow leakage of macromolecules from the capillaries into the surrounding extracellular space, resulting

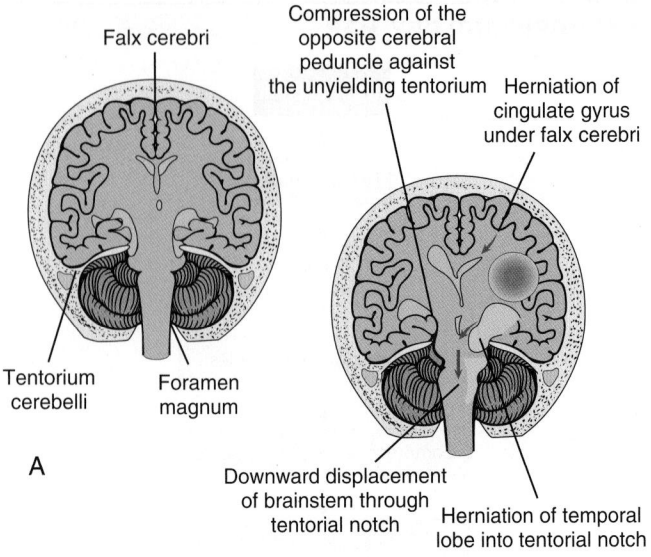

Falx cerebri

Compression of the opposite cerebral peduncle against the unyielding tentorium

Herniation of cingulate gyrus under falx cerebri

Tentorium cerebelli

Foramen magnum

A

Downward displacement of brainstem through tentorial notch

Herniation of temporal lobe into tentorial notch

B

Figure 59-4 Herniation. **A,** Normal relationship of intracranial structures. **B,** Shift of intracranial structures.

Source: Adapted from McCance, K. L., & Huether, S. E. (2010). *Pathophysiology: The biologic basis for disease in adults and children* (6th ed., p. 558, Figure 16-16). St. Louis: Mosby.

Table 59-2 Causes of Cerebral Edema

- Mass lesions
  - Brain abscess
  - Brain tumour (primary or metastatic)
  - Hematoma (intracerebral, subdural, epidural)
  - Hemorrhage (intracerebral, cerebellar, brainstem)
- Head injuries
  - Contusion
  - Diffuse axonal injury
  - Hemorrhage
  - Post-traumatic brain swelling
- Brain surgery
- Cerebral infections
  - Meningitis
  - Encephalitis
- Vascular insult
  - Anoxic and ischemic episodes
  - Cerebral infarction (thrombotic or embolic)
  - Venous sinus thrombosis
- Toxic or metabolic encephalopathic conditions
  - Lead or arsenic intoxication
  - Hepatic encephalopathy
  - Uremia

in an osmotic gradient that favours the flow of water from the intravascular to the extravascular space. A variety of insults, such as brain tumours, head trauma, abscesses, and ingested toxins, may cause an increase in the permeability of the blood–brain barrier and produce an increase in the extracellular fluid volume.

The speed and extent of the spread of the edema fluid are influenced by the systemic BP, the site of the brain injury, and the extent of the blood–brain barrier defect. This edema may produce a continuum of symptoms ranging from focal neurological deficits to disturbances in consciousness, including **coma** (profound state of unconsciousness).

Cytotoxic Cerebral Edema. *Cytotoxic cerebral edema* results from local disruption of the functional or morphological integrity of cell membranes and occurs most often in the grey matter. It develops from destructive lesions or trauma to brain tissue that lead to cerebral hypoxia or anoxia, sodium depletion, and syndrome of inappropriate antidiuretic hormone (SIADH). Cerebral edema results as fluid and protein shift from the extracellular space directly into the cells, with subsequent swelling and loss of cellular function.

Interstitial Cerebral Edema. *Interstitial cerebral edema* is the result of periventricular diffusion of ventricular CSF in a patient with uncontrolled hydrocephalus. It can also be caused by enlargement of the extracellular space as a result of systemic water excess (hyponatremia). Fluid moves into the cells to equilibrate with the hypo-osmotic interstitial fluid. Regardless of the cause of cerebral edema, manifestations of increased ICP result, unless compensation is adequate.

Clinical Manifestations

The clinical manifestations of increased ICP can take many forms, depending on the cause, the location, and the rate at which the pressure increase occurs (Figure 59-5). The earlier the condition is recognized and treated, the better the prognosis. The clinical manifestations of increased ICP are discussed later.

Change in Level of Consciousness. The *level of consciousness* (LOC) is a sensitive and early indicator of the patient's neurological status. Changes in LOC are a result of impaired CBF, which deprives the cells of the cerebral cortex and the reticular activating system (RAS) of oxygen. The RAS is located in the brainstem with neural connections to many parts of the nervous system. An intact RAS can maintain a state of wakefulness even in the absence of a functioning cerebral cortex. Interruptions of impulses from the RAS or alteration of the functioning of the cerebral hemispheres can cause **unconsciousness** (abnormal state of complete or partial unawareness of self or environment).

The patient's state of consciousness is defined by both the behaviour and the pattern of brain activity recorded by an electroencephalogram (EEG). The change in consciousness may be dramatic, as in coma, or subtle, such as a flattening of affect, confusion, or decrease in level of attention. In the deepest state of unconsciousness (i.e., coma), the patient does not respond to painful stimuli. The EEG pattern demonstrates decreased neuronal activity.

Changes in Vital Signs. Changes in vital signs are caused by increasing pressure on the thalamus, the hypothalamus, the pons, and the medulla. Manifestations such as Cushing's triad, consisting of increasing systolic pressure (widening pulse pressure), bradycardia with a full and bounding pulse, and irregular respiratory pattern, may be present but often do not appear until ICP has been increased for some time or suddenly and markedly

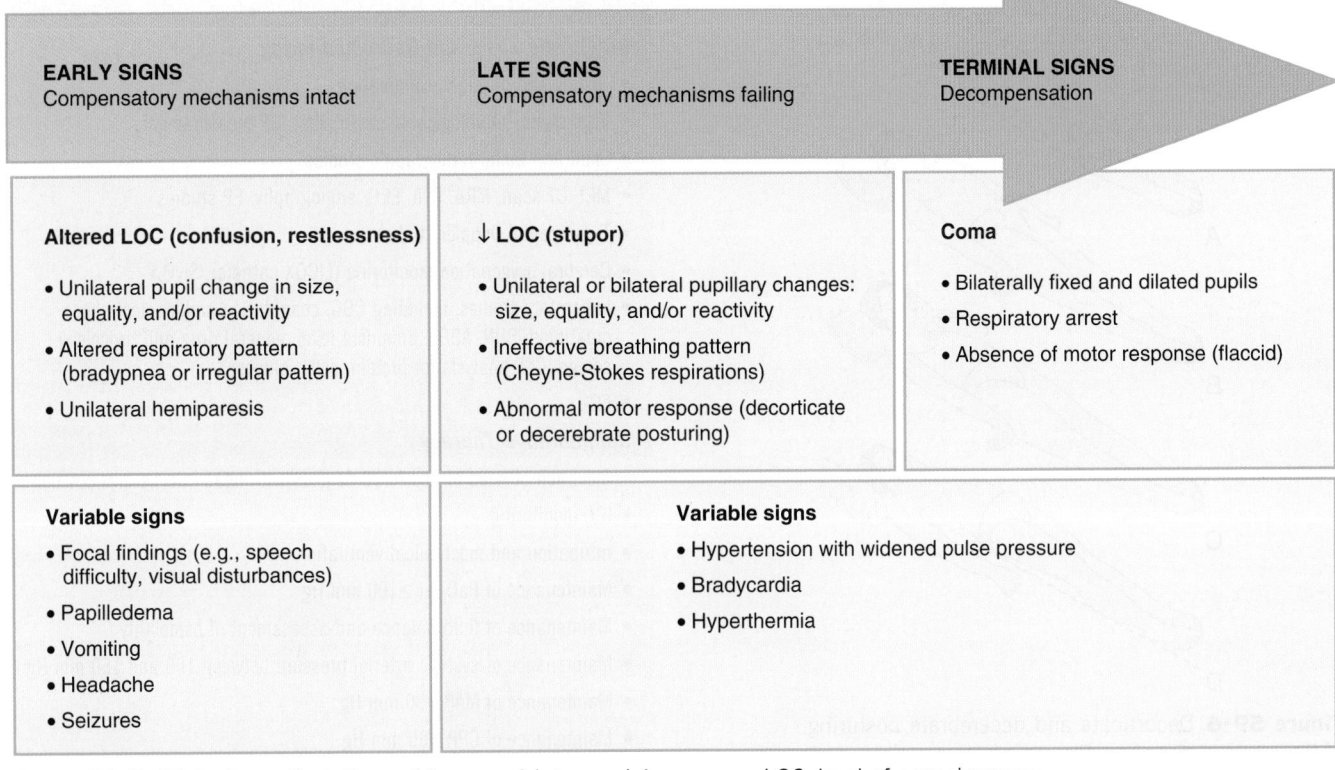

Figure 59-5 Clinical manifestations of increased intracranial pressure. *LOC,* level of consciousness.

increases (e.g., head trauma). A change in body temperature may also be noted and is caused by associated pressure on the hypothalamus.

Ocular Signs. Compression of the oculomotor nerve (cranial nerve [CN] III) results in dilation of the pupil *ipsilateral* to (same side as) the mass or lesion, sluggish or no response to light, inability to move the eye upward, and ptosis of the eyelid. These signs can be the result of a shifting of the brain from the midline, a process that compresses the trunk of CN III, paralyzing the pupil sphincter. A fixed (unresponsive), unilaterally dilated pupil is a neurological emergency that indicates herniation of the brain. Other cranial nerves may also be affected, such as the optic (CN II), trochlear (CN IV), and abducens (CN VI). Signs of dysfunction of these cranial nerves include blurred vision, diplopia, and changes in extraocular eye movements. Central herniation may initially manifest as sluggish but equal pupil responses. Lateral herniation of the uncus, the innermost part of the temporal lobe, may cause a dilated unilateral pupil. *Papilledema,* a choked optic disc seen on retinal examination, is also noted and is a nonspecific sign associated with increased ICP of long standing.

Decrease in Motor Function. As the ICP continues to rise, the patient manifests changes in motor ability. A *contralateral* (opposite side of the mass lesion) hemiparesis or hemiplegia may be seen, depending on the location of the source of the increased ICP. If painful stimuli are used to elicit a motor response, the patient may exhibit localization to the stimuli or a withdrawal from the stimuli. Decorticate (flexor) and decerebrate (extensor)

posturing may also be elicited by noxious stimuli (Figure 59-6). *Decorticate posture* consists of internal rotation and adduction of the arms with flexion of elbows, wrists, and fingers as a result of interruption of voluntary motor tracts. Extension of the legs may also be seen. A *decerebrate posture* may indicate more serious damage and results from disruption of motor fibres in the midbrain and brainstem. In this position, the arms are stiffly extended, adducted, and hyperpronated. There is also hyperextension of the legs with plantar flexion of the feet.

Headache. Although the brain itself is insensitive to pain, compression of other intracranial structures, such as the walls of arteries and veins and the cranial nerves, can produce headache. Headaches associated with increased ICP are often continuous. Straining or movement may accentuate the pain.

Vomiting. Vomiting, usually not preceded by nausea, is often a nonspecific sign of increased ICP. This is related to direct pressure on the vomiting centre located on the floor of the fourth ventricle in the medulla. Vomiting associated with increased ICP is often described as *projectile* owing to the force of vomitus ejection.

Complications

The major complications of uncontrolled, increased ICP are inadequate cerebral perfusion and cerebral herniation (see Figure 59-4). To better understand cerebral herniation, three important structures in the brain must be described. The *falx cerebri* is a thin wall of dura that folds down between the cortex, separating the

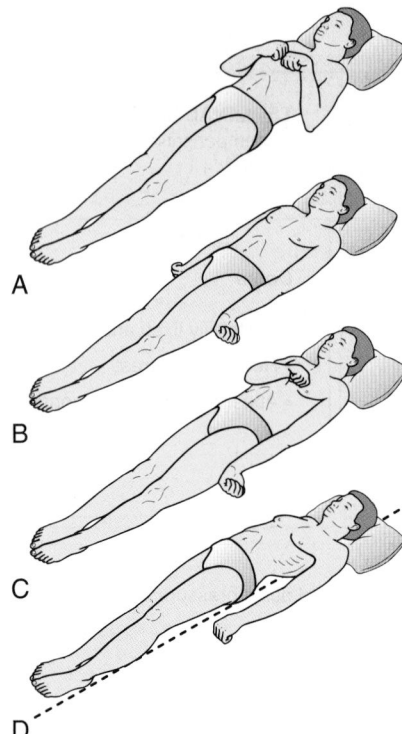

Figure 59-6 Decorticate and decerebrate posturing.
A, Decorticate response. Flexion of arms, wrists, and fingers with adduction in upper extremities. Extension, internal rotation, and plantar flexion in lower extremities.
B, Decerebrate response. All four extremities in rigid extension, with hyperpronation of forearms and plantar flexion of feet.
C, Decorticate response on right side of body and decerebrate response on left side of body. **D,** Opisthotonic posturing.

Source: Adapted from Urden, L. D., Stacy, K. M., & Lough, M. E. (2010). *Critical care nursing: Diagnosis and management* (6th ed., p. 703, Figure 27-1). St. Louis: Mosby.

two cerebral hemispheres. The *tentorium cerebelli* is a rigid fold of dura that separates the cerebral hemispheres from the cerebellum (see Figure 59-4). There is a central opening in the tentorium cerebelli called the *tentorial incisura* from which the brainstem emerges. This is a common site of herniation related to increased ICP.

Cingulate herniation occurs when there is lateral displacement of brain tissue beneath the falx cerebri. *Tentorial herniation* occurs when a mass lesion in the cerebrum forces the brain to herniate downward through the tentorial incisura. *Cerebellar tonsillar herniation* occurs when there is lateral and downward herniation of the cerebellar tonsils through the foramen magnum. This results in medullary compression and is often fatal.

Diagnostic Studies

Diagnostic studies to detect the presence and the underlying cause of increased ICP (Table 59-3) have become increasingly sophisticated. Magnetic resonance imaging (MRI) and computed tomography (CT) have revolutionized the diagnosis of acute intracranial events. Significant technological advancement in these modalities now offers enhanced evaluation of the brain's vasculature utilizing magnetic resonance angiography (MRA) and computed tomography angiography (CTA). All of these tests are

COLLABORATIVE CARE

Table 59-3 Increased Intracranial Pressure

Diagnostic Tests and Neuromonitoring

- History and physical examination
- Vital signs, neurological assessments, ICP measurements
- Skull and facial radiographic studies
- MRI, CT scan, MRA, CTA, EEG, angiography, EP studies
- Transcranial Doppler studies
- Cerebral oxygenation monitoring (LICOX catheter, $SjvO_2$)
- Laboratory studies, including CBC; coagulation profile; electrolytes; creatinine; BUN; ABGs; ammonia level; general drug and toxicology screen; CSF analysis for protein, cells, glucose*
- ECG

Collaborative Therapy

- Elevation of head of bed to 30 degrees with head in a neutral position
- ICP monitoring
- Intubation and mechanical ventilation
- Maintenance of PaO_2 at ≥100 mm Hg
- Maintenance of fluid balance and assessment of osmolality
- Maintenance of systolic arterial pressure between 100 and 160 mm Hg
- Maintenance of MAP >90 mm Hg
- Maintenance of CPP >60 mm Hg
- Reduction of cerebral metabolism (e.g., high-dose barbiturates)
- Drug therapy
  - Osmotic diuretics (mannitol)
  - Antiseizure drugs (e.g., phenytoin [Dilantin])
  - Corticosteroids (dexamethasone) (for brain tumours, bacterial meningitis)
  - Antipyretics
  - Histamine H_2-receptor antagonist (e.g., ranitidine [Zantac]) or proton pump inhibitor (e.g., pantoprazole [Pantoloc]) to prevent gastrointestinal ulcers and bleeding
  - Stool softeners
  - Nutritional support

ABGs, arterial blood gases; *BUN*, blood urea nitrogen; *CBC*, complete blood count; *CPP*, cerebral perfusion pressure; *CSF*, cerebrospinal fluid; *CT*, computed tomography; *CTA*, computed tomography angiography; *ECG*, electrocardiogram; *EEG*, electroencephalogram; *EP*, evoked potential; *ICP*, intracranial pressure; *MAP*, mean arterial pressure; *MRA*, magnetic resonance angiography; *MRI*, magnetic resonance imaging; *PaO₂*, partial pressure of arterial oxygen; *SjvO₂*, jugular venous oxygen saturation.
*CSF sampling via lumbar puncture is contraindicated if there is suspected raised ICP because there is a possibility of cerebral herniation and death.

used to differentiate the many conditions that can cause increased ICP and to evaluate therapeutic options. Other diagnostic tests that may be used include conventional cerebral angiography, EEG, ICP measurement, brain tissue oxygenation measurement via the LICOX catheter (described later), transcranial Doppler studies, and evoked potential studies. In general, a lumbar puncture is not performed when increased ICP is suspected because of the possibility of cerebral herniation from the sudden release of the pressure in the skull from the area above the lumbar puncture.

Neuromonitoring

Measurement of Intracranial Pressure. ICP may become elevated because of head trauma, stroke, subarachnoid haemorrhage, brain tumour, inflammation or infection, hydrocephalus, or brain tissue damage from other causes. Patients with or at risk for elevated ICP usually receive invasive ICP monitoring in a critical care unit (CCU), except those with irreversible problems or advanced neurological disease. Goals for nursing management of an elevated ICP include preservation of cerebral oxygenation and perfusion, early identification of neurological changes, and prevention of complications secondary to intracranial hypertension.

ICP monitoring is used to guide clinical care when the patient is at risk for or has elevations in ICP. ICP should be monitored if patients are admitted with a Glasgow Coma Scale (GCS) score of 8 or less and an abnormal CT scan or MRI (hematomas, contusion, edema, or compressed basal cisterns) (BTF, 2007). (The GCS is presented later in Table 59-5.) Multiple methods and devices are available to monitor ICP (Figure 59-7).

The "gold standard" for monitoring ICP is the *ventriculostomy*, whereby a catheter is inserted into the lateral ventricle and coupled to an external transducer. This technique directly measures the pressure within the ventricles and facilitates removal and/or sampling of CSF. Significant consideration in caring for a patient with a ventriculostomy is the constant positioning of the external transducer relative to the position of the patient's head to maintain consistent measurements. The transducer should be level with the foramen of Monro (intraventricular foramen); the reference point for this on the patient is the tragus of the ear (Figure 59-8, *A*). When repositioning a patient with a ventriculostomy, the system may need to be rezeroed to maintain the level of the transducer. Another device used for the monitoring of ICP is the *fibreoptic catheter*, the tip of which is placed directly into the ventricle or the brain tissue. A sensor transducer located in the catheter tip provides measurement of the pressure in the brain. Lastly, the *subarachnoid bolt* or *screw* may be placed through the skull between the arachnoid membrane and the cerebral cortex

to measure ICP; this method does not allow for drainage of CSF but can be converted into a ventriculostomy if the patient's clinical condition changes to require that intervention.

Infection is a serious consideration with ICP monitoring. Prophylactic systemic antibiotics may be administered to reduce the chances of infection. Factors that contribute to the development of infection include ICP monitoring for longer than 5 days, use of a ventriculostomy, the presence of a CSF leak, a concurrent systemic infection, and improper aseptic technique during manipulation by health care team members. Routine care may include regular diagnostic testing for CSF organism growth.

The ICP waveform is derived from the arterial pulsations of the choroids plexus in the lateral ventricles. A normal ICP waveform has a diastolic and a systolic component and correlates with the cardiac cycle. When the waveform is monitored so that components in synchrony with the cardiac cycle can be visualized, the normal ICP waveform has three phases (Table 59-4).

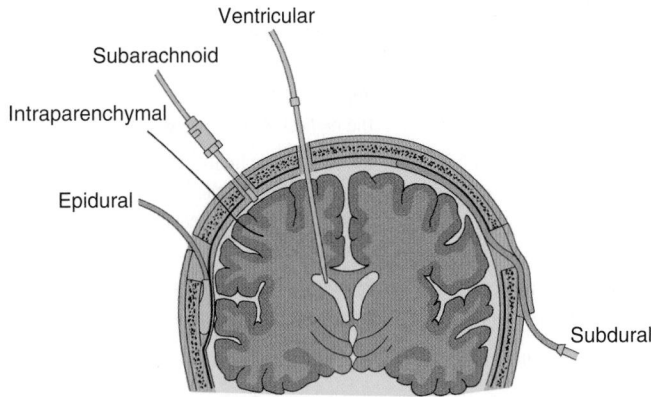

Figure 59-7 Coronal section of the brain shows potential sites for placement of intracranial pressure monitoring devices.

Source: Clochesy, J. M., Breu, C., Cardin, S., Whittaker, A. B., & Rudy, E. B. (1996). *Critical care nursing* (2nd ed.). Philadelphia: Saunders.

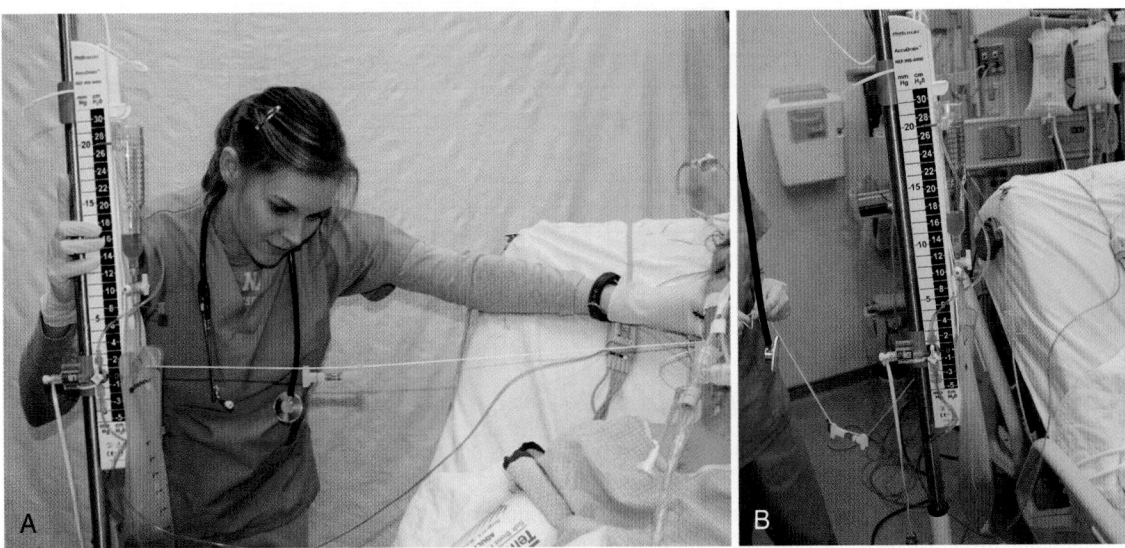

Figure 59-8 A, Levelling a ventriculostomy. **B,** Cerebrospinal fluid is drained into a drainage system.

Source: Courtesy Meg Zomorodi.

It is important to monitor the ICP waveform and the CPP. It has been noted that, when the height of P2 is higher than P1, this represents low *compliance* and the patient is at risk for development of elevated ICP (Figure 59-9). It is important to consider the rate at which changes occur and the patient's clinical condition. Neurological deterioration might not occur until ICP elevation is pronounced and sustained. Any indication of ICP elevation, either as a mean increase in pressure or as an abnormal waveform configuration, should be reported to the physician immediately.

Cerebrospinal Fluid Drainage. With the ventricular catheter and certain fibreoptic systems, it is possible to control elevations in ICP by removing CSF. Using a closed system (Figure 59-10), CSF is removed by gravity drainage and by adjusting the height of the drip chamber and drainage bag relative to the patient's ventricular reference point. Typically a

point 15 cm above the ear is selected (see Figure 59-8, *B*). Raising the system diminishes drainage, whereas lowering the system increases drainage volume. Careful monitoring of the volume of CSF drained is essential, keeping in mind that normal adult CSF production is about 20 to 30 mL/hr, with a total CSF volume of 90 to 150 mL within the ventricles and the subarachnoid space. The level of the ICP indicating that drainage should be initiated, the amount of fluid to be drained, the height of the system, and the frequency of drainage are ordered by the physician. Prevention of infection is imperative by use of strict aseptic technique during dressing changes or sampling of CSF. The system must remain intact to ensure that the ICP readings are accurate because treatment is initiated and evaluated on the basis of the readings.

Complications of this type of drainage system include ventricular collapse, infection, and herniation or subdural hematoma formation from rapid decompression. Although it is generally recognized that CSF removal decreases ICP and improves CPP, guidelines for CSF removal are not universally accepted but are typically based on institution or physician preference.

Cerebral Oxygenation Monitoring. Failure to adequately deliver oxygenated blood to an injured brain is a major contributor to poor outcomes. Critical reliance of the brain on oxygen has prompted significant advances in neuromonitoring related to oxygen delivery and consumption. Readily available now is technology that indirectly measures cerebral oxygenation and cerebral perfusion. Two such devices are currently being used in critical care settings: the *LICOX brain tissue oxygenation catheter* and the *jugular venous bulb catheter*. The LICOX catheter is placed in the frontal white matter of the brain and provides continuous monitoring of the pressure of oxygen in brain tissue ($PbtO_2$); the

Table 59-4 Normal Intracranial Pressure Waveforms*	
WAVEFORM	**MEANING**
P1 Percussion wave	Represents arterial pulsations; normally the highest of the three waveforms.
P2 Rebound wave	Reflects intracranial compliance or relative brain volume. When P2 is higher than P1, intracranial compliance is compromised.
P3 Dicrotic wave	Follows dicrotic notch; represents venous pulsations; normally, the lowest waveform.

*See Figure 59-8.

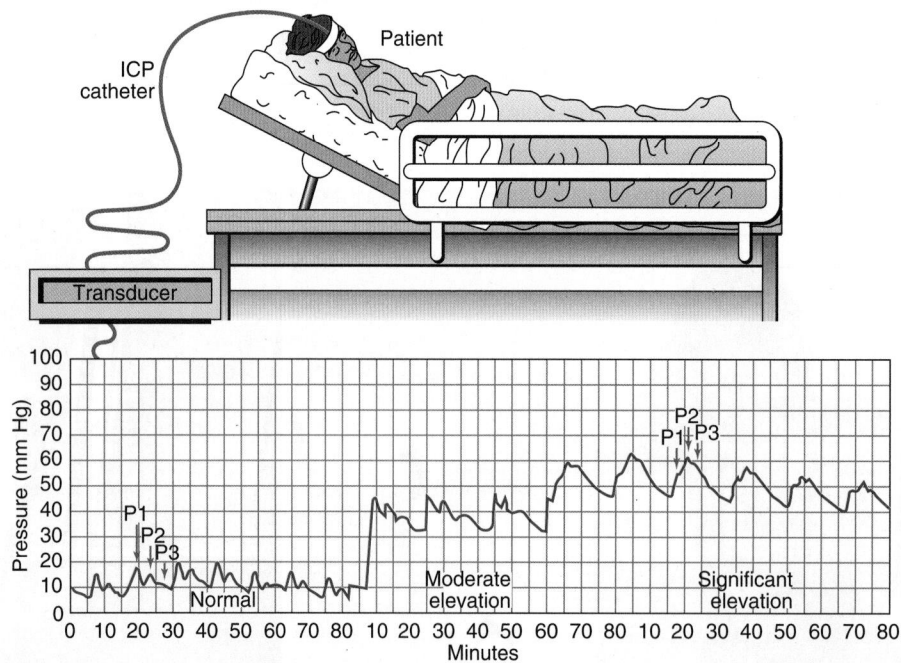

Figure 59-9 Intracranial pressure (ICP) monitoring can be used to continuously measure ICP. The ICP tracing shows normal, elevated, and plateau waves. At high ICP, the P2 peak is higher than the P1 peak, and the peaks become less distinct and plateau.

Source: Copstead-Kirkhorn, L. C., & Banasik, J. L. (2010). *Pathophysiology* (4th ed., p. 1043, Figure 44-7). St Louis: Mosby.

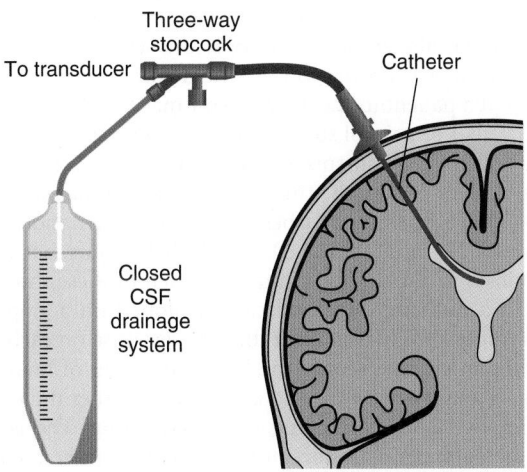

Figure 59-10 Intermittent drainage system. Cerebrospinal fluid (CSF) is drained via a ventriculostomy when intracranial pressure (ICP) exceeds the upper pressure parameter set by the physician. Intermittent drainage involves opening the three-way stopcock to allow CSF to flow into the draining bag for brief periods (≤5 min) until the pressure is below the upper pressure parameters.

Source: Redrawn from Barker, E. (2008). *Neuroscience nursing: A spectrum of care* (3rd ed., p. 321, Figure 10-14, *A*). St. Louis: Mosby.

normal range for PbtO$_2$ is 20 to 40 mm Hg. A lower-than-normal PbtO$_2$ level is indicative of ischemia. The jugular venous bulb catheter is placed in the internal jugular vein and positioned so that the catheter tip is located in the jugular bulb. This catheter provides a measurement of jugular venous oxygen saturation (SjvO$_2$), which indicates total venous brain tissue extraction of oxygen as a measure of cerebral oxygen supply and demand. The normal SjvO$_2$ range is 55 to 75%. Values less than 50% demonstrate impaired cerebral oxygenation. With the use of either device, interventions can be specifically focused to improve brain tissue oxygen levels. The LICOX catheter has the ability to also measure brain temperature; neither device has the capability of monitoring ICP, and therefore, an ICP monitoring device may be placed for this purpose.

Collaborative Care

The goals of collaborative care (see Table 59-3) are to identify and treat the underlying cause of increased ICP and to support brain function. A careful history is an important diagnostic aid that can direct the search for the underlying cause.

Ensuring adequate oxygenation to support brain function is the first step in the management of increased ICP. An endotracheal tube or tracheostomy may be necessary to maintain adequate ventilation. Arterial blood gas (ABG) analysis guides the oxygen therapy. The goal is to maintain the PaO$_2$ at 100 mm Hg or greater. It may be necessary to maintain the patient on a mechanical ventilator to ensure adequate oxygenation.

If the condition is caused by a mass lesion, such as a tumour or hematoma, surgical removal of the mass is the best management (see sections on Brain Tumours and Cranial Surgery later in this chapter). Nonsurgical intervention for the reduction of tissue volume related to cerebral tissue swelling and cerebral edema includes the use of osmotic diuretics, hypertonic saline, and corticosteroids.

Drug Therapy. Drug therapy plays an important role in the management of increased ICP. Mannitol (Osmitrol), an osmotic diuretic given intravenously, is frequently used to decrease the ICP. Mannitol acts to decrease ICP in two ways: plasma expansion and osmotic effect. There is an immediate plasma-expanding effect that reduces the hematocrit and blood viscosity, thereby increasing CBF and cerebral oxygen delivery. A vascular osmotic gradient is created by mannitol. Thus, fluid moves from the tissues into the blood vessels. ICP is reduced by the decrease in the total brain fluid content. Fluid and electrolyte status must be closely monitored when osmotic diuretics are used. Mannitol use may be contraindicated if renal disease is present and if serum osmolality is elevated (Ennis & Brophy, 2010).

There continues to be significant interest in the use of hypertonic saline as an alternative therapy for intracranial hypertension, and it is now routinely used in many institutions. Current research suggests that hypertonic saline offers effective first-line treatment for elevated ICP when compared with mannitol (Kamel, Navi, Nakagawa, Hemphill, & Ko, 2011).

Corticosteroids (e.g., dexamethasone) are thought to control the vasogenic edema surrounding tumours and abscesses but appear to have limited value in the management of head-injured patients; and studies suggest that corticosteroids not be used in patients with head injury because they potentially increase mortality (Alderson & Roberts, 2009). The mode of action of corticosteroids is not completely known. It is theorized that they act by their stabilizing effect on the cell membrane and by inhibiting the synthesis of prostaglandins (see Chapter 14, Figure 14-7), thus preventing the formation of proinflammatory mediators. Corticosteroids are also thought to improve neuronal function by improving CBF and restoring autoregulation.

Complications associated with the use of corticosteroids include hyperglycemia, increased incidence of infections, gastrointestinal (GI) bleeding, and hyponatremia. Fluid intake and sodium and glucose levels should be monitored regularly. Patients receiving corticosteroids should concurrently be given antacids or histamine (H$_2$)-receptor blockers (e.g., ranitidine [Zantac]) or proton pump inhibitors (e.g., omeprazole [Losec], pantoprazole [Pantoloc]) to prevent GI ulcers and bleeding.

Drug therapy for reducing cerebral metabolism may be an effective strategy to control ICP. The reduction of cerebral metabolic rate decreases the CBF and, therefore, the ICP. High-dose barbiturates (e.g., pentobarbital sodium [Somnotol], thiopental sodium [Pentothal]) are used in patients with increased ICP refractory to treatment. Barbiturates dampen the effects of environmental stimuli on patients, thereby decreasing cerebral metabolism and subsequently ICP. A secondary effect is a reduction in cerebral edema and production of a more uniform blood supply to the brain. Capabilities to monitor the patient's ICP, blood flow, EEG, and metabolism should be available when this treatment is used. The physician orders the barbiturate infusion to be administered at a rate that achieves a desired level of brain wave suppression as a means to control ICP. Total burst suppression, recognized by the absence of spikes showing brain activity on the EEG monitor, indicates that maximal therapeutic effect has been achieved. Antiseizure drugs such as phenytoin (Dilantin) may be used because seizures can further increase ICP.

Hyperventilation Therapy. In the past, aggressive hyperventilation (PaCO$_2$ <25 mm Hg) had been a mainstay treatment of elevated ICP. The lowering of the PaCO$_2$ leads to constriction of the cerebral blood vessels, reducing CBF and thereby decreasing the ICP. More recent evidence suggests that aggressive hyperventilation increases the risk of focal cerebral ischemia and may adversely affect outcomes (BTF, 2007). Prolonged aggressive hyperventilation therapy should be avoided in the absence of increased ICP, particularly during the first 24 hours following a head injury or when CBF is low. Brief periods of less aggressive hyperventilation therapy (target PaCO$_2$, 30 to 35 mm Hg) may be useful for refractory intracranial hypertension. However, the effectiveness is time limited and transient.

Nutritional Therapy. All patients must have their nutritional needs met, regardless of their state of consciousness or health. Early feeding following brain injury may improve outcomes (Härtl, Gerber, Ni, & Ghajar, 2008). The patient with increased ICP is in a hypermetabolic and hypercatabolic state that increases the need for glucose to provide the necessary fuel for metabolism of the injured brain. If the patient cannot maintain an adequate oral intake, other means of meeting the nutritional requirements, such as enteral feedings or total parenteral nutrition, should be initiated. Nutritional replacements beginning within 5 days of injury have been shown to decrease mortality (Härtl et al., 2008). Because malnutrition promotes continued cerebral edema, maintenance of optimal nutrition is imperative. (Nutritional therapy is discussed in Chapter 42.) Feedings or supplements should be guided by the patient's fluid and electrolyte status as well as the patient's metabolic needs.

Current therapy is directed at keeping patients normovolemic. Intravenous (IV) 0.45% or 0.9% sodium chloride is the preferred solution for administration of piggyback medications because a lowering of serum osmolarity and an increase in cerebral edema occur if 5% dextrose in water is used. Infusion of hypertonic saline (2 to 7.5%) is another intervention currently used to acutely lower ICP and support intravascular volume. However, long-term patient outcome data are still being investigated.

NURSING MANAGEMENT: INCREASED INTRACRANIAL PRESSURE

▪ Nursing Assessment

Subjective data about the patient with increased ICP can be obtained from the patient or family members or other persons who are familiar with the patient. The nurse must learn appropriate assessment techniques and describe the LOC by noting the specific behaviours observed. When a deviation from the normal state of consciousness occurs, a more structured method of observation should be initiated. This type of systematic approach to nursing assessment is illustrated in eFigure 59-1, available on the Evolve Web site for this chapter, and consists of assessing the LOC by the Glasgow Coma Scale (Table 59-5) and by body functions. Adequate circulation and respiration are the most vital and should always be the first body functions assessed.

▪ Glasgow Coma Scale

The **Glasgow Coma Scale (GCS)**, developed in 1974, is a quick, practical, and standardized system for assessing the degree to

which consciousness is impaired. It provides a universal language for describing altered states of consciousness. The three areas assessed in the GCS correspond to the definition of coma as the inability of a patient to speak, obey commands, or open the eyes when a verbal or painful stimulus is applied (Jennett & Teasdale, 1977). Specific assessments evaluate the patient's response to varying degrees of stimuli. Three indicators of response are evaluated: (1) eye opening, (2) best verbal response, and (3) best motor response (see Table 59-5). Specific behaviours that are seen as responses to the testing stimulus in each of these three areas are given a numeric value and can be plotted on a graph. The nurse's responsibility is to elicit the best response on each of the scales; the higher the scores, the higher the level of brain functioning. A graph can be used to determine whether the patient's condition is stable, improving, or deteriorating. The subscale scores are particularly important if a patient is untestable in one area. For example, severe periorbital edema may make eye opening impossible. The total GCS score is a sum of the numeric values assigned to each of the three areas evaluated. The highest GCS score is 15 for a fully alert person, and the lowest possible score is 3. A GCS score of 8 or less is generally indicative of coma (Teasdale & Jennett, 1974).

The GCS offers several advantages in the assessment of the unconscious patient. It is specific and structured, allowing different health care providers to arrive at the same conclusion regarding the patient's status. It saves time for the assessor because the ratings are done with numbers rather than with lengthy descriptions.

The GCS is also specific enough to discriminate between different or changing states. The GCS is used to assess the arousal aspect of consciousness. Other components of the neurological assessment include pupillary checks, extremity strength testing, vital signs, and if appropriate, testing of the function of specific cranial nerves.

▪ Neurological Assessment

The pupils are compared with one another for size, movement, and response (Figure 59-11). If the oculomotor nerve is compressed, the pupil on the affected side (ipsilateral) becomes

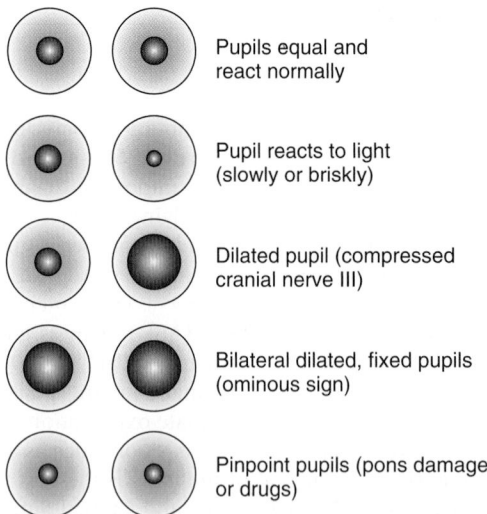

Pupils equal and react normally

Pupil reacts to light (slowly or briskly)

Dilated pupil (compressed cranial nerve III)

Bilateral dilated, fixed pupils (ominous sign)

Pinpoint pupils (pons damage or drugs)

Figure 59-11 Pupillary check for size and response.

Table 59-5 Glasgow Coma Scale

APPROPRIATE STIMULUS	RESPONSE	SCORE
Eyes Open		
Approach to bedside	Spontaneous response	4
Verbal command	Opening of eyes to name or command	3
Pain	Lack of opening of eyes to previous stimuli but opening to pain	2
	Lack of opening of eyes to any stimulus	1
	Untestable (e.g., swollen)	U
Best Verbal Response		
Verbal questioning with maximum arousal	Appropriate orientation, conversant; correct identification of self, place, year, and month	5
	Confusion; conversant, but disorientation in one or more spheres	4
	Inappropriate or disorganized use of words (e.g., cursing), lack of sustained conversation	3
	Incomprehensible words, sounds (e.g., moaning)	2
	Lack of sound, even with painful stimuli	1
	Untestable (e.g., endotracheal tube)	U
Best Motor Response		
Verbal command (e.g., "raise your arm, hold up two fingers")	Obedience of command	6
Pain applied centrally (e.g., sternal rub, pinching of upper third of trapezius, or supraorbital pressure)	Localization of pain, lack of obedience but presence of attempts to remove offending stimulus—purposeful movement	5
	Flexion withdrawal,* flexion of arm in response to pain without abnormal flexion posture—nonpurposeful movement	4
	Abnormal flexion, flexing of arm at elbow and pronation, making a fist	3
	Abnormal extension, extension of arm at elbow usually with adduction and internal rotation of arm at shoulder	2
	Lack of response	1
	Untestable*	U

*Added to the original scale by many centres.

larger until it fully dilates. If ICP continues to increase, both pupils dilate. Pupil size is measured in millimetres before assessing the pupil response to light.

Pupillary reaction is tested with a penlight. The normal reaction is brisk constriction when the light is shone directly into the eye. A consensual response (a slight constriction in the opposite pupil) should also be noted at the same time. A sluggish reaction can indicate early pressure on CN III. A fixed pupil shows no response to light stimulus, which usually indicates increased ICP.

Evaluation of other cranial nerves can be included in the neurological assessment. Eye movements controlled by CNs III, IV, and VI can be examined in the patient who is awake and can be used to assess the function of the brainstem. In the unconscious patient, eye movements can be elicited by reflex with the use of head movements (oculocephalic) and caloric stimulation (oculovestibular) (see Chapters 23 and 24). Testing the corneal reflex provides clinical information regarding the function of CNs V and VII. If corneal reflexes are absent, routine eye care should be initiated to prevent corneal abrasion.

Motor strength is tested by asking the awake patient to squeeze the nurse's hands to compare strength in the hands. The palmar (or pronator) drift test is an excellent measure of strength in the upper extremities. With eyes closed, the patient raises the

arms in front of the body with the palmar surface facing upward. If there is any weakness in the upper extremity, the palmar surface rotates inward and the arm may drift downward. Eyes are closed so that the patient is unable to see the palmar drift and try to correct the rotating hand position. Detection of a palmar drift is an early indicator of corticospinal tract compression and possible increased ICP. Asking the patient to raise the foot from the bed or to bend the knees up in bed is a good assessment of lower extremity strength. All four extremities should be tested for strength and evaluated for any asymmetry in strength or movement.

The motor strength of the unconscious or uncooperative patient can be assessed by observation of spontaneous movement. If no spontaneous movement is possible, a pain stimulus should be applied to the patient, and the response should be noted. Resistance to movement during passive range of motion exercises is another measure of strength.

The vital signs, including BP, pulse, respiratory rate, and temperature, should also be systematically recorded. Cushing's triad is a triad of changes to vital signs (increased BP with a widening pulse pressure, bradycardia, and irregular respiratory pattern). This triad indicates severe increased ICP and impending cerebral herniation. Specific respiratory patterns are associated with severely increased ICP (Figure 59-12).

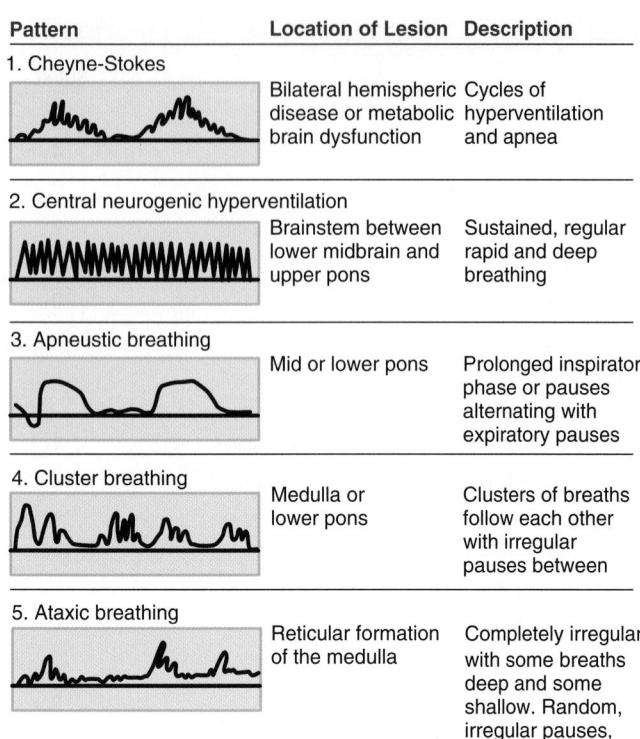

Pattern	Location of Lesion	Description
1. Cheyne-Stokes	Bilateral hemispheric disease or metabolic brain dysfunction	Cycles of hyperventilation and apnea
2. Central neurogenic hyperventilation	Brainstem between lower midbrain and upper pons	Sustained, regular rapid and deep breathing
3. Apneustic breathing	Mid or lower pons	Prolonged inspiratory phase or pauses alternating with expiratory pauses
4. Cluster breathing	Medulla or lower pons	Clusters of breaths follow each other with irregular pauses between
5. Ataxic breathing	Reticular formation of the medulla	Completely irregular with some breaths deep and some shallow. Random, irregular pauses, slow rate

Figure 59-12 Common abnormal respiratory patterns associated with coma.

Nursing Diagnoses

Nursing diagnoses for the patient with increased ICP include, but are not limited to, those presented in Nursing Care Plan (NCP) 59-1.

Planning

The overall goals are that the patient with increased ICP will (1) maintain a patent airway, (2) have ICP and CPP within normal limits, (3) demonstrate normal fluid and electrolyte balance, and (4) have no complications secondary to immobility and decreased LOC.

Nursing Implementation

Acute Intervention

Respiratory Function. Maintenance of a patent airway is critical in the patient with increased ICP and is a primary nursing responsibility. As the LOC decreases, the patient is at increased risk of airway obstruction from the tongue dropping back and occluding the airway or from accumulation of secretions. Altered breathing patterns may become evident. Airway patency can be aided by keeping the patient lying on one side, with frequent position changes. Snoring sounds, which may indicate obstruction, should be noted. Accumulated secretions should be removed by suctioning, as needed. An oral airway

facilitates breathing and provides an easier suctioning route in the comatose patient. Any patient with altered LOC who is unable to maintain a patent airway or effective ventilation requires intubation and mechanical ventilation.

The nurse must use measures to prevent hypoxia and hypercapnia. Proper positioning of the head is important. Elevation of the head of the bed by 30 degrees enhances respiratory exchange and aids in decreasing cerebral edema. Suctioning and coughing can cause transient decreases in the PaO_2 and increases in the ICP. Suctioning should be less than 10 seconds in duration, with administration of 100% oxygen before and after to prevent decreases in the PaO_2. To avoid cumulative increases in the ICP with suctioning, suctioning should be limited to two passes per suction procedure. Patients with elevated ICP are at risk for lower CPP during suctioning (BTF, 2007).

Abdominal distension can interfere with respiratory function and should be prevented. Increased intra-abdominal or intrathoracic pressures can contribute to elevated ICP by impeding cerebral venous drainage. Insertion of a nasogastric tube to aspirate the stomach contents can prevent distension, vomiting, and possible aspiration. However, in patients with facial and skull fractures, a nasogastric tube is contraindicated, and oral insertion of a gastric tube is preferred.

Pain, anxiety, and fear from the initial injury, therapeutic procedures, or noxious stimuli can increase ICP and BP, complicating the management and the recovery of the brain-injured patient. The appropriate choice or combination of sedatives, paralytics, and analgesics for symptom management presents a challenge to the CCU team. Administration of these agents may alter the neurological state, masking true neurological changes. It may be necessary to temporarily suspend pharmacological therapy to appropriately assess neurological status. The choice, the dosage, and the combination of agents may vary depending on the patient's history, neurological state, and overall clinical presentation.

Opioids, such as morphine sulphate and fentanyl, are rapid-onset analgesics with minimal effect on CBF or oxygen metabolism. The IV anaesthetic sedative propofol (Diprivan) has gained popularity in the management of pain and anxiety in the CCU because of its rapid onset, short half-life, and oxygen-saving properties. It has been shown to depress cerebral metabolism and oxygen consumption, offering neuroprotective benefits. Non-depolarizing neuromuscular blocking agents (e.g., cisatracurium [Nimbex]) are useful for ventilatory management and treatment of refractory intracranial hypertension. Because these agents paralyze muscles without blocking pain or noxious stimuli, they are used in combination with sedatives, analgesics, or benzodiazepines. Benzodiazepines, although useful for symptom management and ventilatory support, are often avoided in the management of the patient with increased ICP because of the hypotension effect and long half-life, unless used as an adjunct to neuromuscular blocking agents.

Arterial blood gases should be measured and evaluated regularly (see Chapter 28). The nurse should frequently monitor the arterial blood gas values and maintain the levels within prescribed or acceptable parameters. The appropriate ventilatory support can be ordered on the basis of the PaO_2 and $PaCO_2$ values.

Fluid and Electrolyte Balance. Fluid and electrolyte disturbances can have an adverse effect on ICP. IV fluids should be closely monitored with the use of a limited-volume device or a volume-control apparatus for accuracy. Intake and output, with insensible losses and daily weights taken into account, are important parameters in the assessment of fluid balance.

Electrolyte determinations should be made daily, and any abnormal values should be discussed with the physician. It is especially important to monitor serum glucose, sodium, potassium, and osmolality. Urinary output is monitored to detect problems related to *diabetes insipidus* (DI) (e.g., increased urinary output related to a decrease in antidiuretic hormone secretion); SIADH, which results in decreased urinary output; and cerebral salt wasting, a form of hyponatremia caused by excessive renal sodium excretion associated with cerebral insult. Besides urinary output, the serum and urine sodium and osmolality are also used to diagnose DI, SIADH, and cerebral salt wasting. DI may result

NURSING CARE PLAN 59-1

Increased Intracranial Pressure

NURSING DIAGNOSIS	***Risk for ineffective cerebral perfusion** related to* reduction of venous and/or arterial blood flow and cerebral edema *as evidenced by* CPP <60 mm Hg, altered mental status, changes in motor response, and behavioural changes
Expected Patient Outcome	**Nursing Interventions and *Rationales***
• Maintains cerebral perfusion within normal parameters	**Cerebral perfusion promotion** • Consult with physician *to determine hemodynamic parameters, and maintain within this range.* • Induce hypertension with volume expansion or inotropic or vasoconstrictive agents, as ordered, *to maintain hemodynamic parameters and optimize CPP.* • Consult with physician to determine optimal head of bed placement and monitor patient's responses *to optimize ICP and CPP.* • Monitor determinants of tissue oxygen delivery (e.g., PaCO₂, SaO₂, and hemoglobin levels and cardiac output), if available, *to ensure adequate oxygenation to support brain function.* • Calculate and monitor CPP *to evaluate adequacy of cerebral blood perfusion.* • Monitor neurological status *to determine hemodynamic status.* • Monitor intake and output *to assess effects of diuretic and corticosteroid therapy.*
NURSING DIAGNOSIS	***Decreased intracranial adaptive capacity** related to* decreased cerebral perfusion or sustained increase in ICP *as evidenced by* repeated increases of >10 mm Hg for more than 5 minutes following any of a variety of external stimuli, baseline ICP >20 mm Hg, elevated systolic blood pressure, bradycardia, and widened pulse pressure
Expected Patient Outcomes	**Nursing Interventions and *Rationales***
• Maintains intracranial pressure within normal parameters • Experiences no serious increases in intracranial pressure during or following care activities	**Cerebral edema management** • Monitor vital signs and neurological status closely and compare with baseline *to evaluate patient's response to treatment.* • Monitor respiratory status: rate, rhythm, depth of respirations; PaO₂, PaCO₂, pH, bicarbonate *because low PaO₂ and a high hydrogen ion concentration (acidosis) are potent cerebral blood vasodilators that increase cerebral blood flow and may increase ICP.* • Analyze ICP waveform *to provide an accurate indicator of ICP.* • Position with head of bed up 30 degrees or greater *to promote venous drainage from head, reducing ICP.* • Limit suction passes to <10 seconds *to prevent increased ICP.* • Allow ICP to return to baseline between nursing activities *to prevent sustained increases in ICP.* • Maintain normothermia *because elevated temperature increases cerebral metabolism and causes increased ICP.* • Give sedation *to decrease agitation and hyperactivity that cause increased ICP.* • Decrease stimuli in patient's environment *to prevent increases in ICP.*

CPP, cerebral perfusion pressure; *ICP,* intracranial pressure; *PaCO₂,* partial pressure of carbon dioxide in arterial blood; *PaO₂,* partial pressure of oxygen in arterial blood; *SaO₂,* oxygen saturation of arterial blood.

Continued

NURSING CARE PLAN 59-1

Increased Intracranial Pressure—cont'd

NURSING DIAGNOSIS	**Risk for disuse syndrome** *related to* altered level of consciousness, immobility, altered nutritional intake
Expected Patient Outcome	**Nursing Interventions and *Rationales***
• Experiences no complications of immobility	**Airway management**
	• Position patient to maximize ventilation potential *to prevent aspiration and blocking of airway by tongue.*
	• Remove secretions by encouraging coughing or by suctioning *to remove accumulated secretions, reduce risk of aspiration, and ensure patent airway.*
	• Perform chest physical therapy *to mobilize secretions and prevent pulmonary congestion.*
	Pressure ulcer prevention
	• Use an established risk assessment tool *to monitor individual's risk factors* (e.g., Braden scale [see Chapter 14, Table 14-16]).
	• Inspect skin over bony prominences and other pressure points at least daily when repositioning *to identify potential or actual skin problems and initiate a plan of care.*
	• Turn every 1 to 2 hours as appropriate *because prolonged pressure decreases circulation and leads to tissue ischemia and necrosis.*
	• Turn with care (e.g., avoid shearing) *to prevent injury to fragile skin.*
	• Keep bed linen clean, dry, and wrinkle free *to protect skin.*
	• Use special pressure-reducing or pressure-relieving mattresses *to reduce pressure to bony prominences by distributing body weight evenly.*
	Nutrition therapy
	• Complete a nutritional assessment *to determine current nutritional status and needs.*
	• Determine, in collaboration with the dietitian, the number of calories and the type of nutrients needed to meet nutrition requirements *to assess and make a plan to meet nutritional needs.*
	• Determine need for enteral tube feedings *to meet nutritional needs if patient is unable to ingest foods and fluids.*
	Exercise therapy: joint mobility
	• Perform passive or assisted ROM exercises *to maintain joint ROM and muscle strength.*

ROM, range of motion.

in severe dehydration unless treated. The usual treatment is fluid replacement, vasopressin (Pressyn), or desmopressin acetate (DDAVP). SIADH results in a dilutional hyponatremia that may produce cerebral edema, changes in LOC, seizures, and coma. (Treatment of SIADH is described in Chapter 51.) Treatment of cerebral salt wasting consists of aggressive sodium (Na^+) and volume replacement.

■ **Monitoring Intracranial Pressure.** The measurement of ICP enhances clinical decision making by enabling detection of early signs of intracranial hypertension and response to therapy. ICP monitoring is used in combination with other physiological parameters to guide the care of the patient and assess the patient's response to routine care. Valsalva's manoeuvre, coughing, sneezing, hypoxemia, pain, fever, and environmental stimuli are factors that can increase ICP. Nurses should be alert to these factors and should attempt to keep them to a minimum. Nursing management of the patient with increased ICP is one of the most important aspects of the care provided to these patients.

■ **Body Position.** The patient with increased ICP should be maintained in the head-up position. The nurse must take care to prevent extreme neck flexion, which can cause venous obstruction and contribute to elevated ICP. The body position should be adjusted to decrease the ICP as much as possible and to improve the CPP. Traditional practice has been to elevate the head of the bed to 30 degrees, unless a concurrent cervical neck injury has been identified. Elevation of the head of the bed reduces sagittal sinus pressure, promotes venous drainage from the head via the valveless jugular system, and decreases the vascular congestion that can produce cerebral edema. However, raising the head of the bed above 30 degrees may decrease the CPP. Careful evaluation of the effects of elevation of the head of the bed on both the ICP and the CPP is required. Research now suggests there is an inconsistent response of the ICP and cerebral oxygenation to body position (Ledwith et al., 2010). The bed should be positioned so that it lowers the ICP while maintaining the CPP and other indices of cerebral oxygenation.

Care should be taken to turn the patient with slow, gentle movements because rapid changes in position may increase the

ICP. Caution should be used to prevent discomfort in turning and positioning the patient because pain or agitation also increases ICP. Increased intra-abdominal and intrathoracic pressure contribute to increased ICP by impeding the venous return. Thus, coughing, straining, and the Valsalva manoeuvre should be avoided. Extreme hip flexion should be prevented to decrease the risk of raising the intra-abdominal pressure. The patient should be turned at least every 2 hours.

Decorticate or decerebrate posturing is a reflex response in some patients with increased ICP (see Figure 59-6). Turning, skin care, and even passive range of motion can elicit the posturing reflexes. Attempts should be made to provide needed physical care activities to minimize complications of immobility, such as atelectasis and contractures. In cases of severe posturing reflexes, these activities may have to be done less frequently because posturing can cause increases in ICP.

Protection From Injury.

The patient with increased ICP and a decreased LOC needs protection from self-injury. Confusion, agitation, and the possibility of seizures can put the patient at risk for injury. In these cases, environmental, chemical, or physical restraints may be considered to protect the patient from harm (e.g., removing tubes, wandering). A least-restraint approach should be used and considered only after all possible alternative interventions are exhausted. Specific agency policies and procedures should help guide restraint practice. The need for restraints should be reassessed daily. If restraints are necessary, they should be secure enough to be effective, and the area under the restraints should be observed regularly for skin irritation and adequate blood circulation. Restrained extremities should be assessed at least every 2 hours for colour, warmth, sensation, and movement. Agitation may increase with the use of restraints, which indicates the need for other measures to protect the patient from injury. Light sedation with agents such as haloperidol or lorazepam (Ativan) may be needed. Patient history and clinical presentation may be used to guide drug choice. Having a family member stay with the patient may have a calming effect. For the patient with seizures or the patient at risk for seizure activity, seizure precautions should be instituted. These include padded side rails, an airway at the bedside, accurate and timely administration of antiseizure drugs, and close observation. The patient can benefit from a quiet, nonstimulating environment. The nurse should always use a calm, reassuring approach. Touching and talking to the patient, even one who is in a coma, is always appropriate care. The nurse must create a balance between sensory deprivation and overload for the patient with increased ICP.

Psychological Considerations.

Besides the carefully planned physical care provided patients with increased ICP, the nurse must also be aware of the psychological well-being of patients and their families. Anxiety over the diagnosis and the prognosis for the patient with neurological problems can be distressing to the patient and the family. The nurse's competent and assured manner in performing the care needed by the patient is reassuring to everyone involved. Short, simple explanations are appropriate and allow the patient and the family to acquire the amount of information they desire. There is a need for support, information, and education of patients, families, and caregivers. The nurse should assess the family members' desire to assist in providing care for the patient and allow for their participation as appropriate.

▣ Evaluation

The expected outcomes for the patient with ICP are addressed in NCP 59-1.

Head Injury

Head injury includes any trauma to the scalp, the skull, or the brain. The term *head trauma* is used primarily to signify craniocerebral trauma, which includes an alteration in consciousness, no matter how brief.

Statistics for head injuries are incomplete because many victims die at the scene of the accident or because the condition is considered minor and health care services are not sought. Although the actual incidence and prevalence of traumatic brain injury (TBI) in Canada have not been well documented in any study to date, it is estimated that fewer than 1 in 5 patients seen in emergency departments with TBI is admitted. Since 1994, there has been a 35% decrease in traumatic head injury admissions to hospital in Canada, with 16,811 hospitalizations in 2003 to 2004 (Canadian Institute of Health Information [CIHI], 2006). Although a 20% decline in fatalities related to head injury since 1980 has been estimated, TBI continues to be one of the leading causes of death and the leading cause of disability after trauma. Causes of head injury include motor vehicle accidents, falls, assaults, sports-related injuries, and recreational accidents.

Head trauma has a high potential for poor outcome. Deaths from head trauma occur at three time points after injury: immediately after the injury, within 2 hours after injury, and approximately 3 weeks after injury. Factors that predict a poor outcome include the presence of an intracranial hematoma, increasing age of the patient, abnormal motor responses, impaired or absent eye movements or pupil light reflexes, early sustained hypotension, hypoxemia or hypercapnia, and ICP levels higher than 20 mm Hg (Ramesh, Thirumaran, & Raja, 2008). The majority of deaths after a head injury occur immediately after the injury, either from the direct head trauma or from massive hemorrhage and shock. Deaths occurring within a few hours of the trauma are caused by progressive worsening of the head injury or from internal bleeding. An immediate note of changes in neurological status and surgical intervention are critical in the prevention of deaths at this point. Deaths occurring 3 weeks or more after injury result from multisystem failure. Expert nursing care in the weeks following the injury is crucial in decreasing mortality and optimizing patient outcomes.

Types of Head Injuries

Scalp Lacerations. *Scalp lacerations* are the most minor type of head trauma. Because the scalp contains many blood vessels with poor constrictive abilities, most scalp lacerations are associated with profuse bleeding. The major complications associated with scalp laceration are blood loss and infection.

Skull Fractures. *Skull fractures* frequently occur with head trauma. There are several ways to describe skull fractures: (1) linear or depressed; (2) simple, comminuted, or compound; and (3) closed or open (Table 59-6). Fractures may be closed or open, depending on the presence of a scalp laceration or extension of

Table 59-6 Types of Skull Fractures

DESCRIPTION	CAUSE
Linear	
Break in continuity of bone without alteration of relationship of parts	Low-velocity injuries
Depressed	
Inward indentation of skull	Powerful blow
Simple	
Linear or depressed skull fracture without fragmentation or communicating lacerations	Low-to-moderate impact
Comminuted	
Multiple linear fractures with fragmentation of bone into many pieces	Direct, high-momentum impact
Compound	
Depressed skull fracture and scalp laceration with communicating pathway to intracranial cavity	Severe head injury

Table 59-7 Clinical Manifestations of Different Types of Skull Fractures

LOCATION	CLINICAL MANIFESTATIONS
Frontal fracture	Exposure of brain to contaminants through frontal air sinus, possible association with air in forehead tissue, CSF rhinorrhea, or pneumocranium
Orbital fracture	Periorbital ecchymosis (raccoon eyes), optic nerve injury
Temporal fracture	Boggy temporalis muscle because of extravasation of blood, oval bruise behind ear in mastoid region (Battle's sign), CSF otorrhea, middle meningeal artery disruption, epidural hematoma
Parietal fracture	Deafness, CSF or brain otorrhea, bulging of tympanic membrane caused by blood or CSF, facial paralysis, Battle's sign
Posterior fossa fracture	Occipital bruising resulting in cortical blindness, visual field defects; rare appearance of ataxia or other cerebellar signs
Basilar skull fracture	Otorrhea, bulging of tympanic membrane caused by blood or CSF, Battle's sign, tinnitus or hearing difficulty, rhinorrhea, facial paralysis, conjugate deviation of gaze, vertigo, bilateral raccoon eyes

CSF, cerebrospinal fluid.

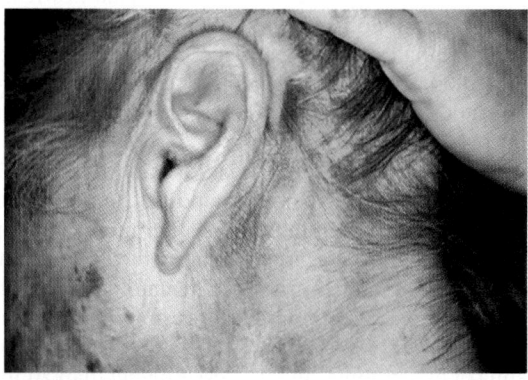

Figure 59-13 Battle's sign.

Source: Bingham, B. J. G., Hawke, M., & Kwok, P. (1992). *Clinical atlas of otolaryngology.* St. Louis: Mosby.

the fracture into the air sinuses or the dura. The type and severity of a skull fracture depend on the velocity, the momentum, the direction of injuring agent, and the site of impact.

The location of the fracture alters the presentation of the manifestations (Table 59-7). For example, a specialized type of linear fracture is seen when the fracture occurs at the base of the skull, a basilar skull fracture. Manifestations include *Battle's sign* (postauricular ecchymosis) (Figure 59-13) and *bilateral periorbital ecchymosis* (raccoon eyes). This fracture generally crosses a sinus and tears the dura (e.g., the frontal or the temporal) and is associated with cranial nerve damage and leakage of CSF. *Rhinorrhea* (CSF leakage from the nose) or *otorrhea* (CSF leakage from the ear) generally confirms that the fracture has traversed the dura (Figure 59-14). The CSF leak places these patients at high risk of meningitis.

Two methods of testing can be used to determine whether the fluid leaking from the nose or ear is CSF. The first method is to test the leaking fluid with a Dextrostix or Tes-Tape strip to determine whether glucose is present. CSF gives a positive reading for glucose. If blood is present in the fluid, testing for the presence of glucose is unreliable because blood contains glucose. In this event, the nurse should look for the *halo* or *ring* sign (see Figure 59-14, *C*). To perform this test, the nurse allows the leaking fluid to drip onto a white pad (4 × 4) or towel and observes the drainage. Within a few minutes, the blood coalesces into the centre, and a yellowish ring encircles the blood if CSF is present. The colour, the appearance, and the amount of leaking fluid must be noted because both tests can give false-positive results.

The major potential complications of skull fractures are intracranial infections and hematoma, as well as meningeal and brain tissue damage.

Mild Brain Injury.
Brain injuries are categorized as being mild, moderate, or severe. An injury resulting in a GCS of 13 to 15 is classified as *mild brain injury.* **Concussion** (a sudden transient mechanical head injury with disruption of neural activity and a change in the LOC) is considered a mild brain injury. The patient may or may not lose total consciousness with this injury.

Signs of concussion include a brief disruption in LOC, amnesia regarding the event (retrograde amnesia), and headache. The manifestations are generally of short duration. If the patient has not lost consciousness, or if the loss of consciousness lasts less than 5 minutes, the patient is usually discharged to the care of a responsible adult with instructions to notify the health care provider if symptoms persist or if behavioural changes are noted.

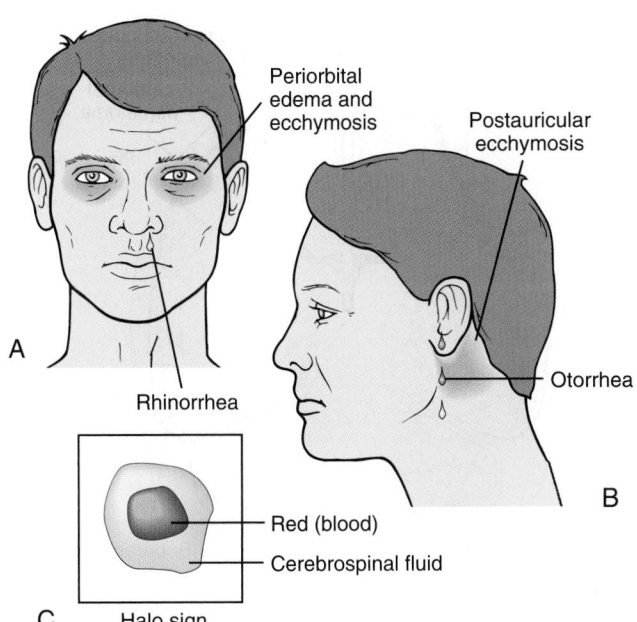

Figure 59-14 A, Raccoon eyes and rhinorrhea. **B,** Battle's sign (postauricular ecchymosis) with otorrhea. **C,** Halo or ring sign (see text).

Source: Redrawn from Barker, E. (2008). *Neuroscience nursing: A spectrum of care* (3rd ed., p. 342, Figure 11-4). St. Louis: Mosby.

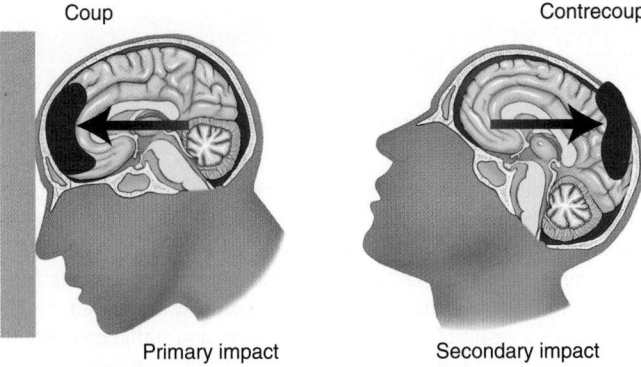

Figure 59-15 Coup-contrecoup injury. After the head strikes the wall, a coup injury occurs as the brain strikes the skull (primary impact). The contrecoup injury (the secondary impact) occurs when the brain strikes the skull surface opposite of the site from the original impact.

Mild TBI is significantly underdiagnosed, and the societal impact is great.

Moderate Brain Injury.
Moderate brain injury, defined as bringing about a GCS of 9 through 12, often necessitates a CT scan and admission to the hospital for close observation. Significant cognitive impairment may exist following moderate brain injury.

The *postconcussion syndrome* is seen anywhere from 2 weeks to 2 months after the concussion. Symptoms include persistent headache, lethargy, personality and behavioural changes, shortened attention span, decreased short-term memory, and changes in intellectual ability. This syndrome can significantly affect the patient's abilities to perform the activities of daily living.

Although concussion is generally considered benign and usually resolves spontaneously, the symptoms may be the beginning of a more serious, progressive problem that can continue for years following the injury. At the time of discharge, it is important to give the patient and the family instructions for observation and accurate reporting of symptoms or changes in neurological status.

Individuals with mild or moderate sports-related concussions are more likely to have future concussive injuries. Recurrent concussions are also associated with slower recovery. Patients should be instructed to avoid contact sports until all symptoms have subsided. In addition, return to play should be gradual.

Severe Brain Injury.
Injury bringing about GCS 3 through 8 is termed *severe brain injury*. Contusions, intracerebral lacerations, and intracranial hemorrhages are associated with closed head injuries.

A **contusion,** frequently occurring near the site of a skull fracture, is the bruising of the brain tissue within a focal area. A contusion often develops areas of hemorrhage, infarction, necrosis, and edema. With contusion, the phenomenon of *coup–contrecoup injury* is often noted (Figure 59-15). Damage from coup–contrecoup injury occurs because of mass movement of the brain inside the skull. Contusions or lacerations occur both at the site of the direct impact of the brain on the skull (*coup*) and at a secondary area of damage on the opposite side away from injury (*contrecoup*), leading to multiple contused areas. Patient prognosis is dependent upon the amount of bleeding around the contusion sites, which can range from minimal to severe. Contusions may continue to bleed or rebleed and appear to evolve on subsequent CT scans of the brain. Contusions that continue to evolve have a poorer prognosis. Neurological assessment demonstrates focal findings and a generalized disturbance in the LOC. Seizures are a common complication of brain contusion.

Lacerations involve actual tearing of the brain tissue and often occur in association with depressed and compound fractures and penetrating injuries. Tissue damage is severe, and surgical repair of the laceration is impossible because of the texture of the brain tissue.

When major head trauma occurs, many delayed responses are seen, including hemorrhage, hematoma formation, seizures, and cerebral edema. Intracerebral hemorrhage is generally associated with cerebral laceration. This hemorrhage manifests as a space-occupying lesion accompanied by unconsciousness, hemiplegia on the contralateral side, and a dilated pupil on the ipsilateral side. As the hematoma expands, symptoms of increased ICP become more severe. Prognosis is generally poor for the patient with a large intracerebral hemorrhage. Subarachnoid hemorrhage and intraventricular hemorrhage can also occur secondary to head trauma. The Ethical Dilemmas box considers a case of brain death due to severe brain injury.

Pathophysiology

Diffuse axonal injury (DAI) is widespread axonal damage occurring after a mild, moderate, or severe TBI. The damage occurs primarily around axons in subcortical white matter of the cerebral hemispheres, the basal ganglia, the thalamus, and the brainstem (Wasserman, 2006). Initially, DAI was believed to occur from the tensile forces of trauma that sheared axons, result-

Brain Death

Situation

The emergency nurse receives a radio call from emergency medical service (EMS) personnel about a young man who has been involved in a motorcycle crash. The patient was not wearing a helmet and has a large open skull fracture with obvious grey matter oozing from the area. Transport from the accident scene was delayed by 45 minutes as a result of a severe thunderstorm and traffic congestion. On the way to the hospital, the patient has fixed, dilated pupils and a cardiac arrest. Estimated arrival at the hospital is still an additional 45 minutes as a result of the severe weather. EMS personnel request permission to stop cardiopulmonary resuscitation (CPR) efforts.

Important Points for Consideration

- Death by neurological criteria occurs when the cerebral cortex stops functioning or is irreversibly destroyed.
- Because technology has been developed that assists in supporting life, controversies have arisen related to an exact definition of death.
- Criteria for brain death include coma or unresponsiveness, absence of brainstem reflexes, and apnea (see Chapter 13). Specific assessments by a physician are required to validate each of the criteria.
- The patient's clinical manifestations indicate that brain death has occurred.
- Although there is a slight chance that the patient's heart function could be resuscitated and supported with mechanical ventilation, there is no obligation to provide medically futile care for a patient with brain death.
- Brain death criteria do not address patients in a permanent vegetative state because the brainstem activity in these patients is adequate to maintain heart and lung function.

Critical Thinking Questions

1. What are the nurse's feelings about cessation of brain function versus cessation of heart and lung function as the criteria for death of a patient?
2. What legislation or practices are there in the nurse's province or territory about stopping CPR efforts by EMS personnel in the field?

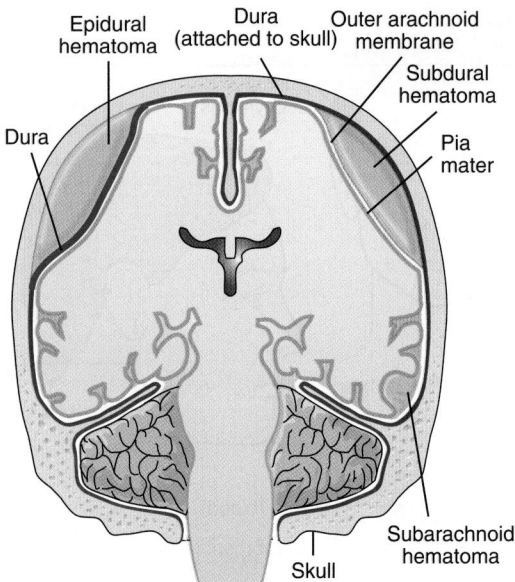

Figure 59-16 Locations of epidural, subdural, and subarachnoid hematomas.

Source: Copstead, L. C., & Banaski, J. L. (2010). *Pathophysiology* (4th ed., p. 1051, Figure 44-13). Philadelphia: Saunders.

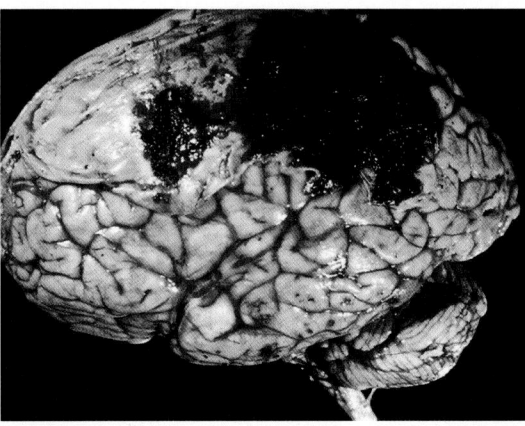

Figure 59-17 Epidural hematoma covering a portion of the dura. Multiple small contusions are seen in the temporal lobe.

Source: Kumar, V., Abbas, A. K., Fausto, N., & Aster, J. C. (2010). *Robbins and Cotran: Pathologic basis of disease* (8th ed., p. 1289, Figure 28-11). Philadelphia: Saunders. Courtesy the late Dr. Raymond D. Adams, Massachusetts General Hospital, Boston.

ing in axonal disconnection. There is increasing evidence that axonal damage is not preceded by an immediate tearing of the axon from the traumatic impact, but rather the trauma changes the function of the axon, resulting in axon swelling (axonal ballooning) and disconnection. This process takes approximately 12 to 24 hours to develop and may persist longer. The clinical signs and symptoms include a decreased LOC, increased ICP, decerebration or decortication, and global cerebral edema. Approximately 90% of patients with severe DAI remain in a persistent vegetative state (Wasserman, 2006).

Complications

Epidural Hematoma. An **epidural hematoma** is a collection of blood that results from bleeding between the dura and the inner surface of the skull (Figure 59-16); it produces compression of the dura mater and thus of the brain. An arterial epidural hematoma is a neurological emergency (Figure 59-17) and is usually associated with a linear fracture to the thin squamous portion of the temporal bone and laceration of the middle meningeal artery or one of its branches. Venous epidural hematomas are less common, are associated with a tear of the dural venous sinus, and develop slowly. Hemorrhage occurs into the epidural space, which lies between the dura and the inner surface of the skull (see Figure 59-16). Epidural hematomas that are a result of a torn artery and are under the influence of a high-pressure arterial system form rapidly. Symptoms typically include unconsciousness at the scene, with a brief lucid interval followed by a decrease in LOC. Other symp-

Table 59-8 Types of Subdural Hematomas		
OCCURRENCE AFTER INJURY	**PROGRESSION OF SYMPTOMS**	**TREATMENT**
Acute		
Up to 48 hr after severe trauma	Immediate deterioration	Craniotomy, evacuation, and decompression
Subacute		
48 hr to 2 wk after severe trauma	Alteration in mental status as hematoma develops; progression dependent on size and location of hematoma	Evacuation and decompression
Chronic		
Weeks, months, usually >20 days after injury; often injury seemed trivial or is forgotten by patient	Nonspecific, nonlocalizing progression; progressive alteration in LOC	Evacuation and decompression, membranectomy

LOC, level of consciousness.

toms may be a headache, nausea and vomiting, or focal findings. Rapid surgical intervention to prevent cerebral herniation dramatically improves outcomes.

Subdural Hematoma. A **subdural hematoma** is a collection of blood that results from bleeding between the dura mater and the arachnoid layer of the meningeal covering of the brain. A subdural hematoma usually results from injury to the brain substance and its parenchymal vessels (see Figure 59-16). The bridging veins that drain from the surface of the brain into the sagittal sinus are the source of most subdural hematomas. Because a subdural hematoma is usually venous in origin, the hematoma is much slower to develop into a mass large enough to produce symptoms. However, a subdural hematoma may also be caused by tearing of small cortical arteries, in which case it develops more rapidly. Subdural hematomas may be acute, subacute, or chronic (Table 59-8).

An *acute subdural hematoma* manifests signs within 48 hours of the injury. The size of the hematoma determines the patient's clinical presentation as well as prognosis. The signs and symptoms are similar to those associated with brain tissue compression in increased ICP and include decreasing LOC and headache. The patient can range from being drowsy and confused to unconscious. The ipsilateral pupil may dilate and become fixed if ICP is sufficiently increased. Acute subdural hematoma is most often associated with traumatic injury, and underlying brain injury may result in cerebral edema worsening the neurological assessment. The subsequent cerebral edema contributes to increased morbidity and mortality despite surgical intervention to evacuate the subdural hematoma.

A *subacute subdural hematoma* usually occurs within 2 to 14 days of the injury. Failure to regain consciousness may point to this possibility. After the initial bleeding, a subdural hematoma may appear to enlarge over time as the breakdown products of the blood draw fluid into the subdural space to reach isotonicity.

A *chronic subdural hematoma* develops over weeks or months after a seemingly minor head injury. The peak incidence of

chronic subdural hematoma occurs to those in their 50s and 60s when a potentially larger subdural space is available as a result of brain atrophy. With atrophy, the brain remains attached to the supportive structures, but tension to the bridging veins is increased and the bridging veins are subject to tearing. The larger size of the subdural space also accounts for the presenting complaint being the focal symptoms, rather than the signs of increased ICP. Chronic alcoholics are also prone to cerebral atrophy and subsequent development of subdural hematoma.

Delay in diagnosis of a subdural hematoma in the older adult can be attributed to symptoms that mimic other health problems in persons of this age group, such as vascular disease and dementia. Somnolence, confusion, lethargy, and memory loss are associated with health problems other than subdural hematoma.

Intraparenchymal Hematoma. Intraparenchymal or **intracerebral hematoma** is a collection of blood within the parenchyma that results from bleeding within the brain tissue itself and occurs in approximately 16% of head injuries. It usually occurs within the frontal and temporal lobes, possibly from the rupture of intracerebral vessels at the time of injury. The size and location of the hematoma are key determinants of patient outcome.

Traumatic Subarachnoid Hemorrhage. This hemorrhage is a result of traumatic forces damaging the superficial vascular structures that exist in the subarachnoid space. The presence of a *traumatic subarachnoid hemorrhage* may predispose the patient to cerebral vasospasm and diminished CBF, increasing the risk of ischemic damage following brain injury.

Diagnostic Studies and Collaborative Care

CT scan is considered the best diagnostic test to determine craniocerebral trauma because it allows for rapid diagnosis and intervention. An MRI scan is more sensitive in detecting small DAI lesions than the CT scan because of the lack of gross pathological changes in brain tissue. Transcranial Doppler studies allow for the measurement of CBF velocity. A cervical spine radiographic study is indicated because cervical spine trauma often occurs concomitantly with head injury. In general, the diagnostic studies are similar to those used for a patient with increased ICP (see Table 59-3). The GCS can be used to classify head injury as mild (score of 13 to 15), moderate (score of 9 to 12), or severe (score of 3 to 8).

Emergency management of the patient with a head injury is presented in Table 59-9. In addition to measures to prevent secondary injury by treating cerebral edema and managing increased ICP, the principal treatment of head injuries is timely diagnosis and surgery if necessary. For the patient with concussion and contusion, observation and management of increased ICP are the primary management strategies.

The treatment of skull fractures is usually conservative. For depressed fractures and fractures with loose fragments, a craniotomy is necessary to elevate the depressed bone and remove the free fragments. If large amounts of bone are destroyed, the bone may be removed (craniectomy) and a cranioplasty will be needed at a later time (see "Cranial Surgery" later in this chapter).

In cases of clinically large subdural and epidural hematomas, or those associated with significant neurological impairment, the blood must be removed surgically through either a craniotomy or a burr-hole approach.

ETIOLOGY	ASSESSMENT FINDINGS	INTERVENTIONS
Blunt	**Surface Findings**	**Initial**
• Motor vehicle collision	• Scalp lacerations	• Ensure patent airway.
• Pedestrian event	• Fracture or depressions in skull	• Stabilize cervical spine.
• Fall	• Bruises or contusions on face, Battle's sign (bruising behind ears)	• Administer O_2 via nasal cannula or non-rebreather mask.
• Assault	• Raccoon eyes (dependent bruising around eyes)	• Establish IV access with two large-bore catheters to infuse normal saline or lactated Ringer's solution.
• Sports injury	**Respiratory**	
Penetrating	• Central neurogenic hyperventilation	• Control external bleeding with sterile pressure dressing.
• High-velocity projectile (e.g., gunshot wound)	• Abnormal respiratory patterns (e.g., Cheyne-Stokes respirations)	• Assess for rhinorrhea, otorrhea, scalp wounds.
• Low-velocity projectile (e.g., knife, bone fragments from skull fracture)	• Decreased O_2 saturation	• Remove patient's clothing.
	• Pulmonary edema	**Ongoing Monitoring**
	Central Nervous System	• Maintain patient warmth using blankets, warm IV fluids, overhead warming lights, warm humidified O_2.
	• Unequal or dilated pupils	• Monitor vital signs, level of consciousness, O_2 saturation, cardiac rhythm, Glasgow Coma Scale score, pupil size and reactivity.
	• Asymmetrical facial movements	
	• Incomprehensible speech, abusive speech	• Anticipate need for intubation for ineffective breathing patterns or absent gag reflex.
	• Confusion	
	• Decreased level of consciousness	• Assume cervical spine injury until proven otherwise.
	• Combativeness	
	• Involuntary movements	• Monitor frequently for signs and symptoms of increased ICP or decreased cerebral perfusion.
	• Seizures	
	• Bowel and bladder incontinence	• Administer fluids cautiously to prevent fluid overload and increasing ICP.
	• Flaccidity	
	• Depressed or hyperactive reflexes	
	• Decerebrate or decorticate posturing	
	• Glasgow Coma Scale score <12	
	• CSF leaking from ears or nose	

CSF, cerebrospinal fluid; *ICP,* intracranial pressure; *IV,* intravenous.

NURSING MANAGEMENT: HEAD INJURY

▪ Nursing Assessment

The patient with a head injury is always considered to have the potential for developing increased ICP. Increased ICP is associated with higher mortality rates and poorer functional outcomes (BTF, 2007). The most important aspects of the objective data are noting the GCS score (see Table 59-5), assessing and monitoring the neurological status (see Figure 59-11), and determining whether a CSF leak has occurred. (Nursing assessment related to increased ICP is presented on pp. 1644-1646).

▪ Nursing Diagnoses

Nursing diagnoses and potential complications for the patient who has sustained a head injury may include, but are not limited to, the following:

• Risk for ineffective cerebral tissue perfusion (cerebral) *related to* interruption of CBF associated with cerebral hemorrhage, hematoma, and edema
• Hyperthermia *related to* increased metabolism, infection, and loss of cerebral integrative function secondary to possible hypothalamic injury
• Acute pain (headache) *related to* trauma and cerebral edema
• Impaired physical mobility *related to* decreased LOC, impaired motor responses, and treatment-imposed bed rest
• Anxiety *related to* abrupt change in health status, hospital environment, and uncertain future
• Potential complication: increased ICP *related to* cerebral edema and hemorrhage

▪ Planning

The overall goals are that the patient with an acute head injury will (1) maintain adequate cerebral perfusion; (2) remain normothermic; (3) be free from pain, discomfort, and infection; and (4) attain maximal cognitive, motor, and sensory function.

Nursing Implementation

Health Promotion

One of the best ways to prevent head injuries is to prevent car and motorcycle accidents. The nurse can be active in campaigns that promote driving safety and can speak to driver education classes regarding the dangers of unsafe driving and of driving after drinking alcohol or using drugs. The use of seat belts in cars and the use of helmets for riding on motorcycles are the most effective measures for increasing survival after accidents (see the Evidence-Informed Practice box). It is also recommended that lumberjacks, construction workers, miners, horseback riders, bicycle riders, snowboarders, and skydivers wear protective helmets. Nurses can become involved with organizations, such as ThinkFirst Foundation of Canada, that attempt to reduce the incidence of traumatic brain and spinal cord injuries among Canadian youth through education, community awareness, and healthy public policy initiatives.

Acute Intervention

Management at the scene of the accident can have a significant impact on the outcome of the head injury. Emergency management of head injury is discussed in Table 59-9. The general goal of nursing management of the head-injured patient is to maintain cerebral oxygenation and perfusion and prevent secondary cerebral ischemia. Surveillance or monitoring for changes in neurological status is critically important because the patient's condition may deteriorate rapidly, necessitating emergency surgery. Appropriate preoperative and postoperative nursing interventions are initiated if surgery is anticipated. Because of the close association between hemodynamic status and cerebral perfusion, the nurse must be aware of any coexisting injuries or conditions. In the acute injury period, treating other life-threatening conditions (i.e., hemorrhage, hypoxia) may take initial priority in nursing care.

The nurse should explain the need for frequent neurological assessments to both the patient and the caregivers. Behavioural manifestations associated with head injury can result in a frightened, disoriented patient who is combative and resists help. The nurse's approach should be calm and gentle. A family member may be available to stay with the patient and thus prevent increasing anxiety and fear. Nursing research also validates that one of the most pressing needs for family members in the acute injury phase of care is for information about the patient's diagnosis, the treatment plan, and the rationale for the interventions (Coco, Tossavainen, Jaaskelainen, & Turunen, 2011). Other teaching points are presented in eTable 59-1, available on the Evolve Web site for this chapter.

The nurse should perform neurological assessments at intervals based on the patient's condition. The GCS is useful in assessing the level of arousal (see Table 59-5). Indications of a deteriorating neurological state, such as a decreasing LOC, increasingly impaired motor strength, or pupillary changes, should be reported to a physician, and the patient's condition should be closely monitored.

The major focus of nursing care for the brain-injured patient relates to increased ICP (see NCP 59-1). However, there may be specific problems that require nursing intervention.

Eye problems may include loss of the corneal reflex, periorbital ecchymosis and edema, and diplopia. Loss of the corneal reflex may necessitate administering lubricating eye drops,

---

EVIDENCE-INFORMED PRACTICE

How Does Helmet Use Affect Mortality and Head Injury in Motorcycle Riders?

Clinical Question

In patients who sustain injury from a motorcycle crash (P), does the wearing of a helmet (I) versus no helmet (C) reduce mortality and head injury (O)?

Best Available Evidence

Systematic review of cohort, case control, and cross-sectional studies

Critical Appraisal and Synthesis of Evidence

- 61 (*n* >72,000) eligible studies were identified that examined helmet use in relation to outcomes of death, head injury, facial injury, neck injury, mortality in various combinations, or independently.
- A subgroup of 19 higher-quality studies that controlled for confounding variables were identified.
- Of this subgroup, 10 studies (*n* = 19,759) examined the outcome of death and 11 (*n* = 5005) examined the outcome of head injury with respect to helmet use.

Conclusions

- Reliance on observational studies was required owing to the inability to study this type of injury ethically.
- In general, the methodological quality of the 61 included studies was poor.
- Despite this, the authors conclude that helmet use has an effect on mortality and head injury in motorcycle riders who crash, with strong estimates that helmets are effective in reducing head injuries in motorcycle riders who crash by 69% and death by 42%.

Implications for Nursing Practice

- This review demonstrates that wearing motorcycle helmets prevents head injury and death in those riders who crash.
- Nurses can use this information to be active in campaigns that promote driver safety.
- Nurses have a role in various injury prevention campaigns that take place in both the community and the acute setting and can make use of quality research in preparation and delivery of education initiatives.

Reference for Evidence

Liu, B. C., Ivers, R., Norton, R., Boufous, S., Blows, S., & Lo, S. K. (2009). Helmets for preventing injury in motorcycle riders [review]. *Cochrane Database of Systematic Reviews, 1,* CD004333. doi:10.1002/14651858.CD004333.pub3

PICO: P, patient population of interest; *I,* intervention or area of interest; *C,* comparison of interest or comparison group; *O,* outcome(s) of interest.

---

taping the eyes shut, or suturing the eyelids closed to prevent abrasion. Periorbital ecchymosis and edema disappear spontaneously, but cold and, later, warm compresses provide comfort and hasten the process. Diplopia can be relieved by use of an eye patch.

Hyperthermia may occur in relation to an infectious process or from injury to or inflammation of the hypothalamus. Elevations in body temperature can result in increased cerebral metabolic rate, CBF, cerebral blood volume, and ICP. Pyrexia increases cerebral metabolic rate, which increases cerebral blood flow, which in turn can further increase ICP. The nurse should attempt to control hyperthermia and maintain normothermia in the head-injured patient.

If CSF rhinorrhea or otorrhea occurs, the nurse should inform the physician immediately. The head of the bed may be raised to decrease the CSF pressure so that a dural tear can seal. A loose collection pad may be placed under the nose or over the ear. No dressing should be placed into the nasal or ear cavities. The patient should be cautioned not to sneeze or blow the nose. Nasogastric tubes should not be used, and nasotracheal suctioning should not be performed on these patients because of the high risk of meningitis.

Nursing measures specific to the care of the immobilized patient, such as those related to bladder and bowel function, skin care, and infection, are also indicated. Nausea and vomiting may be a problem and can be alleviated by antiemetic drugs. Headache can usually be controlled with acetaminophen or small doses of codeine.

If the patient's condition deteriorates, urgent intracranial surgery may be necessary (see "Cranial Surgery" later in this chapter). A burr-hole opening or craniotomy may be indicated, depending on the underlying injury that is causing the symptoms.

The patient is often unconscious before surgery, making it necessary for a family member to sign the consent form for surgery. This is a difficult and frightening time for the patient's family and requires sensitive nursing management. The suddenness of the situation makes it especially difficult for the family to cope.

■ Ambulatory and Home Care

Once the condition has stabilized, the patient is usually transferred for acute rehabilitation management to prepare the patient for re-entry into the community. As with any craniocerebral problem, there may be chronic problems related to motor and sensory deficits, communication, memory, and intellectual functioning. Many of the principles of nursing management of the patient with a stroke are appropriate (see Chapter 60). Conditions that may require nursing and collaborative management include poor nutritional status, bowel and bladder management, spasticity, dysphagia, deep venous thrombosis, and hydrocephalus. The patient's outward appearance is not a good indicator of how well the patient will ultimately function in the home or work environment given recovery time and rehabilitation.

Post-traumatic seizure (PTS) disorders are seen in approximately 5% of patients with a nonpenetrating head injury. The time when the patient is most vulnerable to the development of PTS is during the first week after the head injury. Some patients may not develop a PTS disorder until years after the initial injury. Prophylactic use of anticonvulsants is not recommended for preventing late PTS. Anticonvulsants may be used to decrease the incidence of early PTS, within 7 days of injury (BTF, 2007). Phenytoin (Dilantin) is the antiseizure drug of choice to use with post-traumatic seizure activity.

The mental and emotional sequelae of brain trauma are often the most incapacitating problems. Many patients with head injuries who have been comatose for more than 6 hours undergo some personality change. They may suffer loss of concentration and memory and defective memory processing. Personal drive may decrease; apathy and apparent laziness may increase. Euphoria and mood swings, along with a seeming lack of awareness of the seriousness of the injury, may occur. The patient's behaviour may indicate a loss of social restraint, judgement, tact, and emotional control.

Progressive recovery may continue for 6 months or more before a plateau is reached and a prognosis for recovery can be made. Specific nursing management in the post-traumatic phase depends on specific residual deficits.

In all cases, the family must be given special consideration. They need to understand what is happening and be taught appropriate interaction patterns. The nurse must give guidance and referrals for financial aid, child care, and other personal needs and must assist the family in involving the patient in family activities whenever possible. Community referrals for support should be offered. Assisting the patient and family in developing and maintaining hope and keeping communication open are strategies perceived as supportive by families (Coco et al., 2011).

The family often has unrealistic expectations of the patient as the coma begins to recede. The family expects full return to pre-trauma status. In reality, the patient experiences a reduced awareness and ability to interpret environmental stimuli. The nurse must prepare the family for the emergence of the patient from coma and must explain that the process of awakening often takes several weeks.

When the time for discharge planning arrives, the family and the patient may benefit from very specific posthospital instructions to avoid family–patient friction. Special "no" policies that may be appropriately suggested by the neurosurgeon, neuropsychologist, and nurse include no drinking of alcoholic beverages, no driving, no work with hazardous implements and machinery, and no unsupervised smoking. Family members, particularly spouses, go through role transition as the role changes from one of spouse to that of caregiver.

■ Evaluation

The following are expected outcomes for the patient with a head injury:
- The patient will maintain normal CPP.
- The patient will achieve maximal cognitive, motor, and sensory function.
- The patient will experience no infection or hyperthermia.
- The patient will achieve pain control.

Brain Tumours

It is estimated that 55,000 Canadians are surviving with a brain tumour, and that every day, 27 Canadians are diagnosed (Brain Tumour Foundation of Canada [BTFC], 2011). It was estimated that, in Canada, there would be 1850 deaths related to brain tumours in 2012 (Canadian Cancer Society's Steering Committee on Cancer Statistics, 2012). The brain is a frequent site for metastasis from other sites as well. The 5-year relative survival rate for brain tumours in Canada is approximately 23% (Canadian Cancer Society's Steering Committee on Cancer Statistics, 2011).

Table 59-10 Types of Brain Tumours

TYPE	TISSUE OF ORIGIN	CHARACTERISTICS
Gliomas		
• Astrocytoma	Supportive tissue, glial cells and astrocytes	Can range from low-grade to moderate-grade malignancy.
• Glioblastoma multiforme	Primitive stem cell (glioblast)	Highly malignant and invasive; among the most devastating of primary brain tumours.
• Oligodendroglioma	Oligodendrocytes	Benign (encapsulation and calcification).
• Ependymoma	Ependymal epithelium	Range from benign to highly malignant; most are benign and encapsulated.
• Medulloblastoma	Primitive neuroectodermal cell	Highly malignant and invasive; metastatic to spinal cord and remote areas of brain.
Meningioma	Meninges	Can be benign or malignant; most are benign.
Acoustic neuroma (Schwannoma)	Cells that form myelin sheath around nerves; commonly affects cranial nerve VIII	Many grow on both sides of the brain; usually benign or low-grade malignancy.
Pituitary adenoma	Pituitary gland	Usually benign.
Hemangioblastoma	Blood vessels of brain	Rare and benign; surgery is curative.
Primary central nervous system lymphoma	Lymphocytes	Increased incidence in transplant recipients and acquired immune deficiency syndrome (AIDS) patients.
Metastatic tumours	Lungs, breast, kidney, thyroid, prostate	Malignant.

Types

Brain tumours can occur in any part of the brain or spinal cord. Tumours of the brain may be *primary,* arising from tissues within the brain, or *secondary,* resulting from a metastasis from a malignant neoplasm elsewhere in the body. Secondary brain tumours are the most common type. Brain tumours are generally classified according to the tissue from which they arise. The most common primary brain tumours originate in astrocytes. These tumours are called *gliomas* (astrocytoma, glioblastoma multiforme) and account for 65% of primary brain tumours (Table 59-10). Glioblastoma multiforme is the most common primary brain tumour, followed by meningioma and astrocytoma. More than half of the brain tumours are malignant; they infiltrate the brain parenchyma and are not amenable to complete surgical removal. Other tumours may be histologically benign, but their location is such that complete removal is not possible. Brain tumours are more commonly seen in middle-aged persons, but they may occur at any age.

Unless treated, all brain tumours eventually cause death from increasing tumour volume leading to increased ICP. Brain tumours rarely metastasize outside the central nervous system (CNS) because they are contained by structural (meninges) and physiological (blood–brain) barriers. Table 59-10 compares the major brain tumours. A glioblastoma and a meningioma are depicted in Figure 59-18.

Clinical Manifestations

The clinical manifestations of brain tumours depend mainly on the location, the rate of growth, and the size of the tumour. Figure 59-19 illustrates the functional areas of the cerebral cortex and can be used as a guide to correlate manifestations with the location of the tumour. Some tumours have aggressive mitotic rates and are associated with a rapid onset of symptoms. Tumours such as meningiomas are slow growing and can become quite large before clinical symptoms are noted. The rate of growth depends on the location and size of the tumour and the mitotic rate of the cells of the tissue of origin.

Wide ranges of possible clinical manifestations are associated with brain tumours. Headache is a common problem. Tumour-related headaches tend to be worse at night and may awaken the patient. The headaches are usually dull and constant but occasionally throbbing. Seizures are common in gliomas and brain metastases. Brain tumours can cause nausea and vomiting from increased ICP. Cognitive dysfunction, including memory problems and mood or personality changes, is another common manifestation, especially in patients with brain metastases. Muscle weakness, sensory losses, aphasia, and visuospatial dysfunction are further manifestations of brain tumours. As the brain tumour expands, it may also produce global signs of increased ICP, cerebral edema, or obstruction of the CSF pathways. Manifestations may clearly indicate the location of the tumour by an alteration in the function controlled by the affected area (Table 59-11).

Complications

If the tumour mass obstructs the ventricles or occludes the outlet, ventricular enlargement (hydrocephalus) can occur. Patients may develop manifestations of increased ICP (decreasing LOC, restlessness, headache, blurred vision, or vomiting without nausea). Surgical treatment is necessary to relieve the pressure and involves placement of either an external (temporary) or an internal (ventriculoatrial or ventriculoperitoneal) shunt. An internal shunt is a catheter with one-way valves that is placed in the lateral ventricle and then tunnelled through the skin to drain CSF into the right atrium or the peritoneum. The patient is at risk of shunt failure, which would be evidenced by signs of increased ICP and necessitate immediate attention. Signs of an infected shunt, such as high fever, persistent headache, and a stiff neck, also warrant immediate investigation.

Diagnostic Studies

An extensive history and a comprehensive neurological examination must be done in the workup of a patient with a suspected

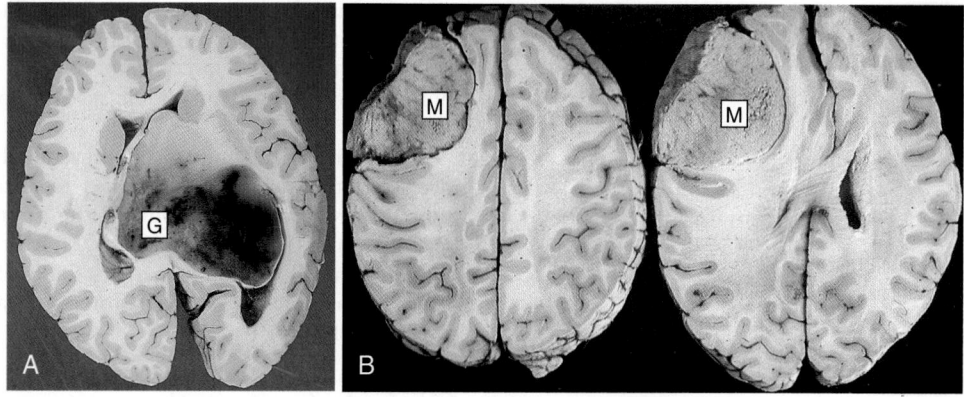

Figure 59-18 A, Glioblastoma. A large glioblastoma (G) arises from one cerebral hemisphere and has grown to fill the ventricular system. **B,** Meningioma. These two different sections from different levels in the same brain show a meningioma (M) compressing the frontal lobe and distorting underlying brain.

Source: Stevens, A., & Lowe, J. (2000). *Pathology: Illustrated review in colour* (2nd ed.). London: Mosby.

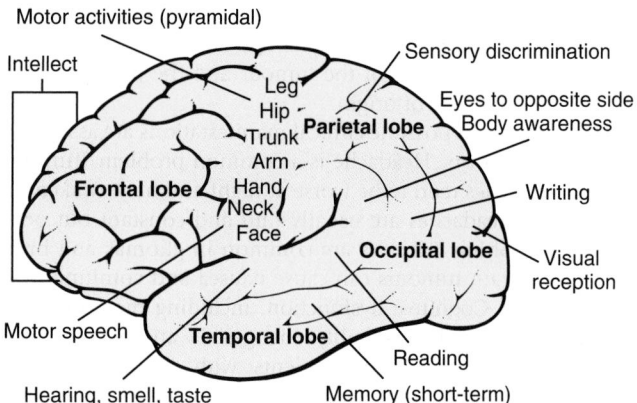

Figure 59-19 Each area of the brain controls a particular activity.

Table 59-11 Brain Tumour Locations and Presenting Manifestations	
TUMOUR LOCATION	**CLINICAL MANIFESTATIONS**
Cerebral hemisphere	
• Frontal lobe (unilateral)	Unilateral hemiplegia, seizures, memory deficit, personality and judgement changes, visual disturbances.
• Frontal lobe (bilateral)	Symptoms associated with unilateral frontal lobe tumours; ataxic gait.
• Parietal lobe	Speech disturbance (if tumour is in the dominant hemisphere: inability to write, spatial disorders, and unilateral neglect).
• Occipital lobe	Vision deficits and seizures.
• Temporal lobe	Few symptoms; seizures, dysphagia.
Subcortical	Hemiplegia; other symptoms may depend on area of infiltration.
Meningeal tumours	Symptoms are associated with compression of the brain and depend on tumour location.
Metastatic tumours	Headache, nausea, or vomiting because of ↑ ICP; other symptoms depend on tumour location.
Thalamus and sellar tumours	Headache, nausea, vision disturbances, papilledema, and nystagmus occur from ↑ ICP; diabetes insipidus may occur.
Fourth ventricle and cerebellar tumours	Headache, nausea, and papilledema from ↑ ICP; ataxic gait and changes in coordination.
Cerebellopontine tumours	Tinnitus and vertigo, deafness.
Brainstem tumours	Headache on awakening, drowsiness, vomiting, ataxic gait, facial muscle weakness, hearing loss, dysphagia, dysarthria, "crossed eyes" or other visual changes, hemiparesis.

ICP, intracranial pressure.

brain tumour. A careful history and physical examination may provide data concerning location. Diagnostic studies are similar to those used for a patient with increased ICP (see Table 59-3). The sensitivity of techniques such as MRI and positron emission tomography allows for detection of very small tumours and may provide more reliable diagnostic information. CT and brain scanning are used to diagnose the location of the lesion. Other tests include magnetic resonance spectroscopy, functional MRI, and single-photon emission computed tomography (SPECT). The EEG is useful but of less importance. A lumbar puncture is seldom diagnostic and carries with it the risk of cerebral herniation. Angiography can be used to determine blood flow to the tumour and further localize the tumour. Other studies are done to rule out a primary lesion elsewhere in the body. Approximately 20 to 40% of all cancer cases develop metastasis to the brain (BTFC, 2011). Endocrine studies are helpful when a pituitary adenoma is suspected (see Chapter 51).

The correct diagnosis of a brain tumour can be made by obtaining tissue for histological study. In most patients, tissue is obtained at the time of surgery. Computer-guided stereotactic biopsy is also an option if surgical intervention does not appear to be the most advantageous treatment option. A smear or frozen section can be performed in the operating room for a preliminary interpretation of the histological type. With this information, the neurosurgeon can make a better decision about the extent of surgery. In some cases, immunohistochemical stains or electron microscopy may be necessary to ascertain the correct diagnosis.

Collaborative Care

Treatment goals are aimed at (1) identifying the tumour type and location, (2) removing or decreasing tumour mass, and (3) preventing or managing increased ICP.

Drug Therapy. Corticosteroids (dexamethasone, prednisone, or methylprednisolone [Solu-Medrol]) are useful in reducing cerebral edema associated with neoplasms. Corticosteroids are often prescribed at diagnosis and continued following surgery until radiation and chemotherapy have been completed. Antiseizure medications are used to prevent seizures. This is necessary only for supratentorial lesions.

Surgical Therapy. Surgical removal is the preferred treatment for brain tumours (see Cranial Surgery later in this chapter). Stereotactic surgical techniques are used with increasing frequency to perform a biopsy and remove small brain tumours. The outcome of surgical therapy depends on the type, size, and location of the tumour. Meningiomas and oligodendrogliomas can usually be completely removed, whereas the more invasive gliomas and medulloblastomas can be only partially removed. Computer-guided stereotactic biopsy, ultrasound, functional MRI, and cortical mapping can be used to localize brain tumours intraoperatively. Complete surgical removal is not always possible because the tumour is not always accessible and sometimes involves vital parts of the brain. Surgery can reduce tumour mass, which decreases ICP and provides relief of symptoms with an extension of survival time. Tumours located in the deep central areas of the dominant hemisphere, the posterior corpus callosum, or the upper brainstem cause extensive neurological damage and are often deemed inoperable.

Radiation Therapy and Radiosurgery. Radiation therapy is commonly used as a follow-up measure after surgery. Radiation seeds can also be implanted into the brain. Cerebral edema and rapidly increasing ICP may be a complication of radiation therapy, but they can be managed with high doses of corticosteroids (dexamethasone, prednisone, or methylprednisolone). (Radiation therapy is discussed in Chapter 18.)

Stereotactic radiosurgery is a method of delivering a high, concentrated dose of radiation precisely directed at a location within the brain. Stereotactic radiosurgery may be used when conventional surgery has failed or is not an option because of the tumour location. (Radiosurgery is discussed on pp. 1660, 1662.)

Chemotherapy. The effectiveness of chemotherapy has been limited by difficulty getting drugs across the blood–brain barrier, tumour cell heterogeneity, and tumour cell drug resistance. A group of chemotherapeutic drugs called the *nitrosoureas* (e.g., carmustine [BiCNU], lomustine [CeeNU]) are particularly effective in treating brain tumours. Normally, the blood–brain barrier prohibits the entry of most drugs into the brain. However, the most malignant tumours cause a breakdown of the blood–brain barrier in the area of the tumour, allowing chemotherapeutic agents to be used to treat the malignancy. Chemotherapy-laden biodegradable wafers (e.g., Gliadel wafer [polifeprosan with

carmustine implant]) implanted at the time of surgery can deliver chemotherapy directly to the tumour site. Other drugs being used include methotrexate and procarbazine (Matulane). Chemotherapeutic drugs can be administered intrathecally via an Ommaya reservoir (see Chapter 18).

Temozolomide (Temodal) is the first oral chemotherapeutic agent found to cross the blood–brain barrier. In contrast with many traditional chemotherapies, which require metabolic activation to exert their effects, temozolomide has the ability to convert spontaneously to a reactive agent that directly interferes with tumour growth. It does not interact with other drugs commonly taken by patients with brain tumours, such as antiseizure medications, corticosteroids, and antiemetics. Concurrent therapy of radiation and temozolomide has demonstrated promising results (Jalali et al., 2007).

Many techniques to control and treat brain tumours are currently under investigation. These include local hyperthermia and biological therapy. Although progress in treatment has increased the length and quality of survival of patients with gliomas, outcomes still remain poor (Preusser et al., 2011).

NURSING MANAGEMENT: BRAIN TUMOURS

▪ Nursing Assessment

The initial assessment should be structured to provide baseline data of the neurological status and the information needed to design a realistic, individualized care plan. Areas to be assessed include the LOC and cognitive function, motor abilities, sensory perception, integrated function (including bowel and bladder function), balance and proprioception, and the coping abilities of the patient and family. Watching a patient perform activities of daily living and listening to the patient's conversation are possible ways to perform part of the neurological assessment. Having the patient or the family explain the problem can be helpful in determining the patient's limitations and can also provide the nurse with information about the patient's insight into the problems. All initial data should be accurately recorded to provide a baseline for comparison to determine whether the patient's condition is improving or deteriorating.

Interview data are as important as the actual physical assessment. Questions concerning medical history, intellectual abilities and educational level, and history of nervous system infections and trauma should be asked. Determination of the presence of seizures, syncope, nausea and vomiting, pain, headaches, and physical limitations is important in planning care for the patient.

▪ Nursing Diagnoses

Nursing diagnoses and potential complications for the patient with a brain tumour may include, but are not limited to, the following:

- Risk for ineffective cerebral tissue perfusion *related to* cerebral edema
- Acute pain (headache) *related to* cerebral edema and increased ICP
- Self-care deficits *related to* altered neuromuscular function secondary to tumour growth or cerebral edema and impaired cognitive function

- Anxiety *related to* diagnosis and treatment
- Potential complication: seizures *related to* abnormal electrical activity of the brain
- Potential complication: increased ICP *related to* presence of tumour and failure of normal compensatory mechanisms

▣ Planning

The overall goals are that the patient with a brain tumour will (1) maintain normal ICP, (2) maximize neurological functioning, (3) be free from pain and discomfort, and (4) be aware of the long-term implications with respect to prognosis and cognitive and physical functioning.

▣ Nursing Implementation

A primary or metastatic tumour of the frontal lobe can cause behavioural and personality changes. Loss of emotional control, confusion, disorientation, memory loss, and depression may be signs of a frontal lobe lesion. These behavioural changes are often not perceived by the patient but can be disturbing and even frightening to the family. These changes can also cause a distancing to occur between the family and the patient. The nurse has an important role in assisting the family in understanding what is happening to the patient and emotionally supporting the family.

The confused patient with behavioural instability can be a challenge. Protecting the patient from self-harm is an important part of nursing care (Catt, Chalmers, & Fallowfield, 2008). At times when the patient manifests rage and aggression, the nurse must also be concerned about self-protection. Close supervision of activity; use of side rails; use of restraints; padding of the rails and the area around the bed; and a calm, reassuring approach to care are all essential techniques for the care of these patients.

Perceptual problems associated with frontal lobe and parietal lobe tumours contribute to a patient's disorientation and confusion. Minimization of environmental stimuli, creation of a routine, and use of reality orientation can be incorporated into the care plan for the confused patient.

Seizures often occur with brain tumours. These are managed with antiseizure drugs. Seizure precautions should be instituted for the protection of the patient. Some behavioural changes seen in the patient with a brain tumour are a result of seizure disorders and can improve with control of the seizures by means of drugs (see Chapter 61).

Motor and sensory dysfunctions are problems that interfere with the activities of daily living (Catt et al., 2008). Alterations in mobility must be managed, and the patient should be encouraged to provide as much self-care as physically possible. Self-image often depends on the patient's ability to participate in care within the limitations of the physical deficits.

Language deficits can also occur in patients with brain tumours. Motor (expressive) or sensory (receptive) aphasia may occur (see Chapter 60). The disturbance in communication can be frustrating for the patient and may interfere with the nurse's ability to meet the patient's needs. Attempts should be made to establish a communication system that can be used by both the patient and the staff.

Nutritional intake may be decreased because of the patient's inability to eat, loss of appetite, or loss of desire to eat. Assessing the nutritional status of the patient and ensuring adequate nutritional intake are important aspects of care. The patient may need encouragement to eat or, in some cases, may have to be fed orally, by gastrostomy or nasogastric tube, or by total parenteral nutrition. The patient with a brain tumour who undergoes cranial surgery requires complex nursing care. This is discussed in the next section.

▣ Evaluation

The following are expected outcomes for the patient with a brain tumour:
- The patient will achieve control of pain, vomiting, and other discomforts.
- The patient will maintain ICP within normal limits.
- The patient will demonstrate maximal neurological function (cognitive, motor, sensory) with regard to the location and extent of the tumour.
- The patient will maintain optimal nutritional status.
- The patient will accept the long-term consequences of the tumour and its treatment.

Cranial Surgery

The cause or indication for cranial surgery may be related to a brain tumour, CNS infection (e.g., abscess), vascular abnormalities, craniocerebral trauma, epilepsy, or intractable pain (Table 59-12).

Types

Various types of cranial surgical procedures are presented in Table 59-13.

Stereotactic Surgery. Stereotactic surgery is a precision apparatus (often computer-guided) that assists the surgeon to target a very precise area of the brain (Figure 59-20).

Stereotactic biopsy can be performed to obtain tissue samples for histological examination. CT scanning and MRI are used to image the targeted tissue. With the patient under general or local anaesthesia, the surgeon drills a burr hole or creates a bone flap for an entry site and then introduces a probe and biopsy needle. Stereotactic procedures are used for removal of small brain tumours and abscesses, drainage of hematomas, ablative procedures for extrapyramidal diseases (e.g., Parkinson's disease), and repair of arteriovenous malformations. A major advantage of the stereotactic approach is a reduction in damage to surrounding tissue.

Stereotactic radiosurgery is a procedure that involves closed-skull destruction of an intracranial target using ionizing radiation focused with the assistance of an intracranial guiding device. A sophisticated computer program is used while the patient's head is held still in a stereotactic frame. Radiosurgical techniques can use linear accelerator or a gamma knife. In the gamma knife procedure, a high dose of cobalt radiation is delivered to precisely targeted tumour tissue. The dose of radiation can be delivered in a few minutes or may take up to an hour or more depending on the size and shape of the tumour. In some situations, tumours are treated over several weeks.

In combination with stereotactic procedures to identify and localize tumour sites, surgical lasers can be used to destroy

Table 59-12 Indications for Cranial Surgery

INDICATION	CAUSE	MANIFESTATIONS	PROCEDURE
Intracranial infection	Bacteria	*Early findings:* stiff neck, headache, fever, weakness, seizures *Later findings:* seizures, hemiplegia, speech disturbances, ocular disturbances, change in LOC	Excision or drainage of abscess
Hydrocephalus	Overproduction of CSF, obstruction to flow, defective reabsorption	*Early findings:* mental changes, disturbances in gait *Later findings:* memory impairment, urinary incontinence, increased tendon reflexes	Placement of ventriculoatrial or ventriculoperitoneal shunt
Brain tumours	Benign or malignant cell growth	Change in LOC, pupillary changes, sensory or motor deficit, papilledema, seizures, personality changes	Excision or partial resection of tumour
Intracranial bleeding	Rupture of cerebral vessels because of trauma or stroke	*Epidural:* momentary unconsciousness; lucid period, then rapid deterioration *Subdural:* headache, seizures, pupillary changes	Surgical evacuation through burr holes or craniotomy
Skull fractures	Trauma to skull	Headache, CSF leakage, cranial nerve deficit	Debridement of fragments and necrotic tissue, elevation and realignment of bone fragments
Arteriovenous (AV) malformation	Congenital tangle of arteries and veins (frequently in middle cerebral artery)	Headache, intracranial hemorrhage, seizures, mental deterioration	Excision of malformation
Aneurysm repair	Dilation of weak area in arterial wall (usually near anterior portion of circle of Willis)	*Before rupture:* headache, lethargy, visual disturbance *After rupture:* violent headache, decreased LOC, visual disturbances, motor deficit	Dissection and clipping or coiling of aneurysm

CSF, cerebrospinal fluid; *LOC,* level of consciousness.

Table 59-13 Types of Cranial Surgery

TYPE	DESCRIPTION
Burr hole	Opening into the cranium made with a drill; used to remove localized fluid and blood beneath the dura
Craniotomy	Opening into the cranium with removal of a bone flap and opening the dura to remove a lesion, repair a damaged area, drain blood, or relieve increased ICP
Craniectomy	Excision into the cranium to cut away a bone flap
Cranioplasty	Repair of a cranial defect resulting from trauma, malformation, or previous surgical procedure; artificial material used to replace damaged or lost bone
Stereotaxis	Precision localization of a specific area of the brain using a frame or a frameless system based on three-dimensional coordinates; procedure is used for biopsy, radiosurgery, or dissection
Shunt procedures	Alternate pathway created to redirect cerebrospinal fluid from one area to another using a tube or implanted device; examples include ventriculoperitoneal shunt and Ommaya reservoir

ICP, intracranial pressure.

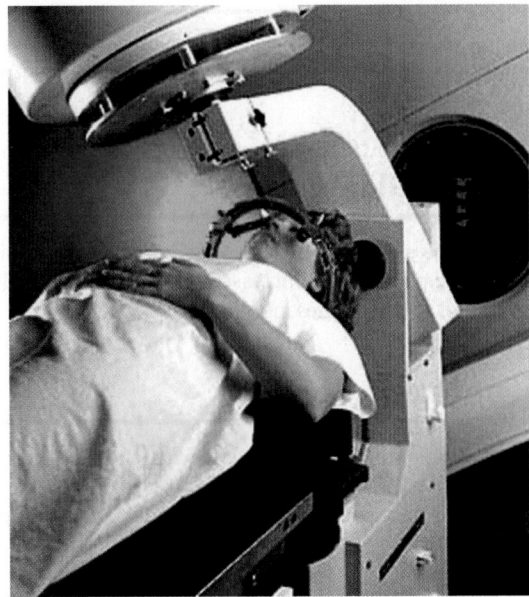

Figure 59-20 Stereotactic frame.

Source: Courtesy Department of Neurological Surgery, Vanderbilt University Medical Center, Nashville, TN.

tumours. Stereotactic procedures are used to identify the tumour site. Three surgical lasers currently used include the carbon dioxide, argon, and neodymium:yttrium–aluminum–garnet (Nd:YAG) lasers. All three work by creating thermal energy, which destroys the tissue on which it is focused. Laser therapy also provides the benefit of reducing damage to surrounding tissue.

Craniotomy. Depending on the location of the pathological condition, a craniotomy may be frontal, parietal, occipital, temporal, or a combination of any of these. A set of burr holes is drilled, and a saw is used to connect the holes to remove the bone flap. Sometimes operating microscopes are used to magnify the site. After surgery, the bone flap is wired or sutured. Sometimes drains are placed to remove fluid and blood. Patients are usually cared for in a CCU until stable.

In certain cases, a tumour may be infiltrating brain tissue that is involved in essential functions such as language. In these cases, an *awake craniotomy* may be performed. The patient is fully anaesthetized during the opening of the cranial vault and then brought to consciousness once the brain is exposed. Relevant areas of the brain are stimulated to assess function and determine what tissue can and cannot be safely resected. Although keeping the patient awake adds to the complexity and length of the surgery, it enhances the safety of the procedure.

NURSING MANAGEMENT: CRANIAL SURGERY

▪ Nursing Assessment

The nursing assessment of the patient undergoing cranial surgery would be similar to that for the patient with increased ICP (see pp. 1644-1646).

▪ Nursing Diagnoses

Nursing diagnoses for the patient with cranial surgery are similar to those for the patient with increased ICP and may include, but are not limited to, those presented in NCP 59-1.

▪ Planning

The overall goals are that the patient with cranial surgery will (1) return to normal consciousness, (2) be free from pain and discomfort, (3) have maximal neuromuscular functioning, and (4) be rehabilitated to maximum ability.

▪ Nursing Implementation

▪ Acute Intervention

Nursing management is presented in NCP 59-1. The patient facing cranial surgery (if conscious and coherent), the caregiver, and the family will be gravely concerned about the potential physical and emotional problems that can result from surgery. The uncertainty regarding prognosis and outcome necessitates compassionate nursing care in the preoperative period.

Preoperative teaching is important in allaying the fears of the patient and the family and also in preparing them for the postoperative period. The patient and the family should be given information regarding the operative procedure and what can be expected immediately after the surgery. Explaining that some hair is shaved to allow for better exposure and prevention of contamination may help alleviate the patient's concern. The family should also be informed that the patient will be taken to a CCU or to a special care unit after the operation.

The primary goal of care after cranial surgery is prevention of increased ICP. (Nursing management of the patient with increased ICP is presented on pp. 1644-1649.) Frequent assessment of the neurological status of the patient is essential during the first 48 hours. In addition to the neurological functions, fluids, electrolyte levels, and osmolality are monitored closely to detect changes in sodium regulation, the onset of diabetes insipidus, or severe hypovolemia. The turning and positioning of the patient sometimes depend on the site of the operation. To lessen postoperative cerebral edema, the patient is nursed with the head of the bed elevated 30 to 45 degrees. Maximum swelling in the operative area usually occurs within 24 to 48 hours after the surgery. If a bone flap has been removed (craniectomy), care should be taken not to have the patient positioned on the operative side. Sutures or staples may be removed after 7 days. Incisions to the posterior fossa require sutures or staples to remain in situ for a minimum of 10 days.

The dressing should be observed for colour, odour, and amount of drainage. The health care provider should be notified immediately of any excessive bleeding or clear drainage. Checking drains for placement and assessing the area around the dressing are also important. Scalp care should include meticulous care of the incision to prevent wound infection. The area should be cleansed and treated in accordance with hospital protocol. Once the dressing is removed, use of an antiseptic soap for washing the scalp may also be beneficial. The psychological impact of hair removal can be alleviated by the use of a wig, a turban, scarves, or a cap after the incision has completely healed. For the patient who is receiving radiation, use of a sunblock and head covering should be advocated if any exposure to the sun is anticipated.

▪ Ambulatory and Home Care

The rehabilitative potential for a patient after cranial surgery depends on the reason for the surgery, the postoperative course, and the patient's general state of health. Nursing interventions must be based on a realistic appraisal of these factors. An overall goal for the nurse is to foster independence for as long as possible and to the highest degree possible.

Specific rehabilitation potential cannot be determined until cerebral edema and increased ICP subside postoperatively. Care must be taken to maintain as much function as possible through measures such as careful positioning, meticulous skin and mouth care, regular range of motion exercises, bowel and bladder care, and adequate nutrition.

Referrals may be made to other specialists on the health care team. For example, the speech therapist may be helpful to the patient who has speech or swallowing deficits or the physiotherapist may provide an exercise plan to regain functional deficits. The needs and problems of each patient should be addressed individually because many variables affect the plan.

The mental and physical deterioration of the patient, including seizures, personality disorganization, apathy, and wasting, is

Withholding Treatment

Situation

A 26-year-old patient in a persistent vegetative state is diagnosed with her fifteenth bladder infection. Her home care nurse must determine whether or not to seek antibiotics for this infection. The family members have expressed a concern that no heroic measures be used to extend the biological life of their daughter and sister, but they have been unwilling to withdraw the existing treatment, which is enteral nutrition through a gastrostomy tube. Should antibiotics be withheld?

Important Points for Consideration

- Patients in a persistent vegetative state do not recover.
- Providing nutrition and hydration, even if by artificial means, can have significant cultural, religious, and psychological meaning to patients and families.
- Clarification with the family about the goals of treatment and the patient's wishes, when she was competent and if they are known, is imperative. It is important to know whether treatment for an infection would be considered heroic based on the family's perspective of what the patient would want.
- The family's concerns about pain, suffering, and quality of life for the patient must be explored within the context of the overall plan of care.
- Withholding treatment is morally acceptable when a competent patient consents to it, if there is no medical benefit to the patient, if the treatment merely prolongs life, or if the burden of treatment outweighs the benefit to the patient.

Clinical Decision-Making Questions

1. How would the nurse approach the patient's family?
2. What might the nurse be feeling about providing nutrition, hydration, and treatments that will prolong life in a patient for whom there is no hope of recovery?
3. What options are available to the family for the care of their daughter once a decision is made about withholding antibiotics?

difficult for both family and health providers to endure. Mental and emotional residual deficits are often more difficult for the patient and the family to accept than are motor and sensory losses. Although progress is continually being made to help the patient with a brain tumour by means of chemotherapy, conventional and interstitial radiation, and biological therapies, prognosis has not changed. The nurse can provide much help and support during the adjustment phase and in long-range planning.

▪ Evaluation

The following are expected outcomes for the patient who has had cranial surgery:

- The patient will regain cognitive, motor, and sensory function to the fullest possible extent.
- The patient will be free of infection.

- The patient will have pain and discomfort alleviated.
- The patient will be free of seizures.
- The patient will have optimal nutritional intake.

Inflammatory Conditions of the Brain

Meningitis, encephalitis, and brain abscesses are the most common inflammatory conditions of the brain and spinal cord. Inflammation can be caused by bacteria, viruses, fungi, and chemicals (e.g., contrast media used in diagnostic tests or blood in the subarachnoid space) (Table 59-14). CNS infections may occur via the bloodstream (e.g., insect bites), by extension from a primary site (e.g., ear infection, sinusitis, open skull fracture), or along cranial, spinal, and peripheral nerves (e.g., rabies). The mortality rate is approximately 2 to 30% in the general population, with higher rates in elderly patients (van de Beek, de Gans, McIntyre, & Prasad, 2007). Up to 40% of those who recover can have long-term neurological deficits (van de Beek et al., 2007).

Bacterial Meningitis

Etiology and Pathophysiology

Meningitis is an acute inflammation of the meningeal tissues (the pia mater and the arachnoid membrane) surrounding the brain and the spinal cord. Meningitis also refers to an infection of the arachnoid mater and CSF. Bacterial meningitis is considered a medical emergency, and untreated meningitis has a mortality rate approaching 100%. The organisms usually gain entry to the CNS through the upper respiratory tract or the bloodstream, but they may enter by direct extension from penetrating wounds of the skull or through fractured sinuses in basal skull fractures. Cases most often occur in infants, older adults, and members of certain high-risk groups.

Meningitis usually occurs in winter or early spring and is often secondary to viral respiratory disease. Older adults and persons who are debilitated are more often affected than the general population. *Streptococcus pneumoniae* (pneumococcus meningitis) and *Neisseria meningitidis* (meningococcal meningitis) are the leading causes of bacterial meningitis. *Haemophilus influenzae* was once the most common cause. However, the use of *H. influenzae* vaccine has resulted in a significant decrease in meningitis related to this organism.

Other causes of meningitis are *Listeria monocytogenes* (commonly called *Listeria*). *Listeria* is a bacteria found in food that can cause a rare and potentially fatal disease called *listeriosis*. Initially presenting as a condition with flulike symptoms, listeriosis can spread to the nervous system and result in a cerebral abscess or meningitis. Those at greatest risk of severe illness or death are older adults or individuals with a weakened immune system. Approximately 20 to 30% of cases in individuals at high risk are fatal. In Canada, listeriosis is a relatively rare disease with only two to three cases reported weekly (Public Health Agency of Canada [PHAC], 2008).

Diagnosis is confirmed by isolation of *L. monocytogenes* bacteria in CSF cultures. The disease can be effectively treated with antibiotics, and early diagnosis is critical to the success of the treatment, especially for those at high risk. At present, there is no vaccine to prevent listeriosis.

Table 59-14 Comparison of Cerebral Inflammatory Conditions

	MENINGITIS	ENCEPHALITIS	BRAIN ABSCESS
Causative organisms	Bacteria (*Streptococcus pneumoniae*, *Neisseria meningitidis*, group B streptococcus, viruses, fungi)	Bacteria, fungi, parasites, herpes simplex virus (HSV), other viruses (e.g., West Nile virus)	Streptococci, staphylococci through bloodstream
CSF			
• Pressure (normal, <20 cm H$_2$O)	Increased	Normal to slight increase	Increased
• WBC count (normal, 0-5 × 10^6/L)	Bacterial: >1000/mcL (mainly PMN) Viral: 25-500/mcL (mainly lymphocytes)	500/mcL, PMN (early), lymphocytes (later)	25-300/mcL (PMN)
• Protein (normal, 0.15-0.45 g/L)	Bacterial: >5 g/L Viral: 0.5-5 g/L	Slight increase	Normal
• Glucose (normal, 2.8-4.2 mmol/L)	Bacterial: decreased Viral: normal or low	Normal	Low or absent
• Appearance	Bacterial: turbid, cloudy Viral: clear or cloudy	Clear	Clear
Diagnostic studies	CT scan, Gram stain, smear, culture, PCR*	CT scan, EEG, MRI, PET, PCR, IgM antibodies to virus in serum or CSF	CT scan, skull radiograph, MRI
Treatment	Antibiotics, dexamethasone, supportive care, prevention of ↑ ICP	Supportive care, prevention of ↑ ICP, acyclovir (Zovirax) for HSV	Antibiotics, incision and drainage Supportive care

CSF, cerebrospinal fluid; *CT*, computed tomography; *EEG*, electroencephalogram; *ICP*, intracranial pressure; *IgM*, immunoglobulin M; *MRI*, magnetic resonance imaging; *PCR*, polymerase chain reaction; *PET*, positron emission tomography; *PMN*, polymorphonuclear cell; *WBC*, white blood cell.
*PCR is used to detect viral RNA or DNA.

The inflammatory response to the infection of the arachnoid mater and CSF (whatever the cause) may increase CSF production, while exudate accumulation leads to blockage of the arachnoid villi, causing obstruction of CSF absorption. The resulting hydrocephalus may cause an increase in ICP. In bacterial meningitis, the purulent secretions that are produced spread quickly to other areas of the brain through the CSF. If this process extends into the brain parenchyma or if concurrent encephalitis is present, cerebral edema and increased ICP become more of a problem. All patients with meningitis must be observed closely for manifestations of increased ICP, which is thought to be a result of swelling around the dura, and increased CSF volume.

Clinical Manifestations

Fever, severe headache, nausea, vomiting, and **nuchal rigidity** (resistance to flexion of the neck) are key signs of meningitis. A positive Kernig sign (flexion of the patient's hip 90 degrees and extension of the knee cause pain), a positive Brudzinski sign (flexion of the patient's neck causes flexion of the patient's hips and knees), photophobia, a decreased LOC, and signs of increased ICP may also be present. Coma is associated with a poor prognosis and occurs in 5 to 10% of patients with bacterial meningitis. Seizures are common in patients with meningitis (Zoons et al., 2008). With meningitis, the headache becomes progressively worse and may be accompanied by vomiting and irritability. If the infecting organism is a meningococcus, early symptoms may include chills, fever, headache, malaise, rash, and petechial hemorrhage on skin and mucous membranes.

Complications

The most common acute complication of bacterial meningitis is increased ICP. Most patients will have increased ICP, and it is the major cause of altered mental status. Another complication of bacterial meningitis is residual neurological dysfunction. Cranial nerve dysfunction often occurs with cranial nerves III, IV, VI, VII, or VIII in bacterial meningitis. The dysfunction usually disappears within a few weeks. However, hearing loss may be permanent after bacterial meningitis.

Cranial nerve irritation can have serious sequelae. The optic nerve (CN II) is compressed by increased ICP. Papilledema is often present, and blindness may occur. When the oculomotor (CN III), trochlear (CN IV), and abducens (CN VI) nerves are irritated, ocular movements are affected. Ptosis, unequal pupils, and diplopia are common. Irritation of the trigeminal nerve (CN V) is evidenced by sensory losses and loss of the corneal reflex, and irritation of the facial nerve (CN VII) results in facial paresis. Irritation of the vestibulocochlear nerve (CN VIII) causes tinnitus, vertigo, and deafness.

Hemiparesis, aphasia, and hemianopsia may also occur. These signs usually resolve over time. If resolution does not occur, the presence of a cerebral abscess, subdural empyema, subdural effusion, or persistent meningitis is suggested. Acute cerebral edema may occur with bacterial meningitis, causing seizures, CN III palsy, bradycardia, hypertensive coma, and death.

A noncommunicating hydrocephalus may occur if the exudate causes adhesions that prevent the normal flow of the CSF from the ventricles. CSF reabsorption by the arachnoid villi may also be obstructed by the exudate. In these cases, surgical implantation of a shunt may be necessary.

Diagnostic Studies

When a patient is seen with manifestations suggestive of bacterial meningitis, a blood culture and CT scan should be done. Diagnosis is usually verified by doing a lumbar puncture and analysis of the CSF. Variations in the CSF depend on the causative organism. Protein levels in the CSF are usually elevated and are higher in bacterial than in viral meningitis. Decreased CSF glucose concentration is common in bacterial meningitis; the glucose level may be normal in viral meningitis. The CSF is purulent and turbid in bacterial meningitis; it may be the same or clear in viral meningitis. The predominant white blood cell type in the CSF during bacterial meningitis is polymorphonuclear cells (see Table 59-14). Specimens of CSF, sputum, and nasopharyngeal secretions are taken for culture before the start of antibiotic therapy to identify the causative organism. A Gram stain is done to detect bacteria.

Radiographic studies of the skull may demonstrate infected sinuses. CT scans and MRI may be normal in uncomplicated meningitis. In other cases, CT scans may reveal evidence of increased ICP or hydrocephalus.

Collaborative Care

Bacterial meningitis is a medical emergency. Rapid diagnosis based on history and physical examination is crucial because the patient is usually in a critical state when health care is sought. When meningitis is suspected, antibiotic therapy is instituted after the collection of specimens for cultures, even before the diagnosis is confirmed (Table 59-15). The fundus of the eye should be examined via ophthalmoscope for papilledema before lumbar puncture for identification of possible increased ICP.

Ampicillin, penicillin, vancomycin, cefuroxime (Ceftin), cefotaxime (Claforan), ceftriaxone, and ceftizoxime (Cefizox) are the drugs of choice for treating meningitis. The corticosteroid dexamethasone may also be prescribed before or with the first dose of antibiotics. Although data are limited, administration of dexamethasone appears to be associated with a lower mortality rate and a reduced incidence of hearing loss in patients with bacterial meningitis (van de Beek et al., 2007).

NURSING MANAGEMENT: BACTERIAL MENINGITIS

Nursing Assessment

Initial assessment should include vital signs, neurological evaluation, assessment of fluid intake and output, and evaluation of the lungs and skin (see Figure 59-10).

Nursing Diagnoses

Nursing diagnoses for the patient with bacterial meningitis may include, but are not limited to, those presented in NCP 59-2.

Planning

The overall goals are that the patient with bacterial meningitis will have (1) return to maximal neurological functioning, (2) resolution of infection, and (3) control of pain and discomfort.

Nursing Implementation

Health Promotion

Prevention of respiratory infections through vaccination programs for pneumococcal pneumonia and influenza should be supported by nurses. A vaccine is available for protection against *N. meningitidis*. Routine vaccination is recommended for children aged 11 or 12, as well as catch-up vaccination for previously unvaccinated teens entering high school and for college students living in dormitories. In addition, early and vigorous treatment of respiratory and ear infections is important. Persons who have close contact with anyone who has bacterial meningitis should be given prophylactic antibiotics. In Canada, cases of pneumococcal meningitis must be reported to the PHAC.

Acute Intervention

The patient with bacterial meningitis is usually acutely ill. The fever is high, and headache is severe. Irritation of the cerebral cortex may result in seizures. The changes in mental status and LOC depend on the degree of increased ICP. Assessment of vital signs, neurological evaluation, monitoring of fluid intake and output, and evaluation of lung fields and skin should be performed at regular intervals based on the patient's condition and recorded carefully.

Head pain and neck pain secondary to movement require attention. Codeine provides some pain relief without undue sedation for most patients. The patient should be assisted to a position of comfort, often curled up with the head slightly extended. The head of the bed should be slightly elevated, when

COLLABORATIVE CARE

Table 59-15 Bacterial Meningitis

Diagnostic	• Codeine for headache
• History and physical examination	• Dexamethasone
• Analysis of CSF for protein, glucose, WBC; Gram stain; culture	• Acetaminophen or aspirin for temperature >38.5°C
• CBC, coagulation profile, electrolyte levels, glucose, platelet count	• Hypothermia
• Blood culture	• Clear liquids as desired or tolerated
• CT scan, MRI	• IV phenytoin (Dilantin)
Collaborative Therapy	• IV furosemide (Lasix) or mannitol (Osmitrol) for diuresis
• Bed rest	
• IV fluids	
• IV antibiotics	
• Ampicillin, penicillin	
• Cephalosporin (e.g., ceftriaxone)	

CBC, complete blood count; *CSF,* cerebrospinal fluid; *CT,* computed tomography; *IV,* intravenous; *MRI,* magnetic resonance imaging; *WBC,* white blood cell.

permitted after lumbar puncture. A darkened room and a cool cloth over the eyes may relieve the discomfort of photophobia.

For the delirious patient, additional low lighting may be necessary to decrease hallucinations. All patients suffer some degree of mental distortion and hypersensitivity and may be frightened and misinterpret the environment. Every attempt should be made to minimize environmental stimuli and prevent injury. The presence of a familiar person at the bedside often has a calming effect. The nurse must be efficient with care but also should project an attitude of caring and of unhurried gentleness. The use of touch and a soothing voice to give simple explanations of activities is helpful. If seizures occur, appropriate observations should be made and protective measures should be taken. Antiseizure drugs such as phenytoin (Dilantin) are administered as ordered. Problems associated with increased ICP are also managed (see "Increased Intracranial Pressure," earlier in this chapter).

Fever must be vigorously managed because it increases cerebral edema and the frequency of seizures. In addition, neurological damage may result from an extremely high temperature over a prolonged time. If the fever is resistant to antipyretics, more vigorous means may be necessary, such as an automatic cooling blanket. Care should be taken not to reduce the temperature too rapidly because shivering may result, causing a rebound effect and increasing the temperature. The extremities should be wrapped in soft towels or covered with a thin blanket to protect them from "frostbite." Skin assessment and care should be meticulous. If a cooling blanket is not available or desirable, tepid sponge baths with water may be effective in lowering the temperature. The skin must be protected from excessive drying and injury.

Because high fever greatly increases the metabolic rate and thus insensible fluid loss, the patient should be assessed for dehydration and adequacy of fluid intake. Diaphoresis further increases fluid losses, which should be estimated and included in an intake and output record. Replacement fluids should be calculated as 800 mL/day for respiratory losses plus 100 mL for each degree of temperature above 38°C. Supplemental feeding to maintain adequate nutritional intake via tube or oral feedings may be necessary. The designated antibiotic schedule must be followed to maintain therapeutic blood levels. Observations should be made for adverse effects of the drugs used.

In most cases, patients with meningitis are placed in respiratory isolation for up to 48 hours of appropriate antibiotic therapy. Meningococcal meningitis is highly contagious, whereas other causes of meningitis may pose minimal to no infection risk with patient contact. Routine practices (also called *standard precautions*) are essential to protect the patient and the nurse.

■ Ambulatory and Home Care

After the acute period has passed, the patient requires several weeks of convalescence before normal activities can be resumed. In this period, good nutrition should be stressed, with an emphasis on a high-protein, high-calorie diet in small, frequent feedings.

Muscle rigidity may persist in the neck and the backs of the legs. Progressive range of motion exercises and warm baths are useful. Activity should be gradually increased as tolerated, but adequate bed rest and sleep should be encouraged.

Residual effects are uncommon in meningococcal meningitis, but pneumococcal meningitis can result in sequelae such as dementia, seizures, deafness, hemiplegia, and hydrocephalus. Vision, hearing, cognitive skills, and motor and sensory abilities should be assessed after recovery, with appropriate referrals as indicated. Meningitis in infancy may have "silent" neurological sequelae, which are manifested as learning and behavioural problems when the child reaches school age.

Throughout the acute and convalescent periods, the nurse should be aware of the anxiety and stress experienced by individuals close to the patient.

■ Evaluation

The expected outcomes for the patient with bacterial meningitis are addressed in NCP 59-2.

Viral Meningitis

The most common causes of viral meningitis are enteroviruses, arboviruses, human immunodeficiency virus (HIV), and herpes simplex virus (HSV). Viral meningitis usually presents as a headache, fever, photophobia, and nuchal rigidity. The fever may be moderate or high. There are usually no symptoms of brain involvement.

The most important diagnostic test is examination of the CSF obtained via a lumbar puncture. The CSF can be clear or cloudy, and the typical finding is lymphocytosis (see Table 59-14). Organisms are not seen on Gram stain or acid-fast smears. Polymerase chain reaction used to detect viral-specific DNA or RNA is a highly sensitive method for diagnosing CNS viral infections. Antibiotics should be administered after the lumbar puncture while awaiting the results of the CSF. Antibiotics are the best defence for bacterial meningitis and can be easily discontinued if the meningitis is found to be viral in nature (Matthews, Miller, & Mott, 2007).

Viral meningitis is managed symptomatically because the disease is self-limiting. Antiviral therapy is not used. Full recovery from viral meningitis is expected. Rare sequelae include persistent headaches, mild mental impairment, and incoordination.

Encephalitis

Etiology and Pathophysiology

Encephalitis, an acute inflammation of the brain, is a serious and sometimes fatal disease. Encephalitis is usually caused by a virus. Many different viruses have been implicated in encephalitis, some associated with seasons of the year or endemic to certain geographic areas. Ticks and mosquitoes transmit epidemic encephalitis. Examples include LaCrosse encephalitis, St. Louis encephalitis, West Nile virus, and Western equine encephalitis. Nonepidemic encephalitis may occur as a complication of measles, chickenpox, or mumps. HSV encephalitis is the most common form of acute nonepidemic viral encephalitis. Cytomegalovirus encephalitis is one of the common complications in patients with acquired immune deficiency syndrome.

West Nile virus was first identified in Uganda in 1937. The first human case of West Nile virus in Canada occurred in summer–fall 2001. By week 46 of 2011, there were 101 reported clinical cases of West Nile virus in Canada (PHAC, 2011a). Advanced age is the primary risk factor for encephalitis and mortality associated with this virus. The incubation period

NURSING CARE PLAN 59-2

Bacterial Meningitis

NURSING DIAGNOSIS	Risk for ineffective cerebral perfusion,* Decreased intracranial adaptive capacity* **Acute confusion** related to impaired cerebral function as evidenced by inaccurate interpretation of environment, fluctuation in cognition and level of consciousness, and misperceptions
Expected Patient Outcomes	**Nursing Interventions and Rationales**
• Demonstrates appropriate cognitive function • Is oriented to person, place, and time	• Monitor neurological status on an ongoing basis to determine extent of problem. • Administer PRN medications for anxiety or agitation to reduce symptoms. • Provide a low-stimulation environment for patient to decrease disorientation caused by overstimulation. • Approach patient slowly and from the front to avoid stimulating or frightening patient. • Provide appropriate level of supervision or surveillance to monitor patient and to allow for therapeutic actions. • Reorient the patient to the health care provider with each contact to assist with orientation and reduce anxiety. • Communicate with simple, direct statements to avoid overstimulation.
NURSING DIAGNOSIS	**Acute pain** related to headache and muscle and joint aches as evidenced by general discomfort of head, joints, and muscles; apathy; and grimacing on movement
Expected Patient Outcomes	**Nursing Interventions and Rationales**
• Reports satisfaction with pain relief • Demonstrates no effects of pain	**Pain management** • Provide patient optimal pain relief with prescribed analgesics to relieve pain. • Select and implement a variety of measures (e.g., pharmacological, nonpharmacological, interpersonal) to facilitate pain relief (e.g., massage, range of motion) to promote comfort and reduce joint stiffness and promote circulation. • Reduce or eliminate factors that precipitate or increase the pain experience (e.g., fear) to promote comfort. • Control environmental factors that may influence the patient's response to discomfort (e.g., room temperature, lighting, noise) because pain can be exhausting to the patient.
NURSING DIAGNOSIS	**Hyperthermia** related to infection and abnormal temperature regulation by hypothalamus from increased ICP as evidenced by increased body temperature
Expected Patient Outcome	**Nursing Interventions and Rationales**
• Maintains normal body temperature	**Fever treatment** • Monitor temperature as frequently as appropriate so that interventions can be initiated immediately. • Monitor blood pressure, pulse, and respirations to evaluate effects of hyperthermia. • Monitor intake and output as increased body temperature increases risk of fluid deficit. • Monitor for decreased levels of consciousness as fever increases brain metabolism. • Encourage increased intake of oral fluids, as appropriate, to replace fluids lost.
Collaborative Problem	
POTENTIAL COMPLICATION	**Seizure activity** related to cerebral irritation
Nursing Goals	**Nursing Interventions and Rationales**
• Monitor for seizure activity • Carry out appropriate medical and nursing interventions • Report and record any seizure activity	• Monitor for seizure activity so that interventions can be initiated immediately. • Keep side rails up and padded to protect patient if a seizure occurs. • Administer sedative and antiseizure drugs as ordered to control or prevent seizure activity. • Carry out interventions to treat underlying causes of inflammatory brain condition to prevent seizure activity.

ICP, intracranial pressure; PRN, as needed.

*Because cerebral edema and increased ICP may occur with bacterial meningitis, see the related nursing care plan, NCP 59-1, on pp. 1647-1648 for nursing interventions and rationales related to these nursing diagnoses.

is from 3 to 14 days. Most cases involve mild, flulike symptoms, but about 1 in 150 will result in severe neurological disease, with encephalitis more commonly seen than meningitis.

Clinical Manifestations and Diagnostic Studies

The onset of infection is typically nonspecific, with fever, headache, nausea, and vomiting. It can be acute or subacute. Signs of encephalitis appear on day 2 or 3 and may vary from minimal alterations in mental status to coma. Virtually any CNS abnormality can occur, including hemiparesis, tremors, seizures, cranial nerve palsies, personality changes, memory impairment, amnesia, and aphasia.

Early diagnosis and treatment of viral encephalitis are essential for favourable outcomes. Diagnostic findings related to viral encephalitis are shown in Table 59-14. Brain imaging techniques include CT, MRI, and PET. Polymerase chain reaction tests for HSV DNA and RNA levels in CSF allow for early detection of HSV viral encephalitis. West Nile virus should be strongly considered in adults older than 50 years who develop encephalitis or meningitis in summer or early fall. The best diagnostic test for West Nile virus is a blood test that detects viral RNA. This test is also used in screening blood, organs, cells, and tissues that have been donated. The clinical distinction between meningitis and encephalitis is based on brain function. Patients with meningitis may be uncomfortable, lethargic, or distracted by headache, but their cerebral function remains normal. In encephalitis, however, abnormalities in brain function are common, including altered mental status, motor or sensory deficits, and speech or movement disorders.

NURSING AND COLLABORATIVE MANAGEMENT: VIRAL ENCEPHALITIS

To prevent encephalitis, mosquito control should be practised, including cleaning rain gutters, removing old tires, draining bird baths, and removing water where mosquitoes can breed. In addition, insect repellent should be used during mosquito season.

Collaborative and nursing management of encephalitis, including West Nile virus infection, is symptomatic and supportive. Treatment for mild cases consists mainly of rest, adequate nutrition and fluids, acetaminophen for fever and headaches, and anticonvulsants for seizures if necessary. Generally, encephalitis does not respond to antiviral medications; however, the HSV and varicella-zoster virus respond to antiviral drugs such as acyclovir (Zovirax) or ganciclovir (Cytovene), and these have been shown to reduce mortality rates. For maximal benefit, antiviral agents should be started before the onset of coma. Current research is investigating the use of interferon therapy as a treatment for encephalitis caused by West Nile and St. Louis viruses; however, more studies are needed. In the initial stages, many patients require intensive care.

Seizure disorders should be treated with antiseizure drugs (see Chapter 61, Table 61-10). Prophylactic treatment with antiseizure drugs may be used in severe cases of encephalitis. Treatment of cytomegalovirus encephalitis in acquired immune deficiency syndrome patients is discussed in Chapter 17.

Rabies

Rabies has been a threat to humans since ancient times. Between 30,000 and 70,000 people die each year from rabies worldwide. Only 23 people have died in Canada from rabies since reporting started in 1924. The most recent death occurred in 2003 (PHAC, 2011b). Louis Pasteur developed the first rabies vaccine in 1885, which drastically reduced the risk of disease transmission from domestic animals to humans, particularly in developed countries where vaccine programs were effectively implemented. Despite the success of vaccines in domestic animals, rabies remains a serious public health concern owing to the presence of the disease in wild animals. Once a human contracts rabies and develops symptoms, the disease almost always ends in death.

The cause of rabies is an RNA virus that produces an acute, progressive viral encephalitis. Although rabies is generally transmitted via saliva from the bite of an infected animal, it can also be spread by scratches, mucous membrane contact with infected secretions, and inhalation of aerosolized virus into the respiratory tract. Any warm-blooded mammal can carry rabies, including livestock. Throughout the world, rabid dogs are the most common disease vector. However, in developed countries, raccoons, skunks, bats, and foxes are the primary animal carriers.

The rabies virus spreads from the contact site through the CNS via peripheral nerve and possibly muscle fibres. During this time (2 to 14 days after exposure), patients experience flulike symptoms, and pain, paresthesias, or numbness at the bite site. An acute neurological syndrome then occurs, 2 to 7 days later and is manifested by agitation, hypersalivation, hydrophobia, dysarthria, vertigo, diplopia, hallucinations, and other neurological sequelae (e.g., hyperactive reflexes, nuchal rigidity, and a positive Babinski sign). Coma develops within 7 to 10 days of the neurological syndrome.

Patients experience flaccid paralysis, apnea, hydrophobia, and seizures. Death ensues as a result of respiratory and cardiovascular collapse within a few days after the onset of coma. Because rabies is nearly always fatal, management efforts are directed at preventing the transmission and onset of the disease. Rabies postexposure prophylaxis involves vaccines that confer passive immunity and active immunity to the disease in the patient. The first vaccine is rabies immune globulin, which confers passive immunity. Rabies immune globulin should be administered to the patient as soon as possible after contact with a rabid animal. Ideally, the entire rabies immune globulin dose is administered via infiltration in and around the bite wound. If the bite wound area is too small, such as a finger, or the contact with rabies occurred via mucous membrane or respiratory tract exposure, the entire dose can be administered intramuscularly, generally in the gluteal site.

Next, a vaccine series to induce active immunity is given. Antibodies take 7 to 10 days to develop. It is essential for the nurse to explain to the patient the need for strict compliance with the rabies vaccine regimen in order to prevent vaccine failure.

Brain Abscess

Brain abscess is an accumulation of pus within the brain tissue that can result from a local or systemic infection. Direct extension from ear, tooth, mastoid, or sinus infection is the primary cause. Other causes for brain abscess formation include spread from a distant site (e.g., pulmonary infection, bacterial endocarditis), skull fracture, and a prior brain trauma or surgery. *Streptococci* and *Staphylococcus aureus* are the primary infective organisms.

Manifestations are similar to those of meningitis and encephalitis and include headache, fever, and nausea and vomiting. Signs of increased ICP may include drowsiness, confusion, and seizures. Focal symptoms may be present and reflect the local area of the abscess. For example, visual field defects or psychomotor seizures are common with a temporal lobe abscess, whereas an occipital abscess may be accompanied by visual impairment and hallucinations. CT and MRI are used to diagnose a brain abscess.

Antimicrobial therapy is the primary treatment for brain abscess. Depending on the size and response of the abscess to antimicrobial treatment, the patient may require surgery to drain or remove the abscess if it is encapsulated. Other manifestations are treated symptomatically. In untreated cases, the mortality rate approaches 100%. Nursing measures are similar to those for management of meningitis or increased ICP. However, the distinct difference is the requirement of longer term (6 weeks or possibly longer) antibiotic therapy (either IV or oral) (Muzumdar, Jhawar, & Goel, 2010). If surgical drainage or removal is the treatment of choice, nursing care is similar to that described under cranial surgery. Some patients may be clinically well enough after the acute surgical phase to be discharged home. The nurse must be aware of the additional discharge planning requirements of a patient going home with IV antibiotic therapy if indicated.

Other infections of the brain include subdural empyema, osteomyelitis of the cranial bones, epidural abscess, and venous sinus thrombosis after periorbital cellulitis.

CLINICAL DECISION-MAKING EXERCISE

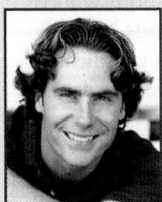

CASE STUDY:
Head Injury
Source: Cora Reed/iStockphoto.

Patient Profile

George Roustas is a 33-year-old White man who was the driver of a motorcycle that ran into an automobile broadside at a high rate of speed. He was sedated, paralyzed, and intubated by emergency medical personnel (EMS) at the scene before transport by helicopter. He was brought to the emergency department with a prehospital report of multiple trauma and an open skull fracture. Paramedics also reported that he was not wearing a helmet.

Subjective Data

He was reportedly unresponsive at the scene with a Glasgow Coma Scale (GCS) score of 3, hypotension, tachycardia, and shallow irregular respirations.

Objective Data

At the Scene
- Unresponsive with obvious deformity to the left side of the skull
- Respirations were shallow and irregular
- O$_2$ saturations ranged from 88 to 90%
- Systolic BP ranged from 50 to 80 mm Hg
- Heart rate ranged from 100 to 130 beats/min

In the Emergency Department
- Right pupil, 4 mm nonreactive; left pupil, 3 mm nonreactive
- GCS score = 3
- Hypotension and tachycardia continued in spite of fluid resuscitation

Diagnostic Studies
- Computed tomography (CT) of the head showed left skull fracture, left subdural hematoma, bilateral intraventricular and subarachnoid hemorrhage, and cerebral edema.
- CT of the abdomen and pelvis showed a lacerated liver, multiple infarcts to the right kidney, fluid around the duodenum and pancreas, and multiple left pelvic fractures.
- C-spine radiograph series was negative.
- Chest radiograph showed a right lung contusion and pneumomediastinum and subcutaneous emphysema.

Discussion Questions

1. What could be the cause of Mr. Roustas' hypoxia, hypotension, and tachycardia?
2. How could the injuries affect his neurological condition?
3. What area of the brain do Mr. Roustas' clinical manifestations suggest may be injured?
4. *Priority Decision:* What are the priority nursing interventions that should be implemented?
5. *Priority Decision:* Based on the assessment data presented, what are the priority nursing diagnoses? Are there any collaborative problems?

evolve *Answers are available at* **http://evolve.elsevier.com/Canada/Lewis/medsurg**

REVIEW QUESTIONS

The number of the question corresponds to the same-numbered objective at the beginning of the chapter.

1. How does vasogenic cerebral edema increase intracranial pressure (ICP)?
   a. By shifting fluid in the grey matter
   b. By altering the endothelial lining of cerebral capillaries
   c. By leaking molecules from the intracellular fluid to the capillaries
   d. By altering the osmotic gradient flow into the intravascular component

2. A patient with ICP monitoring has pressure of 12 mm Hg. What does this pressure reflect?
   a. A severe decrease in cerebral perfusion pressure
   b. An alteration in the production of cerebrospinal fluid (CSF)
   c. The loss of autoregulatory control of ICP
   d. A normal balance between brain tissue, blood, and CSF

3. What is the best way for the nurse to position the patient with increased ICP?
   a. Keep the head of the bed flat.
   b. Elevate the head of the bed to 30 degrees.
   c. Maintain patient on left side with head supported on pillow.
   d. Use a continuous-rotation bed to continuously change patient position.

4. In which of the following situations would the nurse be alert to a possible acute subdural hematoma?
   a. Patient has a linear skull fracture crossing a major artery.
   b. Patient has focal symptoms of brain damage with no recollection of a head injury.
   c. Patient develops decreased level of consciousness and a headache within 48 hours of a head injury.
   d. Patient has an immediate loss of consciousness with a brief lucid interval followed by decreasing level of consciousness.

5. The nurse is admitting a patient with a severe head injury to the emergency department. Which of the following is the nurse's highest priority for assessment?
   a. The patency of the airway
   b. The presence of a neck injury
   c. The neurological status according to the Glasgow Coma Scale
   d. The CSF leakage from the ears or nose

6. A patient is suspected of having an intracranial tumour. The signs and symptoms include memory deficits, visual disturbances, weakness of right upper and lower extremities, and personality changes. The nurse recognizes that the tumour is most likely located in which of the following lobes?
   a. Frontal lobe
   b. Parietal lobe
   c. Occipital lobe
   d. Temporal lobe

7. Which of the following does nursing management of a patient with a brain tumour include?
   a. Discussing with the patient methods to control inappropriate behaviour
   b. Using diversion techniques to keep the patient stimulated and motivated
   c. Assisting and supporting the family in understanding any changes in behaviour
   d. Limiting self-care activities until the patient has regained maximum physical functioning

8. The nurse on the clinical unit is assigned to four patients. Which patient should the nurse assess first?
   a. Patient with a skull fracture whose nose is bleeding
   b. Elderly patient with a stroke who is confused and whose daughter is present
   c. Patient with meningitis who is suddenly agitated and reporting a headache of 10 on a 0-to-10 scale
   d. Patient who had a craniotomy for a brain tumour who is now 3 days postoperative and has had continued emesis

9. Which of the following is a nursing measure that is indicated to reduce the potential for seizures and increased ICP in the patient with bacterial meningitis?
   a. Administering codeine for relief of head and neck pain
   b. Controlling fever with prescribed drugs and cooling techniques
   c. Keeping the room darkened and quiet to minimize environmental stimulation
   d. Maintaining the patient on strict bed rest with the head of the bed slightly elevated

ANSWERS: 1. b; 2. d; 3. b; 4. c; 5. a; 6. a; 7. c; 8. c; 9. b.

REFERENCES

Alderson, P., & Roberts, I. (2009). Corticosteroids for acute traumatic brain injury [review]. *Cochrane Database of Systematic Reviews, 3,* CD000196. doi:10.1002/14651858.CD000196.pub2

Brain Trauma Foundation (BTF). (2007). *Guidelines for the management of severe traumatic brain injury* (3rd ed.). Rolling Meadows, IL: American Association of Neurological Surgeons. Retrieved from *https://www.braintrauma.org/pdf/protectedGuidelines_Management_2007w_bookmarks.pdf*

Brain Tumour Foundation of Canada (BTFC). (2011). *Brain tumour facts.* Retrieved from *http://www.braintumour.ca/2494/brain-tumour-facts*

Canadian Cancer Society's Steering Committee on Cancer Statistics. (2011). *Canadian Cancer Statistics 2011.* Retrieved from *http://www.cancer.ca/~/media/CCS/Canada%20wide/Files%20List/English%20files%20heading/PDF%20-%20Policy%20-%20Canadian%20Cancer%20Statistics%20-%20English/Canadian%20Cancer%20Statistics%202011%20-%20English.ashx*

Canadian Cancer Society's Steering Committee on Cancer Statistics. (2012). *Canadian Cancer Statistics 2012.* Retrieved from *http://www.cancer.ca/~/media/CCS/Canada%20wide/Files%20List/English%20files%20heading/PDF%20-%20Policy%20-%20Canadian%20Cancer%20Statistics%20-%20English/Canadian%20Cancer%20Statistics%202012%20-%20English.ashx*

Canadian Institute for Health Information (CIHI). (2006). *Head Injuries in Canada: A decade of change (1994-1995 to 2003-2004).* Retrieved from *http://secure.cihi.ca/cihiweb/en/downloads/analysis_ntr_2006_e*

Catt, S., Chalmers, A., & Fallowfield, L. (2008). Psychosocial and supportive care needs in high grade glioma. *Lancet Oncology, 9*(9), 884-891. doi:10.1016/S1470-2045(08)70230-4

Coco, K., Tossavainen, K., Jaaskelainen, J. E., & Turunen, H. (2011). Support for traumatic brain injury patients' family members in neurosurgical nursing: A systematic review. *Journal of Neuroscience Nursing, 43*(6), 337-348. doi:10.1097/JNN.0b013e318234ea0b

Cushing, H. (1925). *Studies in intracranial physiology and surgery.* London: Oxford University Press.

Ennis, K. M., & Brophy, G. M. (2010). Management of intracranial hypertension: focus on pharmacologic strategies. *AACN Advanced Critical Care, 22*(3), 177-182. doi:10.1097/NCI.0b013e318214564b

Härtl, R., Gerber, L. M., Ni, Q., & Ghajar, J. (2008). Effect of early nutrition on deaths due to severe traumatic brain injury. *Journal of Neurosurgery, 109*(1), 50-56. doi:10.3171/JNS/2008/109/7/0050

Jalali, R., Basu, A., Gupta, T., Munshi, A., Menon, H., Sarin, R., & Goel, A. (2007). Encouraging experience of concomitant temozolomide with radiotherapy followed by adjuvant temozolomide in newly diagnosed glioblastoma multiforme: Single institution experience. *British Journal of Neurosurgery, 21*(6), 583-587. doi:10.1007/s11060-008-9530-8

Jennett, B., & Teasdale, G. (1977). Aspects of coma after severe head injury. *Lancet, 1*(8017), 878. doi:10.1016/S0140-6736(77)91201-6

Kamel, H., Navi, B. B., Nakagawa, K., Hemphill, C., Ko, N. U. (2011). Hypertonic saline versus mannitol for the treatment of elevated intracranial pressure: A meta-analysis of randomized clinical trials. *Critical Care Medicine, 39*(3), 554-559. doi:10.1097/CCM.0b013e318206b9be

Ledwith, M. B., Bloom, S., Maloney-Wilensky, E., Coyle, B., Polomano, R. S., & LeRoux, P. D. (2010). Effect of body position on cerebral oxygenation and physiologic parameters in patients with acute neurological conditions. *Journal of Neuroscience Nursing, 42*(5), 280-287. doi:10.1097/JNN.0b013e3181ecafd4

Matthews, C., Miller, L., & Mott, M. (2007). Getting ahead of acute meningitis and encephalitis. *Nursing, 37*(11), 36-39. doi:10.1097/01.NURSE.0000298204.31684.c0

Muzumdar, D., Jhawar., S., & Goel, A. (2010). Brain abscess: an overview. *International Journal of Surgery, 9*(2), 136-144. doi:10.1016/j.ijsu.2010.11.005

Preusser, M., de Ribaupierre, S., Wohrer, A., Erridge, S. C., Hegi, M., Weller, M., & Stupp, R. (2011). Current concepts and management of glioblastoma. *Annals of Neurology, 70*(1), 9-21. doi:10.1002/ana.22425

Public Health Agency of Canada (PHAC). (2008). *Listeriosis epidemiological curve.* Retrieved from *http://www.phac-aspc.gc.ca/alert-alerte/listeria/epi-curve-courbe-eng.php*

Public Health Agency of Canada (PHAC). (2011a). *West Nile virus national surveillance reports.* Retrieved from *http://www.phac-aspc.gc.ca/wnv-vwn/mon-hmnsurv-eng.php*

Public Health Agency of Canada (PHAC). (2011b). *Vaccine-preventable disease: Rabies.* Retrieved from *http://www.phac-aspc.gc.ca/im/vpd-mev/rabies-eng.php*

Ramesh, V., Thirumaran, K., & Raja, M. (2008). A new scale of prognostication in head injury. *Journal of Clinical Neuroscience, 15*(10), 1110-1113. doi:10.1016.jocn.2007.08.033

Teasdale, G., & Jennett, B. (1974). Assessment of coma and impaired consciousness. A practical scale. *Lancet, 2*(7872), 81-84. doi:10.1016/S0140-6736(74)91639-0

van de Beek, D., de Gans, J., McIntyre, P., & Prasad, K. (2007). Corticosteroids for acute bacterial meningitis. *Cochrane Database of Systematic Reviews, 1,* CD004405. doi:10.1002/14651858.CD004405.pub2

Wasserman, J. R. (2006). Diffuse axonal injury. *eMedicine Clinical Knowledge Base.* Retrieved from *http://www.emedicine.medscape.com/article/339912-overview*

Zoons, E., Weisfelt, M., de Gans, J., Spanjaard, L., Koelman, J. H. T. M., Reitsma, J. B., & van de Beek, D. (2008). Seizures in adults with bacterial meningitis. *Neurology, 70*(22 pt 2), 2109-2115. doi:10.1212/01.wnl.0000288178.91614.5d

CANADIAN RESOURCES

Acquired Brain Injury Network
http://www.abinetwork.ca
Brain Injury Association of Canada
http://www.biac-aclc.ca
Brain Tumour Foundation of Canada
http://www.braintumour.ca
Canadian Cancer Society
http://www.cancer.ca
ThinkFirst National Brain and Spinal Cord Injury Prevention Foundation
http://www.thinkfirst.ca

RELATED RESOURCES

Encephalitis Global—Support Community
http://www.inspire.com/groups/encephalitis-global/
National Brain Tumor Foundation
http://www.braintumor.org

⊖volve *For additional Internet resources, see the Web site for this book at* **http://evolve.elsevier.com/Canada/Lewis/medsurg**

Written by Meg Zomorodi
Adapted by Jennifer Macauley

LEARNING OBJECTIVES

1. Describe the incidence of and risk factors for stroke.
2. Explain mechanisms that affect cerebral blood flow.
3. Differentiate the etiology and pathophysiology of ischemic and hemorrhagic strokes.
4. Correlate the clinical manifestations of stroke with the underlying pathophysiology.
5. Identify diagnostic studies performed for the patient with a stroke.
6. Describe the collaborative care, drug therapy, and nutritional therapy for a patient with a stroke.
7. Describe the acute nursing management of the patient with a stroke.
8. Discuss the rehabilitative nursing management of the patient with a stroke.
9. Explain the psychosocial impact of a stroke on the patient, caregiver, and family.

KEY TERMS

aneurysm A congenital or acquired weakness and ballooning of vessels, p. 1678

aphasia An abnormal neurological condition in which language function is disordered or absent because of an injury to certain areas of the cerebral cortex; often used interchangeably with *dysphasia*, p. 1679

brain attack Term used to describe a stroke, p. 1673

dysarthria A disturbance in the muscular control of speech, p. 1679

dysphasia Impaired ability to communicate; often used interchangeably with *aphasia*, p. 1679

embolic stroke A stroke that occurs when an embolus lodges in and occludes a cerebral artery, resulting in infarction and edema of the area supplied by the involved vessel, p. 1677

hemorrhagic stroke A stroke that results from bleeding into the brain tissue itself or into the subarachnoid space or the ventricles, p. 1677

intracerebral hemorrhage A type of hemorrhagic stroke in which bleeding occurs within the brain caused by a rupture of a blood vessel, p. 1677

ischemic strokes Strokes that result from inadequate blood flow to the brain from partial or complete occlusion of an artery, p. 1676

stroke Death of brain cells that occurs when there is ischemia to a part of the brain or hemorrhage into the brain, p. 1673

subarachnoid hemorrhage (SAH) A stroke resulting from intracranial bleeding into the cerebrospinal fluid–filled space between the arachnoid and pia mater membranes on the surface of the brain, p. 1678

thrombotic stroke A stroke resulting from thrombosis or narrowing of the blood vessel, p. 1676

transient ischemic attack (TIA) A temporary focal loss of neurological function caused by ischemia of one of the vascular territories of the brain, lasting less than 24 hours and often lasting less than 15 minutes, p. 1676

ELECTRONIC RESOURCES

Supplemental content related to Chapter 60 can be found ...

Evolve Web Site ⊝volve

http://evolve.elsevier.com/Canada/Lewis/medsurg
- Answer Guidelines for Case Study on p. 1697
- Clinical Reference: Laboratory Values
- Content Updates
- Customizable Nursing Care Plan: Stroke

- Electronic Calculators
- Examination Review Questions
- Glossary
- Interactive Case Study: Stroke
- Key Points (Printable and MP3 Download)
- Patient & Caregiver Teaching Guide: Warning Signs of Stroke

---

Stroke occurs when there is *ischemia* (inadequate blood flow) to a part of the brain or hemorrhage into the brain that results in death of brain cells. Functions such as movement, sensation, or emotions that were controlled by the affected area of the brain are lost or impaired. The severity of the loss of function varies according to the location and extent of the brain involved.

The term **brain attack** is increasingly being used to describe stroke. This term communicates the urgency of recognizing the clinical manifestations of a stroke and treating a medical emergency, similar to what would be done with a heart attack. Following the onset of a stroke, immediate medical attention is crucial to reduce disability and death.

Stroke is a major public health concern. More than 50,000 persons in Canada suffer a stroke annually (Canadian Stroke Network [CSN]/Heart and Stroke Foundation of Canada [HSF], 2010). Each year, 14,000 Canadians die from stroke, making it the third most common cause of death in Canada, behind cancer and heart disease (Statistics Canada, 2011). Three hundred thousand Canadians are currently living with the effects of stroke and it is the leading cause of adult disability (CSN/HSF, 2010; HSF, 2012; PHAC, 2009). Common long-term disabilities include hemiparesis, inability to walk, complete or partial dependence in activities of daily living (ADLs), aphasia, and depression. In addition to the physical, cognitive, and emotional impact of stroke on stroke survivors and their families, stroke also has an enormous financial impact. The direct and indirect costs of strokes are estimated to be greater than $3.6 billion per year in Canada (PHAC, 2009).

Pathophysiology of Stroke

Anatomy of Cerebral Circulation

Blood is supplied to the brain by two major pairs of arteries: the internal carotid arteries (anterior circulation) and the vertebral arteries (posterior circulation). The carotid arteries branch to supply most of the frontal, parietal, and temporal lobes; the basal ganglia; and part of the diencephalon (thalamus and hypothalamus). The major branches of the carotid arteries are the middle cerebral and anterior cerebral arteries. The vertebral arteries join to form the basilar artery, which branches to supply the middle and lower part of the temporal lobes, the occipital lobes, the cerebellum, the brainstem, and part of the diencephalon. The main branch of the basilar artery is the posterior cerebral artery. The anterior and posterior cerebral circulation is connected at the circle of Willis by the anterior and posterior communicating arteries (Figure 60-1) (See Chapter 58, Figure 58-14 for an illustration of the arteries at the base of the brain.) Anomalies in this area are common, and all connecting vessels may not be present.

Regulation of Cerebral Blood Flow

The brain requires a continuous supply of blood to provide the oxygen and glucose that neurons need to function. Blood flow

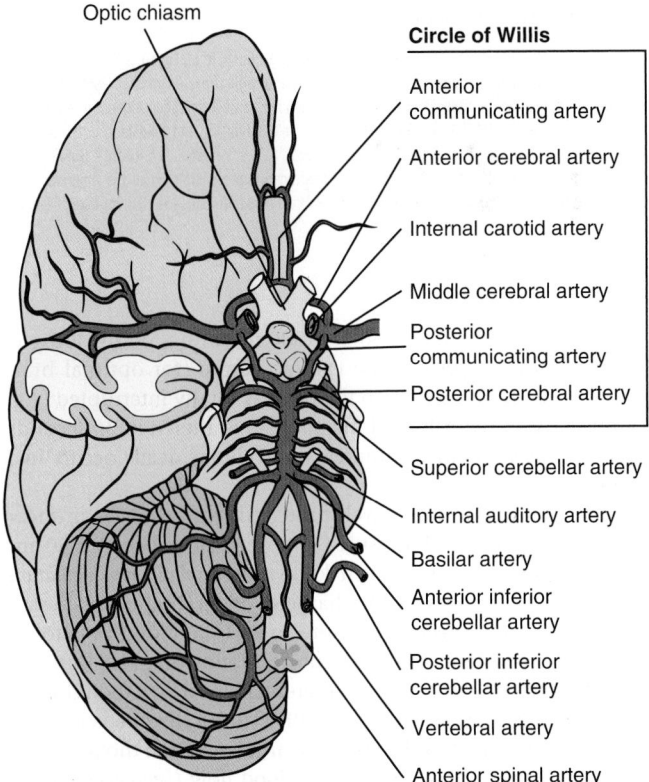

Figure 60-1 Cerebral arteries and the circle of Willis. The tip of the temporal lobe has been removed to show the course of the middle cerebral artery.

DETERMINANTS OF HEALTH
Stroke

Gender

Men

- Stroke is more common in men than in women. Men are more likely to have a thrombotic or embolic stroke, and they have a better chance of surviving.

Women

- Because women live longer than men, more women than men die from strokes.
- Oral contraceptives and hormone replacement therapy contribute to stroke risk. Women are more likely to have a hemorrhagic stroke.

Culture: Biology and Genetic Endowment

- Blacks who have never had a stroke have almost twice the risk of having one as Whites who have never had one.

Social Environment

- Individuals with lower incomes have a higher proportion of risk factors such as obesity, diabetes, smoking, and untreated hypertension, which are all linked to stroke.

Personal Health Practices and Coping Skills

- Over 50% of individuals who experience a TIA fail to report it to health providers.
- Of all stroke survivors, 30% develop depression in the first 3 months following a stroke.

  TIA, transient ischemic attack.

Sources: Furie, K. L., Kasner, S. E., Adams, R. J., Albers, G. W., Bush, R. L., Fagan, S. C., ..., Wentworth, D. (2011). Guidelines for the prevention of stroke in patients with stroke or transient ischemic attack: A guideline for healthcare professionals. From the American Heart Association/American Stroke Association. *Stroke, 42*(1), 227–276. doi:10.1161/STR.0b013e3181f7d043; and Goldstein, L. B., Bushnell, C. D., Adams, R. J., Appel, L. J., Braun, L. T., Chaturvedi, S., ..., Pearson, T. A. (2011). Guidelines for the primary prevention of stroke: A guideline for healthcare professionals. From the American Heart Association/American Stroke Association. *Stroke, 42*(2), 517–584. doi:10.1161/STR.0b013e3181fcb238

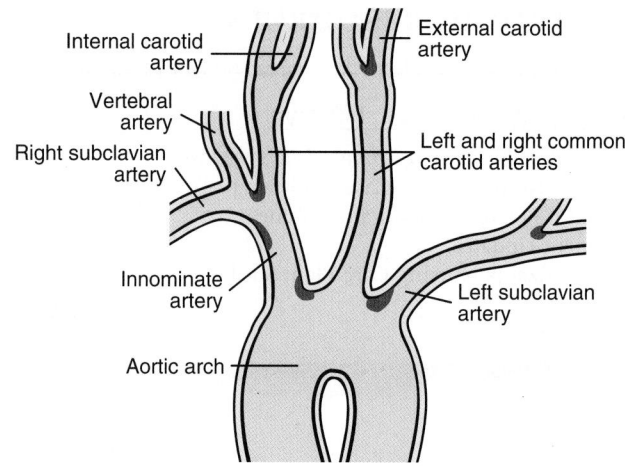

Figure 60-2 Common sites for the development of atherosclerosis in extracranial and intracranial arteries. The main locations are just above the common carotid bifurcation (most common site) and the start of the branches from the aorta and the innominate and subclavian arteries.

must be maintained at 750 to 1000 mL/min (55 mL/100 g of brain tissue), or 20% of the cardiac output, for optimal brain functioning. If blood flow to the brain is totally interrupted (e.g., cardiac arrest), neurological metabolism is altered in 30 seconds, metabolism stops in 2 minutes, and cellular death occurs in 5 minutes.

The brain is normally well protected from changes in mean systemic arterial blood pressure (BP) over a range between 50 and 150 mm Hg by a mechanism known as *cerebral autoregulation.* This involves changes in the diameter of cerebral blood vessels in response to changes in pressure so that the blood flow to the brain stays constant. Cerebral autoregulation may be impaired following cerebral ischemia, and cerebral blood flow then changes directly in response to changes in BP. Carbon dioxide is a potent cerebral vasodilator, and changes in arterial carbon dioxide levels have a dramatic effect on cerebral blood flow (increased carbon dioxide levels increase cerebral blood flow and vice versa). Very low arterial oxygen levels (partial pressure of arterial oxygen <50 mm Hg) or an increase in hydrogen ion concentration also increases cerebral blood flow.

Factors that affect blood flow to the brain include systemic BP, cardiac output, and blood viscosity. During normal activity, oxygen requirements vary considerably, but changes in cardiac output, vasomotor tone, and distribution of blood flow normally maintain adequate blood flow to the head. Cardiac output has to be reduced by one third before cerebral blood flow is reduced. Changes in blood viscosity affect cerebral blood flow, with decreased viscosity increasing flow.

Collateral circulation may develop to compensate for a decrease in cerebral blood flow. Because of the connections between arteries at the circle of Willis, an area of the brain can potentially receive blood supply from another blood vessel if its original blood supply is cut off (e.g., because of thrombosis). Individual differences in collateral circulation partly determine the degree of brain damage and functional loss when a stroke occurs.

Intracranial pressure (ICP) also influences cerebral blood flow (see Chapter 58). Increased ICP causes brain compression and reduced cerebral blood flow.

Atherosclerosis

Atherosclerosis (hardening and thickening of arteries) is a major cause of stroke. It can lead to thrombus formation and contribute to emboli. (The role of atherosclerosis in thrombosis and emboli development is discussed in Chapter 36.) Initially, there is abnormal infiltration of lipids in the intimal layer of the artery. This fatty streak further develops into a plaque. Plaques often develop in areas of increased turbulence of the blood, such as at the bifurcation of an artery or a tortuous area (Figure 60-2). Calcified, brittle plaques may rupture or fissure, which leads to an inflammatory response. Platelet and fibrin are released and stick to the roughened plaque surface. Plaque may narrow or occlude the artery. Also, parts of the plaque or thrombus can break off and travel to a narrower distal artery. Cerebral infarction occurs when a cerebral artery becomes blocked and blood supply to the brain beyond the blockage is occluded.

In response to ischemia, a series of metabolic events, termed the *ischemic cascade,* occur, including inadequate adenosine triphosphate production, loss of ion homeostasis, release of excitatory amino acids (e.g., glutamate), free radical formation, and cell death. Around the core area of ischemia is a border zone of reduced blood flow called the *penumbra*, where ischemia is potentially reversible. If adequate blood flow can be restored early (e.g., within 3 hours) and the ischemic cascade can be interrupted, there may be less brain damage and less neurological function lost. Research is ongoing to identify thrombolytic and neuroprotective therapies to re-establish blood flow and protect neurons from further ischemic damage.

Risk Factors for Stroke

The most effective way to decrease the burden of stroke is prevention. Awareness and control of modifiable risk factors can contribute to reducing the incidence and burden of stroke. Risk factors can be divided into nonmodifiable and modifiable. Stroke risk increases considerably with multiple risk factors.

Nonmodifiable Risk Factors

Nonmodifiable risk factors include age, gender, ethnicity and race, family history and heredity, and low birth weight (Goldstein et al., 2011). Stroke risk increases with age, doubling each decade after 55 years of age. Two thirds of all strokes occur in individuals older than 65 years, but stroke can occur at any age. Strokes are more common in men, but more women than men die from stroke (HSF, 2012). Because women tend to live longer than men, they have more opportunity to suffer a stroke. A family history of stroke, a prior transient ischemic attack (TIA), or a prior stroke also increases the risk of stroke.

Modifiable Risk Factors

Modifiable risk factors are those that can potentially be altered through lifestyle changes and medical treatment, thus reducing the risk of stroke (Table 60-1).

Hypertension is the single most important, well-documented modifiable risk factor for stroke. Five million Canadian adults have diagnosed hypertension, approximately 19% of the population (HSF, 2012). Increases in systolic and diastolic BP independently increase the risk of stroke. Stroke risk can be significantly reduced through the adequate treatment and early diagnosis of hypertension (Goldstein et al., 2011).

Heart disease, including atrial fibrillation (AF), myocardial infarction, cardiomyopathy, carotid stenosis, cardiac valve abnormalities, and congenital defects, is also a risk factor for stroke.

Of these, AF is the most important treatable cardiac-related risk factor (Goldstein et al., 2011). The incidence of AF increases with age. Approximately 25% of strokes in patients older than 80 years are caused by AF (Goldstein et al., 2011). Following myocardial infarction, nearly 8% of men and 11% of women will have a stroke within 6 years.

Diabetes mellitus is a significant risk for ischemic stroke (Goldstein et al., 2011). The risk for stroke in people with diabetes mellitus is four to five times higher than in the general population. Although tight control of hypertension in diabetics significantly decreases stroke risk, achieving a hemoglobin A1C less than or equal to 7% and treatment with a "statin" have been proved to be beneficial (CSN/HSF, 2010).

Increased serum cholesterol is another risk factor for stroke (CSN/HSF, 2010). Smoking nearly doubles the risk of ischemic stroke (Goldstein et al., 2011). Fortunately, the risk associated with smoking decreases over time after quitting smoking and in 5 to 10 years is reduced to that of nonsmokers (Goldstein & Hankey, 2006).

The effect of alcohol on stroke risk appears to depend on the amount consumed. Light to moderate use of alcohol, in particular wine, has been linked to reduced risk of total and ischemic stroke (Goldstein et al., 2011). Heavier use of alcohol does increase risk of stroke. Alcohol consumption of two drinks or fewer per day for men and one drink or fewer per day for nonpregnant women might be reasonable (Goldstein et al., 2011).

Almost 60% of adults ages 18 and older, or 14.1 million Canadians, are overweight or obese (HSF, 2012). Abdominal obesity increases ischemic stroke risk in all ethnic groups. Individuals who are overweight or obese experience a significant decrease in life expectancy. Abdominal obesity in men increases stroke risk, and obesity and weight gain in women increase the risk of ischemic stroke but not hemorrhagic stroke (Air & Kissela, 2007). In addition, obesity is also associated with conditions such as hypertension, high blood glucose, and elevated blood lipid levels, which also increase stroke risk (Goldstein & Hankey, 2006).

An association of physical inactivity and increased stroke risk is present in both men and women, regardless of ethnicity. Benefits of physical activity can occur with even light-to-moderate regular activity and may be in part related to the beneficial effect of exercise on other risk factors. The effect of diet on stroke risk is not clear, although a diet high in saturated fat and low in fibre may increase stroke risk. Illicit drug use, notably cocaine, methamphetamine, and heroin, has been associated with increased stroke risk (Goldstein et al., 2011).

The early forms of birth control pills that contained high levels of progestin and estrogen increased a woman's chance of experiencing a stroke, especially if the woman also smoked heavily. Newer, low-dose oral contraceptives have lower risks for stroke except in those individuals who are hypertensive and smoke (Roederer & Blackwell, 2006). Other conditions that may increase stroke risk include migraines, metabolic syndrome, sleep-disordered breathing, inflammation and infection, hypercoagulability, and hyperhomocysteinemia. Sickle cell disease is another known risk factor for stroke (Goldstein et al, 2011).

Table 60-1 Modifiable Risk Factors for Stroke	
• Asymptomatic carotid stenosis	• Hypertension
• Diabetes mellitus	• Obesity and body fat distribution
• Heart disease; atrial fibrillation	
• Alcohol abuse	• Oral contraceptive use
• Hypercoagulability	• Physical inactivity
• Illicit drugs	• Sickle cell disease
• Dyslipidemia	• Sleep apnea
	• Smoking

Types of Stroke

Strokes are classified as ischemic or hemorrhagic based on the underlying pathophysiological findings (Figure 60-3 and Table 60-2).

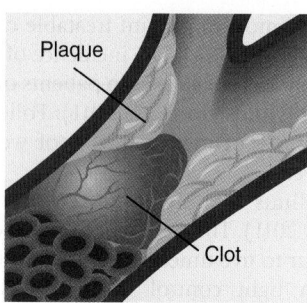

Thrombotic stroke. Cerebral thrombosis is a narrowing of the artery by fatty deposits called *plaque*. Plaque can cause a clot to form, which blocks the passage of blood through the artery.

A

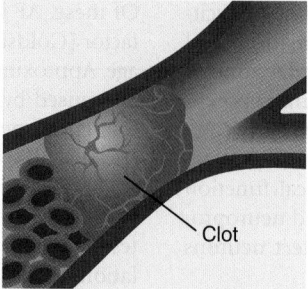

Embolic stroke. An embolus is a blood clot or other debris circulating in the blood. When it reaches an artery in the brain that is too narrow to pass through, it lodges there and blocks the flow of blood.

B

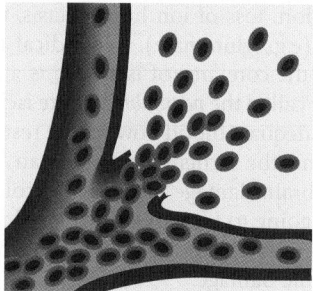

Hemorrhagic stroke. A burst blood vessel may allow blood to seep into and damage brain tissues until clotting shuts off the leak.

C

Figure 60-3 **A** to **C,** Major types of stroke.

Table 60-2 Types of Stroke

GENDER/AGE	WARNING/ONSET	COURSE/PROGNOSIS
Ischemic		
Thrombotic Men more than women. Oldest median age.	*Warning:* TIA (30-50% of cases) *Onset:* Often during or after sleep	Stepwise progression, signs and symptoms develop slowly, usually some improvement, recurrence in 20-25% of survivors
Embolic Men more than women	*Warning:* TIA uncommon *Onset:* Lack of relationship to activity, sudden onset	Single event, signs and symptoms develop quickly, usually some improvement, recurrence common without aggressive treatment of underlying disease
Hemorrhagic		
Intracerebral Slightly higher in women	*Warning:* Headache (25% of cases) *Onset:* Activity (often)	Progression over 24 hr; poor prognosis, fatality more likely with presence of coma
Subarachnoid Slightly higher in women Youngest median age	*Warning:* Headache (common) *Onset:* Activity (often), sudden onset, most commonly related to head trauma	Usually single sudden event, fatality more likely with presence of coma

TIA, transient ischemic attack.

Ischemic Stroke

Ischemic strokes result from inadequate blood flow to the brain from partial or complete occlusion of an artery; these account for approximately 80% of all strokes (HSF, 2012). Ischemic strokes are further divided into thrombotic and embolic. A TIA is usually a precursor to ischemic stroke.

Transient Ischemic Attack. A **transient ischemic attack (TIA)** is a transient episode of neurological dysfunction caused by focal brain, spinal cord, or retinal ischemia, but without acute infarction of the brain. Clinical symptoms typically last less than 1 hour. In the past, TIAs were operationally defined as any focal cerebral ischemic event with symptoms lasting less than 24 hours. However, it has been demonstrated that this arbitrary time threshold was too broad because 30 to 50% of classically defined TIAs show brain injury on magnetic resonance imaging (MRI) (Easton et al., 2009).

Most TIAs resolve. However, patients should be encouraged to go to the emergency department at symptom onset because once a TIA starts, it is not possible to know whether it will persist and become a true stroke or resolve. In general, one third of individuals who experience a TIA will not experience another event, one third will have another TIA, and the remaining third will experience a stroke (Giles & Rothwell, 2009).

TIAs may be caused by microemboli that temporarily block the blood flow. TIAs are a warning sign of progressive cerebrovascular disease (Gao & Jiang, 2009). The signs and symptoms of a TIA depend on the blood vessel that is involved and the area of the brain that is ischemic. If the carotid system is involved, patients may have a temporary loss of vision in one eye *(amaurosis fugax)*, a transient hemiparesis, numbness or loss of sensation, or a sudden inability to speak. Signs of a TIA involving the vertebrobasilar system may include tinnitus, vertigo, darkened or blurred vision, diplopia, ptosis, dysarthria, dysphagia, ataxia, and unilateral or bilateral numbness or weakness.

Thrombotic Stroke. A **thrombotic stroke** occurs from injury to a blood vessel wall and formation of a blood clot (see Figure 60-3, *A*). The lumen of the blood vessel becomes narrowed, and if it becomes occluded, infarction occurs. This is the main difference between TIAs and stroke: in a TIA, ischemia occurs without infarction, but in a stroke, infarction and cell death occur. Thrombosis develops readily where atherosclerotic plaques have already narrowed blood vessels. Thrombotic stroke, which is the result of thrombosis or narrowing of the blood vessel, is the most common cause of stroke, accounting for 60% of strokes (Goldstein et al., 2011). Two thirds of thrombotic strokes are associated with hypertension or diabetes mellitus, both of which accelerate atherosclerosis. In 30 to 50% of individuals, thrombotic strokes have been preceded by a TIA.

The extent of the stroke depends on rapidity of onset, the size of the lesion, and the presence of collateral circulation. Most patients with ischemic stroke do not have a decreased level of consciousness (LOC) in the first 24 hours, unless it is owing to a brainstem stroke or other conditions such as seizures, increased ICP, or hemorrhage. Ischemic stroke symptoms may progress in the first 72 hours as infarction and cerebral edema increase.

A *lacunar stroke* refers to a stroke from occlusion of a small penetrating artery with development of a cavity in the place of the infarcted brain tissue. This most commonly occurs in the basal ganglia, thalamus, internal capsule, or pons. Although many lacunar strokes are asymptomatic, when present, symptoms can cause considerable deficits. These include pure motor hemiplegia, pure sensory stroke (contralateral loss of all sensory modalities), contralateral leg and face weakness with arm and leg ataxia, and isolated motor or sensory stroke. Multiple small vessel infarcts may also result in a decrease in vascular function (i.e., multi-infarct dementia) (See Chapter 62).

Embolic Stroke.

Embolic stroke occurs when an embolus lodges in and occludes a cerebral artery, resulting in infarction and edema of the area supplied by the involved vessel (see Figure 60-3, *B*). Embolism is the second most common cause of stroke, accounting for about 24% of strokes (Goldstein et al., 2011). The majority of emboli originate in the endocardial (inside) layer of the heart, with plaque breaking off from the endocardium and entering the circulation. The embolus travels upward to the cerebral circulation and lodges where a vessel narrows or bifurcates. Heart conditions associated with emboli include valvular heart disease and valvular prosthesis MI, infective endocarditis, rheumatic heart disease, intracardiac congenital defects such as atrial septal defects and patent foramen ovale. In addition, AF is associated with a four- to five-fold increased risk of ischemic stroke owing to embolism of stasis-induced thrombi in the left atrium (Goldstein et al., 2011). Less common triggers of emboli include air and fat from long bone (femur) fractures.

The patient with an embolic stroke commonly has a rapid occurrence of severe clinical symptoms, but warning signs are less common than with thrombotic stroke. The onset of an embolic stroke is usually sudden and may or may not be related to activity. The patient usually remains conscious, and a headache may or may not be present. Prognosis is related to the amount and location of brain tissue deprived of its blood supply. The effects of the emboli are initially characterized by severe neurological deficits, which can be temporary if the clot breaks up and allows blood to flow. Smaller emboli then continue to obstruct smaller vessels, which in turn involve smaller portions of the brain with fewer deficits noted. The embolic stroke often occurs rapidly, and the body does not have time to accommodate by developing collateral circulation. Recurrence of embolic stroke is common unless the underlying cause is aggressively treated.

Hemorrhagic Stroke

Hemorrhagic strokes account for approximately 15% of all strokes; they result from bleeding into the brain tissue itself (intracerebral or intraparenchymal hemorrhage) or into the subarachnoid space or the ventricles (subarachnoid hemorrhage [SAH] or intraventricular hemorrhage) (Goldstein et al., 2011).

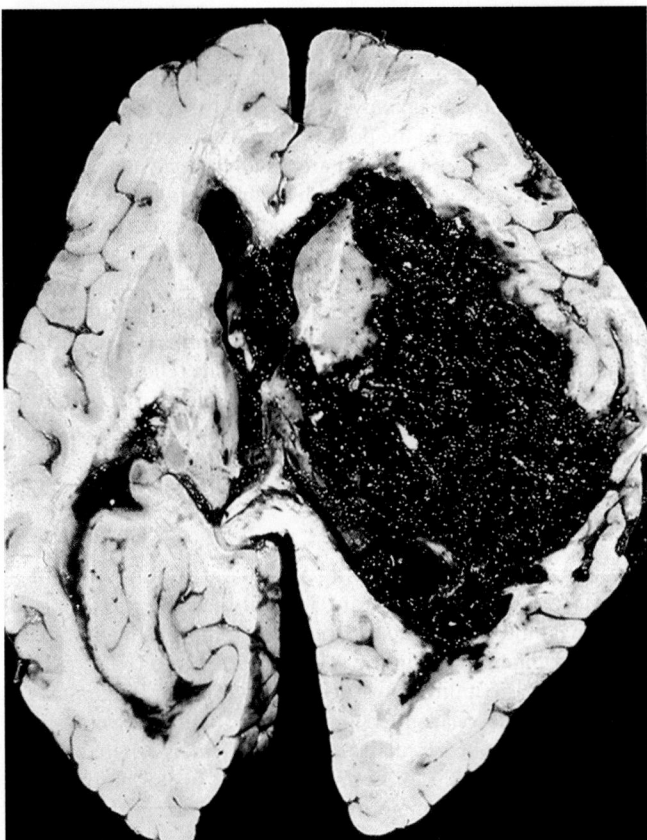

Figure 60-4 Massive hypertensive hemorrhage rupturing into a lateral ventricle of the brain.

Source: Kumar, V., Abbas, A. K., Fausto, N., & Aster, J. (2010). *Robbins and Cotran pathologic basis of disease.* (8th ed. p. 1296, Figure 28-18). Philadelphia: Saunders.

Intracerebral Hemorrhage.

Intracerebral hemorrhage is bleeding within the brain caused by a rupture of a vessel; it accounts for about 10% of all strokes (see Figure 60-3, *C*). Hypertension is the most important cause of intracerebral hemorrhage (Figure 60-4). Other causes include cerebral amyloid angiopathy, vascular malformations, coagulation disorders, anticoagulant and thrombolytic drugs, trauma, brain tumours, and ruptured aneurysms. Hemorrhage commonly occurs during periods of activity. There is most often a sudden onset of symptoms, with progression over minutes to hours because of ongoing bleeding. Symptoms include neurological deficits, headache, nausea, vomiting, decreased LOC (in about 50% of patients), and hypertension. The extent of the symptoms varies depending on the amount and duration of the bleeding. A blood clot within the closed skull can result in a mass that causes pressure on brain tissue, displaces brain tissue, and decreases cerebral blood flow, leading to ischemia and infarction (Nassisi, 2008).

Approximately 50% of intracerebral hemorrhages occur in the putamen and the internal capsule, central white matter, thalamus, cerebellar hemispheres, and pons. Initially, patients experience a severe headache with nausea and vomiting. Clinical manifestations of putaminal and internal capsule bleeding include weakness of one side (including face, arm, and leg), slurred speech, and deviation of the eyes. Progression of symptoms related to a severe hemorrhage includes hemiplegia, fixed and dilated pupils, abnormal body posturing, and coma. Thalamic hemorrhage results in hemiplegia with more sensory than motor loss. Bleeding into the subthalamic areas of the brain leads to problems with vision and eye movement. Cerebellar hemorrhages are characterized by severe headache, vomiting, loss of ability to walk, dysphagia, dysarthria, and eye movement disturbances. Hemorrhage in the pons is the most serious because basic life functions (e.g., respiration) are rapidly affected. Hemorrhage in the pons can be characterized by hemiplegia leading to complete paralysis, coma, abnormal body posturing, fixed pupils (small in size) hyperthermia, and death. The prognosis of patients with intracerebral hemorrhage is poor, with a 30-day mortality rate of 40 to 80% (Goldstein et al., 2011). Over 50% of patients die soon after the initial hemorrhage occurs and only about 20% remain functionally independent at 6 months (Dickerson, Carek, & Quattlebaum, 2007; Goldstein, 2007; Goldstein et al., 2011). Recent studies suggest that most patients present with small intracerebral hemorrhages and that aggressive care of the intracerebral hemorrhage is directly related to mortality for the condition (Morgenstern et al., 2010).

Subarachnoid Hemorrhage.

Subarachnoid hemorrhage (SAH) occurs when there is intracranial bleeding into the cerebrospinal fluid (CSF)–filled space between the arachnoid and the pia mater membranes on the surface of the brain (Kazzi & Ellis, 2009). SAH is commonly caused by rupture of a cerebral **aneurysm** (congenital or acquired weakness and ballooning of vessels). Aneurysms may be saccular or berry aneurysms ranging from a few millimetres to 20 to 30 mm in size, or fusiform atherosclerotic aneurysms. The majority of aneurysms are in the circle of Willis. Other causes of SAH include *arteriovenous malformations* (AVMs), trauma, and illicit drug (cocaine) use. About 40% of people who have a hemorrhagic stroke owing to a ruptured aneurysm die during the first episode; 15% die from subsequent bleeding (Kazzi & Ellis, 2009). The incidence of SAH caused by a ruptured aneurysm increases with age and is higher in women than in men.

The patient may have warning symptoms if the ballooning artery applies pressure to brain tissue, or minor warning symptoms from leaking of an aneurysm before major rupture. Overall, cerebral aneurysms are viewed as a "silent killer" because individuals do not have warning signs of an aneurysm until rupture has occurred.

SAFETY ALERT

Sudden onset of a severe headache that is different from a previous headache and typically the "worst headache of one's life" is characteristic of a ruptured aneurysm.

Loss of consciousness may or may not occur. The patient's LOC may range from alert to comatose, depending on the severity of the bleed. Other symptoms include focal neurological deficits (including cranial nerve deficits), nausea, vomiting, seizures, and stiff neck. Despite improvements in surgical techniques and management, many patients with SAH die. Many are left with significant morbidity, including cognitive difficulties.

Complications of aneurysmal SAH include rebleeding before surgery or other therapy is initiated and cerebral vasospasm (narrowing of the large blood vessels at the base of the brain), which can result in cerebral infarction. Cerebral vasospasm is most likely owing to an interaction between the metabolites of blood and the vascular smooth muscle. During the lysis of subarachnoid blood clots, metabolites are released. These metabolites can cause endothelial damage and vasoconstriction. In addition, release of endothelin (a potent vasoconstrictor) may play a major role in the induction of cerebral vasospasm after SAH. Peak time for vasospasm to occur is 6 to 20 days after the initial bleed.

Clinical Manifestations of Stroke

The neurological manifestations do not significantly differ between ischemic and hemorrhagic stroke. The reason for this is that destruction of neural tissue is the basis for neurological dysfunction caused by both types of stroke. The clinical manifestations are related to location of the stroke. Specific manifestations related to the type of stroke are discussed in the previous section on type of stroke.

The general clinical manifestations of ischemic and hemorrhagic stroke are discussed together in this section. A stroke can have an effect on many body functions, including motor activity, bladder and bowel elimination, intellectual function, spatial–perceptual alterations, personality, affect, sensation, and communication. The functions affected are directly related to the artery involved and the area of the brain it supplies (Table 60-3). Manifestations related to right- and left-brain damage differ somewhat and are shown in Figure 60-5.

Motor Function.

Motor deficits are the most obvious effect of stroke. Motor deficits include impairment of (1) mobility, (2) respiratory function, (3) swallowing and speech, (4) gag reflex, and (5) self-care abilities. Symptoms are caused by the destruction of motor neurons in the pyramidal pathway (nerve fibres from the brain and passing through the spinal cord to the motor cells). The characteristic motor deficits include loss of skilled voluntary movement *(akinesia)*, impairment of integration of movements, alterations in muscle tone, and alterations in reflexes. The initial *hyporeflexia* (depressed reflexes) progresses to *hyperreflexia* (hyperactive reflexes) for most patients.

Motor deficits after a stroke follow certain specific patterns. Because the pyramidal pathway crosses at the level of the medulla, a lesion on one side of the brain affects motor function on the opposite side of the brain (contralateral). The arms and legs of the affected side may be weakened or paralyzed to different degrees depending on which part of and to what extent the cerebral circulation was compromised. A stroke affecting the middle

Table 60-3 Stroke Manifestations Related to Artery Involvement	
ARTERY	**DEFICIT OR SYNDROME**
Anterior cerebral	Motor and/or sensory deficit (contralateral), sucking or rooting reflex, rigidity, and gait problems, loss of proprioception, fine touch
Middle cerebral	*Dominant side:* Aphasia, motor and sensory deficit, hemianopsia
	Nondominant side: Neglect, motor and sensory deficit, hemianopsia
Posterior cerebral	Hemianopsia, visual hallucination, spontaneous pain, motor deficit
Vertebral	Cranial nerve deficits, diplopia, dizziness, nausea, vomiting, dysarthria, dysphagia, and/or coma

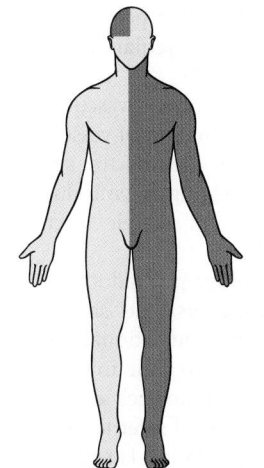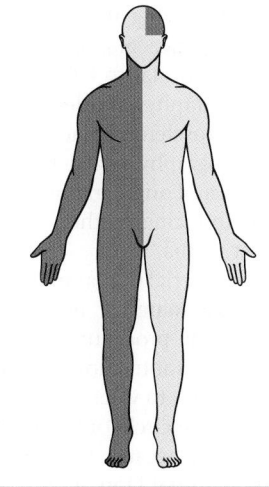

Right-brain damage (stroke on right side of the brain)	**Left-brain damage** (stroke on left side of the brain)
• Paralyzed left side: hemiplegia	• Paralyzed right side: hemiplegia
• Left-sided neglect	• Impaired speech–language (aphasias)
• Spatial–perceptual deficits	• Impaired right–left discrimination
• Tends to deny or minimize problems	• Slow performance, cautious
• Rapid performance, short attention span	• Aware of deficits: depression, anxiety
• Impulsive; safety problems	• Impaired comprehension related to language, math
• Impaired judgement	
• Impaired time concepts	

Figure 60-5 Manifestations of right-brain and left-brain stroke.

cerebral artery leads to a greater weakness in the upper extremity than the lower extremity. The affected shoulder tends to rotate internally and the hip rotates externally. The affected foot is plantar flexed and inverted. An initial period of flaccidity may last from days to several weeks and is related to nerve damage. Spasticity of the muscles follows the flaccid stage and is related to interruption of upper motor neuron influence.

Communication. The left hemisphere is dominant for language skills in right-handed persons and in most left-handed persons. Language disorders involve expression and comprehension of written and spoken words. The patient may experience **aphasia** (total loss of comprehension and use of language or total inability to communicate). It occurs when a stroke damages the dominant hemisphere of the brain. **Dysphasia** refers to impaired ability to communicate. However, in most settings, the terms *aphasia* and *dysphasia* are used interchangeably to mean the same thing, with *aphasia* often being the more common term used.

According to the National Institute of Neurological Disorders and Stroke (NINDS, 2010), there are four categories of aphasia: (1) *Expressive aphasia* (also called *Broca's aphasia*) is difficulty in expressing thoughts through speech or writing. The patient cannot find the words needed but does know what he or she wants to say. The stroke survivor's speech is reduced often to less than four words. (2) *Receptive aphasia* (also called *Wernicke's aphasia*) is difficulty understanding spoken or written language.

These patients are difficult to understand. They speak without hesitation, but words may be used incorrectly and there may be grammatical errors. (3) *Anomic* or *amnesic aphasia* is the least severe form of aphasia and involves problems finding the correct names for specific objects, people, places, or events. (4) *Global aphasia* results in loss of all expressive and receptive function. This is usually caused by a massive stroke. Some aphasic patients are mixed, with impairment in both expression and understanding.

Many stroke patients also experience **dysarthria**, a disturbance in the muscular control of speech. Impairments may involve pronunciation, articulation, and phonation (use of the voice). Dysarthria does not affect the meaning of communication or the comprehension of language, but it does affect the mechanics of speech. Some patients experience a combination of aphasia and dysarthria.

Affect. Patients who have had a stroke may have difficulty controlling their emotions. Emotional responses may be exaggerated or unpredictable. Depression and feelings associated with changes in body image and loss of function can make this worse (Christensen, Mayer, Ferran, & Kissela, 2009). Patients may also be frustrated by mobility and communication problems. Depression is common in the first year following a stroke.

Intellectual Function. Both memory and judgement may be impaired as a result of stroke. These impairments can occur with strokes affecting either side of the brain. A left-brain stroke is more likely to result in memory problems related to language. Patients with a left-brain stroke often are very cautious in making judgements. The patient with a right-brain stroke tends to be impulsive and to move quickly. An example of behaviour with right-brain stroke is the patient who tries to rise quickly from the wheelchair without locking the wheels or raising the foot rests. The patient with a left-brain stroke would move slowly and cautiously from the wheelchair. Patients with either type of stroke may have difficulty making generalizations, which interferes with their ability to learn.

Spatial–Perceptual Alterations. A stroke on the right side of the brain is more likely to cause problems in spatial–perceptual orientation, although this can also occur with left-brain stroke. Spatial–perceptual problems may be divided into four categories. The first is related to the patient's incorrect perception of self and illness. This deficit follows damage to the parietal lobe. Patients may deny their illnesses or their own body parts (*anosognosia*). The second category concerns the patient's erroneous perception of self in space. The patient may neglect all input from the affected side. This may be worsened by *homonymous hemianopsia*, in which blindness occurs in the same half of the visual fields of both eyes. The patient also has difficulty with spatial orientation, such as judging distances. The third spatial–perceptual deficit is *agnosia*, the inability to recognize an object by sight, touch, or hearing. The fourth deficit is *apraxia*, the inability to carry out learned sequential movements on command. Patients may or may not be aware of their spatial–perceptual alterations.

Elimination. Fortunately, most problems with urinary and bowel elimination occur initially and are temporary. When a stroke affects one hemisphere of the brain, the prognosis for normal bladder function is excellent. At least partial sensation for bladder filling remains, and voluntary urination is present.

Initially, the patient may experience frequency, urgency, and incontinence. Although motor control of the bowel is usually not a problem, patients are frequently constipated. Constipation is associated with immobility, weak abdominal muscles, dehydration, and diminished response to the defecation reflex. Urinary and bowel elimination problems may also be related to inability to express needs and to manage clothing.

Diagnostic Studies

When manifestations of a stroke occur, diagnostic studies are done to (1) confirm that it is a stroke and not another brain lesion, such as a subdural hematoma, and (2) identify the likely cause of the stroke (Table 60-4). Tests also guide decisions about therapy to prevent a secondary stroke. The single most important neuroimaging tool for a stroke patient is brain imagining—either MRI or noncontrast computed tomography (CT) scan (CSN/HSF, 2010). The CT scan is quick and easy to access in most facilities. The CT scan should optimally be obtained within 25 minutes and read within 45 minutes of arrival at the emergency department. CT indicates the size and location of the lesion and helps to differentiate between ischemic and hemorrhagic stroke. Serial CT scans may be used to assess the effectiveness of treatment and to evaluate recovery.

Computed tomography angiography (CTA) provides visualization of cerebral vasculature and can be performed after or at the same time as the noncontrast CT scan. CTA can provide an estimate of perfusion and detect defects in the cerebral arteries.

MRI is used to determine the extent of brain injury and has greater specificity in determining the location of vascular lesions and blockages than CT. Patient preparation and access to an MRI scanner can be delayed for many reasons and should not delay

the patient having alternative diagnostic studies performed. Magnetic resonance angiography can detect vascular lesions and blockages, similar to CTA.

Angiography can identify cervical and cerebrovascular occlusion, atherosclerotic plaques, and malformation of vessels. Cerebral angiography is a definitive study to identify the source of SAH. Risks of angiography include dislodging an embolus, vasospasm, inducing further hemorrhage, and allergic reaction to contrast media.

Intra-arterial digital subtraction angiography reduces the dose of contrast material, uses smaller catheters, and shortens the length of the procedure compared with conventional angiography. Digital subtraction angiography involves the injection of a contrast agent to visualize blood vessels in the neck and the large vessels of the circle of Willis. It is considered safer than cerebral angiography because less vascular manipulation is required.

Transcranial Doppler ultrasonography is a noninvasive study that measures the velocity of blood flow in the major cerebral arteries. Transcranial Doppler has been shown to be effective in detecting microemboli and vasospasm and is ideal for the patient suspected of having an SAH. Carotid duplex scanning is used not only to detect the cause of the stroke but also to stratify patients for either medical management or carotid intervention if they have carotid stenoses.

A lumbar puncture may be done to look for evidence of red blood cells in the CSF if an SAH is suspected and the CT does not show hemorrhage. A lumbar puncture is avoided if it is suspected that there is an obstruction in the foramen magnum or other signs of increased ICP because of the danger of herniation of the brain downward, leading to pressure on cardiac and respiratory centres in the brainstem and potentially death.

If the suspected cause of the stroke includes emboli from the heart, diagnostic cardiac tests should be done (see Table 60-4). Blood tests are also done to help identify conditions contributing to stroke and to guide treatment (see Table 60-4).

Collaborative Care

Prevention Therapy. Primary prevention is a priority for decreasing morbidity and mortality from stroke (Table 60-5). The goals of stroke prevention include health management for the well individual and education and management of modifiable risk factors to prevent a primary or secondary stroke. Health management focuses on (1) BP control, (2) blood glucose control, (3) diet and exercise, (4) smoking cessation, (5) limiting alcohol consumption, and (6) routine health assessments. Patients with known risk factors such as diabetes mellitus, hypertension, smoking, high serum lipids, or cardiovascular dysfunction require close management.

Drug Therapy. Measures to prevent the development of a thrombus or embolus are used in patients with TIAs because they are at risk for stroke. Antiplatelet drugs are usually the chosen treatment to prevent stroke in patients who have had a TIA (Healey et al., 2008). Aspirin is the most frequently used antiplatelet agent, commonly at a dose of 81 to 325 mg/day. Other drugs include clopidogrel (Plavix), dipyridamole (Persantine), and combined dipyridamole and aspirin (Aggrenox). Oral anticoagulation using warfarin is the treatment of choice for individuals with AF who have had a TIA (Furie et al., 2011). The CHADS2 score is a clinical prediction rule used to estimate the risk of stroke in patients with AF and to determine the degree of anticoagulation required (Healey et al., 2008).

DIAGNOSTIC STUDIES

Table 60-4 Stroke	
Diagnosis of Stroke (Including Extent of Involvement)	**Additional Studies**
• Computed tomography (CT) scan	• Complete blood count (CBC) including platelets
• CT angiography (CTA)	• Coagulation studies: prothrombin time/international normalized ratio (INR), activated partial thromboplastin time
• Magnetic resonance imaging (MRI)	
• Magnetic resonance angiography (MRA)	
Cerebral Blood Flow	
• Cerebral angiography	• Electrolytes, blood glucose; hemoglobin (Hb) A_{1C}
• Carotid angiography	
• Digital subtraction angiography	
• Transcranial Doppler ultrasonography	• Renal and hepatic studies
• Carotid duplex scanning	• Lipid profile
Cardiac Assessment	• Cerebrospinal fluid analysis*
• Electrocardiogram	
• Chest radiograph	
• Cardiac markers (troponin, creatine kinase-MB)	
• Echocardiography (transthoracic, transesophageal)	

*A lumbar puncture to obtain cerebrospinal fluid is avoided if increased intracranial pressure is suspected.

COLLABORATIVE CARE

Table 60-5 Stroke

Diagnostic (see Table 60-4)	Acute care
• History and physical examination	• Maintenance of airway
Collaborative Therapy	• Fluid therapy
• Prevention	• Treatment of cerebral edema
• Control of hypertension	• DVT prevention with LMWH
• Control of diabetes mellitus	• Prevention of secondary injury
• Treatment of underlying cardiac problem	• Ischemic stroke
• Lifestyle modifications	• Tissue plasminogen activator (tPA)
• Limiting alcohol intake	• MERCI retriever
• Increasing exercise	• Hemorrhagic stroke
• Weight loss to normalize BMI	• Surgical decompression if indicated
• Reduction of sodium intake	• Clipping or coiling of aneurysm
• Smoking cessation	• Embolic stroke
• Drug therapy	• Treatment of underlying cause (usually cardiac related)
• Platelet inhibitors (e.g., aspirin)	
• Anticoagulation therapy for patients with atrial fibrillation (if indicated by use of the CHADS2 classification)	
• Surgical therapy	
• Carotid endarterectomy (see Figure 60-6)	
• Stenting of carotid artery	
• Transluminal angioplasty	
• Extracranial–intracranial bypass	
• Surgical interventions for aneurysms at risk of bleeding	

BMI, body mass index; *CHADS2,* clinical prediction rule used to estimate the risk of stroke in patients with atrial fibrillation and to determine the degree of anticoagulation required; *DVT,* deep venous thrombosis; *LMWH,* low–molecular weight heparin; *MERCI,* mechanical embolus retrieval in cerebral ischemia.

Statins (simvastatin [Zocor], lovastatin [Mevacor]) have also been shown to be effective in the prevention of stroke for individuals who have experienced a TIA in the past (Furie et al., 2011).

SAFETY ALERT

Clopidogrel (Plavix)

- All health care providers and dentists must be informed that drug is being taken, especially before scheduling surgery or major dental procedures.

- Drug may need to be discontinued 10 to 14 days before surgery if antiplatelet effect is not desired.

Surgical Therapy. Surgical interventions for the patient with TIAs from carotid disease are outlined on Table 60-5. Figure 60-6 demonstrates one intervention, carotid endarterectomy.

Transluminal angioplasty is the insertion of a balloon to open a stenosed artery and improve blood flow. The balloon is threaded up to the carotid artery via a catheter inserted in the femoral artery. Stenting involves intravascular placement of a stent in an

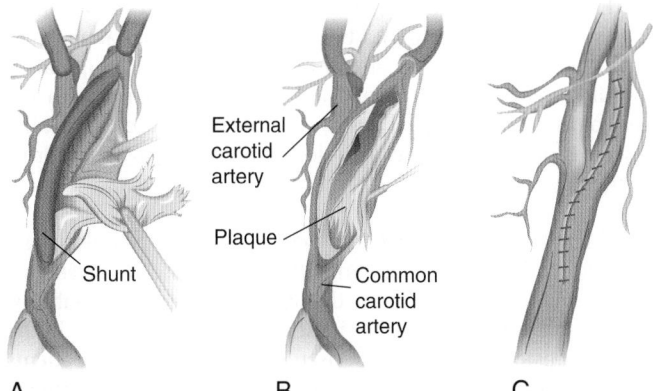

Figure 60-6 Carotid endarterectomy is performed to prevent impending cerebral infarct. **A,** A tube is inserted above and below the blockage to reroute the blood flow. **B,** Atherosclerotic plaque in the common carotid artery is removed. **C,** Once the artery is stitched closed, the tube can be removed. A surgeon may also perform the technique without rerouting the blood flow.

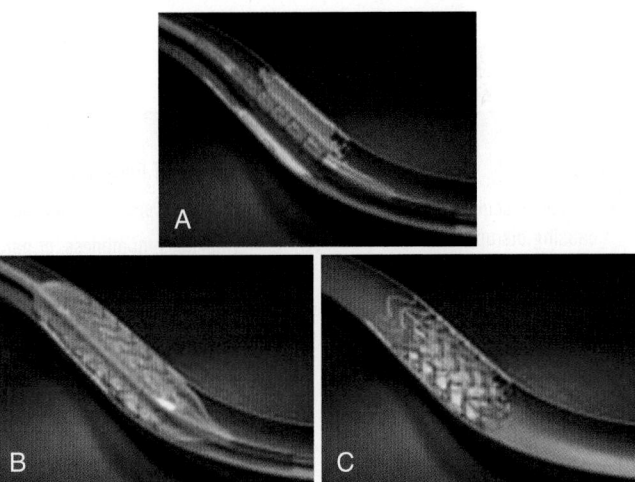

Figure 60-7 Brain stent used to treat blockages in cerebral blood flow. **A,** A balloon catheter is used to implant the stent into an artery of the brain. **B,** The balloon catheter is moved to the blocked area of the artery and then inflated. The stent expands owing to the inflation of the balloon. **C,** The balloon is deflated and withdrawn, leaving the stent permanently in place holding the artery open and improving the flow of blood.

Source: Abbott Vascular, Santa Clara, California.

attempt to maintain patency of the artery (Figure 60-7). The stent can be inserted during an angioplasty. Once in place, the system can be used with a tiny filter that opens like an umbrella. The filter is used to catch and remove the debris that is stirred up during the stenting procedure before it floats to the brain, where it can trigger a stroke. Stenting is a less invasive strategy for revascularization in patients unable to withstand the carotid endarterectomy because of coexisting medical conditions. Initial research has shown the procedure to be as effective as the carotid endarterectomy (Koelemay & Legemate, 2009; Stingele & Ringleb, 2009).

Extracranial-to-intracranial artery bypass involves anastomosing (surgically connecting) a branch of an extracranial artery to an intracranial artery (most commonly, superficial temporal to middle cerebral artery) beyond an area of obstruction with the goal of increasing cerebral perfusion. This procedure is generally reserved for those patients who do not benefit from other forms of therapy.

Collaborative Acute Care for Ischemic Stroke.

The goals for collaborative care during the acute phase are preserving life, preventing further brain damage, and reducing disability. During initial evaluation, the single most important point in the patient's history is the time of onset. Fifty-four percent of patients who seek acute care for stroke present at the emergency department and the rest seek out their primary health care physicians (CSN/HSF, 2010). The current standard for acute care treatment of stroke is that all patients with possible stroke will be assessed, have their acute health needs addressed, undergo diagnostic studies, and receive thrombolytic therapy within 4.5 hours from the onset of their symptoms (CSN/HSF, 2010).

Table 60-6 outlines the emergency management of the patient with a stroke. Acute care begins with managing circulation, airway, and breathing. Patients may have difficulty keeping an open and clear airway because of a decreased LOC or decreased or absent gag and swallowing reflexes. Maintaining adequate oxygenation is important. Both hypoxia and hypercarbia are to be prevented because they can contribute to secondary neuronal injury. Oxygen administration, artificial airway insertion, intubation, and mechanical ventilation may be required. Baseline neurological assessment is carried out, and patients are monitored closely for signs of increasing neurological deficit. About 25% of patients will worsen in the first 24 to 48 hours. It is recommended that acute care facilities have interprofessional stroke teams in place in a geographically dedicated unit, rather than mobile or roving teams, to improve outcomes (CSN/HSF, 2010).

Elevated BP is common immediately after a stroke and may be a protective response to maintain cerebral perfusion. Immediately following ischemic stroke, use of drugs to lower BP is recommended only if BP is markedly increased (mean arterial pressure >130 mm Hg or systolic BP >220 mm Hg). Intravenous antihypertensive drugs such as metoprolol (Lopressor) are used in the acute phase. Although low BP immediately following stroke is uncommon, hypotension and hypovolemia should be corrected if present.

Fluid and electrolyte balance must be controlled carefully. The goal generally is to keep the patient adequately hydrated to promote perfusion and decrease further brain injury. Overhydration may compromise perfusion by increasing cerebral edema.

EMERGENCY MANAGEMENT

Table 60-6 Stroke

ETIOLOGY	ASSESSMENT FINDINGS	INTERVENTIONS
• Sudden vascular compromise causing disruption of blood flow to the brain • Thrombosis • Trauma • Aneurysm • Embolism • Hemorrhage • Arteriovenous malformation	• Altered level of consciousness • Weakness, numbness, or paralysis of portion of body • Speech or visual disturbances • Severe headache • Increased or decreased heart rate • Respiratory distress • Unequal pupils • Hypertension • Facial drooping on affected side • Difficulty swallowing • Seizures • Bladder or bowel incontinence • Nausea and vomiting • Vertigo	**Initial Care** • Ensure patent airway. • Call a stroke code or the stroke team. • Remove dentures. • Perform pulse oximetry. • Maintain adequate oxygenation (SaO_2 >95%) with supplemental O_2, if necessary. • Establish IV access with normal saline. • Maintain BP according to guidelines (e.g., advanced cardiac life support). • Remove clothing. • Obtain CT scan immediately. • Perform baseline laboratory tests (including blood glucose) immediately, and treat if hypoglycemic. • Position head midline. • Elevate head of bed 30 degrees if no symptoms of shock or injury. • Institute seizure precautions. • Anticipate thrombolytic therapy for ischemic stroke. • Keep patient NPO until swallow reflex evaluated. **Ongoing Monitoring** • Monitor vital signs and neurological status, including level of consciousness (e.g., Glasgow Coma Scale or Canadian Neurological Scale or NIH Stroke Scale), motor and sensory function, pupil size and reactivity, SaO_2, and cardiac rhythm. • Reassure patient and family/caregiver.

BP, blood pressure; *CT,* computed tomography; *IV,* intravenous; *NIH,* National Institutes of Health; *NPO,* nothing by mouth; *SaO_2,* arterial oxygen saturation.

Adequate fluid intake during acute care via oral, intravenous (IV), or tube feedings should be 1500 to 2000 mL/day. Urine output is monitored. If secretion of antidiuretic hormone increases in response to the stroke, urine output decreases and fluid is retained. Low serum sodium (hyponatremia) may occur. IV solutions with glucose and water are avoided because they are hypotonic and may further increase cerebral edema and ICP. In addition, hyperglycemia may be associated with further brain damage and should be treated. In general, decisions regarding individualized fluid and electrolyte replacement therapy are based on the extent of intracranial edema, symptoms of increased ICP, central venous pressure levels, laboratory values for electrolytes, and intake and output.

Increased ICP is more likely to occur with hemorrhagic strokes but can occur with ischemic strokes. Increased ICP from cerebral edema usually peaks in 72 hours and may cause brain herniation. Management of increased ICP includes practices that improve venous drainage, such as elevating the head of the bed, maintaining head and neck in alignment, and avoiding hip flexion. Hyperthermia, which is seen commonly following stroke and may be associated with poorer outcome, is prevented if possible (CSN/HSF, 2010). Increased temperature contributes to increased cerebral metabolism. Drug therapies to treat hyperthermia include aspirin or acetaminophen (Tylenol). A temperature elevation of even 1°C can increase brain metabolism by 10% and contribute to further brain damage. Cooling blankets may be used cautiously to lower temperature. Closely monitor the patient's temperature. Aggressive management of temperature during the first 24 hours after a stroke is most effective in preventing detrimental outcomes.

Seizures occur in 5 to 7% of stroke patients in the first 24 hours. Antiseizure drugs, such as phenytoin (Dilantin) or levetiracetam (Keppra), are given if a seizure occurs. Prophylactic use of antiseizure drugs is not recommended for patients who have not had a seizure (Adams et al., 2007).

Other measures include pain management, avoidance of hypervolemia, and management of constipation. CSF drainage may be used in some patients to reduce ICP. Diuretic drugs, such as mannitol (Osmitrol) and furosemide (Lasix), may be used to decrease cerebral edema. The use of mannitol is being re-examined and compared with hypertonic saline and dextran solution infusions for therapeutic treatment of increased ICP. Preliminary findings indicate that hypertonic saline and dextran solution is as effective as mannitol in lowering ICP (Infanti, 2008).

As a last resort in the management of increased ICP, a bone flap may be removed to allow for cerebral edema without increases in ICP. Additional strategies for managing ICP are found in Chapter 59.

Drug Therapy for Ischemic Stroke. Recombinant tissue plasminogen activator (tPA) is administered intravenously to re-establish blood flow through a blocked artery to prevent cell death in patients with the acute onset of ischemic stroke symptoms. Patients are screened carefully before tPA can be given. Screening includes a noncontrast CT or MRI to rule out hemorrhagic stroke; blood tests for coagulation disorders; and screening for recent history of gastrointestinal bleeding, stroke, or head trauma within the past 3 months, or major surgery within 14 days (Adams et al., 2007). Intra-arterial infusion of tPA remains an option for a subgroup of patients with large vessel occlusions primarily in the middle cerebral artery. Thrombolytic drugs, such as tPA, produce localized fibrinolysis by binding to the fibrin in the thrombi. The fibrinolytic action of tPA occurs as the plasminogen is converted to plasmin, whose enzymatic action digests fibrin and fibrinogen and thus lyses the clot. Because it is clot specific in its activation of the fibrinolytic system, tPA is the only treatment indicated for acute ischemic stroke treatment. tPA must be administered within 3 to 4.5 hours of the onset of clinical signs of ischemic stroke (del Zoppo, Saver, Jauch, & Adams, 2009). The door-to-needle time for tPA remains less than 60 minutes whether the patient arrives at the hospital at 3 hours or 1 hour after the onset of clinical signs of stroke. Thrombolytics given in this time frame reduce disability (CSN/HSF, 2012; Hacke et al., 2008), but at the expense of an increase in deaths within the first 7 to 10 days and an increase in intracranial hemorrhage (Goldstein, 2007). (Thrombolytic therapy is further discussed in Chapter 36.)

During infusion of the drug, the patient's vital signs and neurological status are monitored closely to assess for improvement or for potential deterioration related to intracerebral hemorrhage. Control of blood pressure is critical during treatment and for 24 hours afterward. No anticoagulant or antiplatelet drugs are given for 24 hours after tPA treatment.

The use of anticoagulants (e.g., heparin) in the emergency phase following an ischemic stroke is generally not recommended because of the risk for intracranial hemorrhage. Acetylsalicylic acid (aspirin) at a dose of 325 mg may be initiated within 24 to 48 hours after the onset of an ischemic stroke. Complications of aspirin include gastrointestinal bleeding with higher doses. Aspirin administration should be done cautiously if the patient has a history of peptic ulcer disease (Hegge, 2008).

After the patient's condition has stabilized and to prevent further clot formation, patients with stroke caused by thrombi and emboli may also be treated with platelet inhibitors and anticoagulants (see discussion on prevention of stroke earlier in the chapter). Common anticoagulants include warfarin (Coumadin), clopidogrel (Plavix), and dipyridamole (Persantine). In addition, the use of statins has been shown to be effective for the patient with an ischemic stroke.

Surgical Therapy for Ischemic Stroke. The mechanical embolus removal in cerebral ischemia (MERCI) retriever (Figure 60-8) allows physicians to go inside the blocked artery of patients

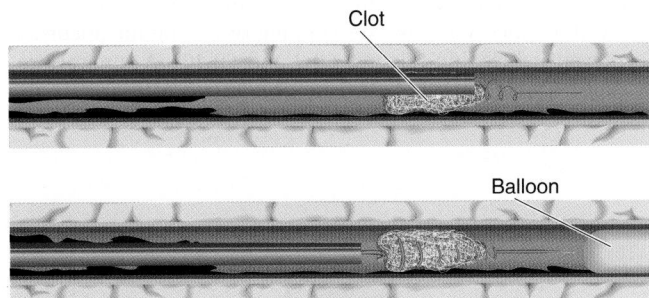

Figure 60-8 The MERCI retriever removes blood clots in patients who are experiencing ischemic strokes. The retriever is a long, thin wire that is threaded through a catheter into the femoral artery. The wire is pushed through the end of the catheter up to the carotid artery. The wire reshapes itself into tiny loops that latch onto the clot and the clot can then be pulled out. To prevent the clot from breaking off, a balloon at the end of the catheter inflates to stop blood flow through the artery.

who are experiencing ischemic strokes. The retriever goes to the artery that is blocked, directly to the site of the problem, and pulls the clot out. The retriever is a tiny corkscrew device that uses a microcatheter inserted through a femoral artery balloon catheter. Once the corkscrew device reaches the clot in the brain, the device penetrates the clot, allowing it to be removed. Under x-ray guidance, the balloon catheter is manoeuvred up to the carotid artery in the neck; a guidewire and the microcatheter are deployed through the balloon catheter and then placed just beyond the clot. The physician then deploys the MERCI retriever device to engage and ensnare the clot. Once the clot is captured, the balloon catheter is inflated to temporarily arrest forward flow while the clot is being withdrawn. The clot is pulled into the balloon catheter and completely out of the body. The balloon is then deflated and blood flow is restored. Research is also being conducted to determine the use of other mechanical thrombectomy devices for the removal of clots and include acute balloon angioplasty and stenting, snare devices, and ultrasonic aspirators.

Collaborative Acute Care for Hemorrhagic Stroke

Drug Therapy. Anticoagulants and platelet inhibitors are contraindicated in patients with hemorrhagic strokes (Broderick et al., 2007).The main drug therapy for patients with hemorrhagic stroke is the management of hypertension. Oral and IV agents may be used to maintain BP within a normal to high-normal range (systolic BP <160 mm Hg).

Seizure prophylaxis in the acute period after intracerebral hemorrhages and SAHs is recommended (Broderick et al., 2007). In these patients, seizure activity may result in further neuronal injury and contribute to coma, although no clinical data support this recommendation.

Surgical Therapy. Surgical interventions for hemorrhagic stroke include immediate evacuation of aneurysm-induced hematomas or cerebellar hematomas larger than 3 cm. Individuals who have an AVM may experience a hemorrhagic stroke if the AVM ruptures. The treatment of AVM is surgical resection and/or radiosurgery (i.e., gamma knife). Both may be preceded by interventional neuroradiology to embolize the blood vessels that supply the AVM.

SAH is usually caused by a ruptured aneurysm. Approximately 20% of patients will have multiple aneurysms. Treatment of an aneurysm involves clipping or coiling the aneurysm to prevent rebleeding (Figures 60-9 and 60-10). A surgical procedure frequently used to prevent rebleeding is clipping of the

aneurysm (see Figure 60-9), but endovascular techniques are also popular. In the procedure known as *coiling*, a metal coil is inserted into the lumen of the aneurysm via interventional neuroradiology (see Figure 60-10). Guglielmi detachable coils provide immediate protection against hemorrhage by reducing the blood pulsations within the aneurysm. Eventually, a thrombus forms within the aneurysm and the aneurysm becomes sealed off from the parent vessel by the formation of an endothelialized layer of connective tissue. Guglielmi detachable coils provide an alternative therapy to traditional surgical clipping of aneurysms.

Goals for managing ICP are the same for patients with SAH as they are for patients dealing with acute stroke. Following aneurysmal occlusion via clipping or coiling, hyperdynamic therapy (hemodilution-induced hypertension using vasoconstricting agents such as phenylephrine or dopamine and hypervolemia) may be instituted in an effort to increase the mean arterial

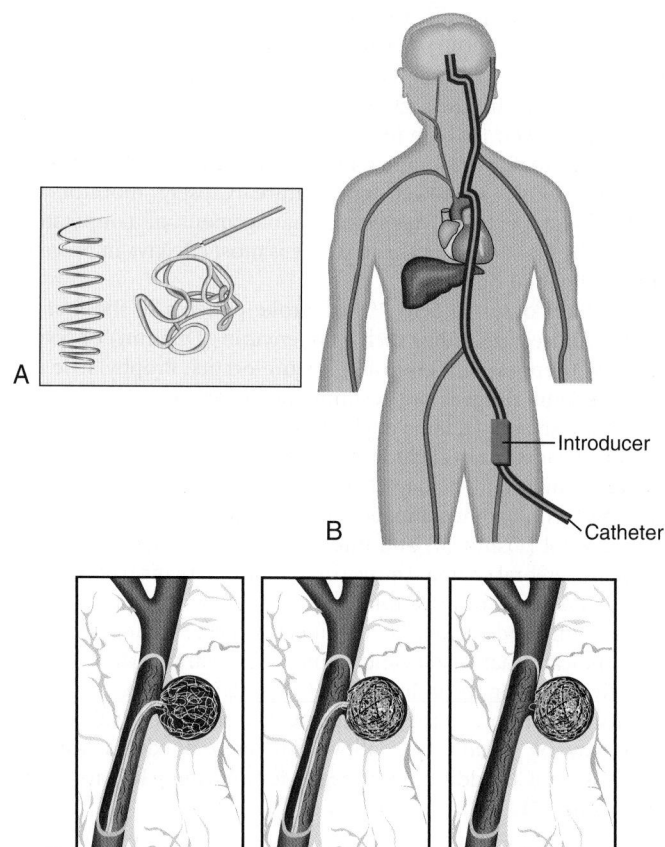

Figure 60-10 Guglielmi detachable coil (GDC). **A,** A coil is used to occlude an aneurysm. Coils are made of soft, springlike platinum. The softness of the platinum allows the coil to assume the shape of irregularly shaped aneurysms while posing little threat of rupture of the aneurysm. **B,** A catheter is inserted through an introducer (small tube) in an artery in the leg. The catheter is threaded up to the cerebral blood vessels. **C,** Platinum coils attached to a thin wire are inserted into the catheter and then placed in the aneurysm until the aneurysm is filled with coils. Packing the aneurysm with coils prevents the blood from circulating through the aneurysm, reducing the risk of rupture.

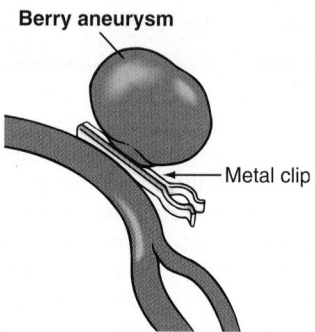

Figure 60-9 Clipping of aneurysms.

pressure and increase cerebral perfusion. Volume expansion is achieved via crystalloid or colloid solution.

Interventions to treat cerebral vasospasm either before or following aneurysm clipping or coiling include administration of the calcium channel blocker nimodipine (Nimotop), which is given to patients with SAH to decrease the effects of vasospasm and minimize cerebral damage. Nimodipine restricts the influx of calcium ions into cells by reducing the number of open calcium channels. Although nimodipine is a calcium channel blocker, its exact mechanism of action in reducing vasospasm is not well understood.

SAFETY ALERT

Nimodipine (Nimotop)
- Assess BP and apical pulses before administration.
- If pulse ≤60 beats/min or systolic BP <90 mm Hg, hold medication and contact physician.

SAH and intracerebral hemorrhage can involve bleeding into the ventricles of the brain. This situation produces hydrocephalus, which further damages brain tissue from increased ICP. Insertion of a ventriculostomy for CSF drainage can result in dramatic improvement in these situations.

Rehabilitation Care. After the acute stroke patient has stabilized for 12 to 24 hours, collaborative care shifts from preserving life to lessening disability and attaining optimal function. The patient may be evaluated by a physiatrist (a physician who specializes in physical medicine and rehabilitation). It is important to remember that some aspects of rehabilitation actually begin in the acute care phase as soon as the patient is stabilized. Depending on the patient's status, other medical conditions, rehabilitation potential, and available resources, the patient may be transferred to a rehabilitation unit. Other options for rehabilitation include outpatient therapy and home care–based rehabilitation (Bottemiller, Bieber, Basford, & Harris, 2006).

As part of the long-term collaborative care after a stroke, various members of the health care team may be involved in the effort to promote optimal function of the patient and family. The composition of the interdisciplinary team depends on patient and family or caregiver needs and rehabilitation facility resources. The Evidence-Informed Practice box discusses how information interventions can affect patient knowledge and mood.

NURSING MANAGEMENT: STROKE

▮ Nursing Assessment

Subjective and objective data that should be obtained from a person who has had a stroke are presented in Table 60-7. Primary assessment is focused on cardiac and respiratory status and neurological assessment. If the patient's condition is stable, the nursing history is obtained as follows: (1) description of the current illness with attention to initial symptoms, including onset and duration, nature (intermittent or continuous), and changes; (2) history of similar symptoms previously experienced; (3)

EVIDENCE-INFORMED PRACTICE
How Can Nurses Support Stroke Patients and Their Caregivers?

Clinical Question
For stroke patients and caregivers (P), do information interventions (I) versus standard care (C) improve knowledge and mood (O)?

Best Available Evidence
Systematic review of randomized controlled trials (RCTs)

Critical Appraisal and Synthesis of Evidence
- 17 RCTs (*n* = 1773 patients and 1058 caregivers) of patients with stroke or transient ischemic attack [TIA]). Stroke knowledge, services, and mood were measured.
- Information given to patient and caregiver improved knowledge and increased patient satisfaction with some information received. Small decrease in patient depression was also noted.
- Information actively involving patient and caregiver (e.g., repeated opportunity for questions) had more effect on improving mood than information given only once.

Conclusion
- Information interventions improved knowledge and mood for patients with stroke and their caregivers.

Implications for Nursing Practice
- Offer patients and families frequent opportunities to ask questions in an unhurried atmosphere. This is most effectively done well in advance of discharge.
- Active patient involvement has greater impact on improving mood than passive receipt of information.

Reference for Evidence
Smith, J., Forster, A., House, A., Knapp, P., Wright, J. J., & Young, J. (2008). Information provision for stroke patients and their caregivers. *Cochrane Database of Systematic Reviews, 2,* CD001919. doi:10.1002/14651858.CD001919.pub2

PICO: P, patient population of interest; *I,* intervention or area of interest; *C,* comparison of interest or comparison group; *O,* outcome(s) of interest.

current medications; (4) history of risk factors and other illnesses such as hypertension; and (5) family history of stroke or cardiovascular diseases. This information is gained through an interview of the patient, family members, significant others, or caregiver.

Secondary assessment should include a comprehensive neurological examination of the patient. This includes (1) LOC, using the Canadian Neurological Scale (Figure 60-11) (or a similar tool), (2) cognition, (3) motor abilities, (4) cranial nerve function, (5) sensation, (6) proprioception, (7) cerebellar function, and (8) deep tendon reflexes. Clear documentation of initial and ongoing neurological examinations is essential to note changes in patient status. The Registered Nurses' Association of Ontario (RNAO, 2005) and the Canadian Stroke Strategy (CSN/ HSF, 2010) have also developed best-practice guidelines and recommendations for stroke care across the continuum.

NURSING ASSESSMENT

Table 60-7 Stroke

Subjective Data

Important Health Information

Past health history: Hypertension; previous stroke, TIA, aneurysm, trauma, cardiac disease (including recent MI), dysrhythmias, heart failure, valvular disease, infective endocarditis, polycythemia dyslipidemia, smoking, kidney disease, diabetes, gout, family history of hypertension, diabetes, stroke, or coronary artery disease

Medications: Use of hormone replacement therapy or oral contraceptives; use of and compliance with antihypertensive and diabetes regimen, antiplatelet therapy, and anticoagulant agents; use of illegal substances and drug use (cocaine)

Symptoms

* Anorexia, nausea, vomiting; dysphagia, altered sensation of taste and smell
* Change in bowel and bladder patterns.
* Loss of movement and sensation; syncope; weakness on one side; mouth droop, half smile; generalized weakness, easy fatigability
* Numbness, tingling of one side of the body; loss of memory; alteration in speech, language, problem-solving ability
* Pain; headache, possibly sudden and severe (hemorrhage); visual disturbances; denial of illness

Objective Data

General

Emotional lability, lethargy, apathy or combativeness, fever

Respiratory

Loss of cough reflex, laboured or irregular respirations, tachypnea, wheezing (aspiration), airway occlusion (tongue), apnea, coughing when eating or delayed coughing

Cardiovascular

Hypertension, tachycardia, carotid bruit

Gastrointestinal

Loss of gag reflex, bowel incontinence, decreased or absent bowel sounds, constipation

Urinary

Frequency, urgency, incontinence

Neurological

Contralateral motor and sensory deficits, including weakness, paresis, paralysis, anaesthesia; unequal pupils, hand grasps; akinesia, aphasia (expressive, receptive, global), dysarthria (slurred speech), agnosias, apraxia, visual deficits, perceptual or spatial disturbances, altered level of consciousness (drowsiness to deep coma) and Babinski's sign, ↓ followed by ↑ deep tendon reflexes, flaccidity followed by spasticity, amnesia, ataxia, personality change, nuchal rigidity, seizures

Possible Findings

Positive CT, CTA, MRI, MRA, or other neuroimaging scans showing size, location, and type of lesion; positive Doppler ultrasonography and angiography indicating stenosis

CT, computed tomography; *CTA,* computed tomography angiography; *MI,* myocardial infarction; *MRA,* magnetic resonance angiography; *MRI,* magnetic resonance imaging; *TIA,* transient ischemic attack.

▪ Nursing Diagnoses

Nursing diagnoses for the person with a stroke may include, but are not limited to, those presented in Nursing Care Plan (NCP) 60-1.

▪ Planning

The patient, the family, and the nurse establish the goals of nursing care in a cooperative manner. Typical goals are that the patient will (1) maintain a stable or improved LOC, (2) attain maximum physical functioning, (3) attain maximum self-care abilities and skills, (4) maintain stable body functions (e.g., bladder control), (5) maximize communication abilities, (6) maintain adequate nutrition, (7) avoid complications of stroke, and (8) maintain effective personal and family coping.

▪ Nursing Implementation

▪ Health Promotion

In any health care setting and for the population as a whole, nurses can play a major role in the promotion of a healthy lifestyle. To reduce the incidence of stroke, the nurse should focus teaching efforts toward stroke prevention, particularly for persons with known risk factors (see Table 60-1). Nursing measures to reduce risk factors for stroke are similar to those for coronary artery disease (see Chapter 36, Table 36-4) and are discussed on p. 899.

One of the nurse's major roles is education about hypertension control and maintaining adherence with antihypertensive medications. Uncontrolled hypertension is the primary cause of stroke.

The nurse needs to be an advocate for the monitoring and management of hypertension, including assessing financial need and prescription coverage. If a person has diabetes, it is very important that the blood glucose level is well controlled. If an individual has AF, an anticoagulant such as warfarin (Coumadin) or aspirin may be used to treat the problem to prevent the risk of stroke. Because smoking is a major risk factor for stroke, the nurse needs to be actively involved in helping patients to stop smoking (see Chapter 11, and eTables 11-1 and 11-2).

Another very important aspect of health promotion is teaching patients and families about early symptoms associated with stroke or TIA. Table 60-8 presents information on when to seek health care for these symptoms.

▪ Acute Intervention for all Stroke Patients

▪ **Respiratory System.** During the acute phase following a stroke, management of the respiratory system is a nursing priority. Stroke patients are particularly vulnerable to respiratory problems (Miller & Mink, 2009). Advancing age and immobility increase the risk for atelectasis and pneumonia.

Risk for aspiration pneumonia may be high because of impaired consciousness or dysphagia. Dysphagia after stroke is common (Palmer & Metheny, 2008). Airway obstruction can occur because of problems with chewing and swallowing, food pocketing (food remaining in the buccal cavity of the mouth),

CANADIAN NEUROLOGICAL SCALE

Assess: Vital Signs and Pupils   **Vital Signs:** BP, Temp, Pulse, Respirations, Oximetry   **Pupils:** Size and reaction to light

Section A: MENTATION: LOC, Orientation, Speech

LEVEL OF CONSCIOUSNESS:
　　CNS (Alert, Drowsy) GCS (Stuporous, Comatose)

ORIENTATION:
　　Place (city or hospital), Time (month and year)
　　*Patient can speak, write, or gesture their responses.
　　SCORE: Patient is Oriented, score 1.0, if they correctly
　　state both place and correct month and year. If
　　dysarthric, speech must be intelligible. If patient cannot
　　state both. Disoriented, score 0.0

SPEECH:
　　RECEPTIVE: Ask patient the following separately
　　(do not prompt by gesturing):

　　1. Close your eyes
　　2. "Does a stone sink in water?"
　　3. Point to the ceiling

　　SCORE: If patient is unable to do all three, Receptive
　　Deficit, score 0.0, go to A2.

EXPRESSIVE:

　　1. Show patient 3 items separately (pencil, watch, key)
　　and ask patient to name each object.

　　2. Ask patient what each object is used for while holding
　　each up again, i.e. "What do you do with a pencil?"

　　SCORE: If patient is able to state the name and use of
　　all 3 objects, Normal Speech, score 1.0.

　　If patient is unable to state the name and use of all
　　3 objects, Expressive Deficit, score 0.5.

　　*If patient answers all questions correctly but speech is
　　slurred and intelligible, score Normal Speech and record
　　"SL" along with the score.

Section A1: MOTOR FUNCTION

NO RECEPTIVE DEFICIT

FACE:　　Ask patient to smile/grin, note weakness in mouth
　　　　or nasal/labial folds.
　　　　SCORE: None/no weakness = 0.5 or Present/
　　　　weakness = 0.0 Test both limbs and always record
　　　　the side with the WORST deficit and indicate side
　　　　by entering a R/L.

None 1.5	no weakness present
Mild 1.0	mild weakness present, full ROM, cannot withstand resistance
Significant 0.5	moderate weakness, some movement, not full ROM
Total 0.0	complete loss of movement, total weakness

SCORE:
Arm: Proximal　Ask patient to lift arm 45-90 degrees. Apply
　　　　　　resistance between shoulder and elbow.
Arm: Distal　Ask patient to make fist and flex wrist backwards,
　　　　　apply resistance between wrist and knuckles.
Leg: Proximal　In supine, ask patient to flex hip to 90 degrees,
　　　　　apply pressure to mid thigh.
Leg: Distal　Ask patient to dorsiflex foot, apply resistance to
　　　　　top of foot.

Section A2: MOTOR RESPONSE

RECEPTIVE DEFICIT PRESENT
FACE:　　Have patient mimic your smile. If unable, note facial
　　　　expression while applying sternal pressure.
ARMS:　　Demonstrate or lift patient's arms to 90 degrees,
　　　　score ability to maintain equal levels (>5 secs).
　　　　If unable to maintain raised arms, apply nail bed
　　　　pressure to assess reflex response.
LEGS:　　Lift patient's hip to 90 degrees, score ability
　　　　to maintain equal levels (>5 secs), If unable to
　　　　maintain raised position, apply nail bed pressure
　　　　to assess reflex response.

Figure 60-11 Canadian Neurological Scale.

Source: Heart and Stroke Foundation, *Stroke Nurse Pocket Guide* (2010), Ottawa.

PATIENT & CAREGIVER TEACHING GUIDE
Table 60-8 Warning Signs of Stroke

Call 911 and get medical help immediately if someone is having one or more of the following signs and symptoms. Also, check the time so the nurse will know when the first symptoms appeared. It is very important to take immediate action.

- Sudden numbness or weakness of the face, arm, or leg, especially on one side of the body
- Sudden confusion, trouble speaking or understanding
- Sudden trouble seeing in one or both eyes
- Sudden trouble walking, dizziness, loss of balance or coordination
- Sudden, severe headache with no known cause

Source: American Heart Association. (2011). Stroke warning signs. Retrieved from *http://www.strokeassociation.org/idc/groups/heart-public/ @wcm/@hcm/documents/downloadable/ucm_434181.pdf*

and the tongue falling back. Some patients with stroke, especially those with brainstem or hemorrhagic stroke, may require endotracheal intubation and mechanical ventilation, initially and/or with increasing cerebral edema or ICP. Enteral tube feedings also place the patient at risk for aspiration pneumonia. All patients should be screened for their ability to swallow and kept on nothing-by-mouth status until dysphagia has been ruled out.

Nursing interventions to support adequate respiratory function are individualized to meet the needs of the patient. An oropharyngeal airway may be used in comatose patients to prevent the tongue from falling back and obstructing the airway and to provide access for suctioning. Alternately, a nasopharyngeal airway may be used to provide airway protection and access. When an artificial airway will be required for a prolonged time,

NURSING CARE PLAN 60-1

Stroke

NURSING DIAGNOSIS	***Decreased intracranial adaptive capacity*** *related to* decreased cerebral perfusion ≤50-60 mm Hg and sustained increase in ICP of 10-15 mm Hg secondary to thrombus, embolus, hemorrhage *as evidenced by* ICP ≥10 mm Hg, elevated blood pressure, bradycardia, widened pulse pressure or decreasing Canadian Neurological Scale score.
Expected Patient Outcome	**Nursing Interventions and *Rationales***
• Demonstrates signs of stable or improved cerebral perfusion	• Monitor neurological status (ICP, LOC) at least hourly initially *to detect changes indicative of worsening or improving condition.* • Calculate and monitor CPP *to detect change in condition.* • Monitor respiratory status (e.g., rate, rhythm, depth of respirations, PaO₂, PaCO₂, pH, and bicarbonate levels) *to assess changes in neurological status.* • Monitor patient's ICP and neurological response to activities *as ICP can increase with changes in positioning and movement.* • Administer and titrate vasoactive drugs (as ordered) *to maintain hemodynamic parameters.* • Avoid neck flexion or extreme hip/knee flexion *to avoid obstruction of arterial and venous blood flow.*
NURSING DIAGNOSIS	***Ineffective airway clearance*** *related to* decreased level of consciousness, decreased or absent gag and swallowing reflexes *as evidenced by* adventitious breath sounds, diminished breath sounds, and ineffective cough
Expected Patient Outcomes	**Nursing Interventions and *Rationales***
• Demonstrates effective coughing and increased air exchange • Maintains a clear airway	• Auscultate breath sounds, noting areas of decreased/absent ventilation, and presence of adventitious sounds *to obtain ongoing data on patient's response to therapy.* • Remove secretions by encouraging coughing or suctioning *to clear airway.* • Encourage slow, deep breathing; turning; and coughing *to increase airway clearance without increasing intracranial pressure.* • Position patient in a sitting position with head slightly flexed, shoulders relaxed, and knees flexed *to maximize ventilation potential.* • Keep patient NPO until swallow evaluation completed *to prevent aspiration.*
NURSING DIAGNOSIS	***Impaired physical mobility*** *related to* neuromuscular and cognitive impairment and decreased muscle strength and control *as evidenced by* limited ability to perform gross and fine motor skills, limited range of motion, and difficulty turning.
Expected Patient Outcomes	**Nursing Interventions and *Rationales***
• Demonstrates increased muscle strength and ability to move • Uses adaptive equipment to increase mobility	• Collaborate with physiotherapist, occupational therapist, and recreational therapist in developing and executing exercise program *to determine extent of problem and plan appropriate interventions.* • Determine patient's readiness to engage in activity or exercise protocol *to assess expected level of participation.* • Apply splints to achieve stability of proximal joints involved with fine motor skills *to prevent contractures.* • Encourage patient to practise range of motion exercises independently, as indicated, *to promote patient's sense of control.* • Provide restful environment for patient after periods of exercise *to facilitate recuperation.*
NURSING DIAGNOSIS	***Impaired verbal communication*** *related to* residual aphasia *as evidenced by* refusal or inability to speak; difficulty expressing thoughts verbally, forming sentences and forming words; and inappropriate verbalization.
Expected Patient Outcomes	**Nursing Interventions and *Rationales***
• Uses effective oral and written communication techniques • Demonstrates congruency of verbal and nonverbal communication	• Listen attentively *to convey the importance of patient's thoughts and to promote a positive environment for learning.* • Provide positive reinforcement and praise, as appropriate, *to build self-esteem and confidence.* • Use simple words and short sentences, as appropriate, *to avoid overwhelming patient with verbal stimuli.* • Use alternative communication aids such as picture boards, as necessary, *to assist patient to express self.* • Provide verbal prompts and reminders (especially if patient is frustrated) *to assist patient to express self.*

CPP, cerebral perfusion pressure; *ICP,* intracranial pressure; *LOC,* level of consciousness; *NPO,* nothing by mouth (nil per os); *PaCO₂,* partial pressure of carbon dioxide in arterial blood; *PaO₂,* partial pressure of oxygen in arterial blood.

NURSING CARE PLAN 60-1

Stroke—cont'd

NURSING DIAGNOSIS	*Unilateral neglect* related to visual field cut and sensory loss on one side of body and brain injury from cerebrovascular problems *as evidenced by* consistent inattention to stimuli on affected side.
Expected Patient Outcomes	**Nursing Interventions and *Rationales***

- Cares for both sides of the body appropriately
- Uses strategies to minimize unilateral neglect

- Monitor for abnormal responses to three primary types of stimuli: sensory, visual, and auditory *to determine the presence of and degree to which unilateral neglect exists* (i.e., inability to see objects on affected side, leaving food on a plate that corresponds to affected side, lack of sensation on affected side).
- Instruct patient to scan from left to right *to visualize the entire environment.*
- Rearrange the environment to use the right or left visual field; position personal items, television, or reading materials within view on unaffected side *to compensate for visual field deficits.*
- Touch unaffected shoulder when initiating conversation *to attract patient's attention.*
- Gradually move personal items and activity to affected side, as patient demonstrates an ability to compensate for neglect, *to further minimize unilateral neglect.*
- Include caregivers in rehabilitation process *to support the patient's efforts and assist with care to promote reintegration with the whole body.*

NURSING DIAGNOSIS	*Impaired urinary elimination* related to impaired impulse to void or inability to reach toilet or manage tasks of voiding *as evidenced by* loss of urinary control and involuntary loss of urine at unpredictable times.
Expected Patient Outcomes	**Nursing Interventions and *Rationales***

- Perceives impulse to void, removes clothing for toileting, and uses toilet
- Demonstrates ability to urinate when the urge arises or with a timed schedule

Urinary habit training

- Keep a continence specification record for 3 days *to establish voiding pattern and plan appropriate interventions.*
- Establish interval of initial toileting schedule, based on voiding pattern and usual routine, *to initiate process of improving bladder functioning and increased muscle tone.*
- Assist patient to toilet or remind patient to void at prescribed intervals *to assist patient in adapting to new toileting schedule.*
- Teach patient to consciously hold urine until the scheduled toileting time *to improve muscle tone.*
- Discuss daily record of continence with staff *to provide reinforcement and to encourage compliance with toileting schedule.*
- Give positive feedback or positive reinforcement to patient when she or he voids at scheduled toileting times, and make no comment when patient is incontinent, *to reinforce desired behaviour.*

NURSING DIAGNOSIS	*Impaired swallowing* related to weakness or paralysis of affected muscles *as evidenced by* drooling, difficulty in swallowing, choking.
Expected Patient Outcome	**Nursing Interventions and *Rationales***

- Demonstrates effective swallowing without choking, coughing, or aspiration

- Collaborate with other members of health care team (i.e., occupational therapist, speech–language pathologist for swallowing assessment, and dietitian) *to provide continuity in patient's rehabilitative plan.*
- Assist patient to sit in an erect position (as close to 90 degrees as possible) for feeding and exercise *to provide optimal position for chewing and swallowing without aspirating.*
- Assist patient to position head in forward flexion ("chin tuck") *to prepare for swallowing and to prevent aspiration.*
- Assist patient to maintain sitting position for 30 minutes after completing meal *to prevent regurgitation of food.*
- Instruct patient and caregiver on emergency measures for choking *to prevent complications in the home setting.*
- Check mouth for pocketing of food after eating, and teach patient and family this technique *to prevent collection and putrefaction of food and/or aspiration.*
- Provide mouth care after meals and as needed *to promote comfort and oral health.*
- Monitor body weight *to determine adequacy of nutritional intake.*

Continued

NURSING CARE PLAN 60-1

Stroke—cont'd

NURSING DIAGNOSIS	*Situational low self-esteem* related to actual or perceived loss of function and altered body image *as evidenced by* refusal to touch or look at affected body parts, refusal to participate in self-care, and expressions of helplessness and uselessness.
Expected Patient Outcomes	**Nursing Interventions and *Rationales***
• Expresses positive feelings of self-worth • Participates in self-care of affected body parts	• Monitor patient's statements of self-worth *to determine effect of stroke on self-esteem.* • Encourage patient to identify strengths *to facilitate patient's recognition of intrinsic value.* • Assist in setting realistic goals *to achieve higher self-esteem.* • Reward or praise patient's progress toward reaching goals *to encourage patient.* • Encourage increased responsibility for self *to promote sense of satisfaction, independence, and control, and to reduce frustrations.* • Monitor levels of self-esteem over time, as appropriate, *to determine stressors or situations that trigger low self-esteem and to teach coping mechanisms.* • Monitor whether patient can look at the changed body part *to determine patient's level of acceptance of new image.* • Help patient to determine the extent of actual changes in the body or its level of functioning *to prevent misperceptions concerning new level of physiological functioning.*

a tracheostomy may be performed. Nursing interventions include frequent assessment of airway patency and function, oxygenation, suctioning, patient mobility, positioning of the patient to prevent aspiration, and encouraging deep breathing. To prevent complications from mechanical ventilation, research has shown that having the nurse provide oral care at a minimum of every 2 hours may reduce the occurrence of ventilator-assisted pneumonia (Muscedere, Dodek, & Keenan, 2008). Patients who have an unclipped or uncoiled aneurysm may experience rebleeding and the possibility of further ICP increases with coughing exercises.

Interventions related to maintenance of airway function are described in NCP 60-1.

■ **Neurological System.** The patient's neurological status must be monitored closely to detect changes suggesting extension of the stroke, increased ICP, vasospasm, or recovery from stroke symptoms. There are many neurological assessment tools, such as the Glasgow Coma Scale (GCS), National Institutes of Health Stroke Scale (NIHSS), and the Canadian Neurological Scale, that can be used to assist in the monitoring of a patient's neurological status. The GCS measures LOC, mental status, pupillary responses, and extremity movement and strength. (The GCS is shown in Chapter 59, Table 59-5.) The GCS might not be sensitive enough for use with stroke patients who have cognitive and communication deficits (rather than impaired LOC) that would not be detected using this scale (RNAO, 2005). The Canadian Neurological Scale was designed specifically for evaluating and monitoring the neurological status of patients with acute stroke (see Figure 60-11) (RNAO, 2005). It is an assessment tool that measures LOC, orientation, speech, and motor responses of the face, arms, and legs.

Additional neurological assessment includes mental status, pupillary responses, and extremity movement and strength. Also closely monitor vital signs. A decreasing LOC may indicate increasing ICP. ICP and cerebral perfusion pressure may be monitored as well if the patient is in a critical care environment. Data from the nursing assessment are recorded on flow sheets to com-

municate evaluation of neurological status to the interdisciplinary team.

■ **Cardiovascular System.** Nursing goals for the cardiovascular system are aimed at maintaining homeostasis. Many patients with stroke have decreased cardiac reserves from the secondary diagnoses of cardiac diseases. Cardiac efficiency may be further compromised by fluid retention, overhydration, dehydration, and/or BP variations. Fluids are retained if there is increased production of antidiuretic hormone and aldosterone secondary to stress. Fluid retention plus overhydration can result in fluid overload. It can also increase cerebral edema and ICP. At the same time, dehydration can add to the morbidity and mortality associated with stroke, especially in the patient with vasospasm. IV therapy should be carefully regulated. The nurse should closely monitor intake and output. Central venous pressure, pulmonary artery pressure, or hemodynamic monitoring may be used as indicators of fluid balance or cardiac function in the critical care unit.

Nursing interventions include (1) monitoring vital signs frequently; (2) monitoring cardiac rhythms; (3) calculating intake and output, noting imbalances; (4) regulating IV infusions; (5) adjusting fluid intake to the individual needs of the patient; (6) monitoring lung sounds for indications of pulmonary congestion; and (7) monitoring heart sounds for murmurs or for third (S3) or fourth (S4) heart sounds. Bedside monitors or telemetry may record cardiac rhythms. Hypertension is sometimes seen following a stroke as the body attempts to increase cerebral blood flow. It is important to monitor for orthostatic hypertension before ambulating the patient for the first time. Neurological changes can occur with a sudden decrease in BP.

After a stroke, the patient is at risk for deep venous thrombosis (DVT), especially in the weak or paralyzed lower extremity. This is related to immobility, loss of venous tone, and decreased muscle pumping activity in the leg. The most effective prevention is to keep the patient moving. Active range of motion exercises should be taught if the patient has voluntary movement in the affected extremity. For the patient with hemiplegia, passive range of motion exercises should be done several times a day. Additional measures to prevent DVT include positioning to minimize the effects of dependent edema and the use of elastic compression gradient stockings or support hose. Sequential compression devices may be ordered for bedridden patients. DVT prophylaxis may include low–molecular weight heparin (e.g., enoxaparin [Lovenox]). The nursing assessment for DVT includes measuring the calf and the thigh daily, observing swelling of the lower extremities, noting unusual warmth of the leg, and asking the patient about pain in the calf.

Musculoskeletal System.

The nursing goal for the musculoskeletal system is to maintain optimal function. This is accomplished by the prevention of joint contractures and muscular atrophy. In the acute phase, range of motion exercises and positioning are important nursing interventions. Passive range of motion exercise is begun on the first day of hospitalization. If the stroke is caused by SAH, the movement is limited to the extremities. The patient is taught to actively exercise as soon as possible. Muscle atrophy secondary to lack of innervation and activity can develop within 1 month following stroke.

The paralyzed or weak side needs special attention when the patient is positioned. Each joint should be positioned higher than the joint proximal to it to prevent dependent edema. Specific deformities on the weak or paralyzed side that may be present in patients with stroke include internal rotation of the shoulder; flexion contractures of the hand, wrist, and elbow; external rotation of the hip; and plantar flexion of the foot. Subluxation of the shoulder on the affected side is common. Careful positioning and moving of the affected arm may prevent the development of a painful shoulder condition; immobilization of the affected upper extremity may precipitate a painful shoulder–hand syndrome.

Nursing interventions to optimize musculoskeletal function include (1) trochanter roll at the hip to prevent external rotation; (2) hand cones (not rolled washcloths) to prevent hand contractures; (3) arm supports with slings and lap boards to prevent shoulder displacement; (4) avoidance of pulling the patient by the arm to avoid shoulder displacement; (5) posterior leg splints, footboards, or high-topped tennis shoes to prevent footdrop; and (6) hand splints to reduce spasticity. Use of a footboard for the patient with spasticity is controversial. Rather than preventing plantar flexion (footdrop), the sensory stimulation of a footboard against the bottom of the foot increases plantar flexion. Likewise, there is disagreement on whether hand splints facilitate or diminish spasticity. The decision regarding the use of footboards or hand splints is made on an individual patient basis.

Integumentary System.

The skin of the patient with stroke is particularly susceptible to breakdown related to loss of sensation, decreased circulation, and immobility. This is compounded by patient age, poor nutrition, dehydration, edema, and incontinence. The nursing plan for prevention of skin breakdown includes (1) pressure relief by position changes, special mattresses, or wheelchair cushions; (2) good skin hygiene; (3) emollients applied to dry skin; and (4) early mobility. The ideal position change schedule is side–back–side with a maximum duration of 2 hours for any position. Nurses should position the patient on the weak or paralyzed side for only 30 minutes. If an area of redness develops and does not return to

normal colour within 15 minutes of pressure relief, the epidermis and dermis are damaged. The damaged area should not be massaged because this may cause additional damage. Pressure relief is the single most important factor in both the prevention and the treatment of skin breakdown. Pillows can be used under lower extremities to reduce pressure on the heels. Vigilance and good nursing care are required to prevent pressure ulcers.

Gastrointestinal System.

The most common bowel problem for the patient who has experienced a stroke is constipation. Patients may be prophylactically placed on stool softeners and/or fibre (psyllium [Metamucil]). The patient who has liquid stools should also be checked for stool impaction. Depending on the patient's fluid balance status and swallowing ability, fluid intake should be 1800 to 2000 mL/day and fibre intake up to 25 g/day. Physical activity also promotes bowel function. Laxatives, suppositories, or additional stool softeners may be ordered if the patient does not respond to increased fluid and fibre. Similarly, enemas are used only if suppositories and digital stimulation are ineffective because they cause vagal stimulation and increase ICP.

Urinary System.

In the acute stage of stroke, the primary urinary problem is poor bladder control, resulting in incontinence. Efforts should be made to promote normal bladder function and avoid the use of indwelling catheters. If an indwelling catheter must be used initially, it should be removed as soon as the patient is medically and neurologically stable. Long-term use of an indwelling catheter is associated with urinary tract infections and delayed bladder retraining. An alternative to intermittent catheterizations is offering the opportunity for frequent toileting to patients with urinary incontinence. Another alternative to intermittent catheterizations is the external catheter for male patients with urinary incontinence.

A bladder retraining program consists of (1) adequate fluid intake with the majority given between 0800 and 1900 hours; (2) scheduled toileting every 2 hours using bedpan, urinal, commode, or bathroom; and (3) noting signs of restlessness, which may indicate the need for urination.

Nutrition.

The nutritional needs of the patient require quick assessment and treatment. The patient may initially receive IV infusions to maintain fluid and electrolyte balance as well as for administration of drugs. Patients with severe impairment may require enteral or parenteral nutrition support. Depending on the severity of the stroke, individual assessment and planning for nutrition are necessary.

SAFETY ALERT

The first oral feeding should be approached carefully because the gag reflex may be impaired owing to dysphagia.

Speech–language pathologists (SLPs) (if available) perform a swallowing evaluation before patients are started on oral intake. The first oral feeding should be approached carefully because the gag reflex may be impaired as a result of dysphagia. The majority of patients will experience dysphagia after a stroke (Palmer & Metheny, 2008). Before initiation of feeding, the gag reflex may be assessed by gently stimulating the back of the throat with a tongue blade. If a gag reflex is present, the patient will gag spontaneously. If it is absent, feeding should be deferred and exercises to stimulate swallowing should be started. The SLP or occupational therapist is usually responsible for designing this program. However, the nurse may be called on to develop the program in some clinical settings.

To screen for swallowing ability, the nurse should elevate the head of the bed to an upright position (unless contraindicated) and do a bedside trial of fluid (e.g., Toronto Bedside Swallowing Screening Test [TOR-BSST] or Burke test), giving the patient at least 3 tsp of water before proceeding to 50 mL of water by cup. Because of the dangers of silent aspiration, the nurse should not use any other liquid but water for this screening. If problems are experienced, the patient is not allowed anything orally and is referred to an SLP. If no problems are experienced, the patient should be placed on a modified diet and monitored during meals.

After careful assessment of swallowing, chewing, gag reflex, and pocketing, oral feedings can be initiated. Mouth care before feeding helps stimulate sensory awareness and salivation and can facilitate swallowing. The patient should remain in a high-Fowler position, preferably in a chair with the head flexed forward for the feeding and for 30 minutes afterward. Various dietary items may be recommended by the SLP. Foods should be easy to swallow and provide enough texture, temperature (warm or cold), and flavour to stimulate a swallow reflex. Crushed ice can be used as a stimulant. The patient should be instructed to swallow and then swallow again. Puréed foods are not usually the best choice because they are often bland and too smooth. Thin liquids are often difficult to swallow and may promote coughing. Thin fluids can be thickened through the use of a commercially available thickening agent (e.g., Thick-It). Milk products should be avoided because they tend to increase the viscosity of mucus and increase salivation.

Food should be placed on the unaffected side of the mouth. The nurse should ensure an unrushed, nonstressful atmosphere. Feedings must be followed by scrupulous oral hygiene because food may collect on the affected side of the mouth.

■ Communication.

During the acute stage of stroke, the nurse's role in meeting the psychological needs of the patient is primarily supportive. An alert patient is usually anxious because of lack of understanding about what has happened and because communication is difficult. The patient is assessed for the ability to both speak and understand. The patient's response to simple questions can give the nurse a guideline for structuring explanations and instructions. If the patient cannot understand words, gestures may be used to support verbal cues. It is helpful to speak slowly and calmly, using simple words or sentences to enhance communication. The nurse must give the patient extra time to comprehend and respond to communication. The stroke patient with aphasia may easily be overwhelmed by verbal stimuli. (Guidelines for communicating with a patient who has aphasia are presented in Table 60-9.) Evaluation and treatment of language and communication deficits are often done by the SLP once the patient has stabilized.

■ Sensory–Perceptual Alterations.

Homonymous hemianopsia (blindness in the same half of each visual field) is a common problem after a stroke (Figure 60-12, *B*). Persistent disregard of objects in part of the visual field should alert the nurse to this possibility. Initially, the nurse helps the patient to compensate by arranging the environment within the patient's perceptual field, such as arranging the food tray so that all foods

Table 60-9 Communication With a Patient With Aphasia
1. Decrease environmental stimuli that may be distracting and disrupting to communication efforts.
2. Look at the patient when speaking because the nurse's facial expression may help the patient with aphasia to understand what the nurse is saying.
3. Speak with normal volume and tone. Speak in a tone of voice suitable for communicating with an adult rather than a child.
4. Present one thought or idea at a time.
5. Write out key words or draw instructions for the patient to follow. Use a thick black marker and big printed letters.
6. Keep questions simple or ask questions that can be answered with "yes" or "no."
7. Let the person speak. Do not interrupt. Allow time for the individual to complete thoughts.
8. Mimic or make use of gestures or demonstration as an acceptable alternative form of communication. Encourage this by saying, "Show me …" or "Point to what you want."
9. Do not pretend to understand the person if you do not. Calmly say you do not understand and encourage the use of nonverbal communication, or ask the person to write out what he or she wants.
10. Give the patient time to process information and generate a response before repeating a question or statement.
11. Allow body contact (e.g., the clasp of a hand, touching) as much as possible. Realize that touching may be the only way the patient can express feelings.
12. Organize the patient's day by preparing and following a schedule (the more familiar the routine, the easier it will be).
13. Do not push communication if the person is tired or upset. Aphasia worsens with fatigue.

are on the right side or the left side to accommodate for field of vision (see Figure 60-12, *B*). Later, the patient learns to compensate for the visual defect by consciously attending or scanning the neglected side (see Figure 60-12, *A*). The weak or paralyzed extremities are carefully checked for adequacy of dressing, for hygiene, and for trauma.

In the clinical situation, it is often difficult to distinguish between a visual field cut and a neglect syndrome. Both problems may occur with strokes affecting either the right or the left side of the brain. A person may be unfortunate enough to have both homonymous hemianopsia and a neglect syndrome, which increases the inattention to the weak or paralyzed side. A neglect syndrome results in decreased safety awareness and places the patient at high risk for injury. Immediately after the stroke, the nurse must anticipate potential safety hazards and provide protection from injury. Safety measures can include close observation of the patient, use of a sitter or family member, lowering the height of the bed, and video monitors. The use of restraints and soft vests is avoided as this may agitate the patient.

Other visual problems may include *diplopia* (double vision), loss of the corneal reflex, and *ptosis* (drooping eyelid), especially if the area of stroke is in the vertebrobasilar distribution. Diplopia is often treated with an eye patch. If the corneal reflex is absent, the patient is at risk for corneal abrasion and should be observed

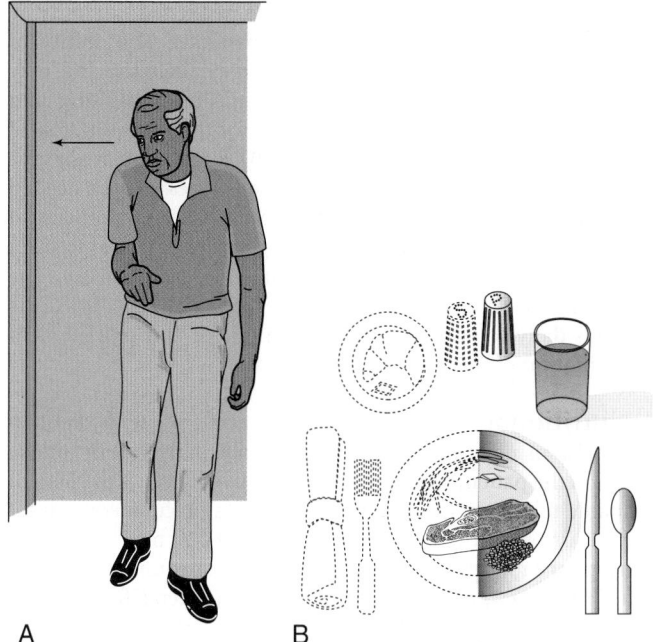

Figure 60-12 Spatial and perceptual deficits in stroke. **A,** The patient is instructed to look toward the affected side when walking, to avoid bumping into things. **B,** With homonymous hemianopia, the patient is unable to see the left side of the tray and may ignore items on that side.

Source: Monahan, F. D., Neighbors, M., Sands, J. K., Marek, J. F., & Green, C. J. (2007). *Phipps' medical-surgical nursing: Health and illness perspectives* (8th ed., p. 1437, Figure 49-10). St. Louis: Mosby.

closely and protected against eye injuries. Corneal abrasion can be prevented with artificial tears or gel to keep the eyes moist and an eye shield (especially at night). Ptosis is generally not treated because it usually does not inhibit vision.

Coping. A stroke is usually a sudden, extremely stressful event for the patient, family members, and significant others. A stroke is often a family disease, affecting the family emotionally, socially, and financially as well as changing roles and responsibilities within the family. An older couple may perceive the stroke as a very real threat to life and to accustomed lifestyle. Reactions to this threat vary considerably but may involve fear, apprehension, denial of the severity of stroke, depression, anger, and sorrow. During the acute phase of caring for the stroke patient and the family, nursing interventions designed to facilitate coping involve providing information and emotional support.

Explanations to the patient about what has happened and about diagnostic and therapeutic procedures should be clear and understandable. Decision making and upholding the patient's wishes during this challenging time are of utmost importance. Advance directives should be honoured and family meetings or updates should be held daily in regard to feeding tube placement or tracheotomy. It is important to give the caregiver and family careful, detailed explanations of what has happened to the patient. However, if the family is extremely anxious and upset during the acute phase, explanations may need to be repeated at a later time. Because family members usually have not had time to prepare for the illness, they may need assistance in arranging care for family members or pets

and for transportation and finances. A social services referral is often helpful.

It is particularly challenging to keep the aphasic patient adequately informed. Tone, demeanour, and touch may also be used to convey support. When communicating with a patient who has a communication deficit, it is important to speak with normal volume and tone, keep questions simple, and present one thought or idea at a time. To decrease frustration, the nurse should always let the patient speak without interruption and make use of gestures. It is important not to forget to make use of writing and communication boards (Gordon, Ellis-Hill, & Ashburn, 2009).

Ambulatory and Home Care: Stroke Recovery

The patient is usually discharged from the acute care setting to home, an intermediate- or long-term care facility, or a rehabilitation facility. Ideally, discharge planning with the patient and family or caregiver starts early in the hospitalization and promotes a smooth transition from one care setting to another. The interdisciplinary team provides the guidance for the appropriate care required after discharge. If the patient requires a short- or long-term health care facility, the team can make appropriate referrals that allow time for the family to select and arrange care. A critical factor in discharge planning is the patient's level of independence in performing ADLs. If the patient is returning home, the team can make referrals for needed equipment and services in preparation for discharge.

Nurses have an excellent opportunity to prepare the patient and family or caregiver for discharge through education, demonstration and return demonstration, practice, and evaluation of self-care skills before discharge. Total care is considered in discharge planning: medications, nutrition, mobility, exercises, hygiene, and toileting. Follow-up care is carefully planned to permit continuing nursing care, physiotherapy, occupational therapy, and speech therapy, as well as medical care. Community resources should be identified to provide recreational activities, group support, spiritual assistance, respite care, adult day care, and home assistance based on the individual patient's needs.

Rehabilitation is the process of maximizing the patient's capabilities and resources to promote optimal functioning related to physical, mental, and social well-being. The goals of rehabilitation are to prevent deformity and maintain and improve function. Regardless of the care setting, ongoing rehabilitation is essential to maximize the patient's abilities. Most patients will see the maximum benefit in the first year of recovery following a stroke (Hoffmann, Bennett, & McKenna, 2009).

Rehabilitation requires a team approach so the patient and family can benefit from the combined, expert care of an interdisciplinary team. The team must communicate and coordinate care to achieve the patient's and family's goals. There is strong evidence that organized postacute, inpatient stroke care delivered within the first 4 weeks by an interdisciplinary team of health care providers can result in a reduction in the number of deaths related to stroke (Miller et al., 2010). The stroke rehabilitation team generally consists of a rehabilitation nurse, neuropsychologist, occupational therapist, certified rehabilitation counsellor, physiotherapist, physician, recreational therapist, social worker, and SLP (Miller et al., 2010). The nurse is in a good position to facilitate rehabilitation and is often key to successful rehabilitation efforts. Physiotherapy focuses on mobility, progressive ambulation, transfer techniques, and equipment needed for mobility. Occupational therapy emphasizes retraining for ADLs such as eating, dressing, hygiene, and cooking. Occupational therapists are also skilled in cognitive and perceptual evaluation and training. Speech–language pathology focuses on speech, communication, cognition, and swallowing abilities.

Many of the nursing interventions outlined in the NCP for the patient with a stroke (see NCP 60-1) are initiated in the acute phase of care and continue throughout rehabilitation. Some of the interventions are independent nursing actions, whereas others involve the entire rehabilitation team.

The rehabilitation nurse assesses the patient, caregiver, and family with attention to the (1) rehabilitation potential of the patient, (2) physical status of all body systems, (3) presence of complications caused by the stroke or other chronic conditions, (4) cognitive status of the patient, (5) family resources and support, and (6) expectations of the patient and family related to the rehabilitation program.

Musculoskeletal Function.

The nurse initially emphasizes the musculoskeletal functions of eating, toileting, and walking for the rehabilitation of the patient. Initial assessment consists of determining the stage of recovery of muscle function. If the muscles are still flaccid several weeks after the stroke, the prognosis for regaining function is poor, and the focus of care is on preventing additional loss. Most patients begin to show signs of spasticity with exaggerated reflexes within 48 hours following the stroke. Spasticity at this phase of the stroke denotes progress toward recovery. As improvement continues, small voluntary movements of the hip or the shoulder may be accompanied by involuntary movements in the rest of the extremity *(synergy)*. The final stage of recovery occurs when the patient has voluntary control of isolated muscle groups.

Interventions for the musculoskeletal system advance in a manner of progressive activity. Balance training is the initial step and begins with the patient sitting up in bed or dangling on the edge of the bed. The nurse evaluates tolerance by noting dizziness or syncope caused by vasomotor instability. Loss of postural stability is common after a stroke. When the nondominant hemisphere is involved, walking apraxia and loss of postural control are usually apparent. Assess if patients autocorrect their posture when sitting on the edge of the bed. If the patient can straighten her or his posture instead of leaning to the weaker side, the patient may be ready for the next step of transferring from bed to chair. The chair is placed beside the bed so that the patient can lead with the stronger arm and leg. The patient sits on the side of the bed, stands, places the strong hand on the far wheelchair arm, and sits down. The nurse may either supervise the transfer or provide minimal assistance by guiding the patient's strong hand to the wheelchair arm, standing in front of the patient blocking the patient's knees with the nurse's knees to prevent knee buckling, and guiding the patient into a sitting position.

In some rehabilitation units, the Bobath approach is used as an approach to mobility. The goal of this approach is to help the patient gain control over patterns of spasticity by inhibiting abnormal reflex patterns. Therapists and nurses use the Bobath approach to encourage normal muscle tone, normal movement, and promotion of bilateral function of the body. An example is to have the patient transfer into the wheelchair using the weak or paralyzed side and the stronger side to facilitate more bilateral functioning.

A more recent approach to stroke rehabilitation is constraint-induced movement therapy. Constraint-induced movement therapy encourages the patient to use the weakened extremity by restricting movement of the normal extremity. The ability of patients to comply with this approach is challenging and may limit its use. Movement training, skill acquisition, splinting, and exercise are additional therapies offered for the rehabilitation of the stroke patient (Hoffmann et al., 2009). Supportive or assistive equipment, such as canes, walkers, and leg braces, may be needed on a short- or long-term basis for mobility. The physiotherapist usually selects the most appropriate supportive device(s) to meet individual needs and instructs the patient regarding use. The nurse should incorporate physiotherapy activities into the patient's daily routine for additional practice and repetition of rehabilitation efforts.

Nutritional Therapy.

After the acute phase, a dietitian can assist in determining the appropriate daily caloric intake based on the patient's size, weight, and activity level. If the patient is unable to take in an adequate oral diet, a percutaneous endoscopic gastrostomy (see Chapter 42, Figure 42-7) may be used for nutritional support if dysphagia persists. Most commercially prepared formulas provide about 1 cal/mL. (Enteral feedings are described in Chapter 42.)

The nurse and the SLP must assess the ability of the patient to swallow solids and fluids and adjust the diet appropriately. The dietitian plans the diet type, texture, calorie count, and fluids to meet the patient's nutritional needs. The occupational therapist and the nurse must evaluate the patient's ability to feed himself or herself and recommend assistive devices to allow for independent eating.

The inability to feed oneself can be frustrating and may result in malnutrition and dehydration. Interventions to promote self-feeding include using the unaffected upper extremity to eat; employing assistive devices such as rocker knives, plate guards, and nonslip pads for dishes (Figure 60-13); removing unnecessary items from the tray or table, which can reduce spills; and providing a nondistracting environment to decrease sensory overload and distraction. The effectiveness of the dietary program is evaluated in terms of maintenance of weight, adequate hydration, and patient satisfaction.

Bowel Function.

A bowel management program is implemented for problems with bowel control, constipation, or incontinence. A high-fibre diet (see Chapter 45, Table 45-9) and adequate fluid intake (2500-3000 mL) are usually recommended. Patients with stroke frequently have constipation, which responds to the following dietary management:

- Fluid intake of 2500 to 3000 mL daily unless contraindicated
- Prune juice (120 mL) or stewed prunes daily
- Cooked vegetables or fruit three times daily
- Whole-grain cereal or bread three to five times daily

The bowel management program for incontinence consists of placing the patient on the bedpan or bedside commode or taking the patient to the bathroom at a regular time daily to re-establish bowel regularity. A good time for the bowel program is 30 minutes after breakfast because eating stimulates the gastrocolic reflex and peristalsis. The time can be adjusted for individual bowel habits and preferred timing. Sitting on the commode or toilet promotes bowel elimination through both gravity and increased abdominal pressure. Stool softeners or suppositories may be ordered if the bowel program is ineffective in re-establishing bowel regularity. A glycerin suppository can be inserted 15 to 30 minutes before evacuation time to stimulate the anorectal reflex. The bisacodyl (Dulcolax) suppository is a chemical stimulant to the bowel and

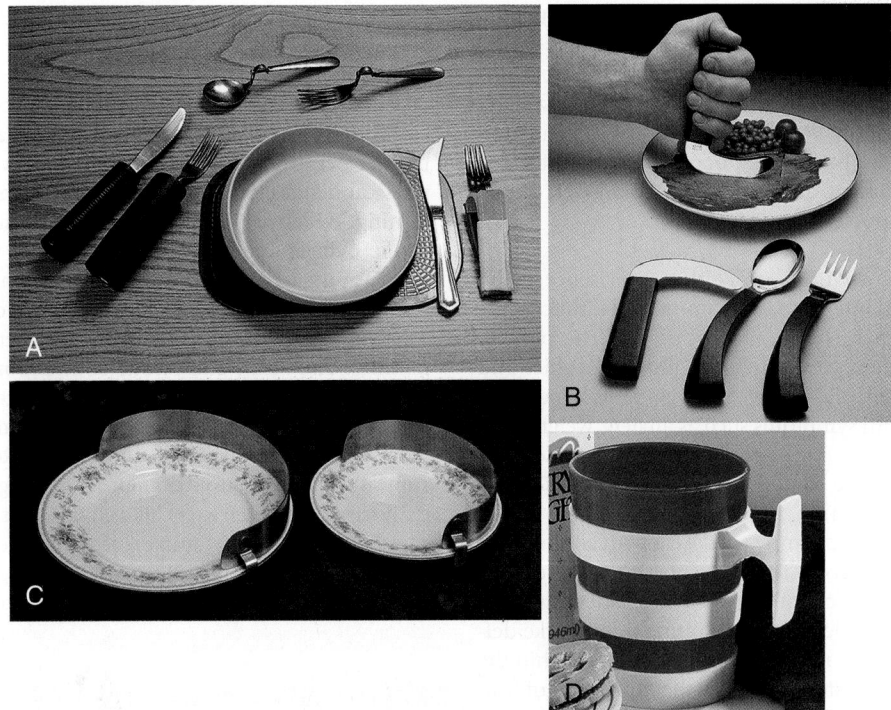

Figure 60-13 Assistive devices for eating. **A,** The curved fork fits over the hand. The rounded plate helps keep food on the plate. Special grips and swivel handles are helpful for some persons. **B,** Knives with rounded blades are rocked back and forth to cut food. The person does not need a fork in one hand and a knife in the other. **C,** Plate guards help keep food on the plate. **D,** Cup with special handle.

Source: Courtesy Sammons Preston, Bolingbrook, Illinois.

is used when other measures are ineffective. Ideally, the suppository use is for short-term management.

■ **Bladder Function.** The nurse often assists the patient with urinary difficulties or incontinence that may follow a stroke. Often the patient with stroke has functional incontinence, which is associated with communication difficulties, mobility problems, and dressing or undressing difficulties. Nursing interventions focused on urinary continence include (1) assessment for bladder distension by palpation; (2) offering the bedpan, urinal, commode, or toilet every 2 hours during waking hours and every 3 to 4 hours at night; (3) focusing the patient on the need to urinate with direct command; (4) assistance with clothing and mobility; (5) scheduling the majority of fluid intake between 0700 and 1900 hours; and (6) encouraging the usual position for urinating (standing for men and sitting for women).

Short-term interventions for urinary incontinence may include indwelling catheters, intermittent catheterization, toileting the patient frequently, or incontinence briefs. These are not long-term solutions for urinary incontinence because complications such as urinary infections or skin irritation may occur.

Assessment of postvoid residual volume is often completed by nurses using bladder ultrasonography. The ultrasonogram measures how much urine is in the bladder after voiding. If urine remains in the bladder, incomplete emptying is a problem and may cause urinary tract infections. A coordinated program by the entire nursing staff is needed to achieve urinary continence.

■ **Sensory–Perceptual Function.** Patients who have had a stroke frequently have perceptual deficits. Patients with a stroke

on the right side of the brain usually have difficulty in judging position, distance, and rate of movement. These patients are often impulsive and impatient and tend to deny problems related to strokes. They may fail to correlate spatial–perceptual problems with the inability to perform activities, such as guiding a wheelchair through the doorway. The patient with a right-brain stroke (left hemiplegia) is at higher risk for injury because of mobility difficulties. Directions for activities are best given verbally for comprehension. The task should be broken down into simple steps for ease of understanding. Environmental control, such as removing clutter and obstacles and providing good lighting, aids in concentration and helps provide safer mobility. Provide nonslip socks at all times. One-sided neglect is common for people with right-brain stroke, so the nurse may assist or remind the patient to dress the weak or paralyzed side or shave the forgotten side of the face.

Patients with a left-brain stroke (right hemiplegia) commonly are slower in organization and performance of tasks. They tend to have impaired spatial discrimination. These patients usually admit to deficits and have a fearful, anxious response to a stroke. Their behaviours are slow and cautious. Nonverbal cues and instructions are helpful for comprehension with patients who have had a left-brain stroke.

■ **Affect.** Patients who have had strokes often exhibit emotional responses that are not appropriate or typical for the situation. Patients may appear apathetic, depressed, fearful, anxious, weepy, frustrated, and angry. Some patients exhibit exaggerated mood swings, especially those with a stroke on the left side of the brain (right hemiplegia). The patient may be unable to control emotions and may suddenly burst into tears or laughter. This behaviour is out of context and often is unrelated to the underlying emotional state of the patient. Nursing interventions for atypical emotional response are to (1) distract the patient who suddenly becomes emotional, (2) explain to the patient and family that emotional outbursts may occur after a stroke, (3) maintain a calm environment, and (4) avoid shaming or scolding the patient during emotional outbursts.

■ **Coping.** The patient with a stroke may experience many losses, including sensory, intellectual, communicative, functional, role behaviour, emotional, social, and vocational. The patient, caregiver, and family often go through the process of grief and mourning associated with the losses. Some patients experience long-term depression with symptoms such as anxiety, weight loss, loss of energy, poor appetite, and sleep disturbances. In addition, the time and energy required to perform previously simple tasks can arouse anger and frustration.

The patient, caregiver, and family need help with coping with the losses associated with stroke. The nurse may assist the coping by (1) supporting communication between the patient and the family; (2) discussing lifestyle changes resulting from stroke deficits; (3) discussing changing roles and responsibilities within the family; (4) being an active listener to allow the expression of fear, frustration, and anxiety; (5) including the family and patient in short- and long-term goal planning and patient care; and (6) supporting family conferences. Maladjusted dependence with inadequate coping occurs when the patient does not maintain optimal functioning for self-care, family responsibilities, decision making, or socialization. This situation can cause resentment from both the patient and the family with a negative cycle of interpersonal dependency and control. *Maladjusted independence* occurs when the patient overestimates personal cognitive or physical capabilities and energy levels. These patients are at risk for injury.

Family members must cope with three aspects of the patient's behaviour: (1) recognition of behavioural changes resulting from neurological deficits that are not changeable, (2) responses to multiple losses by both the patient and the family, and (3) behaviours that may have been reinforced during the early stages of stroke as continued dependency. The patient, caregiver, and family may express feelings of guilt over not living healthy lifestyles or not seeking professional help sooner. Family therapy is a helpful adjunct to rehabilitation. Open communication, information regarding the total effects of stroke, education regarding stroke treatment, and therapy are helpful. Stroke support groups within rehabilitation facilities and in the community are helpful in terms of mutual sharing, education, coping, and understanding.

■ **Sexual Function.** A patient who has had a stroke may be concerned about the loss of sexual function. Many patients are comfortable talking about their anxieties and fears regarding sexual function if the nurse is comfortable and open to the topic. The nurse may initiate the topic with the patient and spouse or significant other. Common concerns of sexual activity involving the patient with a stroke are impotence and the occurrence of another stroke during sex. Nursing interventions for sexual activity include education on (1) optimal positioning of partners,

(2) timing for peak energy times, and (3) patient and partner counselling.

■ **Community Reintegration.** Traditionally, successful community integration following stroke has been difficult for the patient because of persistent problems with cognition, coping, physical deficits, and emotional lability that interfere with functioning. Older patients who have had a stroke often have more severe deficits and frequently experience multiple health problems. Failure to continue the rehabilitation regimen at home may result in deterioration and further complications.

Community resources can be an asset to patients and their families. The Heart and Stroke Foundation of Canada is a great resource for anyone who has been affected by or had a family member affected by a stroke. The Canadian Stroke Network provides newsletters on stroke, and Stroke Recovery Canada offers support to stroke survivors. Other local groups can offer more daily assistance, such as meals and transportation. These resources can be identified by nurse case managers, advanced practice nurses, community health nurses, discharge planners, and social workers. (Resources are listed at the end of the chapter.)

AGE-RELATED CONSIDERATIONS: STROKE

Stroke is a significant cause of death and disability. The highest incidence of stroke occurs among older adults. Stroke can result in a profound disruption in the life of an older person. The magnitude of disability and changes in total function can leave patients wondering if they can ever return to their prestroke life, and loss of independence may be a major concern. It may require many adaptive changes to perform ADLs because of physical, emotional, perceptual, and cognitive deficits. Home management may be a particular challenge if the patient has an elderly spouse caretaker who also has health problems. There may be limited family members (including adult children) living in close proximity to provide help.

The rehabilitative phase and assisting the older patient to deal with the residual deficits of stroke, as well as aging, can provide a challenging nursing experience. Patients may become fearful and depressed because they think they may have another attack or die. The fear can become immobilizing and interfere with effective rehabilitation.

Changes may occur in the patient–spouse relationship. The dependency resulting from a stroke may be threatening to the relationship. The spouse may also have chronic medical problems that affect the ability to take care of the stroke survivor. The patient may not want anyone other than the spouse to provide care, putting a significant burden on the spouse.

The nurse has the opportunity to assist the patient and family in the transition through acute hospitalization, rehabilitation, long-term care, and home care. The needs of the patient and the family require ongoing nursing assessment, and interventions must be adapted in response to changing needs to optimize quality of life for both the patient and the family.

CLINICAL DECISION-MAKING EXERCISE

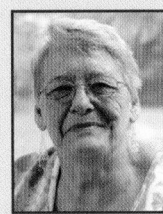

CASE STUDY:
Stroke

Source: © iStockphoto.com/Roberta Osborne.

Patient Profile

Mrs. Hortense Putman, a 66-year-old woman, awoke in the middle of the night and fell when she tried to get up and go to the bathroom. She fell because she was not able to control her left leg. Her husband took her to the hospital, where she was diagnosed with an acute right-sided ischemic stroke (right middle cerebral artery stroke). Because she had awakened with symptoms, the actual time of onset was unknown and she was not a candidate for tissue plasminogen activator (tPA).

Subjective Data

- Left arm, leg, and face are weak and feel numb
- Feeling depressed and fearful
- Requires help with activities of daily living (ADLs)
- Concerned about having another stroke
- Says she has not taken her drugs for high cholesterol for many weeks
- History of a brief episode of left-sided weakness and tingling of face, arm, and hand 3 months earlier, which totally resolved and for which she did not seek treatment

Objective Data

- BP: 180/110 mm Hg
- Left-sided arm weakness (3/5) and leg weakness (4/5)

- Decreased sensation on the left side, particularly the hand
- Left homonymous hemianopsia
- Overweight; body mass index = 27
- Alert, oriented, and able to answer questions appropriately but mild slowness in responding

Discussion Questions

1. How does Mrs. Putman's prior health history put her at risk for a stroke?
2. How can the nurse address Mrs. Putman's concerns regarding having another stroke?
3. Why would Mrs. Putman's ability to drive be affected after the stroke?
4. What strategies might the home health nurse use to help Mrs. Putman and her family cope with her feeling depressed?
5. *Priority Decision:* What priority lifestyle changes should Mrs. Putman make to reduce the likelihood of another stroke?
6. How will homonymous hemianopsia affect Mrs. Putman's hygiene, eating, driving, and community activities?
7. What factors should the nurse assess for related to outpatient rehabilitation for Mrs. Putman?
8. *Priority Decision:* What are the priority nursing interventions for Mrs. Putman?
9. *Priority Decision:* Based on the assessment data provided, what are the priority nursing diagnoses? Are there any collaborative problems?

evolve *Answers are available at* **http://evolve.elsevier.com/Canada/Lewis/medsurg**

REVIEW QUESTIONS

The number of the question corresponds to the same-numbered objective at the beginning of the chapter.

1. Which of the following patients has the highest risk for a stroke?
   a. An obese 45-year-old Aboriginal man
   b. A 35-year-old Chinese Canadian woman who smokes
   c. A 32-year-old White woman taking oral contraceptives
   d. A 65-year-old Black man with hypertension

2. Which of the following factors related to cerebral blood flow most often determines the extent of cerebral damage from a stroke?
   a. Amount of cardiac output
   b. Oxygen content of the blood
   c. Degree of collateral circulation
   d. Level of carbon dioxide in the blood

3. Which of the following pieces of information provided by the patient would help differentiate a hemorrhagic stroke from a thrombotic stroke?
   a. Sensory disturbance
   b. A history of hypertension
   c. Presence of motor weakness
   d. Sudden onset of severe headache

4. A patient with right-sided hemiplegia and aphasia resulting from a stroke most likely has involvement of which of the following?
   a. Brainstem
   b. Vertebral artery
   c. Left middle cerebral artery
   d. Right middle cerebral artery

5. A patient with a stroke is scheduled for angiography. Which of the following can this test detect in stroke patients?
   a. Presence of increased intracranial pressure
   b. Site and size of the infarction
   c. Patency of the cerebral blood vessels
   d. Presence of blood in the cerebrospinal fluid

6. A patient experiencing transient ischemic attacks is scheduled for a carotid endarterectomy. What does the nurse explain to the patient about the purpose of this procedure?
   a. To decrease cerebral edema
   b. To reduce the brain damage that occurs during a stroke in evolution
   c. To prevent a stroke by removing atherosclerotic plaques blocking cerebral blood flow
   d. To provide a circulatory bypass around thrombotic plaques obstructing cranial circulation

7. For a patient who is suspected of having a stroke, what is one of the most important pieces of information that the nurse can obtain?
   a. Time of the patient's last meal
   b. Time at which stroke symptoms first appeared
   c. Patient's hypertension history and management
   d. Family history of stroke and other cardiovascular diseases

8. What does bladder training in a male patient who has urinary incontinence after a stroke include?
   a. Limiting fluid intake
   b. Keeping a urinal in place at all times
   c. Assisting the patient to stand to void
   d. Catheterizing the patient every 4 hours

9. What is the most common response of the stroke patient to the change in body image?
   a. Denial
   b. Depression
   c. Dissociation
   d. Intellectualization

ANSWERS: 1. d; 2. c; 3. d; 4. c; 5. c; 6. c; 7. b; 8. c; 9. b.

REFERENCES

Adams, H., del Zoppo, G., Alberts, M., Bhatt, D. L., Brass, L., Furlan, A., ..., Wijdicks, E. (2007). Guidelines for the early management of adults with ischemic stroke. *Stroke*, *38*(5), 1655-1711. doi:10.1161/STROKEAHA.107.181486

Air, E. L., & Kissela, B. M. (2007). Diabetes, the metabolic syndrome, and ischemic stroke: Epidemiology and possible mechanisms. *Diabetes Care*, *30*(12), 3131-3140. doi:10.2337/dc06-1537

Bottemiller, K. L., Bieber, P. L., Basford, J. R., & Harris, M. (2006). FIM score, FIM efficiency, and discharge disposition following inpatient stroke rehabilitation. *Rehabilitation Nursing*, *31*(1), 22-25.

Broderick, J., Connolly, S., Feldmann, E., Hanley, D., Kase, C., Krieger, D., ..., Zuccarello, M. (2007). Guidelines for the management of spontaneous intracerebral hemorrhage in adults: 2007 update. *Stroke*, *38*(6), 2001-2023. doi:10.1161/STROKEAHA.107.183689

Canadian Stroke Network/Heart and Stroke Foundation of Canada (CSN/HSF). (2010). Canadian Stroke Strategy—Canadian best practices recommendations for stroke care: Update 2010. Retrieved from *http://www.strokebestpractices.ca/wp-content/uploads/2011/04/2010BPR_ENG.pdf*

Christensen, M. C., Mayer, S. A., Ferran, J. M., & Kissela, B. (2009). Depressed mood after intracerebral hemorrhage: The FAST trial. *Cerebrovascular Diseases*, *27*(4), 353-360. doi:10.1159/000202012

del Zoppo, G. J., Saver, J. L., Jauch, E. C., & Adams, H. P., Jr. (2009). Expansion of the time window for treatment of acute ischemic stroke with intravenous tissue plasminogen activator. *Stroke*, *40*(8), 2945-2948. doi:10.1161/STROKEAHA.109.192535

Dickerson, L. M., Carek, P. J., & Quattlebaum, R. G. (2007). Prevention of recurrent ischemic stroke. *American Family Physician*, *76*(3), 383-388. Retrieved from *http://www.aafp.org/afp/2007/0801/p382.html*

Easton, J. D., Saver, J. L., Albers, G. W., Alberts, M. J., Chaturvedi, S., Feldman, E., ..., Sacco, R. L. (2009). Definition and evaluation of transient ischemic attack. *Stroke*, *40*(6), 2276-2293. doi:10.1161/STROKEAHA.108.192218

Furie, K. L., Kasner, S. E., Adams, R. J., Albers, G. W., Bush, R. L., Fagan, S. C., ..., Wentworth, D. (2011). Guidelines for the prevention of stroke in patients with stroke or transient ischemic attack: A guideline for healthcare professionals from the American Heart Association/American Stroke Association. *Stroke*, *42*(1), 227-276. doi:10.1161/STR.0b013e3181f7d043

Gao, F., & Jiang, W. J. (2009). Transient ischemic attack associated with stenosis of accessory middle cerebral artery: A case report. *Clinical Neurology and Neurosurgery*, *111*(7), 588-590. doi:10.1016/j.clineuro.2009.01.006

Giles, M. F., & Rothwell, P. M. (2009). Transient ischaemic attack: Clinical relevance, risk prediction and urgency of secondary prevention. *Current Opinion in Neurology*, *22*(1), 46-53. doi:10.1097/WCO.0b013e32831f1977

Goldstein, L. B. (2007). Acute ischemic stroke treatment in 2007. *Circulation*, *116*(13), 1504-1514. doi:10.1161/CIRCULATIONAHA.106.670885

Goldstein, L. B., Bushnell, C. D., Adams, R. J., Appel, L. J., Braun, L. T., Chaturvedi, S., ..., Pearson, T. A. (2011). Guidelines for the primary prevention of stroke: A guideline for healthcare professionals from the American Heart Association/American Stroke Association. *Stroke*, *42*(2), 517-584. doi:10.1161/STR.0b013e3181fcb238

Goldstein, L. B., & Hankey, G. J. (2006). Advances in primary stroke prevention. *Stroke*, *3*(2), 317-319. doi:10.1161/01.STR.0000200456.43415.11

Gordon, C., Ellis-Hill, C., & Ashburn, A. (2009). The use of conversational analysis: Nurse-patient interaction in communication disability after stroke. *Journal of Advanced Nursing*, *65*(3), 544-553. doi:10.1111/j.1365-2648.2008.04917.x

Hacke, W., Kaste, M., Bluhmki, E., Brozman, M., Davalos, A., Guidetti, D., ..., Toni, D. (2008). Thrombolysis with alteplase 3 to 4.5 hours after acute ischemic stroke. *New England Journal of Medicine*, *359*(13), 1317-1329. doi:10.1056/NEJMoa0804656

Healey, J. S., Hart, R. G., Pogue, J., Pfeffer, M. A., Hohnloser, S. H., De Caterina, R., ..., Connolly, S. J. (2008). Risks and benefits of oral anticoagulation compared with clopidogrel plus aspirin in patients with atrial fibrillation according to stroke risk: The Atrial Fibrillation Clopidogrel Trial with Irbesartan for Prevention of Vascular Events (ACTIVE-W). *Stroke*, *39*(5), 1482-1486. doi:10.1161/STROKEAHA.107.500199

Heart and Stroke Foundation of Canada (HSF). (2012). Statistics: Stroke. Retrieved from *http://www.heartandstroke.com/site/c.ikIQLcMWJtE/b.3483991/k.34A8/Statistics.htm*

Hegge, K. (2008). Antiplatelet agents for recurrent ischemic stroke. *South Dakota Medicine*, *62*(1), 15-17.

Hoffmann, T., Bennett, S., & McKenna, K. (2009). Interventions for stroke rehabilitation: Analysis of the research contained in the OT seeker evidence database. *Topics in Stroke Rehabilitation*, *15*(4), 341-350. doi:10.1310/tsr1504-341

Infanti, J. (2008). Challenging the gold standard: Should mannitol remain our first-line defense against intracranial hypertension? *Journal of Neuroscience Nursing*, *40*(6), 362-368.

Kazzi, A. A., & Ellis, K. (2009). *Subarachnoid hemorrhage.* New York: eMedicine. Retrieved from *http://www.emedicine.com/EMERG/topic559.htm*

Koelemay, M., & Legemate, D. (2009). Carotid artery stenting increased risk for stroke more than carotid endarterectomy in severe symptomatic stenosis. *Annals of Internal Medicine, 150*(4), JC2-JC11.

Miller, E. L., Murray, L., Richards, L., Zorowitz, R. D., Bakas, T., Clark, P., & Billinger, S. A. (2010). Comprehensive overview of nursing and interdisciplinary rehabilitation care of the stroke patient: A scientific statement from the American Heart Association. *Stroke, 41*(10), 2402-2448. doi:10.1161/STR.0b013e3181e7512b

Miller, J., & Mink, J. (2009). Acute ischemic stroke: Not a moment to lose. *Nursing, 39*(5), 36-42. doi:10.1097/01.NURSE. 0000350755.49282.6a

Morgenstern, L. B., Hemphill, J. C., III, Anderson, C., Becker, K., Broderick, J. P., Connolly, E. S., Jr., ..., Tamargo, R. J. (2010). Guidelines for the management of spontaneous intracerebral hemorrhage: A guideline for healthcare professionals from the American Heart Association/American Stroke Association. *Stroke, 41*(9), 2108-2129. doi:10.1161/STR.0b013e3181ec611b

Muscedere, J., Dodek, P., & Keenan, S. (2008). Comprehensive evidence-based clinical practice guidelines for ventilator-associated pneumonia: Prevention. *Journal of Critical Care, 23*(1), 126-137. doi:10.1016/j.jcrc.2007.11.014

Nassisi, D. (2008). Hemorrhagic stroke. *Emedicine.* Retrieved from *http://www.emedicine.com/EMERG/topic557.htm*

National Institute of Neurological Disorders and Stroke (NINDS). (2010). NINDS aphasia information page. Retrieved from *http://www.ninds.nih.gov/disorders/aphasia/aphasia.htm*

Palmer, J. L., & Metheny, N. A. (2008). Preventing aspiration in older adults with dysphagia. *American Journal of Nursing, 108*(2), 40-48. doi:10.1097/01.NAJ.0000308961.99857.33

Public Health Agency of Canada (PHAC). (2009). Tracking heart disease and stroke in Canada. Retrieved from *http://www.phac-aspc.gc.ca/publicat/2009/cvd-avc/index-eng.php*

Registered Nurses' Association of Ontario (RNAO). (2005). Stroke assessment across the continuum of care. *Nursing Best Practice Guidelines.* Retrieved from *http://www.rnao.org/Page.asp?PageID=9 24&ContentID=820*

Roederer, M. W., & Blackwell, J. C. (2006). Risks and benefits of combination contraceptives. *American Family Physician, 74*(11), 1915-1916.

Statistics Canada. (2011). Mortality, summary list of causes 2008. Retrieved from *http://www5.statcan.gc.ca/bsolc/olc-cel/olc-cel?cat no=84F0209X&CHROPG=1&lang=eng*

Stingele, R., & Ringleb, P. (2009). To stent or not to stent: Stent-protected percutaneous angioplasty versus endarterectomy post hoc analyses. *Current Opinion in Neurology, 22*(1), 75-79. doi: 10.1097/WCO.0b013e3283207b1a

CANADIAN RESOURCES

Aphasia Institute
http://www.aphasia.ca
Canadian Association of Neuroscience Nurses (CANN)
http://www.cann.ca
Canadian Diabetes Association
http://www.diabetes.ca/
Canadian Stroke Network & Canadian Stroke Strategy
http://www.canadianstrokenetwork.ca
Heart and Stroke Foundation of Canada
http://www.heartandstroke.com
Hypertension Canada
http://www.hypertension.ca
The Lung Association: Smoking Cessation Resource
http://www.lung.ca/_resources/Making_quit_happen_report.pdf
Montreal Cognitive Assessment (MoCA©)
http://www.mocatest.org/
Registered Nurses' Association of Ontario: Smoking Cessation Resource
http://rnao.ca/bpg/guidelines/integrating-smoking-cessation-daily-nursing-practice
Stroke Recovery Canada
http://www.strokerecoverycanada.com
Thrombosis Interest Group of Canada
http://www.tigc.org

RELATED RESOURCES

American Association of Neuroscience Nurses (AANN)
http://www.aann.org
American Heart Association: Stroke Journal
http://stroke.ahajournals.org/
American Stroke Association
http://www.strokeassociation.org
Association of Rehabilitation Nurses (ARN)
http://www.rehabnurse.org
DASH Diet: DASH Eating Plan
http://www.nhlbi.nih.gov/health/public/heart/hbp/dash/new_dash.pdf
The Internet Stroke Center
http://www.strokecenter.org
National Institute of Neurological Disorders and Stroke
http://www.ninds.nih.gov
National Stroke Association
http://www.stroke.org
Society for Neuroscience
http://www.sfn.org

℮volve *For additional Internet resources, see the Web site for this book at* **http://evolve.elsevier.com/Canada/Lewis/medsurg**

Nursing Management: Chronic Neurological Problems

Written by Cheryl A. Lehman

Adapted by Renee Clarke

LEARNING OBJECTIVES

1. Differentiate between migraine, tension-type, and cluster headaches in terms of etiology, clinical manifestations, diagnosis, collaborative care, and nursing management.
2. Describe the etiology, clinical manifestations, diagnostic studies, collaborative care, and nursing management of seizure disorders, multiple sclerosis, Parkinson's disease, myasthenia gravis, and normal pressure hydrocephalus.
3. Describe the clinical manifestations and the collaborative care of amyotrophic lateral sclerosis and Huntington's chorea.
4. Explain the potential impact of chronic neurological disease on physical, emotional, and psychological well-being.
5. Outline the major goals of treatment for the patient with a chronic, progressive neurological disease.

KEY TERMS

amyotrophic lateral sclerosis (ALS) A rare progressive neurological disorder; characterized by loss of motor neurons and by weakness and atrophy of the muscles of the hands, forearms, and legs, spreading to involve most of the body and the face, p. 1731

epilepsy A condition in which a person has at least two spontaneous seizures more than 24 hours apart; it is caused by a chronic underlying pathology, p. 1707

headache Pain in the head that can arise from many disorders or may be a disorder in and of itself, p. 1701

Huntington's disease (HD) A genetically transmitted, autosomal dominant disorder that affects both men and women of all races; characterized by chronic, devastating loss of all neurological function, resulting in dementia, p. 1731

multiple sclerosis (MS) A chronic, progressive, degenerative disorder of the central nervous system; characterized by disseminated demyelination of nerve fibres of the brain, spinal cord, and optic nerves, p. 1715

myasthenic crisis An acute exacerbation of muscle weakness triggered by infection, surgery, emotional distress, or overdose or inadequate drugs, p. 1728

myasthenia gravis (MG) An autoimmune disease of the neuromuscular junction; characterized by the fluctuating weakness of certain skeletal muscle groups, p. 1727

normal pressure hydrocephalus (NPH) An uncommon disorder characterized by an obstruction in the flow of cerebrospinal fluid, which causes a buildup of this fluid in the ventricles of the brain, p. 1732

Parkinson's disease (PD) A disease of the basal ganglia; characterized by a slowing down in the initiation and execution of movement, increased muscle tone, tremor at rest, and impaired postural reflexes, p. 1722

restless legs syndrome (RLS) Unpleasant sensory and motor abnormalities of one or both legs; characterized by an irritating sensation of uneasiness, tiredness, and itching deep within the muscles of the leg; also known as *Willis-Ekbom disease*, p. 1730

seizure A paroxysmal, uncontrolled electrical discharge of neurons in the brain that interrupts normal function, leading to a sudden, violent involuntary series of contractions of a group of muscles, p. 1706

status epilepticus A state of continuous seizure activity or a condition in which seizures recur in rapid succession without return to consciousness between seizures; a neurological emergency, p. 1708

ELECTRONIC RESOURCES

Supplemental content related to Chapter 61 can be found ...

Evolve Web Site ⊖volve

http://evolve.elsevier.com/Canada/Lewis/medsurg

- Answer Guidelines for Case Study on p. 1732
- Clinical Reference: Laboratory Values
- Content Updates
- Customizable Nursing Care Plans:
  - Headache
  - Multiple Sclerosis
  - Parkinson's Disease
  - Seizure Disorder or Epilepsy

- eFigures:
  - eFigure 61-1: "Peek sign" in Myasthenia Gravis
  - eFigure 61-2: Pathogenesis of Amyotrophic Lateral Sclerosis
- Electronic Calculators
- Examination Review Questions
- Glossary
- Interactive Case Studies:
  - Seizures
  - Parkinson's Disease and Hip Fracture
- Key Points (Printable and MP3 Download)
- Patient & Caregiver Teaching Guide: Headache Management

Headache

Headache is probably the most common type of pain experienced by humans. The majority of people have functional headaches, such as migraine or tension-type headaches that constitute a disorder in and of themselves; the remainder have organic headaches that arise from other disorders and sources, both intracranial and extracranial.

Not all tissues of the cranium are sensitive to pain. The pain-sensitive structures in the head include the venous sinuses, the dura, the cranial blood vessels, the three divisions of the trigeminal nerve (cranial nerve V), the facial nerve (cranial nerve VII), the glossopharyngeal nerve (cranial nerve IX), the vagus nerve (cranial nerve X), and the first three cervical nerves.

Headaches are classified using the International Headache Society (IHS) diagnostic criteria based on the characteristics of the headache and the facial pain. The primary classifications include migraine, tension-type headache, and cluster headaches (Headache Classification Subcommittee of the International Headache Society [HCCIHS], 2004). Characteristics of these headaches are shown in Table 61-1. A patient may have more than one type of headache.

Migraine Headache

Migraine headache (MH) is one of the primary headache classifications of the IHS (HCCIHS, 2004). The effects of MH pain are dramatic, causing both physical and emotional disability. The

Table 61-1 Comparison of Migraine, Tension-Type, and Cluster Headaches

	MIGRAINE HEADACHE	TENSION-TYPE HEADACHE	CLUSTER HEADACHE
Site	Unilateral (in 60%), may switch sides, commonly anterior	Bilateral, bandlike pressure at base of skull, in face, or in both	Unilateral, radiating up or down from one eye
Quality	Throbbing, synchronous with pulse	Constant, squeezing tightness	Severe, "bone-crushing"
Frequency	Periodic; cycles of several months to years	Cycles for several years	May have months or years between attacks; attacks occur in clusters: one to three times a day over a period of 4-8 wk
Duration	Continuous for hours or days	Intermittent for months or years	30-90 min
Time and mode of onset	May be preceded by prodrome; onset after awakening; gets better with sleep	Not related to time	Nocturnal; commonly awakens patient from sleep
Associated symptoms	Nausea or vomiting, edema, irritability, sweating, photophobia, phonophobia, prodrome of sensory, motor, or psychic phenomena; family history (in 65%)	Palpable neck and shoulder muscles, stiff neck, tenderness	Vasomotor symptoms such as facial flushing or pallor, unilateral lacrimation, ptosis, and rhinitis

onset usually occurs in childhood or adolescence with the average Canadian MH patient being older than 40 years and female. MH is likely the most common cause for patient referrals to neurologists in Canada (Jelinski et al., 2006).

Etiology and Pathophysiology

Three theories attempt to explain the etiology of MH. The vascular theory suggests that vasoconstriction followed by vasodilation with resulting changes in blood flow causes the throbbing pain. A second theory proposes that the pain is a result of muscular tension and, thus, is related to tension-type headache. The third theory relates to biochemical changes; changes in the serotonin pathway result in the headache pain (Tfelt-Hansen & Koehler, 2011). Serotonin, a neurotransmitter, is involved in mood, memory, sleep, temperature, and muscle function. During an MH, the serotonin stored in platelets is released into the plasma and becomes inactive, thus altering the serotonin pathway.

MHs may be preceded by prodrome and aura. The *prodrome* (early manifestation of impending symptoms) may precede the headache phase by several hours or days. The *aura* (sensation of light or warmth) of MH is associated with "spreading depression," a wave of *oligemia* (diminished cerebral blood flow) beginning in the occipital lobe and spreading forward in the brain at a rate of 2 to 3 mm/min.

MHs, in many cases, have no known precipitating events. For other patients, the headache may be precipitated or triggered by foods, hormonal fluctuation, head trauma, physical exertion, fatigue, stress, and pharmacological agents (Tfelt-Hansen & Koehler, 2011).

Clinical Manifestations

MHs are subdivided by the IHS into categories including those without aura and those with aura (HCCIHS, 2004). MH without aura is the most common type. MH with aura occurs in only 25% of MH episodes (Loder, 2009). The sharply defined aura may last for 10 to 30 minutes before the start of the headache and may include sensory dysfunction (e.g., visual field defects, tingling or burning sensations, paresthesias), motor dysfunction (e.g., weakness, paralysis), dizziness, confusion, and even loss of consciousness (HCCIHS, 2004; Purdy, 2010).

Clinical manifestations that might occur in MH without and with aura are generalized edema, irritability, pallor, nausea and vomiting, and sweating. In MH without and with aura, the prodrome is not sharply defined. The prodrome can include psychic disturbances, gastrointestinal upset, and changes in fluid balance.

During the headache phase, some patients with MH may tend to seek shelter from noise, light, odours, people, and problems. The headache is described as a steady, throbbing pain that is synchronous with the pulse. However, the presentation of MH is varied in its severity. Although the headache is usually unilateral, it may switch to the opposite side in another episode. Not all MHs are disabling, and many patients do not seek health care treatment for them. In some patients, the symptoms of MHs may become progressively worse over time.

Diagnostic Studies

There are no specific laboratory or radiological tests for MHs. The diagnosis of MH is usually made from the history. Neurological and other diagnostic examinations are often normal.

The 2004 IHS criteria are used as the clinical basis for MH diagnosis. If atypical features are present, secondary headaches must be ruled out. Neuroimaging techniques (such as computed tomography [CT] scan) of head or magnetic resonance imaging (MRI) are not recommended for routine evaluation of headache unless abnormal findings are found on the neurological examination.

Tension-Type Headache

Tension-type headache (TTH) is the second major classification, but the most common type of primary headache. TTH has been called muscle-contraction, stress, psychogenic, and rheumatic headache. TTHs are subcategorized as infrequent episodic, frequent episodic, or chronic.

Etiology and Pathophysiology

It was originally thought that TTHs were the result of sustained and painful contraction of the muscles of the scalp and the neck. However, research has shown it is likely that neurovascular factors similar to those involved in MH play a role in the development of TTH, including central neurological disturbances (Tfelt-Hansen & Koehler, 2011).

Clinical Manifestations

There is no prodrome in TTH. The 2004 IHS classification system defines TTH as involving at least two of the following characteristics: pressure or "bandlike" tightness sensation usually to the temporal area, mild to moderate severity, bilateral location, or worsening with physical activity (HCCIHS, 2004). The headache does not involve nausea or vomiting but may involve sensitivity to light (*photophobia*) or sound (*phonophobia*). The headaches may occur intermittently for weeks, months, or even years. Many patients can have a combination of MH and TTH, with features of both headaches occurring simultaneously. Patients with MH may experience TTHs between MH attacks.

Diagnostic Studies

History taking is the most important diagnostic tool for TTH. If a patient meets TTH criteria, further diagnostic tests are not always conclusive, but they may be done to rule out secondary headache disorders. If TTH is present during physical examination, increased resistance to passive movement of the head and tenderness of the head and neck may be present on palpation (Loder & Rizzoli, 2008).

Cluster Headache

Cluster headaches (CHs) are a rare form of headache characterized by repeated headaches that can occur for weeks to months at a time, followed by periods of remission. It is one of the most severe forms of headache, often occurring without warning (Halker, Vargus, & Dodick, 2010).

Etiology and Pathophysiology

Neither the cause nor the pathophysiological mechanism of CH is fully known. The vasodilation that occurs in the affected part of the face is extracranial. The trigeminal nerve is implicated in the production of pain. CH involves dysfunction of intracranial blood vessels, the sympathetic nervous system, and pain modulation systems. Owing to the circadian rhythmicity of the headaches, the hypothalamus is believed to play a role. A genetic component has been noted in some families. Smoking and alcohol ingestion have been associated with CH (Leroux & Ducros, 2008).

Clinical Manifestations

The pain of CH is described as sharp and stabbing. The CH is one of the most severe forms of headache, with intense pain short in duration (5-180 min). The pain is generally periorbital, radiating to the temple, forehead, cheek, nose, or gums with the pain presenting predominantly unilaterally (Francis, Becker, & Pringsheim, 2010). Other manifestations may include swelling around the eye, lacrimation (tearing), facial flushing or pallor, rhinitis, and constriction of the pupil. During the headache, the patient is often agitated and restless, unable to sit still or relax. The headaches occur with regularity, usually occurring at the same time each day, during the same seasons of the year. Clusters typically last 2 weeks to 3 months, and then go into remission for months to years (HCCIHS, 2004).

Diagnostic Studies

The diagnosis of CH is primarily based on the history. However, CT scan, MRI, or magnetic resonance angiography may be performed to rule out an aneurysm, tumour, or infection.

Other Types of Headaches

The inability to diagnose a headache as MH, TTH, or CH may indicate that the pain is a symptom of a more serious illness. Headache can accompany subarachnoid hemorrhage; brain tumours; other intracranial masses; arteritis; vascular abnormalities; trigeminal neuralgia (tic douloureux); diseases of the eyes, nose, and teeth; and systemic illness (e.g., bacteremia, carbon monoxide poisoning, mountain sickness, polycythemia vera). The symptoms vary greatly. Because of the variety of causes of headache, clinical evaluation must be thorough. It should include an evaluation of personality, life adjustment, environment, and family situation as well as a comprehensive evaluation of neurological and physical status.

Collaborative Care for Headaches

If no systemic underlying disease is found, therapy is directed toward the functional type of headache. Table 61-2 outlines the general workup for a patient with headache to rule out any intracranial or extracranial disease. Table 61-3 summarizes the current therapies for prophylaxis and symptomatic relief of common headaches. These therapies include drugs, meditation, yoga, biofeedback, cognitive–behavioural therapy, and relaxation training. Figure 61-1 shows the location of pain for common headache syndromes.

Drug Therapy

Migraine Headache. Drug treatment of the acute MH attack is aimed at terminating or decreasing the symptoms of the

DIAGNOSTIC STUDIES

Table 61-2 Headaches

- History and physical examination
  - Neurological examination (often negative)
  - Inspection for local infections
  - Palpation for tenderness, bony swellings
  - Auscultation for bruits over major arteries
- Routine laboratory studies
  - CBC
  - Electrolytes
  - Urinalysis
- CT scan of sinuses
- Special studies (e.g., CT scan, angiography, EMG, EEG, MRA, MRI, lumbar puncture)

CBC, complete blood count; *CT,* computed tomography; *EEG,* electroencephalography; *EMG,* electromyography; *MRA,* magnetic resonance angiography; *MRI,* magnetic resonance imaging.

attack. Many people with mild or moderate MH can obtain relief with ibuprofen, acetaminophen, or aspirin. For moderate to severe headaches, the "triptans" have become the first line of therapy. Triptans are drugs that affect selected serotonin receptors and treat the primary cause of MH. These drugs reduce neurogenic inflammation of the cerebral blood vessels and produce vasoconstriction. Because these drugs cause constriction of coronary arteries, they must be avoided in patients with heart disease. Triptans should be taken at the first symptom of TTH.

Tension-type Headache. Drug treatment for TTH usually involves a non-narcotic analgesic (e.g., aspirin, acetaminophen) used alone or in combination with a sedative, caffeine, muscle relaxant, antidepressants, or codeine. However, many of these drugs have serious adverse effects. The patient should be cautioned about the long-term use of aspirin and aspirin-containing drugs because they can cause gastric bleeding and coagulation abnormalities in susceptible patients. Long-term use of Fiorinal (butalbital, caffeine, and aspirin) should be avoided because butalbital is a barbiturate and may be habit forming. Acetaminophen, or drugs containing acetaminophen, can cause kidney damage with chronic use and liver damage when combined with alcohol (Schilling, Corey, Leonard, & Eghtesad, 2011).

Cluster Headache. Because CHs occur suddenly, often at night, and are not long lasting, they are extremely hard to treat. Prophylactic drugs may include verapamil, lithium, divalproex, methysergide, steroids, nonsteroidal anti-inflammatory drugs (NSAIDs), and inhaled dihydroergotamine. Acute treatment of CH is inhalation of 100% oxygen delivered at a rate of 7 to 9 L/min for 15 to 20 minutes, which may relieve headache by causing vasoconstriction (Francis et al., 2010). Patients with frequent headaches may overuse analgesic drugs. Such overuse can lead to chronic daily headache, also called *analgesic rebound headache* or drug-induced headache. Drugs known to cause this problem are acetaminophen, aspirin, NSAIDs (e.g., ibuprofen), butalbital, triptans, and opioids. Treatment can be difficult and involves gradual withdrawal, possible hospitalization, and initiation of prophylactic drugs such as amitriptyline.

COLLABORATIVE CARE

Table 61-3 Headaches

	MIGRAINE HEADACHE	TENSION-TYPE HEADACHE	CLUSTER HEADACHE
Diagnostic	History*	History of neck and head tenderness, resistance to movement	History
Collaborative Therapy			
Symptomatic	Nonopioid analgesics: aspirin, acetaminophen, ibuprofen Serotonin receptor agonists: almotriptan (Axert), eletriptan (Relpax), frovatriptan (Frova), naratriptan (Amerge), rizatriptan (Maxalt), sumatriptan (Imitrex), zolmitriptan (Zomig) Corticosteroids: dexamethasone, prednisone (Apo-Prednisone)	Nonopioid analgesics: aspirin, ibuprofen, acetaminophen, naproxen Analgesic combinations: butalbital, caffeine, and aspirin (Fiorinal) Muscle relaxants	Ergot alkaloids: dihydroergotamine (DHE) via inhalation or IV, ergotamine, sumatriptan (Imitrex), naratriptan (Amerge) Vasoconstrictors Oxygen Anaesthetic: intranasal lidocaine 4% (Xylocaine)
Prophylactic	β-Adrenergic blockers: propranolol (Inderal), metoprolol, timolol Antidepressants: amitriptyline (Elavil), nortriptyline (Aventyl), imipramine Calcium channel blocker: verapamil (Isoptin) Antiseizure: valproate (Depakene), divalproex, gabapentin (Neurontin), topiramate (Topamax) Biofeedback Relaxation therapy Cognitive–behavioural therapy Acupuncture	Tricyclic antidepressants: nortriptyline (Aventyl), amitriptyline (Elavil) Serotonin reuptake inhibitors: fluoxetine (Prozac), sertraline (Zoloft), paroxetine (Paxil) β-Adrenergic blocker: propranolol (Inderal) Biofeedback Psychotherapy Muscle relaxation training Physiotherapy	β-Adrenergic blockers: DHE via inhalation or IV Anticonvulsant: divalproex sodium Serotonin antagonist: methysergide (Sansert) Corticosteroid: prednisone Calcium channel blockers: verapamil (Isoptin), lithium Biofeedback Physiotherapy

*Magnetic resonance imaging (MRI) should be considered in patients with nonacute headache who have unexplained abnormal neurological examination, atypical headache or headache features, or an additional risk factor, such as immune deficiency.

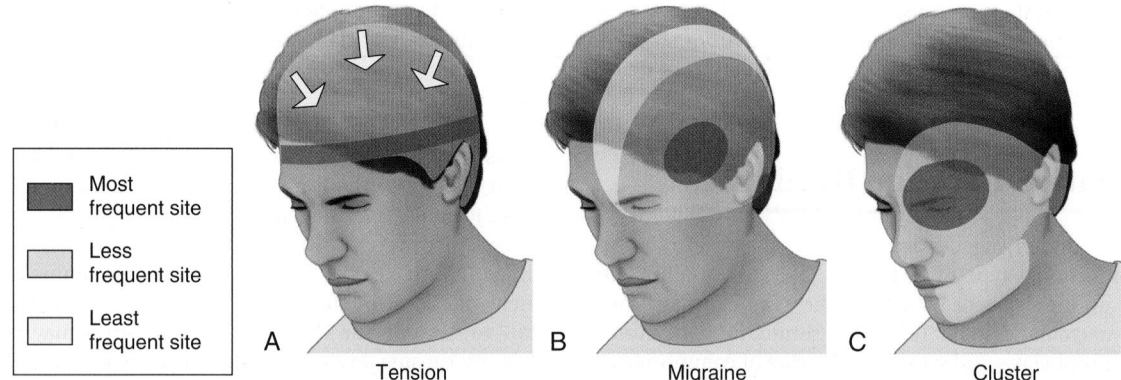

Figure 61-1 Location of pain for common headache syndromes. **A,** Tension headache is often described as feeling of a weight in or on the head and/or a band squeezing the head. **B,** Migraine headache is described as an intense, throbbing, or pounding pain that involves one temple. The pain usually is unilateral (on one side of the head), although it can be bilateral. **C,** Cluster headache pain is focused in and around one eye and is often described as sharp, penetrating, or burning.

NURSING MANAGEMENT: HEADACHES

▪ Nursing Assessment

Subjective and objective data that should be obtained from a patient with headache are presented in Table 61-4. Because the history provides the key to assessment of headache, it should include specific details of the headache itself, such as the location and type of pain, onset, frequency, duration, relation to events (emotional, psychological, physical), and time of day of the occurrence. Information about previous illnesses, surgery, trauma, allergies, family history, and response to medication should also be obtained. The nurse can suggest that the patient keep a diary of headache episodes with specific details. This type of record can be of great help in determining the type of headache and the precipitating events. If the patient has a history of MH, TTH, or CH, it is important to determine whether the character, intensity, or location of the headache has changed. This may be an important clue as to the cause of the headache (Table 61-5).

▪ Nursing Diagnoses

Nursing diagnoses for the patient with headache may include, but are not limited to, those presented in eNCP 61-1, "Patient With Headache," available on the Evolve Web site for this chapter.

▪ Planning

The overall goals are that the patient with a headache will (1) have reduced or no pain, (2) experience increased comfort and decreased anxiety, (3) demonstrate understanding of triggering events and treatment strategies, (4) use positive coping strategies to deal with chronic pain, and (5) experience increased quality of life and decreased disability.

▪ Nursing Implementation

Patients with chronic headache present a challenge to nurses. Headaches may be related to an inability to cope with daily stresses. The most effective therapy may be to help patients examine their lifestyle, recognize stressful situations, and learn to cope with them more appropriately. Encouraging the patient to keep a journal may aid in identifying precipitating factors and develop ways of avoiding them. Daily exercise, relaxation periods, and socializing can be encouraged because each can help decrease the recurrence of headache. The nurse can suggest alternative ways of handling the pain of headache.

In addition to using analgesics and analgesic-combination drugs for the symptomatic relief of headache, the patient should be encouraged to use relaxation techniques because they are effective in relieving TTH and MH. The MH sufferer often needs a quiet, dimly lit environment. Massage and moist hot packs to the neck and head can help a patient with TTH. The patient should learn about the drugs prescribed for prophylactic and symptomatic treatment of headache and should be able to describe the purpose, action, dosage, and adverse effects of the

Table 61-4 Headaches

Subjective Data

Important Health Information

Current health history: Pain assessment including location, characteristics, onset and duration, frequency, quality, intensity or severity of pain, and precipitating factors (nurse should use a pain scale, observation of actions, for cognitively impaired individual); positive family history of headaches; history of ingestion of alcohol, caffeine, cheese, chocolate, monosodium glutamate, aspartame, lunch meats (nitrites in cured meats), sausage, hot dogs, onions, avocados; level of hydration

Past health history: Seizures, cancer, recent fall or trauma, cranial infection, stroke; asthma or allergies; mental illness; relationship of headache to overwork, stress, menstruation, sexual activity, travel, bright lights, disruptions in sleep, or noxious environmental stimuli

Medications: Use of hydralazine, bromides, nitroglycerin, ergotamine (withdrawal), nonsteroidal anti-inflammatory drugs (in high daily doses), estrogen preparations, oral contraceptives, over-the-counter or prescription remedies

Surgery or other treatments: Craniotomy, sinus surgery, facial surgery, dental surgery

Symptoms

- Anorexia, nausea, vomiting (migraine prodrome)
- Vertigo, fatigue, weakness, paralysis, fainting, malaise
- *Migraine:* aura; unilateral, severe, throbbing (possible switching of side) headache; visual disturbances; photophobia; phonophobia; dizziness; tingling or burning sensations
- *Tension-type:* bilateral, bandlike, dull and persistent, base-of-skull headache, neck tenderness
- *Cluster:* unilateral and severe, nocturnal headaches; nasal stuffiness, unilateral lacrimation

Objective Data

General

Anxiety, apprehension

Integumentary

Cluster: Forehead diaphoresis, pallor, unilateral facial flushing with cheek edema, conjunctivitis

Migraine: Generalized edema (prodrome), pallor, diaphoresis

Neurological

Horner's syndrome, restlessness (*cluster*), hemiparesis *(migraine)*

Musculoskeletal

Resistance of head and neck movement, nuchal rigidity *(meningeal, tension-type)*, palpable neck and shoulder muscles *(tension-type)*

Possible Findings

Possible evidence of disease, deformity, or infection on brain imaging (CT, MRI, MRA), cerebral angiogram, lumbar puncture, EEG, EMG; nonspecific brain imaging or laboratory tests

CT, computed tomography; *EEG,* electroencephalography; *EMG,* electromyography; *MRA,* magnetic resonance angiography; *MRI,* magnetic resonance imaging.

Table 61-5 Common Screening Assessment Questions to Determine Type of Headache

- When do the headaches occur?
- How frequent are the headaches?
- What is the duration of the headache(s)?
- Are there any known triggers for the headaches, such as environmental, foods, or alcohol?
- Where is the headache pain felt? Does the pain radiate?
- Are any visual changes such as blurring or diplopia experienced?
- Are any other symptoms experienced such as nausea, vomiting, dizziness, weakness, changes in speech, dysphagia?
- What relieves the headache pain?

PATIENT & CAREGIVER TEACHING GUIDE

Table 61-6 Headaches

1. Keep a diary or calendar of headaches and possible precipitating events.
2. Avoid factors that can trigger a headache:
   - Foods containing amines (cheese, chocolate), nitrites (meats such as hot dogs), vinegar, onions, or monosodium glutamate
   - Fermented or marinated foods
   - Caffeine
   - Nicotine
   - Ice cream
   - Alcohol (particularly red wine)
   - Emotional stress
   - Fatigue
   - Drugs such as those containing ergot and monoamine oxidase inhibitors
3. Describe purpose, action, dosage, and adverse effects of drugs taken.
4. Be able to self-administer sumatriptan (Imitrex) subcutaneously if prescribed.
5. Use stress-reduction techniques such as relaxation.
6. Participate in regular exercise.
7. Contact health care provider if the following occur:
   - Symptoms become more severe, last longer than usual, or are resistant to medication.
   - Nausea and vomiting (if severe or not typical), change in vision, or fever occurs with the headache.

EVIDENCE-INFORMED PRACTICE
Does Acupuncture Help Tension Headaches?

Clinical Question

For patients with tension-type headaches (P), does acupuncture (I) versus sham ("fake") treatment or routine care (C) decrease headaches (O) over 3 mo (T)?

Best Available Evidence

Systematic review of parallel groups design studies.

Critical Appraisal and Synthesis of Evidence

- 11 studies total ($n = 2317$). Six trials compared acupuncture with sham intervention with needles inserted at incorrect points or needles not penetrating the skin. One half of patients receiving true acupuncture reported a decrease in headache days by at least 50% compared with 41% in the sham acupuncture groups.
- Two trials compared acupuncture with acute headache treatment or routine care only. Approximately 47% of patients receiving acupuncture reported a decrease in headache days compared with 16% of patients in the control groups.
- Long-term effects of acupuncture on tension headache were not investigated.

Conclusion

- Acupuncture may decrease patient tension-type headache days over a 3-mo period.

Implications for Nursing Practice

- Patients with frequent tension headaches may have lower quality of life and ability to work productively.
- Counsel patients that acupuncture provided by licensed professionals may decrease tension headaches.

Reference for Evidence

Linde, K., Allais, G., Brinkhaus, B., Manheimer, E., Vickers, A., & White, A. R. (2009). Acupuncture for tension-type headache. *Cochrane Database Systemic Reviews*, 1, CD007587. doi:10.1002/14651858.CD007587

P, patient population of interest; *I*, intervention or area of interest; *C*, comparison of interest or comparison group; *O*, outcome(s) of interest; *T*, timing (see pp. 7-8).

drug. To prevent accidental overdose, the patient should make a written note of each dose of drug taken.

For the patient whose headaches are triggered by food, dietary counselling may be provided. The patient is encouraged to eliminate foods that may provoke headaches. Active challenge and provocative testing with specific foods may be necessary to determine the specific causative agents. However, food triggers may change over time. Patients should avoid smoking and exposure to triggers such as strong perfumes, volatile solvents, and gasoline fumes. CH attacks may occur at high altitudes with low oxygen levels, such as during air travel. Inhaled dihydroergotamine, taken before the plane takes off, may decrease the likelihood of these attacks. A teaching guide for the patient with a headache is presented in Table 61-6. The Evidence-Informed Practice box looks at evidence related to acupuncture for tension headache.

Evaluation

Expected outcomes for the patient with headache are addressed in the Nursing Care Plan "Patient With Headache" (eNCP 61-1 on the Evolve Web site for this chapter).

Chronic Neurological Disorders

Seizure Disorders and Epilepsy

Seizure is a paroxysmal, uncontrolled electrical discharge of neurons in the brain that interrupts normal function (Berg et al.,

2010). Seizures are often symptoms of an underlying illness. They may accompany a variety of disorders, or they may occur spontaneously without apparent cause. Seizures resulting from systemic and metabolic disturbances are not considered epilepsy if the seizures cease when the underlying problem is corrected. In the adult, metabolic disturbances that cause seizures include acidosis, electrolyte imbalances, hypoglycemia, hypoxia, alcohol and barbiturate withdrawal, dehydration, and water intoxication. Extracranial disorders that can cause seizures are heart, lung, liver, or kidney diseases; systemic lupus erythematosus; diabetes mellitus; hypertension; and septicemia.

Epilepsy is a condition in which a person has at least two spontaneous seizures more than 24 hours apart; it is caused by a chronic underlying pathology (Cavazos, 2012). Epilepsy affects approximately 0.6% of Canadians with 75 to 85% of people receiving a diagnosis before age 18. These individuals tend to have low levels of education, income, and employment (Epilepsy Canada, n.d. [a]). Epilepsy is more prevalent in the developing countries. The incidence rates are high during the first year of life, decline through childhood and adolescence, plateau in middle age, and rise sharply again among older adults.

Etiology and Pathophysiology

The most common causes of seizures during the first 6 months of life are severe birth injury, congenital defects involving the central nervous system (CNS), infections, and inborn errors of metabolism. In patients between 2 and 20 years of age, the primary causative factors are birth injury, infection, trauma, and genetic factors. In individuals between 20 and 30 years of age, seizure disorder usually occurs as the result of structural lesions, such as trauma, brain tumours, or vascular disease. After 50 years of age, the primary causes of seizure disorders are cerebrovascular lesions and metastatic brain tumours. Although many causes of seizure disorders have been identified, 70% of all seizure disorder cases cannot be attributed to a specific cause and are considered *idiopathic* (Epilepsy Canada, n.d. [a]).

The role of heredity in the etiology of seizure disorders has been difficult to determine because of the problem of separating hereditary from environmental or acquired influences. In addition, some families carry a predisposition to seizure disorders in the form of an inherently low threshold to seizure-producing stimuli, such as trauma, disease, and high fever. The etiology of recurring seizures (epilepsy) has long been attributed to a group of abnormal neurons (seizure focus) that seem to undergo spontaneous firing. This firing spreads by physiological pathways to involve adjacent or distant areas of the brain. If this activity spreads to involve the whole brain, a generalized seizure occurs. The factor responsible for this abnormal firing is not clear. Any stimulus that causes the cell membrane of the neuron to depolarize induces a tendency to spontaneous firing. Often, the area of the brain from which the epileptic activity arises is found to have scar tissue (gliosis). The scarring is thought to interfere with the normal chemical and structural environment of the brain neurons, making them more likely to fire abnormally. Because epilepsy results from long-lasting changes in the brain, a vigorous attempt must be made to control recurring seizures.

Previously, epilepsy research focused on neuronal causes. However, there is now evidence that astrocytes, or cerebral support cells, may play a key role in recurring seizures. Astrocytes release glutamate, which triggers synchronous firing of neurons. Therefore, drug therapy focused on suppressing astrocyte signalling or

Table 61-7 International Classification of Seizure Disorders	
Generalized Seizures (Nonfocal Origin) • Tonic–clonic seizures • Absence seizures • Myoclonic seizures • Tonic seizures • Atonic seizures • Clonic seizures	**Complex Partial Seizures (Impairment of Consciousness)** • Simple partial onset followed by impaired consciousness • Impairment of consciousness at onset • With automatisms
Partial Seizures (Focal Origin) **Simple Partial Seizures (No Impairment of Consciousness)** • With motor signs • With sensory symptoms • With autonomic symptoms • With psychic symptoms	**Partial Seizures Evolving to Secondary Generalized Seizures** ***Unclassified Epileptic Seizures*** • Epileptic spasms

Source: Adapted from Task Force on Epilepsy Classification and Treatment. (2011). *Epileptic seizure types and precipitating stimuli for reflex seizures.* Brussels: International League against Epilepsy. Retrieved from *http://www.ilae.org/Visitors/Centre/ctf/documents/ClassificationReport_2010_000.pdf*

decreasing glutamate release may be a mechanism to achieve seizure control (Jabs, Seifert, & Steinhauser, 2008).

Clinical Manifestations

The specific clinical manifestations of a seizure are determined by the site of the electrical disturbance. The preferred method of classifying recurring seizures is the International Classification System (Task Force on Epilepsy Classification and Terminology, 2011) (Table 61-7). This system is based on the clinical and electroencephalographic manifestations of seizures. In this system, seizures are divided into two major classes: *generalized* and *partial*. Depending on the type, a seizure may progress through several phases, which include (1) the *prodromal phase* with signs or activities that precede a seizure; (2) the *aural phase* with a sensory warning; (3) the *ictal phase* with full seizure; and (4) the *postictal phase*, which is the period of recovery after the seizure.

Generalized Seizures. *Generalized seizures* are characterized by bilateral synchronous epileptic discharges in the brain from the onset of the seizure. Because the entire brain is affected at the onset of the seizures, there is no warning or aura. In most cases, the patient loses consciousness for a few seconds to several minutes.

Tonic–Clonic Seizures. The most common generalized seizure is the generalized tonic–clonic seizure. *Tonic–clonic seizure* is characterized by loss of consciousness and falling to the ground if the patient is upright, followed by stiffening of the body (tonic phase) for 10 to 20 seconds and subsequent jerking of the extremities (clonic phase) for another 30 to 40 seconds. Cyanosis, excessive salivation, tongue or cheek biting, and incontinence may accompany the seizure.

In the postictal phase, the patient usually has muscle soreness, is very tired, and may sleep for several hours. Some patients may not feel normal for several hours or days after a seizure. The patient has no memory of the seizure.

Typical Absence Seizures. The *absence seizure* usually occurs only in children and rarely continues beyond adolescence. This type of seizure may cease altogether as the child matures, or it may evolve into another type of seizure. The typical clinical manifestation is a brief staring spell that lasts only a few seconds, so it often occurs unnoticed. There may be an extremely brief loss of consciousness. When untreated, the seizures may occur up to 100 times a day.

The electroencephalogram (EEG) demonstrates a 3-Hz (cycles/sec) spike-and-wave pattern that is unique to this type of seizure. Absence seizures can often be precipitated by hyperventilation and flashing lights.

Atypical Absence Seizures. Another type of generalized seizure is *atypical absence seizure*, which is characterized by a staring spell accompanied by other signs and symptoms, including brief warnings, peculiar behaviour during the seizure, or confusion after the seizure. The EEG demonstrates atypical spike-and-wave patterns, usually greater or less than 3 Hz.

Other Types of Generalized Seizures. Other generalized seizures are myoclonic, atonic, tonic, and clonic seizures. A *myoclonic seizure* is characterized by a sudden, excessive jerk of the body or the extremities. The jerk may be forceful enough to hurl the person to the ground. These seizures are very brief and may occur in clusters.

An *atonic* ("drop attack") *seizure* involves either a tonic episode or a paroxysmal loss of muscle tone and begins suddenly with the person falling to the ground. Consciousness usually returns by the time the person hits the ground, and normal activity can be resumed immediately. Patients with this type of seizure are at a great risk of head injury and often have to wear protective helmets. A tonic seizure involves a sudden onset of sustained increased tone in the extensor muscles. These patients often fall. Clonic seizures begin with loss of consciousness and sudden loss of muscle tone, followed by limb jerking that may or may not be symmetrical.

Partial Seizures. *Partial seizures* are the other major class of seizures in the International Classification System. They are also referred to as *partial focal seizures* and are caused by focal irritations. They present with unilateral manifestations that arise from localized brain involvement. Partial seizures begin in a specific region of the cortex, as indicated by the EEG and usually by the clinical manifestations. For example, if the discharging focus is located in the medial aspect of the postcentral gyrus, the patient may experience paresthesias and tingling or numbness in the leg on the side opposite the focus. If the discharging focus is located in the part of the brain that governs a particular function, sensory, motor, cognitive, or emotional manifestations may occur.

Partial seizures may be confined to one side of the brain and remain partial or focal in nature, or they may spread to involve the entire brain, culminating in a generalized tonic–clonic seizure. Any tonic–clonic seizure that is preceded by an aura or warning is a partial seizure that generalizes secondarily. Many tonic–clonic seizures that appear to be generalized from the outset may actually be secondary generalized seizures, but the preceding partial component may be so brief that it is undetected by the patient, by the observer, or even on the EEG. Unlike the primary generalized tonic–clonic seizure, the secondary generalized seizure may result in a transient residual neurological deficit postictally. This is called *Todd's paralysis* (focal weakness), which resolves after varying lengths of time.

Partial seizures are further divided into (1) simple partial seizures (those with simple motor or sensory phenomena) and (2) complex partial seizures (those with complex symptoms).

Simple Partial Seizures. *Simple partial seizures* with elementary symptoms do not involve loss of consciousness and rarely last longer than 1 minute. They may involve motor, sensory, or autonomic phenomena or a combination of these. The terms *focal motor, focal sensory,* and *jacksonian* have been used to describe seizures of the simple partial type.

Complex Partial Seizures. This type of seizure can involve a variety of behavioural, emotional, affective, and cognitive functions. The location of the discharging focus is usually in the temporal lobe, hence the term *temporal lobe seizure*. These seizures usually last longer than 1 minute and are frequently followed by a period of postictal confusion. Complex partial seizures are distinct from simple partial (focal motor, focal sensory) seizures in that they involve alterations in consciousness. The sole manifestation of complex partial seizures may be clouding of consciousness or a confused state without any motor or sensory components. This type of attack is sometimes termed *temporal lobe absence*. There is rarely the complete loss of consciousness that is typical of the generalized absence attack, nor does the patient snap back to the preseizure state as does the patient who has had a generalized absence attack.

The most common complex partial seizure involves lip smacking and *automatisms* (repetitive movements that may not be appropriate). These are often called *psychomotor seizures*. The patient may continue an activity that was initiated before the seizure, such as counting out change or picking items from a grocery shelf, but after the seizure does not remember the activity performed during the seizure. Other automatisms are less organized, such as picking at clothing, fumbling with objects (real or imaginary), or simply walking away.

A variety of psychosensory symptoms may occur during a complex partial seizure, including distortions of visual or auditory sensations and vertigo. There may be alterations in memory, such as a feeling of having experienced an event before (déjà vu), or alterations in thought processes. Alterations in sexual functioning can vary from hyposexuality to hypersexuality. Many patients with temporal lobe seizures have decreased sexual drive or erectile dysfunction. However, some may experience sexual sensations during their seizures. This is because the abnormal electrical activity arises from the brain centres responsible for these sensations. Some experience increased sexual drive just after a seizure. In addition, some antiseizure drugs can cause a decrease in sexual drive because of sedation. Others can cause erectile dysfunction.

Complications

Physical. **Status epilepticus** is a state of continuous seizure activity or a condition in which seizures recur in rapid succession without return to consciousness between seizures. Status epilepticus is a neurological emergency and can involve any type of seizure. During repeated seizures, the brain uses more energy than can be supplied. Permanent brain damage may result. Tonic–clonic status epilepticus is the most dangerous because it can cause ventilatory insufficiency, hypoxemia, cardiac dysrhythmias, hyperthermia, and systemic acidosis, all of which can be fatal. An airway may need to be secured with medical intervention using sedation and endotracheal intubation if necessary to avoid some of these life-threatening complications. Another complication of seizures is severe injury and even death from trauma suffered during a seizure. Patients who lose consciousness during a seizure are at greatest risk. Death can result from head injury incurred in a fall, from drowning, or from severe burns. Seizures occurring throughout pregnancy or during delivery may also pose potential complications to a pregnant woman and her baby (Beghi, 2007).

Psychosocial. Seizure disorders place many limitations on a patient's lifestyle. Epilepsy carries a social stigma because the characteristics of seizures are in conflict with societal values of self-control and independence. Patients diagnosed with seizure disorders may suffer depression, anxiety, or anger, and relationships are often affected. The patient with epilepsy may experience discrimination in employment and educational opportunities. Transportation may be difficult because of legal sanctions against driving, which may require the patient to be seizure free for 6 months before reinstating the licence (Epilepsy Canada, n.d. [a]).

Rates of depression are significantly higher in people with epilepsy than in the general population (Tellez-Zenteno, Patten, Jetté, Williams, & Wiebe, 2007). Not only can depression impair daily functioning, but it can also lead to increased seizure frequency through sleep deprivation and through its role as an emotional stressor. Treatment for depression among epilepsy patients should focus first on seizure control, and if depression persists in spite of good seizure control, antidepressant medication and psychological therapy may be necessary (McLaughlin & McFarland, 2011).

Diagnostic Studies

The most useful diagnostic tools are accurate and comprehensive description of the seizures and the patient's health history (Table 61-8). The EEG is a useful diagnostic adjuvant to the history but only if it shows abnormalities. Abnormal findings help determine the type of seizure and help pinpoint the seizure focus. Unfortunately, only a small percentage of patients with seizure disorders have abnormal findings on the EEG the first time the test is done. EEGs may need to be repeated often, or continuous EEG monitoring may be needed to detect abnormalities. Abnormal discharges may not occur during the 30 to 40 minutes of sampling during EEG, and the test may never indicate an abnormality. It is not a definitive test because some patients who do not have seizure disorders have abnormal patterns on their EEGs, whereas many patients with seizure disorders have normal EEGs between seizures. Magnetoencephalography may be done in conjunction with the EEG. This test has greater sensitivity in detecting small magnetic fields generated by neuronal activity. Video-EEG can give definitive diagnosis of seizures with impairment of consciousness.

A complete blood count, serum chemistries, studies of liver and kidney function, and urinalysis should be done to rule out metabolic disorders. A CT or MRI scan should be done in any new-onset seizure to rule out structural abnormalities (Cavazos,

COLLABORATIVE CARE

Table 61-8 Diagnosis of Seizure Disorders and Epilepsy

History and Physical Examination	Diagnostic Studies
• Birth and development history • Significant illnesses and injuries • Family history • Febrile seizures • Comprehensive neurological assessment	• CBC, urinalysis, electrolytes, creatinine, fasting blood glucose • Lumbar puncture • CT, MRI, MRA, MRS, PET scan • EEG
Seizure History	**Collaborative Therapy**
• Precipitating factors • Antecedent events • Seizure description (including onset, duration, frequency, postictal state)	• Antiseizure drugs (see Table 61-10) • Surgery (see Table 61-11) • Vagal nerve stimulation • Psychosocial counselling

CBC, complete blood count; *CT*, computed tomography; *EEG*, electroencephalography; *MRA*, magnetic resonance angiography; *MRI*, magnetic resonance imaging; *MRS*, magnetic resonance spectroscopy; *PET*, positron emission tomography.

2012). Cerebral angiography, single-photon emission computed tomography, magnetic resonance spectroscopy, magnetic resonance angiography, and positron emission tomography may be used in selected situations.

Collaborative Care

Most seizures do not require professional emergency medical care because they are self-limiting and rarely cause bodily injury. However, if status epilepticus occurs, if significant bodily harm occurs, or if the event is a first-time seizure, medical care should be sought immediately. Table 61-9 summarizes emergency care of the patient with a generalized tonic–clonic seizure, the seizure most likely to warrant professional emergency medical care. The diagnostic studies and collaborative care of seizure disorders are summarized in Table 61-8.

Drug Therapy. Seizure disorders are treated primarily with antiseizure drugs (Table 61-10). Therapy is aimed at preventing seizures because a cure is not possible. Drugs generally act by stabilizing nerve cell membranes and preventing spread of the epileptic discharge. Antiseizure medications offer control in about 50% of patients. Some 30% of patients have reduction in seizure intensity, 30% have a reduction in both intensity and frequency of seizures, and 20% of patients have seizures that are resistant to medication (Epilepsy Ontario, 2011). The primary goal of antiseizure drug therapy is to obtain maximum seizure control with minimal toxic adverse effects. The principle of drug therapy is to begin with a single drug and increase the dosage until seizures are controlled or toxic adverse effects occur (Epilepsy Foundation, 2010). Serum levels of the drug should be monitored if seizures continue to occur, if seizure frequency increases, or if drug compliance is questioned. The therapeutic range for each drug indicates the serum level above which most patients experience toxic adverse effects and below which most continue to have seizures. Therapeutic ranges are only guides for therapy. If the patient's seizures are well controlled with a subtherapeutic level, the drug dose need not be increased. Likewise,

EMERGENCY MANAGEMENT
Table 61-9 Tonic–Clonic Seizures

ETIOLOGY	ASSESSMENT FINDINGS	INTERVENTIONS
Head Trauma	• Aura—peculiar sensations that precede seizure	**Initial**
• Epidural hematoma	• Loss of consciousness	• Ensure patent airway (sedation may be required if teeth are clenched).
• Subdural hematoma	• Bowel and bladder incontinence	• Apply oxygen as needed.
• Intracranial hematoma	• Tachycardia	• Assist ventilations if patient does not breathe spontaneously after seizure. Anticipate need for intubation if gag reflex absent.
• Cerebral contusion	• Diaphoresis	
• Traumatic birth injury	• Warm skin	
Drug-Related Processes	• Pallor, flushing, or cyanosis	• Suction as needed.
• Overdose	• *Tonic phase:* continuous muscle contractions	• Stay with patient until seizure has passed.
• Withdrawal of alcohol, opioids, antiseizure drugs	• *Hypertonic phase:* extreme muscular rigidity lasting 5-15 sec	• Ensure safety at all times and protect patient from injury during seizure. *Do not restrain.* Pad side rails.
• Ingestion, inhalation	• *Clonic phase:* rigidity and relaxation alternate in rapid succession	• Establish IV access.
Infectious Processes	• *Postictal phase:* lethargy, altered level of consciousness	• Anticipate administration of phenobarbital, phenytoin (Dilantin), or benzodiazepines (diazepam [Valium], midazolam [Versed], lorazepam [Ativan]) to control seizures.
• Meningitis	• Confusion and headache	
• Septicemia	• Repeated tonic–clonic seizures for several minutes	• Reposition to side lying position when possible to avoid aspiration if patient vomits.
• Encephalitis		• Remove or loosen tight clothing.
Intracranial Events		**Ongoing Monitoring**
• Brain tumour		• Monitor vital signs, level of consciousness, oxygen saturation, Glasgow Coma Scale, pupil size and reactivity.
• Subarachnoid hemorrhage		
• Stroke		• Reassure and orient the patient after seizure.
• Neurodegenerative diseases		• Never force an airway between a patient's clenched teeth.
• Hypertensive crisis		
• Increased ICP secondary to clogged shunt		• Give IV dextrose for hypoglycemia.
Metabolic Imbalances		
• Fluid and electrolyte imbalance		
• Hypoglycemia		
Medical Disorders		
• Heart, liver, lung, or kidney disease		
• Systemic lupus erythematosus		
Other		
• Cardiac arrest		
• Idiopathic		
• Psychiatric disorders		
• High fever		
• Autoimmune disease		
• Genetic diseases		

ICP, intracranial pressure; *IV*, intravenous.

if a drug level is above the therapeutic range and the patient has good seizure control without toxic adverse effects, the drug dose need not be decreased. Many of the newer drugs do not require drug-level monitoring because the therapeutic range is very large. If seizure control is not achieved with a single drug, the drug dosage or the timing of administration may be changed, or a second drug may be added. About one third of patients require a combination regimen for adequate control (Epilepsy Foundation, 2010). Another consideration that is important when evaluating antiseizure medication is the various hormonal fluctuations in females during puberty, menses, pregnancy, and menopause.

For many years, the primary drugs for treatment of generalized tonic–clonic and partial seizures were sodium channel blockers. Barbiturates, such as phenobarbital, also have a long history of use. Both sodium channel blockers and benzodiazapines are effective in the treatment of absence, akinetic, and myoclonic seizures.

Treatment of status epilepticus requires immediate initiation of a rapid-acting antiseizure drug that can be given intravenously. The drugs most commonly used are lorazepam (Ativan) and diazepam (Valium). Because these are short-acting drugs, they must be followed by administration of long-acting drugs such as phenytoin or phenobarbital (Epilepsy Ontario, 2011).

Table 61-10 Epilepsy

PRODUCT NAME (GENERIC NAME)	AVERAGE ADULT DAILY DOSAGE	POSSIBLE ADVERSE EFFECTS
Depakene (valproic acid)	1750-3000 mg	Upset stomach, altered bleeding time, liver toxicity
Dilantin (phenytoin)	300 mg	Clumsiness, drowsiness, nausea, rash, gum overgrowth, hairiness, thickening of features
Epival (divalproex sodium)	1750-3000 mg	Upset stomach, altered bleeding time, liver toxicity (rare), hair loss, weight gain, tremor
Frisium (clobazam)	30-40 mg	Drowsiness, dizziness, fatigue
Keppra (levetiracetam)	1000-3000 mg	Dizziness, somnolence, asthenia (weakness), low hematocrit and leukocyte count (rare), depression and mood swings
Lamictal (lamotrigine)	100-500 mg	Headache, fatigue, nausea, dizziness, clumsiness, serious and life-threatening rash (rare), double or blurred vision
Primidone (primidone)	250-1000 mg	Clumsiness, dizziness, appetite loss, fatigue, drowsiness, hyperirritability
Neurontin (gabapentin)	900-2400 mg	Somnolence, fatigue, dizziness
Phenobarbital (phenobarbital)	30-600 mg	Drowsiness, irritability, hyperactivity, somnolence
Rivotril (clonazepam)	8-10 mg	Drowsiness, clumsiness, behaviour, changes, tremor, appetite loss
Sabril (vigabatrin)	1000-4000 mg	Drowsiness, weight gain, headache, dizziness, decreased peripheral vision, depression
Topamax (topiramate)	200-600 mg	Drowsiness, dizziness, weight loss, tingling, decreased alertness, kidney stones (rare)
Tegretol (carbamazepine)	800-1200 mg	Dizziness, drowsiness, blurred or double vision, nausea, skin rashes, blood abnormalities
Trileptal (oxcarbazepine)	1200-2400 mg	Somnolence, diplopia, rash, hyponatremia, ataxia and staggering gait
Zarontin (ethosuximide)	500 mg	Appetite loss, nausea, drowsiness, headache, dizziness, fatigue

Source: Adapted from Epilepsy Canada. (1987 [revised 2009]). *Your medication for epilepsy* (pp. 12-13). Toronto: Author. Retrieved from *http://www.epilepsy.ca/App_UserFiles/pdfs/medication-new.pdf*

Current drugs used in seizure management are shown in Table 61-10. Because many of these drugs (e.g., phenytoin, phenobarbital, ethosuximide, lamotrigine, topiramate) have a long half-life, they can be given in once- or twice-daily doses. This increases the patient's compliance with taking the drug by simplifying the drug regimen and avoiding the need to take it at work or school. Antiseizure drugs should not be discontinued abruptly because this can precipitate seizures or status epilepticus and can be life threatening (Epilepsy Canada, n.d. [b]).

Adverse effects of antiseizure drugs primarily involve the CNS and include diplopia, drowsiness, ataxia, and mental slowing. Neurological assessment for dose-related toxicity involves testing the eyes for nystagmus, hand and gait coordination, cognitive functioning, and general alertness.

Idiosyncratic adverse effects involve organs outside the CNS, including skin (rashes), gingiva (hyperplasia), bone marrow (blood dyscrasias), liver, and kidneys. Nurses should be knowledgeable about these adverse effects so that patients can be informed and proper treatment can be instituted. A common adverse effect of phenytoin is gingival hyperplasia (excessive growth of gingival tissue), especially in children and young adults. This can be limited by good dental hygiene, including regular tooth brushing and flossing. If gingival hyperplasia is extensive, the hyperplastic tissue may have to be surgically removed (gingivectomy), and phenytoin may have to be replaced by another drug. Because phenytoin can also cause hirsutism in young people, other drugs are often used first.

Medication nonadherence can be a problem in persons with epilepsy owing to the aforementioned adverse effects. Therefore, measures should be taken to increase patient education and adherence to the prescribed drug regimens. If made aware of the issue, health care providers can work with the patient to find an

Table 61-11 Surgical Procedures for Seizure Disorders and Epilepsy

TYPE OF SEIZURE	SURGICAL PROCEDURE	RESULTS
Complex partial seizure of temporal lobe origin	Resectioning of epileptogenic tissue	Absence of seizures 5 yr postoperatively in 55-70% of patients
Partial seizures of frontal lobe origin	Resectioning of epileptogenic tissue (if in resectable area)	Absence of seizures 5 yr postoperatively in 30-50% of patients
Generalized seizures (Lennox-Gastaut syndrome or drop attacks)	Sectioning of corpus callosum	Persistence of seizures; less violent, less frequent, less disabling events
Intractable unilateral multifocal epilepsy associated with infantile hemiplegia	Hemispherectomy or callosotomy	Reduction in seizure frequency and type, improvement in behaviour

acceptable drug regimen to prevent many of these undesirable adverse effects.

Surgical Therapy. A significant number of patients whose epilepsy cannot be controlled with drug therapy are candidates for surgical intervention to remove the epileptic focus or prevent spread of epileptic activity in the brain (Table 61-11). Surgical interventions include limbic resection, primarily anterior temporal lobe resection; amygdalohippocampectomy; neocortical resection, including extratemporal resection and lesionectomies; hemispherectomies; multilobar resections; and corpus callosum sections (Elger & Schmidt, 2008).

The benefits of surgery include cessation or reduction in frequency of the seizures, but not all types of epilepsy benefit from surgery. An extensive preoperative evaluation is important, including continuous EEG monitoring and other specific tests to ensure precise localization of the focal point. Before surgery is performed, three requirements must be met: (1) the diagnosis of epilepsy must be confirmed; (2) there must have been an adequate trial with drug therapy without satisfactory results; and (3) the electroclinical syndrome (type of seizure disorder) must be defined.

Alternate Therapies. Another treatment for seizure disorders is vagal nerve stimulation. An electrode is surgically placed around the left vagus nerve in the neck. It is connected to a battery placed beneath the skin in the upper chest. The device is programmed to deliver intermittent electrical stimulation to the brain to reduce the frequency and intensity of seizures. The exact mechanism of action is unknown, although it is believed that the stimulation may interrupt synchronization of epileptic brainwave activity. This method is currently used in only a small number of patients (Ramani, 2008).

Among pediatric patients, a ketogenic diet may help to control epilepsy. This is a high-fat, low-protein, and low-carbohydrate diet that has been shown to reduce the incidence of seizure activity by 90% in some individuals (Groesbeck, Bluml, & Kossoff, 2006). The exact mechanism of action is unknown, although patients on this diet need to be monitored closely for signs and symptoms of bleeding if on anticoagulant therapy (Elger & Schmidt, 2008). Studies exploring the effectiveness of ketogenic diets among adults have been rare and inconclusive.

NURSING MANAGEMENT: SEIZURE DISORDERS AND EPILEPSY

■ Nursing Assessment

Subjective and objective data that should be obtained from a patient with a seizure disorder are presented in Table 61-12. Data related to a specific seizure episode can be obtained from a witness.

■ Nursing Diagnoses

Nursing diagnoses for the patient with seizure disorders and epilepsy may include, but are not limited to, those presented in Nursing Care Plan (NCP) 61-1.

NURSING ASSESSMENT

Table 61-12 Seizure Disorders and Epilepsy

Subjective Data	**Cardiovascular**
Important Health Information	Hypertension, tachycardia or bradycardia (ictal)
Past health history: Previous seizures, birth defects, or injuries; anoxic episodes; CNS trauma, tumours, or infections; stroke; metabolic disorders; alcoholism; exposure to metals and carbon monoxide; hepatic or renal failure; fever; pregnancy; systemic lupus erythematosus; positive family history of seizure disorders or epilepsy	**Gastrointestinal**
	Bowel incontinence; excessive salivation
	Urinary
	Incontinence
Medications: Compliance with antiseizure medications; barbiturate or alcohol withdrawal; use of cocaine, amphetamines, lidocaine, theophylline, penicillin, lithium, phenothiazines, tricyclic antidepressants, benzodiazepines	**Neurological**
	Generalized
	Tonic–clonic: Loss of consciousness, muscle tightening, then jerking; dilated pupils; hyperventilation, then apnea; postictal somnolence
Symptoms	*Absence:* Altered consciousness (5-30 sec), minor facial motor activity
• Headaches, aura, mood or behavioural changes before seizure; mentation changes; abdominal pain, muscle pain (postictal)	**Partial**
• Anxiety, depression; loss of self-esteem, social isolation	*Simple:* Aura; consciousness; focal sensory, motor, cognitive, or emotional phenomena (focal motor); unilateral "marching" motor seizure (jacksonian)
• Decreased sexual drive, erectile dysfunction; increased sexual drive (postictal)	*Complex:* Altered consciousness with inappropriate behaviours, automatisms, amnesia of event
Objective Data	**Musculoskeletal**
General	Weakness, paralysis, ataxia (postictal)
Precipitating factors, including severe metabolic acidosis or alkalosis, hyperkalemia, hypoglycemia, dehydration, or water intoxication	**Possible Findings**
Integumentary	Positive toxicology screen or alcohol level; altered serum electrolytes, acidosis or alkalosis, very low blood glucose level, ↑ blood urea nitrogen or creatinine, liver function tests, ammonia; abnormal CT scan or MRI of head, abnormal findings from lumbar puncture; abnormal discharges on EEG
Bitten tongue, soft tissue damage, cyanosis, diaphoresis (postictal)	
Respiratory	
Abnormal respiratory rate, rhythm, or depth; apnea (ictal); absent or abnormal breath sounds, possible airway occlusion	

CNS, central nervous system; *CT,* computed tomography; *EEG,* electroencephalography; *MRI,* magnetic resonance imaging.

NURSING CARE PLAN 61-1

Seizure Disorder or Epilepsy

NURSING DIAGNOSIS	*Ineffective breathing pattern* related to neuromuscular impairment secondary to prolonged tonic phase of seizure or during postictal period *as evidenced by* abnormal respiratory rate, rhythm, or depth
Expected Patient Outcome	**Nursing Interventions and *Rationales***
• Maintains appropriate rate, rhythm, and depth of respirations	• Loosen constrictive clothing *to avoid restricting breathing.* • Assess and document breathing pattern, observing for laboured respiration, tachypnea, bradypnea, dyspnea, and apnea *to determine presence and extent of problem and to initiate appropriate interventions.* • Provide manual ventilation or O₂ when necessary; be prepared to assist with endotracheal intubation *to maintain adequate oxygenation and prevent hypoxia.* • Only after seizure activity has ceased, insert oral airway (if indicated) *to prevent mouth and teeth injury from forcing airway between clamped teeth.*
NURSING DIAGNOSIS	*Risk for injury* related to seizure activity and subsequent impaired physical mobility secondary to postictal weakness or paralysis
Expected Patient Outcomes	**Nursing Interventions and *Rationales***
• Remains free of injury • Verbalizes knowledge of potential for injury during seizure • Arranges environment to minimize risk for injury	• Assess for trauma to mouth, cheek, tongue, lips; abrasions, bruises; broken bones; or burns *because these injuries may occur during seizure activity.* • Assess for weakness, paralysis of one side of body, ataxia, fatigue, and lethargy as potential postictal risks for injury *to plan appropriate interventions.* • If patient anticipates that a seizure may occur, assist to a safe location or position; use seizure precautions as appropriate; remove potentially harmful objects from surrounding area; guide and protect head, arm, or leg movements *to prevent injury during a seizure.* • Refrain from moving or restraining patient during a seizure *to prevent bone or soft tissue injury.* • Assist in determining whether operation of a motor vehicle or dangerous machinery is appropriate for patient *to assist patient in making the appropriate choice about driving.*
NURSING DIAGNOSIS	*Ineffective coping* related to perceived loss of control and denial of diagnosis *as evidenced by* verbalizations about not having epilepsy, lack of truth-telling regarding seizure frequency, noncompliant behaviour
Expected Patient Outcomes	**Nursing Interventions and *Rationales***
• Accepts disorder as evidenced by using the words *seizure disorder or epilepsy* to describe illness • Acknowledges that a seizure has occurred	• Explore reasons for denial *to determine extent of problem and to plan appropriate interventions.* • Implement and individualize teaching plan about causes and mechanisms of seizures, effectiveness of drugs in controlling seizures, inaccuracy of myths about epilepsy, avoidance of precipitating factors, provincial/territorial laws regarding driving, pros and cons of medical identification tags, moderation in drinking and eating, exposure to stress, and avoidance of hazardous activities *to promote effective coping by providing correct information.*
NURSING DIAGNOSIS	*Ineffective self-health management* related to lack of knowledge about management of seizure disorder *as evidenced by* verbalization of lack of knowledge, inaccurate perception of health status, noncompliance with prescribed health behaviour
Expected Patient Outcomes	**Nursing Interventions and *Rationales***
• Maintains therapeutic drug levels of antiseizure medication • Complies with therapeutic regimen	• Provide teaching to patient and family about seizure activity and therapeutic management including diagnosis, treatment, lifestyle adjustments, and community resources *so that patient and family can make necessary lifestyle modifications to manage a chronic disease.*

Planning

The overall goals are that the patient with seizures will (1) be free from injury during a seizure, (2) have optimal mental and physical functioning while taking antiseizure drugs, and (3) have satisfactory psychosocial functioning.

Nursing Implementation

Health Promotion

Many cases of seizure disorders can be prevented by promotion of general safety measures, such as the wearing of helmets in situations involving risk of head injury. Improved perinatal, labour, and delivery care have reduced fetal trauma and hypoxia and thus have reduced brain damage leading to seizure disorders.

The patient with a seizure disorder should practise good general health habits. The patient should be helped to identify events or situations that precipitate the seizures and should be given suggestions for avoiding them or handling them better. Excessive alcohol intake, fatigue, and loss of sleep should be avoided, and the patient should be helped to handle stress constructively.

■ Acute Intervention

The nurse caring for a hospitalized patient with a seizure disorder or a patient who has had seizures as a result of metabolic factors involves several responsibilities, including observation and treatment of the seizure, education, and psychosocial intervention.

When a seizure occurs, the nurse should carefully observe and record details of the event because the diagnosis and subsequent treatment often rest solely on the seizure description. All aspects of the seizure should be noted. What events preceded the seizure? When did the seizure occur? How long did each phase (aural [if any], ictal, postictal) last? What occurred during each phase?

Both subjective data (usually the only type of data in the aural phase) and objective data are important. Objective data should include the exact time of seizure onset; the course and nature of the seizure activity (loss of consciousness, tongue biting, automatisms, stiffening, jerking, total lack of muscle tone); the body parts involved and their sequence of involvement; and the presence of autonomic signs, such as dilated pupils, excessive salivation, altered breathing, cyanosis, flushing, diaphoresis, or incontinence. Assessment of the postictal period should include a detailed description of level of consciousness, vital signs, memory loss, muscle soreness, speech disorders (aphasia, dysarthria), weakness or paralysis, sleep period, and the duration of each sign or symptom.

During the seizure, it is important to maintain a patent airway. This may involve supporting and protecting the head, turning the patient to the side, loosening constrictive clothing, or easing the patient to a lying position on the floor, if seated. The patient should not be restrained, and no objects should be placed in the mouth. After the seizure, the patient may require suctioning, and oxygen may be needed.

A seizure can be a frightening experience for the patient and for others who may witness it. The nurse should assess the level of their understanding and provide information about how and why the event occurred. This is an excellent opportunity for the nurse to dispel many common misconceptions about seizures.

■ Ambulatory and Home Care

Prevention of recurring seizures is the major goal in the treatment of epilepsy. Because many seizure disorders cannot be cured, drugs must be taken regularly, often for life. The nurse should ensure that the patient knows this as well as the specifics of the drug regimen and what to do if a dose is missed. Usually, the dose should be made up if the omission is remembered within 24 hours. The patient should be cautioned not to adjust drug doses without professional guidance because this can increase seizure frequency and even cause status epilepticus. The patient should be encouraged to report any adverse effects and to keep regular appointments with a health care provider.

Nurses play an important role in teaching the patient and caregivers. Guidelines for teaching are shown in Table 61-13. Nurses should teach family members and significant others the emergency management of tonic–clonic seizures (see Table 61-9). They should be reminded that it is not necessary to call an ambulance or send a person to the hospital after a single seizure unless it is the first seizure, it is prolonged, it is immediately followed by another seizure, or extensive injury has occurred.

Patients with a seizure disorder also experience concerns or fears related to recurrent seizures, incontinence, and loss of self-control. The nurse provides support for the patient through education and by helping to identify coping mechanisms.

Perhaps the greatest challenge that a seizure disorder presents to the patient is adjusting to the personal limitations imposed by the illness. Discrimination in employment is the most serious problem facing the person with a seizure disorder. For issues relating to job discrimination, patients can be referred to the Canadian Human Rights Commission through its national or regional offices.

A variety of other resources can be offered to the patient with a seizure disorder who has a specific problem. The patient should be informed that medical alert bracelets, necklaces, and identification cards are available through a number of North American companies specializing in identification devices (e.g., MedicAlert; see Figure 52-11). If the nurse believes that associating with others who have a seizure disorder would be beneficial, the patient can be referred to Epilepsy Canada, a voluntary agency with local members' associations across the country that offer a variety of services to patients with epilepsy. Patients who are eligible veterans can be referred to the Veterans Affairs Canada Health-Care Program to explore services for which they may qualify.

PATIENT & CAREGIVER TEACHING GUIDE

Table 61-13 Seizure Disorders and Epilepsy

The patient should be taught about the following:

1. Drugs must be taken as prescribed. Any and all adverse effects of drugs should be reported to the health care provider. When necessary, blood work may be drawn to ensure that therapeutic drug levels are maintained.

2. Use of nonpharmacological techniques, such as diet and biofeedback training, to potentially reduce the number of seizures.

3. Availability of resources in the community.

4. Need to wear a medical alert bracelet or necklace and carry an identification card.

5. Avoidance of excessive alcohol intake, fatigue, and loss of sleep.

6. Regular meals and snacks in between if feeling shaky, faint, or hungry.

Caregivers should be taught the following:

1. For first aid treatment of tonic–clonic seizure, it is not necessary to call an ambulance or send the patient to the hospital after a single seizure unless the seizure is prolonged, another seizure immediately follows, or extensive injury has occurred.

2. During an acute seizure, it is important to protect the patient from injury. This may involve supporting and protecting the head, turning the patient to the side, loosening constrictive clothing, and easing the patient to a lying position on the floor, if seated.

Social workers and welfare agencies can help with financial problems and living arrangements. Provincial services for individuals with developmental disabilities include assistance with job training and placement for patients whose seizures are not well controlled. Sheltered housing and funding for special needs, such as medical and psychological evaluation and transportation, are also offered. Provincial agencies specializing in vocational rehabilitation services can offer vocational assessment, counselling, funding for training, and assistance with job placement. They can also offer financial assistance for transportation and medical costs that are necessary for vocational rehabilitation or job maintenance. If intensive psychological counselling is needed, the nurse can refer the patient to a community mental health centre.

The patient should be encouraged to learn more about epilepsy through self-education materials. Epilepsy Canada provides information pamphlets and may facilitate support groups. Many agencies that offer services to epileptic patients, as well as many locally based epilepsy associations, have these available.

▪ Evaluation

Expected outcomes for the patient with seizures are addressed in NCP 61-1.

Multiple Sclerosis

Multiple sclerosis (MS) is a chronic, progressive, degenerative, autoimmune disorder of the CNS characterized by disseminated demyelination of nerve fibres of the brain, the spinal cord, and the optic nerves. Canadians have one of the highest rates of MS in the world and an estimated 55,000 to 75,000 Canadians have MS. Across the country, prevalence rates range from 1 MS case per 500 people to 1 in 1000. More than three Canadians a day are diagnosed with MS (Multiple Sclerosis Society of Canada, 2011). On a global scale (Figure 61-2), MS has relatively high prevalence rates (>30 cases/100,000 people) in areas with temperate climates (like those found in large areas of Europe including Russia, Canada, northern United States, southeastern Australia, and New Zealand), and relatively low prevalence rates (<5 cases/100,000 people) in warmer climates (like those found in large areas of Asia, Africa, and northern South America) (Multiple Sclerosis International Federation, 2008). MS is considered a disease of young to middle-aged adults, with the onset usually being between 15 and 50 years of age. Women are affected more often than men with a ratio of 3 : 1 (Multiple Sclerosis Society of Canada, 2011). The variations in incidence of MS suggest that geography, ethnicity, and other factors interact in a very complex way to cause MS (National Multiple Sclerosis Society, n.d.). Chao and colleagues (2011) suggest that MS may be triggered by environmental factors in individuals with genetic susceptibility seen more commonly in females.

Etiology and Pathophysiology

The cause of MS is unknown, although research findings suggest that MS may be related to environmental and infectious (viral) factors, dietary deficiencies (vitamin D deficiency), and immunological and genetic factors and is perpetuated as a result of intrinsic factors (e.g., faulty immunoregulation) (Cohen, 2007). The susceptibility to MS appears to be inherited. First-, second-, and third-degree relatives of patients with MS are at a slightly increased risk. Multiple genes confer susceptibility to MS (Chao et al., 2011; Herrera et al., 2007).

The role of precipitating factors, such as exposure to pathogenic agents, in the etiology of MS is controversial. It is possible that their association with MS is random and that there is no cause-and-effect relationship. Possible precipitating factors include infection, trauma, emotional stress, excessive fatigue, pregnancy, and a state of poor health.

MS is characterized by chronic inflammation, demyelination, and gliosis (scarring) in the CNS. The primary neuropathological

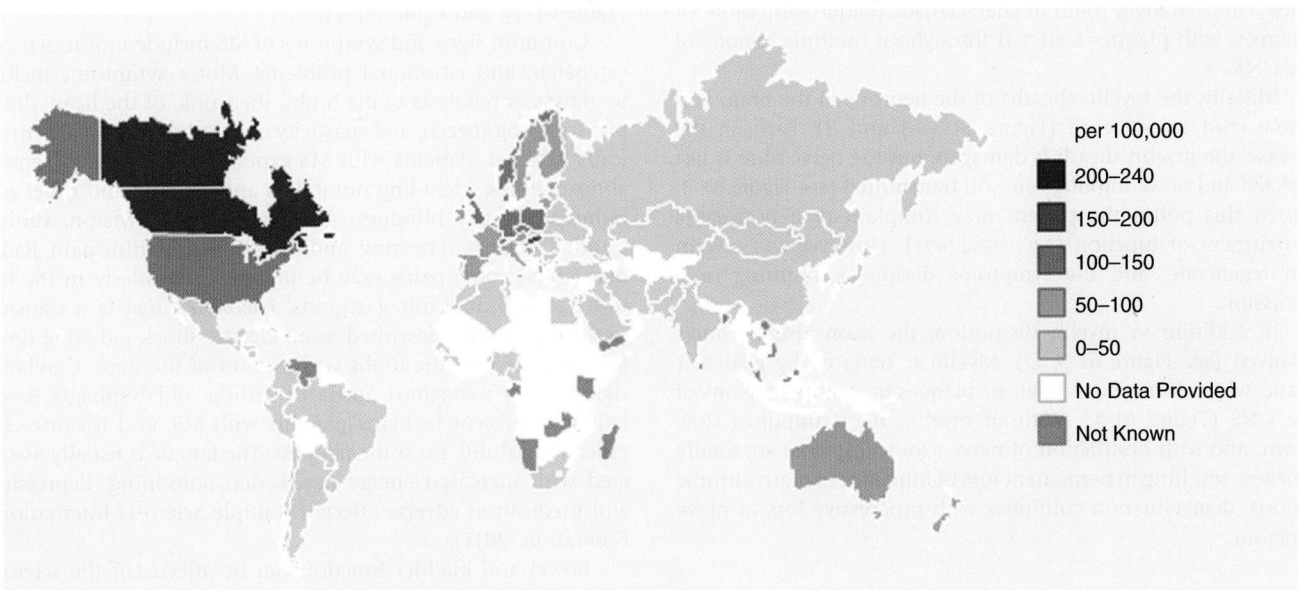

Figure 61-2 Prevalence of multiple sclerosis around the world.

Source: Multiple Sclerosis International Federation. (2008). Retrieved from *http://www.atlasofms.org/query.aspx*. Reprinted with permission.

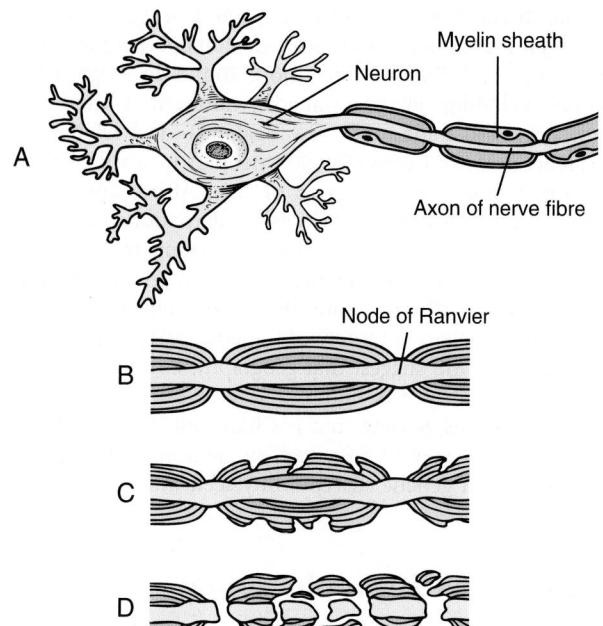

Figure 61-3 Pathogenesis of multiple sclerosis. **A,** Normal nerve cell with myelin sheath. **B,** Normal axon. **C,** Myelin breakdown. **D,** Myelin totally disrupted; axon not functioning.

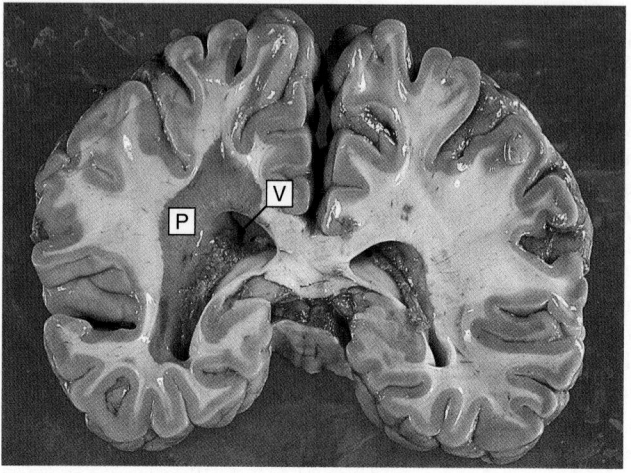

Figure 61-4 Chronic multiple sclerosis. Demyelination plaque (P) at grey-white junction and adjacent partially remyelinated shadow plaque (V).

Source: Stevens, A., & Lowe, J. (2000). *Pathology: Illustrated review in colour* (2nd ed.). London: Mosby.

condition is an autoimmune disease orchestrated by autoreactive T cells (lymphocytes). This process may be initially triggered by a virus in genetically susceptible individuals. The activated T cells in the systemic circulation migrate to the CNS, causing blood–brain barrier disruption. This is likely the initial event in the development of MS. Subsequent antigen–antibody reaction within the CNS results in activation of the inflammatory response and, through multiple effector mechanisms, leads to demyelination of axons. The disease process consists of loss of myelin, disappearance of oligodendrocytes, and proliferation of astrocytes. These changes result in characteristic plaque formation, or sclerosis, with plaques scattered throughout multiple regions of the CNS.

Initially, the myelin sheaths of the neurons in the brain and spinal cord are attacked (Figure 61-3, *A* and *B*). Early in the disease, the myelin sheath is damaged, but the nerve fibre is not affected and nerve impulses are still transmitted (see Figure 61-3, *C*). At this point, the patient may complain of a noticeable impairment of function (e.g., weakness). However, the myelin can regenerate, and the symptoms disappear, resulting in a remission.

In addition to myelin disruption, the axon also becomes involved (see Figure 61-3, *D*). Myelin is replaced by glial scar tissue, which forms hard, sclerotic plaques in multiple regions of the CNS (Figure 61-4). Without myelin, nerve impulses slow down, and with destruction of nerve axons, impulses are totally blocked, resulting in permanent loss of function. In many chronic lesions, demyelination continues with progressive loss of nerve function.

Clinical Manifestations

The onset of MS is often insidious, with vague symptoms that occur intermittently over months or years. As a result, the disease may not be diagnosed until long after the onset of the first symptom. The disease process has a spotty distribution in the CNS, so the signs and symptoms vary over time. MS is characterized by chronic, progressive deterioration in some persons and by remissions and exacerbations in others. With repeated exacerbations, however, progressive scarring of the myelin sheath occurs, and the overall trend is progressive deterioration in neurological function (Tremlett, Zhao, Rieckmann, & Hutchinson, 2010).

The clinical manifestations vary according to the areas of the CNS involved. Some patients have severe, long-lasting symptoms early in the course of the disease. Others may experience only occasional and mild symptoms for several years after onset. A classification scheme that identifies the various courses of MS has been developed (Multiple Sclerosis Society of Canada, 2011) (Table 61-14 and Figure 61-5).

Common signs and symptoms of MS include motor, sensory, cerebellar, and emotional problems. Motor symptoms include weakness or paralysis of the limbs, the trunk, or the head; diplopia; scanning speech; and spasticity of the muscles that are chronically affected. Patients with MS experience a variety of sensory abnormalities, including numbness and tingling and other paresthesias, patchy blindness *(scotomas)*, blurred vision, vertigo, tinnitus, decreased hearing, and chronic neuropathic pain. Radicular (nerve root) pains may be present, particularly in the low thoracic and abdominal regions. *Lhermitte's sign* is a transient sensory symptom described as an electric shock radiating down the spine or into the limbs with flexion of the neck. Cerebellar signs include nystagmus, ataxia, dysarthria, and dysphagia. Severe fatigue is present in many patients with MS, and it causes significant disability for some patients. The fatigue is usually associated with increased energy needs, deconditioning, depression, and medication adverse effects (Multiple Sclerosis International Federation, 2011).

Bowel and bladder function can be affected if the sclerotic plaque is located in areas of the CNS that control elimination. Problems with defecation usually involve constipation rather than fecal incontinence. Urinary problems are variable. A common problem in MS patients is a *spastic* (uninhibited) bladder. This

Table 61-14 Clinical Courses of Multiple Sclerosis

CATEGORY	CHARACTERISTICS
Relapsing–remitting	Clearly defined relapses with full recovery or sequelae and residual deficit on recovery, most common form (75% at time of diagnosis)
Benign	A relapsing-remitting course in which remission after relapses is almost complete with minimal disability (10-20% with retrospective diagnosis)
Primary-progressive	Disease progression from onset with occasional plateaus and temporary minor improvements, no clear relapses or remissions (10-15% at time of diagnosis)
Secondary-progressive	A relapsing-remitting initial course, followed by progression with or without occasional relapses, minor remissions, and plateaus; disability generally accumulates over time
Progressive-relapsing	Progressive disease from onset, with clear acute relapses, with or without full recovery; periods between relapses are characterized by continuing progression

Source: Adapted from Multiple Sclerosis Society of Canada. (2011). *Types of MS.* Retrieved from *http://www.mssociety.ca/en/information/ types.htm*

indicates a lesion above the second sacral nerve, which cuts off suprasegmental inhibiting influences on bladder contractility. As a result, the bladder has a small capacity for urine, and its contractions are unchecked. This is accompanied by urinary urgency and frequency and results in dribbling or incontinence. A *flaccid* (hypotonic) bladder indicates a lesion in the reflex arc governing bladder function. The bladder has a large capacity for urine because there is no sensation or desire to void, no pressure, and no pain. Generally, there is urinary retention, but urgency and frequency may also occur with this type of lesion. Another urinary problem is a combination of the previous two problems. Urinary problems cannot be adequately diagnosed and treated unless urodynamic studies are done.

Sexual dysfunction occurs in many persons with MS. Physiological erectile dysfunction may result from spinal cord involvement in men. Women may experience decreased libido, difficulty with orgasmic response, painful intercourse, and decreased vaginal lubrication. Diminished sensation can prevent a normal sexual response in both sexes. The emotional effects of chronic illness and the loss of self-esteem also contribute to loss of sexual response (Moore, 2007).

MS has no apparent effect on the course of pregnancy, labour, delivery, or lactation. Some women with MS who become pregnant experience remission or an improvement in their symptoms

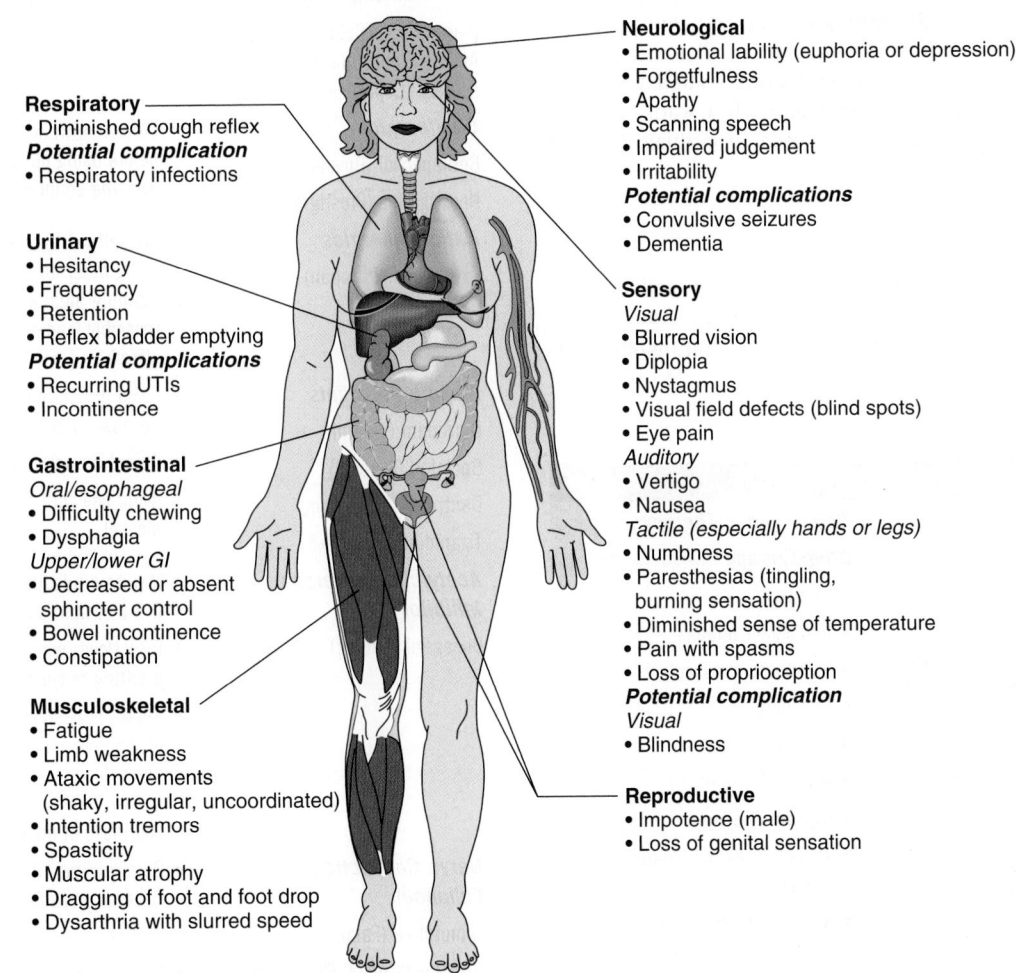

Figure 61-5 Multisystem effects of multiple sclerosis. *UTIs,* urinary tract infections.

Source: Redrawn from LeMone, P., Burke, K. M., & Bauldoff, G. (2011). *Medical surgical nursing: Critical thinking in patient care* (5th ed., p. 1522). Upper Saddle River, NJ: Pearson Prentice Hall.

during the gestation period. The hormonal changes associated with pregnancy appear to affect the immune system. However, during the postpartum period, women are at greater risk for exacerbation of the disease (Moore, 2007).

Although intellectual functioning generally remains intact, emotional stability may be affected. Cognitive sequelae can produce significant disability for some patients with MS. Persons may experience anger, depression, or euphoria. Signs and symptoms of MS are aggravated or triggered by physical and emotional trauma, fatigue, and infection.

The average life expectancy after the onset of symptoms is more than 25 years. Death usually occurs because of infective complications (e.g., pneumonia) of immobility or because of an unrelated disease.

Diagnostic Studies

Because there is no definitive diagnostic test for MS, diagnosis is based primarily on history, clinical manifestations, and the presence of multiple lesions over time as measured by MRI (Table 61-15). Certain laboratory tests are currently used as adjuncts to clinical examination. In some patients, cerebrospinal fluid (CSF) analysis may show an increase in oligoclonal immunoglobulin G. The CSF also contains a high number of lymphocytes and monocytes and protein. Evoked responses are often delayed in persons with MS because of decreased nerve conduction from the eye and the ear to the brain. MRI scan may be helpful because sclerotic plaques as small as 3 to 4 mm in diameter can be detected. Characteristic white-matter lesions scattered through the brain or spinal cord are evident on such a scan. Magnetic resonance spectroscopy may also be used to evaluate patients with MS.

Collaborative Care

Drug Therapy. Because there is no cure for MS, collaborative care is aimed at treating the disease process and providing symptomatic relief (see Table 61-15). The goal of drug therapy is to

decrease the progression of the disease process and control symptoms with a variety of drugs and other forms of therapy. Adrenocorticotropic hormone, methylprednisolone, and prednisone are helpful in treating acute exacerbations of the disease, probably by reducing edema and acute inflammation at the site of demyelination (Table 61-16). These drugs are used in patients with all types of MS. However, they do not affect the ultimate outcome or the degree of residual neurological impairment from the exacerbation. (See Chapter 51 for effects of long-term corticosteroid therapy.)

Immunosuppressive drugs, such as azathioprine (Imuran), methotrexate, and cyclophosphamide (Procytox), have been shown to produce some beneficial effects in patients with progressive-relapsing, secondary-progressive, and primary-progressive MS. However, the potential benefits of these drugs in

COLLABORATIVE CARE

Table 61-15 Multiple Sclerosis

Diagnostic	Collaborative Therapy
• History and physical examination • CSF analysis • Evoked response testing (also called *evoked potential testing*, e.g., somatosensory evoked potential [SSEP], auditory evoked potential [AEP], visual evoked potential [VEP]) • CT scan • MRI, MRS	**Drug Therapy*** • Corticosteroids • Immunomodulators • Immunosuppressants • Cholinergics • Anticholinergics • Muscle relaxants **Surgical Therapy** • Thalamotomy (unmanageable tremor) • Neurectomy, rhizotomy, cordotomy (unmanageable spasticity)

CSF, cerebrospinal fluid; *CT,* computed tomography; *MRI,* magnetic resonance imaging; *MRS,* magnetic resonance spectroscopy.
*See Table 61-16.

DRUG THERAPY

Table 61-16 Multiple Sclerosis

DRUG	PATIENT TEACHING
Corticosteroids ACTH, prednisone, methylprednisolone	• Restrict salt intake. • Do not abruptly stop therapy. • Know drug interactions.
Immunomodulators β-Interferon (Betaseron, Avonex, Rebif) glatiramer acetate (Copaxone)	• Perform self-injection techniques. • Report adverse effects.
Cholinergics Bethanechol (Duvoid) Neostigmine (Prostigmin)	• Consult with health care provider before using other drugs, including over-the-counter drugs.
Anticholinergics Oxybutynin (Ditropan)	• Consult health care provider before using other drugs, especially sleeping aids, antihistamines (possibly leading to potentiated effect).
Muscle Relaxants Diazepam (Valium) Baclofen (Lioresal) Dantrolene (Dantrium) Tizanidine (Zanaflex)	• Avoid driving and similar activities because of sedative effects. • Do not abruptly stop therapy. • Avoid use with tranquilizers and alcohol.
Acetylcholinesterase Inhibitor Donepezil (Aricept)	• Maintain adequate hydration of 2-3 L of fluid/day. • Rise slowly when getting up from a sitting or lying position. • Report persistent abdominal discomfort, increased salivation, unresolved diarrhea, increased muscle pain, visual changes, or shortness of breath.
Nerve Conduction Enhancer Fampridine (Fampyra)	• Be aware that it may cause seizures, especially at higher doses.
Sphingosine-1-Phosphate Receptor Modulators Fingolimod (Gilenya)	• May increase risk of infections.

ACTH, adrenocorticotropic hormone.

patients with MS must be counterbalanced against the potentially serious adverse effects.

Immunomodulator drugs modify the disease process. Interferon β-1b (Betaseron) is used for ambulatory patients with relapsing-remitting MS. Interferon β-1a (Avonex) is similar to interferon β-1b in efficacy and is used in similar patient groups with MS. It is given intramuscularly once a week. Interferon β-1a (Rebif) is administered subcutaneously three times weekly. These drugs have antiviral effects. Glatiramer acetate (Copaxone), formerly known as copolymer-1, is unrelated to interferon. It is given subcutaneously every day in patients with relapsing-remitting MS. Natalizumab (Tysabri), a recombinant monoclonal antibody to a leukocyte adhesion molecule, is a promising new therapy for MS. It works by inhibiting the migration of lymphocytes, thus decreasing the inflammatory process and prevent further damage to the myelin (National Institute for Health and Clinical Excellence [NICE], 2007; Multiple Sclerosis Society of Canada, 2011).

Mitoxantrone is an antineoplastic drug used for the treatment of primary-progressive and progressive-relapsing MS and has some beneficial effects. It is an immunosuppressant drug that reduces both B and T lymphocytes and impairs antigen presentation. Unlike the other disease-modifying drugs, mitoxantrone has a lifetime dose limit because of cardiac toxicity. Therefore, it cannot be used for more than 2 to 3 years.

Many other drugs are used to treat the symptoms of MS. Antispasmodics are used for spasticity. Amantadine and CNS stimulants, such as methylphenidate (Ritalin) and modafinil (Alertec), are used for fatigue. Anticholinergics are used to treat bladder symptoms. Tricyclic antidepressants and antiseizure drugs are used for chronic pain. Erectile dysfunction medication and estrogen creams are used for sexual dysfunction (Moore, 2007). Cannabinoids have also been used to treat both pain and spasticity with mild adverse effects. There remains concern around potential long-term adverse effects, specifically psychiatric and fetal effects of this emerging treatment (Wade, Collin, Stott, & Duncombe, 2010).

Alternate Therapies. A variety of alternate therapies have been utilized aiming to minimize MS symptoms and decrease exacerbations. Surgical intervention may include neurectomy, rhizotomy, cordotomy, dorsal-column electrical stimulation, or use of an intrathecal baclofen (Lioresal) pump may be required to manage spasticity. Tremors that become unmanageable with drugs are sometimes treated by thalamotomy or deep brain stimulation.

Neurological dysfunction may improve with physiotherapy and speech therapy. Exercise improves the daily functioning for patients with MS not experiencing an exacerbation. Exercise decreases spasticity, increases coordination, and retrains unaffected muscles to substitute for impaired ones (Sosnoff, Motl, Snook, & Wynn, 2009). An especially beneficial type of physical therapy is water exercise. Water gives buoyancy to the body and allows the patient to perform activities that would normally be impossible because the patient has more control over the body. Other therapies may include the use of heat therapy, massage, acupuncture, bee stings, and aromatherapy. The effectiveness of these therapies requires more research.

Recent media attention has emerged surrounding the controversial MS treatment of chronic cerebrospinal venous insufficiency (CCSVI). Zamboni and associates (2008) first proposed the theory that CCSVI may be a contributing factor in the pathology of MS. These researchers suggest that MS may be related to an immune or inflammatory reaction to iron accumulation in the CNS relating to drainage impairment of the cerebrospinal vessels. This was detected via the use of ultrasound and cranial ultrasound. MS patients have undergone endovascular CCSVI procedures such as angioplasty or stent placement in jugular and azygos veins to improve venous drainage (Figure 61-6). The safety and efficacy of these procedures is unknown and they are not without risk (Awad, Marder, Milo, & Stuve, 2011; Burton et al., 2011; Lazzaro, Zaidat, Mueller-Kronast, Taqi, & Woo, 2011).

There is inconclusive evidence supporting the CCSVI treatment and further research is needed to determine the best practice. At the time of writing, CCSVI surgery for MS patients was not yet available in Canada (CCSVI Foundation of Canada, 2011).

Nutritional Therapy. Various nutritional measures have been used in the management of MS, including megavitamin therapy (cobalamin [vitamin B_{12}], vitamin C), supplemental vitamin D, and diets consisting of low-fat, gluten-free food and raw vegetables. Particular dietary measures are not widely used owing to insufficient evidence supporting their effectiveness.

A nutritious, well-balanced diet is essential. Although there is no standard prescribed diet, a high-protein diet with supplementary vitamins is often advocated. A diet high in roughage may help relieve constipation. Vitamins are merely supplemental and not curative. Nutrition therapy must be adapted depending on the patient's ability to chew and swallow.

NURSING MANAGEMENT: MULTIPLE SCLEROSIS

Nursing Assessment

Subjective and objective data that should be obtained from a patient with MS are presented in Table 61-17.

Nursing Diagnoses

Nursing diagnoses for the patient with MS may include, but are not limited to, those presented in NCP 61-2.

Planning

The overall goals are that the MS patient will (1) maximize neuromuscular function, (2) maintain independence in activities of daily living for as long as possible, (3) manage disabling fatigue, (4) optimize psychosocial well-being, (5) adjust to the illness, and (6) reduce factors that precipitate exacerbations.

Nursing Implementation

The patient with MS should be aware of triggers that may cause exacerbations or worsening of the disease. Exacerbations of MS are triggered by infection (especially upper respiratory and urinary tract infections), trauma, immunization, childbirth, stress, and change in climate. Each person responds differently to

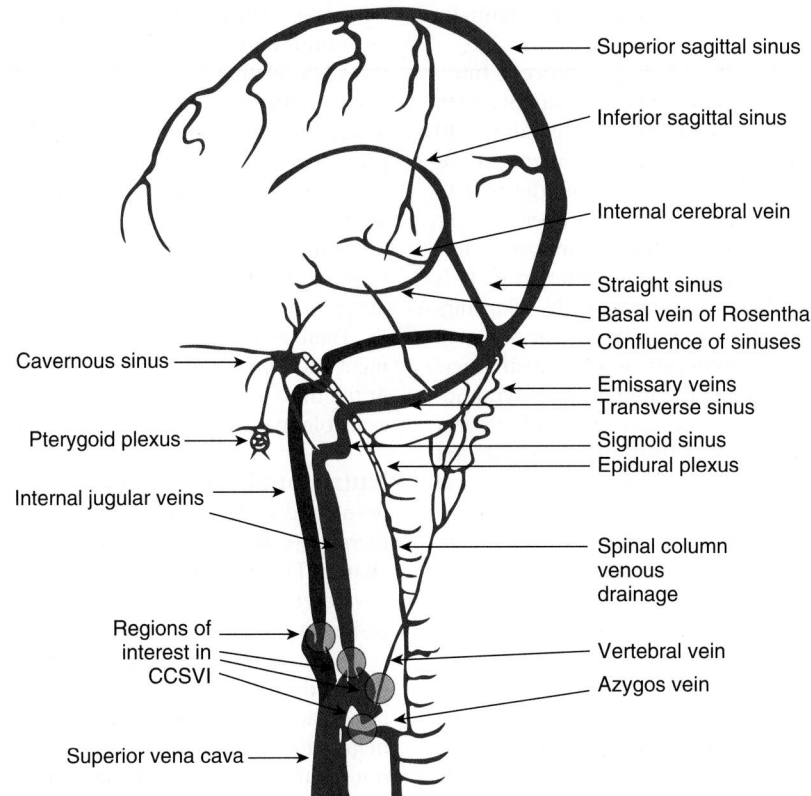

Figure 61-6 Cerebrospinal vessels of interest in chronic cerebrospinal venous insufficiency (CCSVI).

Source: Lazzaro, M. A., Zaidat, O. O., Mueller-Kronast, N., Taqi, M. A., & Woo, D. (2011). Endovascular therapy for chronic cerebrospinal venous insufficiency in multiple sclerosis. *Frontiers in neurology, 2*(Article 44), 1-7. doi:10.3389/fneur.2011.00044

NURSING ASSESSMENT

Table 61-17 Multiple Sclerosis

Subjective Data

Important Health Information

Past health history: Recent or past viral infections or vaccinations, other recent infections, residence in cold or temperate climates, recent physical or emotional stress, pregnancy, exposure to extremes of heat and cold; positive family history

Medications: Use of and compliance in taking corticosteroids, immunomodulators, immunosuppressants, selective adhesion molecule inhibitor cholinergics, anticholinergics, antispasmodics, antivirals

Symptoms

- Weight loss; difficulty chewing, dysphagia
- Urinary frequency, urgency, dribbling or incontinence, retention; constipation
- Generalized muscle weakness, muscle fatigue; tingling and numbness, ataxia (clumsiness), malaise
- Eye, back, leg, joint pain; painful muscle spasms; vertigo; blurred or lost vision; diplopia; tinnitus

- Erectile and sexual dysfunction: decreased libido
- Anger, depression, euphoria, social isolation, cognitive changes, memory loss

Objective Data

General

Apathy, inattentiveness

Neurological

Scanning speech, nystagmus, ataxia, tremor, spasticity, hyperreflexia, decreased hearing

Musculoskeletal

Muscular weakness, paresis, paralysis, spasms, foot dragging, dysarthria (may be unilateral or bilateral changes)

Possible Findings

↓ T suppressor cells, demyelinating lesions on MRI or MRS scans, increased IgG or oligoclonal banding in cerebrospinal fluid, delayed evoked potential

IgG, immunoglobulin G; *MRI*, magnetic resonance imaging; *MRS*, magnetic resonance spectroscopy.

these triggers. The nurse should help the patient identify particular triggers and develop ways to avoid them or minimize their effects.

The most common reasons for hospitalization of the patient with MS are for a diagnostic workup and treatment of an acute exacerbation. During the diagnostic phase, the patient needs reassurance that, even though there is a tentative diagnosis of MS, certain diagnostic studies must be done to rule out other neurological disorders. The nurse should assist the patient in dealing with the anxiety caused by a diagnosis of a disabling

NURSING CARE PLAN 61-2

Multiple Sclerosis

NURSING DIAGNOSIS	**Impaired physical mobility** *related to* muscle weakness or paralysis and muscle spasticity *as evidenced by* inability to ambulate, intermittent muscle spasms, and pain associated with muscle spasms
Expected Patient Outcomes	**Nursing Interventions and *Rationales***
• Demonstrates use of adaptive devices • Maintains or increases strength of limbs • ↓ Muscle spasms	• Use assistive devices as indicated *to decrease fatigue and enhance independence, comfort, and safety.* • Do active range of motion exercises at least twice per day *to prevent contractures and minimize muscle atrophy.* • Encourage and assist with ambulation and transfer as indicated *to maintain mobility, promote independence, and provide for safety.* • Change position of patient (if bedridden) at least q2h *to prevent circulatory problems and pressure ulcers.* • Perform stretching exercises q6-8h *to relieve spasms and contracted muscles.*
NURSING DIAGNOSIS	**Impaired urinary elimination** *related to* sensorimotor deficits, inadequate fluid intake, or both, *as evidenced by* posturination residual volume >50 mL, dribbling, or bladder distension
Expected Patient Outcomes	**Nursing Interventions and *Rationales***
• Residual urine volume <50 mL • Maintains urinary continence	• Administer cholinergic drugs as ordered *to improve the muscle tone of bladder and facilitate bladder emptying.* • Follow intermittent catheterization protocol *to prevent distension or dribbling.* • Use the Credé manoeuvre or reflex stimulation (manual stimulation) *as an alternative method of emptying bladder.* • Maintain fluid intake of 3000 mL/day *to dilute urine and reduce risk of urinary tract infection.* • Teach patient signs and symptoms of urinary tract infection *to ensure early identification and treatment.* • Initiate bladder training program *to help restore adequate bladder function.*
NURSING DIAGNOSIS	**Sexual dysfunction** *related to* neuromuscular deficits *as evidenced by* impotence, verbalization of problem, decreased libido
Expected Patient Outcome	**Nursing Interventions and *Rationales***
• Verbalizes satisfaction with expression of sexuality	• Initiate sexual counselling if indicated *because not all nurses have the education required for this type of counselling.* • Suggest alternative methods of achieving sexual gratification *because sexual intercourse may not be possible as a result of neuromuscular deficits and medication adverse effects.*
NURSING DIAGNOSIS	**Interrupted family processes** *related to* changing family roles, potential financial problems, and fluctuating physical condition *as evidenced by* strained family relations, ineffective communication, verbalization of financial concerns
Expected Patient Outcomes	**Nursing Interventions and *Rationales***
• Open communication between family and patient • Seeks outside assistance when indicated	• Facilitate open communication among patient and family *to promote better interpersonal relationships.* • Promote problem solving *to enable the family to handle the issues of long-term illness.* • Refer for family and financial counselling (if indicated) *to provide additional help in coping with a chronic debilitating disease.* • Educate family regarding fluctuating nature of disease *because lack of knowledge about multiple sclerosis affects ability to cope with the changes.*

illness. The patient with recently diagnosed MS may need assistance with the grieving process.

During an acute exacerbation, the patient may be immobile and bedridden. The focus of nursing intervention at this phase is to prevent major complications of immobility, such as respiratory and urinary tract infections and pressure ulcers.

Patient teaching should focus on building general resistance to illness, including avoiding fatigue, extremes of heat and cold,

and exposure to infection. The last measure involves avoiding exposure to cold climates and to people who are sick as well as vigorous and early treatment of infection when it does occur. It is important to teach the patient to (1) achieve a good balance of exercise and rest, (2) eat nutritious and well-balanced meals, and (3) avoid the hazards of immobility (e.g., contractures, pressure ulcers). Patients should know their treatment regimens, the adverse effects of drugs and how to watch for them, and drug interactions with over-the-counter medications. The patient should consult a health care provider before taking nonprescription drugs.

Bladder control is a major problem for many patients with MS. Although anticholinergics may be beneficial for some patients to decrease spasticity, other patients may need to be taught self-catheterization (see Chapter 48). Bowel problems, particularly constipation, occur frequently in patients with MS. Increasing the dietary fibre intake may help some patients achieve regularity in bowel habits.

The patient with MS and the family must make many emotional adjustments because of the unpredictability of the disease, the need to change lifestyles, and the challenge of avoiding or decreasing precipitating factors. The Multiple Sclerosis Society of Canada and its local chapters can offer a variety of services to meet the needs of MS patients.

▋ Evaluation

Expected outcomes for the patient with MS are addressed in NCP 61-2.

Parkinson's Disease

Parkinson's disease (PD) is a progressive, neurodegenerative disease of the CNS (basal ganglia) characterized by a slowing down in the initiation and the execution of movement *(bradykinesia)*, increased muscle tone (rigidity), tremor at rest, and impaired postural reflexes. It is the most common form of *parkinsonism* (a syndrome characterized by similar symptoms). PD is named after James Parkinson, who in 1817 wrote a classic essay on "shaking palsy," a disease whose cause is still unknown and for which no cure exists.

Etiology and Pathophysiology

In Canada, approximately 100,000 people have PD, a movement disorder and the second most common neurodegenerative disease. This number is expected to rise dramatically with the aging of the population because the average age of diagnosis is 60 years (Parkinson Society Canada, 2011). There is a well-established genetic component to PD, and the field continues to grow and evolve as new genes are identified and mutations in known genes are discovered (Klein & Schlossmacher, 2006). PD is more common in men than women by a ratio of 3:2.

There are many forms of parkinsonism other than PD. Parkinsonism-like symptoms have occurred after intoxication with a variety of chemicals, including carbon monoxide and manganese (among copper miners) and the product of meperidine-analogue synthesis, 1-methyl-4-phenyl-1,2,3,6-tetrahydropyridine (MPTP). Drug-induced parkinsonism can follow reserpine (Serpasil), methyldopa (Aldomet), lithium, haloperidol, and phenothiazine (Thorazine) therapy. Parkinsonism can also be seen following the use of illicit drugs including amphetamine and methamphetamine. Other causes of parkinsonism include encephalitis, meningitis, vascular parkinsonism, progressive supranuclear palsy, multiple system atrophy, and dementia with Lewy bodies (Frank, Pari, & Rossiter, 2006).

The pathological process of PD involves degeneration of the dopamine-producing neurons in the substantia nigra of

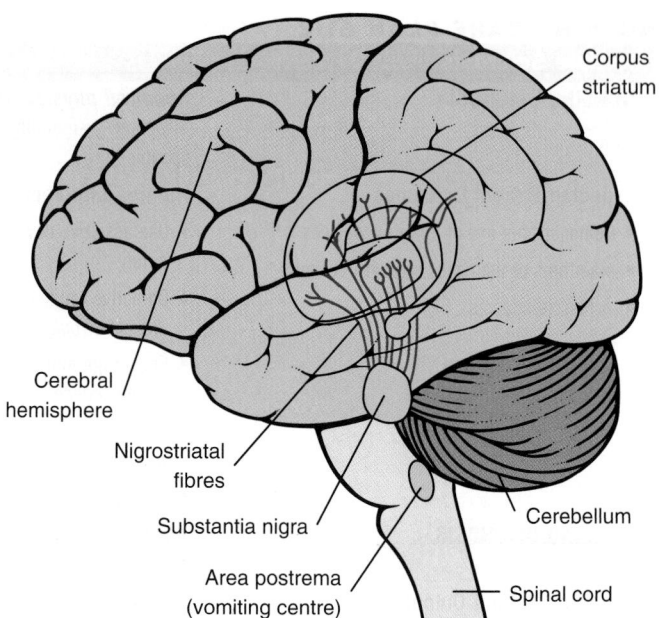

Figure 61-7 Nigrostriatal disorders produce parkinsonism. Left-sided view of the human brain shows the substantia nigra and the corpus striatum *(shaded area)* lying deep within the cerebral hemisphere. Nerve fibres extend upward from the substantia nigra, divide into many branches, and carry dopamine to all regions of the corpus striatum.

the midbrain responsible for controlling voluntary movements (Tugwell, 2008). Lewy bodies are a form of protein deposits that are present in the residual dopaminergic neurons that have been damaged (Figures 61-7 and 61-8). The degeneration disrupts the normal balance between dopamine (DA) and acetylcholine (ACh) in the basal ganglia (Swinn, 2005). DA is an inhibiting neurotransmitter essential for normal functioning of the extrapyramidal motor system, including control of posture, support, and voluntary motion, while ACh is an excitatory neurotransmitter; each is responsible for nerve impulse transmission. PD is characterized by a progressive loss of DA in relation to ACh and results in this imbalance of activity of motor pathways, producing the complex motor clinical manifestations (Swinn, 2005). Symptoms of PD do not occur until 80% of neurons in the substantia nigra are lost or damaged.

Clinical Manifestations

The onset of PD is insidious, with a gradual progression and a prolonged course. PD usually manifests unilaterally with mild symptoms, eventually progressing bilaterally (Tugwell, 2008). In the beginning stages, only a mild tremor, a slight limp, or a decreased arm swing may be evident. Later in the course of the disease, the patient may have a shuffling, propulsive gait with arms flexed and loss of postural reflexes. In some patients, there may be a slight change in speech patterns. None of these alone is sufficient evidence for a diagnosis of the disease (Dickson et al., 2009; Vernon, 2009). The classic triad of symptoms includes tremor, rigidity, and bradykinesia (Figure 61-9).

Tremor. *Tremor*, present in 70 to 100% of patients and often the first sign, may be minimal initially and the patient the only

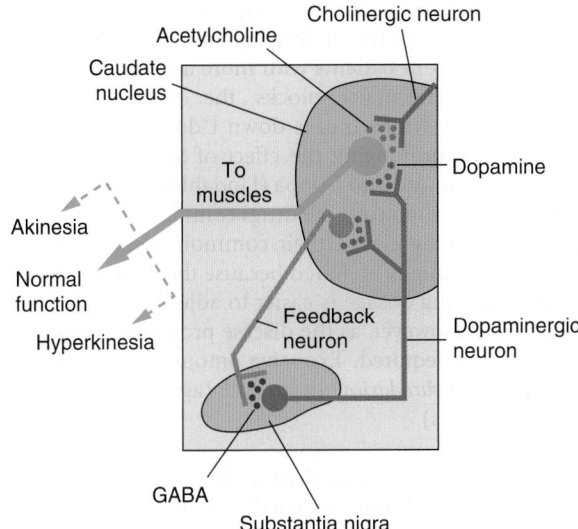

Figure 61-8 Dopaminergic synaptic activity is mediated by dopamine. Cholinergic synaptic activity is mediated by acetylcholine. A balance between the two kinds of activity produces normal motor function. A relative excess of cholinergic activity produces akinesia and rigidity. A relative excess of dopaminergic activity produces involuntary movements. Neurons in the caudate nucleus contain γ-aminobutyric acid (GABA) and possibly control dopaminergic neurons in the substantia nigra through a feedback pathway.

Source: McCance, K. L., & Huether, S. E. (2006). *Pathophysiology: The biologic basis for disease in adults and children* (5th ed., p. 537, Figure 16-23, *B*). St. Louis: Mosby.

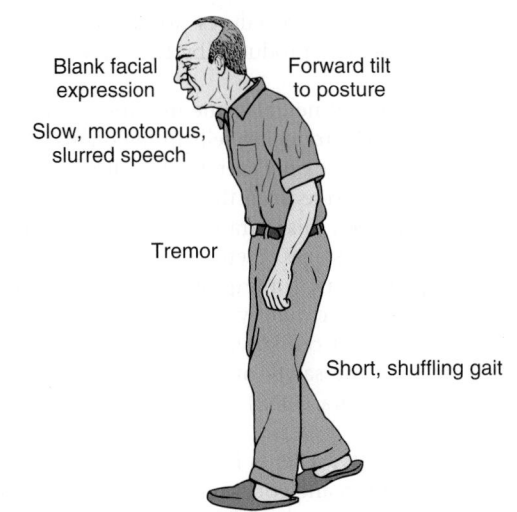

Figure 61-9 Characteristic appearance of a patient with Parkinson's disease.

Source: Redrawn from Rudy, E. (1984). *Advanced neurological and neurosurgical nursing.* St. Louis: Mosby.

one who notices it (Frank et al., 2006). Tremor can affect handwriting, causing it to be small and irregular. Parkinsonian tremor is more prominent at rest and is aggravated by emotional stress or increased concentration. The hand tremor is described as "pill rolling" because the thumb and forefinger appear to move in a rotary fashion as if rolling a pill, coin, or other small object. Tremor can involve the diaphragm, the tongue, the lips, and the

jaw but rarely causes shaking of the head. Unfortunately, in many people, a benign essential tremor has mistakenly been diagnosed as PD. Essential tremor occurs during voluntary movement, has a more rapid frequency than parkinsonian tremor, and is often familial.

Rigidity. *Rigidity,* the second sign of the triad and present in over 90% of patients, is the increased resistance to passive motion when the limbs are moved through their range of motion (Frank et al., 2006). Parkinsonian rigidity is typified by a jerky quality, as if there were intermittent catches in the movement of a cogwheel, when the joint is moved. This is termed *cogwheel rigidity.* The rigidity is caused by sustained muscle contraction and consequently elicits a complaint of muscle soreness; feeling tired and achy; or pain in the head, the upper body, the spine, or the legs. Another consequence of rigidity is slowness of movement because it inhibits the alternating of contraction and relaxation in opposing muscle groups (e.g., biceps and triceps).

Bradykinesia. *Bradykinesia,* present in 80 to 100% of patients, is particularly evident in the loss of automatic movements, which is secondary to the physical and chemical alteration of the basal ganglia and related structures in the extrapyramidal portion of the CNS (Frank et al., 2006). In the unaffected patient, automatic movements are involuntary and occur subconsciously. They include blinking of the eyelids, swinging of the arms while walking, swallowing of saliva, self-expression with facial and hand movements, and minor movement of postural adjustment. The patient with PD does not execute these movements, and there is a lack of spontaneous activity. This accounts for the stooped posture, the masklike face (deadpan expression), the drooling of saliva, and the shuffling gait (festination) that are characteristic of a person with this disease. In addition, there is difficulty in initiating movement.

Complications

In addition to the motor signs of PD, many nonmotor symptoms are common. They include depression, anxiety, apathy, fatigue, pain, constipation, impotence, and short-term memory impairment (Tugwell, 2008). As the disease progresses, complications increase. These include motor symptoms (e.g., dyskinesias [spontaneous, involuntary movements], weakness, akinesia [total immobility]), neurological problems (e.g., dementia), and neuropsychiatric problems (e.g., depression, hallucinations, psychosis) (Backer, 2006). Dementia occurs in approximately 1 in 5 patients with PD (Tugwell, 2008). As swallowing becomes more difficult (dysphagia), malnutrition or aspiration may result. General debilitation may lead to pneumonia, urinary tract infections, and skin breakdown. Orthostatic hypotension may occur in some patients and, along with loss of postural reflexes, may result in falls and injury.

Sleep disorders in patients with PD are common, potentially severe, often underrecognized, and ineffectively treated (Parkinson Society Canada, 2011; Tugwell, 2008). Effective management of sleep disturbances can greatly improve the quality of life for patients with PD.

Diagnostic Studies

Because there is no specific diagnostic test for PD, the diagnosis is based solely on history and clinical features. A firm diagnosis

COLLABORATIVE CARE

Table 61-18 Parkinson's Disease

Diagnostic	Collaborative Therapy
• History and physical examination	• Antiparkinsonian drugs*
• Tremor	• Ablation surgery
• Rigidity	• Deep brain stimulation
• Bradykinesia	
• Positive response to antiparkinsonian drugs*	
• Rule out adverse effects of phenothiazines, reserpine, benzodiazepines, haloperidol	
• MRI	

MRI, magnetic resonance imaging.
*See Table 61-19.

can be made only when at least two of the three characteristic signs of the classic triad are present. Research is ongoing using MRI studies to examine cognitive dysfunction in patients with PD (Vernon, 2009).

Collaborative Care

Because there is no cure for PD, collaborative management (Table 61-18) is focused on symptom management.

Drug Therapy. Drug therapy for PD is aimed at correcting an imbalance of neurotransmitters within the CNS. Antiparkinsonian drugs either enhance the release or supply of DA (dopaminergic) or antagonize or block the effects of the overactive cholinergic neurons in the striatum (anticholinergic). Levodopa (L-dopa) with carbidopa (Sinemet) is often the first drug used. L-Dopa is a precursor of DA and can cross the blood–brain barrier. It is converted to DA in the basal ganglia. Sinemet is the preferred drug because it also contains carbidopa, an agent that inhibits the enzyme dopadecarboxylase in the peripheral tissues. This enzyme breaks down L-dopa before it reaches the brain. The net result of the combination of L-dopa and carbidopa is that more L-dopa reaches the brain, and therefore less drug is needed.

Many patients are given Sinemet early in the disease course. However, some health care providers believe that after a few years of therapy, the effectiveness of Sinemet wears off. Instead, these providers may prefer to initiate therapy with a dopaminergic drug that directly stimulates DA receptors. When more moderate-to-severe symptoms become present, L-dopa with carbidopa (Sinemet) is added to the drug regimen.

Anticholinergic drugs are also used to manage PD. These drugs act by decreasing the activity of ACh, thus providing balance between cholinergic and dopaminergic actions. Antihistamines (e.g., diphenhydramine [Benadryl]) with anticholinergic properties or a β-adrenergic blocker (e.g., propranolol [Inderal]) is used to manage tremors. The antiviral agent amantadine is also an effective antiparkinsonian drug. Although its exact mechanism of action is not known, amantadine promotes the release of DA from neurons.

Selegiline is a monoamine oxidase inhibitor that is sometimes used in combination with Sinemet. By inhibiting monoamine oxidase, the degradative enzyme for DA, levels of DA are increased. Rasagiline (Azilect), a type B monoamine oxidase inhibitor, is used as an initial drug therapy in early PD and as an addition to L-dopa in patients with more advanced disease.

Entacapone (Comtan) blocks the enzyme catechol-O-methyltransferase, which breaks down L-dopa in the peripheral circulation, thus prolonging the effect of Sinemet. These drugs are used only as adjuncts to L-dopa (Lindahl & MacMahon, 2011).

Table 61-19 summarizes the drugs commonly used in PD, the symptoms they relieve, and their common adverse effects. The use of only one drug is preferred because there are fewer adverse effects and the drug dosage is easier to adjust than when several drugs are used. However, as the disease progresses, combination therapy is often required. Excessive amounts of dopaminergic drugs can lead to *paradoxical intoxication* (aggravation rather than relief of symptoms).

Surgical Therapy. Surgical procedures are aimed at relieving symptoms of PD and are usually used in patients who are unresponsive to drug therapy or who have developed severe motor complications. Surgical procedures fall into three categories: ablation (destruction), deep brain stimulation (DBS), and transplantation. *Ablation surgery* involves stereotactic ablation of areas in the thalamus *(thalamotomy)*, globus pallidus *(pallidotomy)*, and subthalamic nucleus *(subthalamic nucleotomy)*. Ablative procedures have been used for PD for over 50 years, but they have been replaced recently by DBS. DBS involves placing an electrode in either the thalamus, the globus pallidus, or the subthalamic nucleus and connecting it to a generator placed in the upper chest (like a pacemaker). The device is programmed to deliver a specific current to the targeted brain location. Unlike ablation procedures, DBS can be adjusted to control symptoms better and is reversible (the device is removable). These ablative and DBS procedures work by reducing the increased neuronal activity produced by DA depletion (Kleiner-Fisman et al., 2006).

Transplantation of fetal neural tissue into the basal ganglia is designed to provide DA-producing cells in the brains of patients with PD. Currently, it is the only therapy that allows patients full functional restoration. Aside from the ethical dilemma of using fetal tissue as a treatment, this therapy has many limitations and is still in experimental stages. Stem cell transplantation is an alternative therapy showing some promise. Both epithelial and bone marrow cells are currently being studied. Limitations include poor rate of graft cell survival and unknown long-term implications, making the safety of this treatment questionable (Singh, Pillay, & Choonara, 2007).

Nutritional Therapy. Diet is important to the patient with PD because malnutrition and constipation can be serious consequences of inadequate nutrition. Patients who have dysphagia and bradykinesia need appetizing foods that are easily chewed and swallowed. The diet should contain adequate roughage and fruit to avoid constipation. Food should be cut into bite-sized pieces before it is served, and it should be served on a warmed plate to preserve its appeal. Eating six small meals a day may be less exhausting than eating three large meals a day. Ample time should be planned for eating to avoid frustration and encourage independence. In addition, absorption of L-dopa can be impaired by ingestion of protein and of vitamin B_6. Some patients are advised to limit their protein intake to the evening meal to decrease this problem and to consult with their health care provider regarding vitamin B_6 in their multivitamins and fortified cereals.

DRUG THERAPY

Table 61-19 Parkinson's Disease

DRUG	SYMPTOMS RELIEVED	ADVERSE EFFECTS AND PRECAUTIONS
Dopaminergic		
Levodopa (L-dopa)	Bradykinesia, tremor, rigidity	Nausea, dyskinesia, hypotension, palpitations, dysrhythmias; agitation, hallucinations, confusion (in older patient)
		Avoidance of multivitamin pills and diet high in vitamin B$_6$ (reversal of effect of levodopa); contraindicated in narrow-angle glaucoma
Levodopa–carbidopa (Sinemet)	Same as above	Less nausea but greater chance of dyskinesia, confusion, hallucinations
		Periodic check of BUN, AST, WBCs, Hct
		Contraindicated in melanoma; narrow-angle glaucoma; combination with MAO inhibitors, reserpine, methyldopa, guanethidine, antipsychotics
Bromocriptine mesylate	Same as above	Orthostatic hypotension, nausea, vomiting, toxic psychosis, limb edema, phlebitis, dizziness, headache, insomnia
Pramipexole (Mirapex)	Same as above	
Ropinirole (Requip)	Same as above	
Amantadine	Rigidity, akinesia	Nervousness, insomnia, confusion, hallucinations, dry mouth, nausea, edema, orthostatic hypotension
Anticholinergic		
Trihexyphenidyl	Tremor	Dry mouth, blurred vision, constipation, delirium, anxiety, agitation, hallucinations
Procyclidine		
Benztropine		Avoidance of drugs with similar actions, including over-the-counter drugs containing scopolamine or antihistamines, antispasmodics (e.g., Bellergal), tricyclic antidepressants (e.g., imipramine, amitriptyline [Elavil])
Antihistamine		
Diphenhydramine (Benadryl)	Tremor, rigidity	Sedation, same precautions as for anticholinergic drugs
Orphenadrine		
Monoamine Oxidase Inhibitor		
Selegiline	Bradykinesia, rigidity, tremor	Similar to dopaminergic drugs
Catechol-O-Methyltransferase (COMT) Inhibitor		
Entacapone (Comtan)	By blocking COMT, this drug slows down the breakdown of levodopa, thus prolonging the action of levodopa	Similar to dopaminergic drugs; works only when used in combination with Sinemet

AST, aspartate aminotransferase; *BUN,* blood urea nitrogen; *Hct,* hematocrit; *MAO,* monoamine oxidase; *WBCs,* white blood cells.

NURSING MANAGEMENT: PARKINSON'S DISEASE

▪ Nursing Assessment

Subjective and objective data that should be obtained from a patient with PD are presented in Table 61-20.

▪ Nursing Diagnoses

Nursing diagnoses for the patient with PD may include, but are not limited to, those presented in NCP 61-3.

▪ Planning

The overall goals are that the patient with PD will (1) experience a lower intensity and frequency of distressing symptoms, (2) maximize neurological function, (3) maintain independence in activities of daily living for as long as possible, and (4) optimize psychosocial well-being.

▪ Nursing Implementation

PD symptoms must be assessed in terms of their intensity, frequency, and duration as well as the distress associated with them. It cannot be assumed that the most frequent symptom is necessarily the most distressing. Therefore, prioritizing interventions should be based on the patient's report of which symptoms are the most troublesome (Backer, 2006).

Promotion of physical exercise and a well-balanced diet are major concerns for nursing care. Exercise can limit the consequences of decreased mobility, such as muscle atrophy, contractures, and constipation. The Parkinson Society Canada (2003)

publishes a brochure called *Exercises for People with Parkinson's* that can be used by caregivers and health care providers (see the link in the Resources section at the end of this chapter.).

A physiotherapist may be consulted to design an exercise program aimed at strengthening and stretching specific muscles. Overall muscle tone, as well as specific exercises to strengthen the

NURSING ASSESSMENT

Table 61-20 Parkinson's Disease

Subjective Data	**Integumentary**
Important Health Information	Seborrhea, dandruff; ankle edema
Past health history: CNS trauma, cerebrovascular disorders, exposure to metals and carbon monoxide, encephalitis; positive family history	**Cardiovascular**
	Postural hypotension
Medications: Use of major tranquilizers, especially haloperidol and phenothiazines, reserpine, methyldopa, amphetamines	**Gastrointestinal**
	Drooling
Symptoms	**Neurological**
• Excessive salivation, dysphagia; weight loss	Tremor at rest, first in hands (pill rolling), later in legs, arms, face, and tongue; aggravation of tremor with anxiety, absence in sleep; poor coordination; subtle dementia, impaired postural reflexes
• Constipation, incontinence; excessive sweating	
• Fatigue, sleep disturbance, difficulty in initiating movements; postural instability; frequent falls; loss of dexterity; micrographia (handwriting deterioration)	**Musculoskeletal**
	Cogwheel rigidity, dysarthria, bradykinesia, contractures, stooped posture, shuffling gait
• Diffuse pain in head, shoulders, neck, back, legs, and hips; muscle soreness and cramping; difficulty concentrating	**Possible Findings**
• Depression, mood swings, hallucinations	Lack of specific tests; diagnosis on basis of history and physical findings and ruling out of other diseases
Objective Data	
General	
Blank (masked) facies, slow and monotonous speech, infrequent blinking	

CNS, central nervous system.

NURSING CARE PLAN 61-3

Parkinson's Disease

NURSING DIAGNOSIS	*Impaired physical mobility related to* rigidity, bradykinesia, and akinesia *as evidenced by* difficulty in initiation of purposeful movements
Expected Patient Outcomes	**Nursing Interventions and *Rationales***
• Ambulates safely	• Assist with ambulation *to assess degree of impairment and to prevent injury.*
• Maintains joint mobility	• Promote stretching and perform active range of motion (ROM) exercises to all extremities *to maintain joint ROM, prevent atrophy and contractures and strengthen muscles.*
	• Consult physiotherapist or occupational therapist for assistive devices *to facilitate activities of daily living and safe ambulation.*
	• Teach techniques to assist with mobility by instructing patient to step over imaginary line, and rock from side to side to initiate leg movements *because these are helpful in dealing with "freezing" (akinesia) while walking.*
NURSING DIAGNOSIS	*Impaired verbal communication related to* dysarthria and tremor or bradykinesia *as evidenced by* decreased amount of communication, slow and slurred speech, inability to move facial muscles, decreased tongue mobility, and micrographia
Expected Patient Outcome	**Nursing Interventions and *Rationales***
• Develops communication method to meet needs	• Allow sufficient time for communication *to reduce patient's frustration.*
	• Encourage deep breaths before speaking.
	• Consult speech therapist *to provide specialized guidance in care of the patient.*
	• Provide alternative communication methods such as picture books or flash cards *because muscle involvement has impaired writing and speaking ability.*
	• Massage patient's facial and neck muscles *to foster relaxation that can facilitate speech.*

NURSING CARE PLAN 61-3

Parkinson's Disease—cont'd

NURSING DIAGNOSIS	**Imbalanced nutrition: less than body requirements** related to dysphagia as evidenced by difficulty in swallowing and chewing, drooling, decreased gag reflex, weight loss
Expected Patient Outcome	**Nursing Interventions and Rationales**
• Maintains satisfactory body weight	• Carefully monitor swallowing ability during drug administration and mealtime to evaluate patient's level of impairment and minimize risk of aspiration.
	• Provide soft-solid and thick-liquid diet because these consistencies are more easily swallowed.
	• Maintain patient in upright position for all meals to reduce risk of aspiration.
	• Consult speech therapist and dietitian because they can provide specific plans to improve swallowing and intake.
	• Have suction available to remove pooled secretions and prevent choking and aspiration.
	• Ensure adequate nutritional intake to meet metabolic needs.
	• Ensure diet includes adequate fiber content to prevent constipation.
NURSING DIAGNOSIS	**Deficient diversional activity** related to inability to perform usual recreational activities as evidenced by boredom, lack of participation, restlessness, depression, or hostility
Expected Patient Outcomes	**Nursing Interventions and Rationales**
• Engages in satisfying diversional activities	• Assess patient's activity to determine physical, emotional, and psychological response to difficulties.
• Expresses acceptance of diminished capabilities	• Determine preferred diversional activities so that individual needs are considered.
	• Adapt difficult activities when possible so that patient is able to continue performing activities.
	• Initiate new activities within patient's capabilities such as reading to replace activities patient can no longer perform.
	• Encourage patient to discuss emotional response to decreasing capabilities to provide opportunity to problem solve and demonstrate a caring attitude.

muscles involved with speaking and swallowing, should be included. Although exercise will not halt the progress of the disease, it will enhance the patient's functional ability. An occupational therapist can also assist the patient with strategies to increase self-care abilities, including eating and dressing.

Because PD is a chronic degenerative disorder with no acute exacerbations, nurses should note that teaching and nursing care are directed toward maintenance of good health, encouragement of independence, and avoidance of complications such as contractures.

Problems secondary to bradykinesia can be alleviated by relatively simple measures. The following are helpful hints for patients who tend to "freeze" while walking: consciously think about stepping over imaginary or real lines on the floor, drop rice kernels and step over them, rock from side to side, lift the toes when stepping, take one step backward and two steps forward. The patient should be assessed for the possibility of L-dopa overdose because it is a common cause of akinesia "freezing." A brief period of dyskinesia, usually *athetosis* (slow, writhing, continuous, and involuntary movement) of the neck, should alert the nurse to this possibility.

Getting out of a chair can be facilitated by using an upright chair with arms and placing the back legs on small 5-cm blocks. Other aspects of the environment can be altered. Rugs and excess furniture can be removed to prevent stumbling. An ottoman can be used to elevate the legs and prevent dependent ankle edema. Clothing can be simplified by the use of slip-on shoes and Velcro hook-and-loop fasteners or zippers on clothing, instead of

buttons and hooks. An elevated toilet seat can facilitate getting on and off the toilet. The nurse should work closely with the patient's family in exploring creative adaptations that allow maximum independence.

▪ Evaluation

Expected outcomes for the patient with PD are addressed in NCP 61-3.

Myasthenia Gravis

Myasthenia gravis (MG) is an autoimmune disease of the neuromuscular junction characterized by fluctuating weakness of certain skeletal muscle groups. No Canadian statistics for this condition are available, but the prevalence of MG in the United States is estimated at 14 to 20 per 100,000 population, approximately 36,000 to 60,000 cases in the United States (Myasthenia Gravis Foundation of America, 2010). However, MG is thought to be underdiagnosed and the prevalence is likely higher. MG can occur at any age but most commonly occurs between the ages of 10 and 65. It most commonly affects women younger than 40 and people older than 60 of either sex, but can affect anyone (National Institute of Neurological Disorders and Stroke [NINDS], 2010). Historically, MG has been more common in

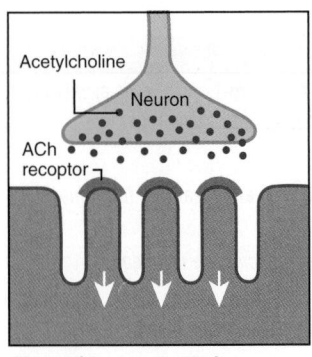
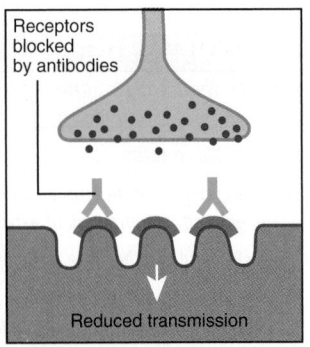

Normal neuromuscular junction

Neuromuscular junction in myasthenia gravis

Figure 61-10 Neuromuscular junction in myasthenia gravis. *ACh*, acetylcholine.

Source: Myasthenia Gravis Coalition of Canada. (2012). *What is MG?* Retrieved from *http://www.mgcc-ccmg.org/about.asp*

women, but as the population ages, both sexes are equally affected (Bershad, Feen, & Suarez, 2008).

Etiology and Pathophysiology

MG is caused by an autoimmune process in which antibodies attack ACh receptors, resulting in a decreased number of ACh receptor sites at the neuromuscular junction (Figure 61-10). This prevents ACh molecules from attaching and stimulating muscle contraction. Nearly all patients will have ocular muscle involvement, and of these, many will have MG symptoms restricted to ocular muscles known as *ocular myasthenia* (Luchanok & Kaminski, 2008). The explanation for muscular weakness in the 10 to 15% of patients who lack autoantibodies to ACh receptors may be related to autoantibodies to muscle-specific receptor tyrosine kinase (Oh, 2009). Thymic tumours or abnormal thymus tissue is found in almost all patients with MG.

Clinical Manifestations and Complications

The primary feature of MG is fluctuating weakness of skeletal muscle. Strength is usually restored after a period of rest. The muscles most often involved are those used for moving the eyes and eyelids, chewing, swallowing, speaking, and breathing. The muscles are generally the strongest in the morning and become exhausted with continued activity. Consequently, by the end of the day, muscle weakness is prominent (Myasthenia Gravis Coalition of Canada, 2011).

The most common symptom of MG is ocular muscle weakness (see eFigure 61-1, the "peek sign" in myasthenia gravis, available on the Evolve Web site for this chapter). Facial mobility and expression can be impaired. There may be difficulty in chewing and swallowing food. Speech is affected, and the voice often fades after a long conversation (Hartl, Leboulleux, Klap, & Schlumberger, 2007). The muscles of the trunk and the limbs are less often affected. Of these, the proximal muscles of the neck, the shoulder, and the hip are more often affected than the distal muscles. No other signs of neural disorder accompany MG; there is no sensory loss, reflexes are normal, and muscle atrophy is rare (Table 61-21).

The course of this disease is variable. Some patients may have short-term remissions, others' conditions may stabilize, and others may have severe, progressive involvement. Restricted

ocular myasthenia, usually seen only in men, has a good prognosis. Exacerbations of MG can be precipitated by stress, pregnancy, menses, secondary illness, trauma, temperature extremes, and hypokalemia. Ingestion of drugs including aminoglycoside antibiotics, β-adrenergic blockers, procainamide, quinidine, and phenytoin can aggravate MG. Psychotropic drugs (e.g., lithium carbonate, phenothiazines, benzodiazepines, tricyclic antidepressants) have also been associated with worsening of myasthenia as have neuromuscular blocking agents (D-tubocurarine, pancuronium, succinylcholine) (Shah, 2006).

Myasthenic crisis is an acute exacerbation of muscle weakness triggered by infection, surgery, emotional distress, or overdose of or inadequate drugs. It generally occurs in the first 2 years after diagnosis. The major complications of MG result from muscle weakness in areas that affect swallowing and breathing, resulting in aspiration, respiratory insufficiency, and respiratory infection (Bershad et al., 2008).

Diagnostic Studies

The diagnosis of MG can be made on the basis of history and physical examination. However, other tests may be used if the diagnosis is still in doubt. Blood tests show that antibodies to ACh receptors are found in 85 to 90% of patients with generalized MG. Repetitive nerve stimulation may show decrements in response to repeated stimulation, indicative of muscle fatigue. Single-fibre electromyography shows the muscles' response to electrical shocks. In the MG patient, jitter is greatest in the weakest muscles and will generally be increased even in muscle of normal strength. Use of drugs may also aid in the diagnosis. The Tensilon test in a patient with MG reveals improved muscle contractility after intravenous injection of the anticholinesterase agent edrophonium chloride (Tensilon). (Anticholinesterase blocks the enzyme acetylcholinesterase.) This test also aids in the diagnosis of cholinergic crisis (secondary to overdose of anticholinesterase drug). In this condition, Tensilon does not improve muscle weakness but may actually increase it. Atropine, a cholinergic antagonist, should be readily available to counteract Tensilon effects when it is used diagnostically (Meriggioli & Sanders, 2005).

Collaborative Care

Drug Therapy. Drug therapy for MG includes anticholinesterase drugs, alternate-day corticosteroids, and immunosuppressants (Table 61-22). Anticholinesterase drugs are aimed at

COLLABORATIVE CARE

Table 61-22 Myasthenia Gravis

Diagnostic	Collaborative Therapy

• History and physical examination
• Fatigability when upward gaze is prolonged (2-3 min)
• Muscle weakness
• EMG
• Tensilon test
• Acetylcholine receptor antibodies
	• Drugs
	   • Anticholinesterase agents
	   • Corticosteroids
	   • Immunosuppressive agents
	• Surgery (thymectomy)
	• Plasmapheresis

EMG, electromyography.

enhancing function of the neuromuscular junction. Acetylcholinesterase is the enzyme that breaks down ACh in the synaptic cleft. Thus, inhibition of this enzyme by an anticholinesterase inhibitor will prolong the action of ACh and facilitate transmission of impulses at the neuromuscular junction. Neostigmine (Prostigmin) and pyridostigmine (Mestinon) are the most successful drugs of this group in treating MG. Tailoring the dose to avoid a myasthenic or cholinergic crisis often presents a challenge. Corticosteroids (specifically prednisone) are used to suppress the immune response. Drugs such as azathioprine (Imuran) and cyclophosphamide (Procytox) may also be used for immunosuppression (Gold & Gold, 2008).

Many drugs are contraindicated for use or must be used with caution in patients with MG. Classes of drug that should be cautiously evaluated before use include anaesthetics, antidysrhythmics, antibiotics, quinine, antipsychotics, barbiturates and sedative-hypnotics, cathartics, diuretics, narcotics, muscle relaxants, thyroid preparations, and tranquilizers (Gold & Gold, 2008).

Surgical Therapy. Because the presence of the thymus gland in the patient with MG appears to enhance the production of ACh receptor antibodies, removal of the thymus gland results in improvement in most patients. Thymectomy is indicated for all patients with thymoma and for patients with generalized MG who are younger than 60 years (Howard, 2006).

Other Therapies. Plasmapheresis can yield a short-term improvement in symptoms and is indicated for patients in crisis or in preparation for surgery when corticosteroids must be avoided. (Plasmapheresis is discussed in Chapter 16.) Intravenous immunoglobulin G (IVIG) has been used with some success and is recommended as a second-line treatment for MG. There is insufficient evidence that IVIG is better than plasmapheresis for treating exacerbations or for moderately severe MG (Gajdos, Chevret, & Toyka, 2006).

NURSING MANAGEMENT: MYASTHENIA GRAVIS

■ Nursing Assessment

The nurse can assess the severity of MG by asking the patient about fatigability, what body parts are affected, and how severely he or she is affected. The patient's coping abilities and understanding of the disorder should also be assessed. Some patients become so fatigued that they are no longer able to ambulate.

Objective data should include respiratory rate and depth, oxygen saturation, arterial blood gas analyses, pulmonary function tests, and evidence of respiratory distress in patients with acute myasthenic crisis. Muscle strength of all face and limb muscles should be assessed, as should swallowing, speech (clarity), voice (volume), cough and gag reflexes, and bladder function.

■ Nursing Diagnoses

Nursing diagnoses for the patient with MG may include, but are not limited to, the following:
- Ineffective breathing pattern *related to* intercostal muscle weakness
- Ineffective airway clearance *related to* intercostal muscle weakness and impaired cough and gag reflex
- Impaired verbal communication *related to* weakness of larynx, lips, mouth, pharynx, and jaw
- Imbalanced nutrition: less than body requirements *related to* impaired swallowing
- Impaired urinary elimination *related to* weakness of pelvic floor muscle
- Disturbed sensory perception (visual) *related to* ptosis, decreased eye movements, and disconjugate gaze
- Activity intolerance *related to* muscle weakness and fatigability
- Disturbed body image *related to* inability to maintain usual lifestyle and role responsibilities

■ Planning

The overall goals are that the patient with MG will (1) have a return of normal muscle endurance, (2) avoid complications, and (3) maintain a quality of life appropriate to disease course.

■ Nursing Implementation

The patient with MG who is admitted to the hospital usually has a respiratory tract infection or is in an acute myasthenic crisis. Nursing care is aimed at maintaining adequate ventilation, continuing drug therapy, and watching for adverse effects of therapy. The nurse must be able to distinguish cholinergic from myasthenic crisis (Table 61-23) because the causes and treatment of the two conditions differ greatly.

As with other chronic illnesses, care focuses on the neurological deficits and their impact on daily living. A balanced diet with food that can be chewed and swallowed easily should be prescribed. Semisolid foods may be easier to eat than solids or liquids. Scheduling doses of drugs so that peak action is reached at mealtime may make eating less difficult. Teaching should focus on the importance of following the medical regimen, potential adverse reactions to specific drugs, planning activities of daily living to avoid fatigue, the availability of community resources, and the complications of the disease and therapy (crisis conditions) and what to do about them. Contact with the Myasthenia Gravis Coalition of Canada or an MG support group may be helpful.

Table 61-23 Comparison of Myasthenic Crisis and Cholinergic Crisis

MYASTHENIC CRISIS	CHOLINERGIC CRISIS
Causes	
Exacerbation of myasthenia following precipitating factors or failure to take drug as prescribed or drug dose too low	Overdose of anticholinesterase drugs resulting in increased ACh at the receptor sites, remission (spontaneous or after thymectomy)
Differential Diagnosis	
Improved strength after IV administration of anticholinesterase drugs; increased weakness of skeletal muscles manifesting as ptosis, bulbar signs (e.g., difficulty in swallowing, difficulty in articulating words), or dyspnea	Weakness within 1 hr after ingestion of anticholinesterase; increased weakness of skeletal muscles manifesting as ptosis, bulbar signs, dyspnea; effects on smooth muscle include papillary miosis, salivation, diarrhea, nausea or vomiting, abdominal cramps, increased bronchial secretions, sweating, or lacrimation

ACh, acetylcholine; *IV*, intravenous.

Evaluation

The following are overall expected outcomes for the patient with MG:

- The patient will maintain optimal muscle function.
- The patient will be free from adverse effects of drugs.
- The patient will not experience complications, in particular myasthenic or cholinergic crises, from the disease.
- The patient will maintain a quality of life appropriate to the disease course.

Restless Legs Syndrome

Etiology and Pathophysiology

Restless legs syndrome (RLS) (also known as *Willis-Ekbom disease*) is characterized by unpleasant sensory (paresthesias) and motor abnormalities of one or both legs as well as an irritating sensation of uneasiness, tiredness, and itching deep within the muscles of the leg. It has an age-dependent prevalence of up to 14%, although the numbers may be higher because the condition is underdiagnosed (Pichler, Hicks, & Pramstaller, 2008). Although the exact cause of RLS is not known, probably more than half of all cases are transmitted in an autosomal dominant pattern. There are two distinct types of RLS: primary (idiopathic) and secondary. The majority of cases are primary, and many patients with this type of RLS report a positive family history. Secondary RLS can be seen in metabolic abnormalities associated with iron deficiency, renal failure, polyneuropathy associated with diabetes mellitus, rheumatic disorders (e.g., rheumatoid arthritis), or pregnancy. Anemia, deficient iron condition, and certain medications can cause or worsen symptoms (Winkelman, 2006; Trotti, Bhadriraju, & Rye, 2008).

Idiopathic RLS may be related to nervous system dysfunction. Although the exact cause remains to be determined, several theories include (1) an alteration in dopaminergic transmission in the basal ganglia, (2) axonal neuropathy, or (3) a brainstem disinhibition phenomenon resulting in motor and sensory disturbances (Trotti et al., 2008).

Clinical Manifestations

The severity of RLS sensory symptoms ranges from infrequent minor discomfort (paresthesias including numbness, tingling, "pins and needles" sensation) to severe pain. Sensory symptoms often appear first and are manifested as an annoying and uncomfortable (but usually not painful) sensation in the legs. The sensation is often compared with the sensation of bugs creeping or crawling on the legs. The leg pain is localized within the calf muscles. Patients can also experience pain in the upper extremities and the trunk. The discomfort occurs when the patient is sedentary and usually occurs in the evening or at night (Restless Legs Syndrome Foundation, 2007).

The pain at night can produce sleep disruptions and is often relieved by physical activity such as walking, stretching, rocking, or kicking. In the most severe cases, patients sleep only a few hours at night, resulting in daytime fatigue and disruption of the daily routine. The motor abnormalities associated with RLS consist of restlessness and stereotyped, periodic, involuntary movements. The involuntary movements usually occur during sleep. Symptoms are aggravated by fatigue. Over time, RLS advances to more frequent and severe episodes (Restless Legs Syndrome Foundation, 2007; Trotti et al., 2008).

Diagnostic Studies

RLS is a clinical diagnosis and is based in large part on the patient's history or the report of the bed partner related to nighttime activities. The International Restless Legs Study Group proposed four minimum diagnostic criteria. They are (1) desire to move the limbs, (2) motor restlessness, (3) symptoms that are worse or exclusively present at rest with at least partial and temporary relief with activity, and (4) symptoms that are worse in the evening or night (Karatas, 2007). Generally, the patient history clearly suggests a diagnosis of RLS (Restless Legs Syndrome Foundation, 2007). The patient's history of diabetes mellitus and its management may provide information to determine whether paresthesias are caused by peripheral neuropathy or RLS.

NURSING AND COLLABORATIVE MANAGEMENT: RESTLESS LEGS SYNDROME

The goal of collaborative management is to reduce patient discomfort and distress and to improve sleep quality. When RLS is secondary to uremia or iron deficiency, correction of these conditions will decrease symptoms. Nonpharmacological approaches to RLS management include establishing regular sleep habits, encouraging exercise, avoiding activities that cause symptoms, and eliminating aggravating factors such as alcohol, caffeine, and certain drugs (i.e., neuroleptics, lithium, antihistamines, and antidepressants) (Restless Legs Syndrome Foundation, 2007).

If nonpharmacological measures fail to provide symptom relief, drug therapy may be started. The main drugs used in RLS are dopaminergic agents, opioids, and benzodiazepines. Dopaminergic agents such as carbidopa–L-dopa (Sinemet) and DA agonists (bromocriptine, pramipexole [Mirapex]) are preferred for treating RLS. These agents are effective in managing sensory and motor symptoms. Dopaminergic agents have a number of adverse effects, including hypotension and gastric irritation (Karatas, 2007).

Other agents that may be used include antiseizure drugs such as gabapentin (Neurontin), divalproex, lamotrigine (Lamictal), and carbamazepine (Tegretol). Clonidine (Catapres) and propranolol (Inderal) are also effective in some patients. Quinine sulphate can be used prophylactically and as a treatment for RLS. Opioids (e.g., oxycodone) are usually reserved for those patients with severe symptoms who fail to respond to other drugs. When used, opioids given in low doses have also been found to be effective in reducing the symptoms associated with RLS.

Amyotrophic Lateral Sclerosis

Amyotrophic lateral sclerosis (ALS) is a rare progressive neurological disorder; it is characterized by loss of motor neurons and by weakness and atrophy of the muscles of the hands, the forearms, and the legs, spreading to involve most of the body and the face. ALS usually leads to death within 2 to 6 years after diagnosis. ALS became known as *Lou Gehrig's disease* when the famous baseball player was stricken with it in the 1940s. ALS has a worldwide incidence of about 1.5 to 2.5 per 100,000 members of the population and a prevalence of 4 to 7 per 100,000 worldwide (Amyotrophic Lateral Sclerosis [ALS] Society of Canada, 2011; Logroscino et al., 2006). Approximately 2500 to 3000 Canadians are currently living with ALS (ALS Society of Canada, 2011). The onset is usually between 40 and 70 years of age and ALS is twice as common in men as in women (ALS Society of Canada, 2011).

For unknown reasons, motor neurons in the brainstem and spinal cord gradually degenerate in ALS (see eFigure 61-2, available on the Evolve Web site for this chapter). Dead motor neurons cannot produce or transport vital signals to muscles. Consequently, electrical and chemical messages originating in the brain do not reach the muscles to activate them.

The typical symptoms are weakness of the upper extremities, dysarthria, and dysphagia. However, weakness may begin in the legs. Muscle wasting and fasciculations result from the denervation of the muscles and lack of stimulation and use. Death usually results from respiratory infection secondary to compromised respiratory function (Logroscino et al., 2006). Unfortunately, there is no cure for ALS. Riluzole (Rilutek) slows the progression of ALS. This drug works to decrease the amount of glutamate (an excitatory neurotransmitter) in the brain. In clinical trials, riluzole has been shown to delay the need for tracheostomy and death by a few months (Miller, Mitchell, Lyon, & Moore, 2008).

The illness trajectory for ALS is devastating because the patient remains cognitively intact while wasting away. The challenge of nursing care is to guide the patient in use of moderate-intensity endurance types of exercises for the trunk and the limbs because this may help to reduce ALS spasticity (Ashworth, Satkunam, & Deforge, 2008). In addition, the nurse must support the patient's cognitive and emotional functions. Nursing interventions may include (1) facilitating communication, (2) reducing risk of aspiration, (3) decreasing pain secondary to muscle weakness, (4) decreasing risk of injury related to falls, (5) providing diversional activities such as reading and human companionship, and (6) helping the patient and family manage the disease process, to include grieving related to loss of motor function and ultimately death.

Huntington's Disease

Huntington's disease (HD) is a genetically transmitted, autosomal dominant disorder that affects both men and women of all races; it is characterized by chronic, devastating loss of all neurological function, resulting in dementia. The offspring of a person with this disease have a 50% risk of inheriting it (see Genetics in Clinical Practice box). The onset of HD is usually between 30 and 50 years of age with an age range of 2 to 80 years (Walker, 2007). Often the diagnosis is made after the affected individual has had children. Approximately 1 in every 10,000 Canadians has HD, and approximately 5 in every 10,000 are at risk for developing it (Huntington Society of Canada, n.d.). Diagnosis in the past was based on family history and clinical symptoms. However, because the gene for HD has been discovered, an individual can now be tested for the presence of the gene. People who are asymptomatic but who have a positive family history of HD face the dilemma of whether or not to get tested. If the test is positive, the person will develop HD, but when and to what extent the disease develops cannot be determined.

GENETICS IN CLINICAL PRACTICE
Huntington's Disease

Genetic Basis
- Autosomal dominant disorder
- Caused by mutation of single gene located on chromosome 4
- Expression similar in homozygotes and heterozygotes

Incidence
- 1 in 10,000
- Higher incidence in people of European ancestry
- With each pregnancy, an affected parent has a 50% chance of having a child with Huntington's disease (HD)

Genetic Testing
- DNA testing is available.
- DNA testing can be done on fetal cells obtained by amniocentesis or chorionic biopsy.
- Genetic testing can determine whether a person is a carrier.
- No test is available to predict when symptoms will develop.

Clinical Implications
- Onset of disease usually occurs between 30 to 50 years of age.
- HD is a progressive, degenerative brain disorder.
- No cure is available.
- Drugs are available to control movements and behavioural problems.
- Genetic counselling may be considered if there is a family history of HD.

Like PD, the pathological process of HD involves the basal ganglia and the extrapyramidal motor system. However, instead of a deficiency of DA, HD involves a deficiency of the neurotransmitters ACh and γ-aminobutyric acid. The net effect is an excess of DA, which leads to symptoms that are the opposite of those of parkinsonism.

The clinical manifestations are characterized by abnormal and excessive involuntary movements (*chorea*) as well as psychiatric abnormalities. These are writhing, twisting movements of the face, the limbs, and the body. The movements worsen as the disease progresses. Facial movements involving speech, chewing, and swallowing are affected and may cause aspiration and malnutrition. The gait deteriorates, and ambulation eventually becomes impossible. Perhaps the most devastating deterioration is in mental functions, which include intellectual decline, emotional lability, and psychotic behaviour. Death usually occurs 10 to 20 years after the onset of symptoms (Huntington Society of Canada, n.d.).

Because there is no cure, collaborative care is palliative. The first drug of any kind approved specifically for HD is tetrabenazine (Nitoman). It is used to treat the chorea, and works to decrease the amount of dopamine available at synapses in the brain and thus decreases the involuntary movements of chorea. Antipsychotic (e.g., haloperidol), antidepressant (fluoxetine [Prozac], sertraline [Zoloft], nortriptyline [Aventyl]), and anti-chorea (clonazepam) drugs are prescribed and provide some benefit. However, they do not alter the course of the disease.

HD presents a great challenge to health care providers. The goal of nursing management is to provide the most comfortable environment possible for the patient and the family by maintaining physical safety, treating physical symptoms, and providing emotional and psychological support. Because of the choreic movements, caloric requirements are high. Patients may require as many as 4000 to 5000 calories per day to maintain body weight. As the disease progresses and the patient has difficulty swallowing and holding the head still, meeting caloric needs becomes an even greater challenge. Depression and mental deterioration can also compromise nutritional intake.

Normal Pressure Hydrocephalus

Normal pressure hydrocephalus (NPH) is an abnormal increase of CSF characterized by an obstruction in the normal flow of CSF throughout the brain, spinal cord, and ventricles. NPH is a relatively uncommon disorder, and symptoms of the condition include mental impairment, dementia, urinary incontinence, and gait and balance disturbances. Meningitis, encephalitis, or head injury may cause the condition. NPH can occur at any age, although it is most common in the elderly. If diagnosed early in the disease, NPH is treatable by surgery that involves a shunt insertion to divert the fluid away from the brain into the abdomen to help resolve symptoms of NPH (NINDS, 2011).

CLINICAL DECISION-MAKING EXERCISE

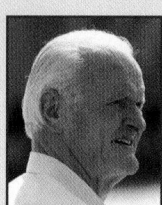

CASE STUDY:
Parkinson's Disease

Source: © iStockphoto.com/Don Bayley.

Patient Profile

Mr. Dufresne, a 79-year-old retiree, was diagnosed with Parkinson's disease 3 years ago after experiencing months of progressive tremor, rigidity, and bradykinesia. He has been taking L-dopa with carbidopa (Sinemet) since then and his symptoms had been improving until recently. When his daughter was visiting, she noticed that Mr. Dufresne had lost considerable weight over the past month, and his speech had become slower and more challenging to understand.

Subjective Data

- Reports increasing difficulty with speech and swallowing
- Dietary intake has decreased
- Reports being constipated for 2 weeks

Objective Data

Physical Examination

- Body weight has decreased by 5 kg in 1 month.
- Gait has developed a mild shuffling and propulsive quality.
- "Pill rolling" motion and tremor are observed in both hands at rest.
- "Cogwheel rigidity" is encountered during passive range of motion exercises.

Discussion Questions

1. What is the pathogenesis of Parkinson's disease?
2. What is the likely explanation for the progression of Mr. Dufresne's condition?
3. What teaching plan should be developed for Mr. Dufresne?
4. *Priority Decision:* What are the priority nursing interventions for Mr. Dufresne?
5. *Priority Decision:* What are the priority nursing diagnoses based on the assessment data presented for Mr. Dufresne?

℮volve *Answers are available at* **http://evolve.elsevier.com/ Canada/Lewis/medsurg**

REVIEW QUESTIONS

The number of the question corresponds to the same-numbered objective at the beginning of the chapter.

1. What of the following is the nurse most likely to recognize as a symptom of a patient with a migraine headache?
   a. Withdraws from stimuli
   b. Acts out with bizarre behaviour
   c. Seeks out the company of others
   d. Experiences painful facial spasms and tearing

2. What are the triad of symptoms the nurse would expect to find during assessment of the patient with Parkinson's disease?
   a. Spasticity, diplopia, tremor
   b. Tremor, rigidity, bradykinesia
   c. Ataxia, drowsiness, dysarthria
   d. Diplopia, tremor, bradykinesia

3. What would the nurse expect to find during an assessment of the patient with amyotrophic lateral sclerosis?
   a. Emotional lability
   b. Mental deterioration
   c. Muscle weakness and wasting
   d. Sensory loss in the extremities

4. What has the greatest impact on emotional response in a patient with a chronic neurological disease?
   a. Symptoms of intellectual deterioration
   b. Cognitive impairment
   c. Physical disability and changes in body image
   d. Family members who provide care

5. What is a major goal of treatment for the patient with a chronic, progressive neurological disease?
   a. Reversal of pathophysiological features
   b. Total remission of the disease
   c. Continuation of usual lifestyle
   d. Adaptation by patient and family to the disease

ANSWERS: 1. a; 2. b; 3. c; 4. c; 5. d.

REFERENCES

Amyotrophic Lateral Sclerosis Society of Canada. (2011). *ALS quick facts.* Retrieved from http://www.als.ca/_media/docs/ALS%20QUICK%20FACTS.pdf

Ashworth, N. L., Satkunam, L. E., & Deforge, D. (2008). Treatment for spasticity in amyotrophic lateral sclerosis/motor neuron disease. *Cochrane Database Systematic Reviews 2008, 1,* CD004156. doi:10.1002/14651858.CD004156.pub3

Awad, A., Marder, E., Milo, R., & Stuve, O. (2011). Multiple sclerosis and chronic cerebrospinal venous insufficiency: a critical review. *Therapeutic Advances in Neurological Disorders, 4*(4), 231-253. doi:10.1177/1756285611405565

Backer, J. H. (2006). The symptom experience of patients with Parkinson's disease. *Journal of Neuroscience Nursing, 38*(1), 51-57. doi:10.1097/01376517-200602000-00010

Beghi, E. (2007). Epilepsy. *Current Opinion in Neurology, 20*(2), 169-174. doi:10.1097/WCO.0b013e3280d646e4

Berg, A., Berkovic, S., Brodie, M., Buchhalter, J., Cross, J. H., van Emde Boas, W., …, Scheffer, I. E. (2010). Revised terminology and concepts for organization of seizures and epilepsies: Report of the ILAE commission on classification and terminology, 2005-2009. *Epilepsia, 51*(4), 676-685. doi:10.1111/j.1528-1167.2010.02522.x

Bershad, E. M., Feen, E. S., & Suarez, J. I. (2008). Myasthenia gravis crisis. *Southern Medical Journal, 101*(1), 63-69. doi:10.1097/SMJ.0b013e31815d4398

Burton, J. M., Alikhani, K., Goyal, M., Costello, F., White, C., Patry, D., …, Hill, M. D. (2011). Complications in MS Patients after CCSVI Procedures Abroad (Calgary, AB). *The Canadian Journal of Neurosciences, 38,* 741-746. Retrieved from http://cjns.metapress.com/content/m2153726237uu554/fulltext.pdf

Cavazos, J. E. (2012). *Epilepsy and seizures.* Retrieved from http://emedicine.medscape.com/article/1184846-overview

CCSVI Foundation of Canada. (2011). About us: Why this foundation exists. Retrieved from http://ccsvifoundationcanada.org/about_us

Chao, M. J., Ramagopalan, S. V., Herrera, B. M., Orton, S. M., Handunnetthi, L., Lincoln, M. R., …, Ebers, G. C. (2011). *Neurology, 76*(3), 242-246. doi:10.1212/WNL.0b013e318207b060

Cohen, B. A. (2007). Evolving views of MS pathogenesis. *International Journal of MS Care, 9*(Suppl 4), 4-10.

Dickson, D., Braak, H., Duda, J., Duyckaerts, C., Gasser, T., Halliday, G. M., …, Litvan, I. (2009). Neuropathological assessment of Parkinson's disease: Refining the diagnostic criteria. *Lancet Neurology, 8*(12), 1150-1157. doi:10.1016/S1474-4422(09)70238-8

Elger, C., & Schmidt, D. (2008). Modern management of epilepsy: a practical approach. *Epilepsy and Behavior, 12*(4), 501-539. doi:10.1016/j.yebeh.2008.01.003

Epilepsy Canada. (n.d. [a]). *Epilepsy facts.* Retrieved from http://www.epilepsy.ca/en-CA/Facts/Types-of-Seizures.html

Epilepsy Canada. (n.d. [b]). *Living with epilepsy.* Retrieved from http://www.epilepsy.ca/en-CA/Coping/Living-with-Epilepsy_/30197/Women.html

Epilepsy Foundation. (2010). *Medications.* Retrieved from http://www.epilepsyfoundation.org/aboutepilepsy/treatment/medications/index.cfm

Epilepsy Ontario. (2011). *Medications for epilepsy.* Retrieved from http://www.epilepsyontario.org/patient/eo/eoweb.nsf/web/Medications

Francis, G., Becker, W., & Pringsheim, T. (2010). Acute and preventive pharmacologic treatment of cluster headache. *Neurology, 75*(5), 463-473. doi:10.1212/WNL.0b013e3181eb58c8

Frank, G., Pari, G., & Rossiter, J. P. (2006). Approach to diagnosis of Parkinson disease. *Canadian Family Physician, 52*(July), 862-868.

Gajdos, P., Chevret, S., & Toyka, K. (2006). Intravenous immunoglobulin for myasthenia gravis. *Cochrane Database Systematic Review, 2,* CD002277. doi:10.1002/14651858.CD002277.pub2

Gold, R., & Gold, C. (2008). Current and future standards in treatment of myasthenia gravis. *Neurotherapeutics, 5*(4), 535-541. doi:10.1016/j.nurt.2008.08.011

Groesbeck, D. K., Bluml, R. M., & Kossoff, E. H. (2006). Long-term use of the ketogenic diet in the treatment of epilepsy. *Developmental Medicine & Child Neurology, 48*(12), 978-981. doi:10.1017/S0012162206002143

Halker, R., Vargus, B., & Dodick, D. (2010). Cluster headache: Diagnosis and treatment. *Seminars in Neurology, 30*(2), 175-184. doi:10.1055/s-0030-1249226

Hartl, D. M., Leboulleux, S., Klap, P., & Schlumberger, M. (2007). Myasthenia gravis mimicking unilateral vocal fold paralysis at presentation. *Journal of Laryngology & Otology, 121*(2), 174-178.

Headache Classification Subcommittee of the International Headache Society. (2004). The International Classification of Headache Disorders (2nd ed.). *Cephalgia, 24*(Suppl 1), 1-152. doi:10.1111/j.1468-2982.2003.00823.x

Herrera, B. M., Ramagopalan, S. V., Orton, S., Chao, M. J., Yee, I. M., Sandovnick, A. D., & Ebers, G. C. (2007). Parental transmission of MS in a population-based Canadian cohort. *Neurology, 69*(12), 1208-1212. doi:10.1212/01.wnl.0000268486.40851.d6

Howard, J. F. (2006). *Myasthenia gravis—A summary.* Retrieved from http://myasthenia.org/hp_clinical_overview.cfm

Huntington Society of Canada. (n.d.). *HSC: We're here to help.* Retrieved from http://www.huntingtonsociety.ca/english/uploads/Were_here_to_Help_final.pdf

Jabs, S., Seifert, G., & Steinhauser, C. (2008). Astrocytic function and its alteration in the epileptic brain. *Epilepsia, 49*(Suppl 2), 3-12. doi:10.1111/j.1528-1167.2008.01488.x

Jelinski, S. E., Becker, W. J., Christie, S. N., Giammarco, R., Mackie, G. F., Gawel, M. J., …, Magnusson, J. E. (2006). Demographics and clinical features of patients referred to headache specialists. *The Canadian Journal of Neurological Sciences. Le Journal Canadien des Sciences Neurologiques, 33*(2), 228-234.

Karatas, M. (2007). Restless legs syndrome and periodic limb movements during sleep: Diagnosis and treatment. *The Neurologist, 13*(5), 294-301. doi:10.1097/NRL.0b013e3181422589

Klein, C., & Schlossmacher, M. G. (2006). The genetics of Parkinson disease: Implications for neurological care. *Nature Clinical Practice Neurology, 2*(3), 136-146. doi:10.1038/ncpneuro0126

Kleiner-Fisman, G., Herzog, J., Fisman, D. N., Tamma, F., Lyons, K. E., Pahwa, R., …, Deuschl, G. (2006). Subthalamic nucleus deep brain stimulation: Summary and metaanalysis of outcomes. *Movement Disorders, 21*(Suppl 14), S290-S304. doi:10.1002/mds.20962

Lazzaro, M., Zaidat, O. O., Mueller-Kronast, N., Taqi, M. A., & Woo, D. (2011). Endovascular therapy for chronic cerebrospinal venous insufficiency in multiple sclerosis. *Frontiers in neurology, 2*(July, Article 44), 1-7. doi:10.3389/fneur.2011.00044

Leroux, E., & Ducros, A. (2008). Cluster headache. *Orphanet Journal of Rare Disorders, 3*, 20. doi:10.1186/1750-1172-3-20

Lindahl, A., & MacMahon, D. (2011). Parkinson's: Treating the symptoms. *British Journal of Nursing, 20*(14), 852-857.

Loder, E. (2009). Migraine with aura and increased risk of ischaemic stroke. *BMJ, 339*(b4380), doi:10.1136/bmj.b4380

Loder, E., & Rizzoli, P. (2008). Tension-type headache. *BMJ, 336*(7635), 88-92. doi:10.1136/bmj.39412.705868.AD

Logroscino, G., Traynor, B. J., Hardiman, O., Chio, A., Couratier, P., Mitchell, J. D., …, EURALS. (2006). Descriptive epidemiology of amyotrophic lateral sclerosis: New evidence and unsolved issues. *Journal of Neurology, Neurosurgery & Psychiatry, 79*(1), 6-11. doi:10.1136/jnnp.2006.104828

Luchanok, U., & Kaminski, H. J. (2008). Ocular myasthenia: Diagnostic and treatment recommendations and the evidence base. *Current Opinion in Neurology, 21*(1), 8-15. doi:10.1097/WCO.0b013e3282f4098e

McLaughlin, D., & McFarland, K. (2011). A randomized trial of a group-based cognitive behavior therapy program for older adults with epilepsy: the impact on seizure frequency, depression and psychosocial well-being. *Journal of Behavioral Medicine, 34*(3), 201-207. doi:10.1007/s10865-010-9299-z

Meriggioli, M. N., & Sanders, D. B. (2005). Advances in the diagnosis of neuromuscular junction disorders. *American Journal of Physical Medicine & Rehabilitation-Association of Academic Physiatrists, 84*(8), 627-638. doi:10.1097/01.phm.0000171169.79816.4c

Miller, R. G., Mitchell, J. D., Lyon, M., & Moore, L. M. (2008). Riluzole for amyotrophic lateral sclerosis (ALS)/motor neuron disease (MND). *Cochrane Database Systematic Reviews, 1*, CD001447. doi:10.1002/14651858.CD001447.pub2

Moore, L. A. (2007). Intimacy and multiple sclerosis. *Nursing Clinics of North America, 42*(4), 605-619. doi:10.1016/j.cnur.2007.07.007

Multiple Sclerosis International Federation. (2008). *Prevalence of MS globally*. Retrieved from *http://www.mssociety.ca/en/pdf/pub_MSl17888Addendum_En.pdf*

Multiple Sclerosis International Federation. (2011). Pharmacological treatments in MS. *MS in Focus, 18*, 1-7.

Multiple Sclerosis Society of Canada. (2011). *Types of MS*. Retrieved from *http://www.mssociety.ca/en/information/types.htm*

Myasthenia Gravis Coalition of Canada. (2011). *Signs and symptoms of MG*. Retrieved from *http://mgcc-ccmg.org/about.asp*

Myasthenia Gravis Foundation of America (2010). *Clinical overview of MG*. Retrieved from *http://www.myasthenia.org/Health Professionals/ClinicalOverviewofMG.aspx*

National Institute for Health and Clinical Excellence (NICE). (2007). *Multiple sclerosis–natalizumab: Appraisal consultation document*. Retrieved from *http://www.nice.org.uk/guidance/index.jsp?action=article&r=true&o=35012*

National Institute of Neurological Disorders and Stroke (NINDS). (2010). *Myasthenia fact sheet*. Retrieved from *http://www.ninds.*

nih.gov/disorders/myasthenia_gravis/detail_myasthenia_gravis.htm?css=print

National Institute of Neurological Disorders and Stroke (NINDS). (2011). *Normal pressure hydrocephalus information page*. Retrieved from *http://www.ninds.nih.gov/disorders/normal_pressure_hydrocephalus/normal_pressure_hydrocephalus.htm*

National Multiple Sclerosis Society. (n.d.). *Who gets MS?* Retrieved from *http://www.nationalmssociety.org/about-multiple-sclerosis/what-we-know-about-ms/who-gets-ms/index.aspx*

Oh, S. (2009). Muscle-specific receptor tyrosone kinase antibody positive myasthenia gravis current status. *Journal of Clinical Neurology, 5*(2), 53-64. doi:10.3988/jcn.2009.5.2.53

Parkinson Society Canada. (2003). *Exercises for people with Parkinson's*. Retrieved from *http://www.parkinson.ca/atf/cf/%7BD40C382A-398D-4841-913A-A1491D9B901F%7D/ExerciseBrochure_Eng.pdf*

Parkinson Society Canada. (2011). *Fact sheet*. Retrieved from *http://www.parkinson.ca/atf/cf/%7B9ebd08a9-7886-4b2d-a1c4-a131e7096bf8%7D/PSCFACTSHEETJUNE2011.PDF*

Pichler, I., Hicks, A. A., & Pramstaller, P. P. (2008). Restless legs syndrome: An update on genetics and future perspectives. *Clinical Genetics, 73*(4), 297-305. doi:10.1111/j.1399-0004.2007.00937.x

Purdy, R. (2010). Migraine is curable. *Neurological Sciences, 31*(1), 141-143. doi:10.1007/s10072-010-0308-3

Ramani, R. (2008). Vagus nerve stimulation therapy for seizures. *Journal of Neurosurgical Anesthesiology, 20*(1), 29-35. doi:10.1097/ANA.0b013e31815b7df1

Restless Legs Syndrome Foundation. (2007). *RLS facts sheet*. Retrieved from *http://www.rls.org//Document.Doc?&id=766*

Schilling, A., Corey, R., Leonard, M., & Eghtesad, B. (2011). Acetaminophen: old drug, new warnings. *Cleveland Clinic Journal of Medicine, 77*(1), 19-27.

Shah, A. K. (2006). *Myasthenia gravis*. Retrieved from *http://www.emedicine.com/neuro/topic232.htm*

Singh, N., Pillay, V., & Choonara, Y. E. (2007). Advances in the treatment of Parkinson's disease. *Progress in Neurobiology, 81*(1), 29-44. doi:10.1016/j.pneurobio.2006.11.009

Sosnoff, J., Motl, R., Snook, E., & Wynn, D. (2009). Effect of a 4-week period of loaded leg cycling exercise on spasticity in multiple sclerosis. *NeuroRehabilitation, 24*(4), 327-331. doi:10.3233/NRE-2009-0486

Swinn, L. (2005). *Parkinson's disease theory and practice for nurses*. Philadelphia: Whurr Publishers.

Task Force on Epilepsy Classification and Terminology. (2011). *Epileptic seizure types and precipitating stimuli for reflex seizures, International League against Epilepsy*. Retrieved from *http://www.ilae-epilepsy.org/Visitors/Centre/ctf/seizure_type.cfm*

Tellez-Zenteno, J. F., Patten, S. B., Jette, N., Williams, J., & Wiebe, S. (2007). Psychiatric comorbidity in epilepsy: A population-based analysis. *Epilepsia 48*(12), 2336-2344. doi:10.1111/j.1528-1167.2007.01222.x

Tfelt-Hansen, P., & Koehler, P. (2011). One hundred years of migraine research: major clinical and scientific observations from 1910 to 2010. *Headache: Journal of Head and Face Pain, 51*(5), 752-778. doi:10.111/j.1526-4610.2011.01892.x

Tremlett, H., Zhao, Y., Rieckmann, P., & Hutchinson, M. (2010). New perspectives in the natural history of multiple sclerosis (Review). *Neurology, 74*, 2004-2015. doi:10.1212/WNL.0b013e3181e3973f

Tugwell, C. (2008). *Parkinson's disease in focus*. London: Pharmaceutical Press.

Trotti, L., Bhadriraju, B., & Rye, B. (2008). An update on the pathophysiology and genetics of restless legs syndrome. *Current neurology and Neuroscience Reports, 8*(4), 281-287. doi:10.1007/s11910-008-0044-8

Vernon, G. (2009). Parkinson disease and the nurse practitioner: Diagnostic and management challenges. *Journal for Nurse Practitioners, 5*(3), 195-206. doi:10.1016/j.nurpra.2008.12.007

Wade, D. T., Collin, C., Stott, C., & Duncombe, P. (2010). Meta-analysis of the efficacy and safety of Sativex (nabiximols) on spasticity in people with multiple sclerosis. *Multiple Sclerosis Journal, 16*(6), 707-714.

Walker, F. O. (2007). Huntington's disease. *Seminars in Neurology, 27*(2), 143-150. doi:10.1055/s-2007-971176

Winkelman, J. W. (2006). Considering the causes of RLS. *European Journal of Neurology, 13*(Suppl 3), 8-14. doi:10.1111/j.1468-1331.2006.01588.x-i1

Zamboni, P., Galeotti, R., Menegatti, E., Malagoni, A., Tacconi, G., Dall'ara, S., ..., Salvi, F. (2008). Chronic cerebrospinal venous insufficiency in patients with multiple sclerosis. *Journal of Neurology, Neurosurgery, and Psychiatry, 80*(4), 392-399. doi:10.1136/jnnp.2008.157164

CANADIAN RESOURCES

Amyotrophic Lateral Sclerosis Society of Canada
http://www.als.ca

Canadian Association of Neuroscience Nurses (CANN)
http://www.cann.ca

Canadian Human Rights Commission
http://www.chrc-ccdp.ca

Canadian Institute of Health Research
http://www.cihr-irsc.gc.ca

CCSVI Foundation of Canada
http://ccsvifoundationcanada.org

Epilepsy Canada
http://www.epilepsy.ca

Huntington Society of Canada
http://www.hsc-ca.org

Multiple Sclerosis Society of Canada
http://www.mssociety.ca

Myasthenia Gravis Coalition of Canada
http://www.mgcc-ccmg.org

Parkinson Society Canada
General: *http://www.parkinson.ca*
Exercises for People with Parkinson's: *http://www.parkinson.ca/atf/cf/%7BD40C382A-398D-4841-913A-A1491D9B901F%7D/ExerciseBrochure_Eng.pdf*

Veterans Affairs Canada
http://www.vac-acc.gc.ca

RELATED RESOURCES

American Council for Headache Education (ACHE)
http://www.achenet.org

Association of Rehabilitation Nurses (ARN)
http://www.rehabnurse.org

Myasthenia Gravis Foundation of America
http://www.myasthenia.org

National Headache Foundation
http://www.headaches.org

National Institute of Neurological Disorders and Stroke (NINDS)
http://www.ninds.nih.gov

Willis-Ekbom Disease Foundation, formerly Restless Legs Syndrome Foundation
http://www.rls.org

⊜volve *For additional Internet resources, see the Web site for this book at* **http://evolve.elsevier.com/Canada/Lewis/medsurg**

Nursing Management: Delirium, Alzheimer's Disease, and Other Dementias

Written by Sharon L. Lewis
Adapted by Lynn McCleary

LEARNING OBJECTIVES

1. Describe the etiology, the pathophysiology, and the clinical manifestations of delirium.
2. Describe the diagnostic studies and the collaborative management of delirium.
3. Define dementia and describe its effect on society.
4. Compare and contrast etiologies of different types of dementia.
5. Describe the clinical manifestations, the diagnostic studies, and the collaborative management of dementia.
6. Describe the clinical manifestations of mild cognitive impairment.
7. Describe the nursing management of patients with dementia.

KEY TERMS

amyloid plaques Clusters of insoluble deposits of β-amyloid protein, other proteins, remnants of neurons, non-nerve cells, and other cells that develop in abnormal quantities in the brains of persons with Alzheimer's disease, p. 1741

Alzheimer's disease (AD) A chronic, progressive, degenerative disease of the brain; the most common form of dementia, p. 1741

behavioural and psychological symptoms of dementia (BPSDs) A term referring to behavioural and psychological manifestations of dementia, caused by a combination of biological factors, environmental factors, and social factors, p. 1744

Confusion Assessment Method A screening instrument that is effective in identifying the presence of delirium, p. 1738

Creutzfeldt-Jakob disease (CJD) A rare and fatal infectious brain disorder thought to be caused by accumulation in the brain of abnormally folded prion protein, p. 1743

delirium A state of acute mental confusion, p. 1737

dementia A collection of symptoms caused by various diseases that affect the brain; impairments typically involve multiple areas of cognitive functioning, including memory, communication, ability to carry out purposeful movements, ability to recognize common objects, judgement, reasoning, mood, and behaviour, p. 1740

dementia with Lewy Bodies (DLB) A condition characterized by the presence of Lewy bodies (intraneural cytoplasmic inclusions) in the brainstem, amygdala, and cortex, p. 1743

familial Alzheimer's disease A form of Alzheimer's disease with a clear pattern of inheritance within a family and onset before the age of 60, p. 1741

frontotemporal dementia (FTD) Dementia characterized by degeneration of the frontal lobe, temporal lobe, or both, p. 1743

mild cognitive impairment (MCI) A state of cognitive decline that is not severe enough to interfere with activities of daily living, p. 1743

neurofibrillary tangles Abnormal collections of twisted protein threads inside nerve cells seen in the areas of the brain most affected by Alzheimer's disease, p. 1741

responsive behaviours Behavioural symptoms of dementia that are often a response to something in the patient's environment, p. 1744

sundowning A pattern of behavioural disturbance that occurs in the late afternoon, p. 1752

vascular dementia The loss of cognitive function resulting from ischemic, ischemic–hypoxic, or hemorrhagic brain lesions caused by cardiovascular disease, p. 1743

ELECTRONIC RESOURCES

Supplemental content related to Chapter 62 can be found...

Evolve Web Site ⊝volve

http://evolve.elsevier.com/Canada/Lewis/medsurg
- Answer Guidelines for Case Study on p. 1755
- Audio Lecture: Alzheimer's Disease
- Clinical Reference: Laboratory Values
- Content Updates
- Customizable Nursing Care Plan: Alzheimer's Disease

- Electronic Calculators
- eNCP 62-1: Caregiver of the Patient With Alzheimer's Disease
- Examination Review Questions
- Glossary
- Interactive Case Study: Alzheimer's Disease
- Key Points (Printable and MP3 Download)
- Patient & Caregiver Teaching Guides:
  - Early Warning Signs of Alzheimer's Disease
  - Managing Alzheimer's Disease

The three most common cognitive problems in adults are delirium, dementia, and depression. These problems often present with overlapping clinical features and may coexist in the older adult (Registered Nurses' Association of Ontario [RNAO], 2003/2010). It is important to be able to identify the distinguishing characteristics because the treatment for each problem is different.

Delirium

Delirium, a state of acute mental confusion, is a medical emergency that occurs frequently in older adults. Although it is one of the most common life-threatening conditions in older individuals, it is preventable in 30 to 40% of cases (Inouye, 2006). Nurses are at the front line for prevention and early detection of delirium. However, like other health providers, nurses often fail to recognize delirium (Steis & Fick, 2008). Prevalence of delirium is highest among hospitalized older adults. More than half of hospitalized older adults develop delirium, with rates of 25 to 50% after fractures or surgery, 70 to 87% in the critical care unit, and 68% among patients with pre-existing dementia (Canadian Coalition for Seniors' Mental Health [CCSMH], 2006; Voyer, Cole, McCusker, & Belzile, 2006). Delirium is associated with longer hospitalizations, loss of functioning, higher rates of institutionalization, and higher rates of mortality (CCSMH, 2006).

Etiology and Pathophysiology

The pathophysiology of delirium is poorly understood and is related to multiple mechanisms. Inflammation, hypoxia, chronic stress, and neurotransmitter imbalance are all hypothesized to contribute to delirium (Inouye, 2006). There is strong evidence implicating cholinergic deficiency (Inouye, 2006), which may, in turn, affect levels of other neurotransmitters such as dopamine, serotonin, and norepinephrine (Hshieh, Fong, Marcantonio, & Inouye, 2008).

Delirium is usually the result of interaction between the patient's underlying condition and a precipitating event. Delirium can occur after a relatively minor insult in a vulnerable patient. For example, patients with underlying health problems such as heart failure, cognitive impairment, or sensory limitations may develop delirium after a relatively minor change (e.g., a single dose of a sleeping medication). In less vulnerable patients,

it may take a combination of factors (e.g., anaesthesia, major surgery, infection, prolonged sleep deprivation) to precipitate delirium (Inouye, 2006). Delirium can also be a symptom of a serious medical illness such as bacterial meningitis.

Knowing which factors increase vulnerability to delirium (predisposing factors) or precipitate delirium (precipitating factors) facilitates prevention of delirium and effective intervention. These factors are listed in Table 62-1.

Delirium occurs in children and adults, but older adults are at higher risk. They are more likely to have one of more of the risk factors for delirium. Normal age-related changes (see Chapter 7) limit older adults' abilities to compensate for physiological insults such as hypoxia, hypoglycemia, and dehydration and increase their susceptibility to medication-induced delirium. Patients with dementia are at risk on two fronts: Their risk for developing delirium is higher, and the probability that the delirium will be identified is lower (Fick & Mion, 2008).

Clinical Manifestations

The core features of delirium are as follows (American Psychiatric Association, 2000, p. 143):

> (A) Disturbance of consciousness (i.e., reduced clarity of awareness of the environment) with reduced ability to focus, sustain or shift attention; (B) a change in cognition (such as memory deficit, disorientation, language disturbance) or the development of a perceptual disturbance that is not better accounted for by a pre-existing, established or evolving dementia; (C) the disturbance develops over a short period of time (usually hours to days) and tends to fluctuate during the course of the day.

There are three subtypes of delirium: hyperactive delirium, which is characterized by restlessness, psychomotor agitation, and hypervigilance; hypoactive delirium, which is characterized by lethargy, drowsiness, and decreased motor activity; and mixed delirium, which has features of both hypoactive and hyperactive delirium. Illusions and hallucinations are present in 30% of all cases (Inouye, 2006). Other common symptoms include disturbed sleep–wake cycle and labile emotional disturbance (i.e., fear, paranoia, anxiety, depressed or euphoric mood, irritability, anger, and apathy; Inouye, 2006).

Hypoactive delirium is more common in older adults and is potentially more serious, inasmuch as this form is often not

Table 62-1 Risk Factors for Delirium

Predisposing Factors	Precipitating Factors
Demographic Characteristics	**Drugs**
• Age of 65 years or older	• Sedative hypnotics
• Male sex	• Narcotics
Cognitive Status	• Anticholinergics
• Dementia	• Treatment with multiple drugs
• Cognitive impairment	• Alcohol or drug withdrawal
• History of delirium	**Neurological Diseases**
• Depression	• Stroke
Functional Status	• Intracranial bleeding
• Functional dependence	• Meningitis or encephalitis
• Immobility	**Surgery**
• Low activity level	• Orthopedic surgery
• History of falls	• Cardiac surgery
Sensory Impairment	• Prolonged cardiopulmonary bypass
Decreased Oral Intake	• Noncardiac surgery
• Dehydration	**Intercurrent Illness**
• Malnutrition	• Infections
Drugs	• Iatrogenic complications
• Treatment with multiple psychoactive drugs	• Severe acute illness
• Treatment with many drugs	• Hypoxia
• Alcohol abuse	• Shock
Coexisting Medical Conditions	• Fever or hypothermia
• Severe illness	• Anemia
• Multiple coexisting conditions	• Dehydration
• Chronic renal or hepatic disease	• Poor nutritional status
• History of stroke	• Low serum albumin level
• Neurological disease	• Metabolic imbalance
• Infection, sepsis	**Environment**
• Fracture or trauma	• Admission to critical care unit
• Terminal illness	• Physical restraints
• Infection with human immunodeficiency virus	• Bladder catheter
	• Multiple procedures
	• Pain
	• Emotional Stress
	Prolonged Sleep Deprivation

Source: Adapted from Inouye, S. K. (2006). Delirium in older persons. *New England Journal of Medicine, 354,* 1157-1168 (Tables 2 and 3). doi:10.1056/NEJMra052321

Table 62-2 Comparison of the Clinical Features of Delirium, Dementia, and Depression

FEATURE	DELIRIUM	DEMENTIA	DEPRESSION
Onset	Acute	Insidious	Variable
Duration	Days to weeks	Months to years	Variable
Course	Fluctuating	Slowly progressive	Diurnal variation (worse in morning, improves during day)
Consciousness	Impaired, fluctuates	Clear until late in the course of the illness	Unimpaired
Attention and memory	Inattentive Poor memory	Poor memory without marked inattention	Difficulty concentrating: memory intact/ minimally impaired
Affect	Variable	Variable	Depressed; loss of interest and pleasure in usual activities

Source: Canadian Coalition for Seniors' Mental Health (CCSMH), (2006). *National guidelines for seniors' mental health: The assessment and treatment of delirium* (Table 1.1, p. 23). Toronto, ON: Author.

Diagnostic Studies

Delirium is diagnosed on the basis of behavioural observation and the results of mental status examination. The **Confusion Assessment Method** is a widely used, validated screening instrument and diagnostic aid that is effective in identifying the presence of delirium. This 5- to 10-minute assessment provides a standardized method of identification of delirium (Inouye et al., 1990). Evaluation with the Confusion Assessment Method can be incorporated into routine nursing assessment. Ratings may be based on findings from a brief mental status assessment such as the Mini-Mental State Examination (MMSE) (Folstein, Folstein, & McHugh, 1975) (see Table 62-7), the Mini Cog (Borson, Scanlan, Brush, Vitallano, & Dokmak, 2000), or the Montreal Cognitive Assessment (MoCA) (Nasreddine et al., 2005). The ConsultGeriRN.org Web site includes brief guides to use of the Confusion Assessment Method and Mini Cog, plus streaming videos demonstrating their use (see the Resources at the end of this chapter.)

It is important to distinguish whether clinical manifestations are new, whether a pre-existing dementia is present, and whether mental status has changed. Collateral information from a reliable informant is needed if the patient is unable to provide it.

When delirium is diagnosed, identification and treatment of the underlying causes is urgent. The patient's history and physical examination findings, medication history, laboratory tests, additional diagnostic investigation as indicated, and environmental risk factors must be evaluated. Usual investigations include complete blood cell count, biochemistry evaluations (measurements of calcium, albumin, magnesium, phosphate, creatinine, urea, electrolytes, and glucose levels; liver function tests), thyroid

identified. It may be overlooked because the patient is quiet, or it may be mistaken for depression. Delirium is often mistaken for dementia (RNAO, 2003/2010). A key distinction between delirium and dementia is the *sudden* development of symptoms of delirium over a short time period. (A comparison of delirium and dementia is presented in Table 62-2.)

When effectively treated, delirium usually resolves within 4 to 7 days. However, it can recur, and it may persist for weeks to months after discharge. Discharge planning should account for the safety of patients who have had an episode of delirium.

function tests, blood culture, oxygen saturation measurement, urinalysis, chest radiography, and electrocardiography (CCSMH, 2006). If meningitis or encephalitis is suspected, a lumbar puncture may be performed (see Chapter 59). If the patient's history includes head injury, appropriate radiographic examinations or scans may be ordered. Brain imaging studies such as computed tomography and magnetic resonance imaging are used only when the patient has a known or suspected head injury or brain lesion.

NURSING AND COLLABORATIVE MANAGEMENT: DELIRIUM

Priorities for nursing care are prevention of delirium and, when it cannot be prevented, identifying and treating underlying cause or causes, maintaining physiological stability, and ensuring the patient's safety (CCSMH, 2006; RNAO, 2004). Prevention involves recognition of patients at high risk for delirium (see Table 62-1) and providing care that targets the individual patient's risk factors. Among older adults, the five precipitating factors that are most predictive of delirium in the first 9 days of hospitalization are influenced by nursing interventions:
- Use of physical restraints
- Low serum albumin levels, indicative of malnutrition
- More than three new medications prescribed
- Use of a urinary catheter
- An iatrogenic event (e.g., cardiopulmonary complications, infections, injury, and complications caused by medications or diagnostic or therapeutic procedures) (Inouye & Charpentier, 1996)

There is strong research evidence that proactive multicomponent interventions reduce incidence of new cases of delirium and improve outcomes for patients with delirium (CCSMH, 2006). The Hospital Elder Life Program (HELP) is a well-researched multicomponent program (see the Resources at the end of this chapter). It has been implemented in more than 600 hospitals, including 10 Canadian hospitals (Agency for Healthcare Research and Quality, 2011). Components of the program are listed in Table 62-3. Details about the program are available on the HELP Web site (see the Resources at the end of this chapter).

Additional strategies to eliminate or minimize risk factors are listed in Table 62-4. Practice guidelines emphasize the need to maintain physiological stability. Many drugs can contribute to delirium. Six categories of drugs to use with caution are anticholinergics, histamine-2–blocking agents, analgesics, sedative hypnotics, antipsychotics, and cardiovascular drugs (RNAO, 2004). The American Geriatrics Society's publication concerning inappropriate use of medication in older patients (American Geriatrics Society 2012 Beers Criteria Update Expert Panel, 2012) is a good tool for reviewing medications. A relevant *Try This* resource is available on the ConsultGeriRN.org Web site (see the Resources at the end of this chapter), with additional resources on the American Geriatrics Society Web page.

Adequate pain management is important because undertreated pain significantly increases risk for delirium. However, analgesics, too, can increase risk for delirium. Thus interventions that minimize the use of opioids are recommended; these interventions include the following:
- Nonpharmacological pain management approaches
- Use of nonnarcotic analgesics as an adjunct to reduce the dose of opioids

Table 62-3 Components of the Hospital Elder Life Program (HELP)

1. Systematic screening to identify patients at risk for developing delirium

2. Tailored interventions developed by an interdisciplinary team consisting of a geriatric nurse specialist, elder life specialist, and trained volunteers. Interventions include:
   - Daily visitor and orientation
   - Sleep deprivation prevention
   - Ambulation three times a day and minimization of immobilizing equipment (e.g., bladder catheters)
   - Visual aids
   - Hearing support
   - Avoiding dehydration
   - Fall prevention

3. Interdisciplinary rounds twice a week

4. Geriatrician and interdisciplinary team consultations

5. Community liaison and postdischarge telephone follow-up

Source: From Agency for Healthcare Research and Quality. (2011). *Hospital-based program proactively identifies, addresses delirium risk factors in elderly, leading to less cognitive/functional decline and lower nursing home costs.* Retrieved from *http://www.innovations.ahrq.gov/ content.aspx?id=2059&tab=1*

Table 62-4 Strategies to Eliminate or Minimize Risk Factors for Delirium

- Judicious use of medication, elimination of nonessential medication, use of the lowest possible dose, avoidance of medications that contribute to delirium
- Prevention and prompt treatment of infections
- Prevention and prompt treatment of dehydration and electrolyte imbalance
- Assessment and treatment of pain
- Maximal oxygen delivery
- Use of sensory aids
- Regulation of bowel and bladder function
- Adequate nutrition

Source: Adapted from Registered Nurses' Association of Ontario. (2004). *Nursing best practice guideline: Caregiving strategies for older adults with delirium, dementia, and depression.* Toronto: Author; and from Tullman, D. F., Mion, L. C., Fletcher, K., & Foreman, M. D. (2008). Delirium: Prevention, early recognition, and treatment. In E. Capezuti, D. Zwicker, M. Mezey, & T. Fulmer (Eds.), *Evidence-based geriatric nursing protocols for best practice* (34th ed., pp. 111-125). New York: Springer.

- When opioids are needed, use of the minimum effective dose for the shortest appropriate time
- Avoidance of meperidine when there is a risk of delirium (CCSMH, 2006)

The *Try This* series on the ConsultGeriRN.org Web site includes tools for pain assessment with older adults and patients who have dementia. See Chapter 10 for information about pain assessment and management.

Strategies to provide a therapeutic environment for patients with delirium or who are at risk for delirium are provided in Table 62-5. In addition, frequent assessment is required. Mental status

Table 62-5 Therapeutic Environment for Patients with Delirium or Risk for Delirium

STRATEGY	EXAMPLES
Foster orientation	• Frequent reassurance and orientation (unless this causes agitation), avoiding confrontation for delusional beliefs • Visible calendars, clocks, and staff identification • Explanation of all activities • Use of hearing aids and glasses
Provide appropriate stimulation	• Quiet room • Adequate light • Noise reduction • One task at a time • Music as preferred by the patient
Facilitate sleep	• Back massage, warm milk, or herbal tea at bedtime • Relaxation music • Noise reduction strategies (e.g., vibrating beepers) • Planning care to avoid waking the patient • Providing light during the day and reducing light at night
Foster familiarity	• Encouraging family or friends to stay with patient • Bringing familiar objects from home • Consistent nursing staff • Minimizing relocation
Maximize mobility	• Avoidance of restraints • Avoidance of bladder catheters • Ambulation or providing range-of-motion exercises three times a day
Communicate clearly	• Simple explanations • One question or direction at a time • Conveying warmth, kindness, and calmness
Reassure and educate patient and family	• Written and verbal education about delirium (e.g., RNAO patient education resources) • Acknowledgement of emotions • Use of distraction • Postdelirium education

Sources: Adapted from Canadian Coalition for Seniors' Mental Health. (2006). *National guidelines for seniors' mental health: The assessment and treatment of delirium.* Toronto: Author; Registered Nurses' Association of Ontario (RNAO). (2004). *Nursing best practice guideline: Caregiving strategies for older adults with delirium, dementia, and depression.* Toronto: Author; and Tullman, D. F., Mion, L. C., Fletcher, K., & Foreman, M. D. (2008). Delirium: Prevention, early recognition, and treatment. In E. Capezuti, D. Zwicker, M. Mezey, & T. Fulmer (Eds.), *Evidence-based geriatric nursing protocols for best practice* (34th ed., pp. 111-125). New York: Springer.

should be assessed every shift for patients with delirium or who are at risk for delirium (Waszynski, 2007). Close observation is required, especially for patients with hyperactive delirium. Invasive procedures should be minimized (Tullman, Mion, Fletcher, & Foreman, 2008).

Drug Therapy

Drug therapy is reserved for patients with severe agitation, especially when agitation interferes with needed medical therapy (e.g., fluid replacement, intubation) or presents a danger. Antipsychotics (neuroleptic agents) are the recommended drug therapy. Haloperidol is the first-line treatment, starting with low doses (0.25 to 0.5 mg once to twice a day) and slow titration upwards if necessary (CCSMH, 2006). In addition to sedation, other adverse effects of haloperidol include hypotension; extrapyramidal drug effects, including tardive dyskinesia (involuntary muscle movements of face, trunk, and arms) and athetosis (involuntary writhing movements of the limbs); muscle tone changes; and anticholinergic effects. Newer antipsychotics, including risperidone (Risperdal), olanzapine (Zyprexa), and quetiapine (Seroquel), may be used. Although these drugs produce fewer adverse effects than does haloperidol, the adverse effects are significant; antipsychotics may worsen the delirium. Close monitoring is needed. Drug therapy should be limited to the shortest time necessary to manage the symptoms. Benzodiazepines (e.g., lorazepam [Ativan]) are contraindicated, except for treatment of delirium caused by withdrawal from alcohol or sedative-hypnotics.

Dementia

Dementia is a collection of symptoms caused by various diseases affecting the brain. Cognitive functioning in multiple areas declines progressively. In addition to impairing memory, dementia affects the individual's ability to communicate, carry out purposeful movements, recognize common objects and familiar people, and judgement and reasoning. Mood and behaviour are commonly affected. Ultimately, these problems lead to inability to work, carry out social and family responsibilities, and perform activities of daily living (ADLs).

In Canada, approximately 500,000 people (1.5% of the population) have dementia, and every year about 104,000 people acquire dementia (Alzheimer Society of Canada, 2010a). Dementia occurs most often in older adults, affecting 2.4% of persons between ages 65 and 74 years, 11.1% of those between ages 75 and 84, and 34.5% of those older than 85 (Canadian Study of Health and Aging Working Group, 1994).

The *Rising Tide* report (Alzheimer Society of Canada, 2010a) provided details of the current and projected costs of dementia in Canada. The cost of dementia is high. Every year, family members and friends provide about 231 million hours of care to people with dementia. The estimated economic value of informal care is almost $6 billion per year. The total direct health care cost of dementia is more than $8 billion per year. The total economic burden of dementia, including the value of informal care, direct health care costs, and indirect costs (e.g., lost wages and lost productivity) is about $15 billion per year. As the average human lifespan increases and the baby-boom generation ages, the number of people affected with dementia is growing. By 2038, over 1.1 million Canadians (2.8% of the population) will have dementia, and more than 257,000 new cases of dementia will be diagnosed each year. By 2038, the total annual cost of dementia is projected to be $152 billion.

The four most common types of dementia are Alzheimer's disease (about 63% of all cases of dementia); vascular dementia (about 20% of cases); dementia with Lewy bodies (about 5% of cases); and frontotemporal dementia (about 5% of cases) (Alzheimer Society of Canada, 2010a; Chertkow, 2008). Mixed dementia, in which more than one type of dementia is present, occurs in about 10% of all cases of dementia (Chertkow, 2008). Dementia is also part of the later stages of Parkinson's disease and Huntington's disease. Moreover, in comparison with the general population, individuals with Down syndrome have higher risk of developing Alzheimer's disease in their 40s and 50s (Alzheimer Society of Canada, 2010b). A fifth type of dementia is caused by Creutzfeldt-Jakob disease, a very rare degenerative brain disorder.

Etiology and Pathophysiology

A small number of cases of dementia are secondary to a treatable condition and are thus potentially reversible if that condition is identified and treated. Potentially reversible dementias are rare, accounting for less than 1% of individuals presenting with dementia symptoms (Clarfield, 2003). Conditions that can result in reversible cognitive impairment include subdural hematoma, cerebral tumours, normal-pressure hydrocephalus, metabolic conditions (e.g., hypothyroidism, vitamin deficiency), heavy metal neurotoxicity, Wilson's disease, and infections such as bacterial meningitis and viral encephalitis.

Dementia is not a normal part of aging. Old age and family history are risk factors for the irreversible dementias (i.e., the four most common types). Etiology and pathophysiology of each type of dementia are described separately as follows.

Alzheimer's Disease. **Alzheimer's disease (AD)** is a chronic, progressive, degenerative disease of the brain. The exact etiology of AD is unknown. As in other forms of dementia, age is the most important risk factor for developing AD. Only a small percentage of people younger than 60 years develop AD.

Having a parent or sibling with AD increases an individual's risk of developing AD by two to three times. Genetics are strongly implicated in a form of AD called **familial Alzheimer's disease** (also known as *early-onset AD*). In this form of AD, there is a clear pattern of inheritance within a family. It develops before the age of 60 and is linked to mutations on the amyloid precursor protein gene, presenilin-1 gene, and presenilin-2 gene. Nonfamilial AD is known as *sporadic AD*. The apolipoprotein E-4 gene has been identified as one of the genes that increases risk for sporadic AD. It is thought that even more genes are linked to increased risk, but they have not yet been identified. The pathogenesis is similar in both forms of AD.

Knowing the modifiable risk factors for AD means that nurses can advise individuals about how to reduce their risk of developing AD (Alzheimer Society of Canada, 2010a). Table 62-6 lists substantiated risk factors for AD. Mild cognitive impairment, discussed later in the chapter, is a risk factor for developing AD. More research is needed about the following possible risk factors: low education, low socioeconomic status, smoking, and excessive alcohol consumption (Alzheimer Society of Canada, 2010a). See the *Brain Health* section of the Alzheimer Society of Canada Web site (listed in the Resources at the end of this chapter) for more information.

Table 62-6 Alzheimer's Disease

MODIFIABLE RISK FACTORS	REDUCING RISK
Medical conditions • Type 2 diabetes • Stroke and transient ischemic attack • Hyperlipidemia • Hypertension • Obesity • Chronic inflammatory conditions (e.g., arthritis)	• Healthy lifestyle choices to reduce the risk of developing these conditions (maintaining healthy weight, regular physical activity, healthy balanced diet, not smoking, stress management) • Appropriate treatment when such conditions are present
Head injury	• Use of recreational/sport helmets
History of clinical depression	• Identification and appropriate treatment of depression • Healthy lifestyle choices and appropriate support for traumatic experiences and stressful life events (may reduce risk for depression)
Inadequate intellectual stimulation	• Active social life • Participation in intellectual activities (reading, playing cards, solving puzzles, playing chess, learning new skills, hobbies)

Sources: Data from Alzheimer Society of Canada. (2010). *Rising tide: The impact of dementia on Canadian society.* Toronto: Author. Retrieved from *http://www.alzheimer.ca/~/media/Files/national/Advocacy/ASC_Rising%20Tide_Full%20Report_Eng.ashx;* and from Alzheimer Society of Canada. (2011). *Brain health.* Retrieved from *http://www.alzheimer.ca/en/About-dementia/About-the-brain/Brain-health*

Characteristic findings of AD are related to changes in the brain's structure and function: (a) amyloid plaques, (b) neurofibrillary tangles, and (c) loss of connections between cells and cell death (National Institute on Aging, 2009). Figure 62-1 shows the pathological changes in AD.

In AD, **amyloid plaques** are present in the brain in abnormal quantities. These plaques consist of clusters of insoluble deposits of a protein called *β-amyloid*, other proteins, remnants of neurons, non-nerve cells such as microglia (cells that surround and digest damaged cells or foreign substances), and other cells, such as astrocytes. β-Amyloid is cleaved from amyloid precursor protein, which is associated with the cell membrane (Figure 62-2). The normal function of amyloid precursor protein is unknown. In AD, plaques develop first in areas of the brain used for memory and cognitive function, including the hippocampus (a structure that is important in forming and storing short-term memories). Eventually, AD attacks the cerebral cortex, especially the areas responsible for language and reasoning.

Neurofibrillary tangles are abnormal collections of twisted protein threads inside nerve cells seen in the areas of the brain most affected by Alzheimer's disease. The main component of these structures is a protein called *tau*. Tau proteins in the central nervous system are involved in providing support for intracellular structure through their support of microtubules. Tau proteins hold the microtubules together in the same way that railroad ties hold railroad tracks together. In AD, the tau protein is altered in

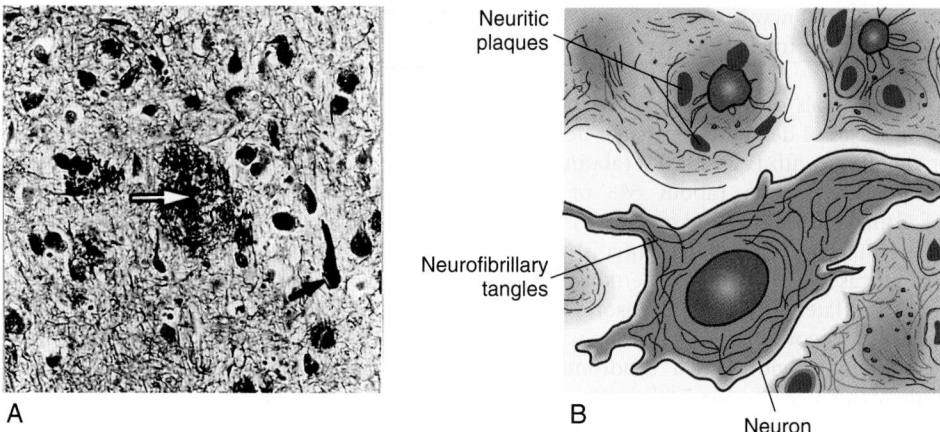

A

B

Figure 62-1 Pathological changes in Alzheimer's disease. **A,** Senile plaque with central amyloid core *(white arrow)* next to a neurofibrillary tangle *(black arrow)* on the histological specimen from a brain autopsy. **B,** Schematic representation of neuritic plaque and neurofibrillary tangle.

Source: **A,** From Damjanov, I., & Linder, J. (Eds.). (1996). *Anderson's pathology* (10th ed.). St. Louis: Mosby.

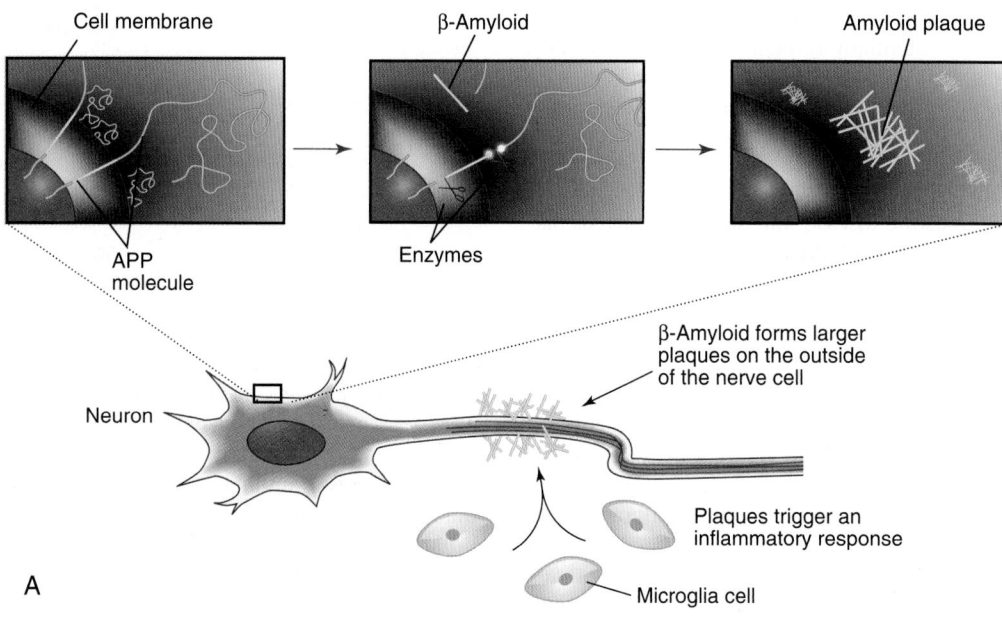

A

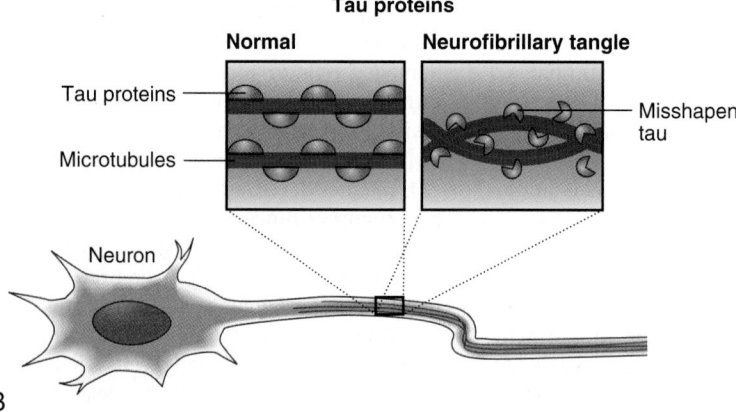

B

Figure 62-2 Current etiological theories for the development of Alzheimer's disease. **A,** Abnormal amounts of β-amyloid are cleaved from the amyloid precursor protein (APP) and released into the circulation. The β-amyloid fragments come together in clumps to form plaques that attach to the neuron. Microglia react to the plaque, and an inflammatory response results. **B,** Tau proteins provide structural support for the neuron microtubules. Chemical changes in the neuron produce structural changes in tau proteins. This results in twisting and tangling (neurofibrillary tangles).

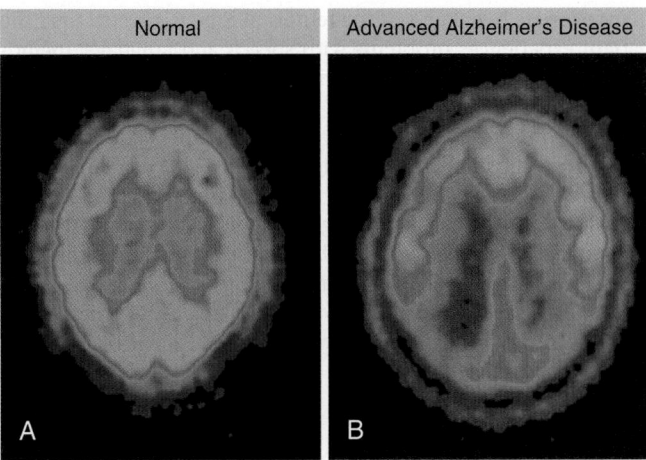

Normal	Advanced Alzheimer's Disease
A	B

Figure 62-3 The effects of Alzheimer's disease on the brain, shown by positron emission tomography (PET). In PET, radioactive fluorine is applied to glucose (fluorodeoxyglucose), and the yellow areas indicate metabolically active cells. **A,** A normal brain. **B,** Advanced AD, recognized by hypometabolism that indicates cell death in many areas of the brain.

Source: From Stuart, G. W. (2009). *Principles and practice of psychiatric nursing* (9th ed., p. 398, Figure 22-4, *A & D*). St. Louis: Mosby.

a way that causes the microtubules to twist together in a helical manner (see Figure 62-2). This twisting ultimately forms the neurofibrillary tangles observed in the neurons of persons with AD.

Plaques and neurofibrillary tangles are not unique to patients with AD. They are also found in the brains of individuals without evidence of cognitive impairment. However, they are more plentiful in the brains of individuals with AD.

The third feature of AD is the gradual loss of connections between neurons. This process leads to damage and then death of the neurons. Affected parts of the brain begin to shrink in a process called *brain atrophy*. By the final state of AD, brain tissue has shrunk significantly (Figure 62-3).

A short video illustrating and explaining the pathology of AD is available on the *Inside the Brain: Unraveling the Mystery of Alzheimer's Disease* section of the National Institute on Aging Web site (see the Resources at the end of this chapter).

Cholinergic neurons are lost in people with AD, particularly in regions essential for memory and cognition. Other neurotransmitter systems, including serotonin and norepinephrine, also show losses over time in patients with AD. Such neurotransmitter changes are the basis of current drug therapies for AD.

Vascular Dementia. **Vascular dementia,** also called *multi-infarct dementia,* results from ischemic, ischemic-hypoxic, or hemorrhagic brain damage caused by cardiovascular disease. When these events occur, blood and oxygen supply to brain tissues is blocked, which results in cell death. Vascular dementia may be caused by a single stroke (infarct) or by multiple strokes. As with AD, risk for vascular dementia increases with older age. Other risk factors are smoking, hypertension, cardiac diseases, diabetes mellitus, hypercholesterolemia, coronary artery disease, and atrial fibrillation.

Dementia with Lewy Bodies. **Dementia with Lewy Bodies (DLB)** is characterized by the presence of Lewy bodies (deposits of α-synuclein protein) in the brainstem, amygdala, and cortex. The α-synuclein protein is also linked to dementia in Parkinson's disease (Alzheimer Society of Canada, 2009a). DLB has features of both AD and Parkinson's disease. There are no known risk factors.

Frontotemporal Dementia. **Frontotemporal dementia (FTD),** previously known as Pick's disease, is characterized by degeneration of the frontal lobe, temporal lobe, or both. Nerve cells die because of abnormal accumulation of proteins in the neurons. The most commonly found proteins are ubiquitin and TDP-43. Tau proteins are present in about 40% of cases. Between 5 and 10% of patients with FTD have an inherited form of the disorder, and 40% have a family history of FTD (University of California, San Francisco, Memory and Aging Center, 2010). Frontotemporal dementia (FTD) tends to strike at a younger age than do the other forms of dementia; the typical age at onset is between 50 and 60 years (Merrilees & Ketelle, 2010).

Creutzfeldt-Jakob Disease. **Creutzfeldt-Jakob disease (CJD)** is a very rare and fatal infectious brain disorder thought to be caused by accumulation in the brain of an abnormally folded prion protein. A prion protein is a normal protein whose function and physiology is poorly understood. The abnormal form is called a *prion*. There are three types of CJD: sporadic, hereditary, and acquired (Hilton, 2006). A variant of CJD (vCJD), first described in the mid-1980s, is linked to eating beef from animals infected with bovine spongiform encephalopathy. vCJD is also known as *mad cow disease*. CJD affects about one per every 1 million people per year worldwide. Since 1999 in Canada, 449 people have contracted CJD, including one case of vCJD. The earliest symptoms of the disease are memory lapses, mood swings, and behaviour changes. The disease progresses rapidly with motor difficulties, involuntary movements, mental deterioration, and eventually coma and death within 1 year of the first symptoms. There is no diagnostic test or treatment for CJD. Only autopsy and examination of brain tissue can confirm the diagnosis. There is no treatment for CJD (Public Health Agency of Canada, 2011).

Clinical Manifestations

The onset of symptoms of dementia is usually insidious and gradual, with progressive deterioration. Vascular dementia, however, may have a sudden onset after a cerebrovascular event. In vascular dementia, mental decline is typically stepwise: Deterioration is followed by stabilization, then deterioration again. The rate of deterioration in AD is highly variable from individual to individual, and the course ranges in duration from 3 to 20 years.

AD may be preceded by **mild cognitive impairment (MCI).** MCI is cognitive decline that is not severe enough to interfere with ADLs (Chertkow et al., 2008). The diagnosis of MCI is made in the presence of several conditions: (a) subjective complaint of memory loss by the patient or a family member; (b) objective evidence of impairment in memory or another cognitive domain; (c) evidence of a decline from previous functioning; (d) retained ability to complete ADLs; and (e) no dementia or medical condition that explains the symptoms (Chertkow et al., 2008). The origin of MCI—whether it is a precursor to AD, a heterogeneous condition with several possible causes, including AD, or a separate clinical condition—is a subject of controversy. About half of patients with MCI develop dementia within 5 years, at a rate of

Table 62-7 The Seven As of Dementia	
Amnesia	• Inability to recall events, especially in new or changing environments
	• Initially loss of recall of recent events but eventually loss of long-term memory
Aphasia	• Loss of ability to express and understand spoken and written language
Agnosia	• Inability to recognize common objects or faces of familiar people (including one's own face), although motor and sensory abilities are normal
Apraxia	• Loss of ability to initiate purposeful movement; inability to perform previously learned tasks; difficulty understanding terms such as *back, front, up,* and *down*
Altered perception	• Misinterpretation of sensory information, loss of depth perception, visual distortions
Apathy	• Loss of drive or initiative
	• Inability to initiate conversation or activities, but participation when invited by someone else
Anosognosia	• Loss of ability to realize that there is a problem with memory and functioning

Source: Adapted from Alzheimer Society of Toronto. (n.d.). *Seven A's of dementia.* Retrieved from *http://www.asmt.org/ad_theSevenAs.htm*; and from Rivard, M., & Puxty, J. (Eds.). (2009). *Introduction to behavioural and psychological symptoms of dementia (BPSD): A handbook for family physicians* (2nd ed.). Kingston, ON: Sagelink.ca; College of Family Physicians, P.I.E.C.E.S. Canada. Retrieved from *http://www.sagelink.ca/sites/default/files/uploads/BPSD_Handbook_2010/201008_e/BPSD-Handbook-All-Chapters.pdf*

between 10 and 15% per year. However, between 20 and 25% return to normal (Rosenberg, Johnston, & Lyketos, 2006).

The symptoms of dementia can be classified according to the *seven A's of dementia* (Alzheimer Society of Toronto, n.d.). These symptoms help the nurse understand why and how dementia affects the patient's ability to function (Table 62-7). These symptoms are common, but patients with dementia do not necessarily experience all of them.

The initial changes of dementia may be difficult to recognize. Many people mistakenly think that they are part of normal aging. It can take up to 4 years after the initial onset of symptoms until patients and their family members seek health care. Reasons for this delay include lack of knowledge about dementia, lack of knowledge about services for dementia, attributing the changes to normal aging, and stigma (McCleary et al., 2012).

As time goes on, more areas of the brain are affected by the dementia. Cognitive abilities and functioning are progressively lost. Clinical manifestations of dementia are classified as mild, moderate, and severe, corresponding to the early, middle, and late stages of the disorder (Table 62-8).

The early clinical manifestations of FTD differ from those of AD because FTD initially affects the frontal lobe, temporal lobe, or both lobes of the brain. Eventually, all areas of the brain are involved diffusely, and the symptoms resemble those of AD. Early in the course of the disorder, social conduct and personality are profoundly altered, but little memory loss is evident (Neary et al., 1998). Behavioural symptoms include personality changes, blunted emotions, lack of insight, apathy, hyperorality, hoarding, compulsions and complex rituals, disinhibition, and socially inappropriate behaviour. If the temporal lobe is affected first, the patient experiences problems with speech and language, including loss of knowledge of the meanings of words and objects (Merrilees & Ketelle, 2010).

Like those of FTD, the early clinical manifestations of DLB differ from those of AD. Patients with DLB have symptoms of Parkinson's disease. In addition to symptoms of dementia, they have least two of the following symptoms: (a) extrapyramidal signs such as bradykinesia, rigidity, and postural instability, but not always a tremor; (b) fluctuating cognitive ability; and (c) hallucinations (McKeith et al., 2005). Swallowing problems can lead to impairment in nutrition. Affected patients are at risk for falls because of impaired mobility and balance. Pneumonia is a common complication.

Behavioural and Psychological Symptoms of Dementia. Some of the clinical manifestations of dementia are called **behavioural and psychological symptoms of dementia (BPSDs).** Behavioural symptoms include pacing, wandering, exit seeking, constant requests for help, grabbing on to people, cursing, screaming, socially inappropriate behaviours, sexual disinhibition, and hoarding. Psychological symptoms include anxiety, depressed mood, psychosis (hallucinations, delusions), and sleep disturbances (Murray Alzheimer Research and Education Program [MAREP] & Alzheimer Societies of Hamilton & Halton, Brant, Haldimand-Norfolk, & Niagara Regions, 2006; National Aging Research Institute, 2009). BPSDs cause distress to patients and negatively affect their functioning (MAREP et al., 2006). BPSDs are caused by a combination of biological factors (e.g., changes in brain functioning, medical conditions, pain, medication adverse effects, hearing or visual impairment), environmental factors (e.g., changes in routine, changes in environment), and social factors (e.g., inadequate support for the patient or family caregiver) (National Aging Research Institute, 2009). Dementia affects patients' abilities to communicate. Sometimes, BPSDs are the only way in which the affected person can communicate an unmet need. The term **responsive behaviours** is an acknowledgement that these behaviours are often a response to something in the patient's environment (MAREP et al., 2006).

SAFETY ALERT

A sudden change in behaviour should trigger a search for underlying causes, including possible delirium.

Diagnostic Studies

The Third Canadian Consensus Conference on the Diagnosis and Treatment of Dementia produced a comprehensive set of recommendations for diagnosis of dementia (Feldman et al., 2008). The process includes making a clinical diagnosis on the basis of the history, interviews with the patient and a caregiver or family member, physical examination findings, and results of brief cognitive tests. The next step in the process is laboratory tests to identify treatable medical conditions. Neuropsychological testing and neuroimaging are used only when certain symptoms are present. Routine laboratory tests include complete blood cell count and measurements of thyroid-stimulating hormone, serum electrolytes, serum calcium, serum fasting glucose, and serum vitamin B_{12} levels. Serum folic acid or red blood cell folate levels are optional. Neuropsychological testing may assist with

Table 62-8 Clinical Manifestations of Dementia

Early (Mild)

- Mild forgetfulness and misplacing items
- Short-term memory impairment, especially for learning new information
- Taking longer than usual to accomplish daily tasks
- Difficulty recognizing what numbers mean, trouble handling money and paying bills
- Loss of initiative and interests
- Poor judgement
- Difficulty finding the right word
- Confusion about location of familiar places (may become lost)
- Anxiety

Middle (Moderate)

- Increasing memory loss, including some loss of remote memory
- Impaired attention
- Anxiety, mood swings, suspiciousness, jealousy, irritability
- Flat affect
- Difficulty recognizing family members and friends
- Difficulty with language and understanding, and problems with reading, writing, and working with numbers
- Difficulty with logic and organizing thoughts
- Difficulty learning new things or coping in new and unexpected situations
- Difficulty completing tasks that involve a sequence of steps; interference with activities of daily living
- Poor insight and decision making, need for supervision and cuing

- Wandering, getting lost
- Loss of remote memory
- Sleep disturbances
- Hallucinations and delusions
- Loss of interest in hygiene
- Loss of impulse control (e.g., undressing at inappropriate times or places, vulgar language)

Late (Severe)

- Loss of most memories, inability to process new information
- Inability to understand words
- Responding to short, simple communication
- Difficulty eating, swallowing
- Repetitious words or sounds
- Inability to perform self-care activities
- Loss of social skills
- Sexual disinhibition
- Hallucinations, delusion, agitation
- Behaviours that may appear aggressive but are communicating a need
- Incontinence
- Loss of appetite and weight loss
- Seizures
- Progression to loss of facial expression, primitive reflexes, loss of voluntary movement, loss of speech, recurrent infections

Source: Adapted from National Institute on Aging. (2011). *Alzheimer's disease: Unraveling the mystery.* Retrieved from *http://www.nia.nih.gov/sites/default/files/alzheimers_disease_unraveling_the_mystery.pdf*; and from Vancouver Health Authority. (2010). *Clinical stages of Alzheimer disease.* Retrieved from *http://geropsychiatriceducation.vch.ca/docs/edu-downloads/dementia/clinical_stages_CPS-MMSE_comparison.pdf*

differentiating between normal aging, mild cognitive impairment, and dementia. Neuroimaging studies (computed tomography or magnetic resonance imaging) are recommended if the patient has one or more of the following characteristics: age younger than 60 years; rapid decline in cognition over 1 to 2 months; less than 2 years' duration of symptoms; recent head trauma; unexplained neurological symptoms; history of cancer that could metastasize to the brain; use of anticoagulants or bleeding disorder; urinary incontinence and gait disorder early in the course of the dementia; localizing neurological signs (e.g., hemiparesis); atypical cognitive symptoms; or gait disturbance. None of the diagnostic procedures can identify whether the underlying pathological change in the brain is present (e.g., plaques and tangles in AD). This determination can be made only by microscopic examination of brain tissue after the person dies. If MCI is diagnosed, annual monitoring of symptoms and functioning is recommended (Chertkow et al., 2008).

Related Assessments. Mental status testing is an important component of assessment. Patients with mild dementia may be able to compensate, which makes it difficult to evaluate cognitive function through conversation alone. Cognitive testing is focused on evaluating memory, attention, ability to perform calculations, language, visuospatial skills, and degree of alertness. The Mini-Mental State Examination (MMSE) (Folstein, Folstein,

& McHugh, 1975) is the most commonly used tool for brief assessment of cognitive functioning (Table 62-9), but it does not diagnose dementia. It is also used to monitor change over time. However, the MMSE is not sensitive to very early stages of dementia and mild cognitive impairment. The Montreal Cognitive Assessment (MoCA) is a brief cognitive screening tool that has good sensitivity for detecting early dementia (Nasreddine et al., 2005).

Additional mental status assessment tools for nurses are available on the ConsultGeriRN.org Web site. This Web site includes two-page *Try This* summaries of research about the tools and copies of the tools, articles about how to use them, and videos that demonstrate and explain how to use them. *Try This* tools include the Mini-Cog (Borson, et al., 2000), which is a brief screening tool for dementia; the Brief Evaluation of Executive Function (Kennedy, 2007); and the Recognition of Dementia in Hospitalized Older Adults tool (Mezey & Maslow, 2007).

Depression is often mistaken for dementia in older adults, and conversely, dementia for depression. Manifestations of depression include excessive sadness, difficulty thinking and concentrating, fatigue, apathy, feelings of despair, and inactivity. When the depression is severe, concentration and attention may be poor, which manifests as memory and functional impairment. When dementia and depression do occur together (which may be the situation in as many as 40% of dementia cases), the

Table 62-9 Mini-Mental State Examination (MMSE): Sample Items

Orientation to Time

"What is the date?"

Registration

"Listen carefully, I am going to say three words. You say them back after I stop. Ready? Here they are...APPLE (pause), PENNY (pause), TABLE (pause). Now repeat those words back to me." (Repeat up to five times, but score only the first trial).

Naming

"What is this?" (Point to a pencil or pen.)

Reading

"Please read this and do what it says."
(Show examinee the words on the stimulus form)
CLOSE YOUR EYES

Source: Reproduced by special permission of the Publisher, Psychological Assessment Resource, Inc., 16204 North Florida Avenue, Lutz, Florida 33549, from the *Mini-Mental State Examination*, by Marshal Folstein and Susan Folstein, Copyright 1975, 1998, 2001, by Mini-Mental, LLC, Inc. Published 2001 by Psychological Assessment Resources, Inc. Further reproduction is prohibited without permission from PAR, Inc. The MMSE can be purchased from PAR, Inc., by calling (813) 968-3003.

DRUG THERAPY
Table 62-10 Alzheimer's Disease

PROBLEM	DRUGS
Decreased memory and cognition	Cholinesterase inhibitors • Donepezil (Aricept) • Rivastigmine (Exelon) • Galantamine (Reminyl) *N*-Methyl-D-aspartate (NMDA) receptor antagonist • Memantine (Ebixa)
Depression	Selective serotonin reuptake inhibitors (SSRIs) • Sertraline (Zoloft) • Citalopram (Celexa) Serotonin modulator • Trazodone
Behavioural symptoms	Atypical antipsychotics (neuroleptic agents) • Risperidone (Risperdal) • Olanzapine (Zyprexa) • Quetiapine (Seroquel) Antiseizure drugs • Carbamazepine (Tegretol) Benzodiazepines • Lorazepam (Ativan)

intellectual deterioration may be more extreme. Depression, alone or in combination with dementia, is treatable. The challenge is to make an early assessment. Information about how to use the Geriatric Depression Scale (Sheikh & Yesavage, 1986), a short screening instrument for depression in older adults, is available in the *Try This* section of the ConsultGeriRN.org Web site.

Risk Modification

Many of the risk factors for AD and vascular dementia are modifiable. Individuals who reduce their risk for cardiovascular disease also reduce their risk for vascular dementia. Table 62-6 presented earlier in the chapter lists strategies to reduce risk for AD. In the report titled *Rising Tide,* the Alzheimer Society of Canada (2010a) showed that national programs to reduce risk of developing dementia are needed. Preventing dementia or delaying its onset would significantly reduce the economic burden of dementia in Canada. Increasing physical activity reduces risk for AD. The *Rising Tide* report demonstrated that a program to increase physical activity in older Canadians would reduce incidence of dementia and reduce the total economic burden of dementia by $5.6 billion over 10 years and $51.8 billion over 30 years. The *Rising Tide* report also recommended implementing a comprehensive prevention program targeting all Canadians aged 65 and older. Such a program could reduce risk of developing dementia by 23%, which would result in fewer new cases of dementia, delayed onset of dementia, and lower prevalence of dementia. It would reduce the economic burden of dementia by $24.2 billion over 10 years and $218.6 billion over 30 years.

Collaborative Care

There is no cure for any of the forms of dementia. The goals of collaborative management of dementia are to slow decline in

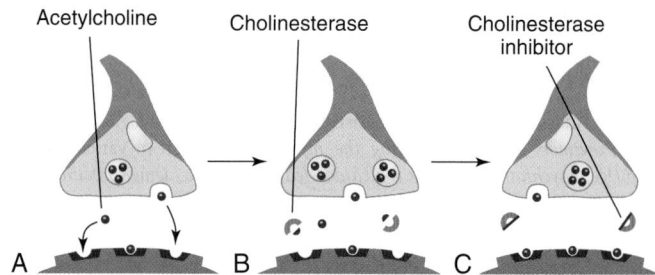

Figure 62-4 Mechanism of action of cholinesterase inhibitors. Acetylcholine **(A)** is released from the nerve synapses and carries a message across the synapse. Cholinesterase **(B)** breaks down acetylcholine. Cholinesterase inhibitors **(C)** block cholinesterase, thus giving acetylcholine more time to transmit the message.

cognition; to maintain and maximize functioning and quality of life of the person with dementia; and to support family caregivers.

Drug Therapy. AD is the only form of dementia for which drugs that affect cognitive decline are available. Drug therapy for AD is listed in Table 62-10. Cholinesterase inhibitors are recommended for treatment of mild, moderate, and severe dementia (Herrmann & Gauthier, 2008; Hogan et al., 2008). They block cholinesterase, the enzyme responsible for the breakdown of acetylcholine in the synaptic cleft (Figure 62-4). Cholinesterase inhibitors include donepezil (Aricept), rivastigmine (Exelon), and galantamine (Reminyl). These drugs improve or stabilize cognitive decline in some people with AD. They can enhance the patient's functional abilities. However, the small benefits from these drugs may not be clinically significant (Hogan et al., 2008). Cholinesterase inhibitors increase risk for bradycardia and syncope—and associated falls. The bradycardia may be difficult to detect because it is often transient. Cardiac monitoring is necessary. The significant risk of death in patients with AD who fall should be considered if cholinesterase inhibitors are prescribed (Gill et al., 2009).

> **SAFETY ALERT**
>
> Fall risk assessment and interventions should be part of care for patients taking cholinesterase inhibitors.

Memantine (Ebixa), an *N*-methyl-D-aspartate (NMDA) receptor antagonist, may be prescribed if cholinesterase inhibitors are ineffective. Memantine appears to protect the brain's nerve cells against excess amounts of glutamate, which is released in large amounts by cells damaged by AD. The attachment of glutamate to NMDA receptors enables calcium to flow freely into the cell, which in turn may lead to cell degeneration. Memantine may prevent this destructive sequence by adjusting the activity of glutamate. Memantine is recommended alone or in combination with a cholinesterase inhibitor in cases of severe AD. It may reduce behavioural and psychological symptoms in later stages of AD. Memantine is not covered by provincial drug plans, except in Quebec. It may be covered by private drug plans. The cost is $5 per day (Alzheimer Society of Canada, 2009b).

Drugs for AD are prescribed until their clinical benefit can no longer be demonstrated. They are discontinued in very late stages of AD, when patients are bedridden, noncommunicative, and cannot perform ADLs (Hogan et al., 2008). Drugs used for AD do not cure or reverse the progression of the disease.

Cholinesterase inhibitors and memantine are not approved for use in other forms of dementia in Canada. Cholinesterase inhibitors might be effective for vascular dementia (Hogan et al., 2008). There are no medications that slow cognitive decline in DLB or FTD. A meta-analysis revealed that ginkgo biloba had small effects on cognition of patients with dementia (Weinmann, Roll, Schwarzbach, Vauth, & Willich, 2010).

Antipsychotic drugs may be used for the management of the BPSDs when nonpharmacological approaches alone are not successful and the patient is experiencing severe psychosis, aggression, or agitation. When pharmacological therapy for BPSDs is used, treatment begins with the lowest possible dose, with slow increases, if necessary. Patients receiving this treatment are monitored carefully for effectiveness and adverse effects, and routine assessment is conducted to taper and discontinue the drug (CCSMH, 2006).

Conventional antipsychotic drugs (e.g., haloperidol) should not be administered because of extrapyramidal and anticholinergic adverse effects. The atypical antipsychotic agents risperidone (Risperdal) and olanzapine (Zyprexa) reduce aggression, and risperidone reduces psychosis. However, these drugs carry significant risks, including 1.5 to 1.7 times increased mortality rate and increased risk of cerebrovascular events. Adverse drug effects include cardiac and metabolic disturbance, extrapyramidal adverse effects, gait disturbance, sedation, and anticholinergic effects. Antipsychotic agents are not used in patients with DLB because they produce severe adverse effects (CCSMH, 2006).

BPSDs without psychosis can be treated with atypical antipsychotic agents and selective serotonin reuptake inhibitors (SSRIs) such as such as sertraline (Zoloft), fluvoxamine (Luvox), and citalopram (Celexa). For severe BPSDs, antiseizure drugs such as carbamazepine (Tegretol) or benzodiazepines may be used. However, benzodiazepines are generally not recommended because they produce such adverse effects as disinhibition and increase the risk for falls. In urgent situations, very low doses of short-acting benzodiazepines such as lorazepam (Ativan) may be used with caution. For patients with FTD, BPSDs may be treated with trazodone or SSRIs (CCSMH, 2006).

> **SAFETY ALERT**
>
> • Do not give antipsychotics to patients with DLB.
> • Psychiatric medications increase the risk of delirium.

For patients who have depression in addition to dementia, the depression should be treated with a combination of pharmacological and nonpharmacological approaches. The first choice of drugs is SSRIs: venlafaxine (Effexor), mirtazapine (Remeron), or bupropion (Wellbutrin) (CCSMH, 2006). Careful monitoring for effectiveness and adverse effects is important.

Scientists are studying other possible treatments for AD: immunization against the formation of β-amyloid plaques, substances to prevent the formation of plaques, substances to prevent tau protein threads from tangling, and substances that reduce inflammatory processes in AD (Mayo Clinic staff, 2010).

NURSING MANAGEMENT: DEMENTIA

Nursing care for patients with dementia is based on four principles (RNAO, 2004):
1. Know the person beyond the symptoms.
2. Recognize retained abilities.
3. Manipulate the social and physical environment to meet the patient's unique needs.
4. Relate effectively, in ways that enable the patient to feel supported, valued, and confident.

Nursing Assessment

Comprehensive assessment is necessary to provide patient-centred care. Assessment should focus on the patient, his or her family or caregivers, and the physical and social environment. Assessment includes mental status, cognition, neurological symptoms, psychiatric symptoms, and functional assessment of ADLs and instrumental ADLs. Lack of awareness of dementia and communication deficits are frequent in dementia. Thus collateral information should be obtained from people who know the patient well. Assessment of communication abilities helps the nurse adapt assessment approaches to the patient's abilities. Objective data from observation are important.

Data that should be obtained are presented in Table 62-11. In addition to cognitive assessment tools described earlier in the chapter, the ConsultGeriRN.org Web site provides standardized assessment tools, including 11 specific to patients with dementia (Table 62-12). The CCSMH's pocket tool for assessment and treatment of behavioural symptoms is useful and can be downloaded from its Web site (see the Resources at the end of this chapter). A number of assessment tools are provided as appendices to the RNAO's (2004) nursing best practice guideline, *Caregiving Strategies for Older Adults with Delirium, Dementia, and Depression*.

NURSING ASSESSMENT

Table 62-11 Patient With Dementia

Subjective Data

Important Information

Past health history: Head trauma, falls, history of previous delirium or psychiatric illness

Medications: All drugs, including cholinesterase inhibitors, psychotropic drugs, and nonprescription drugs

Symptoms

- Mental status examination (mood, perceptions and beliefs, thinking, orientation, memory and recall, concentration, insight, hallucinations, delusions, apathy)
- Instrumental activities of daily living (e.g., managing money, performing household chores, cooking, using transportation)
- Activities of daily living (e.g., dressing, feeding, using the toilet, performing personal hygiene)
- Strength and mobility
- Response to stressful situations
- Symptoms according to mild, moderate, and severe stages of dementia (see Table 62-8)

Objective Data

- Hypotension
- Appearance and behaviour
- Neurological symptoms (tremors, gait, tone, akathisia, dystonia)
- Symptoms according to mild, moderate, and severe stages of dementia

Table 62-12 Standardized Nursing Assessment Tools

- *Try This* tools
- Modified Caregiver Strain Index
- Assessing Family Preferences for Participation in Care in Hospitalized Older Adults
- Preparedness for Caregiving Scale
- Katz Index of Independence in Activities of Daily Living
- The Lawton Instrumental Activities of Daily Living Scale
- Assessing Pain in Persons with Dementia
- Recognition of Dementia in Hospitalized Older Adults
- Wandering in Hospitalized Older Adults
- Communication Difficulties: Assessment and Interventions
- Eating and Feeding Issues in Older Adults with Dementia: Part I: Assessment
- Assessing and Managing Delirium in Persons with Dementia

Source: These tools are available at *http://consultgerirn.org/resources.* This Web site includes demonstrations of how to use many of the tools.

▪ Nursing Diagnoses

Nursing diagnoses for dementia may include, but are not limited to, those presented in Nursing Care Plan 62-1.

▪ Planning

The overall goal is that patients with dementia will have a dignified quality of life. Specific goals are (a) enhancement of ADLs and instrumental ADLs (retaining functional abilities as long as possible), (b) enhancement or stabilization of cognition, (c) elimination of pain, (d) prevention or minimization of behaviours that adversely affect functioning, and (e) enhancement of emotional well-being (RNAO, 2004). The goals for the family caregiver of a patient with dementia are to (1) reduce caregiver stress, and (2) maintain personal health. A nursing goal is to developing partnerships with families (RNAO, 2004).

▪ Nursing Implementation

▪ Health Promotion

Strategies to prevent dementia are described earlier in this chapter. The Alzheimer Society of Canada's *Brain Health* Web page provides helpful information about healthy lifestyle choices for long-term brain health (see the Resources at the end of this chapter).

Dementia must be recognized early so that patients with dementia and their families can have time to make treatment decisions and plan for the future. Sometimes dementia is first identified when patients are admitted to an acute care facility for another condition (McCleary et al., 2012). Nurses who recognize the presence of undiagnosed dementia can help patients access appropriate health care resources. Useful information for patient and family health teaching about early signs of dementia is available on the Alzheimer Society of Canada Web site.

Health promotion can improve quality of life for patients with dementia and for family caregivers. Exercise programs for patients with dementia have positive effects on strength, fitness, cognitive performance, and functioning (Hogan et al., 2008). Yoga, in particular, can improve physical health, mental health, and behaviours for patients with dementia (Fan & Chen, 2011). Exercise also has positive effects for caregivers' physical activity, energy levels, sleep, and well-being (Connell & Janevic, 2009; Hirano et al., 2011).

▪ Acute Intervention

The diagnosis of dementia can be traumatic for both the patient and the family. It is not unusual for patients to respond with depression, denial, anxiety and fear, isolation, and grieving. The nurse is in an important position to assess for depression and suicidal ideation. Antidepressant drugs and counselling may be appropriate interventions. The nurse must assess family members and their abilities to accept and cope with the diagnosis.

Ongoing assessment of the patient and caregiver is required as the dementia progresses and the patient's functioning changes. An important nursing responsibility is to work in partnership with the caregiver to effectively manage clinical manifestations as they change over time. Effective partnership is enhanced when the nurse provides support, education, and collaboration with a focus on enabling meaningful caregiving roles in all settings (RNAO, 2004). The nurse must consider both the patient with dementia and the caregiver as having overlapping but unique problems. To aid in identifying challenges the caregiver may experience, see eNCP 62-1 Caregiver of the Patient with Alzheimer's Disease, available on the Evolve Web site for this chapter.

NURSING CARE PLAN 62-1

Dementia

NURSING DIAGNOSIS	*Impaired memory* related to effects of dementia *as evidenced by* loss of memory and other cognitive deficits
Expected Patient Outcomes	**Nursing Interventions and *Rationale***
• Functions at highest level of cognitive ability • Interacts with others appropriately • Communicates clearly and appropriately for age and ability • Demonstrates attentiveness • Demonstrates recent and remote memory • Processes information • Perceives environment accurately • Experiences cognitive stimulation • Comprehends the meaning of events and situations	• Use standardized diagnostic tools *to establish baseline function.* • Include family members in planning, providing, and evaluating care to the extent desired *to plan appropriate and consistent interventions.* • Identify usual patterns of behaviour for such activities as sleep, elimination, food intake, and self-care *to maintain familiar routines.* • Give one simple direction at a time *to decrease patient's confusion and frustration.* • Provide cues such as familiar events, seasons, names, and locations *to assist patient with orientation, promote memory, and reduce confusion.* • Prepare for interaction with eye contact and touch, as appropriate, *to convey respect for and acceptance of patient.* • Use distraction, rather than confrontation, *to manage patient's behaviour and decrease anxiety.* • Use environmental cues (signs, pictures, clocks, calendars) *to stimulate patient's memory, assist with reorientation, and promote functioning.* • Repeat patient's last expressed thought *to stimulate memory and reduce confusion.*
NURSING DIAGNOSIS	*Self-care deficit (bathing, dressing, toileting)* related to memory deficit and neuromuscular impairment *as evidenced by* inability to independently and appropriately bathe, dress, or toilet
Expected Patient Outcomes	**Nursing Interventions and *Rationale***

• Performs self-care with assistance as needed with dressing
  • Puts on clothing
  • Uses zippers and buttons
  • Ties shoes
	• Monitor patient's ability for independent self-care *to promote retention of abilities.*
	• Be available for assistance in dressing as necessary *to facilitate patient's independence and provide appropriate help.*
	• Provide clothes in accessible area *to facilitate dressing.*

• Performs self-care with assistance as needed with bathing
  • Gets in and out of bathroom
  • Regulates water temperature
  • Washes face
  • Washes upper body
  • Washes lower body
  • Cleans perineal area
  • Dries body
	• Use consistent repetition of daily routines *because cognitive loss impairs ability to plan and complete sequential activities.*
	• Provide familiar personal articles, such as bath soap and hairbrush, *to enhance self-care and minimize distress.*
	• Facilitate patient's bathing of self, as appropriate, *to promote independence, minimize distress, and provide appropriate assistance.*

• Performs self-care with assistance as needed with toileting
  • Gets to and from toilet
  • Removes clothing
  • Empties bladder
  • Empties bowel
  • Wipes self after urinating
  • Wipes self after bowel movement
	• Assist patient in accepting help *to ensure that all needs are met.*
	• Teach family to encourage independence and to intervene only when the patient is unable to perform *to promote independence.*
	• Assist patient to toilet at specified intervals *to promote continence.*
	• Facilitate hygiene after elimination *to prevent discomfort and skin breakdown.*

Continued

NURSING CARE PLAN 62-1

Dementia—cont'd

NURSING DIAGNOSIS	***Risk for injury*** *related to* impaired judgement, possible gait instability, muscle weakness, and sensory–perceptual alteration
Expected Patient Outcomes	**Nursing Interventions and *Rationale***

• Experiences no injury
 • Uses assistive devices appropriately for ambulation and support
 • Fall prevention behaviour
   • Uses assistive devices correctly
   • Controls agitation and restlessness
   • Uses well-fitting, tied shoes
   • Uses vision-correcting devices
	Fall prevention
	 • Identify cognitive or physical deficits that may increase potential for falls in a particular environment *to decrease or prevent injury to patient.*
	 • Provide assistive devices, such as a walker, *to steady patient's gait and provide ambulation support.*
	 • Ensure that patient's shoes fit properly and are secured with nonskid soles *to provide support during ambulation.*
	 • Instruct patient to wear prescription glasses, as appropriate, when out of bed *to allow for proper vision.*

NURSING DIAGNOSIS	***Social isolation*** *related to* dementia progression, alterations in mental status, and unacceptable social behaviour *as evidenced by* feelings of rejection, indifference to other people, hostile behaviour, and isolation from other people
Expected Patient Outcomes	**Nursing Interventions and *Rationale***
• Experiences appropriate social relationships and involvement in the lives of significant others • Identifies feelings about own cognitive changes • Learns effective strategies to combat social isolation	• Appraise the effect of dementia on roles and relationships *to determine extent of understanding of the changes occurring as a result of the disease.* • Identify possible support systems and ability to participate in social activities *to provide pleasurable activities and reduce feelings of isolation.* • Encourage the use of spiritual resources, if desired, *to allow familiarity and provide a sense of calm to the patient.* • Encourage the family to verbalize feelings about the patient and increase communication *to foster mutual understanding among family members.* • Instruct family members about resources in the community *to provide them with adequate support.*
NURSING DIAGNOSIS	***Wandering*** *related to* disease process *as evidenced by* getting lost numerous times a day and patient's statement of "I don't know where I am"
Expected Patient Outcomes	**Nursing Interventions and *Rationale***
• Protects self from injury • Demonstrates minimized wandering behaviour • Is able to ambulate independently within established safe boundaries	• Provide verbal reminders, as necessary, to remain in designated area *to reorient the patient.* • Use a bed alarm to alert caregiver that individual is getting out of bed *to prevent patient from falling.* • Provide safe wandering areas *to prevent patient from being injured and getting lost.* • Use symbols, other than written signs, to assist patient to locate own room, bathroom, or other area *to maintain independence.* • Monitor environment for potential safety hazards *to prevent injury to patient.* • Monitor *patient* for alterations in physical or cognitive function that might lead to unsafe behaviour *to assess any changes that may occur.* • Provide appropriate level of supervision or surveillance *to monitor patient and to allow for therapeutic actions.*

Patients with dementia may be hospitalized for other health care problems. Approximately 25% of older patients in hospitals have dementia. This dementia is not necessarily documented on their health record (Maslow, cited in Mezey & Maslow, 2007). They are at higher risk than other older patients for negative outcomes, including permanent avoidable functional decline (Mezey & Maslow, 2007). Access to rehabilitation after acute care is an issue for patients with dementia. The Evidence-Informed Practice box, "Rehabilitation After Hip Fracture for Patients With Cognitive Impairment," describes a program to improve access to rehabilitation after hip fracture.

SAFETY ALERT

Patients with dementia who are admitted to hospitals are at risk for delirium, falls, dehydration, inadequate nutrition, untreated pain, drug-related problems, wandering, behavioural symptoms, use of restraints, and functional decline.

Patients' inability to communicate symptoms of health problems places the responsibility for assessment and diagnosis on caregivers and health care providers. Patients with dementia who are hospitalized in acute care settings should be observed more closely because of concerns for safety. Consistent assignment of nursing staff, frequent reassurance, and orientation to place and time may reduce anxiety and prevent behavioural symptoms. Pain management is complex. Pain may be communicated through behaviours such as resistance to care, agitation, pacing, and grimacing. If nurses cannot determine the reasons for such behaviours, they should suspect pain and treat with nonpharmacological approaches or regular doses of nonopioid analgesics (RNAO, 2004).

Ambulatory and Home Care

Most persons with dementia live in their homes, supported and cared for by family members or friends. The most typical caregiver is a spouse or an adult daughter. Depending on care needs, safety, availability of family caregivers, finances, and availability of formal programs, patients with dementia may eventually move to retirement homes or long-term care homes.

Patients with dementia progress through the stages at variable rates. Nursing care needs of patients with dementia change as the disease progresses. Thus regular assessment, monitoring, and support are necessary. Regardless of the setting, cognition and functioning decline, and the amount of care required intensifies over time. The specific manifestations of the disease depend on the areas of the brain involved.

In the phase of mild cognitive impairment, memory aids (e.g., calendars) may be beneficial. Patients may develop depression in this phase. Depression may occur because of the neurochemical changes in the brain. Depression may be related to adjusting to a diagnosis of an incurable disorder, as well as the effect of dementia on the person's life (e.g., driving, socializing with friends, participating in hobbies or recreational activities). Drug therapy with cholinesterase inhibitors may be effective. However, adverse effects may deter some people from continuing with the drugs. Adherence to the regimen may be challenging when dementia affects the patient's ability to remember to take drugs.

After the initial diagnosis, patients need to be aware that the progression of the disease is variable. Effective management of

EVIDENCE-INFORMED PRACTICE

Rehabilitation After Hip Fracture for Patients With Cognitive Impairment

Clinical Question

In patients with cognitive impairment, after hip fracture surgery (P), does an interdisciplinary patient-centred model of rehabilitation (I), in comparison with routine rehabilitation (C), improve functional gain, cognitive gain, rehabilitation efficiency, and discharge location (O)?

Best Available Evidence

Longitudinal retrospective feasibility study

Critical Appraisal and Synthesis of Evidence

- Participants were patients with and without cognitive impairment who were admitted to a specialized inpatient rehabilitation unit after hip fracture surgery; their outcomes were compared.
- A new interdisciplinary model provided individualized rehabilitation care on the basis of patient- and family-driven goals, with care strategies to minimize BPSDs.
- Patients who had cognitive impairment ($n = 17$) were compared with patients who did not have cognitive impairment ($n = 14$); average age was 87 years.
- Patients with cognitive impairment had greater functional dependence at baseline.
- Both patients with and without cognitive impairment had significant gains in motor functioning, and 80% were discharged to the community.

Conclusions

- Patients with dementia benefit from rehabilitation after hip fracture.

Implications for Nursing Practice

- Support of staff to provide appropriate individualized care to patients with dementia was an essential part of the program.
- Nursing and interdisciplinary staff should receive education about dementia and effective dementia care strategies.
- A gerontological advanced practice nurse available to staff on all shifts enhanced transfer of learning to practice.
- Consultation from both a geriatrician and psychiatrist supported care.

Reference for Evidence

McGilton, K. S., Mahomed, N., Davis, A. M., Flannery, J., & Calabrese, S. (2009). Outcomes for older adults in an inpatient rehabilitation facility following hip fracture (HF) surgery. *Archives of Gerontology and Geriatrics*, 49, e23-e31. doi:10.1016/j.archger.2008.07.012

BPSDs, behavioural and psychological symptoms of dementia; *PICO: P,* patient population of interest; *I,* intervention or area of interest; *C,* comparison of interest or comparison group; *O,* outcome(s) of interest.

the disease can enhance quality of life of the patient and family and may slow the progress of the disease. Decisions related to care should be made with the patient, family members, and the health care team early in the disease. The nurse has a role in advising the patient and the family to discuss decision making for health care and planning for advanced care while the patient still has the capacity to do so.

Adult day programs are an option for patients with dementia. The goals of day programs are to provide respite for the family and to support the patient's optimal functioning in the community for as long as possible. During the early and middle stages of dementia, the person benefits from therapeutic activities in a safe environment that support functioning. Services that may be provided at adult day programs include assistance with ADLs, therapeutic recreation, cognitive stimulation, and transportation to the program. Patients return home tired, content, less frustrated, and ready to be with the family. The respite from the demands of care allows the caregiver to be more responsive to the patient's needs. Other respite options include home visits from community respite workers, overnight care provided by community nursing services, and short-term (1 to 2 weeks) admission to a respite bed in a long-term care home. In many provinces and territories, this service is subsidized by government funding.

As the disease progresses, the demands on the caregiver may eventually exceed the resources, and the person with dementia may have to move to a long-term care home. Dementia care units are becoming increasingly common in long-term care homes. Patients in the final stages of dementia require total care. Family caregiving responsibility continues when the person moves to a long-term care home. Family caregivers continue to provide personal care, preserve the dignity of the person with dementia, share their unique knowledge of the person with staff, and monitor quality of care (Kellett, 2007).

There are specific issues related to the care of the patient with dementia that span all phases of the disease. Brief, evidence-informed guides to effective nursing intervention help with care planning (Table 62-13). These issues are described in the following sections.

■ **Behavioural Changes.** BPSDs occur in about 50 to 60% of patients with dementia who live in the community (Savva et al., 2009). BPSDs are more common in later stages, and most patients with dementia demonstrate BPSDs at some time. Caregivers need to be aware that these behaviours are not intentional. BPSDs may worsen in acute care settings when behaviour is influenced by delirium, pain, changes in routine, and the unfamiliar environment. BPSDs often contribute to the decision to move patients to a long-term care home.

Behaviours do not occur in a vacuum and are often in response to a precipitating factor (e.g., pain, frustration, temperature extremes, anxiety). The first step is for the nurse to assess the patient's physical status. Physical assessment includes checking for changes in vital signs, urinary and bowel patterns, and pain that could contribute to behavioural changes. Environmental assessment to identify factors that could trigger behaviours is the next step. Extremes in temperature, as well as excessive noise, may result in behaviour change. When the patient is agitated by the environment, either the patient or the stimulus should be moved. The patient can be assisted to call family members if this is reassuring. When a patient resists or pulls at tubes or dressings, these items can be covered with stretch tube gauze or removed from the visual field. The patient should be reassured that the nurse is present to provide safety and protection. Orientation to place and person can be used, depending on the patient's cognitive abilities. Allowing the patient to live in his or her memories is often more appropriate and provides comfort and reassurance. Avoid challenging "why" questions when the patient is anxious or agitated. If the patient cannot verbalize distress, his or her mood should be validated. The patient's statement can be rephrased to validate its meaning. The patient's emotional state should be closely observed.

When nurses communicate effectively with patients during care, patients are less anxious and agitation is reduced. To communicate effectively, it is important that the nurse (a) stay near the patient during the care episode, sit beside the patient, and use touch as appropriate; (b) recognize the patient's rhythm and adapt the pace of care to it; and (c) focus on care beyond the task by acknowledging the personal experience and providing reassurance (RNAO, 2004).

Other strategies to manage behaviour include redirection, distraction, and reassurance. For a patient who is restless or agitated, redirecting would involve changing the patient's focus by having him or her perform activities such as sweeping, raking, or dusting. Effective strategies to distract the agitated patient might include snacks, car rides, favourite music, looking at family photographs, or walking. Repetitive activities, songs, poems, massage, aromas, or a favourite object can be soothing to some patients. (See the Evidence-Informed Practice box, "What Is the Effect of Music on Acute Confusion and Cognition in Surgical Patients?")

When nonpharmacological therapies are ineffective and patient safety is of concern, drugs may be used with caution (see Table 62-10). Adverse effects should be monitored carefully.

Resources about assessment and treatment of behavioural symptoms are available on the CCSMH Web site (see the Resources at the end of this chapter). These resources include a practice guideline (CCSMH, 2006), a guide for patients and families, and a pocket tool for clinicians.

Some patients have a pattern of behavioural disturbance that occurs in the late afternoon. This is often referred to as **sundowning.** However, there is controversy about whether sundowning actually exists. According to some experts, there is no change in behaviour; rather, the behaviour is more disruptive to staff when it occurs in the evening and is thus more noticeable to them. A study revealed, however, that 13% of patients with dementia have more behavioural disturbance in the evening (Bachman & Rabins, 2006). One theory is that sundowning is caused by a disruption of circadian rhythms (with more daytime napping and more nighttime activity) that could be influenced by inadequate daytime exposure to light (Bachman & Rabins, 2006). Other possible causes include fatigue, unfamiliar environment, noise (especially in an acute care setting or during shift changes), medications, reduced lighting, and sleep fragmentation. The behaviour may be

---

Table 62-13 Evidence-Informed Dementia Care Resources: *Try This* **Tools***

- Avoiding Restraints in Patients with Dementia
- Therapeutic Activity Kits
- Wandering in the Hospitalized Older Adult
- Communication Difficulties: Assessment and Interventions
- Working With Families of Hospitalized Older Adults With Dementia
- Eating and Feeding Issues With Older Adults With Dementia: Part II: Interventions

Try This tools are a collaboration of The Hartford Institute for Geriatric Nursing, New York University, College of Nursing, and the Alzheimer's Association, and are available at ConsultGeriRN.org.

What Is the Effect of Music on Acute Confusion and Cognition in Surgical Patients?

Clinical Question

In older adult patients having hip and knee surgery (P), does music therapy (I), in comparison with no music intervention (C), decrease acute confusion and improve cognition postoperatively (O)?

Best Available Evidence

One randomized controlled trial (RCT)

Critical Appraisal and Synthesis of Evidence

- RCT included 22 patients who were undergoing elective hip or knee surgery.
- Subjects were randomly assigned to either listen to music or not during the postoperative recovery period.
- Music therapy consisted of a bedside compact disc (CD) player with various musical choices to be in use for at least 1 hour, four times per day.
- Data on episodes of acute confusion and cognition were collected.

Conclusions

- Patients who listened to music had significantly fewer episodes of acute confusion and better cognition.

Implications for Nursing Practice

- Surgical patients should be given an opportunity to choose and listen to music during their hospitalization.
- Further examination of music therapy as part of multicomponent delirium reduction strategies is warranted.

Reference for Evidence

McCaffrey, R. (2009). The effect of music on the cognition of older adults undergoing hip and knee surgery. *Music and Medicine, 1*(1), 22-28. doi:10.1177/1943862109335215

PICO: P, patient population of interest; I, intervention or area of interest; C, comparison of interest or comparison group; O, outcome(s) of interest.

---

a symptom of mixed delirium. Behaviour should be assessed for underlying cause. Maximizing exposure to light during the day, ensuring quiet and uninterrupted nighttime sleep, implementing other sleep hygiene interventions (see Chapter 9), and engaging the patient in activities during the day may be helpful.

■ **Safety.** The person with dementia is at risk for a number of problems related to personal safety. These problems include injury from falls, wandering in unsafe areas, injury to others and self with sharp objects or from fire and other heat sources, and impaired judgement and decision making. These concerns necessitate careful attention to the home environment to minimize risk and provide supervision. As cognitive function declines over time, patients with dementia may have difficulty navigating physical spaces and interpreting environmental cues. In hospitals, the risk of falling is 2.6 to 6 times higher in patients with

dementia than in patients who do not have dementia (RNAO, 2011). Nursing assessment should include fall risk assessment. Effective fall prevention programs include multiple components such as staff training, environmental modification, and exercises (RNAO, 2011). The Alzheimer Society of Canada Web site (see the Resources at the end of this chapter) has a home safety checklist that nurses can assist families to use. Environmental modifications include improving lighting; removing tripping hazards such as clutter, throw rugs, carpet edges, extension cords, and awkward furniture arrangements; stairway handrails, with the end of rail shaped differently to alert the patient that it is the end of the stairway; wiping wet areas on the floors; removing snow and ice; and grip bars and nonskid surfaces in showers and bathtubs (Alzheimer Society of Canada, 2012a; RNAO, 2011).

Wandering is a major safety concern. Wandering may be the expression of a physical or emotional need or may result from cognitive loss, adverse effects of drugs, restlessness, curiosity, or stimuli that trigger memories of earlier routines. The nurse should observe for factors or events that may precipitate wandering. For example, patients may be sensitive to stress and tension in the environment. In such cases, wandering may reflect an attempt to leave the environment. Patients with dementia can be registered with Safely Home Registry, a nationwide program set up through the Alzheimer Society of Canada in partnership with the Canadian MedicAlert Foundation. The Safely Home Registry includes identification products (e.g., bracelets, necklaces, watches) that allow police and emergency responders to identify the person quickly and return him or her home (Alzheimer Society of Canada, 2012b).

■ **Pain Management.** Because of dementia-associated difficulties with oral and written language, affected patients may have difficulty expressing physical complaints, including pain. The nurse must rely on other clues, including the patient's behaviour. Pain can result in alterations in the patient's behaviour, such as increased vocalization, agitation, withdrawal, and changes in function. Pain should be treated promptly and the patient's response monitored.

■ **Eating and Swallowing Difficulties.** Loss of interest in food and decreased ability to feed oneself *(feeding apraxia)*, as well as comorbid conditions, can result in significant nutritional deficits and possible dehydration for patients with dementia. In long-term care and acute care settings, inadequate assistance with eating may further add to the problem. When patients with dementia are admitted to acute care settings, they tend to lose self-feeding abilities (Amella & Lawrence, 2007).

Individualized nursing interventions should be based on assessment of the patient's needs and abilities (see Table 62-12). Puréed foods, thickened liquids, and nutritional supplements can be used when chewing and swallowing become problematic for patients. Patients may need to be reminded to chew their food and to swallow. A quiet and unhurried environment for eating is essential. Distractions at mealtimes, including television, should be avoided. Creation of a normal social environment for meals provides supportive cues for patients with dementia. If self-feeding is difficult, finger foods, verbal cuing, demonstrating eating motions, and hand-over-hand techniques can initiate self-feeding. Liquids should be offered frequently.

When oral feeding is not possible, alternative routes may be explored. Nutritional support therapies are described in Chapter 42.

■ **Oral Care.** Ability to perform oral self-care declines as dementia progresses. With decreased tooth brushing and flossing, dental problems are likely to occur. Food may become lodged in pockets in the mouth because of swallowing difficulties, which increases the potential for tooth decay. Dental caries and tooth abscesses cause discomfort and pain, potentially increasing responsive behaviours. The mouth should be inspected regularly and mouth care provided for patients unable to perform self-care. Pocket tools about providing oral care to patients with dementia are available in the resources section of the Regional Geriatric Program Central Web site (see the Resource at the end of this chapter).

■ **Infection Prevention.** Urinary tract infection and pneumonia are the most common infections in patients with dementia. Such infections are ultimately the cause of death in many patients with dementia. Patients with dementia are at risk for aspiration pneumonia because of feeding and swallowing problems. See Chapters 30 and 48 for additional information about these infections. Manifestations of infection—including changes in behaviour, delirium, fever, cough (pneumonia), and pain on urination (bladder)—are evaluated and appropriately treated.

■ **Skin Care.** It is important to monitor the patient's skin. Rashes, areas of redness, and skin breakdown should be noted and treated appropriately. In the late stages of dementia, incontinence along with immobility and undernutrition can increase patients' risk for skin breakdown. The skin should be kept dry and clean and the patient's position changed regularly to prevent the creation of pressure areas over bony prominences.

■ **Elimination Problems.** During the middle and late stages of dementia, urinary and fecal incontinence become more common. Multifaceted individualized nursing care to reduce incontinence should include regular toileting (with prompting and reminders if necessary), changing incontinence products, increasing fluid and fibre intake, and ensuring that the toilet is accessible. Drugs for incontinence are unlikely to be effective (Price, 2011).

Constipation is also a common problem. Causes may include immobility, dietary intake (e.g., reduced fibre intake), and decreased fluid intake. Management of constipation is discussed in Chapter 45.

■ **Caregiver Support.** Dementia is a disease that disrupts all aspects of personal and family life. Individuals caring for the person with dementia frequently describe such care as stressful. Caregivers of patients with dementia often experience negative effects on their work and family roles and on their mental and physical health. Caregiver strain is common. Actions that caregivers may take are suggested in Table 62-14. Strategies for reducing caregiver stress are listed in Table 62-15.

As the disease progresses, the relationship of the caregiver to the patient changes. Family roles may be altered or reversed (e.g., child caring for parent). Decisions that must be made include when the patient must stop driving or performing activities that might be dangerous, when to ask for assistance, and when to use respite care services or long-term care homes. With early-onset dementia and FTD, the person is often affected during the most productive working years. The financial consequences can be devastating for the individual and the family.

Sexual relations for couples are also seriously affected by dementia. As dementia progresses, sexual interest may decline

PATIENT & CAREGIVER TEACHING GUIDE

Table 62-14 Dementia Caregiving

1. Confirm the diagnosis. Many treatable (and potentially reversible) conditions can mimic dementia.

2. Adapt communication to the person with dementia's abilities (e.g., read verbal and nonverbal cues, interpret what the person is trying to communicate). Know that communication is possible at all stages of dementia. Nonverbal communication is important in later stages of dementia.

3. Try to remain positive and encouraging. Avoid criticism and corrections. Focus on abilities.

4. Accept the reality of the person with dementia, and interact with him or her in that reality. Do not correct misstatements or faulty memory.

5. Assess and ensure home safety (e.g., tripping hazards, danger from drugs and chemicals, hot water heater temperature, fire hazards from smoking or cooking, exits, lighting, safety in the bathroom).

6. Monitor driving ability and discuss with the person with dementia and health care providers.

7. Encourage activities such as household chores, listening to music, reminiscence, exercising, hobbies, and visiting with friends and relatives.

8. Establish routines and simplify tasks (e.g., wearing clothing that is easy to put on, simplifying the table setting).

9. Register with the Alzheimer Society Safely Home program for individuals who may wander.

Source: Alzheimer Society of Canada. (2010). Alzheimer care. Retrieved from *http://www.alzheimer.ca/en/We-can-help/Education/Education-for-the-caregiver*

Table 62-15 Ten Ways to Reduce Caregiver Stress

1. Learn about the disease.
2. Be realistic about the disease.
3. Be realistic about how much you can do.
4. Accept your feelings.
5. Share information and feelings with others.
6. Be positive.
7. Look for humour.
8. Take care of yourself.
9. Get help, both practical help and support.
10. Plan for the future.

Source: From Alzheimer Society of Canada. (2012). Reducing caregiver stress. Retrieved from *http://www.alzheimer.ca/en/Living-with-dementia/Caring-for-someone/Self-care-for-the-caregiver/Reducing-caregiver-stress*

for both the patient and the partner. A number of reasons account for this, including caregiver fatigue (when the partner is the caregiver), as well as memory impairment, apraxia, and episodes of incontinence in the patient with AD. It is also possible for patients to become sexually disinhibited as the disease progresses.

The nurse should work with the caregiver to identify stressors and determine coping strategies to reduce the burden of caregiving. For example, the nurse should ask which behaviours are most disruptive to family life and remember that this is likely to change over time as the disease progresses. Establishing what the caregiver views as most disruptive or distressful can help in identifying priorities for care. Risk to the safety of the patient and the caregiver is given high priority. It is also important to assess the caregiver's expectations with regard to the patient's behaviour: Are the expectations reasonable in view of the progression of the disease? Working with the caregiver to identify risk factors for complications, including behavioural problems, is an important responsibility of the nurse.

Support groups for caregivers and family members (Figure 62-5) provide emotional support and information about dementia and related topics such as safety, legal, ethical, and financial issues. These groups are often facilitated by nurses, social workers, or occupational therapists. The Alzheimer Society of Canada has many educational and support systems available to help family caregivers. Other strategies related to stress management are discussed in Chapters 8 and 12.

Legal Matters and Personal Care Planning.
In the early stage of dementia, while the patient is still capable of making decisions and signing legal papers, it is important for the patient to be part of the decision making about his or her financial and legal affairs. Some important legal documents that must be put in place as soon as possible are a will; an enduring power of attorney (a document naming a substitute decision maker) for financial and legal matters, as well as for future health care decisions; and an advance directive. The names and the required content of these documents vary among the provinces and territories, and the local chapter of the Alzheimer Society of Canada can help locate this information for persons with dementia and their families. Chapters 7 and 13 provide more information about these documents.

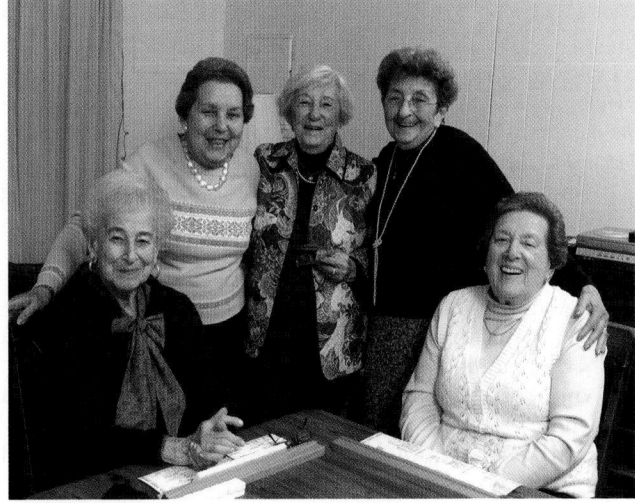

Figure 62-5 Support groups are an effective way to help caregivers cope.

Source: © iStockphoto/Thinkstock.

Evaluation

Expected outcomes for patients with dementia are addressed in Nursing Care Plan 62-1. See eNCP 62-1, available on the Evolve Web site for this chapter, for expected outcomes for the caregiver of a patient with dementia.

CLINICAL DECISION-MAKING EXERCISE

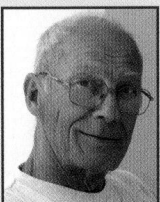

CASE STUDY:
Alzheimer's Disease

Source: © iStockphoto.com/Helle Bro Clemmensen.

Patient Profile

Mr. Yves Bédard, an 80-year-old French Canadian man, received a diagnosis of AD 3 years ago. Today, his 78-year-old wife brings him to the emergency department because he wandered from his home, fell, and injured his left hip.

Subjective Data

- Can state his name
- Is disoriented with regard to place and time
- Cannot recall wandering or falling
- Is agitated, trying to get up
- Denies pain

Objective Data

Physical Examination

- Left leg shorter than right leg
- Patient is tense and anxious
- Grimacing

Diagnostic Studies

- Radiographic study of left hip indicates a fracture.
- Mini-Mental State Examination shows cognitive impairment.

Discussion Questions

1. What is the pathogenesis of AD?
2. What precipitating factors may have resulted in Mr. Bédard's fall?
3. *Priority Decision:* What are the priority nursing interventions for Mr. Bédard?
4. What precautions must be taken regarding the inpatient care of Mr. Bédard?
5. What teaching plan should be developed for Mr. Bédard and his wife?
6. *Priority Decision:* On the basis of the assessment data presented, what are the priority nursing diagnoses? Are there any collaborative problems?

evolve Answers are available at **http://evolve.elsevier.com/ Canada/Lewis/medsurg**

REVIEW QUESTIONS

The number of the question corresponds to the same-numbered objective at the beginning of the chapter.

1. Which of the following patients is most at risk for developing delirium?
   a. A 50-year-old woman with cholecystitis
   b. A 19-year-old man with a fractured femur
   c. A 42-year-old woman having an elective hysterectomy
   d. A 78-year-old man admitted to the medical unit with complications related to congestive heart failure

2. Which of the following symptoms are the hallmarks of delirium?
   a. Inattention, fluctuating course, hyperactivity, and altered level of consciousness
   b. Disorganized thinking, insidious onset, inattention, and altered level of consciousness
   c. Acute onset, fluctuating course, memory loss, and altered level of consciousness
   d. Acute onset, fluctuating course, inattention or disorganized thinking, and altered level of consciousness

3. Which of the following descriptions best characterizes dementia?
   a. Syndrome that results only in memory loss
   b. Disease associated with abrupt changes in behaviour
   c. Disease that is always due to reduced blood flow to the brain
   d. Syndrome characterized by cognitive dysfunction and loss of memory

4. Which of the following is associated with vascular dementia?
   a. Transient ischemic attacks
   b. Bacterial or viral infection of neuronal tissue
   c. Cognitive changes secondary to cerebral ischemia
   d. Abrupt changes in cognitive function that are irreversible

5. On which of the following findings is the clinical diagnosis of dementia based?
   a. Brain biopsy
   b. Electroencephalography
   c. Patient history and cognitive assessment
   d. Computed tomography or MRI

6. Which of the following statements accurately describes mild cognitive impairment?
   a. Always progresses to AD
   b. Caused by variety of factors and may progress to AD
   c. Should be aggressively treated with cholinesterase inhibitor drugs
   d. Caused by vascular infarcts whose treatment, if carried out, will delay progression to AD

7. What is a major goal of treatment for the individual with dementia?
   a. Maintain patient safety
   b. Maintain or increase body weight
   c. Return to a higher level of self-care
   d. Enhance functional ability over time

ANSWERS: 1. d; 2. d; 3. d; 4. c; 5. c; 6. b; 7. a.

REFERENCES

Agency for Healthcare Research and Quality. (2011). *Hospital-based program proactively identifies, addresses delirium risk factors in elderly, leading to less cognitive/functional decline and lower nursing home costs.* Retrieved from *http://www.innovations.ahrq.gov/content.aspx?id=2059&tab=1*

Alzheimer Society of Canada. (2009a). *Lewy body dementia.* Retrieved from *http://www.alzheimer.ca/en/About-dementia/Dementias/Lewy-Body-Dementia*

Alzheimer Society of Canada. (2009b). *Treatment, drug treatments, Ebixa.* Retrieved from *http://www.alzheimer.ca/english/treatment/treatments-ebixa.htm*

Alzheimer Society of Canada. (2010a). *Rising tide: The impact of dementia on Canadian society.* Toronto: Author. Retrieved from *http://www.alzheimer.ca/~/media/Files/national/Advocacy/ASC_Rising%20Tide_Full%20Report_Eng.ashx*

Alzheimer Society of Canada. (2010b). *Down syndrome.* Retrieved from *http://www.alzheimer.ca/en/About-dementia/Dementias/Down-syndrome*

Alzheimer Society of Canada. (2012a). *Maintaining a safe, dementia-friendly environment.* Retrieved from *http://www.alzheimer.ca/en/Living-with-dementia/Day-to-day-living/Safety/Safety%20in%20the%20home*

Alzheimer Society of Canada. (2012b). *MedicAlert® Safely home®.* Retrieved from *http://www.alzheimer.ca/en/Living-with-dementia/Day-to-day-living/Safety/Safely-Home*

Alzheimer Society of Toronto. (n.d.). *Seven A's of dementia.* Retrieved from *http://www.asmt.org/ad_theSevenAs.htm*

Amella, E. J. & Lawrence, J. F. (2007). *Eating and feeding issues in older adults with dementia: Part II: Interventions.* Retrieved from *http://consultgerirn.org/uploads/File/trythis/try_this_d11_2.pdf*

American Geriatrics Society 2012 Beers Criteria Update Expert Panel. (2012). American Geriatrics Society updated Beers criteria for potentially inappropriate medication use in older adults. *Journal of the American Geriatrics Society, 60,* 616-631. doi:10.1111/j.1532-5415.2012.03923.x

American Psychiatric Association. (2000). *Diagnostic and statistical manual of mental disorders, fourth edition, text revision: DSM-IV-TR.* Washington, DC: Author.

Bachman, D., & Rabins, P. (2006). "Sundowning" and other temporally associated agitation states in dementia patients. *Annual Reviews in Medicine, 57,* 499-511. doi:10.1146/annurev.med.57.071604.141451

Borson, S., Scanlan, J., Brush, M., Vitallano, P., & Dokmak, A. (2000). The Mini-Cog: A cognitive "vital signs" measure for dementia screening in multi-lingual elderly. *International Journal of Geriatric Psychiatry, 15,* 1021-1027. doi:10.1002/1099-1166(200011)15:11<1021::AID-GPS234>3.0.CO;2-6

Canadian Coalition for Seniors' Mental Health (CCSMH). (2006). *National guidelines for seniors' mental health: The assessment and treatment of delirium.* Toronto: Author.

Canadian Study of Health and Aging Working Group. (1994). Canadian Study of Health and Aging: Methods and prevalence of dementia. *Canadian Medical Association Journal, 150,* 899-913.

Chertkow, H. (2008). Diagnosis and treatment of dementia: Introduction. *Canadian Medical Association Journal, 178,* 316-321. doi:10.1503/cmaj.070795

Chertkow, H., Massoud, F., Nasreddine, Z., Belleville, S., Joanette, Y., Bocti, C., ..., Bergman, H. (2008). Diagnosis and treatment of dementia: 3. Mild cognitive impairment and cognitive impairment without dementia. *Canadian Medical Association Journal, 178,* 1273-1285. doi:10.1503/cmaj.070797

Clarfield, A. M. (2003). The decreasing prevalence of reversible dementias: An updated meta-analysis. *Archives of Internal Medicine, 163,* 2219-2229. doi:10.1001/archinte.163.18.2219

Connell, C. M., & Janevic, M. R. (2009). Effects of a telephone-based exercise intervention for dementia caregiving wives. *Journal of Applied Gerontology, 28,* 171-194. doi:10.1177/0733464808326951

Fan, J. T. & Chen, K. M. (2011). Using silver yoga exercises to promote physical and mental health of elders with dementia in long-term care facilities. *International Psychogeriatrics, 23,* 1222-1230. doi:10.1017/S1041610211000287

Feldman, H. H., Jacova, C., Robillard, A., Garcia, A., Chow, T., Borrie, M., ..., Chertkow, H. (2008). Diagnosis and treatment of dementia: 2. Diagnosis. *Canadian Medical Association Journal, 178,* 825-836. doi:10.1503/cmaj.070798

Fick, D. M., & Mion, L. C. (2008). Delirium superimposed on dementia. *American Journal of Nursing, 108*(1), 52-60. doi:10.1097/01.NAJ.0000304476.80530.7d

Folstein, M. F., Folstein, S. E., & McHugh, P. R. (1975). "Mini-mental state": A practical method for grading the cognitive state of patients for the clinician. *Journal of Psychiatric Research, 12,* 189-198. doi:10.1016/0022-3956(75)90026-6

Gill, S. S., Anderson, G. M., Fischer, H. D., Bell, C. M., Li, P., Normand, S. L. T., & Rochon, P. A. (2009). Syncope and its consequences in patients with dementia receiving cholinesterase inhibitors: A population-based cohort study. *Archives of Internal Medicine, 169,* 867-873. doi:10.1001/archinternmed.2009.43

Herrman, N., & Gauthier, S. (2008). Diagnosis and treatment of dementia: 6. Management of severe Alzheimer disease. *Canadian Medical Association Journal, 179,* 1279-1287. doi:10.1503/cmaj.070804

Hilton, D. A. (2006). Pathogenesis and prevalence of variant Creutzfeldt-Jakob disease. *Journal of Pathology, 208,* 134. doi:10.1002/path.1880

Hirano, A., Suzuki, Y., Kuzuya, M., Onishi, J., Ban, N., & Umegaki, H. (2011). Influence of regular exercise on subjective sense of burden and physical symptoms in community-dwelling caregivers of dementia patients: A randomized controlled trial. *Archives of Gerontology and Geriatrics, 53,* e153-e158. doi:10.1016/j.archger.2010.08.004

Hogan, D. B., Bailey, P., Black, S., Carswell, A., Chertkow, H., Clarke, B., ..., Thorpe, L. (2008). Diagnosis and treatment of dementia: 5. Nonpharmacologic and pharmacologic therapy for mild to moderate dementia. *Canadian Medical Association Journal, 179,* 1019-1026. doi:10.1503/cmaj.081103

Hshieh, T. T., Fong, T. G., Marcantonio, E. R., & Inouye, S. K. (2008). Cholinergic deficiency hypothesis in delirium: A synthesis of current evidence. *Journal of Gerontology: Medical Sciences, 68A,* 764-772. doi:10.1093/gerona/63.7.764

Inouye, S. K. (2006). Delirium in older persons. *New England Journal of Medicine, 354,* 1157-1165. doi:10.1056/NEJMra052321

Inouye, S. K., & Charpentier, P. A. (1996). Precipitating factors for delirium in hospitalized elderly persons: Predictive model and interrelationship with baseline vulnerability. *JAMA, 275,* 852-857. doi:10.1001/jama.275.11.852

Inouye, S. K., van Dyck, C. H., Alessi, C. A., Balkin, S., Siegal, A. P., & Horwitz, R. L. (1990). Clarifying confusion: The Confusion Assessment Method, a new method for detecting delirium. *Annals of Internal Medicine, 113,* 941-948.

Kellett, U. (2007). Seizing possibilities for positive family caregiving in nursing homes. *Journal of Clinical Nursing, 16,* 1479-1487. doi:10.1111/j.1365-2701.2006.01844.x

Kennedy, G. J. (2007). Brief evaluation of executive dysfunction: An essential refinement in the assessment of cognitive impairment. *Try This,* Issue No. D3. Retrieved from *http://consultgerirn.org/uploads/File/trythis/try_this_d3.pdf*

Mayo Clinic staff. (2010). *Alzheimer's treatments: What's on the horizon?* Retrieved from *http://www.mayoclinic.com/health/alzheimers-treatments/AZ00048*

McCleary, L., Persaud, M., Hum, S., Pimlott, N. J. G., Cohen, C., Koehn, S., ..., Drummond, N. (2012). Pathways to dementia diagnosis among South Asian Canadians. *Dementia: The International Journal of Social Research and Practice.* (April 26). doi:10.1177/1471301212444806

McKeith, I. G., Dickson, D. W., Lowe, J., Emre, M., O'Brien, J. T., Feldman, H., ..., Yamada, M. (2005). Diagnosis and management of dementia with Lewy bodies: Third report of the DLB consortium. *Neurology, 65,* 1863-1872. doi:10.1212/01.wnl.0000187889.17253.b1

Merrilees, J., & Ketelle, R. (2010). Advanced practice nursing: Meeting the caregiving challenges for families of persons with frontotemporal dementia. *Clinical Nurse Specialist, 24*(5), 245-251. doi:10.1097/NUR.0b013e31ecdc32

Mezey, M., & Maslow, K. (2007). Recognition of dementia in hospitalized older adults. *Try This,* Issue D5. Retrieved from *http://consultgerirn.org/uploads/File/trythis/try_this_d5.pdf*

Murray Alzheimer Research and Education Program & Alzheimer Societies of Hamilton & Halton, Brant, Haldimand-Norfolk, & Niagara Regions. (2006). *Managing and accommodating responsive behaviours in dementia care: A resource guide for long-term care.* Waterloo, ON: University of Waterloo.

Nasreddine, Z. S., Phillips, N. A., Bédirian, V., Charbonneau, S., Whitehead, V., Collin, I., ..., Chertkow, H. (2005). The Montreal Cognitive Assessment, MoCA: A brief screening tool for mild cognitive impairment. *Journal of the American Geriatrics Society, 53,* 695-699. doi:10.1111/j.1532-5415.2005.53221.x

National Aging Research Institute. (2009). *Dementia resource guide.* Department of Health and Aging, Government of Australia. Retrieved from *http://www.health.gov.au/internet/publications/publishing.nsf/Content/ageing-dementia-resource-guide-2009-toc.htm*

National Institute on Aging. (2009). *2009 Progress report on Alzheimer's disease: Translating new knowledge.* Retrieved from *http://www.nia.nih.gov/sites/default/files/2009%20AD%20Progress%20Report%20Final%20B.pdf*

Neary, D., Snowden, J. S., Gustafson, D., Passant, U., Stuss, D., Black, S., ..., Benson, D. F. (1998). Frontotemporal lobar degeneration: A consensus on clinical diagnostic criteria. *Neurology, 51,* 1546-1554. doi:10.1212/WNL.51.6.1546

Price, H. (2011). Incontinence in patients with dementia. *British Journal of Nursing, 20,* 721-725.

Public Health Agency of Canada. (2011). *Creutzfeldt-Jakob disease (CJD)/variant Creutzfeldt-Jakob disease (vCJD).* Retrieved from *http://www.phac-aspc.gc.ca/cjd-mcj/*

Registered Nurses' Association of Ontario. (2003/2010). *Nursing best practice guideline: Screening for delirium, dementia, and depression in older adults.* Toronto: Author.

Registered Nurses' Association of Ontario. (2004). *Nursing best practice guideline: Caregiving strategies for older adults with delirium, dementia, and depression.* Toronto: Author.

Registered Nurses' Association of Ontario (RNAO). (2011). *Nursing best practice guideline: Prevention of falls and fall injuries in the older adult.* Toronto: Author.

Rosenberg, P. B., Johnston, D., & Lyketos, C. G. (2006). A clinical approach to mild cognitive impairment. *American Journal of Psychiatry, 163,* 1884-1890. doi:10.1176/appi.ajp.163.11.1884

Savva, G. M., Zaccai, J., Matthews, F. E., Davidson, J. E., McKeith, I., & Brayne, C. (2009). Prevalence, correlates and course of behavioural and psychological symptoms of dementia in the population. *British Journal of Psychiatry, 194,* 212-219. doi:10.1192/bjp.bp.108.049619

Sheikh, J. I., & Yesavage, J. A. (1986). Geriatric Depression Scale (GDS). Recent evidence and development of a shorter version. In T. L. Brink (Ed.), *Clinical gerontology: A guide to assessment and intervention* (pp. 165-173). New York: Haworth.

Steis, M., & Fick, D. (2008). Are nurses recognizing delirium? A systematic review. *Journal of Gerontological Nursing, 34*(9), 40-48. doi:10.3928/00989134-20080901-12

Tullman, D. F., Mion, L. C., Fletcher, K., & Foreman, M. D. (2008). Delirium: Prevention, early recognition, and treatment. In E. Capezuti, D. Zwicker, M. Mezey, & T. Fulmer (Eds.), *Evidence-based geriatric nursing protocols for best practice* (34th ed., pp. 111-125). New York: Springer.

University of California, San Francisco, Memory and Aging Center. (2010). *Frontotemporal dementia.* Retrieved from *http://memory. ucsf.edu/ftd/*

Voyer, P., Cole, M. G., McCusker, J., Belzile, É. (2006). Prevalence and symptoms of delirium superimposed on dementia. *Clinical Nursing Research, 15,* 46-66. doi:10.1177/1054773805282299

Waszynski, C. M. (2007). Detecting delirium. *American Journal of Nursing, 107*(12), 50-59. doi:10.1097/01.NAJ.0000301029. 87489.35

Weinmann, S., Roll, S., Schwarzbach, C., Vauth, C., & Willich, S. N. (2010). Effects of ginkgo biloba in dementia: Systematic review and meta-analysis. *BMC Geriatrics, 10,* 14. doi:10.1186/1471-2318-10-14

CANADIAN RESOURCES

Acute Care Geriatric Nurse Network
http://www.acgnn.ca

Alzheimer Knowledge Exchange
http://www.akeresourcecentre.org/

Alzheimer Society of Canada
http://www.alzheimer.ca

Alzheimer Society of Canada, "Brain Health"
http://www.alzheimer.ca/en/About-dementia/About-the-brain/Brain-health

Alzheimer Society of Canada, Safety in the Home
http://www.alzheimer.ca/en/Living-with-dementia/Day-to-day-living/Safety/Safety%20in%20the%20home

Confusion Assessment Method training manual
http://www.hospitalelderlifeprogram.org/private/cam-disclaimer.php?pageid=01.08.00

Canadian Academy of Geriatric Psychiatry (CAGP)
http://www.cagp.ca

Canadian Association of Retired Persons
http://www.carp.ca

Canadian Caregiver Coalition
http://www.ccc-ccan.ca

Canadian Coalition for Seniors' Mental Health
General website: *http://www.ccsmh.ca*
Pocket card for assessment and treatment of behavioural symptoms: *http://www.ccsmh.ca/pdf/MHI%20in%20LTC%20-%20Final.pdf*

Canadian Geriatrics Society
http://www.canadiangeriatrics.ca

Canadian Gerontological Nursing Association (CGNA)
http://www.cgna.net

Canadian Study of Health and Aging
http://www.csha.ca

National Initiative for the Care of the Elderly (NICE)
http://www.nicenet.ca

Regional Geriatrics Programs of Ontario
http://www.rgps.on.ca
Pocket tools for providing oral care to patients with dementia: *http://www.rgpc.ca/resource/index.cfm*

The Kenneth G. Murray Alzheimer Research & Education Program, University of Waterloo
http://www.marep.uwaterloo.ca

Registered Nurses' Association of Ontario (RNAO)
Nursing Best Practice Guidelines (BPG): *http://www.rnao.org/bestpractices*

Vancouver Island Health Authority
Delirium Resources: *http://www.viha.ca/mhas/resources/delirium/tools.htm*

ADDITIONAL RESOURCES

American Geriatrics Society AGS Updated Beers Criteria for Potentially Inappropriate Medication Use in Older Adults (2012)
http://www.americangeriatrics.org/health_care_professionals/clinical_practice/clinical_guidelines_recommendations/2012

Hartford Institute for Geriatric Nursing: ConsultGeriRN.org
http://www.consultgerirn.org

Hospital Elder Life Program (HELP) at Yale University
http://www.hospitalelderlifeprogram.org/public/public-main.php

National Institute on Aging
http://www.nia.nih.gov
Video, "Inside the Brain: Unraveling the Mystery of Alzheimer's Disease": *http://www.nia.nih.gov/Alzheimers/ADVideo*

National Institute of Neurological Disorders and Strokes
http://www.ninds.nih.gov

ⓔvolve *For additional Internet resources, see the Web site for this book at* **http://evolve.elsevier.com/Canada/Lewis/medsurg**

Nursing Management: Peripheral Nerve and Spinal Cord Problems

Written by Teresa E. Hills

Adapted by Angela Sarro

LEARNING OBJECTIVES

1. Explain the etiology, clinical manifestations, collaborative care, and nursing management of trigeminal neuralgia and Bell's palsy.
2. Explain the etiology, clinical manifestations, collaborative care, and nursing management of Guillain-Barré syndrome, botulism, tetanus, and neurosyphilis.
3. Describe the classification of spinal cord injuries and associated clinical manifestations.
4. Describe the clinical manifestations, collaborative care, and nursing management of spinal cord injury.
5. Explain the correlation between the clinical manifestations of spinal cord injury and the level of disruption and the functional goals for rehabilitation.
6. Describe the nursing management of the major physical and psychological problems of patients with a spinal cord injury.
7. Describe the effects of spinal cord injury on the older adult population.
8. Explain the types, clinical manifestations, collaborative care, and nursing management of spinal cord tumours.
9. Describe the pathophysiology, clinical manifestations, and the nursing and collaborative management of postpolio syndrome.

KEY TERMS

autonomic dysreflexia Massive, life-threatening, uncompensated cardiovascular reaction mediated by the sympathetic nervous system that occurs in response to visceral stimulation, p. 1784

Bell's palsy Disruption of the motor branches of the facial nerve (cranial nerve VII) on one side of the face in the absence of any other disease, p. 1764

botulism A disease caused by the neurotoxin produced by *Clostridium botulinum*; gastrointestinal absorption of the neurotoxin (food poisoning) results in disturbed muscle innervation, p. 1768

Brown-Séquard syndrome Damage to one half of the spinal cord that is characterized by spastic paralysis and loss of proprioception on the body's injured side and by loss of the senses of pain and temperature on the other side of the body, p. 1771

Guillain-Barré syndrome Acute, rapidly progressing, and potentially fatal form of polyneuritis believed to be caused by a cell-mediated immunological reaction directed at the peripheral nerves, p. 1765

neurogenic bladder Bladder dysfunction related to abnormal bladder innervation, or its absence, caused by a spinal cord or cauda equina lesion, p. 1785

neurogenic shock Neurological syndrome caused by the loss of vasomotor tone as a result of spinal cord injury at the fifth thoracic (T5) vertebra or above, p. 1771

neurosyphilis Infection of any part of the nervous system by the organism *Treponema pallidum*, p. 1769

paraplegia Paralysis and loss of sensation in the lower limbs and the trunk, p. 1771

poikilothermism The adjustment of the body temperature to the room temperature, p. 1776

postpolio syndrome (PPS) Recurrence of neuromuscular symptoms of polio in disease survivors as they age, p. 1792

spinal shock Neurological syndrome that is characterized by decreased reflexes, loss of sensation, and flaccid paralysis below the level of the injury, p. 1771

tetanus Lockjaw; an extremely severe polyradiculitis and polyneuritis affecting spinal and cranial nerves that results from the effects of a potent neurotoxin released by the anaerobic bacillus *Clostridium tetani*, p. 1768

tetraplegia Paralysis of the arms, the legs, and the trunk occurring with spinal cord damage at the eighth cervical (C8) vertebra or above; formerly called *quadriplegia*, p. 1770

trigeminal neuralgia Cranial nerve disorder characterized by paroxysms of flashing, stabbing pain radiating along the course of a branch of the trigeminal facial nerve from the angle of the jaw, p. 1760

ELECTRONIC RESOURCES

Supplemental content related to Chapter 63 can be found...

Evolve Web Site ⊖volve

http://evolve.elsevier.com/Canada/Lewis/medsurg
- Answer Guidelines for Case Study on p. 1792
- Clinical Reference: Laboratory Values
- Content Updates
- Customizable Nursing Care Plan: Spinal Cord Injury
- Electronic Calculators

- Examination Review Questions
- Glossary
- Interactive Case Study: Spinal Cord Injury
- Key Points (Printable and MP3 Download)
- Patient & Caregiver Teaching Guides:
  - Autonomic Dysreflexia
  - Bowel Management After Spinal Cord Injury
  - Skin Care for Patient With Spinal Cord Injuries

Cranial Nerve Disorders

Cranial nerve disorders are commonly classified as peripheral neuropathies. The 12 pairs of cranial nerves are considered the peripheral nerves of the brain. The disorders usually involve the motor or sensory (or both) branches of a single nerve *(mononeuropathies)*. Causes of cranial nerve problems include tumours, trauma, infections, inflammatory processes, and idiopathic (unknown) causes. Two cranial nerve disorders are trigeminal neuralgia (tic douloureux) and Bell's palsy (acute peripheral facial paralysis).

Trigeminal Neuralgia

Etiology and Pathophysiology

Trigeminal neuralgia, also known as *tic douloureux,* is a relatively uncommon cranial nerve disorder diagnosed in approximately 1500 Canadians each year (Trigeminal Neuralgia Association of Canada, 2010). However, it is the most commonly diagnosed neuralgic condition. It is diagnosed approximately twice as often in women as in men. The majority of cases (>90%) are diagnosed in individuals older than 40. The trigeminal nerve is the fifth cranial nerve (cranial nerve V) and has both motor and sensory branches (Bennetto, Patel, & Fuller, 2007). In trigeminal neuralgia, the sensory or afferent branches, primarily the maxillary and mandibular branches, are involved (Figure 63-1).

The pathophysiology of trigeminal neuralgia is not fully understood. One theory is that blood vessels, the superior cerebellar artery in particular, are compressed. This results in chronic irritation of the trigeminal nerve at the root entry zone. This irritation results in increased firing of the afferent or sensory fibre. Other factors that may result in neuralgia include herpesvirus infection, infection of gums and jaw, and a brainstem infarct. The

effectiveness of antiseizure drug therapy in reducing pain may be related to the ability of these drugs to stabilize the neuronal membrane and decrease paroxysmal afferent impulses of the nerve (Zakrzewska & McMillan, 2011).

Clinical Manifestations

The classic feature of trigeminal neuralgia is an abrupt onset of paroxysms of flashing, stabbing pain radiating along the course of a branch of the trigeminal facial nerve from the angle of the jaw, described as a burning, knifelike, or lightning-like shock in the lips, the upper or lower gums, the cheek, the forehead, or the side of the nose. Intense pain, twitching, grimacing, and frequent blinking and tearing of the eye occur during the acute attack (hence the term *tic douloureux*). Some patients may experience facial sensory loss. The attacks are usually brief, lasting only seconds to 2 or 3 minutes, and are generally unilateral. Recurrences are unpredictable; they may occur several times a day or weeks or months apart. After the refractory (pain-free) period, a phenomenon known as *clustering* can occur. Clustering is characterized by a cycle of pain and refractoriness that continues for hours.

The painful episodes are usually initiated by a triggering mechanism of light cutaneous stimulation at a specific point *(trigger zone)* along the distribution of the nerve branches. Precipitating stimuli include chewing, brushing teeth, a hot or cold blast of air on the face, washing the face, yawning, and even talking. Touch and tickle seem to predominate as causative triggers, rather than pain or changes in temperature. As a result, the patient may eat improperly, neglect hygienic practices, wear a cloth over the face, and withdraw from interaction with other individuals. The patient may sleep excessively as a means of coping with the pain.

Although this condition is considered benign, the severity of the pain and the disruption of lifestyle can result in almost total physical and psychological dysfunction or even suicide.

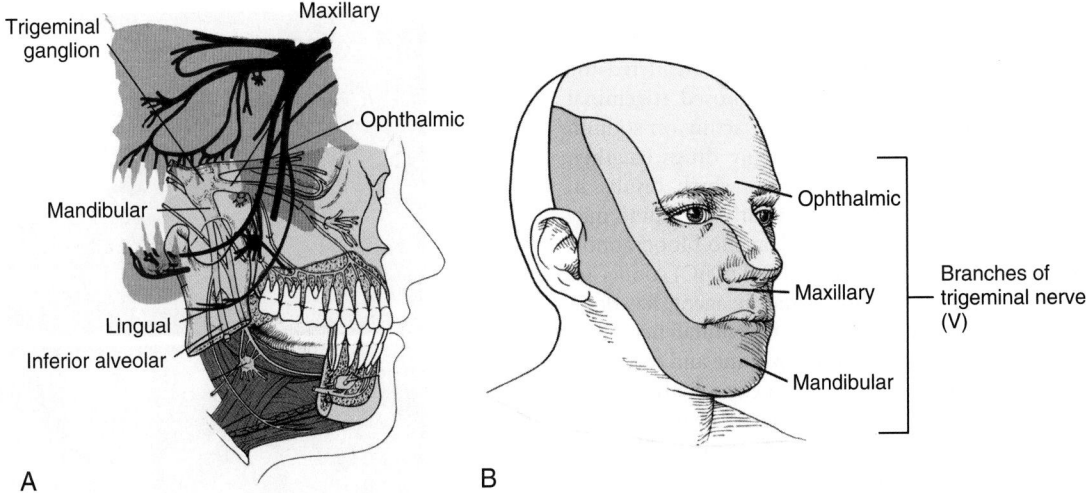

Figure 63-1 A, Trigeminal nerve (fifth cranial nerve) and its three main divisions: the ophthalmic, maxillary, and mandibular nerves. **B,** Cutaneous innervation of the head.

Source: Adapted from Patton, K. T., & Thibodeau, G. A. (2010). *Anatomy and physiology* (7th ed., p. 469, Figure 14-10). St. Louis: Mosby.

COLLABORATIVE CARE

Table 63-1 Trigeminal Neuralgia

Diagnostic

- History and physical examination
- Audiological evaluation
- MRI
- EMG

Collaborative Therapy

- Drug therapy:
  - Phenytoin (Dilantin), carbamazepine (Tegretol), valproate (Depakene), oxcarbazepine (Trileptal), gabapentin (Neurontin), lamotrigine (Lamictal), topiramate (Topamax), pregabalin (Lyrica)
  - Antispasmodic agents: baclofen (Lioresal)
  - Benzodiazepines: clonazepam (Rivotril)
  - Local anaesthetic nerve blocks
- Biofeedback
- Surgical intervention (see Table 63-2)

EMG, electromyography; *MRI,* magnetic resonance imaging.

Diagnostic Studies

It is important to rule out other problems with similar manifestations, such as other forms of facial and cephalic neuralgias and pain arising from the sinuses, the gums, and the jaws. In young adults with bilateral facial pain, magnetic resonance imaging (MRI) is performed to rule out lesions, vascular abnormalities, and multiple sclerosis. A complete neurological assessment is performed, including audiological evaluation, although results are usually normal. Electromyography can be performed to help distinguish between symptomatic and classical trigeminal neuralgia. Once the diagnosis is made, the goal of treatment is relief of pain by either medical or surgical intervention (Tables 63-1 and 63-2).

Table 63-2 Surgical Interventions for Trigeminal Neuralgia

PROCEDURE	TECHNIQUE	OUTCOME
Peripheral		
Glycerol rhizotomy (injection into one or more branches of the trigeminal nerve)	Chemical ablation	Total pain relief with sparing of touch and corneal reflex
Intracranial		
Percutaneous radiofrequency rhizotomy	Destruction of sensory fibres by low-voltage current	Total pain relief, sparing of touch and corneal reflex (increased risk for sensory changes)
Microvascular decompression (Jannetta's procedure)	Lifting of artery pressing on nerve root in posterior fossa with wedge of sponge, leading to removal of pressure at nerve-root entry zone, or removing the involved vessel	Pain relief without loss of sensation
Gamma knife radiosurgery	High doses of radiation focused on the trigeminal nerve root through stereotactic localization	Pain relief 1 day to 4 months after treatment; noninvasive; no loss of sensation
Retrogasserian rhizotomy	Temporal craniotomy (sectioning of sensory root in middle cranial fossa)	Permanent anaesthesia
Suboccipital craniotomy	Sectioning of sensory root of posterior fossa	Permanent anaesthesia

Collaborative Care

Drug Therapy. Carbamazepine (Tegretol) is considered the first-line therapy in patients with newly diagnosed trigeminal neuralgia (Zakrzewska & McMillan, 2011). By acting on sodium channels, carbamazepine and other antiseizure drugs lengthen the time needed for neuron repolarization, which results in decreased neuron firing. Adverse effects of carbamazepine may include bone marrow suppression, which leads to blood abnormalities. Therefore, routine complete blood cell (CBC) counts are required. Baclofen (Lioresal), an antispasmodic agent, has demonstrated efficacy in reducing pain from trigeminal neuralgia. Baclofen works synergistically with carbamazepine and can therefore be used as a monotherapy or in conjunction with carbamazepine if pain relief is incomplete. Other antiseizure medications that may be used in the management of trigeminal neuralgia include oxcarbazepine (Trileptal), gabapentin (Neurontin), lamotrigine (Lamictal), topiramate (Topamax), and pregabalin (Lyrica). These antiseizure drugs may prevent an acute attack or promote a remission of symptoms. Because drug therapy may not provide permanent pain relief, some patients may seek continued help and make numerous visits to otolaryngologists for assessment or may attempt alternative therapies such as acupuncture and megavitamins.

Conservative Therapy.

Local anaesthetics can be used to block nerves. Local nerve blocking results in complete anaesthesia of the area supplied by the injected branches. Relief of pain is temporary, lasting from 6 to 18 months.

Biofeedback is another strategy that may be helpful for some patients. In addition to controlling the pain, the patient may experience a strong sense of personal control by mastering the technique and altering certain body functions. (Biofeedback is discussed in Chapter 12.)

Surgical Therapy.

If a conservative approach, including drug therapy, is not effective, surgical therapy is available. *Glycerol rhizotomy* is a percutaneous procedure that consists of an injection of glycerol through the foramen ovale into the trigeminal cistern (Figure 63-2). Glycerol injections produce immediate pain relief in 90% of patients, but by 5 years, approximately 50% experience recurrence of pain (Zakrzewska & McMillan, 2011).

Percutaneous radiofrequency rhizotomy (electrocoagulation) and microvascular decompression provide the greatest relief of pain. In *percutaneous radiofrequency rhizotomy*, a needle is placed into the trigeminal rootlets that are adjacent to the pons, and the area is destroyed by means of a radiofrequency current. This can result in facial numbness (although some degree of sensation may be retained), corneal anaesthesia, and trigeminal motor weakness. This procedure is easily performed with minimal risk to the patient and essentially exchanges pain for numbness. The procedure is usually performed on an outpatient basis with few complications. It is tolerated well by older adults and avoids a major operative procedure, which is beneficial for patients at high risk for surgical complications (Zakrzewska & McMillan, 2011).

Microvascular decompression of the trigeminal nerve, another commonly used procedure, is accomplished by displacing and repositioning blood vessels that appear to be compressing the nerve at the root entry zone where it exits the pons. This procedure relieves pain without residual sensory loss, but it is potentially dangerous because it is a major neurosurgical procedure involving a craniotomy in the postauricular area. Microvascular decompression has a long-term success rate equal or superior to

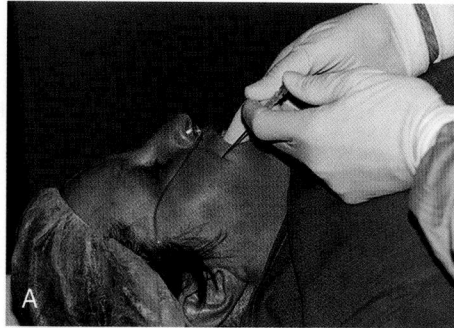
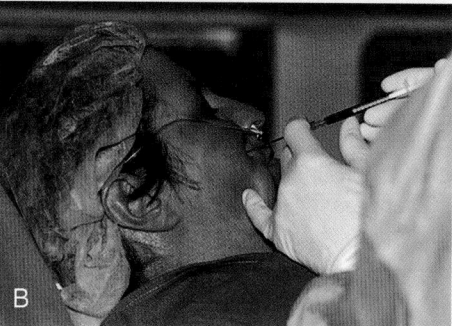

Figure 63-2 Glycerol rhizotomy. **A,** Needle placed in face of patient with trigeminal neuralgia. **B,** Physician injecting glycerol.

Source: Courtesy Joe Rothrock, Media, PA.

that of percutaneous procedures, and the rate of permanent neurological outcomes such as numbness is lower (Zakrzewska & McMillan, 2011).

Gamma knife radiosurgery is another surgical treatment that is used to alleviate trigeminal neuralgia. Radiosurgery with the gamma knife provides precise radiation of the proximal trigeminal nerve identified on high-resolution imaging. This approach has been useful both for patients with persistent pain after other surgical procedures and as a primary surgical option (Zakrzewska & McMillan, 2011) (see Table 63-2).

NURSING MANAGEMENT: TRIGEMINAL NEURALGIA

▪ Nursing Assessment

Assessment of the attacks—including triggering factors, characteristics, frequency, and pain management techniques—helps the nurse plan for patient care. The nursing assessment should include examination of the patient's nutritional status, hygiene (especially oral), and behaviour (including withdrawal). The degree of pain and its effects on the patient's lifestyle, drug history, emotional state, and depression and suicidal ideation are other important factors to assess.

▪ Nursing Diagnoses

Nursing diagnoses for the patient with trigeminal neuralgia include, but are not limited to, the following.

- Acute pain *related to* inflammation or compression of the trigeminal nerve
- Imbalanced nutrition: less than body requirements *related to* fear of triggering pain by eating or chewing
- Anxiety *related to* uncertainty of timing and initiating event of pain and uncertainty regarding effectiveness of pain-relieving treatments
- Impaired oral mucous membrane *related to* unwillingness to practise oral hygiene measures because of their potential for initiating pain
- Social isolation *related to* anxiety over pain attacks and desire to maintain nonstimulating environment

Planning

The overall goals are that the patient with trigeminal neuralgia will (a) be free of pain, (b) maintain adequate nutritional and oral hygiene status, (c) have minimal to no anxiety, and (d) return to normal or previous socialization and occupational activities.

Nursing Implementation

Health Promotion

Because the etiology of trigeminal neuralgia remains unknown, health promotion is directed at reducing recurrent episodes in patients who have trigeminal neuralgia. Awareness and reduction of triggering events may be possible in some patients.

Acute Intervention

Patients with trigeminal neuralgia are usually treated on an outpatient basis. Pain relief is obtained primarily by the administration of the recommended drug therapy. The nurse monitors the patient's response to therapy and notes any adverse effects. Alternative pain relief measures, such as biofeedback, should be explored for patients who are not surgical candidates and whose pain is not controlled by other therapeutic measures. A thorough assessment of pain with a valid and reliable tool, which includes the history of the pain problem and effectiveness of pain relief measures, can assist in selecting appropriate pain management interventions.

Environmental management is essential during an acute period to lessen triggering stimuli. The room should be kept at an even, moderate temperature and free of drafts. A private room is preferred during an acute period. The nurse must use care to avoid touching the patient's face or jarring the bed. Many patients prefer to carry out their own care, fearing that someone else will inadvertently hurt them.

The nurse should review with the patient the importance of nutrition, hygiene, and oral care and teach methods to achieve all of this if neglect is apparent. For cleansing the face, the nurse should provide lukewarm water and soft cloths or cotton saturated with solutions that do not necessitate rinsing. A small, soft-bristled toothbrush or a warm mouthwash assists in promoting oral care. Hygiene activities are best performed when pain is managed and analgesic effectiveness is at its peak.

Food should be high in protein and calories and easy to chew. It should be served lukewarm and offered frequently. When oral intake is sharply reduced and the patient's nutritional status is compromised, a nasogastric tube can be inserted on the unaffected side for enteral feedings.

The patient will probably not engage in extensive conversation during the acute period. Alternative communication methods, such as paper and pencil, should be provided.

The nurse should provide information or instructions related to diagnostic studies used to rule out other problems—such as multiple sclerosis, dental or sinus problems, and neoplasms—and for preoperative teaching if surgery is planned. The nurse may also have to clarify expectations related to postoperative outcomes. Appropriate teaching related to postoperative activities depends on the type of procedure planned (e.g., percutaneous, intracranial). The patient needs to know that he or she will be awake during local procedures so that he or she can cooperate when corneal and ciliary reflexes and facial sensations are checked. Patients are informed about the potential risk of postoperative facial numbness.

After the procedure, the patient's pain is compared with the preoperative level. The corneal reflex, extraocular muscles, hearing, sensation, and facial nerve function are evaluated frequently (see Chapter 58). If the corneal reflex is impaired, special attention must be paid to eye protection. This includes the use of artificial tears or eye shields. General postoperative nursing care after a craniotomy is appropriate if intracranial surgery is performed. (Nursing care related to craniotomy is discussed in Chapter 59.) Caloric intake and ambulation should be increased according to the patient's progress or specific orders.

After a radiofrequency percutaneous electrocoagulation procedure, an ice pack is applied to the jaw on the operative side for 3 to 5 hours. To avoid injuring the mouth, the patient should not chew on the operative side until sensation has returned.

Ambulatory and Home Care

Regular follow-up care should be planned. The patient needs instruction regarding the dosage and adverse effects of medications. Although relief of pain may be complete, the patient should be encouraged to keep environmental stimuli to a moderate level and to use stress-reduction methods. The patient may have developed protective practices to prevent pain and may need counselling or psychiatric assistance in the readjustment, especially in re-establishing personal relationships. Herpes simplex infection (cold sores) can occur as a result of manipulation of the gasserian ganglion. Treatment consists of antiviral agents such as acyclovir (Zovirax) (see Chapter 26).

Long-term management after surgical intervention depends on the residual effects of the type of procedure. If hypoaesthesia (decreased sensitivity to stimulation, excluding the special senses) is present or the corneal reflex is altered, the patient should be taught to (a) chew on the unaffected side; (b) avoid hot foods or beverages, which can burn the mucous membranes; (c) check the oral cavity after meals to remove food particles; (d) practise meticulous oral hygiene and continue with semiannual dental visits; (e) protect the face against extremes of temperature; (f) use an electric razor; and (g) wear a protective eye shield.

Evaluation

The following are expected outcomes for patients with trigeminal neuralgia:
- Relief or decreased pain
- Appearing more comfortable and less anxious

- Normal facial sensation or expected paraesthesias and anaesthesias
- Return to previous socialization, or improved socialization, and occupational activities

Bell's Palsy

Etiology and Pathophysiology

Bell's palsy (peripheral facial paralysis, acute benign cranial polyneuritis) is a disorder characterized by a disruption of the motor branches of the facial nerve (cranial nerve VII) on one side of the face in the absence of any other disease such as a stroke. Bell's palsy is an acute, peripheral facial paresis of unknown cause. Average annual incidence rates of Bell's palsy are fairly similar throughout the world, ranging between 20 and 32.7 per 100,000 (Lockhart, Holland, Swan, & Teixeira, 2011). It can affect any age group, but it is most common among people ages 20 to 60 years.

Although the exact etiology is not known, there is evidence that reactivated herpes simplex virus may be involved in some cases. The reactivation of the herpes simplex virus causes inflammation, edema, ischemia, and eventual demyelination of the nerve, creating pain and alterations in motor and sensory function. Factors that contribute to the incomplete recovery from Bell's palsy include non-ear pain (pain at the back of the head, the cheek, or other area), a history of hypertension, and a history of diabetes (Lockhart et al., 2011).

Bell's palsy is considered benign; the majority of patients make a complete recovery. Improvement in facial function occurs in 85% of people within 3 weeks of onset, but 15% wait 3 to 5 months for any recovery and up to 12 months for the final outcome. Subtle grades of incomplete recovery may have an effect on the individual's quality of life (Lockhart et al., 2011).

Clinical Manifestations

The onset of Bell's palsy is often accompanied by an outbreak of herpes vesicles in or around the ear. Patients may complain of pain around and behind the ear. In addition, manifestations may include fever, tinnitus, and hearing deficit. The paralysis of the motor branches of the facial nerve typically results in flaccidity of the affected side of the face, with drooping of the mouth that is accompanied by drooling (Figure 63-3). Facial weakness is typically maximal within 48 hours of onset and is usually unilateral. An inability to close the eyelid, with an upward movement of the eyeball when closure is attempted, is also evident. A widened *palpebral fissure* (the opening between the eyelids); flattening of the nasolabial fold; and inability to smile or frown on both sides or to whistle are also common. Unilateral loss of taste is common. Decreased muscle movement may alter chewing ability, and although some patients may experience a loss of tearing, many patients complain of excessive tearing. The muscle weakness causes the lower eyelid to turn out, allowing overflow of normal tear production. Pain may be present behind the ear on the affected side, especially before the onset of paralysis.

Complications can include psychological withdrawal because of changes in appearance, malnutrition, dehydration, mucous membrane trauma, corneal abrasions, muscle stretching, and facial spasms and contractures.

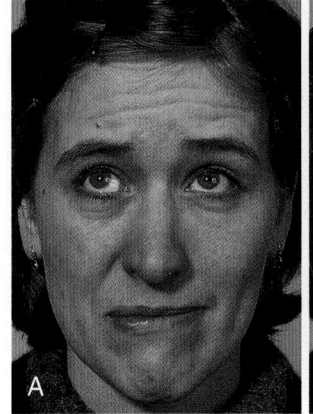 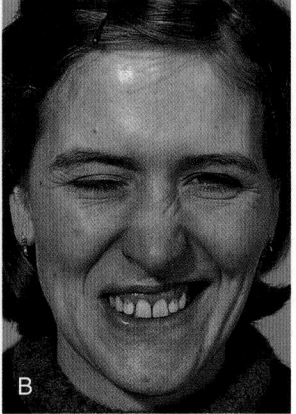

Figure 63-3 Facial characteristics of Bell's palsy. **A,** At rest the face may look almost normal, but the patient is not able to wrinkle her forehead on the affected (right) side, and the right corner of the mouth droops. **B,** When she tries to close her eyes and show her teeth, the differences between the affected and unaffected sides become more obvious.

Source: From Forbes, C. D., & Jackson, W. F. (2003). *Color atlas and text of clinical medicine* (3rd ed., p. 453, Figures 11.15 and 11.16). London: Mosby.

Diagnostic Studies

The diagnosis of Bell's palsy is based on the results of physical examination and is one of exclusion. There is no definitive test. The diagnosis and prognosis are indicated by observation of the typical pattern of onset and signs and by the testing of percutaneous nerve excitability by electromyography. Computed tomography (CT) or MRI may be performed to rule out stroke or other neurological disease (Lockhart et al., 2011).

Collaborative Care

Methods of treatment for Bell's palsy include moist heat, gentle massage, and prescribed exercises. Stimulation may maintain muscle tone and prevent atrophy. Alternative interventions such as aromatherapy, reflexology, and acupuncture can be tried (Haltiwanger, Huber, Chang, & Gonzales-Stuart, 2009). Care is focused primarily on relief of symptoms, prevention of complications, and protection of the eye on the affected side.

Drug Therapy. Treatment with corticosteroids, particularly prednisone, is started immediately and administered over a 3- to 10-day period. The best results are obtained if corticosteroid treatment is initiated before paralysis is complete. When the patient improves to the point that the corticosteroids are no longer necessary, the drugs should be tapered off over a 2-week period. Usually, the corticosteroid treatment decreases the edema and pain, but analgesics can be used if necessary to manage pain. Because herpes simplex virus is implicated in approximately 70% of cases of Bell's palsy, treatment with acyclovir (Zovirax), alone or in conjunction with prednisone, has been used (Lockhart et al., 2011). Combining prednisone with an antiviral agent such as acyclovir or valacyclovir (Valtrex) can improve the rate of recovery (Lockhart et al., 2011). The length of treatment with antiviral medications is usually between 5 and 10 days. Additional antiviral agents, including famciclovir (Famvir), have also been used in the management of Bell's palsy. It is important to review the medications that have been prescribed for the treatment of Bell's palsy with the patient and the family, including any potential adverse effects.

NURSING MANAGEMENT: BELL'S PALSY

▪ Nursing Assessment

Early recognition of the possibility of Bell's palsy is important. Because herpes simplex virus is a possible etiological factor, any person who is prone to herpes simplex should be alerted to seek health care if pain occurs in or around the ear. The facial muscles should be assessed carefully for any signs of weakness; the patient should be asked to close the eyes and show the teeth. Assessment data provide information related to the progress of the syndrome.

▪ Nursing Diagnoses

The nursing diagnoses for the patient with Bell's palsy may include, but are not limited to, the following:
- Acute pain *related to* the inflammation of cranial nerve VII (facial nerve)
- Imbalanced nutrition: less than body requirements *related to* inability to chew, secondary to muscle weakness
- Risk for injury (corneal abrasion) *related to* inability to blink
- Disturbed body image *related to* change in facial appearance secondary to facial muscle weakness

▪ Planning

The overall goals are that the patient with Bell's palsy will (a) be pain free or be able to manage pain, (b) maintain adequate nutritional status, (c) maintain appropriate oral hygiene, (d) not experience injury to the eye, (e) return to normal or previous perception of body image, and (f) be optimistic about disease outcome.

▪ Nursing Implementation

Bell's palsy is treated on an outpatient basis. The following interventions are used throughout the course of the disease. Mild analgesics can relieve pain. Hot wet packs can reduce the discomfort of herpetic lesions, aid circulation, and relieve pain. The face should be protected from cold and drafts because trigeminal *hyperaesthesia* (increased sensitivity to stimulation such as touch) may accompany the syndrome. Maintenance of good nutrition is important. The patient should be taught to chew on the unaffected side of the mouth to avoid trapping food and to enjoy the taste of food. Thorough oral hygiene must be carried out after each meal to prevent the development of parotitis, caries, and periodontal disease from accumulated residual food.

Dark glasses may be worn for protective and cosmetic reasons. Artificial tears (methylcellulose) should be instilled frequently during the day to prevent drying of the cornea. The eye should be inspected for the presence of eyelashes. Ointment and an impermeable eye shield can be used at night to retain moisture. In some patients, taping the lids closed at night may be necessary

to provide protection. The patient is taught to report ocular pain, drainage, or discharge.

A facial sling may be helpful to support affected muscles, improve lip alignment, and facilitate eating. The facial sling is usually made and fitted by a physical or occupational therapist. Vigorous massage can break down tissues, but gentle upward massage has psychological benefits even if physical effects other than the maintenance of circulation are questionable. When function begins to return, active facial exercises are performed several times a day.

The change in physical appearance as a result of Bell's palsy can be devastating. Affected patients must be reassured that a stroke did not occur and that chances for a full recovery are good. A patient's need for privacy should be respected, especially during meals, but the nurse's assistance in the patient's adjustment to the physical changes should not be delayed. Enlisting support from family and friends is important. It is important to inform the patient that most patients with Bell's palsy recover within about 6 weeks of the onset of symptoms.

▪ Evaluation

The following are expected outcomes for the patient with Bell's palsy:
- Freedom from pain
- No complications (e.g., corneal abrasion)
- Appropriate nutritional intake
- Minimal adverse effects associated with corticosteroid treatment
- Return to previous perception of body image

Polyneuropathies

Guillain-Barré Syndrome

Etiology and Pathophysiology

Guillain-Barré syndrome (GBS; also known as *Landry-Guillain-Barré-Strohl syndrome, postinfectious polyneuropathy,* and *ascending polyneuropathic paralysis*) is an acute, rapidly progressing, and potentially fatal form of polyneuritis. GBS affects the peripheral nervous system and results in loss of myelin (segmental demyelination), edema, and inflammation of the affected nerves, which all cause a loss of neurotransmission to the periphery and resultant peripheral neuropathy (McGrogan, Madle, Seaman, & de Vries, 2009). GBS manifests as a symmetrical ascending paralysis. The syndrome affects both sexes in equal percentages and is observed in all age groups, although it is more common in adults. Worldwide, the incidence has varied from 1.3 to 1.9 cases per 100,000 persons per year, with low rates reported in children (<16 years) (Bowyer & Glover, 2010; McGrogan et al., 2009). With adequate supportive care and rehabilitation, 85% of affected patients recover completely from this disorder. However, some patients have ongoing symptoms such as footdrop or paraesthesia that do not interfere with activities of daily living.

The etiology of this disorder is unknown, but it is believed to be a cell-mediated immunological reaction directed at the peripheral nerves. The syndrome is often preceded by infection in two thirds of cases, most frequently respiratory or gastrointestinal infections (McGrogan et al., 2009). Possible links between vaccinations and the occurrence of cases of GBS have been proposed, although the evidence for this link is not strong. *Campylobacter jejuni* is the organism most recognized to be associated with GBS (McGrogan et al., 2009). *C. jejuni*–related gastroenteritis is thought to precede GBS in approximately 30% of cases. Other potential pathogens include *Mycoplasma pneumoniae*, cytomegalovirus, Epstein-Barr virus, varicella-zoster virus, and vaccines (rabies, swine influenza). These stimuli are thought to cause an alteration in the immune system, resulting in sensitization of T lymphocytes to the patient's myelin and, ultimately, myelin damage. Demyelination occurs, and the transmission of nerve impulses is stopped or slowed down. The muscles innervated by the damaged peripheral nerves undergo denervation and atrophy. In the recovery phase, remyelination occurs slowly, and neurological function returns in a proximal-to-distal pattern.

Clinical Manifestations

GBS symptoms range from mild to severe. Symptoms of GBS progress over hours, days, or longer. In most individuals, weakness becomes most severe within the first 2 weeks of symptoms and, in 90%, by the third week of illness (Bowyer & Glover, 2010). Distal muscles are more severely affected. Paraesthesia (numbness and tingling sensation) is frequent, and paralysis usually follows in the extremities. Hypotonia (reduced muscle tone) and areflexia (lack of reflexes) are common, persistent symptoms. Objective sensory loss is variable; deep sensitivity is more affected than are superficial sensations (Bowyer & Glover, 2010).

Four main subtypes of GBS include (a) acute inflammatory demyelinating polyneuropathy, (b) acute motor axonal neuropathy, (c) acute motor and sensory axonal neuropathy, and (d) Miller Fisher syndrome. Miller Fisher syndrome, a rare disorder, is characterized by a triad of symptoms: ataxia, areflexia, and ophthalmoplegia (paralysis of motor nerves of the eye) (McGrogan et al., 2009). In GBS, autonomic nervous system dysfunction results from alterations in both the sympathetic and the parasympathetic nervous systems. Autonomic disturbances are usually observed in patients with severe muscle involvement and respiratory muscle paralysis. The most dangerous autonomic dysfunctions include orthostatic hypotension, hypertension, and abnormal vagal responses (bradycardia, heart block, asystole). Other autonomic dysfunctions include bowel and bladder dysfunction, facial flushing, and diaphoresis (Bowyer & Glover, 2010). Affected patients may also have the syndrome of inappropriate antidiuretic hormone secretion (SIADH, discussed in Chapter 51). Progression of GBS to include the lower brainstem involves the facial, abducens, oculomotor, hypoglossal, trigeminal, and vagus nerves (cranial nerves VII, VI, III, XII, V, and X, respectively). This involvement manifests itself through facial weakness, difficulties with extraocular eye movement, dysphagia, and paraesthesia of the face.

Pain is a common symptom in patients with GBS secondary to the neuropathy that is occurring. Pain can occur in up to 80% of affected patients (Bowyer & Glover, 2010). The pain can be categorized as paraesthesias, muscular aches and cramps, and hyperaesthesias. Pain appears to be worse at night. Pain may lead to a decrease in appetite and may interfere with sleep. Management of pain can include the use of analgesics such as nonsteroidal anti-inflammatory drugs, opioids, and drugs used to treat neuropathic pain (antiseizure type of medications such as gabapentin and carbamazepine) (Bowyer & Glover, 2010). Nonpharmacological measures such as positioning, range-of-motion exercises, massage, and distraction can also be used to help manage pain. Pain management measures should be adapted on the basis of assessment findings and evaluation of the pain management plan.

Complications. The most serious complication of this syndrome is respiratory failure, which occurs as the paralysis progresses to the nerves that innervate the thoracic area. Constant monitoring of the respiratory system by checking respiratory rate, depth, forced vital capacity, and negative inspiratory force provides information about the need for immediate intervention, including intubation and mechanical ventilation. Urinary tract infections (UTIs) or respiratory tract infections may occur. Fever is generally the first sign of infection, and treatment is directed at the infecting organism. Immobility from the paralysis can cause problems such as paralytic ileus, muscle atrophy, contractures, deep venous thrombosis, pulmonary emboli, skin breakdown, orthostatic hypotension, and nutritional deficiencies.

Diagnostic Studies

Diagnosis is based primarily on the patient's history and clinical signs. Cerebrospinal fluid (CSF) is normal or has a low protein content initially, but after 7 to 10 days, the protein level is elevated as high as 7 g/L (normal CSF protein level is 0.15 to 0.45 g/L); however, the cell count is normal. Results of electromyography and nerve conduction studies are markedly abnormal (reduced nerve conduction velocity) in the affected extremities (Bowyer & Glover, 2010).

Collaborative Care

Management is aimed at supportive care, particularly ventilatory support, during the acute phase. Prophylaxis of deep venous thrombosis and pulmonary embolism through anticoagulation with heparin or low-molecular weight heparin (LMWH) is routine. Plasma exchange, or plasmapheresis, is used in the first 2 weeks of GBS. In patients with severe disease who are treated within 2 weeks of onset, there are distinct reductions in the length of hospital stay, length of time on ventilator, and time required to resume walking. Intravenous administration of high-dose immune globulin (IVIG) has also been shown to be as effective as plasma exchange and has the advantage of immediate availability and greater safety. However, patients receiving IVIG need to be well hydrated and have adequate renal function. (Plasmapheresis is discussed in Chapter 16.) Once 3 weeks pass after disease onset, plasma exchange and IVIG therapies have little value. A review of the use of corticosteroids in the treatment of GBS indicated that they do not significantly hasten recovery or affect the long-term outcomes (Hughes & van Doorn, 2012).

Nutritional Therapy. Nutritional intake can be compromised in patients with GBS. During the acute phase, patients may experience difficulty swallowing because of cranial nerve involvement. Mild dysphagia can be managed by placing patients in an upright position and flexing the head forward during feeding. For more severe dysphagia, tube feedings may be required. Patients who experience paralytic ileus or intestinal obstruction may require total parenteral nutrition. Later in the course of the disease, motor paralysis or weakness continues to affect the ability to self-feed. Patients' nutritional status, including body weight, serum albumin levels, and calorie counts, must be evaluated at regular intervals.

NURSING MANAGEMENT: GUILLAIN-BARRÉ SYNDROME

▪ Nursing Assessment

Assessment of patients with GBS is the most important aspect of nursing care during the acute phase. The nurse must monitor the ascending paralysis; assess respiratory function; monitor arterial blood gas (ABG) levels; and assess the gag, corneal, and swallowing reflexes during the routine assessment. Reflexes are usually decreased or absent.

Monitoring blood pressure, cardiac rate, and cardiac rhythm is also important during the acute phase because transient cardiac dysrhythmias may occur as a result of autonomic dysfunction. Orthostatic hypotension secondary to muscle atony may occur in severe cases. Vasopressor agents and volume expanders may be needed to treat the low blood pressure. However, if SIADH is present, fluid restriction may be required.

▪ Nursing Diagnoses

Nursing diagnoses for patients with GBS may include, but are not limited to, the following:
- Impaired spontaneous ventilation *related to* respiratory muscle paralysis that results from progression of disease process
- Risk for aspiration *related to* dysphagia
- Acute pain *related to* paresthaesias, muscle aches and cramps, and hyperaesthesias
- Impaired verbal communication *related to* intubation or paralysis of the muscles of speech
- Fear *related to* uncertain outcome and seriousness of the disease
- Self-care (bathing, dressing, feeding, toileting) deficits *related to* inability to use muscles to accomplish activities of daily living
- Risk for impaired skin integrity *related to* decreased mobility

▪ Planning

The overall goals are that the patient with GBS will (a) maintain adequate ventilation, (b) be free from aspiration, (c) be able to manage pain, (d) maintain an acceptable method of communication, (e) maintain adequate nutritional intake, and (f) return to usual physical functioning.

▪ Nursing Implementation

The objective of therapy is to support body systems until the patient recovers. In the acute phase, patients are often cared for in the critical care unit (CCU). Respiratory failure and infection are serious threats. Monitoring the vital lung capacity and ABG levels is essential. If the vital capacity drops to less than 800 mL (15 mL/kg or two thirds of the patient's normal vital capacity) or the ABG levels deteriorate, endotracheal intubation or tracheostomy may be performed so that the patient can be mechanically ventilated (see Chapter 70). Meticulous suctioning technique is needed to prevent infection if the patient has an endotracheal tube or tracheostomy. Thorough bronchial hygiene and chest physiotherapy help clear secretions and prevent respiratory deterioration. If fever develops, sputum cultures should be obtained to identify the pathogen. Appropriate antibiotic therapy is then initiated.

Fear and anxiety are common feelings for both the patient and the family. These feelings often result from lack of knowledge regarding the disease progression. Answering the patient's and family's questions, clarifying misconceptions, and keeping the patient and the family informed help reduce this fear. Collaboration with other members of the interdisciplinary team, including occupational therapists and speech language pathologists, is essential. At the peak of a severe episode, the patient may be incapable of communicating, and this can add to the patient's fear. A communication system must be established with the use of the patient's available abilities. This is extremely difficult if the disease progresses to involvement of the cranial nerves. The nurse must explain all procedures before performing them and reassure the patient that muscle function will return.

Urinary retention is common for a few days. Intermittent catheterization is preferred to an indwelling catheter to decrease the incidence of UTIs. However, for acutely ill patients receiving a large volume of fluids (>2.5 L/day), indwelling catheterization may be safer because it reduces overdistension of a temporarily flaccid bladder and prevents vesicoureteral reflux. Physiotherapy is indicated early to help prevent problems related to immobility. Passive range-of-motion exercises and attention to body position help maintain function and prevent contractures. Patients who develop facial paralysis must receive meticulous eye care to prevent corneal irritation or damage *(exposure keratitis)*. Artificial tears should be instilled frequently during the day to prevent drying of the cornea. The eyes should be inspected for the presence of eyelashes. Ointment and an impermeable eye shield can be used at night to retain moisture.

Nutritional needs must be met in spite of possible problems associated with delayed gastric emptying, paralytic ileus, and potential for aspiration if the gag reflex is lost. In addition to checking for the gag reflex, nurses should note drooling and other difficulties with secretions, which may be more indicative of an inadequate gag reflex. Initially, tube feedings or parenteral nutrition may be used to ensure adequate caloric intake. Because of delayed gastric emptying, residual volumes of the feedings should be assessed at regular intervals or before feedings (see Chapter 42). Fluid and electrolyte therapy must be monitored carefully to prevent electrolyte imbalances. A bowel program should be initiated because constipation is a common problem related to diet changes, immobility, and decreased gastrointestinal motility.

Pain assessment should be completed at least daily with a valid and reliable tool and the patient's self-report. A method of assessing pain without the patient's self-report may have to be established if the patient is unable to communicate verbally.

Patients with GBS who are experiencing paralysis are prone to skin breakdown as a result of immobility and decreased sensation. Patients should be assisted or encouraged to turn frequently; a turning schedule can be helpful in this regard. Skin and wound assessment should be performed daily. Specialty pressure-relieving beds can be used to decrease the potential for skin breakdown in these patients.

Throughout the course of the illness, the nurse must provide support and encouragement to the family and the patient. Residual problems and relapses are uncommon except in the chronic form of the disease. Complete recovery can be anticipated, although it is generally a slow process that takes months or years.

Evaluation

The following are expected outcomes for the patient with GBS:
• Return to usual level of physical functioning
• Freedom from pain and discomfort
• Maintenance of nutritional status

Botulism

Etiology and Pathophysiology

Botulism is caused by a potent neurotoxin produced by the spore-forming bacterium *Clostridium botulinum*. *C. botulinum* is present naturally throughout the environment and can be found in soil, water, and household dust and on surfaces of many foods (Taillac & Kim, 2010). Foodborne botulism, caused by gastrointestinal absorption of food contaminated with *C. botulinum*, is a potentially life-threatening illness; approximately 1000 annual cases are reported worldwide (Taillac & Kim, 2010). Wound-contaminated botulism occurs when the bacteria produce a toxin that is released into the bloodstream. Infant botulism typically occurs in children younger than 1 year as a result of intestinal colonization. In this age group, normal intestinal flora may not have developed to the degree that prevents colonization of these organisms (Taillac & Kim, 2010). One form of human-made botulism is contracted through inhalation. It is thought that this inhaled form of botulism could be used as a biological weapon. Botulism is a reportable disease. It is thought that the botulism neurotoxin destroys or inhibits the neurotransmission of acetylcholine at the myoneural junction, resulting in disturbed muscle innervation. The classic syndrome of botulism is a symmetrical, descending motor paralysis in an alert patient, with no sensory deficits (Taillac & Kim, 2010).

Clinical Manifestations

Symptoms experienced vary according to the type of botulism and the degree of exposure to the toxin. Symptoms generally appear within 6 to 36 hours for foodborne botulism, within 72 hours for inhalational exposure, and within 4 to 8 days for infection of a wound. Neurological manifestations develop rapidly over 2 to 4 days. Early symptoms for all types of botulism include double or blurred vision, difficulty speaking and swallowing, dry mouth, and fatigue. Symptoms associated with foodborne botulism include nausea, vomiting, and abdominal cramps. Other manifestations include paralytic ileus, mild muscle weakness, seizures, and respiratory symptoms that can rapidly deteriorate to respiratory arrest, cardiac arrest, or both. The course of the disease depends on the amount of toxin absorbed. If only a small amount is absorbed, symptoms are mild and recovery is complete. When large amounts are absorbed, death may occur from circulatory failure, respiratory paralysis, or development of pulmonary complications. The overall fatality rate is approximately 7 to 10%. This rate is doubled among patients older than 60 years (Taillac & Kim, 2010).

Diagnostic Studies and Collaborative Care

Blood cultures and CSF are obtained for studies to rule out other diseases. In patients with botulism, the blood cultures and CSF results are normal.

Drug Therapy. The initial treatment of botulism is intravenous administration of botulinum antitoxin. Before administration of the antitoxin, an intradermal test dose for sensitivity to horse serum is given. If no reactions occur, the test dose is followed by the therapeutic dose of botulism antitoxin, which may be readministered in 2 to 4 hours if symptoms persist and again at 12- to 24-hour intervals if required.

The gastrointestinal tract is purged by high colonic enemas, gastric lavage, and laxatives that do not contain magnesium to decrease the absorption of the toxin. Magnesium is contraindicated because it worsens toxin-induced neuromuscular blockade.

NURSING MANAGEMENT: BOTULISM

Primary prevention of botulism through educating consumers is the goal of nursing management. In particular, attention should be given to avoiding foods with a low acid content, which support germination and the production of botulin, a deadly poison. These foods include fish, vichyssoise, and peppers. Although bacteria and the botulism toxin can be destroyed by boiling foods for 10 minutes, spores are extremely heat resistant and can survive in boiling water for 3 to 5 hours. High-temperature pressure cooking is the only safe method of home canning. Specific suggestions related to the preparation, storage, and use of food include the following:
• In home canning, the equipment manufacturer's directions should be followed. Only fresh fruits and vegetables should be used. All containers and utensils must be cleansed, and the seal on the can or jar must be airtight. Canned foods should be stored in a cool, dry place.
• A can with a swollen end should never be used; the swelling may be caused by gases from *C. botulinum*. This applies to home-canned and commercially prepared products.
• If the food is forcefully expelled when a container is opened, it should be discarded immediately, and the contents should not be tasted.
• If the contents of a can look foul or have a foul smell, they should be discarded, and the contents should not be tasted.

Nursing care during the acute illness is similar to that for GBS. Supportive nursing interventions include rest, activities to maintain respiratory function, adequate nutrition, and prevention of loss of muscle mass. Because the recovery process is slow, patients and their families may experience fear and feelings of helplessness.

Tetanus

Etiology and Pathophysiology

Tetanus (lockjaw) is an extremely severe polyradiculitis (inflammation of the nerve roots) and polyneuritis (inflammation of nerves) affecting spinal and cranial nerves. It results from the effects of a potent neurotoxin produced by *Clostridium tetani* (Parkins, McNeil, & Laupland, 2009). The toxin interferes with the function of the reflex arc by blocking inhibitory transmitters at the presynaptic sites in the spinal cord and the brainstem. The spores of the bacillus are present in soil, garden mould, and manure. Thus *C. tetani* enters the body through contamination of a traumatic wound that provides an appropriate low-oxygen environment for the organisms to mature and produce toxin. Other possible mechanisms of entry include dental infection, chronic otitis media, injections of heroin, human and animal bites, frostbite, compound fractures, and gunshot wounds. The incubation period is usually 7 days but can range from 3 to 21 days; symptoms frequently appear after the original wound is healed. The longer the incubation period, the milder the illness and the better the prognosis.

Worldwide, the number of cases per year is estimated to be 1 million. In Canada, tetanus is a reportable disease, and between 1980 and 2006, an average of four cases per year were reported (Parkins et al., 2009). Risk factors for having inadequate antibody titres include advancing age, female sex, non-White race, and poverty (Parkins et al., 2009). Mortality rates vary according to age; infants and persons older than 50 are most seriously affected.

Clinical Manifestations

Initial manifestations of generalized tetanus include a feeling of stiffness in the jaw (trismus) or the neck, fever, and other symptoms of general infection; these symptoms then descend. Generalized tonic spasms occur because of the lack of reciprocal innervation. As the disease progresses, the neck muscles, the back, the abdomen, and the extremities become progressively rigid. In severe forms, continuous tonic convulsions may occur with *opisthotonos* (extreme arching of the back and retraction of the head). Laryngeal and respiratory spasms cause apnea and anoxia. Additional effects are manifested by overstimulation of the sympathetic nervous system, including profuse diaphoresis, labile hypertension, episodic tachycardia, hyperthermia, and dysrhythmias. The slightest noise, jarring motion, or bright light can set off the seizure. These seizures are agonizingly painful. Mortality rates are highest in infants and older adults, and death is usually attributable to asphyxia or heart failure resulting from constantly recurring spasms. Residual injury—such as vertebral fracture, muscle contracture, and brain damage secondary to hypoxia—may be long-term consequences.

Collaborative Care

Serum electrolyte levels, CBC, albumin level, clotting factors, glucose level, and ABG values are monitored. Cardiac function is monitored by electrocardiography and auscultation. As increasing numbers of nerve cells become involved, their inhibitory control over muscle activity decreases, and symptoms develop.

Drug Therapy. The management of tetanus includes administration of tetanus and diphtheria toxoid booster and tetanus immune globulin (TIG) before the onset of symptoms to neutralize circulating toxins (see Chapter 71, Table 71-6). A much larger dose of TIG is administered to patients with manifestations of clinical tetanus. Control of spasms is essential and is managed by deep sedation and skeletal muscle relaxation, usually with diazepam (Valium), barbiturates, and, in severe cases, neuromuscular blocking agents such as vecuronium that act to paralyze skeletal muscles. Opioid analgesics such as morphine or fentanyl are also indicated for pain management. A 10- to 14-day course of penicillin, metronidazole, tetracycline, or doxycycline is recommended to inhibit further growth of *C. tetani*.

Because of laryngospasm and the potential need for neuromuscular blocking drugs, a tracheostomy is usually performed early, and the patient is maintained on mechanical ventilation.

Sedative agents and opioid analgesics are given concomitantly to all patients who are pharmacologically paralyzed. Any recognized wound should be debrided, and any abscess drained. Antibiotics may be given to prevent secondary infections. Nutrition is maintained through parenteral nutrition or nasogastric feeding. The mortality rate associated with tetanus is declining. However, for patients who recover, convalescence is long and includes extensive physiotherapy.

NURSING MANAGEMENT: TETANUS

Health teaching is aimed at ensuring tetanus prophylaxis, which is the most important factor influencing the incidence of this disease. Tetanus prevention and immunization protocols are summarized in Table 71-6 in Chapter 71. Adults should receive a tetanus and diphtheria toxoid booster every 10 years. The patient should be taught that immediate, thorough cleansing of all wounds with soap and water is important in the prevention of tetanus. If a patient sustains an open wound and has not been immunized within the previous 5 years, the health care provider should be contacted so that the patient can receive a tetanus booster.

If tetanus antitoxin derived from horses (equine tetanus antitoxin) is to be used, the patient should be tested for sensitivity. Administration of equine antitoxin is not recommended if sensitivity occurs; anaphylactic shock is potentially life-threatening, and desensitization is ineffective. The adverse effects of routine administration of the antitoxin are mild and include a sore arm, swelling at the site, and itching. Serious adverse effects rarely occur. Routine administration of a booster shot to an adequately immunized patient can cause arm swelling and lymphadenopathy.

Every patient should receive a written record of immunizations and be encouraged to complete the active immunization schedule. The patient's immunization history should be accurately recorded to legally protect the patient and health care providers.

The acute nursing management of the patient with tetanus is aimed at supportive care based on the treatment of clinical manifestations. The patient should be placed in a quiet, darkened room that is insulated against noise. Sedation should be induced judiciously. Nursing care should be administered with the utmost caution to avoid triggering spasms. For example, the nurse should avoid unnecessary touching, use firm touching when necessary, and maintain a slightly higher than normal ambient temperature to minimize the use of bed linens to cover the patient. Nursing care related to tracheostomy and mechanical ventilation is given as appropriate. An indwelling urinary catheter may be used to prevent bladder distension and urinary reflux in the presence of spasms in the muscles of the pelvic floor. Attention is also given to skin care. The patient needs emotional support during the acute phase because the fear of death is justifiable. The family also needs support and education.

Neurosyphilis

Neurosyphilis is an infection of any part of the nervous system by the organism *Treponema pallidum* (see Chapter 55). The organism can invade the central nervous system within a few months of the original infection, and the disease can be fatal if not treated. Neurosyphilis is often referred to incorrectly as "tertiary syphilis," but it can occur at any time in the course of syphilis and occurs in about 30% of untreated cases (Marra, 2010). Except for causing some changes in the CSF, including increases in the white blood cell count and protein levels and positive serological reaction, *T. pallidum* lies dormant for years. Late neurosyphilis results from degenerative changes in the spinal cord (tabes dorsalis) and the brainstem (general paresis). *Tabes dorsalis* (progressive locomotor ataxia) is characterized by vague, sharp pains in the legs; ataxia; "slapping" gait; loss of proprioception and deep tendon reflexes; and zones of hyperaesthesia. *Charcot's joints*, which are characterized by enlargement, bone destruction, and hypermobility, also occur as a result of joint effusion and edema. Other manifestations of neurosyphilis include seizures and problems with vision and hearing.

Neurological symptoms associated with neurosyphilis are numerous and, in many cases, nonspecific. Neurosyphilis is a differential diagnosis for patients with neurological and psychiatric symptoms. *Dementia paralytica* is an ongoing spirochetal meningoencephalitis that causes a general dissolution of mental and physical capabilities. It may mimic a number of major or minor psychoses. Management includes treatment with penicillin, symptomatic care, and protection from physical injury.

Spinal Cord Problems

Spinal Cord Injury

Spinal cord injuries (SCIs) have a devastating effect on health and well-being. The physical effects of SCI, as well as the complications and comorbid conditions associated with SCI, significantly affect quality of life and can even be life-threatening. Associated economic burdens result not only from health care costs but also from physical morbidity and premature mortality that affect productivity at a societal level.

SCIs occur most frequently in young people between the ages of 15 and 25 years who are otherwise healthy. The male-to-female ratio for SCI is approximately 4:1 (Rowland, Hawryluk, Kwon, & Fehlings, 2008). However, there has been a gradual change in demographics, with the average age at time of injury increasing from 28.7 to 37.6 years and the percentage of SCIs in older adults (>60 years) increasing from 4.7 to 10% (Rowland et al., 2008). Older adults with traumatic injuries experience more complications, are hospitalized longer, and have a higher rate of mortality. Injuries are most common in the cervical spine, and such injuries are associated with the most devastating neurological impairments. In comparison with the general population, an individual with a traumatic SCI has a shorter life expectancy (15 to 30 years less), requires 2.7 times more contact with a physician, requires 30 times more hours of home care services, and is rehospitalized 2.6 times more often (Farry & Baxter, 2010).

The most common causes of premature death in the patient with **tetraplegia** (formerly called *quadriplegia;* paralysis of both arms and legs and the trunk, which occurs with spinal cord damage at C8 or above) are usually related to compromised respiratory function (pneumonia), impaired renal function (UTI) and impaired skin integrity (pressure ulcers). Any combination of these will certainly increase risk of mortality.

Because of the potential for disruption of individual growth and development, altered family dynamics, economic loss in terms of absence from work, and the high cost of rehabilitation and long-term health care, spinal cord trauma is a major problem. The prevalence of individuals living with SCI in Canada ranges from 47,000 to 60,000. Approximately 4100 new SCIs occur each year (Farry & Baxter, 2010). The direct health care costs during the lifetime of each person with SCI, depending on the severity of the injury, vary between $1.6 million for a person with paraplegia and $3 million for a person with tetraplegia. Annual health care costs for Canadians living with traumatic spinal cord injury are $3.6 billion (Rick Hansen Institute, 2012). There are also indirect costs, including lost employment earnings and the resulting lost contributions to the economy and the tax base and the loss of productivity of family caregivers. Although many people with SCIs can care for themselves independently, those with the highest level of injury may require round-the-clock care at home or in a long-term care facility. Between 2000 and 2004, Canadians admitted to inpatient rehabilitation with SCIs stayed an average of 59 days, compared to 35 and 14 days for patients with stroke and those undergoing orthopedic rehabilitation, respectively. Almost 80% of SCI patients receiving inpatient rehabilitation returned to a private residence or apartment after their discharge (Canadian Institute for Health Information, 2006).

Etiology and Pathophysiology

Common causes of SCI include motor vehicle and motorcycle crashes, which account for 50%, and falls and work-related injuries (30%). Other causes include sports injuries, medical conditions, and violence (Rowland et al., 2008).

Initial Injury. SCI can result from cord compression by bone displacement, tumour, or abscess or from interruption of blood supply to the cord. The spinal cord is wrapped in tough layers of dura and is rarely torn or transected by direct trauma. Penetrating trauma, such as gunshot and stab wounds, can result in tearing and transection. The pathophysiology of SCI is best described as biphasic. The initial mechanical injury *(primary injury)* with failure of the spinal column (fracture or dislocation) imparts force to the spinal cord, disrupting axons, blood vessels, and cell membranes. This is followed by a second phase *(secondary injury)* involving vascular dysfunction, edema, ischemia, electrolyte shifts, inflammation, free radical production, and apoptotic cell death (Rowland et al., 2008)

At the molecular level, *apoptosis* (cell death) occurs and may continue for weeks or months after the initial injury. Thus the complete cord damage in severe trauma is related to autodestruction of the cord. This is confirmed by observations that shortly after the injury, petechial hemorrhages are noted in the central grey matter of the cord. This further leads to microvascular disruption and hemorrhage in surrounding white matter. Cord ischemia develops and may extend for many segments above and below the injury (Rowland et al., 2008). By 24 hours or less after injury, the development of edema above and below the level of injury as a result of ischemic damage may cause permanent cord damage. This ongoing destructive process is dominant early on, and it is therefore crucial that the initial care and management of the patient with an SCI limit further activation of these processes.

Figure 63-4 illustrates the cascade of events causing secondary injury after traumatic SCI. The resulting hypoxia reduces the oxygen tension below the level that meets the metabolic needs of the spinal cord. Lactate metabolites and an increase in

PATHOPHYSIOLOGY MAP

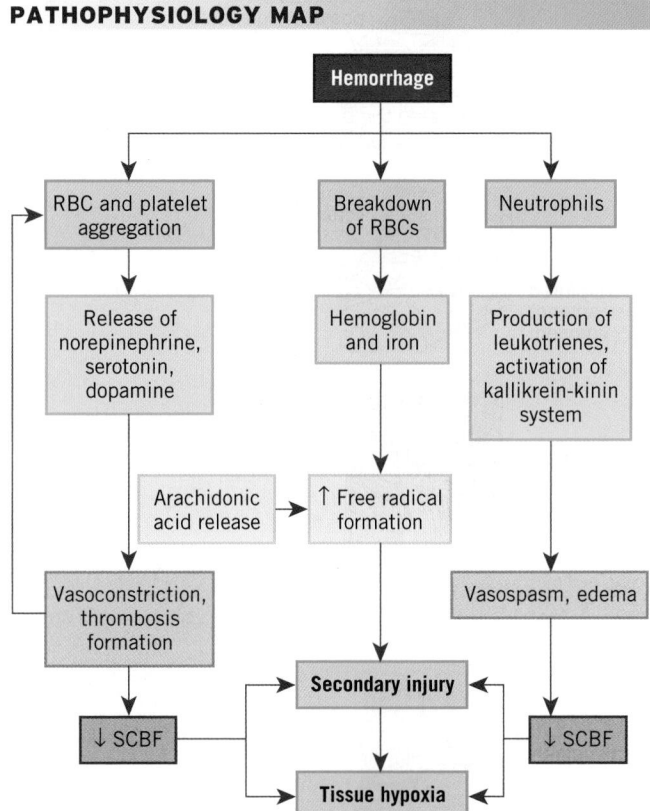

Figure 63-4 Cascade of metabolic and cellular events that leads to spinal cord ischemia and the hypoxia of secondary injury. *RBC*, red blood cell; *SCBF*, spinal cord blood flow.

Source: Redrawn from Marciano, F. F., Greene, K., Apostolides, P. J., Dickman, C. A., & Sonntag, V. (1995). Pharmacologic management of spinal cord injury. *BNI Quarterly, 11*(2), 6; and from McCance, K. L., & Huether, S. E. (2006). *Pathophysiology: The biologic basis for disease in adults and children* (5th ed.). St. Louis: Mosby.

vasoactive substances—including norepinephrine, serotonin, and dopamine—are noted. At high levels, these vasoactive substances cause vasospasms and hypoxia, leading to subsequent necrosis. Unfortunately, the spinal cord has minimal ability to adapt to vasospasm.

The extent of the neurological damage caused by an SCI results both from primary injury or damage (actual physical disruption of axons) and from secondary injury damage (ischemia, hypoxia, microhemorrhage, and edema; Rowland et al., 2008). Because secondary injury processes occur over time, the extent of injury and the prognosis for recovery are most accurately determined at 72 hours or longer after injury.

Spinal and Neurogenic Shock. About 50% of people with acute SCI experience a temporary neurological syndrome known as **spinal shock** that is characterized by decreased reflexes, loss of sensation, and flaccid paralysis below the level of the injury (Dawodu, 2011). This syndrome lasts days to months and may mask postinjury neurological function. Active rehabilitation may begin in the presence of spinal shock.

Neurogenic shock, in contrast, is caused by the loss of vasomotor tone as a result of SCI at the fifth thoracic (T5) vertebra or above in high cervical or thoracic injuries. It is manifested by a triad of hypotension, bradycardia, and hypothermia. Loss of

sympathetic innervation causes peripheral vasodilation, venous pooling, and a decreased cardiac output (Dawodu, 2011).

Classification of Spinal Cord Injury. SCIs are classified according to the mechanism of injury, the skeletal and neurological level of injury, and the completeness or degree of injury.

Mechanisms of Injury. The major mechanisms of injury are flexion, hyperextension, flexion-rotation, extension-rotation, and compression (Figure 63-5). The flexion-rotation injury is the most unstable of all injuries because the ligamentous structures that stabilize the spine are torn. This injury is most often implicated in severe neurological deficits.

Level of Injury. The *skeletal level* of injury is the vertebral level where damage to vertebral bones and ligaments is most extensive. The *neurological level* of injury is the lowest segment of the spinal cord at which sensory and motor function on both sides of the body are normal. The level of injury may be cervical, thoracic, or lumbar. Cervical and lumbar injuries are most common because these levels are associated with the greatest flexibility and movement. If the cervical cord is involved, paralysis of all four extremities (tetraplegia) occurs. If the thoracic cord or conus in the lumbar spine is damaged, the result is **paraplegia** (paralysis and loss of sensation in the lower limbs and the trunk).

Figure 63-6 shows affected structures and functions at different levels of cord injury.

Degree of Injury. The degree of spinal cord involvement may be either complete or incomplete (partial). *Complete cord involvement* (American Spinal Injury Association [ASIA] grade A) results in total loss of sensory and motor function below the level of the lesion (injury). *Incomplete cord involvement* (ASIA grades B-D) results in a mixed loss of motor and sensory function. The degree of sensory and motor loss varies depending on the level of the lesion and reflects the specific nerve tracts damaged. Six syndromes are associated with incomplete lesions: central cord syndrome, anterior cord syndrome, Brown-Séquard syndrome, posterior cord syndrome, cauda equina syndrome, and conus medullaris syndrome.

Central Cord Syndrome. Damage to the central spinal cord is termed *central cord syndrome.* It occurs most commonly in the cervical cord region and is common with hyperextension injuries. Motor weakness and sensory loss are present in both the upper and the lower extremities; the upper extremities are more affected than the lower ones.

Anterior Cord Syndrome. *Anterior cord syndrome* is caused by damage to the anterior spinal artery. It typically results from acute compression of the anterior portion of the spinal cord, often from a flexion injury (see Figure 63-7). Manifestations include motor paralysis and loss of pain and temperature sensation below the level of injury. Because the posterior cord tracts are not injured, sensations of touch, position, vibration, and motion remain intact.

Brown-Séquard Syndrome. Brown-Séquard syndrome is a result of damage to half of the spinal cord (see Figure 63-7). This syndrome is characterized by a loss of motor function (spastic paralysis), sense of position (proprioception), and sense of vibration on the same *(ipsilateral)* side as the lesion. The opposite *(contralateral)* side has loss of pain and temperature sensation below the level of the lesion.

Posterior Cord Syndrome. *Posterior cord syndrome* results from compression or damage to the posterior spinal artery. It is

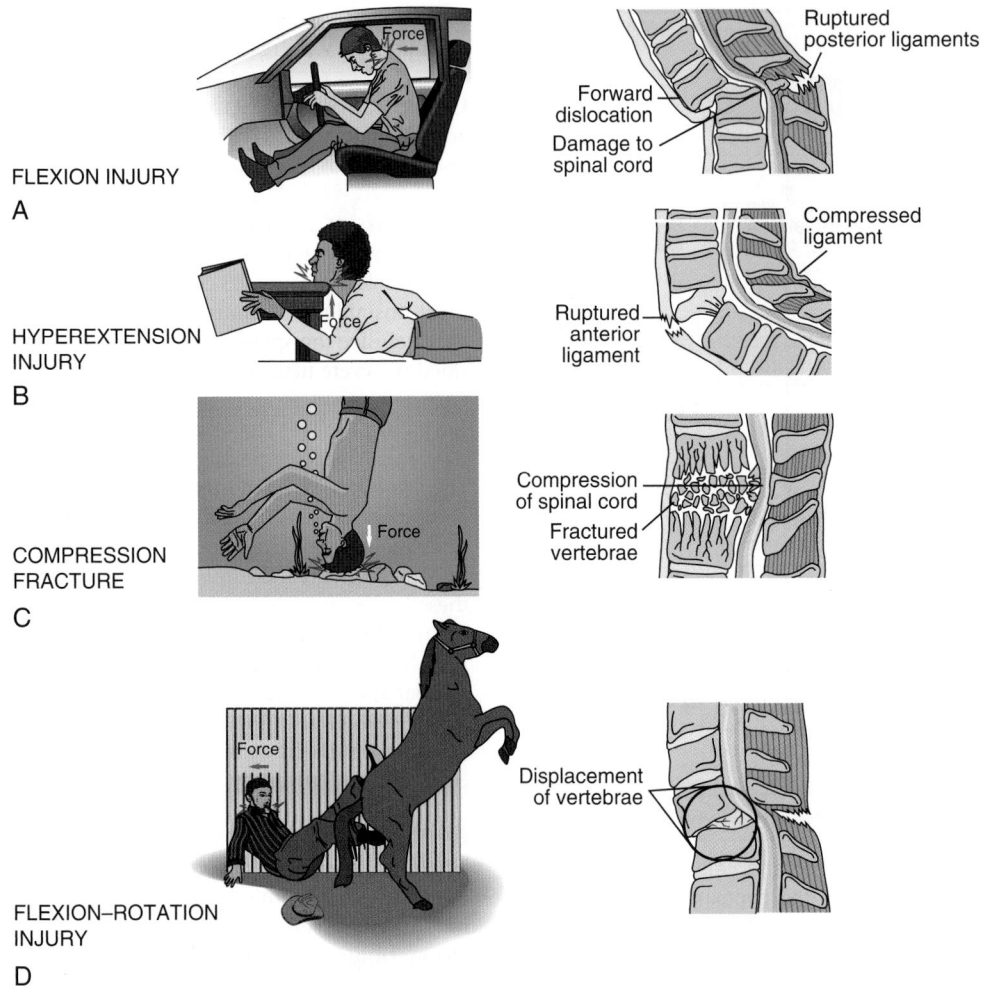

Figure 63-5 Mechanisms of spinal cord injury. Many situations may produce these injuries. This figure shows only some examples. **A,** Flexion injury of the cervical spine ruptures the posterior ligaments. **B,** Hyperextension injury of the cervical spine ruptures the anterior ligaments. **C,** Compression fractures crush the vertebrae and force bony fragments into the spinal canal. **D,** Flexion-rotation injury of the cervical spine often results in tearing of ligamentous structures that normally stabilize the spine.

Source: **A, B,** and **C,** from Copstead-Kirkhorn, L. C., & Banasik, J. L. (2010). *Pathophysiology* (4th ed., p. 1081, Figure 45-12). Philadelphia: W. B. Saunders.

a very rare condition. In general, the dorsal columns are damaged, which results in loss of proprioception. However, pain, temperature sensation, and motor function below the level of the lesion remain intact.

Conus Medullaris Syndrome and Cauda Equina Syndrome. The *conus medullaris syndrome* and the *cauda equina syndrome* result from damage to the very lowest portion of the spinal cord *(conus)* and the lumbar and sacral nerve roots *(cauda equina).* Injury to the conus results in motor and sensory impairment, as well as bladder and bowel dysfunction. Injury to the cauda equina results in nerve root symptoms dependent on the level of the lesion; bowel and bladder function are typically affected.

American Spinal Injury Association Impairment Scale.
The ASIA Impairment Scale is the "gold standard" assessment scale used for classifying the severity of impairment resulting from SCI. It combines assessments of motor and sensory function of various myotomes and dermatomes to determine neurological level and completeness of injury (Figure 63-7) (American Spinal

Injury Association–International Medical Society of Paraplegia, 2004). Muscular strength of key muscle groups is graded on a scale of 0 to 5 and is tested bilaterally. Sensation is documented as *absent, impaired,* or *normal.* An ASIA grade (A-E) is then determined on the basis of the assessment findings (Figure 63-8). This grading establishes whether the findings indicate complete or incomplete SCI or are normal. Various incomplete cord syndromes are also defined with this classification system and have been discussed previously. In addition, this scale is useful for recording changes in neurological status and identifying appropriate functional goals for rehabilitation.

Clinical Manifestations

The manifestations of SCI are generally the direct result of trauma that causes cord compression, ischemia, edema, and possible cord transection. Manifestations of SCI are related to the level and the degree of injury. The patient with an incomplete lesion may demonstrate a mixture of symptoms. The higher the injury, the more serious the sequelae because of the proximity of the

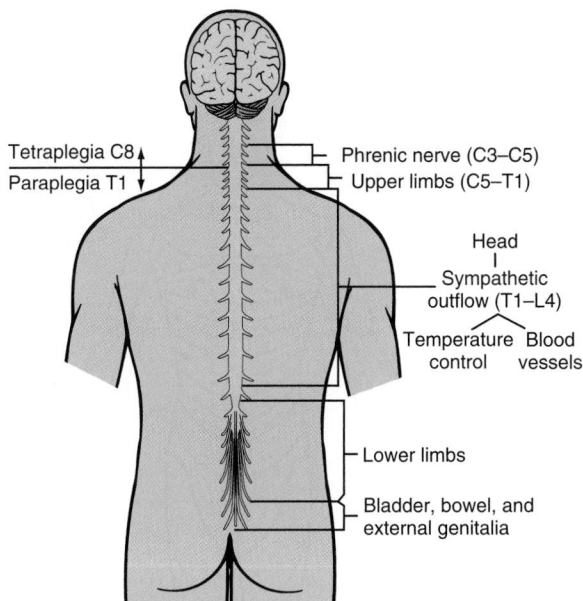

Figure 63-6 Results of spinal cord injury, depending on location. Symptoms, degree of paralysis, and potential for rehabilitation depend on the level of the lesion.

cervical cord to the medulla and the brainstem. Movement and functional goals related to specific locations of the SCI are described in Table 63-3. In general, sensory function closely parallels motor function at all levels.

Immediate postinjury care includes maintaining patency of the airway, adequate ventilation, and adequate circulating blood volume and blood pressure to minimize extension of spinal cord damage (secondary injury).

Respiratory System. Respiratory complications closely correspond to the level of the injury (Schilero, Spungen, Bauman, Radulovic, & Lesser, 2009). Cervical injury above the level of C4 presents special problems because of the total loss of respiratory muscle function. Mechanical ventilation is required to keep the patient alive. At one time, the majority of patients with these injuries died at the scene of the injury, but with improved emergency medical services, more such patients are surviving the initial events of the SCI. Injury or fracture below the level of C4 spares diaphragmatic breathing if the phrenic nerve is functioning. Even if the injury is below C4, spinal cord edema and hemorrhage can affect the function of the phrenic nerve and cause respiratory insufficiency. Hypoventilation almost always occurs with diaphragmatic respirations because of the decrease in vital capacity and tidal volume, which occurs as a result of impairment of the intercostal muscles.

Cervical and thoracic injuries cause paralysis of abdominal muscles and, often, of intercostal muscles. Therefore, the patient cannot cough effectively enough to remove secretions, which leads to atelectasis and pneumonia. An artificial airway such as an endotracheal or tracheostomy tube provides direct access for pathogens; thus bronchial hygiene and chest physiotherapy to reduce infection are extremely important. Neurogenic pulmonary edema may occur secondary to a dramatic increase in sympathetic nervous system activity at the time of injury, which shunts blood to the lungs. In addition, pulmonary edema may occur in response to fluid overload.

ASIA Impairment (AIS) Scale

☐ **A = Complete.** No sensory or motor function is preserved in the sacral segments S4-S5.

☐ **B = Sensory Incomplete.** Sensory but not motor function is preserved below the neurological level and includes the sacral segments S4-S5 (light touch, pin prick at S4-S5: or deep anal pressure [DAP]), AND no motor function is preserved more than three levels below the motor level on either side of the body.

☐ **C = Motor Incomplete.** Motor function is preserved below the neurological level**, and more than half of key muscle functions below the single neurological level of injury (NLI) have a muscle grade less than 3 (Grades 0-2).

☐ **D = Motor Incomplete.** Motor function is preserved below the neurological level**, and *at least half* (half or more) of key muscle functions below the NLI have a muscle grade ≥3.

☐ **E = Normal.** If sensation and motor function as tested with the ISNCSCI are graded as normal in all segments, and the patient had prior deficits, then the AIS grade is E. Someone without an initial SCI does not receive an AIS grade.

**For an individual to receive a grade of C or D, i.e. motor incomplete status, they must have either (1) voluntary anal sphincter contraction or (2) sacral sensory sparing <u>with</u> sparing of motor function more than three levels below the motor level for that side of the body. The Standards at this time allows even non-key muscle function more than 3 levels below the motor level to be used in determining motor incomplete status (AIS B versus C).

NOTE: When assessing the extent of motor sparing below the level for distinguishing between AIS B and C, the *motor level* on each side is used; whereas to differentiate between AIS C and D (based on proportion of key muscle functions with strength grade 3 or greater) the *single neurological level* is used.

Figure 63-7 The American Spinal Injury Association (ASIA) Impairment Scale.

Source: From the American Spinal Injury Association–International Medical Society of Paraplegia. (2011). *International standards for neurological functional classification of spinal cord injury patients* (revised). Chicago: American Spinal Injury Association.

Cardiovascular System. Any cord injury above the level of T6 greatly decreases the influence of the sympathetic nervous system, which results in bradycardia. Peripheral vasodilation results in hypotension. A relative hypovolemia exists because of the increase in venous capacitance. Cardiac monitoring is necessary. In marked bradycardia (heart rate <40 beats/minute), appropriate drugs (atropine) to increase the heart rate are necessary (McKinley, 2011). Peripheral vasodilation reduces the venous return of blood to the heart and subsequently decreases cardiac

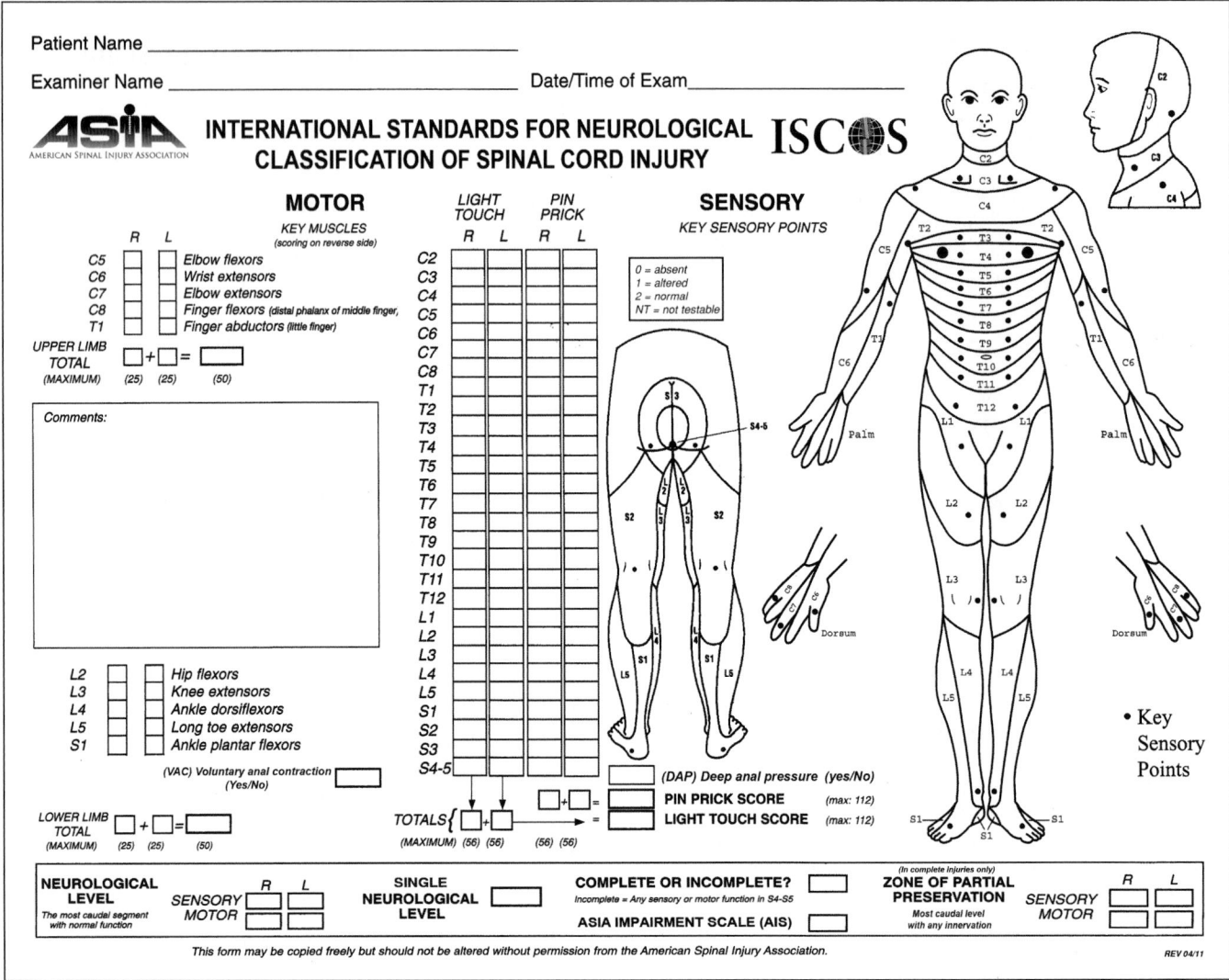

Figure 63-8 International Standards for neurological classification of spinal cord injury.

Source: From American Spinal Injury Association. (2011). *International standards for neurological classification of spinal cord injury.* Retrieved from *http://www.asia-spinalinjury.org/elearning/ISNCSCI_Exam_Sheet_r4.pdf*

output, which results in hypotension. Intravenous fluids or vasopressor drugs may be needed to support blood pressure and maintain a mean arterial pressure of 85 mm Hg to adequately perfuse the spinal cord.

Urinary System. Urinary retention occurs in acute SCIs and spinal shock. During spinal shock, the bladder is atonic and becomes overdistended. An indwelling urinary catheter is inserted to drain the bladder. After the acute phase, the bladder may become hyperirritable, with a loss of inhibition from the brain, which results in reflex emptying. Chronic indwelling catheterization increases the risk of infection. Once the patient is medically and hemodynamically stable and large quantities of intravenous fluids are no longer required, the indwelling catheter should be removed and intermittent catheterization should begin as early as possible. This helps to maintain bladder tone and decrease the risk of infection. (Intermittent catheterization is discussed later on in this chapter and in Chapter 48.)

Gastrointestinal System. If the cord injury has occurred above the level of T5, the primary gastrointestinal problems are related to hypomotility. Decreased gastrointestinal motor activity contributes to the development of paralytic ileus and gastric distension. A nasogastric tube for intermittent suctioning may relieve the gastric distension. Metoclopramide may be used to treat delayed gastric emptying. The development of stress ulcers is common because of excessive release of hydrochloric acid in the stomach. Histamine H_2-receptor blockers (such as ranitidine [Zantac] and famotidine [Pepcid]) and proton pump inhibitors (e.g., omeprazole [Losec] or lansoprazole [Prevacid]) are frequently administered to prevent the occurrence of stress ulcers during the initial phase. Intra-abdominal bleeding may occur and is difficult to diagnose because the patient exhibits no subjective signs such as pain, tenderness, and guarding. Continued hypotension, in spite of vigorous treatment and decreased hemoglobin and hematocrit, may be indications of bleeding. The girth of the abdomen may also expand.

Table 63-3 Functional Goals With Spinal Cord Injury

LEVEL OF INJURY	MOVEMENT REMAINING	FUNCTIONAL GOAL	ASSISTANCE NEEDS
C1-4	Movement in neck and above	Breathing	May necessitate ventilator or other devices
	Loss of innervation to diaphragm	Personal care	Attendant services
	Absence of independent respiratory function	Nutritional needs	Assistance required
		Transfers	Attendant services
		Mobility	Motorized wheelchair
		Environmental control	Devices to control lights, phone, door entry, voice-activated computer
		Housing	Supportive living services
C5	Full neck	Breathing	No assistance needed
	Partial shoulder and biceps	Personal care	Attendant services
	Gross elbow	Nutritional needs	Assistance to meet needs (devices)
	Inability to roll over or use hands	Transfers	Attendant services
	Decreased respiratory reserve	Mobility	Motorized or manual wheelchair
		Environmental control	Devices to control lights, phone, door entry, voice-activated computer
		Housing	Supportive living services
C6	Shoulder and upper back abduction	Personal care	Independent with most activities (eating, washing, dressing upper body)
	Rotation at shoulder		Attendant services for some dressing, toileting
	Full biceps to elbow flexion		Devices to assist sitting up and rolling over in bed
	Wrist extension		
	Weak grasp of thumb	Transfers	Minimal assistance
		Mobility	Independent in manual wheelchair; may be able to drive with adaptation to vehicle
C7	Elbow extension	Personal care	Independent with most self-care activities
	Finger extensors and flexors	Transfers	Independent with transfers
	Good grasp with some decreased strength	Mobility	Independent in wheelchair
C8-T1	Same as for C7	Personal care	Independent with all self-care activities
		Transfers	Independent
		Mobility	Independent
		Driving	Adaptations to vehicle required
		Housing	Independent living
T2-6	Full movement of upper extremities	Personal care	Independent with all self-care activities
	Intrinsic muscles of hand	Mobility	May be able to stand in long leg braces with supports
	Full strength and dexterity of grasp		
	Decreased trunk stability		
T7-12	Full, stable thoracic muscles and upper back	Personal care	Independent with all self-care activities
	Functional intercostal muscles and therefore increased respiratory reserve	Mobility	May walk for limited distances with long leg braces and crutches, using swing-through gait
L1-2	Varying control of legs and pelvis	Personal care	Independent
	Some instability of lower back		May require assistance with bowel and bladder functioning
		Mobility	Good sitting balance
			Independent use of wheelchair
			May walk for limited distances with long leg braces
L3-4	Quadriceps and hip flexors	Personal care	Independent
	Absence of hamstring function	Mobility	Independent ambulation with assistive devices
	Flail ankles		

Source: Adapted from Sarro, A. (2013). Pediatric and adult spine. In *Navigating neuroscience nursing: A Canadian perspective* (Chapter 5). Pembroke, ON: Pappin Communications.

Loss of neurological control over the bowel results in a *neurogenic bowel*. In the early period after injury when spinal shock is present and for patients with an injury level of T12 or below, the bowel is areflexic and sphincter tone is decreased. As reflexes return, the bowel becomes reflexic, sphincter tone is enhanced, and reflex emptying occurs. Both types of neurogenic bowel can be managed successfully with a regular bowel program coordinated with the gastrocolic reflex to minimize untimely incontinence.

Integumentary System. A major consequence of lack of movement is the potential for skin breakdown over bony prominences in areas of decreased or no sensation. Pressure ulcers can occur quickly and can lead to major infection or sepsis. See Chapter 14 for further information on pressure ulcers.

Thermoregulation. **Poikilothermism** is the adjustment of the body temperature to the room temperature. This occurs in SCIs because the interruption of the sympathetic nervous system prevents peripheral temperature sensations from reaching the hypothalamus. The ability to sweat or shiver is also decreased below the level of the lesion, which affects the ability to regulate body temperature. The degree of poikilothermism depends on the level of injury. Patients with high cervical injuries have a greater loss of the ability to regulate temperature than do those with thoracic or lumbar injuries.

Metabolic Needs. Nasogastric suctioning may lead to metabolic alkalosis, and decreases in tissue perfusion may lead to acidosis. Electrolyte levels can be altered by gastric suctioning and must be monitored until suctioning is discontinued and normal nutritional requirements are met. Loss of body weight (10% or more) is common, and nitrogen excretion mirrors weight loss (Thibault-Halman, Casha, Singer, & Christie, 2011). Nutritional needs are much greater than what would be expected for an immobilized person. A positive nitrogen balance, which may not occur for more than 2 months after the injury, and a high-protein diet help prevent skin breakdown and infections and decrease the rate of muscle atrophy.

Peripheral Vascular Problems. Deep venous thrombosis (DVT) is a common problem accompanying SCI during the first 3 months. It is more difficult to detect a DVT in a person with an SCI because the patient does not exhibit the usual signs and symptoms, such as pain and tenderness (Christie, Thibault-Halman & Casha, 2011). Pulmonary embolism is one of the leading causes of death in patients with SCI. Techniques for assessment of DVT include Doppler ultrasound examination and measurement of leg and thigh girth.

Diagnostic Studies

Complete spine radiography may be performed initially to assess for vertebral fracture. However, MRI has become the "gold standard" for imaging neurological tissues, including the spinal cord. It is recommended that MRI be used to direct clinical decision making. An MRI is performed to assess spinal cord compression and damage, ligamentous injury, and soft tissue changes (Bozzo, Marcoux, Radhakrishna, Pelletier, & Goulet, 2011). CT may be used to assess the degree of bony injury and the degree of spinal canal compromise. A comprehensive neurological examination is performed, along with assessment of head, chest, and abdomen for additional injuries or trauma. In patients with cervical injuries who demonstrate altered mental status, vertebral angiography may also be needed to rule out vertebral artery damage.

Collaborative Care

The initial goals for the patient with an SCI are to sustain life and prevent further cord damage. Table 63-4 outlines the emergency management of the patient with an SCI. Systemic and neurogenic shock must be treated to maintain blood pressure. For injury at the cervical level, all body systems must be maintained until the full extent of the damage can be evaluated.

Collaborative care during the acute phase for a patient with a cervical injury is described in Table 63-5. The systemic support required by the patient is less intense for SCIs of the thoracic and lumbar vertebrae. Respiratory compromise is not as severe, and bradycardia is not a problem. Specific problems are treated symptomatically. After stabilization at the injury scene, the patient is transferred to a medical facility where further assessment, both clinical and radiological, is completed. A thorough assessment is performed to specifically evaluate the degree of deficit and to establish the level and the degree of injury. A history is obtained, with emphasis on how the accident occurred and the extent of injury as perceived by the patient immediately after the accident. Assessment involves testing muscle groups rather than individual muscles. Muscle groups should be tested with and against gravity, alone and against resistance, and on both sides of the body. Spontaneous movement should be noted. The patient should be asked to move legs and then hands, spread fingers, extend wrists, and shrug shoulders. After assessment of motor status, a sensory examination, including touch and pain as tested by pinprick, should be carried out, starting at the toes and working upward. If time and conditions permit, position sense and vibration can also be assessed.

The types of injury mechanisms that cause spinal cord trauma, especially those involving the cervical cord, may also result in brain injury. The patient should therefore be assessed for history of unconsciousness, signs of concussion, and increased intracranial pressure (see Chapter 59). In addition, a careful assessment for musculoskeletal injuries and trauma to internal organs should be performed. Because the patient may have no muscle, bone, or visceral sensations, the only clue to internal trauma with hemorrhage may be rapidly falling hematocrit levels or persistent hypotension. Urinary output is examined for volume and hematuria, another indication of internal injuries.

To prevent further injury, the patient must be moved in alignment as a unit, as in log rolling, during transfers and when repositioned. Respiratory, cardiac, urinary, and gastrointestinal functions should be monitored closely. The patient may undergo surgery directly after initial immobilization and stabilization or be taken to the CCU for monitoring and management.

Nonoperative Stabilization. Nonoperative treatments are focused on stabilization and realignment of the injured spinal segment through traction. Stabilization methods eliminate damaging motion at the injury site. They are intended to prevent secondary spinal cord damage caused by repeated contusion or compression (Ahn et al., 2011).

Surgical Therapy. The decision to perform surgery on a patient with an SCI often depends on the preference of the physician and the availability of surgical services. Surgery stabilizes, realigns, and decompresses the spinal column. There is evidence that early surgical intervention is safe and feasible and that it can

EMERGENCY MANAGEMENT
Table 63-4 Spinal Cord Injury

Etiology

Blunt Injury

- Compression, flexion, extension, or rotational injuries to spinal column
- Motor vehicle accidents
- Pedestrian accidents
- Falls
- Diving

Penetrating Injury

- Stretched, torn, crushed, or lacerated spinal cord
- Gunshot
- Stab wounds

Assessment Findings

- Pain, tenderness, deformities, or muscle spasms adjacent to vertebral column
- Numbness, paraesthesias
- Alterations in sensation: temperature, light touch, deep pressure, proprioception
- Weakness or heaviness in limbs
- Weakness, paralysis, or flaccidity of muscles
- Spinal shock
- Cuts; bruises; open wounds over head, face, neck, or back
- Neurogenic shock: hypotension; bradycardia; dry, flushed skin
- Bowel and bladder incontinence
- Urinary retention
- Difficulty breathing
- Priapism
- Diminished rectal sphincter tone

Interventions

Initial

- Ensure patency of airway.
- Stabilize cervical spine with hard collar/sand bags.
- Administer oxygen via nasal cannula or non-rebreathing mask.
- Establish intravenous access with two large-bore catheters to infuse normal saline or lactated Ringer's solution as appropriate.
- Assess for other injuries.
- Control external bleeding.
- Insert Foley catheter.

Ongoing Monitoring

- Monitor vital signs, level of consciousness, oxygen saturation, cardiac rhythm, and urine output.
- Keep patient warm.
- Anticipate need for intubation if gag reflex is absent or respiratory function declines.

COLLABORATIVE CARE
Table 63-5 Cervical Cord Injury

Diagnostic

- History and physical examination, including complete neurological examination
- Arterial blood gas measurements
- Serial bedside pulmonary function testing
- Electrolyte measurements, glucose level, coagulation studies, hemoglobin and hematocrit levels
- Urinalysis
- Anteroposterior, lateral, and odontoid spinal radiographs
- CT, MRI

Collaborative Therapy

Acute Care

- Maintenance of heart rate (e.g., with atropine) and blood pressure (e.g., with dopamine [Intropin])
- High-dose methylprednisolone therapy if ordered
- Insertion of nasogastric tube and attachment to suction
- Intubation if indicated
- Administration of O_2 by high-humidity mask
- Placement of indwelling urinary catheter
- Administration of intravenous fluids
- Placement of halo traction if necessary
- Prophylaxis for stress ulcers
- Prophylaxis for deep venous thrombosis
- Bowel and bladder training
- Pressure-relieving surface

Rehabilitation and Home Care

- Physiotherapy
  - Range-of-motion exercises
  - Chest physiotherapy
  - Mobility training
  - Muscle strengthening
- Occupational therapy (activities of daily living training)
- Bowel and bladder training
- Prevention of autonomic dysreflexia
- Prevention of pressure ulcers
- Recreation therapy
- Patient and caregiver education

CT, computed tomography; *MRI*, magnetic resonance imaging.

improve clinical and neurological outcomes and reduce health care costs (Furlan, Noonan, Cadotte, & Fehlings, 2011) (see the Evidence-Informed Practice box, "What is the Effect of Early Versus Delayed Surgery for Patients with Traumatic Spinal Cord Injury?"). Other criteria used in the decision for early surgery include (a) evidence of cord compression, (b) progressive neurological deficit, (c) compound fracture of the vertebrae, (d) bony fragments (may dislodge and penetrate the cord), and (e) penetrating wounds of the spinal cord or surrounding structures.

The more common surgical procedures include decompression, realignment, and stabilization with instrumentation. These procedures are performed either posteriorly or anteriorly, depending on the level of injury and the area of cord compression (i.e., anterior versus posterior). If instability is considered severe enough, both anterior and posterior stabilization may be considered.

What Is the Effect of Early Versus Delayed Surgery for Patients With Traumatic Spinal Cord Injury?

Clinical Question

What is the effect of early versus delayed surgery for patients with traumatic spinal cord injury?

Best Available Evidence

A multicentre, international, prospective cohort study was conducted in adults ages 16-80 with SCI. Primary outcome was a change in ASIA Impairment Scale grade at the 6-month follow-up visit.

Clinical Appraisal and Synthesis of Evidence

- Results of previous studies in the laboratory supported the theory that decompressive surgery of the spinal cord within 24 hours of SCI reduced secondary injury and improved neurological outcome.
- 313 patients with SCI were enrolled.
- 182 underwent early surgical decompression.
- At 6-month follow-up after the injury, those who underwent early surgery showed a ≥2 grade improvement on the ASIA Impairment Scale.
- Complications occurred in 24.2% of patients who underwent early surgery and in 30.5% of those who underwent late surgery.

Conclusions

Surgical decompression within 24 hours after SCI can be performed safely and is associated with improved neurological outcome. This is defined as at least a 2 grade improvement on the ASIA Impairment Scale at the 6-month follow-up visit.

Implications for Nursing Practice

For nurses working in emergency and acute care, it is important to realize the effect of early surgical treatment for SCI and advocate for the transfer of the patient to a tertiary care facility that offers specialized care in SCI. A change in grade on the ASIA Impairment Scale for patients with SCI can indicate a huge effect on functional gain and can mean the difference between dependence and independence.

Reference for Evidence

Fehlings, M. G., Vaccaro, A., Wilson, J. R., Singh, A., Cadotte, D. W., Harrop, J. S., ..., Rampersaud, R. (2012). Early versus delayed decompression for traumatic cervical spinal cord injury: Results of the surgical timing in acute spinal cord injury study (STASCIS). *PLOS ONE, 7*(2), e32037. doi:10.1371/journal.pone.0032037

Drug Therapy. Clinical trials (National Acute Spinal Cord Injury Studies [NASCIS] I, II, and III) have provided conflicting evidence about steroid treatment in acute SCI (Bracken et al., 1985; Bracken et al., 1997; Tsao, Chen & Tsai, 2009). Steroid therapy is not without risk. Most patients with acute SCI are treated in CCUs, have polytrauma and impaired lung capacity,

and are vulnerable to sepsis. Use of steroids superimposes risks on these compromised patients. The current medical opinion around the use of high-dose steroids is that it should be considered neither a standard treatment nor a guideline for treatment but, rather, a treatment option. If steroid use is considered, the protocol to be followed must be initiated within 8 hours of the SCI. It begins with a loading dose of 30 mg/kg IV over 15 minutes, followed by 5.4 mg/kg IV over the next 23 hours.

Other neuroprotective drugs are being tested, and more treatment options may be available in the near future. Researchers are examining regeneration and repair strategies to induce axonal sprouting and promote remyelination of spared axons. Some of these approaches include anti-Nogo antibodies, a recombinant version of C3 transferase (Cethrin), bone marrow and stem cell implantation, and various cellular approaches (Rowland et al., 2008).

Vasopressor agents such as dopamine and norepinephrine are administered in the acute phase as adjuvants to treatment. These agents are used to maintain the mean arterial pressure at a level greater than 85 mm Hg so that perfusion to the spinal cord is improved.

Pharmacological agents are administered to treat specific autonomic dysfunctions such as bradycardia, orthostatic hypotension, gastrointestinal hypoactivity, inadequate emptying of the bladder, and autonomic dysreflexia. The nurse must know the intended effects of such agents, observe responses, and provide specific interventions when adverse reactions are seen.

NURSING MANAGEMENT: SPINAL CORD INJURY

▮ Nursing Assessment

Subjective and objective data that should be obtained from a patient with a recent SCI are presented in Table 63-6.

▮ Nursing Diagnoses

Nursing diagnoses for patients with an SCI depend on the severity of the injury and the level of dysfunction. The nursing diagnoses for patients with an SCI may include, but are not limited to, those presented in Nursing Care Plan 63-1.

▮ Planning

The overall goals are that the patient with an SCI will (a) maintain optimal level of neurological functioning; (b) have minimal or no complications of immobility; (c) learn new skills, gain new knowledge, and acquire new behaviours to be able to care for self or successfully direct others to do so; and (d) return to home and the community at an optimal level of functioning.

▮ Nursing Implementation

▮ Health Promotion

Nursing interventions for injury prevention include identification of at-risk populations, counselling, and education. Support of

NURSING ASSESSMENT

Table 63-6 Spinal Cord Injury

Subjective Data	Cardiovascular
Important Health Information	Lesions above T5: bradycardia, hypotension, postural hypotension, absence of vasomotor tone
Past health history: Motor vehicle accident, sports injury, industrial accident, gunshot or stabbing injury, falls	**Gastrointestinal**
Current medical history: Use of alcohol or recreational drugs; risk-taking behaviours	Decreased or absent bowel sounds (paralytic ileus in lesions above T5), abdominal distension, constipation, fecal incontinence, fecal impaction
Symptoms	**Urinary**
• Loss of strength, movement, and sensation below level of injury	Retention (for lesions between T1 and L2); flaccid bladder (acute stages); spasticity with reflex bladder emptying (later stages)
• Dyspnea, inability to breathe adequately ("air hunger")	**Reproductive**
• Presence of tenderness, pain at or above level of injury; numbness, tingling sensation, burning sensation, twitching of extremities	Priapism, loss of sexual function
• Fear, denial, anger, depression	**Neurological**
Objective Data	*Complete:* Flaccid paralysis and anaesthesia below level of injury that results in tetraplegia (for lesions above C8) or paraplegia (for lesions below C8); hyperactive deep tendon reflexes; bilaterally positive response to Babinski's test (after resolution of spinal shock)
General	
Poikilothermism (inability to regulate body heat)	*Incomplete:* Mixed loss of voluntary motor activity and sensation
Integumentary	**Musculoskeletal**
Warm, dry, flushed extremities below level of injury (neurogenic shock)	Muscle atony (in flaccid state), contractures (in spastic state)
Respiratory	**Possible Findings**
Lesions at C1-3: apnea, inability to cough	Spinal radiography: location of level and type of bony involvement
Lesions at C4: poor cough, diaphragmatic breathing, hypoventilation	CT: bony destruction and compression
Lesions at C5-T6: decreased respiratory reserve	MRI: lesions and edema

CT, computed tomography; *MRI,* magnetic resonance imaging.

local legislation related to seat belt use in cars, helmets for motorcyclists and bicyclists, child safety seats, and tougher penalties for drunk driving offences is a professional responsibility.

It is important that the nurse emphasize the importance of other health promotion and health screening in addition to SCI care. After injury, health-promoting behaviours can have a significant effect on the health and well-being of the individual with SCI. Nursing interventions include education; counselling and referral to programs such as smoking cessation classes, recreation and exercise programs, and alcohol treatment programs; and maintaining routine physical examinations for non-neurological problems. Outpatient health care requires that screening and prevention programs be accessible to people with SCIs. Nurses in these settings should facilitate the availability of wheelchair-accessible examination rooms, adjustable-height examination tables, and scheduling that allows extra time if needed.

◼ Acute Intervention

Regardless of the mechanism of injury and resultant spinal column damage, care of patients with SCIs is similar. Interventions for care are discussed in this section and may need to be modified on an individual basis.

◼ **Immobilization.** Proper immobilization of the neck involves the maintenance of a neutral position. A blanket or rolled towel, a hard cervical collar, and a backboard can be used to stabilize the neck to prevent lateral rotation of the cervical

spine. The body should always be correctly aligned, and turning should be performed so that the patient is moved as a unit (e.g., log rolling) to prevent movement of the spine. For cervical injuries, cervical traction is used less frequently. Traction should not be used unless the patient can communicate any changes in clinical status during application and subsequent assessments. When cervical traction is used, realignment or reduction of the injury is targeted. Halo traction involves the placement of a halo ring or crown, secured into the skull with four pins, with subsequent additions of weight to aid in spinal realignment. Traction is provided by a rope that is extended from the centre of the halo crown over a pulley and has weights attached at the end. Traction must be maintained at all times. The initial weight is typically 4.5 to 6.8 kg (10 to 15 lb) and thereafter approximately 2.2 kg (5 lb) per level with continual neurological monitoring. Additional weights are added until alignment is achieved, neurological changes occur, or overdistraction within the disc space is noted. Once proper alignment has been established, a halo vest is applied to provide ongoing immobilization of the cervical spine (Sarro, Anthony, Magtoto, & Mauceri, 2010). The halo vest stabilizes the injured area and allows ambulation if the patient is neurologically intact (Figure 63-9). Special care of the halo pin sites and halo vest is important for preventing infection and skin breakdown (Sarro et al., 2010) (Table 63-7).

Infection at the sites of pin insertion is a potential problem. Preventive care includes cleansing the sites twice a day with normal saline solution. The development of redness or crusting could indicate looseness of pins, and the physician or designate

NURSING CARE PLAN 63-1

Spinal Cord Injury

NURSING DIAGNOSIS	*Ineffective breathing pattern related to* respiratory muscle fatigue, neuromuscular paralysis and retained secretions *as evidenced by* decreased vital capacity, alterations in depth of breathing, decreased tidal volume, poor cough, and diminished breath sounds
Expected Patient Outcomes	**Nursing Interventions and *Rationales***
• Experiences no signs of respiratory distress (e.g., lungs sound clear on auscultation, respiratory rate is normal, chest radiograph is normal) • Maintains adequate ventilation	**Respiratory monitoring** • Monitor rate, rhythm, depth, and effort of respirations *to note baseline and changes in status.* • Monitor for diaphragmatic muscle fatigue (paradoxical motion) *to note baseline and changes in status.* • Auscultate breath sounds, noting areas of decreased or absent ventilation and presence of adventitious sounds *to note baseline and changes in status.* • Identify changes in SaO_2, SvO_2, end-tidal CO_2, and ABG values *to identify need for further interventions.* • Monitor PFT values, particularly vital capacity, maximal inspiratory force, and forced expiratory volume, *to identify hypoventilation that necessitates mechanical ventilation.* • Monitor patient's ability to cough effectively *to identify need for suctioning.* **Airway management** • Identify need for actual or potential airway insertion *to ensure timely intervention.* • Perform endotracheal or nasotracheal suctioning *to clear respiratory secretions.*
NURSING DIAGNOSIS	*Impaired skin integrity related to* halo crown placement, immobility, and poor tissue perfusion *as evidenced by* reddened skin over bony prominences and open pin sites
Expected Patient Outcomes	**Nursing Interventions and *Rationales***
• Shows no signs of infection at pin sites • Maintains intact skin over bony prominences	• Monitor skin for areas of redness and breakdown *so that interventions can be initiated promptly if a problem develops.* • Facilitate small shifts of body weight *to relieve pressure without disrupting traction.* • Monitor nutritional intake *to maintain healthy skin's resistance to breakdown.* • Inspect condition of any surgical incision wound *to detect early signs of infection.* • Ensure appropriate wound care technique *to prevent bacterial colonization at pin sites.*
NURSING DIAGNOSIS	*Constipation related to* neurogenic bowel, inadequate fluid intake, low-roughage diet, and immobility *as evidenced by* lack of bowel movement for more than 2 days, decreased bowel sounds, palpable impaction, hard stool, or stool incontinence
Expected Patient Outcomes	**Nursing Interventions and *Rationales***
• Maintains bowel management program based on neurological function and personal preference • Maintains rhythm of a bowel movement at least every other day	• Monitor bowel movements, including frequency, consistency, shape, volume, and colour, *to establish baseline function.* • Monitor bowel sounds at least q4h *to determine whether peristalsis is present.* • Initiate a bowel training program *to establish a bowel routine as quickly as possible.* • Instruct patient regarding increased fluid intake and foods high in fibre *because bulk, fibre, and fluid are necessary for the success of a bowel program.*
NURSING DIAGNOSIS	*Impaired urinary elimination related to* spinal injury and limited fluid intake *as evidenced by* urinary retention, bladder distension, and involuntary emptying of bladder (after spinal shock)
Expected Patient Outcome	**Nursing Interventions and *Rationales***
• Maintains bladder management program based on neurological function, caregiver status, and lifestyle choices	• Monitor intake and output *to evaluate fluid balance.* • Monitor degree of bladder distension by palpation and percussion or use of bladder scanner *because loss of autonomic and reflex control of bladder and sphincter can cause distension.* • Insert urinary catheter *to relieve urinary retention in spinal shock.* • Implement intermittent catheterization after acute phase of spinal cord injury *to maintain bladder tone and prevent infection associated with long-term use of indwelling catheter.* • Refer to urinary continence specialists *to establish long-term bladder management program.*

NURSING CARE PLAN 63-1

Spinal Cord Injury—cont'd

NURSING DIAGNOSIS	*Risk for autonomic dysreflexia* related to reflex stimulation of sympathetic nervous system after spinal shock resolves
Expected Patient Outcomes	**Nursing Interventions and *Rationales***
• Reports no episodes of dysreflexia • Identifies causes, prevention, symptoms, and management of dysreflexia	• Identify and minimize stimuli that may precipitate dysreflexia (bladder distension, renal calculi, infection, fecal impaction, rectal examination, suppository insertion, skin breakdown, and constrictive clothing or bed linen) *to prevent occurrence of dysreflexia.* • Monitor for signs and symptoms of autonomic dysreflexia (paroxysmal hypertension, bradycardia, tachycardia, diaphoresis above the level of injury, facial flushing, pallor below the level of injury, headache, nasal congestion, engorgement of temporal and neck vessels, conjunctival congestion, chills without fever, pilomotor erection, and chest pain) *to prevent a life-threatening situation.* • Place head of bed in upright position if dysreflexia occurs *to reduce blood pressure by allowing blood to pool in the lower extremities.* • Investigate and treat or remove offending cause (e.g., distended bladder, fecal impaction, skin lesions, and constricting bed linens) *to reverse life-threatening situation.* • Stay with patient and monitor status every 3 to 5 minutes if dysreflexia occurs *to ensure timely response to deterioration in patient's condition.* • Administer antihypertensive agents intravenously as ordered *to reduce blood pressure if needed.* • Instruct patient and family/caregivers about causes, symptoms, treatment, and prevention of dysreflexia *to prevent occurrence.*
NURSING DIAGNOSIS	*Ineffective coping* related to loss of control over bodily functions and altered lifestyle secondary to paralysis as evidenced by verbalization of inability to cope, expressions of anger or other negative feelings, or refusal to discuss changes in function and to participate in social contacts
Expected Patient Outcomes	**Nursing Interventions and *Rationales***
• Reports ability to cope with effects of spinal cord injury • Expresses feelings of grief in adapting to losses related to chronic condition	• Appraise patient's adjustment to changes in body image *to determine presence of risk factors for ineffective coping.* • Appraise effect of patient's life situation on roles and relationships *to determine presence of risk factors for ineffective coping.* • Provide an atmosphere of acceptance *to encourage patient to discuss his or her concerns.* • Encourage patient to verbalize feelings, perceptions, and fears *to aid patient in clarifying emotions.* • Provide factual information concerning diagnosis, treatment, and prognosis *because knowledge of expectations can help patient cope with the future.* • Provide patient with realistic choices about certain aspects of care *to enhance patient's sense of control over the situation.* • Encourage family involvement *to enhance patient's sense of worth and value as a person.* • Assist patient to identify positive strategies to deal with limitations and manage needed lifestyle or role changes *to prevent patient from practising ineffective behaviours such as smoking, drinking, or angry outbursts.* • Assist patient to grieve and work through the losses of chronic illness and disability *because spinal cord injury results in a real loss, which requires adjustment through grieving.*

ABG, arterial blood gas; *PFT,* pulmonary function test; *SaO₂,* arterial oxygen saturation; *SvO₂,* venous oxygen saturation.

should be informed. The preventive care of insertion sites may vary, depending on individual hospital standards of care (Sarro et al., 2010).

Special beds are often used in the management of patients with SCIs. Kinetic therapy involves a continual side-to-side slow rotation 62 degrees laterally, with the patient in constant motion. The bed allows turns more than 200 times per day. The bed is used to decrease the likelihood of pressure sores and cardiopulmonary complications. However, in some patients the turning can induce motion sickness and fear of falling out of bed when

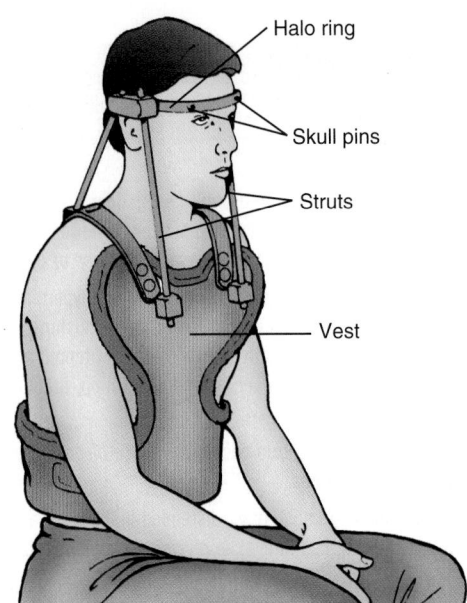

Figure 63-9 Halo vest. The halo traction brace immobilizes the cervical spine, which allows the patient to ambulate and perform self-care.

Source: From Urden, L. D., Stacy, K. M., & Lough, M. E. (2012). *Priorities in critical care nursing* (6th ed., p. 525, Figure 25-6). St. Louis: Mosby.

PATIENT & CAREGIVER TEACHING GUIDE

Table 63-7 Halo Vest Care

The following are teaching guidelines for a patient with a halo vest:

1. Visually inspect the pin sites on the halo ring on a regular basis. Report to the health care provider if pins are loose or if there are signs of infection, including redness, tenderness, swelling, or drainage at the insertion sites.

2. Pin sites are cleansed daily with a clean cotton tip applicator or gauze soaked with normal saline for each individual pin site. If crusting or drainage is present, increase the frequency of cleansing to three times a day or as needed.

3. If crusting is present, wrap the pin site with normal saline–soaked gauze for 15-20 minutes and then remove. Using a gentle rolling motion, the crust can then be removed with a cotton-tipped applicator that has been soaked in normal saline.

4. To provide skin care, have the patient lie down on a bed on his or her side. Loosen one side of the vest, and place a towel against the sheepskin to protect it from getting wet. Assess skin for redness or areas of potential skin breakdown. Wash the patient's chest and back with soap and water. Dry the skin thoroughly, and resecure buckle straps. Do not use lotions or powders underneath the vest. Turn the patient onto the opposite side and repeat the steps.

5. A cotton T-shirt can be worn under the sheepskin for comfort and absorption of perspiration.

6. In case of an emergency, keep a wrench taped to the halo vest at all times.

Source: Modified from Sarro, A., Anthony, T., Magtoto, R., & Mauceri, J. (2010). Developing a standard of care for halo vest and pin site care including patient and family education: A collaborative approach among three Greater Toronto Area teaching hospitals. *Journal of Neuroscience Nursing, 42,* 169-175. doi:10.1097/JNN.0b013e3181d4a3be

turned to the extremes. (Motion sickness is unlikely to occur when automatic rather than manual turning is used.) These devices are rarely used, in view of early surgical interventions that allow for earlier mobilization of these patients.

Cervical collars for postsurgical stabilization are used on the basis of surgeons' preference. With new techniques and better surgical stabilization, a collar is not required postoperatively. Patients with thoracic or lumbar spine injuries are stabilized with a custom thoracolumbar orthosis (TLSO Brace), which controls spinal flexion, extension, and rotation, or with a Jewett brace, which restricts forward flexion.

Immobilization of the neck of a patient with SCI prevents further injury, but the effects of immobility are profound. Meticulous skin care is critical because decreased sensation and circulation render the patient particularly susceptible to skin breakdown. Patients should be removed from backboards as soon as possible to prevent coccygeal and occipital area skin breakdown. Cervical collars should be properly fitted or replaced with other forms of stabilization. It is important that areas under the halo vest, braces, and orthoses be inspected regularly to assess skin condition.

■ **Respiratory Dysfunction.** Patients should be monitored in a special care unit to minimize pulmonary complications. During the first 48 hours after injury, spinal cord edema may increase the level of spinal cord dysfunction, and respiratory distress may occur. If the injury is at or above C3, if the patient is exhausted from laboured breathing, or if ABG levels deteriorate (indicating inadequate oxygenation or ventilation), endotracheal intubation and mechanical ventilation should be initiated. Respiratory arrest is a possibility that necessitates careful monitoring of the respiratory system and prompt action. Pneumonia and atelectasis are potential problems because of reduced vital capacity and the loss of intercostal and abdominal muscle function, which can result in diaphragmatic breathing, pooling of secretions, and ineffectiveness of cough (Casha & Christie, 2011). Predictive factors in addition to the neurologic injury of potential respiratory complications include tachypnea on admission, older age, and previous respiratory disease. Older adults have a more difficult time responding to hypoxia and hypercapnia and are extremely intolerant of hypoxia caused by lack of reserve. Therefore, aggressive chest physiotherapy, adequate oxygenation, and proper pain management are essential for maximizing respiratory function and gas exchange. Other problems include nasal stuffiness and bronchospasm.

The nurse must regularly assess (a) breath sounds, (b) ABG levels, (c) tidal volume, (d) vital capacity, (e) skin colour, (f) breathing patterns (especially the use of accessory muscles), (g) subjective comments about the ability to breathe, and (h) the amount and colour of sputum. Partial pressure of oxygen in arterial blood (PaO_2) above 60 mm Hg and partial pressure of carbon dioxide in arterial blood ($PaCO_2$) below 45 mm Hg are acceptable values in a patient with uncomplicated tetraplegia. A patient who is unable to count to 10 out loud without taking a breath needs immediate attention.

In addition to monitoring, the nurse can intervene in maintaining ventilation. Oxygen is administered until ABG levels stabilize. Chest physiotherapy and assisted coughing facilitate the expulsion of secretions. Assisted coughing simulates the action of the ineffective abdominal muscles during the expiratory phase of a cough. The nurse places the heels of both hands just below the patient's xiphoid process and exerts firm upward pressure to the area, timed with the patient's efforts to cough (see Chapter 70). Tracheal suctioning should be performed if crackles or wheezes are present. Incentive spirometry is an additional technique that can be used to improve the patient's respiratory status.

Cardiovascular Instability.
Because of unopposed vagal response, the heart rate is slowed, often to less than 60 beats per minute. Any increase in vagal stimulation such as turning or suctioning can result in cardiac arrest. Loss of sympathetic tone in peripheral vessels results in chronic low blood pressure with potential postural hypotension. Lack of muscle tone to aid venous return can result in sluggish blood flow and predispose the patient to DVT.

Vital signs should be assessed frequently. If bradycardia is symptomatic, an anticholinergic drug such as atropine is administered. A temporary pacemaker may be inserted. Hypotension is managed with a vasopressor agent, such as dopamine or norepinephrine (Levophed), and fluid replacement.

In older adults, the presence of cardiovascular disease must be considered. The cardiovascular system becomes less able to handle the stress of traumatic injury because heart contractions weaken, and cardiac output is reduced. Maximum heart rate is also reduced.

Compression gradient stockings can be used to prevent thromboemboli and to promote venous return. The stockings must be removed every 8 hours for skin care. The use of pneumatic compression devices for the calves is advocated, and they must be applied as soon as possible after injury and maintained throughout the hospitalization. Venous duplex studies may be performed before compression devices are applied. The nurse should also help the patient perform range-of-motion exercises and stretching regularly. The thighs and calves of the legs should be assessed every shift for signs of DVT.

Administration of LMWH within 72 hours of injury is recommended to minimize the occurrence of DVT. Furthermore, when surgical intervention is required, LMWH therapy should be withheld the morning of surgery and resumed within 24 hours postoperatively (Christie et al., 2011). LMWH is preferable to unfractionated heparin in patients with SCI because of its longer half-life, lower risk of bleeding complications, and more predictable dose effect in comparison with unfractionated heparin (Teasell et al., 2008).

If blood loss has resulted from other injuries, hemoglobin and hematocrit levels should be monitored, and blood should be administered according to protocol. The nurse also should monitor the patient for indications of hypovolemic shock secondary to hemorrhage.

Fluid and Nutritional Maintenance.
During the first 48 to 72 hours after the injury, the gastrointestinal tract may stop functioning (paralytic ileus), and a nasogastric tube must be inserted. Because the patient cannot have oral intake, fluid and electrolyte needs must be carefully monitored. Specific solutions and additives are ordered on the basis of individual requirements. Once bowel sounds are present or flatus is passed, oral food and fluids can gradually be introduced. Because of severe catabolism, a high-protein, high-calorie diet is necessary for energy and tissue repair. In patients with cervical cord injuries, swallowing must be evaluated before oral feedings are started. Enteral feeding is the optimal route after SCI. When oral feeding is not possible, nasogastric, followed by nasojejunal and then percutaneous, endoscopic gastrostomy is suggested. The acute stage of injury is characterized by a reduction in metabolic activity, as well as a negative nitrogen balance that cannot be corrected, even with aggressive nutritional support. Metabolic demands need to be accurately monitored to avoid overfeeding (Thibault-Halman et al., 2011).

Some patients experience anorexia, which can result from psychological depression, boredom with institutional food, or discomfort at being fed. Some patients have a normally small appetite. On occasion, refusal to eat is used as a means of maintaining control over the environment because of diminished or absent body control (see the Ethical Dilemmas box, "Right to Refuse Treatment"). If the patient is not eating adequately, the cause should be thoroughly assessed. On the basis of this assessment, a contract may be made in which the patient and the nurse use mutual goal setting regarding the diet. This gives the patient increased control of the situation and often results in improved nutritional intake. General measures such as providing a pleasant eating environment, allowing adequate time to eat (including any self-feeding that the patient can achieve), encouraging the family to bring in special foods, and planning social rewards for eating may be useful. A calorie count should be kept, and the patient's daily weight recorded as a means of evaluating progress. If feasible, the patient should participate in recording calorie intake. Dietary supplements may be necessary to meet nutritional needs. Increased dietary fibre should be included to promote bowel function. The nurse should avoid allowing the patient's nutritional intake to become a basis for a power struggle.

Bladder and Bowel Management.
Immediately after injury, urine is retained because of the loss of autonomic and reflex control of the bladder and the sphincter. Because the patient has no sensation of fullness, overdistension of the bladder can result in reflux into the kidneys, with eventual renal failure. Bladder distension may even result in rupture of the bladder. Consequently, an indwelling catheter is usually inserted as soon as possible after injury. Its patency must be ensured by frequent inspection and irrigation if necessary. Strict aseptic technique for catheter care is essential to avoid introducing infection.

After patients are stabilized, the best means of managing urinary function is assessed. Usually, an intermittent catheterization program is started. Intermittent catheterization has been shown to reduce UTIs in comparison with use of an indwelling catheter, and it is the safest method of bladder management for protecting the kidneys. Many patients are maintained on fluid restriction of 1800 to 2000 mL/day to facilitate a bladder training program, and urinary output is monitored closely.

UTIs are a common problem. The best method for preventing UTIs is regular and complete bladder drainage. Catheterization should be performed to prevent bladder volume from exceeding 500 mL. A typical regimen would be to catheterize every 4 hours for volumes of 300 to 500 mL, every 3 hours for volumes greater than 500 mL, and every 6 hours for volumes less than 300 mL. Cranberry juice, cranberry extract tablets, or both may be helpful for UTI prevention because there is some evidence that they may prevent bacteria from adhering to the bladder wall. If the appearance or odour of the urine is suspect or if the patient develops symptoms of a UTI (e.g., chills, fever, malaise), a urine specimen is sent for culture.

Age-related changes in renal function should be considered. Older adults are more likely to develop renal calculi, and older men may have prostatic hyperplasia, which may interfere with urinary flow and complicate management of urinary problems.

Constipation is generally a problem during spinal shock because no voluntary or involuntary (reflex) evacuation of the

ETHICAL DILEMMAS
Right to Refuse Treatment

Situation

A 25-year-old man suffered a spinal cord injury (SCI) to C7-8 after a motorcycle accident. Anterior cord syndrome was diagnosed, and he has motor paralysis, which may prevent him from riding motorcycles again. He has become extremely depressed and no longer wishes to live. Because of his emotional state, he is now refusing to eat. Can the patient be forced to receive enteral nutrition (tube feeding)?

Important Points for Consideration

- Withholding treatment in a newly injured but otherwise healthy young adult may present an ethical dilemma for health care professionals.
- Approximately 20 to 30% of people with a new SCI experience a major depressive disorder as a result of the sudden loss of bodily control and feelings of helplessness.
- A thorough mental health and psychological evaluation is warranted; treatment of depression is necessary before determining the patient's capacity to make decisions.
- Most people (more than 90%) with an SCI who receive health care and have access to appropriate resources report a good quality of life. Therefore, requests to withhold treatment soon after SCI should be scrutinized carefully.
- If, after adequate treatment for pain, depression, or other medical conditions, the patient persists in requests to withhold treatment, his ability to make an informed choice must be reassessed.
- A competent adult can decide to withhold treatment. If possible, action on the request should be delayed to ensure adequate informed consent and to determine whether quality of life is adequate.

Clinical Decision-Making Questions

1. What are your feelings about requests to withhold treatment in a young person with a newly acquired disability?
2. What resources are available to help the patient and the staff work through this emotionally charged and ethically complex situation?

bowels occurs. A bowel program should be started during acute care. This consists of a rectal stimulant (suppository or mini-enema) to be inserted daily at a regular time of day, followed by gentle digital stimulation or manual evacuation that is performed by the nurse until evacuation is complete. Initially, the program may be performed in bed in the side-lying position, but as soon as the patient has resumed sitting, it should be performed in the upright position on a padded bedside commode chair.

▌ **Temperature Control.** Temperature control is largely external to the patient because there is no vasoconstriction, piloerection, or heat loss through perspiration below the level of injury. The nurse must monitor the environment closely to maintain an appropriate temperature. Body temperature should be monitored regularly. The patient should not be overloaded with covers or unduly exposed (such as during bathing). If an infection with high fever develops, more extensive means of temperature control, such as a cooling blanket, may be necessary.

▌ **Stress Ulcers.** Stress ulcers are a problem for the patient with an SCI because of the physiological response to severe trauma, psychological stress, and high-dose corticosteroids if used. The incidence of ulcers peaks 6 to 14 days after injury. Histamine H_2-receptor blockers, such as ranitidine and famotidine, or proton pump inhibitors, such as omeprazole or pantoprazole, may be given prophylactically to decrease the secretion of hydrochloric acid.

▌ **Sensory Deprivation.** To prevent sensory deprivation, the nurse must compensate for the patient's absence of sensations by stimulating the patient above the level of injury. Conversation, music, strong aromas, and interesting flavours should be a part of the nursing care plan. Prism glasses are provided so that the patient can read and watch television. Every effort should be made to prevent the patient from withdrawing from the environment.

Patients with SCIs often report altered sensorium and vivid dreams during the acute phase of their treatment. Whether this is caused by drugs used to manage pain and anxiety is not known. Patients may also experience disrupted sleep patterns as a result of the hospital environment or post-traumatic stress disorder.

▌ **Reflexes.** Once spinal cord shock is resolved, the return of reflexes may complicate rehabilitation. In the absence of control from the higher brain centres, reflexes are often hyperactive and responses may be exaggerated. Penile erections can result from a variety of stimuli, causing embarrassment and discomfort. Spasms ranging from mild twitches to convulsive movements below the level of the lesion may also occur. This reflex activity may be interpreted by the patient or family as a return of function, and the nurse must tactfully explain the reason for the activity. The patient may be informed of the positive use of these reflexes in sexual, bowel, and bladder retraining. Spasms may be controlled with the use of antispasmodic drugs. Most commonly prescribed are baclofen (Lioresal), dantrolene (Dantrium), and tizanidine (Zanaflex). Botulism toxin injections may also be given to treat severe spasticity.

▌ **Autonomic Dysreflexia.** The return of reflexes after the resolution of spinal shock means that patients with an injury level at T6 or higher may develop autonomic dysreflexia. **Autonomic dysreflexia** (also known as *autonomic hyperreflexia*) is a massive, uncompensated cardiovascular reaction mediated by the sympathetic nervous system. It occurs in response to visceral stimulation once spinal shock is resolved in patients with spinal cord lesions. This condition is a life-threatening situation that necessitates immediate resolution. If resolution does not occur, this condition can lead to status epilepticus, stroke, myocardial infarction, or even death.

The most common precipitating cause is distension of the bladder or rectum, although any sensory stimulation may cause autonomic dysreflexia. Contraction of the bladder or the rectum, stimulation of the skin, or stimulation of the pain receptors may also cause autonomic dysreflexia. Manifestations include hypertension (up to 300 mm Hg systolic), throbbing headache, marked diaphoresis or flushing of skin above the level of the lesion, bradycardia (30 to 40 beats per minute), piloerection

(erection of body hair) as a result of pilomotor spasm, blurred vision or spots in the visual fields, nasal congestion, anxiety, and nausea. It is important to measure blood pressure when a patient with an SCI complains of a headache (Krassioukov, Warburton, Teasell, & Eng, 2009). A normal blood pressure for a patient with tetraplegic SCI is a systolic blood pressure of 90 to 100 mm Hg. Any pressure higher than this should be considered hypertensive.

The pathology of autonomic dysreflexia involves the stimulation of sensory receptors below the level of the cord lesion. The intact autonomic nervous system below the level of the lesion responds to the stimulation with a reflex arteriolar vasoconstriction that increases blood pressure. Baroreceptors in the carotid sinus and the aorta detect the hypertension and stimulate the parasympathetic system. This results in a decrease in heart rate, but the visceral and peripheral vessels do not dilate because efferent impulses cannot pass through the cord lesion.

In this serious emergency, nursing interventions are elevation of the head of the bed 45 degrees or sitting the patient upright, notification of the physician, and assessment to determine the cause. The most common cause is bladder distention. Immediate catheterization to relieve bladder distension may be necessary. Lidocaine jelly should be instilled in the urethra before catheterization. If a catheter is already in place, it should be checked for kinks or folds. If it is plugged, small-volume irrigation should be performed slowly and gently to open the catheter, or a new catheter may be inserted. Stool impaction can also result in autonomic dysreflexia. A digital rectal examination should be performed only after application of an anaesthetic ointment to decrease rectal stimulation and to prevent an increase of symptoms. If neither bladder or bowel distension is determined to be causative, the nurse should remove all skin stimuli, such as constrictive clothing, tight shoes, and splints. Blood pressure should be monitored frequently during the episode. If symptoms persist after the source has been relieved, an α-adrenergic blocker or an arteriolar vasodilator (e.g., nifedipine) is administered. Careful monitoring must continue until the vital signs stabilize.

The patient and caregivers should be taught the causes and symptoms of autonomic dysreflexia (Table 63-8). They must understand the life-threatening nature of this dysfunction and must know how to relieve the cause.

Rehabilitation and Home Care

The physiological and psychological rehabilitation of patients with SCIs is complex and involved. With physical and psychological care and intensive and specialized rehabilitation, patients with SCIs learn to function at the highest level of wellness. It is recommended that all patients with a new SCI receive comprehensive inpatient rehabilitation in a rehabilitation unit or centre that specializes in spinal cord injuries.

Many of the problems identified in the acute period become chronic and continue throughout life. Rehabilitation focuses on refined retraining of physiological processes and extensive patient and caregiver teaching about how to manage the physiological and life changes resulting from injury.

Rehabilitation is a multidisciplinary endeavour carried out through a team approach. Team members include rehabilitation nurses, physicians, physiotherapists, occupational therapists, speech language pathologists, vocational counsellors, psychologists, therapeutic recreation specialists, prosthetists, orthotists, and dietitians. Rehabilitation care is organized around the

PATIENT & CAREGIVER TEACHING GUIDE

Table 63-8 Autonomic Dysreflexia

The nurse should include the following information in the teaching plan for a patient at risk for autonomic dysreflexia:

1. Signs and symptoms
   - Sudden onset of acute headache
   - Elevation in blood pressure, reduction in pulse rate, or both
   - Flushed face and upper chest (above the level of the lesion) and pale extremities (below the level of the lesion)
   - Sweating above the level of the lesion
   - Nasal congestion
   - Feeling of apprehension

2. Immediate interventions
   - Raise the patient to a sitting position.
   - Remove the stimulus (fecal impaction, distended bladder, tight clothing).
   - Call the health care provider if these actions do not relieve the signs and symptoms.

3. Measures to suppress the incidence of autonomic dysreflexia
   - Maintain regular bladder and bowel function.
   - If manual rectal stimulation is used to promote bowel function, local anaesthetics may prevent autonomic dysreflexia from occurring.
   - Wear a medical alert bracelet indicating a history of autonomic dysreflexia.

individual patient's goals and needs. During rehabilitation, patients are expected to be involved in therapies and learn self-care for several hours each day. Such intensive work at a time when the patient is dealing with the sudden change in health and functional status can be very stressful. Progress may be slow, and frequent encouragement may be required. The rehabilitation nurse has a pivotal role in providing encouragement, specialized nursing care, and patient and caregiver teaching and in helping to coordinate the efforts of the rehabilitation team.

Respiratory Rehabilitation.
The patient with high cervical SCI may have greatly increased mobility with phrenic nerve stimulators or electronic diaphragmatic pacemakers. These devices are not appropriate for all ventilator-dependent patients but may be helpful for those with an intact phrenic nerve. Today, ventilators are also reasonably portable, and ventilator-dependent tetraplegic patients can be mobile and somewhat independent. Patients and caregivers should be taught all aspects of home ventilator care, and referrals should be made to appropriate community agencies. Patients with injuries at the cervical level who are not ventilator dependent should be taught assisted coughing and regular use of incentive spirometry or deep breathing exercises.

Neurogenic Bladder.
A **neurogenic bladder** is any type of bladder dysfunction related to abnormal or absent bladder innervation. After spinal cord shock resolves, depending on the completeness of the SCI, patients usually have some degree of neurogenic bladder. Normal voiding requires nervous system coordination of urethral and pelvic floor relaxation with simultaneous contraction of the detrusor muscle. Depending on the lesion, a neurogenic bladder may have no reflex detrusor contractions (areflexic, flaccid), may have hyperactive reflex

Table 63-9 Types of Neurogenic Bladder

TYPE	CHARACTERISTICS	CAUSES	CLINICAL MANIFESTATIONS
Reflexic (spastic, uninhibited, upper motor neuron)	No inhibitions influence time and place of voiding; bladder empties in response to stretching of bladder wall	Corticospinal tract lesion; observed in spinal cord injury, stroke, multiple sclerosis, brain tumour, brain trauma	Incontinence, frequency, urgency; voiding is unpredictable and incomplete
Areflexic (autonomous, flaccid, lower motor neuron)	Bladder acts as if all motor functions are paralyzed, fills without emptying	Lower motor neuron lesion caused by trauma involving S2-4; observed in lesions of cauda equina, pelvic nerves	If sensory function intact, patient feels bladder distension and hesitancy; no control of micturition results in overdistension of bladder and overflow incontinence
Sensory	Lack of sensation of need to urinate	Damage to sensory limb of bladder spinal reflex arc; observed in multiple sclerosis, diabetes mellitus	Poor bladder sensation, infrequent voiding of large residual volume

COLLABORATIVE CARE

Table 63-10 Neurogenic Bladder

Diagnostic

- History and physical examination, including neurological examination
- Urodynamic testing
- Urine culture

Collaborative Therapy

- Drug therapy
  - Suppression of bladder contractions (anticholinergics)
  - Relaxation of urethral sphincter (α-adrenergic blockers)
  - Suppress pelvic floor spasticity (baclofen [Lioresal])
- Fluid intake of 1800-2000 mL/day
- Urine drainage
  - Voluntary or reflex voiding
  - Intermittent catheterization
  - Indwelling catheter
- Surgery
  - Sphincterotomy
  - Electrical stimulation
  - Urinary diversion

detrusor contractions (hyperreflexic, spastic), or may lack coordination between detrusor contraction and urethral relaxation (dyssynergia). Common problems with a neurogenic bladder include urgency, frequency, incontinence, inability to void, and high bladder pressures that cause reflux of urine into the kidneys.

Neurogenic bladder can be classified according to reflex detrusor activity, intravesical filling pressure, and continence function. Types of neurogenic bladder are outlined in Table 63-9. Diagnostic and collaborative care of neurogenic bladder is described in Table 63-10. Patients with SCI and a neurogenic bladder require a comprehensive program to manage bladder function.

After the patient's overall condition is stable and there is evidence of neurological reflexes, urodynamic testing and a urine culture are performed to aid in determining the type of neurogenic bladder dysfunction experienced. The method used for urinary drainage depends on the type of neurogenic bladder dysfunction, the preference of the patient, and availability of a family member or caregiver, the physician, and the nursing staff. Numerous drainage methods are possible. Surgical options include sphincterectomy, implantation of a functional electrical stimulation device, and urinary diversion.

Many factors are considered when a bladder management strategy is selected: upper extremity function, caregiver burden, and lifestyle choices. The type of bladder dysfunction also defines treatment goals and management options. For a reflexic bladder with detrusor and sphincter dyssynergia, interventions must enable low-pressure storage, low-pressure voiding, and adequate emptying. Anticholinergic drugs (e.g., oxybutynin [Oxytrol], tolterodine [Detrol]) may be used to suppress bladder contraction. α-Adrenergic blockers (e.g., terazosin [Hytrin], doxazosin [Cardura]) may be used to decrease outflow resistance at the bladder neck, and antispasmodic drugs (e.g., baclofen [Lioresal]) may be used to decrease spasticity of pelvic floor muscles.

Drainage options include intermittent catheterization, placement of an external catheter (condom catheter), or placement of an indwelling catheter. A reflexic bladder with detrusor hyperreflexia may be treated with anticholinergic drugs, intravesical capsaicin, or botulinum A toxin. An areflexic bladder is usually managed with intermittent catheterization or an indwelling catheter.

The long-term use of an indwelling catheter should be carefully evaluated because of the associated high incidence of UTI, fistula formation, and diverticula. However, for some patients, this is the best option. Adequate fluid intake and patency of the catheter should be ensured. The frequency of routine catheter changes ranges from 1 week to 1 month, depending on the type of catheter used and institutional policy.

Intermittent catheterization is the most commonly recommended method of bladder management (see Chapter 48). Nursing assessment is important in selecting the time interval between catheterizations. Initially, catheterization is performed every 4 hours. Bladder volume can be assessed with the portable bladder ultrasound machine before catheterization. If less than 200 mL of urine is measured, the time interval may be extended. If 500 mL or more of urine is measured, the time interval is shortened. An overdistended bladder can cause ischemia of the bladder wall, which may predispose tissues to bacterial invasion and infection. Patients often experience diuresis at a regular time during a 24-hour period. The number of intermittent catheterizations per day is usually five or six.

Urinary diversion surgery may be necessary if a patient has repeated UTIs with renal involvement or repeated stones or if therapeutic intervention has been unsuccessful (see Chapter 48). Surgical treatment of neurogenic bladder includes bladder neck revision (sphincterotomy), bladder augmentation (augmentation cystoplasty), penile prosthesis, artificial sphincter, perineal ureterostomy, cystotomy, vesicotomy, and anterior urethral transplantation.

Regardless of which bladder management strategy is selected, the nurse must teach the patient and the family or caregivers about how to accomplish successful self-management. Management techniques, how to obtain necessary supplies, care of supplies and equipment, and when to seek health care must be taught. Resources and referrals for supplies and ongoing care must be arranged.

■ **Neurogenic Bowel.** Careful management of bowel evacuation is necessary in patients with SCIs because voluntary control of this function may be lost. The usual measures for preventing constipation include a high-fibre diet and adequate fluid intake (see Chapter 45, Table 45-9). Patient and caregiver teaching guidelines related to bowel management are presented in Table 63-11. However, these measures by themselves may not be adequate to stimulate evacuation. In addition, suppositories (bisacodyl [Dulcolax] or glycerin) or small-volume enemas and digital stimulation by the nurse or patient may be necessary. In patients with an upper motor neuron lesion, digital stimulation is necessary to relax the external sphincter to promote defecation. A stool softener such as docusate sodium (Colace) can be used to regulate stool consistency. Oral stimulant laxatives should be used only if absolutely necessary for a day or two and not on a regular basis.

Valsalva's manoeuvre and manual stimulation are useful in patients with lower motor neuron lesions. Valsalva's manoeuvre requires intact abdominal muscles, and so it is used in patients with injuries below T12. In general, a bowel movement every other day is considered adequate. However, preinjury patterns should be considered. Incontinence can result from too much stool softener or fecal impaction.

Careful recording of bowel movements, including amount, time, and consistency, is important to overall success. Timing of defecation may also be an important factor. If bowel evacuation is planned for 30 to 60 minutes after the first meal of the day, success may be enhanced by taking advantage of the gastrocolic reflex induced by eating. Again, patient and family education is required to promote successful independent bowel management.

■ **Neurogenic Skin.** Prevention of pressure ulcers and other types of injury to insensitive skin is essential for every patient with SCI. Nurses in rehabilitation are responsible for teaching these skills and providing information about daily skin care. A comprehensive visual and tactile examination of the skin should be performed twice daily, with special attention to areas over bony prominences. The areas most vulnerable to breakdown include the ischia, the trochanters, the heels, and the sacrum. Careful positioning and repositioning should be performed every 2 hours, with gradual increases in the times between turns if no redness over bony prominences is apparent at the time of turning. Pressure-relieving cushions must be used in wheelchairs, and special mattresses may also be needed. Movement during turns

PATIENT & CAREGIVER TEACHING GUIDE

Table 63-11 Bowel Management After Spinal Cord Injury

The following are teaching guidelines for patients with spinal cord injuries:

1. Optimal nutritional intake includes three well-balanced meals each day in accordance with the recommended number of servings from *Eating Well With Canada's Food Guide** (see Chapter 42).

2. Fibre intake should be approximately 20 to 30 g/day. The amount of fibre eaten should be increased gradually over 1 to 2 weeks.

3. Three litres of fluid per day should be consumed, unless contraindicated. Water or fruit juices should be used, and caffeinated beverages such as coffee, tea, and cola should be avoided. Fluid softens hard stools; caffeine stimulates fluid loss through urination.

4. Foods that produce gas (e.g., beans) or upper gastrointestinal upset (spicy foods) should be avoided.

5. *Timing:* A regular schedule for bowel evacuation should be established. A good time is 30 minutes after the first meal of the day.

6. *Position:* If possible, an upright position with feet flat on the floor or on a step stool enhances bowel evacuation. Staying on the toilet, commode, or bedpan for longer than 20 to 30 minutes may cause skin breakdown. Depending on stability, someone may need to stay with the patient.

7. *Activity:* Exercise is important for bowel function. In addition to improving muscle tone, it also increases gastrointestinal transit time and increases appetite. Muscles should be exercised. Exercise includes stretching, range of motion, position changing, and functional movement.

8. *Drug treatment:* Suppositories may be necessary to stimulate a bowel movement. Manual stimulation of the rectum may also be helpful in initiating defecation. Stool softeners and oral laxatives may be used as needed to regulate stool consistency.

*Health Canada. (2011). *Eating Well With Canada's Food Guide.* Retrieved from *http://www.hc-sc.gc.ca/fn-an/alt_formats/hpfb-dgpsa/pdf/food-guide-aliment/view_eatwell_vue_bienmang-eng.pdf*

and transfers should be performed carefully to avoid stretching and folding of soft tissues (shear), friction, or abrasion (Gélis et al., 2009).

Nutritional status should be assessed regularly. Both body weight loss and gain can contribute to skin breakdown. Adequate intake of protein is essential for skin health. Measurement of total protein and albumin can help identify inadequate protein intake. The importance of nutrition to skin health should be stressed to the patient and caregivers.

Protection of the skin also requires avoidance of thermal injury. Burns can be caused by hot food or liquids, bath or shower water that is too warm, radiators, heating pads, and uninsulated plumbing. Thermal injury also can result from extreme cold (frostbite). Injuries may not be noticed until severe damage is done. Anticipatory guidance about potential risks is essential. Patient and caregiver education related to skin care is provided in Table 63-12.

■ **Sexuality.** Knowledge of the level and completeness of injury is needed to understand the male patient's potential for orgasm, erection, and fertility and capacity for sexual satisfaction (Table 63-13). Sexuality is an important issue regardless of the patient's age or sex. To provide accurate and sensitive counselling

Table 63-12 Skin Care for Patients With Spinal Cord Injury

Skin breakdown is a potential problem after spinal cord injury. The following measures are used to decrease this possibility:

Change Position Frequently

- If patient is in a wheelchair, lift self up and shift weight every 15 to 30 minutes.
- If patient is in bed, a regular turning schedule (at least every 2 hours) that includes sides, back, and abdomen is encouraged to change position.
- Use special mattresses and wheelchair cushions.
- Use pillows to protect bony prominences when in bed.

Monitor Skin Condition

- Inspect skin frequently for areas of redness, swelling, and breakdown.
- Keep fingernails trimmed to avoid scratches and abrasions.
- If a wound develops, follow standard wound care management procedures.

Table 63-13 Potential for Sexual Function in Men With Spinal Cord Injury

ERECTION	EJACULATION	ORGASM
Upper Motor Neuron		
Complete		
Frequent (92%), reflexogenic only	Rare (4%)	Rare
Incomplete		
Most frequent (99%); includes reflexogenic (80%) and psychogenic (19%)	Less frequent (32%), after reflexogenic erection (74%), after psychogenic erection (26%)	Present (if ejaculation occurs)
Lower Motor Neuron		
Complete		
Infrequent (26%)	Infrequent (18%)	Present (if ejaculation occurs)
Incomplete		
Psychogenic and reflexogenic	Frequent (70%), after psychogenic and reflexogenic erections	Present (if ejaculation occurs)

and education about sexuality, the nurse must have awareness and an acceptance of personal sexuality, as well as knowledge of human sexual responses. When discussing sexual potential, the nurse should use scientific terminology rather than slang whenever possible.

Reflex sexual function capability is possible if the patient has an upper motor neuron lesion. The presence of tone in the external rectal sphincter indicates an upper motor lesion. The absence of external rectal sphincter tone, bulbocavernosus reflex, or both indicates that the patient has lower motor neuron involvement and may be capable of psychogenic erection but not reflex

erection. If ejaculation occurs, it may be retrograde into the bladder.

The type of lesion determines the physical sexual response. Men with upper motor neuron lesions may have reflexogenic erections that are produced by reflex activity or external stimuli or that occur spontaneously. These spontaneous erections are often short-lived and uncontrolled and cannot be maintained or summoned at the time of coitus. Orgasm and ejaculation are usually not possible for men with a complete upper motor neuron lesion.

Most men with a complete lower motor neuron lesion are unable to have either psychogenic or reflexogenic erections. Men with incomplete lower motor neuron lesions have the highest possibility of successful psychogenic erection with ejaculation, and up to 10% of these patients are fertile.

Treatments for erectile dysfunction include drugs, vacuum devices, and surgical procedures. Sildenafil (Viagra) has become the treatment of choice since several studies documented its effectiveness in men with SCI. Penile injection of vasoactive substances (papaverine, prostaglandin E) is another medical treatment. Risks include *priapism* (prolonged penile erection) and scarring, and so these substances are often considered only after failure of sildenafil. Vacuum suction devices involve the use of negative pressure to encourage blood flow into the penis. Erection is maintained by a constriction band placed at the base of the penis. The main surgical option is implantation of a penile prosthesis. (Erectile dysfunction is discussed in Chapter 57.)

Male fertility is affected by SCI in that sperm quality is poor and ejaculation is dysfunctional. Advances in methods of retrieving sperm (penile vibratory stimulation and electroejaculation), combined with ovulation induction and intrauterine insemination of the female partner, have changed the prognosis for men with SCI to father children from unlikely to a reasonable possibility of successful outcomes.

The effect of SCI on female sexual response is less clear. Lubrication, like erections in men, has reflex and psychogenic components. Women with upper motor neuron injuries may retain the capacity for reflex lubrication, whereas psychogenic lubrication depends on the completeness of injury. Orgasm is reported by about 50% of women with SCI.

Women of childbearing age who have an SCI usually remain fertile. The injury does not affect the ability to become pregnant or to deliver normally through the birth canal. Menses may cease for as long as 6 months after injury. If sexual activity is resumed, protection against an unplanned pregnancy is necessary. A normal pregnancy may be complicated by UTIs, anemia, and autonomic dysreflexia. Because uterine contractions are not felt, a precipitous delivery is always a danger.

Sexual rehabilitation for both men and women should begin informally after the acute phase of the injury has passed. Questions such as "Have you had an erection since your accident?" and "Have your menstrual periods continued since the accident?" are nonthreatening ways to introduce the topic of sexual functioning. The male patient may pose a question such as "Can I ever be a man again?"

Open discussion with the patient is essential. This important aspect of rehabilitation should be handled by someone specially trained in sexual counselling. A nurse or other rehabilitation professional with such expertise works with the patient and partner to provide support with the emphasis on open communication. The nurse's educational role requires respect for every couple's personal standards of religious and cultural beliefs.

Alternative methods of obtaining sexual satisfaction such as oral–genital sex (cunnilingus and fellatio) may be suggested. Explicit video material may also be used, such as a movie demonstrating the sexual activities of a patient with paraplegia with a nondisabled partner. Graphic materials should be used cautiously because they may be too limiting or focus too much on the mechanics of sex rather than on the relationship.

Sexual activities may require more planning and be less spontaneous than before the injury. For example, an attendant may have to undress the patient and remove equipment. A relaxed atmosphere with music and perfume may create an attractive environment. Ample time for caressing, fondling, and kissing is essential. The partners should be encouraged to explore each other's erogenous areas, such as lips, neck, and ears, which can arouse psychogenic erection or orgasm. Few demands should be made initially.

Care should be taken not to dislodge an indwelling catheter during sexual activity. If an external catheter is used, it should be removed before sexual activity, and the patient should refrain from drinking fluids. The bowel program should include evacuation the morning after sexual activity. The partner should be informed that incontinence is always possible. The woman with an SCI may need a water-soluble lubricant to supplement diminished vaginal secretions and facilitate vaginal penetration.

Grief and Depression.

Patients with SCI may feel an overwhelming sense of loss. They may temporarily lose control over everyday life activities and must depend on others for activities of daily living and for life-sustaining measures. Patients may believe that they are useless and burdens to their families. At a stage when independence is often of the greatest importance, they may be totally dependent on others.

The patient's response and recovery differ in some important aspects from those of patients experiencing loss from amputation or terminal illness. First, regression can and does occur at different stages. Working through grief is a difficult, lifelong process for which the patient needs support and encouragement. With advances in rehabilitation, it is usual for the patient to be independent physically and discharged from the rehabilitation centre before completion of the grief process. The goal of recovery is related more to adjustment than to acceptance. Adjustment implies the ability to go on living with certain limitations. Although patients who are cooperative and accepting are easier to treat, the nurse should expect a wide fluctuation of emotions from all patients with SCIs. Depression may not be a component of the recovery process. Societal norms allow depression after severe loss, and persons confronted with death or radical lifestyle changes are almost expected to become depressed. However, not every patient may experience depression.

The nurse's role in grief work is to allow mourning as a component of the rehabilitation process. Table 63-14 summarizes the mourning process and appropriate nursing interventions. Maintaining hope is an important strategy during the grieving process and should not be interpreted as denial (Chevalier, Kennedy, & Sherlock, 2009). During the shock and denial stage, the nurse reassures the patient and stresses the expertise of the entire health care team. During the anger stage, the nurse assists the patient in achieving control over the environment, particularly by allowing the patient's input into the plan of care. The nurse should not respond to anger or manipulation or become involved in a power struggle with the patient. As self-care abilities increase, the patient's independence increases.

Table 63-14 Mourning Process and Nursing Interventions in Spinal Cord Injury	
PATIENT BEHAVIOUR	**NURSING INTERVENTION**
Shock and Denial	
Struggle for survival, complete dependence, excessive sleep, withdrawal, fantasies, unrealistic expectations	• Employ meticulous nursing care. • Provide honest information. • Use simple diagrams to explain injury. • Encourage patient to begin process of recovery. • Establish agreement to use and improve all current abilities while not denying the possibility of future improvement.
Anger	
Refusal to discuss paralysis, decreased self-esteem, manipulation, hostile and abusive language	• Coordinate care with patient and encourage self-care. • Support family members; prevent them from alleviating their guilt by supporting the patient's dependency. • Use humour liberally. • Allow patient outbursts. • Do not allow fixation on injury.
Depression	
Sadness, pessimism, anorexia, nightmares, insomnia, agitation, psychomotor retardation, "blues," suicidal preoccupation, refusal to participate in any self-care activities	• Encourage family involvement and resources. • Plan graded steps in rehabilitation to give success with minimal opportunity for frustration. • Give cheerful and willing assistance with activities of daily living. • Avoid expressing sympathy. • Use firm kindness.
Adjustment	
Planning for future, active participation in therapy, finding of personal meaning in experience and continuation of growth, return to preinjury personality	• Remember that patients have individual personalities. • Balance support systems to encourage independence. • Set goals with the patient's input. • Emphasize potentials.

The patient's caregiver and family also require counselling to avoid promoting dependency in the patient through guilt or misplaced sympathy. The family and caregiver are also experiencing an intense grieving process. A support group of family members and friends of patients with SCIs can help increase family members' knowledge and participation in the grieving process, physical difficulties, the rehabilitation plan, and the meaning of the disability in society (DeSanto-Madeya, 2009).

During the stage of depression, the nurse must be patient and persistent and maintain a sense of humour. Sympathy is not helpful. The patient should be treated in an adult manner and be involved in decision making about care, but the nurse must insist that the care be performed. A primary nurse relationship is helpful. Staff planning and sessions in which staff members can express their feelings are helpful in providing consistency of care. To achieve the stage of adjustment, the patient needs continual support throughout the rehabilitation process in the forms of acceptance, affection, and caring. The nurse must be attentive when the patient needs to talk and sensitive to needs at the various stages of the grief process (Chevalier et al., 2009).

Although the stage of depression during the grief process usually lasts days to weeks, some individuals may become clinically depressed and require treatment for depression. Evaluation by a psychiatric nurse or psychiatrist is recommended. Treatment may include drugs and psychotherapy.

▰ Evaluation

Expected outcomes for patients with SCIs are presented in Nursing Care Plan 63-1 on pp. 1780-1781.

AGE-RELATED CONSIDERATIONS: SPINAL CORD INJURY

The demographics of patients living with SCI are changing. The fact that persons with SCI now have longer lifespans has contributed to the increasing number of older adults living with SCI. Moreover, increasing numbers of older adults sustain SCIs later in life as a result of falls. Aging is also associated with an increased likelihood of other chronic illnesses that may have a serious effect on older adults with SCI. As patients with SCI age, both individual aging changes and duration since injury affect functional ability. For example, bowel and bladder dysfunction can increase with duration and severity of SCI.

Health promotion and screening are important for older patients with SCI. Daily skin inspections, UTI prevention measures, monthly breast examinations for women, and regular prostate cancer screening for men are recommended. Cardiovascular disease is the most common cause of morbidity and mortality among persons with SCIs. The lack of sensation, including that of angina, in patients with high-level injuries may mask acute myocardial ischemia. Altered autonomic nervous system function and decreases in physical activity can increase the risk for cardiovascular problems, including hypertension.

At the same time, because of increased work and recreational activities of older adults, an increasing number of older adults are experiencing SCI. Health promotion to decrease injury risk includes fall prevention strategies (e.g., using a step stool or a grab bar to reach high shelves, handrails on stairs). Rehabilitation for older persons who have SCIs may take longer because of other pre-existing illnesses and poorer health status at the time of the initial injury. Studies show that older persons with SCIs can gain the same degree of neurological recovery as those who are younger at the time of injury, but this does not necessarily translate into meaningful functional outcomes. An interdisciplinary team approach to tailored rehabilitation to match specific needs of older individuals is needed in an effort to maximize their potential for recovery and reintegration into the community (Smith, Purzner, & Fehlings, 2010).

Spinal Cord Tumours

Etiology and Pathophysiology

Spinal cord tumours represent about 5 to 10% of the general population with cancer. About 85% of spinal cord tumours are metastatic in nature; the remainder are primary central nervous system tumours. Metastatic epidural spinal cord compression is a common complication of cancer and occurs in 5 to 14% of patients with cancer (Patchell et al., 2005).

These tumours are classified as primary (arising from some component of the spinal cord, dura, nerves, or vessels) or secondary (from primary growths in breast, thyroid, lung, kidney, prostate and other sites). Spinal cord tumours are further classified as extradural (outside the spinal cord), intradural extramedullary (within the dura but outside the actual spinal cord), and intradural intramedullary (within the spinal cord itself). Intradural intramedullary tumours are usually astrocytomas or ependymomas (Figure 63-10, Table 63-15). Approximately 90% of all spinal tumours are extradural. Extradural tumours are usually metastatic and most often arise in the vertebral bodies. These metastatic lesions can invade intradurally and compress the spinal cord. Spinal intradural extramedullary tumours account for two thirds of all intraspinal neoplasms and consist mainly of meningiomas and schwannomas.

Because many of these tumours are slow growing, their symptoms stem from the mechanical effects of bone destruction, slow compression and irritation of nerve roots, displacement of the cord, or gradual obstruction of the vascular supply. The slow growth does not cause autodestruction (secondary injury), as occurs with traumatic lesions. Therefore, partial to complete functional restoration may be possible when the tumour is removed. Most metastatic tumours are extradural lesions and have metastasized from primary carcinomas such as those of the breast, lung, prostate, and kidney.

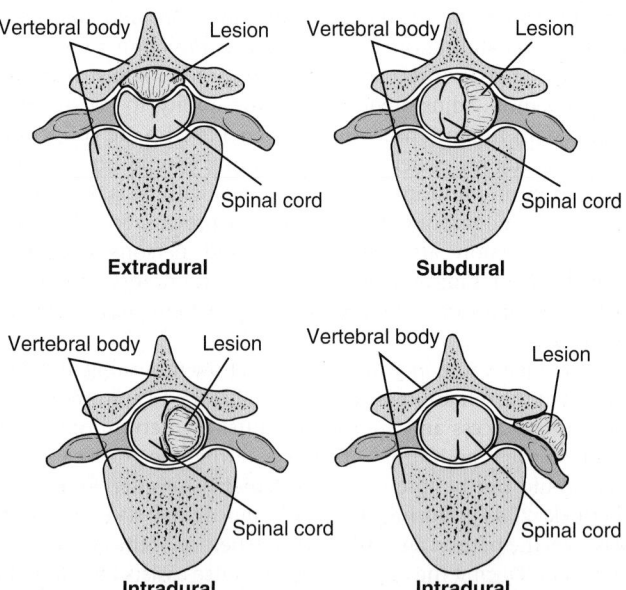

Figure 63-10 Types of spinal cord tumours.

Source: Barker, E. (2008). *Neuroscience nursing: A spectrum of care* (3rd ed., p. 437, Figure 14-1). St. Louis: Mosby.

Table 63-15 Classification of Spinal Cord Tumours			
TYPE	**INCIDENCE**	**TREATMENT**	**PROGNOSIS**
Extradural: from bones of spine, in extradural space, or in paraspinal tissue	20–50% of all intraspinal tumours, mostly malignant metastatic lesions	Relief of cord pressure by surgical laminectomy, radiation, chemotherapy, or combination approach	Dependent on tumour type and stage
Intradural–extramedullary: within dura mater outside spinal cord	Most frequent of intradural tumours (40%), mostly benign meningiomas and neurofibromas	Complete surgical removal of tumour (if possible), partial removal followed by radiation	Usually very good if no damage to cord from compression
Intradural–intramedullary: within spinal cord	Least frequent of intradural tumours (5–10%)	Partial surgical removal, radiation therapy (resulting in only temporary improvement)	Dependent on neurological function before and after decompression

Clinical Manifestations

Both sensory and motor deficits may result; the location and extent of the tumour determine the severity and the distribution of the problem. The most common early symptom of an extradural spinal cord tumour is back pain. Radicular pain may occur as the tumour compresses nerve roots. The location of the pain depends on the level of compression. The pain worsens with activity, coughing, and straining. Some relief may occur with lying down, but there is usually a baseline of pain even in this position secondary to the inflammatory changes within the bone structure. Sensory disruption is manifested by pain, coldness sensation, numbness, and tingling sensation in the dermatomal distribution of the lesion. Motor weakness accompanies the sensory disturbances and consists of slowly increasing clumsiness, weakness, and spasticity, which can lead to paralysis. The sensory and motor disturbances are ipsilateral to the lesion. Bladder dysfunction, if present, is marked by urgency with difficulty in starting the flow and progressing to retention with overflow incontinence (Abrahm, Patchell, & Rades, 2009).

Manifestations of intradural spinal tumours develop as damage to the long spinal tracts progresses, producing paralysis, sensory loss, and bladder dysfunction. Pain can be severe as a result of compression of spinal roots or vertebrae.

NURSING AND COLLABORATIVE MANAGEMENT: SPINAL CORD TUMOURS

Extradural, intradural, and intramedullary tumours are best detected with MRI. CT may be performed to determine amount of bone destruction. More than 85% of primary neoplasms are benign and can be completely resected; 90% of such patients recover without residual problems.

Compression of the spinal cord is an emergency. Relief of the ischemia related to the compression is the goal of therapy. Dexamethasone is usually used to treat edema, often in large doses (100 mg as a bolus dose). Surgical decompression can involve various approaches (anterior, posterior, or combination of both), followed by reconstruction and stabilization. In a randomized control study, Patchell and colleagues (2005) compared direct decompressive therapy followed by radiotherapy with radiotherapy alone; they demonstrated better patient outcomes in regard to neurological recovery, decreased postoperative morbidity, and long-term survival. They concluded that the best treatment for spinal cord compression caused by metastatic cancer is surgery as initial treatment, followed by radiotherapy (Patchell et al., 2005).

Treatment for nearly all spinal cord tumours is surgical removal. The exception is the metastatic tumour that is sensitive to chemotherapy or radiation and that has caused only minimal neurological deficits (e.g., multiple myeloma). In general, extradural and intradural extramedullary tumours can be completely removed surgically. Intradural intramedullary tumours have a less favourable prognosis. However, exploration and removal are usually attempted.

Standard radiation therapy after surgical decompression is considered if the tumour is radiosensitive. Treatment is started approximately 3 to 4 weeks after surgery and usually consists of five doses. In a newer therapy, intensity modulated radiotherapy, higher doses of radiation are delivered to the tumour site, which minimizes injury to surrounding normal spinal and paraspinal tissues. Chemotherapy has also been used in conjunction with radiation therapy for certain tumour types (Abrahm et al., 2009).

Relief of pain and prevention of continued neurological decline are the ultimate goals of treatment. Nurses must be aware of the neurological status of the patient before and after treatment. Ensuring that the patient receives analgesics to manage pain is an important nursing responsibility. Depending on the amount of neurological dysfunction exhibited, the patient may need to be cared for as though he or she were recovering from an SCI. Rehabilitation of patients with spinal cord tumours can increase satisfaction with remaining life and prevent depression and has shown to decrease overall perception of pain (Abrahm et al., 2009).

Postpolio Syndrome

Polio, also known as *poliomyelitis,* is an infectious viral disease transmitted through the oral route by ingestion of contaminated water or food or by contact with infected sources such as unwashed hands. The virus is shed in the feces of infected individuals for as long as 6 weeks. The disease produces a range of manifestations from influenza-like symptoms (abortive poliomyelitis) that resolve in 24 to 36 hours (nonparalytic) to paralytic poliomyelitis that attacks the motor neurons in the anterior horn of the spinal cord, the brainstem, or both. Polio ravaged North American communities during the 1930s, 1940s, and 1950s. Polio was effectively eradicated in North America by the development of the Salk injectable polio vaccine in 1954 and the Sabin oral polio vaccine in 1961. It is still a threat in developing countries because of a lack of effective immunization programs. Polio survivors who recovered from the disease decades ago, notably those who had paralytic poliomyelitis, are now experiencing a recurrence of neuromuscular symptoms as they age. These late effects of polio are collectively referred to as **postpolio syndrome (PPS)**. On the basis of criteria for diagnosis of PPS, the incidence and prevalence can range from 10 to 40% (Gilhus, 2009).

Etiology and Pathophysiology

The etiology of PPS is not completely clear. The most commonly accepted theory is that enlarged distal motor neurons that had recovered after polio degenerate and subsequently begin to fail (Gilhus, 2009). It appears that cellular damage caused by the effects of the polio virus may lead to exhaustion and premature failure of the motor neurons. The result is slowly progressive muscle weakness and fatigue. Factors thought to contribute to PPS include age-related motor neuron loss, musculoskeletal overuse and disuse, weight gain, pain, and other neuromuscular or systemic illnesses. There is no evidence to support the theory that PPS is caused by reactivation of the original polio virus.

Clinical Manifestations and Diagnostic Studies

PPS is manifested by a new onset of joint and muscle weakness, easy fatigability, generalized fatigue, and pain. In uncommon cases, individuals may also exhibit speech, swallowing, and respiratory difficulties. Patients should undergo thorough diagnostic testing to rule out other medical conditions that may produce similar symptoms. Criteria used to establish the diagnosis of PPS include a history of polio in the abortive, nonparalytic, or paralytic forms; recovery from polio; a lengthy period of stability of at least 10 to 20 years' duration; and clinical manifestations of PPS that are not associated with other medical disorders. Disabilities caused by PPS can have a significant effect on the patient's quality of life.

NURSING AND COLLABORATIVE MANAGEMENT: POSTPOLIO SYNDROME

Management approaches for PPS are targeted at controlling symptoms, particularly fatigue, weakness, and pain. An interdisciplinary team approach is essential for management of the patient. The cornerstone of management is lifestyle modification to conserve energy and support performance of activities of daily living.

During the polio epidemic, polio victims were subjected to rigorous therapy to regain muscle function. A particular challenge may be helping the patient understand that aggressive or strenuous therapy to strengthen muscles is now considered counterproductive and that overexertion can worsen fatigue and weakness. It is important to promote pacing of activities to prevent feelings of fatigue. Planning to include rest periods, as well as using assistive devices such as scooters, canes, and wheelchairs, may be beneficial. Adaptive equipment can be helpful to patients who experience difficulty with self-care. Other strategies include arranging for a handicapped licence plate or sticker to facilitate parking close to shops and public buildings, shopping on the Internet to avoid walking, and enlisting the support of family and friends to perform necessary tasks. Physiotherapy can support mobility and fitness in view of the patient's limitations. Weight loss interventions should be considered for affected individuals who are overweight.

Effective pain management through both pharmacological and nonpharmacological approaches with the health care provider or pain management team can enable an individual to remain active and achieve a greater sense of well-being. Nonpharmacological measures include massage, relaxation strategies, and guided imagery (see Chapter 12). Protection from the cold can also aid in pain relief; the individual with PPS may be especially sensitive to a cold environment. For affected individuals with speech, swallowing, or respiratory difficulties, it is important to take measures to prevent aspiration, maintain airway patency, and promote optimal nutrition. Nursing interventions for these problems are similar to those described for patients with GBS and SCI. Experiencing the re-emergence of symptoms related to polio can have a devastating effect on the patient's psychosocial well-being.

Memories of paralysis and the challenges of recovery can cause fear when PPS is diagnosed. Anxiety and depression can occur, as can difficulties with coping. The nurse can assist the individual by actively listening to concerns, providing information about PPS and available resources, and referring the patient to support groups or counselling when necessary. Gaining a sense of control through active participation in lifestyle modifications and therapy may improve the patient's ability to cope with PPS.

CLINICAL DECISION-MAKING EXERCISE

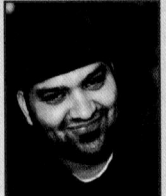

CASE STUDY:
Spinal Cord Injury

Source: © iStockphoto.com/Kevin Russ.

Patient Profile: Acute Phase

Samuel DiMarco, a 24-year-old man, is admitted to the emergency department with the diagnosis of a cervical SCI. Mr. DiMarco was swimming at a neighbour's backyard pool. He dove into the shallow end, striking his head on the bottom of the pool. His friends noticed that he did not resurface. They rescued him and brought him to the side of the pool. They maintained neck immobilization until the rescue crews arrived.

Subjective Data
- Is awake and alert
- Has complaints of neck pain
- Is anxious and asking why he cannot move his legs
- Is asking to see his family

Objective Data
Physical Examination
- Weak biceps movement bilaterally
- No triceps movement bilaterally
- Gross elbow movement present bilaterally

- No movement bilaterally in lower extremities
- Decreased sensation from the shoulders down
- No bladder or bowel control
- BP: 85/50 mm Hg; pulse: 56; respirations: 32 and laboured

Diagnostic Studies
- CT of cervical spine shows subluxation and compression fracture
- MRI of cervical spine shows a severe spinal cord compression at C5-6

Collaborative Care
- Intubated in the emergency department
- Started on mechanical ventilation
- Placed in halo traction on arrival in the CCU

Discussion Questions: Acute Phase

1. *Priority Decision:* What nursing activities would be a priority on Mr. DiMarco's arrival in the CCU?
2. What physiological problems are causing Mr. DiMarco to have hypotension and bradycardia?
3. What would the first line of treatment be for Mr. DiMarco's hypotension and bradycardia?
4. What signs and symptoms would indicate respiratory distress, and what physiological problem would cause respiratory distress in Mr. DiMarco's injury state?
5. What can the nurse do to decrease Mr. DiMarco's anxiety?
6. *Priority Decision:* Based on the assessment data provided, what are the priority nursing diagnoses or problem statements? Are there any collaborative problems?

Patient Profile: Rehabilitation Phase
One month after the injury, Mr. DiMarco is currently at a local inpatient SCI rehabilitation facility. He has since been extubated and uses a wheelchair to mobilize. He eats three meals a day with assistance and is on a strict bowel and bladder program.

Subjective Data
- Awake and alert but anxious
- Complaining of severe headache, blurred vision, and nausea

Objective Data
Physical Examination
- Flushed and diaphoretic above the level of injury
- No bowel movement for 2 days
- BP: 235/107 mm Hg; pulse: 32 beats/min; respirations: 30 breaths/min and laboured

Discussion Questions: Rehabilitation Phase

1. *Priority Decision:* What initial priority nursing interventions would be appropriate?
2. What physiological problem is causing Mr. DiMarco's hypertension and bradycardia?
3. Once the physician has been notified, what other interventions would be appropriate?
4. *Priority Decision:* On the basis of the assessment data provided, what are the priority nursing diagnoses?

evolve *Answers are available at* **http://evolve.elsevier.com/ Canada/Lewis/medsurg**

REVIEW QUESTIONS

The number of the question corresponds to the same-numbered objective at the beginning of the chapter.

1. What should the nurse do during assessment of a patient with trigeminal neuralgia?
   a. Inspect all aspects of the mouth and teeth.
   b. Lightly palpate the affected side of the face for edema.
   c. Test for temperature and sensation perception on the face.
   d. Ask the patient to describe factors that initiate an episode.
2. During routine assessment of a patient with GBS, the nurse finds the patient to be short of breath. What is the cause of the patient's respiratory distress?
   a. Elevated protein levels in the CSF
   b. Immobility resulting from ascending paralysis
   c. Degeneration of motor neurons in the brainstem and the spinal cord
   d. Paralysis ascending to the nerves that stimulate the thoracic area
3. A patient is admitted to the CCU with a C7 SCI, and Brown-Séquard syndrome is diagnosed. What would the nurse probably find on physical examination?
   a. Upper extremity weakness only
   b. Complete motor and sensory loss below C7
   c. Loss of position sense and vibration in both lower extremities
   d. Ipsilateral motor loss and contralateral sensory loss below C7

4. A patient is admitted to the hospital with SCI after an automobile accident. The nurse recognizes that the pathophysiology of secondary SCI involves which of the following?
   a. Initial infarction of the white matter of the spinal cord
   b. Mechanical transection of the cord by the trauma
   c. Necrotic destruction of the cord from hemorrhage and edema
   d. Release of epinephrine leading to massive vasodilation of spinal cord vessels
5. Which of the following would be one of the rehabilitation goals for the patient with an injury at the C5 level?
   a. Feeding self with hand devices
   b. Driving a motorized wheelchair
   c. Assisting with transfer activities
   d. Controlling bowel and bladder functions
6. A patient with a C7 SCI undergoing rehabilitation tells the nurse he must have the flu because he has a bad headache and nausea. What should the nurse's initial action be?
   a. Call the physician.
   b. Check the patient's temperature.
   c. Take the patient's blood pressure.
   d. Elevate the head of the bed to 90 degrees.

7. For a 65-year-old female patient who has lived with a T1 SCI for 20 years, what health teaching information would the nurse emphasize?
   a. A mammogram is needed every 2 years.
   b. Bladder function tends to improve with age.
   c. Heart disease is not common in persons with SCI.
   d. As a person ages, the need to change body position is less important.

8. What is the most common early symptom of a spinal cord tumour?
   a. Urinary incontinence
   b. Back pain that worsens with activity
   c. Paralysis below the level of involvement
   d. Impaired sensation of pain, temperature, and light touch

9. Which of the following descriptions best characterizes PPS?
   a. Autoimmune disease of motor neurons triggered by polio virus
   b. Reactivation of poliomyelitis resulting in acute musculo-skeletal disease
   c. Degeneration of enlarged motor neurons many years after poliomyelitis
   d. Disorder characterized by active viral destruction of the upper motor neurons

ANSWERS: 1. d; 2. d; 3. d; 4. c; 5. b; 6. c; 7. a; 8. b; 9. c.

REFERENCES

Abrahm, J. L., Patchell, R. A., & Rades, D. (2009). Personalized treatment for malignant spinal cord compression: A multidisciplinary approach. In *ASCO's 2009 Educational Book, Patient and Survivor Care* (pp. 555-562). Alexandria, VA: American Society of Clinical Oncology. Retrieved from *http://www.asco.org/ASCOv2/Home/Education%20&%20Training/Educational%20Book/PDF%20Files/2009/09EdBk.PatientCare.04.pdf*

Ahn, H., Singh, J., Nathens, A., MacDonald, R. D., Travers, A., Tallon, J., …, Yee, A. (2011). Pre-hospital care management of a potential spinal cord injured patient: A systematic review of the literature and evidence-based guidelines. *Journal of Neurotrauma, 28*, 1341-1361. doi:10.1089/neu.2009.1168

American Spinal Injury Association–International Medical Society of Paraplegia. (2004). *International standards for neurological functional classification of spinal cord injury patients (revised)*. Chicago: American Spinal Injury Association.

Bennetto, L., Patel, J. K., & Fuller, G. (2007). Trigeminal neuralgia and its management. *BMJ, 334*, 201-205. doi:10.1136/bmj.39085.614792

Bowyer, H. R., & Glover, R. (2010). Guillain-Barré syndrome: Management and treatment options for patients with moderate to severe progression. *Journal of Neuroscience Nursing, 42*, 288-293. doi:10.1097/JNN.0b013e3181ecafa9

Bozzo, A., Marcoux, J., Radhakrishna, M., Pelletier, J., & Goulet, B. (2011). The role of magnetic resonance imaging in the management of acute spinal cord injury. *Journal of Neurotrauma, 28*, 1401-1411. doi:10.1089/neu.2009.1236

Bracken, M. B., Shepard, M. J., Hellenbrand, K. G., Collins, W.F., Leo, L. S., Freeman, D.F., …, Rifkinson, N. (1985). Methylprednisolone and neurological function 1 year after spinal cord injury: Results of the National Acute Spinal Cord Injury Study. *Journal of Neurosurgery, 63*(5), 704-713.

Bracken, M. B., Shepard, M. J., Holford, T. R., Leo-Summers, M. P. H., Aldrich, E. F., Fazl, M., …, Young, W. (1997). Administration of methylprednisolone for 24 or 48 hours or tirilazad mesylate for 48 hours in the treatment of acute spinal cord injury. Results of the Third National Acute Spinal Cord Injury Randomized Controlled Trial. National Acute Spinal Cord Injury Study, *Journal of American Medical Association, 277*(20), 1597-1604.

Canadian Institute for Health Information. (2006). *Life after traumatic spinal cord injury: From inpatient rehabilitation back to the community*. Retrieved from *https://secure.cihi.ca/free_products/life_after_spinal_cord_injury_e.pdf*

Casha, S., & Christie, S. (2011). A systematic review of intensive cardiopulmonary management after spinal cord injury. *Journal of Neurotrauma, 28*, 1479-1495. doi:10.1089/neu.2009.1156

Chevalier, Z., Kennedy, P., & Sherlock, O. (2009). Spinal cord injury, coping and psychological adjustment: a literature review. *Spinal Cord, 47*, 778-782. doi:10.1038/sc.2009.60

Christie, S., Thibault-Halman, G., & Casha, S. (2011). Acute pharmacological DVT prophylaxis after spinal cord injury. *Journal of Neurotrauma, 28*, 1509-1514. doi:10.1089/neu.2009.1155-A

Dawodu, S. T. (2011). Spinal cord injury—Definition, epidemiology, pathophysiology. Retrieved from *http://emedicine.medscape.com/article/322480-overview*

DeSanto-Madeya, S. (2009). Adaptation to spinal cord injury for families post-injury. *Nursing Science Quarterly, 22*(1), 57-66. doi:10.1177/0894318408327295

Farry, A., & Baxter, D. (2010). *The incidence and prevalence of spinal cord injury in Canada. Overview and estimates based on current evidence*. Richmond, BC: Rick Hansen Institute and Urban Futures Institute. Retrieved from *http://fecst.inesss.qc.ca/fileadmin/documents/photos/Lincidenceetlaprevalencedestraumamedullaireau Canada.pdf*

Furlan, J. C., Noonan, V., Cadotte, D. W., & Fehlings, M. G. (2011). Timing of decompressive surgery of spinal cord after traumatic spinal cord injury: An evidence-based examination of pre-clinical and clinical studies. *Journal of Neurotrauma, 28*, 1371-1399. doi:10.1089/neu.2009.1147

Gélis, A., Dupeyron, A., Legros, P., Benaïm, J., Pelissier, J., & Fattal, C. (2009). Pressure ulcer risk factors in persons with SCI: Acute and rehabilitation stages. *Spinal Cord, 47*(2), 99-107. doi:10.1038/sc.2008.107

Gilhus, N. E. (2009). Post-polio syndrome. In R. P. Lisak, D. D. Truong, W. M. Carroll, & R. Bhidayasiri (Eds.), *International neurology: A clinical approach* (Chapter 12, pp. 212-214. Hoboken, NJ: Wiley-Blackwell.

Haltiwanger, E., Huber, T., Chang, J. C., & Gonzales-Stuart, A. (2009). Case study of Bell's palsy applying complementary treatment within an occupational therapy model. *Occupational Therapy International, 16*(1), 71-81. doi:10.1002/oti.267

Hughes, R., & van Doorn, P. A. (2012). Corticosteroids for Guillain-Barré syndrome. *Cochrane Database of Systematic Reviews*, (8), CD001446. doi:10.1002/14651858.CD001446.pub4

Krassioukov, A., Warburton, D. E., Teasell, R., & Eng, J. J. (2009). A systematic review of the management of autonomic dysreflexia after spinal cord injury. *Archives of Physical Medicine and Rehabilitation, 90*, 682-695. doi:10.1016/j.apmr.2008.10.017

Lockhart, P., Holland, N. J., Swan, I., & Teixeira, L. J. (2011). Interventions for Bell's palsy (idiopathic facial paralysis). *Cochrane Database of Systematic Reviews*, (2), CD008974. doi:10.1002/14651858.CD008974

Marra, C. M. (2010). Update on neurosyphilis. *Current Infectious Disease Reports, 11*, 127-134.

McGrogan, A., Madle, G. C., Seaman, H. E., & de Vries, C. S. (2009). The epidemiology of Guillain-Barré syndrome worldwide. *Neuroepidemiology, 32*(2), 150-163. doi:10.1159/000184748

McKinley, W. (2011). Cardiovascular concerns in spinal cord injury. Retrieved from *http://emedicine.medscape.com/article/321771-overview#aw2aab6b3*

Parkins, M. D., McNeil, S. A., & Laupland, K. B. (2009). Routine immunization of adults in Canada: Review of the epidemiology of vaccine-preventable diseases and current recommendations for primary prevention. *Canadian Journal of Infectious Diseases & Medical Microbiology, 20*(3), e81-e90

Patchell, R. A., Tibbs, P. A., Regine, W. F., Payne, R., Saris, S., Kryscio, R. J., …, Young, B. (2005). Direct decompressive surgical resection in the treatment of spinal cord compression caused by metastatic cancer: A randomised trial. *Lancet, 366,* 643-648. doi:10.1016/S0140-6736(05)66954-1

Rick Hansen Institute. (2012). *The high cost of health care in Canada. Case in point: Spinal cord injury.* Retrieved from *http://rickhanseninstitute.org/en/publications*

Rowland, J. W., Hawryluk, G. W. J., Kwon, B., & Fehlings, M. G. (2008). Current status of acute spinal cord injury pathophysiology and emerging therapies: Promise on the horizon. *Neurosurgical Focus, 25*(5), E2. doi:10.3171/FOC.2008.25.11.E2

Sarro, A., Anthony, T., Magtoto, R., & Mauceri, J. (2010). Developing a standard of care for halo vest and pin site care including patient and family education: A collaborative approach among three Greater Toronto Area teaching hospitals. *Journal of Neuroscience Nursing, 42,* 169-175. doi:10.1097/JNN.0b013e3181d4a3be

Schilero, G. J., Spungen, A. M., Bauman, W. A., Radulovic, M., & Lesser, M. (2009). Pulmonary function and spinal cord injury. *Respiratory Physiology & Neurobiology, 166,* 129-141. doi:10.1016/j.resp.2009.04.002

Smith, S. R., Purzner, T., & Fehlings, M. G. (2010). The epidemiology of geriatric spinal cord injury. *Topics in spinal cord injury rehabilitation, 15*(3), 54-64. doi:10.1310/sci1503-54

Taillac, P. P., & Kim, J. (2010). *CBRNE—Botulism.* Retrieved from *http://emedicine.medscape.com/article/829125-overview#a0104*

Teasell, R., Hsieh, J. T. C., Aubut, J., Eng, J. J., Krassioukov, A., & Tu, L. (2008). Venous thromboembolism following spinal cord injury. In J. J. Eng, R. W. Teasell, D. L. Wolfe, & L. Tu (Eds.), *Spinal cord injury rehabilitation evidence* (20th ed., pp. 15.1-15.27). Vancouver: University of British Columbia.

Thibault-Halman, G., Casha, S., Singer, S., & Christie, S. (2011). Acute management of nutritional demands after spinal cord injury. *Journal of Neurotrauma, 28,* 1497-1507. doi:10.1089/neu.2009.1155

Trigeminal Neuralgia Association of Canada. (2010). *About trigeminal neuralgia.* Retrieved from *http://www.tnac.org/abouttn.htm*

Tsao, Y. T., Chen, W. L., & Tsai, W. C. (2009). Steroids for acute spinal cord injury: Revealing silent pathology, *Lancet, 374*(9688), 500. doi:10.1016/S0140-6736(09)60939-9

Zakrzewska, J. M., & McMillan, R. (2011). Trigeminal neuralgia: The diagnosis and management of this excruciating and poorly understood facial pain. *Postgraduate Medical Journal, 87,* 410-416. doi:10.1136/pgmj.2009.080473

CANADIAN RESOURCES

Canadian Association of Neuroscience Nurses (CANN)
http://www.cann.ca
Canadian Paraplegic Association of Alberta
http://www.cpa-ab.org/
Canadian Paraplegic Association of Manitoba
http://www.cpamanitoba.ca/
Canadian Paraplegic Association of Ontario
http://halton.cioc.ca/record/OAK0051
Canadian Paraplegic Association of PEI
http://www.cpapei.org/
Canadian Spinal Research Organization (CSRO)
http://www.csro.com
Canadian Spine Society
http://www.spinecanada.ca/
Rick Hansen Institute *http://www.rickhanseninstitute.org/*
http://parachutecanada.org)
SCI Action Canada
http://www.sciactioncanada.ca/
Spinal Cord Injury Canada
https://www.spinalcordinjurycanada.ca/
Think First Canada (amalgamated with three other Canadian injury prevention groups under the name "Parachute")
http://www.thinkfirst.ca
Trigeminal Neuralgia Association of Canada
http://www.tnac.org

RELATED RESOURCES

Academy of Spinal Cord Injury Nurses
http://www.academyscipro.org/Public/NursesMain.aspx
Christopher and Dana Reeve Foundation
http://www.crpf.org/
Guillain-Barré Syndrome–Chronic Inflammatory Demyelinating Polyneuropathy Foundation International
http://gbs-cidp.org/
National Institute of Neurological Disorders and Stroke (NINDS)
http://www.ninds.nih.gov
National Rehabilitation Information Center (NARIC)
http://www.naric.com

ⓔvolve *For additional Internet resources, see the Web site for this book at* **http://evolve.elsevier.com/Canada/Lewis/medsurg**

Nursing Assessment: Musculoskeletal System

Written by Dottie Roberts
Adapted by Joyce Mammel

LEARNING OBJECTIVES

1. Describe the gross anatomical and microscopic composition of bone.
2. Explain the classification system of joints and movements at synovial joints.
3. Describe the types and structure of muscle tissue.
4. Describe the functions of cartilage, muscles, ligaments, tendons, fascia, and bursae.
5. Describe age-related changes in the musculoskeletal system and differences in assessment findings.
6. Identify the significant subjective and objective data related to the musculoskeletal system that should be obtained from a patient.
7. Describe the appropriate techniques used in the physical assessment of the musculoskeletal system.
8. Differentiate normal from abnormal findings of a physical assessment of the musculoskeletal system.
9. Describe the purpose, significance of results, and nursing responsibilities related to diagnostic studies of the musculoskeletal system.

KEY TERMS

ankylosis Stiffness or fixation of a joint, usually resulting from destruction of articular cartilage and subchondral bone with subsequent scarring; Table 64-6, p. 1805

arthrocentesis Incision or puncture of joint capsule to obtain samples of synovial fluid from within joint cavity or to remove excess fluid, p. 1809

arthroscopy Insertion of an arthroscope into a joint to directly examine or to operate on the interior of the joint cavity; Table 64-7, p. 1807 and p. 1809

atrophy Wasting of muscle, characterized by decreased circumference and flabby appearance, leading to decreased function and tone; Table 64-6, p. 1805

contracture An abnormal, usually permanent condition of a muscle or joint, characterized by flexion and fixation; Table 64-6, p. 1805

crepitation Crackling sound or grating sensation as a result of friction between bones, broken bone, or cartilage bits in joint; Table 64-6, p. 1805

isometric contractions Muscular contractions that increase tension but do not produce movement, p. 1800

isotonic contractions Muscular contraction with shortening that produces movement, p. 1800

kyphosis Forward bending of thoracic spine: exaggerated thoracic curvature; Table 64-6, p. 1805

lordosis Lumbar spinal deformity resulting in exaggerated lumbar curvature; Table 64-6, p. 1805

scoliosis A lateral S-shaped curvature of the thoracic and lumbar spine; p. 1804 and Table 64-6, p. 1805

ELECTRONIC RESOURCES

Supplemental content related to Chapter 64 can be found ...

Evolve Web Site ⊖volve

http://evolve.elsevier.com/Canada/Lewis/medsurg
- Animations:
  - Classification of Joints: Condyloid Joint
  - Classification of Joints: Gliding Joint—Hand
  - Classification of Joints: Hinge Joint
- Assessment Case Study
- Clinical Reference: Laboratory Values
- Content Updates
- Electronic Calculators
- Examination Review Questions
- Glossary
- Key Points (Printable and MP3 Download)

- Physical Examination Video Clips:
  - Neck
  - Upper Extremities
  - Back and Posterior Chest
  - Anterior Chest, Lungs, and Heart
  - Abdominal Reflexes, Abdominal Muscles, and Inguinal Area
  - Feet, Legs, and Hips
  - Musculoskeletal Function
  - Spine
- Video Clips:
  - Inspection: Gait in Older Adult
  - Inspection: General Muscular Strength
  - Inspection and Palpation: Muscular Development

The unique structures of the musculoskeletal system allow human beings to complete complex movements in their interactions with the environment. The dexterity of the upper extremities enables an individual to perform complicated technical tasks, whereas stronger lower extremities allow mobility for varied activities. The musculoskeletal system is composed of voluntary muscle and five types of connective tissue: bones, cartilage, ligaments, tendons, and fascia (Roberts, 2009). Resilient bone and cartilage absorb energy from any impact, minimizing the risk of injury to other body structures. However, this characteristic ability makes the musculoskeletal system itself particularly vulnerable to injury from external forces. Any damage to bone and related soft tissues can cause functional disruption for an individual. Deformity, alteration in body image, alteration in mobility, pain, or permanent disability may result from musculoskeletal injury.

Structures and Functions of the Musculoskeletal System

Bone

Function. The main functions of bone are support, protection of internal organs, voluntary movement, blood cell production, and mineral storage (Altizer, 2007). Bones provide the supporting framework that keeps the body from collapsing and allow the body to bear weight. Bones also protect underlying vital organs and tissues. For example, the skull encloses the brain, the vertebrae surround the spinal cord, and the rib cage contains the lungs and heart. Bones serve as a point of attachment for muscles, which are connected to bones by tendons. Bones act as a lever for muscles, and movement occurs as a result of muscle contractions applied to these levers. Bones contain hematopoietic tissue for the production of red and white blood cells. Bones also serve as a site for storage of inorganic minerals such as calcium and phosphorus.

Bone was previously considered to be a static, inert substance. In reality, it is a dynamic tissue that continually changes form and composition. It contains both organic material (collagen) and inorganic material (calcium, phosphate). The internal and external growth and remodelling of bone are ongoing processes. Bone is classified according to structure as *cortical* (compact and dense) or *cancellous* (spongy).

Microscopic Structure. Cylinder-shaped structural units called *osteons* (haversian systems) fit closely together in compact bone, creating a dense bone structure (Figure 64-1, *B*). Within the systems, the haversian canals run parallel to the bone's long axis and contain the blood vessels that travel to the bone's interior from the periosteum. Surrounding the haversian canals are concentric rings known as *lamellae,* which characterize mature bone. Smaller canals *(canaliculi)* extend from the haversian canals to the *lacunae,* where mature bone cells are embedded. Cancellous (spongy) bone lacks the organized structure of cortical (compact) bone. The lamellae are not arranged in concentric rings but rather along the lines of maximum stress placed on the bone. Networks of bone tissue are filled with red or yellow marrow, and blood reaches the bone cells by passing through spaces in the marrow.

The three types of bone cells are osteoblasts, osteocytes, and osteoclasts. *Osteoblasts* synthesize organic bone matrix (collagen) and are the basic bone-forming cells. *Osteocytes* are the mature bone cells. *Osteoclasts* participate in bone remodelling by assisting in the breakdown of bone tissue. *Bone remodelling* is the removal of old bone by osteoclasts *(resorption)* and the deposition of new bone by osteoblasts *(ossification).* The inner layer of bone is primarily made up of osteoblasts with a few osteoclasts.

Gross Structure. The anatomical structure of bone is best represented by a typical long bone such as the humerus (see Figure 64-1, *A*). Each long bone consists of the epiphysis, the diaphysis, and the metaphysis. The *epiphysis,* the widened area found at each end of a long bone, is composed primarily of cancellous bone. The wide epiphysis allows for greater weight

Humerus

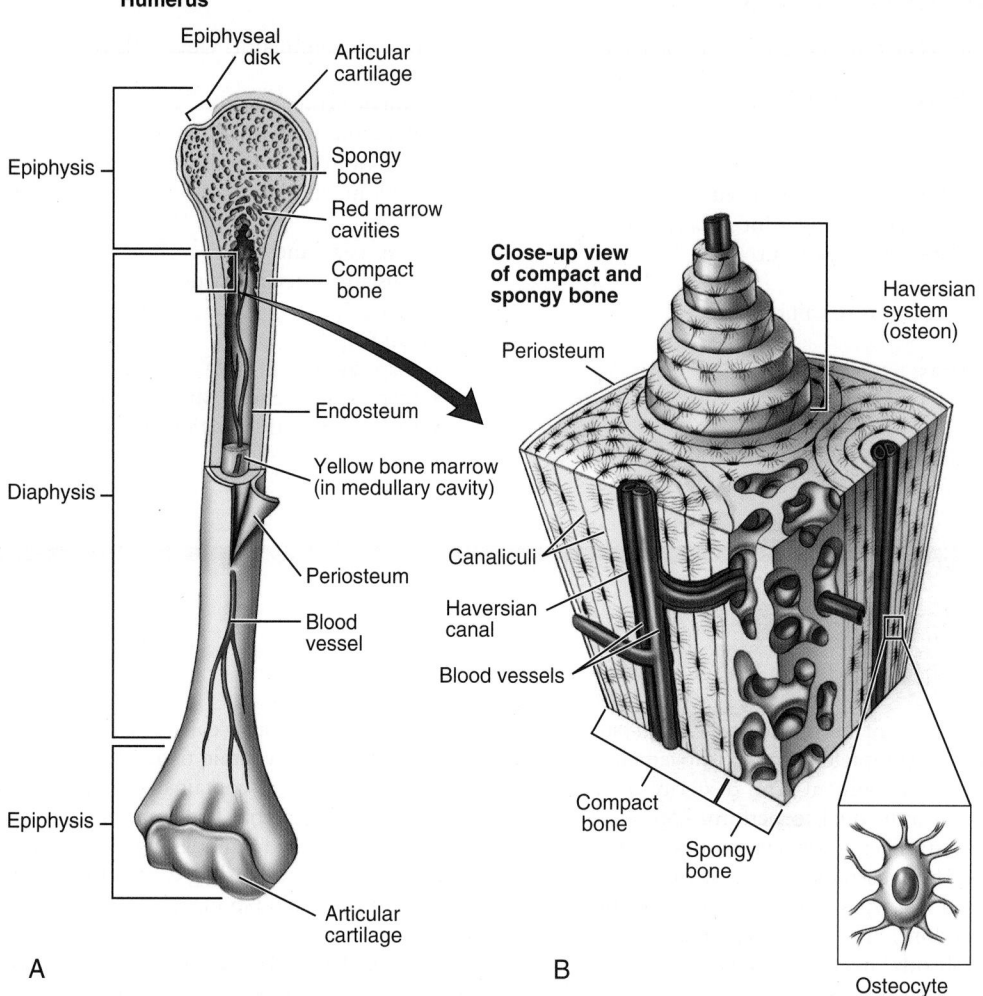

Figure 64-1 Bone structure. **A,** Anatomy of a long bone (humerus) shows cancellous and compact bone. **B,** Cortical (compact) bone shows numerous structural units called *osteons*.

Source: Adapted from Herlihy, B. (2011). *The human body in health and illness* (4th ed., p. 113, Figure 8-3). St. Louis: Elsevier Saunders.

distribution and provides stability for the joint. The epiphysis is also the location of muscle attachment. Articular cartilage covers the ends of the epiphysis to provide a smooth surface for joint movement. The *diaphysis* is the main shaft of the bone. It provides structural support and is composed of compact bone. The tubular structure of the diaphysis allows it to more easily withstand bending and twisting forces. The *metaphysis* is the flared area between the epiphysis and the diaphysis. Like the epiphysis, it is composed of cancellous bone. The *epiphyseal plate,* or growth zone, is the cartilaginous area between the epiphysis and the metaphysis. It actively produces bone to allow longitudinal growth in children. Injury to the epiphyseal plate in a growing child can lead to development of a shorter extremity, which can cause significant functional problems. At age 18 to 25 years, the metaphysis and the epiphysis become joined as this plate hardens to mature bone.

The *periosteum* is composed of fibrous connective tissue that covers the bone. Tiny blood vessels penetrate the periosteum to provide nutrition to underlying bone. Musculotendinous fibres anchor to the outer layer of the periosteum. The inner layer of the periosteum is attached to the bone by bundles of collagen.

No periosteum exists on the articular surfaces of long bones. These bone ends are covered by articular cartilage.

The *medullary* (marrow) cavity is in the centre of the diaphysis and contains either red or yellow bone marrow (Thibodeau & Patton, 2012). In the growing child, *hematopoiesis* (blood cell production) occurs exclusively in red bone marrow. Hematopoiesis in the adult also normally occurs primarily in the red bone marrow of the skull, ribs, sternum, pelvis, vertebrae, and shoulders. However, the medullary cavity of long bones in adults also contains yellow bone marrow, which is mainly adipose tissue. Yellow marrow will be involved in hematopoiesis only in times of great blood cell need.

Types. The skeleton consists of 206 bones, which are classified according to shape as long, short, flat, or irregular.

Long bones are characterized by a central shaft (diaphysis) and two widened ends (epiphyses) (see Figure 64-1, *A*). Examples include the femur, humerus, and radius. *Short bones* are composed of cancellous bone covered by a thin layer of compact bone. Examples include the carpals in the hand and the tarsals in the foot.

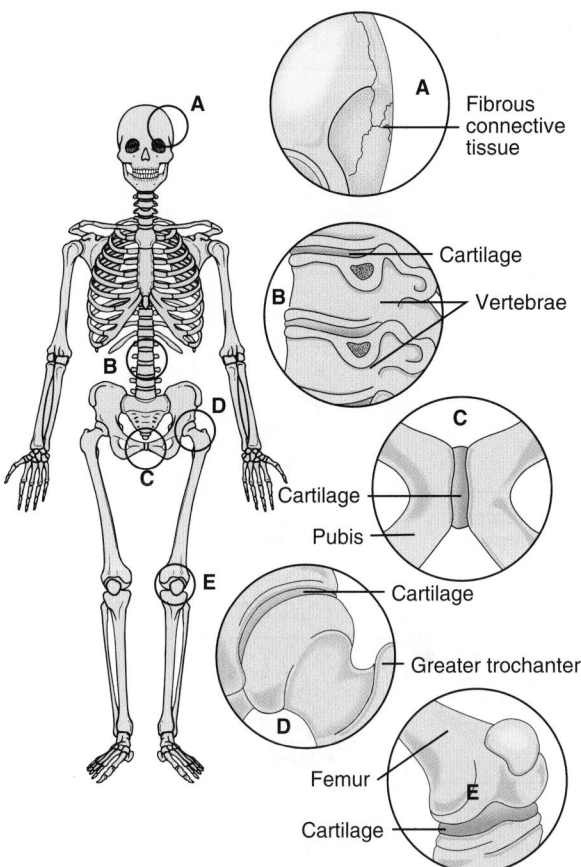

Figure 64-2 Classification of joints. **A** to **C,** Synarthrodial (immovable) and amphiarthrodial (slightly movable) joints. **D** and **E,** Diarthrodial (freely movable) joints.

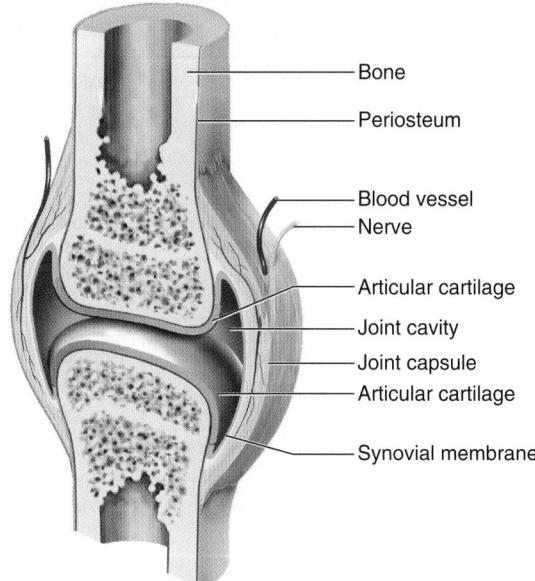

Figure 64-3 Structure of a synovial joint.

Source: Patton, K. T., & Thibodeau, G. A. (2010). *Anatomy and physiology* (7th ed., p. 266, Figure 9-3, *A*). St Louis: Mosby.

Flat bones have two layers of compact bone separated by a layer of cancellous bone. Examples include the ribs, skull, scapula, and sternum. The spaces in the cancellous bone contain bone marrow. *Irregular bones* appear in a variety of shapes and sizes. Examples include the vertebrae, sacrum, and mandible.

Joints

A *joint* (articulation) is a place where the ends of two bones are in proximity and move in relation to each other. Joints are classified according to the degree of movement that they allow (Figure 64-2).

The most common joint is the freely movable *diarthrodial* (synovial) type. Each joint is enclosed in a capsule of fibrous connective tissue that joins the two bones together to form a cavity (Figure 64-3). The capsule is lined by a synovial membrane, which secretes a thick synovial fluid to lubricate the joint and reduce friction. The end of each bone is covered with articular (hyaline) cartilage. Supporting structures (i.e., ligaments, tendons) reinforce the joint capsule and provide limits to joint movement (National Association of Orthopaedic Nurses [NAON], 2007). Types of diarthrodial joints are shown in Figure 64-4.

Cartilage

Cartilage is a rigid connective tissue that serves as a support for soft tissue and provides the articular surface for joint movement.

It protects underlying tissues. The cartilage in the epiphyseal plate is also involved in the growth of long bones before physical maturity is reached. Because articular cartilage is relatively avascular, it must receive nourishment by the diffusion of material from the synovial fluid. The lack of a direct blood supply contributes to the slow metabolism of cartilage cells and explains why cartilage tissue heals slowly.

The three types of cartilage tissue are hyaline, elastic, and fibrous. *Hyaline cartilage*, the most common, contains a moderate amount of collagen fibres. It is found in the trachea, bronchi, nose, epiphyseal plate, and articular surfaces of bones. *Elastic cartilage*, which contains both collagen and elastic fibres, is more flexible than hyaline cartilage. It is found in the ear, epiglottis, and larynx. *Fibrous cartilage* (fibrocartilage) consists mostly of collagen fibres and is a tough tissue that often functions as a shock absorber. It is found between the vertebral discs and also forms a protective cushion between the bones of the pelvic girdle, knee, and shoulder.

Muscle

Types. The three types of muscle tissue are *cardiac* (striated, involuntary), *smooth* (nonstriated, involuntary), and *skeletal* (striated, voluntary) muscle. Cardiac muscle is found in the heart. Its spontaneous contractions propel blood through the circulatory system. Smooth muscle occurs in the walls of hollow structures such as airways, arteries, gastrointestinal tract, urinary bladder, and uterus. Smooth muscle contraction is modulated by neuronal and hormonal influences. Skeletal muscle, which requires neuronal stimulation for contraction, accounts for about half of a human being's body weight. It is the focus of the following discussion.

Structure. The structural unit of muscle is the muscle cell or muscle fibre, which is highly specialized for contraction. Skeletal

Joint	Movement	Examples	Illustration
Hinge joint	Flexion, extension	Elbow joint (shown), interphalangeal joints, knee joint	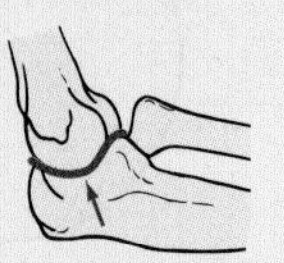
Ball and socket (spheroidal)	Flexion, extension; adduction, abduction; circumduction	Shoulder (shown), hip	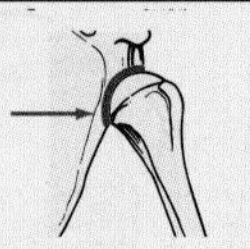
Pivot (rotary)	Rotation	Atlas–axis, proximal radioulnar joint (shown)	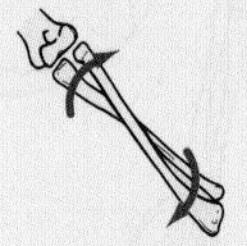
Condyloid	Flexion, extension; abduction, adduction; circumduction	Wrist joint (between radial and carpals) (shown)	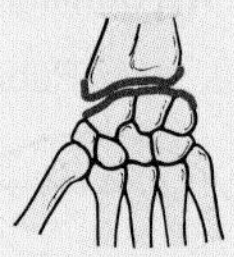
Saddle	Flexion, extension; abduction, adduction; circumduction, thumb–finger opposition	Carpometacarpal joint of thumb	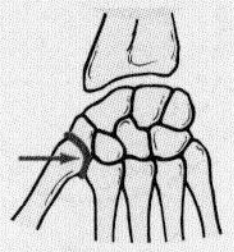
Gliding	One surface moves over another surface	Between tarsal bones, sacroiliac joint, between articular processes of vertebrae, between carpal bones (shown)	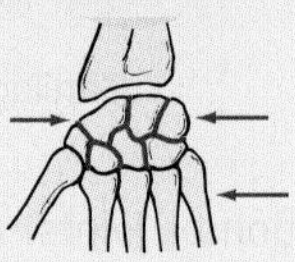

Figure 64-4 Types of diarthrodial (synovial) joints.

muscle fibres are long, multinucleated cylinders that contain many mitochondria to support their high metabolic activity. Muscle fibres are composed of *myofibrils*, which in turn are made up of contractile filaments.

The *sarcomere* is the contractile unit of the myofibrils (McCance & Huether, 2010). Each sarcomere consists of myosin (thick) filaments and actin (thin) filaments. The arrangement of the thick and thin filaments accounts for the characteristic banding of muscle when it is seen under a microscope. Muscle contraction occurs as thick and thin filaments slide past each other, causing the sarcomeres to shorten.

Contractions. Skeletal muscle contractions allow posture maintenance, movement, and facial expressions. **Isometric contractions** increase the tension within a muscle but do not produce movement. Repeated isometric contractions make muscles grow larger and stronger. **Isotonic contractions** shorten a muscle to produce movement. Most contractions are a combination of tension generation (isometric) and shortening (isotonic). Muscular *atrophy* (decrease in size) occurs with the absence of contraction that results from immobility, whereas increased muscular activity leads to *hypertrophy* (increase in size).

Skeletal muscle fibres are divided into two groups based on the type of activity they demonstrate. Slow-twitch muscle fibres support prolonged muscle activity such as marathon running. Because they also support the body against gravity, they assist in posture maintenance. Fast-twitch muscle fibres are used for rapid muscle contraction required for activities such as blinking the eye, jumping, or sprinting.

Neuromuscular Junction. Skeletal muscle fibres require a nerve impulse to contract. A nerve fibre and the skeletal muscle fibres it stimulates are called a *motor end plate*. The junction between the axon of the nerve cell and the adjacent muscle cell is called the *myoneural* or *neuromuscular junction* (Figure 64-5).

Acetylcholine is released from the motor end plate of the neuron and diffuses across the neuromuscular junction to bind with receptors on the muscle fibre. In response to this stimulation, the sarcoplasmic reticulum releases calcium ions into the cytoplasm. The presence of calcium triggers the contraction in the myofibrils. When calcium is low, tetany can occur.

Energy Source. The direct energy source for muscle fibre contractions is adenosine triphosphate. Adenosine triphosphate is synthesized by cellular oxidative metabolism in numerous mitochondria located close to the myofibrils. It is rapidly depleted through conversion to adenosine diphosphate and must be rephosphorylated. Phosphocreatine provides a rapid source for the resynthesis of adenosine triphosphate, but it is in turn converted to creatine and must be recharged. Glycolysis can serve as a source of adenosine triphosphate when the oxygen supply is inadequate for the metabolic needs of the muscle tissue. Glucose

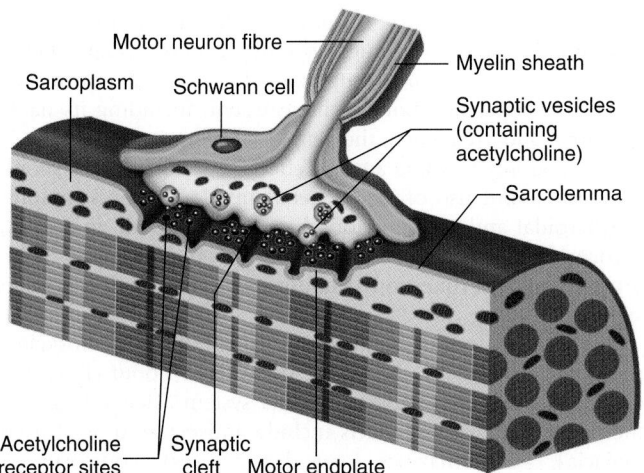

Figure 64-5 Neuromuscular junction.

Source: Adapted from Patton, K. T., & Thibodeau, G. A. (2010). *Anatomy and physiology* (7th ed., p. 345, Figure 11-7, *B*). St. Louis: Mosby.

is broken down to pyruvic acid, which can be further converted to lactic acid to make more oxygen available. An accumulation of lactic acid in tissues leads to fatigue and pain.

Ligaments and Tendons

Ligaments and tendons are both composed of dense, fibrous connective tissue that contains bundles of closely packed collagen fibres arranged in the same plane for additional strength. Tendons attach muscles to bones as an extension of the muscle sheath that adheres to the periosteum. Ligaments connect bones to bones (e.g., tibia to femur at knee joint). They have a higher elastic content than tendons (Herlihy, 2011). Ligaments provide stability while permitting controlled movement at the joint.

Ligaments and tendons have a relatively poor blood supply, usually making tissue repair after injury a slow process. For example, the stretching or tearing of ligaments that occurs with a sprain may require weeks to months to mend.

Fascia

Fascia refers to layers of connective tissue with intermeshed fibres that can withstand limited stretching. Superficial fascia lies immediately under the skin. Deep fascia is a dense, fibrous tissue that surrounds the muscle bundles, nerves, and blood vessels. It also encloses individual muscles, allowing them to act independently and to glide over each other during contraction. In addition, fascia provides strength to muscle tissues.

Bursae

Bursae are small sacs of connective tissue lined with synovial membrane and containing synovial fluid. They are typically located at bony prominences or joints to relieve pressure and prevent friction between moving parts. For example, bursae are found between the patella and the skin *(prepatellar bursa)*, between the olecranon process of the elbow and the skin *(olecranon bursa)*, between the head of the humerus and the acromion process of the scapula *(subacromial bursa)*, and between the greater trochanter of the proximal femur and the skin *(trochanteric bursa)*. *Bursitis* is an inflammation of a bursa sac.

AGE-RELATED CONSIDERATIONS: THE MUSCULOSKELETAL SYSTEM

Many of the functional problems experienced by the aging adult are related to changes of the musculoskeletal system. Although some changes begin in early adulthood, obvious signs of musculoskeletal impairment may not appear until later adult years. Alterations may affect the older adult's ability to complete self-care tasks and pursue other customary activities. Effects of musculoskeletal changes may range from mild discomfort and decreased ability to perform activities of daily living to severe, chronic pain and immobility. The risk for falls also increases in the older adult.

The bone remodelling process is altered in the aging adult. Increased bone resorption and decreased bone formation cause a loss of bone density, contributing to development of osteopenia and osteoporosis (see Chapter 66). Muscle mass and strength also decrease with aging. Tendons and ligaments become less flexible, and movement becomes more rigid. Joints in the aging adult are also more likely to be affected by osteoarthritis (see Chapter 67). The decrease in speed, strength, resistance to fatigue, reaction time, and coordination in the older person is a result of changes in both the musculoskeletal and the nervous systems (Linton & Lach, 2007).

In addition to the usual musculoskeletal assessment with an emphasis on functional and activity status, the nurse should also determine the impact of age-related musculoskeletal changes on the older person's psychosocial well-being and quality of life. Functional limitations that are accepted by older adults as a normal part of aging can often be halted or reversed with appropriate preventive strategies (see Chapter 65, Table 65-1).

Diseases such as osteoarthritis and osteoporosis are not the normal consequences of growing old. The nurse should carefully differentiate between expected changes and the effects of disease in the aging adult. Symptoms of disease can be treated in many cases, helping the older adult to return to a higher functional level. Age-related changes in the musculoskeletal system and differences in assessment findings are presented in Table 64-1.

Assessment of the Musculoskeletal System

Correct diagnosis of any complaint depends on a complete patient history and thorough physical examination. Musculoskeletal assessment focuses on good symptom analyses (e.g., location, quality, timing, severity, intensity of presented symptoms, and precipitating, alleviating, and associating factors), functional assessment (e.g., range of joint motion, muscle strength and tone, self-care deficits), medical history specific to musculoskeletal system (e.g., recent injury, arthritis), family history (e.g., bone cancer, osteoporosis) as well as personal and social history (e.g., dietary intake, exercise habits, sports, work hazards). The most common symptoms of musculoskeletal impairment include pain, weakness, deformity, limitation of movement, stiffness, and joint crepitation. Neurovascular structures are often affected by musculoskeletal problems, and muscular disorders may be manifestations of neurological problems. A neurological system

AGE-RELATED DIFFERENCES IN ASSESSMENT

Table 64-1 Musculoskeletal System

CHANGES	DIFFERENCES IN ASSESSMENT FINDINGS
Muscle	
Decreased number and diameter of muscle cells, replacement of muscle cells by fibrous connective tissue	Decreased muscle strength and bulk, abdominal protrusion, flabby muscle
Loss of elasticity in ligaments and cartilage	Decreased fine motor dexterity, decreased agility
Reduced ability to store glycogen; decreased ability to release glycogen as quick energy during stress	Slowed reaction times and reflexes as a result of slowing of impulse conduction along motor units; earlier fatigue with activity
Joints	
Increased risk for cartilage disruption that contributes to direct contact between bone ends and overgrowth of bone around joint margins	Joint stiffness, possible crepitation on movement; pain with motion, weight bearing, or both
Loss of water from discs between vertebrae, narrowing of intervertebral spaces	Loss of height from disc compression; posture change
Bone	
Decrease in bone density	Loss of height from vertebral compression, back pain; deformity such as dowager's hump (kyphosis) caused by vertebral compression

assessment (discussed in Chapter 58) and head-to-toe assessment are often conducted simultaneously.

Subjective Data

Important Health Information. Appropriate questions to ask during a musculoskeletal assessment are included in Table 64-2.

Past Health History. Because certain illnesses are known to affect the musculoskeletal system either directly or indirectly, question the patient about past medical problems. These include tuberculosis, poliomyelitis, diabetes mellitus, parathyroid problems, hemophilia, rickets, soft tissue infection, and neuromuscular disabilities. In addition, past or developing musculoskeletal problems can affect the patient's overall health. Trauma to the musculoskeletal system is a common reason for seeking medical evaluation. Questions should also focus on symptoms of arthritic and connective tissue diseases (e.g., gout, psoriatic arthritis, systemic lupus erythematosus), osteomalacia, osteomyelitis, and fungal infection of the bones or joints. Ask the patient about possible sources of a secondary bacterial infection, such as the ears, tonsils, teeth, sinuses, lungs, or genitourinary tract. These infections can enter the bones, resulting in osteomyelitis or joint destruction. Obtain a detailed account of the course and treatment of any of these problems.

Medications. The nurse should carefully question the patient regarding prescription drugs, over-the-counter drugs, herbal products, and nutritional supplements. Detailed information should be obtained about each treatment, including its name, the dose and frequency, the length of time it was taken, its effects, and any possible adverse effects. Specific inquiry should be made about use of any skeletal muscle relaxants, opioids, nonsteroidal anti-inflammatory drugs, and systemic and topical corticosteroids. The patient who has taken anti-inflammatory drugs should be questioned about gastrointestinal distress or signs of bleeding.

In addition to drugs taken for treatment of a musculoskeletal problem, the patient should be questioned about drugs that can have detrimental effects on this system. These drugs and their potential adverse effects include antiseizure drugs (osteomalacia), phenothiazines (gait disturbances), corticosteroids (avascular necrosis, decreased bone and muscle mass), and potassium-depleting diuretics (muscle cramps and weakness). Women should be questioned about their menstrual history. Episodes of amenorrhea can contribute to early development of osteoporosis. Questions about the use of hormone replacement therapy and calcium and vitamin D supplements are important for postmenopausal women.

Surgery or Other Treatments. Information should be obtained about past hospitalizations owing to a musculoskeletal problem. The nurse should carefully document the reason for hospitalization, the date and duration, and treatment. Details of emergency treatment for musculoskeletal injuries should also be sought. Specific information should be obtained regarding any surgical procedure and the postoperative course. If the patient experienced a period of prolonged immobilization, the development of osteoporosis and muscle atrophy should be considered.

Objective Data

Physical Examination. Examination of the musculoskeletal system involves observation, palpation, motion, and muscular assessment. Although a general overview will be conducted, data obtained in a careful health history will guide the nurse in choosing areas on which to concentrate the local examination. Specific measurements may be taken as indicated by the local examination.

Inspection. Inspection begins during the nurse's initial contact with the patient. The patient's use of an assistive device such as a walker or cane should be noted. The nurse also observes general body build, muscle configuration, and symmetry of joint movement. If the patient is able to move independently, the nurse should assess posture and gait by watching the patient walk, stand, and sit. Musculoskeletal and neurological problems can result in changes from a normal gait.

A systematic inspection is performed starting at the head and neck and proceeding to the upper extremities, lower extremities, and trunk. A specific order is not required, but the regular use of a systematic approach is important to avoid missing important aspects of the examination. The skin is inspected for general colour, scars, or other overt signs of previous injury or surgery. The nurse notes any swelling, deformity, nodules or masses, and discrepancies in limb length or muscle size. The patient's opposite body part is used for comparison when an abnormality is suspected.

HEALTH HISTORY

Table 64-2 Musculoskeletal System: Questions for Obtaining Subjective Data

Joints

- Any problems with your joints?* Any pain (describe quality, location, onset, timing, frequency)?
- What aggravates or relieves the pain? How do you manage your pain?
- Any stiffness in your joints?*
- Any swelling, heat, redness in any joint?*
- Any limitations in movement or function of any joint?*
- Which activities give you problems?

Muscles

- Any problems with your muscles (pain, cramping)?*
- If in calf muscles: Is the pain with walking? Does it go away with rest?
- Are your muscle aches associated with fever, chills, the "flu"?
- Any weakness?* Where? How long have you noticed the weakness? Do the muscles look smaller there?

Bones

- Any bone pain?* Does movement affect the pain? How? How do you manage the pain?
- Any deformity of any bone or joint? What is the cause? Does it affect range of motion?*
- Any accidents or trauma ever affect your bones or joints? When did this occur? What was the treatment? Any ongoing limitations?*

Functional Assessment (Activities of Daily Living)

- Do your joint, muscle, or bone problems limit any of your usual daily activities?*
- Any problems with bathing (getting in and out of tub, turning faucets)?
- Any problems with toileting (voiding, defecating, able to get on or off toilet, wipe self)?

- Are you able to dress yourself (fastening buttons, zippers, pulling clothes over head, pulling up pants or skirt, tying shoes)?
- Any problems with grooming (shaving, brushing teeth, fixing hair, applying makeup)?
- Are you able to prepare meals (pour liquids, cut up foods, bring food to mouth, drink)?
- Any problems with mobility (are you able to walk up and down stairs, get in and out of bed, get out of the house)?
- Any difficulties with using communication tools (phone, writing, talking)?

Self-Care Behaviours

- Are there any occupational hazards that could affect your muscles and joints? Does your work involve heavy lifting or repetitive motion?*
- Do you use any mechanical assistive devices or prosthetic or orthotic devices?*
- Describe your exercise pattern (frequency, warm-up, type of exercise, any pain).
- Any recent weight gain or loss? What is your usual daily diet? What dietary supplements do you take? (Ask specifically about calcium, vitamin D supplements, and herbal products.)
- Describe how you deal with problems (such as pain or immobility) that have resulted from your musculoskeletal problem.
- How has your illness affected your interaction with friends, family, the way you view yourself?

Additional History for the Aging Adult

- Any change in strength or weakness over the past weeks or months?*
- Any increase in falls or stumbling over the past weeks or months?*
- Do you use any mobility aids to help you get around (cane, walker)?*

*If yes, describe.

Source: Based on Jarvis, C., Browne, A. J., MacDonald-Jenkins, J., & Luctkar-Flude, M. (Eds.). (2009). *Physical examination and health assessment* (1st Canadian ed., pp. 605-608). Toronto: Elsevier.

Palpation. Any area that has aroused concern because of a subjective complaint or appears abnormal on inspection should be carefully palpated. As with inspection, palpation usually proceeds cephalopedally (head to toe) to examine neck, shoulders, elbows, wrists, hands, back, hips, knees, ankles, and feet. Both superficial and deep palpation are usually performed, one after the other. The nurse's hands should be warm to prevent muscle spasm, which can interfere with identification of essential landmarks or soft tissue structures. Palpation allows for evaluation of skin temperature, local tenderness, swelling, crepitation, and presence of nodules. Muscles are palpated during active and passive motion for tone, strength, and ease of movement.

Motion. When assessing the patient's joint mobility, the nurse must carefully evaluate both passive and active range of joint motion. Measurements should be similar for both active and passive range of motion. *Active range of motion* means the patient takes his or her own joints through all movements without assistance. *Passive range of motion* occurs when someone else moves the patient's joints without his or her participation. The nurse should be cautious in performing passive range of motion because of the risk of injury to underlying structures. Manipulation must cease immediately if pain or resistance is

encountered. If deficits in active or passive range of motion are noted, the nurse must also assess functional range of motion to determine whether performance of activities of daily living has been affected by joint changes. This is done by asking the patient whether activities such as eating and bathing must be performed with assistance or cannot be done at all.

Range of motion is most accurately assessed with a goniometer, which measures the angle of the joint (Figure 64-6). Specific degrees of range of motion of all joints are usually not measured unless a musculoskeletal problem has been identified. A less exact but valuable assessment method is to compare the range of motion of one extremity with the range of motion on the opposite side. The most common movements that occur at the synovial joints are described in Table 64-3.

Muscle-strength Testing. The nurse grades the strength of individual muscles or groups of muscles during contraction (Table 64-4). The patient should be instructed to apply resistance to the force exerted by the nurse. For example, the examiner tries to pull the bent arm down while the patient tries to raise it. Muscle strength should also be compared with the strength of the opposite extremity. Subtle variations in muscle strength may be noted when comparing the patient's dominant side with the nondominant side.

Table 64-3 Movement at Synovial Joints

MOVEMENT	DESCRIPTION
Abduction	Movement of part away from midline of body
Adduction	Movement of part toward midline of body
Circumduction	Combination of flexion, extension, abduction, and adduction resulting in circular motion of a body part
Dorsiflexion	Flexing toes and foot upward
Eversion	Turning of sole outward away from midline of body
Extension	Straightening of joint that increases angle between two bones
External rotation	Movement along longitudinal axis away from midline of body
Flexion	Bending of joint that results in decreased angle between two bones
Hyperextension	Extension in which angle exceeds 180 degrees
Internal rotation	Movement along longitudinal axis toward midline of body
Inversion	Turning of sole inward toward midline of body
Plantar flexion	Flexing toes and foot downward
Pronation	Turning of palm downward
Supination	Turning of palm upward

Table 64-4 Muscle Strength Scale

0	No detection of muscular contraction
1	A barely detectable flicker or trace of contraction with observation or palpation
2	Active movement of body part with elimination of gravity
3	Active movement against gravity only and not against resistance
4	Active movement against gravity and some resistance
5	Active movement against full resistance without evident fatigue (normal muscle strength)

Table 64-5 Normal Physical Assessment of the Musculoskeletal System

- Full range of motion of all joints without pain or laxity
- No joint swelling, deformity, or crepitation
- Normal spinal curvatures
- No tenderness on palpation of spine
- No muscle atrophy or asymmetry
- Muscle strength of 5

Measurement. When length discrepancies or subjective problems are noted, the nurse will often obtain limb length and circumferential muscle mass measurements. For example, leg length should be measured when gait disorders are observed. The affected limb is measured between two bony prominences and compared with the similar measurement of the opposite extremity. Muscle mass is measured circumferentially at the largest area of the muscle. When recording measurements, the nurse should document the exact location at which the measurements were obtained (e.g., the quadriceps muscle is measured 15 cm above the patella). This informs the next examiner of the exact area to be measured and ensures consistency during reassessment.

Other. Assessment of reflexes is discussed in Chapter 58. Table 64-5 is an example of how to record a normal physical assessment of the musculoskeletal system. Common abnormal assessment findings of the musculoskeletal system are presented in Table 64-6.

Scoliosis is a lateral S-shaped curvature of the thoracic and lumbar spine (Jarvis, Browne, MacDonald-Jenkins, & Luctkar-Flude, 2009). Unequal shoulder and scapula height is usually noted (Figure 64-7). If the deformity is greater than 45 degrees, lung and cardiac function is generally impaired.

Diagnostic Studies of the Musculoskeletal System

Diagnostic studies provide important objective data that aid the nurse in monitoring the patient's condition and planning appropriate interventions. Table 64-7 contains diagnostic studies common to the musculoskeletal system. Use of studies such as radiographs and magnetic resonance imaging (MRI) has greatly improved orthopedic care. Tests must be carefully chosen to enhance or clarify information gained from the patient's history and physical examination.

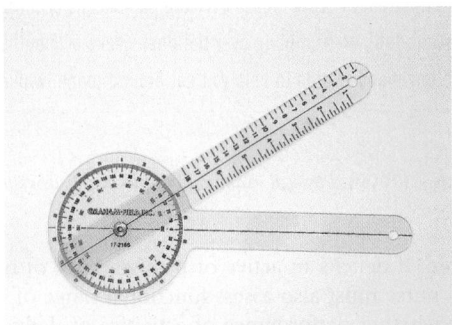

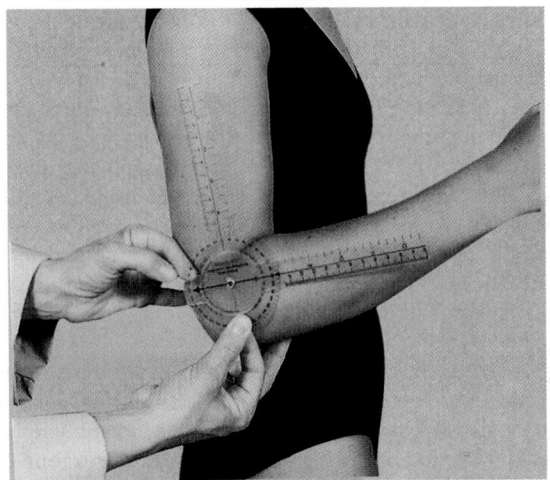

Figure 64-6 Measurement of joint motion with a goniometer.

Source: **A,** Wilson, S. F., & Giddens, J. F. (2009). *Health assessment for nursing practice* (4th ed., p. 38, Figure 4-22). St. Louis: Mosby; **B,** From Patton, K. T., & Thibodeau, G. A. (2010). *Anatomy and physiology* (7th ed., p. 278, Figure 9-15). St. Louis: Mosby.

Text continued on p. 1809

COMMON ASSESSMENT ABNORMALITIES

Table 64-6 Musculoskeletal System*

FINDING	DESCRIPTION	POSSIBLE ETIOLOGY
Achilles tendinitis	Pain in posterior leg when running or walking initially; can progress to pain at rest.	Cumulative stress on Achilles tendon resulting in inflammation.
Ankylosis	Stiffness or fixation of a joint, usually resulting from destruction of articular cartilage and subchondral bone with subsequent scarring.	Chronic joint inflammation.
Antalgic gait	Shortened stride with as little weight bearing as possible on the affected side.	Pain or discomfort in the lower extremity on weight bearing; can be related to trauma or other disorders.
Ataxic gait	Staggering, uncoordinated gait often with sway.	Neurogenic disorders (e.g., spinal cord lesion).
Atrophy	Wasting of muscle, characterized by decreased circumference and flabby appearance, leading to decreased function and tone.	Muscle denervation, contracture, prolonged disuse as a result of immobilization.
Contracture	An abnormal, usually permanent condition of a muscle or joint characterized by flexion and fixation; resistance to movement is a result of fibrosis of supporting soft tissues.	Shortening of muscle or ligaments, tightness of soft tissue, incorrect positioning of immobilized extremity.
Crepitation (crepitus)	Crackling sound or grating sensation as a result of friction between bones, broken bone, or cartilage bits in joint.	Fracture, dislocation, chronic inflammation, osteoarthritis.
Dislocation	Bone is displaced from its normal joint.	Trauma, disorders of surrounding soft tissues.
Hypertrophy	Increase in size of muscle as a result of enlargement of existing cells.	Exercise or other increased stimulation, increased androgens.
Kyphosis (dowager's hump)	Forward bending of thoracic spine: exaggerated thoracic curvature.	Poor posture, tuberculosis, arthritis, osteoporosis, growth disturbance of vertebral epiphyses.
Limited range of motion (ROM)	Joint does not achieve the expected degrees of motion.	Injury, inflammation, contracture.
Lordosis (swayback)	Lumbar spinal deformity resulting in exaggerated lumbar curvature	Secondary to other spinal deformities, muscular dystrophy, obesity, flexion contracture of hip, congenital dislocation of hip.
Muscle spasticity	Increased muscle tone (rigidity) with sustained muscle contractions (spasms); stiffness or tightness may interfere with gait, movement, speech.	Neuromuscular disorders such as multiple sclerosis (MS) or cerebral palsy.
Myalgia	General muscle tenderness and pain.	Chronic rheumatic syndromes (e.g., fibromyalgia).
Paresthesia	Numbness and tingling, often described as a "pins and needles" sensation.	Compromised sensory nerves, often owing to edema in a closed space such as a cast or bulky dressing.
Pes planus (flat foot)	Abnormal flatness of the sole and arch of the foot.	Hereditary, muscle paralysis, mild cerebral palsy, early muscular dystrophy, injury to posterior tibial tendon.
Plantar fasciitis	Burning, sharp pain on sole of foot; worse in the morning.	Chronic degenerative–reparative cycle resulting in inflammation.
Scoliosis	Deformity resulting from lateral S-shaped curvature of the thoracic and lumbar spine (see Figure 64-7).	Idiopathic or congenital condition, fracture or dislocation, osteomalacia.
Subluxation	Partial dislocation of joint.	Instability of joint capsule and supporting ligaments (e.g., trauma, arthritis).
Swan neck deformity	Hyperextension of the PIP joint with flexion of the MCP and DIP joints of the fingers (see Chapter 67, Figure 67-4).	Typical deformity of rheumatoid and psoriatic arthritis caused by contracture of muscles and tendons.
Swelling	Enlargement, often of a joint, owing to fluid collection; generally leads to pain, stiffness.	Trauma or inflammation.
Torticollis (wryneck)	Neck is twisted in unusual position to one side.	Prolonged contraction of neck muscles, congenital or acquired.
Ulnar deviation (ulnar drift)	Fingers drift to ulnar side of forearm (see Chapter 67, Figure 67-4).	Typical deformity of rheumatoid arthritis owing to tendon contracture.
Valgum deformity (knockknees)	When knees are together and there is >2.5 cm space between the medial malleoli.	Poliomyelitis, congenital deformity, arthritis.
Varum deformity (bowlegs)	When the medial malleoli are together, a space of >2.5 cm exists at the knees.	Arthritis, congenital deformity.

DIP, distal interphalangeal; *MCP,* metacarpophalangeal; *PIP,* proximal interphalangeal.
*Boldface entries are Key Terms.

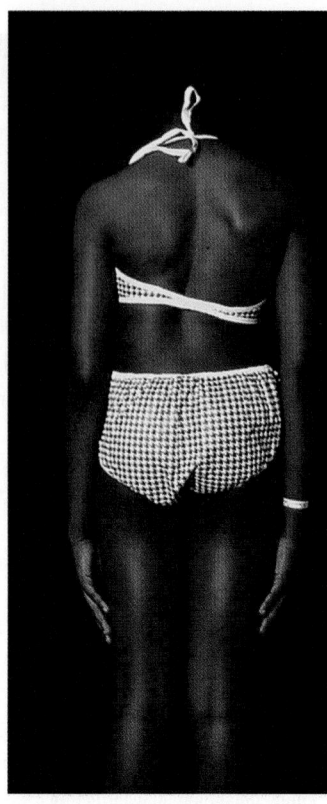

Figure 64-7 Scoliosis in a standing erect posture.

Source: Zitelli, B. J., McIntire, S. C., & Nowalk, A. J. (2012). *Zitelli & Davis' atlas of pediatric physical diagnosis* (6th ed., Figure 21-71, *A*). Philadelphia: Saunders.

FOCUSED ASSESSMENT
Musculoskeletal System

Use this checklist to make sure the key assessment steps have been done.

Subjective
Ask the patient about any of the following and note responses

Joint pain or stiffness	Y	N
Muscle weakness	Y	N
Bone pain	Y	N

Objective: Diagnostic
Check the following laboratory results for critical values

Radiograph results	✓
Bone scans	✓
Erythrocyte sedimentation rate	✓

Objective: Physical Examination
Inspect and Palpate

Skeleton and extremities (and compare sides) for alignment, contour, symmetry, size, and gross deformities	✓
Joints for range of motion, tenderness/pain, heat, crepitus, and swelling	✓
Muscles (and compare sides) for size, symmetry, tone, and tenderness/pain	✓
Bones for tenderness or pain	✓

DIAGNOSTIC STUDIES

Table 64-7 Musculoskeletal System*

STUDY	DESCRIPTION AND PURPOSE	NURSING RESPONSIBILITY
Radiological Studies		
Standard radiograph (x-ray)	An x-ray beam produces an image on photographic film (radiograph), which is used to evaluate structural or functional changes of bones and joints and calcification of soft tissues. Radiographs are two-dimensional, and multiple views may be required to facilitate diagnosis (e.g., anteroposterior, lateral, or oblique view).	Avoid excessive exposure of patient and self to radiation. Before procedure, remove any radiopaque objects that can interfere with results. Explain procedure to patient. Verify patient is not pregnant.
Computed tomography (CT) scan	An x-ray beam is used with a computer to provide a three-dimensional image. It is used to identify soft tissue abnormalities, bony abnormalities, and various musculoskeletal trauma.	Inform patient that procedure is painless. Inform patient of importance of remaining still during procedure.
Magnetic resonance imaging (MRI)	Radiofrequency waves and magnetic field are used to view soft tissue. Study is especially useful in the diagnosis of avascular necrosis, disc disease, tumours, osteomyelitis, ligament tears, and cartilage tears. Patient is placed inside scanning chamber. Gadolinium may be injected into a vein to enhance visualization of the structures. Open MRI does not require the patient to be placed inside a chamber.	Inform patient that procedure is painless. Be aware that it is contraindicated in patients with aneurysm clips, metallic implants, pacemakers, electronic devices, hearing aids, shrapnel, and extreme obesity. Ensure that patient has no metal on clothing (e.g., snaps, zippers, jewellery, credit cards). Inform patient of importance of remaining still throughout examination. Inform patients who are claustrophobic that they may experience symptoms during examination. Administer antianxiety agent if indicated and ordered. Open MRI may be indicated for obese patient or patient with large chest and abdominal girth or severe claustrophobia. Open MRI may not be available at all facilities.

DIAGNOSTIC STUDIES

Table 64-7 Musculoskeletal System—cont'd

STUDY	DESCRIPTION AND PURPOSE	NURSING RESPONSIBILITY
Radiological Studies—cont'd		
Arthrogram	Contrast medium or air is injected into joint cavity, which permits visualization of joint structures. Joint movement is followed with series of radiographic images.	Assess patient for possible allergy to contrast medium. Explain procedure.
Discogram	A radiographic study of cervical or lumbar intervertebral disc is done after injection of contrast dye into nucleus pulposus. Study permits visualization of intervertebral disc abnormalities.	Same as for arthrogram.
Bone Mineral Density (BMD) Measurements		
Dual-energy x-ray absorptiometry (DEXA)	Technique measures bone mass of spine, femur, forearm, and total body. Allows assessment of bone density with minimal radiation exposure; used to diagnose metabolic bone disease and to monitor changes in bone density with treatment. Widely available; free screening test.	Inform patient that procedure is painless.
Quantitative ultrasonography (QUS)	Evaluates density, elasticity, and strength of patella and calcaneus using ultrasound rather than radiation.	Inform patient that procedure is painless.
Radioisotope Studies		
Bone scan	Technique involves injection of radioisotope (usually technetium-99m) that is taken up by bone. Radiation detector (Geiger counter) scans entire body (front and back), and recording is made on paper. Degree of uptake is related to blood flow to bone. Increased uptake is seen in osteomyelitis, osteoporosis, primary and metastatic malignant lesions of bone, and certain fractures. Decreased uptake is seen in areas of avascular necrosis.	Explain that technician gives a calculated dose of radioisotope 2 hr before procedure. Ensure that bladder is emptied before scan. Inform patient that procedure requires 1 hr while patient lies supine and that no pain or harm will result from isotopes. Explain that no follow-up scans are required. Increase fluids after the examination.
Endoscopy		
Arthroscopy	Study involves insertion of arthroscope into joint (usually knee) for visualization of structure and contents. It can be used for exploratory surgery (removal of loose bodies and biopsy) and for diagnosis of abnormalities of meniscus, articular cartilage, ligaments, or joint capsule. Other structures that can be visualized through the arthroscope include shoulder, elbow, wrist, jaw, hip, and ankle.	Inform patient that procedure is performed in operating room with strict asepsis and that either local or general anaesthesia is used. After procedure, cover wound with sterile dressing.
Mineral Metabolism		
Alkaline phosphatase	This enzyme, produced by osteoblasts of bone, is needed for mineralization of organic bone matrix. Elevated levels are found in healing fractures, bone cancers, osteoporosis, osteomalacia, and Paget's disease. *Normal:* 0.5-2.0 mckat (30-120 units/L) (age dependent). Obtain blood samples by venipuncture. Observe venipuncture site for bleeding or hematoma formation.	Inform patient that procedure does not require fasting.
Calcium	Bone is primary organ for calcium storage. Calcium provides bone with rigid consistency. Decreased serum level is found in osteomalacia, renal disease, and hypoparathyroidism; increased level is found in hyperparathyroidism, some bone tumours, varies with albumin. *Normal:* 2.25-2.75 mmol/L (age dependent).	Same as above.
Phosphate (phosphorus)	Amount present is indirectly related to calcium metabolism. Decreased level is found in osteomalacia; increased level is found in chronic renal disease, healing fractures, osteolytic metastatic tumour. *Normal:* 0.97-1.45 mmol/L (age dependent).	Same as above.
Serological Studies		
Rheumatoid factor (RF)	Study assesses presence of autoantibody (RF) in serum. Factor is not specific for rheumatoid arthritis and is seen in other connective tissue diseases, as well as in a small percentage of normal population. *Normal:* negative or <60 units/mL by nephalometric method.	Same as above.
Erythrocyte sedimentation rate (ESR)	Study is nonspecific index of inflammation. Study measures rapidity with which red blood cells settle out of unclotted blood in 1 hr. Results are influenced by physiological factors as well as diseases. Elevated levels are seen with any inflammatory process (especially rheumatoid arthritis, rheumatic fever, osteomyelitis, and respiratory infections). *Normal:* <15-20 mm/hr. Some variation by sex.	Same as above.

Continued

DIAGNOSTIC STUDIES

STUDY	DESCRIPTION AND PURPOSE	NURSING RESPONSIBILITY
Table 64-7 Musculoskeletal System—cont'd		
Serological Studies—cont'd		
Antinuclear antibody (ANA)	Study assesses presence of antibodies capable of destroying nucleus of body's tissue cells. Finding is positive in 95% of patients with systemic lupus erythematosus and may also be positive in individuals with systemic sclerosis (scleroderma) or rheumatoid arthritis and in a small percentage of normal population.	Same as above.
C-reactive protein (CRP)	Study is used to diagnose inflammatory diseases, infections, and active widespread malignancy. CRP is synthesized by the liver and is present in large amounts in serum 18-24 hr after onset of tissue damage. *Normal:* Negative or ≤10 mg/L	Same as above.
Uric acid	End product of purine metabolism is normally excreted in urine. Although not specific, levels are usually elevated in gout. *Normal:* Men 0.24-0.51 mmol/L; women 0.16-0.43 mmol/L (age dependent).	Obtain blood samples by venipuncture. Observe venipuncture site for bleeding or hematoma formation. Inform patient that procedure does not require fasting.
Human leukocyte antigen (HLA)-B27	Antigen present in disorders such as ankylosing spondylitis and rheumatoid arthritis.	Same as above.
Muscle Enzymes		
Creatine kinase (CK)	Highest concentration is found in skeletal muscle. Increased values are found in progressive muscular dystrophy, polymyositis, and traumatic injuries. *Normal:* Men 55-170 units/L; women 30-135 units/L.	Same as above.
Serum potassium (K^+)	Increased values may occur with muscle trauma because cell destruction releases this electrolyte into the serum (depends on renal function). *Normal:* 3.5-5.0 mmol/L.	Monitor trauma patients for cardiac dysrhythmias related to hypokalemia or hyperkalemia.
Invasive Procedures		
Arthrocentesis	A needle is inserted into the joint cavity to aspirate synovial fluid, blood, or pus or to instill medications. Local anaesthesia and aseptic technique are required. Study is useful in diagnosis of joint inflammation, infection, and subtle fractures.	Inform patient that procedure is usually done at bedside or in examination room. Send samples of synovial fluid to laboratory for examination (if indicated). After procedure, apply pressure dressing. Observe for leakage of blood or fluid on dressing.
Electromyogram (EMG)	Study evaluates electrical potential associated with skeletal muscle contraction. Small-gauge needles are inserted into certain muscles. Needle probes are attached to leads that feed information to EMG machine. Recordings of electrical activity of muscle are traced on audiotransmitter, as well as on oscilloscope and recording paper. Study is useful in providing information related to lower motor neuron dysfunction and primary muscle disease.	Inform patient that procedure is usually done in EMG laboratory while patient lies supine on special table. Keep patient awake to cooperate with voluntary movement. Inform patient that procedure involves some discomfort from needle insertion. Avoid administration of stimulants including caffeine and sedatives 24 hr before procedure.
Miscellaneous		
Thermography	Technique uses infrared detector, which measures degree of heat radiating from skin surface. Study is useful in investigation of cause of inflamed joint and in following up patient's response to anti-inflammatory drug therapy.	Inform patient that procedure is painless and noninvasive.
Duplex venous Doppler	Ultrasound of the veins, usually of the lower extremities, to detect blood flow abnormalities that could indicate deep venous thrombosis.	Inform patient that procedure is painless and noninvasive.
Somatosensory evoked potential (SSEP)	Study evaluates evoked potential of muscle contractions. Electrodes are placed on skin and provide recordings of electrical activity of muscle. Study is useful in identifying subtle dysfunction of lower motor neuron and primary muscle disease. SSEP measures nerve conduction along pathways not accessible by EMG. Transcutaneous or percutaneous electrodes are applied to the skin and help identify neuropathy and myopathy.	Inform patient that procedure is similar to EMG but does not involve needles. Electrodes are applied to the skin.

*Boldface entries are Key Terms.

Radiography

The *radiograph*, or x-ray, is the most common diagnostic study used to assess musculoskeletal problems and to monitor the effectiveness of treatment. The x-ray beam produces an image on a photographic film; the image appears dark if the x-rays penetrate the body tissues (e.g., lungs) and white if the transmission is partially blocked (e.g., bones). Radiographs are two-dimensional, and multiple views may be required to facilitate diagnosis (e.g., anteroposterior [front-to-back], lateral [side], oblique [45-degree angle]). Based on the contours and shades of the structures on the radiograph, these images provide useful information such as showing the presence of deformity, joint congruity, calcification in soft tissue, and bone fractures. Radiographs are also useful in the evaluation of hereditary, developmental, infectious, inflammatory, neoplastic, metabolic, and degenerative disorders.

Magnetic Resonance Imaging

MRI can be useful for the early diagnosis of soft tissue disorders, including cartilage or ligament tears and herniated discs, as well as bone disorders such as avascular necrosis, tumours, and multiple myeloma. The body is composed primarily of hydrogen, which possesses magnetic properties that can be scanned by the powerful magnetic fields and radiofrequency waves. Contrast agent may be required to enhance the images. MRI is contraindicated for patients who have implanted metal objects (e.g., pacemaker, aneurysm clips, prosthesis, implanted cardioverter–defibrillator, electronic devices, hearing aids, shrapnel).

Arthroscopy

A small fibreoptic tube called an *arthroscope* is inserted into a joint and used to directly examine or operate on the interior of the joint cavity in a procedure known as **arthroscopy**. Arthroscopy is performed under sterile conditions. After anaesthesia has been administered, a large-bore needle is inserted into the joint, and the joint is distended with fluid or air (Figure 64-8). When the arthroscope is inserted, the surgeon is able to achieve extensive, accurate visualization of the joint cavity. Photographs or videotapes can be made through the scope, and a biopsy of the synovium or cartilage can be obtained. Torn tissue can be repaired through arthroscopic surgery, eliminating the need for a larger incision and greatly decreasing the recovery time. Arthroscopy is a highly cost-effective diagnostic test that is usually done on an outpatient basis.

Arthrocentesis and Synovial Fluid Analysis

An **arthrocentesis** or joint aspiration is an incision or puncture of a joint capsule; it is usually performed to obtain samples of synovial fluid from within the joint cavity for a synovial fluid analysis. It may also be used to instill medications for the patient with septic arthritis or to remove excess fluid from joints to relieve pain. After the skin has been cleaned, a local anaesthetic is instilled. An 18-gauge or larger needle is inserted into the joint, and fluid is withdrawn. The appropriate sterile container should be readily available to receive the aspirated fluid, which must be transported immediately to the laboratory. The fluid will be examined grossly for volume, colour, clarity, viscosity, and *mucin clot formation.* Normal synovial fluid is transparent and colourless or straw-coloured. It should be scant in amount and of low viscosity. Fluid from an infected joint may be purulent and thick or grey and thin. In gout, the fluid may be whitish yellow. Blood may be aspirated

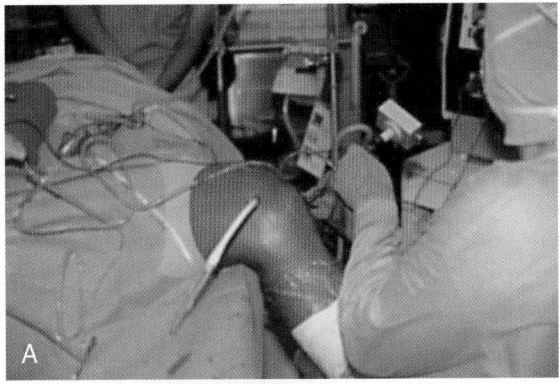

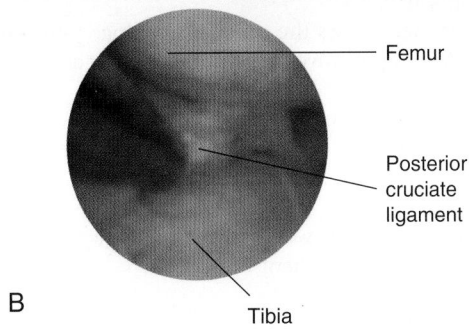

Figure 64-8 Arthroscopy of a knee. **A,** Insertion of a fibreoptic light into a joint. **B,** Internal view of joint.

Source: **A,** Monahan, F. D., Sands, J. K., Neighbors, M., Marek, J. F., & Green-Nigro, C. J. (2007). *Phipps' medical-surgical nursing: Health and illness perspectives* (8th ed., p. 1521, Figure 51-30, *A*). St. Louis: Mosby; **B,** Patton, K. T., & Thibodeau, G. A. (2010). *Anatomy and physiology* (7th ed., p. 287, Figure 9-28, *B*). St. Louis: Mosby.

if there is hemarthrosis because of injury or a bleeding disorder. The mucin clot test indicates the character of the protein portion of the synovial fluid. Normally a white, ropelike mucin clot is formed. In the presence of an inflammatory process, the clot breaks apart easily and fragments. The fluid is examined grossly for floating fat globules, which indicate bone injury.

The fluid is examined microscopically for cell count and identification. Infection would be suspected if the white blood cell count revealed more than 25×10^9/L and more than 25% polymorphonuclear cells. Protein content is elevated, and glucose is considerably decreased in septic arthritis. Presence of uric acid crystals suggests a diagnosis of gout. A Gram stain and culture may also be done of the aspirated fluid.

Muscle Enzymes

Muscle enzymes are released from injured or dead muscle cells. Determinations of muscle enzyme values are used to distinguish between muscle weakness owing to innervation problems and that owing to dystrophic disease of the muscle itself. The level of enzymes reflects the progress of the disorder and the effectiveness of treatment. Creatine kinase is a reliable measure of muscle damage.

Serological Studies

Approximately 80% of people with rheumatoid arthritis and related diseases have an autoantibody known as rheumatoid factor (RF) in their serum. RF is an autoantibody directed against immunoglobulin G. RF titres are higher during periods of increased disease activity. Elevated erythrocyte sedimentation rate and C-reactive protein are nonspecific indicators of active inflammation.

REVIEW QUESTIONS

The number of the question corresponds to the same-numbered objective at the beginning of the chapter.

1. What are the bone cells that function in the breakdown of bone tissue (resorption) called?
   a. Osteoids
   b. Osteocytes
   c. Osteoclasts
   d. Osteoblasts
2. What movements does the nurse put a hinge joint through while performing passive range of motion for a patient?
   a. Rotation.
   b. Flexion and extension
   c. Flexion, extension, abduction, and adduction
   d. Flexion, extension, abduction, adduction, and circumduction
3. Which of the following would prevent muscle atrophy in the immobilized leg of a patient in traction?
   a. Twitch contractions
   b. Tetanic contractions
   c. Isotonic contractions
   d. Isometric contractions
4. A patient with bursitis of the shoulder asks the nurse what the bursa does. What does the nurse tell the patient about the function of the bursa?
   a. Bursae connect bone to bone.
   b. Bursae separate muscle from muscle.
   c. Bursae lubricate joints with synovial fluid.
   d. Bursae relieve friction between moving parts.
5. Why do older adults most likely have an increased risk for falls?
   a. Changes in balance
   b. Decrease in bone mass
   c. Loss of ligament elasticity
   d. Erosion of articular cartilage
6. While obtaining subjective assessment data related to the musculoskeletal system, which of the following conditions requires the nurse to ask about family history?
   a. Osteomyelitis
   b. Osteomalacia
   c. Low back pain
   d. Rheumatoid arthritis
7. When a nurse grades muscle strength with a score of 2, what does that indicate?
   a. Active movement against gravity
   b. A barely detectable flicker of contraction
   c. Active movement with elimination of gravity
   d. Active movement against full resistance without evident fatigue
8. Which of the following is a normal assessment finding of the musculoskeletal system?
   a. Muscle strength of 4
   b. A lateral curvature of the spine
   c. Angulation of bone toward midline
   d. Full range of motion of all joints without pain
9. Which of the following statements best describes an electromyogram?
   a. Placement of thin needles into the muscles
   b. Placement of electrodes on the skin to record electrical activity of muscles
   c. Measurement of the heat of muscle contractions radiating from the skin surface
   d. Administration of a calculated dose of radioisotope 2 hours before the procedure

ANSWERS: 1. c; 2. b; 3. d; 4. d; 5. a; 6. d; 7. c; 8. d; 9. a.

REFERENCES

Altizer, L. (2007). Anatomy and physiology. In *NAON: Core curriculum for orthopaedic nursing* (6th ed.). Boston: Pearson Custom Publishing.

Herlihy, B. (2011). *The human body in health and illness* (4th ed.). St. Louis: Saunders.

Jarvis, C., Browne, A. J., MacDonald-Jenkins, J., & Luctkar-Flude, M. (Eds.). (2009). *Physical examination and health assessment* (1st Canadian ed.). Toronto: Elsevier.

Linton, A. D., & Lach, H. W. (Eds.). (2007). *Matteson & McConnell's gerontological nursing: Concepts and practice* (3rd ed.). St. Louis: Saunders.

McCance, K. L., & Huether, S. E. (2010). *Pathophysiology: The biologic basis for disease in adults and children* (13th ed.). St. Louis: Mosby.

National Association of Orthopaedic Nurses (NAON). (2007). *NAON Core curriculum for orthopaedic nursing* (6th ed.). Boston: Pearson.

Roberts, D. (2009). The musculoskeletal system. In H. Craven (Ed.), *Core curriculum for medical-surgical nursing* (4th ed.), Pitman, NJ: Academy of Medical-Surgical Nurses.

Thibodeau, G. A., & Patton, K. T. (2012). *Structure and function of the body* (14th ed.). St. Louis: Mosby.

RESOURCES

Resources for this chapter are listed in Chapter 65, p. 1852, Chapter 66, p. 1879; and Chapter 67 on p. 1919.

Nursing Management: Musculoskeletal Trauma and Orthopedic Surgery

Written by Kathleen Rourke

Adapted by Maureen A. Barry

LEARNING OBJECTIVES

1. Explain the etiology, pathophysiology, clinical manifestations, and collaborative care of soft tissue injuries, including strains, sprains, dislocations, subluxations, bursitis, repetitive strain injury, carpal tunnel syndrome, and injuries to the rotator cuff, meniscus, and anterior cruciate ligament.
2. Describe the sequential events involved in fracture healing.
3. Compare closed reduction, cast immobilization, open reduction, and traction regarding purpose, complications, and nursing management.
4. Describe a neurovascular assessment for a patient with an injured extremity.
5. Explain common complications associated with a fracture and fracture healing.
6. Describe the collaborative care and nursing management of patients with specific fractures.
7. Describe the indications for and the collaborative care and nursing management of the patient with an amputation.
8. Describe the types of joint replacement surgery associated with arthritis and connective tissue diseases.
9. Identify the preoperative and postoperative management of the patient having joint replacement surgery.

KEY TERMS

arthrodesis Surgical fusion of a joint, p. 1848

arthroplasty Surgical reconstruction or replacement of a joint, p. 1846

avascular necrosis (AVN) Bone cell death as a result of inadequate blood supply, p. 1815

bursitis Inflammation of a bursa, p. 1819

carpal tunnel syndrome (CTS) A condition caused by compression of the median nerve beneath the transverse carpal ligament within the narrow confines of the carpal tunnel located in the wrist, p. 1816

compartment syndrome A condition in which elevated intracompartmental pressure within a confined myofascial compartment compromises the neurovascular function of tissues within that space, p. 1833

dislocation A severe injury of the ligamentous structures that surround a joint resulting in the complete displacement or separation of the articular surfaces of the joint, p. 1815

fat embolism syndrome (FES) Syndrome characterized by the presence of systemic fat globules (from fractures) that are distributed into tissues and organs in a small percentage of patients after a traumatic skeletal injury, p. 1834

fracture A disruption or break in the continuity of the structure of bone, p. 1819

osteotomy Surgery to remove or add a wedge or slice of bone to change alignment (joint and vertebral) and to shift weight bearing, thereby correcting the deformity and relieving pain, p. 1846

phantom limb sensation Phenomenon whereby the patient feels like the amputated limb is still present after surgery, p. 1843

repetitive strain injury (RSI) A cumulative traumatic disorder resulting from prolonged, forceful, or awkward movements that strain tendons, ligaments, and muscles and cause tiny tears that become inflamed, p. 1815

sprain Injury related to the stretching or tearing of ligament tissue surrounding a joint, p. 1813

strain Injury caused by twisting or pulling a muscle or tendon; can range from simple overstretching to a partial or complete tear, p. 1813

subluxation A partial or incomplete displacement of the joint surface, p. 1815

synovectomy Removal of the synovial membrane, often as a prophylactic measure and a palliative treatment of rheumatoid arthritis, p. 1845

traction The application of a pulling force to an injured or diseased part of the body or an extremity while countertraction pulls in the opposite direction, p. 1822

ELECTRONIC RESOURCES

Supplemental content related to Chapter 65 can be found...

Evolve Web Site ⓔvolve

http://evolve.elsevier.com/Canada/Lewis/medsurg
- Answer Guidelines for Case Study on p. 1849
- Clinical Reference: Laboratory Values
- Content Updates
- Customizable Nursing Care Plans:
  - Fracture
  - Orthopedic Surgery

- Electronic Calculators
- Examination Review Questions
- Glossary
- Interactive Case Study: Musculoskeletal Trauma
- Key Points (Printable and MP3 Download)
- Patient & Caregiver Teaching Guides:
  - Care After a Femoral Head Prosthesis
  - Care Following an Amputation
  - Prevention of Musculoskeletal Problems in the Older Adult

The most common cause of musculoskeletal problems is injury from a traumatic event resulting in fracture, dislocation, and associated soft tissue injury. Although most of these injuries are not fatal, the cost in terms of pain, disability, medical expense, and lost wages is enormous. Injury is a serious public health issue with a major impact on the lives of Canadians. In 2009, the most recent date for which data are available, accidents (unintentional injuries) were the leading cause of death for Canadians between the ages of 1 and 34 and the fifth leading cause of death for Canadians of all ages (Statistics Canada, 2012). For all ages, accidents were exceeded only by cancer, heart disease, stroke, and chronic lower respiratory disease as a cause of death (Statistics Canada, 2012).

The nurse has an important role in educating the public about the basic principles of safety and accident prevention. The morbidity associated with accidents can be significantly reduced if people are aware of environmental hazards, use existing safety equipment, and apply safety and traffic rules. In the occupational and industrial setting, the nurse should teach employees and employers about the use of proper safety equipment and avoidance of hazardous working situations.

SAFETY ALERT

- Falls account for many musculoskeletal injuries, particularly in the older adult.
- Provide preventive teaching to high-risk individuals (e.g., people with gait instability or visual or cognitive impairment).
- Stress the importance of wearing shoes with functional soles and heels, avoidance of wet or slippery surfaces, and removing throw rugs from the home.

Ways to prevent common musculoskeletal problems in the older adult are listed in Table 65-1.

Soft Tissue Injuries

Soft tissue injuries include sprains, strains, dislocations, and subluxation. These common injuries are usually caused by trauma. Sprains and strains are the most common injury (51%) with fractures and broken bones accounting for 17% of injuries (Statistics Canada, 2011).

PATIENT & CAREGIVER TEACHING GUIDE

Table 65-1 Prevention of Musculoskeletal Problems in the Older Adult

1. Use ramps in buildings and at street corners instead of steps to prevent falls.
2. Eliminate scatter rugs in the home.
3. Treat pain and discomfort from osteoarthritis.
   - Rest in a reclining position to decrease discomfort.
   - Discuss use of medication for pain with health care provider.
4. Use a walker or cane to help with walking to prevent falls.
5. Eat the amount and the kind of foods needed to prevent excess weight gain because obesity adds stress to joints, which may predispose to osteoarthritis.
6. Get regular and frequent exercise.
   - Activities of daily living provide range of motion exercises.
   - Hobbies (e.g., jigsaw puzzles, needlework, model building) exercise finger joints and prevent stiffness.
   - Performing weight-bearing exercise daily (e.g., walking) is essential and should be done two or three times daily.
7. Use shoes with good support to provide for safety and promote comfort.
8. Gradually initiate activities to promote optimal coordination. Rise slowly to a standing position to prevent dizziness, falls, and fractures.
9. Avoid walking on uneven surfaces and wet floors.

The increase in the number of people who have committed themselves to a regular fitness program or who participate in sports has contributed to the increased incidence of soft tissue injuries. In Canada, 35% of injuries involved participation in sports or exercise (Statistics Canada, 2011). Common sports-related injuries are summarized in Table 65-2.

Sprains and Strains

Sprains and strains are the two most common types of injury affecting the musculoskeletal system. These injuries are usually associated with abnormal stretching or twisting forces that may occur during vigorous activities. These injuries tend to occur around joints and in the spinal musculature.

Table 65-2 Common Sports-Related Injuries

INJURY	DEFINITION	TREATMENT
Impingement syndrome	Entrapment of soft tissue structures under coracoacromial arch of shoulder.	NSAIDs; rest until symptoms decrease, and then gradual ROM and strengthening exercises.
Rotator cuff tear	Tear within muscle or tendinoligamentous structures around shoulder.	If minor tear: rest, NSAIDs, and gradual mobilization with ROM and strengthening exercises. If major tear: surgical repair.
Shin splints	Inflammation along anterior aspect of calf from periostitis caused by improper shoes, overuse, or running on hard pavement.	Rest, ice, NSAIDs, proper shoes; gradual increase in activity. If pain persists, radiographic study to rule out stress fracture of tibia.
Tendinitis	Inflammation of tendon as a result of overuse or incorrect use.	Rest, ice, NSAIDs; gradual return to sport activity; protective brace (orthosis) may be necessary if symptoms recur.
Ligament injury	Tearing or stretching of ligament; usually occurs as a result of inversion, eversion, shearing, or torque applied to a joint. Characterized by sudden pain, swelling, and instability.	Rest, ice, NSAIDs; protection of affected extremity by use of brace. If symptoms persist, surgical repair may be necessary.
Meniscal injury	Injury to fibrocartilage of the knee characterized by popping, clicking, tearing sensation, effusion, and/or swelling.	Rest, ice, NSAIDs; gradual return to regular activities. If symptoms persist, MRI to diagnose meniscal injury and possible arthroscopic surgery.

MRI, magnetic resonance imaging; *NSAIDs,* nonsteroidal anti-inflammatory drugs; *ROM,* range of motion.

A **sprain** is an injury related to the ligamentous structures surrounding a joint, usually caused by a wrenching or twisting motion. Most sprains occur in the ankle and knee joints (Cleveland Clinic, 2008). A sprain is classified according to the degree of tearing in the ligament fibres. A *first-degree (mild) sprain* involves tears in only a few fibres, resulting in mild tenderness and minimal swelling. A *second-degree (moderate) sprain* is a partial disruption of the involved tissue, with more swelling and tenderness. A *third-degree (severe) sprain* is a complete tearing of the ligament in association with moderate to severe swelling. A gap in the muscle may be apparent or palpated through the skin if the muscle is torn. Because areas around joints are rich in nerve endings, the injury can be extremely painful.

A **strain** is an excessive stretching of a muscle, its fascial sheath, or a tendon. Most strains occur in the large muscle groups including the lower back, calf, and hamstrings (Cleveland Clinic, 2008). Strains may also be classified as *first-degree* (mild or slightly pulled muscle), *second-degree* (moderate or moderately torn muscle), and *third-degree* (severely torn or ruptured muscle).

The clinical manifestations of sprains and strains are similar and include pain, edema, decrease in function, and bruising. Pain aggravated by continued use is common. Edema develops in the injured area because of tiny hemorrhages within the disrupted tissues and the ensuing inflammatory response. Usually the patient will recount a history of traumatic injury, possibly of an inversion or twisting nature, or recent exercise activity.

Minor sprains and strains are usually self-limiting, with full function returning within 3 to 6 weeks. A severe sprain can result in an *avulsion fracture,* in which the ligament pulls loose a fragment of bone. Alternatively, the joint structure may become unstable and result in subluxation or dislocation. At the time of injury, *hemarthrosis* (bleeding into a joint space or cavity) or disruption of the synovial lining may occur.

Radiographs of the affected part are usually made to rule out a fracture or widening of the joint structure. However, some health care providers use an assessment protocol called the "Ottawa rules or guidelines" for the examination of an injured ankle or knee before ordering radiographs (Woods, 2011). These rules specify radiographic studies for a patient based on age, capability of flexion, location of tenderness, and ability to bear weight immediately after the injury or when examined. Surgical repair may be necessary if the injury is significant enough to produce severe disruption of ligamentous or muscle structures, fracture, or dislocation.

NURSING MANAGEMENT: SPRAINS AND STRAINS

Nursing Implementation

Health Promotion

Warming up exercises before exercising and vigorous activity followed by stretching significantly reduce the risk of sprains and strains. Strength, balance, and endurance exercises are also important. Strengthening exercises involve working against resistance. These exercises build up muscle strength and bone density. Balance exercises, which may overlap with some strengthening exercises, help to prevent falling. Endurance exercises should start at a low level of effort and progress gradually to moderate level of activities. Patients should try to build up to 30 minutes of moderate-intensity endurance activity on most or all days of the week (National Institute of Aging, 2011). Exercise instructions for these types of physical activity are available online at the National Institute of Aging Web site (see the Resources at the end of this chapter).

The use of elastic support bandages or adhesive tape wrapping before beginning a vigorous activity is thought to reduce the occurrence of sprains and is often used to support an injured joint postinjury while the athlete is competing and training. However,

EMERGENCY MANAGEMENT

Table 65-3 Acute Soft Tissue Injury

ETIOLOGY	ASSESSMENT FINDINGS	INTERVENTIONS
Falls	• Edema	***Initial***
Direct blows	• Ecchymosis/contusion	• Ensure airway, breathing, and circulation.
Crush injury	• Pain, tenderness	• Assess neurovascular status of involved limb.
Motor vehicle collisions	• Decreased sensation with severe edema	• Elevate involved limb.
Sports injuries	• Decreased pulse, coolness, and capillary refill >2 sec	• Apply compression bandage unless dislocation present.
	• Decreased movement	• Apply ice packs to affected area.
	• Pallor	• Immobilize affected extremity in the position found. Do not attempt to realign or reinsert protruding bones.
	• Shortening or rotation of extremity	• Anticipate radiographs of injured extremity.
	• Inability to bear weight when lower extremity involved	• Give analgesia as necessary.
	• Limited or decreased function with upper extremity involvement	• Administer tetanus prophylaxis if skin integrity breached or open fracture.
	• Muscle spasms	• Administer antibiotic prophylaxis for open fracture, large tissue defects, or mangled extremity injury.
		Ongoing Monitoring
		• Monitor for changes in neurovascular status.
		• Eliminate weight bearing when lower extremity involved.
		• Anticipate compartment pressure monitoring if neurovascular status changes and compartment syndrome suspected.

some health care providers do not support preventive wrapping or taping because it may predispose the athlete to injury.

■ Acute Intervention

If an injury occurs, the immediate care focuses on (1) rest and limitation of movement, (2) application of ice to the injured area, (3) compression of the involved extremity, (4) elevation of the extremity, and (5) analgesia, as necessary (Table 65-3).

Rest, ice, compression, and elevation have been found to decrease local inflammation and pain for most musculoskeletal injuries. Movement should be limited and the extremity rested as soon as pain is felt. Unless the injury is severe, prolonged rest is usually not necessary.

Cold *(cryotherapy)* in several forms can be used to produce hypothermia to the involved part. Physiological changes that occur in soft tissue as a result of the use of cold include vasoconstriction and reduction in the transmission and perception of nerve pain impulses. These changes result in analgesia and anaesthesia, reduction of muscle spasm without changes in muscular strength or endurance, and reduction of local metabolic requirements. Cold is most useful when applied immediately after the injury has occurred. Ice applications should not exceed 20 to 30 minutes per application and ice should not be applied directly to the skin.

Compression also helps limit swelling, which, if left uncontrolled, could lengthen healing time. An elastic compression bandage can be wrapped around the injured part. The bandage should be wrapped starting distally (at the point farthest from the midline of the body), and progressing proximally (toward the midline of the body), to encourage fluid return. The bandage is too tight if numbness is felt below the area of compression or if there is additional pain or swelling beyond the edge of the bandage. The bandage can be left in place for 30 minutes and then removed for 15 minutes. However, some elastic bandages are left on during training, athletic, and occupational activities.

The injured part should be elevated above the heart level to help mobilize excess fluid from the area and impede further edema. The injured part should be elevated even during sleep. Mild analgesics such as nonsteroidal anti-inflammatory drugs (NSAIDs) may be necessary to manage patient discomfort.

After the acute phase (usually lasting 24 to 48 hours), warm, moist heat can be applied to the affected part to reduce swelling and provide comfort. Heat applications should not exceed 20 to 30 minutes, allowing a "cool-down" time between applications. NSAIDs may be recommended to decrease edema and pain. The patient is encouraged to use the limb, provided that the joint is protected by means of casting, bracing, taping, or splinting. Movement of the joint improves circulation and resolution of the contusion and swelling.

■ Ambulatory and Home Care

With the exception of treatment in the emergency department following the injury, sprains and strains are treated in the outpatient setting. The patient should be instructed in the use of ice and elevation for 24 to 48 hours after the injury to reduce edema. The use of mild analgesics to promote comfort should be encouraged. Use of an elastic bandage may provide additional support during activity. The patient should learn proper measures of strengthening and conditioning to prevent reinjury.

The physiotherapist may help to provide pain relief by means of modalities such as ultrasonography. The therapist may also teach the patient exercises to perform for flexibility and strength.

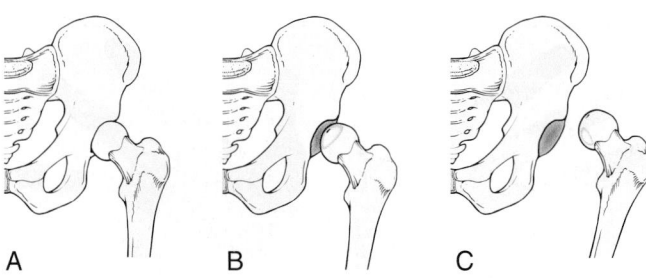

Figure 65-1 Soft tissue injury of the hip. **A,** Normal. **B,** Subluxation (partial dislocation). **C,** Dislocation.

Source: Redrawn from Price, S. A., & Wilson, L. M. (2003). *Pathophysiology: Clinical concepts of disease processes* (6th ed., p. 1029, Figure 68-8). St. Louis: Mosby.

Dislocation and Subluxation

A **dislocation** is a severe injury of the ligamentous structures that surround a joint. Dislocation results in the complete displacement or separation of the articular surfaces of the joint. A **subluxation** is a partial or incomplete displacement of the joint surface. The clinical manifestations of a subluxation are similar to those of a dislocation, but they are less severe. Treatment of subluxation is similar to that of a dislocation, but subluxation may require less healing time.

Dislocations characteristically result from overwhelming forces transmitted to the joint that cause a disruption of the soft tissue support structure surrounding the joint. The joints most frequently dislocated in the upper extremity include the thumb, elbow, and shoulder. In the lower extremity, the hip is vulnerable to dislocation occurring as a result of severe trauma, often associated with motor vehicle accidents (Figure 65-1). The patella may dislocate because of instability of the tendons, ligaments, and muscles surrounding the knee or a sharp blow to the kneecap. Dislocations may also be the result of a congenital anomaly or of a pathological origin. Patellar dislocation has an increased incidence in younger females because the quadriceps muscles are not as strong as in males (Steiner & Parker, 2009).

The most obvious clinical manifestation of a dislocation is deformity. For example, if a hip is dislocated, the limb is shorter and often found externally rotated on the affected side. Additional manifestations include local pain, tenderness, loss of function of the injured part, and swelling of the soft tissues in the region of the joint. The major complications of a dislocated joint are open joint injuries, intra-articular fractures, fractures, **avascular necrosis (AVN)** (bone cell death as a result of inadequate blood supply), and damage to adjacent neurovascular tissue.

Radiographic studies are performed to determine the extent of displacement of the involved structures. The joint may also be aspirated to determine the presence of hemarthrosis or fat cells. Fat cells in the aspirate indicate a probable intra-articular fracture.

NURSING AND COLLABORATIVE MANAGEMENT: DISLOCATION

A dislocation requires prompt attention and is considered an orthopedic emergency. The longer the joint remains unreduced,

the greater the possibility of AVN. Compartment syndrome may also occur after dislocation, and dislocation is often associated with significant vascular injury. The hip joint is particularly susceptible to AVN. Neurovascular assessment is critical (see Neurovascular Assessment on pp. 1825-1826).

The first goal of management is to realign the dislocated portion of the joint in its original anatomical position. This can be accomplished by a closed reduction, which may be performed under local or general anaesthesia or intravenous conscious sedation. Anaesthesia is often necessary to produce muscle relaxation so that the bones can be manipulated. In some situations, surgical open reduction may be necessary. After reduction, the extremity is usually immobilized by bracing, splinting, taping, or using a sling to allow the torn ligaments and capsular tissue time to heal.

Nursing management of subluxation or dislocation is directed toward relief of pain and support and protection of the injured joint. After the joint has been reduced and immobilized, motion is usually restricted. A carefully regulated rehabilitation program can prevent fracture instability and joint dysfunction. Gentle range of motion (ROM) may be started if the joint is stable and the affected joint is well supported. An exercise program slowly restores the joint to its original ROM without causing another dislocation. The patient should gradually return to normal activities.

A patient who has dislocated a joint may be at greater risk for repeated dislocations because of loose ligaments. Activity restrictions of the affected joint may be imposed to decrease the risk of repeatedly dislocating the joint.

Repetitive Strain Injury

Repetitive strain injury (RSI) and *cumulative trauma disorder* are terms used to describe injuries resulting from prolonged force or repetitive movements and awkward postures. RSI is also reported as repetitive trauma disorder, nontraumatic musculoskeletal injury, overuse syndrome (sports medicine), regional musculoskeletal disorder, work-related musculoskeletal disorder, and "nintendinitis" (video game overindulgence). The exact cause of these disorders is unknown. There are no specific diagnostic tests, and diagnosis is often difficult.

Repeated movements strain tendons, ligaments, and muscles, causing tiny tears that become inflamed. If the tissues are not given time to heal properly, scarring can occur. Blood vessels of the arms and hands may become constricted, depriving tissues of vital nutrients and causing an accumulation of lactic acid. Without intervention, tendons and muscles can deteriorate and nerves can become hypersensitive. At this point, even the slightest movement can cause pain.

In 2000 to 2001, 10% of Canadians aged 20 or older, an estimated 2.3 million people, reported having had an RSI owing to work-related activities in the past 12 months (Tjepkema, 2003). In Canada, RSI affects primarily the upper body: 25% occur in the neck or shoulder, 23% in the wrist or hand, 19% in the back, and 16% in the elbow or lower arm (Statistics Canada, 2003).

In addition to the repetitive movements, other factors related to RSI include poor posture and positioning, poor work space ergonomics, badly designed workplace equipment (e.g., computer keyboard), and repetitive lifting of heavy workloads without sufficient muscle rest. The result may be inflammation, swelling,

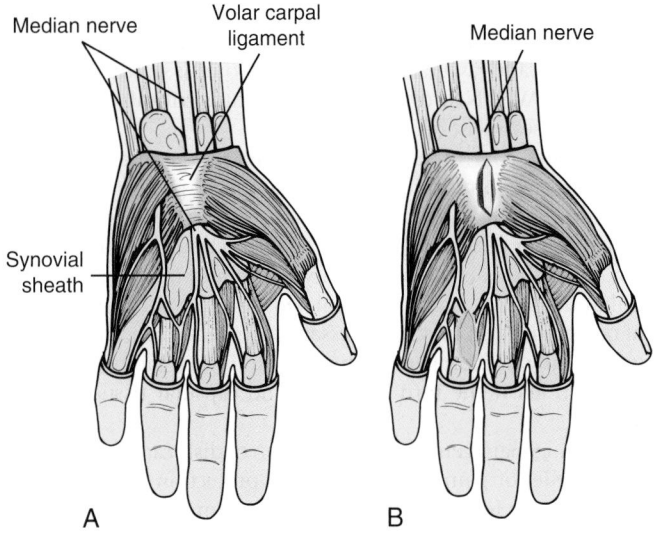

Figure 65-2 A, Wrist structures involved in carpal tunnel syndrome. **B,** Decompression of median nerve by incision through the transverse carpal ligament.

Source: Thompson, J. M., McFarland, G. K., Hirsch, J. E., & Tucker, S. M. (2002). *Mosby's clinical nursing* (5th ed.). St. Louis: Mosby.

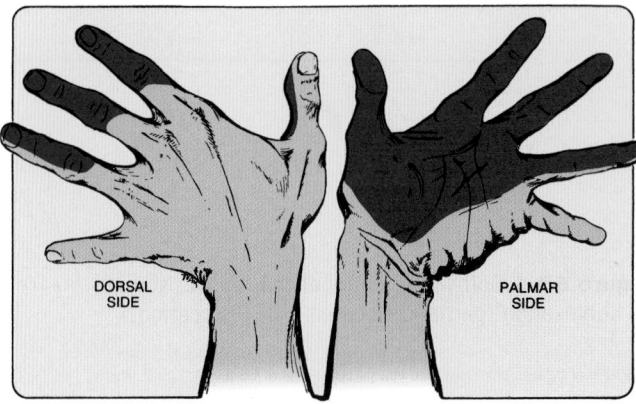

Figure 65-3 Median nerve distribution. *Shaded areas* depict the locations of pain in carpal tunnel syndrome.

Source: *http://www.pinnaclesystems.com*; also in Maher, A. B., Salmond, S. W., & Pellino, T. A. (Eds.). (2002). *Orthopaedic nursing* (3rd ed.). St. Louis: Saunders.

and pain in the muscles, tendons, and nerves of the neck, shoulder, forearm, and hand. Symptoms of RSI include pain, weakness, numbness, or impairment of motor function. Persons most often affected by RSI include musicians, dancers, butchers, grocery clerks, vibratory tool workers, and those frequently using a computer mouse and keyboard.

Competitive athletes and poorly trained athletes may also develop RSI. Swimming, overhead throwing (e.g., baseball), weightlifting, gymnastics, dancing, tennis, skiing, kicking sports (e.g., soccer), and horseback riding require repetitive motion, and overtraining compounds the effects of RSI.

RSI can often be prevented through education and ergonomics (consideration of the interaction of humans and their work environment). A few ergonomic considerations for computer use include keeping the hips and knees flexed to 90 degrees with the feet flat, keeping the wrist straight to type, having the top of the monitor even with the forehead, and taking at least hourly stretch breaks. Once diagnosed, the treatment of RSI consists of identifying precipitating activity, modification of equipment or activity, pain management including heat/cold application, NSAIDs, rest, physiotherapy for strengthening and conditioning exercises, and lifestyle changes.

Carpal Tunnel Syndrome

Carpal tunnel syndrome (CTS) is a condition caused by compression of the median nerve, which enters the hand through the narrow confines of the carpal tunnel (Figure 65-2). The carpal tunnel is formed by ligaments and bones in the wrist. CTS is the most common compression neuropathy in the upper extremity (Walker, 2010). This syndrome is associated with hobbies or occupations that require continuous wrist movement (e.g., butchers, seamstresses, musicians, painters, carpenters, computer operators). This condition often is caused by pressure from trauma or edema caused by inflammation of a tendon (tenosynovitis), neoplasm, rheumatoid arthritis (RA), or soft tissue masses such as

ganglia. Hormones may be involved as initial manifestations often occur during the premenstrual period, pregnancy, and menopause. Persons with diabetes mellitus and hypothyroidism have a higher incidence of CTS. Women are more likely than men to develop CTS, possibly owing to a smaller carpal tunnel.

The clinical manifestations of CTS are weakness (especially of the thumb), burning pain (causalgia) and numbness, or impaired sensation in the distribution of the median nerve and clumsiness in performing fine hand movements (Scanlon & Maffei, 2009). Numbness and tingling may be present, which awaken the patient at night. Shaking the hands will often relieve these symptoms.

Physical signs of CTS include Tinel's sign and Phalen's sign. *Tinel's sign* can be elicited by tapping over the median nerve as it passes through the carpal tunnel in the wrist (Figure 65-3). A positive response is a sensation of tingling in the distribution of the median nerve over the hand. *Phalen's sign* can be elicited by allowing the wrists to fall freely into maximum flexion and maintaining the position for longer than 60 seconds. A positive response is a sensation of tingling in the distribution of the median nerve over the hand. In late stages, there is atrophy of the thenar muscles around the base of the thumb, resulting in recurrent pain and eventual dysfunction of the hand.

NURSING AND COLLABORATIVE MANAGEMENT: CARPAL TUNNEL SYNDROME

Prevention of CTS involves educating employees and employers to identify risk factors. Adaptive devices such as wrist splints may be worn to hold the wrist in slight extension to relieve pressure on the median nerve. Special keyboard pads and mice that help prevent repetitive pressure on the median nerve are available for computer users. Other ergonomic changes include workstation modifications, change in body positions, and frequent breaks from work-related activities.

Collaborative care of the patient with CTS is directed toward relieving the underlying cause of the nerve compression. The early symptoms associated with CTS can usually be relieved by stopping the aggravating movement and by placing the hand and wrist at rest by immobilizing them in a hand splint. Splints worn at night help keep the wrist in a neutral position and may reduce night pain and numbness. Injection of a corticosteroid drug directly into the carpal tunnel may provide short-term relief. Because CTS may result in impaired sensation, the patients should be instructed to avoid hazards such as extreme heat and cold because of the risk of thermal injury. The patient may be required to consider temporary occupational changes because of discomfort and sensory and functional changes.

Carpal tunnel release is generally recommended if symptoms last for more than 6 months. Surgery involves dividing the transverse carpal ligament (the band of tissue around the wrist) to reduce pressure on the median nerve (Huisstede et al., 2010) (see Figure 65-2, B). Surgery is done under local anaesthesia and does not require an overnight hospital stay. The types of carpal tunnel release surgery include open release and endoscopic surgery. In *open release surgery*, an incision is made in the wrist and then the carpal ligament is cut to enlarge the carpal tunnel. *Endoscopic carpal tunnel release* is performed through one or more small puncture incisions in the wrist and palm; a camera is attached to a tube, and the carpal ligament is cut. The endoscopic approach may allow faster functional recovery and less postoperative discomfort than traditional open release surgery.

Although symptoms may be relieved immediately after surgery, full recovery may take months. After surgery, assess the neurovascular status of the hand before discharge. Instruct the patient about wound care and the appropriate assessments to perform at home.

Rotator Cuff Injury

The rotator cuff is a complex of four muscles in the shoulder: the supraspinatus, infraspinatus, teres minor, and subscapularis muscles. These muscles act to stabilize the humeral head in the glenoid fossa while assisting with ROM of the shoulder joint and rotation of the humerus. Degenerative changes of the rotator cuff are associated with normal aging.

A tear in the rotator cuff may occur as a gradual, degenerative process resulting from aging, repetitive stress (especially overhead arm motions), or injury to the shoulder while falling. The rotator cuff can tear as a result of sudden adduction forces applied to the cuff while the arm is held in abduction. In sports, repetitive overhead motions, such as in swimming, racquet sports (tennis, racquetball), football, and baseball (especially pitching), are often activities that initiate injury. Other causative factors include (1) falling onto an outstretched arm and hand, (2) a blow to the upper arm, (3) heavy lifting, or (4) repetitive work motions.

Manifestations of a rotator cuff injury include shoulder weakness and pain and decreased ROM. The patient usually experiences severe pain when the arm is abducted between 60 and 120 degrees (the painful arc). The *drop arm test*, in which the arm falls suddenly after the patient is asked to slowly lower the arm to the side after it has been abducted 90 degrees, is another sign of rotator cuff injury. A radiograph alone is usually not beneficial in the diagnosis of a rotator cuff injury. A tear can be confirmed by magnetic resonance imaging (MRI).

The goal of treatment emphasizes maintaining passive ROM and the return of abduction strength. The patient with a partial tear or cuff inflammation may be treated conservatively with rest, ice and heat, NSAIDs, corticosteroid injections into the joint, and physiotherapy (Smith & Smith, 2010). If the patient does not respond to conservative treatment in 3 to 6 months or if a complete tear is present, a surgical repair may be necessary. Most surgical repairs are performed through an arthroscope (Yadav, Nho, Romeo, & Macgillivray, 2009). If an extensive tear is present, *acromioplasty* (surgical removal of part of the acromion to relieve compression of the rotator cuff during movement) may be necessary. A sling or, more commonly, a shoulder immobilizer may be used immediately after surgery. However, the shoulder should not be immobilized for too long a period because "frozen" shoulder or arthrofibrosis may occur. Pendulum exercises and physiotherapy begin the first postoperative day.

Meniscus Injury

The menisci are crescent-shaped pieces of fibrocartilage in the knee. Menisci are also found in other joints. Meniscus injuries are closely associated with ligament sprains commonly occurring in athletes engaged in sports such as basketball, rugby, football, soccer, and hockey. These activities produce rotational stress when the knee is in varying degrees of flexion and the foot is planted or fixed. A blow to the knee can cause the meniscus to be sheared between the femoral condyles and the tibial plateau, resulting in a torn meniscus. (The knee joint is shown in Figure 65-4.) Individuals who work in occupations that require squatting or kneeling and older adults may be at higher risk for meniscus injuries.

Meniscus injuries alone do not usually cause significant edema because most of the cartilage is avascular. However, an acutely torn meniscus may be suspected when localized tenderness, pain, and effusion are noted (Figure 65-5). Pain is elicited by flexion, internal rotation, and then extension of the knee (called *McMurray's test*). The usual clinical picture is a feeling by the patient that the knee is unstable and a report that the knee

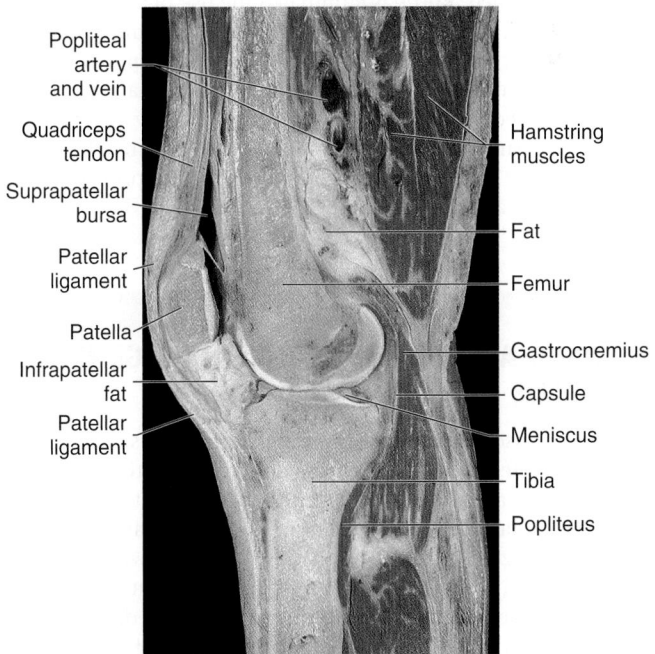

Figure 65-4 Sagittal section through the knee joint.

Source: Patton, K. T., & Thibodeau, G. A. (2010). *Anatomy and physiology* (7th ed., p. 275, Figure 9-11). St. Louis: Mosby.

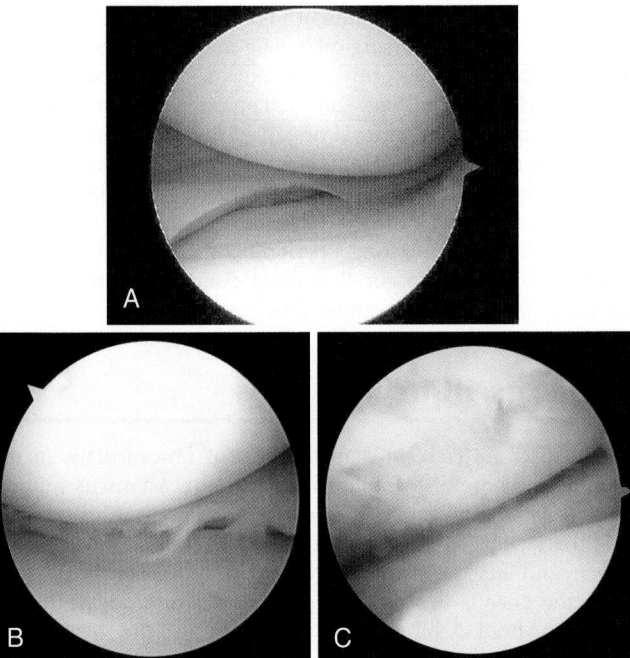

Figure 65-5 Arthroscopic views of the meniscus. **A,** Normal meniscus. **B,** Torn meniscus. **C,** Surgically repaired meniscus.

Source: **A,** David Lintner, MD, Houston. Retrieved from *http://www.drlintner.com*; **B** and **C,** Courtesy Peter Bonner, San Antonio.

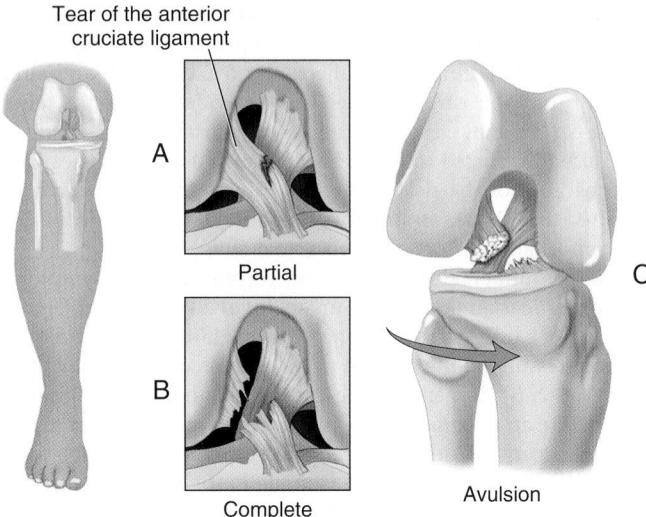

Figure 65-6 Anterior cruciate ligament injury. **A,** Partial tear. **B,** Complete tear. **C,** Avulsion

Figure 65-5). Meniscal surgery is performed by arthroscopy. Pain relief may include NSAIDs or other analgesics. Rehabilitation starts soon after surgery, including quadriceps- and hamstring-strengthening exercises and ROM. When the patient's strength is back to its preinjury level, normal activities may be resumed.

may "click," "pop," "lock," or "give way." Quadriceps atrophy may be evident if the injury has been present for some time. Traumatic arthritis may occur from repeated meniscal injury and chronic inflammation.

MRI is beneficial in confirming the diagnosis before arthroscopy is performed. MRI has eliminated the use of an arthrogram as a diagnostic tool in many cases (Abate, 2008). Surgery may be indicated for a torn meniscus. Meniscal preservation, where possible, is very important because the menisci have an important role in the knee joint and their removal significantly increases the risk of osteoarthritis (OA) (Getgood & Robertson, 2010). The degree of knee pain and dysfunction, occupation, sport activities, and age may affect the patient's decision to have or postpone surgery.

NURSING AND COLLABORATIVE MANAGEMENT: MENISCUS INJURY

Because meniscal injuries are commonly caused by sports-related activity, athletes should be taught to do warm-up activities. Examination of the acutely injured knee should occur within 24 hours of injury. Initial care of this type of injury involves application of ice, immobilization, and partial weight bearing with crutches. Most meniscal injuries are treated in an outpatient setting. Use of a knee brace or immobilizer during the first few days after the injury protects the knee and offers some pain relief.

After acute pain has decreased, physiotherapy can help the patient regain knee flexion and muscle strength to assist the patient to reach full functioning. Surgical repair or excision of part of the meniscus (meniscectomy) may be necessary (see

Anterior Cruciate Ligament Injury

Knee injuries account for over 50% of all sport injuries. The most commonly injured knee ligament is the anterior cruciate ligament (ACL) (Rishiraj et al., 2009). ACL injuries usually occur from noncontact when the athlete pivots, lands from a jump, or slows down when running. Patients often report coming down on the knee, twisting, and hearing a pop, followed by acute knee pain and swelling. Athletes usually cannot continue playing, and the knee may feel unstable. An injury to the ACL can result in a partial tear, a complete tear, or an *avulsion* (tearing away) from the bone attachments that form the knee (Figure 65-6).

Examination of the knee with an ACL tear may produce a positive *Lachman's test.* This test is performed by flexing the knee 15 to 30 degrees and pulling the tibia forward while the femur is stabilized. The test is considered positive for an ACL tear if there is forward motion of the tibia with the feeling of a soft or indistinct end point (Marx, Hockberger & Walls, 2009). Radiographs and MRI are often used to diagnose coexisting conditions including a fracture, meniscus tearing, and collateral ligament injuries.

NURSING AND COLLABORATIVE MANAGEMENT ACL INJURY

Conservative treatment for an intact ACL injury includes rest, ice, NSAIDs, elevation, and ambulation as tolerated with crutches. If there is a tight, painful effusion, it may be aspirated.

A knee immobilizer or hinged knee brace may be helpful in supporting the knee. Physiotherapy often assists the patient in maintaining knee joint motion and muscle tone. Reconstructive surgery is usually recommended in physically active patients who have sustained severe injury to the ligament and meniscus. In reconstruction, the torn ACL tissue is removed and replaced with autologous or allograft tissue. ROM is encouraged soon after surgery and the knee is placed in a brace or immobilizer. Rehabilitation with physiotherapy is critical, with progressive weight bearing determined by the degree of surgical repair. A safe return to the patient's prior level of physical functioning may take 6 to 8 months. Persons with a prior history of ACL injury have a higher risk of developing knee OA later in life (Murray, 2009).

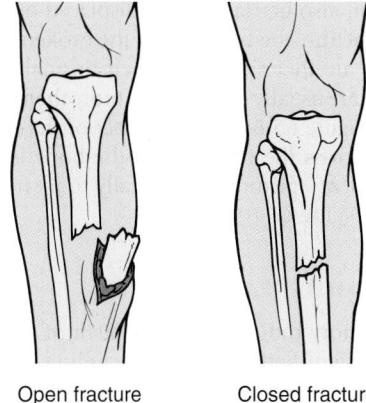

Open fracture   Closed fracture

Figure 65-7 Fracture classification according to communication with the external environment.

Bursitis

Bursae are closed sacs that are lined with synovial membrane and contain a small amount of synovial fluid. They are located at sites of friction, such as between tendons and bones and near the joints. **Bursitis** (inflammation of a bursa) results from repeated or excessive trauma or friction, gout, RA, or infection.

The primary clinical manifestations of bursitis are warmth, pain, swelling, and limited ROM in the affected part. Sites at which bursitis commonly occurs include the hand, knee, greater trochanter of the hip, shoulder, and elbow. Improper body mechanics, repetitive kneeling (e.g., carpet layers, coal miners, and gardeners), jogging in worn-out shoes, and prolonged sitting with crossed legs are common precipitating activities.

Attempts are made to determine and correct the cause of the bursitis. Rest is often the only treatment needed. Icing the area will decrease pain and may reduce inflammation. The affected part may be immobilized in a compression dressing or splint. NSAIDs may be used to reduce inflammation and pain. Aspiration of the bursal fluid and intra-articular injection of a corticosteroid may be necessary. If the bursal wall has become thickened and continues to interfere with normal joint function, surgical excision (bursectomy) may be necessary. Septic bursae usually require surgical incision and drainage.

Fractures

Classification

A **fracture** is a disruption or break in the continuity of the structure of bone. Traumatic injuries account for the majority of fractures, although some fractures are secondary to a disease process (pathological fractures from cancer or osteoporosis).

Fractures can be classified as *open* (formerly called compound) or *closed* (formerly called simple) depending on communication or noncommunication with the external environment (Figure 65-7). In an open fracture, the skin is broken, exposing the bone and causing soft tissue injury. In a closed fracture, the skin has not been ruptured and remains intact. Fractures can also be classified as complete or incomplete. Fractures are termed *complete* if the break is completely through the bone and described as *incomplete* if the fracture occurs partly across a bone shaft but the bone is still in one piece. An incomplete fracture is often the result of bending or crushing forces applied to a bone.

Fractures are also described and classified according to the direction of the fracture line. Types include linear, oblique, transverse, longitudinal, and spiral fractures (Figure 65-8).

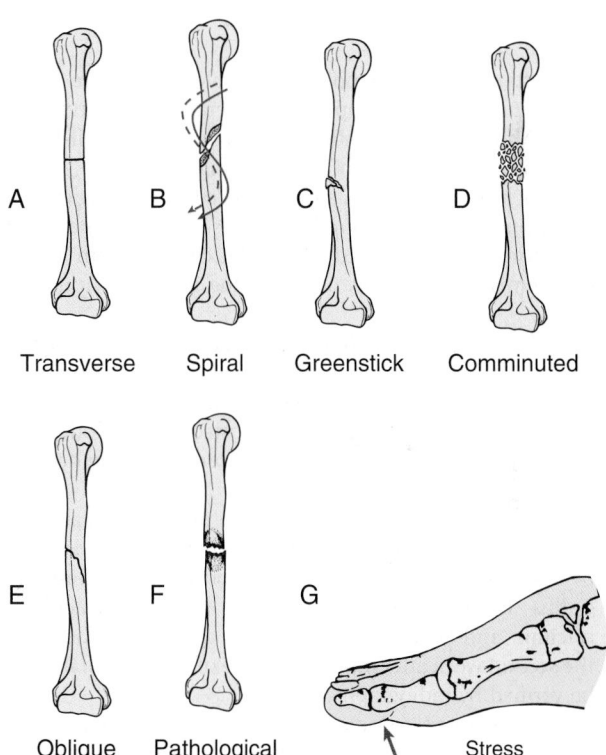

Transverse   Spiral   Greenstick   Comminuted

Oblique   Pathological   Stress

Figure 65-8 Types of fractures. **A,** Transverse fracture is a fracture in which the line of the fracture extends across the bone shaft at a right angle to the longitudinal axis. **B,** Spiral fracture is a fracture in which the line of the fracture extends in a spiral direction along the shaft of the bone. **C,** Greenstick fracture is an incomplete fracture with one side splintered and the other side bent. **D,** Comminuted fracture is a fracture with more than two fragments. The smaller fragments appear to be floating. **E,** Oblique fracture is a fracture in which the line of the fracture extends in an oblique direction. **F,** Pathological fracture is a spontaneous fracture at the site of a bone disease. **G,** Stress fracture is a fracture that occurs in normal or abnormal bone that is subject to repeated stress, such as from jogging or running.

Fractures can also be classified as displaced or nondisplaced. In a *displaced* fracture, the two ends of the broken bone are separated from one another and out of their normal positions. Displaced fractures are usually *comminuted* (more than two fragments) or *oblique* (see Figure 65-8). In a *nondisplaced fracture,* the periosteum is intact across the fracture and the bone is still in alignment. *Nondisplaced* fractures are usually transverse, spiral, or greenstick (see Figure 65-8).

Clinical Manifestations

The patient's history indicates a mechanism of injury associated with numerous signs and symptoms, including immediate localized pain, decreased function, and inability to bear weight on or use the affected part (Table 65-4). The patient guards and protects the extremity against movement. Obvious bone deformity may not be present. If a fracture is suspected, the extremity is immobilized in the position in which it is found. Unnecessary movement increases soft tissue damage and may convert a closed fracture to an open fracture or create further injury to adjacent neurovascular structures.

Fracture Healing

It is important to understand the principles of fracture healing (Figure 65-9) to provide appropriate therapeutic interventions. Bone goes through a remarkable reparative process of self-healing (termed *union*) that occurs in the following stages:

1. *Fracture hematoma.* When a fracture occurs, bleeding creates a hematoma, which surrounds the ends of the fragments. The hematoma is extravasated blood that changes from a liquid to a semisolid clot. This occurs in the initial 72 hours after injury.
2. *Granulation tissue.* During this stage, active phagocytosis absorbs the products of local necrosis. The hematoma converts to granulation tissue. Granulation tissue (consisting of new blood vessels, fibroblasts, and osteoblasts) produces the basis for new bone substance called *osteoid* during days 3 to 14 after injury.
3. *Callus formation.* As minerals (calcium, phosphorus, and magnesium) are deposited in the osteoid, an unorganized network of bone is formed that is woven about the fracture parts. Callus is primarily composed of cartilage, osteoblasts, calcium, and phosphorus. It usually appears by the end of the second week after injury. Evidence of callus formation can be verified by radiography.
4. *Ossification.* Ossification of the callus occurs from 3 weeks to 6 months after the fracture and continues until the fracture has healed. Callus ossification is sufficient to prevent movement at the fracture site when the bones are gently stressed. However, the fracture is still evident on a radiograph. During this stage of *clinical union,* the patient may be allowed limited mobility or the cast may be removed.
5. *Consolidation.* As callus continues to develop, the distance between bone fragments diminishes and eventually closes. During this stage, ossification continues. It can be equated with radiologic union. *Radiologic union* occurs when there is radiographic evidence of complete bony union. This phase can occur up to a year following injury.
6. *Remodelling.* Excess bone tissue is reabsorbed in the final stage of bone healing, and union is completed. Gradual return of the injured bone to its preinjury structural strength and shape occurs. Bone remodels in response to physical loading stress

or Wolf 's law (Boyd, Benjamin, & Asplund, 2009). Weight bearing is gradually introduced. New bone is deposited in sites subjected to stress and resorbed at areas where there is little stress. Radiological union is present.

Many factors, such as age, initial displacement of the fracture, site of the fracture, blood supply to the area, immobilization, implants, infection, and hormones, influence the time required for fracture healing to be complete. Fracture healing may not occur in the expected time *(delayed union)* or may not occur at all *(nonunion).* The ossification process is arrested by causes such as

PATIENT & CAREGIVER TEACHING GUIDE

Table 65-4 Clinical Manifestations of Fracture

MANIFESTATION	SIGNIFICANCE
Edema and Swelling	
Disruption and penetration of bone through skin or soft tissues, or bleeding into surrounding tissues	Unchecked bleeding, swelling, and edema in closed space can occlude circulation and damage nerves (i.e., risk of compartment syndrome).
Pain and Tenderness	
Muscle spasm as a result of involuntary reflex action of muscle, direct tissue trauma, increased pressure on nerves, movement of fracture parts	Pain and tenderness encourage splinting of musculature around the fracture with reduction in motion of injured area.
Muscle Spasm	
Irritation of tissues and protective response to injury and fracture	Muscle spasms may displace nondisplaced fracture or prevent it from reducing spontaneously.
Deformity	
Abnormal position of extremity or part as result of original forces of injury and action of muscles pulling fragment into abnormal position; seen as a loss of normal bony contours	Deformity is cardinal sign of fracture; if uncorrected, it may result in problems with bony union and restoration of function of injured part.
Ecchymosis or Contusion	
Discoloration of skin as a result of extravasation of blood in subcutaneous tissues	Ecchymosis may appear immediately after injury and may appear distal to injury. Reassure patient that process is normal and that discoloration will eventually resolve.
Loss of Function	
Disruption of bone or joint, preventing functional use of limb/part	Fracture must be managed properly to ensure restoration of function to limb/part.
Crepitation	
Grating or crunching together of bony fragments, producing palpable or audible crunching or popping sensation	Crepitation may increase chance for nonunion if bone ends are allowed to move excessively. Micromovement of bone-end fragments (postfracture) assists in osteogenesis (new bone growth).

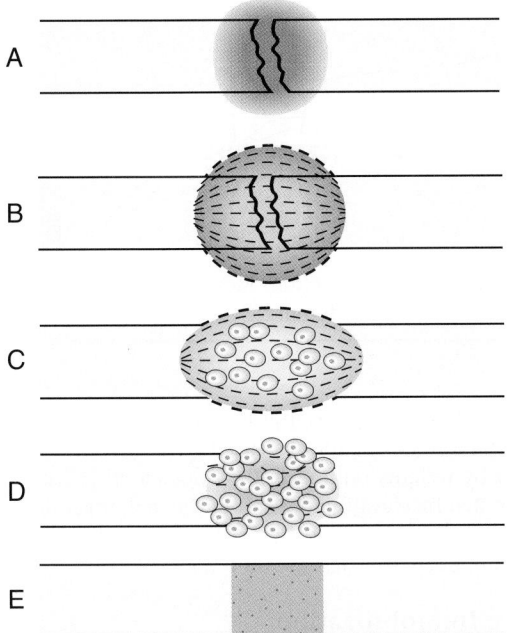

Figure 65-9 Bone healing (schematic representation). **A,** Bleeding at broken ends of the bone with subsequent hematoma formation. **B,** Organization of hematoma into fibrous network. **C,** Invasion of osteoblasts, lengthening of collagen strands, and deposition of calcium. **D,** Callus formation: new bone is built up as osteoclasts destroy dead bone. **E,** Remodelling is accomplished as excess callus is reabsorbed and trabecular bone is laid down.

Source: Monahan, F. D., Neighbors, M., Sands, J. K., Marek, J. F., & Green, C. J. (2007). *Phipps' medical-surgical nursing: Health and illness perspectives* (8th ed., p. 1497, Figure 51-5). St. Louis: Mosby.

Table 65-5 Complications of Fracture Healing	
PROBLEM	**DESCRIPTION**
Delayed union	Fracture healing progresses more slowly than expected; healing eventually occurs.
Nonunion	Fracture fails to heal properly despite treatment; no radiographic evidence of callus formation.
Malunion	Fracture heals in expected time but in unsatisfactory position, possibly resulting in deformity or dysfunction.
Angulation	Fracture heals in abnormal position in relation to midline of structure (type of malunion).
Pseudoarthrosis	Type of nonunion occurring at fracture site in which a false joint is formed with abnormal movement at site.
Refracture	New fracture occurs at original fracture site.
Myositis ossificans	Deposition of calcium in muscle tissue at the site of significant blunt muscle trauma or repeated muscle injury.

COLLABORATIVE CARE

Table 65-6 Fractures		
Diagnostic		**Fracture Immobilization**
• History and physical examination		• Casting or splinting
• Radiographs		• Traction
• CT scan, MRI		• External fixation
		• Internal fixation
Collaborative Therapy		**Open Fractures**
Fracture Reduction		• Surgical debridement and irrigation
• Manipulation		• Tetanus and diphtheria immunization
• Closed reduction		
• Skin traction		• Prophylactic antibiotic therapy
• Skeletal traction		• Immobilization
• Open reduction with internal fixation (ORIF)		

CT, computed tomography; *MRI,* magnetic resonance imaging.

inadequate reduction and immobilization, excess movement of the fracture fragments, infection, poor nutrition, and systemic disease. Healing time for fractures increases with age. For example, an uncomplicated midshaft fracture of the femur heals in 3 weeks in a newborn and in 20 weeks in an adult. Table 65-5 summarizes complications of fracture healing.

Electrical stimulation and pulsed electromagnetic fields can be used to stimulate bone healing in some situations of nonunion or delayed union. The electric current acts by modifying cell mechanisms, causing bone remodelling. The underlying mechanism for electrically induced bone remodelling remains unknown. It is thought to be related to negative electrical fields attracting positive ions such as calcium. The electrodes are placed over the patient's skin or cast and are used 10 to 12 hours each day, usually while the patient is sleeping.

Collaborative Care

The overall goals of fracture treatment are (1) anatomical realignment of bone fragments (reduction), (2) immobilization to maintain realignment, and (3) restoration of normal or near-normal function of the injured part. Table 65-6 summarizes the collaborative care of fractures.

Fracture Reduction

Closed Reduction. Closed reduction is a nonsurgical, manual realignment of bone fragments to their previous anatomical position. Traction and countertraction are manually applied to the bone fragments to restore position, length, and alignment. Closed reduction is usually performed with the patient under local or general anaesthesia. After reduction, traction, casting, external fixation, splints, or orthoses (braces) immobilize the injured part to maintain alignment until healing occurs.

Open Reduction. Open reduction is the correction of bone alignment through a surgical incision. It often includes internal fixation of the fracture with the use of wire, screws, pins, plates, intramedullary rods, or nails. The type and the location of the fracture, the age of the patient, and presence of concurrent disease, as well as the result of attempted closed reduction by means of traction, may influence the decision to use open reduction. The chief disadvantages of this form of fracture management are the possibility of infection, the complications associated with anaesthesia, and the effect of pre-existing medical conditions (e.g., diabetes) in the patient.

If open reduction with internal fixation (ORIF) is used for intra-articular fractures (involving joint surfaces), early initiation of active ROM of the joint is indicated. Machines that provide continuous passive motion to various joints (e.g., knee, shoulder) are now available. Use of these machines can help prevent extra-articular and intra-articular adhesions and result in faster reconstruction of the subchondral (beneath cartilage) bone plate, more rapid healing of the articular cartilage, and possibly decreased incidence of later post-traumatic arthritis. ORIF facilitates early ambulation, which decreases the risk of complications related to prolonged immobility, and promotes fracture healing with gradually increasing increments of stress placed on the affected joint and soft tissue structures.

Traction. **Traction** is the application of a pulling force to an injured or diseased part of the body or extremity while countertraction pulls in the opposite direction. Traction is not used as frequently in adults as it is in children. These days, treatments for fractures and other orthopedic problems in the adult are designed to keep patients more mobile and to discharge them from the hospital faster with fewer complications. Treatment with casts or traction is often preferred over surgery in children to avoid damage to the growth plate.

The purpose of any traction is to (1) prevent or reduce pain and muscle spasm associated with low back pain or cervical sprain (e.g., whiplash), (2) immobilize a joint or part of the body, (3) reduce a fracture or dislocation, and (4) treat a pathological joint condition (e.g., tumour, infection). Traction is also indicated to (1) provide immobilization to prevent soft tissue damage, (2) promote active and passive exercise, (3) expand a joint space during arthroscopic procedures, and (4) expand a joint space before major joint reconstruction.

Traction devices apply a pulling force on a fractured extremity to attain realignment while countertraction pulls in the opposite direction. The two most common types of traction are skin traction and skeletal traction. *Skin traction* is generally used for short-term treatment (48 to 72 hours) until skeletal traction or surgery is possible. Tape, boots, or splints are applied directly to the skin to maintain alignment, assist in reduction, and help diminish muscle spasms in the injured extremity. The traction weights are usually limited to 2.3 to 4.5 kg. Pelvic or cervical skin traction may require heavier weights applied intermittently.

Skeletal traction, generally in place for longer periods than skin traction, is used to align injured bones and joints or to treat joint contractures and congenital hip dysplasia. It provides a long-term pull that keeps the injured bones and joints aligned. To apply skeletal traction, the physician inserts a pin or wire into the bone, either partially or completely, to align and immobilize the injured body part. Weight for skeletal traction ranges from 2 to 20 kg. The use of too much weight can result in delayed union or nonunion. The major disadvantages of skeletal traction are risk for infection in the area of the bone where the skeletal pin has been inserted and the consequences of prolonged immobility.

When traction is used to treat fractures, the forces are usually exerted on the distal fragment to obtain alignment with the proximal fragment. Several types of traction can be used for this purpose. One of the more common types is Buck's traction (Figure 65-10). Fracture alignment depends on the correct positioning and alignment of the patient while the traction forces remain constant. For extremity traction to be effective, forces

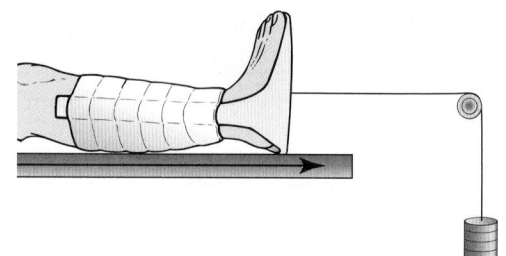

Figure 65-10 Buck's traction. Most commonly used for fractures of the hip and femur.

must be pulling in the opposite direction (countertraction). Countertraction is commonly supplied by the patient's body weight or by weights pulling in the opposite direction and may be augmented by elevating the end of the bed. It is imperative to maintain traction continuously and keep the weights off the floor and moving freely through the pulleys.

Fracture Immobilization

Casts. A cast is a temporary circumferential immobilization device (Boyd et al., 2009). Casting is a common treatment following closed reduction. It allows the patient to perform many normal activities of daily living while providing sufficient immobilization to ensure stability. Cast materials are natural (plaster of Paris) or synthetic acrylic; fibreglass-free, latex-free polymer; or a hybrid of materials. A cast generally incorporates the joints above and below a fracture. Immobilization above and below a joint restricts tendinoligamentous movement, thus assisting with joint stabilization while the fracture heals.

After bony prominences have been padded, plaster of Paris casting material is immersed in water. Then it is wrapped and moulded around the affected part. The number of layers of plaster bandage and the technique of application determine the strength of the cast. The plaster sets within 15 minutes, so the patient may move around without difficulty. However, it is not strong enough for weight bearing until about 24 to 72 hours after application.

A fresh plaster cast should never be covered with a blanket because air cannot circulate and heat builds up in the cast. During the drying period, the cast should be kept dry and clean, and direct pressure should be avoided. Handle the cast gently with an open palm to avoid denting the cast. Once the cast is thoroughly dry, the edges may have to be *petalled* to prevent skin irritation from rough edges and to prevent plaster of Paris debris from falling into the cast and causing irritation or pressure necrosis. Several strips (petals) of tape are placed by the health care provider over the rough areas to ensure a smooth cast edge.

Casts made of fibreglass are being used more than plaster because they are lightweight, stronger, relatively waterproof, stronger and faster-drying than plaster, porous (less risk of skin problems), and allow for almost immediate mobilization (Satryb, Wilson, & Patterson, 2011). Synthetic casting materials (thermolabile plastic, thermoplastic resins, polyurethane, and fibreglass) are activated by submersion in cool or tepid water. Then they are moulded to fit the torso or the extremity.

Types of Casts. Immobilization of an acute fracture or soft tissue injury of the upper extremity is often accomplished by use of (1) the sugar-tong splint, (2) the posterior splint, (3) the short arm cast, or (4) the long arm cast (Figure 65-11). The *sugar-tong splint* is typically used for acute wrist injuries or injuries that may

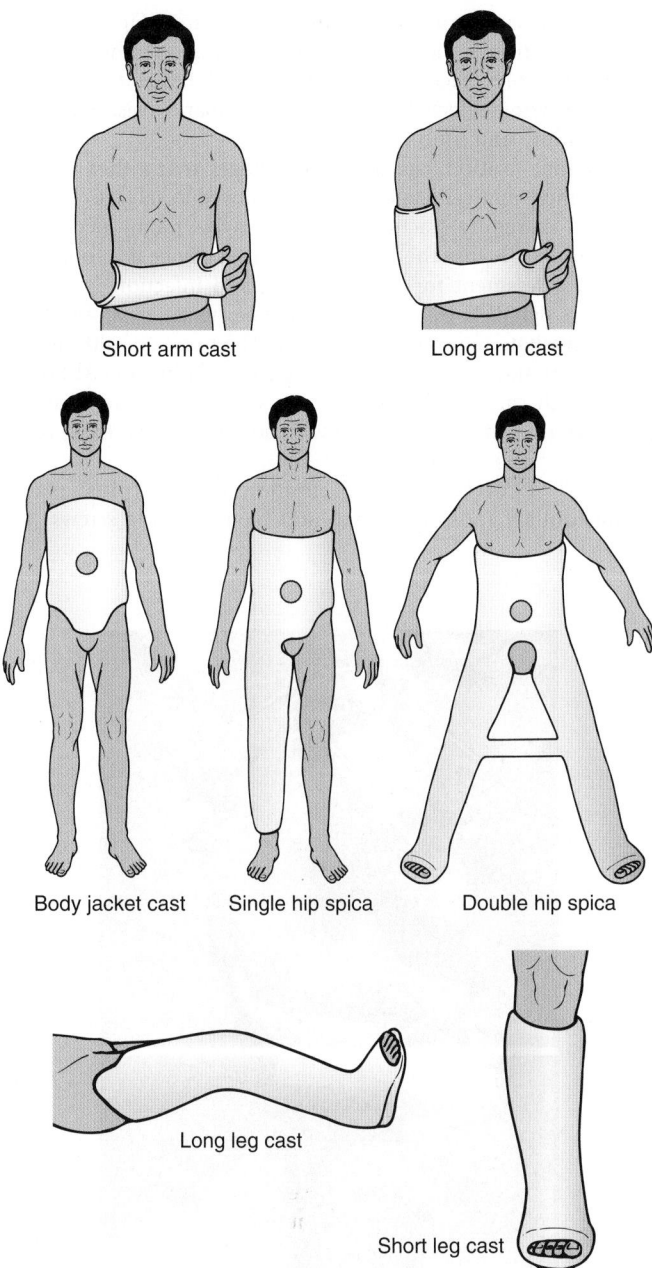

Figure 65-11 Common types of casts.

The *long arm cast* is commonly used for stable forearm or elbow fractures and unstable wrist fractures. It is similar to the short arm cast but extends to the proximal humerus, restricting motion in the wrist and the elbow. Nursing measures should be directed toward supporting the extremity and reducing the effects of edema by maintaining extremity elevation with a sling. However, when a hanging arm cast is used for a proximal humerus fracture, elevation or a supportive sling is contraindicated because hanging provides traction and maintains fracture alignment.

When a sling is used, the nurse must ensure that the axillary area is well padded to prevent skin excoriation and maceration associated with direct skin-to-skin contact. Placement of the sling should not put undue pressure on the posterior neck. Movement of the fingers (unless contraindicated) should be encouraged to enhance the pumping action of vascular and soft tissue structures to decrease edema. The nurse should also encourage the patient to actively move nonimmobilized joints of the upper extremity to prevent stiffness and contractures.

The *body jacket cast* or brace is often used for immobilization and support for stable spine injuries of the thoracic or lumbar spine (Fisher, Williams, & Levine, 2008). This cast is applied around the chest and abdomen and extends from above the nipple line to the pubis. After application of the cast, the nurse must assess the patient for the development of *cast syndrome*. This condition occurs if the body cast is applied too tightly and compresses the superior mesenteric artery against the duodenum. The patient generally complains of abdominal pain, abdominal pressure, nausea, and vomiting. The abdomen should be assessed for decreased bowel sounds (a window may be left over the umbilicus). Treatment includes gastric decompression with a nasogastric tube and suction. The cast may have to be removed or split. Nursing assessment also includes observation of respiratory status, bowel and bladder function, and areas of pressure over the bony prominences, especially the iliac crest.

The *hip spica cast* can also be used for treatment of femoral fractures but is more common in children. The purpose of the hip spica cast is to immobilize the affected extremity and the trunk securely after surgical repair or trauma. It includes two casts joined together: (1) the body jacket cast and (2) the long leg cast. The location of the femoral fracture will determine whether the thigh of the unaffected extremity will have to be immobilized to restrict rotation of the pelvis and possible hip motion on the side of the femur fracture. The hip spica cast extends from above the nipple line to the base of the foot (single spica) and may include the opposite extremity up to an area above the knee (spica and a half) or both extremities (double spica).

Assess the patient with a hip spica cast for the same problems that are associated with the body jacket cast. When the patient is positioned, the support bar joining the thighs must never be used to assist in moving because the bar can break and cause cast disruption. After the cast has dried, turn the patient (with assistance) to the prone position and provide pillow support under the chest and immobilized extremity. Skin care around the cast edges (petalling) is important to prevent pressure sores. Instruct the patient in the positioning activities required to get on and off the bedpan. A fracture bedpan may be used to provide comfort and ease the movement of getting on and off the bedpan. After the hip spica cast has dried sufficiently, the patient may be instructed in ambulation techniques by the physiotherapist.

Injuries to the Lower Extremity. Injuries to the lower extremity are often immobilized by a long leg cast, short leg cast, cylinder cast, Jones dressing, or prefabricated splint or immobilizer. The usual indications for applying a long leg cast are an

result in significant swelling. Plaster splints are applied over a well-padded forearm, beginning at the phalangeal joints of the hand, extending up the dorsal aspect of the forearm around the distal humerus, and then extending down the volar aspect of the forearm to the distal palmar crease. The splinting material is wrapped with either elastic bandage or bias stockinette. The sugar-tong posterior splint accommodates for postinjury swelling in the fractured extremity.

The *short arm cast* is often used for the treatment of stable wrist or metacarpal fractures. An aluminum finger splint can be fabricated into the short arm cast for concurrent treatment of phalangeal injuries. The *short arm cast* is a circular cast extending from the distal palmar area to the proximal forearm. This cast provides wrist immobilization and permits unrestricted elbow motion.

unstable ankle fracture, soft tissue injuries, a fractured tibia, and knee injuries. The cast usually extends from the base of the toes to the groin and the gluteal crease. The short leg cast can be used for a variety of conditions but is primarily used for stable ankle and foot injuries. A cylinder cast is used for knee injuries or fractures. The cast extends from the groin to the malleoli of the ankle. A Jones dressing is composed of bulky padding materials (absorption dressing and cotton sheet wadding), splints, and an elastic wrap or bias-cut stockinette. The Jones dressing, like the sugar-tong splint, is used for knee fractures or surgery when there is a risk of significant edema. After the application of a lower extremity cast or dressing, the extremity should be elevated with pillows above the heart level for the first 24 hours. After the initial phase, the casted extremity should not be placed in a dependent position because of the possibility of excessive edema. Following cast application, the nurse should observe for signs of pressure, especially in the regions of the heel, anterior tibial border, fibular head, and malleoli.

Prefabricated knee and ankle splints and immobilizers are being used in many settings. This type of immobilization is easy to apply and remove, which permits close observation of the affected joint for signs of swelling and skin breakdown (Figure 65-12). Depending on the injury, removal of the splint or immobilizer facilitates ROM of the affected joint and a faster return to function.

External Fixation. An external fixator is a metallic device composed of metal pins that are inserted into the bone and attached to external rods to stabilize the fracture while it heals. It can be used to apply traction or to compress fracture fragments and to immobilize reduced fragments when the use of a cast or other traction is not appropriate. The external device holds fracture fragments in a manner similar to a surgically implanted internal device. The external fixator is attached directly to the bones by percutaneous transfixing pins or wires (Figure 65-13). External fixation is indicated in simple fractures (either open or closed), complex fractures with extensive soft tissue damage, correction of bony defects (congenital), pseudoarthrosis, nonunion or malunion, and limb lengthening.

External fixation has many advantages over other fracture management strategies and is often employed to salvage complex mangled extremity fractures that otherwise might necessitate amputation. Because the use of an external device is a long-term process, assessment for pin loosening and infection is critical. Infection signalled by exudate, erythema, tenderness, and pain may necessitate removal of the device. The nurse should instruct the patient and caregivers about meticulous pin care. Although each health care provider has a protocol for pin care cleaning, half-strength hydrogen peroxide with normal saline is often used.

Internal Fixation. Internal fixation devices (pins, plates, intramedullary rods, and metal and bioabsorbable screws) are

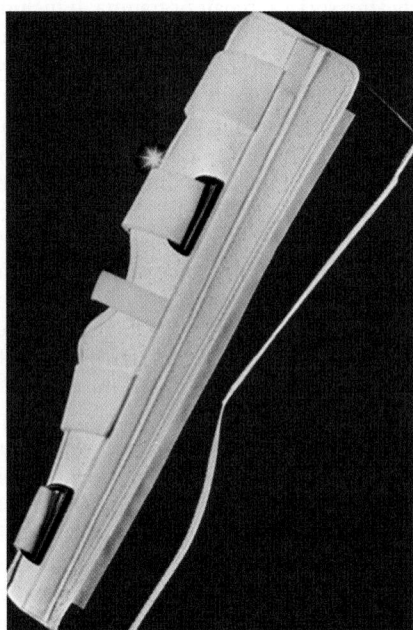

Figure 65-12 Knee immobilizer.

Source: Maher, A., Salmond, S. W., & Pellino, T. A. (Eds.). (2002). *Orthopaedic nursing* (3rd ed.). Philadelphia: Saunders.

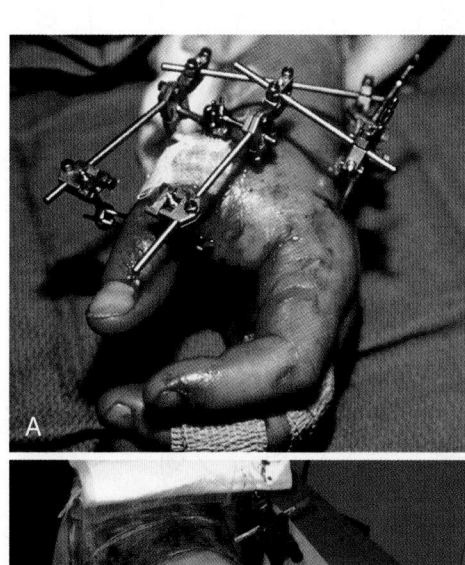

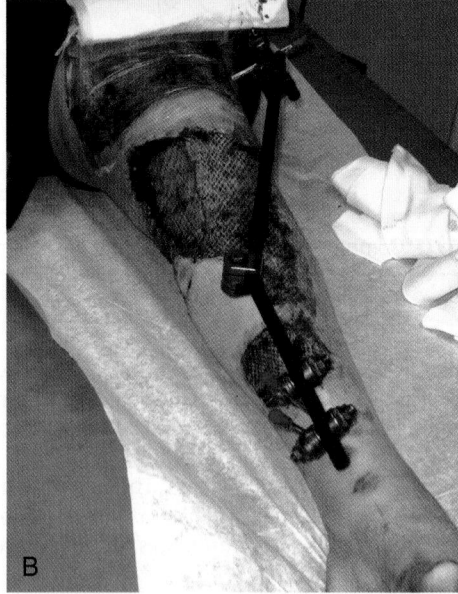

Figure 65-13 External fixators. **A,** Stabilization of a hand injury. **B,** Stabilization of a knee injury with pins in the femur and tibia.

Source: **A,** Courtesy Howmedica, Inc, Allendale, PA; **B,** Browner, B., Jupiter, J. B., Levine, A. M., Trafton, P. G., & Krettek, C. (Eds.). (2008). S*keletal trauma.* (4th ed.). Philadelphia: Saunders.

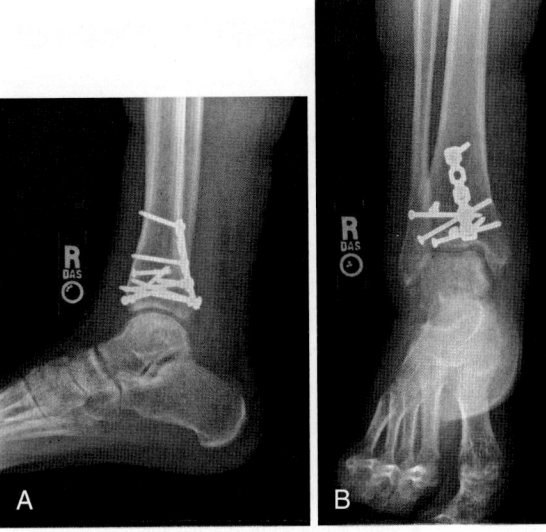

Figure 65-14 Views of internal fixation devices to stabilize a fractured tibia and fibula.

Source: Courtesy Jeremy Lewis, MD.

surgically inserted at the time of realignment (Figure 65-14). Biologically inert metal devices such as stainless steel, Vitallium, or titanium are used to realign and maintain bony fragments. Proper alignment is evaluated by radiographs at regular intervals.

Drug Therapy. Patients with fractures often experience varying degrees of pain associated with muscle spasms. Involuntary reflexes that result from edema following muscle injury cause these spasms. Central and peripheral muscle relaxants, such as cyclobenzaprine or methocarbamol (Robaxin), may be prescribed for relief of pain associated with muscle spasms.

Common adverse effects associated with muscle relaxants are drowsiness, headache, weakness, fatigue, blurred vision, ataxia, and gastrointestinal upset (Hodgson & Kizior, 2011). Hypersensitivity reactions may include skin rash or pruritus. Ingestion of large doses of muscle relaxants may cause hypotension, tachycardia, or respiratory depression.

In an open fracture, the threat of tetanus occurring can be reduced with tetanus and diphtheria toxoid or tetanus immunoglobulin for the patient who has not been previously immunized. Bone-penetrating antibiotics (such as cefazolin) are used prophylactically.

Nutritional Therapy. Proper nutrition is an essential component of the reparative process in injured tissue. An adequate energy source is needed to promote muscle strength and tone, build endurance, and enhance ambulation and gait-training skills. The patient's dietary requirements must include ample protein (e.g., 1 g/kg of body weight), vitamins (especially B, C, and D), and calcium, phosphorus, and magnesium to ensure optimal soft tissue and bone healing. Low serum protein levels and vitamin C deficiencies interfere with tissue healing. Immobility and callus formation increase calcium needs. Three well-balanced meals a day will usually provide the necessary nutrients. The well-balanced meal should be supplemented by a fluid intake of 2000 to 3000 mL/day to promote optimal bladder and bowel function. Adequate fluid and a high-fibre diet with fruits and vegetables will prevent constipation. If immobilized in bed with skeletal traction or in a body jacket or hip spica bandage, the patient should be instructed to eat six small meals so as not to overeat and thus avoid abdominal pressure and cramping.

NURSING MANAGEMENT: FRACTURES

Nursing Assessment

A brief history of the traumatic episode, mechanism of injury, and the position in which the victim was found can be obtained from the patient or witnesses. As soon as possible, the patient should be transported to an emergency department where a thorough assessment and treatment can be initiated (Table 65-7). Subjective and objective data that should be obtained from an individual with a fracture are presented in Table 65-8.

Special emphasis must be placed on the region distal to the site of injury. Clinical findings must be documented before fracture treatment is initiated to prevent doubts about whether a problem discovered later was missed during the original examination or was caused by the treatment.

Neurovascular Assessment

Musculoskeletal injuries have the potential to cause changes in the neurovascular status of an injured extremity. With musculoskeletal trauma, application of a cast or constrictive dressing, poor positioning, and the physiological response to the traumatic injury can cause nerve or vascular damage, usually distal to the injury.

The neurovascular assessment should consist of a *peripheral vascular assessment* (colour, temperature, capillary refill, peripheral pulses, and edema) and a *peripheral neurological assessment* (sensation, motor function, and pain). Throughout the neurovascular assessment, both extremities are compared to obtain an accurate assessment.

An extremity's colour (e.g., pink, pale, cyanotic) and temperature (i.e., hot, warm, cool, cold) in the area of the affected extremity are assessed. Pallor or a cool (or cold) extremity below the injury could indicate arterial insufficiency. A warm, cyanotic extremity could indicate poor venous return. A capillary refill (blanching of the nail bed) of 3 seconds indicates good arterial perfusion. Accurate documentation and ongoing neurovascular assessments are the cornerstones of nursing care for the individual with a musculoskeletal injury.

Pulses on both the unaffected and the injured extremity are compared to identify differences in rate or quality. Pulses are described as strong, diminished, audible by Doppler, or absent. A diminished or absent pulse distal to the injury can indicate vascular dysfunction and insufficiency. However, up to 12% of healthy adults do not have a palpable dorsalis pedis or posterior tibial pulse (Roberts & Hedges, 2010). Peripheral edema is also assessed, and pitting edema may be present with severe injury.

Sensation and motor innervation in the upper extremity are assessed by evaluating the ulnar, median, and radial nerves. Neurovascular status can be assessed by abduction and adduction of the fingers, opposition of the fingers, and supination and pronation of the hand. In the lower extremity, dorsiflexion and plantar flexion provide information about motor function of the peroneal and tibial nerves. Sensory innervation is evaluated for the

EMERGENCY MANAGEMENT

Table 65-7 Fractured Extremity

ETIOLOGY	ASSESSMENT FINDINGS	INTERVENTIONS
Blunt	• Deformity (loss of normal bony contours) or unnatural position of affected limb	**Initial**
• Motor vehicle collision	• Edema and ecchymosis	• Treat life-threatening injuries first.
• Pedestrian event	• Muscle spasm	• Ensure airway, breathing, and circulation.
Falls	• Tenderness and pain	• Control external bleeding with direct pressure or sterile pressure dressing and elevation of the limb.
• Direct blows	• Loss of function	• Splint joints above and below fracture site.
• Forced flexion or hyperextension	• Numbness, tingling, loss of distal pulses	• Check neurovascular status distal to injury before and after splinting.
• Twisting forces	• Grating (crepitus)	• Elevate injured limb if possible.
Penetrating	• Open wound over injured site, exposure of bone	• Do *not* attempt to straighten fractured or dislocated joints.
• Gunshot		• Do *not* manipulate protruding bone ends.
• Blast		• Apply ice packs to affected area.
Other		• Obtain radiographs of affected limb.
• Pathological conditions		• Administer tetanus and diphtheria prophylaxis if skin integrity is violated.
• Violent muscle contractions (seizures)		• Mark location of pulses to facilitate repeat assessment.
• Crush injury		• Splint fracture site, including joints above and below fracture site.
		Ongoing Monitoring
		• Monitor vital signs, level of consciousness, oxygen saturation, peripheral pulses, and pain.
		• Monitor for compartment syndrome characterized by excessive pain, pain with passive stretch of the affected extremity muscles, pallor, paresthesia, and late signs of paralysis and pulselessness.
		• Monitor for signs and symptoms of a fat embolism (e.g., dyspnea, chest pain, temperature elevation).

peroneal nerve on the dorsal part of the foot between the web space of the great and the second toes. Tibial nerve assessment is performed by stroking the plantar surface (sole) of the foot. Contralateral evaluation is critical. Paresthesia (abnormal sensation [e.g., numbness, tingling]) and hyperesthesia (hypersensation), may be reported by the patient. Partial or full loss of sensation (paresis or paralysis) may be a late sign of neurovascular damage. Reduced motion or strength in an injured extremity can alert the nurse to potential limb-threatening complications or disability.

Pain is the final element of the neurovascular assessment. The nurse must carefully assess the location, quality, and intensity of the pain (see Chapter 10). Current best practice in pain management is to ask the patient to rate his or her level of pain on a scale of 0 to 10 with 0 being no pain and 10 being the worst pain ever experienced. Increasing pain unrelieved by drugs and out of proportion to the injury can be an indication of compartment syndrome.

Patients should be instructed to report any changes in their neurovascular status. Patients must verbalize and demonstrate a thorough understanding of all elements before discharge from the treatment setting.

▪ Nursing Diagnoses

Nursing diagnoses for the patient with a fracture may include, but are not limited to, those presented in Nursing Care Plan (NCP) 65-1.

▪ Planning

The overall goals are that the patient with a fracture will (1) have physiological healing with no associated complications, (2) obtain satisfactory pain relief, and (3) achieve maximal rehabilitation potential.

▪ Nursing Implementation

▪ Health Promotion

The public should be taught to take appropriate safety precautions to prevent injuries while at home, at work, when driving,

NURSING ASSESSMENT

Table 65-8 Fracture

Subjective Data

Important Health Information

Past health history: Traumatic injury; long-term repetitive forces (stress fracture); bone or systemic diseases, prolonged immobility (pathological fracture), osteopenia, osteoporosis

Medications: Use of corticosteroids (osteoporotic fractures), analgesics, estrogen replacement therapy, calcium supplementation

Surgery or other treatments: First aid treatment of fracture, previous musculoskeletal surgeries

Symptoms

- Loss of motion or weakness of affected part; muscle spasms
- Sudden and severe pain in affected area; numbness, tingling, loss of sensation distal to injury; chronic pain that increases with activity (stress fracture)

Objective Data

General

Apprehension, guarding of injured site

Integumentary

Skin lacerations, pallor and cool skin or bluish and warm skin distal to injury; ecchymosis, hematoma, edema at site of fracture

Cardiovascular

Reduced or absent pulse distal to injury, decreased skin temperature, delayed capillary refill

Neurological

Paresthesias, decreased or absent sensation, hypersensation

Musculoskeletal

Restricted or lost function of affected part, local bony deformities, abnormal angulation, shortening, rotation, crepitation; muscle weakness

Possible Findings

Localization and extent of fractures on radiograph, bone scans, tomograms, CT scan, or MRI

CT, computed tomography; *MRI,* magnetic resonance imaging.

and when participating in sports. Nurses should be advocates for personal actions known to reduce injuries such as regular use of seat belts, driving within posted speed limits, stretching and warming up muscles before exercise, use of protective athletic equipment (helmets and knee, wrist, and elbow pads), use of safety equipment at work, and not combining drinking and driving.

Individuals (especially older adults) should be encouraged to participate in moderate exercise to aid in the maintenance of muscle strength and balance. To reduce falls, the living environment should be examined so that scatter rugs are removed, adequate footwear and lighting are maintained, and paths to the bathroom are cleared for nighttime use (see also the Evidence-Informed Practice box on falls). The nurse should also stress the importance of adequate calcium and vitamin D intake.

▪ Acute Intervention

Patients with fractures may be treated in an emergency department or a physician's office and discharged to home care, or they may require hospitalization for varying amounts of time. Specific

EVIDENCE-INFORMED PRACTICE

Are Interventions to Reduce the Incidence of Falls in Older Adults Effective?

Clinical Question

In older adults living in nursing care facilities or hospitals (P), are interventions to reduce risk factors for falls (I) more effective than the usual care (C) in reducing the incidence of falls (O)?

Best Available Evidence

Systematic review of randomized controlled trials (RCTs)

Critical Appraisal and Synthesis of Evidence

- 41 RCTs (*n* = 25,422) comparing single intervention programs (e.g., exercise, medication interventions [e.g., vitamin D supplementation, medication review]) and multifactorial interventions.
- Participants were at risk for or had a history of falling and lived in a residential care facility or hospital. Mean age of participants was 83 years, with the majority being female. A large portion of participants in most studies were cognitively impaired.

Conclusions

- In nursing care facilities, interventions found to be beneficial included prescription of vitamin D and possibly a review of medication by a pharmacist. Interventions targeting multiple risk factors were not clearly effective but might be when delivered by multidisciplinary teams. Interventions targeting single risk factors (including exercise programs) were also not effective.
- In hospitals, interventions that targeted multiple risk factors and supervised exercise were effective for patients who were hospitalized for more than a few weeks.

Implications for Nursing Practice

- Falls prevention programs in residential facilities that include exercise should carefully evaluate each person's suitability because exercise programs may increase falls in some older adults.
- Vitamin D supplementation and medication review by a pharmacist should be promoted in nursing care facilities to reduce falls.
- Supervised exercise as well as multifactorial interprofessional programs to reduce falls should be advocated for patients hospitalized for more than a few weeks.
- Future trials need to look at supervised exercise in both residential facilities and hospitals.

Reference for Evidence

Cameron, I. D., Murray, G. R., Gillespie, L. D., Robertson, M. C., Hill, K. D., Cumming, R. G., & Kerse, N. (2010). Interventions for preventing falls in older people in nursing care facilities and hospitals. *Cochrane Database of Systematic Reviews, 1,* CD005465. doi:10.1002/14651858.CD005465.pub2

PICO: P, patient population of interest; *I,* intervention or area of interest; *C,* comparison of interest or comparison group; *O,* outcome(s) of interest.

NURSING CARE PLAN 65-1

Fracture

NURSING DIAGNOSIS	*Impaired physical mobility* *related to* loss of integrity of bone structures, movement of bone fragments, soft tissue injury, and prescribed movement restrictions *as evidenced by* limited joint range of motion, inability to move purposefully, and inability to bear weight
Expected Patient Outcomes	**Nursing Interventions and *Rationales***

Expected Patient Outcomes	Nursing Interventions and Rationales
• Experiences uncomplicated bone healing and return of skeletal function • Uses assistive devices as necessary to increase physical mobility • Experiences no complications of immobility	**Splinting (at time of initial injury)** • Support the affected body part *to avoid fracture displacement and soft tissue injury.* • Move the injured extremity as little as possible *to avoid additional injury.* • Monitor for bleeding at injury site *to plan appropriate intervention.* • Monitor for circulation in the affected part *to detect possible nerve or vascular damage.* **Traction and immobilization care** • Position in proper body alignment *to enhance traction and skeletal function.* • Maintain traction at all times *to prevent misalignment of bone fragments.* • Monitor circulation, movement and sensation of affected extremity *to detect complications of peripheral vascular function.* • Provide trapeze for movement in bed *to reduce complications of immobility.* • Monitor skin and bony prominences *to check for early signs of skin breakdown.* • Administer appropriate skin care at friction and pressure points *to prevent skin breakdown.*

NURSING DIAGNOSIS	*Risk for peripheral neurovascular dysfunction* *related to* vascular insufficiency and nerve compression secondary to edema and mechanical compression of traction, splints, or casts
Expected Patient Outcome	**Nursing Interventions and *Rationales***

Expected Patient Outcome	Nursing Interventions and Rationales
• Experiences no peripheral neurovascular dysfunction	• Perform a comprehensive peripheral vascular assessment (e.g., check peripheral pulses, edema, capillary refill, colour, and temperature of extremity) q4hr and PRN *to monitor for diminished tissue perfusion and plan appropriate intervention.* • Perform a comprehensive peripheral neurological assessment, checking for sensation, motor function, and pain q4h and PRN *to monitor for nerve compression and plan for appropriate interventions.* • Teach patient and caregivers the importance of reporting signs and symptoms of changing neurovascular status immediately *to plan for appropriate interventions as soon as possible.* • Prevent infection in wounds *to prevent further edema and inflammation that can contribute to vascular insufficiency and nerve compression.* • Maintain adequate hydration *to prevent increased blood viscosity.* • Immobilize or support affected body part *to prevent pressure and injury.* • Maintain position and integrity of traction *to prevent compression of blood vessels and nerves.* • Elevate affected limb 20 degrees or greater above the level of the heart *to reduce edema by promoting venous return.*

NURSING DIAGNOSIS	*Acute pain* *related to* edema, movement of bone fragments, and muscle spasm *as evidenced by* pain descriptors, guarding, and crying
Expected Patient Outcome	**Nursing Interventions and *Rationales***

Expected Patient Outcome	Nursing Interventions and Rationales
• Expresses satisfaction with pain-relief measures (pain <3 on 0-10 scale)	• Perform a comprehensive assessment of pain to include location, characteristics, onset/duration, precipitating factors, and intensity or severity of pain using a numeric pain scale (e.g., 0 = no pain and 10 = worst pain) *to plan appropriate interventions and establish a baseline pain level.* • Provide patient optimal pain relief with prescribed analgesics *to relieve pain and promote muscle relaxation.* • Elevate, apply ice (if prescribed), and support affected extremity *to reduce edema and promote comfort.* • Notify physician if measures to relieve pain are unsuccessful or if current pain is a significant change from the patient's past experience of pain *since this might indicate impending compartment syndrome.* • Teach the use of nonpharmacological techniques (e.g., relaxation, guided imagery, hot or cold application, and massage) along with other pain-relief measures *to promote comfort and to help minimize the pain.*

PRN, as needed.

NURSING CARE PLAN 65-1

Fracture—cont'd

NURSING DIAGNOSIS	*Ineffective self-health management* related to lack of knowledge regarding muscle atrophy, exercise program, and cast care *as evidenced by* questions about the long-term effect of immobilization, devices, or activity restrictions
Expected Patient Outcomes	**Nursing Interventions and *Rationales***
• Describes the prescribed activity and its rationale • Demonstrates appropriate care of cast or immobilizer	• Inform patient of the purpose for, and the benefits of, the prescribed activity/exercise to encourage patient *to promote patient compliance.* • Instruct patient how to perform the prescribed activity/exercise. • Provide written instructions/diagrams *for continued reference at home.* • Observe the patient perform the prescribed activity/exercises *to evaluate performance and reinforce the activity.*

nursing measures depend on the type of treatment used and the setting in which patients are placed.

Preoperative Management.
If surgical intervention is required to treat the fracture, patients will need preoperative preparation. In addition to the usual preoperative nursing measures (see Chapter 20), the nurse should inform patients of the type of immobilization and assistive devices that will be used and the expected activity limitations after surgery. Assurance that pain medication will be available, if needed, is often beneficial.

Proper skin preparation is an important part of preoperative preparation. The protocol for skin preparation varies among institutions and may be the nurse's responsibility. The aim of skin preparation is to assist in the cleansing of the skin and to remove debris and hair, thus reducing the possibility of infection. Careful attention to this preoperative treatment can influence the postoperative course.

Postoperative Management.
In general, postoperative nursing care and management are directed toward monitoring vital signs and applying the general principles of postoperative nursing care (see Chapter 22). Frequent neurovascular assessments of the affected extremity are necessary to detect early and subtle neurovascular changes. Any limitations of movement or activity related to turning, positioning, and extremity support should be monitored closely. Pain and discomfort can be minimized through proper alignment and positioning. Dressings or casts should be carefully observed for any overt signs of bleeding or drainage. A significant increase in size of the drainage area should be reported. If a wound drainage system is in place, the patency of the system and the volume of drainage should be regularly assessed and measured. Whenever the contents of a drainage system are measured or emptied, the nurse should use sterile technique to prevent contamination.

Additional nursing responsibilities depend on the type of immobilization used. A blood salvage and reinfusion system that allows for recovery and reinfusion of the patient's own blood may be used. The blood is retrieved from a joint space or cavity, and the patient receives this blood in the form of an autotransfusion. (Autotransfusion is discussed in Chapter 33.) Additional nursing measures for the patient who has had orthopedic surgery are discussed in NCP 65-2 on p. 1830.

Other Measures.
Patients often have reduced mobility as a result of the fracture. The nurse must plan care to prevent the many complications associated with immobility. Constipation can be prevented by activity and maintenance of a high fluid intake (>2500 mL/day unless contraindicated by the patient's health status) and a diet high in bulk and roughage (fresh fruit and vegetables). If these measures are not effective in maintaining the patient's normal bowel pattern, warm fluids, stool softeners, laxatives, or suppositories may be necessary. Maintaining a regular time for elimination aids in promoting regularity.

Renal calculi can develop as a result of bone demineralization. The hypercalcemia from demineralization causes a rise in urine pH and stone formation resulting from the precipitation of calcium. Unless contraindicated, a fluid intake of 2500 mL/day is recommended. Cranberry juice or ascorbic acid (500-1500 mg/day) may be recommended to acidify the urine and prevent calcium precipitation in the urine. (Renal calculi are discussed in Chapter 48.)

Rapid deconditioning of the cardiopulmonary system can occur as a result of prolonged bed rest, resulting in orthostatic hypotension and decreased lung capacity. Unless contraindicated, these effects can be diminished by permitting the patient to sit on the side of the bed, allowing the patient's lower limbs to dangle over the bedside, and having the patient perform standing transfers. When the patient is allowed to increase activity, careful evaluation should be made to assess for orthostatic hypotension. Patients must also be assessed for deep venous thrombosis (DVT) and pulmonary emboli. (DVT and pulmonary embolism are discussed in Chapter 40 and pulmonary embolism is discussed in Chapter 30.)

Traction.
When slings are used with traction, the nurse should inspect exposed skin areas regularly. Pressure over a bony prominence created by the wrinkling of sheets or bedclothes may cause pressure necrosis. Persistent skin pressure may impair blood flow, causing injury to the peripheral neurovascular structures. Skeletal traction pin sites must be observed for signs of infection (Bell, Leader, & Lloyd, 2008). Pin-site care varies but usually includes regular removal of exudates with half-strength hydrogen peroxide, rinsing pin sites with sterile saline, and drying of the area with sterile gauze.

External rotation of the hip can occur when skin traction is used on the lower extremity. The nurse can correct this position by placing a pillow, sandbag, or rolled-up draw sheet (called a *trochanter roll*) along the greater trochanteric region of the femur. Generally, the patient should be in the centre of the bed in a supine position. Incorrect alignment can result in increased pain, nonunion, or malunion.

To offset some of the problems associated with prolonged immobility, the nurse should discuss activity of a specific patient with the health care provider. If exercise is permitted, the nurse

NURSING CARE PLAN 65-2

Orthopedic Surgery*

NURSING DIAGNOSIS	*Acute pain* related to tissue trauma, disruption of skin integrity, and edema *as evidenced by* reluctance to move, guarding of affected area, persistent score of greater than 8 on 10-point pain scale, and facial grimacing
Expected Patient Outcome	**Nursing Interventions and *Rationales***
• Expresses satisfactory relief of pain (<3 on a 10-point scale)	• Encourage patient to monitor own pain and to intervene appropriately *to increase patient's control over pain management.* • Implement use of patient-controlled analgesia (PCA) *to give patient control.* • Medicate before an activity *to decrease discomfort from exercise and increase patient participation.* • Evaluate effectiveness of pain-control measures used through ongoing assessment of pain experience *so that pain relief is in accordance with healing process.* • Position in proper body alignment to reduce pressure on nerves and tissues.
NURSING DIAGNOSIS	*Risk for peripheral neurovascular dysfunction* related to edema, circulatory stasis, or dislocated prosthesis or fixation devices†
NURSING DIAGNOSIS	*Impaired physical mobility* related to pain, stiffness, and physical deconditioning *as evidenced by* limited joint movement, difficulty ambulating, inability to participate in physical rehabilitation, and guarded movement
Expected Patient Outcomes	**Nursing Interventions and *Rationales***
• Participates in exercise therapy to increase joint mobility • Demonstrates ability to transfer, walk with assistive devices, and move with ease	**Exercise therapy: joint mobility** • Determine limitations of joint movement and effect on function *to plan appropriate interventions.* • Assist patient to optimal body position for passive or active joint movement *to prevent dislocation or other complications.* • Initiate pain-control measures before beginning joint exercise *to decrease discomfort from exercise and increase patient participation.* • Perform passive or assisted ROM exercises *to increase joint mobility and prevent contractures.* • Collaborate with physiotherapist in developing and executing an exercise program *to increase patient compliance and promote continuity of exercise.* **Exercise therapy: ambulation** • Assist patient to sit on side of bed *to facilitate postural adjustments.* • Apply or provide assistive device (cane, walker, or wheelchair) for ambulation, if the patient is unsteady, *to prevent falls.* • Assist patient with initial ambulation *to promote mobility according to patient's abilities.* • Consult physiotherapist about ambulation plan *to reinforce plan and to provide unified approach to patient.*
NURSING DIAGNOSIS	*Deficient knowledge* related to lack of exposure to information and resources for follow-up care *as evidenced by* expression of concern with ability to care for self after discharge, frequent questioning about follow-up care, or lack of plan for follow-up care
Expected Patient Outcomes	**Nursing Interventions and *Rationales***
• Describes activities related to treatments, activities of daily living, and obtaining assistance if needed • Verbalizes confidence in ability to follow prescribed discharge plan	**Discharge planning** • Communicate patient's discharge plans (e.g., activity limitations, medications, follow-up visit, signs of infection, dislocation) *to prepare for self-care and decision making.* • Collaborate with the physician, family/caregiver, and other health team members in planning for the supportive environment necessary *to provide patient's posthospital care so appropriate changes can be made.* • Coordinate referrals relevant to linkages among health care providers *to monitor long-term rehabilitation program at home.*

ROM, range of motion.

*This NCP is appropriate for a patient with an open reduction with internal fixation (ORIF) or joint replacement surgery.

†See NCP 65-1 on pp. 1828-1829 for outcomes and interventions.

should encourage participation by the patient in a simple exercise regimen within activity restrictions. Activities that the patient should participate in include frequent position changes, ROM exercises of unaffected joints, deep-breathing exercises, isometric exercises, and use of the trapeze bar (if permitted) to raise oneself off the bed for linen changes and use of the bedpan. These activities should be performed several times each day.

If allowed, active exercises that move uninvolved joints through the ROM are the preferred activity. Frequent exercise of the trunk and the extremities is an excellent stimulus to deep breathing. Active, resistive exercise (isotonic) of uninvolved extremities helps reduce deconditioning from prolonged immobility.

Ambulatory and Home Care

Cast Care.
Because many fractures are treated in an outpatient setting, the patient often requires only a short hospitalization or none at all. Regardless of the type of cast material, a cast can interfere with circulation and nerve function from being applied too tightly or because of excessive edema after application. Thus, frequent neurovascular assessments of the immobilized extremity are critical. The patient must be taught about signs of cast complications so that they can be reported promptly. Elevation of the extremity above the level of the heart to promote venous return and applications of ice to control or prevent edema are measures frequently used during the initial phase. (If compartment syndrome is suspected, do not elevate the extremity above the heart.) The nurse should instruct the patient to exercise joints above and below the cast. Pulling out cast padding and scratching or placing foreign objects inside the cast is forbidden because it predisposes the patient to skin breakdown and infection. For itching, instruct the patient that a hair dryer set on a cool setting can be directed under the cast.

Patient and caregiver teaching is an important nursing responsibility to prevent complications. In addition to specific instructions for cast care and recognition of complications, the nurse should encourage the patient to contact the clinic or care provider if questions arise. Table 65-9 summarizes patient and caregiver instructions for cast care. The nurse should validate the patient's and caregivers' understanding of these instructions before discharge from inpatient and ambulatory settings. Follow-up phone contact is appropriate, and home care nursing visits are warranted, especially with body or spica casts.

Cast removal is done in the outpatient setting. Patients often fear being cut by the oscillating blade of the cast saw. The nurse should reassure the patient. More importantly, the nurse should educate the patient as to the possible alteration in the appearance of the skin that has been beneath the cast. Anxiety may also be present related to weight bearing and continued follow-up care.

Psychosocial Problems.
Short-term rehabilitative goals are directed toward the transition from dependence to independence in performing simple activities of daily living and preserving or increasing strength and endurance. Long-term rehabilitative goals are aimed at preventing problems associated with musculoskeletal injury (Table 65-10). An important part of nursing care during the rehabilitative phase is assisting the patient to adjust to any problems caused by the injury (e.g., separation from family, financial impact of medical care, loss of income from inability to work, potential for lifetime disability).

PATIENT & CAREGIVER TEACHING GUIDE

Table 65-9 Cast Care

Do Not

- Get plaster cast wet.
- Remove any padding.
- Insert any objects inside cast.
- Bear weight on new cast for 48 hr (not all casts are made for weight bearing; check with health care provider when unsure).
- Cover cast with plastic for prolonged periods.

Do

- Apply ice directly over fracture site for first 24 hr (avoid getting cast wet by keeping ice in plastic bag and protecting cast with cloth).
- Check with health care provider before getting fibreglass cast wet.
- Dry cast thoroughly after exposure to water.
  - Blot dry with towel.
  - Use hair dryer on low setting until cast is thoroughly dry.
- Elevate extremity above level of heart for first 48 hr.
- Move joints above and below cast regularly.
- Report signs of possible problems to health care provider.
  - Increasing pain.
  - Swelling associated with pain and discoloration of toes or fingers.
  - Pain during movement.
  - Burning or tingling under cast.
  - Sores or foul odour under cast.
- Keep appointment to have fracture and cast checked.

Ambulation.
The nurse must know the overall goals of physiotherapy in relation to the patient's abilities, needs, and tolerance. Mobility training and instruction in the use of assistive aids (cane, crutches, walker) constitute major areas of responsibility of the physiotherapist. The patient with lower extremity dysfunction is usually started in mobility training when able to sit in bed and dangle the feet over the side. This activity should be done two or three times for 10 to 15 minutes, with the nurse assisting as necessary. Collaboration of the nurse and physiotherapist to coordinate pain management and thus increase patient participation at therapy sessions is critical. As endurance increases, the patient is instructed in the techniques of transferring from bed to chair. Progressive ambulation is usually started with parallel bars and progresses to ambulatory assistive devices.

When the patient begins to ambulate, the nurse must know the weight bearing allowed for the affected extremity and the correct technique if the patient is using an assistive device. There are different degrees of weight-bearing ambulation: (1) non–weight-bearing (no weight borne) ambulation, (2) touch-down, toe-touch, or feather-weight–bearing ambulation (contact with floor but no weight borne), (3) partial weight–bearing ambulation (25 to 50% of patient's weight borne), (4) weight bearing as tolerated (dictated by patient's pain and tolerance), and (5) full weight–bearing ambulation (no limitations) (University of Pittsburgh Medical Center [UPMC], 2012).

Assistive Devices.
Devices for ambulation range from a cane, which can relieve up to 40% of the weight normally borne by a lower limb, to a walker or crutches, which may allow for complete non–weight-bearing ambulation. The decision about

Table 65-10 Problems Associated With Injury of the Musculoskeletal System

PROBLEM	DESCRIPTION	NURSING CONSIDERATIONS
Muscle atrophy	Decreased muscle mass normally occurs as a result of disuse following prolonged immobilization. Loss of nerve innervation can precipitate muscle atrophy.	Isometric muscle-strengthening exercise regimen within the confines of the immobilization device assists in reducing the amount of atrophy. Muscle atrophy interferes with and prolongs the rehabilitation process.
Contracture	Abnormal condition of joint characterized by flexion and fixation. Caused by atrophy and shortening of muscle fibres or by loss of normal elasticity of skin over a joint.	Can be prevented by frequent position change, correct body alignment, and active and passive range of motion exercises several times a day. Intervention requires gradual and progressive stretching of the muscles or ligaments in the region of the joint.
Footdrop	Plantar-flexed position of the foot (footdrop) occurs when the Achilles tendon in the ankle shortens because it has been allowed to assume an unsupported position. Peroneal nerve palsy (a compression neuropathy) also causes footdrop.	Management of the patient with long-term injuries must include supporting the foot in a neutral position. Once footdrop has developed, ambulation and gait training may be significantly hindered. The patient may require a splint to keep the foot/feet in a neutral position. High-top athletic shoes may also help.
Pain	Frequently associated with fractures, edema, and muscle spasm. Pain varies in intensity from mild to severe and is usually described as aching, dull, burning, throbbing, sharp, or deep.	Causes of pain include incorrect positioning and alignment of the extremity, incorrect support of the extremity, sudden movement of the extremity, and immobilization devices that are applied too tightly or in an incorrect position, constrictive dressings, and motion occurring at the fracture site. Causes of pain should be determined so that corrective nursing action can be taken.
Muscle spasms	Caused by involuntary muscle contraction after fracture, muscle strain, or nerve injury, these may last as long as several weeks. Pain associated with muscle spasms is often intense and can last from several seconds to several minutes.	Measures to reduce the intensity of the muscle spasms are similar to the corrective actions for pain control. Do not massage muscle spasms. Thermotherapy, especially heat, may reduce muscle spasm.

which device is appropriate for a patient involves weighing the need for maximum stability and safety versus manoeuvrability, which is required in small spaces such as bathrooms. It is essential to discuss with patients the requirements of their lifestyles and determining the device with which each patient feels most secure and independent.

The technique for using assistive devices varies. The involved limb is usually advanced at the same time or immediately after the advance of the device. The uninvolved limb is advanced last. In almost all cases, canes are held in the hand opposite the involved extremity.

The common gait patterns with assistive devices such as the crutch are the two-point gait, the four-point gait, the swing-to gait, and the swing-through gait:

- *Two-point gait.* Crutch on one side advances simultaneously with the opposite (usually injured) extremity; this gait is also used with cane ambulation.
- *Four-point gait.* A slower version of the two-point gait, in which crutches and legs are advanced separately.
- *Swing-to gait.* Both crutches are advanced together, followed by the lifting of both lower limbs to the same place; this gait is also used with walkers.
- *Swing-through gait.* This gait is similar to the swing-to gait, but the patient swings the body past the crutches. An alternate four-point sweep-through gait for patients with concurrent

visual and neuromuscular disability provides exploration of upcoming terrain by the crutches before they are placed in the traditional position.

A transfer belt can be placed around the patient's waist to provide stability during the learning stages. The nurse should discourage the patient from reaching for furniture or relying on another person for support. When there is inadequate upper limb strength or poorly fitted crutches, the patient bears weight at the axilla rather than at the hands, endangering the neurovascular bundle that passes across the axilla. If verbal coaching does not correct the problem, the patient should be instructed in another form of ambulation until strength is adequate (e.g., platform crutches, walker).

Patients who must ambulate without weight bearing require sufficient upper limb strength to lift their own weight at each step. Because the muscles of the shoulder girdle are not accustomed to this work, they require vigorous and diligent training in preparation for this task. Push-ups, pull-ups using the overhead trapeze bar, and lifting weights develop the triceps and biceps. Straight-leg raises and quadriceps-setting exercises strengthen the quadriceps.

■ **Counselling and Referrals.** During the rehabilitative process, the patient's caregiver assumes an important role in the provision and follow-through of long-term care plans. The caregiver must be instructed in the techniques of strength and endurance exercises, assistance with mobility training, and promoting activities that enhance the quality of daily living. For referral purposes, nurses must know whether any immobilization or support devices are necessary for home use upon discharge.

Patients also need to be evaluated for post-traumatic stress disorder. This is especially important if significant injury to others or fatalities were associated with the patient's injuries.

▪ Evaluation

The expected outcomes for a patient with a fracture are presented in NCPs 65-1 and 65-2.

Complications of Fractures

The majority of fractures heal without complications. If death occurs after a fracture, it is usually the result of damage to underlying organs and vascular structures or from complications of the fracture or immobility. Complications of fractures can be either direct or indirect. *Direct complications* include problems with bone infection, bone union, and AVN. *Indirect complications* are associated with blood vessel and nerve damage that result in conditions such as compartment syndrome, venous thrombosis, rhabdomyolysis, fat embolism, and traumatic or hypovolemic shock. Although most musculoskeletal injuries are not life threatening, open fractures or fractures accompanied by severe blood loss and fractures that damage vital organs (e.g., lung, heart) are medical emergencies requiring immediate attention.

Infection

Open fractures and soft tissue injuries have a high incidence of infection. An open fracture usually results from the impact of severe external forces. Massive or blunt soft tissue injury often has more serious consequences than the fracture. Devitalized and contaminated tissue is an ideal medium for many common pathogens, including gas-forming (anaerobic) bacilli. Treatment of infections is costly in terms of extended nursing and medical care, time for treatment, and loss of patient income. If osteomyelitis (severe infection of the bone, bone marrow, and surrounding soft tissue) develops, healing can take a long time. (See Chapter 66 for discussion of osteomyelitis.)

Collaborative Care. Open fractures necessitate aggressive surgical debridement (Tripuraneni, Ganga, Quinn, & Gehlert, 2008). The wound is initially cleansed with a sterile saline solution via low-pressure lavage in the operating room (Smeltzer, 2010). Gross contaminants are irrigated or mechanically removed from the fracture site. Contused, contaminated, and devitalized tissue such as muscle, subcutaneous fat, skin, and fragments of bone are surgically excised (*debridement*). The extent of the soft tissue damage determines whether the wound will be closed at the time of surgery, whether closed suction drainage may be necessary, and whether skin grafting will be needed. Depending on the location and the extent of the fracture, reduction may be maintained by external fixation or traction. During surgery, the open wound may be irrigated with antibiotic solution. Antibiotic-impregnated beads may also be placed in the surgical site. During the postoperative phase, the patient will have antibiotics administered intravenously for 3 to 7 days. Antibiotics, in conjunction with aggressive surgical management, have greatly reduced the occurrence of infection.

Compartment Syndrome

Compartment syndrome is a condition in which elevated intra-compartmental pressure within a confined myofascial compartment compromises the neurovascular function of tissues within that space (Mamaril, Childs, & Sortman, 2007). Compartment syndrome causes capillary perfusion to be reduced below a level necessary for tissue viability. It is classified as acute, chronic or exertional, or crush syndrome. Thirty-eight compartments are located in the upper and lower extremities. Two basic causes of compartment syndrome are (1) decreased compartment size resulting from restrictive dressings, splints, casts, excessive traction, or premature closure of fascia and (2) increased compartment contents related to bleeding, edema, chemical response to snakebite, or intravenous infiltration. Depending on the patient's age and body mass index, the expected range of intracompartmental readings is 0 to 8 mm Hg. Readings of 30 mm Hg or higher indicate compartment syndrome (Shadgan et al., 2010).

Edema can create sufficient pressure to obstruct circulation and cause venous occlusion, which further increases edema. Eventually arterial flow is compromised, resulting in inadequate arterial circulation *(ischemia)* to the extremity. As ischemia continues, muscle and nerve cells are destroyed over time, and fibrotic tissue replaces the healthy tissue. Contracture, disability, and loss of function can occur. Delay in diagnosis and treatment can result in irreversible muscle and nerve ischemia, resulting in a functionally useless or severely impaired extremity.

Compartment syndrome is associated with trauma, fractures (especially the long bones), extensive soft tissue damage, and crush injury. Fractures of the distal humerus and proximal tibia are the most common fractures associated with compartment syndrome (Malik, Khan, Chaudhry, Ihsan, & Cullen, 2009). Compartment injury can also occur following knee or leg surgery. Prolonged pressure on a muscle compartment may occur when someone is trapped under a heavy object or a person's limb is trapped beneath the body because of an obtunded state such as drug or alcohol overdose. In the upper extremity, this condition is referred to as *Volkmann's ischemic contracture* (Figure 65-15), and in the lower extremity, as *anterior tibial compartment syndrome*, although the underlying pathophysiological mechanism is similar.

Clinical Manifestations and Collaborative Care.
Prompt, accurate diagnosis of compartment syndrome is critical. Prevention or early recognition is the key. Regular neurovascular assessments should be performed and documented on all patients with fractures, but especially those with injury of the distal humerus or proximal tibia or soft tissue disruption in these areas.

Early recognition and effective treatment of compartment syndrome are essential to prevent permanent damage to muscles and nerves. Ischemia can occur within 4 to 8 hours after onset. Compartment syndrome may occur initially from the physiological response of the body or may be delayed for several days from the original insult/injury.

The "six Ps" are a neurovascular assessment mnemonic that can be used to assess for impending compartment syndrome: (1) *paresthesia* (numbness and tingling); (2) *pain* distal to the injury that is not relieved by opioid analgesics and pain on passive stretch of muscle travelling through the compartment; (3) *pressure*

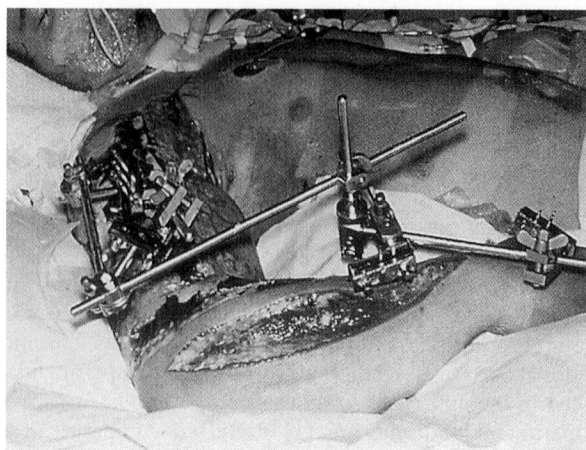

Figure 65-15 Volkmann's ischemic contracture of the forearm following acute compartment syndrome secondary to a supracondylar fracture of the humerus. Note the incision line of an unsuccessful fasciotomy.

Source: Ryan, D. W., & Park, G. R. (1995). *Colour atlas of critical and intensive care: Diagnosis and investigation.* London: Mosby-Wolfe.

increases in the compartment; (4) *pallor,* coolness, and loss of normal colour of the extremity; (5) *paralysis* or loss of function; and (6) *pulselessness* or diminished/absent peripheral pulses (Malik et al., 2009).

Carefully assess the location, quality, and intensity of the pain (see Chapter 10). Evaluate the pain on a scale of 0 to 10. Pain unrelieved by drugs and out of proportion to the level of injury is one of the first indications of impending compartment syndrome. Pulselessness and paralysis (in particular) are later signs of compartment syndrome. Notify the health care provider immediately of a patient's changing condition.

Because of the possibility of muscle damage, assess urine output. Myoglobin released from damaged muscle cells precipitates as a gel-like substance and causes obstruction in renal tubules.

This condition results in acute tubular necrosis and acute kidney injury. Common signs are dark reddish brown urine and clinical manifestations associated with acute kidney injury (see Chapter 49).

Elevation of the extremity may lower venous pressure and slow arterial perfusion; thus, the extremity should not be elevated above heart level. Similarly, the application of cold compresses may result in vasoconstriction and exacerbate compartment syndrome. It may also be necessary to remove or loosen the bandage and bivalve or split the cast in half. A reduction in traction weight may also decrease external circumferential pressures.

Surgical decompression (e.g., fasciotomy) of the involved compartment may be necessary. The fasciotomy site is left open for several days to ensure adequate soft tissue decompression. Infection resulting from delayed wound closure is a potential problem following a fasciotomy. Severe compartment syndrome may require amputation to decrease myoglobinemia or to replace a functionally useless extremity with a prosthesis.

Venous Thromboembolism

The veins of the lower extremities and the pelvis are highly susceptible to thrombus formation after fracture, especially a hip fracture. Venous thromboembolism may also occur after total hip or total knee replacement surgery (Lazo-Langner & Rodger, 2009). In patients with limited mobility, venous stasis is aggravated by inactivity of the muscles that normally assist in the pumping action of venous blood returning to the extremities.

Because of the high risk of venous thromboembolism in the orthopedic surgical patient, prophylactic anticoagulant drugs such as warfarin, low–molecular weight heparin (LMWH) (e.g., enoxaparin [Lovenox]), or fondaparinux (Arixtra) may be ordered. In addition to wearing compression gradient stockings (antiembolism hose) and using sequential compression devices, instruct the patient to move (dorsiflex/plantar flex) the fingers or toes of the affected extremity against resistance and to perform ROM exercises on the unaffected lower extremities. (Assessment and management of venous thromboembolism are discussed in Chapter 40.)

Fat Embolism Syndrome

Fat embolism syndrome (FES) is characterized by the presence of systemic fat globules from fractures that are distributed into tissues and organs after a traumatic skeletal injury. FES is fatal in 5 to 15% of patients (Carlson & Pfadt, 2011). The fractures that most often cause FES are those of the long bones, ribs, tibia, and pelvis. FES has also been known to occur following total joint replacement, spinal fusion, liposuction, crush injuries, and bone marrow transplantation. One theory related to the origin of fat emboli suggests that fat is released from the marrow of injured bone and enters the systemic circulation where the fat embolizes to other organs such as the brain (Galway, Tetzlaff & Helfand, 2009). A second theory postulates that a biochemical change initiated by injury sets up an inflammatory response causing a biochemical injury to the lung parenchyma. The tissues of the lungs, brain, heart, kidneys, and skin are most often affected.

Clinical Manifestations. Early recognition of FES is crucial in preventing a potentially lethal course. Initial manifestations usually occur 24 to 48 hours after the injury. Severe forms have occurred within hours of injury. The fat globules transported to the lungs cause a hemorrhagic interstitial pneumonitis that produces signs and symptoms of acute respiratory distress syndrome, such as chest pain, tachypnea, cyanosis, dyspnea, apprehension, tachycardia, and decreased partial pressure of arterial oxygen (PaO_2). All of these symptoms are caused by poor oxygen exchange. Because they are frequently the first symptoms to manifest, changes in the mental status as a result of hypoxemia are important to recognize. Memory loss, restlessness, confusion, elevated temperature, and headache prompt further investigation so that central nervous system involvement is not mistaken for alcohol withdrawal or acute head injury. The continued change in level of consciousness and petechiae located around neck, anterior chest wall, axilla, buccal membrane, and conjunctiva of the eye helps distinguish fat emboli from other problems. Petechiae result from intravascular thromboses caused by decreased oxygenation.

The clinical course of a fat embolus may be rapid and acute. Frequently, the patient expresses a feeling of impending disaster. In a short time, skin colour changes from pallid to cyanotic, and the patient may become comatose. No specific laboratory examinations are available to aid in the diagnosis. However, certain diagnostic abnormalities may be present. These include fat cells in the blood, urine, or sputum; a decrease of the PaO_2 to less than 60 mm Hg; ST-segment changes on the electrocardiogram; a decrease in the platelet count and hematocrit levels; and a prolonged prothrombin time resulting from hemorrhaging into the lungs. A chest radiograph may reveal areas of pulmonary infiltrate or multiple areas of consolidation. This is sometimes referred to as the "white-out effect."

Collaborative Care. Treatment for fat embolism is directed at prevention. Careful immobilization of a long bone fracture is probably the most important element in the prevention of fat embolism. Management of FES is essentially symptom related and supportive (Galway et al., 2009). Treatment includes fluid resuscitation to prevent hypovolemic shock, correction of acidosis, and replacement blood loss. Coughing and deep breathing should be encouraged. The patient should be repositioned as little as possible before fracture immobilization or stabilization because of the danger of dislodging more fat droplets into the general circulation. Use of corticosteroids to prevent or treat fat embolism is controversial. Oxygen is administered to treat hypoxia. Intubation or intermittent positive-pressure breathing may be considered if a satisfactory PaO_2 cannot be obtained with supplemental oxygen alone. Some patients may develop pulmonary edema, acute respiratory distress syndrome, or both, leading to an increased mortality rate. Most patients survive FES with few sequelae.

Types of Fractures

Colles Fracture

Colles fracture is a fracture of the distal radius and is one of the most common fractures in adults. The styloid process of the ulna may be involved as well. The injury usually occurs when the patient attempts to break a fall with an outstretched hand (Altizer, 2008). This type of fracture most often occurs in women older than age 50 whose bones are osteoporotic.

The clinical manifestations of Colles fracture are pain in the immediate area of injury, pronounced swelling, and dorsal displacement of the distal fragment (silver-fork deformity). This may appear as an obvious deformity on the wrist. The major complication associated with a Colles fracture is vascular insufficiency as a result of edema. CTS can be a later complication.

A Colles fracture is usually managed by closed manipulation of the fracture and immobilization by either a splint or a cast or, if displaced, by external fixation. The wrist must be immobilized to prevent wrist supination and pronation. Nursing management should include frequent neurovascular assessments and measures to prevent or reduce edema. Support and protection of the extremity should be provided, along with encouragement of active movement of the thumb and fingers. This type of movement helps reduce edema and increases venous return. The patient should be instructed to perform active movements of the shoulder to prevent stiffness or contracture.

Fracture of the Humerus

Fractures involving the shaft of the humerus are a common injury among young and middle-aged adults. The prominent clinical manifestations are an obvious displacement of the humerus shaft, shortened extremity, abnormal mobility, and pain (Figure 65-16). The major complications associated with fracture of the humerus are radial nerve injury and vascular injury to the brachial artery as a result of laceration, transection, or muscle spasm.

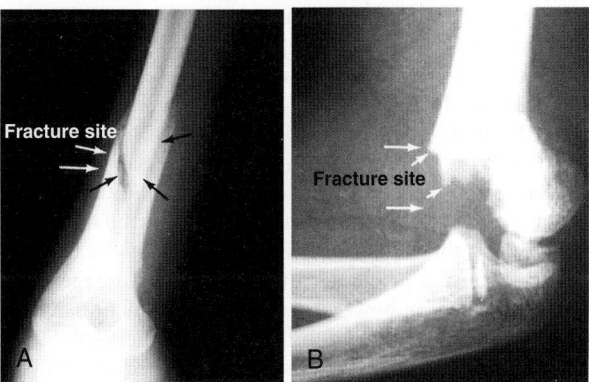

Figure 65-16 A, Supracondylar fracture of the humerus. This type of injury results in the formation of a large hematoma. **B,** Fracture of the distal shaft of the humerus.

The treatment for a fracture of the humerus depends on the location and displacement of the fracture. Nonoperative treatment may include a hanging arm cast, a shoulder immobilizer, or the sling and swathe, which is a type of immobilization that prevents glenohumeral movement. The swathe encircles the trunk and the humerus as an additional binder. It is often used for surgical repairs and shoulder dislocation.

When these devices are used, the head of the bed should be elevated to assist gravity in reducing the fracture. The arm should be allowed to hang freely when the patient is sitting and standing. Nursing care should include measures to protect the axilla and prevent skin maceration by placing lightly powdered absorbable dressing pads in the axilla and changing them twice daily or as needed. Skin or skeletal traction may be used for purposes of reduction and immobilization.

During the rehabilitative phase, an exercise program geared toward improving strength and motion of the injured extremity is extremely important. This should include assisted motion of the hand and fingers. The shoulder can also be exercised if the fracture is stable. This helps to prevent stiffness secondary to frozen shoulder or arthrofibrosis.

Fracture of the Pelvis

Pelvic fractures range from benign to life threatening, depending on the mechanism of injury and associated vascular insult (Bodden, 2009). Although only a small percentage of all fractures are pelvic fractures, this type of injury is associated with the highest mortality rate. Preoccupation with more obvious injuries at the time of a traumatic event may result in an oversight of pelvic injuries. Pelvic fractures may cause serious intra-abdominal injury such as paralytic ileus, hemorrhage, and laceration of the urethra, the bladder, or the colon. Patients may survive the initial pelvic injury, only to die from sepsis, FES, or DVT complications.

Physical examination demonstrates local swelling, tenderness, deformity, unusual pelvic movement, and ecchymosis on the abdomen. The neurovascular status of the lower extremities and manifestations of associated injuries should be assessed. Pelvic fractures are diagnosed by radiography and computed tomography (CT) scan (Walker, 2011).

Treatment of a pelvic fracture depends on the severity of the injury. Stable, nondisplaced fractures such as those sustained in a fall require limited intervention, and early mobilization is encouraged. Bed rest for stable pelvic fractures is maintained from a few days to 6 weeks. More complex fractures may be treated with pelvic sling traction, skeletal traction, hip spica casts, external fixation, open reduction, or a combination of these methods. ORIF of a pelvic fracture may be necessary if the fracture is displaced. Extreme care in handling and moving the patient is important to prevent serious injury from a displaced fracture fragment. Turn the patient only when ordered by the health care provider. Because a pelvic fracture can lead to damage to other organs, assessment of bowel and urinary tract function and distal neurovascular status are important nursing measures. Provide back care while the patient is raised from the bed either by independent use of the trapeze or with adequate assistance. Pelvic fractures can be extremely painful and require the appropriate assessment and management of pain to promote recovery and participation in rehabilitation.

Fracture of the Hip

Hip fractures are common in older adults. In 2005 to 2006, there were approximately 28,200 hospitalizations for hip fractures across Canada, with 88% involving patients aged 65 or older (Canadian Institute for Health Information [CIHI], 2007). Although most hip fractures occur in the community, CIHI reported that nearly 1 in 1000 older persons admitted to a hospital fracture a hip during their stay. Older adult women suffer 80% of broken hips (CIHI, 2009a). Some 70% of hip fractures are related to osteoporosis. Hip fractures require one of the longest hospital stays, averaging more than 19 days. Of older adults hospitalized with hip fracture, 10 to 20% die within 6 months, 50% never walk again without assistance, and 25% need extensive care at home (CIHI, 2009a).

A *fracture of the hip* (Figure 65-17) refers to a fracture of the proximal third of the femur, which extends up to 5 cm below the lesser trochanter. Fractures that occur within the hip joint capsule are called *intracapsular fractures*. Intracapsular fractures (femoral neck) are further identified by a name derived from specific locations: (1) *capital* (fracture of the head of the femur), (2) *subcapital* (fractures just below the head of the femur), and (3) *transcervical* (fractures of the neck of the femur). These fractures are often associated with osteoporosis and minor trauma. *Extracapsular fractures* occur outside the joint capsule. They are termed (1) *intertrochanteric* if they occur in a region between the greater and the lesser trochanter or (2) *subtrochanteric* if they occur in the region below the lesser trochanter. Extracapsular fractures are usually caused by severe direct trauma or a fall.

Clinical Manifestations

The clinical manifestations of hip fractures are external rotation, muscle spasm, shortening of the affected extremity, and severe pain and tenderness in the region of the fracture site. Displaced femoral neck fractures cause serious disruption of the blood supply to the femoral head, which can result in AVN of the femoral head.

Collaborative Care

Surgical repair is the preferred method of managing intracapsular and extracapsular hip fractures. Surgical treatment permits early mobilization of the patient and decreases the risk of major complications. Initially, the affected extremity may be temporarily immobilized by Buck's traction (see Figure 65-10) until the patient's physical condition is stabilized and surgery can be performed. Buck's traction relieves painful muscle spasms and is used for a maximum of 24 to 48 hours.

Intracapsular (femoral neck) fractures are usually repaired with the use of an endoprosthesis to replace the femoral head *(hemiarthroplasty)* (Figure 65-18, *A*). Extracapsular fractures are repaired using sliding hip screws, intramedullary devices, and replacement prostheses (see Figure 65-18, *B*). The principles of patient care for these procedures are similar.

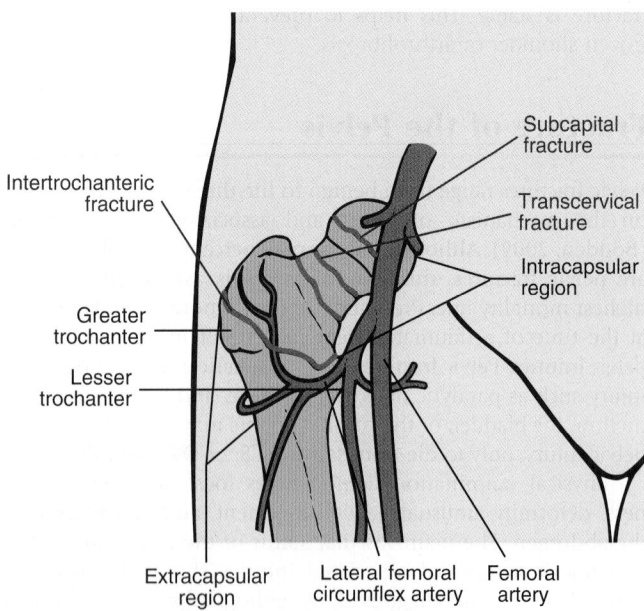

Figure 65-17 Femur with location of various types of fracture.

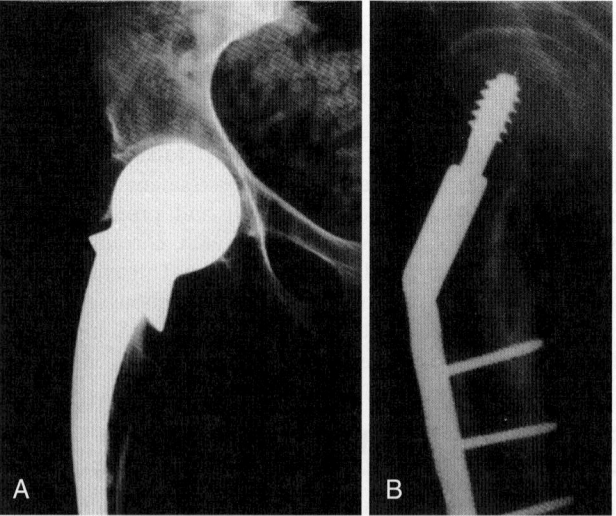

Figure 65-18 Types of internal fixation for a hip fracture. **A,** Femoral head endoprosthesis. **B,** Type of hip compression screw with side plate.

Source: Thompson, J. M., McFarland, G. K., Hirsh, J. E., & Tucker, S. M. (1997). *Mosby's clinical nursing* (4th ed.). St. Louis: Mosby.

NURSING MANAGEMENT: HIP FRACTURE

Nursing Implementation

Preoperative Management

Because older adults are most prone to hip fractures, chronic health problems must often be considered when planning treatment (Auron-Gomez & Michota, 2008). Diabetes mellitus, hypertension, heart failure, pulmonary disease, and arthritis are chronic problems that may complicate clinical status. Surgery may be delayed for a brief time until the patient's general health is stabilized.

Before surgery, severe muscle spasms can increase pain. Appropriate analgesics or muscle relaxants, comfortable positioning unless contraindicated, and properly adjusted traction can help in managing the spasms.

Teaching is often done in the emergency department because quick surgical intervention is the standard of care today. Many patients will not have an overnight preoperative period in which to receive instructions, or the patient may not have the cognitive abilities to retain this important patient education. When possible, the patient can be taught the method and frequency for exercising the unaffected leg and both arms. The patient should also be encouraged to use the overhead trapeze bar and the opposite siderail to assist in changing positions. A physiotherapist can begin to teach out-of-bed and chair transfers. The family/caregiver must also be informed about the patient's weight-bearing status after surgery. Plans for discharge begin as the patient enters the hospital because the length of stay postoperatively will be only a few days.

Postoperative Management

The initial postoperative management of a patient following ORIF of a hip fracture is similar to that for any older adult patient undergoing surgery. The nurse must monitor vital signs, intake, and output; supervise respiratory activities, such as deep breathing and coughing; administer pain medication; and observe the dressing and incision for signs of bleeding and infection. An NCP for the orthopedic surgical patient is presented in NCP 65-2 on p. 1830.

In the early postoperative period, there is a potential for neurovascular impairment. The nurse assesses the patient's extremity for (1) colour, (2) temperature, (3) capillary refill, (4) distal pulses, (5) edema, (6) sensation, (7) motor function, and (8) pain. Edema is alleviated by elevation of the leg whenever the patient is in a chair. The pain resulting from poor alignment of the affected extremity can be reduced by keeping pillows (or an abductor splint) between the knees when the patient is turning to either side. Sandbags, pillows, or a trochanter roll are also used to prevent external rotation. If an endoprosthesis was placed, the patient is at risk for hip dislocation. Hip precautions must be demonstrated and explained to the patient and her or his family or caregiver.

The physiotherapist usually supervises active-assistance exercises for the affected extremity and ambulation when the surgeon permits it. Ambulation usually begins on the first postoperative day. The nurse in collaboration with the physiotherapist monitors the patient's ambulation status for proper crutch walking or use

*For patients having surgery by a posterior approach.

of the walker. For the patient to be discharged home, the patient must be able to safely demonstrate use of crutches or a walker, the ability to transfer into and from a chair and the bed, and the ability to ascend and descend stairs.

Complications associated with femoral neck fracture include nonunion, AVN, dislocation, and degenerative arthritis. As a result of an intertrochanteric fracture, the affected leg may be shortened. A cane or built-up shoe may be required for safe ambulation.

If the hip fracture has been treated by insertion of a femoral head prosthesis with a *posterior approach* (accessing the hip joint from the back), measures to prevent dislocation must always be used (Table 65-11). Avoid extremes in flexion initially after prosthetic replacement from a posterior approach. The patient and the caregiver must be fully aware of positions and activities that predispose the patient to dislocation (>90 degrees of flexion, adduction, or internal rotation). Many daily activities may reproduce these positions, including putting on shoes and socks, crossing the legs or feet while seated, assuming the side-lying position incorrectly, standing up or sitting down while the body is flexed more than 90 degrees relative to the chair, and sitting on low seats, especially low toilet seats. Until the soft tissue surrounding the hip has healed sufficiently to stabilize the prosthesis, usually for at least 6 weeks, these activities must be avoided.

When the hip fracture is accessed during surgery with an *anterior or anterolateral approach* (joint reached from front of body), the hip muscles are left intact. This approach generally results in a more stable hip in the postoperative period with a lower rate of complications (e.g., infection, dislocation) (Ferguson & Eastman, 2011). Precautions for the patient related to motion and weight bearing are few and may include instructions to avoid hyperextension.

Sudden severe pain, a lump in the buttock, limb shortening, and external rotation indicate prosthesis dislocation. This requires a closed reduction with conscious sedation or open reduction to realign the femoral head in the acetabulum. If this occurs (regardless of the setting), keep the patient on nothing-by-mouth status in anticipation of a possible surgical intervention.

In addition to teaching the patient and caregiver how to prevent prosthesis dislocation, the nurse should (1) place a large pillow between the patient's legs when turning, (2) avoid extreme hip flexion, and (3) turn patient only on the side approved by the surgeon. Traditionally, patients were only turned on their unaffected side postoperatively. Some surgeons prefer to turn hip surgery patients on the affected side because there is less chance of the affected leg slipping and causing adduction and, possibly, dislocation. In addition, some health care providers prefer that the patient keep leg abductor splints on except when bathing.

The patient is out of bed on the first postoperative day. Weight bearing on the involved extremity varies. Weight bearing of especially fragile fractures may be restricted until radiography indicates adequate healing, usually at 6 to 12 weeks.

The nurse assists both the patient and the family in adjusting to the restrictions and dependence imposed by the hip fracture. Anxiety and depression can easily occur, but creative nursing care and awareness of the problem can do much to prevent it. The patient and family may need to be informed about community referral services that can assist in the postdischarge rehabilitation phase. Hospitalization averages 4 to 5 days. Patients frequently require care in a subacute unit, at a skilled nursing facility, or in a rehabilitation facility for a few weeks before returning home. More patients are returning directly home (if their home is accessible and they have a caregiver to assist) to be followed by a home care nurse and to attend outpatient physiotherapy.

▪ Evaluation

The expected outcomes for the patient with fracture of the hip are presented in NCP 65-2.

AGE-RELATED CONSIDERATIONS: HIP FRACTURE

Factors that contribute to the occurrence of a hip fracture in older adults include a propensity to fall, inability to correct a postural imbalance, inadequacy of local tissue shock absorbers (e.g., fat, muscle bulk), and underlying skeletal strength. Several factors have been identified in older persons that increase their risk of falling. These include gait and balance problems, decreased vision and hearing, decreased reflexes, orthostatic hypotension, and medication use. Leading hazards of falls are loose rugs and slippery or uneven surfaces. Many falls are associated with getting in or out of a chair or bed. Falls to the side, the most common type in the frail elderly, are more likely to result in a hip fracture than is a forward fall (Centers for Disease Control and Prevention [CDC], 2010). External hip protectors may be helpful in preventing hip fractures in the frail older adult patient who is not taking medication to prevent fractures (Juby, 2009).

Two important factors influencing the amount of force imposed on the hip are the presence of energy-absorbing soft tissue over the greater trochanter and the state of leg muscle contraction at the time of the fall. Because many older adult persons have poor muscle tone, these are important factors in the severity of a fall. Older adult women often have osteoporosis and accompanying low bone density, which increases the risk of hip and other types of fracture.

Targeted interventions to reduce the incidence of hip fractures in the older adult include a variety of strategies. Calcium and vitamin D supplementation, estrogen replacement, and bisphosphonate drug therapy have been shown to decrease bone loss or increase bone density and decrease the likelihood of fracture. (Osteoporosis is discussed in Chapter 66.) Nurses must be vigilant in planning interventions for the older adult that are known to reduce the incidence of falls and hip fractures (Registered Nurses' Association of Ontario [RNAO], 2005, rev. 2011).

Femoral Shaft Fracture

Femoral shaft fracture is a common injury occurring particularly in young adults. Severe direct force is required to produce this injury because the femur can bend slightly before actual fracture occurs. The force exerted to cause the fracture often causes damage to the adjacent soft tissue structures. These injuries may be more serious than the bone injury. Displacement of the fracture fragments often results in open fracture and increased soft tissue damage. This can result in considerable blood loss (1 to 1.5 L).

The clinical manifestations of a fracture of the femoral shaft are usually obvious. They include marked deformity and angulation, shortening of the extremity, inability to move either the hip or the knee, and pain. The common complications associated with fracture of the femoral shaft include fat embolism, nerve and vascular injury, and problems associated with bone union, open fracture, and soft tissue damage.

Initial management is directed toward stabilization of the patient and immobilization of the fracture. Use of prolonged traction is not commonly used as the standard of care. ORIF has become the preferred method to manage a femoral fracture. It is carried out with an intramedullary rod, compression plate, and screws or side plate with an intercondylar nail. Internal fixation is often the preferred treatment because it reduces hospital stay and the complications associated with prolonged bed rest. Other indications for internal fixation are failure to obtain satisfactory reduction by nonsurgical methods and multiple associated injuries. In some instances, the surgically repaired femur may be supported by suspension traction for 3 to 4 days to prevent excessive movement of the extremity and to control rotation. Then non–weight-bearing gait training is begun. Fractures associated with extensive soft tissue injury may be treated with external fixation.

Promotion and maintenance of strength in the affected extremity usually include gluteal and quadriceps isometric exercises. It is important to ensure performance of ROM and strengthening exercises for all uninvolved extremities in preparation for ambulation. The patient may be immobilized in a hip spica cast and gradually progress to an articulating cast brace or may be allowed to begin non–weight-bearing activities with an ambulatory assistive device. Full weight bearing is usually restricted until there is radiographic evidence of union of the fracture fragments.

Fracture of the Tibia

Although the tibia is vulnerable to injury because it lacks anterior muscle covering, strong force is required to produce a fractured tibia. As a result, soft tissue damage, devascularization, and open fracture are frequent. The tibia is one of the more common sites of a stress fracture. Complications associated with tibial fractures are compartment syndrome, FES, problems associated with bony union, and possible infection associated with open fracture. Amputation may be required if adequate muscle and tissue coverage is not achieved following muscle and flap grafts.

The recommended management for closed tibial fracture is closed reduction followed by immobilization in a long leg cast. ORIF with intramedullary rods, plate fixation, or external fixation is indicated for complex fractures and those with extensive soft tissue damage. Locking plates (screw and plate system) is a newer minimally invasive surgical device (Ronga, Shanmugam, Longo, Oliva, & Maffulli, 2009). In both types of reduction, emphasis is placed on maintaining the strength of the quadriceps.

The neurovascular status of the affected extremity must be assessed at least every 2 hours during the first 48 hours. Patients are instructed to perform active ROM exercises with all uninvolved extremities, as well as exercises for the upper extremities, to build the strength required for crutch walking. When the health care provider has determined that the patient is ready for gait training, the patient is instructed in the principles of crutch walking. The patient may be on non–weight-bearing status for 6 to 12 weeks, depending on healing. Home nursing visits can be initiated to augment outpatient appointments and monitor the patient's progress.

Stable Vertebral Fractures

Stable fractures of the vertebral column are usually caused by motor vehicle accidents, falls, diving, or athletic injuries. A stable fracture is one in which the fracture or the fragment is not likely to move or cause spinal cord damage. This type of injury is frequently confined to the anterior element (vertebral body) of the spinal column in the lumbar region and involves the cervical and thoracic regions less frequently. The vertebral bodies are usually protected from displacement by the intact spinal ligaments.

Most patients with spinal fractures have stable fractures and experience only brief periods of disability. However, if the ligamentous structures are significantly disrupted, dislocation of the vertebral structures may occur, resulting in instability and injury to the spinal cord (unstable fracture). These injuries generally necessitate surgery. The most serious complication of vertebral fractures is fracture displacement, which can cause damage to the spinal cord (see Chapter 63). Although stable vertebral fractures are not associated with pathological spinal cord conditions, all spinal injuries should initially be considered unstable and potentially serious until diagnostic tests are done and the physician determines that the fracture is stable.

The patient usually complains of pain and tenderness in the affected region of the spine. Sudden loss of function below the level of fracture indicates severe fracture with spinal cord impingement and paraplegia. Stable compression fractures are associated with a *kyphotic deformity* (flexion angulation of several vertebrae). This deformity may be noted during the physical examination. In patients with a stable vertebral fracture secondary to osteoporosis, several vertebral levels may be involved as evidenced by a *dowager hump* (abnormal curvature of thoracic spine) or *lumbar lordosis* (extreme inward curve). The cervical spine may also be involved. Bowel and bladder dysfunction may be an indication of an interruption of the autonomic nervous system or injury to the spinal cord.

The overall goal in management of stable vertebral fractures is to keep the spine in good alignment until union has been accomplished. Many nursing interventions are aimed at assessing for the possibility of spinal cord trauma. Vital signs and bowel and bladder function should be evaluated regularly. Also monitor the motor and sensory status of the peripheral nerves distal to the injured region. Any deterioration in the patient's neurovascular status should be promptly reported.

Treatment includes support, a short period of rest, and pain medication followed by early mobilization and bracing. If hospitalized, the patient is usually placed in a standard hospital bed with firm support from the mattress or a bed board. The aim is to support the spinal column, relax muscles, and release any compression on nerve roots. When turning, the patient should be taught to keep the spine straight by turning shoulders and pelvis together. Nursing assistance is necessary for the patient to learn the technique of "log rolling" (Figure 65-19). Several days after the initial injury, the physician may apply a specially constructed orthotic device (e.g., Milwaukee, Jewett, or Taylor brace), a jacket cast, or a removable corset if there is no evidence of neurological deficit.

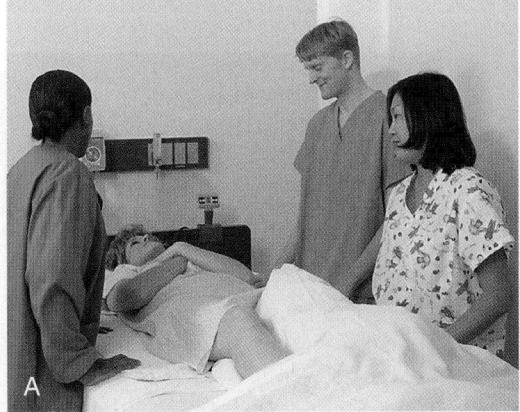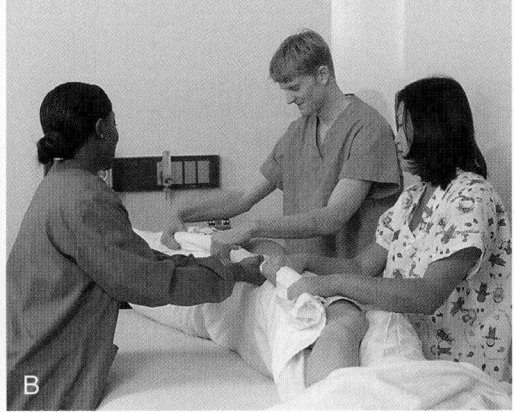

Figure 65-19 Log rolling a patient.

Source: Perry, A. G., & Potter, P. A. (2009). *Clinical nursing skills & techniques* (7th ed., p. 223, Step 6i [3-5]). St. Louis: Mosby.

Vertebral compression fractures (which are often caused by osteoporosis) can be treated with two newer outpatient procedures, vertebroplasty and kyphoplasty. *Vertebroplasty* uses radioimaging to guide the injection of bone cement into the fractured vertebral body. The cement (when hardened) serves to stabilize and prevent further vertebral compression. *Kyphoplasty* initially involves inserting a balloon into the vertebral body and then inflating it. This creates a cavity that is filled with bone cement under low pressure. Kyphoplasty results in a lower leakage of bone cement when compared with vertebroplasty and helps restore the height of the vertebral body (Meade, Malas, Patwardha, & Gavin, 2008). Ongoing clinical trials are mixed as to the effectiveness of these procedures in providing pain relief and improved function (Kallmes et al., 2009; Wilhelm, 2009).

If the fracture is in the cervical spine, a hard cervical collar may be worn by the patient. Some cervical fractures are immobilized by use of a halo vest (see Chapter 63, Figure 63-10). This consists of a plastic jacket or cast fitted about the chest and attached to a halo that is held in place by skeletal pins inserted into the cranium. These devices immobilize the spine in the fracture area but allow patient mobility. The patient is discharged after (1) regaining ambulation skills, (2) learning care of the cast or orthotic device, and (3) learning how to cope with the safety and security imposed by injury and treatment.

Facial Fractures

Any bone of the face can be fractured as a result of trauma. Fractures can occur as a result of collision with another person or object, fighting, or blunt trauma. The primary concern after facial injury is to establish and maintain a patent airway and to provide adequate ventilation by removal of foreign material and blood. Suctioning may be necessary. An alternative airway (tracheostomy) may be needed if a patent airway cannot be maintained. Pressure packing controls hemorrhage. Cervical spine injuries are common. All patients with facial injuries should be treated as if they have a cervical injury until proven otherwise by examination and imaging studies (e.g., CT scan, radiography). Table 65-12 describes the clinical manifestations of common facial fractures.

Concurrent soft tissue injury often makes assessment of a facial injury difficult. Oral and facial examinations should be performed after the patient has been stabilized and any

life-threatening situations have been treated. Careful assessment is made of the ocular muscles and cranial nerve involvement (cranial nerves III, IV, and VI). A radiograph documents the extent of the injury.

CT scanning helps differentiate between bone and soft tissue and gives a more precise view of the fracture.

Injury to the eye must be suspected when a facial injury occurs, particularly if the injury is near the orbit. If an eye-globe rupture is suspected, the examination is stopped and a protective shield is placed over the eye. Signs of globe rupture include the extrusion of vitreous humor or brown tissue (iris or ciliary body) on the surface of the globe or penetrating through a laceration with an eccentric or teardrop-shaped pupil. Specific treatment of a facial fracture depends on the site and the extent of the fracture and the associated soft tissue injury. Immobilization or surgical stabilization may be necessary.

The patient who sustains a facial fracture requires sensitive nursing care because alteration in appearance after the trauma may be drastic. Edema and discolouration subside with time, but concurrent soft tissue injuries may result in permanent scarring. Attention to maintenance of a patent airway and adequate nutrition are ongoing concerns of the nurse throughout the recovery period. Suction should always be available to maintain a patent airway for patients with facial trauma.

Mandible Fracture

A fracture of the mandible may result from trauma to the face or the jaws. Maxillary fractures may also occur, but they are less common than mandibular fractures. The fracture may be simple, with no bone displacement, or it may involve loss of tissue and bone. The fracture may require immediate and sometimes long-term treatment to ensure survival and restore satisfactory appearance and function. Mandibular fracture may also be therapeutically performed to correct an underlying malocclusion problem that cannot be corrected by orthodontic procedures alone. In these conditions, the mandible is resected during surgery and manipulated forward or backward depending on the occlusion problem.

Surgery consists of immobilization, usually by wiring the jaws (*intermaxillary fixation*. Internal fixation may be done with screws and plates. In a simple fracture with no loss of teeth, the lower jaw is wired to the upper jaw. Wires are placed around the teeth, and then cross-wires or rubber bands are used to hold the lower jaw tight against the upper jaw (Figure 65-20). Arch

Table 65-12	Clinical Manifestations of Facial Fractures
FRACTURE	**CLINICAL MANIFESTATION**
Frontal bone	Rapid edema that may mask underlying fractures
Periorbital	Possible frontal sinus involvement, entrapment of ocular muscles
Nasal	Displacement of nasal bones, epistaxis
Zygomatic arch	Depression of zygomatic arch and entrapment of ocular muscles
Maxilla	Segmental motion of maxilla and alveolar fracture of teeth
Mandible	Tooth fractures, bleeding, limited motion of mandible

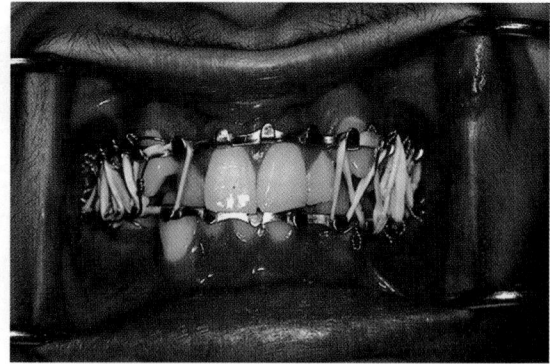

Figure 65-20 Intermaxillary fixation.

Source: Courtesy R. A. Weinstein, Denver.

bars may be placed on the maxillary and mandibular arches of the teeth. Vertical wires are placed between the arch bars holding the jaws together. When teeth are missing or if there is bone displacement, other forms of fixation such as metal arch bars in the mouth or insertion of a pin in the bone may be needed. Bone grafting may also be required. Immobilization is usually necessary for only 4 to 6 weeks because the fractures often heal rapidly.

NURSING MANAGEMENT: MANDIBULAR FRACTURE

■ Nursing Implementation

■ Preoperative Management

The patient should be told preoperatively about the surgical procedure, including what it involves, how the face will look, and alterations caused by the surgery. The patient must be reassured about the ability to breathe normally, speak, and swallow liquids. Usually, hospitalization is brief unless there are other injuries or problems.

■ Postoperative Management

Postoperative care should focus on a patent airway, oral hygiene, communication, and adequate nutrition. Two major potential problems in the immediate postoperative period are airway obstruction and aspiration of vomitus. Because the patient cannot open the jaws, measures to ensure an airway are essential. The nurse must observe for signs of respiratory distress (e.g., dyspnea; alterations in rate, quality, and depth of respirations). The patient should be placed on the side with the head slightly elevated immediately after surgery.

Wire cutters or scissors (for rubber bands) must be taped to the head of the bed and sent with the patient on all appointments and examinations away from the bedside. These may be used to cut the wires or elastic bands in case of an emergency. Once the patient is awake, the wires should be cut only in case of cardiac or respiratory arrest necessitating access to the pharynx or the lungs.

The surgeon should explain, by using a picture, the appropriate wire or wires to cut, and this should be included in the care plan. In some cases, cutting the wires may cause the entire facial and upper jaw structure to collapse and worsen the problem. A tracheostomy tray or an endotracheal tray should always be available.

If the patient begins to vomit or choke, the nurse should try to clear the mouth and airway. Suctioning may be necessary and may be performed by the nasopharyngeal or oral route, depending on the extent of injury and the type of repair. A nasogastric tube may be used for decompression to remove fluids and gas from the stomach in an effort to help prevent aspiration. This technique also helps prevent vomiting. Antiemetic medications may also be administered. The nurse should teach the patient to clear secretions and vomitus.

Oral hygiene is an important part of the nursing care. The mouth should be rinsed frequently, particularly after meals and snacks, to remove food debris. Warm normal saline solution, water, or alkaline mouthwashes may be used. A soft rubber catheter or a Water-Pik is effective for a thorough oral cleansing. The nurse should inspect the mouth several times a day to see that it is clean. A flashlight is necessary, and a tongue depressor is used to retract the cheeks. The lips and corners of the mouth as well as the buccal mucosa should be kept moist.

Communication may be a problem, particularly in the early postoperative period. An effective way of communicating must be established preoperatively (e.g., use of picture board, pad and pencil, small chalkboard). Usually, the patient can speak well enough to be understood, especially after the first few postoperative days.

Ingestion of sufficient nutrients poses a challenge because the diet must be liquid. The patient easily tires of sucking through a straw or laboriously using a spoon. The diet must be planned to include adequate calories, protein, and fluids. Liquid protein supplements may be helpful for improving the nutritional status. The nurse works with the dietitian and the patient to ensure adequate nutrition. The low-bulk, high-carbohydrate diet and the intake of air through the straw create a problem with constipation and flatus. Ambulation, prune juice, and bulk-forming laxatives may help relieve these problems.

The patient is usually discharged with the wires in place. The nurse should allow the patient to verbalize feelings about the altered appearance. Discharge teaching should include oral care, techniques of handling secretions, diet, how and when to use wire cutters, and when to notify the health care provider about concerns and problems.

Amputation

Major advances in surgical amputation techniques, prosthetic design, and rehabilitation programs are enabling amputees to return to productive and satisfying social roles. People in the middle and older age groups have the highest incidence of amputation because of the effects of peripheral vascular disease, atherosclerosis, and vascular changes related to diabetes mellitus. Amputation in the younger population is usually secondary to trauma (e.g., motor vehicle collisions, land mines, farm-related injuries).

Clinical Indications

The clinical indications for an amputation depend on the underlying disease or trauma. Amputation is required more often in persons engaged in hazardous occupations, with a greater incidence in men. Common indications for amputation include circulatory impairment resulting from a peripheral vascular disorder, traumatic and thermal injuries, malignant tumours, uncontrolled or widespread infection of the extremity (e.g., gas gangrene, osteomyelitis), and congenital disorders. These conditions may manifest as loss of sensation, inadequate circulation, pallor, and local or systemic manifestations of infection. Although pain is often present, it is not usually the primary reason for an amputation. Consideration must also be given to the patient's ability to successfully use a prosthetic device.

Diagnostic Studies

The types of diagnostic studies performed depend on the underlying problem that makes the amputation necessary (Table 65-13).

COLLABORATIVE CARE

Table 65-13 Amputation

Diagnostic	Collaborative Therapy
• History and physical examination	**Medical**
• Physical appearance of soft tissues	• Appropriate management of underlying disease
• Skin temperature	• Stabilization of trauma victim
• Sensory function	**Surgical**
• Presence of peripheral pulses	• Selective type of amputation
• Arteriography	• Residual limb management
• Venography	• Immediate prosthetic fitting
• Plethysmography	• Delayed prosthetic fitting
• Transcutaneous ultrasonic Doppler recordings	**Rehabilitation**
	• Coordination of prosthesis-fitting and gait-training activities
	• Coordination of muscle-strengthening and physiotherapy regimens

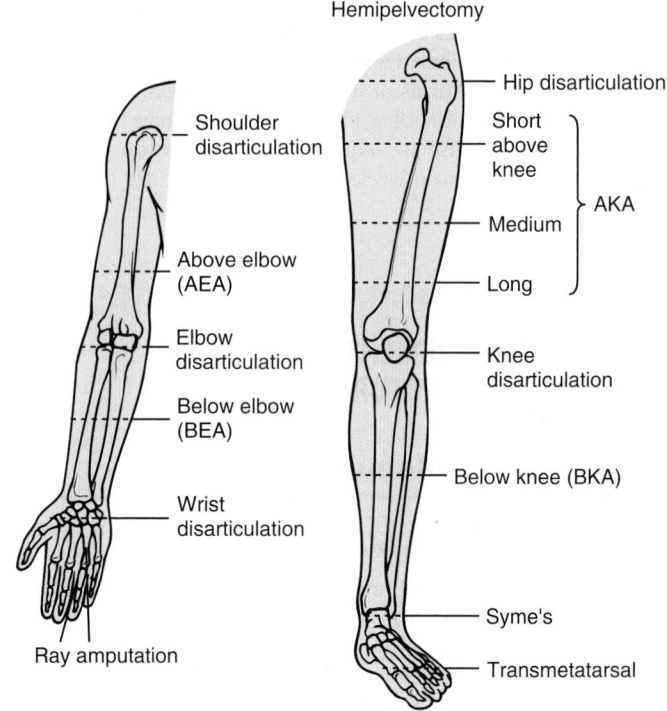

Figure 65-21 Location and description of amputation sites of the upper and lower extremities. *AKA*, above-the-knee amputation.

Test results that show an elevated white blood cell count with abnormal differential may indicate infection. Vascular studies such as arteriography, Doppler studies, and venography provide information about the circulatory status of the extremity.

Collaborative Care

If amputation is to be considered "elective," the patient's general health is carefully assessed. Chronic illnesses and the presence of infection are important considerations. The patient and family should be helped to understand the need for the amputation and be assured that rehabilitation can result in an active, useful life. If the amputation is done on an emergency basis as a result of trauma, the management is physically and emotionally more complicated.

The goal of amputation surgery is to preserve extremity length and function while removing all infected, pathologically compromised, or ischemic tissue. (Levels of amputation of upper and lower extremities are illustrated in Figure 65-21.) The type of amputation depends on the reason for the surgery. A closed amputation is performed to create a weight-bearing *residual limb*. An anterior skin flap with dissected soft tissue padding covers the bony part of the residual limb. The skin flap is sutured posteriorly so that it will not be positioned in a weight-bearing area. Special care is necessary to prevent the accumulation of drainage, which can produce pressure and harbour bacteria that may cause infection.

Disarticulation is an amputation performed through a joint. A *Syme amputation* is a form of disarticulation at the ankle. An open amputation leaves a surface on the residual limb that is not covered with skin. This type of surgery is generally indicated for control of actual or potential infection. The wound is usually closed later by a second surgical procedure or closed by skin traction surrounding the residual limb. This type of amputation is often called a "guillotine amputation."

NURSING MANAGEMENT: AMPUTATION

Nursing Assessment

Pre-existing illnesses must be adequately assessed because most amputations are performed as a result of vascular problems. Assessment of the vascular and neurological status is an important part of this assessment process (see Chapters 34 and 58).

Nursing Diagnoses

Nursing diagnoses for the patient with an amputation may include, but are not limited to, the following:
- Disturbed body image *related to* amputation and impaired mobility
- Impaired skin integrity *related to* immobility and improperly fitted prosthesis
- Chronic pain *related to* phantom limb pain
- Impaired physical mobility *related to* amputation of lower limb

Planning

The overall goals are that the patient with an amputation will (1) have adequate relief from treatment of the underlying health problem, (2) have satisfactory pain control, (3) reach maximum rehabilitation potential with the use of a prosthesis (if indicated),

(4) cope with the body image changes, and (5) make necessary lifestyle adjustments.

Nursing Implementation

Health Promotion

Control of causative illnesses such as peripheral vascular disease, diabetes mellitus, chronic osteomyelitis, and pressure ulcers can eliminate or delay the need for amputation. Patients with these problems should be taught to carefully examine their lower extremities daily for signs of potential problems. If the patient cannot assume this responsibility, a caregiver should be instructed in the procedure. Patients and their caregiver should be instructed to report problems such as change in skin colour or temperature, decrease or absence of sensation, tingling, pain, or the presence of a lesion to the health care provider.

Instruction in proper safety precautions in recreation and in the performance of hazardous work is an important nursing responsibility, especially for occupational health nurses.

Acute Intervention

The nurse must recognize the tremendous psychological and social implications of an amputation for the patient. The disruption in body image caused by an amputation often causes a patient to go through psychological stages similar to the grieving process. Allowing the patient to go through a grieving process or period of depression and recognizing it as a normal consequence may do much to aid the patient's acceptance of the amputation. The patient's family must also be helped to work through the process to arrive at a realistic and positive attitude about the future. The reasons for an amputation and the rehabilitation potential depend on age, diagnosis, occupation, personality, resources, and support systems.

Preoperative Management. Before surgery, the nurse should reinforce information that the patient and family have received about the reasons for the amputation, the proposed prosthesis, and the mobility training program. The patient undergoing an amputation has special education needs. To meet these needs, the nurse must know the level of amputation, the type of postsurgical dressing to be applied, and the type of prosthesis to be utilized. The patient should receive instruction in the performance of upper extremity exercises such as push-ups in bed or the wheelchair to promote arm strength. This instruction is essential for later crutch walking and gait training. General postoperative nursing care should be discussed, including positioning, support, and residual limb care. If a compression bandage is to be used after surgery, the patient should be instructed about its purpose and how it will be applied. If an immediate prosthesis is planned, the general ambulation program should be discussed.

The patient should be warned that she or he may feel as though the amputated limb is still present after surgery. This phenomenon, termed **phantom limb sensation** (any sensation of the missing limb except pain), occurs in 90% of amputees and may cause patients grave concern unless they are forewarned (Hanley et al., 2009). It can take various forms such as the feeling that someone is touching the missing limb, pressure on the missing limb, cold, wetness, itching, tickle, pain, or fatigue (Magee, 2008). Recent studies suggest that 60 to 80% of ampu-

tees may also experience *phantom limb pain* (any painful sensations that are referred to the absent limb), which often begins immediately after surgery. The pain can be described as shooting, burning, crushing, or severe and agonizing (Chapman, 2011). It is more common for the pain to be intermittent with short episodes (seconds to minutes) of severe pain occurring several times a day. There is some evidence that the pain present preoperatively may be mimicked in the phantom limb. Often, the patient may be extremely anxious about this pain because the patient knows the limb is gone but still feels pain in it. As recovery and ambulation progress, phantom limb sensation and pain usually subside, although the pain may become chronic.

Postoperative Management. General postoperative care for the patient who has had an amputation depends largely on the patient's general state of health, the reason for the amputation, and the patient's age. Individuals who undergo amputation as a result of a traumatic injury need to be monitored for post-traumatic stress disorder because they had no time to prepare or perhaps even participate in the decision to have a limb amputated.

Prevention and detection of complications are important nursing responsibilities during the postoperative period. Careful monitoring of the patient's vital signs and dressing can alert the nurse to hemorrhage in the operative area. Careful attention to sterile technique during dressing changes reduces the potential for wound infection.

If an *immediate* postoperative prosthesis has been applied, the nurse must monitor vital signs carefully because the surgical site is heavily covered and may not be visible. A surgical tourniquet must always be available for emergency use. If excessive bleeding occurs, the surgeon should be notified immediately.

The *delayed* prosthetic fitting may be the best choice for patients who have had amputations above the knee or below the elbow, older adults, debilitated individuals, and those with infection (Figure 65-22). The appropriate time for use of a prosthesis

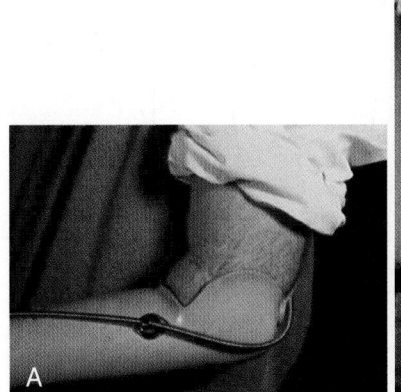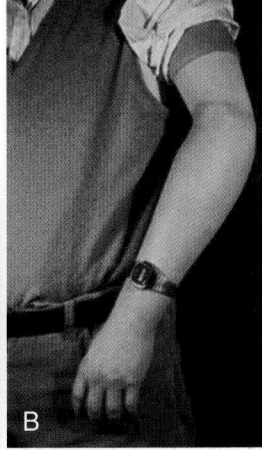

Figure 65-22 Two types of prosthesis. **A,** Traditional fibreglass. **B,** New materials and techniques have made possible the fabrication of prosthetic sockets that are light, soft, flexible, and secure.

Source: Macklin, E. J., Callahan, A., Osterman, A., Skirven, T., Schneider, L., & Hunter, J. (2002). *Hunter, Macklin, and Callahan's rehabilitation of the hand and upper extremity* (vol. 2, 5th ed.). St. Louis: Mosby.

depends on satisfactory healing of the residual limb as well as on the general condition of the patient. A temporary prosthesis may be used for partial weight bearing once the sutures are removed. Barring any problems, patients can bear full weight on permanent prostheses by approximately 3 months after amputation.

Not all patients are candidates for a prosthesis. The seriously ill or debilitated patient may not have the upper body strength and energy required to use a lower extremity prosthesis. Mobility with a wheelchair may be the most realistic goal for patients who are not candidates for prostheses.

Success of the rehabilitative program depends on the physical and emotional health of the patient. Chronic illness and deconditioning complicate aggressive rehabilitation efforts. Both physiotherapy and occupational therapy must be an integral component of the patient's overall plan of care.

Flexion contractures may delay the rehabilitation process. The most common and debilitating contracture is hip flexion. Hip adduction contracture is rare. Patients should avoid sitting in a chair for more than 1 hour with hips flexed, or having pillows under the surgical extremity, to prevent flexion contractures. Unless specifically contraindicated, patients should lie on their abdomen for 30 minutes three to four times each day and position the hip in extension while prone.

Proper residual limb bandaging fosters shaping and moulding for eventual prosthesis fitting (Figure 65-23). The physician usually orders a compression bandage to be applied immediately after surgery to support the soft tissues, reduce edema, hasten healing, minimize pain, and promote residual limb shrinkage and maturation. This bandage may be an elastic roll applied to the residual limb or a residual limb shrinker, which is an elastic stocking that fits tightly over the residual limb and lower trunk area.

The compression bandage is initially worn at all times except during physiotherapy and bathing. The bandage is taken off and reapplied several times daily, and care is taken so that it is applied snugly but not so tightly as to interfere with circulation. Shrinker bandages should be washed and changed daily. After healing has occurred, the residual limb is bandaged only when the patient is not wearing the prosthesis. The patient should be instructed to avoid dangling the residual limb over the bedside to minimize edema formation.

As the patient's overall condition improves, an exercise regimen is normally started under the supervision of the health care provider and the physiotherapist. Active ROM exercises of all joints should be started as soon after surgery as the patient's pain level and medical status permit. In preparation for mobility, the patient should increase triceps and shoulder strength and lower limb support and learn balance of the altered body. The loss of the weight of a limb necessitates adaptation of the patient's proprioceptive mechanisms to prevent falls and frustration.

Crutch walking is started as soon as patients are physically able. After an immediate postsurgical fitting, orders related to weight bearing must be carefully followed to prevent disruption of the skin flap and delay of the healing process. Before discharge, the patient and caregiver need careful instruction related to residual limb care, ambulation, prevention of contractures, recognition of complications, exercise, and follow-up care. Table 65-14 outlines patient and caregiver teaching following an amputation.

▪ Ambulatory and Home Care

When healing has occurred satisfactorily and the residual limb is well moulded, the patient is ready for fitting of a prosthesis. The

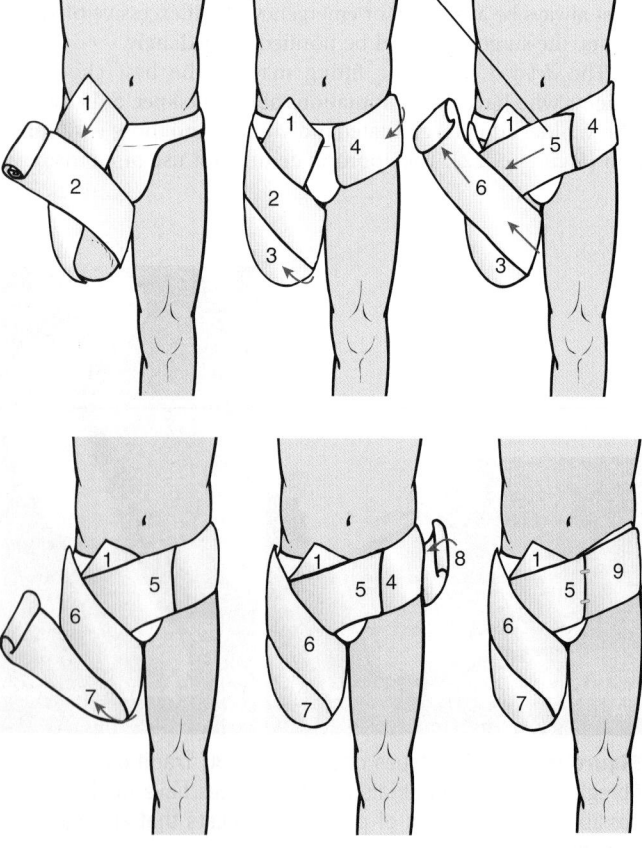

Start of second bandage

Figure 65-23 Bandaging for the above-the-knee amputation residual limb. Figure-of-eight style covers progressive areas of the residual limb. Two elastic wraps are required.

PATIENT & CAREGIVER TEACHING GUIDE

Table 65-14 Following an Amputation
1. Inspect the residual limb daily for signs of skin irritation, especially erythema, excoriation, and odour. Pay particular attention to areas prone to pressure.
2. Discontinue use of the prosthesis if an irritation develops. Have the area checked before resuming use of the prosthesis.
3. Wash residual limb thoroughly each night with warm water and a bacteriostatic soap. Rinse thoroughly and dry gently. Expose the residual limb to air for 20 min.
4. Do not use any substance such as lotions, alcohol, powders, or oil, unless prescribed by the health care provider.
5. Wear only a residual limb sock that is in good condition and supplied by the prosthetist.
6. Change residual limb sock daily. Launder in a mild soap, squeeze, and lay flat to dry.
7. Use prescribed pain management techniques.
8. Perform ROM to all joints daily. Perform general strengthening exercises including the upper extremities daily.
9. Do not elevate the residual limb on a pillow.
10. Lay prone with hip in extension for 30 min three to four times daily.

ROM, range of motion.

prosthetist makes a mould of the residual limb and measures landmarks for the fabrication of the prosthesis. The moulded residual limb socket allows the residual limb to fit snugly into the prosthesis. The residual limb is covered with a stocking to ensure good fit and prevent skin breakdown. The residual limb may continue to shrink, causing a loose fit, in which case a new socket has to be fabricated. The patient may need to have the prosthesis adjusted to prevent rubbing and friction between the residual limb and the socket. Excessive movement of a loose prosthesis can cause severe skin irritation and breakdown.

Artificial limbs become an integral part of the patient's body image. Proper care ensures their long life and useful functioning. The patient should be instructed to clean the prosthesis socket daily with a mild soap and rinse thoroughly to remove irritants. The leather and metal parts of the prosthesis should not get wet. The patient should be encouraged to have regular maintenance of the prosthesis. Consideration of the condition of the shoe is also necessary. A badly worn shoe alters the gait and may cause damage to the prosthesis.

Referral to a community health nurse can foster optimal physical and emotional adjustment. The caregiver should be instructed on ambulation and transfer techniques and proper residual limb care.

▮ Special Considerations in Upper-Limb Amputation

The emotional implications of an upper limb amputation are often more devastating than those for lower limb amputation. The enforced dependency brought about by one-handedness may be both frustrating and humiliating to the patient. Because most upper extremity amputations result from trauma, the patient has not had the opportunity to adjust psychologically to an amputation or to participate in the decision-making process about amputation.

Both immediate and delayed prosthetic fittings are possible for the below-the-elbow amputee. Prosthetic fitting is delayed for the above-the-elbow amputee. The usual functional prosthesis is the arm and hook. A cosmetic hand is available but has limited functional value. As with the lower limb prosthesis, patient motivation and endurance are major factors contributing to a satisfactory outcome.

▮ Evaluation

The expected outcomes are that the patient with an amputation will:
- Accept changed body image and integrate changes into his or her lifestyle.
- Have no evidence of skin breakdown.
- Have reduction or absence of pain.
- Become mobile within limitations imposed by amputation.

AGE-RELATED CONSIDERATIONS: AMPUTATION

If a lower limb amputation has been performed on an older adult, the patient's previous ability to ambulate may affect the extent of recovery. Use of a prosthesis requires a significant amount of energy for ambulation. Walking with a below-the-

knee prosthesis requires 40% additional energy, and an above-the-knee prosthesis requires 60% more energy than walking on two legs. Older adults whose general health is weakened by disorders such as cardiac or pulmonary problems may not be candidates for prosthesis use. This patient's ability to ambulate will be limited. If possible, this should be discussed with the patient and family before surgery so that realistic expectations can be set.

Common Joint Surgical Procedures

Surgery plays an important role in the treatment and rehabilitation of patients with various forms of arthritis, conditions related to trauma, and other painful conditions resulting in functional disability. Joint replacement surgery is the most common orthopedic operation performed on older adults. Significant advances in the field of reconstructive surgery have resulted in improvements in prosthetic design, materials, and surgical techniques that provide significant relief of pain and deformity and improve function and joint motion (Cleveland Clinic, 2010).

Indications for Joint Surgery

Surgery is aimed at relieving chronic pain, improving joint motion, correcting deformity and malalignment, and removing intra-articular causes of erosion. In addition to the effects of chronic pain on the physical and emotional well-being of the patient, any movement of the painful joint is often avoided. If this decreased functional ability is not corrected, contraction with permanent limitation of motion often occurs. Limitation of motion at any joint can be demonstrated on physical examination and by joint-space narrowing on radiological examination.

A slow loss of cartilage in affected joints may also be related to loss of motion. Synovitis can cause tendon damage, resulting in rupture or subluxation of the joint and subsequent loss of function. Continuing disease activity may cause loss of cartilage and bony surface and result in mechanical barriers to movement requiring surgical intervention.

Indications for hip or knee arthroplasty include arthritis, connective tissue disease, failed prior procedures, sepsis, tumours, Paget's disease, congenital hip dysplasia, severe varus or valgus deformity, and spondyloarthropathies.

Types of Joint Surgeries

Synovectomy

Synovectomy (removal of synovial membrane) is used as a prophylactic measure and as a palliative treatment of RA. Removal of the synovial membrane, thought to be the location of the basic pathological changes in joint destruction, helps prevent further progression of joint damage. A synovectomy is best performed early in the disease process to prevent serious destruction of joint surfaces. Removal of the thickened synovium prevents extension of the inflammatory process into the adjacent cartilage, ligaments, and tendons.

It is impossible to surgically remove all the synovium in a joint. The underlying disease process is still present and will again affect the regenerating synovium. However, the disease appears to be milder after synovectomy, and definite improvement in pain, weight bearing, and ROM can be expected. Common sites for this surgery include the elbow, wrist, and fingers. Synovectomy in the knee is done less frequently because knee joint replacement techniques are usually performed.

Osteotomy

An **osteotomy** is performed by removing or adding a wedge or slice of bone to change alignment (joint and vertebral) and to shift weight bearing, thereby correcting deformity and relieving pain. Cervical osteotomy may be used to correct deformity in some patients with ankylosing spondylitis. Halo and body jackets are worn until fusion occurs (at 3-4 months). Subtrochanteric or femoral osteotomy may provide some relief of pain and improve motion in selected patients with hip OA. Osteotomy has proved ineffective in patients with inflammatory joint disease. Osteotomy of the knee (tibia) provides relief of pain in selected patients, but advanced joint destruction is usually corrected by joint replacement surgery.

The postoperative care is similar to the treatment of an internal fixation of a fracture at a comparable site (see pp. 1824-1825). Internal wires, screws, and plates, bone grafts, or an external fixator usually fix the bone in place.

Debridement

Debridement is the removal of degenerative debris such as loose bodies, osteophytes, joint debris, and degenerated menisci from a joint. This procedure is usually performed on the knee or the shoulder using a fibreoptic arthroscope. The procedure is usually done on an outpatient basis. A compression dressing is applied postoperatively. Weight bearing is permitted following knee arthroscopy. Patient education includes monitoring for signs of infection, managing pain, and restricting excessive activity for 24 to 48 hours.

Arthroplasty

Arthroplasty is the reconstruction or replacement of a joint to relieve pain, improve or maintain ROM, and correct deformity. There were 62,196 hip and knee replacements in Canada for 2006 to 2007 (a 10-year increase of 101% and an annual increase of 6%) (CIHI, 2009b). According to 2006 to 2007 data, most Canadians receiving hip or knee arthroplasties were 65 years or older and were obese as measured by body mass index and when compared with the rest of the population (CIHI, 2009b).

The most common uses of arthroplasty are for patients with OA, RA, AVN, congenital deformities or dislocations, and other systemic problems. There are several types of arthroplasty, including replacement of part of a joint *(hemiarthroplasty)*, surgical reshaping of the bones of the joints, and total joint replacement. Replacement arthroplasty is available for elbow, shoulder, phalangeal joints of the fingers, wrist, hip, knee, ankle, and foot. Newer technology and techniques for lumbar disc arthroplasty have also recently shown positive clinical outcomes (Sinigaglia et al., 2009).

Minimally invasive surgery is available in some centres in Canada for hip and knee replacements. Minimally invasive surgery involves less dissection and smaller incisions (5 to 10 cm in the hip and 10 to 12.7 cm in the knee) and a shorter hospital stay. It is technically demanding and requires extra training for the surgeon. There is an initial quicker recovery with less rehabilitation and a quicker return to activities of daily living for the patient. Minimally invasive surgery also results in less blood loss and need for transfusions.

Hip Arthroplasty. Total hip arthroplasty (THA) provides significant relief of pain and improvement of function for patients with OA and RA. Implants are often "cemented" in place with polymethyl methacrylate, which bonds to the bone. With time, femoral components may loosen or become dislocated, which requires revision surgery. Because of this risk, cemented THAs are recommended for less active, older adults with compromised bone strength. Younger individuals receive "cementless" arthroplasties in an effort to prolong the lifetime of the prosthesis. Cementless THAs provide long-term implant stability by facilitating biological ingrowth of new bone tissue into the porous surface coating of the prosthesis (Figure 65-24). Total hip replacements are shown in Figure 65-25.

In posterior approach hip arthroplasties, extremes of internal rotation and 90-degree flexion of the hip must be avoided for 4 to 6 weeks postoperatively. A foam abduction pillow is sometimes placed between the legs to prevent dislocation of the new joint (Figure 65-26).

Following surgery, patients must not allow their hips to be lower than their knees, and elevated toilet seats and chair alterations at home are necessary. When sitting in a regular chair, the patient is advised to use a wedge cushion under the buttocks to ensure hips are flexed less than 90 degrees. Tub baths and driving a car are not allowed for 4 to 6 weeks. An occupational therapist may teach the patient to use assistive devices, such as reach bars ("reachers") to avoid bending over to pick something up off the

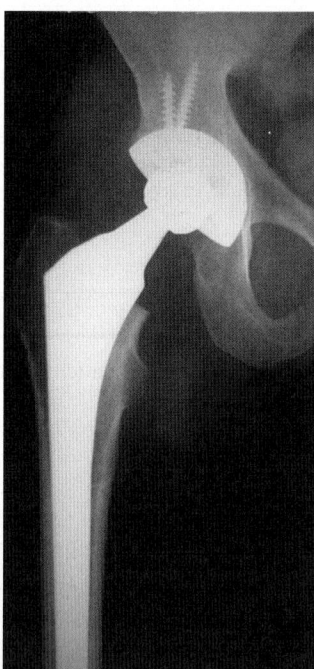

Figure 65-24 Total hip arthroplasty. Porous-coated, noncemented femoral prosthesis of metal alloy with a cemented high-density plastic acetabular socket.

Source: Patton, K. T., & Thibodeau, G. A. (2010). *Anatomy and physiology* (7th ed., p. 286, Box 9-3). St. Louis: Mosby.

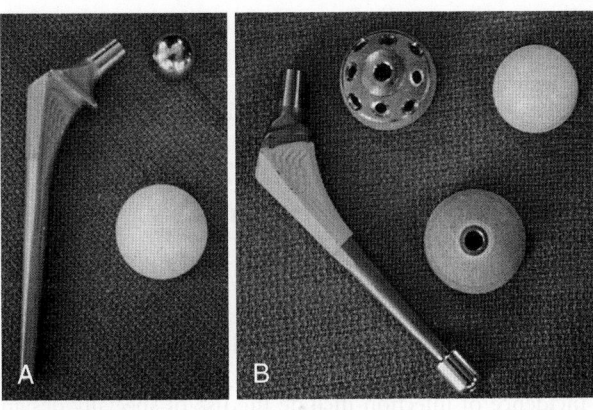

Figure 65-25 Total hip replacements. **A,** Coated cemented components. **B,** Porous cementless components.

Source: Maher, A., Salmond, S. W., & Pellino, T. A. (Eds.). (2002). *Orthopaedic nursing* (3rd ed.). Philadelphia: Saunders.

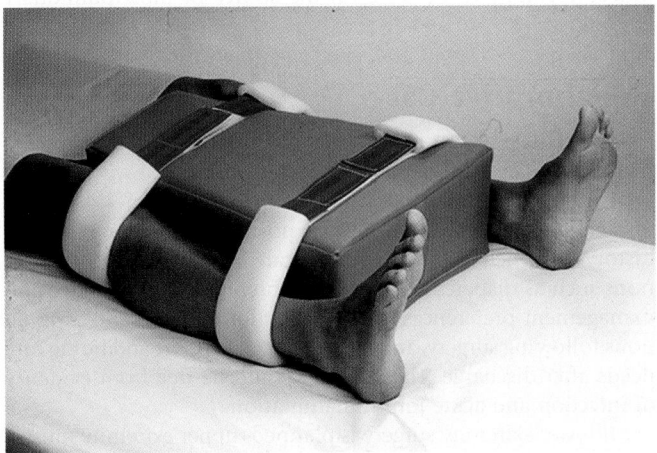

Figure 65-26 Maintaining postoperative abduction following total hip replacement.

Source: Courtesy Zimmer, Inc., Warsaw, IN.

floor, long-handled shoehorns, or sock pullers. The knees must be kept apart and the patient must never cross the legs, twist to reach behind, or twist the operated leg inward or outward. The patient is asked not to bend from the waist more than 90 degrees as well as not to lift the knee on the operated side higher than the hip. Physiotherapy is initiated the first postoperative day with ambulation and weight bearing with a walker for patients with a cemented prosthesis and weight bearing on the operative side for those with a cementless prosthesis.

Exercises are designed to restore strength and muscle tone in the hip muscles essential to improved function and ROM. These include quadriceps setting (e.g., tightening the kneecap), gluteal muscle setting (e.g., tightening the buttocks), leg raises in supine and prone positions, and abduction exercises (e.g., swinging the leg out but never crossing midline) from supine and standing positions. The patient will continue these for many months after discharge, and the caregiver should be well acquainted with the exercise program to offer encouragement at home.

Home care considerations include ongoing assessment of pain management, monitoring for infection, and prevention of DVT. Not all patients will qualify for home care. The incision may be closed with metal staples, which are removed at the surgeon's office. Because of the high risk for DVT, enoxaparin (Lovenox), an LMWH, is commonly administered subcutaneously and can be given at home by the patient or caregiver. An advantage of enoxaparin is that it does not require monitoring of the patient's coagulation status. The patient should also be instructed to use prophylactic antibiotics before dental appointments or surgical procedures that might put the patient at risk for bacteremia.

A physiotherapist will assess ROM, ambulation, and compliance with the exercise regimen. The patient will gradually increase the number of repetitions of exercises, add weights to ankles, swim, and may eventually use a stationary bicycle to tone quadriceps and improve cardiovascular fitness. High-impact exercises and sports, such as jogging and tennis, may loosen the implant and should be avoided. The older adult may require rehabilitation at a subacute or long-term care facility until able to function independently.

Hip Resurfacing. Resurfacing arthroplasty or *hip resurfacing* is another option that does not require removing the head of the femur, like traditional hip replacement. Instead, the head is reshaped and capped with a metal ball. Preserving the top of the femur is an advantage if the hip requires subsequent work. Resurfacing uses a bigger ball, which makes dislocation less likely and gives the joint the ability to handle greater stress. Metal on metal hip resurfacing arthroplasty is recommended as one option for people with advanced hip disease who would otherwise receive, and are likely to outlive, a conventional primary total hip replacement. The use of metal appears to have a lower rate of wear and, thus, the prosthesis may have a longer lifetime. Hip resurfacing is a favourable option for younger, active patients. Resurfacing is a relatively new procedure and does not have the long-term clinical follow-up results that are available for some other types of conventional THA.

Knee Arthroplasty. Unremitting pain and instability as a result of severe destructive deterioration of the knee joint is the main indication for total knee arthroplasty (TKA) or total knee replacement (TKR). The presence of osteoporosis may necessitate bone grafting to augment defects and to correct bone deficiencies. Either part or all of the knee joint may be replaced with a metal and plastic prosthetic device. A compression dressing is used to immobilize the knee in extension immediately after the operation. This is usually removed within 24 hours and may be replaced with a knee immobilizer such as a Zimmer immobilizer splint or posterior plastic shell, which stabilizes the knee and maintains extension during ambulation and at rest for about 4 weeks. Knee immobilizers are removed for various portions of physiotherapy.

Great emphasis is placed on postoperative exercising, and dislocation is not typical with TKA. Isometric quadriceps setting begins the first day after surgery. The patient progresses to straight-leg raises and gentle ROM to increase muscle strength and obtain 90-degree knee flexion. Active flexion exercises or passive flexion exercises through the use of a continuous passive motion machine postoperatively may promote joint mobility. Full weight bearing is begun before discharge. An active home-exercise program involves progressive ROM with muscle strengthening, and flexibility exercises. Following TKA, many older patients with advanced OA have shown significant improvement in mobility, motor function tests, and ability to complete daily tasks (Sloan, Ruiz, & Platt, 2009).

Finger Joint Arthroplasty.

A silicone rubber arthroplastic device is used to help restore function in the fingers of the patient with RA. Ulnar deviation is often present, which results in severe functional limitations of the hand. The goal of hand surgery is primarily to restore function related to grasp, pinch, stability, and strength rather than to correct cosmetic deformity. Before surgery, the patient is instructed in hand exercises, including flexion, extension, abduction, and adduction of the fingers.

Postoperatively, the hand is kept elevated with a bulky dressing in place. Neurovascular assessment is conducted postoperatively, and the nurse assesses for signs of infection. The success of the surgery depends largely on the postoperative treatment plan, which is often carried out under the direction of an occupational therapist. Once the dressing is removed, a guided splinting program is initiated. The patient is discharged with splints to use while sleeping and hand exercises to perform for 10 to 12 weeks at least three or four times a day. The patient is also instructed to avoid lifting heavy objects.

Elbow and Shoulder Arthroplasty.

Although available, total replacement of elbow and shoulder joints is not as common as other forms of arthroplasty. Shoulder replacements are used in patients with severe pain because of RA, OA, AVN, or an old trauma. The shoulder replacement is usually considered if the patient has adequate surrounding muscle strength and bone stock. If joint replacement is necessary for both elbow and shoulder, the elbow is usually done first because a severely painful elbow interferes with the shoulder rehabilitation program.

Significant pain relief has been achieved following arthroplasty, with no pain at rest or minimal pain with activity. Functional improvements have resulted in better hygiene and increased ability to perform activities of daily living in most patients. Rehabilitation is longer and more difficult than with other joint surgeries.

Ankle Arthroplasty.

Total ankle arthroplasty is indicated for RA, OA, and AVN. Although the use of total ankle arthroplasty is not widespread, it is becoming a viable alternative to fusion for the treatment of severe ankle arthritis in selected patients. Devices available include several fixed-bearing devices and a mobile-bearing "cementless" prosthesis. This device more closely imitates natural ankle function.

Ankle fusion is often selected over arthroplasty because the result is more durable. However, the patient is left with a stiff foot and the inability to change heel height. Total ankle arthroplasty is advantageous because a more normal gait pattern can be achieved. Postoperatively, the patient may not bear weight for 6 weeks, must elevate the extremity to reduce and prevent edema, must be extremely careful to prevent postoperative infection, and must maintain immobilization as directed by the physician.

Arthrodesis

Arthrodesis is the surgical fusion of a joint. This procedure is indicated only if articular surfaces are too severely damaged or infected to allow joint replacement or if reconstructive surgery fails. Arthrodesis relieves pain and provides a stable but immobile joint. The fusion is usually accomplished by removal of the articular hyaline cartilage and the addition of bone grafts across the joint surface. The affected joint must be immobilized until bone healing has occurred. Common areas of fusion are wrist, ankle, cervical spine, lumbar spine, and the metatarsophalangeal joint of the great toe.

Complications of Joint Surgery

Infection is a serious complication of joint surgery, particularly joint replacement surgery. The most common causative organisms are Gram-positive aerobic streptococci and staphylococci. Infection almost always leads to pain and loosening of the prosthesis, generally necessitating extensive surgery. Efforts to reduce the incidence of infection include the use of specially designed self-contained operating suites, operating rooms with laminar airflow, and prophylactic antibiotic administration.

Thromboembolism is another potentially serious complication after joint surgeries, particularly those involving the lower extremities. Prophylactic measures such as warfarin, LMWH, and sequential compression devices of the legs are usually instituted. Patients may be followed postoperatively with venous Doppler ultrasonography to detect DVT, the source of most pulmonary emboli.

Collaborative Care

Preoperative Management.

The primary goal of preoperative assessment is to identify risk factors associated with postoperative complications so that nursing strategies can be implemented to promote optimal positive outcomes. A careful history will include previous medical diagnosis and complications such as diabetes and thrombophlebitis, pain tolerance and management preferences, current functional status and expectations following surgery, and level of social support and home care needs after discharge. The patient should be free from evidence of infection and acute joint inflammation.

If lower extremity surgery is planned, upper extremity muscle strength and joint function are assessed to determine the type of assistive devices needed postoperatively for ambulation and activities of daily living. Preoperative teaching informs the patient and family of the expected hospital course and postoperative management at home. In addition, it prepares them to maximize the usefulness and longevity of the prosthesis. Patients also need to realize that recovery is "not going to happen overnight." Both patients and their families or significant others need to speak with individuals who have had a total joint arthroplasty to better understand the reality of rehabilitation (Jacobsen et al., 2008).

Postoperative Management.

Postoperatively, neurovascular assessment is performed to assess nerve function and circulatory status. Anticoagulation therapy, analgesia, and parenteral antibiotics are administered. In general, the affected joint is exercised, and ambulation is encouraged as early as possible to prevent complications of immobility. Specific protocols vary according to patient, type of prosthesis, and surgeon preference. Pain management postoperatively may use epidural or intrathecal analgesia, femoral nerve block (knee only), patient-controlled analgesia, intravenous injections, and oral opioids or NSAIDs.

The hospital stay after arthroplasty is 3 to 4 days for knee replacement and 5 days for hip replacement, depending on the patient's course and need for physiotherapy. Physiotherapy and ambulation enhance mobility, build muscle strength, and reduce the risk of thrombus formation. If the patient is taking warfarin, therapy starts on the day of surgery and continues for 3 weeks with an international normalized ratio (INR) done on a regular basis. For those taking LMWH (e.g., enoxaparin), therapy starts after surgery and continues for 2 weeks postoperatively. Daily monitoring of the patient's coagulation status is not necessary with LMWH. The decision to use warfarin or LMWH depends on many factors including the patient's age and overall state of health.

NURSING MANAGEMENT: JOINT SURGERY

The nursing management of the patient undergoing joint surgery begins with preoperative teaching and realistic goal setting. It is important that the patient understands and accepts the limitations of the proposed surgery and realizes that it will not remove the underlying disease process. Postoperative procedures such as turning, deep breathing, use of bedpan and high bedside commode, and use of abductor pillows should be explained and opportunities for practice provided. The patient should be reassured that pain relief will be available. Patient-controlled analgesia can be helpful. A preoperative visit from a physiotherapist allows practice of postoperative exercises and measurement for crutches or other assistive devices.

Discharge planning begins immediately. The duration of the hospital stay and the expected postoperative events should be discussed because the patient and caregiver must prepare ahead. The home environment must be assessed for safety (e.g., presence of scatter rugs and electrical cords) and accessibility. Are the bathroom and bedroom on the first floor? Are door frames wide enough to accommodate a walker? Social support must also be assessed. Is a friend or family member available to assist the patient in the home, or will the patient need extra assistance? Will the patient require a homemaker or meal services? The older adult patient may need the rehabilitation services of a subacute or long-term care facility for a few weeks postoperatively to progressively develop independent living skills. Specific nursing interventions related to the patient having orthopedic surgery are summarized in NCP 65-2.

Patient teaching includes instructions on reporting complications, including infection (e.g., fever, increased pain, drainage) and dislocation of the prosthesis (e.g., pain, loss of function, shortening or misalignment of an extremity). The home care nurse acts as the liaison between the patient and the surgeon, monitoring for postoperative complications, assessing comfort and ROM, and facilitating improvements in functional performance.

CLINICAL DECISION-MAKING EXERCISE

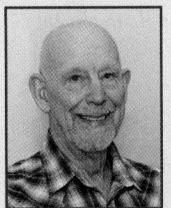

CASE STUDY:
Hip Fracture

Source: © iStockphoto.com/Scott Griessel.

Patient Profile

Gene Wells is an 82-year-old White male admitted to the hospital through the emergency department. He fell on an icy patch outside his home. It appears he may have sustained a fracture to his right hip. He has a history of type 2 diabetes mellitus and has a 40 pack-year smoking history (1 pack/day for 40 years) that is now complicated by chronic obstructive pulmonary disease.

Subjective Data

• Complains of excruciating pain and tenderness in right hip
• Pain not relieved by morphine

Objective Data

Physical Examination
• BP: 166/94 mm Hg
• Diaphoretic and pale skin
• Respiratory rate 36; crackles, expiratory wheeze

Diagnostic Studies
• Radiograph of right hip reveals extracapsular fracture
• Hematocrit 0.3; hemoglobin 150 g/L; white blood cell count 15×10^9/L

Collaborative Care

• Right hip repair with compression plate and bone screws
• Cefazolin 1 g intravenously every 8 hours
• Intake and output for 48 hours postoperatively
• Morphine sulphate per patient-controlled analgesia pump

Discussion Questions

1. How do pre-existing medical conditions predispose Mr. Wells to postoperative complications?
2. What are the most likely postoperative complications that Mr. Wells could develop?
3. *Priority Decision:* What are the priority preoperative and postoperative nursing interventions for Mr. Wells?
4. *Priority Decision:* Based on the assessment data presented, what are the priority nursing diagnoses for an older adult patient with a hip fracture? Are there any collaborative problems?
5. *Priority Decision:* What are the priority teaching interventions that should be done before discharge?

evolve *Answers are available at* **http://evolve.elsevier.com/ Canada/Lewis/medsurg**

REVIEW QUESTIONS

The number of the question corresponds to the same-numbered objective at the beginning of the chapter.

1. When would the nurse suspect an ankle sprain for the patient being seen at the urgent care centre?
   a. Patient was hit by another soccer player on the field.
   b. Patient has ankle pain after sprinting around the track.
   c. Patient dropped a 4.5-kg weight on his lower leg at the health club.
   d. Patient had a twisting injury while running bases during a baseball game.

2. The nurse explains to a patient with a distal tibial fracture returning for a 3-week checkup that healing is indicated by which of the following?
   a. Callus formation
   b. Complete bony union
   c. Hematoma at the fracture site
   d. Presence of granulation tissue

3. A patient with a comminuted fracture of the femur is to have an open reduction with internal fixation (ORIF) of the fracture. In which of the following situations is an ORIF indicated?
   a. The patient is able to tolerate prolonged immobilization.
   b. The patient cannot tolerate the surgery for a closed reduction.
   c. A temporary cast would be too unstable to provide normal mobility.
   d. Adequate alignment cannot be obtained by other nonsurgical methods.

4. Which of the following indicates a neurovascular problem during the nurse's assessment of a patient with a fracture?
   a. Exaggeration of extremity movement
   b. Increased redness and heat below the injury
   c. Decreased sensation distal to the fracture site
   d. Purulent drainage at the site of an open fracture

5. A patient with a stable, closed fracture of the humerus caused by trauma to the arm has a temporary splint with bulky padding applied with an elastic bandage. For which of the following symptoms would the nurse suspect compartment syndrome and notify the physician?
   a. Increasing edema of the limb
   b. Muscle spasms of the lower arm
   c. Rebounding pulse at the fracture site
   d. Pain when passively extending the fingers

6. Which of the following symptoms should the nurse be monitoring for in a patient with pelvic fracture?
   a. Changes in urinary output
   b. Petechiae on the abdomen
   c. A palpable lump in the buttock
   d. Sudden decrease in blood pressure

7. During the postoperative period, what should the patient with an above-the-knee amputation be told about the problem of routinely elevating the residual limb?
   a. The flexed position can promote hip flexion contracture.
   b. This position reduces the development of phantom pain.
   c. This position promotes clot formation at the incision site and thigh.
   d. Unnecessary movement of the extremity can cause wound dehiscence.

8. A patient with rheumatoid arthritis is scheduled for an arthroplasty. Which is the purpose of this procedure?
   a. To fuse a joint and reduce pain
   b. To prevent further joint damage
   c. To assess the extent of joint damage
   d. To replace the joint and improve function

9. What should the nurse teach a patient recovering from a total hip replacement to avoid?
   a. Sleeping on the abdomen
   b. Sitting with the legs crossed
   c. Abduction exercises of the affected leg
   d. Bearing weight on the affected leg for 6 weeks

ANSWERS: 1. d; 2. a; 3. d; 4. c; 5. d; 6. a; 7. a; 8. d; 9. b.

REFERENCES

Abate, J. (2008). Dislocations and soft-tissue injuries of the knee. In B. D. Browner, R. M. Levine, & P. G. Traft, *Skeletal trauma* (4th ed.). Philadelphia: Saunders.

Altizer, L. (2008). Colles' fracture. *Orthopaedic Nursing, 27*(2), 140-145. doi:10.1097/01.NOR.0000315631.30676.2b

Auron-Gomez, M., & Michota, F. (2008). Medical management of hip fracture. *Clinics in Geriatric Medicine, 24*(4), 701-718. doi:10.1016/j.cger.2008.07.002

Bell, A., Leader, M., & Lloyd, H. (2008). Care of pin sites. *Nursing Standard, 22*(33), 44-48.

Bodden, J. (2009). Treatment options in the hemodynamically unstable patient with a pelvic fracture. *Orthopaedic Nursing, 28*(3), 109-114. doi:10.1097/NOR.0b013e3181a469c7

Boyd, A., Benjamin, H., & Asplund, C. (2009). Splints and casts: Indications and methods. *American Family Physician, 80*(5), 491-499.

Canadian Institute for Health Information (CIHI). (2007). *Health indicators 2007*. Ottawa: CIHI.

Canadian Institute for Health Information (CIHI). (2009a). *Health indicators 2009*. Ottawa: CIHI.

Canadian Institute for Health Information (CIHI). (2009b). *Hip and knee replacements in Canada: Canadian Joint Replacement Registry (CJRR) 2008-2009 annual report*. Ottawa: CIHI.

Carlson, D. S., & Pfadt, E. (2011). Action STAT. Fat embolism syndrome. *Nursing, 41*(4), 72. doi:10.1097/01.NURSE.0000395312.91409.7f

Centers for Disease Control and Prevention (CDC). (2010). Hip fractures among older adults. Retrieved from *http://www.cdc.gov/homeandrecreationalsafety/falls/adulthipfx.html*

Chapman, S. (2011). Pain management in patients following limb amputation. *Nursing Standard, 25*(19), 35-40.

Cleveland Clinic. (2008). Sprain vs. strain: Different injuries, same treatment. *Arthritis Advisor, 7*(8). Retrieved from *http://www.arthritis-advisor.com/issues/7_8/features/486-1.html*

Cleveland Clinic. (2010). New materials, improved designs means better hips. *Arthritis Advisor 9*(1). Retrieved from *http://www.arthritis-advisor.com/issues/9_1/features/606-1.html*

Ferguson, T. A., & Eastman, J. A. (2011). Anterior approach hip arthroplasty: A novel technique in the management of femoral neck fractures. *Current Orthopedic Practice, 22*(1), 39-45. doi:10.1097/BCO.0b013e3182059ba6

Fisher, T., Williams, S., & Levine, A. (2008). Spinal orthoses. In B. D. Browner, R. M. Levine, & P. G. Traft (Eds.), *Skeletal trauma* (4th ed.). Philadelphia: Saunders.

Galway, U., Tetzlaff, J. E., & Helfand, R. (2009). Acute fatal fat embolism syndrome in bilateral total knee arthroplasty—A review of the fat embolism syndrome. *The Internet Journal of Anesthesiology, 19*(2).

Getgood, A., & Robertson, A. (2010). Meniscal tears, repairs and replacement—A current concepts review. *Orthopaedics & Trauma, 24*(2), 121-128. doi:10.1016/j.mporth.2010.03.011

Hanley, M., Ehde, D., Jensen, M., Czerniecki, J., Smith, D. G., & Robinson, L. R. (2009). Chronic pain associated with upper-limb loss. *American Journal of Physical Medicine and Rehabilitation, 88*(9), 742-751. doi:10.1097/PHM.0b013e3181b306ec

Hodgson, B. B., & Kizior, R. J. (2011). *Saunders nursing drug handbook.* St. Louis: Saunders.

Huisstede, B., Randsdorp, M., Coert, J., Glerum, S., van Middelkoop, M., & Koes, B. (2010). Carpal tunnel syndrome. Part II: Effectiveness of surgical treatments—A systematic review. *Archives of Physical Medicine & Rehabilitation, 91*(7), 1005-1024. doi:10.1016/j.apmr.2010.03.023

Jacobsen, A., Myerscough, R., DeLambo, K., Fleming, E., Huddleston, A. M., Bright, N., & Varley, J. D. (2008). Patients' perspectives on total knee replacement. *American Journal of Nursing, 108*(5), 54-63.

Juby, A. (2009). The challenges of interpreting efficacy of hip protector pads in fracture prevention in high-risk seniors. *Clinical Rheumatology, 28*(6), 723-727. doi:10.1007/s10067-009-1115-1

Kallmes, D., Comstock, B., Heagerty, P., Turner, J. A., Wilson, D. J., Diamond, T. J., …, Jarvik, J. G. (2009). A randomized trial of vertebroplasty for osteoporotic spinal fractures. *New England Journal of Medicine, 361*(6), 569-579. doi:10.1056/NEJMoa0900563

Lazo-Langner, A., & Rodger, M. (2009). Overview of current venous thromboembolism protocols in hip reconstruction. *Orthopedic Clinics of North America, 40*(3), 427-436. doi:10.1016/j.ocl.2009.02.005

Magee, D. (2008). *Orthopedic physical assessment.* St Louis: Saunders.

Malik, A. A., Khan, W., Chaudhry, A., Ihsan, M., & Cullen, N. P. (2009). Acute compartment syndrome—A life and limb threatening surgical emergency. *Journal of Perioperative Practice, 19*(5), 137-142.

Mamaril, M., Childs, S., & Sortman, S. (2007). Care of the orthopaedic trauma patient. *Journal of PeriAnesthesia Nursing, 22*(3), 184-194. doi:10.1016/j.jopan.2007.03.008

Marx, J., Hockberger, R., & Walls, R. (2009). *Rosen's emergency medicine: Concepts and clinical practice* (7th ed.). Philadelphia: Mosby.

Meade, K. P., Malas, B. S., Patwardha, A. G., & Gavin, T. M. (2008). Orthoses for osteoporosis. In J. D. Hsu, J. W. Michael, & J. R. Fisk. (Eds.), *American Academy of Orthopaedic Surgeons atlas of orthosis and assistive devices* (4th ed.). St. Louis: Mosby.

Murray, M. (2009). Current status and potential of primary ACL repair. *Clinics in Sports Medicine, 28*(1), 51-61. doi:10.1016/j.csm.2008.08.005

National Institute of Aging. (2011). Exercise & physical activity: Your everyday guide from the National Institute on Aging. Retrieved from *http://www.nia.nih.gov/health/publication/exercise-physical-activity-your-everyday-guide-national-institute-aging*

Registered Nurses' Association of Ontario (RNAO). (2005, rev. 2011). Prevention of falls and fall injuries in the older adult. Best Practice Guidelines. Retrieved from *http://www.rnao.org/Page.asp?PageID=924&ContentID=810*

Rishiraj, N., Taunton, J. E., Lloyd-Smith, R., Woollard, R., Regan, W., & Clement, D. B. (2009). The potential role of prophylactic/functional knee bracing in preventing knee ligament injury. *Sports Medicine, 39*(11), 937-960. doi:10.2165/11317790-000000000-00000

Roberts, J., & Hedges, J. (2010). Arterial puncture and cannulation. In J. Roberts & J. Hedges (Eds.), *Roberts: Clinical procedures in emergency medicine* (5th ed.). Philadelphia: Saunders.

Ronga, M., Shanmugam, C., Longo, G., Oliva, F., & Maffulli, N. (2009). Minimally invasive osteosynthesis of distal tibial fractures using locking plates. *Orthopedic Clinics of North America, 40*(4), 499-504. doi:10.1016/j.ocl.2009.05.007

Satryb, S. A., Wilson, T. J., & Patterson, M. M. (2011). Casting: All wrapped up. *Orthopaedic Nursing, 30*(1), 37-41. doi:10.1097/NOR.0b013e31820574f9

Scanlon, A., & Maffei, J. (2009). Carpal tunnel syndrome. *Journal of Neuroscience Nursing, 41*(3), 140-147. doi:10.1097/JNN.0b013e3181a39481

Shadgan, B., Menon, M., Sanders, D., Berry, G., Martin, C., Jr, Duffy, P., …, O'Brien, P. J. (2010). Current thinking about acute compartment syndrome of the lower extremity. *Canadian Journal of Surgery, 53*(5), 329-334.

Sinigaglia, R., Bundy, A., Costantini, S., Nena. U., Finocchiaro, F., & Monterumici, D. A. (2009). Comparison of single-level L4-L5 versus L5-S1 lumbar disc replacement: Results and prognostic factors. *European Spine Journal, 18*(Suppl 1), 52-63. doi:10.1007/s00586-009-0992-y

Sloan, F., Ruiz, D., & Platt, A. (2009). Changes in functional status among persons over age sixty-five undergoing total knee arthroplasty. *Medical Care. 47*(7), 742-748. doi:10.1097/MLR.0b013e31819a5ae3

Smeltzer, M. (2010). Making a point about open fractures. *Nursing, 40*(4), 24-31. doi:10.1097/01.NURSE.0000369860.37315.c6

Smith, M. A. & Smith, W. T. (2010). Rotator cuff tears: An overview. *Orthopaedic Nursing, 29*(5), 319-322. doi:10.1097/NOR.0b013e3181edd8b6

Statistics Canada. (2003). Repetitive strain injury. *The Daily.* Retrieved from *http://www.statcan.ca/Daily/English/030812/d030812b.htm*

Statistics Canada. (2011). Health at a glance. Injuries in Canada: Insights from the Canadian Community Health Survey. Retrieved from *http://www.statcan.gc.ca/pub/82-624-x/2011001/article/11506-eng.htm*

Statistics Canada. (2012). *Table 102-0561—Leading causes of death, total population, by age group and sex, Canada, annual, CANSIM* (database). Retrieved from *http://www5.statcan.gc.ca/cansim/a26?lang=eng&retrLang=eng&id=1020561&paSer=&pattern=&stByVal=1&p1=1&p2=37&tabMode=dataTable&csid=*

Steiner, T., & Parker, R. (2009). Subluxation and dislocation: Patellofemoral instability: Acute dislocation of the patella. In J. DeLee, D. Drez, & M. Miller (Eds.), *DeLee and Drez's orthopaedic sports medicine* (3rd ed.). Philadelphia: Saunders.

Tjepkema, M. (2003). Repetitive strain injury. *Statistics Canada—Health Reports, 14*(11), 11-20. Retrieved from *http://www.statcan.ca/english/studies/82-003/archive/2003/14-4-a.pdf*

Tripuraneni, K., Ganga, S., Quinn, R., & Gehlert, R. (2008). The effect of time delay to surgical debridement of open tibia shaft fractures on infection rate. *Orthopedics, 31*(12), 1195-2000. doi:10.3928/01477447-20081201-27

University of Pittsburgh Medical Center [UPMC]. (2012). Patient education materials: Weight bearing. Retrieved from *http://www.upmc.com/HealthAtoZ/patienteducation/R/Pages/weightbearing.aspx*

Walker, J. A. (2010). Management of patients with carpal tunnel syndrome. *Nursing Standard, 24*(19), 44-48. Retrieved from *http://nursingstandard.rcnpublishing.co.uk/archive/article-management-of-patients-with-carpal-tunnel-syndrome*

Walker, J. A. (2011). Pelvic fractures: Classification and nursing management. *Nursing Standard, 26*(10), 49-57. Retrieved from *http://*

nursingstandard.rcnpublishing.co.uk/archive/article-pelvic-fractures-classification-and-nursing-management

Wilhelm, K. (2009). Kyphoplasty: Better or worse than vertebroplasty? *Neuroradiology Journal, 22*(Suppl 1), 149.

Woods, S. (2011). Sprains and strains. *Practice Nurse, 41*(19), 33-36.

Yadav, H., Nho, S., Romeo, A., & Macgillivray, J. (2009). Rotator cuff tears: Pathology and repair. *Knee Surgery, Sports Traumatology, Arthroscopy, 17*(4), 409-421. doi:10.1007/s00167-008-0686-8

CANADIAN RESOURCES

About Face
http://www.aboutface.ca
Amputee.ca
http://www.amputee.ca/aboutus.htm
The Arthritis Society
http://www.arthritis.ca
Canadian Academy of Sport and Exercise Medicine
http://www.casm-acms.org
Canadian Arthritis Network
http://www.arthritisnetwork.ca
Canadian Centre for Occupational Health and Safety
http://www.ccohs.ca
Canadian Orthopedic Association
http://www.coa-aco.org
Canadian Orthopedic Foundation
http://www.canorth.org
Canadian Orthopedic Nurses Association
http://www.cona-nurse.org
GTA Rehab Network
http://www.gtarehabnetwork.ca/
myJointReplacement.ca
http://myjointreplacement.ca/
Osteoporosis Society of Canada
http://www.osteoporosis.ca

Virtual Knee Replacement Surgery (animation)
http://www.edheads.org/activities/knee/
War Amps of Canada
http://www.waramps.ca/index.html

RELATED RESOURCES

American Academy of Orthopedic Surgeons (AAOS)
http://www.aaos.org
American Association for Hand Surgery
http://www.handsurgery.org
American College of Sports Medicine (ACSM)
http://www.acsm.org
Amputee Coalition of America (ACA)
http://www.amputee-coalition.org
National Amputation Foundation (NAF)
http://www.nationalamputation.org
National Association of Orthopaedic Nurses, Inc. (NAON)
http://www.orthonurse.org
National Center on Physical Activity and Disability (NCPAD)
http://www.ncpad.org
National Institute of Aging: Exercise & Physical Activity: Your Everyday Guide from the National Institute on Aging
http://www.nia.nih.gov/health/publication/exercise-physical-activity-your-everyday-guide-national-institute-aging
National Institute of Arthritis and Musculoskeletal and Skin Diseases (NIAMS)
http://www.nih.gov/niams
OrthoInfo
http://orthoinfo.aaos.org/

evolve *For additional Internet resources, see the Web site for this book at* **http://evolve.elsevier.com/Canada/Lewis/medsurg**

Nursing Management: Musculoskeletal Problems

Written by Colleen R. Walsh
Adapted by Joyce Mammel

LEARNING OBJECTIVES

1. Describe the pathophysiology, clinical manifestations, collaborative care, and nursing management of patients with osteomyelitis.
2. Describe the types, pathophysiology, clinical manifestations, and collaborative care of patients with bone cancer.
3. Differentiate between the causes and characteristics of acute and chronic low back pain.
4. Explain the conservative and surgical therapy of patients with herniated intervertebral disc.

5. Describe the postoperative nursing management of a patient who has undergone spinal surgery.
6. Explain the etiology and the nursing management of patients with common foot disorders.
7. Describe the etiology, pathophysiology, clinical manifestations, and collaborative and nursing management of patients with osteomalacia, osteoporosis, and Paget's disease.

KEY TERMS

degenerative disc disease (DDD) Progressive degeneration that results in intervertebral discs losing their elasticity, flexibility, and shock-absorbing capabilities; thinning of the discs also occurs; a normal process of aging, p. 1865

Ewing's sarcoma family of tumours (ESFT) One of the most common primary malignant neoplasms of bone and soft tissue; characterized by rapid growth within the medullary cavity of long bones, especially femur, humerus, pelvis, and tibia, p. 1858

herniated intervertebral disc Herniation of nuclear material from the intervertebral disc that may compress or place tension on a cervical, lumbar, or sacral spinal nerve root, p. 1865

low back pain A condition most often owing to a musculoskeletal problem caused by (1) acute lumbosacral strain, (2) instability of the lumbosacral bony mechanism, (3) osteoarthritis of the lumbosacral vertebrae, (4) degenerative disc disease, or (5) herniation of an intervertebral disc, p. 1860

osteoclastoma A mostly benign but destructive tumour that arises in the cancellous ends of long bones in young adults, p. 1859

osteomalacia A rare condition of adult bone associated with vitamin D deficiency, resulting in decalcification and softening of bone, p. 1871

osteomyelitis A severe infection of the bone, bone marrow, and surrounding soft tissue, p. 1854

osteoporosis A metabolic bone disease characterized by low bone mass and structural deterioration of bone tissue leading to increased bone fragility and risk of fractures, p. 1871

osteosarcoma A primary neoplasm of bone that is extremely aggressive and is characterized by rapid growth and metastasis, p. 1857

Paget's disease A skeletal bone disorder in which there is excessive bone resorption followed by replacement of normal marrow by vascular, fibrous connective tissue and new bone that is larger, disorganized, and weaker, p. 1875

Osteomyelitis

Etiology and Pathophysiology

Osteomyelitis is a severe infection of the bone, bone marrow, and surrounding soft tissue. The most common infecting microorganism is *Staphylococcus aureus*. A variety of microorganisms can cause osteomyelitis (Berbari, Steckelberg, & Osmon, 2009) (Table 66-1). Aerobic Gram-negative bacteria, alone or mixed with Gram-positive organisms, are often found. The widespread use of antibiotics in conjunction with surgical treatment has significantly reduced the mortality rate and complications associated with osteomyelitis.

The infecting microorganisms can invade by indirect or direct entry. The *indirect entry (hematogenous)* of microorganisms most frequently affects growing bone in boys younger than 12 years old and is associated with their higher incidence of blunt trauma. The most common sites of indirect entry in children are the distal femur, proximal tibia, humerus, and radius (Weichert, Sharland, Clarke, & Faust, 2008). Adults with vascular insufficiency disorders (e.g., owing to diabetes mellitus) and genitourinary and respiratory infections are at higher risk for a primary infection to spread via the blood to the bone. The pelvis and the vertebrae, which consist of vascular-rich bone, are the most common sites of infection.

Direct-entry osteomyelitis can occur at any age when there is an open wound (e.g., fractures, penetrating wounds) and microorganisms gain entry to the body. Osteomyelitis may also occur in the presence of a foreign body such as an implant or an orthopedic prosthetic device (e.g., plate, total joint prosthesis). After gaining entrance to the bone by way of the blood, the microorganisms then lodge in an area of the bone where circulation slows, usually the metaphysis. The microorganisms grow, resulting in an increase in pressure because of the nonexpanding nature of most bone. This increasing pressure within the rigid bone structure leads to ischemia and vascular compromise of the periosteum. Eventually, the infection passes through the bone cortex and the marrow cavity, ultimately resulting in cortical devascularization and necrosis. Once ischemia occurs, the bone dies. The area of devitalized bone eventually separates from the surrounding living bone, forming *sequestra* (sing., *sequestrum*). The part of the periosteum that continues to have a blood supply forms new bone called *involucrum* (Figure 66-1).

Table 66-1 Causative Organisms in Osteomyelitis	
ORGANISM	**POSSIBLE PREDISPOSING PROBLEM**
Staphylococcus aureus	Pressure ulcer, penetrating wound, open fracture, orthopedic surgery, vascular insufficiency disorders (e.g., atherosclerosis; diabetes)
Staphylococcus epidermidis	Indwelling prosthetic devices (e.g., joint replacements, fracture fixation devices)
Streptococcus viridans	Abscessed tooth, gingival disease
Escherichia coli	Urinary tract infection
Mycobacterium tuberculosis	Tuberculosis
Neisseria gonorrhoeae	Gonorrhea
Pseudomonas	Puncture wounds, intravenous drug use
Salmonella	Sickle cell disease
Fungi, Mycobacteria	Immunocompromised host

Once formed, a sequestrum continues to be an infected island of bone surrounded by pus. It is difficult for blood-borne antibiotics or white blood cells to reach the sequestrum. A sequestrum may enlarge and serve as a site for microorganisms that spread to other sites, including the lungs and brain. The sequestrum can move out of the bone and into the soft tissue. Once outside of the bone, the sequestrum may revascularize and then undergo removal by the body's normal immune processes. Another possibility is that the sequestrum can be surgically removed through debridement of the necrotic bone. If the necrotic sequestrum is not resolved naturally or surgically, it may develop a sinus tract, resulting in a chronic, purulent cutaneous drainage (see Figure 66-1).

Chronic osteomyelitis is either a continuous, persistent problem (a result of inadequate acute treatment) or a process of exacerbations and remissions (Figure 66-2). Over time, granulation tissue turns to scar tissue. This avascular scar tissue provides an ideal site for continued microorganism growth and is impenetrable by antibiotics.

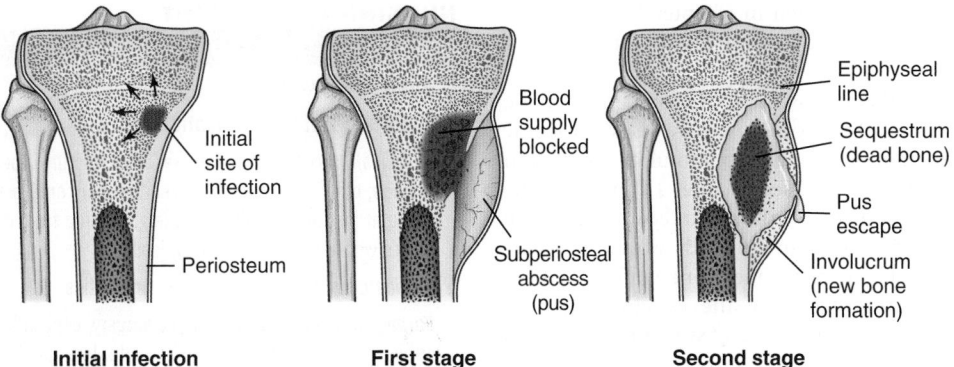

Figure 66-1 Development of osteomyelitis infection with involucrum and sequestrum.

Source: McCance, K. L., & Huether, S. E. (2010). *Pathophysiology: The biologic basis for disease in adults and children* (6th ed., p. 1587, Figure 42-16). St. Louis: Mosby.

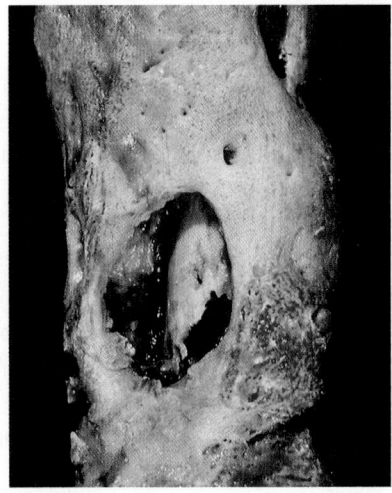

Figure 66-2 Resection of femur owing to osteomyelitis.

Source: Thibodeau, G. A., & Patton, K. T. (2010). *The human body in health and disease* (5th ed., p. 195, Figure 7-34). St. Louis: Mosby.

Clinical Manifestations

Acute osteomyelitis refers to the initial infection or an infection of less than 1 month in duration. The clinical manifestations of acute osteomyelitis are both systemic and local. Systemic manifestations include fever, night sweats, chills, restlessness, nausea, and malaise. Local manifestations include constant bone pain that is unrelieved by rest and worsens with activity; swelling, tenderness, and warmth at the infection site; and restricted movement of the affected part. Later signs include drainage from sinus tracts to the skin or the fracture site.

Chronic osteomyelitis refers to a bone infection that persists for longer than 1 month or an infection that has failed to respond to the initial course of antibiotic therapy. Systemic signs may be diminished; local signs of infection, including constant bone pain and swelling, tenderness, and warmth at the infection site, are more common.

Diagnostic Studies

A bone or soft tissue biopsy is the definitive way to determine the causative microorganism. The patient's blood, wound cultures, or both, are frequently positive for the presence of microorganisms. An elevated white blood cell and erythrocyte sedimentation rate may also be found. Radiological signs suggestive of osteomyelitis usually do not appear until 10 days to weeks after the appearance of clinical symptoms, by which time the disease will have progressed. Radionuclide bone scans (gallium and indium) are helpful in diagnosis and are usually positive in the area of infection. Magnetic resonance imaging (MRI) and computed tomography (CT) scans may be used to help identify the extent of the infection including soft tissue involvement (Averill, Hernandez, Gonzalez, Peña, & Jaramillo, 2009).

Collaborative Care

Vigorous and prolonged intravenous (IV) antibiotic therapy is the treatment of choice for acute osteomyelitis, as long as bone ischemia has not yet occurred. Cultures or a bone biopsy should be done if possible before drug therapy is initiated. If antibiotic therapy is delayed, surgical debridement and decompression are often necessary.

Treatment for osteomyelitis previously involved an extended hospital stay for IV antibiotic treatment. Today, patients are often discharged to home care with IV antibiotics delivered via a central venous catheter or peripherally inserted central catheter. IV antibiotic therapy may initially be started in the hospital and continued in the home for 4 to 6 weeks or as long as 3 to 6 months. A variety of antibiotics may be prescribed depending on the microorganism. These drugs include penicillin, cefazolin (Ancef), gentamicin, and vancomycin.

In adults with chronic osteomyelitis, oral therapy with ciprofloxacin (Cipro) for 6 to 8 weeks may be prescribed instead of IV antibiotics. Oral antibiotic therapy may also be given after acute IV therapy is complete to ensure resolution of the infection. The patient's response to drug therapy is monitored through bone scans and erythrocyte sedimentation rate tests.

Treatment of chronic osteomyelitis includes surgical removal of the poorly vascularized tissue and dead bone and the extended use of antibiotics. Antibiotic-impregnated bead chains may be implanted at this time to aid in combating the infection (Haidar, Der Boghossian, & Atiyeh, 2010). After debridement of the devitalized and infected tissue, the wound may be closed and a suction irrigation system inserted. Intermittent surgical irrigation and debridement of the affected bone may continue. Negative pressure over the site of the infection may be used to draw the wound together (vacuum-assisted closure). (Negative-pressure wound therapy is presented in Chapter 14). The limb or surgical site may be protected with a cast or brace during this time.

Hyperbaric oxygen therapy with 100% oxygen may be administered as an adjunct therapy in refractory cases of chronic osteomyelitis. This therapy is thought to stimulate circulation and healing in the infected tissue (see Chapter 14). Orthopedic prosthetic devices, if a source of chronic infection, must be removed. Muscle flaps or skin grafting provide wound coverage over the dead space (cavity) in the bone. Bone grafts may help to restore blood flow. Amputation of the extremity may be indicated when there is extensive bone destruction and when necessary to preserve the person's life, improve quality of life, or both.

Long-term and mostly rare complications of osteomyelitis include septicemia, septic arthritis, pathological fractures, squamous cell carcinoma, and amyloidosis.

NURSING MANAGEMENT: OSTEOMYELITIS

▥ Nursing Assessment

Subjective and objective data that should be obtained from an individual with osteomyelitis are presented in Table 66-2.

▥ Nursing Diagnoses

Nursing diagnoses for the patient with osteomyelitis may include, but are not limited to, the following:
- Acute pain *related to* inflammatory process secondary to infection
- Impaired physical mobility *related to* pain, immobilization devices, and weight-bearing limitations
- Ineffective self-health management *related to* lack of knowledge regarding long-term management of osteomyelitis

A more complete listing of the nursing diagnoses is presented in eNCP 66-1 on the Evolve website for this chapter.

▥ Planning

The overall goals are that the patient with osteomyelitis will (1) have satisfactory pain and fever control, (2) not experience any complications associated with osteomyelitis, (3) cooperate with the treatment plan, and (4) maintain a positive outlook on the outcome of the disease.

▥ Nursing Implementation

▥ Health Promotion

The control of infections already in the body (e.g., urinary, respiratory tract) is important in preventing osteomyelitis. Adults who are immunocompromised, have orthopedic prosthetic devices, have vascular insufficiencies, or have some combination of these are especially susceptible. These patients should be instructed

NURSING ASSESSMENT

Table 66-2 Osteomyelitis

Subjective Data
Important Health Information
Past health history: Bone trauma, open fracture, open or puncture wounds, other infections (e.g., genitourinary and respiratory infections); vascular insufficiency disorders (e.g., arising from diabetes mellitus); adults who are immunocompromised
Medications: Use of analgesics or antibiotics
Surgery or other treatments: Bone surgery, especially implantation of an orthopedic prosthetic device (e.g., plate, total joint prosthesis)
Symptoms
Constant bone pain that is unrelieved by rest and worsens with activity; restricted movement of the affected part; malaise
Objective Data
General
Restlessness; fever, chills, night sweats
Integumentary
Diaphoresis; erythema, warmth, edema at infected bone
Later signs include drainage from sinus tracts to the skin and/or the fracture site
Musculoskeletal
Restricted movement; wound drainage; spontaneous fractures
Possible Findings
Leukocytosis, positive blood and/or wound cultures, ↑ erythrocyte sedimentation rate; presence of sequestrum and involucrum on radiographs, radionuclide bone scans, CT, and MRI

CT, computed tomography; *MRI,* magnetic resonance imaging.

regarding the local and systemic manifestations of osteomyelitis. Families should also be aware of their role in monitoring the patient's health. Symptoms of bone pain, fever, swelling, and restricted limb movement should be reported immediately to the health care provider.

▥ Acute Intervention

Some immobilization of the affected limb (e.g., splint) is usually indicated to decrease pain. The involved limb should be handled carefully and excessive manipulation avoided because it increases pain and may cause pathological fracture. An important nursing responsibility is to assess the patient's pain. Minor to severe pain with muscle spasms may be experienced. Nonsteroidal anti-inflammatory drugs (NSAIDs), opioid analgesics, and muscle relaxants may be prescribed to provide patient comfort. Non-pharmacological approaches to pain management (e.g., guided imagery, relaxation breathing) should be encouraged by the nurse (see Chapters 10 and 12).

Dressings are used to absorb the exudate from draining wounds. Soiled dressings should be handled carefully to prevent cross-contamination of the wound or spread of the infection to other patients. When the dressing is changed, sterile technique is essential.

The patient is frequently on bed rest in the early stages of the acute infection. Good body alignment and frequent position changes prevent complications associated with immobility and promote comfort. Flexion contracture, especially of the hip or knee, is a common sequel of osteomyelitis of the lower extremity because the patient frequently positions the affected extremity in a flexed position to promote comfort. The contracture may then progress to a deformity. Footdrop can develop quickly if the foot is not correctly supported in the neutral position by a splint or if there is excessive pressure from a splint, which can injure the peroneal nerve. The patient should be instructed to avoid any activities, such as exercise or heat application, that increase circulation and serve as stimuli to the spread of infection. Uninvolved joints and muscles should continue to be exercised.

The patient should also be taught the potential adverse and toxic reactions associated with prolonged and high-dose antibiotic therapy. These reactions include hearing deficit, fluid retention, and neurotoxicity, which can occur with the aminoglycosides (e.g., tobramycin), and jaundice, colitis, and photosensitivity from the extended use of the cephalosporins (e.g., cefazolin). Peak and trough blood levels of most antibiotics must be carefully monitored throughout the course of therapy to prevent these adverse effects. Lengthy antibiotic therapy can also result in an overgrowth of *Candida albicans* and *Clostridium difficile* in the genitourinary and oral cavities, especially in immunosuppressed and older adult patients. The nurse should instruct the patient to report any whitish, yellowish, curdlike lesions or frequent watery diarrhea to the health care provider.

The patient and family are often frightened and discouraged because of the serious nature of the disease, uncertainty of the outcome, and the lengthy course of treatment. Continued psychological and emotional support is an integral part of the nursing management for patients with osteomyelitis.

▮ Ambulatory and Home Care

With the introduction of various intermittent venous access devices, IV antibiotics today can be administered to the patient in his or her home setting. The patient and family must be instructed on the proper care and management of the venous access device. They must also be taught how to administer the antibiotic when scheduled and the need for follow-up laboratory testing. The importance of taking antibiotics even after the symptoms have subsided should be stressed. Periodic home nursing visits provide the family with support, which helps to reduce anxiety. If there is an open wound, dressing changes are often necessary. The patient and family may require supplies and instruction in the technique. Family members also need to understand that the infection is not contagious.

If the osteomyelitis becomes chronic, patients need physical and psychological support for a prolonged period. They may become frustrated, anxious, and angry, especially when treatment plans do not result in a cure. Well-informed patients are better able to participate in decisions and cooperate in treatment plans.

▮ Evaluation

The expected outcomes are that the patient with osteomyelitis will:
- Have satisfactory pain relief.
- Follow the recommended treatment regimen.

- Verbalize confidence in ability to implement treatment regimen at home.
- Demonstrate a consistent increase in mobility and range of motion.

Bone Tumours

Primary benign and malignant bone tumours are rare in adults and occur most often during childhood through young adulthood. Metastatic bone cancer, in which the cancer has spread from another site, is a more common problem. The name given to a bone tumour is based on the area of the bone and surrounding tissue that is affected and on the type of cells forming the tumour (Table 66-3). Primary bone cancer is called *sarcoma*. Sarcomas can also develop in cartilage, muscle fibres, fatty tissue, and nerve tissue (MD Anderson Cancer Center, 2011). The more common types of bone cancer are *osteosarcoma, Ewing's sarcoma, chondrosarcoma,* and *chordoma.*

The main types of benign tumours include *osteoclastoma, osteochondroma,* and *endochroma.* These types of tumours are often cured by surgery and are more common than primary malignant tumours. In 2007, 354 new cases of bone cancer occurred in Canada, and there were 136 deaths (Canadian Cancer Society, Statistics Canada, Provincial/Territorial Cancer Registry, & Public Health Agency of Canada, 2011).

Osteosarcoma

Osteosarcoma is a primary bone tumour that is extremely aggressive and is characterized by rapid growth and metastasis. It usually occurs in the metaphyseal region of the long bones of the extremities, particularly in the regions of the distal femur, proximal tibia, and proximal humerus as well as the pelvis (Figure 66-3). Osteosarcoma is the most common malignant bone tumour affecting children and young adults; the highest incidence is in males in the 10- to 25-year-old age group. Secondary osteosarcoma is known to occur in adults older than age 60 and is most commonly associated with Paget's disease (Kumar, Abbas, Fausto, & Aster, 2010).

Clinical manifestations of osteosarcoma are usually associated with a gradual onset of pain and swelling, especially around the knee. A minor injury does not cause the neoplasm but may bring the pre-existing condition to medical attention. The neoplasm grows rapidly and can restrict joint motion if the tumour is close to a joint structure. The diagnosis is confirmed from tissue biopsy; elevation of serum alkaline phosphatase and calcium levels; and findings on radiographic, CT, or positron emission tomogram scans, and MRI. Metastasis is present in 10 to 20% of individuals on diagnosis, with the lung being the most frequent site.

Canadian Terry Fox was diagnosed with osteosarcoma at 18 years of age and underwent an above-knee amputation in early 1977. Influenced by his experience, Terry decided in 1980 to run across Canada to raise money and awareness about cancer. Since then, more than $550 million has been raised worldwide for cancer research in Terry's name through the annual Terry Fox Run held across Canada and around the world (Terry Fox Foundation, 2011). Fortunately, major advances continue to be made in the treatment of osteosarcoma.

Table 66-3 Types of Primary Bone Cancer	
TYPES	**DESCRIPTION**
Benign	
Osteochondroma	Most common benign bone tumour; frequently located in metaphyseal portion of long bones, particularly leg, pelvis, or scapula; occurs most often in persons ages 10 to 25; malignant transformation may occur. (chondrosarcoma)
Osteoclastoma (giant cell tumour)	Arises in cancellous ends of the arm and leg bones; about 10% are locally aggressive and may spread to lungs; high rate of local recurrence after surgery and chemotherapy
Endochroma	Intramedullary cartilage tumour usually found in cavity of a single hand or foot bone; rare malignant transformation can occur; if tumour becomes painful, a surgical resection is done; peak incidence in persons ages 10 to 20
Malignant	
Osteosarcoma	Most common primary bone cancer; occurs mostly in young males between ages 10 and 25; most often in bones of arms, legs, or pelvis (see Figure 66-3)
Chondrosarcoma	Occurs in cartilage most commonly in arm, leg, and pelvic bones of older adults ages 50-70; can also arise from benign bone tumours (osteochondromas); wide surgical resection is mostly done because tumour rarely responds to radiation and chemotherapy; survival rate depends on stage, size, and grade of tumour
Ewing's sarcoma	Develops in medullary cavity of long bones, especially the femur, humerus, pelvis, and tibia; usually occurs in children and teenagers; use of wide surgical resection, radiation, and chemotherapy has greatly improved the 5-yr survival rate to 60%; occurs most often in White people
Chordoma	Rare tumour that occurs in base of skull and vertebral bones of older adults ages 50-70; wide surgical resection and radiation are difficult because the spinal cord and nerves may also be involved; chemotherapy may be used for late-stage disease; tumour may recur ≥10 yr after treatment

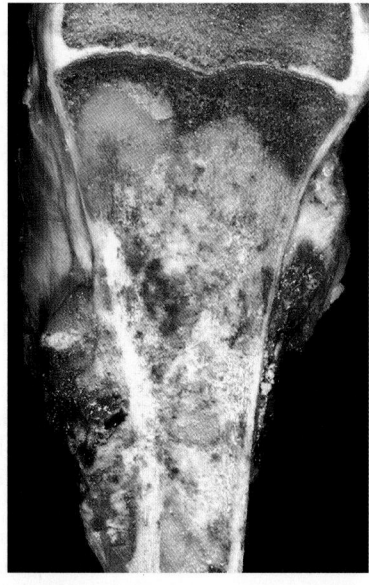

Figure 66-3 Osteosarcoma of the tibia. Tumour has infiltrated the cortex and formed soft tissue masses on both sides of the bone.

Source: Kumar, V., Abbas, A. K., Fausto, N., & Aster, J. (2010). *Robbins and Cotran pathologic basis of disease* (8th ed., p. 1226, Figure 26-22). Philadelphia: Saunders.

Preoperative chemotherapy is used to decrease tumour size, and limb-salvage procedures (e.g., wide surgical resection of the tumour) are being used more often. Limb salvage is contraindicated if there is major neurovascular involvement, pathological fracture, infection, skeletal immaturity, or extensive muscle involvement. Quality-of-life considerations also factor into the decision regarding limb salvage compared with amputation. The introduction of multiagent chemotherapy has improved the outcomes for these patients, and the cure rate for osteosarcoma is currently 60 to 70% (Maki, 2008). Chemotherapeutic agents used include methotrexate, doxorubicin (Adriamycin), cisplatin, cyclophosphamide (Procytox), bleomycin, dactinomycin (Cosmegen), and ifosfamide (Ifex).

Ewing's Sarcoma Family of Tumours

Ewing's sarcoma family of tumours (ESFT) is one of the most common primary malignant neoplasms of bone and soft tissue. It occurs most often in adolescents or young adults, the majority of whom are younger than 30 years of age. There is a slight male predominance, and the disease is most common in Whites (Weiss & Goldblum, 2008).

ESFT is characterized by rapid growth within the medullary cavity of long bones, especially the femur, humerus, pelvis, and tibia. Metastasis occurs early, and the most frequent site is the lungs. Common manifestations are progressive local pain, swelling, palpable soft tissue mass, noticeable increase in size of the affected part, fever, and leukocytosis. Initially, radiographic studies, CT, and MRI show periosteal bone destruction. Bone biopsy confirms the diagnosis. Treatment usually involves radiation therapy and wide surgical resection of the tumour or amputation. Multidrug chemotherapy has improved survival rates. Chemotherapeutic agents commonly used are cyclophosphamide (Procytox), vincristine, ifosfamide (Ifex), doxorubicin (Adriamycin), and etoposide (VePesid). Surgical resection of the tumour has helped decrease the rate of recurrence. The 5-year disease-free survival rate for localized Ewing's sarcoma treated with radiation, surgical resection, and multiagent chemotherapy is 65 to 76%. However, survival is poor in patients with metasta-

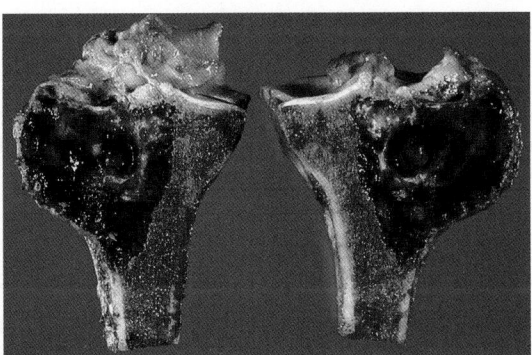

Figure 66-4 Osteoclastoma (giant cell tumour) in a long bone.

Source: Damjanov, I., & Linder, J. (1996). *Anderson's pathology* (10th ed.). St Louis: Mosby.

ses outside the lungs at time of diagnosis and those who have a relapse of Ewing's sarcoma (Balamuth & Womer, 2010).

Osteoclastoma

Osteoclastoma *(giant cell tumour)* is a destructive tumour that arises in the cancellous ends of long bones in young adults. Most (98%) of these variant giant cell tumours are benign, but they can be locally aggressive and spread to the lungs. Giant cell tumours most commonly occur in females between the ages of 20 and 35. Common tumour sites are in the epiphysis of the distal femur, the proximal tibia, and the distal radius (Wheeless, 2011). Clinical manifestations are usually swelling, local pain, and some disturbances in joint function. Radiographic evidence of giant cell tumour is variable, but a radiographic study usually reveals local areas of bone destruction and eventual expansion of the bone ends (Figure 66-4).

Biopsy is used to establish the diagnosis. After diagnosis, surgical curettage of the tumour is usually done, followed by bone grafting. Cryosurgery helps to preserve joint motion and reduce the need for amputation. Complications from cryosurgery include later pathological fracture and delayed union. After treatment, there is a greater than 50% chance of recurrence. Recurrent giant cell tumours may have to be treated with amputation.

Metastatic Bone Cancer

The most common type of malignant bone tumour occurs as a result of metastasis from a primary tumour. Common sites for the primary tumour include breast, prostate, gastrointestinal tract, lungs, kidney, ovary, and thyroid (Coleman & Holen, 2008). The bone is the third most common site for metastatic disease. The metastatic cancer cells travel to other sites from the primary tumour via the lymph and blood supply. The metastatic bone lesion is commonly found in vertebrae, pelvis, femur, humerus, or ribs. Pathological fractures at the site of metastasis are common because of weakening of the involved bone. High serum calcium levels result as calcium is released from damaged bones.

Once a primary lesion has been identified, radionuclide bone scans are often done to detect the presence of metastatic lesions before they are visible on radiography. It is important to note that metastatic bone lesions may occur at any time (even years later) following diagnosis and treatment of the primary tumour. Metastasis to the bone should be suspected in any patient who has local bone pain and a past history of cancer. Treatment may be palliative and consists of pain management and radiation (see Chapter 18). Surgical stabilization of the fracture may be indicated if there is a fracture or pending fracture. Prognosis depends on the extent of metastasis and the location.

NURSING MANAGEMENT: BONE CANCER

◼ Nursing Assessment

The patient with bone cancer should be assessed for the location and severity of pain. Weakness caused by anemia and decreased mobility may also be noted. Swelling at the involved site and decreased joint function, depending on the tumour site, should also be monitored.

◼ Nursing Diagnoses

Nursing diagnoses for the patient with bone cancer may include, but are not limited to, the following:
- Acute pain *related to* the disease process or inadequate pain medication or comfort measures
- Impaired physical mobility *related to* disease process, pain, weakness, and debility
- Disturbed body image *related to* possible amputation, deformity, swelling, and effects of chemotherapy
- Grieving *related to* actual or potential losses and change of body image
- Risk for injury *related to* disease process, possible pathological fracture, or inadequate handling or positioning of affected body part
- Impaired home maintenance *related to* lack of knowledge about care needed at home or how to perform the necessary skills

◼ Planning

The overall goals are that the patient with bone cancer will (1) have satisfactory pain relief; (2) maintain preferred activities as long as possible; (3) demonstrate acceptance of body image changes resulting from chemotherapy, radiation, and surgery; (4) remain free from injury; and (5) verbalize a realistic idea of disease progression and prognosis.

◼ Nursing Implementation

◼ Health Promotion

The nurse should teach the public to recognize the warning signs of bone cancer, including swelling, bone pain of unexplained origin, limitation of joint function, and changes in skin temperature. As with all types of cancer, health promotion should stress the importance of periodic screening and health examinations.

Acute Intervention

Nursing care of the patient with a malignant bone neoplasm does not differ significantly from the care given to the patient with a malignant disease of any other body system (see Chapter 18). However, special attention is required to reduce the complications associated with prolonged bed rest and to prevent falls and pathological fractures. Careful handling and support of the affected extremity and logrolling for those on bed rest are important to prevent pathological fractures (Johnson & Knobf, 2008). The patient is often reluctant to participate in therapeutic activities because of weakness from the disease and treatment and fear of pain. Regular rest periods should be provided between activities.

Ambulatory and Home Care

The nurse must be able to assist the patient and family in accepting the guarded prognosis associated with bone neoplasms. Inability to accomplish age-specific developmental tasks can increase the frustrations with this condition. General principles related to cancer nursing are applicable (see Chapter 18). Special attention is necessary for the problems of pain and disability, chemotherapy, and specific surgery such as spinal cord decompression or amputation.

Evaluation

The following are expected outcomes for the patient with bone cancer:

• The patient will have minimal to no pain.
• The patient will have no falls.
• The patient will have no pathological fractures.
• The patient will accept changes in body image.
• The patient will retain dignity and active participation in treatment decisions.
• The patient will have maximal functional ability.

Low Back Pain

Etiology and Pathophysiology

Low back pain (LBP) is common, and 70 to 85% of the population will experience it at least once during their lifetime (Furlan, Imamura, Dryden, & Irvin, 2010). The incidence of back pain does not differ significantly across social or demographic groups. Back pain continues to be the leading overall cause of lost productivity in the workplace (Ammendolia, Kerr, & Bombardier, 2005; National Institute of Neurological Disorders and Stroke [NINDS], 2011). LBP is a common problem because the lumbar region (1) bears most of the weight of the body, (2) is the most flexible region of the spinal column, (3) contains nerve roots that are vulnerable to injury or disease, and (4) has an inherently poor biomechanical structure.

Several risk factors are associated with LBP, including lack of muscle tone and excess body weight, poor posture, cigarette smoking, and stress. Jobs that require repetitive heavy lifting, operation of vibrating machinery, or prolonged periods of sitting

are also associated with low back pain. **Low back pain** is most often owing to a musculoskeletal problem. The causes of LBP of musculoskeletal origin include (1) acute lumbosacral strain, (2) instability of the lumbosacral bony mechanism, (3) osteoarthritis of the lumbosacral vertebrae, (4) degenerative disc disease (DDD), and (5) herniation of an intervertebral disc.

Acute Low Back Pain

Acute low back pain usually lasts 6 weeks or less. Often, symptoms of LBP do not appear at the time of injury but develop later because of a gradual increase in pressure on the nerve by an intervertebral disc. Few definitive diagnostic abnormalities are present with nerve irritation and muscle strain.

Health care practitioners should not routinely obtain imaging or other diagnostic tests in patients with nonspecific acute back pain (Toward Optimized Practice [TOP], 2009). Diagnostic imaging, including radiography, MRI, and CT scans, are generally not done unless there are red flags such as trauma or systemic disease (e.g., cancer, spinal infection). Most patients self-treat back pain: however, the number seeking medical attention is increasing and is approximately 45% (Wilk, Palmer, Stosic, & McLachlan, 2010).

Collaborative Care

If the acute muscle spasms and accompanying pain are not severe and debilitating, the patient will be treated with analgesics such as NSAIDs or muscle relaxants. Severe pain may require a short course of opioid analgesics. A brief period (1 to 2 days) of rest at home may be necessary for some persons, but most do better with a continuation of their regular activities (Nicholas & George, 2011). Bed rest provides no benefit to patients who have acute LBP with or without sciatica (see Evidence-Informed Practice box on p. 1861). For nonspecific LBP, evidence suggests that to stay active rather than rest in bed means the patient will return to work sooner, improve functional status, and have less pain. Patients who are unable to return to normal activities may have short-term benefits from spinal manipulation, but it may be no more effective than usual care. Multidisciplinary rehabilitation programs in occupational settings may be an option for workers with sick leave of more than 4 to 8 weeks.

The effectiveness of invasive treatments, such as epidural corticosteroid injections and implanted devices that deliver pain medication, remains controversial. The latest research evidence suggests that transcutaneous electrical nerve stimulation and traction are not effective for the treatment of LBP. Although it is important that the patient remains active and fit, the current scientific evidence does not support the use of specific exercises (e.g., strengthening, stretching, flexion, and extension exercises) as a treatment for acute nonspecific LBP (Hayden, van Tulder, Malmivaara, & Koes, 2011). Patients experiencing acute nonspecific LBP should avoid bed rest for prolonged periods and activities that aggravate the pain, including lifting, bending, twisting, and prolonged sitting. Most cases spontaneously improve within 2 to 6 weeks.

Chronic Low Back Pain

Chronic low back pain lasts more than 3 months or is a repeated incapacitating episode. The causes of chronic low back pain

Should Patients With Acute Low Back Pain Stay Active?

Clinical Question

In patients with acute low back pain (P), does staying active (I) or being on bed rest (C) improve recovery (O)?

Best Available Evidence

Systematic review of randomized controlled trials (RCTs)

Critical Appraisal and Synthesis of Evidence

- 10 randomized trials ($n = 1923$); advice to rest in bed was compared with advice to stay active for patients with low back pain (LBP) with or without sciatica.
- Acute LBP was defined as pain lasting <6 wk.
- Staying active involved continuing the daily routine and being mobile at home within the limitations of pain.
- Moderate-quality evidence to show that patients with acute LBP may have small improvements in pain relief and ability to perform daily activities if they stay active as compared with resting in bed.
- Low-quality evidence suggests that patients with sciatica experience little or no difference with the two approaches.

Conclusions

- Staying active while experiencing acute LBP has beneficial results but it is not clear whether this helps patients with sciatica.
- There is no evidence that staying active is harmful.

Implications for Nursing Practice

- Encourage patients with acute LBP to continue daily activities within their limitations of pain.
- Instruct patients on the potential harm of extended bed rest.
- Research on the effects of staying active for chronic LBP is needed.

Reference for Evidence

Dahm, K. T., Brurberg, K. G., Jamtvedt, G., & Hagen, K. B. (2009). Advice to rest in bed versus advice to stay active for acute low-back pain and sciatica. *Cochrane Database of Systematic Reviews*, 6, CD007612. doi:10.1002/14651858. CD007612.pub2

PICO: P, patient population of interest; I, intervention or area of interest; C, comparison of interest or comparison group; O, outcome(s) of interest.

include DDD, lack of physical exercise, prior injury, obesity, structural and postural abnormalities, and systemic disease. Osteoarthritis of the lumbar spine is found in patients older than age 50, whereas chronic back pain in younger patients with osteoarthritis usually involves the thoracic or lumbar spine. Discomfort is increased following periods of inactivity, particularly on awakening or after long periods of sitting.

Spinal stenosis is a narrowing of the vertebral canal or nerve root canals caused by encroachment of bone on the space. The stenosis may be congenital or, more typically, is acquired through degenerative or traumatic changes to the spine. When it occurs in the lumbar area of the spine, it is a common cause of chronic or recurrent LBP. Compression of the nerve roots can result, with subsequent disc herniation. The pain associated with lumbar spinal stenosis often starts in the low back and then radiates to the buttock and the leg (Markham & Gaud, 2008). It worsens with walking and, in particular, standing without walking.

Collaborative Care

Chronic LBP is not a clinical entity but a symptom in patients with very different stages of impairment, disability, and chronicity (Airaksinen et al., 2006). Treatment for chronic LBP is much the same as for acute LBP. Cold, damp weather aggravates the back pain, but this can be relieved with rest and local heat application. Relief of pain and stiffness by the use of mild analgesics, such as NSAIDs, is integral to the daily comfort of the individual with chronic LBP. Weight reduction, sufficient rest periods, local heat or cold application, and exercise and activity throughout the day help to keep the muscles and joints mobilized. Tricyclic antidepressants (e.g., amitriptyline [Elavil]) and selective serotonin reuptake inhibitors (e.g., sertraline) have been shown to improve the chronic symptoms of LBP (Perrot, Javier, Marty, Le Jeune, & Laroche, 2008; Chou, 2010).

Surgical intervention may be indicated in patients with severe chronic LBP who do not respond to conservative care and/or have continued neurological deficits. (Surgery for low back pain is discussed on p. 1867.)

NURSING MANAGEMENT: NONSPECIFIC LOW BACK PAIN

Nursing Assessment

Subjective and objective data that should be obtained from the patient with LBP are summarized in Table 66-4. The initial clinical history taking should aim at identifying red flags of possible serious pathology (Church & Odle, 2007). *Red flags* are risk factors detected in past medical history and symptomatology that are associated with a higher risk of serious disorders. If any of these are present, further investigation may be required to exclude a serious underlying condition (e.g., infection, inflammatory rheumatic disease, or cancer). Examples of red flags are listed in Table 66-5.

Nursing Diagnoses

Nursing diagnoses for the patient with LBP may include, but are not limited to, those presented in Nursing Care Plan (NCP) 66-1.

Planning

The overall goals are that the patient with LBP will (1) have satisfactory pain relief, (2) avoid constipation secondary to medication and immobility, (3) learn back-sparing practices, and (4) return to previous level of activity within prescribed restrictions.

NURSING ASSESSMENT

Table 66-4 Low Back Pain

Subjective Data

Important Health Information

Past health history: Acute or chronic lumbosacral strain/trauma, osteoarthritis, degenerative disc disease, obesity; metabolic, circulatory, gynecological, and urological problems

Occupation requiring heavy lifting, vibrations, or extended driving

Medications: Use of analgesics, muscle relaxants, NSAIDs, corticosteroids, over-the-counter remedies including herbal products and nutritional supplements

Surgery or other treatments: Previous back surgery, epidural corticosteroid injections

Symptoms

- Pain in back, buttocks, or leg associated with walking, turning, straining, coughing, leg raising
- Numbness or tingling of legs, feet, toes; muscle spasms
- Activity intolerance
- Interrupted sleep

Objective Data

General

Guarded movement

Neurological

Depressed or absent Achilles tendon reflex or patellar tendon reflex; positive straight leg–raising test, positive cross-over straight leg–raising test, positive Trendelenburg's test

Musculoskeletal

Tense, tight paravertebral muscles on palpation, decreased range of motion of spine; poor posture

Possible Findings

Localization of site of lesion or disorder on myelogram, CT scan, or MRI; determination of nerve root impingement on electromyography

CT, computed tomography; *MRI,* magnetic resonance imaging; *NSAIDs,* nonsteroidal anti-inflammatory drugs.

Nursing Implementation

Health Promotion

Patients should also be advised to maintain appropriate body weight. Excess body weight places extra stress on the lower back and weakens the abdominal muscles that support the lower back. Flat shoes or shoes with low heels (<2.5 cm) and shock-absorbing shoe inserts are recommended for women.

The position assumed while sleeping is also important in preventing LBP. Sleeping in a prone position should be avoided because it produces excessive lumbar lordosis, placing excessive stress on the lower back. A firm mattress is recommended. The patient should sleep in either a supine or a side-lying position with the knees and hips flexed to prevent unnecessary pressure on support muscles, ligamentous structures, and lumbosacral joints. Patients should be educated about the necessity to avoid or cease smoking. Nicotine has been shown to decrease circulation to the vertebral discs, and a causal relationship exists between

Table 66-5 Red Flags

Red flags are risk factors detected in the patient's past medical history and symptomatology that occur in addition to low back pain. They are indicators of increased risk of serious pathological conditions causing low back pain. These red flags or risk factors include the following:

- A history of cancer
- Unexplained weight loss
- Pain that is insidious in onset, progressive, nonpositional, associated with night pain and systemic symptoms or signs
- Chronic, unremitting pain lasting >6 wk
- History of recent, significant trauma
- Recent mild trauma in patients older than 50 years
- History of osteoporosis
- Patients older than 70 years
- Unexplained fever
- Immunosuppression
- Focal neurological deficit
- Intravenous drug use or prolonged use of corticosteroids

Source: Church, E. J., & Odle, T. G. (2007). Diagnosis and treatment of back pain. *Radiologic Technology, 79*(2), 126-155.

smoking and some types of LBP (Björck-van Dijken, Fjellman-Wiklund, & Hildingsson, 2008).

Acute Intervention

The primary nursing responsibilities in acute LBP are to assist the patient to maintain activity limitations, promote comfort, and educate the patient about the health problem and appropriate exercises. Other nursing interventions are summarized in NCP 66-1. The use of analgesics, NSAIDs, muscle relaxants, and thermotherapy (ice and heat) while avoiding continued bed rest is incorporated into the plan of care.

Muscle stretching and strengthening exercises may be part of the management plan. Exercises can help to strengthen the back as a preventive measure, but there is no evidence to support their effectiveness as treatment for LBP. Although the actual exercises are often taught by the physiotherapist, it is the nurse's responsibility to ensure that the patient understands the type and the frequency of exercise prescribed as well as the rationale for the program.

As a role model, the nurse should use proper body mechanics at all times. The nurse should assess the patient's use of body mechanics and offer advice when activities that could produce back strain are performed (Table 66-6). Exercises to strengthen the back are presented in Table 66-7.

Ambulatory and Home Care

The goal of management is to make an episode of acute LBP an isolated incident. If the lumbosacral mechanism is unstable, repeated episodes can be anticipated. The lumbosacral spine may be unable to meet the demands placed on it without strain because of factors such as obesity, poor posture, poor muscular support, advancing age, or local trauma. Intervention is aimed at strengthening the supporting muscles by exercise. A corset limits extremes of movement and may be useful in decreasing pain and the use of pain medication (Calmels et al., 2009).

NURSING CARE PLAN 66-1

Low Back Pain

Acute Management

NURSING DIAGNOSIS	*Acute pain related to* mechanical disorders or nonmechanical spine diseases and ineffective comfort measures *as evidenced by* verbalization of back pain on movement, guarded movements, palpable muscle spasm, decreased physical activity, and rating of pain as >4 on a 10-point pain scale
Expected Patient Outcomes	**Nursing Interventions and *Rationales***

- Experiences reduction or absence of pain and muscle spasms
- Expresses satisfaction with pain relief (rates pain as <4 on pain scale of 10)

- Perform a comprehensive and ongoing pain assessment to include location, characteristics, onset and duration, frequency, quality, and intensity or severity of pain and precipitating factors *to plan appropriate interventions.*
- Promote adequate rest and sleep *to facilitate pain relief and to reduce paravertebral muscle spasm and resulting pain.*
- Teach the use of nonpharmacological techniques (e.g., relaxation, distraction, hot and cold application, and massage) *to promote muscle relaxation and decrease tension.*
- Provide patient with optimal pain relief with prescribed analgesics *to help decrease pain and inflammation.*
- Ensure that patient receives attentive analgesic care, and evaluate effectiveness *to promote comfort and to assess effectiveness of treatment.*
- Place in the designated therapeutic position (e.g., keep head of bed elevated 20 degrees and knee flexed) *to promote comfort by reducing stress on lower back muscles.*

NURSING DIAGNOSIS	*Impaired physical mobility related to* pain *as evidenced by* limited range of motion (ROM), movement restrictions, or muscle spasms
Expected Patient Outcome	**Nursing Interventions and *Rationales***

- Returns to prior level of mobility within prescribed restrictions

- Determine limitations of joint movement and effect on function *to assess extent of disability.*
- Initiate pain-control measures before beginning joint exercises *to assist in completion of exercises and ROM.*
- Encourage active ROM exercises, according to regular, planned schedule *to maintain all joints in normal ROM.*
- Encourage ambulation *to promote gradual and progressive return to previous mobility level.*
- Provide written discharge instructions for exercise *to help patient to remember what to do at home.*

Chronic Management

NURSING DIAGNOSIS	*Chronic pain related to* progressive degenerative changes of the muscles and skeletal structures of the back *as evidenced by* verbal report of back pain for more than 3 months, fatigue, and protective and guarding behaviours
Expected Patient Outcome	**Nursing Interventions and *Rationales***

- Experiences pain controlled at an acceptable level (<4 on a 10-point scale) with the use of individualized pharmacological and nonpharmacological measures

- Use therapeutic communication strategies *to acknowledge pain experience and convey acceptance of patient's response to pain.*
- Explore with patient factors that relieve or worsen pain *to make adjustments in lifestyle so that pain is reduced.*
- Select and implement a variety of measures (e.g., pharmacological, nonpharmacological) *to facilitate pain relief.*
- Inform other health care providers and family members of nonpharmacological strategies being used by patient *to encourage individualized approaches to pain management.*
- Collaborate with patient, significant other, and other health providers to select and implement nonpharmacological pain-relief measures (e.g., use of heat, transcutaneous electrical nerve stimulation) *to provide information about supplementary methods of pain management.*
- Evaluate effectiveness of pain-control measures used through ongoing assessment of pain experience *to optimize therapy.*

Continued

NURSING CARE PLAN 66-1

Low Back Pain—cont'd

NURSING DIAGNOSIS	*Ineffective coping* related to effects of chronic pain as evidenced by verbalization of hopelessness and inability to cope, irritability, inability to meet role expectations, or ineffective or inappropriate use of coping behaviours
Expected Patient Outcomes	**Nursing Interventions and *Rationales***
• Uses coping behaviours effectively to adapt to effects of chronic pain • Reports a positive sense of control and hope • Reports satisfaction with lifestyle	**Coping enhancement** • Appraise and discuss alternative responses to situation *to assist with coping.* • Assist patient in developing an objective appraisal of the event *to assist with adjustment.* • Seek to understand patient's perception of a stressful situation *to provide patient-centred care.* • Arrange situations that encourage patient's autonomy *to foster effective coping behaviours and adjustments to chronic pain.* • Foster constructive outlets for anger and hostility *to assist with coping.* • Assist patient to identify positive strategies *to deal with limitations and manage needed lifestyle or role changes.*
NURSING DIAGNOSIS	*Ineffective health maintenance* related to knowledge deficit, complexity of therapeutic regimen, or lack of perceived benefits regarding posture, exercises, and body mechanics as evidenced by verbalization that action has not been taken to reduce risk factors for progression of illness and to include treatment regimens in daily routines
Expected Patient Outcomes	**Nursing Interventions and *Rationales***
• Integrates a program of appropriate posture, body mechanics, exercises, and weight management into daily routine • Uses proper body mechanics at all times	• Observe patient perform prescribed activity or exercise *to identify incorrect techniques and intervene appropriately.* • Instruct patient on good posture and body mechanics *to reduce risk of reinjury, provide back support, and maintain proper body alignment.* • Assist patient to incorporate activity and exercise regimen into daily routine or lifestyle *to make desired behaviours a habit.* • Refer patient to physiotherapist, occupational therapist, or exercise physiologist *to develop abdominal and paravertebral muscle strength exercises and to provide increased support.* **Weight management** • Discuss risks associated with being overweight and underweight *because increased abdominal weight alters posture and puts strain on low back.* • Develop with patient a method to keep a daily record of intake, exercise sessions, and/or changes in body weight *to evaluate management of therapeutic regimen.*

PATIENT & CAREGIVER TEACHING GUIDE

Table 66-6 Low Back Problems

The nurse should include the following instructions when teaching the patient how to manage low back problems.

Do Not

• Lean forward without bending knees.

• Lift anything above level of elbows.

• Stand in one position for prolonged time.

• Sleep on abdomen or on back or side with legs out straight.

• Exercise without consulting health care provider, if having severe pain.

• Exceed prescribed amount and type of exercises without consulting health care provider.

Do

• Prevent lower back from straining forward by placing a foot on a step or stool during prolonged standing.

• Sleep in a side-lying position with knees and hips bent.

• Sleep on back with a lift under knees and legs or on back with 25-cm-high pillow under knees to flex hips and knees.

• Exercise 15 minutes in the morning and 15 minutes in the evening regularly; begin exercises with a 2- or 3-minute warm-up period by moving arms and legs; alternate relaxing and tightening muscles; exercise slowly with smooth movements as directed by a physiotherapist.

• Maintain appropriate body weight.

• Use local heat and cold application.

• Use a lumbar roll or pillow for sitting.

• Use proper body mechanics to avoid low back strain (e.g., when lifting objects, bend at the knees, not at the waist, and stand up slowly while holding object close to the body).

Table 66-7 Back Exercises to Promote Back Strength

Knee-to-Chest Lift (To Stretch Hips, Buttocks, Lower Back Muscles) • Lie on back on the floor with knees bent and feet flat on floor. • Draw both knees up to chest. • Place both hands around knees and pull them firmly against chest. Hold for 30 seconds. • Lower legs and return to starting position. • Repeat 5 to 10 times.	**Half Sit-ups (To Strengthen Abdominal Muscles)** • Lie flat on floor on back with knees bent, feet flat on floor, and hands on chest. • Slowly raise head and neck to top of chest. • Reach both hands forward and place them on knees. • Hold for 5 counts. • Return to starting position. • Repeat 5 to 10 times.
Simple Leg Lift • Lie flat on back on floor with left knee bent and left foot flat on floor. • Raise right leg as high as comfortably possible. • Hold for 5 counts. • Slowly return leg to floor. • Bend right knee and put right foot flat on floor. • Raise left leg and hold for 5 counts. • Repeat 5 to 10 times for each leg.	**Elbow Props (To Extend Lower Back)** • Lie face-down with your arms beside your body and your head turned to one side. • Stay in this position for 2 to 5 minutes, making sure that you relax completely. • Remain face-down, and prop yourself on your elbows. • Hold this position for 2 to 3 minutes. • Return to starting position and relax for 1 minute. • Repeat 5 to 10 times.
Double Leg Lift • Lie flat on back. • Slowly lift legs until feet are 30 cm from the floor. • Keep legs straight and hold this position for 10 counts. • Lower legs to floor. • Repeat 5 times.	**Hip Tilts** • Lie flat on back with knees bent. • Slowly bend legs and hips to one side as far as possible. • Bend to other side. • Repeat 5 times.
Pelvic Tilt • Lie flat on back on floor with knees bent and feet flat on the floor. • Firmly tighten your buttock muscles. • Hold for 5 counts. • Relax buttocks. • Repeat 5 to 10 times. • Be sure to keep lower back flat against floor.	**Toe Touches** • Stand straight and relaxed. • Lower head and body and try to touch floor with fingertips. • Keep knees straight. • Do not jerk or lunge toward floor. • Bend only as far as you can. • Repeat 5 times.

Source: From Canobbio, M. M. (2006). *Mosby's handbook of patient teaching* (3rd ed.). St. Louis: Mosby.

Persistent use of poor body mechanics may also result in repeated episodes of LBP. If the strain is work related, occupational counselling may be necessary. The frustration, pain, and disability imposed on the patient with LBP require emotional support and understanding care by the nurse.

▪ Evaluation

The expected outcomes for the patient with LBP are presented in NCP 66-1.

Intervertebral Disc Disease

Etiology and Pathophysiology

An intervertebral disc is interposed between the vertebrae from the cervical axis to the sacrum. Structural degeneration of the lumbar disc is often caused by **degenerative disc disease (DDD)**.

This progressive degeneration is a normal process of aging and results in loss by the intervertebral discs of their elasticity, flexibility, and shock-absorbing capabilities. Thinning of the discs occurs as the nucleus pulposus (gelatinous centre of the disc) starts to dry out and shrink (Fassett, Kurd, & Vaccaro, 2009). Compression of the nerve roots and cord may then occur. Damage to the spine by DDD contributes to osteoarthritis of the spine by the formation of osteophytes (bone spurs).

An acute **herniated intervertebral disc** (slipped disc) can be the result of natural degeneration with age or repeated stress and trauma to the spine. Herniation of the nuclear material from the intervertebral disc may compress or place tension on a cervical, lumbar, or sacral spinal nerve root causing acute back pain (Figure 66-5). The most common sites of rupture are the lumbosacral discs, specifically L4-5 and L5-S1. Disc herniation may also occur at C5-6 and C6-7.

Clinical Manifestations

The most common feature of lumbar disc damage is LBP. Radicular pain that radiates down the buttock and below the knee,

Table 66-8 Clinical Manifestations Based on Level of Disc Herniation*

INTERVERTEBRAL LEVEL	SUBJECTIVE PAIN	AFFECTED REFLEX	MOTOR FUNCTION	SENSATION
L3-4	Back to buttocks to posterior thigh to inner calf	Patellar	Quadriceps, anterior tibialis	Inner aspect of lower leg, anterior part of thigh
L4-5	Back to buttocks to dorsum of foot and big toe	None	Anterior tibialis, extensor hallucis longus, gluteus medius	Dorsum of foot and big toe
L5-S1	Back to buttocks to sole of foot and heel	Achilles	Gastrocnemius, hamstring, gluteus maximus	Heel and lateral foot

*A disc herniation can involve pressure on more than one nerve root.

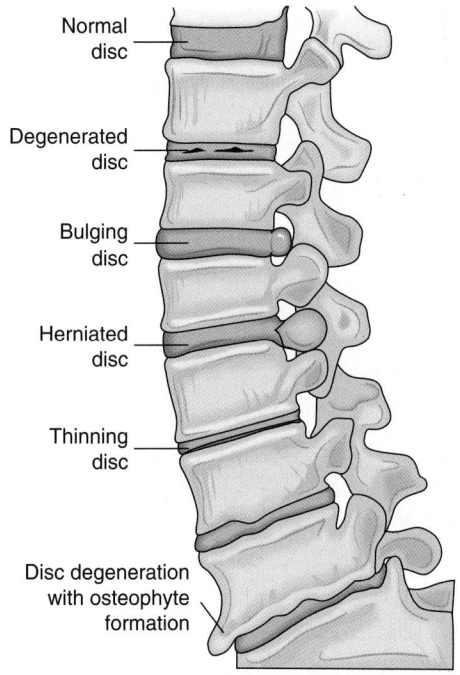

Normal disc

Degenerated disc

Bulging disc

Herniated disc

Thinning disc

Disc degeneration with osteophyte formation

Figure 66-5 Common causes of degenerative disc damage.

Source: Eidelson, S. G., & Spinasanta, S.A. (2005). *Advanced technologies to treat neck and back pain: A patient's guide.* Wheaton, Illinois: SYA Press and Research.

COLLABORATIVE CARE

Table 66-9 Intervertebral Disc Disease

Diagnostic
- History and physical examination
- Radiography
- CT scan
- MRI
- Myelogram
- Discogram
- EMG

Collaborative Therapy

Conservative
- Restricted activity for several days, limit total bed rest
- Medication
  - Analgesics
  - NSAIDs
  - Muscle relaxants

- Local ice or heat
- Physiotherapy
- Epidural corticosteroid injections

Surgical
- Intradiscal electrothermoplasty (IDET)
- Radiofrequency discal nucleoplasty
- Interspinous process decompression system (X Stop)
- Laminectomy with or without spinal fusion
- Discectomy
- Percutaneous laser discectomy
- Artificial disc replacement
- Spinal fusion with (e.g., plates, screws) or without instrumentation

CT, computed tomography; *EMG,* electromyogram; *MRI,* magnetic resonance imaging; *NSAIDs,* nonsteroidal anti-inflammatory drugs.

along the distribution of the sciatic nerve, generally indicates disc herniation. (Specific manifestations for lumbar disc herniation are summarized in Table 66-8.) The straight leg raise test may be positive, indicating nerve root irritation. Back or leg pain may be reproduced by raising the leg and flexing the foot at 90 degrees. LBP from other causes may not be accompanied by leg pain. Reflexes may be depressed or absent, depending on the spinal nerve root involved. Paresthesia or muscle weakness in the legs, feet, or toes may be reported by the patient. Multiple nerve root *(cauda equina)* compression may be manifested as bowel and bladder incontinence or erectile dysfunction.

In cervical disc damage, there is often pain radiating into the arms and hands, following the pattern of the nerve involved. Reflexes may or may not be present, and there is often weakness of the hand grips.

Diagnostic Studies

Radiographic studies are done to note any structural defects. A myelogram, MRI, or CT scan is helpful in localizing the damaged

site. An epidural venogram or discogram may be necessary if other methods of diagnosis are unsuccessful. An electromyogram of the extremities can be performed to determine the severity of nerve irritation or to rule out other pathological conditions such as peripheral neuropathy.

Collaborative Care

The patient with suspected disc damage is usually managed first with conservative therapy (Table 66-9). This includes limitation of extremes of spinal movement (brace, corset, or belt), local heat or ice, ultrasonography and massage, traction, and transcutaneous electrical nerve stimulation. Drug therapy includes NSAIDs, short-term opioids, and muscle relaxants. Epidural corticosteroid injections may be effective in reducing inflammation and relieving acute pain. If the underlying cause remains, the pain tends to recur. Conservative treatment can result in a healing over of the damaged area if not owing to DDD, with a concomitant decrease in pain. Once the symptoms subside, back-strengthening exercises are begun twice a day and are encouraged for a lifetime. The patient should be taught the principles of good body mechanics. Extremes of flexion and torsion are strongly discouraged.

Most patients initially recover with a conservative treatment plan. However, if conservative treatment is unsuccessful, *radiculopathy* (nerve root pain) becomes progressively worse, or loss of bowel or bladder control (cauda equina) is documented, surgery may then be indicated.

Surgical Therapy. Surgery for a damaged disc is generally indicated when diagnostic tests indicate the herniation is not responding to conservative treatment or there is consistent pain, or both consistent pain and a persistent neurological deficit. Surgery should be carefully considered because some patients, for unknown reasons, do not improve and symptoms may actually worsen after surgery. An *intradiscal electrothermoplasty* is a minimally invasive outpatient procedure that may help in treating back and sciatica pain (Cleveland Clinic, 2008). The procedure involves the insertion of a needle into the affected disc with radiological guidance. A wire is then threaded down through the needle and into the disc. The wire is then heated, which denervates the small nerve fibres that have grown into the cracks and have invaded the degenerating disc. The heat also partially melts the annulus, which triggers the body to generate new reinforcing proteins in the fibres of the annulus.

Another outpatient technique is *radiofrequency discal nucleoplasty* (coblation nucleoplasty). A needle is inserted into the disc similar to intradiscal electrothermoplasty. Instead of a heating wire, a special radiofrequency probe is used. The probe generates energy that breaks up the molecular bonds of the gel in the nucleus. The result is that up to 20% of the nucleus is removed, which decompresses the disc and reduces the pressure on both the disc and the surrounding nerve roots. Relief from pain varies among patients.

A third procedure is the use of an *interspinous process decompression system* (X Stop). This device is made of titanium and fits onto a mount that is placed on vertebrae in the lower back.

The X Stop is used in patients with pain owing to lumbar spinal stenosis. The device works by lifting the vertebrae off the pinched nerve. The effect is similar to and less invasive than a laminectomy.

The most common surgical procedure for lumbar disc disease is a *laminectomy*. It involves the surgical excision of part of the posterior arch of the vertebra (referred to as the *lamina*) to gain access to part or all of the protruding disc to remove it. A minimal hospital stay is usually required after the procedure.

A *discectomy* is another common type of surgical procedure that may be performed to decompress the nerve root. Microsurgical discectomy is a version of the standard discectomy in which the surgeon uses a microscope to allow better visualization of the disc and disc space during surgery to aid in the removal of the damaged portion. This helps maintain the bony stability of the spine.

A percutaneous discectomy is an outpatient surgical procedure using a tube that passes through the retroperitoneal soft tissues to the lateral border of the disc with local anaesthesia and the aid of fluoroscopy. A laser is then used on the damaged portion of the disc. Small stab wounds are used, and minimal blood loss occurs during the procedure. The procedure is effective and safe and decreases rehabilitation time.

The *Charité disc* is used in patients with disc damage associated with DDD (Guyer & Roybal, 2008). This artificial disc is made up of a high-density core sandwiched between two cobalt-chromium end plates (Figure 66-6). This device is surgically placed in the spine through a small incision below the umbilicus after the damaged disc is removed. The disc allows for movement at the level of the implant.

A *spinal fusion* may be performed if an unstable bony mechanism is present. The spine is stabilized by creating an *ankylosis* (fusion) of contiguous vertebrae with a bone graft from the patient's fibula or iliac crest or from donated cadaver bone. Metal fixation with rods, plates, or screws may be implanted at the time of spinal surgery to provide more stability and decrease vertebral motion. A posterior lumbar interbody fusion may be performed in patients to provide extra support for bone grafting or a prosthetic device. A more recent device, the InFuse Bone Graft/LT-CAGE, is being used to eliminate the need to use bone from the patient in grafting. The device contains genetically engineered

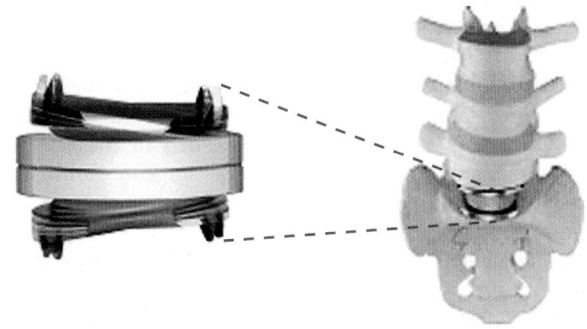

Figure 66-6 The Charité artificial disc used in degenerative disc disease to replace a damaged intervertebral disc. The Charité artificial disc consists of two cobalt-chromium alloy end plates sandwiched around a movable high-density plastic core. The design of the disc helps align the spine and preserve its natural ability to move.

Source: DePuySpine, Inc., Raynham, Massachusetts.

protein that stimulates the body to grow new bone at the spinal fusion site.

NURSING MANAGEMENT: SPINAL SURGERY

Postoperative nursing interventions focus on maintaining proper alignment of the spine at all times until healing has occurred. Depending on the type and extent of surgery, and the surgeon's preference, the patient may be able to dangle the legs at the side of the bed, stand, or even ambulate the first day after surgery.

Pillows can be used under the thighs of each leg when the patient is supine and between the legs when in side-lying positions to provide comfort and ensure alignment. The patient often fears turning or any movement that increases pain by straining the surgical area. The nurse must offer reassurance to the patient that the proper technique is being used to maintain body alignment. Sufficient staff should be available to move the patient without undue pain or strain on staff members or the patient.

Postoperatively, most patients will require opioids such as morphine intravenously for 24 to 48 hours. Patient-controlled analgesia allows for optimal analgesic levels and is the preferred method of continued pain management during this time. Once fluids are being taken, the patient may be switched to oral drugs such as acetaminophen with codeine or oxycodone (Percocet). Medications may be prescribed for muscle relaxation. The nurse should monitor and document pain management and its effectiveness after the surgery.

Because the spinal canal may be entered during surgery, there is potential for cerebrospinal fluid leakage. Severe headache or leakage of cerebrospinal fluid on the dressing should be reported immediately. Cerebrospinal fluid appears as clear or slightly yellow drainage on the dressing. It has a high glucose concentration and will be positive for glucose when a dipstick test is done. The amount, colour, and characteristics of drainage should be noted.

Frequent monitoring of peripheral neurological signs of the extremities is a routine postoperative nursing responsibility after spinal surgery. Movement of the arms and legs and assessment of sensation should be unchanged when compared with the preoperative status. Table 66-10 summarizes a lumbar laminectomy assessment appropriate for the patient who has undergone back surgery. These assessments are repeated every 2 to 4 hours during the first 48 hours after surgery, and findings are compared with the preoperative assessment. Paresthesias, such as numbness and tingling, may not be relieved immediately after surgery. Any new muscle weakness or paresthesias should be documented and reported to the surgeon immediately. Extremity circulation should be assessed by temperature, capillary refill, and pulses.

Paralytic ileus and interference with bowel function may occur for several days and may manifest as nausea, abdominal distension, and constipation. The nurse should assess whether the patient is passing flatus, has bowel sounds in all quadrants, and has a flat, soft abdomen. A bowel protocol should be initiated to prevent constipation.

Adequate bladder emptying may be altered because of activity restrictions, opioids, or anaesthesia. If allowed by the surgeon, men should be encouraged to dangle their legs or stand to urinate. Patients should use the commode or ambulate to the bathroom when allowed to promote adequate emptying of the

Table 66-10 Postoperative Assessment Following Lumbar Surgery
*Sensation**
Assess sensation of extremities for paresthesia in all appropriate dermatomes.
*Movement**
Assess ability to move all extremities.
*Muscle Strength**
Assess for any weakness of the extremities.
Wound
Assess dressing for drainage and note amount, colour, and characteristics.
Pain
• Document location of the pain.
• Ask patient to rate the pain on a scale of 0 to 10, with 0 being no pain and 10 being worst pain.
• Evaluate pain after analgesia has been administered.

*Postoperative findings should be compared with preoperative assessments. It is not unusual for the patient to continue to experience these symptoms after surgery. Symptoms gradually decrease over several months.

bladder. The nurse should ensure that privacy is maintained. It is necessary to clarify whether the patient can be allowed up to go to the bathroom without a corset or brace. Intermittent catheterization or an indwelling catheter may be necessary for patients who have difficulty urinating.

Loss of sphincter tone or bladder tone may indicate nerve damage. Incontinence or difficulty evacuating the bowel or bladder must be monitored closely and reported to the surgeon.

In addition to the nursing care appropriate for a patient who has had a laminectomy, there are other nursing responsibilities if the patient has also had a spinal fusion. Because a bone graft is usually involved, the postoperative healing time is prolonged. Reduced activity for an extended time may be necessary. A rigid orthosis (thoracic–lumbar–sacral orthosis or chairback brace) is often used during this period. Some surgeons require that the patient be taught to put the orthosis on and take it off by logrolling in bed, whereas others allow their patients to apply the brace in a sitting or standing position. The nurse should verify the preferred method before initiating this activity.

In addition to the primary surgical site, the donor site for the bone graft must be regularly assessed. The posterior iliac crest is the most commonly used donor site, although the fibula may also be used. The donor site usually causes greater postoperative pain than the fused area. The donor site is bandaged with a pressure dressing to prevent excessive bleeding. If the donor site is the fibula, neurovascular assessments of the extremity are a postoperative nursing responsibility.

As the bone graft heals, the patient must adjust to the permanent immobility at the graft or fusion site. Instruction in proper body mechanics is essential and should be evaluated during the hospital stay.

The patient should be instructed to avoid sitting or standing for prolonged periods. Activities that should be encouraged include walking, lying down, and shifting weight from one foot to the other when standing. The patient should learn to mentally think through an activity before starting any potentially injurious

Table 66-11 Neck Exercises

- Bend your head backward until you are looking up at the ceiling. Repeat slowly five times. Stop if experiencing dizziness.

- Bring your head forward so that your chin touches your chest and your face is looking down at the floor. Repeat slowly five times.

- Keep your head facing forward, and bend your ear down toward one shoulder. Alternate this movement with your other ear. Repeat slowly five times on each side.

- Turn your head slowly around to one side as far as it will go. Repeat toward the other side. Repeat exercise five times on each side.

- Without tipping your head in any direction, pull your chin and head straight back. Relax the chin forward to its neutral position. Repeat slowly five times.

task such as bending, lifting, or stooping. Any twisting movement of the spine is contraindicated. The thighs and knees, rather than the back, should be used to absorb the shock of activity and movement. A firm mattress or bed board is essential.

Neck Pain

Neck pain may occur almost as frequently as LBP, with 15% of adults experiencing neck pain at any point in time (Hellmann & Stone, 2008). Neck pain may be the result of many conditions, both benign (e.g., poor posture) and serious (e.g., traumatic injury).

Cervical neck sprains and strains occur from hyperflexion and hyperextension injury. Patients have symptoms of stiffness and neck pain and, possibly, pain radiating into the arm and hand. Pain may also radiate into the head, anterior chest, thoracic spine region, and shoulders. Cervical nerve root compression from stenosis, DDD, or herniation may be indicated by weakness or paresthesia of the arm and hand. Diagnosing the cause of neck pain is done by history, physical examination, radiography, MRI, CT scan, and electromyography. An electromyogram of the upper extremities is done to diagnose cervical radiculopathy.

Conservative treatment for neck pain that can commonly occur in patients without an underlying disorder includes head support via soft cervical collars, heat and ice applications, massage, rest until symptoms subside, physiotherapy, ultrasound, and NSAIDs. Most neck pain resolves without surgical intervention. Indications for cervical spine surgery are similar to those for the lower back. Types of surgery are also similar, including discectomy, laminectomy, and spinal fusion. If surgery is done on the cervical spine, the nurse must be alert for symptoms of spinal cord edema such as respiratory distress and a worsening neurological status of the upper extremities. An orthosis or halo may be necessary after surgery depending on the degree of spine stabilization. After surgery, the patient's neck is immobilized in either a soft or a hard cervical collar.

Preventing benign neck pain that occurs owing to everyday activities such as prolonged sitting at a computer or television, sleeping in nonalignment spinal positions, or jarring movements during exercise is important. Preventive strategies can begin by practising good posture and maintaining neck flexibility (Table 66-11).

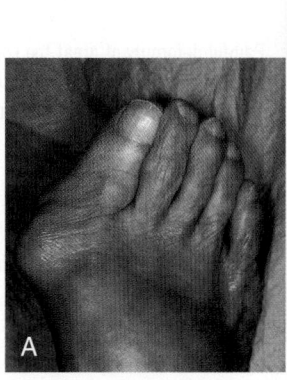
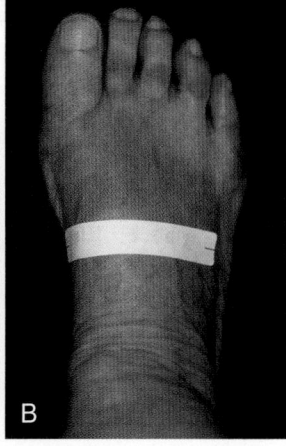

Figure 66-7 A, Severe hallux valgus with bursa formation. **B,** Postoperative correction.

Source: Canale, S., & Beaty, J. (Eds). (2008). *Campbell's operative orthopaedics* (11th ed.). Philadelphia: Saunders.

Foot Disorders

The foot is the platform that provides support for the weight of the body and absorbs considerable shock in ambulation. It is a complicated structure composed of bony structures, muscles, tendons, and ligaments. It can be affected by (1) congenital conditions, (2) structural weakness, (3) traumatic injuries, and (4) systemic conditions such as diabetes mellitus and rheumatoid arthritis. Abnormalities of the foot affect millions of Canadians. Much of the pain, deformity, and disability associated with foot disorders can be directly attributed to or accentuated by improperly fitting shoes, which cause crowding and angulation of the toes and inhibition of the normal movement of foot muscles.

The purposes of footwear are to (1) provide support, foot stability, protection, shock absorption, and a foundation for orthoses; (2) increase friction with the walking surface; and (3) treat foot abnormalities. Table 66-12 summarizes common foot disorders. One of the most common forefoot disorders is a bunion (Figure 66-7). A lateral deviation of the great toe, termed *hallux valgus,* occurs with a bunion (Aly, Mousa, & Elsallakh, 2011).

NURSING MANAGEMENT: FOOT DISORDERS

Nursing Implementation

Health Promotion

Well-constructed and properly fitted shoes are essential for healthy, pain-free feet. Instead of considerations of comfort and support, fashion styles, especially for women, often influence selection of footwear. Patient teaching should stress the importance of having a shoe that conforms to the foot rather than to current fashion trends. The shoe must be long enough and wide enough to prevent crowding of the toes and forcing of the great

Table 66-12 Common Foot Disorders

DISORDER	DESCRIPTION	TREATMENT
Forefoot		
Hallux valgus (bunion)	Painful deformity of great toe consisting of lateral angulation of great toe toward second toe, bony enlargement of medial side of first metatarsal head, swelling of bursa and formation of callus over bony enlargement (see Figure 66-7)	Conservative treatment includes wearing shoes with wide forefoot or "bunion pocket" and use of bunion pads to relieve pressure on bursal sac. Surgical treatment is removal of bursal sac and bony enlargement and correction of lateral angulation of great toe; may include temporary or permanent internal fixation.
Hallux rigidus	Painful stiffness of first MTP joint caused by osteoarthritis or local trauma	Conservative treatment includes intra-articular corticosteroids and passive manual stretching of first MTP joint. A shoe with a stiff sole decreases pain in the joint during walking. Surgical treatment is joint fusion or arthroplasty with silicone rubber implant.
Hammertoe	Deformity of second through fifth toes, including dorsiflexion of MTP joint, plantar flexion of PIP joint, and callus on dorsum of PIP joint and end of involved toe; complaints related to hammertoe include burning on bottom of foot and pain and difficulty in walking when wearing shoes	Conservative treatment consists of passive manual stretching of PIP joint and use of metatarsal arch support. Surgical correction consists of resection of base of middle phalanx and head of proximal phalanx and bringing raw bone ends together. Kirschner wire maintains straight position.
Morton's neuroma (Morton's toe or plantar neuroma)	Neuroma in web space between third and fourth metatarsal heads, causing sharp, sudden attacks of pain and burning sensations	Surgical excision is the usual treatment.
Midfoot		
Pes planus (flatfoot)	Loss of metatarsal arch causing pain in foot or leg	Symptoms are relieved by use of resilient longitudinal arch supports. Surgical treatment consists of triple arthrodesis or fusion of subtalar joint.
Pes cavus	Elevation of longitudinal arch of foot resulting from contracture of plantar fascia or bony deformity of arch	Treatment is manipulation and casting (in patients <6 yr of age); surgical correction is necessary if it interferes with ambulation (in patients >6 yr of age).
Hindfoot		
Painful heels	Complaint of heel pain with weight bearing; common causes include plantar bursitis, plantar fasciitis, or bone spur in adult	Corticosteroids are injected locally into inflamed bursa, and sponge rubber heel cushion is used; surgical excision of bursa or spur is performed. For plantar fasciitis, stretching exercises, NSAIDs, and corticosteroids are used.
Local Problems		
Corn	Localized thickening of skin caused by continual pressure over bony prominences, especially metatarsal head, frequently causing localized pain	Corn is softened with warm water or preparations containing salicylic acid and trimmed with razor blade or scalpel. Pressure on bony prominences caused by shoes is relieved.
Soft corn	Painful lesion caused by bony prominence of one toe pressing against adjacent toe; usual location in web space between toes; softness caused by secretions keeping web space relatively moist	Pain is relieved by placing cotton between toes to separate them. Surgical treatment is excision of projecting bone spur (if present).
Callus	Similar formation to corn but covering of wider area and usual location on weight-bearing part of foot	Same as for corn.
Plantar wart	Painful papillomatous growth caused by virus that may occur on any part of skin on sole of foot	Remedies containing salicylic acid; liquid nitrogen; excision with electrocoagulation or surgical removal; ultrasonography may also be used. Many disappear without treatment.

MTP, metatarsophalangeal; *NSAIDs,* nonsteroidal anti-inflammatory drugs; *PIP,* proximal interphalangeal.

toe into a position of hallux valgus. At the metatarsal head, the width of the shoe should be sufficient to allow free movement of the foot muscles and permit bending of the toes. The shank (narrow part of sole under the instep) of the shoe should be rigid enough to give optimal support. The height of the heel should be realistic in relation to the purpose for which the shoe is worn. Ideally, the heel of the shoe should not rise more than 2.5 cm higher than the forefoot support.

Effective strategies for preventing foot injuries are also required at the workplace. Prolonged standing, especially on hard, unyielding floors, can cause the joints of bones of the feet to become misaligned and inflamed. Special antislip flooring or matting can reduce slipping accidents that can result in sprained ankles or broken foot bones. All jurisdictions in Canada mandate that workers wear adequate protection against workplace hazards. Workers who are exposed to high foot hazard risk (e.g., those in the construction industry) are required to use footwear certified by the Canadian Standards Association.

▪ Acute Intervention

Many foot problems require referral to a podiatrist. Depending on the problem, conservative therapies are usually tried first (see Table 66-12). These therapies include NSAIDs, icing, physiotherapy, alterations in footwear, stretching, warm soaks, orthotics, ultrasonography, and corticosteroid injections. If these methods do not offer relief, surgery may then be recommended.

Depending on the type of surgery, pins or wires (hardware) may extend through the toes or a protective splint that extends over the end of the foot may be in place. The foot is usually immobilized by a bulky dressing, short leg cast, slipper (plaster) cast, or a platform "shoe" that fits over the dressing and has a rigid sole (known as a *bunion boot*). The foot should be elevated with the heel off the bed to help reduce discomfort and prevent edema. The neurovascular status should be assessed frequently during the immediate postoperative period. Care must be taken not to jar any hardware and cause pain. The hardware may interfere with or preclude assessment for movement. The nurse should be aware that sensation may be difficult to evaluate because postoperative pain can interfere with the patient's ability to differentiate pain caused by the surgical procedure from pain resulting from nerve pressure or circulatory impairment.

The type and the extent of surgery determine the degree of ambulation allowed. Crutches, a walker, or a cane may be necessary. The patient may experience pain or a throbbing sensation when starting ambulation. The nurse should reinforce instructions given by the physiotherapist and ensure that the patient does not develop a faulty gait pattern, such as walking on the heels, in an attempt to avoid excessive pain or pressure. The nurse must reinforce the importance of walking with an erect posture and with proper weight distribution. Dysfunction of gait or continued pain should be reported to the physician. The nurse should instruct the patient on the importance of frequent rest periods with the foot elevated.

▪ Ambulatory and Home Care

Foot care should include daily hygienic care and the wearing of clean socks, which should be long enough to prevent wrinkling and the development of pressure areas. Trimming toenails straight across helps prevent ingrown toenails and reduces the possibility of infection. Persons with impaired circulation or diabetes mellitus require detailed instruction to prevent serious complications

associated with blisters, pressure areas, and infections. (See Chapter 52, Table 52-21 for guidelines for foot care.)

Metabolic Bone Diseases

Normal bone metabolism is affected by hormones, nutrition, and hereditary factors. When there is dysfunction in any of these factors, a generalized reduction in bone mass and strength may result. Metabolic bone diseases include osteomalacia, osteoporosis, and Paget's disease.

Osteomalacia

Osteomalacia is an uncommon condition of adult bone associated with vitamin D deficiency, resulting in decalcification and softening of bone. This disease is the same as rickets in children, except that the epiphyseal growth plates are closed in the adult. Vitamin D, with its complex actions and method of synthesis, is required for the absorption of calcium from the intestine. Insufficient vitamin D intake can interfere with the normal mineralization of bone, causing failure or insufficient calcification of bone, which results in bone softening. Etiological factors in the development of osteomalacia include lack of exposure to ultraviolet rays (which is needed for vitamin D synthesis), gastrointestinal malabsorption, extensive burns, chronic diarrhea, pregnancy, kidney disease, and drugs such as phenytoin (Dilantin).

The most common clinical features of osteomalacia are localized bone pain, difficulty rising from a chair, and difficulty walking (Russell, 2010). Other clinical manifestations include LBP and bone pain; progressive muscular weakness, especially in the pelvic girdle; weight loss; and progressive deformities of the spine (kyphosis) or extremities. Fractures are common and demonstrate delayed healing when they occur.

Laboratory findings commonly associated with osteomalacia are decreased serum calcium or phosphorus levels, decreased serum 25-hydroxyvitamin D, and elevated serum alkaline phosphatase. Radiographs may demonstrate the effects of generalized bone demineralization, especially loss of calcium in the bones of the pelvis and the presence of associated bone deformity. Looser's transformation zones (ribbons of decalcification in bone found on radiography) are diagnostic of osteomalacia. However, significant osteomalacia may exist without changes noted on radiography.

Collaborative care of osteomalacia is directed toward correction of the vitamin D deficiency. Vitamin D_3 (cholecalciferol) and vitamin D_2 (ergocalciferol) can be supplemented, and the patient often shows a dramatic response. Calcium salts or phosphorus supplements may also be prescribed. Dietary ingestion of eggs, meat, oily fish, low-fat milk, and breakfast cereals fortified with calcium and vitamin D is encouraged (Prentice, 2008). Exposure to sunlight (and ultraviolet rays) is also valuable, along with weight-bearing exercise.

Osteoporosis

Osteoporosis, or porous bone (Figure 66-8), is a chronic, progressive metabolic bone disease. It is characterized by low bone mass and structural deterioration of bone tissue, leading to increased bone fragility, which predisposes the individual to

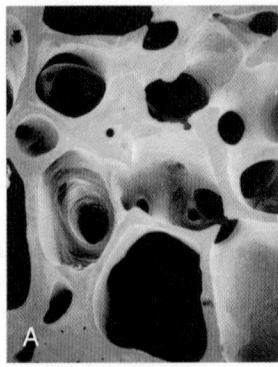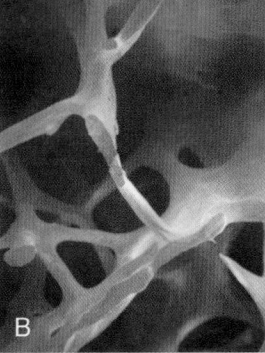

Figure 66-8 A, Normal bone. **B,** Osteoporotic bone.

Source: Patton, K. T., & Thibodeau, G. A. (2010). *Anatomy and physiology* (7th ed., p. 209, Figure 7-22*B* and *C*). St. Louis: Mosby.

Table 66-13 Risk Factors for Osteoporosis

Major Risk Factors

- Age >65 yr
- Family history of osteoporotic fracture (especially maternal hip fracture)*
- Vertebral compression fracture
- Fragility fracture after age 40
- Long-term (>3 mo) use of glucocorticoid therapy
- Malabsorption syndromes such as celiac or Crohn's disease
- Primary hyperparathyroidism
- Tendency to fall
- Osteopenia apparent on radiograph
- Hypogonadism
- Early menopause (<45 yr)

Minor Risk Factors

- Rheumatoid arthritis
- Hyperthyroidism
- Prolonged use of anticonvulsants
- Body weight <57 kg
- Present weight >10% below weight at age 25
- Low calcium intake
- Excessive caffeine intake (consistently more than four cups a day of coffee, tea, or cola)
- Excessive alcohol intake (consistently more than two drinks a day)
- Smoking
- Chronic heparin therapy

*Postmenopausal women are especially at risk (see the Determinants of Health box) because of the important role that estrogen plays in keeping their bones healthy.
Source: Brown, J. P., Fortier, M., Frame, H., Lalonde, A., Papaioannou. A., Senikas, V., . . . , Yuen, C. K. (2006). Canadian Consensus Conference on Osteoporosis, 2006 (update February 2006). SOGC clinical practice guideline. *Journal of Obstetrics and Gynaecology of Canada, 172,* S95-S112. Printed with permission from SOGC. Retrieved from *http://www.sogc.org/guidelines/public/172E-CONS-February2006.pdf*

bone fractures at the hip, wrist, and spine. Osteoporosis is known as the "silent thief" because it slowly and insidiously, over many years, robs the skeleton of its banked resources. Bones can eventually become so fragile that they cannot withstand normal mechanical stress (Al-dabagh, Archer, Newton, Kwagyan, & Nunlee-Bland, 2009).

Osteoporosis affects 1 in 4 Canadian women and 1 in 8 men older than age 50 (Osteoporosis Canada, 2011). With the projected increase in life expectancy, this number is expected to grow. Of all hip fractures, 80% are osteoporosis related. Hip fractures result in death in up to 20% of cases and disability in 50% of those who survive (Osteoporosis Canada, 2011). Osteoporosis-related fractures cause considerable morbidity and an enormous financial burden through the use of health services. According to Osteoporosis Canada (2011), the cost of treating osteoporosis and related fractures is estimated to be $1.9 billion each year in Canada alone.

Osteoporosis is more common in women than in men for several reasons: (1) women tend to have lower calcium intake than men (men between 15 and 50 years of age consume twice as much calcium as women); (2) women have less bone mass because of their generally smaller frame; (3) bone resorption begins at an earlier age in women and is accelerated at menopause; (4) pregnancy and breastfeeding deplete a woman's skeletal reserve unless calcium intake is adequate; and (5) longevity increases the likelihood of osteoporosis, and women live longer than men. Although osteoporosis is more common in women than in men, it is important to realize that men can also develop osteoporosis.

Etiology and Pathophysiology

Risk factors for osteoporosis are listed in Table 66-13. Decreased risk is associated with regular weight-bearing exercise and calcium and vitamin D ingestion (Miller, 2008). Patients who are older than 66 years should be routinely screened for osteoporosis. Postmenopausal women and men older than age 50 with at least one major or two minor risk factors should be evaluated for osteoporosis.

Peak bone mass (maximum bone tissue) is mainly achieved before age 20. It is determined by a combination of four major factors: heredity, nutrition, exercise, and hormone function. Heredity may be responsible for up to 70% of a person's peak bone mass. Bone loss from midlife (age 35 to 40 years) onward

is inevitable, but the rate of loss varies. At menopause, women experience rapid bone loss when the decline in estrogen production is the sharpest. This rate of loss then slows, and eventually matches the rate of bone lost by men 65 to 70 years old.

Bone is continually being deposited by osteoblasts and resorbed by osteoclasts, a process called *remodelling*. Normally, the rates of bone deposition and resorption are equal to each other so that the total bone mass remains constant. In osteoporosis, bone resorption exceeds bone deposition. Although resorption affects the entire skeletal system, osteoporosis occurs most commonly in the bones of the spine, hips, and wrists. Over time, wedging and fractures of the vertebrae produce gradual loss of height and a humped back known as *dowager's hump*, or *kyphosis*. The usual first signs are back pain or spontaneous fractures. The loss of bone substance causes the bone to become mechanically weakened and prone to either spontaneous fractures or fractures from minimal trauma. A person who has one spinal vertebral fracture owing to osteoporosis has a 25% chance of having a second vertebral fracture within 1 year (Freedman et al., 2008).

Specific diseases associated with osteoporosis include inflammatory bowel disease, intestinal malabsorption, kidney disease, rheumatoid arthritis, hyperthyroidism, chronic alcoholism, cirrhosis of the liver, hypogonadism, and diabetes mellitus.

Many drugs can interfere with bone metabolism, including corticosteroids, antiseizure drugs (e.g., phenytoin [Dilantin]), aluminum-containing antacids, heparin, certain cancer treatments, and excessive thyroid hormones (Miller, 2008). At the time a drug is prescribed, the patient should be informed of this possible adverse effect. Long-term corticosteroid use is a major contributor to osteoporosis. When a corticosteroid is taken, there is a disproportionate loss of bone resulting from the inhibition of new bone formation.

Clinical Manifestations

Osteoporosis is often called the "silent disease" because bone loss occurs slowly without symptoms. People may not know they have osteoporosis until their bones become so weak that a sudden strain, bump, or fall causes a hip, vertebra, or wrist fracture. Collapsed vertebrae may initially be manifested as back pain, loss of height, or spinal deformities such as kyphosis or severely stooped posture.

Diagnostic Studies

Osteoporosis often goes unnoticed because it cannot be detected by conventional radiography until more than 25 to 40% of calcium in the bone is lost. Serum calcium, phosphorus, and alkaline phosphatase levels usually are normal, although alkaline phosphatase may be elevated after a fracture.

Bone mineral density (BMD) measurements are typically used to measure bone density. BMD assesses the mass of bone per unit volume, or how tightly the bone is packed. (BMD measurements are presented in Chapter 64, Table 64-7.) Quantitative ultrasonography measures bone density with sound waves in the heel, kneecap, or shin. One of the most common BMD studies is dual-energy x-ray absorptiometry (DEXA), which measures bone density in the spine, hips, and forearm (the most common sites of fractures resulting from osteoporosis). DEXA studies are also useful to evaluate changes in bone density over time and to assess the effectiveness of treatment. DEXA results are frequently reported as T-scores.

Osteoporosis is quantitatively defined as a BMD of at least 2.5 SDs below the mean BMD of young adults. *Osteopenia* is defined as bone loss that is more than normal (a T-score ≤ a range of -1 to -2.5 SDs below the mean), but not yet at the level for a diagnosis of osteoporosis. In addition to the BMD T-score, the patient's risk factors are included in determining a 10-year absolute fracture risk. This risk changes with advancing age and the development of new risk factors. Those patients with low risk are assessed in 5 to 10 years, whereas those with moderate risk are assessed in 1 to 5 years. Quantitative ultrasonography may be considered for fracture risk assessment when DEXA is not available, but it is not precise enough to be used for follow-up BMD testing.

NURSING AND COLLABORATIVE MANAGEMENT: OSTEOPOROSIS

The reduced quality of life for those with osteoporosis is enormous. Osteoporosis can result in disfigurement, lowered self-esteem, reduction or loss of mobility, and decreased independence. Collaborative care of osteoporosis focuses on proper nutrition, calcium supplementation, exercise, prevention of fractures, and medications (Table 66-14). The National Osteoporosis

---

DETERMINANTS OF HEALTH

Osteoporosis

Biology and Genetic Endowment

- White and Native American women are at higher risk of developing osteoporotic fractures than women of other races.*
- Bone mass is greater in Black men, Black women, and White men compared with White women.
- Postmenopausal women are at the highest risk for osteoporosis, regardless of ethnic group.

Sex

Men

- Men are underdiagnosed and undertreated for osteoporosis compared with women.
- One in 8 men older than age 50 will have an osteoporosis-related fracture in their lifetime.

Women

- Osteoporosis is twice as common in women as in men.
- An estimated 1 in 2 women older than age 50 will have an osteoporosis-related fracture in their lifetime.†

*Cauley, J. A. (2011). Defining ethnic and racial differences in osteoporosis and fragility fractures. *Clinical Orthopaedics and Related Research, 469*(7), 1891-1899. doi:10.1007/sl 1999-011-1863-5
†Cohen, K., & Maier, D. (2008). Osteoporosis: Evaluation of screening patterns in a primary group practice. *Journal of Clinical Densitometry, 11*(4), 498-502. doi:10.1016/j.jocd.2008.08.104

COLLABORATIVE CARE

Table 66-14 Osteoporosis

Diagnostic	
Diagnostic	- Bisphosphonates
- History and physical examination	- Alendronate (Fosamax)
- Serum calcium, phosphorus, and alkaline phosphatase levels	- Etidronate (Didrocal)
- Risedronate (Actonel)	
- Bone mineral densitometry	- Zoledronatic Acid (Aclasta)
- Dual-energy x-ray absorptiometry (DEXA)	- Selective estrogen receptor modulator (SERM)
- Quantitative ultrasonography (QUS)	- Raloxifene (Evista)
Collaborative Therapy	- Teriparatide (Forteo)
- Diet high in calcium (see Table 66-15)	- Salmon calcitonin (Calcimar)
- Calcium supplements (see Table 66-16)	
- Vitamin D supplements	
- Exercise program	
- Estrogen replacement therapy	

Foundation (2010) recommends that postmenopausal women and men 50 or older should be considered for treatment of osteoporosis if presenting with any of the following: (1) A hip or vertebral fracture; (2) a DEXA hip (femoral neck) or spine T-score of -2.5 or less; or (3) Low bone mass and a U.S.-adapted World Health Organization 10-year probability of a hip fracture of 3% or greater or a 10-year probability of any major osteoporosis-related fracture of 20% or higher (p. 20).

Prevention and treatment of osteoporosis focus on adequate calcium intake (1000 mg/day in women between the ages 19 and 50 and men between the ages 19 and 70; and 1200 mg in women >50 years of age and men >70 years of age). If dietary intake of calcium is inadequate, supplemental calcium should be taken (Health Canada, 2010). Foods that are high in calcium content include whole and skim milk, yogourt, cottage cheese, ice cream, spinach, almonds, and sardines (Table 66-15). The amount of elemental calcium varies in different calcium preparations (Table 66-16). Calcium supplementation inhibits age-related bone loss; however, it does not stimulate formation of new bone.

Vitamin D is important in calcium absorption and function and may have a role in bone formation. Most Canadians do not get enough vitamin D from the diet or naturally through synthesis in the skin from exposure to sunlight. Supplemental vitamin D (1000-2000 international units) is commonly recommended for older adults, those who are homebound, and those who get minimal sun exposure (Hanley et al., 2010).

Moderate amounts of exercise are important to build up and maintain bone mass. Exercise also increases muscle strength, coordination, and balance. The best exercises are weight-bearing exercises that force an individual to work against gravity. These include walking, hiking, weight training, stair climbing, tennis, and dancing. Walking is preferred to high-impact aerobics or running, both of which may put too much stress on the bones resulting in stress fractures. Walking for 30 minutes, three times a week, is recommended.

Cigarette smoking and excess alcohol intake are risk factors for osteoporosis. Regular consumption of 60 to 90 mL of alcohol a day may increase the degree of osteoporosis, even in young men and women. Patients should be instructed to quit smoking and cut down on alcohol intake to decrease the likelihood of losing bone mass.

Although loss of bone cannot be significantly reversed, further loss can be prevented if the patient follows a regimen of calcium and vitamin D supplementation, exercise, estrogen replacement, and alendronate (Fosamax) or raloxifene (Evista), if indicated. Efforts should be made to keep patients with osteoporosis ambulatory to prevent further loss of bone substance as a result of immobility.

Drug Therapy

Hormone therapy should be considered as first-line therapy for preventing bone loss and fractures in early menopausal women who are symptomatic (e.g., have vasomotor, urogenital, and psychological symptoms). Estrogens are known to have an antiresorptive effect on bone. Estrogen therapy (for women who have had a hysterectomy) and estrogen–progesterone therapy (for women who have not had a hysterectomy) provide significant protection against osteoporotic fractures. Despite earlier concerns raised by a number of studies, it now seems that younger, recently postmenopausal women do not have an increased cardiovascular risk with estrogen or estrogen–progesterone therapy. Considering the benefit-risk profile of hormone therapy, the North American Menopause Society recommends the extended use of hormone therapy is suitable for women at risk of osteoporotic fractures who also have moderate to severe menopausal symptoms. As with any drug therapy, doses and regimens must be individualized according to the patient's needs (Gallagher & Levine, 2011). (See Chapter 56 for further discussion of estrogen replacement therapy.)

Calcitonin is secreted by the thyroid gland and inhibits osteoclastic bone resorption by directly interacting with active osteoclasts. Salmon calcitonin (Calcimar) is available in intramuscular, subcutaneous, and intranasal forms. The nasal form is easy to

NUTRITIONAL THERAPY

Table 66-15 Sources of Calcium

FOOD	CALCIUM (mg)
250 mL (1 cup) milk	
Whole	291
Low-fat	300
Skim	302
30 g (1 oz.) cheese	
Processed cheese	174
Cheddar	130
Cottage	130
Mozzarella	207
Parmesan	390
Swiss	272
250 mL (8 oz) yogourt	415
250 mL (1 cup) ice cream	
Hard ice cream	176
Soft-serve	272
90 g (3 oz) seafood	
Salmon	167
Sardines with bones	372
Shrimp	98
Oysters	113
1 medium stalk cooked broccoli	158
250 g (1 cup) cooked spinach	200
250 g (1 cup) almonds	304

Table 66-16 Elemental Calcium Content of Various Oral Calcium Preparations

CALCIUM PREPARATION	ELEMENTAL CALCIUM CONTENT
Calcium carbonate (Tums 500)	500 mg/tablet
Calcium carbonate + 5 mcg vitamin D_2 (Os-Cal 250)	250 mg/tablet
Calcium gluconate	40 mg/500 mg
Calcium carbonate	400 mg/g
Calcium lactate	80 mg/600 mg
Calcium citrate	40 mg/300 mg

administer, and patients should be taught to alternate nostrils daily. Nasal dryness and irritation are the most frequent adverse effects. Administration of the intramuscular or subcutaneous form of the drug at night has been shown to decrease the adverse effects of nausea and facial flushing. Nausea does not occur with the nasal spray. When calcitonin is used, calcium supplementation is necessary to prevent secondary hyperparathyroidism.

Bisphosphonates inhibit osteoclast-mediated bone resorption, thereby increasing BMD and total bone mass. This group of drugs has been shown to increase BMD by 5%. Common adverse effects are anorexia, weight loss, and gastritis. The most commonly used bisphosphonate drug in treating osteoporosis is alendronate (Fosamax). Patients should be instructed on the proper administration of alendronate to aid in its absorption. It should be taken with a full glass of water after rising in the morning. The patient should not eat or drink anything for 30 minutes after taking it. The patient should also be instructed not to lie down after taking the drug. These precautions have been shown to decrease gastrointestinal adverse effects (especially esophageal irritation) and increase absorption. Alendronate is available as a once-per-week oral tablet. Zoledronatic acid (Aclasta) is approved for a once-yearly IV infusion and can prevent osteoporosis for 2 years after a single infusion. Flulike symptoms may occur for the first few days following administration of the drug (Gnant et al., 2009).

Another type of drug used in treating osteoporosis is selective estrogen receptor modulators, such as raloxifene (Evista). These drugs mimic the effect of estrogen on bone by reducing bone resorption without stimulating the tissues of the breast or uterus. Raloxifene in postmenopausal women significantly increases BMD (Paggiosi et al., 2010). The most commonly reported adverse effects are leg cramps and hot flashes. Teriparatide (Forteo) is used for the treatment of osteoporosis in men and postmenopausal women who are at high risk for fractures. Teriparatide is a recombinant form of human parathyroid hormone and works by increasing the action of osteoblasts. It is the first drug approved for the treatment of osteoporosis that stimulates new bone formation. Most drugs used to treat osteoporosis prevent further bone loss. Teriparatide is administered by subcutaneous injection once a day (Panus et al., 2008).

Medical management of patients receiving corticosteroids includes prescribing the lowest possible dose of the drug, as well as calcium and vitamin D supplementation. If osteopenia is evident on bone densitometry, treatment with bisphosphonate agents, such as alendronate (Fosamax), should be considered.

Paget's Disease

Paget's disease *(osteitis deformans)* is a chronic skeletal bone disorder in which there is excessive bone resorption followed by replacement of normal marrow by vascular, fibrous connective tissue. The new bone is larger, disorganized, and structurally weaker. The regions of the skeleton commonly affected are pelvis, long bones, spine, ribs, sternum, and cranium. The etiology of Paget's disease is unknown, although a viral cause has been proposed. Up to 40% of all patients with Paget's disease have at least one relative with the disorder. Men are affected at a rate of 2:1 compared with women, and Paget's disease is rarely seen in persons younger than 40 years (Sutcliffe, 2009).

In milder forms of Paget's disease, patients may remain free of symptoms, and the disease may be discovered incidentally on radiography or serum chemistry. The initial clinical manifestations are usually insidious development of bone pain (which may progress to severe intractable pain), complaints of fatigue, and progressive development of a waddling gait. Patients may complain that they are becoming shorter or that their heads are becoming larger. Headaches, dementia, visual deficits, and loss of hearing can result with an enlarged, thickened skull. Increased bone volume in the spine can cause spinal cord or nerve root compression. Pathological fracture is the most common complication of Paget's disease and may be the first indication of the disease. Other complications include osteosarcoma, fibrosarcoma, and osteoclastoma (giant cell) tumours.

SAFETY ALERT

Reduce the risk of patient harm resulting from falls:

- Evaluate patients for fall risk.
- Identify high-risk factors, including medications, that increase risk of falls.
- Take action to address any identified risks.
- Encourage at-risk patients to attend fall prevention class.

Serum alkaline phosphatase levels are markedly elevated (indicating high bone turnover) in advanced forms of the disease. Radiographs may demonstrate that the normal contour of the affected bone is curved and the bone cortex is thickened and irregular, especially the weight-bearing bones and cranium. Bone scans using a radiolabelled biphosphate demonstrate increased uptake in the skeletal areas affected.

Collaborative care of Paget's disease is usually limited to symptomatic and supportive care and correction of secondary deformities by either surgical intervention or braces. Bone resorption, relief of acute symptoms, and lowering of the serum alkaline phosphatase levels may be significantly influenced by the administration of human calcitonin, which inhibits osteoclastic activity. It is available as a subcutaneous injection. Salmon calcitonin can also be used as a subcutaneous or intramuscular injection for treating Paget's disease. Salmon calcitonin has a longer half-life and greater milligram potency than human calcitonin. Response to calcitonin therapy is not permanent and often stops when therapy is discontinued. Bisphosphonate drugs are also used to retard bone resorption. Calcium and vitamin D are often given to decrease hypocalcemia, a common adverse effect with these drugs. Drug effectiveness may be monitored by serum alkaline phosphatase levels. Calcitonin therapy is recommended for patients who cannot tolerate bisphosphonate drugs.

Pain from Paget's disease is usually managed by NSAIDs or acetaminophen. Orthopedic surgery for fractures, hip and knee replacements, and knee realignment may be necessary.

A firm mattress should be used to provide back support and to relieve pain. The patient may be required to wear a corset or light brace to relieve back pain and provide support when in the upright position. The patient should be proficient in the correct application of such devices and know how to regularly examine areas of the skin for friction damage. Activities such as lifting and twisting should be discouraged. Physiotherapy may increase muscle strength. Good body mechanics are essential. A properly balanced nutritional program is important in the management of metabolic disorders of bone, especially pertaining to vitamin D, calcium, and protein, which are necessary to ensure the availability of the components for bone formation. Prevention measures such as patient education, use of an assistive device, and environmental changes should be actively pursued to prevent falls and subsequent fractures (Hendriks et al., 2008).

AGE-RELATED CONSIDERATIONS: METABOLIC BONE DISEASES

Osteoporosis and Paget's disease are common in older adults. Patients should be instructed in proper nutritional management to prevent further bone loss such as that occurring from osteoporosis.

Because metabolic bone disorders increase the possibility of pathological fractures, the nurse must use extreme caution when the patient is turned or moved. It is important to keep the patient as active as possible to slow demineralization of bone resulting from disuse or extended immobilization. A supervised exercise program is an essential part of the treatment program. If the patient's condition permits, ambulation without causing fatigue must be encouraged.

Protection from falls is paramount for prevention of osteoporotic fracture among older adults. Osteoporosis-related fractures cause considerable morbidity and an enormous financial burden through the use of health services. In Canada, 1 in 3 older adults will experience a fall each year, and half of those more than once. Forty percent of older adults' falls result in hip fractures, and 20% of injury-related deaths among older adults can be traced back to a fall (Public Health Agency of Canada [PHAC], 2011). The frequency of falls increases dramatically with age, with women more likely to fall than men.

Medical conditions, medications, and environmental factors have been implicated as predisposing factors to injurious falls among the elderly. Best practice guidelines (Registered Nurses' Association of Ontario [RNAO], 2011) should be implemented to prevent falls and fall injuries in older adults, who may already have bone mass below the threshold for fracture. Fall prevention could have a significant impact on the incidence of fracture in this susceptible population.

CLINICAL DECISION-MAKING EXERCISE

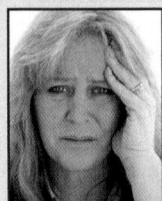

CASE STUDY:
Osteoporosis

Source: © iStockphoto.com/Roberta Osborne.

Patient Profile

Antonija Roncevic is a 56-year-old Croatian Canadian librarian who had a total hysterectomy and salpingo-oophorectomy for removal of a benign ovarian cyst 4 years ago.

Subjective Data

- Experiences chronic, mild lumbar pain and tenderness that radiates to her right hip and the lateral thigh
- Regular walking offers some relief
- Had a stress fracture in wrist 6 months ago
- Reports no noticeable loss of height
- Has maternal history of osteoporosis
- Has been taking corticosteroids for past 6 years for Addison's disease
- Drinks socially—two alcoholic beverages per day
- Dislikes dairy products

Objective Data

- 167 cm (5 ft, 6 in) tall, 53 kg (116 lb)

Diagnostic Studies

- Bone mass measurement tests show decreased bone mineral density at spine and hip.

- Laboratory tests reveal normal serum calcium, phosphorus, and alkaline phosphatase levels.

Collaborative Care

- Premarin 0.625 mg PO daily
- Alendronate (Fosamax) 70 mg once a week
- Calcium supplements 1200 mg PO daily
- High-calcium diet
- Reduce alcohol intake
- Maintain regular exercise program

Discussion Questions

1. What factors place Ms. Roncevic at risk to develop osteoporosis?
2. Why does regular exercise help Ms. Roncevic's symptoms?
3. What are the pros and cons of prescribing estrogen replacement for Ms. Roncevic?
4. *Priority Decision:* What are the priority teaching needs for Ms. Roncevic?
5. What teaching should the nurse provide to Ms. Roncevic regarding alendronate?
6. How might the nurse assist Ms. Roncevic in increasing her intake of calcium?
7. *Priority Decision:* Based on the assessment data presented, what are the priority nursing diagnoses? Are there any collaborative problems?

evolve *Answers are available at* **http://evolve.elsevier.com/Canada/Lewis/medsurg**

REVIEW QUESTIONS

The number of the question corresponds to the same-numbered objective at the beginning of the chapter.

1. A patient with osteomyelitis is treated with intravenous (IV) antibiotics and surgical irrigation and debridement in the operating room. What response should the nurse make to the patient who asks why oral or IV antibiotics cannot be used alone?
   a. "An incision and drainage are necessary to wash out dead tissue and pus from the infected area."
   b. "The microorganisms that cause osteomyelitis often lodge in an area of the bone where circulation slows, so the antibiotics may not reach them through the blood."
   c. "There are no effective oral or IV antibiotics to treat *Staphylococcus aureus*, the most common cause of osteomyelitis."
   d. "An irrigation and debridement can let the surgeon get to the involucrum created by the infection and prevent bacteria from spreading to other tissue."

2. A patient with an osteosarcoma of the left femur has a nursing diagnosis of risk for injury (pathological fracture) related to bone tissue changes. What nursing management for this patient should the nurse implement?
   a. Preventing pain
   b. Relieving edema
   c. Increasing physical mobility
   d. Supporting and positioning the leg

3. Which of the following patients does the nurse identify as having the greatest risk for back injuries and low back pain?
   a. A long-distance truck driver
   b. A 62-year-old widow who walks daily
   c. An aerobics instructor who weighs 45 kg (100 lb)
   d. A 25-year-old nurse who works in a newborn nursery

4. What is the primary nursing responsibility in caring for a patient with acute low back pain associated with pain and muscle spasms?
   a. Teaching exercises such as straight leg raises to decrease pain
   b. Positioning the patient on the abdomen with the legs extended
   c. Providing pain medication and encouraging strict bed rest
   d. Assisting the patient to maintain and gradually increase activity as tolerated

5. What difference would the nurse anticipate in the care of a patient with a spinal fusion as compared with a patient with a simple laminectomy?
   a. Body alignment is maintained by the fusion procedure.
   b. Earlier ambulation is permitted because the spine is more stabilized.
   c. The donor site for the bone graft may be more painful than the spinal incision.
   d. Teaching regarding body mechanics and prevention of future back injuries is not as critical.

6. What instructions should the nurse give the patient who is being discharged from same-day surgery after surgical correction of bilateral hallux valgus?
   a. Rest frequently with the feet elevated.
   b. Soak the feet in warm water several times a day.
   c. Walk primarily on the heels to relieve pressure on the toes.
   d. Expect the feet to be numb for several days postoperatively.

7. What advice should the nurse give to the patient with early osteoporosis?
   a. Lose weight
   b. Stop smoking
   c. Eat a high-protein diet
   d. Start swimming for exercise

ANSWERS: 1. b; 2. d; 3. a; 4. d; 5. c; 6. a; 7. b.

REFERENCES

Airaksinen, O., Brox, J., Cedraschi, C., Hildebrandt, J., Klaber-Moffett, J., Kovacs, F., …, Ursin, H. (2006). Chapter 4: European guidelines for the management of chronic nonspecific low back pain. *European Spine Journal, 15*(Suppl 2), S192-S300. doi:10.1007/s00586-006-1072-1

Al-dabagh, H., Archer, A., Newton, M., Kwagyan, J., & Nunlee-Bland, G. (2009). Osteoporosis awareness protocols for patients with fragility fractures. *Journal of the National Medical Association, 101*(2), 145.

Aly, T. A., Mousa, W., & Elsallakh, S. (2011).Evaluation of scarf osteotomy for management of hallux valgus deformity. *Orthopaedics 34*(2), 95. doi:10.3928/01477447-20101221-08

Ammendolia, C., Kerr, M. S., & Bombardier, C. (2005). Back belt use for prevention of occupational low back pain: A systematic review. *Journal of Manipulative & Physiological Therapeutics, 28*(2), 128-134. doi:10.1016/j.jmpt.2005.01.009

Averill, L. W., Hernandez, A., Gonzalez, L., Peña, A. H., & Jaramillo, D. (2009). Diagnosis of osteomyelitis in children: Utility of fat-suppressed contrast-enhanced MRI. *American Journal of Roentgenology, 192*(5), 1232-1238. doi:10.2214/AJR.07.3400

Balamuth, N. J., & Womer, R. B. (2010). Ewing's sarcoma. *Lancet Oncology, 11*(2), 184-192. doi:10.1016/S1470-2045(09)70286-4

Berbari, E., Steckelberg, J., & Osmon, D. (2009). Osteomyelitis. In G. Mandell (Ed.), *Mandell, Douglas, and Bennett's principles and practice of infectious diseases* (7th ed.). Philadelphia: Churchill Livingstone.

Björck-van Dijken, C., Fjellman-Wiklund, A., & Hildingsson, C. (2008). Low back pain, lifestyle factors and physical activity: A population-based study. *Journal of Rehabilitation Medicine, 40*(10), 864-869. doi:10.2340/16501977-0273

Calmels, P., Queneau, P., Hamonet, C., Le Pen, C., Frederique, M., Lerouvrer, C., & Thoumie, P. (2009). Effectiveness of a lumbar belt in subacute low back pain: An open, multicentric, and randomized clinical study. *Spine, 34*(3), 215-220. doi:10.1097/BRS.0b013e31819577dc

Canadian Cancer Society, Statistics Canada, Provincial/Territorial Cancer Registry, & Public Health Agency of Canada. (2011). Canadian cancer statistics 2011. Retrieved from *http://www.cancer.ca/~/media/CCS/Canada%20wide/Files%20List/English%20files%20heading/PDF%20-%20Policy%20-%20Canadian%20Cancer%20Statistics%20-%20English/Canadian%20Cancer%20Statistics%202011%20-%20English.ashx*

Chou, R. (2010). Pharmacological management of low back pain. *Drugs, 70*(4), 387-402. doi:10.2165/11318690-000000000-00000

Church, E. J., & Odle, T. G. (2007). Diagnosis and treatment of back pain. *Radiologic Technology, 79*(2), 126-155.

Cleveland Clinic. (2008). Breakthroughs in back pain. *Arthritis Advisor, 7*(October), 1. Retrieved from *http://www.arthritis-advisor.com/issues/7_10/features/494-1.html*

Coleman, R. E., & Holen, I. (2008). Bone metastases. In M. Abeloff, J. O. Armitage, J. E. Niederhhuber, M. B. Kastan, & W. G. McKenna (Eds.), *Abeloff's clinical oncology* (4th ed.). New York: Livingstone.

Fassett, D. R., Kurd, M. F., & Vaccaro, A. R. (2009). Biologic solutions for degenerative disk disease. *Journal of Spinal Disorders & Techniques, 22*(4), 297-308. doi:10.1097/BSD.0b013e31816d5f64

Freedman, B., Potter, B., Nesti, L., Giuliani, J. R., Hampton, C., & Kuklo, T. R. (2008). Osteoporosis and vertebral compression fractures—Continued missed opportunities. *Spine Journal, 8*(5), 756-762. doi:10.1016/j.spinee.2008.01.013

Furlan, A. D., Imamura, M., Dryden, T., & Irvin, E. (2010). Massage for low-back pain. *Cochrane Database of Systematic Reviews 2008,* 4, CD001929. doi:10.1002/14651858.CD001929.pub2

Gallagher, J. C., & Levine, J. P. (2011). Preventing osteoporosis in symptomatic postmenopausal women. *Menopause: The Journal of the North American Menopause Society, 18*(1), 109-118. doi:10.1097/gme.0b013e3181e324a6

Gnant, M., Mlineritsch, B., Schippinger, W., Luschin-Ebengreuth G., Pöstlberger, S., Menzel, C., ..., Greil, R. (2009). Endocrine therapy plus zoledronic acid in premenopausal breast cancer. *New England Journal of Medicine, 360*(7), 679-691. doi:10.1056/NEJMoa0806285

Guyer, R. D., & Roybal, R. R. (2008). The Charité study of disc arthroplasty: What does it really mean? In D. K. Resnick, R. W. Haid, & J. C. Wang (Eds.), *Surgical management of low back pain* (2nd ed.). New York: Thieme Medical Publishers.

Haidar, R., Der Boghossian, A., & Atiyeh, B. (2010). Duration of postsurgical antibiotics in chronic osteomyelitis: Empiric or evidence-based? *International Journal of Infectious Disease, 14*(9), e752-e758. doi:10.1016/j.ijid.2010.01.005

Hanley, D. A., Cranney, A., Jones, G., Whiting, S. J., Leslie, W. D., Cole, D. E. C., ..., Rosen, C. (2010). Vitamin D in adult health and disease: A review and guideline statement from Osteoporosis Canada. *Canadian Medical Association Journal, 182*(12), E610-E618. doi:10.1503/cmaj.080663

Hayden, J., van Tulder, M. W., Malmivaara, A., & Koes, B. W. (2011). Exercise therapy for treatment of non-specific low back pain. *Cochrane Back Group Cochrane Database of Systematic Reviews.* 3, CD000335. doi:10.1002/14651858.CD000335.pub2

Health Canada. (2010). Vitamin D and calcium: Updated dietary reference intakes. Retrieved from *http://www.hc-sc.gc.ca/fn-an/nutrition/vitamin/vita-d-eng.php*

Hellmann, D., & Stone, J. (2008). Arthritis and musculoskeletal disorders. In S. J. McPhee, M. A. Papadakis, & L. Tierney (Eds.), *Current medical diagnosis and treatment 2008* (40th ed.). New York: Lange/McGraw-Hill Medical.

Hendriks, M., Bleijlevens, M., van Haastregt, J., de Bruijn, F. H., Diederiks, J. P. M., Mulder, W.J., ..., van Eijk, J. T. M. (2008). A multidisciplinary fall prevention program for elderly persons: A feasibility study. *Geriatric Nursing, 29*(3), 186-196. doi:10.1016/j.gerinurse.2007.10.019

Johnson, S. K., & Knobf, M. T. (2008). Surgical interventions for cancer patients with impending or actual pathologic fractures. *Orthopaedic Nursing, 27*(3), 172-173. doi:10.1097/01.NOR.0000320544.97739.71

Kumar, V., Abbas, A., Fausto, N., & Aster, J. (2010). *Robbins and Cotran pathologic basis of disease* (8th ed.). Philadelphia: Saunders.

Maki, R. (2008). Pediatric sarcomas occurring in adults. *Journal of Surgical Oncology, 97*(4), 360-368. doi:10.1002/jso.20969

Markham, J. D., & Gaud, K. (2008). Lumbar spinal stenosis in older adults: Current understanding and future directions. *Clinics in Geriatric Medicine, 24*(2), 369. doi:10.1016/j.cger.2007.12.007

MD Anderson Cancer Center. (2011). Bone cancer. Retrieved from *http://www.mdanderson.org/patient-and-cancer-information/cancer-information/cancer-types/bone-cancer/index.html*

Miller, C. A. (2008). Mobility and safety. In C. A. Miller (Ed.), *Nursing for wellness in older adults* (5th ed.). Philadelphia: Lippincott Williams & Wilkins.

National Institute of Neurological Disorders and Stroke (NINDS). (2011). Low back pain fact sheet. Retrieved from *http://www.ninds.nih.gov/disorders/backpain/detail_backpain.htm*

National Osteoporosis Foundation. (2010). The clinician's guide to prevention and treatment of osteoporosis. Retrieved from *http://nof.org/files/nof/public/content/file/344/upload/159.pdf*

Nicholas, M. K., & George, S. Z. (2011). Psychologically informed interventions for low back pain: An update for physical therapists. *Physical Therapy, 91*(5), 765-776. doi:10.2522/ptj.20100278

Osteoporosis Canada. (2011). Breaking barriers not bones. Retrieved from *http://www.osteoporosis.ca/index.php/ci_id/5526/la_id/1.htm*

Paggiosi, M. A., Clowes, J. A., Finigan, J., Naylor, K. E., Peel, N. F. A., & Eastell, R. (2010). Performance of quantitative ultrasound measurements of bone for monitoring raloxifene therapy. *Journal of Clinical Densitometry, 13*(4), 441-450. doi:10.1016/j.jocd.2010.06.006

Panus, P., Jobst, E. E., Katzung, B. G., Tinsley, S., Masters, S., & Trevor, A. (2008). *Pharmacology for the physical therapist.* Dubuque, IA: McGraw-Hill.

Perrot, S., Javier, R. M., Marty, M., Le Jeune, C., & Laroche, F. (2008). Antidepressant use in painful rheumatic conditions. *Rheumatic Diseases of North America, 34*(2), 433-453. doi:10.1016/j.rdc.2008.03.004

Prentice, A. (2008). Vitamin D deficiency: A global perspective. *Nutrition Reviews, 66*(Suppl 2), S153-S164. doi:10.1111/j.1753-4887.2008.00100.x

Public Health Agency of Canada (PHAC). (2011). You CAN prevent falls! Retrieved from *222.publichealth.gc.ca/seniors*

Registered Nurses' Association of Ontario (RNAO). (2011). *Prevention of falls and fall injuries in the older adult—Guideline revision 2011. Best Practice Guideline.* Toronto: Author. Retrieved from *http://www.rnao.org/Page.asp?PageID=924&ContentID=810*

Russell, L. A. (2010). Osteoporosis and osteomalacia. *Rheumatic Diseases Clinics of North America, 36*(4), 665-680. doi:10.1016/j.rdc.2010.09.007

Sutcliffe, A. (2009). Paget's disease 1: Epidemiology, causes, and clinical features. *Nursing Times, 105*(6), 14-15. Retrieved from *http://www.nursingtimes.net/nursing-practice-clinical-research/guided-learning-archive/pagets-disease-1-epidemiology-causes-and-clinical-features/1992719.article*

Terry Fox Foundation. (2011). Terry Fox and the Terry Fox Foundation. Retrieved from *http://www.terryfox.org/Foundation/index.html*

Toward Optimized Practice (TOP). (2009). *Guideline for the evidence-informed primary care management of low back pain.* Edmonton: TOP. Retrieved from *http://topalbertadoctors.org/cpgs.php?sid=63&cpg_cats=83*

Weichert, S. M., Sharland, M., Clarke, N. M., & Faust, S. N. (2008). Acute haematogenous osteomyelitis in children: Is there any evidence for how long we should treat? *Current Opinion in Infectious Diseases, 21*(3), 258-262. doi:10.1097/QCO.0b013e3283005441

Weiss, S. W., & Goldblum, J. R. (2008). *Enzinger and Weiss's soft tissue tumors* (5th ed.). Philadelphia: Mosby.

Wheeless, C. R. (2011). Giant-cell tumor of bone. *Wheeless' textbook of orthopedics*. Retrieved from *http://www.wheelessonline.com/ortho/giant_cell_tumor_of_bone*

Wilk, V., Palmer, H. D., Stosic, R. G., & McLachlan, A. J. (2010). Evidence and practice in the self-management of low back pain: Findings from an Australian internet-based survey. *Clinical Journal of Pain, 26*(6), 533-540. doi:10.1097/AJP.0b013e3181dc7abb

CANADIAN RESOURCES

Canadian Academy of Sport Medicine—Academie Canadienne de Médecine du Sport
http://www.casm-acms.org

Canadian Cancer Society, National Office
http://www.cancer.ca/

Canadian Centre for Occupational Health and Safety
http://www.ccohs.ca

The Canadian Orthopaedic Association
http://www.coa-aco.org

The Canadian Orthopaedic Foot & Ankle Society
http://www.coa-aco.org/cofas/cofas-main

Canadian Orthopaedic Nurses Association
http://www.cona-nurse.org/

Canadian Podiatric Medical Association
http://www.podiatrycanada.org

The Easter Seals National Council
http://www.easterseals.ca

Osteoporosis Canada
http://www.osteoporosis.ca

RELATED RESOURCES

National Association of Orthopaedic Nurses (NAON)
http://www.orthonurse.org

NIH Osteoporosis and Related Bone Diseases—National Resource Center
http://www.niams.nih.gov/Health_Info/Bone

Older Women's League
http://www.owl-national.org

The Paget Foundation for Paget's Disease of Bone and Related Disorders
http://www.paget.org

evolve   *For additional Internet resources, see the Web site for this book at* **http://evolve.elsevier.com/Canada/Lewis/medsurg**

Nursing Management: Arthritis and Connective Tissue Diseases

Written by Dottie Roberts
Adapted by Erica Cambly

LEARNING OBJECTIVES

1. Compare and contrast the sequence of events leading to joint destruction in osteoarthritis and rheumatoid arthritis.
2. Describe the clinical manifestations, collaborative care, and nursing management of osteoarthritis and rheumatoid arthritis.
3. Summarize the pathophysiology, clinical manifestations, collaborative care, and nursing management of ankylosing spondylitis, psoriatic arthritis, and reactive arthritis.
4. Describe the pathophysiology, clinical manifestations, and collaborative care of septic arthritis, Lyme disease, and gout.
5. Describe the pathophysiology, clinical manifestations, collaborative care, and nursing management of systemic lupus erythematosus, polymyositis, dermatomyositis, and Sjögren's syndrome.
6. Describe the drug therapy and related nursing management associated with arthritis and connective tissue diseases.
7. Compare and contrast the possible etiologies, clinical manifestations, and collaborative and nursing management of myofascial pain syndrome, fibromyalgia syndrome, and chronic fatigue syndrome.

KEY TERMS

ankylosing spondylitis (AS) A chronic inflammatory disease that primarily affects the axial skeleton, including the sacroiliac joints, intervertebral disc spaces, and costovertebral articulations, p. 1899

arthritis Inflammation of a joint; most prevalent types are osteoarthritis, rheumatoid arthritis, and gout, p. 1881

chronic fatigue syndrome (CFS) A disorder characterized by debilitating fatigue and a variety of associated physical complaints, p. 1916

CREST Acronym used to describe the clinical manifestations of systemic sclerosis (*c*alcinosis, *R*aynaud's phenomenon, *e*sophageal dysfunction, *s*clerodactyly, and *t*elangiectasia), p. 1911

dermatomyositis Diffuse, idiopathic, inflammatory myopathy (see *polymyositis*) that produces bilateral weakness that is usually most severe in the proximal or limb-girdle muscles; characterized by pruritic or eczematous inflammation of the skin and tenderness of the muscles, p. 1913

fibromyalgia syndrome (FMS) A chronic disorder characterized by widespread, nonarticular musculoskeletal pain and fatigue with multiple tender points, p. 1915

gout Condition caused by an increase in uric acid production, underexcretion of uric acid by the kidneys, or increased intake of foods containing purines; joint involvement includes recurrent attacks of acute arthritis, p. 1903

Lyme disease A spirochetal infection caused by *Borrelia burgdorferi* and transmitted by the bite of an infected deer tick; characterized by fever, chills, headache, stiff neck, and migratory joint and muscle pain, p. 1902

myofascial pain syndrome Musculoskeletal pain and tenderness in one anatomical region of the body originating in anterior and posterior trigger points that have developed as a result of muscle trauma, chronic muscle strain, or both, p. 1914

osteoarthritis (OA) A slowly progressive noninflammatory disorder of the diarthrodial (synovial) joints, p. 1881

polymyositis Diffuse, idiopathic, inflammatory myopathy of striated muscle (see *dermatomyositis*); produces bilateral weakness that is usually most severe in the proximal or the limb-girdle muscles; some forms are associated with malignancy, p. 1913

Raynaud's phenomenon An episodic vasospastic disorder of small cutaneous arteries, most frequently involving the fingers and toes; a manifestation of systemic sclerosis, p. 1911

rheumatoid arthritis (RA) A chronic, systemic autoimmune disease characterized by inflammation of connective tissue in the diarthrodial (synovial) joints, typically with periods of remission and exacerbation, p. 1889

septic arthritis An invasion of the joint cavity with microorganisms (also called *infectious* or *bacterial arthritis*), p. 1901

Sjögren's syndrome An autoimmune disease that targets moisture-producing glands, leading to the common symptoms of xerostomia (dry mouth) and keratoconjunctivitis sicca (dry eyes), p. 1914

systemic lupus erythematosus (SLE) A chronic multisystem inflammatory disease of autoimmune origin, p. 1905

systemic sclerosis (SS) A disorder of connective tissue characterized by fibrotic, degenerative, and occasionally inflammatory changes in the skin, blood vessels, synovium, skeletal muscle, and internal organs, p. 1910

ELECTRONIC RESOURCES

Arthritis

Arthritis is the inflammation of a joint and comprises more than 100 different conditions (Arthritis Society, 2011a). It is estimated that by the year 2031, more than 7 million Canadians will be affected by arthritis; more women than men will be affected (Public Health Agency of Canada et al., 2010). The most prevalent types of arthritis are osteoarthritis and rheumatoid arthritis. Another arthritic condition, gout, is described in the Spondyloarthropathies section.

Osteoarthritis

Osteoarthritis (OA), the most common form of joint (articular) disease in North America, is a slowly progressive noninflammatory disorder of the diarthrodial (synovial) joints. Currently, more than 3 million Canadians are affected by OA, and the numbers are expected to increase greatly as the population ages (Arthritis Society, 2011b). Previously identified as *degenerative arthritis,* it is now known to involve the formation of new joint tissue in response to cartilage destruction (Roberts, 2007).

Etiology and Pathophysiology

OA is no longer considered a normal part of the aging process, but growing older continues to be identified consistently as one risk factor for disease development (Arthritis Society, 2011b).

Cartilage destruction can actually begin between ages 20 and 30, but the majority of adults are affected by age 40 (Arthritis Society, 2011b). Few patients experience symptoms until after age 50 or 60, but more than half of those older than 65 years have radiographic evidence of the disease in at least one joint (Public Health Agency of Canada et al., 2010). Women are more often affected than men, and osteoarthritis in women may be more severe (Zhang & Jordan, 2008).

OA may occur as an idiopathic (formerly primary) or secondary disorder. The cause of idiopathic OA is unknown. Secondary OA, on the other hand, is caused by a known event or condition that directly damages cartilage or causes joint instability (Table 67-1).

Researchers have been unable to identify a single cause for OA, but a number of factors have been linked to disease development. The increased incidence of OA in aging women is believed to result from estrogen reduction at menopause. Genetic factors appear to play a significant role in the occurrence of OA. Modifiable risk factors have been identified, including obesity, which contributes to hip and knee OA. Regular moderate exercise, which also helps with weight control, has been shown to decrease the likelihood of disease development and progression. Overuse of knees by strenuous exercise with quick stops and pivoting, as in football and soccer, has been linked to an increased risk of knee OA (Øiestad, Engebretsen, Storheim, & Risberg, 2009).

OA results from cartilage damage that triggers a metabolic response at the level of the chondrocytes (Figure 67-1). Progression of OA causes the normally smooth, white, translucent articular cartilage to become dull, yellow, and granular. Affected

Table 67-1 Causes of Secondary Osteoarthritis

CAUSE	EFFECTS ON JOINT CARTILAGE
Trauma	Dislocations or fractures may lead to avascular necrosis or uneven stress on cartilage.
Mechanical stress	Repetitive physical activities (e.g., sports activities) cause cartilage deterioration.
Inflammation	Release of enzymes in response to local inflammation can affect cartilage integrity.
Joint instability	Damage to supporting structures causes instability, placing uneven stress on articular cartilage.
Neurological disorders	Pain and loss of reflexes from neurological disorders, such as diabetic neuropathy, and in Charcot's joint cause abnormal movements that contribute to cartilage deterioration.
Skeletal deformities	Congenital or acquired conditions such as Legg-Calvé-Perthes disease or dislocated hip contribute to cartilage deterioration.
Hematological or endocrine disorders	Chronic hemarthrosis (e.g., hemophilia) can contribute to cartilage deterioration.
Drugs	Drugs such as indomethacin (Indocin), colchicine, and corticosteroids can stimulate collagen-digesting enzymes in joint synovium.

cartilage gradually becomes softer, less elastic, and less able to resist wear with heavy use. The body's attempts at cartilage repair cannot keep up with the destruction that is occurring. Continued changes in the collagen structure of the cartilage lead to fissuring and erosion of the articular surfaces. As the central cartilage becomes thinner, cartilage and bony growth (*osteophytes*) increase at the joint margins. The resulting incongruity in joint surfaces creates an uneven distribution of stress across the joint and contributes to a reduction in motion.

Although inflammation is not characteristic of OA, a secondary synovitis may result when phagocytic cells try to rid the joint of small pieces of cartilage torn from the joint surface. These inflammatory changes contribute to the early pain and stiffness of OA. The pain of later disease results from contact between exposed bony joint surfaces after the articular cartilage has deteriorated completely.

Clinical Manifestations

Systemic. Systemic manifestations, such as fatigue, fever, and organ involvement, are not characteristic of OA. This is an important distinction between OA and inflammatory joint disorders such as rheumatoid arthritis.

Joints. Manifestations of OA range from mild discomfort to significant disability. Joint pain is the predominant symptom of OA and the typical reason that affected patients seek medical attention. Pain generally worsens with joint use. In the early stages of OA, joint pain is relieved by rest. In advanced disease,

however, patients may complain of pain with rest or experience sleep disruptions caused by increasing joint discomfort. Pain may also become worse as the barometric pressure falls before inclement weather. As OA progresses, increasing pain can contribute significantly to disability and loss of function. The pain of OA may be referred to the groin, the buttock, or the medial side of the thigh or knee. Sitting down becomes difficult, as does rising from a chair when the hips are lower than the knees. As OA develops in the intervertebral (apophyseal) joints of the spine, localized pain and stiffness are common.

Unlike pain, which is typically provoked by activity, joint stiffness occurs after periods of rest or static position. Early-morning stiffness is common but generally resolves within 30 minutes, which is another feature that distinguishes OA from inflammatory arthritic disorders. Overactivity can cause a mild joint effusion that temporarily increases stiffness. *Crepitation*, a grating sensation caused by loose particles of cartilage in the joint cavity, can also contribute to stiffness. Crepitation indicates the loss of cartilage integrity and is present in more than 90% of patients with knee OA.

OA usually affects joints asymmetrically. The most commonly involved joints are the distal interphalangeal (DIP) and proximal interphalangeal (PIP) joints of the fingers, the metacarpophalangeal (MCP) joint of the thumb, weight-bearing joints (hips, knees), the metatarsophalangeal (MTP) joint of the foot, and the cervical and lower lumbar vertebrae (Figure 67-2).

Deformity. Deformity or instability associated with OA is specific to the involved joint. For example, *Heberden's nodes* occur on the DIP joints as an indication of osteophyte formation and loss of joint space (see Figure 67-1). They can appear in patients with OA as early as age 40 and tend to be seen in family members. *Bouchard's nodes* on the PIP joints indicate similar disease involvement. Heberden's and Bouchard's nodes are often red, swollen, and tender. Although these bony enlargements do not usually cause significant loss of function, patients may be distressed by the visible disfigurement.

Knee OA often leads to joint malalignment as a result of cartilage loss in the medial compartment. Affected patients have a characteristic bow-legged appearance, and gait may be altered in response to the obvious deformity. In advanced hip OA, one of the patient's legs may become shorter as a result of a loss of joint space.

Diagnostic Studies

A bone scan, computed tomography (CT) scan, or magnetic resonance imaging (MRI) may be useful for diagnosing OA because of the sensitivity of these tests in detecting early joint changes. Radiological studies are helpful in confirming disease and monitoring the effectiveness of treatment. As OA progresses, radiographs typically show joint space narrowing, bony sclerosis, and osteophyte formation. However, these changes are not always correlated with the degree of pain experienced by patients. Despite significant radiological indications of disease, patients may be relatively free of symptoms. Conversely, another patient may have severe pain with only minimal radiographic changes.

No laboratory abnormalities or biomarkers that are specific diagnostic indicators of OA have been identified. The erythrocyte sedimentation rate (ESR) is normal except in instances of acute synovitis, when elevations may be minimal. Other routine blood tests (e.g., complete blood cell count [CBC], kidney and liver

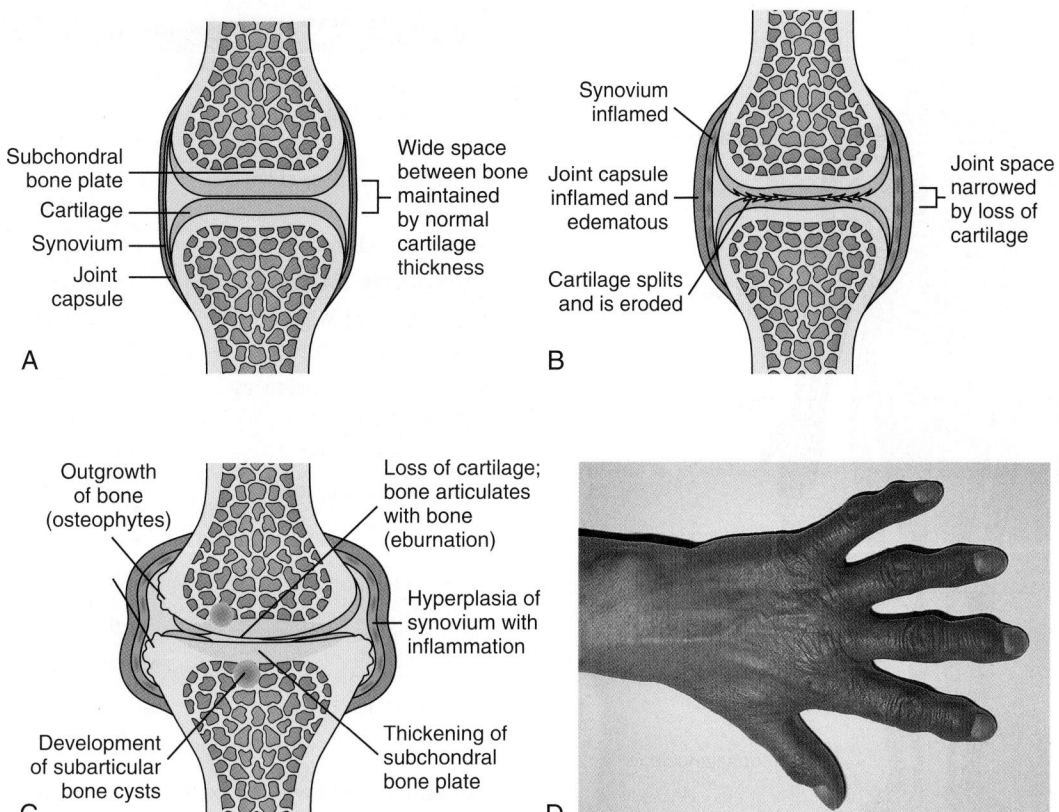

Figure 67-1 Pathological changes in osteoarthritis. **A,** Normal synovial joint. **B,** Early change in osteoarthritis is destruction of articular cartilage and narrowing of the joint space. Inflammation and thickening of the joint capsule and synovium occur. **C,** With time, thickening of subarticular bone is caused by constant friction of the two bone surfaces. Osteophytes form around the periphery of the joint by irregular outgrowths of bone. **D,** In osteoarthritis of the hands, osteophytes on the interphalangeal joints of the fingers, termed *Heberden's nodes*, appear as small nodules.

Source: Stevens, A., & Lowe, J. (2000). *Pathology: Illustrated review in colour* (2nd ed.). London: Mosby.

function tests) are useful only in screening for related conditions or for establishing baseline values before the initiation of therapy. Synovial fluid analysis allows differentiation between OA and other forms of inflammatory arthritis. In the presence of OA, the fluid remains clear yellow with little or no sign of inflammation.

Collaborative Care

Because there is no cure for OA, collaborative care focuses on managing pain and inflammation, preventing disability, and maintaining and improving joint function (Table 67-2). Non-pharmacological interventions are the foundation for OA management and should be maintained throughout a patient's treatment period. Drug therapy serves as an adjunct to nonpharmacological treatments. Symptoms of disease are often managed conservatively for many years, but loss of joint function, unrelieved pain, and diminished ability to perform self-care independently may prompt a recommendation for surgery. Reconstructive surgical procedures are discussed in Chapter 65. In general, arthroscopic surgery with debridement is usually not recommended for OA. However, in 60% of patients with OA, arthroscopic removal of bone bits, cartilage fragments, torn menisci, and osteophytes provides relief from pain for up to 5 years (Arthritis Society, 2011b).

Rest and Joint Protection. The patient with OA must understand the importance of a balance of rest and activity. The affected joint should be rested during any periods of acute inflammation and maintained in a functional position with splints or braces if necessary. However, immobilization should not exceed 1 week because of the risk of joint stiffness with inactivity. Patients may need to modify their usual activities to decrease stress on affected joints. For example, patients with knee OA should avoid prolonged periods of standing, kneeling, or squatting. Using an assistive device such as a cane, a walker, or crutches can also help decrease stress on arthritic joints.

Heat and Cold Applications. Applications of heat and cold may help reduce pain and stiffness. Although ice is not used as often as heat in the treatment of OA, it can be appropriate if patients experience acute inflammation. Heat therapy—including hot packs, whirlpool baths, ultrasound, and paraffin wax baths—is especially helpful for stiffness.

Nutritional Therapy and Exercise. If a patient is overweight, a weight-reduction program is a critical part of the total treatment plan. The nurse should help the patient evaluate the current diet to make appropriate changes. (Chapter 42 describes ways to assist patients in attaining and maintaining a healthy

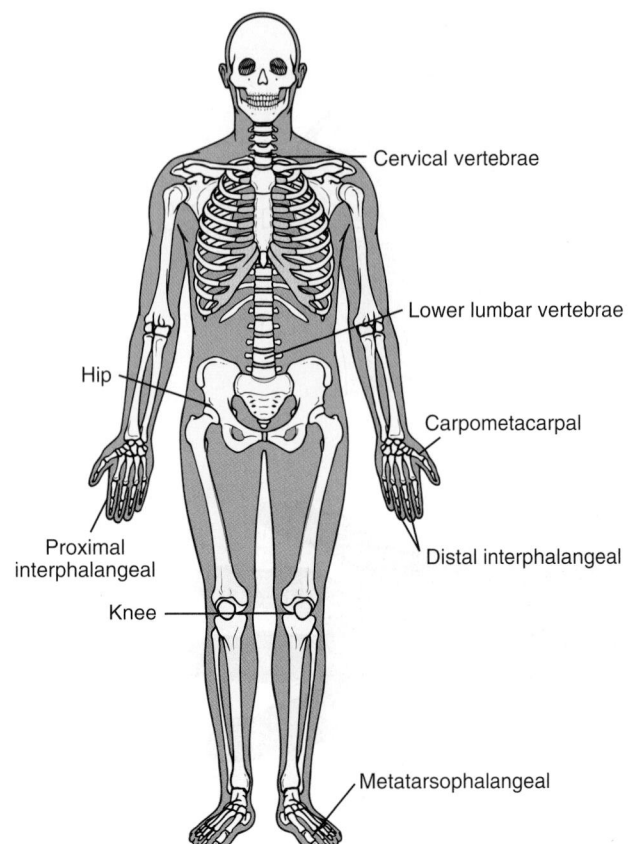

Cervical vertebrae

Lower lumbar vertebrae

Hip

Carpometacarpal

Proximal interphalangeal

Distal interphalangeal

Knee

Metatarsophalangeal

Figure 67-2 Joints most frequently involved in osteoarthritis.

COLLABORATIVE CARE

Table 67-2 Osteoarthritis

Diagnostic

- History and physical examination
- Radiological studies of involved joints
- Synovial fluid analysis

Collaborative Therapy

- Nutritional and weight management counselling
- Rest and joint protection, use of assistive devices
- Therapeutic exercise
- Heat and cold applications

- Complementary and alternative therapies
  - Herbs and nutritional supplements (e.g., glucosamine)
  - Movement therapies (e.g., yoga, Tai Chi)
  - Transcutaneous electrical nerve stimulation (TENS)
  - Acupuncture
- Drug therapy*
  - Acetaminophen
  - Nonsteroidal anti-inflammatory drugs
  - Antibiotics
  - Intra-articular hyaluronic acid
  - Intra-articular corticosteroids
  - Opioid analgesics
- Reconstructive joint surgery

*See Table 67-3.

body weight.) Because the load on the joints and the degree of joint mobilization are essential to the preservation of articular cartilage integrity, exercise is a fundamental part of OA management (Arthritis Society, 2011b). Aerobic conditioning, range-of-motion exercises, and specific programs for strengthening the quadriceps have been beneficial for many patients with knee OA (Fransen & McConnell, 2009).

Complementary and Alternative Therapies. Complementary and alternative therapies for symptom management of arthritis have become increasingly popular with patients who have failed to find relief through traditional medical care. Acupuncture, for example, has been found to be a safe and effective method for arthritis pain management (Manheimer et al., 1996). Other therapies include yoga, massage, guided imagery, and therapeutic touch (see Chapter 12). Nutritional supplements such as glucosamine and chondroitin sulphate may be helpful in some patients for relieving moderate to severe arthritis pain in the knees and improving joint mobility (Towheed et al., 2009).

Drug Therapy. Drug therapy is based on the severity of the patient's symptoms (Table 67-3). Patients with mild to moderate joint pain may receive relief from acetaminophen (Tylenol). A topical agent such as capsaicin cream may also be beneficial, either alone or in conjunction with acetaminophen. It blocks pain by locally interfering with substance P, which is responsible for the transmission of pain impulses. The cream can be applied to affected joints four times daily. The patient should be told that a local burning sensation may accompany initial use. The cream

should not be used with an external heat source such as a heating pad or hot water bottle.

For patients who do not obtain adequate pain management with acetaminophen or for patients with moderate to severe OA pain, a nonsteroidal anti-inflammatory drug (NSAID) may provide greater relief (see the Evidence-Informed Practice box, "Is Acetaminophen or an NSAID More Effective in Treating Osteoarthritis?"). NSAID therapy is typically initiated in low-dose over-the-counter (OTC) strengths (e.g., ibuprofen [Advil]) of 200 mg, up to four times daily, with the dosage increased as the patient's symptoms indicate. If a patient is at risk for or experiences adverse gastrointestinal (GI) effects with a conventional NSAID, supplemental treatment with a protective agent such as misoprostol may be indicated. Arthrotec, a combination of misoprostol and the NSAID diclofenac, is also available.

Because traditional NSAIDs block the production of prostaglandins from arachidonic acid by inhibiting the production of cyclooxygenase-1 (COX-1) and cyclooxygenase-2 (COX-2), the risk for GI erosion and bleeding is increased. Traditional NSAIDs affect platelet aggregation, which prolongs bleeding time. Concerns have also been raised regarding the possible negative effects of long-term NSAID treatment on cartilage metabolism, particularly in older patients, in whom cartilage integrity may already be diminished. As an alternative to traditional NSAIDs, treatment with the COX-2 inhibitor celecoxib (Celebrex) may be considered in selected patients (Arthritis Society, 2011b).

When given in equivalent anti-inflammatory dosages, all NSAIDs are considered comparable in efficacy but vary widely in cost. Individual responses to the NSAIDs are also variable. Aspirin is no longer a common treatment, and it should not be used in combination with NSAIDs because both inhibit platelet function and prolong bleeding time.

Intra-articular injections of corticosteroids may be appropriate for older adults with local inflammation and effusion. When four or more injections do not provide relief, additional

Text continued on p. 1888

DRUG THERAPY

Table 67-3 Arthritis and Connective Tissue Disorders

DRUG	MECHANISM OF ACTION	ADVERSE EFFECTS	NURSING CONSIDERATIONS
Salicylates			
Aspirin, salicylate (acetylsalicylic acid [ASA], Asaphen, Bufferin)	Anti-inflammatory Analgesic Antipyretic Inhibits prostaglandin synthesis	GI irritation (dyspepsia, nausea, ulcer, hemorrhage) Prolonged bleeding time Exacerbation of asthma (aspirin-sensitive asthma) Tinnitus, dizziness with repeated large doses	Administer drug with food, milk, antacids as prescribed, or full glass of water; enteric-coated aspirin may be administered. Report signs of bleeding (e.g., tarry stools, bruising, petechiae, nosebleeds).
Nonsteroidal Anti-Inflammatory Drugs (NSAIDs)			
Ibuprofen (Motrin, Advil) Naproxen (Naprosyn, Anaprox) Ketoprofen (Apo-Keto) Piroxicam (Teva-Pirocam) Indomethacin (Nu-Indo) Sulindac (Teva-Sulindac) Diclofenac (Voltaren) Meloxicam (Mobicox) Celecoxib (Celebrex)	Anti-inflammatory Analgesic Antipyretic Inhibits prostaglandin synthesis	GI irritation (dyspepsia, nausea, ulcer, hemorrhage) Prolonged bleeding time Headache, tinnitus Rash Acute renal insufficiency and other renal medullary changes Exacerbation of asthma (cross-reactivity with aspirin)	Administer drug with food, milk, or antacids as prescribed. Report signs of bleeding (e.g., tarry stools, bruising, petechiae, nosebleeds), edema, skin rashes, persistent headaches, visual disturbances. Monitor BP for elevations related to fluid retention. Drug must be administered regularly for maximal effect.
Antibiotics			
Doxycycline (Vibramycin) Minocycline	Decreases action of enzymes on cartilage degradation Antirheumatic effect, possibly related to immunomodulatory or anti-inflammatory properties	Monilial vaginitis, sensitivity to direct sunlight or ultraviolet light, nonspecific GI irritation GI effects (nausea and vomiting, diarrhea, stomach cramps) Dizziness Photosensitivity (severe)	This is a possible treatment alternative for mild disease.
Topical analgesics			
Capsaicin cream	Depletes substance P from nerve endings, interrupting pain signals to the brain	Rash, urticaria Localized burning sensation, erythema	Drug must be administered regularly over time for maximal effect. Aloe vera cream may modify burning sensation. Advise patient not to use cream with external heat source (heating pad) because of risk of burns. Available in OTC and prescriptive strengths.
Diclofenac diethylamine (Voltaren [Emulgel])	Anti-inflammatory Analgesic	Skin irritation Adverse GI effects similar to those of systemic NSAIDs	Advise patient to avoid sun and ultraviolet exposure. Drug should not be used in combination with other oral NSAIDs or aspirin because of potential for increased adverse effects.
Corticosteroids			
Intra-articular Injections			
Methylprednisolone acetate (Depo-Medrol) Triamcinolone (Aristospan)	Anti-inflammatory Analgesic Inhibit synthesis and release of mediators of inflammation	Local osteoporosis Tendon rupture Neuropathic arthropathy from frequent injection Dermal or subdermal changes leading to depression at injection site Possibility of local infection	Use strict aseptic technique for joint fluid aspiration or corticosteroid injection. Inform patient that joint may feel worse immediately after injection. Inform patient that improvement lasts weeks to months after injection. Advise patient to avoid overusing affected joint after injection.

BP, blood pressure; *GI*, gastrointestinal; *NSAIDs*, nonsteroidal anti-inflammatory drugs; *OTC*, over-the-counter.

Continued

DRUG THERAPY

Table 67-3 Arthritis and Connective Tissue Disorders—cont'd

DRUG	MECHANISM OF ACTION	ADVERSE EFFECTS	NURSING CONSIDERATIONS
Corticosteroids—cont'd			
Systemic			
Hydrocortisone sodium succinate (Solu-Cortef) Methylprednisolone sodium succinate (Solu-Medrol) Dexamethasone (Dexasone) Prednisone	Anti-inflammatory Analgesic Inhibit synthesis and release of mediators of inflammation	Cushing's syndrome (including fluid retention), GI irritation, osteoporosis, insomnia, hypertension, steroid psychosis, diabetes mellitus, acne, menstrual irregularities, hirsutism, risk of antibiotic-resistant infection, bruising	Use only in life-threatening exacerbation or when symptoms persist after treatment with less potent anti-inflammatory drugs. Administer for limited time only, tapering dose slowly. Be aware that symptom exacerbation occurs with abrupt withdrawal of drug. Monitor BP, weight, CBC, and potassium level. Limit sodium intake. Have patient report signs of infection to health care provider.
Disease-Modifying Antirheumatic Drugs (DMARDs)			
Methotrexate	Antimetabolite Inhibits DNA, RNA, and protein synthesis	Hepatotoxicity (occurs more often with frequent small doses than with large intermittent doses); symptoms related to drug's antineoplastic activity (e.g., GI and skin toxicity, bone marrow depression, nephropathy; smaller dose and different administration schedule for RA decrease likelihood that these will develop)	Monitor CBC and hepatic and renal function. Advise patient to report signs of anemia (fatigue, weakness). Keep patient well hydrated. Because of teratogenic potential, drug should not be administered to children or women of childbearing age. Inform patient that contraception should be used during and 3 months after treatment.
Sulphasalazine (Salazopyrin)	Sulphonamide Anti-inflammatory Blocks prostaglandin synthesis	GI effects (anorexia, nausea and vomiting) Bleeding, bruising, jaundice Headache Rash, urticaria, pruritus	Advise patient that drug may cause orange-yellow discoloration of urine or skin. Space doses evenly around the clock, administering drug with 250 mL water after meals. Treatment may be continued even after symptoms are relieved. Monitor CBC.
Leflunomide (Arava)	Anti-inflammatory Immunomodulatory agent that inhibits proliferation of lymphocytes	Hepatotoxicity (especially if patient is also taking methotrexate or has history of prior alcohol abuse) Nausea, diarrhea Respiratory tract infection Alopecia Rash	Evaluate for relief of pain, swelling, stiffness; increase in joint mobility. Advise women of childbearing age to avoid pregnancy.
D-penicillamine (Cuprimine)	Anti-inflammatory Exact mechanism of action in RA unknown, but may suppress cell-mediated immune response	GI irritation (nausea and vomiting, anorexia, diarrhea), reduced or altered taste Rash Proteinuria, hematuria Iron deficiency (especially in menstruating women)	Monitor WBCs, platelets, urinalysis. Advise patient to take medication 1 hr before or 2 hr after meals or at least 1 hr before or after any other drug, food, or milk. Advise women of childbearing age to avoid pregnancy.
Gold compounds			
Parenteral (gold sodium aurothiomalate [Myochrysine]) Oral (auranofin [Ridaura])	Alters immune responses, suppressing synovitis of active RA Antirheumatic	Decreased hemoglobin Leukopenia, thrombocytopenia Proteinuria, hematuria Stomatitis	Rule out pregnancy before beginning treatment. Monitor CBC, urinalysis, and hepatic and renal function. Advise patient that therapeutic response may not occur for 3 to 6 mo. Advise patient to immediately report pruritus, rash, sore mouth, indigestion, or metallic taste.

CBC, complete blood cell count; *RA*, rheumatoid arthritis; *WBC*, white blood cell.

DRUG THERAPY

Table 67-3 Arthritis and Connective Tissue Disorders—cont'd

DRUG	MECHANISM OF ACTION	ADVERSE EFFECTS	NURSING CONSIDERATIONS
Antimalarials			
Hydroxychloroquine (Plaquenil)	Antirheumatic action unknown, but may suppress formation of antigens	Ocular toxicity (retinopathy) may progress even after drug is discontinued Ototoxicity Peripheral neuritis, neuromyopathy, hypotension, electrocardiographic changes with prolonged therapy	Monitor CBC and hepatic function. Advise patient that therapeutic response may not occur for up to 6 mo. Advise patient to immediately report visual difficulties, muscular weakness, and decreased hearing or tinnitus.
Immunosuppressants			
Azathioprine (Imuran) Cyclophosphamide (Procytox)	Inhibit DNA, RNA, and protein synthesis	GI irritation (nausea and vomiting; anorexia with large doses) Rash	Evaluate for relief of pain, swelling, and stiffness and for increase in joint mobility. Advise patient to immediately report unusual bleeding or bruising. Advise patient that therapeutic response may take up to 12 wk. Advise women of childbearing age to avoid pregnancy.
Biological or Targeted Therapy			
Etanercept (Enbrel)	Binds TNF, blocking its interaction with cell surface receptors to decrease inflammatory and immune responses	Injection site reaction including erythema, pain, itching, swelling Abdominal pain, vomiting Dizziness, headache Rhinitis, pharyngitis, cough	Evaluate for relief of pain, swelling, and stiffness and for increase in joint mobility. Advise patient that injection site reaction generally occurs in first month of treatment and decreases with continued therapy. Advise patient not to receive live vaccines during treatment.
Infliximab (Remicade) Adalimumab (Humira)	Monoclonal antibodies that bind to TNF; reduce infiltration of inflammatory cells	Abdominal pain, nausea and vomiting Dizziness, headache Rhinitis, cough, sinusitis, pharyngitis	Evaluate for relief of pain, swelling, and stiffness and for increase in joint mobility.
Anakinra (Kineret)	Blocks the action of interleukin-1 and thus decreases the inflammatory response	Injection site reaction Leukopenia, headache Abdominal pain, rash	Evaluate for relief of pain, swelling, stiffness and for increase in joint mobility. Advise patient that injection site reaction generally occurs during first month of treatment and decreases with continued therapy. Evaluate renal function. Monitor for infection. Do not administer drug with other TNF inhibitors.
Abatacept (Orencia)	Modulates T-cell activation; suppresses immune response	Headache, upper respiratory infection, nausea, sore throat, injection site reaction	Not recommended for concomitant use with TNF inhibitors. Evaluate for relief of pain, swelling, and stiffness and for increase in joint mobility.
Rituximab (Rituxan)	Monoclonal antibody that targets B cells	Dizziness, palpitations, fever, itching, difficulty breathing, sore throat	Administer in combination with methotrexate. Monitor for infection and bleeding. Advise patient to not receive live virus vaccines during treatment. Monitor for low BP if patient is also taking antihypertensives.
Golimumab (Simponi) Certolizumab pegol (Cimzia)	TNF-α blocker; decreases inflammatory response	Upper respiratory tract infection, sore throat, and nasal congestion	Advise patient of increased risk for tuberculosis and invasive fungal infections, which occur with other TNF blockers. Monitor for infection and bleeding. Monitor for the emergence of malignancies with TNF blockers. Advise patient that psoriasis may worsen.
Tocilizumab (Actemra)	Blocks action of interleukin-6	Upper respiratory tract infections, headache, inflammation of nose or nasal passage, ↑ BP, ↑ liver enzyme levels	Administered to patients with RA in whom other therapies have failed. Monitor BP and for infection. Advise patient of adverse GI effects (e.g., perforation). Monitor liver enzyme and LDL levels.

LDL, low-density lipoprotein; *TNF,* tumour necrosis factor; *TNF-α,* tumour necrosis factor α.

Is Acetaminophen or an NSAID More Effective in Treating Osteoarthritis?

Clinical Question

In patients with osteoarthritis (P), is acetaminophen (I) more effective in reducing pain and improving function (O) than NSAIDs (C)?

Best Available Evidence

Systematic review of randomized controlled trials (RCTs)

Critical Appraisal and Synthesis of Evidence

- 15 RCTs (n = 5986 participants); in 7 RCTs, acetaminophen was compared with placebo, and in 10 RCTs, acetaminophen was compared with NSAIDs.
- The safety of acetaminophen was also compared with that of NSAIDs.

Conclusions

- Acetaminophen was superior to placebo in efficacy; no differences in safety were found.
- NSAIDs were superior to acetaminophen for improving knee and hip pain in patients with osteoarthritis.
- NSAIDs were more effective than acetaminophen in reducing overall pain and functional status.
- No significant differences were found overall between the safety of the two drugs, although patients taking NSAIDs were more likely to experience an adverse GI event.
- In patients with moderate to severe pain, NSAIDs appeared to be more effective than acetaminophen.

Implications for Nursing Practice

- Patient care should begin with weight loss, physiotherapy, and occupational therapy before drug therapy is initiated.
- Nurses should assess pain levels, costs and availability, and patient preferences in recommending one treatment over another; surveys have shown patients prefer NSAIDs over acetaminophen.
- Nurses should instruct and monitor patients who are at risk for upper GI bleeding while taking NSAIDs (e.g., patients aged 65 and older, those taking oral corticosteroids or anticoagulants concomitantly with NSAIDs).
- Nurses should inform patients of the increased risk of upper GI problems when they take acetaminophen in doses greater than 2000 mg/day.

Reference for Evidence

Towheed, T. E., Maxwell, L., Judd, M. G., Catton, M., Hochberg, M., & Wells, G. (2009). Acetaminophen for osteoarthritis. *Cochrane Database of Systematic Reviews*, (1), CD004257. doi:10.1002/14651858.CD004257.pub2

GI, gastrointestinal; *NSAIDs*, nonsteroidal anti-inflammatory drugs; *PICO: P*, patient population of interest; *I*, intervention or area of interest; *C*, comparison of interest or comparison group; *O*, outcomes of interest.

intervention is needed. Systemic use of corticosteroids is not indicated and may actually accelerate the disease process.

Another treatment for mild to moderate OA is hyaluronic acid injection, a type of viscosupplementation. Hyaluronic acid is found in normal joint fluid and articular cartilage. It contributes to both the viscosity and the elasticity of synovial fluid, and its depletion can result in joint damage. Synthetic and naturally occurring hyaluronic acid derivatives (Orthovisc, Synvisc, and Hyalgan) are administered in three injections, a week apart, directly into the joint space. These intra-articular injections have been shown to be safe and effective in treating the pain and functional impairment of knee OA (Bellamy et al., 2006).

Medications thought to slow the progression of OA or support joint healing are known as *disease-modifying osteoarthritis drugs (DMOADs)*. A number of drugs are under investigation with mixed results as whether they are effective and safe. Among them is the antibiotic doxycycline (Vibramycin), which may decrease the loss of cartilage in some patients with knee OA (Nüesch, Rutjes, Trelle, Reichenbach, & Jüni, 2009).

NURSING MANAGEMENT: OSTEOARTHRITIS

Nursing Assessment

The nurse should carefully assess and document the type, location, severity, frequency, and duration of the patient's joint pain and stiffness and the extent to which these symptoms affect his or her ability to perform activities of daily living (ADLs). The nurse should note pain-relieving practices and question the patient about the duration and success of each treatment. Physical examination of the affected joint or joints includes assessment of tenderness, swelling, limitation of movement, and crepitation. An involved joint should be compared with the contralateral joint if it is not affected.

Nursing Diagnoses

Nursing diagnoses for patients with OA may include, but are not limited to, the following:

- Acute pain and chronic pain *related to* physical activity and lack of knowledge of pain self-management techniques
- Insomnia *related to* pain
- Impaired physical mobility *related to* weakness, stiffness, or pain on ambulation
- Self-care (bathing, dressing, feeding, toileting) deficits *related to* joint deformity and pain with activity
- Imbalanced nutrition: more than body requirements *related to* intake in excess of energy output
- Chronic low self-esteem *related to* changing physical appearance and social and work roles

Planning

The overall goals are that patients with OA will (a) maintain or improve joint function through a balance of rest and activity, (b) use joint protection measures (Table 67-4) to improve activity tolerance, (c) achieve independence in self-care and maintain

Table 67-4 Joint Protection and Energy Conservation

The following instructions should be included in teaching patients with arthritis to protect joints and conserve energy:

- Maintain appropriate weight.
- Use assistive devices, if indicated.
- Avoid forceful repetitive movements.
- Avoid positions of joint deviation and stress.
- Use good posture and proper body mechanics.
- Seek assistance with necessary tasks that may cause pain.
- Develop organizing and pacing techniques for routine tasks.
- Modify home and work environment to create less stressful ways to perform tasks.

optimal role function, and (d) use pharmacological and non-pharmacological strategies to manage pain satisfactorily.

Nursing Implementation

Health Promotion

Prevention of primary OA is not possible. However, community education should focus on the alteration of modifiable risk factors through weight loss and the reduction of occupational and recreational hazards. Athletic instruction and physical fitness programs should include safety measures that protect the joint structures, as well as reduce trauma to them. Congenital conditions, such as Legg-Calvé-Perthes disease, that are known to predispose a patient to the development of OA should be treated promptly.

Acute Intervention

Patients with OA most often complain of pain, stiffness, limitation of function, and the frustration of coping with these physical difficulties on a daily basis. Older adults may believe that OA is an inevitable part of the aging process and that nothing can be done to ease the discomfort and related disability.

Osteoarthritis is usually treated on an outpatient basis, often by an interdisciplinary team of health care providers that includes a rheumatologist, a nurse, an occupational therapist, and a physiotherapist. Health assessment questionnaires are often used to pinpoint areas of difficulty for patients with arthritis. Questionnaires are repeated at regular intervals to document disease and treatment progression. Treatment goals can be developed on the basis of data from the questionnaires and the physical examination, with specific interventions to target identified problems. Patients are usually hospitalized only if joint surgery is planned (see Chapter 65).

Drugs are administered for the relief of pain and inflammation. Nonpharmacological pain management strategies may include massage, the application of heat (thermal packs) or cold (ice packs), relaxation, and guided imagery. Splints may be prescribed to rest and stabilize painful or inflamed joints. Once an acute flare has subsided, a physiotherapist can provide valuable assistance in planning an exercise program. Therapists may often recommend Tai Chi as a low-impact form of exercise. Tai Chi can

be performed by patients of all ages and may be practised in a wheelchair. The nurse should emphasize the importance of warming up before practice to prevent stretch injuries.

Patient and caregiver teaching related to OA is an important nursing responsibility in any care setting and is the foundation of successful disease management. Teaching should include information about the nature and the treatment of the disease, pain management, correct posture and body mechanics, correct use of assistive devices such as a cane or walker, principles of joint protection and energy conservation (see Table 67-4), nutritional choices and weight management, stress management, and a therapeutic exercise program. Patients should be assured that OA is a localized disease and that severe deforming arthritis is not the usual course. Patients can also obtain support and understanding of the disease process through community resources such as the Arthritis Self-Management Program (ASMP) (Arthritis Society, 2011c).

Ambulatory and Home Care

Chronic pain and a loss of function of the affected joints continue to be primary concerns. Home management goals should be individualized to meet the patient's needs. The caregiver, family members, and significant others should be included in goal setting and teaching. Home and work environment modification is essential for the patient's safety, accessibility, and self-care (Arthritis Society, 2011b). Such modification includes removing scatter rugs, providing rails at the stairs and bathtub, using nightlights, and wearing well-fitting supportive shoes. Assistive devices such as canes, walkers, elevated toilet seats, and grab bars also reduce the load on the joint and promote safety. Patients should be urged to continue all prescribed pharmacological and nonpharmacological therapies at home and also be amenable to the discussion of new approaches to symptom management.

Sexual counselling may help the patient and significant other enjoy physical closeness by introducing the idea of alternative positions and timing for intercourse. Discussion also increases awareness of each partner's needs. The nurse should encourage the patient to take analgesics or a warm bath to decrease joint stiffness before sexual activity.

Evaluation

The expected outcomes for patients with OA are as follows:
- Experience adequate amounts of rest and activity.
- Achieve satisfactory pain management.
- Maintain joint flexibility and muscle strength through joint protection and therapeutic exercise.
- Verbalize acceptance of OA as a chronic disease and collaborate with health care providers in disease management.

Rheumatoid Arthritis

Rheumatoid arthritis (RA) is a chronic, systemic autoimmune disease characterized by inflammation of connective tissue in the diarthrodial (synovial) joints, typically with periods of remission and exacerbation. RA is frequently accompanied by extra-articular manifestations.

RA occurs globally, affecting all ethnic groups. It can occur at any time of life, but in most cases, it develops between the ages of 25 and 50. One percent of Canadians have RA, and two to three times more women than men are affected (Arthritis Society, 2011d).

Etiology and Pathophysiology

The cause of RA is unknown. Older theories notwithstanding, no infectious agent has been cultured from blood and synovial tissue or fluid with enough reproducibility to suggest an infectious cause for the disease. An autoimmune etiology is currently the most widely accepted theory.

Autoimmunity. The autoimmune theory suggests that changes associated with RA begin when a susceptible host experiences an initial immune response to an antigen. The antigen, which is probably not the same in all affected patients, triggers the formation of an abnormal immunoglobulin G (IgG). RA is characterized by the presence of autoantibodies against this abnormal IgG. The autoantibodies, known as *rheumatoid*

factor (RF), combine with IgG to form immune complexes that initially deposit on synovial membranes or superficial articular cartilage in the joints. Immune complex formation leads to the activation of complement, and an inflammatory response results. (Complement activation is discussed in Chapter 14, and immune complex formation is discussed in Chapter 16.) Neutrophils are attracted to the site of inflammation, where they release proteolytic enzymes that can damage articular cartilage and cause the synovial lining to thicken (Figure 67-3). Other inflammatory cells include T helper (CD4) cells, which are the primary orchestrators of cell-mediated immune responses. Activated CD4 cells stimulate monocytes, macrophages, and synovial fibroblasts to secrete the proinflammatory cytokines interleukin-1 (IL-1), interleukin-6 (IL-6), and tumour necrosis factor (TNF). These cytokines are the primary factors that drive the inflammatory response in RA.

Joint changes from chronic inflammation begin when the hypertrophied synovial membrane invades the surrounding cartilage, ligaments, tendons, and joint capsule. *Pannus* (highly

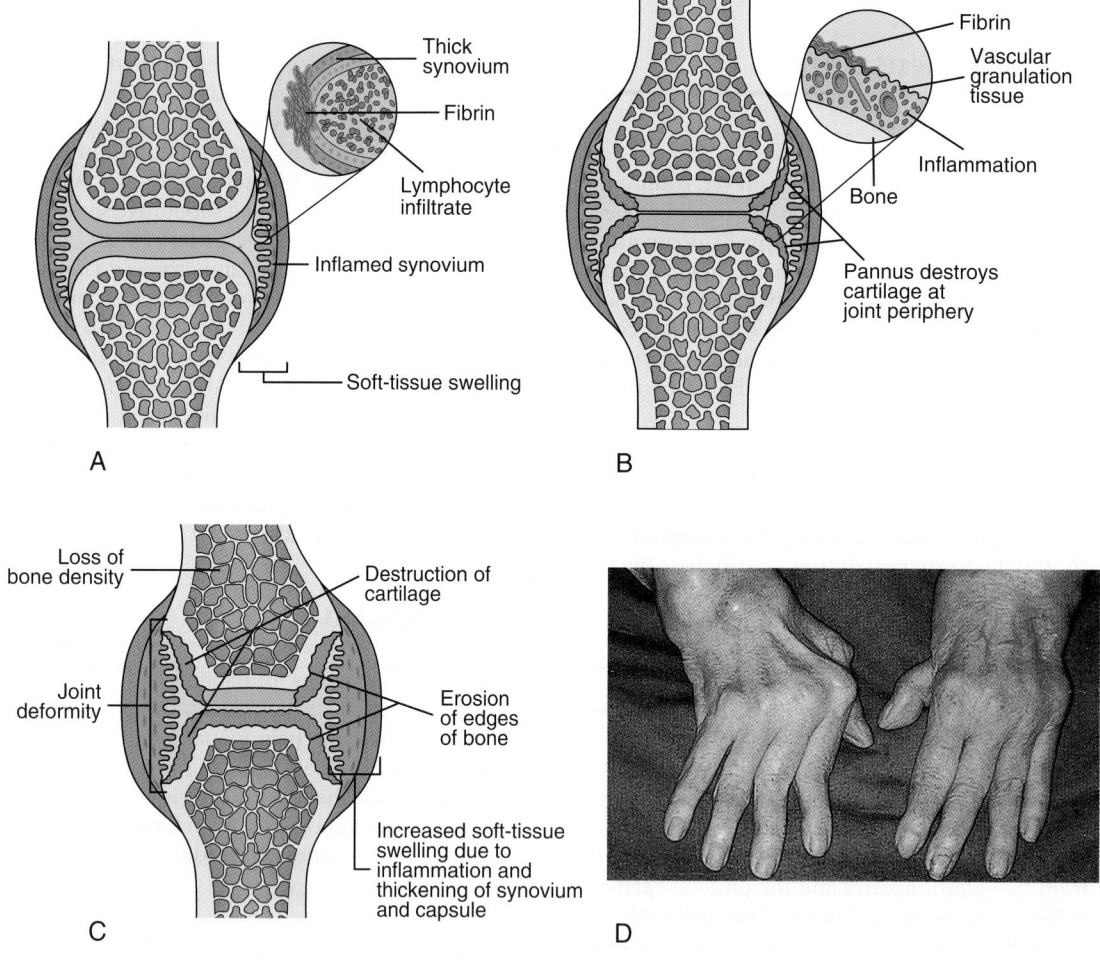

Figure 67-3 Rheumatoid arthritis. **A,** Early pathological change in rheumatoid arthritis is rheumatoid synovitis, characterized by inflammation of the synovium and a great increase in lymphocytes. **B,** With time, articular cartilage is destroyed; vascular granulation tissue grows across the surface of the cartilage (pannus) from the edges of the joint, and the articular surface shows loss of cartilage beneath the extending pannus, most marked at the joint margins. **C,** Inflammatory pannus causes focal destruction of bone. At the edges of the joint, osteolytic destruction of bone is responsible for erosions seen on radiographs. This phase is associated with joint deformity. **D,** Characteristic deformity and soft-tissue swelling associated with long-standing rheumatoid disease of the hands.

Source: Stevens, A., & Lowe, J. (2000). *Pathology: Illustrated review in colour* (2nd ed.). London: Mosby.

Table 67-5 Anatomical Stages of Rheumatoid Arthritis

Table 67-5 Anatomical Stages of Rheumatoid Arthritis

Stage I: Early

No destructive changes visible on radiograph; possible radiographic evidence of osteoporosis

Stage II: Moderate

Radiographic evidence of osteoporosis, with or without slight bone or cartilage destruction; no joint deformities (although possibly limited joint mobility); adjacent muscle atrophy; possible presence of extra-articular soft-tissue lesions (e.g., nodules, tenosynovitis)

Stage III: Severe

Radiographic evidence of cartilage and bone destruction in addition to osteoporosis; joint deformity, such as subluxation, ulnar deviation, or hyperextension, without fibrous or bony ankylosis; extensive muscle atrophy; possible presence of extra-articular soft tissue lesions (e.g., nodules, tenosynovitis)

Stage IV: Terminal

Fibrous or bony ankylosis; stage III criteria

Source: American College of Rheumatology (2008). *ACR classification criteria for determining progression of rheumatoid arthritis.* Retrieved from *http://www.hopkins-arthritis.org/physician-corner/education/acr/acr.html#prog_rheum.* Originally from Steinbrocker, O., Traeger, C. H., & Batterman, R. C. (1949). Therapeutic criteria in rheumatoid arthritis. *JAMA, 140*(8), 659-662.

vascular granulation tissue) forms within the joint. It eventually covers and erodes the entire surface of the articular cartilage. The production of inflammatory cytokines at the pannus–cartilage junction further contributes to cartilage destruction. The pannus also scars and shortens supporting structures such as tendons and ligaments, ultimately causing joint laxity, subluxation, and contracture.

Genetic Factors.

Genetic predisposition appears to be important in the development of RA. For example, the occurrence of the disease has been noted to be more frequent in identical rather than fraternal twins. The strongest evidence for a familial influence is the increased occurrence of a human leukocyte antigen (HLA) known as HLA-DR4 in White patients with RA. Other HLA variants have also been identified in patients from other ethnic groups. (HLAs are discussed in Chapter 16.) Smoking significantly increases the risk of RA for both men and women who are genetically predisposed to the disease (Carmona, Cross, Williams, Lassere, & March, 2010).

The pathogenesis of RA is more clearly understood than its etiology. If unarrested, the disease progresses through four stages, which are identified in Table 67-5.

Clinical Manifestations

Joints.

The onset of RA is typically insidious. Nonspecific manifestations such as fatigue, anorexia, weight loss, and generalized stiffness may precede the onset of arthritic complaints. The stiffness becomes more localized in the following weeks to months. Some patients report a history of a precipitating stressful event such as infection, work stress, physical exertion, childbirth, surgery, or emotional upset. However, researchers have been unable to correlate such events directly with the onset of RA.

Specific articular involvement is manifested clinically by pain, stiffness, limitation of motion, and signs of inflammation such

as heat, swelling, and tenderness (Arthritis Society, 2011d). Joint symptoms occur symmetrically and frequently affect the small joints of the hands (MCP, PIP, and MCP joints) and feet (MTP joints). Larger peripheral joints such as wrists, elbows, shoulders, knees, hips, ankles, and the jaw may also be involved. The cervical spine may be affected, but the axial spine is generally spared. In Table 67-6, the manifestations of RA and OA are compared.

Patients characteristically experience joint stiffness after periods of inactivity. Morning stiffness may last from 60 minutes to several hours or more, depending on disease activity. MCP and PIP joints are typically swollen. In early disease, the fingers may become spindle-shaped from synovial hypertrophy and thickening of the joint capsule (see Figure 67-3). Joints become tender, painful, and warm to the touch. Joint pain increases with motion, varies in intensity, and may not be proportional to the degree of inflammation. Tenosynovitis frequently affects the extensor and flexor tendons around the wrists, producing manifestations of carpal tunnel syndrome and making it difficult for patients to grasp objects.

As disease activity progresses, inflammation and fibrosis of the joint capsule and supporting structures may lead to deformity and disability. Atrophy of muscles and destruction of tendons around the joint cause one articular surface to slip past the other (*subluxation*). Typical distortions of the hand include ulnar drift ("zig-zag deformity"), swan-neck deformity, and boutonnière deformity (Figure 67-4). Subluxation of the metatarsal head and hallux valgus (bunion) in the feet may cause pain and walking disability.

Extra-articular Manifestations.

RA can affect nearly every system in the body. Extra-articular manifestations of RA are depicted in Figure 67-5. The three most common are rheumatoid nodules, Sjögren's syndrome, and Felty's syndrome.

Rheumatoid nodules develop in up to 25% of all patients with RA. Those affected with nodules usually have high titres of RF. Rheumatoid nodules appear subcutaneously as firm, nontender, granuloma types of masses and are usually over the extensor surfaces of joints such as fingers and elbows. Nodules at the base of the spine and the back of the head are common in older adults. Nodules develop insidiously and can persist or regress spontaneously. They are usually not removed because of the high probability of recurrence, but they can easily break down or become infected. Nodules that appear on the sclera or the lungs indicate active disease and a poorer prognosis.

Sjögren's syndrome occurs in 10 to 15% of patients with RA. Sjögren's syndrome can occur as a disease by itself or in conjunction with other arthritic disorders such as RA and systemic lupus erythematosus (SLE). Affected patients have diminished lacrimal and salivary gland secretion, which leads to burning, gritty, and itchy sensations in the eyes. These patients experience decreased tearing and photosensitivity.

Felty's syndrome occurs most commonly in patients with severe, nodule-forming RA. It is characterized by inflammatory eye disorders, splenomegaly, lymphadenopathy, pulmonary disease, and blood dyscrasias (anemia, thrombocytopenia, granulocytopenia).

Complications

Without treatment, joint destruction begins as early as the first year of the disease. Flexion contractures and hand deformities cause grasp strength to diminish and affect the patient's ability to perform self-care tasks. Nodular myositis and muscle fibre

Table 67-6 Comparison of Rheumatoid Arthritis and Osteoarthritis

PARAMETER	RHEUMATOID ARTHRITIS	OSTEOARTHRITIS
Age at onset	Any age but most common between 25-50 years	Usually >40 yr of age
Gender	Female-to-male ratio is 2:1 or 3:1; less marked gender difference after age 60	Before age 50, more men than women; after age 50, more women than men
Weight	Lost or maintained weight	Often overweight
Disease	Systemic disease with exacerbations and remissions	Localized disease with variable, progressive course
Affected joints	Small joints first (PIP, MCP, and MTP joints), wrists, elbows, shoulders, knees; usually bilateral, symmetrical	Weight-bearing joints (knees, hips); MCP, DIP, and PIP joints; cervical and lumbar spine; often asymmetrical
Pain characteristics	Stiffness lasts 1 hr to all day and may decrease with use; pain is variable, may disrupt sleep	Stiffness occurs on arising but usually subsides after 30 min; pain gradually worsens with joint use and time, lessens with rest
Effusions	Common	Uncommon
Nodules	Present, especially on extensor surfaces	Heberden's nodes (DIP joints) and Bouchard's nodes (PIP joints)
Synovial fluid	WBC count > 2 × 10⁹/L with mostly neutrophils	WBC count < 2 × 10⁹/L (mild leukocytosis)
Radiographs	Joint space narrowing, erosion, subluxation with advanced disease; osteoporosis related to corticosteroid use	Joint space narrowing, osteophytes, subchondral cysts, sclerosis
Laboratory findings	RF present in 80% of patients Elevated ESR and CRP level indicative of active inflammation	RF absent Transient elevation in ESR related to synovitis

CRP, C-reactive protein; *DIP*, distal interphalangeal; *ESR*, erythrocyte sedimentation rate; *MCP*, metacarpophalangeal; *MTP*, metatarsophalangeal; *PIP*, proximal interphalangeal; *RF*, rheumatoid factor; *WBC*, white blood cell.

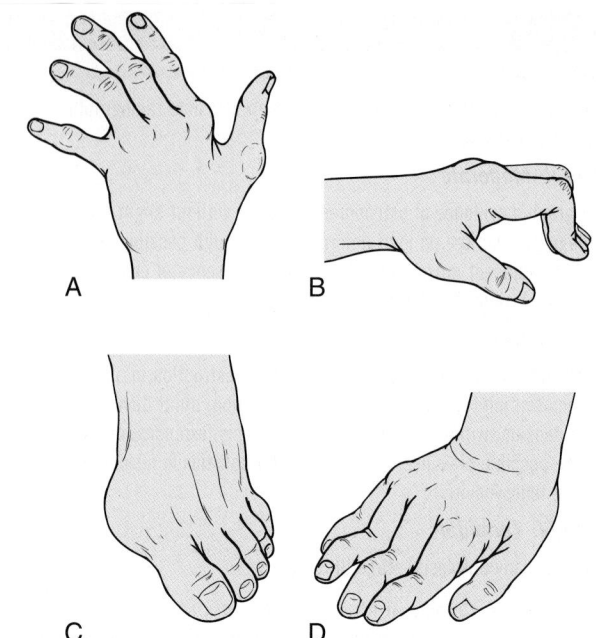

Figure 67-4 Typical deformities of rheumatoid arthritis. **A,** Ulnar drift. **B,** Boutonnière deformity. **C,** Hallux valgus. **D,** Swan-neck deformity.

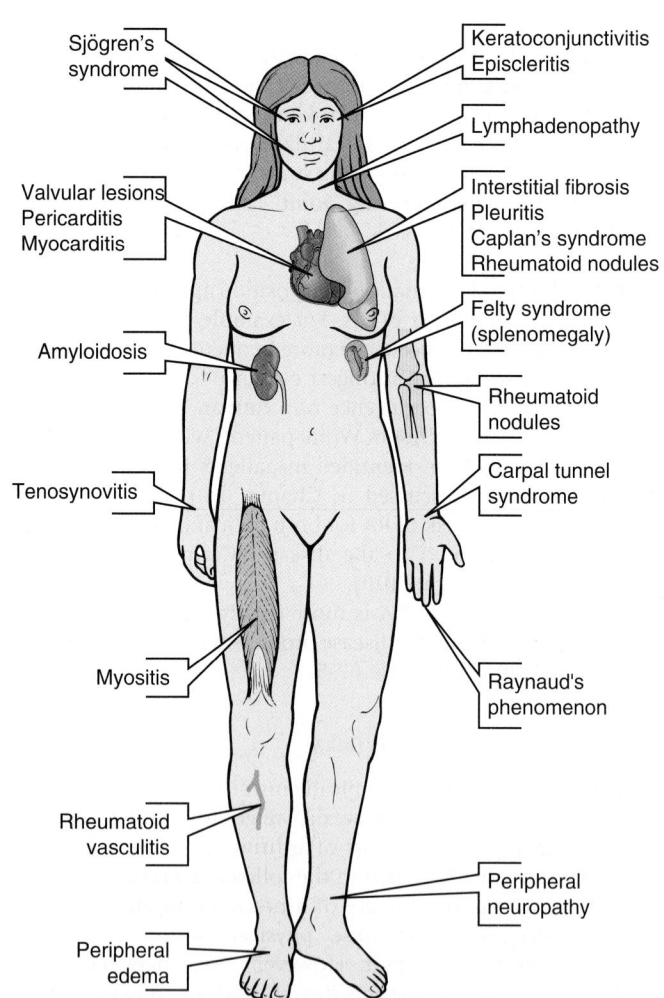

Figure 67-5 Extra-articular manifestations of rheumatoid arthritis.

degeneration can lead to pain similar to that of vascular insufficiency. Cataract development and loss of vision can result from scleral nodules. Complications can also result from rheumatoid nodules. On the skin, these nodules can ulcerate, similar to pressure ulcers. Nodules on the vocal cords lead to progressive hoarseness, and nodules in the vertebral bodies can cause bone destruction. In later disease, cardiopulmonary effects may occur. These may include pleurisy, pleural effusion, pericarditis, pericardial effusion, and cardiomyopathy. Carpal tunnel syndrome of the wrist can result from swelling of the synovial membrane, which causes pressure on the median nerve and results in pain.

Diagnostic Studies

An accurate diagnosis is essential to the initiation of appropriate treatment and the prevention of unnecessary disability. A diagnosis is often based on history and physical findings, but some laboratory tests are useful for confirmation and to monitor disease progression (see Table 67-6). RF is found in approximately 80% of affected patients, and titres rise during active disease. Elevations in ESR and C-reactive protein (CRP) levels are general indicators of active inflammation. Antinuclear antibody (ANA) titres are also present in some patients with RA. Antibodies to cyclic citrulline protein (anti-CCP) are showing important potential as a marker for the early detection of RA, as well as for prediction of the course of the disease (van Venrooij, van Beers, & Pruijn, 2011).

Synovial fluid analysis early in the course of the disease often reveals a straw-coloured fluid with many fibrin flecks. The enzyme MMP-3 is increased in the fluid of patients with RA and may be a marker of progressive damage. The white blood cell (WBC) count of synovial fluid is elevated (up to $25 \times 10^9/L$). Inflammatory changes in the synovium can be confirmed by tissue biopsy.

Radiological studies are not specifically diagnostic of RA. The findings may be inconclusive during early stages of the disease, revealing only soft tissue swelling and possible bone demineralization. In later stages of the disease, narrowing of the joint space, destruction of articular cartilage, erosion, subluxation, and deformity are seen. Malalignment and ankylosis are often evident in advanced disease. Baseline radiographs may be useful in monitoring disease progression and treatment effectiveness. Bone scans are more useful in detecting early joint changes and confirming a diagnosis so that RA treatment can be initiated. Criteria for the diagnosis of RA are described in Table 67-7.

Collaborative Care

Care of patients with RA begins with a comprehensive program of education and drug therapy. Education regarding drug therapy includes correct administration, reporting of adverse effects, and frequent medical and laboratory follow-up visits. Educate patients and caregivers about the disease process and home management strategies. NSAIDs are prescribed to promote physical comfort. Physiotherapy helps patients maintain joint motion and muscle strength. Occupational therapy develops upper extremity function and encourages joint protection through the use of splints or other assistive devices and strategies for activity pacing.

An individualized treatment plan accounts for the nature of the disease activity, joint function, age, sex, family and social roles, and response to previous treatment (Table 67-8). A caring, long-term relationship with an arthritis health care team can promote the patient's self-esteem and positive coping.

Table 67-7 The 2010 American College of Rheumatology/European League Against Rheumatism Classification Criteria for Rheumatoid Arthritis

CRITERION	SCORE
A. Joint Involvement	
1 large joint	0
2–10 large joints	1
1–3 small joints (with or without involvement of large joints)	2
4–10 small joints (with or without involvement of large joints)	3
>10 joints (at least 1 small joint)	5
B. Serology (at Least 1 Test Result is Needed for Classification)	
Negative RF and negative ACPA	0
Low-positive RF or low-positive ACPA	2
High-positive RF or high-positive ACPA	3
C. Acute-Phase Reactants (at Least 1 Test Result is Needed for Classification)	
Normal CRP and normal ESR	0
Abnormal CRP or abnormal ESR	1
D. Duration of Symptoms	
<6 weeks	0
≥6 weeks	1

Patients eligible for classification: at least one joint with definite clinical synovitis (swelling); no alternative diagnosis better explains the synovitis.

Classification criteria: Sum the scores for categories A through D. A score ≥ 6/10 classifies the patient as having definite RA.

Source: Aletaha, D., Neogi, T., Silman, A., Funovits, J., Felson, D. T., Bingham, C. O., ..., Hawker, G. (2010). 2010 rheumatoid arthritis classification criteria. *Arthritis and Rheumatism, 62*, 2569–2581. doi:10.1002/art.27584
ACPA, anticitrullinated peptide antibodies; *CRP,* C-reactive protein; *ESR,* erythrocyte sedimentation rate; *RF,* rheumatoid factor.

Drug Therapy. Drugs remain the cornerstone of RA treatment (see Table 67-3). Instead of administering high doses of aspirin or NSAIDs until radiographs show clear evidence of the disease, health care providers now aggressively prescribe disease-modifying antirheumatic drugs (DMARDs) with the knowledge that irreversible joint changes can occur as early as the first year of RA (Donahue et al., 2008). These drugs have the potential to lessen the permanent effects of RA, such as joint erosion and deformity. The choice of drug is based on disease activity, the patient's level of function, and lifestyle considerations, such as the desire to bear children.

Usually methotrexate is the drug of first choice. The rapid anti-inflammatory effect of methotrexate reduces clinical symptoms in days to weeks. It is inexpensive, and has a lower toxicity compared to other drugs. Adverse effects include bone marrow suppression and hepatotoxicity. Methotrexate therapy necessitates frequent laboratory monitoring, including CBC and chemistry panel. Sulphasalazine (Salazopyrin) and the antimalarial drug hydroxychloroquine (Plaquenil) may be effective DMARDs for mild to moderate disease. They are rapidly absorbed, relatively safe, and well tolerated. The synthetic DMARD leflunomide (Arava) blocks immune cell overproduction. Its efficacy is similar

COLLABORATIVE CARE

Table 67-8 Rheumatoid Arthritis

Diagnostic

- History and physical examination
- Laboratory studies
  - Complete blood cell (CBC) count
  - Erythrocyte sedimentation rate (ESR)
  - Rheumatoid factor (RF)
  - Antinuclear antibody (ANA)
  - C-reactive protein (CRP)
- Radiological studies of involved joints
- Analysis of synovial fluid

Collaborative Therapy

- Nutritional and weight management counselling
- Therapeutic exercise
- Rest, joint protection, and use of assistive devices

- Heat and cold applications
- Complementary and alternative therapies
  - Herbal products
  - Movement therapies
- Drug therapy*
  - Disease-modifying antirheumatic drugs (DMARDs)
  - Intra-articular or systemic corticosteroids
  - Nonsteroidal anti-inflammatory drugs (NSAIDs)
  - Biological or targeted therapy
- Reconstructive surgery
- Implants
- Arthroplasty

*See Table 67-3.

to that of methotrexate and sulphasalazine; adverse effects include hepatotoxicity, diarrhea, and teratogenesis. In women of childbearing age, pregnancy must be ruled out before therapy is initiated.

Biological or targeted drug therapies are also used to slow disease progression in RA. These drugs include etanercept (Enbrel), infliximab (Remicade), adalimumab (Humira), anakinra (Kineret) and abatacept (Orencia). They can be used to treat moderate to severe disease that has not responded to DMARDs or in combination therapy with an established DMARD such as methotrexate.

Etanercept is a biologically engineered (through recombinant DNA technology) copy of the TNF cell receptor. This soluble TNF receptor binds to TNF in circulation before TNF can bind to the cell surface receptor. By thus inhibiting binding of TNF, etanercept inhibits the inflammatory response. This drug is given in doses of 25 mg twice per week, or a once weekly dose of 50 mg in a subcutaneous injection.

Infliximab and adalimumab are monoclonal antibodies against TNF. They bind to TNF, thus preventing it from binding to TNF receptors on cells. Infliximab is given by intravenous (IV) route as an initial dose, followed by additional dosing at 2 and 6 weeks and then every 8 weeks thereafter. It should be given in combination with methotrexate. Adalimumab is administered subcutaneously every other week. If the response is inadequate, dosing can be increased to weekly.

Anakinra is a recombinant version of IL-1 receptor antagonist (IL-1Ra). It blocks the biological activity of IL-1 by competitively inhibiting the binding of IL-1 to the IL-1 receptor. It is given daily in a subcutaneous injection. Anakinra is used to reduce the pain and swelling associated with moderate to severe RA. It can be used in combination with DMARDs but not with TNF inhibitors. Concurrent use of anakinra and TNF inhibitors can cause serious infection and neutropenia.

Abatacept is recommended for patients who have an inadequate response to DMARDs or TNF inhibitors. Abatacept blocks T cell activation and is given by IV infusion. Like anakinra, it should not be used concomitantly with TNF inhibitors.

Rituximab (Rituxan) may be used in combination with methotrexate for patients with moderate to severe RA that does not respond to TNF antagonist therapies (e.g., etanercept, infliximab). This drug therapy is a monoclonal antibody that targets B cells. It is initially given in two IV infusions separated by 2 weeks.

Two newer TNF inhibitors, golimumab (Simponi) and certolizumab pegol (Cimzia), improve symptoms in patients with moderate to severe RA. Both drugs are given in combination with methotrexate. In comparison with other biological agents, certolizumab pegol stays in the system longer and may also produce a more rapid (1 to 2 weeks) and significant reduction in RA symptoms. This drug is also used to treat Crohn's disease.

Tocilizumab (Actemra) is a relatively new drug used to treat patients with moderate-to-severe RA who have not adequately responded to or cannot tolerate other approved drug classes for RA. This drug works by blocking the action of IL-6, a proinflammatory cytokine.

Additional drugs used infrequently for treating RA include antibiotics (minocycline), immunosuppressants (azathioprine [Imuran], D-penicillamine [Cuprimine]), and gold compounds (auranofin [Ridaura], gold sodium thiomalate [Myochrysine]).

Corticosteroid therapy can be used to aid in symptom control. Intra-articular injections may temporarily relieve the pain and inflammation associated with disease flare-ups. Long-term use of oral corticosteroids should not be a mainstay of RA treatment because of the risk of complications, including osteoporosis and avascular necrosis. However, low-dose prednisone may be used for a limited time with select patients to decrease disease activity until a DMARD effect is seen.

Various NSAIDs and salicylates continue to be included in the drug regimen to treat arthritis pain and inflammation. Aspirin is often used in high dosages of 4 to 6 g/day (12 to 18 tablets). Because enteric-coated aspirin is absorbed in the small intestine, it can be prescribed in higher doses than can regular tablets. The ability to measure serum salicylate levels is helpful in developing and evaluating individualized treatment plans.

NSAIDs have anti-inflammatory, analgesic, and antipyretic properties. Although many NSAIDs are potent inhibitors of inflammation, they do not appear to alter the natural history of RA. Some relief may be noted within days of the start of treatment with NSAIDs, but full effectiveness may take 2 to 3 weeks. NSAIDs may be used when patients cannot tolerate high doses of aspirin. Anti-inflammatory drugs that are taken only once or twice a day may improve the patient's ability to follow the treatment regimen (see Table 67-3). A newer generation of NSAIDs, the COX-2 inhibitors, are effective in RA as well as OA. Celecoxib (Celebrex) is currently the only available COX-2 inhibitor.

Nutritional Therapy. Although there is no special diet for RA, balanced nutrition is important. Fatigue, pain, depression, limited endurance, and mobility deficits often accompany RA and may cause a loss of appetite or interfere with the patient's ability to shop for and prepare food. Weight loss may result. An occupational therapist may help the patient modify the home environment and use assistive devices to make food preparation easier.

Corticosteroid therapy or immobility secondary to pain may result in unwanted weight gain. A sensible weight loss program, consisting of balanced nutrition and exercise, reduces stress on arthritic joints. Corticosteroids also increase the appetite, which results in a higher caloric intake. In addition, patients may become distressed as signs and symptoms of Cushing's syndrome—including moon facies and the redistribution of fatty tissue to the trunk—change the physical appearance. Patients must be encouraged to continue a balanced diet and not to alter the corticosteroid dose or stop therapy abruptly. Weight slowly adjusts to normal several months after cessation of therapy.

NURSING MANAGEMENT: RHEUMATOID ARTHRITIS

Nursing Assessment

Subjective and objective data that should be obtained from patients with RA are presented in Table 67-9.

Nursing Diagnoses

Nursing diagnoses for patients with RA may include, but are not limited to, those presented in Nursing Care Plan 67-1.

Planning

The overall goals are that patients with RA will (a) have satisfactory pain relief, (b) have minimal loss of functional ability of the affected joints, (c) participate in planning and following the therapeutic regimen, (d) maintain a positive self-image, and (e) perform self-care to the maximum extent possible.

Nursing Implementation

Health Promotion

RA cannot currently be prevented. However, community education programs should focus on symptom recognition to promote early diagnosis and treatment of RA. The Arthritis Society offers many publications, classes, and support activities (see the Resources at the end of this chapter).

Acute Intervention

The primary goals in the management of RA are reduction of inflammation, management of pain, maintenance of joint function, and prevention or correction of joint deformity. Goals may be met through a comprehensive program of drug therapy, rest, joint protection, heat and cold applications, exercise, and patient and caregiver teaching. The nurse works closely with other health care providers to restore function and to help patients make appropriate lifestyle adjustments to chronic illness.

The patient newly diagnosed with RA is usually treated on an outpatient basis, although hospitalization may be necessary for patients with extra-articular complications or advancing disease that necessitates reconstructive surgery for disabling deformities. Nursing intervention begins with a careful physical assessment (e.g., joint pain, swelling, range of motion [ROM], and general

NURSING ASSESSMENT

Table 67-9 Rheumatoid Arthritis
Subjective Data
Important Health Information
Past health history: Positive family history for rheumatoid arthritis or other autoimmune diseases; presence of precipitating factors such as emotional upset, infections, overwork, childbirth, surgery; pattern of remissions and exacerbations
Medications: Use of aspirin, NSAIDs, corticosteroids, DMARDs
Surgery or other treatments: Any joint surgery
Symptoms
• Symmetrical joint pain and aching that increases with motion or stress on joint; stiffness and joint swelling; muscle weakness, difficulty walking; paraesthesias of hands and feet; numbness, tingling, loss of sensation
• Dry mucous membranes of mouth and pharynx; anorexia, weight loss; fatigue, malaise
Objective Data
General
Lymphadenopathy, fever
Integumentary
Keratoconjunctivitis; subcutaneous rheumatoid nodules on forearm, elbows; skin ulcers; shiny, taut skin over involved joints; peripheral edema
Cardiovascular
Symmetrical pallor and cyanosis of fingers (Raynaud's phenomenon); distant heart sounds, murmurs, dysrhythmias
Respiratory
Chronic bronchitis, tuberculosis, histoplasmosis, fibrosing alveolitis
Gastrointestinal
Splenomegaly (Felty's syndrome)
Musculoskeletal
Symmetrical joint involvement with swelling, erythema, heat, tenderness, and deformities; enlargement of proximal phalangeal and metacarpophalangeal joints; limitation of joint movement; muscle contractures, muscle atrophy
Possible Findings
Positive rheumatoid factor, ↑ ESR, anemia; ↑ C-reactive protein level; ↑ WBC count in synovial fluid; evidence of joint space narrowing and of bone erosion and deformity on radiograph (osteoporosis with advanced disease)

DMARDs, disease-modifying antirheumatic drugs; *ESR,* erythrocyte sedimentation rate; *NSAIDs,* nonsteroidal anti-inflammatory drugs; *WBC,* white blood cell.

health status). The nurse must also evaluate psychosocial needs (e.g., family support, sexual satisfaction, emotional stress, financial constraints, vocational and career limitations) and environmental concerns (e.g., transportation, home or work modifications). After problem identification, a carefully planned program for rehabilitation and education can be coordinated by the nurse for the interdisciplinary health care team.

Suppression of inflammation is achieved most effectively through the administration of NSAIDs, DMARDs, and biological and targeted therapies. Careful attention to timing is crucial for

NURSING CARE PLAN 67-1

Rheumatoid Arthritis

NURSING DIAGNOSIS	**_Chronic pain_** _related to_ joint inflammation, overuse of joint, and ineffective pain or comfort measures _as evidenced by_ (a) communication of pain descriptors, guarding behaviour, and limited joint function and (b) hot, swollen, or painful joints.
Expected Patient Outcomes	**Nursing Interventions and _Rationales_**

- Uses analgesics and nonanalgesic relief measures effectively
- Verbalizes satisfactory pain management

Pain management

- Perform a comprehensive assessment of pain to include location, characteristics, onset and duration, frequency, quality, and intensity or severity of pain and precipitating factors _to establish a pattern and baseline assessment and to plan appropriate interventions._
- Evaluate, with the patient, the family, and the health care team, the effectiveness of past pain control measures that have been used _to assess what has helped and not helped in the past._
- Reduce or eliminate factors that precipitate or increase the pain experience (e.g., fear, fatigue, and lack of knowledge) _to minimize negative stimuli that may increase pain._
- Teach use of nonpharmacological techniques (e.g., relaxation, distraction, hot and cold applications, and massage) before pain occurs or increases _to promote muscle relaxation and decrease tension._
- Provide the patient with optimal pain relief with prescribed analgesics as appropriate _to help decrease pain and inflammation._

NURSING DIAGNOSIS	**_Impaired physical mobility_** _related to_ joint pain, stiffness, and deformity _as evidenced by_ limitation of joint motion, strength and endurance, and inability to perform routine ADLs
Expected Patient Outcomes	**Nursing Interventions and _Rationales_**

- Performs prescribed joint exercises to maintain and improve joint function
- Uses joint protection measures to prevent increased joint inflammation

Exercise therapy: joint mobility

- Determine limitations of joint movement and effect on function _to establish baseline for plan of care._
- Collaborate with physiotherapists in developing and executing an exercise program _to maintain and improve joint function._
- Explain to patient and family the purpose and plan for joint exercises _to provide information and support for patient._
- Initiate pain-control measures (e.g., hot packs, warm shower) before joint exercises begin _to relieve stiffness and increase mobility._
- Assist patient into optimal body position for passive and active joint movement (e.g., with correct application of resting splints, selection of properly fitting footwear, and selection and use of assistive devices) _to prevent or limit joint deformity._

NURSING DIAGNOSIS	**_Disturbed body image_** _related to_ chronic disease activity, long-term treatment, deformities, stiffness, and inability to perform usual activities _as evidenced by_ social withdrawal, flat affect, and altered self-concept
Expected Patient Outcomes	**Nursing Interventions and _Rationales_**

- Discusses feelings about and the meaning of changes in physical appearance
- Verbalizes acceptance of body appearance and function

Body image enhancement

- Identify the effects of the patient's culture, religion, race, gender, and age in terms of body image _to determine extent of problems and plan appropriate interventions._
- Assist patient in discussing changes caused by illness or surgery, as appropriate, _to identify problems and plan appropriate interventions._
- Assist patient in separating feelings about physical appearance from feelings of personal worth _so that a positive body image is fostered despite physical manifestations._
- Facilitate contact with individuals with similar changes in body image _to promote sharing and socialization for patient._

ADLs, activities of daily living.

NURSING CARE PLAN 67-1

Rheumatoid Arthritis—cont'd

NURSING DIAGNOSIS	*Ineffective self-health management* related to complexity of chronic health problem, sense of powerlessness, pain, and decisional conflicts *as evidenced by* questioning management plan, self-doubt about ability to manage disease, and ability to perform activities for only short periods.
Expected Patient Outcomes	**Nursing Interventions and *Rationales***

- Participates in planning and following therapeutic regimen
- Expresses confidence in ability to make treatment decisions

Anticipatory guidance

- Determine the patient's usual method of problem solving *to identify focus of interventions.*
- Provide information on realistic expectations related to patient's behaviour and illness *to ensure correct understanding of disease management.*
- Assist patient in anticipating role changes *to ensure that the patient can adapt to effects of the disease.*
- Refer patient to community agencies (e.g., Meals on Wheels, the Arthritis Society) *to enable patient to meet desired outcomes.*
- Include family and significant others in planning *to increase their sense of involvement and to increase patient's sense of support.*

Pain management

- Determine effects of pain experience on quality of life (e.g., sleep, appetite, activity, cognition, mood, relationships, performance of job, and role responsibilities) *because these are major deterrents to successful disease management and must be addressed.*
- Inform other health care providers/family members about nonpharmacological strategies being used by the patient *to encourage preventive approaches to pain management.*

NURSING DIAGNOSIS	*Self-care (bathing, dressing, feeding, toileting) deficits* related to disease progression, weakness, and contracture *as evidenced by* inability to perform ADLs
Expected Patient Outcomes	**Nursing Interventions and *Rationales***

- Performs ADLs to the maximum extent possible
- Determines when assistance is needed for performance of ADLs

Self-care assistance

- Monitor patient's ability for independent self-care *to plan appropriate interventions.*
- Monitor patient's need for adaptive devices for personal hygiene, dressing, grooming, toileting, and eating *to compensate for contractures and weakness so that patient can perform as many self-care activities as possible.*
- Establish a routine for self-care activities *to foster maximum independence.*
- Assist patient in accepting dependency needs *to ensure that all needs are met.*
- Teach caregivers to encourage independence and to intervene only when the patient is unable to perform ADLs *to promote independence.*

sustaining a therapeutic drug level and reducing early morning stiffness. The nurse should discuss the action and adverse effects of each prescribed drug and the importance of necessary laboratory monitoring. Many patients with RA take several different drugs, and the nurse must make the drug regimen as understandable as possible.

Nonpharmacological relief of pain may include the use of therapeutic heat and cold, rest, relaxation techniques, joint protection (Table 67-10; see also Table 67-4), biofeedback (see Chapter 12), transcutaneous electrical nerve stimulation (TENS; see Chapter 10), and hypnosis. Assessment for individual differences and preferences allows the nurse to help the patient and family choose therapies that promote optimal comfort within the parameters of their lifestyle.

Lightweight splints may be prescribed to rest an inflamed joint and prevent deformity from muscle spasms and contractures. Splints should be removed at regular intervals to give skin care and perform ROM exercises. After assessment has been completed and supportive care has been given, the splints should be reapplied as prescribed. The occupational therapist may help identify additional self-help devices that can assist in ADLs.

Care and procedures should be scheduled around the patient's morning stiffness. Sitting or standing in a warm shower, sitting in a tub with warm towels around the shoulders, or simply soaking the hands in a basin of warm water may help relieve joint stiffness and allow the patient to more comfortably perform ADLs. Gentle skin care should be offered, particularly if a patient is confined to bed.

Table 67-10 Protection of Small Joints

1. Maintain joint in neutral position to minimize deformity.
   - Press water from a sponge instead of wringing.
2. Use strongest joint available for any task.
   - When rising from chair, push with palms rather than fingers.
   - Carry laundry basket in both arms rather than with fingers.
3. Distribute weight over many joints instead of stressing a few.
   - Slide objects instead of lifting them.
   - Hold packages close to body for support.
4. Change positions frequently.
   - Do not hold a book or grip a steering wheel for long periods without resting.
   - Avoid grasping pencils or cutting vegetables with a knife for extended periods.
5. Avoid repetitious movements.
   - Do not knit for long periods.
   - Rest between rooms when vacuuming.
   - Modify home environment to include faucets and doorknobs that are pushed rather than turned.
6. Modify chores to avoid stress on joints.
   - Avoid heavy lifting.
   - Sit on stool instead of standing during meal preparation.

Ambulatory and Home Care

Rest. Alternating scheduled rest periods with activity throughout the day helps relieve fatigue and pain. The amount of rest needed varies according to the severity of the disease and the patient's limitations. Patients should rest before becoming exhausted. Total bed rest is rarely necessary and should be avoided, to prevent stiffness and immobility. However, even a patient with mild disease may require daytime rest in addition to 8 to 10 hours of sleep at night. The nurse should help patients identify ways to modify daily activities to avoid overexertion that can lead to fatigue and an exacerbation of disease activity. For example, a patient may tolerate meal preparation more easily while sitting on a high stool in front of the sink, rather than while standing. Patients should be assisted in pacing activities and setting priorities on the basis of realistic goals.

Good body alignment during rest can be maintained through use of a firm mattress or bed board. Positions of extension should be encouraged, and positions of flexion should be avoided. Splints and casts may be helpful in maintaining proper alignment and promoting rest, especially when joint inflammation is present. Lying prone for half an hour twice daily is also recommended. To decrease the risk of joint contracture, pillows should never be placed under the knees. A small, flat pillow may be used under the head and shoulders.

Joint Protection. Protecting joints from stress is important. The nurse can help patients to identify ways to modify tasks to put less stress on joints during routine activities (see Table 67-10). Energy conservation requires careful planning. The emphasis is on work simplification techniques. Work should be done in short periods with scheduled rest breaks to avoid fatigue (pacing). Work should be spread throughout the week rather than attempted at one time. Activities should be carefully organized to

avoid going up and down stairs repeatedly. Carts should be used to carry supplies, and items that are used often should be stored in a convenient, easily reached area. Time-saving joint protective devices (e.g., electric can opener) should be used whenever possible. Tasks can also be delegated to other family members.

The patient's independence may be increased by occupational therapy training with assistive devices that help simplify tasks, such as built-up utensils, buttonhooks, modified drawer handles, lightweight plastic dishes, and raised toilet seats. Wearing shoes with Velcro fasteners and clothing with snaps or a zipper down the front makes dressing easier. A cane or a walker offers support and relief of pain when walking. A platform-wheeled walker further minimizes strain on the small joints of the hands and wrists.

Heat and Cold Therapy and Exercise. Heat and cold applications can help relieve stiffness, pain, and muscle spasm. Application of ice is especially beneficial during periods of disease exacerbation, whereas moist heat appears to offer better relief of chronic stiffness. The treatment modality should be selected according to disease severity, ease of application, and cost. Superficial heat sources such as heating pads, moist hot packs, paraffin baths, whirlpool baths, and warm baths or showers can relieve stiffness to allow participation in therapeutic exercises. Plastic bags of frozen vegetables (peas or corn), which can easily mould around the shoulder, wrists, or knees, are an easy home treatment. Patients can also use ice cubes or small paper cups of frozen water to massage proximally or distally to a painful joint. Heat and cold can be used as often as desired; however, the heat application should not exceed 20 minutes at one time, and the cold application should not exceed 10 to 15 minutes at one time. The nurse should alert patients to the possibility of a burn and to avoid the use of a heat-producing cream (e.g., capsaicin) with another external heat device.

Individualized exercise is an integral part of the treatment plan (Hurkmans, van der Giesen, Vliet Vlieland, Schoones, & Van den Ende, 2009). Therapeutic exercise programs, usually developed by physiotherapists, include exercises that improve flexibility, strength, and overall endurance. The nurse should reinforce program participation and ensure that the exercises are being performed correctly. Inadequate joint movement can result in progressive joint immobility and muscle weakness, and overaggressive exercise can result in increased pain, inflammation, and joint damage. Emphasize that participating in a recreational exercise program (e.g., walking, swimming) or performing usual daily activities does not eliminate the patient's need for therapeutic exercise to maintain adequate joint motion.

Gentle ROM exercises are usually performed daily to keep the joints functional. Patients should have the opportunity to practise the exercises with supervision. Careful adherence to the prescribed exercise program should be a prime goal of the teaching program. Aquatic exercises in warm water ($25\,°C$ to $30\,°C$) allow easier joint movement because of the buoyancy of the water. At the same time, although movement seems easier, water provides two-way resistance that makes muscles work harder than they would in the air. Aerobic conditioning programs have been shown to improve the physical fitness levels of patients with RA. During acute inflammation, exercise should be limited to one or two repetitions.

Psychological Support. Self-management and adherence to an individualized home treatment program can be accomplished only if the patient has a thorough understanding of RA, the nature and course of the disease, and the goals of therapy. In addition, the patient's value system and perception of the disease must be considered. The patient is constantly challenged by problems of limited function and fatigue, loss of self-esteem, altered body image, and fear of disability and deformity. Discuss alterations in sexuality. Because of chronic pain or loss of function, patients may be vulnerable to injury from unproven or even dangerous remedies through the claims of false advertising. The nurse can help patients recognize fears and concerns that are faced by all people who live with chronic illness.

Evaluation of the family support system is important. Financial planning may be necessary. Community resources such as a home care nurse, homemaker services, and vocational rehabilitation may be considered. Self-help groups are beneficial for some patients.

AGE-RELATED CONSIDERATIONS: ARTHRITIS

The prevalence of arthritis among older adults is high, and the disease is accompanied by problems unique to this age group. The most problematic areas related to connective tissue disease in older adults include the following:

1. Because of the high incidence of OA expected in older adults, health care providers often do not consider the presence of other types of arthritis.
2. Age alone causes changes in serological profiles, which makes interpretation of laboratory values such as RF and ESR more difficult.
3. Polypharmacy in older adults can result in iatrogenic arthritis.
4. Nonorganic musculoskeletal pain syndromes and weakness may be related to depression and physical inactivity.
5. Diseases such as SLE, which commonly occurs in younger adults, can develop in a milder form in older adults.

Aging brings many physical and metabolic changes that may increase older patients' sensitivity to both the therapeutic and the toxic effects of some drugs. The use of NSAIDs with a shorter half-life may necessitate more frequent dosing but may also produce fewer adverse effects in older patients with altered drug metabolism. Older adults who take NSAIDs have an increased risk for adverse effects, particularly GI bleeding and renal toxicity. Because polypharmacy is common among older adults, the addition of drugs for RA treatment is particularly problematic because of the increased likelihood of untoward drug interactions. The drug regimen should be simplified as much as possible to increase older patients' adherence to the regimen (e.g., limited number of drugs with decreased frequency of administration), particularly for patients without regular assistance.

A major concern of treatment in the older patient relates to the use of corticosteroid therapy. Corticosteroid-induced osteopenia can add to the problem of decreased bone density related to age and inactivity. It can also increase the occurrence of pathological fractures, especially compression fractures of vertebrae. Corticosteroid-induced myopathy can be minimized or prevented by an age-appropriate exercise program. Although social networks are important for all age groups, an adequate support system for older adults is a critical factor in their ability to follow a treatment regimen that includes nutritional planning, exercise, general health maintenance, and appropriate pharmacotherapy.

Spondyloarthropathies

The *spondyloarthropathies* are a group of interrelated multisystem inflammatory disorders that affect the spine, the peripheral joints, and periarticular structures. The presence of RF is not a hallmark of these disorders; thus they are often referred to as *seronegative arthropathies*. Inheritance of HLA-B27 is strongly associated with occurrence of these diseases. Both genetic and environmental factors play a role in the development of this group of diseases, which includes ankylosing spondylitis, psoriatic arthritis, and reactive arthritis. (HLAs and their relationship to autoimmune diseases are discussed in Chapter 16.) The spondyloarthropathies share clinical and laboratory characteristics that make it difficult to distinguish among them in early stages of disease. According to the European Spondyloarthropathy Study Group criteria, a spondyloarthropathy is diagnosed when inflammatory spinal pain or asymmetrical synovitis is accompanied by one or more of the following: (a) episodes of alternating buttock pain; (b) radiographic evidence of sacroiliitis; (c) heel enthesopathy (e.g., plantar fasciitis, Achilles tendinitis); (d) positive family history of spondyloarthropathy in a first-degree relative; (e) current or documented history of psoriasis; (f) current or documented history of inflammatory bowel disease; and (g) urethritis, cervicitis, or acute diarrhea that occurred within the month preceding onset of arthritic symptoms (Davis & Mease, 2007; Dougados & Baeten, 2011).

Ankylosing Spondylitis

Ankylosing spondylitis (AS) is a chronic inflammatory disease that affects primarily the axial skeleton, including the sacroiliac joints, the intervertebral disc spaces, and the costovertebral articulations. As many as 150,000 to 300,000 Canadians are affected by AS (Arthritis Society, 2011a). The usual age at onset is 15 to 30 years, and three times more men than women develop AS (Arthritis Society, 2011a).

Etiology and Pathophysiology

The cause of AS is unknown. Genetic predisposition appears to play an important role in the disease pathogenesis, but the precise mechanisms are unknown. The HLA-B27 antigen is found in approximately 90% of people with AS. Individuals with the antigen have a 20 times greater risk of developing a spondyloarthropathy than do those who do not have the HLA-B27 antigen (Arthritis Society, 2011a). Aseptic synovial inflammation in joints and adjacent tissue causes the formation of granulation tissue *(pannus)* and the development of dense fibrous scars that lead to fusion of articular tissues. Extra-articular inflammation can affect the eyes, the lungs, the heart, the kidneys, and the peripheral nervous system.

Clinical Manifestations and Complications

AS is characterized by symmetrical sacroiliitis and progressive inflammatory arthritis of the axial skeleton. Symptoms of inflammatory spine pain are the first clues to the diagnosis. Affected patients typically complain of low back pain, stiffness, and limitation of motion that is worse during the night and in the morning but improves with mild activity. In affected women, early symptoms of disease may be pain and stiffness in the neck

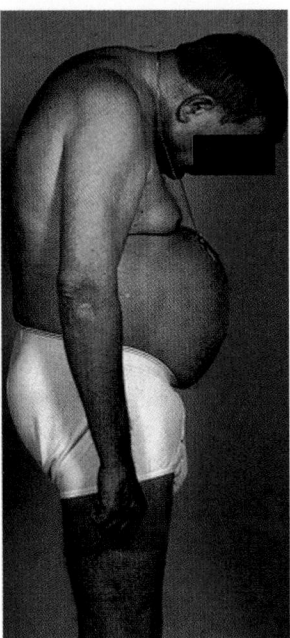

Figure 67-6 Advanced ankylosing spondylitis. Kyphotic posture causes many patients to have a protuberant abdomen secondary to pulmonary restriction.

Source: Kim, D. H., Henn, J., Vaccaro, A. R., & Dickman, C. A. (Eds.). (2006). *Surgical anatomy and techniques to the spine*. Philadelphia: W. B. Saunders.

rather than the lower back. General symptoms such as fever, fatigue, anorexia, and weight loss are rare. Uveitis (intraocular inflammation) is the most common nonskeletal symptom. It can appear as an initial manifestation of the disease years before arthritic symptoms develop. Patients with AS may also experience chest pain and sternal or costal cartilage tenderness that can be distressing.

Severe postural abnormalities and deformity can lead to significant disability for patients with AS (Figure 67-6). Impaired spinal ROM and fixed kyphosis contribute to altered visual function, which raises concerns about safe ambulation. Aortic insufficiency and pulmonary fibrosis are frequent complications. Cauda equine syndrome can also result, contributing to lower extremity weakness and bladder dysfunction. In addition, affected patients are at risk for spinal fracture because of osteoporosis.

Diagnostic Studies

Radiological studies are essential for the diagnosis of AS. Spinal views are seldom useful in initial diagnosis. Instead, pelvic views demonstrate characteristic changes of sacroiliitis that range from subtle erosion to completely fused joints in which joint spaces have been obliterated. Changes on later spinal radiographs include the appearance of "bamboo spine," which is caused by calcifications *(syndesmophytes)* that bridge from one vertebra to another. Laboratory testing is not specific, but ESR may be elevated and mild anemia may be present. When the suspicion of AS is high, the presence of HLA-B27 antigen heightens the likelihood of this diagnosis.

Collaborative Care

AS cannot be prevented. However, families with other diagnosed HLA-B27–positive rheumatic diseases (e.g., acute anterior uveitis, juvenile spondyloarthritis) should be alert to signs of low back pain for early identification and treatment of AS (see the Genetics in Clinical Practice box on ankylosing spondylitis).

Care of the patient with AS is aimed at maintaining maximal skeletal mobility while decreasing pain and inflammation. Heat applications can help in the relief of local symptoms. NSAIDs and salicylates are commonly prescribed. DMARDs such as sulphasalazine (Salazopyrin) or methotrexate have little effect on spinal disease but may be helpful with peripheral joint disease. Local corticosteroid injections may be beneficial in relieving symptoms. Etanercept (Enbrel), a biological/targeted therapy drug, binds TNF and inhibits its action. Levels of TNF, which promotes inflammation, are elevated in the blood and certain tissues of patients with AS. Etanercept has been shown to reduce active inflammation and improve spinal mobility (Widberg, Karimi, & Hafstrom, 2009).

Once pain and stiffness are managed, exercise is essential. Postural control is important for minimizing spinal deformity. The exercise regimen should include back, neck, and chest stretches. Hydrotherapy has also been shown to decrease pain and facilitate spinal extension. Surgery may be indicated for severe deformity and mobility impairment. Spinal osteotomy and total joint replacement are the most commonly performed procedures (see Chapter 65).

NURSING MANAGEMENT: ANKYLOSING SPONDYLITIS

The key nursing responsibility for patients with AS is education about the disease and principles of therapy. The home management program should include regular exercise and attention to posture, local moist heat applications, and knowledgeable use of drugs.

The nurse's baseline ROM assessment should include chest expansion (through breathing exercises). Smoking cessation must be encouraged to decrease the risk for lung complications in patients with reduced chest expansion. Ongoing physiotherapy should include gentle, graded stretching and strengthening exercises to preserve ROM and improve thoracolumbar flexion and extension. The nurse should discourage excessive physical exertion during flare-ups of the disease. Proper positioning at rest is essential. The mattress should be firm, and patients should sleep on the back with a flat pillow, avoiding positions that encourage flexion deformity. Postural training emphasizes avoiding spinal flexion (e.g., leaning over a desk); heavy lifting; and prolonged walking, standing, or sitting. Participation in sports that facilitate natural stretching, such as swimming and racquet games, should be encouraged. Family counselling and vocational rehabilitation are important.

Psoriatic Arthritis

Psoriasis is a common benign, inflammatory skin disorder that appears to have a genetic predisposition (see Chapter 26). Approximately 10 to 30% of people with psoriasis develop psoriatic arthritis (PsA) (Arthritis Society, 2011e). PsA is now recognized as a progressive inflammatory disease that can cause significant disability. The exact cause of PsA is unknown, but a combination of immune, genetic, and environmental factors is suspected. PsA can occur in five forms (National Psoriasis Foundation, 2012):

- Distal interphalangeal predominant arthritis that involves primarily the small joints of the hands and feet
- Asymmetric arthritis that involves few or many joints of the extremities but does not occur in the same joints on both sides of the body
- Symmetric arthritis that resembles RA; affects the same joints on both sides of the body but milder with less deformity than RA
- Spondylitis or inflammation of the spinal column
- Arthritis mutilans, a rare but very deforming and destructive disease that affects the small joints of the hands and feet.

On radiographs, the cartilage loss and erosion resemble those of RA. Many patients with advanced cases of PsA have widened joint spaces, and a "pencil-in-cup" deformity is common at the DIP joints as a result of osteolysis. Elevated ESR, mild anemia, and elevated blood uric acid levels are present in some patients; therefore, gout must be ruled out. Treatment includes splinting, joint protection, and physiotherapy. Intramuscular gold therapy was used to treat PsA in the past with some success but has been replaced by newer DMARDs such as methotrexate, which are effective for both cutaneous and articular manifestations. Sulphasalazine (Salazopyrin) and cyclosporine have also been used with some success in treating PsA. Biological therapy drugs including etanercept, adalimumab, and infliximab, are also being used for the treatment of PsA (Arthritis Society, 2011e).

Reactive Arthritis

Reactive arthritis *(Reiter's syndrome)* more commonly occurs in young men than in young women. The symptom complex includes urethritis, conjunctivitis, and mucocutaneous lesions. In women, symptoms include cervicitis. Although the exact etiology is unknown, reactive arthritis appears to occur after a genitourinary or GI tract infection (Carter & Hudson, 2009). *Chlamydia trachomatis* is most often implicated in sexually transmitted reactive arthritis. Men and women appear to have equal risk for developing dysenteric reactive arthritis, which typically occurs within days or weeks after infection with *Shigella, Salmonella, Campylobacter,* or *Yersinia* organisms. Individuals with inherited HLA-B27 antigen are at increased risk of developing reactive arthritis after sexual contact or exposure to certain enteric pathogens, which supports the likelihood of a genetic predisposition.

Urethritis develops within 1 to 2 weeks after sexual contact or dysentery. Low-grade fever, conjunctivitis, and arthritis may occur over the next several weeks. This type of arthritis tends to be asymmetrical, frequently involving the large joints of the lower extremities and the toes. Lower back pain may occur with severe disease. Mucocutaneous lesions commonly manifest as small, painless, superficial ulcerations on the tongue, the oral mucosa, and the glans penis. Soft-tissue manifestations commonly include enthesopathies such as Achilles tendinitis or plantar fasciitis. Few laboratory findings are abnormal, although the ESR may be elevated.

Prognosis is favourable; most patients recover after 2 to 16 weeks. Because reactive arthritis is often associated with *C. trachomatis* infection, treatment of patients and their sexual partners with doxycycline (Vibramycin), 100 mg twice daily for up to 3 months, is widely recommended. Conjunctivitis and lesions necessitate no treatment, but topical ophthalmic corticosteroids are typically prescribed for treatment of uveitis. Physiotherapy may be helpful during disease recovery.

Joints heal completely, and many patients have complete remission with full joint function. Up to 50% may develop chronic or recurring disease, which can result in major disability. Radiographic changes in chronic disease closely resemble those of AS. Treatment of chronic reactive arthritis is based on symptoms.

Septic Arthritis

Septic arthritis (infectious or bacterial arthritis) is an invasion of the joint cavity with microorganisms. Bacteria can travel through the bloodstream from another site of active infection and hematogenously seed the joint. Organisms can also be introduced directly through trauma or surgical incision. Any bacterium can cause the infection. In immunocompromised patients, even nonpathogenic bacteria can be responsible for development of septic arthritis. *Staphylococcus aureus* is the most common causative organism. *Streptococcus hemolyticus* is also seen. *Neisseria gonorrhoeae* is the most common cause in sexually active young adults. Factors that increase the risk of infection include diseases in which host resistance is decreased, such as leukemia and diabetes mellitus; treatment with corticosteroids or immunosuppressive drugs; and debilitating chronic illness.

Large joints such as the knee and the hip are most frequently involved. Inflammation of the joint cavity causes severe pain, erythema, and swelling. Because infection has often spread from a primary site elsewhere in the body, fever or shaking chills often accompany articular manifestations. Aspiration of the joint (arthrocentesis) and culture of the synovial fluid enables precise diagnosis (Mathews & Coakley, 2008). Blood cultures for aerobic and anaerobic organisms should also be obtained.

Septic arthritis necessitates prompt treatment to prevent joint destruction. Broad-spectrum antibiotics against Gram-negative organisms, pneumococci, and staphylococci are often started before the causative organism is identified. Once the organism is determined, the treatment can become specific. Infections may respond to treatment within 2 weeks or may take as long as 4 to 8 weeks, depending on the causative organism. Local aspiration and surgical drainage may be required. If diagnosis and treatment are delayed, destruction of articular cartilage can occur, followed by loss of joint function. Chronic infection can also develop. Septic arthritis of the hip can contribute to development of avascular necrosis (Chen, Wang, & Juhn, 2008).

Nursing intervention includes assessment and monitoring of joint inflammation, pain, and fever. To achieve immobilization of affected joints to control pain, resting splints or traction should be used. Local hot compresses can also help relieve pain. Gentle ROM exercises should be initiated as soon as tolerated to prevent muscle atrophy and joint contractures. The nurse should explain the need for antibiotics and the importance of their continued use until the infection is resolved. The nurse should offer support to a patient who requires arthrocentesis or operative drainage. Strict aseptic technique should be used in assisting with joint aspiration procedures.

Lyme Disease

Lyme disease is a spirochetal infection caused by *Borrelia burgdorferi* and transmitted by the bite of an infected deer tick. It was first identified in 1975 in Lyme, Connecticut, after an unusual clustering of arthritis in children and is now most common in the northeast and north central regions of North America (Arthritis Society, 2011a). The tick typically feeds on mice, dogs, cats, cows, horses, deer, and humans. Wild animals do not exhibit the illness, but clinical Lyme disease does occur in domestic animals. Person-to-person transmission does not occur. The peak season for infection in humans is summer. The exact number of Canadians with Lyme disease is not known. Ontario has had the largest number of confirmed cases, whereas Newfoundland, Prince Edward Island, the Yukon, and the Northwest Territories have had no confirmed cases (Arthritis Society, 2011f).

Symptoms of Lyme disease can mimic those of other diseases, such as multiple sclerosis, mononucleosis, and meningitis. The most characteristic clinical symptom of early localized disease is erythema migrans (EM), a skin lesion that occurs at the site of the tick bite within 2 to 30 days after exposure (Figure 67-7). The lesion begins as a red macule or papule that slowly expands to form a large round lesion with a bright red border and central clearing. The EM lesion is often accompanied by acute virus-like symptoms, such as fever, chills, headache, stiff neck, fatigue, swollen lymph nodes, and migratory joint and muscle pain. Symptoms usually occur within a week but may be delayed for up to 30 days.

If not treated, the spirochete can disseminate within several weeks or months to the heart, joints, and central nervous system

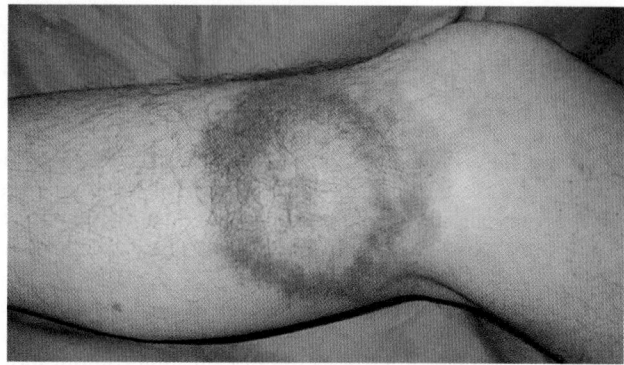

Figure 67-7 Erythema migrans of Lyme disease.

Source: Swartz, M. H. (2010). *Textbook of physical diagnosis: History and examination* (6th ed., p. 186, Figure 8-112). Philadelphia: W. B. Saunders.

(CNS). Carditis may occur with chronic arthritic pain and swelling in the large joints. Nervous system problems may include severe headaches, temporary facial paralysis (e.g., Bell's palsy), or poor motor coordination. One neurological condition, tertiary neuroborreliosis, results in confusion and forgetfulness.

A diagnosis of Lyme disease is often based on clinical manifestations, particularly the EM lesion, and a history of exposure in an endemic area. CBC count and ESR are usually normal. A two-step laboratory testing process is recommended to confirm diagnosis. The first step is the enzyme-linked immunoassay (ELISA), a test that yields positive results for most people with Lyme disease. If the ELISA result is positive or not conclusive, a Western blot test confirms the infection. Cerebrospinal fluid should be examined in individuals with neurological involvement.

Active lesions can be treated with oral antibiotic therapy. Doxycycline (Vibramycin), cefuroxime (Ceftin), and amoxicillin are often effective in early stages of infection and in prevention of later stages of the disease. Doxycycline has also been shown to be very effective in preventing Lyme disease when given within 3 days after the bite of a deer tick. Short-term therapy for 2 to 3 weeks is usually effective for solitary EM, but long-standing infection may necessitate extended parenteral antibiotic therapy. Intravenous ceftriaxone is prescribed for severe cardiac or neurological abnormalities. In most cases, Lyme disease is treated successfully with antibiotics (Girschick, Morbach, & Tappe, 2009).

Reducing exposure to ticks is the best way to prevent Lyme disease. Teaching of patients and caregivers who live in endemic areas is outlined in Table 67-11. Tick bites are discussed in Chapter 71. When teaching patients and caregivers living in endemic areas, the nurse should include instructions for removing ticks (see Chapter 71, Figure 71-5).

HIV-Associated Rheumatic Disease

A variety of rheumatic disorders can develop in the course of human immunodeficiency virus (HIV) infection (Shah, Flanigan, & Lally, 2011). The cause of these disorders in HIV-infected persons is not clearly known. However, an autoimmune process and an inflammatory response may be occurring at the same time in a patient who is immunosuppressed. Up to 70% of HIV-infected patients may develop a rheumatic disease in the later stages of HIV infection. Rheumatic diseases associated with HLA-B27 appear to be more severe in HIV-infected patients.

Table 67-11 Prevention and Early Treatment of Lyme Disease

The nurse should include the following instructions when teaching patients to prevent Lyme disease:

- Avoid wooded and bushy areas with high grass and leaf litter.
- Walk in the centre of trails.
- Wear long pants or nylon tights of tightly woven, light-coloured fabric so that ticks can be easily seen.
- Tuck pants into boots or long socks, tuck long-sleeved shirts into pants, and wear closed shoes when hiking.
- Check often for ticks crawling from pant legs to open skin.
- Bathe or shower as soon as possible after coming indoors, to wash off and more easily find ticks.
- Thoroughly inspect and wash clothes.
- Spray insect repellent containing DEET on skin or apply permethrin to boots and clothes, (especially on lower extremities) and camping gear.
- Have pets wear tick collars, inspect them often, and do not allow pets on furniture or beds.
- Clear tall grasses and brush around homes and at the edge of lawns.
- Place a 1-m–wide barrier of wood chips or gravel between lawns and wooded areas and around patios and play equipment.
- Mow the lawn frequently, keep leaves raked, and stack wood neatly in a dry area.
- See a physician if a rash or fever develops within several weeks of tick removal. Be sure to tell the doctor about the recent tick bite, when the bite occurred, and where the tick was probably acquired.

DEET, N,N-diethyl-meta-toluamide.
Source: Adapted from Centers for Disease Control and Prevention. (2011). *It's spring: Time to prevent Lyme disease.* Retrieved from *http://www.cdc.gov/features/lymedisease*

Conditions typically associated with HIV infection include SLE, reactive arthritis, PsA, Sjögren's syndrome, polymyositis, and fibromyalgia syndrome. The knees and the ankles are generally the most affected joints. Most patients improve with conventional arthritis treatments such as NSAIDs, but patients with reactive arthritis or PsA may not respond as well and may develop progressive deformities. As with other patients, appropriate physiotherapy is recommended.

Gout

Gout is caused by an increase in uric acid production, underexcretion of uric acid by the kidneys, or increased intake of foods containing purines, which are metabolized to uric acid by the body. Characteristic deposits of sodium urate crystals occur in articular, periarticular, and subcutaneous tissues. Joint involvement includes recurrent attacks of acute arthritis. Gout occurs more frequently in men than in women and affects up to 2% of Canadians (Arthritis Society, 2011a).

Gout may be classified as primary or secondary (Hollowell, Thompson, & Pantanowitz, 2008). In *primary gout*, a hereditary error of purine metabolism leads to the overproduction or retention of uric acid. *Secondary gout* may be related to another acquired disorder (see eTable 67-1, available on the Evolve Web site for this chapter) or may be the result of drugs known to inhibit uric acid excretion. Secondary gout may also be caused by drugs that increase the rate of cell death, such as the chemotherapeutic agents used in treating leukemia. Primary gout, which accounts for 90% of cases, occurs predominantly in middle-aged men, with almost no incidence in premenopausal women. Hyperuricemia may also develop in patients taking thiazide diuretics, in postmenopausal women, and in organ transplant recipients who are receiving immunosuppressive agents.

Obesity in men has been shown to increase the risk of gout (Arthritis Society, 2011a). Hypertension and excessive alcohol consumption are additional risk factors. A diet high in purine-rich foods (e.g., shellfish such as crab and shrimp; vegetables such as lentils, asparagus, and spinach; meats such as beef, chicken, and pork) do not cause gout but can trigger an acute attack if a person is susceptible to gout.

Etiology and Pathophysiology

Uric acid is the major end product of purine catabolism and is excreted primarily by the kidneys. Hyperuricemia may be the result of increased purine synthesis, decreased renal excretion, or both. A high dietary intake of purine alone has relatively little effect on uric acid levels. Hyperuricemia may result from prolonged fasting or excessive alcohol drinking because of the increased production of keto acids, which then inhibit uric acid excretion.

Clinical Manifestations and Complications

In the acute phase, gouty arthritis may occur in one or more joints but usually fewer than four. Affected joints may appear dusky or cyanotic and are extremely tender. Inflammation of the great toe (*podagra*) is the most common initial problem. Other affected joints may include the midtarsal area of the foot, the ankle, the knee, and the wrist. Olecranon bursae may also be involved. Acute gouty arthritis is usually precipitated by trigger events such as trauma, surgery, alcohol ingestion, or systemic infection. Symptoms typically begin at night with sudden swelling and excruciating pain, peak within several hours, and are often accompanied by low-grade fever. Individual attacks usually subside, treated or untreated, in 2 to 10 days. The affected joint returns entirely to normal, and patients are often free of symptoms between attacks.

Chronic gout is characterized by multiple joint involvement and visible deposits of sodium urate crystals called *tophi*. These are typically noted in the synovium, subchondral bone, the olecranon bursae, and the vertebrae and along tendons and in the skin and cartilage (Figure 67-8). Tophi are rarely present at the time of the initial attack and are generally noted only many years after the onset of disease.

The severity of gouty arthritis is variable. The clinical course may consist of infrequent mild attacks or multiple severe episodes in association with a slowly progressive disability. In general, the higher the serum uric acid level, the earlier the appearance of tophi and the greater the tendency toward more frequent, severe episodes of acute gout. Chronic inflammation may result in joint deformity, and cartilage destruction may predispose the joint to secondary OA. Large and unsightly tophaceous deposits may perforate overlying skin, producing draining sinuses that often become secondarily infected. Excessive uric acid excretion may lead to kidney or urinary tract stone formation. Pyelonephritis associated with intrarenal sodium urate deposits and obstruction may contribute to renal disease.

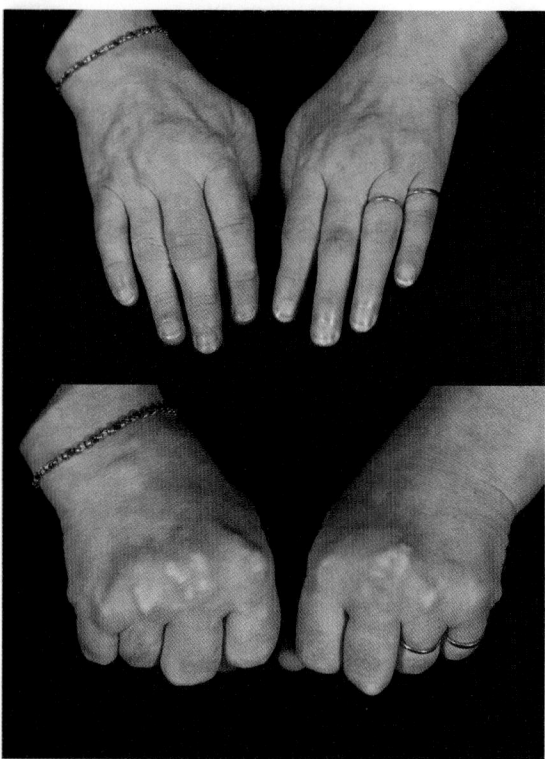

Figure 67-8 Tophi over the dorsum of the hands, accentuated by finger flexion and stretching of overlying skin.

Source: Hochberg, M. C., Silman, A. J., & Smolen, J. S. (2008). *Rheumatology* (4th ed., Figure 175-3). St. Louis: Mosby.

COLLABORATIVE CARE

Table 67-12 Gout

Diagnostic	
• History and physical examination	• Dietary avoidance of food and fluids with high purine content (e.g., anchovies, liver, wine, and beer)
• Family history of gout	• Drug therapy
• Presence of sodium urate crystals in synovial fluid	• Colchicine
• Elevated serum uric acid levels	• Nonsteroidal anti-inflammatory drugs (e.g., naproxen [Naprosyn])
• Elevated uric acid levels in 24-hr urine collection	• Allopurinol (Zyloprim)
• Radiographic studies	• Probenecid (Benuryl)
	• Febuxostat (Uloric)
Collaborative Therapy	• Corticosteroids: oral (prednisone)
• Joint immobilization	• Intra-articular (methylprednisolone acetate)
• Local application of heat or cold	• Adrenocorticotropic hormone (ACTH)
• Joint aspiration and intra-articular corticosteroids	

Diagnostic Studies

Serum uric acid levels are almost always elevated as high as 0.51 mmol/L. However, hyperuricemia is not specifically diagnostic of gout because levels may be increased in relation to a variety of drugs or as a totally asymptomatic abnormality in the general population. Specimens may be obtained for 24-hour urine uric acid levels to determine whether the disease is caused by decreased renal excretion or overproduction of uric acid.

Synovial fluid aspiration is a controversial part of patient evaluation because an accurate diagnosis of gout is possible in 80% of patients on the basis of clinical symptoms alone. However, aspiration may have therapeutic value by decompressing a swollen joint capsule. Joint aspiration is also the only reliable method to distinguish gout from septic arthritis and *pseudogout* (in which the crystals that form are calcium phosphate). Affected fluid characteristically contains needle-like crystals of sodium urate (Malik, Schumacher, Dinnella, & Clayburne, 2009). Radiographic studies appear normal in the early stages of gout; tophi, an indicator of chronic disease, appear as eroded areas in the bone.

Collaborative Care

Goals for care of patients with gout (Table 67-12) include termination of an acute attack through use of an anti-inflammatory agent such as colchicine; NSAIDs are prescribed adjunctively for pain management. Future attacks are prevented by a maintenance dose of allopurinol (Zyloprim) in combination with weight reduction (as needed) and possible avoidance

of alcohol and foods high in purine. Treatment is also aimed at preventing the formation of uric acid kidney stones and the development of associated conditions such as hypertriglyceridemia and hypertension.

Drug Therapy. Acute gouty arthritis is treated with colchicine and NSAIDs. Colchicine has known anti-inflammatory effects but no analgesic properties, and so an NSAID is added to the treatment regimen primarily for pain management. Oral administration of colchicine generally produces a prophylactic, suppressive effect that reduces the incidence of acute attacks and relieves residual pain and mild discomfort within 24 to 48 hours. Colchicine also has diagnostic merit in that a good response to treatment is further evidence for the diagnosis of gout. Recurrent gout may be prevented by combining colchicine with a xanthine oxidase inhibitor such as allopurinol (Zyloprim) or a uricosuric drug such as probenecid (Benuryl). Febuxostat (Uloric), a selective inhibitor of xanthine oxidase, is given for long-term management of hyperuricemia in people with chronic gout (Gray & Walters-Smith, 2011). Corticosteroids, administered either orally or by intra-articular injection, can be helpful in treating acute attacks. Systemic corticosteroids may be used only if routine therapies are contraindicated or ineffective. Adrenocorticotropic hormone (ACTH) may also be used for treating acute gout.

For many years, the standard therapy for hyperuricemia caused by urate underexcretion has been uricosuric drugs such as probenecid, which inhibit renal tubular reabsorption of urates. However, this class of drugs is ineffective when creatinine clearance is reduced, as can occur in patients older than 60. Aspirin inactivates the effect of uricosurics, which results in urate retention, and should be avoided while patients are taking uricosuric drugs. Acetaminophen can be used safely if analgesia is required.

Adequate urine volume with normal renal function (2 to 3 L/day) must be maintained to prevent precipitation of uric acid in the renal tubules. Allopurinol, which blocks the production of uric acid, is particularly useful in patients with uric acid stones or renal impairment, in whom uricosuric drugs may be ineffective or dangerous. The angiotensin II receptor antagonist losartan (Cozaar) may be especially useful in treatment of older adult patients with both gout and hypertension. Losartan, 50 mg daily, promotes urate diuresis and may normalize serum urate levels. Combination therapy with losartan and allopurinol may also be administered. Regardless of which drugs are prescribed, serum uric acid levels must be checked regularly to monitor treatment effectiveness.

Nutritional Therapy. Traditional dietary restrictions include limiting the use of alcohol and the consumption of foods high in purine (see Chapter 48, Table 48-13). However, drugs often control gout without necessitating these changes. Obese patients should be instructed in a carefully planned weight-reduction program.

NURSING MANAGEMENT: GOUT

Nursing interventions for patients with acute gouty arthritis include supportive care for the inflamed joints. The nurse must avoid causing pain to an inflamed joint by careless handling. Bed rest may be appropriate, with affected joints properly immobilized. Involvement of a lower extremity may require use of a cradle or footboard to protect the painful area from the weight of bed linens. The nurse should assess the limitation of motion and degree of pain and document treatment effectiveness.

The nurse should help patients and their families understand that hyperuricemia and gouty arthritis are chronic problems that can be controlled with careful adherence to a treatment program. The importance of drug therapy and the need for periodic determination of serum uric acid levels should be explained thoroughly. Patients should be able to demonstrate knowledge of precipitating factors that may cause an attack, including excessive caloric intake or overindulgence in purine-containing foods and alcohol; starvation (fasting); drug use (e.g., niacin, aspirin, diuretics); and major medical events (e.g., surgery, myocardial infarction).

Systemic Lupus Erythematosus

Systemic lupus erythematosus (SLE) is a chronic, multisystem inflammatory disease of autoimmune origin. It is a complex disorder that results from interactions among genetic, hormonal, environmental, and immunological factors. SLE typically affects the skin, the joints, and serous membranes (pleura, pericardium), along with the renal, hematological, and neurological systems.

SLE affects 17,000 Canadians. Ten times more women than men develop SLE. Most cases occur in women during their child-bearing years (Arthritis Society, 2011a). SLE is characterized by variability within and among persons. Its chronic, unpredictable course is marked by alternating periods of exacerbations and remissions.

Etiology and Pathophysiology

The etiology of the abnormal immune response in SLE is unknown. Because of the high prevalence of SLE among family members, a genetic influence has long been suspected. Multiple susceptibility genes from the HLA complex show associations with SLE, including the gene for HLA-DR3. Hormones are also known to play a role in the etiology of SLE. Onset or exacerbation of disease symptoms sometimes occurs after the onset of menarche, with the use of oral contraceptives, and during and after pregnancy. The disease tends to worsen in the immediate post-partum period.

Environmental factors are believed to contribute to the occurrence of SLE; sun exposure and burns are the most significant environmental triggers. Infectious agents may serve as a stimulus for immune hyperactivity. SLE may also be precipitated or aggravated by certain drugs such as procainamide, hydralazine (Apresoline), and a number of antiseizure agents (Dedeoglu, 2009).

SLE is characterized by the production of a large variety of autoantibodies against nucleic acids (e.g., single- and double-stranded DNA), erythrocytes, coagulation proteins, lymphocytes, platelets, and many other self-proteins. Most characteristically, the autoimmune reactions are directed against constituents of the cell nucleus (ANAs), particularly DNA. Circulating immune complexes containing antibodies against DNA are deposited in the basement membranes of capillaries in the kidneys, the heart, the skin, the brain, and the joints. Complement is activated, and inflammation occurs. The overaggressive antibody response is also related to activation of B and T cells. The specific manifestations of SLE depend on which cell types or organs are involved. SLE is a type III hypersensitivity response (see Chapter 16).

Clinical Manifestations and Complications

The severity of SLE is extremely variable, ranging from relatively mild to rapidly progressive and affecting many organ systems (Figure 67-9). The progressive organ involvement of SLE has no characteristic pattern. Any organ can be affected by an accumulation of circulating immune complexes. The most commonly affected tissues are the skin and muscle, the lining of the lungs, the heart, nervous tissue, and the kidneys. Generalized complaints such as fever, weight loss, arthralgia, and excessive fatigue may precede an exacerbation of disease activity.

Dermatological Manifestations. Cutaneous vascular lesions can appear in any location but are most likely to develop in sun-exposed areas. Severe skin reactions can occur in persons who are photosensitive. The classic so-called butterfly rash over the cheeks and bridge of the nose occurs in 50% of patients with SLE (Figure 67-10). About 20% of patients have *discoid* (round, coin-shaped) lesions. A small number of patients have chronic lesions, photosensitivity, and mild systemic disease in a syndrome referred to as *subacute cutaneous lupus.*

Ulcers of the oral or the nasopharyngeal membranes occur in up to one third of patients with SLE. Transient diffuse or patchy hair loss *(alopecia)* is also common, with or without underlying scalp lesions. The hair may grow back during remission, but hair loss may be permanent over lesions. The scalp becomes dry and scaly, and atrophy of the scalp can occur.

Musculoskeletal Problems. Polyarthralgia with morning stiffness is often the first manifestation of SLE and may precede the onset of multisystem disease by many years. Arthritis occurs in more than 90% of patients with SLE. Diffuse swelling is accompanied by joint and muscle pain, and some stiffness may be experienced. Lupus-related arthritis is generally nonerosive, but it may cause deformities such as swan-neck appearance of the fingers (see Figure 67-4, *D*), ulnar deviation, and subluxation with hyperlaxity of the joints. Patients with SLE are at increased risk for bone loss and fracture.

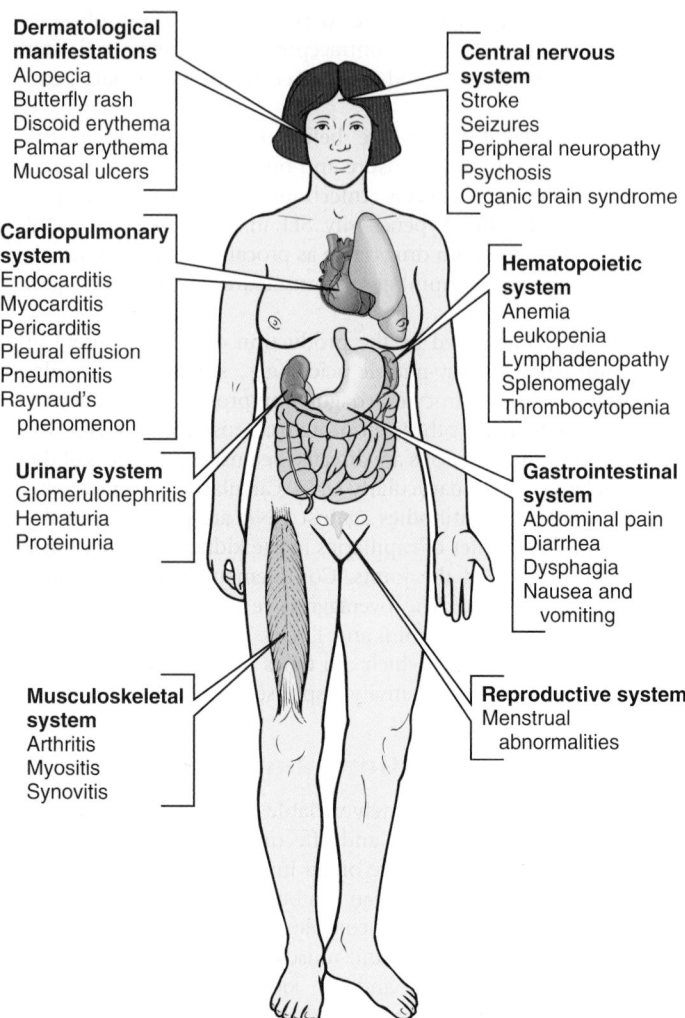

Dermatological manifestations
Alopecia
Butterfly rash
Discoid erythema
Palmar erythema
Mucosal ulcers

Cardiopulmonary system
Endocarditis
Myocarditis
Pericarditis
Pleural effusion
Pneumonitis
Raynaud's
  phenomenon

Urinary system
Glomerulonephritis
Hematuria
Proteinuria

Musculoskeletal system
Arthritis
Myositis
Synovitis

Central nervous system
Stroke
Seizures
Peripheral neuropathy
Psychosis
Organic brain syndrome

Hematopoietic system
Anemia
Leukopenia
Lymphadenopathy
Splenomegaly
Thrombocytopenia

Gastrointestinal system
Abdominal pain
Diarrhea
Dysphagia
Nausea and
  vomiting

Reproductive system
Menstrual
  abnormalities

Figure 67-9 Multisystem involvement in systemic lupus erythematosus.

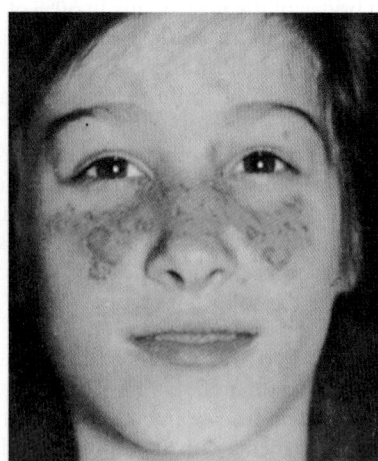

Figure 67-10 Butterfly rash manifestation of systemic lupus erythematosus.

Source: Kliegman, R. M., Stanton, B. F., St. Geme III, J. W., Schor, N. F., & Behrman, R. E. (Eds.). (2011). *Nelson textbook of pediatrics* (19th ed., Figure 152-1, *A*). Philadelphia: W. B. Saunders.

Cardiopulmonary Problems. Tachypnea and cough in patients with SLE are suggestive of restrictive lung disease. Pleurisy with or without pleural effusion is also possible. Cardiac involvement may include dysrhythmias that result from fibrosis of the sinoatrial and atrioventricular nodes. This occurrence is an ominous sign of advanced disease—dysrhythmias contribute significantly to the morbidity and mortality from SLE. Pericarditis can also occur. Clinical factors such as hypertension and hypercholesterolemia necessitate aggressive therapy and careful monitoring. In addition, people with SLE are at risk for secondary antiphospholipid syndrome (APS), a disorder of coagulation that leads to clots in the arteries and veins (Hellman & Imboden, 2008).

Renal Problems. Lupus nephritis (LN) occurs in 50% of patients with SLE (Seshan & Jennette, 2009). Manifestations of renal involvement vary from mild proteinuria to rapid, progressive glomerulonephritis.

The primary goal in treating LN is to slow the progression of nephropathy and preserve renal function by managing the underlying disease. The importance of renal biopsy is controversial, but findings can help guide treatment, which typically includes corticosteroids, cytotoxic agents (cyclophosphamide [Procytox]), and immunosuppressive agents (azathioprine [Imuran], cyclosporine [Neoral]). A newer drug, mycophenolate mofetil [CellCept]), may be more effective and less toxic than cyclophosphamide, which has been the standard of treatment. Oral prednisone or pulsed IV methylprednisolone may also be used as an intervention for LN, especially in the initial treatment period when cytotoxic agents have not had time to take effect.

Nervous System Problems. Along with renal involvement, neuropsychiatric manifestations are the most prevalent problems in SLE. Generalized or focal seizures are the most common manifestation involving the CNS and occur in as many as 15% of patients with SLE by the time of diagnosis. Seizures are generally controlled by corticosteroids or antiseizure drugs. Peripheral neuropathy can also occur, leading to sensory and motor deficits.

Cognitive dysfunction, recognized as a CNS manifestation of SLE, may result from the deposition of immune complexes within brain tissue. It is characterized by disordered thought processes, disorientation, memory deficits, and psychiatric symptoms such as severe depression and psychosis. On occasion, a stroke or aseptic meningitis may be attributable to SLE. Headaches are also common and can become severe during exacerbation of the disease.

Hematological Problems. The formation of antibodies against blood cells (such as erythrocytes, leukocytes, thrombocytes) and against coagulation factors is also a common feature of SLE. Anemia, mild leukopenia, and thrombocytopenia are often present in SLE. Some patients develop a tendency toward coagulopathy, involving either excessive bleeding or blood clot development. A manifestation of antiphospholipid antibody syndrome is a common cause of hypercoagulability in patients with SLE, many of whom benefit from high-intensity treatment with warfarin (Coumadin).

Infection. Patients with SLE appear to have increased susceptibility to infections, possibly in relation to defects in the ability to phagocytize invading bacteria, deficiencies in production of antibodies, and the immunosuppressive effect of many anti-inflammatory drugs. Infection is a major cause of death, pneumonia being the most common infection. Fever should be investigated seriously because it may indicate an underlying infectious process rather than lupus activity alone. Vaccinations are generally safe for patients with SLE. The exception is live virus vaccines, which should be avoided in patients who are being treated with corticosteroids or cytotoxic agents.

Diagnostic Studies

The diagnosis of SLE is based on the presence of distinct criteria revealed through patient history, physical examination, and laboratory findings (Table 67-13). No specific test is diagnostic for SLE, but a variety of abnormalities may be present in the blood. SLE is characterized by the presence of ANA, and identification of ANA establishes the existence of an autoimmune disease. Other antibodies include anti-DNA, antineuronal, anticoagulant, anti-WBC, anti–red blood cell (RBC), antiplatelet, antiphospholipid, and anti–basement membrane antibodies. The tests that are most specific for SLE include titres for anti–double-stranded DNA and anti-Smith (Sm) antibodies. Levels of anti-DNA antibodies are rarely high in any condition other than SLE, and anti-Sm antibody seems to be present almost exclusively in SLE. The lupus erythematosus (LE) cell preparation test is nonspecific for SLE and yields positive results in other rheumatic diseases. ESR and CRP levels are not diagnostic of SLE but may be used to monitor disease activity and effectiveness of therapy.

Table 67-13 Criteria for Diagnosis of Systemic Lupus Erythematosus*
Malar rash
Discoid rash
Photosensitivity
Oral ulcers
Arthritis: nonerosive, involvement of two or more joints characterized by tenderness, swelling, and effusion
Serositis: pleuritis or pericarditis
Renal disorder: persistent proteinuria or cellular casts in urine
Neurological disorder: seizures or psychosis
Hematological disorder: hemolytic anemia, leukopenia, lymphopenia, or thrombocytopenia
Immunological disorder: positive result of LE preparation; anti-DNA antibody or antibody to Sm nuclear antigen; or false-positive result of serological tests for syphilis
Antinuclear antibodies

Sources: Tan, E. M., Cohen, A. S., Fries, J. F., Masi, A. T., McShane, D. J., Rothfield, N. F., …, Winchester, R. J. (1982). The 1982 revised criteria for the classification of systemic lupus erythematosus. *Arthritis and Rheumatism, 25,* 1271-77. doi:10.1002/art.1780251101; and from Hochberg, M. C. (1997). Updating the American College of Rheumatology revised criteria for the classification of systemic lupus erythematosus [Letter]. *Arthritis and Rheumatism, 40,* 1725. doi:10.1002/art.1780400928

LE, lupus erythematosus; *Sm,* Smith.

*SLE is diagnosed if four or more of the criteria are present, serially or simultaneously, during any interval of observation. Revised criteria by a subcommittee of the American College of Rheumatology are used for the purpose of *classification* in population surveys, *not* for the diagnosis in individual patients.

Collaborative Care

A major challenge in treatment of SLE is to manage the active phase of the disease while preventing complications of treatments that cause long-term tissue damage. The improving prognosis in SLE may be the result of earlier diagnosis, prompt recognition of serious organ involvement, and better therapeutic regimens. Survival is influenced by several factors, including age, race, sex, socioeconomic status, the presence of comorbid conditions, and the severity of disease.

Drug Therapy. NSAIDs continue to be an important intervention, especially for patients with mild polyarthralgias or polyarthritis. Because therapy is likely to be prolonged, patients must be monitored carefully for GI effects from NSAID use. Antimalarial agents such as hydroxychloroquine (Plaquenil) are often used to treat fatigue and moderate skin and joint problems. The beneficial effect may not be noticed for several months (Lupus Canada, 2007). Flares may also be prevented with these drugs. Retinopathy can develop with high-dosage use of these drugs, but it generally reverses when they are discontinued. If patients cannot tolerate an antimalarial agent, an antileprosy drug such as dapsone may be used.

Corticosteroid exposure should be limited, but tapering doses of intravenous methylprednisolone may be useful in controlling severe exacerbations of polyarthritis. Steroid-sparing drugs such as methotrexate can serve as an alternative treatment and are prescribed in combination with folic acid to decrease minor adverse effects. However, high doses of corticosteroids may be especially appropriate for patients with very severe cutaneous SLE. Immunosuppressive drugs such as azathioprine (Imuran) and cyclophosphamide (Procytox) may be prescribed to reduce the need for long-term corticosteroid therapy and are also appropriate for treatment of severe organ and systemic disease, especially LN. Close monitoring is necessary to minimize drug toxicity and other adverse effects.

Disease management is most appropriately monitored by serial anti-DNA titres (Table 67-14). Simpler and less costly tests such as ESR or CRP measurement may also help in monitoring

COLLABORATIVE CARE

Table 67-14 Systemic Lupus Erythematosus	
Diagnostic	*Collaborative Therapy*
• History and physical examination	• NSAIDs for mild disease
• Antibody titres (e.g., anti-DNA, anti-Sm, ANA)	• Steroid-sparing drugs (e.g., methotrexate)
• Complete blood cell count	• Antimalarials (e.g., hydroxychloroquine [Plaquenil])
• LE cell preparation	• Corticosteroids for exacerbations and severe disease
• Serum complement levels	
• Urinalysis	• Immunosuppressive drugs (e.g., cyclophosphamide [Procytox], mycophenolate [CellCept])
• Radiographic examination of affected joints	
• Chest radiograph	
• ECG to determine extra-articular involvement	

ANA, antinuclear antibody; *ECG,* electrocardiogram; *LE,* lupus erythematosus; *NSAIDs,* nonsteroidal anti-inflammatory drugs; *Sm,* Smith.

treatment effectiveness. Patient teaching related to prescribed drugs must include their indications for use, proper administration, and possible adverse effects. Patients should understand that abrupt cessation of therapy may precipitate exacerbation of disease activity.

NURSING MANAGEMENT: SYSTEMIC LUPUS ERYTHEMATOSUS

▮ Nursing Assessment

As in the majority of rheumatic diseases, the chronic and unpredictable nature of SLE presents many challenges to patients and caregivers. The physical, psychological, and sociocultural problems associated with the long-term management of SLE necessitate the varied approaches and skills of the multidisciplinary health care team.

Subjective and objective data that should be obtained from patients with SLE are presented in Table 67-15. In particular, the extent to which pain and fatigue influence ADLs must be evaluated. A developmental approach focuses on age-appropriate education and counselling about issues such as personal relationships, family planning, occupational responsibilities, and recreational activities.

▮ Nursing Diagnoses

Nursing diagnoses for patients with SLE may include, but are not limited to, those presented in Nursing Care Plan 67-2.

▮ Planning

As overall disease management goals, patients with SLE will (1) have satisfactory pain management, (2) adhere to the therapeutic regimen to achieve maximum symptom management, (3) demonstrate awareness of and avoid activities that cause disease exacerbation, and (4) maintain optimal role function and a positive self-image.

▮ Nursing Implementation

▮ Health Promotion

SLE currently cannot be prevented. However, education of health care providers and the community should promote a clear understanding of the disease and the need for earlier diagnosis and treatment.

▮ Acute Intervention

During an exacerbation of SLE, a patient may become abruptly and dramatically ill. Nursing interventions include accurately recording the severity of symptoms and documenting the response to therapy. The nurse should assess fever pattern, joint inflammation, limitation of motion, location and degree of discomfort, and fatigability. The nurse should also monitor the patient's weight and fluid intake and output if corticosteroids are

NURSING ASSESSMENT

Table 67-15 Systemic Lupus Erythematosus

Subjective Data

Important Health Information

Past health history: Family history of autoimmune disorders; exposure to ultraviolet radiation, drugs, chemicals, viral infections; stress (physical or psychological); increased estrogen activity (including early onset of menarche; pregnancy and postpartum period); pattern of remissions and exacerbations

Medications: Use of oral contraceptives, procainamide, hydralazine (Apresoline), isoniazid (INH), antiseizure drugs, antibiotics (possibly precipitating symptoms of SLE), corticosteroids, NSAIDs

Symptoms

- Weight loss; nausea and vomiting; xerostomia (salivary gland dryness); oral and nasal ulcers; dysphagia; diarrhea or constipation; decreased urine output
- Morning stiffness; joint pain, swelling and deformity; coldness of fingers with numbness and tingling sensation; photosensitivity with rash; chest pain (pericardial, pleuritic); abdominal pain; shortness of breath, dyspnea
- Visual disturbances; vertigo; headache; excessive fatigue; insomnia
- Amenorrhea; irregular menstrual periods; frequent infections
- Depression, withdrawal

Objective Data

General

Fever, lymphadenopathy, periorbital edema

Integumentary

Alopecia; dry, scaly scalp; keratoconjunctivitis, malar butterfly rash, palmar or discoid erythema, urticaria, periungual erythema, purpura, or petechiae; leg ulcers

Respiratory

Pleural friction rub, decreased breath sounds

Cardiovascular

Vasculitis; pericardial friction rub; hypertension, edema, dysrhythmias, murmurs; bilateral, symmetrical pallor and cyanosis of fingers (Raynaud's phenomenon)

Gastrointestinal

Oral and pharyngeal ulcers; splenomegaly

Neurological

Facial weakness, peripheral neuropathies, papilledema, dysarthria, confusion, hallucination, disorientation, psychosis, seizures, aphasia, hemiparesis

Musculoskeletal

Myopathy, myositis, arthritis

Urinary

Proteinuria

Possible Findings

Presence of anti-DNA, anti-Sm, and antinuclear antibodies; anemia, leukopenia, thrombocytopenia; ↑ ESR; positive result of LE cell preparation; ↑ serum creatinine; microscopic hematuria, cellular casts in urine; pericarditis or pleural effusion evident on chest radiograph

ESR, erythrocyte sedimentation rate; *LE,* lupus erythematosus; *NSAIDs,* nonsteroidal anti-inflammatory drugs; *SLE,* systemic lupus erythematosus; *Sm,* Smith.

NURSING CARE PLAN 67-2

Systemic Lupus Erythematosus

NURSING DIAGNOSIS	***Fatigue*** *related to* chronic inflammation and altered immunity *as evidenced by* lack of energy and inability to maintain usual routine

Expected Patient Outcomes	Nursing Interventions and *Rationales*
• Uses energy conservation techniques • Sets and completes priority activities • Adapts lifestyle to energy level	**Energy management** • Assist patient in assigning priority activities *to accommodate energy levels.* • Assist patient in scheduling rest periods *to temporarily reverse effect of fatigue.* • Teach activity organization and time management techniques *to prevent fatigue.* • Encourage alternating rest and activity periods *to promote recuperation and to foster maximum participation in activities.* • Instruct patient and significant other to recognize signs and symptoms of fatigue *to ensure required reduction in activity.* • Instruct patient and significant other to notify health care provider if signs and symptoms of fatigue persist *to increase patient's support and family's understanding of disease and related problems.*

NURSING DIAGNOSIS	***Acute pain*** *related to* inflammatory process and inadequate comfort measures *as evidenced by* complaints of joint pain, ineffective pain management by current measures, and reduction of activity to avoid exacerbating pain

Expected Patient Outcome	Nursing Interventions and *Rationales*
• Uses analgesics and nonpharmacological measures appropriately to manage pain at an acceptable level	**Pain management** • Perform a comprehensive assessment of pain to include location, characteristics, onset and duration, frequency, quality, intensity, and severity of pain and precipitating factors *to plan appropriate interventions.* • Ensure that patient receives attentive analgesic care *to relieve pain.* • Teach use of nonpharmacological techniques (e.g., relaxation, guided imagery, distraction, and hot and cold application) before pain occurs or increases, and along with other pain relief measures, *to replace or supplement analgesics.*

NURSING DIAGNOSIS	***Impaired skin integrity*** *related to* photosensitivity, skin rash, and alopecia *as evidenced by* rash anywhere on body, butterfly rash on face, hair loss, areas of ulceration on fingertips, complaints of urticaria, and photosensitivity

Expected Patient Outcomes	Nursing Interventions and *Rationales*
• Maintains skin integrity with the use of topical treatments • Prevents exacerbations with the use of sunscreens and by limiting sun exposure	**Skin care: topical treatments** • Inspect skin of patients daily *to assess risk of breakdown.* • Document degree of skin breakdown *to plan appropriate interventions.* • Apply topical anti-inflammatory agent to affected area *to control skin manifestations.* **Teaching: disease process** • Discuss lifestyle changes that may be necessary to prevent future complications and control disease process (e.g., use of sunscreens and sun-protective clothing when outdoors) *to prevent sun exposure from exacerbating manifestations.*

NURSING DIAGNOSIS	***Deficient knowledge*** *related to* lack of exposure to and unfamiliarity with information resources *as evidenced by* questions about SLE, misinterpretation of information, and inaccurate follow-through of instruction

Expected Patient Outcomes	Nursing Interventions and *Rationales*
• Accurately describes the disease process and the rationale for prescribed treatment • Expresses confidence in ability to recognize complications and using precautions to prevent their occurrence	**Teaching: disease process** • Describe disease process *to increase patient's knowledge.* • Discuss therapy and treatment options *to increase probability of success in long-term management.* • Provide family and significant others with information about patient's progress *to provide support during exacerbation and increase their sense of involvement.* • Instruct patient about which signs and symptoms to report to health care providers (e.g., fever, edema, decreased urine output, chest pain, and dyspnea) *to ensure early intervention.* • Refer patient to local community agencies and support groups (e.g., Lupus Canada, the Arthritis Society) *to provide additional sources of information and support.*

SLE, systemic lupus erythematosus.

prescribed because of the fluid-retention effect of these drugs and the possibility of acute kidney injury. Collection of 24-hour urine samples for protein and creatinine clearance may be ordered. The nurse should observe for signs of bleeding that result from drug therapy, such as pallor, skin bruising, petechiae, or tarry stools.

Careful assessment of neurological status includes observation for visual disturbances, headaches, personality changes, seizures, and forgetfulness. Psychosis may indicate CNS disease or may be the effect of corticosteroid therapy. Irritation of the nerves of the extremities (peripheral neuropathy) may produce numbness, tingling sensation, and weakness of the hands and feet.

The nurse should also explain the nature of the disease, modes of therapy, and all diagnostic procedures. Emotional support for the patient and family is essential.

◼ Ambulatory and Home Care

Nursing interventions must emphasize health teaching and the importance of patient cooperation for successful home management. The nurse should help patients understand that even strong adherence to the treatment plan is not a guarantee against exacerbation because the course of the disease is unpredictable but that a variety of factors (such as fatigue, sun exposure, emotional stress, infection, drugs, and surgery) may increase disease activity. Nursing interventions should be directed toward assisting patients and their families in eliminating or minimizing exposure to precipitating factors (Table 67-16).

◼ Lupus and Pregnancy. Because SLE is most common in women of childbearing age, treatment during pregnancy must be considered. The woman's primary health care provider (or rheumatologist) and obstetrician should thoroughly discuss with the woman her desire to become pregnant. Infertility may have already resulted from renal involvement and the use of high-dose corticosteroid and chemotherapy drugs. Patients with SLE should understand that spontaneous abortion, stillbirth, and

intrauterine growth retardation are common problems during pregnancy. They occur because of deposits of immune complexes in the placenta and because of inflammatory responses in the placental blood vessels. The renal, cardiovascular, and pulmonary systems and the CNS may be especially affected during pregnancy. Women who already demonstrate serious SLE involvement in these systems should be counselled against pregnancy.

For the best outcome, pregnancy should be planned at a time when the disease activity is minimal. Exacerbation is common during the postpartum period. Therapeutic abortion offers the same risk of postdelivery exacerbation as does carrying the fetus to term.

In rare cases, neonatal lupus erythematosus (NLE) occurs in infants born to women with SLE. A characteristic skin rash is seen in more than 30% of the cases of NLE.

◼ Psychosocial Issues. Patients with SLE confront many psychosocial issues (Danoff-Berg & Friedberg, 2009). Disease onset may be vague, and SLE may remain undiagnosed for long periods. Supportive therapies may become as important as medical treatment in helping patients cope with the disease. The nurse should inform patients and their families that the prognosis for the majority of people with SLE is good. Families are anxious about hereditary aspects and want to know whether their children will also have SLE. Many couples require pregnancy and sexual counselling. Individuals making decisions about marriage and careers worry about how SLE will interfere with their plans. The nurse may have to educate teachers, employers, and coworkers.

The obvious physical effects of skin rashes, discoid lesions, and alopecia may cause social isolation for a patient with SLE, affecting the individual's self-esteem and body image. However, pain and fatigue are cited most frequently as interfering with quality of life. Friends and relatives are confused by the patient's complaints of transient joint pain and overwhelming fatigue. Pacing techniques and relaxation therapy can help the patient remain involved in day-to-day activities. The nurse should stress the importance of planning both recreational and occupational activities. Young adults find physical limitations and restrictions of sun exposure particularly difficult to handle. Nursing interventions should assist patients in developing and accomplishing reasonable goals for improving or maintaining mobility, energy levels, and self-esteem.

◼ Evaluation

The expected outcomes for patients with SLE are presented in Nursing Care Plan 67-2.

Systemic Sclerosis

Systemic sclerosis (SS), or *scleroderma*, is a disorder of connective tissue characterized by fibrotic, degenerative, and occasionally inflammatory changes in skin, blood vessels, synovium, skeletal muscle, and internal organs. Two types of SS exist: (a) the more common *limited cutaneous disease* (80%) and (b) *diffuse cutaneous disease*. Both forms are systemic, but the degree and type of organ involvement and disease progression are very different (Vincent, 2009). The disease course of SS is variable. SS affects up to five

PATIENT & CAREGIVER TEACHING GUIDE

Table 67-16 Systemic Lupus Erythematosus

Include the following information in the teaching plan for a patient with systemic lupus erythematosus and the caregiver:

1. Disease process
2. Names of drugs, actions, adverse effects, dosage, administration
3. Pain management strategies
4. Energy conservation and pacing techniques
5. Therapeutic exercise, use of heat therapy (for arthralgia)
6. Avoidance of physical and emotional stress
7. Avoidance of exposure to individuals with infection
8. Avoidance of drying soaps, powders, household chemicals
9. Use of sunscreen protection (at least SPF 15), with minimal sun exposure between the hours of 1100 and 1500
10. Regular medical and laboratory follow-up
11. Marital and pregnancy counselling as needed
12. Community resources and health care agencies

SPF, sun protection factor.

COLLABORATIVE CARE

Table 67-17 Systemic Sclerosis

Diagnostic	Collaborative Therapy
• History and physical examination • Antinuclear antibody titre • Anticentromere antibody titre • Microscopic study of nail bed capillaries • Radiographic studies of chest and hands • Skin or visceral biopsy • Urinalysis (proteinuria, hematuria, casts) • Pulmonary function test • Electrocardiography	• Physiotherapy and occupational therapy • Vasoactive agents • Calcium channel blockers (diltiazem [Cardizem], nifedipine [Adalat]) • Angiotensin-converting enzyme (ACE) inhibitors (lisinopril [Prinivil]) • Immunosuppressive drugs (e.g., cyclophosphamide [Procytox]; mycophenolate mofetil [CellCept]) • Corticosteroids

ria, and casts. Serum levels of creatinine may be elevated. Radiographic evidence of subcutaneous calcification, distal esophageal hypomotility, or bilateral pulmonary fibrosis is diagnostic of SS. Pulmonary function studies reveal decreased vital capacity and lung compliance.

Collaborative Care

The collaborative care of SS (Table 67-17) offers no specific long-term treatment. Care is directed toward attempts to prevent or treat secondary complications of involved organs. Physiotherapy helps maintain joint mobility and preserve muscle strength. Occupational therapy assists patients in maintaining functional abilities.

Drug Therapy. No specific drug or combination of drugs has been proven effective in the treatment of SS. Vasoactive agents are often prescribed for early stages of the disease, and calcium channel blockers (nifedipine [Adalat] and diltiazem [Cardizem]) are now a common treatment choice for Raynaud's phenomenon. Losartan (Cozaar), an angiotensin II blocker, may also be used to treat Raynaud's phenomenon. Prazosin (Minipress), an α-adrenergic blocking agent, increases blood flow to the fingers. Bosentan (Tracleer), an endothelin-receptor antagonist, and epoprostenol (Flolan), a vasodilator, may assist in preventing and treating digital ulcers while improving exercise capacity and heart and lung dynamics.

Corticosteroids are generally reserved for patients with significant joint or muscle involvement or severe skin disease with ulcerations. Topical agents may provide some relief from joint pain. Capsaicin cream may be useful not only as a local analgesic but also as a vasodilator. Other therapies are prescribed to address specific systemic problems, such as tetracycline for diarrhea caused by bacterial overgrowth, histamine H_2-receptor blockers (e.g., cimetidine) and proton pump inhibitors (e.g., omeprazole [Losec]) for esophageal symptoms, antihypertensive agents (e.g., captopril, propranolol [Inderal], methyldopa) for hypertension with renal involvement, and immunosuppressive drugs (e.g., cyclophosphamide [Procytox]; mycophenolate mofetil [CellCept]) to suppress the immune system.

NURSING MANAGEMENT: SYSTEMIC SCLEROSIS

Because prevention is not possible, nursing intervention often begins during a hospitalization for diagnostic purposes. The nurse can help patients resolve feelings of helplessness by providing information about the illness and encouraging active participation in planning care. Assess vital signs, weight, intake and output, respiratory and bowel function, and joint ROM at regular intervals as indicated by specific symptoms to plan appropriate care. Emotional stress and cold ambient temperatures may aggravate Raynaud's phenomenon. Patients with SS should not undergo fingerstick blood testing because of compromised circulation and poor healing of the fingers.

Health teaching is an important nursing intervention as patients and their families begin to live with this disease. Obvious changes in the face and the hands often lead to poor self-image and the loss of mobility and function. Patients must actively complete therapeutic exercises at home to prevent skin retraction and promote vascularization. Mouth excursion (opening the mouth widely, as in yawning) is a good exercise to help with temporomandibular joint function. If the patient has arthropathy, isometric exercises are most appropriate because no joint movement occurs. The nurse should encourage the use of moist heat applications or paraffin baths to promote skin flexibility in the hands and feet. Patients should use assistive devices as appropriate and organize activities to preserve strength and reduce disability.

Hands and feet should be protected from cold exposure and possible burns or cuts that might heal slowly. Smoking should be avoided because of its vasoconstricting effect. Signs of infection should be promptly reported. Lotions may help alleviate skin dryness and cracking, but they must be rubbed in for an unusually long time because of the thickness of the skin.

Patients may reduce dysphagia by eating small, frequent meals; chewing carefully and slowly; and drinking fluids. Heartburn may be minimized with the use of antacids 45 to 60 minutes after each meal and by upright sitting for at least 2 hours after eating. Using additional pillows or raising the head of the bed on blocks may help reduce nocturnal gastroesophageal reflux.

Job modifications are often necessary because stair climbing, typing, writing, and cold exposure may pose particular problems. Patients may become socially withdrawn as skin tightening alters the appearance of the face and the hands. Dining out may become a socially embarrassing event because of the patient's restricted opening of the mouth, difficulty swallowing, and reflux. Some individuals with SS wear gloves to protect fingertip ulcers and to provide extra warmth. Sensitive areas on fingertips resulting from ulcers or calcinosis may make padded utensils or special assistive devices necessary to reduce discomfort. Daily oral hygiene must be emphasized; neglect may lead to increased tooth and gingival problems. Patients need a dentist who is familiar with SS and can deal with a small oral aperture. Psychological support reduces stress and may positively influence peripheral motor response. Biofeedback training and relaxation techniques can reduce tension, improve sleeping habits, and raise the temperature of the fingers and toes.

Sexual dysfunction resulting from body changes, pain, muscular weakness, limited mobility, decreased self-esteem, erectile dysfunction, and decreased vaginal secretions may necessitate

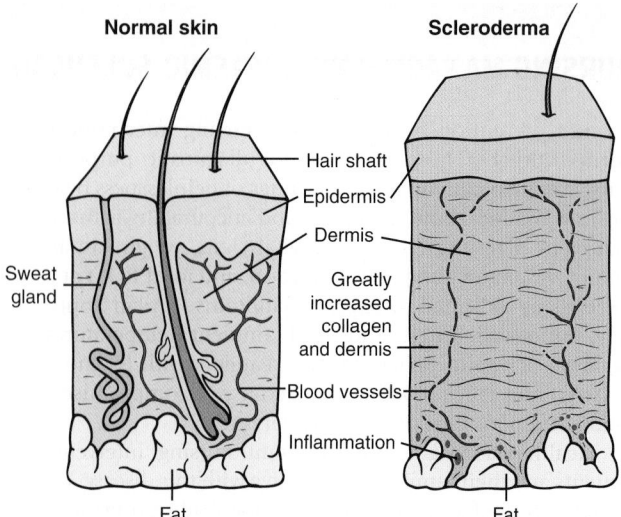

Figure 67-11 Skin changes in systemic sclerosis.

times more women than men. Although symptoms may begin at any time, the usual age at onset is between 30 and 50 years. Overall incidence increases with age. SS affects approximately 16,000 people in Canada (Arthritis Society, 2011a).

Etiology and Pathophysiology

The exact cause of SS remains unknown. Immunological dysfunction and vascular abnormalities are believed to play a role in development of widespread systemic disease. Other risk factors associated with skin thickening include environmental occupational exposure to coal, plastics, and silica dust. In SS, collagen—the protein that gives normal skin its strength and elasticity—is overproduced (Figure 67-11). Disruption of the cell is followed by platelet aggregation and fibrosis. Proliferation of collagen disrupts the normal functioning of internal organs, such as the lungs, the kidneys, the heart, and the GI tract.

Clinical Manifestations

Manifestations of SS range from a diffuse cutaneous thickening with rapidly progressive and widespread organ involvement to the more benign variant of limited cutaneous SS. The signs of limited disease appear on the face and the hands, whereas diffuse disease initially involves the trunk and extremities. Clinical manifestations can be described by the acronym **CREST** (Scleroderma Society of Canada, 2008):

Calcinosis: painful deposits of calcium in the skin

Raynaud's phenomenon: abnormal blood flow in response to cold or stress (Raynaud's phenomenon is described further in Chapter 40)

Esophageal dysfunction: difficulty with swallowing, caused by internal scarring

Sclerodactyly: tightening of the skin on the fingers and toes

Telangiectasia: red spots on the hands, the forearms, the palms, the face, and the lips

Raynaud's Phenomenon. Raynaud's phenomenon (an episodic vasospastic disorder of small cutaneous arteries, most

frequently involving the fingers and toes) is the most co initial complaint in limited disease. Blood flow to the fing toes is diminished on exposure to cold (blanching or phase); this is followed by cyanosis as hemoglobin r oxygen to the tissues (blue phase) and then erythema rewarming (red phase). The colour changes are often ac nied by numbness and tingling. Raynaud's phenomenc precede the onset of systemic disease by months, years, decades.

Skin and Joint Changes. Symmetrical painless swel thickening of the skin of the fingers and hands may prog diffuse scleroderma of the trunk. In limited disease, skin ening does not generally extend above the elbow or abo knee, although in some individuals the face is affected. Ir diffuse disease, the skin loses elasticity and becomes ta shiny, producing the typical expressionless facies with pursed lips. Skin changes in the face may also contrib reduction in ROM in the temporomandibular joint. The may be affected by *sclerodactyly,* in which the fingers ar semiflexed position, with tightened skin up to the wrist. R peripheral joint function may occur as an early sympt polyarthritis.

Internal Organ Involvement. About 20% of peop systemic sclerosis develop secondary Sjögren's syndrome, a tion associated with dry eyes and mouth. Dysphagia, gum and dental caries can result. Frequent reflux of gastric ac result from esophageal fibrosis. If swallowing becomes di patients often decrease food intake and lose weight. Add GI effects include constipation, which results from colonic motility, and diarrhea, caused by malabsorption from ba overgrowth.

Lung involvement includes pleural thickening, pulm fibrosis, and pulmonary function abnormalities. Affected p; develop a cough and dyspnea. Pulmonary artery hyperte may occur in up to 50% of patients with limited SS, and in tial lung disease can occur in addition in another 10% of patients.

Primary heart disease consists of pericarditis, pericardia sion, and cardiac dysrhythmias. Myocardial fibrosis that r in heart failure occurs most frequently in patients with diffu

Renal disease was previously a major cause of death in d SS. Malignant hypertension in association with rapidly pro sive and irreversible renal insufficiency may occur. Early rec tion of renal involvement and initiation of therapy are cri Improvements in dialysis, bilateral nephrectomy in patients uncontrollable hypertension, and kidney transplantation offered some hope to patients with renal failure. In partic angiotensin-converting enzyme (ACE) inhibitors (e.g., lisin [Prinivil]) have markedly improved the treatment of r disease.

Diagnostic Studies

Laboratory findings are relatively normal. Blood studies reveal a mildly elevated ESR and mild hemolytic anemia ; result of RBC damage from diseased small vessels. The scle derma antibody SCL-70 is found in about 30% of patie with diffuse disease, and serum RF is found in 30% of patie affected with either form of SS. An anticentromere antibo is seen in many patients with CREST. If renal involvement present, urinalysis may reveal proteinuria, microscopic hema

sensitive counselling by the nurse. Specific suggestions based on the findings of individual patient assessment should be offered.

Polymyositis and Dermatomyositis

Polymyositis (PM) and dermatomyositis (DM) are diffuse, idiopathic, inflammatory myopathies of the connective tissues, especially striated muscle. They produce bilateral weakness that is usually most severe in the proximal or limb-girdle muscles. These disorders, which are relatively rare, occur in twice as many women as men (Arthritis Society, 2011a) and typically affect adults older than 50. **Dermatomyositis** is characterized by pruritic or eczematous inflammation of the skin and tenderness of the muscles. **Polymyositis** is generally more severe, and some forms of it are associated with malignancy.

Etiology and Pathophysiology

The exact cause of PM and DM is unknown. Putative causes include an infectious agent, neoplasms, drugs or vaccinations, and stress. Because disease severity is not well correlated with altered immune complexes, it is unclear whether the complexes occur as primary or secondary phenomena. Because T cytotoxic cells and macrophages have been found near the damaged muscle fibres of patients with PM, this disease is believed to be caused by cell-mediated injury. In contrast, DM has been associated with B cells (humoral immunity) and destruction of the muscle microvasculature.

Clinical Manifestations and Complications

Muscular. Patients with DM and PM experience weight loss and increasing fatigue with gradually developing weakness of the muscles that leads to difficulty in performing routine activities. The muscles most commonly affected are those of the shoulders, the legs, the arms, and the pelvic girdle. Patients may have difficulty rising from a chair or bathtub, climbing stairs, combing the hair, or reaching into a high cupboard. Neck muscles may become so weak that patients are unable to raise the head from the pillow. Muscle discomfort or tenderness is uncommon. Muscle examination reveals an inability to move against resistance or even gravity. Weakness of the pharyngeal muscles may result in dysphagia and dysphonia (nasal or hoarse voice).

Dermal. Skin changes of DM include a classic violet-coloured, cyanotic, or erythematous symmetrical rash *(heliotrope rash)* with edema around the eyelids. Violet-coloured or erythematous papules (Gottron's papules) and small plaques develop over the DIP or MCP areas and at elbow or knee joints in about 70% of patients with DM. Because of these early skin changes, DM is usually recognized earlier than PM, in which a rash does not appear. Reddened, smooth, or scaly patches appear with the same symmetrical distribution but sparing the interphalangeal spaces (Gottron's sign); they can be confused with psoriasis or seborrheic dermatitis. An erythematous scaling rash (poikiloderma) may develop as a late finding on the back, buttocks, and a V-shaped area of the anterior neck and chest. Hyperemia and telangiectasias are often present at the nail beds. Calcium nodules (calcinosis cutis), which can develop throughout the skin, are especially common in long-standing DM.

Other Manifestations. Joint redness, pain, and inflammation often occur and contribute to limitations in joint ROM in DM and PM. Contractures and muscle atrophy may occur with advanced disease. Weakening of the pharyngeal muscles can lead to a poor cough effort, difficulty swallowing, and increased risk for aspiration pneumonia in both disorders. Interstitial lung disease occurs in up to 65% of all affected patients. People with DM also have an increased risk of an occult malignancy, which may be present at time of diagnosis. Both diseases may be associated with other connective tissue disorders (e.g., systemic sclerosis).

Diagnostic Studies

Diagnosis of DM or PM is confirmed by MRI, electromyographic (EMG) findings, muscle biopsy findings, and serum enzyme levels. Electromyographic findings suggestive of PM reveal bizarre high-frequency discharges and spontaneous fibrillation, with positive spikes at rest. Muscle biopsy reveals necrosis, degeneration, regeneration, and fibrosis with pathological findings distinct for DM or PM. Levels of enzymes such as creatinine kinase and myoglobin are elevated. Elevation of the ESR is also expected with active disease. The skin rash typical of DM is not common in other disorders.

NURSING AND COLLABORATIVE MANAGEMENT: POLYMYOSITIS AND DERMATOMYOSITIS

PM and DM are initially treated with high-dose corticosteroids. Improvement is generally achieved if corticosteroid therapy is promptly instituted, and the dosage can typically be reduced as improvement is noted. Long-term corticosteroid therapy may often be required because relapses are common when the drug is withdrawn. If corticosteroids prove ineffective or organ involvement is occurring (or both), immunosuppressive drugs may be administered (methotrexate, azathioprine [Imuran], or cyclophosphamide [Procytox]) orally or by intermittent IV means. DM has been shown to improve with IV immune globulin when a patient does not respond to corticosteroids. Topical corticosteroids and hydroxychloroquine (Plaquenil) may also be prescribed to treat the skin rash. Biological therapy (e.g., etanercept [Enbrel], infliximab [Remicade]) is being explored for its possible role in the treatment of DM and PM.

Physiotherapy can be helpful and should be tailored to the activity of the disease. Massage and passive movement are appropriate during active disease. More aggressive exercises should be reserved for periods when disease activity is minimal, as evidenced by low serum enzyme levels.

Nursing interventions should include a thorough explanation of the nature of the disease, the prescribed therapies, all diagnostic tests, and the importance of regular medical care. It is important for patients to understand that the benefits of therapy are often delayed. For example, weakness may increase during the first few weeks of corticosteroid therapy. Special attention is paid to patient safety. Use of assistive devices should be encouraged as a fall prevention strategy. To prevent aspiration, patients should be encouraged to rest before meals, maintain an upright position when eating, and choose a diet of easily swallowed foods.

The nurse should assist patients in organizing activities and using pacing techniques to conserve energy. The nurse should encourage the patient to perform daily ROM exercises to prevent contractures. When active inflammation is not evident, muscle-strengthening (repetitive) exercises may be started. Home care and bed rest may become necessary during the acute phase of PM because profound muscle weakness renders patients unable to carry out ADLs.

Mixed (Overlapping) Forms of Connective Tissue Disease

A combination of clinical features of several rheumatic diseases is described as *mixed* or *overlapping connective tissue disease.* Although this combination was originally believed to be a distinct clinical disorder, follow-up revealed that for most affected patients, this disorder is a stage in the progression to a connective tissue disorder such as SLE, SS, or polymyositis (Hellman & Imboden, 2008).

Sjögren's Syndrome

Sjögren's syndrome is a relatively common autoimmune disease that targets moisture-producing glands, leading to the common symptoms of *xerostomia* (dry mouth) and *keratoconjunctivitis sicca* (dry eyes). The nose, the throat, the airways, and the skin can also become dry. The disease can affect other glands as well, including those in the stomach, the pancreas, and the intestines (extraglandular involvement). The disease is usually diagnosed in people older than 40, and 90% of them are women.

In primary Sjögren's syndrome, symptoms can be traced to problems with the lacrimal and the salivary glands. Patients with primary disease are likely to have antibodies against the cytoplasmic antigens SS-A (or RO) and SS-B (or LA), as well as ANA. Patients with secondary Sjögren's syndrome typically have had another autoimmune disease (e.g., RA, SLE) before Sjögren's syndrome develops.

Sjögren's syndrome appears to be caused by genetic and environmental factors. The trigger may be a viral or bacterial infection that adversely stimulates the immune system. In Sjögren's syndrome, lymphocytes attack and damage the lacrimal and salivary glands.

Dry eyes are characterized by decreased tearing, which leads to a "gritty" sensation in the eyes, burning sensation, blurred vision, and photosensitivity (Daniels, 2007). Dry mouth leads to buccal membrane fissures, altered sense of taste, dysphagia, and increased frequency of mouth infections or dental caries. Dryness of the skin and rashes, joint and muscle pain, and thyroid problems may also be present. Other exocrine glands can be affected. For example, vaginal dryness may lead to dyspareunia (painful intercourse). Autoimmune thyroid disorders, including Graves' disease and Hashimoto's thyroiditis, are common with Sjögren's syndrome. Histological study reveals lymphocyte infiltration of salivary and lacrimal glands. The disease may become more generalized and involve the lymph nodes, the bone marrow, and the visceral organs (pseudolymphoma). Lymphoma develops in about 5% of patients with Sjögren's syndrome.

Ophthalmological examination (Schirmer's test), measures of salivary gland function, and lower lip biopsy of minor salivary glands aid in the diagnosis. The treatment is based on symptoms, including (a) instillation of preservative-free artificial tears as necessary to maintain adequate hydration and lubrication, (b)

surgical punctal occlusion, and (c) increased fluids with meals. Dental hygiene is important. Pilocarpine (Salagen) can be used to treat symptoms of dry mouth. Increased humidity at home may reduce respiratory infections. Vaginal lubrication with a water-soluble product may increase comfort during intercourse. Corticosteroids and immunosuppressive drugs are indicated for treatment of pseudolymphoma.

Soft-Tissue Rheumatic Syndromes

Myofascial pain syndrome, fibromyalgia syndrome (FMS), and chronic fatigue syndrome (CFS) are three soft-tissue disease syndromes that have many commonalities and may be related. Research to explore links among these three syndromes is ongoing. A multidisciplinary team approach consisting of a rheumatologist, nurse, mental health care provider, and physiotherapist may be especially helpful for patients with these syndromes, whose disease courses may be chronic.

Myofascial Pain Syndrome

Myofascial pain syndrome is characterized by musculoskeletal pain and tenderness in one anatomical region of the body. The pain has been shown to originate in anterior and posterior trigger points as a result of muscle trauma or chronic muscle strain (e.g., desk or computer work). Regions of pain are often within the taut bands and fascia of skeletal muscles. When activated by pressure, trigger points are thought to activate a characteristic pattern of pain that can be worse with activity or stress (Lavelle, Lavelle, & Smith, 2007). Myofascial pain syndrome occurs most often in middle-aged adults and in more women than men. Affected patients complain of the pain as deep and aching, accompanied by a sensation of burning, stinging, and stiffness. The muscles frequently involved are located in the chest, the neck, the lower back, and the shoulders. Referred pain from these muscle groups can also travel to the buttock, the hand, and the head, causing severe headaches. Additional systemic manifestations have not been reported. Palpation of trigger points reveals induration and frequently a muscle twitch in the area of a trigger point. Once a trigger point is palpated, pain is felt locally and may also be referred to a different region, often some distance away. These findings have also been noted to occur in normal healthy persons and in persons with FMS. Similarities between myofascial pain syndrome and FMS have led to the suggestion that myofascial pain may be a form of or evolve into FMS. The two syndromes are compared in Table 67-18.

Table 67-18 Comparison of Fibromyalgia and Myofascial Pain Syndromes		
VARIABLE	**FIBROMYALGIA**	**MYOFASCIAL PAIN**
Location	Generalized	Regional
Examination findings	Tender points	Trigger points
Response to local therapy	Not sustained	Curative
Gender (female-to-male ratio)	10:1	Equal or unknown

Source: Adapted from McCance, K. L., & Huether, S. E. (2010). *Pathophysiology: The biologic basis for disease in adults and children* (6th ed., p. 1607). St. Louis: Mosby.

Physiotherapy is one treatment used for myofascial pain syndrome. A typical exercise is the "spray and stretch" method, in which the painful area is iced or sprayed with a coolant such as ethyl chloride and then stretched. Positive results have been achieved by injection of the trigger points with a local anaesthetic (e.g., 1% lidocaine). Massage, acupuncture, biofeedback, and ultrasound therapy have also been shown to benefit some patients.

Patient and caregiver teaching is an important nursing responsibility. Instruction should focus on the prevention of muscle tension in work and leisure activities. Good posture and good resting and sleeping positions should also be reviewed. Most patients with myofascial pain syndrome are able to lead a normal and active lifestyle.

Fibromyalgia Syndrome

Fibromyalgia syndrome (FMS) is a chronic disorder characterized by widespread, nonarticular musculoskeletal pain and fatigue with multiple tender points. People with FMS also typically experience nonrestorative sleep, morning stiffness, irritable bowel syndrome, and anxiety. The former name for this disorder, *fibrositis,* implied inflammation of the muscles and soft tissues. However, FMS is now known to be nondegenerative, nonprogressive, and noninflammatory.

Fibromyalgia is a commonly diagnosed musculoskeletal disorder and a major cause of disability that affects 900,000 Canadians (Arthritis Society, 2011a). At least four times more women than men develop fibromyalgia, but it can affect persons of all ages and ethnic groups. FMS and CFS share many commonalities.

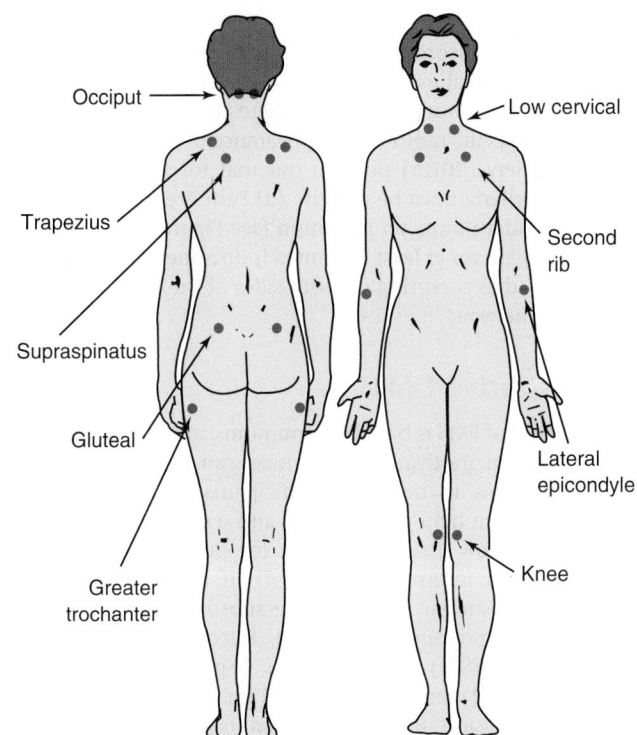

Figure 67-12 Tender points in fibromyalgia syndrome.

Source: Redrawn from Freundlich, B., & Leventhal, L. (1997). The fibromyalgia syndrome. In H. R. Schumacher, Jr., J. H. Klippel, & W. J. Koopman (Eds.), *Primer on the rheumatic diseases* (11th ed.). Atlanta: Arthritis Foundation. Reprinted with permission from The Arthritis Foundation, 1330 W. Peachtree St., Atlanta, GA 30309.

Etiology and Pathophysiology

Research continues to focus on identifying the underlying causes and the pathophysiological mechanisms of FMS. There is general agreement that FMS is a disorder of central processing with neuroendocrine or neurotransmitter dysregulation. The pain amplification experienced by the affected patient is caused by abnormal sensory processing in the CNS. Numerous studies have identified multiple physiological abnormalities in patients with FMS, including increased levels of substance P in the spinal cord, low levels of blood flow to the thalamus, dysfunction of the hypothalamic-pituitary-adrenal (HPA) axis, low levels of serotonin and tryptophan, and abnormalities in cytokine function. Serotonin and substance P play a role in mood regulation, sleep, and pain perception. Changes in the HPA axis can also negatively affect a person's physical and mental health, leading to an increased incidence of depression and a decreased response to stress. A genetic susceptibility for FMS may also exist. A recent viral illness or Lyme disease may serve as an infectious trigger in susceptible persons.

Clinical Manifestations and Complications

Clinical manifestations of FMS overlap with those of CFS (Yunus, 2007). Patients experience a widespread burning pain that worsens and improves through the course of a day. It is often difficult for patients to discriminate whether pain occurs in the muscles, the joints, or soft tissues. Head or facial pain often results from stiff or painful neck and shoulder muscles. It can accompany temporomandibular joint dysfunction, which affects an estimated one third of patients with FMS. Nonrestorative sleep and resulting fatigue are typical.

Physical examination characteristically reveals point tenderness at 11 or more of 18 identified sites (Dell, 2007) (Figure 67-12). However, patients with FMS are sensitive to painful stimuli throughout the body and not merely at the identified tender sites. In addition, point tenderness can vary from day to day. On some occasions, the FMS patient may respond to fewer than 11 tender points; at other times, palpation of all sites may elicit pain.

Cognitive effects range from difficulty concentrating to memory lapses and a feeling of being overwhelmed when dealing with multiple tasks. Many individuals report migraine headaches. Depression and anxiety often occur and may necessitate drug therapy. Numbness or tingling sensation in the hands or feet (paraesthesia) often accompanies FMS. Restless legs syndrome is also typical, with patients describing an irresistible urge to move the legs when at rest or lying down.

Irritable bowel syndrome with manifestations of constipation, or diarrhea, abdominal pain, and bloating (or some combination of these) is common. Patients with FMS may also experience difficulty swallowing, perhaps because of abnormalities in esophageal smooth muscle function. Increased frequency of urination and urinary urgency, in the absence of a bladder infection, are typical complaints. Women with FMS may experience more difficult menstruation, with a worsening of disease symptoms during this time.

Diagnostic Studies

A definitive diagnosis of FMS is often difficult to establish. Lack of knowledge among health care providers may also cause delays in diagnosis and treatment. Laboratory results in most cases serve to rule out other disorders suspected on the basis of the patient's history and physical examination. On occasion, a low ANA titre is present, but it is not considered diagnostic. Muscle biopsy may reveal a nonspecific moth-eaten appearance or fibre atrophy. The Arthritis Society (2011a) pointed out that for FMS to be diagnosed, two criteria must be present: (a) Pain is experienced in 11 of the 18 tender points on palpation (see Figure 67-12) and (b) widespread pain for at least 3 months is documented. *Widespread pain* is defined as occurring on both sides of the body and above and below the waist.

Collaborative Care

The treatment of FMS is based on symptoms, and success depends on high patient motivation. The nurse can play a key role in teaching patients to be active participants in the therapeutic regimen. Rest can help pain, aching, and tenderness. Drug treatment includes low doses of tricyclic compounds such as cyclobenzaprine and amitriptyline (Elavil). If amitriptyline is not well tolerated, similar drugs can be substituted (e.g., doxepin [Sinequan], imipramine, trazodone). Selective serotonin reuptake inhibitor (SSRI) antidepressants (e.g., sertraline [Zoloft], paroxetine [Paxil]) tend to be reserved for affected patients who also have depression. Both antidepressants and muscle relaxants have sedative effects that can help in improving nighttime rest for patients with FMS.

Long-acting opioids are generally not recommended unless FMS is refractory to other therapies. In some patients, pain may be managed with OTC analgesics such as acetaminophen (Tylenol), ibuprofen (Motrin, Advil), or naproxen (Aleve).

Benzodiazepines (e.g., diazepam, alprazolam [Xanax], clonazepam [Rivotril]) are often prescribed with low doses of ibuprofen (Motrin, Advil) to treat anxiety, as well as the muscle spasms that affect many FMS patients.

The antiseizure drugs gabapentin (Neurontin) and pregabalin (Lyrica) are among the newest treatments for FMS. These drugs may help to reduce pain and fatigue and improve sleep and daily functioning.

NURSING MANAGEMENT: FIBROMYALGIA SYNDROME

Because of the chronic nature of FMS and the necessity of maintaining an ongoing rehabilitation program, patients with FMS need consistent support from the nurse and other members of the health care team. Massage is often combined with ultrasound therapy or the application of alternating heat and cold packs to soothe tense, sore muscles and increase blood circulation. Gentle stretching can be performed by a physiotherapist or practised by the patient at home to relieve muscle tension and spasm. Yoga and Tai Chi are often appropriate. Low-impact aerobic exercise such as walking can help prevent muscle atrophy.

Dietitians often urge patients with FMS to limit their consumption of sugar, caffeine, and alcohol because these substances have been shown to be muscle irritants. Vitamin and mineral supplements may be appropriate to combat stress, correct deficiencies, and support the immune system. However, unproven "miracle diets" or supplements should be carefully

investigated by patients and discussed with the health care provider before any of them is used. Patients should understand that some foods and supplements may cause serious or even dangerous adverse effects when taken along with certain drugs.

Pain and the related symptoms of FMS can cause significant stress. There is also some indication that patients with FMS simply do not process stress well. Effective relaxation strategies include biofeedback, guided imagery, and autogenic training. Patients need to receive initial training for these interventions, but they can then continue to practise on their own. Psychological counselling (individual or group) may also prove beneficial for patients. (Stress and stress management are discussed in Chapter 8.)

Chronic Fatigue Syndrome

Chronic fatigue syndrome (CFS), also called *chronic fatigue and immune dysfunction syndrome*, is a disorder characterized by debilitating fatigue and a variety of associated physical complaints. Immune system abnormalities are also frequently present. The prevalence of CFS is difficult to establish because of the lack of validated diagnostic tests. It is more common in women than in men. CFS is a poorly understood condition that can have a devastating effect on the lives of patients and their families. CFS and FMS share some common features.

Etiology and Pathophysiology

Despite numerous attempts to determine the etiology and the pathology of CFS, the precise mechanisms remain unknown. However, there are many theories about the cause of CFS. Neuroendocrine abnormalities that have been implicated involve a hypofunction of the HPA axis and the hypothalamic-pituitary-gonadal (HPG) axis, which together regulate the stress response and reproductive hormone levels (Klimas & Koneru, 2007). Several microorganisms have been investigated as etiological agents, including herpesviruses (e.g., Epstein Barr virus, cytomegalovirus), retroviruses, enteroviruses, *Candida albicans*, and mycoplasma. Because cognitive deficits (e.g., decreased memory, attention, concentration) occur in many affected patients, it has also been proposed that CFS results from changes in the CNS.

Clinical Manifestations

It is often difficult to distinguish between CFS and FMS because many clinical features are similar. In about half the cases, CFS develops insidiously, or patients may have intermittent episodes that gradually become chronic. Incapacitating fatigue is the most common symptom of CFS and causes patients to seek health care. Associated symptoms (Table 67-19) may fluctuate in intensity over time. In other situations, CFS arises suddenly in a previously active, healthy individual. An unremarkable influenza-like illness or other acute stress is often identified as a triggering event.

Patients may become angry and frustrated with the inability of health care providers to diagnose a problem. The disorder may have a major effect on work, family responsibilities, and ADLs.

Table 67-19 Diagnostic Criteria for Chronic Fatigue Syndrome*

Major Criteria

- Unexplained, persistent, or relapsing chronic fatigue is of new and definite onset (not lifelong); is not caused by ongoing exertion; is not substantially alleviated by rest; and results in substantial reduction in occupational, educational, social, or personal activities

Minor Criteria

- Impaired memory or concentration
- Frequent or recurrent sore throat
- Tender cervical or axillary lymph nodes
- Muscle pain
- Multijoint pain without joint swelling or tenderness
- Headaches of a new type, pattern, or severity
- Unrefreshing sleep
- Postexertional malaise

Source: Adapted from Centers for Disease Control and Prevention. (2011). *Chronic fatigue syndrome: Diagnosis.* Retrieved from *http://www.cdc.gov/cfs/diagnosis/index.html*
*For a diagnosis to be made, the patient must demonstrate the major criterion plus four or more of the minor criteria for 6 months or more. These criteria were prepared by the Centers for Disease Control and Prevention, the National Institutes of Health, and the International Chronic Fatigue Syndrome Study Group.

Diagnostic Studies

Physical examination and diagnostic studies can be used to rule out other possible causes of a patient's symptoms. No laboratory test can diagnose CFS or measure its severity. The Centers for Disease Control and Prevention (2011) developed diagnostic criteria based on patients' symptoms (see Table 67-19). In general, CFS remains a diagnosis of exclusion.

NURSING AND COLLABORATIVE MANAGEMENT: CHRONIC FATIGUE SYNDROME

Because there is no definitive treatment for CFS, supportive management is essential. Patients should be informed about what is known about the disease, and all complaints should be taken seriously. NSAIDs can be used to treat headaches, muscle and joint aches, and fever. Because many patients with CFS also have allergies and sinusitis, antihistamines and decongestants can be used to treat allergic symptoms. Tricyclic antidepressants (e.g., doxepin [Sinequan], amitriptyline [Elavil]) and SSRIs (e.g., fluoxetine [Prozac], paroxetine [Paxil]) can improve mood and sleep problems. Clonazepam (Rivotril) can also be used to treat sleep disturbances and panic disorders. The use of low-dose hydrocortisone to decrease fatigue and disability is being studied.

Total rest is not advised because it can potentiate the self-image of being an invalid, and strenuous exertion can exacerbate the exhaustion. Therefore, it is important to plan a carefully graduated exercise program. A well-balanced diet that includes fibre and fresh dark-coloured fruits and vegetables for antioxidant action is essential in treatment. Behavioural therapy may be used to promote a positive outlook, as well as improve overall disability, fatigue, and other symptoms (Centers for Disease Control and Prevention, 2010).

One of the major problems facing many patients with CFS is financial instability. When the illness strikes, they cannot work or must decrease the amount of time spent working. Obtaining disability benefits can be frustrating because of the difficulty in establishing a diagnosis of CFS.

CFS does not appear to progress. Although most patients recover or experience at least gradual improvement over time, some do not show substantial improvement. Recovery is more common in individuals with a sudden onset of CFS. Patients with CFS suffer from substantial occupational and psychosocial impairments and loss, including the social pressure and isolation from being characterized as lazy or crazy.

CLINICAL DECISION-MAKING EXERCISE

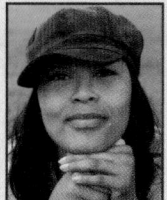

CASE STUDY:
Rheumatoid Arthritis

Source: © iStockphoto.com/Juanmonino.

Patient Profile

Grace Abeda, a 30-year-old married woman, is seen at the rheumatology clinic because she is experiencing swelling and stiffness in the small joints of her hands.

Subjective Data

- Concert pianist
- Experiencing joint pain and stiffness in both hands for the past 6 weeks
- Experiencing fatigue, anorexia, and morning stiffness
- Gave birth to her first child 2 months ago

Objective Data

Physical Examination
- Swelling and tenderness of third and fourth MCP joints of both hands
- Mild pain with neck motion

Diagnostic Studies
- Elevated ESR and positive RF findings
- Evidence of moderate bone demineralization on bilateral hand radiographs

Collaborative Care

- Diagnosis: RA
- Therapy: started on meloxicam (Mobicox), 15 mg daily; hydroxychloroquine (Plaquenil), 400 mg daily; and prednisone, 10 mg daily

Discussion Questions

1. How might the nurse explain the pathophysiology of RA to Ms. Abeda?
2. How might the recent childbirth have influenced the symptoms that she is currently experiencing?
3. What are some home and work modifications that the nurse can suggest to Ms. Abeda that will reduce her symptoms?
4. What suggestions can the nurse make to Ms. Abeda about coping with fatigue?
5. *Priority Decision:* On the basis of the assessment data presented, what are the priority nursing diagnoses? Are there any collaborative problems?

ⓔvolve *Answers are available at* **http://evolve.elsevier.com/ Canada/Lewis/medsurg**

REVIEW QUESTIONS

The number of the question corresponds to the same-numbered objective at the beginning of the chapter.

1. Which of the following would the nurse understand as causing damage to the joints of a patient with rheumatoid arthritis?
   a. The development of Heberden's nodes in the joint capsule
   b. The deterioration of cartilage by the enzyme hyaluronidase
   c. Invasion of pannus into the joint capsule and subchondral bone
   d. Bony ankylosis after inflammation of the joints in HLA-B27–positive individuals
2. Of the following assessment data, which is common in patients with osteoarthritis?
   a. Elevated ESR
   b. Evening but no morning stiffness
   c. Progressive joint pain with activity
   d. Symmetrical swelling of MCP joints
3. Which of the following would the nurse teach to a patient with ankylosing spondylitis?
   a. Avoid extremes in environmental temperatures.
   b. Continue with physical activity during flare-ups.
   c. Apply cool compresses for relief of local symptoms.
   d. Maintain proper posture and engage in regular exercise.
4. When the nurse administers medications to patients with gout, which of the following would the nurse recognize as a treatment for acute disease?
   a. Colchicine
   b. Sulphasalazine
   c. Allopurinol
   d. Cyclosporine
5. The nurse is teaching a patient with SLE about the disorder. The nurse understands that the pathophysiology of SLE includes which of the following?
   a. Circulating immune complexes formed from IgG autoantibodies reacting with IgG.
   b. An autoimmune T cell reaction that results in destruction of the deep dermal skin layer.
   c. Immunologic dysfunction leading to chronic inflammation in the cartilage and bones.
   d. The production of a variety of autoantibodies directed against constituents of the cell nucleus.
6. The nurse is caring for a patient with Sjögren's syndrome. Which of the following autoimmune disorders may the patient also develop?
   a. Uveitis
   b. Ulcerative colitis
   c. Glomerulonephritis
   d. Hashimoto's thyroiditis
7. Which of the following should the nurse understand when teaching a patient with chronic fatigue syndrome about the disorder?
   a. Eliciting pain by palpation of tender points is an indicator of CFS severity.
   b. Many symptoms are similar to those of fibromyalgia syndrome.
   c. Definitive treatment includes low-dose hydrocortisone.
   d. CFS is characterized by progressive memory impairment.

ANSWERS: 1. c; 2. c; 3. d; 4. a; 5. d; 6. d; 7. b.

REFERENCES

Arthritis Society. (2011a). Types of arthritis. Retrieved from *http:// www.arthritis.ca/aboutarthritis*

Arthritis Society. (2011b). Osteoarthritis—Know your options. Retrieved from *http://www.arthritis.ca/document.doc?id=328*

Arthritis Society. (2011c). Arthritis self-management program. Retrieved from *http://www.arthritis.ca/asmp*

Arthritis Society. (2011d). Rheumatoid arthritis—Know your options. Retrieved from *http://www.arthritis.ca/document.doc?id= 336*

Arthritis Society. (2011e). Psoriatic arthritis—Know your options. Retrieved from *http://www.arthritis.ca/document.doc?id=335*

Arthritis Society. (2011f). Lyme disease: How common is Lyme disease? Retrieved from *http://www.arthritis.ca/page.aspx?pid= 926*

Bellamy, N., Campbell, J., Robinson, V., Gee, T., Bourne, R., & Wells, G. (2006). Viscosupplementation for the treatment of osteoarthritis of the knee. *Cochrane Database of Systematic Reviews,* (1), CD005321. doi:10.1002/14651858.CD005321.pub2

Carmona, L., Cross, M., Williams, B., Lassere, M., & March, L. (2010). Rheumatoid arthritis. *Best Practice & Research: Clinical Rheumatology,* 24, 733-745. doi:10.1016/j.berh.2010.10.001

Carter, J., & Hudson, A. (2009). Reactive arthritis: Clinical aspects and medical management. *Rheumatic Disease Clinics of North America,* 35(1), 21-24. doi:10.1016/j.rdc.2009.03.010

Centers for Disease Control and Prevention. (2010). Chronic fatigue syndrome: Management. Retrieved from *http://www.cdc.gov/cfs/ management/index.html*

Centers for Disease Control and Prevention. (2011). Chronic fatigue syndrome: Diagnosis. Retrieved from *http://www.cdc.gov/cfs/ diagnosis/index.html*

Chen, C., Wang, J., & Juhn, R. (2008). Total hip arthroplasty for primary septic arthritis of the hip in adults. *International Orthopaedics, 32,* 573-580. doi:10.1007/s00264-007-0366-1

Daniels, S. (2007). We all need to know about Sjögren's syndrome. *Nursing Times, 103*(42), 15.

Danoff-Berg, S., & Friedberg, F. (2009). Unmet needs of patients with systemic lupus erythematosus. *Behavioral Medicine, 35*(1), 5-13. doi:10.3200/BMED.35.1.5-13

Davis, J., & Mease, P. (2007). Insights into the pathology and treatment of spondyloarthritis: From the bench to the clinic. *Seminars in Arthritis and Rheumatism, 38,* 83-100. doi:10.1016/j.semarthrit.2007.10.007

Dedeoglu, F. (2009). Drug-induced autoimmunity. *Current Opinions in Rheumatology, 21,* 547-551. doi:10.1097/BOR.0b013e32832f13db

Dell, D. (2007). Getting the point about: Fibromyalgia. *Nursing, 37*(2), 61-64.

Donahue, K. E., Gartlehner, G., Jonas, D. E., Lux, L. J., Thieda, P., Jonas, B. L., ..., Lohr, K. N. (2008). Systematic review: Comparative effectiveness and harms of disease-modifying medications for rheumatoid arthritis. *Annals of Internal Medicine, 148,* 124-134.

Dougados, M., & Baeten, D. (2011). Spondyloarthritis. *The Lancet, 377,* 2127-2137. doi:10.1016/S0140-6736(11)60071-8

Fransen, M., & McConnell, S. (2009). Exercise for osteoarthritis of the knee [Review]. *Cochrane Database of Systematic Review, (4),* CD004376. doi:10.1002/14651858.CD004376.pub2

Girschick, H., Morbach., H., & Tappe, D. (2009). Treatment of Lyme borreliosis. *Arthritis Research and Therapy, 11,* 259-268. doi:10.1186/ar2853

Gray, C., & Walters-Smith, N. (2011). Febuxostat for treatment of chronic gout. *American Journal of Health-System Pharmacists, 68,* 389-398. doi:10.2146/ajhp 100394

Hellman, D., & Imboden, J. (2008). Arthritis and musculoskeletal disorders. In S. McPhee, M. Papadakis, & L. Tierney (Eds.), *Current medical diagnosis and treatment* (pp. 725-729). New York: McGraw-Hill.

Hollowell, M., Thompson, L., & Pantanowitz, L. (2008). Gout. *Ear, Nose, & Throat Journal, 87*(3), 132-134.

Hurkmans, E., van der Giesen, F., Vliet Vlieland, T., Schoones, J., & Van den Ende, E. (2009). Dynamic exercise programs (aerobic capacity and/or muscle strength training) in patients with rheumatoid arthritis. *Cochrane Database of Systematic Reviews* (4), CD006853. doi:10.1002/14651858.CD006853.pub2

Klimas, N., & Koneru, A. O. (2007). Chronic fatigue syndrome: inflammation, immune function and neuroendocrine interactions. *Current Rheumatology Reports, 9,* 482-487. doi:10.1007/s11926-007-0078-y

Lavelle, E., Lavelle, W., & Smith, H. (2007). Myofascial trigger points. *Medical Clinics of North America, 91*(2), 22-39. doi:10.1016/j.mcna.2006.12.004

Lupus Canada. (2007). Living well with lupus: An introduction to corticosteroids and anti-malarial drugs. Retrieved from *http://www.lupuscanada.org/english/living/factsheets.html*

Malik, A., Schumacher, H. R., Dinnella, J. E., & Clayburne, G. M. (2009). Clinical diagnostic criteria for gout: Comparison with the gold standard of synovial fluid crystal analysis. *Journal of Clinical Rheumatology, 15,* 22-24. doi:10.1097/RHU.0b013e3181945b79

Manheimer, E., Cheng, K., Linde, K., Lao, L., Yoo, J., Wieland, S., ..., Bouter, L. M. (1996). Acupuncture for peripheral joint osteoarthritis. *Cochrane Database of Systematic Reviews, (1),* CD001977. doi:10.1002/14651858.CD001977.pub2

Mathews, C., & Coakley, G. (2008). Septic arthritis: Current diagnostic and therapeutic algorithm. *Current Opinion in Rheumatology, 20,* 457-462. doi:10.1097/BOR.0b013e3283036975

National Psoriasis Foundation. (2012). Types of psoriatic arthritis. Retrieved from *http://www.psoriasis.org/psoriatic-arthritis/types*

Nüesch, E., Rutjes, A., Trelle, S., Reichenbach, S., & Jüni, P. (2009). Doxycycline for osteoarthritis of the knee or hip. *Cochrane Database of Systematic Reviews* (4), CD007323. doi:10.1002/14651858.CD007323.pub2

Øiestad, B., Engebretsen, L., Storheim, K., & Risberg, M. (2009). Knee osteoarthritis after anterior cruciate ligament injury: A systematic review. *American Journal of Sports Medicine, 37,* 1434-1443. doi:10.1177/0363546509338827

Public Health Agency of Canada, Arthritis Consumer Experts, Arthritis Community Research & Evaluation Unit, Canadian Arthritis Patients Alliance, Canadian Arthritis Network, Canadian Institute for Health Information, ..., The Arthritis Society. (2010). Life with arthritis in Canada: A personal and public health challenge. Retrieved from *http://www.phac aspc.gc.ca/cd-mc/arthritis-arthrite/lwaic-vaaac-10/pdf/arthritis-2010-eng.pdf*

Roberts, D. (2007). Arthritis and connective tissue disorders. In H. M. Taggart (Ed.), *NAON core curriculum for orthopaedic nursing* (6th ed., Chapter 12). Boston: Pearson.

Scleroderma Society of Canada. (2008). What is scleroderma? Retrieved from *http://www.scleroderma.ca/pamphlets.php*

Seshan, S., & Jennette, J. (2009). Renal disease in systemic lupus erythematosus with emphasis on classification of lupus glomerulonephritis: Advances and implications. *Archives of Pathology and Laboratory Medicine, 133,* 233-248.

Shah, D., Flanigan, T., & Lally, E. (2011). Routine screening for HIV in rheumatology practice. *Journal of Clinical Rheumatology, 17,* 154-156. doi:10.1096/RHU.0b013e318214c119

Towheed, T., Maxwell, L., Anastassiades, T., Shea, B., Houpt, J. B., Welch, V., ..., Wells, G. A. (2009). Glucosamine therapy for treating osteoarthritis [Review]. *Cochrane Database of Systematic Reviews,* (2), CD002946. doi:10.1002/14651858.CD002946.pub2

van Venrooij, W., van Beers, J., & Pruijn, G. (2011). Anti-CCP antibodies: the past, the present and the future. *Rheumatology, 7,* 391-398. doi:10.1038/nrrheum.2011.76

Vincent, R. (2009). Scleroderma. *Practice Nurse, 38*(4), 47-52.

Widberg, K., Karimi, H., Hafstrom, I. (2009). Self- and manual mobilization improves spine mobility in men with ankylosing spondylitis—A randomized study. *Clinical Rehabilitation, 23,* 599-608. doi:10.1177/0269215508101748

Yunus, M. B. (2007). Fibromyalgia and overlapping disorders: The unifying concept of central sensitivity syndromes. *Seminars in Arthritis and Rheumatism, 36,* 339-356. doi:10.1016/j.semarthrit.2006.12.009

Zhang, Y., & Jordan, J. (2008). Epidemiology of arthritis. *Rheumatic Diseases Clinics of North America, 34,* 515-529. doi:10.1016/j.rdc.2008.05.007

CANADIAN RESOURCES

Arthritis Research Centre of Canada
http://www.arthritisresearch.ca
The Arthritis Society
http://www.arthritis.ca
Canadian Arthritis Network (CAN)
http://www.arthritisnetwork.ca
Canadian Lyme Disease Foundation (CanLyme)
http://www.canlyme.com
Canadian Organization for Rare Disorders (CORD)
http://www.raredisorders.ca
Canadian Rheumatology Association (CRA)
http://www.rheum.ca
Canadian Spondylitis Association
http://www.spondylitis.ca
Lupus Canada
http://www.lupuscanada.org
National ME/FM Action Network
http://www.mefmaction.net
Scleroderma Society of Canada
http://www.scleroderma.ca

⊜volve *For additional Internet resources, see the Web site for this book at* **http://evolve.elsevier.com/Canada/Lewis/medsurg**

Nursing Care in Specialized Settings

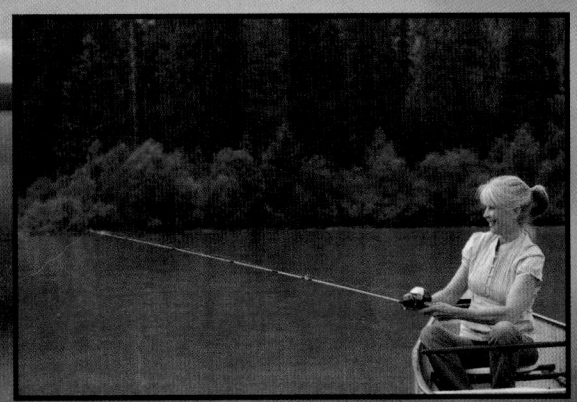

Source: Noel Hendrickson/Photodisc/Thinkstock

SECTION OUTLINE

Nursing Management: Critical Care Environment

Written by Linda Bucher and Maureen A. Seckel

Adapted by Sandra Goldsworthy

LEARNING OBJECTIVES

1. Describe the critical care certification process available to critical care nurses in Canada as well as advanced practice roles such as the clinical nurse specialist and the acute care nurse practitioner.
2. Select appropriate nursing interventions to manage common problems and needs of critically ill patients.
3. Develop effective strategies to manage issues related to the families and caregivers of critically ill patients.
4. Apply the principles of hemodynamic monitoring and the collaborative care and nursing management of the patient receiving this intervention.
5. Differentiate the purpose of, indications for, and function of circulatory-assist devices and related collaborative care and nursing management.
6. Differentiate the indications for and contrast the modes of mechanical ventilation.
7. Select appropriate nursing interventions related to the care of an intubated patient.
8. Relate the principles of mechanical ventilation to the collaborative care and nursing management of patients receiving this intervention.

KEY TERMS

circulatory-assist devices (CADs) Devices that are used to decrease cardiac work and improve organ perfusion in patients with heart failure, p. 1937

continuous positive airway pressure (CPAP) A ventilatory mode used to restore functional residual capacity; delivered during spontaneous breathing, p. 1950

endotracheal (ET) intubation Insertion of a tube into the trachea, bypassing the upper airway and laryngeal structures to create an artificial airway, p. 1941

hemodynamic monitoring Refers to the ongoing measurement of pressure, flow, and oxygenation within the cardiovascular system, p. 1927

intra-aortic balloon pump Device that provides temporary circulatory assistance to the compromised heart by reducing afterload (via reduction in systolic pressure) and augmenting the aortic diastolic pressure, p. 1937

mechanical ventilation The process in which the fraction of inspired oxygen is moved in and out of the lungs by a mechanical ventilator, p. 1946

negative-pressure ventilation Involves the use of chambers that encase the chest or body and surround it with intermittent subatmospheric pressure or negative pressure, p. 1946

phlebostatic axis A landmark used to establish the zero reference point for hemodynamic lines at the level of the atria of the heart; located at the intersection of two imaginary lines intersecting at the fourth intercostal space and at midchest, halfway between the outermost anterior and the outermost posterior surfaces, p. 1929

positive end-expiratory pressure (PEEP) A ventilatory manoeuvre in which positive pressure is applied to the airway during exhalation, p. 1949

positive-pressure ventilation (PPV) A ventilatory mode in which the ventilator pushes air into the lungs under positive pressure; the primary method used with acutely ill patients, p. 1947

pressure ventilation The peak inspiratory pressure is predetermined, and the tidal volume delivered to the patient by the mechanical ventilator varies (see volume ventilation), p. 1947

ventricular assist device (VAD) Provides longer-term support for the failing heart; inserted into the path of flowing blood to augment or replace the action of the ventricle, p. 1940

volume ventilation A predetermined tidal volume is delivered to the patient with each inspiration, and the amount of pressure needed to deliver the breath varies (see pressure ventilation), p. 1947

ELECTRONIC RESOURCES

Supplemental content related to Chapter 68 can be found...

Evolve Web Site ⊜volve

http://evolve.elsevier.com/Canada/Lewis/medsurg
- Answer Guidelines for Case Study on p. 1956
- Clinical Reference: Laboratory Values
- Content Updates
- Electronic Calculators
- eFigure 68-1: Negative-Pressure Ventilator

- eNCP 68-1: Mechanical Ventilation
- eTable 68-1 Abbreviations Commonly Used in the Critical Care Unit
- Examination Review Questions
- Glossary
- Interactive Case Study: Pulmonary Embolism and Respiratory Failure
- Key Points (Printable and MP3 Download)

Critical Care Nursing

Critical Care Units

Critical care nursing is defined as a specialty dealing with human responses to life-threatening problems (American Association of Critical Care Nurses [AACN], 2010). Critical care nurses care for patients with acute and unstable physiological problems, as well as their caregivers. This involves assessing life-threatening conditions, initiating appropriate interventions, and evaluating the outcomes of the interventions.

In many acute care settings, the concept of critical care unit (CCU) care has expanded from delivering care in a standard unit to bringing CCU care to patients wherever they might be. The electronic or virtual CCU is designed to augment the bedside CCU team by monitoring the patient from a remote location (Figure 68-1). Another development is the role of the rapid-response team. The rapid-response team is usually composed of a critical care nurse, a respiratory therapist, and a critical care physician or an advanced practice nurse. The team goes outside the CCU to bring rapid and immediate care to patients in unstable condition in noncritical care units. Research has shown that patients often exhibit subtle early signs of deterioration (e.g., mild confusion) 6 to 8 hours before cardiac or respiratory arrest, and early critical care intervention has made significant contributions to reducing mortality rates in these patients (Jolley, Bendyk, Holaday, Lombardozzi, & Harmon, 2007; Chamberlain & Donley, 2009).

The biotechnology available in the CCU is extensive and always evolving. It is possible to continuously monitor the electrocardiogram (ECG), blood pressure (BP), oxygen (O_2) saturation, cardiac output (CO), intracranial pressure, and temperature. More advanced monitoring devices measure cardiac index (CI), stroke volume (SV), ejection fraction, end-tidal partial pressure of carbon dioxide ($PETCO_2$), and tissue O_2 consumption. Patients may receive ongoing support from mechanical ventilators, intra-aortic balloon pumps (IABPs), circulatory-assist devices (CADs), or dialysis machines. Figure 68-2 shows a typical CCU.

Progressive-care units, also called intermediate-care units or step-down units, provide a transition between the CCU and the general care unit or discharge (Ecklund & Danbaugh, 2009). Generally, progressive-care unit patients are at risk for serious complications, but their risk is lower than that of CCU patients. Examples of patients found in progressive-care units include those scheduled for interventional cardiac procedures (e.g., stent placement), awaiting heart transplant, receiving stable doses of vasoactive intravenous (IV) drugs (e.g., diltiazem [Cardizem]), or

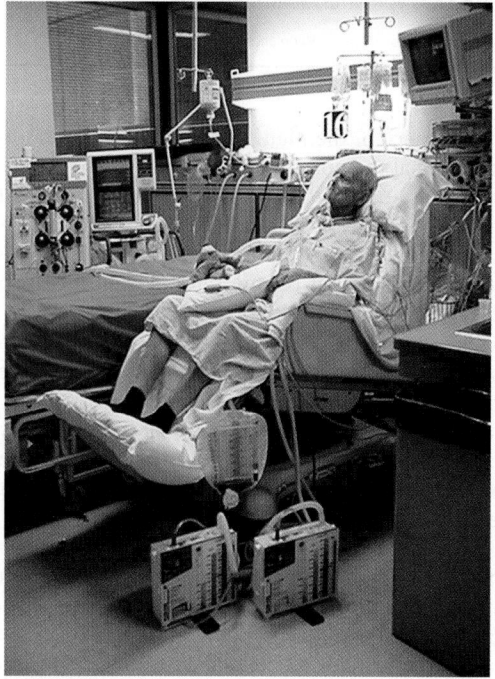

Figure 68-1 Electronic intensive care unit control room.

Source: Frownfelter, D., & Dean, E. (2012). *Cardiovascular and pulmonary physical therapy: Evidence and practice* (5th ed., p. 562, Figure 34-2). St. Louis: Mosby Elsevier.

being weaned from prolonged mechanical ventilation. Some examples of monitoring capabilities in these units include continuous ECG, arterial BP, O_2 saturation, and $PETCO_2$. Patients may be receiving continual support from mechanical ventilators, IABPs, ventricular assist devices, or dialysis machines.

Critical Care Nurse

A critical care nurse has in-depth knowledge of anatomy, physiology, pathophysiology, pharmacology, and advanced assessment skills as well as the ability to use advanced biotechnology. Critical care nurses perform frequent assessments to monitor trends (patterns) in the patient's physiological parameters (e.g., BP, ECG). This allows the nurse to rapidly recognize and manage complications while fostering healing and recovery. The nurse must also provide psychological support to the patient and caregiver(s). To be effective, the critical care nurse must be able to communicate and collaborate with all members of the multidisciplinary health

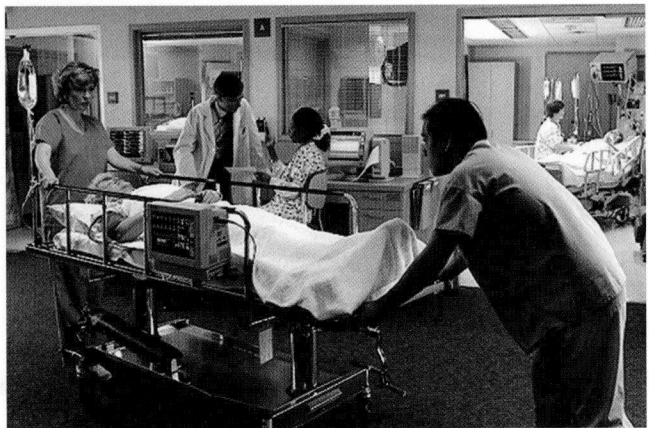

Figure 68-2 Typical critical care unit.

Source: Courtesy Spacelabs Medical, Redmond, Washington.

team (e.g., physician, dietitian, social worker, respiratory therapist, occupational therapist).

Critical care nurses face ethical dilemmas related to the care of patients. Moral distress over perceived issues of delivering futile or nonbeneficial care can lead to emotional exhaustion or burnout. Consequently, it is important that all members of the health team coexist in a healthy work environment.

Specialization in CCU nursing usually initially requires comprehensive theoretical preparation and a preceptored orientation or internship. New innovations for preparing nurses to practise in critical care settings include educational opportunities to participate in simulated cases in the human simulation laboratory that mimic the critical care environment (Durham College Critical Care e-Learning Project, 2012).

The Canadian Nurses Association offers critical care certification, CNCC(C), in critical care nursing. The designation requires that a registered nurse have practice experience in critical care nursing and successfully complete a comprehensive written examination set to national standards. Continued critical care practice and retesting or continuing education is required for recertification. CNCC(C) certification validates knowledge of critical care nursing; it is not the same as advanced practice. In Canada, registered nurses may also choose to complete a Critical Care Certificate through classroom or online education, typically combined with preceptored clinical experience.

Advanced practice critical care nurses have a graduate (master's or doctorate) degree. These nurses are employed in a variety of roles: patient and staff educators, consultants, administrators, researchers, or expert practitioners. The advanced practice critical care nurse who is a clinical nurse specialist typically functions in one or more of these roles. Typically, a clinical nurse specialist has graduate preparation as well as expertise in critical care. Another advanced practice role is the acute care nurse practitioner (ACNP). This ACNP provides comprehensive care to selected critically ill patients and their families. The ACNP conducts comprehensive assessments, orders and interprets diagnostic tests, manages health problems and disease-related symptoms, prescribes treatments, and coordinates care during transitions in settings. The ACNP may practise independently (e.g., providing comprehensive care to the chronically critically ill) or collaboratively (e.g., providing symptom management in conjunction with physicians). In Canada, ACNPs are prepared at the graduate level.

Patient in Critical Care

A patient is generally admitted to the CCU for one of three reasons. First, the patient may be physiologically unstable, requiring advanced and sophisticated clinical judgements by the nurse or physician. Second, the patient may be at risk for serious complications and require frequent and often invasive assessments. Third, the patient may require intensive and complicated nursing support related to the use of IV polypharmacy (e.g., neuromuscular blockade, thrombolytics, drugs requiring titration) and advanced biotechnology (e.g., ventricular assist devices, mechanical ventilation, intracranial pressure monitoring, continuous renal replacement therapy, hemodynamic monitoring).

CCU patients can be clustered by disease condition (e.g., neurology, pulmonary) or age group (e.g., neonatal, pediatrics). CCU patients are sometimes clustered by acuity (e.g., acute and unstable as opposed to technology-dependent but stable). Patients commonly treated in the CCU include those with respiratory distress, myocardial ischemia or infarction, or acute neurological impairment or those receiving care after cardiac surgery or major organ transplantation. The care of the critically injured patient is provided in trauma and burn CCUs. The patient with a medical emergency (e.g., septic shock, drug overdoses, or poisonings or thyroid, adrenal, or hematological crises) is often treated in a medical CCU. The patient who is not expected to recover from an illness is usually not admitted to a CCU. For example, the CCU is not used to manage the patient in a persistent coma or to prolong the natural process of death.

Despite the emphasis on caring for patients who are expected to survive, the incidence of death is higher in CCU patients than in non-CCU patients. Estimates predict that as many as one in five patients die in a CCU. In general, nonsurvivors are older, have co-morbidities (e.g., renal or liver disease, obesity), and experience longer CCU stays (Weigand & Williams, 2009). Consequently, it is essential the nurse be skilled in palliative and end-of-life care (see Chapter 13).

Common Problems of Critical Care Patients. The patient admitted to the CCU is at risk for numerous complications and special problems. Critically ill patients are usually immobile and at risk for venous thromboembolism and skin problems (see Chapter 26). The use of multiple invasive devices predisposes the patient to hospital-acquired infections. Sepsis and multiple organ dysfunction syndrome may follow (see Chapter 69). Adequate nourishment for the critically ill patient is paramount but frequently overlooked. Other special problems for CCU patients relate to anxiety, pain, impaired communication, sensory–perceptual problems, and sleep disorders.

Nutrition. Patients are often admitted to CCUs with conditions that result in either hypermetabolic states (e.g., burns, trauma, sepsis) or catabolic states (e.g., acute renal failure). Other times, patients may be admitted in severely malnourished states, such as those that occur with wasting syndrome and chronic liver disease. In general, malnutrition has been linked to increases in mortality and morbidity.

Determining whom to feed, what to feed, when to feed, and how to feed (e.g., route of administration) are crucial questions that the nurse must ask when caring for a critically ill patient (Stapleton, Jones & Heyland, 2007; Bankhead et al., 2009; see also the Evidence-Informed Practice box "Nutritional Support in Critically Ill Patients"). The nurse must collaborate with the physician and the dietitian to determine how best to meet the nutritional needs of CCU patients.

The primary goal of nutritional support is to prevent or correct nutritional deficiencies. This is usually accomplished by the early provision of enteral nutrition (i.e., delivery of calories via the gastrointestinal [GI] tract) or parenteral nutrition (i.e., delivery of calories intravenously) (McCalve et al., 2009). Enteral nutrition preserves the structure and function of the gut mucosa and prevents the movement of gut bacteria across the intestinal wall and into the bloodstream. In addition, early enteral nutrition is associated with fewer complications and shorter hospital stays and is less expensive than parenteral nutrition (McCalve et al., 2009; Hutchinson, 2009). (Enteral and parenteral nutrition are discussed in Chapter 42.)

Parenteral nutrition is used when the enteral route is unsuccessful in providing adequate nutrition or is contraindicated. Examples of these conditions are paralytic ileus, diffuse peritonitis, intestinal obstruction, pancreatitis, GI ischemia, intractable vomiting, and severe diarrhea.

Anxiety. Anxiety is a common problem for CCU patients. The primary sources of anxiety include the perceived or anticipated threat to physical health, actual loss of control of body functions, and an environment that is foreign. Many patients and caregivers feel uncomfortable in the CCU environment with its complex equipment, high noise and light levels, isolation from family, and intense pace of activity. Pain and sleeplessness enhance anxiety, as do immobilization, loss of control, and impaired communication.

To help reduce anxiety, encourage patients and caregivers to express concerns, ask questions, and state their needs. Include the patient and caregiver in all conversations and explain the purpose of equipment and procedures. Encourage caregivers to bring in photographs and personal items. Judicious use of antianxiety drugs (e.g., lorazepam [Ativan]) and complementary therapies (e.g., guided imagery, massage) may reduce the stress response that can be triggered by anxiety (Woods, 2007).

In one study of over 700 critical care nurses (Gupta, 2007), 71% reported that assessing patients for anxiety was very important. The nurses also identified agitation, increased BP, increased heart rate, patient verbalization of anxiety, and restlessness as the five most important clinical indicators of anxiety. To help reduce anxiety, the nurse should encourage patients and families to express concerns, ask questions, and state their needs. The nurse should include the patient and the family in all conversations and explain the purpose of equipment and procedures. The nurse should also structure the patient's surrounding environment in such a way as to decrease anxiety if possible.

Pain. The control of pain in the CCU patient is paramount. It is reported that as many as 70% of CCU patients recount having moderate to severe unrelieved pain (Garland, 2005). Inadequate pain control is often linked with agitation and anxiety and is known to contribute to the stress response. CCU patients at high risk for pain include patients who (1) have medical conditions that include ischemic, infectious, or inflammatory processes; (2) are immobilized; (3) have invasive monitoring devices, including endotracheal (ET) tubes; and (4) are scheduled for any invasive or noninvasive procedures (Gélinas, 2007).

For some critically ill patients, continuous IV sedation (e.g., propofol [Diprivan]) and an analgesic agent (e.g., fentanyl) are a practical and effective strategy for sedation and pain control. However, patients receiving deep sedation are unresponsive, and

EVIDENCE-INFORMED PRACTICE
Nutritional Support in Critically Ill Patients

Clinical Question
For critical care patients in whom nutritional support is indicated (P), what is the effect of providing enteral nutrition (I) versus parenteral nutrition (C) on patient outcomes (O)?

Best Clinical Practice
- When nutritional support is indicated, enteral nutrition should be preferentially used over parenteral nutrition.
- Parenteral nutrition is not recommended for critically ill patients with an intact gastrointestinal tract.
- In adult surgical patients, the early use of enteral nutrition is associated with a reduction in complications and shorter hospital stay.
- Early use of enteral nutrition is recommended in critically ill surgical patients and should be considered for other critically ill patients.
- Further studies are needed to determine the optimal timing and composition of parenteral nutrition in patients not tolerating enteral nutrition.

Implications for Nursing Practice
- Nurses have a very important role in assessing the nutritional status of critically ill patients.
- Providing nutritional support should be a standard of practice for critically ill patients.

References for Evidence
Jones, N. E., & Heyland, D. K. (2008). Implementing Nutrition Guidelines in the Critical Care Setting: A Worthwhile and Achievable Goal? *JAMA, 300*(23), 2798-2799. doi:10.1001/jama.2008.814; Heyland, D. K. (2000). Parenteral nutrition in the critically ill patient: More harm than good? *Proceedings of the Nutrition Society, 59*(3), 457-66; and Jones, N. E., Suurdt, J., Ouellette-Kuntz, H., & Heyland, D. K. (2007). Implementation of the Canadian Clinical Practice Guidelines for Nutrition Support: A multiple case study of barriers and enablers. *Nutrition in Clinical Practice, 22*(4), 449-457.

P, patient population of interest; *I,* intervention or area of interest; *C,* comparison of interest or comparison group; *O,* outcome(s) of interest.

this prevents the nurse and other health care providers from properly assessing the patient's neurological status. To address this limitation, guidelines that include a daily, scheduled interruption of sedation, or "drug holiday," have been developed. Daily sedative interruption allows the patient to awaken and the health care provider to conduct a neurological examination and assess readiness for weaning from the mechanical ventilator (Safer Health Care Now, 2012). (Chapter 10 has more detailed information on pain management.)

Impaired Communication. Inability to communicate is a distressing problem for the patient who may be unable to speak because of the use of sedative and paralyzing drugs or an ET tube. As part of any procedure the nurse should explain what will happen or is happening to the patient. When the patient cannot speak, the nurse should explore alternative methods of communication, including the use of devices such as picture boards, notepads, magic slates, or computer keyboards. When speaking with the patient, the nurse should look directly at the patient and use hand gestures when appropriate. For patients who do not speak English, the use of an approved interpreter is required (see Chapter 2, Tables 2-5 and 2-6).

Nonverbal communication is important. High levels of procedure-related touch and lower levels of comfort-related touch often characterize the CCU environment. Patients have different levels of tolerance for being touched, usually related to cultural background and personal history. It may be appropriate to provide comforting touch with ongoing evaluation of the patient's response. If appropriate, encourage caregivers to touch and talk with the patient even if the patient is unresponsive or comatose.

Sensory–Perceptual Problems. Acute and reversible sensory–perceptual changes are common in CCU patients. The combination of alterations in mentation (e.g., delusions, short attention span, loss of recent memory), psychomotor behaviour (e.g., restlessness, lethargy), and sleep–wake cycle (e.g., daytime sleepiness, nighttime agitation) has been inappropriately labelled "CCU psychosis." The patient experiencing these alterations is not psychotic but is suffering from delirium. It is estimated that the prevalence of delirium in CCU patients is as high as 80% (Ouimet, Cavanagh, Gottfried, & Skrobik, 2007).

Demographic factors predisposing the patient to delirium include advanced age, pre-existing cognitive impairment (e.g., dementia), vision or hearing impairments, and a history of drug or alcohol use. Environmental factors that can contribute to delirium include sleep deprivation, anxiety, sensory overload, and immobilization. Physical conditions such as hemodynamic instability, hypoxemia, hypercarbia, electrolyte disturbances, and severe infections can precipitate delirium. Last, certain drugs (e.g., sedatives [benzodiazepines], furosemide [Lasix], antimicrobials [aminoglycosides]) have been associated with the development of delirium (Devlin et al., 2008). (Delirium is discussed in Chapter 62.)

The nurse should monitor the patient for delirium and mental clarity. Tools to assess for delirium include the Confusion Assessment Method for the CCU and the Intensive Care Delirium Screening Checklist (Sona, 2009; see the Resources at the end of the chapter.) It is critical that physiological factors be addressed (e.g., correction of oxygenation, perfusion, and electrolyte problems). The use of clocks and calendars can help orient the patient. In addition, the presence of a caregiver may help orient the patient and reduce agitation.

Sensory overload can also result in patient distress and anxiety. Environmental noise levels are particularly high in the CCU (Friese, 2008). The nurse can limit noise and assist the patient in understanding noises that cannot be prevented. Conversation is a particularly stressful noise, especially when the discussion concerns the patient and is held in the presence of, but without participation from, the patient. The nurse can eliminate this source of stress by finding suitable places for patient-related discussions and, when possible, include the patient in the discussion.

The nurse can also limit noise levels directly by muting phones, setting alarms appropriate to the patient's condition, and eliminating unnecessary alarms. For example, the nurse can silence the BP alarms when manipulating invasive lines and then reactivate the alarms when done. Similarly, the nurse can silence ventilator alarms during ET suctioning. Finally, the nurse can limit overhead paging and all unnecessary noise in patient care areas.

Sleep Problems. Nearly all CCU patients experience sleep disturbances. Patients may have difficulty falling asleep or have disrupted sleep because of noise, anxiety, pain, frequent monitoring, or treatment procedures. Sleep disturbance is a significant stressor in the CCU, contributing to delirium and possibly affecting recovery (Friese, 2008). The nurse can structure the environment to promote the patient's sleep–wake cycle. Strategies include clustering activities, scheduling rest periods, dimming lights at nighttime, opening curtains during the daytime, obtaining physiological measurements without disturbing the patient, limiting noise, and providing comfort measures (e.g., back rubs). If necessary, pharmacological therapy may be needed to induce and maintain sleep. (Sleep and sleep disorders are discussed in Chapter 9.)

Issues Related to Caregivers. When someone becomes critically ill, care extends beyond the patient to the patient's caregivers because they are intimately involved. Caregivers play a valuable role in the patient's recovery and are members of the health care team. They contribute to the patient's well-being by:
1. Providing a link to the patient's personal life (e.g., news of family, job)
2. Advising the patient in health care decisions or functioning as the decision maker when the patient cannot
3. Helping with activities of daily living (e.g., bathing, oral suctioning)
4. Providing positive, loving, and caring support

To be effective in caring for their loved one, caregivers need the nurse's guidance and support. The experience of having a friend or family member as a patient in the CCU is physically and emotionally difficult, often to the point of exhaustion. Anxiety regarding the patient's condition and prognosis and concerns regarding the patient's pain and other discomforts are some of the issues caregivers confront. In addition, it is common for caregivers to experience anxiety regarding the financial issues related to the provision of care during a critical illness. Consulting with the case manager or social worker is helpful in these instances.

Caregivers typically experience disruption of their daily routines to support the patient. They may be far from their own home and supportive friends and family members. Ultimately, caregivers of the critically ill are considered to be in crisis, and family-centred care is essential. To provide family-centred care effectively, the nurse must be skilled in crisis intervention. The nurse should conduct a family assessment and intervene as necessary. Interventions can include active listening, reduction of anxiety, and support of those who become upset or angry (Davidson, 2009).

The nurse should acknowledge the caregivers' feelings and accept and support their decisions. The nurse should consult other health care team members (e.g., chaplains, psychologists, patient representatives) as necessary to assist caregivers to adjust. The extent to which family-centred care is provided can affect the patient's clinical course in the CCU.

The major needs of caregivers of critically ill patients include informational needs, reassurance needs, and convenience needs (Leske & Pasquale, 2007). Lack of information is a major source of anxiety for the caregivers. The nurse should assess the caregiver's understanding of the patient's status, treatment plan, and prognosis and provide information as appropriate. The nurse can identify a spokesperson for the family so that information between the health care team and the family is coordinated.

The caregiver needs reassurance regarding the way in which the patient's care is managed and decisions are made. The nurse should provide the caregiver with the opportunity to participate in decision making. If the patient has an advance directive or a living will, the caregiver will need to see that the patient's wishes are followed. When patients are incapable of making their own health care decisions, they may have designated a durable power of attorney for health care, and this person should be involved in the patient's plan of care. The nurse can invite the caregiver to meet the health care team members. The nurse should evaluate the appropriateness of including caregivers in multidisciplinary rounds and patient care conferences.

It helps caregivers to accept and cope with problems if they observe that the health care team is hopeful, caring, and competent; decisions are deliberate; and their input is valued. Caregivers of critically ill patients need the convenience of access to the patient. Limiting visitation does not protect the patient from adverse physiological consequences (Davidson, 2009; Leske & Pasquale, 2007). Strict visitation policies in CCUs should be reviewed. AACN strongly recommends a move toward less restrictive, individualized visiting policies (Redekopp & Leske, 2007). This is accomplished by assessing the patient's and caregiver's needs and preferences and incorporating these into the plan of care.

Research has demonstrated that families of critically ill patients need the convenience of access to the patient and that limiting family visitation does not protect that patient from adverse physiological consequences (Gonzalez, Carroll, Elliott, Fitzgerald, & Vallent, 2004). Rigid visitation policies in CCUs should be reviewed, and a move toward less restrictive, individualized visiting policies is strongly recommended by the AACN (2010). This can be accomplished by assessing the patient's and family or caregivers' needs and preferences and incorporating these into the plan of care.

The first time that caregivers visit it is important for the nurse to prepare them for the experience by briefly describing the patient's appearance and the physical environment (e.g., equipment, noise) (Society of Critical Care Medicine, n.d.). The nurse should accompany the caregivers as they enter the room and observe the responses of both the patient and the caregivers. The nurse should invite them to participate in the patient's care if they desire. In some CCUs, visitation includes animal-assisted therapy or pet visitation. The positive benefits of these interventions (e.g., decreases in BP and anxiety) far outweigh the risks (e.g., transmission of infection from animal to patient) and they should be a part of the visitation policy.

In addition to traditional visiting, research has shown that caregivers of patients undergoing invasive procedures (e.g., central line insertion) and cardiopulmonary resuscitation want the option of being present at the bedside during these events. Even when the outcomes were not favourable, being present helped caregivers remove doubts about the patient's condition, decreased their anxiety and fear, facilitated the need to be together and to support their loved one, and facilitated the grief process when death occurred. The Canadian Association of Critical Care Nurses (CACCN) encourages ICUs to develop policies and procedures that provide for the option of family presence during invasive procedures and cardiopulmonary resuscitation (CACCN, 2005).

CULTURALLY COMPETENT CARE: CRITICAL CARE PATIENTS

Providing culturally competent care to critically ill patients and families is challenging. Often, the nurse is focused on meeting the physiological needs of the patient and may not appreciate the influence of the patient's culture on the illness experience. The cultural dimensions of the meaning of sickness and health, pain, dying and death, and grief need to be considered when caring for critically ill patients and their families. (Chapter 2 discusses cultural issues.)

Cultural perspectives on dying and death are complex. Telling some patients that they are dying as a way of letting them prepare for death may be considered an infringement on the role of the family. Others view a discussion about advance directives as a legal device to deny care. Customs surrounding dying and death vary widely, from leaving a window open to allow the spirit of the dead person to leave to providing the final bath for the deceased. The nurse caring for the dying patient must make every attempt to understand and accommodate the family's cultural traditions. The expressions of grief that follow the loss of a loved one are highly individualized and influenced by several variables. These include the relationship between the grieving person and the deceased, whether the loss is sudden or anticipated, the support systems available to the grieving person, past experiences with loss, and the person's religious and cultural beliefs. It is of utmost importance that the critical care nurse proceed cautiously when approaching patients facing death and their families. Asking patients, "What do you want to know?" and "Who do you want with you when discussing options?" are good starting points (Gries, Curtis, Wall, & Engelberg, 2008). (Chapter 13 provides additional information about end-of-life care.)

Hemodynamic Monitoring

Hemodynamic monitoring refers to ongoing measurement of pressure, flow, and oxygenation within the cardiovascular system. Both invasive (internally placed devices) and noninvasive (external devices) hemodynamic measurements are made in the CCU. Values commonly measured include systemic arterial pressure and pulmonary artery pressure (PAP), central venous pressure (CVP), pulmonary artery occlusive pressure (PAOP), CO and CI, SV and stroke index, and oxygen saturation of the hemoglobin of arterial blood (SaO_2) and mixed venous blood (SvO_2). From these measurements, the clinician calculates several values, including the resistance of the systemic and pulmonary arterial vasculature as well as oxygen content, delivery, and consumption. When these data are integrated with clinical assessment data, the nurse can derive a picture of the patient's hemodynamic status and the effect of therapy. It is important that all measures be made with attention to technical accuracy. False or inaccurate data are potentially misleading and thus dangerous.

Hemodynamic Terminology

Cardiac Output and Cardiac Index. *Cardiac output* (CO) is the volume of blood pumped by the heart in 1 minute. *Cardiac index* (CI) is the measurement of the CO adjusted for body size, and it is a more precise measurement of the efficiency of the pumping action of the heart. Although minor beat-to-beat changes may occur, generally the left and right ventricles pump the same volume. The volume pumped with each heartbeat is the SV. Like CI, stroke volume index (SVI) is the measurement of SV adjusted for body size. CO and the forces opposing blood flow determine BP, the force exerted by blood on the vessel wall. The opposition to blood flow offered by the vessels is called

Table 68-1 Hemodynamic Parameters at Rest

INDICATORS	NORMAL RANGE
Preload	
Right atrial pressure (RAP) or central venous pressure (CVP)	2-8 mm Hg
Pulmonary artery occlusive pressure (PAOP)—wedge or left atrial pressure (LAP)	6-12 mm Hg
Pulmonary artery diastolic pressure (PADP)	4-12 mm Hg
Afterload	
Pulmonary vascular resistance (PVR) = (pulmonary artery mean pressure [PAMP] − PAOP) × 80/cardiac output (CO)	<250 dynes/sec/cm^{-5}
Pulmonary vascular resistance index (PVRI) = (PAMP − PAOP) × 80/cardiac index (CI)	160-380 dynes/sec/cm^{-5}/m^2
Systemic vascular resistance (SVR) = (mean arterial pressure [MAP] − CVP) × 80/CO	800-1200 dynes/sec/cm^{-5}
Systemic vascular resistance index (SVRI) = (MAP − CVP) × 80/CI	1970-2390 dynes/sec/cm^{-5}/m^2
*Mean arterial pressure (MAP) = systolic blood pressure + 2(diastolic blood pressure)/3	70-105 mm Hg
*Pulmonary artery mean pressure (PAMP) = pulmonary artery systolic pressure (PASP) + 2PADP/3	10-20 mm Hg
Other	
Stroke volume (SV) = CO/Heart rate	60-150 mL/beat
Stroke volume index (SVI) = CI/heart rate (HR)	30-65 mL/beat/m^2
HR	60-100 beats/min
CO = SV × HR	4-8 L/min
CI = CO/body surface area (BSA)	2.2-4 L/min/m^2
Arterial hemoglobin oxygen saturation	95-99%
Mixed venous hemoglobin oxygen saturation	60-80%

*These formulas are approximations because they do not take into consideration the heart rate. The monitor looks at the area under the pressure curve, as well as the heart rate, to calculate MAP and PAMP.

systemic vascular resistance (SVR) or *pulmonary vascular resistance*. Preload, afterload, and contractility (see Chapter 34) determine SV (and thus CO and BP). Understanding these concepts and relationships is essential for the critical care nurse. In addition, the nurse must understand the effects of manipulation of each of these variables. The formulas and normal values for common hemodynamic parameters are given in Table 68-1.

Preload. *Preload* is the volume within a cardiac chamber at the end of diastole. Unfortunately, chamber volume measurements are difficult to obtain. Instead, various pressures are used to estimate volume. Left ventricular preload is called *left ventricular end-diastolic pressure*. PAOP, a measure of pulmonary occlusive

pressure, reflects left ventricular end-diastolic pressure under normal conditions (i.e., when there is no mitral valve pathological condition, intracardiac defect, or dysrhythmia). CVP, measured in the right atrium or in the vena cava close to the heart, is the right ventricular preload or right ventricular end-diastolic pressure when there is no tricuspid valve pathological condition, intracardiac defect, or dysrhythmia.

The effects of preload are explained by *Starling's law*, which states that the more a myocardial fibre is stretched during filling, the more it shortens during systole and the greater the force of the contraction to a physiological limit. As preload increases, force generated in the following contraction increases; thus, SV and CO increase. The greater the preload, the greater the myocardial (heart muscle) stretch and the greater the oxygen requirement of the myocardium. Hence, increases in CO via increased preload require increased delivery of oxygen to the myocardium. It should be remembered that the change in SV with preload comes about because of stretching of the heart muscle. However, the clinical measurement made is not a direct measurement of the muscle length; the measurement made is pressure at the time of the peak stretch (end diastole) (see Table 68-1). This pressure indirectly indicates the amount of stretch and the volume. This pressure is also important because it indicates pressure in the blood vessels of the lung or in the blood returning to the heart. Preload can be increased by fluid administration and decreased by diuresis.

Afterload. *Afterload* refers to the forces opposing ventricular ejection. These forces include systemic arterial pressure, the resistance offered by the aortic valve, and the mass and density of the blood to be moved. Clinically, although the measures fail to include all the components of afterload, SVR and arterial pressure are indexes of left ventricular afterload. Similarly, pulmonary vascular resistance and PAP are indexes of right ventricular afterload. Increased afterload often results in a decreased CO. CO can be restored by decreasing afterload (i.e., decreasing forces opposing contraction). When afterload is reduced, myocardial oxygen needs are decreased. Thus, when CO is increased, myocardial oxygen requirements are decreased. Drug therapy directed at reducing afterload (e.g., nitroglycerin or nitroprusside) is often used in the management of heart failure (see Chapter 37).

Vascular Resistance. *Systemic vascular resistance* (SVR) is the resistance of the systemic vascular bed. *Pulmonary vascular resistance* is the resistance of the pulmonary vascular bed. Both of these measures reflect afterload as described earlier and can be adjusted for body size (see Table 68-1).

Contractility. *Contractility* describes the strength of contraction. Contractility is said to increase when preload is not changed yet the heart contracts more forcefully. Epinephrine, norepinephrine, isoproterenol (Isuprel), dopamine, dobutamine, digitalis-like drugs, calcium, and milrinone (Primacor) increase contractility. These agents are termed *positive inotropes*. Contractility is diminished by *negative inotropes*, such as acidosis and certain drugs (e.g., barbiturates, alcohol, procainamide [Pronestyl], calcium channel blockers, β-adrenergic blockers). Increased contractility results in increased SV and increased myocardial oxygen requirements. There are no direct clinical measures of cardiac contractility. To indirectly determine contractility, the nurse measures the patient's preload (PAOP or wedge) and CO and graphs the results. If preload, heart rate, and afterload remain constant yet CO changes, contractility is altered. Contractility is diminished in the failing heart.

Principles of Invasive Pressure Monitoring

Invasive lines are commonly used in the CCU to measure systemic and pulmonary BPs. Components of a typical invasive arterial pressure monitoring system are illustrated in Figure 68-3. Catheter, pressure tubing, flush system, and usually the transducer are disposable.

To accurately measure pressure, equipment must be referenced and zero-balanced, and dynamic response characteristics

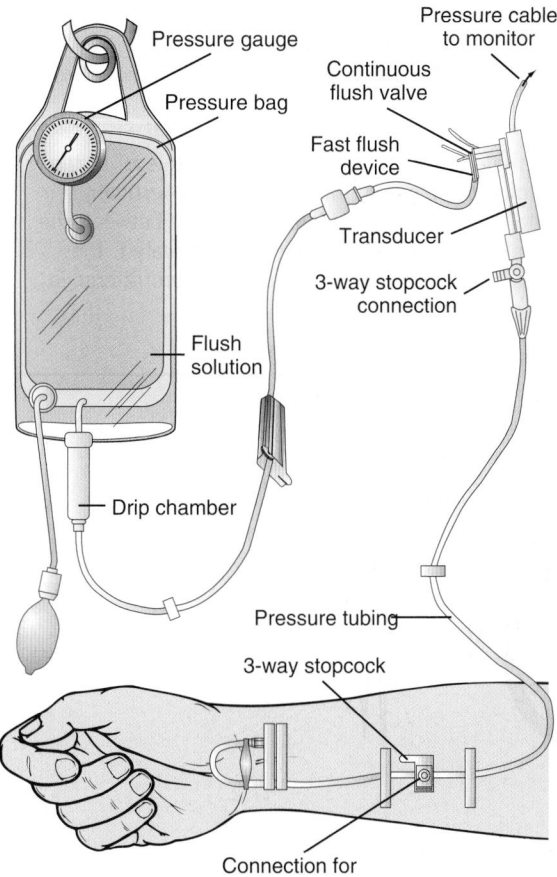

Figure 68-3 Components of a pressure monitoring system. The cannula, shown entering the radial artery, is connected via pressure (nondistensible) tubing to the transducer. The transducer converts the pressure wave into an electronic signal. The transducer is wired to the electronic monitoring system, which amplifies, conditions, displays, and records the signal. Stopcocks are inserted into the line for specimen withdrawal and for referencing and zero-balancing procedures. A flush system, consisting of a pressurized bag of intravenous fluid, tubing, and a flush device, is inserted into the line. The flush system provides continuous slow (~3 mL/hr) flushing and provides a mechanism for fast flushing of lines. Commonly, all items except the electronic monitoring system are disposable equipment.

Source: Redrawn from Gardner, P. E. (1994). *Hemodynamic pressure monitoring*. Redmond, Washington: Spacelabs Medical.

optimized. *Levelling* means positioning the transducer so that the zero reference point is at the level of the atria of the heart. The stopcock nearest the transducer is usually the zero reference for the transducer. To place this level with the atria, the nurse uses an external landmark, the phlebostatic axis. To identify the **phlebostatic axis,** two imaginary lines are drawn with the patient supine (Figure 68-4, *A*). The first line, a horizontal line, is drawn through the midchest, halfway between the outermost anterior and the outermost posterior surfaces. The second line, a vertical line, is drawn through the fourth intercostal space at the sternum. The phlebostatic axis is the intersection of the two imaginary lines. Once the phlebostatic axis is identified, it should be marked on the patient's chest with a permanent marker. The port of the stopcock nearest the transducer must be positioned level with the phlebostatic axis.

Zeroing confirms that when pressure within the system is zero, the equipment reads zero. This is accomplished by opening the reference stopcock to room air and observing the monitor for a reading of zero. Most transducers in current use are disposable and have little zero drift. Zeroing the transducer is recommended during initial setup, immediately after insertion of the arterial line, when the transducer has been disconnected from the pressure cable or the pressure cable has been disconnected from the monitor, and when the accuracy of the measurements is questioned, and it should be done according to the manufacturer's guidelines. Optimizing dynamic response characteristics involves checking that the equipment reproduces without distortion a signal that changes rapidly. A *dynamic response test (square wave test)* is performed every 8 to 12 hours and when the system is opened to air, or if the accuracy of the measurements is questioned. It involves checking that the equipment reproduces a distortion-free signal (Figure 68-5).

Steps in obtaining BP measurements with an invasive line are given in Table 68-2. Pressure measurements can be obtained from both digital and printed analogue outputs, but accurate readings are best obtained from a printed pressure tracing at the end of expiration. Initial readings are made with the patient flat. Unless the patient's BP is extremely sensitive to orthostatic changes, values at modest degrees of backrest elevation (≤45 degrees) are generally equivalent to measurements with the patient flat. Studies have not demonstrated the accuracy of readings obtained for patients in the lateral position but do support the accuracy of readings in the prone position (Nohrenberg, Moselely, & Sole, 2009). It is not necessary to reposition the patient for each pressure reading. However, it is necessary to move the zero reference stopcock to keep it positioned at the phlebostatic axis (see Figure 68-4, *B*).

Types of Invasive Pressure Monitoring

Arterial Blood Pressure. Continuous arterial pressure monitoring is indicated for patients in many situations, including acute hypertension and hypotension, respiratory failure, shock, neurological injury, coronary interventional procedures, continuous infusion of vasoactive drugs, and frequent arterial blood gas (ABG) sampling. A 20-gauge, 5.1-cm, nontapered Teflon cannula-over-the-needle is typically used to cannulate a peripheral artery, such as the radial, brachial, or femoral, using a percutaneous approach. It is important that the insertion site be immobilized so that the catheter line is not dislodged and lines do not become kinked.

Measurements. The nurse can use the arterial line to obtain systolic, diastolic, and mean BPs (Figure 68-6). High- and

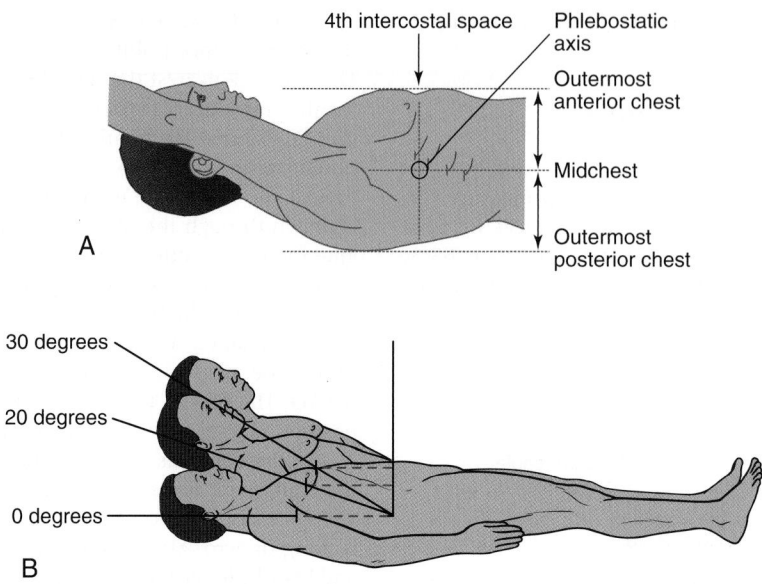

Figure 68-4 Identification of phlebostatic axis. **A,** Phlebostatic axis is an external landmark used to identify the level of the atria in the supine patient. The phlebostatic axis is defined as the intersection of two imaginary lines: one drawn vertically through the fourth intercostal space at the sternum and another drawn horizontally through the midchest, halfway between the outermost anterior and the outermost posterior points of the chest. **B,** As the backrest of the supine patient is elevated, the phlebostatic axis remains at the same anatomical location, becoming progressively elevated from the floor. The zero reference point must be repositioned with changes in backrest elevation to keep it at the phlebostatic level.

Source: Redrawn from Flynn, J. B. M., & Bruce, N. P. (1993). *Introduction to critical care skills.* St. Louis: Mosby.

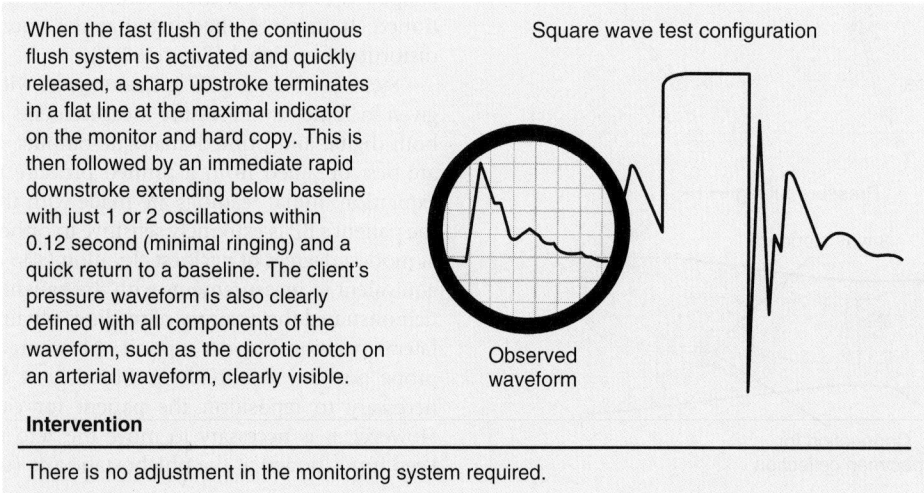

When the fast flush of the continuous flush system is activated and quickly released, a sharp upstroke terminates in a flat line at the maximal indicator on the monitor and hard copy. This is then followed by an immediate rapid downstroke extending below baseline with just 1 or 2 oscillations within 0.12 second (minimal ringing) and a quick return to a baseline. The client's pressure waveform is also clearly defined with all components of the waveform, such as the dicrotic notch on an arterial waveform, clearly visible.

Square wave test configuration

Observed waveform

Intervention

There is no adjustment in the monitoring system required.

Figure 68-5 Optimally damped system. Dynamic response test (square wave test) using the fast flush system: normal response.

Source: Darovic, G. O. (1995). *Hemodynamic monitoring* (2nd ed.). Philadelphia: Saunders.

low-pressure alarms should be set, based on the patient's current status, and activated. Measurements are obtained at end-expiration to limit the effect of the respiratory cycle on arterial pressure (Shaffer, 2005). In heart failure, the systolic upstroke may be slower. In volume depletion, systolic pressure varies greatly with mechanical ventilation, diminishing during inspiration. In severe congestive heart failure, systolic amplitude does not vary with ventilation. With dysrhythmias, it is useful to observe simultaneous ECG and pressure tracings. Dysrhythmias that significantly diminish arterial pressure are more urgent than those that cause only a slight decrease in systolic amplitude.

Complications. Arterial lines carry the risk of hemorrhage, infection, thrombus formation, and neurovascular impairment. Hemorrhage is most likely to occur when the catheter becomes dislodged or the line becomes disconnected. To avoid this serious complication, the nurse uses Luer-Lok connections and always checks the arterial waveform and that the alarms are activated. If the pressure in the line falls (e.g., when the line is disconnected), the low-pressure alarm sounds immediately, allowing prompt correction of the problem. Pressure is always monitored when an arterial line is in place, even if the line was placed for ABG sampling.

Infection is a risk with any invasive line. The nurse should inspect the insertion site for local signs of inflammation and monitor the patient for signs of systemic infection. To limit the risk of contamination and catheter-related infection, the pressure tubing and transducer should be changed every 72 hours. The pressure bag should be changed every 24 hours.

Circulatory impairment can result from formation of a thrombus around the catheter, release of an embolus, spasm, or occlusion of the circulation by the catheter. Before inserting a line

into the radial artery, an Allen test should be performed to confirm that ulnar circulation is sufficient to sustain the hand. In this test, pressure is applied to the radial and ulnar arteries simultaneously. The patient is instructed to open and close the hand repeatedly. The hand should blanch. The nurse then releases the pressure on the ulnar artery while compressing the radial artery. If pinkness fails to return within 6 seconds, the ulnar artery is insufficient, indicating that the radial artery should not be used for line insertion.

To maintain line patency and limit thrombus formation, assess the continuous flush system every 1 to 4 hours to determine that the (1) pressure bag is inflated to 300 mm Hg, (2) flush bag contains fluid, and (3) system is delivering 3 to 6 mL/hr. Owing to the risk of heparin-induced thrombocytopenia, heparinized saline should not be routinely used for the flush solution (Nohrenberg, Moseley, & Sole, 2009). Once the catheter is inserted, evaluate the neurovascular status distal to the arterial insertion site hourly. The limb with compromised arterial flow will be cool and pale, with capillary refill time longer than 3 seconds. There may be symptoms of neurological impairment (e.g., paresthesia, pain, paralysis). Neurovascular impairment can result in loss of a limb and is an emergency.

Pulmonary Artery Flow–Directed Catheter. PAP monitoring is used to guide acute-phase management of patients with complicated cardiac, pulmonary, and intravascular volume problems (Table 68-3). PA diastolic pressure and PAOP are sensitive indicators of fluid volume status and cardiac function. PA diastolic pressure and PAOP are increased in fluid volume overload and heart failure. They are decreased with volume deficit. Fluid therapy based on PAP allows restoration of fluid balance while avoiding overcorrection of the problem. Monitoring PAPs can allow precise therapeutic manipulation of preload, which

---

Table 68-2 Measurement of Blood Pressure With Invasive Lines

1. Explain the procedure to the patient.

2. Position the patient supine and flat or, if appropriate, with the head of the bed elevated up to 45 degrees.

3. Confirm that the zero reference (port of the stopcock nearest the transducer) is placed at the level of the phlebostatic axis (see Figure 68-4). If the reference stopcock is not taped to the patient's chest, a carpenter's level should be used to position the stopcock on a bedside pole at the point level with the phlebostatic axis.

4. Observe the monitor tracing and assess the quality of the tracing. Perform a dynamic response test (see Figure 68-5).

5. Obtain an analogue printout, if available, and measure the systolic and diastolic pressures at end-expiration (see Figure 68-6). If no printout is available, freeze the tracing on the oscilloscope screen, and use the cursor to measure the pressures at end-expiration.

6. Record the pressure measurements promptly, including (if available) the printout marked to identify the points read.

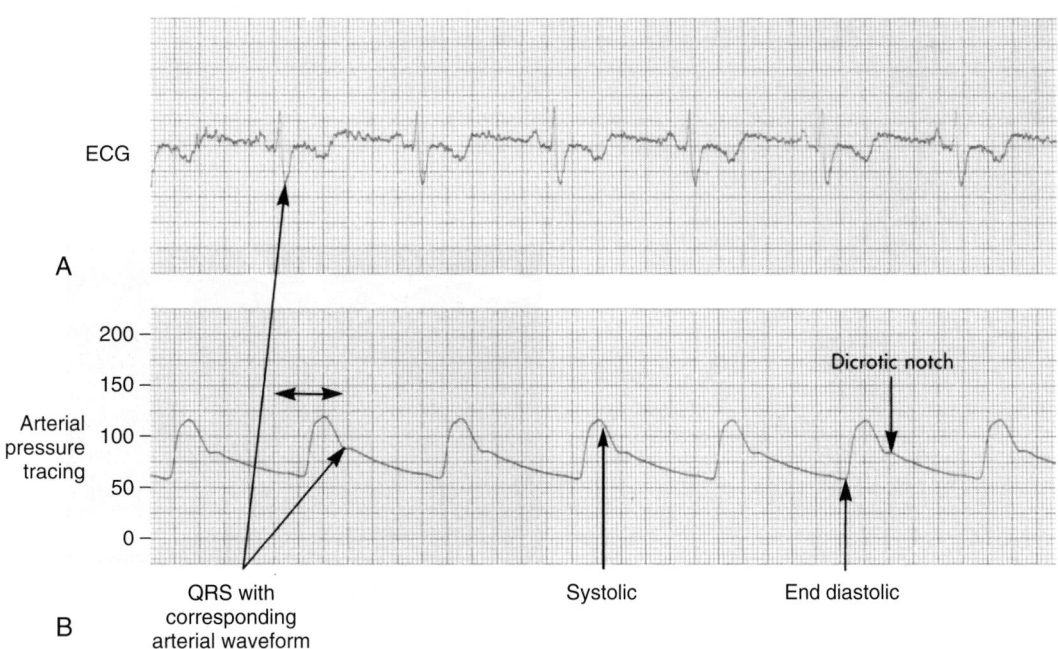

Figure 68-6 Simultaneously recorded electrocardiogram (ECG) tracing **(A)** and systemic arterial pressure tracing **(B).** Systolic pressure is the peak pressure. The dicrotic notch indicates aortic valve closure. Diastolic pressure is the lowest value before contraction. Mean pressure is the average pressure over time calculated by the monitoring equipment.

Source: Adapted from Urden, L. D., Stacy, K. M., & Lough, M. E. (2010). *Critical care nursing: Diagnosis and management* (6th ed., p. 333, Figure 18-8). St. Louis: Mosby.

allows CO to be maintained without placing the patient at risk for pulmonary edema.

A PA flow–directed catheter is used to measure PAPs, including PAOP. The standard PA catheter is number 7.5 French, 110 cm long, with four or five lumens (Figure 68-7). When properly positioned, the distal lumen port (catheter tip) is within the PA (Figure 68-8). This port is used to monitor PAPs and withdraw mixed venous blood specimens (e.g., to evaluate oxygen saturation). A balloon connected to an external valve via the second lumen surrounds the distal lumen port. Balloon inflation has two purposes: (1) to allow moving blood to float the catheter forward and (2) to allow PAOP measurement. There will be one or two proximal lumens, with exit ports in the right atrium (if only one) or the right atrium and the right ventricle (if two). The right

atrium port is used for measurement of CVP, injection of fluid for CO determination, and withdrawal of blood specimens. If a second proximal port is available, it is used for infusion of fluids and drugs or blood sampling. A thermistor lumen port located near the distal tip is wired to an external connector. This port is used for monitoring blood or core temperature and in the thermodilution method of measuring CO.

In addition to these standard features, PA catheters with specialized features are available. One modification is the inclusion of an atrial electrode, useful in recording the atrial ECG or pacing the heart. Another common modification is inclusion of a fibre-optic sensor in the distal tip that detects SvO_2. Another type of PA catheter provides continuous measurement of right ventricular volume and ejection fraction, and some catheters provide continuous CO monitoring. The PA catheter sheath (introducer) usually has a side port that serves as a large-bore IV line. Most catheters have a plastic "sleeve" connected to the sheath. This allows the catheter to be advanced or pulled back while maintaining sterility. The physician or other qualified health care provider (e.g., ACNP) usually manipulates the PA catheter, but this practice varies by institution.

Pulmonary Artery Catheter Insertion. Before PA catheter insertion, note the patient's electrolyte, acid–base, oxygenation, and coagulation status. Imbalances such as hypokalemia, hypomagnesemia, hypoxemia, or acidosis can make the heart more irritable and increase the risk of ventricular dysrhythmia during catheter insertion. Coagulopathy increases the risk of the monitor, cables, and infusion and pressurized flush solutions. The system is zero referenced to the phlebostatic axis. The physician or other health care provider explains the procedure to the patient and obtains informed consent. The patient is positioned supine and flat. The PA catheter is inserted through a sheath percutaneously into the internal jugular, subclavian, antecubital, or femoral vein using surgical asepsis. Venous cut-down is rarely required. The catheter is advanced through the venous system to the right side of the heart.

Table 68-3 Clinical Indications for Pulmonary Artery Catheterization

- Acute respiratory distress syndrome
- Acute respiratory failure in patients with chronic obstructive pulmonary disease
- Cardiac tamponade
- Complex fluid imbalance (e.g., trauma, burns, sepsis)
- Evaluation of circulatory syndromes (e.g., heart failure, mitral valve regurgitation, intraventricular shunts)
- Intra-aortic balloon pump therapy
- Myocardial infarction with complications (e.g., left ventricular failure, cardiogenic shock, ventricular septal rupture)
- Perioperative fluid imbalance in high-risk patients (e.g., cardiac history)
- Shock states (e.g., cardiogenic, septic, hypovolemic)
- Vasoactive drug therapy support

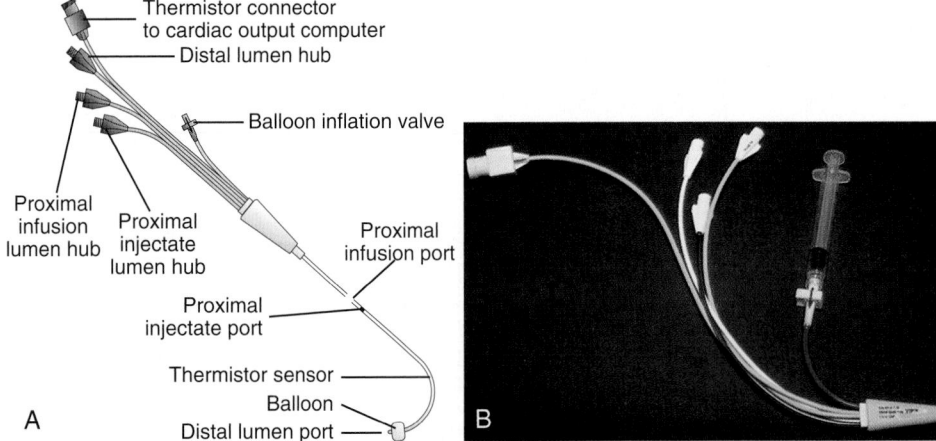

Figure 68-7 Pulmonary artery (PA) catheter. **A,** Illustrated catheter has five lumens. When properly positioned, the distal lumen port is in the PA, and the proximal lumen ports are in the right atrium and the right ventricle. The distal and one of the proximal ports are used to measure PA and central venous pressures, respectively. A balloon surrounds the catheter near the distal end. The balloon inflation valve is used to inflate the balloon with air to allow reading of the pulmonary artery wedge pressure. A thermistor located near the distal tip senses PA temperature and is used to measure thermodilution cardiac output when solution cooler than body temperature is injected into a proximal port. **B,** Photograph of a catheter.

Source: Courtesy Edwards Critical Care Division, Baxter Healthcare Corporation, Santa Ana, California.

Flow-directed catheter

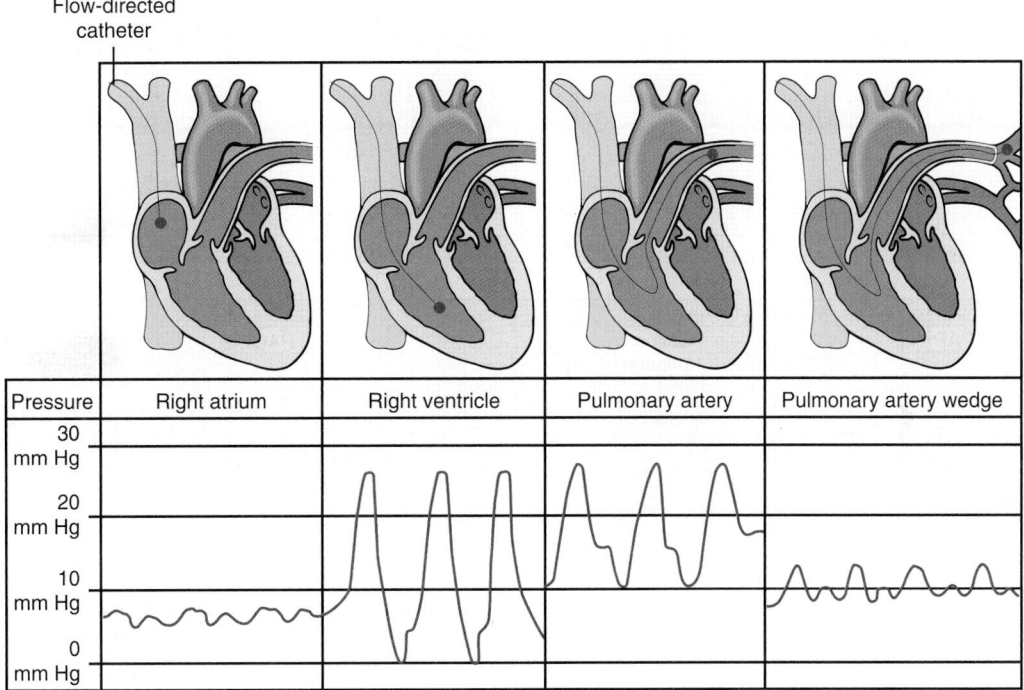

Pressure	Right atrium	Right ventricle	Pulmonary artery	Pulmonary artery wedge
30 mm Hg				
20 mm Hg				
10 mm Hg				
0 mm Hg				

Figure 68-8 Position of the pulmonary artery flow-directed catheter during progressive stages of insertion with corresponding pressure waveforms.

Source: Adapted from Urden, L. D., Stacy, K. M., & Lough, M. E. (2010). *Critical care nursing: Diagnosis and management* (6th ed., p. 348, Figure 18-18). St. Louis: Mosby.

Continuously observe the characteristic waveforms on the monitor as the catheter is moved through the heart to the PA (see Figure 68-8). When the tip reaches the right atrium, the balloon is inflated. Inflation of the balloon should not exceed the balloon's capacity (usually 1-1.5 mL of air). The catheter is then "floated" through the tricuspid valve into the right ventricle and then through the pulmonic valve to the PA. It is necessary to monitor the ECG continuously during insertion because of the risk for dysrhythmias, particularly when the catheter reaches the right ventricle. Once a typical pulmonary artery occlusive pressure (PAOP) tracing is observed, the balloon is deflated, and the PA waveform should return on the monitor. Following insertion, a chest radiograph confirms the catheter's position. To maintain the catheter in its proper position, it is secured at the point of entry into the skin. Note and record the measurement at the exit point. Finally, apply an occlusive dressing, and then change it according to institution policy.

Pulmonary Artery Pressure Measurements. Systolic, diastolic, and mean pressures are routinely monitored. PA systolic is the peak pressure point and PA diastolic is the lowest pressure point on the PA waveform. Mean PA pressure is the time-weighted average. Because PA ports are in the chest, intrathoracic pressures alter PAP. To produce accurate data, PA measurements are obtained at the end of expiration.

The measurement of PAOP or wedge is obtained by slowly inflating the balloon with air (not to exceed balloon capacity) until the PA waveform changes to a PAOP waveform (Figure 68-9). Before inflation, the PAP tracing on the monitor looks like an arterial tracing, with a systolic peak, dicrotic notch, and then the diastolic low point. As the waveform becomes "wedged," the tracing changes shape and amplitude. Generally, the PAOP wave-

form is characterized by two small positive waves, the *a* and *v* waves. The *a* wave indicates atrial contraction, and it is followed by the *x* descent, indicating atrial relaxation. At times, a *c* wave may be seen following the *a* wave and indicates closure of the mitral valve. The *v* wave is seen during the interval between the T and the P waves of the ECG. The *v* wave indicates inflow into the left atrium when the mitral valve is closed and the ventricle is contracting. The *v* wave is followed by the *y* descent, indicating the emptying of the left atrium when the mitral valve opens and the ventricle fills.

When measuring the wedge, the balloon should be inflated for no more than four respiratory cycles or 8 to 15 seconds. There is danger of rupture of the PA if the catheter migrates distally into a smaller vessel or if the balloon is overinflated. This is suspected when less than 1 mL is needed to wedge the tracing or an "over-wedge" tracing is obtained (Figure 68-10). Readings should be acquired from an analogue strip pressure recording, and the strip should be placed into the patient's record. If a printout of the tracing is not available, the readings can be taken from the monitor using the cursor.

Central Venous or Right Atrial Pressure Measurement. CVP is a measurement of right ventricular preload. It can be measured with a PA catheter using one of the proximal lumens or with a central venous catheter placed in the internal jugular or subclavian vein. CVP is measured as a mean pressure at the end of expiration. CVP waveforms (Figure 68-11) are similar to PAOP waveforms. Although the PA diastolic pressure and the wedge pressure are more sensitive indicators of fluid volume status, CVP also reflects fluid volume problems. An elevated CVP indicates right ventricular failure or volume overload. A low CVP indicates hypovolemia.

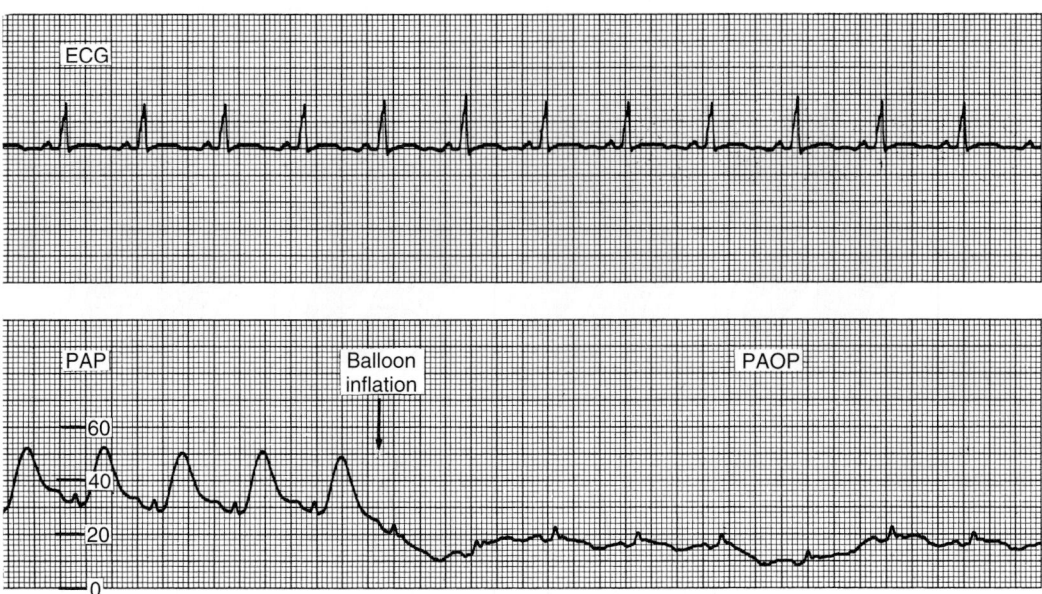

Figure 68-9 Change in pulmonary artery pressure (PAP) waveform to pulmonary artery occlusive pressure (PAOP) waveform with balloon inflation. The balloon is inflated while observing the bedside monitor for change in the waveform. Balloon inflation *(arrow)* in a patient with a normal pulmonary artery occlusive pressure (PAOP). *ECG*, electrocardiogram.

Source: Wiegand, D. L. (2011). *AACN procedure manual for critical care* (6th ed., p. 635, Figure 73-10). Philadelphia: Saunders.

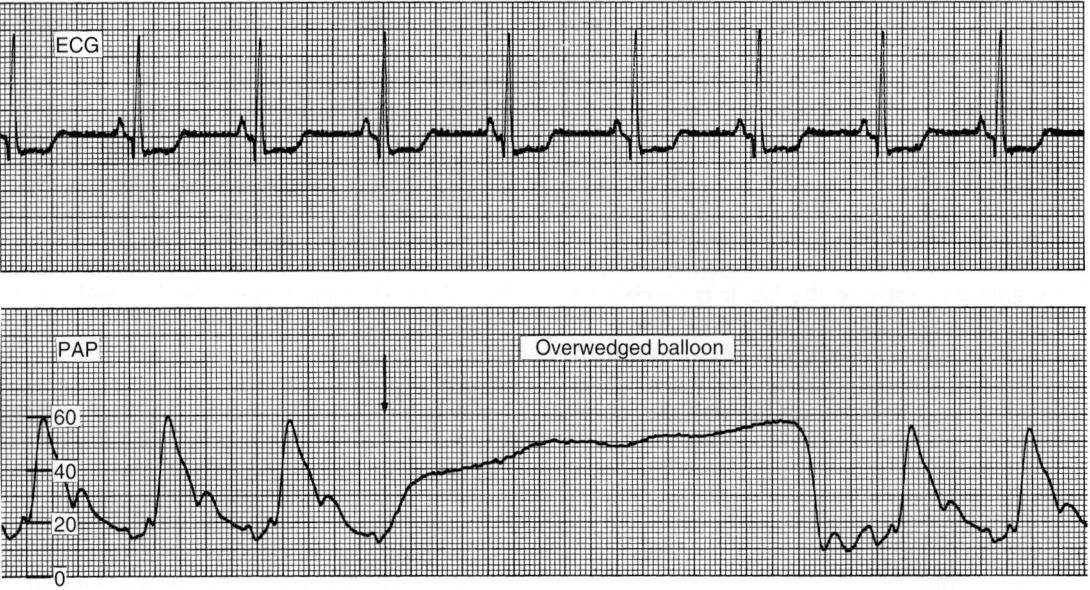

Figure 68-10 Balloon inflation *(arrow)* in patient with elevated wedge pressure. Overwedging of balloon (balloon has been overinflated). The danger of overinflating the balloon is that the pulmonary artery vessel may rupture from the pressure of the balloon. *ECG*, electrocardiogram; *PAP*, pulmonary artery pressure.

Source: Wiegand, D. L. (2011). *AACN procedure manual for critical care* (6th ed., p. 656, Figure 75-1). Philadelphia: Saunders.

Invasive Cardiac Output Measurement Techniques. CO is frequently monitored in patients with hemodynamic instability. Normal resting CO is 4 to 8 L/min and varies with body size. CI accounts for variations in body size and is normally 2.2 to 4 L/min/m². CO is decreased in conditions such as hypovolemia, cardiogenic shock, and heart failure. Under normal conditions, CO increases with exercise. Increases in CO at rest indicate a hyperdynamic state seen with fever or sepsis.

The PA catheter is commonly used to measure CO via the intermittent bolus *thermodilution cardiac output* (TDCO) method or the *continuous cardiac output* (CCO) method. With the TDCO method, a fixed volume (5 to 10 mL) of 5% dextrose solution (or saline, if dextrose is contraindicated) at room temperature (or iced for patients with low or high COs) is injected rapidly (≤4 sec) and smoothly into the proximal lumen port of the PA catheter (Nohrenberg, Moseley, & Sole, 2009). The thermistor lumen port

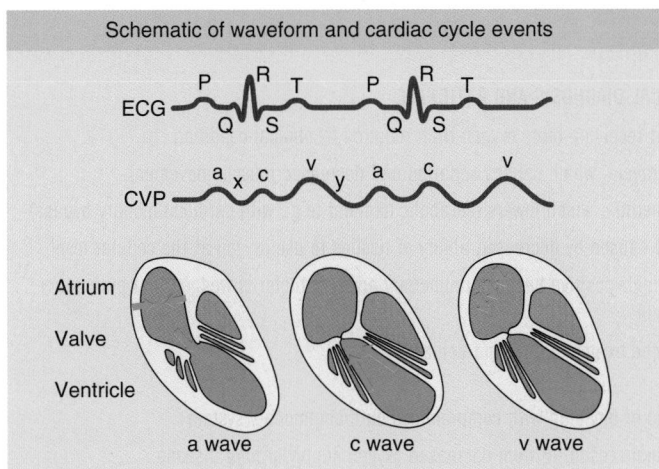

Schematic of waveform and cardiac cycle events

Figure 68-11 Cardiac events that produce the central venous pressure (CVP) waveform with *a*, *c*, and *v* waves. *a* wave represents atrial contraction. *x* descent represents atrial relaxation. *c* wave represents the bulging of the closed tricuspid valve into the right atrium during ventricular systole. *v* wave represents atrial filling. *y* descent represents opening of the tricuspid valve and filling of the ventricle. *ECG*, electrocardiogram.

Source: Adapted from Urden, L. D., Stacy, K. M., & Lough, M. E. (2010). *Critical care nursing: Diagnosis and management* (6th ed., p. 338, Figure 18-11). St. Louis: Mosby.

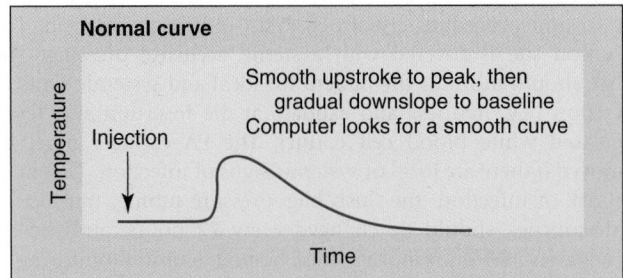

Figure 68-12 Normal cardiac output curve. Cardiac output is calculated from the temperature change in the pulmonary artery when a fixed volume and known temperature of a solution is injected into the proximal port in the right atrium. The nurse should observe the curve during injection to make sure that it is smooth.

located near the distal tip of the PA catheter detects the drop in blood temperature. The CO is mathematically calculated from the area under the temperature curve by the computer. The larger the area under the curve, the smaller the CO, and conversely, the smaller the area under the curve, the larger the CO (Figure 68-12). This procedure is repeated three times, with each measurement 1 to 2 minutes apart. Any CO measurement that does not have a normal curve is discarded. An average of three acceptable measurements is calculated to determine the CO.

The CCO method uses a heat-exchange CO catheter. This PA catheter contains a thermal filament that is located in the right atrium. This filament emits a pulsed signal every 30 to 60 seconds that allows for the mixing of blood with heat as it passes through the right ventricle. The thermistor lumen port detects the change

in temperature. A bedside computer displays digital measurements every 30 to 60 seconds that reflect the average CO for the past 3 to 6 minutes. The CCO method eliminates the need for fluid boluses, reduces the risk of contamination, and permits ongoing evaluation (or trending) of the CO. Comparisons of the TDCO method with the CCO method have shown the CCO method to be reliable (Urden, Stacy, & Lough, 2010).

SVR, SVR index, SV, and SVI can be calculated each time that CO is measured. The formulas for calculating these parameters are shown in Table 68-1. Increased SVR (>1200 dynes/sec/cm^{-5}) indicates vasoconstriction from shock, increased release or administration of epinephrine or norepinephrine, or left ventricular failure. A low SVR (>800 dynes/sec/cm^{-5}) indicates vasodilation, which may occur during sepsis, septic shock, or neurogenic shock or with drugs that reduce afterload. Changes in SV are rapidly becoming more important indicators of the pumping status of the heart. High SV may be seen in bradycardia and exercise and with the use of positive inotropes (e.g., milrinone). Low SV is seen with tachydysrhythmias, extreme vasodilation, and cardiac tamponade.

Minimally Invasive Cardiac Output Monitoring. Advances in hemodynamic monitoring have led to the development of a minimally invasive approach for determining CO. This technology involves the use of a specialized sensor that attaches to a standard arterial pressure line and a monitor. CCO/CCI (continuous cardiac index), SV/SVI, and SV variation are measured every 20 seconds. More research is needed to determine whether this technology will replace hemodynamic monitoring using the PA catheter.

Noninvasive Hemodynamic Monitoring: Impedance Cardiography. Impedance cardiography (ICG) is a continuous or intermittent, noninvasive method of obtaining CO and assessing thoracic fluid status. Based on the concepts of impedance (the resistance to the flow of electric current [Ω]), ICG uses four sets of external electrodes to deliver a high-frequency, low-amplitude current similar to that used in apnea monitors. Blood is an excellent conductor of electricity (lower impedance), and pulsatile blood flow generates electrical impedance changes. ICG measures the change in impedance (dΩ) in the ascending aorta and left ventricle over time (dt) and is represented as dΩ/dt. Ωo is the measurement of the average impedance of the fluid in the thorax. Impedance-based hemodynamic parameters (CO, SV, and SVR) are calculated from Ωo, dΩ/dt, mean arterial pressure, CVP, and the ECG.

Major indications for ICG include early signs and symptoms of pulmonary or cardiac dysfunction, differentiation of cardiac or pulmonary cause of shortness of breath, evaluation of etiology and management of hypotension, monitoring after discontinuing a PA catheter or justification for insertion of a PA catheter, evaluation of pharmacotherapy, and diagnosis of rejection following cardiac transplantation. ICG is not recommended in patients who have generalized edema or third spacing because the excess volume interferes with accurate signals.

Mixed Venous Oxygen Saturation. PA catheters can include sensors to measure oxygen saturation of hemoglobin of PA blood. This value is the *mixed venous oxygen saturation* (SvO$_2$), and it is useful in determining the adequacy of tissue oxygenation. SvO$_2$ reflects the dynamic balance between oxygenation of the arterial blood, tissue perfusion, and tissue oxygen consumption. SvO$_2$, when considered in conjunction with the SaO$_2$, is useful

Table 68-4 Clinical Interpretation of SvO₂ Measurements

SVO₂ MEASUREMENT	PHYSIOLOGICAL BASIS FOR CHANGE IN SVO₂	CLINICAL DIAGNOSIS AND RATIONALE
High SvO₂ (80-95%)	Increased oxygen supply	Patient receiving more oxygen than required by clinical condition
	Decreased oxygen demand	Anaesthesia, which causes sedation and decreased muscle movement
		Hypothermia, which lowers metabolic demand (e.g., with cardiopulmonary bypass)
		Sepsis caused by decreased ability of tissues to use oxygen at the cellular level
		False high-positive because pulmonary artery catheter is wedged in a pulmonary capillary
Normal SvO₂ (60-80%)	Normal oxygen supply and metabolic demand	Balanced oxygen supply and demand
Low SvO₂ (<60%)	Decreased oxygen supply caused by:	Anemia or bleeding with compromised cardiopulmonary system
	Low hemoglobin	Hypoxemia resulting from decreased oxygen supply or lung disease
	Low arterial saturation (SaO₂)	Cardiogenic shock caused by left ventricular pump failure
	Low cardiac output	Metabolic demand exceeds oxygen supply in conditions increasing metabolic rate, including physiological states such as shivering, seizures, and hyperthermia and nursing interventions, such as obtaining bed scale weight and repositioning, that increase muscle movement
	Increased oxygen consumption (VO₂)	

Source: Urden, L. D., Stacy, K. M., & Lough, M. E. (2010). *Critical care nursing: Diagnosis and management* (6th ed., p. 362, Table 18-8). St. Louis: Mosby.

in analyzing hemodynamic status and response to treatments or activities (Table 68-4). Normal SvO₂ at rest is 60 to 80%.

Sustained decreases and increases in SvO₂ must be analyzed carefully. Decreased SvO₂ may indicate decreased arterial oxygenation, low CO, low hemoglobin, or increased oxygen consumption. If the SvO₂ falls, the nurse determines which of these four factors has changed. The nurse observes for changes in arterial oxygenation by monitoring pulse oximetry results or ABGs. By noting any changes in level of consciousness, strength and quality of peripheral pulses, urine output, and skin colour and temperature, the nurse can grossly assess CO and tissue perfusion. If arterial oxygenation, CO, and hemoglobin are unchanged, a fall in SvO₂ indicates increased oxygen consumption, which could result from an increased metabolic rate, pain, movement, or fever. If oxygen consumption increases without a comparable increase in oxygen delivery, more oxygen is extracted from the blood, and SvO₂ will continue to fall.

Increased SvO₂ is also clinically significant and may indicate a clinical improvement (e.g., increased SaO₂, improved perfusion, decreased metabolic rate) or problems (e.g., sepsis, ventricular septal defect). In sepsis, oxygen may not be extracted properly at the tissue level, resulting in increased mixed venous oxygen saturation.

Nursing interventions may be guided by changes in SvO₂. The nurse might note that the patient's heart rate increased moderately during repositioning but that the SvO₂ remained stable. In this case, the nurse might conclude that the position change was tolerated. If the SvO₂ had dropped, this would be an indication to stop the activity until the SvO₂ returns to the previous level.

In many cases, as activity or metabolism increases, heart rate and CO increase, and SvO₂ remains constant or varies slightly. However, it is not uncommon for critically ill patients to have conditions that prevent substantial increases in CO. For example, this could occur in the patient with heart failure, shock, dysrhythmias, or cardiac transplantation. In these cases, SvO₂ can provide a useful indicator of the balance between oxygen delivery and consumption.

Complications With PA Catheters. Infection and sepsis are serious problems associated with PA catheters. Careful surgical asepsis for insertion and maintenance of the catheter and tubing line is mandatory to prevent infection. The skin is cleaned according to unit procedure, usually with an iodine preparation. The insertion site is covered with a sterile occlusive dressing. The nurse should monitor the patient for local and systemic signs of infection (e.g., redness and exudate at the insertion site, fever, increased white blood cell count). The PA catheter must be removed if there are local or systemic signs of infection. To reduce the risk of infection, the flush bag, pressure tubing, transducer, and stopcock should be changed every 72 hours, and the PA catheter should be removed once hemodynamic monitoring is no longer needed.

Air embolus is another risk associated with PA catheters. Air embolus can be caused by injection of air into the lumen of a ruptured balloon or by balloon rupture. The nurse decreases the risk of air embolus by first aspirating to check for the absence or presence of blood and by injecting only the prescribed volume of air into the balloon before obtaining the PAOP. Catheters are also checked for balloon leak before insertion; defective catheters are not used. If the nurse aspirates blood from the balloon port or observes that injected air does not flow back into the syringe, the catheter should be so labelled and the physician notified. Air can also be introduced into the system if connections are not tight, and Luer-Lok connections should be used on all pressure lines. In addition, the low-pressure alarm is activated for all pressure lines to signal any substantial drop in the pressure. Any time the line has to be disconnected to change the apparatus, the nurse closes the line to the patient via clamping or stopcocks.

The patient with a PA catheter is at risk for pulmonary infarction or PA rupture from the following causes: (1) the balloon may rupture, releasing fragments that could embolize; (2) prolonged balloon inflation may obstruct blood flow; (3) the catheter may advance into a wedge position, obstructing blood flow; and (4) a thrombus could form and embolize. To reduce the risk of pulmonary infarction and rupture, the balloon must never be inflated beyond the balloon's capacity (usually 1 to 1.5 mL of air). The balloon must not be left inflated for more than four breaths (except during insertion) or 15 seconds. PAP waveforms are monitored continuously for evidence of catheter occlusion, dislocation, or spontaneous wedging. The pressure tracing will be blunted if the catheter starts to be occluded. The pressure tracing will appear wedged if the PA catheter advances and becomes spontaneously wedged. In each of these cases, the catheter must be immediately repositioned. Ventricular dysrhythmias can occur during PA catheter insertion or removal or if the tip migrates back from the PA to the right ventricle and irritates the ventricular wall. In addition, the nurse may observe that the PA catheter cannot be wedged. In these situations, the catheter may have to be repositioned by the physician or a qualified nurse.

Noninvasive Arterial Oxygenation Monitoring.

Pulse oximetry is a noninvasive and continuous method of determining arterial oxygenation (SpO_2), and monitoring SpO_2 may reduce the frequency needed of ABG sampling (see Chapter 28). SpO_2 is normally 95 to 100%. A common use for pulse oximetry is to evaluate the effectiveness of oxygen therapy. Decreased SpO_2 indicates inadequate oxygenation of the blood in the pulmonary capillaries. This may be corrected by increasing the fraction of inspired oxygen (FiO_2) and evaluating the patient's response. Similarly, the nurse uses SpO_2 to monitor how the patient tolerates decreases in FiO_2 and responds to changes in position and treatments. For example, the nurse might note that SpO_2 falls when the patient is positioned in a left lateral recumbent position. The nurse could then plan position changes that pose less risk for the patient.

Accurate SpO_2 measurements may be difficult to obtain on patients who are hypothermic, receiving IV vasopressor therapy (e.g., norepinephrine [Levophed]), or experiencing hypoperfusion (e.g., shock). Usual locations for placement of the oximetry probe are the fingers; alternate locations for probe placement may have to be considered (e.g., forehead, earlobe) during periods of hypoperfusion.

NURSING MANAGEMENT: HEMODYNAMIC MONITORING

Assessment of hemodynamic status requires integration of data from many sources and comparison of the data over time. Thorough, basic nursing observations provide important clues about the patient's hemodynamic status. The nurse should begin by obtaining baseline data regarding the patient's general appearance, level of consciousness, skin colour and temperature, vital signs, peripheral pulses, and urine output. Does the patient appear tired, weak, exhausted? There may be too little cardiac reserve to sustain even minimum activity. Pallor, cool skin, and diminished pulses may indicate decreased CO. Changes in mental clarity may reflect problems with cerebral perfusion or oxygenation. Monitoring urine output reflects the adequacy of perfusion to the kidneys. The patient with diminished perfusion to the GI tract may develop hypoactive or absent bowel sounds. If the patient is bleeding and developing shock, BP might initially be relatively stable, yet the patient may become increasingly pale and cool from peripheral vasoconstriction. Conversely, the patient experiencing septic shock may remain warm and pink yet develop tachycardia and blood pressure instability. Although heart rates of 100 beats/min are common among stressed, compromised,

critically ill patients, sustained tachycardia greatly increases myocardial oxygen demand and may result in diminished CO.

The critical care nurse correlates observational data with data obtained from biotechnology (e.g., ECG; arterial pressure, PAP, PAOP; SvO_2). Single hemodynamic values are rarely significant. The nurse must evaluate the whole clinical picture with the goals of recognizing early clues and intervening before problems escalate.

Circulatory-Assist Devices

Mechanical **circulatory-assist devices (CADs),** such as the IABP and the left ventricular assist device (VAD), are used to decrease cardiac work and improve organ perfusion in patients with heart failure when conventional drug therapy is no longer adequate. The type of device used depends on the extent and the nature of the myocardial problem and the capabilities of the institution and staff. CADs provide interim support in three types of situations: (1) the left ventricle requires support while recovering from acute injury; (2) the heart requires surgical repair (e.g., a ruptured septum), but the patient's condition must be stabilized; and (3) the heart has failed, and the patient is awaiting cardiac transplantation. All CADs decrease left ventricular workload, increase myocardial perfusion, and augment circulation. The most commonly used CAD is the IABP. Several types of VADs are available, and additional devices are under development.

Intra-Aortic Balloon Pump

The **intra-aortic balloon pump** (IABP) provides temporary circulatory assistance to the compromised heart by reducing afterload (via reduction in systolic pressure) and augmenting the aortic diastolic pressure. Table 68-5 lists clinical conditions for which the IABP is used. The IABP consists of a sausage-shaped balloon, a pump that inflates and deflates the balloon, control devices for synchronizing the balloon inflation to the cardiac cycle, and fail-safe devices (Figure 68-13). Under strict aseptic technique, the balloon is inserted percutaneously or surgically into the femoral artery, advanced toward the heart, and positioned in the descending thoracic aorta just below the left subclavian artery (Figure 68-14). Following placement, the position is confirmed radiologically. A pneumatic device cyclically fills the balloon with helium at the start of diastole (immediately after aortic valve closure) and deflates it just before systole. The ECG is the primary trigger used to initiate the deflation on the R wave (of the QRS) and the inflation on the T wave, and the dicrotic notch of the arterial pressure tracing is used to refine timing (Figure 68-15, A). IABP support is referred to as *counterpulsation* because the timing of balloon inflation is opposite to ventricular contraction. The IAPB assist ratio is 1:1 in the acute phase of treatment, that is, one IABP cycle of inflation and deflation for every heartbeat.

Effects of Counterpulsation.

In late diastole when the balloon is totally inflated, blood is forcibly displaced distally to the extremities and proximally to the coronary arteries and the main branches of the aortic arch. Diastolic arterial pressure rises (diastolic augmentation), increasing coronary artery perfusion pressure and perfusion of vital organs. The rise in coronary artery perfusion pressure causes an increase in blood flow to the myocardium. The balloon is rapidly deflated just before systole. The

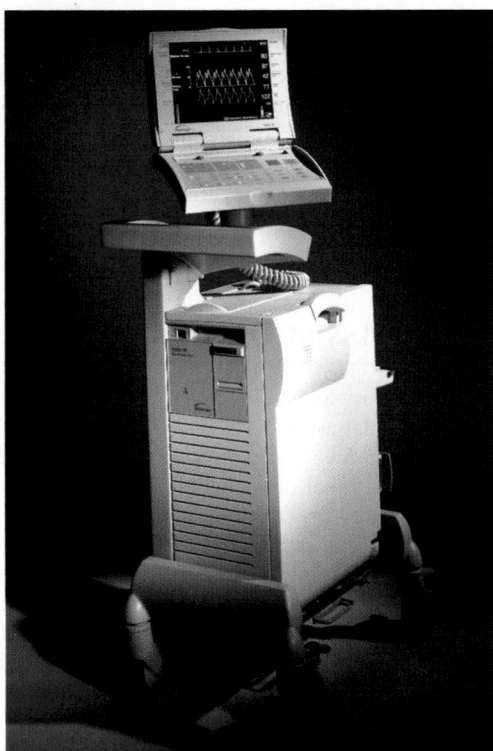

Figure 68-13 Intra-aortic balloon pump machine.

Source: Courtesy Datascope Corporation, Fairfield, New Jersey.

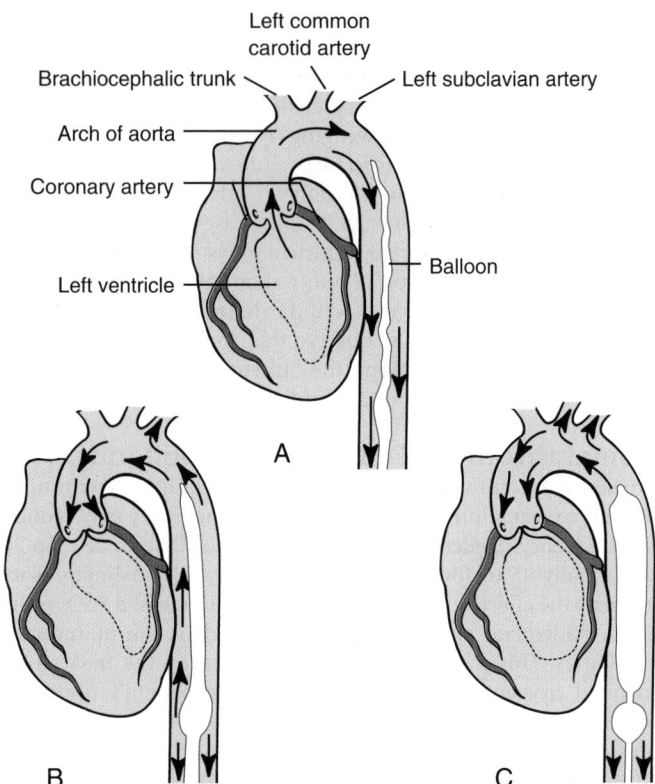

Figure 68-14 Intra-aortic balloon pump. **A,** During systole, the balloon is deflated, which facilitates ejection of the blood into the periphery. **B,** In early diastole, the balloon begins to inflate. **C,** In late diastole, the balloon is totally inflated, which augments aortic pressure and increases the coronary perfusion pressure, with the end result of increased coronary and cerebral blood flow.

Table 68-5 Indications and Contraindications for the Intra-Aortic Balloon Pump

Indications

- Refractory unstable angina (when drugs have failed)
- Short-term bridge to cardiac transplantation
- Acute myocardial infarction with any of the following:*
  - Ventricular aneurysm accompanied by ventricular dysrhythmias
  - Acute ventricular septal defect
  - Acute mitral valve dysfunction
  - Cardiogenic shock
  - Recurrent chest pain with or without ventricular dysrhythmias
  - Preoperative, intraoperative, and postoperative cardiac surgery (e.g., prophylaxis before surgery, failure to wean from cardiopulmonary bypass, left ventricular failure after cardiopulmonary bypass)
  - High-risk interventional cardiology procedures

Contraindications

- Irreversible brain damage
- Terminal or untreatable diseases of any major organ system
- Abdominal aortic and thoracic aneurysms
- Moderate to severe aortic insufficiency
- Generalized peripheral vascular disease†

*Allows time for emergent angiography and corrective cardiac surgery to be performed.
†May inhibit placement of balloon and is considered a relative contraindication; sheathless insertion may be used.

suddenly created vacuum causes aortic pressure to drop. With aortic resistance to left ventricular ejection reduced (reduced afterload), the left ventricle empties more easily and completely. As with other types of afterload reduction, the SV increases, yet the myocardial oxygen consumption decreases. Hemodynamic effects of the IABP are summarized in Table 68-6.

Complications With Intra-Aortic Balloon Pumps.

Complications are common with the IABP (Table 68-7). Vascular injuries such as dislodging of plaque, aortic dissection, and compromised distal circulation are common, occurring in 3 to 65% of cases. Thrombus and embolus formation add to the risk of circulatory compromise to the extremity. Peripheral nerve damage can occur, particularly when a cut-down is performed for insertion. To reduce these risks, cardiovascular, neurovascular, and hemodynamic assessments are necessary every 15 to 60 minutes, depending on the patient's status. The action of the balloon pump can cause physical destruction of platelets, and thrombocytopenia is common. Coagulation profiles must be monitored, and the patient must be assessed for evidence of systemic bleeding. Displacement of the balloon can occlude the left subclavian, renal, or mesenteric arteries and can result in diminished or absent radial pulse, decreased urine output, and diminished or absent bowel sounds. Patients receiving IABP therapy are

Table 68-6 Hemodynamic Effects of Intra-Aortic Balloon Pumps

Effects of Inflation During Diastole

- Increased diastolic pressure (may exceed systolic pressure)
- Increased pressure in the aortic root during diastole
- Increased coronary perfusion pressure
- Improved oxygen delivery to the myocardium
  - Decreased angina pain
  - Decreased electrocardiographic evidence of ischemia
  - Decreased ventricular ectopy

Effects of Deflation During Systole

- Decreased afterload
- Decreased peak systolic pressure
- Decreased myocardial oxygen consumption
- Increased stroke volume, possibly associated with the following:
  - Improved sensorium
  - Warmed skin
  - Increased urine output
  - Decreased heart rate
- Increased forward flow of blood, decreasing preload
  - Decreased PA pressures, including PAOP
  - Decreased crackles

PA, pulmonary artery; PAOP, pulmonary artery occlusive pressure.

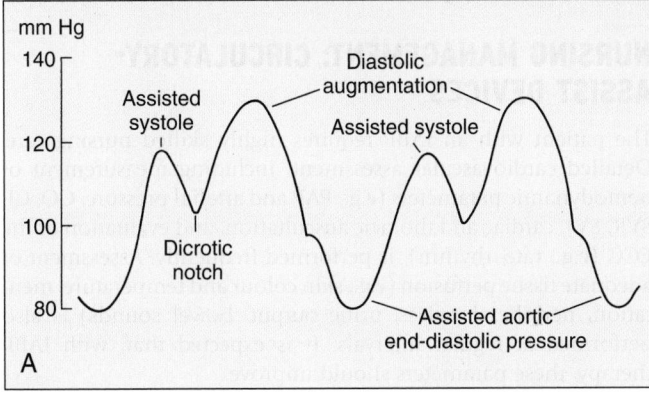

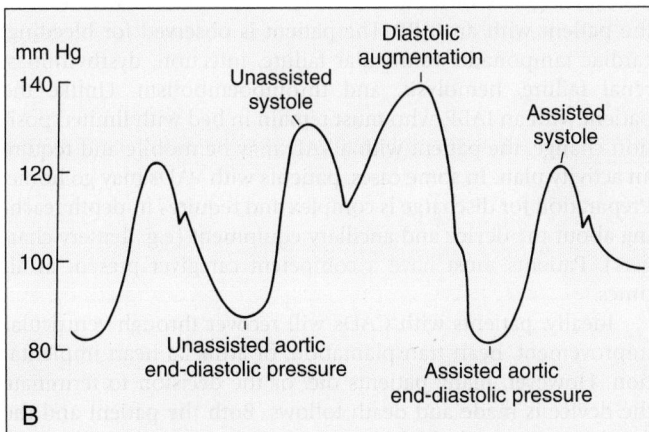

Figure 68-15 A, Correct 1:1 intra-aortic balloon pump frequency. **B,** Correct 1:2 intra-aortic balloon pump frequency.

Source: Courtesy Datascope Corporation, Montvale, New Jersey.

Table 68-7 Nursing Management: Potential Complications of the Intra-Aortic Balloon Pump

POTENTIAL COMPLICATION	NURSING MANAGEMENT
Site infection from invasive lines	Use strict aseptic technique for insertion and dressing changes for all lines. Cover all insertion sites with occlusive dressings. Administer prescribed prophylactic antibiotic for entire course of therapy.
Pneumonia associated with immobilization	Reposition patient q2h, being careful not to displace balloon. If patient with pneumonia requires physical therapy of the chest, avoid introducing an ECG artifact.
Arterial trauma caused by insertion or displacement of balloon	Evaluate and mark peripheral pulses before insertion of balloon to use as baseline for assessing pulses after insertion. After insertion of balloon, evaluate perfusion to both extremities at least every hour. Measure urine output at least every hour (occlusion of renal arteries causes severe decrease in urine output). Observe arterial waveforms for sudden changes. Keep head of bed <45 degrees. Do not flex cannulated leg at the hip. Immobilize cannulated leg to prevent flexion using a draw sheet tucked under the mattress, soft ankle restraint, or knee immobilizer.
Thromboembolism caused by trauma, balloon obstruction of blood flow distal to catheter	Administer prophylactic heparin if ordered. Evaluate pulses, urine output, and level of consciousness at least every hour. Check circulation, sensation, and movement in both legs at least every hour.
Hematological complications caused by platelet aggregation along the balloon (decrease in platelets possible)	Administer Rheomacrodex (low–molecular weight dextran) if ordered. Monitor coagulation profiles, hematocrit, and platelet count.
Hemorrhage from insertion site	Check site for bleeding at least every hour. Observe vital signs for hypovolemia with each check of vital signs.

ECG, electrocardiogram.

prone to infection, and local or systemic signs of infection necessitate catheter removal.

Mechanical complications are rare but may occur. Improper timing of balloon inflation may cause increased afterload, decreased CO, myocardial ischemia, and increased myocardial oxygen use and must be immediately recognized by the nurse. If the balloon develops a leak, the catheter must be changed immediately to avoid a helium gas embolus. Signs of a leak include less effective augmentation, repeated alarms for gas loss, and blood backing up into the catheter. A malfunction of the balloon or the console triggers fail-safe alarms and automatic shutdown of the unit.

The patient with an IABP is relatively immobile and limited to side-lying or supine positions with the head of the bed elevated less than 45 degrees. The leg in which the catheter is inserted must not be flexed at the hip. The patient may be receiving ventilatory support and will likely have multiple invasive lines that increase the challenge of comfortable positioning. The patient may experience sleeplessness and anxiety. Adequate sedation, pain relief, skin care, and comfort measures are required. IABP therapy is weaned as the patient improves; that is, circulatory support provided by the IABP is gradually reduced. Weaning involves reducing the IABP assist ratio from 1:1 to 1:2 and assessing the patient's response (see Figure 68-15, B). If hemodynamic parameters remain stable, the ratio can be changed, going from 1:3 to 1:8 until the IABP catheter is removed. Even if the patient is stable without IABP, pumping is continued until the line is removed. This reduces the risk of thrombus formation around the catheter. Frequent hemodynamic assessment continues to be required during the weaning phase.

Ventricular Assist Devices

The **ventricular assist device (VAD)** provides short- and longer-term support for the failing heart and allows more mobility than the IABP. VADs are inserted into the path of flowing blood to augment or replace the action of the ventricle. Some VADs are implanted internally (e.g., peritoneum), and others are positioned externally. A typical VAD shunts blood from the left atrium or ventricle to the device and then to the aorta. Some VADs provide right or biventricular support (Figure 68-16). Failure to wean from cardiopulmonary bypass after surgery is a primary indicator for VAD support. VADs are also used to support patients with ventricular failure caused by myocardial infarction and patients awaiting cardiac transplantation. A VAD is a temporary device with the capability to partially or totally support circulation until the heart recovers or a donor heart can be obtained. Cannula sites depend on the type of device used. For support of the right side of the heart, the right atrium and PA are cannulated. The left ventricular apex can be cannulated for left VADs. Direct

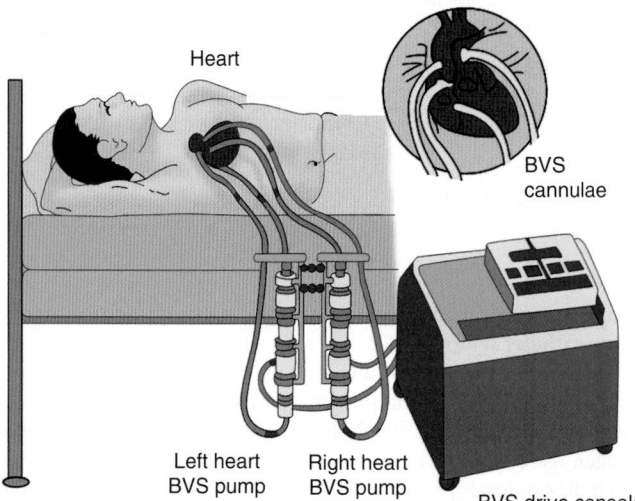

Figure 68-16 Schematic diagram of a biventricular assist device. *BVS*, biventricular support.

Labels: Heart; BVS cannulae; Left heart BVS pump; Right heart BVS pump; BVS drive console

Source: Jett, G. K. (2000). In D. J. Goldstein & M. C. Oz (Eds.), *Cardiac assist devices*. Armonk, NY: Futura.

cannulation of the atria and great vessels occurs in the operating room through a sternotomy.

Appropriate patient selection for VAD therapy is critical. Indications include (1) failure to wean from cardiopulmonary bypass or postcardiotomy cardiogenic shock, (2) a bridge to recovery or cardiac transplantation, and (3) patients with New York Heart Association Classification IV (see Table 37-4) who have failed medical therapy. Relative contraindications for VAD therapy include (1) body surface area less than manufacturer's limit (e.g., 1.3 m²), (2) renal or liver failure unrelated to a cardiac event, and (3) co-morbidities that would limit life expectancy to less than 3 years (Puhlman & Hargraves, 2011).

Implantable Artificial Heart

In Canada in 2010, 167 heart transplants were performed (Heart and Stroke Foundation of Canada, 2010). Research on mechanical CADs has led to the development of a fully implantable artificial heart that can sustain the body's circulatory system. This device is designed not only to extend life but also to provide a satisfactory quality of life for the thousands of patients with irreversible heart disease who never receive a donor heart. One major anticipated advantage of the artificial heart compared with heart transplantation is decreased costs for implantation and drug therapies. Patients will not require immunosuppression therapy, nor will they experience the inevitable, long-term effects of this therapy. However, patients will require life-long anticoagulation (Abiomed, 2007).

NURSING MANAGEMENT: CIRCULATORY-ASSIST DEVICES

The patient with an IABP requires highly skilled nursing care. Detailed cardiovascular assessment, including measurement of hemodynamic parameters (e.g., PAP and arterial pressure, CO, CI, SVR, SV), cardiac and thoracic auscultation, and evaluation of the ECG (e.g., rate, rhythm), is performed frequently. Assessment of adequate tissue perfusion (e.g., skin colour and temperature, mentation, peripheral pulses, urine output, bowel sounds) is also performed at regular intervals. It is expected that, with IABP therapy, these parameters should improve.

Nursing care of the patient with a VAD is similar to that of the patient with an IABP. The patient is observed for bleeding, cardiac tamponade, ventricular failure, infection, dysrhythmias, renal failure, hemolysis, and thromboembolism. Unlike the patient with an IABP, who must remain in bed with limited position change, the patient with a VAD may be mobile and require an activity plan. In some cases, patients with VADs may go home. Preparation for discharge is complex and requires in-depth teaching about the device and ancillary equipment (e.g., battery chargers). Patients must have a competent caregiver present at all times.

Ideally, patients with CADs will recover through ventricular improvement, heart transplantation, or artificial heart implantation. However, many patients die, or the decision to terminate the device is made and death follows. Both the patient and the family require psychological support. Nursing care should include the family as much as possible. Other members of the health care team, such as social workers or clergy, should be consulted as needed.

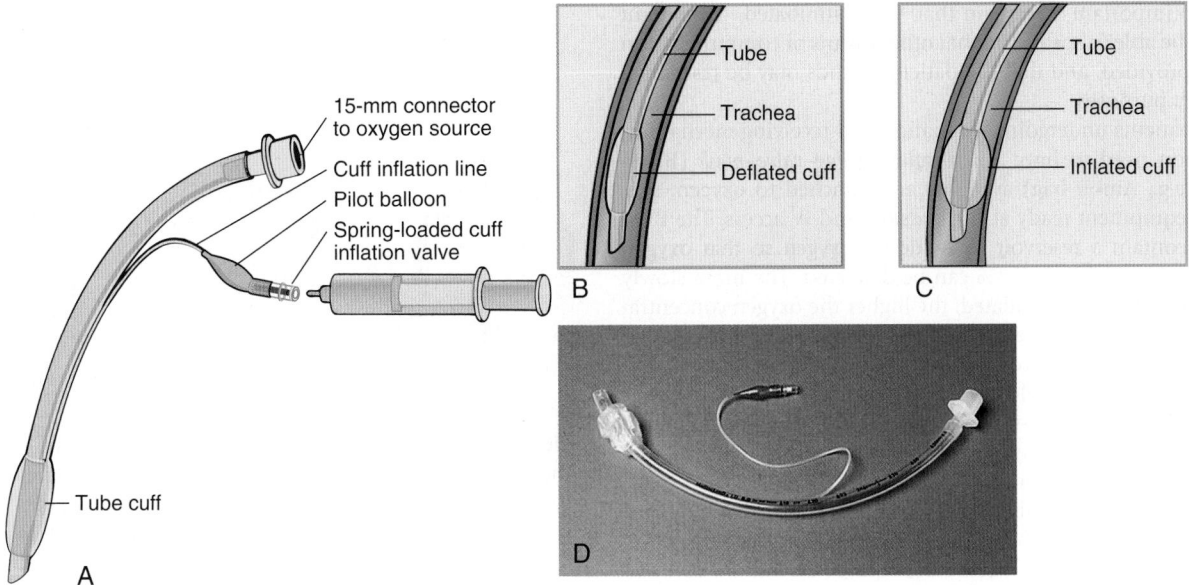

Figure 68-17 Endotracheal tube. **A,** Parts of an endotracheal tube. **B,** Tube in place with the cuff deflated. **C,** Tube in place with the cuff inflated. **D,** Photograph of the tube before placement.

Source: Beare, P. G., & Myers, J. L. (1998). *Adult health nursing* (3rd ed.). St. Louis: Mosby.

Artificial Airways

The patient in the CCU often requires mechanical assistance to maintain airway patency. Inserting a tube into the trachea, bypassing upper airway and laryngeal structures, creates an artificial airway. The tube is placed into the trachea via the mouth or the nose past the larynx (**endotracheal [ET] intubation**) or through a stoma in the neck (tracheostomy). ET intubation is more common in CCU patients. It can be performed quickly and safely at the bedside. Indications for ET intubation include (1) upper airway obstruction (e.g., secondary to burns, tumour, bleeding), (2) apnea, (3) high risk of aspiration, (4) ineffective clearance of secretions, and (5) respiratory distress. ET tubes are illustrated in Figure 68-17.

A tracheotomy is a surgical procedure that is performed when the need for an artificial airway is expected to be long term. There is ongoing debate regarding the timing of a tracheotomy in the patient requiring an ET tube. Research has suggested that early tracheotomy (2 to 10 days) may have advantages over delayed tracheotomy, particularly when mechanical ventilation is predicted to be needed for longer than 10 to 14 days (Hsu et al., 2005). The situation varies with the patient, the physician, and the institution. Tracheostomy tubes and related nursing management are discussed in Chapter 29.

Endotracheal Tubes

In oral intubation, the ET tube is passed through the mouth, past the vocal cords, and into the trachea with the aid of a laryngoscope or bronchoscope. In nasal ET intubation, the ET is placed blindly (i.e., without visualizing the larynx) through the nose and the nasopharynx, and past the vocal cords. Oral ET intubation is the procedure of choice for most emergencies because the airway can be secured rapidly. Compared with the nasal route, a larger-diameter tube can be used for oral intubation. With a larger-bore

ET tube, work of breathing (WOB) is reduced because there is less airway resistance. It is easier to remove secretions and perform fibreoptic bronchoscopy if needed. Nasal ET intubation is indicated when head and neck manipulation is risky.

There are risks associated with oral ET intubation. It may be difficult to place an oral tube if head and neck mobility is limited (e.g., suspected spinal cord injury). Teeth can be chipped or inadvertently dislodged during the procedure. Salivation is increased, and swallowing is difficult. Often, a patient will obstruct the ET tube by biting down on it. A bite block or oropharyngeal airway can be used to prevent this, along with sedatives. The ET tube and the bite block (if used) should be secured (separately) to the face. Mouth care is a challenge owing to the limitations of space in the oral cavity but can be achieved with smaller or pediatric-sized oral products for toothbrushing, cleaning, and suctioning.

Nasal intubation is contraindicated in patients with facial fractures, suspected fractures at the base of the skull, and postoperatively after cranial surgeries. The nasal tube may be uncomfortable for some patients because it presses on the septum, whereas others may prefer it because there is no need for a bite block and mouth care is more easily accomplished. However, nasal ET tubes are more subject to kinking than oral tubes; the WOB is greater because the longer, narrower tube offers more airflow resistance; and suctioning and secretion removal are more difficult. Finally, nasal tubes have been linked with an increased incidence of sinus infection and ventilator-associated pneumonia (American Thoracic Society and the Infectious Diseases Society of America, 2005).

Endotracheal Intubation Procedure

Unless ET intubation is emergent, consent for the procedure should be obtained. The patient and the family should be told the reason for ET intubation, the steps that will occur in the procedure, and the patient's role in the procedure (if indicated).

It is also important to explain that, while intubated, the patient will not be able to speak, but that other means of communication will be provided, and that the patient's hands may be restrained for safety purposes.

All patients undergoing intubation and receiving mechanical ventilation need to have a self-inflating *bag–valve–mask* (BVM) device (e.g., Ambu bag) available and attached to oxygen, suctioning equipment ready at the bedside, and IV access. The BVM should contain a reservoir to sequester oxygen so that oxygen concentrations of 90 to 95% can be delivered. The more slowly the bag is deflated and inflated, the higher the oxygen concentration that will be delivered. The nurse assembles and checks the equipment to be used, removes the patient's dentures or partial plates, or both (for oral intubation), and administers drugs as ordered. Premedication varies, depending on the patient's level of consciousness (e.g., awake, obtunded) and the nature of the procedure (e.g., emergent, nonemergent).

Rapid-sequence intubation is the rapid, concurrent administration of both a paralytic and a sedative agent during emergency airway management to decrease the risks of aspiration, combativeness, and injury to the patient. Rapid-sequence intubation is not indicated in patients who are comatose or in cardiac arrest (Mace, 2008). A sedative–hypnotic–amnesic (e.g., midazolam) is used if the patient is agitated, disoriented, or combative. A rapid-onset opioid (e.g., fentanyl) is used to blunt the pain of laryngoscopy and intubation. A paralytic drug (e.g., succinylcholine) is used to produce skeletal muscle paralysis. Atropine may be used to limit secretions. Monitor the patient's oxygenation status during the procedure with pulse oximetry.

For oral intubation, place the patient supine with the head extended and the neck flexed ("sniffing position"). This position allows for visualization of the vocal cords by aligning the axes of the mouth, pharynx, and trachea. For nasal intubation, it may be necessary to spray the nasal passages with a local anaesthetic and vasoconstrictor (e.g., lidocaine [Xylocaine] with epinephrine) to decrease trauma and bleeding. Before intubation is attempted, preoxygenate the patient using a self-inflating BVM and 100% O_2 for 3 to 5 minutes. Each intubation attempt is limited to less than 30 seconds. Ventilate the patient between successive attempts using the BVM and 100% O_2.

Following intubation, inflate the cuff and confirm the placement of the ET tube while the patient is manually ventilated using the BVM with 100% O_2. Use a $PETCO_2$ detector to confirm proper placement by measuring the amount of exhaled CO_2 from the lungs. Place the detector between the BVM and the ET tube and observe for either a colour change (indicating the presence of CO_2) or a number. If no CO_2 is detected, the tube is in the esophagus and needs to be reinserted (Nagler & Krauss, 2008). Auscultate the lung bases and apices for bilateral breath sounds and the epigastrium for the absence of air insufflations. Observe the chest for symmetrical chest wall movement. In addition, SpO_2 should be stable or improved. If the evidence supports proper ET tube placement, connect the tube to an O_2 source and secure per institution policy (Figure 68-18). Suction the ET tube and the pharynx and insert a bite block as needed. Arrange for a portable chest radiograph immediately to confirm tube location (3-5 cm above the carina in the adult). This position allows the patient to move the neck without dislodging the tube or causing it to enter the right mainstem bronchus. Once proper positioning is confirmed with radiography, record and mark the position of the tube at the lip or teeth (usually 21 cm for women and 23 cm for men) or nose ("exit mark") (St. John & Seckel, 2006). Excess tubing is cut to reduce dead space.

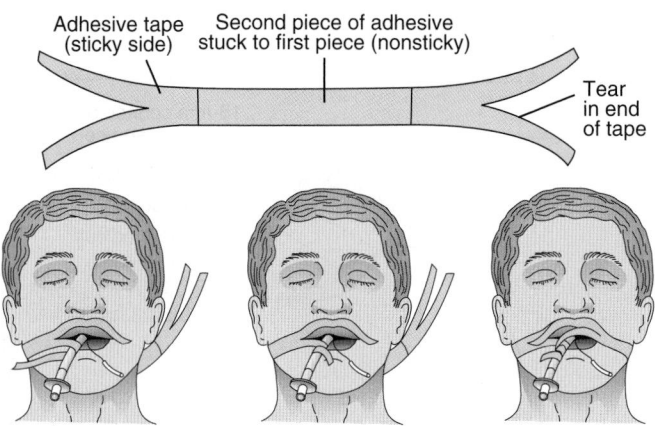

Figure 68-18 Example of protocol for securing an endotracheal tube using adhesive tape:
1. Clean the patient's skin with mild soap and water.
2. Remove oil from the skin with alcohol and allow to dry.
3. Apply a skin adhesive product to enhance tape adherence. (When tape is removed, an adhesive remover will be necessary.)
4. Place a hydrocolloid membrane over the cheeks to protect friable skin.
5. Secure with adhesive tape as shown.

Source: Henneman, E., Ellstrom, K., & St. John, R. E. (1999). *AACN protocols for practice: Care of the mechanically ventilated patient series*. Aliso Viejo, CA: American Association of Critical Care Nurses.

The ET tube is connected to either humidified air, O_2, or a mechanical ventilator. Obtain ABGs within 25 minutes after intubation to determine oxygenation and ventilation status. ABG values are reviewed and used to guide oxygenation and ventilation changes. Continuous pulse oximetry monitoring provides a valuable estimate of arterial oxygenation.

NURSING MANAGEMENT: ARTIFICIAL AIRWAY

Nursing responsibilities for the patient with an artificial airway include (1) maintaining correct tube placement, (2) maintaining proper cuff inflation, (3) monitoring oxygenation and ventilation, (4) maintaining tube patency, (5) assessing for complications, (6) providing oral care and maintaining skin integrity, and (7) fostering comfort and communication (see eNCP 68-1, available on the Evolve Web site for this chapter).

Maintaining Correct Tube Placement

The nurse must monitor the patient with an ET tube for proper placement at least every 2 to 4 hours. If the tube is dislodged, it could terminate in the pharynx or enter the esophagus or the right mainstem bronchus (thus ventilating only the right lung). The nurse maintains proper tube position by confirming that the exit mark on the tube remains constant while at rest, during patient care, repositioning, and patient transport. The nurse observes for symmetrical chest wall movement and auscultates to confirm bilateral breath sounds. It is an emergency if the ET tube is not positioned properly. The nurse stays with the patient, maintains the airway, supports ventilation, and secures the appropriate assistance to immediately reposition the tube. It may be necessary to ventilate the patient with a BVM. If a malpositioned tube is not repositioned, minimal or no oxygen will be delivered to the lungs or the entire tidal volume (V_T) will be delivered to one lung, placing the patient at risk for pneumothorax.

■ Maintaining Proper Cuff Inflation

The cuff is an inflatable, pliable sleeve encircling the outer wall of the ET tube (see Figure 68-17). The high-volume, low-pressure cuff stabilizes and "seals" the ET tube within the trachea and prevents escape of ventilating gases. However, the cuff can damage the trachea. To avoid this, inflate the cuff with air and measure and monitor the cuff pressure. Normal arterial tracheal perfusion is estimated at 30 mm Hg. To ensure adequate tracheal perfusion, maintain cuff pressure at 20 to 25 mm Hg (St. John & Seckel, 2006). Measure and record cuff pressure after intubation and on a routine basis (e.g., q8h) using the minimal occluding volume technique or the minimal leak technique.

The steps in the minimal occluding volume technique for cuff inflation are (1) for the mechanically ventilated patient, place a stethoscope over the trachea and inflate the cuff to the minimal occluding volume by adding air until no air leak is heard at peak inspiratory pressure (end patient, inflate until no sound is heard after a deep breath or after inhalation with a BVM; (3) use a manometer to verify that cuff pressure is between 20 and 25 mm Hg; and (4) record cuff pressure in the chart. If adequate cuff pressure cannot be maintained or larger volumes of air are needed to keep the cuff inflated, the cuff could be leaking or there could be tracheal dilation at the cuff site. In these situations, notify the physician to reposition or change the ET tube.

The procedure for the minimal leak technique is similar with one exception. Remove a small amount of air from the cuff until a slight air leak is auscultated at peak inflation. Both techniques aim to prevent the risks of tracheal damage due to high cuff pressures.

■ Monitoring Oxygenation and Ventilation

The patient with an ET tube is vigilantly monitored for adequate oxygenation by assessing clinical findings, ABGs, SpO_2, and SvO_2 or central venous oxygen saturation ($ScvO_2$). The nurse must assess for clinical signs of hypoxemia such as a change in mental status (e.g., confusion), anxiety, dusky skin, and dysrhythmias. Periodic ABGs (specifically partial pressure of oxygen in arterial blood [PaO_2]) and continuous SpO_2 provide objective data regarding oxygenation. Lower values are expected in patients with some disease states, such as chronic obstructive pulmonary disease (COPD). PA or CVP catheters with SvO_2 or $ScvO_2$ capability also can give an indirect indication about the patient's oxygenation status (see Table 68-4).

Indicators of ventilation include assessment of clinical findings, partial pressure of carbon dioxide in arterial blood ($PaCO_2$), and continuous $PETCO_2$. The patient's respirations should be assessed for rate and rhythm and use of accessory muscles. The patient who is hyperventilating will be breathing rapidly and

deeply and may experience circumoral and peripheral numbness and tingling. The patient who is hypoventilating will be breathing shallowly or slowly and may appear dusky. $PaCO_2$ is the best indicator of alveolar hyperventilation (e.g., decreased $PaCO_2$, increased pH indicate respiratory alkalosis) or hypoventilation (e.g., increased $PaCO_2$, decreased pH indicate respiratory acidosis).

$PETCO_2$ monitoring is done by analyzing exhaled gas directly at the patient–ventilator circuit (mainstream sampling) or by transporting a sample of gas via a small-bore tubing to a bedside monitor (sidestream sampling). Continuous $PETCO_2$ monitoring can be used to assess the patency of the airway and the presence of breathing. In addition, gradual changes in $PETCO_2$ values may accompany an increase in CO_2 production (e.g., sepsis, hypoventilation, neuromuscular blockade) or a decrease in CO_2 production (e.g., hypothermia, decreased CO, metabolic acidosis). In patients with normal ventilation–perfusion ratios (see Chapter 70), $PETCO_2$ can be used as an estimate of $PaCO_2$, with $PETCO_2$ generally 1 to 5 mm Hg lower than $PaCO_2$. However, in patients with unusually large dead space or serious mismatch between ventilation and perfusion, $PETCO_2$ is not a reliable estimate of $PaCO_2$ (Nagler & Krauss, 2008).

■ Maintaining Tube Patency

The patient should be assessed routinely to determine a need for suctioning, but the patient should not be suctioned routinely. Indications for suctioning include (1) visible secretions in the ET tube; (2) sudden onset of respiratory distress; (3) suspected aspiration of secretions; (4) increase in peak airway pressures; (5) auscultation of adventitious breath sounds over the trachea, the bronchi, or both; (6) increase in respiratory rate, sustained coughing, or both; and (7) sudden or gradual decrease in PaO_2, SpO_2, or both. Two recommended suctioning methods, the *closed-suction technique* (CST) and the *open-suction technique* (OST), are described in Table 68-8. The CST uses a suction catheter that is enclosed in a plastic sleeve connected directly to the patient–ventilator circuit (Figure 68-19). With the CST, oxygenation and ventilation are maintained during suctioning, and exposure to the patient's secretions is reduced. The CST should be considered for patients who require high levels of positive end-expiratory pressure (PEEP) (>7-8 cm H_2O), who have bloody or infected pulmonary secretions, who require frequent suctioning, and who experience clinical instability with the OST (St John & Seckel, 2006).

Potential complications associated with suctioning include hypoxemia, bronchospasm, increased intracranial pressure, dysrhythmias, hypertension, hypotension, mucosal damage, pulmonary bleeding, and infection (Arroyo-Novoa et al., 2008). The nurse must closely assess the patient before, during, and after the suctioning procedure. If the patient does not tolerate suctioning (e.g., decreased SpO_2, increased or decreased BP, sustained coughing, development of dysrhythmias), the procedure is halted, and the patient is manually hyperventilated with 100% oxygen or, if performing CST, hyperoxygenated until equilibration occurs and before another suction pass is attempted.

Hypoxemia is prevented by hyperoxygenating the patient before and after each suctioning pass and limiting each suctioning pass to 10 seconds or less (see Table 68-8). Research has shown that there are no differences in outcomes between the use of hyperventilation or hyperoxygenation to prevent suction-induced hypoxia (Oh & Seo, 2003). If SvO_2 or $ScvO_2$ and/or SpO_2

Table 68-8 Suctioning Procedures for a Patient on a Mechanical Ventilator

General Measures

1. Gather all equipment.
2. Wash hands and don personal protective equipment.
3. Explain procedure and patient's role in assisting with secretion removal by coughing.
4. Monitor patient's cardiopulmonary status (e.g., vital signs, SpO_2, SvO_2, $ScvO_2$, ECG, level of consciousness) before, during, and after the procedure.
5. Turn on suction and set vacuum to 100 to 120 mm Hg.
6. Pause ventilator alarms.

Open-Suction Technique

1. Open sterile catheter package using the inside of the package as a sterile field. *Note:* Suction catheter should be no wider than half the diameter of the ET tube (e.g., for a 7-mm ET tube, select a 10-French suction catheter).
2. Fill the sterile solution container with sterile normal saline or water.
3. Don sterile gloves.
4. Pick up sterile suction catheter with the dominant hand. Using the nondominant hand, secure the connecting tube (to suction) to the suction catheter.
5. Check equipment for proper functioning by suctioning a small volume of sterile saline solution from the container. (Go to step 7.)

Closed-Suction Technique

6. Connect the suction tubing to the closed-suction port.
7. Hyperoxygenate the patient for 30 sec using one of the following methods:
   - Activate the suction hyperoxygenation setting on the ventilator using the nondominant hand.
   - Increase FiO_2 to 100%. *Note:* FiO_2 must be returned to baseline level at the completion of the procedure.

- Disconnect the ventilator tubing from the ET tube and manually ventilate the patient with 100% O_2 using a BVM device.* Administer 5 or 6 breaths over 30 sec. *Note:* Use of a second person to deliver the manual breaths will significantly increase the tidal volume delivered.

8. With suction off, gently and quickly insert the catheter using the dominant hand. When resistance is met, pull back ½ inch.
9. Apply continuous or intermittent suction using the nondominant thumb. Rotate the catheter between the dominant thumb and the dominant forefinger and withdraw the catheter over 10 sec or less.
10. Hyperoxygenate for 30 sec as described in step 7.
11. If secretions remain and the patient has tolerated the procedure, two to three suction passes may be performed as described in steps 8 and 9. *Note:* Rinse the suction catheter with sterile saline solution between suctioning passes as needed.
12. Reconnect patient to ventilator (open-suction technique).
13. At the completion of ET tube suctioning, rinse the catheter and connecting tubing with the sterile saline solution.
14. Suction nasal and/or oral pharynx. *Note:* A separate catheter must be used for this step when using the closed-suction technique.
15. Discard the suction catheter, and rinse the connecting tubing with the sterile saline solution (open-suction technique).
16. Reset FiO_2 (if necessary) and ventilator alarms.
17. Reassess patient for signs of effective suctioning.

BVM, bag–valve–mask; *ECG*, electrocardiogram; *ET*, endotracheal; *FiO₂*, fraction of inspired oxygen; *PEEP*, positive end-expiratory pressure; *SpO₂*, oxygen saturation; *SvO₂*, venous oxygen saturation.
*Attach a PEEP valve to the BVM for patients on >5 cm H_2O PEEP.
Source: Adapted from Chulay, M. (2011). Suctioning: Endotracheal or tracheostomy tube. In D. L. Wiegand (Ed.), *AACN procedure manual for critical care* (6th ed., Procedure 12). St. Louis: Mosby.

is used, trends should be assessed throughout the suctioning procedure. Causes of dysrhythmias during suctioning include hypoxemia resulting in myocardial hypoxia; vagal stimulation caused by tracheal irritation; and sympathetic nervous system stimulation caused by anxiety, discomfort, or pain. Dysrhythmias include tachydysrhythmias and bradydysrhythmias, premature beats, and asystole. Suctioning should be halted if any new dysrhythmias develop. Excessive suctioning should be avoided in patients with severe hypoxemia or bradycardia.

Tracheal mucosal damage may occur because of excessive suction pressures (>120 mm Hg), overly vigorous catheter insertion, and the characteristics of the suction catheter itself. The presence of blood streaks or tissue shreds in aspirated secretions may indicate that mucosal damage has occurred. Mucosal damage increases the risk of infection and bleeding, particularly if the patient is receiving anticoagulants. Trauma to the mucosa can be prevented by following the steps described in Table 68-8.

Secretions may be thick and difficult to suction because of inadequate hydration, inadequate humidification, infection, or inaccessibility of the left mainstem bronchus or the lower airways. Adequately hydrating the patient (e.g., oral or IV fluids) and providing supplemental humidification of inspired gases may assist in thinning secretions. Instillation of normal saline into the ET tube is discouraged. SpO_2 has been shown to decrease during suctioning with instillation of normal saline (Akgül & Akyolcu, 2002). If infection is the cause of thick secretions, the patient should be given appropriate antibiotics. Postural drainage, percussion, and turning the patient every 2 hours may help move secretions into larger airways.

Providing Oral Care and Maintaining Skin Integrity

When an oral ET tube is in place, the patient's mouth is always open, and the lips, tongue, and mouth should be moistened with saline or water swabs to prevent mucosal drying. Oral care

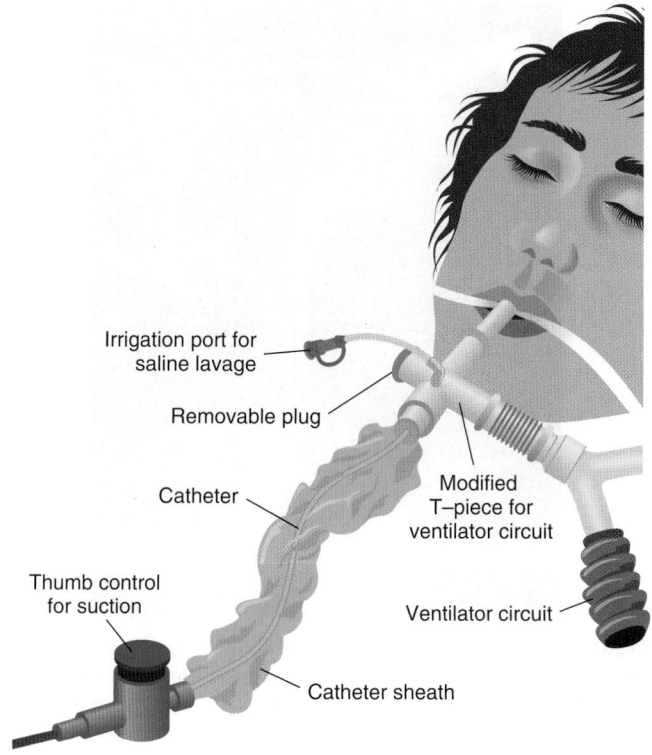

Figure 68-19 labels:
- Irrigation port for saline lavage
- Removable plug
- Catheter
- Modified T–piece for ventilator circuit
- Thumb control for suction
- Ventilator circuit
- Catheter sheath
- To vacuum source

Figure 68-19 Closed tracheal suction system.

Sources: Adapted from Sills, J. R. (1991). *Respiratory care certification guide: The complete review resource for the entry-level exam* (2nd ed.). St Louis: Mosby; Urden, L. D., Stacy, K. M., & Lough, M. E. (2010). *Critical care nursing: Diagnosis and management* (6th ed., p. 651, Figure 25-6). St Louis: Mosby.

Table 68-9 Oral Care Procedures for a Patient on a Mechanical Ventilator General Measures
1. Gather all equipment.
2. Wash hands and don personal protective equipment.
3. Explain procedure to the patient and the family, if present.
4. Perform oral care using pediatric or adult soft toothbrushes at least twice a day by gently brushing to clean and remove plaque.
5. Use oral swabs with a 1.5% hydrogen peroxide solution q2-4h.   *Note:* Postoperative cardiac surgery patients are the only population in which use of 2% chlorhexidine gluconate is recommended twice a day.
6. Apply a mouth moisturizer to oral mucosa and lips with each cleaning.
7. Suction oral cavity and pharynx frequently. See Figure 68-20 for an example of an endotracheal tube that can provide continuous subglottic suctioning.

Note

- All oral suction equipment and suction tubing should be changed q24h.
- Nondisposable oral suction apparatus should be rinsed with sterile normal saline after each use and placed on a dry paper towel.

Source: Adapted from Vollman, K. M., & Sole, M. L. (2011). Endotracheal tube and oral care. In D. L. Wiegand (Ed.), *AACN procedure manual for critical care* (6th ed., pp. 33-37). St. Louis: Mosby.

should include toothbrushing twice a day along with use of moistened mouth swabs and oral or pharyngeal suctioning every 2 to 4 hours and as needed to provide comfort and to prevent injury to the gums and plaque accumulation (Table 68-9). Meticulous care is required to prevent skin breakdown on the face, lips, tongue, and nares as a result of pressure from the ET tube or bite block or from the method used to secure the ET tube to the patient's face. The ET tube should be repositioned and retaped every 24 hours and as needed. Repositioning and retaping of the ET tube may be shared practice between nursing and respiratory therapy or limited to respiratory therapy.

If the patient is nasally intubated, the nurse should remove the old tape or ties and clean the skin around the ET tube with saline-soaked gauze or cotton swabs. If the patient is orally intubated, the nurse should remove the bite block (if present) and the old tape or ties. Oral hygiene should be provided, and the ET tube should be repositioned to the opposite side of the mouth. The nurse replaces the bite block (if appropriate) and reconfirms proper cuff inflation and tube placement. The ET tube is resecured per institutional policy (see Figure 68-18). If a manufactured tube holder is used, the straps can be loosened, the area under the straps massaged, and the straps reapplied. If the patient is anxious or uncooperative, it is recommended that two nurses perform the repositioning procedure to prevent accidental dislodgement. The patient should be monitored for any signs of respiratory distress throughout the procedure.

Fostering Comfort and Communication

Patients have reported that intubation is a major stressor in the CCU (Lusk & Lash, 2005). The intubated patient may experience anxiety because of the inability to communicate and not knowing what to expect. Communicating with the intubated patient can be a frustrating experience for the patient, the family, and the nurse. To communicate more effectively, the nurse should employ a variety of methods (see Common Problems of Critical Care Patients earlier in this chapter) (Happ, Tuite, Dobbin, DiVirgilio-Thomas, & Kitutu, 2004).

The physical discomfort associated with ET intubation and mechanical ventilation often necessitates sedating the patient and administering an analgesic until the ET tube is no longer required. The patient may require morphine, lorazepam (Ativan), propofol, or other sedatives to blunt the anxiety and discomfort related to intubation. The nurse should evaluate the effectiveness of the drugs used to achieve an acceptable level of patient comfort. In addition, the nurse should consider initiating alternative therapies (e.g., music therapy, guided imagery) to complement drug therapy.

Complications of Endotracheal Intubation

Two major complications of ET intubation are unplanned (inadvertent) extubation and aspiration. Unplanned *extubation* (i.e., removal of the ET tube from the trachea) can be a catastrophic event and usually complicates the patient's recovery. Unplanned extubations can be caused by patient removal of the ET tube or accidental (i.e., result of movement or procedural-related) removal. Usually, the unplanned extubation is obvious (the patient is holding the ET tube). Other times, the tip of the ET tube is in the hypopharynx or the esophagus and the extubation is not so obvious.

SAFETY ALERT

Unplanned Extubation

• Observe for signs of unplanned extubation, which can be a life-threatening event:

  • Patient speaking

  • Activation of the low-pressure ventilator alarm

  • Diminished or absent breath sounds

  • Respiratory distress

  • Gastric distension

The nurse is responsible for preventing unplanned extubation by ensuring adequate securing of the ET tube and observation and support of the ET tube during repositioning, procedures, patient transfer, and so on. In addition, immobilizing the patient's hands through the use of soft wrist restraints and providing sedation and analgesia as ordered may be needed. The nurse should provide explanations to the patient and the family when restraints are used for patient safety. Reassessment for continued need of restraints is done per institution policy.

Should an unplanned extubation occur, the nurse should stay with the patient and call for help. Interventions are directed at maintaining the patient's airway, supporting ventilation (usually by manually ventilating the patient with 100% oxygen), securing the appropriate assistance to immediately re-intubate the patient (if necessary), and providing psychological support to the patient.

Aspiration is a potential hazard for the patient with an ET tube. The ET tube passes through the epiglottis, splinting it in an open position. Thus, the intubated patient cannot protect the airway from aspiration. The high-volume, low-pressure ET or tracheal cuff cannot totally prevent the trickle of oral or gastric secretions into the trachea. Furthermore, secretions accumulate above the cuff. When the cuff is deflated, those secretions can move into the lungs. Some ET tubes provide continuous suctioning of secretions above the cuff (Figure 68-20).

Oral intubation increases salivation, yet swallowing is difficult, so the mouth must be suctioned frequently. This may be performed with a Yankauer (tonsil-tip) suction catheter or a sterile single-use catheter. Other contributing factors to aspiration include improper cuff inflation, patient positioning, and tracheo-esophageal fistula. The patient with an ET tube is at risk for aspiration of gastric contents. Even when the cuff is properly inflated, the nurse must take precautions to prevent emesis, which can lead to aspiration. Frequently, an orogastric or nasogastric tube is inserted and connected to low, intermittent suction when a patient is intubated. Preference should be given to placement of an orogastric tube to reduce the risk of sinusitis. All intubated patients and patients receiving enteral feedings should have the head of the bed elevated a minimum of 30 to 45 degrees unless medically contraindicated (AACN, 2008).

Mechanical Ventilation

Mechanical ventilation is the process by which the FiO_2 is at 21% (room air) or greater and moved into and out of the lungs by a

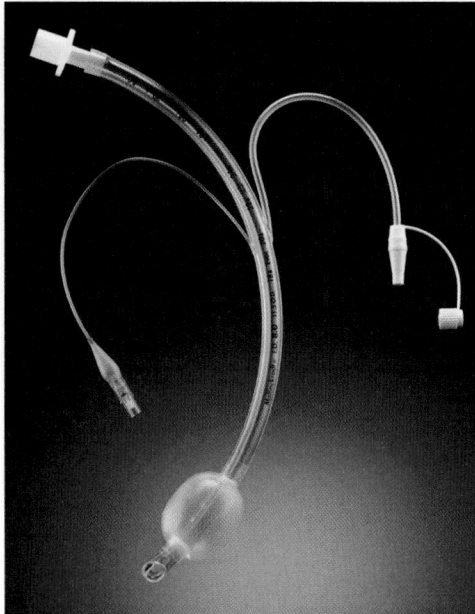

Figure 68-20 Continuous subglottal suctioning can be provided by the Hi Lo Evac Tube. A dorsal lumen above the cuff allows for suctioning of secretions from the subglottic area.

Source: Reprinted by permission of Nellcor Puritan Bennett, Inc., Pleasanton, California.

---

mechanical ventilator. Mechanical ventilation is not curative. It is used as a means of supporting patients until they recover the ability to breathe independently, as a bridge to long-term mechanical ventilation, or until a decision is made to withdraw ventilatory support. Indications for mechanical ventilation include (1) apnea or impending inability to breathe, (2) acute respiratory failure (generally defined as pH ≤7.25 with a $PaCO_2$ ≥50 mm Hg), (3) severe hypoxia, and (4) respiratory muscle fatigue (Burns, 2008; Pierce, 2007). Patients with chronic pulmonary disease and their families should be given the opportunity to decide the issue of mechanical ventilation before terminal respiratory disease develops. All patients, particularly those with grave or chronic illnesses, should also be encouraged to discuss the subject with their families and health care providers along with formalizing the results of that discussion in an advance directive. The decision to use, withhold, or withdraw mechanical ventilation must be made carefully, respecting the informed wishes of the patient and the family.

Types of Mechanical Ventilation

The two major types of mechanical ventilation are negative-pressure and positive-pressure ventilation (PPV).

Negative-Pressure Ventilation. **Negative-pressure ventilation** involves the use of chambers that encase the chest or body and surround it with intermittent subatmospheric or negative pressure. The "iron lung" was the first form of negative-pressure ventilation that developed during the polio epidemic. Intermittent negative pressure around the chest wall causes the chest to be pulled outward. This reduces intrathoracic pressure. Air rushes in via the upper airway, which is outside the sealed chamber.

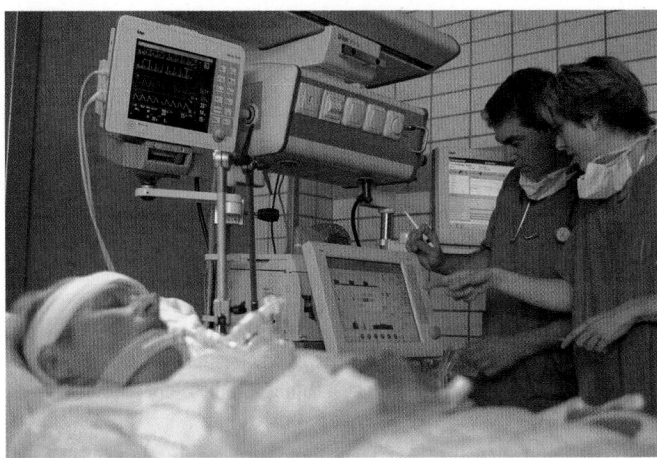

Figure 68-21 Patient receiving mechanical ventilation.

Source: Courtesy Draeger Medical.

Expiration is passive; the machine cycles off, allowing chest retraction. This type of ventilation is similar to normal ventilation in that decreased intrathoracic pressures produce inspiration and expiration is passive. Negative-pressure ventilation delivers non-invasive ventilation and does not require an artificial airway (see eFigure 68-1, available on the Evolve Web site for this chapter). Negative-pressure ventilators are not used extensively for acutely ill patients.

Positive-Pressure Ventilation. **Positive-pressure ventilation (PPV)** is the primary method used with acutely ill patients (Figure 68-21). During inspiration, the ventilator pushes air into the lungs under positive pressure. Unlike spontaneous ventilation, intrathoracic pressure is raised during lung inflation rather than lowered. Expiration occurs passively as in normal expiration. Modes of PPV are categorized into two groups: volume and pressure ventilation.

Volume Ventilation. With **volume ventilation**, a predetermined V_T is delivered with each inspiration, and the amount of pressure needed to deliver the breath varies based on the compliance and resistance factors of the patient–ventilator system. Consequently, the V_T is consistent from breath to breath, but airway pressures will vary.

Pressure Ventilation. With **pressure ventilation**, the peak inspiratory pressure is predetermined, and the V_T delivered to the patient varies based on the selected pressure and the compliance and resistance factors of the patient–ventilator system. With this understanding, careful attention must be given to the V_T to prevent unplanned hyperventilation or hypoventilation. For example, when the patient breathes out of synchrony with the ventilator, the pressure limit may be reached quickly, and the volume of gas delivered may be small. Initially, pressure ventilation was used only in patients in stable condition being weaned from the ventilator. Today, pressure ventilation is frequently selected to treat critically ill patients (Burns, 2008; Pierce, 2007).

Settings of Mechanical Ventilators

Mechanical ventilator settings regulate the rate, the depth, and other characteristics of ventilation (Table 68-10). Settings are

Table 68-10 Settings of Mechanical Ventilation

PARAMETER	DESCRIPTION
Respiratory rate (f)	Number of breaths the ventilator delivers per minute; usual setting is 6-20 breaths/min
Tidal volume (V_T)	Volume of gas delivered to patient during each ventilator breath; usual volume is 6-10 mL/kg
Oxygen concentration (FiO_2)	Fraction of inspired oxygen (FiO_2) delivered to patient; may be set between 21% (essentially room air) and 100%; usually adjusted to maintain PaO_2 level >60 mm Hg or SpO_2 level >90%
Positive end-expiratory pressure (PEEP)	Positive pressure applied at the end of expiration of ventilator breaths; usual setting is 5 cm H_2O
Pressure support	Positive pressure used to augment patient's inspiratory pressure; usual setting is 6-18 cm H_2O
I:E ratio	Duration of inspiration (I) to duration of expiration (E); usual setting is 1:2 to 1:1.5 unless IRV is desired
Inspiratory flow rate and time	Speed with which the V_T is delivered; usual setting is 40-80 L/min and time is 0.8-1.2 sec
Sensitivity	Determines the amount of effort the patient must generate to initiate a ventilator breath; it may be set for pressure triggering or flow triggering; usual setting for a pressure trigger is 0.5-1.5 cm H_2O below baseline pressure and for a flow trigger is 1-3 L/min below baseline flow
High pressure limit	Regulates the maximal pressure the ventilator can generate to deliver the V_T; when the pressure limit is reached, the ventilator terminates the breath and spills the undelivered volume into the atmosphere; usual setting is 10-20 cm H_2O above peak inspiratory pressure

IRV, inverse ratio ventilation.

Source: Urden, L. D., Stacy, K. M., & Lough, M. E. (2010). *Critical care nursing: Diagnosis and management* (6th ed., p. 655, Table 25-6). St. Louis: Mosby.

based on the patient's status (e.g., ABGs, body weight, level of consciousness, muscle strength). The ventilator is tuned as finely as possible to match the patient's ventilatory pattern. Settings are evaluated and adjusted frequently until the patient achieves optimal ventilation. Some settings serve as a fail-safe mechanism, alerting staff to problems with ventilation. It is important that the nurse ensure that all ventilator alarms are on at all times. Alarms alert the staff of potentially dangerous situations such as mechanical malfunction, apnea, or patient asynchrony with the ventilator. On many ventilators, the alarms can be temporarily suspended or silenced for up to 2 minutes for suctioning or testing. After that time, the alarm system automatically becomes functional again.

Modes of Volume Ventilation

The variable methods by which the patient and the ventilator interact to deliver effective ventilation are called modes. The selected ventilator mode is based on how much WOB the patient ought to or can perform and is determined by the patient's ventilatory status, respiratory drive, and ABGs. WOB refers to the inspiratory effort needed to overcome the elasticity and viscosity of the lungs along with the airway resistance. Generally, ventilator modes are controlled or assisted. With controlled ventilatory support, the ventilator does all of the WOB, and with assisted ventilatory support, the ventilator and the patient share the WOB. Historically, volume modes such as controlled mandatory ventilation (CMV), assist-control ventilation (ACV), and synchronized intermittent mandatory ventilation (SIMV) have been used to treat critically ill patients. More recently, pressure modes such as pressure-support ventilation (PSV) and pressure-controlled inverse ratio ventilation (PC-IRV) have become more widespread (Burns, 2008; Pierce, 2007). These modes are described in Table 68-11.

Controlled Mandatory Ventilation.

With *controlled mandatory ventilation* (CMV), breaths are delivered at a set rate per minute and at a set V_T, which are independent of the patient's ventilatory efforts. Although CMV is used infrequently, it is used when the patient has no drive to breathe (e.g., the anaesthetized patient) or is unable to breathe spontaneously (e.g., the paralyzed patient). In contrast, ACV can achieve similar results and not "lock out" the patient's inspiratory efforts. In the CMV mode, the patient performs no WOB and cannot adjust respirations to meet changing demands.

Assist-Control Mechanical Ventilation.

With *assist-control ventilation* (ACV), the ventilator delivers a preset V_T at a preset frequency, but when the patient initiates a spontaneous breath, the preset V_T is delivered. The ventilator senses a decrease in intrathoracic pressure and then delivers the preset V_T. The patient can breathe more quickly than the preset rate but not more slowly. This mode has the advantage of allowing the patient some control over ventilation while providing some assistance. ACV is used in patients with a variety of conditions, including neuromuscular disorders (e.g., Guillain-Barré syndrome), pulmonary edema, and acute respiratory failure. In the ACV mode, the patient has the potential for hypoventilation and hyperventilation. The spontaneously breathing patient can easily be overventilated, resulting in hyperventilation. If the volume or the minimum rate is set low and the patient is apneic or weak, the patient will be hypoventilated. Thus, these patients require vigilant assessment and monitoring of ventilatory status, including respiratory rate, ABGs, SpO_2, and SvO_2 or $ScvO_2$. It is also important that the sensitivity or amount of negative pressure required to initiate a breath is appropriate to the patient's condition. For example, if it is too difficult for the patient to initiate a breath, the WOB is increased and the patient may tire and/or develop ventilator asynchrony (i.e., the patient "fights" the ventilator).

Synchronized Intermittent Mandatory Ventilation.

With *synchronized intermittent mandatory ventilation* (SIMV), the ventilator delivers a preset V_T at a preset frequency in synchrony with the patient's spontaneous breathing. Between ventilator-delivered breaths, the patient is able to breathe spontaneously through the ventilator circuit. Thus the patient receives the preset FiO_2 concentration during the spontaneous breaths but self-regulates the rate and volume of those breaths. This mode of

Table 68-11 Modes of Mechanical Ventilation

Volume Modes

Control Ventilation (CV) or Controlled Mandatory Ventilation (CMV)

With this mode, the ventilator provides all of the patient's minute ventilation. The clinician sets rate, tidal volume (V_T), inspiratory time, and positive end-expiratory pressure (PEEP). Generally, this term is used to describe those situations in which the patient is chemically relaxed or is paralyzed from a spinal cord or neuromuscular disease and is therefore unable to initiate spontaneous breaths. The ventilator mode setting may be set on CMV, assist-control (AC), or synchronized intermittent mandatory ventilation (SIMV) because all these options provide volume breaths at the clinician-selected rate.

Assist-Control (AC) or Assisted Mandatory Ventilation (AMV)

This option requires that a rate, V_T, inspiratory time, and PEEP be set for the patient. The ventilator sensitivity is also set, and when the patient initiates a spontaneous breath, a full-volume breath is delivered.

Intermittent Mandatory Ventilation (IMV) and Synchronized Intermittent Mandatory Ventilation (SIMV)

This mode requires that rate, V_T, inspiratory time, sensitivity, and PEEP are set by the clinician. In between "mandatory breaths," patients can spontaneously breathe at their own rates and V_T. With SIMV, the ventilator synchronizes the mandatory breaths with the patient's own inspirations.

Pressure Modes

Pressure-Support Ventilation (PSV)

This mode provides an augmented inspiration to a spontaneously breathing patient. With PSV, the clinician selects an inspiratory pressure level, PEEP, and sensitivity. When the patient initiates a breath, a high flow of gas is delivered to the preselected pressure level, and pressure is maintained throughout inspiration. The patient determines the parameters of V_T, rate, and inspiratory time.

Pressure-Controlled Inverse Ratio Ventilation (PC-IRV)

This mode combines pressure-limited ventilation with an inverse ratio of inspiration to expiration. The clinician selects the pressure level, the rate, the inspiratory time (1:1, 2:1, 3:1, 4:1), and the PEEP level. With the prolonged inspiratory times, auto-PEEP may result. The auto-PEEP may be a desirable outcome of the inverse ratios. Some clinicians use PC without IRV. Conventional inspiratory times are used, and rate, pressure level, and PEEP are selected.

Positive End-Expiratory Pressure (PEEP) and Continuous Positive Airway Pressure (CPAP)

PEEP

This ventilatory option creates positive pressure at end-exhalation. PEEP restores functional residual capacity (FRC). The term *PEEP* is used when end-expiratory pressure is provided during ventilator positive-pressure breaths.

CPAP

Similar to PEEP, CPAP restores FRC. This pressure is continuous during spontaneous breathing; no positive-pressure breaths are present.

Source: Burns, S. M. (2011). Ventilatory management: Volume and pressure modes. In D. L. Wiegand (Ed.), *AACN procedure manual for critical care* (6th ed., p. 266, Table 35-2). St. Louis: Mosby.

ventilation differs from ACV, in which all breaths are of the same preset volume. It is used during continuous ventilation and during weaning from the ventilator. SIMV may also be combined with PSV (described later). Potential benefits of SIMV include improved patient–ventilator synchrony, lower mean airway pressure, and prevention of muscle atrophy as the patient takes on more of the WOB.

There are disadvantages with SIMV. If spontaneous breathing decreases when the preset rate is low, ventilation might not be adequately supported. Low-rate SIMV should be used only in patients with regular, spontaneous breathing. Weaning with SIMV demands close monitoring and may take longer because the rate of breathing is gradually reduced. Patients being weaned with SIMV may also have increased muscle fatigue associated with spontaneous breathing efforts.

Modes of Pressure Ventilation

Pressure-Support Ventilation. With *pressure-support ventilation* (PSV), positive pressure is applied to the airway only during inspiration and is used in conjunction with the patient's spontaneous respirations. The patient must be able to initiate a breath in this modality. A preset level of positive airway pressure is selected so that the gas flow rate is greater than the patient's inspiratory flow rate. As the patient initiates a breath, the machine senses the spontaneous effort and supplies a rapid flow of gas at the initiation of the breath and variable flow throughout the breath. With PSV, the patient determines inspiratory length, V_T, and respiratory rate. V_T depends on the pressure level and airway compliance. PSV is used with continuous ventilation and during weaning. PSV may also be used with SIMV during weaning. PSV is not used as a sole ventilatory support during acute respiratory failure because of the risk of hypoventilation. Advantages to PSV include increased patient comfort, decreased WOB (because inspiratory efforts are augmented), decreased oxygen consumption (because inspiratory work is reduced), and increased endurance conditioning (because the patient is exercising respiratory muscles).

Pressure-Controlled Inverse Ratio Ventilation. *Pressure-controlled inverse ratio ventilation* (PC-IRV) combines pressure-limited ventilation with an inverse ratio of inspiration (I) to expiration (E). Some clinicians use PC without IRV. The I/E ratio is the ratio of duration of inspiration (I) to the duration of expiration (E). This value is normally a ratio of 1:2. With IRV, a prolonged positive pressure is applied, increasing inspiratory time; the I/E ratio begins at 1:1 and may progress to 4:1. IRV progressively expands collapsed alveoli. The short expiratory time has a PEEP-like effect, preventing alveolar collapse. Because IRV imposes a nonphysiological breathing pattern, the patient requires sedation with or without paralysis. PC-IRV is indicated for patients with acute respiratory distress syndrome (ARDS) who continue to have refractory hypoxemia despite high levels of PEEP. Not all patients with poor oxygenation respond to PC-IRV.

Airway Pressure-Release Ventilation. *Airway pressure-release ventilation* permits spontaneous breathing at any point during the respiratory cycle with a preset continuous positive airway pressure (CPAP) with short timed pressure releases. The CPAP level (pressure high, pressure low) is adjusted to maintain oxygenation goals while the timed releases (time high, time low) are increased or decreased to meet ventilation goals. V_T is not a set variable and is dependent on the CPAP level, the patient's

compliance and resistance, and spontaneous breathing effort. The mode is designed for patients with ARDS who require high pressure levels for alveolar recruitment. One advantage of this mode is the ability to permit spontaneous respirations. This may reduce the need for deep sedation or paralytics.

Other Modes. Increases in ventilator technology have led to the development of additional pressure modes. However, owing to the nonstandardization of these options, the names and features are manufacturer specific. The superiority of these modes has not been established. Some examples include volume-assured pressure ventilation and adaptive support ventilation.

Other Ventilatory Manoeuvres

Positive End-Expiratory Pressure. *Positive end-expiratory pressure* (PEEP) is a ventilatory manoeuvre in which positive pressure is applied to the airway during exhalation. Normally during exhalation, airway pressure drops to zero, and exhalation occurs passively. With PEEP, exhalation remains passive, but pressure falls to a preset level greater than zero, often 3 to 20 cm H_2O. With PEEP, lung volume during expiration and between breaths is greater than normal. Thus, PEEP increases functional residual capacity (FRC), and this often improves oxygenation with restoration of lung volume that normally remains at the end of passive exhalation. The mechanisms by which PEEP increases FRC and oxygenation include increased aeration of patent alveoli, aeration of previously collapsed alveoli, and prevention of alveolar collapse throughout the respiratory cycle. PEEP is titrated to the point that oxygenation improves without compromising hemodynamics. This is termed *best or optimal PEEP*. Often, 5 cm H_2O PEEP (referred to as *physiological PEEP*) is used prophylactically to replace the glottic mechanism, help maintain a normal FRC, and prevent alveolar collapse. PEEP of 5 cm H_2O is also used for patients with a history of alveolar collapse during weaning. PEEP has demonstrated improvements in gas exchange, vital capacity, and inspiratory force when used during weaning.

In contrast, auto-PEEP is not purposely set on the ventilator but is a result of inadequate exhalation time. Auto-PEEP is additional PEEP over what is set by the clinician and can be measured at the end-expiratory hold button located on most ventilators. This additional PEEP may result in increased WOB, barotrauma, and hemodynamic instability. However, during some ventilator modes (PC-IRV), auto-PEEP may be desirable. Interventions to limit auto-PEEP include sedation and analgesia, large-diameter ET tube, bronchodilators, short inspiratory times, decreased respiratory rates, and reducing water accumulation in the ventilator circuit by frequent emptying or use of heated circuits. In patients with short exhalation times and early airway closure (e.g., COPD, asthma), setting PEEP can offset auto-PEEP by splinting the airway open during exhalation and preventing "air trapping." In general, the major purpose of PEEP is to maintain or improve oxygenation while limiting risk of oxygen toxicity. FiO_2 can often be reduced when PEEP is used. PEEP is thought to be useful in pulmonary edema, providing a counterpressure opposing fluid extravasation. PEEP is indicated in lungs with diffuse disease, severe hypoxemia unresponsive to FiO_2 greater than 50%, and loss of compliance or stiffness. The classic indication for PEEP therapy is ARDS (see Chapter 70). PEEP is generally contraindicated or used with extreme caution in patients with highly compliant lungs (e.g., COPD), unilateral or nonuniform disease, hypovolemia, and low CO. In these situations, the adverse effects of PEEP may outweigh any benefits.

Continuous Positive Airway Pressure. **Continuous positive airway pressure (CPAP)** restores FRC and is similar to PEEP. However, the pressure in CPAP is delivered continuously during spontaneous breathing, thus preventing the patient's airway pressure from falling to zero. For example, if CPAP is 5 cm H_2O, airway pressure during expiration is 5 cm H_2O. During inspiration, 1 to 2 cm H_2O of negative pressure is generated, thus reducing airway pressure to 3 or 4 cm H_2O. The patient receiving SIMV with PEEP receives CPAP when breathing spontaneously. CPAP is commonly used in the treatment of obstructive sleep apnea. CPAP can be administered noninvasively by a tight-fitting mask or with an ET or a tracheal tube. CPAP increases WOB because the patient must forcibly exhale against the CPAP and so must be used with caution in patients with myocardial compromise.

Bilevel Positive Airway Pressure. *Bilevel positive airway pressure* provides two levels of positive-pressure support, higher inspiratory positive airway pressure and lower expiratory positive airway pressure, along with oxygen. It is a noninvasive modality and is delivered through a tight-fitting face mask, nasal mask, or nasal pillows. Similarly to PSV that is delivered through an artificial airway, the patient must be able to spontaneously breathe and cooperate with this treatment. Indications include acute respiratory failure in patients with COPD and heart failure, and sleep apnea. Bilateral positive airway pressure may also be used after extubation to avert the need for re-intubation. Patients with shock, altered mental status, or increased airway secretions are not candidates for bilateral positive airway pressure (Burns, 2008).

High-Frequency Ventilation. High-frequency ventilation involves delivery of a small V_T (usually 1-5 mL/kg of body weight) at rapid respiratory rates (100 to 300 breaths/min) in an effort to recruit and maintain lung volume and reduce intrapulmonary shunting. One benefit of high-frequency ventilation may be the ability to support gas exchange while minimizing the risk of volutrauma. High-frequency ventilation has been widely accepted in neonatal and pediatric CCUs. Its use in adults is still considered investigational and limited to patients with ARDS (Rose, 2008). Patients receiving high-frequency ventilation must be paralyzed to suppress spontaneous respiration. In addition, patients must receive concurrent sedation and analgesia as necessary adjuncts when inducing paralysis (see Chapter 70).

Nitric Oxide. Nitric oxide is a gaseous molecule that is made intravascularly and participates in the regulation of pulmonary vascular tone. Inhibition of nitric oxide production results in pulmonary vasoconstriction, and administration of continuous inhaled nitric oxide results in pulmonary vasodilation. Administration of nitric oxide may be given through an ET tube or a tracheostomy or via a face mask. Currently, nitric oxide is used in ARDS, as a diagnostic screening tool for pulmonary hypertension during a cardiac catheterization, and during or after cardiac surgery.

Prone Positioning. Prone positioning is the repositioning of a patient from a supine or lateral position to a prone (on the stomach with face down) position. This repositioning improves lung recruitment through various mechanisms. Gravity reverses the effects of fluid in the dependent parts of the lungs as the patient is moved from supine to prone. In this position, the heart rests on the sternum, away from the lungs, contributing to an overall uniformity of pleural pressures. The prone position is a relatively safe (although nurse-intensive) supportive therapy used in critically ill patients with acute lung injury or ARDS to improve oxygenation (Abroug, Ouanes-Besben, Elatrous, & Brouchard, 2008).

Extracorporeal Membrane Oxygenation. Extracorporeal membrane oxygenation is an alternative form of pulmonary support for the patient with severe respiratory failure. It is used more frequently in the pediatric and neonatal populations but is increasingly being used in adults. ECMO is a modification of cardiac bypass and involves partially removing blood from a patient with large-bore catheters, infusing O_2, removing CO_2, and returning the blood back to the patient. This intensive therapy requires systemic anticoagulation and is a time-limited intervention. A skilled team of specialists including a perfusionist is required continuously at the bedside.

Complications of Positive-Pressure Ventilation

Although mechanical ventilation may be essential to maintain ventilation and oxygenation, it can cause adverse effects. It is often difficult to distinguish complications of mechanical ventilation from the underlying disease.

Cardiovascular System. PPV can affect circulation because of the transmission of increased mean airway pressure to the thoracic cavity. With increased intrathoracic pressure, thoracic vessels are compressed. This results in decreased venous return to the heart, decreased left ventricular end-diastolic volume (preload), decreased CO, and hypotension. Mean airway pressure is further increased if PEEP is titrated (>5 cm H_2O) to improve oxygenation.

If the lungs are noncompliant (as in ARDS), airway pressures are not as easily transmitted to the heart and the blood vessels. Thus, the effects of PPV on CO are reduced. Conversely, with compliant lungs (e.g., emphysema), there is increased danger of transmission of high airway pressures and negative effects on hemodynamics.

Compromise of venous return by PPV is exaggerated by hypovolemia (e.g., hemorrhage, multiple trauma) and decreased venous tone (e.g., sepsis, spinal shock). Restoration and maintenance of the circulating blood volume are important in minimizing cardiovascular complications.

Pulmonary System
Barotrauma. As lung inflation pressures increase, risk of barotraumas increases. Patients with compliant lungs (e.g., COPD) are at greater risk for barotrauma because the increased airway pressure readily distends the lungs and may rupture alveoli or emphysematous blebs. Patients with stiff lungs (e.g., ARDS) who are given high inspiratory pressures and high levels of PEEP (>5 cm H_2O) and patients with suppurative lung abscesses resulting from necrotizing organisms (e.g., staphylococci) are also susceptible to barotrauma.

Air can escape into the pleural space from alveoli or interstitium, accumulate, and become trapped. Pleural pressure increases and collapses the lung, causing pneumothorax. (Clinical manifestations of pneumothorax are discussed in Chapter 30.) The lung receives air during inspiration but cannot expel it during expiration. Respiratory bronchioles are larger on inspiration than expiration. They may close on expiration, and air becomes trapped. With PPV, a simple pneumothorax can become a life-threatening tension pneumothorax. With tension pneumothorax, the mediastinum and contralateral lung are compressed, compromising CO. Immediate treatment of the pneumothorax is required. For some patients, chest tubes may be placed prophylactically.

Pneumomediastinum usually begins with rupture of alveoli into the lung interstitium; progressive air movement then occurs into the mediastinum and subcutaneous neck tissue. This is commonly followed by pneumothorax. Occurrence of new, unexplained subcutaneous emphysema is an indication for immediate chest radiographic examination. Pneumomediastinum and subcutaneous emphysema in the neck may be too small to be detected radiographically or clinically before the development of a pneumothorax.

Volutrauma. The concept of volutrauma in PPV relates to the lung injury that occurs when large V_Ts are used to ventilate noncompliant lungs (e.g., ARDS). Volutrauma results in alveolar fractures and movement of fluids and proteins into the alveolar spaces. The ARDS Network Study demonstrated a change in mortality rate of patients with ARDS by using smaller V_T of 6 mL/kg. The use of low-volume ventilation rather than pressure ventilation is the suggested strategy for lung protection in ARDS patients.

Alveolar Hypoventilation. Hypoventilation can be caused by inappropriate ventilator settings, leakage of air from the ventilator tubing or around the ET tube or tracheostomy cuff, lung secretions or obstruction, and low ventilation–perfusion ratio. Low V_T or respiratory rate decreases minute ventilation, causing hypoventilation. A leaking cuff or tubing that is not secured may cause air leakage, lowering the delivered V_T. Too low an SIMV rate in a patient who is unable to produce adequate spontaneous respirations causes hypoventilation, respiratory acidosis, and additional problems related to acidosis such as cardiac dysrhythmias. Excess lung secretions can cause hypoventilation. Turning the patient every 1 to 2 hours, providing chest physical therapy to lung areas with increased secretions, encouraging deep-breathing and coughing, and suctioning as needed may alleviate this. Atelectasis may develop. Increasing the V_T, adding small increments of PEEP, and adding a preset number of sighs to the ventilator settings lessen the likelihood of atelectasis.

Alveolar Hyperventilation. Respiratory alkalosis can occur if the respiratory rate or the V_T is set too high (mechanical overventilation) or if the patient receiving assisted ventilation is hyperventilating. It is easy to overventilate a patient on PPV. Particularly at risk are patients with chronic alveolar hypoventilation and CO_2 retention (e.g., patients with COPD). The patient with COPD may have a chronic $PaCO_2$ elevation (acidosis) and compensatory bicarbonate retention by the kidneys. When the patient is ventilated, the patient's "normal baseline" rather than the standard normal values should be the therapeutic goal. If the COPD patient is returned to a standard normal $PaCO_2$, the patient will develop alkalosis because of the retained bicarbonate. Such a patient could move from compensated respiratory acidosis to serious metabolic alkalosis. The presence of alkalosis makes weaning from the ventilator difficult. Alkalosis, especially if the onset is abrupt, can have additional serious consequences, including hypokalemia, hypocalcemia, and dysrhythmias. Neuromuscular irritability, seizures, coma, and death can occur. Usually, the patient with COPD who is supported on

the ventilator does better with a short inspiratory and longer expiratory time.

If hyperventilation is spontaneous, it is important to determine the cause and treat it. Causes might include hypoxemia, pain, fear, anxiety, or compensation for metabolic acidosis. Patients who fight the ventilator or breathe out of synchrony may be anxious or in pain. If the patient is anxious and fearful, sitting with the patient and verbally coaching the patient to breathe with the ventilator may help. If these measures fail, manually ventilating the patient slowly with a 100% oxygen source may slow breathing enough to bring it in synchrony with the ventilator.

Ventilator-Associated Pneumonia. The risk for hospital-acquired pneumonia is highest in patients requiring mechanical ventilation because the ET or tracheostomy tube bypasses normal upper airway defences. In addition, poor nutritional state, immobility, and the underlying disease process (e.g., immunosuppression, organ failure) make the patient more prone to infection. Ventilator-associated pneumonia (VAP) is defined as a pneumonia that occurs 48 hours or more after ET intubation (American Thoracic Society, Infectious Diseases Society of America, 2005; Safer Health Care Now, 2012). VAP occurs in 9 to 27% of all intubated patients, with 50% of the occurrences developing within the first 4 days of mechanical ventilation. In addition, patients who develop VAP have significantly longer hospital stays and higher mortality rates than those who do not develop VAP.

In patients with early VAP (within 96 hours of mechanical ventilation), sputum cultures often grow Gram-negative bacteria such as *Escherichia coli*, *Klebsiella*, *Proteus*, *Streptococcus pneumoniae*, *Haemophilus influenzae*, and oxacillin-sensitive *Staphylococcus aureus*. Organisms associated with late VAP include antibiotic-resistant organisms such as *Pseudomonas aeruginosa* and oxacillin-resistant *S. aureus*. These organisms can be abundant in the hospital environment and the patient's GI tract. Organisms can spread in a number of ways, including contaminated respiratory equipment, inadequate handwashing, adverse environmental factors such as poor room ventilation and high traffic flow, and decreased patient ability to cough and clear secretions. Colonization of the oropharynx tract by Gram-negative organisms is a predisposing factor in the development of Gram-negative pneumonia.

Clinical evidence suggesting VAP includes fever, elevated white blood cell count, purulent sputum, odorous sputum, crackles or rhonchi on auscultation, and pulmonary infiltrates noted on chest radiograph. The patient is treated with antibiotics after appropriate cultures are taken by tracheal suctioning or bronchoscopy and when infection is evident.

Guidelines on VAP prevention include (1) head of bed elevation at a minimum of 30 to 45 degrees unless medically contraindicated, (2) no routine changes of the patient's ventilator circuit tubing, and (3) the use of an ET tube with a dorsal lumen above the cuff to allow continuous suctioning of secretions in the subglottic area (see Figure 68-20). Prevention also includes effective and frequent handwashing before and after suctioning, whenever ventilator equipment is touched, and after contact with any respiratory secretions (see Nursing Management: Artificial Airway earlier in this chapter). The nurse should wear gloves when in contact with the patient and change gloves between activities (e.g., bathing the patient, administering an IV drug).

Sodium and Water Imbalance. Progressive fluid retention often occurs after 48 to 72 hours of PPV, especially PPV with PEEP. It is associated with decreased urinary output and increased sodium retention. Fluid balance changes may be caused by decreased CO, which in turn results in diminished renal perfusion. Consequently, renin release is stimulated with subsequent production of angiotensin and aldosterone (see Chapter 47, Figure 47-6). This results in sodium and water retention. It is also possible that pressure changes within the thorax are associated with decreased release of atrial natriuretic peptide, which also causes sodium retention. Mild water retention is also associated with PPV. There is less insensible water loss via the airway because ventilated delivered gases are humidified with body-temperature water. In addition, as a part of the stress response, release of antidiuretic hormone and cortisol may be increased, contributing to sodium and water retention.

Neurological System.

In patients with head injury, PPV, especially with PEEP, can impair cerebral blood flow. This is related to increased intrathoracic positive pressure impeding venous drainage from the head as evidenced by jugular venous distension. As a result of the impaired venous return and increase in cerebral volume, the patient may exhibit increases in intracranial pressure. Elevating the head of the bed and keeping the patient's head in alignment may decrease the deleterious effects of PPV on intracranial pressure.

Gastrointestinal System.

Patients receiving PPV are often stressed because of serious illness, immobility, and discomforts associated with the ventilator. Thus, the ventilated patient is at risk for developing stress ulcers and GI bleeding. Patients with a pre-existing ulcer or those receiving corticosteroid therapy are at an especially increased risk. Any kind of circulatory compromise, including reduction of CO caused by PPV, may contribute to ischemia of the gastric and intestinal mucosa and possibly increase the risk of translocation of GI bacteria (Metheny, Schallom, & Edwards, 2004).

Peptic ulcer prophylaxis includes the administration of histamine H_2-receptor blockers (e.g., ranitidine [Zantac]), proton pump inhibitors (e.g., omeprazole [Prilosec]), and tube feedings to decrease gastric acidity and diminish the risk of stress ulcer and hemorrhage. Although the research regarding the use of H_2-receptor blockers or proton pump inhibitors is conflicting, guidelines support the use of routine peptic ulcer prophylaxis in patients who are mechanically ventilated to decrease the risk of VAP.

Gastric and bowel dilation may occur as a result of gas accumulation in the GI tract from swallowed air. The irritation of an artificial airway may cause excessive air swallowing and subsequent gastric dilation. Gastric or bowel dilation may put pressure on the vena cava, decrease CO, and prohibit adequate diaphragmatic excursion during spontaneous breathing. Elevation of the diaphragm as a result of paralytic ileus or bowel dilation leads to compression of the lower lobes of the lungs, which may cause atelectasis and compromise respiratory function. Decompression of the stomach can be accomplished by the insertion of a nasogastric or an orogastric tube.

Immobility, sedation, circulatory impairment, decreased oral intake, use of opioid pain medications, and stress contribute to decreased peristalsis. The patient's inability to exhale against a closed glottis may make defecation difficult. As a result, the ventilated patient could be predisposed to constipation.

Musculoskeletal System.

Maintenance of muscle strength and prevention of the problems associated with immobility are important. Exercise tolerance is enhanced by adequate analgesia

and adequate nutrition. Progressive ambulation of patients receiving long-term PPV can be attained without interruption of mechanical ventilation. The ventilator can be pushed around the room, or the patient can be manually ventilated with a BVM while ambulating. Passive and active exercises, consisting of movements to maintain muscle tone in the upper and lower extremities, should be done in bed. Simple manoeuvres such as leg lifts, knee bends, quadriceps setting, or arm circles are appropriate. Prevention of contractures, pressure ulcers, footdrop, and external rotation of the hip and legs by proper positioning is important.

Psychosocial Needs.

The patient receiving mechanical ventilation may experience physical and emotional stress. In addition to the problems related to critical care patients discussed at the beginning of this chapter, the patient supported by a mechanical ventilator is unable to speak, eat, move, or breathe normally. Tubes and machines may cause pain, fear, and anxiety. Ordinary activities of daily living such as eating, elimination, and coughing are extremely complicated.

In studying the psychosocial needs of CCU patients, one researcher (Hupcey, 2000) discovered that feeling safe was an overpowering need of CCU patients. Four related needs that were identified were the need to know (information), the need to regain control, the need to hope, and the need to trust. Patients reported that when these needs were met, they felt safe. The nurse should work to strengthen the various factors that affect feeling safe. Communication must be creative in the case of the intubated patient, and information must be given in a forthright manner. Patients should be involved in decision making as much as possible.

Patients receiving PPV usually require some type of sedation (e.g., propofol) or analgesia (e.g., fentanyl), or both to facilitate optimal ventilation. Before initiating sedation or analgesia in the mechanically ventilated patient who is agitated or anxious, it is important to assess for the cause of distress. Common problems that can result in patient agitation or anxiety include PPV, nutritional deficits, pain, hypoxemia, hypercapnia, drugs, and environmental stressors (e.g., sleep deprivation). It is important to note that delirium is an acute change in mental status and is a marker of cerebral insufficiency with associated longer hospital stays and a higher mortality rate. CCU patients are particularly vulnerable to delirium, and every effort should be made to assess and treat it (Ely et al., 2004).

At times, the decision is made to paralyze the patient with a neuromuscular blocking agent (e.g., pancuronium) to provide more effective synchrony with the ventilator and increased oxygenation. If the patient is paralyzed, the nurse should remember that the patient can hear, see, think, and feel. IV sedation and analgesia must always be administered concurrently when the patient is paralyzed. Assessment of the patient should include train-of-four peripheral nerve stimulation, physiological signs of pain or anxiety (changes in heart rate and BP), and ventilator synchrony. The train-of-four assessment involves the use of a peripheral nerve stimulator to deliver four successive stimulating currents to elicit muscle twitches (Figure 68-22). The number of twitches will vary with the percentage of neuromuscular blockade; the usual goal is one or two twitches out of four. Excessive administration of neuromuscular blocking agents may predispose the patient to prolonged paralysis and muscle weakness even after these agents are discontinued. Many patients have few memories of their time in the CCU, whereas others remember vivid details. Although appearing to

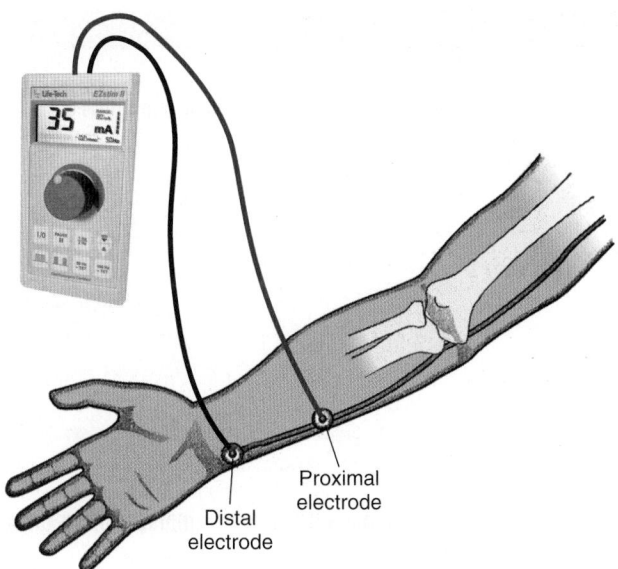

Figure 68-22 Placement of electrodes along the ulnar nerve.

Source: Wiegand, D. L. (2011). *AACN procedure manual for critical care* (6th ed., p. 310, Figure 38-1). Philadelphia: Saunders.

be asleep, sedated, or paralyzed, patients may be aware of their surroundings and should always be addressed as if they are awake and alert.

Nutritional Therapy: Patient Receiving Positive-Pressure Ventilation

PPV and the hypermetabolism associated with critical illness can contribute to inadequate nutrition. Presence of an ET tube eliminates the normal route for eating. A patient with a tracheostomy may be able to eat normally once the stoma has healed and swallowing has been assessed via a speech therapy consultation. When eating with a tracheostomy tube in place, the patient should tilt the head slightly forward to facilitate swallowing and to prevent aspiration. Diet may be restricted to soft foods (e.g., puddings, ice cream) and thickened liquids.

For patients likely to be without food for 3 to 5 days, a nutritional program should be initiated. Inadequate nutrition makes the patient receiving prolonged mechanical ventilation more prone to poor oxygen transport secondary to anemia and to poor tolerance of minimal exercise. Poor nutrition and the disuse of respiratory muscles contribute to decreased respiratory muscle strength. In addition, the hypermetabolism associated with critical illness, trauma, and surgery and the presence of anxiety, pain, and increased WOB greatly increase caloric expenditure. Serum protein levels (e.g., albumin, prealbumin, transferrin, total protein) are usually decreased. Inadequate nutrition can delay weaning, decrease resistance to infection, and decrease the speed of recovery. Enteral feeding via a small-bore feeding tube is the preferred method to meet caloric needs of ventilated patients (see Chapter 42 for discussion of enteral feeding). There is no evidence to support gastric feedings over small bowel feedings in ventilated patients (Metheny et al., 2004).

Verification of feeding tube placement includes (1) radiological confirmation before initial use, (2) marking and ongoing assessment of the tube's exit site, and (3) ongoing review of routine radiographs and aspirate (AACN, 2006). The auscultatory method of assessment (i.e., listening for air after injection) is not a reliable method for verifying placement of feeding tubes. A concern regarding the nutritional support of patients receiving PPV is the carbohydrate content of the diet. Metabolism of carbohydrates may contribute to an increase in serum CO_2 levels. The resulting CO_2 load results in a higher minute ventilation requirement. This, in turn, can cause an increase in WOB. Limiting carbohydrate content in the diet may lower CO_2 production. The dietitian should be consulted to determine the caloric and nutrient needs of these patients.

Weaning From Positive-Pressure Ventilation and Extubation

The process of reducing ventilator support and resuming spontaneous ventilation is termed *weaning*. The weaning process differs for patients requiring short-term ventilation (≤3 days) as opposed to long-term ventilation (>3 days). Patients requiring short-term ventilation (e.g., after cardiac surgery) will experience a linear weaning process. Patients likely to require prolonged PPV (e.g., patients with COPD who develop respiratory failure) will most likely experience a weaning process that consists of peaks and valleys. In principle, preparation for weaning should begin when PPV is initiated and should involve a team approach (e.g., nurse, physician, patient, family, respiratory therapist, dietitian, physical therapist).

Weaning can be viewed as consisting of three phases. The preweaning or assessment phase determines the patient's ability to breathe spontaneously. Assessment in this phase depends on a combination of respiratory (Table 68-12) and nonrespiratory factors. Weaning assessment parameters should include criteria to assess muscle strength (negative inspiratory force) and endurance (spontaneous V_T, vital capacity, minute ventilation, and rapid shallow breathing index [RSBI]). In addition, the patient's lungs should be reasonably clear on auscultation and chest radiograph. Nonrespiratory factors include the assessment of the patient's neurological status, hemodynamics, fluid and electrolytes and acid–base balance, nutrition, and hemoglobin. It is important to have an alert, well-rested, and well-informed patient relatively free from pain and anxiety who can cooperate with the weaning plan. Evidence-informed clinical guidelines recommend a spontaneous breathing trial (SBT) in patients who demonstrate weaning readiness. Tolerance of the trial may lead to extubation. Failure to tolerate an SBT should prompt a search for reversible or complicating factors and a return to a nonfatiguing ventilator modality for the patient. The SBT should be reattempted the next day.

In addition, the use of a standard approach for weaning or weaning protocols has been shown to decrease ventilator days. The components of the protocol are not as important as the use of a protocol to prevent delays in weaning. All methods can be delivered with the patient remaining connected to the ventilator circuit. The patient receiving SIMV can have the ventilator breaths gradually reduced as the patient's ventilatory status permits. CPAP or PSV can be added to SIMV. Another method involves PSV, CPAP, or both delivered without SIMV. PSV is thought to provide gentle, slow respiratory muscle conditioning and may be especially beneficial for patients who are deconditioned or have cardiac problems. Some patients may be weaned by simply providing humidified oxygen (*T*-piece or flow-by method).

Weaning is usually carried out during the day, with the patient ventilated at night in a rest mode. The rest mode should be a stable, nonfatiguing, and comfortable form of support for the

Table 68-12 Indicators for Weaning

Weaning Readiness

Patients receiving mechanical ventilation for respiratory failure should undergo a formal assessment of weaning potential if the following are satisfied:*

1. Reversal of the underlying cause of respiratory failure

2. Adequate oxygenation:
   - PaO_2 >80-100
   - PEEP ≤5-8 cm H_2O
   - FiO_2 ≤40-50%
   - pH ≥7.25

3. Hemodynamic stability:
   - Absence of myocardial ischemia
   - Absence of clinically significant hypotension (no vasopressor therapy or low dose)

4. Patient ability to initiate an inspiratory effort

Weaning Assessment

MEASUREMENT	SIGNIFICANCE	NORMAL VALUES	INDICES FOR WEANING
Spontaneous respiratory rate (f)	Respiratory rate and frequency >1 min	12-20 min	<38 min
Spontaneous tidal volume (V_T)	Amount of air exchanged during normal breathing at rest; measure of muscle endurance	7-9 mL/kg	≥5 mL/kg
Minute ventilation (V_E)	Tidal volume multiplied by respiratory rate over 1 min For example: 0.350 (V_T) × 28 (f) = 8.8 L/min	5-10 L/min	≤10 L/min
Negative inspiratory force (NIF) or pressure (NIP)	Amount of negative pressure that a patient is able to generate to initiate spontaneous respirations. Measured by clinician: After complete occlusion of inspiratory valve, a pressure manometer is attached to airway or mouth for 10-20 sec while negative inspiratory efforts are noted.	−75 to −100 cm H_2O	>−20 cm H_2O The more negative the number, the better indication for weaning.
Positive expiratory pressure (PEP)	Measure of expiratory muscle strength and ability to cough. Measured by clinician: After complete occlusion of expiratory valve, a pressure manometer is attached to the airway or mouth for 10-20 sec while positive expiratory efforts are noted.	60-85 cm H_2O	≥30 cm H_2O
Compliance, rate, oxygenation, and pressure (CROP) index	Combined index that is complex to calculate. C_{Dyn} = Compliance C_{Dyn} × NIF × (PaO_2/PAO_2)/f PaO_2/PAO_2 = Oxygenation ratio of arterial O_2/alveolar O_2	Not applicable	>13
Rapid shallow breathing index (f/V_T)	Spontaneous respiratory rate over 1 min divided by tidal volume (in L). Easier calculation and more widely used. For example: 30(f)/0.400(V_T) = 75/L	60-105/L	<105/L
Vital capacity (VC)	Maximum inspiration and then measurement of air during maximal forced expiration; measure of respiratory muscle endurance or reserve or both; requires patient cooperation.	65-75 mL/kg	≥10-15 mL/kg

*The decision to use these criteria must be individualized to the patient.

Sources: Adapted from MacIntyre, N. R., Cook, D. J., Ely E. W., Jr., Epstein, S. K., Fink, J. B., Heffner, J. E., . . ., American College of Critical Care Medicine. (2001). Evidence-based guidelines for weaning and discontinuing ventilatory support. *Chest, 120* (6 Suppl), 375S-395S; and Burns, S. M. (2011). Weaning process. In D. L. Wiegand (Ed.), *AACN procedure manual for critical care* (6th ed., pp. 291-300). St. Louis: Mosby.

patient. Regardless of the weaning mode selected, all team members should be familiar with the weaning plan. Furthermore, regardless of the method used, it is important to permit the patient's respiratory muscles to rest between weaning trials. Once the respiratory muscles become fatigued, they may require 12 to 24 hours to recover.

The patient being weaned and the family should be provided ongoing psychological support. The weaning process should be explained, and the patient and family informed of progress. The patient should be placed in a sitting or semirecumbent position and made comfortable. Baseline vital signs and respiratory parameters are measured. During the weaning trial, the patient must be monitored closely and noninvasively for criteria that may signal intolerance and result in cessation of the trial (e.g., tachypnea, dyspnea, tachycardia, dysrhythmias, sustained desaturation [SpO_2 <91%], hypertension or hypotension, agitation, diaphoresis, anxiety, sustained V_T <5 mL/kg, changes in level of consciousness). Documentation of the patient's tolerance throughout the weaning process is important and should include statements regarding the patient's and the family's perceptions.

The weaning outcome phase refers to the period when weaning stops and the patient is extubated or weaning is stopped because no further progress is being made. The patient who is ready for extubation should receive hyperoxygenation and suctioning (e.g., oropharynx, ET tube). The patient should be instructed to take a deep breath, and at the peak of inspiration, the cuff should be deflated and the tube removed in one motion. After removal, the patient should be encouraged to deep breathe and cough, and the pharynx should be suctioned as needed. Supplemental oxygen should be applied and naso-oral care provided. The nurse must carefully monitor the patient's vital signs, respiratory status, and oxygenation immediately following extubation, within 1 hour, and per institutional policy. If the patient cannot tolerate extubation, immediate re-intubation may be necessary.

Chronic Mechanical Ventilation

Mechanical ventilators are no longer limited to the CCU but are now a part of long-term and home care. In some instances, terminally ill, ventilated patients may be discharged to hospice. The emphasis on controlling hospital health care costs has increased the early discharge of patients and the need to provide highly technical care such as mechanical ventilation in home settings (Ecklund, 2006). The success of home mechanical ventilation will depend, in part, on careful predischarge assessment and planning for both the patient and the caregivers.

Both negative-pressure and positive-pressure ventilators can be used in the home. Negative-pressure ventilators do not require an artificial airway and may be less complicated to use. Several types of small, portable (battery-powered) positive-pressure ventilators are available and can be attached to a wheelchair or placed on a bedside table. Settings and alarms on these ventilators are simpler to use than the standard CCU ventilators.

Home mechanical ventilation has advantages and disadvantages. Having the patient in the home eliminates the strain that the hospital setting may impose on family dynamics. The feeling of helplessness by family members when they first hear about the necessity for long-term mechanical ventilation is frequently countered by the ability of the family to participate fully in the patient's care in the home setting. At home, the patient may be able to participate more in activities of daily living around a more individualized schedule and, because of the smaller size of the home ventilator, may be more mobile. Another advantage of home mechanical ventilation is the reduction in the patient's risk of hospital-acquired infection.

Disadvantages of home mechanical ventilation include problems related to reimbursement, equipment, caregiver stress and fatigue, and the complex needs of these patients. Ventilated patients are usually dependent, requiring extensive nursing care, at least initially. Disposable products may not be reimbursable. Financial resources must be carefully assessed when arranging home mechanical ventilation, and a meeting with the discharge team should be scheduled before initiating a teaching plan for discharge. Another disadvantage of home mechanical ventilation is its potential impact on the family. Family members may seem enthusiastic about caring for their loved one in the home but may be motivated by numerous, complex factors. They may lack understanding of the potential sacrifices they may have to make financially and in personal time and commitment. Families should be encouraged to consider respite care to periodically relieve caregiver stress and fatigue.

NURSING MANAGEMENT: MECHANICAL VENTILATION

Nursing

A nursing care plan (eNCP 68-1) for the patient receiving mechanical ventilation is available on the Evolve Web site for this chapter.

Other Critical Care Content

Table 68-13 lists additional critical care content presented in other chapters of this book.

Table 68-13 Cross-References to Other Critical Care Content	
TOPIC	**DISCUSSED IN CHAPTER**
Acute congestive heart failure	37
Acute respiratory distress syndrome	70
Acute respiratory failure	70
Advanced cardiac life support	38
Burns	27
Cardiac dysrhythmias	38
Cardiac pacemakers	38
Cardiac surgery	37
Cardiopulmonary resuscitation	38
Emergencies	71
Enteral nutrition	42
Head injury, including ICP monitoring	59
Multiple organ dysfunction syndrome	69
Myocardial infarction	36
Oxygen delivery	31
Pulmonary edema	37
Renal dialysis, including renal replacement therapy	49
Shock	69
Systemic inflammatory response syndrome	69
Total parenteral nutrition	42
Tracheostomy	29
Trauma	71

ICP, intracranial pressure.

CLINICAL DECISION-MAKING EXERCISE

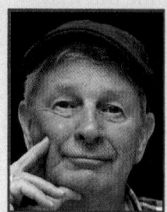

CASE STUDY:
Critical Care and Mechanical Ventilation

Source: © iStockphoto.com/Barbara Helgason

Patient Profile

Richard Kincaid is a 72-year-old White man who collapsed on the street. He was unresponsive on admission and remains unresponsive. He has an oral endotracheal (ET) tube in place and is receiving mechanical ventilation. He weighs 90 kg. A subclavian central line was placed to monitor central venous pressure (CVP) and administer fluids.

Subjective Data

None; patient is unresponsive to painful stimuli.

Objective Data

Physical Examination
- Noninvasive blood pressure (BP) is 100/75 mm Hg; heart rate is 128 (atrial fibrillation with a rapid ventricular response); temperature is 38.8°C; arterial oxygenation (SpO$_2$) is 98%
- Purulent secretions from ET tube
- Breath sounds: rhonchi bilaterally, decreased breath sounds on the right

Diagnostic Studies
- Chest radiography reveals right lower lung consolidation.
- Arterial blood gases (ABGs): pH 7.48; arterial partial pressure of oxygen (PaO$_2$) 94 mm Hg; arterial partial pressure of carbon dioxide (PaCO$_2$) 30 mm Hg; bicarbonate (HCO$_3$) 34 mEq/L.
- Computed tomography (CT) scan is positive for massive cerebrovascular accident.

Collaborative Care
- Positive-pressure ventilation settings: assist-control mode
- Settings: fraction of inspired oxygen (FiO$_2$) 70%, tidal volume (V$_T$) 700 mL, respiratory rate 16 breaths/min, positive end-expiratory pressure (PEEP) 5 cm H$_2$O
- Enteral feeding at 25 mL/hr via small-bore feeding tube
- Indwelling urinary catheter to bedside drainage

- Head of bed elevated at 40 degrees.
- Change position every 2 hours.
- Perform chest physical therapy every 2 to 4 hours.
- Azithromycin (Zithromax) 500 mg intravenously q24h
- Cefotaxime (Claforan) 2 g intravenously q6h
- Five percent dextrose in normal saline (D5NS) with potassium chloride (KCl) 20 mEq/L at 100 mL/hr

Discussion Questions

1. Identify two reasons for intubating and providing mechanical ventilation for Mr. Kincaid
2. What do Mr. Kincaid's ABGs indicate, and which ventilator setting(s) should be changed?
3. What is his PaO$_2$/FiO$_2$ ratio and what does it signify?
4. Mr. Kincaid's BP drops to 80 mm Hg, and he remains in atrial fibrillation with a ventricular rate of 158. A pulmonary artery (PA) catheter is inserted for further hemodynamic monitoring. What would be the purpose of hemodynamic monitoring (in addition to CVP monitoring) in this patient?
5. *Priority Decision:* What are the two priority nursing considerations for a patient with a PA catheter?
6. Mr. Kincaid's initial pulmonary artery occlusive pressure (PAOP) is 14 mm Hg, cardiac index (CI) is 2 L/min/m^2, and systemic vascular resistance index (SVRI) is 2667 dynes/sec/cm^{-5}/m^2. How would the nurse interpret these values? What medical interventions would the nurse anticipate?
7. Mr. Kincaid's pulmonary condition deteriorates. PaO$_2$ drops to 70 mm Hg, and SpO$_2$ is 89%. PEEP is increased to 7.5 cm H$_2$O. What implications does this have for Mr. Kincaid given his hemodynamic status?
8. Based on the data presented, what are the actual and potential problems that the nurse can identify with this patient?
9. After 4 days, Mr. Kincaid remains unresponsive and has developed renal failure. The physician believes the patient will not recover and wishes to discuss goals of care with the patient's caregiver. What would be the nurse's role in this meeting?

evolve   *Answers are available at* **http://evolve.elsevier.com/Canada/Lewis/medsurg**

REVIEW QUESTIONS

The number of the question corresponds to the same-numbered objective at the beginning of the chapter.

1. What does a certification in critical care by the Canadian Nurses Association indicate?
   a. Has earned a master's degree in the field of providing advanced critical care nursing
   b. Is an advanced practice nurse in the care of acutely ill patients
   c. May practise independently to provide symptom management for the critically ill
   d. Has practised in critical care and successfully completed a test of critical care knowledge

2. What is the most appropriate intervention for a patient with delirium in the critical care unit (CCU)?
   a. Use tranquillizers to establish normal sleep patterns.
   b. Identify the factors contributing to the patient's confusion and irritability.
   c. Silence all alarms, overhead paging, and conversations around the patient.
   d. Sedate the patient with psychotropic drugs to protect the patient from harmful behaviours.

3. What is the most ideal plan for family involvement in the CCU?
   a. A family member at the bedside at all times
   b. Allowing family at the bedside at present, brief intervals
   c. An individually devised plan with family involved with care and comfort measures
   d. Restriction of visiting in the CCU because the environment is overwhelming to visitors

4. In hemodynamic monitoring, what does zeroing refer to, and which one of the following does the nurse zero to?
   a. Cardiac output (CO) monitoring system to the level of the left ventricle
   b. Pressure monitoring system to the level of the catheter tip located in the patient
   c. Pressure monitoring system to the level of the atrium, identified as the midaxillary line
   d. Pressure monitoring system to the level of the atrium, identified as the phlebostatic axis

5. What hemodynamic changes should the nurse expect to find after successful initiation of intra-aortic balloon pump use in a patient in cardiogenic shock?
   a. Decreased wedge and increased CO
   b. Decreased systemic vascular resistance (SVR) and decreased stroke volume (SV)
   c. Increased diastolic blood pressure (BP) and decreased systolic BP
   d. Decreased central venous pressure (CVP) and increased right atrial pressure

6. What nursing management should be included in the patient with an artificial airway?
   a. Routine suctioning of the tube at least every 2 hours
   b. Observing for cardiac dysrhythmias during suctioning
   c. Maintaining endotracheal (ET) tube cuff pressure at 30 cm H_2O
   d. Preventing tube dislodgement by limiting mouth care to lubrication of the lips

7. What is the purpose of adding positive end-expiratory pressure (PEEP) to positive-pressure ventilation?
   a. Increase functional residual capacity and improve oxygenation.
   b. Increase fraction of inspired oxygen (FiO_2) in an attempt to wean the patient and avoid oxygen toxicity.
   c. Determine whether the patient is able to be weaned and avoid the risk of pneumomediastinum.
   d. Determine whether the patient is in synchrony with the ventilator or needs to be paralyzed.

8. For what should the nurse monitor the patient with positive-pressure mechanical ventilation?
   a. Paralytic ileus because pressure on the abdominal contents affects bowel motility
   b. Diuresis and sodium depletion because of increased release of atrial natriuretic peptide
   c. Signs of cardiovascular insufficiency because pressure in the chest impedes venous return
   d. Respiratory acidosis in a patient with chronic obstructive pulmonary disease (COPD) because of alveolar hyperventilation and increased arterial partial pressure of oxygen (PaO_2) levels

ANSWERS: 1. d; 2. b; 3. c; 4. d; 5. a; 6. b; 7. a; 8. c.

REFERENCES

Abiomed. (2007). AbioCor FAQs. Retrieved from *http://www.abiomed.com/products/faqs.cfm*

Abroug, F., Ouanes-Besbens, L., Elatrous, S., Brouchard, L. (2008). The effect of prone positioning in acute respiratory distress syndrome or acute lung injury: a meta-analysis. Areas of uncertainty and recommendations for research, *Intensive Care Medicine, 34*(6), 1002. doi:10.1007/s00134-008-1062-3

Akgül, S., & Akyolcu, N. (2002). Effects of normal saline on endotracheal suctioning. *Journal of Clinical Nursing, 11*(6), 826. doi:10.1046/j.1365-2702.2002.00655.x

American Association of Critical-Care Nurses. (2010). AACN practice alert: Family presence during CPR and invasive procedures. Retrieved from *http://www.aacn.org/wd/practice/docs/practicealerts/family%20presence%2004-2010%20final.pdf*

American Association of Critical Care Nurses (AACN). (2006). AACN practice alert: Verification of feeding tube placement. Retrieved from *http://www.aacn.org/AACN/practiceAlert.nsf/Files/VOTP/$file/Verification%20of%20Feeding%20Tube%20Placement%2005-2005.pdf*

American Association of Critical-Care Nurses. (2008). AACN practice alert: Ventilator-associated pneumonia. Retrieved from *http://www.aacn.org/WD/Practice/Docs/PracticeAlerts/Ventilator%20Associated%20Pneumonia%201-2008.pdf*

American Association of Critical Care Nurses (AACN). (2010). About critical care nursing. Retrieved from *http://www.aacn.org/WD/PressRoom/Content/aboutcriticalcarenursing.cms?pid=1&&menu*

American Thoracic Society, Infectious Diseases Society of America. (2005). Guidelines for the management of adults with hospital-acquired, ventilator-associated, and healthcare-associated pneumonia. *American Journal of Respiratory and Critical Care Medicine, 171*(4), 388. doi:10.1164/rccm.200405-644ST

Arroyo-Novoa, C. M., Figueroa-Ramos, M. L., Puntillo, K. A., Stanik-Hutt, J., Thompson, C. L., White, C. & Rietman Wild, L. (2008). Pain related to tracheal suctioning in awake acutely and critically ill adults: a descriptive study, *Intensive and Critical Care Nursing, 24*(1), 20-27. doi:10.1016/j.iccn.2007.05.002

Bankhead, R., Boullata, J., Brantley, S., Corkins, M., Guenter, P., Krenitsky, J., ..., A.S.P.E.N. Board of Directors. (2009). Enteral nutrition practice recommendations. *Journal of Parenteral and Enteral Nutrition, 33*: 122-67. doi:10.1177/0148607108330314

Burns, S. M. (2008). Pressure modes of mechanical ventilation: The good, the bad, and the ugly. *AACN Advanced Critical Care, 19*, 399-411. doi:10.1097/01.AACN.0000340721.78495.25.

Canadian Association of Critical Care Nurses (CACCN). (2005). Position statement of family presence at cardiac arrests. Retrieved from *http://www.caccn.ca.vsd20.korax.net/en/publications/position_statements/ps2005.html*

Chamberlain, B., & Donley, K. (2009). Patient outcomes using a rapid response team. *Clinical Nurse Specialist, 23*(1), 11-12. doi:10.1097/01.NUR.0000343071.34967.89

Davidson, J. (2009). Family-centered care. Meeting the needs of patients' families and helping families adapt to critical illness. *Critical Care Nurse, 29*(3), 28. doi:10.4037/ccn2009611

Devlin, J. W., Fong, J. J., Howard, E. P., Skrobik, Y., McCoy, N., Yasuda, C., & Marshall, J. (2008). Assessment of delirium in the intensive care unit: Nursing practices and perceptions. *American Journal of Critical Care, 17*(6), 6.

Durham College Critical Care e-Learning Program (2012). Critical care simulation. Retrieved from *http://www.durhamcollege.ca/criticalcare*

Ecklund, M. M. (2006). Beyond the ICU, homecare management of patients receiving mechanical ventilation. In S. M. Burns (Ed.), *Protocols for practice: Care of the mechanically ventilated client* (2nd ed.). Sudbury, MA: Jones & Bartlett.

Ecklund, M. M., & Danbaugh, L. A. (2009). Alternative settings for critical care. In K. K. Carlson (Ed.), *Advanced critical care nursing*. St. Louis: Saunders.

Ely, E., Shintani, A., Truman B., Speroff, T., Gordon, S. M., Harrell, F., Jr., ..., Dittus, R. S. (2004). Delirium as a predictor of mortality in mechanically ventilated clients in the intensive care unit. *Journal of the American Medical Association, 291*(14), 1753-1762. doi:10.1001/jama.291.14.1753

Friese, R. (2008). Sleep and recovery from critical illness and injury: A review of theory, current practice, and future directions. *Critical Care Medicine, 36*(3), 697. doi:10.1097/CCM.0b013e31818726b1

Garland, A. (2005). Improving the ICU. *Chest, 127*(6), 2151-2176.

Gélinas, C. (2007). Pain issues in the critical care unit. In R. Kaplow & S. Hardin (Eds.), *Primer of critical care nursing: A synergistic approach* (pp. 41-50). Sudbury, MA: Jones & Bartlett Publishers.

Gonzalez, C. E., Carroll, D. L., Elliott, J. S., Fitzgerald, P. A., & Vallent, H. J. (2004). Visiting preferences of patients in the intensive care unit and in a complex care medical unit. *American Journal of Critical Care, 13*(4), 194-198.

Gries, C., Curtis, J., Wall, R., & Engelberg, R. (2008). Family member satisfaction with end of life decision making in the ICU. *Chest, 133*(3), 704-712. doi:10.1378/chest.07-1773

Gupta, P. (2007). Managing sedation in intensive care. *Journal of Anesthesiology Clinical Pharmacology, 23*(3), 241-247.

Happ, M., Tuite, P., Dobbin, K., DiVirgilio-Thomas, D., & Kitutu, J. (2004). Communication ability, method, and content among nonspeaking nonsurviving patients treated with mechanical ventilation in the intensive care unit. *American Journal of Critical Care, 13*(3), 210-220.

Heart and Stroke Foundation of Canada. (2010). Statistics. Retrieved from *http://www.heartandstroke.com/site/c.ikIQLcMWJtE/b.3483991/k.34A8/Statistics.htm*

Hsu, C., Chen, K., Chang, C., Jerng, J., Yu, C., & Yang, P. (2005). Timing of tracheostomy as a determinant of weaning success in critically ill patients: A retrospective study. *Critical Care, 9*(1), R46-R52. doi:10.1186/cc3018

Hupcey, J. (2000). Feeling safe: The psychosocial needs of ICU Patients. *Journal of Nursing Scholarship, 32*, 361-367.

Hutchinson, M. (2009). Nutritional support. In M. Sole, D. Klein, & M. Moseley (Eds.), *Introduction to critical care nursing* (5th ed.). St. Louis: Saunders.

Jolley, J., Bendyk, H., Holaday, B., Lombardozzi, K. A., & Harmon, C. (2007). Rapid response teams: Do they make a difference? *Dimensions of Critical Care Nursing, 26*(6), 253-260. doi:10.1097/01.DCC.0000297401.67854.78

Leske, J., & Pasquale, M. (2007). Family needs, interventions and presence. In N. Molter (Ed.), *Protocols for practice: creating healing environments* (2nd ed.). Sudbury, MA: Jones & Bartlett.

Lusk, B., & Lash, A. (2005). The stress response. Psychoneuroimmunology and stress among ICU patients. *Dimensions in Critical Care Nursing, 24*(1), 25-31. doi:10.1097/00003465-200501000-00004

Mace, S. (2008). Challenges and advances in intubation: Rapid sequence intubation. *Emergency Medicine Clinics of North America, 26*(4), 1043. doi:10.1016/j.emc.2008.10.002

McCalve, S., Martindale, R., Vanek, V., McCarthy, M., Roberts, P., Taylor, B., ..., The American College of Critical Care Medicine. (2009). Guidelines for the provision and assessment of nutrition support therapy in the adult critically ill patient. *Journal of Parenteral and Enteral Nutrition, 33*(3), 277. doi:10.1177/0148607109335234

Metheny, N. A., Schallom, M., & Edwards, S. J. (2004). Effect of gastrointestinal motility and feeding tube site on aspiration risk in critically ill patients: A review. *Heart & Lung, 33*(3), 131-145. doi:10.1016/j.hrtlng.2004.02.001

Nagler, J., & Krauss, B. (2008). Capnography: A valuable tool for airway management. *Emergency Medicine Clinics of North America, 26*(4), 881. doi:10.1016/j.emc.2008.08.005

Nohrenberg, J., Moseley, M., & Sole, M. (2009). Hemodynamic monitoring. In M. Sole, D. Klein, & M. Moseley (Eds.), *Introduction to Critical Care Nursing* (5th ed., pp. 141-172). St. Louis: Saunders.

Oh, H., & Seo, W. (2003). A meta-analysis of the effects of various interventions in preventing endotracheal suction-induced hypoxia. *Journal of Clinical Nursing, 12*(6), 912-924. doi:10.1046/j.1365-2702.2003.00796.x

Ouimet, S., Kavanagh, B. P., Gottfried, S. B., & Skrobik, Y. (2007). Incidence, risk factors, and consequences of ICU delirium. *Intensive Care Medicine, 33*(1), 66. doi:10.1007/s00134-006-0399-8

Pierce, L. N. (2007). Management of the mechanically ventilated patient (2nd ed.) St Louis: Saunders.

Puhlman, M., & Hargraves, J. (2011). Ventricular assist devices. In D. Wiegand (Ed.), *AACN procedure manual for critical care* (6th ed.). St. Louis: Saunders.

Redekopp, M. A., & Leske, J. S. (2007). Family visitation and partnership. In N. C. Molter (Ed.), *Protocols for practice: Creating healing environments* (2nd ed.). Sudbury, MA: Jones & Bartlett.

Rose, L. (2008). High-frequency oscillatory ventilation in adults. *AACN Advanced Critical Care 19*(4), 412. doi:10.1097/01.AACN.0000340722.72657.f2

Safer Health Care Now! (2012). Prevent ventilator associated pneumonia: Getting started kit. Retrieved from *http://www.saferhealthcarenow.ca/EN/Interventions/VAP/Documents/VAP%20Getting%20Started%20Kit.pdf*

Shaffer, R. B. (2005). Arterial catheter insertion (assist), care, and removal. In D. J. Lynn-McHale & K. K. Carlson (Eds.), *AACN procedure manual for critical care* (5th ed.). Philadelphia: Saunders.

Society of Critical Care Medicine. (n.d.). Patient and family resources: ICU issues and answers brochures. Retrieved from *http://www.myicucare.org/Support _Brochures /Pages/default.aspx*

Sona, C. (2009). Assessing delirium in the intensive care unit. *Critical Care Nurse, 29*(2), 103. doi:10.4037/ccn2009329

St. John, R., & Seckel, M. (2006). Airway management. In S. Burns (Ed.), *Protocols for practice: Care of the mechanically ventilated patient* (2nd ed.). Sudbury, MA: Jones & Bartlett.

Stapleton, R., Jones, N., & Heyland, D. (2007). Feeding critically ill patients: What is the optimal amount of energy? *Critical Care Medicine, 35*(9 Suppl), S535. doi:10.1097/01.CCM.0000279204.24648.44

Urden, L. D., Stacy, K. M., & Lough, M. E. (2010). *Critical care nursing* (6th ed.). St Louis: Elsevier.

Weigand, D. J. L., & Williams, L. D. (2009). End of Life Care. In K. K. Carlson (Ed.), *Advanced Critical Care Nursing* (pp. 1507-1526). St. Louis: Mosby.

Woods, S. (2007). Spiritual and complementary therapies to promote healing and reduce stress. In C. Molter (Ed.), *Protocols for practice: Creating healing environments* (2nd ed.). Sudbury, MA: Jones & Bartlett.

CANADIAN RESOURCES

Canadian Association of Critical Care Nurses (CACCN)
http://www.caccn.ca
Canadian Critical Care Society
http://www.canadiancriticalcare.org/
Safer Health Care Now
http://www.saferhealthcarenow.ca

RELATED RESOURCES

American Association of Critical Care Nurses (AACCN)
http://www.aacn.org
Australian College of Critical Care Nurses
http://www.acccn.com.au
Confusion Assessment Method for the ICU
http://www.mc.vanderbilt.edu/icudelirium/assessment.html
Intensive Care Delirium Screening Checklist
http://www.mc.vanderbilt.edu/icudelirium/docs/ICDSC.pdf
Society of Critical Care Medicine (SCCM)
http://www.sccm.org

evolve *For additional Internet resources, see the Web site for this book at* **http://evolve.elsevier.com/Canada/Lewis/medsurg**

Nursing Management: Shock, Systemic Inflammatory Response Syndrome, and Multiple-Organ Dysfunction Syndrome

Written by Maureen A. Seckel

Adapted by Janet A. Piper

LEARNING OBJECTIVES

1. Define shock.
2. Differentiate the two major classifications of shock: low blood flow and maldistribution of blood flow.
3. Describe the pathophysiology and the clinical manifestations of the different types of shock.
4. Compare and contrast the effects of shock, systemic inflammatory response syndrome, and multiple organ dysfunction syndrome on the major body systems.
5. Compare the collaborative care, the drug therapy, and the nursing management of different types of shock.
6. Describe the nursing management of multiple organ dysfunction syndrome.

KEY TERMS

anaphylactic shock An acute and life-threatening hypersensitivity (allergic) reaction to a sensitizing substance, such as a drug, chemical, vaccine, food, or insect venom, p. 1962

cardiogenic shock Shock occurring when either systolic or diastolic dysfunction of the pumping action of the heart results in compromised cardiac output, p. 1960

hypovolemic shock Shock that is caused by a loss of intravascular fluid volume, p. 1961

multiple-organ dysfunction syndrome (MODS) The failure of two or more organ systems in an acutely ill patient to such a degree that homeostasis cannot be maintained without intervention, p. 1983

neurogenic shock A hemodynamic syndrome of massive vasodilation without compensation that results from the loss of sympathetic nervous system vasoconstrictor tone, caused by spinal cord injury at the fifth thoracic (T5) vertebra or above; characterized by hypotension and bradycardia, p. 1962

sepsis A systemic inflammatory response to infection, p. 1965

septic shock The presence of sepsis with hypotension despite adequate fluid resuscitation, along with the presence of tissue perfusion abnormalities, p. 1965

shock A syndrome characterized by decreased tissue perfusion and impaired cellular metabolism that results in an imbalance between the supply of and the demand for oxygen and nutrients, p. 1960

systemic inflammatory response syndrome (SIRS) A systemic inflammatory response to a variety of insults, including infection, ischemia, infarct, and injury, p. 1982

ELECTRONIC RESOURCES

Supplemental content related to Chapter 69 can be found...

Evolve Web Site ⊘volve

http://evolve.elsevier.com/Canada/Lewis/medsurg
• Answer Guidelines for Case Study on p. 1986
• Clinical Reference: Laboratory Values
• Content Updates

• Customizable Nursing Care Plan: Shock
• Electronic Calculators
• Examination Review Questions
• Glossary
• Interactive Case Study: Cardiogenic Shock
• Key Points (Printable and MP3 Download)

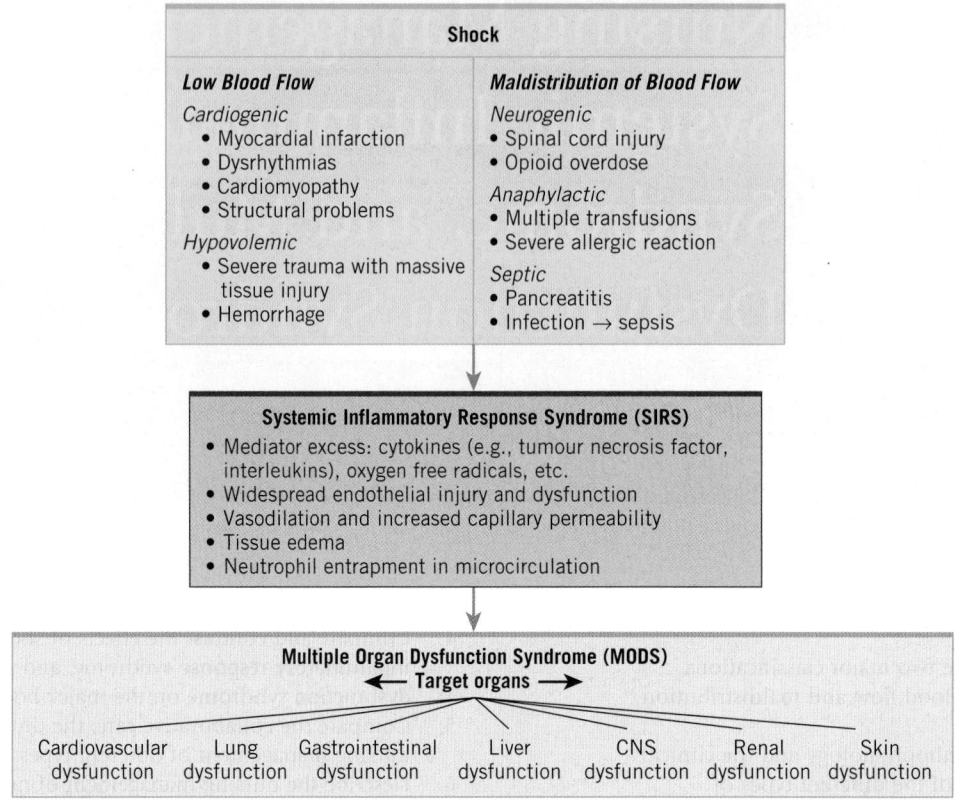

Figure 69-1 Relationship of shock, systemic inflammatory response syndrome, and multiple-organ dysfunction syndrome. *CNS*, central nervous system.

Shock, systemic inflammatory response syndrome (SIRS), and multiple-organ dysfunction syndrome (MODS) are serious and interrelated problems. Figure 69-1 shows the relationship among shock, SIRS, and MODS. Shock is a complex process that often leads to the development of SIRS and MODS. This chapter provides an overview of shock, SIRS, and MODS.

Shock

Shock is a syndrome characterized by decreased tissue perfusion and impaired cellular metabolism. This condition results in an imbalance between the supply of and the demand for oxygen and nutrients. The exchange of oxygen and nutrients at the cellular level is essential for life. When a cell is in a state of hypoperfusion, the demand for oxygen and nutrients exceeds the supply.

Classification of Shock

Although the cause, the initial presentation, and the management strategies of the various types of shock differ, the physiological responses of the cell to hypoperfusion are similar. For the purposes of discussion, shock is classified as low blood flow (cardiogenic and hypovolemic shock) or maldistribution of blood flow (septic, anaphylactic, and neurogenic shock; Lawrence, 2011; Thibodeau & Patton, 2007). Classification details are listed in Table 69-1.

Shock Caused by Low Blood Flow

Cardiogenic Shock. **Cardiogenic shock** occurs when either systolic or diastolic dysfunction of the pumping action of the heart results in compromised cardiac output (CO). The heart's inability to pump the blood forward is classified as systolic dysfunction. Systolic dysfunction affects primarily the left ventricle because systolic pressure and tension are greater in the left chambers of the heart. When systolic dysfunction affects the right chambers of the heart, blood flow through the pulmonary circulation is compromised. Precipitating causes of systolic dysfunction include myocardial infarction (MI), cardiomyopathies, blunt cardiac injury, severe systemic or pulmonary hypertension, and myocardial depression caused by metabolic problems. Extensive left ventricular infarction and subsequent ventricular failure account for more than 75% of all cases of cardiogenic shock, and the prognosis is extremely poor (Topalian, Ginsberg, & Parrillo, 2008). Diastolic dysfunction is impairment of the ability of the right or left ventricle to fill during diastole. Decreased filling of the ventricle results in decreased stroke volume. Precipitating causes of diastolic dysfunction include cardiac tamponade and cardiomyopathy.

Figure 69-2 describes the pathophysiology of cardiogenic shock. Whether the initiating event is myocardial dysfunction, a structural problem (e.g., valvular abnormality, ventricular septal rupture, tension pneumothorax), or dysrhythmias, the physiological responses are similar: Both tissue perfusion and cellular metabolism are impaired.

The early clinical presentation of a patient with cardiogenic shock is similar to that of a patient with acute decompensated

Table 69-1 Classification of Shock and Precipitating Factors

Low Blood Flow

Cardiogenic Shock

- Systolic dysfunction: inability of the heart to pump blood forward (e.g., myocardial infarction, cardiomyopathy)
- Diastolic dysfunction: inability of the heart to fill during diastole (e.g., pericardial tamponade)
- Dysrhythmias
- Structural factors: valvular abnormality (e.g., stenosis or regurgitation), ventricular septal rupture, tension pneumothorax

Hypovolemic Shock

Absolute Hypovolemia

- External loss of whole blood (e.g., through hemorrhage from trauma, surgery, GI bleeding)
- Loss of other body fluids (e.g., through vomiting, diarrhea, excessive diuresis, diabetes insipidus, diabetes mellitus)

Relative Hypovolemia

- Pooling of blood or fluids (e.g., from bowel obstruction)
- Fluid shifts (e.g., from burn injuries, ascites)
- Internal bleeding (e.g., from fracture of long bones, ruptured spleen, hemothorax, severe pancreatitis)
- Massive vasodilation (e.g., from sepsis)

Maldistribution of Blood Flow

Neurogenic Shock

- Hemodynamic consequence of injury, disease, or both to the spinal cord at or above T5
- Spinal anaesthesia
- Vasomotor centre depression (e.g., severe pain, drugs, hypoglycemia, injury)

Anaphylactic Shock

- Contrast media, blood or blood products, drugs, insect bites, anaesthetic agents, foods or food additives, vaccines, environmental agents, latex

Septic Shock

- Infection (e.g., urinary, respiratory, invasive procedures, and indwelling devices)
- At-risk patients: according to CIHI (2009), older adults >60 years and infants <1 year (incidence is higher in men [54.6%] than in women [45.4%]); immunosuppressed/immunocompromised patients; malnourished or debilitated patients, many with comorbid conditions, most common of which are diabetes mellitus and cancers (CIHI, 2009) but also chronic kidney disease, and heart failure
- Gram-negative bacteria most common; also Gram-positive bacteria, viruses, fungi, and parasites; of special concern are methicillin-resistant organisms and endemic or pandemic outbreaks (WHO, 2010)

CIHI, Canadian Institute for Health Information; *GI*, gastrointestinal; *WHO*, World Health Organization.

PATHOPHYSIOLOGY MAP

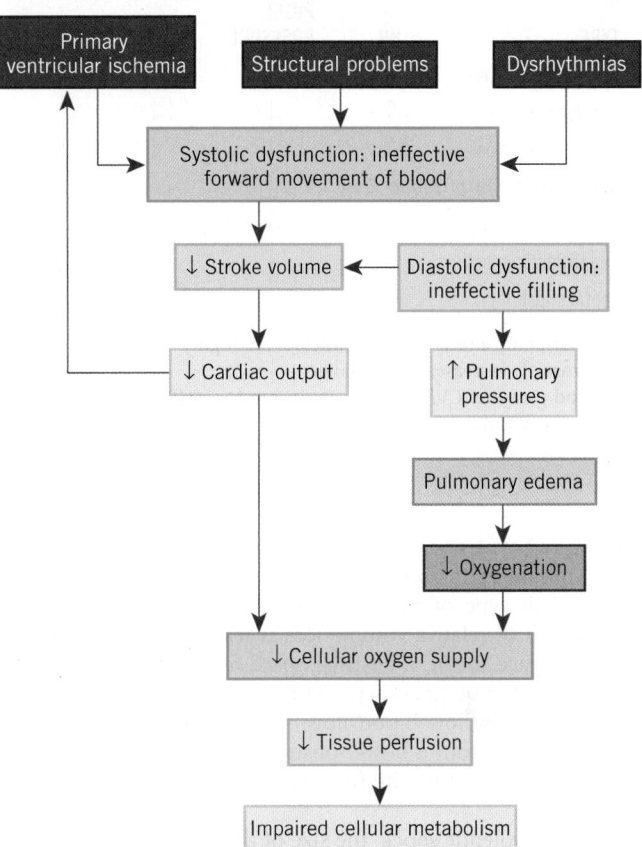

Figure 69-2 The pathophysiology of cardiogenic shock.

Source: Urden, L. D., Stacy, K. M., & Lough, M. E. (2010). *Critical care nursing: Diagnosis and management* (6th ed., p. 984, Figure 39-2). St. Louis: Mosby.

blood forward results in low CO (<4 L/min) and low cardiac index (<2.1 L/min/m²). On examination, the patient appears tachypneic, and pulmonary congestion is evidenced by the presence of crackles. The hemodynamic profile demonstrates increases in the pulmonary artery occlusive (or wedge) pressure (PAOP) and pulmonary vascular resistance (Table 69-2). Signs of peripheral hypoperfusion (e.g., cyanosis, pallor, cool and clammy skin, decreased capillary refill time) are apparent. Decreased renal blood flow results in sodium and water retention and decreased urine output. Anxiety, confusion, and agitation may develop as cerebral perfusion is impaired. Studies that may be helpful in diagnosing cardiogenic shock include laboratory studies (e.g., cardiac enzymes, troponin levels), electrocardiography (ECG), chest radiography, and echocardiography (Table 69-3). The overall clinical presentation of a patient with cardiogenic shock is described in Table 69-4.

Hypovolemic Shock. The second type of shock caused by low blood flow is hypovolemic shock. **Hypovolemic shock** occurs when intravascular fluid volume is lost. In hypovolemic shock, the volume is inadequate to fill the vascular space. The volume loss may be either an absolute or a relative volume loss. Absolute hypovolemia results when fluid is lost through hemorrhage, gastrointestinal (GI) loss (e.g., through vomiting, diarrhea), fistula drainage, diabetes insipidus, hyperglycemia, or diuresis. In

heart failure (see Chapter 37). The patient's response to low blood flow may include tachycardia, hypotension, and a narrowed pulse pressure. An increase in systemic vascular resistance (SVR) increases the workload of the heart, thus increasing the myocardial oxygen consumption. The heart's inability to pump

Table 69-2 Effects of Shock on Hemodynamic Parameters*

TYPE	HR	PULSE PRESSURE	BP	SVR	PVR	CVP	PAP	PAOP	CO	SVO₂/SCVO₂
Low Blood Flow										
Cardiogenic shock	↑	↓	↓	↑	↑	≈, ↑	↑	↑	↓	↓
Hypovolemic shock	↑	↓	↓	↑	↑	↓	↓	↓	↓	↓
Maldistribution of Blood Flow										
Neurogenic shock	↓	↓	↓	↓	≈	↓	↓	↓	↓	↓
Anaphylactic shock	↑	↓	↓	↓	≈, ↑	↓	↓	↓	↓	↓
Septic shock	↑	↓	↓	↓	≈, ↑	↓	↑, ≈, ↓	↓	↑, ≈, ↓	↑, ≈, ↓

*Hemodynamic effects in some illnesses are highly variable.
↓, decrease; ↑, increase; ≈, no change.
BP, blood pressure; *CVP*, central venous pressure; *HR*, heart rate; *PAOP*, pulmonary artery occlusive pressure; *PAP*, pulmonary artery pressure; *PVR*, pulmonary vascular resistance; *ScvO₂*, central venous oxygen saturation; *SvO₂*, venous oxygen saturation; *SVR*, systemic vascular resistance.

relative hypovolemia, fluid volume moves out of the vascular space into the extravascular space (e.g., interstitial or intracavitary space). This type of fluid shift is called "third spacing." One mechanism of relative volume loss is leakage of fluid from the vascular space to the interstitial space from increased capillary permeability, as occurs in sepsis. Table 69-1 provides examples of shock caused by low blood flow, such as confinement of fluid into the colon from a bowel obstruction, ascites, loss of blood volume into a fracture site (e.g., pelvic fracture), and burns (see Chapter 27).

In hypovolemic shock, the size of the vascular compartment remains unchanged, but the volume of blood or plasma decreases. Whether the loss of intravascular volume is absolute or relative, the physiological consequences are similar. A reduction in intravascular volume results in a decreased venous return to the heart, decreased preload, decreased stroke volume, and decreased CO (see Table 69-2). A cascade of events results in decreased tissue perfusion and impaired cellular metabolism, the hallmarks of shock (Figure 69-3).

A patient's response to low blood flow as a result of acute volume loss is dependent on a number of factors, including extent of injury or insult, the patient's age, and general state of health; however, the clinical presentations of hypovolemic shock are similar (see Table 69-4). An overall assessment of physiological reserves may indicate the patient's ability to compensate. A patient may compensate for a loss of up to 15% of the total blood volume (approximately 750 mL). Further loss of volume (15 to 30%) results in a sympathetic nervous system (SNS)–mediated response. This response results in increases in heart rate, CO, and respiratory rate and depth. The stroke volume and PAOP are decreased because of the decreased circulating blood volume. The patient may appear anxious, and urine output begins to decrease. If hypovolemia is corrected by crystalloid fluid replacement at this time, tissue dysfunction is generally reversible. If volume loss is greater than 30%, compensatory mechanisms may begin to fail, and replacement with blood or blood products should be initiated immediately. With loss of more than 40% of the total blood volume, autoregulation in the microcirculation is lost, and irreversible tissue destruction occurs (Guyton & Hall, 2011). Laboratory studies that may be helpful include serial measurements of hemoglobin and hematocrit levels, urine specific gravity, serum electrolytes, blood gases, and lactic acid (see Table 69-3).

Shock Caused by Maldistribution of Blood Flow

Neurogenic Shock. **Neurogenic shock** is a hemodynamic phenomenon that can occur within 30 minutes of a spinal cord injury at the fifth thoracic (T5) vertebra or above and lasts up to 6 weeks. The injury results in a massive vasodilation without compensation that is caused by the loss of SNS vasoconstrictor tone. This massive vasodilation leads to a pooling of blood in the blood vessels, tissue hypoperfusion, and, ultimately, impairment of cellular metabolism (Figure 69-4).

Like spinal cord injury, spinal anaesthesia can block transmission of impulses from the SNS. Depression of the vasomotor centre of the medulla from drugs (e.g., benzodiazepines, opioids) also can result in decreased vasoconstrictor tone of the peripheral blood vessels, which leads to neurogenic shock (see Table 69-1).

The most important clinical manifestations in neurogenic shock are hypotension (from the massive vasodilation) and bradycardia (from unopposed parasympathetic stimulation (Hickey, 2009). A patient in neurogenic shock may be unable to regulate temperature. The inability to regulate temperature, in combination with massive vasodilation, promotes heat loss. Initially, the patient's skin is warm as a result of the massive dilation without compensation. As the heat dissipates, the patient is at risk for hypothermia. Later, the patient's skin may be cool or warm, depending on the ambient temperature (*poikilothermia*, the taking on the temperature of the environment). In either case, the skin is usually dry. Tables 69-2, 69-3, and 69-4 further describe the clinical presentation of a patient with neurogenic shock.

Although spinal shock and neurogenic shock often occur in the same patient, they are not the same disorder. Spinal shock is a transient condition that is present after an acute spinal cord injury (see Chapter 63). A patient with spinal shock experiences the absence of all voluntary and reflex neurological activity below the level of the injury (Hickey, 2009).

Anaphylactic Shock. **Anaphylactic shock** is an acute and life-threatening hypersensitivity (allergic) reaction to a sensitizing substance (e.g., drug, chemical, vaccine, food, insect venom). Usually an immediate reaction causes massive vasodilation, release of vasoactive mediators, and an increase in capillary permeability. As capillary permeability increases, fluid leaks from the vascular space into the interstitial space. Affected patients are anxious and have a sense of impending doom. Anaphylactic

DIAGNOSTIC STUDIES

Table 69-3 Laboratory Abnormalities in Shock

LABORATORY STUDY	FINDING	SIGNIFICANCE OF FINDING
Blood		
RBC count, hematocrit, hemoglobin	Normal	Remains within normal limits (a) in shock because of relative hypovolemia and pump failure and (b) in hemorrhagic shock before fluid resuscitation
	Decreased	In hemorrhagic shock, decreases after fluid resuscitation when fluids other than blood are used
	Increased	In nonhemorrhagic shock, increases as a result of actual hypovolemia because fluid lost does not contain erythrocytes
DIC screen		Acute DIC can develop within hours to days after an initial assault on the body (e.g., shock)
Fibrin split products	Increased	
Fibrinogen level	Decreased	
Platelet count	Decreased	
PTT and INR	Prolonged	
Thrombin time	Increased	
D-dimer	Increased	
Creatine kinase	Increased	In trauma and myocardial infarction, increases in response to cellular damage or hypoxia
Troponin	Increased	In myocardial infarction
BUN	Increased	Indicates impaired kidney function as a result of hypoperfusion caused by severe vasoconstriction, or occurs secondary to catabolism of cells (e.g., in trauma, infection)
Creatinine	Increased	Indicates impaired kidney function as a result of hypoperfusion caused by severe vasoconstriction; is more sensitive indicator of renal function than BUN
Glucose	Increased	In early shock, increases because of release of liver glycogen stores in response to sympathetic nervous system stimulation and cortisol; insulin insensitivity develops
	Decreased	Decreases because of depleted glycogen stores with hepatocellular dysfunction as shock progresses
Serum Electrolytes		
Sodium	Increased	In early shock, increases because of increased secretion of aldosterone, causing renal retention of sodium
	Decreased	May occur iatrogenically when excessive hypotonic fluid is administered after fluid loss
Potassium	Increased	Increases when cellular death liberates intracellular potassium; in acute kidney injury; and in the presence of acidosis
	Decreased	In early shock, decreases because of increased secretion of aldosterone, which causes renal excretion of potassium
Arterial blood gases	Respiratory alkalosis	In early shock, occurs secondary to hyperventilation
	Metabolic acidosis	In later shock, occurs when organic acids, such as lactic acid, accumulate in blood as a result of anaerobic metabolism
Base deficit	≥6	Indicates acid production secondary to hypoxia
Blood cultures	Growth of organisms	May occur in patients who are in septic shock
Lactic acid	Increased	Usually increases once significant hypoperfusion and impaired oxygen use at the cellular level have occurred; by-product of anaerobic metabolism
Liver enzymes (ALT, AST, GGT)	Increased	Elevations indicate liver cell destruction in progressive stage of shock
Urine		
Specific gravity	Increased	Occurs secondary to the action of ADH
	Fixed at 1.010	Occurs in renal failure

ADH, antidiuretic hormone; *ALT,* alanine aminotransferase; *AST,* aspartate aminotransferase; *BUN,* blood urea nitrogen; *DIC,* disseminated intravascular coagulation; *GGT,* γ-glutamyl transferase; *INR,* international normalized ratio; *PTT,* partial thromboplastin time; *RBC,* red blood cell.

Table 69-4 Clinical Presentation in the Major Types of Shock

	LOW BLOOD FLOW	MALDISTRIBUTION OF BLOOD FLOW		
CARDIOGENIC SHOCK	**HYPOVOLEMIC SHOCK**	**NEUROGENIC SHOCK**	**ANAPHYLACTIC SHOCK**	**SEPTIC SHOCK**
Cardiovascular (see Table 69-2 for complete hemodynamic profile)				
↓ Capillary refill time ↑ MVO$_2$ Chest pain may or may not be present	↓ Preload ↓ Stroke volume ↓ Capillary refill time	↓ or ↑ Temperature Bradycardia	Chest pain Third spacing of fluid	↓ or ↑ Temperature Biventricular dilation: ↓ ejection fraction
Pulmonary				
Tachypnea Cyanosis Crackles Wheezes	Tachypnea, progressing to bradypnea (late)	Dysfunction related to level of injury	Swelling of lips and tongue Shortness of breath Edema of larynx and epiglottis Wheezing Rhinitis Stridor	Hyperventilation Respiratory alkalosis, progressing to respiratory acidosis Hypoxemia Respiratory failure ARDS Pulmonary hypertension Crackles
Renal				
↑ Na$^+$ and H$_2$O retention ↓ Renal blood flow ↓ Urine output	↓ Urine output	Bladder dysfunction		↓ Urine output
Skin				
Pallor Cool, clammy	Pallor Cool, clammy	↓ Skin perfusion Cool or warm Dry	Flushing Pruritus Urticaria Angioedema	Warm and flushed (early), becoming cool and mottled (late)
Neurological				
↓ Cerebral perfusion: anxiety, confusion, agitation	Anxiety Confusion Agitation	Flaccid paralysis below level of lesion Loss of reflex activity	Anxiety Sensation of impending doom Confusion ↓ LOC Metallic taste	Alteration in mental status (e.g., confusion) Agitation Coma (late)
Gastrointestinal				
↓ Bowel sounds Nausea and vomiting	Absence of bowel sounds	Bowel dysfunction	Cramping Abdominal pain Nausea Vomiting Diarrhea	GI bleeding Paralytic ileus
Other Diagnostic Findings (also see Table 69-3)				
↑ Cardiac markers ↑ Blood glucose ↑ BUN Electrocardiographic (e.g., dysrhythmias) Echocardiographic (e.g., left ventricular dysfunction) Chest radiographic (e.g., pulmonary infiltrates)	↓ Hematocrit ↓ Hemoglobin ↑ Lactate ↑ Urine specific gravity Changes in electrolytes		Sudden onset History of allergies Exposure to contrast media	↑ or ↓ WBC count ↓ Platelets ↑ Lactate ↑ Glucose ↑ Urine specific gravity ↓ Urine Na$^+$ Positive blood cultures

ARDS, acute respiratory distress syndrome; *BUN*, blood urea nitrogen; *GI*, gastrointestinal; *LOC*, level of consciousness; *MVO$_2$*, myocardial oxygen consumption; *WBC*, white blood cell.

PATHOPHYSIOLOGY MAP

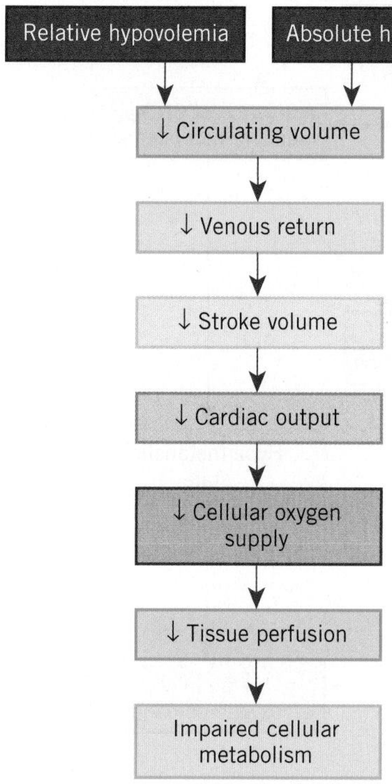

Figure 69-3 The pathophysiology of hypovolemic shock.

Source: Urden, L. D., Stacy, K. M., & Lough, M. E. (2010). *Critical care nursing: Diagnosis and management* (6th ed., p. 982, Figure 39-1). St. Louis: Mosby.

PATHOPHYSIOLOGY MAP

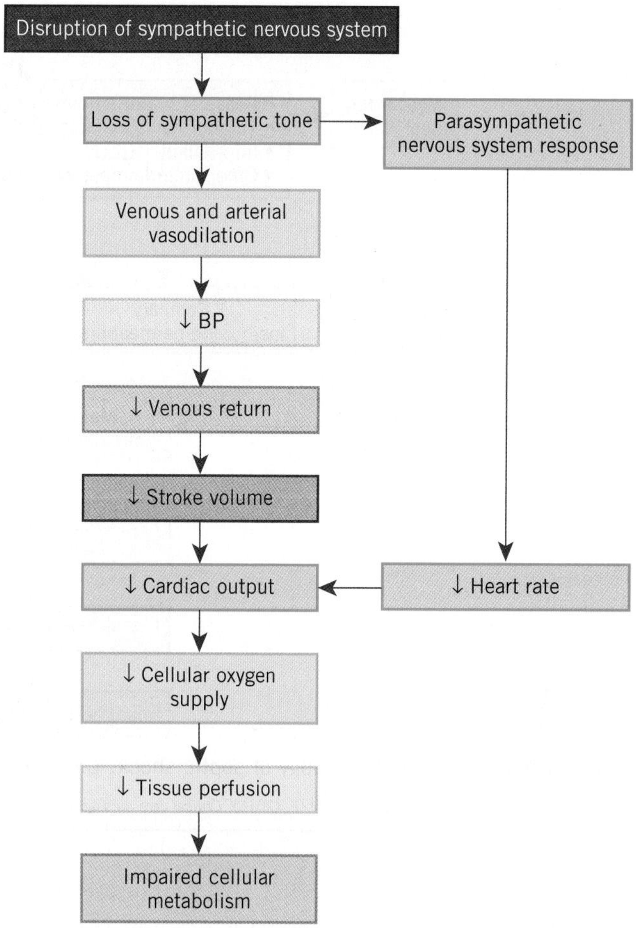

Figure 69-4 The pathophysiology of neurogenic shock. *BP*, blood pressure.

Source: Urden, L. D., Stacy, K. M., & Lough, M. E. (2010). *Critical care nursing: Diagnosis and management* (6th ed., p. 990, Figure 39-4). St. Louis: Mosby.

shock can lead to airway swelling (pharyngeal/laryngeal edema, stridor, hoarse voice), breathing problems (shortness of breath, increased respirations, fatigue, confusion as a result of hypoxia), and circulation problems (hypotension; tachycardia; pale, clammy skin; faintness; and even loss of consciousness). If it is not treated, respiratory or cardiac arrest may develop (Resuscitation Council [UK], 2008). A patient can develop a severe allergic reaction, which possibly leads to anaphylactic shock, after contact, inhalation, ingestion, or injection with an antigen (allergen) to which the person has previously been sensitized (see Table 69-1). Parenteral administration of the antigen (allergen) is the route most likely to cause anaphylaxis; however, oral, topical, and inhalation routes can also cause anaphylactic reactions. Tables 69-2, 69-3, and 69-4 describe the clinical presentation of anaphylactic shock. Quick and decisive action by the nurse is crucial for preventing the progression of an anaphylactic reaction to anaphylactic shock. (Anaphylaxis is discussed in Chapter 16.)

Septic Shock. **Sepsis** is a systemic inflammatory response to a documented or suspected infection (Canadian Institute for Health Information, 2009). In as many as 30% of patients with sepsis, the causative organism is not identified. *Severe sepsis* is defined as sepsis complicated by organ dysfunction, hypoperfusion or hypotension (Johnson & Henry, 2009). In **septic shock,** the patient has hypotension that cannot be reversed with fluid resuscitation and tissue perfusion abnormalities are present (Dellinger et al., 2008; Johnson & Henry, 2009). In the United States, sepsis is diagnosed in more than 750,000 patients per year, and mortality rates are as high as 50% (60% for septic shock; Powers & Burchell, 2010). In Canada, mortality rates in the period 2008

to 2009 were 30% among patients with sepsis, 45.2% among patients with severe sepsis, and 20.9% among patients in whom sepsis did not worsen from the initial state (Canadian Institute for Health Information, 2009). The primary organisms that cause sepsis are Gram-negative and Gram-positive bacteria. The morbidity and mortality rates from infections with Gram-negative organisms are higher than those with Gram-positive organisms. Parasites, fungi, and viruses can also lead to the development of sepsis and septic shock (Canadian Institute for Health Information, 2009). The pathogenesis of septic shock is complex (Figure 69-5).

When an antigen (microorganism) enters the body, the normal immune or inflammatory cascade responses are initiated and work together to destroy the antigen; however, in severe sepsis and septic shock, the response initiated by the body to an antigen is exaggerated. Inflammation and coagulation are increased, and fibrinolysis is decreased. Endotoxins from the microorganism cell wall stimulate the release of cytokines, including tumour necrosis factor (TNF) and interleukin-1 (IL-1), and other proinflammatory mediators that act through secondary mediators such as platelet-activating factor, interleukin-6, and interleukin-8 (Bridges & Dukes, 2005). (See Chapter 14 for a

PATHOPHYSIOLOGY MAP

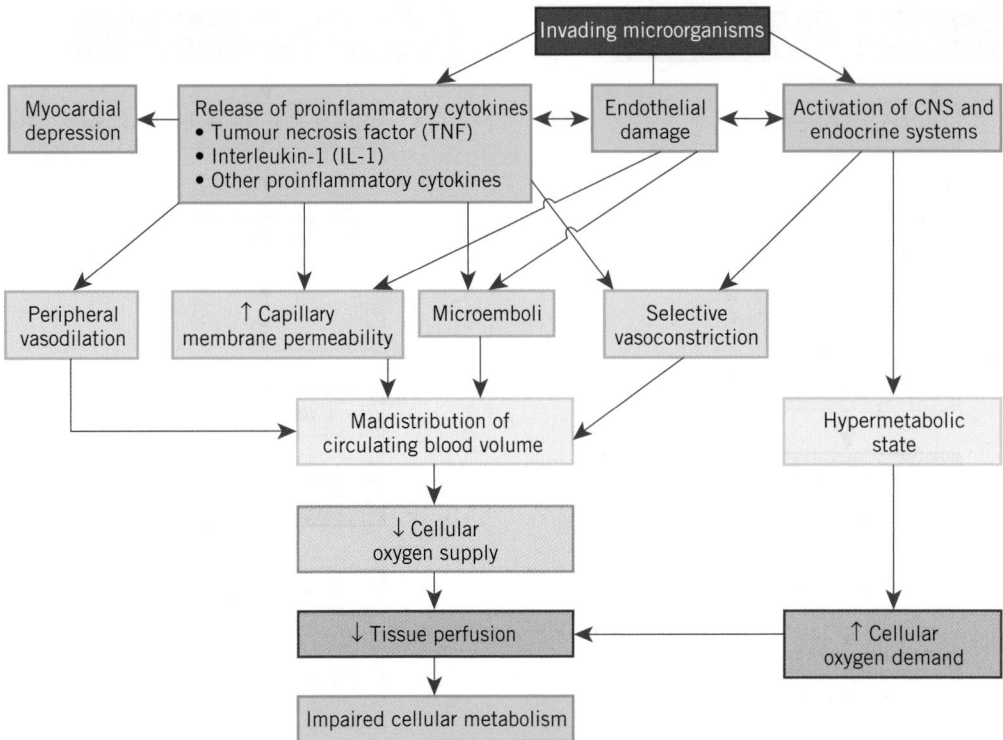

Figure 69-5 The pathophysiology of septic shock. *CNS*, central nervous system.

Source: Urden, L. D., Stacy, K. M., & Lough, M. E. (2010). *Critical care nursing: Diagnosis and management* (6th ed., p. 992, Figure 39-5). St. Louis: Mosby.

discussion of the inflammatory response.) The release of platelet-activating factor results in the formation of microthrombi and obstruction of the microvasculature. The combined effects of the mediators result in damage to the endothelium, vasodilation, increased capillary permeability, and neutrophil and platelet aggregation and adhesion to the endothelium.

The clinical presentation of sepsis is complex, and no single symptom or group of symptoms is specific to the diagnosis (Table 69-5). Affected patients usually experience an initial hyperdynamic state characterized by increased CO and decreased SVR (Bridges & Dukes, 2005). Despite this, the combination of TNF and IL-1 is thought to have a role in sepsis-induced myocardial dysfunction. The ejection fraction is decreased for the first few days after the initial insult. Because of a decreased ejection fraction, the ventricles dilate in order to maintain the stroke volume. The ejection fraction typically improves, and the ventricular dilation resolves over 7 to 10 days. Persistence of high CO and low SVR beyond 24 hours is an ominous finding and is often associated with an increased development of hypotension and MODS. Coronary artery perfusion and myocardial oxygen metabolism are not primarily altered in septic shock (Bridges & Dukes, 2005).

In addition to the cardiovascular dysfunction that accompanies sepsis, respiratory failure is common. Affected patients initially hyperventilate as a compensatory mechanism, which results in respiratory alkalosis. Once the patient can no longer compensate, respiratory acidosis develops. Respiratory failure develops in 85% of patients with sepsis, and acute respiratory distress syndrome (ARDS) develops in 40%. Other clinical signs of septic shock include alteration in neurological status, decreased urine

output, and GI dysfunction, such as GI bleeding and paralytic ileus. Tables 69-2 and 69-4 further delineate the clinical presentation of septic shock.

Stages of Shock

The health care provider must understand the underlying pathogenesis of the type of shock the client is experiencing, but monitoring and management are also guided by knowing which stage of the shock "continuum" the patient is in. This continuum begins with the initial stage of shock, which occurs at a cellular level and is usually not clinically apparent. Metabolism changes at the cellular level from aerobic to anaerobic, causing lactic acid build-up. Lactic acid is a waste product and must be removed by the liver. However, this process requires oxygen, which is unavailable because of the decrease in tissue perfusion. This stage is followed by the three clinically apparent but overlapping stages of shock: the compensatory stage, the progressive stage, and the refractory (irreversible) stage (Guyton & Hall, 2011).

Compensatory Stage. In the compensatory stage, the body activates neural, hormonal, and biochemical compensatory mechanisms in an attempt to overcome the increasing consequences of anaerobic metabolism and to maintain homeostasis (Figure 69-6). The patient's clinical presentation begins to reflect the body's responses to the imbalance in oxygen supply and demand (Table 69-6).

One of the first clinical signs of shock is hypotension, which occurs because of a decrease in cardiac output and a narrowing

Table 69-5 Diagnostic Criteria for Sepsis

Infection, documented or suspected, and some of the following:

General Variables

- Fever (temperature >38.3°C)
- Hypothermia (core temperature <36°C)
- Heart rate >90 beats/min
- Tachypnea
- Altered mental status
- Significant edema or positive fluid balance (>20 mL/kg over 24 hr)
- Hyperglycemia (blood glucose level >7.77 mmol/L) in the absence of diabetes

Inflammatory Variables

- Leukocytosis (WBC count >12.0 × 10⁹/L)
- Leukopenia (WBC count <4.0 × 10⁹/L)
- Normal WBC count with >10% immature forms
- Elevated C-reactive protein
- Elevated procalcitonin level

Hemodynamic Variables

- Arterial hypotension (SBP <90 mm Hg, MAP <70 mm Hg, or a decrease in SBP of >40 mm Hg)

Organ Dysfunction Variables

- Arterial hypoxemia (PaO₂ <85)
- Acute oliguria (urine output <0.5 mL/kg/hr for at least 2 hr despite adequate fluid resuscitation)
- Serum creatinine increase >44.2 micromol/L
- Coagulation abnormalities (INR >1.5 or PTT >60 sec)
- Ileus (absence of bowel sounds)
- Thrombocytopenia (platelet count <1.0 × 10⁹/L)
- Hyperbilirubinemia (total bilirubin level >68.4 micromol/L)

Tissue Perfusion Variables

- Hyperlactatemia
- Decreased capillary refill or mottling

Source: Dellinger, R. P., Levy, M. M., Carlet, J. M., Bion, J., Parker, M. M., Jaeschke, K. R., ..., World Federation of Societies of Intensive and Critical Care Medicine. (2008). Surviving Sepsis Campaign: International guidelines for management of severe sepsis and septic shock. *Critical Care Medicine, 36*, 296-327. doi:10.1097/01. CCM.0000298158.12101.41

FiO₂, fraction of inspired oxygen; *INR*, international normalized ratio; *MAP*, mean arterial pressure; *PaO₂*, partial pressure of arterial oxygen; *PTT*, partial thromboplastin time; *SBP*, systolic blood pressure; *WBC*, white blood cell.

---

of the pulse pressure. The baroreceptors in the carotid and aortic bodies immediately respond by activating the SNS. The SNS stimulates vasoconstriction and the release of the potent vasoconstrictors epinephrine and norepinephrine. Blood flow to the most vital organs (the heart and the brain) is maintained, whereas blood flow to the nonvital organs, such as the kidneys, the GI tract, the skin, and the lungs, is diverted or shunted (Guyton & Hall, 2011).

Decrease in blood flow to the kidneys activates the renin–angiotensin system. Renin is released, which activates angiotensinogen to produce angiotensin I, which is then converted to angiotensin II (see Chapter 47, Figure 47-6). Angiotensin II is a potent vasoconstrictor that causes both arterial and venous vasoconstriction. The net result is an increase in venous return to the heart and an increase in blood pressure (BP). Angiotensin II also stimulates the adrenal cortex to release aldosterone, which results in sodium and water reabsorption and in potassium excretion by the kidneys. The increase in sodium reabsorption raises the serum osmolality and stimulates the release of antidiuretic hormone (ADH) from the posterior pituitary gland. ADH works by increasing water reabsorption by the kidneys, thus further increasing blood volume. The increase in total circulating volume results in increases in CO and BP (Guyton & Hall, 2011).

The shunting of blood from other organ systems also results in clinically important changes. The decrease in blood flow to the GI tract results in impairment of motility and a slowing of peristalsis, which increase the risk for developing a paralytic ileus. When blood flow to the skin is decreased, the patient's skin feels cool and clammy, except in early septic shock, when the patient's skin feels warm and appears flushed, as a result of a hyperdynamic state (Bridges & Dukes, 2005).

Shunting blood away from the lungs has an important clinical effect in the patient in shock. The decrease in blood flow to the lungs increases the patient's physiological dead space: the amount of air that does not reach gas-exchanging units and any inspired air that cannot participate in gas exchange. The clinical result of an increase in dead space is a ventilation–perfusion mismatch. Some areas of the lungs participating in ventilation are not perfused because of the decrease in blood flow to the lungs. Arterial oxygen levels decrease, and the rate and depth of respirations increase to compensate.

The myocardium responds to the SNS stimulation and the increase in oxygen demand by increasing the heart rate and contractility. However, increased contractility increases myocardial oxygen consumption (MVO₂). The coronary arteries dilate in an attempt to meet the increased oxygen demands of the myocardium.

A multisystem response to decreasing tissue perfusion is initiated in the compensatory stage of shock. At this stage, the body is able to compensate for the changes in tissue perfusion. If the perfusion deficit (and, it is hoped, the cause of the shock) is corrected, the patient recovers with few or no residual sequelae. If the perfusion deficit is not corrected and the body is unable to compensate, the patient enters the progressive stage of shock.

Progressive Stage. The progressive stage of shock begins as compensatory mechanisms fail (Figure 69-7). In this stage, aggressive interventions are necessary to prevent the development of MODS. Continued decreased cellular perfusion and resulting altered capillary permeability are the distinguishing features of this stage. As a result of altered capillary permeability, fluid and protein leak out of the vascular space into the surrounding interstitial space. In addition to the decrease in circulating volume, systemic interstitial edema increases. The patient may have *anasarca* (diffuse profound edema). Fluid leakage from the vascular space also affects the solid organs (e.g., liver, spleen, GI tract, lungs) and peripheral tissues by further decreasing perfusion.

The pulmonary system is often the first system to display signs of critical dysfunction. During the compensatory stage, blood flow to the lungs is already reduced. In response to the decreased blood flow and the SNS stimulation, the pulmonary arterioles constrict, resulting in increased pulmonary artery (PA) pressure. As the pressure within the pulmonary vasculature increases, blood flow to the pulmonary capillaries decreases, and

Text continued on p. 1971

PATHOPHYSIOLOGY MAP

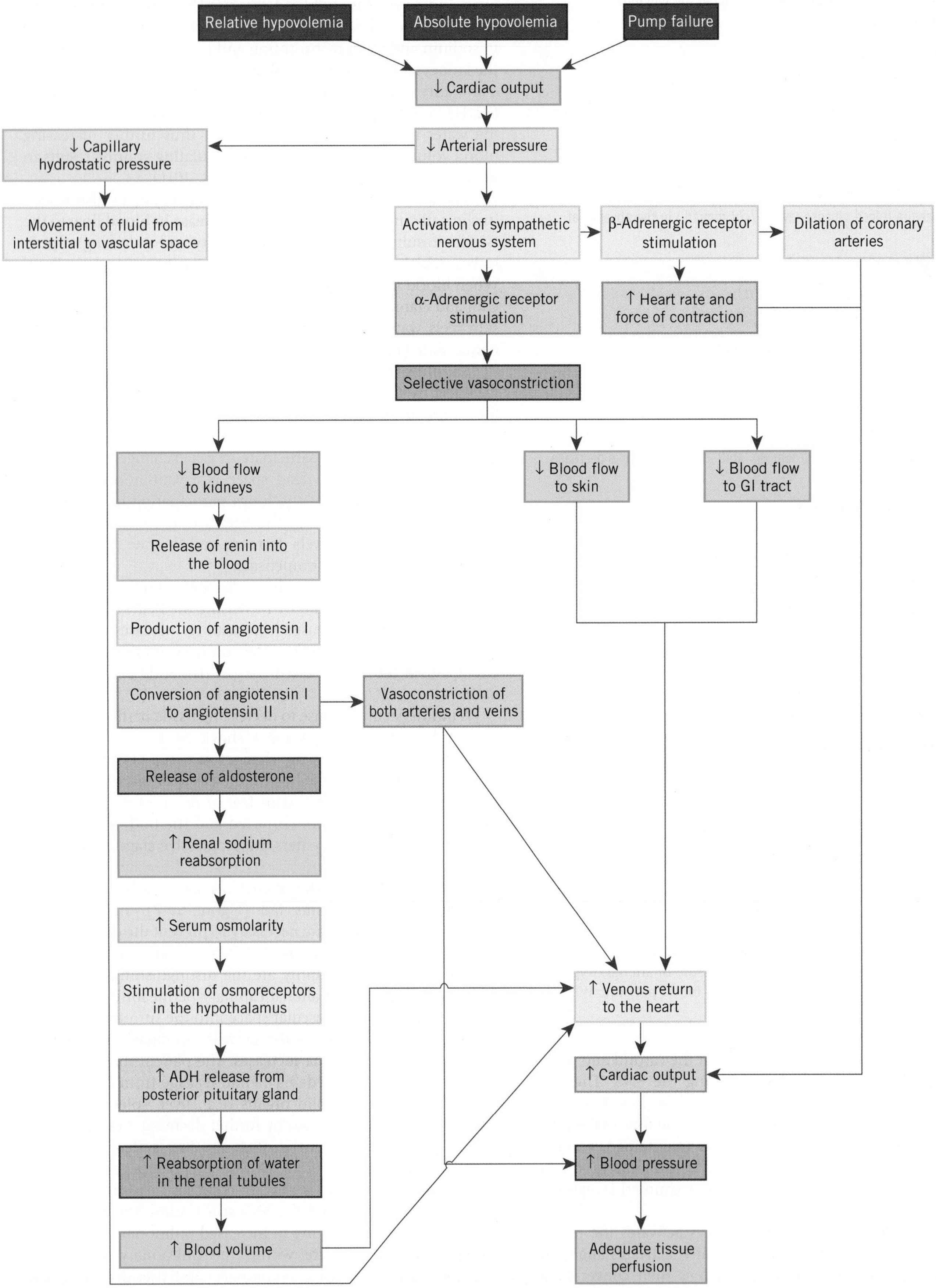

Figure 69-6 Compensatory stage of shock: reversible stage during which compensatory mechanisms are effective and homeostasis is maintained. *ADH,* antidiuretic hormone, *GI,* gastrointestinal.

Table 69-6 Clinical Manifestations of the Stages of Shock

SYSTEM	COMPENSATORY STAGE	PROGRESSIVE STAGE	REFRACTORY STAGE
Neurological	Oriented to person, place, time Restless, apprehensive, confused Change in level of consciousness Changes in Glasgow Coma Scale score	↓ Cerebral perfusion pressure ↓ Cerebral blood flow Listless or agitated ↓ Responsiveness to stimuli	Unresponsive Areflexia (loss of reflexes) Pupils unreactive and dilated
Cardiovascular	Sympathetic nervous system response: • Release of epinephrine and norepinephrine, which promotes vasoconstriction • ↑ MVO_2 • ↑ Contractility • ↑ HR Coronary artery dilation Narrowed pulse pressure BP adequate to perfuse vital organs (heart, brain)	Loss of autoregulation in microcirculation ↑ Capillary permeability → systemic interstitial edema ↓ Cardiac output → ↓ BP and ↑ HR MAP <60 mm Hg (or 40 mm Hg drop in BP from baseline) ↓ Coronary perfusion → • Dysrhythmias • Myocardial ischemia • Myocardial infarction • Myocardial dysfunction → impaired cardiac output ↓ Peripheral perfusion → ischemia of distal extremities, diminished pulses, ↓ capillary refill	Profound hypotension ↓ Cardiac output Bradycardia; irregular rhythm ↓ BP inadequate to perfuse vital organs
Respiratory	↓ Blood flow to the lungs ↑ Physiological dead space ↑ Ventilation–perfusion mismatch Hyperventilation ↑ Minute ventilation (V_E)	Acute respiratory distress syndrome (ARDS) • ↑ Capillary permeability • Pulmonary vasoconstriction • Pulmonary interstitial edema • Alveolar edema • Diffuse infiltrates • ↑ Respiratory rate • ↓ Compliance Moist crackles	Severe refractory hypoxemia Respiratory failure
Gastrointestinal	↓ Blood supply Hypoactive bowel sounds Possible ileus	Vasoconstriction and ↓ perfusion → ischemic gut (e.g., stomach, small and large intestines, gallbladder, pancreas) • Erosive ulcers • GI bleeding • Translocation of GI bacteria • Impaired absorption of nutrients	Ischemic gut
Renal	↓ Renal blood flow ↑ Renin level, resulting in release of angiotensin II (vasoconstrictor) ↑ Aldosterone level, resulting in Na^+ and H_2O reabsorption ↑ Antidiuretic hormone level, resulting in H_2O reabsorption	Renal tubules become ischemic → acute tubular necrosis ↓ Urine output ↑ BUN/creatinine ratio ↑ Urine Na^+ ↓ Urine osmolarity and specific gravity ↓ Urine K^+ Metabolic acidosis	Anuria
Hepatic	—	Failure to metabolize drugs and waste products Jaundice (decreased clearance of bilirubin) ↑ NH_3 and lactate	Metabolic changes from accumulation of waste products (e.g., NH_3, lactate, CO_2)
Hematological	—	DIC • Thrombin clots in microcirculation • Consumption of clots in microcirculation	DIC

BP, blood pressure; *BUN*, blood urea nitrogen; *DIC*, disseminated intravascular coagulation; *GI*, gastrointestinal; *HR*, heart rate; *K⁺*, potassium ions; *MAP*, mean arterial pressure; *MVO₂*, myocardial oxygen consumption; *Na⁺*, sodium ions; *NH₃*, ammonia.

Continued

Table 69-6 Clinical Manifestations of the Stages of Shock—cont'd

SYSTEM	COMPENSATORY STAGE	PROGRESSIVE STAGE	REFRACTORY STAGE
Temperature	Normal or abnormal	Hypothermia Sepsis: hypothermia or hyperthermia	Hypothermia
Skin	Pale and cool or warm and flushed (early onset of septic shock)	Cold and clammy	Mottled, cyanotic
Key laboratory findings	↑ Blood glucose ↑ pH ↓ PaO₂ ↓ PaCO₂	↑ Liver enzymes: ALT, AST, GGT ↑ Bleeding times Thrombocytopenia	↓ Blood glucose ↑ NH₃, lactate, and K⁺ Metabolic acidosis

ALT, alanine aminotransferase; *AST,* aspartate aminotransferase; *GGT,* γ-glutamyl transferase; *PaO₂,* partial pressure of arterial oxygen; *PaCO₂,* partial pressure of arterial carbon dioxide.

PATHOPHYSIOLOGY MAP

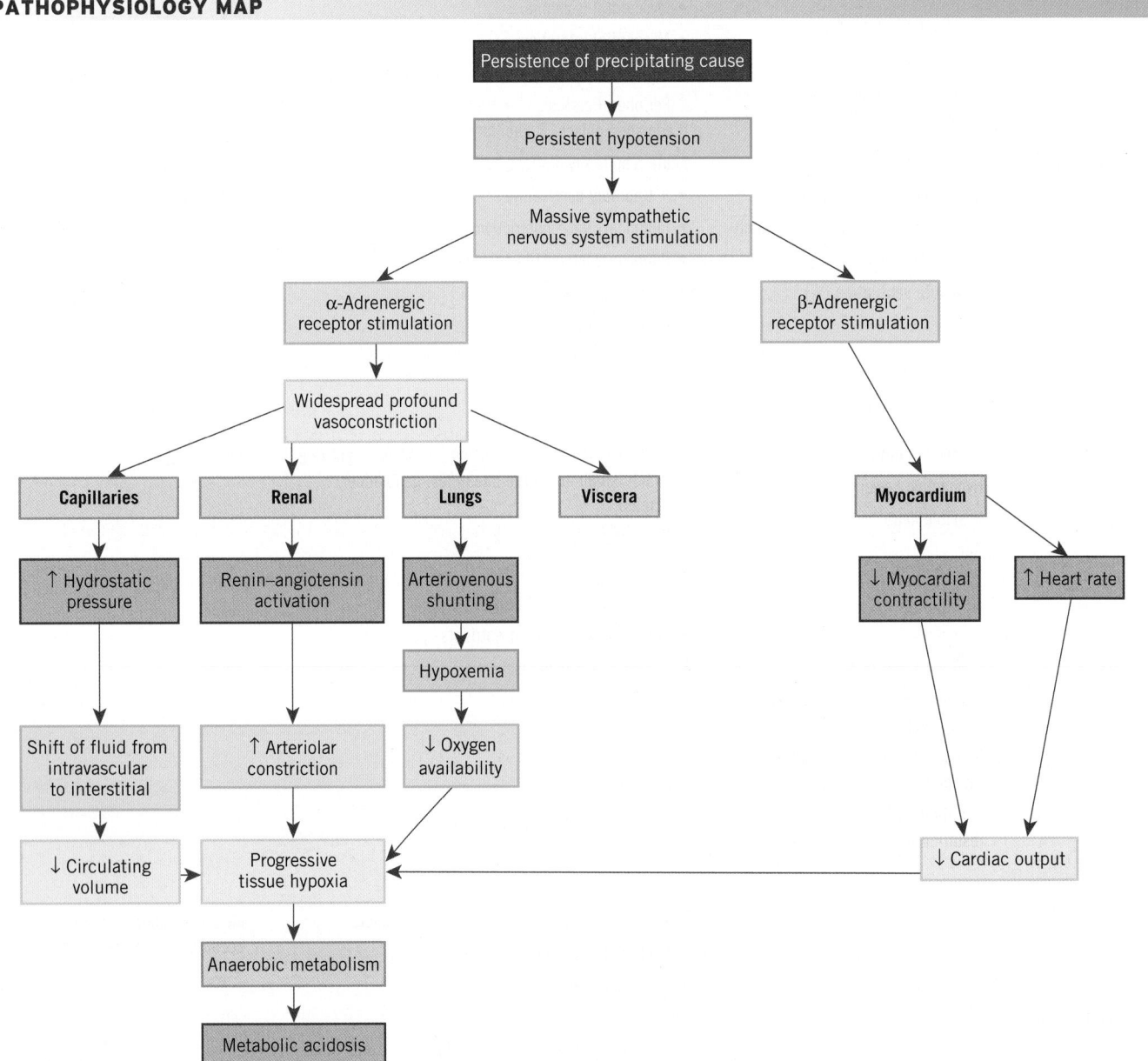

Figure 69-7 Progressive stage of shock: compensatory mechanisms are becoming ineffective and fail to maintain perfusion to vital organs.

ventilation–perfusion mismatch worsens. Another key response in the lungs is the movement of fluid from the pulmonary vasculature into the interstitial space. As capillary permeability increases, the movement of fluid to the interstitial spaces results in interstitial edema, bronchoconstriction, and a decrease in functional residual capacity. With further increases in capillary permeability, the fluid moves to the alveoli, with resultant alveolar edema and a decrease in surfactant production. The combined effects of pulmonary vasoconstriction and bronchoconstriction are impaired gas exchange, decreased compliance, and worsening ventilation–perfusion mismatch. Clinical manifestations are tachypnea, crackles, and an overall increased work of breathing.

The cardiovascular system is profoundly affected. CO begins to fall, with resultant decreases in BP and in coronary artery, cerebral, and peripheral perfusion. Changes in the patient's mental status are important findings in this stage. Capillary permeability continues to increase, enhancing the movement of fluid from the vascular space into the interstitial space. Sustained hypoperfusion results in weakening of peripheral pulses and ischemia of the distal extremities. Myocardial dysfunction from decreased perfusion results in dysrhythmias, myocardial ischemia, and potentially MI. The effect of prolonged hypoperfusion on the kidneys is renal tubular ischemia. The resulting acute tubular necrosis (ATN) may lead to the development of acute kidney injury, which can be worsened by nephrotoxic drugs, including certain antibiotics, anaesthetics, and diuretics (see Chapter 49). Renal function is markedly impaired during the progressive stage of shock. The urine output is decreased, and BUN and creatinine (Cr) levels are elevated. Metabolic acidosis results from an inability to excrete acids and reabsorb bicarbonate.

The GI system is also affected as the blood supply to the GI tract is decreased. The normally protective mucosal barrier becomes ischemic. This ischemia predisposes the patient to erosive ulcers and GI bleeding, thus increasing the potential risk of bacterial translocation from the GI tract to the blood. The decrease in perfusion to the GI tract also leads to a decrease in the ability to absorb nutrients (McClave & Heyland, 2009).

Other systems are also affected by the sustained hypoperfusion in the progressive stage of shock. The loss of the functional ability of the liver leads to a failure of the liver to metabolize drugs and waste products such as ammonia (NH_3) and lactate. Jaundice results from an accumulation of bilirubin. As the liver cells die, enzyme levels become elevated, particularly alanine aminotransferase (ALT), aspartate aminotransferase (AST), and γ-glutamyl transferase (GGT). The liver also loses its ability to function as an immune organ. Bacteria that may translocate from the GI system cannot be scavenged by Kupffer's cells. Instead, they are released into the bloodstream, which increases the possibility of the development of bacteremia (Cheek, Rodgers, & Schulman, 2009).

Dysfunction of the hematological system adds to the complexity of the clinical picture. The patient is at risk for the development of disseminated intravascular coagulation (DIC). In DIC, the platelets and the clotting factors are consumed, and secondary fibrinolysis develops. This situation results in clinically significant bleeding from many orifices, including, but not limited to, the GI tract, the lungs, and puncture sites (see Chapter 33). Altered laboratory values in DIC include decreases in platelets, prolonged prothrombin time, prolonged partial thromboplastin time, decreases in fibrinogen, elevated levels of D-dimer fragments, and increased levels of fibrin degradation products (Wada & Hatada, 2008; see Tables 69-3 and 69-6).

Refractory Stage. In the final stage of shock, the refractory stage, decreased perfusion from peripheral vasoconstriction and decreased CO exacerbate anaerobic metabolism (Figure 69-8). The accumulation of lactic acid contributes to an increased capillary permeability and dilation of the capillaries. Because capillary permeability is increased, fluid and plasma proteins leave the vascular space and move to the interstitial space. Blood pools in the capillary beds as a result of constriction of the venules and dilation of the arterioles. The loss of intravascular volume worsens hypotension and tachycardia and decreases coronary blood flow. Decreases in coronary blood flow lead to worsening myocardial depression and a further decline in CO. Cerebral blood flow cannot be maintained, and cerebral ischemia results.

Patients in this stage of shock demonstrate profound hypotension and hypoxemia. The failure of the liver, the lungs, and the kidneys results in an accumulation of waste products, such as lactate, urea, ammonia, and carbon dioxide. The failure of one organ system has an effect on several other organ systems. In this final stage, recovery is unlikely. The organs are in failure, and the body's compensatory mechanisms are overwhelmed (see Table 69-6).

Diagnostic Studies

There is no single diagnostic study to determine whether a patient is in shock. The process of establishing a diagnosis begins with physical examination and a thorough history, documented from the patient, the family, or friends. The patient's medical and surgical history and a history of recent events (e.g., upper respiratory tract infection, surgery, chest pain, trauma) provide valuable data.

Decreased tissue perfusion in shock initially leads to an elevation of lactate levels (>4 mmol/L) and a high base deficit (the amount needed to bring the pH back to normal). These laboratory changes reflect an undesirable increase in anaerobic metabolism. Other laboratory values found in shock are summarized in Table 69-3.

Additional diagnostic studies include 12-lead ECG, continuous cardiac monitoring, chest radiography, continuous pulse oximetry, and hemodynamic monitoring (e.g., arterial pressure monitoring, central venous or PA pressure monitoring). (See Chapter 68 for information on hemodynamic monitoring.)

Collaborative Care: General Measures

Critical factors in the successful management of a patient experiencing shock are the early recognition and prompt intervention in the early stages. Astute assessment skills and urgent communication with a rapid response team (RRT) may prevent the decline to the progressive or the refractory stage. Successful management of the patient in shock probably requires quick transfer to a critical care unit; however, nurses in non–critical care settings may institute physician's orders and care bundles early on, such as the "sepsis six," a protocol developed in the United Kingdom stemming from the 2008 Surviving Sepsis Campaign guidelines (SSG) (Dellinger et al., 2008) (Table 69-7). Other nursing considerations directly related to the SSG were developed internationally through the World Federation of Critical Care Nurses (Aitken et al., 2011). They also included the sepsis six.

Table 69-8 provides an overview of the initial assessment findings and interventions for the emergency care of patients in shock (Dellinger et al., 2008; Robson & Daniels, 2008). The nurse must ensure that the patient's airway is patent. Once the airway is established, either as a natural airway or with an endotracheal

PATHOPHYSIOLOGY MAP

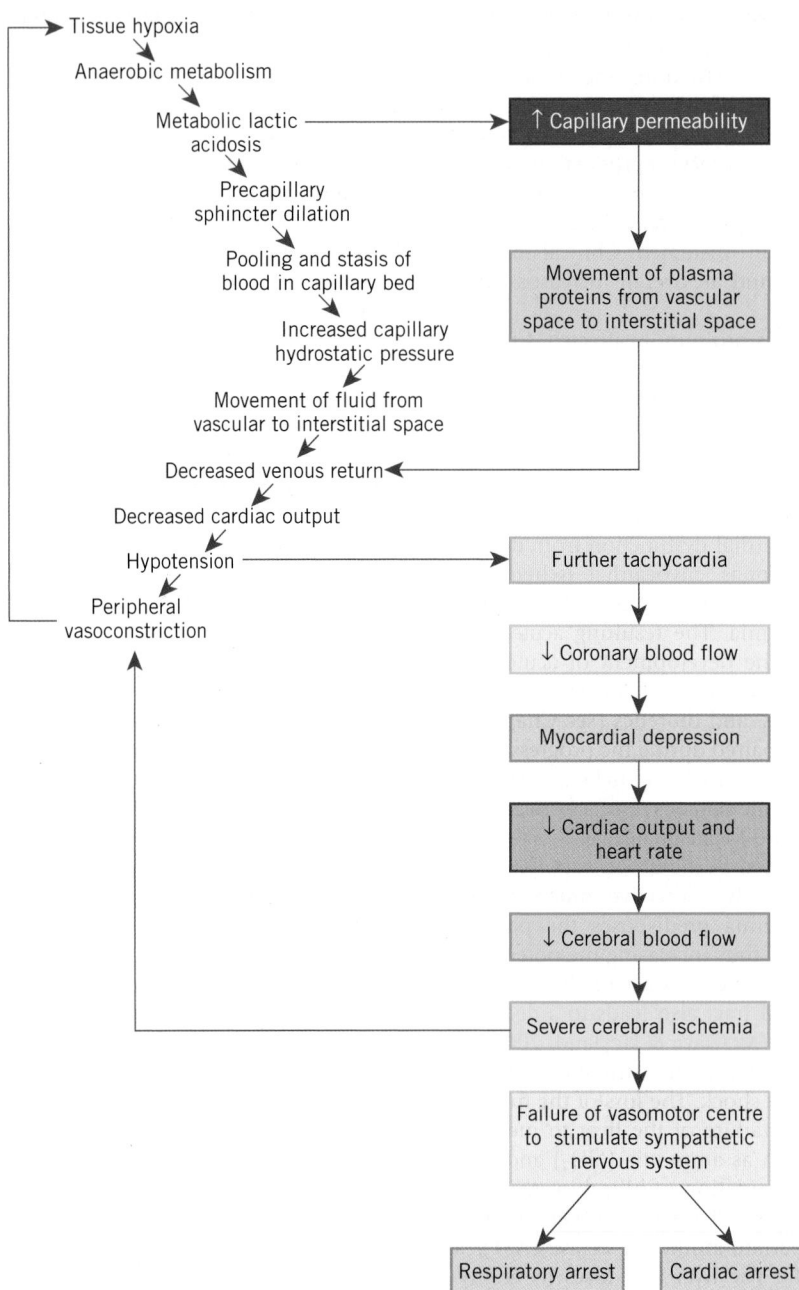

Figure 69-8 Irreversible or refractory stage of shock: compensatory mechanisms are not functioning or are totally ineffective, and multiple-organ dysfunction syndrome (MODS) results.

tube, oxygen should be delivered to maintain an arterial oxygen saturation (SaO_2) of 90% or higher (partial pressure of arterial oxygen [PaO_2] > 60 mm Hg) to avoid hypoxemia (see Chapter 68). Mechanical ventilation may be necessary. The mean arterial pressure and the circulating blood volume are optimized with fluid replacement and drug therapy.

Oxygen and Ventilation. Oxygen delivery is dependent on CO, available hemoglobin, and SaO_2. Methods to optimize oxygen delivery are directed at increasing supply and decreasing demand. Supply can be increased by (a) optimizing the CO with

drug therapy or fluid replacement, (b) increasing the hemoglobin by the transfusion of blood or packed red blood cells (RBCs), (c) increasing the SaO_2 with supplemental oxygen and mechanical ventilation, or some combination of these.

Care must be planned so as not to disrupt the balance of oxygen supply and demand. Activities that increase oxygen consumption (e.g., endotracheal suctioning, position changes) should be appropriately spaced for oxygen conservation. Continuous monitoring of central venous oxygen saturation ($ScvO_2$) by a central venous catheter or of mixed venous oxygen saturation (SvO_2) by a PA catheter is helpful. Both values reflect the dynamic balance between oxygen supply and demand. These values are considered in conjunction with the SaO_2, CO, hemoglobin, and oxygen consumption to evaluate the patient's response to treatments or activities (see Chapter 68).

Fluid Resuscitation.

Except for cardiogenic and neurogenic shock, all other classifications of shock involve decreased circulating blood volume. The cornerstone of therapy for septic, hypovolemic, and anaphylactic shock is volume expansion with the

administration of the appropriate fluid. Before fluid resuscitation begins, two large-bore intravenous catheters must be inserted, preferably into the antecubital veins. Both crystalloids and colloids may have a role in fluid resuscitation (Table 69-9; see Chapter 19). Initial fluid amounts administered for resuscitation are 1.5 to 4.5 L of crystalloids (isotonic or hypertonic) or 300 to 500 mL of colloids over 30 minutes. More rapid and larger volumes may be used for severe hypoperfusion, even as much as 200 mL/kg, but 40 to 60 mL/kg is average (Dellinger et al., 2008). Lactated Ringer's solution should be used cautiously in all shock situations because the failing liver cannot convert lactate to bicarbonate, and thus the serum lactate levels would increase. In some cases, hypertonic saline may be administered to expand plasma volume and reduce risk for mortality (Bulger, 2011). Colloids, although costly, are effective volume expanders because the size of their molecules keeps them in the vascular space for a longer time, and less volume is required (Dellinger et al., 2008).

Serial blood pressure measurements with an automatic BP cuff or an intra-arterial catheter can be used to monitor the patient's response. An indwelling bladder catheter to monitor urine output also assists in monitoring the patient's fluid status.

When large amounts of fluids are required, the patient must be protected against complications. Two major complications are hypothermia and coagulopathy. The patient can be protected from hypothermia by warming both crystalloid and colloid solutions used during massive fluid resuscitation. If the patient is

---

Table 69-7 The Sepsis Six: What You Can Do Within the First Hour and for at Least 6 Hours

1. Give 100% oxygen.
2. Take blood cultures to help determine antibiotic therapy.
3. Give IV antibiotics.
4. Give IV fluid therapy.
5. Measure lactate and hemoglobin.
6. Insert catheter, and monitor urine output.

IV, intravenous.
Source: Adapted from Robson, W. P., & Daniels, R. (2008). The sepsis six: Helping patients to survive sepsis. *British Journal of Nursing*, 17(1), 20.

EMERGENCY MANAGEMENT

Table 69-8 Shock

ETIOLOGY*	ASSESSMENT FINDINGS	INTERVENTIONS
Surgical	• Restlessness	**Initial**
• Postoperative bleeding	• Confusion	• Establish and maintain patency of airway.
• Rupture of organ or vessel	• Anxiety	• Administer humidified high-flow oxygen (100%) by non-rebreather mask or bag–valve–mask device.
• Gastrointestinal bleeding	• Sensation of impending doom	• Anticipate need for intubation and mechanical ventilation.
• Aortic dissection	• Decreased level of consciousness	• Stabilize cervical spine as appropriate.
• Vaginal bleeding	• Weakness	• Establish IV access with two large-bore catheters, and begin fluid resuscitation with isotonic or hypertonic crystalloids (e.g., normal saline solution).
• Rupture from ectopic pregnancy or of ovarian cyst	• Rapid, weak, thready pulses	• Collect blood for laboratory studies (e.g., blood cultures, lactate measurement, WBC count).
Medical	• Dysrhythmias	• Control any external bleeding with direct pressure or pressure dressing.
• Myocardial infarction	• Hypotension	• Assess for life-threatening injuries (e.g., pericardial tamponade, liver laceration, tension pneumothorax).
• Dehydration	• Narrowed pulse pressure	• Consider vasopressor therapy only after hypovolemia has been corrected.
• Addisonian crisis	• Cool, clammy skin (warm skin in early stages of septic and neurogenic shock)	• Insert an indwelling bladder catheter and nasogastric tube.
• Diabetes insipidus		• Institute antibiotic therapy if sepsis is suspected.
• Sepsis	• Tachypnea, dyspnea, or shallow, irregular respirations	• Treat dysrhythmias.
• Diabetes mellitus	• Decreased O_2 saturation	**Ongoing Monitoring**
• Pulmonary embolus	• Extreme thirst	• Level of consciousness
Trauma	• Nausea and vomiting	• Vital signs, including pulse oximetry, peripheral pulses, capillary refill
• Rupture or laceration of vessel or organ (e.g., spleen)	• Chills	• Respiratory status
	• Pallor	• Cardiac rhythm
• Fractures, spinal injury	• Cyanosis	• Urine output
• Multisystem or multiorgan injury	• Obvious hemorrhage or injury	
• Burns	• Temperature dysregulation	

*See Table 69-1 for additional causes of shock.
IV, intravenous; *WBC*, white blood cell.

Table 69-9 Fluid Therapy for Shock

FLUID TYPE	MECHANISM OF ACTION	TYPE OF SHOCK	NURSING IMPLICATIONS
Crystalloids			
Isotonic			
• 0.9% NaCl (NSS) • Lactated Ringer's solution	Fluid remains primarily in the intravascular space, increasing intravascular volume.	Used cautiously for initial volume replacement in most types of shock	Monitor patient closely for circulatory overload. Lactated Ringer's solution should not be administered to patients with liver failure.
Hypertonic			
1.8%, 3%, or 5% NaCl	Fluid remains in the intravascular space, producing rapid volume expansion.	May be used for initial volume expansion in hypovolemic shock	Monitor patient closely for signs of hypernatremia (e.g., disorientation, convulsions).
Blood/Blood Products			
• Whole blood or packed RBCs • Fresh-frozen plasma	These replace blood loss and increase oxygen-carrying capability. They also replace coagulation factors.	All types of shock if hemoglobin is <120 g/L or if the patient does not respond to crystalloids	Use same precautions as for any blood administration (see Chapter 33).
Colloids			
• Hetastarch	This is made from starch and acts as volume expander; it is at least as effective as albumin; it can exert osmotic effect for up to 36 hr.	All types of shock except cardiogenic and neurogenic shock	This may be 50% less costly than albumin. Use cautiously in patients with heart failure, renal failure, or bleeding disorders (because of antiplatelet effect).
• Human serum albumin (5%, 25%), plasma protein fraction (5% albumin in 500 mL of NSS)	This can increase plasma colloid osmotic pressure and produces rapid volume expansion.	All types of shock except cardiogenic and neurogenic shock	Monitor patient for circulatory overload. Mild adverse effects of chills, fever, and urticaria may develop. This product is more expensive than other colloids.
• Dextran; dextran 40; dextran 70	This is a hyperosmotic glucose polymer; similar degrees of volume expansion are achieved with dextran, dextran 40, and dextran 70; duration of action is longer with dextran 70.	Limited use because of adverse effects, including reducing platelet adhesion, diluting clotting factors	This product increases risk of bleeding. Patient must be monitored for allergic reactions and acute renal failure.

NSS, normal saline solution; *RBCs,* red blood cells.

receiving large volumes of packed RBCs, it is important to remember that they do not contain clotting factors. Therefore, clotting factors must be replaced on the basis of the clinical situation and results of blood studies. If the patient has chronic hypotension after adequate fluid resuscitation, a vasopressor (e.g., dopamine, norepinephrine [Levophed]) or an inotrope (e.g., dobutamine) may be added. The goal of fluid resuscitation remains the restoration of tissue perfusion. Thus decisions about which agent to use should be based on the physiological goal. Although BP helps determine whether the patient's CO is adequate, an assessment of end-organ perfusion (e.g., urine output, neurological function, peripheral pulses) provides information that is more relevant.

Drug Therapy. The primary goal of drug therapy for shock is the correction of decreased tissue perfusion. Medications are administered intravenously via an infusion pump, ideally via a central venous catheter. One of the key reasons for administration of these medications via a central catheter is that many of the medications that have vasoconstrictor properties may cause extravasation if administered peripherally (Table 69-10).

Sympathomimetic Drugs. Many of the drugs used in the treatment of shock have an effect on the SNS. Drugs that mimic the action of the SNS are termed *sympathomimetic.* The effects of these drugs are mediated through their binding to α-adrenergic or β-adrenergic receptors. The various drugs have different relative α-adrenergic and β-adrenergic effects. (See Chapter 35, Table 35-2, for a discussion of adrenergic receptors.) Many of the sympathomimetic drugs cause peripheral vasoconstriction and are referred to as *vasopressor drugs* (e.g., epinephrine [Adrenalin], norepinephrine). These drugs have the potential to cause severe peripheral vasoconstriction and an increase in SVR. This further jeopardizes tissue perfusion, either directly or indirectly. The increased SVR increases the workload of the heart and can be detrimental to a patient in cardiogenic shock by causing further myocardial damage. Use of vasopressor drugs is generally reserved for patients who have been unresponsive to other therapies. Adequate fluid resuscitation must be achieved before the use of any vasopressor because peripheral vasoconstrictor effects in patients with low blood volume cause further reduction in tissue perfusion.

DRUG THERAPY

Table 69-10 Shock*

MECHANISM OF ACTION	HEMODYNAMIC EFFECTS	TYPE OF SHOCK	NURSING IMPLICATIONS
Dobutamine			
↑ Myocardial contractility ↓ Ventricular filling pressures	↓ SVR and PAOP ↑ CO, stroke volume, and CVP ↑↓ HR	Used for cardiogenic shock with severe systolic dysfunction Used for septic shock with normal CO that is not meeting metabolic demands	Correct hypovolemia. Do not administer in same catheter with NaHCO$_3$. Administration via central catheter is recommended (infiltration leads to tissue sloughing). Monitor HR and BP (hypotension may worsen, necessitating addition of a vasopressor). Monitor for tachydysrhythmias.
Dopamine			
Precursor to epinephrine and norepinephrine Hemodynamic effects from release of norepinephrine Positive inotropic effects: • ↑ Myocardial contractility • ↑ Automaticity • ↑ Atrioventricular conduction Low doses: ↑ blood flow to renal, mesenteric, and cerebral circulation High doses: can cause progressive vasoconstriction	↑ HR ↑ CO ↑ BP	Cardiogenic shock: • ↑ Mean arterial pressure • ↑ HR • ↑ MVO$_2$	Correct hypovolemia. Administer via central catheter (infiltration leads to tissue sloughing); do not administer in same catheter with NaHCO$_3$. Monitor for tachydysrhythmias. Monitor for peripheral vasoconstriction at moderate to high doses (e.g., paraesthesias, coldness in extremities).
Epinephrine (Adrenalin)			
Low doses: β-adrenergic agonist (cardiac stimulation, bronchial dilation, peripheral vasodilation)	↑ HR, contractility, and CO ↓ SVR	Cardiogenic shock combined with afterload reduction Anaphylactic shock	Correct hypovolemia if necessary. Monitor for HR >110 beats/minute. Monitor for dyspnea and pulmonary edema.
High doses: α-adrenergic agonist (peripheral vasoconstriction)	↑ Stroke volume ↑ SVR ↑ Systolic BP, ↓ diastolic BP, widened pulse pressure ↑ CVP, PAOP	Cardiac arrest, pulseless ventricular tachycardia, ventricular fibrillation, asystole	Monitor for renal failure secondary to ischemia. Monitor for chest pain, dysrhythmias secondary to ↑ MVO$_2$.
Hydrocortisone (Solu-Cortef)			
Decreases inflammation; reverses increased capillary permeability	↑ BP, HR	Septic shock necessitating vasopressor therapy, despite fluid resuscitation, to maintain adequate BP Anaphylactic shock if hypotension persists past initial therapy	Monitor for hypokalemia and hyperglycemia.
Norepinephrine (Levophed)			
β$_1$-Adrenergic agonist (cardiac stimulation) α-Adrenergic agonist (peripheral vasoconstriction) Renal and splanchnic vasoconstriction	↑ BP, MAP ↑ CVP, PAOP ↑ SVR ↑ or ↓ CO	Cardiogenic shock after myocardial infarction Septic shock: works by increasing vascular tone	Used for hypotension unresponsive to adequate fluid resuscitation. Administer via a central catheter (infiltration leads to tissue sloughing). Monitor for dysrhythmias secondary to ↑ MVO$_2$ requirements.

BP, blood pressure; *CO*, cardiac output; *CVP*, central venous pressure; *HR*, heart rate; *MAP*, mean arterial pressure; *MVO$_2$*, myocardial oxygen consumption; *PAOP*, pulmonary artery occlusive pressure; *SVR*, systemic vascular resistance.

Continued

Table 69-10 Shock—cont'd

MECHANISM OF ACTION	HEMODYNAMIC EFFECTS	TYPE OF SHOCK	NURSING IMPLICATIONS
Phenylephrine (Neo-Synephrine)			
α-Adrenergic agonist Vasoconstriction: renal, mesenteric, splanchnic, cutaneous, and pulmonary vessels	↑ HR ↑ BP ↑ SVR ↑↓ CO	Neurogenic shock	Monitor for reflex bradycardia, headache, restlessness. Monitor for renal failure secondary to ↓ renal blood flow. Administer via central catheter (infiltration leads to tissue sloughing).
Nitroglycerin			
Venodilation Dilates coronary arteries ↓ Preload ↓ MVO₂	↓ SVR ↓ BP	Cardiogenic shock	Continuously monitor BP and for reflex tachycardia. Use glass bottles for storage of drug.
Sodium Nitroprusside (Nipride)			
Arterial and venous vasodilation ↓ Preload, afterload	↓ CVP, PAOP ↑↓ CO ↓ BP	Cardiogenic shock with ↑ SVR	Continuously monitor BP. Protect solution from light; wrap infusion bottle with opaque covering. Administer with D₅W only. Monitor for cyanide toxicity (e.g., tinnitus, hyperreflexia, confusion, seizures).
Vasopressin (Pressyn)			
Antidiuretic hormone, nonadrenergic vasoconstrictor	↑ MAP ↑ Urine output ↓ Need for other vasopressors	Shock states (most commonly septic shock) refractory to other vasopressors	Usually administer low dose. Monitor hemodynamic pressures and urine output.

*Consult individual facility's guidelines, pharmacist, pharmacology references, and drug manufacturer's administration materials for additional information and dosage recommendations.

D_5W, 5% dextrose in water; *INR*, international normalized ratio; *PTT*, partial thromboplastin time.

The goals of vasopressor therapy are to achieve and maintain a mean arterial pressure of at least 65 mm Hg (Dellinger et al., 2008). The nurse must continuously monitor end-organ perfusion (e.g., urine output, SvO_2, serum lactate levels) to ensure that tissue perfusion is adequate.

Vasodilator Drugs. Some patients in shock show evidence of excessive vasoconstriction and poor tissue perfusion in spite of fluid replacement and normal or even high systemic BP. This is especially true of patients in cardiogenic shock. Although generalized sympathetic vasoconstriction is a useful compensatory mechanism for maintaining systemic pressure, excessive constriction can reduce tissue blood flow and increase the workload of the heart. The rationale for using vasodilator therapy for a patient in shock is to break the deleterious cycle in which widespread vasoconstriction causes a decrease in cardiac output and BP, resulting in further SNS-induced vasoconstriction.

The goal of vasodilator therapy, as in vasopressor therapy, is to maintain a MAP of 60 to 65 mm Hg or higher. It is also important to closely monitor PA pressures along with MAP so that fluid administration can be increased or the dose of the vasodilator decreased if CO or BP falls dramatically. The vasodilator agent most often used for the patient in cardiogenic shock is nitroglyc-

erin. Vasodilation may be enhanced with nitroprusside (Nipride) in noncardiogenic shock.

Nutritional Therapy. Protein–calorie malnutrition is one of the primary manifestations of hypermetabolism in shock. Nutrition is vital in decreasing morbidity. Enteral nutrition should be initiated within the first 24 hours (Aitken et al., 2011; Dellinger, et al., 2008). A continuous drip of very small amounts of enteral feedings is started early on to enhance perfusion of the GI tract and help maintain the integrity of the gut mucosa.

Parenteral nutrition may be required when enteral nutrition is contraindicated; however, it must be used with caution because the dextrose can cause hyperglycemia and the lipids can have an immunosuppressive effect (McClave & Heyland, 2009). (Parenteral nutrition and enteral tube feedings are discussed in Chapter 42.)

A patient in shock should be weighed daily on the same scale at the same time of day. If the patient exhibits a significant weight loss, dehydration should be ruled out before additional calories are provided. Large weight gains are common because of third spacing of fluids. Therefore, daily weight measurements may function better as an indicator of fluid status than do caloric needs and balance. Serum protein, nitrogen balance, BUN, serum glucose level, and serum electrolyte values are all used to assess nutritional status.

Collaborative Care: Specific Measures

Cardiogenic Shock. For a patient in cardiogenic shock, the overall goal is to restore blood flow to the myocardium by restoring the balance between oxygen supply and demand. Definitive measures to restore blood flow include thrombolytic therapy, angioplasty with stent implantation, emergency revascularization, and valve replacement (see Chapter 36). Cardiac catheterization should be performed as soon as possible after the initial insult. Coronary angioplasty with or without stent implantation may be performed during the cardiac catheterization. Until these interventions can be performed, stroke volume and CO must be optimized in an effort to facilitate optimal perfusion (Table 69-11; see also Table 69-10).

Treatment measures of a patient in cardiogenic shock are geared toward reducing the workload of the heart through reperfusion, drug therapy, or mechanical interventions. Early

COLLABORATIVE CARE

Table 69-11 Specific Strategies for the Treatment of Shock

CARDIOGENIC SHOCK	HYPOVOLEMIC SHOCK	SEPTIC SHOCK	NEUROGENIC SHOCK	ANAPHYLACTIC SHOCK
Oxygenation				
• Provide supplemental O₂ (e.g., via nasal cannula, non-rebreather mask) • Initiate intubation and mechanical ventilation, if necessary • Monitor SvO₂ or ScvO₂	• Provide supplemental O₂ • Monitor SvO₂ or ScvO₂	• Provide supplemental O₂ • Initiate intubation and mechanical ventilation, if necessary • Monitor SvO₂ or ScvO₂	• Maintain patency of airway • Provide supplemental O₂ • Initiate intubation and mechanical ventilation, if necessary	• Maintain patency of airway • Optimize oxygenation with supplemental O₂ • Initiate intubation and mechanical ventilation, if necessary
Circulation				
• Restore blood flow with thrombolytics, angioplasty with stent implantation, emergency coronary revascularization • Reduce workload of the heart with circulatory assist devices (IABP, VAD)	• Restore fluid volume (e.g., blood or blood products, crystalloids) • Provide rapid fluid replacement via two large-bore (14- to 16-gauge) peripheral IV lines • Accomplish end points of fluid resuscitation: • CVP of 15 mm Hg • PAOP of 10-12 mm Hg	• Provide aggressive fluid resuscitation • Accomplish end points of fluid resuscitation: • CVP of 15 mm Hg • PAOP of 10-12 mm Hg	• Administer fluids with caution	• Provide aggressive fluid resuscitation with colloids
Drug Therapies				
• Nitrates (e.g., nitroglycerin) • Inotropes (e.g., dobutamine) • Diuretics (e.g., furosemide) • β-Adrenergic blockers (contraindicated with ↓ ejection fraction)	No specific drug therapies	• Antibiotics as ordered • Vasopressors (e.g., dopamine) • Inotropes (e.g., dobutamine) • Anticoagulants (e.g., low-molecular weight heparin)	• Vasopressors (e.g., phenylephrine) • Atropine (for bradycardia)	• Antihistamines (e.g., diphenhydramine) • Epinephrine (subQ, IV, with nebulizer) • Bronchodilators: with nebulizer (e.g., albuterol) • Corticosteroids (if hypotension persists)
Supportive Therapies				
• Correct dysrhythmias	• Correct the cause (e.g., stop bleeding, GI losses) • Use warmed fluids	• Obtain cultures (e.g., blood, wound) before beginning antibiotics • Monitor temperature • Control blood glucose level • Prevent stress ulcers	• Minimize spinal cord trauma with stabilization • Monitor temperature	• Identify and remove offending cause • Prevent by avoidance of known allergens • Premedicate according to history of prior sensitivity (e.g., contrast media)

CVP, central venous pressure; *GI*, gastrointestinal; *IABP*, intra-aortic balloon pump; *IV*, intravenously; *PAOP*, pulmonary artery occlusive pressure; *subQ*, subcutaneously; *ScvO₂*, central venous oxygen saturation; *SvO₂*, venous oxygen saturation; *VAD*, ventricular assist device.

recognition and prompt revascularization by means of percutaneous coronary intervention or coronary artery bypass graft (CABG) substantially improves survival rates. Fibrinolytic therapy is another option for reperfusion. Inotropes and vasopressors in low doses are effective pharmacological agents. Dopamine is the first drug of choice because it is both an inotrope and a vasopressor. Dobutamine is an effective inotrope for patients with mild hypotension and can improve cardiac output when combined with a vasopressor, such as norepinephrine or vasopressin. Patients with pulmonary edema should receive diuretics. Aspirin is given to patients with acute MI. Amiodarone is used to treat arrhythmias. β-Blockers and nitrates should be given with caution and avoided in the acute stage (Reynolds & Hochman, 2008; Topalian et al., 2008).

Patients may also benefit from a circulatory assist device such as an intra-aortic balloon pump (IABP) or a ventricular assist device (VAD) (see Chapter 68). The IABP is a circulatory assist device that is inserted into the femoral artery and placed in the aorta just distal to the aortic arch. The goal of this intervention is to increase coronary blood flow and thus decrease left ventricular workload. The VAD is used when cardiogenic shock is refractory to the IABP or fibrinolytic therapy. It is a temporary measure for patients who are in cardiogenic shock or awaiting cardiac transplantation. Cardiac transplantation is an option for a small and select group of patients with cardiogenic shock.

Hypovolemic Shock.
The underlying principles of managing patients with hypovolemic shock focus on stopping the loss of fluid and restoring the circulating volume. Fluid resuscitation in hypovolemic shock initially is calculated according to a 3:1 rule (3 mL of isotonic crystalloid for every 1 mL of estimated blood loss). Table 69-9 delineates the different types of fluid used for volume resuscitation, the mechanisms of action, and specific nursing implications for each fluid type.

Septic Shock.
Patients in septic shock require large amounts of fluid replacement, sometimes as much as 6 to 10 L of isotonic crystalloids and 2 to 4 L of colloids (Dellinger et al., 2008). Predetermined end points of fluid resuscitation are suggested in Table 69-11. To optimize and evaluate large-volume fluid resuscitation, hemodynamic monitoring with a PA catheter or central venous catheter and arterial pressure monitoring may be necessary. The overall goal of fluid resuscitation is to restore perfusion. If that cannot be accomplished with IV fluids, vasopressor drug therapy may be added. Vasodilation and low CO, or vasodilation alone, can cause low BP in spite of adequate volume resuscitation. Vasopressin (Pitressin) may be given for patients whose condition is refractory to vasopressor therapy (Bridges & Dukes, 2005; Dellinger et al., 2008). Exogenous vasopressin is used to replace the stores of physiological vasopressin that are often depleted in septic shock.

Vasopressor drugs may increase BP but may also result in a decrease in stroke volume. An inotropic agent (e.g., dobutamine) is often added to offset the decrease in stroke volume (see Table 69-10). In addition, IV corticosteroids are recommended for patients who require vasopressor therapy, despite fluid resuscitation, to maintain adequate BP (Dellinger et al., 2008). In an attempt to meet the increasing tissue demands coupled with a low SVR, the patient initially demonstrates normal or high CO. If the patient is unable to achieve and maintain adequate CO and has unmet tissue oxygen demands, CO may have to be increased through drug therapy (e.g., dobutamine; Dellinger et al., 2008). The adequacy of CO can be assessed with SvO_2 monitoring. The

SvO_2 (normal, 65-75%) is a reflection of the balance between oxygen delivery and consumption (see Chapter 68). If the balance is maintained, the tissue demands are met.

Antibiotics are an important and early component of therapy. Outcomes are improved if administered within the first 6 hours (Dellinger, et al., 2008; Francis, Rich, Williamson, & Peterson, 2010). Before definitive treatment for the infection begins, the cause of the infection must be identified. Cultures (e.g., blood, wound exudate, urine, stool, sputum) are obtained before antibiotics are started. Broad-spectrum antibiotics are given initially, followed by antibiotics that are more specific once the organism has been identified (Dellinger et al., 2008).

Drotrecogin alfa (Xigris), a recombinant form of activated protein C, has provided treatment of patients with severe sepsis through producing an anti-inflammatory effect. Activated protein C is a naturally occurring substance in the body but is found in subnormal levels in patients with sepsis. Drotrecogin interrupts the body's response to severe sepsis, including bleeding and clotting abnormalities. Experts reported a significant decrease in mortality rate when it was used for patients with severe sepsis and septic shock (Dellinger et al., 2008; Tazbir, 2004). However, it was withdrawn from the market in October 2011 and removed from the International Guidelines for management of severe sepsis and septic shock (Dellinger et al., 2008) by the Surviving Sepsis Campaign executive committee because it failed to demonstrate a statistical reduction in mortality during the PROWESS-SHOCK study (Surviving Sepsis Campaign, 2011).

Glucose levels should be maintained at less than 8.33 mmol/L (Dellinger et al., 2008). Research has shown improved survival rates when continuous infusions of insulin and glucose are used to keep glucose levels between 4.44 and 6.11 mmol/L (Dellinger et al., 2008). Therefore, frequent monitoring of glucose levels of all patients in septic shock is necessary. Stress ulcer prophylaxis with histamine H_2-receptor blockers (e.g., famotidine [Pepcid]) and deep venous thrombosis prophylaxis with low-dose unfractionated heparin or low-molecular weight heparin (e.g., enoxaparin [Lovenox]) are also recommended for these patients (Dellinger et al., 2008).

Neurogenic Shock.
The specific treatment of neurogenic shock is dependent on the cause. If the cause is spinal cord injury, general measures to promote spinal stability (e.g., spinal precautions, cervical stabilization with a collar) are initially used. Once the spine is stabilized, definitive treatment of the hypotension and bradycardia is essential to prevent further spinal cord damage. Hypotension, which occurs as a result of a loss of sympathetic tone, is associated with peripheral vasodilation and decreased venous return. Treatment involves the use of vasopressors (e.g., phenylephrine [Neo-Synephrine]) to maintain BP and organ perfusion (see Table 69-10). Bradycardia may be treated with atropine. Fluids are administered cautiously because the cause of the hypotension is not related to fluid loss (Carlson, 2010).

The patient with a spinal cord injury also needs to be monitored for hypothermia because of hypothalamic dysfunction (see Table 69-11). Although corticosteroids do not have an effect in neurogenic shock, methylprednisolone (Solu-Medrol) is used for patients with a spinal cord injury to prevent secondary spinal cord damage caused by the release of chemical mediators (see Chapter 63).

Anaphylactic Shock.
The first strategy in managing patients at risk for anaphylactic shock is prevention. A thorough history is key in avoiding the risk factors for anaphylaxis (see Table 69-1).

The clinical presentation of anaphylactic shock is dramatic, and immediate intervention is required. Epinephrine remains the first line of treatment for anaphylactic shock (East, 2010). It causes peripheral vasoconstriction and bronchodilation and opposes the effect of histamine. Diphenhydramine (Benadryl) is administered to block the massive release of histamine from the allergic reaction.

Maintaining patency of the airway is important because the patient can quickly develop airway compromise from laryngeal edema or bronchoconstriction. Nebulized bronchodilators are highly effective. Aerosolized epinephrine can also be used to treat laryngeal edema. Endotracheal intubation or cricothyroidotomy may be necessary to secure and maintain airway patency (Resuscitation Council [UK], 2008).

Hypotension results from leakage of fluid out of the intravascular space into the interstitial space as a result of increased vascular permeability and vasodilation. Aggressive fluid resuscitation, predominantly with colloids, is necessary. Intravenous corticosteroids may be helpful in anaphylactic shock if significant hypotension persists after 1 to 2 hours of aggressive therapy (see Tables 69-10 and 69-11).

NURSING MANAGEMENT: SHOCK

Nursing Assessment

The role of the nurse is vital in the care of patients who are at risk for developing shock or are in a state of shock. The initial assessment should be geared toward the ABCs: *a*irway, *b*reathing, and *c*irculation. Further assessment should focus on the assessment of tissue perfusion and includes evaluation of vital signs, level of consciousness, peripheral pulses, capillary refill, skin (e.g., temperature, colour, moisture), and urine output. As shock progresses, the patient's skin becomes cooler and mottled, urine output decreases, peripheral pulses diminish, and neurological status continues to deteriorate.

To understand the complexity of the patient's clinical status, the nurse must integrate all the assessment data. As care is initiated (see Tables 69-7 and 69-11), it is essential for the nurse to obtain a brief history from the patient or another knowledgeable person. This information should include a description of the events leading to the shock condition, time at onset and duration of symptoms, and a health history (e.g., medications, allergies, date of last tetanus vaccination). In addition, details regarding any care that the patient received before hospitalization are also important.

Nursing Diagnoses

The main nursing diagnosis for the patient with shock is presented in Nursing Care Plan 69-1. Many other diagnoses are relevant, and examples appear in other chapters.

Planning

The overall goals for patients in shock include (a) assurance of adequate tissue perfusion, (b) restoration of normal or baseline BP, (c) return or recovery of organ function, and (d) avoidance of complications from prolonged states of hypoperfusion.

Nursing Implementation

Health Promotion

It is important for nurses to become involved in the prevention of shock. To prevent shock, the nurse must identify patients at risk. In general, patients who are older, those with debilitating illnesses, and those who are immunocompromised are at increased risk. Any person who sustains surgical or accidental trauma is at high risk for shock as a result of hemorrhage, spinal cord injury, and other conditions (see Table 69-1). Any patient who is at risk for decreased oxygen delivery or tissue hypoxia is also at risk for the development of shock. Planning is essential to help prevent shock after a susceptible individual has been identified. For example, a person with an MI, especially an anterior wall MI, is at risk for cardiogenic shock. The primary goal in this scenario is to limit the size of the infarction. The infarct size can be limited by restoring coronary blood flow through thrombolytic therapy, percutaneous coronary intervention, or surgical revascularization. Rest, analgesics, sedatives, and judicious use of paralytic agents (if the patient is intubated) can reduce the myocardial demand for oxygen. The nurse can modify the patient's environment to provide care at intervals that do not increase the patient's oxygen demand. For example, if the patient becomes anxious with bathing, that activity can be planned at a time so as not to interfere with radiographic examinations or other activities that may also increase oxygen demand.

A person with a severe allergy to such substances as drugs, shellfish, and insect bites is at increased risk for developing anaphylactic shock. The risk of anaphylactic shock can be decreased if the patient is carefully questioned about allergies before a drug is administered (even if the patient has received this drug in the past) or before the patient undergoes diagnostic procedures involving the use of contrast media. If a patient's condition warrants receiving a medication to which he or she is at high risk for an allergic reaction (e.g., contrast media), the patient should receive a premedication such as diphenhydramine or methylprednisolone. Patients with severe allergies should wear a medical alert tag that identifies their allergies. The patient and those close to them should always have an epinephrine autoinjector (EpiPen) ready. They should know how to safely administer this autoinjector intramuscularly into the vastus lateralis site (Resuscitation Council [UK], 2008).

Careful monitoring of fluid balance can help prevent hypovolemic shock. Ongoing monitoring of intake and output and daily weight measurements are important. In addition, monitoring of the patient's clinical status is essential because trends in clinical findings are more meaningful than any single piece of clinical information.

All patients must be carefully monitored for the development of infection. Progression from an infection to sepsis and septic shock is dependent on the patient's host defence mechanisms. Patients who are immunocompromised or immunosuppressed are at especially high risk for developing an opportunistic infection. Interventions to decrease the risk of infection in hospitalized patients include decreasing the number of indwelling catheters (e.g., central lines, urinary catheters), using aseptic technique during invasive procedures, and paying strict attention to handwashing. In addition, all equipment must be changed according to institutional policy or thoroughly cleaned or discarded (if disposable) before use in another patient.

NURSING CARE PLAN 69-1

Shock*

NURSING DIAGNOSIS	***Ineffective tissue perfusion: Renal, cerebral, cardiopulmonary, gastrointestinal, hepatic, and peripheral*** related to low blood flow or maldistribution of blood *as evidenced by* the following possible findings:
	• Renal: urinary output <0.5 mL/kg/hr; ↑ BUN, ↑ plasma creatinine, ↑ BUN/creatinine ratio, ↑ urine specific gravity
	• Cerebral: anxiety, confusion, agitation, altered mentation, ↓ LOC, ↑ or ↓ temperature
	• Cardiopulmonary: ↓ BP, orthostatic hypotension, tachycardia; dysrhythmias, ↓ CVP and PAOP; weak, thready pulses; flat neck veins; tachypnea, ↓ SpO₂; crackles; ↑ ventilation–perfusion mismatch, refractory hypoxemia, respiratory failure
	• Gastrointestinal: ↓ bowel sounds, paralytic ileus, hyperglycemia or hypoglycemia
	• Hepatic: ↑ liver enzymes (e.g., ALT, AST, GGT), ↑ NH₃ and lactate
	• Peripheral: ↓ peripheral pulses, cool and clammy skin, decreased capillary refill, pallor or cyanosis

Expected Patient Outcomes	Nursing Interventions and *Rationales*
• Experiences adequate tissue perfusion with restoration of normal blood pressure • Recovers normal organ function with no complications from hypoperfusion	**Shock management** • Monitor vital signs, orthostatic blood pressure, mental status, and urinary output *to assess trends in patient's condition and evaluate patient's response to treatment.* • Monitor trends in hemodynamic parameters (e.g., CVP, PAP, PAOP) *to assess patient's status and detect fluid deficits or excesses and to evaluate patient's response to treatment.* • Administer fluids *to maintain blood pressure and cardiac output.* • Monitor laboratory evidence of inadequate tissue perfusion (e.g., increased lactic acid levels, decreased arterial pH levels) *to assess trends in patient's status and evaluate patient's response to treatment.* • Monitor determinants of tissue oxygen delivery (e.g., PaO₂, SpO₂, ScvO₂, SvO₂, hemoglobin levels, cardiac output) *to assess trends in patient's status and evaluate patient's response to treatment.* • Monitor for symptoms of respiratory failure (e.g., low PaO₂, elevated PaCO₂, respiratory muscle fatigue) *to plan respiratory interventions.* • Monitor fluid status, including hourly intake and output, *to evaluate response to treatment.* • Monitor renal function (e.g., BUN, creatinine levels) *to evaluate response to treatment.* • Provide oxygen therapy, mechanical ventilation, or both *to maximize oxygenation and keep SpO₂ at >90% to maintain normal levels.* **Cardiac management** • Monitor for symptoms of inadequate coronary artery perfusion (e.g., ST changes on ECG or angina) *to assess cardiac function.* • Promote optimal preload *to improve contractility while minimizing heart failure (e.g., administer nitroglycerin and maintain PAOP within prescribed range).* • Promote coronary artery perfusion (e.g., maintain mean arterial pressure at >60 mm Hg and control tachycardia) *to prevent myocardial ischemia.* **Vasogenic management** • Remove stimuli precipitating neurogenic reaction *to control symptoms.* • Administer antibiotics, antihistamines, epinephrine, and anti-inflammatory drugs, if appropriate, *to control symptoms.* **Volume management** • Monitor the patient closely for hemorrhage. • Note hemoglobin and hematocrit levels before and after blood loss *to evaluate patient's response to treatment.* • Administer blood products (e.g., platelets or fresh-frozen plasma) *to replace lost volume.*

ALT, alanine aminotransferase; *AST,* aspartate aminotransferase; *BP,* blood pressure; *BUN,* blood urea nitrogen; *CVP,* central venous pressure; *ECG,* electrocardiography; *GGT,* γ-glutamyl transferase; *LOC,* level of consciousness; *PAP,* pulmonary artery pressure; *PaCO₂,* partial pressure of arterial carbon dioxide; *PaO₂,* partial pressure of arterial oxygen; *PAOP,* pulmonary artery occlusive pressure; *ScvO₂,* central venous oxygen saturation; *SpO₂,* percentage of oxygen saturation of hemoglobin measured by pulse oximetry; *SvO₂,* venous oxygen saturation.

*The outcomes and related interventions are not all-inclusive and vary according to the type of shock that the patient is experiencing.

Acute Intervention

The role of the nurse in the treatment of shock involves (a) monitoring the patient's ongoing physical and emotional status to detect subtle changes in the patient's condition, (b) planning and implementing nursing interventions and therapy, (c) evaluating the patient's response to therapy, (d) providing emotional support to the patient and family, and (e) collaborating with other members of the health team to coordinate care (see Nursing Care Plan 69-1).

Neurological Status.

Neurological status, including orientation and level of consciousness, should be assessed every hour or more often. The patient's neurological status is the best indicator of cerebral blood flow. The nurse should be aware of the clinical manifestations that may indicate neurological involvement, such as changes in behaviour, restlessness, hyperalertness, blurred vision, confusion, and paraesthesias. The nurse must also be alert to any subtle changes in the neurological status (e.g., mild agitation).

Attempts should be made to orient the patient to time, place, person, and events. If the patient is in a critical care unit, orientation to the environment is particularly important. Measures such as minimizing noise and light levels should be taken to control sensory input. A day–night cycle of activity and rest should be maintained as much as possible. Sensory overload and disruption of the patient's diurnal cycle may contribute to delirium.

Cardiovascular Status.

Most therapy for shock is based on information about the patient's cardiovascular status. If the patient is unstable, the heart rate, the BP, the central venous pressure, and the PA pressures, including continuous cardiac output (if available), should be assessed at least every 15 minutes. PAOP should be measured every 1 to 2 hours. (Hemodynamic monitoring is discussed in Chapter 68.) Monitoring trends in hemodynamic parameters yields more important information than individual numbers. Integration of hemodynamic data with physical assessment data is essential in planning strategies to manage the patient with shock.

Patients in shock often have hypotension, a critical factor in increased mortality rates. A retrospective cohort study performed between July 1989 and June 2004 in Canada and the United States revealed that if antimicrobial administration was initiated within the first hour of the onset of hypotension, mortality rates were markedly improved (Kumar et al., 2006).

The patient's ECG should be monitored continuously. Heart sounds should be assessed for the presence of an S_3 or S_4 sound or new murmurs. The presence of an S_3 sound in an adult may indicate heart failure. The frequency of monitoring is decreased as the patient's condition improves.

In addition to monitoring the patient's cardiovascular status, the nurse must administer the prescribed therapy that is designed to correct the dysfunctions of the cardiovascular system. The patient's response to fluid and medication administration is assessed as often as every 10 to 15 minutes. Appropriate adjustments (e.g., medication titration) should be made as needed. Once tissue perfusion is restored and the patient is stabilized, the frequency of monitoring is decreased, and the patient is slowly weaned off medications that support BP and tissue perfusion.

Respiratory Status.

The respiratory status of the patient in shock must be frequently assessed to ensure adequate oxygenation, detect complications early, and provide data regarding the patient's acid–base status. The rate, the depth, and the rhythm of respirations are initially monitored as frequently as every 15 to 30 minutes. Increased rate and depth provide information regarding the patient's attempts to correct metabolic acidosis. Breath sounds should be assessed every hour for any changes that may indicate fluid overload or accumulation of secretions.

Pulse oximetry is used to continuously monitor oxygen saturation. Pulse oximetry with a patient's finger or toe may not be accurate in an advanced shock state because of poor peripheral circulation. In this situation, the probe should be attached to the nose, the ear, or the forehead (according to the manufacturer's guidelines) to increase accuracy. Levels of arterial blood gases (ABGs) provide definitive information on ventilation and oxygenation status and acid–base balance. Initial interpretation of ABGs is often the nurse's responsibility. A PaO_2 below 60 mm Hg (in the absence of chronic lung disease) indicates the presence of hypoxemia and the need for the administration of higher oxygen concentrations or for a different mode of oxygen administration. Low partial pressure of arterial carbon dioxide ($PaCO_2$) in the presence of a low pH and low bicarbonate level may indicate that the patient is attempting to compensate for a metabolic acidosis. A rising $PaCO_2$ in the presence of a persistently low pH and PaO_2 may indicate the need for intubation and mechanical ventilation.

Most patients in shock are intubated and on mechanical ventilation. Maintaining airway patency and monitoring for ventilator-related complications are critical. (Artificial airways and mechanical ventilation are discussed in Chapter 68.)

Renal Status.

Hourly measurements of urinary output are essential in assessment of the adequacy of renal perfusion. An indwelling bladder catheter is inserted to facilitate measurements. Urine output of less than 0.5 mL/kg/hr may indicate inadequate perfusion of the kidneys. BUN and serum creatinine values are additional indicators used to assess renal function. Serum creatinine is a better indicator of renal function because BUN levels can be influenced by the catabolic state of the patient.

Body Temperature and Skin Changes.

When temperature is elevated or subnormal, tympanic or pulmonary arterial temperatures should be measured hourly. If normal, the temperature should be monitored every 4 hours. The patient should be kept comfortably warm with the use of light covers and the control of environmental temperature. If the patient's temperature rises above 38.6°C and the patient becomes uncomfortable or experiences cardiovascular compromise, the fever may be managed with nonsteroidal anti-inflammatory drugs (e.g., ibuprofen [Motrin]), with acetaminophen (Tylenol), or by removal of some of the patient's covers.

The patient's skin should be monitored for temperature, pallor, flushing, cyanosis, diaphoresis, and piloerection. In addition, capillary refill should be assessed as an indicator of peripheral perfusion.

Gastrointestinal Status.

Bowel sounds should be auscultated at least every 4 hours, and abdominal distension should be assessed. If a nasogastric tube is inserted, drainage should be measured and checked for occult blood. Stools should also be checked for occult blood.

Personal Hygiene.

Hygiene is especially important for patients in shock because impaired tissue perfusion predisposes the skin to breakdown and infection. However, bathing and other nursing measures must be carried out judiciously because a patient in shock is experiencing problems with oxygen delivery to tissues. The nurse must use clinical judgement in determining priorities of care in order to limit the demands for increased oxygen.

Oral care for patients in shock is essential because mucous membranes may become dry and fragile in the state of volume depletion. In addition, intubated patients usually have difficulty swallowing, which results in pooled secretions in the mouth. A water-soluble lubricant applied to the lips prevents drying and cracking. Moist swabbing of the tongue and oral mucosa with saline solution or diluted mouthwash is also beneficial. Lemon glycerin swabs should not be used because they can cause further drying of the mucosa.

Passive range of motion should be performed three to four times per day to maintain joint mobility. The patient should be turned at least every 1 to 2 hours and positioned in good body alignment to help prevent pressure ulcers. A pressure-relieving mattress or a specialty bed may also be needed. If possible, oxygen consumption (e.g., SvO_2 or $ScvO_2$) should be monitored during all nursing interventions to monitor the patient's tolerance of activity.

▪ Emotional Support and Comfort.

The nurse must recognize that the patient and the family are faced with a critical, life-threatening situation. The nurse should address any anxiety, fear, or pain because such symptoms may aggravate respiratory distress and increase the release of catecholamines. Medications to decrease anxiety and pain are common modes of therapy. Continuous infusions of a benzodiazepine (e.g., lorazepam [Ativan]), an opioid or anaesthetic (e.g., morphine, propofol [Diprivan]), and occasionally a neuromuscular blocking agent (e.g., cisatracurium [Nimbex]) are extremely helpful in decreasing anxiety, pain, and oxygen demand.

The nurse should talk to the patient and encourage the family to talk to the patient, even if the patient is intubated, is sedated, or appears comatose. Hearing is often the last sense to be diminished, and even if the patient cannot respond, he or she may still be able to hear. If the intubated patient is capable of writing, a "magic slate" or a pencil and paper should be provided. Alphabet boards or signboards with common requests (e.g., "turn," "fan," "lights") are also useful. The patient should also receive simple explanations of procedures before they are carried out, as well as information regarding the current plan of care and its rationale. Advanced directives should be discussed and documented. Questions by the patient and the family about progress and prognosis must be answered in a very compassionate manner. It is important for the nurse to provide culturally sensitive care (College of Nurses of Ontario, 2009) in whatever way does not compromise patient safety. This may include notifying an interpreter or non-traditional clergy if the patient wishes.

Family and significant others can have a therapeutic effect on the patient. To perform this role, they need to be supportive and comforting. Family and significant others (a) link the patient to the outside world, (b) facilitate decision making and advise the patient, (c) assist with activities of daily living, (d) act as liaisons to advise the health care team of the patient's wishes for care, and (e) provide safe, caring, familiar relationships for the patient. The family primarily needs to be kept informed of the patient's condition. If possible, the same nurses should continuously care for the patient to decrease anxiety, limit contradictory information, and increase trust. Should the prognosis become increasingly grave, the patient's family should be given support when making difficult decisions regarding continuation of life support. The nursing staff must support the family's decisions and facilitate realistic expectations and outcomes. It is important for the nurse

to remember that compassionate understanding is as essential as scientific and technical expertise in the total care of a patient and family (Maxwell, Stuenkel, & Saylor, 2007).

Family time with the patient should be facilitated, provided that the patient perceives this time as comforting. The nurse should explain in simple terms the purpose of tubes and equipment surrounding the patient, and the family should be informed of what they may and may not touch. If possible, the patient's hands and arms can be kept outside the sheets to encourage therapeutic touch. If desired, the family may be encouraged to perform simple comfort measures. Privacy should be provided as much as possible, but the patient and family should be assured that assistance is readily available if it is required. The call bell should be in reach at all times.

▪ Ambulatory and Home Care

Rehabilitation of the patient who has experienced critical illness must be monitored for indications of complications throughout the recovery period. Complications may include decreased range of motion, decreased physical endurance, renal failure after acute tubular necrosis, and the development of fibrotic lung disease as a result of ARDS (see Chapters 49 and 70). Thus patients recovering from shock may require diverse services on discharge. These can include admission to transitional care units (e.g., for weaning from mechanical ventilation), rehabilitation centres (inpatient or outpatient), or home health care agencies. The nurse should begin to anticipate and facilitate a safe transition from the hospital to home when the patient is admitted.

▪ Evaluation

Expected outcomes for the patient with shock are addressed in Nursing Care Plan 69-1.

Systemic Inflammatory Response Syndrome and Multiple-Organ Dysfunction Syndrome

Etiology and Pathophysiology

Systemic inflammatory response syndrome (SIRS) is a systemic inflammatory response to a variety of insults, including infection, ischemia, infarction, and injury (see Table 69-5). SIRS is characterized by at least two of the following: fever, edema, hypotension, tachycardia, impaired oxygenation, and elevated white blood cell count (Cheek et al., 2009).

A systemic inflammatory response can be triggered by many mechanisms. Examples are as follows:

- Mechanical tissue trauma: burns, crush injuries, surgical procedures
- Abscess formation: intra-abdominal, on extremities
- Ischemic or necrotic tissue: pancreatitis, vascular disease, myocardial infarction
- Microbial invasion: bacteria, viruses, fungi, parasites
- Endotoxin release: Gram-negative bacteria
- Global perfusion deficits: after cardiac resuscitation, in shock states
- Regional perfusion deficits: distal perfusion deficits

Multiple-organ dysfunction syndrome (MODS) is the failure of two or more organ systems in an acutely ill patient to such a degree that homeostasis cannot be maintained without intervention. MODS is a progression from SIRS. The mortality rate is 54% when two organs fail and 100% with five failing organs (Cheek et al., 2009; see Figure 69-1).

Organ and Metabolic Dysfunction. When the inflammatory response is not controlled, the consequences that occur include activation of inflammatory cells and release of mediators, direct damage to the endothelium, and hypermetabolism. Vasodilation becomes excessive and leads to decreased SVR and hypotension. In addition, vascular permeability increases, which allows mediators and protein to leak out of the endothelium and into the interstitial space. The white blood cells begin to phagocytize the foreign debris, and the coagulation cascade is activated (see Chapter 32). Organ perfusion may be compromised because of hypotension, decreased perfusion, microemboli, and redistributed or shunted blood flow.

The respiratory system is most commonly affected in MODS (Nguyen & Nguyen, 2009). Inflammatory mediators have a direct effect on the pulmonary vasculature. The endothelial damage from the release of inflammatory mediators results in an increase in capillary permeability and facilitates movement of proteinaceous fluid from the pulmonary vasculature into the pulmonary interstitial spaces. The fluid then moves to the alveoli, causing alveolar edema. Type I pneumocytes (alveolar cells) are destroyed. Type II pneumocytes become dysfunctional, and surfactant production decreases. The alveoli collapse, which leads to an increase in shunt (blood flow to the lungs that does not participate in gas exchange) and a worsening of the ventilation–perfusion mismatch. The end result is ARDS. Patients with ARDS require aggressive pulmonary management with mechanical ventilation. (See Chapter 70 for a complete discussion of ARDS.)

Cardiovascular changes in MODS include myocardial depression and massive vasodilation in response to increasing tissue demands. Vasodilation results in decreases in SVR and BP. The baroreceptor reflex causes release of inotropic factors (which increase force of contraction) and chronotropic factors (which increase heart rate) that enhance CO. To compensate for hypotension, CO rises by means of an increase in heart rate and stroke volume. Increases in capillary permeability cause a shift of albumin and fluid out of the vascular space, further diminishing venous return and thus preload. The patient becomes warm and tachycardic with a high CO and a low SVR. Other signs of MODS include decreased capillary refill, skin mottling, increases in central venous pressure and PAOP, and dysrhythmias. SvO$_2$ may be abnormally high because areas not consuming much oxygen (e.g., skin, nonworking muscle) are being perfused but other areas may have blood shunted away from them. Eventually, either perfusion of vital organs becomes insufficient, or the cells are unable to use oxygen and their function is further compromised.

Neurological dysfunction commonly manifests as mental status changes with SIRS and MODS. Acute alteration in mental status can be an early sign of MODS. The patient may become confused and agitated, combative, disoriented, lethargic, or comatose. These changes may be caused by hypoxemia, the direct effect of the inflammatory mediators, or impaired perfusion (Krau, 2007). Acute kidney injury is frequent in SIRS and MODS. Acute kidney injury can be caused not only by hypoperfusion but also by the effects of the mediators. When kidney perfusion is decreased, the SNS and the renin–angiotensin system are acti-

vated. The stimulation of the renin–angiotensin system results in systemic vasoconstriction and aldosterone-mediated sodium and water reabsorption. Another risk factor for the development of acute kidney injury is the use of nephrotoxic drugs. Antibiotics commonly used to treat Gram-negative bacteria, such as aminoglycosides, can be nephrotoxic. Careful monitoring of drug levels is essential to avoid the nephrotoxic effects.

The GI tract also plays a key role in the development of MODS. GI motility is often decreased in critical illness, and this results in abdominal distension and paralytic ileus. In the early stages of SIRS and MODS, blood also is shunted away from the GI mucosa; thus the mucosa is highly vulnerable to ischemic injury. Decreased perfusion leads to a breakdown of this normally protective mucosal barrier, thus increasing the risk for ulceration and GI bleeding. The breakdown of the mucosal barrier of the gut increases the potential for bacterial translocation from the GI tract into the systemic circulation, which provides a pathway to the lungs, liver, and kidneys (McClave & Heyland, 2009). Metabolic changes are pronounced in SIRS and MODS. Both syndromes trigger a hypermetabolic response. Glycogen stores are rapidly converted to glucose (glycogenolysis). Once glycogen is depleted, amino acids are converted to glucose (gluconeogenesis), which reduces protein stores. Fatty acids are mobilized for fuel. Catecholamines and glucocorticoids are released and result in hyperglycemia and insulin resistance. The net result is a catabolic state, and lean body mass (muscle) is lost.

The hypermetabolism that is associated with SIRS and MODS may last for several days and results in liver dysfunction. Liver dysfunction in MODS may exist long before it is clinically evident. Protein synthesis is impaired. The liver is unable to synthesize albumin, one of the key proteins that has an essential role in maintaining plasma oncotic pressure. Consequently, plasma oncotic pressure is altered, and fluid and protein leak from the vascular spaces to the interstitial space. Administration of albumin does not normalize oncotic pressure in this situation.

As the state of hypermetabolism persists, the patient is unable to convert lactate to glucose, and lactate accumulates (lactic acidosis). Despite increases in glycogenolysis and gluconeogenesis, the liver eventually becomes unable to maintain a glucose level, and the patient becomes hypoglycemic.

Failure of the coagulation system manifests as DIC. DIC results in simultaneous microvascular clotting and bleeding because of the depletion of clotting factors and platelets in addition to excessive fibrinolysis. (DIC is discussed in Chapter 33.) Electrolyte imbalances, which are common, are related to hormonal and metabolic changes and fluid shifts. These changes exacerbate mental status changes, neuromuscular dysfunction, and dysrhythmias. The release of antidiuretic hormone and aldosterone results in sodium and water retention. Aldosterone increases urinary potassium loss, and catecholamines cause potassium to move into the cell, which results in hypokalemia. Hypokalemia is associated with dysrhythmias and muscle weakness. Metabolic acidosis results from impairment in tissue perfusion, hypoxia, and a shift to anaerobic metabolism with a resultant increase in hydrogen ion production. Progressive renal dysfunction also contributes to metabolic acidosis. Hypocalcemia, hypomagnesemia, and hypophosphatemia are common.

Clinical Manifestations

The clinical manifestations of MODS are presented in Table 69-12.

Table 69-12 Multiple-Organ Dysfunction Syndrome: Clinical Manifestations and Management

SYSTEM	CLINICAL MANIFESTATIONS OF ORGAN FAILURE	MANAGEMENT
Respiratory	Development of ARDS (see Chapter 70): • Severe dyspnea • PaO$_2$/FiO$_2$ ratio <200 • Bilateral fluffy infiltrates on chest radiograph • PAOP <18 mm Hg • Ventilation–perfusion mismatch • Pulmonary hypertension • Increased minute ventilation • Increased respiratory rate • Decreased compliance • Refractory hypoxemia	Prevention Optimizing oxygen delivery, minimizing oxygen consumption Mechanical ventilation (see Chapter 68) • Positive end-expiratory pressure • Lung protective modes (e.g., pressure control or inverse ratio ventilation, low tidal volumes) • Permissive hypercapnia Positioning (e.g., continuous lateral rotation therapy, prone positioning)
Renal	Prerenal: renal hypoperfusion • BUN/creatinine ratio >20 : 1 • ↓ Urine Na$^+$ level to <40 mmol/L • ↑ Urine specific gravity to >1.020 • ↑ Urine osmolality Intrarenal: acute tubular necrosis • BUN/creatinine ratio <10 : 1-15 : 1 • ↑ Urine Na$^+$ level to >40 mmol/L • ↓ Urine osmolality • Urine specific gravity (≈1.010)	Diuretics • Loop diuretics (e.g., furosemide [Lasix]) • May need to increase dose owing to ↓ glomerular filtration rate Dopamine (Intropin) • Enhances renal blood flow • Improves renal perfusion • Increases urine output (if volume resuscitated) • May work synergistically with diuretics Continuous renal replacement therapy (see Chapter 49)
Hepatic	Bilirubin >34 micromol/L ↑ Liver enzymes (ALT, AST, GGT) ↑ Serum NH$_3$ ↓ Serum albumin, prealbumin, transferrin Jaundice Hepatic encephalopathy	Maintenance of adequate tissue perfusion Nutritional support (e.g., enteral feedings) Judicious use of hepatically metabolized drugs
Gastrointestinal	Mucosal ischemia • ↓ Intramucosal pH • Potential translocation of gut bacteria Hypoperfusion → ↓ peristalsis, paralytic ileus Mucosal ulceration on endoscopy GI bleeding	Stress ulcer prophylaxis • Antacids (e.g., Maalox) • Histamine H$_2$-receptor blockers (e.g., famotidine [Pepcid]) • Proton pump inhibitors (e.g., omeprazole) • Sucralfate Dietary consultation Enteral feedings • Stimulate mucosal activity • Provide essential nutrients and optimal calories
Central nervous	Acute change in neurological status Fever Hepatic encephalopathy Seizures Confusion, disorientation Failure to wean, prolonged rehabilitation	Evaluation for hepatic and metabolic encephalopathy Optimization of cerebral blood flow ↓ Cerebral oxygen requirements Prevention of secondary tissue ischemia • Calcium channel blockers (reduce cerebral vasospasm) Prevention of further compromise

ALT, alanine aminotransferase; *ARDS*, acute respiratory distress syndrome; *AST*, aspartate aminotransferase; *BUN*, blood urea nitrogen; *FiO₂*, fraction of inspired oxygen; *GGT*, γ-glutamyl transferase; *GI*, gastrointestinal; *PaO₂*, partial pressure of arterial oxygen; *PAOP*, pulmonary artery occlusive pressure.

Table 69-12 Multiple-Organ Dysfunction Syndrome: Clinical Manifestations and Management—cont'd

SYSTEM	CLINICAL MANIFESTATIONS OF ORGAN FAILURE	MANAGEMENT
Cardiovascular	Myocardial depression Biventricular failure Systolic, diastolic dysfunction ↑ HR, CO, SVR ↓ Stroke volume ↓ MAP ↓ Ejection fraction, contractility	Volume management • Pulmonary artery catheter for hemodynamic monitoring • ↑ Preload via volume replacement • Maximizing myocardial function • Maintaining CO • Arterial pressure monitoring • Maintaining MAP of >60 mm Hg Vasopressors Continuous SvO₂ monitoring; balance O₂ supply and demand Continuous electrocardiographic monitoring Circulatory assist devices • Intra-aortic balloon pump • Ventricular assist device
Hematological	↑ Bleeding times, ↑ PT, ↑ PTT, ↑ INR ↓ Platelet count (thrombocytopenia) ↑ Fibrin split products ↑ D-dimer test results	Observation for bleeding from obvious and occult sites Replacement of factors being lost (e.g., platelets) Minimizing traumatic interventions (e.g., intramuscular injections, multiple venipunctures)
Endocrinological	Hyperglycemia → hypoglycemia	Continuous infusion of insulin and glucose to maintain blood glucose at <8.33 mmol/L

CO, cardiac output; *HR,* heart rate; *INR,* international normalized ratio; *MAP,* mean arterial pressure; *PT,* prothrombin time; *PTT,* partial thromboplastin time; *SvO₂,* venous oxygen saturation; *SVR,* systemic vascular resistance.

NURSING AND COLLABORATIVE MANAGEMENT: SIRS AND MODS

MODS is an end-stage consequence that has been described as a "death" process (Papathanassoglou, Bozas, & Giannakopoulou, 2008). The most important goals are (a) to prevent the progression of SIRS to MODS and (b) strict adherence to prompt and supportive management (Krau, 2007).

A critical component of the nursing role is vigilant assessment and ongoing monitoring to detect early signs of deterioration or organ dysfunction. Collaborative care for patients with MODS focuses on (a) prevention and treatment of infection, (b) maintenance of tissue oxygenation, (c) nutritional and metabolic support, and (d) appropriate support of individual failing organs. Table 69-12 summarizes the management for patients with MODS.

■ Prevention and Treatment of Infection

Aggressive infection control strategies are essential to decrease the risk for hospital-acquired infections. Despite aggressive strategies, host dysfunction may lead to the development of an infection. Once an infection is suspected, interventions to control the source must be instituted. Appropriate cultures should be performed, and broad-spectrum antibiotic therapy should be initi-

ated. Early, aggressive surgery is recommended to remove necrotic tissue (e.g., early debridement of burn tissue) that may provide a culture medium for microorganisms. Once a specific organism is identified, therapy should be modified if necessary. Aggressive pulmonary management, including early ambulation, can reduce the risk of infection. Strict asepsis can decrease infections related to intra-arterial lines, endotracheal tubes, urinary catheters, IV lines, and other invasive devices or procedures.

■ Maintenance of Tissue Oxygenation

Hypoxemia frequently occurs in patients with SIRS and MODS. These patients have greater oxygen needs and decreased oxygen supply to the tissues. Interventions that decrease oxygen demand and increase oxygen delivery are essential. Sedation, mechanical ventilation, analgesia, paralysis, and rest may decrease oxygen demand and should be considered. Oxygen delivery may be optimized by maintaining normal levels of hemoglobin (e.g., transfusion of packed RBCs) and PaO₂ (80 to 100 mm Hg), using individualized tidal volumes with positive end-expiratory pressure (PEEP), increasing preload or myocardial contractility to enhance CO, or reducing afterload to increase CO.

■ Nutritional and Metabolic Needs

Hypermetabolism in SIRS or MODS can result in profound weight loss, cachexia, and further organ failure. Protein–calorie malnutrition is one of the primary manifestations of hypermetabolism and MODS. Total energy expenditure is often increased to 1.5 to 2.0 times the normal metabolic rate. Because of their relatively short half-life, plasma transferrin and prealbumin levels are monitored to assess hepatic protein synthesis.

The goal of nutritional support is to preserve organ function. Providing early and optimal nutrition decreases morbidity and mortality rates in patients with SIRS and MODS (Dellinger et al., 2008). The use of the enteral route is preferable to parenteral nutrition. If the enteral route cannot be used or cannot meet the caloric needs, parenteral nutrition should be initiated or added (McClave & Heyland, 2009). (Enteral and parenteral nutrition are discussed in Chapter 42.) Attention to tight glycemic control (blood glucose level of <8.33 mmol/L) with the use of insulin protocols is important in these patients (Dellinger et al., 2008).

Support of Failing Organs

Support of any failing organ is a primary goal of therapy. For example, the patient with ARDS requires aggressive oxygen therapy and mechanical ventilation (see Chapter 70). DIC should be treated appropriately (e.g., blood products; see Chapter 33). Renal failure may necessitate dialysis. Continuous renal replacement therapy (CRRT) is better tolerated than hemodialysis, especially in a patient with hemodynamic instability (see Chapter 49).

CLINICAL DECISION-MAKING EXERCISE

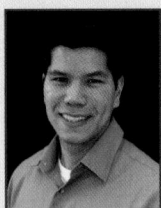

CASE STUDY:
Shock

Source: © iStockphoto.com/Yvonne Chamberlain.

Patient Profile

Mr. Lui, a 25-year-old Asian Canadian, was not wearing his seat belt when he was the driver involved in a motor vehicle collision. The windshield was broken, and Mr. Lui was found 4 metres from his car. He was face-down, conscious, and moaning. His wife and daughter were found in the car with their seat belts on. They sustained no obvious injuries but were very upset. All passengers were taken to the emergency department. The following information pertains to Mr. Lui.

Subjective Data

- States, "I can't breathe."
- Cries out when abdomen is palpated.

Objective Data

Physical Examination

- Cardiovascular: BP 80/56 mm Hg; apical pulse 135 but no radial or brachial pulses palpable; carotid pulse present but weak
- Lungs: respiratory rate 35 breaths/minute; laboured breathing with severe respiratory distress; asymmetrical chest wall movement; absence of breath sounds on left side
- Trachea deviated slightly to the right

- Abdomen: slightly distended and painful on palpation
- Musculoskeletal: open compound fracture of the lower left leg

Diagnostic Studies

- Chest radiograph: hemopneumothorax and rib fractures on left side
- Hematocrit: 28%

Collaborative Care

- In the emergency department, placement of left chest tube, which drained bright red blood

Surgical Procedure

- Splenectomy
- Repair of torn intercostal artery
- Repair of compound fracture

Discussion Questions

1. What type of shock was present in Mr. Lui? What clinical manifestations did he display?
2. What were the causes of Mr. Lui's shock? What are other causes of this type of shock?
3. *Priority Decision:* What are the priority nursing responsibilities for Mr. Lui?
4. *Priority Decision:* What ongoing nursing assessment parameters are essential for this patient?
5. What are his potential complications?
6. *Priority Decision:* On the basis of the assessment data presented, what are the priority nursing diagnoses?

ℰvolve *Answers are available at* **http://evolve.elsevier.com/ Canada/Lewis/medsurg**

REVIEW QUESTIONS

The number of the question corresponds to the same-numbered objective at the beginning of the chapter.

1. How is shock best defined?
   a. Cardiovascular collapse
   b. Loss of sympathetic tone
   c. Inadequate tissue perfusion
   d. Blood pressure less than 90 mm Hg systolic

2. A patient has a spinal cord injury at T4. Vital signs include a falling blood pressure with bradycardia. What type of shock is the patient probably experiencing?
   a. Relative hypervolemia
   b. Absolute hypovolemia
   c. Neurogenic shock from low blood flow
   d. Neurogenic shock from a maldistribution of blood flow

3. What early effect does shock have on the body?
   a. Sympathetic nervous system activation that results in stimulation of adrenergic receptors
   b. Massive vasoconstriction in the heart and brain that causes stimulation of the renin–angiotensin system
   c. Decreased tissue perfusion that results in anaerobic metabolism, leading to the development of lactic acidosis
   d. Heart rate that is usually slow and irregular in the compensatory stage because of parasympathetic nervous stimulation

4. A 78-year-old man is exhibiting confusion and a temperature of 40°C. He has diabetes and has purulent drainage from his right great toe. His assessment findings are as follows: BP, 84/40 mm Hg; heart rate, 110/minute; respiratory rate, 42/minute and shallow; cardiac output, 8 L/min; and PAOP, 4 mm Hg. What is this patient probably experiencing?
   a. Sepsis
   b. Septic shock
   c. Multiple organ dysfunction syndrome
   d. Systemic inflammatory response syndrome

5. What treatment modalities would be included in the management of cardiogenic shock?
   a. Dobutamine to increase myocardial contractility
   b. Vasopressors to increase SVR
   c. Corticosteroids to stabilize the cell wall in the infarcted myocardium
   d. Plasma volume expanders such as albumin to decrease an elevated preload

6. What are the most accurate assessment parameters for the nurse to use to determine adequate tissue perfusion in a patient with MODS?
   a. Blood pressure, pulse, and respirations
   b. Breath sounds, blood pressure, and body temperature
   c. Pulse pressure, level of consciousness, and pupillary response
   d. Level of consciousness, urine output, skin colour, and temperature

ANSWERS: 1. c; 2. d; 3. a; 4. b; 5. a; 6. d.

REFERENCES

Aitken, L. M., Williams, G., Harvey, M., Blot, S., Kleinpell, R., Labeau, S., …, Ahrens, T. (2011). Nursing considerations to complement the Surviving Sepsis Campaign guidelines. *Critical Care Medicine, 39,* 1800-1817.

Bridges, E. J., & Dukes, S. (2005). Cardiovascular aspects of septic shock: Pathophysiology, monitoring and treatment. *Critical Care Nurse, 25,* 14-24.

Bulger, E. (2011). 7.5% Saline and 7.5% saline/6% dextran for hypovolemic shock. *Journal of Trauma: Injury, Infection, and Critical Care, 70*(5), S27-S29. doi:10.1097/TA.0b013e31821a559a

Canadian Institute for Health Information. (2009). *In focus: A national look at sepsis.* Ottawa: Author. Retrieved from *https://secure.cihi.ca/free_products/HSMR_Sepsis2009_e.pdf*

Carlson, B. A. (2010). Shock. In L. D. Urden, K. M. Stacy, & M. E. Lough (Eds.), *Critical care nursing: Diagnosis and management* (6th ed., p. 990). St. Louis: Mosby.

Cheek, D. J., Rodgers, S. C., & Schulman, C. S. (2009). Systemic inflammatory response syndrome and multiorgan dysfunction syndrome. In K. K. Carlson (Ed.), *AACN advanced critical care nursing* (p. 1189). St. Louis: Saunders/Elsevier.

College of Nurses of Ontario. (2009). *Practice guideline: Culturally sensitive care.* Toronto: Author. Retrieved from *http://www.cno.org/Global/docs/prac/41040_CulturallySens.pdf*

Dellinger, R. P., Levy, M. M., Carlet, J. M., Bion, J., Parker, M. M., Jaeschke, K. R., …, World Federation of Societies of Intensive and Critical Care Medicine. (2008). Surviving Sepsis Campaign: International guidelines for management of severe sepsis and septic shock. *Critical Care Medicine, 36,* 296-327. doi:10.1097/01.CCM.0000298158.12101.41

East, L. (2010). Acute emergency situations. In F. Creed & C. Spiers (Eds.), *Care of the acutely ill adult: An essential guide for nurses* (pp. 385-425). New York: Oxford University Press.

Francis, M., Rich, T., Williamson, T., & Peterson, D. (2010). Effect of an emergency department sepsis protocol on time to antibiotic in severe sepsis. *Canadian Journal of Emergency Medicine, 12,* 303-310.

Guyton, A. C., & Hall, J. E. (2011). *Textbook of medical physiology* (12th ed.). Philadelphia: W. B. Saunders.

Hickey, J. V. (2009). *The clinical practice of neurological and neurosurgical nursing* (6th ed.). Philadelphia: Wolters Kluwer Health/Lippincott Williams & Wilkins.

Johnson, K. L., & Henry, K. (2009). Shock, systemic inflammatory response syndrome, and multiple organ dysfunction syndrome. In P. G. Morton & D. K. Fontaine (Eds.), *Critical care nursing: A holistic approach* (9th ed., pp. 1379-1407). Philadelphia: Wolters-Kluwer Health/Lippincott Williams & Wilkins.

Krau, S. D. (2007). Making sense of multiple organ dysfunction syndrome. *Critical Care Nursing Clinics of North America, 19,* 87-97. doi:10.1016/j.ccell.2006.11.002

Kumar, A., Roberts, D., Wood, K. E., Light, B., Parrillo, J. E., Sharma, S., …, Cheang, M. (2006). Duration of hypotension before initiation of effective antimicrobial therapy is the critical determinant of survival in human septic shock. *Critical Care Medicine, 34*(6), 1589-1596. doi:10.1097/01.CCM.0000217961.75225.E9

Lawrence, K. (2011). Pediatric sepsis and multiorgan dysfunction syndrome: Progress and continued challenges. *Critical Care Nursing Clinics of North America, 23,* 323-337. doi:10.1016/j.ccell.2011.02.005

Maxwell, K. E., Stuenkel, D., & Saylor, C. (2007). Needs of family members of critically ill patients: A comparison of nurse and family perceptions. *Heart & Lung, 36,* 367-376. doi:10.1016/j.hrtlng.2007.02.005

McClave, S. A., & Heyland, D. K. (2009). The physiologic response and associated clinical benefits from provision of early enteral nutrition. *Nutrition in Clinical Practice, 24,* 305-315. doi:10.1177/0884533609335176

Nguyen, L. N., & Nguyen, T. G. (2009). Characteristics and outcomes of multiple organ dysfunction syndrome among severe-burn patients. *Burns, 35,* 937-941. doi:10.1016/j.burns.2009.04.015

Papathanassoglou, E. D., Bozas, E., & Giannakopoulou (2008). Multiple organ dysfunction syndrome pathogenesis and care: A complex systems' theory perspective. *Nursing in Critical Care, 13,* 249-259. doi:10.1111/j.1478-5153.2008.00289.x

Powers, K. A., Burchell, P. L. (2010). Sepsis alert: Avoiding the shock. *Nursing, 40*(4):34-38.

Resuscitation Council (UK). (2008). *Emergency treatment of anaphylactic reactions: Guidelines for healthcare providers.* London: Working

Group of the Resuscitation Council (UK). Retrieved from *http://www.resus.org.uk/pages/reaction.pdf*

Reynolds, H. R., & Hochman, J. S. (2008). Cardiogenic shock: Current concepts and improving outcomes. *Circulation, 117,* 686-697. doi:10.1161/CIRCULATIONAHA.106.613596

Robson, W. P., & Daniels, R. (2008). The sepsis six: Helping patients to survive sepsis. *British Journal of Nursing, 17*(1), 16-21.

Surviving Sepsis Campaign. (2011). Surviving Sepsis Campaign guidelines. Retrieved from *http://www.survivingsepsis.org/guidelines/Pages/default.aspx*

Tazbir, J. (2004). Sepsis and the role of activated protein C. *Critical Care Nurse, 24,* 40-45.

Thibodeau, G. A., & Patton, K. T. (2007). *Anatomy and physiology* (6th ed.). St. Louis, MO: Mosby.

Topalian, S., Ginsberg, F., & Parrillo, J. E. (2008). Cardiogenic shock. *Critical Care Medicine, 36*(1), S66-S74. doi:10.1097/01.CCM.0000296268.57993.90

Wada, H., & Hatada, T. (2008). Pathophysiology and diagnostic criteria for disseminated intravascular coagulation associated with sepsis. *Critical Care Medicine, 36*(1), 348-349. doi:10.1097/01.CCM.0000295274.74280.00

World Health Organization. (2010). *Clinical management of adult patients with complications of pandemic influenza A (H1N1) 2009: Emergency guidelines for the management of patients with severe respiratory distress and shock in district hospitals in limited-resource settings.* Retrieved from *http://whqlibdoc.who.int/publications/2010/9789241599610_eng.pdf*

RESOURCES

Additional resources for this chapter are listed in Chapter 71, p. 2034.

Nursing Management: Respiratory Failure and Acute Respiratory Distress Syndrome

Written by Richard B. Arbour
Adapted by Debbie Rickeard

LEARNING OBJECTIVES

1. Compare the pathophysiological mechanisms that result in hypoxemic and hypercapnic respiratory failure.
2. Differentiate between early and late clinical manifestations of acute respiratory failure.
3. Describe the nursing and collaborative management of the patient with hypoxemic or hypercapnic respiratory failure.
4. Relate the pathophysiological mechanisms that result in acute respiratory distress syndrome (ARDS) to the clinical manifestations.
5. Describe the nursing and collaborative management of the patient with acute respiratory distress syndrome (ARDS).
6. Identify complications that may result from acute respiratory failure or acute respiratory distress syndrome (ARDS) and measures to prevent or reverse these complications.

KEY TERMS

acute respiratory distress syndrome (ARDS) A sudden and progressive form of acute respiratory failure in which the alveolar–capillary membrane becomes damaged and more permeable to intravascular fluid, p. 2004

alveolar hypoventilation A decrease in ventilation that results in an increased arterial carbon dioxide pressure ($PaCO_2$), p. 1993

diffusion limitation Occurs when gas exchange across the alveolar–capillary membrane is compromised by processes that thicken or destroy the membrane, p. 1993

hypercapnia Greater than normal amounts of carbon dioxide in the blood; also called *hypercarbia*, p. 1990

hypercapnic respiratory failure A condition in which the $PaCO_2$ is elevated in combination with acidemia, p. 1990

hypoxemia A condition that is manifested by a decrease in partial pressure of oxygen in arterial blood (PaO_2) and a decrease in arterial oxygen saturation (SaO_2), p. 1990

hypoxemic respiratory failure A condition in which the PaO_2 is 60 mm Hg or less when the patient is receiving inspired oxygen at a fractional concentration (FiO_2) of 60% or greater, p. 1990

hypoxia The state in which the PaO_2 has fallen sufficiently to cause signs and symptoms of inadequate oxygenation, p. 1995

refractory hypoxemia Hypoxemia unresponsive to increasing concentrations of oxygen, p. 2006

ELECTRONIC RESOURCES

Supplemental content related to Chapter 70 can be found…

Evolve Web Site evolve

http://evolve.elsevier.com/Canada/Lewis/medsurg
• Answer Guidelines for Case Study on p. 2010
• Clinical Reference: Laboratory Values
• Content Updates
• Customizable Nursing Care Plan: Acute Respiratory Failure

• Electronic Calculators
• Examination Review Questions
• Glossary
• Interactive Case Studies:
  • Acute Respiratory Failure
  • Pulmonary Embolism and Respiratory Failure
• Key Points (Printable and MP3 Download)

The normal function of the respiratory system is to facilitate gas exchange. Without an adequate exchange of oxygen (O_2) and carbon dioxide (CO_2), the metabolic demands of the tissues would not be met and body systems would begin to rapidly fail. The management of the patient in acute respiratory distress or failure revolves around the improvement of oxygenation and ventilation, treatment of the underlying disease state, reduction of anxiety, prevention, and management of complications. Acute respiratory failure and acute respiratory distress syndrome (ARDS) represent an important and costly public health problem. In a recent multicentre prospective cohort study, the incidence of acute lung injury (ALI) was 79 per 100,000 person-years, yielding more than 26,000 cases per year when applied to the Canadian population; of these, more than 45% will die (Lamontagne et al., 2010). These patients require critical nursing assessments and collaborative management to improve their outcomes, which will be the focus of this chapter.

Acute Respiratory Failure

The major function of the respiratory system is gas exchange, which involves the transfer of O_2 and CO_2 between the atmosphere and the blood (Figure 70-1) (Urden, Stacy, & Lough, 2010). *Respiratory failure* results when one or both gas-exchanging functions are inadequate, either insufficient O_2 is transferred to the blood or inadequate CO_2 is removed from the lungs. Clinical states that interfere with O_2 transfer result in **hypoxemia**, which is manifested by a decrease in partial pressure of oxygen in arterial blood (PaO_2; also called oxygen *tension*) and a decrease in arterial oxygen saturation as measured by arterial blood gases (SaO_2). Insufficient CO_2 removal results in **hypercapnia**, the presence of greater than normal amounts of CO_2 in the blood; also called *hypercarbia*, it is manifested by an increase in partial pressure (or tension) of carbon dioxide in arterial blood ($PaCO_2$) (Brashers, 2010). Arterial blood gases (ABGs) can be used to intermittently assess changes in pH, PaO_2, $PaCO_2$, bicarbonate, and SaO_2; and pulse oximetry can be applied to intermittently or continuously assess arterial oxygen saturation (SpO_2). Pulse oximetry offers advantages of noninvasiveness and real-time values; however, accurate readings depend on correct application of the sensor to a well-perfused digit, usually a middle or ring finger. When the SpO_2 is 90%, the PaO_2 is approximately 60 mm Hg, if factors such as temperature, $PaCO_2$ and pH are normal (Brashers, 2010). Data should be interpreted alongside clinical assessment findings and the patient's baseline values. For example, an individual with chronic lung disease may have a baseline $PaCO_2$ higher than what is considered the "normal" range. (To assist the reader, Table 70-1 summarizes abbreviations used in this chapter.)

Respiratory failure is not a disease; it is a condition that occurs as a result of one or more diseases involving the lungs or other body systems (Tables 70-2 and 70-3). It is classified as hypoxemic or hypercapnic (Figure 70-2). *Hypoxemic respiratory failure* is also referred to as *oxygenation failure* because the primary problem is inadequate O_2 transfer between the alveoli and the pulmonary capillary bed (Anderson & Spencer, 2009). Although no universal definition exists, **hypoxemic respiratory failure** is commonly defined as a PaO_2 of 60 mm Hg or less when the patient is receiving inspired oxygen at a fractional concentration (FiO_2) of 60% or greater. This definition incorporates two important concepts: (1) the PaO_2 level indicates inadequate O_2 saturation of hemoglobin; and (2) this PaO_2 level exists despite administration of supplemental O_2 at a percentage (60%) that is three times that in room air (21%). Disorders that interfere with O_2 transfer into the blood include pneumonia, pulmonary edema, pulmonary emboli, alveolar injury related to inhalation of toxic gases (e.g., smoke inhalation), and ventilator-induced lung injury. In addition, states of low cardiac output (e.g., congestive heart failure, shock) can also cause hypoxemic respiratory failure (Urden et al., 2010).

Hypercapnic respiratory failure is referred to as *ventilatory failure* because the primary problem is insufficient CO_2 removal. **Hypercapnic respiratory failure** is commonly defined as a $PaCO_2$

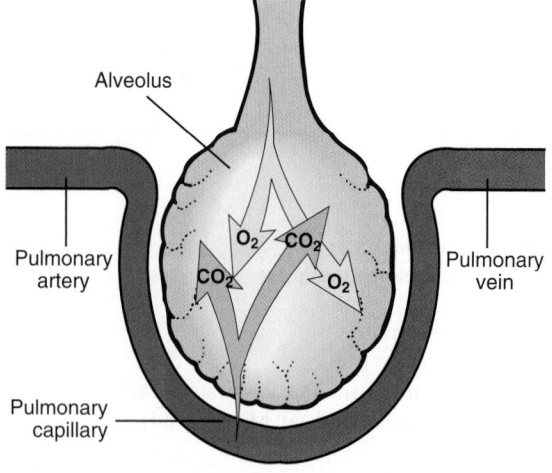

Figure 70-1 Normal gas-exchange unit in the lung.

Table 70-1 Glossary of Abbreviations	
Arterial Blood Monitoring	
ABGs	Arterial blood gases
pH	Negative log of the free hydrogen ion [H⁺]
PaO_2	Partial pressure of oxygen in arterial blood
$PaCO_2$	Partial pressure of carbon dioxide in arterial blood
SaO_2	Oxygen saturation in arterial blood as measured by ABGs
SpO_2	Oxygen saturation in arterial blood as measured by pulse oximetry
Oxygen and Lung Function Monitoring	
FiO_2	Fraction of inspired oxygen concentration
FRC	Functional residual capacity (volume of air in lung at end of expiration)
PEEP	Positive end-expiratory pressure (pressure in lungs at end of expiration)
PEFR	Peak expiratory flow rate (maximum airflow during a forced expiration)
$\dot{V}/\dot{Q}$	Ventilation–perfusion ratio (relationship of ventilation to perfusion in the lungs)
V_E	Minute ventilation (tidal volume × respiratory rate)
V_T	Tidal volume (volume of air inspired with each breath)

Table 70-2 Types of Respiratory Failure and Common Causes*

Hypoxemic Respiratory Failure	Chest Wall
Respiratory System	• Thoracic trauma (e.g., flail chest)
• ARDS	• Kyphoscoliosis
• Pneumonia	• Pain
• Toxic inhalation (smoke inhalation)	• Massive obesity
• Hepatopulmonary syndrome (low resistance flow state, $\dot{V}/\dot{Q}$ mismatch)	**Neuromuscular System**
	• Myasthenia gravis
• Massive pulmonary embolism (e.g., thrombus emboli, fat emboli)	• Critical illness polyneuropathy
	• Acute myopathy
Cardiac System	• Toxic ingestion (tree tobacco)
• Anatomical shunt (e.g., ventricular septal defect)	• Amyotrophic lateral sclerosis
	• Phrenic nerve injury
• Cardiogenic pulmonary edema	• Guillain-Barré syndrome
• Shock (decreasing blood flow through pulmonary vasculature)	• Poliomyelitis
	• Muscular dystrophy
Hypercapnic Respiratory Failure	• Multiple sclerosis
Respiratory System	
• Asthma	
• COPD	
• Cystic fibrosis	
Central Nervous System	
• Brainstem infarction	
• Sedative and narcotic overdose	
• Spinal cord injury	
• Severe head injury	

ARDS, acute respiratory distress syndrome; *COPD,* chronic obstructive pulmonary disease.
*This list is not all-inclusive.

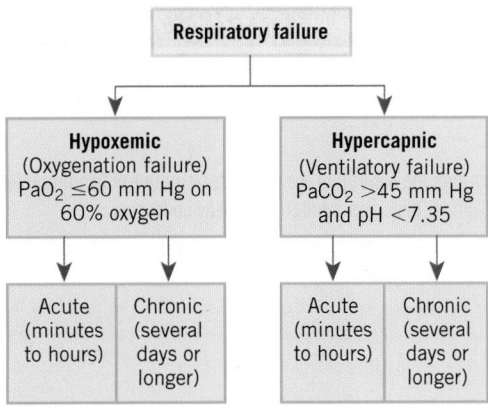

Figure 70-2 Classification of respiratory failure. *PaCO₂*, partial pressure of carbon dioxide in arterial blood; *PaO₂*, partial pressure of oxygen in arterial blood.

above normal (>45 mm Hg) in combination with academia (arterial pH <7.35). This definition incorporates three important concepts: (1) the $PaCO_2$ is higher than normal; (2) there is evidence of the body's inability to compensate for this increase (acidemia); and (3) the pH is at a level at which a further decrease may lead to severe acid–base imbalance. (See Chapter 19 for a discussion of acid–base balance.) Disorders that compromise lung ventilation and subsequent CO_2 removal include drug overdoses with central nervous system (CNS) depressants, neuromuscular diseases (e.g., myasthenia gravis), and trauma or diseases involving the spinal cord and its role in lung ventilation. Many patients experience both hypoxemic and hypercapnic respiratory failure.

Etiology and Pathophysiology

Hypoxemic Respiratory Failure. Common diseases and conditions that cause hypoxemic respiratory failure are listed in Table 70-2. Four physiological mechanisms may cause

hypoxemia and subsequent hypoxemic respiratory failure: (1) mismatch between ventilation ($\dot{V}$) and perfusion ($\dot{Q}$), commonly referred to as $\dot{V}/\dot{Q}$ mismatch; (2) shunt; (3) diffusion limitation; and (4) hypoventilation. The most common causes are $\dot{V}/\dot{Q}$ mismatch and shunt (Urden et al., 2010).

Ventilation–Perfusion ($\dot{V}/\dot{Q}$) Mismatch. In the normal lung, the volume of blood perfusing the lungs each minute (4 to 5 L) approximates the amount of fresh gas that reaches the alveoli each minute (4 to 5 L). In a perfectly matched system, each portion of the lung would receive about 1 mL of air for each 1 mL of blood flow. This match of ventilation and perfusion would result in a $\dot{V}/\dot{Q}$ ratio of 1 : 1 (e.g., 1 mL of air per 1 mL of blood), which is expressed as $\dot{V}/\dot{Q} = 1$. Ventilation is ideally matched with perfusion. Although this example implies that ventilation and perfusion are ideally matched in all areas of the lung, this situation does not normally exist. In reality, there is some regional mismatch even under normal conditions. At the lung apex, $\dot{V}/\dot{Q}$ ratios are greater than 1 (more ventilation than perfusion). At the lung base, $\dot{V}/\dot{Q}$ ratios are less than 1 (less ventilation than perfusion). Because changes at the lung apex balance changes at the base, the net effect is a close overall match (Figure 70-3).

Many diseases and conditions alter overall $\dot{V}/\dot{Q}$ matching and thus cause $\dot{V}/\dot{Q}$ mismatch (Figure 70-4). The most common are those in which increased secretions are present in the airways (e.g., chronic obstructive pulmonary disease [COPD]) or the alveoli (e.g., pneumonia) and when bronchospasm is present (e.g., asthma). $\dot{V}/\dot{Q}$ mismatch may also result from alveolar collapse (atelectasis) or from pain. Uncontrolled pain interferes with chest and abdominal wall movement, compromising lung ventilation. In addition, pain increases muscle and motor tension, producing generalized muscle rigidity; causes systemic vasoconstriction and activation of the stress response; and increases O_2 consumption and CO_2 production (Brashers, 2010). All of these conditions may increase both metabolic (O_2) and ventilatory demands and, at the same time, result in limited airflow (ventilation) to alveoli. Because no effect on blood flow (perfusion) to the gas-exchange units is exerted to balance the equation, the consequence is $\dot{V}/\dot{Q}$ mismatch. A pulmonary embolus affects the perfusion portion of the $\dot{V}/\dot{Q}$ relationship. The embolus limits blood flow but has no effect on airflow to the alveoli, again causing $\dot{V}/\dot{Q}$ mismatch (see Figure 70-4).

Table 70-3 Predisposing Factors for Acute Respiratory Failure

PREDISPOSING FACTORS	MECHANISMS OF RESPIRATORY FAILURE
Airways and Alveoli	
ARDS	Fluid enters the interstitial space and the alveoli, markedly impairing gas exchange. The result is an initial $\downarrow$ in PaO_2 and a later $\uparrow$ in $PaCO_2$. A low-flow state to pulmonary capillaries can result in ischemic injury to lung tissues with loss of integrity of the alveolar–capillary membrane.
Direct lung injury: Aspiration; severe, disseminated pulmonary infection; near-drowning; toxic gas inhalation; airway contusion	
Indirect lung injury: Sepsis or septic shock, severe nonthoracic trauma, cardiopulmonary bypass	
Asthma	Bronchospasm escalates in severity rather than responding to therapy. Bronchospasm, edema of the bronchial mucosa, and plugging of small airways with secretions greatly reduce airflow.
	Work of breathing increases, causing respiratory muscle fatigue. $\downarrow PaO_2$ and $\uparrow PaCO_2$. (See Chapter 31.)
COPD	Alveoli are destroyed by protease–antiprotease imbalance or respiratory infection, or an exacerbation of COPD escalates in severity rather than responding to therapy. Secretions obstruct airflow. Work of breathing increases and causes respiratory muscle fatigue. $\downarrow PaO_2$ and $\uparrow PaCO_2$.
Cystic fibrosis	Abnormal Na^+ and Cl^- transport produces secretions that are viscous, poorly cleared, and therefore foci for infection. Over time, the airways become clogged with copious, purulent sputum. Secretions obstruct airflow. Repeated infections destroy alveoli. Work of breathing increases, causing respiratory muscle fatigue. $\downarrow PaO_2$ and $\uparrow PaCO_2$.
Central Nervous System	
Narcotic or other drug overdose with CNS depressant	Respirations are slowed by drug effect. Insufficient CO_2 is excreted, resulting in $\uparrow PaCO_2$.
Brainstem infarction, head injury	Medulla cannot alter respiratory rate in response to changes in $PaCO_2$.
Chest Wall	
Severe soft tissue injury, flail chest, rib fracture, pain	Structural dysfunction and pain prevent normal rib cage expansion, resulting in inadequate gas exchange.
Kyphoscoliosis	Change in spinal configuration compresses the lungs and prevents normal expansion of the chest wall, resulting in inadequate gas exchange.
Morbid obesity	Weight of the chest and abdominal contents prevents normal rib cage movement, resulting in inadequate gas exchange.
Neuromuscular Conditions	
Cervical cord injury, phrenic nerve injury	Neural control is lost, preventing use of the diaphragm, the major muscle of respiration. Consequently, the patient inspires a smaller tidal volume, which predisposes to an $\uparrow$ in $PaCO_2$.
Amyotrophic lateral sclerosis (ALS), Guillain-Barré syndrome, muscular dystrophy, multiple sclerosis, poliomyelitis, myasthenia gravis, myopathy, critical illness polyneuropathy, prolonged use of neuromuscular blocking agents	Respiratory muscle weakness or paralysis occurs, preventing normal CO_2 excretion. Dysfunction may be progressive (muscular dystrophy, multiple sclerosis), progressive with no potential of recovery (ALS), rapid with good expectation of recovery (Guillain-Barré), or stable for extended periods (poliomyelitis, myasthenia gravis).

ARDS, acute respiratory distress syndrome; *CNS,* central nervous system; *COPD,* chronic obstructive pulmonary disease; *PaCO₂,* partial pressure of carbon dioxide in arterial blood; *PaO₂,* partial pressure of oxygen in arterial blood.

O_2 therapy is an appropriate first step to reverse hypoxemia caused by $\dot{V}/\dot{Q}$ mismatch because not all gas-exchange units are affected. O_2 therapy increases the PaO_2 in blood leaving normal gas-exchange units, thus causing a higher than normal PaO_2. The well-oxygenated blood mixes with poorly oxygenated blood, raising the overall PaO_2 of blood leaving the lungs. Optimal treatment for hypoxemia caused by $\dot{V}/\dot{Q}$ mismatch is directed at the cause.

Shunt. Shunt occurs when blood exits the heart without having participated in gas exchange. A shunt can be viewed as an extreme

$\dot{V}/\dot{Q}$ mismatch (see Figure 70-4). There are two types of shunt: anatomical and intrapulmonary. An *anatomical shunt* occurs when blood passes through an anatomical channel in the heart (e.g., ventricular septal defect), bypassing the lungs. An *intrapulmonary shunt* occurs when blood flows through the pulmonary capillaries without participating in gas exchange. Intrapulmonary shunt is seen in conditions in which alveoli fill with fluid (e.g., ARDS, pneumonia, pulmonary edema). O_2 therapy alone may not effectively increase the PaO_2 in hypoxemia due to shunt because (1) blood passes from the right to the left heart without passing through the lungs (anatomical shunt) or (2) the alveoli are filled

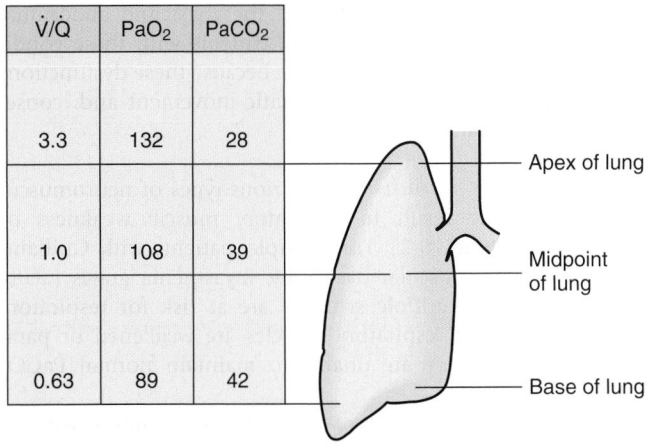

$\dot{V}/\dot{Q}$	PaO_2	$PaCO_2$
3.3	132	28
1.0	108	39
0.63	89	42

Apex of lung
Midpoint of lung
Base of lung

Figure 70-3 Regional ventilation–perfusion ($\dot{V}/\dot{Q}$) differences in the normal lung. At the lung apex, the $\dot{V}/\dot{Q}$ ratio is 3.3, at the midpoint 1.0, and at the base 0.63. This difference causes the arterial partial pressure of oxygen (PaO_2) to be higher at the apex of the lung and lower at the base. Values for arterial partial pressure of carbon dioxide ($PaCO_2$) are the opposite (i.e., lower at the apex and higher at the base). Blood that exits the lung has a mixture of these values.

with fluid, which prevents gas exchange (intrapulmonary shunt). Patients with shunt are usually more hypoxemic than patients with $\dot{V}/\dot{Q}$ mismatch, and they may require both mechanical ventilation (MV) and a high FiO_2 to improve gas exchange.

Diffusion Limitation. **Diffusion limitation** occurs when gas exchange across the alveolar–capillary membrane is compromised by processes that thicken or destroy the membrane (Figure 70-5). Conditions that affect the pulmonary vascular bed, such as severe emphysema or recurrent pulmonary emboli, can worsen diffusion limitation. Some diseases (e.g., pulmonary fibrosis, interstitial lung disease, ARDS) cause the alveolar–capillary membrane to become thicker (fibrotic), which slows gas transport. Diffusion limitation is more likely to cause hypoxemia during exercise than at rest. During exercise, blood moves more rapidly through the lungs. Because the transit rate is increased, red blood cells are in the lungs for a shorter time, shrinking the window of opportunity for diffusion of O_2 across the alveolar–capillary membrane. The classical sign of diffusion limitation is hypoxemia that is present during exercise but not at rest.

Alveolar Hypoventilation. **Alveolar hypoventilation** refers to a decrease in ventilation that results in an increased $PaCO_2$ and a consequent decrease in PaO_2. Alveolar hypoventilation may result from restrictive lung disease, CNS disease, chest wall dysfunction, or neuromuscular disease. Although primarily a mechanism of hypercapnic respiratory failure, alveolar hypoventilation is mentioned here because it also causes hypoxemia.

Interrelationship of Mechanisms. Frequently, hypoxemic respiratory failure is caused by a combination of two or more of the following: $\dot{V}/\dot{Q}$ mismatch, shunting, diffusion limitation, and hypoventilation. The patient with acute respiratory failure secondary to pneumonia may have a combination of $\dot{V}/\dot{Q}$ mismatch and shunt because inflammation, edema, and the hypersecretion

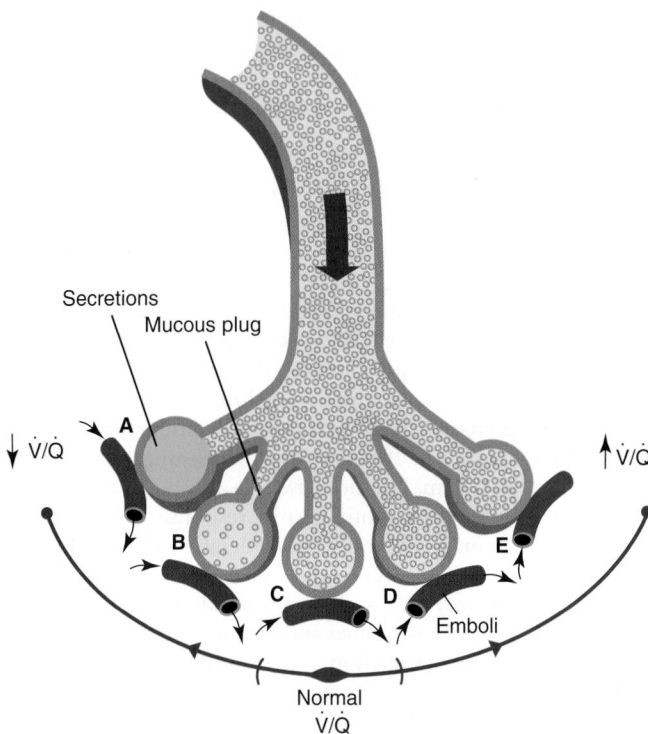

Secretions
Mucous plug
$\downarrow \dot{V}/\dot{Q}$
A
B
C
D
E
Emboli
$\uparrow \dot{V}/\dot{Q}$
Normal $\dot{V}/\dot{Q}$

Figure 70-4 Range of ventilation to perfusion ($\dot{V}/\dot{Q}$) relationships. **A,** Absolute shunt, no ventilation as a result of fluid filling the alveoli. **B,** $\dot{V}/\dot{Q}$ mismatch, ventilation partially compromised by secretions in the airway. **C,** Normal lung unit. **D,** $\dot{V}/\dot{Q}$ mismatch, perfusion partially compromised by emboli obstructing blood flow. **E,** Dead space, no perfusion as a result of obstruction of the pulmonary capillary.

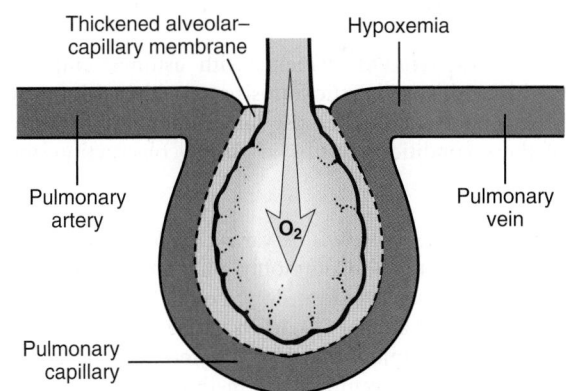

Thickened alveolar–capillary membrane
Hypoxemia
Pulmonary artery
Pulmonary vein
O_2
Pulmonary capillary

Figure 70-5 Diffusion limitation. Exchange of CO_2 and O_2 cannot occur because of the thickened alveolar–capillary membrane.

of exudate within the bronchioles and the terminal respiratory units obstruct the airways ($\dot{V}/\dot{Q}$ mismatch) and fill the alveoli with exudate (shunt). In addition, shunt may be increased because of improper positioning (affected lung down). The patient with cardiogenic pulmonary edema or ARDS may have a combination of shunt and $\dot{V}/\dot{Q}$ mismatch because some alveoli are completely filled with fluid from edema (shunt) and others are partially filled with fluid ($\dot{V}/\dot{Q}$ mismatch).

Hypoxemia resulting from shunting does not respond to increases in supplemental oxygen because the capillary bed surrounding the affected alveoli is never exposed to oxygen-rich gas. This makes hypoxemia owing to shunting difficult to treat (Brashers, 2010).

Hypercapnic Respiratory Failure. Hypercapnic respiratory failure results from an imbalance between ventilatory supply and demand. *Ventilatory supply* is the maximum ventilation (gas flow in and out of the lungs) that the patient can sustain without developing respiratory muscle fatigue. *Ventilatory demand* is the amount of ventilation needed to keep the $PaCO_2$ level normal. Normally, ventilatory supply far exceeds ventilatory demand. As a consequence, individuals with normal lung function can engage in strenuous exercise, which increases CO_2 production without an elevation in $PaCO_2$. Patients with pre-existing lung disease (e.g., severe emphysema) do not have this advantage and cannot effectively increase lung ventilation in response to exercise or metabolic demands. Typically, considerable dysfunction is present before ventilatory demand exceeds supply.

When ventilatory demand does exceed supply, a normal $PaCO_2$ level cannot be sustained and hypercapnia occurs, reflecting substantial lung dysfunction. Hypercapnic respiratory failure is sometimes called *ventilatory failure* because it represents primarily an inability of the respiratory system to clear sufficient CO_2 and maintain a normal $PaCO_2$

The associated respiratory acidosis that accompanies hypercapnia can result in dysrhythmias, somnolence, and even coma. There are changes in intracranial pressure associated with high levels of CO_2. Hypoventilation may be overlooked because the ventilator rate and pattern may appear normal initially (Brashers, 2010).

Diseases involving respiratory failure can be grouped into four categories: (1) abnormalities of the airways and alveoli, (2) abnormalities of the CNS, (3) abnormalities of the chest wall, and (4) neuromuscular conditions (see Table 70-3).

Airways and Alveoli. Patients with asthma, emphysema, chronic bronchitis, and cystic fibrosis are at high risk for hypercapnic respiratory failure because the underlying pathophysiology of these conditions results in airflow obstruction and air trapping.

Central Nervous System. A variety of problems may suppress the drive to breathe. Commonly, a narcotic or other respiratory depressant drug overdose decreases CO_2 reactivity in the brainstem, allowing arterial CO_2 levels to rise. A brainstem infarction or severe head injury may also interfere with normal function of the respiratory centre in the medulla. These patients are at risk for respiratory failure because the medulla does not alter the respiratory rate in response to changes in $PaCO_2$. Independent of direct brainstem dysfunction, brain injury resulting in significant depression or loss of consciousness may impair the patient's ability to protect the airway. CNS dysfunction may also include high-level spinal cord injuries that limit innervation to the respiratory muscles.

Chest Wall. Various conditions prevent normal chest wall movement, thereby limiting lung expansion. In patients with flail chest, the rib cage cannot expand normally because of painful fractures, mechanical restriction, and muscle spasm. In patients with kyphoscoliosis, changes in spinal configuration compress the lungs, preventing normal chest wall expansion. In patients with massive obesity, the weight of the chest and abdominal contents may limit lung expansion. Patients with these conditions are at risk for respiratory failure because these dysfunctions limit lung expansion or diaphragmatic movement and, consequently, gas exchange.

Neuromuscular Conditions. Various types of neuromuscular diseases may result in respiratory muscle weakness or paralysis (see Table 70-2). For example, patients with Guillain-Barré syndrome, muscular dystrophy, myasthenia gravis (acute exacerbation), or multiple sclerosis are at risk for respiratory failure because the respiratory muscles are weakened or paralyzed. Therefore, they are unable to maintain normal $PaCO_2$ levels.

Note that respiratory failure occurs in three of these categories (CNS, chest wall, neuromuscular conditions) despite normal lungs. The patient may have no damage to lung tissue but is unable to inspire sufficient tidal volume to expel CO_2 from the lungs.

Tissue Oxygen Needs. Even though PaO_2 and $PaCO_2$ determine the definition of respiratory failure, the major threat is the inability of the lungs to meet the oxygen demands of the tissues, whether as a result of inadequate O_2 delivery or because the tissues are unable to use the O_2 delivered to them. It may also occur as a result of the stress response and dramatic increases in tissue oxygen consumption (Brashers, 2010). Tissue O_2 delivery is determined by the amount of O_2 carried in the hemoglobin as well as cardiac output. Therefore, respiratory failure places the patient at greater risk if there are coexisting cardiac problems or anemia. Failure of O_2 utilization most commonly occurs as a result of septic shock. In this situation, adequate O_2 may be delivered to the tissues, but an abnormally high amount of O_2 returns in the venous blood, indicating that it is not being extracted and used at the tissue level. (Shock is discussed in Chapter 69.) Acid–base alterations (e.g., alkalosis, acidosis) may also interfere with oxygen delivery to peripheral tissues (see Chapter 28).

Clinical Manifestations

Respiratory failure may develop suddenly or gradually over several days or longer. A sudden decrease in PaO_2 or a rapid rise in $PaCO_2$ implies a serious condition, which can rapidly become a life-threatening emergency. An example is the patient with asthma who develops severe bronchospasm and a marked decrease in airflow, resulting in respiratory arrest. A more gradual change in PaO_2 and $PaCO_2$ is better tolerated because compensation can occur. An example is the patient with COPD who develops a progressive increase in $PaCO_2$ over several days following the onset of a respiratory infection. Because the change occurred gradually over several days, there is time for renal compensation (e.g., retention of bicarbonate), which will minimize the change in arterial pH. The patient has compensated respiratory acidosis (Urden et al., 2010). (See Chapter 19 for a discussion of renal compensation for acid–base disorders.)

Manifestations of respiratory failure are related to the extent of change in PaO_2 or $PaCO_2$, the rapidity of change (acute versus chronic), and the ability to compensate or overcome this change. When the patient's compensatory mechanisms fail, respiratory failure occurs. Because clinical manifestations are variable, it is important to monitor trends in ABGs and pulse oximetry to evaluate the extent of change. These measurements cannot substitute for clinical assessment and should be interpreted within the context of clinical assessment findings. Frequently, the initial indication of respiratory failure is a change in the patient's mental status. The cerebral cortex is very sensitive to variations in oxygenation and acid–base balance, and mental status changes will occur early and frequently before ABG results are obtained. Restlessness, confusion, agitation, and combative behaviour suggest inadequate delivery of O_2 to the brain and should be investigated.

The nurse may detect manifestations of respiratory failure that are specific (arise from the respiratory system) or nonspecific (arise from other body systems) (Table 70-4). An understanding of these manifestations is critical for detecting the onset of respiratory failure and effective treatment.

Tachycardia and mild hypertension can also be early signs of respiratory failure. They may indicate an attempt by the heart to compensate for decreased O_2 delivery. A severe morning headache may suggest that hypercapnia occurred during the night, increasing cerebral blood flow by vasodilation. At night, the respiratory rate is slower and the lungs of patients at risk for respiratory failure may remove less $PaCO_2$. Rapid, shallow breaths suggest that the tidal volume may be inadequate to remove CO_2 from the lungs. Cyanosis is an unreliable indicator of hypoxemia and is a late sign of respiratory failure because it does not occur until hypoxemia is severe ($PaO_2 \leq 45$ mm Hg).

Consequences of Hypoxemia and Hypoxia.
Hypoxemia occurs when the amount of O_2 in arterial blood is less than the normal value (see Chapter 28). **Hypoxia** occurs when the PaO_2 has fallen sufficiently to cause signs and symptoms of inadequate oxygenation (see Table 70-4). Hypoxemia can lead to hypoxia if not corrected. If hypoxia or hypoxemia is severe, cell metabolism shifts from aerobic to anaerobic. Anaerobic metabolism uses more fuel and produces less energy and is less efficient than aerobic metabolism. The waste product of anaerobic metabolism, lactic acid, is more difficult to remove from the body than CO_2 because lactic acid must be buffered with sodium bicarbonate. When the body does not have adequate sodium bicarbonate to buffer the lactic acid produced by anaerobic metabolism, metabolic acidosis and cell death may result.

Hypoxia and metabolic acidosis have adverse effects on the vital organs and systems, especially the heart and the CNS. The heart tries to compensate for decreased O_2 in the blood by increasing the heart rate and cardiac output. A cardiovascular hyperdynamic state may also occur as a result of catecholamine release associated with the physiological stress response. This can be a fairly rapidly occurring response. As the PaO_2 decreases and acidosis increases, the heart muscle may become dysfunctional and cardiac output may decrease. In addition, angina and dysrhythmias may occur. All of these consequences result in a further decrease in oxygen delivery. Permanent brain damage may occur because of O_2 deprivation. Renal function may also be impaired, and sodium retention, edema formation, acute tubular necrosis, and uremia may occur. Gastrointestinal system alterations include tissue ischemia, increased permeability of the intestinal wall, and possible translocation of bacteria from the gastrointestinal tract into the circulation.

Specific Clinical Manifestations.
The patient in respiratory failure may have several clinical findings indicating distress, such as rapid, shallow breathing or a respiratory rate slower than normal. Both changes predispose to insufficient CO_2 removal. The patient may increase the respiratory rate in an effort to blow

Table 70-4 Clinical Manifestations of Hypoxemia and Hypercapnia*	
SPECIFIC	**NONSPECIFIC**
Hypoxemia	
Respiratory	*Cerebral*
Dyspnea	Agitation
Tachypnea	Disorientation
Prolonged expiration (I:E = 1:3, 1:4)	Delirium
Intercostal muscle retraction	Restlessness, combativeness
Use of accessory muscles in respiration	Confusion
$\downarrow$ SpO$_2$ (<80%)	$\downarrow$ Level of consciousness
Paradoxical chest or abdominal wall movement with respiratory cycle (late)	Coma (late)
Cyanosis (late)	*Cardiac*
	Tachycardia
	Hypertension
	Skin cool, clammy, and diaphoretic
	Dysrhythmias (late)
	Hypotension (late)
	Other
	Fatigue
	Unable to speak without pausing to breathe
Hypercapnia	
Respiratory	*Cerebral*
Dyspnea	Morning headache
$\downarrow$ Respiratory rate or $\uparrow$ rate with shallow respirations	Disorientation
$\downarrow$ Tidal volume	Progressive somnolence
$\downarrow$ Minute ventilation	Coma (late)
	Cardiac
	Dysrhythmias
	Hypertension
	Tachycardia
	Bounding pulse
	Neuromuscular
	Muscle weakness
	$\downarrow$ Deep tendon reflexes
	Tremor, seizures (late)
	Other
	Pursed-lip breathing

I:E, ratio of inspirations to expirations; *SpO$_2$*, oxygen saturation in arterial blood as measured by pulse oximetry.
*This list is not all-inclusive.

off accumulated CO_2. This breathing pattern requires a substantial amount of work and predisposes to respiratory muscle fatigue. A change from a rapid rate to a slower rate in a patient in acute respiratory distress suggests extreme fatigue and possible impending respiratory arrest.

The position that the patient assumes is an indication of the effort associated with breathing. The patient may be able to lie down (mild distress), be able to lie down but prefer to sit (moderate distress), or be unable to breathe unless sitting upright (severe distress). A common position is to sit with the arms propped on the overbed table. This position, called the *tripod position*, helps decrease the work of breathing because propping the arms increases the anterior–posterior diameter of the chest and changes pressure in the thorax. Pursed-lip breathing may be seen (see Chapter 31) because it increases SaO_2 by slowing respirations, allowing more time for expiration, and preventing the small bronchioles from collapsing, thus facilitating air exchange. Another assessment parameter is the number of pillows the patient requires to breathe comfortably when resting. This is termed *orthopnea*, referring to the degree of dyspnea when lying flat, documented as one-, two-, three-, or four-pillow orthopnea.

A person experiencing dyspnea is working hard to breathe and may be able to speak only a few words between breaths. The degree to which the patient is able to speak without pausing to breathe is an indication of the severity of dyspnea. The patient may speak in sentences (mild or no distress), phrases (moderate distress), or words (severe distress). The patient may have "two-word" or "three-word" dyspnea, signifying that only two or three words can be said before pausing to breathe. There may also be earlier onset of fatigue with walking. An additional assessment parameter is how far the patient is able to walk without stopping to rest.

There may be a change in the *inspiratory (I) to expiratory (E) (I:E) ratio*. Normally, the I:E ratio is 1:2, meaning expiration is twice as long as inspiration. In respiratory distress, the ratio may increase to 1:3 or 1:4, signifying airflow obstruction, with more time required to empty the lungs.

The nurse may observe *retraction* (inward movement) of the intercostal spaces or the supraclavicular area and use of the accessory muscles during inspiration or expiration, signifying moderate distress. Paradoxical breathing indicates severe distress. Normally, the thorax and the abdomen move outward on inspiration and inward on exhalation. During *paradoxical breathing*, the abdomen and the chest move in the opposite manner—outward during exhalation and inward during inspiration. Paradoxical breathing results from maximal use of the accessory muscles of respiration. The patient may also be diaphoretic from the work associated with breathing.

Auscultation should be performed in order to assess the patient's baseline breath sounds as well as any changes from baseline. The nurse should note the presence and the location of any adventitious breath sounds. Crackles and wheezes may indicate pulmonary edema or emphysema. Absent or diminished breath sounds may indicate atelectasis or pleural effusion. Bronchial breath sounds over the lung periphery often result from lung consolidation, as seen with pneumonia. A pleural friction rub may also be heard in the presence of pneumonia that has involved the pleura.

A thorough nursing assessment may result in early detection of manifestations associated with respiratory insufficiency, allowing therapy to be instituted before the patient experiences respiratory failure. Patients with end-stage (severe) chronic lung disease may have low PaO_2 values or elevated $PaCO_2$ levels and crackles as their "normal" baseline. It is especially important to monitor specific and nonspecific signs of respiratory failure in patients with COPD or other pre-existing chronic diseases because a small change can cause significant decompensation (see Table 70-4). Any deterioration in mental status, such as agitation, combative behaviour, confusion, or decreased level of consciousness, should be reported immediately because this may indicate deterioration in clinical status and the need for MV.

Diagnostic Studies

After physical assessment, the most common diagnostic studies used to determine respiratory failure are ABG analysis and chest radiographic studies. ABGs are used to determine the levels of $PaCO_2$, PaO_2, bicarbonate, and pH. An indwelling catheter may be inserted into a peripheral artery for monitoring systemic blood pressure (BP) and obtaining ABGs. Pulse oximetry is used for monitoring oxygenation but tells little about ventilation. In respiratory failure, ABGs are necessary to obtain both oxygenation (PaO_2) and ventilation ($PaCO_2$) status as well as information related to acid–base balance (Lynn-McHale Weigand, 2011). Chest radiographic examination helps identify possible causes of respiratory failure (e.g., atelectasis, pneumonia). In patients of lower acuity, pulmonary function tests may be performed.

Other diagnostic studies that may be done include complete blood count (CBC), serum electrolytes, urinalysis, and electrocardiogram (ECG). Sputum and blood cultures are obtained if infection is likely. If pulmonary embolus is suspected, a $\dot{V}/\dot{Q}$ lung scan or pulmonary angiography may be done. For the patient requiring endotracheal intubation, end-tidal CO_2 is used to assess tube placement immediately following intubation and during ventilator management to assess trends in lung ventilation based on expired CO_2.

In severe respiratory failure, a pulmonary artery catheter may be inserted to measure heart pressures and cardiac output, as well as mixed venous oxygen saturation. This information is helpful in determining the adequacy of tissue perfusion and the patient's response to treatment. Pulmonary artery, pulmonary artery wedge (occlusion), and left atrial pressures are monitored to determine whether the accumulation of fluid in the lungs is the result of cardiac or pulmonary problems. These parameters are also monitored to determine the response of the lung and heart to hypoxemia and the patient's response to therapy. Pulmonary arterial pressure monitoring can also provide feedback on the physiological effects of MV on hemodynamic status. (See Chapter 68 for a discussion of hemodynamic monitoring.)

NURSING AND COLLABORATIVE MANAGEMENT: ACUTE RESPIRATORY FAILURE

Because many different problems cause respiratory failure, care of these patients varies. This section discusses general assessment and collaborative treatments that apply to patients with acute respiratory failure. In acute care settings, there is often an overlap of function between nursing and other members of the health care team. This also includes the family members who play a valuable role in the patient's care and recovery. Further discussion of issues related to the family and caregivers can be found in Chapter 68.

▪ Nursing Assessment

Subjective and objective data that should be obtained from the patient with acute respiratory failure are presented in Table 70-5.

NURSING ASSESSMENT

Table 70-5 Acute Respiratory Failure

Subjective Data	Respiratory
Important Health Information	Shallow, increased respiratory rate progressing to decreased rate; use of accessory muscles with evidence of retractions, altered I:E ratio; increased diaphragmatic excursion or asymmetrical chest expansion; asynchronous respirations; tactile fremitus, crepitus, or deviated trachea on palpation; resonant, hyperresonant, or dull percussion note; absent, diminished, or adventitious breath sounds; bronchial or bronchovesicular sounds heard in other than normal location, inspiratory stridor, pleural friction rub

Subjective Data

Important Health Information

Past health history: Chronic lung disease; potential occupational exposures to lung toxins; smoking (pack-years); childhood illnesses, previous hospitalizations related to lung disease; thoracic or spinal cord trauma; extreme obesity; altered consciousness; age (physiological and chronological); use or abuse of alcohol, other drugs; drug allergies, recent travel, SARS

Medications: Use of oxygen, inhalers (bronchodilators), home nebulization, over-the-counter medications; immunosuppressant (corticosteroid) therapy, CNS depressants; vitamin and herbal supplements

Surgery or other treatments: Previous intubation and mechanical ventilation; recent thoracic or abdominal surgery

Symptoms

- Anorexia, bloatedness, heartburn; weight gain or loss; decreased appetite
- Fatigue, dizziness; diaphoresis
- Dyspnea at rest or with activity, wheezing, cough (productive or nonproductive); sputum (volume, colour, viscosity)
- Palpitations, swollen feet
- Changes in sleep pattern
- Headache, chest pain or tightness
- Anxiety, depression

Objective Data

General

Restlessness, agitation

Integumentary

Pale, cool, clammy skin or warm flushed skin; peripheral and central cyanosis; peripheral dependent edema

Respiratory

Shallow, increased respiratory rate progressing to decreased rate; use of accessory muscles with evidence of retractions, altered I:E ratio; increased diaphragmatic excursion or asymmetrical chest expansion; asynchronous respirations; tactile fremitus, crepitus, or deviated trachea on palpation; resonant, hyperresonant, or dull percussion note; absent, diminished, or adventitious breath sounds; bronchial or bronchovesicular sounds heard in other than normal location, inspiratory stridor, pleural friction rub

Cardiovascular

Tachycardia progressing to bradycardia, dysrhythmias, extra heart sounds (S3, S4); bounding pulse; hypertension progressing to hypotension; pulsus paradoxus; jugular vein distension; pedal edema

Gastrointestinal

Abdominal distension with tympany; ascites, epigastric tenderness, hepatojugular reflex

Neurological

Somnolence, confusion, slurred speech, restlessness, delirium, agitation, tremors, seizures, coma; asterixis, decreased deep tendon reflexes; papilledema

Possible Laboratory Findings

$\uparrow$ or $\downarrow$ pH, $\uparrow$ or $\downarrow$ $PaCO_2$, $\downarrow$ PaO_2, $\uparrow$ or $\downarrow$ bicarbonate, $\downarrow$ SaO_2, $\downarrow$ PEFR, $\downarrow$tidal volume, $\downarrow$ forced vital capacity, $\downarrow$ minute ventilation, $\downarrow$ negative inspiratory force; altered serum electrolyte values, hemoglobin, white blood cells, and hematocrit; abnormal findings on chest radiograph; abnormal pulmonary artery and pulmonary artery wedge pressures

CNS, central nervous system; *I:E*, inspiratory:expiratory; *PaCO₂*, partial pressure of carbon dioxide in arterial blood; *PaO₂*, partial pressure of oxygen in arterial blood; *PEFR*, peak expiratory flow rate; *SARS*, severe acute respiratory syndrome; *SaO₂*, oxygen saturation in arterial blood as measured by arterial blood gases.

Nursing Diagnoses

Nursing diagnoses for the patient with acute respiratory failure include, but are not limited to, those presented in Nursing Care Plan (NCP) 70-1.

Planning

The overall goals for the patient in acute respiratory failure are to restore baseline (1) ABG values, (2) breath sounds, (3) breathing patterns, and (4) ability to clear secretions.

Prevention

Prevention and early recognition of respiratory distress are important aspects of care for any patient at risk for respiratory failure. Prevention involves a thorough physical assessment and history (to identify the patient at risk for respiratory failure) followed by appropriate nursing interventions. For example, a patient at risk for respiratory failure should receive teaching regarding cough-

ing, deep breathing, incentive spirometry, and ambulation as appropriate. Prevention of atelectasis, pneumonia, and complications of immobility, as well as optimizing hydration and nutrition, can potentially decrease the risk of respiratory failure in acute or critically ill patients.

Respiratory Therapy

The major goals of care for acute respiratory failure include maintaining adequate oxygenation and ventilation. This is accomplished by collaboration among the nursing, medical, and respiratory care teams. The interventions used include O_2 therapy, mobilization of secretions, and positive pressure ventilation (Table 70-6).

Oxygen Therapy

The primary goal of O_2 therapy is to correct hypoxemia. If hypoxemia is secondary to $\dot{V}/\dot{Q}$ mismatch, supplemental O_2 administered at 1 to 3 L/min by nasal cannula or 24 to 32% by simple face mask or Venturi mask should improve the PaO_2 and

NURSING CARE PLAN 70-1

Acute Respiratory Failure*

NURSING DIAGNOSIS	**Ineffective airway clearance** *related to* excessive secretions, ↓ level of consciousness, presence of an artificial airway, neuromuscular dysfunction, and pain *as evidenced by* difficulty in expectorating sputum, presence of wheezes or crackles, and ineffective or absent cough
Expected Patient Outcomes	**Nursing Interventions and *Rationales***

• Has no abnormal breath sounds (e.g., wheezes, crackles) • Has normal baseline breath sounds • Able to cough effectively • Able to expectorate sputum effectively	• Assess patient's ability to cough *to determine need for assistance in secretion removal.* • Implement deep-breathing or coughing exercises, assistive coughing strategies, and incentive spirometry *to promote secretion removal.* • Position patient with head of bed elevated at least 45 degrees, or in the tripod position, *to promote maximal chest expansion and cough efforts.* • Humidify O₂ if >3 L/min *to prevent drying of the mucosa.* • Perform tracheobronchial suctioning if cough is ineffective or if artificial airway is present *to remove secretions and improve oxygenation.* • Perform chest physiotherapy *to enhance removal of secretions.* • Splint abdominal or chest incision with pillow *to reduce pain and allow for improved inspiratory efforts.* • Turn q2h *to prevent stasis of secretions and promote optimal ventilation.* • Ensure adequate fluid intake of 2 to 3 L/day *to liquefy secretions.* • Administer prescribed regimen and as needed of bronchodilator and mucolytic medications *to promote better airflow and secretion removal.*

NURSING DIAGNOSIS	**Ineffective breathing pattern** *related to* neuromuscular impairment of respirations, pain, anxiety, ↓ level of consciousness, respiratory muscle fatigue, and bronchospasm *as evidenced by* respiratory rate <12 or >24 breaths/min, altered I:E ratio, irregular breathing pattern, use of accessory muscles, asynchronous thoracoabdominal movement, wheezing, and apnea
Expected Patient Outcomes	**Nursing Interventions and *Rationales***

• Experiences restored baseline respiratory rate, depth, and rhythm • Has synchronous thoracoabdominal movement • Has accessory muscle use appropriate for level of activity	• Monitor for ↑ or ↓ respiratory rate, periods of apnea, and ↓ inspiratory depth between chest and abdomen *to assess for presence of inability to sustain ventilation.* • Position patient with head of bed elevated at least 45 degrees or in a tripod position *to promote diaphragmatic excursion.* • Place oral or nasal airway and Ambu bag at the bedside *because airway support may be needed in the event of severely impaired ventilation or apnea.* • Provide comfort measures (e.g., analgesics, positioning) *to reduce anxiety and promote patient cooperation.* • Anticipate the need for application of NIPPV or intubation with mechanical ventilation *to maintain adequate oxygenation and ventilation.*

NURSING DIAGNOSIS	**Risk for imbalanced fluid volume** *related to* ↑ in peripheral or pulmonary fluid
Expected Patient Outcomes	**Nursing Interventions and *Rationales***

• Has normal breath sounds • Has decreased or absent peripheral edema • Has normal pulmonary artery or pulmonary artery wedge (occlusion) pressures	• Assess for manifestations of fluid overload such as abnormal breath sounds (crackles), dyspnea, jugular venous distension, and peripheral or sacral edema. • Monitor intake and output, daily weights, pulmonary artery or pulmonary artery wedge pressures, and central venous pressure *to monitor for changes in systemic fluid volume.* • Restrict fluid intake and administer diuretics as ordered *to prevent or reduce fluid overload.*

NURSING DIAGNOSIS	**Anxiety** *related to* dyspnea, intubation, severity of illness, loss of control, and uncertain outcome *as evidenced by* ↑ heart rate, respiratory rate, and blood pressure; agitation, restlessness; and verbalization of anxiety
Expected Patient Outcomes	**Nursing Interventions and *Rationales***

• Reports reduced feelings of anxiety • Maintains relaxed demeanour • Has increased sense of control	• Perform interventions in a calm, assured manner *to decrease patient's anxiety.* • Reassure patient *to encourage relaxation.* • Answer questions simply and honestly *to provide patient with information for decision making.* • Teach and demonstrate relaxation techniques, slow pursed-lip breathing, and guided imagery *to promote restoration of control over breathing.* • Administer and evaluate patient's response to prescribed antianxiety medication *to determine efficacy.*

NURSING CARE PLAN 70-1

Acute Respiratory Failure—cont'd

NURSING DIAGNOSIS	*Impaired gas exchange* related to alveolar hypoventilation, intrapulmonary shunting, V̇/Q̇ mismatch, and diffusion impairment *as evidenced by* hypoxemia or hypercapnia
Expected Patient Outcomes	**Nursing Interventions and *Rationales***
• Maintains ABG values within normal ranges for patient • Has normal breath sounds	• Monitor for clinical manifestations of hypoxemia and hypercapnia *to detect systemic manifestations of* ↓ O_2 and ↑ CO_2. • Administer O_2 as ordered *to* ↑ PaO_2 and SaO_2 levels. • Monitor ABGs for PaO_2 <60 mm Hg, SaO_2 <90%, and $PaCO_2$ >50 mm Hg *to assess pulmonary gas exchange.* • Place the patient on continuous pulse oximetry *to assess for* ↑ *or* ↓ *in blood O_2 saturation levels.* • Monitor apical–radial heart rate for irregular rhythm, tachycardia, bradycardia, and cardiac dysrhythmias on the cardiac monitor *because hypoxemia may precipitate cardiac dysrhythmias.* • Teach and encourage pursed-lip breathing *to improve gas exchange.* • Anticipate the need for ventilatory support *to improve oxygenation and ventilation status.* • Withhold sedative drugs unless discussed with physician *because they can depress respirations.*
NURSING DIAGNOSIS	*Imbalanced nutrition: less than body requirements* related to poor appetite, shortness of breath, presence of artificial airway, reduced energy level, and increased caloric requirements *as evidenced by* weight loss, weakness, muscle wasting, dehydration, poor muscle tone, and poor skin integrity
Expected Patient Outcomes	**Nursing Interventions and *Rationales***
• Maintains weight or weight gain • Has serum albumin and protein levels within normal ranges	• Provide oral, enteral, or parenteral nutritional as ordered *to meet nutritional requirements.* • If oral nutrition tolerated, provide six small meals daily *to* ↓ O_2 *energy expenditure* with between-meal supplements *to maintain adequate caloric intake.* • Maintain the ordered O_2 delivery device during meals *to prevent shortness of breath and blood oxygen desaturation while eating.* • Monitor for signs of ↑ CO_2 with parenteral nutrition *because carbohydrates may* ↑ CO_2 *levels in patients with hypercapnia.*

ABG, arterial blood gases; *I:E,* inspiratory:expiratory; NIPPV, noninvasive positive-pressure ventilation; *PaCO₂,* partial pressure of carbon dioxide in arterial blood; *PaO₂,* partial pressure of oxygen in arterial blood; *SaO₂,* oxygen saturation in arterial blood as measured by ABGs; V̇/Q̇, ventilation–perfusion ratio.
*The nursing care for the patient on mechanical ventilation is presented in eNCP 68-1 and discussed in Chapter 68.

SaO_2. Hypoxemia secondary to an intrapulmonary shunt is usually not responsive to high O_2 concentrations, and the patient will usually require positive-pressure ventilation (PPV). PPV offers a means of providing O_2 therapy and humidification, decreasing the work of breathing, and reducing respiratory muscle fatigue. In addition, the positive pressure may assist in opening collapsed airways and decreasing shunt. PPV may be provided via an endotracheal tube (most frequently) or noninvasively by means of a tight-fitting mask (Peñuelas, Frutos-Vivar, & Esteban, 2007). (See Chapter 68 for a detailed discussion of mechanical ventilation.)

The type of O_2 delivery system chosen for the patient in acute respiratory failure should (1) be tolerated by the patient, because feelings of claustrophobia related to the face mask may prompt the patient to remove it, and (2) maintain PaO_2 at 55 to 60 mm Hg or more and SaO_2 at 90% or more at the lowest O_2 concentration possible. High O_2 concentration is associated with adverse patient effects. Intubated patients who receive greater than 50% FiO_2 for more than 24 hours are at greatest risk to develop O_2 toxicity (Urden et al., 2010). Although toxic O_2 free radicals are a metabolite of O_2 metabolism, in the setting of extended exposure to high concentrations, the supply of enzymes responsible for neutralizing those radicals is exhausted, resulting in ALI. Absorption atelectasis can also occur when excess O_2 displaces the nitrogen

normally present in alveoli, causing alveolar collapse (Brashers, 2010). The effects of prolonged exposure to high levels of O_2 include increased pulmonary microvascular permeability, decreased surfactant production and surfactant inactivation, and fibrotic changes in the alveoli. (O_2 delivery devices are discussed in Chapter 31.)

Additional risks of O_2 therapy are specific to the patient with chronic hypercapnia such as the patient with COPD. Chronic hypercapnia may blunt the response of chemoreceptors in the medulla. In this situation, respirations are stimulated by hypoxia. If the PaO_2 is suddenly increased, the patient will no longer be hypoxemic, will have a decreased stimulus to breathe, and may experience a respiratory arrest. Patients with chronic hypercapnia should receive O_2 through a low-flow device such as a nasal cannula at 1 to 2 L/min or a Venturi mask at 24 to 28%. Close monitoring for changes in mental status and respiratory rate and ABG results is essential until PaO_2 levels have reached their baseline value.

▪ Mobilization of Secretions

Retained pulmonary secretions may cause or exacerbate acute respiratory failure by blocking movement of O_2 into the alveoli and the pulmonary capillary blood and removal of CO_2 during

COLLABORATIVE CARE

Table 70-6 Acute Respiratory Failure

Diagnostic	Drug Therapy
• History and physical examination	• Relief of bronchospasm (e.g., salbutamol)
• ABGs	• Reduction of airway inflammation (corticosteroids)
• O₂ saturation	
• Chest radiograph	• Reduction of pulmonary congestion (e.g., furosemide [Lasix])
• CBC	
• Serum electrolytes and urinalysis	• Treatment of pulmonary infections (e.g., antibiotics)
• ECG	• Reduction of anxiety and restlessness (e.g., lorazepam [Ativan])
• Blood and sputum cultures (if indicated)	
• PAP, PAOP, LAP	**Medical Supportive Therapy**
Collaborative Therapy	• Management of the underlying cause of respiratory failure
Respiratory Therapy	
• O₂ therapy	• Maintenance of adequate cardiac output
• Mobilization of secretions	• Maintenance of adequate hemoglobin concentration
• Effective coughing	
• Incentive spirometry	**Nutritional Therapy**
• Hydration and humidification	• Parenteral nutrition support
• Chest physiotherapy	• Enteral nutrition support
• Airway suctioning	
• Positive-pressure ventilation	
• Noninvasive positive-pressure ventilation	
• Intubation with mechanical ventilation	

ABGs, arterial blood gases; *CBC,* complete blood count; *ECG,* electrocardiogram; *LAP,* left atrial pressure; *PAP,* pulmonary artery pressure; *PAOP,* pulmonary artery occlusive (wedge) pressure.

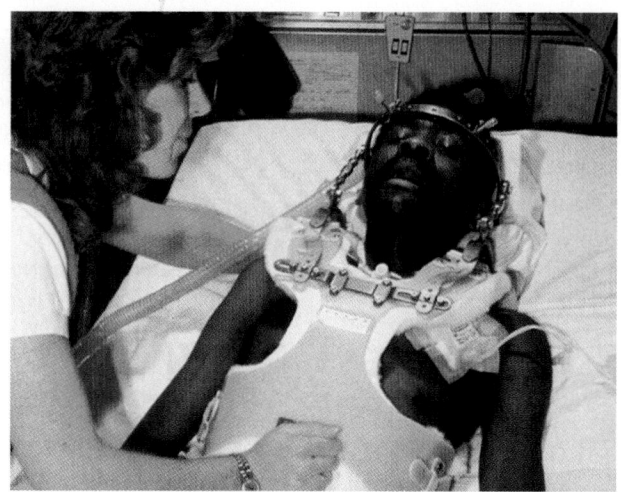

Figure 70-6 Augmented coughing is performed by placing the palm of the hand on the abdominal musculature below the xiphoid process. As the patient ends a deep inspiration and begins the expiration, the hand should be moved forcefully downward, increasing abdominal pressure, resulting in a forceful cough.

Source: Richmond T. S. (1985). The patient with a cervical spinal cord injury: A critical care challenge. *Focus on Critical Care, 12*(2), 23-33 (p. 27).

the respiratory cycle. Secretions can be mobilized through effective coughing, adequate hydration and humidification, chest physiotherapy, and tracheal suctioning.

▌ Effective Coughing and Positioning.

If secretions are obstructing the airway, the patient should be encouraged to cough. The patient with a neuromuscular weakness from a disease or exhaustion may not be able to generate sufficient airway pressures to produce an effective cough. *Augmented coughing (quad coughing)* may be of benefit to these patients. Augmented coughing is performed by placing the palm of the hand or hands on the abdomen below the xiphoid process (Figure 70-6). As the patient ends a deep inspiration and begins the expiration, the hands should be moved forcefully downward, increasing abdominal pressure and facilitating the cough. This measure helps increase expiratory flow and thereby facilitates secretion clearance.

Some patients may benefit from therapeutic cough techniques. *Huff coughing* is a series of coughs performed while saying the word "huff." This technique prevents the glottis from closing during the cough. Patients with COPD generate higher flow rates with a huff cough than is possible with a normal cough. The huff

cough is effective in clearing only the central airways, but it may assist in moving secretions upward. The *staged cough* also assists secretion mobilization. To perform the staged cough, the patient sits in a chair, breathes three or four times in and out through the mouth, and coughs while bending forward and pressing a pillow inward against the diaphragm.

Positioning the patient either by elevating the head of the bed at least 45 degrees or by using a reclining chair or chair bed may help maximize thoracic expansion, thereby decreasing dyspnea and improving secretion mobilization. A sitting position improves pulmonary function and assists in venous pooling in dependent body areas such as the lower extremities. When lungs are upright, ventilation and perfusion are best in the lung bases. Lateral or side-lying positioning, termed *good lung down,* may be used in patients with disease involving only one lung and allows for improved V̇/Q̇ matching in the affected lung. Pulmonary blood flow and ventilation are optimal in dependent lung areas. This positioning also allows for secretions to drain out of the affected lung to the point where they may be removed by suctioning. For example, in patients with a significant right-sided pneumonia, optimal positioning would be to place them on their left side to maximize ventilation and perfusion in the "good" lung and facilitate secretion removal from the affected lung (postural drainage). All patients should be side-lying if there is any possibility that the tongue will obstruct the airway or that aspiration may occur. An oral or nasal airway should be kept at the bedside for use if necessary.

▌ Hydration and Humidification.

Thick and viscous secretions should be thinned to facilitate removal. Adequate fluid intake (2 to 3 L/day) is necessary to keep secretions thin and easy to expel. If the patient is unable to take sufficient fluids orally, intravenous (IV) hydration will be used. Thorough assessment of the patient's cardiac and renal status determines whether he or she can tolerate the intravascular volume and avoid congestive heart failure and pulmonary edema. Assessment for signs of fluid overload (e.g., crackles, dyspnea, and increased central venous pressure) at regular intervals is essential. These considerations would also apply to the patient with renal dysfunction.

An appropriate humidification device is an adjunct in secretion management. Aerosols of sterile normal saline, administered by a nebulizer, may be used to liquefy secretions. O_2 may also be administered by aerosol mask to thin secretions and facilitate their removal. Aerosol therapy may induce bronchospasm and severe coughing, causing a decreased PaO_2. As such, frequent assessment of patient tolerance to therapy is paramount (Sims, 2011). Mucolytic agents such as nebulized acetylcysteine (Mucomyst) mixed with a bronchodilator may be used to thin secretions but, as an adverse effect, may also cause airway erythema and bronchospasm. Therefore, it is used only in special situations (e.g., during bronchoscopy to remove thick, copious secretions).

Chest Physiotherapy.

Chest physiotherapy is indicated in patients who produce more than 30 mL of sputum per day or have evidence of severe atelectasis or pulmonary infiltrates. If tolerated, postural drainage, percussion, and vibration to the affected lung segments may assist in moving secretions to the larger airways where they may be removed by coughing or suctioning. Because positioning may affect oxygenation, patients may not tolerate head-down or lateral positioning because of extreme dyspnea or hypoxemia caused by $\dot{V}/\dot{Q}$ mismatch. (Chest physiotherapy is discussed in Chapter 31.)

Airway Suctioning.

If the patient is unable to expectorate secretions, nasopharyngeal, oropharyngeal, or nasotracheal suctioning (blind suctioning without a tracheal tube in place) is indicated. Suctioning through an artificial airway, such as endotracheal or tracheostomy tubes, may also be performed (see Chapters 29 and 68). A mini-tracheostomy (or "mini-trach") may be used to suction patients who have difficulty mobilizing secretions and when blind suctioning is difficult or ineffective. The *mini-trach* is a 4 mm indwelling plastic cuffless cannula inserted through the cricothyroid membrane. It is used to instill sterile normal saline solution to elicit a cough and to perform suctioning using a size 10 or less French catheter. Contraindications for a mini-trach include an absent gag reflex, history of aspiration, and the need for long-term MV.

Positive-Pressure Ventilation

If intensive measures fail to improve ventilation and oxygenation and the patient continues to exhibit acute respiratory failure, ventilatory assistance may be initiated. PPV may be provided invasively through endotracheal or nasotracheal intubation or noninvasively through a nasal or face mask. Patients who require PPV are typically cared for in a critical care unit. (See Chapter 68 for a discussion of artificial airways and mechanical ventilation.)

Noninvasive positive-pressure ventilation (NIPPV) may be used to treat patients with acute or chronic respiratory failure. During NIPPV, a mask is placed over the patient's nose or nose and mouth while the patient breathes spontaneously (Figure 70-7). With NIPPV, it is possible to decrease the work of breathing without using invasive endotracheal intubation. Bilevel positive airway pressure ventilation is a form of NIPPV in which different positive-pressure levels are set for inspiration and expiration (see Figure 70-7). Continuous positive airway pressure is

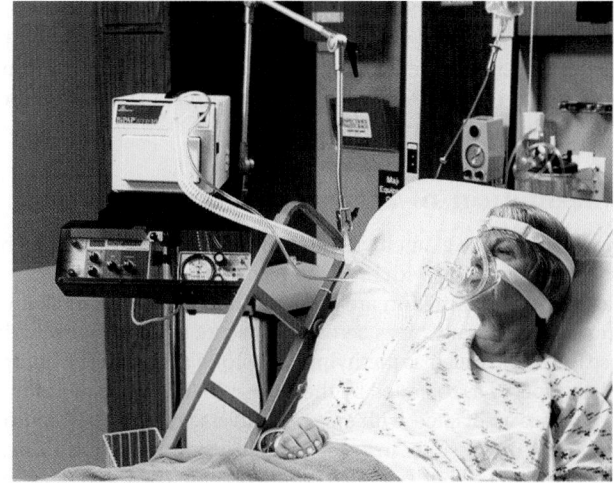

Figure 70-7 Noninvasive bilevel positive-pressure ventilation. A mask is placed over the nose or the nose and mouth. Positive pressure from a mechanical ventilator assists the patient's breathing efforts, decreasing the work of breathing.

Source: Courtesy Respironics, Inc., Pittsburgh, PA.

another form of NIPPV in which a constant positive pressure is delivered to the airway during inspiration and expiration (Urden et al., 2010).

NIPPV is most useful in managing chronic respiratory failure in patients with chest wall and neuromuscular disease (see Table 70-3). NIPPV has been used in patients with hypoxemic respiratory failure (e.g., ARDS, cardiogenic pulmonary edema), but with less success (Nava, Schreiber, & Domenighetti, 2011). NIPPV may also be used for patients who refuse endotracheal intubation but still desire some palliative ventilatory support (e.g., patients with end-stage COPD). NIPPV is not appropriate for the patient who has absent respirations, excessive secretions, and decreased level of consciousness, high O_2 requirements, facial trauma, or hemodynamic instability (Urden et al., 2010).

Drug Therapy

Goals of drug therapy for patients in acute respiratory failure include relief of bronchospasm, reduction of airway inflammation and pulmonary congestion, treatment of pulmonary infection, and reduction of severe anxiety and restlessness.

Relief of Bronchospasm

Alveolar ventilation will be increased with relief of bronchospasm. Short-acting *bronchodilators*, such as fenoterol hydrobromide and salbutamol are frequently administered to reverse bronchospasm using either a handheld nebulizer or a metered-dose inhaler with a spacer (Simon, 2011). In acute bronchospasm, these drugs may be given at 15- to 30-minute intervals until a response can be determined. If severe bronchospasm continues, IV aminophylline may be administered. The bronchodilator effects of all of these medications can sometimes cause a worsening of arterial hypoxemia by redistributing the inspired gas to areas of decreased perfusion. Administering the bronchodilator with an O_2-enriched gas mixture usually alleviates this effect (Sims, 2011). (See Chapter 31 for nursing management related to bronchodilators.) In addition to bronchodilators, IV magnesium sulphate may be beneficial in cases of severe asthma and asthma refractory to conventional treatment (Jones & Goodacre, 2009; Urden et al., 2010).

Reduction of Airway Inflammation

Corticosteroids (e.g., methylprednisolone [Solu-Medrol]) may be used in conjunction with bronchodilating agents when bronchospasm and inflammation are present. They may be administered intravenously, orally, or as aerosols. In acute exacerbations, high-dose IV steroids such as methylprednisolone are used. The dosage is then tapered as tolerated by the patient. Because long-term oral steroids are associated with systemic adverse effects, they should be avoided if possible. Instead, inhaled steroids such as fluticasone (Flovent) or budesonide (Pulmicort) are used to reduce the risk of those systemic adverse effects (Fisher, Charlebois, Tribble, & Merrel, 2009).

Reduction of Pulmonary Congestion

Pulmonary interstitial fluid can accumulate as a consequence of direct or indirect injury to the alveolar capillary membrane (e.g., ARDS) or from right- or left-sided heart failure and, therefore, can be either cardiac or noncardiac in origin. The result is decreased alveolar ventilation and hypoxemia. IV diuretics (e.g., furosemide [Lasix]) and nitroglycerin are used to decrease the pulmonary congestion caused by heart failure. If atrial fibrillation is also present, calcium channel blockers (e.g., diltiazem) and β-adrenergic blockers (e.g., metoprolol) may be used to decrease heart rate and improve cardiac output. (See Chapter 37 for discussion of heart failure.)

Treatment of Pulmonary Infections

Pulmonary infections (pneumonia, acute bronchitis) result in excessive mucus production, fever, increased oxygen consumption, and inflamed, fluid-filled, or collapsed alveoli. Alveoli that are fluid filled or collapsed cannot participate in gas exchange. Pulmonary infections can either cause or exacerbate acute respiratory failure. IV antibiotics, such as vancomycin (Vancocin) or ceftriaxone, are frequently administered to inhibit bacterial growth. Chest radiographic examinations are performed to determine the location and the extent of a suspected infectious process. Sputum cultures are used to determine the type of organisms causing the infection and their sensitivity to antimicrobial medications.

Reduction of Severe Anxiety, Pain, and Agitation

Anxiety, restlessness, and agitation result from cerebral hypoxia. In addition, fear caused by the inability to breathe and a sense of loss of control may exacerbate anxiety. Anxiety, pain, and agitation increase O_2 consumption, which may worsen the degree of hypoxemia. Increase in anxiety and agitation can affect ventilator management. Administration of sedatives, narcotics, or muscle relaxants may be necessary to provide adequate oxygenation and ventilation. Several nursing strategies can assist the patient in reducing the level of anxiety and pain (see NCP 70-1).

Sedation and analgesia with drug therapy such as benzodiazepines (e.g., lorazepam [Ativan], midazolam) and narcotics (e.g., morphine, fentanyl) may decrease anxiety, agitation, and pain. Continued agitation will increase the patient's work of breathing, O_2 consumption, CO_2 production, and risk of injury (e.g., accidental extubation). In the critical care setting, sedation and analgesia are commonly used, and patients must be monitored closely for cardiovascular and respiratory depression. It is important to note that agitation is best characterized as a symptom and may be caused by pain, hypoxemia, electrolyte imbalance, evolution of structural or metabolic brain injury, and adverse drug reactions. As such, assessment and treatment of potentially reversible causes should always be undertaken. Sedative and analgesic agents may have prolonged duration of action in critically ill patients. This may contribute to increased length of stay and prolonged ventilator days (Mehta et al., 2008). Patients receiving these agents are best managed using a research-based, protocol-driven plan of care (Mehta et al., 2008) (see the Nursing Research box on this page).

Sedation protocols can be used to guide the level of sedation. Most patients who are difficult to oxygenate require heavy sedation (4 to 5 on the Richmond Agitation Sedation Scale). Patients who breathe asynchronously with MV may also benefit from titration of ventilator settings as well as addressing underlying causes of agitation.

Once complete sedation is achieved, if the patient is still hypoxic, the use of neuromuscular blockade (NMB) may be indicated with agents such as vecuronium or cisatracurium (Nimbex). These NMB agents produce skeletal muscle relaxation and synchrony with MV. NMB may also decrease the patient's risk of lung injury related to excessive intrathoracic pressures and promote optimal ventilatory support. Patients receiving NMB should receive sedation and analgesia to the point of unconsciousness for comfort, elimination of patient awareness, and prevention of the terrifying experience of being awake and in pain while paralyzed (Papazian et al., 2010). The level of pharmacological paralysis is monitored using a peripheral nerve stimulator and clinical correlation to achieve absence of respiratory effort. Daily interruption of sedative drug infusions (DI) decreases the duration of MV and length of stay in the critical care unit and shows a reduction in 1-year mortality (Girard et al., 2008).

Medical Supportive Therapy

Interventions to maximize O_2 delivery and treat the underlying cause of respiratory failure are essential to improving the patient's oxygenation and ventilation status. The primary goal is to treat the underlying cause of the respiratory failure. Other goals include maintaining an adequate cardiac output and hemoglobin concentration.

Treating the Underlying Cause

Interventions are directed toward reversing the disease process that resulted in the development of acute respiratory failure. Patients with hypoventilation can be diagnosed and treated rapidly. Patients with $\dot{V}/\dot{Q}$ mismatch, shunting, or diffusion limitation are managed differently depending on the underlying cause. In all patient situations, monitoring treatment effects, including trends in ABGs and changes in respiratory status, is a continuous process.

NURSING RESEARCH
Sedation Practices in Critical Care

Citation

Mehta, S., Burry, L., Martinez-Motta, J., Stewart, T., Hallett, D., McDonald, E., . . ., Cook, D. (2008). A randomized trial of daily awakening in critically ill patients managed with a sedation protocol: A pilot trial. *Critical Care Medicine*, *36*(7), 2092-2099. doi:10.1097/CCM.0b013e31817bff85

Purpose

Protocolized sedation (PS) and daily sedative interruption (DI) in critically ill patients have both been shown to shorten the durations of mechanical ventilation (MV) and critical care unit (CCU) stay. The objective of this study was to determine the safety and feasibility of a randomized trial to determine whether adults managed with both PS + DI have a shorter duration of MV than patients managed with PS alone.

Methods

This was a randomized, multicentre pilot trial that took place in three university-affiliated medical–surgical CCUs. The sample included 65 adults who required MV for greater than 48 hours and were receiving sedation/analgesic infusions. Patients were randomized to PS alone or to PS + DI. PS was implemented by bedside nurses; sedatives/analgesics were titrated to achieve Sedation Agitation Score of 3 to 4. The PS + DI group also had infusions interrupted daily until the patients awoke.

Results

The median duration of MV in the PS and PS + DI groups was 8.0 and 10.5 days, respectively, and CCU stay was 10.0 and 13.0 days, respectively. The Sedation Agitation Score was within target range (3 to 4) in 59% of 9611 measurements, and within an acceptable range (2 to 5) in 86% of measurements. Self-assessed nursing and respiratory therapist workload was low in the majority of the cohort. Adverse events were similar in both groups. This pilot trial comparing PS vs. PS + DI confirmed the safety and acceptability of the sedation protocol and DI and guided important modifications to the protocol, thus enhancing the feasibility of a future multicentre trial.

Implications for Nursing Practice

Barriers to the use of DI include a lack of nursing acceptance and concerns regarding patient removal of invasive devices, patient discomfort, respiratory compromise, and withdrawal syndromes. The development of evidence-informed sedation protocols that are multidisciplinary affect ventilator length of stay in addition to time spent on the ventilator. DI has been found to limit oversedation in the CCU without compromising patient comfort or safety and should be incorporated into the routine care of mechanically ventilated patients.

Maintaining Adequate Cardiac Output

Cardiac output reflects the blood flow reaching the tissues. BP and mean arterial pressure are important indicators of the adequacy of cardiac output and should be interpreted within the context of the overall assessment indicating adequacy of cardiac output and tissue perfusion. Usually, a systolic BP of 90 mm Hg or higher and a mean arterial pressure of 60 mm Hg or higher is adequate to maintain perfusion to the vital organs; therefore, changes in mental status can usually be attributed to the level of O_2 and CO_2, rather than decreased cerebral perfusion, when these pressures are maintained. Patients with chronic, uncontrolled hypertension may require higher systemic arterial pressures and mean arterial pressures to prevent episodes of brain ischemia.

Decreased cardiac output is treated by administration of IV fluids, medications, or both. (See Chapter 69 for a discussion of drugs used to treat decreased cardiac output and shock.) Cardiac output may also be decreased by changes in intrathoracic or intrapulmonary pressures from PPV. Patients experiencing exacerbation of COPD or asthma and those receiving controlled ventilation are at risk of alveolar hyperinflation, increased right ventricular afterload, and excessive intrathoracic pressures. These alterations in thoracic pressure dynamics may cause increased right ventricular afterload, which limits blood flow from the right side of the heart through the pulmonary vasculature to the left side of the heart; this may potentially result in dramatic hemodynamic compromise. In addition, blood return from the systemic circulation to the right side of the heart may be impaired, decreasing preload (Urden et al., 2010). Each of these physiological consequences can potentially compromise hemodynamics. Consequently, clinical indicators of adequate cardiac output and tissue perfusion should be monitored alongside initiation or titration of MV by mask or endotracheal intubation.

Maintaining Adequate Hemoglobin Concentration

Hemoglobin is the primary carrier when delivering O_2 to the tissues. If the patient is anemic, tissue O_2 delivery will be compromised. A hemoglobin concentration of 6 mmol/L or greater typically ensures adequate O_2 saturation of the hemoglobin. The patient should be monitored for sites of blood loss and transfused with packed red blood cells if an adequate hemoglobin concentration cannot be maintained.

Nutritional Therapy

Maintenance of protein and energy stores is especially important in patients with acute respiratory failure because nutritional depletion causes loss of muscle mass, including the respiratory muscles, and may prolong recovery. During the acute manifestations of respiratory failure, the risk of aspiration typically prevents oral intake; therefore, enteral or parenteral nutrition may be administered until symptoms subside and the patient tolerates oral intake. A multitude of nutritional supplements are available (Pontes-Arruda, Demichele, Seth, & Singer, 2008). Although controversial, a high-carbohydrate diet may be avoided in patients who retain CO_2 because carbohydrates metabolize into CO_2, further increasing CO_2 load. In addition, the hypermetabolic state encountered in critical illness can dramatically increase caloric requirements.

Evaluation

The expected outcomes for the patient with acute respiratory failure are presented in NCP 70-1.

AGE-RELATED CONSIDERATIONS: RESPIRATORY FAILURE

The older adult population is the fastest growing age group in North America, a trend that is reflected within acute and critical care settings. Importantly, older adults are more vulnerable to delirium, hospital-acquired infections, and medication effects. Multiple factors contribute to an increased risk of respiratory failure in older adults, including the reduction in ventilatory capacity that accompanies aging, especially if risk factors are present. Physiological aging of the lung may produce alveolar dilation, diminished elastic recoil within the airways, decreased chest wall compliance, and decreased respiratory muscle strength. In older adults, the PaO_2 falls further and the $PaCO_2$ rises to a higher level before the respiratory system is stimulated to alter the rate and the depth of breathing. This delayed response can contribute to the development of respiratory failure. In addition, smoking is a risk factor that accelerates age-related respiratory changes. Poor nutritional status predisposes to decreased muscle mass, and less physiological reserve in cardiovascular, respiratory, and autonomic nervous systems increases the risk of additional diseases such as pneumonia and cardiac disease that may compromise respiratory function and precipitate respiratory failure (Delerme & Ray, 2008; Urden et al., 2010).

Assessment parameters should be adjusted for age. For example, heart rate and BP generally increase with age and changes in the cardiovascular system. Therefore, determination of the patient's baseline vital signs and using them as a basis for comparison of physical assessment findings is most appropriate in evaluating changes in cardiopulmonary function in the older adult.

Acute Respiratory Distress Syndrome

Acute respiratory distress syndrome (ARDS) is a sudden and progressive form of acute respiratory failure in which the alveolar–capillary membrane becomes damaged and more permeable to intravascular fluid (Figure 70-8). The alveoli fill with fluid, resulting in severe dyspnea, hypoxemia refractory to supplemental O_2, reduced lung compliance, and diffuse pulmonary infiltrates (Leaver & Evans, 2007; Brashers, 2010; Urden et al., 2010). ARDS has been the focus of extensive clinical research which has not significantly improved survival rates (Bosma, Taneja, & Lewis, 2010). Despite supportive therapy, the mortality rate from ARDS is approximately 50% (Koutsogiannidis, Ampatzidou, Ananiadou, Karaiskos, & Drossos, 2012). Patients who have both gram-negative septic shock and ARDS have a significantly higher mortality (Chau-Chyun et al., 2010).

Etiology and Pathophysiology

Table 70-7 lists conditions that predispose patients to the development of ARDS. The most common cause of ARDS is sepsis. Patients with multiple risk factors are three to four times more likely to develop ARDS.

Direct lung injury may cause ARDS (Figure 70-9) or ARDS may develop as a consequence of the systemic inflammatory response syndrome (SIRS) (see Chapter 69, Figure 69-1). SIRS may have an infectious or a noninfectious etiology and is

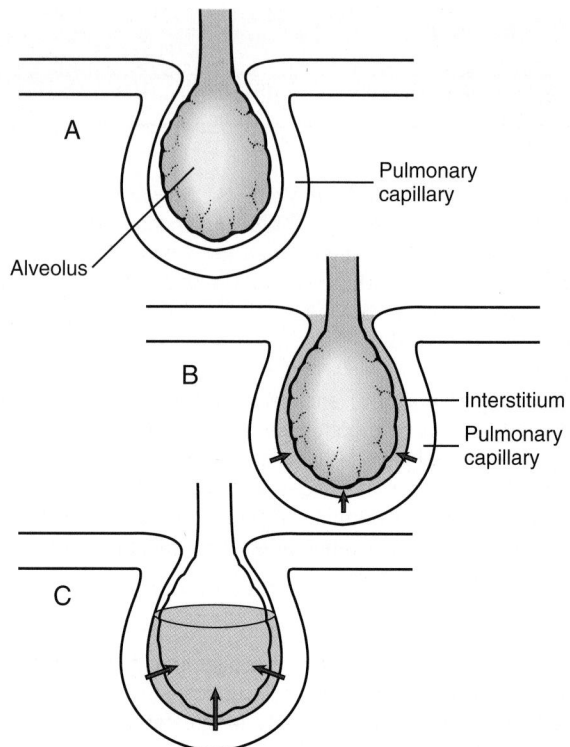

Figure 70-8 Stages of edema formation in acute respiratory distress syndrome. **A,** Normal alveolus and pulmonary capillary. **B,** Interstitial edema occurs with increased flow of fluid into the interstitial space. **C,** Alveolar edema occurs when the fluid crosses the blood–gas barrier.

Table 70-7 Conditions Predisposing to Acute Respiratory Distress Syndrome	
DIRECT LUNG INJURY	**INDIRECT LUNG INJURY**
Common Causes	
• Aspiration • Viral or bacterial pneumonia	• Sepsis (especially Gram-negative infection) • Severe massive trauma
Less Common Causes	
• Chest trauma • Embolism: fat, air, amniotic fluid • Inhalation of toxins • Near-drowning • O_2 toxicity • Radiation pneumonitis	• Acute pancreatitis • Anaphylaxis • Blood transfusions • Cardiopulmonary bypass • Disseminated intravascular coagulation • Narcotic overdose (e.g., heroin) • Nonpulmonary systemic diseases • Severe head injury • Shock

characterized by widespread inflammation or clinical responses to inflammation following a variety of physiological insults, including severe trauma, gut ischemia, lung injury, and sepsis (Urden et al., 2010). ARDS may also develop as a consequence of multiple organ dysfunction syndrome (MODS). MODS results

PATHOPHYSIOLOGY MAP

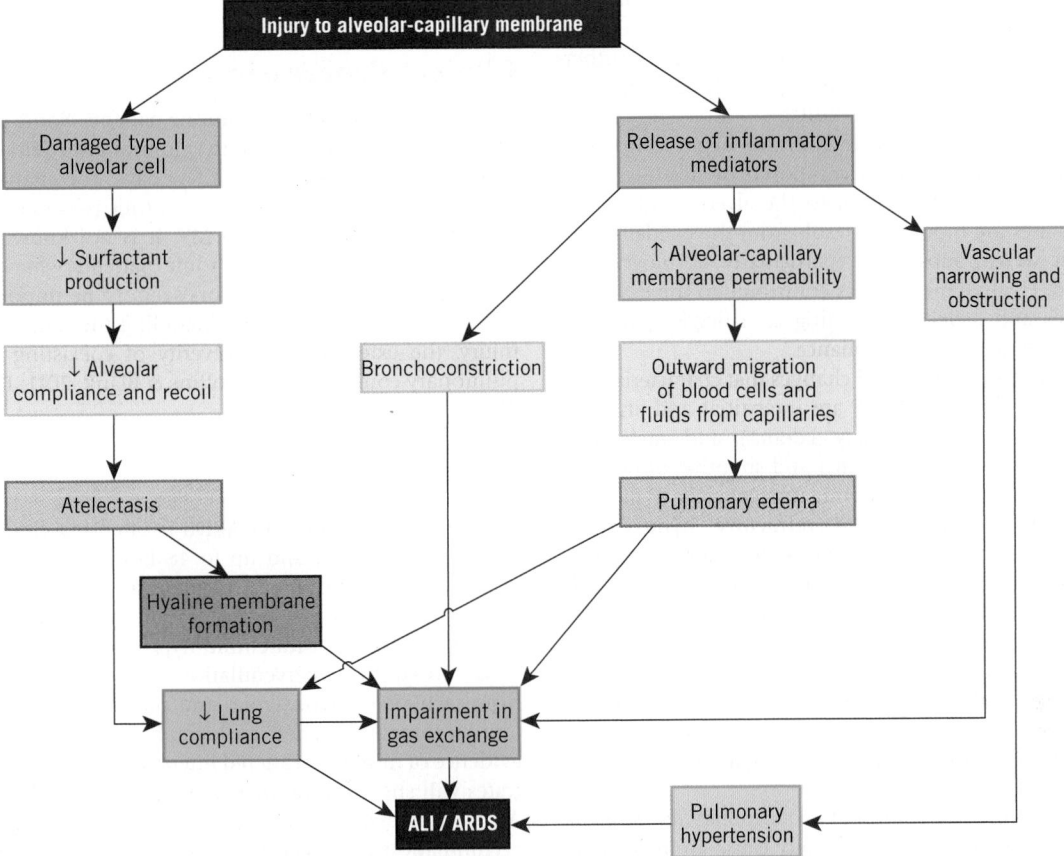

Figure 70-9 Pathophysiology of acute respiratory distress syndrome (ARDS). *ALI,* acute lung injury.

from organ system dysfunction that progressively increases in severity and ultimately results in multisystem organ failure. (SIRS and MODS are discussed in Chapter 69.)

The initial injury to the lungs damages the alveolar–capillary membrane. This activates complement and stimulates platelet aggregation and intravascular thrombus formation. Platelets release substances that attract and activate neutrophils (Brashers, 2010). The neutrophils cause a release of biochemical, humoral, and cellular mediators (Table 70-8) that produce changes in the lung, including increased pulmonary capillary membrane permeability, destruction of elastin and collagen, formation of pulmonary microemboli, and pulmonary artery vasoconstriction (see Figure 70-9). (Mediators are discussed in Chapters 14 and 16.) The pathophysiological changes in ARDS are divided into three phases: (1) injury or exudative phase, (2) reparative or proliferative phase, and (3) fibrotic phase.

Injury or Exudative Phase.
The *injury or exudative phase* occurs approximately 1 to 7 days (usually 24 to 48 hours) after the initial direct lung injury or host insult. Neutrophils adhere to the pulmonary microcirculation, causing damage to the vascular endothelium and increased capillary permeability. In the earliest phase of injury, there is engorgement of the peribronchial and perivascular interstitial space, which produces interstitial edema. Next, fluid from the interstitial space crosses the alveolar epithelium and enters the alveolar space. Intrapulmo-

Table 70-8 Mediators of Acute Lung Injury

- Complement component C5a
- Neutrophil products, including proteases and O_2 radicals
- Monocyte and macrophage products, including tumour necrosis factor, interleukin-1, and colony-stimulating factor
- Arachidonic acid metabolites, including prostaglandins and leukotrienes
- Coagulation products, including kallikreins, kinins, fibrin degradation products, and plasminogen-activating factor
- Histamine
- Serotonin
- Endotoxin
- Elastase
- Collagenase

nary shunt develops because the alveoli fill with fluid, and blood passing through them cannot be oxygenated (see Figures 70-4 and 70-7).

Alveolar type 1 and type 2 cells (which produce surfactant) are damaged by the changes caused by ARDS. This damage, in addition to further fluid and protein accumulation, results in surfactant dysfunction. The function of *surfactant* is to maintain alveolar stability by decreasing alveolar surface tension and preventing alveolar collapse. Decreased synthesis of surfactant and inactivation of existing surfactant cause the alveoli to become unstable and collapse (atelectasis). Widespread atelectasis further decreases lung compliance, compromises gas exchange, and contributes to hypoxemia (Urden et al., 2010).

Also during this stage, hyaline membranes begin to line the alveoli. The hyaline membrane is composed of necrotic cells, protein, and fibrin and lies adjacent to the alveoli wall. These hyaline membranes are thought to result from the exudation of high–molecular weight substances (particularly fibrinogen) in the edema fluid. Hyaline membranes contribute to the development of fibrosis and atelectasis, leading to a decrease in gas-exchange capability and lung compliance.

The primary pathophysiological changes that characterize the injury or exudative phase of ARDS are interstitial and alveolar edema (noncardiogenic pulmonary edema) and atelectasis (Brashers, 2010). Severe $\dot{V}/\dot{Q}$ mismatch and shunting of pulmonary capillary blood result in hypoxemia unresponsive to increasing concentrations of O_2 (termed **refractory hypoxemia**). Diffusion limitation, caused by hyaline membrane formation, further contributes to the severity of the hypoxemia. As the lungs become less compliant because of decreased surfactant, pulmonary edema, and atelectasis, the patient must generate higher airway pressures to inflate "stiff" lungs. Reduced lung compliance greatly increases the patient's work of breathing. During ventilator management at this stage, a progressive increase in plateau and inspiratory pressures may be noted as lung compliance worsens.

Hypoxemia and the stimulation of juxtacapillary receptors in the stiff lung parenchyma (J reflex) initially cause an increase in respiratory rate and decrease in tidal volume. This breathing pattern increases CO_2 removal, producing respiratory alkalosis. Cardiac output increases in response to hypoxemia, a compensatory effort to increase pulmonary blood flow. However, as atelectasis, pulmonary edema, and pulmonary shunt increase, compensation fails, and hypoventilation and decreased cardiac output and tissue O_2 perfusion eventually occur.

Reparative or Proliferative Phase. The *reparative or proliferative phase* of ARDS begins 1 to 2 weeks after the initial lung injury. During this phase, there is an influx of neutrophils, monocytes, and lymphocytes, together with fibroblast proliferation, as part of the inflammatory response. The injured lung has an immense regenerative capacity after ALI. The proliferative phase is complete when the diseased lung becomes characterized by dense, fibrous tissue. Increased pulmonary vascular resistance and pulmonary hypertension may occur in this stage because fibroblasts and inflammatory cells destroy the pulmonary vasculature. Lung compliance continues to decrease as a result of interstitial fibrosis. Hypoxemia worsens because of the thickened alveolar membrane, causing diffusion limitation and shunting. If the reparative phase persists, widespread fibrosis results. If the reparative phase is arrested, the lesions resolve (Brashers, 2010; Urden et al., 2010).

Fibrotic Phase. The *fibrotic phase* of ARDS, also called chronic or late phase, occurs approximately 2 to 3 weeks after the initial lung injury. The lung is now completely remodelled by sparsely collagenous and fibrous tissues. Diffuse scarring and fibrosis further decrease lung compliance. In addition, the surface area for gas exchange is significantly reduced because the interstitium is fibrotic, and therefore, hypoxemia continues. Pulmonary hypertension results from pulmonary vascular destruction and fibrosis.

Clinical Progression

Progression of ARDS varies among patients. Some people survive the acute phase of lung injury; pulmonary edema resolves and complete recovery occurs in a few days. The chance for survival is poor in patients who enter the fibrotic (chronic or late) phase, which necessitates long-term MV. It is not known why injured lungs repair and recover in some patients whereas, in others, ARDS progresses. Several factors seem to be important in determining the course of ARDS, including the nature of the initial injury, the extent and the severity of coexisting diseases, and pulmonary complications (Collins & Blank, 2011; Herridge et al., 2011).

Clinical Manifestations

The initial presentation of ARDS is often insidious. At the time of the initial injury, and up to 48 hours afterward, the patient may exhibit only dyspnea, tachypnea, cough, and restlessness. Chest auscultation may be normal or reveal fine, scattered crackles. ABGs usually indicate mild hypoxemia and respiratory alkalosis caused by hyperventilation. Respiratory alkalosis results from tachypnea, hypoxemia, and the stimulation of juxtacapillary receptors. The chest radiograph may be normal or exhibit evidence of minimal scattered interstitial infiltrates. Bilateral infiltrates will show on the chest radiograph as ARDS progresses. As ARDS progresses, symptoms worsen because of increased fluid accumulation and decreased lung compliance. Respiratory distress becomes evident as the work of breathing increases. Tachypnea and intercostal and suprasternal retractions may be present. Pulmonary function tests in ARDS reveal decreased compliance and decreased lung volumes, particularly a decreased functional residual capacity. Tachycardia, diaphoresis, changes in sensorium with decreased mentation, cyanosis, and pallor may be present. Chest auscultation usually reveals scattered to diffuse crackles and wheezes. The chest radiograph demonstrates diffuse and extensive bilateral interstitial and alveolar infiltrates. A pulmonary artery catheter may be inserted. Pulmonary artery wedge pressure does not increase in ARDS because the cause is noncardiogenic (not related to cardiac function).

Hypoxemia and a PaO_2/FiO_2 ratio below 200 despite increased FiO_2 by mask, cannula, or endotracheal tube are hallmarks of ARDS. ABGs may initially demonstrate a normal or decreased $PaCO_2$ despite severe dyspnea and hypoxemia. Hypercapnia signifies that hypoventilation is occurring and the patient is no longer able to maintain the level of ventilation needed to provide optimum gas exchange.

As ARDS progresses, it is associated with profound respiratory distress necessitating endotracheal intubation and PPV. The chest radiograph (Figure 70-10) shows what is often termed *whiteout* or *white lung*, because consolidation and coalescing infiltrates are widespread throughout the lungs, leaving few recognizable air spaces. Pleural effusions may also be present. Severe hypoxemia, hypercapnia, and metabolic acidosis, with symptoms of target organ or tissue hypoxia, may ensue if prompt therapy is not instituted.

No precise criteria define ARDS. ARDS is considered to be present if the patient has (1) refractory hypoxemia, (2) a chest radiograph with new bilateral interstitial or alveolar infiltrates,

Table 70-9 Diagnostic Findings in Acute Respiratory Distress Syndrome

Refractory Hypoxemia

PaO_2 <50 mm Hg on FiO_2 >40% with PEEP >5 cm H_2O

PaO_2/FiO_2 ratio <200

Chest Radiograph

New bilateral interstitial and alveolar infiltrates

Pulmonary Artery Wedge Pressure

≤18 mm Hg and no evidence of heart failure

Predisposing Condition

Identification of a predisposing condition for ARDS within 48 hours of clinical manifestations

ARDS, acute respiratory distress syndrome; *FiO₂,* fraction of inspired oxygen; *PaO₂,* partial pressure of oxygen in arterial blood; *PEEP,* positive end-expiratory pressure.

Table 70-10 Complications Associated With Acute Respiratory Distress Syndrome

Infection

- Catheter-related infection
- Hospital-acquired pneumonia
- Sepsis (bacteremia)

Respiratory Complications

- O_2 toxicity
- Pulmonary barotraumas (e.g., pneumothorax, pneumomediastinum, subcutaneous emphysema)
- Pulmonary emboli
- Pulmonary fibrosis
- Ventilator-associated pneumonia

Gastrointestinal Complications

- Paralytic ileus
- Pneumoperitoneum
- Stress ulceration and hemorrhage
- Hypermetabolic state, dramatically increased nutritional requirements

Renal Complications

- Acute renal failure

Cardiac Complications

- Dysrhythmias
- Decreased cardiac output

Hematological Complications

- Anemia
- Disseminated intravascular coagulation
- Thrombocytopenia

ET Intubation Complications

- Laryngeal ulceration
- Tracheal malacia
- Tracheal stenosis
- Tracheal ulceration

ET, endotracheal.

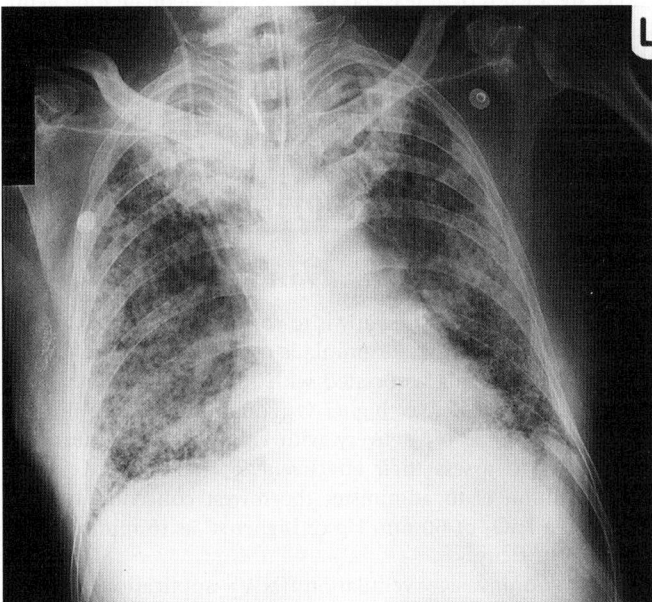

Figure 70-10 Chest radiograph of a patient with acute respiratory distress syndrome. The image shows new, bilateral diffuse, homogeneous pulmonary infiltrates without cardiac failure, fluid overload, chest infection, or chronic lung disease.

Source: Cohen, J., & Powderly, W. G. (2004). *Infectious diseases* (2nd ed.). St. Louis: Mosby.

(3) a pulmonary artery wedge pressure of 18 mm Hg or less and no evidence of heart failure, and (4) a predisposing condition for ARDS within 48 hours of clinical manifestations (Table 70-9).

Complications

Complications may develop as a result of ARDS or its treatment. (Table 70-10 lists the common complications of ARDS.) The major cause of death in ARDS is multiple organ dysfunction syndrome, often accompanied by sepsis. The vital organs most commonly involved are the kidneys, liver, and heart. The organ systems most often involved are the CNS and the hematological and gastrointestinal systems.

Hospital-Acquired Pneumonia. A frequent complication of ARDS is hospital-acquired pneumonia, occurring in as many as 68% of patients with ARDS. Risk factors include impaired host defences, contaminated medical equipment, invasive monitoring devices, aspiration of gastrointestinal contents, and prolonged MV as well as colonization of the respiratory tract. Strategies to prevent hospital-acquired pneumonia include infection control measures (e.g., strict handwashing and sterile technique during endotracheal suctioning) and elevating the head of the bed 45 degrees or more to prevent aspiration (Bream-Rouwenhorst, Beltz, Ross, & Moores, 2008; Urden et al., 2010). (See Chapter 30 for discussion of pneumonia.)

Barotrauma. *Barotrauma* may result from rupture of overdistended alveoli during MV. The high airway pressures required to ventilate patients with ARDS predispose to this complication. Barotrauma results in the presence of alveolar air in locations where it is not usually found. This can lead to pulmonary interstitial emphysema, pneumothorax, subcutaneous emphysema, pneumoperitoneum, pneumomediastinum, and tension pneumothorax. (See Chapter 30 for discussion of pneumothorax.)

To avoid barotrauma, patients with ARDS are ventilated with smaller tidal volumes. Different approaches to lung-protective ventilation are in current clinical use. Ventilation protocol include the use of small tidal volumes (e.g., 6 mL/kg) and varying amounts of positive end-expiratory pressure (PEEP) while allowing the $PaCO_2$ to gradually rise above normal *(permissive hypercapnia)* with the pH supported at 7.2 to 7.25 or above (Mulligan, 2011). High-frequency oscillation uses a constant mean airway pressure to maintain the alveoli in a recruited state while low tidal volumes are oscillated at a fast rate. Ventilation is achieved by the generation of extremely rapid pressure oscillations, usually in the range of 300 to 900 cycles/min (Putensen, Theuerkauf, Zinserling, Wrigge, & Pelosi, 2009; Collins & Blank, 2011).

Volutrauma. *Volutrauma*, or *volupressure trauma*, can occur in patients with ARDS when large tidal volumes (10 to 15 mL/kg) are used to ventilate noncompliant lungs. Volutrauma results in alveolar fractures and movement of fluids and proteins into the alveolar spaces. To limit this complication, it is recommended that smaller tidal volumes or pressure ventilation be used in patients with ARDS (Nelles & Gentile, 2007) (see Chapter 68).

Stress Ulcers. Critically ill patients with acute respiratory failure are at high risk for stress ulcers. Bleeding from stress ulcers occurs in 30% of patients with ARDS who require PPV, a higher incidence than other causes of acute respiratory failure. Management strategies include correction of predisposing conditions such as hypotension, shock, and acidosis. Prophylactic management includes antiulcer agents (e.g., famotidine [Pepcid], omeprazole [Losec], sucralfate [Sulcrate]) and early initiation of enteral nutrition (see Chapters 42 and 68).

Renal Failure. Renal failure results from decreased renal tissue oxygenation owing to hypotension, hypoxemia, or hypercapnia and from administration of nephrotoxic drugs (e.g., aminoglycosides).

NURSING AND COLLABORATIVE MANAGEMENT: ACUTE RESPIRATORY DISTRESS SYNDROME

The collaborative care for acute respiratory failure (see Table 70-6) and the NCP for acute respiratory failure (see NCP 70-1) are applicable to ARDS. The following section discusses additional collaborative care measures for the patient with ARDS (Table 70-11). Patients with ARDS are commonly cared for in critical care units.

COLLABORATIVE CARE

Table 70-11 Acute Respiratory Distress Syndrome

Diagnostic	*Supportive Therapy*
• See Table 70-9.	• Identification and treatment of underlying cause
Collaborative Therapy	• Hemodynamic monitoring
Respiratory Therapy	• Inotropic or vasopressor medications
• O₂ administration	• Dopamine
• Prone positioning	• Dobutamine
• Lateral rotation therapy	• Diuretics
• Mechanical ventilation with PEEP	• IV fluid administration (fluid resuscitation early and less fluids later)
• High-frequency oscillation	

IV, intravenous; *PEEP*, positive end-expiratory pressure.

Nursing Assessment

Because ARDS causes acute respiratory failure, the subjective and objective data that should be obtained from a person with ARDS are the same as that for acute respiratory failure (see Table 70-5). Abnormal findings on physical examination are indications that ARDS has progressed beyond the initial stages.

Nursing Diagnoses

Nursing diagnoses for the patient with ARDS may include, but are not limited to, those described for acute respiratory failure (see NCP 70-1).

Planning

With appropriate therapy, the overall goals for the patient with ARDS are a PaO₂ of at least 60 mm Hg and adequate lung ventilation to maintain normal pH. Following recovery from ARDS, the patient will have (1) PaO₂ within normal limits for age or baseline values on room air (FiO₂ of 21%), (2) SaO₂ greater than 90%, (3) patent airway, and (4) clear lungs on auscultation.

Respiratory Therapy

Oxygen Administration

The primary goal of O₂ therapy is to correct hypoxemia. Use of a simple face mask or nasal cannula is usually inadequate to treat refractory hypoxemia associated with ARDS. Masks with high-flow systems that deliver higher O₂ concentrations are initially used to maximize O₂ delivery with continuous O₂ saturation monitoring to assess their effectiveness. The standard for O₂ administration is to administer the lowest concentration that results in a PaO₂ of 60 mm Hg or higher so as to minimize the risk of O₂ toxicity.

Early noninvasive ventilation (NIV) application may be extremely helpful in immunocompromised patients with pulmonary infiltrates, in whom intubation dramatically increases the risk of infection, pneumonia, and death. Overall, the high rate of NIV failure suggests a cautious approach to NIV use in patients with ALI/ARDS, including early initiation, intensive monitoring, and prompt intubation if signs of NIV failure emerge (Nava et al., 2011). Patients with ARDS commonly need intubation with MV because the PaO₂ cannot otherwise be maintained at acceptable levels.

Mechanical Ventilation

Endotracheal intubation and MV provide additional respiratory support. However, it may still be necessary to administer FiO₂ of 50% or greater to maintain the PaO₂ at 60 mm Hg or higher. During MV, it is common to apply PEEP at 5 cm H₂O to compensate for loss of glottic function caused by the presence of the endotracheal tube. In patients with ARDS, higher levels of PEEP (e.g., 10 to 20 cm H₂O) may be used to increase functional residual capacity and recruit (open up) collapsed alveoli. PEEP is typically applied in 3- to 5-cm H₂O increments until oxygenation is adequate with FiO₂ of 60% or lower. PEEP may improve $\dot{V}/\dot{Q}$

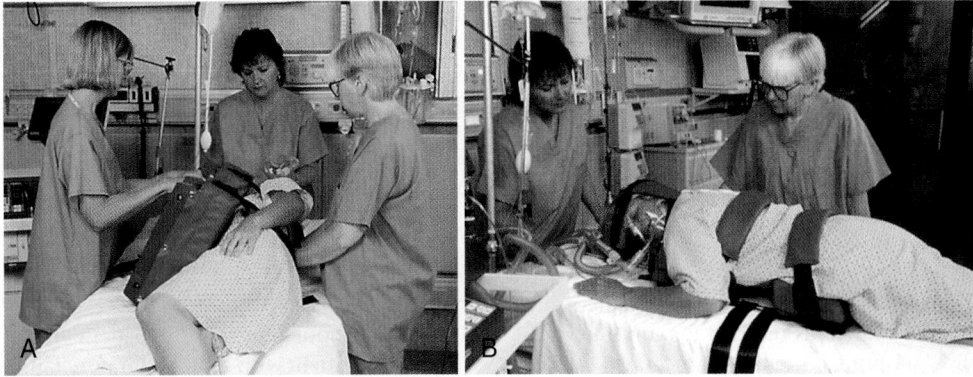

Figure 70-11 A, Turning a patient prone on the Vollman Prone Positioner. **B,** A patient lying prone on the Vollman Prone Positioner.

in respiratory units that collapse at low airway pressures, thus allowing the FiO_2 to be lowered.

However, PEEP is not a benign therapy. The additional intrathoracic and intrapulmonic pressures can compromise venous return to the right side of the heart, thereby decreasing preload, cardiac output, and BP. PEEP can also cause hyperinflation of the alveoli, compression of the pulmonary capillary bed, a reduction in blood return to the left side of the heart, and a dramatic reduction in BP. In addition, PEEP and excessive inspiratory pressures can contribute to barotrauma and volutrauma (Malhotra, 2007).

If hypoxemia persists despite high PEEP, alternative modes and therapies may be used. These include pressure-support ventilation, pressure-release ventilation, pressure-control ventilation, inverse ratio ventilation, high-frequency oscillation, and permissive hypercapnia. (Additional information on mechanical ventilation and PEEP is provided in Chapter 68.)

Extracorporeal membrane oxygenation and extracorporeal carbon dioxide removal pass blood across an external gas-exchanging membrane and return oxygenated blood back to the body. Although extracorporeal membrane oxygenation has not clearly been demonstrated to be better than the standard of care for ARDS, referral to a specialized centre with extracorporeal membrane oxygenation experience should be considered early after the initiation of high-level ventilator support (Valenza, 2009).

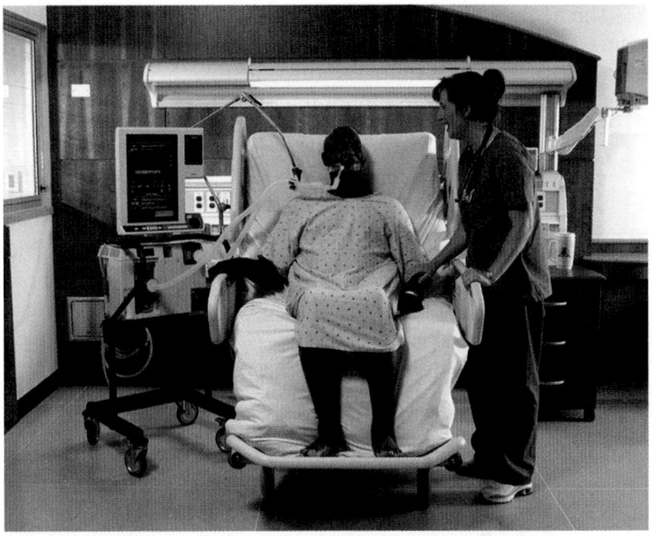

Positioning Strategies

Some patients with ARDS demonstrate an improvement in PaO_2 when turned from supine to prone position with no change in FiO_2 (Figure 70-11). The response may be sufficient to allow a reduction in FiO_2 or PEEP.

In early ARDS, fluid moves freely throughout the lung. Because of gravity, this fluid pools in dependent lung regions such that some alveoli are fluid filled (dependent areas) whereas others are air filled (nondependent areas). In addition, when the patient is supine, the mediastinal contents place more pressure on the lungs than in the prone position, which changes pleural pressure and predisposes to atelectasis. If the patient is turned to prone position, air-filled, nonatelectic alveoli in the ventral (anterior) lung become dependent. Perfusion may be better matched to ventilation, causing less $\dot{V}/\dot{Q}$ mismatch. Prone positioning is typically reserved for patients with refractory hypoxemia, but not

Figure 70-12 TotalCare SpO_2RT® Bed System offers continuous lateral rotation therapy and percussion and vibration therapies. Patients can easily and quickly be repositioned.

all respond with an increase in PaO_2. When prone positioning is used, there must be a plan for immediate repositioning for cardiopulmonary resuscitation in the event of a cardiac arrest (Collins & Blank, 2011).

Other positioning strategies used in ARDS are lateral rotation therapy and kinetic therapy (Fessler & Talmor, 2010). The purpose of this therapy is to provide continuous, slow, side-to-side turning of the patient by rotating the bed frame. Lateral movement of the bed is maintained for 18 hours daily to simulate postural drainage and help mobilize secretions. In addition, the bed may also contain a vibrator pack that can provide chest physiotherapy to further assist with secretion removal (Figure 70-12). Assessment of the patient's pulmonary status (e.g., respiratory rate and rhythm, breath sounds, ABGs, SpO_2) should be obtained before initiation of the therapy and continued throughout.

Medical Supportive Therapy

Maintenance of Cardiac Output and Tissue Perfusion

Patients on PPV and PEEP frequently experience decreased cardiac output related to impaired contractility, decreased preload, decreased venous return, or some combination, as a result of PEEP-induced increases in intrathoracic pressure. Continuous hemodynamic monitoring is essential to detect changes and titrate therapy. An arterial catheter is inserted for continuous BP monitoring and ABG sampling. A pulmonary artery catheter permits monitoring of pulmonary artery pressures, pulmonary artery wedge pressures (which reflect the fluid status of the left side of the heart), mixed venous oxygen saturation, and cardiac output. If the cardiac output falls, it may be necessary to administer fluids or to lower the PEEP. Use of inotropic drugs such as dobutamine or dopamine may also be necessary. (See Chapter 68 for discussion of hemodynamic monitoring.)

The hemoglobin is usually kept above 6 mmol/L with an O_2 saturation of 90 or higher (when $PaO_2 \geq 60$ mm Hg). Packed red blood cells may be administered to increase hemoglobin and, thus, the O_2-carrying capacity of the blood.

Maintenance of Nutrition and Fluid Balance

Maintenance of nutrition and fluid balance is challenging in patients with ARDS. Nutrition consultations determine optimal caloric needs. Attaining access and initiating enteral nutrition should be considered as soon as fluid resuscitation is completed and the patient is hemodynamically stable. A "window of opportunity" exists in the first 24 to 72 hours following admission or the onset of a hypermetabolic insult. Research has shown that enteral formulas enriched with omega-3 fatty acids may improve the clinical outcomes of patients with ARDS (McClave et al., 2009).

Increased pulmonary capillary permeability results in pulmonary edema. Yet the patient may be volume depleted, hypotensive, and prone to decreased cardiac output from MV and PEEP. Pulmonary artery wedge pressures, daily weights, and intake and output are monitored to assess fluid status. Fluid replacement with crystalloids versus colloids is controversial. Critics of colloids believe that proteins in colloid solutions leak into the pulmonary interstitium, exacerbating the movement of proteinaceous fluid into the alveoli (Brodie & Bacchetta, 2011). Advocates of colloids as replacement believe that colloids help keep fluid from leaking into the alveoli (Brodie & Bacchetta, 2011). The pulmonary artery wedge pressure is kept as low as possible without impairing cardiac output in order to limit pulmonary edema. The patient is usually mildly fluid restricted with diuretic use as needed (Urden et al., 2010).

Evaluation

The expected outcomes for the patient with ARDS are similar to those for a patient with acute respiratory failure and are presented in NCP 70-1.

Severe Acute Respiratory Syndrome

Severe acute respiratory syndrome (SARS) is a serious, acute respiratory infection caused by a coronavirus (CoV). The virus spreads by close contact between people. SARS-CoV is most likely spread via droplets in the air. It is possible that SARS-CoV may also be spread more broadly through the air or from touching contaminated objects.

The vast majority of patients with SARS-CoV will have a history of exposure to a SARS patient or to a setting in which SARS-CoV transmission is occurring and will develop pneumonia (Schub & Ciasulli, 2012). In general, SARS begins with a fever greater than 38°C. Other manifestations may include sore throat, headache, chills, generalized discomfort, and muscle aches. After 2 to 7 days, SARS patients may develop a dry cough and dyspnea.

Because the disease is severe, treatment is started based on symptoms and immediately, before the illness is confirmed. First, suspected SARS patients should be placed in isolation to protect others. Although there is no definitive treatment for SARS, antiviral medications (such as ribavirin) and corticosteroids may be used. Although antibiotics will not help with SARS (because it is believed to be caused by a virus), they may be used in cases in which the person also has a bacterial infection.

About 80 to 90% of infected people start to recover after 6 to 7 days. However, 10 to 20% go on to develop severe breathing problems and may need MV. The risk of death is higher for this group and appears to be linked to the person's pre-existing health condition. People older than age 40 are more likely to develop severe breathing problems (Cleri, Ricketti, & Vernaleo, 2010).

CLINICAL DECISION-MAKING EXERCISE

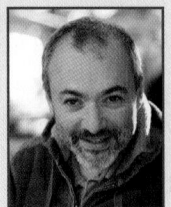

CASE STUDY:
Acute Respiratory Distress Syndrome

Source: © iStockphoto.com/Galina Barskaya.

Patient Profile

Mr. Habib is a 55-year-old man who was admitted to a surgical critical care unit (CCU) 72 hours ago after bowel resection. The surgery was extensive to repair a perforated colon, irrigate the abdominal cavity, and provide hemostasis. During surgery, his systolic blood pressure (BP) dropped to 70 mm Hg. Seven units of packed red blood cells and 4 L of normal saline were administered to restore blood loss and circulating volume. He is currently receiving 60% FiO_2 through an aerosol face mask and has continuous cardiac monitoring and O_2 saturation in place. He is receiving 0.9% normal saline at 125 mL/hr through a central line. A urinary catheter is in place.

Subjective Data

- He complains of shortness of breath, inability to lie flat, and diffuse abdominal pain.

- His wife and two adult children are at the bedside voicing concerns and asking questions about his condition.

Objective Data

Physical Assessment

- General: Alert, well nourished, appears restless and anxious; head of bed elevated 30 degrees; skin cool, moderate diaphoresis
- Respiratory: No accessory muscle use, retractions, or paradoxical breathing; rate 28 breaths/min; arterial oxygen saturation measured by pulse oximetry (SpO_2) 85%; fine crackles at lung bases
- Cardiovascular: BP 90/60 mm Hg; sinus tachycardia at 130 beats/min, equal apical–radial pulse; temperature 38°C orally
- Gastrointestinal: No bowel sounds heard; surgical dressing dry and intact
- Urological: Catheter draining concentrated urine at <30 mL/hr

Diagnostic Findings

- Arterial blood gas (ABG) results: pH 7.35, partial pressure of oxygen in arterial blood (PaO_2) 55 mm Hg, partial pressure of carbon dioxide in arterial blood ($PaCO_2$) 27 mm Hg, bicarbonate 16 mmol/L, arterial oxygen saturation measured by ABGs (SaO_2) 86%

- Chest radiograph: new scattered interstitial infiltrates compatible with acute respiratory distress syndrome (ARDS)

Discussion Questions

1. How does the pathophysiology of ARDS predispose to the development of refractory hypoxemia?
2. What clinical manifestations does Mr. Habib exhibit that support a diagnosis of ARDS?
3. What are the possible causes of ARDS in Mr. Habib?
4. What are the possible complications that Mr. Habib is at risk for developing secondary to ARDS?
5. *Priority Decision:* What priority interventions should be implemented to improve Mr. Habib's respiratory status and hypoxemia?
6. *Priority Decision:* Based on the assessment data presented, what are the priority nursing diagnoses?
7. What information should the nurse provide to the caregiver(s) given Mr. Habib's decline in cardiopulmonary function?

evolve *Answers are available at* **http://evolve.elsevier.com/ Canada/Lewis/medsurg**

REVIEW QUESTIONS

The number of the question corresponds to the same-numbered objective at the beginning of the chapter.

1. What is the cause of hypercapnic respiratory failure?
   a. Acute respiratory distress syndrome (ARDS)
   b. Asthma
   c. Pneumonia
   d. Pulmonary emboli
2. What is an early sign of acute respiratory failure?
   a. Coma
   b. Cyanosis
   c. Restlessness
   d. Paradoxical breathing
3. Which type of oxygen delivery system should be chosen for patients in acute respiratory failure?
   a. Should always be a low-flow device, such as a nasal cannula
   b. Should correct the partial pressure of oxygen in arterial blood (PaO_2) to a normal level as quickly as possible
   c. Should administer positive-pressure ventilation to prevent CO_2 narcosis
   d. Should maintain the PaO_2 at 60 mm Hg or higher at the lowest fraction of inspired oxygen (FiO_2) possible

4. What are the early clinical manifestations of ARDS?
   a. Dyspnea and tachypnea
   b. Cyanosis and apprehension
   c. Hypotension and tachycardia
   d. Respiratory distress and frothy sputum
5. How is fluid balance maintained in the patient with ARDS?
   a. Hydration using colloids
   b. Administration of surfactant
   c. Mild fluid restriction and diuretics as necessary
   d. Keeping the hemoglobin at levels of 9.5 mmol/L (15 g/dL)
6. Which of the following is designed to prevent barotrauma in the patient with ARDS?
   a. Increasing positive end-expiratory pressure (PEEP)
   b. Increasing the tidal volume
   c. Permissive hypercapnia
   d. Pressure support ventilation

ANSWERS: 1. b; 2. c; 3. d; 4. a; 5. c; 6. c.

REFERENCES

Anderson, S., & Spencer, D. (2009). Common respiratory disorders. In P. G. Morton & D. K. Fontaine (Eds.), *Critical care nursing: A holistic approach* (9th ed., pp. 660-661). Philadelphia: Wolters Kluwer Health.

Bosma, K., Taneja, R., & Lewis, J. (2010). Pharmacotherapy for prevention and treatment of acute respiratory distress syndrome: Current and experimental approaches. *Drugs, 70*(10), 1255-1282. doi:10.2165/10898570-000000000-00000

Brashers, V. (2010). Alterations of pulmonary function. In K. L. McCance & S. E. Huether (Eds), *Pathophysiology: The biologic basis for disease in adults and children* (6th ed., pp. 1242-1307). St. Louis: Elsevier Mosby.

Bream-Rouwenhorst, H., Beltz, E., Ross, M., & Moores, K. (2008). Recent developments in the management of acute respiratory distress syndrome in adults. *American Journal of Health-System Pharmacy, 65*(1), 29-36. doi:10.2146/ajhp060530

Brodie, D., & Bacchetta, M. (2011). Extracorporeal membrane oxygenation for ARDS in adults. *New England Journal of Medicine, 365*(20), 1905-1914. doi:10.1056/NEJMct1103720

Chau-Chyun, S., Gong, M. N., Rihong, Z., Feng, C., Bajwa, E. K., Clardy, P. F., ..., Christiani, D. C. (2010). Clinical characteristics and outcomes of sepsis-related vs non-sepsis-related ARDS. *Chest, 138*(3), 559-567. doi:10.1378/chest.09-2933

Cleri, D., Ricketti, A., & Vernaleo, J. (2010). Severe acute respiratory syndrome (SARS). *Infectious Disease Clinics, 24*(1), 175-202. doi:10.1016/j.idc.2009.10.005

Collins, S. R., & Blank, R. S. (2011). Approaches to refractory hypoxemia in acute respiratory distress syndrome: Current understanding, evidence, and debate. 26th New Horizons Symposium, "ARDS Update," at the 56th International Respiratory Congress of the American Association for Respiratory Care, held December 6-9, 2010, Las Vegas, NV. *Respiratory Care, 56*(10), 1573-1582. doi:10.4187/respcare.01366

Delerme, S., & Ray, P. (2008). Acute respiratory failure in the elderly: Diagnosis and prognosis. *Age and Ageing, 37*(3), 251-257. doi:10.1093/ageing/afn060

Fessler, H., & Talmor, D. (2010). Should prone positioning be routinely used for lung protection during mechanical ventilation? Includes discussion. *Respiratory Care, 55*(1), 88-99.

Fisher, C., Charlebois, D. L., Tribble, S. S., Merrel, P. K. (2009). In P. G. Morton & D. K. Fontaine (Eds.), *Critical care nursing: A holistic approach* (9th ed., p. 588). Philadelphia: Wolters Kluwer Health.

Girard, T. D., Kress, J. P., Fuchs, B. D., Thomason, J. W., Schweickert, W. D., Pun, B. T., ..., Ely, E. W. (2008). Efficacy and safety of a paired sedation and ventilator weaning protocol for mechanically ventilated patients in intensive care (Awakening and Breathing Controlled trial): A randomised controlled trial. *Lancet, 371*: 126–134. doi:10.1016/S0140-6736(08)60105-1

Herridge, M., Tansey, C., Matté, A., Tomlinson, G., Diaz-Granados, N., Cooper, A., ..., Cheung, A. (2011). Functional disability 5 years after acute respiratory distress syndrome. *New England Journal of Medicine, 364*(14), 1293-1304. doi:10.1056/NEJMoa1011802

Jones, L., & Goodacre, S. (2009). Magnesium sulphate in the treatment of acute asthma: Evaluation of current practice in adult. *Emergency Medicine Journal, 26*(11), 783-785. doi:10.1136/emj.2008.065938

Koutsogiannidis, C. C., Ampatzidou, F. C., Ananiadou, O. G., Karaiskos, T. E., & Drossos, G. E. (2012). Noninvasive ventilation for post-pneumonectomy severe hypoxemia. *Respiratory Care, 57*(9), 1514-1516. doi:10.4187/respcare.01493

Lamontagne, F., Briel, M., Guyatt, G., Cook, D., Bhatnagar, N., & Meade, M. (2010). Corticosteroid therapy for acute lung injury, acute respiratory distress syndrome, and severe pneumonia: A meta-analysis of randomized controlled trials. *Journal of Critical Care, 25*(3), 420-435. doi:10.1016/j.jcrc.2009.08.009

Leaver, S. K., & Evans, T. W. (2007). Acute respiratory distress syndrome. *British Medical Journal, 335*(7616), 389-394.

Lynn-McHale Weigand, D. J. (Ed.). (2011). *AACN procedure manual for critical care* (6th ed.). St. Louis: Elsevier Saunders.

Malhotra, A. (2007). Low-tidal-volume ventilation in the acute respiratory distress syndrome. *New England Journal of Medicine, 357*(11), 1113-1120. doi:10.1056/NEJMct074213

McClave, S., Martindale, R., Vanek, V., McCarthy, M., Roberts, P., Taylor, B., ..., Cresci, G. (2009). Guidelines for the provision and assessment of nutrition support therapy in the adult critically ill patient: Society of Critical Care Medicine (SCCM) and American Society for Parenteral and Enteral Nutrition (A.S.P.E.N.). *JPEN Journal of Parenteral & Enteral Nutrition, 33*(3), 277-316. doi:10.1177/0148607109335234

Mehta, S., Burry, L., Martinez-Motta, J., Stewart, T., Hallett, D., McDonald, E., ..., Cook, D. (2008). A randomized trial of daily awakening in critically ill patients managed with a sedation protocol: A pilot trial. *Critical Care Medicine, 36*(7), 2092-2099. doi:10.1097/CCM.0b013e31817bff85

Mulligan, M. (2011). Permissive hypercapnia: Finding its place in clinical care. *MLO: Medical Laboratory Observer, 43*(1), 26-28.

Nava, S., Schreiber, A., & Domenighetti, G. (2011). Noninvasive ventilation for patients with acute lung injury or acute respiratory distress syndrome. 26th New Horizons Symposium, "ARDS Update," at the 56th International Respiratory Congress of the American Association for Respiratory Care, held December 6-9, 2010, Las Vegas, NV. *Respiratory Care, 56*(10), 1583-1588. doi:10.4187/respcare.01209

Nelles, S. M., & Gentile, M. A. (2007). Specialized techniques in mechanical ventilation. In L. N. B. Pierce (Ed), *Management of the mechanically ventilated patient* (2nd ed., pp. 406-456). St. Louis: Saunders.

Papazian, L., Forel, J., Gacouin, A., Penot-Ragon, C., Perrin, G., Loundou, A., ..., Roch, A. (2010). Neuromuscular blockers in early acute respiratory distress syndrome. *New England Journal of Medicine, 363*(12), 1107-1116. doi:10.1056/NEJMoa1005372

Peñuelas, O., Frutos-Vivar, F., & Esteban, A. (2007). Non-invasive positive-pressure ventilation in acute respiratory failure. *Canadian Medical Association Journal, 177*(10), 1211-1218. doi:10.1503/cmaj.060147

Pontes-Arruda, A., Demichele, S., Seth, A., & Singer, P. (2008). The use of an inflammation-modulating diet in patients with acute lung injury or acute respiratory distress syndrome: A meta-analysis of outcome data. *JPEN Journal of Parenteral & Enteral Nutrition, 32*(6), 596-605. doi:10.1177/0148607108324203

Putensen, C., Theuerkauf, N., Zinserling, J., Wrigge, H., & Pelosi, P. (2009). Meta-analysis: Ventilation strategies and outcomes of the acute respiratory distress syndrome and acute lung injury. *Annals of Internal Medicine, 151*(8), 566-576.

Schub, T., & Ciasulli, K. (2012). Severe acute respiratory syndrome (SARS). [serial online]. May 11, 2012. Available from: CINAHL Plus with Full Text, Ipswich, MA.

Simon, E. (2011). *Critical care nursing practice guide: A road map for students and new graduates.* Sudbury, MA: Jones & Bartlett Learning.

Sims, M. (2011). Aerosol therapy for obstructive lung diseases: Device selection and practice management issues. *Chest, 140*(3), 781-788. doi:10.1378/chest.10-2068

Urden, L. D., Stacy, K. M., & Lough, M. E. (2010). *Critical care nursing: Diagnosis and management* (6th ed.). St. Louis: Mosby.

Valenza, T. (2009). The CESAR trial: ECMO versus conventional ventilation. Conventional versus ECMO for severe adult respiratory failure. *RT: The Journal for Respiratory Care Practitioners, 22*(5), 30-32. Retrieved from *http://www.rtmagazine.com/issues/articles/2009-05_05.asp*

RESOURCES

Resources for this chapter are listed in Chapter 71, p. 2034.

Nursing Management: Emergency Care Situations

Written by Linda Bucher

Adapted by Lynne Thibeault

LEARNING OBJECTIVES

1. Apply the sequential steps in the primary and the secondary survey to assess a patient in an emergency situation.
2. Describe the pathophysiology, the assessment, and the collaborative care of select environmental emergencies, including hyperthermia, hypothermia, submersion injury, bites, and stings.
3. Discuss the assessment and the collaborative care of select toxicological emergencies.
4. Develop an awareness of organ donation and mandatory reporting of various forms of abuse and weapon-related injuries.
5. Develop an awareness of domestic violence, and the nurse's role in assessing and caring for victims in the ED.

KEY TERMS

domestic violence A pattern of coercive behaviour in a relationship that involves fear; humiliation; intimidation; neglect; intentional physical, emotional, financial, or sexual injury or assault; or a combination of these, p. 2030

frostbite True tissue freezing, which results in the formation of ice crystals in the tissues and cells, p. 2024

heat cramps Severe cramps in large muscle groups fatigued by heavy work, p. 2022

heat exhaustion A clinical syndrome characterized by fatigue, light-headedness, nausea, vomiting, diarrhea, and a sensation of impending doom, caused by prolonged exposure to heat over hours or days, p. 2022

heat stroke The most serious form of heat stress; results from failure of the central thermoregulatory mechanisms, p. 2022

hypothermia Core temperature lower than 36°C; occurs when heat produced by the body cannot compensate for heat lost to the environment, p. 2024

jaw-thrust manoeuvre A technique for establishing a clear airway, in which the rescuer uses forearms to stabilize the patient's head (while avoiding neck hyperextension) and then applies pressure with the index fingers to push the patient's jaw forward, p. 2015

pneumatic antishock garment (PASG) A three-chambered suit that increases peripheral resistance in the lower extremities, thus elevating blood pressure and working to control pelvic fracture–related bleeding, p. 2016

primary survey A systematic approach to emergency assessment that focuses on airway, breathing, circulation, and disability (ABCDs) and serves to identify life-threatening conditions, p. 2015

rapid-sequence intubation Preferred procedure for securing an unprotected airway; involves the use of sedation and paralysis to facilitate intubation while the risk of aspiration and airway trauma is minimized, p. 2015

secondary survey A brief, systematic process that is aimed at identifying all injuries (follows primary survey and lifesaving interventions), p. 2017

submersion injury Injury resulting when a person becomes hypoxic as a result of submersion in a substance, usually water, p. 2025

triage system A process of identifying and sorting patients' conditions so that those in most critical condition are treated first, p. 2014

ELECTRONIC RESOURCES

Supplemental content related to Chapter 71 can be found ...

Evolve Web Site ⊖volve

http://evolve.elsevier.com/Canada/Lewis/medsurg
- Answer Guidelines for Case Study on p. 2032
- Clinical Reference: Laboratory Values

- Content Updates
- Electronic Calculators
- Examination Review Questions
- Glossary
- Interactive Case Study: Musculoskeletal Trauma
- Key Points (Printable and MP3 Download)

Most patients with life-threatening problems arrive at the hospital through the emergency department (ED). According to the National Trauma Registry of the Canadian Institute for Health Information (CIHI), there were 14,065 major-injury cases in 2008 and 2009. The leading causes of injury were motor vehicle collisions, which were responsible for almost 41% of the cases. Of these patients, 11% died as a result of their injuries. Blunt trauma was the most common injury in 93% of those who died, followed by penetrating injuries (5%) and burn injuries (2%; CIHI, 2011). Many patients report to the ED for less urgent conditions, often because they do not have access to a health care provider. Emergency nurses care for patients of all ages and with a variety of problems, especially in the areas of health promotion and prevention and chronic disease management. Some EDs specialize in certain patient populations, such as pediatric patients, or certain conditions, such as trauma.

The National Emergency Nurses Affiliation (NENA) is the Canadian specialty nursing organization aimed at advancing emergency nursing practice. NENA publishes standards of care for nurses working in the ED and endorses the Canadian Nurses Association's (CNA) certification process to become a certified emergency nurse, ENC(C). This certification validates the knowledge and skills that a nurse needs to provide competent care in emergency settings (Canadian Nurses Association, 2011; NENA, 2011).

Specific emergency management of patients with various medical, surgical, and traumatic emergencies is described throughout this book (Table 71-1).

This chapter focuses on initial assessment and management of patients with trauma and emergency conditions not addressed elsewhere in this book, including heat- and cold-related emergencies, submersion injuries, bites, stings, poisonings, abuse, and violence.

EMERGENCY MANAGEMENT

Table 71-1 Emergency Management Tables

SUBJECT	CHAPTER
Abdominal trauma	45
Acute abdominal pain	45
Acute soft-tissue injury	65
Anaphylactic shock	16
Chemical burns	27
Chest pain	36
Chest trauma	30
Cocaine and amphetamine toxicity	11
Depressant drugs, overdose of	11
Diabetic ketoacidosis	52
Electrical burns	27
Eye injury	24
Fractured extremity	65
Head injury	59
Hyperthermia	71
Hypothermia	71
Inhalation injury	27
Sexual assault	56
Shock	69
Spinal cord injury	63
Stroke	60
Submersion injuries	71
Thermal burns	27
Thoracic injuries	30
Tonic–clonic seizures	61

Care of the Emergency Patient

A **triage system** identifies and categorizes patients' conditions so that those in most critical condition are treated first. The process is based on the premise that patients who have a threat to life, limb, or vision should be treated before other patients. The Canadian Triage and Acuity Scale (CTAS) is used in the ED and by community paramedics to define the urgency of the patient's presenting problem (Bullard, Unger, Spence, Grafstein, & The CTAS National Working Group, 2008).

The CTAS is a five-level scale consisting of the following categories: resuscitation, emergency, urgent, less urgent, and nonurgent (Table 71-2). Patients who are assigned to a high triage level (level I: resuscitation) are allocated the most health care resources and are assessed immediately. Those assigned to a low triage level (e.g., level V: nonurgent) wait longer for nurse and physician assessment, unless there is deterioration in clinical status while they wait (Canadian Association of Emergency Physicians, 2008). The CTAS has four major components: (a) five

Table 71-2 The Canadian Emergency Department Triage and Acuity Scale

CONSIDERATION	RESUSCITATION (LEVEL I)	EMERGENCY (LEVEL II)	URGENT (LEVEL III)	LESS URGENT (LEVEL IV)	NONURGENT (LEVEL V)
Condition	Threat to life or limb; immediate assessment required	Potential threat to life, limb, or function	Potential to progress to serious problem	May progress to urgent status	Acute or chronic but nonurgent
Time to nurse and physician assessment	Immediate	15 min	30 min	60 min	120 min
Recommended re-evaluation	Continuous	Every 15 min	Every 30 min	Every 60 min	Every 120 min

Source: Adapted from Bullard, M. J., Unger, B., Spence, J., Grafstein, E., & The CTAS National Working Group. (2008). Revisions to the Canadian Triage and Acuity Scale (CTAS) adult guidelines. *Canadian Journal of Emergency Medicine, 10*(2), 137.

triage levels (ranging from nonurgent to resuscitation); (b) a *time to nurse and physician assessment,* which is based on the assigned triage level; (c) *usual presentation of the patient* (e.g., head injury, alert, with no vomiting; sore throat with no respiratory symptoms), which is based on the patient's complaints and presentation; and (d) a *sentinel diagnosis* (e.g., head injury; upper respiratory infection; Canadian Association of Emergency Physicians, 2008).

The emergency nurse must complete an initial assessment to determine the presence of actual or potential threats to life and then rapidly initiate interventions appropriate for the patient's condition. A history is obtained simultaneously. A systematic approach to the initial assessment of the patient decreases the time required to identify potential threats and keeps to a minimum the risk of missing a life-threatening condition. Two systematic approaches initially developed for use with patients with trauma, a primary and a secondary survey, can be applied to emergency assessment.

Primary Survey

The **primary survey** (Table 71-3) focuses on *a*irway, *b*reathing, *c*irculation, and *d*isability (ABCDs) and serves to identify life-threatening conditions so that appropriate interventions can be initiated. Life-threatening conditions related to airway, breathing, circulation, and disability (Table 71-4) may be identified during the primary survey, and the nurse starts interventions immediately before proceeding to the next step of the survey.

A = Airway With Cervical Spine Stabilization or Immobilization

Nearly all immediate deaths from trauma occur because of airway obstruction. Saliva, bloody secretions, vomitus, laryngeal trauma, facial trauma, fractures, and the tongue can obstruct the airway. Medical patients at risk for airway compromise include those who have seizures, near-drowning, anaphylaxis, foreign body obstruction, or cardiopulmonary arrest. If an airway is not maintained, airflow is obstructed, and hypoxia, acidosis, and death result.

Primary signs and symptoms in a patient with a compromised airway include dyspnea, inability to vocalize, presence of a foreign body in the airway, and trauma to the face or neck. Airway maintenance should progress rapidly from the least to the most invasive method. One treatment method is to open the airway by means of the **jaw-thrust manoeuvre,** in which the rescuer uses forearms to stabilize the patient's head (while avoiding neck hyperextension) and then applies pressure with the index fingers to push the patient's jaw forward (Figure 71-1). Other treatment methods include suctioning and removal of foreign bodies; insertion of a nasopharyngeal or oropharyngeal airway (which causes a conscious patient to gag); and endotracheal intubation. If the patient cannot be intubated because of airway obstruction, an emergency cricothyroidotomy or tracheotomy should be performed (Chapter 29). Patients should be ventilated with 100% oxygen through a bag–valve–mask (BVM) device before intubation or cricothyroidotomy (Bair, Walls, & Grayzel, 2011).

Rapid-sequence intubation is the preferred procedure for securing an unprotected airway in the ED. It involves the use of a rapid-acting sedative (e.g., etomidate) and a paralyzing neuromuscular blocking agent (e.g., succinylcholine) to facilitate intubation and minimize the risk of aspiration and airway trauma (Bair, Walls, & Grayzel, 2011).

In any patient with significant injuries to the upper torso or trauma to the face, head, or neck, cervical spine trauma should always be suspected. The cervical spine must be stabilized with the head immobilized in a neutral position. At the scene of the injury, the spine is immobilized with a rigid cervical collar or an immobilization device such as head blocks or towel rolls that are secured to a backboard on either side of the head. Finally, the patient's forehead is taped to the backboard.

B = Breathing

Adequate airflow through the upper airway does not ensure adequate ventilation. Breathing alterations are caused by many conditions, including fractured ribs, pneumothorax, penetrating injuries, allergic reactions, pulmonary emboli, and asthma attacks. Patients may exhibit a variety of signs and symptoms, including dyspnea (e.g., pulmonary emboli), stridor, accessory muscle use, paradoxical or asymmetrical chest wall movement (e.g., flail chest), decreased or absent breath sounds on the affected side (e.g., pneumothorax), visible wound to chest wall (e.g., penetrating injury), cyanosis (e.g., asthma), tachycardia, and hypotension.

Every critically injured or ill patient has increased metabolic and oxygen demands and should receive supplemental oxygen. High-flow oxygen (100%) should be administered via a nonrebreather mask and the patient's response monitored. Life-

Table 71-3 Primary Survey of a Patient in an Emergency

ASSESSMENT	INTERVENTIONS
Airway With Simultaneous Cervical Spine Stabilization and Immobilization	
• Clear and open airway. • Assess for obstruction of airway. • Assess for respiratory distress. • Check for loose teeth and foreign objects. • Assess for bleeding, vomitus, or edema.	• Use suction. • Perform jaw-thrust manoeuvre. • Assess nasal or oral airway, endotracheal tube, or cricothyroidotomy. • Immobilize cervical spine with collar, backboard, or soft rolls; tape forehead to board.
Breathing	
• Assess ventilation. • Look for paradoxical movement of the chest wall during inspiration and expiration. • Note use of accessory muscles or abdominal muscles. • Listen for air being expelled through nose and mouth. • Feel for air being expelled. • Observe and count respiratory rate. • Note colour of nail beds, mucous membranes, and skin. • Auscultate lungs. • Assess for jugular venous distension and position of trachea.	• Ventilate with bag–valve–mask device with 100% O_2. • Prepare to intubate if respiratory arrest occurs. • Have suction available. • Administer supplemental O_2 via appropriate delivery system. • If breath sounds are absent, prepare for needle thoracostomy and chest tube insertion.
Circulation	
• Check carotid or femoral pulse. • Palpate pulse for quality and rate. • Assess colour, temperature, and moisture of skin. • Check capillary refill. • Assess for external bleeding. • Auscultate blood pressure.	• If pulse is absent, initiate cardiopulmonary resuscitation and advanced life support measures. • If shock symptoms are present or patient is hypotensive, insert two large-bore (14- to 16-gauge) intravenous catheters and initiate infusions of normal saline or lactated Ringer's solution. • Administer blood products, if ordered. • Consider autotransfusion if chest trauma is isolated. • Consider use of a pneumatic antishock garment in the presence of pelvic fracture. • Obtain blood samples for typing and crossmatching. • Control bleeding with direct pressure.
Disability: Brief Neurological Assessment	
• Assess level of consciousness by determining response to verbal stimuli, painful stimuli, or both. • Assess pupils for size, shape, equality, and response to light.	• Periodically reassess level of consciousness. • Consider the possibility of hyperventilation if signs of brain herniation are present (e.g., motor posturing).

threatening conditions, such as tension pneumothorax and flail chest, can severely compromise ventilation. Interventions in these situations include BVM ventilation with 100% oxygen, intubation, and treatment of the underlying cause. In patients with established chronic obstructive pulmonary disease, carbon dioxide retention and level of consciousness must be monitored.

C = Circulation

An effective circulatory system includes the heart, intact blood vessels, and adequate blood volume. Uncontrolled internal or external bleeding increases the risk for hemorrhagic shock (Chapter 69). A central pulse (e.g., carotid) should be checked because peripheral pulses may be absent as a result of direct injury or vasoconstriction. If a pulse is palpated, the quality, the rate, and the regularity are assessed. Skin should be assessed for colour, temperature, and moisture. Capillary refill delayed longer

than 3 seconds and altered mental status are the most significant signs of shock. Care must be taken when capillary refill is evaluated in cold environments because the cold can cause vasoconstriction, which delays refill.

Intravenous (IV) catheters are inserted into veins in the upper extremities unless this is contraindicated, as in a massive fracture or an injury that affects limb circulation. Two large-bore (14- to 16-gauge) IV catheters should be inserted and aggressive fluid resuscitation initiated with lactated Ringer's solution or normal saline. Direct pressure with a sterile dressing should be applied to obvious bleeding sites. Blood samples are obtained for typing to determine ABO and Rh group. Type-specific packed red blood cells should be administered if needed. In an emergency (life-threatening) situation, blood that is not crossmatched may be given if immediate transfusion is warranted.

The **pneumatic antishock garment (PASG)** is a temporary strategy that has been used for hemorrhage. Blood is shunted

Table 71-4 Causes of Life-Threatening Conditions Identified During the Primary Survey*

Airway	Circulation
• Inhalation injury	• Direct cardiac injury (e.g., myocardial infarction, trauma)
• Obstruction, partial or complete, by foreign bodies, debris (e.g., vomitus), or tongue	• Pericardial tamponade
• Penetrating wounds, blunt trauma, or both to the upper airway structures	• Shock (e.g., massive burns)
	• Uncontrolled external hemorrhage
	• Hypothermia
Breathing	**Disability**
• Anaphylaxis	• Head injury
• Flail chest with pulmonary contusion	• Stroke
• Hemothorax	
• Open pneumothorax	
• Tension pneumothorax	

* This list is not all-inclusive.

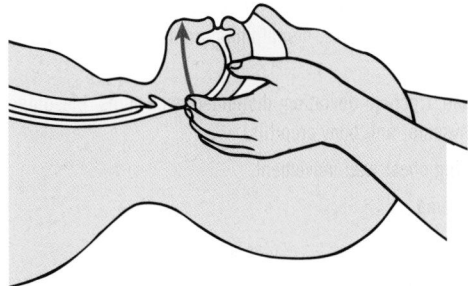

Figure 71-1 The jaw-thrust manoeuvre is the only widely recommended procedure for use on an unconscious patient with possible neck or spinal injuries. The patient should be lying supine, and the rescuer should kneel at the top of the patient's head. The rescuer carefully reaches forward and gently places one hand on each side of the patient's chin at the lateral angles of the lower jaw. The patient's head should be stabilized with the rescuer's forearms; then the rescuer applies pressure with the index fingers to push the patient's jaw forward.

from the lower limbs and abdomen to the vital organs by means of an inflated three-chambered suit. The use of PASG is controversial (Miller, Martin, & Morris, 2008).

D = Disability

A brief neurological examination completes the primary survey. The degree of disability is measured by level of consciousness, which is assessed by determining the patient's alertness and response to verbal and painful stimuli with the following scale:

A Alert
V Responsive to voice
P Responsive to pain
U Unresponsive

The Glasgow Coma Scale (GCS) and the Canadian Neurological Scale are used to further assess the arousal aspect of the patient's consciousness (Chapter 59). Pupils should be also assessed for size, shape, equality, and response or reactivity to light.

Secondary Survey

After each step of the primary survey is addressed and any necessary lifesaving interventions are initiated, the secondary survey begins. The **secondary survey** is a brief, systematic process that is aimed at identifying *all* injuries and continues the ABCD mnemonic through EFGHI: *e*xposure and *e*nvironmental control; *f*ull set of vital signs–*f*ive interventions–*f*acilitating family presence; *g*iving comfort measures; *h*istory and *h*ead-to-toe assessment; and *i*nspection of the posterior surfaces (Table 71-5).

E = Exposure and Environmental Control

Any patient who has suffered trauma should have clothes removed so that a thorough physical assessment can be performed. Once the patient is exposed, it is important to limit heat loss and prevent hypothermia by using warming blankets, overhead warmers, and warmed IV fluids. The nurse should observe for medical alert bracelets or necklaces, tattoos, or wallet cards for ongoing health illnesses. Any faith-based objections to blood transfusions should be ascertained.

F = Full Set of Vital Signs/Five Interventions/Facilitate Family Presence

A complete set of vital signs, including blood pressure, heart rate, respiratory rate, and temperature, should be measured after the patient's clothes are removed. Blood pressure should be obtained in both arms if the patient has sustained or is suspected of having chest trauma.

At this point, it must be determined whether to proceed with the secondary survey or to perform additional interventions. The availability of other team members often influences this decision. For patients who have sustained significant trauma and have required lifesaving interventions during the primary and secondary surveys, the following five interventions should be performed next:

First, the patient should be monitored by electrocardiography for heart rate and rhythm. Second, pulse oximetry and oxygen saturation monitoring are initiated. Third, an indwelling catheter should be inserted to monitor urine output and to check for hematuria, unless a urethral tear is suspected. Patients with pelvic injuries or blood at the meatus, and men with a high-riding prostate gland (detected on digital rectal examination), are at risk for a urethral tear or transection. Urethrography should be performed before a catheter is inserted. Fourth, an orogastric or nasogastric tube should be inserted to provide gastric decompression and emptying to reduce the risk of aspiration and to test contents for blood. A nasogastric tube should not be placed in the nares in a patient suspected of having facial fractures or a basilar skull fracture because the tube could enter the brain through the cribriform plate; it should be placed orally. Fifth, laboratory studies for typing and crossmatching, hematocrit, hemoglobin, blood urea nitrogen, creatinine, blood alcohol, toxicology screening, arterial blood gases (ABGs), electrolytes,

Table 71-5 Secondary Survey of a Patient in an Emergency

PARAMETER	ASSESSMENT
Exposure and environmental control	Remove clothing for adequate examination; keep patient warm with blankets, IV fluids, and overhead lights.
Full set of vital signs	Obtain vital signs: temperature, heart rate, respiratory rate, and blood pressure bilaterally.
Five interventions	Monitor and record heart rhythm; monitor O_2 saturation; insert a urinary catheter (if not contraindicated) and gastric tube; and obtain specimens for laboratory studies.
Facilitate family presence	Determine family's desire to be present during resuscitation.
Giving comfort measures	Address patient's level of pain and anxiety.
History and head-to-toe assessment	
History	Document details of the incident or illness, mechanism and pattern of injury, length of time since incident occurred, injuries suspected, treatment provided and patient's response, and patient's level of consciousness.
	Assess for allergies.
	Document medication history.
	Document past health history (e.g., pre-existing medical conditions, most recent menstrual period).
	Determine the patient's most recent meal.
	Document events and environment preceding illness or injury.
Head, neck, face	Note general appearance, skin, and colour.
	Examine face and scalp for lacerations, bone or soft tissue deformity, tenderness, bleeding, and foreign bodies.
	Examine eyes, ears, nose, and mouth for bleeding, foreign bodies, drainage, pain, deformity, ecchymosis, and lacerations.
	Examine head for depressions of cranial or facial bones, contusions, hematomas, areas of softness, and bony crepitus.
	Examine neck for stiffness, pain in cervical vertebrae, tracheal deviation, distended neck veins, bleeding, edema, difficulty swallowing, bruising, subcutaneous emphysema, and bony crepitus.
Chest	Observe rate, depth, and effort of breathing, including chest wall movement.
	Palpate for bony crepitus and subcutaneous emphysema.
	Observe for use of accessory muscles.
	Auscultate breath sounds.
	Obtain ECG.
	Document external signs of injury: petechiae, bleeding, cyanosis, bruises, abrasions, lacerations, or scars.
Abdomen and flanks	Assess symmetry of external abdominal wall and bony structures.
	Observe for external signs of injury: bruising, abrasions, lacerations, or punctures.
	Assess for masses, note guarding, and check femoral pulses.
	Document type and location of pain, rigidity, or distension of abdomen.
	Assess bowel sounds.
Pelvis and perineum	Assess genitalia for blood at meatus and for priapism, ecchymosis, rectal bleeding, and anal sphincter tone.
Extremities	Document signs of external injury: deformity, ecchymosis, abrasions, lacerations, or swelling.
	Assess for pain.
	Evaluate movement and strength in arms and legs.
	Assess sensation in each limb.
	Evaluate colour of skin.
	Document presence and quality of peripheral pulses.
Posterior surfaces	Logroll patient, and inspect and palpate back for deformity, bleeding, lacerations, or bruising.

ECG, electrocardiogram; *IV*, intravenous.

coagulation profile, liver enzymes, cardiac enzymes, and pregnancy should be performed.

Facilitating *family presence* completes this step of the secondary survey. Although research findings support the positive benefits of family presence during invasive procedures and cardiopulmonary resuscitation (CPR), it is not a widely accepted practice (Cox, 2007; NENA, 2010). The most significant barrier to family presence during CPR was the concern that conflicts may occur within the emergency team. If family presence during CPR is allowed, written policies, guidelines, and education on the practice need to be developed (Cox, 2007; Madden & Condon, 2007). It is essential that a member of the team explain to the family the care delivered and be available to answer their questions.

G = Give Comfort Measures

Provision of comfort measures is of paramount importance during care for patients in the ED. It has been reported that pain (both acute and chronic) is the primary complaint of all patients who come to the ED (Motov & Khan, 2009).

Pain management strategies should include a combination of pharmacological (e.g., narcotics) and nonpharmacological (e.g., imagery) measures (National Opioid Use Guideline Group, 2010). Emergency nurses play a pivotal role in pain management because of their frequent contact with patients. General comfort measures such as verbal reassurance, listening, reducing stimuli (e.g., dimming lights), and developing a trusting relationship with the patient and family should be provided in the ED.

Positioning on a spinal board for long periods often causes pain and discomfort. Spinal immobilization on a hard board can lead to decubitus ulcers, headaches, respiratory compromise, and difficulties with radiological imaging. To prevent these complications, spinal boards should be removed as soon as possible, ideally after the primary and resuscitation phases.

H = History and Head-to-Toe Assessment

The history of the incident, injury, or illness provides clues to the cause of the crisis and suggests specific assessment and intervention needs. The patient may be unable to provide a history; however, family, friends, witnesses, and personnel involved before arrival at the hospital can frequently provide important information. Prehospital information should focus on the mechanism and the pattern of injury, injuries suspected, vital signs, treatment initiated, and the patient's responses.

Details of the incident are extremely important because the mechanism of injury and injury patterns can help predict specific injuries. For example, a front-seat passenger with a seat belt may have a head injury from hitting the steering wheel; knee, femur, or hip fractures or dislocation from striking the dashboard; and an abdominal injury from the seat belt. If other victims were dead at the scene, the patient has a high chance of significant injury.

Patients who jump from buildings or bridges may have bilateral calcaneal (heel) fractures, wrist fractures, or lumbar spine compression fractures, and they may be at risk for aortic tears. In older patients who have climbed ladders and fallen, a stroke or myocardial infarction may have led to the fall.

Prehospital personnel often provide a detailed description of the patient's general condition, level of consciousness, and apparent injuries. An experienced ED team can complete a history within 5 minutes of the patient's arrival. If the patient's condition is classified by triage as resuscitative, a thorough history is obtained from family or friends after the patient is taken to the treatment area. The history should include the following questions:

1. What is the chief complaint? What caused the patient to seek attention?
2. What are the patient's subjective complaints?
3. What is the patient's description of pain (e.g., location, duration, quality, character)?

4. What are witnesses' (if any) descriptions of the patient's behaviour since the onset?
5. What is the patient's health care history? The mnemonic *AMPLE* helps:
   A   Allergies
   M   Medication history
   P   Past health history (e.g., pre-existing medical conditions, previous hospitalizations and surgeries, smoking history, recent use of drugs or alcohol, tetanus immunization, most recent menstrual period)
   L   Last meal
   E   Events or environment preceding illness or injury

Head, Neck, and Face.   The patient should be assessed for general appearance, skin colour, and temperature. The eyes should be evaluated for extraocular movements. A disconjugate gaze is an indication of neurological damage. Periorbital ecchymosis ("raccoon eyes") is usually caused by a basilar skull fracture. The tympanic membranes and the external canals are checked for blood and cerebrospinal fluid. Cerebrospinal fluid is allowed to flow freely because the leak usually resolves in 2 to 10 days (Chapter 59).

The airway is assessed for foreign bodies, bleeding, edema, and loose or missing teeth. The nurse should assess for difficulty swallowing, movement of the palate, and ability to open the mouth. The neck should be examined for bruising, edema, bleeding, pain, or distended neck veins. The trachea is palpated and visualized to determine whether it is in the midline. A deviated trachea may signal a life-threatening tension pneumothorax. Subcutaneous emphysema may indicate laryngotracheal disruption. A stiff or painful cervical spine area may signify a fracture of a cervical vertebra. The cervical spine must be protected with a rigid collar and supine positioning. Patients with cervical spine injuries must be logrolled when movement is necessary.

Chest.   The chest is examined for paradoxical chest movements and large, sucking chest wounds. The sternum, the clavicles, and the ribs are palpated for deformity and point tenderness. The chest is assessed for pain on palpation, respiratory distress, decreased breath sounds, distant or muffled heart sounds (e.g., pericardial tamponade), and distended neck veins. In addition to tension and open pneumothorax, the patient should be evaluated for rib fractures, pulmonary contusion, blunt cardiac injury, and simple pneumothorax. A 12-lead ECG should be obtained, particularly for an older patient or a patient with suspected heart disease. ECG should be performed to detect dysrhythmias and evidence of ischemia or infarction.

Abdomen and Flanks.   Assessment of the abdomen and the flanks is more difficult. Frequent evaluation for subtle changes in the abdominal examination is essential. Motor vehicle collisions and assaults can cause blunt trauma. Penetrating trauma tends to injure specific organs. Decreased bowel sounds may indicate a temporary paralytic ileus. Bowel sounds in the chest may indicate a diaphragmatic rupture. The abdomen is percussed for distension (e.g., tympany [excessive air] and dullness [excessive fluid]) and palpated for peritoneal irritation.

If intra-abdominal hemorrhage is suspected, diagnostic peritoneal lavage may be performed to determine the presence of blood in the peritoneal space (hemoperitoneum). Before the procedure, a gastric tube and a bladder catheter must be inserted to decompress these organs and reduce the possibility of perforation. An alternative to diagnostic peritoneal lavage that is gaining support is bedside ultrasonography: *focused abdominal sonography for trauma* (FAST). This procedure is noninvasive and can be performed quickly.

Pelvis and Perineum. The pelvis is gently palpated. If pain is elicited, the patient may have a pelvic fracture. The genitalia are inspected for bleeding and obvious injuries. A rectal examination is performed to check for blood, a high-riding prostate gland, and loss of sphincter tone. The examiner should assess for bladder distension, hematuria, dysuria, or the inability to void.

Extremities. The upper and the lower extremities are assessed. Injured extremities are splinted above and below the injury to decrease the occurrence of further soft tissue injury and pain. Grossly deformed, pulseless extremities should be realigned and splinted. Pulses are checked before and after movement or splinting. A pulseless extremity represents a time-critical vascular or orthopedic emergency.

The extremities are palpated for point tenderness, crepitus, and abnormal movements. Injured extremities should be elevated, and ice applied. Fractures necessitate splinting, and patients may need pain control with analgesics (MacDonald & Burgess, 2010). Prophylactic antibiotics are administered for open fractures.

I = Inspect the Posterior Surfaces

All patients who have suffered trauma should be turned using spinal precautions to inspect the posterior surfaces. The back is inspected for ecchymosis, abrasions, puncture wounds, cuts, and obvious deformities. The entire spine is palpated for misalignment, deformity, and pain.

Intervention and Evaluation

Once the secondary survey is complete, all findings are recorded. Patients should be evaluated to determine their need for tetanus prophylaxis. It is not uncommon for older adults to have an outdated tetanus status. Information is needed about previous vaccinations and the condition of any wounds to make an appropriate decision (Table 71-6).

Regardless of the patient's chief complaint, ongoing monitoring and evaluation are critical in an emergency situation. The nurse is responsible for providing appropriate interventions and assessing the patient's response. The evaluation of airway patency and the effectiveness of breathing always assumes highest priority. The nurse monitors O_2 saturation and ABGs to help determine the patient's progress. Level of consciousness, vital signs, quality of peripheral pulses, urine output, and skin temperature, colour, and moisture provide key information about circulation and perfusion.

Depending on the patient's injuries or illness, the patient may be (a) transported for diagnostic tests such as a computed tomography (CT), radiography, or magnetic resonance imaging (MRI); (b) admitted to a general or critical care unit; or (c) transferred to another facility. The emergency nurse is responsible for monitoring the patient during transport and notifying the team if the patient's condition changes from baseline. Nurses accompanying critically ill patients must be competent in advanced life support measures.

Table 71-6 Prophylaxis Against Tetanus in Wound Management

HISTORY OF TETANUS TOXOID (DOSES)	TYPE OF WOUND			
	TETANUS-PRONE WOUND		CLEAN MINOR WOUND	
	TD	TIG*	TD	TIG
Unknown or fewer than three	Yes	Yes	Yes	No
Three or more†	No‡	No	No§	No

TD, tetanus-diphtheria toxoid absorbed (adult use); *TIG*, tetanus immune globulin (human).
*When TIG and TD are administered concurrently, separate sites must be used.
†If only three doses of fluid toxoid have been received, a fourth dose of toxoid, preferably absorbed toxoid, should be administered.
‡Yes, if more than 5 years since most recent dose. More frequent boosters are not needed and can accentuate adverse effects.
§Yes, if more than 10 years since most recent dose.

Mandatory Reporting of Gunshot and Stab Wounds

Most provinces have legislation that requires mandatory reporting of gunshot and stab wounds by health care agencies (MacDonald & Burgess, 2010). Emergency staff must be familiar with their specific provincial law.

Reporting Abuse of Children

All provinces have laws requiring the mandatory reporting of suspected child abuse or maltreatment. The Ontario Association of Children's Aid Societies and the College of Nurses of Ontario mandate that nurses be vigilant and accountable in reporting abuse concerns:
1. If the nurse suspects that a child is being abused or neglected, it is the nurse's legal duty to report the situation to the local Children's Aid Society.
2. Maltreatment may be in the form of physical or sexual abuse. It can also be in the form of neglect: failure to meet a child's basic needs for food, clothing, shelter, sleep, medical attention, education, and protection from harm.
3. Unexplained injuries, fear of a specific adult, difficulty trusting others or making friends, sudden changes in eating or sleeping patterns, poor hygiene, secrecy, and inappropriate sexual behaviour may be signs of abuse.

Death in the Emergency Department

Unfortunately, a number of patients in the ED do not survive, despite the skill, expertise, and technology available in the ED. It is important for the emergency nurse to be able to deal with feelings about sudden death so that the nurse can help families and significant others begin the grieving process. The nurse may also require debriefing when dealing with traumatic deaths.

The emergency nurse should recognize the importance of rituals in preparing the bereaved to grieve, such as multicultural differences, collecting belongings, coroner considerations, arranging for autopsy, viewing the body, and making mortuary arrangements. The emergency nurse plays a significant role in providing comfort to and advocacy for the surviving loved ones after a death. Collaborations with clergy and social workers are valued enhancements to the team's crisis management and grief work.

Organ and Tissue Donation

Transplantation is a critical component of the health care system. Many patients who die in the ED are potential candidates for tissue and organ donation. Certain tissues and organs such as corneas, heart valves, skin, bone, and kidneys can be harvested from patients after death. Solid-organ procurement includes retrieval of heart, lungs, liver, pancreas, and kidney. According to the Trillium Gift of Life Network (2011), everyone is a potential donor, regardless of age, if the organs and the tissue are healthy at the time of death. Organ and tissue recovery is carried out with confidentiality, respect, and dignity and does not interfere with funeral practices.

Approaching families about donation after an unexpected death is distressing to both the staff and the family. For many families, however, the act of donation may be the first positive step in the grieving process. Studies show that donating the organs and tissue of a loved one who has died can provide immediate comfort and lasting consolation to family members in their grieving (Trillium Gift of Life Network, 2011). Before families are made aware of the option for donation, they must be told that the patient has died and they must accept the fact that death has occurred. Once the family has accepted the patient's death, then the nurse can provide the family with the choice to donate, provide information, and support the family's decision.

Careful assessment of patients with standardized criteria is necessary to make an accurate determination of death. Neurological determination of death is defined as "a permanent loss of all brain function" (Trillium Gift of Life Network, 2011). Once this determination is complete, the donor is screened to ensure that only viable organs are recovered for transplantation. *Organ donor coordinators* are available in most institutions to assist in the process of screening potential donors, counselling donor families, obtaining informed consent, and retrieving organs from patients who have died in the ED. (Organ donation is discussed in Chapter 16.)

The organ donor who is on a mechanical ventilator is often hemodynamically unstable, with many fluid and electrolyte imbalances. The nurse carries out interventions to attempt to stabilize the patient's condition until the organs can be retrieved. Nursing care may consist of administration of fluids (crystalloids and colloids), medications (vasopressors and hormones), promotion of normothermia, maintenance of ventilation and oxygenation through ventilator manipulation, and review of laboratory values such as electrolytes, blood urea nitrogen, creatinine, hematological studies, ABGs, liver function studies, and cardiac enzymes. (Transplantation is discussed in Chapter 16.)

Emergency Department Wait Times. In the period 2010 to 2011, Canadians made more than 15 million visits to EDs (CIHI, 2012). Of these visits, 21.7% were for trauma (CIHI, 2012). People were more likely to visit EDs between 0800 and 2000 hours; morning was the peak arrival time. The median length of stay in EDs, measured from the time of registration or triage to the time of ED discharge, was approximately 2 hours (CIHI, 2012). The amount of time that people spent in the ED varied according to the severity of their illness, the patient's age, how many other patients were being cared for, and the time of the day the visit took place.

AGE-RELATED CONSIDERATIONS: EMERGENCY CARE

The proportion of the population older than 65 is growing; most older adults lead active lives. Regardless of a patient's age, aggressive interventions are warranted for all injuries or illnesses, unless the patient is known to have a pre-existing terminal illness, an extremely low probability of survival, or an advance directive indicating a different course of action.

The older population is at high risk for injury because of many anatomical and physiological changes that occur with aging (e.g., reduced visual acuity, limited neck rotation, slower gait, reduced reaction time).

Of the injury-related admissions of people aged 65 or older, many are for fractures resulting from falls. Age-related decline in balance and gait stability, as well as in cardiovascular function, increase the risk of falling (Kiel, 2011). When assessing a patient who has experienced a fall, the nurse must determine whether the physical findings may have actually caused the fall or may be caused by the fall itself. For example, a patient may exhibit acute confusion (delirium). The confusion may be the result of an acute myocardial infarction that caused the patient to lose consciousness and fall, or the patient may have suffered a head injury as a result of a fall from tripping.

Knowledge of the concepts of aging improves the care delivered to older adults in the ED (Chapter 7). Older adults and their conditions must be fully investigated because of atypical presentations and comorbid conditions. The expertise of advanced practice nurses, such as nurse practitioners or clinical nurse specialists, should be put to use in caring for this complex population to improve access to care. In Ontario, geriatric emergency medicine (GEM) nurse clinicians target the older population in the ED and have been found to improve care and clinical outcomes (Regional Geriatric Program of Toronto, 2011).

The Triage Risk Screening Tool is a brief screening tool that can identify older patients as being at high risk and can predict adverse health outcomes; the results enable GEM nurses to deliver targeted interventions. It is a risk stratification tool used to predict functional decline. The six-item questionnaire is completed by registered nurses to identify older patients at risk for repeat ED visits, hospitalization, and nursing home placement after an index ED visit. Risk factors include being 75 years of age or older when discharged home; having cognitive impairment; living alone; having difficulty transferring or a history of falling; taking five or more medications (polypharmacy); and having used the ED recently (previous 30 days) or having been hospitalized recently (previous 90 days). Other risk factors are identified by registered nurses' recommendation for issues such as malnutrition, depression, and failure to cope. Patients are considered at high risk if cognitive impairment or two or more other risk factors are present, and the GEM nurse is consulted (Hustey, Mion, & Connor, 2007).

Environmental Emergencies

Increased interest in outdoor activities such as running, hiking, cycling, skiing, sailing, and swimming has raised the number of environmental emergencies seen in the ED. Illness or injury may be caused by the activity, exposure to weather, or attack from various animals or humans. Specific environmental emergencies discussed in this section include heat-related emergencies, cold-related emergencies, submersion injuries, bites, and stings.

Heat-Related Emergencies

Brief exposure to intense heat or prolonged exposure to less intense heat leads to heat stress. Thermoregulatory mechanisms such as sweating, vasodilation, and increased respirations cannot compensate for such exposure to increased ambient temperatures (Flarity, 2007). Ambient temperature is a product of environmental temperature and humidity. Strenuous activities in hot or humid environments, clothing that interferes with perspiration, high fevers, and pre-existing illnesses predispose individuals to heat stress (Table 71-7). Effects can be mild (heat rash and heat edema) or severe (heat exhaustion and heat stroke). The management of heat-related emergencies is summarized in Table 71-8.

Heat rash (miliaria or prickly heat) is a fine, red, papular rash that occurs on the torso and the neck and in skinfolds. The rash occurs when sweat ducts are obstructed and become inflamed so that sweat excretion does not occur. The rash usually occurs in warm weather, but it has also been reported in cold weather as a result of clothing.

Heat syncope is associated with prolonged standing and heat exposure. Manifestations include dizziness, orthostatic hypotension, and syncope. Inadequate vasomotor tone associated with aging increases older adults' risk for heat syncope.

Heat edema is characterized by swelling of the hands, the feet, and the ankles, usually in nonacclimatized individuals as a result of prolonged standing or sitting. Swelling usually resolves in days with rest, elevation, and support hose. Diuretics are not recommended because this condition is self-limiting and necessitates no additional treatment.

Heat Cramps

Heat cramps are severe cramps in large muscle groups fatigued by heavy work. Cramps are brief and intense and tend to occur during rest after exercise or heavy labour. Nausea, tachycardia, pallor, weakness, and profuse diaphoresis are often present. The condition occurs most often in healthy, acclimated athletes with inadequate fluid intake. Cramps resolve rapidly with rest and oral or parenteral replacement of sodium and water. Elevation, gentle massage, and analgesia keep pain to a minimum. The patient should avoid strenuous activity for at least 12 hours after the development of heat cramps. Education should emphasize salt replacement during strenuous exercise in hot, humid environments. Commercially prepared electrolyte solutions and sports drinks are recommended.

Heat Exhaustion

Prolonged exposure to heat over hours or days leads to **heat exhaustion,** a clinical syndrome characterized by fatigue, light-headedness, nausea, vomiting, diarrhea, and the sensation of impending doom (see Table 71-8). Tachypnea, hypotension, tachycardia, elevated body temperature, dilated pupils, mild confusion, ashen colour, and profuse diaphoresis are also present. Hypotension and mild to severe temperature elevation (37.5 to 40°C) are caused by dehydration (Flarity, 2007). Heat exhaustion usually occurs in individuals engaged in strenuous activity in hot, humid weather, but it also occurs in sedentary individuals.

Treatment begins with placing the patient in a cool area and removing constrictive clothing. The patient is monitored for airway, breathing, and circulation (ABCs), including cardiac dysrhythmias. Oral and parenteral fluid replacement should correspond to clinical and laboratory parameters. Salt tablets are not recommended because of potential gastric irritation and hypernatremia. A 0.9% normal saline solution is initiated intravenously when oral solutions are not tolerated. An initial fluid bolus may be used to correct hypotension. Admission is considered for affected older adults, chronically ill patients, and those whose condition does not improve within 4 hours.

Heat Stroke

Heat stroke, the most serious form of heat stress, results from failure of the central thermoregulatory mechanisms and is considered a medical emergency. Table 71-7 lists risk factors for heat-related emergencies. Increased sweating, vasodilation, and increased respiratory rate, which occur in an attempt to lower temperature, deplete fluids and electrolytes. Eventually, sweat glands stop functioning, and so core temperature increases rapidly. The patient exhibits a core temperature higher than 40°C, altered mentation, absence of perspiration, and circulatory collapse. The skin is hot, dry, and ashen. Because the brain is extremely sensitive to thermal injuries, a range of neurological symptoms occur, such as hallucinations, combativeness, and loss of muscle coordination. Cerebral edema and hemorrhage may occur as a result of direct thermal injury to the brain and decreased cerebral blood flow.

Table 71-7 Risk Factors for Heat-Related Emergencies	
Age	***Prescription Drugs***
• Older age	• Anticholinergics
• Extreme young age	• Antihistamines
Environmental Conditions	• Antiparkinsonian drugs
• High environmental temperature	• Antispasmodics
• High relative humidity	• β-Adrenergic blockers
• Low wind	• Butyrophenones
Pre-existing Illness	• Diuretics
• Cardiovascular disease	• Phenothiazines
• Cystic fibrosis	• Tricyclic antidepressants
• Diabetes	***Street Drugs***
• Obesity	• Amphetamines
• Previous stroke or other central nervous system lesion	• Jimson weed
• Skin disorders (e.g., large burn scars)	• Lysergic acid diethylamide (LSD)
	• Phencyclidine (PCP)
	• 3,4-Methylenedioxymethamphetamine (MDMA, Ecstasy)
	Alcohol

Source: Emergency Nurses Association. (2010). *Sheehy's emergency nursing: Principles and practice* (6th ed., p. 537, Box 40-1) (L. Newberry, Ed.). St. Louis: Mosby.

EMERGENCY MANAGEMENT
Table 71-8 Hyperthermia

ETIOLOGY	ASSESSMENT FINDINGS	INTERVENTIONS
Environmental	**Heat Cramps**	**Initial**
• Lack of acclimatization	• Severe muscle contractions in muscles subjected to exertion	• Manage and maintain ABCs.
• Prolonged exposure to extreme temperatures	• Excessive thirst	• Provide high-flow O_2 via non-rebreather mask or BVM device.
• Physical exertion, especially during hot weather	**Heat Exhaustion**	• Establish IV access, and begin fluid replacement for significant heat injury.
Trauma	• Pale, ashen complexion	• Place patient in a cool environment.
• Head injury	• Fatigue, weakness	• For patient with heat stroke, initiate rapid cooling measures: remove patient's clothing, place wet sheets over patient, and place patient in front of fan; immerse in ice water bath; administer cool IV fluids or perform lavage with cool fluids.
• Spinal cord injury	• Profuse sweating	
Metabolic	• Altered mental status (e.g., irritable)	
• Dehydration	• Hypotension	
• Thyrotoxicosis	• Tachycardia	
• Diabetes	• Weak, thready pulse	• Obtain ECG.
Drugs	• Temperature >37.8°C but <40°C	• Obtain blood specimens for electrolytes and CBC.
• Phenothiazines	**Heat Stroke**	• Insert urinary catheter.
• Tricyclic antidepressants	• Hot, dry skin	**Ongoing Monitoring**
• Diuretics	• Altered mental status (e.g., ranging from confusion to coma)	• Monitor ABCs, vital signs, level of consciousness.
• Cocaine	• Hypotension	• Monitor cardiac rhythm, O_2 saturation, electrolyte levels, and urinary output.
• Ethanol	• Tachycardia	• Monitor urine for development of myoglobinuria.
• Antihistamines	• Weakness	• Monitor clotting studies for development of disseminated intravascular coagulation.
	• Temperature >40°C	

ABCs, airway, breathing, and circulation; *BVM*, bag–valve–mask; *CBC*, complete blood cell count; *ECG*, electrocardiogram; *IV*, intravenous.

The development of heat stroke is directly related to the amount of time that the patient's body temperature remains elevated (Crawford Mechem, 2010). Prognosis is related to age, baseline health status, and length of exposure. Older adults and individuals with diabetes mellitus, chronic renal disease, cardiovascular disease, pulmonary disease, or other physiological compromise are vulnerable.

Collaborative Care. Treatment of heat stroke focuses on stabilizing the patient's ABCs and rapidly reducing the core temperature. Administration of 100% O_2 compensates for the patient's hypermetabolic state. Ventilation with a BVM device or intubation and mechanical ventilation may be required. Fluid and electrolyte imbalances are corrected, and continuous cardiac monitoring for dysrhythmias is initiated.

Various cooling methods are available, such as removal of clothing, covering with wet sheets, and placing the patient in front of a large fan (evaporative cooling); providing an ice water bath (conductive cooling); and administering cool fluids or performing lavage with cool fluids (Crawford Mechem, 2010). Whatever method is selected, the nurse is responsible for closely monitoring the patient's temperature and controlling shivering. Shivering increases core temperature and is associated with heat generated by muscle activity, which complicates cooling efforts. Chlorpromazine, diazepam or lorazepam may be used to suppress shivering (Crawford Mechem, 2010). Aggressive temperature reduction should continue until core temperature reaches 38.9°C. Antipyretics are not recommended because they have no effect on the nonfunctioning thermoregulatory mechanisms.

The patient is also monitored for signs of *rhabdomyolysis*, a fatal disease characterized by the breakdown of skeletal muscle. Muscle breakdown leads to myoglobinuria, which increases the risk for acute kidney failure. Therefore, urine should be carefully monitored for colour, amount, pH, and myoglobin. Finally, clotting studies are performed to monitor the patient for signs of disseminated intravascular coagulation (Chapter 33).

Patient and caregiver teaching focuses on how to avoid future problems. Essential information regarding proper hydration during hot weather and physical exercise is imperative. Patients should also be instructed on the early signs of and interventions for heat-related stress.

Cold-Related Emergencies

Cold-related injuries may be localized (frostbite) or systemic (hypothermia). Contributing factors include age, duration of exposure, environmental temperature, homelessness, pre-existing conditions (e.g., diabetes), medications that suppress shivering (narcotics, heroin, psychotropic agents, and antiemetics), and alcohol intoxication, which causes peripheral vasodilation, increases sensations of warmth, and depresses shivering. People who smoke have an increased risk of cold-related injury as a result of the vasoconstrictive effects of nicotine.

Frostbite

Frostbite can be described as "true tissue freezing," which results in the formation of ice crystals in the tissues and cells. Peripheral vasoconstriction is the initial response to cold stress and results in a decrease in blood flow and vascular stasis. As cellular temperature decreases and ice crystals form in intracellular spaces, intracellular sodium and chloride levels increase, the cell membrane is destroyed, and organelles are damaged. These alterations result in edema. The depth of frostbite is the result of ambient temperature, length of exposure, type and condition of clothing (wet or dry), and contact with metal surfaces. Other factors that affect severity include skin colour (dark-skinned people are more prone to frostbite), lack of acclimatization, previous episodes, exhaustion, and poor peripheral vascular status.

Superficial frostbite involves skin and subcutaneous tissue, usually the ears, the nose, the fingers, and the toes. The skin appearance ranges from pale and blue to mottled, and the skin feels crunchy and frozen. The patient may complain of tingling, numbness, or a burning sensation. Injured tissue is easily damaged, and so the area should be handled carefully and never squeezed, massaged, or scrubbed. Clothing and jewellery should be removed because they may constrict the extremity and decrease circulation. The affected area should be immersed in a water bath of 37°C to 39°C (Crawford Mechem & Zafren, 2010). Warm soaks may be used for the face. The patient often experiences a warm, stinging sensation as tissue thaws. Blisters form within a few hours (Figure 71-2). Nonhemorrhagic blisters should be drained, debrided, and covered with a sterile dressing. Heavy blankets and clothing should be avoided because friction and weight can lead to sloughing of damaged tissue. Rewarming is extremely painful. Residual pain may last weeks or even years. Analgesics should be administered, and tetanus prophylaxis should be provided as appropriate (see Table 71-6). The patient should be evaluated for systemic hypothermia.

Deep frostbite involves muscle, bone, and tendon. The skin is white, hard, and insensitive to touch and involves complete tissue necrosis. The area has the appearance of deep thermal injury with mottling gradually progressing to gangrene (see Figure 14-1, p. 251). Significant edema may begin within 3 hours, with blistering in 6 hours to days. Intravenous analgesia is always required in severe frostbite because of the pain associated with tissue thawing. Tetanus prophylaxis should be given (see Table 71-6), and the patient should be evaluated for systemic hypothermia. Amputation may be required if the injured area is untreated or if

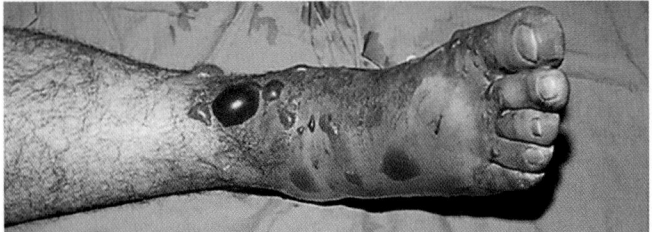

Figure 71-2 Edema and blister formation 24 hours after frostbite injury occurring in an area covered by a tightly fitted boot.

treatment is unsuccessful. Thrombolytic agents have been shown to reduce the need for amputation when used within the first 24 hours of injury. The use of thrombolytic agents may be considered if there are no contraindication (Crawford Mechem & Zafren, 2010). The patient may be admitted to the hospital, with bed rest and elevation of the injured part. Prophylactic antibiotics are used if the wound is at risk for infection.

Hypothermia

Hypothermia, defined as a core temperature lower than 36°C, occurs when heat produced by the body cannot compensate for heat lost to the environment. Up to 60% of all body heat is lost as radiant energy; the loss is greatest from the head, the thorax, and the lungs (with each breath). Wet clothing increases evaporative heat loss five times greater than normal; immersion in cold water (e.g., near-drowning) increases evaporative heat loss 25 times greater than normal. Environmental exposure to freezing temperatures, cold winds, and wet, damp terrain in the presence of physical exhaustion, inadequate clothing, or inexperience predisposes individuals to hypothermia (Crawford Mechem & Zafren, 2010). Near-drowning and water immersion are also associated with hypothermia.

Older adults are more prone to hypothermia because of decreased body fat, diminished energy reserves, decreased basal metabolic rate, decreased shivering response, decreased sensory perception, chronic medical conditions, and medications that alter body defences. In addition, certain drugs, alcohol, and diabetes are considered risk factors for hypothermia.

Hypothermia mimics cerebral or metabolic disturbances, causing ataxia, confusion, and withdrawal, and so the condition may be misdiagnosed. Peripheral vasoconstriction is the body's first attempt to conserve heat. As cold temperatures persist, shivering and movement are the body's only mechanisms for producing heat. Death usually occurs when core temperature falls below 25.6°C.

Core temperature below 30.6°C is severe and potentially life-threatening. Assessment findings in hypothermia are variable and dependent on core temperature (Table 71-9). Patients with *mild hypothermia* (32° to 36°C) exhibit shivering, increased heart rate, slurred speech, and incoordination. *Moderate hypothermia* (28-32°C) causes decreased shivering, bradycardia, slowed respiratory rate, and lethargy. *Severe hypothermia* (less than 28°C) causes coma, hypotension, arrhythmias, and muscle rigidity (Crawford Mechem & Danzl, 2011).

As core temperature drops, basal metabolic rate decreases to 50% or 25% of normal. The cold myocardium is extremely irritable, making it vulnerable to dysrhythmias (e.g., atrial and ventricular fibrillation). Decreased renal blood flow decreases glomerular filtration rate, which impairs water reabsorption and leads to dehydration. Hematocrit increases as intravascular volume decreases. Cold blood becomes viscous and acts as a thrombus, increasing the patient's risk for stroke, myocardial infarction, pulmonary emboli, acute tubular necrosis, and renal failure. Decreased blood flow leads to lactic acid accumulation from anaerobic metabolism and subsequent metabolic acidosis.

In *severe hypothermia* (<28°C), the person appears dead. Metabolic rate, heart rate, and respirations are so slow that they may be difficult to detect. Reflexes are absent, and the pupils are fixed and dilated. Profound bradycardia, asystole, or ventricular fibrillation may be present. Every effort is made to warm the patient to at least 32°C before the person is pronounced dead. The cause of death is usually refractory ventricular fibrillation.

EMERGENCY MANAGEMENT
Table 71-9 Hypothermia

ETIOLOGY	ASSESSMENT FINDINGS	INTERVENTIONS
Environmental	• Core body temperature:	**Initial**
• Prolonged exposure to cold	• Mild hypothermia: 32° to 36°C	• Remove patient from cold environment.
• Prolonged submersion	• Moderate hypothermia: 28° to <32°C	• Manage and maintain ABCs.
• Inadequate clothing for environmental temperature	• Severe hypothermia: <28°C	• Provide high-flow O_2 via non-rebreather mask or BVM device.
	• Shivering (diminished or absent at core body temperature ≤33.3°C)	• Anticipate intubation if gag reflex is diminished or absent.
	• Hypoventilation	• Rewarm patient:
	• Hypotension	• *Passive external warming:* Remove wet clothing, apply dry clothing and warm blankets, and administer warm fluids.
	• Altered mental status (ranging from confusion to coma)	• *Active external warming:* Use body-to-body contact; apply heating devices (e.g., air-filled warming blankets) or radiant lights.
	• Areflexia (absence of reflexes)	• *Active core warming:* Administer warmed IV fluids; heated, humidified O_2; and peritoneal, gastric, or colonic lavage with warmed fluids.
	• Pale, cyanotic skin	• Anticipate the need for hemodialysis or cardiopulmonary bypass.
	• Blue, white, or frozen extremities	• Warm central trunk first in patients with moderate, severe, or profound hypothermia to prevent aftershock.
	• Dysrhythmias: bradycardia, atrial fibrillation, ventricular fibrillation, asystole	• Establish IV access with two large-bore catheters for fluid resuscitation.
	• Fixed, dilated pupils	• Assess for other injuries.
		• Keep patient's head covered with warm, dry towels, or stocking cap, to limit loss of heat.
		• Treat patient gently to avoid increased cardiac irritability.
		Ongoing Monitoring
		• Monitor ABCs, level of consciousness, temperature, and vital signs.
		• Monitor O_2 saturation and cardiac rhythm.
		• Monitor electrolyte and glucose levels.

ABCs, airway, breathing, and circulation; *BVM,* bag–valve–mask; *IV,* intravenous.

Collaborative Care. Treatment of hypothermia focuses on managing and maintaining ABCs, rewarming the patient, correcting dehydration and acidosis, and treating cardiac dysrhythmias. Passive or active external rewarming is used for mild hypothermia. *Passive external rewarming* involves moving the patient to a warm, dry place; removing damp clothing; and placing warm blankets on the patient. Gentle handling is essential to prevent stimulation of the cold myocardium. *Active external rewarming* involves body-to-body contact (when the patient cannot access health care), fluid- or air-filled warming blankets, or radiant heat lamps. The patient should be closely monitored for marked vasodilation and hypotension during rewarming.

Active core rewarming is used for moderate to profound hypothermia and involves heat applied directly to the core. Techniques include heated, humidified oxygen; warmed intravenous fluids; and peritoneal, gastric, or colonic lavage with warmed fluids. Hemodialysis or cardiopulmonary bypass may also be considered for profound hypothermia (Flarity, 2007).

Core temperature should be carefully monitored during rewarming procedures. Warming places the patient at risk for *afterdrop,* a further drop in core temperature, which occurs when cold peripheral blood returns to the central circulation. Rewarming shock can produce hypotension and dysrhythmias. Thus, in patients with moderate to profound hypothermia, the core should be warmed before the extremities.

Patient teaching should focus on how to avoid future cold-related problems. Essential education includes dressing in layers for cold weather, covering the head, carrying high-carbohydrate foods for extra calories, and developing a plan for survival should an injury occur.

Submersion Injuries

Submersion injury results when a person becomes hypoxic as a result of submersion in a substance, usually water. The primary risk factors for submersion injury include inability to swim, risk taking, inadequate adult supervision, use of alcohol or drugs, trauma, seizures, and hypothermia (Chandy & Weinhouse, 2012).

Drowning is death from suffocation after submersion in water or other fluid medium. *Near-drowning* is defined as survival from potential drowning. *Immersion syndrome* occurs with immersion in cold water, which leads to stimulation of the vagus nerve and potentially fatal dysrhythmias (e.g., bradycardia).

Death from a submersion injury is caused by hypoxia secondary to aspiration and swallowing of fluid. Swallowed water may cause vomiting and additional aspiration. The majority of all drowning victims aspirate water into the pulmonary tree and develop pulmonary edema. Victims who do not aspirate fluid develop intense laryngospasm and airway obstruction; the cause of death is "dry drowning." The osmotic gradient that results from aspirated fluid causes fluid imbalances. Hypotonic freshwater is rapidly absorbed into the circulatory system through the alveoli. Freshwater may be contaminated with chlorine, mud, and algae, which cause the breakdown of lung surfactant, fluid seepage, and pulmonary edema. Hypertonic saltwater draws protein-rich fluid from the vascular space into the alveoli, impairing alveolar ventilation and resulting in hypoxia. Figure 71-3 shows the pulmonary effects of saltwater and freshwater aspiration.

The body attempts to compensate for hypoxia by shunting blood to the lungs. This results in increased pulmonary pressures and deteriorating respiratory status. Blood is shunted through the alveoli; however, it is not adequately oxygenated, and so the hypoxemia worsens. Anaerobic metabolism occurs, which leads to lactic acidosis.

The assessment findings of a patient with a submersion injury are listed in Table 71-10. Aggressive resuscitation efforts and the mammalian diving reflex improve survival of near-drowning victims even after submersion in cold water for long periods (Chandy & Weinhouse, 2012). Cold water lowers the body's metabolic rate and oxygen demand. The mammalian diving reflex causes apnea, bradycardia, and peripheral vasoconstriction and further decreases the metabolic rate. Blood flow is redistributed to the most vital organs (i.e., heart, lungs, and brain).

Collaborative Care

Treatment of submersion injuries includes aggressive resuscitation efforts that focus on correcting hypoxia and acid–base and fluid imbalances; supporting basic physiological functions; and rewarming when hypothermia is present. Initial evaluation and interventions involve assessment of airway, cervical spine, breathing, and circulation (see Table 71-10).

Mechanical ventilation with positive end-expiratory pressure or continuous positive airway pressure may be used to improve

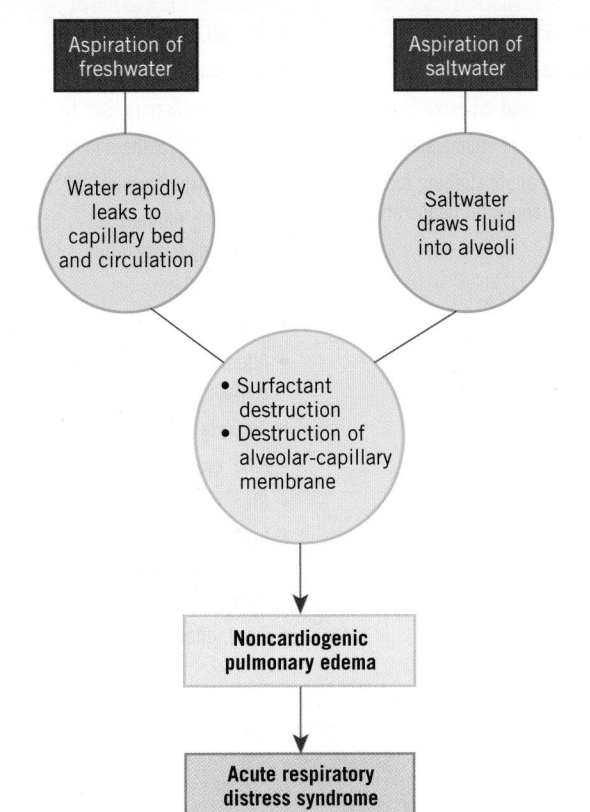

PATHOPHYSIOLOGY MAP

Figure 71-3 Pathophysiology of submersion injury.

EMERGENCY MANAGEMENT

Table 71-10 Submersion Injuries

ETIOLOGY	ASSESSMENT FINDINGS	INTERVENTIONS
• Inability to swim or exhaustion while swimming	*Pulmonary*	*Initial*
• Entrapment in or entanglement with objects in water	• Ineffective breathing	• Manage and maintain ABCs.
	• Dyspnea	• Assume cervical spine injury in all drowning victims, and stabilize or immobilize cervical spine.
• Loss of ability to move secondary to trauma, stroke, hypothermia, acute myocardial infarction	• Respiratory distress	• Provide 100% O_2 via non-rebreather mask or BVM device.
	• Respiratory arrest	• Anticipate need for intubation if gag reflex is absent.
• Poor judgement as a result of alcohol or drugs	• Crackles, wheezes	• Establish IV access with two large-bore catheters for fluid resuscitation and infuse warmed fluids if appropriate.
• Seizure while in water	• Cough with pink, frothy sputum	• Assess for other injuries.
	Other	• Remove wet clothing and cover with warm blankets.
	• Cyanosis	• Measure temperature, and begin rewarming if needed.
		• Obtain cervical spine and chest radiographs.
		• Insert gastric tube.
		Ongoing Monitoring
		• Monitor ABCs, vital signs, and level of consciousness.
		• Monitor O_2 saturation and cardiac rhythm.
		• Monitor temperature, and maintain normothermia.
		• Monitor for signs of acute respiratory failure.

ABCs, airway, breathing, and circulation; *BVM,* bag–valve–mask; *IV,* intravenous.

gas exchange across the alveolar–capillary membrane when significant pulmonary edema is present. Ventilation and oxygenation are the primary techniques used to treat acidosis. Mannitol or furosemide (Lasix) may be used with caution to decrease the amount of free water and treat cerebral edema.

Deterioration of neurological status is suggestive of cerebral edema, increased hypoxia, or profound acidosis. Near-drowning victims may also have head injuries that cause prolonged alterations in level of consciousness. All victims of near-drowning should be observed in a hospital for a minimum of 4 to 6 hours. Delayed pulmonary edema *(secondary drowning)*, aspiration pneumonia, and cerebral edema have been reported in patients who were essentially free of symptoms immediately after the near-drowning episode (Chandy & Weinhouse, 2012).

Teaching should focus on water safety and minimizing the risks for drowning. Swimming pool gates should be locked; life jackets should be used on all water craft and tubes; and learning water survival skills (i.e., swimming lessons and the buddy system) should be a priority. The dangers of combining alcohol and drugs with swimming and other water sports should be emphasized.

Bites and Stings

Animals, spiders, and insects cause injury and even death by biting or stinging. Morbidity is a result of either direct tissue damage or lethal toxins. Direct tissue damage is a result of animal size, characteristics of the animal's teeth, and strength of the jaw. Tissue may be lacerated, crushed, or chewed, and toxins that are released through teeth, fangs, stingers, spines, or tentacles provoke local or systemic effects. Death associated with animal bites is caused by blood loss, allergic reactions, or lethal toxins. Injuries caused by insects, spiders, ticks, snakes, dogs, cats, rodents, and humans are described as follows.

Hymenopteran Stings

The Hymenoptera order includes bees, yellow jackets, hornets, and wasps. Stings can cause reactions ranging from mild discomfort to life-threatening anaphylaxis (Chapters 16 and 69). Venom may be cytotoxic, hemolytic, allergenic, or vasoactive. Symptoms may begin immediately or may be delayed up to 48 hours. Reactions are more severe with multiple stings. Most hymenopterans sting repeatedly. However, the honeybee stings only once, usually leaving the stinger in the skin so that release of venom continues. A scraping motion with a fingernail, knife, or needle is recommended for removing the stinger. Tweezers squeeze the stinger and may cause more venom release. However, the fastest method of removing the stinger is ultimately the best, so if tweezers are available, they can be used.

Manifestations vary and range from stinging, burning sensation, swelling, and itching to edema, headache, fever, syncope, malaise, nausea, vomiting, wheezing, bronchospasm, laryngeal edema, and hypotension. Treatment depends on the severity of the reaction. Mild reactions are treated with elevation, cool compresses, antipruritic lotions, and oral antihistamines. Rings, watches, and restrictive clothing are removed. More severe reactions necessitate intramuscular or intravenous antihistamines (diphenhydramine [Benadryl]), subcutaneous epinephrine, and corticosteroids. Allergic reactions and anaphylaxis are discussed in Chapter 16.

Spider Bites (Arachnid)

Although there are 20,000 species of venomous spiders in the world, only 50 species cause illness. The venomous black widow spider is found in southern parts of Canada and also has been found in imported grapes. The venom can provoke responses ranging from a localized reaction to systemic anaphylaxis. Tarantulas look more dangerous than they actually are; their bite causes only localized stinging and pain. Other types of spiders release venom when they bite and may cause allergic reactions in some individuals, but they are not considered poisonous.

Black Widow Spiders. Black widow spiders are the most feared of all spiders. The female's venom is especially poisonous. Both the female and the male are black. The fully grown female is about 1.2 cm long and is jet black, with an hourglass-shaped red mark on the underside of the abdomen (Figure 71-4). Males are only about half as long and usually have four pairs of red dots along the sides of the abdomen. Males are rarely seen and are generally harmless. The female rarely leaves the web, biting defensively if disturbed. Black widow spiders are found among fallen branches, firewood, and under objects such as furniture, outhouse seats, and garbage.

The black widow spider venom is neurotoxic. When bitten, the patient feels a pinprick-like sensation, and a tiny, red bite mark appears. Approximately 15 to 60 minutes later, the patient experiences severe pain that increases over the next 12 to 48 hours. Systemic symptoms develop 30 minutes after *envenomation* (introduction of poisonous venom into the body by a bite or sting). These symptoms can include nausea, vomiting, abdominal cramping, hypertension, dyspnea, paraesthesias, and tachycardia. Symptoms usually peak 2 to 3 hours after onset; however,

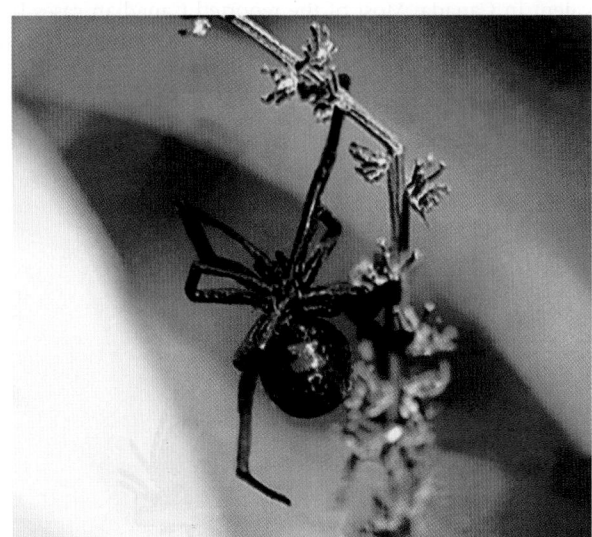

Figure 71-4 Female black widow spider. The fully grown female is about 1.2 cm (0.5 in) long and is jet black with an hourglass-shaped red mark on the underside of the abdomen. The female's sting is poisonous to humans. Males are only about half as long and usually have four pairs of red dots along the sides of the abdomen. Males are rarely seen and are generally harmless.

Source: Auerbach, P. S., Donner, H. J., & Weiss, E. A. (2003). *Field guide to wilderness medicine* (2nd ed.). St. Louis: Mosby.

muscle spasms and hypertension can recur for 12 to 24 hours. Chest and abdominal pain, seizures, and shock can also occur. Bites on the lower body cause abdominal rigidity, whereas bites on the upper body lead to chest, back, and shoulder rigidity. A black widow spider bite is not prominent and can be easily missed. In patients not aware of the bite, the envenomation can be misdiagnosed because symptoms mimic those of a perforated ulcer, appendicitis, pancreatitis, or other abdominal emergency.

Treatment includes IV access and oxygen administered as needed. The wound should be cleaned and tetanus prophylaxis given as appropriate. Muscle spasms are treated with benzodiazepines such as lorazepam. Pain medication may be required either orally or parentally. Antivenin may be used to reduce the duration of symptoms (Vetter, Swanson, & White, 2011).

Tick Bites

Ticks are found in various parts of Canada. Emergencies associated with tick bites include Rocky Mountain spotted fever, Lyme disease, and tick paralysis. Disease is caused by an infected tick or by the release of neurotoxin. Ticks release a neurotoxic venom as long as the tick head is attached to the body (Ogden et al., 2010). Removal of the attached tick is essential for effective treatment. Forceps may be used to safely remove the tick by grasping at the point of entry and pulling upward in a steady motion (Figure 71-5). Covering the tick with alcohol, mineral oil, petroleum jelly, or ether causes the tick to release because the tick breathes through the skin in which it is embedded.

Rocky Mountain spotted fever caused by *Rickettsia rickettsii* has an incubation period of 2 to 14 days. A pink, macular rash appears on palms, wrists, soles, feet, and ankles within 10 days of exposure. Other symptoms include fever, chills, malaise, myalgias, and headache. Treatment is antibiotic therapy.

Lyme disease, an arthropod-borne disease, is becoming more prevalent in Canada. Most of the reported Canadian cases have occurred in Ontario and Quebec (Canadian Centre for Occupational Health and Safety, 2008). Symptoms appear within 4 to 20 days of a bite from the *Ixodes* tick and result from exposure to the spirochete *Borrelia burgdorferi*, which is found on the tick. The initial stage of this disease is characterized by nonspecific influenza-like symptoms (e.g., headache, stiff neck, fatigue) and a characteristic bull's-eye rash—an expanding circular area of redness that is 5 cm in diameter or more. Symptoms disappear in 2 weeks if not treated. Monoarticular arthritis, meningitis, and neuropathies occur days or weeks after the initial symptoms. Chronic arthritis and myocarditis characterize the later stage of the disease, which can develop several months to 2 years after the initial skin lesion. Treatment includes antibiotic therapy (Chapter 67).

Tick paralysis occurs 5 to 7 days after exposure to the wood or dog tick. Classic symptoms are flaccid ascending paralysis, which develops over 1 to 2 days. Without tick removal, the patient dies as respiratory muscles become paralyzed. Tick removal leads to return of muscle movement, usually within 48 to 72 hours.

Snakebite

Only 375 of the 3000 species of snakes in the world are poisonous. Poisonous snakes indigenous to Canada are members of the Crotalidae (pit viper) family. There are only two types of these poisonous snakes, and they are found in the Western provinces (western rattlesnake) and Ontario (massasauga). Figure 71-6 highlights differences between snakes.

Venom from the pit viper is hemolytic. Envenomation occurs in approximately 75 to 80% of all snakebites. If swelling does not occur within 30 minutes after the bite, envenomation is unlikely to have occurred. Local reaction is characterized by one

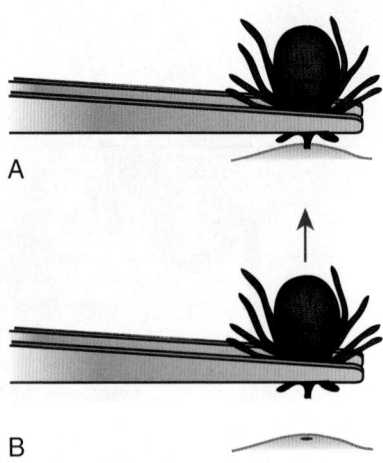

Figure 71-5 Tick removal. **A,** Use tweezers to grasp the tick close to the skin. **B,** With a steady motion, pull the tick's body away from the skin. Do not be alarmed if the tick's mouth parts remain in the skin. Once the mouth parts are removed from the rest of the tick, it can no longer transmit disease.

Source: Courtesy Centers for Disease Control and Prevention, Division of Vital and Rickettsial Diseases. Retrieved from *http://www.cdc.gov/lyme/removal/index.html*

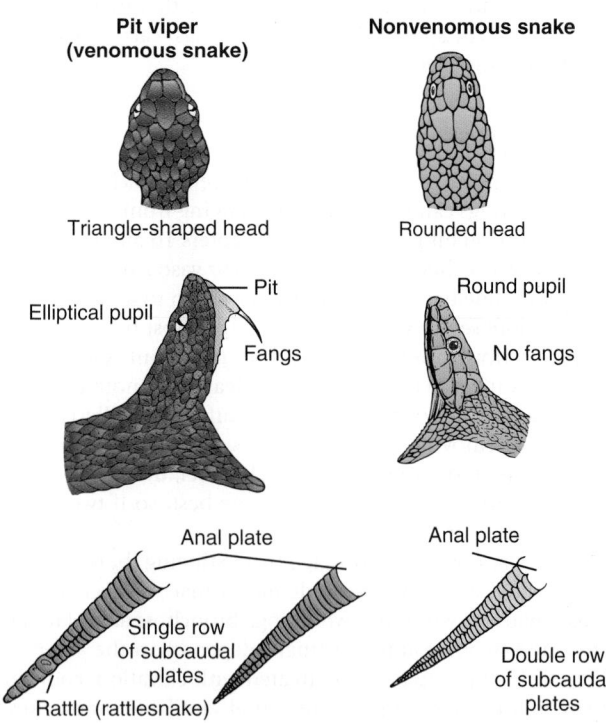

Figure 71-6 Comparison of pit viper (venomous snake) and nonvenomous snake.

Source: Redrawn from Rosen, P. (1988). *Emergency medicine* (2nd ed., Vol. 1). St. Louis: Mosby.

or two fang marks associated with pain, bruising, edema, petechiae, ecchymosis, and erythema within 36 hours of injury. Loss of function and necrosis of the affected limb may occur 16 to 36 hours after the bite. Systemic reactions include nausea and vomiting, dizziness, tachycardia, muscle fasciculations, gastrointestinal bleeding, and respiratory problems. The patient may experience a metallic or rubber taste. Neurological symptoms such as constricted pupils, drowsiness, weakness, fasciculations, muscle weakness, and seizures occur with neurotoxic venom. Life-threatening problems associated with systemic envenomation include severe hemorrhage, renal failure, and hypovolemic shock.

Treatment focuses on preventing the spread of venom. Rings, watches, and restrictive clothing should be removed, and then the affected limb should be immobilized at the level of the heart. The use of ice is contraindicated because it is associated with tissue necrosis, and tourniquets are not recommended because they may impede arterial flow. Incision of the wound is controversial. If done within 3 minutes of injury with the appropriate device (e.g., a Sawyer extractor), 25 to 30% of the venom may be removed. Caffeine, alcohol, and smoking increase the spread of venom and should be avoided.

ED management includes vascular access with a large-bore (14- to 16-gauge) catheter and administration of crystalloids to maintain blood pressure. Diagnostic tests include complete blood cell count, urinalysis, coagulation studies, and measurements of blood urea nitrogen, creatinine, creatine kinase, and electrolytes. Extremity swelling must be assessed, usually through documentation of circumference every 30 to 60 minutes. Pain should be treated with acetaminophen; aspirin and nonsteroidal anti-inflammatory drugs should be avoided because they may exacerbate bleeding, and narcotics may cause respiratory depression. Tetanus prophylaxis should be administered as needed (see Table 71-6). Secondary infection caused by microorganisms in the snake's mouth or other contaminants may necessitate antibiotic therapy. Debridement or fasciotomy (Chapter 27) is necessary in some patients. Antivenin therapy (polyvalent Crotalidae antivenin ovine Fab [CroFab]) is used in mild to moderate reactions; the amount of antivenin required depends on the timing, the type, and the severity of envenomation (Table 71-11). Insufficient dosage is the most common cause of treatment failure.

Animal and Human Bites

Children are at greatest risk for animal bites. The most significant problems associated are infection and mechanical destruction of skin, muscle, tendons, blood vessels, and bone. The bite may cause a simple laceration or be associated with a crush injury, puncture wound, or tearing or avulsion of tissue. The severity of injury depends on animal size, victim size, and anatomical location of the bite. Animal bites from cats and dogs are common; dog bites account for the majority of the bite injuries that are treated in the ED. Wild or domestic rodents are ranked behind dogs and cats as the third most frequent offenders in reported animal bites (Ricci & Rizzolo, 2011). All animal bites should be reported to the local public health unit.

Dog bites usually occur on the extremities; however, facial bites are common in small children. Most victims own the dogs that bite them. Dog bites may involve significant tissue damage, and fatalities have been reported, usually in children. Skull fractures with intracranial injury and death may occur in children younger than 2 years. Disfiguring wounds of the face should be evaluated by a plastic surgeon.

Table 71-11 Antivenin* Snakebite Treatment		
ENVENOMATION	**SIGNS AND SYMPTOMS**	**NUMBER OF VIALS OF ANTIVENIN†**
None	Fang marks, no local swelling, hemorrhage, or paraesthesia	No antivenin Tetanus prophylaxis and observation
Mild to moderate	*Mild:* Fang marks, local swelling of hands or feet, pain, no systemic reactions	*Initial dosage:* 4-6 vials (3000-4500 mg) infused over 1 hr; infusion should be initiated slowly for the first 10 min to detect any allergic reactions; if initial control of symptoms is not achieved, dose may be repeated once
	Moderate: Fang marks, progressive swelling beyond bite, mild systemic reaction (e.g., nausea, vomiting, paraesthesias, hypotension)	*Additional regimen:* 2 vials every 6 hr for 18 hr

*Polyvalent Crotalidae antivenin ovine Fab (CroFab).
†For Crotalidae envenomation (e.g., rattlesnakes, copperheads).

Cat bites cause deep puncture wounds that can involve tendons and joint capsules and result in a greater incidence of infection (Enzler, Berbari, & Osmon, 2011). The most common causative organisms of infections from cat and dog bites are from species of the genus *Pasteurella* (e.g., *P. canis*). This organism is found in the mouths of most healthy cats and dogs (Ricci & Rizzolo, 2011). Septic arthritis, osteomyelitis, and tenosynovitis have been reported in cat bites.

Human bites also cause puncture wounds or lacerations and carry a high risk of infection from oral bacterial flora, most commonly *Staphylococcus aureus*, streptococci, and hepatitis virus. The hands, fingers, ears, nose, vagina, and penis are the most common sites of human bites and are frequently a result of violence or sexual activity. Boxer's fracture of the fifth metacarpal is often associated with an open wound when knuckles strike teeth. The human jaw has great crushing ability, causing laceration, puncture, crush injury, soft tissue tearing, and even amputation. More than 40 potential pathogens found in the human mouth account for an infection rate of approximately 50% in cases in which victims did not seek medical intervention within 24 hours of injury.

Collaborative Care. Initial treatment for animal and human bites includes cleaning with copious irrigation, debridement, tetanus prophylaxis, and analgesics as needed. Prophylactic antibiotics are used for animal and human bites at risk for infection such as wounds over joints, wounds more than 6 to 12 hours old, puncture wounds, and bites of the hand or foot. Individuals at greatest risk of infection are infants, older adults, immunosuppressed patients, alcoholic patients, diabetic patients, and people taking corticosteroids (Ricci & Rizzolo, 2011).

Puncture wounds are left open, whereas lacerations are loosely sutured. Wounds over joints are splinted. Initial closure is reserved only for facial wounds. The patient may require intravenous antibiotic therapy when an infection is present because of an increased incidence of cellulitis, osteomyelitis, and septic arthritis.

Consideration of rabies prophylaxis is an essential component in management of animal bites. A neurotoxic virus found in the saliva of some mammals causes rabies. If untreated, the condition is fatal in humans. Rabies exposure should be considered if an animal attack was not provoked, involved a wild animal, or involved a domestic animal not immunized against rabies. Rabies prophylaxis is always given when the animal cannot be found or when a carnivorous wild animal causes the bite. The prophylaxis regimen begins with an injection of rabies immune globulin to provide passive immunity. This is followed by a series of five injections of human diploid cell vaccine on days 0, 3, 7, 14, and 28 to provide active immunity. Dosage is based on the patient's weight.

Poisonings

A poison is any chemical that harms the body. Poisonings can be accidental, occupational, recreational, or intentional. Natural or manufactured toxins can be ingested, inhaled, injected, splashed in the eye, or absorbed through the skin. Common poisons are reviewed in Table 71-12. Other poisonings related to the use of illegal drugs such as amphetamines, narcotics, and hallucinogens are discussed in Chapter 11. Poisoning may also be caused by toxic plants or contaminated foods. (Food poisoning is discussed in Chapter 44.)

The severity of the poisoning depends on type, concentration, and route of exposure. Toxins can affect every tissue of the body, and so symptoms can be manifested by any body system. Specific management of toxins involves decreasing absorption, enhancing elimination, and implementation of toxin-specific interventions. Local poison control centres are available 24 hours a day and should be consulted for the most current treatment-specific protocols.

Options for decreasing absorption of poisons include emesis, gastric lavage, activated charcoal, dermal cleansing, and eye irrigation. Gastric lavage involves oral insertion of a large-diameter (36- to 40-French) gastric tube for instillation of copious amounts of saline. The head of the bed should be elevated or the patient placed in the side-lying position to prevent aspiration. Patients with an altered level of consciousness or diminished gag reflex are intubated before lavage. Lavage is contraindicated in patients who ingested caustic agents, sharp objects, or nontoxic substances. Otherwise, gastric lavage must be performed within 2 hours of ingestion of most poisons to be effective (Burns, 2006; Lehne, 2007). Problems associated with lavage include epistaxis, esophageal perforation, and aspiration.

The most effective intervention for management of poisonings is administration of activated charcoal orally or via a gastric tube. Toxins adhere to charcoal and are excreted through the gastrointestinal (GI) tract rather than absorbed into the portal circulation. Adults receive 50 to 100 g of charcoal. Activated charcoal can absorb a number of poisons from the GI tract, but it does not absorb ethanol, alkali, iron, boric acid, lithium, methanol, or cyanide. For some toxins (e.g., phenobarbital), multiple doses of charcoal may be required (Burns, 2006; Lehne, 2007). Contraindications to charcoal administration are diminished bowel sounds, ileus, ingestion of a substance poorly absorbed by charcoal, or previous administration of *N*-acetylcysteine (Muco-

myst) because charcoal inactivates oral *N*-acetylcysteine, the antidote used for acetaminophen toxicity.

Skin and ocular decontamination involves removal of toxins with copious amounts of water or saline. With the exception of mustard gas, most toxins can be safely removed with water or saline (Burns, 2006). Water mixes with mustard gas and releases chlorine gas. As a general rule, dry substances should be brushed from the skin and clothing before water is used. Powdered lime should not be removed with water; it should just be brushed off. Health care providers should wear personal protective equipment (gloves, gowns, goggles, and respirators) for decontamination to prevent secondary exposure. Decontamination procedures are usually performed by professionals specially trained in hazardous material decontamination before the patient arrives at the hospital. Decontamination takes priority over all interventions except basic life support techniques. Resources such as the Workplace Hazardous Materials Information System are part of mandatory orientation.

Elimination of poisons is increased through administration of cathartics, whole-bowel irrigation, hemodialysis, hemoperfusion, urine alkalinization, chelating agents, and antidotes. Cathartics such as sorbitol, magnesium citrate, and magnesium sulphate are administered with activated charcoal to stimulate intestinal motility and increase elimination. The use of cathartics is controversial, and multiple doses should be avoided because they can induce potentially fatal electrolyte abnormalities. Whole-bowel irrigation is controversial and involves administration of a nonabsorbable bowel evacuant solution (e.g., GoLYTELY). The solution is administered every 4 to 6 hours until stools are clear. This process can be effective for swallowed objects such as cocaine-filled balloons or condoms. There is a high risk for electrolyte imbalance from fluid and electrolyte losses with this intervention (Burns, 2006).

Hemodialysis and hemoperfusion are reserved for patients who develop severe acidosis from ingestion of toxic substances (e.g., aspirin). Other interventions include alkalinization and chelation therapy. Sodium bicarbonate administration raises the pH (to >7.5), which is particularly effective for phenobarbital and salicylate poisoning. Vitamin C may be added to IV fluids to enhance excretion of amphetamines and quinidine. Chelation therapy may be considered for heavy-metal poisoning (e.g., edetate calcium disodium [calcium EDTA] for lead poisoning). A limited number of true antidotes are available, and many are themselves toxic (Lehne, 2007).

Education for toxic emergencies focuses on how the poisoning occurred. Patients who experience poisoning because of a suicide attempt or related to substance abuse should be evaluated by a mental health care provider and referred for alcohol or drug detoxification if required. Patients should be made aware of Canadian Centre for Occupational Safety and Health measures for a safe work environment.

Domestic Violence

Domestic violence is a pattern of coercive behaviour in a relationship that involves fear; humiliation; intimidation; neglect; intentional physical, emotional, financial, or sexual injury or assault; or a combination of these (see Chapter 56 for a discussion of sexual assault). It occurs in all professions, cultures, and socioeconomic groups; people of all ages and of either gender may be victims. Although men can be victims of domestic violence, most victims are women, children, and older adults.

Table 71-12 Common Poisons

SUBSTANCE	MANIFESTATIONS	TREATMENT
Acetaminophen (Tylenol)	*Phase 1* (within 24 hr of ingestion): malaise, diaphoresis, nausea, and vomiting *Phase 2* (24-28 hr): right upper quadrant pain, decreased urine output, diminished nausea; LFTs demonstrate rise *Phase 3* (72-96 hr): nausea and vomiting; malaise; jaundice; hypoglycemia; enlarged liver; possible coagulopathies, including DIC *Phase 4* (7-8 days after ingestion): recovery, resolution of symptoms; results of LFTs return to normal	Activated charcoal, *N*-acetylcysteine (oral form may cause vomiting, IV form available in Canada)

Acids and alkalis
  Acids: toilet bowl cleaners, antirust compounds
  Alkalis: drain cleaners, dishwashing detergents, ammonia
	Excess salivation, dysphagia, epigastric pain, pneumonitis; burns of mouth, esophagus, and stomach	Immediate dilution (water, milk); corticosteroids (for alkali burns)
		
		Induced vomiting is contraindicated

Aspirin and aspirin-containing medications	Tachypnea, tachycardia, hyperthermia, seizures, pulmonary edema, occult bleeding or hemorrhage, metabolic acidosis	Gastric lavage, activated charcoal, urine alkalinization, hemodialysis for severe acute ingestion, intubation and mechanical ventilation, supportive care
Bleaches	Irritation of lips, mouth, and eyes; superficial injury to esophagus; chemical pneumonia and pulmonary edema	Washing of exposed skin and eyes, dilution with water and milk, gastric lavage, prevention of vomiting and aspiration
Carbon monoxide	Dyspnea, headache, tachypnea, confusion, impaired judgement, cyanosis, respiratory depression	Removal from source; administration of 100% O_2 via non-rebreather mask, BVM device, or intubation and mechanical ventilation; consider hyperbaric oxygen therapy
Cyanide	Almond odour to breath, headache, dizziness, nausea, confusion, hypertension, bradycardia followed by hypotension and tachycardia, tachypnea followed by bradypnea and respiratory arrest	Amyl nitrate (nasally), IV sodium nitrate, IV sodium thiosulphate, supportive care
Ethylene glycol	Sweet aromatic odour to breath, nausea and vomiting, slurred speech, ataxia, lethargy, respiratory depression	Gastric lavage, activated charcoal, supportive care
Iron	Vomiting (often bloody), diarrhea (often bloody), fever, hyperglycemia, lethargy, hypotension, seizures, coma	Gastric lavage, chelation therapy (deferoxamine [Desferal])
Nonsteroidal anti-inflammatory drugs	Gastroenteritis, abdominal pain, drowsiness, nystagmus, hepatic and renal damage	Gastric lavage, activated charcoal, cathartics, supportive care
Tricyclic antidepressants (e.g., amitriptyline [Elavil])	In low doses: anticholinergic effects, agitation, hypertension, tachycardia In high doses: central nervous system depression, dysrhythmias, hypotension, respiratory depression	Multidose activated charcoal, gastric lavage, serum alkalinization with sodium bicarbonate, intubation and mechanical ventilation, supportive care Never induce vomiting
Alcohol, barbiturates, benzodiazepines, cocaine, hallucinogens, stimulants	See Chapter 11	See Chapter 11

BVM, bag–valve–mask; *DIC*, disseminated intravascular coagulation; *IV*, intravenous; *LFTs*, liver function tests.

Domestic violence is often hidden and undiagnosed (Sillman, 2010).

It is recommended that all patients arriving at the ED should be screened to determine whether they are victims of domestic violence. Barriers to conducting effective screening include limited privacy for screening, lack of time, and lack of knowledge about how to inquire about domestic violence. The development and implementation of policies, procedures, and education programs can improve the practices of ED staff in screening for domestic violence. Screening should begin by creating a safe and supportive environment in which to talk with the patient. Privacy must be provided, and the patient should not be questioned in the presence of the possible abuser. Several instruments have been developed for screening, but research has shown that a few short questions are the most realistic for health care providers (Cherniak, Grant, Mason, Moore, & Pellizzari, 2005). The Partner Violence Screen includes the following three questions:

1. Have you been hit, kicked, punched, or otherwise hurt by someone within the past year? If so, by whom?
2. Do you feel safe in your current relationship?
3. Is there a partner from a previous relationship who is making you feel unsafe?

In addition to questioning the patient, it is important for the nurse to assess for risk factors such as injuries consistent with abuse; fearfulness of caregivers, including health care providers; withdrawn behaviour; regular ED use; and mental health and sleep disorders (Sillman, 2010). If the assessment reveals physical and behavioural findings suggestive of abuse, a more detailed assessment should be completed. A caring, nonjudgemental, and respectful approach should be used to facilitate patient disclosure. Detailed documentation and preservation of forensic evidence may be necessary, and appropriate interventions should be initiated, such as making referrals, providing emotional support, and informing victims about their options (e.g., safe plan, safe house, legal rights). Some EDs have affiliated Sexual Assault Care Centre/Domestic Violence centres to facilitate ED and community referrals and linkages and to support discharges into the community.

CLINICAL DECISION-MAKING EXERCISE

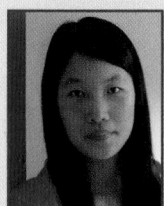

CASE STUDY:
Trauma
Source: © iStockphoto.com/Eva Serrabassa.

Patient Profile
Lian Wu, a 20-year-old woman, is brought to the ED in an ambulance. She was the driver in a motor vehicle collision and was not wearing a seat belt. Two children in the car were pronounced dead at the scene. The paramedics stated that there was significant damage to the car on the driver's side.

Subjective Data
- Ms. Wu asks, "What happened? Where are the children?"
- Complains of shortness of breath and abdominal pain

Objective Data
Physical Examination
- One 4-cm head laceration
- Badly deformed right lower leg with a pedal pulse detectable only by Doppler ultrasonography
- Glasgow Coma Score of 14; unequal pupils

- Decreased breath sounds on left side of chest
- Asymmetrical chest movement
- Vital signs: blood pressure, 90/40 mm Hg; heart rate, 130 beats/min; respiratory rate, 36 breaths/min
- O$_2$ saturation, 82%

Discussion Questions
1. What life-threatening injury does Ms. Wu probably have?
2. *Priority Decision:* What is the priority of care for Ms. Wu?
3. *Priority Decision:* What interventions are needed immediately?
4. What other interventions should the nurse consider?
5. Several family members have arrived in the ED, including the mother of one of the children who died. The second child who died was Ms. Wu's child. How should the nurse approach the family of the first child?
6. *Priority Decision:* On the basis of the assessment data presented, what are the priority nursing diagnoses? Are there any collaborative problems?

evolve *Answers are available at* **http://evolve.elsevier.com/ Canada/Lewis/medsurg**

REVIEW QUESTIONS

The number of the question corresponds to the numbered objectives at the beginning of the chapter.

1. An older man arrives at the ED disoriented and breathing rapidly. He has hot, dry skin. What is the priority for treatment at this point?
   a. To assess his airway, breathing, and circulation
   b. To obtain a detailed medical history from his family
   c. To determine that he has his health card before treating him
   d. To start oxygen administration and have the ED physician see him

2. A patient has a core temperature of 32°C. Which of the following is the most appropriate rewarming technique?
   a. Passive rewarming with body-to-body contact
   b. Active core rewarming using warmed IV fluids
   c. Passive rewarming using air-filled warming blankets
   d. Active external rewarming by submersing in a warm bath

3. What is the most effective intervention in decreasing absorption of an ingested poison?
   a. Ipecac syrup
   b. Milk dilution
   c. Gastric lavage
   d. Activated charcoal

4. Of patients who die in the ED, whom should the nurse regard as potential organ donors?
   a. Those who were young and strong
   b. Victims of accidents who were otherwise disease free
   c. Patients who can be kept on life support until the transplantation team is ready
   d. Anyone whose organs and tissues were healthy at the time of death

5. An older adult patient arrives in the ED with his son. The older man is in no apparent physical distress, although his clothes are soiled with urine and feces and he is tearful. Which of the following should the nurse should consider?
   a. Cancer
   b. Stroke
   c. Neglect
   d. Depression

ANSWERS: 1. a; 2. b; 3. d; 4. d; 5. c.

REFERENCES

Bair, A. E., Walls, R. M., & Grayzel, J. (2011). *Rapid sequence intubation in adults*. Retrieved from *http://www.uptodate.com/contents/rapid-sequence-intubation-in-adults*

Bullard, M., Unger, B., Spence, J., Grafstein, E., & The CTAS National Working Group. (2008). Revisions to the Canadian Triage and Acuity Scale (CTAS) adult guidelines. *Canadian Journal of Emergency Medicine, 10*, 136-151.

Burns, M. J. (2006). *General approach to drug poisoning in adults*. Retrieved from *http://www.uptodate.com/contents/general-approach-to-drug-poisoning-in-adults*

Canadian Association of Emergency Physicians. (2008). The Canadian Triage and Acuity Scale: Implementation guidelines. Retrieved from *http://caep.ca/resources/ctas/implementation-guidelines#level5*

Canadian Centre for Occupational Health and Safety. (2008). *What is Lyme disease?* Retrieved from *www.ccohs.ca/oshanswers/diseases/lyme.html*

Canadian Institute for Health Information. (2011). *National Trauma Registry 2011 report: Hospitalizations for major injury in Canada, 2008-2009 data.* Ottawa: Author. Retrieved from *https://secure.cihi.ca/free_products/NTR_CDS_2008_2009_Annual_Report.pdf*

Canadian Institute for Health Information. (2012). *Highlights of 2010-2011 inpatient hospitalizations and emergency department visits.* Retrieved from *https://secure.cihi.ca/free_products/DAD-NACRS_Highlights_2010-2011_EN.pdf*

Canadian Nurses Association. (2011). *Specialties/Areas of Nursing Practice.* Retrieved from *http://www.cna-aiic.ca/en/professional-development/specialty-certification/what-is-certification/specialtiesareas-of-nursing-practice/*

Chandy, D., & Weinhouse, G. (2012). *Drowning: Submersion injuries.* Retrieved from *http://www.uptodate.com/contents/drowning-submersion-injuries*

Cherniak, D., Grant, L., Mason, R., Moore, B., & Pellizzari, R. (2005). Intimate partner violence consensus statement. *Journal of Obstetrics and Gynaecology Canada, 157* (April), 365-388.

Cox, B. (2007). Family presence during CPR and invasive procedures. *American Journal of Critical Care, 16*(3), 283. Retrieved from *http://ajcc.aacnjournals.org/content/16/3/283.full*

Crawford Mechem, C. (2010). *Severe hyperthermia (heat stroke) in adults.* Retrieved from *http://www.uptodate.com/contents/severe-hyperthermia-heat-stroke-in-adults*

Crawford Mechem, C., & Danzl, D. (2011). *Accidental hypothermia in adults.* Retrieved from *http://www.uptodate.com/contents/accidental-hypothermia-in-adults*

Crawford Mechem, C., & Zafren, K. (2010). *Frostbite.* Retrieved from *http://www.uptodate.com/contents/frostbite*

Enzler, M., Berbari, E., & Osmon, D. (2011). Antimicrobial prophylaxis in adults. *Mayo Clinic Proceedings, 86*, 686-701. doi:10.4065/mcp.2011.0012

Flarity, K. (2007). Environmental emergencies. In K. S. Hoyt & J. Selfridge-Thomas (Eds.), *Emergency nursing: Core curriculum* (6th ed., pp. 310-348). St. Louis: W. B. Saunders.

Hustey, F., Mion, L., & Connor, J., Emmerman, C. L., Campbell, J., & Palmer, R. M. (2007). A brief risk stratification tool to predict functional decline in older adults discharged from emergency departments. *Journal of the American Geriatrics Society, 55*(8), 1269-1274. doi:10.1111/j.1532-5415.2007.01272.x

Kiel, D. (2011). *Falls in older persons: Risk factors and patient evaluation.* Retrieved from *http://www.uptodate.com/contents/falls-in-older-persons-risk-factors-and-patient-evaluation*

Lehne, R. A. (2007). *Pharmacology for nursing care* (6th ed.). St. Louis: Elsevier.

MacDonald, R., & Burgess, R. (2010). *Nancy Caroline's emergency care in the streets (Canadian ed.).* Toronto: Jones & Bartlett.

Madden, E., & Condon, C. (2007). Emergency nurses' current practices and understanding of family presence during CPR. *Journal of Emergency Nursing, 33*, 433-440. doi:10.1016/j.jen.2007.06.024

Miller, S., Martin, H., & Morris, J. (2008). Pneumatic antishock garment. *Best Practice & Research Clinical Obstetrics & Gynaecology, 22*(6), 1057-1074. doi:10.1016/j.bpobgyn.2008.08.008

Motov, S. M., Khan, A. N. (2009). Problems and barriers of pain management in the emergency department: Are we ever going to get better? *Journal of Pain Research, 2*:5-11.

National Emergency Nurses Affiliation (NENA). (2010). *Position statement: Family-PSU presence during resuscitation.* Retrieved from *http://nena.ca/public/b/about/archive/2010/01/11/position-statement-family-psu-presence-during-resuscitation.aspx*

National Emergency Nurses Affiliation (NENA). (2011). *Certification.* Retrieved from *http://nena.ca/*

National Opioid Use Guideline Group. (2010). *Canadian guideline for safe and effective use of opioids for chronic non-cancer pain. Part A: Executive summary and background.* Retrieved from *http://nationalpaincentre.mcmaster.ca/documents/opioid_guideline_part_a_v4_5.pdf*

Ogden, N., Bouchard, C., Kurtenbach, K., Margos, G., Lindsay, R., Trudel, L., …, Milord, F. (2010). Active and passive surveillance and phylogenetic analysis of *Borrelia burgdorferi* elucidate the process of Lyme disease risk in Canada. *Environmental Health Perspectives, 118*, 909-914. doi:10.1289/ehp.0901766

Regional Geriatric Program of Toronto. (2011). *Frequently asked questions about the Regional Geriatric Program of Toronto.* Retrieved from *http://rgp.toronto.on.ca/files/RGP%20FAQ%20-%20updated%20Dec%202011.pdf*

Ricci, N., & Rizzolo, P. (2011). Laceration repair: Avoid infection, optimize healing, minimize scarring. *Journal of the American Academy of Physician Assistants, 24*(9), 29-33.

Sillman, J. (2010). *Diagnosing, screening and counselling for domestic violence.* (January). Retrieved from *http://www.uptodate.com.normedproxy.lakeheadu.ca.ezproxy.lakeheadu.ca/contents/diagnosing-screening-and-counseling-for-domestic-violence?source=search_result&search=DOMESTIC+VIOLENCE&selectedTitle=1%7E67*

Trillium Gift of Life Network. (2011). *Organ and tissue donation.* Retrieved from *http://www.giftoflife.on.ca/page.cfm?id=313B576D-E970-4CBE-B946-49A4B3F306D8*

Vetter, R., Swanson, D., & White, J. (2011). *Bites of widow spiders.* Retrieved from *http://www.uptodate.com/contents/bites-of-widow-spiders?source=search_result&search=SPIDER+BITES&selectedTitle=3~26*

CANADIAN RESOURCES

Canadian Association of Emergency Physicians
http://www.caep.ca
Canadian Centre for Abuse Awareness (CCAA)
http://www.ccfaa.com/
Canadian Centre for Occupational Health and Safety
http://www.ccohs.ca
Canadian Institute for Health Information
http://www.cihi.ca/
Canadian Nurses Association
http://www.cna-aiic.ca/
Canadian Association of Poison Control Centres
http://www.capcc.ca/
Canadian Red Cross
http://www.redcross.ca
Canadian Society for the Investigation of Child Abuse (CSICA)
http://www.csicainfo.com/
Centre for Research & Education on Violence Against Women & Children
http://www.crvawc.ca/
Health Canada
http://www.hc-sc.gc.ca/english/contact
National Clearinghouse on Family Violence
http://www.phac-aspc.gc.ca/ncfv-cnivf/index-eng.php
National Emergency Nurses Affiliation (NENA)
http://www.nena.ca
National Trauma Registry
http://www.cihi.ca/cihi-ext-portal/internet/en/document/ types+of+care/specialized+services/trauma+and+injuries/ services_ntr

Parks Canada National Office
http://www.pc.gc.ca/index_e.asp
Public Health Agency of Canada
http://www.phac-aspc.gc.ca/index-eng.php
Parachute: Preventing Injuries, Saving Lives
http://parachutecanada.org/
Safe Kids Canada
http://www.safekidscanada.ca/
St. John Ambulance Canada
http://www.sja.ca
Trauma Association of Canada
http://www.traumacanada.org

RELATED RESOURCES

Centers for Disease Control and Prevention: Emergency Preparedness and Response
http://www.bt.cdc.gov
Wilderness Medicine Institute
http://wmi.nols.edu

evolve *For additional Internet resources, see the Web site for this book at* **http://evolve.elsevier.com/Canada/Lewis/medsurg**

Written by **Karen Baguley**

LEARNING OBJECTIVES

1. Differentiate between an emergency and a disaster situation.
2. Identify the roles and responsibilities of individuals, communities, and select provincial or territorial and federal agencies in emergency planning and disaster management.
3. Define and describe the characteristics of disaster nursing.
4. Outline the components of a comprehensive emergency management program.
5. Describe the four phases of disaster management and the nursing role in each phase.
6. Describe the differences between daily emergency department triage and triage in emergency and disaster situations.
7. Classify the major types of disasters based on their characteristics and describe their consequences.
8. Identify those agents most likely to be used in a terrorist attack and their health impact.
9. Describe key differences between chemical, biological, radiological, nuclear, and explosive (CBRNE) events and the relevance of casualty decontamination in health care settings.
10. Describe the difference between epidemics and pandemics and discuss the importance of pandemic planning.

KEY TERMS

bioterrorism The deliberate spreading of microbes or toxins with the intent of causing disease or death in animals, plants, or humans, p. 2045

CBRNE event An acronym used to describe exposure to chemical, biological, radioactive, nuclear, or explosive substances, p. 2045

critical incident stress management (CISM) or debriefing An approach to preventing and managing the emotional trauma that can be a result of involvement in a disaster response, p. 2044

disaster The outcome of a natural hazard (e.g., hurricane, flood, earthquake, snowstorm) or a result of human action or error, whether malicious (e.g., terrorist attacks, use of biological warfare) or unintentional (e.g., accidental chemical spill), p. 2037

disaster nursing The provision of nursing care, advocacy, and health promotion within the context of a disaster situation, p. 2053

emergency Any situation that requires a rapid and skilled response and that can be typically managed by a community's existing resources, p. 2036

emergency and disaster management A process that includes a series of steps from anticipation of a hazardous event, to minimizing the risks from such an event, to preparing for and recovering from an emergency or disaster, p. 2038

epidemic When the number of cases of a communicable disease exceeds the normal expected occurrence during a given period, p. 2050

hazards Anything that has the potential to cause harm or loss. Hazards can be substances, human activities, or conditions that may cause injury or loss of life, threaten the delivery of critical services, cause social and economic disruption and/or environmental damage, p. 2037

outbreak management Strategies used to prevent the spread of communicable disease among a cluster of people, p. 2050

pandemic When a communicable disease is widespread affecting large numbers of people globally, p. 2050

pandemic influenza Highly infectious outbreak of influenza that spreads rapidly around the world, with much more serious consequences than the usual effects of seasonal influenza, p. 2051

quarantine The isolation of people who have been exposed to infection but who are not yet sick or showing any signs of infection, p. 2051

terrorism Overt actions that are committed to cause fear, panic, destruction, injury, and death with the intent to intimidate the public or a particular segment of the public

or to compel a specific person, government, or international organization, p. 2045

triage A system used to identify and categorize casualties and prioritize health care needs and allocation of resources, p. 2043

ELECTRONIC RESOURCES

Supplemental content related to Chapter 72 can be found …

Evolve Web Site ⊝volve

http://evolve.elsevier.com/Canada/Lewis/medsurg
- Answer Guidelines for Case Study on p. 2054
- Clinical Reference: Laboratory Values

- Content Updates
- Electronic Calculators
- eTable 72-1: Acute Radiation Syndrome
- Examination Review Questions
- Glossary
- Key Points (Printable and MP3 Download)

Emergencies, often referred to as "disasters," are a worldwide occurrence. Global media coverage has allowed us to witness disaster events firsthand. Impact may be localized, affecting a single geographic community, or of such a large scale that the event affects a country or countries around the globe. Disasters are caused by natural hazards (e.g., weather, floods, earthquakes), disease outbreaks, and human actions (e.g., accidents, acts of aggression). Although humans have always been subject to the forces of nature, illness and other humans, we have learned over time to better adapt to our environment and have developed strategies to reduce the impact. Although natural hazards like Hurricane Katrina (2005), the Haiti earthquake (2010), and the Great East Japan earthquake (2011) are often better predicted than they once were, human-caused disasters and disease outbreaks raise additional challenges. Images of the September 11th terrorist attacks in New York City (2001), the 2010 oil spill in the Gulf of Mexico, and the severe acute respiratory syndrome (SARS) outbreak in Canada (2003) had effects far beyond their immediate borders.

War, terrorism, violence, famine, epidemics, globalization, environmental degradation, and climate change all have profound consequences for populations worldwide. There has been a steady increase in the number of disasters occurring globally over the last several decades. According to the United Nations–UN News Centre (2011), 2010 was one of the deadliest years for disasters, reflecting the need for better planning and preparation. Although we often think of disasters as occurring suddenly, without warning, and with the outcome beyond our control, harm to individuals, property, and the environment can be mitigated or the impact reduced. Although each disaster situation varies in its severity and consequences, the use of appropriate emergency management systems, before, during, and after events, will ultimately result in better outcomes. Owing to the increasing incidence of disaster situations globally and because nurses make up the largest sector of the health care workforce in Canada, many nurses can expect to be confronted by an emergency or disastrous event at some point in their careers. Disaster nursing is a growing

practice specialty for nurses. Nurses who work in acute and long-term care settings and within the community play a key role in emergency planning and response, protecting the public from harm (Canadian Nurses' Association [CNA], 2007, p. 1). Today, it is an expectation that all nurses demonstrate an awareness of the impact of emergency planning on disaster response and work collaboratively to implement strategies to prevent illness and injuries that are a result of community disasters and global health issues (College of Nurses of Ontario [CNO], 2008; World Health Organization and International Council of Nurses [WHO & ICN, 2009]).

Emergency Preparedness and Disaster Planning

Emergency preparedness and disaster planning involves advanced preparation for a variety of potential situations, ranging in scale from mass casualty incidents, to natural events, to conflicts and acts of terrorism (Veenema, 2007a). Planning, when done in a comprehensive and diligent manner, decreases the impact that an emergency or disaster has on individuals, organizations, and communities.

When discussing emergency preparedness and disaster planning, it is important to differentiate between the terms *emergency* and *disaster*. According to the WHO and ICN (2009), no single agreed-upon definition of the term *disaster* exists (p. 3). Disasters are often defined by governments, humanitarian groups, and other agencies, reflecting the mission and needs of that agency. Although events are typically labelled as "disasters" by the communities affected and by the media, many events may be more accurately classified as an "emergency." An **emergency** may be described as an event that requires a rapid and skilled response to protect the health, safety, and wellness of individuals and to limit damage to property. Emergency situations are typically able to be quickly managed without requiring the support and resources of other communities (Powers, 2010a), but require urgent intervention to prevent worsening of the situation. A **disaster** is the outcome of a natural hazard or event (e.g., hurricane, flood, earthquake) or a result of human action or error, whether malicious (e.g., terrorist attacks, use of biological warfare) or unintentional (e.g., an accidental chemical spill), that seriously disrupts the functioning of a community or society (Noji, 1996; WHO, 2007). Disasters typically occur suddenly and can result in mass casualties (i.e., large numbers of people injured), loss of human life, materials, and significant destruction of the environment and critical infrastructure (e.g., government, water, power, food supply) (UNISDR, 2009; WHO, 2007). A disaster, owing to its scale and impact, exceeds the capacity of a community to respond with existing resources requiring "outside" assistance from trained responders, government and non-government organizations, humanitarian relief agencies, or some combination of all of these.

Two approaches are used in emergency preparedness and disaster planning initiatives: an *agent-specific approach*, in which planning efforts are directed at those threats most likely to take place within a single geographical location (e.g., earthquakes in California) (Veenema, 2007a); and more commonly, an *all-hazards approach*, a comprehensive disaster management strategy, where all hazards are considered to be potential possibilities even if they have never happened or are unlikely to ever occur. **Hazards** are defined as anything that has the potential to cause harm or loss. Hazards can be substances, human activities or conditions that may cause injury or loss of life, threaten the delivery of critical services, cause social and economic disruption, and/or environmental damage (UNISDR, 2009, p. 17). Emergencies and disasters occur when a hazard interacts with a vulnerable area to produce adverse consequences that may exceed a community or society's ability to cope. An all-hazards approach to emergency preparedness and disaster planning helps ensure that managing one type of risk does not increase vulnerability to other risks (Public Safety Canada [PSC], 2009a). Emergency planning in Canada includes broad strategies aimed at maintaining public safety and civil defence from all potential hazards or emergency and disaster situations (PSC, 2009a).

Individual, Local–Municipal, Provincial–Territorial, and Federal Responsibilities

In order to be successful, emergency and disaster planning initiatives must be done at a variety of levels, specifically, the individual/family, the local community or municipal, the provincial–territorial, and the federal levels.

Emergency preparedness involves having plans of action, supplies, and resources in place to respond in a timely and efficient manner to inevitable emergency events. Emergency preparedness begins at an individual level and requires that individuals and families assume responsibility for taking appropriate steps to ensure that they have the "basics" of what might be required for short-term survival following an emergency or disaster situation (PSC, 2010). This level of preparation requires stockpiling items that would be needed to be self-sufficient for a period of at least 72 hours and a detailed plan, considering risks to the region, knowledge of safe exits from a neighbourhood, advanced identification of emergency contacts and meeting places for reunification, and awareness of household fire extinguishers, water and gas valves, and electrical control panels (Canadian Red Cross, 2010a; PSC, 2010). Emergency workers focus on community members with the most urgent needs, and search and rescue

efforts for casualties take precedence in the first 72 hours of an emergency event. Critical infrastructure (e.g., water and power) could potentially be interrupted for an extended period of time, reflecting the need for advanced planning and availability of basic survival resources. Table 72-1 details items that should be included in an individual or a family emergency preparedness kit.

According to the Government of Canada (2008, p. 1), "Every disaster is a local disaster." Accountability for emergency planning and response in Canada is held by individual municipalities, the underlying principle being that communities possess the greatest knowledge of their individual needs and, thus, are in a

---

Table 72-1 Individual or Family Emergency Preparedness Kit

Basic Emergency Kit Items to Include

Food and Drinking Water: Have at least a 3-day (72-hr) supply of food and water on hand

Food—Ready-to-eat foods that will not spoil such as canned food, energy bars, and dried foods.

Drinking Water—Two litres of water per person per day (include small water bottles)

Equipment for Emergency Survival

☐ Wind-up or battery-powered flashlight (with extra batteries)

☐ Wind-up or battery-powered radio (with extra batteries)

☐ First-aid kit

☐ Extra keys for car and house

☐ Cash (include smaller bills, such as $10 bills and change for pay phones)

Additional Supplies That Should Be Considered:

☐ Additional bottles of water (2 L/person) for cooking and cleaning

☐ Candles; matches or lighter

☐ Change of clothing and footwear (one change of clothes/person)

☐ Blankets or sleeping bags for each household member

☐ Utensils, disposable cups and plates

☐ Toiletries, hand sanitizer

☐ Manual can opener, bottle opener

☐ Small fuel-operated stove and fuel

☐ Garbage bags

☐ Important papers (identification, personal documents)

☐ Backpack or duffel bag (in case of evacuation)

☐ Whistle (to attract attention)

☐ Duct tape and basic tools (hammer, pliers, wrench, screwdrivers, pocket knife)

☐ Playing cards and games

Any Special Needs Family Members Might Have

☐ Personal prescription medications

☐ Infant formula, diapers

☐ Pet food

☐ Equipment for people with disabilities

Source: Public Safety Canada. (2012). Your emergency preparedness guide. 72 hours: Is your family prepared? Retrieved from *http://www.getprepared.gc.ca/cnt/rsrcs/pblctns/yprprdnssgd/yprprdnssgd-eng.pdf*. Reproduced with the permission of the Minister of Public Works and Government Services Canada, 2012.

strategic position to most effectively plan for and manage local emergency events. Local *first responders* (fire, police, and paramedics) are typically the first to respond to an emergency, assuming responsibility for local events as a component of the municipal emergency plan. Most emergency situations can be effectively handled by a community, with different levels of organizations being introduced progressively if the situation escalates and additional help and resources are needed. When a community is unable to provide required response efforts because of the scope of the situation or inadequate personnel or equipment, a "community emergency" is declared and the province or territory is contacted for support. All provinces and territories have an *Emergency Management Organization* (EMO) that is responsible for developing, coordinating, training, and response operations in their jurisdiction. EMOs typically manage large-scale emergencies, providing assistance to municipal or community response teams (Government of Canada, 2008). Recognizing the potential for emergencies and disasters to rapidly escalate in scope and severity, cross jurisdictional lines, and have an international impact (PSC, 2011a, p. 1), the provincial–territorial EMO will notify the federal government for further assistance when required. Federal assistance is most commonly dispatched in disaster situations, for example, in those involving mass casualties or in areas under federal authority such as nuclear safety, national defence, and border security (Government of Canada, 2008).

Public Safety Canada (PSC) is the department of the federal government accountable for Canadian safety and protection. This Department was created after the events of September 11, 2001, with the goal of ensuring peace and safety in this country. PSC plays a role in the development of national policy, response systems, and standards and is responsible for providing guidance to federal government institutions on the development of emergency management plans. This approach strengthens the Canadian Government's capacity to prevent, protect against, respond to, and recover from major disasters and other emergencies (PSC, 2011a). PSC also plays a critical role by establishing partnerships across sectors with key organizations, like the provincial–territorial EMOs, Canadian Security Intelligence Services, the Royal Canadian Mounted Police, and the U.S. Department of Homeland Security, as a means of managing national risks, reducing vulnerabilities to hazards, and strengthening the resiliency of critical infrastructure (PSC, 2011b). *Critical infrastructure* consists of physical and information technology facilities, networks, services, and assets that are considered to be essential to the health, safety, security, and economic well-being of Canadians and to the continued functioning of the country as a whole. Examples of critical infrastructure include power, water, government, and sewage services (PSC, 2011b). Several federal departments work alongside PSC to provide emergency response resources. For example, Health Canada plays a role in implementing strategies aimed at reducing risks to individual health and the overall environment. The Department of National Defence administers the Canadian Forces Disaster Assistance Response Team (DART), which provides purified drinking water, engineering capabilities, and supportive medical services following a disaster (National Defence Canada, 2005).

Nongovernment organizations (NGOs) are an important component of the emergency response system. These nonprofit, nongovernment organizations offer assistance with disaster prevention and preparedness, response, and recovery. The Canadian Red Cross, St. John Ambulance, and the Salvation Army are examples of NGOs providing resources that include emergency response

support (equipment, supplies, and human resources) and that address basic human needs (food, clothing, shelter, emotional support, and family reunification) in times of disaster (Canadian Red Cross, 2010b; St. John Ambulance, 2011; The Salvation Army, 2011).

Emergency and Disaster Management

Emergency and disaster management is a process that includes a series of steps from anticipation of a hazardous event, to minimizing the risks from such an event, to preparing for and recovering from an emergency or disaster. When an emergency or disaster strikes, individuals and communities are at risk. The *Emergency Management Act* (EMA) was developed with the goal of strengthening emergency management efforts in this country. The Act sets out clear roles and responsibilities for emergency management and is directed at ensuring that Canada and its jurisdictions are prepared to prevent or mitigate, prepare for, respond to, and recover from natural and human-caused hazards. The Act also focuses on the protection of critical infrastructure with the goal of ensuring the safety and the security of all Canadians (PSC, 2009b).

Emergencies and disasters are best considered as distinct phases, as opposed to a single point in time, each of which requires action in order to decrease the impact of the situation. The *disaster management continuum* is accepted globally as the method for addressing all aspects of a disaster (WHO & ICN, 2009, p. 39) (Figure 72-1). This approach emphasizes a continuous emergency planning process aimed at reducing harm to populations and critical infrastructure and building community resilience. In this sense, emergency planning includes a chain of activities or series of steps related to each phase of a disaster. Although a range of models exists with varied terminology to explain the phases and activities, all describe a system of continuous and connected activities, some of which occur concurrently. The phases outlined in the disaster management continuum are related to the timeline of a disaster: preincident/preimpact; incident/impact; and postincident/postimpact (Veenema, 2007a; WHO & ICN, 2009). Within each disaster phase are activities that include: (1) preincident: activities designed to prevent or mitigate and plan for the potential impact of an emergency or disaster; (2) incident: all activities involved in the response to an emergency or disaster situation; and (3) postincident: recovery or rehabilitation from said situation (WHO & ICN, 2009). The use of an all-hazards approach to planning, multilevel partnerships to respond to emergency and disaster situations, and integration of the activities outlined in each phase together comprise a *comprehensive emergency and disaster management program* (PSC, 2011a).

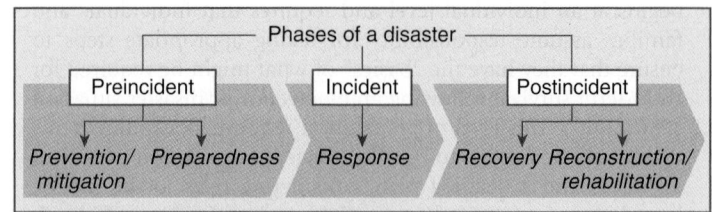

Figure 72-1 Disaster management continuum.

Source: World Health Organization and International Council of Nurses (2009). *ICN Framework of Disaster Nursing Competencies* (p. 40, Figure 1). Retrieved from http://www.icn.ch/images/stories/documents/networks/DisasterPreparednessNetwork/Disaster_Nursing_Competencies_lite.pdf

Mitigation

Mitigation, also called *prevention*, is a critical first step in emergency management and is done in the preincident phase before an emergency or disaster occurs, through the anticipation of potential risks. A *risk* is defined as the combination of the likelihood that a hazard, or event, will occur and the consequences that may result if it does (UNISDR, 2009). Emergency management is a *risk-based* process, meaning decisions and activities are to be based on an assessment of hazards, risks, and vulnerabilities. *Vulnerabilities* are conditions that increase the susceptibility of organizations and communities to negative impact by a hazard. Examples of vulnerabilities include poor construction and design of buildings, lack of public information, and inadequate preparedness measures (UNISDR, 2009). Mitigation, therefore, involves the identification of potential hazards faced by an organization or a community and the minimization of possible consequences from those hazards.

The goal of mitigation is to identify and implement long-term strategies to reduce, deflect, or altogether avoid the consequences a hazard might have on human health, organizational or community function, and critical infrastructure (PSC, 2009c; UNISDR, 2009). Examples of mitigation strategies within the community include flood mapping and the use of water-resistant building materials to decrease the effects of floods and hurricanes; another example is the development of public warning systems to assist with evacuation in times of emergency (Federal Emergency Management Agency [FEMA], 2010). Implementing these strategies in advance will have the potential of reducing risks (e.g., number of injuries and deaths) to a community when faced by these hazards. In the hospital setting, mitigation might include ensuring the availability of essential equipment (e.g., portable medical gases) that does not require the use of electricity, or availability of backup emergency generators for critical equipment, thereby decreasing the risk and impact on patients should critical infrastructure fail. Nurses play a pivotal role in mitigation activities. Nurses' knowledge of community needs, available resources, populations at risk, and workforce issues is essential in preparing an organization or a community for emergency situations (WHO & ICN, 2009).

Preparedness

Preparedness is a proactive activity that also occurs in the preincident phase. Preparedness involves preplanning for emergencies and disasters that could occur within an organization, a community, or a jurisdiction. Preparedness is closely tied to emergency response, as the delineation of "what should happen, when" and "who does what, where" when an emergency occurs. Preparedness includes the knowledge and capacity developed by individuals, organizations, communities, governments, and response organizations to anticipate, respond to, and recover from the impact of a hazard (PSC, 2011a; UNISDR, 2009). Nurses play an important role in preparedness by educating communities on disaster preparedness; working to reduce hazards in the home, work settings, and within communities; participating in drills and training exercises; and through the development of emergency operations plans (EOPs) and protocols (WHO & ICN, 2009). Within the hospital setting, the nursing role is one of leadership and advocacy through participation on unit and corporate-based committees and task forces and in the development of disaster plans and exercises.

Health Care Emergency Operations Plans. An *emergency operations plan* (EOP) is a document that describes strategies and frameworks for how emergencies will be planned for and managed and delineates training and exercise requirements with the goal of increasing disaster resiliency (Andress, 2010a). Plans and processes are detailed through the EOP that should be implemented almost automatically in an emergency or disaster situation. Health care facilities and community agencies are required under Accreditation Canada to have policies and processes in place to manage all types of internal emergencies (e.g., fires, bomb threats, unmanageable or hazardous spills) as well as those arising external to the organization (e.g., mass casualty incidents) that, owing to their size and impact, have the potential of affecting day-to-day operations and patient care (Veenema, 2007a).

Internal and External Disasters. *Internal disasters* refer to any situation that threatens or disrupts the daily, routine services of a health care facility. These situations present a potential danger to patients and staff and may or may not occur at the same time as an external event. Internal disasters have the potential to result in a series of outcomes, including patient and staff evacuation, decreased levels of service, diversion of transportation (e.g., ambulance and air transport), and reallocation of patient care (Veenema, 2007a). Causes of internal disasters include bomb threats, chemical or radiological accidents, spills, power and water loss, unavailability of staff, outbreaks of communicable disease, and violence (Qureshi & Gebbie, 2007; Veenema 2007a). Health care facilities must develop internal disaster plans to address all scenarios that have the potential to affect patient care.

External disasters are a result of events that originate outside of a health care organization. This type of disaster has the potential to threaten a facility when the consequences of the event create a demand for service that exceeds what is routinely available (Qureshi & Gebbie, 2007). Examples of external disasters include *mass casualty incidents* that precipitate the arrival of large numbers of trauma patients or the presentation of victims from exposure to a hazardous material incident called a *chemical-biological-radiological-nuclear-explosive* (CBRNE) *event*.

Combined external–internal disasters are a result of external conditions that trigger a response within the internal environment of a health care facility (Qureshi & Gebbie, 2007). In Canada, severe weather conditions (e.g., snowstorms) can result in a combined external–internal disaster. For example, the inability of staff to travel to work, coupled with an increased volume of trauma patients, can precipitate a staffing crisis in the hospital setting. Consequently, remaining staff resources may be unable to address demands owing to increased patient volumes and acuity levels of those needing care (Qureshi & Gebbie, 2007).

Contents of Health Care Emergency Operations Plans. In Canada, most disaster response activities typically occur in hospital, necessitating a comprehensive EOP. Whereas hospitals must be prepared for a variety of potential events, most disasters place similar demands necessitating the use of an all-hazards approach to planning. This approach allows for a flexible and scaleable response and focuses on commonalities among different types of potential disasters that could occur in that area (Andress, 2010a; California Emergency Medical Services Authority [CEMSA], 2006a). Supplements are included for those events needing a specific action.

A health care EOP outlines how an emergency situation is identified, initiated, managed, and terminated within the health care setting. This extensive document starts with a needs assessment. Resources and supplies are identified that are considered to be essential. Stockpiles of medications (e.g., analgesics, sedatives, and antidotes), required personal protective equipment (PPE) (e.g., masks, splash suits, chemical-resistant gloves), and medical supplies (e.g., stretchers, ventilators, bandages, dressings) to support patient care should be identified and processes for acquiring needed supplies and equipment considered. Information technology requirements may include computers (for documentation and patient registration), televisions and radios (to receive external coverage of the emergency event), telephones, walkie-talkies, and fax machines (Veenema, 2007a). Space and needed resources for emergency response (e.g., emergency operations centre, media centre, staffing and patient–family information centres, patient surge locations) should also be included in the plan. Basic human-needs requirements (e.g., nonperishable food, water, accommodations, rest areas) for staff and family members who stay for prolonged periods should be identified as essential resources.

Numerous challenges have been identified in the management of emergency and disaster situations. These include communication difficulties; lack of leadership, planning, and clear lines of accountability; inadequate surge capacity, casualty triage, transportation, and evacuation processes; poor safety, security, and control of entry points; patient identification and data tracking processes; management of resources; and resistance to planning initiatives (Andress, 2010a; CEMSA, 2006a; Landesman, 2001). Addressing these challenges in the EOP will facilitate effective management of the situation. Components of an EOP in a health care setting is as follows:

1. *Activation of Emergency Status.* The EOP should outline how notification is received of an emergency or disaster situation. In the case of an external disaster, notification may come from emergency medical services or the media, whereas initial notification of an internal event typically comes from an inpatient unit or department (e.g., in the case of a bomb threat or fire). The EOP must describe how notification of other departments and escalation of the situation occurs, when and to whom.

2. *Communication Plan.* Although communication is essential to successful emergency response, it often represents a challenge. A *communication plan* provides details highlighting internal and external communication processes that should take place between first responders and the hospital; between staff members (front-line and management); and between the hospital and family members of casualties. Communication with the public must also be taken into consideration through the development of a *media communication plan.* Documentation tools and tracking forms are often of assistance in enhancing communication between departments and with family members. Communication of decisions made, requests for support, and initiation and setup of emergency response centres follow a hierarchical process and is a component of the incident management system (IMS) (CEMSA, 2006a; Qureshi & Gebbie, 2007).

3. *Plan for the Coordination of Patient Care.* This portion of the EOP outlines processes for managing patient care with a specific focus on the area most affected by the emergency event; this might be the emergency department as the portal of entry for those injured in an external disaster or, in the case of an internal disaster, those areas directly affected by the emer-

gency situation. *Surge capacity,* a calculation of the number of available beds (including possible transfers and discharges), and the availability of multidisciplinary staff and supplies (e.g., ventilators, medications) should be included (Lentz, Reid, Rera, & Kehoe, 2007). A process for the suspension of normal daily services (e.g., elective surgeries, outpatient clinics) should be provided and triggers for that eventuality identified.

4. *Staffing Plan.* A staffing plan provides a detailed process for calling in additional staff when required (called *fan-out*) to support patient care as well as for reassigning staff to areas with the highest volume, acuity level, and patient concentration (Qureshi & Gebbie, 2007). An outline of skill sets of staff across the facility assists with this process. Reassignment of staff is typically coordinated via the facility's emergency operations centre through the use of a *labour pool and staffing centre.*

5. *Equipment and Supply Plan.* This plan includes detailed lists of the equipment and supplies that will be needed in an emergency situation. Storage for the stockpiling of equipment and supplies should be arranged in advance and a process outlined for accessing additional resources from suppliers (including contact numbers) (Veenema, 2007a). This is of particular importance in situations involving chemical or other hazardous material exposure because safe patient care cannot be provided without immediate access to specific PPE. The availability and functional status of equipment called for in an emergency situation must be evaluated on a regular basis (Veenema, 2007a). A process for monitoring expiration dates and ensuring circulation of supplies before their expiration should be considered as a component of planning activities.

6. *Security Plan.* A security plan outlines procedures for ensuring a safe work and patient care environment. This includes procedures for instating *lockdown status* within the organization. Lockdown, a process that involves limiting access to entry points to a health care facility, should ideally be an instantaneous process (CEMSA, 2006a). This is of particular importance in situations that pose a potential or real threat to staff and patients. For example, in cases in which there is chemical, biological, radiological, or nuclear exposure, lockdown will assist in redirecting contaminated patients to a single designated point of entry where decontamination can occur before common areas are entered. Security plans must also detail processes aimed at ensuring "crowd control" and access to entry points during a disaster (CEMSA, 2006a).

7. *Documentation and Data Management Strategy.* A documentation and data management strategy outlines how patients will be rapidly identified (also called *banded*) and tracked when moving within and across departments or institutions (Veenema, 2007a). Consistent documentation of care delivered is essential in an emergency situation and for follow-up after the event. Owing to the potential for loss of critical infrastructure (e.g., power, communication) during an emergency, backup paper-based systems should be created.

8. *Deactivation and Recovery Process.* A deactivation and recovery process should be outlined in the EOP highlighting processes for terminating emergency status. Clear delineation should be provided of those who are able to deactivate disaster response activities, how this is to be done, and when.

9. *Postincident Debriefing Plan.* This plan provides guidelines as to when debriefing of those people involved in emergency response initiatives will occur and in what format. Postinci-

dent debriefing not only assists in improving components of the emergency plan and future response activities but also allows staff to discuss and cope with events that took place during the disaster response (Grigg & Hughes, 2010).

10. *Educational Plan.* An educational plan for emergency drills and training exercises should be outlined in the EOP and include dates, times, frequency, and format for testing the plan (Andress, 2010a; WHO, 2009).

Testing of Emergency Plans. Organizations and staff respond to and recover from emergency and disaster situations based on their level of preparation, the culture of the organization, past experience in dealing with emergencies, and the nature or scale of the situation (Veenema, 2007a). Emergency exercises are conducted in the preincident, preparedness phase to promote staff preparation, evaluate the organization's level of readiness, and assist in training staff in emergency management roles (Chaffee & Oster, 2006).

The maintenance and testing of health care EOPs is a requirement of Accreditation Canada. Several methods may be used to exercise the plan, the most effective being its use in an actual disaster situation (Veenema, 2007a). The use of a variety of strategies including traditional educational formats, like lectures and case studies, and alternate methods, including tabletop exercises, computer simulations, role play, operational or mock disaster drills, will enhance the disaster response (Andress, 2010a; Silenas, Akins, Parrish, & Edwards, 2008). Staff responders require not only the clinical skills to respond to an emergency event but also an understanding of the core competencies of emergency preparedness, incident command, and risk communication and a clear understanding of roles in relation to other participants in the disaster response (Markenson, DiMaggio, Redlener, 2005).

Response

The third phase of emergency and disaster management, response, occurs in the incident phase of the disaster management continuum. Response can be enacted either upon impact (e.g., explosion, fire) of an emergency event or upon an imminent event (e.g., hurricane, tornado). The EOP is critical in this stage because it provides details and resource information as to how response initiatives should occur. *Response* is the execution phase in which trained and exercised staff are in place, possessing the knowledge of where they need to be and the skill to do what they need to do when confronted with an emergency situation. The goal of response is to save lives, reduce health impacts, ensure public safety, and meet the needs of individuals affected by the event (UNISDR, 2009). It is in the response phase that the IMS is enacted and triage of patients occurs.

The nursing role is most visible in the response phase of a disaster. Nurses provide care in a variety of areas including patient triage, emergency and trauma care, critical care, infection control and occupational health and safety, supportive and palliative care, and public health. Nurses in acute care inpatient settings are also pivotal in disaster response because they receive the casualties who may require care on a longer-term basis as they recover from their injuries. Nurses may be required to work in a variety of alternate settings during the response phase, such as emergency aid shelters, homes, mass immunization sites, shelters, mortuaries, or makeshift clinics (WHO & ICN, 2009).

The Incident Management System. The IMS used in Canada is based on the incident command system that was devel-

oped as a result of mass wildfires that took place in California in the 1970s. These incidents were poorly managed owing to competition for supplies and equipment between response agencies, precipitating the need for a systematic and coordinated process to manage communication and response initiatives (CEMSA, 2006a). IMS is used by police, fire, emergency medical services, health care organizations, hydro, and government agencies, as well as in many areas of the private sector.

IMS is an integrated and flexible framework that clearly identifies disaster response roles (Figure 72-2). The goal of the IMS structure is to ensure that effective communication, incident command, and control are maintained during disaster response initiatives (Emergency Management Ontario [EMO], 2009; Ontario Ministry of Health and Long-Term Care [MoHLTC], 2008). Communication and teamwork between groups of people and departments (e.g., fire, police, paramedics, other health care facilities) that do not usually work together is emphasized (CEMSA, 2006a). IMS in the hospital setting, also referred to as the *hospital incident command system*, enables quick action, provides access to needed resources, and ensures continuation of essential services through all phases of a disaster (Qureshi & Gebbie, 2007; DeAtley, 2010).

IMS is a modular organizational structure that can be used in small- and large-scale emergency situations. All directives, information, and requests flow up or down the hierarchical structure through a chain of command. Under this management system, problems are identified and plans of action developed and coordinated by delegated positions. Resources and responsibilities are assigned to meet identified needs for response (CEMSA, 2006a; DeAtley, 2010; Qureshi & Gebbie, 2007). Each position in the IMS structure has an accompanying job action, accountabilities, and set of tasks and responsibilities that must be fulfilled. Typically, the role of *incident manager* is held by an individual with sound knowledge of the organization and of disaster management processes. The incident manager is in charge of the mission, directs the response process, and monitors and oversees any deviations from the EOP. The incident manager appoints other command staff and establishes the emergency operations centre, which serves as the control point for management of the disaster (DeAtley, 2010; Qureshi & Gebbie, 2007).

IMS command roles are filled by individuals possessing knowledge of the tasks required to successfully address the emergency situation. These individuals include (1) a *public information officer*, who is responsible for coordinating and overseeing public affairs. This includes providing information to the public and the media, helping to create media releases, coordinating interviews and media tours, and developing question-and-answer sheets as required; (2) a *safety officer*, whose role is to ensure the safety of staff, patients, visitors, and the facility during the emergency operation; (3) a *liaison officer*, who serves as a link to external agencies and emergency response services, and (4) a *medical–technical specialist*, who possesses the specific knowledge required (e.g., legal affairs, risk management, ethics, infectious diseases) to guide decision making and response actions (CEMSA, 2006b; DeAtley, 2010).

Additional positions in the IMS structure include (1) a *logistics section chief*, who ensures that resources, including staff, fuel, and services to support staff (equipment, supplies, and food), are available as needed; (2) a *finance section chief*, whose role is to monitor financial assets used; (3) a *planning section chief*, who is accountable for gathering information (data and research) and assisting with planning decisions; and (4) an *operations section chief*, who directs patient care activities and is responsible for

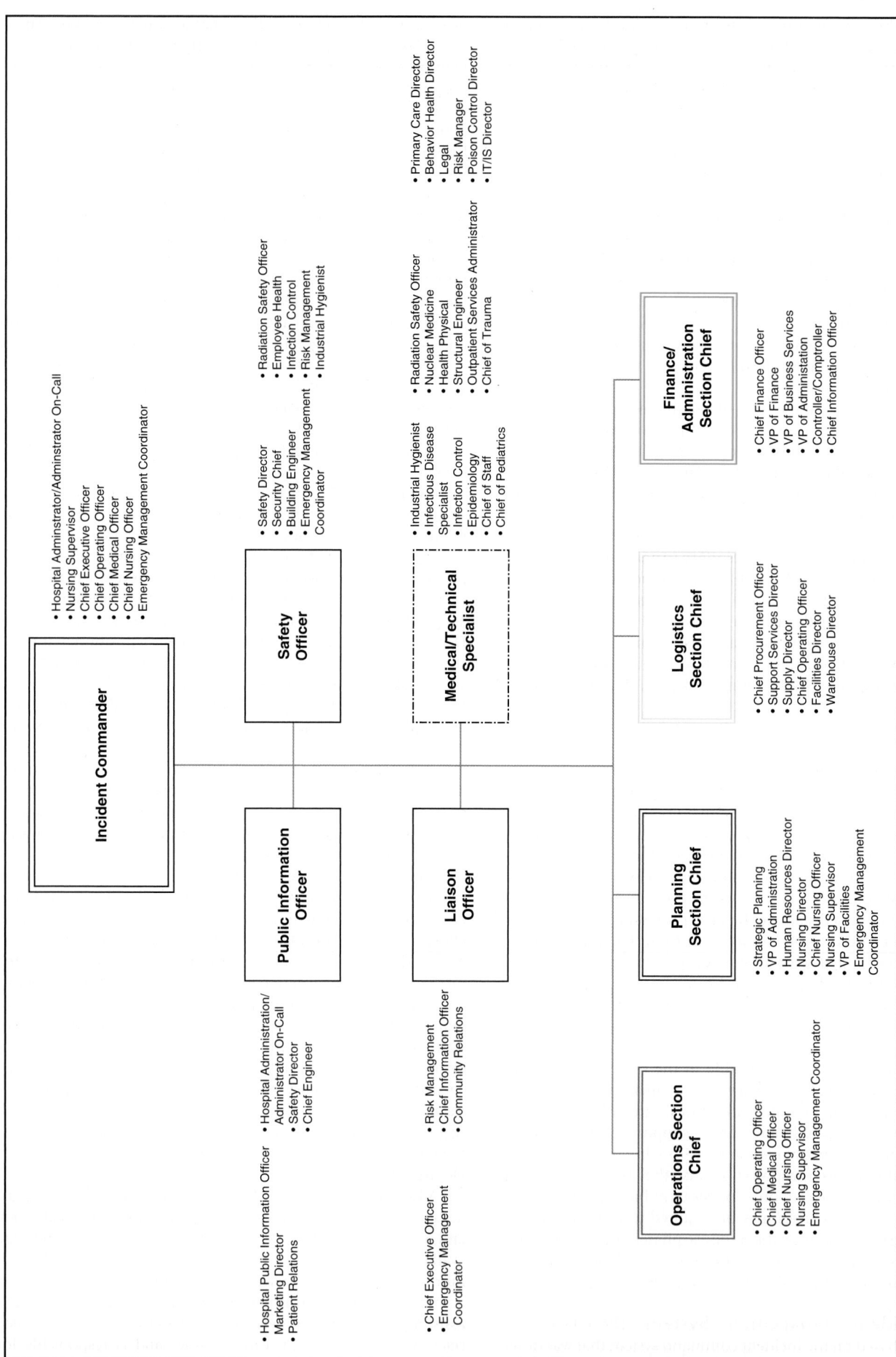

Figure 72-2 Incident management system. *IS,* information services; *IT,* information technology; *VP,* vice president.

Source: California Emergency Medical Services Authority. (2006). *Hospital incident command system guidebook* (Appendix F, p. 466). Retrieved from *http://www.emsa.ca.gov/HICS/files/Appendixes.pdf*

work direction of staff at the scene of the incident (CEMSA, 2006a, 2006b; DeAtley, 2010; Qureshi & Gebbie, 2007). Unit-specific supervisors oversee activities at the ground or unit level and are required to report progress and difficulties in emergency response activities to people in the IMS structure if and when these arise.

Triage. Triage (a French word meaning "sorting") involves the sorting or ranking of casualties to prioritize health care needs and to allocate resources (e.g., staff, treatment areas). The Canadian Triage and Acuity Scale (CTAS) is used in emergency departments (EDs) in nonemergency or nondisaster situations (see Chapter 71, Table 71-2). Using this five-level triage scale, health care workers assign high priority to those who are most critically ill according to the seriousness of their presenting condition, reported signs, and symptoms (Bullard, Unger, Spence, Grafstein, & The CTAS National Working Group, 2008). Daily ED triage is described with greater detail in Chapter 71.

Triage in Disaster Situations. Triage is a critical skill. Effective and timely prehospital triage is pivotal to population survival, helping to ensure equitable distribution to appropriate services/facilities through the health system (Bullard et al., 2008). Although several mass casualty triage systems exist, one of the more common, *simple triage and rapid treatment* (START), offers a systematic approach to triage that may be used to rank the seriousness of casualty injuries in a disaster situation (Table 72-2). This process, used at the disaster scene by first responders, involves rapid assessment and sorting of casualties by a *triage officer.* The START system is based on five clinical observations: (1) the person's ability to ambulate; (2) the presence of spontaneous breathing; (3) the respiratory rate (greater or less than 30/min); (4) perfusion and circulation (i.e., palpable radial pulse or visible capillary refill rate); and (5) mental status (i.e., as assessed by an ability to obey commands) (U.S. Department of Health and Human Services [USDHHS], 2011a). Triage is followed by tagging and transportation to a medical facility or the provision of lifesaving interventions (e.g., intubation, defibrillation) by members of the first-response team. *Patient tagging* involves a system of

coloured tags that are used to designate both the seriousness of the injury and the likelihood of survival (Qureshi & Veenema, 2007; USDHHS, 2011a). A green tag using the START approach indicates a *minor* injury (e.g., sprains, lacerations). Patients assigned a green tag may be able to assist with their own care and are considered "walking wounded." A yellow tag indicates a non–life-threatening injury, suggesting that casualty transport can be delayed (e.g., open fractures, soft tissue wounds). A red tag is used to indicate a life-threatening injury requiring immediate intervention (e.g., shock, airway obstruction, unstable wounds). Patients with a red tag require immediate intervention and transport for survival. A black tag is used to identify those casualties who are deceased or who are unlikely to survive as a result of their injuries, the level of care available to the casualty, or a combination of both (e.g., massive head trauma, profound shock with multiple injuries) (USDHHS, 2011a). Triage of children, or people who look like children, is done using the *JumpSTART* framework. This framework addresses the physiological differences between children and adults (USDHHS, 2011b; Romig, 2008).

Disaster Triage in the Hospital Setting. The triage of casualties in a disaster situation differs from the routine emergency triage process. What is a disaster for one facility might not be so for another. Disaster response is dependent on the size of the organization, the number of staff and resources available, and past experience in dealing with large-scale emergency events. All health care organizations must be able to implement disaster triage with minimal notice (Qureshi & Veenema, 2007).

When an emergency occurs in the community, hospitals are typically notified by emergency medical services in the field, and preparation for a potential influx of patients is done. This preparation includes gathering necessary equipment, including first-aid supplies, personal protective gear, and medications (e.g., analgesics, antidotes). As patients are triaged, they are assigned a pre-designated medical record number, and thus, care can be provided immediately without waiting for the formal registration process (Qureshi & Veenema, 2007). Disaster charts should include a prestamped triage slip, a patient identification band, medical and nursing documentation forms, and laboratory and radiographic

Table 72-2 Simple Triage and Rapid Treatment (START)			
START CATEGORY/ TRIAGE TAG COLOUR	**TYPE OF INJURY**	**PATIENT CONDITION AND EXAMPLES OF PRESENTING FEATURES**	**CLINICAL INDICATORS**
Green "MINOR"	MINOR injuries Walking wounded; minor injuries	Sprains Lacerations	Able to ambulate
Yellow "DELAYED"	DELAYED Transport can be delayed; non–life threatening	Open fractures Soft tissue wounds	Respiration rate: <30 breaths/min Perfusion: <2 sec Mental status: Obeys commands
Red "IMMEDIATE"	Unstable; immediate transport needed; life-threatening requiring immediate intervention	Shock Airway obstruction Unstable wounds	Respiration rate: >30 breaths/min Perfusion: capillary refill >2 sec Mental status: Does not obey commands
Black "EXPECTANT"	Deceased or expected to die owing to injuries	Massive head trauma Profound shock with multiple injuries	Respirations/ spontaneous breathing: Not breathing/apnea

Source: Adapted from Hogan, D. E., & Lairet, J. L. (2007). Triage. In D. E. Hogan & J. L. Burstein (Eds.), *Disaster medicine* (2nd ed., pp. 12-28). Philadelphia: Lippincott Williams & Wilkins; Qureshi, K., & Veenema, T. G. (2007). Disaster triage. In T. G. Veenema (Ed.), *Disaster nursing and emergency preparedness for chemical, biological, and radiological terrorism and other hazards* (2nd ed., pp. 162-176). New York: Springer; and U.S. Department of Health and Human Services (USDHHS). (2011). *START adult triage algorithm.* Retrieved from *http://www.remm.nlm.gov/startadult.htm*

examination requisitions and labels. Chart numbers should be entered onto a tracking form upon entry to the ED so patient allocation and destination can be monitored (Qureshi & Veenema, 2007).

As patients enter the ED, they are greeted by a triage team. In mass-casualty incidents, several triage teams may be used. These teams typically include one to two experienced triage nurses, a physician (the triage officer), a porter (who assists with patient transportation), and a registration clerk (who assists with patient banding and data entry on the tracking form) (Qureshi & Veenema, 2007). Disaster triage in the hospital setting must be rapid and should be conducted in less than 15 seconds. Following this rapid assessment, patients assigned with higher levels of acuity are directed to a treatment location in the ED. In situations in which patient volume is high and ED space limited, another predesignated area of the facility to accommodate surge may be used for the care of less-acute casualties.

Recovery and Rehabilitation

Recovery and rehabilitation takes place in the postincident phase of the disaster continuum (WHO & ICN, 2009) and is the process through which staff, an organization, a community, or some combination of these regains the ability to function after a disaster. Services have typically been disrupted during the disaster response, and the goal is to return to a state of "normal." This includes ensuring the restoration of vital services normally provided by an organization, within a community, or by local government, rebuilding infrastructure, and meeting the needs of the population served (WHO & ICN, 2009). Nurses are critical in the recovery and rehabilitation phase and in re-establishing health care infrastructure. Nurses must consider the psychosocial impact of a disaster on its survivors—individuals, groups, and communities. Nursing functions related to the care and coordination of health care services, case management, identification, and implementation of casualty referrals (e.g., social services) are essential for the return of individuals to normal activities (WHO & ICN, 2009). Nurses play a key role in the documentation, review, and evaluation of the disaster response as well as in championing changes both to the EOPs and to corporate, municipal, and provincial policy (WHO & ICN, 2009).

Critical Incident Stress Management. The massive effort put forth by health care workers in response to a catastrophic event is critical to a community's recovery. Health care workers, who are already at risk for experiencing high levels of stress and burnout, are at increased risk following participation in a disaster event (Public Health Agency of Canada [PHAC], 2011). A *critical incident* is a situation faced by individuals involved in a disaster, or a disaster response, that causes them to experience strong emotional reactions that have the potential to interfere with their ability to return to their normal state of functioning at work and at home during or after an event (McMahon, 2010; PHAC, 2011). Multiple deaths; inadvertent exposure to hazardous materials or substances; exposure to shocking sights, sounds, or smells; and incidents with high media coverage are examples of critical incidents. Challenging triage decisions, the volume of seriously injured, limitations in needed resources, ethical issues that accompany disasters, concern for personal safety and liability, lack of sleep, heavy workload, time pressures and unmet basic needs, political and organizational pressures, also significantly contribute to the stress and an individual's resilience in the aftermath of a disaster event (McMahon, 2010; PHAC, 2011).

All disasters have the potential to cause psychological stress to the individuals involved. This stress can persist for an extended period and is influenced in part by the nature of the event, the individual's age, pre-existing coping mechanisms, role in the event, and prior medical and psychological history (Plum & Veenema, 2007). Although the psychological trauma that is a result of involvement in a critical incident varies, common symptoms range from insomnia to excessive sleeping, loss of appetite to overeating, and a loss of interest in activities normally considered pleasurable (PHAC, 2011). Most individuals experience relief from these symptoms 4 to 6 weeks after the incident. However, when symptoms persist longer, a mental health consultation may be necessary. Unresolved critical incident stress may have a variety of consequences including *post-traumatic stress disorder,* a severe reaction to the incident that severely affects an individual's ability to function at a normal level (McMahon, 2010; Plum & Veenema). Post-traumatic stress disorder is a condition that requires ongoing psychological counselling, psychiatric support, or both.

Critical incident stress management (CISM) or debriefing is an approach to preventing and managing the emotional trauma that can be a result of involvement in a disaster response (McMahon, 2010). Crisis intervention is the mainstay of postdisaster management and can be initiated by individuals with the knowledge and skill to actively listen to survivors and assist with problem solving (Mitchell, Sakraida, & Zalice, 2005). CISM is most effective when it is done at the scene of the incident. In the health care setting, initial support involves brief, short-term interventions such as ensuring that staff are taking breaks and that their physical needs are being met. *Defusing sessions* occur within a few hours of the incident and are typically offered as staff are going off duty. This process involves brief discussion of the incident and assistance with stress management. Debriefing, a group process led by specially trained personnel, is critical to recovery and should be done within 24 to 72 hours after the event and repeated a couple of weeks following the event.

The Role of Nursing Leadership in Disaster Preparedness and Response

Leadership at all levels is essential for a positive outcome after a disaster event. However, nurses who hold formal leadership roles have extended responsibilities to ensure the delivery of safe care at all stages of the disaster continuum. Proactive planning and support of staff education and training are critical to an effective disaster response (Fahlgren & Drenkard, 2002). Leadership in times of disaster involves recognition of the uncertainty created during such events requiring open, consistent communication; flexibility; and creative problem-solving (Druce, 2009). Clear communication of expectations and goals, and a commitment to cause with an expectation of success, is an antecedent to a positive outcome. Nursing leadership plays a role in advocating for individual and community needs and services in the recovery/rehabilitation stage and is essential for ensuring that staff have the emotional support that is needed (Deeny & McFetridge, 2005; Druce, 2009). At the executive level, nurse leaders play a key role in ensuring health care organizations are prepared for response, providing oversight for recovery processes, the creation of safe work environments, and assuming a role as a member of the Command Team. Nursing executives have a role in influencing policy and financial decisions and creating an environment that offers needed supports before, during, and following a disaster event (Fahlgren & Drenkard, 2002).

Natural Hazards and Human-Made Disasters

A *disaster* can be defined in numerous ways, but the term is generally interpreted to mean a destructive event that disrupts the functioning of a community (Veenema, 2007a). There are two general classifications of disasters: *natural* and *human-made*. Disease outbreaks and epidemics are usually considered to be "natural" events, but they can also be classified as "human-made" disasters when disease-causing organisms are used as an agent of terrorism with the goal of inducing large-scale epidemics. Because of these variations, disease outbreaks and epidemics are described in a separate section of this chapter. Table 72-3 presents a timeline of notable disasters in Canadian history.

Natural Disasters and Hazards

Natural disasters, also referred to as *natural hazards*, are caused by nature or the environment, are often unpredictable, and can happen at a rapid or slow rate. Natural disasters include forest fires, avalanches, landslides and mudslides, blizzards, ice storms, cold or heat waves, hurricanes, tornadoes, cyclones, hailstorms, tsunamis, floods, drought, earthquakes, and volcanic eruptions (PSC, 2011c). Today, communities are built in well-known tornado "alleys," on river flood plains, and on mountainous or hillside terrain, leaving them at risk for possible forest fires, volcanic eruptions, and the ravages of water, snow, ice, and mud. Human-caused damage to the environment and the resultant climate change has also altered the intensity, pattern, and distribution of natural forces, contributing to an increase in the number of natural disasters (Veenema, 2007a).

Human-Made Disasters

Human-made disasters can be accidental or deliberate and can cause injuries, deaths, and long-term consequences for individuals and communities. *Accidental human-made disasters* include industrial accidents, chemical spills, inadvertent release of nuclear energy, explosions (e.g., from hazardous materials such as chemicals, nuclear materials, fuel), contamination, fires, structural collapse, large transportation accidents, and power outages. *Deliberate human-made disasters* include conventional warfare, unconventional warfare (e.g., nuclear and chemical), civil unrest, and acts of terrorism. Computer viruses or cyber attacks are classified as human-made disasters because of their cost and potential impact on critical infrastructure.

Terrorism. September 11, 2001, marks a tragic day of death and destruction, when two hijacked planes hit the Twin Towers in New York City, precipitating their collapse a short time after. Since that time, terrorism has become a main focus of emergency planning in Canada and worldwide.

Terrorism involves intentional and overt actions that are committed to cause fear, panic, destruction, injury, and death in service of political, religious, or ideological goals. The intent of a terrorist event is to intimidate the public or a particular segment of the public or to compel a specific person, government, or international organization to take specific action. Terrorist events include threats, assassinations, kidnappings, hijackings, bomb scares and bombings, and computer cyber attacks (Langan, 2005). **Bioterrorism,** a type of terrorist event, involves the deliberate spreading of microbes or toxins with the intent of causing disease or death in animals, plants, or humans (Christopher, Eitzen, Kortepeter, & Rowe, 2007). Plans for dealing with each type of terrorist event with consideration of advanced training exercises is essential to a safe, expedient response.

Chemical–Biological–Radiological–Nuclear–Explosive Events. A *CBRN event* refers to any situation in which weapons of a *chemical, biological, radiological,* or *nuclear* nature are used with the goal of causing harm. A CBRN event can also be the result of a civilian or military accident. More recently, the term **CBRNE event** has been used, with "E" representing situations in which an *explosive or incendiary device* is used. A CBRNE event may be the result of a terrorist event or an industrial accident. *Weapons of mass destruction* refers to a broad range of weapons, including CBRNE weapons, that have the potential to affect the health and the well-being of a large population (Callaway, 2007).

Victims of CBRNE exposure may arrive at health care facilities in large or small numbers and without advanced notice. Consequently, these events have significant implications to the health and safety of those who come into contact with them. Early identification, diagnosis, and treatment of victims exposed to such substances is essential to preventing secondary injury and avoiding contamination of the public, staff and the health care facility (Veenema, 2007b). Individuals with CBRN contamination require appropriate decontamination *before* any medical care or surgical intervention is provided. *Decontamination* is the process of removing or neutralizing a hazardous agent from the environment, from property or equipment, or from a life form (Koenig et al., 2008; Veenema, 2007b). Decontamination is an essential process because it accomplishes the following: (1) decreases further absorption and toxicity of the agent; (2) reduces contamination of other people and equipment by substances on the casualties' clothing or belongings; and (3) prevents potential closure of portions of a health care organization where contaminated victims may seek care (Koenig et al., 2008).

Victims of chemical, biological, and radiological exposure will often use health care facilities as their first point of contact, bypassing community resources (Koenig et al., 2008). Other challenges include patients who do not proceed to hospital until they become symptomatic or who proceed to hospital as information is shared about potential exposure through such venues as the media (Crowe, 2010). For this reason, the use of PPE is essential not only for first responders in the field but also for health care workers in hospital settings.

The degree of casualty contamination is affected by four factors: (1) the contact time with the agent; (2) the concentration of the agent; (3) temperature, which affects the agent's permeative characteristics; and (4) the physical state of the agents (i.e., liquids, solids, vapours) (Koenig et al., 2008). Ideally, patients will be decontaminated at the site before arrival at the hospital. This may be difficult when the exposure is a result of a terrorist event because casualties may flee the site and go directly to EDs, potentially not knowing they have been contaminated and the risk they pose to others. In the hospital setting, decontamination is typically a multidisciplinary initiative that might include participation from a team of nursing and intraprofessional staff, security and housekeeping, engineering and occupational health and safety, and porters. Participation in casualty decontamination requires significant education and training before a potential event on the safe use of the necessary PPE, decontamination equipment assembly and use, setup of decontamination areas, and the decontamination process. Decontamination should be completed only by trained staff members, and training should be

Table 72-3 Best-Known and Worst Canadian Disasters

YEAR	DISASTER AND PLACE	APPROXIMATE NUMBER OF CANADIAN DEATHS*	YEAR	DISASTER AND PLACE	APPROXIMATE NUMBER OF CANADIAN DEATHS*
1825	Forest fire, Miramichi, New Brunswick	160	1987	Tornado, Edmonton, Alberta	27
1851	Sinking ship, Prince Edward Island	300	1992	Westray mining accident, Plymouth, Nova Scotia	26
1862	Smallpox epidemic (nationwide)	20,000	1996	Floods, Saguenay, Province of Quebec	10
1885	Smallpox epidemic, Montreal, Province of Quebec	6000	1997	Bus crash, St. Joseph de la Rive, Province of Quebec	43
1903	Rock slide in town of Frank (Frank slide), Turtle Mountain, Alberta	70	1998	Plane crash, Peggy's Cove, Nova Scotia	230
1910	Avalanche, Rogers Pass, Bear Creek, British Columbia	62	1998	Ice storm, eastern Ontario, Province of Quebec, Maritimes	35
1912	Tornado, Regina, Saskatchewan	30	2000	Contaminated water, Walkerton, Ontario	7
1917	Harbour explosion, Halifax, Nova Scotia	2000	2000	Tornado, Pine Lake, Alberta	16
1918	Spanish influenza pandemic (Spanish flu)	30,000-50,000	2003	Severe acute respiratory syndrome (SARS), Toronto, Ontario	44
1922	Wildfire, Timiskaming District, Ontario	43	2003	Hurricane Juan, Halifax, Nova Scotia, and Charlottetown, Prince Edward Island	8
1929	Tsunami, Burin Peninsula, Newfoundland	30			
1942	Building fire, Knights of Columbus hostel, St. John's, Newfoundland	100	2005	Outbreak of Legionnaire's disease, Toronto, Ontario	21
1947	Train derailment, Dugald, Manitoba	40	2006	De la Concorde overpass collapse, Laval, Quebec	5
1954	Hurricane Hazel, Ontario	81	2008	Outbreak of Listeriosis, Toronto, Ontario	20
1958	Mining accident, Springhill, Nova Scotia	75	2008	Motor vehicle accident/van collision, Bathurst, New Brunswick	8
1974	Bus crash, St. Joseph de la Rive, Province of Quebec	13	2009	Cougar Helicopters Flight 91 crash, off of Newfoundland.	17
1974	Airplane crash, Rea Point, Northwest Territories	32	2010	Hurricane Igor, Cape Race, Newfoundland	1
1978	Soviet satellite, COSMOS 954, comes down in the Northwest Territories, scattering 65 kg of radioactive material over a wide area	0	2011	Slave Lake Wildfire, Slave Lake, Alberta	1
1985	Airplane crash (plane from Toronto, Ontario, crashed in the North Atlantic off Ireland's coast)	280	2011	First Air Flight 6560 crash, near Resolute Bay, Nunavut	12
1986	Train derailment, Hinton, Alberta	23	2011	Tornado, Goderich, Ontario	0

*Twenty-five Canadians died in the September 11, 2001, terrorist attack in New York City.
Sources: Adapted from Stanhope, M., Lancaster, J., Jessup-Falcioni, H., & Viverais-Dressler, G. (2011). *Community health nursing in Canada* (Table 16-2, p. 506). Toronto: Mosby; and PSC (2011). *Canadian disaster database*. Retrieved from *http://www.publicsafety.gc.ca/prg/em/cdd/index-eng.aspx*

completed on annual basis to ensure competence (Koenig et al., 2008).

Crowd control and safety is of primary concern in CBRN situations. First responders, health care workers, and other patients who have physical contact with contaminated casualties, their belongings, or both without appropriate protection may also require decontamination (Koenig et al., 2008). Lockdown of all entry points to a health care facility, with the exception of a single designated access point for those who require decontamination, is one strategy to prevent inadvertent exposure of patients and staff to the contaminant.

Triage will require, when possible, identification of the contaminant and an assessment of the degree of contamination and the level of casualty distress (Koenig et al., 2008). Triage will also help to identify the potential for secondary contamination of others and to assign treatment interventions and decontamination protocols (Koenig et al., 2008). Information about the event will have to be provided to the person in charge using the hospital IMS.

Hospitals are required to have policies and procedures in place to manage CBRN exposure and to complete casualty decontamination. Casualties should be segregated from other patient populations until appropriate decontamination takes place. This requires a designated decontamination area that is external to the ED. Some facilities have constructed showers outside of ED points of entry, where ambulatory patients may shower and scrub to remove hazardous material from their bodies, once contaminated clothing has been removed. Decontamination trailers or tents with "conveyor belts" are an option for nonambulatory patients: As they are moved along on a belt, these patients may be scrubbed by trained staff and rinsed with water from hoses. The use of heaters is necessary in cold weather. Decontamination depends on the type of contaminant but is typically done by the use of high-volume dilution with water. Mild soaps may be required if the substance is oily and hard to remove (Koenig et al, 2008).

The health and safety of health care providers is essential in a CBRN event. A comprehensive combination of respirators and protective gear (goggles, boots, full-facepiece respirators, protective suits, chemically resistant gloves) must be used (Veenema, 2007b). Because of the equipment that is required to be worn, workers must undergo medical screening or surveillance (including a full set of vital signs) before donning and after removing protective gear. Staff also need to be monitored by a designated surveyor while involved in the decontamination process (Koenig et al., 2008). Staff who have higher-than-normal blood pressure; rashes, open sores, or wounds; previous history of nausea, vomiting, or diarrhea; upper respiratory infection or history of respiratory illness (i.e., asthma); allergies; sensitivities or phobias (i.e., claustrophobia); or who are potentially or known to be pregnant may not participate in the decontamination process. Time in decontamination gear is typically limited to 30 minutes or less because extreme heat, poor ventilation, and the heavy weight of the suit cause fatigue and other common adverse effects (Veenema, 2007b). These risks also make it necessary to monitor hydration status before and after protective gear is donned. Once casualties have been decontaminated, they may be cared for with other patients in the ED.

Biological Agents of Terrorism. Terrorist attacks using biological agents represent challenges for health care providers because they can be difficult to detect and can have a prolonged impact on health care facilities (Crowe, 2010). Biological contaminants can range from accidental releases of biohazardous waste to intentional exposure from bioweapons (Koenig et al., 2008). Table 72-4 summarizes general information regarding biological agents of terrorism. The pathogens most likely to be used as biological weapons include anthrax, smallpox, botulism, plague, tularemia, and hemorrhagic fever. Anthrax, plague, and tularemia can be treated effectively with antibiotics if the organisms are not resistant and if there is an available and sufficient quantity of the appropriate drug. Smallpox can be prevented or ameliorated by vaccination, even when it is first given after initial exposure. Botulism can be treated with antitoxin. In most cases, supportive treatment is the primary mode of care for viruses that cause hemorrhagic fever (Borio, Inglesby, & Peters, 2009).

Chemical Agents of Terrorism. Certain chemicals may be used as agents of terrorism because their toxic properties produce significant physiological and psychological effects. Chemical agents have the potential for rapidly spreading and contaminating staff and other patients (Koenig et al., 2008). Chemically exposed individuals are more likely to seek health care in large numbers and to have early, external evidence of contamination (Powers, 2010b). Chemical agents are categorized according to

their target organ or effect (Andress, 2010b). For example, sarin, a highly toxic nerve gas that enters the body through the eyes and the skin, acts by paralyzing the respiratory muscles, potentially causing death within minutes of exposure. Phosgene, a colourless gas normally used in chemical manufacturing, can cause severe respiratory distress, pulmonary edema, and death when it is inhaled at high concentrations for a long enough time (Andress, 2010b). Mustard gas, an agent used during World War I, is yellow to brown in colour and has a garlic-like odour and acts by irritating the eyes and causing skin burns and blisters. Protocols to treat victims with chemical exposure are varied but are specific for the causative agent (Veenema, Benitez, & Benware, 2007). Table 72-5 details the effects chemical agents have on various human organs.

Radiological and Nuclear Agents of Terrorism. Radiological and nuclear substances can also be categorized as agents of terrorism. Radiological dispersal devices (RDDs), or "dirty bombs," consist of a mix of explosives and radioactive material. When an RDD is detonated, the blast scatters radioactive dust, smoke, and other material into the surrounding environment, causing radioactive contamination (CDC, 2006). Uranium and iodine-131, the radioactive materials used in RDDs, typically generate only enough radiation to cause immediate serious illness to those in close proximity to the explosion. The main danger of an RDD results from the explosion itself. Patients with a traumatic injury combined with significant exposure of radiation have substantially worse prognosis (Military Medical Operations [MMO], 2010). Because radiation cannot be seen, has no scent, and is unable to be felt or tasted, measures to limit contamination, like covering the patient's nose and mouth and prompt decontamination (e.g., through the use of a decontamination shower), are best initiated in a timely manner (CDC, 2006). Ionizing radiation, which comes from a nuclear bomb or damage to a nuclear reactor, represents a serious threat to the health and safety of casualties and the environment (see eTable 72-1, available on the Evolve Web site for this chapter). Although exposure to ionizing radiation may or may not include skin contamination, decontamination procedures should be initiated immediately in circumstances in which radioactive contaminants are present (Andress, 2010b).

Explosive Agents of Terrorism. Explosive devices (e.g., TNT, dynamite) that are used as agents of terrorism result in one or more of the following types of injuries: blast, crush, or penetrating injuries. *Blast injuries* occur from the supersonic overpressurization shock wave that results from the explosion, having the potential to cause mass injury to multiple body systems (Plurad, 2011). This shock wave primarily causes damage to the lungs, gastrointestinal tract, and middle ear. Blast injuries are also a result of the blast wind that causes injury owing to casualties being blown against objects and structures (MMO, 2010). *Crush injuries* (i.e., blunt trauma) often ensue from explosions that occur in confined spaces and result from structural collapse (e.g., falling debris). Some explosive devices contain materials that are projected during the explosion (e.g., shrapnel) leading to *penetrating injuries* (Plurad, 2011; FEMA, 2008).

Epidemics and Pandemics

Nurses are required to have an understanding of the etiology and impact of communicable disease, whether the diseases are a con-

Table 72-4 Biological Agents of Terrorism

PATHOGEN AND DESCRIPTION	CLINICAL MANIFESTATIONS	TRANSMISSIBILITY	TREATMENT
Anthrax (Bacillus anthracis)			
Inhalation			
• Bacterial spores multiply in the alveoli • Toxins cause hemorrhage and destruction of lung tissue • High mortality rate	• Incubation period: 1-2 days to 6 wk • Abrupt onset • Dyspnea • Diaphoresis • Fever • Cough • Chest pain • Septicemia • Shock • Meningitis • Respiratory failure • Widened mediastinum (seen on chest radiograph) • Incubation period: ≤12 days	• No person-to-person spread • Found in nature; most commonly infects wild and domestic hoofed animals • Spread through direct contact with bacterium and its spores • Spores are dormant, encapsulated bacteria that become active when they enter a living host	• Antibiotics prevent systemic manifestations • Effective only if treated early • Ciprofloxacin (Cipro) is the treatment of choice • Penicillin • Doxycycline • Postexposure prophylaxis for 30 days (if vaccine available) or 60 days (if vaccine not available) • Vaccine has limited availability
Cutaneous			
• 95% of anthrax infections • Least lethal form • Spores enter skin through cuts or abrasions • Handling of contaminated animal skin products • Toxins destroy surrounding tissue	• Small papule resembles an insect bite • Advances to a depressed, black ulcer • Swollen lymph nodes in adjacent areas • Edema	—	—
Gastrointestinal			
• Ingestion of contaminated, undercooked meat • Intestinal lesions in ileum or cecum • Acute inflammation of intestines	• Nausea • Vomiting • Anorexia • Hematemesis • Diarrhea • Abdominal pain • Ascites • Sepsis	—	—
Smallpox (Variola Major and Minor Viruses)			
• Canada ended routine vaccination in 1972 • Global eradication declared in 1980	• Incubation period: 7-17 days • Sudden onset of symptoms • Fever • Headache • Myalgia • Lesions that progress from macules to papules to pustular vesicles • Malaise • Back pain	• Highly contagious • Direct person-to-person spread • Transmitted in air droplets • Transmitted by handling contaminated materials	• No known cure • Cidofovir (Vistide) under testing • Isolation for containment • Vaccine available for those exposed • Vaccinia immune globulin (VIG) available

Table 72-4 Biological Agents of Terrorism—cont'd

PATHOGEN AND DESCRIPTION	CLINICAL MANIFESTATIONS	TRANSMISSIBILITY	TREATMENT
Botulism (Clostridium botulinum)			
• Spore-forming anaerobe • Found in soil • Seven different toxins • Lethal bacterial neurotoxin • Can die within 24 hr	• Incubation period: 12-36 hr • Abdominal cramps • Diarrhea • Nausea • Vomiting • Cranial nerve palsies (diplopia, dysarthria, dysphonia, dysphagia) • Skeletal muscle paralysis • Respiratory failure	• Spread through air or food • No person-to-person spread • Improperly canned foods • Contaminated wound	• Induce vomiting • Enemas • Antitoxin • Mechanical ventilation • Penicillin • No vaccine available • Toxin can be inactivated by heating food or drink to 100°C for at least 10 min
Plague (Yersinia pestis)			
• Bacteria found in rodents and fleas **Forms** • Bubonic (most common) • Pneumonic • Septicemic (most deadly)	• Incubation period: 2-4 days • Hemoptysis • Cough • High fever • Chills • Myalgia • Headache • Respiratory failure • Lymph node swelling	• Direct person-to-person spread • Transmitted through flea bites • Ingestion of contaminated meat	• Antibiotics only effective if administered immediately • Drug of choice: streptomycin or gentamicin • Vaccine under development • Hospitalization • Isolation for containment
Tularemia (Francisella tularensis)			
• Bacterial infectious disease of animals • Mortality rate about 35% without treatment	• Incubation period: 3-10 days • Sudden onset • Fever • Swollen lymph nodes • Fatigue • Sore throat • Weight loss • Pneumonia • Pleural effusion • Ulcerated sore from tick bite	• No person-to-person spread • Aerosol or intradermal route • Spread by rabbits and ticks • Contaminated food, air, water	• Gentamicin treatment of choice • Streptomycin, doxycycline, and ciprofloxacin are alternatives • Vaccine in developmental stage
Hemorrhagic Fever			
• Caused by several viruses, including Marburg, Ebola, Lassa fever, yellow fever, and Rift Valley fever	• Fever • Conjunctivitis • Headache • Malaise • Prostration • Hemorrhage of tissues and organs • Nausea • Vomiting • Hypotension • Organ failure	• Carried by rodents and mosquitoes • Direct person-to-person spread by body fluids • Virus can be aerosolized	• No intramuscular injections • No anticoagulants • Isolation for containment • Ribavirin (Virazole) effective in some cases • Supportive treatment only for most • Vaccine available for yellow fever only

Source: Adapted from Lewis, S. L., Heitkemper, M. M., Dirksen, S. R., O'Brien, P. G., & Bucher, L. (2011). *Medical-surgical nursing: Assessment and management of clinical problems.* St. Louis: Mosby.

Table 72-5 Chemical Agents of Terrorism by Target Organ or Effect

NERVE	BLOOD	PULMONARY	BLISTER OR VESICANTS
• Sarin (isopropyl methylphosphonofluoridate) • Tabun (ethyl *N,N*-dimethylphosphoramidocyanidate) • Soman (pinacolyl methylphosphonofluoridate) • GF (cyclohexylmethylphosphonofluoridate) • VX (O-ethyl S-[2-diisopropylaminoethyl] methylphosphonothiolate)	• Hydrogen cyanide • Cyanogen chloride	• Phosgene • Chlorine • Vinyl chloride	• Nitrogen and sulphur mustards • Lewisite (an aliphatic arsenic compound, 2-chlorovinyldichloroarsine) • Phosgene oxime

sequence of a natural disaster (e.g., contaminated water during flooding) or are human-made and the result of a deliberate act (e.g., a result of bioterrorism) (CNA, 2007). Morbidity, mortality, and disruption from an infectious disease epidemic overwhelm a community and its infrastructure. In Canada and Asia, the 2003 SARS outbreak demonstrated the enormous toll an infectious disease could have on individuals, communities, and health care workers, highlighting the need for diligent advance planning for managing future communicable illnesses.

Communicable diseases may occur in an individual or a group of individuals. When diseases occur among a cluster of individuals, it is classified as an *outbreak* (Whitney, Marchant-Short, & Yiu, 2008). When the number of cases of a communicable disease exceeds the normal expected occurrence during a given period, it is referred to as an **epidemic**. If transmission of the disease is widespread and affects large numbers of people across several countries, continents, or globally, it is considered to be a **pandemic** (Slepski, 2010).

Severe Acute Respiratory Syndrome

Severe acute respiratory syndrome, also known as *SARS*, refers to an outbreak that occurred primarily in Canada and Asia in 2003. SARS is a contagious severe febrile respiratory illness caused by a coronavirus and characterized by a fever of 38°C or higher, myalgia, headache, malaise, chills, a dry nonproductive cough, and shortness of breath (Farquharson & Baguley, 2003; McFee, 2008). The illness is spread through close contact with someone who is infected with the virus, such as those living in the same household, providing unprotected care to someone with SARS, or having direct contact with respiratory secretions of someone affected by SARS (Health Canada, 2004). The *incubation period*, the time from exposure to the virus to the onset of symptoms, ranges from 2 to 10 days (Health Canada, 2004). SARS is discussed in Chapter 30.

The SARS outbreak was a critical juncture in Canadian emergency management because it demonstrated all too vividly the tremendous impact a communicable disease outbreak could have on individuals, communities, and the economy. The effects of SARS were felt globally. In Canada, there were over 252 cases of SARS and 44 deaths, including 2 nurses and a physician; globally, there were 8098 cases and 774 deaths (National Advisory Committee on SARS and Public Health, 2003). SARS cost billions of dollars across Asia and Canada as a result of its impact on health care, critical infrastructure, trade, and tourism.

SARS served as a wake-up call for health care institutions, governments, and health care providers, highlighting Canada's inadequacies in responding to public health threats. Since 2003, our country has recognized the central role of health care services

in disaster mitigation and response, resulting in enhanced planning initiatives. Stockpiles of medications, PPE, and mobile hospital response teams have been put in place in anticipation of future outbreaks (Amaratunga et al., 2008).

Outbreak Management

Studies of the SARS outbreak across numerous countries have provided insight into the need for diligent infection control practices and disease monitoring. The effects of globalization and the ease of air travel has led not only to the "shrinking" of the world but also to the global mobility of people, food, viruses, and bacteria. In the Middle Ages, cities and towns could close their gates and erect high walls to keep out disease; now, our global problems demand a global response. The strategies used to prevent and contain communicable diseases are fundamental and nurses play an essential role in understanding common outbreak management strategies. This knowledge helps nurses working in acute and chronic care and within community settings to implement containment interventions and to understand how best to protect themselves and their patients.

Outbreak Management Strategies. **Outbreak management** refers to the strategies used to prevent the spread of communicable disease among clusters of people. Management of outbreaks within health care facilities must begin with recognition of potentially exposed patients by trained staff or through public health notification. Case-finding, early-detection, and treatment strategies not only improve the health of the infected individuals but also prevent transmission to others.

Surveillance is the ongoing and systematic process of gathering, analyzing, and disseminating data on communicable diseases or events to detect changes in trends or distribution of diseases (Greenough & Burkle, 2007). Simply put, surveillance processes gather the *"who, when, where, and what"* to answer *"why"* (Stanhope, Lancaster, Jessup-Falcioni, & Viverais-Dresler, 2011, p. 539). Since the events of September 11, 2001, and the 2003 SARS outbreak, there have been major efforts to develop and strengthen these early-warning mechanisms at the local and global levels. The Centre for Infectious Disease Prevention and Control, a component of the Public Health Agency of Canada (PHAC), operates a number of national surveillance systems on health problems that range from chronic diseases and congenital anomalies to the *Respiratory Virus Detection Surveillance System* and *FluWatch*. These latter two systems are in place to observe and scrutinize changes in the number of febrile and respiratory illnesses across the country.

Many communicable diseases are considered reportable or notifiable diseases. *Reportable diseases* are those that must be

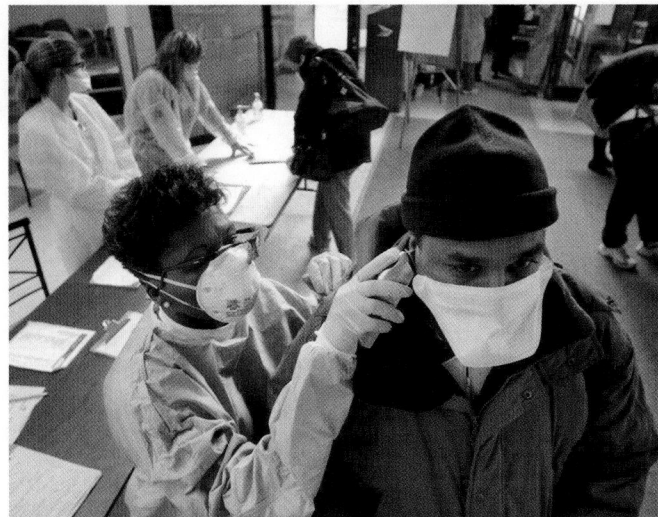

Figure 72-3 A critical strategy in managing the severe acute respiratory syndrome (SARS) outbreak was screening patients for possible signs of the disease.

Source: CP/J. P. Moczulski.

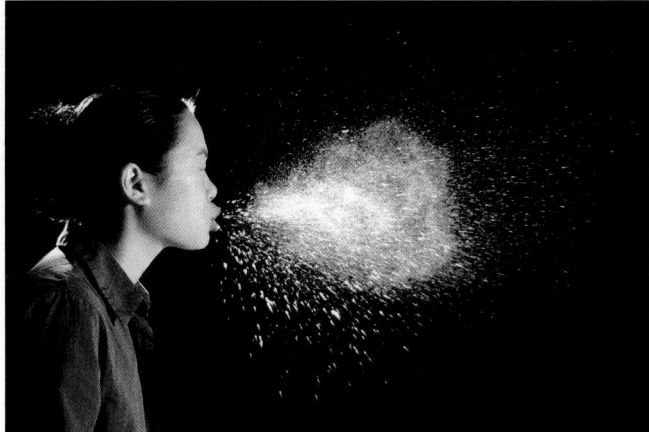

Figure 72-4 Particle mist created upon sneezing.

Source: Photo by Andrew Davidhazy/RIT.

reported to the local public health unit (PHAC, 2005). Nurses are often involved, both formally and informally, in different levels of the surveillance system. Nurses are often the first to detect an outbreak when they observe abnormal clusters of illness in a patient population or a group such as in a school setting.

Isolation is an outbreak management strategy that separates infected people from those assumed to be unaffected during a period of the disease's communicability (Whitney et al., 2008) (Figure 72-3). In Toronto, the SARS epidemic demonstrated how rapidly airborne diseases can spread through crowded spaces, emergency departments, or shared rooms (Varia et al., 2003). Infected individuals may be confined to a hospital room or unit or to their home. There are varying types of isolation depending on the disease, its route of transmission, and the period of communicability.

Quarantine is the isolation of people who have been exposed, or potentially exposed, to an infection or contagious disease but who are not yet sick or showing signs of illness (Richter, 2010). These people are assumed to be incubating the disease and may be infectious to other people before they display symptoms. The quarantine period is the longest usual incubation period for the disease. During the SARS outbreak in Canada, thousands of people, mostly in the Toronto area, were quarantined at home for 10-day periods, the incubation period for SARS (Ontario MoHLTC, 2004). Although most people complied voluntarily during the SARS event, all provinces have public health legislation that enforces compliance with a quarantine order. Owing to circumstances and the number of staff potentially infected with the virus, a special form of quarantine, called *work quarantine,* was used for health care workers during the SARS outbreak. This level of quarantine allowed health care workers who may have been exposed to SARS to continue working as long as they followed certain requirements including wearing N95 mask at work and on any public commute; home confinement when not at work; and self-monitoring for temperature and signs and symptoms of SARS (City of Toronto, 2003).

Pandemic Planning

Pandemic influenza is a highly infectious outbreak of influenza that spreads rapidly around the world, with much more serious consequences than the usual effects of seasonal influenza (Toronto Academic Health Sciences Network [TAHSN], 2006). There are two primary routes by which the influenza virus exits the respiratory tract of an infected person: (1) expulsion of the virus into the air through sneezing (Figure 72-4), coughing, speaking, or breathing, or through aerosol-generating medical procedures and (2) by direct transfer of respiratory secretions to another person or surface (Expert Panel on Influenza and Personal Protective Respiratory Equipment, 2007). Coupled with the short incubation period (from 1 to 3 days) and the fact that the virus can be transmitted before an infected person is symptomatic, it is essential that nurses use appropriate infection control techniques to prevent the spread of influenza (see the Evidence-Informed Practice box "Influenza Transmission and the Role of Personal Protective Respiratory Equipment").

In June 2009, the beginning of a global influenza pandemic was confirmed as the illness was identified across 74 countries, raising the WHO alert from a "5" (widespread human transmission) to a "6" (pandemic phase) (Slepski, 2010). Although there is no way to predict the length or severity of the next pandemic, the WHO is predicting a second wave of global pandemic, and consequently, planning is taking place to prepare for the next occurrence. Owing to this concern and the need for vigilant monitoring of this illness in humans, the WHO monitors the risk as determined by its experts and an analysis of the situation in countries around the world. For further information, follow the WHO link at the end of the chapter for the current phase of pandemic influenza alert and a detailed explanation of the phases of pandemic alert.

Faced with the demands of a novel H1N1 pandemic, hospitals and communities have shifted much of their focus in emergency planning to pandemic planning over the last several years. In the hospital setting, inpatient areas and critical services are key to an effective pandemic response (Hota, Fried, Burry, Stewart, & Christian, 2010). The duration and acuity of patient illness, impact on hospital systems, and prior experiences with the H1N1 pandemic reflect a need for advanced surge capacity planning across clinical settings. H1N1 brings a surge in patient volume,

EVIDENCE-INFORMED PRACTICE

Influenza Transmission and the Role of Personal Protective Respiratory Equipment: An Assessment of the Evidence

The following are the consensus findings of the Expert Panel on Influenza and Personal Protective Respiratory Equipment (PPRE) (see Reference for Evidence).

Conclusions on the Modes of Influenza Transmission

1. Ballistic-, nasopharyngeal-, tracheobronchial-, and alveolar-sized particles are all emitted from the human respiratory tract.
2. Evidence about the relative contributions of the different modes of transmission to the spread of influenza is sparse and inconclusive.
3. There is evidence that influenza is transmitted primarily at short range.
4. There is evidence that influenza can be transmitted via inhalation of tracheobronchial- and alveolar-sized particles at short range.
5. There is evidence that deposition of nasopharyngeal-sized particles in the upper respiratory tract can cause infection.
6. There is evidence that contact transmission can occur. The current weight of evidence suggests that transmission of influenza by inhalation is more probable than by indirect contact.
7. The evidence is lacking to determine whether long-range transmission of influenza occurs, but it cannot be ruled out.

Conclusions on Protective Measures Against Influenza Transmission

1. The primary elements of protection against influenza transmission are engineering and administrative controls. When exposure to an infected person is required or unavoidable, PPRE is the final layer of protection.

2. N95 respirators protect against the inhalation of nasopharyngeal-, tracheobronchial-, and alveolar-sized particles.
3. Surgical masks worn by an infected person may play a role in the prevention of influenza transmission by reducing the amount of infectious material that is expelled into the environment.
4. Both surgical masks and N95 respirators offer a physical barrier to contact with contaminated hands and ballistic trajectory particles.
5. The efficiency of the filters of surgical masks to block penetration of alveolar- and tracheobronchial-sized particles is highly variable. When combined with the inability of these masks to ensure a sealed fit, these factors suggest that surgical masks offer no significant protection against the inhalation of alveolar- and tracheobronchial-sized particles.
6. The efficiency of the filters of surgical masks to block penetration of nasopharyngeal-sized particles is unknown. The lack of a sealed fit on a surgical mask will allow for the inhalation of an unknown quantity of nasopharyngeal-sized particles.

Reference for Evidence

Expert Panel on Influenza and Personal Protective Respiratory Equipment. (2007). *Influenza transmission and the role of personal protective respiratory equipment (PPRE): An assessment of the evidence* (pp. 3-4). Ottawa: Council of Canadian Academies. Retrieved from *http://www.scienceadvice.ca/uploads/eng/assessments%20and%20publications%20and%20news%20releases/flu/(2007-12-19)_influenza_ppre_final_report.pdf*

---

affecting a younger population of individuals, many with severe lung injury as a result of the illness. Prolonged ventilation resulting in an extended surge situation has a significant impact on the health care system as a whole (Hota et al., 2010). With a pandemic wave that typically lasts 8 to 10 weeks, consideration of staff, patient triage, equipment and supplies, space to accommodate patients, and systems to respond to the pandemic event are key to preparedness and response activities (Hota et al., 2010; Frolic, Kata, & Kraus, 2009).

Ethical Issues During a Disaster or Pandemic. Either in connection with experiences with SARS or in anticipation of a major health disaster such as a pandemic, nurses have raised tough ethical questions. These include who gets access to critical care unit services, ventilators, and respiratory support in hospital and which sectors of the population should be given priority to receive vaccines and antivirals during a pandemic. During a disaster situation, the primary health focus shifts from obtaining the best possible health outcomes for the individual patient to protecting the health and safety of the population as a whole, which is both the moral and the legal mandate of public health (Gostin, Bayer, & Fairchild, 2003; Kotalik, 2005). Many of these ethical dilemmas are about balancing the best interests of the

entire population, which is referred to as the "public good," with the rights of the individual. For example, putting an individual in quarantine, even though the individual may not yet be ill or may not become ill, could be considered an infringement of the individual's rights, but at the same time, this action may prevent further transmission of the disease to others (CNA, 2006). The other major ethical dilemma is the duty to provide care, especially during a pandemic or disaster situation (CNA, 2008a, 2008b) (see the Ethical Dilemmas box). Nurses and other health care workers have expressed the conflict they feel between their professional and legal obligations to their patients and their responsibilities to themselves and their family (Chaffee, 2006; CNA, 2008b; Olsen, 2006; Ovadia, Gazit, Silner, & Kagan, 2005; Reid, 2005; see also the Nursing Research box "Caring for Nurses in Public Health Emergencies"). Since the SARS outbreak, there have been a number of ethical frameworks, articles, and resources created to provide guidance for nurses, health care workers, and decision makers in health care and government settings. Many of these can be found in the reference list at the end of this chapter.

Vulnerable Individuals and Populations. Special attention, in all the phases of a disaster or emergency, must be given to vulnerable individuals and marginalized groups. Failure to address the physical and psychological impact of a disaster in a timely and comprehensive manner can lead to long term challenges and mental health issues. Individuals with pre-existing health conditions, disabilities, and mental health issues; women; the frail; homeless, recent immigrants; children; and the elderly are among the more vulnerable of the population and are at higher risk for the negative impacts of a disaster (Milligan &

McGuinness, 2009; Saunders, 2007; WHO & ICN, 2009; Slepski, 2010). Where possible, these populations should be pre-identified as a part of emergency preparation, with the creation of specific plans addressing their unique needs. Vulnerable populations have limited resources, and their ability to recover is affected by their culture, support systems, gender, and previous experiences. In the aftermath of a disaster, nurses are key to offering reassurance, education, and referral to needed resources to these higher risk populations. An understanding of stress and the impact of stress, while offering strategies to cope, is a key component of the nursing role.

Disaster Nursing

With an increasing number of global disasters has come recognition of the need for increased health care preparedness. **Disaster nursing** involves the provision of nursing care, advocacy, and health promotion within the context of a disaster situation. Nurses, owing to their position and numbers, are essential in

---

NURSING RESEARCH

Caring for Nurses in Public Health Emergencies

Amaratunga, C., Carter, M., O'Sullivan, T., Thille, P., Phillips, K., & Saunders, R. (2008). *Caring for nurses in public health emergencies: Enhancing capacity for gender-based support mechanisms in emergency preparedness planning.* Ottawa: Canadian Policy Research Networks. Retrieved from *http://www.cprn.org/documents/49473_EN.pdf*

Purpose

- To provide a summary of the key findings and recommendations from a research project that explored limitations in support systems for nurses during public health threats and emergencies
- To identify how to better support nurses and other health care workers during public health emergencies

Methods

A multi-strategy approach included focus groups of nurses and nurse managers working in emergency departments, critical care, and infection control; a Web-based survey of emergency and critical care nurses about the psychosocial, family, and health impacts of emergencies and disasters; a qualitative content analysis of pandemic plans; a gender-based analysis of public health personnel policy and decision-making capacity; and dissemination of study findings to policy audiences.

Results and Conclusions

Nurses do not feel adequately prepared, nor do they have confidence in the system to react promptly and appropriately to large-scale disasters. Nurses described many challenges related to surge capacity during a disaster, threats to infection control, and problematic risk communication.

"Conflicts between professional and family responsibilities are often reported by women health care workers, and public health emergencies can greatly exacerbate the stress of these conflicts. This is especially true when occupational responsibilities jeopardize the health and safety of vulnerable dependent family members, a valid concern during an infectious disease outbreak or other biohazard event. Many respondents reported that family concerns may prevent them from reporting for work if another highly contagious disease outbreak occurs in the future."

Implications for Nursing Practice

The authors recommend that support mechanisms for nurses that acknowledge traditional gender roles and work–family conflict are urgently needed.

ETHICAL DILEMMAS

Duty to Provide Care During a Pandemic

Situation

You are a senior undergraduate nursing student in the last semester of your program. The Centre for Emergency Preparedness and Response, part of the Public Health Agency of Canada, has declared that areas in your province are in the midst of the initial wave of a pandemic influenza. Because the university you attend is in a city that has not yet had any reported cases of pandemic influenza, your university is open, and both your classes and your clinical practice placements are continuing. Your parents are worried about your safety and are urging you to return home to your rural community, 200 miles north of the city. You do not know what to do because you want to finish your program.

Important Points for Consideration

There will be a massive need for health care workers during a pandemic owing to the number of ill and in need of care; health care workers will also be ill. Many provincial pandemic influenza plans discuss the utilization of health science students in response to the overwhelming health human resource requirements. Universities are preparing pandemic influenza plans and have developed contingency plans for students who live in residence or cannot travel to their home communities during a pandemic. Nursing programs have begun developing specific guidelines and decision-making protocols for use during a pandemic because nursing students participate in the health care system.

Clinical Decision-Making Questions

1. What guidance is provided by the Canadian Nurses Association (CNA) Code of Ethics to help nurses address their ethical dilemmas about providing care during a pandemic?
2. You are not yet a registered nurse. What are the legal obligations for you, as a student, during a pandemic?
3. What are your feelings about registered nurses' duty to provide care during a pandemic? What are your ethical considerations?

disaster mitigation, preparedness, response, and recovery (CNA, 2007). Nurses fill a variety of roles through the disaster management continuum. Eric Laroch, WHO Assistant Director General for Health Action in Crises, states, "Nurses are often the first medical personnel on-site after disaster strikes. In disaster situations, nurses are called upon to take roles as first responder, direct care provider, on-site coordinator of care, information provider or educator, mental health counsellor or triage officer" (WHO & ICN, 2009, pp. 5-6). Therefore, the need for nurses to develop competencies in this growing field is vital.

When disaster strikes, the demand for nurses is much greater than for other health care providers (Lavin, 2006). Opportunities for nursing abroad in countries affected by disaster also exist through humanitarian networks and volunteer agencies. Disaster nursing, irrespective of the location of the disaster, requires application of basic nursing knowledge and skills in difficult environments with scarce resources, rapidly changing conditions, and large volumes of patients. Disaster nursing involves collaboration with other health care providers, first responders, and individuals not commonly worked with, requiring an ability to shift focus in care, while working within the parameters of the laws in place in the area of work (WHO & ICN, 2009). The International Council of Nurses [ICN] has a mission to advance nurses and to bring nursing together worldwide (ICN, 2007). Recognizing the valuable role that nurses play in disaster responses, the ICN believes that "nurses with their technical skills and knowledge of epidemiology, physiology, pharmacology, cultural familial structures, and psychological issues can assist in disaster preparedness programmes, as well as during disasters" (ICN, 2006, p. 2). The *ICN Framework of Disaster Nursing Competencies* (WHO & ICN, 2009) was created as an underpinning for the development of additional advanced competencies among nurses globally. These competencies have been included in the reference section at the end of this chapter.

CLINICAL DECISION-MAKING EXERCISE

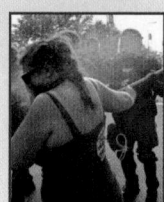

CASE STUDY:
Pepper Spray

Source: AP Photo/Matt Rourke.

Profile

It is 1636 hours on a Thursday in the month of May, and you are working as the triage nurse in the emergency department of a downtown hospital in a major Canadian city. It has been an extremely busy day, and you are currently working with the corridors fully occupied by patients, many of whom have been waiting a day or longer for inpatient beds. Several ambulances are waiting to off-load their patients from stretchers. You receive a call from emergency medical services informing you of the need to be prepared for the potential arrival of patients from a nearby protest rally. You are told that the protesters breached the security fences and the police intervened by using significant amounts of pepper spray. On-site first responders (emergency medical services) have conducted some decontamination on site; however, many of the protesters fled on foot before decontamination.

Subjective Data

Patients arrive within 6 minutes with the following complaints:
- Eye burning; some patients have temporary blindness
- "Skin is burning" complaints

Objective Data

- Severe coughing; some patients with shortness of breath
- Runny nose and watery eyes
- High levels of panic and anxiety

Collaborative Care

Decontamination shower and scrubbing ordered before any medical intervention.

Discussion Questions

1. What risk factors do patients who require decontamination pose to an emergency department?
2. *Priority Decision:* Identify priority actions you will need to take in order to prepare for potential patient arrival.
3. Who will you inform regarding the potential arrival of these patients?
4. What actions must be taken to manage patients who have been contaminated?
5. What equipment might be needed to care for contaminated patients?
6. *Priority Decision:* What are your primary concerns as a triage nurse?
7. What information will you need to obtain from contaminated patients?
8. What actions will you take to ensure the safety of staff and patients currently in the emergency department?

evolve *Answers are available at* **http://evolve.elsevier.com/ Canada/Lewis/medsurg**

REVIEW QUESTIONS

The number of the question corresponds to the same-numbered objective at the beginning of the chapter.

1. A chemical spill has occurred at a nearby industrial site. The first responders report that approximately 20 victims need to be transported to the emergency department after decontamination at the site. What is this an example of?
   a. An emergency
   b. A natural disaster or hazard
   c. A human-made disaster
   d. An emergency response plan

2. Individuals and families must assume responsibility for taking appropriate steps for ensuring that they have the basics of what might be required following an emergency or disaster. Which list of items should be included in an individual emergency preparedness kit?
   a. Batteries, fresh fruit and vegetables, cups and plates
   b. Canned soups and stews, can opener, 2 L of water/day/person
   c. Fresh bread, frozen vegetables, lighter or matches
   d. 1 L of water/day/person, utensils, blankets and sleeping bags

3. Which of the following statements *best* describes disaster nursing?
   a. Provision of nursing care, advocacy, and health promotion
   b. Provision of medical care and teaching
   c. Development and review of emergency operations plan and policy
   d. Provision of nursing care and coordination of health care interventions

4. Which of the following is a component of a comprehensive emergency operations plan?
   a. A closure strategy
   b. A documentation and data management strategy
   c. A pandemic plan
   d. A transfer policy

5. Which activity is correlated with the recovery/rehabilitation phase?
   a. Development of an emergency plan
   b. Conducting emergency exercises and drills
   c. Conducting critical incident stress debriefing with responders
   d. Completing construction to build a flood-resistant emergency department

6. Which of the following statements related to disaster triage in hospitals is correct?
   a. Hospital and emergency department disaster triage is conducted by first responders.
   b. The Canadian Triage and Acuity Scale was specifically designed for disaster triage.
   c. Disaster triage should be done in 2 minutes or less.
   d. Disaster triage involves a triage team composed of one to two nurses, a physician, a porter, and a registration clerk.

7. Which of the following is an example of a human-made disaster?
   a. A terrorist attack
   b. A pandemic
   c. A hurricane
   d. A severe ice storm

8. Which of the following biological agents of bioterrorism has no effective treatment?
   a. Anthrax
   b. Botulism
   c. Smallpox
   d. Hemorrhagic fever

9. Which of the following situations is an example of a chemical-biological, radiological, nuclear (CBRN) event?
   a. Dissemination of anthrax spores to a department in an office building
   b. A train derailment
   c. An outbreak of seasonal influenza
   d. Forest fires

10. Which of the following examples meet the criteria for a pandemic?
    a. A cluster of patients on an inpatient unit with diarrhea
    b. Acquired immune deficiency syndrome (AIDS)
    c. A school that has been closed as a result of flulike symptoms in children in three classrooms
    d. Sudden acute respiratory syndrome (SARS) in Asia and Toronto

ANSWERS: 1. c; 2. b; 3. a; 4. b; 5. c; 6. d; 7. a; 8. d; 9. a; 10. b.

REFERENCES

Amaratunga, C., Carter, M., O'Sullivan, T., Thille, P., Phillips, K., & Saunders, R. (2008). *Caring for nurses in public health emergencies: Enhancing capacity for gender-based support mechanisms in emergency preparedness planning.* Ottawa: Canadian Policy Research Networks. Retrieved from *http://www.cprn.org/documents/49473_EN.pdf*

Andress, K. (2010a). Healthcare facility preparedness. In R. Powers & E. Daly (Eds.), *Disaster nursing international* (pp. 13-28). Cambridge, UK: Cambridge University Press.

Andress, K. (2010b). Nuclear, biologic and chemical agents of mass destruction. In P. K. Howard & R. A. Steinmann (Eds.), *Sheehy's emergency nursing* (6th ed.). St. Louis: Mosby.

Borio, L., Inglesby, T., & Peters, C. J. (2009). Hemorrhagic fever viruses as biological weapons: Medical and public health management. *Journal of the American Medical Association, 287*(18), 2391-2405. doi:10.1001/jama/287.18.2391

Bullard, U. M. J., Unger, B., Spence, J., Grafstein, E., & The CTAS National Working Group (2008). Revisions to the Canadian emergency department triage and acuity scale. *Canadian Journal of Emergency Medicine, 10*(2), 136-142. Retrieved from *http://www.cjem-online.ca/v10/n2/p136*

California Emergency Medical Services Authority (CEMSA). (2006a). *Hospital incident command guidebook.* Retrieved from *http://www.emsa.ca.gov/HICS/default.asp*

California Emergency Medical Services Authority (CEMSA). (2006b). *Hospital incident command system guidebook* (Appendix F). Retrieved from *http://www.emsa.ca.gov/HICS/files/Appendixes.pdf*

Callaway, D. (2007). Tactical emergency services. In D. E. Hogan & J. L. Burstein (Eds.), *Disaster medicine* (2nd ed., pp. 431-443). Philadelphia: Lippincott Williams & Wilkins.

Canadian Nurses Association (CNA). (2006). *Ethics in practice: Public health nursing practice and ethical challenges.* Retrieved from *http://www.cna-aiic.ca/cna/documents/pdf/publications/Ethics_in_Practice_Jan_06_e.pdf*

Canadian Nurses Association (CNA). (2007). *Position statement: Emergency preparedness and response.* Retrieved from *http://www.cna-nurses.ca/CNA/documents/pdf/publications/PS91_Emergency_e.pdf*

Canadian Nurses Association (CNA). (2008a). Code of ethics for registered nurses. Retrieved from *http://www.cna-aiic.ca/CNA/practice/ethics/code/default_e.aspx*

Canadian Nurses Association (CNA). (2008b). *Ethics in practice: Nurses' ethical considerations in a pandemic or other emergency.* Retrieved from *http://www.cna-aiic.ca/CNA/practice/ethics/inpractice/default_e.aspx*

Canadian Red Cross (2010a). *Make a plan.* Retrieved from *http://www.redcross.ca/article.asp?id=33845&tid=001*

Canadian Red Cross (2010b). *How we help.* Retrieved from *http://www.redcross.ca/article.asp?id=000014&tid=020*

Centers for Disease Control and Prevention (CDC). (2006). *Frequently asked questions (FAQs) about dirty bombs.* Retrieved from *http://www.bt.cdc.gov/radiation/dirtybombs.asp*

Chaffee, M. W. (2006). Making the decision to report to work in a disaster: Nurses may have conflicting obligations. *American Journal of Nursing, 106*(9), 54-57. doi:10.1097/00000446-200609000-00027

Chaffee, M. W., & Oster, N. S. (2006). The role of hospitals in disaster. In G. R. Ciottone (Ed.), *Disaster medicine* (3rd ed., pp. 34-42). Philadelphia: Mosby.

Christopher, G. W., Eitzen, E. M., Kortepeter, M. G., & Rowe, J. R. (2007). In D. E. Hogan & J. L. Burstein (Eds.), *Disaster medicine* (2nd ed., pp. 412-430). Philadelphia: Lippincott Williams & Wilkins.

City of Toronto (2003). *Fact sheet: Work quarantine.* Retrieved from *http://www.health.gov.on.ca/english/providers/program/pubhealth/sars/docs/docs2/com_052803_a1.pdf*

College of Nurses of Ontario (CNO). (June 2008). *National competencies in the context of entry-level Registered Nurse practice.* Retrieved from *http://www.cno.org/Global/docs/reg/41037_EntryToPracitic_final.pdf*

Crowe, A. (2010). Biological preparedness and response. In R. Powers & E. Daly (Eds.), *Disaster nursing international* (pp. 199-215). Cambridge, UK: Cambridge University Press.

DeAtley, C. (2010). Healthcare facilities incident command. In R. Powers & E. Daly (Eds.), *Disaster nursing international* (pp. 165-182). Cambridge, UK: Cambridge University Press.

Deeny, P., & McFetridge, B. (2005). The impact of disaster on culture, self, and identity: Increased awareness by health care professionals is needed. *Nursing Clinics of North America, 40*(3), 431-440, vii

Druce, S. (2009). Leadership and management in a disaster. In D. S. Adelman & T. J. Legg (Eds.), *Disaster nursing: A handbook for practice* (pp. 37-49). Sudbury, MA: Jones & Bartlett.

Emergency Management Ontario (EMO). (2009). *About IMS.* Retrieved from *http://www.emergencymanagementontario.ca/english/IMS/about_ims/about_ims.html*

Expert Panel on Influenza and Personal Protective Respiratory Equipment. (2007). *Influenza transmission and the role of personal protective respiratory equipment (PPRE): An assessment of the evidence* (pp.

3-4). Ottawa: Retrieved from *http://www.scienceadvice.ca/uploads/eng/assessments%20and%20publications%20and%20news%20releases/flu/(2007-12-19)_influenza_ppre_final_report.pdf*

Fahlgren, T. L., & Drenkard, K. N. (2002). Healthcare system disaster preparedness, part 2: Nursing executive role in leadership. *Journal of Nursing Administration, 32*(1), 531-537.

Farquharson, C., & Baguley, K. (2003). Responding to the severe acute respiratory (SARS) outbreak: Lessons learned in a Toronto emergency department. *Journal of Emergency Nursing, 29*(3), 222-228. doi:10.1067/men.2003.109

Federal Emergency Management Agency (FEMA). (2008). *Explosions.* Retrieved from *http://www.fema.gov/hazard/terrorism/exp/index.shtm*

Federal Emergency Management Agency (FEMA). (2010). Hazard mitigation planning risk assessment. Retrieved from *http://www.fema.gov/plan/mitplanning/risk.shtm*

Frolic, A., Kata, A., & Kraus, P. (2009). Development of a critical care triage protocol for pandemic influenza: Integrating ethics, evidence and effectiveness. *Healthcare Quarterly, 12*(4), 56-64.

Gostin, L. O., Bayer, R., & Fairchild, A. L. (2003). Ethical and legal challenges posed by SARS: Implications for the control of severe infectious disease threats. *Journal of the American Medical Association, 290*(24), 3229-3237. doi:10.1001/jama.290.24.3229

Government of Canada (2008). Who does what in an emergency? Retrieved from *http://www.getprepared.gc.ca/knw/wh/wh-eng.aspx*

Greenough, P. G., & Burkle, F. M. (2007). Surveillance. In D. E. Hogan & J. L. Burstein (Eds.), *Disaster medicine* (2nd ed., pp. 255-259). Philadelphia: Lippincott Williams & Wilkins.

Grigg, M., & Hughes, F. (2010). Disaster mental health. In R. Powers & E. Daly (Eds.), *Disaster nursing international* (pp. 449-472). Cambridge, UK: Cambridge University Press.

Health Canada (2004). SARS: It's your health. Retrieved from *http://www.hc-sc.gc.ca/hl-vs/iyh-vsv/diseases-maladies/sars-sras-eng.php#ho*

Hota, S., Fried, E., Burry, L., Stewart, T. E., & Christian, M. D. (2010). Preparing your intensive care unit for the second wave of H1N1 and future surges. *Critical Care Medicine, 38*(4), e110-e115. doi:10.1097/CCM.0b013e3181c66940

International Council of Nurses (ICN). (2007). *About ICN.* Retrieved from *http://www.icn.ch/about-icn/about-icn/*

International Council of Nurses (ICN). (2006). *Position statement: Nurses and disaster preparedness.* Retrieved from *http://www.icn.ch/images/stories/documents/publications/position_statements/A11_Nurses_Disaster_Preparedness.pdf*

Koenig, K. L., Boatright, C. J., Hancock, J. A., Denny, F. J., Teeter, D. S., Kahn, C. A., & Schultz, C. A. (2008). Health care facility-based decontamination of victims exposed to chemical, biological and radiological materials. *American Journal of Emergency Medicine, 26*(1), 71-80. doi:10.1016/j.ajem.2007.07.004

Kotalik, J. (2005). Preparing for an influenza pandemic: Ethical issues. *Bioethics, 19*(4), 422-431. doi:10.1111/j.1467-8519.2005.00453.x

Landesman, L. Y. (2001). Essentials of disaster planning. In L. Y. Landesman (Ed.), *Public health management of disasters: The practice guide* (pp. 109-119). Washington, DC: American Public Health Association.

Langan, J. C. (2005). Disasters: A basic overview. In J. C. Langan & D. C. James (Eds.), *Preparing nurses for disaster management* (pp. 1-16). Upper Saddle River, NJ: Pearson.

Lavin, R. P. (2006). HIPAA and disaster research: Preparing to conduct research. *Disaster Management and Response, 4*(2), 32-36.

Lentz, C., Reid, D., Rera, B., & Kehoe, K. (2007). Management of burn mass casualty incidents. In T. G. Veenema (Ed.), *Disaster nursing and emergency preparedness for chemical, biological, and radiological terrorism and other hazards* (2nd ed., pp. 221-236). New York: Springer.

Markenson, D., DiMaggio, C., & Redlener, I. (2005). Preparing health professions students for terrorism, disaster and public health emergencies: Core competencies. *Academic Medicine, 80*(6), 517-526. doi:10.1097/00001888-200506000-00002

McFee, R. (2008). SARS: Severe acute respiratory syndrome. In R. B. McFee & J. B. Leikin (Eds.), *Toxico-terrorism: Emergency response and clinical approach to chemical, biological, and radiological agents* (pp. 13-18). New York: McGraw-Hill Medical.

McMahon, M. M. (2010). Hospital impact: Emergency Department. In R. Powers & E. Daly (Eds.), *Disaster nursing international* (pp. 81-100). Cambridge, UK: Cambridge University Press.

Military Medical Operations (MMO). (2010). *Medical management of radiological casualties* (on-line 3rd ed.). Armed Forces Radiobiology Research Institute. Retrieved from *http://www.afrri.usuhs.mil*

Milligan, G., & McGuinness, T. M. (2009). Mental health needs in a post-disaster environment. *Journal of Psychosocial Nursing, 47*(9), 23-30. doi:10.3928/02793695-20090731-01

Mitchell, A. M., Sakraida, T. J., & Zalice, K. K. (2005). Disaster care: Psychological considerations. *Nursing Clinics of North America, 40*(3), 535-550. doi:10.1016/j.cnur.2005.04.006

National Advisory Committee on SARS and Public Health. (2003). *Learning from SARS: Renewal of public health in Canada (Naylor report)*. Ottawa: Health Canada. Retrieved from *http://www.phac-aspc.gc.ca/publicat/sars-sras/naylor/index.html*

National Defence Canada (2005). *National Defence and the Canadian Forces*. Retrieved from *http://comfec-cefcom.forces.gc.ca/pa-ap/nr-sp/doc-eng.asp?id=301*

Noji, E. K. (1996). Disaster epidemiology. *Emergency Medicine Clinics of North America, 14*(2), 289-300. doi:10.1016/S0733-8627(05)70252-2

Olsen, D. P. (2006). The ethical dilemma: Questions to consider when deciding whether to show up for work in a disaster. *American Journal of Nursing, 106*(9), 57. doi:10.1097/00000446-200609000-00028

Ontario Ministry of Health and Long-Term Care (MoHLTC). (2004). *SARS: Severe acute respiratory syndrome*. Retrieved from *http://www.health.gov.on.ca/english/public/updates/archives/hu_03/hu_sars.html*

Ontario Ministry of Health and Long Term Care (MoHLTC). (2008). *Introduction to the incident management system for Ontario* (on-line presentation). Retrieved from *http://www.emergencymanagement ontario.ca/english/emcommunity/professionaldevelopment/Training/ims100/ims100.html*

Ovadia, K. L., Gazit, I., Silner, D., & Kagan, I. (2005). Better late than never: A re-examination of ethical dilemmas in coping with SARS. *Journal of Hospital Infection, 61*(1), 75-79. doi:10.1016/j.jhin.2004.12.018

Plum, K. C., & Veenema, T. G. (2007). Management of psychosocial effects. In T. G. Veenema (Ed.), *Disaster nursing and emergency preparedness for chemical, biological, and radiological terrorism and other hazards* (2nd ed., pp. 254-271). New York: Springer.

Plurad, D. S. (2011). Blast injury. *Military Medicine, 176*(3), 276-282.

Powers, R. (2010a). Introduction to disasters and disaster nursing. In R. Powers & E. Daly (Eds.), *Disaster nursing international* (pp. 2-11). Cambridge, UK: Cambridge University Press.

Powers, R. (2010b). Decontamination. In R. Powers & E. Daly (Eds.), *Disaster nursing international* (pp. 265-287). Cambridge, UK: Cambridge University Press.

Public Health Agency of Canada (PHAC). (2005). *National notifiable diseases on-line*. Retrieved from *http://dsol-smed.phac-aspc.gc.ca/dsol-smed/ndis/list-eng.php*

Public Health Agency of Canada (PHAC). (2011). *Self-care for caregivers*. Retrieved from *http://www.phac-aspc.gc.ca/publicat/oes-bsu-02/caregvr-eng.php*

Public Safety Canada (PSC). (2009a). *About disaster mitigation*. Retrieved from *http://www.publicsafety.gc.ca/prg/em/ndms/aboutsnac-eng.aspx#all*

Public Safety Canada (PSC). (2009b). *Emergency Management Act*. Retrieved from *http://www.publicsafety.gc.ca/media/nr/2007/bk20070807-eng.aspx*

Public Safety Canada (PSC). (2009c). *About disaster mitigation*. Retrieved from *http://www.publicsafety.gc.ca/prg/em/ndms/aboutsnac-eng.aspx*

Public Safety Canada (PSC). (2010). *Get an emergency kit. Start today!* Retrieved from *http://www.getprepared.gc.ca/_fl/pub/mrgnc-kt-eng.pdf*

Public Safety Canada (PSC). (2011a). *Emergency management planning*. Retrieved from *http://www.publicsafety.gc.ca/prg/em/emp/index-eng.aspx*

Public Safety Canada (PSC). (2011b). *Critical infrastructure partners*. Retrieved from *http://www.publicsafety.gc.ca/prg/ns/ci/prtn-eng.aspx*

Public Safety Canada (PSC). (2011c). *Canadian disaster database*. Retrieved from *http://www.publicsafety.gc.ca/prg/em/cdd/index-eng.aspx*

Qureshi, K., & Gebbie, G. M. (2007). Disaster management. In T. G. Veenema (Ed.), *Disaster nursing and emergency preparedness for chemical, biological, and radiological terrorism and other hazards* (2nd ed., pp. 138-159). New York: Springer.

Qureshi, K., & Veenema, T. G. (2007). Disaster triage. In T. G. Veenema (Ed.), *Disaster nursing and emergency preparedness for chemical, biological, and radiological terrorism and other hazards* (2nd ed., pp. 162-176). New York: Springer.

Reid, L. (2005). Diminishing returns? Risk and the duty to care in the SARS epidemic. *Bioethics, 19*(4), 348-361. doi:10.1111/j.1467-8519.2005.00448.x

Richter, J. E. V. (2010). Public health response. In R. Powers & E. Daly (Eds.), *Disaster nursing international* (pp. 385-396). Cambridge, U.K: Cambridge University Press.

Romig, L. (2008). *The JumpSTART pediatric MCI triage tool: Principles of multicasualty triage*. Retrieved from *http://www.jumpstarttriage.com/JumpSTART_and_MCI_Triage.php*

Salvation Army. (2011). *Emergency disaster services*. Retrieved from *http://www.salvationarmy.ca/eds/*

Saunders, J. M. (2007). Vulnerable populations in an American Red Cross shelter after Hurricane Katrina. *Perspectives in Psychiatric Care, 43*(1), 30-37. doi:10.1111/j.1744-6163.2007.00103.x

Silenas, R., Akins, R., Parrish, A. R., & Edwards, J. C. (2008). Developing disaster preparedness competence: An experiential learning exercise for multiprofessional education. *Teaching and Learning in Medicine, 20*(1), 62-68. doi:10.1080/10401330701798311

Slepski, L. A. (2010). Pandemic planning. In R. Powers & E. Daly (Eds.), *Disaster nursing international* (pp. 397-426). Cambridge, UK: Cambridge University Press.

St. John Ambulance. (2011). *Emergency preparedness information*. Retrieved from *http://www.sja.ca/Canada/CommunityServices/Pages/EmergencyPreparednessInformation.aspx*

Stanhope, M., Lancaster, J., Jessup-Falcioni, H., & Viverais-Dresler, G. L. (2011). *Community health nursing in Canada*. Toronto: Mosby.

Toronto Academic Health Sciences Network (TAHSN). (2006). *TAHSN pandemic influenza planning guideline*. Retrieved from *http://sunnybrook.ca/uploads/TAHSNManualMay2006.pdf*

UNISDR. (2009). *Terminology on disaster risk reduction*. Retrieved from *http://www.unisdr.org/files/7817_UNISDRTerminologyEnglish.pdf*

United Nations–UN News Centre. (2011). *UN: 2010 among deadliest years for disasters, urges better preparedness*. Retrieved from *http://www.un.org/apps/news/story.asp?NewsID=37357&Cr=disaster+reduction&Cr1*

U.S. Department of Health and Human Services (USDHHS). (2011a). *START adult triage algorithm*. Retrieved from *http://www.remm.nlm.gov/startadult.htm*

U.S. Department of Health and Human Services (USDHHS). (2011b). *JumpSTART pediatric triage algorithm*. Retrieved from *http://www.remm.nlm.gov/startpediatric.htm*

Varia, M., Wilson, S., Sarwal, S., McGeer, A., Gournis, E., Galanis, E., …, Hospital Outbreak Investigation Team. (2003). Investigation of a nosocomial outbreak of severe acute respiratory syndrome (SARS) in Toronto, Canada. *Canadian Medical Association Journal, 169*(4), 285-292.

Veenema, T. G. (2007a). Essentials of disaster planning. In T. G. Veenema (Ed.), *Disaster nursing and emergency preparedness for chemical, biological, and radiological terrorism and other hazards* (2nd ed., pp. 2-23). New York: Springer.

Veenema, T. G. (2007b). Mass casualty decontamination. In T. G. Veenema (Ed.), *Disaster nursing and emergency preparedness for chemical, biological, and radiological terrorism and other hazards* (2nd ed., pp. 505-519). New York: Springer.

Veenema, T. G., Benitez, J., & Benware, S. (2007). In T. G. Veenema (Ed.), *Disaster nursing and emergency preparedness for chemical, biological, and radiological terrorism and other hazards* (2nd ed., pp. 483-502). New York: Springer.

Whitney, L., Marchant-Short, S., & Yiu, L. (2008). In L. L. Stamler & L. Yiu (Eds.), *Community health nursing: A Canadian perspective* (2nd ed., pp. 142-161). Toronto: Pearson.

World Health Organization (WHO). (2007). *Risk reduction and emergency preparedness: WHO six-year strategy for the health sector and community capacity development.* Retrieved from *http://www.who.int/ hac/techguidance/preparedness/emergency_preparedness_eng.pdf*

World Health Organization (WHO). (2009). *Call to protect hospitals, schools from impact of disasters.* Retrieved from *http://www.who.int/ mediacentre/news/releases/2009/disaster_risk_reduction_20090618/ en/index.html*

World Health Organization and International Council of Nurses (WHO & ICN) (2009). *ICN framework of disaster nursing competencies.* Retrieved from *http://www.icn.ch/images/stories/documents/ networks/DisasterPreparednessNetwork/Disaster_Nursing_ Competencies_lite.pdf*

CANADIAN RESOURCES

Canadian Centre for Emergency Preparedness
http://www.ccep.ca
Canadian Disaster Database (Public Safety Canada)
http://www.publicsafety.gc.ca/prg/em/cdd/index-eng.aspx
Canadian Pandemic Influenza Plan for the Health Sector
http://www.phac-aspc.gc.ca/cpip-pclcpi/
Canadian Red Cross
http://www.redcross.ca
Government of Canada
http://www.GetPrepared.ca

Government of Canada—Emergency Management Organizations
http://www.getprepared.gc.ca/cnt/rsrcs/mrgnc-mgmt-rgnztns-eng.aspx
Health Canada, Emergencies and Disasters
http://www.hc-sc.gc.ca/hc-ps/ed-ud/index-eng.php
Ministry of Health and Long-Term Care
Ontario Health Plan for an Influenza Pandemic 2008:
http://www.health.gov.on.ca/english/providers/program/emu/pan_flu/ pan_flu_plan.html
Public Health Agency of Canada
http://www.publichealth.gc.ca
Public Health Agency of Canada
Chemical, Biological, Radiological and Nuclear Resource Links:
http://www.phac-aspc.gc.ca/cepr-cmiu/ophs-bssp/links_index_e.html
Public Safety Canada
http://www.publicsafety.gc.ca/
Salvation Army
http://www.SalvationArmy.ca
St. John Ambulance
http://www.sja.ca
http://www.sja.ca/Canada/CommunityServices/Pages/ EmergencyPreparednessInformation.aspx

OTHER RESOURCES

Centers for Disease Control and Prevention
http://www.cdc.gov/
Federal Emergency Management Agency (FEMA)
http://www.fema.gov/
START Triage
http://www.start-triage.com/
World Health Organization
http://www.who.int/en/
World Health Organization and International Council of Nurses
Framework of Disaster Nursing Competencies:
http://www.icn.ch/images/stories/documents/networks/ DisasterPreparednessNetwork/Disaster_Nursing_Competencies_ lite.pdf

ℰvolve *For additional Internet resources, see the Web site for this book at* **http://evolve.elsevier.com/Canada/Lewis/medsurg**

Domain 1: Health Promotion

Class 1: Health Awareness
Deficient Diversional Activity (00097)
Sedentary Lifestyle (00168)

Class 2: Health Management 153
Deficient Community Health (00215)*
Risk-Prone Health Behavior (00188)†
Ineffective Health Maintenance (00099)
Readiness for Enhanced Immunization Status (00186)
Ineffective Protection (00043)
Ineffective Self-Health Management (00078)
Readiness for Enhanced Self-Health Management (00162)†
Ineffective Family Therapeutic Regimen Management (00080)

Domain 2: Nutrition

Class 1: Ingestion
Insufficient Breast Milk (00216)*
Ineffective Infant Feeding Pattern (00107)
Imbalanced Nutrition: Less Than Body Requirements (00002)
Imbalanced Nutrition: More Than Body Requirements (00001)
Readiness for Enhanced Nutrition (00163)
Risk for Imbalanced Nutrition: More Than Body Requirements (00003)
Impaired Swallowing (00103)

Class 2: Digestion
Class 3: Absorption
Class 4: Metabolism
Risk for Unstable Blood Glucose Level (00179)
Neonatal Jaundice (00194)
Risk for Neonatal Jaundice (00230)*
Risk for Impaired Liver Function (00178)

Class 5: Hydration
Risk for Electrolyte Imbalance (00195)
Readiness for Enhanced Fluid Balance (00160)
Deficient Fluid Volume (00027)
Excess Fluid Volume (00026)
Risk for Deficient Fluid Volume (00028)
Risk for Imbalanced Fluid Volume (00025)

Domain 3: Elimination and Exchange

Class 1: Urinary Function
Functional Urinary Incontinence (00020)
Overflow Urinary Incontinence (00176)
Reflex Urinary Incontinence (00018)
Stress Urinary Incontinence (00017)
Urge Urinary Incontinence (00019)
Risk for Urge Urinary Incontinence (00022)
Impaired Urinary Elimination (00016)
Readiness for Enhanced Urinary Elimination (00166)
Urinary Retention (00023)

Class 2: Gastrointestinal Function
Constipation (00011)
Perceived Constipation (00012)
Risk for Constipation (00015)
Diarrhea (00013)
Dysfunctional Gastrointestinal Motility (00196)
Risk for Dysfunctional Gastrointestinal Motility (00197)
Bowel Incontinence (00014)

Class 3: Integumentary Function
Class 4: Respiratory Function
Impaired Gas Exchange (00030)

Domain 4: Activity/Rest

Class 1: Sleep/Rest
Insomnia (00095)
Sleep Deprivation (00096)
Readiness for Enhanced Sleep (00165)
Disturbed Sleep Pattern (00198)

Class 2: Activity/Exercise
Risk for Disuse Syndrome (00040)
Impaired Bed Mobility (00091)
Impaired Physical Mobility (00085)
Impaired Wheelchair Mobility (00089)
Impaired Transfer Ability (00090)
Impaired Walking (00088)

Class 3: Energy Balance
Disturbed Energy Field (00050)
Fatigue (00093)
Wandering (00154)

Class 4: Cardiovascular/Pulmonary Responses
Activity Intolerance (00092)
Risk for Activity Intolerance (00094)
Ineffective Breathing Pattern (00032)
Decreased Cardiac Output (00029)
Risk for Ineffective Gastrointestinal Perfusion (00202)
Risk for Ineffective Renal Perfusion (00203)
Impaired Spontaneous Ventilation (00033)
Ineffective Peripheral Tissue Perfusion (00204)
Risk for Decreased Cardiac Tissue Perfusion (00200)†
Risk for Ineffective Cerebral Tissue Perfusion (00201)
Risk for Ineffective Peripheral Tissue Perfusion (00228)*
Dysfunctional Ventilatory Weaning Response (00034)

Class 5: Self-Care
Impaired Home Maintenance (00098)
Readiness for Enhanced Self-Care (00182)
Bathing Self-Care Deficit (00108)
Dressing Self-Care Deficit (00109)†
Feeding Self-Care Deficit (00102)
Toileting Self-Care Deficit (00110)
Self-Neglect (00193)†

Domain 5: Perception/Cognition

Class 1: Attention
Unilateral Neglect (00123)

Class 2: Orientation
Impaired Environmental Interpretation Syndrome (00127)

Class 3: Sensation/Perception
Class 4: Cognition
Acute Confusion (00128)
Chronic Confusion (00129)
Risk for Acute Confusion (00173)
Ineffective Impulse Control (00222)*
Deficient Knowledge (00126)
Readiness for Enhanced Knowledge (00161)
Impaired Memory (00131)

Class 5: Communication
Readiness for Enhanced Communication (00157)
Impaired Verbal Communication (00051)

Domain 6: Self-Perception

Class 1: Self-Concept
Hopelessness (00124)
Risk for Compromised Human Dignity (00174)
Risk for Loneliness (00054)
Disturbed Personal Identity (00121)
Risk for Disturbed Personal Identity (00225)*
Readiness for Enhanced Self-Concept (00167)

Class 2: Self-Esteem
Chronic Low Self-Esteem (00119)
Situational Low Self-Esteem (00120)
Risk for Chronic Low Self-Esteem (00224)*
Risk for Situational Low Self-Esteem (00153)

Class 3: Body Image
Disturbed Body Image (00118)

Domain 7: Role Relationships

Class 1: Caregiving Roles
Ineffective Breastfeeding (00104)
Interrupted Breastfeeding (00105)
Readiness for Enhanced Breastfeeding (00106)*
Caregiver Role Strain (00061)
Risk for Caregiver Role Strain (00062)
Impaired Parenting (00056)
Readiness for Enhanced Parenting (00164)
Risk for Impaired Parenting (00057)

Class 2: Family Relationships
Risk for Impaired Attachment (00058)*
Dysfunctional Family Processes (00063)†
Interrupted Family Processes (00060)
Readiness for Enhanced Family Processes (00159)

Class 3: Role Performance
Ineffective Relationship (00223)*
Readiness for Enhanced Relationship (00207)

Risk for Ineffective Relationship (00229)*
Parental Role Conflict (00064)
Ineffective Role Performance (00055)
Impaired Social Interaction (00052)*

Domain 8: Sexuality

Class 1: Sexual Identity
Class 2: Sexual Function
Sexual Dysfunction (00059)
Ineffective Sexuality Pattern (00065)

Class 3: Reproduction
Ineffective Childbearing Process (00221)*
Readiness for Enhanced Childbearing Process (00208)
Risk for Ineffective Childbearing Process (00227)*
Risk for Disturbed Maternal–Fetal Dyad (00209)

Domain 9: Coping/Stress Tolerance

Class 1: Post-Trauma Responses
Post-Trauma Syndrome (00141)
Risk for Post-Trauma Syndrome (00145)
Rape-Trauma Syndrome (00142)
Relocation Stress Syndrome (00114)
Risk for Relocation Stress Syndrome (00149)

Class 2: Coping Responses
Ineffective Activity Planning (00199)
Risk for Ineffective Activity Planning (00226)*
Anxiety (00146)
Defensive Coping (00071)
Ineffective Coping (00069)
Readiness for Enhanced Coping (00158)
Ineffective Community Coping (00077)
Readiness for Enhanced Community Coping (00076)
Compromised Family Coping (00074)
Disabled Family Coping (00073)
Readiness for Enhanced Family Coping (00075)
Death Anxiety (00147)
Ineffective Denial (00072)
Adult Failure to Thrive (00101)
Fear (00148)
Grieving (00136)
Complicated Grieving (00135)
Risk for Complicated Grieving (00172)
Readiness for Enhanced Power (00187)
Powerlessness (00125)
Risk for Powerlessness (00152)
Impaired Individual Resilience (00210)
Readiness for Enhanced Resilience (00212)
Risk for Compromised Resilience (00211)
Chronic Sorrow (00137)
Stress Overload (00177)

Class 3: Neurobehavioral Stress
Autonomic Dysreflexia (00009)
Risk for Autonomic Dysreflexia (00010)
Disorganized Infant Behavior (00116)
Readiness for Enhanced Organized Infant Behavior (00117)
Risk for Disorganized Infant Behavior (00115)
Decreased Intracranial Adaptive Capacity (00049)

Domain 10: Life Principles

Class 1: Values
Readiness for Enhanced Hope (00185)

Class 2: Beliefs
Readiness for Enhanced Spiritual Well-Being (00068)

Class 3: Value/Belief/Action Congruence
Readiness for Enhanced Decision-Making (00184)
Decisional Conflict (00083)
Moral Distress (00175)
Noncompliance (00079)
Impaired Religiosity (00169)
Readiness for Enhanced Religiosity (00171)
Risk for Impaired Religiosity (00170)
Spiritual Distress (00066)
Risk for Spiritual Distress (00067)

Domain 11: Safety/Protection 415

Class 1: Infection 417
Risk for Infection (00004)

Class 2: Physical Injury 421
Ineffective Airway Clearance (00031)
Risk for Aspiration (00039)
Risk for Bleeding (00206)
Impaired Dentition (00048)
Risk for Dry Eye (00219)*
Risk for Falls (00155)
Risk for Injury (00035)
Impaired Oral Mucous Membrane (00045)
Risk for Perioperative Positioning Injury (00087)
Risk for Peripheral Neurovascular Dysfunction (00086)
Risk for Shock (00205)
Impaired Skin Integrity (00046)
Risk for Impaired Skin Integrity (00047)
Risk for Sudden Infant Death Syndrome (00156)
Risk for Suffocation (00036)
Delayed Surgical Recovery (00100)
Risk for Thermal Injury (00220)*
Impaired Tissue Integrity (00044)
Risk for Trauma (00038)
Risk for Vascular Trauma (00213)

Class 3: Violence 447
Risk for Other-Directed Violence (00138)
Risk for Self-Directed Violence (00140)
Self-Mutilation (00151)
Risk for Self-Mutilation (00139)
Risk for Suicide (00150)

Class 4: Environmental Hazards 454
Contamination (00181)
Risk for Contamination (00180)
Risk for Poisoning (00037)

Class 5: Defensive Processes 461
Risk for Adverse Reaction to Iodinated Contrast Media (000218)*
Latex Allergy Response (00041)
Risk for Allergy Response (00217)*
Risk for Latex Allergy Response (00042)

Class 6: Thermoregulation 467
Risk for Imbalanced Body Temperature (00005)
Hyperthermia (00007)
Hypothermia (00006)
Ineffective Thermoregulation (00008)

Domain 12: Comfort

Class 1: Physical Comfort
Class 2: Environmental Comfort
Class 3: Social Comfort
Impaired Comfort (00214)
Readiness for Enhanced Comfort (00183)
Nausea (00134)
Acute Pain (00132)
Chronic Pain (00133)
Social Isolation (00053)

Domain 13: Growth/Development

Class 1: Growth
Risk for Disproportionate Growth (00113)

Class 2: Development
Delayed Growth and Development (00111)
Risk for Delayed Development (00112)

Retired Diagnoses

Disturbed Sensory Perception
Disturbed Thought Process
Effective Breastfeeding
Effective Health Management
Effective Self-Health Management
Effective Therapeutic Regimen Management
Health-Seeking Behaviors
Ineffective Activity Planning
Ineffective Community Therapeutic Regimen Management
Ineffective Tissue Perfusion
Rape-Trauma Syndrome: Compound Syndrome
Rape-Trauma Syndrome: Silent Reaction
Risk for Impaired Parent/Infant/Child Attachment
Risk for Ineffective Cardiac Tissue Perfusion
Total Urinary Incontinence

Data from *Nursing Diagnoses—Definitions and Classification 2012-2014.* ©2012, 2009, 2007, 2005, 2003, 2001, 1998, 1996, 1994 NANDA International. Used by arrangement with Wiley-Blackwell Publishing, a company of John Wiley and Sons, Inc.
In order to make safe and effective judgments using NANDA-I nursing diagnoses, it is essential that nurses refer to the definitions and defining characteristics of the diagnoses listed in this work.
*Diagnosis new to North American Nursing Diagnosis Association. (2012). *NANDA-I nursing diagnoses: Definitions and classification 2012-2014.* Philadelphia: Author.
†Diagnosis retired from North American Nursing Diagnosis Association. (2009). *NANDA-I nursing diagnoses: Definitions and classification 2009-2011.* Philadelphia: Author.

Laboratory Values

Adapted by Jennifer E. Cooke

The tables in this appendix list some of the most common tests, their normal values, and possible etiologies of abnormal values. Laboratory values are expressed in the Système International d'Unités (SI units) that are used in Canada. Conventional units, used in the United States, are presented after the SI units in parentheses. Laboratory values may vary with different techniques or different laboratories. Possible etiologies are presented in alphabetical order. Abbreviations appearing in the tables are defined as follows:

<	=	less than
>	=	greater than
≥	=	greater than or equal to
≤	=	less than or equal to
AU	=	arbitrary unit
dL	=	decilitre
EU	=	Ehrlich unit
fL	=	femtolitre
g	=	gram
IU	=	international unit
kPa	=	kilopascal
L	=	litre
mcg	=	microgram (one millionth of a gram) (10^{-6})
mckat	=	microkatal
mcL	=	microlitre

mcmol	=	micromole
mcU	=	microunit
mEq	=	milliequivalent
mg	=	milligram (10^{-3})
mL	=	millilitre
mm	=	millimetre
mm Hg	=	millimetre of mercury
mmol	=	millimole
mOsm	=	milliosmole
nmol	=	nanomole
ng	=	nanogram (one billionth of a gram) (10^{-9})
pg	=	picogram (one trillionth of a gram) (10^{-12})
pmol	=	picomole
U	=	unit

Table B-1 Serum, Plasma, and Whole Blood Chemistries

TEST	NORMAL VALUES SI UNITS (CONVENTIONAL UNITS)	POSSIBLE ETIOLOGY HIGHER	LOWER
Acetone		Diabetic ketoacidosis, high-fat diet, low-carbohydrate diet, starvation	—
Quantitative	<200 mcmol/L (<1.16 mg/dL)		
Qualitative	Negative (negative)		
Alanine aminotransferase (ALT) (formerly serum glutamate pyruvate transferase [SGPT])	4-36 U/L (same as SI units)	Liver disease, shock	—
Albumin	35-50 g/L (3.5-5 g/dL)	Dehydration	Burns, chronic liver disease, malabsorption, malnutrition, nephrotic syndrome, pregnancy
Aldolase	22-59 mU/L (3-8.2 Sibley-Lehninger U/dL)	Infection, muscle trauma, skeletal muscle disease	Late muscular dystrophy, renal disease
α_1-Antitrypsin	0.85-2.13 g/L (85-213 mg/dL)	Acute and chronic inflammation and infection, arthritis, malignancy, stress syndrome, thyroid infections	Chronic lung disease (early onset of emphysema), malnutrition, nephrotic syndrome
α_1-Fetoprotein	<40 mcg/L (<40 ng/mL)	Cancers of testes and ovaries, carcinoma of liver, neural tube defects or multiple pregnancies in pregnant women	In pregnant women, trisomy 21 or fetal distress/death
Ammonia	6-47 mcmol/L (10-80 mcg/dL)	GI bleeds, hepatic encephalopathy, portal hypertension, severe liver disease	—

Continued

Table B-1 Serum, Plasma, and Whole Blood Chemistries—cont'd

TEST	NORMAL VALUES SI UNITS (CONVENTIONAL UNITS)	POSSIBLE ETIOLOGY	
		HIGHER	LOWER
Amylase	30-220 U/L (60-120 Somogyi units/dL)	Acute and chronic pancreatitis, mumps (salivary gland disease), perforated ulcers	Acute alcoholism, cirrhosis of liver, extensive destruction of pancreas
Ascorbic acid	23-85 mcmol/L (0.4-1.5 mg/dL)	Excessive ingestion of vitamin C	Connective tissue disorders, hepatic disease, renal disease, rheumatic fever, vitamin C deficiency
Aspartate aminotransferase (AST) (formerly serum glutamic oxaloacetic transferase [SGOT])	0-35 U/L (same as SI units)	Acute hepatitis, liver disease, myocardial infarction (MI), pulmonary infarction	—
B-type (or brain) natriuretic peptide	<100 ng/L (<100 pg/mL)	Congestive heart failure, MI, hypertension, cor pulmonale	—
Bicarbonate	21-28 mmol/L (21-28 mEq/L)	Chronic use of loop diuretics, compensated respiratory acidosis, metabolic alkalosis	Acute renal failure, compensated respiratory alkalosis, diarrhea, metabolic acidosis
Bilirubin		Biliary obstruction, hemolytic anemia, impaired liver function, pernicious anemia, prolonged fasting	—
Total	5.1-17 mcmol/L (0.3-1.0 mg/dL)		
Indirect	3.4-12 mcmol/L (0.2-0.8 mg/dL)		
Direct	1.7-5.1 mcmol/L (0.1-0.3 mg/dL)		
Blood gases*			
Arterial pH	7.35-7.45 (same as SI units)	Alkalosis	Acidosis
Venous pH	7.31-7.41 (same as SI units)	Alkalosis	Acidosis
$PaCO_2$	35-45 mm Hg (same as SI units)	Compensated metabolic alkalosis, respiratory acidosis	Compensated metabolic acidosis, respiratory alkalosis
PaO_2	80-100 mm Hg (same as SI units)	Administration of high concentration of oxygen	Chronic lung disease, decreased cardiac output
Venous PO_2	40-50 mm Hg (same as SI units)		
Calcium	2.25-2.75 mmol/L (9-10.5 mg/dL)	Acute osteoporosis, hyperparathyroidism, multiple myeloma, vitamin D intoxication	Acute pancreatitis, hypoparathyroidism, liver disease, malabsorption syndrome, renal failure, vitamin D deficiency
Calcium, ionized	1.05-1.30 mmol/L (4.5-5.6 mg/dL)	—	—
Carbon dioxide (CO_2 content)	21-28 mmol/L (21-28 mEq/L)	Same as bicarbonate	—
β-Carotene	1.4-4.7 mcmol/L (75-253 mcg/dL)	Cystic fibrosis, hypothyroidism, pancreatic insufficiency	Dietary deficiency, malabsorption disorders
Chloride	98-106 mmol/L (98-106 mEq/L)	Corticosteroid therapy, dehydration, excessive infusion of normal saline, metabolic acidosis, respiratory alkalosis, uremia	Addison's disease, congestive heart failure, diarrhea, metabolic alkalosis, overhydration, respiratory acidosis, SIADH (syndrome of inappropriate antidiuretic syndrome), vomiting
Cholesterol	<5 mmol/L (<200 mg/dL) age dependent	Biliary obstruction, cirrhosis hypothyroidism, hyperlipidemia, idiopathic hypercholesterolemia, renal disease, uncontrolled diabetes	Corticosteroid therapy, extensive liver disease, hyperthyroidism, malnutrition
HDL (high-density lipoproteins)	>1.55 mmol/L (>40 mg/dL)		
LDL (low-density lipoproteins)	<2.59 mmol/L (<100 mg/dL)		
Cholinesterase (RBC)	5-10 U/L (same as SI units)	Exercise, sickle cell disease	Acute infections, insecticide intoxication, liver disease, muscular dystrophy
Copper	11-22 mcmol/L (70-140 mcg/dL)	Cirrhosis, contraceptive use by female patient	Wilson's disease

*Because arterial blood gases are influenced by altitude, the value for PO_2 decreases as altitude increases. The lower value is normal for an altitude of 1 mile.

Table B-1 Serum, Plasma, and Whole Blood Chemistries—cont'd

TEST	NORMAL VALUES SI UNITS (CONVENTIONAL UNITS)	POSSIBLE ETIOLOGY HIGHER	LOWER
Cortisol	8 A.M.: 138-635 nmol/L (5-23 mcg/dL) 8 P.M.: < 83-359 nmol/L (3-13 mcg/dL)	Adrenal adenoma, Cushing's syndrome, hyperthyroidism, pancreatitis, stress	Addison's disease, adrenal insufficiency, hypopituitary states, hypothyroidism, liver disease
Creatine	15.3-76.3 mcmol/L (0.2-1.0 mg/dL)	Active rheumatoid arthritis, biliary obstruction, hyperthyroidism, renal disorders, severe muscle disease	Diabetes mellitus
Creatine kinase (CK) Male Female	55-170 U/L (same as SI units) 30-135 U/L (same as SI units)	Brain damage, exercise, musculoskeletal injury or disease, MI, numerous intramuscular injections, severe myocarditis	—
CK-MB (CK-2)	Male: 2-6 mcg/L (2-6 ng/mL) Female: 2-5 mcg/L (2-5 ng/mL)	Acute MI	—
CK mass fraction	<0.05 fraction of total CK	—	—
Creatinine Male Female	53-106 mcmol/L (0.6-1.2 mg/dL) 44-97 mcmol/L (0.5-1.1 mg/dL)	Severe renal disease	Diseases with decreased muscle mass (e.g. muscular dystrophy, myasthenia gravis)
Ferritin (serum) Male Female	12-300 ng/L (12-300 ng/mL) 10-150 ng/L (10-150 ng/mL)	Anemia of chronic disease (infection, inflammation, liver disease), sideroblastic anemia	Iron-deficiency anemia, severe protein deficiency
Folic acid (folate)	11-57 mmol/L (5-25 ng/mL)	Hypothyroidism, pernicious anemia	Alcoholism, hemolytic anemia, inadequate diet, malabsorption syndrome, malnutrition, megaloblastic anemia
γ-Glutamyltranspeptidase (GGT)	8-38 IU/L (same as SI units)	Cholestasis, cytomegalovirus infection, Epstein-Barr, liver disease, MI, pancreatitis	—
Glucose, fasting	4-6 mmol/L (70-110 mg/dL)	Acute stress, cerebral lesions, Cushing's syndrome, diabetes mellitus, hyperthyroidism, pancreatic insufficiency	Addison's disease, hepatic disease, hypothyroidism, insulin overdosage, pancreatic tumour, pituitary hypofunction, postdumping syndrome
2-Hr oral glucose tolerance testing (OGTT) Fasting 1 hr 2 hr	4-6 mmol/L (70-110 mg/dL) <11.1 mmol/L (<200 mg/dL) <7.8 mmol/L (<140 mg/dL)	Diabetes mellitus	Hyperinsulinism
Haptoglobin	0.5-2.2 g/L (50-220 mg/dL)	Acute MI, infectious and inflammatory processes, malignant neoplasms	Chronic liver disease, hemolytic anemia, mononucleosis, systemic lupus erythematosus, toxoplasmosis, transfusion reactions
Homocysteine	4-14 mcmol/L (0.54-1.9 mg/L)	Cardiovascular disease, cerebrovascular disease, peripheral vascular disease, cystinuria, vitamin B_6 or B_{12} deficiency, folate deficiency, malnutrition	—
Insulin	43-186 pmol/L (6-26 mcU/mL)	Acromegaly, adenoma of islet cells, obesity, untreated mild case of type 2 diabetes	Diabetes mellitus, obesity
Iron Male Female	14-32 mcmol/L (80-180 mcg/dL) 11-29 mcmol/L (60-160 mcg/dL)	Excessive red blood cell destruction, hemochromatosis, massive transfusion	Anemia of chronic disease, iron-deficiency anemia

Continued

Table B-1 Serum, Plasma, and Whole Blood Chemistries—cont'd

TEST	NORMAL VALUES SI UNITS (CONVENTIONAL UNITS)	POSSIBLE ETIOLOGY HIGHER	LOWER
Total iron-binding capacity (TIBC)	45-82 mcmol/L (250-460 mcg/dL)	Iron deficient state, oral contraceptive use, polycythemia	Cancer, chronic infections, pernicious anemia, uremia
Lactic acid	0.6-2.2 mmol/L (5-20 mg/dL)	Acidosis, congestive heart failure, severe liver disease, shock, tissue ischemia	—
Lactic dehydrogenase (LDH)	100-190 U/L (same as SI units)	Congestive heart failure, hemolytic disorders, hepatitis, metastatic cancer of liver, MI, pernicious anemia, pulmonary embolus and infarction, skeletal muscle damage	—
Lactic dehydrogenase isoenzymes			
LDH$_1$	0.17-0.27 (17-27%)	MI, pernicious anemia, strenuous exercise	—
LDH$_2$	0.27-0.37 (27-37%)	Exercise, pulmonary embolus, sickle cell crisis	—
LDH$_3$	0.18-0.25 (18-25%)	Malignant lymphoma, pulmonary embolus	—
LDH$_4$	0.03-0.08 (3-8%)	Systemic lupus erythematosus, pancreatitis, pulmonary infarction, renal disease	—
LDH$_5$	0.0-0.05 (0-5%)	Congestive heart failure, hepatitis, pulmonary embolus and infarction, skeletal muscle damage, strenuous exercise	—
Lipase	0-160 U/L (same as SI units)	Acute and chronic pancreatitis, hepatic disorders, pancreatic disorder (cancer, pseudocyst), perforated peptic ulcer, salivary gland inflammation or tumour	—
Magnesium	0.65-1.05 mmol/L (1.3-2.1 mEq/L)	Addison's disease, hypothyroidism, renal failure	Chronic alcoholism, hyperparathyroidism, hyperthyroidism, hypoparathyroidism, malnutrition, severe malabsorption
Myoglobin	<90 mcg/L (same as SI units)	MI, myositis, malignant hyperthermia, muscular dystrophy, skeletal muscle ischemia or trauma, rhabdomyolysis, seizures	Polymyositis
Osmolality	285-295 mmol/kg (285-295 mOsm/kg) H$_2$0	Chronic renal disease, dehydration, diabetes mellitus, hypernatremia, shock	Addison's disease, diuretic therapy, hyponatremia, overhydration
Oxygen saturation		Increased inspired oxygen, polycythemia vera	Anemia, cardiac decompensation, decreased inspired oxygen, respiratory disorders
Arterial	≥95% (same as SI units)		
Venous	60-80% (same as SI units)		
pH	*See* Blood gases		
Phenylalanine	0-121 mcmol/L (0-2 mg/dL)	Phenylketonuria	
Phosphatase, acid	2.2-10.5 U/L (0.13-0.63 U/L–Roy, Brower, Hayden 37°C)	Advanced Paget's disease, cancer of prostate, hyperparathyroidism	—

Table B-1 Serum, Plasma, and Whole Blood Chemistries—cont'd

TEST	NORMAL VALUES SI UNITS (CONVENTIONAL UNITS)	POSSIBLE ETIOLOGY HIGHER	LOWER
Phosphatase, alkaline (ALP)	35-120 U/L (0.5-2.0 mckat/L)	Bone diseases, cirrhosis, malignancy of liver/bone, marked hyperparathyroidism, obstruction of biliary system, rickets	Excessive vitamin D ingestion, hypothyroidism, milk-alkali syndrome
Phosphorus, phosphate	0.97-1.45 mmol/L (3.0-4.5 mg/dL)	Bone metastasis, healing fractures, hypoparathyroidism, hypocalcemia, renal disease, vitamin D intoxication	Chronic alcoholism, diabetes mellitus, hypercalcemia, hyperparathyroidism, vitamin D deficiency
Potassium	3.5-5.0 mmol/L (3.5-5.0 mEq/L)	Acute or chronic renal failure, Addison's disease, dehydration, diabetic ketosis, excessive dietary/IV intake, massive tissue destruction, metabolic acidosis	Burns, Cushing's syndrome, deficient dietary or IV intake, diarrhea (severe), diuretic therapy, GI fistula, insulin administration, pyloric obstruction, starvation, vomiting
Prostate-specific antigen (PSA)	<4 mcg/L (<4 ng/mL)	Benign prostatic hypertrophy, prostate cancer, prostatitis	—
Proteins		Burns, cirrhosis (globulin fraction), dehydration	Congenital agammaglobulinemia, increased capillary permeability, inflammatory disease, liver disease, malabsorption, malnutrition
Total	64-83 g/L (6.4-8.3 g/dL)		
Albumin	35-50 g/L (3.5-5 g/dL)		
Globulin	23-34 g/L (2.3-3.4 g/dL)		
Albumin/globulin ratio	1.5:1-2.5:1 (same as SI units)	Multiple myeloma (globulin fraction), shock, vomiting	Malnutrition, nephrotic syndrome, proteinuria, renal disease, severe burns
Pseudocholinesterase (serum)	8-18 U/mL (same as SI units)	—	—
Renin		Renal hypertension, salt-losing GI disease (vomiting/diarrhea), volume decrease (e.g., hemorrhage)	Increased salt intake, primary aldosteronism
Upright position	0.03-1.2 ng/L/sec (0.1-4.3 mg/mL/hr)		
Sodium	135-145 mmol/L (135-145 mEq/L)	Corticosteroid therapy, dehydration, impaired renal function, increased sodium intake in diet/IV, primary aldosteronism	Addison's disease, decreased sodium intake in dietary or IV intake, diabetic ketoacidosis, diuretic therapy, excessive loss from GI tract, excessive perspiration, water intoxication
Testosterone		Adrenal hyperplasia, adrenal or pituitary tumours, testicular tumours	Hypofunction of testes
Male	9.75-38 nmol/L (280-1080 ng/dL)		
Female	0.52-2.43 nmol/L (<70 ng/dL)	Polycystic ovary, virilizing tumours	—
T_4 (thyroxine), total	64-154 nmol/L (5-12 mcg/dL)	Hyperthyroidism, thyroiditis	Cretinism, hypothyroidism, myxedema
T_4 (thyroxine), free	10-36 pmol/L (0.8-2.8 ng/dL)	Hyperthyroidism, metastatic neoplasms	Hypothyroidism, pregnancy
T_3 uptake	24-34 AU (24-34%)	—	—
T_3 (triiodothyronine)	1.2-3.4 nmol/L (70-205 ng/dL)	Hyperthyroidism	Hypothyroidism
Thyroid-stimulating hormone (TSH)	2-10 mU/L (2-10 mcU/L)	Graves' disease, myxedema, primary hypothyroidism	Secondary hypothyroidism
Triglycerides		Diabetes mellitus, hyperlipidemia, hypothyroidism, liver disease	Hyperthyroidism, malabsorption syndrome, malnutrition
Male	0.45-1.81 mmol/L (40-160 mg/dL)		
Female	0.40-1.52 mmol/L (35-135 mg/dL)		
Troponin T (cTnT)	<0.2 mcg/L (<0.2 ng/mL)	Cardiac muscle damage, (MI, myocarditis or pericarditis), chronic renal failure, multiorgan failure, severe heart failure	—
Troponin I (cTnI)	<0.03 mcg/L (<0.3 ng/mL)		—

Continued

Table B-1 Serum, Plasma, and Whole Blood Chemistries—cont'd

TEST	NORMAL VALUES SI UNITS (CONVENTIONAL UNITS)	POSSIBLE ETIOLOGY HIGHER	LOWER
Urea nitrogen, blood (blood urea nitrogen [BUN], serum urea nitrogen)	3.6-7.1 mmol/L (10-20 mg/dL)	Burns, dehydration, GI bleeds, increase in protein catabolism (fever, stress), renal disease, shock, urinary tract infection	Fluid overload, malnutrition, severe liver damage, SIADH
Uric acid Male Female	0.24-0.51 mmol/L (4.0-8.5 mg/dL) 0.16-0.43 mmol/L (2.7-7.3 mg/dL)	Alcoholism, eclampsia, gout, gross tissue destruction, high-protein weight reduction diet, leukemia, multiple myeloma, renal failure	Administration of uricosuric drugs
Vitamin A	0.52-2.09 mcmol/L (15-60 mcg/dL)	Excess ingestion of vitamin A	Vitamin A deficiency
Vitamin B_{12}	118-701 pmol/L (160-950 pg/mL)	Chronic myeloid leukemia	Malabsorption syndrome, pernicious anemia, strict vegetarianism, total or partial gastrectomy
Zinc	11.5-18.5 mcmol/L (75-120 mcg/dL)	—	Alcoholic cirrhosis

Table B-2 Hematology

TEST	NORMAL VALUES SI UNITS (CONVENTIONAL UNITS)	POSSIBLE ETIOLOGY HIGHER	LOWER
Bleeding time (IVY)	1-9 min	Aspirin ingestion, clotting factor deficiency, defective platelet function, thrombocytopenia, vascular disease, von Willebrand's disease	—
Activated partial thromboplastin time (aPTT)	30-40 sec* (same as SI units)	Deficiency of Factors I, II, V, VIII, IX and X, XI, XII; hemophilia; heparin therapy; liver disease	—
Partial thromboplastin time (PTT)	28-35 sec (same as SI units)	Same etiology as for aPTT	—
Activated coagulation time or automated clotting time (ACT)	70-120 sec (same as SI units)	Same etiology as for aPTT	—
Prothrombin time (Protime, PT)	11-12.5 sec* (same as SI units)	Deficiency of Factors I, II, V, VII, and X; liver disease; vitamin K deficiency; warfarin therapy	—
International normalized ratio (INR)	0.81-1.2 (same as SI units)	Same etiology as for PT	—
Thrombin time	8-12 sec (same as SI units)	Disseminated intravascular coagulation (DIC), increased tendency to bleed	—
Fibrinogen	2-4 g/L (200-400 mg/dL)	Burns (after first 36 hr), inflammatory disease	Burns (during first 36 hr), DIC, severe liver disease
Fibrin split (degradation) products	<10 mg/L (<10 mcg/mL)	Acute DIC, massive hemorrhage, massive trauma, primary fibrinolysis	—
D-Dimer	<250 mcg/L (<250 ng/mL)	Deep vein thrombosis, DIC, myocardial infarction, unstable angina	—

*Patients receiving anticoagulant therapy:
aPTT: 1.5-2.5 times control value in seconds.
PT: 1.5-2.0 times control value in seconds.

Table B-2 Hematology—cont'd

TEST	NORMAL VALUES SI UNITS (CONVENTIONAL UNITS)	POSSIBLE ETIOLOGY	
		HIGHER	LOWER
Erythrocyte count† Red blood cell count [RBC count] (altitude dependent)		Dehydration, high altitudes, polycythemia vera, severe diarrhea	Anemia, leukemia, post hemorrhage
Male	$4.7\text{-}6.1 \times 10^{12}/L$ $(4.7\text{-}6.1 \times 10^6/mcL)$		
Female	$4.2\text{-}5.4 \times 10^{12}/L$ $(4.2\text{-}5.4 \times 10^6/mcL)$		
Mean corpuscular volume (MCV) [Hct/RBC]	80-95 fL (80-95 mm^3)	Folic acid and vitamin B_{12} deficiency, liver disease, macrocytic anemia	Microcytic anemia
Mean corpuscular hemoglobin (MCH) [Hb/RBC]	27-31 pg (same as SI units)	Macrocytic anemia	Microcytic anemia
Mean corpuscular hemoglobin concentration (MCHC)	32-36 g/dL or 32-36%	Intravascular hemolysis, spherocytosis	Hypochromic anemia
Erythrocyte sedimentation rate (ESR), Westergren		*Moderate increase:* acute hepatitis, myocardial infarction, rheumatoid arthritis	Malaria, severe liver disease, sickle cell anemia
Male	≤15 mm/hr (same as SI units)	*Marked increase:* acute and severe bacterial infections, malignancies, pelvic inflammatory disease	
Female	≤20 mm/hr (same as SI units)		
Hematocrit (altitude dependent)†		Dehydration, high altitudes, polycythemia	Anemia, bone marrow failure, hemorrhage, leukemia, overhydration
Male	0.42-0.52 volume fraction (42-52%)		
Female	0.37-0.47 volume fraction (37-47%)		
Hemoglobin (altitude dependent)†		Chronic obstructive pulmonary disease, high altitudes, polycythemia	Anemia, hemorrhage
Male	140-180 mmol/L (14-18 g/dL)		
Female	120-160 mmol/L (12-16 g/dL)		
Hemoglobin, glycosylated or glycated (HbA1c [A1c])	<6% (adult without diabetes)	Nondiabetic hyperglycemia, poorly controlled diabetes mellitus	Chronic blood loss, chronic renal failure, pregnancy, sickle cell anemia
Red cell distribution width (RDW)	11-14.5% (same as SI units)	—	Anisocytosis, macrocytic anemia, microcytic anemia
Platelet count (thrombocytes)	$150\text{-}400 \times 10^9/L$ (150,000-400,000 mm^3)	Acute infections, chronic granulocytic leukemia, chronic pancreatitis, cirrhosis, collagen disorders, polycythemia, post splenectomy	Acute leukemia, cancer chemotherapy, DIC, hemorrhage, infection, systemic lupus erythematosus, thrombocytopenic purpura
Reticulocyte count (manual)	0.5-2% of RBC (same as SI units)	Hemolytic anemia, polycythemia vera	Hypoproliferative anemia, macrocytic anemia, microcytic anemia
White blood cell (WBC) count†	$5\text{-}10 \times 10^9/L$ (5000-10,000 mm^3)	Inflammatory and infectious processes, leukemia	Aplastic anemia, autoimmune diseases, overwhelming infection, side effects of chemotherapy and irradiation

†Components of complete blood count (CBC).

Continued

Table B-2 Hematology—cont'd

TEST	NORMAL VALUES SI UNITS (CONVENTIONAL UNITS)	POSSIBLE ETIOLOGY HIGHER	LOWER
WBC differential			
Segmented neutrophils	$2.5-7.5 \times 10^9$/L (62-68%)	Bacterial infections, collagen diseases, Hodgkin's disease	Aplastic anemia, viral infections
Band neutrophils	$0-1 \times 10^9$/L (0-9%)	Acute infections	—
Lymphocytes	$0.1-0.4 \times 10^9$/L (1000-4000 mm^3) (20-40%)	Chronic infections, lymphocytic leukemia, mononucleosis, viral infections	Corticosteroid therapy, whole body irradiation
Monocytes	$0.02-0.07 \times 10^9$/L (100-700 mm^3) (2-8%)	Acute infections, chronic inflammatory disorders, Hodgkin's disease, malaria, monocytic leukemia	—
Eosinophils	$0.01-0.04 \times 10^9$/L (50-100 mm^3) (1-4%)	Allergic reactions, eosinophilic and chronic granulocytic leukemia, Hodgkin's disease, parasitic disorders	Corticosteroid therapy
Basophils	$0-0.01 \times 10^9$/L (25-100 mm^3) (0.5-1%)	Hypothyroidism, myeloproliferative diseases, ulcerative colitis	Hyperthyroidism, stress
Sickle cell solubility	Negative (negative)	Sickle cell anemia	—

Table B-3 Serology-Immunology

TEST	NORMAL VALUES SI UNITS (CONVENTIONAL UNITS)	POSSIBLE ETIOLOGY HIGHER	LOWER
Antinuclear antibody (ANA)	Negative at 1:40 dilution (same as SI units)	Chronic hepatitis, rheumatoid arthritis, scleroderma, systemic lupus erythematosus (SLE)	—
Anti-DNA antibody	Negative <70 U/mL (same as SI units)	SLE	—
Anti-RNP (ribonucleoprotein)	Negative (negative)	Mixed connective tissue disease, scleroderma, rheumatoid arthritis, Sjögren's syndrome, SLE	—
Anti-Sm (Smith)	Negative (Negative)	SLE	—
Antistreptolysin-O (ASO)	≤160 Todd units/mL (same as SI units)	Acute glomerulonephritis, rheumatic fever, streptococcal infection	—
C-reactive protein(CRP)	<10 mg/L (<1.0 mg/dL)	Acute infections, any inflammatory condition (e.g., acute rheumatic fever/arthritis), widespread malignancy	—
Carcinoembryonic antigen (CEA)	5 mcg/L (5 ng/mL)	Carcinomas of colon, liver, pancreas; chronic cigarette smoking; inflammatory bowel disease; other cancers	—
Complement assay components	—		Acute glomerulonephritis, rheumatoid arthritis, serum sickness, subacute bacterial endocarditis, SLE
Total	75-160 k/units/L (75-160 U/mL)		
C3	0.55-1.2 g/L (55-120 mg/dL)		
C4	0.2-0.5 g/L (20-50 mg/dL)		
Direct antihuman globulin test (DAT) or direct Coombs' test	Negative (negative) (no agglutination)	Acquired hemolytic anemia, drug reactions, hemolytic disease of the newborn, transfusion reactions	

Table B-3 Serology-Immunology—cont'd

TEST	NORMAL VALUES SI UNITS (CONVENTIONAL UNITS)	POSSIBLE ETIOLOGY HIGHER	LOWER
Fluorescent treponemal antibody absorption (FTAAbs)	Negative (nonreactive)	Syphilis	—
Hepatitis A antibody	Negative (negative)	Hepatitis A	—
Hepatitis B surface antigen (HBsAg)	Negative (negative)	Hepatitis B	—
Hepatitis C antibody	Negative (negative)	Hepatitis C	—
Immunoglobulins			
IgA	0.85-3.85 g/L (85-385 mg/dL)	Autoimmune disorders, chronic infection, chronic liver disease, IgA myeloma, rheumatoid arthritis	Burns, hereditary telangiectasia, malabsorption syndromes
IgD	Minimal	Chronic infection, connective tissue disease	—
IgE	Minimal	Anaphylactic shock, atopic disease (allergies), parasite infections	—
IgG	5.65-17.65 g/L (565-1765 mg/dL)	Hepatitis, IgG monoclonal gammopathy, infections—acute and chronic, SLE	Acquired deficiencies, burns, congenital deficiencies, immunosuppression, nephrotic syndromes
IgM	0.55-3.75 g/L (55-375 mg/dL)	Acute infections, liver disease, rheumatoid arthritis	Congenital and acquired antibody deficiencies, lymphocytic leukemia, protein-losing enteropathies
Monospot or Mono-Test	Negative (<1:28 titre)	Infectious mononucleosis	—
Rheumatoid factor (RA factor)	Negative or <60 units/mL by nephelometric method	Rheumatoid arthritis, Sjögren's syndrome, SLE	—
RPR (rapid plasma reagin) test	Negative or nonreactive (same as SI units)	Febrile diseases, IV drug abuse, leprosy, malaria, rheumatoid arthritis, syphilis, SLE	—
VDRL (Venereal Disease Research Laboratory) test	Negative or nonreactive (same as SI units)	Syphilis	—
Thyroid antibodies	Titre <1:100 (same as SI units)	Early hypothyroidism, Graves' disease, Hashimoto's thyroiditis, pernicious anemia, SLE, thyroid carcinoma	—

Table B-4 Urine Chemistry

TEST	SPECIMEN	NORMAL VALUES SI UNITS (CONVENTIONAL UNITS)	POSSIBLE ETIOLOGY HIGHER	LOWER
Acetone (ketones)	Random	Negative (negative)	Diabetes mellitus, high-fat and low-carbohydrate diets, starvation states	—
Aldosterone	24 hr	6-72 nmol/24 hr (2-26 mcg/24 hr) (depends on urinary sodium)	*Primary aldosteronism:* Adrenocortical tumours *Secondary aldosteronism:* Cardiac failure, cirrhosis, large dose of ACTH, salt depletion	Adrenocorticotropic hormone (ACTH) deficiency, Addison's disease, corticosteroid therapy
Amylase	24 hr	≤5000 Somogyi units/24 hr OR 6.5-48.1 units/hr	Acute pancreatitis	—

Continued

Table B-4 Urine Chemistry—cont'd

		NORMAL VALUES		POSSIBLE ETIOLOGY	
TEST	**SPECIMEN**	**SI UNITS (CONVENTIONAL UNITS)**		**HIGHER**	**LOWER**
Bence Jones protein	Random	Negative (negative)		Biliary duct obstruction, multiple myeloma	—
Bilirubin	Random	Negative (negative)		Hepatitis	—
Calcium	24 hr	6.2 mmol/day (<250 mg/day)		Bone tumour, hyperparathyroidism, milk-alkali syndrome	Hypoparathyroidism, malabsorption of calcium and vitamin D
Catecholamines	24 hr			Heart failure, pheochromocytoma, progressive muscular dystrophy	
Epinephrine		<109 nmol/day (<20 mcg/day)			
Norepinephrine		<590 nmol/day (<100 mcg/day)			
Chloride	24 hr	110-250 mmol/day (110-250 mEq/day)		Addison's disease	Burns, diarrhea, excess perspiration, menstruation, vomiting
		<0.5 mcmol/day (<30 mcg/day)			
Copper	24 hr	0.6 mcmol/day (<40 mcg/day)		Cirrhosis, Wilson's disease	—
Coproporphyrin	24 hr	<300 nmol/day (<200 mcg/day)		Lead poisoning, oral contraceptive use, poliomyelitis	—
Creatine	24 hr			Addison's disease, burns, carcinoma of liver, diabetes, hyperthyroidism, infections, muscular dystrophy, skeletal muscle atrophy	Hypothyroidism
Male		<300 mcmol/day (<60 mg/day)			
Female		<600 mcmol/day (<80 mg/day)			
Creatinine	24 hr	7.1-17.7 mmol/day (0.8-2 g/day)		Anemia, leukemia, muscular atrophy, salmonellosis	Renal disease
Creatinine clearance	24 hr	1.42-2.25 mL/sec (85-135 mL/min)		—	Renal disease
Male		1.78-2.32 mL/sec (107-139 mL/min)			
Female		1.45-1.78 mL/sec (87-107 mL/min)			
Estriol	24 hr			Gonadal or adrenal tumour	
Female					Agenesis of ovaries, endocrine disturbance, menopause, ovarian dysfunction
• Ovulation peak		104-370 nmol/day (28-100 mcg/day)			
• Luteal peak		81-296 nmol/day (22-80 mcg/day)			
• Pregnancy		≤166,455 nmol/day (≤45,000 mcg/day)			
• Menopause		5.2-72.5 nmol/day (1.4-19.6 mcg/day)			
Male		18-67 nmol/day (5-18 mcg/day)		—	—
Glucose	Random	Negative (negative)		Diabetes mellitus, low renal threshold for glucose resorption, physiological stress, pituitary disorders	—
Hemoglobin	Random	Negative (negative)		Extensive burns, glomerulonephritis, hemolytic anemias, hemolytic transfusion reaction	—
5-Hydroxyindole-acetic acid (5-HIAA)	24 hr	10-40 mcmol/day (2-8 mg/24 hr)		Malignant carcinoid syndrome	—

Table B-4 Urine Chemistry—cont'd

TEST	SPECIMEN	NORMAL VALUES SI UNITS (CONVENTIONAL UNITS)	POSSIBLE ETIOLOGY HIGHER	LOWER
Ketone bodies	Random	Negative (negative)	Alcoholism, fasting, high-protein diets, marked ketonuria, poorly controlled diabetes mellitus, starvation	—
Lead	24 hr	<0.40 mcmol/day (<80 mcg/day)	Lead poisoning	—
Metanephrine	24 hr	<7 mcmol/day (<1.3 mg/day)	Pheochromocytoma	—
Myoglobin	Random	Negative (negative)	Crushing injuries, electric injuries, extreme physical exertion	—
pH	Random	4.6-8 (same as SI units) Average: 6	Chronic renal failure, compensatory phase of alkalosis, salicylate intoxication, vegetarian diet	Compensatory phase of acidosis, dehydration, emphysema
Phenylpyruvic acid	Random	Negative (negative)	Phenylketonuria	—
Phosphorus, inorganic	24 hr	29-42 mmol/day (0.9-1.3 g/day)	Fever, hypoparathyroidism, nervous exhaustion, rickets, tuberculosis	Acute infections, nephritis
Porphobilinogen	Random 24 hr	Negative (negative) <8.8 mcmol/day (<2 mcg/day)	Acute intermittent porphyria, liver disorders	—
Potassium	24 hr	25-100 mmol/day (25-100 mEq/day)	Chronic renal failure, starvation, Cushing's syndrome, hyperaldosteronism, alkalosis, diuretic therapy	Reduced intake, dehydration, Addison's disease, malnutrition, vomiting, diarrhea, acute renal failure
Protein (dipstick)	Random	Negative (negative)	Congestive heart failure, nephritis, nephrosis, physiological stress	—
Protein (quantitative) At rest During exercise	24 hr	<0.15 g/day (<150 mg/day) 0.05-0.08 g/day (<50-80 mg/day) <0.25 g/day (<250 mg/day)	Cardiac failure, inflammatory processes of urinary tract, nephritis, nephrosis, toxemia of pregnancy	—
Sodium	24 hr	40-250 mmol/day (40-250 mEq/day)	Acute tubular necrosis	Hyponatremia
Specific gravity	Random	1.005-1.030 (same as SI units)	Albuminuria, dehydration, fever, GI losses (vomiting/diarrhea), glycosuria, syndrome of inappropriate antidiuretic hormone (SIADH)	Diabetes insipidus, diuresis, overhydration
Titratable acidity	24 hr	20-50 mEq/day (same as SI units)	Metabolic acidosis	Metabolic alkalosis
Uric acid	24 hr	1.48-4.43 mmol/day (250-750 mg/24 hr)	Gout, leukemia	Nephritis
Urobilinogen	24 hr Random	0.0-6.8 mcmol/day (0.0-4.0 mg/24 hr) <0.01-1 EU (same as SI units)	Hemolytic disease, hepatic parenchymal cell damage, liver disease	Complete obstruction of bile duct
Uroporphyrins Male Female	24 hr	4-46 mcg/day (same as SI units) 3-22 mcg/day (same as SI units)	Lead poisoning, liver disease, porphyria	—
Vanillylmandelic acid	24 hr	<35 mcmol/day (<6.8 mg/day)	Pheochromocytoma, neuroblastomas	—

Table B-5 Gastric Analysis

TEST	NORMAL VALUES SI UNITS (CONVENTIONAL UNITS)	POSSIBLE ETIOLOGY	
		HIGHER	LOWER
Basal			
Free hydrochloric acid	0.3 mmol/L (0.3 mEq/L)	Hypermotility of stomach	Pernicious anemia
Total acidity	15-45 mmol/L (15-45 mEq/L)	Gastric and duodenal ulcers, Zollinger-Ellison syndrome	Gastric carcinoma, severe gastritis
Poststimulation			
Free hydrochloric acid	10-130 mmol/L (10-130 mEq/L)	—	—
Total acidity	20-150 mmol/L (20-150 mEq/L)	—	—

Table B-6 Fecal Analysis

TEST	NORMAL VALUES SI UNITS (CONVENTIONAL UNITS)	POSSIBLE ETIOLOGY	
		HIGHER	LOWER
Fecal fat	7.21 mmol/day (2-6 g/day)	Chronic pancreatic disease, cystic fibrosis, malabsorption syndrome, obstruction of common bile duct, short gut syndrome	—
Urobilinogen	51-372 mcmol/100 g of stool (30-220 mg/100 g of stool)	Hemolytic anemias	Complete biliary obstruction
Mucus	Negative (negative)	Mucous colitis, spastic constipation	—
Pus	Negative (negative)	Chronic bacillary dysentery, chronic ulcerative colitis, localized abscesses	—
Blood*	Negative (negative)	Anal fissures, hemorrhoids, inflammatory bowel disease, malignant tumour, peptic ulcer	—
Colour			
Brown		Various colours depending on diet	—
Clay		Biliary obstruction or presence of barium sulphate	—
Tarry		More than 100 mL of blood in GI tract	—
Red		Blood in large intestine	—
Black		Blood in upper GI tract or iron medication	—

*Ingestion of meat may produce false-positive results. Patient may be placed on a meat-free diet for 3 days before the test.

Table B-7 Cerebrospinal Fluid Analysis

TEST	NORMAL VALUES SI UNITS (CONVENTIONAL UNITS)	POSSIBLE ETIOLOGY	
		HIGHER	LOWER
Pressure	<20 cm H_2O (same as SI units)	Hemorrhage, intracranial tumour, meningitis	Head injury, spinal tumour, subdural hematoma
Blood	Negative (negative)	Intracranial hemorrhage	—
Cell count (age dependent)			
WBCs (white blood cells)	0-5 × 10^6/L (0-5 cells/mcL)	Inflammation or infections of central nervous system (CNS)	—
RBCs (red blood cells)	Negative (negative)		—
Chloride	115-130 mmol/L (115-130 mEq/L)	Uremia	Bacterial infections of CNS (meningitis, encephalitis)
Glucose	2.8-4.2 mmol/L (50-75 mg/dL)	Diabetes mellitus, viral infections of CNS	Bacterial infections and tuberculosis of CNS
Protein			
Lumbar	0.15-0.45 g/L (15-45 mg/dL)	Guillain-Barré syndrome, poliomyelitis, traumatic tap	—
Cisternal	0.15-0.25 g/L (15-25 mg/dL)	Syphilis of CNS	
Ventricular	0.05-0.15 g/L (5-15 mg/dL)	Acute meningitis, brain tumour, chronic CNS infections, multiple sclerosis	

Index

Page numbers followed by b, f, or t indicate boxes, figures, and tabular material,
respectively.

Special Features

Boxes

EVIDENCE-INFORMED PRACTICE

FOCUSED ASSESSMENT

GENETICS IN CLINICAL PRACTICE

Tables

AGE-RELATED DIFFERENCES IN ASSESSMENT

TABLE TITLE	TABLE NUMBER	PAGE
Age-Related Changes and Associated Clinical Manifestations	Table 7-2	103-106
Auditory System	Table 23-7	494
Cardiovascular System	Table 34-1	848
Cognitive Functioning, Effects of Aging on	Table 7-3	107
Endocrine System	Table 50-5	1380
Gastrointestinal System	Table 41-5	1048
Hematological Studies, Effects of Aging on	Table 32-4	771
Immune System, Effects of Aging on	Table 16-6	293
Integumentary System	Table 25-1	543
Musculoskeletal System	Table 64-1	1802
Nervous System	Table 58-5	1620
Nutritional Intake in Older Adults, Factors Affecting	Table 42-6	1075
Respiratory System	Table 28-4	617
Urinary System	Table 47-2	1273
Visual System	Table 23-1	485

DIAGNOSTIC STUDIES

TABLE TITLE	TABLE NUMBER	PAGE
Auditory System	Table 23-12	500
Cardiovascular System	Table 34-5	854-859
Endocrine System	Table 50-8	1385-1391
Gastrointestinal (GI) System	Table 41-12	1055-1060
Headaches	Table 61-2	1703
Hematological System	Table 32-12	782
Integumentary System	Table 25-10	550
Laboratory Abnormalities in Shock	Table 69-3	1963
Liver Function Tests	Table 41-13	1062
Male and Female Reproductive Systems	Table 53-12	1487
Musculoskeletal System	Table 64-7	1806-1808
Nervous System	Table 58-9	1629-1630
Respiratory System	Table 28-11	626-627
Stroke	Table 60-4	1680
Urinary System	Table 47-8	1279-1281
Venous Thromboembolism	Table 40-8	1025
Visual System	Table 23-6	492

COMMON ASSESSMENT ABNORMALITIES

TABLE TITLE	TABLE NUMBER	PAGE
Auditory System	Table 23-11	498
Breast	Table 53-9	1484
Cardiovascular System	Table 34-3	851-852
Endocrine System	Table 50-7	1383-1384
Female Reproductive System	Table 53-10	1485
Fluid and Electrolyte Imbalances	Table 19-19	410
Gastrointestinal System	Table 41-11	1054-1055
Hematological System	Table 32-7	777-778
Integumentary System	Table 25-9	549
Male Reproductive System	Table 53-11	1485
Musculoskeletal System	Table 64-6	1805
Nervous System	Table 58-8	1628
Respiratory System	Table 28-9	623-624
Urinary System	Table 47-7	1278
Visual System	Table 23-5	488-489

HEALTH HISTORY

TABLE TITLE	TABLE NUMBER	PAGE
Auditory System	Table 23-8	495
Cardiovascular System	Table 34-2	849
Endocrine System	Table 50-6	1381
Gastrointestinal System	Table 41-8	1050
Hematological System	Table 32-5	772
Integumentary System	Table 25-3	545
Musculoskeletal System	Table 64-2	1803
Nervous System	Table 58-6	1622
Patient About to Undergo Surgery	Table 20-3	427
Reproductive System	Table 53-6	1481
Respiratory System	Table 28-5	618
Urinary System	Table 47-4	1275
Visual System	Table 23-2	486

DRUG THERAPY